# BIRTH DEFECTS
## ❖ ENCYCLOPEDIA ❖

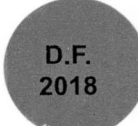

# BIRTH DEFECTS
# ❖ ENCYCLOPEDIA ❖

*The Comprehensive, Systematic, Illustrated Reference Source*
*for the Diagnosis, Delineation, Etiology, Biodynamics,*
*Occurrence, Prevention, and Treatment of Human Anomalies*
*of Clinical Relevance*

## Mary Louise Buyse, M.D.

Editor-in-Chief

CENTER FOR BIRTH DEFECTS INFORMATION SERVICES, INC.

Dover Medical Building     30 Springdale Avenue     Box 1776     Dover, MA 02030     U.S.A.

Tel. (508) 785-2525          **BDFax** (508) 785-BDIS                    Fax. (508) 785-2526

The **BIRTH DEFECTS ENCYCLOPEDIA**
is a service of the
**Center for Birth Defects Information Services, Inc.**
Dover Medical Building
30 Springdale Avenue   Box 1776
Dover, MA   02030   U.S.A.

Published in association with
**Blackwell Scientific Publications**
Three Cambridge Center, Suite 208,
   Cambridge, Massachusetts 02142, USA
Osney Mead, Oxford OX2 0EL, England
25 John Street, London, WC1N 2BL, England
23 Ainslie Place, Edinburgh, EH3 6AJ, Scotland
54 University Street, Carlton, Victoria 3053, Australia

Distributors:

USA and Canada
   Mosby–Year Book Medical Publishers
   11830 Westline Industrial Drive
   St. Louis, Missouri 63146-3313
   (Orders: Telephone: 1-800-633-6699)

Australia
   Blackwell Scientific Publications (Australia) Pty Ltd
   54 University Street
   Carlton, Victoria 3053
   (Orders: Telephone: 03-347-0300)

Outside North America and Australia
   Blackwell Scientific Publications, Ltd.
   Osney Mead
   Oxford OX2 0EL
   England
   (Orders: Telephone: 011-44-865-240201)

Typeset by The William Byrd Press
Printed and bound by Arcata/Kingsport

Blackwell Scientific Publications, Inc.
© 1990 by The Center for Birth Defects Information Services, Inc.
Printed in the United States of America
90  91  92  93  5  4  3  2  1

Library of Congress Cataloging in Publication Data

Birth defects encyclopedia : the comprehensive, systematic,
   illustrated reference source for the diagnosis, delineation,
   etiology, biodynamics, occurrence, prevention, and treatment of
   human anomalies of clinical relevance / Mary Louise Buyse,
   editor-in-chief.
      p.   cm.
   Includes index.
   ISBN 0-86542-088-2 : $195.00
   1. Abnormalities, Human—Dictionaries.   I. Buyse, Mary Louise.
   [DNLM: 1. Abnormalities—encyclopedias.   QS 13 B619]
QM690.B57   1990
616'.043—dc20
DNLM/DLC
for Library of Congress                        90-522
                                                CIP

# ACKNOWLEDGEMENTS

The Center for Birth Defects Information Services, and this *Birth Defects Encyclopedia*, would not be possible without the efforts, support, and encouragement of thousands of people from around the world.

The contributions of over a thousand authors, editors, and illustrators are reflected in the over two-thousand articles and 1,700 illustrations which appear on the following pages. Countless other contributors prepared, reviewed, and edited articles which, although not published here in their original form, contributed to the accuracy, richness, and depth of this volume. Similarly, it required the effort and consideration of thousands of patients, families, and scientists to assemble the tens of thousands of photographs which made it possible to determine and select for publication in this edition those which would most contribute to the volume's research, educational, and clinical objectives.

We are greatly indebted to Prof. Victor A. McKusick for his help and encouragement, and particularly for his permission to reprint gene map pictorials from *Mendelian Inheritance in Man*. Human Gene Map 10 data and symbol names were made available through the kind collaboration of the Human Gene Mapping Library, and are reprinted by the kind permission of *Cytogenetics and Cell Genetics*.

The Center for Birth Defects Information Services, Inc. gratefully acknowledges the support and effort of the March of Dimes Birth Defects Foundation in the creation of this publication.

The Center is particularly indebted to the people of Dover, Massachusetts, and to the New England high-technology community for their special interest in and support of the work of the Center.

Everyone connected with the Center also wishes to express their thanks and offer tribute to the many hundreds of patients and families whose encouragement, stories, queries, and support helped us to define our mission and to see its impact in very human terms. These often touching letters and calls, from around the world, were our most sincere reward. This book is for you.

The Center for Birth Defects Information Services, Inc. is an independent, non-profit, international scientific collaborative incorporated in the State of Massachusetts, U.S.A., and operating under Section 501(c)(3) of the U.S. Internal Revenue Service Code. The research and publications of the Center would not be possible without the tax-deductible contributions of friends and supporters. In particular, the *Birth Defects Encyclopedia* has been made possible by the help and support of:

Automation Graphics, Inc.
Eric H. Boehm
The Estate of Drew H. Bone
The Estate of Ruth L. Born
F. Gorham Brigham, Jr.
Coopers & Lybrand
Copia International, Ltd.
Copley Systems
Elizabeth A. Coughlin
Debevoise & Plimpton
Dover Country Properties
Dover Law Offices
Dunn Copy Products, Inc.
Eastman Kodak Company
Everex Systems, Inc.
Expert Computer Services
Foley, Hoag & Eliot
Fordham & Starrett
Four Oaks Research Institute
James Goodale, Esq.
Thomas M.S. Hemnes, Esq.
Steve A. Hersee
Jay Hughes
Andrew Langowitz
Brian W. LeClair, Esq.
Dr. Franklin M. Loew
Luttazi Realty Trust
Margulies, Wind, Herrington & Katz
MEDx Systems, Ltd.
MICROSELL
The MITRE Corporation
J. Lincoln Passmore, Esq.
The Permanent Endowment for Research in Birth Defects
Smith, Teuber & Hansen
Spectrum Enterprises, Inc.
Hon. Paul E. Tsongas
Tweeter etc.
Voice Systems
James Andrew Weisman, Esq.

# TABLE OF CONTENTS

ACKNOWLEDGEMENTS . . . . . . . . . . . . . . . . . . . . . . . . . . . . . . . . . . . . . . . . . . . . . . . . . . . . . . . . vi

PREFACE . . . . . . . . . . . . . . . . . . . . . . . . . . . . . . . . . . . . . . . . . . . . . . . . . . . . . . . . . . . . . . . . . . ix

BOARD OF TRUSTEES . . . . . . . . . . . . . . . . . . . . . . . . . . . . . . . . . . . . . . . . . . . . . . . . . . . . . . xiii

ADVISORY BOARD . . . . . . . . . . . . . . . . . . . . . . . . . . . . . . . . . . . . . . . . . . . . . . . . . . . . . . . . . xiv

EDITORIAL BOARD . . . . . . . . . . . . . . . . . . . . . . . . . . . . . . . . . . . . . . . . . . . . . . . . . . . . . . . . . xv

TOPIC EDITORS . . . . . . . . . . . . . . . . . . . . . . . . . . . . . . . . . . . . . . . . . . . . . . . . . . . . . . . . . . . xvii

CONTRIBUTING EDITORS . . . . . . . . . . . . . . . . . . . . . . . . . . . . . . . . . . . . . . . . . . . . . . . . . . . xx

CONTRIBUTORS . . . . . . . . . . . . . . . . . . . . . . . . . . . . . . . . . . . . . . . . . . . . . . . . . . . . . . . . . . . xxi

## PART I

HOW TO USE THIS ENCYCLOPEDIA . . . . . . . . . . . . . . . . . . . . . . . . . . . . . . . . . . . . . . . . liii

   RELATED SERVICES . . . . . . . . . . . . . . . . . . . . . . . . . . . . . . . . . . . . . . . . . . . . . . . . . . lxxi

     **BDFax** . . . . . . . . . . . . . . . . . . . . . . . . . . . . . . . . . . . . . . . . . . . . . . . . . . . . . . . . . . lxxi

     BIRTH DEFECTS ENCYCLOPEDIA *Online* . . . . . . . . . . . . . . . . . . . . . . . . . . . . . . . . . lxxii

     BIRTH DEFECTS INFORMATION SYSTEM ( **BDIS** ) . . . . . . . . . . . . . . . . . . . . . . . . . . lxxiii

     DYSMORPHOLOGY AND CLINICAL GENETICS . . . . . . . . . . . . . . . . . . . . . . . . . . . . . lxxvii

     RESEARCH, EDUCATION, AND PUBLIC INFORMATION . . . . . . . . . . . . . . . . . . . . . . lxxviii

HOW TO PARTICIPATE IN THE WORK OF THE CENTER . . . . . . . . . . . . . . . . . . . . . . . lxxviii

   HOW TO COMMUNICATE WITH THE CENTER . . . . . . . . . . . . . . . . . . . . . . . . . . . . . . lxxx

## PART II

MASTER INDEX AND ARTICLES . . . . . . . . . . . . . . . . . . . . . . . . . . . . . . . . . . . . . . . . . . . . 1

   GENE MAP TABLE BY SYMBOL NAME . . . . . . . . . . . . . . . . . . . . . . . . . . . . . . . . . . . . 1809

   GENE MAP PICTORIALS BY CHROMOSOME . . . . . . . . . . . . . . . . . . . . . . . . . . . . . . . . 1821

   BIRTH DEFECT-NUMBER-TO-PRIME NAME INDEX . . . . . . . . . . . . . . . . . . . . . . . . . . 1833

   MIM-NUMBER-TO-PRIME-NAME INDEX . . . . . . . . . . . . . . . . . . . . . . . . . . . . . . . . . . . 1851

   POSSUM-NUMBER-TO-PRIME-NAME INDEX . . . . . . . . . . . . . . . . . . . . . . . . . . . . . . . 1869

   CDC-NUMBER-TO-PRIME-NAME INDEX . . . . . . . . . . . . . . . . . . . . . . . . . . . . . . . . . . . 1877

ILLUSTRATION CREDITS BY PUBLISHER . . . . . . . . . . . . . . . . . . . . . . . . . . . . . . . . . . . . 1883

ILLUSTRATION CREDITS BY CONTRIBUTOR . . . . . . . . . . . . . . . . . . . . . . . . . . . . . . . . . 1887

# ❖ PREFACE ❖

Birth defects are involved in about half of all pediatric hospital admissions, and next to accidents are the leading cause of death in children. As many as sixteen percent of all deliveries involve birth defects. Birth defects that can have an impact on function occur in a little over seven percent of deliveries, or about 250,000 births per year in the United States alone. The number of practitioners, researchers, and students who come in contact with the more than ten million American men and women with birth defects reaches into the hundreds of thousands. Involving all medical specialties and crossing all human organ systems, birth defects are extraordinary in scope and present a worldwide medical challenge.

While our understanding of birth defects, and our ability to treat them effectively, have increased rapidly over the past few decades, birth defects can still be viewed as a vast array of possibly linked but nevertheless distinct conditions. While at least two thousand of these conditions are now well-enough delineated to be named and described, more than a third of the complex cases seen in specialty centers around the world do not fit any established diagnoses. Often these are one-of-a-kind conditions or anomalies that are confined to a single family.

Yet information on each affected individual is critical, not only for the patient and family searching for a probable prognosis and optimum treatment, but for the research community, which now has powerful new technologies for the study and classification of underlying genetic, structural, and biomedical mechanisms. Both of these objectives must contend, however, with the vast diversity and geographic dispersion of individual conditions. The situation is much like a massive puzzle for which the pieces, and the clues, are scattered around the globe, typically known only to a handful of clinicians who may never see more than one or two examples of a given rare condition in their entire careers.

Even the definition of birth defects has been the topic of debate. The term itself would imply a *congenital* anomaly or defect; one present at birth, yet many of the best-known birth defects do not manifest until the fourth or fifth decade of life. Other observers equate birth defects with genetic or inherited anomalies, but of the many thousands of inherited human conditions classified to date, most are traits or variations such as eye color that are not of clinical significance. In fact, U.S. government figures suggest that as few as twenty percent of birth defects are inherited in the classic sense, despite the increasing recognition that genetic or chromosomal factors play at least some role in most medical conditions.

Transplacental infections directly account for some two to three percent of the conditions commonly termed birth defects, and may play a role in additional defects. A similar percentage can be attributed to teratogens: chemicals, drugs, or other substances taken by the mother during pregnancy. Mechanical deformations and poor maternal health are also implicated in a small percentage of birth defects. Other defects appear to be multifactorial, being influenced by combinations of these multiple, complex etiologies. In most instances of birth defects, however, the precise etiology is still undetermined, or at best our knowledge is incomplete.

Attempts to define birth defects by such factors as

etiology or age of detectability have, therefore, been of limited help to the people who care for children and families with birth defects. While such classifications are useful to scientists seeking to direct the most appropriate research expertise to particular diagnoses, individuals with birth defects usually come to the attention of the medical community without an exact diagnosis, motivated instead by concern for an unusual feature, sign, or symptom, or by the developmental disabilities that often accompany physical anomalies. Often the family itself can recognize that the source of concern is not a simple variation of normal human traits, and the primary practitioner rules out disease or injury. That which remains, which may or may not be recognized as a birth defect, almost certainly consists of one or more human anomalies of clinical relevance. It is these anomalies of clinical relevance which typically bring the patient to the attention of a specialist, and which perhaps best define the conditions and syndromes that are commonly called birth defects.

The significance of these anomalies, and the accurate diagnosis of individual conditions or of complex syndromes composed of multiple anomalies, are often difficult to determine. Many conditions simply do not look like their textbook definitions, or actually appear to be something else. Yet accurate diagnosis is critical to prognosis and treatment.

For example, some children have a facial muscle problem which seems to give them an uneven or lopsided smile. Sometimes this goes unnoticed. In other cases it is seen as a neurological problem associated with weak facial muscles. In still other cases, however, it is a component of a cardiofacial syndrome characterized not only by the asymmetric facies resulting from the absence of a facial muscle, but by an associated congenital heart defect.

Even within birth defects, things are not always as they appear. Severe limb defects are known to be caused by the drug Thalidomide. However, limb defects of this type have always existed and still do despite the lack of use of Thalidomide. Most limb defects result from various prenatal factors, but others are due to inherited malformation syndromes where the limb defects are seen in combination with other anomalies such as congenital heart disease. This is but one instance in which similar presenting problems have very different causes. Among the mucopolysaccharidoses, for example, conditions that look very different share common mechanisms of action, while others that seem to look alike have very different underlying mechanisms.

Since minor anomalies may serve as a clue to more serious problems, accurate and timely diagnosis is of vital concern to both parents and practitioners. This concern is felt not only by birth defect specialists, but by clinicians in the full range of specialties including cardi-

ologists, neurologists, orthopedic surgeons, and gastroenterologists, all of whom must consider possible birth defects in formulating diagnoses and interventions, and must also take into account the possibility that their treatment interventions may mask potential clues to more serious underlying conditions.

But even when a diagnosis can be established, prognosis and treatment can be hampered by a lack of information on the natural history of the diagnosed condition. This is particularly true of new or rare conditions for which few if any affected individuals have been available for follow-up study throughout the course of their lives. Since individual birth defect conditions tend to occur across time and with great geographic dispersion, a clinician trying to determine the prognosis and optimum treatment for a given patient may need to know the outcomes for all of the dozen or so similar patients seen throughout history in all corners of the globe.

While the dozen affected individuals in the above example are united in a concern which may be basic to the length and quality of their lives, gathering the needed data may pose an insurmountable task. Even if each of the dozen cases were accurately diagnosed and reported in the literature, it is highly probable that these reports will appear not only in different languages, but will define the condition in different ways using different names and with an emphasis on different aspects of the condition. While some reports would appear in medical journals, others may appear in basic science publications, public health reports, epidemiologic articles, or in other forms not even indexed as part of the medical literature. Since the condition has no consistent name, or is simply known by the names of the various people who reported the condition in different parts of the world, there may be no medical indexing terms that could unite the different reports.

Even if another clinician, faced with an earlier patient, had succeeded in bringing together most of the published reports, the nature of the medical literature makes it unlikely that subsequent cases would find their way into print. As ten separate reports of "new" conditions, each case could be accepted for publication, but the eleventh case of a defined rare condition would be of little interest to most journals, as in fact would all subsequent cases until such time as the condition became recognized as common enough to appear in epidemiologic studies or until there was a significant advance in knowledge about the condition. Since birth defects are both numerous and diverse, the majority of the individual conditions are uncommon and tend to fall between the focus of the various components of the established medical literature. But without some means of scientific communication about birth defects, it is difficult to make the progress that is needed both for individual patient care and for the advancement of medical knowledge.

Given the current state of medical science and technology, that potential progress can be highly significant, not only to individuals affected by a given condition but for the health sciences as a whole. The past few decades have been marked by two significant developments. First is the conceptual realization that all living things are united by common or complementary physiologic elements and by a corresponding biodynamic interdependence. This has been the driving force behind such major trends as the ecology movement, multidisciplinary research, and integrated health sciences education. The second development has been the rapid advance of biomedical technologies such as gene mapping and diagnostic imaging that hold the potential of creating a new and massive knowledgebase against which we can test and confirm our conceptual beliefs and theories about the basic nature of life itself.

Birth defects are our clearest examples of variation in the basic building blocks of life. The application of gene mapping and other advanced technologies to clearly delineated birth defect conditions can provide the key which unlocks our understanding of specific building blocks, not only as they apply to the condition in question, but as they affect all human beings and potentially all living things. Progress in the clinical diagnosis and treatment of individual patients with birth defects continues to be hampered by the lack of this basic information, yet the advancement of basic science research into the building blocks of life requires that clinicians be able to delineate human anomalies in a way which will make them amenable to basic science research.

More than a decade ago, these realizations made it clear to both the clinical and basic science communities that the then-fragmented approach to birth defects information and research would have to be supplemented by a set of permanent, ongoing, integrated services operated in support of international birth defects research, teaching, and clinical practice. A worldwide survey resulted in the election of an Advisory Board which would represent the interests of the contributors to and users of such services. This Board, which continues today, developed a foundation for the organization and programs that would follow.

While several governments expressed interest in and support of the objectives formulated by the Advisory Board, none could guarantee the continuity of participation or long-term support essential for such an undertaking. Similarly, individual universities and foundations offered to host the program, but it soon became clear that the effort would require the combined collaboration of institutions around the world. A consensus soon emerged that, in an age of competing political and economic interests, the only way to assure the independence, direction, and long-range future of such an ambitious undertaking would be through operation by and for the larger scientific community that it would serve.

The result was creation of the Center for Birth Defects Information Services, Inc. as an independent, non-profit international scientific collaborative. Every center of relevant expertise in the world was invited to collaborate in the work of the Center, and this invitation met with unanimous participation and support. From that point on, the strength of the Center has always been its network of participating experts who have devoted tens of thousands of hours to the missions of the Center, and whose scientific curiosity, humor, and dedication have made possible not only the success of the Center but the creation of an intellectual environment that transcends traditional physical boundaries and unites medical scientists in a spirit of cooperative determination and good will.

The basic concept was very simple. The leading experts in each topic or birth defect condition would prepare and continually update a structured article on their subject of expertise. The resulting combined literature would be made universally available. Every expert would have ongoing access to the work of all of the other contributors, thus assuring maximum information exchange and minimum duplication of effort. Other interested parties, including basic scientists and individuals with a direct professional or personal interest in birth defects, would have ongoing access to the knowledgebase and could share information that otherwise would not appear in the literature or would be communicated only indirectly or with considerable delay.

While the concept was simple, its implementation created unprecedented challenges. New birth defect conditions are delineated at a rate of about two per week, while significant advances are made in our understanding of over twenty percent of the known birth defects each year. Additional information on undiagnosed cases and new case reports of established conditions result in an enormous volume of information. Creation of this edition of the *Birth Defects Encyclopedia* alone would require author and editor review of over 100,000 pages of text. While new information technologies such as the personal computer, CD-ROM, Fax, and the laser printer would be enlisted in the service of the Center's missions, the sheer volume of data would stretch both technical and human limits. Computer storage requirements simply for active electronic communications (digitized incoming and outgoing fax and telephone messages), for example, would exceed half a gigabyte, a volume comparable to a full year of MEDLINE.

The nature and volume of the data placed particular

demands on the editorial staff, and on managing editorial operations which had to assure that the right information was routed to the right people in the right form at the right time. Ultimately, some sixty editors would be required to provide the necessary breadth of expertise and to deal with the quantity of information. Since scientific progress requires a constant cycle of obtaining new information, searching for patterns, sharing results with colleagues throughout the discipline, and once again collecting new information to be tested against current theories and assumptions, management and presentation of the evolving knowledgebase had to support this process. In addition, new information had to be processed quickly. Acceleration in the rate of scientific progress is not possible without a corresponding increase in the speed of the information assimilation cycle, while a cycle which falls behind the rate of new information production is of little more than archival value.

In addressing these issues, the Center was fortunate in being able to draw upon the services of a Board of Trustees who brought with them world-class expertise in the management of high-technology-based information management ventures. Its first focus, however, was not upon information hardware but upon the unique legal, intellectual property, and governance issues confronting this first-of-its-kind undertaking. Since centers of expertise shift, author and editor agreements had to be created that would protect the interests of both initial and subsequent contributors, and deal with the legal realities that result from new combinations of international print and electronic information delivery. In order to assure quality control and maintain prompt and appropriate access to the Center's knowledgebases, new types of publishing contracts had to be negotiated under which the Center would act as publisher while still being able to take advantage of the distribution and support services available only through collaboration with major international medical publishers.

The support of the high-technology community did provide early access to an expanding array of processing hardware, and the Center became the site of some the first applications for such diverse technologies as PC laser printers, the i486 computer chip, multiple access CD-ROM disk readers, and digital illustration processing. This facilitated, in turn, the Center's active program of software development, which included creation of the first computer-based medical diagnostic support system in general use by practicing clinicians, as well as special software for editorial operations support on for the electronic development, editing, storage, and multiple-media distribution of text-based knowledge. These technologies were developed to assure accurate, comprehensive, and timely access to an evolving knowledgebase that reflects the unique human expertise of the authors and editors who ultimately make it possible for the Center to implement its services and programs.

In the pages that follow, the Center's current services and programs are described in detail. We see these not as the culmination of our work, but as its beginning. We invite every reader of this *Encyclopedia* to join us in the continuing mission of the Center, and welcome your suggestions, comments, and participation.

# BOARD OF TRUSTEES

# ADVISORY BOARD

# TOPIC EDITORS

## CARDIOVASCULAR

**James J. Nora, M.D.**
Professor of Genetics
Preventive Medicine and Pediatrics
UNIVERSITY OF COLORADO MEDICAL CENTER
4200 East Ninth Avenue Container A-007
Denver, CO 80262

**Audrey H. Nora, M.D., M.P.H.**
Assistant Surgeon General
Public Health Service
HEALTH AND HUMAN SERVICES
1961 Stout Street
Denver, CO 80294

## CENTRAL NERVOUS SYSTEM

**William DeMyer, M.D.**
Professor of Child Neurology
Pediatric Neurology
INDIANA UNIVERSIRT - RILEY HOSPITAL
Room N-125
1100 W. Michigan Street
Indianapolis, IN 46223

## CHROMOSOMAL

**Jean de Grouchy, M.D.**
Directeur de Recherche au CNRS
Laboratoire de Cytogenetique Humaine
HOPITAL NECKER ENFANTS MALADES
149, rue de Sevres,
75743 Paris Cedex 15,
FRANCE

**Jean-Pierre Fryns, M.D.**
Head of Clinical Genetics
Division of Human Genetics
U.Z. GASTHUISBERG
Herestraat, 49
B-3000 Leuven,
BELGIUM

## CRANIOFACIAL

**Ronald J. Jorgenson, D.D.S., Ph.D.**
Department of Pediatric Dentistry
UNIVERSITY OF TEXAS HEALTH SCIENCE CENTER
7703 Floyd Curl Drive
San Antonio, TX 78284 7888

**Hermine Pashayan, M.D.** ‡
TUFTS UNIVERSITY SCHOOL OF MEDICINE
131 Harrison Avenue
Boston, MA 02111

**Jaime L. Frias, M.D.**
Professor and Chairman
Department of Pediatrics
UNIVERSITY OF NEBRASKA MEDICAL CENTER
42nd & Dewey Avenue
Omaha, NE 68105

‡ Deceased

## DERMATOLOGY

**Lawrence Solomon, M.D.**
Professor and Head
Department of Dermatology
UNIVERSITY OF ILLINOIS COLLEGE OF MEDICINE
P.O. Box 6998
Chicago, IL 60680

**Joseph Alper, M.D.**
Associate Professor of Medicine
Division of Dermatology
ROGER WILLIAMS GENERAL HOSPITAL
825 Chalkstone Avenue
Providence, RI 02908

## ENDOCRINOLOGIC

**R. Neil Schimke, M.D.**
Professor Internal Medicine/Pediatrics
UNIVERSITY OF KANSAS MEDICAL CENTER
39th and Rainbow Blvd, 413-C
Kansas City, KS 66103

## EAR, NOSE AND THROAT

**Charles M. Myer, III, M.D.**
Department of Pediatric Otolaryngology
CHILDREN'S HOSPITAL MEDICAL CENTER
Elland & Bethesda Avenues
Cincinnati, OH 45229 2899

## GASTROINTESTINAL

**Peter F. Whitington, M.D.**
Director, Gastroenterology
Department of Pediatrics
UNIVERSITY OF CHICAGO PRITZKER SCHOOL OF MEDICINE
5825 South Maryland Avenue Box 107
Chicago, IL 60637

**Marvin Ament, M.D.**
Chief, Division of Pediatric Gastroenterology
UNIVERSITY OF CALIFORNIA SCHOOL OF MEDICINE
MDCC 22-340 PS 62
Los Angeles, CA 90024

## GENITOURINAL

**Alan B. Retik, M.D.**
Chief, Division of Urology
BOSTON CHILDRENS HOSPITAL
300 Longwood Avenue
Boston, MA 02115

## HEMATOLOGY

**George R. Honig, M.D., Ph.D.**
Professor and Head
Department of Pediatrics (M/C 856)
THE UNIVERSITY OF ILLINOIS AT CHICAGO
840 South Wood Street
Box 6998
Chicago, IL 60680

## IMMUNOLOGY

**Stanley A. Schwartz, M.D., Ph.D.**
Director, Clinical Immunology Section
Department of Pediatrics
UNIVERSITY OF MICHIGAN
109 Observatory Street Room 3073
Ann Arbor, MI 48109

**Richard A. Gatti, M.D.**
Department of Pathology
UNIVERSITY OF CALIFORNIA SCHOOL OF MEDICINE
10833 Le Conte Avenue
Los Angeles, CA 90024-1732

## METABOLIC/AMINO ACID DEFECTS

**William L. Nyhan, M.D.**
Department of Pediatrics (M-009-A)
U.C.S.D. SCHOOL OF MEDICINE
La Jolla, CA 92093 0609

## METABOLIC/CARBOHYDRATE DEFECTS

**Edward R.B. McCabe, M.D., Ph.D.**
Director, R.J. Kleberg Jr. Center
Institute for Molecular Genetics
BAYLOR COLLEGE OF MEDICINE
One Baylor Plaza T-526
Houston, TX 77030

**James B. Sidbury, Jr., M.D.**
Senior Scientist
NATIONAL INSTITUTE OF CHILD HEALTH AND HUMAN DEVELOPMENT
Building 10, 8C311
Bethesda, MD 20205

## METABOLIC/LIPID DEFECTS

**Hugo Moser, M.D.**
Professor of Neurology and Pediatrics
Johns Hopkins University and President
J.F. KENNEDY INSTITUTE FOR HANDICAPPED CHILDREN
707 North Broadway
Baltimore, MD 21205

## METABOLIC/OTHER DEFECTS

**William L. Nyhan, M.D.**
Department of Pediatrics (M-009-A)
U.C.S.D. SCHOOL OF MEDICINE
La Jolla, CA 92093 0609

## METABOLIC/RENAL TRANSPORT

**Charles R. Scriver, M.D.**
Professor, Center for Human Genetics
McGILL UNIVERSITY-MONTREAL CHILDREN'S HOSPITAL
2300 Tupper Street
Montreal H3H 1P3,
CANADA

## MYOPATHY

**Victor Ionasescu, M.D.**
Professor of Pediatrics
THE UNIVERSITY OF IOWA
University of Iowa Hospitals and Clinics
Iowa City, IA 52242

## NEUROLOGY

**Raymond S. Kandt, M.D.**
Associate Professor
Pediatric Neurology
DUKE UNIVERSITY
Box 3533
Durham, NC 27710

## ORAL AND DENTAL PATHOLOGY

**David Bixler, D.D.S., Ph.D.**
Professor of Oral-Facial Genetics
INDIANA UNIVERSITY - PURDUE UNIVERSITY
Ball Residence, Room 026
1226 West Michigan Street
Indianapolis, IN 46223

## OPHTHALMOLOGY

**Bernard Becker, M.D.**
Professor and Head
Department of Ophthalmology
WASHINGTON UNIVERSITY SCHOOL OF MEDICINE
660 South Euclid Avenue
Box 8096
St. Louis, MO 63110

**Elias Traboulsi, M.D.**
5550 Columbia Pike No. 702
Arlington, VA 22204

## PULMONARY DEFECTS

**Samuel T. Giammona, M.D.**
Chairman and Professor
Department of Pediatrics
CHILDREN'S HOSPITAL OF SAN FRANCISCO
3700 California Street
San Francisco, CA 94119

## SKELETAL AND CONNECTIVE TISSUE DEFECTS

**William A. Horton, M.D.**
Professor of Pediatrics and Medicine
UNIVERSITY OF TEXAS MEDICAL SCHOOL
P.O. Box 20708
Houston, TX 77225

**Peter Beighton, M.D., Ph.D.**
Professor of Human Genetics
MEDICAL SCHOOL, UNIVERSITY OF CAPE TOWN
Observatory
Cape Town, 7925
SOUTH AFRICA

## SPECIAL SYNDROMES

**Frank Greenberg, M.D.**
Birth Defects Genetics Clinic
BAYLOR COLLEGE OF MEDICINE
Texas Medical Center
6621 Fannin
Houston, TX 77030

## TERATOGENS

**Franz W. Rosa, M.D., M.P.H.**
FOOD AND DRUG ADMINISTRATION
Room 15 B-07
HFN-733
5600 Fishers Lane
Rockville, MD 20852

**Sidney Q. Cohlan, M.D.**
Department of Pediatrics
NEW YORK UNIVERSITY MEDICAL CENTER
530 First Avenue Suite 3A
New York, NY 10016

## RHEUMATIC AND JOINT DISEASES

**Balu H. Athreya, M.D.**
Pediatric Rheumatology Center
UNIVERSITY OF PENNSYLVANIA
One Children's Center
34th Street & Civic Center Boulevard
Philadelphia, PA 19104

**Don C. Van Dyke, M.D.**
Department of Pediatrics
UNIVERSITY OF IOWA HOSPITALS AND CLINICS
213 University Hospital School
Iowa City, IA 52242

## HEARING DISORDERS

**Frederick R. Bieber, Ph.D.**
Department of Pathology
BRIGHAM AND WOMEN'S HOSPITAL
75 Francis Street
Boston, MA 02115

## GENETIC ONCOLOGY

**John J. Mulvihill, M.D.**
Director, NIH Center Institute
Medical Genetics Program
NATIONAL CANCER INSTITUTE
National Institutes of Health
Executive Plaza North, Room 400
Bethesda, MD 20892

## NEW SYNDROMES

**Helga Toriello, Ph.D.**
Genetics Services
BUTTERWORTH HOSPITAL
21 Michigan Street Suite 350
Grand Rapids, MI 49503

## SKELETAL DYSPLASIAS

**William A. Horton, M.D.**
Professor of Pediatrics and Medicine
UNIVERSITY OF TEXAS MEDICAL SCHOOL
P.O. Box 20708
Houston, TX 77225

## REPRODUCTIVE SYSTEM DEFECTS

**Joe Leigh Simpson, M.D.**
Faculty Professor and Chairman
Department of Obstetrics and Gynecology
UNIVERSITY OF TENNESSEE, MEMPHIS
853 Jefferson Avenue
Memphis, TN 38163

# CONTRIBUTING EDITORS

**Frank Greenberg, M.D.**
Birth Defects Genetics Clinic
BAYLOR COLLEGE OF MEDICINE
Texas Medical Center
6621 Fannin
Houston, TX 77030


**Ronald J. Jorgenson, D.D.S., Ph.D.**
Department of Pediatric Dentistry
UNIVERSITY OF TEXAS HEALTH SCIENCE CENTER
7703 Floyd Curl Drive
San Antonio, TX 78284 7888


**Marta Pinheiro, D.Sc.**
Department of Genetics
FEDERAL UNIVERSITY OF PARANA
Caixa Postal 19071
81504 Curitiba
Parana
BRAZIL


**Franz W. Rosa, M.D., M.P.H.**
FOOD AND DRUG ADMINISTRATION
Room 15 B-07 HFN-733
5600 Fishers Lane
Rockville, MD 20852


**Helga Toriello, Ph.D.**
Genetics Services
BUTTERWORTH HOSPITAL
21 Michigan Street Suite 350
Grand Rapids, MI 49503


**Catherine Turleau, M.D.**
Directeur de Recherche au C.N.R.S.
Laboratoire de Cytogenetique Humaine
HOPITAL NECKER ENFANTS MALADES
Unite 173 INSERM
75743 Paris Cedex 15
FRANCE

# CONTRIBUTORS

**Dagfinn Aarskog, M.D.**
Professor of Pediatrics
Haukeland Hospital
UNIVERSITY OF BERGEN
N-5021 Bergen
NORWAY

**Jon M. Aase, M.D.**
Department of Pediatrics
UNIVERSITY OF NEW MEXICO SCHOOL OF MEDICINE
Albuquerque, NM 87131

**Donald C. Aberfeld, M.D.**
870 United Nations Plaza 14-F
New York, NY 10017

**Dianne Abuelo, M.D.**
Director
Genetic Counseling Center
R.I. HOSPITAL
593 Eddy Street
Providence, RI 02902

**Hugo Aebi, M.D.** ‡
Medizinisch-Chemisches Institut
UNIVERSITAT BERN
Buhlstrasse 28
CH-3000
Bern 9
SWITZERLAND

**Peter Agre, M.D.**
Associate Professor of Medicine
JOHNS HOPKINS HOSPITAL
725 North Wolfe Street Hunterian 103
Baltimore, MD 21205

**Luke P. Akard, M.D.**
Assistant Professor of Medicine
Division of Hematology/Oncology
INDIANA UNIVERSITY SCHOOL OF MEDICINE
Clinical Building, Room 379
541 Clinical Drive
Indianapolis, IN 46223

**S.A. Al-Awadi, M.D.**
Maternity Hospital
KUWAIT MEDICAL GENETICS CENTRE
P.O. Box 4080 Code 13041
Safat
KUWAIT

**Mark J. Alberts, M.D.**
Assistant Professor
Division of Neurology, Dept. of Medicine
DUKE UNIVERSITY MEDICAL CENTER
P.O. Box 2900
Durham, NC 27710

**Deborah Alcorn, M.D.**
The Wilmer Ophthalmological Institute
THE JOHNS HOPKINS HOSPITAL
Maumenee Building Room 321
600 North Wolfe Street
Baltimore, MD 21205

**Kirk Aleck, M.D.**
VIVIGEN, INC.
435 St. Michael's Drive
Santa Fe, NM 87501

**Judith Allanson, M.D.**
Division of Clinical Genetics
CHILDREN'S HOSPITAL OF EASTERN ONTARIO
401 Smyth
Ottawa K1H 8L1 ONT
CANADA

**Richard Allen, M.D.**
Pediatric Neurology
UNIVERSITY OF MICHIGAN MEDICAL CENTER
Box 0800 C7123 O.P.D.
1500 East Medical Drive
Ann Arbor, MI 48109 0800

**Estella M. Alonso, M.D.**
Research Fellow
Pediatric Gastroenterology
UNIVERSITY OF CHICAGO PRITZKER SCHOOL OF MEDICINE
5825 South Maryland Avenue Box 107
Chicago, IL 60637

**R. Stephan S. Amato, M.D., Ph.D.**
Prof. and Director of Medical Genetics
Department of Pediatrics
WEST VIRGINIA UNIVERSITY MEDICAL CENTER
Morgantown, WV 26506

**Arthur J. Ammann, M.D.**
Director
Collaborative Medical Research Program
GENENTECH, INC.
460 Point San Bruno Boulevard
South San Francisco, CA 94080

**Mary Ampola, M.D.**
Acting Director, Clinical Genetics
Department of Pediatrics
NEW ENGLAND MEDICAL CENTER
750 Washington Street
Boston, MA 02111

**Eva Andermann, M.D., Ph.D.**
Department of Neurology
MONTREAL NEUROLOGICAL HOSPITAL / McGILL UNIVERSITY
3801 University Street
Montreal PQ H3A 2B4
CANADA

**Frederick Andermann, M.D.**
Department of Neurology
MONTREAL NEUROLOGICAL HOSPITAL / McGILL UNIVERSITY
3801 University Street
Montreal PQ H3A 2B4
CANADA

**David E. Anderson, Ph.D.**
Ashbel Smith Professor of Genetics
M.D. ANDERSON CANCER CENTER
1515 Holcombe Blvd. HMB Box 209
Houston, TX 77030

**Ray M. Antley, M.D.**
Department of Radiology
GRACE HOSPITAL, INC.
2201 South Sterling Street
Morganton, NC 28655

**Rene A. Arcilla, M.D.**
Depts. of Cardiology and Genetics
UNIVERSITY OF CHICAGO PRITZKER SCHOOL OF MEDICINE
950 East 59th Street
Chicago, IL 60637

**Holly Hutchison Ardinger, M.D.**
Assistant Professor
Department of Pediatrics
Box 777
UNIVERSITY OF ROCHESTER
601 Elmwood Avenue
Rochester, NY 14642

**Fernando Arena, M.D., Ph.D.**
Genetics Division
MAILMAN CENTER FOR CHILD DEVELOPMENT
University of Miami
P.O. Box 016820
Miami, FL 33101

‡ Deceased

**Frank C. Arnett, M.D.**
Prof. of Internal Medicine
Division of Rheumatology
UNIVERSITY OF TEXAS HEALTH SCIENCE CENTER
Houston, TX 77225

**Keith W. Ashcraft, M.D.**
CHILDREN'S MERCY HOSPITAL
24th at Gillham Road
Kansas City, MO 64108

**Balu H. Athreya, M.D.**
Pediatric Rheumatology Center
UNIVERSITY OF PENNSYLVANIA
One Children's Center
34th Street & Civic Center Boulevard
Philadelphia, PA 19104

**Joan F. Atkin, M.D.**
Department of Pediatrics
UNIVERSITY OF VIRGINIA HOSPITAL
P.O. Box 386
Charlottesville, VA 22908

**Thomas Aufdemorte, D.M.D.**
Division of Oral Pathology
School of Dentistry
UNIVERSITY OF TEXAS HEALTH SCIENCE CENTER
7703 Floyd Curl Drive
San Antonio, TX 78284

**Pertti P. Aula, M.D.**
Associate Professor of Medical Genetics
Institute of Biomedicine
UNIVERSITY OF TURKU
Kiinamyllynkatu 10
SF-20520 Turku
FINLAND

**James H. Austin, M.D.**
Professor and Chairman
Department of Neurology
UNIVERSITY OF COLORADO SCHOOL OF MEDICINE
Denver, CO 80220

**Paula D. Awrich**
Department of Human Genetics
MEDICAL COLLEGE OF VIRGINIA
Box 33 - MCV Station
Richmond, VA 23298

**Richard Ashley Axtell, M.D.**
Assistant Professor of Hematology
UNIVERSITY OF MICHIGAN MEDICAL CENTER
Mott Hospital Box 0238
Ann Arbor, MI 48109

**Arthur S. Aylsworth, M.D.**
Division of Genetics & Metabolism
Department of Pediatrics
UNIVERSITY OF NORTH CAROLINA SCHOOL OF MEDICINE
C.B. No. 7250 - B.S.R.C.
Chapel Hill, NC 27599-7250

**Segolene Marie Ayme, M.D.**
Director of Research
Centre de Genetique Medicale
INSERM U 242
Hopital de la Timone
Marseille 13385
FRANCE

**A. Aynsley-Green, D.Phil.**
James Spence Professor of Child Health
Department of Child Health
UNIVERSITY OF NEWCASTLE UPON TYNE MEDICAL SCHOOL
Framlington Place
NE2 4HH
Newcastle Upon Tyne
ENGLAND

**Biagio Azzarelli, M.D.**
Associate Professor of Pathology
INDIANA UNIVERSITY SCHOOL OF MEDICINE
Medical Science Building A142
635 Barnhill Drive
Indianapolis, IN 46223

**Patricia A. Baird, M.D.**
Professor of Medical Genetics
UNIVERSITY OF BRITISH COLUMBIA
Westbrook Building
Room 222
Vancouver V6T 1W5 BC
CANADA

**Mark Ballow, M.D.**
Department of Pediatrics
UNIVERSITY OF CONNECTICUT HEALTH CENTER
Farmington, CT 06032

**I. Hussain Bangash, M.R.C.P.**
Fellow in Pediatric Neurology
DUKE UNIVERSITY MEDICAL CENTER
Box 3533
Durham, NC 27710

**Betty Banker, M.D.**
Professor of Pathology
DARTMOUTH MEDICAL SCHOOL
Remsen 236
Hanover, NH 03756

**Agnes Bankier, M.D.**
Department of Genetics
ROYAL CHILDREN'S HOSPITAL
Flemington Road
Parkville
Victoria 3052
AUSTRALIA

**Michael Baraitser, M.D.**
Clinical Genetics Unit
INSTITUTE OF CHILD HEALTH
30 Guilford Street
London WC1N 1EH
ENGLAND

**Amin Y. Barakat, M.D.**
Clinical Professor of Nephrology
GEORGETOWN UNIVERSITY MEDICAL CENTER
107 North Virginia Avenue
Falls Church, VA 22046

**Kristine K. Barlow, Ph.D.,B.Sc.**
COMMONWEALTH INSTITUTE OF HEALTH
University of Sydney A27
N.S.W 2006
Sydney
AUSTRALIA

**Bruce A. Barshop, M.D., Ph.D.**
Department of Medicine (M-0131)
U.C.S.D. SCHOOL OF MEDICINE
La Jolla, CA 92093

**James A. Bartley, M.D., Ph.D.**
Department of Pediatrics
LOMA LINDA UNIVERSITY SCHOOL OF MEDICINE
11370 Anderson Street, Suite B-100
Loma Linda, CA 92354

**Louis E. Bartoshesky, M.D., M.P.H.**
708 Coverdale Road
Wilmington, DE 19805

**Harold N. Bass, M.D.**
Clinical Professor, U.C.L.A
Director of Genetic Services
KAISER-PERMANENTE MEDICAL CENTER
13652 Cantara Street
Panorama City, CA 91402 5497

**J. Bronwyn Bateman, M.D.**
Assistant Professor
Jules Stein Eye Institute
U.C.L.A. MEDICAL SCHOOL
Los Angeles, CA 90024

**Mark L. Batshaw, M.D.**
Physician-in-Chief
CHILDREN'S SEASHORE HOUSE
3400 Civic Center Blvd.
Philadelphia, PA 19104

**R. Beals, M.D.**
Division of Orthopedics and Rehab.
OREGON HEALTH SCIENCES UNIVERSITY OP 13B
3181 S.W. Sam Jackson Park Road
Portland, OR 97201

**Michael Beck, M.D.**
Children's Hospital
UNIVERSITY OF MAINZ
Langenbeckstrasse 1
65 Mainz
WEST GERMANY

**Frits A. Beemer, M.D., Ph.D.**
KLINISCH GENETISCH CENTRUM UTRECHT
Postbus 18009
3501 CA Utrecht
THE NETHERLANDS

**Peter Beighton, M.D., Ph.D.**
Professor of Human Genetics
MEDICAL SCHOOL, UNIVERSITY OF CAPE TOWN
Observatory
Cape Town 7925
SOUTH AFRICA

**Merrill D. Benson, M.D.**
Professor of Medical Genetics
INDIANA UNIVERSITY SCHOOL OF MEDICINE
Medical Research Building IB 130
Indianapolis, IN 46223

**Donald R. Bergsma, M.D.**
L.S.U. EYE CENTER
2020 Gravier Street Suite B
New Orleans, LA 70112 2234

**LaVonne Bergstrom, M.D.**
Professor of Surgery
Division of Head and Neck Surgery
UNIVERSITY OF CALIFORNIA AT LOS ANGELES
1000 Veteran Avenue
Room 31-24 Rehab.
Los Angeles, CA 90024

**Michael A. Berman, M.D.**
Professor of Pediatrics
UNIVERSITY OF MARYLAND
225 Greene Street, Room S-1011
Baltimore, MD 21201

**Renee Bernstein, M.D.**
Director of the Cytogenetic Laboratory
Division of Human Genetics
UNIVERSITY OF CALIFORNIA IRVINE MEDICAL CENTER
Medical Center Building 27, Route 81
101 City Drive South
Orange, CA 92668

**Arthur S. Besser, M.D.**
Asso. Prof. of Surgery and Pediatrics
UNIVERSITY OF CHICAGO WYLER CHILDREN'S HOSPITAL
5841 South Maryland Avenue
Box 163
Chiacgo, IL 60637

**Diana W. Bianchi, M.D.**
Division of Genetics
CHILDREN'S HOSPITAL MEDICAL CENTER
300 Longwood Avenue
Boston, MA 02115

**Frederick R. Bieber, Ph.D.**
Department of Pathology
BRIGHAM AND WOMEN'S HOSPITAL
75 Francis Street
Boston, MA 02115

**Robert M. Bilenker, M.D.**
Head, Comprehensive Care Program
Department of Pediatrics
METROHEALTH MEDICAL CENTER
3395 Scranton Road
Cleveland, OH 44109

**Nesrin Bingol, M.D.**
Director of Clinical Genetics
Department of Pediatrics & Obstetrics
NEW YORK MEDICAL COLLEGE / LINCOLN HOSPITAL
234 East 149th Street
Bronx, NY 10451

**Thomas Bird, M.D.**
Department of Neurology
UNIVERSITY OF WASHINGTON MEDICAL CENTER
Seattle, WA 98195

**David Bixler, D.D.S., Ph.D.**
Professor of Oral-Facial Genetics
INDIANA UNIVERSITY - PURDUE UNIVERSITY
Ball Residence, Room 026
1226 West Michigan Street
Indianapolis, IN 46223

**Dennis D. Black, M.D.**
Division of Gastroenterology
UNIVERSITY OF CHICAGO PRITZKER SCHOOL OF MEDICINE
5825 South Maryland Avenue Box 107
Chicago, IL 60637

**Will Blackburn, M.D.**
Professor and Director
Perinatal-Pediatric Pathology
UNIVERSITY OF SOUTH ALABAMA COLLEGE OF MEDICINE
2451 Fillingim Street
Mobile, AL 36617

**John P. Blass, M.D.**
THE BURKE REHABILITATION CENTER
785 Mamaroneck Avenue
White Plains, NY 10605

**E.M. Bleeker-Wagemakers, M.D., Ph.D.**
Prof. of Ophthalmogenetics
Department of Ophthalmogenetics
THE NETHERLANDS OPHTHALMIC RESEARCH INSTITUTE
Meibergdreef 9
P.O. Box 12141
1100 AC Amsterdam
THE NETHERLANDS

**Robert M. Blizzard, M.D.**
Professor and Chairman
Department of Pediatrics
UNIVERSITY OF VIRGINIA SCHOOL OF MEDICINE
Charlottesville, VA 22901

**Joseph R. Bloomer, M.D.**
Head, Division of Gastroenterology
Department of Medicine
UNIVERSITY OF MINNESOTA MEDICAL SCHOOL
Mayo Box 36
Minneapolis, MN 55455

**Jan A. Book, M.D., Ph.D.**
Clinical Genetics
LE HAMEAU DU CHATEAU
23 Rue de la cour
F-74000
Annecy-Le-Vieux
FRANCE

**Digamber S. Borgaonkar, Ph.D.**
Director, Cytogenetics Lab
MEDICAL CENTER OF DELAWARE
P.O. Box 6001
Wilmington, DE 19718

**Zvi Borochowitz, M.D.**
Director
Genetics Institute
BNAI-ZION MEDICAL CENTER
P.O. Box 4940
Haifa 31048
ISRAEL

**Carla Borrone, Primario**
Head, II Divisione Pediatria
INST GIANNINA GASLINI
Largo G. Gaslini 1
16148 Genova Quarto
ITALY

**Valerie L. Boswell, M.D.**
Department of Otolaryngology
UNIVERSITY OF TORONTO
7-219 Eaton North
200 Elizabeth Street
Toronto M5G 2C4 ON
CANADA

**Sylvia S. Bottomley, M.D.**
Hematology Section
(111J)
V. A. MEDICAL CENTER
921 N.E. 13th Street
Oklahoma City, OK 73104

**Rose-Mary N. Boustany, M.D.**
Associate Professor of Medicine
Division of Pediatric Neurology
DUKE UNIVERSITY MEDICAL CENTER
Box 3533
Durham, NC 27710

**Peter A. Bowen, M.D.** ‡
Department of Pediatrics
UNIVERSITY OF ALBERTA
Edmonton AL T6G 2B7
CANADA

**Barbara Bowman, Ph.D.**
Department of Cellular and Structural Biology
UNIVERSITY OF TEXAS HEALTH SCIENCE CENTER
7703 Floyd Curl Drive
San Antonio, TX 78284

**Laurence A. Boxer, M.D.**
Section on Pediatric Hematology-Oncology
Department of Pediatrics Room F6515
MOTT CHILDREN'S HOSPITAL
Box 0238
Ann Arbor, MI 48109 0238

**Walter Bradley, M.D.**
Chairman
Department of Neurology
UNIVERSITY OF VERMONT MEDICAL CENTER
One South Prospect Street
Burlington, VT 05405

**Elizabeth A. Braunlin, M.D.**
Pediatric Cardiology
UNIVERSITY OF MINNESOTA
420 Delaware Street, S.E.
Box 94
Minneapolis, MN 55455

**W. Roy Breg, M.D.**
Professor of Human Genetics
YALE UNIVERSITY SCHOOL OF MEDICINE
333 Cedar Street
New Haven, CT 06510 8005

**David A. Brenner, M.D.**
Department of Medicine
(M-023-D)
U.C.S.D. SCHOOL OF MEDICINE
La Jolla, CA 92093

**Joel I. Brenner, M.D.**
Associate Professor of Pediatrics
UNIVERSITY OF MARYLAND SCHOOL OF MEDICINE
22 South Greene Street
Baltimore, MD 21201

**Jan L. Breslow, M.D.**
ROCKEFELLER UNIVERSITY
1230 York Avenue
New York, NY 10021 6399

**J. Timothy Bricker, M.D.**
Associate in Pediatric Cardiology
Pediatric Cardiology
TEXAS CHILDREN'S HOSPITAL
6621 Fannin Street
Houston, TX 77030

**Diane L. Broome, M.D.**
4100 Locust
Long Beach, CA 90807

**W. Ted Brown, M.D., Ph.D.**
Chief, Division of Human Genetics
NORTH SHORE UNIVERSITY HOSPITAL
300 Community Drive
Manhasset, NY 11030

**Christine Bryke, M.D.**
Fellow in Genetics
Department of Medical Genetics
YALE UNIVERSITY
P.O. Box 3333
I-310 SHM
New Haven, CT 06510 8062

**Richard L. Bucciarelli, M.D.**
3531 NW 30th Boulevard
Gainesville, FL 32607

**Janet A. Buchanan, Ph.D.**
Postdoctoral Fellow
Department of Genetics
HOSPITAL FOR SICK CHILDREN
555 University Avenue
Toronto M5G 1X8
CANADA

**Rebecca H. Buckley, M.D.**
J. Buren Sidbury Professor
Depts. of Pediatrics and Immunology
DUKE UNIVERSITY MEDICAL CENTER
Box 2898
Durham, NC 27710

**Bruce A. Buehler, M.D.**
Director
Center for Human Genetics
UNIVERSITY OF NEBRASKA MEDICAL CENTER
42nd Street and Dewey Avenue
Omaha, NE 68105

**Neil R.M. Buist, M.B., Ch.B.**
Prof. of Pediatrics and Medical Genetics
Department of Pediatrics - Genetics
THE OREGON HEALTH SCIENCES UNIVERSITY L473
3181 S.W. Sam Jackson Park Road
Portland, OR 97201

**Marilyn J. Bull, M.D.**
Riley Hospital for Children Room S139
INDIANA UNIVERSITY SCHOOL OF MEDICINE
702 Barnhill Drive
Indianapolis, IN 46202 5200

**Randall W. Burt, M.D.**
Associate Professor of Medicine
Division of Gastroenterology Room 4R118
UNIVERSITY OF UTAH MEDICAL CENTER
Salt Lake City, UT 84132

**Merlin G. Butler, M.D., Ph.D.**
Division of Genetics
Department of Pediatrics
VANDERBILT COLLEGE OF MEDICINE
Medical Center North Room T2404
Nashville, TN 37232

**Mary Louise Buyse, M.D.**
Director
CENTER FOR BIRTH DEFECTS INFORMATION SERVICES, INC.
Dover Medical Building Box 1776
Dover, MA 02030

**L. Katie Byrd, M.D.**
MEDICAL COLLEGE OF GEORGIA
1120 15th Street
Augusta, GA 30912

**Jose-Maria Cantu, M.D.**
INSTITUTO MEXICANO DEL SEGURO SOCIAL
Ap. Postal 1-3838
Guadalajara
MEXICO

**Mary Esther Carlin, M.D.**
Assistant Professor, Pediatrics
Division of Genetics
UNIVERSITY OF MIAMI
School of Medicine
P.O. Box 016820
Miami, FL 33101

**J. Aidan Carney, M.D., Ph.D.**
Department of Pathology
MAYO CLINIC AND FOUNDATION
200 S.W. First Street
Rochester, MN 55905

**Nancy J. Carpenter, Ph.D.**
CHILDREN'S MEDICAL CENTER
5300 East Skelly Drive
P.O. Box 35648
Tulsa, OK 74153

**Sandra Ann Carson, M.D.**
Assistant Professor of OB/GYN
Division of Reproductive Endocrinology
UNIVERSITY OF TENNESSEE HEALTH SCIENCES CENTER
Coleman Building D-324
956 Court Avenue
Memphis, TN 38163

**Anthony C. Casamassima, M.D.**
Associate Director of Medical Genetics
WESTCHESTER COUNTY MEDICAL CENTER
Valhalla, NY 10595

**Suzanne B. Cassidy, M.D.**
Associate Professor of Pediatrics
Division of Genetics and Dysmorphology
UNIVERSITY OF ARIZONA HEALTH SCIENCES CENTER
1501 North Campbell Avenue
Tucson, AZ 85724

**Stephen D. Cederbaum, M.D.**
Mental Retardation Unit
Neuropsychiatric Institute
U.C.L.A. CENTER FOR HEALTH SCIENCES
760 Westwood Plaza
Los Angeles, CA 90024

**Jaroslav Cervenka, M.D., Ph.D.**
Professor and Director Cytogenetics
Department of Oral Pathology & Genetics
UNIVERSITY OF MINNESOTA
MOOS Health Sci. Tower-16-144
515 Delaware Street, S.E.
Minneapolis, MN 55455

**Philip F. Chance, M.D.**
Division of Genetics
VANDERBILT UNIVERSITY SCHOOL OF MEDICINE
Nashville, TN 37232

**Catherine E. Charman, R.N., B.S.N.**
Nurse Coordinator
Clinical Genetics Program
DARTMOUTH MEDICAL SCHOOL
Hanover, NH 03756

**Juan Chemke, M.D.**
Division of Medical Genetics
THE MONTREAL CHILDREN'S HOSPITAL
2300 Tupper
Montreal H3H 1P3 PQ
CANADA

**Harold Chen, M.D.**
Director
Medical Genetics / Birth Defects
CHILDREN'S MEDICAL CENTER
One Children's Plaza
Dayton, OH 45404

**Russell Wallace Chesney, M.D.**
3321 Waynoka Avenue
Memphis, TN 38111

**Jayanta Roy Chowdhury, M.D.**
Professor of Medicine
Liver Research Center
ALBERT EINSTEIN COLLEGE OF MEDICINE
Ullman Building Room 605
1300 Morris Park Avenue
Bronx, NY 10461

**Joe C. Christian, M.D., Ph.D**
Professor and Chairman
Department of Medical Genetics
INDIANA UNIVERSITY MEDICAL CENTER
702 Barnhill Drive RR 129
Indianapolis, IN 46223

**George P. Chrousos, M.D.**
Senior Investigator
Developmental Endocrinology Branch
N.I.C.H.D.
NATIONAL INSTITUTES OF HEALTH
Bethesda, MD 20892

**Georgia A. Chrousos, M.D.**
Center for Sight
GEORGETOWN UNIVERSITY MEDICAL CENTER
3800 Reservoir Road, N.W.
Washington, DC 20007

**Krysztyna Chrzanowska, M.D.**
Center for Human Genetics
U.Z. GASTHUISBERG
Herestraat, 49
B-3000 Leuven
BELGIUM

**Fred Chu, M.D.**
Pediatric Ophthalmology
ST. LOUIS CHILDREN'S HOSPITALS
Eye Clinic
400 South King's Highway
St. Louis, MO 63110

**Albert E. Chudley, M.D.**
Associate Professor
Child Health and Human Genetics
CHILDREN'S HOSPITAL
840 Sherbrook Street FE231 C.S.B.
Winnipeg R3A 1S1 MB
CANADA

**G. Gregory Clark, M.D.**
Clinical Instructor
INDIANA UNIVERSITY MEDICAL CENTER
50 East 91st Street, Suite 104
Indianapolis, IN 46240

**Robin Dawn Clark, M.D.**
Division of Genetics
Department of Pediatrics
LOMA LINDA UNIVERSITY SCHOOL OF MEDICINE
Loma Linda, CA 92350

**Sterling K. Clarren, M.D.**
Professor of Pediatrics
Head, Division of Congenital Defects
UNIVERSITY OF WASHINGTON
Children's Hospital Medical Center
4800 Sand Point Way, N.E.
Seattle, WA 98105

**H. William Clatworthy, Jr., M.D.**
Professor Emeritus of Pediatric Surgery
Ohio State University College of Medicine
COLUMBUS CHILDREN'S HOSPITAL
17th and Livingston
Columbus, OH 43205

**C. Carlyle Clawson, M.D.**
Professor of Pediatrics
UNIVERSITY OF MINNESOTA
Box 742 U.M.H.C.
516 Delaware Street, S.E.
Minneapolis, MN 55455

**Hartwig Cleve, M.D.**
Department of Anthropology
UNIVERSITY OF MUNICH
Richard-Wagner-Strasse 10/I
D-8000 Munchen 2
FED REP OF GERMANY

**Paul M. Coates, Ph.D.**
Research Professor
Division of Gastroenterology & Nutrition
CHILDREN'S HOSPITAL OF PHILADELPHIA
34th Street and Civic Center Blvd.
Philadelphia, PA 19104

**David Cogan, M.D.**
Senior Medical Officer
Clinical Branch
NATIONAL EYE INSTITUTE
NIH Room 10C205
Bethesda, MD 20014

**Alan Cohen, M.D.**
Chief of Medicine
BOSTON CITY HOSPITAL
Thorndike 314
818 Harrison Avenue
Boston, MA 02118

**David E.C. Cole, M.D., Ph.D.**
I.W. KILLAM CHILDREN'S HOSPITAL
5850 University Avenue Room 415
P.O. Box 3070
Halifax B3J 3G9 NS
CANADA

**Mary Coleman, M.D.**
321 West 13th Street 5C
New York, NY 10011 1242

**David E. Comings, M.D.**
Department of Medical Genetics
CITY OF HOPE MEDICAL CENTER
1500 East Duarte Road
Duarte, CA 91010

**Mike Conneally, Ph.D.**
Distinguished Professor
Medical Genetics and Neurology
INDIANA UNIVERSITY MEDICAL SCHOOL
975 West Walnut Street
Indianapolis, IN 46202 5251

**J. Michael Connor, M.D.**
Professor of Medical Genetics
DUNCAN GUTHRIE INSTITUTE OF MEDICAL GENETICS
Yorkhill
Glasgow G3 8SJ
SCOTLAND

**William J. Conte, M.D.**
1580 West El Camino Real Suite Two
Mountain View, CA 94040

**Brian Cook, M.D.**
Dermatology Resident
Department of Dermatology
UNIVERSITY OF ILLINOIS COLLEGE OF MEDICINE
P.O. Box 6998
Chicago, IL 60680

**Linda F. Cooper, M.S.**
Genetic Counselor
Department of Pediatric Genetics
THE JOHNS HOPKINS SCHOOL OF MEDICINE
Blalock 1008
600 North Wolfe Street
Baltimore, MD 21205

**Louis Z. Cooper, M.D.**
Professor and Director
Department of Pediatrics
ST. LUKES - ROOSEVELT HOSPITAL
Amsterdam Avenue at 114th Street
New York, NY 10025

**Enrique Corona-Rivera, M.D.**
Clinica de Asesoramiento Genetico CAGUG
Laboratorio de Genetica Humana
UNIVERSIDAD DE GUADALAJARA
Apartado Postal 2-298
Guadalajara, Jalisco
MEXICO

**James J. Corrigan, M.D.**
Professor of Pediatrics
UNIVERSITY OF ARIZONA HEALTH SCIENCES CENTER
1501 North Campbell Avenue
Tucson, AZ 85724

**Xavier Cortada, M.D.**
GENETIC SERVICES OF TAMPA BAY
2901 St. Isabel Street Suite F
Tampa, FL 33607

**Maria P. de A. Coutinho, M.D.**
Chefe de Servico de Neurologia
Departamento de Doencas Neurologicas
HOSPITAL GERAL DE SANTO ANTONIO
Lg. Abel Salazar
4000 Porto
PORTUGAL

**F. Susan Cowchock, M.D.**
Department of Medicine
JEFFERSON MEDICAL COLLEGE
408 Curtis
Philadelphia, PA 19107

**Barbara Crandall, M.D.**
Department of Psychiatry and Pediatrics
NEUROPSYCHIATRIC INSTITUTE
University of California at Los Angeles
Los Angeles, CA 90024

**John Currah Crawhall, M.D., Ph.D.**
Director of Clinical Biochemistry
ROYAL VICTORIA HOSPITAL
687 Pine Avenue West
Montreal H3A 1A1
CANADA

**Cor W.R.J. Cremers, M.D.**
Department of Otorhinolaryngology
UNIVERSITY OF NIJMEGEN
St. Radboud Hospital P.O. Box 9101
Nijmegen
THE NETHERLANDS

**Carlo Croce, M.D.**
WISTAR INSTITUTE
3601 Spruce Street
Philadelphia, PA 19104

**Carl J. Crosley, M.D.**
Department of Neurology
UPSTATE MEDICAL CENTER
750 East Adams Street
Syracuse, NY 13210

**Harold E. Cross, M.D., Ph.D.**
2375 North Wyatt Drive No. 101
Tucson, AZ 85712

**Floyd L. Culler, M.D.**
Pediatric Endocrinologist
THE WHITTIER INSTITUTE
9894 Genesee Avenue
La Jolla, CA 92037

**Charlotte Cunningham-Rundles, M.D., Ph.D.**
Department of Medicine
MT. SINAI MEDICAL CENTER
Fifth Avenue & 100th Street Box 1089
New York, NY 10029

**John Curnutte, M.D., Ph.D.**
Associate Member, Div. of Biochemistry
Molecular and Experimental Medicine
SCRIPPS CLINIC AND RESEARCH FOUNDATION
10666 North Torrey Pines Road
La Jolla, CA 92037

**Cynthia J. Curry, M.D.**
Director
Medical Genetics and Prenatal Detection
VALLEY CHILDREN'S HOSPITAL
3151 North Millbrook
Fresno, CA 93703

**Ernest Cutz, M.D.**
Department of Pathology
HOSPITAL FOR SICK CHILDREN
555 University Avenue
Toronto M5G 1X8
CANADA

**Andrew Czeizel, M.D.**
Depts. of Human Genetics & Teratology
WHO CENTER FOR COMMUNITY CONTROL OF HEREDITARY DISEASES
National Institute of Hygiene
Gyali ut 2-6
Budapest, IX H-196 6
HUNGARY

**Bernard D'Souza, M.D.**
Chief, Division of Pediatric Neurology
Pediatric Neurology, Box 3533
DUKE UNIVERSITY SCHOOL OF MEDICINE
Durham, NC 27710

**Elias O. da-Silva, M.D.**
Servico de Genetica Medica
INSTITUTO MATERNO-INFANTIL DE PERNAMBUCO (IMIP)
Rua dos Coelhos 300
Boa Vista
50000 Recife, P.E.
BRAZIL

**Albert A. Dahlberg, D.D.S.**
Research Associate Professor
Department of Anthropology
UNIVERSITY OF CHICAGO
Chicago, IL 60637

**Joseph Dancis, M.D.**
Department of Pediatrics
NEW YORK UNIVERSITY MEDICAL CENTER
560 First Avenue
New York, NY 10016

**Margaret Davee, M.S.**
Department of Medical Genetics
INDIANA UNIVERSITY SCHOOL OF MEDICINE
James Whitcomb Riley Hospital RR129
702 Barnhill Drive
Indianapolis, IN 46223

**Sandra L.H. Davenport, M.D.**
5801 Southard Drive
Bloomington, MN 55437 1739

**Murray Davidson, M.D.**
Department of Pediatrics
QUEENS HOSPITAL CENTER
82-68 164 Street
Jamaica, NY 11432

**N.K. Day, Ph.D.**
Professor of Pediatrics
ALL CHILDREN'S HOSPITAL
801 6th Street South
St. Petersburg, FL 33701

**Jean-Pierre de Chadarevian, M.D.**
Professor and Chief
Department of Anatomical Pathology
ST. CHRISTOPHER'S HOSPITAL FOR CHILDREN
Fifth Street & Lehigh Avenue
Philadelphia, PA 19133

**Jean de Grouchy, M.D.**
Directeur de Recherche au CNRS
Laboratoire de Cytogenetique Humaine
HOPITAL NECKER ENFANTS MALADES
149, rue de Sevres
75743 Paris Cedex 15
FRANCE

**Monte A. Del Monte, M.D.**
Skillman Professor
Pediatric Ophthalmology
UNIVERSITY OF MICHIGAN / W.K. KELLOGG EYE CENTER
1000 Wall Street
Ann Arbor, MI 48105

**William DeMyer, M.D.**
Professor of Child Neurology
Pediatric Neurology
INDIANA UNIVERSITY - RILEY HOSPITAL
Room N-125
1100 W. Michigan Street
Indianapolis, IN 46223

**Joao Monteiro de Pina-Neto, M.D.**
Department of Genetics
UNIVERSITY OF SAO PAULO
Faculty of Medicine of Ribeirao Preto
14.049 Ribeirao Preto
San Paulo
BRAZIL

**Vazken M. Der Kaloustian, M.D.**
Professor of Pediatrics, McGill Univ.
Director, Division of Medical Genetics
THE MONTREAL CHILDREN'S HOSPITAL / McGILL UNIVERSITY
2300 Tupper Street
Montreal, PQ H3H 1P3
CANADA

**Eugene L. Derlacki, M.D.**
OTOLOGIC PROFESSIONAL ASSOCIATES, S.C.
55 East Washington Street
Chicago, IL 60602

**Robert J. Desnick, Ph.D., M.D.**
Professor and Chief
Medical and Molecular Genetics
MT. SINAI SCHOOL OF MEDICINE
Fifth Avenue at 100th Street
New York, NY 10029

**Curtis K. Deutsch, Ph.D.**
Associate Scientist
SHRIVER CENTER
200 Trapelo Road
Waltham, MA 02254

**John H. DiLiberti, M.D.**
Professor and Director
Department of Pediatrics
SAINT FRANCIS HOSPITAL AND MEDICAL CENTER
114 Woodland Street
Hartford, CT 06105 1299

**Gary R. Diamond, M.D.**
Division of Ophthalmology
CHILDREN'S HOSPITAL OF PHILADELPHIA
One Children's Center
34th Street & Civic Center Boulevard
Philadelphia, PA 19104

**Louis K. Diamond, M.D.**
Department of Pediatrics
250
U.C.S.F. SCHOOL OF MEDICINE
San Francisco, CA 94143

**Stephen Robert Dlouhy, Ph.D.**
Postdoctoral Fellow
Department of Medical Genetics
INDIANA UNIVERSITY SCHOOL OF MEDICINE
702 Barnhill Drive
Indianapolis, IN 46223

**George N. Donnell, M.D.**
CHILDREN'S HOSPITAL OF LOS ANGELES
4650 Sunset Boulevard
Los Angeles, CA 90027

**Alan E. Donnenfeld, M.D.**
Assistant Professor
Section on Genetics, Dept. OB/GYN
PENNSYLVANIA HOSPITAL
Eighth & Spruce Streets
Philadelphia, PA 19107

**Craig Douglas, M.D.**
6E Suburban Medical Plaza
4001 Dutchman's Lane
Louisville, KY 40207

**Peter A. Duncan, M.D.**
Medical Genetics Unit
WESTCHESTER COUNTY MEDICAL CENTER
New York Medical College
Valhalla, NY 10595

**Paolo Durand, M.D.**
Direttore Scientifico
Scientific Division 1st G. Gaslini
GIANNINA GASLINI INSTITUTE
via 5 - Maggio 39
16148 Genova-Quarto
ITALY

**Nancy Lorraine Earl, M.D.**
Assistant Professor of Medicine
Division of Neurology
THE J. & K. BRYAN ALZHEIMER'S DISEASE RESEARCH CENTER
725 Broad Street
Durham, NC 27705

**Charles Eil, M.D., Ph.D.**
Director, Clinical Research Center
ROGER WILLIAMS GENERAL HOSPITAL
825 Chalkstone Avenue
Providence, RI 02908

**B. Rafael Elejalde, M.D.**
Prof. of OB/GYN
Head, Genetics Section
UNIVERSITY OF WISCONSIN MEDICAL SCHOOL
Mount Sinai Medical Center Box 342
950 North 12th Street
Milwaukee, WI 53201

**Maria Mercedes Elejalde, R.N.**
Genetics Section
UNIVERSITY OF WISCONSIN MEDICAL SCHOOL
Mount Sinai Medical Center Box 342
950 North 12th Street
Milwaukee, WI 53201

**Sami B. Elhassani, M.D.**
751 North Church Street
Spartanburg, SC 29303

**Larry P. Elliott, M.D.**
Chairman
Department of Radiology
GEORGETOWN UNIVERSITY MEDICAL CENTER
3800 Reservoir Road, NW
Washington, DC 20007

**Robert M. Ellsworth, M.D.**
Professor
Department of Ophthalmology
NEW YORK HOSPITAL CORNELL MEDICAL SCHOOL
515 East 71st Street
New York, NY 10021

**Nabil I. Elsahy, M.D.**
Plastic & Reconstructive Surgeon
6524 Professional Place, Suite A
Riverdale, GA 30274

**Louis J. Elsas, II, M.D.**
Department of Pediatrics
EMORY UNIVERSITY SCHOOL OF MEDICINE
2040 Ridgewood Drive
Atlanta, GA 30322

**Beverly S. Emanuel, Ph.D.**
Associate Professor
The Clinical Cytogenetics Laboratory
CHILDREN'S HOSPITAL OF PHILADELPHIA
34th Street and Civic Center Boulevard
Philadelphia, PA 19104

**Andrew G. Engel, M.D.**
Department of Neurology
THE MAYO CLINIC
Rochester, MN 55905

**Gerald M. English, M.D.**
COLORADO OTOLARYNGOLOGY, P.C.
601 East Hampden Avenue Suite 390
Denver, CO 80110

**Ervin H. Epstein, Jr., M.D.**
Clinical Professor of Dermatology
SAN FRANCISCO GENERAL HOSPITAL
Room 269, Building 100
1001 Potero Avenue
San Francisco, CA 94110

**John B. Erich, M.D.**
MAYO CLINIC
716 10th Street, S.W.
Rochester, MN 55901

**Marianne P. Eronen, M.D.**
Children's Hospital
UNIVERSITY OF HELSINKI
Helsinki SF-00290
FINLAND

**Theresa J. Escalante, M.D.**
21851 Drexel Way
El Toro, CA 92630

**Luis F. Escobar, M.D.**
Department of Oral Facial Genetics
INDIANA UNIVERSITY SCHOOL OF DENTISTRY
Ball Residence 026
1226 West Michigan Street
Indianapolis, IN 46223

**Victor Escobar, D.D.S., Ph.D.**
1364 Overbacker Court
Louisville, KY 40208

**John R. Esterly, M.D. ‡**
UNIVERSITY OF TENNESSEE CENTER FOR HEALTH SCIENCES
Perinatal Pathology
858 Madison Avenue
Memphis, TN 38163

**Carla Evans, D.D.S.**
Dental Clinic
BOSTON CHILDREN'S HOSPITAL
300 Longwood Avenue
H-4
Boston, MA 02115

**David A. Price Evans, M.D., Ph.D.**
Hon. Professor and Director
Department of Medicine
RIYADH ARMED FORCES HOSPITAL
P.O. Box 7897
Riyadh 11159
SAUDI ARABIA

**Jane A. Evans, Ph.D.**
Department of Human Genetics
UNIVERSITY OF MANITOBA
250-770 Bannatyne Avenue
Winnipeg MB R3E 0W3
CANADA

**Talaat I. Farag, D.C.H.**
Senior Clinical and Community Geneticist
KUWAIT MEDICAL GENETICS CENTRE
P.O. Box 31145
Sulibikhat 90802
KUWAIT

**Anwar I. Farhood, M.D.**
Assistant Professor of Pathology
METHODIST HOSPITAL
6565 Fannin
Houston, TX 77030

**Moshe Feinmesser, M.D.**
E.N.T. Department
HADASSAH UNIVERSITY HOSPITAL
Hadassah, Ein Karem
Jerusalem 91120
ISRAEL

**Gerald Feldman, M.D., Ph.D.**
Fellow, Institute for Molecular Genetics
BAYLOR COLLEGE OF MEDICINE
One Baylor Plaza
Houston, TX 77054

**Malcolm A. Ferguson-Smith, M.D.**
Professor of Pathology
Center for Medical Genetics
UNIVERSITY OF CAMBRIDGE
Tennis Court Road
Cambridge CB2 1QP
ENGLAND

**Judith A. Ferry, M.D.**
Department of Pathology
MASSACHUSETTS GENERAL HOSPITAL
Fruit Street
Boston, MA 02114

**Cheryl Fialkoff, M.D.**
Department of Dermatology (M/C 624)
UNIVERSITY OF ILLINOIS COLLEGE OF MEDICINE AT CHICAGO
Box 6998
Chicago, IL 60680

**G. Filippi, M.D.**
Istituto per l'Infanzia
Cattedra di Genetica Medica
UNIVERSITA DI TRIESTE
Trieste 34137
ITALY

**Ben S. Fine**
5409 Surrey Street
Chevy Chase, MD 20815

**Robert Fineman, M.D., Ph.D.**
Department of Pediatrics
UNIVERSITY OF UTAH COLLEGE OF MEDICINE
50 North Medical Drive
Salt Lake City, UT 84132

**Janice Finkelstein, M.D.**
Pediatric Genetics Center
THE JOHNS HOPKINS CHILDREN'S CENTER
CMSC 1004
Baltimore, MD 21205

**Wayne H. Finley, Ph.D., M.D.**
Director
Laboratory of Medical Genetics
UNIVERSITY OF ALABAMA BIRMINGHAM
University Station
Birmingham, AL 35294

**Mark H. Fishbein, M.D.**
Research Fellow
Pediatric Gastroenterology
UNIVERSITY OF CHICAGO PRITZKER SCHOOL OF MEDICINE
5825 South Maryland Avenue Box 107
Chicago, IL 60637

**William N. Fishbein, M.D., Ph.D.**
Chief, Biochemistry Division
ARMED FORCES INSTITUTE OF PATHOLOGY
14th Street & Alaska Avenue, N.W.
Washington, DC 20306

**Delbert A. Fisher, M.D.**
Professor of Pediatrics and Medicine
Harbor General Hospital
U.C.L.A. SCHOOL OF MEDICINE
1000 W. Carson Street
Torrance, CA 90509

**Naomi Fitch, M.D., Ph.D.**
Lady Davis Institute
JEWISH GENERAL HOSPITAL
3755 Cote St. Catherine Road
Montreal, Quebec H3T1E 2
CANADA

**J.S. Fitzsimmons, M.D.**
Clinical Genetics
NOTTINGHAM HEALTH AUTHORITY
City Hospital
Hucknall Road
Nottingham NG5 1PD
ENGLAND

**David B. Flannery, M.D.**
Director, Division of Medical Genetics
Department of Pediatrics
MEDICAL COLLEGE OF GEORGIA
Augusta, GA 30912 3770

**Ellen Fleischnick, M.D.**
19 Copley Street
Brookline, MA 02146

**Gordon M. Folger, Jr., M.D.**
Director, Pediatric Cardiology
HAMAD GENERAL HOSPITAL
P.O. Box 3050
Doha
QATAR

**David J. Forster, M.D.**
Center for Sight
GEORGETOWN UNIVERSITY MEDICAL CENTER
3800 Reservoir Road, N.W.
Washington, DC 20007

**Ruben Fragoso, M.D.**
INSTITUTO MEXICANO DEL SEGURO SOCIAL
Ap. Postal 1-3838
Guadalajara
MEXICO

**Piergiorgio Franceschini, M.D.**
Professore Associato
Servizio di Genetica Clinica
INSTITUTO DI DISCIPLINE PEDIATRICHE
Piazza Polonia 94
10126 Torino
ITALY

**Clair A. Francomano, M.D.**
Assistant Professor
Pediatric Genetics
JOHNS HOPKINS HOSPITALS
CSMC Room 8-108
Baltimore, MD 21205

**Donald Fraser, M.D.**
Professor of Pediatrics and Physiology
UNIVERSITY OF TORONTO
555 University Avenue
Room 5128B
Toronto ON M5G-1
CANADA

**F. Clarke Fraser, Ph.D., M.D.**
Emeritus Professor Biology & Pediatrics
Center for Human Genetics
McGILL UNIVERSITY
Stewart Biology Building
1205 rue docteur Penfield
Montreal H3A 1B1 PQ
CANADA

**G. R. Fraser, M.D., Ph.D.**
Cancer Epidemiology Clinical Trials Unit
Imperial Cancer Research Fund
UNIVERSITY OF OXFORD
Gibson Building
The Radcliffe Infirmary
Oxford OX2 6HE
ENGLAND

**Joseph F. Fraumeni, Jr., M.D.**
Epidemiology and Biostatistics Program
NATIONAL CANCER INSTITUTE
Landow Bldg., Room 4C03
Bethesda, MD 20892

**Bruce Fredrickson, M.D.**
550 Harrison Center Suite 100
Syracuse, NY 13202

**Bishara J. Freij, M.D.**
Assistant Professor of Pediatrics
Division of Infectious Diseases
GEORGETOWN UNIVERSITY SCHOOL OF MEDICINE
3800 Reservoir Road, N.W.
Washington, DC 20007

**Ademar Freire-Maia, Ph.D.**
Professor of Genetics
UNIVERSIDADE ESTADUAL PAULISTA (UNESP)
Rubiao Jr.
18600 Botucatu, SP
BRAZIL

**Newton Freire-Maia, D.Sc.**
Professor Emeritus of Genetics
FEDERAL UNIVERSITY OF PARANA
P.O. Box 19071
81504 Curitiba
BRAZIL

**Jaime L. Frias, M.D.**
Professor and Chairman
Department of Pediatrics
UNIVERSITY OF NEBRASKA MEDICAL CENTER
42nd & Dewey Avenue
Omaha, NE 68105

**J.M. Friedman, M.D., Ph.D.**
Associate Professor of Medical Genetics
Clinical Genetics Unit (UBC)
GRACE HOSPITAL
4490 Oak Street
Vancouver V6H 3V5 BC
CANADA

**William F. Friedman, M.D.**
Chairman, Department of Pediatrics
U.C.L.A. SCHOOL OF MEDICINE
412 2-2
Los Angeles, CA 90024

**E. Rudolf Froesch, M.D.**
Professor of Medicine
STOFFWECHSELLABOR UNIVERSITY HOSPITAL
Ramistr. 100
8091 Zurich
SWITZERLAND

**Moshe Frydman, M.D.**
Genetics Clinic
Department of Pediatrics
GOLDA MEDICAL CENTER
Hasharon Hospital P.O. Box 121
7 Keren Kayemet
Petah-Tiqva 49100
ISREAL

**Jean-Pierre Fryns, M.D.**
Head of Clinical Genetics
Division of Human Genetics
U.Z. GASTHUISBERG
Herestraat, 49
B-3000 Leuven
BELGIUM

**Magdalena Fuchs, M.D.**
Associate Professor of Pediatrics
METROPOLITAN HOSPITAL
1901 First Avenue
New York, NY 10029

**Atsuko Fujimoto, M.D., Ph.D.**
Chief, Genetics Division
L.A. COUNTY - U.S.C. MEDICAL CENTER
1129 North State Street Room 1G-24
Los Angeles, CA 90033

**Diana Garcia-Cruz**
Division of Genetics
UNIDAD DE INVESTIGACION BIOMEDICA
Centro Medico de Occidente
Apartado Postal 1-3838
Guadalajara Jalisco
MEXICO

**Bhuwan P. Garg, M.D.**
Associate Professor
Department of Neurology
INDIANA UNIVERSITY SCHOOL OF MEDICINE
Riley Hospital
702 Barnhill Drive
Indianapolis, IN 46202 5200

**Ellen Garibaldi, M.D.**
Allergy Division, Department of Medicine
ST. LOUIS UNIVERSITY HOSPITALS
1402 South Grand
St. Louis, MO 63104

**Arthur R. Garrett, M.D., Ph.D.**
Associate Professor
Department of Pediatrics
QUILLEN-DISHNER COLLEGE OF MEDICINE
Professional Building, Suite 400
Johnson City, TN 37601

**Richard A. Gatti, M.D.**
Department of Pathology
U.C.L.A. SCHOOL OF MEDICINE
Center for the Health Sciences
10833 Le Conte Avenue
Los Angeles, CA 90024 1732

**Mark C. Gebhardt, M.D.**
Assistant Professor of Orthopaedic Surg.
Department of Orthopaedic Surgery
MASSACHUSETTS GENERAL HOSPITAL
Gray Building Six
Boston, MA 02114

**Robert N. Gebhart, M.D.**
DESERT EAR, NOSE AND THROAT MEDICAL GROUP, INC.
39000 Bob Hope Drive
Rancho Mirage, CA 92270

**William C. Gentry, Jr., M.D.**
Department of Dermatology
UNIVERSITY OF MINNESOTA
Box 98 Mayo
Minneapolis, MN 55455

**James German, M.D.**
Director, Laboratory of Human Genetics
THE NEW YORK BLOOD CENTER
310 East 67th Street
New York, NY 10021

**Ira H. Gessner, M.D.**
Chief, Division of Cardiology
Department of Pediatrics
UNIVERSITY OF FLORIDA COLLEGE OF MEDICINE
Box J-296, Shands Teaching Hospital
Gainesville, FL 32610

**Ruby Ghadially, M.B., Ch.B.**
Fellow in Dermatology
Dermatology Service UCSF 190
V.A. MEDICAL CENTER
4150 Clement Street
San Francisco, CA 94121

**H. Ghadimi, M.D.**
1757 Merrick Avenue
North Merrick, NY 11566

**Kenneth Michael Gibson, Ph.D.**
Senior Research Scientist
Metabolic Disease Center
BAYLOR UNIVERSITY MEDICAL CENTER
3500 Gaston Avenue
Dallas, TX 75246

**Ronald E. Gier, D.M.D.**
Professor & Chairman
Department of Oral Diagnosis
UNIVERSITY OF MISSOURI-KANSAS CITY
650 East 25th Street
Kansas City, MO 64108 2795

**Enid F. Gilbert-Barness, M.D.**
Professor of Pathology and Pediatrics
Center for Health Sciences
UNIVERSITY OF WISCONSIN-MADISON
600 Highland Avenue - E5/326
Madison, WI 53792

**Herbert Gilmore, M.D.**
Pediatric Neurology Department
NEW ENGLAND MEDICAL CENTER HOSPITALS
750 Washington Street Box 394
Boston, MA 02111

**Richard Gitzelmann, M.D.**
Professor of Pediatrics
Division of Metabolism
KINDERSPITAL - UNIVERSITY OF ZURICH
Steinwiesstrasse 75
CH-8032 Zurich
SWITZERLAND

**Mahin Golabi, M.D., M.P.H.**
Division of Genetics
Department of Pediatrics
UNIVERSITY OF CALIFORNIA MEDICAL CENTER
250 Room U-100A
San Francisco, CA 94143 0706

**Morton F. Goldberg, M.D.**
Director and Ophthalmologist-in-Chief
Wilmer Eye Institute
JOHNS HOPKINS MEDICAL INSTITUTIONS
Baltimore, MD 21205

**Rosalie B. Goldberg, B.S., M.S.**
Coordinator / Genetic Counselor
Department of Pediatrics
MONTEFIORE MEDICAL CENTER
111 East 210 Street
Bronx, NY 10467

**J. Goldblatt, M.D.**
Director, Genetic Services
PRINCESS MARGARET HOSPITAL FOR CHILDREN
Box D184
GPO Perth 6001
AUSTRALIA

**Lawrence I. Goldblatt, D.D.S., M.S.D**
Professor of Oral Pathology
INDIANA UNIVERSITY SCHOOL OF DENTISTRY
1121 West Michigan Street
Indianapolis, IN 46202

**Donald Goldsmith, M.D.**
Associate Professor of Pediatrics
Pediatric Rheumatology Center
CHILDREN'S HOSPITAL OF PHILADELPHIA
Children's Seashore House
One Civic Center Boulevard
Philadelphia, PA 19104

**Stanley Goldstein, M.D.**
Director, Pediatrics & Ped. Cardiology
ST. ELIZABETH HOSPITAL MEDICAL CENTER
1044 Belmont Avenue
Youngstown, OH 44501 1790

**Thomaz Rafael Gollop, Ph.D.**
Director, Servico de Genetica
Associacao Maternidade de Sao Paulo
DA MATERNIDADE DE SAO PAULO
Rua Ofelia, 248 - Jardim Paulistano
Sao Paulo 05423
BRAZIL

**Robert Goltz, M.D.**
Adjunct Professor Medicine/Dermatology
Division of Dermatology (H-811J)
UNIVERSITY OF CALIFORNIA SAN DIEGO MEDICAL CENTER
225 Dickinson Street
San Diego, CA 92103

**Edward Gomperts, M.D.**
Director, Hemophilia Comp. Care Center
Division of Hematology/Oncology
CHILDRENS HOSPITAL OF LOS ANGELES
4650 Sunset Boulevard
P.O. Box 54700
Los Angeles, CA 90054 0700

**Robert A. Good, M.D.**
Physician-in-Chief
Department of Pediatrics
ALL CHILDREN'S HOSPITAL
801 6th Street South
St. Petersburg, FL 33701

**Richard M. Goodman, M.D. ‡**
Professor of Human Genetics
Department of Genetics
CHAIM SHEBA MEDICAL CENTER
Tel-Hashomer 52621
ISRAEL

**Stephen I. Goodman, M.D.**
Department of Pediatrics
UNIVERSITY OF COLORADO HEALTH SCIENCES CENTER
4200 East 9th Avenue, Box C-233
Denver, CO 80262

**Paul Goodyer, M.D.**
Associate Professor of Pediatrics
Division of Nephrology
MONTREAL CHILDREN'S HOSPITAL
2300 Tupper Street
Montreal H3H 1P3
CANADA

**Robert J. Gorlin, D.D.S.**
Regent's Professor and Chairman
Dept. of Oral Pathology and Genetics
UNIVERSITY OF MINNESOTA SCHOOL OF DENTISTRY
16-206 HS Unit A
515 Deleward Street, S.E.
Minneapolis, MN 55455

**W. Lea Gorsuch, M.D.**
808 Middleford Road
Seaford, DE 19973

**John M. Graham, Jr., M.D., Sc.D.**
Director
Division of Clinical Genetics
CEDARS - SINAI MEDICAL CENTER
444 South San Vicenti Blvd.
Los Angeles, CA 90048

**Thomas P. Graham, Jr., M.D.**
Professor
Division of Pediatric Cardiology
VANDERBILT UNIVERSITY MEDICAL CENTER
Nashville, TN 37232

**Harvey R. Gralnick, M.D.**
Chief, Hematology Service, CPD
NATIONAL INSTITUTES OF HEALTH
Building 10, Room 2C-390
9000 Rockville Pike
Bethesda, MD 20892

**Elizabeth Gray, M.B., F.R.C.**
Department of Pathology
UNIVERSITY OF ABERDEEN MEDICAL SCHOOL
University Medical Buildings
Aberdeen AB9 2ZD
SCOTLAND

**David A. Greenberg, Ph.D.**
Department of Psychiatry
THE MOUNT SINAI MEDICAL CENTER
One Gustav Levy Place
New York, NY 10029 6574

**Frank Greenberg, M.D.**
Birth Defects Genetics Clinic
BAYLOR COLLEGE OF MEDICINE
Texas Medical Center
6621 Fannin
Houston, TX 77030

**Alice Greene, Ph.D.**
Department of Pediatrics (M-009-F)
U.C.S.D. SCHOOL OF MEDICINE
La Jolla, CA 92093

**Gisele A. Greenhaw, M.D.**
Fellow in Medical Genetics
Department of Pediatrics
UNIVERSITY OF TEXAS MEDICAL SCHOOL
6431 Fannin
Houston, TX 77030

**May L. Griebel, M.D.**
Fellow in Child Neurology
DUKE UNIVERSITY MEDICAL CENTER
Box 31124
Durham, NC 27710

**Arthur W. Grix, Jr., M.D.**
Assistant Professor
Department of Pediatrics
UNIVERSITY OF CALIFORNIA, DAVIS
1625 Alhambra Plaza Suite 2901
Sacramento, CA 95816

**Jay L. Grosfeld, M.D.**
Professor and Chairman
Department of Surgery
INDIANA UNIVERSITY MEDICAL CENTER
J.W. Riley Hospital for Children K-21
Indianapolis, IN 46223

**Michael Grunebaum, M.D.**
Professor of Pediatric Radiology
BEILINSON MEDICAL CENTER
Petah Tikva 49100
ISRAEL

**Ralph Gruppo, M.D.**
Division of Hematology/Oncology
CHILDREN'S HOSPITAL MEDICAL CENTER
Elland & Bethesda Avenues
Cincinnati, OH 45229 2899

**Christian Guilleminault, M.D.**
Professor
Sleep Disorders Center
STANFORD UNIVERSITY SCHOOL OF MEDICINE
701 Welch Road
Palo Alto, CA 94304

**Sudhir Gupta, M.D.**
Department of Medicine
UNIVERSITY OF CALIFORNIA
Medical Science I
Irvine, CA 92717

**Alan E. Guttmacher, M.D.**
VERMONT REGIONAL GENETICS CENTER
96 Colchester Avenue
Burlington, VT 05401

**Barrett G. Haik, M.D.**
Professor of Ophthalmology
TULANE UNIVERSITY MEDICAL SCHOOL
1430 Tulane Avenue
New Orleans, LA 70112

**Fahed Halal, M.D.**
Department of Pediatrics
HOPITAL NOTRE-DAME
1560 Est. Sherbrooke
Montreal H2L 4M1 PQ
CANADA

**Judith G. Hall, M.D.**
Director, Clinical Genetics Service
Clinical Genetics Unit (UBC)
UNIVERSITY HOSPITAL - SHAUGHNESSY SITE
4500 Oak Street
Vancouver V6H 3N1 BC
CANADA

**Jerome S. Haller, M.D.**
Director, Section on Child Neurology
ALBANY MEDICAL CENTER
New Scotland Avenue
Albany, NY 12208

**Michael T. Halpern, B.A.**
Graduate Fellow
UNIVERSITY OF MICHIGAN
109 South Observatory 3073 SPH I
Ann Arbor, MI 48109 2029

**Stanley R. Hamilton, M.D.**
Associate Professor of Pathology
Department of Pathology
THE JOHNS HOPKINS UNIVERSITY
600 North Wolfe Street
Baltimore, MD 21205

**James W. Hanson, M.D.**
Division of Medical Genetics
Z944
UNIVERSITY OF IOWA
Hospital and Clinics
Iowa City, IA 52242

**B. Hardcastle, M.D.**
7019 N.W. 11th Place
Gainesville, FL 32605

**David J. Harris, M.D.**
Chief, Section of Genetics
CHILDREN'S MERCY HOSPITAL
Twenty-Fourth at Gillham Road
Kansas City, MO 64108

**James K. Hartsfield, Jr., D.M.D.**
Asst. Prof. Pediatrics and Genetics
Department of Pediatrics
UNIVERSITY OF SOUTH FLORIDA
12901 Bruce B. Downs Blvd.
Tampa, FL 33612 4799

**Robert H.A. Haslam, M.D.**
Professor and Chairman of Pediatrics
HOSPITAL FOR SICK CHILDREN
555 University Avenue
Toronto ONT MS9 1X8
CANADA

**W. Allen Hauser, M.D.**
Prof. Neurology and Public Health
G.S. Sergievsky Center
COLUMBIA UNIVERSITY COLLEGE OF PHYSICIANS AND SURGEONS
630 West 168th Street
New York, NY 10032

**Irvin F. Hawkins, Jr., M.D.**
Department of Radiology
CHANDS TEACHING HOSPITAL
Gainesville, FL 32610

**Pamela Hawks Arn, M.D.**
Postdoctoral Fellow in Genetics
Department of Pediatrics
THE JOHNS HOPKINS SCHOOL OF MEDICINE
Baltimore, MD 21205

**Alberto Hayek, M.D.**
THE WHITTIER INSTITUTE
9894 Genesee Avenue
La Jolla, CA 92037

**James R. Hayward, D.D.S.**
Oral and Maxillofacial Consultant
1029 Lincoln
Marquette, MI 49866

**Gregory S. Heard, Ph.D.**
Assistant Professor of Human Genetics
MEDICAL COLLEGE OF VIRGINIA
MCV Station Box 169
Richmond, VA 23298 0169

**Barbara Kaiser Hecht, Ph.D.**
The Genetics Center
SOUTHWEST BIOMEDICAL RESEARCH INSTITUTE
6401 East Thomas Road
Scottsdale, AZ 85251

**Frederick Hecht, M.D.**
4134 McGirtz Blvd.
Jacksonville, FL 32210

**Jacqueline Hecht, Ph.D.**
Department of Pediatrics
UNIVERSITY OF TEXAS HEALTH SCIENCE CENTER
P.O. Box 20708
Houston, TX 77225

**Douglas Heiner, M.D.**
Director, Pediatric Allergy/Immunology
HARBOR GENERAL HOSPITAL
1000 West Carson Street
Torrance, CA 90509

**William E. Hellenbrand, M.D.**
Asso. Prof. Pediatrics and Imaging
Department of Pediatrics
YALE UNIVERSITY SCHOOL OF MEDICINE
333 Cedar Street
New Haven, CT 06510

**Alejandro Hernandez, M.D.**
INSTITUTO MEXICANO DEL SEGURO SOCIAL
Ap. Postal 1-3838
Guadalajara
MEXICO

**Jurgen Herrmann, M.D.**
GREAT LAKES GENETICS CENTER
2323 North Mayfair Road
Milwaukee, WI 53226

**Joseph H. Hersh, M.D.**
Department of Pediatrics
CHILD EVALUATION CENTER
334 East Broadway
Louisville, KY 40202

**Riitta Herva, M.D.**
Department of Pathology
UNIVERSITY OF OULU
Kajaanintie 52 D
SF-90220 Oulu 22
FINLAND

**Gene Higashi, M.D.**
Department of Epidemiology
UNIVERSITY OF MICHIGAN
109 Observatory SPH-I
Ann Arbor, MI 48109 2029

**James V. Higgins, Ph.D.**
MICHIGAN STATE UNIVERSITY
B 240 Life Sciences Building
East Lansing, MI 48824

**M.E. Hodes, M.D., Ph.D.**
Professor of Medical Genetics
INDIANA UNIVERSITY SCHOOL OF MEDICINE
975 West Walnut Street
Indianapolis, IN 46202 5251

**Ronald Hoffman, M.D.**
Professor of Medicine
Chief, Division of Hematology/Oncology
INDIANA UNIVERSITY SCHOOL OF MEDICINE
Clinical Building, Room 379
541 Clinical Drive
Indianapolis, IN 46223

**Georg Hoffmann, M.D.**
Abt. fur Neuropadiatrie
Ruprecht-Karls-Universitat Heidelberg
UNIVERSITATS-KINDERKLINIK
Im Neuenheimer Feld 150
WEST GERMANY

**Thomas M. Holder, M.D.**
Pediatric Surgeon
THE CHILDREN'S MERCY HOSPITAL
2415 Locust St.
Kansas City, MO 64108

**David W. Hollister, M.D.**
Prof. Pediatric Pathology & Medicine
Munroe Center for Human Genetics
UNIVERSITY OF NEBRASKA MEDICAL CENTER
444 44th Street
Omaha, NE 68198 5440

**Kenneth Holmes, M.D.**
DUKE UNIVERSITY MEDICAL CENTER
Durham, NC 27710

**Lewis B. Holmes, M.D.**
Embryology - Teratology Unit
MASSACHUSETTS GENERAL HOSPITAL
32 Fruit Street
Boston, MA 02114

**John Harry Holtkamp, M.D.**
Fellow in Pediatric Neurology
DUKE UNIVERSITY MEDICAL CENTER
Box 31026
Durham, NC 27710

**George R. Honig, M.D., Ph.D.**
Professor and Head
Department of Pediatrics (M/C 856)
THE UNIVERSITY OF ILLINOIS AT CHICAGO
840 South Wood Street
Box 6998
Chicago, IL 60680

**Jean Hood, M.D.**
Assistant Professor
Department of Pediatrics
UNIVERSITY OF TEXAS MEDICAL SCHOOL
6431 Fannin
Houston, TX 77030

**Lili Kawaharada Horton, M.D., S.M.**
1521 South King Street Suite 307
Honolulu, HI 96826

**William A. Horton, M.D.**
Professor of Pediatrics and Medicine
UNIVERSITY OF TEXAS MEDICAL SCHOOL
P.O. Box 20708
Houston, TX 77225

**Judith Howard, M.D.**
Intervention Program
UNIVERSITY OF CALIFORNIA AT LOS ANGELES
1000 Veteran Avenue
Room 23-10
Los Angeles, CA 90024

**James B. Howell, M.D.**
Wadley Tower Suite 862
3600 Gaston
Dallas, TX 75246

**H. Eugene Hoyme, M.D.**
Chief, Genetics and Dysmorphology
Department of Pediatrics
UNIVERSITY OF ARIZONA COLLEGE OF MEDICINE
2504 East Elm
Tucson, AZ 85724

**Richard Hubbell, M.D.**
Assistant Professor
Division of Pediatric Otolaryngology
VERMONT MEDICAL CENTER
One South Prospect Street
Burlington, VT 05405

**Alasdair G.W. Hunter, M.D.**
Chief, Division of Genetics
CHILDREN'S HOSPITAL OF EASTERN ONTARIO
401 Smyth Road
Ottawa K1H 8L1
CANADA

**Lee R. Hunter, M.D.**
Fellow, Pediatric Ophthalmology
CHILDREN'S HOSPITAL NATIONAL MEDICAL CENTER
111 Michigan Avenue, N.W.
Washington, DC 20010

**Carol A. Huseman, M.D.**
Director, Pediatric Endocrinology
Department of Pediatrics
UNIVERSITY OF NEBRASKA MEDICAL CENTER
42nd Street and Dewey Avenue
Omaha, NE 68105

**Leonard C. Hymes, M.D.**
Department of Pediatrics
EMORY UNIVERSITY SCHOOL OF MEDICINE
2040 Ridgewood Dr., N.E.
Atlanta, GA 30322

**A. Kimberly Iafolla, M.D.**
Clinical Genetics and Child Development
Dept. of Maternal and Child Health
DARTMOUTH MEDICAL SCHOOL
Hanover, NH 03756

**Juhana Idanpaan-Heikkila, M.D., Docent**
Chief Medical Officer for Pharmacology
NATIONAL BOARD OF HEALTH
00530 Helsinki
FINLAND

**Victor Ionasescu, M.D.**
Professor of Pediatrics
THE UNIVERSITY OF IOWA
University of Iowa Hospitals and Clinics
Iowa City, IA 52242

**Mira Irons, M.D.**
PRENATAL DIAGNOSTIC CENTER
80 Hayden Avenue
Lexington, MA 02173

**Harry Israel, D.D.S., Ph.D.**
Director of Dental Research
Dental Department
CHILDREN'S MEDICAL CENTER
One Children's Plaza
Dayton, OH 45404

**Mohammad S. Jaafar, M.D.**
Department of Ophthalmology
CHILDREN'S HOSPITAL NATIONAL MEDICAL CENTER
111 Michigan Avenue, N.W.
Washington, DC 20010

**Douglas A. Jabs, M.D.**
Associate Professor of Ophthalmology
Wilmer Ophthalmological Institute
THE JOHNS HOPKINS UNIVERSITY SCHOOL OF MEDICINE
550 North Broadway Suite 700
Baltimore, MD 21205

**Ethylin Wang Jabs, M.D.**
Assistant Professor
Center for Medical Genetics
THE JOHNS HOPKINS CHILDREN'S CENTER
600 North Wolfe Street Room 10-04
Baltimore, MD 21205

**R. Kirk Jackson, M.D.**
Department of Pediatric Otolaryngology
CHILDREN'S HOSPITAL MEDICAL CENTER
Elland & Bethesda Avenues
Cincinnati, OH 45229 2899

**Jerry C. Jacobs, M.D.**
BABIES HOSPITAL
3959 Broadway Room 106N
New York, NY 10032

**Larry S. Jefferson, M.D.**
Medical Director
Pediatric Intensive and Intermed. Care
TEXAS CHILDREN'S HOSPITAL
6621 Fannin
Houston, TX 77030

**Egil Jellum, M.D.**
Institute of Clinical Biochemistry
Rikshospitalet
UNIVERSITY OF OSLO
Oslo 1
NORWAY

**Jan E. Jirasek, M.D.**
Institute of Clinical Biochemistry
INSTITUTE FOR THE CARE OF MOTHER AND CHILD
Nabrezi Karla Marxe 157
147 10 Praha 4
Podoli
CZECHOSLOVAKIA

**Clinton C. Johnson, D.D.S.**
4429 Buckingham Drive
El Paso, TX 79902

**John P. Johnson, M.D.**
Department of Genetics
CHILDREN'S HOSPITAL OAKLAND
747 52nd Street
Oakland, CA 94609

**Virginia P. Johnson, M.D.**
Professor of Medical Genetics
OB/GYN, Pediatric and Laboratory Medicine
UNIVERSITY OF SOUTH DAKOTA
414 East Clark Street
Vermillion, SD 57069

**Waine C. Johnson, M.D.**
Professor of Dermatology
DERMATOLOGY ASSOCIATES OF GRADUATE HOSPITAL
Pepper Pavilion Suite #805
One Graduate Plaza
Philadelphia, PA 19146

**Paul W. Johnston, M.D.**
Associate Clinical Professor of Surgery
Children's Hospital of Los Angeles
UNIVERSITY OF SOUTHERN CALIFORNIA SCHOOL OF MEDICINE
50 Bellefontaine Street Suite 303
Pasadena, CA 91105

**Ronald J. Jorgenson, D.D.S., Ph.D.**
Department of Pediatric Dentistry
UNIVERSITY OF TEXAS HEALTH SCIENCE CENTER
7703 Floyd Curl Drive
San Antonio, TX 78284 7888

**Richard C. Juberg, M.D., Ph.D.**
Professor of Pediatrics and OB-GYN
Biological Sciences
2511 South Patterson Blvd.
Kettering, OH 45409

**Stephen G. Kahler, M.D.**
Department of Pediatrics
DUKE UNIVERSITY MEDICAL CENTER
Box 3028
Durham, NC 27710

**Muriel Kaiser-Kupfer, M.D.**
National Eye Institute
NATIONAL INSTITUTES OF HEALTH
Building 10, Room 10N226
9000 Rockville Pike
Bethesda, MD 20892

**Ilkka I. Kaitila, M.D.**
Department of Clinical Genetics
HELSINKI UNIVERSITY CENTRAL HOSPITAL
Tukholmankatu 8 F
SF-00290 Helsinki
FINLAND

**Stephen G. Kaler, M.D.**
National Institutes of Health
DEPARTMENT OF HEALTH AND HUMAN SERVICES
Building 10, Room 8C 429
Bethesda, MD 20205

**Hans Kalmus, Ph.D.**
Galton Laboratory - Genetics & Biometry
University College
UNIVERSITY OF LONDON
London NW1 2HE
ENGLAND

**Raymond S. Kandt, M.D., Ph.D.**
Associate Professor of Pediatric Neurology
DUKE UNIVERSITY MEDICAL CENTER
Box 3533
Durham, NC 27710

**Bernard S. Kaplan, M.D.**
Director of Nephrology
CHILDREN'S HOSPITAL OF PHILADELPHIA
34th and Civic Center Boulevard
Philadelphia, PA 19104

**Frederick Kaplan, M.D.**
Chief, Metabolic Bone Diseases
HOSPITAL OF THE UNIVERSITY OF PENNSYLVANIA
34th & Spruce Street
Philadelphia, PA 19104

**Joseph Kaplan, M.D.**
Department of Pediatrics
WAYNE STATE UNIVERSITY SCHOOL OF MEDICINE
Children's Hospital of Michigan
3901 Beaubien Blvd.
Detroit, MI 48201

**Paige Kaplan, M.D.**
Division of Metabolism
CHILDREN'S HOSPITAL OF PHILADELPHIA
34th and Civic Center Boulevard
Philadelphia, PA 19104

**James R. Kasser, M.D.**
CHILDREN'S HOSPITAL
300 Longwood Avenue
Boston, MA 02115

**Hassan M. Kattan, M.D.**
Center for Sight
GEORGETOWN UNIVERSITY MEDICAL CENTER
3800 Reservoir Road, N.W.
Washington, DC 20007

**Donald Kaufman, M.D.**
Professor of Pediatrics
MICHIGAN STATE UNIVERSITY
Life Sciences Building Room B240
East Lansing, MI 48824

**Celia I. Kaye, M.D., Ph.D.**
Clinical Associate Professor
Department of Pediatrics
UNIVERSITY OF TEXAS HEALTH SCIENCE CENTER
7703 Floyd Curl Drive
San Antonio, TX 78006 4829

**James P. Keating, M.D., M.Sc.**
Professor of Pediatrics
ST. LOUIS CHILDREN'S HOSPITAL
400 South Kings Highway
P.O. Box 14871
St. Louis, MO 63178

**Harris J. Keene, D.D.S.**
Oral Oncology
UNIVERSITY OF TEXAS HEALTH SCIENCE CENTER
Dental Branch Dental Science Institute
P.O. Box 20068
Houston, TX 77225

**Thaddeus E. Kelly, M.D.**
Director, Division of Medical Genetics
UNIVERSITY OF VIRGINIA
University Hospital Box 386
Charlottesville, VA 22908

**Nancy G. Kennaway, D. Phil.**
Assistant Director
Pediatric Metabolic Laboratory
THE OREGON HEALTH SCIENCES UNIVERSITY
3181 S.W. Sam Jackson Park Road
Portland, OR 97201

**Janice D. Key, M.D.**
Pediatric Teaching Service
MOSES H. CONE MEMORIAL HOSPITAL
1200 North Elm Street
Greensboro, NC 27401

**Richard Allen King, M.D., Ph.D.**
Professor of Medicine
Dept. of Medicine, Genetics Section
UNIVERSITY OF MINNESOTA
Box 485 Mayo Memorial Building
University of Minnesota Hospital
Minneapolis, MN 55455

**Smita Kittur, M.D.**
Gerontology Research Center
NATIONAL INSTITUTE ON AGING
4940 Eastern Avenue
Baltimore, MD 21224

**Jane Kivlin, M.D.**
Department of Ophthalmology
MEDICAL COLLEGE OF WISCONSIN
8700 West Wisconsin Avenue
Milwaukee, WI 53226

**Alice Kleczkowska, M.D., Ph.D.**
Center for Human Genetics
U.Z. GASTHUISBERG
Herestraat, 49
B-3000 Leuven
BELGIUM

**Gordon K. Klintworth, M.D.**
Department of Ophthalmology 3802-200
DUKE UNIVERSITY MEDICAL CENTER
Durham, NC 27710

**Marion A. Koerper, M.D.**
Associate Clinical Professor
Department of Pediatrics M650
UNIVERSITY OF CALIFORNIA
San Francisco, CA 94143 0106

**Maurice D. Kogut, M.D.**
Professor and Chairman
Department of Pediatrics
WRIGHT STATE UNIVERSITY SCHOOL OF MEDICINE
The Children's Medical Center
One Children's Plaza
Dayton, OH 45404

**Alfried Kohlschutter, M.D.**
Professor of Pediatrics
UNIVERSITATSKINDERKLINIK
Martinistr 52
D-2000 Hamburg 20
WEST GERMANY

**Roger Kohn, M.D.**
Clinical Professor
Department of Ophthalmology
U.C.L.A. SCHOOL OF MEDICINE
1009 Las Palmas Drive
Santa Barbara, CA 93110

**Edwin H. Kolodny, M.D.**
EUNICE KENNEDY SHRIVER CENTER
200 Trapelo Road
Waltham, MA 02154

**Bruce Korf, M.D., Ph.D.**
Division of Genetics
CHILDREN'S HOSPITAL
300 Longwood Avenue
Boston, MA 02115

**Boris G. Koussef, M.D.**
Director, Medical Genetics
UNIVERSITY OF SOUTH FLORIDA
Medical Center
12901 Bruce B. Downs Blvd. Box 15-G
Tampa, FL 33612

**Frederick K. Kozak, M.D.**
Faculty of Medicine
Department of Otolaryngology
ST. PAUL'S HOSPITAL
1081 Burrard Street
Vancouver V5Y 1W3 BC
CANADA

**K.S. Kozlowski, M.D.**
Staff Radiologist
ROYAL ALEXANDRA HOSPITAL FOR CHILDREN
Camperdown N.S.W.
Sydney 2050
AUSTRALIA

**Kenneth H. Kraemer, M.D.**
Laboratory of Molecular Carcinogenesis
NATIONAL CANCER INSTITUTE
Building 37, RM 3E16
Bethesda, MD 20892

**Celeste M. Krauss, M.D.**
Division of Medical Genetics
HARVARD COMMUNITY HEALTH PLAN
147 Milk Street
Boston, MA 02109

**Dhavendra Kumar, M.D.**
Center for Human Genetics
UNIVERSITY OF SHEFFIELD
Sheffield
ENGLAND

**Jurgen Kunze, M.D.**
Institute of Human Genetics
Department of Pediatrics
FREE UNIVERSITY OF BERLIN
Heubnerweg 6
1000 Berlin 19
WEST GERMANY

**Peter Kwiterovich, Jr., M.D.**
Department of Pediatrics
JOHNS HOPKINS UNIVERSITY SCHOOL OF MEDICINE
600 North Wolfe Street
Baltimore, MD 21205

**Michael Edison Labhard, M.D.**
13375 S.W. Peters Road
Lake Oswego, OR 97035

**Richard J. Labotka, M.D.**
Head, Division of Hematology/Oncology
Department of Pediatrics (M/C 856)
UNIVERSITY OF ILLINOIS SCHOOL OF MEDICINE AT CHICAGO
840 South Wood Street P.O. Box 6998
Chicago, IL 60680

**Ralph S. Lachman, M.D.**
Prof. of Radiology and Pediatrics
LOS ANGELES COUNTY HARBOR - UCLA MEDICAL CENTER
1000 West Carson Street
Box 27
Torrance, CA 90509

**Roger L. Ladda, M.D.**
Chief, Division of Genetics
THE PENNSYLVANIA STATE UNIVERSITY
College of Medicine
P.O. Box 850
Hershey, PA 17033

**Stephan K. Ladisch, M.D.**
Professor of Pediatrics
Division of Hematology/Oncology
U.C.L.A. MEDICAL CENTER
10833 Le Conte Avenue
Los Angeles, CA 90024 1752

**Charlotte Z. Lafer, M.D.**
Chief, Division of Medical Genetics
NEMOURS CHILDREN'S CLINIC
Laurette Howard Building Suite 713
P.O. Box 5720
Jacksonville, FL 32247

**Peter A. Lane, M.D.**
Assistant Professor of Pediatrics
UNIVERSITY OF COLORADO SCHOOL OF MEDICINE
Box C-222, UCHSC
4200 East 9th Avenue
Denver, CO 80262

**Leonard O. Langer, Jr., M.D.**
Clinical Professor
Department of Radiology
UNIVERSITY OF MINNESOTA MEDICAL SCHOOL
1235 Yale Place, 710
Minneapolis, MN 55403

**Stephen J. Lanspa, M.D.**
Assistant Professor of Medicine
Department of Gastroenterology
AMI/SAINT JOSEPH HOSPITAL
601 North 30th Street
Omaha, NE 68131

**Renata Laxova, M.D., Ph.D.**
Professor and Director
Wisconsin Clinical Genetics Center
UNIVERSITY OF WISCONSIN
1500 Highland Avenue
Madison, WI 53706

**James E. Lee, M.D.**
Department of Psychiatry
DUKE UNIVERSITY MEDICAL CENTER
Box 3825
Durham, NC 27710

**Woon K. Lee, M.B., B.S.**
ALL CHILDREN'S HOSPITAL
801 Sixth Street South
St. Petersberg, FL 33701

**Alan R. Lehmann, Ph.D.**
Section Head, Molecular Biology
MRC Cell Mutation Unit
UNIVERSITY OF SUSSEX
Falmer Brighton
Sussex BN1 9RR
ENGLAND

**Michael A. Lemp, M.D.**
Center for Sight
GEORGETOWN UNIVERSITY MEDICAL CENTER
3800 Reservoir Road, N.W.
Washington, DC 20007

**L. Stefan Levin, D.D.S.,M.S.D.**
Associate Professor
Department of Otolaryngology
THE JOHNS HOPKINS HOSPITAL
Osler 425
600 N. Wolfe Street
Baltimore, MD 21205 9977

**Harvey L. Levy, M.D.**
Amino Acid Lab
MASSACHUSETTS GENERAL HOSPITAL
Boston, MA 02114

**Raymond C. Lewandowski, M.D.**
CENTER FOR GENETIC SERVICES
1415 Third Street Suite 505
Corpus Christi, TX 78463 0584

**Richard Alan Lewis, M.D., M.S.**
Associate Professor
Cullen Eye Institute
BAYLOR COLLEGE OF MEDICINE
Baylor Plaza Ste. NC-206
Houston, TX 77030

**Raymond M. Lewkonia, M.B., Ch.B.**
Clinical Genetics Unit
ALBERTA HEREDITARY DISEASES PROGRAM
Alberta Children's Hospital
1820 Richmond Road, S.W.
Calgary T2T 5C7
CANADA

**Frederick P. Li, M.D.**
Div. of Biostatistics and Epidemiology
DANA FARBER CANCER CENTER
44 Binney Street
Room 1110
Boston, MA 02115

**Henry J. Lin, M.D.**
Associate Director
Division of Medical Genetics
CEDARS-SINAI MEDICAL CENTER
8700 Beverly Blvd.
Los Angeles, CA 90048

**Leonard M. Linde, M.D.**
Professor of Pediatrics (Cardiology)
Department of Pediatric Cardiology
U.S.C. SCHOOL OF MEDICINE
Children's Hospital
4650 Sunset Blvd.
Los Angeles, CA 90027

**D. Lindhout, M.D., Ph.D.**
Department of Clinical Genetics
ERASMUS UNIVERSITY
P.O. Box 1738
3000 DR Rotterdam
THE NETHERLANDS

**Martha S. Linet, M.D.**
Analytic Studies Section, Biostatistics
Epidemiology & Biostatistics Program
NATIONAL CANCER INSTITUTE
Division of Cancer Etiology
Executive Plaza North, Room 415B
Bethesda, MD 20892

**David A. Link, M.D.**
Chief, Department of Pediatrics 5W
THE CAMBRIDGE HOSPITAL
1493 Cambridge Street
Cambridge, MA 02139

**Elaine Louie, Ph.D.**
WISTAR INSTITUTE
3601 Spruce Street
Philadelphia, PA 19103

**R.B. Lowry, M.D.**
Director, Medical Genetics Clinic
ALBERTA CHILDREN'S HOSPITAL
1820 Richmond Road, S.W.
Calgary T2T 5C7 AB
CANADA

**John P. Lubicky, M.D.**
Chief of Staff
Chicago Unit
SHRINERS HOSPITAL FOR CRIPPLED CHILDREN
2211 North Oak Park Avenue
Chicago, IL 60635

**Bertram Lubin, M.D.**
Director of Medical Research
CHILDREN'S HOSPITAL OAKLAND
747 52nd Street
Oakland, CA 94609

**Mark Lubinsky, M.D.**
Human Genetics Center
UNIVERSITY OF NEBRASKA MEDICAL CENTER
Hattie B. Monroe Center
4402 Dewey
Omaha, NE 60105

**Herbert A. Lubs, M.D.**
Director, Genetics Division
UNIVERSITY OF MIAMI SCHOOL OF MEDICINE
Mailman Center for Child Development
P.O. Box 016820
Miami, FL 33101

**Russell V. Lucas, M.D.**
Pediatric Cardiology
UNIVERSITY OF MINNESOTA
Mayo Memorial Building Box 94
420 Delaware Street, S.E.
Minneapolis, MN 55455

**Henry T. Lynch, M.D.**
Professor and Chairman
Preventive Medicine/Public Health
CREIGHTON UNIVERSITY SCHOOL OF MEDICINE
California at 24th Street
Omaha, NE 68178

**Ghodsi Madani, M.D.**
Fellow, Pediatric Allergy/Immunology
HARBOR GENERAL HOSPITAL
3200 Larotonda Drive No. 305
Rancho Palos Verde, CA 90274

**R. Ellen Magenis, M.D.**
Profesor of Medical Genetics and Director
Clinical Genetics Program
OREGON HEALTH SCIENCES UNIVERSITY
707 S.W. Gaines Road
Portland, OR 97201

**Robert W. Mahley, M.D., Ph.D.**
Director, Gladstone Laboratories
UNIVERSITY OF CALIFORNIA
P.O. Box 40608
San Francisco, CA 94140

**Joe Malouf, M.D.**
KING FAHAD HOSPITAL
Riyadh
SAUDI ARABIA

**A.J. Man in 't Veld, M.D.**
Department of Internal Medicine
ERASMUS UNIVERSITEIT ROTTERDAM
Postbus 1738
3000 DR Rotterdam
THE NETHERLANDS

**James Mandell, M.D.**
Division of Urology
BOSTON CHILDREN'S HOSPITAL
300 Longwood Avenue
Boston, MA 02115

**Philip M. Marden, M.D.**
340 E. Summit Avenue
Oconomowoc, WI 53066

**Robert W. Marion, M.D.**
Associate Professor of Pediatrics
ALBERT EINSTEIN COLLEGE OF MEDICINE
Montefiore Medical Center
111 East 210 Street
Bronx, NY 10461

**Pierre Maroteaux, M.D.**
Directeur de Recherche au C.N.R.S.
Clinique Maurice Lamy
HOPITAL DES ENFANTS-MALADES
149, Rue de Sevres
75734 Paris Cedex 15
FRANCE

**Deborah L. Marsden, M.D.**
Fellow in Biochemical Genetics
Department of Pediatrics
UNIVERSITY OF CALIFORNIA AT SAN DIEGO
La Jolla, CA 92093 0609

**Laura S. Martin, M.D.**
Postdoctoral Fellow in Genetics
Department of Pediatrics
THE JOHNS HOPKINS SCHOOL OF MEDICINE
Baltimore, MD 21205

**John T. Martsolf, M.D.**
Director, Division of Medical Genetics
UNIVERSITY OF NORTH DAKOTA SCHOOL OF MEDICINE
501 Columbia Rd.
Grand Forks, ND 58203

**Bartholomew Martyak, M.D.**
Center for Sight
GEORGETOWN UNIVERSITY MEDICAL CENTER
3800 Reservoir Road, N.W.
Washington, DC 20007

**Janice M. Massey, M.D.**
Assistant Professor of Neurology
DUKE UNIVERSITY MEDICAL CENTER
Box 3403
Durham, NC 27710

**Irene H. Maumenee, M.D.**
Associate Professor of Ophthalmology
THE JOHNS HOPKINS HOSPITAL
Maumenee Building Room 321
601 North Broadway
Baltimore, MD 21205

**Emeran A. Mayer, M.D.**
Division of Gastroenterology
U.C.L.A. HARBOR MEDICAL CENTER
1000 West Carson Street C-1 Trailer
Torrance, CA 90509

**Edward R.B. McCabe, M.D., Ph.D.**
Director, R.J. Kleberg Jr. Center
Institute for Molecular Genetics
BAYLOR COLLEGE OF MEDICINE
One Baylor Plaza T-526
Houston, TX 77030

**Catherine McKeon, Ph.D.**
Senior Staff Fellow
Diabetes, Digestive & Kidney Diseases
NATIONAL INSTITUTES OF HEALTH
Building 10-8N250
Bethesda, MD 20892

**David H. McKibben, Jr., D.M.D.**
Associate Prof. of Pediatric Dentistry
School of Dental Medicine
UNIVERSITY OF PITTSBURGH
Children's Hospital of Pittsburgh
3705 Fifth Avenue at DeSoto Street
Pittsburgh, PA 15213

**Ross Erwin McKinney, Jr., M.D.**
Department of Pediatrics
DUKE UNIVERSITY MEDICAL CENTER
Box 3461
Durham, NC 27710

**Victor A. McKusick, M.D.**
Department of Medicine
THE JOHNS HOPKINS UNIVERSITY SCHOOL OF MEDICINE
Baltimore, MD 21205

**D. Ross McLeod, M.D.**
Division of Medical Genetics
ALBERTA CHILDREN'S HOSPITAL
1820 Richmond Road, S.W.
Calgary T2T 5C7
CANADA

**Dan G. McNamara, M.D.**
Pediatric Cardiology
TEXAS CHILDREN'S HOSPITAL
6621 Fannin Street
Houston, TX 77030

**Roland S. Medansky, M.D.**
7447 West Talcott
Chicago, IL 60631

**Peter Meinecke, M.D.**
Abt. fur Medizinische Genetik
ALTONAER KINDERKRANKENHAUS
Bleickenallee 38
2000 Hamburg 50
WEST GERMANY

**Heirie M.M. Mendez, M.D., Ph.D.**
FFFCMPA
Rua Sarmento Leite, 245
90050 Porto Alegre
Porto Alegre RS
BRAZIL

**Marvin C. Mengel, M.D.**
Clinical Assistant Professor of Medicine
UNIVERSITY OF FLORIDA
1200 East Hillcrest
Orlando, FL 32803

**William C. Mentzer, Jr., M.D.**
Professor of Pediatrics
Department of Pediatrics, U.C.S.F.
SAN FRANCISCO GENERAL HOSPITAL
1001 Potrero Avenue 6J5
San Francisco, CA 94110

**Thomas J. Merimee, M.D.**
Professor and Chief
Department of Medicine
UNIVERSITY OF FLORIDA SCHOOL OF MEDICINE
J.H.M.H.C. Box J-226
Gainesville, FL 32610 0277

**Paul Merlob, M.D.**
Head, Neonatal Department
Beilinson Medical Center
SACKLER SCHOOL OF MEDICINE
49100 Petah-Tikva
ISRAEL

**David F. Merten, M.D.**
Professor of Radiology and Pediatrics
UNIVERSITY OF NORTH CAROLINA SCHOOL OF MEDICINE
Department of Radiology
Old Clinic Building Campus Box #7510
Chapel Hill, NC 27599 7510

**Louise Brearley Messer, D.D.S.**
Professor
UNIVERSITY OF MINNESOTA
6-150, Unit A
Health Sciences Building
Minneapolis, MN 55455

**Marilyn Baird Mets, M.D.**
Assistant Professor of Ophthalmology
Eye Research Laboratories
UNIVERSITY OF CHICAGO
939 East 57th Street
Chicago, IL 60637

**Irving Meyer, D.M.D., D.Sc.**
50 Maple Street
Suite 209
Springfield, MA 01103 1974

**Paul A. Meyers, M.D.**
Assistant Attending
Department of Pediatrics
MEMORIAL SLOAN KETTERING CANCER CENTER
1275 York Avenue
New York, NY 10021

**Giuseppe Micali, M.D.**
Clinica Dermatologica
UNIVERSITA DI CATANIA
Piazza S. Agata La Vetere, 6
Catania
ITALY

**Virginia V. Michels, M.D.**
Department of Medical Genetics
THE MAYO CLINIC
East 7B
Rochester, MN 55905

**Bruce Middleton, Ph.D.**
Department of Biochemistry
UNIVERSITY OF NOTTINGHAM MEDICAL SCHOOL
Queen's Medical Center
Clifton Boulevard
Nottingham NG7 2UH
ENGLAND

**George R. Mikhail, M.D.**
Department of Dermatology
HENRY FORD HOSPITAL
2799 West Grand Boulevard
Detroit, MI 48202

**Samuel Milham, Jr., M.D., M.P.H.**
Chronic Disease Epidemiologist
WASHINGTON STATE DEPARTMENT OF SOCIAL AND HEALTH SERVICES
E.T. - 13
Olympia, WA 98504

**B. Lynn Miller, M.D.**
610 S.W. First Avenue
Williston, FL 32696

**Michael E. Miller, M.D.** ‡
Professor and Chairman
Department of Pediatrics
UNIVERSITY OF CALIFORNIA, DAVIS
4301 X Street Trailer 1528
Sacramento, CA 95817

**Robert H. Miller, M.D.**
Division of Pediatric Cardiology
UNIVERSITY HOSPITAL OF JACKSONVILLE
655 West Eighth Street
Jacksonville, FL 32209

**Robert W. Miller, M.D., Dr. P.H**
Chief, Clinical Epidemiology Branch
NATIONAL CANCER INSTITUTE
National Institutes of Health
Executive Plaza North, Room 400
Bethesda, MD 20892

**Stephen H. Miller, M.D.**
Chief, Div. Plastic & Reconst. Surgery
THE OREGON HEALTH SCIENCES UNIVERSITY
3181 S.W. San Jackson Park Road
Portland, OR 97201

**Henry G. Mishalany, M.D.**
Department of Surgery (Pediatric)
CHILDREN'S HOSPITAL OF LOS ANGELES
4650 Sunset Boulevard
Los Angeles, CA 90027

**Joyce A. Mitchell, Ph.D.**
Associate Professor
Medical Genetics Unit
UNIVERSITY OF MISSOURI HEALTH SCIENCE CENTER
One Hospital Drive
Columbia, MO 65212

**Donald I. Moel, M.D.**
Division of Pediatric Nephrology
CHILDREN'S MEMORIAL HOSPITAL
2300 Children's Plaza
Chicago, IL 60614

**John B. Moeschler, M.D.**
Director, Child Development Program
Dept. of Maternal and Child Health
DARTMOUTH-HITCHCOCK MEDICAL CENTER
Butler Building #2
Hanover, NH 03756

**James H. Moller, M.D.**
Professor of Pediatrics (Cardiology)
UNIVERSITY OF MINNESOTA
420 Delaware St. S.E. Box 288
Minneapolis, MN 55455

**Peggy Smith Monahan, M.D.**
Fellow, Developmental Pediatrics
J.F. KENNEDY INSTITUTE FOR HANDICAPPED CHILDREN
707 North Broadway
Baltimore, MD 21205

**Arnold S. Monto, M.D.**
Professor of Epidemiology
UNIVERSITY OF MICHIGAN
SPH1 Room 2010
Ann Arbor, MI 48109 2029

**Cynthia A. Moore, M.D.**
Clinical Lecturer in Medical Genetics
INDIANA UNIVERSITY SCHOOL OF MEDICINE
975 West Walnut Street IB130
Indianapolis, IN 46202

**Patrick S. Moore, M.D.**
Meningitis and Special Pathogens Branch
Division of Bacterial Diseases
CENTERS FOR DISEASE CONTROL CO-9
Atlanta, GA 30336

**Regan Lynn Moore, D.D.S., M.S.D**
Assistant Professor, Periodontics
Director of Periodontal Research
UNIVERSITY OF LOUISVILLE
Louisville, KY 40292

**Jesus S. Mora, M.D.**
Service of Neurology
CLINICA PUERTA DE HIERRO
San Martin De Porres, 4
28035 Madrid
SPAIN

**Merle E. Morris, M.D.**
School of Dentistry
UNIVERSITY OF CALIFORNIA
25 Robert Road
Orinda, CA 94563

**Gabriel Mortimer, M.D.**
Consultant Histopathologist
Department of Histopathology
UNIVERSITY COLLEGE HOSPITAL
Galway
IRELAND

**Hugo Moser, M.D.**
Professor of Neurology and Pediatrics
Johns Hopkins University, and President
J.F. KENNEDY INSTITUTE FOR HANDICAPPED CHILDREN
707 North Broadway
Baltimore, MD 21205

**David B. Mosher, M.D.**
20 Pickering Street
Needham, MA 02192

**Thomas J. Muckle, M.D.**
Director, Dept. of Laboratories
Chedoke Division
CHEDOKE-McMASTER HOSPITALS
P.O. Box 2000, Station A
Hamilton ONT L8N 3Z5
CANADA

**Sigfrid A. Muller, M.D.**
Department of Dermatology
THE MAYO CLINIC
200 First Street S.W.
Rochester, MN 55905

**Charles E. Mullins, M.D.**
Associate Director
Section of Pediatric Cardiology
TEXAS CHILDREN'S HOSPITAL
6621 Fannin Street MS 1-105
Houston, TX 77030

**John J. Mulvihill, M.D.**
Director, NIH Center Institute
Medical Genetics Program
NATIONAL CANCER INSTITUTE
National Institutes of Health
Executive Plaza North, Room 400
Bethesda, MD 20892

**Michele Munoz, M.D.**
Jules Stein Eye Institute
UNIVERSITY OF CALIFORNIA SCHOOL OF MEDICINE
Los Angeles, CA 90024

**Jeff Murray, M.D.**
Department of Pediatrics
UNIVERSITY OF IOWA HOSPITAL
Iowa City, IA 52242

**Charles M. Myer, III, M.D.**
Department of Pediatric Otolaryngology
CHILDREN'S HOSPITAL MEDICAL CENTER
Elland & Bethesda Avenues
Cincinnati, OH 45229 2899

**Terry L. Myers, M.D., Ph.D.**
Head, Division of Clinical Genetics
Department of Pediatrics
TEXAS TECH UNIVERSITY HEALTH SCIENCES CENTER
Lubbock, TX 79430

**Madhavan Nair, Ph.D.**
Department of Pediatrics
UNIVERSITY OF MICHIGAN MEDICAL CENTER
Box 56, Kregg II-R6048
Ann Arbor, MI 48109

**Jennifer Lee Najjar, M.D.**
Instructor, Department of Pediatrics
Division of Pediatric Endocrinology
VANDERBILT UNIVERSITY SCHOOL OF MEDICINE
DD-2205
Nashville, TN 37232

**Samir S. Najjar, M.D.**
Division of Endocrinology
BOSTON CHILDREN'S HOSPITAL
300 Longwood Avenue
Boston, MA 02115

**Victor A. Najjar, M.D.**
Chairman, Department of Protein Chemistry
TUFTS UNIVERSITY SCHOOL OF MEDICINE
133 Harrison Avenue
Boston, MA 02111

**Walter Nance, M.D.**
Department of Human Genetics
MEDICAL COLLEGE OF VIRGINIA
Box 33 MCV Station
Richmond, VA 23298

**Karin B. Nelson, M.D.**
Perinatal Collaborative Study
Neuroepidemiology Branch
NATIONAL INSTITUTES OF HEALTH
Federal Building Room 804
7550 Wisconsin Avenue
Bethesda, MD 20892

**Giovanni Neri, M.D.**
Instituto di Genetica Umana
UNIVERSITA CATTOLICA DEL SACRO CUORE
Via della Pineta Sacchetti 644Largo A. G
Largo A. Gemelli, 8
00168 Roma
ITALY

**Gerhard Neuhauser, M.D.**
Professor
Neuropadiat. Abt.
UNIVERSITATS-KINDERKLINIK
Feulgenstrasse 12
D-6399 Giessen-Lahn
WEST GERMANY

**Won Gin Ng, Ph.D.**
Associate Professor of Research, U.S.C.
Division of Medical Genetics
CHILDREN'S HOSPITAL OF LOS ANGELES
P.O. Box 54700
Los Angeles, CA 90054 0700

**Buford L. Nichols, M.D.**
BAYLOR COLLEGE OF MEDICINE
6621 Fannin Street
C.N.C.R.
Houston, TX 77030

**Pat Nichols, M.S.**
Genetic Associate
Department of Pediatrics
UNIVERSITY OF SOUTH FLORIDA
12901 North 30th Street Box 15-G
Tampa, FL 33612 4799

**Michael R. Nihill, M.B.,B.S.**
Associate Professor of Pediatrics
Pediatric Cardiology
TEXAS CHILDREN'S HOSPITAL
6621 Fannin Street
Houston, TX 77030

**Norio Niikawa, M.D., Ph.D.**
Professor and Director
Department of Human Genetics
NAGASAKI UNIVERSITY SCHOOL OF MEDICINE
Nagasaki 852
JAPAN

**Audrey H. Nora, M.D., M.P.H.**
Assistant Surgeon General
Public Health Service
HEALTH AND HUMAN SERVICES
1961 Stout Street
Denver, CO 80294

**James J. Nora, M.D.**
Professor of Genetics
Preventive Medicine and Pediatrics
UNIVERSITY OF COLORADO MEDICAL CENTER
4200 East Ninth Avenue Container A-007
Denver, CO 80262

**Richard E. Nordgren, M.D.**
Associate Professor Clinical Medicine
Department of Neurology
DARTMOUTH-HITCHCOCK MEDICAL CENTER
Hanover, NH 03756

**Arthur L. Norins, M.D.**
Professor of Dermatology
Regenstrief Health Center 524
INDIANA UNIVERSITY SCHOOL OF MEDICINE
1100 West Michigan Street
Indianapolis, IN 46223

**Kaare R. Norum, M.D., Ph.D.**
Professor
UNIVERSITY OF OSLO SCHOOL OF MEDICINE
P.O. Box 1046 Blindern
0316 Oslo 3
NORWAY

**Fiorella Nuzzo, Ph.D.**
Professor in Human Genetics
ISTITUTO DI GENETICA BIOCHIMICA ED EVOLUZIONISTICA C.N.R.
Via Abbiategrasso 207
Pavia I-27100
ITALY

**William L. Nyhan, M.D.**
Department of Pediatrics (M-009-A)
U.C.S.D. SCHOOL OF MEDICINE
La Jolla, CA 92093 0609

**Jane O'Brien, M.D.**
NATIONAL BIRTH DEFECTS CENTER
30 Warren Street
Brighton, MA 02135

**John S. O'Brien, M.D.**
Department of Neurosciences M-008
U.C.S.D. SCHOOL OF MEDICINE
La Jolla, CA 92093

**Geoffrey J. O'Neill, Ph.D.**
The Blood Bank
AMERICAN RED CROSS
1675 Northwest 9th Avenue Box 013201
Miami, FL 33101

**Gilbert S. Omenn, M.D., Ph.D.**
Professor and Dean
Public Health and Community Med. SC-30
UNIVERSITY OF WASHINGTON
Seattle, WA 98195

**Jose M. Ordovas, Ph.D.**
Lipid Metabolism Laboratory
HUMAN NUTRITION RESEARCH CENTER AT TUFTS
711 Washington Street
Boston, MA 02111

**Peter Orobello, M.D.**
Resident in Otolaryngology
CHILDREN'S HOSPITAL MEDICAL CENTER
Elland and Bethesda Avenues
Cincinnati, OH 45229 2899

**Eduardo Orti, M.D.**
Associate Professor of Pediatrics
S.U.N.Y. DOWNSTATE MEDICAL CENTER
450 Clarkson Avenue
Box 49
Brooklyn, NY 11203 2098

**A. Lee Osterman, M.D.**
Department of Orthopaedic Surgery
UNIVERSITY OF PENNSYLVANIA HOSPITAL
Silverstein Pavilion Second Floor
3400 Spruce Street
Philadelphia, PA 19104

**Rajendra H. Pahwa, M.D.**
ALL CHILDREN'S HOSPITAL
801 Sixth Street South # 795
P.O. Box 31020
St. Petersburg, FL 33731 8920

**Savita G. Pahwa, M.D.**
Chief, Immunology Division
Department of Pediatrics
NORTH SHORE UNIVERSITY HOSPITAL
300 Community Drive
Manhasset, NY 11030

**G. Shashidhar Pai, M.D.**
Director, Genetics-Birth Defects Center
Department of Pediatrics
MEDICAL UNIVERSITY OF SOUTH CAROLINA
171 Ashley Avenue
Charleston, SC 29425 2248

**Philip D. Pallister, M.D., D.Sc.**
Box 86
Boulder, MT 59632

**Stephen M. Paridon, M.D.**
Fellow in Pediatric Cardiology
TEXAS CHILDREN'S HOSPITAL
6621 Fannin
Houston, TX 77030

**Michael W. Partington, M.D., Ph.D.**
Regional Medical Genetics Unit
WESTERN SUBURBS HOSPITAL
P.O. Box 21
Newcastle, NSW 2298
AUSTRALIA

**Steven Pascucci, M.D.**
Center for Sight
GEORGETOWN UNIVERSITY MEDICAL CENTER
3800 Reservoir Road, N.W.
Washington, DC 20007

**Hermine Pashayan, M.D. ‡**
TUFTS UNIVERSITY SCHOOL OF MEDICINE
131 Harrison Avenue
Boston, MA 02111

**Eberhard Passarge, M.D.**
INSTITUTE FOR HUMANGENETIK
Hufelandstr 55
D4300 Essen
WEST GERMANY

**Raj A. Patel, D.D.S., M.S.**
Department of Oral-Facial Genetics
INDIANA UNIVERSITY SCHOOL OF DENTISTRY
10999 Windjammer Trace
Indianapolis, IN 46256

**A. D. Patrick, M.D.**
Institute of Child Health
UNIVERSITY OF LONDON
30 Guilford Street
London WC1N 3JH
ENGLAND

**David Pauls, Ph.D.**
Associate Professor
Child Study Center
YALE UNIVERSITY SCHOOL OF MEDICINE
333 Cedar Street
P.O. Box 3333
New Haven, CT 06510

**Sergio D.J. Pena, M.D., Ph.D.**
NUCLEO DE GENETICA MEDICA DE MINAS GERAIS (GENE/MG)
Caixa Postal 3396
CEP 30112
Belo Horizonte MG
BRAZIL

**Myles L. Pensak, M.D.**
Associate Professor and Director
Division of Otology/Neurotology
UNIVERSITY OF CINCINNATI COLLEGE OF MEDICINE
Cincinnati, OH 45267

**Jay S. Pepose, M.D., Ph.D.**
Department of Ophthalmology
WASHINGTON UNIVERSITY SCHOOL OF MEDICINE
660 South Euclid Avenue Box 8096
St. Louis, MO 63110

**Frederick A. Pereira, M.D.**
5114 Kissena Blvd.
Flushing, NY 11355 4163

**Angel R. Perez, M.D.**
Clinical Fellow
Division of Cardiology
CHILDREN'S HOSPITAL
Elland and Bethesda Avenues
Cincinnati, OH 45229 2899

**James C. Perry, M.D.**
Assistant Professor
Pediatric Cardiology
TEXAS CHILDREN'S HOSPITAL
6621 Fannin
Houston, TX 77030

**Rudolf A. Pfeiffer, M.D.**
Institut fur Humangenetik
UNIVERSITAT ERLANGEN-NURNBERG
Schwabachanlage 10
Erlangen 8520 D-852
WEST GERMANY

**Michel Philippart, M.D.**
Neuropsychiatric Institute
UNIVERSITY OF CALIFORNIA AT LOS ANGELES
760 Westwood Plaza
Los Angeles, CA 90024

**John A. Phillips, III, M.D.**
Professor of Pediatrics and Biochemistry
VANDERBILT UNIVERSITY SCHOOL OF MEDICINE
Room T-2404 Medical Center North
Nashville, TN 37232

**Claus A. Pierach, M.D.**
ABBOTT NORTHWEST HOSPITAL
800 East 28th Street
Minneapolis, MN 55407

**Marta Pinheiro, D.Sc.**
Department of Genetics
FEDERAL UNIVERSITY OF PARANA
Caixa Postal 19071
81504 Curitiba
Parana
BRAZIL

**Leonard Pinsky, M.D.**
Cell Genetics Laboratory
LADY DAVIS INSTITUTE FOR MEDICAL RESEARCH
3755 Chemin Cote Ste-Catherine
Montreal H3T 1E2 PQ
CANADA

**Guillem Pintos-Morell, M.D.**
Post-doctoral Fellow
Div. of Pediatric Metabolism (M-009-F)
U.C.S.D. MEDICAL CENTER
La Jolla, CA 92093 0609

**Sergio Piomelli, M.D.**
Director, Pediatric Hematology/Oncology
COLUMBIA UNIVERSITY COLLEGE OF PHYSICIANS AND SURGEONS
630 West 168th Street
New York, NY 10032

**Barbara R. Pober, M.D., M.P.H.**
Division of Genetics
BOSTON CHILDREN'S HOSPITAL
300 Longwood Avenue
Boston, MA 02115

**Joel M. Pokorny, Ph.D.**
Eye Research Laboratory
UNIVERSITY OF CHICAGO
939 East 57th Street
Chicago, IL 60637

**Robert C. Polomeno, M.D.**
Associate Professor of Ophthalmology
MONTREAL CHILDREN'S HOSPITAL OF McGILL UNIVERSITY
2300 Tupper Street
Montreal, PQ H3H 1P3
CANADA

**Andrew E. Poole, D.D.S., Ph.D.**
Professor, Pediatric Dentistry
Director, Craniofacial Team
UNIVERSITY OF CONNECTICUT HEALTH CENTER
Farmington, CT 06032

**Ian Porter, M.D.**
New York State Birth Defects Institute
ALBANY MEDICAL CENTER
I-309
New Scotland Avenue
Albany, NY 12208

**Scott L. Portnoy, M.D.**
L.S.U. EYE CENTER
2020 Gravier Street Suite B
New Orleans, LA 70112 2234

**Andrew K. Poznanski, M.D.**
Radiologist-in-Chief
Department of Radiology
CHILDREN'S MEMORIAL HOSPITAL
2300 Children's Plaza
Chicago, IL 60614

**Marilyn Preus, Ph.D.**
Center for Human Genetics
McGILL UNIVERSITY
Stewart Biology Building
1205 Rue Docteur Penfield
Montreal, QB H3A 1B1
CANADA

**Visnja Milavec Puretic, M.D.**
Dermatovenerologist
Hospital for Skin and Venereal Diseases
MEDICAL UNIVERSITY OF ZAGREB
Petrova 90
41000 Zagreb
YUGOSLAVIA

**Zvonimir Puretic, M.D.**
Head, Pediatric Dialysis Unit
Department of Urology
UNIVERSITY OF ZAGREB MEDICAL SCHOOL
Petrova 90
41000 Zagreb 41000
YUGOSLAVIA

**David T. Purtilo, M.D.**
Department of Pathology-Microbiology
UNIVERSITY OF NEBRASKA MEDICAL CENTER
42nd and Dewey Avenues
Omaha, NE 68105

**Reed E. Pyeritz, M.D., Ph.D.**
Associate Professor & Clinical Director
Center for Medical Genetics
JOHNS HOPKINS UNIVERSITY SCHOOL OF MEDICINE
Blalock 1012
Baltimore, MD 21205

**Qutub H. Qazi, M.D., Ph.D.**
Professor of Clinical Pediatrics
STATE UNIVERSITY OF NEW YORK HEALTH SCIENCE CENTER
450 Clarkson Avenue Box 49
Brooklyn, NY 11203

**Stephen J. Qualman, M.D.**
Department of Laboratory Medicine
CHILDREN'S HOSPITAL
700 Children's Drive
Columbus, OH 43205

**Leslie J. Raffel, M.D.**
Assistant Professor of Pediatrics
Division of Human Genetics
UNIVERSITY OF MARYLAND SCHOOL OF MEDICINE
Bressler Research Building
655 West Baltimore Street
Baltimore, MD 21201

**Elsa K. Rahn, M.D.**
363 Hempstead Avenue
Rockville Center, NY 11570

**Maria Lourdes Ramirez, M.D.**
CENTRO ESTUDIO Y TERAPIAS ESPECIALES
Sistema DIF Jalisco
Apartado Postal 1-1781
Jalisco
MEXICO

**Maria A. Ramos-Arroyo, M.D.**
Associate Researcher
Facultad de Medicina
UNIVERSIDAD COMPLUTENSE
ECEMC, Catedra de Anatomia II
Madrid 28040
SPAIN

**Sonja Rasmussen, M.S.**
Division of Genetics
Department of Pediatrics
UNIVERSITY OF FLORIDA
J-296, JHMHC
Gainesville, FL 32610

**Dietz Rating, M.D.**
Professor
Abteilung Neuropadiatrie
UNIVERSITATS-KINDERKLINIK
Robert-Koch Str. 40
D-3400 Gottingen
GERMANY

**Yaddanapudi Ravindranath, M.B., B.S.**
Department of Pediatrics
WAYNE STATE UNIVERSITY SCHOOL OF MEDICINE
3901 Beaubien Blvd.
Detroit, MI 48201

**B. Eileen Rawnsley, B.S.N.**
Clinical Coordinator
Maternal and Child Health
DARTMOUTH-HITCHCOCK MEDICAL CENTER
Hanover, NH 03755

**Robert S. Redman, D.D.S., Ph.D.**
Chief, Oral Pathology Research (151-I)
V.A. MEDICAL CENTER
50 Irving Street, N.W.
Washington, DC 20422

**Helena Reece, M.D.**
Assistant Professor of Pediatrics
THE MONTREAL CHILDREN'S HOSPITAL OF McGILL UNIVERSITY
2300 Tupper Street
Montreal PQ H3H 1P3
CANADA

**Theresa Greene Reed, M.D., M.P.H.**
Acting Group Leader
Division of Anti-infective Drug Products
CENTER FOR DRUG EVALUATION AND RESEARCH
Food and Drug Administration
5600 Fishers Lane
Rockville, MD 20857

**Samuel Refetoff, M.D.**
Professor of Medicine and Pediatrics
Thyroid Study Unit Box 138
THE UNIVERSITY OF CHICAGO
5841 South Maryland Avenue
Chicago, IL 60637

**Philip R. Reilly, J.D., M.D.**
Executive Director
SHRIVER CENTER, INC.
200 Trapelo Road
Waltham, MA 02254

**Salomon H. Reisner, M.B., Ch.B.**
Head, Neonatal Department
BEILINSON MEDICAL CENTER
Petach Tikvah
ISRAEL

**Martin Renlund, M.D.**
Visting Scientist
N.I.C.H.D.
NATIONAL INSTITUTES OF HEALTH
Building 10, Room 10N-320
Bethesda, MD 20892

**James F. Reynolds, M.D.**
Director, Medical Division
Department of Medical Genetics
SHODAIR HOSPITAL
P.O. Box 5539
Helena, MT 59604

**Martha Celina Reynoso, M.D.**
INSTITUTO MEXICANO DEL SEGURO SOCIAL
Apartado Postal 1-3838
Guadalajara Jalisco
MEXICO

**William J. Rhead, M.D., Ph.D.**
Professor of Pediatrics
UNIVERSITY OF IOWA
Iowa City, IA 52242

**J. Marc Rhoads, M.D.**
Department of Pediatrics
UNIVERSITY OF NORTH CAROLINA
Clinical Sciences Building CB No. 7220
Chaple Hill, NC 27599

**Arthur R. Rhodes, M.D., M.P.H.**
Associate Professor of Dermatology
UNIVERSITY OF PITTSBURGH SCHOOL OF MEDICINE
3601 Fifth Avenue
Pittsburgh, PA 15213

**Vincent M. Riccardi, M.D.**
THE GENETICS INSTITUTE
11 West Del Mar Blvd.
Pasadena, CA 91105

**S.S. Rich, Ph.D.**
Associate Professor
Laboratory Medicine and Pathology
UNIVERSITY OF MINNESOTA SCHOOL OF MEDICINE
Box 511 Mayo Memorial Building
420 Delaware Street, S.E.
Minneapolis, MN 55455

**Thomas A. Riemenschneider, M.D.**
Associate Dean, School of Medicine
CASE WESTERN RESERVE UNIVERSITY
2119 Abington Road
Cleveland, OH 44106

**Harris D. Riley, Jr., M.D.**
Distinguished Professor of Pediatrics
Children's Memorial Hospital
UNIVERSITY OF OKLAHOMA HEALTH SCIENCES CENTER
Post Office Box 26901
Oklahoma City, OK 73190

**David L. Rimoin, M.D.**
Medical Genetics - Birth Defects Center
CEDARS - SINAI MEDICAL CENTER
8700 Beverly Blvd.
Los Angeles, CA 90048

**Richard E. Ringel, M.D.**
Assistant Professor
Division of Pediatric Cardiology
UNIVERSITY OF MARYLAND SCHOOL OF MEDICINE
22 South Greene Street
Baltimore, MD 21202

**Fernando Rivas, M.D.**
INSTITUTO MEXICANO DEL SEGURO SOCIAL
Ap. Postal 1-3838
Guadalajara
MEXICO

**Horacio Rivera, M.D.**
INSTITUTO MEXICANO DEL SEGURO SOCIAL
Ap. Postal 1-3838 ·
Guadalajara
MEXICO

**Charles C. Roberts, M.D.**
Chief, Pediatric Gastroenterology
CHILDREN'S MERCY HOSPITAL
24th at Gillham Road
Kansas City, MO 64108

**Richard M. Roberts, M.D., Ph.D.**
Director, Genetics Services
T.C. Thompson Children's Hospital
ERLANGER MEDICAL CENTER
910 Blackford Street
Chattanooga, TN 37403

**Meinhard Robinow, M.D.**
Director
Birth Defects, Genetics, Dysmorphology
CHILDREN'S MEDICAL CENTER
129 Grant Street
Dayton, OH 45404

**Luther K. Robinson, M.D.**
Director, Dysmorphology/Clinical Genetics
Department of Pediatrics
CHILDREN'S HOSPITAL OF BUFFALO
219 Btyant Street
Buffalo, NY 14222

**Walter Rogan, M.D.**
Epidemiology Branch
NATIONAL INSTITUTE OF ENVIRONMENTAL HEALTH SCIENCES
Research Triangle Park
P.O. Box 12233
Triangle Park, NC 27709

**Beverly R. Rollnick, Ph.D.** ‡
Director, Genetic Counseling
Center for Craniofacial Anomalies
UNIVERSITY OF ILLINOIS
College of Medicine
P.O. Box 6998
Chicago, IL 60680

**Allen Root, M.D.**
Department of Pediatrics
UNIVERSITY OF SOUTH FLORIDA
12901 North 30th Street Box 15
Tampa, FL 33612

**Franz W. Rosa, M.D., M.P.H.**
FOOD AND DRUG ADMINISTRATION
Room 15 B-07
HFN-733
5600 Fishers Lane
Rockville, MD 20852

**Leon E. Rosenberg, M.D.**
Chief, Department of Human Genetics
YALE UNIVERSITY
333 Cedar Street
New Haven, CT 06510 8055

**David S. Rosenblatt, M.D.**
Director, Division of Medical Genetics
ROYAL VICTORIA HOSPITAL
687 Pine Avenue Room H5-63
Montreal H3A 1A1 PQ
CANADA

**Sally Shulman Rosengren, M.D.**
Assistant Professor of Pediatrics
Division of Human Genetics
UNIVERSITY OF CONNECTICUT HEALTH CENTER
School of Medicine
Farmington, CT 06032 9984

**Jerome I. Rotter, M.D.**
Director, Division of Medical Genetics
CEDARS - SINAI MEDICAL CENTER
8700 West Beverly Blvd.
Los Angeles, CA 90048 0750

**Nathaniel H. Rowe, D.D.S.**
Professor of Oral Pathology
School of Dentistry
THE UNIVERSITY OF MICHIGAN
4223 Schools of Dentistry and Medicine
Ann Arbor, MI 48109 1078

**Carlos Ruiz, M.D.**
INSTITUTO MEXICANO DEL SEGURO SOCIAL
Apartado Postal 1-3838
Guadalajara Jalisco
MEXICO

**Laura Russell, M.D.**
Department of Pediatrics
CHILD EVALUATION CENTER
334 East Broadway
Louisville, KY 40202

**Barry S. Russman, M.D.**
Clinical Director of Pediatric Neurology
NEWINGTON CHILDREN'S HOSPITAL
181 East Cedar Street
Newington, CT 06111

**Joe C. Rutledge, M.D.**
Associate Professor
Department of Laboratories
CHILDREN'S HOSPITAL AND MEDICAL CENTER
P.O. Box C5371
Seattle, WA 98105

**Stephen G. Ryan, M.D.**
Chief, Pediatric Neurology
Depts. of Pediatrics and Medicine
UNIVERSITY OF TEXAS HEALTH SCIENCE CENTER
7703 Floyd Curl Drive
San Antonio, TX 78284 7814

**Howard Saal, M.D.**
Division of Clinical Genetics
CHILDREN'S HOSPITAL NATIONAL MEDICAL CENTER
111 Michigan Avenue, N.W.
Washington, DC 20010

**George H. Sack, Jr., M.D., Ph.D.**
Associate Professor of Medicine
Department of Medical Genetics
THE JOHNS HOPKINS HOSPITAL
Blalock 1008
Baltimore, MD 21205

**Raymond Saddi, M.D.**
Maitre de Recherche CNRS
INSTITUT DE PATHOLOGIE MOLECULAIRE
24 Rue du Faubourg-Saint Jacques
Paris 75014
FRANCE

**Vicki L. Sadewitz**
Research Associate and Coordinator
Congenital Disorder Unit, Dept. Otolary.
MONTEFIORE MEDICAL CENTER
111 East 210th Street
Bronx, NY 10467

**Adele D. Sadovnick, Ph.D.**
Research Associate
Department of Medical Genetics
UNIVERSITY OF BRITISH COLUMBIA
226 - 6174 University Boulevard
Vancouver V6T 1W5 BC
CANADA

**Inge Sagel, M.D.**
Associate Professor of Pediatrics
WESTCHESTER COUNTY MEDICAL CENTER
Valhalla, NY 10595

**Sudha S. Saksena, Ph.D.**
Research Scientist
Department of Oral-Facial Genetics
INDIANA UNIVERSITY MEDICAL CENTER
Ball Residence 026
1226 West Michigan Street
Indianapolis, IN 46223

**Gerald Salen, M.D.**
Professor of Medicine
Division of Gastroenterology
NEW JERSEY MEDICAL SCHOOL
100 Bergen Street
Newark, NJ 07103

**Carlos F. Salinas, D.M.D.**
Associate Professor
Div. Craniofacial Genetics BSB 332
MEDICAL UNIVERSITY OF SOUTH CAROLINA
171 Ashley Avenue
Charleston, SC 29425

**Riitta Salonen, M.D.**
Laboratory of Prenatal Genetics
Dept. of Obstetrics and Gynecology
HELSINKI UNIVERSITY CENTRAL HOSPITAL
Helsinki SF-00290
FINLAND

**Jose Sanchez-Corona, M.D.**
Division of Genetics
INSTITUTO MEXICANO DEL SEGURO SOCIAL
Apartado Postal 1-3838
Guadalajara, Jalisco
MEXICO

**Avery A. Sandberg, M.D.**
Director, The Cancer Center
SOUTHWEST BIOMEDICAL RESEARCH INSTITUTE
6401 East Thomas Road
Scottsdale, AZ 85251

**Warren G. Sanger, Ph.D.**
Director, Human Genetics
HATTIE B. MUNROE CENTER FOR HUMAN GENETICS
4420 Dewey Avenue
Omaha, NE 68105

**Joel R. Saper, M.D.**
Director
MICHIGAN HEAD PAIN AND NEUROLOGICAL INSTITUTE
3120 Professional Drive
Ann Arbor, MI 48104

**John J. Sauk, Jr., D.D.S.**
Department of Oral Pathology
UNIVERSITY OF MARYLAND AT BALTIMORE
College of Dental Surgery
Baltimore, MD 21201 1586

**Robert A. Saul, M.D.**
GREENWOOD GENETIC CENTER
One Gregor Mendel Circle
Greenwood, SC 29646

**Christina M. Sax, Ph.D.**
Lab. of Molecular & Development. Biology
NATIONAL EYE INSTITUTE
Building 6, Room 203
National Institutes of Health
Bethesda, MD 20892

**Burhan Say, M.D.**
Director
H. Allen Chapman Research Institute
CHILDREN'S MEDICAL CENTER
5300 East Skelly Drive
P.O. Box 35648
Tulsa, OK 74135

**Thomas Scanlin, M.D.**
Director, Cystic Fibrosis Center
Division of Pulmonary Medicine
CHILDREN'S HOSPITAL OF PHILADELPHIA
34th and Civic Center Blvd.
Philadelphia, PA 19104

**Paula R. Scarbrough, M.D.**
306 Poinciana Drive
Birmingham, AL 35209

**Ernst J. Schaefer, M.D.**
Lipid Metabolism Laboratory
U.S.D.A. HUMAN NUTRITION RESEARCH CENTER ON AGING
Tufts University and N.E. Medical Center
711 Washington Street
Boston, MA 02111

**Georges Schapira, M.D.**
Institute de Pathologie Moleculaire
UNIVERSITE DE PARIS
24 Rue de Faubourg-Saint Jacques
Paris 75014
FRANCE

**Richard K. Scher, M.D.**
Professor of Clinical Dermatology
COLUMBIA-PRESBYTERIAN MEDICAL CENTER
630 West 168th Street
New York, NY 10032

**Gerold L. Schiebler, M.D.**
Associate V.P. for Health Affairs
Department of Pediatrics
UNIVERSITY OF FLORIDA COLLEGE OF MEDICINE
J 296-JHMHC
Gainesville, FL 32610

**R. Neil Schimke, M.D.**
Professor Internal Medicine/Pediatrics
UNIVERSITY OF KANSAS MEDICAL CENTER
39th and Rainbow Blvd, 413-C
Kansas City, KS 66103

**Detlev Schindler, M.D.**
Department of Human Genetics
UNIVERSITY OF WUERZBURG
Koellikerstrasse 2
D-8700 Wuerzburg
WEST GERMANY

**Albert A.G.L. Schinzel, M.D.**
Professor
Institute for Medical Genetics
UNIVERSITY OF ZURICH MEDICAL SCHOOL
Ramistrasse 74
8001 Zurich
SWITZERLAND

**Bruce M. Schnall, M.D.**
Department of Ophthalmology
CHILDREN'S HOSPITAL NATIONAL MEDICAL CENTER
111 Michigan Avenue, N.W.
Washington, DC 20010

**Jerry A. Schneider, M.D.**
Professor of Pediatrics
Department of Pediatrics (M-009-F)
U.C.S.D. SCHOOL OF MEDICINE
La Jolla, CA 92093

**Craig M. Schramm, M.D.**
Division of Pulmonary Medicine
CHILDREN'S HOSPITAL OF PHILADELPHIA
34th and Civic Center Blvd.
Philadelphia, PA 19104

**H.W. Schroeder, M.D.**
UNIVERSITY OF WASHINGTON SCHOOL OF MEDICINE
Seattle, WA 98195

**Richard J. Schroer, M.D.**
GREENWOOD GENETIC CENTER
One Gregor Mendel Circle
Greenwood, SC 29646

**Joseph D. Schulman, M.D.**
GENETICS AND LVF INSTITUTE
3020 Javier Road
Fairfax, VA 22031

**Stanley A. Schwartz, M.D., Ph.D.**
Director, Clinical Immunology Section
Department of Pediatrics
UNIVERSITY OF MICHIGAN
109 Observatory Street Room 3073
Ann Arbor, MI 48109

**Mary E. Schwind, D.D.S.**
UNIVERSITY OF MINNESOTA SCHOOL OF DENTISTRY
6-150 Health Sciences Unit A
515 Delaware Street S.E.
Minneapolis, MN 55455

**C. Ronald Scott, M.D.**
Professor
Department of Pediatrics RD-20
UNIVERSITY OF WASHINGTON SCHOOL OF MEDICINE
Seattle, WA 98105

**Nina Scribanu, M.D.**
Center for Genetic Counseling
GEORGETOWN UNIVERSITY MEDICAL CENTER
3800 Reservoir Road, N.W.
Washington, DC 20007

**Charles R. Scriver, M.D.**
Professor
Center for Human Genetics
McGILL UNIVERSITY-MONTREAL CHILDREN'S HOSPITAL
2300 Tupper Street
Montreal H3H 1P3
CANADA

**John H. Seashore, M.D**
Department of Surgery
YALE UNIVERSITY SCHOOL OF MEDICINE
333 Cedar Street
P.O. Box 3333
New Haven, CT 06510 8062

**Heddie O. Sedano, D.D.S.**
Division of Oral Pathology
UNIVERSITY OF MINNESOTA SCHOOL OF DENTISTRY
515 Delaware Street, S.E.
Minneapolis, MN 55455

**Ruth Andrea Seeler, M.D.**
Professor of Pediatrics
Department of Pediatrics (M/C 856)
UNIVERSITY OF ILLINOIS SCHOOL OF MEDICINE AT CHICAGO
840 South Wood Street
Chicago, IL 60612

**Victor J. Selmanowitz, M.D.**
395 South End Avenue
No. 18J
New York, NY 10280

**Jorge Sequeiros, M.D.**
Assistant Professor of Medical Genetics
Instituto de Ciencias Biomedicas
UNIVERSITY OF PORTO
Lg. Prof. Abel Salazar, 2
4000 Porto
PORTUGAL

**John L. Sever, M.D., Ph.D.**
Chief, Infectious Diseases Branch
Neurological and Communicative Disorders
NATIONAL INSTITUTES OF HEALTH
Building 36, Room 5 D 06
Bethesda, MD 20892

**Douglas R. Shanklin, M.D.**
Chief, Perinatal Pathology
Department of Pathology
UNIVERSITY OF TENNESSEE CENTER FOR HEALTH SCIENCES
899 Madison Avenue
Memphis, TN 38163

**Bruce K. Shapiro, M.D.**
Director
Center for Learning and Its Disorders
J.F. KENNEDY INSTITUTE FOR HANDICAPPED CHILDREN
707 North Broadway
Baltimore, MD 21205

**Kenneth Shapiro, M.D.**
MONTEFIORE MEDICAL CENTER
111 East 210th Street
Bronx, NY 10467

**Lawrence R. Shapiro, M.D.**
Professor and Director
Medical Genetics Unit
WESTCHESTER COUNTY MEDICAL CENTER/
   NEW YORK MEDICAL COLLEGE
Valhalla, NY 10595

**Bruce I. Sharon, M.D.**
Department of Pediatrics (M/C 856)
THE UNIVERSITY OF ILLINOIS AT CHICAGO
840 South Wood Street Box 6998
Chicago, IL 60680

**Kathleen Shaver Arnos, Ph.D.**
Director, Genetic Services Center
GALLAUDET UNIVERSITY RESEARCH INSTITUTE
Kendall Green
800 Florida Avenue, N.E.
Washington, DC 20002

**Carol S. Shear, M.D.**
6181 S.W. 102 Street
Miami, FL 33156

**Vivian E. Shih, M.D.**
Director, Amino Acid Disorder Laboratory
Neurology Service
MASSACHUSETTS GENERAL HOSPITAL
149 13th Street Sixth Floor West
Boston, MA 02129 2000

**Henry R. Shinefield, M.D.**
THE PERMANENTE MEDICAL GROUP, INC.
2200 O'Farrell Street
San Francisco, CA 94119 3394

**Mordechai Shohat, M.D.**
Department of Pediatrics / Genetics
CEDARS - SINAI MEDICAL CENTER
8700 Beverly Blvd.
Los Angeles, CA 90048 1869

**Stephen B. Shohet, M.D.**
Director, Cancer Research Institute
MOFFITT HOSPITAL OF THE UNIVERSITY OF CALIFORNIA
San Francisco, CA 94143

**Sally R. Shott, M.D.**
Dept. Pediatric Otolaryngology
CHILDREN'S HOSPITAL MEDICAL CENTER
Elland & Bethesda Avenues
Cincinnati, OH 45229 2899

**Robert J. Shprintzen, Ph.D.**
Director
Center for Craniofacial Disorders
MONTEFIORE MEDICAL CENTER
111 East 210th Street
Bronx, NY 10467

**Margaret Siber, M.D.**
Birth Defects Unit
TUFTS - NEW ENGLAND MEDICAL CENTER
171 Harrison Avenue, Box 50
Boston, MA 02111

**James B. Sidbury, Jr., M.D.**
Senior Scientist
NATIONAL INSTITUTE OF CHILD HEALTH AND HUMAN DEVELOPMENT
Building 10, 8C311
Bethesda, MD 20205

**Teepu Siddique, M.D.**
Assistant Professor of Neurology
Department of Medicine
DUKE UNIVERSITY MEDICAL CENTER
Box 2900
Durham, NC 27710

**William K. Sieber, M.D.**
Webster Hall
4415 Fifth Avenue
Pittsburgh, PA 15213 3263

**M. Cirillo Silengo, M.D.**
Servizio di Genetica Clinica Infantile
ISTITUTO DI DISCIPLINE PEDIATRICHE
Universita di Torino
Torino
ITALY

**David O. Sillence, M.D.**
Professor of Medical Genetics
Medical Genetics and Dysmorphology Unit
CHILDREN'S HOSPITAL
P.O. Box 34
Campertown N.S.W. 2050
AUSTRALIA

**Henry K. Silver, M.D.**
Department of Pediatrics
Box C218
UNIVERSITY OF COLORADO HEALTH SCIENCES CENTER
4200 E. Ninth Avenue
Denver, CO 80262

**Frederic N. Silverman, M.D.**
Professor Emeritus
Departments of Radiology and Pediatrics
STANFORD UNIVERSITY MEDICAL CENTER
Stanford, CA 94305

**Olli G. Simell, M.D.**
Professor and Chairman
Department of Pediatrics
UNIVERSITY OF TURKU
SF-20520 Turku 52
FINLAND

**Joe Leigh Simpson, M.D.**
Faculty Professor and Chairman
Department of Obstetrics and Gynecology
UNIVERSITY OF TENNESSEE, MEMPHIS
853 Jefferson Avenue
Memphis, TN 38163

**Dharmdeo N. Singh, Ph.D.**
Professor of Pediatrics & Psychiatry
MEHARRY MEDICAL COLLEGE
1005 D.B.Todd Blvd.
Nashville, TN 37208

**Herbert B. Slade, M.D.**
Department of Pediatrics
UNIVERSITY OF MICHIGAN SCHOOL OF MEDICINE
109 Observatory Street Room 3073
Ann Arbor, MI 48109

**William S. Sly, M.D.**
Chairman, Department of Biochemistry
ST. LOUIS UNIVERSITY SCHOOL OF MEDICINE
1402 South Grant
St. Louis, MO 63104

**Kent W. Small, M.D.**
North Carolina Macular Dystrophy
DUKE UNIVERSITY
Box 2900
Durham, NC 27710

**Ann C.M. Smith, M.A.**
Clinical Director
Division of Genetics
THE CHILDREN'S HOSPITAL
1056 East 19th Avenue
Denver, CO 80218

**Margaret Smith, Ph.D.**
Department of Pediatrics M-009-F
U.C.S.D. SCHOOL OF MEDICINE
La Jolla, CA 92093

**Morton E. Smith, M.D.**
Department of Ophthalmology
WASHINGTON UNIVERSITY SCHOOL OF MEDICINE
Box 8096
St. Louis, MO 63110

**Shelley D. Smith, Ph.D.**
Associate Professor
Hereditary Communication Disorders
BOYS TOWN NATIONAL INSTITUTE
555 N. 30th Street
Omaha, NE 68131

**Thomas F. Smith, M.D.**
Department of Pediatrics
EMORY UNIVERSITY SCHOOL OF MEDICINE
69 Butler Street, S.E.
Atlanta, GA 30303

**Vivianne C. Smith, Ph.D.**
Professor of Ophthalmology
Department of Ophthalmology
UNIVERSITY OF CHICAGO
939 East 57th Street
Chicago, IL 60637

**Allan D. Sniderman, M.D.**
Professor of Medicine
Director, Cardiology Division
ROYAL VICTORIA HOSPITAL OF McGILL UNIVERSITY
687 Pine Avenue West
Montreal H3A 1A1 PQ
CANADA

**Selma E. Snyderman, M.D.**
Professor of Pediatrics
Department of Pediatrics
NEW YORK UNIVERSITY SCHOOL OF MEDICINE
550 First Avenue
New York, NY 10016

**Joseph J. Sockalosky, M.D.**
Director, Pediatric Endocrinology
ST. PAUL RAMSEY MEDICAL CENTER
640 Jackson Street
St. Paul, MN 55101

**Lawrence Solomon, M.D.**
Professor and Head
Department of Dermatology
UNIVERSITY OF ILLINOIS COLLEGE OF MEDICINE
P.O. Box 6998
Chicago, IL 60680

**William Solomon, M.D.**
Division of Allergy
Department of Internal Medicine
UNIVERSITY OF MICHIGAN SCHOOL OF MEDICINE
Taubman Center Room 3918
Ann Arbor, MI 48109 0380

**Annemarie Sommer, M.D.**
Associate Professor
Department of Pediatrics
CHILDREN'S HOSPITAL
700 Children's Drive
Columbus, OH 43205

**Mark A. Sperling, M.D.**
Chairman, Department of Pediatrics
CHILDREN'S HOSPITAL OF PITTSBURGH
3705 Fifth Avenue at DeSoto Street
Pittsburgh, PA 15213 2583

**Jurgen W. Spranger, M.D.**
Professor of Pediatrics
Department of Pediatrics
UNIVERSITY OF MAINZ MEDICAL SCHOOL
Langenbeckstrasse 1
D-6500 Mainz
WEST GERMANY

**F. Bruder Stapleton, M.D.**
Professor and Chairman
Department of Pediatrics
STATE UNIVERSITY OF NEW YORK AT BUFFALO
219 Bryant Street
Buffalo, NY 14222

**Mark W. Steele, M.D.**
Director of Clinical Genetics
UNIVERSITY OF PITTSBURGH CHILDREN'S HOSPITAL
125 DeSoto Street
Pittsburgh, PA 15213

**Fernando Stein, M.D.**
Deputy Director
Pediatric Intensive Care
TEXAS CHILDREN'S HOSPITAL
6621 Fannin
Houston, TX 77030

**Arthur G. Steinberg, Ph.D.**
Department of Biology
CASE WESTERN RESERVE UNIVERSITY
Cleveland, OH 44106

**Daniel Steinberg, M.D., Ph.D.**
Professor of Medicine
Division of Metabolic Disease M013D
U.C.S.D. SCHOOL OF MEDICINE
La Jolla, CA 92093

**Roger E. Stevenson, M.D.**
Director
GREENWOOD GENETIC CENTER
One Gregor Mendel Circle
Greenwood, SC 29646

**Janet M. Stewart, M.D.**
Department of Pediatrics
UNIVERSITY OF COLORADO
Health Sciences Center
4200 East Ninth Avenue
Denver, CO 80262

**John A. Stith, M.D.**
Assistant Professor and Director
Pediatric Otolaryngology
ST. LOUIS UNIVERSITY MEDICAL CENTER
1465 South Grand Blvd. Suite 325
St. Louis, MO 63104 1095

**Hartmut Stoess, M.D.**
Pathologisches Institut
UNIVERSITAT ERLANGEN-NURNBERG
Krankenhausstrasse 8-10
D-8520 Erlangen
WEST GERMANY

**Sheldon S. Stoffer, M.D.**
OAKLAND INTERNISTS ASSOCIATES
28625 Northwestern Highway Suite 200
Southfield, MI 48034

**Claude Stoll, M.D.**
Professor of Genetics
Institut de Puericulture
HOSPICES CIVILS De STRASBOURG
23, Rue de la Porte de l'Hopital
Strasbourg 67000
FRANCE

**Orville J. Stone, M.D.**
Clinical Professor of Dermatology
CALIFORNIA COLLEGE OF MEDICINE
18700 Main Street
No. 201
Huntington Beach, CA 92648

**Stephen M. Strakowski, B.S.E.**
Senior Medical Student
VANDERBILT UNIVERSITY SCHOOL OF MEDICINE
T-2404 Medical Center North
Nashville, TN 37232

**Gerald G. Striph, M.D.**
The Wilmer Institute
Maumenee B-107
THE JOHNS HOPKINS HOSPITAL
601 North Broadway
Baltimore, MD 21205

**Charles Strom, M.D., Ph.D.**
Department of Pediatrics
UNIVERSITY OF CHICAGO
5825 South Maryland Avenue Box 413
Chicago, IL 60637

**Joel Sugar, M.D.**
Professor of Ophthalmology
UNIVERSITY OF ILLINOIS COLLEGE OF MEDICINE
1855 West Taylor Street
Chicago, IL 60612

**Robert L. Summitt, M.D.**
Provost and Dean
College of Medicine
UNIVERSITY OF TENNESSEE, MEMPHIS
Three North Dunlap
Memphis, TN 38163

**Kunihiko Suzuki, M.D.**
Professor and Director
Biological Sciences Research Center
UNIVERSITY OF NORTH CAROLINA SCHOOL OF MEDICINE
CB #7250 311 B.S.R.C.
Chapel Hill, NC 27599 7250

**Tomas Sveger, M.D.**
Department of Pediatrics
UNIVERSITY OF LUND
Malmo General Hospital
S-214 01 Malmo
SWEDEN

**Lawrence Sweetman, Ph.D.**
Department of Pediatrics (M-009)
U.C.S.D. SCHOOL OF MEDICINE
La Jolla, CA 92093

**Ann E. Swinford, M.S.**
College of Human Medicine
MICHIGAN STATE UNIVERSITY
5525 Kaynorth # 12
Lansing, MI 48911

**Chester A. Swinyard, M.D.**
Two White Oak Court
Menlo Park, CA 94025

**Virginia P. Sybert, M.D.**
Division of Medical Genetics
CHILDREN'S ORTHOPEDIC HOSPITAL
4800 Sand Point Way, N.E. Box 3C5371
Seattle, WA 98105

**Norman S. Talner, M.D.**
Department of Pediatrics
YALE UNIVERSITY SCHOOL OF MEDICINE
333 Cedar Street
New Haven, CT 06510

**Lloyd Tani, M.D.**
Fellow in Pediatric Cardiology
TEXAS CHILDREN'S HOSPITAL
6621 Fannin
Houston, TX 77030

**A.S. Teebi, M.D.**
Maternity Hospital
KUWAIT MEDICAL GENETICS CENTRE
P.O. Box 4080 Code 13041
Safat
KUWAIT

**Samia A. Temtamy, M.D., Ph.D.**
Head, Human Genetics Department
NATIONAL RESEARCH CENTER
El Tahrir Street, El Dokki
Cairo
EGYPT

**George Thomas, M.D.**
J.F. KENNEDY INSTITUTE FOR HANDICAPPED CHILDREN
707 North Broadway
Baltimore, MD 21205

**Theodore F. Thurmon, M.D.**
Department of Pediatrics
LOUISIANA STATE UNIVERSITY SCHOOL OF MEDICINE
1501 Kings Highway
Shreveport, LA 71130

**Kathleen E. Toomey, M.D., J.D.**
Assistant Professor of Pediatrics
ST. CHRISTOPHER'S HOSPITAL FOR CHILDREN
Philadelphia, PA 19133

**Helga Toriello, Ph.D.**
Genetics Services
BUTTERWORTH HOSPITAL
21 Michigan Street Suite 350
Grand Rapids, MI 49503

**Robert J. Touloukian, M.D.**
Department of Surgery
YALE UNIVERSITY SCHOOL OF MEDICINE
333 Cedar Street
136 FMB
New Haven, CT 06510 8062

**Oscar Touster, Ph.D.**
Department of Molecular Biology
VANDERBILT UNIVERSITY
Box 1820 Station B
Nashville, TN 37235

**Jeffrey A. Towbin, M.D.**
Fellow in Pediatric Cardiology
TEXAS CHILDREN'S HOSPITAL
6621 Fannin
Houston, TX 77030

**Elias Traboulsi, M.D.**
5550 Columbia Pike No. 702
Arlington, VA 22204

**Jeffrey Trent, Ph.D.**
Arizona Cancer Center
UNIVERSITY OF ARIZONA
1515 North Campbell Avenue Room 3945
Tucson, AZ 85724

**John N. Trodahl, D.D.S.**
V.A. CENTRAL OFFICE
(161)
810 Vermont Avenue, N.W.
Washington, DC 20420

**Carlos Trujillo-Botero, M.D.**
Department of Genetics
INSTITUTO DE CIENCIAS DE LA SALUD (C.E.S.)
Carrera 35 # 8 A 58
A.A. 2055
Medellin
COLOMBIA

**Margaret A. Tucker, M.D.**
Chief, Family Studies Section
Environmental Epidemiology Branch
NATIONAL CANCER INSTITUTE
Landow Building, Room 3C19
Bethesda, MD 20892

**Gordon Tuffli, M.D.**
MADISON MEDICAL CENTER
20 South Park Street
Suite 303
Madison, WI 53715 2389

**Sheila Marie Tunnell, M.D.**
Associate Clinical Professor
Department of Pediatrics
UNIVERSITY OF COLORADO MEDICAL CENTER
13853 East Hamilton Drive
Aurora, CO 80014

**Catherine Turleau, M.D.**
Directeur de Recherche au CNRS
Laboratoire de Cytogenetique Humaine
HOPITAL NECKER ENFANTS MALADES
Unite 173 INSERM
75743 Paris Cedex 15
FRANCE

**Robert A. Ulstrom, M.D.**
Professor of Pediatrics
UNIVERSITY OF MINNESOTA HOSPITALS
Box 391 Mayo
Minneapolis, MN 55455

**Susonne A. Ursin, M.D.**
Assistant Professor of Pediatrics
Pediatrics, Genetics Section
LOUISIANA STATE UNIVERSITY SCHOOL OF MEDICINE
1501 Kings Highway
Shreveport, LA 71130

**Constance M. Vadheim, Ph.D.**
Medical Genetics - Birth Defects Center
CEDARS - SINAI MEDICAL CENTER
8700 Beverly Blvd.
Los Angeles, CA 90048 0750

**William Valentine, M.D.**
Professor Emeritus
Department of Medicine
U.C.L.A. CENTER FOR THE HEALTH SCIENCES
Room 42-121
Los Angeles, CA 90024 1736

**David L. Valle, M.D.**
Professor of Pediatrics
Pediatrics, Molecular Biology, Genetics
JOHNS HOPKINS UNIVERSITY SCHOOL OF MEDICINE
P.C.T.B. Room 802
725 North Wolfe Street
Baltimore, MD 21205

**Daniel L. Van Dyke, Ph.D.**
Director of Cytogenetics
Medical Genetics and Birth Defects Center
HENRY FORD HOSPITAL
Detroit, MI 48202

**Don C. Van Dyke, M.D.**
Department of Pediatrics
UNIVERSITY OF IOWA HOSPITALS AND CLINICS
213 University Hospital School
Iowa City, IA 52242

**L. H. S. Van Mierop, M.D.**
Professor and Chairman
Department of Pediatrics
UNIVERSITY OF FLORIDA COLLEGE OF MEDICINE
Box J-296 JHMHC
Gainesville, FL 32610 0296

**Paul R. Vandersteen, M.D.**
Department of Dermatology
FARGO CLINIC
737 Broadway, Box 2067
Fargo, ND 58102

**V. Vedanarayanan, M.D.**
Box 3533
DUKE UNIVERSITY MEDICAL CENTER
Durham, NC 27710

**Michel Vekemans, M.D.**
Associate Professor
Dept. Pathology / Cytogenetics
MONTREAL CHILDREN'S HOSPITAL
2300 Tupper Street
Montreal PQ H3H 1P3
CANADA

**A. Verloes, M.D.**
CENTRE DE GENETIQUE HUMAINE DE L' UNIVERSITE DE LIEGE
Pathologie B 23
C.H.U. Sart-Tilman
(B) 4000 Liege
BELGIUM

**B. E. Victorica, M.D.**
Professor
Department of Pediatrics (Cardiology)
UNIVERSITY OF FLORIDA COLLEGE OF MEDICINE
Box J-296
Gainesville, FL 32610

**Jaclyn M. Vidgoff, Ph.D.**
Medical and Biochemical Geneticist
EMANUEL HOSPITAL AND HEALTH CENTER
2801 North Gantenbein Avenue
Portland, OR 97227

**Denis Viljoen, M.D.**
Department of Human Genetics
UNIVERSITY OF CAPE TOWN MEDICAL SCHOOL
Observatory
Cape Town
SOUTH AFRICA

**Per Erik Waaler, M.D.**
Professor of Pediatrics
Haukeland Hospital
UNIVERSITY OF BERGEN
N-5021 Bergen
NORWAY

**Auguste Wackenheim, M.D.**
Professor and Chairman
Department of Radiology
UNIVERSITY OF STRASBOURG MEDICAL SCHOOL
CHR de Strasbourg
BP No. 426
67091 Strasbourg
FRANCE

**William B. Wadlington, M.D.**
2614 Old Lebanon Road
Nashville, TN 37214

**Renata Wajsman, M.D.**
Division of Gastroenterology
MOUNT SINAI SERVICES AT ELMHURST HOSPITAL
79-01 Broadway
Elmhurst, NY 11373

**Thomas A. Waldmann, M.D.**
Chief, Metabolism Branch
NATIONAL INSTITUTES OF HEALTH
Building 10, Room 4N110
Bethesda, MD 20892

**Charles A. Waldron, D.D.S., M.S.D**
Professor Emeritus of Oral Pathology
EMORY UNIVERSITY SCHOOL OF POSTGRADUATE DENTISTRY
1197 Hunter's Drive
Stone Mountain, GA 30083

**Paul O. Walker, D.D.S., M.S.D**
Associate Professor
School of Dentistry
UNIVERSITY OF MINNESOTA
6-150 Health Sciences Unit A
515 Delaware Street S.E.
Minneapolis, MN 55455

**Margaret R. Wallace, Ph.D.**
Associate
Howard Hughes Medical Institute
UNIVERITY OF MICHIGAN
4562 M.S.R.B. II
1150 West Medical Center Drive
Ann Arbor, MI 48109 0650

**Silas Wallk, M.D.**
2434 West Pederson Street
Chicago, IL 60659

**I.S. Wallman, M.D.**
111 Barker Road
Subiaco 6008
AUSTRALIA

**Diane W. Wara, M.D.**
Department of Pediatrics
U.C.S.F. SCHOOL OF MEDICINE
San Francisco, CA 94143

**Dorothy P. Warburton, Ph.D.**
Professor of Human Genetics
COLUMBIA UNIVERSITY COLLEGE OF PHYSICIANS AND SURGEONS
630 West 168th Street
New York, NY 10032

**Josef Warkany, M.D.**
Professor of Research Pediatrics
Department of Pediatrics
THE CHILDREN'S HOSPITAL RESEARCH FOUNDATION
Elland Avenue and Bethesda
Cincinnati, OH 45229

**Edward Wasserman, M.D.**
Chairman of Pediatrics
NEW YORK MEDICAL COLLEGE
Munger Pavillion
Valhalla, NY 10595

**John Waterson, M.D., Ph.D.**
Medical Geneticist
Genetics Center of Akron
CHILDREN'S HOSPITAL MEDICAL CENTER
281 Locust Street
Akron, OH 44308

**David Watkins, Ph.D.**
Post-Doctoral Fellow
Division of Medical Genetics
MONTREAL GENERAL HOSPITAL
1650 Cedar Avenue Room 4849
Montreal H3G 1A4 PQ
CANADA

**David G. Watson, M.D.**
Division of Pediatric Cardiology
UNIVERSITY OF MISSISSIPPI MEDICAL CENTER
2500 North State Street
Jackson, MS 39216

**David D. Weaver, M.D.**
Department of Medical Genetics
INDIANA UNIVERSITY SCHOOL OF MEDICINE
James Whitcomb Riley Hospital RR129
702 Barnhill Drive
Indianapolis, IN 46223

**William B. Weil, Jr., M.D.**
Department of Human Development
MICHIGAN STATE UNIVERSITY
B 240 Life Sciences
East Lansing, MI 48824 1317

**Bernd Weinberg, M.D.**
Audiology and Speech Sciences
PURDUE UNIVERSITY
Heavilon Hall
West Lafayette, IN 47907

**Avery Weiss, M.D.**
Department of Ophthalmology
UNIVERSITY OF SOUTH FLORIDA EYE INSTITUTE
13131 Magnolia Drive
Tampa, FL 33612

**Robert A. Weiss, M.D.**
Assistant Professor of Ophthalmology
NEW YORK HOSPITAL - CORNELL MEDICAL CENTER
525 East 68th Street No. K-809
New York, NY 10021

**Richard G. Weleber, M.D.**
Professor
Ophthalmology and Medical Genetics
OREGON HEALTH SCIENCES UNIVERSITY
3181 Southwest Sam Jackson Park Road
Portland, OR 97201

**Franz Wenger, M.D.**
Emeritus Professor
ZULIA UNIVERSITY MEDICAL SCHOOL
Edificio El Saman - 80
Calle 73A, No. 2B-45
Maracaibo
VENEZUELA

**Martha Werler, M.P.H.**
Slone Epidemiology Unit
BOSTON UNIVERSITY SCHOOL OF MEDICINE
1371 Beacon Street
Brookline, MA 02146

**Wladimir Wertelecki, M.D.**
Department of Medical Genetics
UNIVERSITY OF SOUTH ALABAMA MEDICAL CENTER
2451 Fillingim Street
Mobile, AL 36617

**James G. White, M.D.**
Department of Pediatrics
UNIVERSITY OF MINNESOTA MEDICAL SCHOOL
Box 490 Mayo Memorial Building
420 Delaware Street, S.E.
Minneapolis, MN 55455

**Peter F. Whitington, M.D.**
Director, Gastroenterology
Department of Pediatrics
UNIVERSITY OF CHICAGO PRITZKER SCHOOL OF MEDICINE
5825 South Maryland Avenue Box 107
Chicago, IL 60637

**Chester B. Whitley, Ph.D., M.D.**
Assistant Professor of Pediatrics
Institute for Human Genetics
UNIVERSITY OF MINNESOTA
Box 446
Minneapolis, MN 55455

**Brian Jeffrey Wiatrak, M.D.**
Chief Resident
Otolaryngology and Maxillofacial Surgery
UNIVERSITY OF CINCINNATI MEDICAL CENTER
231 Bethesda Avenue
Cincinnati, OH 45267

**Peter Wieacker, M.D.**
UNIVERSITATS-FRAUENKLINIK FREIBURG
Hugstetter Strasse 55
D-7800 Freiburg
GERMANY

**Hans-Rudolph Wiedemann, M.D.**
Professor Emeritus
DER UNIVERSITATS-KINDERKLINIK I.R.
Caprivi Strastross 26
D-2300 Kiel
WEST GERMANY

**Charles A. Williams, M.D.**
Associate Professor
Division of Genetics
UNIVERSITY OF FLORIDA
Box J-296, J.H.M.H.C.
Gainesville, FL 32610 0296

**Mary L. Williams, M.D.**
Associate Professor
Dermatology Service
190
V.A. MEDICAL CENTER
4150 Clement Street
San Francisco, CA 94121

**R.S. Wilroy, Jr., M.D.**
Department of Pediatrics
UNIVERSITY OF TENNESSEE CENTER FOR THE HEALTH SCIENCES
523 Child Development Center
711 Jefferson Avenue, Room 523
Memphis, TN 38163

**Charles J. Wilson, M.D.**
200 University Boulevard
Suite 834
Galveston, TX 77550

**Dana E. Wilson, M.D.**
Professor of Internal Medicine
VETERANS ADMINISTRATION MEDICAL CENTER (111E)
500 Foothill Drive
Salt Lake City, UT 84148

**Golder N. Wilson, M.D., Ph.D.**
Department of Pediatrics
UNIVERSITY OF TEXAS SOUTHWESTERN MEDICAL CENTER
5323 Harry Hines Blvd.
Dallas, TX 75235 9063

**A.M. Winchester, Ph.D.**
7830 East Camelback No. 211
Scottsdale, AZ 85251

**Jeffrey Winn, D.D.S.**
Department of Medical Genetics
INDIANA UNIVERSITY SCHOOL OF MEDICINE
James Whitcomb Riley Hospital RR 129
702 Barnhill Drive
Indianapolis, IN 46223

**Ingrid Winship, MB, ChB, M.D.**
Department of Human Genetics
UNIVERSITY OF CAPE TOWN MEDICAL SCHOOL
Observatory
Cape Town
SOUTH AFRICA

**Robin M. Winter, M.D.**
Consultant Clinical Geneticist
Kennedy Galton Centre
NORTHWICK PARK HOSPITAL
Watford Road, Level 8
Harrow
ENGLAND

**Susan C. Winter, M.D.**
Director, Medical Genetics / Metabolism
VALLEY CHILDREN'S HOSPITAL
3151 North Millbrook
Fresno, CA 93711

**Carl J. Witkop, Jr., D.D.S., M.S.**
Professor of Human & Oral Genetics
UNIVERSITY OF MINNESOTA
Moos H.S.T. 16-262
515 Delaware Street, S.E.
Minneapolis, MN 55455

**David R. Witt, M.D.**
Genetics Department
THE PERMANENTE MEDICAL GROUP, INC.
260 International Circle
San Jose, CA 95119

**Ehrenfried O. Wittig, M.D.**
Prof. of Internal Medicine (Neurology)
Hospital de Clinicas
UNIVERSIDADE FEDERAL DO PARANA
80.069 Curitiba PR
BRAZIL

**Andrew Wiznia, M.D.**
Pediatrics / Genetic Counseling
ALBERT EINSTEIN COLLEGE OF MEDICINE
Kennedy Building, Room 211
1300 Morris Park Avenue
Bronx, NY 10461

**Barry Wolf, M.D., Ph.D.**
Professor
Depts. of Human Genetics & Pediatrics
MEDICAL COLLEGE OF VIRGINIA
Richmond, VA 23298

**Mitchel L. Wolf, M.D.**
Director of Ophthalmology
THE JEWISH HOSPITAL OF ST. LOUIS
4910 Forest Park Suite 220
St. Louis, MO 63108

**Gerhard Wolff, M.D.**
Medical Genetics and Psychotherapy
Institute for Human Genetics
ALBERT LUDWIGS UNIVERSITY
Albertstrasse 11
D-7800 Freiburg
WEST GERMANY

**Morton M. Woolley, M.D.**
Surgeon-in-Chief
CHILDREN'S HOSPITAL OF LOS ANGELES
4650 Sunset Boulevard
P.O. Box 54700
Los Angeles, CA 90054 0700

**Janet Wright, Ph.D.**
Department of Biology
DICKENSON COLLEGE
Carlisle, PA 17013

**Gloria Wu, M.D.**
JOSLIN CLINIC
One Joslin Place
Boston, MA 02215

**Herman E. Wyandt, Ph.D.**
Director, Cytogenetic Laboratory
DANBURY HOSPITAL
24 Hospital Avenue
Danbury, CT 06810

**Sonja R. Wyss, B.S.**
Research Assistant
Institut fur Biochemie und Molekularbiol
UNIVERSITAT BERN
Buhlstrasse 28
CH-3000 Bern 9
SWITZERLAND

**Yoshifumi Yamamoto, M.D.**
Department of Pediatrics
JICHI MEDICAL SCHOOL
Minamikawachi-machi
Kawachi-gun
Tochigi-ken 329-04
JAPAN

**Tatsuhiko Yuasa, M.D.**
Associate Professor
Department of Neurology
NIIGATA UNIVERSITY
Brain Research Institute
Asahimachi-dori
Niigata City
951
JAPAN

**Elaine H. Zackai, M.D.**
Associate Professor of Clinical Genetics
THE CHILDREN'S HOSPITAL OF PHILADELPHIA
Room 7076
34th Street & Civic Center Blvd.
Philadelphia, PA 19104

**Ismail Zayid, M.D.**
Professor of Pathology
Director of Anatomic Pathology
DALHOUSIE UNIVERSITY AND VICTORIA GENERAL HOSPITAL
5788 University Avenue
Halifax B3H 1V8 NS
CANADA

**Israel Zelikovic, M.D.**
Assistant Professor
Department of Pediatrics RD-20
UNIVERSITY OF WASHINGTON SCHOOL OF MEDICINE
Seattle, WA 98195

**Hans Zellweger, M.D.**
Division of Medical Genetics
Department of Pediatrics
UNIVERSITY OF IOWA HOSPITALS
Iowa City, IA 52242

**William H. Zinkham, M.D.**
Rainey Professor of Pediatric Hematology
THE JOHNS HOPKINS SCHOOL OF MEDICINE
Brady 208
Baltimore, MD 21205

**Arthur B. Zinn, M.D., Ph.D.**
Department of Pediatrics
RAINBOW CHILDREN'S HOSPITAL
2101 Adelbert Road
Cleveland, OH 44106

**Janice Zunich, M.D.**
Assistant Professor of Medical Genetics
INDIANA UNIVERSITY SCHOOL OF MEDICINE
Northwest Center for Medical Education
3400 Broadway
Gary, IN 46408

**Susan Zunt, D.D.S.**
Department of Oral Pathology
UNIVERSITY OF INDIANA SCHOOL OF DENTISTRY
Indianapolis, IN 46223

# Part I

# ❖ HOW TO USE THIS ENCYCLOPEDIA ❖

The *Birth Defects Encyclopedia* is a comprehensive, systematic, illustrated knowledgebase of the biomedical sciences as they relate to human anomalies of clinical relevance, with special attention to the application of that knowledge to patient care. To most effectively serve its mission, the *Encyclopedia* has been designed to contain the maximum information in the least space, in a format and organization which assures readability, uniformity, and ease of use. A true encyclopedia, it contains encyclopedia headings at the top of each page, and extensive cross-referencing, including Master Index cross-referencing for conditions that are known by more than one name.

The heart of the *Encyclopedia* consists of over two thousand articles on specific birth defect conditions and complex syndromes, arranged alphabetically under some ten thousand established names and terms. Each article follows a specific format, with consistent elements arranged in a consistent order.

While the *Encyclopedia* is accessed in a variety of print and non-print forms, it is assembled and maintained in a single computer-based "generic" format which allows both for direct typesetting with the many special characters and symbols seen in this print edition, as well as for rapid distribution through paper and electronic forms which may be limited to the most basic display character sets.

In every case, however, creation of an article begins with authors and editors assembling and examining information on each of the thirty sections, or elements, that make up each *Birth Defects Encyclopedia* article:

**1. Birth Defect Number** is a unique four-digit number assigned to each article. Printed to the right and just below the **Article Title**, the Birth Defect Number is a constant, unique identifier assigned to each article by the Center. An example of a Birth Defect Number, and of other article elements described below, is illustrated in Fig. 1. Birth Defect Numbers 1 through 1005 have been assigned to articles that correspond to articles of the same number that appeared in the *Birth Defects Compendium, Second Edition* (New York: Alan R. Liss, 1979), although the **Article Titles** may have been changed to reflect more recent findings or to conform to established naming conventions.

Articles may be located by Birth Defect Number by consulting the BIRTH DEFECT-NUMBER-TO-PRIME-NAME INDEX which appears after the Master Index and Articles, and the Gene Map Table and Pictorials, at the back of this edition of the *Encyclopedia*. Birth Defect Numbers are listed in numeric order and cross-referenced to prime Article Name (see **Article Title** below), which can then be easily located in the alphabetical Master Index that contains the actual articles.

The reader will notice that not all numbers in a numeric sequence have corresponding articles in this edition of the *Encyclopedia*. This results from the fact that, during the editorial process, articles originally thought to present different medical conditions were found to in fact describe a common condition, in which case the contents of the different articles may be merged into a common article, and the number(s) of the article(s) merged into a different article were discontinued so as to avoid any future confusion. However, since all of the names under which the merged articles were known will appear in the final combined article, the article can still be easily located in the Master Index.

X-linked mental retardation, Fitzsimmons type
*See HYPERKERATOSIS PALMOPLANTARIS-SPASTIC PARAPLEGIA-RETARDATION*

**Master Index Cross-Reference**

3. **Article Title**

**X-LINKED MENTAL RETARDATION, FRAGILE X SYNDROME**

(2073)

1. **Birth Defect Number**

**Includes:**
Chromosome, Marker X
Fragile X chromosome
Martin-Bell X-linked mental retardation
Mental retardation, X-linked-marXq28
X-linked fragile site
X-linked mental retardation-macroorchidism
X-linked mental retardation with fragile X

4. **Includes Term(s)/ Other Title(s)**

**Excludes:**
X-linked mental retardation, Renpenning type (2920)
X-linked mental retardation without the fragile X chromosome

5. **Excludes Term(s)/ Differential Diagnoses**

**Excludes cross-reference shown in bold type**

**Major Diagnostic Criteria:** The definitive diagnosis depends upon finding the fragile X chromosome. Males with the fragile X

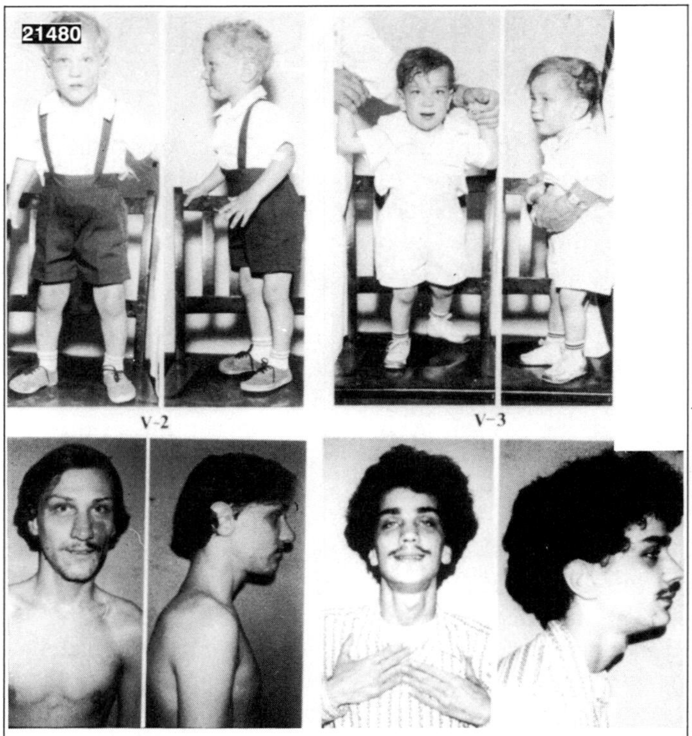

6. **Illustration(s)**

6A. **Article Number**

6B. **Frame Letter**

6C. **Illustration Number**

2073A 21480: Original siblings with fragile X described by Lubs (1969). Sib 1 on left at age 3 and 18. Sib 2 at right at 18 mo. and age 17. Both had low set, posteriorly angulated and slightly large ears and broadly based stance. Heads in both at age 17 and 18 are narrower than their normal brother's and father's (not shown). Ears and jaws have changed little in 15

6D. **Legend**

Fig. 1. Portion of *X-linked mental retardation, Fragile X syndrome* article.

Similarly, an article thought at one point to describe a single condition may be found, upon further study, to in fact contain information on two or more distinct entities. In such cases, the information that best fits the condition originally described in the article is left in the original article with its original number, while a new article(s) with a new number(s) is created for the newly defined additional entitie(s). Again, the Master Index permits

6. **Illustrations**

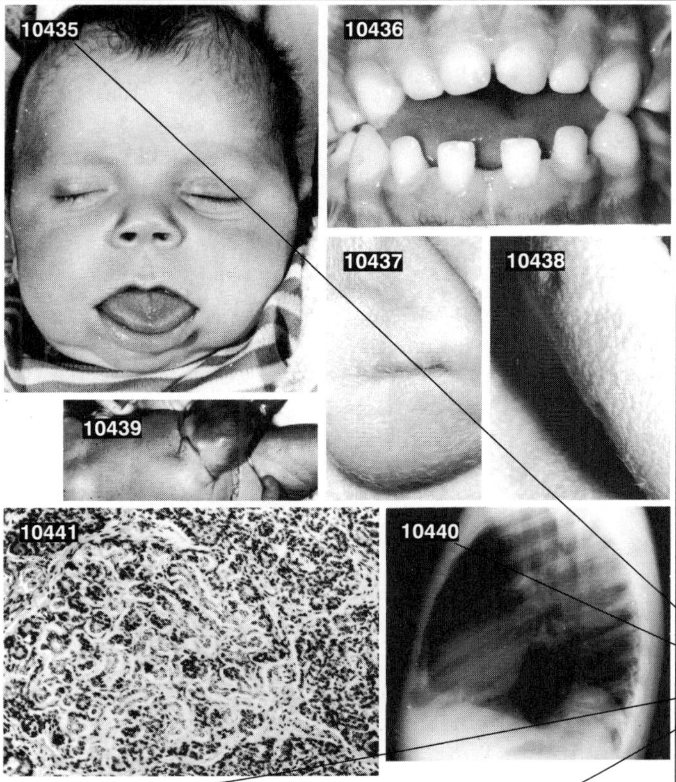

6A. **Article Number**

6C. **Illustration Number(s)**

0104-10435: Macroglossia. 10436: Anterior open bite. 10439: Omphalocele. 10437: Ear lobe groove. 10438: Circular depression on posterior rim of helix. 10441: Hyperplasia of the ducts and acini in pancreas. 10440: Diaphragmatic eventration.

Fig. 2. Composite illustration frame with several illustration components from *Beckwith-Wiedemann syndrome* article.

7. **Major Diagnostic Criteria**

8. **Clinical Findings**

**Major Diagnostic Criteria:** Clinical findings may be quite variable, but the diagnosis should be considered in an infant with **Macroglossia and Omphalocele** or umbilical anomaly. **Hypoglycemia, familial neonatal** may be present and ear lobe grooves or circular depressions on the posterior helices, when present, are especially significant for diagnosis.

**Text Cross-Reference**

**Clinical Findings:** The frequency of clinical features in 248 Beckwith-Wiedemann syndrome patients from the literature was recently summarized by Pettenati et al. (1986). These findings include macroglossia (98%), visceromegaly [nephromegaly (97%), splenomegaly (82%), heptomegaly (73%)], somatic gigantism (average birth weight and birth length for both sexes greater than the 90th percentile), midface hypoplasia (81%), cryptorchidism (81%), omphalocele (76%), prominent occiput (72%), ear anomalies (pits

Fig. 3. Portion of *Beckwith-Wiedemann syndrome* article.

quick and easy location of the appropriate article, and this is usually supplemented by additional cross-referencing as needed.

Birth Defect Numbers are, however, the most succinct and consistent way to identify a given article and the condition it describes, and are usually the fastest way to obtain an article through non-print information services. For this reason, we encourage the use of Birth

Defect Numbers and their inclusion in all editorial correspondence and other communication with the Center.

**2. Creation/Revision Date** is the last date on which the article was updated or reviewed and found to be current. Most updating is done by the author(s) of the individual article, but this is supplemented by editorial review and by information provided to the Center by other scientists, support groups, and qualified experts. While the publication dates of the **References** provide one clue to the currentness of an article, some articles describe conditions delineated decades ago on which there have been no significant publications in many years, while articles describing other conditions under active study may have very recent references and still be outdated.

Articles in this print edition can be assumed to be current as of the date of publication, so Creation/Revision Date is not shown. However, when accessing articles in the *Encyclopedia* knowledgebase through some of our other services, particularly through the electronic services designed to provide article updates between print editions, this information can be important. For example, when searching the *Birth Defects Online* version of the *Encyclopedia* through **BRS** ^ , you can specify a search that will *only* display articles updated since your last search.

**3. Article Title** is the name or Title under which an article appears in the alphabetic listing of the print *Encyclopedia*'s Master Index. Since the condition described in the article may be known under several additional names (see **Includes Terms** below), the article title is also known as the *prime* name. This Article Title or prime name is shown in all capital letters, and appears at the very top of the article.

Since the basic structure of the *Encyclopedia* is anatomically and biochemically based, eponyms are avoided in prime names. Instead, Article Titles are selected to best describe the condition to a reader unfamiliar with the eponyms, abbreviations, and colloquialisms of the medical specialties. If an article describes a syndrome made up of a few known conditions, the prime name can simply be a list of those conditions in order of predominance, separated by dashes. In other instances, however, the syndrome is simply too complicated to describe in this way, and use of an eponym may be the only recourse. In no case, however, should an "s" appear after a person's name when used in the name of a condition or the title of an article; a condition can be called the "Smith syndrome", but it would not be "Smith's syndrome".

**4. Includes Term(s)**, in some instances also referred to simply as **Other Title(s)**, provides an alphabetical list of the other names under which the condition or syndrome may be known. These appear in upper and lower case, with only the first word and proper names capitalized.

Eponyms *do* appear in the Includes, as well as common non-English names (although not simple translations of English names into other languages). All names are listed according to standard indexing conventions, with key word first and adjectives following in a decending hierarchy; thus "neonatal familial hypoglycemia" becomes "Hypoglycemia, familial neonatal".

Similarly, "hypertelorism of the eyes" (often shortened simply to "hypertelorism" in clinical use, although strictly defined this means simply "abnormally increased distance between two organs or parts") becomes "Eye, hypertelorism". Words such as "familial", "genetic", "inherited", and "congenital" are used to begin a name or descriptive term only in special instances, since they would have little indexing value in a reference work of this type.

Outdated names, if still in use, are listed but are followed by the word "obsolete" in parenthesis. The word "pejorative" may also appear in parenthesis, and while this does not necessarily imply that there is a consensus that the term is depreciatory, it does indicate that objections to its use have been noted.

As with **Article Titles**, an Includes Term can describe a syndrome through a list of known conditions linked by dashes. Here the dash can be read as "accompanied by", an established convention in the birth defect specialties. Similarly, a slash is occasionally used to designate "or", so a Term that appears as "Ear abnormalities-short stature-elbow/hip dislocation" should be read as "A patient with ear abnormalities accompanied by short stature and either elbow or hip dislocation".

Since syndromes which consist of a few established conditions may be known by different compound names differing only in the order in which the component conditions are listed, the above example may also appear as "Stature, short-ear abnormalities-elbow/hip dislocation". There are, however, component conditions that are avoided as the first term of an indexed Article Title or Includes Term. These are conditions which occur as components of syndromes with such a high frequency as to give them little utility as an index term. Mental retardation, for example, occurs in about half of the established syndromes, and therefore appears as the first part of a syndrome name only when the retardation is of special significance. When a frequent condition has distinct sub-types, the sub-type is the preferred index term (all variants of X-linked mental retardation, for example, appear not under mental retardation but under "X-linked mental retardation").

A dash may aso, of course, link proper names in a compound eponym (as in "Beckwith-Wiedeman"), or serve simply as a dash in normal usage, or even as a negative sign, although these instances should be clear by their context. For readability, as well as for standardization and use in computer-based text processing and retrieval systems, all titles and naming terms, including Includes and **Excludes Terms**, are limited to 66 characters in length, including blanks and special characters.

All Includes Terms, since they constitute different ways of identifying conditions and syndromes covered in *Encyclopedia* articles, appear both in the Includes term list in the article itself *and* in the Master Index where they appear in alphabetical order as a **Master Index Cross-Reference**.

Figs. 1 and Fig. 6 each contain examples from the **Master Index Cross-Reference**. Note that cross-references appear in upper and lower case bold type, and when referring to a prime name in the Master Index, show the prime name (Article Title) in all upper case type as it appears at the head of the article which it identifies and that can be found in its own alphabetical sequence in the Master Index.

While Includes Terms are often thought of as synonyms for the prime Article Title, it is more precise to regard them as topics included in the article. While most articles describe a single diagnostic entity, many conditions and syndromes have one or more variants, and there is frequently disagreement as to whether these variants constitute a separate condition. Also, on occasion, brief mention is made of another condition that may be important to the understanding of the article's central topic, but which is nevertheless acknowledged to be different yet not in itself sufficient to justify an article of its own. In such cases, Includes Terms that are *not* synonyms for the prime article title appear in the text in *italics*, along with any necessary additional elaboration which may be necessary to place the term in proper context.

**5. Excludes Terms** are an alphabetical list of conditions *not* described in the article. Typically, these are potential differential diagnoses, and Excludes can therefore be read as "not to be confused with" or "see also and rule out the following".

Usually **Excluded** conditions are similar in their presenting clinical pictures, but conditions can also appear in an Excludes list because they have similar names, or are related in such a way as make knowledge of one condition helpful in the understanding or treatment of the other.

Excludes lists also contain a second form of cross-referencing: the **Excludes Cross-Reference**. As shown in Fig. 1, an Excludes Cross-Reference appears in bold type, but in this case the cross-reference is to a *prime* **Article Title**. This tells the reader that the Excluded condition is covered in another *Encyclopedia* article, and that this article can be found sequentially in the alphabetical Master Index under the prime Article Title shown in bold. In addition, for those accessing articles through

one of our electronic services, the **Birth Defect Number** also appears in parentheses after the **Article Title**.

In some instances, a number may not appear in parentheses after an Excludes in bold, and the reader should note that in these instances the cross-reference is to a *class* of articles. For example, a cross-reference to **Oro-facio-digital syndrome** refers the reader to this entry in the Master Index, under which appear a number of articles on different variants of this condition.

Excludes terms that do not appear in bold generally describe well-known conditions that do not meet the criteria for inclusion in this *Encyclopedia*, or which are otherwise self-explanatory. Any exceptions should be brought to the attention of the Center, and we welcome new authors of articles on any topic appropriate to the mission of the *Encyclopedia*.

**6. Illustrations** are an important feature of the *Encyclopedia*, and appear throughout this volume. Illustrations include both photographs and other graphic material such as diagrams. Since photographs are most helpful in illustrating conditions in which dysmorphology is a presenting feature, there has been no attempt to illustrate every condition in this Book, but to instead concentrate the illustrations among those articles which most benefit from visual supplements.

In instances where a syndrome is made up of several component conditions, illustrations of the respective conditions may appear not only in the article describing the syndrome, but in articles on the respective conditions, which may be located through cross-references or in the Master Index.

Examples of illustrations appear in Figs. 1 and 2. The illustration in Fig. 1 is actually a composite made up of eight photographs illustrating fragile X in two siblings at different ages. An illustration appearing alone and a composite of illustrations within a common border with common legend text are each referred to as a single "frame", and this illustration frame can be confirmed as being associated with article 2073 by the article number which always appears as the first four digits of the illustration legend (see **6A. Article Number** in Figs 1 and 2).

In Fig. 1, the article number 2073 is followed by the Frame Letter "A" (see **6B. Frame Letter** in Fig. 1). Frame letters are used only when the same article is illustrated by two or more illustration frames, and in this case indicates the first of two or more frames illustrating article 2073.

The Article Number, and Frame Letter if present, are then followed by a dash and a five digit Illustration Number, in the case of article 2073's frame A, illustration number 21480 (see **6C. Illustration Number** in Fig. 1). Note that while Frame 2073A contains eight pictures, it has only one illustration number. This is because the eight pictures in the frame, reprinted from a 1969 journal article, are in a single negative. This frame therefore follows the same illustration numbering conventions that would be used if the frame contained a single picture, and the Center files, preserves, and retrieves the entire contents of this frame as it would a single picture.

Fig. 2, on the other hand, shows another composite in which the various pictures in the composite have been assembled at the Center. This composite illustrates article 0104, and since there is no frame letter we know that article 0104 is illustrated only by the seven pictures in this composite. The reader will note that each of the seven individual pictures has its own illustration number, and that the legend provides a separate description of the contents of each picture by illustration number.

The Center serves as a central depository for illustrations of birth defect conditions, and is often authorized to grant permission for the re-publication of illustrations in its care. Interested parties should refer to specific Illustration Numbers in communications regarding illustrations and their use.

Credits for illustrations that appear in this edition of the *Encyclopedia* are listed at the back of the Book in two parts. The first, ILLUSTRATION CREDITS BY PUBLISHER, shows the publications, by publisher, in which each respective illustration first appeared. This listing is by illustration number within publisher, with publishers listed alphabetically. A typical entry for an academic journal shows the year of publication, the volume number, the page number(s), and finally the five-digit Illustration Number.

ILLUSTRATION CREDITS BY CONTRIBUTOR, at the back of the Book, lists the scientists and photographers who have contributed to the Center illustrations that appear in this edition of the *Encyclopedia*. Their names are listed in alphabetical order, followed by a numeric listing by Illustration Number of their contributions.

**7. Major Diagnostic Criteria** consists of a brief statement of all clinical features and laboratory tests needed to establish or strongly suggest the diagnosis. In effect, this is a sentence or brief paragraph which defines the condition.

An example of a Major Diagnostic Criteria, in this case that of **Beckwith-Wiedemann syndrome**, is shown in Fig. 3. This example also illustrates the third and final type of cross-referencing: the **Text Cross-Reference**. **Beckwith-Wiedemann syndrome** includes among its Major Diagnostic Criteria three conditions which are in themselves the topics of other *Encyclopedia* articles. These conditions appear in the text of this section in bold type, indicating not only that the condition is among this syndrome's Major Diagnostic Criteria, but that further information on the condition can be found in another article, and

that this article can be found alphabetically in the Master Index under the Title shown in bold.

**Text Cross-Reference**s can be found throughout the text sections of *Encyclopedia* articles. Because of their hierarchical structure, as prime names, many cross-reference terms contain commas. If read as normal text, these can sound stilted or awkward. Instead, these should be read and understood as cross-references to specific article titles, and as such quickly become a confortable and useful reference convention. When appearing in a continuous list, text cross-references are separated by semicolons.

**8. Clinical Findings** is a succinct descriptive summary of the clinical features associated with the condition or syndrome described in the article. This usually includes information on the natural history, course, and progression; as well as intra-familial variability and general variations in expressivity. Clinical and laboratory findings should be discussed, providing a clear picture of the condition and its progression and outcome. If information on the frequency of individual clinical findings is available, these should be cited as frequency (3/11), percentage (30%), or as ranges (25–40%). Examples of Clinical Findings are presented in Figs. 3 and 4.

**9. Complications** provides a list of any conditions, findings, or consequence that may result from the primary defect(s). Again, frequency information should be quantified if at all possible. This discussion explains the biodynamics of the complications, if known, as well as any appropriate preventive measures that can be taken. This and the following ten article sections are illustrated in Fig. 4.

**10. Associated Findings** are developmental anomalies or birth defects and conditions that have a frequency of association greater than expected by chance, but nevertheless do not appear to be caused by or are a complication of the primary condition(s). Usually the findings listed here occur in ten percent or less of those affected by the primary condition or syndrome, although Associated Findings occasionally do occur with greater frequency.

**11. Etiology** summarizes the known or hypothesized intrinsic or extrinsic cause(s) of the condition or syndrome presented in the article.

If the condition is genetic, etiology consists of the mode(s) of inheritance, if known. For further reference, the definitive resource and an exhaustive bibliography on Mendelian disorders can be found in Victor A. McKusick's *Mendelian inheritance in man: catalogs of autosomal dominant, autosomal recessive, and X-linked phenotypes* published in Baltimore and London by Johns Hopkins University Press (in its eighth edition at press time).

If the condition results from exposure to a teratogen (a term taken from the Greek word for both marvel and

and/or creases - 66%), facial nevus flammeus (62%), neonatal hypoglycemia (61%), polyhydramnios (51%), **Hernia, umbilical** (49%), cardiac defects (34%), hemihypertrophy (33%), diastasis recti (33%), clitoromegaly (16%), and malignant tumors (e.g., Wilms) in approximately 5% of the patients. Other reported findings include microcephaly, polycythemia, advanced bone age, prematurity, mental retardation, diaphragmatic eventration (occasionally diaphragmatic hernia), **Hypospadias**, bicornuate uterus, intestinal malrotation, enlarged labia, hypercalcemia, hyperlipemia, hypercholesterolemia, and hypocalcemia.

Neonatal hypoglycemia occurs in about 60% or more of the infants. This hypoglycemia is due to relative hyperinsulinemia (leucine sensitive) associated with pancreatic islet hyperplasia (nesidioblastosis) and is most common in Beckwith-Wiedemann infants with high birth weight (>4000 g). The hypoglycemia tends to be severe and resists simple treatment (frequent feedings, intravenous glucose). A nonketogenic diet high in calories and low in protein (leucine) may be helpful. Diazoxide, long-acting epinephrine, corticosteroids, ACTH, or a partial pancreatectomy may be necessary.

**9. Complications**

**Complications:** Mental retardation may result from undetected or untreated neonatal hypoglycemia. In light of the recently reported chromosome 11p abnormalities in patients with this syndrome, high-resolution chromosome studies should be carried out on any child with this syndrome, particularly with unexplained mental retardation.

**10. Associated Findings**

**Associated Findings:** Wilms tumor and adrenal cortical carcinoma occur in about 5% of reported cases. Hepatoblastoma, glioma, embryonal rhabdomyosarcoma, carcinoid tumor, myxoma, and fibroma have been noted rarely. There also appears to be an increased risk of malignancies in those patients with hemihypertrophy. Gonadal interstitial cell hyperplasia occurs in males and may be due to elevated serum gonadotropin levels. Seizures can also occur in children with this syndrome.

**Etiology:** Although most cases (85%) are sporadic, familial cases have been reported. Affected sibs appear occasionally, and consanguinity has been reported. Based on familial cases, autosomal recessive, autosomal dominant, multifactorial, and autosomal dominant sex-dependent inheritance have been proposed. Recent segregation analysis is most consistent with autosomal dominant inheritance with incomplete penetrance. Etiologic heterogeneity is possible with recent reports of patients with features of Beckwith-Wiedemann syndrome and a chromosome 11p abnormality, usually a duplicaion.

**11. Etiology**

**12. Pathogenesis**

**Pathogenesis:** Altered placental endocrine physiology may play a role in producing many of the features found during the neonatal period. Omphalocele, anomalies of intestinal rotation and fixation, and diaphragmatic eventration may be secondary to early visceromegaly. A possible reason for somatic gigantism may be due to increased levels of growth hormone, including insulin and/or insulin-like growth factors.

**13A. MIM Number**

**13. Classification Codes**

MIM No.: *13065

POS No.: 3036

CDC No.: 759.870

**13B. POSSUM Number**

**13C. CDC Number**

**14. Sex Ratio**

**Sex Ratio:** M1:F1

**Occurrence:** Undetermined; 1:13,700 live births in the West Indies.

**15. Occurrence**

**16. Risk of Recurrence for Siblings**

**Risk of Occurence for Patient's Sib:**
See Part I, *Mendelian Inheritance.* Recurrence risk low, but not negligible in sporadic instances.

**17. Risk of Recurrence for Child**

**Risk of Recurrence for Patient's Child:**
See Part I, *Mendelian Inheritance.*

**Age of Detectability:** At birth by clinical evaluation.

**18. Age of Detectability**

**19. Gene Mapping and Linkage**

**Gene Mapping and Linkage:** BWS (Beckwith-Wiedemann syndrome) has been mapped to 11pter-p15.4.

Fig. 4. Continuation of *Beckwith-Wiedemann syndrome* article.

monster, and currently used to describe drugs, chemicals, or other environmental agents that cause malformations), any known significant information regarding the exact composition of the teratogen, threshold dosages, and critical periods for exposure should be presented. Since most teratogens act on the unborn fetus, most articles on teratogens can be found in the Master Index under "Fetal" or "Fetal effects". Perhaps the best known of recent teratogens is thalidomide, which can be found under "Fetal thalidomide syndrome". For the definitive reference source and comprehensive bibliography in this field see Thomas H. Shepard's *Catalog of teratogenic agents* also published in Baltimore and London by Johns Hopkins University Press (in its sixth edition at press time).

If the condition results from a chromosomal anomaly, the exact nature of the anomaly or variant is described here. All chromosome conditions described in the *Encyclopedia* are listed in the Master Index under "Chromosome", in order by chromosome number. Usually the prime Article Title itself describes the nature of the anomaly. Although a number of outstanding references are available on chromosomal anomalies, notably Jean de Grouchy and Catherine Turleau's *Clinical atlas of human chromosomes* (New York: John Wiley & Sons), an exhaustive bibliography can be found in Digamber S. Borgaonkar's *Chromosomal variation in man: a catalog of chromosomal variants and anomalies* published in New York by John Wiley & Sons (in its fifth edition at press time).

Finally, if the condition is known to result from some form of fetal trauma, compression, infection, or other biodynamic event or sequence, this is described.

**12. Pathogenesis** consists of a short summary of the known or theorized sequence of cellular or biodynamic events, reactions, or other pathologic mechanisms occurring in the development, course, and natural history of the condition or syndrome. Discussions of inborn errors of metabolism should designate amino acid sequences and positional changes when known. While most of the literature on the pathogenesis of human anomalies is highly dispersed and often obscure, we are fortunate in having a definitive single-source reference on inborn errors of metabolism in the Charles R. Scriver, Arthur L. Beaudet, William S. Sly, and David Valle's two-volume *The metabolic basis of inherited disease* published in New York by McGraw-Hill (in its sixth edition at press time).

**13. Classification Codes** are unique numbers assigned to medical conditions or syndromes by various authors, agencies, or sources of reference materials. As with the *Encyclopedia*'s own **Birth Defect Numbers**, these are unique identification codes that can be used to access or classify conditions and related informational resources. While creators of these various codes may not always share the same definition of a given condition or syndrome, and may group or separate entities in different ways, Classification Codes facilitate cross-reference between different informational resources concerning the same or related conditions. In a field in which there is little agreement on the names given to conditions and syndromes, these Codes can have considerable utility.

This edition of the *Encyclopedia* presents, where applicable, three different Classification Codes:

**MIM Numbers** are the unique numbers assigned to conditions by Victor A. McKusick in his *Mendelian inheritance in man*. While McKusick has recently expanded the number of digits in his code to accomodate the rapid growth of the discipline, this edition of the *Encyclopedia* shows the five-digit code (now prefix) used in the print version of *Mendelian inheritance in man* (MIM) in use at press time. The first of these five digits serves to designate the mode of Mendelian inheritance; one for autosomal dominant, two for autosomal recessive, and three for X-linked (it should be noted that other, more complex, models of human inheritance have also been reported, some only recently). An asterisk before the number indicates that the mode of inheritance, in McKusick's judgment, has been established, while a lack of asterisk designates a possible mode of inheritance.

Since August of 1987, a computerized version of the **MIM** knowledgebase has also been available online under the designation **OMIM; Online Mendelian Inheritance in Man**. This service supports a number of complex search and retrieval options that greatly expand the utility of the **MIM** knowledgebase. Updated versions of specific **MIM** articles can be accessed through **OMIM** by the **MIM** classification code number.

Users of **MIM** and **OMIM** can quickly locate *Encyclopedia* articles corresponding to specific **MIM** numbers through the MIM-NUMBER-TO-PRIME-NAME INDEX which follows the BIRTH DEFECT-NUMBER-TO-PRIME-NAME-INDEX in the back portion of this *Encyclopedia*. **MIM** numbers are listed in numeric order and cross-referenced to *Encyclopedia* prime Article Names, which can then be easily located in the Master Index.

For further information on **OMIM** contact:

Richard E. Lucier, M.L.S., M.P.H.
Associate Director for Academic Information
 Systems, Research, and Services
THE WELCH MEDICAL LIBRARY
1900 East Monument Street
Baltimore, MD 21205
U.S.A.

Tel. (301) 955-9637

**POS** (POSSUM) **Number**s are the four-digit unique syndrome identification numbers used by the **P**ictures **O**f **S**tandard **S**yndromes and **U**ndiagnosed **M**alformations videodisk reference system. The videodisk used by **POSSUM** contains over 18,000 illustrations of patients from the clinics of the Royal Children's Hospital, Melbourne, Australia, as well as photographs contributed by colleagues from other facilities. Most of these illustrations are in color.

Data in the **POSSUM** System is cross-referenced by *Birth Defects Encyclopedia* number so that **POSSUM** users can quickly locate corresponding *Encyclopedia* articles. Prime Article Titles can also be located by **POSSUM** number in the POSSUM-NUMBER-TO-PRIME-NAME-INDEX which appears following the MIM-NUMBER-TO-PRIME-NAME-INDEX in the back portion of this *Encyclopedia*.

Further information on **POSSUM** can be obtained from:

Dr. Agnes Bankier, M.D.
P.O.S.S.U.M. Project
Department of Genetics
ROYAL CHILDREN'S HOSPITAL
Flemington Road
Parkville, Victoria 3052
AUSTRALIA

Tel. (03) 345-5522

**CDC Number**s, also referred to as the MACDP six-digit code, are code numbers assigned to reportable congenital anomalies adapted from World Health Organization (WHO) and U.S. Department of Health and Human Services International Classification of Diseases (ICD) codes by the Division of Birth Defects and Developmental Disabilities, Center for Environmental Health, Centers for Disease Control, Atlanta, GA 30333. The full code consists of six digits plus a period between the third and fourth digit, although not all conditions have been assigned a full seven-place code.

The CDC/MACDP codes are often required when completing government reports, and are useful in conducting and interpreting various research studies. The prime Article Names of *Encyclopedia* articles corresponding to the various CDC/MACDP codes can be identified through use of the CDC-NUMBER-TO-PRIME-NAME-INDEX which appears following the POSSUM-NUMBER-TO-PRIME-NAME-INDEX in the back portion of the *Encyclopedia*. CDC numbers are listed in numeric order and are cross-referenced to prime Article Names, which can then be easily located in the Master Index.

The CDC/MACDP Codes are revised on an ongoing basis and planned revisions in selected portions of the Code are in testing at press time, so users should ensure that they are working with the most current version. For further information on the CDC/MACDP Codes and their use contact:

Mr. Larry Edmonds, M.S.P.H., Chief
Surveillance Section
Birth Defects & Genetic Diseases Branch
CENTERS FOR DISEASE CONTROL
Atlanta, GA 30333
U.S.A.

Tel. (404) 488-4717

A given classification code can be cross-referenced to more than one *Encyclopedia* article, so when checking the classification code Indexes at the back of this volume check to see if the code you are interested in appears more than once. Similarly, the classification code listings in *Encyclopedia* articles can refer to more than one code. Finally, it is possible to cross-reference from one classification code to another. For example, if you wish to know the **CDC** code corresponding to a given **MIM** number, first locate the article corresponding to the **MIM** number, then check the **CDC** code listed in that article.

**14. Sex Ratio** indicates the distribution of affected individuals by sex. The usual format is "Mn:Fn" where "n" is a number. For conditions with an equal distribution, as would be expected in most autosomal dominant and autosomal recessive conditions, this is usually "M1: F1". When mode of inheritance has not been determined with certainty, or the number of known cases is small, the sex ratio of the known cases may be given in place of or in addition to the expected ratio; for example "Presumably M1:F1, M5:F3 observed".

**15. Occurrence** should consist of a concise statement of the incidence and prevalence of the condition, e.g. "5:10,000 live births, 20:100,000 general population", would indicate that out of every ten thousand live births five have this condition, while twenty of every one hundred thousand people in the general population have the condition. Since affected individuals may have different expectations for survival from other members of the general population, both figures are necessary in order to appreciate the occurrence or frequency of the condition.

While these statistical conventions work well for the more frequent conditions, particularly if evenly distributed geographically and over time, and well studied as part of large, systematic epidemiological research programs, few birth defects have met these exacting requirements. Most first appear in particular regions, populations, or ethnic groups. Some tend to remain within these groups where they occur with disproportionate frequency, or move to new geographic areas as members of the group relocate (or even with a single member to whom a large number of cases in a given area can be traced—a "founder effect"). In such cases, occurrence rates may be known for one geographic area but not for the general population.

In the case of rare conditions, there may be no reliable occurrence figures at all, and "rare" in and of itself has little meaning since there is no true agreement on the definition of "rare". In such cases, Occurrence should specify any factual information that *is* known, e.g. "five cases have been reported in the literature; one in Sweden, two in the American mid-west in children of Swedish extraction, and two Japanese siblings".

Unfortunately, even this detailed information may not provide a conclusive indication of occurrence, and in fact occurrence data on birth defects is very limited and often poor. This is particularly true for conditions that have been reported a few times in the literature, as could be the case in the above example, but are not common enough or well-enough delineated to be studied in large-scale epidemiological research. After a given condition has been reported in the literature, few academic journals are willing to publish new cases unless these cases are in some way unusual. However, since the condition is still poorly defined, it is not easy to know what is "usual" for this particular condition. While it could be of great value to conduct systematic research on a defined population with the condition, including the use of technologies such as gene mapping which could have benefits well beyond the affected population, there is no simple way to further delineate the condition or define the population.

Support groups can often play a significant role since they can function to bring together individuals with a given condition, acting both as research advocates and an informal case registry. Again, however, unless the condition is clearly delineated and the number of families with affected members reaches a critical number, a support group for that condition is unlikely to emerge. Support groups are, however, one source of information on occurrence, and tend to report both numbers of affected individuals and occurrence rates which are higher than those confirmed by academic and government research statistics. This may be due in part to the fact that families with members affected by related or similar conditions, particularly if they have not been conclusively diagnosed, join established support groups out of their need for services which support groups are uniquely prepared to provide.

Given these problems, and the fact that occurrence figures are not only central to the determination of present and future need for services, but an integral part of our ability to place the full spectrum of birth defects within reach of available research technologies that can benefit the entire society, the Center for Birth Defects Information Services has designated Occurrence and Delineation as major research and service priorities. In addressing this initiative the Center has:

• Established a registry for clinical cases, both diagnosed and undiagnosed, which would otherwise not appear in the medical literature or be included in existing academic research programs.

• Implemented an editorial policy at its official journal *Dysmorphology and Clinical Genetics* which will allow and facilitate publication of clinical cases which further the objectives of diagnostic classification and delineation, but which otherwise would not be published in the scientific literature.

• Implemented, in conjunction with its computerized **Birth Defects Information System** (BDIS), both an undiagnosed case registry and a full spectrum of computer-based statistical and analytic resources directed to meeting the goals of this special initiative.

• Established a program to work with support groups on issues of common concern related to the objectives of this initiative.

• Formed a special international multidisciplinary Task Force on Occurrence and Delineation to examine the unique challenges of birth defect epidemiology and to formulate and implement recommendations for successfully meeting these challenges. This Task Force, under the Chairmanship of Dr. Jose F. Cordero, Deputy Chief of the Birth Defects and Genetic Diseases Branch of the U.S. Centers for Disease Control, includes among its members Professors Michael Baraitser of the University of London, England; F. Clarke Fraser of McGill University, Canada; Frank Greenberg of Baylor College of Medicine; Richard A. Lewis of Baylor College of Medicine; and Helga Rehder of the Medical University of Lubeck, West Germany.

### 16. Risk of Recurrence for Patient's Sib and
### 17. Risk of Recurrence for Patient's Child

The above two sections deal with the probability, by sex of an affected individual, of the condition recurring in that individual's siblings and offspring respectively. These questions are obviously of great interest to family members, and in some instances the risks can be explained in a simple statement.

Most frequently the text contains the words "See Part I, *Mendelian Inheritance*, which should refer the reader to the following explanation.

**Mendelian Inheritance** refers to the principle in genetics credited to the work of the Austrian botanist and monk Gregor Mendel in the late nineteenth century and studied by most school children as "Mendel's law". Mendel's interest was agriculture, and while his "law" is easily demonstrated in a corn field, the basic concepts also apply to many human traits as well. Table 1 presents the classic summary of Mendelian inheritance as it has been applied to recurrence risks and sex ratios

**Table 1**
**Modes of Mendelian Inheritance, Related Sex Ratios, and Risks of Recurrence**

| Code | Mode of transmission | Sex ratio | Risk of recurrence for | |
|---|---|---|---|---|
| AR | Autosomal recessive | M1:F1 | Patient's sib: | 1 in 4 (25%) for each to be affected |
| | | | Patient's child: | Not increased unless mate is carrier or homozygote |
| AD | Autosomal dominant | M1:F1 | Patient's sib: | If parent is affected 1 in 2 (50%) for each to be affected; otherwise not increased |
| | | | Patient's child: | 1 in 2 (50%) |
| AD-85% ± penetrance | Autosomal dominant with about 85% penetrance | M1:F1 | Patient's sib: | If parent is affected <1 in 2 (<50%) for each to be affected |
| | | | Patient's child: | <1 in 2 (50%) |
| AD-60% ± penetrance | Autosomal dominant with about 60% penetrance | M1:F1 | Patient's sib: | If parent is affected 1 in 3 ($\approx$30%) for each to be affected, 1 in 2 for inheriting mutant gene |
| | | | Patient's child: | 1 in 3 ($\approx$30%) for each to be affected, 1 in 2 for inheriting mutant gene |
| AD-possibly | Autosomal dominant possibly | M1:F1 probable | Patient's sib: | ? If parent is affected 1 in 2 (50%) for each to be affected; otherwise not increased |
| | | | Patient's child: | ? 1 in 2 (50%) |
| X-linked R | X-linked recessive | M1:F0 | Patient's sib: | If mother is a carrier 1 in 2 (50%) for each brother to be affected and 1 in 2 (50%) for each sister to be a carrier |
| | | | Patient's child: | 1 in 1 (100%) for carrier daughters; not increased for sons unless wife is a carrier |
| X-linked D | X-linked dominant | M1:F2 | Patient's sib: | If affected parent is female 1 in 2 (50%) for each sib to be affected. If affected parent is male 1 in 1 (100%) for each sister to be affected; not increased for brothers |
| | | | Patient's child: | If patient is female 1 in 2 (50%) for each offspring to be affected; if patient is male 1 in 1 (100%) for daughters; not increased for sons |

in humans. The information in this Table appears here, in part, to save repetition throughout the *Encyclopedia*, but also because interpretation of this sometimes oversimplified law is not always as easy as it may seem.

The reference to Mendelian inheritance is made only in the Recurrence Risk sections of articles in which the **Etiology** section contains at least the suggestion that some cases of the condition in question *may* follow a Mendelian mode of inheritance—one or more of the "modes of transmission" described in the second column of Table 1. The information in the corresponding row of the Table provides the sex ratio of affected individuals (information which is usually consistent with that seen under **Sex Ratio**), as well as the recurrence risks for the patient's sib (siblings; brothers and sisters) and child (or offspring in general regardless of number). Interpretation of this information must be tempered by at least two considerations.

First, there are few diagnoses in which the etiology of the condition in all affected individuals can be attributed

to a single Mendelian mode of transmission. Often some percentage of the cases are *sporadic*—have occurred in isolation in individuals with no family history of the condition. In other instances more than one mode of inheritance has been suggested. Which, if any apply? Could more than one apply? How do you determine which applies in a given instance? Other articles talk of "etiologic heterogeneity", suggesting that different cases have different causes. Others speak of "multifactorial" etiology or inheritance, suggesting that inheritance plays a role, perhaps as a necessary but not sufficient factor, which requires some other factor such as a trigger or environmental event for the condition to be expressed. What is the additional factor? How can you determine if it is applicable in a given instance? Furthermore, some conditions simply seem to have different degrees of "penetrance", or do not appear in a family as often as their mode of transmission would predict; while others have reduced "expressivity", suggesting that while they may be inherited with the predicted frequency, not all of those who have the condition show all of its signs and symptoms.

While the study of this interplay of often complex considerations in even one medical condition can be the focus of entire careers, interpretation is further complicated by the problems inherent in the application of mathematics developed for large-number settings such as agriculture to the small numbers involved in estimating who may or may not be affected among the members of one generation of a modern family. These potential interpretation errors, usually of the type referred to as "gambler's fallacies" by professional statisticians, can complicate the interpretation of any data based on small numbers, including those inherent in the study of rare medical conditions.

For these reasons, great care must be taken to avoid drawing the wrong conclusion from recurrence risk information. Clinical geneticists and genetic counselors receive years of preparation before they confront these issues, and anyone who becomes involved with the topic would benefit from familiarity with at least a sound introductory text on the subject such as:

Nora JJ and Fraser FC: *Medical genetics: principles and practice, 3rd ed*. Philadelphia: Lea & Febiger, 1989.

or

Thompson MW: *Genetics in medicine, 4th ed*. Philadelphia: W.B. Saunders, 1986.

**18. Age of Detectability** indicates the earliest age at which the condition can be diagnosed in an affected individual, as well as the method or methods which can be used to make that diagnosis. This varies widely from condition to condition.

In many instances the diagnosis can be made before birth, and a very useful supplementary reference on this subject can be found in David D. Weaver's *Catalog of prenatally diagnosed conditions* published in Baltimore and London by Johns Hopkins University Press (in its first 1989 edition at press time). This book includes the **MIM** number of each listed condition (when applicabel), and includes some seventy pages of references.

Since this Age of Detectability section, combined with the information listed under Major Diagnostic Criteria, tells how to diagnose the condition in question, their contents can be important and detailed. It is necessary to remember, however, that diagnostic technologies are in a period of rapid advancement, and this affects both the speed with which specific information will be outdated and the interpretation of specific terminology and nomenclature.

For example, amniocentesis is a frequently mentioned procedure, but this is being increasingly superceded by chorionic villus sampling, with corresponding reduc-

tions in the age of the fetus at which diagnosis can be made. Similarly, submicroscopic DNA analysis has proven capable of detecting abnormalities beyond the scope of standard cytogenetic analysis, and is consequently gaining wider acceptance.

Advances in medical imaging have produced a succession of new technologies, replacing X-rays with ultrasound and with still newer methods that are increasingly effective and less invasive. At one point the Center experimented with substituting the general term "medical imaging" for the current technology of choice, but has found no truly satisfactory solution to the rapid outdating produced by this explosion in technology.

This acceleration in technology need not, however, be matched by a corresponding advance in the basic science of diagnosis, and even when outdated by new technologies, basic principles of diagnosis, once discovered, can remain state-of-the-art for many years. When selecting a specific procedure it is always wise to consult with experts in the appropriate sub-specialty in order to determine current practices and assess the implications of any recent advances.

**19. Gene Mapping and Linkage** has been accomplished on some ten percent of the conditions listed in this edition of the *Encyclopedia*, with significant research findings reported on an additional ten percent. Chromosome plotting is among the most rapidly advancing areas of human biomedical research. Gene mapping, as a technical procedure, can be applied in any instance where there is an available research population with a clearly delineated condition which distinguishes the members of that research group from the general population. Given the scientific breakthrough inherent in the gene mapping of a medical condition or syndrome, and the potential benefits that can result not only for individuals affected by that condition but to medical science in general, it is not surprising that the newest gene mapping technologies are being steadily applied to an expanding array of human anomalies.

This flurry of worldwide activity has produced major advances, but also its share of false starts. A significant proportion of the reported findings have failed to be replicated, or have subsequently been withdrawn. In part this points to the critical need for clear delineation of the medical conditions under study, since failure to replicate findings in a different sample with the "same" condition is often attributable to the recognition that the two samples are not truly affected by the "same" entity. In other instances failure to replicate has helped to point out the complexity of the relationship between chromosomes and human diversity, and the likelihood that some conditions, both medical and psychiatric, may be related to more than one gene locus.

To help bring order to this process, a series of Human Gene Mapping Workshops were instituted in the early

1970s. Among the first steps taken by the Workshops was the formation of a Human Gene Mapping Library (HGML) based in New Haven, CT. Operated in conjunction with the Howard Hughes Medical Institute and Yale University, the HGML works with the Workshops in documenting Workshop-approved gene map symbol names and chromosome plots. Most scientists accept the HGML as the authority of record in the field of human gene mapping and linkage.

The Gene Mapping and Linkage information presented in this edition of the **Encycopedia** has been cross-referenced against, and is consistent with, the HGML's Human Gene Map 10 (HGM10), and reflects the conclusions of the most recent Human Gene Mapping Workshop, 10, as published in *Cytogenetics and Cell Genetics*, volume 51, 1989.

An example of the format in which this Gene Mapping and Linkage data is presented is shown in Fig. 4. The first item is the official Symbol Name (in this case "BWS") approved by the Workshop and used in all HGML databases. These symbols do change over time, and a current symbol name is key to accessing current data.

This is followed in parentheses by the Marker Name (in this example, "Beckwith-Wiedemann syndrome") also approved by the Workshop; the HGML's full text description of the mapped condition (the Center has taken the liberty of shortening a few extremely long marker names to accomodate the space requirements of presentation formats). This may or may not correspond directly with the Article Title or an Includes Term.

The third item indicates the Workshop's level of confidence in the mapping. The words "has been mapped to" (as seen in the example) indicate that the Workshop agrees that mapping has been accomplished. Otherwise a wording such as "has been tentatively mapped to" or "has been inconsistently mapped to" reflect the view of the Workshop.

Finally, the map location is provided (in this example, "11pter–p15.4"). This standard format may be followed by other text information provided by the article's author. The standardized information provides a quick summary of the condition's gene map status (although not necessarily the opinion of the article's author), and allows for quick cross-reference to HGML databases and the general literature.

The *Encyclopedia* also provides two other means of accessing gene map data. Both of these are through tables which appear directly after the Master Index.

The GENE MAP TABLE BY SYMBOL NAME lists all of the gene mapped conditions *described in this edition of the Encyclopedia* by gene map Symbol name. The Symbol appears in the first column, followed by Marker Name, Map Location, *Encyclopedia* Birth Defect Number, and finally *Encyclopedia* prime Article Title as the article on

the condition appears in the Master Index. This Table allows anyone starting with a HGML Symbol name to quickly determine if the condition is described in this edition of the *Encyclopedia*, and if so to go directly to the actual article which describes the condition.

The GENE MAP PICTORIALS BY CHROMOSOME, which follows the GENE MAP TABLE BY SYMBOL NAME, presents actual pictorials of the chromosomes, as well as the Symbol, Marker Name, Map Location, and *Encyclopedia* Birth Defect Number and prime Article Title, all arranged in order by chromosome and chromosome location. This is an important reference for readers interested in specific chromosomes, allowing quick identification of the conditions *described in this edition of the Encyclopedia* by chromosome, and direct access to the respective articles as they appear in the Master Index.

Because gene mapping is in itself a rapidly moving discipline, the *Encyclopedia* does not list references related to gene mapping unless they contain information which the HGM Workshop has not yet had an opportunity to review. For those who require more in-depth access to the gene mapping literature, a number of excellent sources are available.

The Human Gene Mapping Library serves users in 41 countries with a range of print and online services including its *Chromosome plotbooks* which summarize Workshop conclusions, and a 24-hour electronic database consisting of five cross-linked components: *MAP* contains an entry for each of more than 5,500 mapped loci; *PROBE* contains more than 10,000 unique entries for DNA probes and clones, PCR primers, and ASOs pertinent to mapping; *RFLP* describes more than 3,500 polymorphic systems at over 2,000 loci; *LIT* contains some 14,000 full citations to the gene mapping literature; and *CONTACT* contains the names, addresses, telephone, fax, and electronic mail addresses of some 5,000 people involved or interested in gene mapping. The **OMIM** database can also be accessed directly through the Library, and staff are available to provide additional services.

Interested researchers are invited to become HGML subscribers. Registration and user materials can be obtained at no cost by contacting:

HUMAN GENE MAPPING LIBRARY
25 Science Park
New Haven, CT 06511

Tel. (203) 786-5515
Fax. (203) 786-5534

In addition, the Office of Health and Environmental Research of the U.S. Department of Energy and the National Center for Human Genome Research of the U.S. National Institutes of Health jointly sponsor a

Human Genome Management Information System which publishes the bimonthly *Human Genome News* and also operates the **Human Genome Information Database**. Its regular mailings and special services are helpful to researchers, and also a great help in keeping track of the acronyms, activities, and players in this major research initiative. To subscribe to the *News* and be placed on the mailing list, contact:

> Betty K. Mansfield
> HUMAN GENOME MANAGEMENT
>      INFORMATION SYSTEM
> Oak Ridge National Laboratory
> P.O. Box 2008
> Oak Ridge, TN 37831-6050
>
> Tel. (615) 576-6669
> Fax. (615) 574-9888

**20. Prevention** outlines any steps that can be taken, if known, to prevent the condition or syndrome described in the article. Rubella vaccine in the case of **Fetal rubella syndrome** would be one example. Another example is shown in Fig. 5, which also provides examples of the next seven Article sections.

Unfortunately, there is no known prevention for most birth defects. In such cases, the articles read "None known", often followed by "Genetic counseling is indicated". This latter term is *not* intended to necessarily suggest that the condition in question is inherited, or to imply any particular course of action. Instead, it is simply a reminder that the Article contains information regarding recurrence risks which may be of interest to affected individuals and their families. This information may, in fact, help to reassure interested parties that a fear of recurrence may not be warranted.

**21. Treatment** outlines any known treatment or corrective measures. Experimental or controversial treatments, when included, should be identified.

**22. Prognosis** indicates the usual course of the condition or syndrome, including any factors that may affect anticipated life span, any functional impairments, or relevant areas known not to be impaired (such as intelligence). Variations in the usual course (between or within families) should be noted, along with any factors that may explain such variation.

**23. Detection of Carrier** describes any methods of detection which may be available, with their degree of accuracy and diagnostic limitations where applicable.

**24. Special Considerations** is an optional section which can be used to present information of importance to the reader which would not be appropriate if included in any other section of the Article. This could include but is not limited to facts of historical interest, theories, work in progress, relevant animal models, case registries, and comments regarding nomenclature.

**25. Support Groups** are listed in this section when such groups are known to exist for the condition or syndrome discussed in the article. Since names of contact persons, addresses, and telephone numbers change frequently, only the name of the organization is shown, preceded by the name of the city in which the group is listed and a semicolon. If the city is not easily recognized, it may be preceded by the state zip code abbreviation and semicolon. If the organization or group is not in the United States, these are preceded by the name of the country in capital letters and a colon. If an organization may not be listed in the telephone directory of the indicated city, a post office address is provided.

Support groups play a vital role in providing affected individuals and family members with a forum in which they can exchange information, share concerns, and obtain help. In addition, support groups can play an important role in research designed to understand, treat, and possibly even prevent or cure the condition. We encourage all support groups to provide the Center with any new or updated information which will help to keep this feature of the *Encyclopedia* as accurate, complete, and current as possible, and help us to facilitate research programs of mutual interest.

Support groups prepared to work with complex malformation syndromes can often be found by consulting the *Encyclopedia* articles on the individual conditions which make up the syndrome. However, support groups in two areas have *not* been listed throughout this Encyclopedia—those dealing with general hearing disorders and mental retardation. The reason for this is two-fold. First, these symptoms occur in a very high percentage of conditions covered in this Volume. Second, since the conditions are also frequent in the general population, most regions have support groups in these areas. If it becomes necessary to locate such an organization, however, help is available from a number of sources.

Since there is a great deal of activity and evolution surrounding support groups, practitioners have an ongoing need for current directories and related information. Perhaps the best single source is the National Center for Education in Maternal and Child Health (NCEMCH). This organization publishes both *A guide to selected national genetic voluntary organizations* and *Reaching out: a directory of national organizations related to maternal and child health*. These provide current addresses for most of the support groups listed in this *Encyclopedia*, as well as information of related interest. In addition, NCEMCH published *Starting early: a guide to Federal resources in maternal and child health* which contains information of interest to both

20. **Prevention**

**Prevention:** Avoiding contaminated needles and drug administration materials, and avoiding sexual exposure to HIV-infected sex partners. Identifying infections in high risk women, with avoidance of pregnancies, where this is an acceptable choice.

21. **Treatment**

**Treatment:** Many treatments for the complicating infections and other manifestation are available, but none curative of the primary infection. Specific therapies may modify or alleviate specific secondary infections. Maintenance therapy with intravenous gamma globulin has been reported to modify secondary disease symptoms. Steroids are used as therapy for LIP. Azidothymidine (AZT) is the first agent approved for specific treatment by the Food and Drug Administration, but the duration of experience is limited. Trials in the pediatric age group are underway. AZT treatment of pediatric AIDS appears to be particularly effective, especially against the prevalent neurological findings, but not curative. AZT trials are being initiated in pregnant women. Other treatments are under exploration.

22. **Prognosis**

**Prognosis:** Once congenital AIDS is established, diminishing health until death is inexorable, although treatment may alleviate specific infections. Recurrence of infections is the rule. Death often occurs in a few months, although some cases have survived for several years. In general the earlier the onset, the more fulminating the course. *Pneumocystis caranii* pneumonia in infants is the main contributor to early mortality. In cases where this is avoided, survival is longer.

23. **Detection of Carrier**

**Detection of Carrier:** HIV infection can be determined by isolation of the virus in blood or body tissues, antigen detection in blood or body tissues, presence of HIV antibody as indicated by repeated reactive screening test (e.g., enzyme immunoassay), plus a positive confirmatory test (e.g., Western blot, immunoflourescence assay).

24. **Special Considerations**

**Special Considerations:** Pediatric AIDS cases do not require isolation, as the risk of transmission is very low. The usual precautions should be observed, however, in wearing gloves and avoiding finger pricks when exposed to possibly infected blood.

All health care personnel are encouraged to report AIDS cases to their public health departments. Report AZT pregnancy exposures to the manufacturer, Burrough's Welcome; a registry of these exposures is being followed to assess effects.

25. **Support Groups**

**Support Groups:** Los Angeles; World Hemophilia AIDS Center

26. **Acknowledgements**

*The authors wish to thank Janine M. Jason, Chief of Epidemiology Studies Section, Division of Host Factors, Centers for Disease Control, and Susan Mankoff of the CDC's AIDS Program, for their assistance in the preparation of this article. Nothing in this article, however, represents an official statement of the United States Government or of any employee or branch thereof.*

27. **References**

**References:**
Marion RW, et al.: Human T-cell lymphotropic virus type III (HTLV-III) embryopathy: a new dysmorphic syndrome associated with intrauterine HTLV-III infection. Am J Dis Child 1986; 140:638–640. †
Barbour SD: Acquired immunodeficiency syndrome of childhood Pediatric Clinics of North America 1987; 2:247–268 *
Borkowsky W, et al.: Human-immunodeficiency-virus infections in infants negative for anti-HIV by enzyme-linked immunoassay. Lancet 1987; I:1168–1170.
Centers for Disease Control: Classification system for human immunodeficency virus infection in children under 13 years of age. Morbidity and Mortality Weekly Rep. 1987; ?; ?5–235

**Illustrated Reference indicated by a dagger**

**Prime Reference indicated by asterisk**

Fig. 5. Portion of *Fetal acquired immune deficiency syndrome (AIDS) infection* article.

professionals and support groups. Finally, for a $10.00 fee, this organization publishes *Genetic support groups: volunteers and professionals as partners*.

In addition to issuing these publications on a regular basis, NCEMCH maintains an in-house computerized database of support groups and can quickly respond to special needs. For further information contact:

Olivia Pickett, M.L.S., Librarian
NATIONAL CENTER FOR EDUCATION IN
   MATERNAL AND CHILD HEALTH
   (NCEMCH)
38th and R Street, N.W.
Washington, DC 20057

Tel. (202) 625-8400
Fax. (202) 625-8404

Another organization that can provide or help to locate support services for individuals and families with rare conditions and syndromes is the National Organization for Rare Disorders (NORD). For further information contact:

Abbey S. Meyers, Executive Director
NATIONAL ORGANIZATION FOR RARE
   DISORDERS (NORD)
P.O. Box 8923
New Fairfield, CT 06812

Tel. (203) 746-6518

Under certain circumstances, it may be appropriate to consider formation of a new support group, in which case additional help and information may be obtained by contacting:

Frank Riessman, Director
NATIONAL SELF-HELP CLEARINGHOUSE
25 West 43rd Street Room 620
New York, NY 10036

Tel. (212) 642-2944

**26. Acknowledgements** is an additional optional section which appears in italics without a heading. As the name suggests, it is used to acknowledge colleagues for their help in preparing the article, acknowledge sources of funding, and to otherwise state essential notices and disclaimers.

**27. References** are presented in chronological order with the earliest appearing first, thus providing a quick history of the development of the literature on the condition or syndrome. It is not the role or objective of the *Encyclopedia* to present an exhaustive bibliography, but instead to identify key sources while providing an appropriate entry point into the complete literature on the subject. This can generally be accomplished with between three and seven citations, although some conditions have only been reported once or twice in the literature. Other conditions may have a complex, fragmented literature without a good recent review article, and these could require a somewhat longer list of references.

Primary sources are preferable, and an ideal list includes the *first publication* to describe and delineate the condition, the most *recent review article* providing a comprehensive review, synthesis, and bibliography of the complete literature, and, if appropriate, a *well-illustrated* reference containing a comprehensive selection of photographs of representative affected individuals.

Because illustrations are important for most conditions and syndromes, particularly those involving dysmorphology, the author may draw attention to **illustrated references** by placing a dagger (†) after the reference. In addition, authors are encouraged to indicate their **prime reference** by placing an asterisk (*) after the reference, indicating that a reader wishing an overview of the topic could start with this citation (see Fig. 5).

With few exceptions, references follow the format recommended by the American Medical Association in its *Manual for authors and editors*. Most journal title abbreviations follow the rules of the *American National Standard for Abbreviation of Titles of Periodicals* as used by *Index Medicus* and *MEDLINE*, although some acronyms such as **JAMA** are replaced by the long form *J Am Med Assoc* for the convenience of readers who may not be familiar with the acronym form. The full page range is provided for the convenience of users who may be considering the ordering of copies and wish to estimate costs.

In the interest of space, the *Encyclopedia* shows the names of authors only when a reference has a single author or no more than *two* authors. References with three or more authors show only the first author followed by *et al*. We would prefer to see **all** authors properly acknowledged, and regret this concession which must be made in the name of brevity.

When references are cited from within the text, the *Encyclopedia* shows the the author name(s) and year of publication, rather than the reference numbers popular in most medical journals. Unlike journal articles, *Encyclopedia* articles are constantly updated, creating an ongoing potential for introducing and overlooking errors in numbered references. We also find that most readers prefer citations in the full name format. We do not, however, place the customary period after *et al* when part of a reference citation from text; it is easily confused with periods used for other purposes, and most readers know that *et al* is not a person's name.

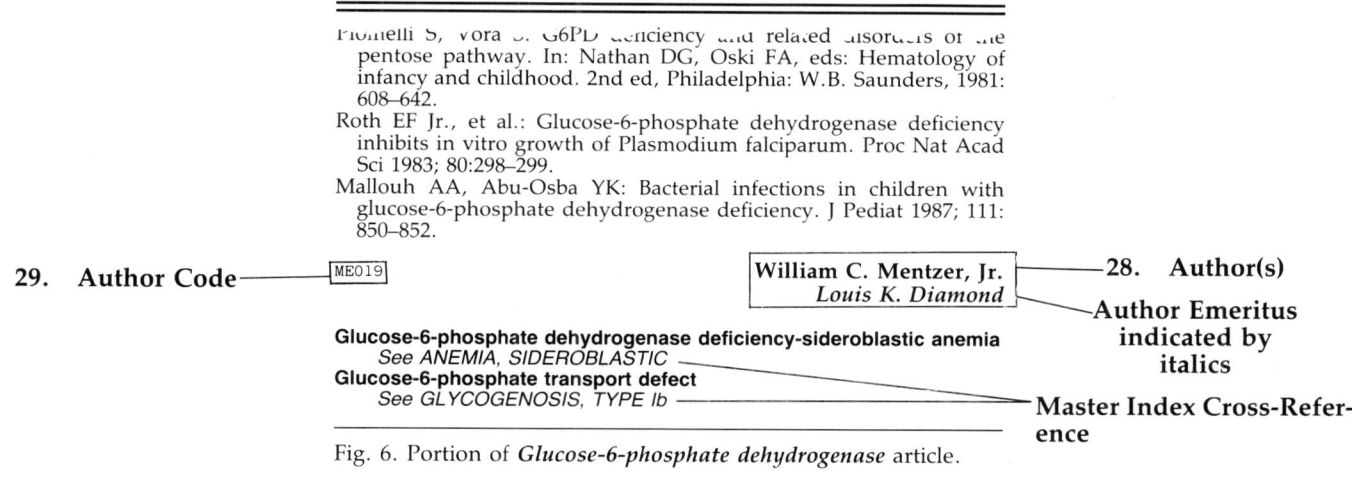

29. Author Code ── ME019        William C. Mentzer, Jr. ── 28. Author(s)
                                 *Louis K. Diamond*       Author Emeritus
                                                          indicated by
                                                          italics

Glucose-6-phosphate dehydrogenase deficiency-sideroblastic anemia
  *See ANEMIA, SIDEROBLASTIC*
Glucose-6-phosphate transport defect                     Master Index Cross-Refer-
  *See GLYCOGENOSIS, TYPE Ib*                             ence

Fig. 6. Portion of *Glucose-6-phosphate dehydrogenase* article.

**28. Author(s)** of each article appear at the end of the article on the right side of the column (see Fig. 6). Degrees and other titles are not shown here, but *do* appear, along with addresses, in the list of CONTRIBUTORS in the front of the *Encyclopedia*.

When the name of an author appears in *italics*, this indicates that the author is **emeritus**. It is the nature of rare medical conditions that they are often first documented by the clinician or scientist who first recognizes the condition as new or unique. This author becomes, if only by default, the world's "expert". If subsequent cases are found in another part of the world, a new expert may emerge, if only to understand the condition well enough to treat the new patients effectively. This continual shifting of centers of expertise, combined with normal retirements and life changes, made it necessary to develop a way of acknowledging major contributions while allowing new authors to assume responsibility for existing articles.

By contract with the Center, all authors accept that articles may be reassigned as needed, and that former authors who have made significant contributions which remain through subsequent revision(s) may, at the option of the Center, be designated as *emeritus*. Often reassignments are made at the request of an original author, at retirement or for any reason that the author may feel such a change would be in the interest of *Encyclopedia* readers. Emeritus authors are *not* responsible for the contents of the article, but are acknowledged as recognized experts and past contributors to an article which has continued as the foundation upon which others have built.

**29. Author Code** appears to the left of an author's name, next to the left side of the column. With thousands of authors affiliated with the Center, similar names are inevitable. For the Center's operations to function effectively, however, it is essential that its

continual flow of communications reach the right person as quickly as possible. To this end, Author Codes serve two purposes. First, they are a unique identifier which allows positive identification of one specific individual. Second, they are also a kind of mailbox number, electronically linked to a current mailing address, telephone number, and fax number. Messages identified by Author Code can be instantly routed by the fastest method, and assure the most efficient possible communications.

An Author Code is not shown for authors emeritus, since they do not normally receive copies of communications regarding the topic of the article. However, in order to assure the most efficient communication, all correspondence with the Center regarding a given article or a condition described in an *Encyclopedia* article, delivered by mail, telephone, fax, or any other method, should **indicate both the Birth Defect Number and the Author Code(s) as shown.**

**30. Agreements, Consents, and Releases**, while not shown in the published article, are essential elements of any *Encyclopedia* contribution, and no article can reach publication without them. All Authors must sign a model **Contributor Agreement** developed to both meet the requirements inherent in all publishing relationships and to address issues unique to ongoing medical knowledgebases distributed through both print and electronic media. Copies of this **Agreement** are available upon request.

Illustrations cannot appear in the knowledgebase unless accompanied by the necessary **Consent** and **Release** documents. The Center worked for several years with the legal, medical and photography communities in order to develop a model **Consent** form to be signed by subjects or guardians prior to the taking of medical illustrations. The resulting form protects the interest of all parties, and the Center encourages its use, along with basic photographic procedures and standards (including the use of grids or uniform references to scale) in documenting clinical cases.

An **Illustration Release Form** must be signed by submitting scientists, and often the photographer or artist, in order for the Center to distribute submitted illustrations through any of its publications or services. Again, the Center has developed a model Form, which also allows, at the submitter's option, for the Center to retain, digitize, preserve, and authorize the re-publication of the illustrations as appropriate.

Copies of the **Illustration Release Form** and **Consent for Taking and Publication of Photographs** appear in the *Author's Guide* to the Center's official journal *Dysmorphology and Clinical Genetics*, available at no charge from the Center or by writing to:

DCG Guide
BLACKWELL SCIENTIFIC PUBLICATIONS, INC.
Three Cambridge Center   Suite 208
Cambridge, MA 02142
U.S.A.

**Core Articles**. While most of the articles in the *Encyclopedia* deal with a single condition or syndrome, many of these single conditions are members of a larger class or group of conditions; for example the **Amyloidoses**. Repetition of basic information on the amyloidoses in each amyloidosis article would not only be redundant and space consuming, but could not do justice to the overall, or "core", material on the topic. In order to deal with this reality, a limited number of "Core" articles are included in this print edition of the *Encyclopedia*. Core articles often have a simpler format than regular articles, and may not have or need each of the normal article elements. In addition, Core articles can be easily recognized by their Birth Defect Number which always begins with "15", for example 1502 in the case of **Amyloidoses**.

The actual text within all *Encyclopedia* articles follows most accepted conventions and is largely self-explanatory. Specialized terms are defined in the text, and other terms should be easily located in standard or medical dictionaries. Few abreviations are used, but these do include MCA for Multiple Congenital Amonalies; MR for Mental Retardation; and CNS for Central Nervous System. As is common practice, EKG is used to designate electrocardiogram since the technically correct "ECG" can be confused with "EEG".

**Foreign language accent marks** may seem to appear inconsistently within articles, and this results in part from a compromise with an evolving technology. While we respect the use of accent marks which remind us of the history of our field and literature, and of our debt to a rich range of diverse languages, the use of accent marks can create problems with the use of computers in

text searching and management. While we are able to handle accent marks, Greek letters, and special symbols, we have had to avoid their use in sections of the articles which are routinely searched and indexed by computer. This includes any of the items which are alphabetized in the Master Index, or which appear in the back matter of the *Encyclopedia*. In other cases, we have tried to accomodate the wishes of the authors and the conventions of their sub-discipline. We were able to do this in the case of author name (as it appears in the article but not in the list of Contributors) because authors can be searched by Author Code. Even when accent marks have been preserved in this print edition, however, it may be impossible to preserve them in versions of the *Encyclopedia* distributed over electronic systems which must accomodate very limited character sets.

**Copyrights and Trademarks** also present problems, not only with computers but when used in the context of the small type required in reference books. The trademark abbreviation "TM" and the trademark and copyright registration symbols are only clearly recognized in fairly large type, and even then can not be easily searched out by computer. Consequently the *Encyclopedia* has adopted an emerging standard by using the caret symbol ($\wedge$; ASCII character 94) to designate a proper name for a product or service protected by special legal status. For example, Netromycin$^{\wedge}$ is the name used by Schering Corporation for its trade version of the generic drug netilmicin sulfate. The $\wedge$ designation not only identifies trademarks and special status, but directs readers to the correct section of the *PDR* and otherwise assists in further research.

**Ratios and mathematical notation**. As demonstrated by **Risk of Recurrence**, care must be taken in the interpretation of statistics and other mathematical data, particularly when underlying assumptions vary, or the magnitude of the numbers involved differ from the intended mathematical application. Furthermore, even the use of mathematical notation may not be consistent.

As a case in point, the recurrence risks shown in Table 1 (1 in 4; 1 in 2, etc.) are usually expressed by geneticists as ratios (1:4; 1:2, etc.) where the colon is intended to mean "in" or "of". **Sex Ratios** also use a colon in their notation (M1:F1), but here the colon is intended to mean "versus" or "to each" as in "one male to each female". The notation "M1:F6 observed" is unlikely to be interpreted as "of the six females born, one of them was a male".

Interpretation of the same colon in **Occurrence** may not be as unambiguous. Does "1:13,700" mean "one affected child *versus* 13,700 unaffected children" or "one of the 13,700 children born was affected"? While the practical difference in this case may not seem great, the reality is that the notation is not used with great consistency. As a convention, use of the notation for incidence or prevalence *should* be the same as that for recurrence risk; 1:10,000 should mean "of every 10,000, one is affected".

In most instances, intent is clear from the context, and *Encyclopedia* editors do their best to query and clarify anything that could be misinterpreted. However, because inconsistent use of notation is common throughout the medical literature, it is important that *all* statistics and mathematical expressions be interpreted with great care.

## RELATED SERVICES

While the print editions of the *Birth Defects Encyclopedia* are a cornerstone of the Center's services and programs, its pages nevertheless represent simply a snapshot of one moment in the evolution of a rapidly changing and expanding knowledgebase. Print editions of the *Encyclopedia* are comprehensive and current at publication, and as they are superseded become building blocks and mileposts in the history of our collective disciplines. But most of life, its excitement of discovery, crises of patient care, quiet search for truth and progress, and the ongoing task of educating new scientists and practitioners, takes place between the print editions of the reference works that mark our daily progress.

In recognition of this reality, the Center provides a number of related services which allow *Encyclopedia* readers and contributors to participate in the ongoing events of the knowledgebase, both as contributors to its evolution and as beneficiaries of its growth. These services provide continual access to updated articles, support specialized research activities, assist in clinical diagnosis, facilitate and conduct research and information exchange, provide a forum for discussion and debate, and assist in public and professional education.

# BDFax

The Center's **BDFax**^ service allows anyone in the world to call the Center from any Fax (facsimile) machine equipped with a **Touch-tone**^ telephone, and to request a *current, updated version* of *any* article then in the *Encyclopedia* knowledgebase. To request the article, simply enter the four-digit **Birth Defect Number** as it appears in the version of the article in the current print edition of the *Encyclopedia*. The **Birth Defect Number** is entered with the buttons on your Fax machine's **Touch-tone**^ pad. The updated article you request will be instantly and automatically transmitted directly to the Fax machine you are using.

**BDFax**^ can be used to confirm that you have the very

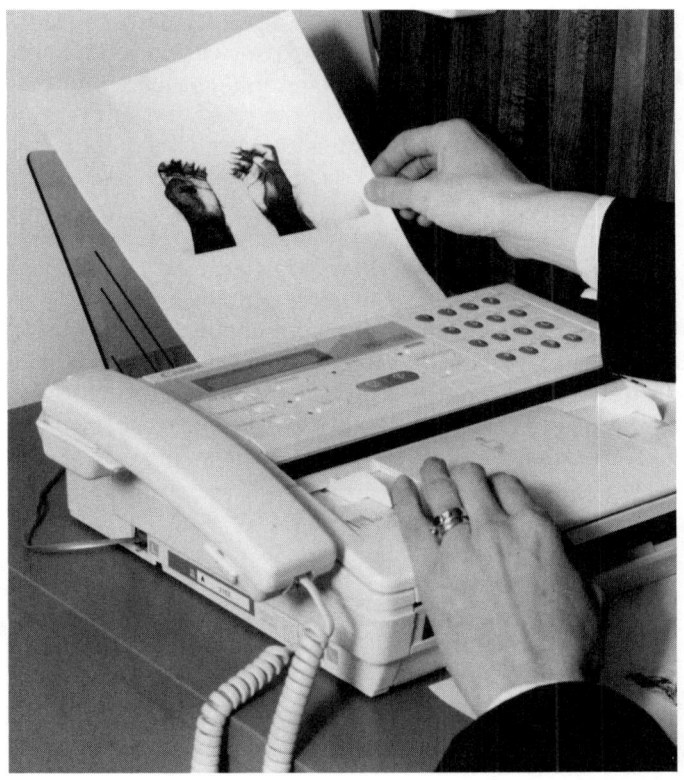

latest information on any condition or syndrome. It can be used to get a copy of vital information when you are away from your office, or to obtain extra copies of current articles for students or patients. *Encyclopedia* authors and editors use **BDFax**^ to check articles that they are updating or editing, or to check on the current status of conditions that may be appropriate for listing in the **Excludes** section of their own articles. Support groups and the media use **BDFax**^ to remain current on conditions and syndromes of interest, and scientists and researchers consult the service to assure that they are working with up-to-date facts and references.

If an article has been deleted from the *Encyclopedia* knowledgebase, **BDFax**^ will tell you why. If an article has been merged into a different article, **BDFax**^ will automatically give you the new article. If an article has been divided into two or more new articles, **BDFax**^ will give you access to the new articles. Finally, you can obtain a list of articles and illustrations added to the *Encyclopedia* since the last print edition by requesting document 9550 just as you would an article. Copies of these articles *and* illustrations can then be requested directly through **BDFax**^. General information on the Center can be obtained by requesting **BDFax**^ document 9500.

To reach the **BDFax**^ service, simply call (508) 785-BDIS (508-785-2347) from your touch-tone^ Fax, 24-

hours a day, year-round[1]. **BDFax** ^ will answer with a voice message and instructions. You will then be asked to enter the number of the document(s) you are requesting. If you make a mistake, simply press the star (*) key to start over. You can request several documents by pressing the pound (#) key between each four-digit document request.

Articles in the **BDFax** ^ knowledgebase are updated on a daily basis, but contain only articles which have been subjected to peer-review and approved by the Editorial Board. As a reader convenience, however, new **References** may be added to an article while the article is undergoing update and editorial review but before its contents have been fully integrated into the peer-reviewed article.

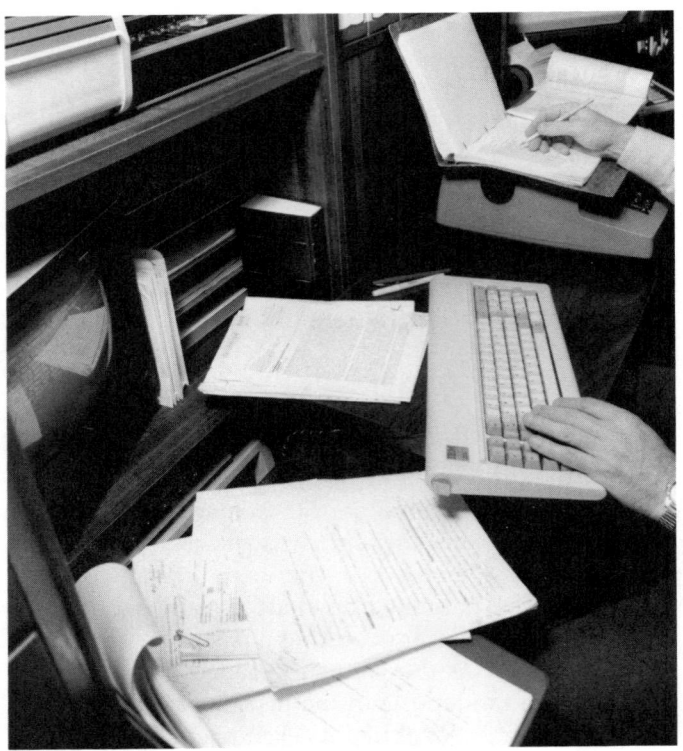

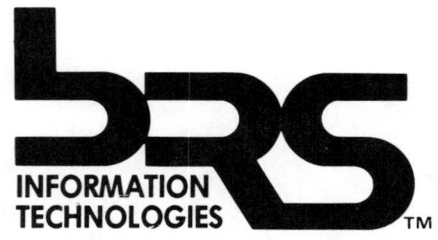

The BIRTH DEFECTS ENCYCLOPEDIA *Online* (**BDEO**^) database makes the full text of all updated *Birth Defects Encyclopedia* articles available for online search and retrieval through the services of BRS Information Technologies, a division of Maxwell Online. One of the online industry's premier information retrieval services, **BRS**^ makes the **BDEO**^ database available through both its **BRS/Search Services**, available through most medical libraries, and through its special end-user biomedical service **BRS Colleague**^.

While **BDFax**^'s strength is its ability to quickly provide updated articles on known topics, **BDEO**^ provides a unique ability to search a continually updated version of the *Encyclopedia* for articles and conditions which meet specific clinical or research criteria. Any combination of *Encyclopedia* article elements or sections can be searched, with any combination of boolean logic. The availability of this service provides every reader of the *Encyclopedia* with the same search and retrieval capabilities contained in the powerful Editorial Workstations used by Center staff and editors.

For example, it would be possible to obtain a list of articles, or the actual articles, describing all non-Mende-

lian conditions involving cardiac defects which occur in males in the United States with an incidence of more than 1:100,000 live births. Or, it is possible to request a listing of the **Occurrence**, by **Article Title**, of all Mendelian conditions which affect both males and females, and include among their **Clinical Findings** microcephaly accompanied by dental defects but not by hearing disorders.

Using **BDEO**^ through **BRS**^ also allows you to request Selective Dissemination of Information (**SDI**) according to your own specifications, with the results to be sent, in printed form, directly to you. For example, a dentist specializing in restorative surgery can enter an **SDI** request that all new or updated *Encyclopedia* articles involving craniofacial defects with dental anomalies be mailed directly to his or her office as they are released by the Center. A similar **SDI** can be developed by pediatric orthopedic surgeons, or any other subspecialty practitioner whose practice involves human anomalies of clinical relevance.

For more information, or to sign up for BIRTH DEFECTS ENCYCLOPEDIA *Online* (**BDEO**^) through the services of **BRS**^, call toll-free from the United States and Canada (800) 955-0906. From Europe, call the London office at (081) 993-9962, or toll-free (within the U.K.) at (0800) 289512. From the Australasian region, you can call the office in Sydney at (02) 360-2691 or toll-free (within Australia) at (008) 22-6474. Written correspondence may be directed to:

---

[1] **BDFax** ^ operates under the **FaxFacts** ^ software system developed and distributed by Copia International Ltd. of Wheaton, IL 60187. The Center is grateful to **Copia** ^ for helping to make this important service available to *Encyclopedia* readers.

MAXWELL ONLINE, INC.
8000 Westpark Drive
McLean, VA 22102

Fax. (703) 893-4632

For updated information on the BIRTH DEFECTS ENCYCLO-PEDIA *Online* (**BDEO**^) service, request **BDFax**^ document 9600.

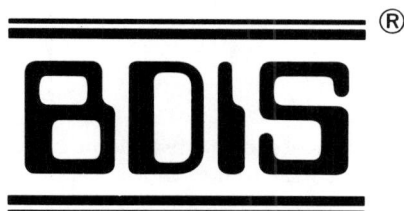

## BIRTH DEFECTS INFORMATION SYSTEM

While the Center's various text-based services are very effective in providing systematic, succinct descriptions of known conditions and syndromes, and at guiding the reader to and through the salient literature, the task of matching these established conditions and syndromes to new clinical cases, or even comparing them to each other, poses challenges of a special magnitude. Although single conditions, or even syndromes consisting of up to about three individual component conditions, are fairly easily located in the Master Index, the complex malformation syndromes that make up more than half of the entries in this edition of the *Encyclopedia* average more than seven components, and can easily contain thirty or more.

While the Master Index has been designed to help the reader match patient clinical findings to appropriate articles, and to help the Center locate possible duplicate articles or identical conditions known under different names, the nature of complex syndromes imposes unique demands that push the task well beyond the scope of paper-based information systems. Not only are the number of syndrome components too great to manage either cognitively or procedurally, but the number of components in each half of a potential match tend to be different. Furthermore, even the reported component configurations tend to be variable, since the pivotal diagnostic skill is an ability to accurately search out and recognize signs and symptoms which comes chiefly from experience.

Over the years, a number of methodologies have been developed to examine clusters of data and to simulate clinical decision making[2]. Each approach presented its own difficulties. Simple systems have proven ineffective, but as systems become increasingly complex their conclusions become harder to replicate and clinicians find it increasingly difficult to understand or explain why particular results are achieved. For a system to work and be accepted, it must be able to easily adapt to a continually evolving knowledgebase while at the same time presenting results that can be explained without mystery and interpreted as easily as using a reference book[3].

The Center, faced with the enormous task of creating the *Encyclopedia* and applying its knowledgebase to real-life clinical and research challenges, had a practical need for such a system and made its development an initiative effort for the mid-1980s. The result was the Birth Defects Information System (**BDIS**^), a sophisticated computer-based profile matching system that reduced the research and diagnostic assistance tasks associated with complex syndromes to computer profile displays that can be evaluated in much the same way that less complex conditions are evaluated by browsing through the *Encyclopedia*'s Master Index.

With the advent of increasingly powerful personal computers, the Center was able to introduce *Micro BDIS*^, a system-on-a-diskette that clinicians and researchers could use on their own computers, thus avoiding modem connections to a central computer and gaining the rapid, detailed displays so essential for quick and easy use. Still, *Micro BDIS*^ was kept simple enough to use on portable PCs without special graphics or color monitors, yet powerful enough to contain an **Unknowns Registry** through which cases can be confidentially submitted to the Center and shared among colleagues in the further search for a match or diagnosis[4].

The article reprinted on the following pages describes the 1987 release of *Micro BDIS*^ as used in clinics and research centers worldwide in the late 1980s.

[2] Edwards CN: Information management in the health industries. *Information Management Review* 1985; 1:65-75.
[3] Edwards CN: Expert systems and the advancement of the scientific knowledgebase. Paper Presented at the First International Conference on Artificial Intelligence and its Impacts in Biology and Medicine, Montpellier, France, September 29, 1986.
[4] *Micro BDIS* was produced in the MEDx^ software language developed and distributed by MEDx System, Ltd., Dover, MA 02030. The Center is grateful to MEDx^ for helping to make **BDIS**^ available to *Encyclopedia* readers.

## THE BIRTH DEFECTS INFORMATION SYSTEM‡

### A Computer-based Information Resource for Diagnostic Support, Education, and Research

Mary Louise Buyse, M.D. and Carl N. Edwards

By design, the Birth Defects Information System is a comprehensive database and knowledgebase management system for human genetics. Clinical case information can be collected, stored, and managed in *Micro BDIS*. In addition, the center provides a number of knowledgebases that contain models of potential diagnostic candidates. These knowledgebases cover such diagnostic categories as complex malformation syndromes, local and familial conditions, and chromosome diagnoses, as well as research knowledgebases containing cases with unknown diagnoses, and new provisional diagnoses that have been observed with sufficient frequency to justify their consideration as possible new birth defect syndromes.

Clinical genetics is a rapidly changing discipline. About one-third of all clinical cases do not fit an established diagnostic classification. Yet new syndromes are being discovered every day. Syndromes that once were thought to be very different and were consequently classified separately emerge as different manifestations of the same condition or as the same condition at different points in its natural history. At the same time, conditions that appear the same are found to have very different underlying dynamics and prognoses. The field demands an information technology that can adapt to rapid change, and actually support this research and classification process.

The Birth Defects Information System is designed to help the clinician by providing a quick and easy-to-use case management, recordkeeping, and report generating capability, while at the same time integrating clinical practice with the ongoing identification and delineation of new birth defect conditions and syndromes. By improving diagnostic capabilities, clinicians are better able to advise patients and families about prognosis and further risk of inheritance.

As part of an international network of cooperating scientists,[1] subscribers can help to discover and prevent new causes of birth defects. More than a standard of care, *Micro BDIS* is a critical research and communication tool through which clinicians and researchers can work together to expand the scientific frontiers of their discipline.

### DEVELOPING A CLINICAL CASE PROFILE

A major challenge in clinical genetics information involved the development of a standardized language for case description. *Micro BDIS* not only provides such a language, but its data-driven design allows rapid and convenient update of the descriptive language and System's content.

Upon logging on to *Micro BDIS*,[2] the clinician is presented with the main menu (Table 1). Any option on this or any other menu can be selected easily by moving a pointer with the cursor keys. When entering a new case, the clinician first answers a few standard descriptive questions such as age and

‡ First published in the *American Journal of Perinatology*, 1987; 4:8–11. Reprinted by permission of Thieme Medical Publisher, 381 Park Avenue South, New York, NY 10016.

**TABLE BDIS-1.**
**Birth Defects Information System (*Micro BDIS*) Main Menu**

**Main Menu**

→ Enter a new case
  Update an existing case
  Enter a new search
  Update an existing search
  Run a diagnostic evaluation
  Run a search
  Display evaluation or search results, or profile
  Create 'search' criteria from a candidate
  File maintenance
  Alter/review default settings
  Review documentation
  Exit *Micro BDIS*™

sex, and is then presented with a menu of major diagnostic sections (Table 2). Any section can be selected by setting the pointer on the desired section and pressing the enter key. The section will then expand and the screen will display a menu of groups under the selected section. Selected groups, in turn, expand to display menus of specific conditions within the selected group. An example of the over 800 terms is shown in a portion of the directory listing (Table 3).

A section, group, or condition can be designated as *present* in the case by pressing the enter key, at which point the text is *highlighted* on the screen. Pressing the backspace key designates the descriptor as *not present*, at which point the text is presented in *reverse video*. The clinician can move through the menus rapidly, in any order, and can change or update information at any time. Any information that cannot be expressed through use of the standard terms can be entered in English text through a built-in word processor.

The listing of a sample testcase (Table 4) demonstrates not only the selected descriptive terms, but the standardized background information and free text as well. In this listing, which may be entered in the patient's record, the asterisk

**TABLE BDIS-2.**
**Case Description Main Section Menu**

\*Case: Testcase Doe, John J., III  Age: 1 .10  Sex: M

→ HISTORY
  DEFECT OF EYE AND VISION
  DEFECT OF EAR AND HEARING
  DEFECT OF FACE AND NECK
  DEFECT OF ORAL CAVITY OR NASOPHARYNX
  DEFECT OF TOOTH
  RESPIRATORY OR SPEECH DEFECT
  DEFECT OF CARDIOVASCULAR SYSTEM
  SKELETAL DEFECT
  MUSCLE DEFECT
  DEFECT OF NERVOUS SYSTEM
  DEFECT OF GASTROINTESTINAL SYSTEM
  DEFECT OF GENITOURINARY SYSTEM
  DEFECT OF SKIN, HAIR OR NAILS
  HEMATOLOGIC IMMUNE OR ENDOCRINE SYSTEM
    DEFECT

**TABLE BDIS-3.**
**Portion of Directory Listing**

DEFECT OF FACE AND NECK
  Onset and distribution of facial defect
    face or neck defect at birth (congenital)
    facial or neck defect starting in infancy or childhood
    bilaterial distribution of facial or neck defect
    unilateral distribution of facial or neck defect
  Defect of facial size, shape or appearance
    round facies (moon-face, broad)
    long facies
    triangular facies (fetal)
    craniofacial disproportion
    asymmetric facies
    flat facies (Potter facies; not mid-facial hypoplasia)
    masklike facies (lack expression, immobile)
    coarse facial features
    facial bone defect
    aged facies (senile appearance, wrinkled)
    other defect of facial size, shape or appearance
  Defect of upper face, forehead or frontal zone
    broad forehead (wide)
    high forehead
    frontal bossing (prominent)
    defect of frontal bone
    supraorbital ridge defect
    other defect of upper face, forehead or frontal bone

**TABLE BDIS-4.**
**Listing of Testcase**

*Case: Testcase Doe, John J., III Age: 1 .10 Sex: M

    ***Start of list***
    HISTORY
      Prenatal and perinatal history
(*)     birthweight low (small for gestational age)
      Postnatal history
*       early death (infancy or early childhood)
(*) DEFECT OF EYE AND VISION
(*) DEFECT OF EAR AND HEARING
      Onset, distribution or progression of ear or hearing defect
*       hearing defect at birth or during infancy
(*)     unilateral ear or hearing defect
*       bilateral ear or hearing defect
      Defect of inner ear or labyrinth
*       defect of cochlea, organ of Corti or cochlear nerve
      Hearing loss or deafness
(*) conductive hearing loss
*     sensorineural hearing loss
    DEFECT OF CARDIOVASCULAR SYSTEM
*     Defect of heart or pericardium
    DEFECT OF NERVOUS SYSTEM
      Onset and progression of neurologic defect
*       neurologic defect onset in infancy or childhood
      Defect of cerebral function, consciousness or mentation
*       fainting (syncope)
    DEFECT OF SKIN, HAIR OR NAILS
(*)   Skin lesions (nonvascular)
    HEMATOLOGIC IMMUNE OR ENDOCRINE SYSTEM
      DEFECT
*     Defect of hematologic system
    ***End of List***

***Summary***
Facility: American Journal of Perinatology
Clinician: MLB
Date Case Entered: 860501   Date Diagnosed: 860505
***Unknowns Registry Information***
Patient's date of birth 06/27/83
Patient's first name John, III
Patient's birth place Los Angeles, CA
Age of mother: 18   Age of father: 21
Race of mother: Native American
Race of father: Black
Ancestry of mother: S.W. USA Tribes
Ancestry of father: South Africa

before selected descriptive terms is shown in parentheses for those terms designated as *not present or ruled out*.

## DIAGNOSTIC EVALUATION

In formulating a differential diagnosis, the clinician may request that a case be compared against the diagnostic models on any one or a combination of knowledgebases provided by the Center. A typical evaluation takes about 2 minutes and provides a list (Table 5), ranked according to criteria selected by the clinician, of candidate diagnoses showing the best matches.

The clinician can then select a Diagnostic Profile of the case against any of the candidate diagnoses. A profile of testcase against its highest scoring candidate diagnosis (Table 6) shows where testcase and the cardioauditory syndrome from the complex malformations knowledgebase "Syndinfo" do and do not correspond. Descriptive terms preceded by an asterisk were selected in the case description; those preceded by a greater than sign appear in the model. Those in parenthesis are ruled out or contraindicated. Matching items are highlighted, with an equal sign in the first column if a positive match and a number sign if negative in both the case and the model. Conflicts between the case and the model are indicated by a minus sign, and partial matches by a percent sign.

The clinician can scan profiles of the case against any of the diagnostic candidates at the press of a key. In this same way, potential diagnoses can be selected or rejected, and information can be entered into the patient record and printed for future reference or for use by family or referring physician.

## UNKNOWNS REGISTRY

By pressing a single key, a case diagnosis also can be designated as Unknown. An additional single keystroke trans-

fers Unknown cases, with personal identifiers removed, to a diskette for mailing to the Center's Unknowns Registry.

If a clinician submits a case to the Registry that matches another Unknown, or is considered a potential case contribution to a scientific discovery or professional publication, the clinician is notified. Knowledgebases of cases submitted to the Unknowns Registry also are made available for research applications.

## ADVANCED FEATURES

Because *Micro BDIS* is a modular knowledgebase management system, subscribers can display a wide range of reports and profiles. The actual weights of each candidate model are displayed easily, and score calculations can be traced easily. *Micro BDIS* contains its own online documentation, which can be displayed or printed. Most options can be user-defined, and each installation can be custom-configured.

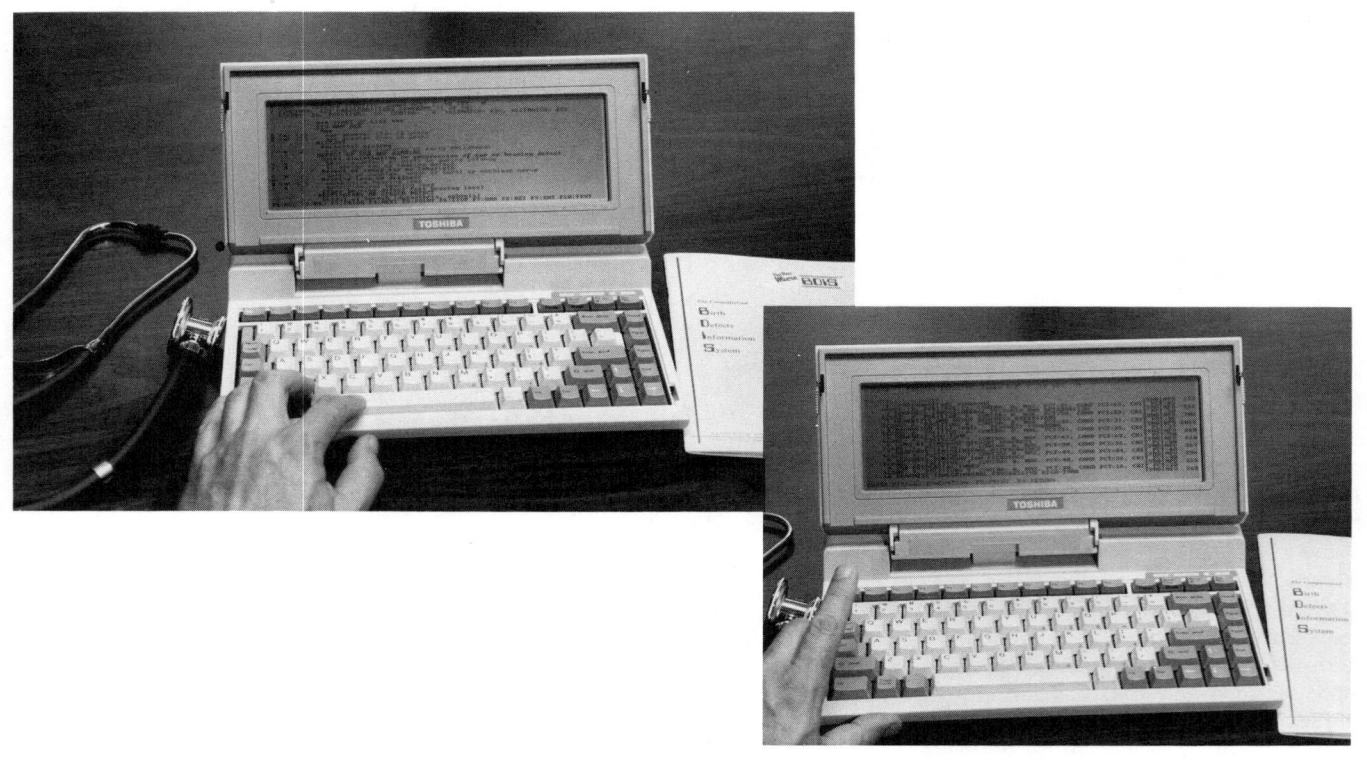

**TABLE BDIS-5.**
Listing of Ranked Candidate Diagnoses

*Case: Testcase Doe, John J., III Age: 1 .10 Sex: M

→ Cardioauditory syndrome
    score = 15, positive = 15, contra = 0, max. pct = 85, cand
    pct = 65, crit pct = 85
  2 Deafness-sensorineural, dystonia and retardation
    score = 8, positive = 8, contra = 0, max. pct = 50, cand
    pct = 25,   crit pct = 50
  3 Nephritis and nerve deafness, hereditary
    score = 8, positive = 8, contra = 0, max. pct = 45, cand
    pct = 31, crit pct = 45
  4 Bjornstad pili torti—deafness syndrome
    score = 8, positive = 8, contra = 0, max. pct = 33, cand
    pct = 25, crit pct = 33
  5 Deafness, low-tone
    score = 7, positive = 7, contra = 0, max. pct = 63, cand
    pct 63, crit pct 50
  6 Long QT syndrome without deafness
    score = 7, positive = 7, contra = 0, max. pct = 50, cand
    pct = 36, crit pct = 50
  7 Deafness-sensorineural, midfrequency
    score = 7, positive = 7, contra = 0, max. pct = 44, cand
    pct = 44, crit pct = 40
  8 Deafness, dominant low-frequency
    score = 7, positive = 7, contra = 0, max. pct = 40, cand
    pct = 36, crit pct = 40
  9 Ear dysplasias, inner
    score = 7, positive = 7, contra = 0, max. pct = 30, cand
    pct = 16, crit pct = 30
 10 Deafness-sensorineural, progressive high-tone
    score = 6, positive = 6, contra = 0, max. pct = 50, cand
    pct = 26, crit pct = 50

In addition to clinical applications, *Micro BDIS* is designed to run search procedures that can prepare lists of conditions that meet specified criteria and serve other research and educational objectives. Subscribers can build their own knowledgebases and participate in the development and updating of birth defect models. Versions of the system are available in language other than English, and international subscribers are located worldwide.

### ADDITIONAL INFORMATION

Other services provided by the Center include its official journal *Dysmorphology and Clinical Genetics*, as well as its text reference services, available in print and online electronic versions, that provide standardized, comprehensive summaries describing all known birth defects and syndromes.

The Birth Defects Information System will operate on any IBM or compatible personal computer, and is available under license to qualified clinical, research, and educational institutions.

### REFERENCES

1. Edwards CN, Buyse ML: Building a computerized international network for medical expertise: The birth defects information system. *Proceedings of the Fifth National Congress of the American Association for Medical Systems and Informatics.* Anaheim, CA, May 8–10, 1986
2. *Subscriber's Guide to the Computerized Birth Defects Information System,* Dover, MA: Center for Birth Defects Information Services, Inc, 1985

**TABLE BDIS-6.**
Diagnostic Profile

*Case: Testcase Doe, John J., III Age: 1 .10 Sex: M
>Syndinfo 123 Cardioauditory syndrome (1 of 20)
  Score = 15, Positive = 15, Contra = 0
>SSTMatch = 65%, *SSTMatch = 85%

    ***Start of list***
    SEX AND AGE
      Age
#(*)(>)    **age greater than 10 years**
#(*)(>)    **age greater than 18 years**
    HISTORY
      Postnatal history
= * >    **early death (infancy or early childhood)**
    DEFECT OF EAR OR HEARING
      Onset, distribution or progression of ear or hearing defect
= * >    **hearing defect at birth or during infancy**
= * >    **bilateral ear or hearing defect**
      Defect of inner ear or labyrinth
= * >    **defect of cochlea, organ of Corti or cochlear nerve**
% >    Hearing loss or deafness
#(*)(>)    **conductive hearing loss**
= * >    **sensorineural hearing loss**
  >    Other hearing defect (not hearing loss)
    RESPIRATORY OR SPEECH DEFECT
  >    Defect of speech (dysarthria, aphonia)
    DEFECT OF CARDIOVASCULAR SYSTEM
% *    Defect of heart or pericardium
= >    **heart failure**
    DEFECT OF NERVOUS SYSTEM
      Onset and progression of neurologic defect
= * >    **neurologic defect onset in infancy or childhood**
      Defect of cerebral function, consciousness or mentation
= * >    **fainting (syncope)**
  >    other defect of cerebral function or mentation
    DEFECT OF SKIN, HAIR OR NAILS
%(*)    Skin lesions (nonvascular)
- >    pigmented skin lesion (eg, nevi, cafe-au-lait spots)
    HEMATOLOGIC, IMMUNE OR ENDOCRINE SYSTEM DEFECT
% *    Defect of hematologic system
= >    **anemia**
    ***End of List***

The Center continues to issue new releases of *Micro BDIS*^ to keep pace with the expanding knowledgebase and new generations of personal computers. For information on the current release, as well as information on how you can subscribe or submit a clinical case to a licensed subscriber for analysis, request **BDFax**^ document 9700.

## DYSMORPHOLOGY AND CLINICAL GENETICS

The Center's official journal, *Dysmorphology and Clinical Genetics*, was designed specifically to address the needs of the international birth defects community.

DCG^ is a comprehensive scholarly forum for the presentation of current clinical findings in human dysmorphology, and for the systematic analysis of rare and emerging birth defects as well as known and documented conditions and syndromes. The pages of DCG^ feature:

• **Clinical Reports**: well-illustrated case presentations of patients with unusual birth defects and complex malformation syndromes. These reports help to identify and share information about new birth defect syndromes and to prompt recognition of patients with similar findings.

• **Original Articles** delineating new conditions and syndromes, illustrating clinical variability, and documenting the natural history of birth defects.

• **Feature Articles** providing in-depth discussions of special topics such as problems in diagnosis, descriptions of physical findings, difficult counseling problems, and controversial issues.

• **Nomenclature and Classification** serving as an ongoing forum for discussion and debate on problems and controversies in nomenclature and classification.

• **Photo Essays** presenting excellent photographic illustrations accompanied by brief explanatory text to provide an in-depth pictorial review of a particular defect or syndrome.

• **Statistical and Descriptive Reports** of new findings and patterns in birth defects drawn from analyses of clinical case data submitted to the *Unknowns Registry Facility* of the **Birth Defects Information System (BDIS^)**.

• **Reports and Photographic Illustrations** designed to serve as updates and supplements to the *Birth Defects Encyclopedia*.

*Dysmorphology and Clinical Genetics* is an ongoing forum through which readers can share in and shape the evolution of the discipline. For further information, request **BDFax**^ document 9800.

## RESEARCH, EDUCATION, AND PUBLIC INFORMATION

The Center for Birth Defects Information Services operates a number of ongoing research, professional

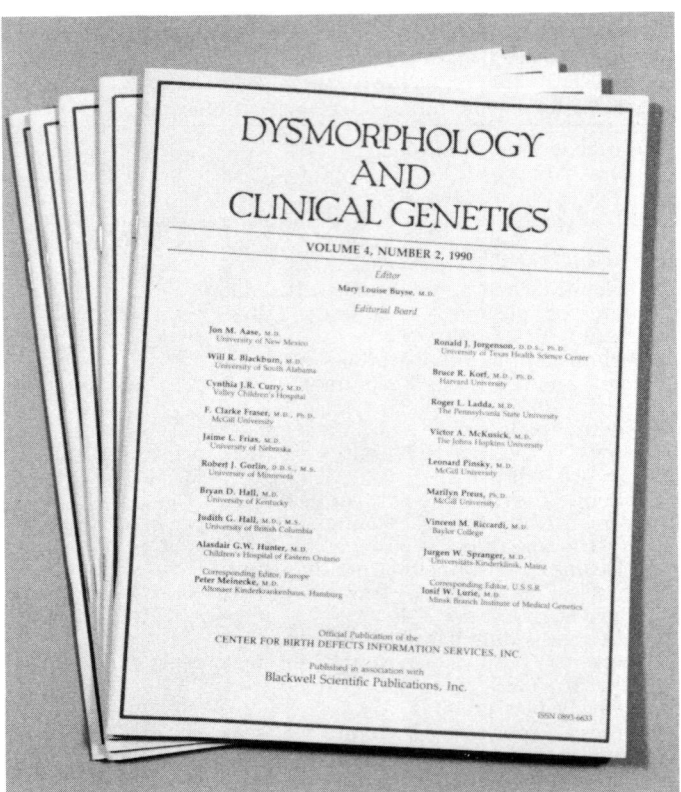

education, and public information programs. Several of these are discussed in Part I of this *Encyclopedia*.

In addition, the power and compactness of the Center's information services have made them particularly popular in emerging nations where medical services are desperately needed but library facilities are extremely limited. The participation of emerging nations in the research and information reporting activities of the Center is furthermore vital to the true understanding of the nature and distribution of human anomalies. For these reasons, the Center has introduced a Grant-in-Aid program where corporate sponsors underwrite specific facilities in designated countries. These awards are granted on the basis of proposals outlining need and the intended use of the facilities. For further information, request **BDFax**^ document 9950.

For general information on current research and education programs, request **BDFax**^ document 9900.

# ❖ HOW TO PARTICIPATE IN THE WORK OF THE CENTER ❖

The programs and services provided by the Center reflect a diversity of technologies, delivery options, and goals designed to assure an integrated, comprehensive response to a critical information need. All of these programs and services do, however, share one thing in common. Each is part of an ongoing, collective commitment to the search for still-undiscovered answers to a vast puzzle as basic as life itself. Each of the tens of thousands of pieces of that puzzle, like the tens of thousands of article elements throughout this *Encyclopedia*, helps to form a completed picture in which every man, woman, and child ultimately shares a vital stake.

This is a pursuit which never ends, and which requires the collective observation and participation of every scientist, clinician, researcher, support group, parent and patient who may ever have reason to be interested in the pages of this book. Clues to the puzzle we all seek to solve are scattered to every corner of the globe, and can only form a picture when gathered together, sifted through, and arranged in successive configurations, in open forum, until yet another pattern is added to the larger whole.

Your role is important, and may prove critical. We welcome your participation, and particularly urge you to:

*Inform* the Center of any error or omission which you may notice in any Center publication or service. Everything from typographical errors to overlooked findings is important, particularly if it can improve the service or make it easier for a future user.

*Observe* differences between published information and conditions as they actually appear in life. The history of the discipline is filled with accounts of people who noticed that their observations did not match those in the literature, but failed to report the differences because they assumed that their experiences were the exception. Report your findings to the Center. Together with those of other observers, they may change the direction of our assumptions.

*Photograph* features which may be noteworthy. Once lost, the opportunity to take a picture may never be regained. But do take the time to learn the basics of good clinical photography, including the use of standards of scale (such as grids and rulers), lighting, and multiple points of view. Also, **do** obtain the necessary legal paperwork. Photographs which show individual identity can NOT be shown if you do not have an accompanying **Consent Form** (in a language understood by the signer) signed by the subject or guardian. While many

forms meet this requirement, a model Form developed by the Center and discussed earlier is recommended and is available in the DCG^ *Author's Guide* or by requesting **BDFax**^ document 9850.

*Submit* illustrated cases to the Center. This is particularly important in the case of rare conditions or syndromes, or when the case can help to clarify the actual Occurence of the condition. Diagnosed or undiagnosed cases are best submitted in the standardized, systematic format of the *Micro BDIS* **Unknowns Registry** facility, but cases in any well-documented form will be accepted. Manuscripts which meet the editorial criteria for *Dysmorphology and Clinical Genetics* are always welcome. In addition, the Center will review and welcomes unsolicited articles submitted to the *Birth Defects Encyclopedia* (in fact, evaluation of possible new *Encyclopedia* entries usually cannot be made without completed manuscripts).

*Donate Illustrations* for preservation by the Center. Each year thousands of irreplaceable clinical photographs are destroyed or lost forever as researchers move, retire, or clean out old files. Many are thrown away on the assumption that journal publishers retain master copies, but most publishers also regularly destroy their back files. With few exceptions, there has never been a systematic program to preserve and catalog vital birth defect illustrations. It was for these reasons that the Center opened its Illustration Library. Through modern digital technologies, illustrations can now be preserved, enhanced, reproduced and transfered entirely through electronic means. Film and prints, which quickly deteriorate, can then be archived for maximum preservation. **Contributors retain legal rights** in the illustrations, but are relieved from the task of filling requests for copies and otherwise preserving and storing their illustrations. All quality illustrations with adequate documentation (including necessary Consents and Releases) are eligible for submission.

*Request information* from the Center when that information can assist in your own work or improve the accuracy and detail of reports which you may later submit to the Center. Most information requests can be handled quickly and easily through **BDFax**^ at any hour of the day or night. Special requests will be directed to the most appropriate specialist.

*Volunteer* to prepare submissions for Center publications, to serve on Boards and Committees, and to otherwise play an active role in the Center's programs

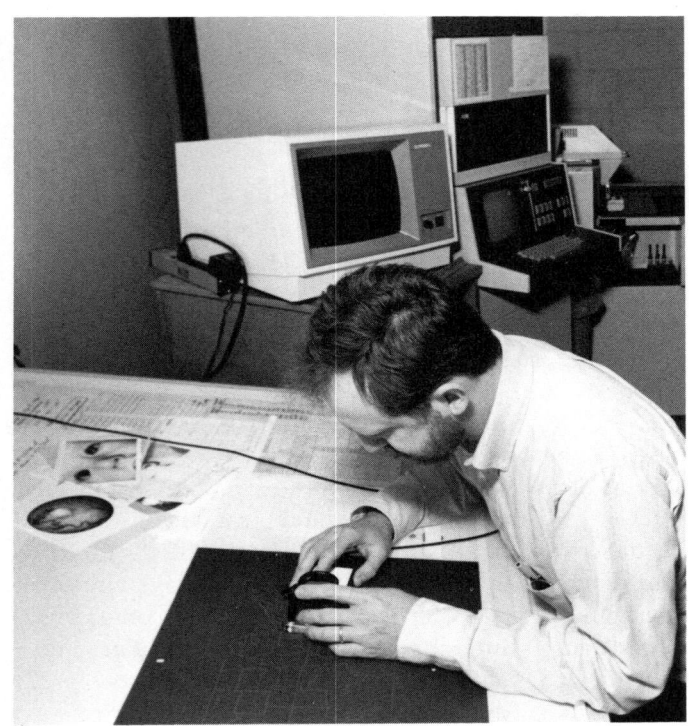

and services. The Center is *your* organization, operated by and for the community which it serves.

*Suggest* new programs or directions, and otherwise share your opinions about the Center and its operations. These can be directed either to the Center directly, or shared in confidence through any member of the Advisory Board.

*Support* the Center. Most of the professional work of the Center is done by volunteers, but the support services and technology needed to maintain an operation of the Center's size and scope are both labor and capital intensive. As a non-profit international scientific collaborative, the Center is entirely dependent upon the generosity of private donors. If you know of anyone who may be interested in contributing to either the operations of the Center as a whole or any of its specific programs through a tax-deductible cash or in-kind donation, please contact the Development Office at (508) 785-2525 Extension 103.

## HOW TO COMMUNICATE WITH THE CENTER

Success of the Center's mission is largely attributable to an efficient network of authors, editors, and other professional specialists united and served by a modern computer-based information processing, communications, and messaging system. Operating around the clock, this system permits the rapid evaluation of incoming communications, and speeds queries, manuscripts,

revisions, and reviews to their most appropriate destination. Most communications are transferred electronically, by fax or modem, across time zones and hemispheres, transcending seasons and oblivious to the rising and setting sun. Yet every year countless communications are lost to us forever because we have no way of knowing who they are from, who they are for, or what they intended to say.

By far the best way to communicate with the Center is in writing. There are very few things that can be acted upon until we have them in writing, so the best way to bring them to the attention of the Center in the first place is *in* writing. Recently, the most popular and effective way to do this has become by *facsimile*. Fax combines the immediacy of the telephone with the detail and permanence of writing at a cost competitive with mail. In addition, the Center's all-electronic paperless fax systems permit quick re-routing of communications to their appropriate destination.

Large manuscripts and illustrations may require delivery by mail or overnight express. Even in these cases, a fax alerting the Center that the package is on its way allows us to prepare reviewers and ensure that the package arrives. Always keep a copy of **anything** you send, and retain negatives and masters of illustrations.

If you do telephone the Center, your incoming call will be processed by an electronic messaging center. This voice mail system allows us to process telephone messages much the way that faxes are processed. Touch-tone^ menus will guide you to answers to common questions or help to route your message. Be prepared to leave a complete detailed message, just as you would if you were dictating a letter.

Unexplained call-back requests can be honored *only* on a time-available basis, and cause needless delay. This is particularly true in view of the fact that most communications involve different time zones, and usually require additional research and possibly consultation within the Center before a proper reply can be formulated. Furthermore, most voice messages can only be acted on *after* they are confirmed in writing.

Submission of manuscripts and reports in machine-readable form is always appreciated, and the Center has both modem facilities and the ability to convert text from most word-processor formats. However, for greatest efficiency it is still fastest if you *fax* a copy of the document followed up by a paper copy **and** diskette version by overnight mail.

**Regardless of your method of communication**, there is some key information that you must **always provide**. In addition to your full **name, degrees, title, affiliation, and complete mailing address**, we also need your **telephone number and fax number**. If you have an **Author Code** including this will help to speed your communication. Finally, if you are communicating about a specific article, you must **indicate the Birth Defect Number or DCG Manuscript Number**.

If you are **responding to a query** RETURN THE ORIGINAL QUERY WITH YOUR REPLY. Unaccompanied notes or messages saying simply ''No'' or ''That's O.K. by me'' are a never-ending source of mystery!

PROOF AND RETURN ALL REVIEW COPIES PROMPTLY. The speed of today's information handling no longer permits the leisure once inherent in print publishing, nor can we assume that unseen eyes will ferret out our oversights, misspellings, and typographical errors. Send all materials in their *final* version, and assume that they are being released to the world.

If you are **suggesting a change** in an *Encyclopedia* entry MARK THE SUGGESTED CHANGE OR REVISION ON THE ARTICLE ITSELF. Provide the *entire* article, showing the Title and Birth Defect Number. If there may be any chance that the version you are working with is out of date, request a current version through **BDFax**^ .

**Please TYPE** everything. The biggest problem in medical publishing is still unreadable handwriting! This not only creates the danger of errors, but it can bring progress to a halt as queries are exchanged and interpretations approved. If your secretary tells you he or she has no trouble with your handwriting, have *them* TYPE it for you or put it on a diskette. Then *proof* their work.

**Request and use Author Guides**. The HOW TO USE THIS ENCYCLOPEDIA section is a good guide to preparing *Encyclopedia* articles. For a *Dysmorphology and Clinical Genetics* **Author's Guide**, which contains copies of the Center's illustration **Consent** and **Release** forms, write

to DCG Guide, Blackwell Scientific Publications, Three Cambridge Center, Suite 208, Cambridge, MA 02142 U.S.A.

**Submit all required Consent, Release, and Agreement documents**. Manuscripts or submissions cannot be processed until these are received at the Center.

**Direct all business correspondence to the appropriate party**. While the Center appreciates hearing about any problems you may have with the Center's publishers or distributors, and will do its best to help in resolving them, **do NOT send order or fulfillment correspondence to the Center** if your business is with a publisher or distributor. Correspondence regarding orders for this *Encyclopedia* should be sent to the appropriate address listed on the copyright page of this book. Correspondence regarding orders or **Author Guide**s for *Dysmorphology and Clinical Genetics* should be directed to the Cambridge office of Blackwell Scientific Publications. Directing these business affairs through the Center will only contribute to their delay. **All manuscripts and editorial correspondence, however, should be sent directly to the Center at:**.

CENTER FOR BIRTH DEFECTS INFORMATION SERVICES, INC.
Dover Medical Building   Box 1776
30 Springdale Avenue
Dover, MA 02030
U.S.A.

Tel. (508) 785-2525
Fax. (508) 785-2526

**Part II**

❖ MASTER INDEX AND ARTICLES ❖

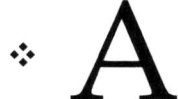

**A Beta-2-microglobulin**
*See AMYLOIDOSIS, HEMODIALYSIS-RELATED*
**A-P window**
*See AORTICO-PULMONARY SEPTAL DEFECT*
**A2m antigens**
*See SERUM ALLOTYPES, HUMAN*
**Aagenaes syndrome**
*See CHOLESTASIS-LYMPHEDEMA, AAGENAES TYPE*
**Aarskog lipodystrophy syndrome**
*See LIPODYSTROPHY-RIEGER ANOMALY-SHORT STATURE-DIABETES*

## AARSKOG SYNDROME                                   0001

**Includes:**

Aarskog-Scott syndrome
Digito-facio-genital syndrome
Facio-digito-genital dysplasia
Faciogenital dysplasia
Genito-facio-digital syndrome
Hypertelorism
Shawl scrotum

**Excludes:** Noonan syndrome (0720)

**Major Diagnostic Criteria:** A male child of short stature who has the major facial features and a "shawl" scrotum. Observation of the characteristic positions of the interphalangeal joints when the fingers are extended might be helpful in establishing the diagnosis.

**Clinical Findings:** Based upon more than 100 reported cases, the principal features of the syndrome are short stature (90%), and facial, digital, and genital malformations.

The birth weight is usually normal for gestational age. In cases in which the growth pattern could be evaluated, the growth deficiency was evident during the first year of life. From 2–4 years of age, growth usually parallels the normal growth curve but remains at or below the third percentile until puberty. Bone age is retarded and corresponds roughly to height age. Endocrine studies, including measurement of serum growth hormone levels, have been normal. One patient showed no response to a therapeutic trial with human growth hormone.

The major facial features include widow's peak (60%), hypertelorism (90%), broad nasal bridge (85%), short nose with anteverted nostrils (90%), and long philtrum (85%). Eyelid ptosis has occurred in about one-half of the cases and usually is pronounced because of the associated antimongoloid obliquity of the palpebral fissures. Ophthalmoplegia, strabismus, hyperopic astigmatism, and large corneas may be additional ophthalmic features. Anomalies of the auricles have been noted in 75% of reported cases.

The limb manifestations consist of short and broad hands (80%), short fifth finger with/without single flexion crease (70%), mild cutaneous **Syndactyly** (60%), and simian line (70%). When the fingers are extended at the metacarpophalangeal joints there is marked hyperextensibility of the proximal interphalangeal joints, with concomitant flexion of the distal joints. This sign seems to be

fairly characteristic of this syndrome. Broad feet with bulbous toes have been encountered in 75% of cases.

The most characteristic genital manifestation consists of a scrotal fold extending dorsally surrounding the base of the penis (80%). Cryptorchidism has been noted in 75% of cases and inguinal hernia in 60%.

Skeletal features include **Pectus excavatum** (60%), metatarsus adductus, and joint laxity.

Although most of the children have normal intelligence (90%), mild mental retardation or learning difficulties apparently occur more often in this group of children than in the general population.

**Complications:** Unknown.

**Associated Findings:** None known.

**Etiology:** Most probably X-linked recessive inheritance.

**Pathogenesis:** Unknown.

**MIM No.:** 10005, *30540

**POS No.:** 3001

**Sex Ratio:** M1:F0

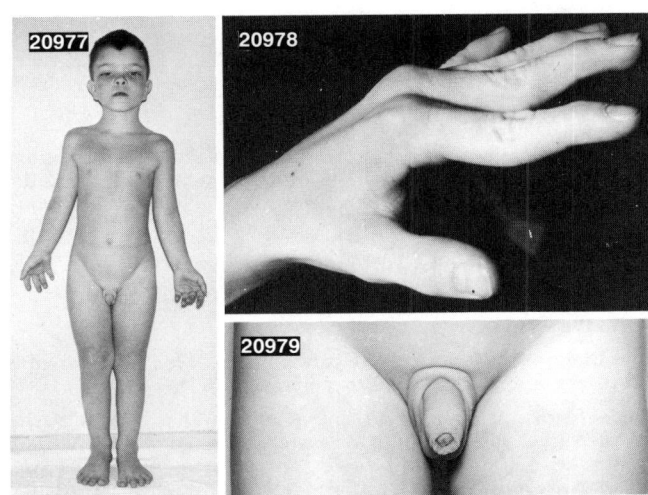

**0001-20977:** Aarskog syndrome; note widow's peak, hypertelorism, mild ptosis, short nose with anteverted nostrils, long philtrum, broad hands and feet, and scrotal fold. **20978:** Hand shows hyperextension at proximal interphalangeal joint and flexion at the distal interphalangeal joints. **20979:** Typical genital morphology demonstrating the scrotal fold encircling the base of the penis.

**Occurrence:** Undetermined; some 100 cases identified.

**Risk of Recurrence for Patient's Sib:**
See Part I, *Mendelian Inheritance.*

**Risk of Recurrence for Patient's Child:**
See Part I, *Mendelian Inheritance.*

**Age of Detectability:** At birth.

**Gene Mapping and Linkage:** FGDY (faciogenital dysplasia (Aarskog syndrome)) has been mapped to Xq13.

**Prevention:** None known. Genetic counseling indicated.

**Treatment:** Surgical treatment of possible cryptorchidism and inguinal hernia.

**Prognosis:** Bone age is delayed. Growth might continue into the late teenage years. Puberty is delayed, but is otherwise normal and is accompanied by a growth spurt. With the exception of affected males in one French-Canadian family, the reported final adult heights have been above 158 cm. The life span appears normal.

**Detection of Carrier:** Varying degrees of short stature and minor facial and digital anomalies may occur in mothers and sisters of affected boys.

**References:**
Aarskog D: A familial syndrome of short stature associated with facial dysplasia and genital anomalies. J Pediatr 1970; 77:856–861. *
Furukawa CT, et al.: The Aarskog syndrome. J Pediatr 1972; 81:1117–1122. *
Berman MB, et al.: The inheritance of the Aarskog facial-digital-genital syndrome. J Pediatr 1975; 86:885–891.
Grier RE, et al.: Autosomal dominant inheritance of the Aarskog syndrome. Am J Med Genet 1983; 15:39–46.
Bawle E, et al.: Aarskog syndrome: full male and female expression associated with an X-autosome translocation. Am J Med Genet 1984; 17:595–602.
van den Bergh, P, et al.: Anomalous cerebral venous draining in Aarskog syndrome. Clin Genet 1984; 25:288–294.

AA002                                    **Dagfinn Aarskog**

**Aarskog-Scott syndrome**
*See AARSKOG SYNDROME*
**Aase syndrome**
*See ANEMIA, HYPOPLASTIC-TRIPHALANGEAL THUMBS, AASE-SMITH TYPE*

---

## AASE-SMITH SYNDROME                          3029

**Includes:**
  Cleft palate-joint contractures-Dandy-Walker malformation
  Dandy-Walker malformation-joint contractures-cleft palate
  Joint contractures-cleft palate-Dandy-Walker malformation

**Excludes:**
  **Arthrogryposis, distal types** (2280)
  **Camptodactyly-trismus syndrome** (0882)
  **Joubert syndrome** (2908)
  **Walker-Warburg syndrome** (2869)

**Major Diagnostic Criteria:** The combination of joint contractures, **Cleft palate**, and Dandy-Walker malformation.

**Clinical Findings:** Joint contractures and cleft hard or soft palate. Dandy-Walker malformation was present in three patients, and oculomotor palsy was present in one. Joint contractures were variable, involving elbows, knees, wrists, and fingers in more severe cases, with **Foot, talipes equinovarus (TEV)** only occurring in less severe cases. Absent finger flexion creases and abnormal fingertip dermal ridge patterns are usually present. Facial features are described as including a broad, prominent forehead with a short nose and micrognathia in infancy and a broad forehead, short palpebral fissures, and ptosis in adulthood.

**Complications:** Unknown.

**Associated Findings:** One individual also had multiple **Ventricular septal defect** and a single sternal ossification center. One had early neuroblastoma. One had strabismus.

**Etiology:** Autosomal dominant inheritance is suggested by the occurrence of the condition in multiple generations, with male-to-male transmission occurring.

**Pathogenesis:** Unknown.

**MIM No.:** *14780

**POS No.:** 3829

**Sex Ratio:** M1:F1

**Occurrence:** Five patients from two families have been reported in detail, although isolated patients described as having Dandy-Walker with other anomalies may also represent this condition.

**Risk of Recurrence for Patient's Sib:**
See Part I, *Mendelian Inheritance.*

**Risk of Recurrence for Patient's Child:**
See Part I, *Mendelian Inheritance.*

**Age of Detectability:** At birth, although prenatal diagnosis by ultrasound may be possible.

**Gene Mapping and Linkage:** Unknown.

**Prevention:** None known. Genetic counseling indicated.

**Treatment:** Treatment of joint contractures and correction of talipes and cleft palate are indicated.

**Prognosis:** Variable, in that one child was stillborn and two died in the neonatal period, whereas two other affected individuals were adults at the time they were reported. The intellect in the two adults was normal in one and borderline normal in the other.

**Detection of Carrier:** Unknown.

**References:**
Aase JM, Smith DW: Dysmorphogenesis of joints, brain and palate: a new dominantly inherited syndrome. J Pediatr 1968; 73:606–609.
Patton MA, et al.: The Aase-Smith syndrome. Clin Genet 1985; 28:521–525.

T0007                                    **Helga V. Toriello**

**Abdominal muscles, absence-urinary tract anomaly-cryptorchidism**
  *See PRUNE-BELLY SYNDROME*
**Abdominal musculature, agenesis, congenital**
  *See PRUNE-BELLY SYNDROME*
**Abdominal wall defect**
  *See GASTROSCHISIS*
**Abducens palsy-skeletal dysplasia-mental retardation**
  *See X-LINKED MENTAL RETARDATION-SKELETAL DYSPLASIA*
**Abductor vocal cord paralysis**
  *See LARYNGEAL PARALYSIS*
**Aberfeld syndrome**
  *See CHONDRODYSTROPHIC MYOTONIA, SCHWARTZ-JAMPEL TYPE*

---

## ABETALIPOPROTEINEMIA                          0002

**Includes:**
  Acanthocytosis
  Apolipoprotein B deficiency
  Bassen-Kornzweig syndrome
  Betalipoprotein deficiency

**Excludes:**
  **Analphalipoproteinemia** (0048)
  **Ophthalmoplegia, progressive external** (0752)

**Major Diagnostic Criteria:** A patient with malabsorption, diffuse CNS signs, and acanthocytes should be studied for this syndrome. A serum immunoelectrophoresis showing absent or greatly reduced betalipoprotein confirms the diagnosis.

**Clinical Findings:** Acanthocytes are found in the blood smear. The primary clinical findings are diarrhea, steatorrhea, ataxia, tremor, muscle weakness and an atypical retinal pigmentation. The intestinal symptoms are the earliest and most consistent (>90%). The neurologic signs and symptoms tend to occur later and are less frequent, though progressive. Of these, areflexia, proprioceptive changes and cerebellar symptoms are the most notable, with muscle weakness and sensory changes less prominent. **Retinitis pigmentosa** eventually occurs in about 50% of the patients. Associated laboratory abnormalities include reduced serum cholesterol and triglycerides. RBC phosphatidyl choline and linoleic acid are reduced, while RBC sphingomyelin is often increased. The red cell peroxide hemolysis test for vitamin E deficiency is positive. Recently, a rare case presenting as vitamin K deficiency with hemorrhage was reported.

**Complications:** A progressive neurologic handicap develops, reflecting damage to the cerebellum, basal ganglia and posterior columns. Blindness can also develop if the retinopathy involves the macula.

**Associated Findings:** $^{51}$Cr RBC survival may be somewhat shortened, but clinical hemolytic anemia does not occur.

**Etiology:** Autosomal recessive inheritance of reduced betalipoprotein synthesis (referable to the deficiency of the principal apoprotein in the low-density lipoproteins). Possibly a variant of abetalipoproteinemia is due to autosomal dominant mode of transmission; *familial hypobetalipoproteinemia.*

**Pathogenesis:** Possibly the malabsorption results from defective chylomicron synthesis (normally dependent upon betalipoprotein), or there may be an intrinsic defect in the small intestine mucosal cell membrane. The low levels of circulating apolipoprotein have been shown to be due to reduced synthesis rather than increased catabolism or redistribution between vascular and extravascular compartments. A basic abnormality in the red blood cell membrane is presumably responsible for the shortened cell survival; defective phospholipid and cholesterol renewal and increased vulnerability to oxidative stress are both suggested as the background for the membrane defect. Reduced erythrocyte levels of vitamin E, secondary to malabsorption, are probably responsible for the abnormal sensitivity of the red cells to exposure to peroxide. The mechanism of the neurologic changes remains puzzling; a defect in myelin membrane function has been suggested.

**MIM No.:** *20010

**POS No.:** 4318

**Sex Ratio:** M1:F1

**Occurrence:** About 40 cases have been published in the literature.

**Risk of Recurrence for Patient's Sib:**
See Part I, *Mendelian Inheritance.*

**Risk of Recurrence for Patient's Child:**
See Part I, *Mendelian Inheritance.*

**Age of Detectability:** Probably at birth or early infancy (blood smear, immunoelectrophoresis).

**Gene Mapping and Linkage:** APOB (apolipoprotein B (including Ag(x) antigen)) has been mapped to 2p24-p23.

**Prevention:** None known. Genetic counseling indicated.

**Treatment:** Infusions of betalipoprotein preparations have not been of value. K.J. Isselbacher has had some success with a diet substituting medium chain length fatty acids in triglycerides. It is assumed that lipid of this sort can be absorbed without the need for chylomicron formation. Although weight gain and reduction in steatorrhea has occurred, the red blood cell and neurologic changes have not been reversed. Parenteral vitamin E or massive oral vitamin E may inhibit erythrocyte peroxide sensitivity in vitro. Though clinical usefulness has not been definitively established, long-term vitamin E therapy seems reasonable, and has been tried in a few instances.

Other therapy should be administered as required for progressive ataxia and other neurologic manifestations.

**Prognosis:** Up to this time deaths have been rare, and patients are known who have survived to the fourth decade.

**Detection of Carrier:** In the variant with autosomal dominant mode of transmission "familial hypobetalipoproteinemia," the parents of patients with homozygous abetalipoproteinemia are heterozygous carriers with reduced levels of lipoproteins.

**Special Considerations:** This rare disorder has special interest because of the multiple systems involved. The common denominator for all of the manifestations appears to be cell membrane deficiencies. Nerve cells, retinal pigment cells, red blood cells, and intestinal mucosa cells are all affected. The possibility that the membranes of these cells are handicapped because of a lack of lipid-carrying protein is intriguing. It does not seem unreasonable that membrane renewal and maintenance could be partially dependent upon such a protein.

**References:**
Bassen FA, Kornzweig AL: Malformation of erythrocytes in a case of atypical retinitis pigmentosa. Blood 1950; 5:381–387.
Isselbacher KJ, et al.: Congenital beta-lipoprotein deficiency; an hereditary disorder involving a defect in the absorption and transport of lipids. Medicine 1964; 43:347–361.
Gotto AM, et al.: On the protein defect in abetalipoproteinemia. New Engl J Med 1971; 284:813.
Biemer JJ, McCammon RE: The genetic relationship of abetalipoproteinemia and hypobetalipoproteinemia: a report of the occurrence of both diseases within the same family. J Lab Clin Med 1976; 85:556.
Azizi E, et al.: Abetalipoproteinemia treated with parenteral and oral vitamins A and E, and with medium chain triglycerides. Acta Paediatr Scand 1978; 67:797–801.
Caballero FM, Buchanan GR: Abetalipoproteinemia presenting as severe vitamin K deficiency. Pediatrics 1980; 65:161.
Muller DPR, et al.: The role of vitamin E in the treatment of the neurological features of abetalipoproteinaemia and other disorders of fat absorption. J Inherit Metab Dis 1985; (Suppl. 1):88–92.
Lackner KJ, et al.: Analysis of the apolipoprotein B gene and messenger ribonucleic acid in abetalipoproteinemia. J Clin Invest 1986; 78:1707–1712.

GA018
SH035

**Bhuwan P Garg
Stephen B. Shohet**

**Abetalipoproteinemia, hereditary**
*See ANEMIA, HEMOLYTIC, RED CELL MEMBRANE DEFECTS*
**Abiotrophic ophthalmoplegia externa**
*See EYE, FIBROSIS OF THE EXTRAOCULAR MUSCLES, GENERALIZED*
*also OPHTHALMOPLEGIA, PROGRESSIVE EXTERNAL*
**Abiotrophies of inner ear**
*See EAR, INNER DYSPLASIAS*
**Ablepharon**
*See EYE, CRYPTOPHTHALMOS WITH OTHER MALFORMATIONS*

---

**ABLEPHARON-MACROSTOMIA**       **2777**

**Includes:** Macrostomia-ablepharon

**Excludes:** Fraser syndrome (2271)

**Major Diagnostic Criteria:** The combination of ablepharon, macrostomia, sparse hair, thickened skin, absent or small nipples, and genital anomalies.

**Clinical Findings:** The three reported cases had absent eyebrows, upper and lower eyelids and eyelashes; macrostomia caused by a lip fusion defect; small, hypoplastic teeth; low-set, abnormal ears; absent or small nipples; ambiguous genitalia (male); dry, coarse, thickened skin; sparse, thin hair; and proximal syndactyly with fingers held in flexion by tight skin over the joints. One child had normal intelligence at age 12 years; the other two were mentally retarded. None had renal or laryngeal anomalies, which are common in **Fraser syndrome**. CT scan in one child demonstrated an absent zygomatic arch.

**Complications:** Corneal irritation and dryness due to lack of eyelids.

**Associated Findings:** One affected child had a ventral hernia with small omphalocele and aberrant urethral bud.

**Etiology:** Possibly autosomal or X-linked recessive inheritance.

**Pathogenesis:** A defect of programmed cell death, as suggested for **Fraser syndrome**, may account for some of the findings.

**MIM No.:** 20011

**POS No.:** 3919

**Sex Ratio:** M3:F0 (observed).

**Occurrence:** Three unrelated male children have been reported.

**Risk of Recurrence for Patient's Sib:**
See Part I, *Mendelian Inheritance*.

**Risk of Recurrence for Patient's Child:**
See Part I, *Mendelian Inheritance*.

**Age of Detectability:** At birth, by physical examination.

**Gene Mapping and Linkage:** Unknown.

**Prevention:** None known. Genetic counseling indicated.

**Treatment:** Reconstructive surgery is indicated, particularly for the eyelid defect.

**Prognosis:** Intellectual development can be normal to mildly retarded; life span is undetermined, although it may be normal.

**Detection of Carrier:** Unknown.

**References:**
McCarthy GT, West CM: Ablepharon macrostomia syndrome. Dev Med Child Neurol 1977; 19:659–672. * †
Hornblass A, Reifler DM: Ablepharon macrostomia syndrome. Am J Ophthal 1985; 99:552–556.
Thomas IT, et al.: Isolated and syndromic cryptophthalmos. Am J Med Genet 1986; 25:85–98.
Jackson IT, et al.: A new feature of the ablepharon macrostomia syndrome: zygomatic arch absence. Br J Plast Surg 1988; 41:410–416. †

T0007                                      **Helga V. Toriello**

## ABRUZZO-ERICKSON SYNDROME                     2365

**Includes:**
Cleft palate-multiple anomalies, Abruzzo-Erickson type
Cleft palate, X-linked

**Excludes:**
**Arthro-ophthalmopathy, hereditary, progressive, Stickler type** (0090)
**Hypertelorism-hypospadias syndrome** (0505)

**Major Diagnostic Criteria:** Cleft palate, coloboma, deafness, hypospadias, radial synostosis, and short stature.

**Clinical Findings:** Birth weight in the affected individuals is within normal limits. Among four affected individuals, including three males and one female, the findings were as follows: malar flatness (4); large ears (4); esotropia (3); coloboma of iris and/or retina (3); epicanthal folds (1); highly arched or cleft palate (3); bifid uvula (1); neurosensory ± conductive deafness (3); **Atrial septal defects** (1); **Kidney, horseshoe** (1); cryptorchidism (1); hypospadias (3); radial synostosis (2); widely spaced second and third fingers (3); ulnar deviation of the second finger (2); small hands and feet (1); short stature (3); and frequent infections (1).

**Complications:** Increased tendency for otitis media, secondary to the **Cleft palate.**

**Associated Findings:** None known.

**Etiology:** X-linked inheritance seems likely in that the anomalies are more severe in males than in females, and all the affected males were related through females, although an autosomal dominant trait with milder expression in females cannot be ruled out.

**Pathogenesis:** Unknown.

**POS No.:** 4057

**Sex Ratio:** M3:F1 (observed)

**Occurrence:** One kinship has been reported.

**Risk of Recurrence for Patient's Sib:**
See Part I, *Mendelian Inheritance.*

**Risk of Recurrence for Patient's Child:**
See Part I, *Mendelian Inheritance.*

**Age of Detectability:** At birth, if cleft palate, coloboma, or hypospadias is present.

**Gene Mapping and Linkage:** Unknown.

**Prevention:** None known. Genetic counseling indicated.

**Treatment:** Surgical correction of palatal cleft, heart defect, and/or hypospadias if indicated; ventilation tube placement for recurrent ear infections; and hearing aids for neurosensory hearing loss.

**Prognosis:** Life span appears to be normal, and intellectual development appears to be within normal limits.

**Detection of Carrier:** If condition is X-linked, mild manifestations of the syndrome in females may indicate carrier status.

**Special Considerations:** Weinstein and Cohen (1966) described a family in which cleft palate, strabismus, low-set, posteriorly rotated ears, and urethral obstruction occurred in an X-linked pattern. It is not known, however, whether this represents the same condition.

**References:**
Weinstein E, Cohen MM: Sex-linked cleft palate: report of a family and review of 77 kindreds. J Med Genet 1966; 3:17–22.
Abruzzo MA, Erickson RP: A new syndrome of cleft palate associated with coloboma, hypospadias, deafness, short stature, and radial synostosis. J Med Genet 1977; 14:76–80.

T0007                                      **Helga V. Toriello**

**Absence defects of limbs, scalp, and skull**
*See LIMB AND SCALP DEFECTS, ADAMS-OLIVER TYPE*
**Absence of intrinsic factor, congenital**
*See ANEMIA, PERNICIOUS CONGENITAL*
**Absence seizures**
*See SEIZURES, CENTRALOPATHIC*
**Acanthocytosis**
*See ANEMIA, HEMOLYTIC, RED CELL MEMBRANE DEFECTS
also ABETALIPOPROTEINEMIA*
**Acanthocytosis-hypobetalipoproteinemia**
*See HYPOBETALIPOPROTEINEMIA*

## ACANTHOCYTOSIS-NEUROLOGIC DEFECTS          2398

**Includes:**
Amyotrophic chorea with acanthocytosis, familial
Choreoacanthocytosis
Levine-Critchley syndrome
Neuroacanthocytosis

**Excludes:**
**Abetalipoproteinemia** (0002)
Acanthocytosis, benign
**Chorea, benign familial** (2306)
**Huntington disease** (0478)
**Lesch-Nyhan syndrome** (0588)

**Major Diagnostic Criteria:** Progressive chorea associated with facial tics, depressed tendon reflexes, muscle atrophy and red cell acanthocytosis with normal amounts of betalipoprotein.

**Clinical Findings:** Usually onset of subtle chorea and facial tics in young adulthood which slowly progress over a period of years and develop into severe truncal and limb chorea with oral-facial dyskinesia and frequent tongue-biting. Mental status generally remains normal, although difficult to evaluate in the late stages of the disorder. Intellectual deterioration has been noted in a few patients. Generalized seizures may occur. Decreased tendon reflexes and later onset of distal muscle weakness and atrophy are common. Ten percent to fifty percent of peripheral red blood cells are acanthocytes. Serum lipids may sometimes be in the low normal range, but betalipoprotein is normal. Creatine kinase is frequently elevated. Electromyogram is often abnormal, showing fasciculations, positive waves, fibrillations, and other signs compatible with neurogenic disease. Nerve conduction velocities are usually normal. EEG may be normal or abnormal, with diffuse slow waves or seizure activity.

**Complications:** Chorea and oral-facial dyskinesias may become severely handicapping requiring wheelchair, restraint, or bed rest. Eating may become difficult. Generalized seizures occur in one-half of the patients. Mental deterioration is reported but uncommon.

**Associated Findings:** A Parkinsonian syndrome with rigidity has been described. Muscle biopsy may show neurogenic atrophy. Computed tomographic (CT) scan or magnetic resonance imaging (MRI) may demonstrate caudate atrophy.

**Etiology:** The history of most families is compatible with autosomal recessive inheritance, and several examples of parental consanguinity are reported. A New England family reported by Estes and Levine (1968) showed probable autosomal dominant inheritance and raises the likelihood of genetic heterogeneity. The autosomal recessive variety seems to be most common.

**Pathogenesis:** Low fluidity of erythrocyte membranes has been reported, but the basic etiology and pathogenesis are unknown. Presumably there is some defect common to erythrocyte and neuronal membranes. Post-mortem examination has shown marked neuronal loss and gliosis of caudate and putamen, with normal activities of glutamic acid decarboxylase and choline acetyl transferase.

**MIM No.:** *20015, *10050

**POS No.:** 4364

**Sex Ratio:** M1:F1

**Occurrence:** At least nine families with two or more affected members have been documented. Cases have been reported from the United States, Great Britain, Japan, and Finland.

**Risk of Recurrence for Patient's Sib:**
See Part I, *Mendelian Inheritance.*

**Risk of Recurrence for Patient's Child:**
See Part I, *Mendelian Inheritance.*

**Age of Detectability:** Typically in the third or fourth decade, but earlier onset has been reported. Red cell acanthocytosis may precede clinical symptoms, but this has not been well-documented.

**Gene Mapping and Linkage:** Unknown.

**Prevention:** None known. Genetic counseling indicated.

**Treatment:** Dopamine-blocking agents such as haloperidol have been of some modest benefit in treating the chorea. Anticonvulsants should be used for seizures.

**Prognosis:** Life span is shortened, and functional impairment from the movement disorder may become severe. Death in the fifth or sixth decade has been reported.

**Detection of Carrier:** Some asymptomatic sibs, parents, and other blood relatives have been noted to have low levels of red cell acanthocytosis (a finding of one percent acanthocytes is normal). The significance of this finding is unclear. It could identify heterozygotes with an autosomal recessive gene, or the very mild expression of an autosomal dominant gene.

**References:**
Critchley EMR, et al.: Acanthocytosis and neurological disorder without abetalipoproteinemia. Arch Neurol 1968; 18:134–140.
Levine IM, et al.: Hereditary neurological disease with acanthocytosis. Arch Neurol 1968; 19:403–409.
Bird TD, et al.: Familial degeneration of the basal ganglia with acanthocytosis: a clinical, neuropathological, and neurochemical study. Ann Neurol 1978; 3:253–258.
Sakai T, et al.: Choreoacanthocytosis. Arch Neurol 1981; 38:335–338.
Gross KB, et al.: Familial amyotrophic chorea with acanthocytosis. Arch Neurol 1985; 42:753–756.
Oshima M, et al.: Erythrocyte membrane abnormalities in patients with amyotrophic chorea with acanthocytosis. J Neuro Sci 1985; 68:147–160.
Spitz MC, et al.: Familial tic disorder, parkinsonism, motor neuron disease, and acanthocytosis. Neurology 1985; 35:366–370.
Vance JM, et al.: Chorea-acanthocytosis: a report of three new families and implications for genetic counseling. Am J Med Genet 1987; 28:403–410.
Villegas A, et al.: A new family with hereditary chorea-acanthocytosis. Acta Haemat 1987; 77:215–219.

BI019 **Thomas D. Bird**

**Acanthosis nigricans**
*See SKIN, ACANTHOSIS NIGRICANS*

## ACATALASEMIA 0006

**Includes:**
> Acatalasemia, type I (Japanese variant of low specific activity)
> Acatalasemia, type II (Swiss variant of low stability)
> Acatalasia
> Takahara syndrome

**Excludes:**
> Allocatalasia
> Other catalase variants with approximately normal activity

**Major Diagnostic Criteria:** Progressive gangrenous lesions of gingiva suggest this condition. Diagnosis confirmed by demonstration that catalase in blood is virtually absent.

**Clinical Findings:** Clinical evidence of acatalasemia (Takahara syndrome) occurs in the mouth only when the hydrogen peroxide concentration in the mucosa is persistently and sufficiently high to injure exposed cells. Progressive gangrenous lesions may involve the gingiva and alveolar bone with loss of teeth.

Catalase activity is almost completely absent in the blood of homozygotes. The level of catalase in tissues is also reduced, but apparently to a variable degree. The red cells have a high sensitivity to reagent-$H_2O_2$, to agents generating peroxides, and to X-irradiation. Detection of homozygous and heterozygous individuals can be accomplished only by screening.

Absence of catalase in blood can be proved by adding a drop of blood to 2 ml of 2% $H_2O_2$. If the sample contains a normal amount of catalase, there is immediate foaming, but no change in color. If the sample contains less than about 5% of the normal catalase concentration, no foaming occurs; however, the color rapidly changes to brown and then to white due to hemoglobin oxidation. Leukocytes and cultured skin fibroblasts are also deficient in catalase.

**Complications:** A special form of gangrene similar to noma affecting about 50% of Japanese homozygotes. Children are especially affected.

**Associated Findings:** None known.

**Etiology:** Autosomal dominant inheritance of an enzyme defect. Also occurs in mice and guinea pigs.

**Pathogenesis:** Deficiency of catalase in blood and tissue. Instead of the normal enzyme, a variant of very low specific activity (type I) or an unstable variant (type II) are synthesized. Oral organisms produce $H_2O_2$, which accumulates and injures exposed tissues by oxidation.

**MIM No.:** *11550

**Sex Ratio:** M1:F1

**Occurrence:** The genes responsible for acatalasemia are rare but highly variable in occurrence, e.g., in a screening covering 73,661 individuals in Switzerland three homozygotes were detected. From this figure an average gene frequency of 0.0064 was calculated. No homozygote has been reported from the United States.

Large-scale screening in East Asia revealed considerable variation as to frequency of heterozygotes for acatalasemia type I, namely 1:77 in North Korea, 1:115 in North China, 1:323 in Taiwan, and 1:400 in Japan. Based on these data a total average gene frequency of 0.00083 was calculated.

**Risk of Recurrence for Patient's Sib:**
See Part I, *Mendelian Inheritance.*

**Risk of Recurrence for Patient's Child:**
See Part I, *Mendelian Inheritance.*

**Age of Detectability:** Unknown.

**Gene Mapping and Linkage:** CAT (catalase) has been mapped to 11p13.

**Prevention:** Careful oral and dental hygiene, good nutrition.

**Treatment:** Excision of oral gangrenous lesions, extraction of involved teeth, and systemic antibiotic treatment. (Healing capability of tissue is normal.)

**Prognosis:** Normal life span unless sepsis is untreated.

**Detection of Carrier:** The heterozygote carrier state for acatalasemia can be detected by measuring catalase activity in blood (type I) or by means of heat stability and electrophoretic mobility tests (Type II). Depending on the type of acatalasemia, the level of activity in blood of heterozygotes varies between 35% and 60% (type I) or 60% and 100% (type II).

**Special Considerations:** There are now 96 individuals known to be homozygous for acatalasemia (84 in Japan, 11 in Switzerland, and 1 in Israel). Heterogeneity must be assumed because several types of acatalasemia can be distinguished. Variations are found in the level of residual catalase activity in blood of homozygotes and heterozygotes, in cellular distribution of residual activity among the red cell population, in the frequency of Takahara syndrome, and, finally, in combination with another enzyme deficiency (e.g., G6PD).

In allocatalasia a normal level of catalase activity in blood is associated with an unusually fast electrophoretic mobility of the enzyme. Here, apparently, a variant catalase exerting normal activity and stability is synthesized. Detection and investigation of more individuals homozygous for acatalasemia are desirable for practical reasons. Most likely catalase-deficient cells (notably erythrocytes) have an increased sensitivity toward X-irradiation or toward certain drugs producing oxidizing radicals, e.g., hydrazine derivatives. On the other hand, their ability to oxidize methanol is probably reduced.

**References:**
Aebi H, et al.: Heterogeneity of erythrocyte catalase. Eur J Biochem 1974; 48:137 and 1976; 69:603. *
Wyss SR, Aebi H: Properties of leukocyte catalase in Swiss type acatalasemia: a comparative study of normals, heterozygotes and homozygotes. Enzyme 1975; 20:257.
Aebi H, et al.: Properties of erythrocyte catalase from homozygotes and heterozygotes for Swiss-type acatalasemia. Biochem Genet 1976; 14:791. *
Matsunaga T, et al.: Congenital acatalasemia: a study of neutrophil functions after provocation with hydrogen peroxide. Pediat Res 1985; 19:1187–1190.
Eaton JW: Acatalasemia. In: Scriver CR, et al, eds: The metabolic basis of inherited disease, 6th ed. New York: McGraw-Hill, 1989:1551–1563.

WY003

**Sonja R. Wyss**
*Hugo Aebi*

**Acatalasemia, type I (Japanese variant of low specific activity)**
*See ACATALASEMIA*
**Acatalasemia, type II (Swiss variant of low stability)**
*See ACATALASEMIA*
**Acatalasia**
*See ACATALASEMIA*
**ACC**
*See SKIN, LOCALIZED ABSENCE OF*
**Accelerated AV conduction**
*See ARRHYTHMIA, WOLFF-PARKINSON-WHITE TYPE*
**Accelerated skeletal maturation syndrome**
*See MARSHALL-SMITH SYNDROME*
**Accessory hepatic lobes**
*See LIVER, ACCESSORY LOBE*
**Accessory lung arising from bronchial tree, esophagus, and stomach**
*See LUNG, ABERRANT LOBE*
**Accessory lung with foregut communication**
*See LUNG, ABERRANT LOBE*
**Accutane^, fetal effects of**
*See FETAL RETINOID SYNDROME*
**Acetaldehyde dehydrogenase-2 (ALDH2) deficiency**
*See ALCOHOL INTOLERANCE*
**Acetyl CoA:alpha-glucosaminide N-acetyltransferase deficiency**
*See MUCOPOLYSACCHARIDOSIS III*

**Acetylator phenotype, slow**
*See NEUROPATHY, HERITABLE ISONIAZIDE TYPE (INH)*

## ACETYLATOR POLYMORPHISM 0007

**Includes:**
Hyperacetylation
Hypoacetylation
Isoniazid inactivation
Rapid isoniazid (INH) inactivation

**Excludes:** N/A

**Major Diagnostic Criteria:** Plasma isoniazid half-life after intravenous dose of isoniazid and after oral isoniazid.

Plasma concentration isoniazid, e.g., 6 hours after 10 mg oral isoniazid per kilogram of body weight, > about 2.5 $\mu$g/ml = slow acetylation, whereas < 2.5 $\mu$g/ml = rapid acetylation.

Ratio urinary acetylisoniazid to acid-labile isoniazid in urine, e.g., 3 hours after 5 mg/kg intravenously.

Percentage sulfamethazine in the acetylated form in 1) 1-hour urine collection 5 to 6 hours after drug ingestion, and 2) serum collected 6 hours after ingestion of 40 mg sulfamethazine per kilogram of metabolically active mass (= weight to the power of 0.7). Doses vary between 500 and 1,000 mg. Analyses can be automated. Sulfapyridine can be used instead of sulfamethazine. All these procedures give a bimodal frequency distribution (or a 2-cloud scatterogram) separating persons into rapid and slow acetylators. It is also possible to perform phenotyping using dapsone and by estimating the ratio of 5-acetylamino-6-amino-3-methyl uracil (the deformylated derivative of 5-acetyl amino-6-formyl amino-3-methyl uracil) to 1-methyl xanthine in the urine after the subject has ingested a cup of coffee.

**Clinical Findings:** This genetic polymorphism, like the ABO blood groups and other polymorphisms, occurs in normal healthy persons. The medical importance of this polymorphism lies first in its influence on the outcome of medical treatments and second, on the fact that it is becoming increasingly likely that different phenotypes are more prone to certain common spontaneous disorders.

The existence of polymorphic acetylation has been demonstrated for isoniazid, hydralazine, salicylazosulfapyridine, dapsone, sulfamethazine, procainamide, aminoglutethimide, and the amino metabolites of nitrazepam and clonazepam.

Slow acetylators are more prone than rapid acetylators to peripheral neuropathy on conventional doses of isoniazid; phenytoin toxicity when also on isoniazid; various adverse reactions when under treatment with hydralazine, dapsone, and salicylazosulfapyridine; and hepatotoxicity when rifamyicin and isoniazid are used in combination.

Rapid acetylators 1) have less favorable results when open tuberculosis is treated with a once-weekly isoniazid dosage regime and 2) require higher doses of hydralazine to control hypertension, and of dapsone to control dermatitis herpetiformis.

Recent publications report associations between phenotypes and spontaneous disorders: 1) slow acetylation is associated with bladder cancer, bronchial cancer, Gilbert disease, leprosy in Chinese, and an earlier age of onset of Graves disease; and 2) rapid acetylation is associated with diabetes mellitus in Europeans and with breast cancer.

**Complications:** Drug toxicity or therapeutic ineffectiveness.

**Associated Findings:** None known.

**Etiology:** Autosomal recessive inheritance. Populations are polymorphic for acetylation. Individuals are either slow or rapid acetylators using conventional phenotyping tests. Slow acetylators are recessive homozygotes. The dominant rapid acetylator includes both heterozygous and homozygous rapid acetylator genotypes. A rather more elaborate test using sulphamethazine may be successful in separating the three genotypes.

**Pathogenesis:** Unknown.

**MIM No.:** *24340

**Sex Ratio:** M1:F1

**Occurrence:** About 35–50% of Caucasian and African populations and about 90% of the Japanese are rapid acetylators.

**Risk of Recurrence for Patient's Sib:**
See Part I, *Mendelian Inheritance*.

**Risk of Recurrence for Patient's Child:**
See Part I, *Mendelian Inheritance*.

**Age of Detectability:** Difficult below 4 or 5 years with most of the above phenotyping procedures.

**Gene Mapping and Linkage:** Unknown.

**Prevention:** None known. Genetic counseling indicated.

**Treatment:** Adjustment or substitution of therapeutic agents, use of plasma drug levels, and use of pyridoxine, with isoniazid if possible.

**Prognosis:** It has been suggested that slow acetylators are more prone than rapid acetylators to develop spontaneous lupus erythematosus. Further surveys now show that this is unlikely to be true.

**Detection of Carrier:** Unknown.

**References:**

Evans DAP, et al.: Genetic control of isoniazid metabolism in man. Br Med J 1960; 2:485–491.

Evans DAP, White TW: Human acetylation polymorphism. J Lab Clin Med 1964; 63:394–403.

Karim AKMB, et al.: Human acetylator polymorphism: estimate of allele frequency in Libya and details of global distribution. J Med Genet 1981; 18:325–330.

Evans DAP: Survey of the human acetylator polymorphism in spontaneous disorders. J Med Genet 1984; 21:243–253.

Weber WW, Hein DW: N-Acetylation pharmacogenetics. Pharmacol Rev 1985; 37:25–79. *

Tang BK, Zubovits T, Kalow W: Determination of acetylated caffeine metabolites by high-performance exclusion chromatography. J Chromatog 1986; 375:170–173.

EV000                                          **David A. Price Evans**

**Acetylcholine receptor, defect in**
*See MYASTHENIC SYNDROME, FAMILIAL INFANTILE TYPE*
**Achalasia, esophageal**
*See ESOPHAGUS, ACHALASIA*
**Acheiropodia**
*See ACHEIROPODY*

---

## ACHEIROPODY                                 2486

**Includes:**
    Acheiropodia
    Brazilian type acheiropody
    Footless and handless families of Brazil
    Handless and footless families of Brazil

**Excludes:**
    **Hypoglossia-hypodactylia** (0451)
    Peromelia

**Major Diagnostic Criteria:** Congenital absence of hands, feet, forearms, and fists, followed by atrophy of arms and legs; a very specific anomaly that should not be confused with similar cases.

**Clinical Findings:** Relatively uniform anomaly in its general anatomic and morphologic aspects. Characterized by the presence of the shoulder joint and humerus, the almost uniform absence of the humerus-radius-ulnar joint, absence of the forearm and hand, reduction of the tibia to its proximal two-thirds, and absence of the fibula and foot. Some variations, including length of the remaining parts and thickness of the stumps, can be found both between individuals and between the two sides of the same affected person. In some but not all of the affected individuals, an elongated small bone (Bohomoletz bone) has been detected in the distal part of the upper stump, parallel to the humerus axis. In other cases, the presence of a finger or fingers has been described. This bone and vestigial finger(s) may have the same origin and represent osteogenic nuclei of the forearm and carpal bones.

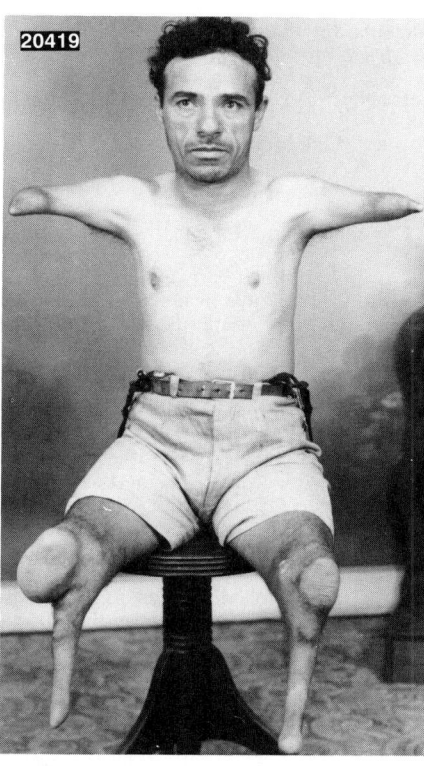

2486-20419: Acheiropody; note the hypertrophy in the knee was due to an accident.

In a search for possible pleiotropic effects of the gene, laboratory analyses were performed, with negative results. Clinical and X-ray examinations of the acheiropods failed to show involvement of other organs. X-ray analyses of the limbs of some of the heterozygous parents of the acheiropods were performed, and the results were normal. No evidence of a chromosomal abnormality has been found. No recognizable dermatoglyphic pattern was found.

**Complications:** Eventual hypertrophy (of a functional nature) of the knees.

**Associated Findings:** Possible presence of a finger or fingers, with or without nail, or a small bone in the upper stumps.

**Etiology:** Autosomal recessive inheritance, with full penetrance and some variability in expression. Consanguinity was found in some 82% of parents.

**Pathogenesis:** Unknown. The absence of large vessels in the legs of one acheiropod beyond the knees has been reported. Whether this is a cause or effect of the basic pathogenetic disturbance remains unknown.

**MIM No.:** *20050

**Sex Ratio:** M1:F1

**Occurrence:** Apparently the anomaly has thus far been detected only in Brazil, in families with Portuguese ancestry. The prevalence in Brazil has been tentatively estimated as 3:10,000,000, with at least 22 identified sibships. It is suggested that all Brazilian acheiropods can be traced to a single mutation. A conservative estimate of the number of acheiropods to appear in the future in Brazil is 14,000, with an extinction time of no less than 2,300 generations, or almost 70,000 years.

**Risk of Recurrence for Patient's Sib:**
See Part I, *Mendelian Inheritance*.

**Risk of Recurrence for Patient's Child:**
See Part I, *Mendelian Inheritance.*

**Age of Detectability:** At birth, or prenatally by ultrasound.

**Gene Mapping and Linkage:** Unknown.

**Prevention:** None known. Genetic counseling indicated.

**Treatment:** Prosthetic replacement.

**Prognosis:** Normal stillbirth rate. Higher infant mortality rate, particularly in the first 10 days of life. Physical handicaps lead to a change in lifestyle, but patients adapt well to the use of prosthetic devices. Fertility is diminished due to the cosmetic effects. Intelligence is normal.

**Detection of Carrier:** Unknown.

**Special Considerations:** Cases that do not conform strictly to published criteria should not be classified as acheiropody.

No evidence has been found for the existence of an appreciable number of recessive lethal mutations in the vicinity of the acheiropody locus. Dermal ridges were not found on the tips of the stumps, but an atypical dermatoglyphic configuration was documented on the hypoplastic digits found at the tips of the limbs of two acheiropods; one apparently normal brother of acheiropods had an abnormal pattern found in only 1–2% of the general population. Results of routine and hormonal laboratory tests, excretory urography, EKG, visual acuity, and Ishihara tests were normal. The acheiropody genotype is under the action of strong reproductive selection (s = 0.83). The frequency of consanguineous marriages among the parents of the acheiropods (more than 82%) is one of the highest found thus far in a genetic disorder. No evidence for a birth-order effect was found. The mean sibship size of the acheiropods is twice as great as that of other mean sibship sizes in their families (8 vs. 4), and correction for ascertainment bias did not greatly diminish the difference.

The estimated proportion of sporadic cases in the total population of cases was not significantly different from zero. Although acheiropods have the enormous handicap of being born without hands and feet, in large part they are able to overcome their difficulties; they can therefore be used in genetic counseling as a vivid example that there are few incapable people, just people with different capacities for different jobs.

**References:**
Toledo SPA, et al.: Handless and footless families of Brazil (acheiropody): cytogenetics, dermatoglyphics and laboratory aspects. Proc 13th Int Congr Pediatr 1971; II:477–480.
Freire-Maia A, et al.: Genetics of acheiropodia (the handless and footless families of Brazil). VI: formal genetic analysis. Am J Hum Genet 1975; 27:521–527.
Freire-Maia A, et al.: Genetics of acheiropodia (the handless and footless families of Brazil). X: roentgenologic study. Am J Med Genet 1978; 2:321–330.
Marçallo FA, et al.: Genetics of acheiropodia (the handless and footless families of Brazil). XI: pathologic aspects. Am J Med Genet 1979; 4:287–291.
Freire-Maia A: The extraordinary handless and footless families of Brazil: 50 years of acheiropodia. Am J Med Genet 1981; 9:31–41. *
Morton NE, Barbosa CAA: Age, area, and acheiropody. Hum Genet 1981; 57:420–422.
Grimaldi A, et al.: Variable expressivity of the acheiropodia gene. (Letter) Am J Med Genet 1983; 16:631–634.

FR036                                              **Ademar Freire-Maia**

**Achondrogenesis (McKusick type 1B)**
*See ACHONDROGENESIS, LANGER-SALDINO TYPE*
**Achondrogenesis (Whitley & Gorlin type II)**
*See ACHONDROGENESIS, LANGER-SALDINO TYPE*
**Achondrogenesis (Whitley & Gorlin type III)**
*See ACHONDROGENESIS, LANGER-SALDINO TYPE*
**Achondrogenesis (Whitley & Gorlin type IV)**
*See ACHONDROGENESIS, LANGER-SALDINO TYPE*

**Includes:**
   Achondrogenesis, type I
   Achondrogenesis, type IA
**Excludes:**
   **Achondrogenesis** (other)
   **Grebe syndrome** (0445)
   **Thanatophoric dysplasia** (0940)
   **Thanatophoric dysplasia, Glasgow type** (2821)

**Major Diagnostic Criteria:** Lethal neonatal dwarfism with characteristic clinical, X-ray, and histopathologic features.

**Clinical Findings:** This disorder is a form of neonatal dwarfism associated with second trimester polyhydramnios, prematurity, fetal hydrops, and death either *in utero* or shortly thereafter. The head may be soft; however, its size is accurate for gestational age. The neck is shortened, trunk is barrel-shaped, and there is extreme shortening of the limbs. On X-ray, there is poorly ossified skull and complete lack of ossification of the vertebral bodies. The ribs are very short, cupped, and flared, with multiple fractures. The pelvis ossifies poorly, with an arched configuration to the ilia. The ischium is very hypoplastic. The long tubular bones are extremely short, with metaphyseal changes on both proximal and distal ends. The femur has a wedge-like configuration. The tibia, fibulae, radii, and ulnae are ossified, even though short, in all patients.

**Complications:** Intrauterine or neonatal death.

**Associated Findings:** None known.

**Etiology:** Autosomal recessive inheritance.

**Pathogenesis:** A distinct abnormal pattern of chondro-osseous morphology is present. The resting chondrocytes lie in a large lacunae, with a round, centrally located nucleus giving rise to a "bull's eye" appearance and containing unusual cytoplasmic inclusion bodies.

**MIM No.:** *20060, *20061

**Sex Ratio:** Presumably M1:F1, although observed cases show a male predominance.

**Occurrence:** At least two families have been described.

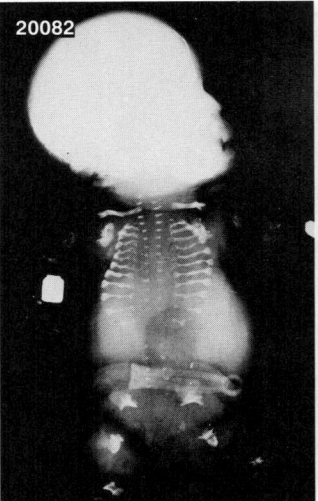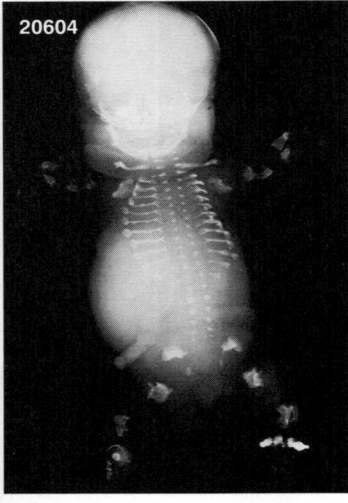

**2870-20082:** X-ray of a stillborn infant shows short ribs without fractures, ossified posterior pedicles of the spine and short stellate long bones. The ilium is crenated; the ischium is unossified. **20604:** Short ribs, ossified posterior pedicles of the spine and short, stellate long bones.

**Risk of Recurrence for Patient's Sib:**
See Part I, *Mendelian Inheritance.*

**Risk of Recurrence for Patient's Child:**
See Part I, *Mendelian Inheritance.* Affected individuals are not expected to survive to reproduce.

**Age of Detectability:** At birth. Prenatal diagnosis through midtrimester (14–16 weeks gestation) by ultrasound is potentially available.

**Gene Mapping and Linkage:** Unknown.

**Prevention:** None known. Genetic counseling indicated.

**Treatment:** Unknown.

**Prognosis:** Fatal in the neonatal period.

**Detection of Carrier:** Unknown.

**References:**
Harris R, et al.: Pseudo-achondrogenesis with fractures. Clin Genet 1972; 3:435–441.
Houston CS, et al.: Fetal neonatal dwarfism. J Can Radiol 1972; 23:45–61.
Rimoin DL: The chondrodystrophies. Adv Hum Genet 1975; 5:10–118.
Borochowitz Z, et al.: Achondrogenesis type I: delineation of further heterogeneity and identification of two distinct subgroups. J Pediatr 1988; 112:23–31.

B0025                                      **Zvi Borochowitz**

## ACHONDROGENESIS, LANGER-SALDINO TYPE     0008

**Includes:**
Achondrogenesis (McKusick type 1B)
Achondrogenesis, type II
Achondrogenesis (Whitley & Gorlin type II)
Achondrogenesis (Whitley & Gorlin type III)
Achondrogenesis (Whitley & Gorlin type IV)
Chondrogenesis imprefecta
Langer-Saldino achondrogenesis

**Excludes:**
**Achondrogenesis, Houston-Harris type** (2870)
**Achondrogenesis, Parenti-Fraccaro type** (0009)
**Grebe syndrome** (0445)

**Major Diagnostic Criteria:** Lethal neonatal dwarfism with short trunk and very short limbs; decreased ossification of lumbar vertebrae and absent ossification of sacrum and pubis. Skull is enlarged but ossification is normal.

**Clinical Findings:** This form of neonatal dwarfism is often associated with prematurity and hydrops. It is characterized by a very large head and severe shortening of the limbs, neck, and trunk which is often square in shape. On X-ray, there are short ribs, hypoplastic iliac wings, flat acetabular roofs, short broad femora and metaphyseal irregularities. The pedicles are ossified, but there is variable ossification of the vertebral bodies. At the severe end of the spectrum the entire spine and sacrum are unossified. Less severely affected cases show ossification defects only of the cervical vertebrae and sacrum.

**Complications:** Intrauterine or neonatal death.

**Associated Findings:** None known.

**Etiology:** Autosomal recessive and probably autosomal dominant inheritance.

**Pathogenesis:** The characteristic histopathologic abnormalities at the growth plate, ie hypertrophic chondrocytes with little intervening matrix, and presence of type I rather than type II collagen in epiphyseal cartilage suggest a defect in synthesis or secretion of cartilage matrix.

**MIM No.:** *20061

**POS No.:** 3004

**Sex Ratio:** M1:F1

**Occurrence:** Undetermined but infrequent.

**Risk of Recurrence for Patient's Sib:**
See Part I, *Mendelian Inheritance.*

**Risk of Recurrence for Patient's Child:** Affected individuals are not expected to survive to reproduce.

**Age of Detectability:** At birth. Prenatal diagnosis is potentially available in midtrimester by ultasonography.

**Gene Mapping and Linkage:** Unknown.

**Prevention:** None known. Genetic counseling indicated.

**Treatment:** Unknown.

**Prognosis:** Fatal in neonatal period, except for mildest case who may survive a few weeks.

**Detection of Carrier:** Unknown.

**Special Considerations:** There is wide variation in severity ranging from severely affected cases who were previously considered typical achondrogenesis (Langer-Saldino) to milder cases that were previously labeled hypochondrogenesis. Cases of intermediate severity have been reported suggesting a continuous spectrum of severity. Biochemical and histologic studies of growth cartilage show the same changes throughout the spectrum supporting this view but not excluding the possibility of several allelic disorders with overlapping phenotypes. The nomenclature is confusing because Whitley and Gorlin have suggested the designations achondrogenesis type II-IV, McKusick has used the designation 1B, and others have employed achondrogenesis type II (Langer-Saldino) for the entire spectrum.

**References:**
Saldino RM: Lethal short-limbed dwarfism: achondrogenesis and thanatophoric dwarfism. Am J Roentgen 1971; 112:185–197.
Spranger JW, et al.: Bone dysplasias: an atlas of constitutional disorders of skeletal development. Philadelphia, WB Saunders, 1974:26.

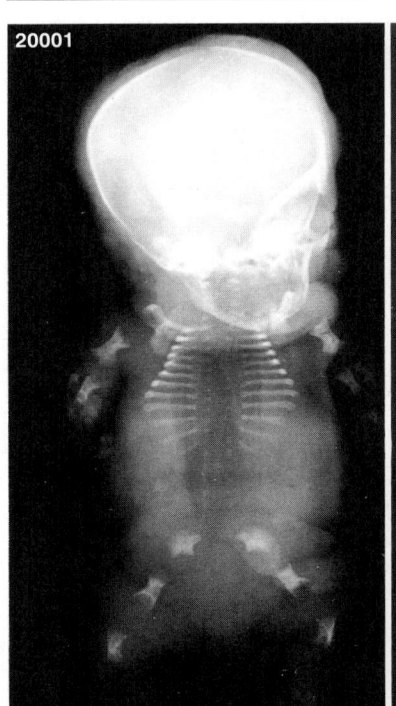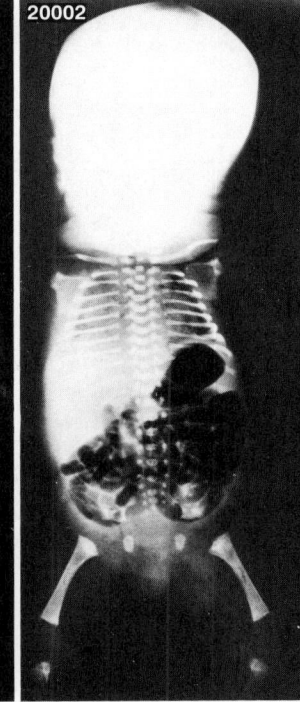

**0008A-20001:** Achondrogenesis, Langer-Saldino type: X-ray of a severely affected infant showing short long bones with severe metaphyseal changes and almost unossified vertebral bodies. **20002:** Moderately affected infant with better ossified vertebral bodies and long bones without metaphyseal irregularities.

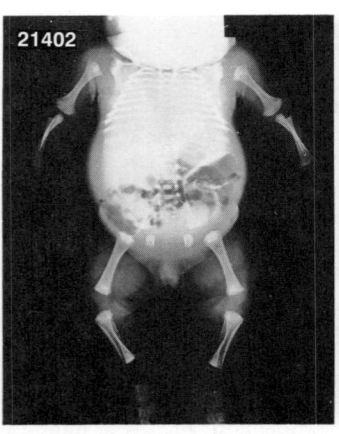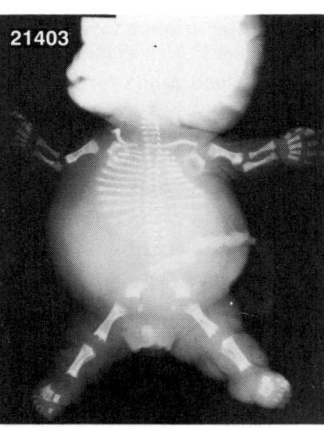

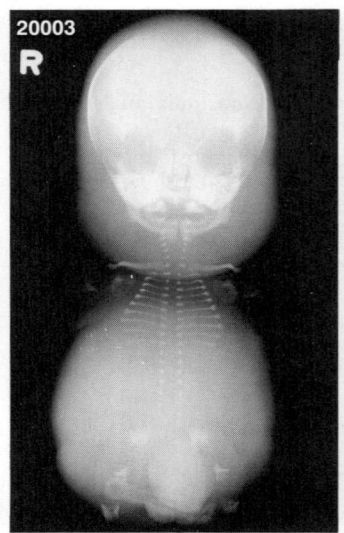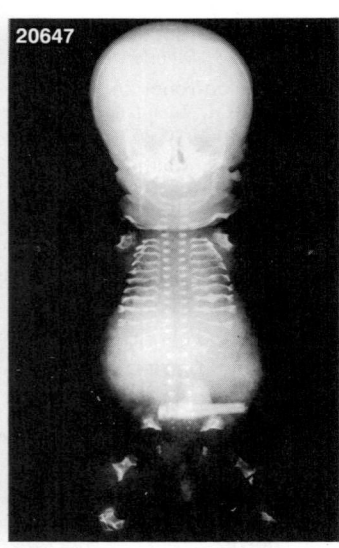

**0008B-21402:** X-ray of mildly affected infant; note the degree of ossification of the vertebral bodies, the better modeled femora with no metaphyseal irregularities, and the larger ischium. These changes are similar to those seen in cases of spondyloepiphyseal dysplasia congenita at birth. **21403:** X-ray of a more severely affected infant shows short femora with severe metaphyseal irregularities of the distal and proximal ends and the almost unossified vertebral bodies. The ischium is not ossified.

**0009-20003:** X-ray of a still born infant showing short fractured ribs with unossified spine and short long bones. The ilium is arched and the ischium hypoplastic. **20647:** Absent ossification of the vertebral bodies, short ribs with multiple fractures, small and square iliac wings, marked shortness of the tubular bones with concave ends.

Chen H, et al.: Achondrogenesis: a review with special considerations of achondrogenesis type II (Langer-Saldino). Am J Med Genet 1981; 10:379–394.
Whitley CB, Gorlin RJ: Achondrogenesis, new hosology with evidence of genetic heterogeneity. Radiology 1983; 148:693–698.
Borochowitz Z, et al.: Achondrogenesis II - Hypochondrogenesis, variability, versus heterogeneity. Am J Med Genet 1986; 24:273–288.
Horton WA, et al.: Achondrogenesis type II, abnormalities of extracellular matrix. Pediatr Res 1987; 22:324–329.

H0033
H0025                                                      **William A. Horton**
                                                           **O.J. Hood**

## ACHONDROGENESIS, PARENTI-FRACCARO TYPE          0009

**Includes:**
   Achondrogenesis, type I
   Achondrogenesis, type IA

**Excludes:**
   **Achondrogenesis, Houston-Harris type** (2870)
   **Achondrogenesis, Langer-Saldino type** (0008)
   **Grebe syndrome** (0445)
   **Thanatophoric dysplasia** (0940)

**Major Diagnostic Criteria:** Lethal neonatal dwarfism with characteristic clinical, X-ray and histopathologic features.

**Clinical Findings:** This disorder is a form of neonatal dwarfism associated with prematurity, fetal hydrops, and death either in utero or shortly thereafter. The clinical presentation is indistinguishable from **Achondrogenesis, Houston-Harris type.** The head is soft, but its size is accurate for gestational age. The neck is shortened, the trunk is barrel-shaped, and there is extreme shortening of the limbs. On X-ray there is poorly ossified skull, and the vertebral bodies are not ossified; however, some punctate posterior pedicles are seen. The ribs are very short, with cupped and flared ends, but lack fractures. The ilia is crenated, and the ischium is not ossified. The long bones are stellate in configuration.

**Complications:** Intrauterine or neonatal death.

**Associated Findings:** None known.

**Etiology:** Autosomal recessive inheritance.

**Pathogenesis:** A distinct abnormal pattern of chondro-osseous morphology is present, with an abnormal matrix devoid of collagen fibrils and a dense ring of collagen fibrils that surrounds the chondrocytes and fills in the lacunar space. The chondrocytes do not contain inclusion bodies.

**MIM No.:** *20060

**POS No.:** 3004

**Sex Ratio:** Presumably M1:F1, although reported cases have shown a slight predominance of females.

**Occurrence:** Some 15 cases documented in the literature.

**Risk of Recurrence for Patient's Sib:**
   See Part I, *Mendelian Inheritance.*

**Risk of Recurrence for Patient's Child:**
   See Part I, *Mendelian Inheritance.* Affected individuals are not expected to survive to reproduce.

**Age of Detectability:** At birth. Prenatal diagnosis through midtrimester (14–16 weeks gestation) by ultrasound is potentially available.

**Gene Mapping and Linkage:** Unknown.

**Prevention:** None known. Genetic counseling indicated.

**Treatment:** Unknown.

**Prognosis:** Fatal in neonatal period.

**Detection of Carrier:** Unknown.

**References:**
Parenti GC: La anosteogenesi. Pathologica 1936; 28:447–462.
Rimoin DL: The chondrodystropies. Adv Hum Genet 1975; 5:1–118.
Smith WL, et al.: In utero diagnosis of achonodrogenesis, type I. Clin Genet 1981; 19:51–54.
Borochowitz Z, et al.: Achondrogenesis type I. Delineation of further heterogeneity and identification of two distinct sub groups. J Pediatr 1988; 112:23–31.

B0025                                                      **Zvi Borochowitz**

**Achondrogenesis, type I**
   *See ACHONDROGENESIS, PARENTI-FRACCARO TYPE*
   *also ACHONDROGENESIS, HOUSTON-HARRIS TYPE*

**Achondrogenesis, type IA**
*See ACHONDROGENESIS, HOUSTON-HARRIS TYPE
also ACHONDROGENESIS, PARENTI-FRACCARO TYPE*
**Achondrogenesis, type II**
*See ACHONDROGENESIS, LANGER-SALDINO TYPE*
**Achondrogenesis, type II (McKusick)**
*See GREBE SYNDROME*

## ACHONDROPLASIA                                    0010

**Includes:**
 Chondrodystrophia
 Chondrodystrophy
**Excludes:**
 **Dwarfism** (other short-limb)
 **Hypochondroplasia** (0510)
 Pseudoachondroplasia
 **Thanatophoric dysplasia** (0940)

**Major Diagnostic Criteria:** Although X-ray findings are pathognomonic for achondroplasia, at any age, the diagnosis is suggested by the following physical findings: (1) Disproportionately large head, prominent forehead, depressed nasal bridge. (2) Rhizomelic micromelia - relatively shorter proximal segments of extremities as compared to middle and distal segments - especially of upper extremities. Small stature with usual length at birth 46–48 cm. Decreased range of motion at elbows. (3) Increased pelvic tilt producing protuberant abdomen and prominent buttocks; (4) Trident hand - inability to approximate, in extension, the sides of distal fingers.

**Clinical Findings:** Since the physical findings are frequently subtle in the newborn period, radiographic evidence is helpful: (1) Skull is large with frontal, parietal, and occipital prominence; foramen magnum and base of skull are small; (2) Lack of normal increase in interpedicular distance from upper to lower lumbar spine; pedicles, on lateral view, are short; (3) Flat, squared iliac wings with absent iliac flaring; small sacrosciatic notches; (4) Tubular bones display shortening at all ages. Particular to infancy are radiolucent areas in the proximal humerus and femur caused by decreased anteroposterior diameter of these regions.

In childhood and adulthood, the tubular bones take on a massive appearance secondary to disproportion between shortened length and normal width (metaphyses appear flared and diaphyses appear wide) The humeri are most markedly shortened, while fibulae appear disproportionately lengthened.

**Complications:** Spinal cord compression at the foramen magnum is a well known problem with new implications. Patients with apnea, and sudden unexpected death, mimicking sudden infant death syndrome, have been described. Necropsy revealed gross and/or microscopic changes at the medulla through $C_2$ cord range consistent with chronic compression. It is speculated that involuntary respiratory center fibers, originating at the level of the medulla, may become dysfunctional and/or cervical cord compression causes lateral pyramidal tract dysfunction with decreased diaphragmatic and intercostal muscle function. Other authors report cystic necrosis, cavitation, and glioma of the spinal cord secondary to presumed chronic compression at the level of foramen magnum.

There can also be lower spinal stenosis with associated symptomatology. Risk of disk herniation and osteophyte formation increases with age.

Other respiratory complications include obstructive sleep apnea (related to general facial hypoplasia, flat nasal bridge, decreased muscle tone), chronic hypoxemia (related to decreased functional residual capacity with atelectasis), cor pulmonale, and recurrent pulmonary infiltrate.

Obesity may also be an early complicating factor, and may contribute to problems associated with lumbar canal stenosis, arthralgias in weight bearing joints, and early cardiovascular failure.

**Associated Findings:** Recurrent otitis media, conductive or sensorinural deafness. Possibly psychologic problems related to body image.

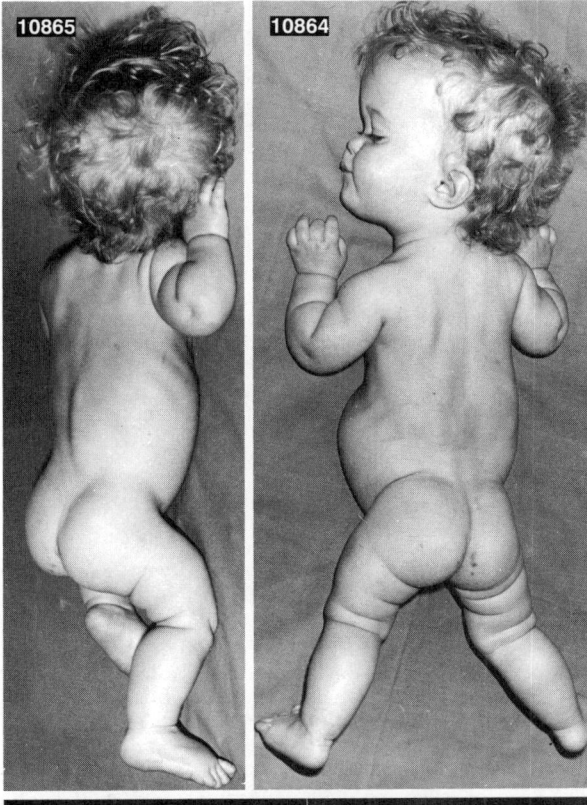

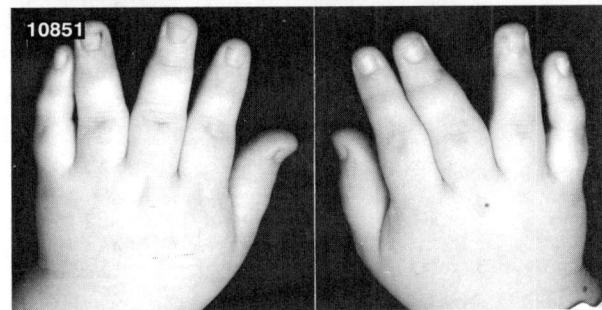

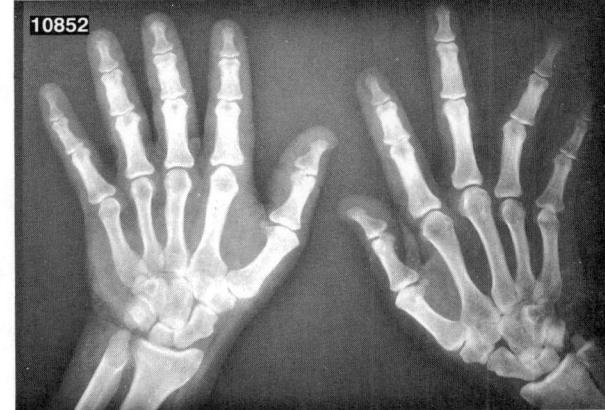

**0010**-10865–64: Note large head, depressed nasal bridge, short limbs and lumbar kyphosis. 10851: Hands in classic achondroplasia showing trident hands and short metacarpals. 10852: X-ray of hands shows achondroplastic changes in the right hand but the metacarpals and phalanges of the 2nd-5th digits of the left hand appear normal.

**Etiology:** Autosomal dominant inheritance with complete penetrance. However, 80% of cases represent fresh mutation. The mutation rate for achondroplasia has been estimated to be 1.72 to 5.57 x 10$^{-5}$. Familial recurrences of presumed mutations are reported. Germinal mosaicism, malsegregation, unequal crossing over, unstable premutation, and insertion of transposable elements have all been postulated as explanations for familial recurrences. Incidence of new mutations significantly increases with paternal age, especially at or above 40 years of age.

**Pathogenesis:** Decreased rate of endochondral ossification with normal membranous ossification leading to the short, squat long bones and disproportion between the base of the skull and the calvaria. Recent studies demonstrate abnormalities of the mitochondrial oxidative energy systems in patients with achondroplasia. Investigators suggest that this defect, when specifically expressed in the growth plate of long bones where oxygen tension is low despite active proliferation, may result in poor cell growth ultimately producing the achondroplastic phenotype.

**MIM No.:** *10080

**POS No.:** 3006

**CDC No.:** 756.430

**Sex Ratio:** M1:F1

**Occurrence:** The most common skeletal dysplasia, at between 5–15:100,000 live births.

**Risk of Recurrence for Patient's Sib:**
See Part I, *Mendelian Inheritance*. For sporadic case, the risk is usually considered equal to the mutation rate. With continued reports of familial recurrences, however, this may eventually prove to be an underestimation.

**Risk of Recurrence for Patient's Child:**
See Part I, *Mendelian Inheritance*. If both parents are achondroplastic, 25% of offspring will be normal, 50% will be typical heterozygous achondroplastic while 25% will be homozygous for the achondroplasia gene. Homozygous achondroplasia is usually lethal, but there are reports of homozygous achondroplasts surviving as long as 37 months. Homozygous expression shows more pronounced X-ray changes, severe psychomotor development, and early onset of medical complications.

**Age of Detectability:** At birth. Prenatal diagnosis is possible. In utero, ultrasound has shown initially normal femur length that progressively decreases in growth, falling below the 99% confidence limits by 30 weeks gestation. Biparietal diameter may be large compared with limb lengths.

**Gene Mapping and Linkage:** Unknown.

**Prevention:** None known. Genetic counseling indicated.

**Treatment:** Since cord compression, both at the level of foramen magnum and lower, is associated with significant complications, early monitoring with brainstem and somatosensory evoked potentials, polysomnography, and radiographic data may be useful.

Suboccipital craniotomies and laminectomies as indicated. Osteotomies for leg lengthening and bowleg deformity when indicated. Appropriate treatment of recurrent otitis media and associated conductive hearing loss. Cesarean sections are indicated for delivering mothers with achondroplasia. Support groups, such as Little People of America are helpful for affected individuals and their families.

**Prognosis:** Normal life span for heterozygous individuals if serious complications can be avoided. Average final adult height 130 cm for males, 123 cm for females. Prognosis for homozygous achondroplasts may be enhanced by early surgical intervention.

**Detection of Carrier:** By clinical examination.

**Special Considerations:** Since achondroplastic children have delayed motor milestones secondary to their particular body morphology, it is more appropriate to compare development of these children to their achondroplastic peers. Standard growth curves and confidence bands for head circumference in achondroplastic children are available. These are useful in evaluating macrocephaly in these children, since megalencephaly and true hydrocephalus can develop in childhood.

**Support Groups:**
MD; Bethesda; Human Growth Foundation (HGF)
CA; San Bruno; Little People of America, Inc. (LPA)

**References:**
Spranger, et al: Bone dysplasias: an atlas of constitutional disorders of skeletal development. Philadelphia: W.B. Saunders Company, 1974: 55–61. *
Horton DV, et al: Standard growth curves for achondroplasia. J Pediatr 1978; 93:435–438. *
Dawson DV: Confidence bands for the growth of head circumference in achondroplastic children during the first year of life. Am J Med Genet 1980; 7:529–532. *
Todorov AB, et al: Developmental Screening Tests in Achondroplastic Children. Am J Med Genet 1981; 9:19–23.
Pauli RM, et al: Homozygous achondroplasia with survival beyond infancy. Am J Med Genet 1983; 16:459–473.
Hecht JT, et al: Long - term neurological sequelae in achondroplasia. Europ J Pediatr 1984; 143:58–60. *
Pauli RM, et al: Apnea and sudden unexpected death in infants with achondroplasia. J Pediatr 1984; 104:342–348.
Hoegerman SF, et al: Speculation on the role of transposable elements in human genetic disease with particular attention to achondroplasia and the fragile X syndrome. Am J Med Genet 1986; 23:685–699.
Orioli IM, et al.: The birth prevalence rates for the skeletal dysplasias. J Med Genet 1986; 23:19–22.
Dodinval P, LeMarec B: Genetic counseling in unexpected familial recurrence of achondroplasia. Am J Med Genet 1987; 28:949–954.
Pyeritz RE, et al.: Thoracolumbosacral laminectomy in achondroplasia: long-term results in 22 patients. Am J Med Genet 1987; 28:433–444.
Hecht JT, et al.: Obesity in achondroplasia. Am J Med Genet 1988; 31:597–602.
Mackler B, Shepard TH: Human achondroplasia: defective mitochondrial oxidative energy metabolism may produce the pathophysiology. Teratology 1989; 40:571–582.

BY006
FL001

**Katie Byrd**
**David B. Flannery**

**Achondroplasia, so-called, and Swiss-type agammaglobulinemia**
*See METAPHYSEAL CHONDRODYSPLASIA WITH THYMOLYMPHOPENIA*

---

## ACHOO SYNDROME                    3229

**Includes:**
Compelling helio-ophthalmic outburst syndrome
Helio-ophthalmic outburst syndrome
Peroutka sneeze
Photic sneeze reflex
Sneezing from light exposure

**Excludes:** N/A

**Major Diagnostic Criteria:** Multiple sneezes on exposure to bright light from lowered ambient light, i.e. bright sunlight, slit lamp or ophthalmoscopic examination. In a few subjects, the sneezing response may be induced by eyebrow plucking or rubbing the inner canthus.

**Clinical Findings:** The number of sneezes is usually two or three, but as many as 43 have been reported. Normal neurologic exam; no allergic or other otorhinolaryngeal diseases.

**Complications:** Unknown.

**Associated Findings:** None known.

**Etiology:** Possibly autosomal dominant inheritance.

**Pathogenesis:** Unknown.

**Sex Ratio:** Presumably M1:F1.

**Occurrence:** Presumed frequency in the white population has been estimated at 2–30%. Apparently uncommon in Blacks.

**Risk of Recurrence for Patient's Sib:**
See Part I, *Mendelian Inheritance*.

**Risk of Recurrence for Patient's Child:**
See Part I, *Mendelian Inheritance.*

**Age of Detectability:** As early as one month of age.

**Gene Mapping and Linkage:** Unknown.

**Prevention:** None known. Genetic counseling indicated.

**Treatment:** Dark sunglasses.

**Prognosis:** A benign condition with no impact on life span.

**Detection of Carrier:** Unknown.

**References:**

Everett HC: Sneezing in response to light. Neurology 1964; 14:483–490.
Collie WR, et al.: ACHOO syndrome (Autosomal Dominant Compelling Helio-Ophthalmic Outburst Syndrome) BD:OAS XIV(6B). New York: March of Dimes Birth Defects Foundation, 1978:361–363.
Peroutka SJ, Peroutka LA: Autosomal dominant trasmissions of the "Photic Sneeze Reflex" (letter) New Engl J Med 1984; 310:599–600.
Morris HH: ACHOO syndrome prevalence and inheritance. Cleve Clin J Med 1987; 54:431–433.

HA015                                       **Jerome S. Haller**

**Achromatism**
*See COLOR BLINDNESS, TOTAL*
**Achromatopsia, incomplete**
*See COLOR BLINDNESS, TOTAL*
**Achromatopsia, X-chromosomal linked incomplete**
*See COLOR BLINDNESS, BLUE MONOCONE-MONOCHROMATIC*
**Achromatopsia-amblyopia**
*See COLOR BLINDNESS, TOTAL*
**Achromia, primary**
*See SKIN, VITILIGO*
**Acid beta-glucosidase deficiency**
*See GAUCHER DISEASE*
**Acid cholesteryl ester hydrolase deficiency, type 2**
*See CHOLESTERYL ESTER STORAGE DISEASE*
**Acid maltase deficiency, adult onset**
*See GLYCOGENOSIS, TYPE IIb*
**Acid maltase deficiency, childhood onset**
*See GLYCOGENOSIS, TYPE IIb*
**Acid maltase deficiency, infant onset**
*See GLYCOGENOSIS, TYPE IIa*
**Acidemia, 2-Methyl-3-hydroxybutyric acidemia**
*See ACIDEMIA, 3-KETOTHIOLASE DEFICIENCY*

---

## ACIDEMIA, 2-OXOGLUTARIC            2565

**Includes:**
Hyper-2-oxoglutaric aciduria
Two-oxoglutaric aciduria
Transsuccinylase (E2) deficiency

**Excludes:**
Aciduria, fumaric (2599)
Dihydrolipoyl dehydrogenase (E3) deficiency
Organoacidopathies with concomitant 2-oxoglutaric aciduria, other
Two-oxoglutaric aciduria, transient in infancy

**Major Diagnostic Criteria:** Slowly progressive nervous disorder, primarily involving the extrapyramidal system. Loss of motor and language skills, muscular rigidity, and intention tremor. Mental and emotional development may be normal. Some patients with milder hyper-2-oxoglutaric aciduria present with **Deafness-onycho-osteo-dystrophy-retardation-seizures (DOORS)** syndrome or mental retardation.

2-Oxoglutaric acidemia is a frequent finding when patients are screened for organoacidopathies. Other primary organoacidopathies can be differentiated by the pattern of metabolites, which are excreted in the urine. Concomitant lactic acidemia points toward different defects of the carbohydrate and energy metabolism, e.g., combined deficiency of pyruvic and 2-oxoglutarate dehydrogenase due to dihydrolipoyl dehydrogenase (E3) deficiency.

**Clinical Findings:** Clinical signs vary widely, probably corresponding to the residual enzyme activity and genetic heterogeneity.

A partial deficiency of the transsuccinylase (E2) component within the 2-oxoglutarate dehydrogenase complex was proven only in two sibs of a consanguineous marriage presenting with a slowly progressive neurodegenerative disorder and gross 2-oxoglutaric aciduria (Kohlschütter et al, 1982). Initially both children had normal psychomotor development with acquisition of gait and speech. At about age two years, athetoid movements were noticed, followed by loss of all motor and language skills. There was severe rigidity and intention tremor. Mental and emotional development appeared to be normal. A similar case with failure to thrive and severe progressive ataxia was reported by Chalmers et al. (1980).

Milder 2-oxoglutaric acidemia in 21 patients was reported from a study on unselected retarded individuals by Hoffmann et al (1986) and in patients with **Deafness-onycho-osteo-dystrophy-retardation-seizures (DOORS)** syndrome by Patton et al (1987). In both reports, there were strong indications for citric acid cycle defects; however, enzymatic studies have not yet been reported. Clinical findings were heterogenous, but there was an increased incidence of affected sibs, cerebellar atrophy, seizure disorders, and cerebral palsy.

2-Oxoglutaric acid is highly elevated in the urine. Plasma 2-oxoglutaric acid is only slightly elevated as are plasma pyruvic and citric acids. There is no elevated anion gap or metabolic acidosis.

**Complications:** Seizures and possibly cerebellar atrophy. The cerebellum appears to be especially sensitive to disturbances of the carbohydrate and energy metabolism.

**Associated Findings:** None known.

**Etiology:** Autosomal recessive inheritance.

**Pathogenesis:** A partial deficiency of 2-oxoglutarate dehydrogenase may have severe effects on metabolic compartmentation and fluxes of metabolites and neurotransmitters in the CNS. Some patient with milder 2-oxoglutaric acidemia presented with seizures, which is a leading symptom of citric acid cycle inhibition due to fluorocitrate intoxication.

**Sex Ratio:** M1:F1

**Occurrence:** Undetermined, but presumed rare.

**Risk of Recurrence for Patient's Sib:**
See Part I, *Mendelian Inheritance.*

**Risk of Recurrence for Patient's Child:**
See Part I, *Mendelian Inheritance.*

**Age of Detectability:** Increased levels of 2-oxoglutaric acid may already be present prenatally in the amniotic fluid. In affected children, 2-oxoglutaric acidemia precedes neurologic symptoms and is present from birth.

**Gene Mapping and Linkage:** Unknown.

**Prevention:** None known. Genetic counseling indicated.

**Treatment:** Unknown. Therapeutic trials with thiamine, lipoic acid, and pyridoxine did not improve the neurologic symptoms or the biochemical abnormality.

**Prognosis:** Depends on the degree of enzyme deficiency. Some patients may encounter a halt in their neurodegenerative disease and subsequently suffer from a stationary extrapyramidal syndrome or mental handicap. One patient with concomitant failure to thrive died at age three years.

**Detection of Carrier:** Unknown.

**Special Considerations:** 2-Oxoglutaric acidemia is frequently encountered when patients are screened for organoacidopathies. Neonates and young infants often excrete increased amounts of 2-oxoglutaric acid with or without increased 3-hydroxy-3-methylglutaric acid, citric acid, or both. These abnormalities are frequently associated with prolonged jaundice and may be due to functional immaturity of hepatic enzymes. Furthermore, 2-oxoglutaric aciduria of bacterial origin is frequently seen in urinary tract infections. Therefore, 2-oxoglutaric acidemia in very young infants should be followed up until about age two years, and urinary tract infection should be excluded before further investigations are initiated.

Genetic heterogeneity in 2-oxoglutaric acidemia can be expected, because 2-oxoglutaric acid excretion is closely linked with gluconeogenesis and the operation rate of the citric acid cycle. 2-Oxoglutaric acidemia is found in many organic acidopathies and appears to be a sensitive pointer toward disturbances of carbohydrate and energy metabolism.

**Support Groups:** KS; Kansas City; The Organic Acidemia Association

**References:**

Chalmers RA, et al.: Screening for organic acidurias and amino acidopathies in newborns and children. J Inherit Metab Dis 1980; 3:27–43.

Kohlschütter A, et al.: A familiar progressive neurodegenerative disease with 2-oxoglutaric aciduria. Eur J Pediatr 1982; 138:32–37. * †

Hoffmann G, et al.: Hyper-2-oxoglutaric aciduria in long-term mental handicap. J Ment Defic Res 1986; 30:251–260. *

Patton MA, et al.: DOOR syndrome (deafness, onychoosteodystrophy and mental retardation): elevated plasma and urinary 2-oxoglutarate in three unrelated patients. Am J Med Genet 1987; 26:207ff.

H0051 **Georg Hoffmann**

---

## ACIDEMIA, 3-HYDROXY-3-METHYLGLUTARIC     2114

**Includes:**

Aciduria, 3-hydroxy-3-methylglutaric
HMG-CoA lyase deficiency
Hydroxy methylglutaric aciduria
Leucine metabolism, defect in

**Excludes:** Reye syndrome

**Major Diagnostic Criteria:** Clinical signs include those normally seen in hypoglycemia and acidosis. Patients are characteristically hypoketotic. Urine organic acids have a characteristic pattern and confirm the diagnosis.

**Clinical Findings:** Onset, often in infancy, of episodes of severe illness in which acidosis and hypoglycemia may lead to deep coma. Persistent vomiting may be the first symptom, often complicating an intercurrent infection. Patients then develop lethargy progressive to coma, pallor, hypotonia, dehydration, and apnea. In the absence of artificial ventilation death ensues. Some patients have had convulsions. Most, but not all, patients have hepatomegaly.

Hypoglycemia may be impressive. In the first three patients blood sugars of 5,4 and 7 mg/dl were recorded, and one of these patients died in a second episode in which the blood sugar was less than 1.8 mg/dl. Metabolic acidosis is prominent in these episodes of illness. Plasma concentrations of bicarbonate reported have ranged from 11 to 15.6 mEq/l, and the pH from 7.11 to 7.29. Three patients have had hyperammonemia, and in our patient the blood concentration of ammonia was 1370 μM/l at five days of age. Liver function tests may be abnormal. The clinical manifestations and the laboratory findings may lead to confusion with the Reye syndrome.

Patients do not develop ketonuria. The pattern of excretion of organic acids is characteristic. The hallmark compound which accumulates in large amounts is 3-hydroxy-3-methylglutaric acid. In addition, there are large amounts of 3-methylglutaconic acid, 3-methylglutaric acid, and 3-hydroxyisovaleric acid. There may be large amounts of lactic acid in blood and urine during episodes of clinical illness. Moderately elevated amounts of adipic, suberic, and 3-hydroxybutyric acids may be found.

Defective activity of 3-hydroxy-3-methylglutaryl CoA lyase can be demonstrated in cultured fibroblasts in leukocytes or in liver.

**Complications:** Brain damage, cerebral atrophy, and death.

**Associated Findings:** None known.

**Etiology:** Autosomal recessive inheritance.

**Pathogenesis:** Deficiency of 3-hydroxy-3-methylglutaryl CoA lyase. This is consistent with the absence of ketonuria because the lyase catalyzes the conversion of 3-hydroxy-3-methylglutaryl CoA to acetylCoA and acetoacetic acid, the source of the ketones. Interference with the formation of acetyl CoA could adversely affect gluconeogenesis and lead to hypoglycemia. Hyperammonemia might be the result of the inhibition of acetylglutamate synthetase by the CoA derivatives that accumulate as has been shown for propionyl CoA.

**MIM No.:** *24645

**Sex Ratio:** M1:F1

**Occurrence:** Thirteen patients have been reported in the literature, and additional cases have been studied.

**Risk of Recurrence for Patient's Sib:**
See Part I, *Mendelian Inheritance.*

**Risk of Recurrence for Patient's Child:**
See Part I, *Mendelian Inheritance.*

**Age of Detectability:** Should be diagnosable prenatally.

**Gene Mapping and Linkage:** Unknown.

**Prevention:** None known. Genetic counseling indicated.

**Treatment:** Protein restriction in order to minimize the intake of extra leucine appears prudent. Avoidance of fasting, especially under circumstances of intercurrent illness is important. Frequent high carbohydrate feedings are important, as is the use of intravenous solutions of glucose when the oral route is not tolerated. Lipid restriction may also be required.

**Prognosis:** Guarded. While a number of patients recently reported have been doing well with treatment, death and severe retardation have been known.

**Detection of Carrier:** Analysis of the activity of 3-hydroxy-3-methylglutaryl CoA lyase in leukocytes and in cultured fibroblasts show intermediate levels diagnostic of heterozygosity.

**Support Groups:** KS; Kansas City; The Organic Acidemia Association

**References:**

Faull KF, et al.: The urinary organic acid profile associated with 3-hydroxy-3-methylglutaric aciduria. Clin Chim Acta 1976; 73:553–559.

Divry P, et al.: 3-hydroxy-3-methylglutaric aciduria combined with 3-methylglutaconic aciduria: a new case. J Inherited Metab Dis 1981; 4:173–174.

Francois B, et al.: Glucose metabolism in a child with 3-hydroxy-3-methylglutaryl-coenzyme A lyase deficiency. J Inherited Metab Dis 1981; 4:163-164.

Gibson KM, et al.: 3-Hydroxy-3-methylglutaric aciduria: a new assay of 3-hydroxy-3-methylglutaryl-CoA lyase using high performance liquid chromatography. Clin Chim Acta 1982; 126:171–181.

Greene C, et al.: 3-Hydroxy-3-methylglutaric aciduria. J Neurogenet 1984; 1:165–173.

Gibson KM, et al.: 3-Hydroxy-3-methylglutaryl-coenzyme A lyase deficiency. J Inherited Metab Dis 1988; 11:76–87.

NY000 **William L. Nyhan**

---

## ACIDEMIA, 3-KETOTHIOLASE DEFICIENCY     0040

**Includes:**

Acidemia, 2-Methyl-3-hydroxybutyric acidemia
Alpha-methylacetoacetic aciduria
Beta-ketothiolase deficiency
Mitochondrial acetoacetyl-CoA thiolase deficiency

**Excludes:**

Cytoplasmic acetoacetyl-CoA thiolase deficiency
Peroxisomal thiolase deficiency
Pseudo-Zellweger syndrome

**Major Diagnostic Criteria:** Severe episodic ketoacidosis with elevated urinary 2-methyl-3-hydroxybutyric acid, 2-methylacetoacetic acid, tiglycylglycine, and 3-hydroxybutyric and acetoacetic acids. Enzymic assay shows very low or nondetectable β-ketoacyl-

CoA thiolase activity toward 2-methylacetoacetyl-CoA measured in skin fibroblasts or leukocytes.

**Clinical Findings:** Severe episodic ketoacidosis is the most frequent clinical sign. It is triggered by catabolic states, infections, fasting, or a high protein diet. Recurrent headaches have been reported  Onset is usually within 6–20 months of age, with one neonatal case and three reports of onset above the age of four years. Psychomotor development in most subjects is normal, but in three patients occasional abnormalities have been described.

During attacks blood lactate, ammonia, and amino acid levels are generally normal, as are blood glucose concentrations, although two cases of hyper- and hypoglycemia have been reported. The high concentrations of acetoacetate in blood and urine during attacks can simulate salicylism (two cases) on routine testing. With one exception, all patients showed greatly increased excretion of 2-methyl-3-hydroxybutyric acid and tiglycylglycine in urine, although the absolute and relative amounts may vary greatly between subjects. These acids are sometimes accompanied by the less stable 2-methylacetoacetic acid or its breakdown product butanone. Detection of 2-methylacetoacetic acid and 2-methyl-3-hydroxybutyric acid can be complicated by the large amounts of acetoacetic and 3-hydroxybutyric acids present during attacks.

Between attacks, the excretion of these abnormal urinary acids depends on the protein intake. They can usually be detected following an isoleucine load, although this has precipitated an attack in one case. Physical and mental development are normal between attacks, which respond well to treatment and which only occur in childhood. When untreated, attacks can lead to neurologic damage (three cases) or death: Five family histories reveal previous sibs who died in infancy of the disease.

Since 1982, when the direct enzyme assay was developed, all reported patients have shown very low or undetectable β-ketoacyl-CoA thiolase activity toward 2-methylacetoacetyl-CoA in extracts of cultured skin fibroblasts.

**Complications:** Consequent to untreated ketoacidosis, acidotic coma can develop, with subsequent neurologic damage or death. One child, diagnosed at age 12 weeks, developed congestive cardiomyopathy at age eight years and died.

**Associated Findings:** None known.

**Etiology:** Autosomal recessive inheritance. Lack of β-ketoacyl-CoA thiolase, which is active with 2-methylacetoacetyl-CoA and acetoacetyl-CoA. Clinical expression is variable.

**Pathogenesis:** Two mitochondrial β-ketoacyl-CoA thiolases are known. Type I, EC 2.3.1.16, has wide chain-length specificity for 3-ketoacyl-CoA substrates. Type II, EC 2.3.1.9, is only active with acetoacetyl- and 2-methylacetoacetyl-CoA and requires $K^+$ ions. In fibroblast and leukocyte extracts from patients with this disorder, type II β-ketoacyl-CoA thiolase activity is very low or nondetectable. Absence of this enzyme prevents: (a) extrahepatic breakdown of isoleucine beyond 2-methylacetoacetyl-CoA, and (b) extrahepatic metabolism of acetoacetate beyond acetoacetyl-CoA. This single enzyme deficiency causes accumulation of the organic acids 2-methylacetoacetic, 2-methyl-3-hydroxybutyric, and tiglycylglycine from isoleucine as well as acetoacetic and 3-hydroxybutyric acids from the block in ketone body utilization. Any stress or condition leading to ketoacidosis or accelerated isoleucine catabolism in the normal child should cause a ketoacidotic crisis in homozygotes for this disorder.

The mutation must only affect the extrahepatic type II β-ketoacyl-CoA thiolase, because the liver contains another isoenzyme involved in the synthesis of acetoacetyl-CoA for ketogenesis. This is unaffected by the mutation.

The nature and site of the mutation is not known, but Yamaguchi et al (1988) report a defective enzyme synthesis resulting in lack of immunoreactive type II β-ketoacyl-CoA thiolase in extrahepatic cells.

**MIM No.:** *20375

**Sex Ratio:** M1:F1

**Occurrence:** Twenty-two cases have been reported.

**Risk of Recurrence for Patient's Sib:** See Part I, *Mendelian Inheritance*.

**Risk of Recurrence for Patient's Child:** See Part I, *Mendelian Inheritance*.

**Age of Detectability:** Detectable in the neonate. Prenatal diagnosis possible.

**Gene Mapping and Linkage:** Unknown.

**Prevention:** None known. Genetic counseling indicated.

**Treatment:** Acidotic episodes are treated with bicarbonate and glucose infusion. Occurrence of further attacks is reduced by avoiding starvation and low-calorie or high-protein diets.

**Prognosis:** Probable normal life span, but limited data are available. One patient developed congestive cardiomyopathy and died at age eight years.

**Detection of Carrier:** By examination of β-ketoacyl-CoA thiolase activity with 2-methylacetoacetyl-CoA in extracts of cultured skin fibroblasts of relatives.

**Special Considerations:** The involvement of the liver in isoleucine catabolism may explain the very variable clinical severity and excretion of isoleucine metabolites found in urine during attacks. One homozygote showed none of these metabolites in urine either during attacks or when given an oral load of isoleucine. In liver mitochondria of rats the enzyme affected in this disorder (type II β-ketoacyl-CoA thiolase, EC 2.3.1.9) appears in two isoenzyme forms. Both have identical substrate specificity and can therefore metabolize 2-methylacetoacetyl-CoA. It is not known whether these enzymes are absent from liver mitochondria of homozygous patients. It is presumed that at least one isoenzyme must be present, since hepatic ketogenesis is very active in affected patients. Absence of the extrahepatic isoenzyme alone would leave ketogenesis unaffected, and intermediates of isoleucine breakdown in liver would not accumulate. This could reduce the amounts of urinary isoleucine breakdown products without decreasing the severity of the ketoacidosis.

**Support Groups:** KS; Kansas City; The Organic Acidemia Association

**References:**

Daum RS, et al.: An inherited disorder of isoleucine catabolism causing accumulation of α-methylacetoacetate and α-methyl-β-hydroxybutyrate and intermittent metabolic acidosis. Pediatr Res 1973; 7:149–160. *

Robinson BH, et al.: Acetoacetyl-CoA thiolase deficiency: a cause of severe ketoacidosis in infancy simulating salicylism. J Pediatr 1979; 95:228–233.

Schutgens RBH, et al.: Beta-ketothiolase deficiency in a family confirmed by in vitro enzymatic assays in fibroblasts. Eur J Pediatr 1982; 139:39–42.

Middleton B, Bartlett K: The synthesis and characterisation of 2-methylacetoacetyl-coenzyme A and its use in the identification of the site of the defect in 2-methylacetoacetic and 2-methyl-3-hydroxybutyric aciduria. Clin Chim Acta 1983; 128:291–305. *

Leonard JV, et al.: Acetoacetyl-CoA thiolase deficiency as ketotic hypoglycaemia. Pediatr Res 1987; 21:211–213.

Saudubray JM, et al.: Hyperketotic states due to inherited defects of ketolysis. Enzyme 1987; 38:80–90.

Yamaguchi S, et al.: Defect in the biosythesis of acetoacetyl-CoA thiolase in cultured fibroblasts from a boy with 3-ketothiolase deficiency. J Clin Invest 1988; 81:813–817.

MIO40                                               **Bruce Middleton**

**Acidemia, 4-aminobutyrate aminotransferase deficiency**
*See GAMMA-AMINOBUTYRIC ACID (GABA) TRANSAMINASE DEFICIENCY*
**Acidemia, 4-hydroxybutyric**
*See ACIDEMIA, GAMMA-HYDROXYBUTYRIC*

## ACIDEMIA, ETHYLMALONIC-ADIPIC          **2377**

**Includes:**

Aciduria, ethylmalonic-adipic
Electron transfer flavoprotein (ETF), partial deficiencies of
ETF dehydrogenase, partial deficiencies of
Ethylmalonic-adipic aciduria
Glutaric aciduria type IIB (mild and/or adult variants)
Multiple Acyl-CoA Dehydrogenation (MAD) disorders, mild variants
ETF:ubiquinone oxidoreductase, partial deficiencies of

**Excludes:**

Acidemia, glutaric acidemia I (0421)
Acidemia, glutaric acidemia II, neonatal onset (2289)
Acyl-CoA dehydrogenase deficiency, long chain type (2228)
Acyl-CoA dehydrogenase deficiency, medium chain type (2324)
Acyl-CoA dehydrogenase deficiency, short chain type (2323)
Carnitine deficiency, systemic (2121)
Dicarboxylic aciduria due to any other cause
Glycogenosis, type Ia (0425)
Hypoglycin A intoxication (Jamaican vomiting sickness)
Viscera, fatty metamorphosis (0990)

**Major Diagnostic Criteria:** Urinary excretion of $C_6$-$C_{10}$-dicarboxylic acids, ethylmalonic, methylsuccinic, isovaleric, $\alpha$-methylbutyric, isobutyric, and glutaric acids, sarcosine, and/or dimethylglycine. Defective oxidation of short-, medium- and long-chain fatty acids, branched-chain amino acids, and lysine in fibroblasts. For riboflavin-responsive variants, there is exaggeration of these oxidative defects after culture of fibroblasts in a riboflavin-free medium. Partial deficiencies of electron transfer flavoprotein or electron transfer flavoprotein dehydrogenase.

**Clinical Findings:** Episodic hypoketotic hypoglycemia, lethargy, Reye syndrome-like episodes, coma, hypotonia, hepatomegaly, fatty liver, lipomyopathy, lipocardiomyopathy, and hepatic dysfunction. Development ranges from normal to moderately delayed, generally, but not always, correlated with the severity and frequency of metabolic crises. The age of presentation ranges from birth to early adult life. Ethylmalonic and adipic excretions are relatively more elevated than those of the branched-chain amino acid metabolites and glutarate. Total plasma carnitines are often below the normal range, with an elevated esterified fraction.

**Complications:** Variable; including developmental delay and sudden death.

**Associated Findings:** None known.

**Etiology:** Autosomal recessive inheritance. Partial deficiencies of electron transfer flavoprotein or its dehydrogenase (generally 5–50% of control) have been found in a number of patients. Defects in riboflavin transport, flavin adenine dinucleotide (FAD) synthesis, maintenance of intramitochondrial FAD levels, or apoenzyme FAD binding could explain the riboflavin-responsive phenotype(s). While the degree of enzymatic deficiency roughly correlates with clinical severity, clinical and biochemical heterogeneity is marked.

**Pathogenesis:** The enzymatic deficiencies indicated above globally interrupt intramitochondrial acyl-CoA dehydrogenation, blocking catabolism of short-, medium- and long-chain fatty acids, branched-chain amino acids, lysine, sarcosine and dimethylglycine. The accumulated acyl-CoAs are oxidized to other metabolites, such as straight-chain dicarboxylic acids and ($\Omega$-1)- hydroxy acids. Butyryl-CoA is converted to ethylmalonyl-CoA and methylsuccinate following carboxylation by propionyl-CoA carboxylase. The short- and medium-chain fatty acids may interfere with mitochondrial ATP production and pyruvate oxidation. The acyl-CoAs are also converted to their acyl-glycine and/or acyl-carnitine derivatives; sequestration of CoA and carnitine as acyl derivatives may interfere with other aspects of intermediary metabolism, including ketogenesis, gluconeogenesis, and glycogenolysis. In fasting or catabolic states, glucose production is either impaired by accumulated metabolites or is insufficient to meet energy demands in the absence of normal $\beta$-oxidation and ketogenesis. In some patients, the inability to oxidize fatty acids apparently produces muscle weakness, cardiomyopathy and/or hepatic deposition of fat. Systemic carnitine deficiency may result from increased excretion of the accumulated acyl-carnitines and/or an unproven depression of carnitine synthesis.

**MIM No.:** *23168

**Sex Ratio:** Presumably M1:F1.

**Occurrence:** About two-dozen documented cases have been reported.

**Risk of Recurrence for Patient's Sib:**
See Part I, *Mendelian Inheritance.*

**Risk of Recurrence for Patient's Child:**
See Part I, *Mendelian Inheritance.*

**Age of Detectability:** Highly variable. Prenatal diagnosis may be feasible in given families, once the metabolic and/or enzymatic defect is defined in the proband. Urinary organic acid analysis should detect most affected individuals, especially if they are in a catabolic state or challenged with precursor loads.

**Gene Mapping and Linkage:** ETFA (electron transfer flavoprotein, alpha polypeptide (glutaric aciduria II)) has been provisionally mapped to 15q23-q25.

**Prevention:** None known. Genetic counseling indicated. Hypoglycemia and metabolic crisis might be prevented by avoiding fasting and providing a low fat and protein diet.

**Treatment:** Treatment is experimental, but is similar to regimens developed for other inborn errors of amino and/or fatty acid metabolism. Parenteral glucose, fluids and electrolytes should be provided during acidotic and/or hypoglycemic episodes. Carnitine and/or glycine administration might promote conjugation and excretion of acyl-moieties and raise free carnitine and CoA. While untested, riboflavin supplementation should be safe and may reveal riboflavin-responsive variants. Oral cornstarch therapy (1.75–2.5 gm/kg every six hours) may prevent hypoglycemia during fasting.

**Prognosis:** Variable, depending on the frequency and severity of metabolic crises.

**Detection of Carrier:** Unknown. Dicarboxylic acid excretion after a medium-chain triglyceride challenge (150–500 mg/kg) might be informative, as well as biochemical studies in fibroblasts of presumed carriers. Ideally, both prenatal diagnosis and carrier detection require a specific enzymatic diagnosis in the proband.

**Special Considerations:** As the name implies, patients with ethylmalonic-adipic aciduria appear to have defective oxidation of only short- to medium-chain length fatty acids. However, impairment of multiple acyl-CoA dehydrogenase dependent pathways distinguishes ethylmalonic-adipic aciduria and the other multiple acyl-Coa dehydrogenation disorders from deficiencies of any single acyl-CoA dehydrogenase. The full spectrum of phenotypes in this disorder has not been defined, with the clinical and biochemical manifestations ranging from those of **Acidemia, glutaric acidemia II, neonatal onset**, to milder cases resembling **Acyl-CoA dehydrogenase deficiency, medium chain type**. Other patients have had cardiomyopathy, similar to that seen in **Acyl-CoA dehydrogenase deficiency, long chain type**. To date, many patients identified with ethylmalonic-adipic aciduria have not had biochemical studies performed in tissues or fibroblasts. The diagnosis should always be confirmed by finding deficient oxidation of fatty acids, branched-chain amino acids and/or lysine in fibroblasts or other tissues, generally no lower than 15% of control values. When feasible, electron transfer flavoprotein and its dehydrogenase should be assayed directly in all suspected patients or the enzyme defect assigned by complementation analysis. Riboflavin responsive variants are identified clinically by unequivocal response to vitamin therapy and biochemically by worsening of the metabolic defect after fibroblast culture in riboflavin free medium.

**Support Groups:** KS; Kansas City; The Organic Acidemia Association

**References:**

Mantagos S, et al.: Ethylmalonic-adipic aciduria. J Clin Invest 1979; 64:1580–1589.

Gregersen N: The acyl-CoA dehydrogenation deficiencies. Scand J Clin Lab Invest 1985; 45(Suppl 174):11–60.

Amendt BA, Rhead WJ: The multiple acyl-coenzyme A dehydrogenation disorders, glutaric aciduria type II and ethylmalonic-adipic aciduria. J Clin Invest 1986; 78:205–213.

DiDonato S, et al.: Systemic carnitine deficiency due to lack of electron transfer flavoprotein: ubiquinone oxidoreductase. Neurology 1986; 36:957–963.

Moon A, Rhead WJ: Complementation analysis of fatty acid oxidation disorders. J Clin Invest 1987; 79:59–64.

Rhead WJ, et al.: Clinical and biochemical variation and family studies in the multiple acyl-CoA dehydrogenation disorders. Pediatr Res 1987; 21:371–376.

Frerman FE, Goodman SI: Glutaric acidemia type II and defects of the mitochondrial respiratory chain. In: Scriver CR, et al, eds: The metabolic basis of inherited disease, 6th ed. New York: McGraw-Hill, 1989:915–932.

RH000                                                    **William J. Rhead**

## ACIDEMIA, GAMMA-HYDROXYBUTYRIC                    2113

**Includes:**

Acidemia, 4-hydroxybutyric
GABA metabolic defect
Gamma-hydroxybutyric aciduria
Hydroxybutyric aciduria
Succinic semialdehyde dehydrogenase deficiency

**Excludes:**

**Ataxia-telangiectasia** (0094)
**Dysequilibrium syndrome** (2421)

**Major Diagnostic Criteria:** Persistently elevated concentrations of 4-hydroxybutyric acid in urine, blood, and cerebrospinal fluid.

**Clinical Findings:** The clinical picture is that of mild psychomotor retardation (6/6), mild-to-marked muscular hypotonia (5/6), and a nonprogressive truncal and appendicular ataxia (4/6). Seizures have been documented (2/6). Ocular manifestations have been variable. Mild ocular apraxia has been observed in conjunction with normal vision (1/6). Conjunctival vascular changes (2/6) and retardation of language development (4/6) have been noted.

There is a wide range of excretion of 4-hydroxybutyric acid in body fluids. Reported values include urine, 35–2,120 $\mu$mol/mol creatinine (6/6 measured); plasma, 15–1,010 $\mu$mol/liter (5/5 measured); and cerebrospinal fluid, 245–600 $\mu$mol/liter (3/3 measured). Increased urinary levels of succinic semialdehyde and glycolic acid have been observed (2/6). In normal human body fluids, 4-hydroxybutyric acid and succinic semialdehyde are not detectable. Elevated levels of 3,4-dihydroxybutyric acid have been identified (2/6), and an approximately fourfold elevation of GABA (4-aminobutyric acid) was documented in the cerebrospinal fluid of the index case.

Four of six patients have been followed approximately two years following initial examination. Two were found to be stable, with no progression. Two patients showed significant improvement of ataxia and speech; both displayed only a slight truncal and appendicular ataxia, and in one only a mild ocular dyspraxia remained. In all four there was a continued fall in the plasma concentration of 4-hydroxybutyric acid.

**Complications:** Ataxia may be severe enough to cause inability to stand or walk.

**Associated Findings:** In individual cases, the following manifestations have been documented: moderate cerebral atrophy, abnormal EEG, dysarthric speech, mild autistic features associated with mild hyporeflexia, extreme hyperkinesia, retarded bone age, marked perspiration upon minimal exertion in the neonatal period, and increased urinary and plasma concentrations of glycine. These findings may or may not be related to the biochemical defect.

**Etiology:** Autosomal recessive inheritance.

**Pathogenesis:** In mammalian liver and central nervous system, the inhibitory neurotransmitter GABA is converted into succinic semialdehyde by GABA-transaminase (E.C.2.6.1.19). Succinic semialdehyde is further oxidized to succinic acid by succinic semialdehyde dehydrogenase (E.C.1.2.1.24), permitting entry into the citric acid cycle. Succinic semialdehyde may also be reduced to 4-hydroxybutyric acid by 4-hydroxybutyrate dehydrogenase (E.C.1.1.1.61). In normal mammalian brain the oxidation of succinic semialdehyde to succinic acid is the dominant reaction. Succinic semialdehyde dehydrogenase deficiency has been documented in extracts of lymphocytes and sometimes in lymphoblasts derived from all six patients described. The result is a significant conversion of accumulated succinic semialdehyde into 4-hydroxybutyric acid.

4-Hydroxybutyric acid has been known to have neuropharmacologic and neurophysiologic activity for many years. More recent data demonstrating a specific transport mechanism and regional binding sites in mammalian brain strongly suggest a role for 4-hydroxybutyric acid as a neurotransmitter. The neurologic abnormalities associated with 4-hydroxybutyric aciduria are consistent with the pharmacologic effects of the compound. In animals, 4-hydroxybutyric acid has been observed to produce changes in the EEG associated with a trance-like state at blood levels similar to those found in patients. Higher concentrations render the animal unresponsive to stimuli and induce focal and generalized seizures.

**MIM No.:** *27198

**Sex Ratio:** Expected, M1:F1; observed, M5:F8.

**Occurrence:** Of the six reported cases, one was of Turkish descent, two sibs in an unrelated family were Lebanese, one was Mexican, and the two remaining patients were of Algerian and Maltese descent, respectively. Details on seven additional patients have not yet been published. Deficient succinic semialdehyde dehydrogenase activity has been documented in extracts of lymphocytes and sometimes lymphoblasts obtained from five of these patients.

**Risk of Recurrence for Patient's Sib:**
See Part I, *Mendelian Inheritance.*

**Risk of Recurrence for Patient's Child:**
See Part I, *Mendelian Inheritance.*

**Age of Detectability:** Four of six patients manifested symptoms in the neonatal period, although in one patient early motor milestones were normal. Prenatal diagnosis can be made by assaying succinic semialdehyde dehydrogenase activity in ammiocytes and in chorionic villus cells, and probably by direct assey of 4-hydroxybutyric acid in amniotic fluid by gas chromatography-mass spectrometry.

**Gene Mapping and Linkage:** Unknown.

**Prevention:** None known. Genetic counseling indicated.

**Treatment:** No treatment employed has significantly altered the clinical status or the urinary excretion of 4-hydroxybutyric acid.

**Prognosis:** Undetermined, although some degree of permanent psychomotor deficit appears probable. There may be clinical improvement with age.

**Detection of Carrier:** Levels of enzyme activities of succinic semialdehyde dehydrogenase consistent with heterozygosity have been documented in extracts of lymphocytes and lymphoblasts obtained from the parents and sibs of four patients.

**Special Considerations:** There may be considerable heterogeneity in 4-hydroxybutyric aciduria. It may not be sufficient to assay for 4-hydroxybutyric acid in body fluids of patients presenting with ataxia and convulsions. Rather, it may be of value to recommend urinary organic acid analysis in patients presenting with psychomotor delay and hypotonia.

**Support Groups:** KS; Kansas City; The Organic Acidemia Association

**References:**

Jakobs C, et al.: Urinary excretion of gamma-hydroxybutyric acid in a patient with neurological abnormalities: the probability of a new inborn error of metabolism. Clin Chim Acta 1981; 111:169–178.

Gibson KM: 4-Hydroxybutyric aciduria. Bioassays 1984; 1:110–113. *

Rating D, et al.: 4-Hydroxybutyric aciduria: a new inborn error of metabolism. J Inherited Metab Dis 1984; 7(suppl. 1):90–92. *

Haan EA, et al.: Succinic semialdehyde dehydrogenase deficiency: a further case. J Inherited Metab Dis 1986; 8:99 only.

Roesel RA, et al.: 4-Hydroxybutyric aciduria and glycinuria in two siblings. (Abstract) Am J Hum Genet 1987; 41:A16 only.

De Vivo DC, et al.: 4-Hydroxybutyric acidemia: clinical features, pathogenetic mechanisms, and treatment strategies. (Abstract) Ann Neurol 1988; 24:304A only.

Gibson KM, et al.: 4-Hydroxybutyric aciduria in a patient without ataxia and convulsions. Eur J Pediatr 1988; 147:529–531.

Gibson KM, et al.: Succinic semialdehyde dehydrogenase deficiency associated with combined 4-hydroxybutyric and dicarboxylic acidurias. J Pediatr 1989; 114:607–610.

GI019
H0051
RA024

**Kenneth M. Gibson**
**Georg Hoffmann**
**D. Rating**

## ACIDEMIA, GLUTARIC ACIDEMIA I  0421

**Includes:**

Aciduria, glutaric
Glutaric aciduria type I
Glutaryl-CoA dehydrogenase deficiency

**Excludes:**

**Acidemia, ethylmalonic-adipic** (2377)
**Acidemia, glutaric acidemia II, neonatal onset** (2289)
**Acidemia** (others)
**Aciduria** (others)
**Viscera, fatty metamorphosis** (0990)

**Major Diagnostic Criteria:**  Elevated concentrations of glutaric acid in blood and urine; deficiency of glutaryl-CoA dehydrogenase in tissues (white blood cells, fibroblasts, and the like).

**Clinical Findings:**  Patients appear normal at birth, but episodes of hypotonia, vomiting, and metabolic acidosis appear in the first year of life. The chronic picture is dominated by dystonic posturing, involuntary movements, and usually mental retardation.

Urinary excretion of glutaric acid may be in excess of 1 gm/day. This compound is normally found in urine only in ketosis, and even then in amounts less than 0.1 mg/mg creatinine. β-Hydroxyglutaric acid is usually found in the urine; glutaconic acid is found on occasion, usually during ketosis. Glutaric acid concentrations are also elevated in serum, CSF, and tissues.

**Complications:**  Death, mental retardation, choreoathetosis, and neuronal degeneration in putamen and caudate.

**Associated Findings:**  Dystonia, frontotemporal atrophy.

**Etiology:**  Autosomal recessive inheritance.

**Pathogenesis:**  Deficient activity of glutaryl-CoA dehydrogenase. Striatal necrosis probably due to accumulation of glutaric acid in brain.

**MIM No.:**  *23167

**Sex Ratio:**  M1:F1

**Occurrence:**  More than 35 cases have been documented.

**Risk of Recurrence for Patient's Sib:**
See Part I, *Mendelian Inheritance.*

**Risk of Recurrence for Patient's Child:**  Affected individuals are not expected to survive to reproduce.

**Age of Detectability:**  Presumably at birth, by demonstrating glutaric aciduria or glutaryl-CoA dehydrogenase deficiency in cord blood leukocytes. Detection in utero possible by enzyme assay in cultured amniotic cells and by demonstrating glutaric acid accumulation in amniotic fluid.

**Gene Mapping and Linkage:**  Unknown.

**Prevention:**  None known. Genetic counseling indicated.

**Treatment:**  The usefulness of dietary restriction of glutarigenic amino acids (lysine, hydroxylysine, tryptophan) is unknown. Acute episodes of acidosis and dehydration should be treated with fluids and bicarbonate. Lioresal may be helpful in treatment of the movement disorder.

**Prognosis:**  Most patients are retarded and incapacitated by the movement disorder. Death during acute episodes is common.

**Detection of Carrier:**  Demonstration of reduced activity (about 25% of normal) of glutaryl-CoA dehydrogenase in peripheral leukocytes.

**Support Groups:**  KS; Kansas City; The Organic Acidemia Association

**References:**

Goodman SI, et al.: Glutaric aciduria; a 'new' disorder of amino acid metabolism. Biochem Med 1975; 12:12–21.

Goodman SI, et al.: Glutaric aciduria: biochemical and morphologic considerations. J Pediatr 1977; 90:746–750.

Brandt NJ, et al: Treatment of glutaryl-CoA dehydrogenase deficiency (glutaric aciduria): experience with diet, riboflavin and GABA analogue. J Pediatr 1979; 94:669–673.

Goodman SI, et al.: Antinatal diagnosis of glutaic acidemia. Am J Hum Genet 1980; 32:695–699.

Bennett MJ, et al.: Glutaric aciduria type I: biochemical investigations and postmortem findings. Europ J Pediat 1986; 145:403–405.

Amir N, et al.: Glutaric aciduria type I: clinical heterogeneity and neuroradiologic feature. Neurology 1987; 37:1654–1657.

G0025

**Stephen I. Goodman**

## ACIDEMIA, GLUTARIC ACIDEMIA II  2289

**Includes:**

Acyl-Coenzyme A dehydrogenase, multiple
Electron transfer flavoprotein (ETF) deficiency
Electron transfer flavoprotein, alpha subunit, deficiency of
ETF:ubiquinone oxidoreductase (ETF:QO) deficiency
Glutaric aciduria type IIA, neonatal form
Multiple acyl-CoA dehydrogenation deficiency (MADD)
Multiple acyl-CoA dehydrogenation deficiency, severe variants

**Excludes:**

**Acidemia, ethylmalonic-adipic** (2377)
**Acidemia, glutaric acidemia I** (0421)
**Acyl-CoA dehydrogenase deficiency, long chain type** (2228)
**Acyl-CoA dehydrogenase deficiency, medium chain** (2324)
**Viscera, fatty metamorphosis** (0990)

**Major Diagnostic Criteria:**  Elevated urine concentrations of metabolites of substrates of mitochondrial flavoprotein dehydrogenases, including glutaric acid, ethylmalonic acid, 3-hydroxyisovaleric acid, isovalerylglycine, 2-hydroxyglutaric acid, and sarcosine.

Deficiency of electron transfer flavoprotein (ETF) or electron transfer flavoprotein:ubiquinone oxidoreductase (ETF:QO) in cultured skin fibroblasts.

**Clinical Findings:**  Glutaric acidemia type II is characterized clinically by nonketotic hypoglycemia, metabolic acidosis, and (occasionally) a "sweaty feet" odor and pathologically by fatty degeneration of the liver, kidney, and myocardium. Patients usually fall into one of three groups, each consistent within a family.

*Neonatal-onset glutaric acidemia type II with congenital anomalies:* Symptoms develop during the first few days of life, and patients die within the first week. The kidneys show multiple cysts and dysplastic changes. Intrauterine growth retardation, hypotonia, Potter facies, high-arched palate, and anomalies of the abdominal wall and external genitalia may be present.

*Neonatal-onset glutaric acidemia type II without congenital anomalies:* These children have a similar onset and clinical course as the first group, with cardiomyopathy as an important part of the terminal event.

*Later onset glutaric acidemia type II* (see **Acidemia, ethylmalonic-adipic**).

**Complications:**  The neonatal-onset forms have been uniformly fatal, with death usually being due to a cardiomyopathy.

**Associated Findings:** None known.

**Etiology:** Autosomal recessive inheritance.

**Pathogenesis:** The disease can be caused by deficiency of ETF or ETF:QO, both enzyme deficiencies are inherited as autosomal recessive traits. All infants with anomalies studied to date have had defects in ETF:QO. The defect in electron transfer causes failure of ketone body and energy production from fatty acid oxidation, possibly causing cardiomyopathy, and the loss of organic acids in the urine as carnitine esters leads to tissue deficiency of carnitine.

**MIM No.:** *30595

**Sex Ratio:** M1:F1

**Occurrence:** More than a dozen cases have been documented in the literature.

**Risk of Recurrence for Patient's Sib:**
See Part I, *Mendelian Inheritance.*

**Risk of Recurrence for Patient's Child:**
See Part I, *Mendelian Inheritance.*

**Age of Detectability:** Several affected fetuses have been identified by the presence of glutaric acid and other organic acids in the amniotic fluid.

**Gene Mapping and Linkage:** ACAD (acyl-Coenzyme A dehydrogenase, multiple) has been provisionally mapped to X.

**Prevention:** None known. Genetic counseling indicated.

**Treatment:** Therapy with carnitine and riboflavin.

**Prognosis:** Usually fatal in the first week to several weeks of life, often because of cardiomyopathy.

**Detection of Carrier:** May be possible by assaying fibroblast extracts for activities of ETF and ETF:QO.

**Special Considerations:** One pedigree in which inheritance appeared to be X-linked (Coude et al, 1981) involved male deaths which were probably due to **Ornithine transcarbamylase deficiency**.

**Support Groups:** KS; Kansas City; The Organic Acidemia Association

**References:**
Coude FX, et al.: Neonatal glutaric aciduria type II: an X-linked recessive inherited disorder. Hum Genet 1981; 59:263–265.
Goodman SI, Frerman FE: Glutaric acidemia type II (multiple acyl-CoA dehydrogenation deficiency). J Inherited Metab Dis 1984; 7(Suppl 1):33–37.
Frerman FE, Goodman SI: Deficiency of electron transfer flavoprotein or electron transfer flavoprotein:ubiquinone oxidoreductase in glutaric acidemia type II fibroblasts. Proc Natl Acad Sci USA 1985; 82:4517–4520. *
Amendt BA, Rhead WJ: The multiple acyl-coenzyme A dehydrogenation disorders, glutaric aciduria type II and ethylmalonic-adipic aciduria: mitochondrial fatty acid oxidation, acyl-coenzyme A dehydrogenase, and electron tranfer flavoprotein activities in fibroblasts. J Clin Invest 1986; 789:205–213.
Frerman FE, Goodman SI: Glutaric acidemia type II and defects of the mitochondrial respiratory chain. In: Scriver CR, et al, eds: The metabolic basis of inherited disease, 6th ed. New York: McGraw-Hill, 1989:915–932. * †
Wilson GN, et al.: Glutaric aciduria type II: review of the phenotype and report of an unusual glomerulopathy. Am J Med Genet 1989; 32:395–401.

LA008
G0025

**Charlotte Z. Lafer**
**Stephen I. Goodman**

**Acidemia, Hawkinsinuria type**
*See HAWKINSINURIA*
**Acidemia, hyperpipecolic**
*See CEREBRO-HEPATO-RENAL SYNDROME*

---

**ACIDEMIA, ISOVALERIC**      **0547**

**Includes:**
Isovaleric acid CoA dehydrogenase deficiency
Isovaleric acidemia
IVD deficiency
Sweaty feet syndrome

**Excludes:** N/A

**Major Diagnostic Criteria:** Increased concentrations of isovaleric acid are demonstrated in serum by gas phase chromatography. In the urine, isovalerylglycine is identifiable by simple chromatographic techniques. A deficiency in isovaleryl coenzyme A (CoA) dehydrogenase is observed in leukocytes or skin fibroblasts.

**Clinical Findings:** Onset is usually acute, often within the first days of life with vomiting, acidosis, rapidly progressive neurological signs and possibly death. The only distinctive clinical sign is the characteristic "sweaty feet" odor of isovaleric acid. Survivors frequently have acute relapses that decrease in frequency with age. Mental retardation is common (IQ of 50–80). Onset of symptoms may be delayed until the patient is weeks or months old.

There is no aminoacidemia or ketoaciduria so that the common diagnostic procedures for metabolic disease are not informative. The extreme elevations of isovaleric acid are evident only during the acute attacks, but isovalerylglycine can be commonly demonstrated in the urine even when the patient is clinically normal. The enzyme defect in leukocytes and fibroblasts is constant.

**Complications:** Mental retardation has been common in the early-onset disease. The frequency of this serious condition may be reduced with early diagnosis and aggressive treatment.

**Associated Findings:** Bone marrow depression, particularly with leukopenia and thrombocytopenia, is common.

**Etiology:** Autosomal recessive inheritance of a deficiency in isovaleryl-CoA dehydrogenase.

**Pathogenesis:** The degradation of leucine proceeds through α-ketoisocaproic acid to isovaleric acid to β-methylcrotonic acid. A deficiency in isovaleryl-CoA dehydrogenase reduces the efficiency of the last metabolic, step resulting in increases in isovaleric acid. Conjugation with glycine and excretion as isovalerylglycine protects the patient against minor increases in isovaleric acid. Excesses above this cause the described symptomatology. The unidirectional action of the branched-chain keto acid decarboxylase prevents retrograde elevations of the respective keto acid and amino acid (leucine).

**MIM No.:** *24350

**Sex Ratio:** M1:F1

**Occurrence:** About 40 cases reported in the literature.

**Risk of Recurrence for Patient's Sib:**
See Part I, *Mendelian Inheritance.*

**Risk of Recurrence for Patient's Child:**
See Part I, *Mendelian Inheritance.*

**Age of Detectability:** Enzyme defect should be demonstrable at birth.

**Gene Mapping and Linkage:** IVD (isovaleryl Coenzyme A dehydrogenase) has been mapped to 15q14-q15.

**Prevention:** None known. Genetic counseling indicated.

**Treatment:** The acute episodes are treated aggressively to correct dehydration and acidosis, with glucose as a source of calories. This approach is usually adequate. Patients are maintained on a low protein diet (1.5–2 gm per kg). Glycine supplements have been used to facilitate excretion of isovalerylglycine.

**Prognosis:** The prognosis is influenced by the age of onset (better in late onset cases), and by the rapidity with which the diagnosis is made and treatment instituted.

**Detection of Carrier:** Unknown.

**Support Groups:** KS; Kansas City; The Organic Acidemia Association

**References:**
Efron ML: Isovaleric acidemia. Am J Dis Child 1967; 113:74–76.
Ando T, Nyhan WL: A simple screening method for detecting isovaleric acidemia. Clin Chem 1970; 16:420–422.
Shih VE, et al.: Diagnosis of isovaleric acidemia in cultured fibroblasts. Clin Chim Acta 1973; 48:473–479.
Kelleher JFL, et al.: The pancytopenia of isovaleric acidemia. Pediatrics 1980; 65:1023–1027.
Rhead WJ, Tanaka K: Demonstration of a specific mitochondrial isovaleryl-CoA dehydrogenase deficiency in fibroblasts from patients with isovaleric acidemia. Proc Natl Acad Sci USA 1980; 77:580–583.
Tanaka K, Rosenberg LE: Isovaleric acidemia. In: Stanbury JB, et al., eds: The metabolic basis of inherited disease, ed 5. New York: McGraw-Hill, 1983:457–461. *
de Sousa C, et al.: The response to L-carnitine and glycine therapy in isovaleric acidemia. Eur J Pediatr 1986; 144:451–456.

DA003                                                          **Joseph Dancis**

## ACIDEMIA, METHYLMALONIC                                           0658

**Includes:**
 B(12)-responsive forms of methylmalonic acidemia
 Methylmalonic acidemia
 Methylmalonic aciduria

**Excludes:**
 **Acidemia, propionic** (0826)
 **Anemia, pernicious congenital** (2656)

**Major Diagnostic Criteria:** Early onset of lethargy or coma; episodic ketoacidosis. Elevation of the concentration of methylmalonic acid in blood or urine.

**Clinical Findings:** Onset early in life of life-threatening illness. Repeated episodes of ketoacidosis may lead to coma and may be fatal. Neutropenia is prominent, and osteoporosis and thrombocytopenia may occur. Infections are common and may precipitate life-threatening ketoacidosis. Mental retardation may occur in those surviving early infancy, but with treatment, normal mental development is achievable. Growth retardation is striking. Convulsions and EEG abnormalities may be seen. Some patients have had chronic monilial infections. Red cells are normal, and megaloblastosis is absent.

Concentrations of methylmalonic acid in the plasma are elevated; they tend to approximate 10 mg/dl. Urinary excretion of methylmalonic acid may be over 500 mg per day. This compound is not normally detectable in blood or urine. It has even been found in the cerebrospinal fluid and in tissues of patients dying of the disease. Increased quantities of glycine are found in the blood and urine. Normal concentrations of glycine are also found frequently in patients who manifest elevations at other times. Concentrations of $B_{12}$ in the blood are not low.

**Complications:** Death, mental retardation, pathological fractures.

**Associated Findings:** None known.

**Etiology:** Autosomal recessive inheritance.

**Pathogenesis:** Enzymatic site of the defect is in methylmalonyl CoA mutase. This may be primary, or may be secondary to a defect in $B_{12}$ metabolism. Genetic heterogeneity has been established in that there are now a number of distinct forms of methylmalonic acidemia, some of which represent abnormalities in the metabolism of $B_{12}$. In one of these disorders there is associated homocystinuria and cystathionuria. Routine screening of newborns or sibs of affected patients has identified eight children with an apparently benign clinical variant of this disorder.

**MIM No.:** *25100
**POS No.:** 3781
**Sex Ratio:** M1:F1

**Occurrence:** More than fifty cases reported.
**Risk of Recurrence for Patient's Sib:**
 See Part I, *Mendelian Inheritance.*
**Risk of Recurrence for Patient's Child:**
 See Part I, *Mendelian Inheritance.*
**Age of Detectability:** Detectable in the fetus by assay of methylmalonic or methylcitric acid in amniotic fluid, or by assay of propionate metabolism or methylmalonyl CoA mutase activity in cultured amniocytes.
**Gene Mapping and Linkage:** MUT (methylmalonyl Coenzyme A mutase) has been mapped to 6p21.
**Prevention:** Prenatal treatment has been successful in $B_{12}$-responsive methylmalonic acidemia.
**Treatment:** $B_{12}$ should be used in those patients who are sensitive to the vitamin. Diets low in isoleucine, valine, threonine, and methionine are effective therapy for those who are not $B_{12}$-responsive, but management is demanding. Avoidance of exposure to and prompt treatment of infection is important. Deletion of protein-containing foods and substitution of electrolyte and glucose-containing fluids should be instituted in the presence of ketosis.
**Prognosis:** Most patients have died very early in infancy.
**Detection of Carrier:** Unknown.
**Support Groups:** KS; Kansas City; The Organic Acidemia Association

**References:**
Matsui SM, et al.: The natural history of the inherited methylmalonic acidemias. New Eng J Med 1983; 308:857–861.
Ledley FD, et al.: Benign methylmalonic aciduria. New Eng J Med 1984; 311:1015–1018.
Ney DN, et al.: An evaluation of protein requirements in methylmalonic acidemia. J Inherited Metab Dis 1985; 8:132–142.
Nyhan WL: Diagnostic recognition of genetic disease. Philadelphia: Lea and Febiger, 1987:42–50. *

NY000                                                     **William L. Nyhan**

## ACIDEMIA, MEVALONIC                                               2564

**Includes:**
 Mevalonate kinase deficiency
 Mevalonic aciduria

**Excludes:**
 **Ataxia**
 **Muscular dystrophy** (1515)
 **Peroxisomal disorders** (1533)

**Major Diagnostic Criteria:** Psychomotor retardation, recurrent diarrhea, severe failure to thrive, ataxia, anemia, hepatosplenomegaly, and dysmorphic features. Elevated creatine kinase. Urinary and plasma levels of mevalonic acid are grossly elevated. Mevalonate kinase activity is deficient in amniocytes, fibroblasts, lymphoblasts, lymphocytes, and liver.

**Clinical Findings:** Six patients have been reported. Clinical manifestations include psychomotor retardation (6/6), recurrent diarrhea (5/6), severe failure to thrive (3/6), and dysmorphic features (3/6). The course of the disease was progressive in four out of the six patients; two of them died within the first two years of life.

Clinical presentation is variable. More severely affected patients present in the neonatal period with severe failure to thrive, developmental delay, and gastroenteropathies, which resemble cow's milk intolerance. Fat is poorly tolerated. Further clinical findings are seizures, hypotonia, hepatosplenomegaly, and lymphadenopathy. Dysmorphic features include **Microcephaly;** dolichocephaly; wide fontanels with irregular borders; third fontanel; blue sclera; bilateral central cataracts; a triangular face; down-slanted eyes; and large, posteriorly rotated, low-set ears. X-rays show a severely retarded bone age and a CT scan a generalized atrophy of the brain. The pathobiochemical effects of mevalonic acidemia may severely compromise normal intrauter-

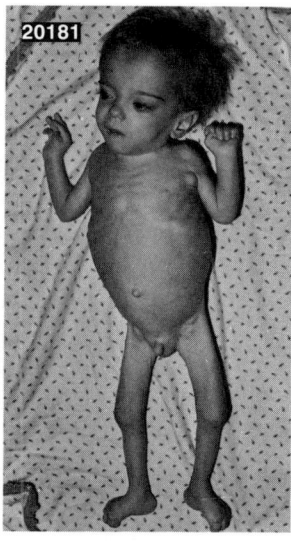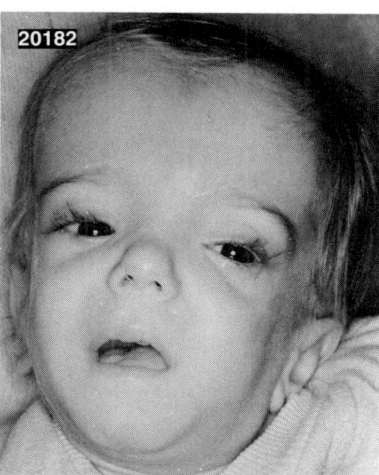

**2564**-20181: Infant with failure to thrive and hepatosplenomegaly from mevalonic acidemia. 20182: Note triangular facies, down slanted palpebral fissures and large, posteriorly rotated ears.

ine development. Two other pregnancies in a family of a severely affected patient ended with stillbirth at 26 weeks' gestation (the fetus showed micrognathia and hand and foot abnormalities) and with spontaneous abortion, respectively.

One patient, a six year old boy, presented only with a slight developmental delay and ataxia. His urinary excretion of mevalonic acid was lower than in the severely affected patients, and serum cholesterol levels were higher. However, mevalonate kinase activity was less than 5% of control means in all patients.

Mevalonic acid is excreted several thousand-fold above normal. Plasma mevalonic acid is also highly elevated (100–500 $\mu$mol/l), but does not lead to metabolic acidosis or an elevated anion gap. Standard clinical chemical investigations reveal a strikingly elevated creatine kinase. Serum cholesterol levels are normal or slightly reduced. Serum alanine and aspartate aminotransferases are concomitantly elevated. There may be severe iron deficient anemia.

**Complications:** Malabsorption, probably due to diminished pool of bile acids. Secondary carnitine deficiency.

**Associated Findings:** None known.

**Etiology:** Autosomal recessive inheritance.

**Pathogenesis:** Symptoms are thought to be due to an underproduction of the end products of the biosynthetic pathway of cholesterol and nonsterol isoprenes, e.g., lack of bile acids leads to severe malabsorption and failure to thrive. In the affected fetus the highest level of mevalonic acid was detected in the brain. This may reflect a particular need for cholesterol in brain development and is consistent with the severe developmental delay of patients with mevalonic aciduria. Central cataracts, minor anomalies, and deranged liver functions are known side effects of high doses of drugs interfering with cholesterol biosynthesis. Some clinical features may also be due to a thus far unknown toxicity of high plasma levels of mevalonic acid.

**MIM No.:** *25117

**POS No.:** 4366

**Sex Ratio:** M1:F1

**Occurrence:** Six cases have been reported in the literature.

**Risk of Recurrence for Patient's Sib:**
See Part I, *Mendelian Inheritance.*

**Risk of Recurrence for Patient's Child:**
See Part I, *Mendelian Inheritance.*

**Age of Detectability:** Prenatal diagnosis is possible by assaying mevalonate kinase activity in amniocytes and in chorionic villus cells and by direct assay of mevalonic acid in amniotic fluid by gas chromatography-mass spectrometry. After birth, affected children excrete large amounts of mevalonic acid in the urine.

**Gene Mapping and Linkage:** Unknown.

**Prevention:** None known. Genetic counseling indicated.

**Treatment:** Unknown. Dietary supplementations of bile acid, cholesterol and other nonsterol isoprenes may be beneficial.

**Prognosis:** Varies, depending on the degree of enzyme deficiency. In most patients, the course of the disease has been progressive.

**Detection of Carrier:** Possible through optimized assay of mevalonate kinase in lymphoblasts. Among 17 members of the index patient's family, heterozygotes and homozygous normals could be distinguished. Heterozygotes were also found to show a significantly increased excretion of mevalonic acid in their urine by means of a stable isotope dilution assay with capillary gas chromatography-mass spectrometry. It would probably be preferential to determine the exceedingly low levels of mevalonic acid by an enzymatic assay.

**Special Considerations:** Mevalonic aciduria is the first described defect of cholesterol and nonsterol isoprene biosynthesis in humans. In contrast to patients with metabolic defects in catabolic pathways, mevalonic aciduria does not lead to recurrent acidosis triggered by excess of dietary nutrients or catabolic crises, but to a chronic multisystemic disease. Enormous amounts of mevalonic acid are constantly produced and excreted efficiently into the urine. This would be consistent with a diminution in the feedback inhibition of HMG-CoA reductase resulting from diminished production of end products. Even a more than 95% reduction in the enzyme activity of mevalonate kinase only moderately reduces the flow through the entire cholesterol pathway. The enzyme deficiency appears to be balanced in the cell by expression of a high activity of HMG-CoA reductase, which markedly increases the concentration of mevalonic acid, the substrate for the deficient enzyme.

Other defects of the biosynthesis of cholesterol and nonsterol isoprenes are likely to be discovered in the near future. If a more distant enzyme would be affected, there may be no organic acidemia. These children would present with hypocholesterolemia and chronic multisystemic disease.

**Support Groups:** KS; Kansas City; The Organic Acidemia Association

**References:**
Berger R, et al.: Mevalonic aciduria: an inborn error of cholesterol biosynthesis? Clin Chim Acta 1985; 152:219–222.
Hoffmann G, et al.: Mevalonic aciduria: an inborn error of cholesterol and nonsterol isoprene biosynthesis. New Engl J Med 1986; 1610–1614. *
Mol MJTM, et al.: Effects of synvinolin (MK-733) on plasma lipids in familial hypercholesterolaemia. Lancet 1986; II:936–939.
Gibson KM, et al.: Mevalonic aciduria: family studies in mevalonate kinase deficiency: an inborn error of cholesterol biosynthesis. J Inherit Metab Dis 1987; 10(suppl 2):282–285.
Hoffmann G, et al.: Mevalonic aciduria: pathobiochemical effects of mevalonate kinase on cholesterol metabolism and cellular growth in intact fibroblasts. J Inherited Metab Dis 1988; 2(suppl 11):229–232.
de Klerk, et al.: A patient with mevalonic aciduria presenting with hepatosplenomegaly, congenital anaemia, thrombocytopenia and leukocytosis. J Inherited Dis 1988; 2(suppl 11):233–236.

**Georg Hoffmann**

## ACIDEMIA, OROTIC 0772

**Includes:**
Orotate phosphoribosyltransferase-omp decarboxylase deficiency
Orotic acidemia
Orotic aciduria
Orotidylic decarboxylase deficiency
Orotidylic pyrophosphorylase-orotidylic decarboxylase deficiency
Ump synthase deficiency

**Excludes:**
Acquired orotic aciduria produced by 6-azauridine
Arginase deficiency or other urea cycle abnormalities
**Argininemia** (0086)
**Ornithine transcarbamylase deficiency** (3023)

**Major Diagnostic Criteria:** The diagnosis is suggested by megaloblastic anemia unresponsive to $B_{12}$ or folic acid and confirmed by the documentation of orotic acid in large amounts in the urine. Erythrocytes and fibroblasts in cell culture are deficient in both orotidylic pyrophosphorylase and orotidylic decarboxylase.

**Clinical Findings:** Patients with orotic aciduria have a megaloblastic anemia which is unresponsive to treatment with $B_{12}$ or folic acid. They also have growth retardation. They excrete large amounts of orotic acid in the urine and may present with crystalluria. One patient has been reported as having only a deficiency of orotidylic decarboxylase (OMP-DC), with an increased activity of orotidylic pyrophosphorylase (OMP-PP). Two surviving patients are mentally retarded.

**Complications:** The first patient described died of generalized varicella, suggesting that resistance to infectious disease may be abnormal.

**Associated Findings:** None known.

**Etiology:** Autosomal recessive inheritance.

**Pathogenesis:** Deficiency of OMP-PP and OMP-DC suggests gene linkage or that one defect is secondary. 5-Azaorotic acid or dihydro-orotic acid induces higher levels of both enzymes, thus providing evidence for post-translational change. The pathogenesis of the clinical findings is unknown.

**MIM No.:** *25890, 25892

**Sex Ratio:** Presumably M1:F1

**Occurrence:** Undetermined but presumed rare.

**Risk of Recurrence for Patient's Sib:**
See Part I, *Mendelian Inheritance.*

**Risk of Recurrence for Patient's Child:**
See Part I, *Mendelian Inheritance.*

**Age of Detectability:** Presumably at birth, by enzyme assay of erythrocytes or fibroblasts.

**Gene Mapping and Linkage:** UMPS (uridine monophosphate synthetase) has been provisionally mapped to 3cen-q21.

**Prevention:** None known. Genetic counseling indicated.

**Treatment:** Partial remissions have been observed with glucocorticoid administration. Replacement therapy with a mixture of yeast nucleotides led to a complete remission and a decrease in urinary orotic acid. This preparation was poorly tolerated. Surviving patients are being successfully maintained on oral uridine therapy.

**Prognosis:** Unknown.

**Detection of Carrier:** Assay of OMP-DC in the erythrocyte or fibroblast.

**Support Groups:** KS; Kansas City; The Organic Acidemia Association

**References:**
Fox FM: Hereditary orotic aciduria: differing enzyme patterns. Am J Med 1969; 47:332–336.
Fox FM, et al.: Hereditary orotic aciduria: types I and II. Am J Med 1973; 55:791–798.
Harden KK, Robinson JL: Deficiency of UMP synthase in dairy cattle: a model for hereditary orotic aciduria. J Inherited Metab Dis 1987; 10:201–209.
Suttle DP, et al.: Hereditary orotic aciduria and other disorders of pyrimidine metabolism. In: Scriver CR, et al, eds: The metabolic basis of inherited disease, 6th ed. New York: McGraw-Hill, 1989: 1095–1128.

NY000 **William L. Nyhan**

## ACIDEMIA, PROPIONIC 0826

**Includes:**
Glycinemia, ketotic, I
Hyperglycinemia-ketoacidosis-leukopenia, type I
Hyperglycinemia, ketotic
Ketotic hyperglycinemia I
PCCA Complementation group
Propionic acidemia
Propionicacidemia I
Propionyl-CoA-carboxylase deficiency, type I

**Excludes:**
**Acidemia, methylmalonic** (0658)
Glycinuria without hyperglycinemia
**Glucoglycinuria** (0418)
**Hyperglycinemia, nonketotic** (0492)

**Major Diagnostic Criteria:** Identification of methylcitric acid in urine, increased concentrations of glycine in the blood, recurrent episodes of ketoacidosis, and elevated concentrations of propionate in the serum. Definitive diagnosis requires the determination that propionyl-CoA-carboxylase activity is deficient in fibroblasts, leukocytes, and tissue.

**Clinical Findings:** Onset early in life of vomiting, acidosis, and ketonuria. Episodes of ketoacidosis are recurrent; they lead to coma and often to death in infancy. Mental retardation and variable neurologic findings may be observed in those surviving early infancy, but this may be a function of the severity of complications, such as shock and hypoxemia, and especially of early neonatal hyperammonemia, rather than an inherent consequence of the metabolic defect. Neutropenia and thrombocytopenia occur, as do frequent infections and transient purpura. Osteoporosis may be followed by pathologic fractures.
Plasma concentrations of glycine are usually greater than 5 mg/dl, and tend to approximate 10 mg/dl. Normal mean concentrations approximate 1 mg/dl. Mean urinary excretion of glycine, even in a patient less than three years of age, was over 400 mg/dl, or 5.5 mg of glycine/mg creatinine. Glycine excretion in controls was 0.2 mg/mg of creatinine. Glycine concentration in the cerebrospinal fluid is also elevated. Concentrations of propionic acid in the blood are high. Even remission levels approximate 10–20 $\mu$M. In relapse they may be 100 times that. These patients have sizeable amounts of methylcitrate and hydroxypropionate in the urine; methylcitrate is found in concentrations of 2–6 $\mu$M/mg creatinine.

**Complications:** Mental retardation and early death.

**Associated Findings:** None known.

**Etiology:** Autosomal recessive inheritance of a deficiency of propionyl-CoA-carboxylase.

**Pathogenesis:** Accumulation of propionyl Co has a number of direct effects on other systems. Hyperammonemia results from inhibition of acetylglutamate synthetase. Ketosis results from inhibition of citric acid cycle enzymes and the formation of massive amounts of acetoacetate. The compound inhibits granulocyte, T cell and B cell development, and specifically interferes with T cell responses to Candida.

**MIM No.:** *23200

**Sex Ratio:** M1:F1

**Occurrence:** Undetermined but presumed rare.

**Risk of Recurrence for Patient's Sib:**
See Part I, *Mendelian Inheritance.*

**Risk of Recurrence for Patient's Child:**
See Part I, *Mendelian Inheritance*. Affected individuals are not expected to survive to reproduce.

**Age of Detectability:** Birth to seven days of age, by quantitative assay of the plasma concentration of glycine or propionate and urinary methylcitrate. Prenatal diagnosis may be made by assay of propionyl-CoA-carboxylase in cultured amniocytes. The diagnosis can be made more rapidly by assay of the amniotic fluid for methylcitrate.

**Gene Mapping and Linkage:** PCCA (propionyl Coenzyme A carboxylase, alpha polypeptide) has been mapped to 13q22-q34.

**Prevention:** None known. Genetic counseling indicated.

**Treatment:** For these patients, the essential amino acids isoleucine, threonine, valine, and methionine are toxic. Patients have been successfully treated with low-protein diets in which the relevant amino acids are kept at levels of intake just sufficient to meet anabolic needs and no more. Such diets must be fashioned individually. Avoidance of exposure to, and prompt treatment of, infection. Deletion of protein-containing foods, and the use of electrolyte-containing solutions in the presence of ketosis.

**Prognosis:** The majority of patients have died very early in life. The prognosis for those surviving early childhood should be improved.

**Detection of Carrier:** Unknown.

**Support Groups:** KS; Kansas City; The Organic Acidemia Association

**References:**
Ando T, et al.: Propionic acidemia in patients with ketotic hyperglycinemia. J Pediatr 1971; 78:827–834.
Ando T, et al.: Isolation and identification of methylcitrate, a major metabolic product of propionate in patients with propionic acidemia. J Biol Chem 1972; 247:2200–2204.
Sweetman L, et al.: Prenatal diagnosis of propionic and methylmalonic acidemia by stable isotope dilution analysis of methylcitric and methylmalonic acids in amniotic fluids. In: Schmidt H-L, et al, eds: Stable isotopes. Amsterdam: Elsevier Scientific Publishing, 1982:287–293.
Ney D, et al.: An evaluation of protein requirements in methylmalonic acidemia. J Inherited Metab Dis 1985; 8:132–142. *
Nyhan WL: Disorders of propionate metabolism. In: Bickel H, Wachtel U, eds: Inherited diseases of amino acid metabolism. Stuttgart: Georg Thiem Verlag Thieme, 1985:363–382. *
Nyhan WL: Propionic acidemia. In Nyhan WL, ed: Diagnostic recognition of genetic disease. Philadelphia: Lea & Febiger, 1987:36–41.

NY000                                          **William L. Nyhan**

---

## ACIDEMIA, PYROGLUTAMIC                          0849

**Includes:**
Five-oxoprolinuria
Glutathione synthetase deficiency
Pyroglutamic acidemia

**Excludes:**
Gamma-glutamyl-cysteine synthetase deficiency
**Glutathionuria** (0422)
Prolinemia

**Major Diagnostic Criteria:** The finding of large amounts of pyroglutamic acid (5-oxoproline) in the urine.

**Clinical Findings:** Onset is early in life. The 12 patients described have shown variable signs and symptoms. Severe and chronic metabolic acidosis was seen in 10/12. Neonatal jaundice and episodes of hemolytic anemia also occurred in most. The only adult patient had an episode of jaundice in the newborn period, but has since had no signs of hemolytic anemia. Four of the 12 have retarded psychomotor development and neurologic symptoms.

The first described patient died at 28 years of age. Mental retardation, cerebellar ataxia, spastic tetraparesis, intention tremor, seizures, and frequent episodes of vomiting were the major manifestations. Progressive tremor, movement disorder, and ataxia complicated the last decade of his life. The immediate cause of death was a leg vein thrombosis with pulmonary embolism. The main autopsy findings were cerebellar atrophy of the granular layer, patchy loss of neurons in a laminar pattern in the visual cortex, and focal lesions in the central region and the thalami. In addition, there were two cystic cavities, indicating old cerebral infarctions. The brain alterations may have been due to oxidative damage because of lack of glutathione in the brain.

Plasma concentrations of pyroglutamic acid are usually about 50 mg/100 ml (4 mmol/liter), and the urinary excretion of the metabolite is about 0.5 gm (4 mmol)/kg body weight/24 hours. The urinary excretion of urea and the concentration of potassium in serum may be reduced. The erythrocyte glutathione level in the 12 patients has ranged from not detectable to 25% of the normal values (normal value is about $2.0 \pm 0.5$ $\mu$mole/gm of wet cells). There may be cyclic variations in the erythrocyte glutathione content, and only when the level is very low (not detectable) there may be an increased content of amino acids in the erythrocytes. Analysis of biopsy/autopsy material indicates that all organs are deficient in glutathione, and all contain increased amounts of pyroglutamic acid, with a particularly high content (11–19 $\mu$mol/gm of wet tissue) in the kidney, brain, and lungs. The level of the enzyme glutathione synthetase was low (1–4% of controls) in all organs of the dead patient. The erythrocytes of all patients are deficient in the enzyme (0–2% of normal). The pattern of amino acids in serum and cerebrospinal fluid are normal, except for elevation of proline (3 times normal in the adult patient). Only one patient showed generalized amino aciduria.

**Complications:** Metabolic acidosis.

**Associated Findings:** Hemolytic anemia, mental retardation, cerebellar ataxia, and probably increased tendency for thrombosis and cerebellar atrophy.

**Etiology:** Autosomal recessive inheritance.

**Pathogenesis:** All patients described to date have a defect in the ability to synthesize glutathione synthetase. The last enzyme needed in the glutathione pathway, catalyzing the conversion of $\gamma$-glutamylcysteine to glutathione, is deficient. Production of pyroglutamic acid is secondary to the glutathione synthetase deficiency. The synthetic defect also causes the marked deficiency in glutathione that is needed to maintain hemoglobin in its reduced form and to maintain the red cell membrane. The glutathione deficiency presumably contributes to hemolysis.

**MIM No.:** *26613

**Sex Ratio:** M1:F1

**Occurrence:** About a dozen cases documented in the literature.

**Risk of Recurrence for Patient's Sib:**
See Part I, *Mendelian Inheritance*.

**Risk of Recurrence for Patient's Child:**
See Part I, *Mendelian Inheritance*.

**Age of Detectability:** Neonatal period to adult years, by detection of elevated amounts of pyroglutamic acid in the urine; or metabolic acidosis (acid-base status) and reduced excretion of urea in the urine. There is always a low content of glutathione and glutathione synthetase in the erythrocytes.

**Gene Mapping and Linkage:** Unknown.

**Prevention:** None known. Genetic counseling indicated.

**Treatment:** Treatment with bicarbonate to compensate for the metabolic acidosis. The patients should not be given amino acids intravenously, and should not be given large amounts of ascorbic acid or drugs known to precipitate hemolysis.

Substitution with an antioxidant, e.g., cysteine, penicillamine, mercaptopyridoxal, or vitamin E to prevent the cerebellar atrophy has not been tried but might be useful.

**Prognosis:** Ten of the 12 patients detected to date are still alive. One patient died at the age of six months (diagnosed post mortem) and the other died at 28 years of age. It is unknown whether the affected children treated with bicarbonate, who do not now have neurologic symptoms, will develop them over time.

**Detection of Carrier:** Fibroblast assay of glutathione synthetase activity in first degree relatives.

**Support Groups:** KS; Kansas City; The Organic Acidemia Association

**References:**

Jellum E, et al.: Pyroglutamic aciduria: a new inborn error of metabolism. Scand J Clin Lab Invest 1970; 26:327–335.

Wellner VP, et al.: Glutathione synthetase deficiency, an inborn error of metabolism involving the γ-glutamyl cycle in patients with 5-oxoprolinuria (pyroglutamic aciduria). Proc Natl Acad Sci (USA) 1974; 71:2505–2509.

Marstein S, et al.: Biochemical studies of erythrocytes in a patient with pyroglutamic acidemia (5-oxoprolinemia). New Engl J Med 1976; 295:406–412.

Skullerud K, et al.: The cerebral lesions in a patient with generalized glutathione deficiency and pyroglutamic aciduria (5-oxoprolinuria). Acta Neuropathol (Berl) 1980; 52:235–238.

Marstein S, et al.: Biochemical investigations of biopsied brain tissue and autopsied organs from a patient with pyroglutamic acidemia (5-oxoprolinemia). Clin Chim Acta 1981; 11:219–228.

Larsson A, et al.: Ophthalmological, psychometric and therapeutic investigation in two sisters with hereditary glutathione synthetase deficiency (5-oxoprolinuria). Neuropediatrics 1985; 16:131–136.

Meister A, Larsson A: Glutathione synthetase deficiency and other disorders of the γ-glutamyl cycle. In: Scriver CR, et al, eds: The metabolic basis of inherited disease, 6th ed. New York: McGraw-Hill, 1989:855–868.

HA041

**David J. Harris**
*Egil Jellum*

## ACIDEMIA, TRIHYDROXYCOPROSTANIC      3275

**Includes:**
Coprostanic acidemia
Trihydroxycoprostanic acidemia

**Excludes:**
**Arterio-hepatic dysplasia** (2084)
**Cerebro-hepato-renal syndrome** (0139)
**Jaundice, intrahepatic cholestatic, Byler type** (2371)
Non-syndromic ductular hypoplasia

**Major Diagnostic Criteria:** Increased content of trihydroxycoprostanic acid in biological fluids (bile, serum and urine) in association with chronic, progressive intrahepatic cholestasis.

**Clinical Findings:** The disease presents with cholestasis (elevated serum total bilirubin, conjugated bilirubin, and alkaline phosphatase) and hepatomegaly during infancy. Liver biopsy has demonstrated a decreased number of interlobular bile ducts. Liver disease progresses rapidly, with cirrhosis and liver failure developing during the first year of life.

**Complications:** All of the complications of chronic cholestatic liver disease, including malabsorption of fat and fat-soluble vitamins, pruritus, hypercholesterolemia, xanthomatosis, and growth failure, and cirrhosis, including portal hypertension, hypersplenism, ascites, porto-systemic encephalopathy, esophageal varices, etc.

**Associated Findings:** None known.

**Etiology:** Presumably autosomal recessive inheritance; one report described two affected siblings.

**Pathogenesis:** Trihydroxycoprostanic acid is a metabolic precursor in the production of cholic acid. This metabolite can be found in meconium from normal newborns and in small amounts in biological fluids from children and adults with other forms of cholestasis. It is the principal bile acid of the American alligator. The mitochondrial enzyme responsible for the reduction of the terminal aliphatic carbon chain of trihydroxycoprostanic acid is absent or decreased in affected individuals. Trihydroxycoprostanic acid is thought to be poorly transported by the human hepatocyte so it accumulates within the liver, where it acts as a detergent and disrupts membranes. Its accumulation in bile epithelial cells may cause obliteration of bile ducts, which results in a decreased number of interlobular bile ducts as observed in histological specimens.

**MIM No.:** *21495, 27565

**Sex Ratio:** Presumably M1:F1.

**Occurrence:** Fewer than ten cases have been documented in the literature.

**Risk of Recurrence for Patient's Sib:**
See Part I, *Mendelian Inheritance.*

**Risk of Recurrence for Patient's Child:**
See Part I, *Mendelian Inheritance.*

**Age of Detectability:** During early infancy.

**Gene Mapping and Linkage:** Unknown.

**Prevention:** None known. Genetic counseling indicated.

**Treatment:** Replacement of the bile acid pool with ursodeoxycholic acid has theoretical advantage, but has not been used in this disease. Orthopic liver transplantation would be curative.

**Prognosis:** Death has occurred before one year of age in all reported cases.

**Detection of Carrier:** Unknown.

**References:**

Hanson R, et al.: The metabolism of 3-alpha, 7-alpha, 12-alpha-trihydroxy-five-beta-cholestan-26-oic acid in two siblings with cholestasis due to intrahepatic bile duct anomalies. J Clin Invest 1975; 56:577–578.

Freese D, Hanson R: Neonatal cholestatic syndromes associated with alterations in bile acid synthesis. J Pediatr Gastro Nutr 1983; 2:374–380.

FI035
AL037

**Mark Fishbein**
**Estella M. Alonso**

**Aciduria, 3-hydroxy-3-methylglutaric**
*See ACIDEMIA, 3-HYDROXY-3-METHYLGLUTARIC*
**Aciduria, 3-methylglutaconic**
*See ACIDURIA, 3-METHYLGLUTACONIC TYPE II*

## ACIDURIA, 3-METHYLGLUTACONIC TYPE I      2967

**Includes:** Aciduria, 3-methylglutaconyl-coenzyme A hydratase

**Excludes:**
**Aciduria, 3-methylglutaconic type II** (2968)
**Aciduria** (other)
Inborn errors of metabolism (other)

**Major Diagnostic Criteria:** Excessive urinary excretion of 3-methylglutaconic, 3-methylglutaric, and 3-hydroxyisovaleric acids without elevated urinary levels of 3-hydroxy-3-methylglutaric acid.

**Clinical Findings:** In two male sibs, the only clinical abnormality was a retardation of speech development. In both sibs the approximate levels of the relevant organic acids excreted in the urine were (mmol/mol creatinine) 3-methylglutaconic acid, 780; 3-hydroxyisovaleric acid, 204; and 3-methylglutaric acid, 9.

**Complications:** Unknown.

**Associated Findings:** One of two sibs was reported to be slow in motor development, having first walked at age two years. At age one year this patient had had an attack of unconsciousness lasting for almost 24 hours. He was further reported to have a short attention span.

**Etiology:** Presumably autosomal recessive inheritance.

**Pathogenesis:** In both patients, a severe deficiency of 3-methylglutaconyl-coenzyme A hydratase (approximating less than 5% of control activity), an enzyme on the leucine catabolic pathway, was documented in extracts of cultured skin fibroblasts. The result is a massive urinary excretion of 3-methylglutaconic and 3-methylglutaric acid. The presence of 3-methylglutaric acid is probably the result of the action of a specific or nonspecific oxidoreductase on accumulated 3-methylglutaconic acid. Increased urinary levels of 3-hydroxyisovaleric acid may arise from the hydration of increased concentrations of 3-methylcrotonyl-coenzyme A, the penultimate metabolite to 3-methylglutaconyl-coenzyme A in the leucine degradative pathway. The similar clinical course of the two sibs suggests that this is the clinical presentation of 3-methylglutaconyl-coenzyme A hydratase deficiency.

**MIM No.:** *25095

**Sex Ratio:** Presumably M1:F1

**Occurrence:** Two male sibs of Moroccan descent have been documented.

**Risk of Recurrence for Patient's Sib:**
See Part I, *Mendelian Inheritance*.

**Risk of Recurrence for Patient's Child:**
See Part I, *Mendelian Inheritance*.

**Age of Detectability:** Most likely at a chronologic age at which speech development can be tested.

**Gene Mapping and Linkage:** Unknown.

**Prevention:** None known. Genetic counseling indicated.

**Treatment:** Restriction of protein intake, especially leucine.

**Prognosis:** Favorable in view of the mild clinical course.

**Detection of Carrier:** Unknown.

**Special Considerations:** It may be of value to analyze urinary organic acids in patients presenting with delayed speech development. It should be noted, however, that increased urinary concentrations of 3-methylglutaconic and 3-methylglutaric acids may be nonspecific indicators of deranged metabolism and may not correlate with a defect in the leucine catabolic pathway. On the other hand, quantitative or qualitative enzyme assays of 3-methylglutaconyl-coenzyme A hydratase are warranted when the excretion of these two organic acids are elevated in the urine in conjunction with increased amounts of 3-hydroxyisovaleric acid.

**References:**
Duran M, et al.: Inherited 3-methylglutaconic aciduria in two brothers: another defect of leucine metabolism. Pediatrics 1982; 101:551–554. *
Hammond J, Wilcken B: 3-Hydroxy-3-methylglutaric, 3-methylglutaconic and 3-methylglutaric acids can be non-specific indicators of metabolic disease. J Inherited Metab Dis 1984; 7(suppl 2):117–118.
Narisawa K, et al.: Deficiency of 3-methylglutaconyl-coenzyme A hydratase in two siblings with 3-methylglutaconic aciduria. J Clin Invest 1986; 77:1148–1152. *

GI019
H0051

**Kenneth M. Gibson**
**Georg Hoffmann**

## ACIDURIA, 3-METHYLGLUTACONIC TYPE II            2968

**Includes:** Aciduria, 3-methylglutaconic

**Excludes:**
   **Aciduria, 3-methylglutaconic type I** (2967)
   **Aciduria** (other)
   Inborn errors of metabolism (other)

**Major Diagnostic Criteria:** Persistently elevated urinary concentrations of 3-methylglutaconic and 3-methylglutaric acids without elevated 3-hydroxy-3-methylglutaric acid. Parallel quantitative or qualitative enzyme studies in leukocytes or cultured fibroblasts or studies monitoring the conversion of $^{14}C$-leucine or isovaleric acid to $^{14}CO_2$ indicate normal functioning of 3-methylglutaconyl-coenzyme A hydratase in the leucine catabolic pathway.

**Clinical Findings:** The clinical picture is one of profound psychomotor retardation (13/15), spasticity with or without hypertonicity (11/15), neurologic deterioration (9/15), and hypotonia (8/15). Other less frequent manifestations have included failure to thrive (7/15), optic atrophy with or without chorioretinal degeneration (6/15), seizures (5/15), choreoathetosis with or without dystonia (4/15), abnormalities of the EEG (4/15), and damage or degeneration of hepatic tissue (4/15). Hypodense areas with or without cerebral atrophy with enlarged ventricles have been documented by CT scan or pneumoencephalography (4/15), and at least three patients were noted to be microencephalic. Hepatomegaly and hepatosplenomegaly were observed in two patients.

The excretion of 3-methylglutaconic acid in the urine has ranged from 52 to 1,600 mmol/mol creatinine, with the excretion of 3-methylglutaric acid being as low as 5 and as high as 215 mmol/mol creatinine. While the excretion of 3-methylglutaconic acid in these patients is lower in some cases and comparable in others in comparison to patients with a known deficiency of 3-methylglutaconyl-coenzyme A hydratase, the excretion of urinary 3-methylglutaric acid appears generally higher. Interestingly, two of the patients with the lowest excretion in the urine (40–80 mmol/mol creatinine, both acids) were reported to have dementia. Two patients had elevated urinary 3-hydroxyisovaleric acid at 46 and 100 mmol/mol creatinine, the latter value being about 50% of the concentration of the same compound in patients with defective 3-methylglutaconyl-coenzyme A hydratase. Elevated citric acid cycle intermediates have also been remarked on in the urine of patients. In one the excretion of 2-oxoglutaric acid was approximately 2,500 mmol/mol creatinine, and other compounds such as succinic, fumaric, citric, isocitric, malic, and cis-aconitic acids were highly elevated. Two other patients had increased urinary 2-oxoglutaric acid, and another patient excreted excessive amounts of succinic acid in the urine. Dicarboxylic aciduria, including glutaric, adipic, and suberic acids, may or may not be present.

**Complications:** Death has been recorded for six patients as early as ages 28 days and up to 48 months. The onset of neurologic symptoms has generally ranged from the neonatal period up to the first 12 months of life. Neurogenic hearing loss or impairment was mentioned in three patients, and three patients were reported to be blind. For the surviving patient, psychomotor retardation is expected to be extreme.

**Associated Findings:** Manifestations in various patients have included myoclonus, ataxia, cyanotic and breath-holding spells, and right-sided pyelonephritis. One patient, who appeared to have a transient 3-methylglutaconic aciduria, displayed self-mutilative behavior, while another patient displayed dysmorphic features of the face, clinodactyly of both index fingers, hypospadias, undescended testes, talipes equinovarus, and umbilical and inguinal hernias. Metabolic acidosis has been documented in many cases, and the plasma concentration of lactic and pyruvic acids may be increased.

**Etiology:** Presumably autosomal recessive inheritance, as patients from both sexes have been reported and parental consanguinity was reported in two families.

**Pathogenesis:** It is probable that the combined 3-methylglutaconic and 3-methylglutaric aciduria observed in these patients is secondary to another metabolic derangement. Normal activity for 3-methylglutaconyl-coenzyme A hydratase in extracts of leukocytes or cultured fibroblasts obtained from five patients has been documented.

**MIM No.:** *25095

**Sex Ratio:** Presumably M1:F1; observed, M7:F8

**Occurrence:** Of 15 patients, five were of Caucasian ancestry; two were Swedish, two Turkish, one Yugoslavian, one black, one German, and another was of North African descent.

**Risk of Recurrence for Patient's Sib:**
See Part I, *Mendelian Inheritance*.

**Risk of Recurrence for Patient's Child:**
See Part I, *Mendelian Inheritance*.

**Age of Detectability:** In most cases, from the first few days of life up to several months. The potential for in utero detection by stable-isotope dilution analysis of 3-methylglutaconic acid in amniotic fluid using combined gas chromatography-mass spectrometry remains to be assessed.

**Gene Mapping and Linkage:** Unknown.

**Prevention:** None known. Genetic counseling indicated.

**Treatment:** Unknown.

**Prognosis:** Extremely guarded. Six patients have died, whereas others have survived to adolescence.

**Detection of Carrier:** Unknown.

**Special Considerations:** It may be wise to recommend urinary organic acid analysis on patients who present with psychomotor deficit, spasticity or hypertonicity, neurologic impairment, and hypotonia. It is clear that the urinary accumulation of 3-methylglutaconic and 3-methylglutaric acids may be nonspecific manifestations of metabolic derangement. However, it remains prudent to assess the activity of the leucine catabolic pathway in tissues derived from patients in whom these metabolites accumulate in body fluids either in the presence or absence of 3-hydroxyisovaleric and 3-hydroxy-3-methylglutaric acids.

**References:**

Greter J, et al.: 3-Methylglutaconic aciduria: report on a sibship with infantile progressive encephalopathy. Eur J Pediatr 1978; 129:231–238. *

Hagberg B, et al.: 3-Methylglutaconic aciduria in two infants. Clin Chim Acta 1983; 134:59–67. *

Hammond J, Wilcken B: 3-Hydroxy-3-methylglutaric, 3-methyl-glutaconic and 3-methylglutaric acids can be non-specific indicators of metabolic disease. J Inherited Metab Dis 1984; 7(suppl 2):117–118.

Lehnert W, et al.: 3-Methylglutaconic and 3-methylglutaric aciduria in a patient with suspected 3-methylglutaconyl CoA hydratase deficiency. Eur J Pediatr 1985; 143:301–303.

Gibson KM, et al.: 3-methylglutaconic aciduria: a phenotype in which activity of 3-methylglutaconyl-coenzyme A hydratase is normal. Europ J Pediatr 1988; 148:76–82.

GI019                                   **Kenneth M. Gibson**
H0051                                    **Georg Hoffmann**

**Aciduria, 3-methylglutaconyl-coenzyme A hydratase**
*See ACIDURIA, 3-METHYLGLUTACONIC TYPE I*

---

## ACIDURIA, ARGININOSUCCINIC             0087

**Includes:** Argininosuccinic aciduria

**Excludes:** Urea cycle defects (other)

**Major Diagnostic Criteria:** Elevation of urinary argininosuccinic acid (ASA) level; lesser accumulations in cerebrospinal fluid and blood.

**Clinical Findings:** The acute neonatal form is manifested shortly after feedings are begun, with poor sucking, vomiting, lethargy, and often hepatomegaly. These findings rapidly progress to seizures, coma, apnea, and death if untreated.

In some patients, the disorder is manifested later, with episodic ataxia, vomiting, and often hepatomegaly. They may also have friable hair, which has the microscopic features of trichorrhexis nodosa, and seizures; progressive mental retardation is usual.

If the patient with either the acute neonatal or later-onset form survives the initial insult, recurrent crises occur, precipitated by intercurrent infection or by excessive protein intake. Each is potentially life-threatening.

During any acute episode, the plasma ammonia level is several times normal, with values over 1,000 mg/dl (normal for neonates is less than 100). Secondary increases in glutamine, alanine, and lysine are seen. Blood ASA levels rise to 10–50 mg/dl in severely affected newborns and to 3–4 mg/dl in older patients (normally only trace amounts are present). Urinary excretion may reach several grams per day. Serum arginine is low, and the BUN may be low or normal.

**Complications:** Most surviving patients have a significant degree of mental retardation. Recurrent bouts of hyperammonemia are usual.

**Associated Findings:** None known.

**Etiology:** Autosomal recessive inheritance.

**Pathogenesis:** Deficiency of argininosuccinate lyase (AL; argininosuccinase) enzyme, which mediates the reversible breakdown of argininosuccinate to arginine and fumarate. The enzyme is detectable in erythrocytes and in liver and fibroblast tissues.

**MIM No.:** *20790

**POS No.:** 3028

**CDC No.:** 270.600

**Sex Ratio:** M1:F1

**Occurrence:** Undetermined but presumed rare.

**Risk of Recurrence for Patient's Sib:**
See Part I, *Mendelian Inheritance.*

**Risk of Recurrence for Patient's Child:**
See Part I, *Mendelian Inheritance.*

**Age of Detectability:** Elevated urinary ASA levels after protein-containing infant feedings.
*Prenatal diagnosis:* Enzymatic analysis of cultured amniotic fluid cells will detect the defect. Increase in ASA content has also been found in amniotic fluid.

**Gene Mapping and Linkage:** ASL (argininosuccinate lyase) has been mapped to 7pter-q22.

**Prevention:** None known. Genetic counseling indicated.

**Treatment:** *Acute:* Hemodialysis or peritoneal dialysis to help clear ammonia; high-caloric, nonnitrogenous intravenous fluids help to minimize tissue catabolism. Arginine stimulates step 1 of the urea cycle, encouraging protein synthesis and nitrogen elimination via pyrimidines. Nitrogen excretion is enhanced by sodium benzoate (conjugates with glycine, excreted as hippuric acid) and sodium phenylacetate (conjugates with glutamine, excreted as phenylacetylglutamine).
*Chronic:* Dietary protein restriction with high-caloric intake. Supplementary arginine as needed.

**Prognosis:** Most patients who live beyond the neonatal period are mentally retarded. There is a good correlation between the duration of the neonatal hyperammonemic coma and the severity of both mental retardation and brain CT abnormalities (increase in ventricular and sulcus size, and in areas of low density). In one series, eight surviving patients aged 30 ± 4 months had IQs that measured 37 ± 10 (mean ± SEM).

**Detection of Carrier:** Intermediate levels of AL enzyme have been found in the fibroblasts of parents of affected children.

**Special Considerations:** Fasting blood ammonia levels may be normal. If a urea cycle defect is suspected and the fasting level is normal, a protein load of 1.5 g of protein per kilogram is given, by nasogastric tube if necessary. The ammonia determination, made about 2 hours afterward, will reveal a severalfold increase.

**References:**

Brusilow SW, et al.: Neonatal hyperammonemic coma. Adv Pediatr 1982; 29:69–103. *

Brusilow SW, et al.: Treatment of episodic hyperammonemia in children with inborn errors of urea synthesis. New Engl J Med 1984; 310:1630–1634.

Msall M, et al.: Neurologic outcome in children with inborn errors of urea synthesis. New Engl J Med 1984; 310:1500–1505. *

Vimal CM, et al.: Prenatal diagnosis of argininosuccinicaciduria by analysis of cultured chorionic villi. Lancet 1984; II:521–522.

Hyman SL, et al.: Anorexia and altered serotonin metabolism in a patient with argininosuccinic aciduria. J Pediatr 1986; 108:705–709.

Simard L, et al.: Argininosuccinate lyase deficiency: evidence for heterogeneous structural gene mutations by immunoblotting. Am J Hum Genet 1986; 39:38–51.

Brusilow SW and Horwich AL: Urea cycle enzymes. In: Scriver CR, et al.: The metabolic basis of inherited disease, 6th ed. New York: McGraw-Hill, 1989:629–664.

AM004                                      **Mary G. Ampola**

## ACIDURIA, BETA-MERCAPTOLACTATE-CYSTEINE DISULFIDURIA    0106

**Includes:** Beta-mercaptolactate-cysteine disulfiduria

**Excludes:** N/A

**Major Diagnostic Criteria:** Urine is positive by the nitroprusside test. Chromatography of the urinary amino acids shows the presence of a characteristic spot, which can be revealed by the following reagents: ninhydrin, iodoplatinic acid, and cyanide-nitroprusside.

**Clinical Findings:** Five patients have been identified. The first was a 46-year-old American male with severe, lifelong mental retardation. The parents were sibs. The second and third patients were two Swiss female sibs identified by a screening program. They were mentally and physically normal. The parents were unrelated. The fourth patient was a 16-year-old Scottish male with severe mental retardation. The parents were first cousins. The fifth patient was a Swedish female who had ulcerative colitis and autoimmune hemolytic anemia. Her intelligence was normal.

**Complications:** Unknown.

**Associated Findings:** Mental retardation (two cases). Chronic otitis media with subsequent deafness (one case). Obesity, hypogonadism, valgus deformity of both knees, severe pes planus, bilateral congenital cataract with nystagmus (one case). Ulcerative colitis and autoimmune hemolytic anemia (one case).

**Etiology:** Probably autosomal recessive inheritance.

**Pathogenesis:** A deficiency of the enzyme $\beta$-mercaptopyruvate sulfur transferase (MST) has been identified in the erythrocytes of the first and fifth patients described.

**MIM No.:** *24965

**Sex Ratio:** M2:F3 observed

**Occurrence:** Rare. Five known cases.

**Risk of Recurrence for Patient's Sib:**
See Part I, *Mendelian Inheritance.*

**Risk of Recurrence for Patient's Child:**
See Part I, *Mendelian Inheritance.*

**Age of Detectability:** Has been detected in childhood and adult life. Probably present from infancy.

**Gene Mapping and Linkage:** Unknown.

**Prevention:** None known. Genetic counseling indicated.

**Treatment:** Unknown.

**Prognosis:** Life span may be normal, but mental retardation appears to be unchanged through life.

**Detection of Carrier:** No carriers identified. MST has been described in small quantities in the urine of normal people. Erythrocyte MST activity is reduced in the father, mother, and sibs of the fifth patient, with some increase of the urinary disulfide.

**Special Considerations:** On the basis of the five patients currently known, it is not possible to be certain that the metabolic abnormality and the mental retardation are causally related.

**References:**
Ubuka T, et al.: S-(2-hydroxy-2-carboxyethylthio) cysteine and S-(carboxymethylthio) cysteine in human urine. Biochim Biophys Acta 1968; 158:493–495.
Ampola MG, et al.: Mental deficiency and a new aminoaciduria. Am J Dis Child 1969; 117:66–70.
Crawhall JC, et al.: $\beta$-mercaptolactate cysteine disulfide in the urine of a mentally retarded patient. Am J Dis Child 1969; 117:71–82.
Niederwieser A, et al.: $\beta$-mercaptolactate cysteine disulfiduria in two normal sisters. Isolation and characterization of $\beta$-mercaptolactate cysteine disulfide. Clin Chim Acta 1973; 43:405–416. *
Law EA, Fowler B: $\beta$-mercaptolactate cysteine disulphiduria in a mentally retarded Scottish male. J Ment Defic Res 1976; 20:99–104.
Shih VE, et al.: $\beta$-mercaptopyruvate sulfur transferase deficiency. The enzyme defect in $\beta$-mercaptolactate-cysteine disulfiduria. Pediatr Res 1977; 11:464.
Hannestad U, et al.: 3-mercaptolactate cysteine disulfiduria: biochemical studies on affected and unaffected members of a family. Biochem Med 1981; 26:106–114. *

CR006                                               **John C. Crawhall**

## ACIDURIA, BETA-METHYL-CROTONYL-GLYCINURIA    0107

**Includes:**
Beta-hydroxyisovaleric acidemia
Beta-methylcrotonylglycinurie
Three methylcrotonyl-CoA carboxylase deficiency, isolated
Three-methylcrotonylglycinuria

**Excludes:**
Carboxylase deficiency, holocarboxylase deficiency type (2006)
Acidemia, isovaleric (0547)

**Major Diagnostic Criteria:** Lethargy, hypotonia, and feeding difficulties with or without acidosis in the absence of ketosis may indicate this disorder. One patient had severe muscle atrophy and fibrillations of the tongue. One patient had hair loss and another severe hypoglycemia. An odor similar to that of tomcat's urine and elevated $\beta$-hydroxyisovaleric acid and $\beta$-methylcrotonylglycine or $\beta$-methylcrotonic acid indicates this disorder.

**Clinical Findings:** Onset and clinical signs vary widely. The initial patient (female) had feeding difficulties at two weeks and had clinical signs similar to infantile spinal muscular atrophy with severe hypotonia, atrophy of muscle, tongue fibrillations, and absence of deep tendon reflexes without ketosis or acidosis at 4 1/2 months. The urine had an odor similar to that of cat's urine or black currant leaves. The patient excreted up to 560 mg per day of $\beta$-hydroxyisovaleric acid and 140 mg per day of $\beta$-methylcrotonyl-glycine. The second patient (female) developed normally until 5 weeks of age, then developed increasing irritability, drowsiness, feeding difficulties and vomiting. By 11 weeks of age infantile spasms and metabolic acidosis without ketosis occurred. The urine contained large amounts of $\beta$-hydroxyisovaleric acid and (alpha)-ketoglutaric acid but not $\beta$-methylcrotonylglycine. The third and fourth patients, a brother and sister, were Vietnamese refugees and were asymptomatic for 5–6 years, presumably because of a low protein diet. With a higher protein diet the male vomited and became acidotic and comatose. The fifth patient (female) had recurrent otitis media, and presented at 22 months of age with hypotonia, coma, apnea, severe hypoglycemia and mild metabolic acidosis. The last three patients all excreted large amounts of 3-hydroxyisovaleric acid and 3-methylcrotonylglycine, which was unresponsive to treatment with 15–30 mg of biotin per day.

**Complications:** Retardation of motor development occurred in the first case and death at an early age in the first two cases but the last three patients are clinically normal with a restricted protein diet.

**Associated Findings:** One patient excreted large amounts of $\alpha$-ketoglutaric acid, and one patient had life-threatening hypoglycemia.

**Etiology:** Probably autosomal recessive inheritance. Deficient activity of $\beta$-methylcrotonyl-CoA carboxylase demonstrated in four patients. Multiple carboxylase deficiency was not completely excluded in first two patients but was excluded in the last three patients.

**Pathogenesis:** The defect is in the metabolism of leucine involving the carboxylation of $\beta$-methylcrotonyl-CoA to $\beta$-metylglutaconyl-CoA. Accumulated $\beta$-methylcrotonyl-CoA is metabolized to $\beta$-methylcrotonylglycine and $\beta$-hydroxyisovaleric acid and excreted. The relation of the laboratory findings to clinical features is unknown.

**MIM No.:** *21020, 21021

**Sex Ratio:** M1:F3

**Occurrence:** Rare; five cases reported in the literature.

**Risk of Recurrence for Patient's Sib:**
See Part I, *Mendelian Inheritance.*

**Risk of Recurrence for Patient's Child:**
See Part I, *Mendelian Inheritance.*

**Age of Detectability:** At birth and by prenatal diagnosis.

**Gene Mapping and Linkage:** Unknown.

**Prevention:** None known. Genetic counseling indicated.

**Treatment:** In one case restriction of isoleucine intake significantly reduced the excretion of β-hydroxyisovaleric acid but had no effect on the clinical course. Biotin (up to 30 mg per day) is of no therapeutic value. The last three patients are clinically normal on diets with protein restricted to 1.9–2.0 g/kg body weight per day.

**Prognosis:** Uncertain; two patients died, three are doing well.

**Detection of Carrier:** May be detectable by assay of 3-methylcrotonyl-CoA carboxylase in leucocytes and fibroblasts.

**Special Considerations:** Patients initially described as biotin-responsive β-methylcrotonylglycinuria have a defect in biotin metabolism which affects at least 3 carboxylases and are now identified as having **Carboxylase deficiency, holocarboxylase deficiency type** and have a good clinical prognosis. All patients with suspected β-methylcrotonylglycinuria should have propionyl-CoA, pyruvate, and β-methylcrotonyl-CoA carboxylases assayed and should be treated with 10 mg or more of biotin per day to distinguish the 2 disorders.

**Support Groups:** KS; Kansas City; The Organic Acidemia Association

**References:**
Stokke O, et al.: Beta-methylcrotonyl-CoA carboxylase deficiency: a new metabolic error in leucine degradation. Pediatrics 1972; 49:726–735.
Finnie MDA, et al.: Massive excretion of 2-oxoglutaric acid and 3-hydroxyisovaleric acid in a patient with a deficiency of 3-methyl-crotonyl-CoA carboxylase. Clin Chim Acta 1976; 73:513–519.
Beamer FA, et al.: Isolated biotin-resistant 3-metylcrotonyl-CoA carboxylase deficiency in two sibs. Eur J Pediatr 1982; 138:351–354. *
Bartlett K, et al.: Isolated biotin-resistant 3-metylcrotonyl-carboxylase deficiency presenting with life-threatening hypoglycemia. J Inher Metab Dis 1984; 7:182. *
Sweetman L, Nyhan WL: Inheritable biotin-treatable disorders and associated phenomena. Ann Rev Nutr 1986; 6:317–343.

SW002                                          **Lawrence Sweetman**

---

### ACIDURIA, DICARBOXYLIC AMINOACIDURIA        0294

**Includes:** Glutamate-aspartate transport defect

**Excludes:** Dicarboxylic aciduria

**Major Diagnostic Criteria:** Selective excess of L-glutamate and L-aspartate in urine (dicarboxylic monoamino acids), identifiable by partition chromatography, electrophoresis, or elution chromatography on ion-exchange resin columns. The corresponding plasma concentrations are normal. Endogenous renal clearance of both dicarboxylic amino acids are elevated and can exceed creatinine clearance.

**Clinical Findings:** Incidental finding by urine amino acid screening in two infants. A tendency toward fasting hypoglycemia, coupled with the presence of increased serum ketone bodies and low plasma bicarbonate without a defect in ammoniagenesis with modest hyperprolinemia ($< 1$ mM; $< 11.5$ mg/dl) was observed by Teijema et al. (1974). Similar findings were absent in the study by Melancon et al. (1977).

**Complications:** Hypoglycemia after mild fasting; ketosis; impaired bicarbonate conservation (probably renal).

**Associated Findings:** None known.

**Etiology:** Presumably autosomal recessive inheritance of a homozygous phenotype involving either a defect in selective membrane transport system for dicarboxylic monoamino acids or intracellular transamination to keto acids during transepithelial movement.

**Pathogenesis:** Simple defect in uptake from tubule lumen will not explain $C_{glu}$ and $C_{asp}$ greater than $C_{creatinine}$; therefore, impaired intracellular metabolism of amino acid to keto-acid, with intracellular accumulation and reflux, is a possible explanation. Intestinal uptake defect was also suspected by Teijema et al; pathogenesis (and etiology) of the intestinal defect was presumed to be similar to the renal defect.

**MIM No.:** 22273

**Sex Ratio:** M1:F1

**Occurrence:** 1:28,000 (Quebec); $<10^{-5}$ elsewhere.

**Risk of Recurrence for Patient's Sib:**
See Part I, *Mendelian Inheritance.*

**Risk of Recurrence for Patient's Child:**
See Part I, *Mendelian Inheritance.*

**Age of Detectability:** Presumably in newborn period.

**Gene Mapping and Linkage:** Unknown.

**Prevention:** None known. Genetic counseling indicated.

**Treatment:** Frequent feeding of L-glutamine has been demonstrated to prevent hypoglycemia.

**Prognosis:** Unknown.

**Detection of Carrier:** Parents of proband have normal urine and plasma amino acid concentration and renal clearance of glutamate and aspartate (Melançon SB, personal communication, May 1983).

**Special Considerations:** Selective dicarboxylic monoamino aciduria fulfills prediction from **Hartnup disorder** that there is a separate transepithelial transport system for these anionic amino acids. Phenotype is apparently benign in over 30 unreported patients (S. Melançon, pers. comm.).

**References:**
Teijema HL, et al.: Dicarboxylic amino aciduria: an inborn error of glutamic and aspartic transport with metabolic implications, in combination with a hyperprolinemia. Metabolism 1974; 23:115–123.
Melançon SB, et al.: Dicarboxylic aminoaciduria: an inborn error of amino acid conservation. J Pediatr 1977; 91:422–427.

SC050                                        **Charles R. Scriver**

**Aciduria, dicarboxylic due to LCAD**
*See ACYL-CoA DEHYDROGENASE DEFICIENCY, LONG CHAIN TYPE*
**Aciduria, dicarboxylic due to MCAD**
*See ACYL-CoA DEHYDROGENASE DEFICIENCY, MEDIUM CHAIN TYPE*
**Aciduria, ethylmalonic-adipic**
*See ACIDEMIA, ETHYLMALONIC-ADIPIC*

---

### ACIDURIA, FUMARIC                          2599

**Includes:**
Fumarase deficiency
Fumaric acidemia

**Excludes:**
Acidemia, 2-oxoglutaric (2565)
Other lactic acidemias with concomitant fumaric aciduria

**Major Diagnostic Criteria:** A progressive nervous disorder, presenting in early infancy with failure to thrive, developmental delay, hypotonia, cerebral atrophy, **Microcephaly**, liver disease, and mild lactic acidemia. Mildly affected patients present with mental retardation and speech impairment.

**Clinical Findings:** Clinical signs vary widely, probably corresponding to the residual enzyme activity and possibly genetic heterogeneity.

Fumaric aciduria due to fumarase deficiency has been established in three patients presenting in early infancy with failure to thrive, developmental delay, hypotonia, poor feeding, and mild lactic acidemia (Zinn et al, 1986; Petrova-Benedict et al, 1987; Walker et al, 1988). In one patient, cerebral malformations and liver disease were present from birth; the others suffered from a progressive cerebral atrophy leading to **Microcephaly** within a few months. The disease progressed quickly in one boy; with increasing irritability and opisthotonic posturing. This infant died at eight months of age during an episode of otitis media.

Fumaric acid is highly elevated in the urine. There are variable elevations of citric acid, 2-oxoglutaric acid, and succinic acid. Plasma fumaric acid is only marginal elevated, as are plasma lactic and pyruvic acid, and an intermittently elevated lactate-to-pyruvate ratio; however, there is no elevated anion gap or metabolic acidosis. Transient hyperammonemia and mildly elevated liver transaminases are found. Both the cytosolic and the mitochondrial forms of fumarase are severely deficient. Histochemical and ultrastructural studies of liver are normal, whereas an increased number of mitochondria is observed in skeletal muscle, consistent with a mitochondrial myopathy.

Milder fumaric aciduria in two siblings (a male aged 19 years, and a female aged 25 years) was reported by Whelan et al (1983). These sibs presented with severe mental retardation, especially speech impairment. Computerized tomography of the brain showed internal obstructive **Hydrocephaly** in both cases.

Fumaric aciduria due to fumarase deficiency may have been the underlying biochemical defect in another boy, who died at the age of 3 1/2 years with a progressive encephalomyelopathy suffering from psychomotor retardation, hemiparesis, hypotonia, myoclonic contractions, and seizures (Prick et al 1982). On autopsy, a diagnosis of **Alpers disease** was made.

**Complications:** Seizures. Secondary carnitine deficiency.

**Associated Findings:** None known.

**Etiology:** Autosomal recessive inheritance.

**Pathogenesis:** Mitochondrial fumarase is a component of the tricarboxylic acid cycle. A deficiency may have severe effects on metabolic compartmentation and fluxes of metabolites and neurotransmitters in the CNS. The accumulation of fumarate in the mitochondrium can be anticipated to inhibit succinate dehydrogenase and glutamate dehydrogenase. These pathways are differently regulated in different organs, which may account for tissue-specific consequences in fumarase deficiency.

**MIM No.:** *13685, 13686

**Sex Ratio:** M1:F1

**Occurrence:** Three cases have been fully documented.

**Risk of Recurrence for Patient's Sib:**
See Part I, *Mendelian Inheritance.*

**Risk of Recurrence for Patient's Child:**
See Part I, *Mendelian Inheritance.*

**Age of Detectability:** Increased levels of fumaric acid may be present prenatally in the amniotic fluid. Prenatal diagnosis may be possible by direct assay of fumaric acid in amniotic fluid by gas chromatography-mass spectrometry and/or by assaying fumarase activity in amniocytes and in chorionic villus cells. In affected children, fumaric aciduria probably preceeds neurological symptoms and is present from birth.

**Gene Mapping and Linkage:** FH (fumarate hydratase) has been mapped to 1q42.1.

**Prevention:** None known. Genetic counseling indicated.

**Treatment:** Unknown.

**Prognosis:** The clinical course is one of rapid deterioration, leading to death in early childhood. Mildly affected patients suffer from a non-progressive mental handicap.

**Detection of Carrier:** Unknown.

**Special Considerations:** Metabolic diseases due to disturbances in the tricarboxylic acid cycle have been virtually unknown. They could be expected to produce catastrophic physiological and clinical consequences. However, the few known cases presented with progressive neurological disease or non-progressive mental retardation. There has been no elevated anion gap or metabolic acidosis. As in the only other known defect of the tricarboxylic acid cycle, **Acidemia, 2-oxoglutaric,** fumaric aciduria due to fumarase deficiency causes highly elevated excretions of tricarboxylic acids in the urine, but only insignificant elevations in plasma or cerebrospinal fluid.

Plasma tricarboxylic acids are actively and specifically taken up by the kidney from the blood as well as from the tubules. They share the same carrier systems and are excreted in response to changes in energy metabolism. These characteristics are probably responsible for the observed pathobiochemical effects of enzyme deficiencies of the tricarboxylic acid cycle.

McKusick lists a condition (MIM numbers *13685, 13686), in which rare individuals have an increased number of electrophoretically different forms of fumarases. In these cases, which are inherited in an autosomal dominant way, fumarase activity is reduced (Edwards and Hopkinson, 1979). In contrast, in fumarase deficiency leading to fumaric aciduria all forms of fumarases are virtually absent.

**References:**
Edwards YH, Hopkinson DA: Further characterisation of the human fumarase variant FH 2–1. Ann Hum Genet 1979; 43:103–108.
Kohlschütter A, et al.: A familiar progressive neurodegenerative disease with 2-oxoglutaric aciduria. Eur J Pediatr 1982; 138:32–37.
Prick MJJ, et al.: Progressive infantile poliodystrophy (Alpers' Diesease) with a defect in citric acid cycle activity in liver and fibroblasts. Neuropediat 1982; 13:108–111.
Whelan DT, et al.: Fumaric Aciduria: a new organic aciduria, associated with mental retardation and speech impairment. Clin Chim Acta 1983; 132:301–308. *
Hoffmann G, et al.: Hyper-2-oxoglutaric aciduria in long-term mental handicap. J Ment Defic Res 1986; 30:251–260.
Zinn AB, et al.: Fumarase deficiency: a new cause of mitochondrial encephalomyopathy. New Engl J Med 1986; 315:469–475. *
Petrova-Benedict R, et al.: Deficient fumarase activity in an infant with fumaricacidemia and its distribution between different forms of the enzyme seen on isoelectric focusing. Am J Hum Genet 1987; 40:257–266. *
Walker V, et al.: Fumarase deficiency: neonatal presentation with cerebral malformation and liver disease. (Abstract) 26th Symp Society for the Study of Inforn Errors of Metabolism, Glasgow, September 6–9, 1988:87.

H0051          **Georg Hoffmann**
ZI002          **Arthur B. Zinn**

**Aciduria, glutaric**
*See ACIDEMIA, GLUTARIC ACIDEMIA I*
**Aciduria, hyperdibasic aminoaciduria**
*See HYPERDIBASIC AMINOACIDURIA*

---

## ACIDURIA, SULFITE OXIDASE DEFICIENCY      0921

**Includes:** Sulfocysteinuria

**Excludes:**
    Homocystinuria (0474)
    Molybdenum co-factor deficiency (2412)

**Major Diagnostic Criteria:** Mental retardation with progressive cerebral palsy occurs in infancy with ectopia lentis. Abnormally large urinary excretion of S-sulpho-L-cysteine, sulfite and thiosulfate. Very reduced urinary excretion of sulfate.

**Clinical Findings:** Of the three cases documented, the first was a male with progressive cerebral palsy until decerebrate, who died at the age of two years. Dislocated ocular lenses were also present. The second patient was a male who developed myoclonic jerks and ataxic gait at 24 months; later seizures and choreiform movements developed. At four years, the child had subluxation of both lenses and bilateral spastic paresis. The latter case report (Shih et al, 1977) referred to a third male patient in Belgium with similar findings. The report was referred to as a personal communication to Dr. Shih. It is believed that these two patients may not have had as complete an enzyme defect as the first case, which may affect the course of the disease.

Similar clinical findings have also been observed in **Molybdenum co-factor deficiency**, although in the latter condition both sulfite oxidase and xanthine oxidase are deficient.

**Complications:** Progressive cerebral dysfunction and early death.

**Associated Findings:** None known.

**Etiology:** Autosomal recessive inheritance.

**Pathogenesis:** Deficiency of sulfite oxidase (sulfite: oxygen oxido reductase E.C.1.8.3.1.) in liver, brain, and kidney obtained at autopsy. In the second patient, skin fibroblasts grown in supplemented culture medium showed approximately 20% of the enzyme activity found in normal control fibroblasts. The enzymes require molybdenum as a cofactor. Studies of the liver obtained from the first patient showed that molybdenum levels were normal, but the crossreacting protein corresponding to sulfite oxidase was absent.

**MIM No.:** *27230

**Sex Ratio:** Presumably M1:F1, although the reported cases have been male.

**Occurrence:** Three patients have been reported.

**Risk of Recurrence for Patient's Sib:**
See Part I, *Mendelian Inheritance.*

**Risk of Recurrence for Patient's Child:**
See Part I, *Mendelian Inheritance.* No known patient has survived to reproduce.

**Age of Detectability:** As a neonate, by clinical findings and by finding S-sulfocysteine in the urine. Increased quantities of sulfite, thiosulfate, and taurine are also found with reduced quantities of sulfate in the urine.

**Gene Mapping and Linkage:** Unknown.

**Prevention:** None known. Genetic counseling indicated.

**Treatment:** Diet low in sulfur-containing amino acids may modify the course of the disease.

**Prognosis:** The first reported patient died at 32 months. Three of seven sibs died in infancy with pertinent data not recorded. The second patient was alive at 6 1/2 years of age, although with a severe neurological handicap. He was the first child of a 22-year-old mother who had two previous abortions.

**Detection of Carrier:** Unknown. Abnormality was not present in the urine of a clinically normal parent. Sulfite oxidase activity was reduced in cultured skin fibroblasts of both parents.

**References:**
Irreverre F, et al.: Sulfite oxidase deficiency: studies of a patient with mental retardation, dislocated ocular lenses, and abnormal urinary excretion of S-sulfo-L-cysteine, sulfite and thiosulfate. Biochem Med 1967; 1:187–199.
Mudd SH, et al.: Sulfite oxidase deficiency in man: demonstration of the enzymatic defect. Science 1967; 156:1599–1602.
Johnson JL, Rajagopalan KV: Human sulfite oxidase deficiency: characterization of the molecular defect in a multicomponent system. J Clin Invest 1976; 58:551–556.
Shih VE, et al.: Sulfite oxidase deficiency: biochemical and clinical investigations of a hereditary metabolic disorder in sulfur metabolism. New Engl J Med 1977; 297:1022–1028.
Shih VE, et al.: A simple screening test for sulfite oxidase deficiency: detection of urinary thiosulfate by a modification of Sorbo's method. Clin Chim Act 1979; 95:143–145.
Crawhall JC: A review of the clinical presentation and laboratory findings in two uncommon hereditary disorders of sulfur amino acid metabolism, beta-mercaptolactate cysteine disulfideuria and sulfite oxidase deficiency. Clin Biochem Rev 1987; 1:21–31.

CR006                                                    **John C. Crawhall**

**Ackerman syndrome**
*See DENTO-FACIO-SKELETAL DEFECTS, ACKERMAN TYPE*
**Acordia**
*See UMBILICAL CORD, SHORT UMBILICAL CORD SYNDROME*

---

## ACOUSTIC NEUROMATA                                          0012

**Includes:**
  Acoustic schwannomas, bilateral
  Bilateral acoustic neuromas
  Central neurofibromatosis
  Neurofibromatosis 2
**Excludes:**
  Acoustic neuromas, isolated unilateral
  **Neurofibromatosis** (0712)

**Major Diagnostic Criteria:** Bilateral acoustic neuromas or unilateral acoustic neuromas and subcapsular cataract and/or paraspinal neurofibromas and/or first-degree relative with verified acoustic neuroma.

**Clinical Findings:** Early symptoms are referable to abnormalities of auditory or vestibular function: hearing loss, tinnitus, imbalance and, less commonly, vertigo. Relatively early mild cerebellar ataxia and corneal reflex depression are seen. Spinal tumors appear, in most patients, before the acoustic neuromas. Other complaints may be facial weakness, pain or numbness; headache; nausea and vomiting; visual loss; diplopia; emotional or mental changes; progressing to blindness, emotional or mental change; dysphagia; and dysarthria. Paraspinal neurofibromas are common, and often associated with lower cervical and/or upper thoracic kyphoscoliosis. Cafe-au-lait spots and skin neurofibromas are not consistent findings. Other nervous tumors (e.g. intracranial meningiomas, or spinal meningiomas, astrocytomas, or schwannomas) will be present in many cases. Increased symptomatology or precipitation of symptoms is often noted during late pregnancy. At onset, symptoms may occur unilaterally, and involvement of the opposite side will appear within 2 years. Brainstem auditory evoked response studies can be of diagnostic value, as is plain tomography of the internal auditory meatus. However, NMR scan is the diagnostic test of choice. Subcapsular cataracts are distinctive features.

**Complications:** Profound deafness, due the tumors themselves and/or to surgical intervention. Hydrocephalus is not an uncommon complication. Brain tumors may cause an early death or lead to other serious problems, including hemiplegia, and similar neurologic problems. Facial paralysis may result from the tumors themselves and/or surgical intervention.

**Associated Findings:** Fatal accidents and drowning have been reported.

**Etiology:** Autosomal dominant inheritance with high penetrance. Bilateral acoustic neuromas appear to be distinct from unilateral acoustic neuromas, which are generally sporadic, occur later, and have a more rapid course.

**Pathogenesis:** Unknown.

**MIM No.:** *10100

**Sex Ratio:** M1:F1

**Occurrence:** More than 30 kindreds and 130 cases have been reported. Eight percent of CNS tumors are acoustic neuromas; 5% of them being bilateral.

**Risk of Recurrence for Patient's Sib:**
See Part I, *Mendelian Inheritance.*

**Risk of Recurrence for Patient's Child:**
See Part I, *Mendelian Inheritance.*

**Age of Detectability:** At about 20 years of age by symptoms; earlier by brain stem auditory evoked response (BAER) and/or magnetic resonance imaging (MRI).

**Gene Mapping and Linkage:** NF2 (neurofibromatosis 2 (bilateral acoustic neuroma)) is 22q11-q13.1.

**Prevention:** None known. Genetic counseling indicated.

**Treatment:** Surgery and possibly radiotherapy.

**Prognosis:** Rate of progression is variable. Severe problems, such as deafness and paralysis or more likely than not. Survival after onset of symptoms ranges from 2–40 years with an average of about 20 years.

**Detection of Carrier:** Possibly through genetic linkage studies.

**Support Groups:** PA; Carlisle; Acoustic Neuroma Association (ANA)

**References:**
Moyes PD: Familial bilateral acoustic neuromas affecting 14 members from four generations. J Neurosurg 1968; 29:78–82.
Perez Demoura LF, et al.: Bilateral acoustic neurinoma and neurofibromatosis. Arch Otolaryngol 1969; 90:28–34.
Rouleau GA, et al.: Genetic linkage of bilateral acoustic neurofibromatosis to a DNA marker on chromosome 22. Nature 1987; 329:246–248.
Martuza RL, Eldridge R: Neurofibromatosis 2 (bilateral acoustic neurofibromatosis). New Engl J Med 1988; 318:684:688.
Wertelecki W, et al.: Neurofibromatosis 2: clinical and DNA linkage studies of a large kindred. New Engl J Med 1988; 319:278–283.

RI000

**Vincent M. Riccardi**
*Cor W.R.J. Cremers*

**Acoustic schwannomas, bilateral**
*See ACOUSTIC NEUROMATA*
**Acoustic-cervico-oculo syndrome**
*See CERVICO-OCULO-ACOUSTIC SYNDROME*
**'Acquired' agammaglobulinemia with thymoma**
*See AGAMMAGLOBULINEMIA-THYMOMA SYNDROME*
**Acral dysostosis-facial and genital abnormalities**
*See ROBINOW SYNDROME*
**Acrania**
*See ANENCEPHALY*

## ACRO-FRONTO-FACIO-NASAL DYSOSTOSIS          2779

**Includes:**
   Cleft lip/palate-frontonasal dysplasia-postaxial polysyndactyly
   Polysyndactyly, postaxial-frontonasal dysostosis-cleft lip/palate

**Excludes:**
   **Face, median cleft face syndrome** (0635)
   **Oro-facio-digital syndrome, Mohr type** (0771)
   **Oto-palato-digital syndrome, II** (2258)

**Major Diagnostic Criteria:** The combination of frontonasal dysplasia with skeletal anomalies and **Polydactyly** in a severely retarded child.

**Clinical Findings:** Craniofacial anomalies were numerous and included mental retardation, **Eye, hypertelorism**, S-shaped palpebral fissures, ptosis, long eyelashes, broad and notched nasal tip, bilateral cleft lip/palate, hypoplastic midface, macrostomia, prominent lower lip, mild retrognathia, and anteverted auricles with prominent tragus and lobule. Both affected sibs also had hypoplastic distal phalanges, **Camptodactyly**, brachymetacarpia, hypoplastic toenails, equinovarus or equinovalgus, and short legs. One sib also had postaxial **Polysyndactyly** and lumbar lordosis. X-ray anomalies were numerous and included brachycephaly, hypoplastic facial bones, midline gap in upper maxilla, fusion between hamate and capitate, disorganized carpal bones, iliac hypoplasia, hip dislocation, fibular hypoplasia, short and broad metatarsal and proximal phalanx I, tibiotalar dislocation, and hypoplasia/agenesis of distal phalanges of toes. CT examination in one child showed mild cortical atrophy. Chromosome studies were normal.

**Complications:** Unknown.

**Associated Findings:** None known.

**Etiology:** Autosomal recessive inheritance is strongly suggested by the presence of the condition in sibs of each sex, born to unaffected consanguineous parents.

**Pathogenesis:** Unknown.

**MIM No.:** 20118

**POS No.:** 3695

**Sex Ratio:** M1:F1 (observed).

**Occurrence:** Reported in one pair of siblings from Brazil.

**Risk of Recurrence for Patient's Sib:**
   See Part I, *Mendelian Inheritance.*

**Risk of Recurrence for Patient's Child:**
   See Part I, *Mendelian Inheritance.*

**Age of Detectability:** At birth, by physical examination.

**Gene Mapping and Linkage:** Unknown.

**Prevention:** None known. Genetic counseling indicated.

**Treatment:** Unknown.

**Prognosis:** Intellectual retardation is severe. Prognosis for life span is undetermined, but may not be affected.

**Detection of Carrier:** Unknown.

**References:**
Richieri-Costa A, et al.: A previously undescribed autosomal recessive multiple congenital anomalies/mental retardation (MCA/MR) syndrome with fronto-nasal dysostosis, cleft lip/palate, limb hypoplasia, and postaxial poly-syndactyly: acro-fronto-facio-nasal dysostosis syndrome. Am J Med Genet 1985; 20:631–638.

T0007

**Helga V. Toriello**

**Acro-osteolysis without neuropathy**
*See ACRO-OSTEOLYSIS, DOMINANT TYPE*

## ACRO-OSTEOLYSIS, DOMINANT TYPE          0021

**Includes:** Acro-osteolysis without neuropathy

**Excludes:**
   Dactylolysis spontanea
   **Fibromatosis, juvenile hyaline** (0411)
   **Hajdu-Cheney syndrome** (2022)
   **Hyperparathyroidism, familial** (0499)
   Leprosy
   **Oculo-auriculo-vertebral anomaly** (0735)
   **Osteolysis, carpal-tarsal and chronic progressive glomerulopathy** (0128)
   **Osteolysis, recessive carpal-tarsal** (0129)
   **Pyknodysostosis** (0846)
   **Raynaud disease** (2115)
   Sclerodactyly
   ''Vinyl chloride'' acro-osteolysis

**Major Diagnostic Criteria:** Osteolysis of phalanges, especially in the distal phalanges, with a compatible clinical course and absence of sensory deficits, cutaneous changes, vertebral, skull, or mandibular skeletal defects, osteoporosis or osteosclerosis, abnormal facies, or exposure to the vinyl chloride polymerization process.

**Clinical Findings:** The term ''acro-osteolysis'' is used to designate a variety of syndromes that have as a prominent feature osteolysis of the distal bones of a limb. ''Acro-osteolysis'' in the present usage refers to osteolysis predominantly involving, but not necessarily limited to, the phalanges without neuropathic changes.
   The following clinical description is based on two cases reported by Lamy and Maroteaux (1961).
   Beginning in early childhood, essentially asymptomatic osteolysis of the distal phalanges of the fingers and toes develops. Insidious shortening of the digits occurs without functional disability, loss of sensation, or cutaneous ulceration or atrophy. The nails are present, although somewhat shortened and elliptical in shape. There are no associated skeletal deformities and the facies is normal.
   Osteolysis of the phalangeal tufts with subsequent extension to the diaphyses of the terminal phalanges is seen on X-ray. The distal phalanx of the thumb is also involved. In the fourth and fifth digits of the hands and feet, however, the osteolytic process may commence in the proximal or middle phalanges, leaving the terminal phalanx intact.
   The osteolysis is a chronic, slowly progressive affliction; in the most advanced case (age 34) there was significant shortening of

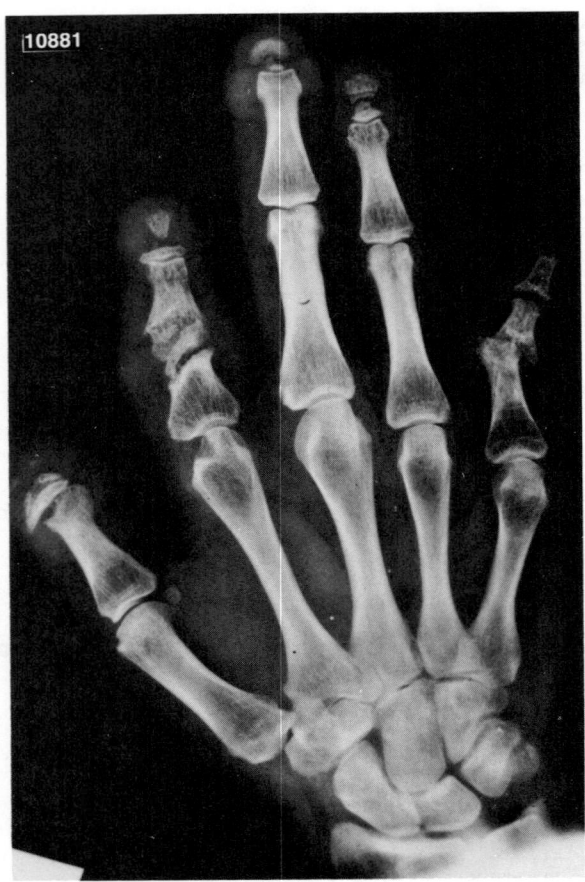

0021-10881: Acro-osteolysis at multiple sites is demonstrated in right hand.

**Risk of Recurrence for Patient's Child:**
See Part I, *Mendelian Inheritance.*

**Age of Detectability:** Early-to-late childhood by clinical and X-ray examination.

**Gene Mapping and Linkage:** Unknown.

**Prevention:** None known. Genetic counseling indicated.

**Treatment:** Unknown.

**Prognosis:** Apparently good for life span, apparently normal for intelligence, with mild-to-moderate manual disability.

**Detection of Carrier:** Unknown.

**Special Considerations:** Differentiation of dominant acro-osteolysis from the many syndromes in which acro-osteolysis is a prominent feature requires thorough clinical and laboratory evaluation. Absence of sensory deficits and cutaneous ulcerations or atrophy tends to rule out leprosy, sclerodactyly, Raynaud disease, and the sensory neuropathy-acro-osteolysis syndromes. An X-ray survey disclosing normal carpal-tarsal bones, long tubular bones, vertebrae, skull, and mandible without osteoporosis or osteosclerosis rules out the **Fibromatosis, juvenile hyaline, Hajdu-Cheney syndrome, Pyknodysostosis,** and various carpal-tarsal osteolysis syndromes. Normal facies without eye or ear malformations or vertebral defects rules out **Oculo-auriculo-vertebral anomaly.** The pattern of bone resorption, absence of other skeletal changes, and lack of alterations in calcium and phosphorus metabolism separates this syndrome from advanced hyperparathyroidism. Dactylolysis spontanea (ainhum) affects a limited number of digits of the feet only. "Vinyl chloride" acro-osteolysis has been confined to individuals employed in cleaning polymerization vats; there is a notable lack of this problem in individuals participating in the further manufacture of polyvinyl chloride products.

**References:**
Lamy M, Maroteaux P: Acro-osteolyse dominante. Arch Fr Pediatr 1961; 18:693–702.
Harris DK, Adams WGF: Acro-osteolysis occurring in men engaged in the polymerization of vinyl chloride. Brit Med J 1967; 3:712–714.

B0025

**Zvi Borochowitz**
*David L. Rimoin*

the digits, some of which were reduced to wrinkled nubbins of tissue, especially those digits with more proximal osteolysis.

The distal phalanges were either absent or reduced to small fragments on X-ray. Occasionally, the lytic process extended past the proximal interphalangeal joint to involve the adjacent middle phalanx. Those digits involved in the more proximal osteolysis exhibited variable loss of all phalanges with marked tapering and shortening of adjacent metacarpals and metatarsals ("sucked candy" appearance). Lateral erosion of the bases of metacarpals and metatarsals was evident with moderate irregularity and loss of outline of carpal and tarsal bones.

No pathologic examination of affected tissues was reported.

The laboratory examination was completely normal, including normal calcium, phosphorus, and alkaline phosphatase. Calcium balance studies were normal.

**Complications:** Mild-to-moderate manual disability secondary to loss of finger length.

**Associated Findings:** None known.

**Etiology:** Autosomal dominant inheritance.

**Pathogenesis:** Unknown.

**MIM No.:** 10240

**POS No.:** 3013

**Sex Ratio:** Presumably M1:F1

**Occurrence:** Rare. Only one pedigree known.

**Risk of Recurrence for Patient's Sib:**
See Part I, *Mendelian Inheritance.*

---

## ACRO-OSTEOLYSIS, NEUROGENIC     3052

**Includes:**
Feet, ulceration and loss of sensation
Giaccai type acroosteolysis

**Excludes:**
Acro-osteolysis, dominant type (0021)
Brain, spongy degeneration (0115)
Hajdu-Cheney syndrome (2022)
Osteolysis, essential (2596)

**Major Diagnostic Criteria:** Ulceration of the feet with loss of sensation and positive family history are suggestive of the diagnosis.

**Clinical Findings:** In the reported sibs, ulceration of the feet began between ages 7–13 years. Pieces of bone were discharged from the ulcerations, with subsequent healing and thickening of the soft tissues. The toes underwent a destructive process, which was reflected as acro-osteolysis of the phalanges, more severe distally. Loss of sensation then developed, with loss of sensation occurring in the hands as well. However, although foot X-rays revealed acro-osteolysis, hand X-rays were normal.

**Complications:** Unknown.

**Associated Findings:** None known.

**Etiology:** Autosomal recessive inheritance.

**Pathogenesis:** Unknown.

**MIM No.:** *20130

**Sex Ratio:** M1:F1

**Occurrence:** One family of four sibs from Lebanon has been reported.

**Risk of Recurrence for Patient's Sib:**
See Part I, *Mendelian Inheritance.*

**Risk of Recurrence for Patient's Child:**
See Part I, *Mendelian Inheritance.*

**Age of Detectability:** Between 7–13 years of age.

**Gene Mapping and Linkage:** Unknown.

**Prevention:** None known. Genetic counseling indicated.

**Treatment:** Supportive; antibiotics if infection occurs.

**Prognosis:** Life span and intellectual development are apparently normal.

**Detection of Carrier:** Unknown.

**Special Considerations:** Sirinavin et al (1982) reported a girl with acro-osteolysis of the fingers and toes; however, onset of symptoms was at age seven months and, in addition to the acro-osteolysis, she had hyperhidrosis of hands and feet, osteoporosis, and soft tissue thickening. This child likely has a different condition.

**References:**
Giaccai L: Familial and sporadic neurogenic acro-osteolysis. Acta Radiol 1952; 38:17–29.
Sirinavin C, et al.: Digital clubbing, hyperhidrosis, acroosteolysis and osteoporosis: a case resembling pachydermoperiostosis. Clin Genet 1982; 22:83–89.

T0007                                        **Helga V. Toriello**

**Acro-osteolysis-osteoporosis-changes in skull and mandible**
*See HAJDU-CHENEY SYNDROME*
**Acro-renal syndrome, Sofer type**
*See RADIAL-RENAL SYNDROME*

---

## ACRO-RENAL-MANDIBULAR SYNDROME          2778

**Includes:**
Foot (split)-mandibular hypoplasia-renal anomalies
Mandibular-acro-renal syndrome
Renal-acro-mandibular syndrome
Split hand and split foot with mandibular hypoplasia

**Excludes:** Radial-renal syndrome (2771)

**Major Diagnostic Criteria:** Split foot with or without split hand; polycystic dysplastic kidneys or renal agenesis; severe mandibular hypoplasia.

**Clinical Findings:** Described in two sisters who died in the neonatal period from severe renal malformations. Patient A was born by cesarean section five weeks before term and weighed 2,000 g. She had an extremely hypoplastic mandible, absent left 5th metacarpal, enlarged abdomen, and bilateral split foot anomaly. She died 32 hours after birth. Autopsy showed hyaline membrane disease and bilateral type 3 dysplastic, polycystic kidneys.
Patient B was born by cesarean section four weeks before term and weighed 1,300 g. She died a few minutes after birth. Severe intrauterine growth retardation and oligohydramnios were shown on serial echograms during the pregnancy. She had a severely hypoplastic mandible, right split hand, and bilateral split foot. Autopsy showed bilateral renal agenesis with absent ureters.

**Complications:** Uterus didelphys (separate uterine cavities leading to the same cervix) in patient A. Uterus unicornis (absence of one uterine horn) in patient B. Since genital defects are frequently observed in severe renal anomalies, they can be considered manifestations of the primary defect or as part of a single acro-renal (genital) developmental field defect.

**Associated Findings: Pectus carinatum; Diaphragmatic hernia;** large cervical spine; 13 pairs of irregular, thin ribs; thoracolumbar scoliosis; a hemivertebra at $L_2$.

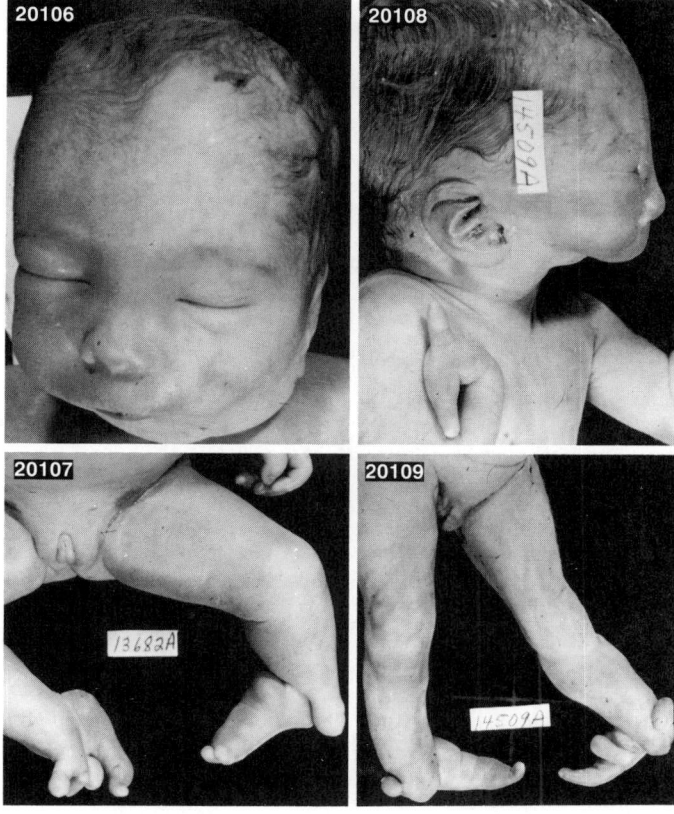

**2778-20106:** Patient 1: Note severe mandibular hypoplasia. **20107:** Bilateral split foot in patient 1. **20108:** Patient 2; Severely hypoplastic mandible, apparently low-set, posteriorly angulated ear, and right split hand anomaly. **20109:** Bilateral split foot in patient 2.

---

**Etiology:** Possibly autosomal recessive inheritance. Parents of two reported cases were second cousins.

**Pathogenesis:** Unknown.

**MIM No.:** 20098

**POS No.:** 3819

**Sex Ratio:** MO:F2 (observed).

**Occurrence:** Reported in two sisters.

**Risk of Recurrence for Patient's Sib:**
See Part I, *Mendelian Inheritance.*

**Risk of Recurrence for Patient's Child:**
See Part I, *Mendelian Inheritance.* Affected individuals are not expected to survive to reproduce.

**Age of Detectability:** During the prenatal period, by ultrasonography.

**Gene Mapping and Linkage:** Unknown.

**Prevention:** None known. Genetic counseling indicated.

**Treatment:** Unknown.

**Prognosis:** Syndrome has been lethal.

**Detection of Carrier:** Unknown.

**Special Considerations:** The mother of the reported cases had a septate uterus and a normal IVP. IVP in the only living female sib showed a duplication of the right collecting system. Whether these findings are coincidental or are a heterozygous expression of a gene responsible for the complete manifestation of the syndrome in the homozygote is undetermined. Results of chromosome studies (G-banding) in both patients were normal.

**References:**
Halal F, et al.: Acro-renal-mandibular syndrome. Am J Med Genet 1980; 5:277–284.

HA074                                                                **Fahed Halal**

**Acro-renal-ocular syndrome**
*See RADIAL-RENAL-OCULAR SYNDROME*

## ACROCALLOSAL SYNDROME, SCHINZEL TYPE          2263

**Includes:**
  Hallux duplication-postaxial polydactyly-absent corpus
    callosum
  Schinzel type acrocallosal syndrome

**Excludes:**
  **Oro-facio-digital syndrome, Mohr type** (0771)
  **Polysyndactyly-dysmorphic craniofacies, Greig type** (2925)

**Major Diagnostic Criteria:** A combination of absence or hypoplasia of the corpus callosum; **Megalencephaly**; prominent forehead, **Eye, hypertelorism**, epicanthic folds, strabismus, depressed nasal bridge, short nose and upper lip; duplication or partial duplication of the big toe phalanges; postaxial **Polydactyly** of fingers and/or toes; bifid terminal phalanges of thumbs; **Syndactyly** between fingers and toes, particularly between the duplicated first toe phalanges and second and third toes; mental retardation, usually severe; and hypotonia.

**Clinical Findings:** Pregnancies may be complicated by polyhydramnios and abnormal fetal presentation. Birth weight and

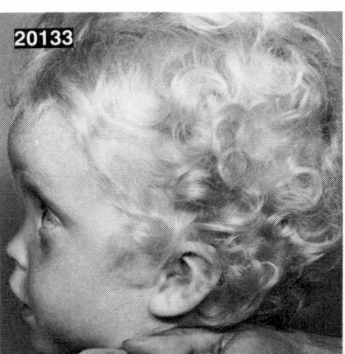

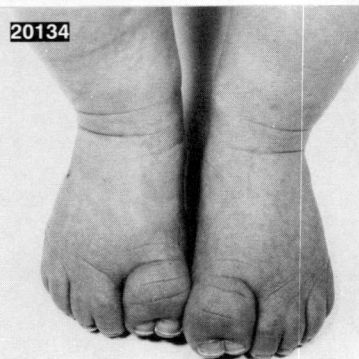
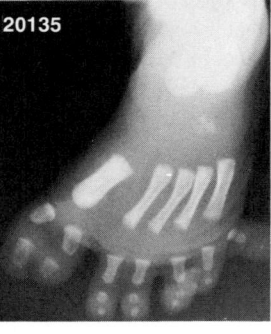

**2263-20132:** Facies at 4 years; note prominent forehead and hypertelorism.   **20133:** Lateral view of the face demonstrates the depressed nasal bridge, short nose and short upper lip. **20134–35:** Note duplicated great toes and postaxial polydactyly. X-ray was obtained in the newborn period.

length are normal, but head circumference is increased. The majority of patients are short at age two years. Hypoxia frequently occurs in the neonatal period, and the early postnatal course is complicated by feeding difficulties, frequent respiratory infections, and seizures.

**Complications:** Derived from the brain malformations: seizures, **Hydrocephaly**, increased intracranial pressure.

**Associated Findings:** Based on eight published cases and another seven observed patients: *Brain*: cerebellar hypoplasia (3), abnormal respiration (1), seizures of various types (3); *Facies*: Up or downslanting palpebral fissures (8/8), preauricular skin tags (2), ear creases (2), **Cleft lip** with (1) or without (1) **Cleft palate**, gingival cysts and/or frenula (1); *Trunk*: accessory nipples (1), umbilical, inguinal, epicastric hernias (5), cryptorchidism (2), renal dysplasia (unilateral, 1), X-ray vertebral and rib anomalies (2); *Extremities*: multiple joint dislocation or restricted movements(2), hypoplasia of femora (1); duplication of tarsal and metatarsal bones (1); high degree of **Polydactyly** of toes/fingers (hepta-to dekadactyly, 2).

**Etiology:** While this was initially thought to be a dominant condition, the occurrence of this syndrome in one pair of sibs, in first cousins, and in two instances with parental consanguinity is consistent with autosomal recessive inheritance.

**Pathogenesis:** Unknown.

**MIM No.:** 20099

**POS No.:** 3555

**Sex Ratio:** Presumably M1:F1.

**Occurrence:** Some fifteen known cases.

**Risk of Recurrence for Patient's Sib:**
  See Part I, *Mendelian Inheritance*.

**Risk of Recurrence for Patient's Child:**
  See Part I, *Mendelian Inheritance*.

**Age of Detectability:** By ultrasound or fetoscopy during the second trimester of gestation (macrocephaly with midbrain defects; pre-, post-axial polydactyly), at birth by clinical features.

**Gene Mapping and Linkage:** Unknown.

**Prevention:** None known. Genetic counseling indicated.

**Treatment:** Shunt operation of secondary **Hydrocephaly**, amputation of supernumerary digits.

**Prognosis:** A minority of patients (1/15) died during the first years of life from complications of their brain malformations. The oldest known child is now over ten years of age. All known patients were mentally retarded, with the majority showing severe intellectual deficit. Shortness of stature is very common in this condition.

**Detection of Carrier:** Unknown.

**Special Considerations:** It is possible that **Oro-facio-digital syndrome, Mohr type** and this syndrome are different expressions of the same genetic entity with preservation of the corpus callosum in the former.

**References:**
Schinzel A, Schmid W: Hallux duplication, postaxial polydactyly, absence of the corpus callosum, severe mental retardation and additional anomalies in two unrelated patients: a new syndrome. Am J Med Genet 1980; 6:241–249. * †
Nelson MM, Thomson AJ: The acrocallosal syndrome. Am J Med Genet 1982; 12:195–199.
Legius E, et al.: Schinzel acrocallosal syndrome: a variant example of the Greig syndrome? Ann Genet (Paris) 1985; 28:239–240.
Sanchis A, et al.: Duplication of hands and feet, multiple joint dislocations, absence of the corpus callosum and hypsarrhythmia: acrocallosal syndrome? Am J Med Genet 1985; 20:123–130.
Schinzel A, Kaufmann U: The acrocallosal syndrome in sisters. Clin Genet 1986; 30:399–405. * †
Schinzel A: The acrocallosal syndrome in first cousins: widening of the spectrum of clinical features and further support for autosomal recessive inheritance. J Med Genet 1988; 25:332–336.

Moeschler JB, et al.: Acrocallosal syndrome: new findings. Am J Med Genet 1989; 32:306–310.

SC017 **Albert A.G.L. Schinzel**

## ACROCEPHALOPOLYDACTYLOUS DYSPLASIA 2528

**Includes:**
>   Elejalde acrocephalopolydactylous dysplasia
>   Macrosomia associated with polydactyly and
>       craniosynostosis
>   Renal dysplasia, Elejalde type

**Excludes:**
>   **Acrocephalopolysyndactyly**
>   **Acrocephalosyndactyly**
>   **Beckwith-Wiedemann syndrome** (0104)
>   **Cebebral gigantism** (0137)
>   Fetal macrosomia associated with maternal diabetes
>       mellitus
>   **Hemihypertrophy** (0458)
>   **Osteodystrophy-mental retardation, Ruvalcaba type** (2076)
>   **Weaver syndrome** (2036)

**Major Diagnostic Criteria:** Craniosynostosis producing turricephaly and macrosomia are the most noticeable signs at first inspection; patients also have hypertelorism; epicanthal folds; hypoplastic nose; redundant skin all over, but most noticeably on the neck; short limbs; polydactyly; omphalocele; lung hypoplasia; cystic renal dysplasia; sponge kidneys; and redundant overgrowth of the connective tissue in the skin and viscera growing between normal structures of the organ. Perivascular nerve fibers proliferate more than normal in many of the tissues.

**Clinical Findings:** The most noticeable observation is gigantism, which is noted early in the pregnancy and could be detected by sonographic examination of the developing fetus, which will show an abnormally thick skin with normal or delayed skeletal growth. The infants have severe respiratory distress syndrome at birth due to the severe pulmonary hypoplasia, in part due to the absence of amniotic fluid, caused by the renal dysplasia and the anuria that it produces. None have been successfully resuscitated or have survived the first moments of life. Renal lesions are very severe and are incompatible with adequate urine production.

The condition should be considered in all those macrosomic infants who have very thick skin, severe lung hypoplasia, and renal dysplasia. It is probable that these are the minimal manifestations of the condition. Definite diagnosis can be established only by histologic demonstration of the overgrowth of the connective tissue in different organs.

It is likely that there is much variation in the manifestation of the syndrome and that **Craniosynostosis**, **Polydactyly**, and **Syndactyly** may be present in only a few of those with the syndrome.

The possibility that milder forms of the condition are compatible with life should be considered, since the renal dysplasia, which is the most important lesion in regard to infant survival, could be less severe than is observed in our patients and consequently will allow for the formation of adequate amniotic fluid and lung maturation. Thus, the minimal diagnostic criterion is the demonstration of excessive growth of connective tissue in different organs and tissues.

**Complications:** Depend on the severity of the condition. The severity of the renal dysplasia will be the determining factor of the ability of the fetus to survive. It is possible that survivors have many other problems, including diabetes mellitus due to the abnormalities seen in the fetal pancreas, where the islets are surrounded by bundles of connective tissue.

If the fetus is affected by premature craniosynostosis, one of the major complications will be the craniostenosis produced by the early closure of the sutures, and a craniotomy should be considered to prevent damage to the CNS.

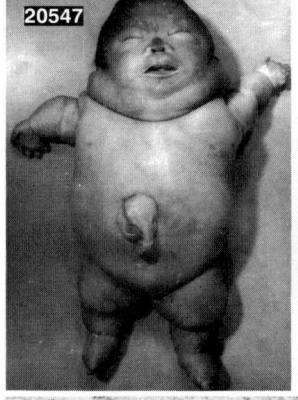
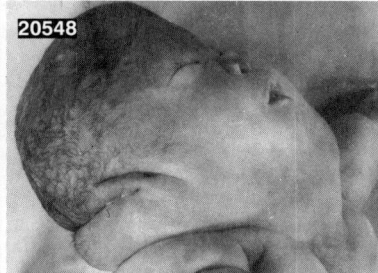
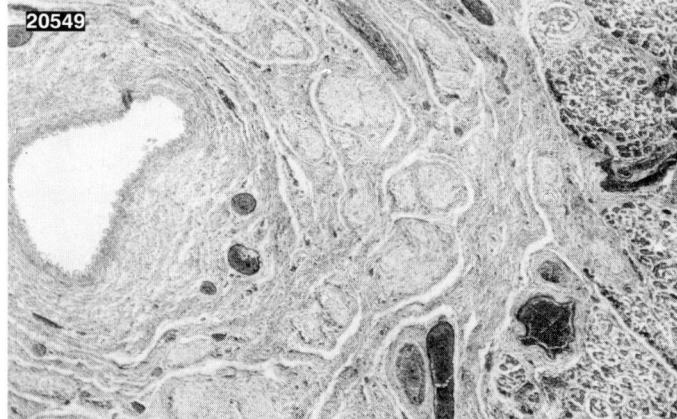
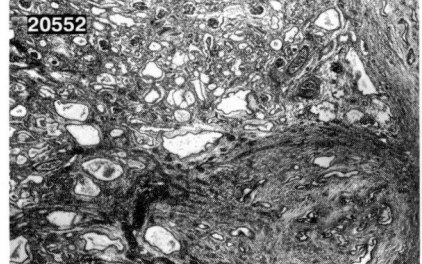
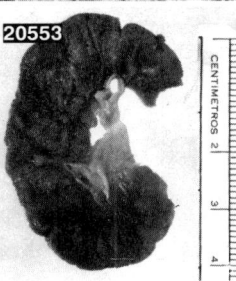

**2528-20547:** Acrocephalopolydactylous dysplasia in an affected newborn; note the turricephaly, the broad short and small nose, the thick upper lip, the redundant skin, the upper limb polydactyly, and the small omphalocele. **20548:** Lateral view shows the abnormal head shape, the hypoplastic nose, and the large amount of redundant tissue over the neck which deforms the ear. **20549:** Micrograph of a section of pancreas shows the proliferation of connective tissue and nerve fibers around one artery. **20552:** Micrograph of a section of the kidney shows the scarcity of glomeruli, the multicystic dysplasia, and the marked proliferation of connective tissue surrounding the tubuli and producing their dilatation. **20553:** Kidney sectioned midway in the coronal plane; note the spongy appearance of the renal tissue.

It is likely that if the renal dysplasia is not incompatible with life at birth, it may produce chronic renal failure later in life.

**Associated Findings:** Oligohydramnios is generally a common observation in all who are severely affected, and it should be a sign to suspect the condition during pregnancy. Cryptorchidism and dry, thick skin have been observed, probably as abnormalities not primarily due to the defect causing the condition, but secondary to the oligohydramnios.

**Etiology:** Probably autosomal recessive inheritance. This hypothesis is supported by the consanguinity of the two families that produced affected children. Fibroblasts and perhaps other cells of the connective tissue complete the cell cycle in 63% of the time of other cells from the same fetus. The exact gene or the product they code for has not been isolated.

**Pathogenesis:** The lesions observed in these fetuses are due to two basic defects: 1) the rapid proliferation of the connective tissue and 2) the overgrowth of the perivascular nerve fibers.

The growth of connective tissue between the elements of the glomeruli and proximal and distal tubules produces their obstruction and dilation with retrograde retention of urine and complete damage of the glomeruli. This obstruction and dilation of the renal system produces the "sponge kidney" recognizable by microscopic examination.

The proliferation of the same tissue in excessive amounts accounts for the thickening of the skin and subdermic tissues and for the changes seen both in the lung, where the thick interalveolar connective tissue does not allow for the expansion of the alveoli and for its normal growth and development, and in the pancreas, where it impedes the normal development of the different pancreatic elements, mostly of the islets.

Proliferation of biliary canaliculi was observed in the liver of both infants, probably due to the same factors that accelerated the cycle of the connective tissue.

This condition and its manifestations are a good example of the pleiotropic effects of a gene in the development of different tissues and organs.

**Sex Ratio:** M2:F1

**Occurrence:** Two consanguineous related families have been reported. One of them has two affected children, and the other has two males and one female affected members.

**Risk of Recurrence for Patient's Sib:**
See Part I, *Mendelian Inheritance.*

**Risk of Recurrence for Patient's Child:**
See Part I, *Mendelian Inheritance.* Affected individuals are not expected to survive to reproduce.

**Age of Detectability:** At birth. The condition appears to be detectable by sonography, probably during the second trimester. Mild cases may be very difficult to detect and may not be typical enough to be recognized during the neonatal period or early childhood.

**Gene Mapping and Linkage:** Unknown.

**Prevention:** None known. Genetic counseling indicated.

**Treatment:** In the severe cases, none possible. In the mild cases, resuscitation and kidney transplantation.

**Prognosis:** Very poor in severe cases, since the lesions are incompatible with life.

**Detection of Carrier:** Unknown.

**Special Considerations:** It is possible that mild forms of the condition, not having all the manifestations seen in reported cases, are not recognized. Careful examination of the tissue of macrosomic stillbirths and fetuses may reveal the redundant, rapidly grown connective tissue diagnostic of the condition. The condition should be considered in the differential diagnosis of fetuses affected by polycystic kidney disease involving both kidneys.

**References:**
Elejalde BR, et al.: Acrocephalopolydactylous dysplasias. BD:OAS XIII(3B). New York: March of Dimes Birth Defects Foundation, 1977:53:67.
Cohen MM: The Elejalde syndrome. In: Cohen MM, ed: The child with multiple birth defects. New York: Raven Press, 1982:109–111.

EL002
EL014
IA001

**B. Rafael Elejalde**
**Maria Mercedes de Elejalde**
**A. Kimberly Iafolla**

## ACROCEPHALOPOLYSYNDACTYLY 0013

**Includes:**
    Acrocephalopolysyndactyly (ACPS), types I, II, III, and IV
    Carpenter syndrome
    Goodman syndrome
    Noack syndrome
    Pfeiffer acrocephalopolysyndactyly
    Sakati syndrome
    Sakati-Nyhan syndrome
    Summitt syndrome

**Excludes:**
    **Acrocephalosyndactyly type I** (0014)
    **Acrocephalosyndactyly type III** (0229)
    **Acrocephalosyndactyly type V** (2284)
    **Polysyndactyly-dysmorphic craniofacies, Greig type** (2925)

**Major Diagnostic Criteria:** Acrocephaly, with polysyndactyly of hands, feet, or both.

**Clinical Findings:** It is generally accepted that ACPS, type I (Noack syndrome), is not a distinct entity and that patients previously described as having this condition most probably have **Acrocephalosyndactyly type V** (Pfeiffer syndrome).

ACPS, type II (Carpenter syndrome), is characterized by acrocephaly and by facial and limb abnormalities. The acrocephaly, usually severe, results from premature synostosis of the coronal, sagittal, and lambdoidal sutures. The hypoplastic supraorbital ridges, lateral displacement of the medial canthi, downslanting palpebral fissures, epicanthic folds, flat nasal bridge, relatively low-set ears, broad cheeks, and hypoplastic mandible give the facies a characteristic appearance. The hands are characterized by brachydactyly, clinodactyly, soft tissue syndactyly, and, occasionally, postaxial polydactyly. The proximal phalanx of the thumb commonly has two ossification centers, resulting in duplication of the phalanx. Syndactyly and preaxial polydactyly of the feet are usually present. Other features include mild-to-moderate obesity, hypogonadism, congenital heart disease and abdominal hernias.

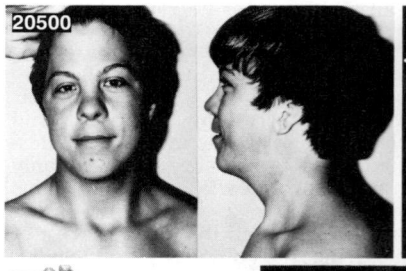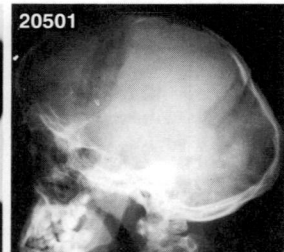
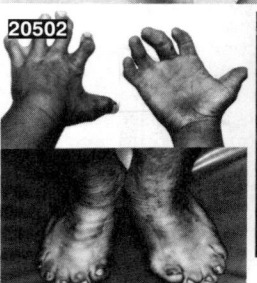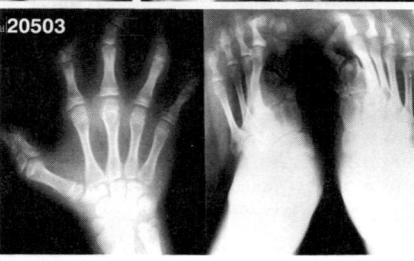

**0013-20500:** Acrocephalopolysyndactyly type II: note acrocephaly, hypoplastic orbital ridges, downslanting palpebral fissures, flat nasal bridge, and low-set ears. **20501:** Skull X-ray; note craniosynostosis. **20502:** Note digital defects: polydactyly, syndactyly, brachydactyly and camptodactyly. **20503:** X-ray of digital defects; note the duplication of the proximal phalanx of the thumb among other digital defects.

Coxa valga, genu valgum, and pes varus have also been described. Although mental retardation was considered a constant feature of Carpenter syndrome in early reports, several patients with normal intelligence have been described in the last few years.

The main features of ACPS, type III (Sakati-Nyhan syndrome), are acrocephaly, polydactyly and syndactyly of the feet, brachydactyly and polydactyly of the hands, and defects of the lower limbs. Large deformed ears, alopecia, and congenital heart disease are also seen. Facial features are unusual, with shallow orbits, protruding eyes, elongated, beak-like nose, and prominent forehead. Both upper and lower limbs are short. Defects in the lower limbs include bowed femurs, hypoplastic tibias, and posterior displacement of the fibulas. Intelligence is usually within normal limits.

ACPS, type IV (Goodman syndrome), is characterized by marked acrocephaly, congenital heart disease, postaxial polydactyly and soft tissue syndactyly of the hands, and syndactyly of the feet. Additional hand abnormalities include clinodactyly and camptodactyly of the fifth digits, with ulnar deviation of the fingers. Genu valgum may also be present. Dysmorphic facial features include high-arched eyebrows, prominent nose, epicanthal folds, mild upslanting palpebral fissures, and large, protruding ears. Normal intelligence has been the rule. Clinical distinction between ACPS, type II (Carpenter syndrome), and ACPS, type IV, is difficult, and it is not possible at this time to determine if these two conditions are variations in the expression of a single gene or discrete entities with phenotypic overlap.

Summitt (1969) described two brothers with craniosynostosis and syndactyly. Both were obese with normal intelligence. Cohen et al (1987) have concluded that Summitt and Goodman syndromes are variants of Carpenter syndrome.

**Complications:** Neurologic, orthopedic, and psychologic problems may result from the skeletal abnormalities and the altered self-image.

**Associated Findings:** None known.

**Etiology:** ACPS, type II (Carpenter syndrome); autosomal recessive inheritance.
ACPS, type III, (Sakati-Nyhan syndrome); undetermined.
ACPS, type IV (Goodman syndrome); autosomal recessive inheritance.
Summitt syndrome; autosomal recessive inheritance.

**Pathogenesis:** Unknown.

**MIM No.:** *20100, *10160, 10112, 20102, 27235

**POS No.:** 3054, 4132, 3010, 3818, 3008

**Sex Ratio:** M1:F1

**Occurrence:** ACPS, type II, approximately 30 patients have been described in the medical literature.
ACPS, type III, only one patient has been reported.
ACPS, type IV, three patients within one family have been documented.

**Risk of Recurrence for Patient's Sib:**
See Part I, *Mendelian Inheritance.*

**Risk of Recurrence for Patient's Child:**
See Part I, *Mendelian Inheritance.*

**Age of Detectability:** At birth.

**Gene Mapping and Linkage:** Unknown.

**Prevention:** None known. Genetic counseling indicated.

**Treatment:** Surgical correction of the craniosynostosis may help prevent mental retardation and improve the appearance of the child. Further craniofacial surgery and repair of the polydactyly and syndactyly are recommended for cosmetic purposes. Environmental support and stimulation to achieve maximum potential are also very important.

**Prognosis:** The practitioner must assess each case individually and establish a prognosis based on the type and severity of the malformations present in the patient. The observation of normal intelligence in the Goodman syndrome and in several patients with Carpenter syndrome must be kept in mind. The skull &

skeletal defects should not affect life-span, but congenital heart defects, if present, may do so (ACPS II).

**Detection of Carrier:** Unknown.

**References:**
Summitt RL: Recessive acrocephalosyndactyly with normal intelligence. BD:OAS; V(3). New York: March of Dimes Birth Defects Foundation, 1969:35–38.
Sakati N, et al.: A new syndrome with acrocephalopolysyndactyly, cardiac disease, and distinctive defects of the ear, skin, and lower limbs. J Pediatr 1971; 79:104–109.
Robinow M, Sorauf TJ: Acrocephalopolysyndactyly, type Noack, in a large kindred. BD:OAS XI(5) New York: March of Dimes Birth Defects Foundation, 1975:99–106.
Frias JL, et al.: Normal intelligence in two children with Carpenter syndrome. Am J Med Genet 1978; 2:191–199.
Goodman RM, et al.: Acrocephalopolysyndactyly type IV: a new genetic syndrome in 3 sibs. Clin Genet 1979; 15:209–214.
Hall JG, et al.: Autosomal recessive acrocephalosyndactyly revisited. Am J Med Genet 1980; 5:423–424.
Robinson LK, et al.: Carpenter syndrome: natural history and clinical spectrum. Am J Med Genet 1985; 20:461–469.
Cohen DM, et al.: Acrocephalopolysyndactyly type II - Carpenter syndrome: clinical spectrum and an attempt at unification with Goodman and Summitt syndromes. Am J Med Genet 1987; 28:311–324.

RA025                                      **S.A. Rasmussen**
FR016                                      **Jaime L. Frias**

**Acrocephalopolysyndactyly (ACPS), types I, II, III, and IV**
*See ACROCEPHALOPOLYSYNDACTYLY*
**Acrocephalopolysyndactyly type I**
*See ACROCEPHALOSYNDACTYLY TYPE V*
**Acrocephalosynankie**
*See ANTLEY-BIXLER SYNDROME*

## ACROCEPHALOSYNDACTYLY TYPE I                 0014

**Includes:**
Acrocephalosyndactyly type II
Apert-Crouzon disease (Acrocephalosyndactyly type II)
Apert syndrome
Vogt cephalosyndactyly

**Excludes:**
Acrocephalopolysyndactyly (0013)
Acrocephalosyndactyly type III (0229)
Acrocephalosyndactyly type V (2284)
Contractures, Herrmann-Opitz arthrogryposis type (0470)
Craniofacial dysostosis (0225)

**Major Diagnostic Criteria:** Craniosynostosis and severe syndactyly of the hands and feet.

**Clinical Findings:** Acrocephalosyndactyly type I (Apert syndrome) is characterized by craniosynostosis, and abnormalities of the face, hands and feet. The degree of craniosynostosis is variable, although most commonly the coronal sutures are involved. The resulting skull is acrocephalic, with a shortened antero-posterior diameter, a high prominent forehead and a flattened occiput. In rare instances, the cloverleaf skull anomaly (Kleeblattschadel) has been observed.

Abnormalities of the face include ocular hypertelorism, downslanting of the palpebral fissures, depressed nasal bridge and hypoplastic midface. The face is often asymmetric. A supraorbital horizontal groove is observed in some patients. The corners of the mouth are characteristically down-turned, and the mandible is prominent. The palate is high-arched, and shows median furrowing in some cases. Cleft of the soft palate occurs in about 30 percent of patients. The upper teeth are frequently crowded. The ears have been described as low-set in some patients, and congenital hearing loss is a frequent finding.

The malformation of the hands ranges from partial to complete fusion of the digits. Most often digits 2, 3 and 4 are involved, although the thumb and fifth digit may also be involved. The

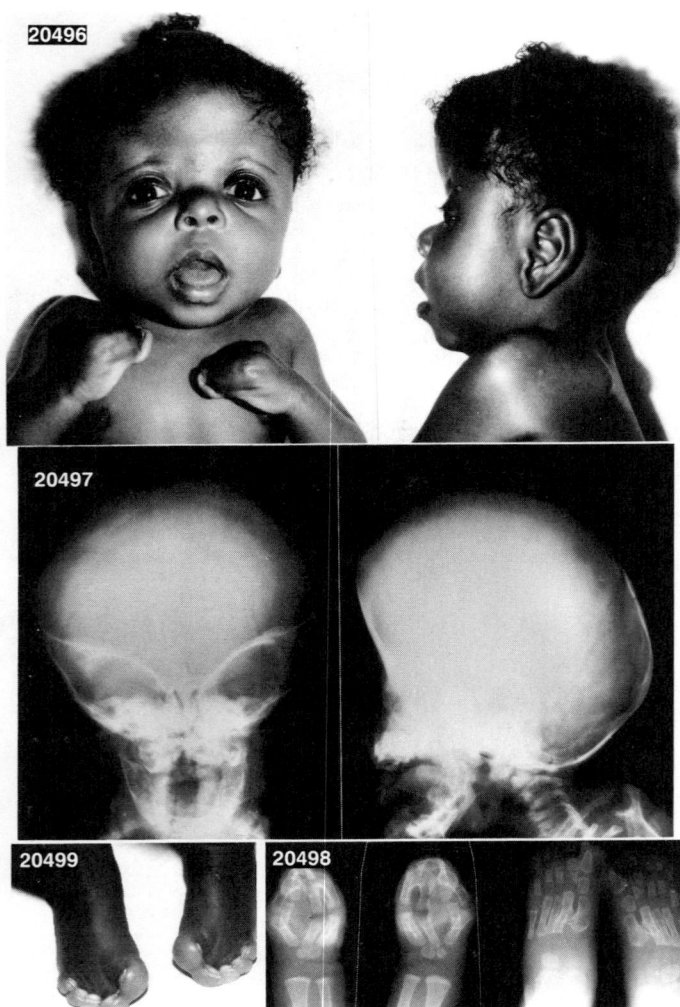

**0014-20496:** Acrocephalosyndactyly I; note acrocephaly, prominent forehead, depressed upper midface and digital fusion. **20497:** Craniosynostosis, acrocephaly and short AP diameter. **20499:** Stocking type syndactyly. **20498:** Digital defects.

**Complications:** Hydrocephalus has been described in several patients. In some instances, the hydrocephalus was not associated with the common indicators of ventricular dilatation such as increased head circumference, increased cerebrospinal fluid pressure or changes in the optic fundi.

**Associated Findings:** Extensive acne is common in adolescents and young adults.

**Etiology:** Autosomal dominant inheritance. Few parent child transmissions have been reported, although Rollnick (1988) described a case of male transmission. Increased parental age has been demonstrated.

**Pathogenesis:** Unknown.

**MIM No.:** *10120

**POS No.:** 3007

**CDC No.:** 756.055

**Sex Ratio:** M1:F1

**Occurrence:** Estimates vary from 1:100,000 - 1:160,000 births.

**Risk of Recurrence for Patient's Sib:**
See Part I, *Mendelian Inheritance.*

**Risk of Recurrence for Patient's Child:**
See Part I, *Mendelian Inheritance.* Reduced fertility has been a feature of this condition.

**Age of Detectability:** At birth.

**Gene Mapping and Linkage:** Unknown.

**Prevention:** None known. Genetic counseling indicated.

**Treatment:** Surgical correction of the craniosynostosis may help prevent mental retardation. Repair of the severe syndactyly of the hands and feet are recommended for functional and cosmetic reasons. The detection of hydrocephalus, present in a number of patients, may be difficult since the usual signs of hydrocephalus are not always present. Therefore, careful evaluation for other signs, such as developmental regression and increased tone in the lower limbs, is essential.

**Prognosis:** Depends on the severity of the malformations, specifically those affecting the central nervous system.

**Detection of Carrier:** Unknown.

**References:**
Blank CE: Apert's syndrome (a type of acrocephalosyndactyly): observations on a British series of thirty-nine cases. Ann Hum Genet 1960; 24:151–164.
Hogan GR, Bauman ML: Hydrocephalus in Apert's syndrome. J Pediatr 1971; 79(5):782–787.
Temtamy SA, McKusick VA: The genetics of hand malformations. BD:OAS. 1978:XIV(3):328–350.
Maroteaux P, Fonfria Marie C: Apparent Apert syndrome with polydactyly. Am J Med Genet 1987; 28:153–158.
Rollnick BR: Male transmission of Apert syndrome. Clin Genet 1988; 33:87–90.
Cohen MM, Jr., Kreiborg S: The central nervous system in Apert syndrome. Am J Med Genet 1990; 35:36–45.

RA025
FR016

S.A. Rasmussen
Jaime L. Frias

fusion usually involves the soft tissue only, but osseous fusion may occur. Maroteaux and Fonfria (1987) reported two patients with duplication of the fifth finger and of the first metacarpal. A single continuous nail is frequently observed. The thumb, when separate from the other fingers, is short and deviates radially. Brachydactyly has also been described.

A similar type of malformation is observed in the feet. The toenails are usually separate, but may be continuous.

Aplasia or ankyloses of joints, most commonly the shoulder, hip and elbow, may be present.

Mental retardation has been noted in many patients, although individuals of normal intelligence have been reported.

In I (Vogt cephalodactyly or Apert-Crouzon disease), the hand and foot malformations characteristic of Apert syndrome are combined with facial characteristics of **Craniofacial dysostosis** (Crouzon syndrome), caused by a very hypoplastic maxilla. Syndactyly is usually less severe, and the thumbs and little fingers free. Most authorities consider this to be simply a variant of Acrocephalosyndactyly type I with unusually marked facial features.

**Acrocephalosyndactyly type II**
*See ACROCEPHALOSYNDACTYLY TYPE I*

## ACROCEPHALOSYNDACTYLY TYPE III    0229

**Includes:**
Acrocephaly-skull asymmetry-mild syndactyly
Chotzen syndrome
Cranio-oculo-dental syndrome
Dentocranioocular syndrome
Oculocraniodental syndrome
Saethre-Chotzen syndrome

**Excludes:**
**Acrocephalopolysyndactyly** (0013)
**Acrocephalosyndactyly** (all others)
**Contractures, Herrmann-Opitz arthrogryposis type** (0470)
**Craniofacial dysostosis** (0225)
**Craniosynostosis** (all forms)
**Oculo-dento-osseous dysplasia** (0737)
**Oro-facio-digital syndrome** (all forms)

**Major Diagnostic Criteria:** Craniosynostosis, low anterior hair line, deviated nasal septum, brachydactyly, syndactyly between fingers 2 and 3, and ptosis of eyelids.

**Clinical Findings:** Acrocephalosyndactyly type III (Saethre-Chotzen syndrome) is characterized by craniosynostosis and facial and digital abnormalities. The degree of craniosynostosis is mild, usually involving the coronal sutures, or sphenobasilar sutures and acrocephaly and brachycephaly are most often observed. Head circumference is decreased in some patients. The fusion of the sutures is often asymmetric, producing plagiocephaly and facial asymmetry.

The low frontal hairline, broad forehead, ptosis of the eyelids, downslanting of palpebral fissures, dystopia canthorum, depressed nasal bridge, parrot-beaked nose, flat midface and maxillary hypoplasia give the facies a recognizable appearance. Strabismus and lacrimal duct stenosis have been documented in some cases. In many patients, deviation of the nasal septum occurs. The palate is usually high-arched and intact, but cleft palate has been noted occasionally. Dental findings include peg-shaped, missing, or anomalous maxillary lateral incisors and supernumerary teeth.

The ears may be low-set, posteriorly rotated, or malformed. A minor degree of hearing loss is a common finding.

Partial cutaneous syndactyly occurs in most patients, frequently between fingers 2 and 3. Clinodactyly of the 5th fingers and brachydactyly may be present. The thumbs may appear finger-like.

Syndactyly of the toes usually involves partial soft tissue fusion between the second and third toes, although other toes may be involved. The great toes may be broad, and hallux valgus has been noted in some instances. Simian creases are present in more than half of affected individuals. The ridge count is low, peculiar thenar and hypothenar loop and whorl patterns have been demonstrated.

The majority of individuals with Saethre-Chotzen syndrome are of normal intelligence; however, mild to moderate mental retardation has been reported in some cases.

**Complications:** Early closure of cranial sutures may lead to optic nerve atrophy. Tear duct stenosis leads to decreased tearing and susceptibility to eye infection.

**Associated Findings:** Epilepsy, cryptorchism, and renal anomalies. Cryptorchidism, renal anomalies, imperforate annus, enlarged sella turcica and congenital heart disease have been reported in a few patients with acrocephalosyndactyly type III.

**Etiology:** Autosomal dominant inheritance with a wide range in expressivity and high degree of penetrance. A paternal age effect has been suggested.

**Pathogenesis:** Unknown.

**MIM No.:** *10140

**POS No.:** 3010

**CDC No.:** 756.056

**Sex Ratio:** M1:F1

**Occurrence:** Given the relatively minor findings of acrocephalosyndactyly type III, many cases may go unrecognized. Therefore, the incidence and prevalence are difficult to estimate.

**Risk of Recurrence for Patient's Sib:**
See Part I, *Mendelian Inheritance.*

**Risk of Recurrence for Patient's Child:**
See Part I, *Mendelian Inheritance.*

**Age of Detectability:** At birth.

**Gene Mapping and Linkage:** Unknown.

**Prevention:** None known. Genetic counseling indicated.

**Treatment:** Craniotomy and prevention of closure of cranial sutures. Surgery for ptosis and tear duct anomalies. Correction of septum deviation may be necessary.

**Prognosis:** Excellent in general, since most patients are mildly affected.

**Detection of Carrier:** Unknown.

**References:**
Bartsocas CS, et al.: Acrocephalosyndactyly type III: Chotzen's syndrome. J Pediatr 1970; 77:267–272.
Pantke OA, et al.: The Saethre-Chotzen syndrome. Birth Defects 1975; 11(2):190–225. * †
Pantke OA, et al.: The Saethre-Chotzen syndrome. BD:OAS; XI(2). New York: March of Dimes Birth Defects Foundation, 1975:191–225.
Pruzansky S, et al.: Roentgencephalometric studies of the premature craniofacial synostoses: report of a family with the Saethre-Chotzen syndrome. Birth Defects 1975; 11(2):226–237.
Friedman JM, et al.: Saethre-Chotzen syndrome: a broad and variable pattern of skeletal malformations. Pediatrics 1977; 91(6):929–933.
Kopysc Z, et al.: The Saethre-Chotzen syndrome with partial bifid of the distal phalanges of the great toes. Hum Genet 1980; 56:195–204.
Thompson EM, et al.: Parietal foramina in Saethre-Chotzen syndrome. J Med Genet 1984; 21:369–372.
Bianchi E, et al.: A family with Saethre-Chotzen syndrome. Am J Med Genet, 1985; 22:649–658.

FR016                  **Jaime L. Frias**
RA025            **S.A. Rasmussen**
J0027       **Ronald J. Jorgenson**

## ACROCEPHALOSYNDACTYLY TYPE V    2284

**Includes:**
Acrocephalopolysyndactyly type I
Noack syndrome
Pfeiffer syndrome

**Excludes:**
**Acrocephalopolysyndactyly** (0013)
**Acrocephalosyndactyly type I** (0014)
**Acrocephalosyndactyly type III** (0229)
**Acrocephalosyndactyly type V** (2284)
**Brain, Arnold-Chiari malformation** (2944)
**Craniofacial dysostosis** (0225)

**Major Diagnostic Criteria:** **Craniosynostosis** and malformations of the thumb and great toe.

**Clinical Findings:** Craniosynostosis and facial and digital abnormalities. The craniosynostosis, usually involving the coronal sutures, results most commonly in a turribrachycephalic skull. The degree of craniosynostosis is, however, quite variable. At the severe end of the spectrum, a few patients with **Craniosynostosis, Kleeblattschadel type** have been described, while at the mild end, patients may have minimal or no craniosynostosis.

Abnormal facies includes a high forehead, **Eye, hypertelorism,** flattened nasal bridge, prominent eyes with a slight downward slant, beaked nose, maxillary hypoplasia, and relative mandibular prognathism. The palate is high arched, and the teeth may be crowded.

Broad, short thumbs with radial deviation is a characteristic feature of Pfeiffer syndrome. X-ray evaluation demonstrates either a trapezoidal or triangular-shaped proximal phalanx of the thumb. The distal phalanx of the thumb may be bifid. The hands also

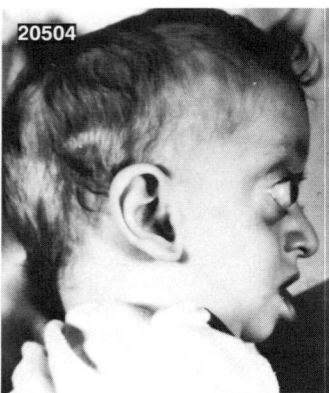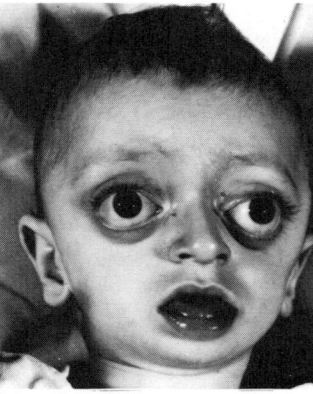

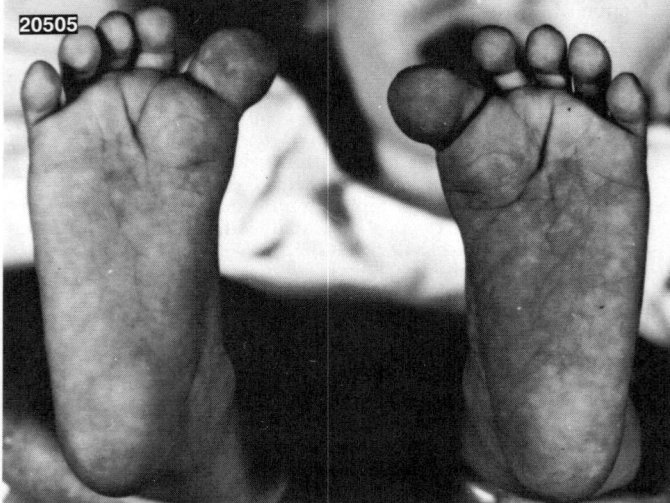

**2284-20504:** Abnormal cranial configuration, proptosis, hypoplastic midface and low-set ears. **20505:** Broad hallux with varus deviation.

---

show brachymesophalangy (see **Brachydactyly**). Soft tissue **Syndactyly** may occur, usually involving digits 2 and 3.

Similar malformations are found in the feet. The great toes are broad, and the proximal phalanx of the great toe is often malformed, being rudimentary, triangular, or trapezoidal in shape, or duplicated or absent. Hallux varus, brachymesophalangy, and partial cutaneous syndactyly, usually involving the second and third toes, are commonly present. Other skeletal malformations that have been described include radioulnar and radiohumeral synostosis and fused cervical and lumbar vertebrae.

Intelligence has been described as normal in the majority of patients. **Hydrocephaly**, seizures, and the combination of anencephaly and spina bifida have been observed in a few cases. Rate of growth is normal. Mild hearing loss has been present in some patients.

**Complications:** The potential for increased intracranial pressure as a consequence of craniosynostosis and hydrocephaly must be kept in mind. Proptosis, resulting from the shallow orbits, may require surgical intervention.

**Associated Findings:** Hearing loss.

**Etiology:** Autosomal dominant inheritance.

**Pathogenesis:** Unknown.

**MIM No.:** *10160

**POS No.:** 3008

**CDC No.:** 756.057

**Sex Ratio:** M1:F1

**Occurrence:** Some seven kindreds have been documented.

**Risk of Recurrence for Patient's Sib:**
See Part I, *Mendelian Inheritance.*

**Risk of Recurrence for Patient's Child:**
See Part I, *Mendelian Inheritance.*

**Age of Detectability:** At birth.

**Gene Mapping and Linkage:** Unknown.

**Prevention:** None known. Genetic counseling indicated.

**Treatment:** Early surgical correction of the craniosynostosis may be necessary to prevent complications and for cosmetic reasons. Further plastic surgery may be considered to improve the appearance of the child. Repair of the hand malformation to enhance function may be indicated.

**Prognosis:** Difficult to define due to variability of the phenotype. In severe cases, neurologic abnormalities may affect function and life span.

**Detection of Carrier:** Unknown.

**Special Considerations:** The concomitant observation of patients with characteristics of this condition and **Acrocephalosyndactyly type I** within the same pedigree have led some authors to believe that these syndromes could be caused by a single mutant gene. It appears more likely that this condition is a separate entity, but with a great degree of variability in expression. This variable expressivity must be considered when counseling families with apparently sporadic cases, since parents have been described with only minor manifestations of the condition.

**References:**
Martsolf JT, et al.: Pfeiffer syndrome: an unusual type of acrocephalosyndactyly with broad thumbs and great toes. Am J Dis Child 1971; 121:257–262.
Cohen MM Jr: An etiologic and nosologic overview of craniosynostosis syndromes. BD:OAS XI(2). New York: March of Dimes Birth Defects Foundation, 1975:137–188.
Escobar V, Bixler D: Are the acrocephalosyndactyly syndromes variable expressions of a single gene defect? BD:OAS XIII(3C). New York: March of Dimes Birth Defects Foundation, 1977:139–154.
Baraitser M, et al.: Pitfalls of genetic counseling in Pfeiffer's syndrome. J Med Genet 1980; 17:250–256.
Kroczek RA, et al.: Cloverleaf skull associated with Pfeiffer syndrome: pathology and management. Europ J Pediat 1986; 145:442–445.
Rasmussen SA, Frias JL: Mild expression of Pfeiffer syndrome. Clin Genet 1988; 33:5–10.

RA025
FR016

**S.A. Rasmussen**
**Jaime L. Frias**

**Acrocephalosyndactyly, Robinow-Sorauf type**
*See CRANIOSYNOSTOSIS-FOOT DEFECTS, JACKSON-WEISS TYPE*
**Acrocephaly-skull asymmetry-mild syndactyly**
*See ACROCEPHALOSYNDACTYLY TYPE III*
**Acrodental dysostosis of Weyers**
*See ACROFACIAL DYSOSTOSIS*
*also ACROFACIAL SYNDROME, CURRY-HALL TYPE*

---

**ACRODERMATITIS ENTEROPATHICA**                    **0015**

**Includes:**
Brandt syndrome
Danbolt-Close syndrome
Danbolt syndrome

**Excludes:**
Chronic monilial granuloma
**Gluten sensitive enteropathy** (0423)
Lerner disease
Staphylococcal scalded skin syndrome

**Major Diagnostic Criteria:** Clinical symptoms include vesiculopustular eruptions, alopecia, and severe diarrhea due to deficient zinc absorption.

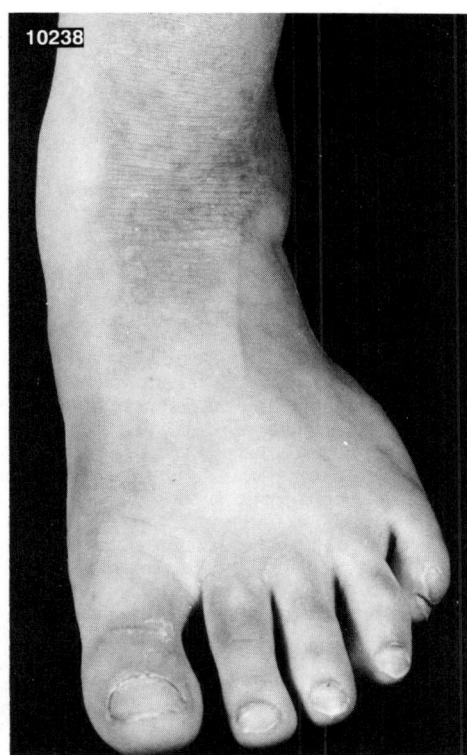

**0015-10238:** Skin changes in acrodermatitis enteropathica.

**Clinical Findings:** The skin eruption consists of lesions varying from bullae to verrucous plaques and has a predilection for the distal portions of the limbs, the perioral region, and the perineum. One hundred percent of the patients have skin lesions, 90% have diarrhea, and 98% have alopecia. Patients may also have glossitis and stomatitis, photophobia, conjunctivitis, paronychia, dystrophy of the nails, perleche, irritability, and emotional disturbances, as well as frequent secondary infection of the skin and mucous membrane with *Candida albicans*, bacteria, or both.

Infants who are destined to have the disease rarely give evidence of an abnormality at birth. The first indication of the disease is usually the appearance of a skin eruption, localized to the body orifices and limbs, which is accompanied by or followed shortly afterward by alopecia and GI symptoms. The sequence of appearance of symptoms is not consistent. The alopecia is usually total, although in 13% of cases it has been diffuse but not total. The diarrhea may be severe or mild, and in 10% of cases it has not been a prominent feature of the disease. The primary skin lesions are usually vesiculobullous in type. They appear in groups and are located symmetrically about the body orifices, eyes, occiput, elbows, knees, hands, and feet. The lesions are prone to occur around the nails and between the fingers and toes. The trunk is usually not involved. After a time the lesions begin to dry and crust. With the occurrence of lamellar scaling they develop a psoriasiform appearance. Lesions in various stages of development may be present simultaneously, and the appearance may be further altered by the occurrence of bacterial infection, monilial infection, or both, common features of this condition. Any stage of development may predominate and in many instances the vesicular phase is not observed at all. The heavily scaled psoriasiform lesions seem to dominate the picture in many instances. Resolution of the skin lesions leaves no scarring or atrophy. In general the baldness, skin eruption, and dejected attitude of affected children produce a striking uniformity of appearance. If unrecognized or untreated, the disease follows an intermittent but relentlessly progressive course that may lead to death because of general debility, intercurrent infection, or both. Short-lived spontaneous remissions are followed by relapses that are increasingly more severe and in many instances are related to intercurrent infection.

**Complications:** Intercurrent infection, particularly of the respiratory tract; general debility, if untreated.

**Associated Findings:** Secondary infections.

**Etiology:** Autosomal recessive inheritance. This heritable disease of zinc deficiency can also be induced in patients maintained on total parenteral nutrition (TPN) without adequate zinc supplementation. These patients develop the classic signs of acrodermatitis enteropathica, which are reversed by zinc supplementation.

**Pathogenesis:** It has been suggested that absence of a low-molecular-weight zinc-binding factor may be the cause of deficient zinc absorption. This binding factor is produced by the pancreas, binds dietary zinc, and transports it into epithelial cells. The binding factor is present in human breast milk, which has been known to ameliorate acrodermatitis enteropathica.

**MIM No.:** *20110

**Sex Ratio:** M1:F1

**Occurrence:** Undetermined but appears to affect all regions and ethnic groups.

**Risk of Recurrence for Patient's Sib:**
See Part I, *Mendelian Inheritance.*

**Risk of Recurrence for Patient's Child:**
See Part I, *Mendelian Inheritance.*

**Age of Detectability:** The disorder begins insidiously between the ages of three weeks and 10 years, with an average age of onset of nine months, frequently at the time of weaning.

**Gene Mapping and Linkage:** Unknown.

**Prevention:** None known. Genetic counseling indicated.

**Treatment:** The standard, effective, simple, and innocuous treatment at present consists of the oral administration of zinc sulfate, 50 mg three times daily, in the form of tablets or powder dissolved in fruit juice. The response to this treatment is clinically noticeable within 3–4 days. Usually there is complete healing of the skin lesions and disappearance of all signs and symptoms within one month after the start of treatment.

**Prognosis:** Excellent, if the treatment is continued indefinitely.

**Detection of Carrier:** Unknown.

**References:**
Idriss ZH, Der Kaloustian VM: Acrodermatitis enteropathica. Clin Pediatr 1973; 12:393–395.
Moynahan EJ: Acrodermatitis enteropathica: a lethal inherited human zinc deficiency disorder. Lancet 1974; II:399–400.
Der Kaloustian VM, et al.: Oral treatment of acrodermatitis enteropathica with zinc sulfate. Am J Dis Child 1976; 130:421–423. †
Evans GW, Johnson PE: Zinc-binding factor in acrodermatitis enteropathica (letter). Lancet 1976; II:1310.
Gordon EF, et al.: Zinc metabolism: basic, clinical and behavioral aspects. J Pediat 1981; 99:341–349.

DE030                                    **Vazken M. Der Kaloustian**

| **ACRODYSOSTOSIS** | **0016** |
|---|---|

**Includes:**
Dysostosis, peripheral-nasal hypoplasia-mental retardation (PNM)
Nasal hypoplasia-peripheral dysostosis-mental retardation

**Excludes:**
**Acromicric dysplasia** (2716)
**Brachydactyly** (0114)
**Parathormone resistance** (0830)
**Tricho-rhino-phalangeal syndrome, type I** (0966)
**Tricho-rhino-phalangeal syndrome, type II** (0967)

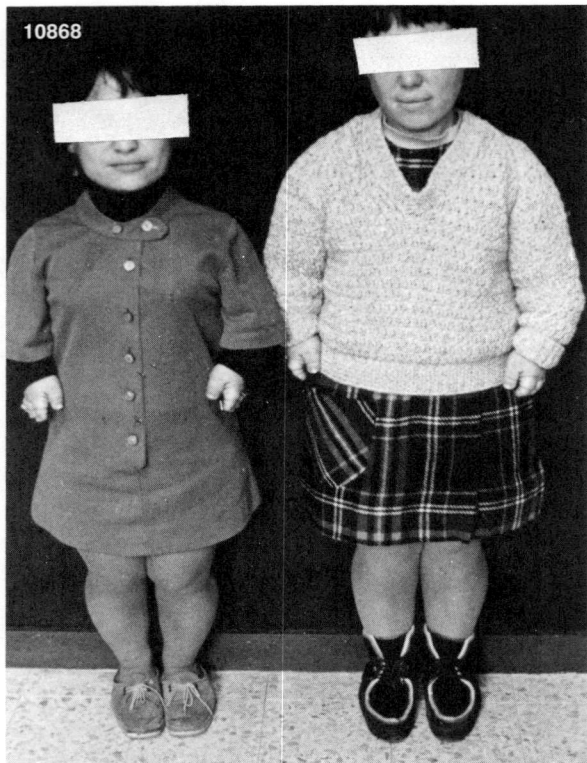

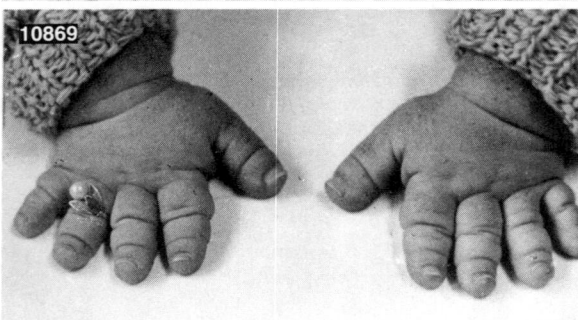

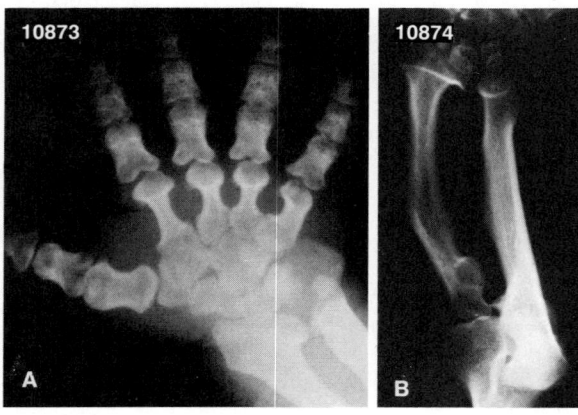

**0016-10868:** Stature is very short with a semiflexed arm position and short limbs with an extremely short acral segment. **10869:** Hands have very short, broad digits and short nails. **10873:** X-ray of the hand shows extremely short metacarpals, cone-shaped epiphyses of the phalanges and flaring of the distal metaphyseal portion of the radius. **10874:** Bowed radius.

Tricho-rhino-phalangeal syndrome, type III (2847)
Other forms of acrodysplasia
Other forms of peripheral dysostosis

**Major Diagnostic Criteria:** The diagnosis of this syndrome depends on clinical and X-ray criteria. Peripheral dysostosis, nasal hypoplasia, and mental retardation are found in almost all cases; at least two of these features should be present to make a diagnosis. This syndrome must be distinguished from other disorders included in the heterogeneous group of "peripheral dysostosis," i.e., those with short and deformed bones of the hands and feet. Lack of alterations in calcium and phosphorus metabolism and the presence of generalized brachymetacarpaly with severely shortened phalanges distinguishes this syndrome from Albright osteodystrophy.

**Clinical Findings:** The major features of this syndrome are peripheral dysostosis, nasal hypoplasia, mental retardation, and short stature. The hands and feet are short with stubby fingers and toes and broad, short nails. These patients are short at birth, and growth retardation is progressive. This shortening is acromesomelic with short forearms and limitation of motion at the elbows. The facies is characteristic, having marked nasal hypoplasia: a low nasal bridge, a flat and short nose, a broad and somewhat dimpled nasal tip with anteverted nostrils, and a long philtrum. Maxillary hypoplasia, hypertelorism, epicanthal folds, and malocclusion are often present. Almost all of the reported patients have had some degree of mental retardation.

Severe shortening of the metacarpals and phalanges is seen on X-ray. The epiphyses are deformed in the metacarpals and cone-shaped in the phalanges. The carpal bones may be small, and the distal radius and ulna are often malformed. There is premature fusion of the epiphyses of the hands, feet, and elbows. Changes in the feet are comparable to those of the hands. X-ray changes suggestive of juvenile spondylitis have been described in several cases. The skull is usually brachycephalic and may show thickening of the calvaria, but is not small.

**Complications:** Difficulty with manual skills due to shortened fingers and limitation of motion in the elbows and spine. Arthritic symptoms in the hands and feet may occur with age.

**Associated Findings:** None known.

**Etiology:** Undetermined. Most reported cases to date have been sporadic, although autosomal dominant inheritance has been reported. No parental consanguinity has been reported, but advanced paternal age has been noted.

**Pathogenesis:** Undetermined. Premature epiphyseal fusion may partially account for the severe shortening of the hands and feet, but there is also generalized growth retardation involving many bones whose epiphyses are normal on X-ray.

**MIM No.:** 10180

**POS No.:** 3011

**Sex Ratio:** M1:F2

**Occurrence:** Rare. More than 20 cases have been reported in the literature.

**Risk of Recurrence for Patient's Sib:** Undetermined. Most reported cases were sporadic.

**Risk of Recurrence for Patient's Child:** None of the reported cases have reproduced.

**Age of Detectability:** Usually detectable at birth or early infancy by the clinical features.

**Gene Mapping and Linkage:** Unknown.

**Prevention:** None known. Genetic counseling indicated.

**Treatment:** Plastic surgery may be required in severe cases to improve the facial appearance.

**Prognosis:** Apparently normal for life span and poor for intelligence and, with reduced function of hands, feet, and elbows.

**Detection of Carrier:** Unknown.

**Special Considerations:** This syndrome must be differentiated from other disorders that are associated with "peripheral dysostosis," a descriptive term that simply refers to shortening and deformity of the bones of the hands and feet. This can be found in pseudohypoparathyroidism, the **Tricho-rhino-phalangeal syndrome** as part of the various **Brachydactyly** syndromes, and as an isolated phenomenon. Bachman and Norman (1967) have described peripheral dysostosis in a woman and her two children, but these patients did not have the peculiar facial appearance and were mentally normal, ruling out acrodysostosis. A number of experts in the field now feel that acrodysostosis may be simply a form of pseudohypoparathyroidism, although studies of the N-protein system will be required to confirm this hypothesis.

**References:**
Bachman RK, Norman AP: Hereditary peripheral dysostosis (3 cases). Proc R Soc Med 1967; 60:21–25.
Maroteaux P, Malamut G: L'Acrodysostose. Presse Med 1968; 76:2189–2192.
Robinow M, et al.: Acrodysostosis. A syndrome of peripheral dysostosis, nasal hypoplasia, and mental retardation. Am J Dis Child 1971; 121:195–203.
Butler MG, et al.: Acrodysostosis: report of a 13-year-old boy with review of literature and metacarpophalangeal pattern profile analysis. Am J Med Genet 1988; 30:971–980. †

B0025                                              **Zvi Borochowitz**
                                                   *David L. Rimoin*

**Acrodysplasia with exostoses**
*See TRICHO-RHINO-PHALANGEAL SYNDROME, TYPE II*

## ACROFACIAL DEFECTS, EMERY-NELSON TYPE          2100

**Includes:**
   Emery-Nelson syndrome
   Faces (flat) with hand and foot deformity
   Foot and hand deformity with flat facies
   Hand and foot deformity with flat facies

**Excludes:**
   **Acrodysostosis (0016)**
   **Arthro-ophthalmopathy, hereditary, progressive, Stickler type (0090)**
   **Cranio-carpo-tarsal dysplasia, whistling face type (0223)**

**Major Diagnostic Criteria:** The combination of short stature, flat facies, and flexion contractures of fingers and toes.

**Clinical Findings:** In the reported mother and daughter, congenital hypotonia/muscular weakness (1); developmental delay (1); short stature (2); short extremities (2); high forehead (1); small nose with anteverted nares (2); flattened malar region (2); high-arched palate (1); long philtrum (2); dry, coarse hair (1); flexion contractures of fingers and toes (2); and pes cavus (2) were present.
   No other anomalies were evident on X-ray. Metabolic studies and chromosome analysis were normal. The joint contractures were flexion contractures of the metacarpophalangeal joints of the fingers and extension "deformities" of the thumbs. The toes were described as "clawed."

**Complications:** Unknown.

**Associated Findings:** Possible mild mental retardation.

**Etiology:** Probably autosomal dominant inheritance, although X-linked dominant inheritance cannot be ruled out.

**Pathogenesis:** Unknown.

**MIM No.:** 13975

**POS No.:** 3213

**Sex Ratio:** M0:F2 (Observed).

**Occurrence:** A mother and daughter in one family have been reported.

**Risk of Recurrence for Patient's Sib:**
   See Part I, *Mendelian Inheritance.*

**Risk of Recurrence for Patient's Child:**
   See Part I, *Mendelian Inheritance.*

**Age of Detectability:** Possibly at birth by clinical examination. The contractures of fingers and toes were not noticed until the age of two years in the propositus.

**Gene Mapping and Linkage:** Unknown.

**Prevention:** None known. Genetic counseling indicated.

**Treatment:** If indicated, surgery for the joint contractures.

**Prognosis:** Although the proband was mildly mentally retarded, the proband's affected mother was described as very intelligent. Life span is unlikely to be affected.

**Detection of Carrier:** Unknown.

**References:**
Emery AEH, Nelson MM: A familial syndrome of short stature, deformities of the hands and feet, and an unusual facies. J Med Genet 1970; 7:379–382.

T0007                                              **Helga V. Toriello**

## ACROFACIAL DYSOSTOSIS                            0017

**Includes:**
   Acrodental dysostosis of Weyers
   Acrofacial postaxial defect syndrome
   Curry-Hall syndrome
   Dysostosis, acrofacial
   Weyers acrofacial dysostosis

**Excludes:**
   **Acrofacial dysostosis, Nager type (2167)**
   **Acrofacial dysostosis, postaxial type (2126)**
   **Clefts, lower median lip, mandible and tongue (0636)**
   **Oro-facio-digital syndrome, Mohr type (0771)**
   Other syndromes with **polydactyly**

**Major Diagnostic Criteria:** Postaxial hexadactyly and bony cleft of mandibular symphysis or anomalies of lower central incisors.

**Clinical Findings:** Postaxial hexadactyly of both hands and feet with synostosis of the fifth and sixth metacarpals (metatarsals) have been observed in all reported cases. Bony cleft of mandibular symphysis, anomalies of lower central incisors ranging from peg-shaped teeth to complete aplasia especially in the permanent dentition, and peg-shaped or missing lateral incisors have also been noted frequently.
   The oral vestibule is absent in the anterior mandibular region. Occasionally this feature is present also in the anterior maxillary region often associated with persistent folds at the borders of the premaxilla.

**Complications:** Early loss of malformed teeth leading to malocclusion.

**Associated Findings:** Dysplastic nails and short stature.

**Etiology:** Autosomal dominant inheritance with variable expressivity and incomplete penetrance.

**Pathogenesis:** Limb abnormalities and mandibular clefting arise during the fifth and sixth week of embryogenesis.

**MIM No.:** *19353

**POS No.:** 3283, 3012, 3610, 3143, 3487

**Sex Ratio:** Presumably M1:F1

**Occurrence:** Approximately one dozen reported cases.

**Risk of Recurrence for Patient's Sib:**
   See Part I, *Mendelian Inheritance.*

**Risk of Recurrence for Patient's Child:**
   See Part I, *Mendelian Inheritance.*

**Age of Detectability:** At birth by clinical evaluation (including X-ray examination of mandible).

**Gene Mapping and Linkage:** Unknown.

**Prevention:** None known. Genetic counseling indicated.

**Treatment:** Excision of extra digits, surgical repair of mandibular symphysial cleft, prosthodontic treatment for missing or malformed teeth, surgical correction of fused vestibular mucosa.

**Prognosis:**  Good. Impact upon longevity is undetermined.

**Detection of Carrier:**  Unknown.

**References:**

Weyers H: Hexadactylie, unterkieferspalt und oligodontie, ein neuer symptomenkomplex. Dysostosis acro-facialis. Ann Paediatr (Basel) 1953; 181:45–60.

Weyers H: Zur kenntnis der chondroektodermaldysplasie (Ellis-van Creveld); bericht über 2 beobachtungen. Z Kinderheilkd 1956; 78:111–129.

Curry CJR, Hall BD: Polydactyly, conical teeth, nail dysplasia and short limbs: a new autosomal dominant malformation syndrome. BD:OAS XV(5B). New York: March of Dimes Birth Defects Foundation, 1979:253–263.

Roubicek M, Spranger J: Weyers acrodental dysostosis in a family. Clin Genet 1984; 26:587–590.

Shapiro SD, Jorgenson RJ, Salinas CF: Curry-Hall syndrome. Am J Med Genet 1984; 17:579–583.

SE007                                                    **Heddie O. Sedano**

## ACROFACIAL DYSOSTOSIS, NAGER TYPE          2167

**Includes:**

    Mandibulofacial dysostosis, Treacher-Collins type-limb anomalies

    Nager acrofacial dystosis

    Split hand deformity-mandibulofacial dysostosis

**Excludes:**

    **Acrofacial dysostosis, postaxial type** (2126)

    **Anus-hand-ear syndrome** (0072)

    Hemifacial microsomia/Goldenhar syndrome with radial ray defects

    **Mandibulofacial dysostosis** (0627)

**Major Diagnostic Criteria:**  Includes abnormalities of the craniofacial structures of the Treacher-Collins type, with radial ray defects. Absent eyelashes in the medial third of the lower lids; mandibular and malar hypoplasia; dysplastic ears with external ear canal defect; macrostomia; cleft palate; tongue shaped extension of the hair on the upper cheek; and downward slanting palpebral fissures.

**Clinical Findings:**  Antimongoloid palpebral fissures (85%), malar hypoplasia (85%), mandibular hypoplasia (76%), lower lid coloboma (19%), partial to total absence of lower lid eyelashes (60%), malformation of the auricles (85%), external ear canal defects (70%), conductive hearing loss (60%), cleft palate (57%), and projection of scalp hair onto lateral cheek (14%).

    Limb defects are radial and include thumb hypoplasia to complete absence of the thumb (preaxial radial ray defect). Radiographs show hypoplasia of aplasia of the radial bones bilaterally or unilaterally (symmetry is not necessary).

    Other findings include **Camptodactyly**; simian crease; **Syndactyly** of toes 2 and 3; rib, vertebral, pulmonary and upper airway anomalies.

**Complications:**  Developmental delay may be observed during the first two years of life. This delay is usually due to feeding difficulty, hearing loss, and surgical procedures to correct ear and palate anomalies. There is a high rate of prematurity and perinatal mortality.

**Associated Findings:**  None known.

**Etiology:**  Most cases have been sporadic, but autosomal dominant and autosomal recessive inheritance has been suggested. At least four families with apparent autosomal recessive inheritance have been documented.

**Pathogenesis:**  Unknown.

**MIM No.:**  15440, 18370

**POS No.:**  3143

**Sex Ratio:**  M1:F1

**Occurrence:**  Unknown. Extensive literature.

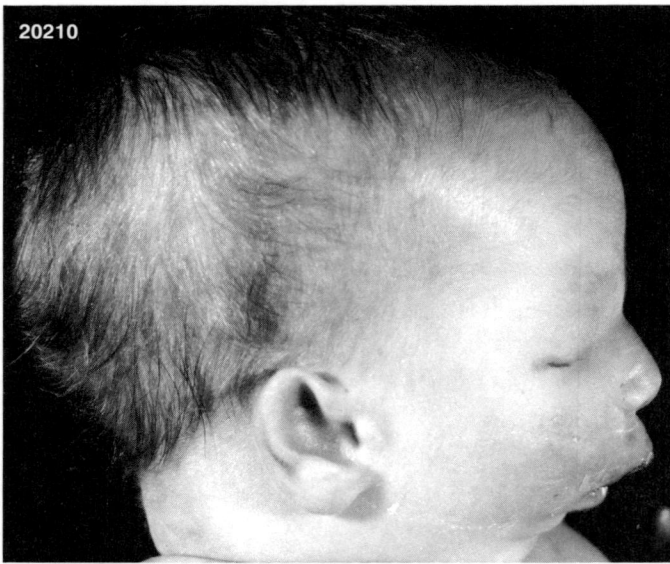

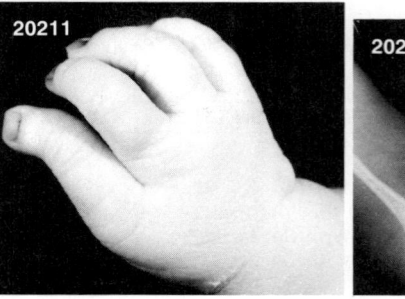 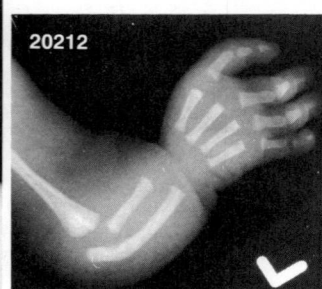

2167-20210:  Simple, apparently low-set and posteriorly rotated ear and severe micrognathia.  20211:  Note 4 digit hand, absent thumb and camptodactyly of the first digit.  20212:  Note 3 phalanges in each digit, hypoplastic radius and bowed ulna. The thumb is absent.

**Risk of Recurrence for Patient's Sib:**

    See Part I, *Mendelian Inheritance.*

**Risk of Recurrence for Patient's Child:**

    See Part I, *Mendelian Inheritance.*

**Age of Detectability:**  At birth. Prenatal diagnosis by ultrasound has been achieved at 19 weeks gestation.

**Gene Mapping and Linkage:**  Unknown.

**Prevention:**  None known. Genetic counseling indicated.

**Treatment:**  Close surveillance at birth due to prematurity, upper airway obstruction, and feeding problems. Hearing should be assessed as soon as possible, and, remediation offered where this is necessary.

**Prognosis:**  Unknown.

**Detection of Carrier:**  Unknown.

**References:**

Bowen P, Harley F: Mandibulofacial dysostosis with limb malformations (Nager's acrofacial dysostosis). BD:OAS X(5). New York: March of Dimes Birth Defects Foundation, 1974:109–115.

Burton BK, Nadler HL: Nager acrofacial dysostosis: report of a case. J Pediatr 1977; 91:84–86.

Lowry RB: The Nager syndrome (acrofacial dysostosis): evidence for autosomal dominant inheritance. BD:OAS XIII(3C). New York: March of Dimes Birth Defects Foundation, 1977:195.

Meyerson MD, et al.: Nager acrofacial dysostosis: early intervention and long term planning. Cleft Palate J 1977; 14:35–40.

Halal F, et al.: Differential diagnosis of Nager acrofacial dysostosis syndrome. Am J Med Genet 1983; 14:209–224.

Krauss CM, et al.: Additional clinical anomalies in an infant with Nager acrofacial dysostosis syndrome. Am J Med Genet 1985; 21:761–764.

Hecht JT, et al.: The Nager syndrome. Am J Med Genet 1987; 27:965–969.

Chemke J, et al.: Autosomal recessive inheritance of Nager acrofacial dysostosis. J Med Genet 1988; 25:230–232.

Goldstein DJ, Mirkin LD: Nager acrofacial dysostosis: evidence for apparent heterogeneity. Am J Med Genet 1988; 30:741–746.

KR005                                         **Celeste M. Krauss**

## ACROFACIAL DYSOSTOSIS, POSTAXIAL TYPE          2126

**Includes:**

Postaxial acrofacial dysostosis syndrome (POADS)
Acrofacial dysostosis, type Genee-Wiedemann
Genee-Wiedemann syndrome
Miller syndrome

**Excludes:**

**Acrofacial dysostosis, Nager type** (2167)
**Acrofacial dysostosis** (other)
**Cleft palate-micrognathia-glossoptosis** (0182)
**Clefting-ectropion-conical teeth** (2759)
**Mandibulofacial dysostosis, Treacher-Collins type, recessive** (2802)

**Major Diagnostic Criteria:**  First branchial arch anomalies of variable expression combined with predominantly postaxial defects of upper and lower limbs including mesomelic shortening.

**Clinical Findings:**  Newborn infants present with variable degrees of first branchial arch anomalies: malar hypoplasia, downward slanting of palpebral fissures, ± lower lid coloboma (in some patients in severe expression as seen in **Mandibulofacial dysostosis**), microretrognathia, **Cleft palate**, and small, not well differentiated, typically protruding ("cupped") ears. Anatomical changes and functional symptoms can resemble those in the so-called Robin complex. Short, in some patients upslanting, palpebral fissures and/or dacryostenosis were repeatedly observed.

Limb anomalies typically consist of bilateral absence of the fifth ray of hands and feet (including metacarpals and metatarsals). In some patients there was only hypoplasia of one fifth finger or toe while the other was absent. As an exception, also the fourth and even the third ray can be affected. In addition, **Syndactyly** of fingers or toes and malposition of toes were described in some patients.

Most of the patients showed also shortened forearms due to short, sometimes severely deformed ulna and less affected radius. Radioulnar synostosis was also seen in a few cases.

Though postaxial defects represent a leading feature, also preaxial involvement in variable degrees (rarely absent first ray) with short and proximally placed thumbs is apparently the rule.

**Complications:**  Early complications can arise from severe glossoptosis with its functional sequelae (respiratory distress, swallowing difficulties, and failure to thrive). Dacryostenosis and/or lower lid coloboma/ectropion are often complicated by chronic eye infection. Cleft palate often leads to speech impairment and sometimes hearing deficit due to chronic middle ear infections.

**Associated Findings:**  Among the not regularly observed findings are extra nipples, congenital heart defects, renal anomalies,

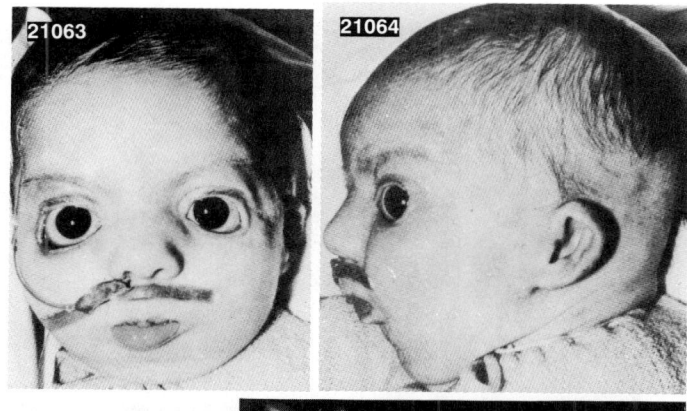

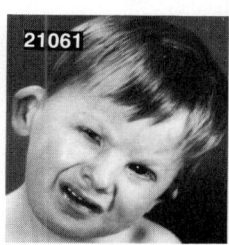

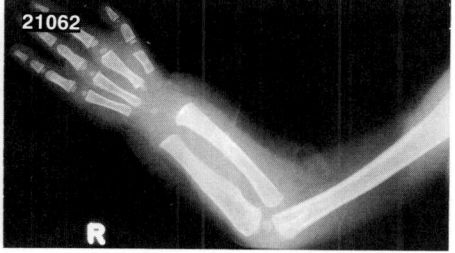

**2126A-21063–64:**  7-month-old with lower lid colobomas, downward slanting of the palpebral fissures, microretrognathia, malar hypoplasia and cupped ears.    21061: Older child with less severe facial expression; note micrognathia, malar hypoplasia and cupped ears.    21062: Mesomelic shortening of the forearm, absent fifth ray and slightly hypoplastic 1st ray in the same child as shown in 21061.

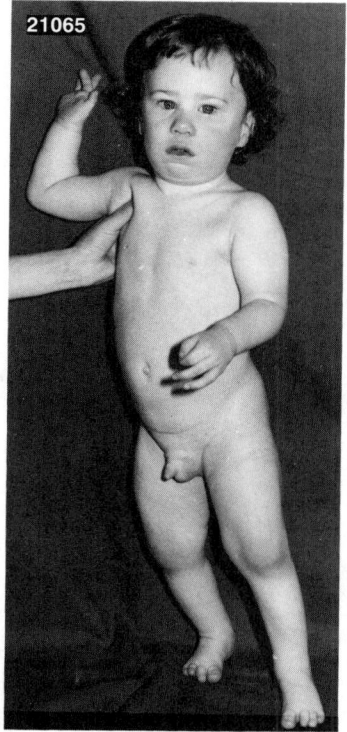

**2126B-21065:**  Robin anomaly, hypotelorism, short upslanted palpebral fissures, malar hypoplasia, and retrognathia with oligodactyly.

micropenis, and cryptorchidism. Mental retardation typically is not a feature of this syndrome, although it was observed in a few otherwise well documented cases.

**Etiology:** Probably autosomal recessive inheritance (two well documented instances of affected sibs of opposite sex). Genetic heterogeneity cannot yet be excluded.

**Pathogenesis:** Undetermined, but possibly the homozygous gene (if autosomal recessive) is affecting a still hypothetical "acrofacial developmental field".

**MIM No.:** 26375

**POS No.:** 3487

**Sex Ratio:** M15:F9 (in published cases).

**Occurrence:** At least two dozen cases have been reported.

**Risk of Recurrence for Patient's Sib:**
See Part I, *Mendelian Inheritance.*

**Risk of Recurrence for Patient's Child:**
See Part I, *Mendelian Inheritance.*

**Age of Detectability:** At birth.

**Gene Mapping and Linkage:** Unknown.

**Prevention:** None known. Genetic counseling indicated.

**Treatment:** Early monitoring and treatment as in isolated cases of Robin complex if functional symptoms are present. Later surgical repair of cleft palate including velopharyngeal plastic surgery and speech therapy. Surgical repair of ectropion/coloboma of lower lid for functional and cosmetic reasons. In some instances plastic surgery and orthopedic means will be required for improvement of limb function.

**Prognosis:** Life span generally not reduced.

**Detection of Carrier:** Unknown.

**Special Considerations:** In spite of the considerable clinical variability, mental retardation obviously is not a characteristic in this type of acrofacial dysostosis. But if present, it could have been an independently segregating feature which is possibly true for the case reported by Wiedemann (1973). Brain damage due to hypoxia as a preventable feature of the Robin complex is also thought to be a plausible explanation for rarely observed mental retardation and/or seizures in this syndrome. Heterogeneity may exist.

**References:**
Genée E: Une forme extensive de dysostose mandibulo-faciale. J Génét hum 1969; 17:45–52.
Wiedemann HR: Missbildungs-Retardierungs-Syndrom mit Fehlen des 5. Strahls an Händen und Füssen, Gaumenspalte, dysplastischen Ohren und Augenlidern und radioulnarer Synostose. Klin Pädiat 1973; 185:181–186.
Miller M, et al: Postaxial acrofacial dysostosis syndrome. J Pediatr 1979; 95:970–975. * †
Donnai D, et al: Postaxial acrofacial dysostosis (Miller) syndrome. J Med Genet 1987; 24:422–425. * †
Opitz JM, Stickler GB: Genée-Wiedemann syndrome: an acrofacial dysostosis - Further observation. Am J Med Genet 1987; 27:971–975.
Meinecke P, Wiedemann HR: Robin sequence and oligodactyly in mother and son: probably a further example of the postaxial acrofacial dysostosis syndrome. Am J Med Genet 1987; 27:953–956. †

ME008
WI003
Peter Meinecke
Hans-Rudolf Wiedemann

**Acrofacial dysostosis, type Genée-Wiedemann**
*See ACROFACIAL DYSOSTOSIS, POSTAXIAL TYPE*

## ACROFACIAL DYSOSTOSIS-CLEFT LIP/PALATE-TRIPHALANGEAL THUMB
**3197**

**Includes:**
Cleft lip/palate-acrofacial dysostosis-triphalangeal thumb
Thumb, triphalangeal-acrofacial dysostosis-cleft lip/palate
**Excludes:**
**Acrofacial dysostosis** (other)
**Oro-facio-digital syndrome, Mohr type** (0771)
**Oto-palato-digital syndrome, II** (2258)

**Major Diagnostic Criteria:** The combination of **Mandibulofacial dysostosis**, **Cleft lip**, **Cleft palate**, hypoplastic **Thumb, triphalangeal**, and normal intellect.

**Clinical Findings:** Facial anomalies are numerous and included **Eye, hypertelorism**, S-shaped palpebral fissures, malar and mandibular hypoplasia, downward obliquity of palpebral fissures, partial absent eyelashes, high nasal bridge, rudimentary ears, absent external auditory meatus, extension of the hair on the upper check, cleft lip/palate, hypoplastic triphalangeal thumbs, hypoplastic first metacarpals, and lack of mental retardation. X-ray anomalies included hypoplastic triphalangeal thumbs, hypoplastic first metacarpal bones, and hypoplastic zygomatic, malar and mandibular bones. Dermatoglyphic studies showed increased atd angle and a longitudinal tendency of the main lines.

**Complications:** Unknown.
**Associated Findings:** None known.
**Etiology:** Possibly autosomal recessive inheritance. The condition has been observed in sibs, born to unaffected nonconsanguineous parents.
**Pathogenesis:** Unknown.
**Sex Ratio:** Presumably M1:F1.
**Occurrence:** Reported in one pair of sibs from Brazil.

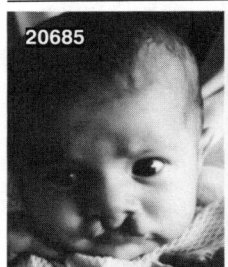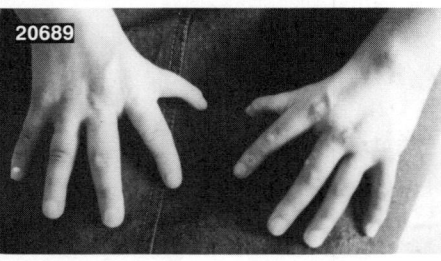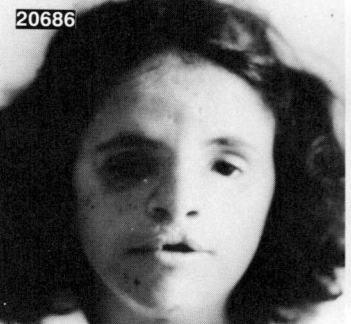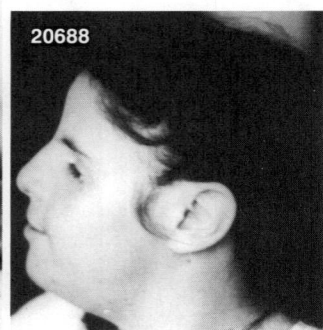

**3197-20685:** Affected infant proband; note hypertelorism, partial absence of eyelashes, high nasal bridge and bilateral cleft lip and palate. **20689:** Bilateral triphalangeal thumbs. **20686–88:** Affected older sister has hypertelorism, "S"-shaped palpebral fissures, ptosis, partial absence of eyelashes, repaired cleft lip and palate, small mid-face, and extension of hair onto the upper cheek.

**Risk of Recurrence for Patient's Sib:**
See Part I, *Mendelian Inheritance.*

**Risk of Recurrence for Patient's Child:**
See Part I, *Mendelian Inheritance.*

**Age of Detectability:** At birth, by physical examination.

**Gene Mapping and Linkage:** Unknown.

**Prevention:** None known. Genetic counseling indicated.

**Treatment:** Unknown.

**Prognosis:** Life span undetermined, but may not be affected.

**Detection of Carrier:** Unknown.

**References:**
Richieri-Costa A, et al: Syndrome of acrofacial dysostosis, cleft lip/palate, and triphalangeal thumb in a Brazilian Family. Am J Med Genet 1983; 14:225–229.

G0044

**Thomaz R. Gollop**

**Acrofacial dysplasia**
*See GELEOPHYSIC DWARFISM*
**Acrofacial postaxial defect syndrome**
*See ACROFACIAL DYSOSTOSIS*

## ACROFACIAL SYNDROME, CURRY-HALL TYPE     2273

**Includes:**
Acrodental dysostosis of Weyers
Polydactyly-conical teeth-nail dysplasia-short limbs
Teeth (conical)-polydactyly-nail dysplasia-short limbs
Weyers acrofacial dysostosis

**Excludes:**
Chondroectodermal dysplasia (0156)
Nail-patella syndrome (0704)
Onychodystrophy-coniform teeth-sensorineural hearing loss (2034)

**Major Diagnostic Criteria:** Conical teeth, hypodontia, onychodysplasia, polydactyly, and short stature.

**Clinical Findings:** The teeth may be reduced in size (conical) or absent; these two traits are thought to be variable manifestations of a single developmental flaw, whether they exist as isolated traits or as parts of a syndrome. There is no pattern to the hypodontia, but its presence may result in malocclusion or deficient midfacial growth. Some or all nails of the fingers and toes may be affected. The nails are foreshortened and may split easily. They may also be ridged. The **Polydactyly** is postaxial and may involve from one to four limbs. Stature is not markedly reduced; affected individuals are between the 10th and 25th percentiles for age-adjusted height.

**Complications:** Malocclusion.

**Associated Findings:** Short, upturned nasal tip; obliteration of the oral vestibule by mucosal bands from the lip to the alveolus; and prominant anthelix of the ears.

**Etiology:** Autosomal dominant inheritance.

**Pathogenesis:** Unknown.

**MIM No.:** *19353

**POS No.:** 3632

**Sex Ratio:** M1:F1

**Occurrence:** Four kinships have been documented, with backgrounds including Spanish-Mexican, Cherokee, Irish, and German.

**Risk of Recurrence for Patient's Sib:**
See Part I, *Mendelian Inheritance.*

**Risk of Recurrence for Patient's Child:**
See Part I, *Mendelian Inheritance.*

**Age of Detectability:** At birth.

**Gene Mapping and Linkage:** Unknown.

**Prevention:** None known. Genetic counseling indicated.

**Treatment:** Surgical removal of extra fingers; orthodontics and prosthodontics for conical and malaligned teeth.

**Prognosis:** Normal life span.

**Detection of Carrier:** Unknown.

**References:**
Weyers H: Hexadactylie, Unterkieferspalt und Oligodontie, ein neuer Symptomenkomplex: dysostosis acro-facialis. Ann Padiatr (Basel) 1953; 181:45–60.
Curry CJR, Hall BD: Polydactyly, conical teeth, nail dysplasia, and short limbs: a new autosomal dominant malformation syndrome. BD:OAS XV(5B). New York: March of Dimes Birth Defects Foundation, 1979:253–263.
Roubichek M, Spranger J: Weyers acrodental dysostosis in a family. Clin Genet 1984; 26:587–590.
Shapiro SD, et al.: Curry-Hall syndrome. Am J Med Genet 1984; 17:579–583.

J0027

**Ronald J. Jorgenson**

**Acrogeria**
*See PROGERIA*

## ACROKERATOELASTOIDOSIS     3068

**Includes:**
AKE
Collagenous plaques of the hands
Elastodosis marginalis
Hands, collagenous plaques of

**Excludes:**
Collagenous plaques of the hands, degenerative
Keratoelastoidosis marginalis
Palmoplantar xanthomas

**Major Diagnostic Criteria:** Typical skin lesions of the hands and feet beginning in childhood or early adult life without any apparent inciting event.

**Clinical Findings:** The skin lesions consist of small, symmetric, round or oval, firm papules usually over the dorsal aspects of the hands, at the interphalangeal and metacarpophalangeal joints, in the interdigital spaces, and along the lateral margins of the hands and wrists. Lesions may also be seen over the knuckles and over the nailbeds. Similar lesions occur along the margins of the soles of the feet. Occasionally these lesions may be present on the lower two-thirds of the anterior surfaces of the legs. Clinically the papules may appear yellowish with a smooth and shiny surface resembling corneous, keratotic, or umbilicated pearls. The lesions are asymptomatic and slowly progressive. However, rapid extension of the lesions during pregnancy has been reported. Hyperhidrosis has frequently been seen, but does not seem to be a constant finding.

To make a diagnosis of acrokeratoelastoidosis (AKE), the skin lesions must have the characteristic aspects and distribution. Also, there should be no history of chronic trauma or chronic sun exposure. The typical histologic pattern must be present, showing epidermal hypertrophy with acanthosis and marked hyperkeratosis and coarse, scattered, and fragmented fibers in the reticular dermis, being most marked in the deeper layers. Electron microscopic studies showed abnormalities in the appearance and shape of the elastic fibers and the presence of dense granules in or near the plasma membrane of the fibroblasts, suggesting a disturbance of the secretion or excretion of elastic tissue.

**Complications:** Unknown.

**Associated Findings:** None known.

**Etiology:** Autosomal dominant inheritance, although sporadic cases have been reported.

**Pathogenesis:** Unknown.

**MIM No.:** *10185

**Sex Ratio:** M1:F1, although several reports describe predominantly female patients.

**Occurrence:** Several kindreds have been reported in the literature.

**Risk of Recurrence for Patient's Sib:**
See Part I, *Mendelian Inheritance.*

**Risk of Recurrence for Patient's Child:**
See Part I, *Mendelian Inheritance.*

**Age of Detectability:** Usually during the second or third decade of life, but sometimes in early childhood.

**Gene Mapping and Linkage:** Unknown.

**Prevention:** None known. Genetic counseling indicated.

**Treatment:** The lesions are asymptomatic. Treatment with liquid nitrogen and preparations containing keratolytic agents have been unsuccessful.

**Prognosis:** Good. The disorder runs a benign course.

**Detection of Carrier:** Unknown.

**Special Considerations:** Degenerative, *collagenous plaques of the hands,* or *elastodosis marginalis,* which clinically resemble AKE but occur on the hands of aged Caucasian patients exposed to chronic sun rays or trauma, with histological evidence of such, must be differentiated from the form described by Costa (1953). An additional form, called *focal acral hyperkeratosis,* that shows the same clinical lesions as AKE, but lacking the collagen or elastic degeneration, has been described. It is still in debate whether or not this condition should be differentiated from AKE. Recently it has been suggested to consider AKE as a syndrome with a broad spectrum of clinical and histologic abnormalities.

**References:**
Costa OG: Akrokerato-elastoidosis: a hitherto undescribed skin disease. Dermatologica 1953; 107:164–167.
Rahbari H: Acrokeratoelastoidosis and keratoelastoidosis marginalisany relation? J Am Acad Dermatol 1981; 5:348–350.
Highet AS, et al.: Acrokeratoelastoidosis. Br J Dermatol 1982; 106:337–344.
Dowd PM, et al.: Focal acral hyperkeratosis. Br J Dermatol 1983; 109:97–103.
Greiner J, et al.: A linkage study of acrokeratoelastoidosis: possible mapping to chromosome 2. Hum Genet 1983; 63:222–227.
Saruk M, et al.: Acrokeratoelastoidosis. Cutis 1983; 32:250–251.
de Boer EM, van Dijk E: Acrokeratoelastoidosis: a spectrum of diseases. Dermatologica 1985; 171:8–11.
Korc A, et al.: Acrokeratoelastoidosis of Costa in North America: a report of two cases. J Am Acad Dermatol 1985; 12:832–836.

MI038                                          **Giuseppe Micali**

## ACROKERATOSIS VERRUCIFORMIS                    3256

**Includes:**
Acrokeratosis verruciformis of Hopf
Hopf disease
Skin, acrokeratosis verruciformis

**Excludes:**
**Darier disease** (2865)
Epidermodysplasia verruciformis
Keratosis follicularis

**Major Diagnostic Criteria:** Skin-colored verrucous papules on hands and feet. Histology-showing hyperkeratosis, an increased granular layer, and acanthosis. Papillomatosis of a pointed nature is said to resemble church spires.

**Clinical Findings:** Skin colored verrucous papules usually occurring on hands or feet, but may occur on the knees, elbows, or forearms. Other skin findings may include punctate keratones of palms and soles, and occasionally nail dystrophy.

**Complications:** Unknown.

**Associated Findings:** Similar papular lesions on the extremities may occur in patients with **Darier disease**. However, in most pedigrees, these appear to be separate entities.

**Etiology:** Autosomal dominant inheritance.

**Pathogenesis:** Unknown.

**MIM No.:** *10190

**Sex Ratio:** M1:F2

**Occurrence:** Undetermined but presumed rare.

**Risk of Recurrence for Patient's Sib:**
See Part I, *Mendelian Inheritance.*

**Risk of Recurrence for Patient's Child:**
See Part I, *Mendelian Inheritance.*

**Age of Detectability:** Usually appears at birth or early childhood.

**Gene Mapping and Linkage:** Unknown.

**Prevention:** None known. Genetic counseling indicated.

**Treatment:** Superficial destruction; e.g., surgical excision or curettage and electrodessication.

**Prognosis:** Lesions persist throughout life. No serious sequelae. Lesions may become darker after sun-exposure.

**Detection of Carrier:** Unknown.

**References:**
Hofp G: Ober eine bisher nicht beschriebene disseminierte Keratose Akrokeratosis verruciformis. Dermat Zeitschr 1931; 60:227–250.
Waisman M: Verruciform manifestations of keratosis follicularis. Arch Dermatol 1960; 81:1–14.
Niedelman ML, McKusick VA: Acrokeratosis verruciformis (Hofp). Arch Dermatol 1962; 86:779.

GH001                                          **Ruby Ghadially**

**Acrokeratosis verruciformis of Hopf**
*See ACROKERATOSIS VERRUCIFORMIS*
**Acrokeratotic poikiloderma, hereditary**
*See POIKILODERMA, HEREDITARY ACROKERATOTIC, KINDLER-WEARY TYPE*
**Acromandibular dysplasia**
*See MANDIBULOACRAL DYSPLASIA*

## ACROMEGALOID FACIAL APPEARANCE SYNDROME      2756

**Includes:**
Face, acromegaloid appearance
Lips, thick-oral mucosa
Thick lips-oral mucosa

**Excludes:**
Acromegaly
**Blepharochalasis-double lip-nontoxic goiter** (0111)
Multiple neuroma syndrome
**Pachydermoperiostosis** (0788)

**Major Diagnostic Criteria:** The presence of a progressive acromegaloid facial appearance without endocrine defects or increased frequency of malignancies.

**Clinical Findings:** Clinical findings in a five generation kindred were limited to face and hands. Facial features included progressively thickened periorbital skin, lips, and intraoral mucosa; bulbous nose; and furrowed tongue. The hands were described as large and having a doughy consistency to the skin as well as hyperextensible metacarpophalangeal and interphalangeal joints. X-rays of the hands sometimes showed distal phalangeal tufting.

**Complications:** Narrow palpebral fissures secondary to thickened skin around the eyes.

**Associated Findings:** One affected individual had a grand mal seizure at age two years.

**Etiology:** Autosomal dominant inheritance with virtually complete penetrance.

**Pathogenesis:** Unknown. Histologic studies of the skin were not performed.

**MIM No.:** *10215

**POS No.:** 3661

**Sex Ratio:** M1:F1

**Occurrence:** One family from Canada has been documented in the literature.

**Risk of Recurrence for Patient's Sib:**
See Part I, *Mendelian Inheritance.*

**Risk of Recurrence for Patient's Child:**
See Part I, *Mendelian Inheritance.*

**Age of Detectability:** Although the disorder is progressive, with onset in childhood, one individual was identified at age six months by the presence of intraoral mucosal thickening.

**Gene Mapping and Linkage:** Unknown.

**Prevention:** None known. Genetic counseling indicated.

**Treatment:** Cosmetic surgery may be indicated.

**Prognosis:** Life span and intellectual development are normal.

**Detection of Carrier:** Unknown.

**References:**
Hughes HE, et al.: An autosomal dominant syndrome with "acromegaloid" features and thickened oral mucosa. J Med Genet 1985; 22:119–125.

T0007                                                      **Helga V. Toriello**

## ACROMEGALOID PHENOTYPE-CUTIS VERTICIS GYRATA-CORNEAL LEUKOMA                              **0018**

**Includes:**
Corneal leukoma-acromegaloid phenotype-cutis verticis
Cutis verticis-gyratacorneal leukoma-acromegaloid phenotype

**Excludes:**
**Acromegaloid facial appearance syndrome** (2756)
**Acromegaloid phenotype-cutis verticis gyrata-corneal leukoma** (0018)

**Major Diagnostic Criteria:** Progressive leukoma formation and gyrate convolutions of the scalp in association with acromegaly-like features.

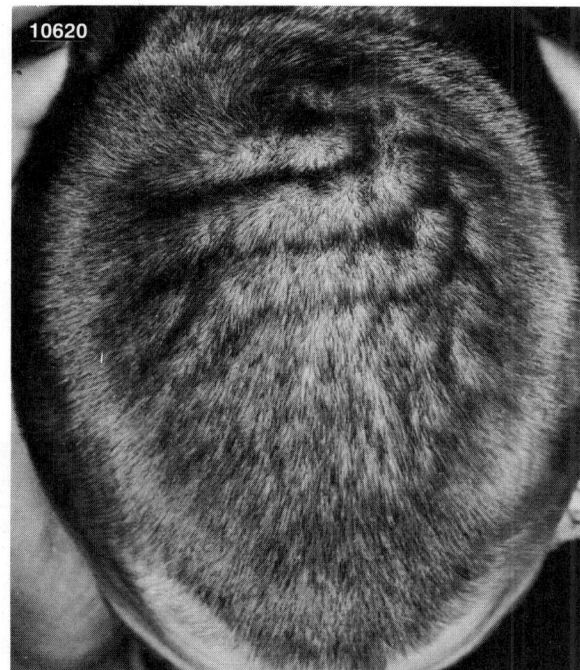

**0018-10620:** Gyrate scalp folds—cutis verticis gyrata.

**Clinical Findings:** Acromegaloid features include large bones, e.g. the jaw, but the sella turcica is normal in size. The lateral half of the supraorbital arch of the frontal bone is particularly enlarged. The scalp is also enlarged, causing gyrus-like formations of skin over the surface of the skull. There is longitudinal splitting of dermal ridges in the palms. During the first decade of life, unilateral or bilateral progressive opacification of the cornea occurs. It characteristically begins in the inferonasal quadrant of the corneal epithelium as a flat, then raised, leukoma, which subsequently becomes slightly elevated (about 1/2 mm) and considerably more widespread, leading to blindness. The peripheral 1 mm of the cornea is usually spared.

**Complications:** Blindness due to corneal opacification.

**Associated Findings:** None known.

**Etiology:** Autosomal dominant inheritance.

**Pathogenesis:** Unknown.

**MIM No.:** *10210

**POS No.:** 3839

**Sex Ratio:** Presumably M1:F1

**Occurrence:** Reported in 13 members of four generations of a Lousiana Black family.

**Risk of Recurrence for Patient's Sib:**
See Part I, *Mendelian Inheritance.*

**Risk of Recurrence for Patient's Child:**
See Part I, *Mendelian Inheritance.*

**Age of Detectability:** At birth.

**Gene Mapping and Linkage:** Unknown.

**Prevention:** None known. Genetic counseling indicated.

**Treatment:** Optical iridectomy.

**Prognosis:** Normal life expectancy, with poor vision and questionably normal intelligence.

**Detection of Carrier:** Unknown.

**References:**
Rosenthal JW, Kloepfer HW: An acromegaloid cutis verticis gyrata, corneal leukoma syndrome. A new medical entity. Arch Ophthalmol 1962; 68:722–726.
Harbison JB, Nice CM: Familial pachydermoperiostosis presenting as an acromegaly-like syndrome. Am J Roentgen 1971; 112;532–536.

SU001                                                         **Joel Sugar**
G0006                                                   **Morton F. Goldberg**

**Acromesomelic dwarfism**
*See ACROMESOMELIC DYSPLASIA, MAROTEAUX-MARTINELLI-CAMPAILLA TYPE*

## ACROMESOMELIC DYSPLASIA, CAMPAILLA-MARTINELLI TYPE                                    **0019**

**Includes:**
Campailla-Martinelli acromesomelic dysplasia
Dwarfism, acromesomelic, Campailla-Martinelli type
Mesomelic dwarfism of Campailla and Martinelli
Micromesomelia, Campailla-Martinelli

**Excludes:**
**Acrodysostosis** (0016)
**Acromesomelic dysplasia, Maroteaux-Martinelli-Campailla type** (0020)
**Chondroectodermal dysplasia** (0156)
**Dyschondrosteosis** (0308)
All forms of mesomelic dysplasia

**Major Diagnostic Criteria:** Marked short stature with short middle segments of the limbs and short distal parts of the fingers and toes. Characteristic X-ray findings.

**Clinical Findings:** Disproportionate short stature with marked shortening of the forearms and mild shortening of the lower legs. The digits are stubby and foreshortened but nails are normal. The

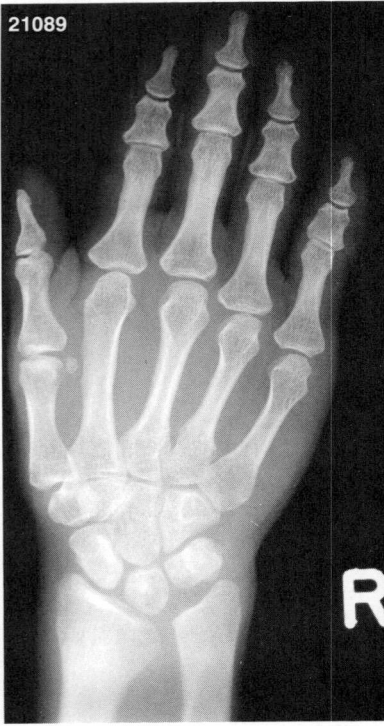
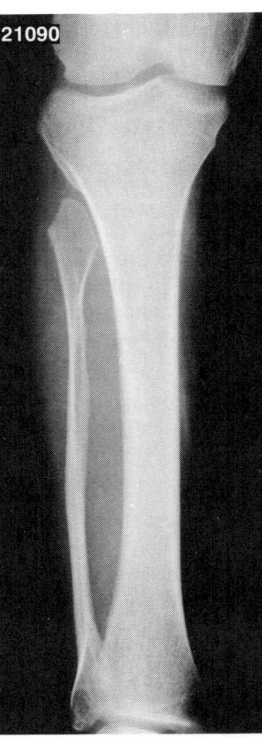

0019-21089: The tubular bones are shortened and hypoplastic. There is a Madelung deformity at the wrist joint. 21090: The fibula is shortened and dysplastic.

trunk is normal or sturdy. There may be mild limitation of extension and pronation-supination of the elbows. The lower extremities are straight but there may be pes planus and hallux valgus. Mild thoraco-lumbar kyphoscoliosis and increased lumbar lordosis may be present. The head is normal or macrocephalic, and the face is normal. Adult height varies between 126 and 137 cm, arm span 115 to 125 cm, and the upper-lower segment ratio is about 1.15. Skeletal X-rays show somewhat short and thick ulna, radius and tibia with hypoplasia of the proximal radius and the distal ulna. The radius is laterally curved, and there is Madelung deformity at the wrists. The fibula is short and hypoplastic. Metacarpals and the proximal phalanges are only slightly shortened whereas the middle phalanges and particularly the terminal phalanges are short and severely dysplastic. At the wrists there may be fusion of the capitate and hamate bones. The fourth and fifth metatarsals may be short. Kyfoscoliosis may be associated with mild vertebral dysplasia and anterior wedging of the Th X and Th XI.

**Complications:** Mild scoliosis.

**Associated Findings:** None known.

**Etiology:** Autosomal recessive inheritance.

**Pathogenesis:** Disturbed development and growth of the vertebra and tubular bones, particularly at the distal digits.

**MIM No.:** *20125

**POS No.:** 3014

**Sex Ratio:** Presumably M1:F1; M1:F6 observed.

**Occurrence:** Two affected siblings reported in one family, while five of eight siblings in a second reported family were affected.

**Risk of Recurrence for Patient's Sib:**
See Part I, *Mendelian Inheritance.*

**Risk of Recurrence for Patient's Child:**
See Part I, *Mendelian Inheritance.*

**Age of Detectability:** At infancy.

**Gene Mapping and Linkage:** Unknown.

**Prevention:** None known. Genetic counseling indicated.

**Treatment:** Physiotherapy. Orthopedic surgery may be needed for correction of hallux valgus.

**Prognosis:** A normal life span is probable with no major physical handicaps except the short stature.

**Detection of Carrier:** Unknown.

**References:**
Campailla E, Martinelli B: Deficit staturale con micromesomelia. Minerva Ortop 1971; 22:180–184.
Beighton P: Autosomal recessive inheritance in the mesomelic dwarfism of Campailla and Martinelli. Clin Genet 1974; 5:363–367.
Kaitila II, et al.: Mesomelic skeletal dysplasias. Clin Orthop 1976; 114:94–106.
Langer LO, et al.: Acromesomelic dwarfism: manifestations in childhood. Am J Med Genet 1977; 1;87–100.

KA004                                              **Ilkka I. Kaitila**

## ACROMESOMELIC DYSPLASIA, MAROTEAUX-MARTINELLI-CAMPAILLA TYPE                    0020

**Includes:**
Acromesomelic dwarfism
Dysostosis, peripheral
Maroteaux-Martinelli-Campailla acromesomelic dysplasia

**Excludes:**
**Acrodysostosis** (0016)
**Acromesomelic dysplasia, Campailla-Martinelli type** (0019)
**Chondroectodermal dysplasia** (0156)
**Dyschondrosteosis** (0308)
All forms of mesomelic dysplasia

**Major Diagnostic Criteria:** Disproportionate progressive short stature with relatively large head, short forearms, small hands and feet, short fingers, general loose-jointedness except at elbows, radial head dislocation, and normal intelligence. Characteristic skeletal X-rays.

**Clinical Findings:** Mild short limbed short stature. Short hands and feet are often observed at birth. These features, and bowing of the forearms and limitation of elbow extension become more obvious during the first years of life. The head appears disproportionately large, and due to frontal, and possibly parietal and occipital bossing, scaphocephaly, poor head control and delayed motor development, hydrocephalus has been suspected. The midface may be slightly flattened and the nose is short. Low thoracic kyphosis may develop. In childhood, the fingers and the toes become very short, have redundant and loose skin, and a marked ligamentous laxity of the fingerjoints. The nails are short and broad but not dysplastic. The limitations of pronation-supination and extension at the elbows are due to posterior subluxation or dislocation of the radial head. Legs are straight but lower

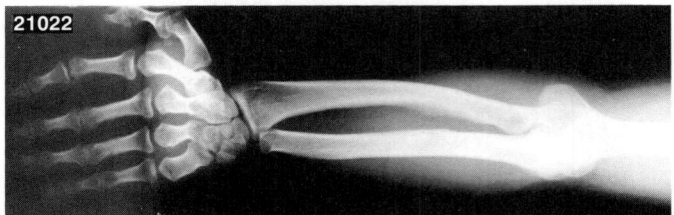

0020-21022: Acromesomelic dysplasia, Maroteaux type; note short long bones, curved radius and short, boxy metacarpals.

legs are short. Feet are short, flat and square with stubby toes; the great toe being relatively large. The thorax is small with flaring of the costal margins and Harrison grooves. The clavicles are superiorly curved, and their medial portions are high in position. The thoracolumbar kyphosis may be severe, and it may be associated with loss of normal kyphosis or actual lordosis in the thoracic region. Adult height ranges from 94 to 123 cm.

In infancy, X-rays show short tubular bones with about normal shape. With age the skeletal abnormalities become more obvious. During the first year of life the metacarpals and the phalanges progressively become shorter and broader, and at about two years of age there is a generalized early cone-shaped epiphysis formation, and later a premature growth plate fusion. There is relative metaphyseal flaring of all long tubular bones, and exaggeration of outlines, particularly at the sites of muscular attachments. The distal ulna may be severely hypoplastic, and its midshaft may be curved. The radius is shortened, often bent, and the proximal head is posteriorly subluxated or dislocated. The vertebra are oval shaped in infancy, have an anterior central protrusion in childhood, and become slightly flattened. In adults, one or more vertebral bodies at the thoracolumbar junction may be anteriorly hypoplastic, and the adjacent vertebra may appear posteriorly wedged or concave. In childhood, relative hypoplasia of the basilar portion of the ilia and irregular ossification of the lateral superior acetabula may be observed.

**Complications:** Pain at the low back requiring laminectomy has been reported in one case. Pain at the elbow region has also been associated with subluxation or dislocation of the radial head has been observed in several cases.

**Associated Findings:** Delayed sexual maturation has been observed in some patients. Corneal opacities have been reported in two cases.

**Etiology:** Autosomal recessive inheritance.

**Pathogenesis:** Disturbed growth of the vertebral and tubular bones associated with the early fusion of the growth plates in the phalanges, metacarpals and metatarsals. Growth hormone excretion normal.

**MIM No.:** *20125

**POS No.:** 3015

**Sex Ratio:** M1:F1

**Occurrence:** Over 30 cases from some 18 families reported world-wide.

**Risk of Recurrence for Patient's Sib:**
See Part I, *Mendelian Inheritance.*

**Risk of Recurrence for Patient's Child:**
See Part I, *Mendelian Inheritance.*

**Age of Detectability:** By six months of age.

**Gene Mapping and Linkage:** Unknown.

**Prevention:** None known. Genetic counseling indicated.

**Treatment:** Physiotherapy and orthopedic procedures may be required to relieve pain at the low back and elbow.

**Prognosis:** Probably normal life span.

**Detection of Carrier:** Unknown.

**References:**
Hall JG: Peripheral dysostosis. BD:OAS 1969; V(4):371–372.
Maroteaux P, et al.: Le nanisme acromésomélique. Presse Méd. 1971; 79:1839.
Goodman RM, et al.: Peripheral dysostosis: an autosomal recessive form. BD:OAS 1974; X(12):137–146.
Langer LO, et al.: Acromesomelic dwarfism: manifestations in childhood. Am J Med Genet 1977; 1:87–100.
Raes M, et al.: A boy with Acromesomelic dysplasia: growth course and growth hormone release. Helv Paediat Acta 1985; 40:415–420.

**Ilkka I. Kaitila**

## ACROMICRIC DYSPLASIA 2716

**Includes:** Skeletal dysplasia, acromicric

**Excludes:**
   **Aarskog syndrome** (0001)
   **Acrodysostosis** (0016)
   **Geleophysic dwarfism** (2020)
   Pseudo-pseudohypoparathyroidism

**Major Diagnostic Criteria:** Markedly shortened hands and feet, mild facial anomalies, growth retardation.

**Clinical Findings:** The dwarfism is variable but always notable. Besides a relative micromelia, the shortness and the stockiness of the hands and feet are striking. Peculiar facial manifestations are present: narrowness of the palpebral fissures and short, stubby nose with anteverted nostrils. No cutaneous, visceral, genital, or ocular abnormalities have been noted with the exception of an atrial defect in one patient.

On X-ray, the metacarpals are short, with a mild pointing of the proximal portion of the last four and a notch medial on the fifth and lateral on the second. A round-shaped pseudoepiphysis at the distal end of the first metacarpal has been noted. There is generalized shortening and broadening of the first and second phalanges of all fingers, with a delay of maturation of the carpal bones. The bones of the feet are short and stocky, and the phalanges have a cone epiphyses. The long bones are short, but their shape is normal. In some patients, the femoral head is slightly deformed with a notched inside border.

**Complications:** The dwarfism is often marked, and a femoral osteochondritis was noted in a 14-year-old patient (Legg-Perthes-Calve disease).

**Associated Findings:** An **Atrial septal defect** was found in one patient.

**Etiology:** Probably autosomal dominant inheritance.

**Pathogenesis:** Study of the growth cartilage shows the disorganization of the growth zone, with a round or ovalar group of

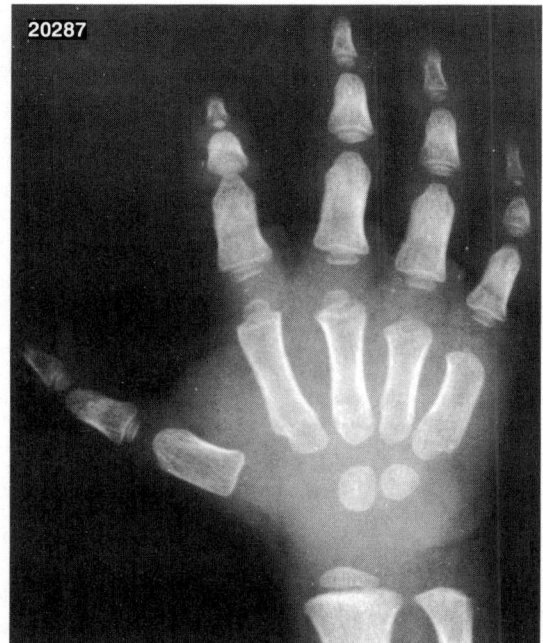

**2716-20287:** Acromicric dysplasia; hand X-ray of 7-year-old male, note short phalanges and metacarpals with pointing of the proximal portion of the last four.

chondrocytes instead of columns and thick and irregular primary trabeculae. A relatively high number of cells shows signs of degeneration; the organization of collagen is abnormal around the cells' lacunae, and in the interterritorial matrix. A large accumulation of glycogen is noted in most cells, even in the provisional calcification area. This accumulation may be the consequence of cell degeneration, or may indicate an initial disorder of carbohydrate metabolism or oxidative phosphorylation.

**MIM No.:** 10237

**POS No.:** 3872

**Sex Ratio:** Presumably M1:F1.

**Occurrence:** Eight cases have been reported in the literature.

**Risk of Recurrence for Patient's Sib:**
See Part I, *Mendelian Inheritance.*

**Risk of Recurrence for Patient's Child:**
See Part I, *Mendelian Inheritance.*

**Age of Detectability:** Growth is usually normal during the first months of life. Growth delay is noted after age two years.

**Gene Mapping and Linkage:** Unknown.

**Prevention:** None known. Genetic counseling indicated.

**Treatment:** Unknown. Regular X-ray examination of the hips is advised because of the risk of osteochondritis.

**Prognosis:** Dwarfism is always significant (adult height, 121–138 cm).

**Detection of Carrier:** Clinical examination.

**References:**
Maroteaux P, et al.: Acromicric dysplasia. Am J Med Genet 1986; 24:447–459. *

MA034                                          **Pierre Maroteaux**

**Acroosteolysis**
*See OSTEOLYSIS, ESSENTIAL*
**Acroosteolysis-osteoporosis-skull and mandible changes**
*See OSTEOLYSIS, ESSENTIAL*

---

## ACROPECTOROVERTEBRAL DYSPLASIA                    0022

**Includes:** F syndrome

**Excludes:**
Syndactyly (0923)
Synostosis, multiple synostosis syndrome (2312)

**Major Diagnostic Criteria:** Hypoplasia of first digits, partial webbing of first and second digits, carpal and tarsal synostoses.

**Clinical Findings:** The syndrome affects the hands and feet most conspicuously. Major anomalies include extensive carpal and tarsal synostoses, prominence of the sternum with a more or less extensive pectus excavatum component, and spina bifida occulta of L5 or S1. Characteristically, the broad, short, and malformed thumbs show incipient distal phalangeal duplication and are, to a variable degree, webbed with the index finger, which is radially deviated, particularly when the webbing is extensive. An extra bone may be present in the web; it seems to be derived from thumb phalanges and is associated with the formation of a bony bridge between the tip of the thumb and a radial projection from the distal end of the first phalanx of the index finger. When the web between the first two fingers is complete, the two distal phalanges of the index finger are hypoplastic and form part of a bony "chain" connecting the tips of the thumb and index finger. The capitate and hamate are fused; other carpals may also be incorporated into the fusion. Clinodactyly of the fifth finger commonly occurs.

The first two toes generally consist of two phalanges; they are more or less webbed and are associated with a single broad and short metatarsal. One accessory bone, which extends laterally from the tip of the "common metatarsal" to the proximal end of the adjacent first phalanx, is frequently present and may perhaps represent the head of an incompletely formed second metatarsal.

Camptodactyly, partial or complete postaxial polydactly, polysyndactyly, or syndactyly occur infrequently in other toes. The two lateral metatarsals are always fused at their base, and the three lateral metatarsals are proximally fused when the "third" metatarsal is involved in the synostotic process, or when one of the two lateral metatarsals is partially duplicated distally. Extensive tarsal fusion never involves the first cuneiform bone.

Minor craniofacial anomalies (highly arched palate with or without broad alveolar ridges, highly bridged nose, long and broad uvula) and apparent predisposition to middle ear infection may be manifestations or coincidental findings in the one known family. Affected individuals generally obtained lower mean scores on tests of psychometric intelligence, academic achievement, and psychomotor and motor proficiency than their unaffected relatives.

**Complications:** Inability to use hands properly; difficulties in fitting shoes; at times pain in walking.

**Associated Findings:** Possibly reduced intelligence.

**Etiology:** Autosomal dominant inheritance with complete penetrance and variable expressivity.

**Pathogenesis:** Unknown.

**MIM No.:** *10251

**POS No.:** 3016

**Sex Ratio:** M1:F1

**Occurrence:** Reported in eight members from four generations of one kindred.

**Risk of Recurrence for Patient's Sib:**
See Part I, *Mendelian Inheritance.*

**Risk of Recurrence for Patient's Child:**
See Part I, *Mendelian Inheritance.*

**Age of Detectability:** At birth.

**Gene Mapping and Linkage:** Unknown.

**Prevention:** None known. Genetic counseling indicated.

**Treatment:** Unknown.

**Prognosis:** Functional impairment of hand and fine motor activities may occur.

**Detection of Carrier:** Unknown.

The author is indebted to John M. Opitz, who prepared the original version of this article.

**Special Considerations:** The term "F" syndrome takes its name from the first letter of the surname of the affected kindred.

*The author is indebted to John M. Opitz who prepared the original version of this article.*

**References:**
Grosse FR, et al.: The *F*-form of acro-pectoro-vertebral dysplasia: The *F*-syndrome. In: Bergsma D, ed: Part III. Limb malformations. BD:OAS 1969; V(3):48–63. White Plains: The National Foundation-March of Dimes.
Trites RL, Matthews CG: Psychological test findings in the *F*-form of acro-pectoro-vertebral dysplasia: The *F*-syndrome. In: Bergsma D, ed: Part III. Limb Malformation. BD:OAS 1969; V(3):64–67. White Plains: The National Foundation-March of Dimes.

MY001                                          **Terry L. Myers**

**Acrorenal field defect-ectodermal dysplasia-lipoatrophic diabetes**
*See AREDYLD SYNDROME*
**ACTH deficiency, isolated**
*See ADRENOCORTICOTROPIC HORMONE DEFICIENCY, ISOLATED*
**Acute anterior poliomyelitis**
*See POLIO, SUSCEPTIBILITY TO*
**Acute lymphocytic leukemia (ALL)**
*See LEUKEMIA, ACUTE LYMPHOCYTIC, FAMILIAL*
**Acyl-CoA dehydrogenase deficiency (some)**
*See VISCERA, FATTY METAMORPHOSIS*

## ACYL-COA DEHYDROGENASE DEFICIENCY, LONG CHAIN TYPE 2228

**Includes:**

Aciduria, dicarboxylic due to LCAD
Dicarboxylic aciduria due to LCAD
Hypoglycemia, nonketotic, due to LCAD
Long-chain acyl-CoA dehydrogenase deficiency (LCAD)
Palmityl-CoA dehydrogenase deficiency

**Excludes:**

**Acidemia, ethylmalonic-adipic** (2377)
**Acidemia, glutaric acidemia I** (0421)
**Acidemia, glutaric acidemia II, neonatal onset** (2289)
**Acyl-CoA dehydrogenase deficiency, medium chain type** (2324)
**Acyl-CoA dehydrogenase deficiency, short chain type** (2323)
**Carnitine deficiency, systemic** (2121)
Dicarboxylic aciduria due to any other cause
**Glycogenosis, type Ia** (0425)
Hypoglycin A intoxication (Jamaican vomiting sickness)

**Major Diagnostic Criteria:** Decreased plasma carnitine (10–28 $\mu$mole/l; normal, 40–60) with 48–100% esterified (normal, 10–20%) during attacks. Urinary excretion of medium-chain and long-chain dicarboxylic acids. Impaired $\beta$-oxidation of long-chain fatty acids by fibroblasts. Definitive diagnosis of enzyme deficiency can be made in fibroblasts and leukocytes.

**Clinical Findings:** Episodic hypoketotic hypoglycemia, systemic carnitine deficiency, dicarboxylic aciduria, hepatomegaly and fatty infiltration of liver, hypertrophic cardiomyopathy, hypotonia in three infants (see below for details of two sibs identified as teenagers). Pregnancy and delivery are normal, and birth weight is appropriate for gestational age. The first few weeks of life may be complicated by poor feeding, poor weight gain, and frequent emesis. Recurrent episodes of persistent vomiting with or without fever or diarrhea in the first few months of life may lead to obtundation, lethargy, and hypotonia. Episodes are characterized by hypoglycemia with no or little ketosis, dicarboxylic aciduria, cardiomegaly, cardiomyopathy, and a variable response to intravenous glucose. These episodes may be confused with those of Reye syndrome.

**Complications:** Developmental delay, chronic muscle weakness, cardiorespiratory arrest, respiratory arrest, death (in one of three infants).

**Associated Findings:** None known.

**Etiology:** Autosomal recessive inheritance.

**Pathogenesis:** A deficiency of long-chain acyl-CoA dehydrogenase (< 10% of normal in fibroblasts and leukocytes). Inability to $\beta$-oxidize long-chain fatty acyl-CoA in mitochondria of liver results in failure of fasting adaptation and ketogenesis. Accumulation of long-chain acyl-CoA in mitochondria alters acyl-CoA/CoASH ratios, presumably disturbing other metabolic pathways, such as glycogenolysis and gluconeogenesis. Inability of muscle (both skeletal and cardiac) to $\beta$-oxidize long-chain fatty acyl-CoA results in muscle weakness and cardiomyopathy. Accumulated long-chain acyl-CoAs are excreted in urine as medium- and long-chain ($C_6$-$C_{12}$) dicarboxylic acids and as long-chain acyl carnitines.

**MIM No.:** *20146

**Sex Ratio:** M1:F4 (observed).

**Occurrence:** Five cases from two families have been documented.

**Risk of Recurrence for Patient's Sib:**
See Part I, *Mendelian Inheritance.*

**Risk of Recurrence for Patient's Child:**
See Part I, *Mendelian Inheritance.*

**Age of Detectability:** At birth. Prenatal diagnosis is feasible.

**Gene Mapping and Linkage:** ACADL (acyl-Coenzyme A dehydrogenase, long chain) is unassigned.

**Prevention:** None known. Genetic counseling indicated.

**Treatment:** Affected fetus and newborn should be managed as being at risk from birth. Episodes might be prevented by avoiding fasting, maintaining low-fat diet, and using medium-chain triglycerides to bypass the metabolic block. Oral cornstarch therapy during fasting or viral illness (1.75–2.5 g/kg every six hours) may prevent hypoglycemia. Sibs of affected patients should be tested.

Glucose infusion and management of complications, as necessary for the treatment of short- and medium-chain acyl-CoA dehydrogenase deficiencies. While no vitamin-responsive variants have been identified *in vivo*, oral riboflavin therapy should be safe and may reveal vitamin-responsive patients.

**Prognosis:** Of the first three known affected infants, one died in the first year of life; the others survived the first year, but with chronic muscle weakness and developmental delay. Two other patients (sibs H.C. and J.C., in Naylor et al., 1980), in whom the enzyme diagnosis was made as teenagers, appear to be in good health without cardiac dysfunction, but H.C. has episodes of poor exercise tolerance and recurrent rhabdomyolysis. J.C. has had no episodes of overt illness referable to her enzyme deficiency.

**Detection of Carrier:** Carriers have long-chain acyl-CoA dehydrogenase activity 50% of normal, as measured in leukocytes or fibroblasts.

**References:**

Naylor EW, et al.: Intermittent non-ketotic dicarboxylic aciduria in two siblings with hypoglycemia: an apparent defect in the $\beta$-oxidation of fatty acids. J Inherited Metab Dis 1980; 3:19–24.
Hale DE, et al.: Long-chain acyl-CoA dehydrogenase deficiency: an inherited cause of non-ketotic hypoglycemia. Pediatr Res 1985; 19:666–671.
Amendt BA, et al.: Long-chain acyl-coenzyme A dehydrogenase deficiency: biochemical studies in fibroblasts from three patients. Pediatr Res 1988; 23:603–605.
Roe CR, Coates PM: Acyl-CoA dehydrogenase deficiencies. In: Scriver CR, et al, eds: The metabolic basis of inherited disease, 6th ed. New York: McGraw-Hill, 1989:889–914.

C0063 **Paul M. Coates**
RH000 **William J. Rhead**

## ACYL-COA DEHYDROGENASE DEFICIENCY, MEDIUM CHAIN TYPE 2324

**Includes:**

Aciduria, dicarboxylic due to MCAD
Hypoglycemia, nonketotic and/or carnitine deficiency due to MCAD
Medium-chain acyl-CoA dehydrogenase deficiency (MCAD)
Octanoyl-CoA or general acyl-CoA dehydrogenase deficiency
Reye-like syndrome, recurrent, due to MCAD
Straight-chain C6-C10-omega-dicarboxylic aciduria
Suberylglycinuria
Systemic carnitine deficiency due to MCAD

**Excludes:**

**Acidemia, glutaric acidemia I** (0421)
**Acidemia, glutaric acidemia II, neonatal onset** (2289)
**Acidemia, ethylmalonic-adipic** (2377)
**Acyl-CoA dehydrogenase deficiency, long chain type** (2228)
**Acyl-CoA dehydrogenase deficiency, short chain type** (2323)
Dicarboxylic aciduria due to any other cause
**Glycogenosis, type Ia** (0425)
Hypoglycin A intoxication (Jamaican vomiting sickness)
**Viscera, fatty metamorphosis** (0990)

**Major Diagnostic Criteria:** Episodic hypoketotic hypoglycemia may occur with or without mild metabolic acidosis, vomiting, coma, variable hepatomegaly, mild hepatic dysfunction, and hepatic lipid deposition, suggesting recurrent Reye syndrome. Excretion of $C_6$-$C_{10}$-$\Omega$-dicarboxylic acids, hexanoyl-, 3-phenylpropionyl-, and suberyl-glycine, octanoyl-carnitine, and low circulating carnitine levels with elevated acyl-carnitine/carnitine ratios are highly suggestive. Medium-chain acyl-CoA dehydrogenase deficiency in liver, fibroblasts, or leukocytes is diagnostic.

**Clinical Findings:** Medium-chain acyl-CoA dehydrogenase activity is severely deficient (less than 10% of that seen in normal controls) in liver, leukocytes, and fibroblasts from affected patients. The degree of enzymatic deficiency does not predict clinical severity, and no biochemical heterogeneity has been identified to date.

Clinical findings range from asymptomatic to occasional hypoglycemic episodes to severe recurrent hypoglycemia and possibly sudden death. Episodes of lethargy are often noted during viral illnesses. The association of vomiting, coma, hypoglycemia, hepatomegaly, hepatic dysfunction and steatosis, and mild hyperammonemia suggests Reye syndrome. The metabolic acidosis and hyperammonemia are variable and rarely severe. Total plasma carnitines are usually below the normal range; several patients previously diagnosed as having systemic carnitine deficiency have medium-chain acyl-CoA dehydrogenase deficiency. Ketosis during illness or fasting is characteristically low or absent. Glucose loading and glucagon tests are normal. In general, the hypoglycemia responds quickly to intravenous glucose administration. Recurrences during childhood range from none to ten, with most individuals having fewer than five. Urinary organic acid analysis characteristically shows excretion of adipic, suberic, and sebacic acids (hexane-, octane-, and decanedioic acids), hexanoyl-, 3-phenylpropionyl-, and suberyl-glycine, and octanoyl-carnitine.

**Complications:** Hypoglycemia and sudden death occurred after 39 hours of fasting in one child, while several other patients have died during metabolic crises. The majority of surviving patients display normal intellectual and motor development and muscle strength. Cardiomyopathy has not been demonstrated. All patients should have extended follow-up until the nature and extent of more subtle complications are delineated.

**Associated Findings:** None known.

**Etiology:** Autosomal recessive inheritance.

**Pathogenesis:** Medium-chain acyl-CoA dehydrogenase deficiency interrupts β-oxidation of medium-chain fatty acids. During fasting or catabolic states, glycogen utilization and gluconeogenesis are either impaired by the accumulated metabolites or are insufficient to meet energy demands in the absence of normal β-oxidation and ketogenesis.

The accumulated acyl-CoAs are omega-oxidized to dicarboxylic acids and/or converted to their acyl-glycine/-carnitine derivatives. While little studied, medium-chain fatty acids may interfere with mitochondrial ATP production and pyruvate oxidation. Sequestration of CoA and carnitine as their medium-chain acyl derivatives may interfere more generally with mitochondrial metabolism. Systemic carnitine deficiency may result from increased excretion of accumulated acyl-carnitines and/or an unproven depression of carnitine synthesis. The metabolic consequences of this enzymatic defect may be lessened by the peroxisomal β-oxidation and microsomal omega-oxidation of medium-chain length fatty acids.

**MIM No.:** *20145

**Sex Ratio:** M1:F1

**Occurrence:** More than 75 cases have been documented worldwide. Homozygotes may have mild disease and remain undetected.

**Risk of Recurrence for Patient's Sib:**
See Part I, *Mendelian Inheritance.*

**Risk of Recurrence for Patient's Child:**
See Part I, *Mendelian Inheritance.*

**Age of Detectability:** Affected homozygotes may have few or no symptoms and excrete few metabolites. However, urinary organic acid analysis should identify most affected individuals, especially if hexanoyl-, 3-phenylpropionyl, and suberyl-glycine or octanyl-carnitine are found. Enzymatic assays or complementation analysis will clearly demonstrate the defect in leukocytes or fibroblasts. Prenatal diagnosis is theoretically possible using the same assays in amniocytes.

**Gene Mapping and Linkage:** ACADM (acyl-Coenzyme A dehydrogenase, C-4 to C-12 straight-chain) has been provisionally mapped to 1p31.

**Prevention:** None known. Genetic counseling indicated.

**Treatment:** Treatment is experimental but modeled on regimens developed for other inborn errors of amino and/or fatty acid metabolism. A low-fat diet should be prescribed; fasting and other catabolic states should be avoided. Parenteral glucose, fluids, and electrolytes should be provided during acidotic/hypoglycemic episodes. While untested, glycine and/or carnitine administration might promote conjugation and excretion of acyl moieties and permit repletion of carnitine stores. Cautious trials of riboflavin supplementation should be safe and may reveal vitamin-responsive variants. Oral cornstarch (1.75–2.5 gm/kg every 6 hours) may prevent hypoglycemia during periods of fasting.

**Prognosis:** Presumably good. Individuals with frequent and/or severe hypoglycemic crises may be more likely to suffer long-term sequelae.

**Detection of Carrier:** Parents of affected patients have half-normal enzymatic activity in fibroblasts and leukocytes. While enzymatic assays in leukocytes or fibroblasts will detect carriers reliably, routine organic acid analyses have been largely uninformative.

**References:**

Divry P, et al.: Dicarboxylic aciduria due to medium-chain acyl-CoA dehydrogenase defect. Acta Pediatr Scand 1983; 72:943–949.

Rhead WJ, et al.: Dicarboxylic aciduria: deficient [1–$^{14}$C]octanate oxidation and medium-chain acyl-CoA dehydrogenase activity in fibroblasts. Science 1983; 221:73–75.

Stanley CA, et al.: Medium-chain acyl-CoA dehydrogenase deficiency in children with non-ketotic hypoglycemia and low carnitine levels. Pediatr Res 1983; 17:877–884.

Coates PM, et al.: Genetic deficiency of medium-chain acyl-CoA dehydrogenase: studies in cultured skin fibroblasts and peripheral mononuclear leukocytes. Pediatr Res 1985; 19:671–676.

Roe CR, et al.: Diagnostic and therapeutic implications of medium-chain acyl-carnitine in the medium-chain acyl-CoA dehydrogenase deficiency. Pediatr Res 1985; 19:459–465.

Bennett MJ, et al.: Prenatal diagnosis of medium-chain acyl-coenzyme A dehydrogenase deficiency. Prenatal Diag 1987; 7:135–141.

Taubman B, et al.: Familial Reye-like syndrome: a presentation of medium-chain acyl-coenzyme A dehydrogenase deficiency. Pediatrics 1987; 79:382–385.

Rinaldo P, et al.: Medium-chain acyl-CoA dehydrogenase deficiency: diagnosis by stable-isotope dilution measurement of urinary n-hexanoylglycine and 3-phenylpropionylglycine. New Engl J Med 1988; 319:1308–1313.

Roe CR, Coates PM: Acyl-CoA dehydrogenase deficiencies. In: Scriver CR, et al, eds: The metabolic basis of inherited disease, 6th ed. New York: McGraw-Hill, 1989:889–914.

RH000                                            **William J. Rhead**

---

## ACYL-COA DEHYDROGENASE DEFICIENCY, SHORT CHAIN TYPE                                    2323

**Includes:**
    Butyryl-CoA dehydrogenase deficiency
    Ethylmalonic aciduria due to SCAD
    Lipid-storage myopathy secondary to SCAD
    Short chain acyl-CoA dehydrogenase deficiency (SCAD)

**Excludes:**
    **Acidemia, glutaric acidemia I** (0421)
    **Acidemia, glutaric acidemia II, neonatal onset** (2289)
    **Acidemia, ethylmalonic-adipic** (2377)
    **Acyl-CoA dehydrogenase deficiency, long chain type** (2228)
    **Acyl-CoA dehydrogenase deficiency, medium chain type** (2324)
    Dicarboxylic aciduria due to any other cause
    **Glycogenosis, type Ia** (0425)
    Hypoglycin A intoxication (Jamaican vomiting sickness)
    **Viscera, fatty metamorphosis** (0990)

**Major Diagnostic Criteria:** The clinical features vary and are not fully defined. In infancy, they may include signs and symptoms of metabolic acidoses, possibly recurrent hypoketotic hypoglycemia, or in older patients, myopathy. Laboratory findings may include lipid storage myopathy, excretion of ethylmalonic, methylsuccinic, or butyric acids and their acyl-glycine or carnitine derivatives, elevated acyl-carnitine/carnitine ratios in muscle, plasma, and urine. Short-chain acyl-CoA dehydrogenase deficiency in liver, fibroblasts, leukocytes, or muscle is diagnostic.

**Clinical Findings:** Short-chain acyl-CoA dehydrogenase activity is low (25% and 50% of normal in muscle and fibroblasts, respectively), inhibiting β-oxidation of butyryl- and hexanoyl-CoAs.

Metabolic acidosis was prominent in three neonates with SCAD, with one dying in the neonatal period. Hyperammonemia was also noted in this patient. Another child survived and was asymptomatic at two years of age on a normal diet, while a third survived and had muscle weakness and fatty infiltration of muscle and liver.

Another patient presented in the fifth decade with proximal muscle weakness, lipid deposition in type I skeletal muscle fibers, and no antecedent history. This patient had low short-chain acyl-CoA dehydrogenase activity in muscle, but normal activity in fibroblasts. All patients excreted predominantly ethylmalonic, methylsuccinic, and/or butyric acids with variable low excretion of glutaric, isovaleric, and/or lactic acids.

**Complications:** Muscle weakness and lipomyopathy may result from chronic acidosis, interruption of fatty acid β-oxidation, and/or secondary carnitine deficiency.

**Associated Findings:** None known.

**Etiology:** Autosomal recessive inheritance.

**Pathogenesis:** Short-chain acyl-CoA dehydrogenase deficiency produces intramitochondrial accumulation of butyryl-CoA, which is carboxylated by propionyl-CoA carboxylase to form ethylmalonyl-CoA. This latter compound is either hydrolyzed to ethylmalonic acid or converted to methylsuccinyl-CoA. Related short-chain organic acids interfere with mitochondrial pyruvate oxidation, ATP production, electron transport, and ureagenesis. Generalized inhibition of fatty acid β-oxidation and ketogenesis could also result from sequestration of coenzyme A and carnitine as their short-chain acyl derivatives and subsequent excretion of acyl-carnitines with whole body carnitine depletion.

**MIM No.:** *20147

**Sex Ratio:** M0:F4 (observed).

**Occurrence:** Four cases have been documented.

**Risk of Recurrence for Patient's Sib:**
See Part I, *Mendelian Inheritance.*

**Risk of Recurrence for Patient's Child:**
See Part I, *Mendelian Inheritance.*

**Age of Detectability:** Ethylmalonic acid excretion might presumably be elevated at or shortly after birth. Prenatal diagnosis is theoretically possible.

**Gene Mapping and Linkage:** ACADS (acyl-Coenzyme A dehydrogenase, C-2 to C-3 short chain) has been provisionally mapped to 12q22-qter.

**Prevention:** None known. Genetic counseling indicated.

**Treatment:** Treatment is experimental but modeled on regimens developed for other inborn errors of amino and/or fatty acid metabolism. A low-fat diet should be prescribed; fasting and other catabolic states should be avoided. Parenteral glucose, fluids, and electrolytes should be provided during acidotic/hypoglycemic episodes. While untested, glycine and/or carnitine administration might promote conjugation and excretion of acyl moieties and permit repletion of carnitine stores. Cautious trials of riboflavin supplementation should be safe and may reveal vitamin-responsive variants. Oral cornstarch (1.75–2.5 gm/kg every 6 hours) may prevent hypoglycemia during periods of fasting.

**Prognosis:** Presumably related to frequency and severity of clinically significant crises and/or lipid accumulation in striated muscle.

**Detection of Carrier:** Ethylmalonic acid excretion after a medium-chain triglyceride load (150-500 mg/kg) might be informative, as well as enzymatic assays in fibroblasts or other tissues of presumed carriers.

**Special Considerations:** The range of clinical phenotypes in this disorder has not been fully defined. Even if short-chain acyl-CoA dehydrogenase activity is completely absent, butyryl-CoA dehydrogenation will not be totally deficient, since the substrate specificities of short- and medium-chain acyl-CoA dehydrogenases overlap, thus confusing clinical and biochemical analysis. Although we cannot exclude the existence of multiple tissue-specific isozymes of short-chain acyl-CoA dehydrogenase in man, this is not the case in the mouse model for SCAD. While ethylmalonic acid excretion is prominent in patients lacking this enzyme, its excretion is also high in individuals with mild variants of multiple acyl-CoA dehydrogenation disorder (ethylmalonic-adipic aciduria) due to deficiencies of electron transferring flavoprotein (ETF) or its dehydrogenase. For these reasons, all three straight-chain acyl-CoA dehydrogenases, ETF, and ETF dehydrogenase should be assayed in patients with a clinical phenotype and organic aciduria suggesting an isolated defect in short-chain fatty acid β-oxidation.

**References:**
Turnbull DM, et al.: Short chain acyl-CoA dehydrogenase deficiency associated with a lipid-storage myopathy and secondary carnitine deficiency. New Engl J Med 1984; 311:1232–1236.
Amendt BA, et al.: Short-chain acyl-coenzyme A dehydrogenase deficiency: clinical and biochemical studies in two patients. J Clin Invest 1987; 79:1303–1309.
Coates PM, et al.: Genetic deficiency of short-chain acyl-coenzyme A dehydrogenase in cultured fibroblasts from a patient with muscle carnitine deficiency and severe skeletal muscle weakness. J Clin Invest 1988; 81:171-175.
Roe CR, Coates PM: Acyl-CoA dehydrogenase deficiencies. In: Scriver CR, et al, eds: The metabolic basis of inherited disease, 6th ed. New York: McGraw-Hill, 1989:889–914.
Wood PA, et al.: Short-chain acyl-coenzyme A dehydrogenase deficiency in mice. Pediatr Res 1989; 25:38–43.

RH000                                                 **William J. Rhead**

**Acyl-Coenzyme A dehydrogenase, multiple**
  *See ACIDEMIA, GLUTARIC ACIDEMIA II*
**Acylcholine acyl-hydrolase EC 3.1.1.8**
  *See CHOLINESTERASE, ATYPICAL*
**ADA deficiency**
  *See IMMUNODEFICIENCY, ADENOSINE DEAMINASE DEFICIENCY*
**ADAM complex**
  *See AMNIOTIC BANDS SYNDROME*
**Adams-Oliver syndrome**
  *See LIMB AND SCALP DEFECTS, ADAMS-OLIVER TYPE*
**Addison disease, X-linked**
  *See ADRENAL HYPOPLASIA, CONGENITAL*
**Addison disease-cerebral sclerosis**
  *See ADRENOLEUKODYSTROPHY, X-LINKED*
**Addison-Schilders**
  *See ADRENOLEUKODYSTROPHY, X-LINKED*
**Adducted thumb syndrome**
  *See THUMB, ADDUCTED THUMB SYNDROME*
**Adducted thumb-mental retardation**
  *See X-LINKED MENTAL RETARDATION-CLASPED THUMB*
**Adducted thumbs**
  *See THUMB, CLASPED*
**Adductor vocal cord paralysis**
  *See LARYNGEAL PARALYSIS*

## ADENINE PHOSPHO-RIBOSYL-TRANSFERASE (APRT) DEFICIENCY 3104

**Includes:** Urolithiasis, 2,8-dihydroxyadenine (DHA)

**Excludes:**
    **Gout** (0441)
    **Lesch-Nyhan syndrome** (0588)

**Major Diagnostic Criteria:** Characteristic renal lithiasis with DHA calculi, raised urinary adenine levels, and deficient APRT activity in erythrocyte lysates.

**Clinical Findings:** The clinical symptoms are secondary to urolithiasis and present a wide spectrum, including dysuria, hematuria, abdominal colic, and urinary tract infections. Urinary tract obstruction may be associated with acute or chronic renal insufficiency. The age of presentation in Caucasian patients is usually during infancy and childhood. However, there is evidence of clinical heterogeneity. Some excrete gravel from birth, while others are asymptomatic adult homozygotes. Gault et al. (1981) described an adult female homozygote who first presented symptoms of urolithiasis at age 42 years. The stones are structurally and biochemically "uric acid-like" when analyzed by conventional colorimetric or thermogravimetric methods. Also, DHA and uric acid stones are both radiolucent, but they can be differentiated from each other by UV, infrared, or X-ray diffraction and mass spectrometry. Heterozygotes do not excrete detectable amounts of adenine or DHA.

**Complications:** Chronic obstruction of the urinary tract may lead to recurrent urinary tract infections, interstitial nephritis, and chronic renal failure.

**Associated Findings:** None known.

**Etiology:** Autosomal recessive inheritance. The defect is a consequence of a mutation in the gene coding for APRT.

**Pathogenesis:** APRT normally catalyzes the conversion of adenine to adenylic acid (AMP). The deficiency of this purine salvage enzyme leads to the accumulation of adenine and its oxidation by xanthine oxidase to DHA. The endogeneous sources of adenine include the polyamine pathway.

**MIM No.:** *10260

**Sex Ratio:** M1:F1

**Occurrence:** Thirty-four patients have been reported; 21 of them Japanese. Prevalence of heterozygosity has been established from four different Caucasian populations to be 0.41–1.1%, giving an estimation of homozygosity of 1:100,000 or greater.

**Risk of Recurrence for Patient's Sib:**
See Part I, *Mendelian Inheritance.*

**Risk of Recurrence for Patient's Child:**
See Part I, *Mendelian Inheritance.*

**Age of Detectability:** From birth. A screening method has been developed using a dry blood sample technique. The condition should be diagnosable prenatally.

**Gene Mapping and Linkage:** APRT (adenine phosphoribosyltransferase) has been mapped to 16q24.
This gene has been cloned and the nucleotide sequence determined.

**Prevention:** None known. Genetic counseling indicated.

**Treatment:** A low-purine diet to decrease the amount of exogenous adenine and allopurinol (xanthine oxidase inhibitor). A large fluid intake is recommended for those with intact renal function and history of lithiasis. In contradistinction to the management of uric acid calculi, alkali therapy is not useful or even contraindicated.

**Prognosis:** Depends on renal complications at the time of diagnosis.

**Detection of Carrier:** APRT activity in erythrocyte lysates from Caucasian heterozygotes usually range between 25 and 30% of normal. Heterozygotes for the Japanese APRT mutant cannot be easily distinguished from the normal population, since they show 49 to 66% of normal activity.

**Special Considerations:** Early diagnosis and proper differentiation from uric acid lithiasis may help to avoid complications. A blood transfusion shortly before determination of APRT activity in erythrocytes can cause a false result. A different mutant enzyme has been described in Japanese patients, 79% of whom present a partial deficiency leading to DHA urolithiasis, unlike Caucasian patients in whom symptomatology is always associated with a total APRT deficiency.

**References:**

Kelley WN, et al.: Adenine phosphoribosyltransferase deficiency: a previously undescribed genetic defect in man. J Clin Invest 1968; 47:2281–2289.

Cartier P, et al.: Une nouvelle maladie metabolique: le deficit complet en adenine phosphoribosyltransferase avec lithiase de 2,8-dihydroxyadenine. CR Acad Sci [D] (Paris) 1974; 279:883–886.

Gault MH, et al.: Urolithiasis due to 2,8-dihydroxyadenine in an adult. New Engl J Med 1981; 305:1570–1572.

Fratini A, et al.: A new location for the human adenine phosphoribosyltransferase gene (APRT) distal to the haptoglobin (HP) and fra(16)(q23)(FRA16D) loci. Cytogenet Cell Genet 1986; 43:10–13.

Kamatani N, et al.: Genetic and clinical studies on 19 families with adenine phosphoribosyltransferase deficiencies. Hum Genet 1987; 75:163–168.

PI011                         **Guillem Pintos-Morell**

**Adenocarcinoma of the kidney**
   *See CANCER, RENAL CELL CARCINOMA*
**Adenocarcinoma of the pancreas**
   *See CANCER, PANCREAS, FAMILIAL ADENOCARCINOMA OF*
**Adenocarcinoma of the vagina, fetal DES effects**
   *See FETAL DIETHYLSTILBESTROL (DES) EFFECTS*
**Adenolipomatosis**
   *See NECK/FACE, LIPOMATOSIS*
**Adenoma sebaceum-seizures-mental retardation**
   *See TUBEROUS SCLEROSIS*
**Adenoma, hereditary pleomorphic salivary**
   *See SALIVARY GLAND, MIXED TUMOR*
**Adenomatous polyposis coli**
   *See INTESTINAL POLYPOSIS, TYPE I*
**Adenomatous polyposis, familial**
   *See INTESTINAL POLYPOSIS, TYPE I*
**Adenosine aminohydrolase deficiency (ADA)**
   *See IMMUNODEFICIENCY, ADENOSINE DEAMINASE DEFICIENCY*
**Adenosine deaminase**
   *See IMMUNODEFICIENCY, ADENOSINE DEAMINASE DEFICIENCY*
**Adenosine deaminase deficiency**
   *See METAPHYSEAL CHONDRODYSPLASIA WITH THYMOLYMPHOPENIA*
**Adenylate kinase (AK) deficiency**
   *See ANEMIA, ADENYLATE KINASE DEFICIENCY*
**Adenylate kinase, soluble**
   *See ANEMIA, ADENYLATE KINASE DEFICIENCY*

## ADENYLOSUCCINATE MONOPHOSPHATE LYASE DEFICIENCY 3113

**Includes:**
    Autism, succinylpurinemic type
    Purine autism

**Excludes:**
    **Autism, infantile** (2128)
    **Rett syndrome** (2226)

**Major Diagnostic Criteria:** Decreased activity of adenylosuccinase (adenylosuccinate monophosphate lyase E.C.4.3.2.2) in liver and kidney. Other tissues (fibroblasts, lymphocytes, and skeletal muscle) are variably deficient. Presence of succinyladenosine and succinylamino-imidazole carboxamide riboside in urine (large amounts; trace amounts present in controls), plasma, and cerebrospinal fluid.

**Clinical Findings:** Normal pregnancy and delivery followed by severe psychomotor retardation and autistic behavior. At ages 20–44 months, the three affected children reported by Jaeken and Van den Berghe (1984) had no speech, were at developmental ages of 2–6 months, and had gross motor development of 2–9 months. Their behavior was characterized by wandering gaze and poor eye contact, hypokinesia, and stereotyped behaviors (rubbing hands and feet, clapping hands, moving hands before eyes, grimacing, crying, and intermittent laughing). Axial hypotonia with normal deep tendon reflexes was present; placing and equilibrium reactions were absent. Heterogeneity was suggested later (Van den Berghe and Jaeken, 1986) after finding progressive muscle wasting in two sibs who had deficient enzyme activity in skeletal muscle. These patients also had progressive growth failure.

Four patients reported by Wadman et al. (1986) were not described as autistic. Hypertonicity, spastic tetraplegia, dystonia, motoric unrest, involuntary movements, and severe retardation were the main features. Epilepsy and diminished responsiveness to light and noise were each present in a single patient.

Cranial CT scan findings include hypoplasia of the cerebellum, especially the vermis (4/7), widened ventricles or basal cisterns (2/7), severe **Hydrocephaly** (1/7), and normal CT scan (done at six months; 1/7). Other laboratory findings include low CSF protein, normal plasma uric acid and urine uric acid/creatinine ratio, and normal urine amino acids, organic acids, and acid mucopolysaccharides.

**Complications:**  Unknown.

**Associated Findings:**  None known.

**Etiology:**  Presumably autosomal dominant or recessive inheritance. Affected sibs and consanguinuity has been reported.

**Pathogenesis:**  The enzyme adenylosuccinase participates in two steps in the de novo synthesis of purines: formation of AICAR (5'-aminoimidazole carboxamide ribotide) from SAICAR (succinyl AICAR) and formation of adenosine monophosphate (AMP) from adenylosuccinate. Dephosphoraylation of the precursors (by cytoplasmic 5'-nucleotidase) would account for the presence of the two signal metabolites found in the patients. Normal levels of enzyme in erythrocytes, granulocytes, and muscle (some patients) suggest the presence of isozymes. Total body impairment of purine synthesis would probably be lethal early in development, as intake and the purine salvage pathway would be unable to meet the demand for purine metabolites. Despite the impairment of adenylosuccinase in the liver, a major site of purine synthesis, there did not seem to be a diminution of total-body purine production. The role purines play in brain function is well known from the **Lesch-Nyhan syndrome**, but the specific pathogenetic mechanisms are not yet understood.

**MIM No.:**  *10305

**Sex Ratio:**  M3:F4 (observed).

**Occurrence:**  Seven cases have been reported. The incidence of the disorder has not been established through screening of retarded and autistic children.

**Risk of Recurrence for Patient's Sib:**
See Part I, *Mendelian Inheritance.*

**Risk of Recurrence for Patient's Child:**
See Part I, *Mendelian Inheritance.* Reproduction is precluded in this disorder as currently delineated. Mild cases have not been reported.

**Age of Detectability:**  Presumably at birth. Prenatal diagnosis has not been reported, but may be feasible.

**Gene Mapping and Linkage:**  ADSL (adenylosuccinate lyase) has been provisionally mapped to 22.

**Prevention:**  None known. Genetic counseling indicated.

**Treatment:**  Unknown. Allopurinol and sodium benzoate are ineffective.

**Prognosis:**  Poor.

**Detection of Carrier:**  Unknown.

**Support Groups:**
NY; Albany; National Society for Autistic Children
DC; Washington; National Society for Children and Adults with Autism

**References:**
Jaeken J, Van den Berghe G: An infantile autistic syndrome characterised by the presence of succinylpurines in body fluids. Lancet 1984; II:1058-1061.
Laikind PK, et al.: Detection of 5;pr-phosphoribosyl-4-(N-succinylcarboxamide)-5-aminoimidazole in patients' urine by use of the Bratton-Marshall reaction: identification of patients deficient in adenylosuccinate lyase activity. Anal Biochem 1986; 156:81–90.
Van den Berghe G, Jaeken J: Adenylosuccinase deficiency. Adv Exp Biol Med 1986; 195A:27–33.
Van Keuren ML, et al.: Human chromosome 22 corrects the defect in the CHO mutant (Ade-I) lacking adenylosuccinase activity. Am J Hum Genet 1986; 39:A172.
Wadman SK, et al.: Detection of inherited adenylosuccinase deficiency by two dimensional thin layer chromatography of urinary imidazoles. Adv Exp Med Biol 1986; 195A:21–25.
Van Keuren ML, et al.: A somatic cell hybrid with a single human chromosome 22 corrects the defect in the CHO mutant (Ade-I) lacking adenylosuccinase activity. Cytogenet Cell Genet 1987; 44: 142–147.

KA002  **Stephen G. Kahler**

**Adrenal 18-hydroxylase deficiency**
*See STEROID 18-HYDROXYLASE DEFICIENCY*
**Adrenal 18-hydroxysteroid dehydrogenase deficiency**
*See STEROID 18-HYDROXYSTEROID DEHYDROGENASE DEFICIENCY*
**Adrenal aplasia**
*See ADRENAL HYPOPLASIA, CONGENITAL*
**Adrenal cyst-ectodermal dysplasia**
*See ECTODERMAL DYSPLASIA-ADRENAL CYST*
**Adrenal hyperplasia I**
*See STEROID 20-22 DESMOLASE DEFICIENCY*
**Adrenal hyperplasia II**
*See STEROID 3 BETA-HYDROXYSTEROID DEHYDROGENASE DEFICIENCY*
**Adrenal hyperplasia III**
*See STEROID 21-HYDROXYLASE DEFICIENCY*
**Adrenal hyperplasia IV**
*See STEROID 11 BETA-HYDROXYLASE DEFICIENCY*
**Adrenal hyperplasia V**
*See STEROID 17 ALPHA-HYDROXYLASE DEFICIENCY*
**Adrenal hyperplasia-1, congenital virilizing**
*See STEROID 21-HYDROXYLASE DEFICIENCY*

---

**ADRENAL HYPOALDOSTERONISM OF INFANCY, TRANSIENT ISOLATED**  0023

**Includes:**
Adrenocortical insufficiency of infancy, transient
Steroid 18-oxidation, delayed biochemical maturation of

**Excludes:**
Adrenal hypoplasia, congenital (0024)
Salt-losing adrenal hyperplasia, congenital
**Steroid 18-hydroxylase deficiency (0905)**
**Steroid 18-hydroxysteroid dehydrogenase deficiency (0906)**
**Steroid 21-hydroxylase deficiency (0908)**

**Major Diagnostic Criteria:**  Clinical features of aldosterone deficiency confirmed by appropriate studies of plasma or urine. Adrenal secretion of other steroids and response to ACTH must be normal. A deficiency of 18-hydroxylase or 18-OH dehydrogenase cannot be excluded initially but should not persist beyond the early childhood years to fulfill the criterion of transience.

**Clinical Findings:**  This syndrome is characterized by renal salt-wasting, hyponatremia, hyperkalemia, vomiting, dehydration and failure to thrive in infancy. Urinary excretion of aldosterone is negligible and does not increase following salt deprivation or the administration of ACTH. However, urinary excretion of 17-ketosteroids and 17-hydroxycorticosteroids is normal and rises significantly following ACTH. The external genitalia are normal in males and females, thereby excluding defects early in steroidogenesis. There is an excellent response to salt-retaining steroids such as deoxycorticosterone (DOC) and supplemental salt. As affected infants grow, the symptoms spontaneously ameliorate, so that therapy may gradually be diminished and may frequently be discontinued in the second year of life. Reinvestigation of an affected infant at age 5 years revealed normal secretion rates of cortisol and aldosterone and an appropriate response to administration of ACTH and salt deprivation. Definitive steroid studies have not been performed; consequently a maturational defect or an enzyme block in the final two steps of aldosterone biosynthesis have not been excluded. One report concerned sibs, raising the possibility of an inherited enzyme defect.

**Complications:** These are a function of the degree of electrolyte disturbance and dehydration; all are avoidable by recognition of the disorder and therapy with supplemental salt and mineralocorticoids.

**Associated Findings:** None known.

**Etiology:** It is not entirely clear whether this is a separate entity representing maturational delay in aldosterone biosynthesis, or poorly documented enzyme deficiencies. Since affected sibs have been described, the possibility of an autosomal recessively inherited enzyme defect affecting aldosterone biosynthesis cannot be excluded.

**Pathogenesis:** In all forms of aldosterone deficiency, there is a tendency for the severity of symptoms and urinary salt-wasting to improve with increasing age. Thus, the transient nature of this disorder of hypoaldosteronism in infancy may represent the amelioration of an inadequately documented enzyme deficiency in aldosterone biosynthesis. Alternatively, the syndrome may represent a true maturational delay in the zona glomerulosa of the adrenal, or a delay in the biochemical maturation of the final two enzyme steps of aldosterone biosynthesis; namely 18-hydroxylase and 18-OH-dehydrogenase. Apart from these 2 enzyme deficiencies, affecting aldosterone synthesis only, all other adrenal enzyme deficiencies and diseases involving the entire adrenal cortex also affect some steps in glucocorticoid or sex steroid synthesis, a useful point in differential diagnosis.

**Sex Ratio:** M1:F1

**Occurrence:** Unknown.

**Risk of Recurrence for Patient's Sib:**
See Part I, *Mendelian Inheritance.*

**Risk of Recurrence for Patient's Child:**
See Part I, *Mendelian Inheritance.*

**Age of Detectability:** Neonatal period. Symptoms and signs ameliorate after the second year and the affected individual may return to normal by the fifth year.

**Gene Mapping and Linkage:** Unknown.

**Prevention:** None known. Genetic counseling indicated.

**Treatment:** Recognition of aldosterone deficiency with salt and mineralocorticoid supplementation is essential. Other enzyme deficiencies must be ruled out.

**Prognosis:** Normal for life and intelligence if recognized and treated in the neonatal period. In addition, the transience of the disorder assures an excellent prognosis in later life.

**Detection of Carrier:** Unknown.

**References:**
Russell A, et al.: A reversible salt-wasting syndrome of the newborn and infant: possible infantile hypoaldosteronism. Arch Dis Child 1963; 38:313–325.
Visser HKA: Hypoadrenocorticism. In: Gardner LI, ed: Endocrine and genetic diseases of childhood, ed. 2.. Philadelphia: W.B. Saunders, 1975: 513–538.
Ulick S: Diagnosis and nomenclature of the disorders of the terminal portion of the aldosterone biosynthetic pathway. J Clin Endocrinol Metab 1976; 43:92–96.
Honour JW, et al.: Analysis of steroids in urine for differentiation of pseudohypoaldosteronism and aldosterone biosynthetic defect. J Clin Endocrinol Metab 1982; 54:325–331. *

SP004                                    **Mark A. Sperling**

## ADRENAL HYPOPLASIA, CONGENITAL                    0024

**Includes:**
> Addison disease, X-linked
> Adrenal aplasia
> Adrenal hypoplasia, congenital, autosomal recessive
> Adrenal hypoplasia, congenital, X-linked
> Cytomegalic adrenocortical hypoplasia
> Hypoadrenocorticism, familial
> Pituitary gland hypoplasia-adrenal hypoplasia, congenital

**Excludes:**
> **Adrenocortical unresponsiveness to acth, hereditary** (0025)
> Enzyme defects in adrenal steroid biosynthesis
> **Steroid 20–22 desmolase deficiency** (0907)

**Major Diagnostic Criteria:** Vomiting, cyanosis, apneic spells, hypoglycemia, seizures and vascular collapse in the neonatal period, accompanied by hyponatremia and hyperkalemia, are the usual presenting manifestations. Biochemical features of adrenal insufficiency, with low plasma or urinary concentrations of all adrenal steroids and no response to administered ACTH confirm the diagnosis. A family history is helpful in suspecting the diagnosis, particularly when affecting males. Adrenal hemorrhage, calcification or cysts can be excluded by X-ray and/or ultrasonagraphy. Definitive diagnosis may require arteriography. Gonadal function and external genitalia are normal.

**Clinical Findings:** This is a disorder in which there is hypoplasia or aplasia of the adrenal glands. The clinical features result from the deficiency of glucocorticoids and mineralocorticoids and may include cyanosis, apneic spells, hypoglycemia, vascular collapse, and seizures shortly after birth. Death may occur within 72 hours; electrolyte disturbances consisting of hyponatremia and hyperkalemia may be profound, reflecting the deficiency of mineralocorticoids. However, affected individuals have been known to survive and to present later in infancy or childhood with feeding difficulties, vomiting, growth retardation, hypoglycemia, and pigmentation of the skin.

Laboratory findings reveal low or undetectable plasma concentrations or urinary excretion of cortisol, 17-hydroxycorticosteroids, 17 ketosteroids and aldosterone. In patients without pituitary hypoplasia there is no response to stimulation by ACTH, dietary manipulation of sodium, and changes in posture. Pituitary ACTH and growth hormone secretion in response to insulin-induced hypoglycemia were reported to be normal in affected identical twins. However, gonadotropin deficiency, clinically manifested by delayed pubertal development at adolescence or by cryptorchidism in younger boys, is now increasingly recognized, and has been attributed to the deletion of two genes on the X chromosome in the region of Xp21.

**Complications:** Those associated with the degree of electrolyte disturbance and dehydration.

**Associated Findings:** An association with **Glycerol kinase deficiency** been reported in cases of gene deletions in the region of Xp21.

**Etiology:** Most cases are sporadic but solid evidence exists for autosomal recessive and X-linked recessive forms of inheritance. The basic defect in embryogenesis is unknown. Adrenal hypoplasia associated with pituitary hypoplasia suggests that ACTH may be important in determining fetal adrenal growth. Pituitary hypoplasia has also been described in familial aggregates.

**Pathogenesis:** Undetermined. In those cases with pituitary hypoplasia and in the autosomal recessive form the adrenal histology is of the immature adult type, with a well-differentiated permanent cortex and diminished or absent fetal cortex. In contrast, in the X-linked form, the adrenal cortex is disorganized and composed of large cells resembling those of the fetal cortex. Occasionally, adrenal tissue has been identified in conjunction with the ovary or testis, or diffusely scattered throughout the retroperitoneum; rarely, no adrenal tissue is found.

**MIM No.:** *30020, *24020

**CDC No.:** 759.110

**Sex Ratio:** M3:F1

**Occurrence:** Rare.

**Risk of Recurrence for Patient's Sib:**
See Part I, *Mendelian Inheritance.*

**Risk of Recurrence for Patient's Child:**
See Part I, *Mendelian Inheritance.*

**Age of Detectability:** May be detected from birth to adult life with the most frequent age of detection birth to two years.

**Gene Mapping and Linkage:** AHC (adrenal hypoplasia, congenital) has been mapped to Xp21.3-p21.2.
See also **Glycerol kinase deficiency.**

**Prevention:** None known. Genetic counseling indicated.

**Treatment:** Prompt recognition of adrenal insufficiency and appropriate replacement with gluco- and mineralocorticoids will prevent death and can result in normal growth and development. Lifelong treatment is essential to ensure normal growth and development; surgical or other stress may require additional supplemental steroids to prevent collapse from adrenal insufficiency. If associated with pituitary hypoplasia, and pituitary hormone insufficiency is confirmed, replacement with thyroid, growth hormone and sex steroids or chorionic gonadotropin is indicated.

**Prognosis:** Excellent if condition is recognized and treated.

**Detection of Carrier:** Unknown.

**Special Considerations:** Steroid 20–22 desmolase deficiency will mimic all the biochemical features discussed above, but in that condition the adrenals are large and lipid laden, with the defect also involving the gonads, thus causing genital ambiguity in males.

**References:**
Sperling MA, et al.: Congenital adrenal hypoplasia: an isolated defect of organogenesis. J Pediatr 1973; 82:444–449.
Pakravan P, et al.: Familial congenital absence of adrenal glands; evaluation of glucocorticoid, mineralocorticoid, and estrogen metabolism in the perinatal period. J Pediatr 1974; 84:74–78.
Zachmann M, et al.: Gonadotropin deficiency and cryptorchidism in three prepubertal brothers with congenital adrenal hypoplasia. J Pediatr. 1980; 97:255–257.
Bartley JA, et al.: Concordance of X-linked glycerol kinase deficiency with X-linked congenital adrenal hypoplasia. Lancet 1981; 2:733–736.
Kruse K, et al.: Hypogonadism in congenital adrenal hypoplasia: Evidence for a hypothalamic origin. J Clin Endocrinol Metab 1984; 58:12–17.
Dunger DB, et al.: Deletion of the X chromosome detected by direct DNA analysis in one of two unrelated boys with glycerol kinase deficiency, adrenal hypoplasia and Duchenne muscular dystrophy. Lancet 1986; 1:585–587.
Burke BA, et al.: Congenital adrenal hypoplasia and selective absence of pituitary luteinizing hormone. Am J Med Genet 1988; 31:75–97.

SP004 **Mark A. Sperling**

**Adrenal hypoplasia, congenital, autosomal recessive**
See *ADRENAL HYPOPLASIA, CONGENITAL*
**Adrenal hypoplasia, congenital, X-linked**
See *ADRENAL HYPOPLASIA, CONGENITAL*
**Adrenal hypoplasia-glycerol kinase deficiency**
See *GLYCEROL KINASE DEFICIENCY*
**Adrenocortical insufficiency of infancy, transient**
See *ADRENAL HYPOALDOSTERONISM OF INFANCY, TRANSIENT ISOLATED*
**Adrenocortical nodular dysplasia-Cushing syndrome-cardiac myxomas**
See *NEVI-ATRIAL MYXOMA-MYXOID NEUROFIBROMAS-EPHELIDES*

## ADRENOCORTICAL UNRESPONSIVENESS TO ACTH, HEREDITARY    0025

**Includes:**
Glucocorticoid deficiency, familial isolated
Migeon syndrome

**Excludes:**
Addison disease-multiple endocrine deficiency-autoantibodies
**Adrenal hypoplasia, congenital** (0024)
**Steroid 3 beta-hydroxysteroid dehydrogenase deficiency** (0909)
**Steroid 11 beta-hydroxylase deficiency** (0902)

**Major Diagnostic Criteria:** In infants or young children, lethargy, feeding problems, hyperpigmentation of skin or gums, and recurrent episodes of hypoglycemia and seizures, which may result in intellectual deficit. Genitalia are normal. Documented glucocorticoid deficiency is unresponsive to ACTH administration, with normal serum electrolytes and normal aldosterone secretion as reflected by plasma concentration and urinary excretion, and renal conservation of salt during a low-sodium diet.

**Clinical Findings:** This inherited defect affects one of the sites of ACTH action on glucocorticoid biosynthesis. However, mineralocorticoids, produced in the zona glomerulosa, are not affected, suggesting a normal adrenocortical response to angiotensin. A lack of feedback inhibition by cortisol leads to high levels of ACTH. Symptoms and signs are related to severe cortisol deficiency and the melanocyte-stimulating hormone-like activity inherent in ACTH, without disturbances in serum electrolytes. Affected individuals commonly are discovered in late infancy or early childhood with lethargy, feeding problems, hyperpigmentation of the skin or gums, and recurrent episodes of hypoglycemia. Seizures of the grand mal or minor motor type may occur during the hypoglycemia episodes and may result in permanent impairment of brain function. Thus, developmental milestones may be delayed, and seizures may continue in the absence of hypoglycemia. Occasionally blood glucose concentration is normal, while cerebrospinal fluid glucose concentration is clearly in the hypoglycemic range. Despite glucocorticoid deficiency, growth and weight gain are frequently normal or above normal, and bone age is appropriate for chronologic age. Pulse, blood pressure, and degree of hydration remain normal. If unrecognized and untreated, sudden death can occur during periods of stress such as infection or surgery; a history of sudden death in one or more sibs has been recorded. Laboratory investigation reveals normal serum concentrations of electrolytes. Plasma cortisol concentration and production rate are low or undetectable, while aldosterone, deoxycorticosterone, and corticosterone levels and production rates are normal or high. Similarly, urinary excretion of 17-hydroxycorticosteroids, 17-ketosteroids, and pregnanetriol is low or undetectable, while aldosterone excretion is normal or high. Endogenous plasma ACTH concentration is strikingly elevated, and there is no response in plasma or urinary cortisol, 17-OHCS, or 17-KS to acute or prolonged administration of ACTH in pharmacologic doses. Similarly, aldosterone levels fail to rise with ACTH infusion if the patient remains recumbent, so that renin levels do not change. However, renal conservation of sodium is demonstrable following the institution of a salt-restricted diet or of erect posture. Antibodies to adrenal tissue are not present in affected patients. A variant of this syndrome affecting siblings of both sexes is associated with achalasia of the cardia and deficient tear production.

**Complications:** Hypoglycemic seizures may lead to permanent impairment of brain function, resulting in persistence of seizure activity or psychomotor retardation.

**Associated Findings:** None known.

**Etiology:** Autosomal recessive or X-linked recessive inheritance.

**Pathogenesis:** The adrenal glands are usually small, and histologically show marked atrophy of the adrenal cortex but relative sparing of the zona glomerulosa. The high endogenous ACTH concentration and lack of response to administered ACTH, with normal mineralocorticoid production by the zona glomerulosa, clearly implicate unresponsiveness of the zona fasciculata and reticularis to the action of ACTH. The mechanism of action of ACTH has been reviewed recently; it involves attachment of ACTH to a specific cell membrane receptor, activation of cyclic 3'5'-adenosine monophosphate (cAMP) and a subsequent series of intracellular events. Theoretically, a defect in any of these sites is possible; however, in vitro incubation of adrenal slices from an affected individual in the presence of added cAMP produced no change in cortisol production but did increase corticosterone synthesis. Thus in this instance the defect in cortisol synthesis resided in steps beyond the membrane activation of cAMP. Investigation of parents and sibs suggests potential for recognizing the heterozygote by virtue of low-normal plasma cortisol and subnormal cortisol response following ACTH.

Glucocorticoid deficiency is responsible for the hypoglycemia by virtue of cortisol's effect on gluconeogenesis.

**MIM No.:** *20220, *30025

**Sex Ratio:** Males predominate because of the X-linked form.

**Occurrence:** About a dozen kindreds have been documented.

**Risk of Recurrence for Patient's Sib:**
See Part I, *Mendelian Inheritance.*

**Risk of Recurrence for Patient's Child:**
See Part I, *Mendelian Inheritance.*

**Age of Detectability:** Birth to adult life with most frequent presentation from 6 months to 5 years of age.

**Gene Mapping and Linkage:** Unknown.

**Prevention:** None known. Genetic counseling indicated. Intrauterine diagnosis is not currently feasible.

**Treatment:** Replacement with cortisol (15 mg/m²/day) results in disappearance of hypoglycemia and reduction of pigmentation. Salt and mineralocorticoid replacement is not required.

**Prognosis:** Excellent if treated with glucocorticoids before permanent CNS sequelae result from hypoglycemia.

**Detection of Carrier:** Potentially feasible by plasma cortisol and response to ACTH.

**Special Considerations:** In the deceased sib of one well-documented case of adrenocortical unresponsiveness to ACTH, in which enzyme deficiency early in adrenal steroid biosynthesis was excluded, the adrenals were large, hyperplastic, and lipid-laden. Thus, there is heterogeneity in this syndrome with regard to the effects of ACTH on steroidogenesis and adrenal growth-promoting activity. Further evidence for heterogeneity comes from genetic analyses of affected pedigrees, suggesting that the inheritance of the disorder may be either autosomal recessive or X-linked recessive.

**References:**
Migeon CJ, et al.: The syndrome of congenital adrenocortical unresponsiveness to ACTH: report of six cases. Pediatr Res 1968; 2:501–513. *
Franks RC, Nance WE: Hereditary adrenocortical unresponsiveness to ACTH. Pediatrics 1970; 45:43–48.
Gill GM: Mechanism of ACTH action. Metabolism 1972; 21:571-588.
Kelch RP, et al.: Hereditary adrenocortical unresponsiveness to adrenocorticotropic hormone. J Pediatr 1972; 81:726–736.
Spark RF, Etzkorn JR: Absent aldosterone response to ACTH in familial glucocorticoid deficiency. N Engl J Med 1977; 297:917–920. *
Allgrove J, et al.: Familial glucocorticoid deficiency with achalasia of the cardia and deficient tear production. Lancet 1978; I:1284.

**Mark A. Sperling**

## ADRENOCORTICOTROPIC HORMONE DEFICIENCY, ISOLATED      **0026**

**Includes:** ACTH deficiency, isolated

**Excludes:**
**Adrenal hypoplasia, congenital** (0024)
**Adrenocortical unresponsiveness to acth, hereditary** (0025)
**Dwarfism, panhypopituitary** (0303)
**Steroid 3 beta-hydroxysteroid dehydrogenase deficiency** (0909)
**Steroid 11 beta-hydroxylase deficiency** (0902)
**Steroid 17 alpha-hydroxylase deficiency** (0903)
**Steroid 20–22 desmolase deficiency** (0907)
**Steroid 21-hydroxylase deficiency** (0908)

**Major Diagnostic Criteria:** Weight loss, anorexia, weakness, nausea and vomiting with evidence of ACTH deficiency, i.e. low serum cortisol and urinary 17-hydroxy steroids confirmed by abnormal metapyrone test with otherwise normal pituitary function. Undetectable plasma ACTH.

**Clinical Findings:** Clinical features of isolated adrenocorticotropic hormone (ACTH) deficiency are those of adrenal insufficiency with weight loss, anorexia, weakness, nausea with vomiting and hypotension. Hypoglycemia, hyponatremia, and hyperkalemia often occur. Although males have a normal hair pattern, females have very little pubic or axillary hair. Skin pigmentation is usually decreased but may be normal. Although most cases have been seen in adults, a few cases have been diagnosed in childhood. Specific endocrine abnormalities include a low circulating cortisol concentration, low urinary 17-hydroxy- and 17-ketosteroids, lack of normal response to metapyrone and undetectable circulating levels of ACTH.

**Complications:** Unknown.

**Associated Findings:** None known.

**Etiology:** All cases appear to be sporadic.

**Pathogenesis:** Possibly defects in the hypothalamic-pituitary axis.

**MIM No.:** 20140

**Sex Ratio:** M1:F1

**Occurrence:** Rare. About a half-dozen cases have been reported.

**Risk of Recurrence for Patient's Sib:** Probably negligible since most cases appear to have been sporadic. In a case reported by Ichiba & Goto (1983), a deceased sibling may have had the same same disorder.

**Risk of Recurrence for Patient's Child:** Negligible.

**Age of Detectability:** Usually not suspected until adulthood but prenatal diagnosis has been reported (Malpuech et al, 1988).

**Gene Mapping and Linkage:** Pro-opiomelanocortin gene has been localized to chromosome 2p23.

**Prevention:** None known. Genetic counseling indicated.

**Treatment:** Replacement with cortisone.

**Prognosis:** Probably normal life span with therapy.

**Detection of Carrier:** Unknown.

**References:**
O'Dell WD: Isolated deficiencies of anterior pituitary hormones. JAMA 1966; 197:1006–1016.
Hung W, Migeon CJ: Hypoglycemia in a two-year-old boy with adrenalcortiocotropic hormone (ACTH) deficiency (probably isolated) and adrenal medullary unresponsiveness to insulin-induced hypoglycemia. J Clin Endocrinol Metab 1968; 28:146–152.
Rimoin DL, Schimke RN: Genetic disorders of the endocrine gland. St. Louis: CV Mosby, 1971: 11–65.
Aynsley-Green A, et al.: Isolated ACTH deficiency: metabolic and endocrine studies in a 7-year-old boy. Arch Dis Child 1978; 53:499–502.
Ichiba Y, Goto T: Isolated corticotropin deficiency. Am J Dis Child 1983; 137: 202–1203.
Malpuech G, et al.: Isolated familial adrenocorticotropin deficiency:

prenatal diagnosis by maternal plasma estriol assay. Am J Med Genet 1988; 29:125–130.

H0033
H0025

William A. Horton
O.J. Hood

**Adrenogenital syndrome with hypertension**
*See STEROID 11 BETA-HYDROXYLASE DEFICIENCY*
**Adrenoleukodystrophy, neonatal**
*See CEREBRO-HEPATO-RENAL SYNDROME*
**Adrenoleukodystrophy, neonatal (some forms)**
*See PHYTANIC ACID OXIDASE DEFICIENCY, INFANTILE TYPE*

## ADRENOLEUKODYSTROPHY, X-LINKED 2533

**Includes:**

> Addison disease-cerebral sclerosis
> Addison-Schilders
> Adrenomyeloneuropathy
> Bronze Schilder disease
> Melanodermic leukodystrophy
> Orthochromatic leukodystrophy
> Siemerling-Creutzfeldt disease

**Excludes:**

> **Adrenal hypoplasia, congenital** (0024)
> **Alexander disease** (2712)
> **Brain, spongy degeneration** (0115)
> Brain tumor
> Central pontine myelinolysis
> **Cerebro-hepato-renal syndrome** (0139)
> **Glycerol kinase deficiency** (2310)
> **Leukodystrophy, globoid cell type** (0415)
> Leukoencephalopathy, subacute sclerosing
> **Metachromatic leukodystrophies** (0651)
> **Multiple sclerosis, familial** (2598)
> **Pelizaeus-Merzbacher syndrome** (0803)
> **Phytanic acid oxidase deficiency, infantile type** (2278)
> **Phytanic acid storage disease** (0810)

**Major Diagnostic Criteria:** *Childhood form:* Beginning at 3–8 years of age; hyperactivity, emotional lability, dementia, impaired auditory discrimination, impaired vision, seizures, paralysis, and ataxia. White matter lesions are seen in the posterior part of the brain on CT or MRI. Impaired adrenal function in 85%.

*Adult form:* Progressive spastic paraparesis, urinary disturbance, impotence, peripheral neuropathy, impaired adrenal function in 60%, dementia or psychosis in 20–30%.

*All forms:* Elevated levels of very-long-chain fatty acids (VLCFA) in plasma, red cells, or cultured skin fibroblasts.

**Clinical Findings:** There is a wide range of phenotypes, even within a kindred. The *childhood form* is most common (60%), with a mean age of onset of 7.2 years ± 1.7 years. Cerebral symptoms include hyperactivity, emotional lability, impaired vision and auditory discrimination, weakness, ataxia, seizures, progressing to vegetative state in 1.9 ± two years, and death in 2.8 ± two years (range 0.75–11 years).

The *adult form*, adrenomeyloneuropathy, is second in frequency (21%). Its slowly progressive paraparesis begins at age 29 ± seven years, accompanied by rinary incontinence or retention, impotence, and peripheral neuropathy mainly in the legs. Dementia or psychosis occurs in 20–30%. Impaired adrenal function is present in 85% of children and 70% of adults.

*Rarer forms* include 1) adrenal insufficiency without neurological involvement; 2) psychotic or dementing illness in adulthood; 3) localized cerebral defect presenting as a mass lesion which may be mistaken for brain tumor even after cerebral biopsy; and 4) Of those adrenoleukodystrophy (ADL) cases with a biochemical defect, 5–10% remain asymptomatic even in adulthood.

**Complications:** *Childhood form:* severe behavioral disturbance; seizures; progressive neurological deficits lead to vegetative state requiring total support.

*Adult form:* progressive paraparesis leading to gait disturbance.

Need for crutches or wheelchair; urinary disturbance possibly leading to retention, infections, or the need for a catheter.

*Adrenal insufficiency* may lead to hypoglycemia and weakness.

**Associated Findings:** Impotence, pigmentations, and abnormally thin or sparse hair. Color vision defects may be linked to the fact that adrenoleukodystrophy and red/green color blindness are both mapped to the X chromosome at Xq28.

**Etiology:** X-linked recessive inheritance. Of the female heterozygotes, (20–30%) show neurological deficit with progressive paraparesis.

**Pathogenesis:** The primary defect is impaired oxidation of very-long-chain-fatty-acids (VLCFA), probably due to deficiency of lignoceroyl-CoA ligase; a reaction that normally takes place in the peroxisome (see **Peroxisomal disorders**).

**MIM No.:** *30010

**Sex Ratio:** M1:F0. Twenty to thirty percent of female heterozygotes have a milder neurological deficit (progressive paraparesis).

**Occurrence:** More than 1,000 cases from over 400 kindreds have been documented. All races are affected. With application of new diagnostic assays, particularly VLCFA levels and CT scan, it now appears that the disorder is not uncommon. Estimated incidence is 1–2:100,000.

**Risk of Recurrence for Patient's Sib:**
See Part I, *Mendelian Inheritance.*

**Risk of Recurrence for Patient's Child:**
See Part I, *Mendelian Inheritance.*

**Age of Detectability:** At birth. Prenatal diagnosis by elevated VLCFA levels in cultured amniocytes or cultured chorion villus samples.

**Gene Mapping and Linkage:** ALD (adrenoleukodystrophy) has been mapped to Xq28.
The locus of lignoceroyl CoA ligase is unassigned.

**Prevention:** None known. Genetic counseling indicated.

**Treatment:** Steroid replacement for adrenal insufficiency. Experimental dietary therapy consisting of a diet restricted in VLCFA, and oral administration of glycerol trioleate and glycerol trierucate oil. These diets hormalize levels of saturated VLCFA. Therapeutic trials are in progress.

**Prognosis:** *Childhood form:* Vegetative state in 1.9 ± two years, and death in 2.8 ± two years (range 0.75–11 years) from the first neurologic symptom.

*Adrenomyeloneuropathy:* Serious motor disability 5–20 years after onset. Mental impairment or psychosis in 20–30%.

Ten to twenty percent of patients have adrenal insufficiency only, or remain asymptomatic.

**Detection of Carrier:** Most carriers (80–90%) show elevated levels of VLCFA in plasma and/or cultured skin fibroblasts. Use of linkage studies with St-14 DNA probe, in combination with fatty acid studies, may approach 100% accuracy in carrier detection in families in which affected and unaffected members are available for study.

**Special Considerations:** X-linked adrenoleukodystrophy (ADL) must be distinguished from neonatal ALD, which has an autosomal recessive mode of inheritance and resembles **Cerebro-hepato-renal syndrome**.

**Support Groups:**
MD; Baltimore; JFK Institute for Handicapped Children ALD Project
IL; Sycamore; United Leukodystrophy Foundation

**References:**
Siemerling E, Creutzfeldt HC: Bronzekrankheit und skleroriesende Encephalomyelitis (diffuse Sclerose). Arch Psychiatr 1923; 68:217–244.
Schaumburg HH, et al.: Adrenoleukodystrophy: a clinical and pathological study of 17 cases. Arch Neurol 1975; 32:577–591.
Griffin JW, et al.: Adrenomyeloneuropathy: a probable variant of adrenoleukodystrophy. Neurology (MN) 1977; 27:1107–1113.

Moser HW, et al.: Adrenoleukodystrophy: survey of 303 cases: biochemistry, diagnosis and therapy. Ann Neurol 1984; 16:628–641.

Aubourg PR, et al.: Linkage of adrenoleukodystrophy to a polymorphic DNA probe. Ann Neurol 1987; 21:349–352.

Moser AB, et al.: A new dietary therapy for adrenoleukodystrophy: biochemical and preliminary clinical results in 36 patients. Ann Neurol 1987; 21:240–249.

Aubourg PR, et al.: Frequent alterations of visual pigment genes in adrenoleukodystrophy. Am J Hum Genet 1988; 42:408–413.

Lazo O, et al.: Peroxisomal lignoceroyl-CoA ligase deficiency in childhood adrenoleukodystrophy and adrenoueyeloueuropathy. Proc Nat Acad Sci USA 1988; 85:7647–7651.

Wanders, RJA, et al.: Direct demonstration that the deficient oxidation of very long chain fatty acids in X-linked adrenoleukodystrophy is due to impaired ability of peroxisomes to activate very long chain fatty acids. Biochem Biophys Res Commun 1988; 153:618–623.

Moser HW, Moser AB: Adrenoleukodystrophy (X-linked). In: Scriver CR, et al, eds: The metabolic basis of inherited disease, 6th ed. New York: McGraw-Hill, 1989:1511–1532.

Rizzo WB, et al.: Dietary erucic acid therapy for X-linked adrenoleukodystrophy. Neurology 1989; 39:1415–1422.

M0038                                                    **Hugo Moser**

**Adrenomyeloneuropathy**
  See ADRENOLEUKODYSTROPHY, X-LINKED
**Adult Fanconi syndrome**
  See RENAL TUBULAR SYNDROME, FANCONI TYPE
**Adult non-nephropatic cystinosis**
  See CYSTINOSIS
**Adult polycystic kidney disease (APKD)**
  See KIDNEY, POLYCYSTIC DISEASE, DOMINANT
**Adult-onset leukodystrophy, hereditary**
  See LEUKODYSTROPHY, ADULT ONSET PROGRESSIVE
    DOMINANT TYPE
**Adynamia episodica hereditaria**
  See PARALYSIS, HYPERKALEMIC PERIODIC
**Affective personality disorders**
  See MOOD AND THOUGHT DISORDERS
**Afibrinogenemia, primary**
  See AFIBROGINEMIA, CONGENITAL

## AFIBROGINEMIA, CONGENITAL                          2661

**Includes:**  Afibrinogenemia, primary

**Excludes:**

  Afibrinogenemia, secondary
  **Coagulation defect, familial multiple factors** (2674)
  **Fibrinogens, abnormal congenital** (0004)
  **Hemophilia**

**Major Diagnostic Criteria:**  Congenital absence of circulating fibrinogen associated with a lifelong bleeding disorder. Coagulation tests, which are dependent on the presence of fibrinogen, are incoagulable. Fibrinogen is absent or may be present in trace amounts when measured by sensitive immunologic methods.

**Clinical Findings:**  Affected individuals have a hemorrhagic tendency, which is particularly severe during childhood. In two-thirds of reported cases manifestations began in the first few days of life and included bleeding from the umbilicus, melena, vomiting blood, hematomas from forceps application, bleeding from injection sites, and bleeding from circumcision. Exsanguination has occurred in the absence of appropriate replacement therapy. Later hemorrhagic problems have included excessive bleeding from even minor lacerations, bleeding with loss of deciduous teeth, subcutaneous hematoma formation from minor trauma, and prolonged bleeding following dental extractions or surgery. Hemarthrosis has occurred in 20% of cases, but has been infrequent. Epistaxis and gastrointestinal bleeding may be present. Menses may be normal or associated with heavy or prolonged bleeding. Life-threatening bleeding episodes have included cerebral hemorrhage, hemothorax, rupture of an ovarian luteal cyst, and spontaneous splenic rupture. Coagulation tests, dependent for an endpoint on the formation of a fibrin clot (whole blood clotting time, partial thromboplastin time, prothrombin time, thrombin clotting time, and snake venom clotting time), are

abnormal. In afibrinogenemia various techniques for the measurement of fibrinogen, such as heat or salt precipitation, measurement of clottable fibrinogen, and electrophoresis, all fail to detect fibrinogen. In some instances, trace amounts of fibrinogen (less than 10 mg/dl) are detectable when using sensitive immunologic techniques. The bleeding time has been reported to be prolonged in more than 50% of cases. Reports of platelet function studies in congenital afibrinogenemia have shown variable results. Reduced adhesion to glass surfaces and impaired (but not absent) aggregation in response to ADP, collagen, epinephrine, and thrombin have been reported. These abnormalities are correctable by the addition of fibrinogen.

**Complications:**  Complications are primarily the result of bleeding. Death from catastrophic hemorrhage, particularly cerebrovascular hemorrhage, is not uncommon. Chronic blood loss may lead to iron deficiency anemia. Since intramuscular and joint hemorrhage is much less common than in **Hemophilia**, the chronic musculoskeletal changes associated with hemophilia are not usually seen in afibrinogenemia.

Skeletal changes as a result of hemorrhages into bone have been reported. Juxtatrabecular hemorrhages occurring mainly in the metaphyses may lead to the formation of intraosseous cysts or pseudotumor formation. Clinical reports suggest that afibrinogenemia is associated with recurrent abortions and premature separation of the placenta. Venous thrombosis, pulmonary embolism, myocardial infarct, and cerebral arterial thrombosis have been reported in association with fibrinogen infusions. Antibodies to fibrinogen have been reported in two cases, rendering effective replacement therapy impossible and resulting in severe reactions and death. Hepatitis B, non A, non B hepatitis, and human immunodeficiency virus (HIV) may be acquired as a consequence of transfusion therapy.

**Associated Findings:**  Mild thrombocytopenia (rarely below 100,000/mm³) may be observed in 25% of cases.

**Etiology:**  Possibly autosomal recessive inheritance. A high frequency of consanguinity (50%) has been noted, as well as the presence of affected sibs in reported cases. In some cases the fibrinogen levels in one or both parents have been found to be low.

**Pathogenesis:**  Appears to reflect a decreased or absent protein synthesis of fibrinogen. There is no evidence of increased fibrinolysis or intravascular coagulation. The survival of transfused fibrinogen is normal. Bleeding manifestations are due to the absence of fibrinogen and the inability of blood to form a clot. The binding of fibrinogen to the platelet membrane is also necessary for normal platelet aggregation. To what extent impaired platelet function contributes to the bleeding manifestations is not clear, since reports of platelet function studies in afibrinogenemia have shown variable results. Perhaps related to the platelet function defect is the observation that platelet fibrinogen content is abnormally low in congenital afibrinogenemia. Fibrinogen is synthesized in the intracellular pool of the platelet and is present within the alpha granules. Amino acid sequencing suggests that platelet-associated fibrinogen is identical to plasma fibrinogen, suggesting that the two proteins are products of the same gene.

**MIM No.:**  20240, *13482, *13483, *13485

**Sex Ratio:**  M1:F1

**Occurrence:**  More than 130 cases have been described.

**Risk of Recurrence for Patient's Sib:**
  See Part I, *Mendelian Inheritance.*

**Risk of Recurrence for Patient's Child:**
  See Part I, *Mendelian Inheritance.* Due to spontaneous early abortions, full-term pregnancy with a successful outcome has been reported in only one instance. The infant had a fibrinogen concentration of 55 mg/dl from umbilical venous blood.

**Age of Detectability:**  Since the concentration of fibrinogen in the plasma of normal newborn infants is within the normal adult range, afibrinogenemia is detectable at birth. Prenatal detection has not been reported.

**Gene Mapping and Linkage:** FGA (fibrinogen, A alpha polypeptide) has been mapped to 4q28.

FGB (fibrinogen, B beta polypeptide) has been mapped to 4q28.

FGG (fibrinogen, gamma polypeptide) has been mapped to 4q28.

Fibrinogen is composed of three nonidentical chains (A$\alpha$, B$\beta$, and $\gamma$) that are synthesized under the direction of three different and coordinately expressed RNAs. Recent structural analysis of chromosomes from somatic cell hybrids has established that mammalian fibrinogen is composed of three coding sequences for A$\alpha$, B$\beta$, and $\gamma$ linked in a small portion of the long arm of chromosome 4. Restriction endonuclease analysis of the DNA in two patients with congenital afibrinogenemia using specific cDNA probes for each fibrinogen-constitutive chain was unable to detect an abnormality in the A$\alpha$, B$\beta$, and $\gamma$ genes.

**Prevention:** None known. Genetic counseling indicated.

**Treatment:** Bleeding episodes can be treated with cryoprecipitate or fibrinogen concentrates. Until hepatitis-free fibrinogen concentrates are available, cryoprecipitate is preferred. Sufficient cryoprecipitate should be given to raise the plasma fibrinogen level to about 100 mg/dl (normal 200 to 400 mg/dl). The biological half-life of infused fibrinogen is 4–5 days. Prophylactic infusions of cryoprecipitate administered every 7–10 days has been reported to be effective in preventing hemorrhage. Because of the possibility of antibody formation, prophylactic therapy to prevent bleeding episodes is probably not generally warranted.

**Prognosis:** Due to the risk of life-threatening hemorrhages, prognosis through adulthood was guarded in the past. With appropriate replacement therapy for bleeding episodes, however, the expectation for reaching adult life should be similar to that for hemophilia.

**Detection of Carrier:** Although in some families studied the fibrinogen levels in known heterozygotes (carriers) are lower than normal, the overlap with normal fibrinogen levels makes the accurate detection of the carrier state impossible.

**Special Considerations:** To establish the diagnosis of afibrinogenemia versus hypofibrinogenemia, it is important to consider the techniques for the determination of fibrinogen. Immunologic techniques are the most sensitive, and it is common to detect traces of fibrinogen in homozygous afibrinogenemic patients. As a practical consideration, fibrinogen levels of less than 15 mg/dl measured by immunologic means can be considered to be consistent with the definition of afibrinogenemia. In congenital hypofibrinogenemia, fibrinogen levels are decreased from normal, but not absent. This condition probably represents a heterogeneous population of patients, two types of autosomal transmission having been observed. In some families, absence of consanguinity between parents, a low fibrinogen level in one parent, and symptoms of a hemorrhagic disorder in one parent suggest autosomal dominant transmission. In other families, consanguinity between parents, low fibrinogen levels in both parents, and lack of clinical symptoms in both parents suggest recessive transmission. It is not clear whether the dominant inherited form of hypofibrinogenemia represents a "symptomatic carrier" form of afibrinogenemia.

**References:**

Rabe F, Salomon E: Über Faserstoffmangel im Blute bei einem Fall von Hämophilie. Dtsch Arch Klin Med 1920; 132:240–244.

Mammen EF: Fibrinogen abnormalities. Semin Thromb Hemostas 1983; 9:1–9.

Ménaché D: Congenital fibrinogen abnormalities. Ann NY Acad Sci 1983; 408:121–130.

Uzan G, et al.: Analysis of fibrinogen genes in patients with congenital afibrinogenemia. Biochem Biophys Res Commun 1984; 120:376–83.

Inamoto Y, Terao T: First report of a case of congenital afibrinogenemia with successful delivery. Am J Obstet Gynecol 1985; 153:803–804.

Cattaneo M, et al.: Fibrinogen-independent aggregation and deaggregation of human platelets: studies in two afibrinogenemic patients. Blood 1987; 70:221–226.

Cronin C, et al.: Multiple pulmonary emboli in a patient with afibrinogenaemia. Acta Haemat 1988; 79:53–54.

Rodriguez R, et al.: Prophylactic cryoprecipitate in congenital afibrinofenemia. Clin Pediatr 1988; 27:543–545.

GR036                               **Ralph A. Gruppo**

**African Burkitt lymphoma**
   *See LYMPHOMA, BURKITT TYPE*
**African cardiopathy**
   *See VENTRICLE, ENDOMYOCARDIAL FIBROSIS OF RIGHT*
   *also VENTRICLE, ENDOMYOCARDIAL FIBROSIS OF LEFT*
**AGA deficiency**
   *See N-ACETYLGLUTAMATE SYNTHETASE DEFICIENCY*
**Agammaglobulinemia, acquired**
   *See IMMUNODEFICIENCY, COMMON VARIABLE TYPE*
**Agammaglobulinemia, adult**
   *See IMMUNODEFICIENCY, COMMON VARIABLE TYPE*
**Agammaglobulinemia, alymphocytotic type**
   *See IMMUNODEFICIENCY, SEVERE COMBINED*
**Agammaglobulinemia, late-onset**
   *See IMMUNODEFICIENCY, COMMON VARIABLE TYPE*
**Agammaglobulinemia, Swiss type**
   *See IMMUNODEFICIENCY, SEVERE COMBINED*
**Agammaglobulinemia, variant form of Swiss type**
   *See METAPHYSEAL CHONDRODYSPLASIA WITH THYMOLYMPHOPENIA*
**Agammaglobulinemia, X-linked recessive lymphopenic type**
   *See IMMUNODEFICIENCY, X-LINKED SEVERE COMBINED*
**Agammaglobulinemia, X-linked Swiss-type**
   *See IMMUNODEFICIENCY, X-LINKED SEVERE COMBINED*
**Agammaglobulinemia, X-linked, infantile**
   *See IMMUNODEFICIENCY, AGAMMAGLOBULINEMIA, X-LINKED, INFANTILE*
**Agammaglobulinemia-beta-2 macroglobulinemia**
   *See IMMUNODEFICIENCY, X-LINKED WITH HYPER IgM*
**Agammaglobulinemia-lymphopenia-dwarfism**
   *See METAPHYSEAL CHONDRODYSPLASIA, TYPE McKUSICK*

## AGAMMAGLOBULINEMIA-THYMOMA SYNDROME      0944

**Includes:**

   "Acquired" agammaglobulinemia with thymoma

   Good syndrome

   Hypogammaglobulinemia-thymoma syndrome

   Immunodeficiency-thymoma syndrome

   Thymoma-agammaglobulinemia syndrome

   Thymoma with "acquired" combined immunodeficiency

**Excludes:** Immunodeficiency without thymoma

**Major Diagnostic Criteria:** Anterior mediastinal mass on X-ray and low immunoglobulin levels.

**Clinical Findings:** Adults (20–77 years of age) with recurrent chronic bronchitis and bronchopneumonia, weight loss, weakness, diarrhea, stomatitis, sinusitis, GU infections, skin infections, septicemia, splenomegaly, anemia, and bleeding tendencies. Thymoma and immunodeficiency may be present, simultaneously or there may be a delay of as long as ten years before the appearance of immunodeficiency. Serum IgG is always low, or absent. Other immunoglobulins may be normal, low or absent. Antibody responses to typhoid, paratyphoid, and diphtheria antigens are usually deficient. Impaired cell-mediated immunity in some patients, e.g., poor response of lymphocytes to phytohemagglutinin, concanavalin A, and a variety of antigens; inability to demonstrate delayed cutaneous hypersensitivity to a variety of ubiquitous antigens; and sensitization with 2,4-dinitrochlorobenzene. T-lymphocyte numbers are usually normal, but may be decreased. Absence of OKT4 epitope on peripheral blood T cells and thymocytes has been observed in a patient with Good syndrome associated with red cell aplasia. Circulating B lymphocytes are usually absent. Pre-B cells are also lacking in the bone marrow. Antinuclear antibody and antistriated muscle antibody may be present. X-ray of chest reveals an anterior mediastinal mass. Thymoma is usually benign (75% spindle cells) but may occasionally be malignant.

**Complications:** The epiphenomenon includes overwhelming pulmonary infections (cytomegalovirus, *Pneumocystis carinii*), and diarrhea (possibly secondary to low IgA levels on mucosal surface, deficient T lymphocytes, and infestation with *Giardia*).

**Associated Findings:** Myasthenia gravis, aregenerative anemia, thrombocytopenia, agranulocytosis, absence of eosinophils and basophils in the blood and bone marrow, eosinophilia, **Inflammatory bowel disease**, pernicious anemia, astrocytoma, **Amyloidosis**, **Lupus erythematosis, systemic**, pulmonary tuberculosis, Cushing syndrome, dermatomyositis, **Sjogren syndrome**, Waldenström macroglobulinemia, **Anemia, hemolytic**, **Arthritis, rheumatoid**, an unusual form of diabetes mellitus, pemphigus, exudative enteropathy, chronic hepatitis, adrenal gland atrophy, selective IgA deficiency, and cytomegalovirus encephalites.

**Etiology:** Unknown. One Greek sibship has been reported with familial thymoma without agammaglobulinemia (Matani and Dristsas, 1973).

**Pathogenesis:** Undetermined. Neither the appearance of the tumor, nor its removal, correlates well with the appearance or disappearance of any of the clinical findings, except in some cases associated with aregenerative anemia, which may be cured by thymectomy. Early in the clinical course, when myasthenia gravis is present, thymectomy results in a cure of the myasthenia, but not of the immunodeficiency. Recently, increased "suppressor" cell activity for immunoglobulin synthesis and secretions by B cells and plasma cells, as well as for the proliferation of pre-B cells, have been reported. Furthermore, increased suppressor T cell activity both for immunoglobulin production by B lymphocytes and erythroid differentiation has been reported in two patients with thymoma and hypogammaglobulinemia, one of whom had red cell agenesis as well. An increased incidence of autoimmunity has been found in several family members. Antoreactive erythroid progenitor T suppressor cells have been reported in a patient with Good syndrome and pure red cell aplasia. In one family, thymomas were found in the propositus, and a maternal uncle.

**MIM No.:** 27423

**Sex Ratio:** M1:F2

**Occurrence:** Undetermined but presumed rare.

**Risk of Recurrence for Patient's Sib:** Unknown.

**Risk of Recurrence for Patient's Child:** Unknown.

**Age of Detectability:** Twenty years of age or older, usually between the fourth and seventh decades.

**Gene Mapping and Linkage:** Unknown.

**Prevention:** None known. Genetic counseling indicated.

**Treatment:** Excision and removal of thymoma. No improvement in immunodeficiency; however, in some cases aregenerative anemia and myasthenia gravis are cured. Gamma globulin replacement therapy may be of benefit for control of the recurrent infections, particularly for chronic diarrhea.

**Prognosis:** An interval of 12 years has been reported between the appearance of the thymoma and immunodeficiency; however, overall prognosis is poor. Once the first symptoms of recurrent infection appear, there is usually a progressive deterioration of immunologic competence. Death usually results from infection, but may be related to the development of associated disorders, such as thrombocytopenia or diabetes. Only one patient is known to have died with metastases.

**Detection of Carrier:** Unknown.

**References:**
Matini A, Dristsas C: Familial occurrence of thymoma. Arch Path 1973; 95:90–91.
Hayward AR, et al.: Pre-B cell suppression by thymoma patient lymphocyte. Clin Exp Immunol 1982; 48:437–442.
Brenner MK, et al.: Thymoma and hypogammaglobulinemia with and without T suppressor cells. Clin Exp Immunol 1984; 58:619–624.
Levinson AI, et al.: Absence of the OKT4 epitope on blood T cells and thymus cells in a patient with thymoma, hypogammaglobulinemia, and red blood cell aplasia. J Allergy Clin Immunol 1985; 76:433–439.
Mamgan KF, et al.: Autoreactive erythroid progenitor T-suppressor cells in the pure red cell aplasia associated with thymoma and hypogammaglobulinemia. Am J Hematol 1986; 23:167–173.

GU004                                                    **Sudhir Gupta**

**Aganglionic megacolon**
    *See COLON, AGANGLIONOSIS*
**Aganglionic megalcolon-albanism**
    *See ALBINISM, WAARDENBURG TYPE-HIRSCHSPRUNG AGANGLIONOSIS*
**Agenesis of corpus callosum**
    *See CORPUS CALLOSUM AGENESIS*
**Agenesis of corpus callosum, partial**
    *See CORPUS CALLOSUM AGENESIS*
**Agenesis of corpus callosum-chorioretinal abnormality**
    *See AICARDI SYNDROME*
**Agenesis of corpus callosum-infantile spasms-ocular anomalies**
    *See AICARDI SYNDROME*
**Agenesis of inner ear**
    *See EAR, LABYRINTH APLASIA*
**Agenesis of paranasal sinuses, unilateral**
    *See SINUS, ABSENT PARANASAL*
**Agenesis of pericardium**
    *See HEART, PERICARDIUM AGENESIS*
**Agenesis of the corpus callosum-anterior horn cell disease**
    *See CORPUS CALLOSUM AGENESIS-SENSORIMOTOR NEUROPATHY, FAMILIAL*
**Agenesis of the salivary gland**
    *See SALIVARY GLAND, AGENESIS*
**Agenesis of the temporal lobe**
    *See BRAIN, ARACHNOID CYSTS*
**Aging, accelerated**
    *See PROGERIA*
**Aging, premature (one form)**
    *See WERNER SYNDROME*
**Aglossia congenita**
    *See HYPOGLOSSIA-HYPODACTYLIA*
**Aglossia-adactylia syndrome**
    *See HYPOGLOSSIA-HYPODACTYLIA*
**Aglycogenosis**
    *See GLYCOGEN SYNTHETASE DEFICIENCY*

---

## AGNATHIA-HOLOPROSENCEPHALY                          2780

**Includes:** Holoprosencephaly-agnathia

**Excludes:**
    **Agnathia-microstomia-synotia** (0028)
    **Holoprosencephaly** (0473)

**Major Diagnostic Criteria:** Coexistence of aplasia or hypoplasia of the mandible and holoprosencephaly.

**Clinical Findings:** Affected individuals have any of the variable features of agnathia and holoprosencephaly. The former include absence of the mandible or small mandible with variable degrees of fusion of the ears, although the ears may be only low set in some cases. External ear structures are generally well formed, while ossicles of the middle ear are often defective. The mouth is small and the tongue is small or absent. The oral cavity may be a blind-ended pouch. Muscles of facial expression and salivary glands are affected to variable degrees. Any of the features of holoprosencephaly may be present.

**Complications:** Respiratory distress leading to neonatal death is universal in affected individuals. Polyhydramnios may result from persistence of the oropharyngeal membrane.

**Associated Findings:** Congenital heart defects, particularly **Heart, tetralogy of Fallot**; fused cervical vertebrae; and absence of distal limb muscles may be seen.

**Etiology:** Possibly autosomal recessive inheritance.

**Pathogenesis:** Possibly a defect in the inductive capability of prechordal mesoderm that leads to agnathia by an abnormal migration of neural crest cells to the ventral portions of the first branchial arch and second pharyngeal pouch, and to holoprosencephaly by a failure of neural crest cell stimulation of the neural tube.

**MIM No.:** 20265

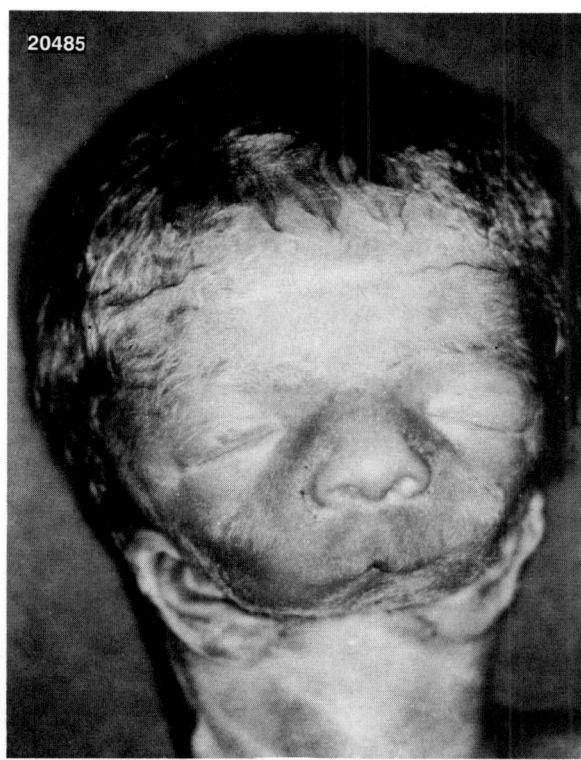

**2780**-20485:  Agnathia-holoprosencephaly in this 27-week still-born fetus; note agnathia with normal upper facial form. There is extreme microstomia with a 2.5 cm oral opening. The ears are malformed, ventrally placed and posteriorly rotated.

**POS No.:**  3478

**Sex Ratio:**  M1:F1

**Occurrence:**  About a half-dozen cases been reported.

**Risk of Recurrence for Patient's Sib:**
See Part I, *Mendelian Inheritance.*

**Risk of Recurrence for Patient's Child:**
See Part I, *Mendelian Inheritance.* Affected individuals are not expected to survive to reproduce.

**Age of Detectability:**  Prenatal diagnosis by ultrasonography is possible.

**Gene Mapping and Linkage:**  Unknown.

**Prevention:**  None known. Genetic counseling indicated.

**Treatment:**  Unknown.

**Prognosis:**  Invariably lethal.

**Detection of Carrier:**  Unknown.

**Special Considerations:**  The similarities in clinical features suggest that agnathia and holoprosencephaly may constitute a continuum of a specific developmental field defect. Clinical and genetic heterogeneity of these overlapping disorders is likely.

**References:**
Pauli RM, et al.: Familial agnathia-holoprosencephaly. Am J Med Genet 1983; 14:677–698. * †
Bixler D, et al.: Agnathia-holoprosencephaly: a developmental field complex involving face and brain: report of 3 cases. J Craniofac Genet Dev Biol 1985; 1(suppl.):241–249.
Machin GA, et al.: Monozygotic twin aborted fetuses discordant for holoprosencephaly/synotia. Teratology 1985; 31:203–215.

**Ronald J. Jorgenson**

## AGNATHIA-MICROSTOMIA-SYNOTIA          0028

**Includes:**
Ears (low-set)-reduced mouth and jaws
Jaws/mouth (small or absent)-low set ears
Microstomia-agnathia-synotia
Otocephaly
Synotia-agnathia-microstomia

**Excludes:**
**Agnathia-holoprosencephaly** (2780)
**Cyclopia** (0234)
Mandible, cleft
**Cleft palate-micrognathia-glossoptosis** (0182)

**Major Diagnostic Criteria:**  Agnathia, low-set ears, and microstomia.

**Clinical Findings:**  The mandible may be completely absent, but small fragments of mandibular bone are usually present at the midline. The ears are low-set and may be fused at their lower borders in the area usually occupied by the mandible. The oral cavity is usually a cul-de-sac with no connection to the pharynx. The tongue may be absent or small.

**Complications:**  Deformities of the auditory ossicles, temporal bones, palate, maxilla, and sphenoid bones may occur.

**Associated Findings:**  Transposition of the viscera, congenital heart defects and anomalies of the ribs may occur.

**Etiology:**  Unknown.

**Pathogenesis:**  Incomplete development of the mandibular process of the first branchial arch.

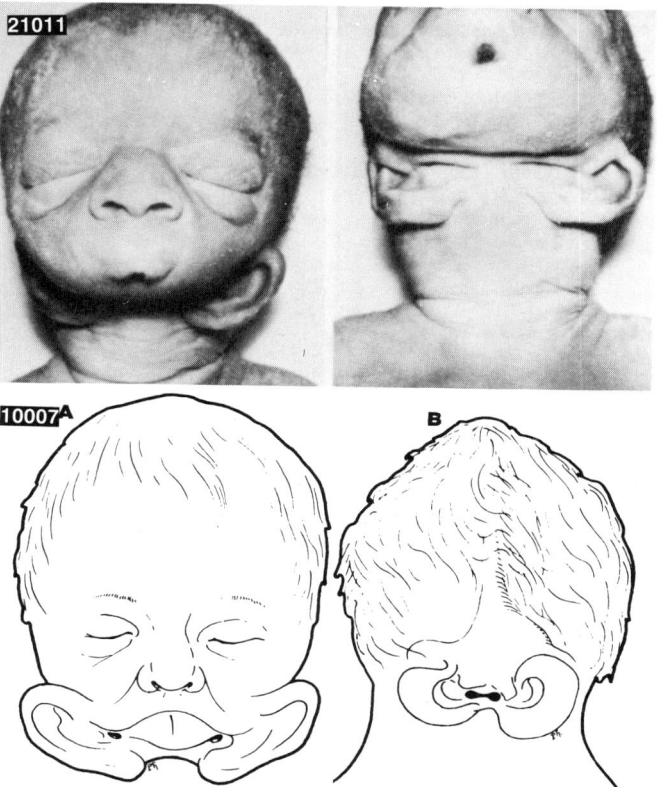

**0028**-21001:  Agnathia, microstomia and synotia; note the low placement of the ears.  10007: Otocephaly: A) moderate; B) marked.

**POS No.:** 3478

**Sex Ratio:** Presumably M1:F1

**Occurrence:** Rare.

**Risk of Recurrence for Patient's Sib:** Unknown.

**Risk of Recurrence for Patient's Child:** Affected individuals are not expected to survive to reproduce.

**Age of Detectability:** At birth by clinical evaluation.

**Gene Mapping and Linkage:** Unknown.

**Prevention:** None known. Genetic counseling indicated.

**Treatment:** Unknown.

**Prognosis:** Condition is incompatible with life.

**Detection of Carrier:** Unknown.

**References:**

Keen JA: A case of agnathia with a note on the development of the maxillary process. S Afr J Lab Clin Med 1955; 1:197–202.

Altman F: The ear in severe malformations of the head. Arch Otolaryngol 1957; 66:7–25.

Johnson WW, Cook JB: Agnathia associated with pharyngeal isthmus atresia and hydramnios. Arch Pediatr 1961; 78:211–217.

J0027                     **Ronald J. Jorgenson**

**Agoitrous cretinism**
*See THYROID, DYSGENESIS*
**Agoitrous hypothyroidism**
*See THYROID, DYSGENESIS*

## AGONADIA            0029

**Includes:**

Anorchia, familial
Gonadal agenesis
Testicular regression, embryonic
Testicular regression syndrome
True agonadism
XY gonadal agenesis syndrome

**Excludes:**

Anorchia (0068)
Chromosome mosaicism, 45x/46,xy type (0173)
Gonadal dysgenesis, XY type (0437)
Gonadotropin deficiencies (0438)
Sertoli cell-only syndrome (3163)
All forms of male pseudohermaphroditism

**Major Diagnostic Criteria:** Surgically verified absence of gonads in a 46,XY individual with abnormal external genitalia and absence of all but rudimentary müllerian or wolffian derivatives.

**Clinical Findings:** Individuals with agonadia have abnormal external genitalia, rudimentary müllerian and wolffian derivatives, and no detectable gonads. Mental retardation may coexist with craniofacial, vertebral, and dermatoglyphic anomalies. External genitalia usually consist of a small phallus about the size of a clitoris, underdeveloped labia majora, and usually almost complete fusion of the labioscrotal folds. The sex of rearing is usually female. By definition, no gonadal tissue is present. Sex steroid secretion is thus decreased, and gonadotropin secretion is increased. Although neither normal müllerian nor normal wolffian derivatives are present, structures resembling a rudimentary fallopian tube, an epioophoron, or an epididymis may be present along the lateral pelvic wall. Affected individuals are either ascertained at birth because of genital ambiguity or at puberty because secondary sexual development fails to occur.

**Complications:** Lack of secondary sexual development; infertility.

**Associated Findings:** Craniofacial anomalies, ptosis, highly arched palate, esotropia, epicanthal folds, and possibly mental retardation.

**Etiology:** Undetermined. In several kindred multiple sibs were affected, suggesting autosomal recessive inheritance.

**Pathogenesis:** Any explanation for agonadia must account not only for the absence of gonads but also for abnormal genital development and lack of normal internal ductal derivatives. The fetal testes might have functioned long enough to inhibit müllerian development, yet not sufficiently long to produce genital virilization. Teratogenic factors or defective connective tissue could also play roles. These hypotheses are consistent with the presence of H-Y antigen, which is documented.

**MIM No.:** 27325

**Sex Ratio:** M1:F0

**Occurrence:** About 25 cases have been reported.

**Risk of Recurrence for Patient's Sib:**
See Part I, *Mendelian Inheritance*. Possibly as high as 25% for 46,XY sibs and (12.5%) for all sibs.

**Risk of Recurrence for Patient's Child:** Affected individuals are infertile.

**Age of Detectability:** Usually at birth because of genital ambiguity, but sometimes not until puberty.

**Gene Mapping and Linkage:** Unknown.

**Prevention:** None known. Genetic counseling indicated.

**Treatment:** Hormone replacement. Surgical creation of vagina. Detection and treatment of craniofacial and other somatic abnormalities.

**Prognosis:** Normal life span provided associated somatic abnormalities are not serious.

**Detection of Carrier:** Unknown.

**Special Considerations:** This condition should be distinguished from **Anorchia**; a condition in which gonads are also absent but well-differentiated male external genitalia are present. In addition, at least two 46,XX individuals have shown features of agonadism.

**References:**

Sarto GE, Opitz JM: The XY gonadal agenesis syndrome. J Med Genet 1973; 10:288–293.

Simpson JL: Disorders of sexual differentiation: etiology and clinical delineation. New York: Academic, 1976.

Coulam CB: Testicular regression syndrome. Obstet Gynecol 1979; 53:44–49.

Kinoshita K, et al.: Agonadism with positive H-Y antigen. Clin Genet 1984; 26:61–64.

Rosenberg C, et al.: Testicular regression in a patient with virilized female phenotype. Am J Med Genet 1984; 19:183–188.

de Grouchy J, et al.: Embryonic testicular regression syndrome and severe mental retardation in sibs. Ann Genet 1985; 28:154–160.

SI018                    **Joe Leigh Simpson**

**Agranulocytosis, infantile Kostmann type**
*See IMMUNODEFICIENCY, AGRANULOCYTOSIS, INFANTILE KOSTMANN TYPE*
**AHF deficiency**
*See HEMOPHILIA A*
**AHG deficiency**
*See HEMOPHILIA A*
**Ahotutuo**
*See ANEMIA, SICKLE CELL*
**AI apolipoprolipoprotein variants**
*See HYPOALPHALIPOPROTEINEMIA*

## AICARDI SYNDROME           2320

**Includes:**

Agenesis of corpus callosum-chorioretinal abnormality
Agenesis of corpus callosum-infantile spasms-ocular anomalies
Corpus callosum, agenesis of-chorioretinal abnormality

**Excludes:**

Corpus callosum agenesis (0220)
Fetal cytomegalovirus syndrome (0381)
Fetal rubella syndrome (0384)
Fetal toxoplasmosis syndrome (0387)

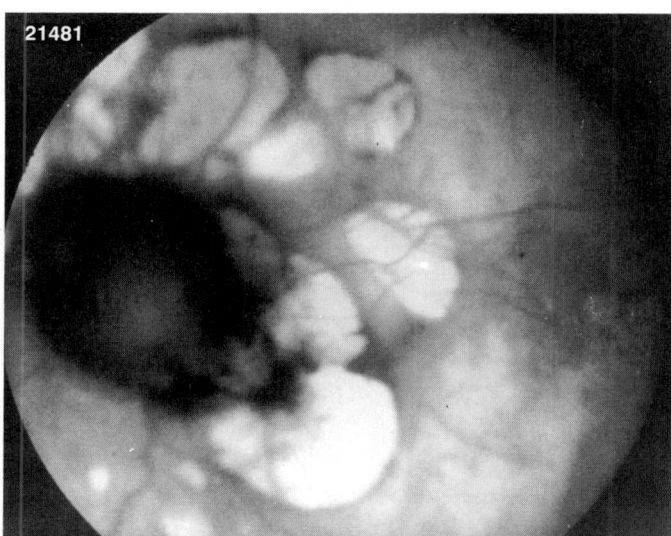

**2320A**-21481: Chorioretinal lacunar lesions have sharply defined borders with little pigmentary change in the surrounding retina. A partial optic nerve coloboma is also noted.

**FG syndrome, Opitz-Kaveggia type** (0754)
**Spastic ataxia, Charlevoix-Saguenay type** (2566)
**Tuberous sclerosis** (0975)

**Major Diagnostic Criteria:** Infantile flexor spasms with characteristic EEG abnormalities, agenesis of the corpus callosum, chorioretinal lacunae, and psychomotor retardation, usually in a female.

**Clinical Findings:** Myoclonic seizures (flexor spasms) beginning within the first few months is the usual initial feature. The EEG

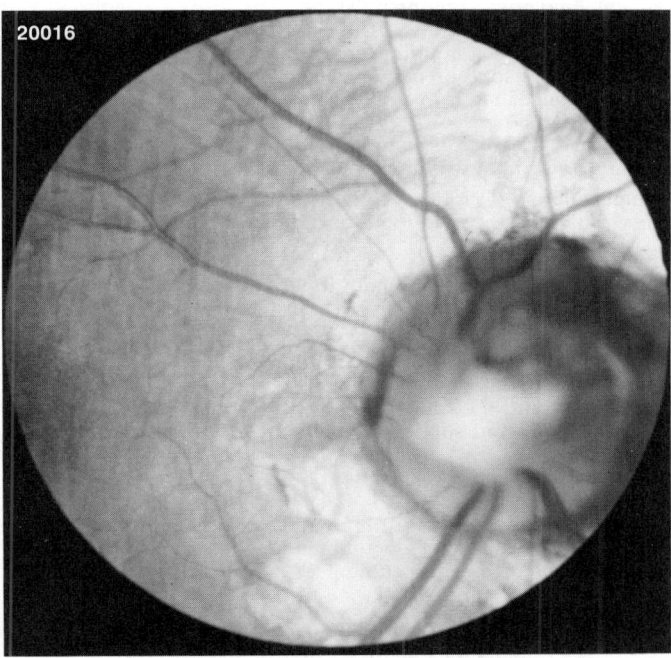

**2320B**-20016: Chorioretinal lacunae.

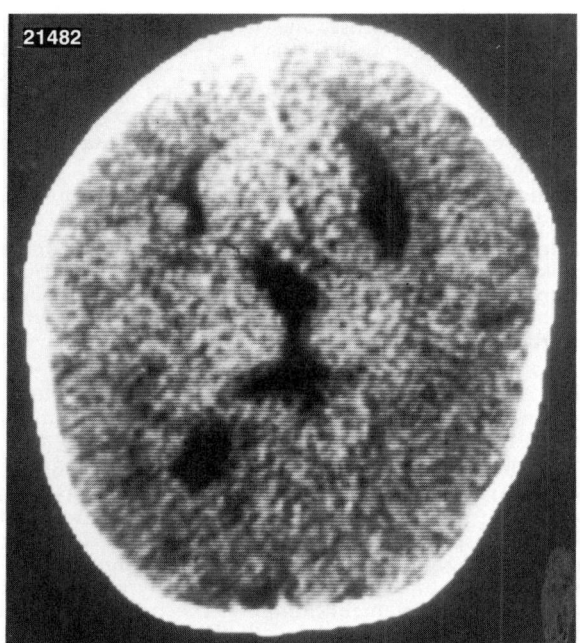

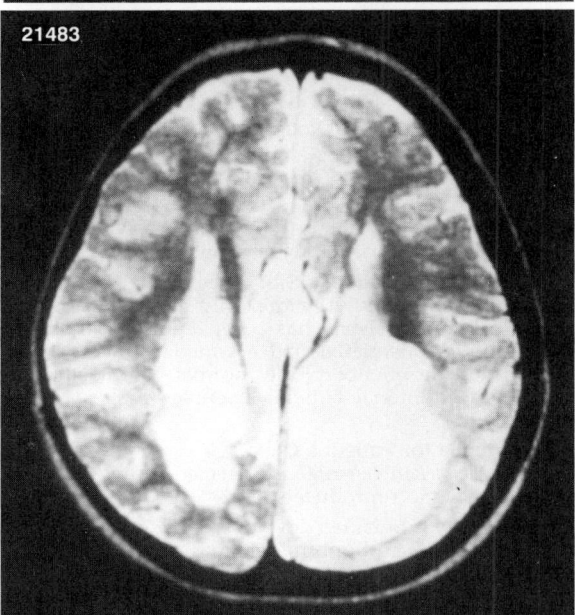

**2320C**-21482: CT scan of the brain in Aicardi syndrome; note the high-rising third ventricle in the same plane as the lateral ventricles, indicating agenesis of the corpus callosum. 21483: Magnetic resonance imaging of the brain shows asymmetric ventriculomegaly of the lateral ventricles, a high-rising third ventricle and agenesis of the corpus callosum.

typically shows periodic asynchronous discharges from the right and left hemispheres, without true hypsarrhythmia. Complete or partial absence of the corpus callosum and cortical heterotopia are demonstrable by computerized cranial tomography or magnetic resonance imaging (MRI). Psychomotor development is markedly delayed.

The pathognomonic ocular finding is a striking lacunar chorioretinopathy, which may be accompanied by unilateral or bilateral microphthalmia, a persistent pupillary membrane, and colobomas of the optic nerve and choroid. The circular or ovoid chorioretinal lacunae vary in size from less than one to several optic disk diameters.

Hemivertebrae, fused vertebrae, scoliosis, and rib abnormalities often are present.

Except for one girl with an apparently balanced X/3 translocation, chromosomes have been normal.

**Complications:** Blindness, intractable seizures, respiratory infections, and early death.

**Associated Findings:** Hypotonia, oral clefting, hand deformities, **Microcephaly**, **Plagiocephaly**, facial asymmetry, porencephalic cysts, papillomas of the choroid plexus, Dandy-Walker malformation, and hepatoblastoma. At autopsy, lissencephaly, polymicrogyria, cortical ectopia, and absence of the pineal gland have been found.

**Etiology:** Although no familial cases have been reported, the striking female preponderance (only one male with Aicardi syndrome has been described) suggests the possibility of X-linked dominant inheritance with lethality in the hemizygous male.

**Pathogenesis:** Aicardi (1965) and Dennis and Bower (1970) have proposed an insult prior to 16 weeks of gestation, at which time the corpus callosum, retina, and choroid should be well formed. The precise timing, however, has not been determined.

The choroidal lacunae consist of regions of hypopigmentation, with a variable rim of pigment clumping. The grossly undisturbed choroidal vasculature visible beneath the lesions and the fine perilacunar pigmentation serve to differentiate these findings from those of congenital toxoplasmosis.

**MIM No.:** 30405

**POS No.:** 3018

**Sex Ratio:** M0:F1 (M1:F >100 observed).

**Occurrence:** Except for one 46, XY male, whose diagnosis has been disputed on the basis of fundoscopic findings, and another with 47, XXY, all of the more than 100 patients thus far described have been girls. The great majority of reports have originated in France, Great Britain, Japan, and the United States.

**Risk of Recurrence for Patient's Sib:**
See Part I, *Mendelian Inheritance*. Only a single familial case involving two Spanish sisters has been reported (Molina et al, 1989). The authors postulated that a gonadal mutation had occurred in one of the phenotypically normal parents' X chromosomes. Lack of additional familial examples makes recurrence very unlikely.

**Risk of Recurrence for Patient's Child:**
See Part I, *Mendelian Inheritance*. Affected individuals are not expected to survive to reproduce.

**Age of Detectability:** Seizures develop during early infancy, and the characteristic EEG and ophthalmic findings should alert physicians to the diagnosis. Microphthalmia and cerebral malformations may be detectable by prenatal ultrasound after 16 weeks gestation.

**Gene Mapping and Linkage:** AIC (Aicardi syndrome) has been provisionally mapped to Xp22.

**Prevention:** None known. Genetic counseling indicated.

**Treatment:** Anticonvulsants, although seizures may prove difficult to control. There is no known treatment for the ocular abnormalities or psychomotor retardation.

**Prognosis:** Guarded. Many patients succumb to respiratory infections by age five years.

**Detection of Carrier:** Unknown.

**References:**
Aicardi J, et al.: A new syndrome: spasm in flexion, callosal agenesis, ocular abnormalities. Electroencephalogr Clin Neurophysiol 1965; 19:609–610.
Dennis J and Bower BD: The Aicardi syndrome. Dev Med Child Neurol 1970; 14:382–390.
Hoyt CS, et al: Ocular features of Aicardi's syndrome. Arch Ophthalmol 1978; 96:291–295. * †

Curtaolo P, et al.: Aicardi syndrome in a male infant. J Pediatr 1980; 96:286–287.
Ropers HH, et al: Agenesis of corpus callosum, ocular, and skeletal anomalies (X-linked dominant Aicardi's syndrome) in a girl with balanced X/3 translocation. Hum Genet 1982; 61:364–368.
McMahon RG, et al: Aicardi's syndrome: a clinicopathologic study. Arch Ophthalmol 1984; 102:250–253.
Yamamoto N, et al: Aicardi syndrome: report of 6 cases and a review of Japanese literature. Brain Dev 1985; 7:443–449.
Donnenfeld AE, et al.: Clinical, cytogenetic, and pedigree findings in 18 cases of Aicardi syndrome. Am J Med Genet 1989; 32:461–467. * †
Molina JA, et al.: Aicardi syndrome in two sisters. J Pediatr 1989; 115:282–283.

BA041                                                    **Harold N. Bass**

**AIDS, perinatal**
*See FETAL ACQUIRED IMMUNE DEFICIENCY SYNDROME (AIDS) INFECTION*
**Aka pygmy growth deficiency**
*See GROWTH DEFICIENCY, AFRICAN PYGMY TYPE*
**AKE**
*See ACROKERATOELASTOIDOSIS*

---

## ALACRIMA-APTYALISM                                    2604

**Includes:**
Lacrimal puncta, absence of
Parotid aplasia or hypoplasia
Salivary glands and lacrimal puncta, absence of

**Excludes:**
Alacrimia, congenita
**Dysautonomia I, Riley-Day type** (0307)
**Ectodermal dysplasia**
Glucocorticoid deficiency-achalasia
**Neuropathy, congenital sensory with anhidrosis** (2390)
**Palsy, congenital facial** (0377)
**Salivary gland, agenesis** (2722)
**Sjogren syndrome** (2101)

**Major Diagnostic Criteria:** Variable xerostomia with absent Stensen foramina; absent or hypoplastic salivary glands; absent or hypoplastic lacrimal puncta; and hypoplastic or atretic nasolacrimal canaliculi.

**Clinical Findings:** Epiphora is frequent during childhood but may also be seen in adults. Ocular injection and mucoid conjunctival secretion are common. Xerophthalmia does not occur. Xerostomia may be total or partial. Dental decay with yellow-brown discoloration of teeth occurs early in life, and the patient may become edentulous.

Clinical variability is common. Some individuals have mild salivary or lacrimal dysfunction.

**Complications:** Epiphora, conjunctivitis, xerostomia with deglutitory difficulties of solid food, and dental decay.

**Associated Findings:** Dextrocardia was seen in one individual.

**Etiology:** Autosomal dominant inheritance with complete penetrance and variable expressivity. New mutations have not been documented.

**Pathogenesis:** Failure of canalization of lacrimal and salivary ducts at approximately eight weeks gestation. Lacrimal and parotid glands and their ducts are derived from ectoderm, whereas submandibular and sublingual ducts are endodermic.

**MIM No.:** *18092

**Sex Ratio:** M1:F1

**Occurrence:** Incidence is unknown partly because of the variable expressivity and lack of documentation of the disorder. A few dozen cases have been documented, all in Caucasians.

**Risk of Recurrence for Patient's Sib:**
See Part I, *Mendelian Inheritance*.

**Risk of Recurrence for Patient's Child:**
See Part I, *Mendelian Inheritance*.

**Age of Detectability:** During infancy.

**Gene Mapping and Linkage:** Unknown.

**Prevention:** None known. Genetic counseling indicated.

**Treatment:** Massaging of lacrimal puncta may bring temporary relief of epiphora in cases of obstructed hypoplastic puncta or nasolacrimal ducts; probing or surgery may be needed. Dental capping or prosthestics may be necessary.

**Prognosis:** Normal intelligence and life span.

**Detection of Carrier:** By physical examination. CT scanning, scintigraphy, or both can document absence of lacrimal and salivary glands.

**Special Considerations:** It is not clear if familial absence of the salivary glands and alacrima-aptyalism are the same condition, as suggested by the study of Hughes and Syrop (1959). Ocular examination of individuals with absent salivary glands and their relatives is indicated.

**References:**
Blackmar FB: Congenital atresia of all lacrimal puncta with absence of salivary glands. Am J Ophthalmol 1925; 8:139–140.
Hughes RD, Syrop HW: A familial study of the agenesis of the parotid gland duct. Xth International Congress on Genetics, Montreal, 1958. Toronto: University of Toronto Press, 1959:128 only.
Vogel C, Reichart P: Parotid and submandibular gland aplasia with atresia of the lacrimal canaliculi [in German]. Dtsch Zahnarztl Z 1978; 33:415–417.
Caccamise WC, Townes PL: Congenital absence of the lacrimal puncta associated with alacrima and aptyalism. Am J Ophthalmol 1980; 89:62–65.
Cortada X, et al.: Alacrima-aptyalism: an autosomal dominant condition. (Abstract). Am J Hum Genet 1986; 39:A57 only.
Higashino H, et al.: Congenital absence of lacrimal puncta and of all major salivary glands: case report and literature review. Clin Pediat 1987; 26:366–368.

XA001                                               **Xavier Cortada**

**Alactasia, congenital**
See LACTASE DEFICIENCY, CONGENITAL
**Alactasia, early onset**
See LACTASE DEFICIENCY, CONGENITAL
**Alactasia, late-onset**
See LACTASE DEFICIENCY, PRIMARY
**Alagille syndrome**
See ARTERIO-HEPATIC DYSPLASIA
**Aland Island disease**
See FORSIUS-ERIKSSON SYNDROME
**Alanine 60 amyloidosis**
See AMYLOIDOSIS, APPALACHIAN TYPE
**Alaninemia, hyperbeta**
See HYPERBETA-ALANINEMIA
**Alaninuria**
See PYRUVATE DEHYDROGENASE DEFICIENCY
**Albers-Schonberg**
See DYSOSTEOSCLEROSIS
**Albers-Schonberg disease**
See OSTEOPETROSIS, MALIGNANT RECESSIVE
also OSTEOPETROSIS, BENIGN DOMINANT

**ALBINISM**                                           **1516**

**Includes:**
Melanin formation, reduction or absence
Ocular albinism
Oculocutaneous albinism

**Major Diagnostic Criteria:** Foveal hypoplasia, reduced visual acuity that cannot be corrected to normal, reduced pigment in the retinal pigment epithelium, and misrouting of the retinal ganglion fibers at the optic chiasm are the cardinal features of all types of albinism. Mild-to-total reduction of melanin pigment in the skin, hair, and irides are features of oculocutaneous albinism. Minimal to no reduction of melanin pigment in the skin and hair, with varying degrees of iris pigment, are features of ocular albinism.

**Clinical Findings:** Albinism refers to a group of inherited disorders of the melanin pigment system in which there is a congenital reduction or an absence of melanin formation. Types of albinism not associated with other metabolic defects include all types of oculocutaneous and ocular albinisms. Types of albinism associated with other metabolic defects include the **Albinism, oculocutaneous, Hermansky-Pudlak type** and **Chediak-Higashi syndrome**. **Prader-Willi syndrome** is considered a form of hypomelanosis and does not represent a true type of albinism.

The ocular features are most constant and are necessary to make the diagnosis of albinism. Foveal hypoplasia with an associated reduction in visual acuity that cannot be corrected to normal must be present. The retina will show generalized hypopigmentation to a variable degree, and the underlying choroidal vessels are usually present, but the amount of retinal pigment may be similar to that of a normally pigmented blond individual. Nystagmus is also a constant feature of albinism and is usually present within the first year of life. Onset of nystagmus six or more weeks after birth is well described, and nystagmus is generally less severe with age, such that adults with albinism may appear to have little or no nystagmus. The hypopigmentation usually affects the iris, particularly in the oculocutaneous types of albinism, resulting in iris translucency, while the types of albinism that are predominantly ocular may have a translucent or a normally dense iris. The iris may be blue, gray, hazel, brown, or mixed (pigmented in the inner one-third to one-half), and globe transillumination will demonstrate pigment when present. The existence of clinically significant congenital retinal hypopigmentation correlates with misrouting of the retinal ganglion fibers, with an excess of optic fibers from 20 degrees or more of the temporal retina crossing to the contralateral hemisphere instead of projecting to the ipsilateral hemisphere. A functional consequence of the optic tract misrouting is an alternating strabismus, which is found in the majority of individuals with albinism.

The skin and hair changes are more variable in oculocutaneous and ocular albinism. **Albinism, oculocutaneous, tyrosinase negative** is the only type in which there is no formation of melanin during life. Melanin is present at birth or develops with time in all other types of albinism. The skin and hair are involved in the oculocutaneous types, and this is clinically obvious when the ethnic background of the affected individual is considered. Skin and hair involvement may not be as apparent in the types that are predominantly ocular in involvement, but examination of the skin melanocytes in **Albinism, Ocular late onset-sensorineural deafness, X-linked** shows large melanosomes (macromelanosomes, melanin macroglobules), demonstrating cutaneous involvement, and affected individuals are often fair or have hypopigmented macules. It is likely that all types of albinism with predominant eye involvement also have cutaneous involvement.

Evaluation of an individual with albinism should include a complete ophthalmologic examination and hairbulb analysis. Freshly plucked anagen hairbulbs are a readily accessible source of melanocytes for study. Hairbulb tyrosinase activity can be quantitated with a tritiated tyrosine assay, and the presence or absence of melanin can be qualitatively determined by dissecting microscopic evaluation of a hairbulb after incubation in tyrosine and dopa. Tyrosinase activity is low or absent in **Albinism, oculocutaneous, tyrosinase negative**; **Albinism, oculocutaneous, yellow mutant**; **Albinism, oculocutaneous, minimal pigment type** and in most individuals with **Albinism, oculocutaneous, Hermansky-Pudlak type**. Tyrosinase activity is normal in all other types of oculocutaneous and ocular albinism.

**Complications:** The foveal hypoplasia and the misrouting of the optic fibers are thought to be the results of hypopigmentation of the retina during development. The reduced amount of melanin in the skin is associated with an increased sensitivity to the UV radiation of the sun, and prolonged exposure will lead to the development of thickening of the skin (pachydermia), solar keratoses, and skin cancer.

**Etiology:** All types of albinism not associated with other metabolic defects are autosomal recessive in inheritance except for **Albinism, Ocular late onset-sensorineural deafness, X-linked**.

**Pathogenesis:**   All types of albinism are thought to be the result of different mutations involving the melanin synthesis pathway, and most are probably due to an enzyme abnormality. Two enzymes in the pathway are currently known, and tyrosinase is the only enzyme that has been shown to produce albinism when deficient (tyrosinase-negative, yellow, and minimal pigment types).

**Occurrence:   Albinism, oculocutaneous, tyrosinase negative** and **Albinism, oculocutaneous, tyrosinase positive** are the most common types, and all other types are considerably less frequent.

**Age of Detectability:**   Usually evident at birth or in the first three months of life.

**Prevention:**   None known. Genetic counseling indicated.

**Treatment:**   All individuals with albinism should have regular ophthalmologic care, including yearly examinations while in school. Sensitive skin should be protected with a sun screen (No. 15 or higher), long sleeves, and a hat with a brim.

**Prognosis:**   Normal life span except for **Albinism, oculocutaneous, Hermansky-Pudlak type.** Vision is stable and does not progress in severity. Individuals with albinism are not blind, even though their best corrected vision is within the legal definition of blindness, and they usually require glasses to achieve their best vision. Their close vision (six feet and closer) is good, and affected individuals can expect to be able to work in most professions. It may be difficult to get a driver's licence.

**Support Groups:**   Philadelphia; National Organization for Albinism and Hypopigmentation (NOAH)

**References:**
Kinnear PE, et al.: Albinism. Surv Ophthalmol 1983; 30:75–101.
King RA: Albinism. In: Gomez MR (ed): Neurocutaneous diseases. Stoneham, MA: Butterworths, 1987:311–325.
Witkop CJ, et al.: Albinism. In: Scriver CR, et al, eds: The metabolic basis of inherited disease, 6th ed. New York: McGraw-Hill, 1989: 2905–2947.

KI007                                                          **Richard A. King**

**Albinism and immunodeficiency**
*See* HYPOPIGMENTATION-IMMUNE DEFECT, GRISCELLI TYPE
**Albinism oculocutaneous, type IA**
*See* ALBINISM, OCULOCUTANEOUS, TYROSINASE NEGATIVE

## ALBINISM, CUTANEOUS                                           0031

**Includes:**
   Cutaneous albinism without deafness
   Piebaldism with white forelock
   Piebaldness
   Piebaldness-deafness
   Piebalds
   Forelock (whit) without deafness
   Wolff syndrome
   Zypokowski-Margolis syndrome

**Excludes:**
   **Albinism, cutaneous-deafness** (0030)
   Heterochromia, isolated
   **Skin, vitiligo** (0993)
   **Waardenburg syndromes** (0997)

**Major Diagnostic Criteria:**   Albinism restricted to the ventral portions of the body with normal pigmentation of the mid-dorsal surfaces of the back and neck, present since birth.

**Clinical Findings:**   Absence of skin pigmentation primarily on the ventral surfaces of the body. This includes such characteristics as a frontal blaze of white hair (white forelock), absence of pigmentation of the central portion of the forehead, the medial portion of the eyebrows, and portions of the nose and chin, and to a variable degree the ventral portion of the chest, abdomen, and ventral surfaces of arms and legs. The wrists, hands, ankles, and feet are often fully pigmented. The occiput, back of the neck, and mid-dorsal surface of the trunk are fully pigmented. Islands of pig-

mentation may occur within the nonpigmented areas. The borders between normally pigmented and nonpigmented skin are usually hyperpigmented. Heterochromia is occasionally present.

**Complications:**   Unknown.

**Associated Findings:**   *Wolff syndrome* (Wolff et al, 1965) and *Zypokowski-Margolis syndrome* (Zipokowsky et al, 1962; Margolis, 1962) combine partial albinism with hearing and speech disorders.

**Etiology:**   Autosomal dominant inheritance.

**Pathogenesis:**   Electron microscopy of the affected skin shows an absence of melanoblasts but presence of Langerhans cells. The defect could be explained by incomplete migration of melanoblasts to the ventral midline or by a defect in differentiation of ventral melanoblasts. The relationship between Langerhans cells and melanoblasts, the similarity in the electron microscopic picture with that of acquired vitiligo, and transplantation studies of piebald spotting in mice all suggest that an inherited defect in melanoblast differentiation is the most likely cause.

**MIM No.:**   *17280

**CDC No.:**   270.200

**Sex Ratio:**   M1:F1

**Occurrence:**   Established literature.

**Risk of Recurrence for Patient's Sib:**
   See Part I, *Mendelian Inheritance.*

**Risk of Recurrence for Patient's Child:**
   See Part I, *Mendelian Inheritance.*

**Age of Detectability:**   At birth.

**Gene Mapping and Linkage:**   PBT (piebald trait) has been tentatively mapped to 4q12-q21.

**Prevention:**   None known. Genetic counseling indicated.

**Treatment:**   For cosmetic problems, hair dye and skin cosmetics may be used.

**Prognosis:**   Normal life span.

**Detection of Carrier:**   Penetrance is high.

**Support Groups:**   Philadelphia; National Organization for Albinism and Hypopigmentation (NOAH)

**References:**
Cooke JV: Familial white skin spotting (piebaldness) ("partial albinism") with white forelock. J Pediatr 1952; 41:1.
Margolis E: A new hereditary syndrome: sex linked deaf-mutism associated with total albinism. Acta Genet (Basel) 1962; 12:12–19.
Zipokowsky L, et al.: Partial albinism and deaf-mutism due to a recessive sex-linked gene. Arch Dermat 1962; 86:530–539.
Wolff CM, et al.: Congenital deafness associated with piebaldness. Arch Otolaryng 1965; 82:244–250.
Comings DE, Odland GF: Partial albinism. J Am Med Asso 1966; 195:510–523.
Hoo, JJ, et al.: Tentative assignment of piebald trait gene to chromosome band 4q12. Human Genet 1986; 73:230–231.
Hulten MA, et al.: Homozygosity in piebald trait. J Med Genet 1987; 24:568–571.

C0030                                                        **David E. Comings**

## ALBINISM, CUTANEOUS-DEAFNESS                                     0030

**Includes:**
   Cutaneous albinism-deafness
   Deafness-cutaneous albinism

**Excludes:**
   **Albinism, cutaneous** (0031)
   **Albinism, Ocular late onset-sensorineural deafness, X-linked** (2824)
   **Albinism, Waardenburg type-hirschsprung aganglionosis** (2823)
   **Waardenburg syndromes** (0997)

**Major Diagnostic Criteria:**   Sensorineural deafness, areas of hypomelanosis and hypermelanosis of skin in a symmetric distribution.

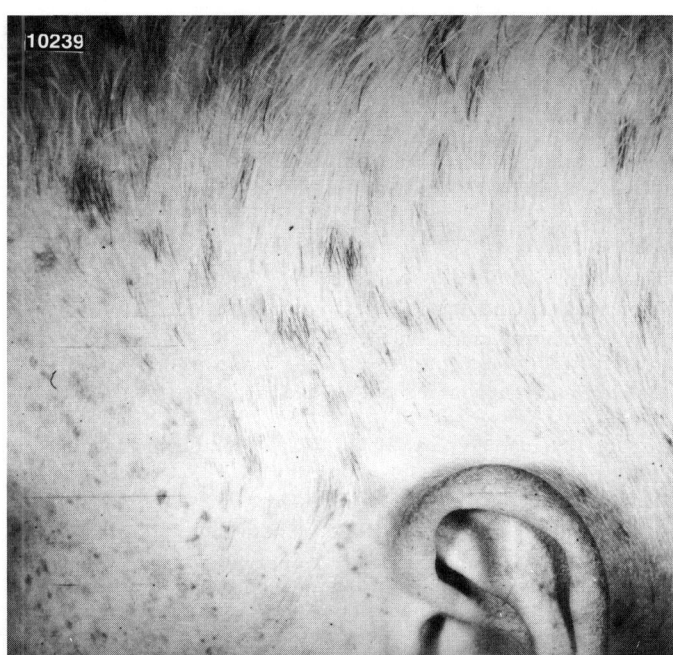

0030-10239: Cutaneous albinism-hyperpigmentation-deafness syndrome; scalp hair is white with patchy pigmentation.

**Clinical Findings:** Pigmentation of genital and scrotal regions. Scalp hair white, sometimes with patches of pigmentation. Few show heterochromia of iris.

**Complications:** Unknown.

**Associated Findings:** None known.

**Etiology:** X-linked inheritance.

**Pathogenesis:** Disturbance of melanocyte migration to skin and ear.

**MIM No.:** *30070

**POS No.:** 4120

**Sex Ratio:** M1:F0

**Occurrence:** About six kinships reported. A six-generation Sephardic Jewish family was reported.

**Risk of Recurrence for Patient's Sib:**
See Part I, *Mendelian Inheritance.*

**Risk of Recurrence for Patient's Child:**
See Part I, *Mendelian Inheritance.*

**Age of Detectability:** Neonatal period.

**Gene Mapping and Linkage:** ADFN (albinism-deafness syndrome) has been mapped to Xq25-q27.

**Prevention:** None known. Genetic counseling indicated.

**Treatment:** Hearing aid and special training.

**Prognosis:** Unknown.

**Detection of Carrier:** Undetermined. Some carriers may have hearing loss.

**Support Groups:** Philadelphia; National Organization for Albinism and Hypopigmentation (NOAH)

**References:**
Margolis, E: A new hereditary syndrome: sex linked deaf-mutism associated with total albinism. Acta Genet 1962; 12:12–19.
Ziprkowski L, et al.: Partial albinism and deaf-mutism due to a recessive sex-linked gene. Arch Dermatol 1962; 86:530–539. *

Reed WB, et al.: Pigmentary disorders in association with congenital deafness. Arch Dermatol 1967; 95:176–186.
Fried K, et al.: Hearing impairment in female carriers and the sex-linked syndrome of deafness with albinism. J Med Genet 1969; 6:132–134. *

HA041 **David J. Harris**

**Albinism, incomplete oculocutaneous**
*See CHEDIAK-HIGASHI SYNDROME*

## ALBINISM, OCULAR  0032

**Includes:**
Nettleship-Falls ocular albinism
Ocular albinism

**Excludes:**
**Albinism, cutaneous** (0031)
Albinism, ocular-lentisines-deafness
**Albinism, ocular, autosomal recessive type** (2010)
**Albinism, oculocutaneous**
**Albinoidism** (2359)
**Chediak-Higashi syndrome** (0143)
**Forsius-Eriksson syndrome** (3183)
**Waardenburg syndromes** (0997)

**Major Diagnostic Criteria:** Deficiency of uveal pigmentation with photophobia, nystagmus, and decreased vision in males and variable coarse mottling and stippled appearance of ocular fundus in female carriers.

**Clinical Findings:** Photophobia, nystagmus, and decreased vision are usually present in males. The degree of pigmentation present is variable. In infants the iris is light grey and in adults blue-grey and translucent. A red pupil glow may be present. The fundus is bright red-orange with prominent vessels and the macula is pink and often devoid of yellow pigment. Retinal pigment is usually completely absent and uveal pigment variable. In Negroes more pigmentation may be present. Central scotomas and poor visual acuity relate to the amount of pigmentation and development of the fovea centralis. Laboratory tests are normal except for presence of macromelanosomes on skin biopses.

**Complications:** Foveal aplasia, decreased visual acuity, nystagmus, head nodding, strabismus, poor pupillary responses may be present.

**Associated Findings:** Partial aniridia, ocular colobomas, astigmatism.

**Etiology:** X-linked recessive inheritance.

**Pathogenesis:** While it appears that the ocular form may also have skin involvement, there is less information available on the ocular form than for generalized albinism. In the latter case melanocytes are present and the defect is metabolic not structural. Serum tyrosine is normal but melanocytes produce less than normal amounts of melanin either due to a deficiency of the enzyme tyrosinase or insufficient amounts of tyrosine locally.

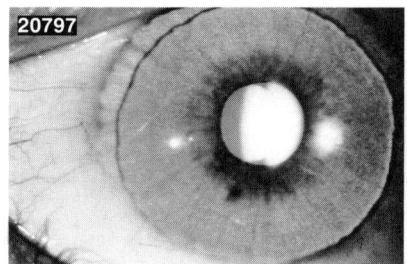 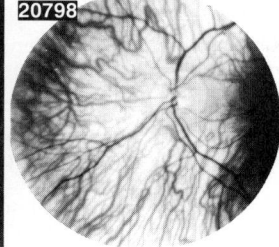

0032-20797: Note iris translucency; the lens margin is visible.
20798: Hypopigmentation of the fundus in ocular albinism.

Therefore, in the generalized forms, there is a reduced amount of melanin in each melanosome. In the ocular form, there is a reduced number of melanosomes and macromelanosomes seen in skin biopsy.

**MIM No.:** *30050

**CDC No.:** 270.200

**Sex Ratio:** M1:F0. Rare homozygous females have been reported.

**Occurrence:** Undetermined; established literature.

**Risk of Recurrence for Patient's Sib:**
See Part I, *Mendelian Inheritance.*

**Risk of Recurrence for Patient's Child:**
See Part I, *Mendelian Inheritance.*

**Age of Detectability:** At birth.

**Gene Mapping and Linkage:** OA1 (ocular albinism 1 (Nettleship-Falls)) has been mapped to Xp22.3.

**Prevention:** None known. Genetic counseling indicated.

**Treatment:** Colored glasses, artificial pupil, scleral contact lenses and corneal tattooing have been employed.

**Prognosis:** Normal life span but poor visual prognosis.

**Detection of Carrier:** Although variably affected and usually functionally normal, the female heterozygote has a translucent iris, coarse pigment stippling of the macula and islands of brown pigment clusters alternating with deep depigmentation in the near periphery. In known pedigrees, some carriers can be identified by determination of their Xg status, since this locus is closely linked to that of the ocular albinism locus.

**Support Groups:** Philadelphia; National Organization for Albinism and Hypopigmentation (NOAH)

**References:**
Falls HF: Sex-linked ocular albinism displaying typical fundus changes in female heterozygote. Am J Ophthalmol 1951; 34 (part 2):41.
O'Donnell FE, et al.: X-linked ocular albinism. Arch Ophthalmol 1976; 94:1883–1892.
O'Donnell FE, Green RW: The eye in albinism. In: Duane TD, ed: Clinical Ophthalmology, Vol 4, New York: Harper & Row, 1984.
Kinnear PR, et al.: Albinism. Survey Ophthalmol 1985; 30:75–101.

ME032
CR012
**Marilyn B. Mets**
**Harold E. Cross**

## ALBINISM, OCULAR, AUTOSOMAL RECESSIVE TYPE     2010

**Includes:** Ocular albinism

**Excludes:**
   Albinism (1516)
   Albinism, ocular (0032)
   Albinism, oculocutaneous, tyrosinase negative (0034)
   Albinism, oculocutaneous, tyrosinase positive (0035)
   Chediak-Higashi syndrome (0143)
   Waardenburg syndromes (0997)

**Major Diagnostic Criteria:** Deficiency in uveal pigmentation with nystagmus, photophobia and decreased acuity in males and females.

**Clinical Findings:** Generalized hypopigmentation at birth with darkening of skin and hair usually noted as patients grow older. Infants may be erroneously diagnosed as having oculocutaneous albinism. Pigmented nevi or freckles are usually present. Patients may tan lightly but usually sunburn easily. The uvea may contain some pigmentation especially at the macula with streaks of choroidal pigmentation in the periphery but iris, retina and choroid remain abnormally hypopigmented throughout life. Foveal reflexes are absent and perifoveal retinal vessels may appear abnormally straight.

**Complications:** Poor visual acuity, strabismus, photophobia and nystagmus.

**Associated Findings:** Sunburn easily, iris transillumination and extreme generalized hypopigmentation at birth.

**Etiology:** Autosomal recessive inheritance.

**Pathogenesis:** Unknown. No melanosome alterations have been found in skin or hairbulbs. Hairbulb incubation in tyrosine yields normal pigmentation. Electrophysiologic tests do not provide diagnostic information.

**MIM No.:** *20331

**CDC No.:** 270.200

**Sex Ratio:** M1:F1

**Occurrence:** Undetermined but presumed rare.

**Risk of Recurrence for Patient's Sib:**
See Part I, *Mendelian Inheritance.*

**Risk of Recurrence for Patient's Child:**
See Part I, *Mendelian Inheritance.*

**Age of Detectability:** At Birth. May resemble oculocutaneous albinism in first year of life.

**Gene Mapping and Linkage:** Unknown.

**Prevention:** None known. Genetic counseling indicated.

**Treatment:** Although the defect cannot be reversed, visual comfort and function may be improved to some extent through tinted glasses or contacts. Cosmetic defect may be corrected with surgery for the strabismus.

**Prognosis:** Life span is normal, but visual handicap remains.

**Detection of Carrier:** Unknown.

**Special Considerations:** In families with affected males only, light and electron microscopy may be necessary to distinguish X-linked ocular albinism (with macromelanosomes in the skin) from autosomal recessive ocular albinism (normal melanosomes).

**Support Groups:** Philadelphia; National Organization for Albinism and Hypopigmentation (NOAH)

**References:**
O'Donnell FE, et al.: Autosomal recessively inherited ocular albinism: a new form of ocular albibism affecting females as severely as males. Arch Ophthalmol 1978; 96:1621–1625.
Witkop CF, Jr., et al.: Albinism. In: Scriver CR, et al, eds: The metabolic basis of inherited disease, 6th ed. New York: McGraw-Hill, 1989:2905–2948.

CR012
**Harold E. Cross**

**Albinism, ocular, Forsius-Eriksson type**
*See FORSIUS-ERIKSSON SYNDROME*

## ALBINISM, OCULAR-LATE-ONSET-SENSORINEURAL DEAFNESS, X-LINKED     2824

**Includes:**
Deafness (sensorineural) with X-linked ocular albinism
Ocular albinism-sensorineural deafness (OASD)

**Excludes:**
   Albinism, cutaneous-deafness (0030)
   Albinism, ocular (0032)
   Forsius-Eriksson syndrome (3183)

**Major Diagnostic Criteria:** Ocular albinism, normal cutaneous pigmentation, late-onset sensorineural deafness, macromelanosomes, and X-linked inheritance.

**Clinical Findings:** *Affected males:* The classic signs of ocular albinism are seen, notably, in early childhood, pale blue irides, which are translucent on slit-lamp examination; nystagmus; poor visual acuity, and retinal hypopigmentation. In the fourth decade, onset of progressive perceptive deafness. Skin biopsy showing macromelanosomes (giant melanin globules) within the melanocytes.

*Female heterozygotes:* The findings are pale blue eyes, translucent irides patchy hypopigmentation of fundi, and macromelanosomes on skin biopsy.

**Complications:** Visual acuity deteriorates, culminating in blindness. Profound deafness ensues, progressive with age.

**Associated Findings:** None known.

**Etiology:** Presumably X-linked recessive inheritance.

**Pathogenesis:** Unknown.

**MIM No.:** 30065

**POS No.:** 4120

**Sex Ratio:** M1:F0. Males are affected; females are carriers.

**Occurrence:** One large kindred has been reported in South Africa, with seven affected males and 11 carrier females.

**Risk of Recurrence for Patient's Sib:**
See Part I, *Mendelian Inheritance.*

**Risk of Recurrence for Patient's Child:**
See Part I, *Mendelian Inheritance.*

**Age of Detectability:** Prenatal diagnosis may be possible by fetal skin sampling via fetoscopy to find macromelanosomes, or clinically during infancy.

**Gene Mapping and Linkage:** Uninformative linkage studies with XgA + G6PD. (No linkage with color blindness.)

**Prevention:** None known. Genetic counseling indicated.

**Treatment:** Symptomatic.

**Prognosis:** Life span and intelligence are not affected.

**Detection of Carrier:** Manifesting heterozygotes have translucent irides, retinal hypopigmentation, and macromelanosomes on skin biopsy.

**Support Groups:** Philadelphia; National Organization for Albinism and Hypopigmentation (NOAH)

**References:**
Winship I, et al.: X-linked inheritance of ocular albinism with late-onset sensorineural deafness. Am J Med Genet 1984; 19:797–803.

WI055                                                    **Ingrid M. Winship**

## ALBINISM, OCULOCUTANEOUS, BROWN TYPE          2357

**Includes:**
Albinism, oculocutaneous, type IV
Brown albino

**Excludes:**
Albinism, oculocutaneous, Rufous type (2358)
Albinism, oculocutaneous, tyrosinase positive (0035)
Albinism, oculocutaneous, yellow mutant (0036)

**Major Diagnostic Criteria:** Light brown hair and skin. Blue-gray to light brown irides. Ocular features of albinism, including nystagmus, reduced visual acuity, reduced retinal pigment, and foveal hypoplasia. Thus far, this condition has only been reported in blacks of African origin.

**Clinical Findings:** At birth, the hair and the skin are light brown, and the irides are gray to tan. With age there is some increase in the hair and iris pigment, but little change in the skin. A slight tan develops on sun exposure, and the skin is resistant to the acute effects of sun exposure (does not burn). Pigmented nevi, lentigines, or freckles are uncommon. The ocular features indicate the diagnosis of albinism. Nystagmus is present throughout life, often being less obvious with age. Photophobia is not a major problem. Strabismus is alternating. Visual acuity is reduced to 20/60 to 20/150. The iris shows moderate translucency on globe transillumination, and the fovea is hypoplastic with a muted foveal light reflex. Retinal pigment is present but reduced in amount.

Quantitative hairbulb tyrosinase activity is normal. Hairbulbs and skin melanocytes have normal morphology, but the melanosomes are not fully melanized and are small in skin melanocytes.

**Complications:** Nystagmus, reduced visual acuity, and an alternating strabismus are thought to be the result of reduced melanin in the optic system during development. Chronic sun exposure does not damage the skin.

**Associated Findings:** None known.

**Etiology:** Autosomal recessive inheritance.

**Pathogenesis:** Brown oculocutaneous albinism is thought to be the result of a block in the eumelanin pathway. The defective enzyme is unknown. It is possible that **Albinism, ocular, autosomal recessive type** is the same condition in Caucasians.

**MIM No.:** *20329

**POS No.:** 3536

**CDC No.:** 270.200

**Sex Ratio:** M1:F1

**Occurrence:** Brown oculocutaneous albinism has only been described in blacks of African origin. The incidence is unknown. Twenty-three of 79 (29%) Nigerian albinos had this condition, and seven affected individuals were identified in Houston over a three-year period.

**Risk of Recurrence for Patient's Sib:**
See Part I, *Mendelian Inheritance.*

**Risk of Recurrence for Patient's Child:**
See Part I, *Mendelian Inheritance.*

**Age of Detectability:** At birth.

**Gene Mapping and Linkage:** Unknown.

**Prevention:** None known. Genetic counseling indicated.

**Treatment:** Yearly ophthalmologic evaluation through school, then ophthalmologic care as needed. Sun screens are generally not necessary.

**Prognosis:** Normal life span.

**Detection of Carrier:** Unknown.

**Support Groups:** Philadelphia; National Organization for Albinism and Hypopigmentation (NOAH)

**References:**
King RA, et al.: Albinism in Nigeria with delineation of new recessive oculocutaneous type. Clin Genet 1980; 17:259–270.
King RA, et al.: Brown oculocutaneous albinism. Ophthalmology 1985; 92:1496–1505.
King RA, et al.: Brown oculocutaneous albinism: clinical, ophthalmological, and biochemical charcterization. Ophthalmology 1986; 92:1496–1505.
King RA, Rich SS: Segregation analysis of brown oculocutaneous albinism. Clin Genet 1986; 29:496–501.

KI007                                                    **Richard A. King**

## ALBINISM, OCULOCUTANEOUS, HERMANSKY-PUDLAK TYPE          0033

**Includes:**
Albinism-hemorrhagic diathesis-pigmented
  reticuloendothelial cells
Albinism, oculocutaneous, type VI
Delta-storage pool disease
Hermansky-Pudlak syndrome

**Excludes:**
Albinism, oculocutaneous, tyrosinase negative (0034)
Albinism, oculocutaneous, tyrosinase positive (0035)
Albinism, oculocutaneous, yellow mutant (0036)
Chediak-Higashi syndrome (0143)
Other storage pool deficient platelet disorders

**Major Diagnostic Criteria:** A tyrosinase-positive deficiency of pigment of eyes and skin accompanied by a bleeding diathesis due to storage pool deficient platelets and the presence of a granular pigment that fluoresces bright yellow under UV light and is present in urine or bone marrow.

**Clinical Findings:** This form of albinism was originally described by Hermansky and Pudlak as albinism with a hemorrhagic diathesis due to a vascular hemophilia and storage of ceroid in reticuloendothelial cells of lung, liver, bone marrow, lymph nodes, and kidney. The condition is now known to consist of the triad of a tyrosinase-positive form of oculocutaneous albinism; storage pool-deficient platelets with a marked decreased in dense bodies, adenosine diphosphate, and serotonin; and accumulation of a yellow granular substance in reticuloendothelial cells, kidney, tubular epithelium, cardiac muscle, lung, colonic mucosa, circulating macrophages, urine sediment, and oral mucosal cells. Phenotypically, patients may resemble any type of oculocutaneous or ocular albinism depending upon the racial and pigmentary background of the parents. Patients have moderate-to-severe photophobia, nystagmus, and decreased visual acuity; about 30% have strabismus. With increasing age, some pigment accumulates at the limbus and pupillary border, giving a cartwheel effect on transillumination of the irides.

Hair color may vary from white to reddish-brown, the latter in patients from darkly pigmented populations. Pigmented nevi may be frequent. Patients usually give a history of mild-to-moderate bleeding episodes (but fatal hemorrhage has occurred), easy bruisability, epistaxis, and prolonged bleeding following tooth extraction or delivery. With few exceptions, menses have not been unusual. Bleeding time may be prolonged or fall within the upper limits of normal. Aspirin may prolong bleeding, usually for several minutes. Chest X-rays of older patients frequently show diffuse streaking and dense nodular radiopaque areas due to storage material. Some patients over 3 or 4 years of age develop restrictive lung disease and ulcerative colitis that is refractory to nonsurgical treatment. Patients over age 30 years frequently also develop granulomatous colitis. Many over age 35 develop tubular kidney disease. Small papules with white centers resembling gouty tophi may be found on the palate in older patients. The storage material is not ceroid. It is found in bone marrow, lung, liver, cardiac muscle, spleen, colonic mucosa, kidney, bladder, urine sediment, and oral epithelium as a yellow granular pigment that fluoresces bright yellow under UV light.

**Complications:** Death may occur from hemorrhage, especially in patients taking aspirin or aspirin-like drugs that block prostaglandin synthesis following minor surgery such as tooth extraction or delivery. Several patients have developed a severe fatal colitis, especially after taking a proprietary antacid containing aspirin. Older patients have died from kidney failure and degenerative cardiac muscle disease. Gastric bleeding is frequent following aspirin ingestion. Severe sunburn following solar exposure may occur. Degenerative skin changes, solar keratoses, and basal cell and squamous cell carcinomas occur in patients over 30 years of age following prolonged solar exposure.

**Associated Findings:** None known.

**Etiology:** Autosomal recessive inheritance.

**Pathogenesis:** Undetermined. Probably represents the pleiotropic effect of a gene involving a metabolic step affecting pigmentation, the platelet storage pool, and accumulation of an unidentified storage material. Ultramicroscopic specimens of hairbulbs show pheomelanosomes with uneven pigmentation but tyrosinase activity in the Golgi apparatus. Hairbulbs incubated in l-tyrosine or l-dopa show increased pigmentation, and tyrosinase assay falls within normal limits. Platelet-rich plasma exposed to aggregating agents such as collagen and epinephrine show lack of secondary aggregation on nephalometry, have less than 1 dense body per 70 platelets (normal 1.4 dense bodies per platelet), have less than 10% normal levels of ADP and serotonin, but have a normal prostaglandin endoperoxide-generating system. Serotonin uptake by platelets is initally normal but is rapidly lost. The storage material is not ceroid, does not increase in urine following ingestion of a high polyunsaturated fat diet, and does not have an elemental analysis compatible with a lipid. Vitamins C and E levels in serum are normal. Circulating macrophages contain two types of inclusions, the yellow granular UV fluorescing material and a membrane-bound particle with a dense core and radiating fibrillar material similar to a pterydine pigment described in a species of tree frogs. Dermal melanocytes may contain macromelanosomes.

**MIM No.:** *20330

**POS No.:** 3245

**CDC No.:** 270.200

**Sex Ratio:** M1:Fl

**Occurrence:** Reported or observed in over 100 patients. All Puerto Rican albinos except two tested to date have this disorder. In the Arecibo-Aguadilla area of Puerto Rico, incidence is about 1:2,000. Occurs with high frequency in residents and families who trace ancestry to Appledorn, Holland or Madras, India.

**Risk of Recurrence for Patient's Sib:**
See Part I, *Mendelian Inheritance.*

**Risk of Recurrence for Patient's Child:**
See Part I, *Mendelian Inheritance.*

**Age of Detectability:** Childhood.

**Gene Mapping and Linkage:** Unknown.

**Prevention:** None known. Genetic counseling indicated.

**Treatment:** Avoid drugs that inhibit prostaglandin synthesis, such as aspirin and indomethacin. *Fatal bleeding has occurred after use of aspirin.* Platelet transfusion for surgery. Avoidance of sun exposure and use of sunscreens and visual aids are important.

**Prognosis:** With avoidance of solar exposure and aspirin-like drugs and treatment of premalignant skin lesions, prognosis is fair for a normal life span.

**Detection of Carrier:** Obligate heterozygotes have statistically significant lower levels of serotonin in platelets. The test is not reliable, however, because about 40% overlap the lower range of normal.

**Special Considerations:** The majority of retinofugal optic neurons that in normals arise in the temporal retina and course to the same side of the brain as the eye of origin do not do so in these patients but cross to the opposite side. They tend to have a completely crossed optic neuronal system. The geniculocortical tracts are rearranged, and optic tracts show a decussation defect at the superior olive. They lack the mechanism for binocular vision and do not benefit from early strabismus surgery, which in pigmented persons preserves a degree of binocularity of vision.

**Support Groups:** Philadelphia; National Organization for Albinism and Hypopigmentation (NOAH)

**References:**
Hermansky F, Pudlak P: Albinism associated with hemorrhagic diathesis and unusual pigmented reticular cells in the bone marrow: report of two cases with histochemical studies. Blood 1959; 14:162–169.
Garay SM, et al.: Hermansky-Pudlak syndrome: pulmonary manifestations of a ceroid storage disorder. Am J Med 1979; 66:737–747.
Schinella RA: Hermansky-Pudlak syndrome with granulomatous colitis. Ann Intern Med 1980; 92:20–23.
Witkop CJ Jr, et al.: Albinism and other disorders of pigment metabolism. In: Stanbury JB et al., eds: The metabolic basis of inherited disease, 5th ed. New York: McGraw-Hill, 1983:301.
Depinho RA, Kaplan KL: The Hermansky-Pudlak syndrome. Medicine 1985; 64:192–202.
Takahashi A, Yokoyama T: Hermansky-Pudlak syndrome with special reference to lysosomal dysfunction. Virchows Arch Path Anat 1984; 402:247–258.
Kinnear PE, Tuddenham EGD: Albinism with haemorrhagic diathesis. Brit J Ophthal 1985; 69:904–908.

WH004
WI043

James G. White
Carl J. Witkop, Jr.

## ALBINISM, OCULOCUTANEOUS, MINIMAL PIGMENT TYPE      2711

**Includes:**
> Albinism, oculocutaneous, type III
> Minimal pigment albanism

**Excludes:**
> **Albinism, oculocutaneous, Brown type** (2357)
> **Albinism, oculocutaneous, tyrosinase negative** (0034)
> **Albinism, oculocutaneous, tyrosinase positive** (0035)
> **Albinism, oculocutaneous, yellow mutant** (0036)
> **Albinism, oculocutaneous** (other)

**Major Diagnostic Criteria:** Extreme hypopigmentation of the hair, skin, and eyes at birth. Ocular features of albinism with nystagmus, reduced visual acuity, and foveal hypoplasia with no retinal pigment. Iris pigment develops in the first decade.

**Clinical Findings:** At birth, affected individuals have white hair, white skin with no pigmented birth marks, and very light blue irides. Nystagmus is present at birth or develops in the first three months of life, and bright light may be uncomfortable. The irides are translucent on globe transillumination. Visual acuity is reduced, which may result in poor fixation early in life or in holding objects close to the face for recognition. An alternating strabismus is usually present. The amount of retinal pigment is markedly reduced, and the choroidal vessels are visible throughout the retina, except for the perimacular region. The fovea is hypoplastic, and a normal foveal light reflex is absent.

Children with this condition appear to have **Albinism, oculocutaneous, tyrosinase negative** (type 1A) at birth. During the first decade, sparse-to-dense iris pigment develops, and the iris translucency may be reduced. The hair remains white or develops a faint yellow tint. The skin remains white and does not tan or freckle.

Clinical variability is demonstrated in the amount of iris pigment present. The first individual who was recognized with this type of oculocutaneous albinism developed a thin ring of pigment at the pupillary border and small clumps of pigment at the periphery of the iris at about age seven years. There are two affected third cousins in this family. One had dense iris pigment at age 21 months, while the other had no iris pigment at age six months.

This type of oculocutaneous albinism is recognized because of the clinical features and the results of the quantitative hairbulb tyrosinase activity assay. Affected individuals have very low or absent tyrosinase activity (mean, $0.02 \pm 0.03$ pmole of tyrosinase oxidized per 120 minutes per hairbulb). Parental values are characteristic. One parent will have very low tyrosinase activity (mean, $0.06 \pm 0.07$) and the other parent will have tyrosinase activity in the normal range (mean, $1.20 \pm 0.61$). With **Albinism, oculocutaneous, tyrosinase negative** (type 1B) or **Albinism, oculocutaneous, yellow mutant**, both parents will have very low or absent activity.

**Complications:** Photophobia, nystagmus, reduced visual acuity, and alternating strabismus are thought to be results of reduced melanin in the optic system during development. The skin is sensitive to ultraviolet radiation and burns on sun exposure. Cutaneous malignancy may develop with chronic sun exposure.

**Associated Findings:** None known.

**Etiology:** Autosomal recessive inheritance.

**Pathogenesis:** Thought to be the expression of two separate alleles affecting tyrosinase. The hypothesis is that the parent with the low hairbulb tyrosinase activity has one normal tyrosinase allele and one allele for **Albinism, oculocutaneous, tyrosinase negative** ($c^a/c^+$), while the parent with the activity in the normal range has one normal allele and one allele for minimal pigment oculocutaneous albinism ($c^{mp}/c^a$). The biochemical or molecular abnormality for the minimal pigment allele is unknown. The affected individual would be a genetic compound ($c^a/c^{mp}$).

**MIM No.:** 20328

**CDC No.:** 270.200

**Sex Ratio:** M1:F1

**Occurrence:** Five Caucasian families from Minnesota have been reported.

**Risk of Recurrence for Patient's Sib:**
See Part I, *Mendelian Inheritance.*

**Risk of Recurrence for Patient's Child:**
See Part I, *Mendelian Inheritance.*

**Age of Detectability:** At birth, using parental hairbulb tyrosinase assay.

**Gene Mapping and Linkage:** Unknown.

**Prevention:** None known. Genetic counseling indicated.

**Treatment:** Yearly ophthalmologic evaluation through school, then ophthalmologic care as needed. Skin protection with hats, long-sleeved shirts, and sun screen (No. 15 or greater).

**Prognosis:** Normal life span expected. Most likely will not have the vision required to be able to drive a car.

**Detection of Carrier:** Quantitative hairbulb tyrosinase activity assay for relatives of parent with low activity. None available for relatives of parent with activity in the normal range.

**Support Groups:** Philadelphia; National Organization for Albinism and Hypopigmentation (NOAH)

**References:**
King RA, et al.: Minimal pigment: a new type of oculocutaneous albinism. Clin Genet 1986; 29:42–50.

KI007      **Richard A. King**

**Albinism, oculocutaneous, red type**
*See ALBINISM, OCULOCUTANEOUS, RUFOUS TYPE*

## ALBINISM, OCULOCUTANEOUS, RUFOUS TYPE      2358

**Includes:**
> Albinism, oculocutaneous, red type
> Albinism, oculocutaneous, type V
> Rufous albinism
> Xanthism
> "Xanthous negros"

**Excludes:**
> **Albinism, oculocutaneous, Brown type** (2357)
> **Albinism, oculocutaneous, tyrosinase positive** (0035)
> **Albinism, oculocutaneous, yellow mutant** (0036)

**Major Diagnostic Criteria:** White skin. Red to red-brown hair. Hazel to brown irides with patchy transillumination, especially basal, and the ocular features of albinism including nystagmus, reduced visual acuity, reduced retinal pigment, and foveal hypoplasia.

**Clinical Findings:** Clinical features have been incompletely described in only a few individuals. In affected Caucasian individuals, the skin is white at birth. Freckles and lentigines develop on sun-exposed surfaces with time, and a minimal tan develops. The hair is light red at birth, turning bright red and then red-brown (auburn) usually in postadolescence. The irides are hazel-green at birth, turn hazel to brown with time, and show moderate transillumination defects. Retinal pigment is reduced, especially in the periphery, and the fovea is hypoplastic. Corrected visual acuity is reduced (20/60 to 20/200). The phenotype in blacks has not been adequately described; biochemical or morphologic studies are not available.

**Complications:** Nystagmus, reduced visual acuity, and an alternating strabismus are thought to be the results of a reduced amount of melanin in the optic system during development. The skin burns after sun exposure, and may be more susceptible to the development of skin cancer with age.

**Associated Findings:** None known.

**Etiology:** Probably autosomal recessive inheritance.

**Pathogenesis:** Unknown.

**MIM No.:**  27840

**POS No.:**  3536

**CDC No.:**  270.200

**Sex Ratio:**  Presumably M1:F1.

**Occurrence:**  Undetermined but presumed rare.

**Risk of Recurrence for Patient's Sib:**
See Part I, *Mendelian Inheritance.*

**Risk of Recurrence for Patient's Child:**
See Part I, *Mendelian Inheritance.*

**Age of Detectability:**  At birth.

**Gene Mapping and Linkage:**  Unknown.

**Prevention:**  None known. Genetic counseling indicated.

**Treatment:**  Yearly ophthalmologic evaluation and refractive correction (probably with bifocals and sometimes low vision magnification) through school, then ophthalmologic care as appropriate. Skin protection with sun screens, long sleeves, and hats.

**Prognosis:**  Normal life span.

**Detection of Carrier:**  Unknown.

**Special Considerations:**  The term *red* or *rufous* oculocutaneous albinism should be limited to an individual with hypopigmented skin, red or red-brown hair, and all of the ocular features of albinism.

A form of congenital nystagmus associated with red skin has been described in the Eastern Highlands population of New Guinea. Approximately 1.5–2.0% of the population had bronze-red skin, and 58% of those with red skin had nystagmus. Hair color ranged from light brown to black rather than being red or auburn. Visual acuity was normal, as was retinal pigment and foveal development. The red skin was inherited as an autosomal recessive trait. Individuals with red skin, described as *xanthous negros*, have also been described in Africa in the older literature. Red skin with or without congenital nystagmus does not appear to represent a type of albinism, because the visual acuity and the fovea are normal.

**Support Groups:**  Philadelphia; National Organization for Albinism and Hypopigmentation (NOAH)

**References:**
Pearson K, et al.: The rufous albino. In: A monograph on albinism. Draper's Company Research Memoirs, Biometric Series VIII. London: Dulau, 1913:329–333.
Barnicot NA: Human pigmentation. Man 1957; 57:114–120.
Walsh RJ: A distinctive pigment of the skin in New Guinea indigenes. Ann Hum Genet 1971; 34:379–385.
Hornabrook RW: Congenital nystagmus among the red-skins of the Highlands of Papua, New Guinea. Br J Ophthalmol 1980; 64:375–380.

KI007                                                        **Richard A. King**
LE039                                                    **Richard Alan Lewis**

**Albinism, oculocutaneous, type IB**
*See ALBINISM, OCULOCUTANEOUS, YELLOW MUTANT*
**Albinism, oculocutaneous, type II**
*See ALBINISM, OCULOCUTANEOUS, TYROSINASE POSITIVE*
**Albinism, oculocutaneous, type III**
*See ALBINISM, OCULOCUTANEOUS, MINIMAL PIGMENT TYPE*
**Albinism, oculocutaneous, type IV**
*See ALBINISM, OCULOCUTANEOUS, BROWN TYPE*
**Albinism, oculocutaneous, type V**
*See ALBINISM, OCULOCUTANEOUS, RUFOUS TYPE*
**Albinism, oculocutaneous, type VI**
*See ALBINISM, OCULOCUTANEOUS, HERMANSKY-PUDLAK TYPE*

## ALBINISM, OCULOCUTANEOUS, TYROSINASE NEGATIVE                                0034

**Includes:**
Albinism oculocutaneous, type IA
Albinism, tyrosinase negative, oculocutaneous
Tyrosinase negative oculocutaneous albinism

**Excludes:**
**Albinism, cutaneous** (0031)
**Albinism, ocular** (0032)
**Albinism, oculocutaneous, Hermansky-Pudlak type** (0033)
**Albinism, oculocutaneous, tyrosinase positive** (0035)
**Albinism, oculocutaneous, yellow mutant** (0036)
**Chediak-Higashi syndrome** (0143)

**Major Diagnostic Criteria:**  Absent pigmentation of all of the skin, hair, and eyes with nystagmus, photophobia, and a red reflex in a patient whose hairbulbs do not form pigment when incubated in l-tyrosine solution.

**Clinical Findings:**  A severe lack of pigmentation is found in the skin, hair, and eyes. Nystagmus, photophobia, and a prominent red reflex occur because of the lack of pigmentation. There is no visible pigment in these structures, the fundus is unpigmented, and the iris diaphanous is without a cartwheel effect on transillumination. Iris color is blue to gray-blue in oblique light but may have a pinkish color when viewed in light reflected from the fundus. Hair, skin, and eye color is the same in all racial backgrounds and does not change with age. Hair is dead white but may have a light yellow cast after exposure to sunlight. Skin is pink-red and shows no tanning. A prominent red reflex is present and does not vary with age or race of the subject. Pigmented nevi and freckles are absent. Nystagmus and photophobia are severe. Visual acuity is impaired for both near and far vision, usually 20/200 or worse, and does not improve with age. Other eye abnormalities occur, but their exact frequency in the ty-neg albino must be reevaluated. (See **Albinism, oculocutaneous, tyrosinase positive [0035]**.) The macular reflex is absent. This

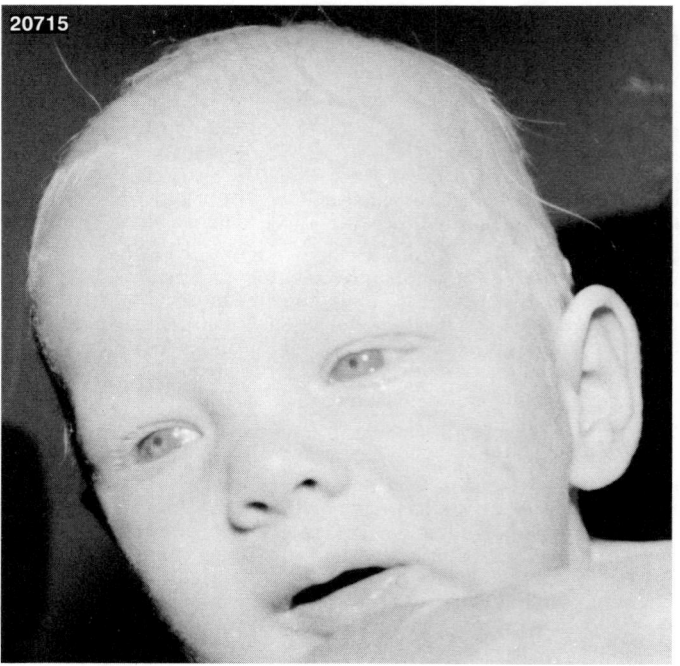

**0034-20715:**  Albinism, oculocutaneous tyrosinase negative; note white hair and translucent, pink irides.

phenotype cannot always be distinguished from some Caucasian ty-pos albinos by clinical criteria. Patients lack binocular vision.

**Complications:**    Increased susceptibility to skin cancer (basal cell, squamous cell or basosquamous carcinoma).

**Associated Findings:**    Albinos have been reported with a number of anomalies such as cleft palate, pretragal ear pits, deafness, and oligophrenia, or have developed malignant melanomas, but these traits either segregate separately in kindreds or do not appear in albinos in a frequency greater than chance expectation.

**Etiology:**    Autosomal recessive inheritance.

**Pathogenesis:**    Absence of the enzyme tyrosinase in melanocytes causing a block in the pathway for melanogenesis at the steps l-tyrosine→l-dopa→dopaquinone and from 5,6-dihydroxy-indole→indole-5,6-quinone, which results in the production of unpigmented premelanosomes (premelanosomes stage II) but none beyond this stage. Stage II unpigmented premelanosomes are passed to keratinocytes but are not effective in increasing protective pigmentation.

**MIM No.:**    *20310

**POS No.:**    3536

**CDC No.:**    270.200

**Sex Ratio:**    M1:F1

**Occurrence:**    Caucasians, 1:39,000; American blacks, 1:28,000. Not observed to date in American Indians.

**Risk of Recurrence for Patient's Sib:**
See Part I, *Mendelian Inheritance.*

**Risk of Recurrence for Patient's Child:**
See Part I, *Mendelian Inheritance.* (Chances 1:99 for Caucasian, 1:84 for American black.)

**Age of Detectability:**    At birth by physical examination, hairbulb incubation test, and tyrosinase assay.

**Gene Mapping and Linkage:**    ATN (albinism, tyrosinase-negative (?=TYR)) is ULG5.

TYR (tyrosinase) has been provisionally mapped to 11q14-q21.

Tyrosinase-negative oculocutaneous albinism (OCA) is allelic with yellow-mutant OCA.

**Prevention:**    None known. Genetic counseling indicated.

**Treatment:**    Avoidance of exposure to sunlight, protective clothing, and sun screen lotions. Tinted glasses or contact lenses and low-vision aids may be needed.

**Prognosis:**    Is compatible with long life, but longevity is probably reduced somewhat in general due to susceptibility to skin cancer and higher risk for accidents due to poor vision. Most are legally blind with visual acuity 20/200 or worse.

**Detection of Carrier:**    Tyrosinase activity in hairbulbs is essentially zero in heterozygotes by the King method.

**Special Considerations:**    Oculocutaneous albinos of all types have absent or decreased ipsilateral retinogeniculate nerve tracts, reorganization of geniculocortical tracts, and decussation defect in auditory tract at the superior olive. Binocular vision is absent or decreased.

**Support Groups:**    Philadelphia; National Organization for Albinism and Hypopigmentation (NOAH)

**References:**

Witkop CJ Jr, et al.: Autosomal recessive oculocutaneous albinism in man: evidence for genetic heterogeneity. Am J Hum Genet 1970; 22:55.

Creel D, et al.: Asymmetric visually evoked potentials in various types of human oculocutaneous albinos: evidence for anatomic abnormalities of the optic tract. Invest Ophthalmol 1974; 13:430–440.

King RA, Witkop CJ Jr: Detection of heterozygotes for tyrosinase-negative oculocutaneous albinism by hairbulb tyrosinase assay. Am J Hum Genet 1977; 29:164–168.

Creel D, et al.: Auditory brainstem anomalies in human albinos. Science 1980; 209:1253–1255.

Witkop CJ Jr: Inherited disorders of pigmentation. Clinics in dermatology, vol. 3. Philadelphia: Lippincott 1985:70–134. †

Witkop CJ Jr, et al.: Albinism. In Scriver CR, et al. (eds): The Metabolic Basis of Inherited Disease. 6th ed, New York: McGraw-Hill, 1988, chapter 118. *

WI043                                                                **Carl J. Witkop, Jr.**

## ALBINISM, OCULOCUTANEOUS, TYROSINASE POSITIVE                                        0035

**Includes:**

Albinism, oculocutaneous, type II
Albinism, tyrosinase positive oculocutaneous
Tyrosinase positive oculocutaneous albinism

**Excludes:**

**Albinism, cutaneous** (0031)
**Albinism, ocular** (0032)
**Albinism, oculocutaneous, Hermansky-Pudlak type** (0033)
**Albinism, oculocutaneous, tyrosinase negative** (0034)
**Albinism, oculocutaneous, yellow mutant** (0036)
**Chediak-Higashi syndrome** (0143)
**Chediak-Higashi syndrome** (0143)

**Major Diagnostic Criteria:**    Decreased pigment throughout the skin, hair, and eyes, with nystagmus and photophobia in a patient whose hairbulbs form pigment when incubated in tyrosine solution.

**Clinical Findings:**    Decreased pigment is found throughout the skin, hair, and eyes in a patient with nystagmus and photophobia. The amount of visible pigment in this type of albino varies with age and race. The clinical pigment characteristics overlap those of **Albinism, oculocutaneous, tyrosinase negative** (ty-neg) on the one hand and **Albinism, oculocutaneous, yellow mutant** and normal lightly pigmented individuals on the other. There is a gradual accumulation of pigment with age so that the patient may give a history of a change in eye color from blue to yellow-hazel or brown, and in hair color from white to cream, tan, or light brown. Nystagmus and photophobia are marked but less severe than in the ty-neg type. In all infants a red reflex is easily elicited, which is lost in older children from deeply pigmented populations but may be retained in adult Caucasians. Funduscopically the retina of infants, children, and adult Caucasians appears to have no pigment, but in older children and adults from deeply pigmented populations appears typically blond. Diaphanous irides are present in all patients, and on transillumination, a cartwheel effect may be noted due to pigment at the pupil border and limbus. Visual acuity is decreased usually 20/200 or worse in children but may improve with age so adults may have 20/100 or better.

Increased frequency of eye defects is found in this type: absent or markedly diminished foveal reflex (98%); mesodermal remnants on anterior suface of iris and posterior suface of corneal (25%); strabismus, usually esotropia (60%); high-grade myopia (30%); pigmented nevi and freckles (60%); absent binocular vision (100%).

**Complications:**    Susceptibility to skin neoplasia and basal cell, squamous cell, and basosquamous carcinomas.

**Associated Findings:**    Albinos have been reported with a number of other anomalies such as cleft palate, pretragal ear pits, deafness, sickle cell trait, and oligophrenia, or have developed malignant melanomas. These traits either segregate in kindreds or do not appear in albinos in a frequency greater than chance expectation.

**Etiology:**    Autosomal recessive inheritance.

**Pathogenesis:**    Undetermined. Melanocytes can utilize tyrosine to form normal-appearing pigment in vitro. Serum tyrosine levels are normal. Hairbulb tyrosinase levels are either normal or markedly elevated, suggesting heterogeneity. Site of the block is unknown.

**MIM No.:**    *20320

**POS No.:**    3536

**CDC No.:**    270.200

**Sex Ratio:**    M1:F1

**Occurrence:** Caucasian, 1:37,000; American black, 1:15,000; American Indian varies by tribe from 1:85 to 1:6500 at birth in Southern and Southwestern tribes. Nigerians (Ibo) 1:1,200.

**Risk of Recurrence for Patient's Sib:**
See Part I, *Mendelian Inheritance.*

**Risk of Recurrence for Patient's Child:**
See Part I, *Mendelian Inheritance.*

**Age of Detectability:** At birth to neonatal period by clinical examination and hairbulb incubation test.

**Gene Mapping and Linkage:** Undetermined. Matings of tyrosinase-negative and tyrosinase-positive albinos, as well as of tyrosinase-positive and Hermansky-Pudlak albinos, are each complementary. The gene loci are different.

**Prevention:** None known. Genetic counseling indicated.

**Treatment:** Avoidance of exposure to sunlight. Protective skin creams and clothing. Tinted glasses or contact lenses with tinted iris. Low vision aids.

**Prognosis:** Good. Most are legally blind, exceeding 20/200, in childhood but may improve with age. Longevity probably somewhat reduced by susceptibility to skin cancer and accidents secondary to poor vision.

**Detection of Carrier:** Undetermined. Obligate carriers as a group do not have a higher frequency of diaphanous irides on transillumination than controls. Tyrosinase values in hairbulbs fall within the normal ranges for hair color.

**Special Considerations:** Oculocutaneous albinos of all types have absent or decreased ipsilateral retinogeniculate nerve tracts, reorganization of geniculocortical tracts, and a decussation defect in otic tracts at the level of the superior olive. Binocular vision is decreased or absent.

**Support Groups:** Philadelphia; National Organization for Albinism and Hypopigmentation (NOAH)

**References:**

Witkop CJ Jr, et al.: Autosomal recessive oculocutaneous albinism in man: evidence for genetic heterogeneity. Am J Hum Genet 1970; 22:55–74.

Creel D, et al.: Asymmetric visually evoked potentials in various types of human oculocutaneous albinos: evidence for anatomic abnormalities of the optic tract. J Invest Ophthalmol 1974; 13:430–440.

Guillery RW, et al.: Abnormal visual pathways in the brain of a human albino. Brain Res 1975; 96:373–377.

Creel D, et al.: Auditory brainstem anomalies in human albinos. Science 1980; 209:1253–1255.

Witkop CJ Jr: Inherited disorders of pigmentation. Clinics in dermatology, vol. 3. Philadelphia: Lippincott 1985:70–134. †

Witkop CJ Jr, et al.: Albinism. In Scriver CR, et al. (eds): The Metabolic Basis of Inherited Disease. 6th ed, New York: McGraw-Hill, 1988, chapter 118. *

WI043                              **Carl J. Witkop, Jr.**

---

## ALBINISM, OCULOCUTANEOUS, YELLOW MUTANT     0036

**Includes:**
Albinism, oculocutaneous, type IB
Albinism, yellow mutant oculocutaneous
Amish albinism
Yellow mutant oculocutaneous albinism

**Excludes:**
**Albinism, ocular** (0032)
**Albinism, oculocutaneous, Hermansky-Pudlak type** (0033)
**Albinism, oculocutaneous, tyrosinase negative** (0034)
**Albinism, oculocutaneous, tyrosinase positive** (0035)
**Chediak-Higashi syndrome** (0143)
**Gingival fibromatosis-depigmentation-microphthalmia** (0413)

**Major Diagnostic Criteria:** All of the skin, hair, and eyes are depigmented. Patients have a weak but distinct tanning on exposure to sunlight. Adult hair color is yellow to yellow-red. Nystagmus and photophobia are present. The hairbulbs contain

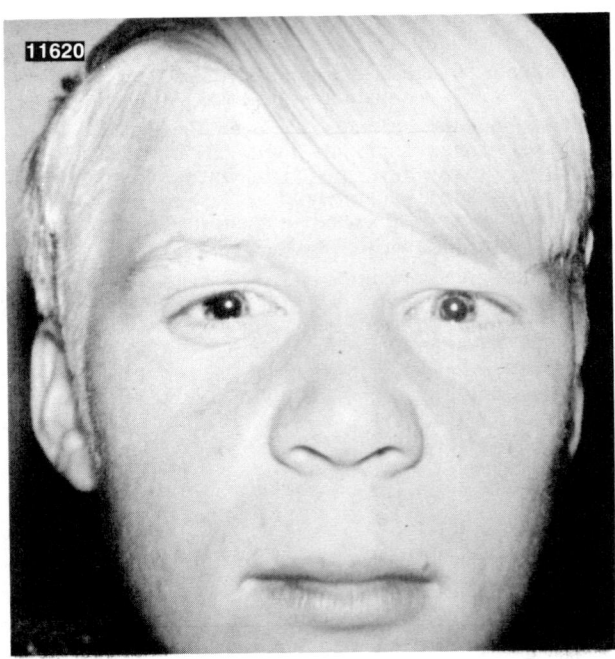

0036-11620: Pale yellow hair and light irides in a male with yellow mutant albinism.

some pigment but they do not increase in pigment upon incubation in l-tyrosine solution. Pheomelanin is increased when incubated with l-tyrosine and l-cysteine.

**Clinical Findings:** Depigmentation of all the skin, hair, and eyes occurs with nystagmus and photophobia. At birth, children have snow-white hair, pink skin, gray-blue translucent irides, a prominent red reflex, and a pigment-free fundus. At this time, they have a marked photophobia and nystagmus. During the first few months of life there is a gradual increase in pigment so that by 2 years of age the hair is flaxen yellow to bright yellow-brown, often with a red tint. Older children have a mild-to-moderate horizontal or rotary nystagmus, profound retinal depigmentation, and a prominent red reflex. The eye color darkens with age, so adults may have dark blue irides. Skin tanning occurs after 2 years of age but is less than that of most normal red-haired individuals. Skin sensitivity to actinic radiation is not a marked feature of this type. Visual acuity is markedly defective usually from 20/100 to 20/400. Black children have very light yellow-brown hair at birth, which rapidly becomes cream-brown to light reddish brown by 1 year of age. Older black children and adults have brown eyes with diaphanous irides, moderate nystagmus and photophobia, and light brown skin. Older children and adults are frequently mistaken for ocular albinos. Absent or markedly decreased binocular vision is found.

**Complications:** Undetermined. Probably susceptibility to skin cancer, but not enough subjects have been observed to substantiate this.

**Associated Findings:** Probably none; 1 of 22 subjects had a ventricular septal defect.

**Etiology:** Autosomal recessive inheritance.

**Pathogenesis:** Essentially unknown. Patients have peripheral melanocytes, which appear to be normal in number and distribution. Melanocytes contain numerous round-to-ovoid and few elongated stage III premelanosomes, which show irregular pigmentation of matrix resembling that seen in normal yellow and red hair. Hairbulbs do not form black eumelanin when incubated with various combinations of tyrosine, dopa, or copper. When cysteine and tyrosine are added, there is an intensification of yellow color. Hairbulb tyrosinase varies from zero to 0.10 pm/120 min/hairbulb.

**MIM No.:** 20332

**POS No.:** 3536

**CDC No.:** 270.200

**Sex Ratio:** M1:F1

**Occurrence:** Rare; by indirect estimates 1:125,000. High frequency among Amish.

**Risk of Recurrence for Patient's Sib:**
See Part I, *Mendelian Inheritance.*

**Risk of Recurrence for Patient's Child:**
See Part I, *Mendelian Inheritance.*

**Age of Detectability:** At birth by physical examination, hairbulb incubation test, and tyrosinase assay.

**Gene Mapping and Linkage:** Allelic with tyrosinase-negative OCA.

**Prevention:** None known. Genetic counseling indicated.

**Treatment:** Tinted glasses or contact lenses and low vision aids may be recommended.

**Prognosis:** It is essentially unknown; probably slight reduction in longevity. Most patients are legally blind, 20/200 or worse.

**Detection of Carrier:** Abnormal iris translucency not found in majority of heterozygotes. Ym is allelic with ty-neg. Carriers have low values of tyrosinase activity using the King method of tyrosinase assay.

**Special Considerations:** Oculocutaneous albinos of all types have absent or decreased ipsilateral retinogeniculate nerve tracts, reorganization of geniculocortical tracts, and a defect in otic tracts at the level of the superior olive. Binocular vision is decreased or absent. Ym albinism is allelic with ty-neg albinism.

**Support Groups:** Philadelphia; National Organization for Albinism and Hypopigmentation (NOAH)

**References:**
Nance WE, et al.: Amish albinism: a distinctive autosomal recessive phenotype. Am J Hum Genet 1970; 22:579–586.
Creel D, et al.: Asymmetric visually evoked potentials in various types of human oculocutaneous albinos: evidence for anatomic abnormalities of the optic tract. Invest Ophthalmol 1974; 13:430–440.
Creel D, et al.: Auditory brainstem anomalies in human albinos. Science 1980; 209:1253–1255.
Hu F, et al.: Yellow mutant albinism: cytochemical, ultrastructural, and genetic characterization suggesting multiple allelism. Am J Hum Genet 1980; 32:387–395.
Witkop CJ Jr: Inherited disorders of pigmentation. Clinics in dermatology, vol. 3. Philadelphia: Lippincott 1985:70–134. †
Witkop CJ Jr, et al.: Albinism. In Scriver CR, et al. (eds): The Metabolic Basis of Inherited Disease. 6th ed, New York: McGraw-Hill, 1988, chapter 118. *

WI043                                                          **Carl J. Witkop, Jr.**

**Albinism, partial**
*See ALBINOIDISM*
**Albinism, tyrosinase negative, oculocutaneous**
*See ALBINISM, OCULOCUTANEOUS, TYROSINASE NEGATIVE*
**Albinism, tyrosinase positive oculocutaneous**
*See ALBINISM, OCULOCUTANEOUS, TYROSINASE POSITIVE*

## ALBINISM, WAARDENBURG TYPE-HIRSCHSPRUNG AGANGLIONOSIS                                          2823

**Includes:**
Aganglionic megalcolon-albanism
Albinism-Hirschsprung agangliosis
Colon, aganglionosis-pigmentary anomaly
Hirschsprung agangliosis-albinism
Pigmentary anomaly-colon, aganglionosis
Shah-Waardenburg syndrome
Waardenburg-Shah syndrome
Waardenburg syndrome variant

**Excludes:** Waardenburg syndromes (0997)

**Major Diagnostic Criteria:** The combination of congenital white forelock, heterochromia irides, and long-segment Hirschsprung disease (see **Colon, aganglionosis**) helps to distinguish this condition from similar disorders.

**Clinical Findings:** In one report, all affected infants had white forelock, white eyebrows, and white eyelashes. Intestinal obstruction occurred neonatally, caused by long-segment Hirschsprung disease. Heterochromia irides was present in more than 50% of affected infants. However, dystopia canthorum and broad nasal root were not present in any of the examined infants. One child in another family had white forelock, telecanthus, mild deafness, and Hirschsprung disease; another child had white forelock, **Eye, hypertelorism**, pale irides, Hirschsprung disease, and suspected deafness; and a pair or sibs had bicolor irides and Hirschsprung disease only.

**Complications:** Failure of the ileostomy, leading to death.

**Associated Findings:** None known.

**Etiology:** The presence of consanguinity in three families suggests autosomal recessive inheritance.

**Pathogenesis:** The basic defect is likely one of neural crest cell migration.

**MIM No.:** 27758

**POS No.:** 4100

**Sex Ratio:** Presumably M1:F1.

**Occurrence:** Reported in 12 members of five families from India, and in at least four other families from other parts of the World.

**Risk of Recurrence for Patient's Sib:**
See Part I, *Mendelian Inheritance.*

**Risk of Recurrence for Patient's Child:**
See Part I, *Mendelian Inheritance.*

**Age of Detectability:** In the neonatal period by the presence of Hirschsprung disease.

**Gene Mapping and Linkage:** Unknown.

**Prevention:** None known. Genetic counseling indicated.

**Treatment:** Unknown. Surgical intervention has usually not been effective.

**Prognosis:** Variable for life span, although most affected infants have died within a few months of birth.

**Detection of Carrier:** Unknown.

**Special Considerations:** Shah et al (1981) reported five families; all delineated by the presence of one infant with a white forelock, heterochromia irides, and **Colon, aganglionosis**. However, although in one family there is no other history of similarly affected individuals, in two there is a history of heterochromia irides in a parent and others and in two others the pattern of affected relatives is more consistent with autosomal dominant inheritance and thus a diagnosis of **Waardenburg syndromes**. Therefore, the existence of an autosomal recessive condition characterized by white forelock, heterochromia irides, and Hirschsprung disease should be viewed as tentative.

**Support Groups:** Philadelphia; National Organization for Albinism and Hypopigmentation (NOAH)

**References:**
Branski D, et al.: Hirschsprung's disease and Waardenburg's syndrome. Pediatrics 1979; 63:803–804.
Shah KN, et al.: White forelock, pigmentary disorder of irides, and long segment Hirschsprung disease: possible variant of Waardenburg syndrome. J Pediatr 1981; 99:432–435.
Ambani LM: Waardenburg and Hirschsprung syndromes. J Pediatr 1983; 102:802 only.
Farrdon PA, Bianchi A: Waardenburg's syndrome associated with total agangliosis. Arch Dis Child 1983; 58:932–933.
Liang JC, et al.: Bilateral bicolored irides with Hirschsprung's disease: a neural crest syndrome. Arch Ophthal 1983; 101:69–73.

T0007                                    **Helga V. Toriello**

---

**Albinism, yellow mutant oculocutaneous**
*See ALBINISM, OCULOCUTANEOUS, YELLOW MUTANT*

---

## ALBINISM-BLACK LOCKS-DEAFNESS                    2356

**Includes:**
   BADS syndrome
   Deafness-albinism-block locks
   Ermine phenotype
   Hair (black)-albinism-deafness

**Excludes:**
   Albinism, cutaneous-deafness (0030)
   Albinism, Ocular late onset-sensorineural deafness, X-linked (2824)
   Waardenburg syndromes (0997)

**Major Diagnostic Criteria:** White skin, white hair with patches of black hair, ocular features of albinism, and deafness. Intellectual development normal or delayed.

**Clinical Findings:** The skin, hair, and eyes are similar to **Albinism, oculocutaneous, tyrosinase negative,** except for the presence of one or more patches of pigmented hair on the scalp and light café-au-lait spots on the extremities and trunk, which develop after birth. The hypopigmented hair and skin are white. Blue, translucent irides are associated with nystagmus, photophobia, reduced visual acuity, foveal hypoplasia, and no retinal pigment. Profound congenital sensorineural hearing loss and poor speech development are present. Intellectual development is normal or delayed, and the delay may be secondary to severe sensory deprivation and isolation rather than a primary developmental defect. No biochemical or morphologic studies have been published.

**Complications:** Nystagmus, reduced visual acuity, and foveal hypoplasia are thought to be the result of a reduced amount of melanin in the optic system during development. The skin burns after sun exposure and may be more susceptible to the development of skin cancer with time.

**Associated Findings:** None known.

**Etiology:** Probably autosomal recessive inheritance.

**Pathogenesis:** Unknown.

**CDC No.:** 270.200

**Sex Ratio:** Presumably M1:F1.

**Occurrence:** Undetermined but presumably rare. The original case described by Pearson et al. (1911). Brief descriptions of several other cases have been published (Witkop, 1985). One family was evaluated by King (unpublished) in Minnesota.

**Risk of Recurrence for Patient's Sib:**
   See Part I, *Mendelian Inheritance.*

**Risk of Recurrence for Patient's Child:**
   See Part I, *Mendelian Inheritance.*

**Age of Detectability:** At birth to the first few months of life.

**Gene Mapping and Linkage:** Unknown.

**Prevention:** None known. Genetic counseling indicated.

**Treatment:** Regular ophthalmologic evaluation. Skin protection with long sleeves, hats, and sun screen (No. 15 and above). Speech therapy. Special education for developmental delay.

**Prognosis:** Unknown. Physical and developmental handicaps will alter life-style.

**Detection of Carrier:** Unknown.. One heterozygote had irregular iris translucency with irregular areas of fundus hypo- and hyper-pigmentation. Hairbulb tyrosinase activity is normal, with pigmented hairs from obligate heterozygotes.

**Special Considerations:** Witkop (1985) has reported that melanocytes are absent from the white skin and hairbulbs, while the pigmented skin and hairbulbs contain melanocytes. He hypothesized that this condition is the result of abnormal melanocyte migration or survival. The normal tyrosinase activity in the obligate heterozygote hairbulbs supports this hypothesis, since heterozygotes for the types of albinism that are the result of abnormal tyrosinase function have low hairbulb tyrosinase activity.

**Support Groups:** Philadelphia; National Organization for Albinism and Hypopigmentation (NOAH)

**References:**
Pearson K, et al.: A monograph on albinism in man. Draper's Company Research Memoirs, Biometric Series VI. London: Dulan, 1911.
Witkop CJ, Jr.: Inherited disorders of pigmentation. Clin Dermatol 1985; 3:70–134.
O'Doherty NJ, Gorlin RJ: The ermine phenotype: pigmentary-hearing loss heterogeneity. Am J Med Genet 1988; 30:945–952.

KI007                                    **Richard A. King**

---

**Albinism-hemorrhagic diathesis-pigmented reticuloendothelial cells**
*See ALBINISM, OCULOCUTANEOUS, HERMANSKY-PUDLAK TYPE*
**Albinism-Hirschsprung agangliosis**
*See ALBINISM, WAARDENBURG TYPE-HIRSCHSPRUNG AGANGLIONOSIS*

---

## ALBINISM-MICROCEPHALY-DIGITAL DEFECTS          2781

**Includes:**
   Digital defects-albinism-microcephaly
   Microcephaly-albinism-digital defects

**Excludes:**
   Albinism, oculocutaneous, tyrosinase negative (0034)
   Albinism, oculocutaneous, tyrosinase positive (0035)
   Coffin-Siris syndrome (2025)
   Oro-cranio-digital syndrome (0769)

**Major Diagnostic Criteria:** The combination of **Albinism, Microcephaly,** and digital anomalies.

**Clinical Findings:** Affected children have normal birth weight, but congenital **Microcephaly.** Albinism is of the oculocutaneous type. Digital anomalies consist of hypoplasia or aplasia of the distal phalanges. In addition, micrognathia is present, and tone is increased. CT scans demonstrate cortical atrophy.

**Complications:** Unknown.

**Associated Findings:** None known.

**Etiology:** Possibly autosomal recessive inheritance.

**Pathogenesis:** Unknown.

**MIM No.:** 20334

**POS No.:** 3805

**Sex Ratio:** M1:F1

**Occurrence:** Reported in a brother and sister.

**Risk of Recurrence for Patient's Sib:**
   See Part I, *Mendelian Inheritance.*

**Risk of Recurrence for Patient's Child:**
   See Part I, *Mendelian Inheritance.*

**Age of Detectability:** At birth, by physical examination.

**Gene Mapping and Linkage:** Unknown.

**Prevention:** None known. Genetic counseling indicated.

**Treatment:** Unknown.

**Prognosis:** One sib died at age one month; the other had severe mental retardation when examined at age four months.

**Detection of Carrier:** Unknown.

**Support Groups:** Philadelphia; National Organization for Albinism and Hypopigmentation (NOAH)

**References:**
Castro-Gago M, et al.: Sindrome familiar de microcefalia con albinismo oculocutaneo y anomalias digitales. An Esp Pediatr 1983; 19:128–131.

T0007                                       **Helga V. Toriello**

## ALBINOIDISM                               2359

**Includes:**
> Albinism, partial
> Cutaneous albinism
> Cutaneous hypomelanosis
> Cutaneous hypopigmentation
> Dilution, pigmentary
> Hypopigmentation
> Oculocutaneous albinoidism

**Excludes:**
> **Albinism, cutaneous** (0031)
> **Albinism, oculocutaneous** (all forms)
> **Skin, vitiligo** (0993)

**Major Diagnostic Criteria:** Congenital reduction in melanin pigment in the hair and skin in the absence of ocular features of albinism.

**Clinical Findings:** Generalized hypopigmentation of the skin and hair is present throughout life and is often obvious only after comparison with normally pigmented family members. There may be an increase of skin and hair pigment with time. Hair color ranges from light blond to brown. The skin is fair and will burn on sun exposure. A minimal tan may develop. Iris and retinal pigment are normal or reduced, and the iris may be translucent, but the ocular features of albinism, including nystagmus, photophobia, reduced visual acuity, and foveal hypoplasia, are absent. It is sometimes hard to distinguish hypopigmentation from the normal familial variation in pigmentation.

**Complications:** Sunburn on exposure to the sun. Probable increased risk for skin cancer with prolonged sun exposure.

**Associated Findings:** None known.

**Etiology:** At least two families with autosomal dominant albinoidism have been reported. One family with autosomal dominant albinoidism associated with deaf-mutism has been described (Tietz, 1963), but the true phenotype of this family has been disputed (Reed et al., 1967). Sporadic cases of unknown etiology have been reported.

**Pathogenesis:** It is possible that albinoidism is a defect in melanin formation limited to the neural crest-derived melanocytes (skin, hair follicle, iris stroma, choroid), without involvement of the neuroectodermally derived melanocytes (retinal pigment epithelium, ciliary body).

**MIM No.:** 12607

**Sex Ratio:** Presumably M1:F1.

**Occurrence:** Undetermined but presumed rare.

**Risk of Recurrence for Patient's Sib:**
See Part I, *Mendelian Inheritance.*

**Risk of Recurrence for Patient's Child:**
See Part I, *Mendelian Inheritance.*

**Age of Detectability:** At birth or within the first decade of life. Hypopigmentation may not be obvious until the normal onset of mature pigmentation, which usually occurs after ages 3–5 years, or after adequate sun exposure reveals reduced tanning.

**Gene Mapping and Linkage:** Unknown.

**Prevention:** None known. Genetic counseling indicated.

**Treatment:** Skin protection with sun screen (No. 15 and above); long sleeves and hats if sensitive to the UV radiation of the sun.

**Prognosis:** Normal life span.

**Detection of Carrier:** Unknown.

**Special Considerations:** *Albinoidism* is a poorly defined term and should only be used in cases of cutaneous hypopigmentation after a complete ophthalmologic examination has shown normal foveal development and normal corrected visual acuity. Biochemical quantitation of melanin pathway components may be necessary to characterize this condition.

**References:**
Cockayne EA: Inherited abnormalities of the skin and its appendages. Oxford: University Press, 1933.
Tietz W: A syndrome of deaf-mutism associated with albinism showing dominant autosomal inheritance. Am J Hum Genet 1963; 15:259–264.
Reed WB, et al.: Pigmentary disorders in association with congenital deafness. Arch Dermatol 1967; 95:176–186.
Donaldson DD: Transillumination of the iris. Trans Am Ophthalmol Soc 1974; 72:89–106.
Fitzpatrick TB, et al.: Dominant oculo-cutaneous albinism. Br J Dermatol (suppl 10) 1974; 91:23 only.
Ortonne JP, et al.: Vitiligo and other hypomelanoses of hair and skin. New York: Plenum, 1983:89.

KI007                                     **Richard A. King**

**Albopapuloid dominant dystrophic epidermolysis bullosa**
*See EPIDERMOLYSIS BULLOSUM, TYPE III*
**Albrecht syndrome**
*See DEAFNESS (SENSORINEURAL), PROGRESSIVE HIGH-TONE*
**Albright hereditary osteodystrophy**
*See PARATHYROID HORMONE RESISTANCE*
**Albright syndrome**
*See FIBROUS DYSPLASIA, POLYOSTOTIC*
**Albumin**
*See ANALBUMINEMIA*

## ALCOHOL INTOLERANCE                          3074

**Includes:**
> Acetaldehyde dehydrogenase-2 (ALDH2) deficiency
> Alcohol sensitivity
> ALDH, liver mitochondrial
> ALDH1 deficiency
> ALDH2/2 variant
> Mitochondrial ALDH deficiency

**Excludes:** Chlorpropamide-alcohol flushing

**Major Diagnostic Criteria:** Affected individuals have elevated plasma acetaldehyde levels (35 ± 13 $\mu$mole/liter compared with controls: 2 ± 1.7 $\mu$mole/liter) and absence of a faster migrating isozyme of acetaldehyde dehydrogenase-2 (ALDH2) in liver samples (by starch gel electrophoresis) and in hair roots (by isoelectric focusing). The most reliable diagnostic criterion is identification of the variant gene by hybridization of leukocyte DNA with one of two synthetic oligonucleotide probes.

**Clinical Findings:** Facial flushing, muscle weakness, and tachycardia occur soon after alcohol ingestion.

**Complications:** Unknown.

**Associated Findings:** Differential incidence of alcoholism.

**Etiology:** Possibly by autosomal dominant inheritance, although it is common enough in the affected groups that there may be a significant number of homozygous individuals.

**Pathogenesis:** Alcohol is dehydrogenated by alcohol dehydrogenase to form acetaldehyde. In the absence of functional liver ALDH2, which has a low Km for acetaldehyde, acetaldehyde accumulates until ALDH1, with a lower affinity for this substrate, becomes effective. There is a point mutation in ALDH2, changing amino acid residue number 487 from Glu in the usual gene product (ALDH1$_2$) to a Lys in the atypical gene product (ALDH2$_2$). Since the first step in alcohol metabolism, catalyzed by alcohol dehydrogenase (ADH), is the rate limiting step, polymorphism in ADH3 and particularly ADH2 may modulate expression of symptoms. There is a nonsignificant increase in the variant ADH2$_2$ in Oriental populations. The variant enzyme has greater activity than the usual ADH1$_2$, so the aldehyde intermediate is synthesized more rapidly. The combination of excessive ADH activity and attenuated ALDH activity augments the levels of the acetaldehyde. The rate of regeneration of NAD$^+$, a cofactor for both ADH and ALDH, is critical and is probably regulated by many genetic factors.

**MIM No.:** *10065, 10370, 10372, 10373, 10375

**Sex Ratio:** M1:F1

**Occurrence:** This condition is rare in Caucasians and Western Europeans. About 50% of Orientals lack functional ALDH2 and exhibit clinical expression after alcohol exposure.

**Risk of Recurrence for Patient's Sib:**
See Part I, *Mendelian Inheritance.*

**Risk of Recurrence for Patient's Child:**
See Part I, *Mendelian Inheritance.*

**Age of Detectability:** Symptomatically, this condition is detectable when the patient is old enough to consume alcohol. Presymptomatically, the genotype can be detected by characterizing leukocyte DNA with oligonucleotide probes.

**Gene Mapping and Linkage:** ALDH2 (aldehyde dehydrogenase 2, mitochondrial) has been mapped to 12q24.2.
ADH1 (alcohol dehydrogenase (class I), alpha polypeptide) has been mapped to 4q21-q23.
ADH2 (alcohol dehydrogenase (class I), beta polypeptide) has been mapped to 4q21-q23.
ADH3 (alcohol dehydrogenase (class I), gamma polypeptide) has been mapped to 4q21-q23.

**Prevention:** The environmental agent responsible for induction of symptoms can be avoided.

**Treatment:** Abstinence from alcohol intake.

**Prognosis:** Excellent with abstinence from alcohol intake.

**Detection of Carrier:** The least invasive and most reliable method of genotype identification is hybridization of leukocyte DNA with oligonucleotide probes.

**Special Considerations:** The nomenclature derived from electrophoretic forms is ALDHII and ALDHI for ALDH1 and ALDH2, respectively.
There have been suggestions that a variant alcohol dehydrogenase, ADH2, with an altered ratio of activity at two pH values and an excessive activity, causes more rapid oxidation of alcohol. This proposes enhanced synthesis of acetaldehyde as opposed to slower metabolism of that intermediate; this is more compatible with autosomal dominant inheritance. The gene for ADH2 and its isozymes has been regionalized to 4q21 to 4q25. Isozymes 1, 4, and 5, also called alpha, pi, and chi, respectively, do not exist in polymorphic forms. An ADH3 has been reported.
Since the genetic role, if any, in **Fetal alcohol syndrome** and alcoholism is not yet understood, possibly the role of various combinations of these polymorphisms and others not yet identified may help us to understand the mechanisms for these conditions.

**References:**
Stamatoyannopoulos G, et al.: Liver alcohol dehydrogenase in Japanese: high population frequency of atypical form and its possible role in alcohol sensitivity. Am J Hum Genet 1975; 27:789–796.
Goodwin D: Is alcoholism hereditary? New York: Oxford University Press, 1976.
Harada S, et al.: Liver alcohol dehydrogenase and aldehyde dehydrogenase in the Japanese: isozyme variation and its possible role in alcohol intoxication. Am J Hum Genet 1980; 32:8–15.
Smith M, et al.: Assignment of ADH1, ADH2 and ADH3 genes (class I ADH) to human chromosome 4q21–4q25, through use of DNA probes. Cytogenet Cell Genet 1985; 40:784A.
Hsu LC, et al.: Chromosomal assignment of the genes for human aldehyde dehydrogenase 1 and aldehyde dehydrogenase 2. Am J Hum Genet 1986; 38:641–648.
Goedde HW, Agarwal DP: Polymorphism of aldehyde dehydrogenase and alcohol sensitivity. Enzyme 1987; 37:29–44.
Hsu LC, et al.: Direct detection of usual and atypical alleles on the human aldehyde dehydrogenase-2 (ALDH2) locus. Am J Hum Genet 1987; 41:996–1001.
Shibuya A, Yoshida A: Genotypes of alcohol-metabolizing enzymes in Japanese with alcohol liver diseases: a strong association of the usual Caucasian-type aldehyde dehydrogenase gene (ALDH1$_2$) with the disease. Am J Hum Genet 1988; 43:744–748.

VI006
**Jaclyn M. Vidgoff**

**Alcohol sensitivity**
*See ALCOHOL INTOLERANCE*
**Alcohol, fetal effects of**
*See FETAL ALCOHOL SYNDROME*
**Aldehyde oxidase/sulfite oxidase/xanthine dehydrogenase deficiency**
*See MOLYBDENUM CO-FACTOR DEFICIENCY*
**ALDH, liver mitochondrial**
*See ALCOHOL INTOLERANCE*
**ALDH1 deficiency**
*See ALCOHOL INTOLERANCE*
**ALDH2/2 variant**
*See ALCOHOL INTOLERANCE*
**Aldolase B deficiency**
*See FRUCTOSE-1-PHOSPHATE ALDOLASE DEFICIENCY*
**Aldolase-A deficiency, erythrocyte**
*See ERYTHROCYTE ALDOLASE-A DEFICIENCY*
**Aldosterone deficiency I**
*See STEROID 18-HYDROXYLASE DEFICIENCY*
**Aldosterone deficiency II**
*See STEROID 18-HYDROXYSTEROID DEHYDROGENASE DEFICIENCY*

## ALDOSTERONE RESISTANCE 0829

**Includes:**
Aldosterone-receptor deficiency
Aldosterone unresponsiveness
Hyperkalemia-hyperchloremic acidosis-hypertension-hyporeninemia
Mineralocorticoid-receptor deficiency
Pseudohypoaldosteronism
Pseudohypoaldosteronism, Persian-Jewish type

**Excludes:**
**Adrenal hypoaldosteronism of infancy, transient isolated** (0023)
**Adrenal hypoplasia, congenital** (0024)
Renal diseases with salt wasting
**Steroid 3 beta-hydroxysteroid dehydrogenase deficiency** (0909)
**Steroid 18-hydroxylase deficiency** (0905)
**Steroid 18-hydroxysteroid dehydrogenase deficiency** (0906)
**Steroid 21-hydroxylase deficiency** (0908)
**Steroid 20–22 desmolase deficiency** (0907)

**Major Diagnostic Criteria:** Failure to thrive, anorexia, vomiting, dehydration, and circulatory collapse in an infant with hyponatremia, hyperkalemia, and urinary salt-wasting in the absence of renal or adrenal disease, and in the presence of high aldosterone concentration in plasma and/or urine.

**Clinical Findings:** Pseudohypoaldosteronism is a term applied to a salt-wasting syndrome of infancy and early childhood in which there appears to be renal tubular unresponsiveness to the metabolic effects of aldosterone. In addition, unresponsiveness to mineralocorticoid is present in the colon and in the sweat and salivary glands, all of which manifest sodium-wasting despite high plasma concentrations and urinary excretion of aldosterone. Failure to thrive, anorexia, lethargy, vomiting, dehydration, and circulatory collapse are almost universal findings in early infancy. The external genitalia are normal. Hyponatremia, often severe, hyperkalemia, and urinary sodium-wasting are also characteristic. Renal function is otherwise normal, as is adrenal function determined by cortisol levels, which are normal or high and respond appropriately to administration of ACTH. Plasma aldosterone concentrations and secretion rate are markedly elevated to ten-fold normal levels, and plasma renin concentrations are also extraordinarily high. There is no correction of urinary salt loss following administration of mineralocorticoids such as deoxycorticosterone or 9α-fluorohydrocortisone. A variant of this syndrome, in which plasma aldosterone levels are normal or modestly elevated, and in which there is a clinical response to salt-retaining steroids, has also been described. In this latter form parental consanguinity has been prominent in the families of affected individuals. Re-evaluation of these affected individuals, however, has documented that they have deficiency of the final enzymatic step in aldosterone biosynthesis (see **Steroid 18-hydroxysteroid dehydrogenase deficiency**) rather than pseudohypoaldosteronism. There is a tendency for spontaneous amelioration of salt loss with increasing age in both syndromes, so that treatment sometimes may be discontinued in the second or third year of life.

**Complications:** Related to degree of electrolyte disturbance and dehydration.

**Associated Findings:** None known.

**Etiology:** The majority of cases previously described have been sporadic in nature, although autosomal dominant or autosomal recessive inheritance has been noted in about one-third of reported cases.

**Pathogenesis:** The syndrome can be explained on the basis of renal tubular and other tissue unresponsiveness to the action of aldosterone and secondary homeostatic adjustments due to salt loss and dehydration in stimulating the renin-angiotensin-aldosterone system. As such, the syndrome would represent a further example of end-organ unresponsiveness to a hormone, akin to pseudohypoparathyroidism and nephrogenic diabetes insipidus. Patients with this syndrome lack type I or "mineralocorticoid-like" receptors. However, complete unresponsiveness is unlikely, since in some of the reported cases an aldosterone inhibitor, spironolactone, aggravated salt loss, and a partial response to high doses of mineralocorticoids have been observed. The defect may also reside at a post-receptor step as suggested by the finding of absent or low Na-K ATPase activity in microdissected nephrons from an affected patient. Alternatively, the clinical findings could be due to a defect in salt reabsorption in the proximal renal tubule or ascending limb of the Henle loop, thus flooding the distal renal tubule with sodium beyond its reabsorptive capacity and resulting in secondary hyperaldosteronism with some response to mineralocorticoids.

**MIM No.:** *17773, *26435

**Sex Ratio:** M1:F1

**Occurrence:** Undetermined but presumed rare. Extensive literature. A number of cases have been described in Persian Jews.

**Risk of Recurrence for Patient's Sib:**
See Part I, *Mendelian Inheritance.*

**Risk of Recurrence for Patient's Child:**
See Part I, *Mendelian Inheritance.*

**Age of Detectability:** Usually in the neonatal period, or during the first three years of life.

**Gene Mapping and Linkage:** MLR (mineralocorticoid receptor (aldosterone receptor)) has been mapped to 4q31.

**Prevention:** None known. Genetic counseling indicated.

**Treatment:** In most cases, supplemental salt intake of up to 5 gm daily corrects the electrolyte disturbance and restores growth to normal. Some patients may respond to mineralocorticoids with appropriate reduction in salt intake. A potassium exchange resin has been necessary in one case to correct severe hyperkalemia.

**Prognosis:** With correction of electrolyte disturbance, the prognosis appears to be very good for growth and development.

**Detection of Carrier:** Clinical and laboratory examination of first degree relatives.

**References:**
Roy C: Familial pseudohypoaldosteronism (a series of 5 cases). Arch Franc Pediatr 1977; 34:37–54.
Oberfield S, et al.: Pseudohypoaldosteronism: multiple target organ unresponsiveness to mineralocorticoid hormones. J Clin Endocrinol Metab 1979; 48:228–232.
Rösler A: The natural history of salt-wasting disorders of adrenal and renal origin. J Clin Endocrinol Metab 1984; 59:689–700.
Armamim D, et al.: Aldosterone-receptor deficiency in pseudohypoaldosteronism. New Engl J Med 1985; 313:1178–1181.
Bosson D, et al.: Generalized unresponsiveness to mineralocorticoid hormones: familial recessive pseudohypoaldosteronism due to aldosterone-receptor deficiency. Acta Endocr 1986; 112(suppl. 279): 376–380.
Speiser PW, et al.: Pseudohypoaldosteronism. In: Chrousos GP, et al, eds: Steroid hormone resistance: mechanisms and clinical aspects. New York: Plenum Press, 1986:173–195.
Arriza JL, et al.: Cloning of human mineralocorticoid receptor complementary DNA: structural and functional kinship with the glucocorticoid receptor. Science 1987; 237:268–275.

SP004                        **Mark A. Sperling**

**Aldosterone unresponsiveness**
See ALDOSTERONE RESISTANCE
**Aldosterone-receptor deficiency**
See ALDOSTERONE RESISTANCE
**Aldosteronism, sensitive to dexamethasone**
See HYPERALDOSTERONISM, FAMILIAL GLUCOCORTICOID SUPPRESSIBLE
**Aldrich syndrome**
See IMMUNODEFICIENCY, WISKOTT-ALDRICH TYPE
**Aleukia, congenital**
See IMMUNODEFICIENCY, SEVERE COMBINED

---

## ALEXANDER DISEASE            2712

**Includes:**

Dysmyelinogenic leukodystrophy
Fibrinoid leukodystrophy
Hyaline panneuropathy
Leukodystrophy, Alexander disease

**Excludes:**
**Brain, spongy degeneration** (0115)
**Multiple sclerosis, familial** (2598)
**Neuronal ceroid-lipofuscinoses (NCL)** (0713)
Neuronal sphingolipidoses

**Major Diagnostic Criteria:** *In infants:* psychomotor regression, **Megalencephaly**, spasticity, seizures. *In juveniles:* cranial nerve dysfunction, spasticity, intact mental status. *In adults:* may have normal neurologic exam or may have intermittent cerebellar signs, paraparesis, quadriparesis.

Pathologically, Rosenthal fibers are present throughout the central nervous system; especially in subpial, subependymal and perivascular regions.

**Clinical Findings:** *In infants:* psychomotor regression, **Megalencephaly**, spasticity, seizures and progressive neurologic deterioration. The age of onset is from birth to two years of age with a mean of six months of age. The average duration of illness in this group has been 28 months, with a range of two months to seven-and-one-half years. As of 1976, there were 11 patients in this subgroup, ten male and one female.

*In juveniles:* dysphagia, dysarthria, respiratory difficulty with inability to cough, vomiting, and spastic quadriparesis. Mental status may not be significantly affected. The average age of onset is nine-and-one-half years, with a range of seven to fourteen years. The average duration of the illness is eight years, with a range of fifteen months to twelve years.

*In adults:* The seven known patients in this subgroup can be further divided into two subcategories. In one (three cases), there is no neurologic dysfunction until the terminal phase. The average age of onset is 27 years of age with a range of 19 to 43 years of age. The average duration of illness is one year. The sex ratio is M1:F2.

Adults in the second subcategory present with stuttering,

followed by slow progression and increasing disability consisting of paraparesis or quadriparesis and bulbar signs. Clinically, the condition resembles classic **Multiple sclerosis, familial**. The average age of onset is 34 years of age with a range of 32 to 44 years. The mean duration of illness is nine-and-one-half years with a range of six to seventeen years. There is no male or female preponderance.

Sensory exam is normal in all patients.

*Laboratory findings*: Brain CT scan shows mild to marked ventriculomegaly with diffuse, low attenuation of the white matter which is markedly pronounced in the frontal regions. The CT scan may also show enhancement of the caudate nuclei, ventricular margins and gyri. Routine blood count and chemistries, liver enzymes, urinalysis, electromyography and nerve conduction studies, CSF exam and leukocyte enzyme assays are normal.

**Complications:** Aspiration pneumonia, failure to thrive or weight loss, and pressure sores and contractures, may occur in any group. In the juvenile and adult onset types, urinary tract infection may be a problem.

**Associated Findings:** None known.

**Etiology:** Possibly autosomal recessive inheritance. Most reported cases have been sporadic.

**Pathogenesis:** The pathological hallmark, irrespective of age of onset, is the accumulation of Rosenthal fibres in relation to astrocytes throughout the central nervous system, and which are concentrated predominantly in the subpial, subependymal and perivascular regions. There is extensive demyelination in the infantile cases, less severe in the juvenile group and variable in adults. Neurons are invariably preserved. There is consensus of opinions that Alexander disease represents a non-neoplastic disease of astrocytes, but it is not known which of the numerous functions of astrocytes is impaired, or how. It is assumed that early in the course of the illness there is proliferation of atypical astrocytes which may be the cause of **Megalencephaly**, followed by astrocyte death, leaving a normocellular neuropil with abundant Rosenthal fibres. While the chemical composition of Rosenthal fibres is not known, they consist of electron-dense masses with irregular but distinct margins and no limiting membrane. These masses are always associated with bundles of glial filaments which appear to enter and exit from them.

**MIM No.:** 20345

**Sex Ratio:** Presumably M1:F1, although this has appeared to vary with the age group.

**Occurrence:** More than two dozen cases have been documented, including two black brothers.

**Risk of Recurrence for Patient's Sib:** Unknown.

**Risk of Recurrence for Patient's Child:** Unknown.

**Age of Detectability:** Can occur at any age.

**Gene Mapping and Linkage:** Unknown.

**Prevention:** None known. Genetic counseling indicated.

**Treatment:** Prevention of aspiration pneumonia, other infections, malnutrition, contractures, and pressure sores as indicated. Anti-seizure medications may be required.

**Prognosis:** Variable.

**Detection of Carrier:** Unknown.

**Special Considerations:** Alexander disease is generally regarded as a leukodystrophy because of variable demyelination present in pathologic specimen. However, the most conspicuous pathologic feature is the accumulation of Rosenthal fibres throughout the central nervous system, which may be more numerous in the grey matter than is white matter, particularly basal ganglia, thalamus and brainstem. Generally the severity of demyelination is proportional to the degree of accumulation of Rosenthal fibres. Areas of extensive deposition of Rosenthal fibres without any significant demyelination may be found.

**References:**
Alexander WS: Progressive fibrinoid degeration of fibrillary astrocytes, associated with mental retardation. Brain 1949; 72:373–381.
Russo LS, et al.: Alexander's disease: a report and reappraisal. Neurology 1976; 26:607–614.
Holland IM, Kendall BE: CT in Alexander's disease. Neuroradiology 1980; 20:103–106.
Borrett D, Becker LE: Alexander's disease. Brain 1985; 108:367–385.

BA061          **I. Hussain Bangash**
KA008          **Raymond S. Kandt**

**Alkaline phosphatase, liver/bone/kidney type**
 *See* HYPOPHOSPHATASIA
**Alkalosis with diarrhea**
 *See* DIARRHEA, CONGENITAL CHLORIDE

## ALKAPTONURIA                                    0037

**Includes:**
 Homogentisic acid oxidase deficiency
 Homogentisic aciduria
 Ochronosis
 Ochronotic arthritis

**Excludes:**
 Acquired ochronosis from exogenous chemicals or drugs
 **Arthritis, rheumatoid** (2517)
 Osteoarthritis

**Major Diagnostic Criteria:** Homogentisic acid can be documented by paper chromatography; alkalinization of the urine results in the appearance of black pigment.

**Clinical Findings:** Children and young adults usually have no symptoms. The urine is usually clear when passed but on standing or alkalinization it turns brown or black. Patients may never have recognized this. The urine is also positive for reducing substance and reacts with ferric chloride. With age, patients develop pigmentation of the sclerae, cartilages, or other fibrous tissue. The sweat may be dark, and the cerumen is often brown or black. There may be widespread dusky pigmentation of the skin, particularly over the cheeks, forehead, axillae, and genital regions. The buccal mucosa and nails may be brown. Marked darkening of tissues is seen on exposure to air at surgery. Later the patients develop an arthritis that resembles osteoarthritis but has some inflammatory features resembling rheumatoid arthritis. Some degree of limitation of motion is usually the ultimate result, and complete ankylosis is common.

**Complications:** Ruptured intervertebral disk.

**Associated Findings:** Cardiovascular disease, prostatitis, and renal stones are probably unrelated.

**Etiology:** Autosomal recessive inheritance of enzyme defect.

**Pathogenesis:** Deficiency of hepatic homogentisic acid oxidase.

**MIM No.:** *20350

**Sex Ratio:** M1:F1

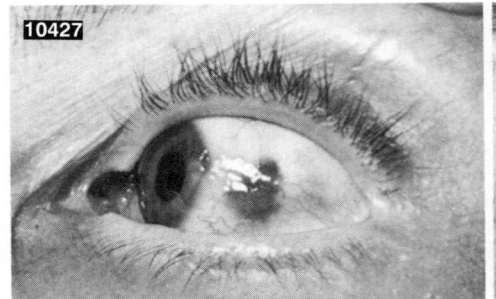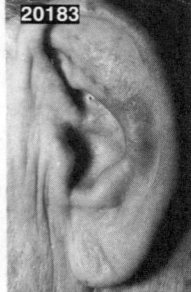

**0037-10427:** Note dark pigmentation of the sclera. **20183:** Dark pigmentation of the auricle.

**Occurrence:** One of the first discovered inborn errors of metabolism classified as Mendelian ( in 1902). Hundreds of documented cases. Most frequent in Dominican Republic, Czechoslovakia and Germany.

**Risk of Recurrence for Patient's Sib:**
See Part I, *Mendelian Inheritance.*

**Risk of Recurrence for Patient's Child:**
See Part I, *Mendelian Inheritance.*

**Age of Detectability:** At birth.

**Gene Mapping and Linkage:** Unknown.

**Prevention:** None known. Genetic counseling indicated.

**Treatment:** Dependent on arthritic condition.

**Prognosis:** Normal for life span and intelligence, but function may be reduced because of arthritis.

**Detection of Carrier:** Unknown.

**References:**
Garrod AE: The incidence of alkaptonuria: a study in chemical individuality. Lancet 1902; II:1616–1620.
Garrod AE: Inborn Errors of Metabolism. London: Oxford University Press, 1923.
LaDu BN, et al.: The nature of the defect in tyrosine metabolism in alcaptonuria. J Biol Chem 1958; 230:251–260.
O'Brien WM, et al.: Biochemical, pathologic and clinical aspects of alcaptonuria, achronosis and ochronotic arthropathy: review of the world literature (1584–1962). Am J Med 1963; 34:813–838.
Nyhan WL: Alkaptonuria. In Nyhan WL: Diagnostic Recognition of Genetic Disease. Philadelphia: Lea and Febiger, 1987.

NY000                                      **William L. Nyhan**

**Allan-Herndon-Dudley (limber neck) mental retardation**
*See X-LINKED MENTAL RETARDATION-MUSCULAR WEAKNESS-AWKWARD GAIT*
**Allergic diathesis**
*See SKIN, ATOPY, FAMILIAL*
**Allergic rhinitis**
*See SKIN, ATOPY, FAMILIAL*
**Alloimmune hemolytic disease of the newborn**
*See ERYTHROBLASTOSIS FETALIS*
**Allotypes, antibodies to human**
*See ANTIBODIES TO HUMAN ALLOTYPES*
**Alopecia areata**
*See HAIR, ALOPECIA AREATA*
**Alopecia totalis**
*See HAIR, ALOPECIA AREATA*
**Alopecia universalis**
*See HAIR, ALOPECIA AREATA*
**Alopecia, chronic diffuse**
*See HAIR, BALDNESS, COMMON*
**Alopecia, congenital**
*See HAIR, ATRICHIA CONGENITA*
**Alopecia, male or female pattern**
*See HAIR, BALDNESS, COMMON*
**Alopecia, partial-hypogonadism**
*See HYPOGONADISM-PARTIAL ALOPECIA*

## ALOPECIA-ANOSMIA-DEAFNESS-HYPOGONADISM, JOHNSON TYPE                                2765

**Includes:**
Johnson neuroectodermal syndrome
Neuroectodermal syndrome, Johnson type

**Excludes:**
Ear, microtia-atresia (0664)
Neuroectodermal syndrome, Flynn-Aird type (2173)

**Major Diagnostic Criteria:** Alopecia and hyposmia or anosmia plus other frequently associated conditions such as ear anomaly with conductive deafness, hypogonadotrophic hypogonadism, and a tendency to dental caries.

**Clinical Findings:** Alopecia (16/16), total (12/16) or partial (4/16); anosmia/hyposmia (3/3); ear abnormality (6/7); microtia (2/5); atresia of the auditory canal (3/6); asymmetric or prominent ears

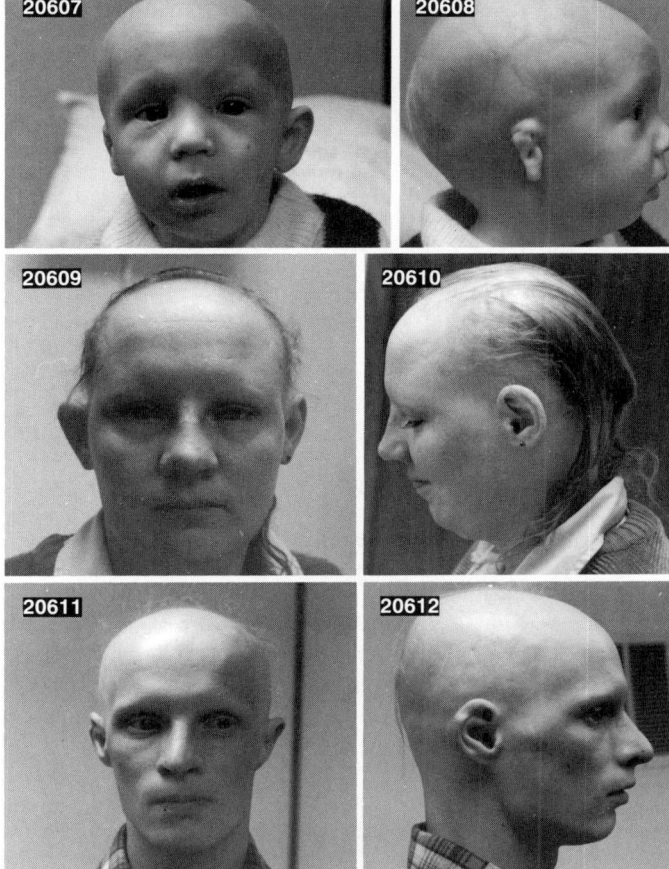

2765-20607–12: Alopecia-anosmia-deafness-hypogonadism, Johnson type; note the partial to complete alopecia, microtia or asymmetric ears in the proband son, mother and uncle.

(5/6); conductive hearing loss (7/8); dental caries/dentures (7/9); retro/micrognathia (4/4); hypogonadism, LH deficiency (3/10); and mild facial asymmetry (5/6).

The alopecia consists of practically total baldness among males and very sparse hair among females, which microscopically was normal although narrow. The ear anomalies range from severe microtia and atresia of the auditory canals to asymmetric or prominent ears with variable conductive hearing loss. Other facial features include variable micrognathia or retrognathia and facial asymmetry with mild facial nerve weakness. The hypogonadism was secondary to an FSH and LH deficiency. The inability to smell was total or partial, and present in all those tested. Dental caries was common, with several individuals wearing dentures by their second to third decade.

**Complications:** Dental caries, failure of sexual maturation among cases with hypogonadism. Mild mental retardation was occasionally present.

**Associated Findings:** Mental retardation (3/7); **Ventricular septal defect** (1/6); **Cleft palate** (1/7); choanal stenosis (1/1); and bilateral cervical ribs. Scholastic failure or speech delay and impairment secondary to an undiagnosed conductive hearing loss; emotional and behavioral problems secondary to the striking alopecia or failure to mature sexually at puberty.

**Etiology:** Autosomal dominant inheritance with variable expressivity.

**Pathogenesis:** Virtually all of the facial and branchial arch structures are derived from the neural crest. The first and second branchial arches contribute to the hillocks of His, ossicles, and trigeminal and facial nerves. The mesoderm that invades the palatal shelves is neuroectoderm from the lateral and ventral aspects of the neural crest. The olfactory bulb consists of epithelium from the nasal placodes and neural extension from the telencephalon. The pituitary/hypothalamic axis arises from an outpocketing of the ventral neural ridge, Rathke pouch, and infundibular portion of the diencephalon. The apparently disparate clinical findings involving hair, ears, palate, facial nerve olfactory bulb, hypothalamic/pituitary axis find common ground if assumed secondary to a genetic mutation of an ectodermal/neuroectodermal origin.

**MIM No.:** 14777

**POS No.:** 3595

**Sex Ratio:** M10:F6 (observed).

**Occurrence:** One kindred with 16 affected individuals in three generations, and one sporadic case, have been reported in the literature.

**Risk of Recurrence for Patient's Sib:**
See Part I, *Mendelian Inheritance.*

**Risk of Recurrence for Patient's Child:**
See Part I, *Mendelian Inheritance.*

**Age of Detectability:** At birth.

**Gene Mapping and Linkage:** Unknown.

**Prevention:** None known. Genetic counseling indicated.

**Treatment:** Hormonal replacement for hypogonadism, dental care.

**Prognosis:** Normal life span.

**Detection of Carrier:** Unknown.

**References:**
Johnson VP: A newly recognized neuroectodermal syndrome of familial alopecia, anosmia, deafness and hypogonadism. Am J Med Genet 1983; 15:497–506.
Johnston K, et al.: Alopecia-anosmia-deafness-hypogonadism syndrome revisited: report of a new case. Am J Med Genet 1987; 26:925–927.

J0010         **Virginia P. Johnson**

**Alopecia-deafness-hypogonadism**
*See CRANDALL SYNDROME*

---

## ALOPECIA-EPILEPSY-OLIGOPHRENIA, MOYNAHAN TYPE          0670

**Includes:**
Moynahan alopecia syndrome
EEG (unsual)-alopecia-epilepsy-mental retardation

**Excludes:**
Oculo-mandibulo-facial syndrome (0738)
Progeria (0825)
Alopecia-mental retardation (2783)
Alopecia-seizures-mental retardation, shokeir type (3031)

**Major Diagnostic Criteria:** EEG shows absence of alpha rhythm and slow activity at 1–4 cycles per second mixed with occasional low amplitude fast activity. Large stature, delayed bone development, grand mal convulsions at 2–3 week intervals, sparce or absent hair. Marked developmental delay.

**Clinical Findings:** Hairless at birth. Very scanty, lanugo type hair and eyelashes may appear later. Grand mal convulsions form a prominent part of the symptomology usually at intervals of 2 to 3 weeks. Status epilepticus may supervene. There is a marked delay in the milestones; patient takes little interest in his surroundings or food until well into the 3rd year. Talking is delayed and speech limited to a few words. Features include large stature, gross features, short lanugo scalp hair, no eyebrows and few eyelashes.

Skeletal changes include delay in bone development. EEG shows gross abnormality of unusual kind, with absence of alpha rhythm and generalized slow activity between 1 and 4 cycles per second, mixed with a small amount of low amplitude fast activity. No differences between anterior and posterior halves of the head and no spikes or complex wave forms have appeared at any time. Lumbar puncture reveals normal CSF pressure and protein, no cells; urine contains no abnormal amino acids. Blood chemistry is normal.

Biopsy of scalp shows scanty hair follicles, some of which contain a rim of keratin.

**Complications:** Unknown.

**Associated Findings:** None known.

**Etiology:** Possibly autosomal recessive inheritance.

**Pathogenesis:** Ultraphysiology studies have revealed a developmental anomaly involving both cerebral hemispheres, but there are other metabolic changes, such as delay in bone development as well as the absence or deficiency of hair follicles, which remain unexplained.

**MIM No.:** 20360

**POS No.:** 3304

**Sex Ratio:** M1:F1

**Occurrence:** Eight cases reported in three families.

**Risk of Recurrence for Patient's Sib:**
See Part I, *Mendelian Inheritance.*

**Risk of Recurrence for Patient's Child:**
See Part I, *Mendelian Inheritance.*

**Age of Detectability:** Probably at birth or early infancy.

**Gene Mapping and Linkage:** Unknown.

**Prevention:** None known. Genetic counseling indicated.

**Treatment:** For epilepsy, as indicated.

**Prognosis:** The mental deficit is severe enough to possibly require life-long care. At times the child may be difficult to restrain.

**Detection of Carrier:** By clinical examination. Alopecia has been noted in parents and siblings.

*The author wishes to thank Edmund J. Moynahan for his contribution to a previous version of this article.*

**References:**
Moynahan EJ: Familial congenital alopecia, epilepsy, mental retardation with unusual electroencephalograms. Proc Roy Soc Med 1962; 55:411–412.
Mosavy SH: Universal alopecia and microcephaly in 4 siblings. S Afr Med J 1975; 49:172 only.
Pfeiffer RA, Volklein J: Congenital universal alopecia, and microcephaly in two sibs. J Med Genet 1982; 19:388–389.

GR011         **Frank Greenberg**

**Alopecia-growth retardation-pseudoanodontia**
*See GROWTH RETARDATION-ALOPECIA-PSEUDOANODONTIA-OPTIC ATROPHY*

---

## ALOPECIA-MENTAL RETARDATION          2783

**Includes:**
Hair (absence)-microcephaly-developmental delay
Mental retardation-alopecia

**Excludes:**
Atrichia with papular lesions
Alopecia-epilepsy-oligophrenia, Moynahan type (0670)
Alopecia-seizures-mental retardation, shokeir type (3031)
Trichothiodystrophy (2559)

**Major Diagnostic Criteria:** Alopecia, mental retardation, **Microcephaly**.

**Clinical Findings:** There is total lack of hair from birth. Some lanugo is present but little permanent hair after that. Very

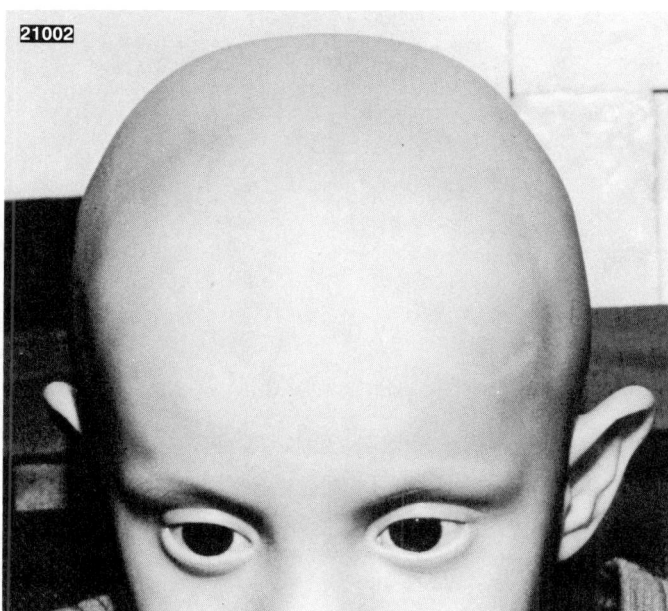

2783-21002: Alopecia-mental retardation; note total lack of scalp hair, brows and lashes.

occasionally single strands appear on the scalp, but the histology of these is normal. The lack of hair growth involves both eyebrows and eyelashes. **Microcephaly** is present from birth. The face is not dysmorphic, and seizures are not usually a feature. Birth weight is usually below the 3rd percentile, and developmental milestones are delayed.

**Complications:** Mental retardation.

**Associated Findings:** One sib in the Pfeiffer and Volklein (1982) report had a **Ventricular septal defect**.

**Etiology:** Autosomal recessive inheritance. Three cousins in one in-bred pedigree the condition (Baraitser et al, 1983). The report by Pfeiffer and Volklein (1982) involved affected sibs.

**Pathogenesis:** Unknown.

**MIM No.:** *20365

**POS No.:** 3549

**Sex Ratio:** Presumably M1:F1.

**Occurrence:** About a dozen cases have been reported.

**Risk of Recurrence for Patient's Sib:**
See Part I, *Mendelian Inheritance.*

**Risk of Recurrence for Patient's Child:**
See Part I, *Mendelian Inheritance.* No affected individuals are known to have reproduced.

**Age of Detectability:** At birth. Hair fails to grow after lanugo falls out.

**Gene Mapping and Linkage:** Unknown.

**Prevention:** None known. Genetic counseling indicated.

**Treatment:** Unknown.

**Prognosis:** Life span not affected.

**Detection of Carrier:** Unknown.

**References:**
Pfeiffer RA, Volklein J: Congenital universal alopecia, mental deficiency and microcephaly in two sibs. J Med Genet 1982; 19:388–389.
Baraitser M, et al.: A new alopecia/mental retardation syndrome. J Med Genet 1983; 20:64–75.
Benke PJ, Hajianpour MJ: Alopecia universalis-mental retardation is an autosomal recessive syndrome disorder. (Abstract) Am J Hum Genet 1985; 37:A44 only.

BA058                                            **Michael Baraitser**

**Alopecia-odonto-onychodysplasia**
 *See ODONTO-ONYCHODYSPLASIA-ALOPECIA*
**Alopecia-polyposis-pigmentation-nail defects**
 *See POLYPOSIS-ALOPECIA-PIGMENTATION-NAIL DEFECTS*
**Alopecia-rickets syndrome**
 *See RESISTANCE TO 1,25 DIHYDROXY VITAMIN D*

## ALOPECIA-SEIZURES-MENTAL RETARDATION, SHOKEIR TYPE                                    3031

**Includes:**
   Epilepsy-alopecia-pyorrhea-mental retardation
   Pyorrhea-epilepsy-alopecia-mental retardation
   Seizures-mental retardation-alopecia
   Shokeir syndrome

**Excludes:**
   **Alopecia-mental retardation** (2783)
   **Alopecia-epilepsy-oligophrenia, Moynahan type** (0670)

**Major Diagnostic Criteria:** Alopecia universalis and pyorrhea, with or without mild mental retardation, and psychomotor epilepsy occurring in an autosomal dominant pattern.

**Clinical Findings:** Universal alopecia and pyorrhea are apparently constant findings, with mild mental deficiency (the reported IQ in one individual was 72) and psychomotor seizures occurring in 8/12 affected individuals in the reported family. Microscopic examination of scalp hairs demonstrated that they were thin with beading.

**Complications:** Premature loss of teeth secondary to pyorrhea can occur.

**Associated Findings:** None known.

**Etiology:** The occurrence of the disorder in four generations, with male-to-male transmission, confirms autosomal dominant inheritance.

**Pathogenesis:** Unknown. A defect in the ectoderm has been postulated.

**MIM No.:** *10413

**Sex Ratio:** M1:F1

**Occurrence:** Documented in 12 members from four generations of one Canadian family.

**Risk of Recurrence for Patient's Sib:**
   See Part I, *Mendelian Inheritance.*

**Risk of Recurrence for Patient's Child:**
   See Part I, *Mendelian Inheritance.*

**Age of Detectability:** Presumably during infancy by the presence of alopecia.

**Gene Mapping and Linkage:** Unknown.

**Prevention:** None known. Genetic counseling indicated.

**Treatment:** Dental treatment is indicated the pyorrhea.

**Prognosis:** Life span appears normal; intellectual impairment, when present, is mild.

**Detection of Carrier:** Unknown.

**Special Considerations:** **Alopecia-epilepsy-oligophrenia, Moynahan type** is similar in that affected individuals have seizures, mental retardation, and alopecia. However, it differs in that the seizures are of the grand mal type, and inheritance is either autosomal or X-linked recessive.

**References:**
Shokeir MHK: Universal permanent alopecia, psychomotor epilepsy, pyorrhea, and mental subnormality. Clin Genet 1977; 11:13–17.

**Helga V. Toriello**

## ALOPECIA-SKELETAL ANOMALIES-SHORT STATURE-MENTAL RETARDATION 2782

**Includes:**

Ectodermal dysplasia-skeletal anomalies-growth/mental retardation
Mental retardation, ACD type
Mental retardation-alopecia-skeletal anomalies-short stature
Short stature-alopecia-skeletal anomalies-mental retardation
Skeletal anomalies-short stature-mental retardation-alopecia
Van Gelderen syndrome

**Excludes:**

**Seckel syndrome** (0881)
**Dwarfism, osteodysplastic primordial, Majewski-Winter type** (2581)

**Major Diagnostic Criteria:**  1) Short stature of prenatal onset; 2) congenital **Microcephaly** and severe mental deficiency; 3) sparse hair, alopecia; 4) multiple joint contractures; and 5) fusions of various bones, particularly in elbows, carpals, metacarpals and spine.

**Clinical Findings:**  The pregnancies of the two affected patients were normal, but a striking pattern of abnormalities was reported at birth. One patient was short and underweight at birth; measurements of the other patient were not recorded. Clinical findings include the following (in both patients unless otherwise indicated): *Hair, scalp, and skin* showed total alopecia of scalp, eyebrows, and lashes; follicular hyperkeratosis; and normal perspiration. *Skull* showed severe **Microcephaly** and turricephaly. *Facies* had upslanting palpebral fissures (one); short palpebral fissures (one); relatively large, beaked nose; large, poorly modeled, and posteriorly rotated ears. *Skeletal defects* included kyphoscoliosis, hip dislocation, and vertebral fusions. *Extremities* had restricted movements in various joints (contractures), humeroradial synostosis, short midphalanges, fusions between carpal bones (one) and between 4th and 5th metacarpals, complete cutaneous **Syndactyly** between toes 4 and 5 (one), hypoplastic distal phalanges with excess of arches on fingertips, and hypoplastic toenails. *Sexual development*: there was a lack of sexual development in the 16-year-old boy; sparse pubic and absent axillary hair but normal menstruation in the 18-year-old girl.

**Complications:**  Unknown.

**Associated Findings:**  None known.

**Etiology:**  Possibly autosomal recessive inheritance is suggested by parental consanguinity in the history of one of the two observed patients.

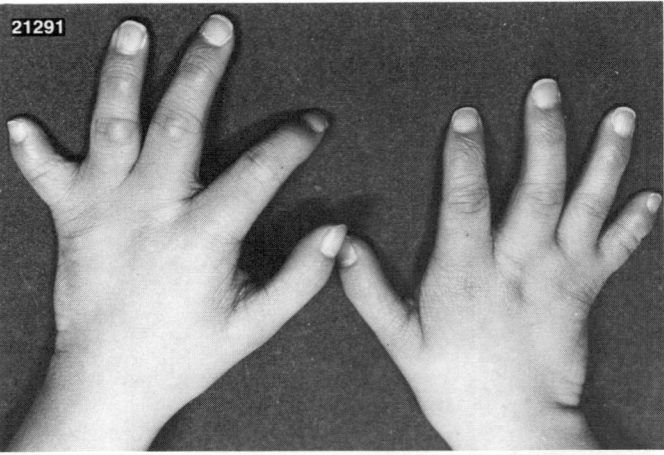
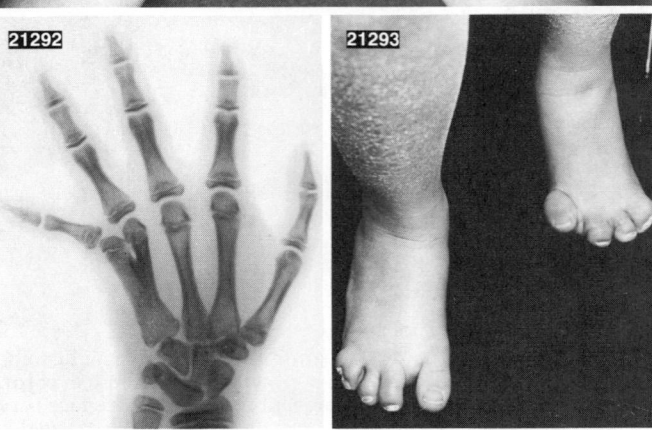

**2782B**-21291:  Narrow hands with short index and little fingers. 21292:  X-ray of the hand shows fusion between lunate and triquetal bones, proximal Y-shaped synostosis between fourth and fifth metacarpals and short midphalanges.  21293:  Hyperkeratosis of lower legs, left hammer toe, broad gap between first and second toes, complete cutaneous syndactyly between fourth and fifth toes.

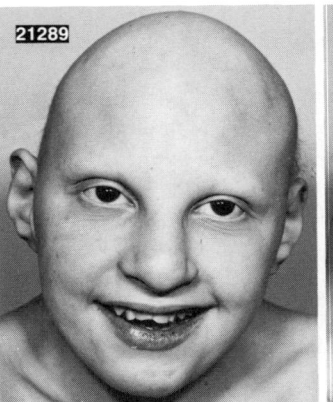
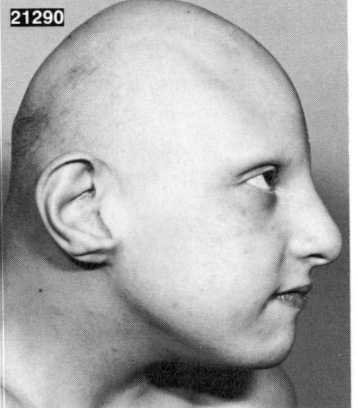

**2782A**-21289–90:  Facies show alopecia with absent scalp hair, eyebrows and lashes, large prominent nose, upslanting palpebral fissures, short upper lip, and large poorly formed ears.

**Pathogenesis:**  Unknown.

**MIM No.:**  20355

**POS No.:**  3562

**Sex Ratio:**  Presumably M1:F1.

**Occurrence:**  Four cases have been observed; one male and one female case have been reported in the literature.

**Risk of Recurrence for Patient's Sib:**
See Part I, *Mendelian Inheritance.*

**Risk of Recurrence for Patient's Child:**
See Part I, *Mendelian Inheritance.* Due to severe mental deficiency, affected probands will normally not reproduce.

**Age of Detectability:**  By ultrasound or fetoscopy possibly during the second trimester of gestation (intrauterine growth retardation, microcephaly, limited excursions in elbows and sometimes in other joints) or by histologic examination of a skin biopsy specimen from the skull (absence or gross reduction in number of hair follicles). At birth or later on the basis of clinical features.

**Gene Mapping and Linkage:**  Unknown.

**Prevention:**  None known. Genetic counseling indicated.

**Treatment:**  Unknown.

**Prognosis:** Life span is probably not affected; both reported patients were adolescents. The patients were severely mentally retarded.

**Detection of Carrier:** Parents of affected individuals will usually be carriers, although there is no way to demonstrate heterozygosity by clinical or other examinations.

**References:**

Schinzel A: A case of multiple skeletal anomalies, ectodermal dysplasia, and severe growth and mental retardation. Helv Paediatr Acta 1980; 35:243.

Van Gelderen HH: Syndrome of total alopecia, multiple skeletal anomalies, shortness of stature, and mental deficiency. Am J Med Genet 1982; 13:383.

SC017                          **Albert A.G.L. Schinzel**

## ALOPECIA-SKIN ATROPHY-ANONYCHIA-TONGUE DEFECT       2842

**Includes:**

    Anonychia-skin atrophy-alopecia-tongue defect
    Dermatitis, congenital erosive and vesicular
    Sequeiros-Sack syndrome
    Skin atrophy, linear
    Skin, atrophy-anonychia-alopecia-tongue defect

**Excludes:**

    Anetoderma
    Atrophoderma
    **Dermal hypoplasia, focal** (0281)

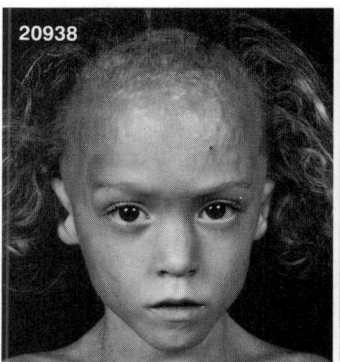
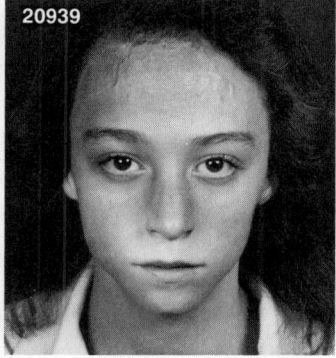
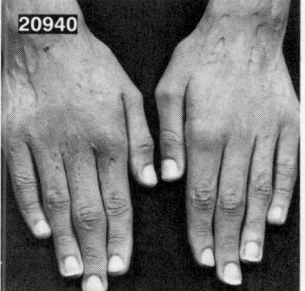
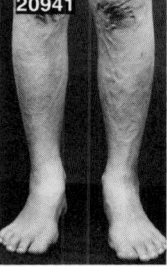
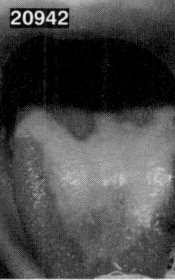

**2842-20938:** Anterior scarring and alopecia at age 5 years. **20939:** Hair growth and smoothing of the lesions is apparent at age 13 years. **20940:** Linear reticular lesions of forearm and hand with some smoothing and pitting. **20941:** Skin lesions on the legs appear in a reticulated pattern; nails were absent on the halluces and the fourth right toe. **20942:** Whitish, depapillated, raised area of geographic outline is in the anterior two-thirds of the tongue.

**Epidermolysis bullosum**
**Hair, alopecia areata** (0038)
**Skin, localized absence of** (0608)
**Tongue, geographic** (0954)

**Major Diagnostic Criteria:** Congenital atrophy of skin with linear depressed scars alternating with ridges of nearly normal skin. Lesions progress from friable skin with vesicular-bullous eruptions to scabs and scars but no new lesions develop. Toenails may be absent. A scar-like lesion has been found on the tongue.

**Clinical Findings:** Birth is premature. The lesions are erythematous with bullae; these heal slowly to depressed scars without dermal appendages. Heat intolerance may be present in infancy, but gradually lessens. The possibility of intrauterine infection has been suggested by elevated immunoglobulin levels in some but diagnostic antibody titers have not been found. The lesions become less prominent with age and new ones do not develop but appendages do not appear.

Biopsy of affected areas shows no appendages. Elastic fiber size and number are occasionally reduced.

**Complications:** Permanent loss of dermal appendages can cause alopecia, anonychia and scars. Febrile convulsions may develop in infancy.

**Associated Findings:** One case was a member of a pair of monozygotic twins.

**Etiology:** Sporadic event; may reflect intrauterine infection or inflammation.

**Pathogenesis:** Early inflammation from any potentially scarring agent could disrupt the skin and exposed mucous membranes.

**Sex Ratio:** M1:F2 (observed).

**Occurrence:** Three cases have been documented.

**Risk of Recurrence for Patient's Sib:** No affected sibs are known, including a monozygotic twin.

**Risk of Recurrence for Patient's Child:** Unknown.

**Age of Detectability:** At birth.

**Gene Mapping and Linkage:** Unknown.

**Prevention:** None known. Genetic counseling indicated.

**Treatment:** Supportive care while lesions heal. Hair transplantation has been successful.

**Prognosis:** Good; lesions become less prominent with age. Intelligence is unaffected.

**Detection of Carrier:** Unknown.

**Special Considerations:** *Atrophy* best describes the cutaneous findings. *Poikiloderma*, *atrophoderma*, and *anetoderma* are terms that may be used both descriptively and as distinct clinical entities. The absence of full expression of typical color changes (hypo- and hyperpigmentation and telangiectases) precludes the use of the term poikiloderma. *Atrophoderma* describes several different conditions characterized by depressed lesions without induration, wrinkles, or protrusions, and with little alteration in the elastica; its main characteristic is pigmentation. *Anetoderma* is localized skin atrophy with thinning and fine wrinkling, involving mainly the elastica; it varies from the more typical macular pseudotumoral form to depressed bizarrely shaped lesions. Though the age of onset and location of the lesions are unusual, some of the dermal changes observed here resemble anetoderma.

**References:**

Sequeiros J, Sack GH Jr: Focal dermal hypoplasia in one of a pair of MZ twins. (Abstract) Am J Hum Gen 1983; 35:116A only.

Cohen BA, et al.: Congenital erosive and vesicular dermatosis healing with reticulated supple scarring. Arch Dermatol 1985; 121:361–367. †

Sequeiros J, Sack GH Jr: Linear skin atrophy, scarring alopecia, anonychia, and tongue lesion: a "new" syndrome? Am J Med Gen 1985; 21:669–680. * †

SA005                          **George H. Sack, Jr.**
SE020                          **Jorge Sequeiros**

## ALPERS DISEASE                                    3261

**Includes:**

Christensen Krabbe disease
Liver disease-neuronal degeneration of childhood
Neuronal degeneration of childhood-liver disease,
    progressive
Poliodystrophica cerebri dystrophica
Sclerosing poliodystrophy, progressive
Spongy glioneuronal dystrophy

**Excludes:**

Encephalopathy secondary to hypoxic-ischemic insult
Encephalopathy secondary to acid metabolism anomalies
**Hepatolenticular degeneration** (0469)
**Menkes syndrome** (0643)
**Rett syndrome** (2226)

**Major Diagnostic Criteria:** Psychomotor retardation usually starts in infancy after an otherwise normal pregancy and early development. As the condition progresses, intractable seizures, **Microcephaly**, progressive spasticity, optic atrophy, deafness and ataxia develop. The disease always ends in death, although some patients may be in a vegetative state for a prolonged period of time.

Imaging studies demonstrate marked cortical atrophy; EEG is abnormal, and CSF may show elevated protein. Diagnosis is established by pathologic examination of brain which shows diffuse neuronal loss with glial proliferation in cerebral cortex and to lesser extent in cerebellum, brain stem and basal ganglia.

**Clinical Findings:** Alpers (1931) described a three-month-old girl with acute onset of seizures, rigidity, and unconsciousness; pathology of brain showed degeneration of cortical neurons. The illness is variable in onset, but usually starts with developmental delay between the ages of 3–12 months. Later, regression of development progresses to a chronic vegetative state or death. Seizures generally appear after the onset of developmental delay and are of multiple types: generalized tonic-clonic, focal motor, myoclonic seizures and infantile spasms. Status epilepticus is frequent and seizures become medically intractable. Motor involvement includes rigidity, spasticity, hemiparesis and quadriparsis or plegia. Choreiform movements (12%) and ataxia (7%) also occur. Blindness and optic atrophy are present and may be associated with abnormal or absent visual evoked responses (VERs.) Deafness with abnormal brainstem auditory evoked responses (BAERs) may also occur.

The duration of the illness is 1–4 years, and most affected children die within 2–6 years. Infections often precipitate acute deterioration in clinical condition, often resulting in status epilepticus.

A *juvenile form* with onset around 4–10 years and death around 12–20 years has been reported. Klein and Dichgans (1969) reported a case with focal and myoclonic seizures, visual disturbance, and elevated CSF protein which started at age 25 years and showed changes similar to Alpers on autopsy.

Neuroimaging study reveals diffuse atrophy of the brain, more marked in cerebral cortex, and at times atrophy may be asymmetric involving one hemisphere more than the other. EEG demonstrates severe generalized slowing with generalized and focal epileptiform discharges. Slowed nerve conduction velocities and denervation changes in muscles have been reported in some cases.

**Complications:** Unknown.

**Associated Findings:** An association with cirrhosis of liver has been reported by Blackwood et al (1963). Subsequently several reports have corroborated this association. The changes in liver are those of subacute hepatitis with massive fatty accumulation in hepatocytes, loss of hepatocytes, bile duct proliferation and fibrous scarring. The cirrhosis is of the micronodular type.

**Etiology:** Alpers disease is not a distinct clinicopathological entity, but rather a clinical syndrome caused by a variety of etiological factors or agents. While in the majority of cases the etiology is unknown, three distinct etiologic associations have been described.

*Associated with hepatic cirrhosis*: more than 15 cases have been reported with this association. A single etiologic factor has been postulated as causing injury to brain and liver. Familial cases have been reported, and an autosomal recessive inheritance has been suggested for this entity.

*Associated with abnormality of energy metabolism*: a second subset of Alpers associated with deficiency of pyruvate dehydrogenase in brain was reported by Prick et al (1981). Prick and Gabreels reported a total of 11 cases associated with defects in citric acid cycle and electron transport chain: two cases had decreased activity in cytochrome aa3 complex, b and c in one, and b alone in another, decreased pyruvate carboxylase and pyruvate dehydrogenase were seen in one each. Two patients had "ragged red fibers" on muscle biopsy and one other had abnormality in citric acid cycle before fumarate.

*Associated with* **Creutzfeldt-Jakob disease** *(CJD)-like transmissible agent*: Manuelidis & Rorke (1989) have reported that they were able to serially pass a transmissible agent in hamsters' brains from the brain of a child who had Alpers disease. The changes in hamster's brains were reminiscent of CJD.

**Pathogenesis:** Unknown.

**MIM No.:** *20370

**Sex Ratio:** M1:F1

**Occurrence:** More than 70 cases have been reported.

**Risk of Recurrence for Patient's Sib:**
See Part I, *Mendelian Inheritance.*

**Risk of Recurrence for Patient's Child:**
See Part I, *Mendelian Inheritance.*

**Age of Detectability:** Usually during infancy. Juvenile forms have a later onset.

**Gene Mapping and Linkage:** Unknown.

**Prevention:** None known. Genetic counseling indicated.

**Treatment:** Evaluation to rule out other causes of seizures and developmental delay: congenital infections, inborn errors of metabolism. Antiepileptic drug (AED) therapy. The ketogenic diet may occasionally stop seizures refractory to the usual AEDS.

**Prognosis:** All know patients have died.

**Detection of Carrier:** Unknown.

**References:**

Alpers BJ: Diffuse progressive degenration of the gray matter of the cerebrum, Arch Neurol Psychiat 1931; 25:469–505.
Blackwood W, et al.: Diffuse cerebral degeneration in infancy: Alpers disease. Arch Dis Childh 1963; 38:193–204.
Klein H, Dichgans J: Familiare juvenile gilo-neurale dystrophie: akut beginnende progressive encephalopathic mit rechtsseitigen occipito-parietalen Herdsymptomen und status epilepticus. Archiv für Psychiatrie und Nervenkrankeiten 1969; 212:400–422.
Prick M, et al.: Pyruvate dehydrogenase deficiency restricted to brain. Neurology 1981; 31:398–404.
Prick MJJ, et al.: Progressive poliodystrophy (Alpers disease) with a defect in cytochrome aa3 in muscle: a report of two unrelated patients. Clin Neurol Neurosurg 1983; 85:57–70.
Gabreels FMJ, et al.: Defects in citric acid cycle and the electron transport chain in progressive poliodystrophy. Acta Neurol Scand 1984; 70:145–154.
Harding BN, et al.: Progressive neuronal degeneration of childhood with liver disease. Brain 1986; 109:181–206. *
Manuelidis EE, Rorke LB: Transmission of Alpers disease (chronic progressive encephalopathy) produces experimental Creutzfeldt Jakob disease in hamsters. Neurology 1989; 39:615–621.

VE011                                                    **V.V. Vedanarayanan**
KA008                                                    **Raymond S. Kandt**

**Alpha 1,4-glucosidase deficiency**
    *See GLYCOGENOSIS, TYPE IIa*
**Alpha and Beta LCAT deficiency**
    *See LECITHIN-CHOLESTEROL ACYL TRANSFERASE DEFICIENCY*

**Alpha LCAT deficiency**
*See LECITHIN-CHOLESTEROL ACYL TRANSFERASE DEFICIENCY*

## ALPHA(1)-ANTITRYPSIN DEFICIENCY       0039

**Includes:**
> Antitrypsin
> Cholestasis, neonatal
> Cirrhosis, juvenile (some)
> Emphysema, familial
> Hepatitis, neonatal (some)
> Jaundice, prolonged obstructive
> Liver fibrosis and cirrhosis, adult
> Lung disease, familial chronic obstructive
> Pi phenotype ZZ, SZ, Z- and --
> Protease inhibitor

**Excludes:**
> **Alpha-1-antichymotrypsin deficiency (3279)**
> **Bile ducts, interlobular, nonsyndromic paucity (3277)**
> Pulmonary obstructive disease, nonfamilial idiopathic chronic

**Major Diagnostic Criteria:** Clinical presentation is variable, including early onset hepatitis, cirrhosis, or emphysema. Low serum concentrations of $\alpha_1$ AT may occur with the clinical disease or in an asymptomatic individual. Pi typing is necessary to onfirm the phenotype, and other Pi phenotypes with slightly decreased or normal levels of $\alpha$-antitrypsin serum content of $\alpha_1$-antitrypsin ($\alpha_1$AT) levels should be excluded.

**Clinical Findings:** The natural history of $\alpha_1$ AT deficiency is not known.
*Lung Disease:* In adult PiZZ individuals a characteristic form of emphysema may occur by the 3rd or 4th decade of life. The presenting symptom is often shortness of breath. The chest x-ray shows overinflation of the lungs with diffuse loss of vascular markings over the lower lung fields. Lung scanning confirms a bilateral decrease in lower zone profusion. In younger PiZZ subjects the lung function may be normal or near normal. The median age at onset of dyspnea is about 40 years in PiZZ smokers compared with about 55 years in nonsmokers. Clinical manifestations of lung disease in childhood is exceptionally rare. Pi--subjects acquire severe emphysema early in life. PiSZ individuals are at moderately increased risk of chronic obstructive pulmonary disease (COPD) but the natural history of lung disease in this type of $\alpha_1$ AT deficiency is not completely known.
*Liver disease:* Neonatal cholestasis appears during the first months of life in about 10% of the PiZZ infants. About one-half of the apparently healthy PiZZ infants have abnormal liver tests. Usually the cholestatic symptoms subside within weeks or months. The development of cirrhosis may be noted in about one-fourth of the PiZZ children who suffered neonatal liver disease after a variable time interval. PiSZ children have no increased risk of liver disease. Cirrhosis and liver carcinoma have been observed in about 10% of the PiZZ adults above 50–60 years of age.

**Complications:** Respiratory failure, heart failure, cirrhosis, and liver failure.

**Associated Findings:** Minimal glomerular lesions, peptic ulcer, and possibly rheumatoid arthritis.

**Etiology:** The levels of $\alpha_1$ AT are genetically determined by more than 30 autosomal codominant alleles. Important Pi alleles have the following production rates of $\alpha_1$ AT compared with PiM 1.0: PiS 0.60, PiP 0.25, PiZ 0.15, and Pinull 0. Substitution of one glutamic acid in the M protein by lysine and valine in the Z and S proteins, respectively, has been found.

**Pathogenesis:** The major biological function of $\alpha_1$AT is the inactivation of proteases released mainly intercellularly by the granulocytes. The lungs are an important site of granulocyte destruction and subsequent release of proteolytic enzymes. Another source of proteases are the alveolar macrophages. The lung tissue, especially elastin, is attacked by free proteolytic enzymes, which may result in a degradation of the elastin leading to disturbed physiologic function and lung disease. In smokers both the number and activity of granulocytes and macrophages are increased, and the proteolytic-inhibiting capacity of $\alpha_1$AT is decreased. Cigarette smokers develop symptoms of lung disease roughly 15 years earlier than PiZZ non-smokers. The pathogenesis of liver disease is unknown.

**MIM No.:** *10740

**CDC No.:** 277.620

**Sex Ratio:** M1:F1

**Occurrence:** $\alpha$ AT deficiency occurs with various incidence in different countries. The PiZ gene frequency is 0.026 in Sweden and Norway, 0.013 in the United States, and 0.006 in France.
   Prevalence varies from country to country. In the Scandinavian population 1:1500 has the PiZZ and 1:750 the PiSZ phenotype.

**Risk of Recurrence for Patient's Sib:** 1 in 4 (25%) for each sibling to be affected (PiZZ) if parents are Pi MZ heterozygotes.

**Risk of Recurrence for Patient's Child:** Not increased unless mate is heterozygote or has $\alpha_1$-antitrypsin deficiency.

**Age of Detectability:** An mass-screening method for the detection of PiZZ subjects is available. Prenatal diagnosis is possible.

**Gene Mapping and Linkage:** PI (alpha-1-antitrypsin (protease inhibitor)) has been mapped to 14q32.1.

**Prevention:** Avoid environmental pollutants, especially cigarette smoke. Genetic counseling is indicated.

**Treatment:** Substitution therapy with $\alpha_1$ AT is available (Prolastin R, Cutter Biological) for patients with $\alpha_1$AT deficiency and emphysema. The $\alpha_1$AT-concentrate from human plasma is infused once weekly and establishes a normal elastase-antielastase balance in the lower respiratory tract. on an experimental basis. Treatment of liver and lung disease is mainly supportive and symptomatic. Liver transplantation has been done in some subjects.

**Prognosis:** About 10% of PiZZ children develop neonatal cholestasis with an about 25% risk of juvenile cirrhosis. Another 10% suffer cirrhosis or liver cancer after 50 years of age. About 50–80% of the PiZZ subjects get symptoms of COPD in mid-life, smokers roughly 15 years earlier than non-smokers.

**Detection of Carrier:** Different Pi alleles are expressed in the Pi pattern using preferentially the electrofocusing technique.

**Special Considerations:** Since $\alpha_1$-antitrypsin deficiency and smoke combine in an additive manner to produce premature emphysema, firm advice on the dangers of smoking and certain occupational pollutants should be given at an early age. Screening for $\alpha_1$-antitrypsin deficiency should be considered in countries with high frequencies of the deficiency alleles. Prenatal diagnosis may be indicated in families who already have had a PiZZ child with liver cirrhosis.

**References:**
Larsson C: Natural history and life expectancy in severe $\alpha_1$-antitrypsin deficiency, PiZ. Acta Med Scand 1978; 204:345–351.
Sveger T: Prospective study of children with $\alpha_1$-antitrypsin deficiency. J Pediatr 1984; 104:91–94.
Carrell RW: $\alpha_1$-antitrypsin: molecular pathology, leucocytes, and tissue damage. J Clin Invest 1986; 78:1427–1431.
Cohen AB: The clinical usefulness of different forms of $\alpha_{-1}$-protease inhibitor. Am Rev Resp Dis 1986; 133:349.
Eriksson S, et al.: Risk of cirrhosis and primary liver cancer in $\alpha_1$-antitrypsin deficiency. New Eng J Med 1986; 314:736–739.
Nukiwa T, et al: Identification of a second mutation in the protein-coding sequence of the Z type $\alpha_1$-antitrypsin gene. J Biol Chem 1986; 261:15989–15994.
Cox DW, Mansfield T: Prenatal diagnosis of $\alpha_1$-antitrypsin deficiency and estimates of fetal risk for disease. J Med Genet 1987; 24:52-59.
Wewers MD, et al,: Replacement therapy for $\alpha_1$-antitrypsin deficiency associated with emphysema. New Eng J Med 1987; 316:1055–1062.

SV000                                                   **T. Sveger**

## ALPHA-1-ANTICHYMOTRYPSIN DEFICIENCY    3279

**Includes:** Alpha-1-antichymotrypsin deficiency, primary

**Excludes:**
**Alpha(1)-antitrypsin deficiency** (0039)
Alpha-1-antichymotrypsin deficiency, secondary and acquired

**Major Diagnostic Criteria:** Serum deficiency of alpha-1-antichymotrypsin, as defined by a serum level below 50% of normal, in the absence of other disease that could cause a secondary deficiency in the first criterion. Identification of affected family members confirms the disease.

**Clinical Findings:** Among subjects with serum deficiency of alpha-1-antichymotrypsin, the majority have no evidence of organ disease, while a minority have liver and/or lumg involvement. Symptoms of liver and lung disease have been identified only in the population over 25 years of age. Liver involvement ranges from no clinical signs of liver disease with subtle biochemical abnormalities to to a disease resembling chronic active hepatitis. Hepatomegaly may be present. Liver biopsy in one subject revealed steatosis and fibrosis. One case with liver failure and hepatic coma has been reported, and another case has been reported where cirrhosis developed.

Lung involvement varies from reversible airway obstruction (asthmalike disease) to more chronic destructive brocho-alveolar disease, with decreased lung compliance and/or increased residual volumes.

**Complications:** *Hepatic*: Presumably all of the complications of chronic parenchymal liver disease, including portal hypertension, hypersplenism, ascites, porto-systemic encephalopathy, esophageal varices, and related signs and symptoms.
*Pulmonary*: Emphysema, recurrent pneumonia, pulmonary insufficiency.

**Associated Findings:** None known.

**Etiology:** Autosomal dominant inheritance with variable phenotypic expression.

**Pathogenesis:** Possibly a deletion of one of two alleles in the gene for alpha-1-antichymotrypsin. Subnormal alpha-1-antichymotrypsin levels may be inadequate to inhibit the action of protcases released during inflammatory responses, which results in exaggerated local tissue destruction.

**MIM No.:** *10728

**Sex Ratio:** Presumably M1:F1.

**Occurrence:** A study in Sweden estimated the frequency at 0.7%.

**Risk of Recurrence for Patient's Sib:**
See Part I, *Mendelian Inheritance.*

**Risk of Recurrence for Patient's Child:**
See Part I, *Mendelian Inheritance.*

**Age of Detectability:** Presumably at birth. Clinical disease can be detected in patients twenty-five years of age or older.

**Gene Mapping and Linkage:** AACT (alpha-1-antichymotrypsin) has been mapped to 14q32.1.

**Prevention:** None known. Genetic counseling indicated.

**Treatment:** Unknown.

**Prognosis:** Variable.

**Detection of Carrier:** Measuring plasma level of alpha-1-antichymotrypsin.

**References:**
Eriksson S, et al.: Familial alpha-1-antichymotrypsin deficiency. Acta Med Scand 1986; 220:447–453.

FI035
AL037

**Mark Fishbein**
**Estella M. Alonso**

**Alpha-1-antichymotrypsin deficiency, primary**
*See ALPHA-1-ANTICHYMOTRYPSIN DEFICIENCY*

**Alpha-antitrypsin deficiency and connective tissue defect**
*See CUTIS LAXA*
**Alpha-galactosidase A deficiency**
*See FABRY DISEASE*
**Alpha-galactosidase B deficiency**
*See ALPHA-N-ACETYLGALACTOSAMINIDASE DEFICIENCY*
**Alpha-interferon deficiency**
*See INTERFERON DEFICIENCY*
**Alpha-L-fucosidase deficiency**
*See FUCOSIDOSIS*
**Alpha-L-iduronidase deficiency**
*See MUCOPOLYSACCHARIDOSIS I-H*
**Alpha-mannosidosis**
*See MANNOSIDOSIS*
**Alpha-methylacetoacetic aciduria**
*See ACIDEMIA, 3-KETOTHIOLASE DEFICIENCY*

## ALPHA-N-ACETYLGALACTOSAMINIDASE DEFICIENCY    3254

**Includes:**
Alpha-galactosidase B deficiency
Glycoaminoacid storage disease-angiokeratoma corporis diffusion
Neuroaxonal dystrophy, infantile (one form)
Schindler disease

**Excludes:**
Angiokeratoma mibelli
**Fabry disease** (0373)
**Fucosidosis** (0398)
**Galactosialidosis** (3110)
**Neuroaxonal dystrophy, infantile** (2701)
**Telangiectasia, Osler hemorrhagic** (2021)

**Major Diagnostic Criteria:** Children with the infantile-onset subtype develop normally for the first six to twelve months of life and then experience a rapid neurodegenerative course characteristic of **Neuroaxonal dystrophy, infantile.** Pathologically, dystrophic axonal swellings or "spheroids" can be found in the cortical brain, and dystrophic axons are present in the myenteric plexus in rectum. Individuals with the adult-onset subtype have angiokeratoma corporis diffusum as the major manifestation of the disease and do not have neurologic symptoms. In both subtypes, the abnormal urinary excretion of O-linked glycopeptides and sialoglycopeptides can be detected. The diagnosis of either subtype requires the demonstration of deficient $\alpha$-N-acetylgalactosaminidase activity in plasma, leukocytes or cultured cells.

**Clinical Findings:** Two subtypes of $\alpha$-N-acetylgalactosaminidase deficiency have been described. Clinical onset in the infantile subtype occurs in the first year of life when developmental delay and retrogression of developmental milestones are noted. Subsequently, patients experience a rapid neurodegenerative course with loss of all previously acquired mental and motor skills. Grand-mal seizures, muscular weakness, incoordination, strabismus, and nystagmus are early manifestations. Later neurological signs include spastic quadriplegia, cortical blindness, deafness, myoclonus, rigidity, immobility, and a decorticate state with little, if any, contact with the environment. Imaging studies reveal generalized atrophy of the brain, especially of the cerebellum and brainstem. The clinical course is identical to that seen in **Neuroaxonal dystrophy, infantile.**

In marked contrast, the adult-onset form is characterized by the development of telangiectasia (angiokeratoma corporis diffusum), which appear in the second or third decade of life and progressively become more dense and disseminated. These cutaneous lesions are distributed from the chest to the perineum, and are similar in appearance to those observed in affected males with **Fabry disease.** In addition, the only adult-onset patient described to date had mild shortness of stature and slightly coarse facial features.

**Complications:** Frequent and severe respiratory tract infections may occur in the infantile-onset subtype. Angina pectoris may occur in the adult-onset subtype.

**Associated Findings:** None known.

**Etiology:** Autosomal recessive inheritance of lysosomal α-N-acetylgalactosaminidase deficiency.

**Pathogenesis:** The enzyme deficiency in both subtypes results in the lysosomal and urinary accumulation of O-linked glycopeptides and oligosaccharides with terminal and internal α-N-acetylgalactosaminyl residues. The enzyme defect in the infantile-onset subtype causes the neuropathologic abnormalities characteristic of **Neuroaxonal dystrophy, infantile.** However, studies of six patients with biopsy-proven **Neuroaxonal dystrophy, infantile** did not have α-N-acetylgalactosaminidase deficiency or glycopeptiduria. The pathophysiologic events leading to either neuroaxonal dystrophy or to angiokeratoma corporis diffusum have not been identified. In contrast, the adult-onset form is characterized by lysosomal accumulation, particularly in blood vessels leading to a disseminated angiokeratoma similar to that observed in hemizygotes with **Fabry disease.** The nervous system was not clinically involved in the one adult-onset patient described to date.

**MIM No.:** *10417

**Sex Ratio:** M1:F1

**Occurrence:** Two male siblings with the infantile-onset subtype have been described. They are Caucasian of German origin, the offspring of a fourth cousin mating. The only adult-onset patient identified is a 46 year old Japanese female, the product of a first cousin mating.

**Risk of Recurrence for Patient's Sib:**
See Part I, *Mendelian Inheritance.* Two in three (67%) for each normal sibling to be a carrier.

**Risk of Recurrence for Patient's Child:**
See Part I, *Mendelian Inheritance.* Affected individuals with the infantile-onset subtype do not reproduce. All offspring of affected individuals with the adult-onset disease will be carriers.

**Age of Detectability:** For either subtype, the biochemical diagnosis can be accomplished by demonstrating the deficient activity of α-N-acetylgalactosaminidase in plasma, leukocytes, or cultured cells at any age of life. As the enzyme is expressed in chorionic villi and amniocytes, prenatal diagnosis is possible for families at risk.

**Gene Mapping and Linkage:** NAGA (acetylgalactosaminidase, alpha-N-) has been mapped to 22q13-qter.

**Prevention:** None known. Genetic counseling indicated.

**Treatment:** Unknown. Physical therapy and supportive care in the infantile-onset form to facilitate patient comfort.

**Prognosis:** Infantile-onset patients are severely retarded and debilitated by five years of age, and are subject to life-threatening aspirations and intercurrent infections. The only adult-onset patient has survived into the fifth decade without serious health complications.

**Detection of Carrier:** Carriers can be identified by their intermediate levels of α-N-acetylgalactosaminidase activity in plasma, leukocytes or cultured cells.

**Special Considerations:** Infants diagnosed as having **Neuroaxonal dystrophy, infantile** by demonstration of the characteristic morphologic alterations in biopsied tissues, as well as patients who have angiokeratoma corporis diffusum but normal α-galactosidase, α-L-fucosidase, β-galactosidase and sialidase activity, should be investigated for increased urinary glycopeptide excretion and deficient α-N-acetylgalactosaminidase activity in plasma or leukocytes.

**References:**
Van Diggelen OP, et al.: Lysosomal α-N-acetylgalactosaminidase deficiency: a new inherited metabolic disease. (Letter) Lancet 1987; II:804.
Schindler D, et al.: Neuroaxonal dystrophy due to lysosomal α-N-galactosaminidase deficiency. New Eng J Med 1989; 320:1735–1740. *
Desnick RJ, Bishop DF: Fabry disease: α-galactosidase deficiency; Schindler disease: α-N-acetylgalactosaminidase deficiency. In: Scriver CR, et al, eds: The metabolic basis of inherited disease, 6th ed. New York: McGraw-Hill, 1989:1751–1796. †
Kanzaki T, et al.: Novel lysosomal glycoaminoacid storage disease with angiokeratoma corporis diffussum. Lancet 1989; I:875–877.

DE024
SC076

Robert J. Desnick
Detlev Schindler

**Alphalipoprotein deficiency**
See ANALPHALIPOPROTEINEMIA
**Alport syndrome**
See NEPHRITIS-DEAFNESS (SENSORINEURAL), HEREDITARY TYPE
**Alport syndrome-like hereditary nephritis**
See NEPHRITIS-DEAFNESS (SENSORINEURAL), HEREDITARY TYPE
**Alprazolam, fetal effects**
See FETAL BENZODIAZEPINE EFFECTS
**ALS**
See AMYOTROPHIC LATERAL SCLEROSIS
also AMYOTROPHIC LATERAL SCLEROSIS, FAMILIAL ADULT AND JUVENILE TYPES
**ALS-PD**
See AMYOTROPHIC LATERAL SCLEROSIS, GUAM TYPE

---

**ALSTROM SYNDROME**      0041

**Includes:** Alstrom-Hallgren syndrome

**Excludes:**
**Bardet-Biedl syndrome** (2363)
**Biemond I syndrome** (3034)
**Biemond II syndrome** (2169)
Klein syndrome
Weiss syndrome

**Major Diagnostic Criteria:** Diffuse retinitis of early childhood onset leading to functional blindness by adolescence, with development of cataracts in early adulthood. Sensory neural hearing loss gradualy develops in later childhood and progresses to clinical deafness in adolescence. Moderate obesity is associated with glucose intolerance or manifest diabetes mellitus, and is usually controlled by diet. Hypogenitalism is present in 50% of reported cases. There is normal intelligence and stature but no polydactyly.

**Clinical Findings:** In ten documented cases, pre and post-natal history were normal and visual imparment occurred by age one year (8/10) followed by gradual onset of moderate neural hearing loss (10/10). All cases have had cataracts, usually of the posterior capsule. Other ophthalmologic abnormalities observed are: glaucome (2/10), dislocated lens (1/10), and vitreous fibrosis (1/10).

Glucose intolerance or diabetes mellitus had early adulthood onset (8/10), but few patients required insulin (2/10). Renal function was impaired due to a chronic nephropathy (6/8). Hyalinized or sclerosed glomeruli and tubules resembling nephronophithisis were observed on kidney biopsies from two patients.

The four females reported have had onset of menses between age 9 and 14 years. Males have had small testes (5/6) and biopsy in three of them demonstrated reduced germinal cells, tubular sclerosis, and well developed Leydig cells. Development of secondary sex characteristics was normal in all patients.

Intelligence has been normal in all cases, and most patients (9/10) have had normal stature. Karotypes in 2 males and 1 female were normal. Other observations include acanthosis nigricans (4/10), mild scalp hair loss (6/6), and amino aciduria (4/7).

**Complications:** Chronic nephropathy with or without diabetes mellitus can lead to renal failure. Hair loss usually produces receding temporal hairline but has rarely resulted in generalized scalp alopecia. Since no patient has reproduced, infertility may be presumed as a complication.

**Associated Findings:** None known.

**Etiology:** Autosomal recessive inheritance. No vertical transmission reported, and both male and female sibs have been affected.

**Pathogenesis:** Unknown.

**MIM No.:** *20380

**POS No.:** 3020

**Sex Ratio:** M6:F4

**Occurrence:** Rare; ten cases reported in four families.

**Risk of Recurrence for Patient's Sib:**
See Part I, *Mendelian Inheritance.*

**Risk of Recurrence for Patient's Child:**
See Part I, *Mendelian Inheritance.*

**Age of Detectability:** Retinopathy commonly occurs in first year and obesity is present in early childhood. Visual impairment, and hearing loss are usually evident by age 20 years. Age range of all reported cases is 16 to 36.

**Gene Mapping and Linkage:** Unknown.

**Prevention:** None known. Genetic counseling indicated.

**Treatment:** Effects of hearing loss may be ameliorated by hearing aids. Where mild retinopathy and cataracts exists, removal of cataracts may improve vision. Treatment of diabetes may decrease risk of renal disease. Renal failure may necessitate dialysis.

**Prognosis:** Two reports of death were at age 16 and 32, and due to renal failure. Concurrence of blindness, deafness, diabetes mellitus, and nephropathy probably shorten life span but degree is unknown. Intelligence appears normal.

**Detection of Carrier:** Alstrom reported impaired glucose tolerance in both parents of a proband, but otherwise, no carrier detection is possible.

**References:**

Alstrom CH, et al: Retinal degeneration combined with obesity, diabetes mellitus and neurogenous deafness: A specific syndrome (not hitherto described): Distinct from the Laurence-Moon-Bardet-Biedl syndrome. A clinical, endocrinological and genetic examination basd on a large pedigree. Acta Psychiat Neurol Scand (Suppl 129) 1959; 34:1–35.

Klein D, Ammann F: the syndrome of Laurence-Moon-Bardet-Biedl and allied diseases in Switzerland: clinical, genetic and epidemiological studies. J Neurol Sci 1969; 9:479.

Weinstein RL, et al: Familial syndrome of primary testicular insufficiency with normal virilization, blindness, deafness, and metabolic abnormalities. New Eng J Med 1969; 281:969–977.

Goldstein JL, Fialkow PJ: The Alstrom syndrome. Report of three cases with further delineation of the clinical, pathophysiological, and genetic aspects of the disorder. Medicine 1973; 52:53–71.

Schachat AP, Maumenee IH: Bardet-Biedl syndrome and related disorders. Arch Ophthalmol 1982; 100:285–288.

WI049
FR016

**Charles A. Williams**
**Jaime L. Frias**

**Alstrom-Hallgren syndrome**
*See ALSTROM SYNDROME*

## ALVEOLAR RIDGES, LYMPHANGIOMA                0613

**Includes:** Lymphangioma of alveolar ridges

**Excludes:**
Eruption cysts
**Inclusion cysts of the oral mucosa in the newborn** (3236)
Mucous retention cysts
**Teeth, epulis, congenital** (0360)

**Major Diagnostic Criteria:** Lymphangioma on the alveolar ridges of newborns, confirmed histologically.

**Clinical Findings:** These lymphangiomas are seen on the maxillary or mandibular alveolar ridges of newborn infants. When on the maxillary ridge, they are on the crest at the site where the first molars are expected to erupt. When on the mandibular ridge, they are on the lingual surface at a site homologous to those on the maxillary ridge. The tongue may have to be displaced to see those on the mandibular ridge. The lymphangiomas may be solitary (26%) or multiple (74%). They are frequently bilateral (55%) and may exist in all four quadrants simultaneously. They are fluid-filled, and their surfaces vary from being slightly raised above adjacent mucosa to being raised 3–4 mm above adjacent mucosa. Their diameters vary from < 1 mm to several millimeters.

**Complications:** The lesions appear to bother infants during nursing.

**Associated Findings:** None known.

**Etiology:** Undetermined. All affected infants have been black. The racial predilection and symmetric distribution of alveolar ridge lymphangiomas suggest the possibility of a developmental, perhaps genetic, etiology.

**Pathogenesis:** Undetermined. The histologic appearance of some biopsied lesions is similar to that of hemangioma, but the majority resemble lymphangioma. The lesions are composed of soft tissue, with numerous endothelial-lined vascular channels. They collapse when biopsied and discharge a thin, clear fluid. No teeth are evident in the tissue under the lesions.

**Sex Ratio:** M3:F2

**Occurrence:** Approximately 1:25 among blacks (4%). Not reported among non-blacks. Prevalence not reported for older children.

**Risk of Recurrence for Patient's Sib:** Unknown.

**Risk of Recurrence for Patient's Child:** Unknown.

**Age of Detectability:** At birth.

**Gene Mapping and Linkage:** Unknown.

**Prevention:** None known. Genetic counseling indicated.

**Treatment:** None needed in most cases. Occasionally surgical excision may be necessary.

**Prognosis:** Good. Since these lesions have not been reported in older children, it could be assumed that they regress prior to intraoral examination by a physician or dentist. Several cases that were followed showed variable changes in the lesions. In some, the lesions became smaller with time. In others, the lesions remained the same size, but changed color and surface character. In still others, the lesions became fibrotic masses. The longest follow-up was 6 1/2 months.

**Detection of Carrier:** Unknown.

**References:**

Levin LS, et al.: Lymphangiomas of the alveolar ridges in neonates. Pediatrics 1976; 58:881–884.

Jorgenson RJ, et al.: Intraoral findings and anomalies in neonates. Pediatrics 1982; 69:577–582.

J0027
LE028

**Ronald J. Jorgenson**
**L. Stefan Levin**

**Alymphocytosis**
*See IMMUNODEFICIENCY, X-LINKED SEVERE COMBINED*
**Alymphocytosis, pure**
*See IMMUNODEFICIENCY, NEZELOF TYPE*
**Alymphopenic immunologic deficiency, Gitlin form**
*See IMMUNODEFICIENCY, X-LINKED SEVERE COMBINED*

## ALZHEIMER DISEASE, FAMILIAL                2354

**Includes:**
Amyloid beta A4 precursor protein
Amyloid of aging and Alzheimer disease
Cerebral vascular amyloid peptide
Presenile dementia, familial
Senile dementia of the Alzheimer's type
Senile dementia, familial

**Excludes:**
**Creutzfeldt-Jakob disease** (3244)
**Leukodystrophy, adult onset progressive dominant type** (2975)
Multi-infarct dementia
**Pick disease of the brain** (3243)
Progressive dementia not of the Alzheimer type
Subcortical arteriosclerotic encephalopathy

**Major Diagnostic Criteria:** The slow and insidious onset of a progressive memory disturbance accompanied by deficits in cognitive functions. There is a lack of focal neurologic signs such as hemiparasis and hemisensory loss. A computed tomography (CT) scan or magnetic resonance image (MRI) often show cerebral atrophy and ventricular enlargement. The diagnosis is confirmed by postmortem (or occasional biopsy) examination of the brain which shows gross cortical atrophy and microscopic changes consisting of neuronal loss, senile plaques, and neurofibrillary tangles. There is no reliable diagnostic laboratory test to confirm the diagnosis.

**Clinical Findings:** Symptoms usually begin after 60 years of age with progressive forgetfulness. Names and words are forgotten and recent conversations are not remembered. The deficits include disturbances in judgment, language, calculation, visuospatial functions, and personality. Patients have difficulty finding correct words in speaking and writing. Patients may become lost while driving or walking in a familiar neighborhood. Difficulty occurs in performing motor tasks (motor apraxia) and patients eventually cannot perform the activities of daily living. Patients may exhibit paranoia or unusual behavior.

Early in the illness patients attempt to circumvent minor deficits through the use of list making and the transfer of responsibilities. As the disease progresses these mechanisms are unable to compensate for the deficits and patients may become withdrawn, hostile, or restless. In later stages frontal release signs (grasp, suck reflex) may appear, incontinence develops, and patients develop an unsteady gait with occasional falls. Hypokinesia progresses to akinesia and mutism. The disease progresses for 5–10 years until the patient becomes bedridden and expires from an intercurrent infection or other medical problem.

There is a marked lack of focal motor, sensory, or visual signs such as hemiplegia or visual field deficits. Myoclonic jerks or generalized motor seizures may develop in as many as 10% of patients, especially in younger cases.

Routine laboratory studies are normal. Vitamin B12 and folate deficiency, neurosyphilis and hypothyroidism should always be excluded as reversible causes of dementia. Neuroimaging studies such as head computed tomography (CT) or magnetic resonance imaging (MRI) often show cerebral atrophy and ventricular enlargement. Similar, though less severe changes are also seen in aged non-demented patients. Head CT and MRI are also useful for excluding other causes of dementia such as multiple infarcts, tumors, and normal pressure hydrocephalus. In addition, single photon emission computer tomography (SPECT) has proven useful in identifying those cases in which depression mimics early dementia (Kirn, 1989). The EEG may show slowing of the background rhythm. Neuropsychiatric evaluation using the Mini-Mental State test and Dementia Rating Scale are useful for characterizing the cognitive deficits and quantifying changes as the disease progresses. The recently described Alz-50 antibody assay detects a specific antigen in the CSF of patients. The sensitivity and specificity of this antibody are being investigated.

**Complications:** Pulmonary, urinary, and skin infections caused by a bedridden state often occur in the latter stages of the illness. Malnutrition and dehydration may occur due to poor oral intake.

**Associated Findings:** In patients with Alzheimer disease (A.D.) an excess of thyroid disease and head trauma have been reported in some studies. An increased incidence of **Chromosome 21, trisomy 21** was reported in the close relatives of the probands with a frequency between 3.6–8.3:1,000 relatives. Although one study found an increased incidence of hematologic cancers in relatives of probands, other studies have not confirmed this finding.

**Etiology:** Autosomal dominant inheritance with age-dependent penetrance.

**Pathogenesis:** Numerous theories have been advanced, including viruses, toxins, and genetic abnormalities. Aluminum has been implicated as a possible cause, but while aluminum and other metals may accumulate in the brain as part of a non-specific response to brain degeneration, there is no evidence of a causal relationship.

A genetic factor is supported by several lines of evidence. People over the age of 35 with **Chromosome 21, trisomy 21** almost always develop progressive mental deterioration with pathologic changes identical to those seen in A.D. There is an increased

incidence of **Chromosome 21, trisomy 21** in relatives of probands with A.D. Several recent studies have found evidence for a gene locus on chromosome 21 that may be responsible for some cases of Alzheimer disease. The gene locus for late onset familial Alzheimer disease appears not to be on chromosome 21, although controversy continues to surround this issue.

Masters et al (1985) have purified and characterized a cerebral amyloid protein (amyloid beta (A4) protein) that forms in the plaque core in Alzheimer disease and in aged persons with **Chromosome 21, trisomy 21**.

**MIM No.:** *10430, 10476

**Sex Ratio:** M1:F1.5. Most studies have found a higher overall prevelance ratio and age-specific incidence rates for females.

**Occurrence:** Since the diagnosis of A.D. can only be confirmed by pathologic examination, most epidemiologic studies can only approximate the true incidence and prevalence of A.D. The incidence and prevalence of clinically diagnosed A.D. increases with age. The average annual incidence rate is 2.4:100,000 populations between 40 and 60 years, but increases to 127:100,000 after 60 years. The prevalence is between 1.9–5.8:100 population aged 65 or greater.

Studies of autopsy-proven cases of Alzheimer disease found the cumulative incidence of secondary cases of dementia at age 74 in siblings and parents of probands to be 7.7 and 11.8%, respectively. The risk of secondary cases of dementia at age 85 or more increased to 19.5 and 22.7% in the two groups. One study found that sibs of probands with onset of dementia before age 70 with an affected parent had almost a 50% risk of developing dementia. This age effect was not confirmed in a later study. Despite these differences, it is clear that an individual's risk of developing A.D. increases if other family members are affected.

**Risk of Recurrence for Patient's Sib:**
See Part I, *Mendelian Inheritance*. Probably 1:2 by age 90 in well-documented familial cases with apparent autosomal dominant inheritance (i.e. sib and parent affected).

**Risk of Recurrence for Patient's Child:**
See Part I, *Mendelian Inheritance*. This risk has not been adequately studied. While one might assume a maximum risk of 50% in well-documented pedigrees with apparent autosomal dominant inheritance, reliable data is not available to permit accurate predictions.

**Age of Detectability:** Symptoms may begin after 60 years of age; however there is convincing evidence for age-dependent penetrance, as evidenced by increasing incidence with advancing age.

**Gene Mapping and Linkage:** AD1 (Alzheimer disease) has been mapped to 21q21-q22.1.

APP (amyloid beta (A4) protein) has been mapped to 21q21.

AD1 may only apply to early onset AD. Studies using chromosome 21 DNA markers have linked several families with early onset familial AD to chromosome 21, close to the centromere. While the beta-amyloid gene is close to this region on chromosome 21, linkage studies have found cross-overs between A.D. and the beta-amyloid gene, thus indicating that amyloid is not the primary gene responsible for A.D. Two recent studies have examined late onset familial AD and have failed to detect linkage to the chromosome 21q21-q22 region. This may indicate genetic heterogeneity in the pathogenesis of familial AD.

**Prevention:** None known. Genetic counseling indicated.

**Treatment:** Regimens using cholinomimetic agents and cholinesterase inhibitors have not yielded encouraging results. Trials of the acetylcholine precursors choline and lecithin failed to demonstrate any improvement in memory. Some studies of the cholinesterase inhibitor physostigmine demonstrated marginal and short term memory improvement. However the short half-life of physostigmine and its side effects limit its usefulness. Supportive medical care, family support groups, and symptomatic treatment of complications (infections, nutritional support) may provide short-term comfort.

**Prognosis:** The disease progresses over five to ten years. Decreased life expectancy is observed, with approximately 75% of patients dying within ten years after onset of the disease.

**Detection of Carrier:** Careful neurologic and psychologic assessments may detect individuals early in the course of the disease. Pedigree analysis may allow detection of families and individuals at high risk.

**Special Considerations:** Controversy exists regarding the percentage of Alzheimer's Disease (A.D.) cases that are familial. It now appears that from 40% to 90% of Alzheimer disease cases are familial. It has been argued that most cases are hereditary but the gene is not fully penetrant until age 90. Some cases thought to be sporadic may be familial, but family members die from other causes before they express the disease. However, several large families have been studied in which members at risk lived into their 90s without evidence of dementia. While a positive family history may help distinguish familial from sporadic cases, a negative family history may not rule out familial A.D. due to its age-dependent penetrance.

The differentiation of familial from non-familial A.D. may not be possible based on an isolated clinical examination of the patient. One study found that the presence of aphasia or agraphia in a proband increased the risk for developing A.D. among sibs and children to 55%. However, these findings have not been confirmed in several other studies. Until a reliable genetic marker is identified, only careful pedigree analysis can provide convincing evidence of the familial form of A.D.

**Support Groups:**
Chicago; Alzheimer's Disease and Related Disorders Association (ADRDA)
CANADA: Ontario; Toronto; Alzheimer Society

**References:**
Heston LL, et al.: Dementia of the Alzheimer type: clinical genetics, natural history, and associated conditions. Arch Gen Psychiatry 1981; 38:1085–1090. *

Heyman A, et al.: Alzheimer's disease: genetic aspects and associated clinical disorders. Ann Neurol 1983; 14:507–515.

Masters CL, et al.: Amyloid plaque core protein in Alzheimer disease and Down syndrome. Proc Nat Acad Sci 1985; 82:4245–4249.

Katzman R: Alzheimer's disease. New Engl J Med 1986; 314:964–973. *

Rocca WA, et al.: Epidemiology of clinically diagnosed Alzheimer's disease. Ann Neurol 1986; 19:415–424.

Whitehouse PJ: Understanding the etiology of Alzheimer's disease: current approaches. In: Hutton JT, ed: Neurologic clinics, dementia, Vol 14(2). Philadelphia: W.B. Saunders, 1986:427–438.

Delabar JM, et al.: β-amyloid gene duplication in Alzheimer's disease and karyotypically normal Down's syndrome. Science 1987; 235:1390–1393.

St. George-Hyslop PH, et al.: Absence of duplication of chromosome 21 genes in familial and sporadic Alzheimer's disease. Science 1987; 238:664–666.

St. George-Hyslop PH, et al.: The genetic defect causing familial Alzheimer's disease maps on chromsome 21. Science 1987; 235:885–890.

Mark JL: Evidence uncovered for a second Alzheimer's gene. Science 1988; 241:1432–1433.

Pericak-Vance MA, et al.: Genetic linkage studies in Alzheimer disease families. Exp Neurol 1988; 102:271–279.

Schellenberg GD, et al.: Absence of linkage chromosome 21q21 markers to familial Alzheimer's disease. Science 1988; 241:1507–1510.

Goate AM, et al.: Predisposing locus for Alzheimer's disease on chromosome 21. Lancet 1989; I:352–355.

Joachim CL, et al.: Amyloid beta-protein deposition in tissues other than brain in Alzheimer's disease. Nature 1989; 341:226–230.

Kirn TF: Dementias appear to have individual profiles in single photon emission computed tomography. J Am Med Asso 1989; 261:965–968.

AL026                                        **Mark J. Alberts**

**Amastia, breast**
*See BREAST, AMASTIA*
**Amaurosis congenita of Leber, types I and II**
*See RETINA, AMAUROSIS CONGENITA, LEBER TYPE*

**Amaurosis of retinal origin, congenital**
*See RETINA, AMAUROSIS CONGENITA, LEBER TYPE*
**Amaurotic familial idiocy**
*See NEURONAL CEROID-LIPOFUSCINOSES (NCL)*
**Amegakaryocytic thrombocytopenia-bilateral absence of the radii**
*See THROMBOCYTOPENIA-ABSENT RADIUS*
**Amelia**
*See LIMB REDUCTION DEFECTS*

---

## AMELO-CEREBRO-HYPOHIDROTIC SYNDROME        0044

**Includes:**
Epilepsy-amelogenesis
Epilepsy-yellow teeth
Kohlschutter syndrome
Teeth, hypoplastic enamel

**Excludes:**
**Amelo-onycho-hypohidrotic syndrome** (0045)
**Ectodermal dysplasia, Christ-Siemens-Touraine type** (0333)

**Major Diagnostic Criteria:** Thin hypoplastic enamel occurs on all teeth in a patient with seizures, spasticity, progressive oligophrenia and hypohidrosis.

**Clinical Findings:** The syndrome is characterized by thin hypoplastic enamel on teeth of both dentitions, severe epileptiform seizures usually appearing between 11 months and 4 years of age, muscle spasticity, progressive mental retardation, and hypohidrosis. Peripheral nerve conduction velocities and nerve biopsy are normal and EEG is diffusely abnormal. Decreased numbers of sweat and sebaceous glands, and increased sweat potassium have been found. Brain histology shows diminished number of neurons, small glial cells, ballooning of axons and lipid-filled pericytes.

**Complications:** Sensitivity of teeth to thermal changes. Psychosocial changes with oligophrenia. The mental retardation, muscle spasticity, and microcephaly occur after the onset of seizures. In one studied case, head circumference was normal (at 50th percentile) before the onset of seizures at 11 months of age, but subsequent to onset of seizures showed little further growth and was below the 3rd percentile at two years of age.

**Associated Findings:** None known.

**Etiology:** Undetermined. All affected patients have been male. Autosomal recessive or X-linked recessive inheritance is possible.

**Pathogenesis:** Unknown.

**MIM No.:** 22675

**POS No.:** 3021

**Sex Ratio:** Undetermined. M1:F0 observed.

**Occurrence:** Rare. Occurs in isolates in Switzerland and Germany. Four kindreds known with 11 males affected.

**Risk of Recurrence for Patient's Sib:**
See Part I, *Mendelian Inheritance.*

**Risk of Recurrence for Patient's Child:**
See Part I, *Mendelian Inheritance.*

**Age of Detectability:** For tooth defect: at time of eruption of primary teeth (6 months-1 year). For spasticity: 11 months-4 years.

**Gene Mapping and Linkage:** Unknown.

**Prevention:** None known. Genetic counseling indicated.

**Treatment:** Crowning and reconstruction of teeth; prevention of seizures by anticonvulsant drugs.

**Prognosis:** Guarded. Most affected males have died in first decade.

**Detection of Carrier:** Unknown.

**Support Groups:** MD; Landover; Epilepsy Foundation of America

**References:**
Kohlschütter A, et al.: Familial epilepsy and yellow teeth - a disease of the CNS associated with enamel hypoplasia. Helv Paediatr Acta 1974; 29:283–294. *

Witkop CJ Jr, Sauk JJ Jr.: Defects of enamel. In: Stewart RE, Prescott GH, eds: Oralfacial genetics. St. Louis: CV Mosby Co, 1976:200–202.

WI043
K0005

**Carl J. Witkop, Jr.**
**Alfried Kohlschütter**

**Amelo-onycho-dyshidrotic syndrome**
*See AMELO-ONYCHO-HYPOHIDROTIC SYNDROME*

## AMELO-ONYCHO-HYPOHIDROTIC SYNDROME    0045

**Includes:**
> Amelo-onycho-dyshidrotic syndrome
> Amelo-onycho-lyticdyshidrotic syndrome
> Enamel hypocalcification-onycholysis-hypohidrosis
> Hypohidrosis-onycholysis-enamel hypocalcification
> Onycholysis-hypohidrosis-enamel hypocalcification

**Excludes:**
> Anhidrosis and neurolabyrinthitis
> **Ectodermal dysplasia, Christ-Siemens-Touraine type** (0333)
> Onycholysis
> **Teeth, amelogenesis imperfecta** (0046)
> **Tricho-dento-osseous syndrome** (0965)

**Major Diagnostic Criteria:**  Hypoplastic enamel, elevation of nails from nail bed, deficiency of sweating, seborrhea of scalp and dry, rough skin. In one kindred all 12 affected members had all five signs. In another kindred, four affected patients lacked seborrheic dermatitis of scalp.

**Clinical Findings:**  The condition is characterized by the association of five distinctive features:
1.) A hypocalcified-hypoplastic enamel that is brown, pitted, thin, and soft. Many teeth fail to erupt in the permanent dentition and undergo resorption of enamel of the occlusal edges. Enamel at the cervical of the crown is usually better formed, approaching normal thickness and mineralization.
2.) Onycholysis of finger and toenails involve from 1/4 to 1/2 of the distal portion of the nail, separating the nail from the nail bed with a thin layer of subungual hyperkeratosis. The surface of the nail is smooth.
3.) Hypohidrosis. The number of sweat gland openings on dermal ridges is normal, but the response of the glands to heat by secreting sweat is markedly diminished. Rectal temperatures may be slightly elevated.
4.) Skin is rough and dry, particularly on the volar surfaces, back, and upper arm.
5.) Seborrheic dermatitis of scalp.

**Complications:**  Premature loss of teeth, impacted teeth with radiolucent lesions of jaws, and intra-alveolar resorption of teeth.

**Associated Findings:**  None known.

**Etiology:**  Autosomal dominant inheritance .

**Pathogenesis:**  Undetermined. Possibly a defect in keratin-producing cells

**MIM No.:**  *10457

**POS No.:**  3022

**Sex Ratio:**  M1:F1

**Occurrence:**  Rare; three kindreds reported.

**Risk of Recurrence for Patient's Sib:**
> See Part I, *Mendelian Inheritance.*

**Risk of Recurrence for Patient's Child:**
> See Part I, *Mendelian Inheritance.*

**Age of Detectability:**  Six to 12 months of age with eruption of teeth. Nail and skin involvement become apparent later at 2–3 years of age.

**Gene Mapping and Linkage:**  Unknown.

**Prevention:**  None known. Genetic counseling indicated.

**Treatment:**  Dental restoration.

**Prognosis:**  Does not appear to reduce longevity or fertility. Premature loss of teeth.

**Detection of Carrier:**  Unknown.

**References:**
Witkop CJ Jr, et al.: Hypoplastic enamel, onycholysis and hypohidrosis inherited as an autosomal dominant trait. A review of the ectodermal dysplasia syndromes. Oral Surg 1975; 39:71–86. *
Witkop CJ Jr., Sauk JJ Jr.: Heritable defects of enamel. In Stewart RE, Prescott GH, eds: Oral facial genetics. St Louis: C.V. Mosby, 1976:194–197.

WI043

**Carl J. Witkop, Jr.**

**Amelo-onycho-lyticdyshidrotic syndrome**
*See AMELO-ONYCHO-HYPOHIDROTIC SYNDROME*
**Amelogenesis imperfecta, hypocalcification type**
*See TEETH, AMELOGENESIS IMPERFECTA*
**Amelogenesis imperfecta, hypomaturation type**
*See TEETH, AMELOGENESIS IMPERFECTA*
*also TEETH, SNOW-CAPPED*
**Amelogenesis imperfecta, hypoplastic type**
*See TEETH, AMELOGENESIS IMPERFECTA*
**Amelogenesis imperfecta, pigmented hypomaturation type**
*See TEETH, AMELOGENESIS IMPERFECTA*
**Amikacin, fetal effects**
*See FETAL AMINOGLYCOSIDE OTOTOXICITY*
**Amikin^, fetal effects**
*See FETAL AMINOGLYCOSIDE OTOTOXICITY*
**Aminoglycoside, fetal effects**
*See FETAL AMINOGLYCOSIDE OTOTOXICITY*
**Aminopterin syndrome without aminopterin (ASSA)**
*See PSEUDOAMINOPTERIN SYNDROME*
**Aminopterin, fetal effects of**
*See FETAL AMINOPTERIN SYNDROME*
**Aminorex, effects of**
*See PULMONARY HYPERTENSION, PRIMARY*
**Amish albinism**
*See ALBINISM, OCULOCUTANEOUS, YELLOW MUTANT*
**Amish brittle hair syndrome**
*See TRICHOTHIODYSTROPHY*
**Amniotic band syndrome, sequence, or disruption complex**
*See AMNIOTIC BANDS SYNDROME*
**Amniotic bands complex**
*See LIMB AND SCALP DEFECTS, ADAMS-OLIVER TYPE*

## AMNIOTIC BANDS SYNDROME    0874

**Includes:**
> ADAM complex
> Amniotic band syndrome, sequence, or disruption complex
> Amniotic deformities, adhesion, mutilation complex (ADAM)
> Annular grooves
> Amputation, congenital
> Constricting bands, congenital
> Streeter bands
> Transverse terminal defects of limb

**Excludes:**
> **Brachydactyly** (type B)
> Constrictions, ainhum or postnatally appearing
> **Hypoglossia-hypodactylia** (0451)
> Peromelia, familial
> **Schisis association** (2249)
> Vascular occlusion, prenatal

**Major Diagnostic Criteria:**  Ideally, documentation of actual bands or of the presence of an amputated part at delivery. Can be presumed with evidence of amputation with scarring, interruption of dermatoglyphics, constrictive bands, distal syndactyly, or mutilations that do not fit normal embryologic patterns.

**Clinical Findings:**  Extremely varied, depending on the time of band formation and the areas involved. Early bands can cause multiple, often bizarre, disruptions of fetal development and are frequently associated with stillbirths. Findings can include calvarial defects (anencephaly or encephalocele), gastroschisis, omphalocele, ectopia cordis, facial clefts, and ''nonanatomic'' defects such as gastropleuroschisis. Internal anomalies may even result, including hydrocephalus. Later bands are more likely to

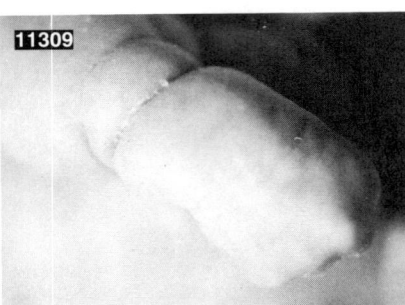

**0874-11307—09:** Ring constrictions and amputations.

cause only limb abnormalities, characteristically ring constrictions or amputations. These may involve arms, legs, or digits, either singly or multiply. The constrictions are indentations with scar tissue, and distal lymphedema is often seen. Amputations typically leave scars and disruptions of dermatoglyphics, sometimes with distal fusion of affected fingers. Other findings may include short umbilical cord, scoliosis, and growth deficiency. Usually the diagnosis can be made without difficulty if it is considered, but it is easily overlooked in a hasty examination. Occasionally other disorders may mimic the "typical" findings, particularly of the limbs, and thus can be very difficult to differentiate. The range and diversity of findings with amniotic bands are extensive.

**Complications:** With severe cases, miscarriage is frequent. There may be a transient oligohydramnios prenatally. Postnatal problems with neuromuscular function secondary to scarring in constrictions, as well as lymphedema and compromised vascularity can be seen. **Hydrocephaly** may develop in patients in whom there have been early effects on the midface. Other malformations not obviously caused by the direct influence of bands have been seen in some cases.

**Associated Findings:** None known.

**Etiology:** Most cases lack any apparent predisposing cause. A history of significant abdominal trauma seems more frequent than chance alone would allow, and would be a reasonable cause in some cases. The incidence of discontinuance of oral contraceptives within one month of conception was increased in one study. Genetic factors may be operating in some rare families, but even in these the risk seems low. Connective tissue abnormalities may predispose to bands, as in **Epidermolysis bullosum** and possibly other conditions, such as **Ehlers-Danlos syndrome**. **Arthrogryposes** with stiff, immobile limbs may result in disruption of the amnion and late band formation.

**Pathogenesis:** A primary cellular defect in the fetus was once suggested, and this may occur in some instances. However, most cases are now thought to be derived from the effects of tissue bands that form from the fetal membrane. A variety of injuries to the fetus can result. Early bands may interfere with the normal sequence of embryonic development through adhesion or pressure. Mechanical effects can also occur. There may be a transient oligohydramnios as the exposed chorion increases reabsorption of amniotic fluid, crowding, or tethering from a band. Rarely, mechanical distortion of fetal parts may even produce internal anomalies or unusual findings such as polydactyly. Later bands can disrupt already formed structures.

**MIM No.:** 21710

**POS No.:** 3621

**CDC No.:** 658.800

**Sex Ratio:** M1:F1

**Occurrence:** About 1:1,300 live births. Increased in miscarriages.

**Risk of Recurrence for Patient's Sib:** In the absence of a connective tissue disorder, risk seems minimal and even low in the rare familial cases.

**Risk of Recurrence for Patient's Child:** Unknown.

**Age of Detectability:** Prenatal bands and their effects can be seen with ultrasound prenatally, and some may cause early increases in maternal serum alpha-fetoprotein.

**Gene Mapping and Linkage:** Unknown.

**Prevention:** None known. Genetic counseling indicated.

**Treatment:** Deep constrictions should be released early by Z-plasty.

**Prognosis:** Generally depends on the structures involved. If the central nervous system is not involved, intelligence would be expected to be normal. If the thumb is preserved, manual function may be excellent even with what appear to be major digital amputations.

**Detection of Carrier:** Unknown.

**References:**
Torpin R: Fetal malformations caused by amnion rupture during gestation. Springfield: Charles C Thomas, 1968.
Ossipoff V, Hall BD: Etiologic factors in the amniotic band syndrome: a study of 24 patients. BD:OAS XIII(3D). New York: March of Dimes Birth Defects Foundation, 1977:117.
Keller H, et al: "ADAM complex" (amniotic deformity, adhesions, mutilations): a pattern of craniofacial and limb defects. Am J Med Genet 1978; 2:81–98.
Higginbottom MC, et al.: The amniotic band disruption complex: timing of amniotic rupture and variable spectra of consequent defects. J Pediatr 1979; 95:544.
Lubinsky M, et al.: Familial amniotic bands. Am J Med Genet 1983; 14:81–87.
Herva R, Karkinen-Jaaskelainen M: Amniotic adhesion malformation syndrome: fetal and placental pathology. Teratology 1984; 29:11.
Hunter AGW, Carpenter BF: Implications of malformations not due to amniotic bands in the amniotic band sequence. Am J Med Genet 1986; 24:691.

LU001                                                            **Mark Lubinsky**

**Amniotic deformities, adhesion, mutilation complex (ADAM)**
  *See* AMNIOTIC BANDS SYNDROME
**Amputation, congenital**
  *See* AMNIOTIC BANDS SYNDROME
  also LIMB REDUCTION DEFECTS
**Amylo-1,6-glucosidase deficiency**
  *See* GLYCOGENOSIS, TYPE III
**Amyloid arthropathy of chronic hemodialysis**
  *See* AMYLOIDOSIS, HEMODIALYSIS-RELATED
**Amyloid beta A4 precursor protein**
  *See* ALZHEIMER DISEASE, FAMILIAL
**Amyloid corneal dystrophy, Japanese type**
  *See* AMYLOIDOSIS, CORNEAL
**Amyloid cranial neuropathy-lattice corneal dystrophy**
  *See* AMYLOIDOSIS, FINNISH TYPE
**Amyloid of aging and Alzheimer disease**
  *See* ALZHEIMER DISEASE, FAMILIAL
**Amyloid polyneuropathy, type I**
  *See* AMYLOIDOSIS, TRANSTHYRETIN METHIONINE-30 TYPE
**Amyloid polyneuropathy, type II**
  *See* AMYLOIDOSIS, INDIANA TYPE

## AMYLOIDOSES                                                   1502

**Includes:**
  Familial Amyloidotic Polyneuropathy (FAP)
  Transthyretin amyloidoses

The hereditary amyloidoses are a group of adult-onset autosomal dominant syndromes that are associated with deposition of fibrillar protein material in body tissues. These insoluble protein deposits cause illness by the displacement of normal tissue structures. Depending on which organs are involved, a person with amyloidosis may have neuropathy, blindness, cardiomyopathy, nephropathy, autonomic nervous dysfunction, or bowel dysfunction. Age of onset and clinical findings can vary widely between families, but are usually fairly consistent within each family. Although no cure or prevention exists for this condition, treatment of symptoms can often prolong the lives of patients. Colchicine is an experimental treatment that is sometimes used because it has been found to be effective in preventing the reactive (AA protein) amyloidosis of **Fever, familial mediterranean (FMF)**, but there is no evidence of its efficacy in hereditary amyloidosis.

A number of kindreds with hereditary amyloidosis have been described, with most cases being recognized by the presence of a symmetric peripheral neuropathy. The first and most prevalent hereditary amyloidosis was reported in a northern Portuguese population. These patients had a very profound peripheral and autonomic neuropathy, often leading to paralysis and severe bowel and bladder dysfunction. Varying degrees of kidney and heart involvement were also noted. This syndrome was called *Familial Amyloidotic Polyneuropathy (FAP)*, Type I. Two other large kindreds with amyloid neuropathy were described in the United States, one in Maryland and Pennsylvania (of German descent) and a second in Indiana (of Swiss descent). Members of these kindreds had as a prominent feature the carpal tunnel syndrome, and to distinguish them from the Portuguese patients, this was designated *Familial Amyloidotic Polyneuropathy (FAP)*, Type II. Another kindred from Iowa, which was of English and Scottish origin, had peripheral neuropathy with very prominent renal involvement. This was called FAP, Type III. FAP, Type IV refers to patients originally described in Finland who had as prominent features lattice corneal dystrophy and cranial neuropathy with varying degrees of systemic involvement with amyloid deposition. Many of the current individual amyloidoses are subsets of the classic FAP classifications, and a number of other families have since been reported with varying degrees of neuropathy, nephropathy, or cardiomyopathy due to amyloid deposition.

Many of these conditions have now been shown to be associated with variant molecules of plasma transthyretin (the term *transthyretin* has been introduced as a replacement for the term "prealbumin" which had often been confused with albumin). Transthyretin is synthesized mainly in the liver but also in the choroid plexus of the central nervous system. It has two known functions: 1) to transport thyroid hormone (thyroxine), and 2) to transport the retinol binding protein/vitamin A complex. The transthyretin (prealbumin) variants have been found to be the major amyloid proteins in affected families. This has led to the model that patients are heterozygous at the transthyretin locus, producing normal or variant proteins with the variant molecule being predisposed toward amyloid formation.

In FAP, Type I, a valine at position 30 of the transthyretin molecule has been replaced with methionine. In FAP, Type II, an isoleucine at position 84 has been replaced by serine. Other types of amyloidosis have been found in which there are substitutions at positions 33, 60, or 77 of the transthyretin molecule. It would appear that there are other kindreds with amyloidosis associated with as yet undescribed transthyretin variants. Thus far, all have been the result of single nucleotide changes in the transthyretin gene. There is only one gene for transthyretin, and this is located on the proximal long arm of chromosome 18.

In addition to the transthyretin amyloidoses, preliminary work with the Iowa type (FAP, Type III) suggests that the amyloid fibrils are composed of apolipoprotein A1. Also, hereditary cerebral hemorrhage with amyloidosis (HCHWA), originally described in families from Iceland, has vascular amyloid composed of a variant of cystatin C (γ-trace protein). Most likely, other types of hereditary amyloidosis exist that are associated with other plasma proteins as well.

With the discovery of mutations in the transthyretin molecule associated with hereditary amyloidosis it has been possible to develop a number of DNA tests (using Southern blot or RFLP analysis) that directly detect the mutations. This technique has allowed the identification of gene carriers prior to the onset of the disease. In this way, kindreds are now being classified, and presymptomatic diagnosis is possible.

**Support Groups:**
WI; Wausau (c/o Donald Rasmussen, 602 Bernard St.); Amyloidosis Network

**References:**
Benson MD, Wallace MR: Amyloidosis. In: Scriver CR, et al, eds: The metabolic basis of inherited disease, 6th ed. New York: McGraw-Hill, 1989:2439–2462.

BE045                                                          **Merrill D. Benson**
WA048                                                        **Margaret R. Wallace**

**Amyloidosis type VIII**
*See AMYLOIDOSIS, FAMILIAL VISCERAL*

---

## AMYLOIDOSIS, APPALACHIAN TYPE          2881

**Includes:**

    Alanine 60 amyloidosis
    Amyloidosis, transthyretin (prealbumin) Ala-60
    Appalachian amyloid polyneuropathy, familial
    Prealbumin (TTR) Ala-60 amyloidosis
    Transthyretin (prealbumin) Ala-60 amyloidosis

**Excludes:   Amyloidosis (other)**

**Major Diagnostic Criteria:**   Adult onset of cardiomyopathy and autonomic dysfunction; positive family history (dominant inheritance); histologically proven amyloidosis; and biochemical proof of Ala-60 transthyretin (prealbumin) variant or DNA analysis showing the Ala-60 transthyretin (prealbumin) gene.

**Clinical Findings:**   Cardiomyopathy is a major feature. Some patients may initially show other symptoms common to other forms of hereditary amyloidosis, such as gastrointestinal disturbances and peripheral neuropathy (including carpal tunnel syndrome).

**Complications:**   After a number of years, patients deteriorate and are usually bedridden in the final stages of the disease. Complications of heart failure often occur.

**Associated Findings:**   None known.

**Etiology:**   Autosomal dominant inheritance with adult onset and high penetrance.

**Pathogenesis:**   The interstitial amyloid deposits accumulate and interfere with functioning of surrounding tissue. The amyloid fibrils consist primarily of variant transthyretin (prealbumin) molecules containing an alanine-for-threonine substitution at position 60. The tissues most heavily infiltrated are the heart and nerves.

**MIM No.:**   10490, 17630

**Sex Ratio:**   M1:F1

**Occurrence:**   Based on the original family described, which is part of an extensive American kindred, this disorder may be one of the most prevalent forms in the United States. The gene in this family has been traced to a couple from the 1700s, from whom over 1,000 individuals have descended. Laboratory identification has also been made of the gene in six other apparently unrelated families. No cases have yet been reported outside the United States, but it is believed that the gene originated in Europe.

**Risk of Recurrence for Patient's Sib:**
See Part I, *Mendelian Inheritance.*

**Risk of Recurrence for Patient's Child:**
See Part I, *Mendelian Inheritance.*

**Age of Detectability:**   This form seems to have an unusually late onset, after age 50 years, but in some cases not until the 60s or 70s.

**Gene Mapping and Linkage:**   PALB (prealbumin [transthyretin]) has been mapped to 18q11.2-q12.1.

**Prevention:**   None known. Genetic counseling indicated.

**Treatment:**   No treatment can reduce the deposits; however, colchicine is sometimes administered since it appears to slow amyloid formation in **Fever, familial mediterranean (FMF)** (associated with amyloid A protein). Treatment of symptoms may bring some relief and prolong the lives of patients.

**Prognosis:**   Most patients die of complications of heart failure. This disorder has a fairly slow progression, with duration often

10–15 years or more. One gene carrier is still leading a functional life at age 83 and apparently has only cardiac symptoms.

**Detection of Carrier:** The Ala-60 variant can be detected by biochemical means. The Ala-60 transthyretin (prealbumin) gene can be detected by a standard Southern analysis (DNA test, RFLP) with the restriction enzyme PvuII and transthyretin (prealbumin) cDNA or gene probe, and also by polymase chain reaction amplification of exam 3 and RFLP.

**Special Considerations:** This disease may go unrecognized or misdiagnosed because patients may simply die of heart problems at an advanced age. Primary amyloidosis, senile cardiac amyloidosis, and **Amyloidosis, Danish cardiac type** (transthyretin (prealbumin) Met-111) hereditary amyloidosis are other syndromes characterized by severe cardiac amyloidosis. Family medical history can thus be misleading, and gene carriers may also have died prior to onset of symptoms. It may be more difficult to establish a positive family history in this form than in others. New mutations are considered very unlikely for this and other transthyretin (prealbumin) variants.

**References:**
Wallace MR, et al.: Biochemical and molecular genetic characterization of a new variant prealbumin associated with hereditary amyloidosis. J Clin Invest 1986; 78:6–12.
Benson MD, et al.: Hereditary amyloidosis: description of a new American kindred with late onset cardiomyopathy. Arthritis Rheum 1987; 30:195–200.

WA048                                 **Margaret R. Wallace**
BE045                                 **Merrill D. Benson**

---

## AMYLOIDOSIS, ASHKENAZI TYPE             2880

**Includes:**
    Isoleucine 33 amyloidosis
    Israeli hereditary amyloidosis
    Jewish amyloidosis
    Polish hereditary amyloidosis
    Prealbumin (TTR) Ile-33 and/or Gly-49
    Transthyretin (prealbumin) Ile-33 and/or Gly-49

**Excludes: Amyloidosis** (other)

**Major Diagnostic Criteria:** Adult onset of lower limb neuropathy and autonomic dysfunction; positive family history (dominant inheritance); histologically proven amyloidosis; and biochemical proof of Isoleucine-33 (Ile-33) and/or Gly-49 transthyretin (prealbumin) variant.

**Clinical Findings:** One family (Jewish, of Polish origin) has been described, with two patients (a father and son). These men developed symptoms betwen ages 25 and 30 years. The symptoms included neuropathy (initially in the lower limbs), diarrhea, impotence, and vitreous deposits. The father died of gastric bleeding. Autopsy results from both patients revealed amyloid deposits throughout the body and in all major organs, particularly in the thyroid, kidneys, spleen, and nerves.

**Complications:** Weight loss, recurrent urinary tract infections, incontinence, and visual impairment caused by the vitreous deposits.

**Associated Findings:** None known.

**Etiology:** Presumably autosomal dominant inheritance with early adult onset.

**Pathogenesis:** Like the other hereditary amyloidoses, amyloid accumulation causes deterioration of surrounding tissues, resulting in the clinical findings. One group of investigators originally analyzed amyloid fibrils from one patient's thyroid and spleen and found a variant transthyretin (prealbumin) containing a glycine-for-threonine substitution at position 49. However, another group sequenced the same protein and found transthyretin (prealbumin) with an isoleucine-for-phenylalanine change at position 33, with 49 being normal. The substitution at 49 would require a double-nucleotide change in the 49 codon of the transthyretin (prealbumin) gene, whereas the Ile-33 variant can be

explained by a single base change. Another report stated that the glycine at 49 could be explained by modification of the protein after amyloid formation. It would thus appear that the Ile-33 is more likely to be the true variant, although the Gly-49 may also be present. The Ile-33 mutation has been established by Southern analysis.

**MIM No.:** 17630

**Sex Ratio:** M2:F0 (observed). While the only two patients have been male, the transmission is clearly dominant, so the expected ratio is M1:F1

**Occurrence:** One small Jewish family of Polish origin has been documented. However, since clinically this form is similar to other types of hereditary amyloidosis, biochemical analysis is necessary to distinguish among the types and determine prevalence.

**Risk of Recurrence for Patient's Sib:**
    See Part I, *Mendelian Inheritance.*

**Risk of Recurrence for Patient's Child:**
    See Part I, *Mendelian Inheritance.*

**Age of Detectability:** Onset between ages 25 and 30 years.

**Gene Mapping and Linkage:** PALB (prealbumin [transthyretin]) has been mapped to 18q11.2-q12.1.

**Prevention:** None known. Genetic counseling indicated.

**Treatment:** There is no effective treatment to eliminate the amyloid deposits; however, colchicine is sometimes administered since it appears to slow amyloid formation associated with **Fever, familial mediterranean (FMF)** (in which the amyloid protein is the A protein). Treatment of symptoms may bring some relief and prolong the lives of patients.

**Prognosis:** One patient died seven years after onset of symptoms. The other patient died of unrelated causes four years after onset, at which time he had severe manifestations of the disease.

**Detection of Carrier:** The transthyretin (prealbumin) variants have been detected in amyloid fibrils by biochemical means and presumably could be detected in plasma transthyretin (prealbumin). A DNA test has yet to be reported.

**References:**
Nakazato M, et al.: Revised analysis of amino acid replacement in a prealbumin variant (SKO-III) associated with familial amyloidotic polyneuropathy of Jewish origin. Biochem Biophys Res Commun 1984; 123:921–928.
Gafni J, et al.: Amyloidotic polyneuropathy in a Jewish family: evidence for the genetic heterogeneity of the lower limb familial amyloidotic neuropathies. Quart J Med 1985; NS55:33–43.

WA048                                 **Margaret R. Wallace**
BE045                                 **Merrill D. Benson**

**Amyloidosis, cerebral, with spongiform encephalopathy**
*See GERSTMANN-STRAUSSLER SYNDROME*

---

## AMYLOIDOSIS, CORNEAL               2147

**Includes:**
    Amyloid corneal dystrophy, Japanese type
    Corneal dystrophy, gelatinous drop-like
    Gelatinous drop-like corneal dystrophy

**Excludes:**
    **Amyloidosis, Finnish type** (2145)
    Corneal amyloid, acquired
    **Corneal dystrophy, lattice type** (0211)

**Major Diagnostic Criteria:** 1) Absence of previous ocular trauma; 2) absence of symptoms until about age eight years, then foreign body sensation with possible decreased acuity; 3) bilateral, symmetric nodular, diffuse subepithelial eosinophilic deposits in corneas; 4) microscopic absence of Bowman membrane with possible extension of nodules into stroma, thinned overlying epithelium; 5) positive staining of deposits with Congo red, exhibits green birefringence and dichroism.

**Clinical Findings:** Visual history normal until 8–10 years of age when signs and symptoms of punctate keratitis develop. Acuity may be decreased at this time. Slit lamp examination shows multiple diffuse bilateral subepithelial nodular deposits which appear opaque on direct focal illumination and translucent on retroillumination. Two reported cases (sibs) had anterior and posterior lenticular opacities, both requiring cataract extraction. The remainder of the eye and systemic examinations are unremarkable and the disorder appears progressive.

**Complications:** Recurrent corneal erosions with tearing, pain and photophobia; decreased visual acuity requiring lamellar or penetrating keratoplasty; bilateral cataracts, possibly requiring extraction.

**Associated Findings:** Anterior and posterior cortical cataracts, in one reported sibship.

**Etiology:** Autosomal recessive inheritance.

**Pathogenesis:** Possibly an abnormal accumulation of material normally present in extracellular spaces in very small amounts, an abnormal protein produced by genetically-defective cells under chronic stress, or a fragment of a normal constituent.

**MIM No.:** *20487

**POS No.:** 3959

**Sex Ratio:** M1:F1

**Occurrence:** At least three kindreds have been reported.

**Risk of Recurrence for Patient's Sib:**
See Part I, *Mendelian Inheritance.*

**Risk of Recurrence for Patient's Child:**
See Part I, *Mendelian Inheritance.*

**Age of Detectability:** Undetermined. The corneal lesion may be present at birth.

**Gene Mapping and Linkage:** Unknown.

**Prevention:** None known. Genetic counseling indicated.

**Treatment:** For corneal abrasions, standard measures consisting of ointments, patching and cycloplegia as necessary. For visually significant opacities, lamellar or penetrating keratoplasty. For visually significant cataracts, extraction.

**Prognosis:** Presumably progressive, although the rate of progression is unknown. Modern techniques of corneal and lens surgery can yield good visual results. Amblyopia may be a consideration in patients under nine years of age.

**Detection of Carrier:** Unknown.

**Special Considerations:** Sporadic cases resembling the above have been reported; these may represent index case of familial disorder. The relationship of lens opacities to this entity is unclear; the lenses removed have not contained amyloid. Occasional case reports of lattice corneal dystrophy possess nodular subepithelial opacities, suggesting similar mechanisms of amyloid deposit.

**References:**
Stafford WR, et al.: Amyloidosis of the cornea. Br J Ophthalmol 1969; 53:73–78.
Akiya S, et al.: Gelatinous drop-like dystrophy of the cornea. Jpn J Ophthalmol 1972; 26:815–822.
Ramsey MS, et al.: Localized corneal amyloidosis. Am J Ophthalmol 1972; 73:560–565.
Kirk HQ, et al.: Primary familial amyloidosis of the cornea. Am Acad Ophthalmol Otolaryngol 1973; 77:411–416.
Stock EL, et al.: Primary familial amyloidosis of the cornea. Am J Ophthalmol 1976; 82:266–271.
Weber SM, et al.: Gelatinous drop-like dystrophy. Arch Ophthalmol 1980; 98:149–153.
Fujiki K, et al.: Gelatinous drop-like corneal dystrophy in a Japanese population. (Abstract) 7th Int Cong Hum Genet., Berlin, 1986:248–249.

DI014                                            **Gary R. Diamond**

**Amyloidosis, corneal, lattice**
*See CORNEAL DYSTROPHY, LATTICE TYPE*

## AMYLOIDOSIS, DANISH CARDIAC TYPE                    2143

**Includes:**
   Amyloidosis, prealbumin met-111
   Amyloidosis, type III
   Cardiac type amyloidosis
   Danish type amyloidosis
   Methionine 111 amyloidosis
   Prealbumin met-111 amyloidosis
   Transthyretin (prealbumin) met-111 amyloidosis

**Excludes:**
   **Amyloidosis** (other)
   Amyloidosis, sporadic
   Primary amyloidosis (immunoglobulin)
   Secondary (reactive) amyloidosis (amyloid A protein)

**Major Diagnostic Criteria:** Adult onset of cardiomyopathy and heart failure; positive family history (dominant inheritance); histologically proven amyloidosis; biochemical proof of Met-111 transthyretin (prealbumin) in plasma or amyloid.

**Clinical Findings:** Although traces of amyloid can be found throughout the body of these patients, the primary organ involved is the heart. Symptoms begin in adulthood and include cardiomyopathy and heart failure. No neuropathy, vitreal amyloid, renal, or gastrointestinal dysfunction is evident.

**Complications:** Those associated with heart failure.

**Associated Findings:** None known.

**Etiology:** Autosomal dominant inheritance with adult onset.

**Pathogenesis:** Transthyretin (prealbumin) molecules containing a methionine-for-leucine substitution at position 111 were identified in amyloid fibrils. The pathogenesis is considered to be similar to that of other hereditary amyloidoses, which are associated with transthyretin (prealbumin) variants.

**MIM No.:** 10500, 17630

**Sex Ratio:** M1:F1

**Occurrence:** All patients identified thus far are members of Danish families. A few families outside of Denmark have been described with similar findings, but the Met-111 variant has not yet been demonstrated in these families.

**Risk of Recurrence for Patient's Sib:**
See Part I, *Mendelian Inheritance.*

**Risk of Recurrence for Patient's Child:**
See Part I, *Mendelian Inheritance.*

**Age of Detectability:** In most patients, the illness begins near age 40 years.

**Gene Mapping and Linkage:** PALB (prealbumin) has been mapped to 18q11.2-q12.1.

**Prevention:** None known. Genetic counseling indicated.

**Treatment:** There is no treatment that affects the amyloid deposits; however, colchicine is sometimes prescribed since it appears to slow amyloid formation in **Fever, familial mediterranean (FMF)** (in which the amyloid consists of amyloid A protein). Treatment of the symptoms may provide relief and prolong the lives of patients.

**Prognosis:** Most patients have died within 3–6 years of onset of cardiac problems. Mental capacity is reported to be unaffected.

**Detection of Carrier:** The Met-111 transthyretin (prealbumin) variant can be detected biochemically in plasma or amyloid fibrils. As yet there is no report of a DNA test for this variant transthyretin (prealbumin) gene.

**Special Considerations:** Other forms of hereditary amyloidosis, such as the transthyretin (prealbumin) Ala-60 form, may be clinically similar. Senile systemic (cardiac) amyloidosis (SSA) is characterized by cardiac amyloid; however, it may have such a late onset that patients die of old age before showing symptoms. Until recently SSA was thought to be a sporadic form of amyloidosis. However, since transthyretin (prealbumin) has been found in the amyloid of SSA, it too may be another hereditary form.

**References:**
Frederiksen T, et al.: Familial primary amyloidosis with severe amyloid heart disease. Am J Med 1962; 33:328–348.
Husby G, et al.: The amyloid in familial amyloid cardiomyopathy of Danish origin is related to prealbumin. Clin Exp Immunol 1985; 60:207–216.
Husby G, Sletten K: Chemical and clinical classification of amyloidosis 1985. Scand J Immunol 1986; 23:253–265.

WA048
BE045

**Margaret R. Wallace**
**Merrill D. Benson**

## AMYLOIDOSIS, FAMILIAL CUTANEOUS       2250

**Includes:** Amyloidosis, X-linked cutaneous

**Excludes:**
    **Amyloidosis, corneal** (2147)
    **Amyloidosis, familial lichen** (2851)
    **Amyloidosis, familial visceral** (2150)
    **Deafness-triphalangeal thumbs-onychodystrophy** (2151)
    **Incontinentia pigmenti** (0526)

**Major Diagnostic Criteria:** The patient's pedigree should be consistent with X-linkage. Although the histologic findings in the skin lesions of the two sexes are identical, the clinical manifestations in males and females are quite different.

*In females*: 1) spots, streaks or whorls of brown pigmentation of the skin of the trunk and limbs similar in color, appearance, and distribution to that of Stage III **Incontinentia pigmenti**; no history of preceding eruptions or verrucous lesions; and 2) absence of ocular, dental, or neurologic abnormalities.

*In males*: 1) severe colitis starting in the neonatal period; 2) recurrent respiratory infections starting in infancy; 3) photopho-

bia; and 4) sheets of reticular brown skin pigmentation on the inner thighs and posterior arms starting in the third year of life.

Adults of both sexes have similar histologic changes in the skin, i.e., demonstration of amyloid deposits in the papillary dermis, increased melanin in the basal layer, and slight hyperkeratosis of the pigmented skin.

**Clinical Findings:** Females may show no unusual skin pigmentation, or small (3 cm) linear streaks of pigmentation, or extensive pigmentation covering 10% of the trunk and running in linear streaks down the long axes of the limbs.

In males, bloody diarrhea may start in the first week of life and may be severe. The mucosal appearance on sigmoidoscopy and by biopsy mimics ulcerative colitis. The clinical course may be less acute, with loose stools and failure to thrive. If the child lives, bowel symptoms subside in late infancy. Recurrent respiratory infections may start in infancy; discrete episodes of pneumonia may or may not be interspersed with wheezing. The longest-lived male died at the age of 50 from pneumonia; autopsy showed diffuse interstitial pneumonitis. One 22-year-old adult has had no respiratory symptoms.

Skin hyperpigmentation starts in childhood and progresses slowly as reticular sheets on the inner thighs and backs of the arms. It may spread to the trunk and cover most of the skin, including the hands. Photophobia may be marked. The hair may be somewhat thin and fair with a frontal upsweep.

**Complications:** In females, the only complication so far recognized has been dystrophic changes in the nails (2) when there is linear pigmentation on the adjoining skin. In males, neonatal colitis led to a colectomy at age two months with death postoperatively (1). In another infant, seizures, hemiplegia, and mild mental retardation followed severe electrolyte disturbances. One boy died from recurrent pneumonia at three years of age. The skin lesions may lead to severe cracking and exudation on the fingers. In one male, amyloid deposition in the cornea led to blindness, which responded poorly to corneal transplants.

**Associated Findings:** In females, talipes equinovarus (1) and **Horner syndrome** (1). In males, recurrent **Hernia, inguinal** and urethral stenosis (1), and moderate sensorineural deafness (1).

**Etiology:** X-linked semidominant inheritance.

**Pathogenesis:** Undetermined. The manifestation common to both sexes is amyloid deposition in the skin. Amyloid accumulations have not been found in the internal organs.

**MIM No.:** *30122

**Sex Ratio:** M1:F1

**Occurrence:** One Canadian family with nine males and ten females (three of whom were unaffected obligate heterozygotes) has been documented.

**Risk of Recurrence for Patient's Sib:**
    See Part I, *Mendelian Inheritance.*

**Risk of Recurrence for Patient's Child:**
    See Part I, *Mendelian Inheritance.*

**Age of Detectability:** In females, sometime in childhood. In males, blood may be found in the stools on the third day of life; chronic diarrhea appears some weeks later. Recurrent respiratory infections start in infancy and pigmentation develops in the third year of life.

**Gene Mapping and Linkage:** Unknown.

**Prevention:** None known. Genetic counseling indicated.

**Treatment:** Symptomatic. In one infant, neonatal colitis subsided promptly when Nutramigen was substituted for breast-feeding. Many of the attacks of pneumonia appear to be bacterial, as indicated by the satisfactory response to antibiotics. In one male, long-term cortisone did not improve the skin lesions, nor did it prevent recurrence of corneal lesions or pneumonia.

**Prognosis:** Normal life span in females. In males, death may occur in infancy from colitis or respiratory infection. Recurrent respiratory infections may lead to functional impairment. Longest-lived male died at age 50 years.

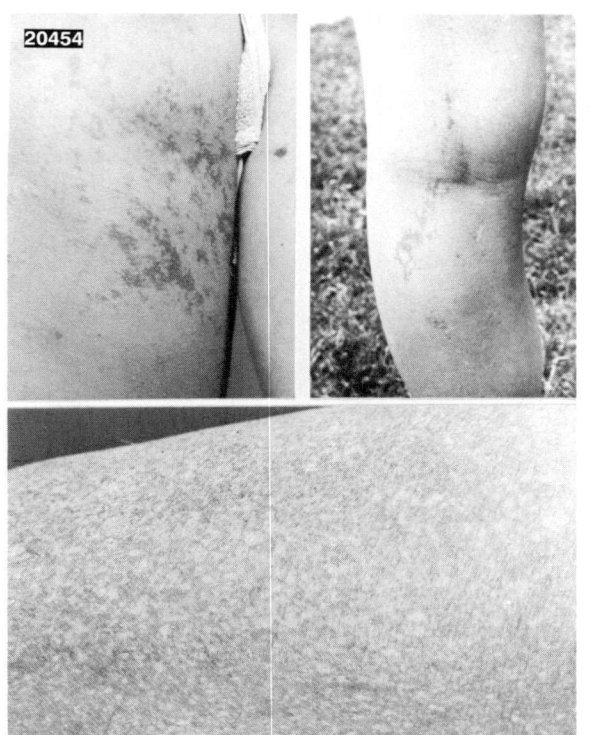

**2250-20454:** Skin pigmentation in familial cutaneous amyloidosis in 2 females (upper) and a male (lower).

**Detection of Carrier:** All daughters of an affected male are carriers whether skin pigmentation is present or not. Skin pigmentation with the characteristic histologic changes in a mother of a boy with neonatal colitis would be presumptive evidence of the carrier state.

**Special Considerations:** Before this type of X-linked cutaneous amyloidosis was recognized as a discrete entity, affected individuals in the family had received various diagnoses. Females had been diagnosed as having **Incontinentia pigmenti** and the males, icthyosis, Salzmann nodular degeneration of the cornea, infantile ulcerative colitis, and **Cystic fibrosis**. It is possible that this disease is "private" to the one family described.

**References:**
Partington MW, et al.: Familial cutaneous amyloidosis with systemic manifestations in males. Am J Med Genet 1981; 10:65–75. * †
Partington MW, Prentice RSA: X-linked cutaneous amyloidosis: further clinical and pathological observations. Am J Med Genet 1989; 32:115–119.

PA026                                              **M.W. Partington**

## AMYLOIDOSIS, FAMILIAL LICHEN                    2851

**Includes:**
    Amyloidosis, primary cutaneous
    Amyloidosis, type IX
    Cutaneous amyloidosis, familial, dominant type

**Excludes:**
    **Amyloidosis, familial cutaneous** (2250)
    **Amyloidosis** (other)

**Major Diagnostic Criteria:** Development of amyloid-containing skin lesions, usually on extremities, and positive family history.

**Clinical Findings:** Although this appears to be a heterogeneous group of disorders, the following findings are common to most reports in the literature. In most cases the skin lesions are pruritic papules, which may be hyperkeratotic (pigmented), or nodules. The lesions most commonly occur on the extremities, especially legs, but may appear on the trunk. The dermal papillae contain amyloid deposits, and the epidermis over these may be hyperplastic or may become thin and fragile. Patients show no signs of systemic amyloidosis, and there have been no reports of amyloid located anywhere except the skin. The skin findings may begin in childhood. In advanced cases the lesions may form confluent plaques. Although pruritis is often seen in the initial stages, it tends to lessen with age.

**Complications:** Complications such as infection can occur when lesions are open (for example, from being scratched). Otherwise the lesions do not compromise health or ability to function.

**Associated Findings:** Hypopigmented regions may be present, especially after the lesions have been treated and regressed.

**Etiology:** Autosomal dominant inheritance, with variable penetrance in some families. Another form, **Amyloidosis, familial cutaneous**, is X-linked.

**Pathogenesis:** The skin lesions are probably the result of an inflammatory response to the amyloid deposits. The skin or its blood vessels may also become fragile because of amyloid infiltration. The biochemical nature of the amyloid is unknown. However, in nonfamilial lichen amyloidosis, the amyloid deposits contain disulfide bonds and react with antikeratin.

**MIM No.:** *10525

**Sex Ratio:** Presumably M1:F1, but may vary because of penetrance.

**Occurrence:** This disorder has been identified in families in Asia, Russia, Europe, and North and South America. Hereditary cases may not be recognized because of variable penetrance and expression.

**Risk of Recurrence for Patient's Sib:**
See Part I, *Mendelian Inheritance.*

**Risk of Recurrence for Patient's Child:**
See Part I, *Mendelian Inheritance.*

**Age of Detectability:** Some cases begin in childhood, and others may not begin for several decades. Onset does appear to be fairly consistent in each family.

**Gene Mapping and Linkage:** Unknown. One small study suggested a possible relationship to HLA-B allele 4c.

**Prevention:** None known. Genetic counseling indicated.

**Treatment:** The papules and nodules often regress in response to topical application of corticosteroids and/or dimethyl sulfoxide. The lesions have been known to disappear completely, leaving only a depigmented area; however, they usually recur if treatment is discontinued. Notably, the actual amyloid deposits are not affected by this treatment.

**Prognosis:** Life span is unaffected.

**Detection of Carrier:** Unknown.

**Special Considerations:** The type and extent of the skin findings varies between families. One family was reported with small hypopigmented macules instead of papules, and in a Russian family the lesions occurred only on the back. These forms may have different genetic or biochemical bases, and environment may be a factor in expression of the disorder. This set of disorders is distinct from the systemic amyloidoses, which may also have skin findings.

**References:**
Sagher F, Shanon J: Amyloid cutis: familial occurrence in three generations. Arch Dermatol 1963; 87:171–175.
Rajagopalan K, Tay CH: Familial lichen amyloidosis: report of 19 cases in four generations of a Chinese family in Malaysia. Br J Dermatol 1972; 87:123–129.
Eng AM, et al.: Familial generalized dyschromic amyloidosis cutis. J Cutan Pathol 1976; 3:102–108.
DePietro WP: Primary familial cutaneous amyloidosis. Arch Dermatol 1981; 117:639–642.
Kyle RA: Amyloidosis. Int J Dermatol 1981; 20:75–80.
Ozaki M: Familial lichen amyloidosis. Int J Dermatol 1984; 23:190–193.
Breathnach SM: The cutaneous amyloidoses. Arch Dermatol 1985; 121:470–475.
Newton JA, et al.: Familial primary cutaneous amyloidosis. Br J Dermatol 1985; 112:201–208.

WA048                                        **Margaret R. Wallace**
BE045                                           **Merrill D. Benson**

**Amyloidosis, familial renal**
*See AMYLOIDOSIS, FAMILIAL VISCERAL*

## AMYLOIDOSIS, FAMILIAL VISCERAL                  2150

**Includes:**
    Amyloidosis type VIII
    Amyloidosis, familial renal
    German type amyloidosis
    Ostertag type amyloidosis, familial
    Renal type amyloidosis

**Excludes:**
    **Amyloidosis** (other)
    Amyloidosis, sporadic
    Primary amyloidosis (immunoglobulin)
    Secondary (reactive) amyloidosis (amyloid A protein)

**Major Diagnostic Criteria:** Adult onset of nephropathy; positive family history; and histologically proven amyloidosis in kidneys and possibly other tissues.

**Clinical Findings:** The clinical findings are almost exclusively confined to renal failure and associated complications. The kidneys, adrenals, and spleen usually contain significant amyloid deposits. Neuropathy is not a finding in this disorder.

**Complications:** The complications, such as hypertension, edema, proteinuria, hematuria, and uremia, can be attributed to the renal failure.

**Associated Findings:** It is difficult to be certain that all reports of familial renal amyloidosis represent the identical syndrome and defect. In these reports have been mention of additional findings such as hepatomegaly and left ventricular hypertrophy. Amyloid has never been found in the peripheral nerves and has been reported only in minute trace amounts in nonvisceral tissues. One patient was reported to have glomerular giant cells. In a couple of families, patients had persistent fevers throughout their lives.

**Etiology:** Probably autosomal dominant inheritance.

**Pathogenesis:** Renal amyloid deposits result in progressive kidney failure. The biochemical nature of the amyloid has not been identified. However, in one Irish-American family, amyloid deposits failed to react with antisera for amyloid A protein, kappa and lambda immunoglobulin light chains, and transthyretin (prealbumin).

**MIM No.:** *10520

**Sex Ratio:** M1:F1

**Occurrence:** Amyloidosis limited to the kidneys has been reported in several American families and in families from Germany, Sweden, and Canada (of Polish descent).

**Risk of Recurrence for Patient's Sib:**
See Part I, *Mendelian Inheritance.*

**Risk of Recurrence for Patient's Child:**
See Part I, *Mendelian Inheritance.*

**Age of Detectability:** Age of onset is fairly consistent within each family and is usually in the third or fourth decade of life. One at-risk individual died at age 13 years of renal failure. Because there are no pathologic data on this patient, it is unknown if he had amyloidosis (Weiss and Page, 1973).

**Gene Mapping and Linkage:** Unknown.

**Prevention:** None known. Genetic counseling indicated.

**Treatment:** There is no treatment to eliminate the amyloid deposits. Dialysis or renal transplantation may extend the lives of patients, although donor kidneys may also develop amyloid and fail.

**Prognosis:** The literature indicates that most patients die within 0–20 years after detection of the disorder.

**Detection of Carrier:** Unknown.

**Special Considerations:** These families must be distinguished from other forms of systemic amyloidosis with severe renal involvement (see **Amyloidosis, transthyretin methionine-30 type** and **Amyloidosis, Illinois type**). This can be difficult because of the possibility of variable expressivity. Renal amyloidosis is also found in noninherited conditions. Systemic amyloidosis in which the deposits contain beta-2-microglobulin has been shown to develop in dialysis patients. In some of the reported families the inheritance is inferred from medical history only, and it is possible that there may be other causes of the renal problems in those people presumed to be affected.

**References:**
Weiss SW, Page DL: Amyloid nephropathy of Ostertag with special reference to renal glomerular giant cells. Am J Pathol 1973; 72:447–456.
Alexander F, Atkins EL: Familial renal amyloidosis: case reports, literature review and classification. Am J Med 1975; 59:121–128.
Mornaghi R, Rubinstein P, Franklin EC: Familial renal amyloidosis: case reports and genetic studies. Am J Med 1982; 73:609–614.
Libbey CA, Talbert ML: A 43-year-old woman with hepatic failure after renal transplantation because of amyloidosis. New Engl J Med 1987; 317:1520–1531.

WA048
BE045

**Margaret R. Wallace**
**Merrill D. Benson**

**Includes:**
Amyloid cranial neuropathy-lattice corneal dystrophy
Amyloidosis, type V
Finnish amyloidosis with lattice corneal dystrophy
Meretoja-type amyloidosis

**Excludes:**
**Amyloidosis** (other)
**Amyloidosis, corneal** (2147)
Amyloidosis, sporadic
**Corneal dystrophy, lattice type** (0211)
Primary amyloidosis (immunoglobulin)
Secondary (reactive) amyloidosis (amyloid A protein)

**Major Diagnostic Criteria:** Adult onset of cranial neuropathy, lattice corneal dystrophy, and skin changes; positive family history (dominant inheritance); and histologically proven amyloidosis.

**Clinical Findings:** The disease first manifests with lattice dystrophy of the cornea, which appears as spider-web-like lines radiating toward the center of the cornea. In the next several decades skin changes become evident, particularly thickening of the skin on the forehead and back. Following this, most patients develop facial paralysis as the amyloid affects the cranial nerves, and the skin then becomes lax and atrophic.

**Complications:** As the facial nerves become involved, patients may exhibit symptoms such as ptosis and drooling. The lattice dystrophy generally does not interfere with vision until very late in the disease. Involvement in peripheral nerves may result in neuropathy, and renal amyloid may cause nephropathy.

**Associated Findings:** The skin changes can be quite variable, and in some patients may include lichenoid formations. Some patients have exhibited gastrointestinal disorders. Renal amyloid has been severe enough in some cases to cause kidney failure. Two cases have been reported in which the patient was suspected to have been a homozygote for the amyloidosis gene. Both of these patients had unusually severe forms of this disease.

**Etiology:** Autosomal dominant inheritance with adult onset and high penetrance.

**Pathogenesis:** The syndrome is caused by the accumulation of amyloid deposits, which compromise the functioning of surrounding tissues. The amyloid fibril protein has not yet been biochemically characterized.

**MIM No.:** *10512

**POS No.:** 3959

**Sex Ratio:** M1:F1

**Occurrence:** Although almost all of the cases have occurred in Finland, there are reports of patients with similar syndromes in Holland, Czechoslovakia, and the United States.

**Risk of Recurrence for Patient's Sib:**
See Part I, *Mendelian Inheritance.*

**Risk of Recurrence for Patient's Child:**
See Part I, *Mendelian Inheritance.*

**Age of Detectability:** In the fourth or fifth decade of life.

**Gene Mapping and Linkage:** Unknown.

**Prevention:** None known. Genetic counseling indicated.

**Treatment:** No treatment is known to affect the amyloid deposits; however, colchicine is sometimes administered in hereditary amyloid cases as an experimental treatment because it appears to inhibit amyloid formation associated with **Fever, familial mediterranean (FMF)** (in which the fibrils consist of amyloid A protein). Treatment of clinical symptoms may provide relief and, in some cases, prolong lives.

**Prognosis:** Since this disorder generally proceeds very slowly, patients may live normal life spans if they do not have severe autonomic dysfunction or nephropathy.

**Detection of Carrier:** Unknown.

**References:**

Meretoja J: Familial systemic paramyloidosis with lattice dystrophy of the cornea, progressive cranial neuropathy, skin changes and various internal symptoms. Ann Clin Res 1969; 1:314–324.

Meretoja J: Genetic aspects of familial amyloidosis with corneal lattice dystrophy and cranial neuropathy. Clin Genet 1973; 4:173–185.

Sack GH, et al.: Three forms of dominant amyloid neuropathy. Johns Hopkins Med J 1981; 149:239–247.

Darras BT, et al.: Familial amyloidosis with cranial neuropathy and corneal lattice dystrophy. Neurology 1986; 36:432–435.

WA048                                                    **Margaret R. Wallace**
BE045                                                    **Merrill D. Benson**

---

## AMYLOIDOSIS, HEMODIALYSIS-RELATED                    3106

**Includes:**

A Beta-2-microglobulin
Amyloid arthropathy of chronic hemodialysis
Beta-2-microglobulin
B2M amyloidosis
Carpal tunnel amyloid of chronic hemodialysis
Dialysis-associated amyloidosis
Hemodialysis-related amyloidosis

**Excludes:**

**Alzheimer disease, familial** (2354)
Amyloid renal disease
Amyloidosis, acquired
**Amyloidosis** (other)
**Fever, familial mediterranean (FMF)** (2161)

**Major Diagnostic Criteria:** Biopsy-proven (green birefringence on polarization microscopy after Congo red stain) amyloid in musculoskeletal system of patients on chronic hemodialysis (5–10 or more years) for chronic renal failure. The lesions are found in the carpal tunnel lesions, synovia, tendons, ligaments, joints, and bone.

**Clinical Findings:** Patients with any type of chronic renal disease usually on long-term cupraphane membrane hemodialysis most commonly develop, after 8–10 years, a carpal tunnel syndrome characterized by numbness and tingling in the median nerve distribution. On biopsy, deposits staining as amyloid are found. Shoulder pain is not uncommon. The frequency increases with duration of hemodialysis and can lead to an increasingly destructive arthritis and arthropathy. On very long-term hemodialysis the possibility of more extensive internal organ deposits of beta-2-microglobulin (B2M) amyloid has been reported. Bone and joint pain increases in time and causes increasing disability.

**Complications:** Weak grip, paresthesias, pain in and about joints, gait difficulties due to amyloid in and about hips, bone fractures possible due to cystic B2M amyloid bone lesions.

**Associated Findings:** B2M amyloid in synovial fluid. Also B2M kidney stones have been reported in chronic uremic patients.

**Etiology:** No specific inheritance pattern has been established. It now appears that most individuals on chronic hemodialysis and perhaps also peritoneal dialysis are susceptible to this type of amyloidosis. No mutation of B2-microglobulin has been documented in patients with this condition.

**Pathogenesis:** Current theory postulates that as opposed to other amyloid lesions that develop from enzymatic digestion of precursor molecules, B2M chronic hemodialysis amyloid may be due to the physicochemical effect of the strikingly elevated serum B2M levels and the polymerization of such molecules either spontaneously or due to interaction with connective tissue elements such as glycosaminoglycans.

**MIM No.:** *10970

**Sex Ratio:** Presumably M1:F1.

**Occurrence:** Depends on type of dialysis membrane (B2M levels stay higher with cupraphane as opposed to polysulfone membranes), duration of hemodialysis, level of B2M, and as yet unknown factors.

**Risk of Recurrence for Patient's Sib:** None unless on chronic hemodialysis.

**Risk of Recurrence for Patient's Child:** None unless on chronic hemodialysis.

**Age of Detectability:** After a minimum of five years, and more likely ten years, of chronic hemodialysis.

**Gene Mapping and Linkage:** B2M (beta-2-microglobulin) has been mapped to 15q21-q22.2.

B2M is the small subunit or light chain of histocompatibility (HLA) antigens. It may have a common evolution from the precursor gene that gave rise to immunoglobulin light and heavy chains.

**Prevention:** Avoidance of chronic elevation of beta-2-microglobulin levels by using hemodialysis membranes that prevent its accumulation. Preliminary data suggest that polysulfone membranes are better in this respect than are cupraphane membranes.

**Treatment:** Attempt to lower B2M levels by changing hemodialysis membrane. Always define the presence of amyloid by special stains and then the specificity of the lesion with specific anti-B2M antibodies to avoid confusion with other possible types of amyloid.

**Prognosis:** Increasing musculoskeletal difficulty after ten years with potential for systemic involvement. Possible improvement with new dialysis membranes.

**Detection of Carrier:** Unknown.

**References:**

Cunningham BA: Structure and significant of B2-microglobulin. Fed Proc 1976; 35:1171–1176.

Bardin T, et al.: Synovial amyloidosis in patients undergoing long-term hemodialysis. Arthritis Rheum 1985; 28:1052–1058.

Connors LH, et al.: In vitro formation of amyloid fibrils from intact beta-2-microglobulin. Biochem Biophy Res Commun 1985; 131: 1063–1068.

Geyjo F, et al.: A new form of amyloid protein associated with chronic hemodialysis was identified as B2-microglobulin. Biochem Biophys Res Commun 1985; 129:701–706.

Shirahama T, et al.: Histochemical and immunohistochemical characterization of amyloid associated with chronic hemodialysis as B₂-microglobulin. Lab Invest 1985; 53:705–709.

Geyjo F, et al.: Beta-2-microglobulin: a new form of amyloid protein associated with chronic hemodialysis. Kidney Int 1986; 30:385–390.

Bardin T, et al.: Hemodialysis-associated amyloidosis and beta-2-microglobulin. Clinical and immunohistochemical study. Am J Med 1987; 83:419–424.

Cohen AS, et al.: Beta-2 microglobulin amyloidosis. In Isobe T, et al, eds: Amyloid and amyloidosis. New York: Plenum Press, 1988:605–610.

Benson MD, Wallace MR: Amyloidosis. In: Scriver CR, et al, eds: The metabolic basis of inherited disease, 6th ed. New York: McGraw-Hill, 1989:2439–2461.

C0071                                                         **Alan S. Cohen**

---

## AMYLOIDOSIS, ICELANDIC TYPE                         2146

**Includes:**

Amyloidosis, type VI
Cystatin C
Cerebral arterial amyloidosis
Cerebral amyloid angiopathy, familial
Cerebral hemorrhage, familial
Gamma-trace, defect in metabolism of
Hereditary cerebral hemorrhage with amyloidosis (HCHWA)
Icelandic type amyloidosis

**Excludes:**

**Amyloidosis** (other)
Amyloidosis, sporadic
Primary amyloidosis (immunoglobulin)
Secondary (reactive) amyloidosis (amyloid A protein)

**Major Diagnostic Criteria:** Adult onset of central nervous system hemorrhage and damage; positive family history (dominant inheritance); histologically proven amyloidosis; demonstration of gamma trace protein (cystatin C) in amyloid deposits; and extremely low levels of gamma trace in cerebrospinal fluid.

**Clinical Findings:** Patients suffer from episodes of cerebral bleeding because of weakening of cerebral arterial walls caused by amyloid infiltration. The symptoms can vary, depending on location and severity of bleeding. Some patients may die suddenly without having exhibited any prior symptoms. Other patients may have many non fatal episodes and suffer significant impairment for years before death. There are very few noncerebral findings in this disorder, since the amyloid is primarily restricted to cerebral blood vessel walls.

**Complications:** Those associated with intracranial hemorrhages.

**Associated Findings:** Patients have extremely low levels of gamma trace in the cerebrospinal fluid. This has also been found in some young at-risk individuals.

**Etiology:** Autosomal dominant inheritance with adult onset and high penetrance.

**Pathogenesis:** A large degradative product of gamma trace protein (cystatin C), lacking the first ten residues, has been found in the amyloid deposits. In addition, the amyloid protein (the gamma trace fragment) has a glutamine at position 58, which is a previously unreported variant (normal gamma trace has leucine at position 58). The amyloid weakens the vessel walls, making them prone to rupture.

**MIM No.:** *10515

**Sex Ratio:** M1:F1

**Occurrence:** Originally identified in one geographical area in Iceland. However, several Dutch families have a clinically similar syndrome. Immunohistochemical studies of Dutch-type amyloid showed only a weak reaction to antigamma trace, and, in addition, the gamma trace levels in the CSF were normal. Thus, the Dutch form is probably related but not identical to the Icelandic form.

**Risk of Recurrence for Patient's Sib:**
See Part I, *Mendelian Inheritance.*

**Risk of Recurrence for Patient's Child:**
See Part I, *Mendelian Inheritance.*

**Age of Detectability:** In the patients second and third decade of life, although the disease may not be evident prior to the patient's death.

**Gene Mapping and Linkage:** Unknown.

**Prevention:** None known. Genetic counseling indicated.

**Treatment:** There is no treatment that can reduce the deposits or prevent further amyloid formation.

**Prognosis:** Nearly all of the Icelandic patients have died by age 40 years. The Dutch patients have lived beyond age 40 years.

**Detection of Carrier:** Low gamma trace levels in the CSF may identify presymptomatic gene carriers, but this has not yet been established. The Gln-58 gamma trace variant can be identified by biochemical means; however, it has not been shown that this variant is indeed the cause of the disorder.

**Special Considerations:** Although the Gln-58 variant was found in the amyloid, the gamma trace in the plasma and CSF was not studied. Thus it is unclear if the patients were heterozygous for this protein. Since the amyloid is formed from a degraded gamma trace, it is possible that the pathogenesis is an abnormal metabolism of gamma trace and that the Gln-58 variant is insignificant and does not contribute to amyloid formation. Another possibility is that the transport of this protein is altered (as the low CSF gamma trace concentrations might indicate), which may involve catabolism or the amino acid substitution.

Senile plaques (containing amyloid), neurofibrillary tangles, and long-term dementia are not characteristic of this condition. Therefore, this disorder is considered to be separate from sporadic cerebral amyloid angiopathy (often found in elderly demented

patients) and Alzheimer disease (hereditary or sporadic forms). There have been several reports of dominant "congophilic angiopathy," but these families have different histologic and clinical findings. Apparently a number of distinct disorders demonstrate amyloid in cerebral blood vessels.

**References:**
Gudmundsson G, et al.: Hereditary cerebral hemorrhage with amyloidosis. Brain 1972; 95:387–404.
Griffiths RA, et al.: Congophilic angiopathy of the brain: a clinical and pathological report on two siblings. J Neurol Neurosurg Psychiatry 1982; 45:396–408.
Wattendorf AF, et al.: Familial cerebral amyloid angiopathy presenting as recurrent cerebral hemorrhage. J Neurol Sci 1982; 55:121–135.
Cohen DH, et al.: Amyloid fibril in hereditary cerebral hemorrhage with amyloidosis (HCHWA) is related to the gastroentero-pancreatic neuroendocrine protein, gamma trace. J Exp Med 1983; 158:623–628.
Grubb A, et al.: Abnormal metabolism of gamma trace alkaline microprotein: the basic defect in hereditary cerebral hemorrhage with amyloidosis. New Engl J Med 1984; 311;1547–1549.
Hochwald GM, Thorbecke GJ: Abnormal metabolism or reduced transport of CSF gamma trace microprotein in hereditary cerebral hemorrhage with amyloidosis. New Engl J Med 1985; 312:1127–1128.
Ghiso J, et al.: Hereditary cerebral amyloid angiopathy: the amyloid fibrils contain a protein which is a variant of cystatin C, an inhibitor of lysosomal cysteine proteases. Biochem Biophys Res Commun 1986; 136:548–554.
Jensson O, et al.: Hereditary cystatin C (gamma trace) amyloid angiopathy of the central nervous system causing cerebral hemorrhage. Acta Neurol Scand 1986; 73:308–320.

WA048
BE045
**Margaret R. Wallace**
**Merrill D. Benson**

---

## AMYLOIDOSIS, ILLINOIS TYPE                                        2882

**Includes:**
Amyloidosis, prealbumin Tyr-77
German amyloidosis
Illinois amyloidosis
Prealbumin Tyr-77 amyloidosis
Transthyretin (prealbumin) Tyr-77 amyloidosis
Tyrosine 77 amyloidosos

**Excludes:** Amyloidosis (other)

**Major Diagnostic Criteria:** Adult onset of lower limb neuropathy and GI dysfunction; positive family history (dominant inheritance); histologically proven amyloidosis; and biochemical proof of Tyrosine-77 (Tyr-77) transthyretin (prealbumin) in plasma or amyloid or DNA analysis showing the Tyr-77 transthyretin (prealbumin) gene.

**Clinical Findings:** In the single family described, the proband developed lower limb neuropathy at age 51 years, followed by intermittent diarrhea. The proband, still living at age 57 years, has normal renal function thus far. However, his father, who was an obligate carrier, reportedly had the same symptoms and died of renal failure. Kidney involvement may be a major finding in this form.

**Complications:** Those of neuropathy and autonomic dysfunction, such as incontinence.

**Associated Findings:** None known.

**Etiology:** Autosomal dominant inheritance with adult onset.

**Pathogenesis:** Variant transthyretin (prealbumin) molecules, containing a tyrosine-for-serine substitution at position 77, were found in the proband's plasma. Immunohistochemistry demonstrated transthyretin (prealbumin) in his amyloid deposits (from biopsy). It is assumed that the pathogenesis is similar to other forms of hereditary amyloidosis, with the amyloid consisting primarily of the Tyr-77 transthyretin (prealbumin) molecules.

**MIM No.:** 17630

**Sex Ratio:** Presumably M1:F1.

**Occurrence:** One United States family (of German descent) has been documented, and the gene has been found in six unrelated families. Hereditary amyloidosis has been reported in German families, and may represent the same variant.

**Risk of Recurrence for Patient's Sib:**
See Part I, *Mendelian Inheritance.*

**Risk of Recurrence for Patient's Child:**
See Part I, *Mendelian Inheritance.*

**Age of Detectability:** The proband had onset at age 51 years, and his father, whose medical history indicates that he was affected, had onset in his early 50s.

**Gene Mapping and Linkage:** PALB (prealbumin [transthyretin]) has been mapped to 18q11.2-q12.1.

**Prevention:** None known. Genetic counseling indicated.

**Treatment:** There is no treatment that affects the amyloid deposits; however colchicine, is sometimes administered since it appears to slow amyloid formation in **Fever, familial mediterranean (FMF)** (in which the amyloid fibrils consist of the A protein). Treatment of the symptoms may bring some relief and prolong the lives of patients.

**Prognosis:** The proband is still alive and doing well six years after onset. The exact duration of his father's disease is unknown, but appears to have been at least five years. Renal failure was the cause of death in the father. Mental capacity is not impaired.

**Detection of Carrier:** The Tyr-77 transthyretin (prealbumin) variant can be identified in the plasma by biochemical methods. In addition, Southern analysis of DNA can detect the Tyr-77 transthyretin (prealbumin) gene by use of the enzyme SspI and a transthyretin (prealbumin) gene fragment as probe. Also, RFLP analysis of PCR amplified DNA has been reported.

**Special Considerations:** The symptoms in this disease mimic those in other forms of transthyretin (prealbumin) hereditary amyloidosis, such as **Amyloidosis, transthyretin methionine-30 type.** Biochemical or DNA methods are required to distinguish among these clinically similar syndromes.

**References:**
Wallace MR, et al.: Identification of a new prealbumin variant, Tyr-77, associated with autosomal dominant amyloidosis. Am J Hum Genet 1986; 39:A22 only.

WA048
BE045

**Margaret R. Wallace**
**Merrill D. Benson**

**Amyloidosis, Indiana type**
*See AMYLOIDOSIS, INDIANA TYPE*

## AMYLOIDOSIS, INDIANA TYPE                 2142

**Includes:**
Amyloid polyneuropathy, type II
Amyloidosis, Indiana type
Amyloidosis, type II
Indiana type hereditary amyloidosis
Prealbumin-84 isoleucine-to-serine
Rukavina type hereditary amyloidosis
Serine 84 amyloidosis
Swiss type hereditary amyloidosis
Transthyretin-84 isoleucine-to-serine

**Excludes:**
**Amyloidosis** (other)
Amyloidosis, sporadic
Primary amyloidosis (immunoglobulin)
Secondary (reactive) amyloidosis (amyloid A protein)

**Major Diagnostic Criteria:** Adult onset of carpal tunnel syndrome and peripheral neuropathy, vitreous deposits, and cardiomyopathy; positive family history (dominant inheritance); histologically proven amyloidosis; and biochemical proof of Ser-84 transthyretin (prealbumin) variant or DNA analysis showing gene for Ser-84 transthyretin (prealbumin).

**Clinical Findings:** This syndrome usually begins with carpal tunnel syndrome around age 40 years. Patients suffer from vitreous deposits, cardiomyopathy, cardiomegaly, and progressive neuropathy in both upper and lower extremities. Some patients have gastrointestinal disturbances, which may result in malnutrition.

**Complications:** Practically all patients develop deposits of amyloid in the vitreous, which may lead to blindness. The complications of heart failure are common, and many of these patients eventually require pacemakers.

**Associated Findings:** Gene carriers (both affected and presymptomatic) have been shown to have significantly reduced retinol-binding protein (RBP) concentrations in their serum. This is not thought to have any effect on the health of the patient, but is most likely a result of a decreased capacity of the Ser-84 transthyretin (prealbumin) to bind RBP.

**Etiology:** Autosomal dominant inheritance, with adult onset and very high penetrance.

**Pathogenesis:** A variant of plasma transthyretin (prealbumin), containing a serine at position 84 in place of the normal isoleucine, has been implicated in this disease. While the Ser-84 transthyretin (prealbumin) is most likely the determining factor in expression of this disease, both variant and normal transthyretin (prealbumin) molecules are incorporated into the fibril deposits. This suggests that the fibrils are constructed by aggregation of dimers or tetramers (containing at least one Ser-84 molecule) of circulating transthyretin (prealbumin), which is normally tetrameric. The amyloid deposits interfere with functioning of the surrounding tissues. For example, the heart muscle becomes thick and stiff because of amyloid infiltration and loses the ability to contract efficiently.

**MIM No.:** 10490, 17630

**Sex Ratio:** M1:F1

**Occurrence:** The Ser-84 transthyretin (prealbumin) variant has been identified in only one family, a large Indiana kindred of Swiss descent originally described by Rukavina. However the disease in a large Maryland kindred is clinically very similar to that in the Indiana family. Biochemical or DNA analysis remains to be done to determine if the Maryland family has the Ser-84 variant. No other families have been reported with this clinical form of amyloidosis.

**Risk of Recurrence for Patient's Sib:**
See Part I, *Mendelian Inheritance.*

**Risk of Recurrence for Patient's Child:**
See Part I, *Mendelian Inheritance.*

**Age of Detectability:** Onset is usually between ages 35 and 45 years.

**Gene Mapping and Linkage:** PALB (prealbumin) has been mapped to 18q11.2-q12.1.

**Prevention:** None known. Genetic counseling indicated.

**Treatment:** No effective treatment exists that affects amyloid deposition. Colchicine is sometimes administered in hereditary amyloid cases as an experimental treatment, because it appears to inhibit amyloid formation in familial Mediterranean fever (in which the amyloid fibrils consist of amyloid A protein, not transthyretin (prealbumin)). Treatment of symptoms may bring some relief and prolong the lives of patients. Vitrectomy and carpal tunnel decompression are common procedures among these patients.

**Prognosis:** The duration of the disease is generally 8–15 years, with death resulting most often from heart failure. Mental capacity is not impaired.

**Detection of Carrier:** The Ser-84 variant can be detected in blood by biochemical methods, and the corresponding variant transthyretin (prealbumin) gene can be identified by an RFLP (DNA) test using the enzyme AluI and a specific transthyretin (prealbumin) gene fragment as probe.

**Special Considerations:** Although vitreous deposits are often considered a hallmark of this disorder, this finding has been seen in other forms of hereditary amyloidosis. Furthermore, carpal tunnel syndrome and cardiomyopathy are not unique to this form.

### References:
Rukavina JG, et al.: Primary systemic amyloidosis: a review and an experimental, genetic, and clinical study of 29 cases with particular emphasis on the familial form. Medicine 1956; 35:239–334.

Schlesinger AS, et al.: Peripheral neuropathy in familial primary amyloidosis. Brain 1962; 85:357–370.

Mahloudji M, et al.: The genetic amyloidoses, with particular reference to hereditary neuropathic amyloidosis, type II (Indiana or Rukavina type). Medicine 1969; 48:1–37.

Benson MD, Dwulet FE: Prealbumin and retinol binding protein serum concentrations in the Indiana type hereditary amyloidosis. Arthritis Rheum 1983; 26:1493–1498.

Dwulet FE, Benson MD: Characterization of a transthyretin (prealbumin) variant associated with familial amyloidotic polyneuropathy type II (Indiana/Swiss). J Clin Invest 1986; 78:880–886.

WA048                                    **Margaret R. Wallace**
BE045                                       **Merrill D. Benson**

## AMYLOIDOSIS, IOWA TYPE                                          2144

### Includes:
> Amyloidosis, type IV
> Iowa type amyloidosis
> Van Allen type amyloidosis

### Excludes:   Amyloidosis (other)

**Major Diagnostic Criteria:**   Adult onset of lower limb neuropathy, gastric ulcers, and renal failure; positive family history (dominant inheritance); and histologically proven amyloidosis.

**Clinical Findings:**   The initial symptom is neuropathy in the lower extremities. As the disease progresses, additional findings include renal failure and gastric and peptic ulcers.

**Complications:**   Patients may suffer from gastrointestinal bleeding because of the ulcers and may have other complications of autonomic dysfunction, such as incontinence.

**Associated Findings:**   In one Iowa family, a number of patients have had hearing impairment and cataracts. These findings may or may not be related to the amyloidosis syndrome.

**Etiology:**   Autosomal dominant inheritance with adult onset.

**Pathogenesis:**   Preliminary studies in an Iowa patient have found a degradative product of a variant form of apoliprotein A1 in the amyloid deposits. The amyloid deposits, which are interstitial, destroy the integrity of the surrounding tissues, resulting in the clinical findings.

**MIM No.:**   *10510

**Sex Ratio:**   M1:F1

**Occurrence:**   This disease was found in an Iowa family of English/Irish/Scottish descent. The prevalence of this form of amyloidosis is unknown. One other family, from Spain, was classified as having the Iowa-type amyloidosis based on clinical data.

**Risk of Recurrence for Patient's Sib:**
See Part I, *Mendelian Inheritance.*

**Risk of Recurrence for Patient's Child:**
See Part I, *Mendelian Inheritance.*

**Age of Detectability:**   Average age of onset is reported to be 35 years.

**Gene Mapping and Linkage:**   Unknown.

**Prevention:**   None known. Genetic counseling indicated.

**Treatment:**   There is no known treatment to eradicate or prevent amyloid deposits, but colchicine is sometimes administered in hereditary amyloidosis because it appears to slow amyloid formation in **Fever, familial mediterranean (FMF)** (in which the amyloid fibril contains amyloid A protein). Treatment of the symptoms may bring relief and prolong the lives of patients.

**Prognosis:**   In the Iowa family the patients survived an average of 12 years after onset. Mental capacity is not affected.

**Detection of Carrier:**   Unknown.

**Special Considerations:**   There is some confusion in the literature as to nomenclature, because the Iowa type has been referred to as both amyloidosis, type III and amyloidosis, type IV, while the Danish cardiac type has also been called type III.

### References:
Van Allen MW, et al.: Inherited predisposition to generalized amyloidosis: clinical and pathological studies of a family with neuropathy, nephropathy and peptic ulcer. Neurology 1968; 19:10–25.

Gimeno A, et al.: Amyloidotic polyneuritis of type III (Iowa-Van Allen). Eur Neurol 1974; 11:46–57.

Nichols W, et al.: Apoliprotein A1 in Iowa type hereditary amyloidosis (FAP type IV). (Abstract) Clin Res 1987; 35:595A only.

WA048                                    **Margaret R. Wallace**
BE045                                       **Merrill D. Benson**

**Amyloidosis, Japanese type**
*See AMYLOIDOSIS, TRANSTHYRETIN METHIONINE-30 TYPE*

## AMYLOIDOSIS, OHIO TYPE                                          2149

### Includes:
> Amyloidosis, type VII
> Oculoleptomeningeal type amyloidosis
> Ohio type amyloidosis

### Excludes:
> **Amyloidosis** (other)
> Amyloidosis, sporadic
> Primary amyloidosis (immunoglobulin)
> Secondary (reactive) amyloidosis (amyloid A protein)

**Major Diagnostic Criteria:**   Adult onset of central nervous system and ocular dysfunction; positive family history; and histologically proven amyloidosis.

**Clinical Findings:**   This form has been reported in only one family, from Ohio, of German origin. In the seven patients, the symptoms included dementia, seizures, strokes, coma, abnormal gait, vitreous deposits, and other signs of central nervous system (CNS) dysfunction.

**Complications:**   Most patients had CNS complications such as those listed above, and hemiparesis and hemihyperesthesia were found as well. Several patients had to be institutionalized because of dementia, and most were bedridden or wheelchair-bound for some time prior to their deaths.

**Associated Findings:**   Two patients were noted to have hearing loss. Amyloid was found in the rectal biopsy specimen of one patient, but not in specimens from two other patients. Postmortem studies of five patients revealed amyloid in the CNS, particularly leptomeninges and subarachnoid vessels. Amyloid was also found in small amounts in the internal organs. Only traces of amyloid were found in the peripheral nerves and skeletal muscles.

**Etiology:**   Presumably autosomal dominant inheritance, although the seven pathologically established cases were all from one generation.

**Pathogenesis:**   This is a systemic form of amyloidosis; however, the CNS is most severely affected. Other systems generally are not involved enough to suffer impairment of function. The pathogenesis appears to be decreased blood supply to (and perhaps small hemorrhages in) the brain because of amyloid infiltration of the blood vessel walls. The biochemical nature of the amyloid fibril has not been investigated, but both transthyretin (prealbumin) and gamma trace protein have been found in CNS amyloid in other families that show different symptoms.

**MIM No.:**   *10521

**Sex Ratio:**   M1:F1

**Occurrence:**   Only one family (seven affected members), living in Ohio and of German descent, has been reported.

**Risk of Recurrence for Patient's Sib:**
See Part I, *Mendelian Inheritance*.

**Risk of Recurrence for Patient's Child:**
See Part I, *Mendelian Inheritance*.

**Age of Detectability:**  Earliest symptoms were reported between the ages of 30 and 56 years of age.

**Gene Mapping and Linkage:**  Unknown.

**Prevention:**  None known. Genetic counseling indicated.

**Treatment:**  No treatment can reduce or prevent amyloid deposition. Vitrectomy might improve the eyesight of patients with vitreal deposits.

**Prognosis:**  Appears to be fatal, as are most systemic amyloidoses. Six of the patients died between ages 46 and 60 years, with the seventh still alive as of 1980 at age 57.

**Detection of Carrier:**  Unknown.

**Special Considerations:**  It may be difficult to diagnose this disorder by biopsy, because the most accessible sites, such as rectum or skin, may be negative even though amyloid is present in the CNS. In two patients, amyloid was identified in vitreous material.

**References:**
Goren H, et al.: Familial oculoleptomeningeal amyloidosis. Brain 1980; 103:473–495.

WA048
BE045

Margaret R. Wallace
Merrill D. Benson

**Amyloidosis, Portuguese type**
*See AMYLOIDOSIS, TRANSTHYRETIN METHIONINE-30 TYPE*
**Amyloidosis, prealbumin met-111**
*See AMYLOIDOSIS, DANISH CARDIAC TYPE*
**Amyloidosis, prealbumin Tyr-77**
*See AMYLOIDOSIS, ILLINOIS TYPE*
**Amyloidosis, primary cutaneous**
*See AMYLOIDOSIS, FAMILIAL LICHEN*
**Amyloidosis, Swedish type**
*See AMYLOIDOSIS, TRANSTHYRETIN METHIONINE-30 TYPE*
**Amyloidosis, transthyretin (prealbumin) Ala-60**
*See AMYLOIDOSIS, APPALACHIAN TYPE*

---

## AMYLOIDOSIS, TRANSTHYRETIN METHIONINE-30 TYPE                              2141

**Includes:**
Amyloid polyneuropathy, type I
Amyloidosis, Japanese type
Amyloidosis, Portuguese type
Amyloidosis, Swedish type
Amyloidosis, type I
Japanese-type hereditary amyloidosis
Methionine 30 amyloidosis
Portuguese (Andrade)-type hereditary amyloidosis
Prealbumin defect
Swedish-type hereditary amyloidosis
Transthyretin abnormality

**Excludes:**
Amyloidosis (other)
Amyloidosis, sporadic
Primary amyloidosis (immunoglobulin)
Secondary (reactive) amyloidosis (amyloid A protein)

**Major Diagnostic Criteria:**  Adult onset of lower limb neuropathy, bowel dysfunction; positive family history (dominant inheritance); histologically proven amyloidosis (e.g., rectal biopsy); and biochemical proof of Methionine-30 ("Met"-30) transthyretin (prealbumin) variant or DNA analysis showing the gene for Met-30 transthyretin (prealbumin).

**Clinical Findings:**  Lower limb neuropathy and autonomic dysfunction are nearly universal and are often the first symptoms. The autonomic involvement is usually manifested as recurrent diarrhea, which may alternate with constipation. Sexual impo-

tence is common as well. Those patients with vitreal amyloid may suffer from significantly reduced vision. Renal failure, if the kidneys are involved, may become evident in the later stages of the disease. As the disease progresses over several years, patients lose weight and mobility. Incontinence is common, and patients become cachectic and bedridden. Mental function is generally not affected, but amyloid may be present in the central nervous system.

**Complications:**  Because of paresis and paresthesia in the lower (and sometimes upper) limbs, decubitus ulcers are common and often fail to heal because patients unknowingly reinjure the sites. Amyloid in the nerves of the intestinal tract causes peristalsis to slow, leading to overgrowth of intestinal flora and malabsorption. Blindness may occur from deposits of amyloid in the vitreous or as a complication of vitrectomy.

**Associated Findings:**  In one United States family with this defect, the heart was severely affected and cardiomyopathy resulted. In one Japanese family, central nervous system dysfunction also occurred in some patients, although it is not clear whether this is part of the amyloid syndrome.

**Etiology:**  Autosomal dominant inheritance, with adult onset and very high penetrance.

**Pathogenesis:**  Variant transthyretin (prealbumin) molecules (containing a methionine in place of the normal valine at amino acid 30) circulate and deposit systemically as amyloid. These deposits, more prevalent in certain tissues such as nerve and kidney, interfere with the functioning of these tissues.

**MIM No.:**  *10480, 10527, 17630

**Sex Ratio:**  M1:F1

**Occurrence:**  Appears to be the most widespread type of hereditary amyloid. The Met-30 transthyretin (prealbumin) variant has been described in families of Japanese, Swedish, Portuguese, Greek, and English descent. Prevalence rates for this or other types of hereditary amyloid have not been estimated, but the frequency of the disease (all hereditary forms) would appear to be in excess of 1:1,000,000 in the United States. New mutations are thought to be quite rare.

**Risk of Recurrence for Patient's Sib:**
See Part I, *Mendelian Inheritance*.

**Risk of Recurrence for Patient's Child:**
See Part I, *Mendelian Inheritance*.

**Age of Detectability:**  Onset of the disease has been reported between the ages of 13 and 70 years, but is usually within a fairly close range in each family.

**Gene Mapping and Linkage:**  PALB (prealbumin) has been mapped to 18q11.2-q12.1.

**Prevention:**  None known. Genetic counseling indicated.

**Treatment:**  No effective treatment exists that affects amyloid deposition; however, colchicine is sometimes administered since it appears to slow amyloid formation associated with familial Mediterranean fever (in which the amyloid consists of amyloid A protein, not transthyretin (prealbumin)). Treatment of symptoms may bring some relief and prolong the lives of patients.

**Prognosis:**  Death inevitably occurs, usually 5–15 years after onset of symptoms.

**Detection of Carrier:**  Several biochemical methods can detect the Met-30 transthyretin (prealbumin), which is present in the blood starting before birth. As well, a DNA test has been developed to detect the variant transthyretin (prealbumin) gene. This is a standard RFLP (Southern analysis) test using the restriction enzymes NsiI or BalI and a transthyretin (prealbumin) cDNA or gene probe.

**Special Considerations:**  Because this syndrome's features may be very similar to those of other forms of hereditary amyloid, biochemical or DNA testing must be done to demonstrate this particular (Met-30) form. Several other transthyretin (prealbumin) variants have been found in association with this set of disorders, and clinical findings may overlap. In addition, family histories are not always reliable, since this disorder may be misdiagnosed or gene carriers may have died before expressing the disease. It is extremely important to discriminate between hereditary and acquired amyloid in new patients with a "negative" family history. A number of Swedish families have been described that have not been tested for the Met-30 variant, so other forms may exist in the Swedish population. Apparently most, if not all, Japanese and Portuguese families have the Met-30 form.

**References:**
Andrade C: A peculiar form of peripheral neuropathy. Brain 1952; 75:408–426.
Araki S, et al.: Polyneuritic amyloidosis in a Japanese family. Arch Neurol 1968; 18:593–602.
Andersson R: Hereditary amyloidosis with polyneuropathy. Acta Med Scand 1970; 188:85–94.
Costa PP, et al.: Amyloid fibril protein related to prealbumin in familial amyloidotic polyneuropathy. Proc Natl Acad Sci USA 1978; 75:4499–4503.
Dwulet FE, Benson MD: Polymorphism of human plasma thyroxine binding prealbumin. Biochem Biophys Res Commun 1983; 114:657–662.
Saraiva MJM, et al.: Amyloid fibril protein in familial amyloidotic polyneuropathy, Portuguese type. J Clin Invest 1984; 74:104–119.
Sasaki H, et al.: Diagnosis of familial amyloidotic polyneuropathy by recombinant DNA techniques. Biochem Biophys Res Commun 1984; 125:636–642.
Wallace MR, et al.: Molecular detection of carriers of hereditary amyloidosis in a Swedish-American family. Am J Med Genet 1986; 25:335–341.
Yoshioka K, et al.: Structure of the mutant prealbumin gene responsible for familial amyloidotic polyneuropathy. Mol Biol Med 1986; 3:319–328.
Ikeda S-I, et al.: Hereditary generalized amyloidosis with polyneuropathy: clinicopathological study of 65 Japanese patients. Brain 1987; 110:315–337.

WA048
BE045

**Margaret R. Wallace
Merrill D. Benson**

**Amyloidosis, type I**
*See AMYLOIDOSIS, TRANSTHYRETIN METHIONINE-30 TYPE*
**Amyloidosis, type II**
*See AMYLOIDOSIS, INDIANA TYPE*
**Amyloidosis, type III**
*See AMYLOIDOSIS, DANISH CARDIAC TYPE*
**Amyloidosis, type IV**
*See AMYLOIDOSIS, IOWA TYPE*
**Amyloidosis, type V**
*See AMYLOIDOSIS, FINNISH TYPE*
**Amyloidosis, type VI**
*See AMYLOIDOSIS, ICELANDIC TYPE*
**Amyloidosis, type VII**
*See AMYLOIDOSIS, OHIO TYPE*
**Amyloidosis, type IX**
*See AMYLOIDOSIS, FAMILIAL LICHEN*
**Amyloidosis, X-linked cutaneous**
*See AMYLOIDOSIS, FAMILIAL CUTANEOUS*
**Amyloidosis-deafness-urticaria**
*See URTICARIA-DEAFNESS-AMYLOIDOSIS*
**Amylopectinosis**
*See GLYCOGENOSIS, TYPE IV*
**Amyotrophic chorea with acanthocytosis, familial**
*See ACANTHOCYTOSIS-NEUROLOGIC DEFECTS*

## AMYOTROPHIC LATERAL SCLEROSIS    2067

**Includes:**
ALS
Aran-Duchenne disease
Bulbar palsy, progressive
Gehrig's disease
Lou Gehrig's disease
Motor neuron disease, juvenile and adult
Muscular atrophy, progressive

**Excludes:**
**Amyotrophic lateral sclerosis, familial adult and juvenile types** (2069)

**Amyotrophic lateral sclerosis, Guam type** (2068)
Amyotrophy in multisystem disease
**Arthrogryposes** (0088)
**Arthrogryposis, amyoplasia type** (2281)
**G(M2)-gangliosidosis with hexosaminidase A deficiency** (0434)
Motor neuron disorders due to endocrinopathies
Motor neuron disorders due to intoxicants
Motor neuron disorders due to physical agents
Motor neuron disorders due to plasma cell disorders
Neuraxonal dystrophy
**Palsy, progressive bulbar of childhood** (2045)
Poliomyelitis or postpolio syndrome
**Spinal muscular atrophy** (0895)
Viral infections

**Major Diagnostic Criteria:** Weakness of spinal and cranial nerve innervated voluntary muscles. Absence of clinically detectable sensory or autonomic dysfunction. Upper motor neuron signs in the presence of muscle wasting, weakness, and fasciculations. EMG and histologic evidence of denervation and reinnervation in a diffuse manner. Normal motor and sensory nerve conduction studies. A combination of brisk deep tendon reflexes and extensor plantar response in a setting of muscle weakness, wasting, and fasciculations with preserved sensation helps make the diagnosis.

**Clinical Findings:** Clinical signs may become evident at almost any age, though they are more commonly seen in the fifth and sixth decades. There is progressive weakness and wasting of voluntary muscles usually accompanied by fasciculations and upper motor neuron signs. The clinical picture depends on the part of the nervous system that bears the brunt of the disease. A majority of patients present with the clinical picture of both upper and lower motor neuron involvement (typical ALS), about one-third with predominantly bulbar signs (progressive bulbar palsy), and less than 10% with lower motor neuron signs only (progressive muscular atrophy or Aran-Duchenne disease); however, pathologic evidence of upper motor neuron involvement is usually found in all types.

The early symptoms may reflect patchy distribution of weakness that is usually distal, but can be proximal. If the upper extremities are initially involved there may be clumsiness in the performance of fine tasks. Lower extremity weakness may give rise to tripping while walking or to other subtle gait problems. Bulbar involvement may lead to complaints of food sticking during eating, choking spells due to pooling of saliva and sometimes hoarseness, or a hyperactive cough reflex. In many instances, the earliest symptom may be cramping of muscles, usually of the lower extremities, especially during sleep. Upper motor neuron involvement, besides giving rise to bulbar symptoms and signs, may lead to a feeling of heaviness or clumsiness of the extremities and occasionally clonus. Facial weakness may be seen, but the extraocular muscles are usually spared. There is no manifest loss of sensory or autonomic function. Deterioration of speech is usually due to a combination of upper and lower motor neuron involvement.

The natural history of the disease is a progressive and unremitting course of global muscular weakness ultimately leading to failure of speech, swallowing, and respiration and resulting in death. With time the patient becomes increasingly helpless, being confined to a wheelchair within 12–18 months. Most patients (90% in one series) die within six years. A small number (10%) with a very slow progress of the disease may survive longer, perhaps as long as 10 to 20 years or even longer.

The creatinine kinase may be elevated two-to-three-fold in some patients and the CSF protein may also be elevated, but neither of these findings are helpful. Needle EMG examination may pick up evidence of diffuse denervation and reinnervation in extremities that may not be clinically involved and in this way help to differentiate diffuse lower motor neuron disorders, such as ALS from focal ones. ALS may also present as focal weakness.

**Complications:** Weakness of muscles leads to progressive helplessness in activities of daily living and in essential functions such as swallowing, breathing, and speech. Aspiration pneumonia or bronchospasm and respiratory failure are usual end-stage complications. Even though many of the patients are eventually bedridden, decubitus ulcers are unusual.

**Associated Findings:** Extraocular muscle weakness and ptosis may be rarely seen. There is occasional association with Parkinson disease and with dementia. ALS has also been reported with *dementia* in several families, including two Old Order Armish sibships and two Canadian families. An association with *polyglucosan bodies* was reported in four children, including two sisters.

**Etiology:** Various etiologies have been postulated, including infection with a slow virus, autoimmune disorder, absence of an essential neuronal trophic factor, accelerated aging of neurons due to DNA repair defect, and environmental toxins. Up to ten percent of cases are thought to be inherited, and in many families inheritance follows an autosomal dominant or autosomal recessive pattern. See **Amyotrophic lateral sclerosis, familial adult and juvenile types**.

**Pathogenesis:** Progressive loss of specific neuronal populations such as the alpha motor neurons in the spinal cord and brain stem pyramidal cells in the motor cortex and cells of Clarke nucleus due to one or more of the etiologies speculated above.

**MIM No.:** *10540, 10555, *20510, *20520, 20525

**Sex Ratio:** M1.8:F1

**Occurrence:** Incidence is 1–2: 100,000, which is similar to that of multiple sclerosis. The prevalence is 2–7: 100,000; 90 to 95% of ALS is sporadic and about 5–10% familial. Foci of high incidence of ALS exist in the Western Pacific (see **Amyotrophic lateral sclerosis, Guam type**).

**Risk of Recurrence for Patient's Sib:** Unknown.

**Risk of Recurrence for Patient's Child:** Not increased unless familial type.

**Age of Detectability:** ALS may occur at any age, but patients over age 60 years and under age 30 years account for less than 10% of the total.

**Gene Mapping and Linkage:** ALS (amyotrophic lateral sclerosis) is UNASSIGNED.

**Prevention:** None known. Genetic counseling indicated.

**Treatment:** Many drugs, including thyrotropin-releasing hormone, have been tried without success, and no specific treatment is known to halt, prevent, or reverse the course of the disease. Supportive physical treatment such as braces, walkers, grab bars, and other physical aids are used to assist in the activities of daily living as required. Later in the course of the disease page turners and appropriate communication measures may have to be devised. Physical therapy should be used to keep joints mobile and to prevent the pain of frozen shoulder. Quinine, Phenytoin, Carbamazepine or diazepam is used to prevent nocturnal muscle cramps and spasms. Anticholinesterase inhibitors in small doses may prevent or postpone fatigue in some cases. Gastrostomy or other such measures are usually required for appropriate nutrition and prevention of aspiration pneumonia. Suction devices are employed to remove pooled saliva from the mouth and throat. Ventilatory support may be provided, but the relevant social, economic and quality of life problems that its institution may produce should be discussed with the patient and the family early in the course of illness.

**Prognosis:** Mean survival is about three years, with 90% dying within six years. Ten percent may live longer, sometimes even 20 years or more. Physical handicap due to muscle weakness eventually leads to total physical dependence. Speech may be totally lost or reduced to a moan. Swallowing difficulties may result in malnutrition and aspiration pneumonia. Ventilatory assistance may be required to prevent terminal respiratory failure. Mental faculties usually remain intact until death.

**Detection of Carrier:** As 5–10% of the ALS is familial and no clinical test differentiates it from the sporadic form of the diseases, a careful inquiry into the family history is important.

**Special Considerations:** In all cases of ALS, abnormalities of calcium and phosphate metabolism should be ruled out. In addition, plasma cell dyscrasias in the form of circulating gamma globulins should be ruled out by serum protein electrophoresis and serum immune electrophoresis. ALS-like syndromes associated with gammopathy usually involve the lower motor neuron. The circulating gamma globulin is directed against GM(1) gangliosides, and is treatable with immunosuppression. Nerve conduction studies demonstrate conduction block, and will usually rule out this entity.

A recent study of incidence of ALS is suggestive of an increasing incidence with age. This study is based on small numbers, but is suggestive of a genetic influence that may become operative with increasing age. The occurrence of ALS many years later in three unrelated football players who were members of the same team at the same time is very intriguing. Such a clustering is suggestive of a toxic environmental factor acting in the presence of an existing predisposition that may have progressively impaired a maintenance system specific and essential for motor neuron survival.

ALS is perhaps best known in the minds of the American public as the condition responsible for the death of New York Yankees baseball player Henry Louis Gehrig.

**Support Groups:**
New York; Muscular Dystrophy Association of America
CA; Woodland Hills; Amyotrophic Lateral Sclerosis Association (ALSA)
Il; Highland Park (P.O. Box 1465); Families of Spinal Muscular Atrophy

**References:**
Norris FH, Kurland LT: Motor neuron diseases. New York: Grune & Stratton, 1969.
Rowland LP, ed: Human motor neuron diseases. New York: Raven Press, 1982.
Engel WK, et al.: Effect on weakness and spasticity in amyotrophic lateral sclerosis and thyrotropin-releasing hormone. Lancet 1983; II:73–75.
Tandan R, Bradley WG: Amyotrophic lateral sclerosis: part 1. Clinical features, pathology, and ethical issues in management. Ann Neurol 1985; 18:271–280.
Tandan R, Bradley WG: Amyotrophic lateral sclerosis: part 2. Etiopathogenesis. Ann Neurol 1985; 18:419–431.
Brooke MB: Diseases of the motor neurons. In: Brooke MB, ed: A clinician's view of neuromuscular diseases, ed 2. Baltimore: Williams & Wilkins, 1986:53–69.
Pestronk A, et al.: A treatable multifocal motor neuropathy with antibodies to GM1 ganglioside. Ann Neurol 1988; 24:73–78.

SI032                                           **Teepu Siddique**

---

## AMYOTROPHIC LATERAL SCLEROSIS, FAMILIAL ADULT AND JUVENILE TYPES                 2069

**Includes:**
ALS
Amyotrophic lateral sclerosis, juvenile-dementia
Amyotrophic lateral sclerosis-polyglucosan bodies
Aran-Duchenne disease
Bulbar palsy, progressive
Gehrig's disease
Lou Gehrig's disease
Motor neuron disease, juvenile and adult
Muscular atrophy, progressive

**Excludes:**
**Amyotrophic lateral sclerosis** (2067)
**Amyotrophic lateral sclerosis, Guam type** (2068)
Amyotrophy in multisystem disease
**Arthrogryposes** (0088)
**Arthrogryposis, amyoplasia type** (2281)
**G(M2)-gangliosidosis with hexosaminidase A deficiency** (0434)
Motor neuron disorders due to endocrinopathies
Motor neuron disorders due to intoxicants
Motor neuron disorders due to physical agents
Motor neuron disorders due to plasma cell disorders
Neuraxonal dystrophy
**Palsy, progressive bulbar of childhood** (2045)

Poliomyelitis or postpolio syndrome
**Spinal muscular atrophy** (0895)
Viral infections

**Major Diagnostic Criteria:** Weakness of spinal and cranial nerve innervated voluntary muscles. Absence of clinically detectable sensory and autonomic dysfunction. Upper motor neuron signs in the presence of muscle wasting, weakness, and fasciculations. EMG and histologic evidence of denervation and reinnervation in a diffuse manner. Normal motor and sensory nerve conduction studies.

**Clinical Findings:** *Adult onset:* In 82% of familial cases, clinical signs become evident by age 55 years, whereas clinical signs are evident by this age in 43% of sporadic cases. There is progressive weakness and wasting of voluntary muscles usually accompanied by fasciculations and upper motor neuron signs. There is an earlier age of onset, a shorter duration of illness (an average of 18 months longer in sporadic cases), and a 1:1 male to female ratio in the familial form of the disease. Except for these differences, there is no clinical or laboratory test that will differentiate the adult onset form of familial ALS from the sporadic variety. However, differences in pathology are noted.

Clinical and EMG findings are detailed under Amyotrophic Lateral Sclerosis. Though the disease may first appear in any part of the body, in a majority it appears in the legs (48.2% as opposed to 31.9% in the sporadic forms), followed by arms (35.0% vs. 41.7% in sporadic forms) and bulbar muscles (16.8% vs. 20.4% in sporadic forms). There is apparent heterogeneity, and Horton et al. (1976) have divided adult-onset familial ALS into three groups on the basis of duration of illness and pathologic findings: two with a relatively short course (one with degeneration of the posterior columns, but no sensory loss in life; the other purely motor in pathology) and one with a longer course. Duration may vary within a single family.

*Juvenile onset:* Data on 43 affected individuals in ten families reported in the literature were consistent with an autosomal recessive trait in five families and with an autosomal dominant trait in the other five. The duration of illness is much longer in the juvenile-onset familial cases than in those with adult onset. In one series, 85.7% presented with leg weakness and 14.3% with arm involvement, and none presented with bulbar involvement. The mean age of onset is earlier in recessive cases. Bulbar symptoms eventually occurred in more than 80% of recessive cases, but only rarely in dominant cases.

**Complications:** Muscle weakness leads to progressive helplessness in the activities of daily living and in essential functions such as swallowing, breathing, and speech. Aspiration pneumonia or bronchospasm and respiratory failure are usual end-stage complications. Even though many of the patients are bedridden, decubitus ulcers are unusual.

**Associated Findings:** There is occasional association with Parkinson disease and with dementia. ALS has also been reported with *dementia* in several families, including two Old Order Amish sibships and two Canadian families. An association with *polyglucosan bodies* was reported in four children, including two sisters.

**Etiology:** Autosomal dominant and autosomal recessive inheritance.

**Pathogenesis:** Cell death of specific populations of neurons such as the alpha motor neurons in the spinal cord and brain stem and pyramidal cells in the motor cortex by an unknown genetic mechanism. Posterior columns and spinocerebellar tracts may be involved, but no clinical signs pertaining to their dysfunction are elicited.

**MIM No.:** *10540, 10555, *20510, *20520, 20525

**Sex Ratio:** M1:F1

**Occurrence:** The incidence of all forms of ALS is 1–2:100,000; 5–10% of cases are familial. Juvenile onset of familial ALS is rare.

Foci of high incidence of ALS exist in the Western Pacific (see **Amyotrophic lateral sclerosis, Guam type**).

**Risk of Recurrence for Patient's Sib:**
See Part I, *Mendelian Inheritance.*

**Risk of Recurrence for Patient's Child:**
See Part I, *Mendelian Inheritance.*

**Age of Detectability:** At any age, but most patients are diagnosed after thirty and under sixty years of age.

**Gene Mapping and Linkage:** ALS (amyotrophic lateral sclerosis) is UNASSIGNED.

**Prevention:** None known. Genetic counseling indicated.

**Treatment:** No specific treatment is known that will halt, prevent, or reverse the course of the disease. Supportive treatment such as physical aids in the form of braces, walkers, and so forth. Aids to assist in the activities of daily living are required. Later in the course of the disease page turners and appropriate communication measures may have to be devised. Physical therapy to keep joints mobile and to prevent the pain of frozen shoulder. Quinine or diazepam to prevent nocturnal muscle cramps and spasms. Gastrostomy, esophagostomy, or cricopharyngeal myectomy may be required for appropriate nutrition and prevention of aspiration pneumonia. Suction device to remove pooled saliva from the mouth. Ventilatory support, especially if requested by the patient.

**Prognosis:** Mean survival is about three years, and is 18 months longer in adult-onset sporadic ALS. Some families are long-lived. There may be variation within families. Physical handicap due to muscle weakness eventually leads to total physical dependence. Speech may be lost or reduced to a moan. Swallowing difficulties may result in malnutrition and aspiration pneumonia. Ventilatory assistance may be required to prevent terminal respiratory failure. Mental faculties usually remain intact until death.

**Detection of Carrier:** As 5–10% of ALS is familial and no clinical test differentiates it from sporadic ALS, a careful family history is important.

**Special Considerations:** A majority of adult-onset familial ALS appears to be an autosomal dominant trait, but heterogeneity is very likely based on short-lived and long-lived families and on posterior columns and spinocerebellar tract involvement on pathologic examination of the CNS in some families. Linkage techniques using the sibship-pair method and the likelihood methods may in the near future establish linkage and clarify the problem of clinical heterogeneity. Some cases of **Palsy, progressive bulbar of childhood** may be classified as juvenile-onset familial amyotrophic lateral sclerosis.

**Support Groups:**
New York; Muscular Dystrophy Association of America
CA; Woodland Hills; Amyotrophic Lateral Sclerosis Association (ALSA)
Il; Highland Park (P.O. Box 1465); Families of Spinal Muscular Atrophy

**References:**
Norris FH, Kurland LT, eds: Motor neuron diseases. New York: Grune & Stratton, 1969.
Horton WA, et al.: Familial motor neuron disease: evidence for at least three different types. Neurology 1976; 26:460–465.
Emery EH, Holloway S: Familial motor neuron diseases. In: Rowland, LP ed: Human motor neuron diseases. New York: Raven, 1982:139–147.
Tandan R, Bradley WG: Amyotrophic lateral sclerosis: Part 1. Clinical features, pathology, and ethical issues in management. Ann Neurol 1985; 18:271–280.
Tandan R, Bradley WG: Amyotrophic lateral sclerosis: Part 2. Etiopathogenesis. Ann Neurol 1985; 18:419–431.
Mulder DW, et al.: Familial adult motor neuron disease: amyotrophic lateral sclerosis. Neurology 1986; 36;511–517.

**Teepu Siddique**

## AMYOTROPHIC LATERAL SCLEROSIS, GUAM TYPE     2068

**Includes:**
> ALS-PD
> Amyotrophic lateral sclerosis-Parkinsonism/dementia complex
> Cycad nut, effects of
> Cycas circinalis (cycad nut), effects of
> Guam disease
> Lytico-bodig

**Excludes:**
> **Amyotrophic lateral sclerosis** (2067)
> **Amyotrophic lateral sclerosis, familial adult and juvenile types** (2069)
> Amyotrophy in multisystem disease
> **Arthrogryposes** (0088)
> **Arthrogryposis, amyoplasia type** (2281)
> **G(M2)-gangliosidosis with hexosaminidase A deficiency** (0434)
> Motor neuron disorders due to endocrinopathies
> Motor neuron disorders due to intoxicants
> Motor neuron disorders due to physical agents
> Motor neuron disorders due to plasma cell disorders
> Neuraxonal dystrophy
> **Palsy, progressive bulbar of childhood** (2045)
> Poliomyelitis or postpolio syndrome
> **Spinal muscular atrophy** (0895)
> Viral infections

**Major Diagnostic Criteria:** The Guam type of ALS occurs in high incidence in isolated populations of East Asia and the Western Pacific. Filipino migrants to Guam and Guamanian migrants to the United States are also affected. There is a high incidence of parkinsonism-dementia in the same populations. Weakness of spinal and cranial nerve innervated voluntary muscles. Absence of clinically detectable sensory and autonomic dysfunction. Upper motor neuron findings in the presence of muscle wasting, weakness, and fasciculations. EMG and histologic evidence of denervation and reinnervation in a diffuse manner. Normal or near-normal motor and normal sensory nerve conduction studies.

**Clinical Findings:** Clinical signs may become evident earlier in Guamanian ALS than in sporadic ALS. There is progressive weakness and wasting of voluntary muscles, accompanied by signs of upper motor neuron involvement. Except for an earlier onset and longer duration of the illness, especially in women, the clinical and electromyographic findings in Guamanian ALS are similar to the sporadic form of ALS (see **Amyotrophic lateral sclerosis**). Neurofibrillary tangles are seen in brains and spinal cords of Guamanians with the ALS-parkinsonism-dementia complex, and even in the nonsymptomatic population of Guam, but are unusual in sporadic ALS.

**Complications:** Weakness of muscles leads to progressive helplessness in activities of daily living and compromises essential functions such as swallowing, breathing, and speech. Aspiration pneumonia or bronchospasm and respiratory failure are usual end-stage complications. Even though many of the patients may become bedridden, decubitus ulcers are unusual.

**Associated Findings:** Neurofibrillary tangles are seen on pathologic examination, a finding not present in the CNS of patients with sporadic ALS. Parkinsonism-dementia complex coexists in high prevalence in the populations with high incidence of Guamanian ALS. Patients with parkinsonism-dementia complex may develop signs of amyotrophy, but not vice versa.

**Etiology:** Environmental toxins are suspected. The following two theories of environmental toxicity are favored: 1) prolonged toxicity from amino acids such as $\alpha$-amino-$\beta$-methylaminopropionic acid and $\beta$-N-methylamino-L-alanine (L-BMAA) in the cycad nut, which was used as a staple diet prior to the diet changes introduced by external cultural impact. L-BMAA is thought to be a toxin and may act as an excitatory amino acid on the glutamate-type receptors on the motor neurons (Spencer et al, 1987); and 2) low calcium and magnesium levels and high aluminum, manganese, and iron levels in the soil, water, and vegetation of these communities are suspected to lead to mineral imbalance and deposition of hydroxyapatite in neurons. These theories explain both the decline in the incidence of ALS in Guam, where cultural and dietary changes have occurred, and the lack of change in incidence in Western New Guinea, where use of cycad as a poultice, and traditional food sources, are still dominant.

**Pathogenesis:** Cell death of specific populations of neurons, such as the alpha motor neurons in the spinal cord and brain stem and pyramidal cells in the motor cortex, probably due to an environmental toxin or mineral imbalance in the setting of an appropriate genetic substrate.

**MIM No.:** *10540

**Sex Ratio:** M2:F1

**Occurrence:** The incidence of ALS in Guam, Rota, and Tinian Islands of Marianas chain (in Micronesia) was 50 times higher than the 1–2:100,000 found in the continental United States when first described. It has declined, now being two to three times higher. The highest incidence of ALS is seen among the Auyu and Jakai peoples of West New Guinea, where the incidence is 100-fold higher than in the rest of the world and has not declined. Other pockets of high incidence include the Kii Peninsula of Japan centered around the relatively isolated areas of Hobara and Kazagawa on the main island of Honshu. All these foci of high incidence are marked by typically low calcium and magnesium levels and high aluminum and manganese levels in the water and soil.

**Risk of Recurrence for Patient's Sib:** Unknown.

**Risk of Recurrence for Patient's Child:** There is a familial incidence of 14% without any particular pattern of inheritance. The disease probably occurs because of environmental factors interacting with an abnormal gene substrate.

**Age of Detectability:** The mean age of onset of symptoms has steadily increased in Guam from 47.6 to 51.9 years in men and from 42.1 to 52.5 years in women when the decades of 1950s and 1970s are compared. No patient of either sex has had onset before age 30 years since 1970.

**Gene Mapping and Linkage:** Unknown.

**Prevention:** None known. Avoidance of toxic foods and correction of any mineral imbalance may be beneficial.

**Treatment:** No specific treatment is known that will halt, prevent, or reverse the course of the disease. Supportive treatment in the form of braces, walkers, and other physical aids to assist in the activities of daily living is required. Later in the course of the disease page turners and appropriate communication measures may have to be devised. Physical therapy to keep joints mobile and to prevent the pain of frozen shoulder. Quinine, Phenytoin, Carbamazepine, or diazepam to prevent nocturnal muscle cramps and spasms. Gastrostomy or other such measures for appropriate nutrition and prevention of aspiration pneumonia. Suction device to remove pooled saliva from the mouth and throat. Ventilatory support may have to be instituted in consultation with the patient and his family.

**Prognosis:** Whereas the mean age of onset of symptoms has steadily increased, the mean duration of symptoms has decreased. When comparing the decade of 1951–1959 to that of 1970–1979, the mean duration of illness has decreased from 5.5 to 3.4 years in men and from 8 to 3.9 years in women. Physical handicap eventually leads to total physical dependence. Speech may be lost or reduced to a moan. Swallowing difficulties lead to malnutrition and aspiration pneumonia. Ventilatory assistance may be required to prevent terminal respiratory failure. Mental faculties usually remain intact until death.

**Detection of Carrier:** Unknown.

**Special Considerations:** Guamanians who have spent their childhood and adolescence in Guam and then migrated to the United States carry a higher risk for acquiring ALS. In addition to the foci of high incidence of ALS mentioned here, there are other foci of high incidence of chronic neurologic disease, often with associated signs of upper motor neuron with or without lower motor neuron involvement: 1) Australian aborigines in Groote

Eylandt and the adjacent coastal Arnhem Land in the Gulf of Carpentaria; 2) Iakut people in the Viliui River Valley of Iakut, Autonomous Soviet Socialist Republic, in Siberia; 3) Filipino immigrants to Guam and Hawaii, mostly from Ilocos Sur and Ilocos Norte provinces; 4) tropical spastic paraplegia on the Pacific Coast of Columbia; 5) tropical spastic paraplegia in the South of India; 6) progressive muscular atrophy in Northern India; 7) progressive muscular atrophy in Zaire; and 8) progressive muscular atrophy in Mozambique.

The Guamanian disease is probably different from ALS elsewhere, not only on the basis of factors discussed above, but by virtue of its long duration of illness and the propensity of affected individuals to develop decubitus ulcers, in contast to other ALS patients in which such ulcers are uncommon.

**Support Groups:**
New York; Muscular Dystrophy Association of America
CA; Woodland Hills; Amyotrophic Lateral Sclerosis Association (ALSA)

**References:**
Arnold A, et al.: Amyotrophic lateral sclerosis: fifty cases observed on Guam. J Nerv Ment Dis 1953; 117:135–139.
Mulder DW, Espinosa RE: Amyotrophic lateral sclerosis: comparison of the clinical syndrome in Guam and the United States. In: Norris FH, Kurland LT, eds: Motor neuron diseases. New York: Grune & Stratton, 1969:12–19.
Yase Y: ALS in the Kii Peninsula: one possible etiological hypothesis. In: Tsubaki T, Toyokura Y, eds: Amyotrophic lateral sclerosis. Tokyo: University of Tokyo Press, 1979:307–318.
Giajdusek DC: Foci of motor neuron disease in high incidence in isolated populations of East Asia and the Western Pacific. In: Rowland LP, ed: Human motor neuron diseases. New York: Raven, 1982:363–393.
Garruto RM, et al.: Disappearance of high-incidence amyotrophic lateral sclerosis and parkinsonism-dementia on Guam. Neurology 1985; 35:193–198.
Rodgers-Johnson P, et al.: Amyotrophic lateral sclerosis and parkinsonism-dementia of Guam: a 30-year evaluation of clinical and neuropathological trends. Neurology 1986; 36:7–13. *
Spencer PS, et al.: Guam amyotrophic lateral sclerosis-parkinsonism-dementia linked to plant excitant neurotoxin. Science 1987; 237:517–522.

SI032                                              **Teepu Siddique**

**Amyotrophic lateral sclerosis, juvenile-dementia**
*See AMYOTROPHIC LATERAL SCLEROSIS, FAMILIAL ADULT AND JUVENILE TYPES*
**Amyotrophic lateral sclerosis-Parkinsonism/dementia complex**
*See AMYOTROPHIC LATERAL SCLEROSIS, GUAM TYPE*
**Amyotrophic lateral sclerosis-polyglucosan bodies**
*See AMYOTROPHIC LATERAL SCLEROSIS, FAMILIAL ADULT AND JUVENILE TYPES*
**Anal aganglionosis**
*See COLON, AGANGLIONOSIS*
**Anal atresia or stenosis**
*See ANORECTAL MALFORMATIONS*
**Anal atresia-iris coloboma**
*See CAT EYE SYNDROME*
**Anal membrane**
*See ANORECTAL MALFORMATIONS*

## ANALBUMINEMIA                                    0047

**Includes:**
Albumin
Dysalbuminemic hyperthyroxinemia
Proalbumin Christchurch
**Excludes:**
Exudative enteropathy
**Nephrosis, congenital** (0709)
**Nephrosis, familial type** (0710)
Protein-losing gastroenteropathy
**Major Diagnostic Criteria:** Plasma albumin concentration is less than 100 mg/dl. Cholesterol concentrations in the blood may be elevated and the erythrocyte sedimentation accelerated.

**Clinical Findings:** The critical finding is a virtually complete absence of albumin in the plasma. The typical concentration lies between 4 and 100 mg/dl. Small amounts of globulin may remain unprecipitated in precipitation methods which would lead to falsely high albumin values in this disease. Immunochemical methods are more reliable. Traces of immunologically normal serum albumin have been demonstrated in one family. Edema may occur, especially in female patients and then mostly in the premenstrual period. In other cases no edema has ever been observed. No evidence of exercise intolerance has been observed even in the presence of only 10 mg/dl of albumin. The sedimentation rate of erythrocytes is always much accelerated. The concentrations of calcium and bilirubin may be abnormally low. The cholesterol and transferrin values are always distinctly higher than normal. Elevated levels of thyroxine may be seen in completely euthyroid patients, especially those with an abnormal albumin variant that binds abnormally to thyroxine. Pterygia and pinquecula may be seen in the conjunctiva.

**Complications:** Unknown.

**Associated Findings:** None known.

**Etiology:** Autosomal recessive inheritance, although a dominant variant has been reported.

**Pathogenesis:** Analbuminemia is generally found in adults. It is not known to cause illness. There is an analbuminemic rat in which mRNA precursors for albumin are found in nuclei but not in cytoplasm, suggesting a mutation interfering with mRNA maturation.

**MIM No.:** *10360, *20530

**Sex Ratio:** M1:F1

**Occurrence:** Unclear since most individuals are not recognized. Some 11 patients with analbuminemia have been reported.

**Risk of Recurrence for Patient's Sib:**
See Part I, *Mendelian Inheritance.*

**Risk of Recurrence for Patient's Child:**
See Part I, *Mendelian Inheritance.*

**Age of Detectability:** Presumably after two months. It is improbable that in the first weeks of life the analbuminemia is already present because no instances of bilirubin intoxication and kernicterus have been observed.

**Gene Mapping and Linkage:** ALB (albumin) has been mapped to 4q11-q13.

**Prevention:** None known. Genetic counseling indicated.

**Treatment:** Not clearly indicated. Human albumin can be infused intravenously. Caution should be exercised about the administration of drugs which generally bind to serum albumin such as sulphonamides, suramin, tolbutamides and coumarin derivatives. A slow IV infusion of albumin might be prudent in order to prevent overabundant supply of active drug to the tissues.

**Prognosis:** Excellent.

**Detection of Carrier:** Heterozygotes have normal concentration of immunochemical identical albumin.

**Special Considerations:** There is other evidence of variation of the gene locus for albumin. In addition to the analbuminemia variant a number of other variants have been described. In one, first referred to as bis-albuminemia, heterozygotes have two albumin proteins, one normal and the other more rapidly migrating in electrophoresis. A number of other electrophoretic variants have been described. Variants are particularly common in American Indians. There is no evidence that any of these variants lead to any human illness, even in homozygotes.

One albumin variant binds thyroxine preferentially so that individuals with this protein have high levels of thyroxine in blood, but they are euthyroid. In another family an albumin variant was reported as related to a connective tissue disorder, but a true relationship appears unlikely.

## References:

Bennhold H, Kallee E: Comparative studies on the half-life of I (131) labelled albumins and non radioactive human serum albumin in a case of analbuminemia. J Clin Invest 1959; 38:863–872.

Laurel CB, Nilehn JE: A new type of inherited serum albumin anomaly. J Clin Invest 1966; 45:1935–1945. *

Boman H, et al: Analbuminemia in an American Indian Girl. Clin Genet 1976;9:513–526. *

Harper ME, Saunders GF: Chromosomal localization of human insulin gene, placental lactogen-growth hormone genes and other single copy genes by in situ hybridization. (Abs) Am J Hum Genet 1981; 33:105A.

Kao FT, et al: Assignment of the structural gene coding for albumin to human chromosome 4. Hum Genet 1982; 62:337–341.

Murray JC, et al: Molecular genetics of human serum albumin: restriction enzyme fragment length polymorphisms and analbuminemia. Proc Nat Acad Sci 1983; 80:5951–5955.

Murray JC et al: Linkage disequilibrium and evolutionary relationships of DNA variants (restriction enzyme fragment length polymorphisms) at the serum albumin locus. Proc Nst Acad Sci 1984; 81:3486–3490.

NY000

**William L. Nyhan**

## Analgesia, familial
*See NEUROPATHY, CONGENITAL SENSORY WITH ANHIDROSIS*

## ANALPHALIPOPROTEINEMIA                                    0048

**Includes:**

Alphalipoprotein deficiency
Apolipoprotein A deficiency
Lipoprotein deficiency, familial high-density
Tangier disease

**Excludes:**

**Apolipoprotein A-I and C-III deficiency states** (3165)
**Hypoalphalipoproteinemia** (3096)
**Lecithin-cholesterol acyl transferase deficiency** (0580)

**Major Diagnostic Criteria:** Enlarged, orange-colored tonsils are usually present. Orange spots are seen on rectal mucosa. Plasma cholesterol is low and $\alpha$ or high-density lipoproteins (HDL) are nearly absent. Triglycerides are normal or high. Cholesteryl ester storage is demonstrable in tonsils, histiocytes, and other reticuloendothelial tissues. Apolipoprotein A1 concentration is markedly reduced. Apolipoprotein A2 concentration is also reduced.

**Clinical Findings:** Clinically the patients have large, orange-colored tonsils. Mild lymphadenopathy and hepatosplenomegaly may be present. Orange-colored spots on the rectal mucosa are present. There may be mild corneal opacification. Almost one-half of the patients have had relapsing neuropathy. A clinical syndrome resembling syringomyelia, with dissociated loss of pain and temperature sensation associated with muscle weakness, has been described but appears to be very rare. There is accumulation of cholesteryl esters in reticuloendothelial and Schwann cells. In the peripheral nerves, the unmyelinated and the small myelinated axons appear to be more vulnerable than the large myelinated axons. Plasma cholesterol level is low, and there is near absence of high-density lipoproteins (HDL). Apolipoprotein A1 is nearly absent, and there is a marked reduction of apolipoprotein A2. Deposition of cholesteryl ester is seen on skin biopsy, and foam cells are present in the bone marrow. Incidence of vascular disease in the fourth decade and beyond is increased.

**Complications:** Almost one-half of the reported patients have had recurrent peripheral neuropathy. A syringomyelia-like syndrome has been described but appears to be very rare. Hypersplenism is occasionally seen. Accelerated atherosclerosis may possibly be associated.

**Associated Findings:** Hypersplenism and anemia may occur.

**Etiology:** Autosomal recessive inheritance. There is a deficiency of apolipoprotein A1 (apo A1). There appears to be normal synthesis. It has been postulated that there is a faulty conversion of pro-apo A1 to mature apo A1 because of either a defective converting enzyme activity or a structurally abnormal apo A1. This defect in apo A1 posttranslational modification may result in enhanced apo A1 catabolism. There is little normal HDL, and a small amount of HDL particle-containing apo A2 circulates in the plasma. There is a deficiency of C-apolipoproteins for which the HDL normally provide a reserve pool. The concentration of low-density lipoproteins (LDL) is therefore also reduced, and abnormal chylomicrons and triglyceride-rich particles are seen in the plasma after meals.

**Pathogenesis:** The defect is not known, but affected individuals do have marked hypercatabolism of HDL constituents to account for their HDL deficiency. The circulating chylomicrons are abnormal with altered metabolism. Storage of nonlysosomal-bound cholesteryl esters occurs by phagocytosis of these abnormal particles. Lipid storage occurs in Schwann cells. Normal clearance of histiocyte cholesterol by HDL is impaired, resulting in progressive accumulation. The accelerated atherosclerosis may be modified by the associated subnormal levels of the low-density lipoproteins.

**MIM No.:** *20540

**Sex Ratio:** M1:F1

**Occurrence:** Less than 30 cases have been reported.

**Risk of Recurrence for Patient's Sib:**
See Part I, *Mendelian Inheritance.*

**Risk of Recurrence for Patient's Child:**
See Part I, *Mendelian Inheritance.*

**Age of Detectability:** Probably at birth by measurement of the plasma apo A1 concentration.

**Gene Mapping and Linkage:** APR (apolipoprotein receptor) has been provisionally mapped to 12q13-q14.

**Prevention:** None known. Genetic counseling indicated.

**Treatment:** No definite treatment. Low fat diet may possibly minimize lipid storage. Splenectomy may be indicated for hypersplenism.

**Prognosis:** Good. Incidence of atherosclerosis is high in the fourth decade and beyond. Severe accelerated atherosclerosis appears not to occur possibly because of low LDL.

**Detection of Carrier:** Heterozygotes have approximately one-half the normal plasma concentration of apo A1.

**Special Considerations:** While only a few of the patients with this condition have come from Tangier Island, the name Tangier disease is used because the original two patients came from this small Chesapeake Bay fishing community in the eastern United States.

## References:

Frederickson DS, et al.: Tangier disease. Ann Intern Med 1961; 55:1016–1031.

Engel WK, et al.: Neuropathy in Tangier disease. Alpha-lipoprotein deficiency manifesting as familial recurrent neuropathy and intestinal lipid storage. Arch Neurol 1967; 17:1–9.

Ferrans VJ, Frederickson DS: The pathology of Tangier disease. Am J Pathol 1975; 78:101–158.

Assmann G, et al.: Isolation and characterization of an abnormal high density lipoprotein in Tangier disease. J Clin Invest 1977; 60:242–252.

Schaefer EJ, et al.: Coronary heart disease prevalence and other clinical features in familial high density lipoprotein deficiency (Tangier disease). Ann Intern Med 1980; 93:261–266.

Herbert PN, et al.: Familial lipoprotein deficiency. In: Stanbury JB, et al., eds: The metabolic basis of inherited disease, ed 5. New York: McGraw-Hill, 1983:589.

Pietrini V, et al.; Neuropathy in Tangier disease: a clinicopathologic study and a review of the literature. Acta Neurol Scand 1985; 72:495–505.

GA018

**Bhuwan P. Garg**

**Ancell-Spiegler-Brooke cylindromas**
*See EPITHELIOMAS, HEREDITARY MULTIPLE CYSTIC*
**Andermann syndrome**
*See CORPUS CALLOSUM AGENESIS-SENSORIMOTOR NEUROPATHY, FAMILIAL*

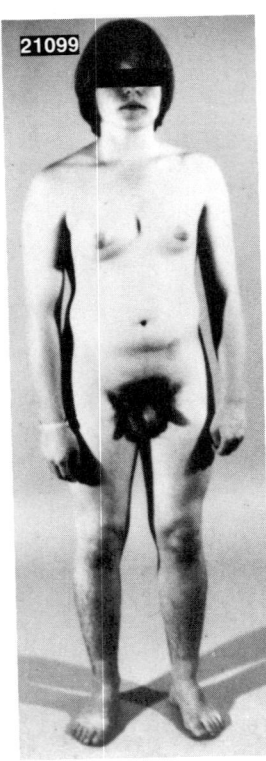

**2954-21099:** A 14-year-old boy with minimal androgen resistance. The body shape, muscularity, penis, and pubic hair are normal male, despite appreciable, persistent, bilateral gynecomastia that required reduction mammoplasty.

**Andersen disease**
*See GLYCOGENOSIS, TYPE IV*
**Anderson disease**
*See LIPID TRANSPORT DEFECT OF INTESTINE*
**Andre syndrome**
*See OTO-PALATO-DIGITAL SYNDROME, II*

## ANDROGEN INSENSITIVITY (RESISTANCE), MINIMAL    2954

**Includes:**
Micropenis, isolated
Oligoazoospermia, idiopathic
Penis, micropenis
Puberty, incoordinate pattern of in adult male

**Excludes:**
**Androgen insensitivity syndrome, complete** (0049)
**Androgen insensitivity syndrome, incomplete** (0050)
**Gynecomastia due to increased aromatase activity, familial** (2308)
Primary hypothalamic-pituitary dysfunction

**Major Diagnostic Criteria:** *Male external genital phenotype*: penis, possibly small, without hypospadias; scrotum, possibly with prominent raphe as minimal expression of bifidity; testes, usually descended; prostate size may be reduced; wolffian duct derivatives are normal; müllerian duct derivatives are absent; puberty is masculine, but may be late or incomplete generally or focally (incoordinate) with persistent gynecomastia; 46,XY karyotype; plasma testosterone and luteinizing hormone are normal or elevated; androgen-receptor activity in genital skin fibroblasts may be deficient or defective.

**Clinical Findings:** Except for possible micropenis and minimal scrotal bifidity, external genital morphogenesis is unambiguously male. Puberty is predominantly masculine, but may be delayed or terminally incomplete, generally or selectively, the latter yielding a pattern that is incoordinate. Thus, an otherwise normal affected man may first come to medical attention when he is investigated for infertility and found to have "idiopathic" oligoazoospermia. Persistent (postpubertal) gynecomastia may be present. However, spermatogenesis may be adequate, and gynecomastia may not develop or persist postpubertally in a subject who lacks one or more of the other components of normal male puberty; for example, normal skeletal muscularity, facial and body hair, and pitch of the voice. Pubic and leg hair are usually normal; axillary hair may be normal as well. In some families with incomplete androgen insensitivity syndrome, the range of intrafamilial expressivity may include affected individuals who meet the diagnostic criteria for minimal androgen insensitivity syndrome.

**Complications:** The psychologic consequences of gynecomastia or other expressions of subnormal virilization and masculinity.

**Associated Findings:** None known.

**Etiology:** Those individuals with deficient or defective androgen-receptor activity in their genital skin fibroblasts very likely have mutations at the X-linked locus that encodes the androgen receptor protein. This interpretation is compatible with the pattern of transmission in two affected families. Some individuals probably have postreceptor defects in the intracellular androgen-response apparatus. Defects in parareceptor "factors" that affect the quality of otherwise normal androgen receptors are possible as well. Nothing is known about the genetic identity of such post- or parareceptor defects.

**Pathogenesis:** A mildly deficient or defective androgen-receptor activity, or a mild disability in another portion of the androgen-response apparatus, supplies sufficient androgen sensitivity to support normal male internal and external genital morphogenesis, but an insufficient degree of sensitivity to support androgen-dependent pubertal development. Selective failure of male puberty presumably reflects differential thresholds of various pubertal target organs for normal androgen sensitivity.

**MIM No.:**   31230, *31370

**Sex Ratio:**   M1:F0

**Occurrence:** Unknown. Several families, one set of twins, and sporadic cases have been reported. In some, deficient or defective androgen-receptor activity has been identified; in others, the diagnosis has rested on clinical and endocrine criteria of androgen insensitivity. A series of studies from one center indicated that 40% of males with idiopathic oligoazoospermia have deficient or defective androgen-receptor activity in their genital skin fibroblasts. Two other studies have yielded much lower estimates of androgen receptor involvement in men with idiopathic oligoazoospermia: One was based on pubic skin fibroblasts; both used different, perhaps less sensitive, criteria than the first. In one study on alveolar and pubic skin fibroblasts from 12 men with postpubertal gynecomastia, no abnormalities in androgen-receptor number or equilibrium binding affinity were discovered. It remains to be established whether other indices of androgen-receptor quality or detection of post- or parareceptor defects will incriminate focal expression of androgen resistance as a cause of isolated gynecomastia (macromastia) in some men.

**Risk of Recurrence for Patient's Sib:** For androgen-receptor defects, if the mother is an obligate heterozygote, 50% for each XY sib and 25% for all sibs.

**Risk of Recurrence for Patient's Child:** Recurrence is possible since oligoazoospermia is not obligatory. For androgen-receptor defects, 0% for an XY child and 50% that an XX child will be a carrier.

**Age of Detectability:** In the absence of micropenis and minimal scrotal bifidity, the phenotype is not expressed until puberty.

**Gene Mapping and Linkage:** AR (androgen receptor (dihydrotestosterone receptor; testicular feminization)) has been mapped to Xq12.

**Prevention:** None known. Genetic counseling indicated.

**Treatment:** For those with congenital micropenis, a course of intramuscular testosterone ester therapy may be tried in early infancy, if adequate precautions are taken to avoid the toxic effects of androgen excess on parts of the body that are normally androgen sensitive. If the penile growth response is inadequate, some advocate a female sex-of-rearing despite the attendant need for multistaged reconstructive surgery. Reduction mammoplasty is indicated for adult males with appreciable macromastia. For men with generalized or incoordinate undervirilization, intramuscular androgen may be efficacious objectively or subjectively, but the cost may be reduced spermatogenesis in those with normal androgen sensitivity of the hypothalamic-pituitary axis.

A report of improved spermatogenesis after treatment with the antiestrogen tamoxifen in a man with **Androgen insensitivity syndrome, incomplete** (Gooren, 1989) suggests that the same treatment should be tried in infertile men with the present condition.

**Prognosis:** Good.

**Detection of Carrier:** If a qualitative androgen-receptor defect has been identified in an affected XY relative, cellular (clonal) mosaicism of the mutant phenotype may be demonstrable in genital skin fibroblasts of a possible carrier. Direct or indirect detection of the heterozygous state by recombinant DNA techniques will very likely be possible soon.

**Special Considerations:** Unlike individuals with **Androgen insensitivity syndrome, complete** or **Androgen insensitivity syndrome, incomplete**, who often have high plasma levels of testosterone (T) or luteinizing hormone (LH), those with androgen insensitivity, minimal, often have normal levels of T and LH. This indicates normal androgen sensitivity of their hypopituitary-pituitary axes. The T x LH product has been proposed as a clinical endocrine screening test for androgen insensitivity, minimal, but it has low sensitivity, and its positive predictive value has not been assessed. To maximize the chance of finding elevated plasma T or LH, multiple determinations should be done during one day, taking into account physiologic fluctuation or pulsation in the secretory rates of these hormones.

**References:**
Larrea F, et al.: Gynecomastia as a familial incomplete male pseudohermaphroditism type I: a limited androgen resistance syndrome. J Clin Endocrinol Metab 1978; 46:961–970.
Aiman J, Griffin JE: The frequency of androgen receptor deficiency in infertile men. J Clin Endocrinol Metab 1982; 54:725–732. *
Schulster A, et al.: Frequency of androgen insensitivity in infertile phenotypically normal men. J Urol 1983; 130:699–701.
Migeon CJ, et al.: A clinical syndrome of mild androgen insensitivity. J Clin Endocrinol Metab 1984; 59:672–678. * †
Pinsky L, et al.: Human minimal androgen insensitivity with normal dihydrotestosterone-binding capacity in cultured genital skin fibroblasts: evidence for an androgen-selective qualitative abnormality of the receptor. Am J Hum Genet 1984; 36:965–978. * †
Smallridge RC, et al.: Androgen receptor abnormalities in identical twins with oligospermia. Am J Med 1984; 77:1049–1054.
Cundy TF, et al.: Mild androgen insensitivity presenting with sexual dysfunction. Fertil Steril 1986; 46:721–723.
Morrow AF, et al.: Variable androgen receptor levels in infertile men. J Clin Endocrinol Metab 1987; 64:1115–1121.
Grino PB, et al.: A mutation of the androgen receptor associated with partial androgen resistance, familial gynecomastia, and fertility. J Clin Endocrinol Metab 1988; 66:754–761.
Pinsky L, et al.: Impaired spermatogenesis is not an obligate expression of receptor-defective androgen resistance. Am J Med Genet 1989; 32:100–104. * †
Brown CJ, et al.: Androgen receptor locus on the X chromosome: regional localization to Xq11–12 and description of a DNA polymorphism. Am J Hum Genet 1989; 44:264–269.
Gooren L: Improvement of spermatogenesis after treatment with the antiestrogen tamoxifen in a man with incomplete androgen insensitivity syndrome. J Clin Endocrinol Metab 1989; 68:1207–1210.

**Leonard Pinsky**

**Includes:**
>   Androgen resistance syndrome, complete
>   Dihydrotestosterone receptor deficiency
>   Feminizing testes syndrome, complete
>   Testicular feminization, complete

**Excludes:**
>   **Androgen insensitivity syndrome, incomplete** (0050)
>   Enzymatic defects in testosterone biosynthesis
>   **Gonadal dysgenesis, XX type** (0436)
>   **Gonadal dysgenesis, XY type** (0437)
>   **Leydig cell hypoplasia** (2298)

**Major Diagnostic Criteria:** 46,XY karyotype; female external genitalia, including separate urinary and vaginal orifices; bilateral testes; absent or rudimentary Müllerian and Wolffian duct derivatives; normal or elevated levels of plasma luteinizing hormone (LH) deficient or defective androgen-receptor activity in cultured genital skin fibroblasts.

**Clinical Findings:** The phenotype is age-dependent. During infancy, the only reason for suspecting the diagnosis is surgical exploration of a female with inguinal hernia(e) that reveals gonads whose identity as testes is confirmed histologically. At this age, diagnostic confirmation can be provided by imaging techniques that reveal an absent or rudimentary uterus (a müllerian duct derivative). It can also be provided by measurements of plasma testosterone and LH that reveal normal or elevated levels basally or normal increments of their levels in response to stimulation·by human chorionic gonadotropin (hCG) or by gonadotropin-releasing hormone (Gn-RH), respectively. If the testes are intra-abdominal, the diagnosis is not suspected until the onset of puberty, when the pattern of feminization appears to be disordered: Breast

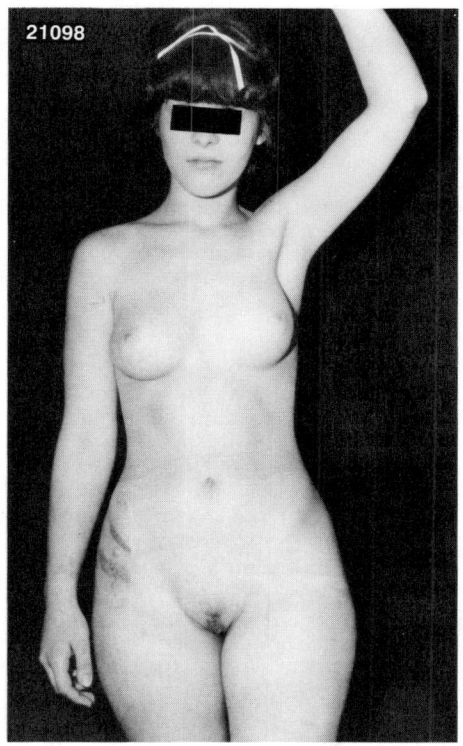

**0049-21098:** A young adult (46,XY) with complete androgen resistance. Note the absent axillary hair, very sparse pubic hair, and female habitus.

development and female fat deposition occur before pubarche. After puberty is established, the full extent of the abnormal phenotype becomes obvious: There are no menses, and pubic and axillary hair remain absent or scanty.

**Complications:** There are two major complications: emotional problems, stemming from primary amenorrhea and sterility, and the possibility of gonadal neoplasia, which is probably attributable to the basic risk of neoplasia in any ectopic (cryptorchid) testis.

**Associated Findings:** Possibly secondary 17-ketosteroid reductase and (peripheral) 5α-reductase deficiency.

**Etiology:** Pedigree analysis indicates maternal transmission to XY offspring and is compatible with X-linked recessive or male-limited autosomal dominant inheritance. The androgen receptor locus is X-linked in man and mouse, and a homologous disorder occurs in the latter species. In individuals with deficient or defective androgen-receptor activity in their genital skin fibroblasts, a mutation at the androgen receptor locus is very likely. In those patients who meet the clinical and endocrine criteria for complete androgen resistance, yet do not appear to have abnormal androgen receptor activity by current tests, androgen resistance may be due to faulty post- or parareceptor factors, still unidentified, that are encoded by loci still unknown, whether X-linked or autosomal.

**Pathogenesis:** Normal morphogenesis of the internal and external male genitalia is androgen-dependent. Hence, complete androgen resistance will preclude differentiation of the vasa deferentia, seminal vesicles, and epididymes from the bilateral wolffian ducts; of the prostate from a portion of the urogenital sinus; and of the penis and scrotum from the bipotential neutral external genital primordia. In the absence of normal androgen sensitivity, the external genital primordia develop in a normal female way autonomously. Regression of the müllerian ducts, hence prevention of their differentiation into the oviducts, uterus, cervix, and upper vagina, is dependent on secretion of a glycoprotein hormone from the Sertoli cells of the ipsilateral testis that acts in a paracrine fashion. This process is intact in affected individuals. At puberty, resetting of the hypothalamic-pituitary gonadostat is expressed by increased levels of LH (and possibly other pituitary hormones) that result in increased secretion of testicular and adrenal androgens. Indeed, resistance of the hypothalamic-pituitary axis to the normal feedback effect of circulating androgens may result in levels of LH and testosterone that are higher than normal for age-matched males. In either event, complete androgen resistance prevents the changes of pubertal virilization that are seen in normal males. Furthermore, estrogen normally secreted by the testes of affected individuals, and that produced by peripheral aromatization of circulating androgen, conspire to yield a feminizing puberty that, if anything, is accentuated in the absence of any androgenic opposition.

**MIM No.:** *31370

**CDC No.:** 257.800

**Sex Ratio:** M1:F0

**Occurrence:** Relatively rare; 1:50,000 live born males or less. Negative family histories are common, in keeping with the sterility (genetic lethality) of affected males.

**Risk of Recurrence for Patient's Sib:**

See Part I, *Mendelian Inheritance.* If mother is proven or obligate carrier and the gene mutation is known to be X-linked, 1:2 for 46,XY sib and 1:4 for all sibs.

**Risk of Recurrence for Patient's Child:** Affected individuals do not reproduce.

**Age of Detectability:** In the absence of a positive family history: in infancy, if an inguinal hernia(e) and testes are discovered; otherwise, at asymmetric puberty. In the presence of a positive family history: in utero by recombinant DNA techniques; after birth, by karyotyping and follow-up of XY females.

**Gene Mapping and Linkage:** AR (androgen receptor (dihydrotestosterone receptor; testicular feminization)) has been mapped to Xq12.

**Prevention:** None known. Genetic counseling indicated.

**Treatment:** Herniorraphy for inguinal hernia. Vaginal dilation, or surgical vaginoplasty if necessary, when vaginal length is too short for painless coitus. Gonadectomy, before or immediately after completion of puberty, to avoid gonadal neoplasia; if before, exogenous estrogen is necessary to cause development of female secondary sexual characteristics; if after, estrogen replacement is indicated to avoid menopausal complaints. Supportive counseling should be available for the emotional costs of amenorrhea, sterility, and perhaps vaginal surgery.

**Prognosis:** The subject is reared as a female and develops female sexual identity and orientation. Libido is grossly normal and normal sexual activity is possible if vaginal length is adequate. Life span is normal in those with no systemic consequences of gonadal malignancy.

**Detection of Carrier:** XX female carriers may exhibit delayed menarche or delayed, sparse, asymmetric pubic/axillary hair, presumably due to random X-chromosome inactivation of the androgen receptor locus. Clonal mosaicism of their genital skin fibroblasts is demonstrable if a decisive marker of the responsible mutation is available. For some families indirect detection of the carrier state is imminent by linkage of one or more informative RFLPs that are linked closely to the androgen receptor locus on the X chromosome. In other families direct detection of the carrier state will likely be possible when direct probes for the androgen receptor locus are available. When a marker of deficient or apparently defective androgen receptor activity is not available, despite a pattern of inheritance that is compatible with X linkage, a search for such linkage may be rewarding.

**Special Considerations:** *Differential diagnosis*: Some affected persons have rudimentary epididymes and vasa deferentia, implying that wolffian duct differentiation is partly androgen-independent. Likewise, some persons have a rudimentary uterus, suggesting that Müllerian duct regression is not entirely androgen-independent. Rudimentary Wolffian duct derivatives are also found in XY individuals who develop female external genitalia due to Leydig cell agenesis or severe degrees of deficiency for several enzymatic steps in testosterone biosynthesis. Among the latter are several that also interfere with adrenocorticosteroid synthesis. The differential diagnosis among these disorders is made easily on clinical, genetic, endocrine, and, if necessary, histopathologic grounds. A rudimentary uterus is also found in apparently nonmosaic XY females who have pure gonadal dysgenesis or mixed gonadal dysgenesis. Again, the differential diagnosis among the latter disorders is easily made on the grounds given above.

*Hormone profiles*: In theory, all persons with complete androgen resistance should have elevated plasma levels of testosterone and LH. However, measurements of testosterone on random single specimens are often normal, and those of LH may be normal as well. Three plasma samples, taken 0.5 hour apart and pooled, will often yield an elevated LH level and may do so for testosterone as well. In fact, the plasma level of δ⁴-androstenedione is more likely to be elevated than is that of testosterone, suggesting that there may be some degree of secondary 17-ketosteroid reductase deficiency among persons with complete androgen resistance. Such a secondary enzyme deficiency has been reported in the rat model of androgen resistance. In addition, those with complete androgen resistance may have secondary 5α-reductase deficiency, presumably a reflection of the fact that peripheral (vs. hepatic) steroid 5α-reductase is androgen-inducible by a receptor-dependent mechanism.

*Use of cultured skin fibroblasts*: Genital skin fibroblasts have more androgen receptor activity than do nongenital skin fibroblasts; pubic skin fibroblasts have intermediate levels. Therefore, labium majus skin fibroblasts are the preferred vehicle for assessing the androgen receptor system in suspects for complete androgen resistance. The 5α-reductase activity of pubic skin fibroblasts has been reported to be androgen-inducible. Hence, when a direct marker of deficient or defective androgen receptor activity is lacking, they may be useful for documenting receptor-dependent androgen resistance in vitro.

*Possible causes of androgen resistance*: The concentration of androgen receptor activity in labium majus skin fibroblasts of persons with complete androgen resistance may be essentially absent, deficient, or normal. If deficient, it is most likely also to be qualitatively defective to account for the clinical phenotype. If normal in concentration, the clinical phenotype may be purely due to a qualitative receptor defect. However, when a qualitative receptor defect cannot be found, the androgen resistance may result from a defect in a para- or postreceptor factor that is essential for normal integrity of the androgen-response system within an androgen target cell, tissue, or organ.

**References:**

Meyer WJ III, et al.: Locus on human X chromosome for dihydrotestosterone receptor and androgen insensitivity. Proc Natl Acad Sci USA 1975; 72:1469–1472.

Boyar RM, et al.: Studies of gonadotropin-gonadal dynamics in patients with androgen insensitivity. J Clin Endocrinol Metab 1978; 47:1116–1122.

Schwartz M, et al.: Male pseudohermaphroditism secondary to an abnormality in Leydig cell differentiation. J Clin Endocrinol Metab 1981; 52:123–127.

Imperato-McGinley J, et al.: Hormonal evaluation of a large kindred with complete androgen insensitivity: evidence for secondary 5α-reductase deficiency. J Clin Endocrinol Metab 1982; 54:931–941.

Saenger P: Abnormal sex differentiation. J Pediatr 1984; 100:1–17. *

Ulloa-Aguirre A, et al.: The presence of müllerian remnants in the complete androgen insensitivity syndrome: a steroid-mediated effect? Fertil Steril 1986; 45:302–305.

Pinsky L, Kaufman M: The genetics of steroid receptors and their disorders. Adv Hum Genet 1987; 16:299–472. *

Wieacker P, et al.: Linkage analysis with RFLPs in families with androgen resistance syndromes: evidence for close linkage between the androgen receptor locus and the DXS1 segment. Hum Genet 1987; 76:248–252.

PI005                                            **Leonard Pinsky**

---

**ANDROGEN INSENSITIVITY SYNDROME, INCOMPLETE    0050**

**Includes:**

Androgen receptor deficiency
Dihydrotestosterone receptor deficiency
Feminizing male pseudohermpahroditism (Jones)
Gilbert-Dreyfus syndrome
Incomplete feminizing testes syndrome
Incomplete male pseudohermaphroditism, type 1 (Wilson & Goldstein)
Incomplete testicular feminization syndrome
Lubs syndrome
Pseudohermaphroditism, incomplete male, type I
Reifenstein syndrome
Rosewater syndrome
Testicular feminization, incomplete type

**Excludes:**

**Androgen insensitivity (resistance), minimal** (2954)
**Androgen insensitivity syndrome, complete** (0049)
**Chromosome mosaicism, 45x/46,xy type** (0173)
**Mullerian derivatives in males, persistent** (0683)
**Steroid 3 beta-hydroxysteroid dehydrogenase deficiency** (0909)
**Steroid 5 alpha-reductase deficiency** (3062)
**Steroid 17-ketosteroid reductase deficiency** (2299)
**Steroid 17 alpha-hydroxylase deficiency** (0903)
**Steroid 17,20-desmolase deficiency** (0904)
**Steroid 20–22 desmolase deficiency** (0907)

**Major Diagnostic Criteria:** Male pseudohermaphroditism in which the phenotype includes intersex external genitalia (clitoromegaly with varying degrees of labioscrotal fusion), normal sized intraabdominal or inguinal testes, a 46,XY karyotype (rarely 47,XXY or 47,XYY), absent or hypoplastic wolffian duct derivatives, absent müllerian duct derivatives, and breast development with variably defective virilization at puberty. Plasma testosterone is normal, and no error in androgen biosynthesis is demonstrable. The administration of androgens in doses that ordinarily produce normal adult plasma testosterone levels fails to induce virilization

**0050-21100:** The ambiguous external genitalia of a 12-year-old boy with partial androgen resistance. During his 13th year, the conjunction of spontaneous puberty with pharmacologic doses of intramuscular testosterone generated sufficient phallic and scrotal growth to facilitate satisfactory surgical design of male external genitalia. Ideally, however, the sex-of-rearing should be chosen and appropriate surgical reconstruction performed in early life.

---

or nitrogen retention. An attempt should be made in every suspected case to demonstrate a defect in androgen receptor protein in cultured genital skin fibroblasts. The demonstration of a defect in androgen receptor protein in cultured genital fibroblasts from an affected patient strongly supports the diagnosis.

Androgen hyposensitivity should be demonstrated either clinically, by showing deficient nitrogen retention following androgen administration, or biochemically by demonstration of a defect in androgen receptor protein activity. Individuals who on the basis of the external appearance could be said to have the incomplete androgen insensitivity syndrome may actually represent a heterogeneous sample.

**Clinical Findings:** Certain 46,XY individuals with testes who feminize at puberty have been shown to have partial or incomplete androgen insensitivity (androgen hyposensitivity). Such patients have intersex external genitalia characterized by phallic enlargement (clitoromegaly) and partial labioscrotal fusion. Somatic anomalies are absent. This incomplete androgen insensitivity syndrome shares the following features with the complete androgen insensitivity syndrome: bilateral testes with similar histologic features, absence of müllerian duct derivatives, absence or hypoplasia of wolffian duct derivatives, pubertal breast development, defective pubertal virilization, normal male plasma testosterone levels, normal response to HCG and ACTH, and failure to show an anabolic response (eg nitrogen retention) following testosterone administration in usual doses. Testes are usually cryptorchid (intraabdominal) or in inguinal canals; pubic hair is present. The incomplete and complete androgen insensitivity syndromes differ only in that in the incomplete androgen insensitivity syndrome, the external genitalia show partial labioscrotal fusion and clitoromegaly. Some individuals with the incomplete androgen insensitivity syndrome have wolffian duct derivatives, namely epididymides and vasa deferentia; however, such derivatives are not consistently present. No evidence of enzymatic deficiency in testosterone biosynthesis or conversion of testosterone to dihydrotestosterone is present in these individuals, although they may show an abnormality of the target-cell receptor protein for androgens (androgen cytosol receptor protein).

**Complications:** Neoplastic transformation of cryptorchid or inguinal testes; infertility.

**Associated Findings:** None known.

**Etiology:** X-linked recessive inheritance.

**Pathogenesis:** Target cell hyporesponsiveness to testosterone and dihydrotestosterone. In all or virtually all cases of **Androgen insensitivity syndrome, complete**, a defect in the receptor protein that binds testosterone and dihydrotestosterone to target cells and transports these androgens to the nuclei has been demonstrated. Available data further suggest that similar but less severe defects are responsible for at least some cases of the incomplete androgen insensitivity syndrome. Whether this mechanism explains all such cases remains to be determined.

**MIM No.:** 31210, 31230, *31370

**Sex Ratio:** M1:F0

**Occurrence:** Rare. Many affected kindreds have been reported, but in most, defects in testosterone biosynthesis or its conversion to dihydrotestosterone were not excluded.

**Risk of Recurrence for Patient's Sib:** 1:2 (50%) for each 46,XY sib to be affected; 1:4 (25%) for all sibs, assuming the mother is heterozygous for the responsible mutant allele.

**Risk of Recurrence for Patient's Child:** Affected individuals are infertile.

**Age of Detectability:** Usually at birth because of genital ambiguity, but occasionally not until puberty because of primary amenorrhea.

Prenatal diagnosis may be possible on the basis of the demonstration of an androgen cytosol binding protein defect in cultured amniotic cells.

**Gene Mapping and Linkage:** AR (androgen receptor (dihydrotestosterone receptor; testicular feminization)) has been mapped to Xq12.

**Prevention:** None known. Genetic counseling indicated.

**Treatment:** Assignment of a female sex of rearing with orchiectomy and surgical construction of female external genitalia. Construction of an artificial vagina may be necessary, but this is preferably performed in the second decade of life. Estrogen substitution therapy should be initiated in the second decade of life and continued until the usual age of menopause.

**Prognosis:** Presumably normal lifespan, provided neoplastic transformation of testes does not occur.

**Detection of Carrier:** The locus for the human androgen receptor gene has been sequenced, potentially allowing heterozygote detection by RFLP analysis. Receptor protein deficiency had earlier been reported in a proportion of cloned fibroblasts from an obligate heterozygous female.

**Special Considerations:** Individuals said to have the Reifenstein syndrome differ in no important way from patients with the incomplete androgen insensitivity syndrome. As appropriate studies are performed on more patients heretofore said to have the Reifenstein syndrome, hyposensitivity to androgen will probably be demonstrated. The same is probable for the so-called Lubs syndrome and the so-called syndrome of Gilbert-Dreyfus. Prior to puberty individuals with **Steroid 5 alpha-reductase deficiency** may be clinically indistinguishable from those with incomplete androgen insensitivity. Finally, to prevent nosologic confusion, it should be mentioned that Wilson et al (1974) reported a family in which there appeared to be segregating a variably expressed X-linked recessive or male-limited autosomal dominant gene capable of producing phenotypes consistent with either the incomplete androgen insensitivity syndrome or the Reifenstein syndrome; those authors concluded that both conditions resulted from a single mutant gene, and designated the condition, "incomplete male pseudohermaphroditism, type 1." Affected individuals in the kindred reported by Wilson et al have the incomplete androgen insensitivity syndrome, and in 3 members of that family

a defect has been demonstrated in the binding of dihydrotestosterone to cultured genital skin fibroblasts. The family reported by Wilson et al demonstrates the clinical variablity possible in a single kindred in which the incomplete androgen insensitivity syndrome is segregating.

**References:**

Wilson JD, et al.: Familial incomplete male pseudohermaphroditism, type 1. New Engl J Med 1974; 290:1097–1103. * †
Griffin JE, et al.: Dihydrotestosterone binding to cultured human fibroblasts: comparison of cells from control subjects and from patients with hereditary male pseudohermaphroditism due to androgen resistance. J Clin Invest 1976; 57:1342–1351.
Simpson JL: Male pseudohermaphroditism: genetics and clinical delineation. Hum Genet 1978; 44:1
Griffin JE, Wilson JD: The syndromes of androgen resistance. New Engl J Med 1980; 302:198–209.
Pinsky L, et al.: Congenital androgen insensitivity due to a qualitatively abnormal androgen receptor. Am J Med Genet 1981; 10:91–99.
Summitt RL: Abnormalities of sex differentiation. In: Givens JR, Anderson GD eds: Endocrinology of pregnancy. Chicago: Year Book Publishers. 1981:279.
Pinsky L, et al.: Reduced affinity of the androgen receptor for 5α-dihydrotestosterone but not methyltrienolone in a form of partial androgen resistance. J Clin Invest 1985; 75:1291–1296.
Pinsky L, et al.: Partial androgren resistance due to a distinctive qualitative defect of the androgen receptor. Am J Med Genet 1987; 27:459–466. *
Gooren L: Improvement of spermatogenesis after treatment with the antiestrogen tamoxifen in a man with the incomplete androgen insensitivity syndrome. J Clin Endocrinol Metab 1989; 68:1207–1210.

SU008           **Robert L. Summitt**
SI018           **Joe Leigh Simpson**

**Androgen insensitivity syndrome, incomplete (some)**
    *See GERM CELL APLASIA*
**Androgen receptor deficiency**
    *See ANDROGEN INSENSITIVITY SYNDROME, INCOMPLETE*
**Androgen resistance syndrome, complete**
    *See ANDROGEN INSENSITIVITY SYNDROME, COMPLETE*
**Androgen, fetal effects**
    *See FETAL EFFECTS FROM MATERNAL EXTRINSIC ANDROGENS*
**Androgen-genetic regional alopecia**
    *See HAIR, BALDNESS, COMMON*
**Androgenetic alopecia**
    *See HAIR, BALDNESS, COMMON*
**Androgenic substance, maternal exposure and fetal virilization**
    *See FETAL EFFECTS FROM MATERNAL EXTRINSIC ANDROGENS*
**Anectine apnea**
    *See CHOLINESTERASE, ATYPICAL*
**Anemia falciforme**
    *See ANEMIA, SICKLE CELL*
**Anemia with multinucleated erythroblasts**
    *See ANEMIA, DYSERYTHROPOIETIC, TYPE III*

## ANEMIA, ADENYLATE KINASE DEFICIENCY       2660

**Includes:**

Adenylate kinase (AK) deficiency
Adenylate kinase, soluble
Deficiency of ATP:AMP phosphotransferase (E.C.2.7.4.3)

**Excludes:** Adenosine kinase deficiency

**Major Diagnostic Criteria:** Decreased activity of adenylate kinase in the erythrocytes.

**Clinical Findings:** Adenylate kinase (AK) catalyzes the equilibrium between ATP, ADP, and AMP in the following reaction:

ATP + AMP AK/<--> 2 ADP

The first case of erythrocyte AK deficiency was discovered by Szeinberg et al (1969) in an Arab youngster in Israel during a population survey. The male child was known to have hemolytic anemia (Hb, 6.5–7.1 g/dl; reticulocytes, 8.4–12%) from birth. He also had glucose-6-phosphate dehydrogenase (G6PD) deficiency and was transfusion dependent. An older male sib who was known to have hemolytic anemia and G6Pd deficiency died at age

7 years. A female sib had AK deficiency, normal G6PD activity, and only mild anemia (Hb, 8.5–9.0 g/dl; reticulocytes, 2.0–3.2%). Three other families have been described since then, with a total of four affected individuals. The clinical findings in these families are varied and raise doubts as to whether the apparently associated hemolytic anemia in AK-deficient individuals is indeed due to AK deficiency. Boivin et al (1971) reported the case of a 14-year-old French boy who had hemolytic anemia since age 3 years, thrombocytopenia of 31,000/mm³, splenomegaly, and mental retardation. The erythrocyte AK activity was between one and 13% of normal. The relationship of thrombocytopenia and AK deficiency to mental retardation was not clear. Miwa et al (1983) described a 10-year-old Japanese girl with erythrocyte AK activity of 44% who had mild hemolytic anemia (Hb, 9.6 g/dl; reticulocyte count, 7.2%; MCV, $\mu^3$), hepatosplenomegaly, and reduced red cell life span ($^{51}$Cr half-life of 16 days). Most revealing was the report of Beutler et al (1983), who noted severe erythrocyte AK deficiency in two Black children, one of whom had mild hemolytic anemia (Hb, 8.4–9.6 g/dl; reticulocytes, 5.2–10.9%), but the other showed no evidence of hemolysis (Hb, 11.9–12/8 g/dl; reticulocyte count, 0.8–0.9%). In all these cases adenosine triphosphate levels were normal or increased except in the two boys described by Beutler et al who had a slightly decreased level (2,920 $\mu$mol/g Hb compared with a normal of 3,530 ± 300).

**Complications:** Possibly hemolytic anemia, although this is now in doubt.

**Associated Findings:** Of six children with AK deficiency, one had coexistent **Glucose-6-phosphate dehydrogenase deficiency** (G6PD), one had possible mild **Pyruvate kinase deficiency**, and one had thrombocytopenia and mental retardation.

**Etiology:** Autosomal recessive inheritance.

**Pathogenesis:** It was anticipated that AK deficiency leads to hemolysis by depletion of ATP. However, in four of six children described, ATP levels were higher than normal; in the other two patients the ATP levels were only slightly reduced. Moreover, the severity of anemia did not correlate with the residual enzyme activity; in one patient there was no evidence of hemolytic anemia, and in one patient coexistent G6PD deficiency may be contributing to the hemolytic anemia. Paglia and Valentine (1981) hypothesized that AK deficiency may lead to gradual depletion of ATP as the red cells become older, but in the one patient in whom this was studied (Miwa et al, 1983) there was no difference in the ATP levels in density-separated reticulocyte-rich and reticulocyte-poor red cell fractions. Beutler et al (1983) recently showed that despite the small amount of residual AK activity (1/2,000 of normal), the red cells had the capacity to generate AMP, ADP, and ATP. Beutler et al concluded that AK deficiency is another example of an erythrocyte enzyme defect without clinical consequences. The associated hemolytic anemia may be due to an unrelated enzyme defect (G6PD deficiency, as in one patient) or to the interaction of another unidentified defect with AK deficiency.

**MIM No.:** *10300, *10302, *10303

**Sex Ratio:** M1:F1 for any expression of the gene; observed, M4:F2

**Occurrence:** Only four families have been described to date, with a total of six affected individuals. Families included Arab, black, and Japanese ancestories.

**Risk of Recurrence for Patient's Sib:**
See Part I, *Mendelian Inheritance.*

**Risk of Recurrence for Patient's Child:**
See Part I, *Mendelian Inheritance.*

**Age of Detectability:** At birth.

**Gene Mapping and Linkage:** AK1 (adenylate kinase 1) has been mapped to 9q34.1-q34.2.
AK2 (adenylate kinase 2) has been mapped to 1p34.
AK3 (adenylate kinase 3) has been mapped to 9p24-p13.
Only AK₁ has been identified in erythrocytes.

**Prevention:** None known. Genetic counseling indicated.

**Treatment:** AK deficiency does not appear to be associated with any clinical consequences.

Other coexistant potential causes of hemolytic anemia should be thoroughly investigated and appropriate therapy instituted.

**Prognosis:** Depends on the severity of associated hemolytic anemia.

**Detection of Carrier:** Measurement of AK activity.

**References:**
Szeinberg A, et al.: Hereditary deficiency of adenylate kinase in red blood cells. Acta Haematol 1969; 42:111–126.
Boivin P, et al.: Une nouvelle erythroenzymopathie: anemie hemolytique congenitale non spherocytaire et deficit hereditaire en adenylate-kinase erythrocytaire. Presse Med 1971; 79:215–218.
Paglia DE, Valentine WN: Haemolytic anaemia associated with disorders of the purine and pyrimidine salvage pathways. Clin Haematol 1981; 10:81–98. *
Beutler E, et al.: Metabolic compensation for profound erythrocyte adenylate kinase deficiency. A hereditary enzyme defect without hemolytic anemia. J Clin Invest 1983; 72:648–655. *
Miwa S, et al.: Red cell adenylate kinase deficiency associated with hereditary nonspherocytic hemolytic anemia: clinical and biochemical studies. Am J Hematol 1983; 14:325–333.

RA022                                    **Yaddanapadi Ravindranath**

## ANEMIA, CONGENITAL SIDEROBLASTIC, NOT B(6) RESPONSIVE                    2659

**Includes:**
  Hypochromic anemia, congenital
  Sideroblastic anemia, congenital hereditary
  Sideroblastic anemia, hereditary X-linked
  Sideroblastic hypochromic aplastic anemia, congenital

**Excludes:**
  Anemia, sideroblastic, acquired
  **Anemia, dyserythropoietic, type II** (2652)
  **Anemia, dyserythropoietic** (other)

**Major Diagnostic Criteria:** Microcytic anemia or dimorphic population of red cells, bone marrow erythroid hyperplasia with numerous (greater than 10%) ringed sideroblasts, diminished reticulocytes, increased iron stores, no evidence for hemolysis, no evidence for abnormal myelopoiesis or megakaryopoiesis.

**Clinical Findings:** Clinical signs may become manifest any time during the first three or four decades of life. Pallor, fatigue, and dyspnea may be present if anemia is significant. There are case reports of delayed physical and sexual maturation. Hepatomegaly and splenomegaly are common. The degree of anemia is variable, ranging from severe to mild, with an average hemoglobin of 7.0 g/dl. Anisocytosis, poikilocytosis, target cells, and basophilic stippling are seen on the blood smears. Transferrin saturation and iron stores are increased. Jaundice is unusual.

Free erythrocyte protoporphyrin levels are low or low normal. Free erythrocyte coproporphyrin levels are normal or elevated. Occasional patients (under 20%) have improved anemia during pyridoxine treatment, although the marrow and erythroid morphologic abnormalities persist despite therapeutic improvement.

**Complications:** Excessive iron loading, especially in multiply transfused patients, can result in hemochromatosis with cardiac dysrhythmias, liver damage, skin hyperpigmentation, and diabetes.

**Associated Findings:** None known.

**Etiology:** X-linked recessive inheritance. Most female carriers are not anemic, but have evidence of abnormal red cell morphology and can have elevated iron stores. There are a number of case reports of female children in whom autosomal recessive inheritance seems likely.

**Pathogenesis:** When studied, most cases have shown defective heme synthesis. There is decreased formation of delta-aminolevulinic acid (ALA) by the pyridoxine cofactor-requiring enzyme ALA synthase, which is located in mitochondria. Several different mechanisms of decreased ALA synthase activity have been proposed, including decreased affinity for pyridoxine cofactor and increased sensitivity to inactivation of the apoenzyme by a mitochondrial protease. More than one mechanism is likely to play a role in different patients.

**MIM No.:**  20595

**Sex Ratio:**  M>15:F1.

**Occurrence:**  About 200 cases have been documented. Reports originate from all races and different locations around the world.

**Risk of Recurrence for Patient's Sib:**
See Part I, *Mendelian Inheritance.*

**Risk of Recurrence for Patient's Child:**
See Part I, *Mendelian Inheritance.*

**Age of Detectability:**  Usually present before age 30 years and may be seen before age one year.

**Gene Mapping and Linkage:**  Unknown.

**Prevention:**  None known. Genetic counseling indicated.

**Treatment:**  A trial of pyridoxine is likely to be beneficial in less than 20% of cases. Red cell transfusions are restricted to symptomatic patients. Iron therapy is contraindicated. Long-term iron chelation therapy may play a role in preventing hemochromatosis.

**Prognosis:**  Most patients have normal or near-normal life spans and do not develop hematologic malignancies. The development of hemochromatosis will decrease life span.

**Detection of Carrier:**  Examination of relatives for abnormal red cell morphology, anemia, and free erythrocyte protoporphyrin.

**Special Considerations:**  In the past, congenital sideroblastic anemia was classified into two groups: pyridoxine responsive and pyridoxine nonresponsive. This classification is artificial and probably does not separate two distinct pathologic or clinical entities.

**References:**
Seip M, et al.: Congenital sideroblastic anemia in a girl. Scand J Haematol 1971; 8:505–512.
Mollin DL, MacGibbon BH: Sideroblastic and megaloblastic anemias. Br J Haematol (suppl) 1972; 23:147–158.
White JM, Ali MAM: Globin synthesis in sideroblastic anemia. Br J Haematol 1973; 24:481–484.
Konopka L, Hoffbrand AV; Haem synthesis in sideroblastic anemia. Br J Haematol 1979; 42:73–83.
Manabe Y, et al.: A study of a female with congenital sideroblastic anemia. Am J Hematol 1982; 12:63–67.

AK000                                                    **Luke Akard**
H0052                                                  **Ronald Hoffman**

---

## ANEMIA, DYSERYTHROPOIETIC, TYPE I                              2651

**Includes:**
CDA (congenital dyserythropoietic anemia) I
Dyserythropoietic anemia, type I

**Excludes:**
**Anemia, congenital sideroblastic, not B(6) responsive** (2659)
Anemia, dyserythropoietic (other)

**Major Diagnostic Criteria:**  Moderate macrocytic anemia with inappropriately low reticulocyte count. The bone marrow demonstrates ineffective erythropoiesis with marked erythroid hyperplasia, megaloblastoid erythroblasts, some of which have binuclearity or internuclear chromatin bridging that connects two cells, and no evidence of red cell membrane abnormalities or red cell enzymopathies causing hemolysis or ineffective erythropoiesis.

**Clinical Findings:**  Usually manifests in the first two decades of life with pallor, weakness, and fatigue. Low birth weights are reported. Typically patients present with hyperbilirubinemia, macrocytic anemia, and splenomegaly. Hepatomegaly occurs less often. Some patients develop evidence of iron overload as adults, with skin, endocrine, and liver abnormalities.

Laboratory evaluation shows macrocytosis and anisopoikilocytosis of red cells, the reticulocyte count is normal or minimally elevated, and the bone marrow evaluation demonstrates that most

erythroblasts have abnormal morphology with the characteristics listed above. Ferrokinetic studies demonstrate ineffective erythropoiesis with increased red cell iron turnover. There is increased bone marrow iron, and the ferritin level is elevated.

**Complications:**  Iron overload with evidence of hemochromatosis (in approximately 20% of described cases).

**Associated Findings:**  Two case reports of skeletal anomalies (brachydactyly of digits). Short stature in two case reports. Four cases of membranous **Syndactyly.**

**Etiology:**  Autosomal recessive inheritance.

**Pathogenesis:**  Altered deoxynucleoprotein metabolism in erythroblasts has been suggested to result in early intramedullary death of these cells in some studies. Whether altered DNA synthesis impairs hemoglobin formation, red cell membrane function, or some other functional structure in red cells is unknown.

**MIM No.:**  *22412

**Sex Ratio:**  M1:F1

**Occurrence:**  About 40 cases have been documented from all races.

**Risk of Recurrence for Patient's Sib:**
See Part I, *Mendelian Inheritance.*

**Risk of Recurrence for Patient's Child:**
See Part I, *Mendelian Inheritance.*

**Age of Detectability:**  Usually identified after infancy but before adulthood. Many cases are not identified until late adulthood.

**Gene Mapping and Linkage:**  Unknown.

**Prevention:**  None known. Genetic counseling indicated.

**Treatment:**  Unknown. In some cases splenectomy has decreased transfusion requirements. Anemia is generally mild, and avoidance of transfusions to prevent iron overload is preferred. Iron is contraindicated. Careful attention to iron accumulation is necessary to prevent hemochromatosis. Iron chelation therapy is likely to be beneficial in those patients with iron overload.

**Prognosis:**  Variable. Many patients have normal life spans. Patients with a greater degree of dyserythropoiesis have a greater likelihood of developing iron overload or complications from anemia.

**Detection of Carrier:**  Unknown. Parents have had normal red cell morphology.

**Special Considerations:**  *Congenital dyserythropoietic anemia* (CDA) is the term used to describe a family of hereditary anemias that exhibit chronic hemolysis and ineffective erythropoiesis. The anemias are generally classified into three groups based on red blood cell morphologic and serologic criteria. Some authors recognize a fourth group. CDA I is the second most common of the three groups. CDA II is the most common and is characterized by marrow erythroblastic multinuclearity associated with a positive acidified serum test (HEMPAS). CDA III is the least frequent in reported occurrence and is characterized by numerous erythrocytic gigantoblasts. If a bone marrow examination is not performed, CDA I might be confused with **Hyperbilirubinemia, unconjugated** or one of the thalassemic syndromes.

**References:**
Heimpel H, Wendt F: Congenital dyserythropoietic anemia with karyorrhexis and multinuclearity of erythroblasts. Helv Med Acta 1968; 34:103.
Lewis SM, et al.: Clinical and ultrastructural aspects of congenital dyserythropoietic anemia type I. Br J Haematol 1972; 23:113–119.
Heimpel H: Congenital dyserythropoietic anemia type I. In: Lewis SM, Verwilghen RL, eds: Dyserythropoiesis. London: Academic, 1977:55–70.
Holmberg L, et al.: Type I congenital dyserythropoietic anemia with myelopoietic abnormalities and hand malformations. Scand J Haematol 1978; 21:72–79.
Vainchenker W, et al.: Congenital dyserythropoietic anaemia type I: absence of clonal expression in the nuclear abnormalities of cultured erythroblasts. Br J Haematol 1980; 46:33–37.

Mori PG, et al.: Congenital dyserythropoietic anemia type I: report of a pair of siblings. Acta Haematol 1986; 75:219–223.

AK000
H0052

**Luke Akard
Ronald Hoffman**

## ANEMIA, DYSERYTHROPOIETIC, TYPE II  2652

**Includes:**
CDA (congenital dyserythropoietic anemia) II
Dyserythropoietic anemia, HEMPAS type
Erythroblastic endopolyploidy-multinucleated normoblasts
HEMPAS

**Excludes:**
**Anemia, congenital sideroblastic, not B(6) responsive** (2659)
Anemia, dyserthropoietic (other)

**Major Diagnostic Criteria:** Mild-to-severe anemia characteristic of peripheral hemolysis and ineffective erythropoiesis. The bone marrow late erythroblasts demonstrate two or more nuclei or lobulated nuceli (10–30%), and Gaucher-like cells may be observed due to phagocytosis of erythroblasts by macrophages. Characteristic serologic features include lysis of red cells by certain group-compatible sera at acidic pH (6.8), strong agglutinability by anti-i, and weakly increased lysis by anti-I.

**Clinical Findings:** Patients usually have mild-to-moderate anemia with few anemic symptoms. The diagnosis is often suspected based on finding evidence for red cell destruction, including jaundice (40%), hepatosplenomegaly (35%), and occasionally evidence for iron overload with cirrhosis or hemosiderosis of the liver (under 10%). Laboratory evaluation demonstrates anisopoikilocytosis and occasional hypochromic and microcytic cells on the peripheral smear. The absolute reticulocyte count tends to be normal. The bone marrow is markedly hypercellular with erythrocytic hyperplasia and the findings listed above. Unconjugated bilirubin is increased in almost all patients. Serum lipid and vitamin E levels tend to be decreased. Iron turnover is increased, with decreased iron utilization typical of ineffective erythropoiesis. Red cell survival time is diminished so that increased peripheral red cell destruction plays a part in the development of anemia.

About 30% of group-compatible sera results in a positive acidified serum test (discussed above). Unlike paroxysmal nocturnal hemoglobinuria (PNH), the cells are not lysed by their own acidified serum.

**Complications:** Nearly 10% of reported cases have developed clinical signs of iron overload leading to hemochromatosis. There is an increased likelihood of developing gallstones. Patients treated by splenectomy have had an increased incidence of septicemia.

**Associated Findings:** None known.

**Etiology:** Autosomal recessive inheritance.

**Pathogenesis:** A failure in glycosylation of erythrocyte lactosaminoglycan proteins caused by lowered N-acetylglucosaminyltransferase II. The condition is unique among inborn errors of metabolism in that it is a defect in biosynthesis of a glycoprotein.

It is thought that the major defect is in the red cell membrane. Several groups of researchers have reported abnormal membrane glycoprotein glycosylation or glycosphingolipid composition from erythrocytes. These abnormalities are thought to result in abnormal erythroblast maturation and the development of alloantibodies that cause shortened red cell survival once they are released into the circulation.

**MIM No.:** *22410

**Sex Ratio:** M1:F1

**Occurrence:** Unknown. The most common of the congenital dyserythropoietic anemias. Nearly all reported patients have been Caucasians, with a geographic distribution in Italy, northwest Europe, and North Africa.

**Risk of Recurrence for Patient's Sib:**
See Part I, *Mendelian Inheritance.*

**Risk of Recurrence for Patient's Child:**
See Part I, *Mendelian Inheritance.*

**Age of Detectability:** Most patients are detected in the first two decades of life when anemia and evidence of ineffective erythropoiesis are found. However, many cases are mild and go undiagnosed until adulthood.

**Gene Mapping and Linkage:** Unknown.

**Prevention:** None known. Genetic counseling indicated.

**Treatment:** Unknown. Blood transfusions should be limited to correcting severe anemia. Iron therapy is contraindicated. Splenectomy has improved the anemia in fewer than ten case reports. Careful attention to iron loading must be made to avoid the development of hemochromatosis.

The development of hemochromatosis is the most serious result of CDA II. Iron chelation therapy has been used in a number of patients, as has phlebotomy, with varying degrees of success.

**Prognosis:** Most patients have a near-normal life span unless complications from iron overload or splenectomy develop.

**Detection of Carrier:** Unaffected parents and sibs have had typical serologic findings with red cell lysis by anti-i and anti-I in a few case reports. This is not a consistent finding, however.

**Special Considerations:** HEMPAS has been used as an acronym for Hereditary Erythroblastic Multinuclearity associated with a Positive Acidified Serum test

**References:**
Crookston JH, et al.: Hereditary erythroblastic multinuclearity associated with a positive acidified-serum test: a type of congenital dyserythropoietic anaemia. Br J Haematol 1969; 17:11–26.
Verwilghen RL, et al.: HEMPAS: congenital dyserythropoietic anaemia (type II). Quart J Med 1973; 42:257–278.
Punt K, et al.: Congenital dyserythropoietic anemia type II (HEMPAS). In: Lewis SM, Verwilghen RL, eds: Dyserythropoiesis. London: Academic, 1977:71–81.
Fukuda MN, et al.: Defect in glycosylation of erythrocyte membrane proteins in congenital dyserythropoietic anaemia type II (HEMPAS). Br J Haematol 1984; 56:55–68.
Bouhours JF, et al.: Abnormal fatty acid composition of erythrocyte glycosphingolipids in congenital dyserythropoietic anemia type II. J Lipid Res 1985; 26:435–441.
Ucci G, et al.: Proliferation kinetics of bone marrow cells in congenital dyserythropoietic anemia type II. Blut 1985; 50:219–224.
Fukuda MN, et al.: Primary defect of congenital dyserythropoietic anemia type II: failure in glycosylation of erythrocyte lactosaminoglycan proteins caused by lowered N-acetylglucosaminyltransferase II. J Biol Chem 1987; 262:7195–7206.

AK000
H0052

**Luke Akard
Ronald Hoffman**

## ANEMIA, DYSERYTHROPOIETIC, TYPE III  2650

**Includes:**
Anemia with multinucleated erythroblasts
CDA (congenital dyserythropoietic anemia) III
Dyserythropoietic anemia, type III
Erythroid multinuclearity, familial
Erythroreticulosis, hereditary benign

**Excludes:**
**Anemia, congenital sideroblastic, not B(6) responsive** (2659)
Anemia, dyserythropoietic (other)
**Thalassemia** (0939)
**Vitamin B(12) malabsorption** (0992)

**Major Diagnostic Criteria:** Hereditary refractory anemia with ineffective erythropoiesis and characteristic morphologic abnormalities of marrow erythroblasts.

**Clinical Findings:** The onset of mild-to-moderate anemia generally occurs between infancy and adolescence. Occasionally, there is mild or moderate hepatosplenomegaly, splenomegaly, and mild hyperbilirubinemia. The bone marrow shows erythroid hyperplasia, but there is relative reticulocytopenia. Three distinct types of congenital dyserythropoietic anemia have been defined on the basis of morphologic abnormalities of marrow erythroblasts, serologic characteristics, and mode of genetic transmission.

Bone marrow examination under the light miscroscope shows distinctive "gigantoblasts," which are multi-nucleated erythroblasts containing up to 12 nuclei. The erythroblasts are found to have nuclear clefts and blebs when viewed with the electron microscope. The peripheral red blood cells are macrocytic, with anisocytosis and poikilocytosis. Limited experience suggests that there is increased agglutination with anti-i, and increased lysis with anti-I; the acidified serum test is negative.

**Complications:** Hepatosplenomegaly may be present; hemosiderosis and hepatic cirrhosis are rare complications. Clinically significant hemochromatosis may result from excessive red cell transfusions or unwarranted iron therapy, but more commonly is noniatrogenic in origin; it is probably due to excessive absorption of iron from the gastrointestinal tract. Those who are most severely affected by chronic anemia may suffer its consequences, while patients who receive frequent red cell transfusions are exposed to its attendant risks.

**Associated Findings:** Mental retardation has been reported in one case but this observation lacked specific detail.

**Etiology:** Autosomal dominant inheritance with complete penetrance.

**Pathogenesis:** Unknown.

**MIM No.:** *10560

**Sex Ratio:** M1:F1

**Occurrence:** Less than 30 cases have been reported. Based on the origin of case reports, there appears to be a predominance in northwestern Europe and in India. This is the least common of the three types of dyserythropoietic anemia.

**Risk of Recurrence for Patient's Sib:**
See Part I, *Mendelian Inheritance.*

**Risk of Recurrence for Patient's Child:**
See Part I, *Mendelian Inheritance.*

**Age of Detectability:** Symptomatology may be evident in infancy, and it is likely that at least some characteristic abnormalities should be detectable at that time. However, it is far more common for definitive diagnosis to be made in later childhood, or even adulthood.

**Gene Mapping and Linkage:** Unknown.

**Prevention:** None known. Genetic counseling indicated.

**Treatment:** There is no definitive therapy. Periodic red cell transfusions may be beneficial in cases of severe anemia, but should be minimized to decrease the likelihood of developing hemosiderosis. Splenectomy may help to improve red cell survival and thereby decrease the transfusion requirement. Limited phlebotomy and chelating agents have been tried, but their efficacy has not been critically evaluated. Traditional hematinics are generally not useful.

**Prognosis:** Long-term prognosis appears favorable, except in the minority of cases in which severe complications intervene.

**Detection of Carrier:** Unknown.

**References:**
Wolff JA, Van Hofe FH: Familial erythroid multinuclearity. Blood 1951; 6:1274–1283.
Bergström I, Jacobsson L: Hereditary benign erythroreticulosis. Blood 1962; 19:296–303.
Heimpel H, Wendt F: Congenital dyserythropoietic anemia with karyorrhexis and multinuclearity of erythroblasts. Helv Med Acta 1968; 34:103–115. *
Goudsmit R, et al.: Congenital dyserythropoietic anaemia, type III. Br J Haematol 1972; 23:97–105. †
Björkstén B, et al.: Congenital dyserythropoietic anaemia type III: an electron microscopic study. Br J Haematol 1978; 38:37–42. †
Choudhry VP, et al.: Congenital dyserythropoietic anaemias: splenectomy as a mode of therapy. Acta Haematol 1981; 66:195–201.

SH052

**Bruce I. Sharon**

## ANEMIA, GLUCOSE PHOSPHATE ISOMERASE DEFICIENCY 2750

**Includes:**
D-glucose-6-phosphate ketol isomerase (E.C.5.3.1.9), deficiency of
Glucosephosphate isomerase, deficiency of
Hexosephosphate isomerase, deficiency of
Phosphoglucose isomerase, deficiency of
Phosphohexose isomerase, deficiency of

**Excludes:**
**Anemia** (other)
Enzyme deficiencies (other)

**Major Diagnostic Criteria:** Chronic nonspherocytic hemolytic anemia is present from the neonatal period or from early childhood. Diagnosis is confirmed by demonstration of severely reduced activity of erythrocyte glucose phosphate isomerase (GPI), and exclusion of other causes of hemolytic anemia.

**Clinical Findings:** Glucose phosphate isomerase catalyzes the reversible interconversion of glucose-6-phosphate and fructose-6-phosphate at the second step in the Embden-Meyerhof pathway of anaerobic glycolysis. The deficiency of erythrocyte GPI causes a chronic hemolytic anemia usually manifest in infancy and early childhood. The severity of anemia is variable, with some patients requiring monthly transfusions while in others the hemolytic anemia is well compensated. Hemolysis may be severe enough to cause neonatal jaundice sometimes necessitating exchange transfusions. Hydrops fetalis resulting in either fetal loss or neonatal death has been observed in two families. Slight-to-moderate splenomegaly and jaundice is usually present, and sometimes gallstones and hepatomegaly are present in early childhood.

Hematologic features reflect the variable clinical severity. Reported values for mean hemoglobin values range from 6.0 to 12.5 g/dl, and for reticulocytes from 7 to 72%. Peripheral smears invariably show anisopoikilocytosis and polychromasia. Nucleated erythrocytes, target cells, burr cells, erythrocytes with scalloped margins, dense spiculated microspherocytes, basophilic stippling, Pappenheimer bodies, and Howell-Jolly bodies (in splenectomized patients) may be present in small numbers. These findings are common to most erythroenzymopathies and are not specific for GPI deficiency.

**Complications:** A characteristic finding is the occurrence of acute hemolytic crises, often in association with intercurrent infections. Aplastic crises have also been observed. As is the case with most hemolytic anemias, occurrence of gallstones has been reported.

All tissues possess the same isozyme of GPI. Thus, in all but two cases, deficiency of GPI has been noted in leukocytes and, when appropriate studies have been done, in platelets and fibroblasts as well. Despite this, other organ involvement has been infrequent. Only one case showed mental retardation (GPI-Utrecht), and in the same child hepatomegaly was determined to be due to excessive glycogen storage. The enlarged liver could be reduced by balanced carbohydrate diet. Priapism attributed to increased blood viscosity was reported in one child. Others have reported decreased filterability of erythrocytes deficient in GPI. This latter finding may be nonspecific in that erythrocytes deficient in pyruvate kinase (PK) and glucose-6-phosphate dehydrogenase (G6PD) have also been found to exhibit decreased filterability.

**Associated Findings:** Deficiency of GPI and coexistent glucose-6-phosphate dehydrogenase has been reported, and in these cases 1) the hemolytic anemia was milder, and 2) episodic hemolysis associated with exposure to oxidant drugs was observed.

Elliptocytosis with hemolytic anemia has been found in combination with partial (50%) GPI deficiency in a young girl and her mother. Other family members with either trait alone were hematologically normal.

**Etiology:** Autosomal recessive inheritance. About one-half of the reported cases are true homozygotes, and the remaining cases are either heterozygotes or heterozygous for two different GPI mutants (compound heterozygotes).

**Pathogenesis:** In the majority of cases the mutant GPI was noted to be thermolabile compared with the normal enzyme. It has recently been suggested but not yet established that severity of hemolysis in GPI deficiency parallels the thermal instability of the defective mutant enzyme. Unstable mutant enzymes may be inactivated *in vivo* with progressively more serious effects on cellular metabolism. As in pyruvate kinase (PK) deficiency, selective reticulocyte destruction by splenic macrophages has been shown.

**MIM No.:** *17240

**Sex Ratio:** M1:F1

**Occurrence:** Ranks among the four most common erythroenzymopathies, including those of glucose-6-phosphate dehydrogenase, pyruvate kinase, and pyrimidine nucleotidase. Since the first description of GPI deficiency in 1968, over 40 cases have been reported with a worldwide distribution. Gene frequency remains undefined. Paglia and Valentine (1974) observed two incidental heterozygotes in approximately 1,000 selected individuals (excluding families with known GPI deficiency cases but including normal controls) referred to their laboratory. Several normally occurring electrophoretic variants have been described, with only the type 3 variant having a polymorphic frequency of greater than 1% in certain ethnic groups in Northern India.

**Risk of Recurrence for Patient's Sib:**
See Part I, *Mendelian Inheritance.*

**Risk of Recurrence for Patient's Child:**
See Part I, *Mendelian Inheritance.*

**Age of Detectability:** GPI deficiency is detectible by intrauterine diagnosis. Whitelaw et al (1979) observed normal electrophoretic mobility and thermal stability of GPI from both parents' erythrocytes and paternal leukocytes. Maternal leukocytes, however, contained the normal isozyme and a variant isozyme with thermal instability and altered electrophoretic pattern. GPI extracted from the placenta of the first child (who died of hydrops) possessed the abnormal isozyme. Antenatal diagnosis was established in the second child at 28 weeks gestation on the basis of marked thermal instability of the isomerase isozyme extracted from cultured amniotic fluid cells. In this case and in a family reported by Ravindranath et al (1987), the pregnancy was successfully managed by early intervention based on fetal activity and amniotic fluid bilirubin levels.

**Gene Mapping and Linkage:** GPI (glucose phosphate isomerase) has been mapped to 19q13.1.

**Prevention:** None known. Genetic counseling indicated.

**Treatment:** Splenectomy remains the primary treatment. In all cases but one, splenectomy resulted in amelioration of anemia and reduction or elimination of transfusion requirements. Despite this improvement there is frequently an increase in reticulocyte counts and further shortening of radiochromium half-lives following splenectomy. The same paradoxic phenomenon was observed in PK deficiency and presumably reflects labeling and rapid demise of markedly deficient cells that would not have survived long enough to be present in a presplenectomy blood specimen.

Alternative approaches to treatment with infusion of inorganic phosphate to stimulate glycolysis and mannose have yielded mixed results and should be considered investigational.

The potential for postsplenectomy sepsis should be recognized. The fear of postsplenectomy complications, however, should not be the reason for delaying splenectomy for patients encumbered by symptoms, transfusion requirements, or frequent or severe episodes of acute hemolysis.

All patients undergoing splenectomy should receive polyvalent pneumococcal vaccine prior to splenectomy and penicillin prophylaxis for at least 2–3 years following splenectomy.

**Prognosis:** Prognosis for life appears to be good.

**Detection of Carrier:** By direct assay of enzyme activity in erythrocytes through standard methods.

**References:**
Baughan MA, et al.: Hereditary hemolytic anemia with associated glucosephosphate isomerase (GPI) deficiency-a new enzyme defect of human erythrocytes. Blood 1968; 32:236–249.
Paglia DE, Valentine WN: Hereditary glucosephosphate isomerase deficiency: a review. Am J Clin Pathol 1974; 62:740–751. †
van Biervliet JPGM et al.: A new variant of glucosephosphate isomerase deficiency (GPI-Utrecht). Clin Chim Acta 1975; 65:157–166.
Arnold H: Inherited glucosephosphate isomerase deficiency: a review of known variants and some aspects of the pathomechanism of the deficiency. Blut 1979; 39:405–417.
Whitelaw AGL, et al.: Congenital haemolytic anaemia resulting from glucose phosphate isomerase deficiency: genetics, clinical picture, and prenatal diagnosis. J Med Genet 1979; 16:189–196. †
Ravindranath Y, et al.: Glucose phosphate isomerase deficiency as a cause of hydrops fetalis. New Engl J Med 1987; 316:258–261.

RA022                                    **Yaddanapudi Ravindranath**

---

**ANEMIA, HEINZ BODY**       **2647**

**Includes:**
   Heinz body anemia
   Hemoglobin variants, unstable with inclusion body formation

**Excludes:**
   **Glucose-6-phosphate dehydrogenase deficiency** (0420)
   Hexose monophosphate shunt enzyme deficiencies (other)
   Thalassemia syndromes
   Toxic Heinz-body anemia

**Major Diagnostic Criteria:** Heinz-bodies are demonstrable in the erythrocytes of affected individuals when the cells are stained with oxidant supravital stains such as methyl violet. A structurally altered hemoglobin, the underlying abnormality in these conditions, can be detected by laboratory tests (heat stability, isopropanol stability) which detect the presence of an unstable hemoglobin fraction. Some, but not all of these abnormal hemoglobins exhibit altered mobility in hemoglobin electrophoresis or isoelectric focusing. Hemolytic anemia is often present in affected

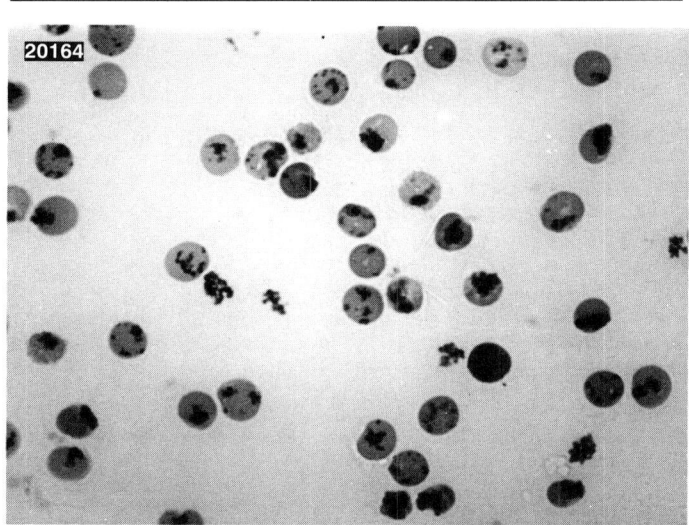

**2647-20164:** Note Heinz bodies in these stained erythrocytes from a patient with severe hemolytic anemia associated with Hb Abraham Lincoln (β 32 Leu→Pro).

individuals, and may range from very severe chronic hemolytic disease (e.g., Hb Abraham Lincoln, Hb Köhn, Hb Mizuho) to mild or inapparent hemolysis. Others of these hemoglobin variants typically cause only mild hemolytic manifestations under normal circumstances, but produce severe hemolytic episodes with exposure to oxidant drugs and chemicals, or in association with infections. Hb Zürich and Hb Hasharon exhibit this phenotype.

**Clinical Findings:** The clinical manifestations of Heinz-body anemia may be apparent at birth when the molecular abnormality involves the $\alpha$ or $\gamma$ chains of hemoglobin; in the latter case the hemolytic disease characteristically disappears as $\beta$ chain synthesis replaces that of the $\gamma$ chains. Abnormal clinical findings may include anemia, jaundice and splenomegaly. The anemia is often well-compensated, with superimposed acute hemolytic episodes precipitated by exposure to oxidant drugs and chemicals or infections. Some forms of Heinz-body anemia are accompanied by "dipyrolluria," with excretion of darkly pigmented substances, especially in association with acute hemolytic episodes.

**Complications:** Oxidant drugs and chemicals, generally those known to initiate hemolysis in **Glucose-6-phosphate dehydrogenase deficiency** individuals, may precipitate severe hemolytic episodes and must be carefully avoided.

**Associated Findings:** Gall-stone formation, in some cases with secondary liver disease, and cardiac complications of chronic anemia may accompany more severe forms of these conditions.

**Etiology:** Autosomal dominant inheritance; among the clinically severe forms, a substantial number appear to have arisen as new mutations, with neither parent exhibiting the abnormality.

**Pathogenesis:** Most of the hemoglobin variants which give rise to the Heinz-body anemia phenotype contain a single amino acid substitution in one of the globin chains. In most of the remaining variants in this group, one or more amino acids have been shown to be deleted from the affected globin chains. The molecular instability which results from these structural changes appears to promote the initiation of an oxidative pathway within the erythrocytes of these individuals, resulting ultimately in hemoglobin denaturation and the intracellular precipitation of the hemoglobin to produce the Heinz-body inclusions. This process is initiated by the oxidation of oxyhemoglobin to produce ferrihemoglobin ($Fe^{+3}$) with the release of superoxide ($O_2^-$). Subsequent oxidation of the hemoglobin leads to the formation of internally-bonded denaturation intermediates termed hemichromes, which undergo precipitation and become bound to the erythrocyte membrane. This process, as well as oxidative injury to the cell membrane due to the action of superoxide, are believed to be the major causes of the hemolytic manifestations.

**MIM No.:** 14070

**Sex Ratio:** M1:F1

**Occurrence:** Hb Hasharon ($\alpha$47 Asp → His) is an uncommon abnormality, confined mainly to Ashkenazi Jews and Northern Italians. All of the other forms are undetermined and presumed rare.

**Risk of Recurrence for Patient's Sib:**
See Part I, *Mendelian Inheritance*.

**Risk of Recurrence for Patient's Child:**
See Part I, *Mendelian Inheritance*.

**Age of Detectability:** Most of the severe forms of Heinz-body anemia involve the $\beta$ chains of hemoglobin, and may become clinically apparent as early as 4–6 months of age.

**Gene Mapping and Linkage:** See **Thalassemia.**

**Prevention:** None known. Genetic counseling indicated.

**Treatment:** Folic acid supplements have been recommended to meet increased need for the vitamin due to the hemolytic anemia. Splenectomy has been beneficial in some patients with splenomegaly when there have been associated hypersplenic changes, but the hemolytic disease is seldom improved following the surgery.

**Prognosis:** Most of the unstable hemoglobin syndromes have a relatively benign clinical course, even those producing chronic

hemolytic disease. In the more severe forms, life span may be affected by long-term organ damage related to chronic hemolysis and possibly from consequences of severe acute hemolytic episodes.

**Detection of Carrier:** With only rare exceptions, affected individuals are heterozygotes, with carriers of the condition therefore exhibiting full expression of the abnormality. Examples have been reported, however, of unstable $\alpha$-chain variants occurring in combination with $\alpha$-thalassemia, or $\beta$-chain variants in combination with $\beta$-thalassemia. In both of these circumstances the compound heterozygotes are usually more severely affected than are heterozygous carriers. In all cases, however, tests for an unstable hemoglobin fraction, particularly the isopropanol stability test, will allow the abnormality to be detected.

**References:**
Dacie JV, et al.: Hereditary Heinz-body anaemia. a report of studies on five patients with mild anaemia. Br J Haematol 1964; 10:388–402.
White JM: The unstable haemoglobin disorders. Clin Haematol 1974; 3:333–356.
Winterbourn CC, Carrell RW: Studies of hemoglobin denaturation and Heinz body formation in unstable hemoglobins. J Clin Invest 1974; 54:678–689.
Stamatoyannopoulos G, et al.: De novo mutations producing unstable hemoglobins or hemoglobins M. Hum Genet 1981; 58:396–404.
Honig GR, Adams JG III: Human hemoglobin genetics. Vienna: Springer-Verlag, 1986:186–190.

H0024                                                        **George R. Honig**

**Anemia, hemolytic**
*See ERYTHROBLASTOSIS FETALIS*
**Anemia, hemolytic pyruvate kinase type**
*See PYRUVATE KINASE DEFICIENCY*
**Anemia, hemolytic, due to triose isomerase deficiency**
*See ERYTHROCYTE TRIOSEPHOSPHATE ISOMERASE DEFICIENCY*

---

## ANEMIA, HEMOLYTIC, ERYTHROCYTE HEXOKINASE DEFICIENCY                                           2678

**Includes:**
Erythrocyte hexokinase deficiency hemolytic anemia
Hexokinase deficiency hemolytic anemia

**Excludes:**
**Anemia, hemolytic** (other)
**Pancytopenia syndrome, Fanconi type** (2029)

**Major Diagnostic Criteria:** Erythrocyte hexokinase activity is normally greatly increased in reticulocytes. In severe deficiency, activities are far below those of reticulocyte-rich blood present with hemolytic anemia.

**Clinical Findings:** Diagnosis rests on enzyme assay of the red cell enzyme. Chronic nonspherocytic hemolytic anemia of variable severity and splenomegaly are present.

**Complications:** Transfusion requirements in some cases. Early development of cholelithiasis in some cases.

**Associated Findings:** None known.

**Etiology:** Usually autosomal recessive inheritance. In two cases there has been evidence of dominant inheritance.

**Pathogenesis:** Defective glycolysis leading to metabolic depletion in the glycolytic-dependent erythrocyte.

**MIM No.:** 23570, *14260

**Sex Ratio:** Presumably M1:F1

**Occurrence:** Over a dozen cases have been documented.

**Risk of Recurrence for Patient's Sib:**
See Part I, *Mendelian Inheritance*.

**Risk of Recurrence for Patient's Child:**
See Part I, *Mendelian Inheritance*.

**Age of Detectability:** At birth if appropriate studies are done.

**Gene Mapping and Linkage:** HK1 (hexokinase 1) has been mapped to 10q22.

**Prevention:** None known. Genetic counseling indicated.

**Treatment:** Supplements of folate are indicated. Splenectomy confers partial benefits, but hemolysis continues unabated. Reserved for cases with ongoing transfusion requirements.

**Prognosis:** Aside from complications of chronic hemolysis (anemia, cholelithiasis, and transfusion requirements) subjects appear to have a fair prognosis.

**Detection of Carrier:** Heterozygotes are asymptomatic and often have red cell hexokinase activities in the low normal range. Difficult to detect other than the obligate heterozygote.

**References:**

Valentine WN, et al.: Hereditary hemolytic anemia with hexokinase deficiency. Role of hexokinase in erythrocyte aging. New Engl J Med 1967; 276:1–11.

Newman P, et al.: Non-spherocytic haemolytic anaemia in mother and son associated with hexokinase deficiency. Br J Haematol 1980; 46:537–547.

Jansen G, et al.: Characteristics of hexokinase, pyruvate kinase, and glucose-6-phosphate dehydrogenase during adult and neonatal reticulocyte maturation. Am J Hematol 1985; 20:203–218.

Valentine WN, et al.: Pyruvate kinase and other enzyme deficiency disorders of the erythrocyte. In: Scriver CR, et al, eds: The metabolic basis of inherited disease, 6th ed. New York: McGraw-Hill, 1989: 2341–2366.

VA024                                          **William N. Valentine**

## ANEMIA, HEMOLYTIC, ERYTHROCYTE PHOSPHOGLYCERATE KINASE DEFICIENCY          2657

**Includes:**
> Erythrocyte phosphoglycerate kinase deficiency
> Phosphoglycerate kinase (PGK) deficiency, erythrocyte

**Excludes:  Anemia** (other)

**Major Diagnostic Criteria:** In males, chronic nonspherocytic hemolytic anemia, severely defective red cell phosphoglycerate kinase by specific assay, and neurologic or myopathic features.

**Clinical Findings:** In 12 reduced activity variants about half have had varied neurologic and behavioral aberrations ranging from near normality to variable mental retardation, seizures, extrapyramidal tract disease, and even coma and hemiplegia during neurologic crisis, which may accompany exacerbations of the hemolytic syndrome. Two cases have had myopathy without hemolysis. Females in this X-linked disorder have a mosaic of normal and deficient cells. Depending on the size of the latter clone, they may exhibit hemolysis alone or may be virtually undetectable by laboratory parameters. Neurologic complications in females have not been reported.

**Complications:** Early cholelithiasis and transfusion requirements in some.

**Associated Findings:** None known.

**Etiology:** X-linked recessive inheritance, with some cases by apparent autosomal recessive inheritance.

**Pathogenesis:** Hemolysis is presumably secondary to defective glycolysis and metabolic depletion. The exact mechanism of neurologic dysfunction is unknown, but the enzyme deficiency in brain and other tissues in autopsy tissue has been documented. Myopathy and rhabdomyolysis with exercise presumably result from impaired glycolysis in muscle.

**MIM No.:** *31180, 26170

**Sex Ratio:** M1:F<1; rare affected females are thought to be heterozygotes.

**Occurrence:** About a dozen cases have been documented.

**Risk of Recurrence for Patient's Sib:**
> See Part I, *Mendelian Inheritance.*

**Risk of Recurrence for Patient's Child:**
> See Part I, *Mendelian Inheritance.*

**Age of Detectability:** At birth if requisite studies are done. Heterozygous females, being mosaic, are sometimes nearly undetectable by red cell assay.

**Gene Mapping and Linkage:** PGK1 (phosphoglycerate kinase 1) has been mapped to Xq13.

**Prevention:** None known. Genetic counseling indicated.

**Treatment:** Supplements of folate, transfusions when necessary, and avoidance of severe exertion if rhabdomyolysis has been documented.

**Prognosis:** Variable in hemizygous males, depending on the severity of clinical findings. Good in heterozygous females. Neurologic complications can be fatal.

**Detection of Carrier:** By specific enzyme assay.

**References:**

Valentine WN, et al.: Hereditary hemolytic anemia associated with phosphoglycerate kinase deficiency in erythrocytes and leukocytes. A probable X-chromosome-linked syndrome. New Engl J Med 1969; 280:528–534.

Chen S-H, et al.: Phosphoglycerate kinase: X-linked polymorphism in man. Am J Hum Genet 1971; 23:87–91.

Huang I-Y, et al.: Structure and function of normal and variant human phosphoglycerate kinase. Hemoglobin 1980; 4:601–609.

Svirklys LG, O'Sullivan WJ: Tissue levels of glycolytic enzymes in phosphoglycerate kinase deficiency. Clin Chim Acta 1980; 108:309–315.

Guis MS, et al.: Phosphoglycerate kinase San Francisco: a new variant associated with hemolytic anemia but not with neuromuscular manifestations. Am J Hemat 1987; 25:175–182.

VA024                                          **William N. Valentine**

## ANEMIA, HEMOLYTIC, ERYTHROCYTE PHOSPHOLIPID DEFECT          2667

**Includes:**
> High phosphatidylcholine hemolytic anemia (HPCHA)
> Red cell membrane phosphatidylcholine hemolytic anemia

**Excludes:**
> **Elliptocytosis** (2665)
> Hemoglobinopathies
> High red cell membrane phosphatidylcholine, acquired
> **Lecithin-cholesterol acyl transferase deficiency** (0580)
> Red cell enzyme deficiencies
> Red cell hydration disorders with normal membrane
>     phospholipids
> **Spherocytosis** (0892)

**Major Diagnostic Criteria:** Chronic, nonspherocytic hemolytic anemia. Red cells have excess phosphatidylcholine. Variable degrees of anemia, macrocytosis, reticulocytosis, hyperbilirubinemia, and splenomegaly.

**Clinical Findings:** Jaundice, hemolytic anemia, splenomegaly. The clinical findings in patients are variable.

**Complications:** Those associated with chronic hemolytic anemia: splenomegaly, gallstones.

**Associated Findings:** None known.

**Etiology:** Probably autosomal dominant inheritance.

**Pathogenesis:** Red cells are characterized by an increase in phosphatidylcholine. Plasma lipids are usually normal, and other cells are not known to be affected. In one family, the abnormal erythrocyte membrane phospholipid content was attributed to a defect in the conversion of phosphatidylcholine to phosphatidylethanolamine. The membrane lipid defect is accompanied by increased cation permeability, which results in an increased intracellular sodium content and decreased intracellular potassium content, with a variable degree of cellular dehydration. A loss of erythrocyte deformability may explain the shortened cell survival. No qualitative abnormalities of membrane proteins have been detected, and the molecular defect responsible for the disorder remains to be identified.

**MIM No.:** *17970

**Sex Ratio:** M1:F1

**Occurrence:** Undetermined but presumably rare.

**Risk of Recurrence for Patient's Sib:**
See Part I, *Mendelian Inheritance.*

**Risk of Recurrence for Patient's Child:**
See Part I, *Mendelian Inheritance.*

**Age of Detectability:** Variable depending upon presenting clinical findings.

**Gene Mapping and Linkage:** Unknown.

**Prevention:** None known. Genetic counseling indicated.

**Treatment:** No specific treatment is usually required. Splenectomy has been performed in some cases, but is usually to no benefit.

**Prognosis:** Expected life span is normal, with no associated abnormalities.

**Detection of Carrier:** Unknown.

**References:**
Jaffe ER, Gottfried EL: Hereditary nonspherocytic hemolytic disease associated with an altered phospholipid composition of the erythrocytes. J Clin Invest 1968; 47:1375–1388.
Lane P, et al.: Characterization of high Na+ low K+ red blood cells (RBC) in a family with hereditary high phosphatidylcholine (PC) hemolytic anemia. Blood 1968; 86(suppl 1):56a (abstr).
Shohet SB, et al.: Hereditary hemolytic anemia associated with abnormal membrane lipids: mechanism of accumulation of phosphatidylcholine. Blood 1971; 38:445–456.
Clark MR, et al.: Effects of abnormal cation transport on deformability of disiccacytes. J Supramol Struct 1978; 8:521–532.
Godin DV, et al.: Study of erythrocytes in a hereditary hemolytic syndrome (HHS): comparison with erythrocytes in lecithin:cholesterol acyltransferase (LCAT) deficiency. Scand J Haematol 1980; 24:122–130.
Yawata T, et al.: Lipid analyses and fluidity studies by electron spin resonance of red cell membranes in hereditary high red cell membrane phosphatidylcholine hemolytic anemia. Blood 1984; 64:1129–1134.
Butikofer P, et al.: Erythrocyte phospholipid organization and vesiculation in hereditary high red cell membrane phosphatidylcholine hemolytic anemia. J Lab Clin Med 1989; 113:278–284.

LU013
LA043
**Bertram H. Lubin**
**Peter A. Lane**

---

## ANEMIA, HEMOLYTIC, GAMMA-GLUTAMYL/CYSTEINE SYNTHETASE DEFICIENCY    3221

**Includes:** Gamma-glutamyl cysteine synthetase deficiency

**Excludes: Anemia, hemolytic** (others)

**Major Diagnostic Criteria:** Demonstration of absence, or near absence, of glutathione (GSH) in erythrocytes, and severe deficiency of gamma-glutamyl cysteine synthetase activity.

**Clinical Findings:** In the index case, the clinical phenotype was characterized by nonspherocytic hemolytic anemia and adult onset spinocerebellar ataxia. In a second kindred, the propositus in her twenties lacked neurologic manifestations. Although undocumented, the severe deficiency of erythrocyte GSH is also expected to be associated with exacerbations of hemolysis potentially occurring on ingestion of oxidant-producing medications and stresses producing hemolytic exacerbations in G6PD deficiency.

**Complications:** Since only two kindreds are currently recognized, in one of which two members exhibited spinocerebellar ataxia, it cannot be stated with certainty that neurologic manifestations share a common etiology with hemolytic anemia. This is likely to be the case in some kindreds, however.

**Associated Findings:** Neurologic dysfunctions.

**Etiology:** Autosomal recessive inheritance. Heterozygotes are phenotypically normal but have partial deficiencies in the activity of gamma-glutamyl cysteine synthetase.

**Pathogenesis:** Reduced GSH is essential in protecting the erythrocyte against many forms of oxidant damage, and in the enzymatic destruction of harmful peroxides. Its multiple roles in other body tissues such as the nervous system are difficult to define, but serves as a major reductant.

**MIM No.:** *23045

**Sex Ratio:** M1:F1

**Occurrence:** Two kinships have been reported.

**Risk of Recurrence for Patient's Sib:**
See Part I, *Mendelian Inheritance.*

**Risk of Recurrence for Patient's Child:**
See Part I, *Mendelian Inheritance.*

**Age of Detectability:** The hemolytic anemia is presumably detectable at birth. Neurologic abnormalities, where detected, have been of adult onset (third and fourth decade of life).

**Gene Mapping and Linkage:** Unknown.

**Prevention:** None known. Genetic counseling indicated.

**Treatment:** Oxidant producing medications and agents known to provoke hemolytic exacerbations in subjects with G6PD deficiency should be avoided. Closer monitoring of hemoglobin levels is indicated under conditions of potential stress, e.g., surgery, infection, pregnancy.

**Prognosis:** In the rare cases recognized, reported hemolytic anemia has been definite, but moderate in degree.

**Detection of Carrier:** Heterozygotes are phenotypically normal but have about half-normal enzyme activities by specific assay.

*The author wishes to thank E. Beutler, R. Moroose, L. Kramer, T. Gelbart, and L. Forman for their help in the preparation of this article.*

**References:**
Konrad PN, et al.: Gamma-glutamyl-cysteine synthetase deficiency: a cause of hereditary hemolytic anemia. New Eng J Med 1972; 286:557–561.
Meister A: The gamma-glutamyl cycle: diseases associated with specific enzyme deficiencies. Ann Intern Med 1974; 81:247–253.
Richards F, et al.: Familial spinocerebellar degeneration, hemolytic anemia, and glutathione deficiency. Arch Intern Med 1974; 134:534–537.

VA024
**William N. Valentine**

---

## ANEMIA, HEMOLYTIC, GLUTATHIONE REDUCTASE DEFICIENCY    2676

**Includes:**
Glutathione reductase deficiency, hemolytic anemia due to
Hemolytic anemia due to glutathione reductase deficiency

**Excludes: Anemia, hemolytic** (other)

**Major Diagnostic Criteria:** This inherited severe deficiency must be diagnosed by a specific apoenzyme assay, taking care to exclude noninherited deficiency due to the insufficient cofactor flavin adenine dinucleotide (FAD). The latter insufficiency is secondary to nutritional insufficiency of riboflavin or to its defective metabolism. Noninherited deficiency may also be induced by chemotherapy with 1,3-bis(2-chlorethyl)-1-nitrosourea (BCNU).

**Clinical Findings:** Symptoms have been lacking except for episodes of hemolysis following fava bean ingestion in one subject, and cataracts in two sibs, possibly, but not conclusively, secondary to the deficiency.

**Complications:** Unknown.

**Associated Findings:** Possibly cataracts.

**Etiology:** Autosomal recessive inheritance.

**Pathogenesis:** Glutathione reductase is necessary to maintain glutathione in the reduced state and to cycle reduced nicotinamide adenine dinucleotide phosphate (NADPH) to NADP. It, like **Glucose-6-phosphate dehydrogenase**, is a component of the pentose phosphate shunt, which affords protection from oxidant stresses.

**MIM No.:** 23180, *13830

**Sex Ratio:** Presumably M1:F1

**Occurrence:** One kindred has been fully documented.

**Risk of Recurrence for Patient's Sib:**
See Part I, *Mendelian Inheritance.*

**Risk of Recurrence for Patient's Child:**
See Part I, *Mendelian Inheritance.*

**Age of Detectability:** Probably dependent on occurrence of a hemolytic episode and on a specific enzyme assay being done by a specialized research laboratory.

**Gene Mapping and Linkage:** GSR (glutathione reductase) has been mapped to 8p21.1.

**Prevention:** None known. Genetic counseling indicated.

**Treatment:** Avoidance of oxidant stresses such as those producing hemolysis in subjects with **Glucose-6-phosphate dehydrogenase deficiency.**

**Prognosis:** As far as is known, this is a mild disorder unlikely to influence survival.

**Detection of Carrier:** Depends on a specific apoenzyme assay showing partial deficiency.

**Special Considerations:** A wide diversity of syndromes have been reported to be associated with glutathione reductase deficiency, but virtually all patients have been shown to suffer from inadequate synthesis of FAD or its defective metabolism and not from an inherited defective apoenzyme. BCNU, employed chemotherapeutically, specifically inhibits glutathione reductase and is another cause of noninherited deficiency.

**References:**
Waller HD: Glutathione reductase deficiency. In: Beutler E, ed: Hereditary disorders of erythrocyte metabolism. New York: Grune & Stratton, 1968:185–208.
Beutler E: Effect of flavin compounds on glutathione reductase acitivity: in vivo and in vitro studies. J Clin Invest 1969; 48:1957–1966.
Beutler E: Glutathione reductase: stimulation in normal subjects by riboflavin supplementation. Science 1969; 165:613–615.
Loos H, et al.: Familial deficiency of glutathione reductase in human blood cells. Blood 1976; 48:53–62.
Frischer H, Ahmad T: Severe generalized glutathione reductase deficiency after antitumor chemotherapy with BCNU (1,3-bis[2-chloroethyl]-1-nitrosourea). J Lab Clin Med 1977; 89:1080–1091.

VA024                                      **William N. Valentine**

## ANEMIA, HEMOLYTIC, GLUTATHIONE SYNTHETASE DEFICIENCY                                 2677

**Includes:**
Glutathione synthetase deficiency, hemolytic anemia due to
Hemolytic anemia due to glutathione synthetase deficiency
Five-Oxoprolinuria
Pyroglutamic aciduria

**Excludes:** **Anemia, hemolytic** (other)

**Major Diagnostic Criteria:** The diagnosis requires demonstration of absent or near-absent glutathione (GSH) in erythrocytes and severe deficiency of glutathione synthetase. One form of the deficiency also requires the demonstration of metabolic acidosis and the accumulation of pyroglutamic acid in blood and urine (5-oxoprolinuria). The Heinz body test in erythrocytes is positive.

**Clinical Findings:** One phenotype of the disorder is characterized by nonspherocytic hemolytic anemia alone with hemolytic exacerbations potentially occurring on ingesting oxidant medications such as those causing hemolysis in **Glucose-6-phosphate dehydrogenase deficiency**. A second phenotype involves multisystem disease with metabolic acidosis, massive 5-oxoprolinuria, and often variably severe neurologic dysfunction.

**Complications:** The generalized syndrome in the index case was associated with selective atrophy of the granular cell layer of the cerebellum and focal lesions in the frontoparietal cortex, visual cortex, and thalamus.

**Associated Findings:** In the severest form, neurologic dysfunction can be associated with mental retardation, progressive neurologic deterioration from severe organic brain disease, and even death.

**Etiology:** Autosomal recessive inheritance. Depending on the characteristics of the mutant gene product, effects may be generalized or confined to the erythrocyte, which, unlike nucleated tissues, is devoid of the ability to synthesize any new protein enzymes to renew losses of activity due to enhanced lability of the variant gene product.

**Pathogenesis:** Reduced GSH is essential to protect the erythrocyte from oxidant damage to Hb and to participate in the destruction of harmful peroxides. Its role in the central nervous system is less clear, and it is difficult to differentiate damage due to deficiency of GSH per se and that due to the severe metabolic acidosis that accompanies it. 5-Oxoproline is an intermediate in the metabolism of GSH. It is produced in great excess from γ-glutamyl cysteine, the immediate precursor of GSH, when the latter is lacking. GSH normally controls its own synthesis by inhibiting the synthesis of its immediate precursor. Unimpeded synthesis of γ-glutamyl cysteine results in subsequent excess of 5-oxoproline so massive that it overwhelms the enzymatic conversion to glutamate by 5-oxoprolinase. The accumulation of 5-oxoproline is the cause of the severe metabolic acidosis.

**MIM No.:** *23190

**Sex Ratio:** M1:F1

**Occurrence:** Some six kinships have been documented.

**Risk of Recurrence for Patient's Sib:**
See Part I, *Mendelian Inheritance.*

**Risk of Recurrence for Patient's Child:**
See Part I, *Mendelian Inheritance.*

**Age of Detectability:** Hemolytic anemia is detectable at birth. Neurologic manifestations, when present, appear at an early age and progress, but precise onset is not well documented.

**Gene Mapping and Linkage:** Unknown.

**Prevention:** None known. Genetic counseling indicated.

**Treatment:** Control of metabolic acidosis by administration of bicarbonate is important in the phenotype in which pyroglutamic aciduria is present.

It is not known for certain, but early diagnosis and control of metabolic acidosis by administration of bicarbonate may mitigate neurologic deterioration. Those medications and ingestion of fava beans known to induce hemolysis in **Glucose-6-phosphate dehydrogenase deficiency** should be avoided.

**Prognosis:** Guarded where severe neurologic function exists. The first reported case died at age 28 years.

**Detection of Carrier:** Heterozygotes are asymptomatic, have normal concentrations of red cell GSH, but about half-normal GSH synthetase activity by enzyme assay.

**References:**
Oort M, et al.: Hereditary absence of reduced glutathione in the erythrocytes: a new clinical and biochemical entity. Vox Sang 1961; 6:370–373.
Prins HK, et al.: Congenital nonspherocytic hemolytic anemia, associated with glutathione deficiency of the erythrocytes: hematologic, biochemical and genetic studies. Blood 1966; 27:145–166.
Jellum E, et al.: Pyroglutamic aciduria: a new inborn error of metabolism. Scand J Clin Lab Invest 1970; 26:327–335.
Mohler DN, et al.: Glutathione synthetase deficiency as a cause of hereditary hemolytic disease. New Engl J Med 1970; 283:1253–1257.
Beutler E, et al.: Erythrocyte glutathione synthetase deficiency leads not only to glutathione but also to glutathione-S-transferase deficiency. J Clin Invest 1986; 77:38–41.
Meister A, Larsson A: Glutathione synthetase deficiency and other disorders of the γ-glutamycycle. In: Scriver CR, et al, eds: The

metabolic basis of inherited disease, 6th ed. New York: McGraw-Hill, 1989:855–868.

VA024 **William N. Valentine**

## ANEMIA, HEMOLYTIC, GLUTATIONINE PEROXIDASE DEFICIENCY 2675

**Includes:**
Glutathione peroxidase deficiency, hemolytic anemia due to
Hemolytic anemia due to glutathione peroxidase deficiency

**Excludes: Anemia, hemolytic** (others)

**Major Diagnostic Criteria:** By specific erythrocyte enzyme assay and characterization.

**Clinical Findings:** While partial deficiency of erythrocyte glutathione peroxidase has been documented in conjunction with otherwise unexplained hemolytic syndromes, this could represent fortuitous association with a common variant in many healthy persons. In many Jews and persons with ethnic origins around the Mediterranean Sea, half-normal activity of the enzyme is a common finding and without a clinical counterpart. The role of the enzyme in producing a clinical hemolytic syndrome is therefore unsettled.

**Complications:** Unknown.

**Associated Findings:** None known.

**Etiology:** Autosomal recessive inheritance.

**Pathogenesis:** This selenoenzyme simultaneously oxidizes glutathione and converts harmful peroxides to water and alcohols. Its putative role in producing hemolysis when deficient is presumed to reflect impaired detoxification of harmful peroxides capable of producing oxidant damage in the red cell and its hemoglobin.

**MIM No.:** *23170

**Sex Ratio:** Presumably M1:F1.

**Occurrence:** Undetermined, and confounded by racial and geographic variations in "normal" findings.

**Risk of Recurrence for Patient's Sib:**
See Part I, *Mendelian Inheritance.*

**Risk of Recurrence for Patient's Child:**
See Part I, *Mendelian Inheritance.*

**Age of Detectability:** During the newborn period.

**Gene Mapping and Linkage:** KRT19 (keratin 19) has been provisionally mapped to 17q21-q23.
GPX1 (glutathione peroxidase 1) has been mapped to 3q11-q12.

**Prevention:** None known. Genetic counseling indicated.

**Treatment:** Vitamin E, an antioxidant, has been recommended.

**Prognosis:** Unknown.

**Detection of Carrier:** Demonstration of defective enzyme variants is theoretically required but rendered relatively ineffective by virtue of wide variations in enzyme activity in healthy populations.

**References:**
Cohen G, Hochstein P: Glutathione peroxidase: the primary agent for the elimination of hydrogen peroxide in erythrocytes. Biochemistry 1963; 2:1420–1428.
Paglia DE, Valentine WN: Studies on the quantitative and qualitative characterization of erythrocyte glutathione peroxidase. J Lab Clin Med 1967; 70:158–169.
Necheles TF, et al.: Erythrocyte glutathione-peroxidase deficiency. Br J Haematol 1970; 19:605–612.
Steinberg MH, et al.: Acute hemolytic anemia associated with erythrocyte glutathione-peroxidase deficiency. Arch Intern Med 1970; 125:302–303.
Beutler E, Matsumoto F: Ethnic variation in red cell glutathione peroxidase activity. Blood 1975; 46:103–110.
Rea HM, et al.: Relation between erythrocyte selenium and glutathione peroxidase (E.C.1.11.1.9) activities of New Zealand residents and visitors to New Zealand. Br J Nutr 1979; 42:201–208.
Meera Khan P, et al.: Electrotypes and formal genetics of red cell

glutathione peroxidase (GPX1) in the Djuka of Surinam. Am J Hum Genet 1986; 38:712–723.
Takahashi K, et al.: Glutathione peroxidase protein: absence in selenium deficiency states and correlation with enzymatic activity. J Clin Invest 1986; 77:1402–1404.

VA024 **William N. Valentine**

**Anemia, hemolytic, phosphofructokinase deficiency**
*See GLYCOGENOSIS, TYPE VII*

## ANEMIA, HEMOLYTIC, RED CELL MEMBRANE DEFECTS 2646

**Includes:**
Abetalipoproteinemia, hereditary
Acanthocytosis
Anemia, high red cell phosphatidylcholine hemolytic
Apolipoprotein B deficiency
ATPase deficiency
Bassen-Kornzweig syndrome
Beta-LCAT deficiency
Blood, red cell membrane defects
Desiccacytosis, hereditary
Dyserythropoietic anemia, type II (HEMPAS)
Elliptocytosis, hereditary
Elliptocytosis with transverse siltlike changes
Erythrocyte membrane defects
Gerbich-negative phenotype
Glycophorin deficiency
Hydrocytosis, hereditary
Kell blood group precursor substance
LCAT deficiency
Leaky red cell syndrome
Lecithin-cholesterol acyl transferase (LCAT) deficiency
McLeod phenotype
Minkowski-Chauffard syndrome (obsolete)
Norum disease
Phosphatidylcholine red cell membrane disorder
Potassium-sodium disorder of erythrocyte
Pyropoikilocytosis, hereditary
Red cell membrane defects
Red cell permeability defect
Red cell phospholipid defect-hemolysis
Rh null syndrome
Spherocytosis, hereditary
Stomatocytosis, hereditary
Xerocytosis, hereditary

**Excludes:**
Erythrocyte cytosolic enzyme defects
Hemoglobinopathies
Red cell defects, morphologic due to acquired liver disease
Red cell defects, morphologic due to mechanical trauma
Red cell defects, morphologic due to toxins
Red cell membrane defects, acquired
Thalassemias

**Major Diagnostic Criteria:** In general, congenital red cell membrane disorders lead to hemolytic anemias, whose mechanisms of hemolysis depend on the site of the membrane lesion: lipid bilayer, transmembrane proteins and ionic transporters, or cytoskeletal structural proteins. Typically, affected individuals have chronic hemolytic anemias with blood smears exhibiting morphologic red cell abnormalities (spherocytes, elliptocytes, stomatocytes, acanthocytes, and so forth) characteristic of a given disorder. The severity of the hemolysis varies among the membrane abnormalities. The hemolytic process characteristically leads to increased indirect acting bilirubin formation and reticulocytosis. Sensitivity of the erythrocytes to hypotonic lysis (osmotic fragility) is increased in disorders characterized by decreased surface: volume ratio or markedly increased cation permeability (spherocytosis, some forms of elliptocytosis, and stomatocytosis) and decreased in disorders of increased surface: volume ratio (xerocytosis, acanthocytosis). Passive Na$^+$/K$^+$ fluxes, active Na$^+$/K$^+$ transport, and total cell cation content are measured when stomatocytosis, xerocytosis, and other disorders of cation permeability are suspected. Acanthocytes indicate abnormalities in membrane lipid distribution and often result from abnormalities in serum lipids and serum lipoproteins, such as liver disease, hereditary abetalipoproteinemia, and anorexia nervosa. Membrane lipid content can be measured, but measurement of lipid distribution between inner and outer leaflets is available only experimentally.

**Clinical Findings:** Pallor, jaundice, and often splenomegaly. Hemolytic facies is only found in the severely affected individual. Hemolytic jaundice is not uncommon in neonates with membrane disorders, and infants often have more severe anemia than older patients. With increasing age, the incidence of gallbladder disease and leg ulcers increases. Patients with otherwise relatively mild anemias may be asymptomatic and undiagnosed until they experience an acute exacerbation of the anemia. Such exacerbations include aplastic crises, characterized by rapidly falling hematocrit and absence of reticulocytes. Bone marrow aspiration reveals severe depression of erythroid activity. These crises are often viral-associated, particularly with human parvovirus. The aplasia resolves spontaneously in 1 to 2 weeks. Hyperhemolytic events occur, often in conjunction with other viral illnesses and sometimes associated with signs of hypersplenism: enlarging spleen, leukopenia, thrombocytopenia, falling hematocrit, and increasing reticulocyte count. Occasionally, the morphologic red cell abnormality is associated with a systemic disorder. One example is hereditary abetalipoproteinemia, an autosomal recessive disorder, in which there is absence of low density lipoproteins. These individuals present with retarded growth, progressive neurologic deterioration, retinitis pigmentosa, and malabsorption. The erythrocytes characteristically are acanthocytic. Another systemic disorder associated with acanthocytosis is the McLeod red cell phenotype seen in chronic granulomatous disease, an X-linked disorder of granulocyte function, presenting with severe and repeated bacterial and fungal infections.

Red cell membrane protein electrophoresis (SDS-PAGE) is available experimentally in a variety of laboratories and can form the initial basis for the workup of suspected membrane protein abnormalities. When approaching the diagnosis of chronic hemolytic anemia, consideration should be given to hemoglobinopathies and cytosolic enzyme defects. Moreover, acquired hemolytic processes such as antibody-mediated (autoimmune) and microangiopathic anemias may give rise to abnormal erythrocyte morphology and must be excluded.

**Complications:** Unknown.

**Associated Findings:** None known.

**Etiology:** Autosomal dominant disorders include most forms of spherocytosis, elliptocytosis, stomatocytosis, and xerocytosis. Homozygosity may be lethal or associated with severe anemia. Rare recessive forms of spherocytosis are reported. Hereditary pyropoikilocytosis may represent homozygosity for elliptocytosis or a compound heterozygosity for two membrane defects. Abetalipoproteinemia is autosomal recessive. The inheritance of ATPase deficiency and lecithin-cholesterol acyl transferase deficiency appears to be variable. The McLeod phenotype is X-linked.

**Pathogenesis:** In any congenital membrane abnormality, the process whereby a given defect will result in hemolytic anemia depends on the role that component plays in the organization and function of the membrane. The red cell membrane is organized into three major domains: the membrane lipid bilayer, transmembrane proteins, and the membrane cytoskeleton.

As in all cell membranes, the lipid bilayer is composed of cholesterol and phospholipids. Interestingly, the phospholipids are asymmetrically distributed between inner and outer leaflets so that choline lipids (phosphatidyl choline and sphingomyelin) predominate in the outer leaflet, while amino lipids (phosphatidylcholine and phosphatidylethanolamine) predominate in the inner leaflet. It has been speculated that the inward-facing amino lipids serve to provide charged residues that stabilize the attachment of the submembrane cytoskeleton to the membrane inner surface by electrostatic attraction. Loss of phospholipid asymme-

try has been found in the membrane lesion associated with the sickling process in sickle cell anemia, and abnormal phospholipid distribution is seen in hereditary spherocytosis, although its role in hemolysis in uncertain. Congenital systemic lipid abnormalities such as hereditary abetalipoproteinemia, in which there is an absence of low density lipoproteins, lead to a decrease in membrane phosphatidylcholine, with relatively high levels of cholesterol and sphingomyelin. The deficiency of membrane lipid selectively occurs at the inner leaflet, leading to deformation of the cell membrane, known as *acanthocytosis*, in which the cell exhibits a small number (five to ten) of broad projections. Despite the morphologic abnormality, hemolytic anemia tends to be mild or absent. Inherited deficiency of the serum enzyme lecithin-cholesterol acyl transferase (LCAT) also leads to accumulation of neutral cholesterol in the outer leaflet of the cell membrane and acanthocyte formation. Inheritance is codominant, with heterozygotes mildly affected. Elevation of bile salts in liver disease also inhibits this enzyme, and thus acanthocytes are often seen in individuals with congenital or acquired liver pathology. Another congenital disorder in which acanthocytosis occurs is known as the *McLeod phenotype*, characterized by absence of the Kx (Kell) antigen in male patients. This disorder has been associated with chronic granulomatous disease, with which it is closely linked on the Xp21 chromosome region.

The transmembrane proteins include several sialoglycoproteins (the glycophorins), enzymes such as acetylcholinesterase, cation transport proteins (Na$^+$/K$^+$ ATPase and others), and the anion exchange protein "band 3." The glycophorins serve to supply much of the negative electric charge of the red cell membrane, as well as provide an attachment for the submembrane cytoskeleton. Loss of sialic acid groups with cell aging has been postulated to be one mechanism for the recognition of senescent red cells by the reticuloendothelial system. Interestingly, erythrocytes congenitally deficient in glycophorins A (En[a-] cells) or B (S-s-U- and S-s-U+ cells) show considerable resistance to invasion by *Plasmodium falciparum* merozoites. These proteins may form recognition sites for protozoal invasion. The glycophorins have also recently been found to form an attachment site for the submembrane cytoskeleton. It is not surprising, therefore, that absence of glycophorin C (Ge-; Gerbich-negative red cells) has been associated with instability of red cell shape and in some cases, elliptocytic morphology.

To maintain high intracellular K$^+$, low intracellular Na$^+$, and Ca2$^+$, the membrane contains cation transport proteins (ATPase) that transport these ions against concentration gradients, driven by the hydrolysis of ATP. For the most part, specific defects in these proteins have yet to be related to hemolytic anemias. In 1964 Harvald et al. reported a family with mild hemolytic anemia associated with a decrease in membrane Na$^+$-K$^+$ ATPase (Quabain-sensitive) activity. Other reports of ATPase deficiency have suggested both dominant and recessive inheritance patterns, but these have not been well characterized. However, a variety of disorders have been described in which the major red cell abnormalities are related to cation and water content. These appear to result from increased permeability of the membrane to specific cations. Hereditary xerocytosis is an autosomal disorder characterized by hemolytic anemia, splenomegaly, and erythrocyte morphology dominated by echinocytes and target cells. Coupled with a *decrease* in osmotic fragility, these cells appear to have increased surface:volume ratio due to loss of cell water. Total cation content is decreased, with decreased K$^+$ concentration, and (to a lesser extent) increased Na$^+$ concentration. The membrane defect is not yet identified, although the increase in K$^+$ permeability is thought to exceed that for Na$^+$. In contrast, hereditary stomatocytosis is caused by a variety of membrane abnormalities characterized by increased cation content and membrane surface area. Increased membrane lipids, particularly phosphatidylcholine, are often seen, and the activity of the Na$^+$-K$^+$ ATPase has been described as normal or increased, although there is one report of abnormal Na$^+$-K$^+$ stoichiometry for ouabain-sensitive Na$^+$-K$^+$ ATPase. Total cell water and cation content may be increased (hydrocytosis) or decreased (desiccacytosis), depending on whether the Na$^+$ leak or the K$^+$ leak predominates. Both dominant and recessive forms of stomatocytosis have been reported, and at least one kindred has been found to have a deficiency of membrane protein band 7. The Rh null phenotype has been associated with a hemolytic anemia characterized by stomatocytosis, dehydrated cells, and, paradoxically, increased osmotic fragility, with no apparent membrane protein or glycophorin abnormality. Hemolytic anemia associated with deficiency of membrane acetocholinesterasel has not been reported, although deficiency of this enzyme occurs in an acquired clonal membrane abnormality known as *paroxysmal nocturnal hemoglobinuria* (PNH). However, the hemolytic process in PNH is due to an abnormal sensitivity of the cell to lysis by complement, and not to cholinesterase deficiency.

The anion transport protein (band 3; MW 90–100 kd) is responsible for the extremely rapid, electrically neutral exchange of $HCO_3^-$ for $Cl^-$ in opposite directions across the membrane in the respiratory cycle of the red cell. This transport allows about 50% of $CO_2$ produced in the body to be transported as plasma bicarbonate, through the action of the red cell enzyme carbonic anhydrase. Unlike cation transport, anion transport is driven along concentration gradients and does not consume ATP. What role abnormal anion transport function might play in congenital hemolytic anemias is not yet certain. An abnormal band 3 molecule, with rapid movement on gel electrophoresis, has been described in congenital dyserythropoietic anemia type II (HEMPAS), a disorder in which the red cells lyse readily in the presence of complement (acidified serum test). Band 3 contains the major blood group antigens ABO and possibly some of the Rh and Kell determinants, although this matter is unresolved. This protein has an additional function in that its cytoplasmic domain is highly charged, and it forms an attachment site for the submembrane cytoskeleton as well as for several glycolytic enzymes and possibly hemoglobin. An atypical form of hereditary elliptocytosis may be due to an altered binding of the band 3 protein to ankyrin (vide infra). Abnormal association of sickle hemoglobin to this protein may contribute to the multitude of membrane abnormalities seen in sickle cell anemia.

The red cell cytoskeleton is a network of insoluble proteins that confers flexibility and strength to the cell. The major structural proteins are the spectrins (alpha and beta: bands 1 and 2), which account for 75% of the cytoskeletal mass. Alpha-spectrin (MW 240 kd) has five rigid alpha helical regions joined by flexible regions; beta-spectrin (MW 220 kd) has only four rigid alpha helical regions. These two proteins spontaneously associate to form heterodimers, and these dimers are capable of forming a head-to-head tetramer. In the cell, spectrin oligomers are joined by actin (band 5) and band 4.1. Another protein, ankyrin (band 2.1), serves to join the cytoskeleton to the membrane by attaching beta-spectrin to the anion transport protein. Membrane glycophorins also serve to attach the cytoskeleton to the membrane by binding to band 4.1. A variety of qualitative and quantitative spectrin abnormalities may be responsible for hereditary sperhocytosis (HS), spectrin abnormalites may be responsible for hereditary speherocytosis (HS), and abnormal spectrin-spectrin or spectrin-band 4.1 interactions may account for most forms of hereditary elliptocytosis (HE) and pyropoikilocytosis.

**MIM No.:** *10927, *13045, *13050, *13060, *17965, *17970, *18290, *18500, *18501, *19438, *20010, 2254

**Sex Ratio:** M1:F1 for most known variants.

**Occurrence:** For the more common disorders such as spherocytosis and elliptocytosis, the reader is referred to specific articles on these subjects. The true incidence of many of the rarer membrane defects are undetermined.

**Risk of Recurrence for Patient's Sib:**
See Part I, *Mendelian Inheritance.*

**Risk of Recurrence for Patient's Child:**
See Part I, *Mendelian Inheritance.*

**Age of Detectability:** At birth in most instances.

**Gene Mapping and Linkage:** EPB3 (erythrocyte surface protein band 3) has been provisionally mapped to 17q21-qter.

EL1 (elliptocytosis 1 (Rh-linked); band 4.1 protein) has been mapped to 1pter-p34.

SPH1 (spherocytosis 1 (clinical type II)) has been mapped to 8p21.1-p11.22.

ANK (ankyrin) has been provisionally mapped to 8p21-p11.

APOB (apolipoprotein B (including Ag(x) antigen)) has been mapped to 2p24-p23.

LCAT (lecithin-cholesterol acyltransferase) has been mapped to 16q22.1.

XK (Kell blood group precursor (McLeod phenotype)) has been mapped to Xp21.1.

**Prevention:** None known. Genetic counseling indicated.

**Treatment:** Hemolytic anemia associated with a variety of congenital membrane disorders may respond to splenectomy: spherocytosis, hemolytic forms of elliptocytosis, pyropoikilocytosis, and some forms of stomatocytosis. Other anemias may not improve with splenectomy. For many membrane disorders, no specific therapy is available. Severe anemias may require transfusion therapy, while milder anemias often require no therapy. Aplastic and hyperhemolytic crises may necessitate red cell transfusion. Transient folate deficiency may occur during recovery from aplastic crises and responds to folic acid therapy. Acanthocytosis in nutritional, malabsorptive, and lipid disorders is occasionally related to vitamin E deficiency and may respond to vitamin E therapy.

Because splenectomy carries a risk for potentially fatal bacterial infections, chiefly by pneumococcus, the decision to perform splenectomy must be based on several factors: a diagnosis in which the response to splenectomy is known, symptoms sufficiently severe to require intervention, and the ability to deliver effective prophylaxis against septicemia (pneumococcal vaccine, prophylactic penicillin therapy, prompt hospitalization for febrile illnesses, and so forth).

**Prognosis:** Varies with specific condition.

**Detection of Carrier:** In some instances, by hematologic examination.

**Special Considerations:** The first congenital membrane lesion to be recognized as a clinical entity was hereditary spherocytosis. In fact, this was the first hereditary hemolytic anemia of any kind to be described. In 1871, Vanlair and Masius reported a young woman with repeated attacks of abdominal pain over the spleen, associated with prostration and jaundice. The blood smear, with characteristic spherocytes, was described as containing "microcytes." Hereditary spherocytosis was at one time known as the *Minkowski-Chauffard syndrome.* In 1900, Oskar Minkowski provided the clinical descriptions of eight affected members within three generations of one family. In 1907, Anatole Chauffard discovered a major pathologic feature of spherocytosis, namely, the increased sensitivity to lysis of erythrocytes in hypotonic media. This test, the osmotic fragility test, remains the principal diagnostic procedure to date for spherocytosis. Chauffard also accurately implicated spleen as the culprit in the hemolytic process. Splenectomy for this disorder may date as far back as 1887. Differentiation between hereditary spherocytosis and "hereditary nonspherocytic anemias" was first made by Hayden in 1947. However, it was not until 1954 that Selwyn and Dacie concluded that some of these anemias were due to defective glucose utilization. Affected individuals had increased spontaneous hemolysis upon in vitro incubation of their red cells (autohemolysis), which, unlike spherocytosis, was not improved by incubation in the presence of glucose. An exciting discovery that for a while was thought to be responsible for the spherocyte formation in hereditary spherocytosis was the observation by Jacob and Jandl in 1964 that these erythrocytes had a marked increase in permeability to cations. Although abnormal cation permeability is a consistent feature of this disorder, this feature is not affected by splenectomy, despite the resolution of the hemolytic anemia. A major breakthrough in the study of the biochemistry of membrane disorders was the description by Fairbanks et al. in 1971, of the major polypeptide constituents of the red cell membrane using a sodium dodecyl sulfate polyacrylamide gel electrophoresis technique. The last two decades have seen an explosion in the knowledge of the structure and function of this intriguing membrane, and the natures of the molecular defects in many of these disorders are now being investigated.

**References:**
Biemer JJ: Acanthocytosis: biochemical and physiological considerations. Ann Clin Lab Sci 1980; 10:238–249.
Wintrobe MM: Blood, pure and eloquent. New York: McGraw Hill, 1980.
Baines AJ, et al.: Red cell membrane protein anomalies in congenital dyserythropoietic anaemia, type II (HEMPAS). Br J Haematol 1982; 50:563–574.
Frolich J, et al.: Lecithin:cholesterol acyl transferase (LCAT). Clin Biochem 1982; 15:269–278.
Lande WM, et al.: Missing band 7 membrane protein in two patients with high Na, low K erythrocytes. J Clin Invest 1982; 70:1273–1280.
Facer CA: Erythrocyte sialoglycoproteins and *Plasmodium falciparum* invasion. Trans R Soc Trop Med Hyg 1983; 77:524–530.
Knowles W, et al.: Spectrin: structure, function, and abnormalities. Semin Hematol 1983; 20:159–174.
Palek J, Lux SE: Red cell membrane skeletal defects in hereditary and acquired hemolytic anemias. Semin Hematol 1983; 20:189–224.
Ballas SK, et al.: Red cell membrane and cation deficiency in Rh null syndrome. Blood 1984; 63:1046–1055.
Fairbanks G, et al.: Passive cation transport in hereditary xerocytosis. Prog Clin Biol Res 1984; 159:205–217.
Kruckeberg WC, et al. (eds): Erythrocyte membranes 3: recent clinical and experimental advances. New York: Alan R. Liss, 1984.
Francke U, et al.: Minor Xp21 chromosome deletion in a male associated with expression of Duchenne muscular dystrophy, chronic granulomatous disease, retinitis pigmentosa, and McLeod syndrome. Am J Hum Genet 1985; 37:250–267.
Low PS: Structure and function of the cytoplasmic domain of band 3: center of erythrocyte membrane-peripheral protein interactions. Biochim Biophys Acta 1986; 864:146–167.
Kay MMB, et al.: Molecular anatomy of an anemia (Abstract) Clin Res 1987; 35:599A only.
Kuczmarski CA, et al.: Instability of red cell shape associated with the absence of membrane glycophorin C. Vox Sang 1987; 52:36–42.

LA041                                         **Richard J. Labotka**

**Anemia, high red cell phosphatidylcholine hemolytic**
  *See ANEMIA, HEMOLYTIC, RED CELL MEMBRANE DEFECTS*
**Anemia, hypochromic**
  *See ANEMIA, SIDEROBLASTIC*

---

## ANEMIA, HYPOPLASTIC CONGENITAL                       0051

**Includes:**
  Aregenerative anemia, chronic congenital
  Blackfan-Diamond syndrome
  Diamond-Blackfan syndrome
  Erythroid hypoplastic anemia, congenital
  Erythrogenesis imperfecta
  Estren-Dameshek variant of Fanconi anemia
  Hypoplastic anemia, congenital
  Red cell aregenerative anemia, congenital

**Excludes:**
  **Anemia, hypoplastic-triphalangeal thumbs, Aase-Smith type**
    (2028)
  Aplastic anemia with leukopenia or thrombocytopenia
  Aplastic phase of hemolytic anemia
  **Pancytopenia syndrome, Fanconi type** (2029)
  Secondary or transient hypoplastic anemia

**Major Diagnostic Criteria:**  Moderate to severe anemia with reticulocytopenia beginning in early infancy and without serious leukopenia or thrombocytopenia. Red cells are generally macrocytic. Bone marrow cytology shows normal white cell and megakaryocyte production with virtual absence of recognizable erythroid elements.

**Clinical Findings:**  Moderate to severe anemia is manifested by gradual onset of pallor generally before age three months. Sometimes the onset is shortly after birth, or it may rarely occur after six

to 12 months of age. The pulse becomes rapid as anemia increases, and cardiac enlargement and dilatation may develop. Heart failure and secondary pneumonia may ensue as the anemia becomes profound. A preagonal level as low as 1 gm/dl hemoglobin has been seen. The white cells are not affected and usually respond normally to infections. Platelets elevated are petechiae, ecchymoses, and free bleeding with trauma do not ordinarily occur. The plasma immunoglobulins are normal and no circulating antibodies against red cell elements are found. The spleen and liver are usually not enlarged except in association with hemosiderosis after years of multiple transfusions in the patients unresponsive to corticosteroids. Growth retardation of varying severity, from severe to relatively mild, is frequent. This is probably associated with the congenital nature of this disorder but may be augmented if there is chronic and recurrent anemia and particularly if corticosteroids must be given in large doses for long periods. Birth weights are low in over one-third of the recorded cases. The red cells show a distinct macrocytosis with mean cell volumes usually over 90 femtoliters and reaching 110 or more in some patients. This macrocytosis persists even during remissions. Reticulocytes are few or absent as are the recognizable erythroid elements in bone marrow. A few clusters of small cells resembling lymphocytes, not "blast-forms" but possibly erythroid precursors may be present. Red cell survival in the circulation is usually normal or only slightly shortened. The percent of fetal hemoglobin is characteristically elevated in most cases. Other evidences of fetal type of erythropoiesis are the presence of little "i" antigens on the red cell surface and higher levels of activity of red cell enzymes such as transaminase and glutathione peroxidase.

**Complications:**  Generalized hemosiderosis involving the skin and viscera can be caused by repeated transfusions. The liver, kidneys, spleen, and heart are early sites of excessive iron pigment deposits from the destruction of infused red cells and have storage lesions of varying severity. Continued transfusions may lead to allosensitization against red cell antigens (blood groups) foreign to the patient. Also, white cell, platelet, and even plasma factors may initiate antibody responses and cause subsequent troublesome transfusion reactions. In such cases, washed red cells may be required for each transfusion. Cirrhosis and liver failure as well as potentially fatal heart disease can result from the increasing iron accumulation. Chronic chelation therapy in transfusion-dependent patients may reduce the total body iron burden. Viral hepatitis may occur in patients receiving multiple blood transfusions and complicate the course of the disease. Growth retardation occurs in the multitransfused patients, possibly as a result of a combination of chronic anemia, liver insufficiency, and unknown metabolic derangements.

**Associated Findings:**  One or more associated congenital anomalies are found in about 20% of the patients. An unusual frequency of accessory or triphalangeal thumbs are also noted among these. Another abnormality of note is the presence of a short, webbed neck as seen in **Turner syndrome**. No abnormal karyotypes have been demonstrated.

**Etiology:**  Probably autosomal recessive inheritance although in rare cases there may be an autosomal dominant mode of transmission. Two affected sibs occur in about one-quarter of the families. Usually other relatives with the same condition are not found (3–4 possible cases) and related blood dyscrasias rarely occur in family members in contrast to **Pancytopenia syndrome, Fanconi type**. Parental consanguinity has been noted. Recently, however, a few families with possible affected persons in two or three generations are reported. These may have an autosomal dominant variant.

**Pathogenesis:**  The disorder probably is due to an end-organ failure of erythrogenesis beginning late in fetal life or early in infancy. The severity varies considerably but usually is alike in sibs. An enzymatic abnormality or defect is suggested by the corrective effect of adrenal corticosteroid therapy in most patients when it is begun early. No proof of this has been definitely found. On the other hand, there is some evidence that the erythroid stem cells in the bone marrow may be less numerous and relatively unresponsive to erythropoietin. Corticosteroids may induce more responsiveness and progression to normal growth and maturity. In most of these children the sensitivity of erythrogenesis to small changes, even 2.5-5 mg/week in prednisone dosage, is extraordinary. Spontaneous remissions occur, usually after puberty, even after years of transfusion therapy.

**MIM No.:**  20590, 10565

**Sex Ratio:**  M1:F1

**Occurrence:**  About 200 verified cases reported or recognized since first described in 1938. No racial or ethnic association.

**Risk of Recurrence for Patient's Sib:**
See Part I, *Mendelian Inheritance.*

**Risk of Recurrence for Patient's Child:**
See Part I, *Mendelian Inheritance.*

**Age of Detectability:**  Usually before six months of age.

**Gene Mapping and Linkage:**  Unknown.

**Prevention:**  None known. Genetic counseling indicated.

**Treatment:**  As soon as diagnosis is established by blood and bone marrow examinations, and exclusion of other causes, adrenal corticosteroid therapy should be started in order to increase the likelihood of a favorable response. Most infants under 4 months of age have shown rapid restoration of red cell levels whereas only one-half of those who have been treated by transfusions for a year or more have responded to corticosteroids thereafter. Usually oral prednisone is given 2–3 mg/kg/day for 7–10 days. Responders will show an increase in erythroblasts and normoblasts in bone marrow aspirates within 4–5 days and fairly brisk reticulocytosis in the peripheral blood shortly thereafter with a rise in hemoglobin or hematocrit levels following. If there is no response within 3–4 weeks, it is wiser to stop the drug lest its side effects become troublesome, and to delay another drug trial for a few months, using red cell transfusion when necessary. It has been recommended in such cases that corticosteroid be tried in large doses by parenteral routes, especially intravenously.

In the responders, the hemoglobin is brought to a normal level of 11–12 g/dl or more, using intermittent corticosteroid therapy (every other day or 3 consecutive days per week, etc). The dosage is then slowly diminished on a weekly basis until the hemoglobin value levels off at about 11 g/dl. Corticosteroid responsiveness generally continues even if the drug is stopped for a time and then resumed. In only a few cases have the patients become refractory to adrenal corticosteroid for no known reason. Any infection, overt or occult, may produce exacerbation of erythroid hypoplasia with recurrence of anemia requiring a temporary increase in corticosteroid dosage and possibly transfusion until the marrow recovers. When the disorder is unresponsive to adrenal corticosteroids, transfusions must be given every 4–6 weeks. The recently tested hepatitis B vaccine should be given to these patients.

**Prognosis:**  If treatment with corticosteroid is successful, the patient's health seems to be unimpaired except for possible growth retardation. Remission with no further need for therapy may occur within a few years of beginning treatment or more commonly by early adolescence. Relapses have occurred in some patients particularly following nonspecific viral infections, often of the mildest form. Usually resumption of corticosteroid treatment for a few weeks or months may be necessary if the anemia does not improve spontaneously. There have been rare reports of patients who developed complete aplastic anemia with leukopenia and thrombopenia after having become refractory to corticosteroid. Bone marrow transplantation may then become necessary. Also, at least five cases of leukemia have been reported after patients have had complete remissions.

**Detection of Carrier:**  Unknown.

**References:**
Diamond LK, et al.: Congenital hypoplastic anemia. In: Schulman I, ed: Advances in pediatrics, vol. 22. Chicago: Year Book Medical Publishers, 1976:349–378.

Alter BP: Childhood red cell aplasia. Am J Pediat Hematol/Oncol 1980; 2:221. Freedman MH: Congenital failure of hematopoiesis in the newborn infant. Clinics in Perinatology 1984; 11:417.

Szsoylu S: High-dose intravenous corticosteroid for a patient with Diamond-Blackfan syndrome refractory to classical prednisone treatment. Acta Haematologica 1984; 71:207.

Nowell P, et al.: Progressive preleukemia with a chromosomally abnormal clone in a kindred with the Estren-Dameshek variant of Fanconi's anemia. Blood 1984; 64:1135–1138.

Viskochil DH, et al.: Congenital hypoplastic (Diamond-Blackfan) anemia in seven members of one kindred. Am J Med Genet 1990; 35:251–256.

K0003                                         Marion A. Koerper
                                              *Louis K. Diamond*

---

## ANEMIA, HYPOPLASTIC-TRIPHALANGEAL THUMBS, AASE-SMITH TYPE                                    2028

**Includes:**
Aase syndrome
Thumbs, triphalangeal-hypoplastic anemia

**Excludes:**
**Anemia, hypoplastic congenital** (0051)
**Heart-hand syndrome** (0455)
**Pancytopenia syndrome, Fanconi type** (2029)
**Thrombocytopenia-absent radius** (0941)

**Major Diagnostic Criteria:**  Triphalangeal (finger-like) thumbs and pure red cell anemia without leukopenia or thrombocytopenia.

**Clinical Findings:**  Triphalangeal thumbs with hypoplasia of the thenar muscles; moderate-to-severe anemia with low reticulocyte count.

**Complications:**  If repeated transfusions are necessary, complications of this treatment may be seen, including hypersplenism with secondary thrombocytopenia, hemosiderosis, transfusion reactions, and growth retardation.

**Associated Findings:**  Narrow shoulders, cleft lip/palate, vertebral anomalies, and **Ventricular septal defect**.

**Etiology:**  Autosomal recessive inheritance.

**Pathogenesis:**  Unknown.

**MIM No.:**  20560

**POS No.:**  3829

**Sex Ratio:**  M1:F1

**Occurrence:**  About 20 cases reported in the literature.

**Risk of Recurrence for Patient's Sib:**
See Part I, *Mendelian Inheritance.*

**Risk of Recurrence for Patient's Child:**
See Part I, *Mendelian Inheritance.*

**Age of Detectability:**  At birth for thumb abnormalities; in infancy for anemia.

**Gene Mapping and Linkage:**  Unknown.

**Prevention:**  None known. Genetic counseling indicated.

**Treatment:**  In several instances, the anemia has responded to steroid therapy. Prednisone in appropriate dosage should be tried, and some patients have achieved apparently permanent remission of their anemia after cessation of therapy.

**Prognosis:**  Normal life span; anemia may persist if unresponsive to steroids, and periodic transfusions may be necessary.

**Detection of Carrier:**  Unknown.

**Special Considerations:**  Some authors have suggested that this condition is simply a variant of the Blackfan-Diamond syndrome (see **Anemia, hypoplastic congenital**), and indeed, 1:30 patients in the original description of that disorder had triphalangeal thumbs, and 6:133 cases in a later review were similarly affected. However, the Blackfan-Diamond syndrome appears to be a heterogeneous category with examples of both autosomal dominant and autosomal recessive inheritance patterns. Reports of affected sibs with the Aase syndrome would indicate that the condition "breeds true" within families. This could be explained by: 1) variability of expression for the Blackfan-Diamond gene in those families; 2) close linkage between the Blackfan-Diamond locus and one for triphalangeal thumbs; or 3) a unique gene mutation that produces both the cardinal features of the syndrome. While the last seems the most likely possibility, final reconciliation of the controversy will depend upon delineation of further families with multiple affected members, and future gene linkage analysis and/or gene mapping.

**References:**
Diamond LK, et al.: Congenital (erythroid) hypoplastic anemia. Am J Dis Child 1961; 102:403–415.
Aase JM, Smith DW: Congenital anemia and triphalangeal thumbs: a new syndrome. J Pediatr 1969; 74:471–474. * †
Alter BP: Thumbs and anemia. Pediatrics 1978; 62:613–614.
Higginbottom MC, et al.: The Aase syndrome in a female infant. J Med Genet 1978; 15:484–486.
Pfeiffer RA, Ambs A: Das Aase-syndrom: autosomal-rezessiv vererbte, konnatal insuffiziente Erythropoese und triphalangie der daumen. Monatsschr Kinderheilk 1983; 131:235–237.
Muis N, et al.: The Aase syndrome: case report and review of the literature. Europ J Pediatr 1986; 145:153–157.

AA003                                              **Jon M. Aase**

---

## ANEMIA, PERNICIOUS CONGENITAL                        2656

**Includes:**
Absence of intrinsic factor, congenital
Intrinsic factor, abnormal
Pernicious anemia, due to defect in intrinsic factor

**Excludes:**
Pernicious anemia (others)
**Vitamin B(12) malabsorption** (0992)

**Major Diagnostic Criteria:** Megaloblastic anemia, irritability, and failure to thrive are the presenting clinical features. The diagnosis is confirmed by the demonstration of low serum vitamin $B_{12}$, an abnormal Schilling test, absent gastric secretion of intrinsic factor, normal gastric acidity, and absence of antibodies directed against intrinsic factor or gastric parietal cells.

**Clinical Findings:** The great majority of patients present before age three years, but sporadic cases have been diagnosed as late as the second or third decade. At presentation children demonstrate megaloblastic anemia with macrocytic red cells and hypersegmented neutrophils. Some patients are irritable and fail to thrive. Bone marrow aspiration usually reveals a hypercellular marrow with megaloblastic changes in all the hematopoietic lineages.
Serum vitamin $B_{12}$ levels are low. Schilling test reveals almost complete failure to absorb an orally administered dose of radioactive cobalamin. The malabsorption can be completely corrected by concomitant oral administration of intrinsic factor.
In distinction to classic addisonian pernicious anemia, gastric acidity is normal; the gastric mucosa is normal without atrophy; there are no serum antibodies to intrinsic factor or to gastric parietal cells. Gastric contents contain no immunologically detectable intrinsic factor. One patient has been described with immunologically recognizable intrinsic factor that bound cobalamin but could not bind to the terminal ileum, the site of absorption of cobalamin-intrinsic factor complex. Other patients have been described with intrinsic factor that was unusually susceptible to breakdown by acid and proteolytic enzymes.

**Complications:** Administration of folate may ameliorate the anemia but can exacerbate neurologic deficits.

**Associated Findings:** None known.

**Etiology:** Autosomal recessive inheritance.

**Pathogenesis:** Alleles that do not code for immunologically or functionally recognizable intrinsic factor.

**MIM No.:** *26100

**Sex Ratio:** M1:F1

**Occurrence:** Several dozen cases have been described. Many, but not all, occur in large, consanguineous kinships.

**Risk of Recurrence for Patient's Sib:**
See Part I, *Mendelian Inheritance.*

**Risk of Recurrence for Patient's Child:**
See Part I, *Mendelian Inheritance.*

**Age of Detectability:** Usually presents between ages four and 28 months of age, but could theoretically be diagnosed at birth.

**Gene Mapping and Linkage:** Unknown.

**Prevention:** None known. Genetic counseling indicated.

**Treatment:** Parenteral administration of cyanocobalamin or hydroxycobalamin is curative. Lifetime administration is required.

**Prognosis:** Normal life span.

**Detection of Carrier:** Unknown.

**References:**
McIntyre OR, et al.: Pernicious anemia in childhood. New Engl J Med 1965; 273:432–438.
Miller DR, et al.: Juvenile "congenital" pernicious anemia. New Engl J Med 1966; 275:978–983.
McNicholl B, Egan B: Congenital pernicious anemia: effects on growth, brain, and absorption of B12. Pediatrics 1968; 42:149–156.
Katz M, et al.: Vitamin B(12) malabsorption due to biologically inert intrinsic factor. New Engl J Med 1972; 287:425–429.
Heisel MA, et al.: Congenital pernicious anemia: report of seven patients, with studies of the extended family. J Pediatr 1984; 105:564–568.
Yang Y, et al.: Cobalamin malabsorption in three siblings due to an abnormal intrinsic factor that is markedly susceptible to acid and proteolysis. J Clin Invest 1985; 76:2057–2065.

ME040                                              **Paul Meyers**

**Anemia, pernicous, juvenile**
*See VITAMIN B(12) MALABSORPTION*

---

## ANEMIA, SICKLE CELL                                    0886

**Includes:**
Ahotutuo
Anemia falciforme
Chwechweechwe
Drepanocytic anemia
Homozygous sickle hemoglobinopathy
Lakuregebee
Nuidudui
Orengua
Sickle cell anemia

**Excludes:**
Sickle beta-thalassemia
Sickle cell trait (sickle hemoglobin heterozygosity)

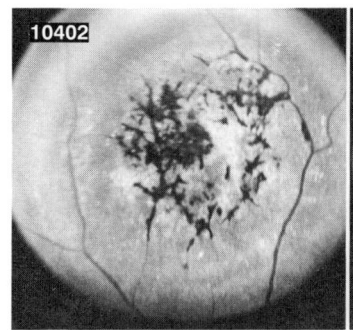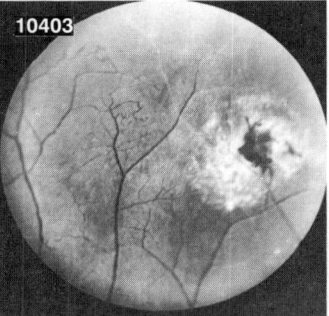

**0886**-10402–03: Examples of black sunburst in sickle cell anemia.

**Table 0886-1**  Sickle Cell Syndromes Associated with Significant Clinical Disease

| Sickle Cell Disorder | Hemoglobin Composition | Hb A₂ level | Erythrocyte Volume (MCV) | Clinical Severity | Clinical Features |
|---|---|---|---|---|---|
| Hb SS | Hb S: 80–95%<br>Hb F: 2–20% | normal | normal | ++ to ++++ | (see text) |
| Hb S β⁰ thal. | Hb S: 75–90%<br>Hb F: 5–25% | increased | decreased | ++ to ++++ | Generally indistinguishable from SS |
| Hb S β⁺ thal. | Hb S: 55–85%<br>Hb A: 10–30%<br>Hb F: 5–10% | increased | decreased | + to +++ | Generally milder than SS |
| Hb S δβ thal. | Hb S: 60–80%<br>Hb F: 15–40% | normal | decreased | + to ++ | Mild sickle cell disease |
| Hb SS with α thal. trait (α,-/α,-) | Hb S: 80–90%<br>Hb F: 10–20% | normal | decreased | ++ to ++++ | May be milder than SS |
| Hb SC | Hb S: 45–50%<br>Hb C: 45–50%<br>Hb F: 2–5% | normal | normal | + to +++ | Generally milder than SS; higher frequency of bone infarcts and proliferative retinal disease |
| Hb SO-Arab | Hb S: 50–55%<br>Hb O: 40–45%<br>Hb F 2–15% | normal | normal | ++ to ++++ | Generally indistinguishable from SS |
| Hb SD-Los Angeles | Hb S: 45–50%<br>Hb D: 30–40%<br>Hb F: 5–20% | normal | normal | ++ to ++++ | May be as severe as SS |
| Hb SC-Harlem | Hb S: 45–50%<br>Hb C_H: 45–50%<br>Hb F: 5–10% | normal | normal | ++ to ++++ | Similar to SS |

Sickle hemoglobin with other structurally abnormal hemoglobins

**Major Diagnostic Criteria:** Chronic hemolytic anemia with intermittant episodes of "pain crises" with pallor, fever, swelling of extremities, and red blood cells showing sickle shape when deoxygenated. Hemoglobin electrophoresis demonstrates sickle hemoglobin, with an absence of hemoglobin A or other structurally abnormal hemoglobins. Variable quantities of hemoglobin F (fetal hemoglobin) may be present. The presence of β-thalassemia, hereditary persistence of fetal hemoglobin, and other abnormal hemoglobins with electrophoretic mobility similar or identical with that of hemoglobin S, may require additional studies for exclusion. The presence of hemoglobin S demonstrated in each parent, and confirmed by a sickling test, provides the most reliable means for establishing the diagnosis.

**Clinical Findings:** The earliest manifestation of sickle cell anemia is often a dactylitis of the phalanges of the hands and feet presenting in infancy as a swelling of the affected areas, and associated with fever and irritability. In the older child and adult, the *pain crisis* is the most characteristic clinical expression. In relatively younger children, pain most commonly occurs in the limbs; painful episodes involving the back, thorax, abdomen, and head occur more often in older children and adults. Acidosis, dehydration, and fever, frequently associated with intercurrent infections, often precipitate these episodes of pain crisis. Clinical features associated with chronic hemolysis are present, including pallor, jaundice, an increase in the reticulocyte count, and erythroid hyperplasia of the bone marrow. Stained smears of peripheral blood demonstrate polychromatophilia and target cells, and frequently include sickled erythrocytes. Howell-Jolly bodies are often present in peripheral blood erythrocytes in the older child and adult. Hyposthenuria, or the inability to concentrate urine, is a constant feature in the adult.

**Complications:** *Ischemia:* Occlusion of major blood vessels by masses of sickled cells may produce gross infarction leading to major degrees of organ dysfunction. Ischemia of bone may lead to avascular necrosis. Massive liver necrosis and kidney failure may develop. Major insults to the central nervous system (CNS) are

frequent, and severe sequelae, including hemiparesis, have been described in up to 25% of reported cases.

*Splenic enlargement* is often present in younger children, and may produce the hematologic picture of hypersplenism. In the older child, the pattern of blood circulation through the spleen is altered so as to shunt the circulating blood away from the active follicles. The result of this alteration is a "functional asplenia"; a change that helps to explain the increased susceptibility of these patients to pneumococcal and *H. influenzae* infections. "Autosplenectomy" is common in adults, resulting from a process of involution attributable to repeated episodes of splenic infarction.

*Osteomyelitis:* For reasons that are poorly understood, children with sickle cell anemia have an unusual predisposition to develop osteomyelitis, most commonly due to *Salmonella* and other enteropathic organisms.

*Gallstones* are related to the chronic hemolytic process, and while uncommon in younger children, occur with a substantial, increasing frequency in teenagers and adults.

*Aplastic crisis* is seen in all forms of chronic hemolytic anemia, and results from a transient period of erythroid aplasia in the bone marrow. These episodes have been shown to be related to parvovirus infections. Rapidly increasing anemia, sometimes life-threatening, is accompanied by an absence or major reduction in the reticulocyte count.

*Acute Splenic Sequestration crisis* occurs almost exclusively in infants and young children, and presents as a sudden onset of severe anemia accompanied by an acutely enlarged spleen. Transfusions may be life-saving.

*Priapism* is relatively uncommon and results from pooling of sickle cells in the corpora cavernosa causing obstruction of the venous outflow.

*Leg ulcers*, although unusual in children, occur frequently in adults. Blood stasis, perhaps accompanied by trauma, is assumed responsible.

**Associated Findings:** Sexual maturation is often delayed. Adults frequently exhibit increased height, with long limbs and a decrease in the upper-to-lower segment ratio.

Three major "haplotypes" of Hb S alleles, i.e., linked sets of restriction fragment length polymorphisms, have been identified, and have been shown to be associated with greater or lesser degrees of disease severity in homozygotes. One of the less severe alleles has been shown to exist in linkage with a gene that promotes a higher level of Hb F production.

**Etiology:** Autosomal recessive inheritance of a substitution of valine for glutamate at position number 6 of the hemoglobin beta chains.

**Pathogenesis:** As a consequence of the structural abnormality of the hemoglobin in this condition, under conditions of deoxygenation a process of molecular aggregation of the hemoglobin occurs, resulting in the formation of rigid fiber-like structures. This change imparts a major distortion to the red blood cell, causing it to assume an elongated shape and rigid, brittle properties. Under circumstances of deoxygenation, primarily involving the venous side of the circulation, masses of these sickled cells bring about varying degrees of vascular obstruction. Conditions of acidosis, dehydration, and hypoxia all may potentiate this process.

The high prevalence of the Hb S allele in various subtropical regions is believed to represent a "balanced polymorphism", with its deleterious effect in the homozygote being offset by its protective effect in heterozygotes against *falciparum* malaria (Honig and Adams, 1986).

**MIM No.:** *14190

**CDC No.:** 282.600

**Sex Ratio:** M1:F1

**Occurrence:** An estimated 1:625 births in the American black population. A considerably higher risk has been established in certain areas of West Africa. Other populations of substantial risk include areas of Greece, Italy, several Mid-Eastern populations, Southern Turkey, and certain populations of Southern India. Prevalence estimated to be 1:1,875 in the American black population.

**Risk of Recurrence for Patient's Sib:**
See Part I, *Mendelian Inheritance.*

**Risk of Recurrence for Patient's Child:**
See Part I, *Mendelian Inheritance.*

**Age of Detectability:** Clinically, at about three to six months of age. Can be detected at birth, and prenatally in the first or second trimester fetus by special studies. Neonatal screening programs for sickle cell disease have been established in many parts of the United States.

**Gene Mapping and Linkage:** HBB (hemoglobin, beta) has been mapped to 11p15.5.

**Prevention:** None known. Genetic counseling indicated.

**Treatment:** Many complications are not presently preventable. However, a generally less severe clinical course is observed in patients who receive good nutrition and prompt treatment of intercurrent infections, dehydration, and related problems. Oral penicillin prophylaxis in infants and young children has been shown to be very effective in preventing serious pneumococcal infections.

Specific forms of therapy are not available. Transfusions often provide a major temporary supportive role when various complications of this disease occur. Bone marrow transplantation has been carried out in selected patients, and when successful is curative. Experimental treatment using 5-azacytidine and hydroxyurea has provided symptomatic benefit in some patients, due to a resulting elevation of their levels of hemoglobin F.

**Prognosis:** The clinical course is extremely variable and often unpredictable. Patients having access to adequate medical care often survive into adulthood, and lead productive lives.

**Detection of Carrier:** The heterozygous carrier can be readily identified by any of a variety of sickling tests. A positive test requires confirmation by hemoglobin electrophoresis.

**Special Considerations:** Of major diagnostic importance is the need to distinguish this condition from a variety of phenotypically similar sickling syndromes. Many of these are indistinguishable from sickle cell anemia by application of usual hematologic studies, and in some cases can be identified only by family studies and other special forms of testing. Some of the known phenocopies of sickle cell anemia carry strikingly different implications for treatment and prognosis, and for this reason need to be distinguished from sickle cell anemia. In general, if both parents are available for study, the finding in each parent of a positive sickling test, and an electrophoresis study consistent with sickle trait, will allow the diagnosis to be established with certainty.

**Support Groups:**
Los Angeles; National Association for Sickle Cell Diseases (NASCD)
　Chicago; Midwest Association for Sickle Cell Anemia (MASCA)
　DC; Washington; Center for Sickle Cell Disease
　TX; Houston; National Sickle Cell Clinics Foundation
　CANADA: Ontario; Toronto; The Canadian Sickle Cell Society

**References:**
Motulsky AG: Frequency of sickling disorders in U.S. blacks. New Engl J Med 1973; 288:31–33.
Nagel RL, et al.: Hematologically and genetically distinct forms of sickle cell anemia in Africa. New Engl J Med 1985; 312:880–884.
Serjeant GR: Sickle cell disease. New York; Oxford University Press, 1985.
Gaston M, et al.: Prophylaxis with oral penicillin in children with sickle cell anemia. New Engl J Med 1986; 314:1593–1599.
Honig GR, Adams JG III: Human hemoglobin genetics. Vienna: Springer-Verlag, 1986.
Vermylen C, et al.: Bone marrow transplantation in five children with sickle cell anemia. Lancet 1988; II:1427–1428.
Vichinsky E, et al.: Newborn screening for sickle cell disease: effect on mortality. Pediatrics 1988; 81:749–755.
Newborn screening for sickle cell disease and other hemoglobinopathies. Pediatrics 1989; 83:813–914.

H0024 　　　　　　　　　　　　　　　　　　**George R. Honig**

---

## ANEMIA, SIDEROBLASTIC 　　　　　　　　　　　1518

**Includes:**
　　Anemia, hypochromic
　　Factor IX defeciency-sideroblastic anemia
　　Glucose-6-phosphate dehydrogenase deficiency-
　　　sideroblastic anemia
　　Iron-loading anemia
　　Sideroblastic anemia, autosomal recessive
　　Sideroblastic anemia-exocrine pancreatic dysfunction
　　Sideroblastic anemia-glucose-6-phosphate dehydrogenase
　　　deficiency
　　Sideroblastic anemia-Xg(a) blood group antigen
　　Sideroblastic anemia, X-linked
　　Sideroblastic anemia, X-linked-ataxia
　　Spinocerebellar ataxia-sideroblastic anemia

**Excludes:** Acquired sideroblastic anemias

**Major Diagnostic Criteria:** Variably severe hypochromic-microcytic anemia with or without siderocytes in the blood is present at birth. In the X-linked type, female carriers are usually not anemic, the MCV is often normal, but a microcytic erythrocyte population is detected on the blood smear or by automated cell size distribution analysis. Ring sideroblasts in the Prussian blue-stained bone marrow aspirate confirm the diagnosis. The serum iron profile (serum iron, transferrin saturation, and ferritin) may be normal or reflect iron overload even before transfusions have been given.

**Clinical Findings:** Symptoms and signs of variable anemia may be present at birth; sometimes it may be noted only in adulthood or not at all. Hepatosplenomegaly may occur. Depending on the severity of the defect, the condition tends to be stable, and progression to an iron overload state with organ damage is gradual unless regular transfusions are given.

**Complications:** The principal complication is a slowly progressive iron overload in most cases. The iron overload produces micronodular cirrhosis, heart failure and arrhythmias, and im-

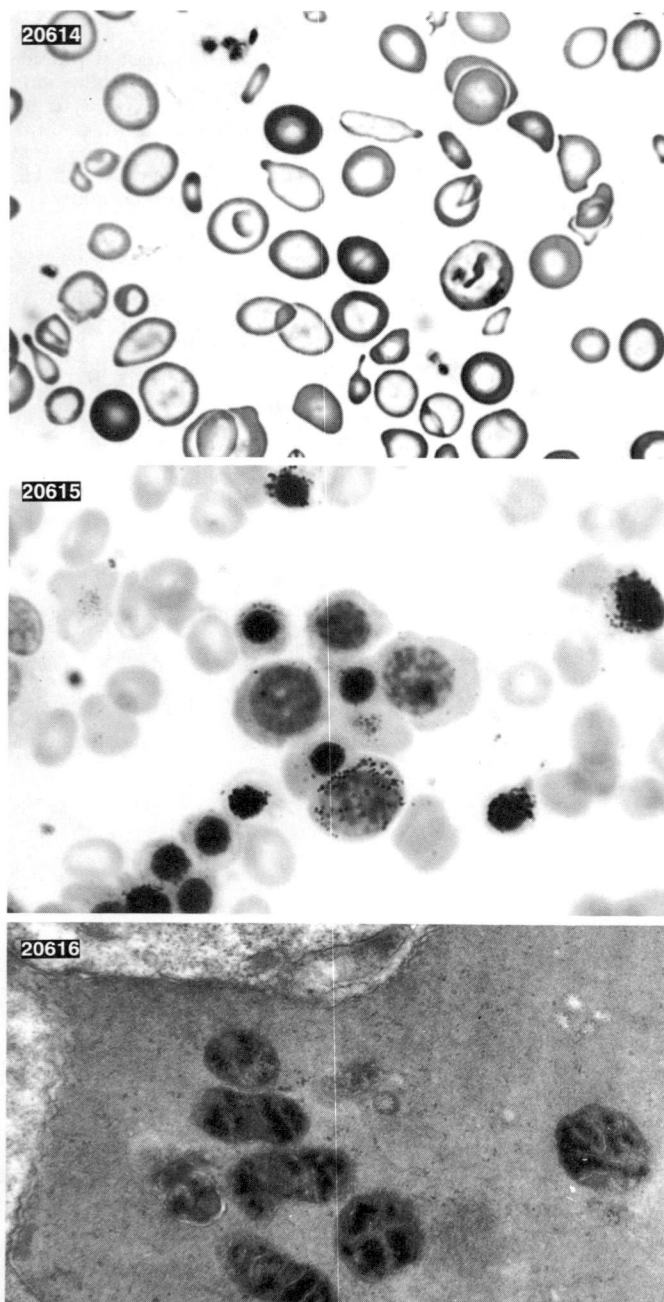

**1518-20614:** Anemia, sideroblastic, congenital; note peripheral smear (Wright's stain × 1200) showing marked hypochromia, microcytosis and poikilocytosis. **20615:** Bone marrow smear (Prussian blue stain × 1500), showing ring sideroblasts. **20616:** Electron micrograph of a portion of an erythroblast with numerous iron-laden mitochondria, × 33,000.

pairs normal growth and endocrine functions if not controlled by iron chelation therapy or, in less anemic cases, phlebotomy. Transfusion therapy predictably accelerates any iron overload state and introduces the risk of transfusion-associated viral illnesses.

**Associated Findings:** In some kindreds the anemia is very responsive to pharmacologic doses of vitamin $B_6$, and the hemoglobin is often restored to normal. However, the abnormal red cell morphology persists.

Several individual kindreds with the X-linked type have been described in which another X-linked trait segregated with the erythroid defect. In one, but not in others examined, affected female heterozygotes expressed the $Xg^a$ antigen on the abnormal erythrocyte population, while males in this family may have succumbed to the defect *in utero*. In another family, the sideroblastic anemia defect and **Glucose-6-phosphate dehydrogenase deficiency** segregated in affected males, and female carriers exhibited only the mild morphologic abnormalities. In two further kindreds, sideroblastic anemia and a nonprogressive spinocerebellar ataxia syndrome segregated in an X-linked recessive manner. In these the anemia was mild; iron overload was not yet evident in the very young affected males, but the free erythrocyte protoporphyrin (FEP) was raised. Some heterozygous females expressed the erythroid defect by having only a hypochromic red cell population, a raised FEP, and marrow ring sideroblasts, but no anemia or neurologic deficit.

**Hemophilia B** and sideroblastic anemia occurred in a Swedish family. Using the Factor IX deficiency as an X-chromosome marker, the sideroblastic trait appeared to be an autosomal transmission.

In five unrelated infants, moderate-to-severe congenital sideroblastic anemia was associated with variable exocrine pancreatic dysfunction and in some with extensive fibrosis of the pancreas. The anemia was normocytic to macrocytic and was accompanied by variable pancytopenia and marked vacuolization of erythroid and myeloid precursor cells in the bone marrow. The milder affected patients experienced apparent spontaneous improvement; the severe affected ones died early from complicating medical illnesses.

**Etiology:** X-linked and autosomal recessive forms have been identified. Others occur as isolated congenital types.

**Pathogenesis:** Experimental models of vitamin $B_6$ depletion and crude enzyme assays of bone marrow 5-aminolevulinic acid (ALA) synthase in a few cases support an abnormality of the ALA synthase enzyme, catalyzing the initial step of heme biosynthesis. When measured, the enzyme activity has been uniformly reduced and was variably enhanced by its coenzyme pyridoxal-phosphate, apparently stabilizing a labile enzyme or enhancing coenzyme affinity for the enzyme. These findings in part explain why supraphysiologic supply of the coenzyme *in vivo* can enhance ALA synthase activity sufficiently to restore effective erythropoiesis and correct the hemoglobin values (pyridoxine-responsive anemia) in some cases.

Recent work has demonstrated two genes for ALA synthase; a housekeeping gene and an erythroid-specific gene that is coexpressed with the former only in erythroid cells but to a much greater extent. While the human liver ALA synthase gene is on chromosome 3, the erythroid gene maps to the X chromosome, suggesting that a defect(s) in this gene may underlie X-linked sideroblastic anemia(s).

**MIM No.:** *30130, 30131

**Sex Ratio:** M1:F0 for full expression in X-linked cases; otherwise, theoretically, M1:F1

**Occurrence:** Unknown.

**Risk of Recurrence for Patient's Sib:**
See Part I, *Mendelian Inheritance.*

**Risk of Recurrence for Patient's Child:**
See Part I, *Mendelian Inheritance.*

**Age of Detectability:** Usually evident at birth or in early childhood; mild forms and female heterozygotes may only be detected by analysis of red cell and bone marrow morphology, iron status, and occasionally the FEP.

**Gene Mapping and Linkage:** ASB (anemia, sideroblastic/hypochromic) has been mapped to X.

Recent work has demonstrated two genes for ALA synthase, a housekeeping gene and an erythroid-specific gene that is coexpressed with the former only in erythroid cells but to a much greater extent. While the human liver ALA synthase gene is on chromosome 3, the erythroid gene maps to the X chromosome, suggesting that the defect(s) in this gene may underlie X-linked sideroblastic anemia(s).

**Prevention:** None known. Genetic counseling indicated.

**Treatment:** Therapeutic trial with vitamin $B_6$ at diagnosis. Transfusion and iron chelation therapy as indicated.

**Prognosis:** Good for mild cases; guarded in more severe cases.

**Detection of Carrier:** By analysis of blood smear, cell size and FEP in some cases; by bone marrow examination in others.

**Special Considerations:** An intrinsic mitochondrial defect impairing heme biosynthesis, specifically, the function of ALA synthase possibly through altered handling of iron or its toxicity, cannot be excluded in etiology or pathogenesis. The raised FEP and impaired ferrochelatase in occasional cases could also result from such alternative mechanisms. Even the limited data available suggest considerable heterogeneity in the fundamental mechanisms of hereditary sideroblastic anemia. The associated X-linked defects noted in the X-linked forms may relate to mutations of either closely linked loci or pleiotropic effects of an altered allele.

**References:**
Pearson HA, et al.: A new syndrome of refractory sideroblastic anemia with vacuolization of marrow precursors and exocrine pancreatic dysfunction. J Pediatr 1979; 95:976–984.

Bottomley SS: Sideroblastic anaemia. In: Jacob A, Worwood M, eds: Iron in biochemistry and medicine II. London: Academic Press, 1980:363–392.

Buchanan GR, et al.: Bone marrow delta-aminolaevulinate synthase deficiency in a female with congenital sideroblastic anemia. Blood 1980; 55:109–115.

Hast R, et al.: Hereditary ring sideroblastic anaemia and Christmas disease in a Swedish family. Scand J Haematol 1983; 30:444–450.

Pagon RA, et al.: Hereditary sideroblastic anaemia and ataxia: an X-linked recessive disorder. J Med Genet 1985; 22:267–273.

Sutherland GR, et al.: 5-Aminolevulinate synthase is at 3p21 and thus not the primary defect in X-linked sideroblastic anemia. Am J Hum Genet 1988; 43:331–335.

Cox TC, et al.: Erythroid 5-aminolevulinate synthase is located on the X chromosome. Am J Hum Genet 1990; 46:107–111.

B0050                                    **Sylvia S. Bottomley**

**Anemia, spherocytic, congenital**
*See SPHEROCYTOSIS*

---

## ANENCEPHALY                                              0052

**Includes:**
    Acrania
    Anencephaly-spina bifida
    Arnold-Chiari malformation
    Craniorachischisis
    Exencephaly
    Hemicrania
    Neural tube defects, X-linked

**Excludes:**
    **Brain, Arnold-Chiari malformation** (2944)
    **Hydranencephaly** (0480)
    **Schisis association** (2249)

**Major Diagnostic Criteria:** Absence or deficiency of a major portion of the cranial vault at birth. Anencephaly should be suspected when hydramnios develops during the pregnancy.

**Clinical Findings:** The cranial vault is deficient with frontal, parietal, and occipital bones present only in their basal portions. The basal bones are abnormal with small orbits causing protrusion of the eyes. Exposed neural tissue is pervaded by an angiomatous stroma filling the open cranial defect, usually covered by a thin membrane (possibly arachnoid) continuous with surrounding hair-bearing skin. The child is generally stillborn or short-lived.

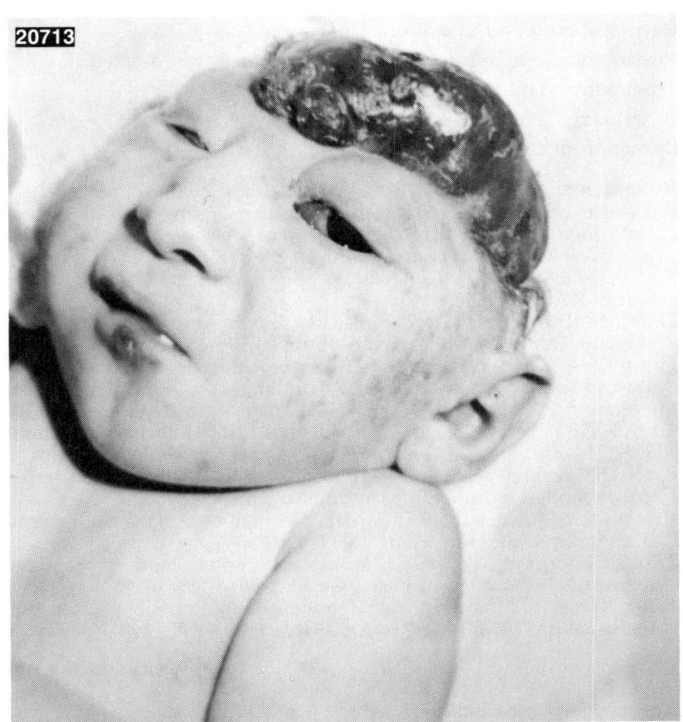

0052-20713: Anencephaly; note deficient cranial vault, protruding eyes and unilateral microphthalmia.

---

**Complications:** Unknown.

**Associated Findings:** Ganglia cells of the retina are absent. The pituitary gland is represented by the anterior lobe only. Other findings include an adrenal cortex of adult type with high pressor amine content, amyelia, and spina bifida.

**Etiology:** In doubt, but appears to be multifactorial. Genetic factors seem important by the familial incidence, while geographic variation suggests an environmental cause. Causative factors act on the developing embryo between the 16th and 26th day after conception. Concordance and discordance have occurred in monozygous twins.

**Pathogenesis:** Secondary necrosis of developing cerebral hemispheres.

**MIM No.:** 20650, 20795, 30141

**POS No.:** 3720

**CDC No.:** 740.0

**Sex Ratio:** M1:F3–7

**Occurrence:** Variable; 1:1000 live births to as high as 1:105 births in South Wales. Increasing risk is associated with birth order.

**Risk of Recurrence for Patient's Sib:** 1:20 (5%); a second affected sib raises risk to 13%.

**Risk of Recurrence for Patient's Child:** Unknown.

**Age of Detectability:** At birth or prenatally, may be detected by maternal serum and amniotic fluid alpha-fetoprotein (AFP) testing, which yields increased fibrin/fibrinogen degradation products; increased acetylcholinesterase, cholinesterase in amniotic fluid; decreased glucose; rapidly adherent neural cells in 20-hour culture of amniotic fluid cells; smear of uncultured amniotic fluid cells shows increased proportions of macrophages and elongated cells. Also detected by in utero ultrasound.

**Gene Mapping and Linkage:** Unknown.

**Prevention:** None known. Genetic counseling indicated.

**Treatment:** Unknown.

**Prognosis:** Stillborn or death at birth.

**Detection of Carrier:** Unknown.

**References:**
Carter CO, et al.: The genetics of the major central nervous system malformations, based on the South Wales socio-genetic investigation. Dev Med Child Neurol (Suppl.) 1967; 13:30.
Yen S, MacMahon B: Genetics of anencephaly and spina bifida? Lancet II 1968; 623–626.
Laurence KM: The recurrence risk in spina bifida cystica and anencephaly. Dev Med Child Neurol (Suppl.) 1969; 20:23.
Fuhrmann W, et al.: Apparently monogenic inheritance of anencephaly and spina bifida in a kindred. Humangenetik 1971; 13: 241–243.
Lindenberg R, Walker BA: Arnold-Chiari malformation in sibs. BD: OAS VII(1). New York: March of Dimes Birth Defects Foundation, 1971:234–236.
Brock DJH, et al.: Prenatal diagnosis of anencephaly through maternal serum-alphafetoprotein measurement. Lancet 1973; 2:923.
Imaizumi Y: Anencephaly in Japan: paternal age, maternal age and birth order. Ann Hum Genet 1979; 42:445.
Toriello HV, et al.: Possible X-linked anencephaly and spina bifida: report of a kindred. Am J Med Genet 1980; 6:119–121.
Farag TI, et al.: Nonsyndromal anencephaly: possible autosomal recessive trait. Am J Med Genet 1986; 24:461–464.

SH007                                    **Kenneth Shapiro**

**Anencephaly-spina bifida**
    See ANENCEPHALY
    also BRAIN, ARNOLD-CHIARI MALFORMATION
**Anesthesia, malignant hyperthermia susceptibility**
    See MYOPATHY, MALIGNANT HYPERTHERMIA
**Anetodermia-exostoses-brachydactyly type E**
    See EXOSTOSES-ANETODERMIA-BRACHYDACTYLY TYPE E
**Aneuploidy, chromosomal**
    See CHROMOSOME X, TRIPLO-X
    also CHROMOSOME X, POLY-X
**Aneurysm of aortic sinus of Valsalva**
    See AORTIC SINUS OF VALSALVA, ANEURYSM
**Aneurysm of membranous septum with one or more perforations**
    See VENTRICULAR SEPTAL DEFECT
**Aneurysm of middle ear**
    See EAR, ANEURYSM OF INTERNAL CAROTID ARTERY
**Aneurysm serpentina of external ear**
    See EAR, ARTERIOVENOUS FISTULA
**Aneurysm, congenital left ventricular**
    See VENTRICLE, DIVERTICULUM
**Angeborene lues**
    See FETAL SYPHILIS SYNDROME
**Angeborene Toxoplasmose**
    See FETAL TOXOPLASMOSIS SYNDROME
**Angel dust, fetal effects**
    See FETAL EFFECTS FROM ANGEL DUST (PHENCYCLIDINE OR PCP)
**Angel's kiss**
    See NEVUS FLAMMEUS
**Angelman puppet syndrome**
    See ANGELMAN SYNDROME

## ANGELMAN SYNDROME                                    2086

**Includes:**
    Angelman puppet syndrome
    Happy puppet syndrome (obsolete, pejorative)

**Excludes:**
    Ataxia and mental retardation associated with cerebral palsy
    Epilepsy, gelastic
    **Prader-Willi syndrome** (0823)

**Major Diagnostic Criteria:** Mental retardation with absence of speech, characteristic ataxic gait, microcephaly with flat occiput, mandibular prognathism, protruding tongue, paroxysms of laughter and diffusely abnormal EEG with or without seizures.

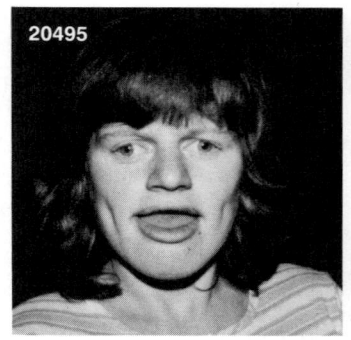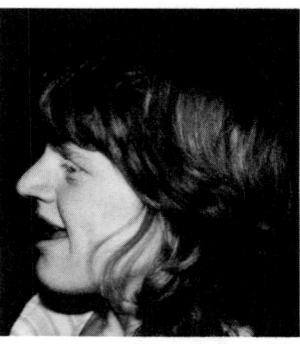
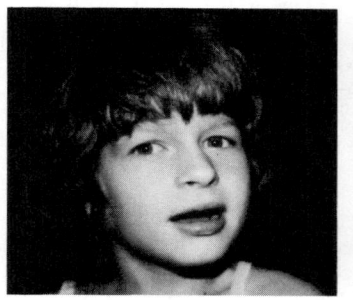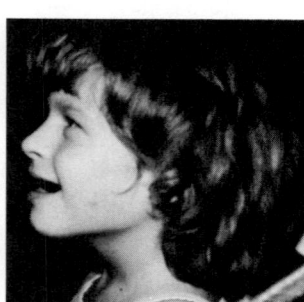

**2086-20495:** Angelman syndrome; note typical facial appearance in these two unrelated females with relative prognathism and macrostomia.

**Clinical Findings:** The diagnosis is usually not evident at birth. **Microcephaly** develops during infancy, and is often associated with poor feeding, abnormal sleep patterns, and hyperactivity. In early childhood, severe developmental delay, ataxia and jerky arm movements resembling a puppet gait are distinctive characteristics. Patients also have an apparent happy disposition and may have paroxysms of inappropriate laughter. This laughter is not epileptogenic but may be a reflexive motor phenomenon. Severe or profound mental retardation is the rule. All reported patients are functionally mute but receptive intelligence may allow them to understand simple commands.

The EEG is abnormal and usually shows generalized high amplitude spike and slow waves at 2–3 cps. Most patients develop seizures in infancy or early childhood but the type of seizure is variable. Early onset of severe seizures often delays full expression of the puppet-like phenotype until later childhood. CT and MRI scans may show mild cortical atrophy or mild, generalized ventricular enlargement but the posterior fossa is usually normal.

Microbrachycephaly is consistently present. The cranium may have a pronounced horizontal, occipital groove. Additional craniofacial abnormalities include midface retrusion, relative prognathism, macrostomia, wide-spaced teeth and protruding tongue (especially during laughter). Decreased pigmentation of choroid and iris is frequent.

**Complications:** Injuries related to seizures or ataxia; acquired orthopedic deformities due to ataxic gait.

**Associated Findings:** None known.

**Etiology:** Unknown. As many as 40% of cases demonstrate, using high resolution chromosome study, a deletion in region q11–13 of chromosome 15 (Pembrey et al, 1989; Williams et al, 1989). In **Prader-Willi syndrome** chromosomal deletion in the region 15q11-q13 has been shown to be paternally derived in almost every case. When the same or similar deletion is in the maternally derived chromosome it has been associated with the Angelman syndrome phenotype. Among those patients with Prader-Willi syndrome who do not have a cytogenetically detectable deletion, some have no detectable paternal contribution but have both maternal contributions in the 15q11-q13 region (maternal hetero-disomy; see Nicholls et al, 1989). These unique findings suggest that genes arising from different sex parents are modified differently prior to conception, and are expressed differently in their offspring (genetic imprinting).

Most patients have apparently represented sporadic occurrences although affected siblings have been reported on at least five occasions. Deletion positive patients have not been reported in cases of sibling recurrence. Although recurrence in siblings suggests autosomal recessive inheritance, the preponderance of sporadic cases, and the recent observations of a chromosome deletion in many patients, suggests that genetic heterogeneity is present.

**Pathogenesis:** Phenotype analysis suggests that the majority of clinical findings can be attributed to a primary CNS defect. The microbrachycephaly, midface retrusion, and relative mandibular prognathism are probably the result of decreased brain growth. Ataxia, excessive laughter, absent speech, abnormal EEG, and seizure disorder also reflect disorganized CNS function. Accordingly, this syndrome might be viewed as a pleiotropy of a mutation primarily affecting the CNS.

**MIM No.:** 23440

**POS No.:** 3462

**Sex Ratio:** M1:F1

**Occurrence:** About 80 cases have been reported in the literature.

**Risk of Recurrence for Patient's Sib:** The empiric recurrence risk has been estimated by Willems et al (1987) to be 1–2% based on study of 48 cases.

**Risk of Recurrence for Patient's Child:** No patient is known to have reproduced.

**Age of Detectability:** Late infancy and early childhood.

**Gene Mapping and Linkage:** ANCR (Angelman syndrome chromosome region) has been mapped to 15q11-q12.

**Prevention:** None known. Genetic counseling indicated.

**Treatment:** Control of seizures and correction of orthopedic deformities to improve gait. Early education and training to ameliorate effects of mental retardation; sign language training and augmented non-verbal techniques may be of benefit.

**Prognosis:** Severity of seizures may decrease with advancing age. Prognosis for verbal communication is extremely poor. Most affected persons achieve ambulation and continued training in basic self-care skills are needed throughout adulthood. Most reach adulthood.

**Detection of Carrier:** Unknown.

**Special Considerations:** The deletion of the q11–13 region on chromosome 15 appears cytogenetically similar to that observed in the **Prader-Willi syndrome** (PWS), but the clinical phenotypes of PWS and Angelman syndrome are easily distinguishable in later childhood. Absence of the deletion in a child with the classic clinical picture does not exclude the diagnosis of Angelman syndrome. Presence of the deletion in neonates and young infants indicates high risk for subsequent development of either a PWS or Angelman syndrome phenotype. No information is available yet on prenatal diagnosis, but high resolution chromosome studies may prove useful for selected families. The *de novo* deletion is of maternal origin in Angelman syndrome, but of predominant paternal origin in PWS (Knoll et al, 1989). Identification of the parental origin of the deleted chromosome 15 is highly predictive of subsequent phenotype development.

**References:**

Angelman H: "Puppet" children: a report on three cases. Dev Med Child Neurol 1965; 7:681–688.

Williams CA, Frias JL: The Angelman ("happy puppet") syndrome. Am J Med Genet 1982; 11:453–460.

Willems RJ, et al.: Recurrence risk in the Angelman ("Happy puppet") syndrome. Am J Med Genet 1987; 27:773–780.

Knoll JHM, et al.: Angelman and Prader-Willi syndromes share a common chromosome 15 deletion but differ in parental origin of the deletion. Am J Med Genet 1989; 32:285–290.

Nicholls RD, et al.: Genetic imprinting suggested by maternal hetero-disomy in non-deletion Prader-Willi syndrome. Nature 1989; 342: 281–285.

Pembrey M, et al.: The association of Angelman's syndrome with deletions within 15q11–13. J Med Genet 1989; 26:73–77.

Williams CA, et al.: Incedence of 15q deletions in the Angelman syndrome: a survey of 12 affected persons. Am J Med Genet 1989; 32:339–345.

WI049
FR016

**Charles A. Williams**
**Jaime L. Frias**

## ANGIO-OSTEOHYPERTROPHY SYNDROME          0055

**Includes:**

> Hemangiectatic hypertrophy
> Klippel-Trenaunay-Weber syndrome (KTW)
> Nevus varicosus osteohypertrophicus
> Parkes-Weber syndrome

**Excludes:**

> **Enchondromatosis and hemangiomas** (0346)
> **Hemihypertrophy** (0458)
> **Neurofibromatosis** (0712)
> **Nevus flammeus** (0715)
> **Proteus syndrome** (2382)
> **Sturge-Weber syndrome** (0915)

**Major Diagnostic Criteria:** Hemihypertrophy, varicose veins, and cutaneous hemangiomatous lesions constitute the classic triad of signs. Arteriovenous fistulae are further components of the syndrome not always expressed in affected individuals. When arteriovenous fistulae are present, some clinicians refer to the condition as Parkes-Weber syndrome.

**Clinical Findings:** Cutaneous hemangiomatous lesions are usually extensive and may comprise capillary **Nevus flammeus** or

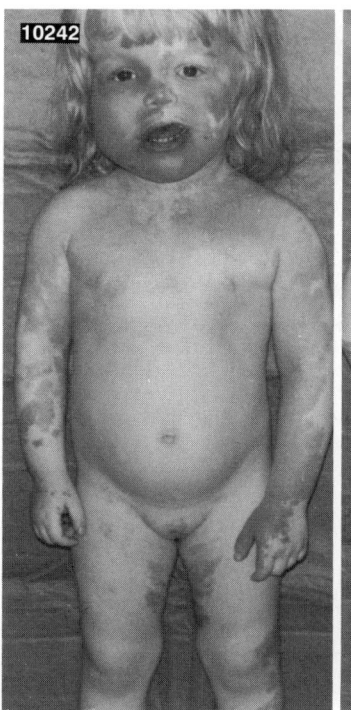 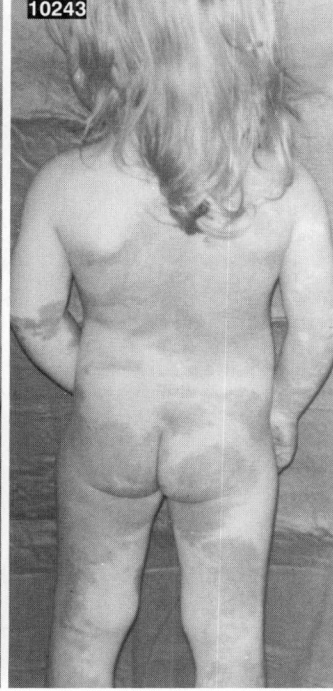

**0055A-10242–43:** Extensive hemangiomas and facial asymmetry; Sturge-Weber syndrome is present here as part of the complex.

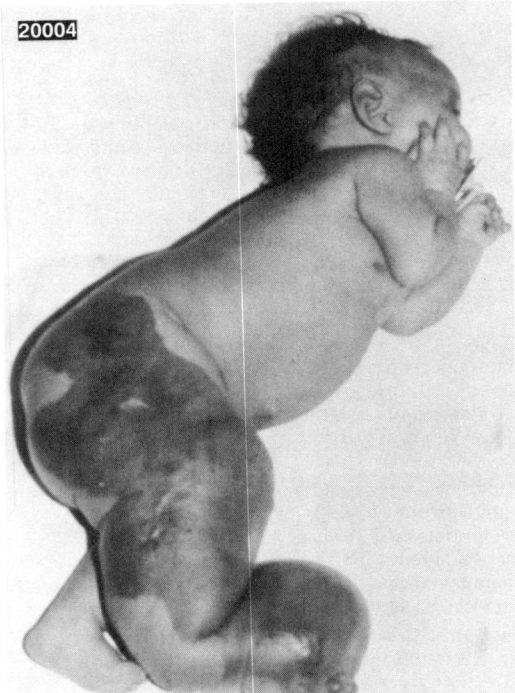

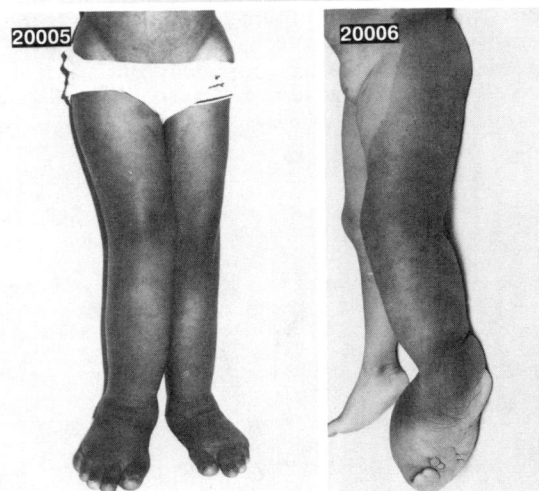

**0055B-20004:** Severe hemihypertrophy of the right leg because of capillary and cavernous hemangiomatous infiltration. Amputation of this limb was eventually necessary. 20005: Hypertrophy of the right leg and both feet. 20006: Hemihypertrophy affecting the left leg with distortion of the foot and toes. A capillary nevus extends to the left thigh.

cavernous elements. Any part of the body, but especially the limbs and trunk, may be involved. Capillary hemangiomas can occur in the distribution of the fifth cranial nerve in KTW syndrome but associated intracerebral vascular anomalies should be sought and, if present, would suggest concomitant expression of **Sturge-Weber syndrome** and KTW syndrome in one individual. Hemangiomas occur in the lung, bowel, liver, and tongue. Other reported skin manifestations are telangiectasia, **Cutis marmorata**, pigmented streaks, aseptic cellulitis, and varicose ulcers.

**Hemihypertrophy** usually involves all the unilateral tissue components, but overgrowth may extend across the midline contralat-

erally. Polydactyly or syndactyly with accompanying isolated macrodactyly may be present. Hemihypertrophy usually, but not always, occurs in the limbs manifesting hemangiomas. Varicose veins, which may only become evident after the onset of walking in the infant, probably result in increased blood flow through valveless, superficial veins consequent upon an atretic or hypoplastic deep venous system. Arteriovenous fistulae, either microscopic or of substantial caliber, are present in a minority of individuals.

**Complications:** Aseptic cellulitis and varicose ulcer formation occur as a result of venous stasis in abnormal vessels. These indolent lesions are difficult to treat and become secondarily infected. If significant arteriovenous fistulae are present, signs of high-output cardiac failure may result. Hemorrhage has been reported from gut hemangiomas, and thrombocytopenia may result from sequestration in large visceral lesions.

**Associated Findings:** Rarely, protein-losing enteropathy is associated with intestinal lymphangiectasia. Mental retardation has been occasionally reported.

**Etiology:** Unknown. Most cases appear to be sporadic, but familial cases have been reported.

**Pathogenesis:** Hypertrophy has been attributed to increased vascular supply, but, in view of the discordance between the location of arteriovenous malformations and areas of hypertrophy, this seems unlikely. Abnormalities in the regulation of tissue growth factors have been postulated as a possible cause.

**MIM No.:** 14900

**POS No.:** 3273

**CDC No.:** 759.840

**Sex Ratio:** M1:F1

**Occurrence:** Undetermined, but Servelle (1985) reported on some 768 operated cases.

**Risk of Recurrence for Patient's Sib:** Unknown.

**Risk of Recurrence for Patient's Child:** Unknown.

**Age of Detectability:** Hemangiomas and signs of overgrowth are present from birth, while varicosities may only develop in early childhood.

**Gene Mapping and Linkage:** Unknown.

**Prevention:** None known. Genetic counseling indicated.

**Treatment:** Some arteriovenous fistulae are amenable to surgery. Problematic varicose ulcers may necessitate intensive medical treatment. Stripping of varicose veins is contraindicated because of the lack of a deep venous plexus. Elastic stockings are recommended to prevent dependent edema. Persistent, severe ulceration and secondary infection may eventually necessitate limb amputation.

**Prognosis:** Depends on the type and extent of involvement.

**Detection of Carrier:** Unknown.

**References:**
Weber FP: Angioma formation in connection with hypertrophy of limbs and hemihypertrophy. Br J Dermatol 1907; 19:231–235.
Lindenauer MS: Congenital arterio-venous fistula and the Klippel-Trenaunay syndrome. Ann Surg 1971; 174:248–263.
Smith DW: Recognizable patterns of human malformation. Philadelphia: WB Saunders 1982:382–383. *
Servelle M: Klippel and Trenaunay's syndrome: 768 operated cases. Ann Surg 1985; 201:365–373.
Viljoen D, et al.: The cutaneous manifestations of the Klippel-Trenaunay-Weber syndrome. Clin Expt Derm 1987; 12:12–17. †

**Denis L. Viljöen**

## ANGIOEDEMA, HEREDITARY                    0054

**Includes:**
  Angioneurotic edema, hereditary
  Autoimmune disease, deficiency of regulatory component C1
  Complement C1 esterase inhibitor deficiency
  Complement C1 esterase inhibitor dysfunction
  Complement component C1, regulatory components, deficiency of

**Excludes:**
  Acquired C1 esterase inhibitor deficiency
  Angioedema, nonhereditary
  Angioedema, secondary to other disorders.

**Major Diagnostic Criteria:** History of recurrent self-limiting episodes of edema or abdominal pain. Demonstration of either the deficiency of the C1 esterase inhibitor in serum or the presence of a nonfunctional $C_1$ inhibitor immunochemically identical with the normal inhibitor.

**Clinical Findings:** Usually a family history or individual history of recurrent episodes of localized peripheral subcutaneous edema, usually without apparent precipitating event, although sometimes associated with menses, extremes of temperature, and physical trauma or emotional distress. Any area of the body may be affected. Attacks are self-limiting lasting 6 to 72 hours; recurrent episodes of self-limited abdominal pain and vomiting, episodes of pharyngeal and laryngeal edema. Peripheral edema may involve any part of the body and is noninflammatory, nonpitting, and usually nonpruritic and nonpainful. During episodes of abdominal pain, the abdomen may be diffusely tender, but no localization is apparent. The abdomen may be distended.

This clinical picture may be confused with other causes of acute abdominal pain. Facial edema may progress to involve mucosa of the mouth, the soft palate, epiglottis, and larynx. This has led to fatality in 10–30% of affected individuals. Patients with hereditary angioedema could present with epiglottitis. Attacks are occasionally preceded by or associated with a transient salmon-pink serpiginous skin eruption. Hereditary angioedema has been associated with pregnancy. Although the disease follows a benign course, maternal mortality has been noted. Coronary arteritis associated with hereditary angioedema, manifesting as substernal chest pain, has been described. The only primary abnormality is deficiency (quantitative or functional) of the C1 esterase inhibitor, an $\alpha_2$-globulin which normally prevents formation of C1 esterase and the reaction with its natural substrates. The lower than anticipated levels of C1 inhibitor in hereditary angioedema with low antigen concentration (type 1) appears to results from: (1) the single functional gene and (2) increased catabolism of protein; perhaps related to activation of C1 or other proteases. Modified inactive first component of complement inhibitor has been found in patients with hereditary angioedema.

*Secondary depletion of serum C4 and C4.* C4 titers are consistently depressed, becoming more so during the symptomatic period. However, C2 titers are sometimes normal in the intervals between attacks of angioedema. Decreased high molecular weight (HMW)-Kininogen levels, increased Factor XII activity, and slightly lower plasma kallikrein levels have been observed. Intrinsic coagulation and fibrinolytic systems do not appear to be involved. X-rays reveal persistent narrowing of lumen of small bowel segment presumably due to mucosal edema; during abdominal pain distended loops of intestine and increased thickness of the intestinal wall have been reported.

**Complications:** Death from laryngeal edema in approximately 10–30% of affected individuals. Unnecessary abdominal surgery. Pulmonary edema.

**Associated Findings:** None known.

**Etiology:** Autosomal dominant inheritance of biochemical deficiency. Although this deficiency of C1 esterase inhibitor (an $\alpha_2$-globulin, an inhibitor of the esterase activity of the first component of serum complement, which also inhibits other factors that affect vascular permeability) is present continuously

through life, the symptoms often become more frequent and severe at adolescence, are episodic in nature, and are self-limiting. The exact relationship of the biochemical deficiency to the symptoms has not been clarified.

**Pathogenesis:** It is believed, though not substantiated, that the edema in these patients results from an uninhibited enzyme activity leading directly or indirectly to the release of permeability factors from complement components, kinin precursors, or other similar substances. It is reported that the ultimate mediation of the symptoms in angioedema is probably perpetrated by a vasoactive, kinin-like peptide, probably derived from C2 and not by bradykinin. The resulting edema may be due to increased vascular permeability at the time of enhanced enzyme activity.

**MIM No.:** *10610

**Sex Ratio:** M1:F1

**Occurrence:** Undetermined. This disorder has been observed in a large number of ethnic groups. Affected kindreds have been found to originate in Northern Europe, the Mediterranean area, and Africa.

**Risk of Recurrence for Patient's Sib:**
  See Part I, *Mendelian Inheritance.*

**Risk of Recurrence for Patient's Child:**
  See Part I, *Mendelian Inheritance.*

**Age of Detectability:** In infancy by deficiency of C1 esterase inhibitor. Subsides in the fifth decade.

**Gene Mapping and Linkage:** C1NH (complement component 1 inhibitor (angioedema, hereditary)) has been mapped to 11q12-q13.1.

**Prevention:** None known. Genetic counseling indicated.

**Treatment:** (1) There is some recent evidence that epsilon aminocaproic acid may reduce the frequency of attacks of edema. (2) An analog, tranexamic acid, has proven effective in aborting attacks of angioedema. The drug has not yet been released by the F.D.A. (3) Recently danazol, a derivative of ethinyltestosterone, has been shown to prevent attacks of hereditary angioedema and it acts to correct the underlying biochemical abnormality. Side effects are weight gain and depression. (4) Although controversial, transfusion of fresh frozen plasma is another alternative. (5) If possible, affected members should carry information indicating the nature of their disease in order to avoid unnecessary abdominal surgery and to alert physicians of the possible need for tracheotomy when edema of the face and oral mucosa occurs.

Careful observation in hospital, if possible, during episodes of facial and oral edema since swelling can extend to the larynx rapidly. Tracheotomy is often necessary; the need should be anticipated.

Analgesia may be helpful if abdominal pain is severe. Hospitalization and intavenous fluid therapy may be necessary if vomiting is excessive.

There is some suggestion that administration of fresh plasma may stop progress of the edema and perhaps prevent the need for tracheotomy or terminate abdominal pain in selective instances. This effect is thought to be dependent upon replacement of C1 esterase inhibitor by plasma; however, its value is questionable.

**Prognosis:** The degree of disruption of normal daily living depends on the frequency of attacks. Some individuals have one attack of peripheral edema in a lifetime. Others are troubled by frequent episodes of peripheral edema or abdominal pain, which may cause frequent work loss, and some individuals have had repeated tracheotomies. Deaths from respiratory obstruction secondary to laryngeal edema occur in 10–30% of affected individuals in different reported series.

**Detection of Carrier:** Clinical anf laboratory examination.

**References:**
Landerman MS: Hereditary angioneurotic edema. I. Case reports and review of the literature. J Allergy 1962; 33:330–341.
Rosen FS, et al.: Hereditary angioneurotic edema: two genetic variants. Science 1965; 148:957–958.

Donaldson VH, Rosen FS: Hereditary angioneurotic edema: a clinical survey. Pediatrics 1966; 37:1017–1027.

Gelfand JA, et al.: Treatment of hereditary angioedema with danazol. N Engl J Med 1976; 295:1444–1448. *

Gadek JE, et al.: Replacement therapy in hereditary angioedema: successful treatment of acute episodes of angioedema with partly purified C1 inhibitor. N Engl J Med 1980; 302:542–546.

Donaldson VH, et al.: Variability in purified dysfunctional C1-inhibitor proteins from patients with hereditary angioneurotic edema: functional and analytic gel-studies. J Clin Invest 1985; 75:124–132. *

Dalmasso AP: Complement in the pathophysiology and diagnosis of human disease. CRC Crit Rev Clin Lab Sci 1986; 24:123.

Zuraw BL, Curd JG: Demonstration of modified inactive first component of complement C1 inhibitor in the plasmas of C1 inhibitor-deficient patients. J Clin Invest 1986; 78:567–575.

Cicardi M, et al.: Molecular basis for the deficiency of complement 1 inhibitor in type I hereditary angioneurotic edema. J Clin Invest 1987; 79:698–702.

Stoppa-Lyonnet D, et al: Altered C1 inhibitor genes in type I hereditary angioedema. N Eng J Med 1987; 317:1–6

GU004                                            **Sudhir Gupta**

**Angioid streaks with skin changes**
*See PSEUDOXANTHOMA ELASTICUM*
**Angiokeratoma, diffuse**
*See FABRY DISEASE*
**Angiolipoma, infiltrating**
*See ANGIOLIPOMATOSIS*
**Angiolipoma, microthromboticum**
*See ANGIOLIPOMATOSIS*
**Angiolipomata, multiple**
*See ANGIOLIPOMATOSIS*

---

## ANGIOLIPOMATOSIS                            3033

**Includes:**
  Angiolipoma, infiltrating
  Angiolipoma, microthromboticum
  Angiolipomata, multiple
  Angiolipomatosis, familial
  Angiolipomatosis microthromoticum
  Hapnes-Boman-Skeie syndrome
  Hemangiolipomatosis

**Excludes:**
  Angiomatosis
  **Neurofibromatosis** (0712)

**Major Diagnostic Criteria:** The presence of one or more angiolipomas (tumors consisting of fat tissue and blood vessels, with the vascular component comprising more than 15% of the tumor).

**Clinical Findings:** It is likely that at least three types of conditions with this appellation exist. In the form called *multiple angiolipomata*, tumors are multiple, occur subcutaneously, preferentially on upper extremities and trunk, and are small and encapsulated. They appear in the second and third decades. The second condition is called *infiltrating angiolipoma*, in which tumors are often solitary and occur largely within the skeletal muscle. They are moderate to large in size, occur more often on the lower extremities or dorsal trunk, and lack a capsule. The third type of condition has only been reported in one pair of sibs. This form was termed *familial angiolipomatosis* and was characterized by multiple subcutaneous angiolipomas, occurring at wrist, knee, and ankle joints. The tumors were moderate in size and lacked a capsule. In addition, both sibs had mild osteoporosis; one also had muscular hypotrophy. Onset of the condition was in childhood.

**Complications:** Chronic synovitis following surgery occurred in one case.

**Associated Findings:** None known.

**Etiology:** Infiltrating angiolipomas have not occurred in families; rather, they have been sporadic cases. Multiple angiolipomas may be heterogeneous in that pedigrees compatible with both recessive and dominant inheritance have been reported. Familial angiolipomatosis is likely autosomal recessive.

**Pathogenesis:** Unknown.

**MIM No.:** 20655

**POS No.:** 3673

**Sex Ratio:** M1:F1

**Occurrence:** Angiolipomas are not uncommon, although the exact occurrence rate is unknown.

**Risk of Recurrence for Patient's Sib:**
  See Part I, *Mendelian Inheritance.*

**Risk of Recurrence for Patient's Child:**
  See Part I, *Mendelian Inheritance.*

**Age of Detectability:** Dependent on the type: ages 20–30 for multiple angiolipomas or infiltrating angiolipomata, and early childhood for familial angiolipomatosis.

**Gene Mapping and Linkage:** Unknown.

**Prevention:** None known. Genetic counseling indicated.

**Treatment:** Surgical removal of the angiolipoma may be indicated.

**Prognosis:** With proper treatment, life span and intellect are not affected.

**Detection of Carrier:** Unknown.

**Special Considerations:** Although Kumar et al (1989) has described a pedigree of what thay termed *familial angiolipomatosis*, the described condition is likely multiple angiolipomatosis, and distinct from that described by Hapnes et al (1980).

**References:**
Klem KK: Multiple lipoma-angiolipomas. Acta Chir Scand 1949; 97: 527–532.

Gonzalez-Crussi F, et al.: Infiltrating angiolipoma. J Bone Joint Surg 1966; 48A:1111–1124.

Hapnes SA, et al.: Familial angiolipomatosis. Clin Genet 1980; 17:202–208.

Kumar R, et al.: Autosomal dominant inheritance in familial angiolipomatosis. Clin Genet 1989; 35:200–204.

T0007                                        **Helga V. Toriello**

**Angiolipomatosis microthromoticum**
*See ANGIOLIPOMATOSIS*
**Angiolipomatosis, familial**
*See ANGIOLIPOMATOSIS*
**Angioma cavernosum of external ear**
*See EAR, ARTERIOVENOUS FISTULA*
**Angioma pigmentosum et atrophicum**
*See XERODERMA PIGMENTOSUM*
**Angiomas (cavernous) of CNS and retina**
*See RETINA, CAVERNOUS HEMANGIOMA*
**Angioneurotic edema, hereditary**
*See ANGIOEDEMA, HEREDITARY*
**Anhidrosis-mental retardation-eye and skeletal defects**
*See VAN DEN BOSCH SYNDROME*

---

## ANIRIDIA                                    0057

**Includes:**
  Aniridia-absent patella
  Hypoplasia of iris with rudimentary root
  Iris coloboma, atypical
  Iris, congenital absence
  Lens, aniridia
  Wilms tumor-aniridia syndrome

**Excludes:**
  **Aniridia-cerebellar ataxia-mental deficiency** (3235)
  **Eye, microphthalmia/coloboma** (0661)

**Major Diagnostic Criteria:** Congenital absence of all or part of iris.

**Clinical Findings:** In aniridia a rudimentary stump of iris, often visible only on slit-lamp examination, is usually present at birth. The anomaly is generally bilateral (50:1). On examination the pupil is large and the lens edge, zonules and ciliary body may be visible. Photophobia, poor vision and nystagmus are very com-

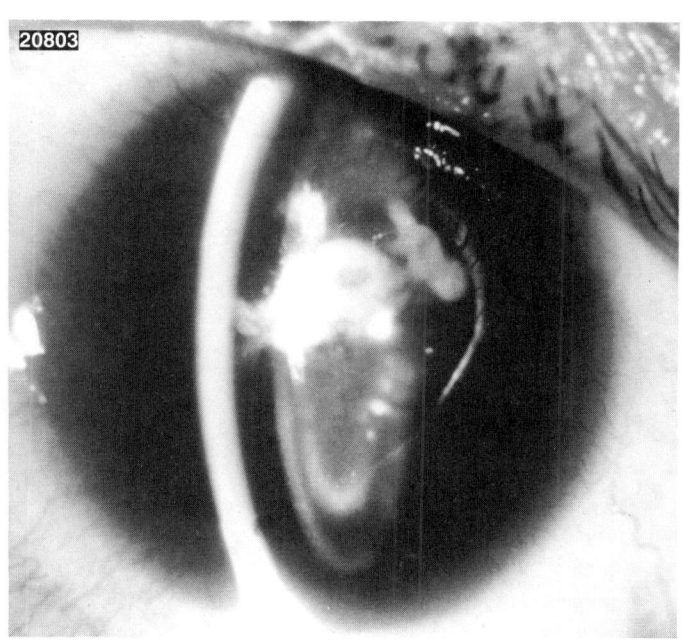

**0057-20803:** Aniridia, total with cataractous lens.

mon, with frequencies over 50%. Cataracts are said to be present in about 66% of cases, but may not be present at birth. A secondary glaucoma due to structural angle changes is frequently seen. Structural deformities of the cornea and progressive opacification are frequently present. Atypical colobomata and slit-like defects of the iris stroma may be partial expressions.

**Complications:** Glaucoma, cataracts, corneal pannus, and foveal hypoplusia.

**Associated Findings:** Microphthalmia, ectopia lentis, coloboma of lens and choroid, persistence of pupillary membrane. Mirkinson and Mirkinson (1975) reported a family where a boy, his father, and his maternal grandmother had aniridia and hypoplastic or absent patella.

**Etiology:** Autosomal dominant inheritance with about 85% penetrance. Heterogeneity exists. Aniridia in combination with cerebellar ataxia and mental deficiency (Gillespie (1965) could be autosomal recessive. Care must also be taken to distinguish this disorder from sporadic cases of aniridia associated with Wilms tumor, hemihypertrophy, GU tract anomalies, mental retardation and skeletal malformations. Only one familial case of aniridia with Wilms tumor has been reported.

**Pathogenesis:** Theories suggested are defective neural ectoderm development and aberrant or persistent vascular mesoderm of the lens tunica vasculosa at the anterior optic cup preventing the normal growth of the iris.

**MIM No.:** *10620, *10621, 10622, 19407

**CDC No.:** 743.420

**Sex Ratio:** M1:F1

**Occurrence:** 1:100,000 to 1:200,000.

**Risk of Recurrence for Patient's Sib:**
See Part I, *Mendelian Inheritance.* In one series the ratio was 38:62 affected to normal children in segregating sibships).

**Risk of Recurrence for Patient's Child:**
See Part I, *Mendelian Inheritance.*

**Age of Detectability:** Usually at birth

**Gene Mapping and Linkage:** AN1 (aniridia 1) has been provisionally mapped to 2p.

AN2 (aniridia 2 without Wilms' tumor, GU abnormalities, and M.R.) has been mapped to 11p13.

WAGR (Wilms tumor, aniridia, genitourinary abnormalities, and MR) has been mapped to 11p13.

**Prevention:** None known. Genetic counseling indicated.

**Treatment:** Cataract extraction and glaucoma therapy as indicated; some evidence for the beneficial use of artificial pupil contact lenses.

All sporadic cases should have evaluation for Wilms tumor and other malformations.

**Prognosis:** Life span and intelligence normal; ocular prognosis generally poor.

**Detection of Carrier:** Unknown.

**Special Considerations:** Simple or atypical iris colobomas (not embryonic fissure derived) are very common congenital abnormalities that occur in all sectors of the iris, complete or incomplete, total or partial. These are also autosomal dominant. The theories of formation are the same as those for aniridia.

Six cases of aniridia among 440 patients with Wilms tumor emphasize this recently described association. Two of the children had residual iris tags visible on external examination, four had cataract and 1 glaucoma. Ear deformities were present in three. None had a parent with aniridia. Nonocular associated defects are more common in those patients with aniridia and Wilms tumor.

**References:**
Shaw MW et al.: Congenital aniridia. Am J Hum Genet 1960; 12:389–415.
Fraumeni JF, Jr: The aniridia - Wilms' tumor syndrome. BD:OAS V(2). New York: March of Dimes Birth Defects Foundation, 1969:198–201.
Mirkinson AE, Mirkinson NK: A familial syndrome of aniridia and absence of the patella. BD:OAS vol XI, no 5. New York: The National Foundation-March of Dimes, 1975:129–131.
Elsas FJ et al.: Familial aniridia with preserved ocular function. Am J Opthal 1977; 83:718–724.
Riccardi V, et al.: Wilms tumor with anaridia/iris dysplasia and apparently normal chromosomes. J Pediat 1982; 100:574–577.

ME032                                 **Marilyn B. Mets**
CR012                                 **Harold E. Cross**

**Aniridia, partial-unilateral renal agenesis-retardation**
*See ANIRIDIA-CEREBELLAR ATAXIA-MENTAL DEFICIENCY*
**Aniridia, type II**
*See CHROMOSOME 11, PARTIAL MONOSOMY 11p*
**Aniridia-absent patella**
*See ANIRIDIA*
**Aniridia-ambiguous genitalia-mental retardation (AGR triad)**
*See CHROMOSOME 11, PARTIAL MONOSOMY 11p*

---

## ANIRIDIA-CEREBELLAR ATAXIA-MENTAL DEFICIENCY      3235

**Includes:**
    Aniridia, partial-unilateral renal agenesis-retardation
    Gillespie syndrome
    Oligophrenia-aniridia-cerebellar ataxia

**Excludes:**
    **Aniridia** (0057)
    **Cancer, Wilms tumor** (2742)
    **Marinesco-Sjogren syndrome** (2031)
    **Optic atrophy, infantile heredofamilial** (0755)

**Major Diagnostic Criteria:** Partial aniridia, cerebellar ataxia, and mental deficiency.

**Clinical Findings:** In addition to partial aniridia, cerebellar ataxia, and mental deficiency, the patients so far described in the literature have shown palpebral ptosis, convergent strabismus, hypermetropia, photophobia, partial remains of the Wachendorf membrane, absence of pupillary sphincter, absence of border in the pupillary margin, mydriasis, hypoplasia of cerebellum (particularly of the vermis), transpalmar crease, fusion of vertebral C1 + C2, valvar pulmonary stenosis, and delayed developmental milestones.

**Complications:**  Ataxic gait; difficulty in walking; poor school performance; vision impairment.

**Associated Findings:**  Cardiac malformations, systolic murmurs, equinovarus deformity, and pes planus.

**Etiology:**  Probably autosomal recessive inheritance, although no case of consanguineous parents has been reported. The possibility of an autosomal dominant gene with low penetrance has not been excluded. G-banded chromosomes have been normal.

**Pathogenesis:**  Unknown.

**MIM No.:**  20670, 20675

**Sex Ratio:**  M6:F3

**Occurrence:**  Nine affected persons have been reported as occurring in six sibships from five families.

**Risk of Recurrence for Patient's Sib:**
See Part I, *Mendelian Inheritance.*

**Risk of Recurrence for Patient's Child:**
See Part I, *Mendelian Inheritance.*

**Age of Detectability:**  During childhood.

**Gene Mapping and Linkage:**  Unknown.

**Prevention:**  None known. Genetic counseling indicated.

**Treatment:**  Special education; physiotherapy.

**Prognosis:**  Probably normal for life span.

**Detection of Carrier:**  Unknown. The mother of the patients described by Wittig et al (1988) presented moderately oval pupil in both eyes with smaller pigmentary border in the lower portion, as well as reduced reaction of the photomotor reflex.

**Special Considerations:**  A brother and sister reported by Sommer et al (1974) had *partial aniridia, unilateral renal agenesis, and mild psychomotor retardation.* The condition reported by De Hauwere et al (1973) was similar.

**References:**
Gillespie FD: Aniridia, cerebellar ataxia, and oligophrenia in siblings. Arch Ophthal 1965; 73:338–341.
Sarsfield JK: The syndrome of congenital cerebellar ataxia, aniridia and mental retardation. Develop Med Child Neurol 1971; 13:508–511.
De Hauwere RC, et al.: Iris dysplasia, orbital hypertelorism, and psychomotor retardation: a dominantly inherited developmental syndrome. J Pediatr 1973; 82:679–681.
Sommer A, et al.: A syndrome of partial aniridia, unilateral renal agenesis, and mild psychomotor retardation in siblings. (Letter) J Pediatr 1974; 85:870–872.
Crawfurd Md'A, et al.: Nonprogressive cerebellar ataxia, aplasia of pupillary zone of iris, and mental subnormality (Gillespie's syndrome) affecting three members of a nonconsanguineous family in two generations. J Med Genet 1979; 16:373–378.
Lechtenberg R, Ferreti C: Ataxia with aniridia of Gillespie: a case report. Neurol 1981; 31:95–97.
Wittig EO, et al.: Partial aniridia, cerebellar ataxia and mental deficiency (Gillespie syndrome) in two brothers. Am J Med Genet 1988; 30:703–708.

FR033
PI008
WI065

Newton Freire-Maia
Marta Pinheiro
Ehrenfried O. Wittig

**Aniridia-Robin sequence-growth delay**
See RAG SYNDROME
**Aniridia-Wilms tumor association (AWTA)**
See CHROMOSOME 11, PARTIAL MONOSOMY 11p
**Aniridia-Wilms tumor-gonadoblastoma**
See CHROMOSOME 11, PARTIAL MONOSOMY 11p
**Anisocoria**
See PUPIL, ANISOCORIA
**Anisomaltasia**
See SUCRASE-ISOMALTASE DEFICIENCY
**Anisometropia**
See EYE, ANISOMETROPIA
**Anisospondylic camptomicromelic dwarfism**
See DWARFISM, DYSSEGMENTAL, ROLLAND-DESBUQUOIS TYPE
**Anisospondylic camptomicromelic dwarfism, lethal**
See DWARFISM, DYSSEGMENTAL, SILVERMAN-HANDMAKER TYPE

**Ankyloblepharon filiforme adnatum**
See EYELID, ANKYLOBLEPHARON
**Ankyloblepharon filiforme adnatum-cleft palate**
See CLEFT LIP/PALATE-FILIFORM FUSION OF EYELIDS
**Ankyloblepharon, external**
See EYELID, ANKYLOBLEPHARON
**Ankyloblepharon, internal**
See EYELID, ANKYLOBLEPHARON
**Ankyloblepharon-curly hair-nail dysplasia syndrome**
See CHANDS
**Ankyloblepharon-ectodermal defects-cleft lip and palate (AEC)**
See ECTODERMAL DYSPLASIA, HAY-WELLS TYPE
**Ankylodontia, multiple heritable type**
See TEETH, ANKYLODONTIA, MULTIPLE HERITABLE TYPE
**Ankyloglossia**
See TONGUE, ANKYLOGLOSSIA
**Ankyloglossum superior syndrome**
See HYPOGLOSSIA-HYPODACTYLIA
**Ankylosed teeth**
See TEETH, ANKYLOSED

## ANKYLOSING SPONDYLITIS 2516

**Includes:**
Arthropathies of ulcerative colitis
Bechterew syndrome
Marie-Strumpell spondylitis
Pelvospondylitis ossificans
Psoriatic arthritis
Reactive arthritis
Reiter syndrome
Spondylitis deformans
von Bechterew disease

**Excludes:**
**Arthritis, rheumatoid (2517)**
Degenerative spondyloses
Diffuse idiopathic skeletal hyperostosis (DISH)
**Hallervorden-Spatz disease (2526)**

**Major Diagnostic Criteria:**  Based on the New York Criteria of 1966. *Clinical:* 1) Limitation of motion of the lumbar spine in all three planes-anterior flexion, lateral flexion, and extension; 2) History or presence of pain in the dorsolumbar junction or lumbar spine; 3) Limitation of chest expansion to one inch (2.5 cm) or less measured at the fourth intercostal space.
*Definite ankylosing spondylitis* 1) Grade 3–4 bilateral sacroiliitis with at least one clinical criterion; 2) grade 3–4 unilateral or grade 2 bilateral sacroiliitis with clinical criterion 1 or with clinical criteria 2 and 3.
*Probable ankylosing spondylitis* 1) Grade 3–4 bilateral sacroiliitis with no clinical criteria.

**Clinical Findings:**  Clinical symptoms and signs appear in the second and third decades of life. Chronic low back pain and stiffness are the initial symptoms in the majority of patients; however, some, especially women and children, will present with an inflammatory peripheral lower limb arthritis, typically involving a hip or knee. The disease usually begins in the sacroiliac joints and progressively ascends into lumbar, dorsal, and cervical spines, causing fusion. Normal lumbar lordosis becomes flattened, dorsal kyphosis accentuated, and chest expansion restricted. Spinal mobility is lost in all segments, including the neck, which becomes fixed in a flexed position. A forward "stooped" posture results, requiring compensatory flexion of the knees to maintain a center of gravity. There is great variability in clinical expression, even in families. Some patients develop only sacroiliitis, and others progress to fusion of the entire spine.

Pathologically, inflammatory lesions, composed primarily of mononuclear cells, are found affecting cartilage, subchondral bone, and bony periosteum. Sites of attachment for tendons and fascia are prominently involved (enthesopathy). The inflammatory lesions promote prominent fibrosis and new bone growth, resulting in bony or periarticular fusion of spinal articulations. Hips and sometimes shoulders are similarly involved in over 50% of patients, but other peripheral joints are infrequently damaged.

X-ray changes are virtually pathognomonic. Sacroiliac joints show sclerosis and erosion early but eventually become completely fused. Spinal apophyseal, facet, and costovertebral joints also show bony fusion. Inflammatory erosions at the vertebral body margins results in a "squared" appearance. Ossified ligamentous structures bridging intervertebral disks (syndesmophytes) are characteristically found at multiple spinal levels.

Laboratory studies show elevation of the erythrocyte sedimentation rate with or without other acute phase reactants in the majority of patients. Serum alkaline phosphatase is elevated in approximately 50%. Serum rheumatoid factor and other autoantibodies are not found. The histocompatibility class I antigen HLA-B27 is present in over 90% of patients.

**Complications:** Episodes of acute anterior uveitis occur in 25% of patients. Inflammatory lesions of the aortic root and valve, as well as adjacent AV nodal tissue, result in aortic regurgitation and sometimes heart block in approximately 5% of patients. Amyloidosis eventually emerges in 4%. Cervical fractures of the brittle spine, often after trivial trauma, may result in neurologic catastrophes (quadriplegia or sudden death). Cauda equina syndrome from a chronic arachnoiditis around exiting sacral nerves is a rare complication.

Additional features are rare in primary ankylosing spondylitis, but occur more predictably in related conditions. *Reiter syndrome* is primarily a peripheral arthritis manifesting a variety of mucocutaneous lesions, including nongonococcal urethritis, conjunctivitis, keratodermia blennorrhagicum (pustular psoriasis), circinate balanitis, painless oral ulcers, and dystrophy of the nails. Sacroiliitis with or without spondylitis occurs in approximately 20% of patients. *Psoriatic arthritis* complicates cutaneous psoriasis vulgaris in 5–7% of patients, of which 20% will have spinal involvement. A *spondylitis* indistinguishable clinically and on X-ray from ankylosing spondylitis develops in 10% of patients with ulcerative colitis and Crohn disease (see **Inflammatory bowel disease**). All of these conditions show variable and weaker associations with HLA-B27 than does primary ankylosing spondylitis.

**Associated Findings:** Excess frequencies of **Multiple sclerosis, familial** and IgA nephropathy have been reported.

**Etiology:** Autosomal dominant inheritance with incomplete penetrance. The condition is always associated with HLA-B27 allele in multiplex families; however, only 25% of B27-positive relatives will be affected. Discordance in 30% of monozygotic twins suggests a nongermline effect.

**Pathogenesis:** Current knowledge suggests class I molecule (B27) interaction with certain infectious agents, i.e., *Klebsiella pneumoniae, Yersinia enterocolitica,* and others, yielding an autoimmune cytotoxic T-cell response. Sequence homology of HLA-B27 amino acid residues 72–77 and *Klebsiella* outer membrane protein residues 188–193 suggest molecular mimicry.

**MIM No.:** *10630

**Sex Ratio:** M3:F1

**Occurrence:** The prevalence rate in different populations parallels the frequency of HLA-B27. In Caucasian populations, HLA-B27 occurs with frequencies ranging from 6–14%. Approximately 2% of random B27-positive individuals develop disease. Estimated prevalence in Caucasians is 0.2%. Disease prevalence in American blacks is undetermined, but B27 occurs in 2–3%. Ankylosing spondylitis is rare in pure African blacks and in Japanese, in whom the B27 gene frequency is exceedingly low. Certain American Indian tribes have high disease and B27 frequencies, i.e., Haida, Pima, Navajo, and Chippewa.

**Risk of Recurrence for Patient's Sib:**
See Part I, *Mendelian Inheritance.*

**Risk of Recurrence for Patient's Child:**
See Part I, *Mendelian Inheritance.*

**Age of Detectability:** Usually before age 35 years.

**Gene Mapping and Linkage:** Linked to the HLA-B27 allele of the major histocompatibility complex on the short arm of chromosome 6.

**Prevention:** None known. Genetic counseling indicated.

**Treatment:** Anti-inflammatory drugs to suppress inflammation and relieve symptoms. Physical therapy to maintain normal posture and joint mobility and to prevent deformity.

**Prognosis:** Normal life span in 95%. Physical handicaps leading to major changes in life-style or to occupational disability in less than 20%.

**Detection of Carrier:** Determination of HLA-B27 and X-rays of sacroiliac joints.

**References:**
Carette S, et al.: The natural disease course of ankylosing spondylitis. Arthritis Rheum 1983; 26:186–190.
van der Linden S, et al.: Evaluation of diagnostic criteria for ankylosing spondylitis. Arthritis Rheum 1984a; 27:361–368.
van der Linden SM, et al.: The risk of developing ankylosing spondylitis in HLA-B27 positive individuals. Arthritis Rheum 1984b; 27:241–249.
Arnett FC: Seronegative spondyloarthropathies. Bull Rheum Dis 1987; 37:1–12.

AR008 **Frank C. Arnett**

**Ankylosis of teeth**
*See TEETH, MOLAR REINCLUSION*
**Annular corneal dystrophy**
*See CORNEAL DYSTROPHY, REIS-BUCKLERS TYPE*
**Annular grooves**
*See AMNIOTIC BANDS SYNDROME*
**Annular pancreas**
*See PANCREAS, ANNULAR*
**Annulus migrans**
*See TONGUE, GEOGRAPHIC*
**Anodontia-hypotrichosis syndrome**
*See OCULO-OSTEO-CUTANEOUS SYNDROME, TOUMAALA-HAAPANEN TYPE*
**Anogenital warts, congenital**
*See PAPILLOMA VIRUS, CONGENITAL INFECTION*
**Anomalous atrioventricular (AV) conduction**
*See ARRHYTHMIA, WOLFF-PARKINSON-WHITE TYPE*
**Anomalous muscle bundle of the right ventricle**
*See VENTRICLE, DOUBLE CHAMBERED RIGHT*
**Anomalous right ventricular muscles**
*See VENTRICLE, DOUBLE CHAMBERED RIGHT*
**Anonychia**
*See NAILS, ANONYCHIA, HEREDITARY*
**Anonychia-ectrodactyly**
*See ECTRODACTYLY-ANONYCHIA*
**Anonychia-fibular dysplasia**
*See OTO-ONYCHO-PERONEAL SYNDROME*
**Anonychia-onychodystrophy**
*See NAIL-PATELLA SYNDROME*
**Anonychia-skin atrophy-alopecia-tongue defect**
*See ALOPECIA-SKIN ATROPHY-ANONYCHIA-TONGUE DEFECT*
**Anoperineal fistula**
*See ANORECTAL MALFORMATIONS*
**Anophthalmia, clinical**
*See EYE, ANOPHTHALMIA*
**Anophthalmia, recessive Waardenburg type**
*See ANOPHTHALMIA-LIMB ANOMALIES*
**Anophthalmia-hand-foot defects-mental retardation**
*See ANOPHTHALMIA-LIMB ANOMALIES*

---

## ANOPHTHALMIA-LIMB ANOMALIES 2784

**Includes:**

Anophthalmia, recessive Waardenburg type
Anophthalmia-hand-foot defects-mental retardation
Fingers, "crooked fingers syndrome"
Ophthalmo-acromelic syndrome
Syndactyly-anophthalmos
Waardengurg anophthalmia syndrome

**Excludes:**

**Charge association** (2124)
**Chromosome 13, trisomy 13** (0168)
**Eye, anophthalmia** (0067)
**Lenz microphthalmia syndrome** (3171)
**Walker-Warburg syndrome** (2869)

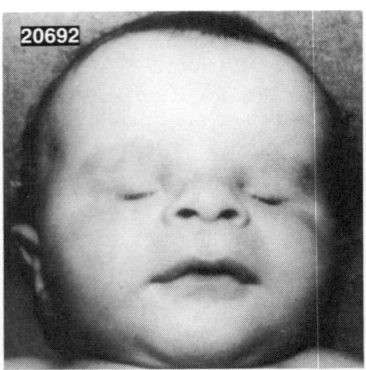
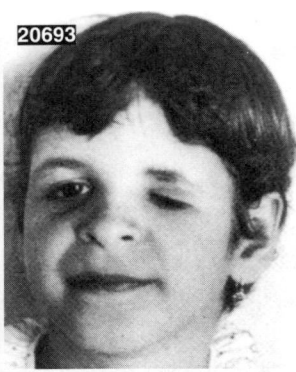
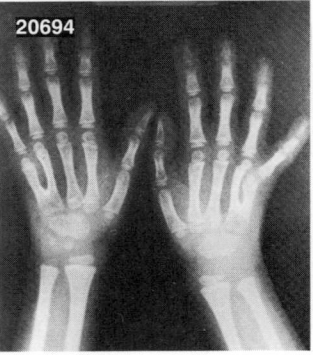
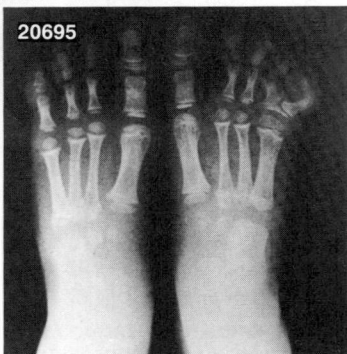

**2784-20692:** Anophthalmos-limb defects, Waardenburg type; note bilateral anophthalmos. **20693:** Unilateral anophthalmos. **20694–95:** X-rays show bony fusions and absence defects.

**Major Diagnostic Criteria:** Unilateral or bilateral clinical anophthalmia with **Syndactyly** or other deformities of the hands and/or feet. Other congenital anomalies may be present. Mental retardation may occur.

**Clinical Findings:** Absence of one or both globes is noted at birth along with digital and/or toe abnormalities usually in the form of soft tissue and bony syndactylism. The distal limb abnormalities include bifid thumbs, enlarged big toes, digital **Syndactyly** with or without oligodactyly, **Brachydactyly**, fusion or enlargement of metacarpals/metatarsals 4 and 5, fusion of other wrist or ankle bones, hypoplasia, and clinodactyly of the fifth finger. All four distal limbs are usually, though not always, affected, but not necessarily with equal severity. Other skeletal abnormalities are not likely. Dermatoglyphics and palmar creases are reported to be abnormal.

Other concomitant abnormalities include **Cleft lip** and/or **Cleft palate**, widely-spaced nipples, simian crease, absent prepuce, and mental retardation. A maternal history of spontaneous abortions of similarly affected fetuses may be present. Parental consanguinity was present in the families reported by Waardenburg (1935), Richieri-Costa et al (1983), and Traboulsi et al (1983). The karyotype is normal.

**Complications:** Severely affected fetuses are aborted. Orthopedic problems among survivors.

**Associated Findings:** None known.

**Etiology:** Presumably autosomal recessive inheritance.

**Pathogenesis:** Clinical anophthalmia results from failure of the optic vesicle to develop either primarily or secondary to a complex developmental error of forebrain development. In true anophthalmia, no ocular tissue is found on histopathologic sectionning of the orbit; in clinical anophthalmia or extreme microphthalmos ocular tissue can be identified histologically. In *Waardenburg anophthalmia* the type of anophthalmia is not known and is therefore referred to as clinical anophthalmia.

It is hypothesized that normal embryogenesis of the eyes and distal limbs require temporal synchronization and sequential progression of two distinct developmental fields. These morphogenic programs are controlled in part by many interacting genes, some of which induce a similar sequential event in each field. Consequently, if one such inducing gene is abnormal, dysmorphogenesis can occur in different developmental fields, such as those of the eyes and distal limbs.

**MIM No.:** 20692

**Sex Ratio:** M1:F1

**Occurrence:** Some 21 cases from several unrelated families, from different countries, have been reported; including one set of twins.

**Risk of Recurrence for Patient's Sib:**
See Part I, *Mendelian Inheritance.*

**Risk of Recurrence for Patient's Child:**
See Part I, *Mendelian Inheritance.*

**Age of Detectability:** At birth, and possibly prenatally by ultrasound starting in the second trimester.

**Gene Mapping and Linkage:** Unknown.

**Prevention:** None known. Genetic counseling indicated.

**Treatment:** Surgical correction of digital and cleft lip abnormalities.

**Prognosis:** Poor for vision. Good for life if no major abnormalities of brain or internal organs are found. Mental retardation is not a consistent finding.

**Detection of Carrier:** Unknown.

**Special Considerations:** The twins and isolated case reported by Pallota (1983) probably have this condition.

Several chromosomally normal newborns and children have been observed with microphthalmos and/or anophthalmos with or without mental retardation or other congenital anomalies that appear to be sporadic cases in otherwise normal, unrelated, and nonconsanguinous families. However, in each case one parent had significant clinodactyly with or without **Camptodactyly** of one or more fingers, unilaterally or bilaterally. In some of the families these *crooked fingers* segregated through several generations, with instances of male-to-male transmission suggesting autosomal dominant inheritance with low penetrance for the eye defects or other congenital anomalies. Two unrelated male newborns with eye abnormalities had fathers with "crooked fingers". These two fathers were otherwise normal.

**References:**
Waardenburg PJ: Autosomally-recessive anophthalmia with malformations of the hands and feet. In: Waardenburg PJ, et al., eds: Genetics and Ophthalmology, Vol 1. Assen, The Netherlands: Royal Van Gorcum, 1961:773.
Richieri-Costa A, et al.: Autosomal recessive anophthalmia with multiple congenital abnormalities: type Waardenburg. Am J Med Genet 1983; 14:607–615. †
Pallota R, Dallapiccola B: A syndrome with true anophthalmia, hand-foot defects and mental retardation. Ophthalmol Paediatr Genet 1984; 4:19–23. †
Traboulsi EI: Letter to the Editor. Ophthalmol Paediatr Genet 1984; 4:203.
Traboulsi EI, et al.: Waardenburg's recessive anophthalmia syndrome. Ophthalmol Paediatr Genet 1984; 4:13–18. †
Le Merrer M, et al.: Ophthalmo-acromelic syndrome. Annales de Genetique 1988; 31:226–229.

ST008
TR009

**Mark W. Steele**
**Elias I. Traboulsi**

**Anophthalmos with associated anomalies**
*See LENZ MICROPHTHALMIA SYNDROME*
**Anophthalmos, true or primary**
*See EYE, ANOPHTHALMIA*

## ANORCHIA                                             0068

**Includes:**

> Testicular regression, embryonic
> Testicular regression syndrome
> Testes, congenital absence of
> XY gonadal agenesis syndrome

**Excludes:**

> **Agonadia** (0029)
> **Gonadal dysgenesis, XY type** (0437)
> **Gonadotropin deficiencies** (0438)
> **Hypogonadotropic hypogonadism** (2300)
> **Kallmann syndrome** (2301)
> **Sertoli cell-only syndrome** (3163)
> All forms of male pseudohermaphroditism

**Major Diagnostic Criteria:** Surgically verified absence of testes in a 46,XY individual with well-differentiated male external genitalia.

**Clinical Findings:** Males with anorchia have well-differentiated male external genitalia and normal wolffian derivatives, but absent müllerian derivatives and absent testes. No somatic anomalies are present. To verify the diagnosis, a surgeon should explore the scrotum, inguinal canal, and entire path along which the testes descend during embryogenesis. Splenic gonadal fusion should be excluded. Vasa deferentia terminate blindly, often at the same location as spermatic vessels. Individuals with anorchia appear normal at birth except for absence of scrotal testes, and during the first decade development is completely normal. Anorchia may be unilateral or bilateral; the latter is much rarer. The diagnosis of congenital anorchia may not be made until virilization fails to occur at puberty, despite androgen sensitivity; unilateral anorchia may not be recognized until later in life.

**Complications:** If bilateral, lack of secondary sexual development and infertility.

**Associated Findings:** A virilized female prototype was reported in one case (Rosenberg et al, 1984), and mental retardation has been reported in sibs (de Grouchy, 1985).

**Etiology:** The etiology is uncertain, although familial tendencies exist. Monozygotic twins concordant for anorchia have been reported, and in several kindreds other family members (sibs, father, son) were affected. In still other families, one sib had bilateral anorchia and another sib had unilateral anorchia. On the other hand, monozygotic twins are not always concordant for anorchia, indicating that genetic factors are not operative in all cases.

**Pathogenesis:** In anorchic individuals the fetal testes presumably secreted hormones necessary for external genital virilization, wolffian differentiation, and müllerian inhibition. Testicular tissue thus probably persisted until at least 14–20 weeks of embryonic development, after which time the fetal testes could have undergone atrophy to produce the anorchic phenotype.

**MIM No.:** 27325

**CDC No.:** 752.800

**Sex Ratio:** M1:F0

**Occurrence:** Over 100 cases of bilateral anorchia have been reported; unilateral anorchia is more common.

**Risk of Recurrence for Patient's Sib:** Presumably zero for 46,XX sibs; increased to a small but unknown magnitude in 46,XY sibs.

**Risk of Recurrence for Patient's Child:** Patients with bilateral defect are sterile; possibly increased to a small degree for offspring of fathers with unilateral defect.

**Age of Detectability:** During infancy because of absence of testes or at puberty because of lack of secondary sexual development (bilateral cases). Variable for unilateral defects.

**Gene Mapping and Linkage:** Unknown.

**Prevention:** None known. Genetic counseling indicated.

**Treatment:** Treatment of hypogonadism in bilateral cases; none for unilateral cases.

**Prognosis:** Presumably normal life span; infertility in bilateral but not in unilateral anorchia.

**Detection of Carrier:** Unknown.

**Special Considerations:** Anorchia should be distinguished from **Agonadia**, a condition in which not only are gonads absent but genital and ductal differentiation is abnormal.

**References:**

Simpson JL, et al.: Bilateral anorchia: discordance in monozygotic twins. In: BD:OAS 1971; 196–200. Baltimore: Williams and Wilkins.
Hall JG, et al.: Familial congenital anorchia. In: BD:OAS 1975; 115–118. New York: Alan R. Liss.
Simpson JL: Disorders of sexual differentiation: etiology and clinical delineation. New York: Academic, 1976.
Rosenberg C, et al.: Testicular regression in a patient with virilized female phenotype. Am J Med Genet 1984; 19:183–188.
de Grouchy J, et al.: Embryonic testicular regression syndrome and severe mental retardation in sibs. Ann Genet 1985; 28:154–160.

SI018                                          **Joe Leigh Simpson**

**Anorchia, familial**
*See AGONADIA*

## ANORECTAL MALFORMATIONS                              0069

**Includes:**

> Anal atresia or stenosis
> Anal membrane
> Anoperineal fistula
> Ectopic anus
> Imperforate anus, "high" and "low"
> Perineal anus
> Rectoperineal fistula

**Excludes:** Colon, atresia or stenosis (0193)

**Major Diagnostic Criteria:** The external opening of the terminal bowel is (1) normal in location but smaller than normal in size, or (2) occupies an ectopic site in the perineum, scrotum, vulva, vestibule, or vagina, or 3) is not visible on examination. Signs of low intestinal obstruction may occur in newborn period. Diagnosis is made by inspection and digital exam.

**Clinical Findings:** Imperforate anus is the traditional descriptive term for a large number of anorectal malformations resulting from a defect in the embryologic development of the terminal portion of

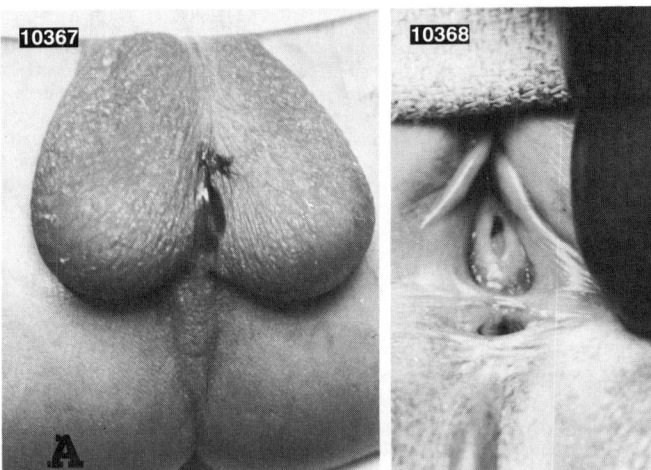

**0069**-10367: Covered anus in newborn male with meconium in the scrotal raphe. 10368: Anterior perineal anus in newborn female.

the hindgut. The majority of infants with anorectal malformations will show signs of low intestinal obstruction within 24 hours of birth because of the incomplete evacuation of meconium. In the male, pneumaturia or the passage of meconium in the urine indicates a rectourinary fistula. Constipation is the first symptom, developing several days or weeks after birth if the external opening is of nearly normal size. The diagnosis in these patients is evident by digital examination of the anus.

An international classification that integrates the clinical and anatomical features of all anorectal anomalies previously described has been proposed. In 41.3% of males, the bowel traversed the puborectalis sling of the levator ani muscle, and an external opening was present at the normal anal site (10.3%) or in the perineum (31%). In 51.2% of male patients the termination of the bowel was above the puborectalis sling, ending with a urinary fistula to the posterior urethra or bladder in 40.3% of cases. The bowel terminated in an intermediate position between the supralevator and infralevator groups in the remaining 7.5% of male patients. The bowel terminated below the puborectalis sling in 59.4% of female patients, and an external opening was identified at the normal anal site (4.7%), in the perineum (26.6%), or at the vulva (28.1%). Supralevator anomalies were less common in females (17.8%) than in males (51.2%). In 19.0% of the remaining 22.8% of female patients, the bowel terminated in an intermediate position with an external opening in the vestibule or the lower portion of the vagina.

**Complications:** The untreated patient who has an external opening of inadequate size gradually develops signs of low intestinal obstruction or constipation. Rectal bleeding from fissuring of the anal canal, buttock and perineal excoriation from paradoxical diarrhea with fecal impaction, and acquired megacolon are findings secondary to constipation in patients having an external orifice.

**Associated Findings:** Anomalies occur in 48% of all patients with anorectal malformation. These are subclassified as (1) skeletal (30%), usually lumbosacral (agenesis; dysplasia; hemivertebrae; malsegmentation), (2) GU (38%) renal agenesis and ectopia, vesicoureteral reflux and obstruction, (3) esophageal atresia with tracheoesophageal fistula (9.6%), (4) CNS (9.0%), (5) cardiovascular (5.6%), (6) other GI (4.7%), and (7) miscellaneous (13%). See also **Vater association.**

**Etiology:** Anorectal malformations are chance occurrences in the great majority of cases. Autosomal recessive inheritance is strongly suggested in studies of seven of ten families having more than one offspring with an anorectal malformation.

**Pathogenesis:** Anorectal malformations result from a defect or arrest in the embryologic development of the terminal hindgut (1) during the initial cloacal stage, or (2) when the cloaca is separated into a urogenital sinus and rectum by the urorectal septum, (3) during the posterior migration of the rectum, or (4) at the final stage of anal perforation. Infants with anorectal agenesis and urinary, cloacal, or high vaginal fistulae have anomalies related to the first and second stage of hindgut development. Infants having an abnormal external opening in the perineum, scrotum, vulva, vestibule, or lower vagina manifest an arrest in posterior migration of the rectum and belong to the intermediate or infralevator group of anorectal malformations. Completely covered anus and anal stenosis are examples of abnormalities in anal perforation.

**MIM No.:** 20750, 30180

**CDC No.:** 751.240, 751.230

**Sex Ratio:** M6:F4

**Occurrence:** 1:5,000 live births (in the United States). No racial or ethnic predilection is known.

**Risk of Recurrence for Patient's Sib:**
See Part I, *Mendelian Inheritance.*

**Risk of Recurrence for Patient's Child:**
See Part I, *Mendelian Inheritance.*

**Age of Detectability:** At birth.

**Gene Mapping and Linkage:** Unknown.

**Prevention:** None known. Genetic counseling indicated.

**Treatment:** Operative treatment of the newborn is directed to adequate decompression of the colon either by (1) dilation of the external orifice, (2) enlargement of the external orifice by anoplasty procedure, or (3) temporary defunctionalizing double-barrelled colostomy in infants without a visible external orifice or when an external opening is present but anoplasty procedure is not suitable. Definitive operative treatment by perineal anoplasty or by combined abdominoperineal pull-through or sacroabdominal pull-through is deferred until 1 year of age.

**Prognosis:** The overall mortality rate varies from 9.1% to 30% in reported cases. Over 90% of the deaths were attributed to major associated anomalies; these occurred more commonly in the group with supralevator anorectal malformations. The functional results are related to the inherent sensory neural and motor components left undisturbed by the embryologic defects as well as to the expertise of the anorectal reconstruction. Impairment of normal defecation occurs in approximately 50% of the supralevator group following anorectal reconstruction.

**Detection of Carrier:** Unknown.

**Special Considerations:** Dilation of anal stenosis constitutes complete treatment. Dilation of ectopic anal openings to allow decompression may precede definitive anoplasty procedures in selected patients. The risk of constipation in this group is high. Anoplasty procedures, usually by the "cut-back" techniques, are performed when the ectopic external opening is in the perineum, scrotum, vulva, or vestibule. If the external opening is in the vagina, colostomy is recommended. An adequate perineal body must be constructed during the definitive perineal anoplasty procedure. Transverse or sigmoid colostomy should be performed promptly in all newborn infants without a visible external opening instead of attempting anoplasty by perineal exploration since the risk of recurrent fistulae, undetected fistulae, nerve injury, anal stenosis, and fecal incontinence is increased by this treatment. Definitive anorectal reconstruction for infants not having a visible external opening and those infants with a vaginal orifice should be deferred until approximately 1 year of age. Male patients in this group require combined abdominoperineal pull-through operation with special attention directed to division of the existing urinary communications, preservation of the pelvic parasympathetic nerve plexus, precise placement of the rectum through the puborectalis sling, and creation of a skin-lined anal orifice surrounded by external sphincter muscle.

**References:**

Bill AH Jr, Johnson RJ: Failure of migration of the rectal opening as a cause for most cases of imperforate anus. Surg Gynecol Obstet 1958; 106:643.
Cozzi F, Wilkinson AW: Familial incidence of congenital anorectal anomalies. Surgery 1968; 64:669–671.
Santulli TV, et al.: Ano-rectal anomalies: a suggested international classification. J Pediatr Surg 1970; 5:281–287.
de Vries PA, Pena A: Posterior sagittal ano-rectoplasty: Important technical considerations and new applications. J Pediatr Surg 1982; 17:796–811.
Japan Study Group of Ano-rectal Anomalies: A group study for the classification of anorectal anomalies in Japan with comments to the international classification (1970). J Pediatr Surg 1982; 17:302–308.

T0009 **Robert J. Touloukian**

---

**ANOSMIA, CONGENITAL** 0070

**Includes:**
Anosmia, isolated
Anosmia, selective
Hyposmia
Olfaction loss, congenital
Smelling loss, congenital

**Excludes:**
Acquired anosmia
Hyposmia or anosmia associated with various syndromes

**Major Diagnostic Criteria:** Congenital anosmia and hyposmia include a group of individuals with an inability to smell certain or all odors. Formal diagnostic criteria are not yet established for hyposmia or anosmia; the mercaptans and potassium cyanide have been most commonly used in the past as olfactory stimulants. Delineation of hyposmic entities has been presented by Henkin (1968).

**Clinical Findings:** Except for the group with congenital craniofacial defects and those with endocrinologic disabilities such as pseudohypoparathyroidism and hypogonadotropic hypogonadism, most people with isolated anosmia are detected by clinical surveys.

It has been noted that certain individuals are anosmic to certain odors of which most persons are aware. However, the same patients are acutely sensitive to other odors, thus suggesting a selective anosmia or hyposmia. Such patients have not been found in the previously mentioned craniofacial or endocrine categories. Perhaps, because the above information is relatively new, they were not studied for these abnormalities.

**Complications:** Unknown.

**Associated Findings:** Findings include hypogonadotropic hypogonadism, pseudohypoparathyroidism, craniofacial defects, **Usher syndrome** and **Phytanic acid storage disease**.

**Etiology:** Undetermined. Many accept that anosmia and hyposmia are developmental abnormalities when trauma, neoplasia, inflammation, hypovitaminosis A can be ruled out. There are numerous examples in the literature of isolated familial anosmia: Anosmia, Congenital (MIM No. 10720), Anosmia for Isobutyric Acid (20700), Isovaleric Acid, Inability to Smell (24345), Musk, Inability to Smell (*25415), Anosmia (30170), and Cyanide, Inability to Smell (30430).

**Pathogenesis:** Agenesis of the olfactory system, especially in the region of the olfactory bulb.

**MIM No.:** 10720, 20700, 24345, *25415, 30170, 30430

**Sex Ratio:** Undetermined. Documentation is very limited.

**Occurrence:** Unknown.

**Risk of Recurrence for Patient's Sib:**
See Part I, *Mendelian Inheritance*.

**Risk of Recurrence for Patient's Child:**
See Part I, *Mendelian Inheritance*.

**Age of Detectability:** In childhood, dependent upon subject communication.

**Gene Mapping and Linkage:** Unknown.

**Prevention:** None known. Genetic counseling indicated.

**Treatment:** It appears that specific therapy for endocrine abnormalities does not alter the olfactory function.

**Prognosis:** Normal for life span and intelligence.

**Detection of Carrier:** Unknown.

**Special Considerations:** In the early 1900s, when investigation was first recorded on this subject, flowers, such as verbena, were used to differentiate between normal function, anosmia, or hyposmia. Later multiple substances such as hydrogen cyanide, alcohol, ether, chloroform, isobutyric acid, thymol, heliotrope, methyl salicilate, many of the mercaptans, especially butyl mercaptan (skunk), pyridine, and thiophene have been used as olfactory stimuli for purposes of differentiation.

Much recent interest in and development of theories of chemoreception have made feasible experimentation into hyposmia and anosmia. Amoore has described 7 basic molecular configurations that stimulate a particular subjective olfactory response. He has further demonstrated combinations of these as producing another specific response. The responses are dependent upon morphologic character of the molecule and, hence, increase the potential objectivity of studies into this field.

**References:**
Amoore JE: Specific anosmia: a clue to the olfactory code. Nature 1967; 214:1095–1098.
Henkin RI: Impairment of olfaction and of the tastes of sour and bitter in pseudohypoparathyroidism. J Clin Endocrinol 1968; 28:624–628.

Lygonis CS: Familial absence of olfaction. Hereditas 1969; 61:413–423.
Singh N, Grewal MS, Austin JH: Familial anosmia. Arch Neurol 1970; 22:40–45.
Whissell-Buechy D, Amoore JE: Odour-blindness to musk: simple recessive inheritance. Nature 1973; 242:271–273.
Kalmus H, Seedburgh D: Correlated odour threshold bimodality of two out of three synthetic musks. Ann Hum Genet 1975; 38:495–499.
Anholt RRH: Primary events in olfactory reception. Trends Biochem 1987; 12:58–62.
Lancet D, Pace U: The molecular basis of odor recognition. Trends Biochem 1987; 12:63–66.

BE028                                                **LaVonne Bergstrom**

**Anosmia, isolated**
    *See ANOSMIA, CONGENITAL*
**Anosmia, selective**
    *See ANOSMIA, CONGENITAL*
**Anotia**
    *See EAR, MICROTIA-ATRESIA*
**Anotopol disease**
    *See GLYCOGENOSIS, TYPE IId*
**Anterior chamber cleavage syndrome**
    *See EYE, ANTERIOR SEGMENT DYSGENESIS*
**Anterior duodenal portal vein**
    *See LIVER, VENOUS ANOMALIES*
**Anterior megalophthalmos**
    *See CORNEA, MEGALOCORNEA*
**Anterior nasal atresia**
    *See NOSE, ANTERIOR ATRESIA*
**Anterior nasal stenosis**
    *See NOSE, ANTERIOR STENOSIS*
**Anterior tunica vasculosa lentis persistence**
    *See EYE, PUPILLARY MEMBRANE PERSISTENCE*
**Anterolateral diaphragmatic hernia**
    *See DIAPHRAGMATIC HERNIA*
**Anthelix, prominent**
    *See EAR, PROMINENT ANTHELIX*

## ANTIBODIES TO HUMAN ALLOTYPES                         0071

**Includes:**
    Allotypes, antibodies to human
    Rheumatoid agglutinators (Raggs)
    Serum normal agglutinants (SNaggs)

**Excludes:** N/A

**Major Diagnostic Criteria:** Ability of the serum to cause red blood cells coated with an appropriate immunoglobulin (Ig) to agglutinate and for the agglutinating activity to be inhibitable by some serum samples and not others.

**Clinical Findings:** Ragg antibodies against gamma globulin (Gm) antigens are frequently found in the serum of patients with rheumatoid arthritis. These antibodies are carried by IgM, ie, the same molecules that carry the rheumatoid factor. Ragg antibodies almost invariably act against two or more of the Gm antigens. While they generally have a high titer, they are difficult to use because they are inhibited by all serum samples if the samples are not diluted more than 1/4, hence the difference between a positive serum and a negative serum is one of titer. Furthermore, it is a common finding that the specificity of the antibody varies during the course of the patient's disease. Thus far no Ragg antibody against the Inv antigens has been found. SNagg (from the French, *Serum Normal agglutinant*) antibodies against Gm and Inv(km) antigens are found in the serum of healthy individuals. Although these antibodies are almost invariably IgM they are, with rare exceptions, unspecific. While they are generally of low titer they have the great virtue of not reacting with negative serum samples even when the samples are undiluted. In the majority of cases SNagg antibodies seem to result from an immune reaction by the fetus against the mother's IgG when the latter carries an antigen not present in the genotype of the fetus. The frequency with which these antibodies are detected in healthy individuals depends upon the IgG employed to coat the red blood cells used in the test and upon the age of the donors being tested. In 1 study, 11% of children between 6 months and 5 years of age were found to have antibodies, while older children and adults had antibodies in approximately 5% of the cases. SNagg antibodies may be induced by repeated transfusions. Antibodies against Gm antigens have been raised in many kinds of animals, including rabbits and rhesus monkeys. Antibodies against Inv(km) have been raised in rabbits.

Antibodies against alpha globulin allotypes (Am) have been found in patients who have experienced transfusion reactions. These antibodies, unlike those against the Gm and Inv allotypes, are IgG.

**Complications:** Gm and Inv antibodies: No complications are ordinarily associated with the presence of antibodies against the Gm or Inv allotypes. However, one volunteer in whom an antibody had been induced by repeated transfusions showed a reaction to a massive infusion of incompatible plasma, and a patient with a presumably normally induced antibody has been reported to have suffered a transfusion reaction.

Am antibodies: As indicated above, antibodies against the Am allotypes are IgG and may cause transfusion reactions.

**Associated Findings:** None known.

**Etiology:** Antigen-antibody interaction.

**Pathogenesis:** Unknown.

**Sex Ratio:** M1:F1

**Occurrence:** High (>50%) when the fetus is exposed to an foreign antigen. The frequency of exposure depends on the frequency of the allele in the population.

**Risk of Recurrence for Patient's Sib:** Unknown.

**Risk of Recurrence for Patient's Child:** Unknown.

**Age of Detectability:** Detectable with special care at birth; easily observed after six months of age.

**Gene Mapping and Linkage:** The Gm and Am antigens are located at chromosome 14q32. Inv (km) is located on 2p.

**Prevention:** None known. Genetic counseling indicated.

**Treatment:** Unknown.

**Prognosis:** Normal for life span, intelligence, and function.

**Detection of Carrier:** Unknown.

**References:**
Giblett ER: Genetic Markers in Human Blood. Philadelphia: FA Davis Co, 1969.
Steinberg AG: Globulin polymorphism in man. Ann Rev Genet 1969; 3:25–52.
Vyas GN, Fudenberg HH: Immunobiology of human anti-IgA: a serologic and immunogenetic study of immunization to IgA in transfusion and pregnancy. Clin Genet 1970; 1:45–64.
Steinberg AG, Cook CE: The distribution of the human Immunoglobulin allotypes. Oxford: Oxford University Press, 1981.

ST013                                          **Arthur G. Steinberg**

**Antibody deficiencies, partial**
*See IMMUNODEFICIENCY, IgG SUBCLASS DEFICIENCIES*
**Antibody deficiency-beta-2 macroglobulinemia**
*See IMMUNODEFICIENCY, X-LINKED WITH HYPER IgM*
**Anticoagulant, oral, embryopathy**
*See FETAL WARFARIN SYNDROME*
**Antiepileptic drugs (some), fetal effects**
*See FETAL BARBITURATE EFFECTS*
**Antimongolism**
*See CHROMOSOME 21, MONOSOMY 21*

---

## ANTITHROMBIN III DEFICIENCY                          3066

**Includes:**
    AT III deficiencies
    Heparin cofactor deficiency
    Thrombophilia due to deficiency of AT III, hereditary

**Excludes:** Antithrombin III deficiency, acquired

**Major Diagnostic Criteria:** Less than 60–75% of the normal biologic activity of antithrombin III (AT III), often demonstrated by measuring the inhibitory effect of the test plasma on thrombin's ability to convert a chromogenic substrate. Normal individuals usually have 85–115% activity compared with normal reference plasma. Such tests must be interpreted with caution prior to age six months. Differentiation between the inherited and acquired forms of AT III deficiency rely on clinical and laboratory criteria.

**Clinical Findings:** The major clinical manifestation of AT III deficiency is an increased propensity toward venous thrombosis, especially in adulthood. Less than 10% of AT III-deficient individuals younger than age 15 years suffer a thrombotic event, but the risk increase markedly thereafter; by age 55 years, 85% will have had a clinically obvious thrombotic event. The median age for first thrombosis is 24 years. In 40% of patients the first thrombotic event is spontaneous, but in the remainder it develops in association, with conditions known to predispose to thrombosis, including pregnancy, delivery, surgery and trauma, and ingestion of oral contraceptives. The most common sites of thrombosis are the deep leg and iliac embolism occurs in 40% of affected patients. Thrombosis of the mesenteric veins occurs in only 8% of affected individuals, but this complication is nearly unique to AT III-deficient patients. Almost 60% of those with AT III deficiency suffer from recurrent thromboses. There is substantial heterogeneity of disease expression not only between, but even within, families.

**Complications:** Venous thrombosis at various sites. It does not appear that deficiency of AT III predisposes to arterial thrombosis.

**Associated Findings:** None known.

**Etiology:** Autosomal dominant inheritance with complete penetrance.

**Pathogenesis:** Both deletional and nondeletional DNA mutations affecting the AT III gene have been demonstrated to be causes of AT III deficiency; both types of mutations have been associated with the most common ("classical") type of AT III deficiency.

**MIM No.:** *10730

**Sex Ratio:** M1:F1

**Occurrence:** The prevalence of congenital AT III deficiency is approximately 1:2,000–5,000. No racial predilection has been reported.

**Risk of Recurrence for Patient's Sib:**
    See Part I, *Mendelian Inheritance.*

**Risk of Recurrence for Patient's Child:**
    See Part I, *Mendelian Inheritance.*

**Age of Detectability:** It is highly unusual for children to be clinically affected, and typically the diagnosis is made in early adulthood. However, diminished AT III activity should be demonstrable even in infancy. It should be noted that "normal" adult levels of activity are not achieved until age six months, even in unaffected individuals. In those rare families in which the molecular defect has been characterized, prenatal diagnosis is theoretically achievable. Furthermore, a common DNA polymorphism has been described within the AT III gene, and thus family studies may prove informative and permit early diagnosis.

**Gene Mapping and Linkage:** AT3 (antithrombin III) has been mapped to 1q23-q25.1.
Linkage has been established between AT III and the Duffy blood group locus.

**Prevention:** None known. Genetic counseling indicated.

**Treatment:** Treatment of venous thromboses in patients with AT III deficiency is often similar to that generally used for thrombotic events, i.e., acute heparin administration followed by long-term oral anticoagulant treatment. While resistance to heparin is occasionally encountered, oral anticoagulants are much more consistently helpful. Alternative acute therapy includes fresh frozen plasma or AT III concentrate with or without concomitant heparin administration.

**Prognosis:** The prognosis generally worsens with advancing age, as the risk of thrombosis increases. It may also worsen in the presence of predisposing prothrombotic conditions, e.g., pregnancy, surgery, and so forth. The range of severity is large; a fortunate few escape without any clinical sequelae, whereas in others severe thrombotic events may prove fatal.

**Detection of Carrier:** Clinical and laboratory examinations.

**Special Considerations:** By definition, all patients with AT III deficiency demonstrate reduced biologic activity of AT III; variants may be classified on the basis of whether there is concordant diminution of AT III antigen as determined by immunoassay and whether the heparin or thrombin binding activity is predominantly affected. Type I ("classical") is most common and refers to quantitative diminution in the amount of AT III molecule synthesized; activity and level of antigen are reduced concordantly. (In type Ib, a rare subtype, patients demonstrate these characteristics, but the molecule has abnormal electrophoretic mobility in the presence of heparin). Type II patients synthesize sufficient antigen, but the molecule carries a mutation in the thrombin binding region, causing reduced plasma antithrombin activity. Type III patients also synthesize sufficient antigen, but carry a mutation in the heparin binding region. Their AT III can slowly inhibit thrombin, but the rate of inhibition is not accelerated by heparin (i.e., reduced heparin cofactor activity). The following variants have been described:

AT III Budapest (Sas et al., 1974);
AT III Basel (Tran et al., 1980);
AT III Aalborg (Søorensen et al., 1980);
AT III Chicago (Ashenhurst et al., 1981);
AT III Vicenza (Barbui and Rodeghiero, 1981);
AT III Paris (Wolf et al., 1982);
AT III Toyama (Sakuragawa et al., 1983);
AT III Roma (Leone et al., 1983);
AT III Padua (Girolami et al., 1983a);
AT III Padua-2 (Girolami et al., 1983b);
AT III Tours (Chasse et al., 1984);
AT III Hvidovre (Jorgensen et al., 1984);
AT III Trento (Girolami et al., 1984);
AT III Charleville (Aiach et al., 1985);
AT III Milano (Wolf et al., 1985);
AT III Malmo (Tengborn et al., 1985);
AT III Alger (Fischer et al., 1986);
AT III Denver (Sambrano et al., 1986);
AT III Fontainebleau (Boyer et al., 1986);
AT III Milano 2 (Tripodi et al., 1986);
AT III Northwick Park (Lane et al., 1987a);
AT III Dublin (Daly et al., 1987);
AT III Geneva (deMoerloose et al., 1987);
AT III Rouen-I (Owen et al., 1987).
AT III Glasgow (Lane et al., 1987b);
AT III Clichy (Aiach et al., 1987).
AT III Avranches (Aiach et al., 1988).
AT III Barcelona (Grau et al., 1988).
AT III Hamilton (Devraj-Kizuk et al., 1988).
AT III Rouen-II (Borg et al., 1988).
AT III Utah (Bock et al., 1988).
AT III Kumamoto (Okajima et al., 1989).
AT III Sheffield (appears to be the same as AT III Glasgow) (Lane et al., 1
AT III Pescara (Lane et al., 1989b).

**References:**
Egeberg O: Inherited antithrombin deficiency causing thrombophilia. Thromb Diath Haemorrh 1965; 13:516–530. *
Sas G, et al.: Abnormal antithrombin III (antithrombin III "Budapest") as a cause of a familial thrombophilia. Thromb Diath Haemorrh 1974; 32:105–115.
Søorensen PJ, et al.: Familial functional antithrombin III deficiency. Scand J Haematol 1980; 24:105–109.
Tran TH, et al.: Purification and partial characterization of a hereditary abnormal antithrombin III fraction of a patient with recurrent thrombophlebitis. Thromb Haemost 1980; 44:87–91.
Ashenhurst JB, et al.: Antithrombin III (AT) "Chicago": a congenital defect in the heparin-dependent allosteric mechanism of antithrombin. Blood (suppl 1) 1981; 58:229a.
Barbui T, Rodeghiero F: Hereditary dysfunctional antithrombin III (AT-III Vicenza). Thromb Haemost 1981; 45:97.
Thaler E, Lechner K: Antithrombin III deficiency and thromboembolism. Clin Haematol 1981; 10:369–390. *
Wolf M, et al.: A new familial variant of antithrombin III: "Antithrombin III Paris." Br J Haematol 1982; 51:281–295.
Girolami A, et al.: Antithrombin III Padua: a "new" congenital antithrombin III abnormality with normal or near normal activity, normal antigen, abnormal migration and no thrombotic disease. Folia Haematol (Leipz) 1983a; 110:98–111.
Girolami A, et al.: Antithrombin III (AT III) Padua₂: a "new" congenital abnormality with defective heparin co-factor activities but no thrombotic disease. Blut 1983b; 47:93–103.
Leone G, et al.: Antithrombin III Roma: a familial quantitative-qualitative AT-III deficiency identifiable by crossed immunoelectrofocusing and by crossed immunoelectrophoresis. Haematologica 1983; 68:765–774.
Prochownik EV, et al.: Molecular heterogeneity of inherited antithrombin III deficiency. New Engl J Med 1983; 308:1549–1552.
Sakuragawa N, et al.: Antithrombin III Toyama: a hereditary abnormal antithrombin III of a patient with recurrent thrombophlebitis. Thromb Res 1983; 31:305–317.
Chasse JF, et al.: An abnormal plasma antithrombin with no apparent affinity for heparin. Thromb Res 1984; 34:297–302.
Girolami A, et al.: Antithrombin III Trento. Acta Haemat 1984; 72:73–82.
Jorgensen M, et al.: Purification and characterization of hereditary abnormal antithrombin III with impaired thrombin binding. J Lab Clin Med 1984; 104:245–256.
Aiach M, et al.: A functional abnormal antithrombin III (AT III) deficiency: AT III Charleville. Thromb Res 1985; 39:559–570.
Bock SC, et al.: Assignment of the human antithrombin III structural gene to chromosome 1q23–25. Cytogenet Cell Genet 1985; 39:67–69. *
Rosenberg RD, et al.: Antithrombin III: the heparin-antithrombin system. J Med 1985; 16:351–416. *
Tengborn L, et al.: A Swedish family with abnormal antithrombin III. Scand J Haematol 1985; 34:412–416.
Wolf M, et al.: Antithrombin Milano: a new variant with monomeric and dimeric inactive antithrombin III. Blood 1985; 65:496–500.
Boyer C, et al.: Homozygous variant of antithrombin III: AT III Fontainebleau. Thromb Haemost 1986; 56:18–22.
Fischer AM, et al.: Antithrombin III Alger: a new homozygous AT III variant. Thromb Haemost 1986; 55:218–221.
Sambrano JE, et al.: Abnormal antithrombin III with defective serine protease binding (antithrombin III "Denver"). J Clin Invest 1986; 77:887–893.
Tripodi A, et al.: Characterization of an abnormal antithrombin (Milano 2) with defective thrombin binding. Thromb Haemost 1986; 56:349–352.
Aiach M, et al.: An abnormal antithrombin III (AT III) with low heparin affinity: AT III Clichy. Br J Haematol 1987; 66:515–522.
Daly M, et al.: Identification and characterization of a new antithrombin III familial variant (AT Dublin) with possible increased frequency in children with cancer. Br J Haematol 1987; 65:457–462.
deMoerloose PA, et al.: Antithrombin III Geneva: a hereditary abnormal antithrombin III with defective heparin cofactor activity. Thromb Haemost 1987; 57:154–157.
Lane DA, et al.: Antithrombin III Northwick Park: demonstration of an inactive high MW complex with increased affinity for heparin. Br J Haematol 1987a; 65:451–456.
Lane DA, et al.: Antithrombin III Glasgow: a variant with increased heparin affinity and reduced ability to activate thrombin, associated with familial thrombosis. Br J Haematol 1987b; 66:523–527.
Owen MC, et al.: Heparin binding defect in a new antithrombin III variant: Rouen, 47 Arg to His. Blood 1987; 69:1275–1279.
Aiach M, et al.: Antithrombin III Avranches, a new variant with

defective serine-protease inhibition: comparison with Antithrombin III Charleville. Thromb Haemost 1988; 60:94–96.

Bock SC, et al.: Antithrombin III Utah: Proline-407 to leucine mutation in a highly conserved region near the inhibitor reactive site. Biochemistry 1988; 27:6171–6178.

Borg JY, et al.: Proposed heparin binding site in antithrombin based on arginine 47; a new variant Rouen-II, 47 arg to ser. J Clin Invest 1988; 81:1292–1296.

Devraj-Kizuk R, et al.: Antithrombin-III-Hamilton: a gene with a point mutation (guanine to adenine) in codon 382 causing impaired serine protease reactivity. Blood 1988; 72:1518–1523.

Grau E, et al.: AT III Barcelona: a familial quantitative-qualitative AT III deficiency. Thromb Haemost 1988; 59:13–17.

Lane DA, et al.: Antithrombin Sheffield: amino acid substitution at the reactive site (Arg 393 to His) causing thrombosis. Brit J Haematol 1989a; 71:91–96.

Lane DA, et al.: A novel amino acid substitution in the reactive site of a congenital variant antithrombin; Antithrombin Pescara, arg [393] to pro caused by a CGT to CCT mutation. J Biol Chem 1989b; 264:10200–10204.

Okajima K, et al: Homozygous variant of antithrombin III that lacks affinity for heparin, AT III Kumamoto. Thromb Haemost 1989; 61:20–24.

SH052                              **Bruce I. Sharon**

**Antithyroid drug goiter**
*See GOITER, GOITROGEN INDUCED*
**Antithyroid fetal effects, scalp and urachal**
*See FETAL EFFECTS FROM METHIMAZOLE AND CARBIMAZOLE*
**Antitrypsin**
*See ALPHA(1)-ANTITRYPSIN DEFICIENCY*
**Antiviral interferon deficiency**
*See INTERFERON DEFICIENCY*

---

## ANTLEY-BIXLER SYNDROME                2125

**Includes:**
    Acrocephalosynankie
    Multisynostotic osteodysgenesis-long bone fractures
    Osteodysgenesis, multisynostotic, with fractures
    Trapezoidocephaly-synostosis syndrome

**Excludes:**
    **Acrocephalopolysyndactyly**
    **Acrocephalosyndactyly**

**Major Diagnostic Criteria:** Craniostenosis (100%); severe midface hypoplasia (100%); proptosis (100%); dysplastic ears (100%); camptodactyly (100%); radiohumeral synostosis (100%); femoral bowing/fractures (100%); choanal stenosis/atresia (44%).

**Clinical Findings:** Based on nine reported cases, prenatal and postnatal growth have been normal. Normal neonatal adaptation

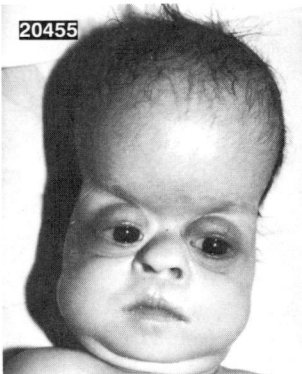
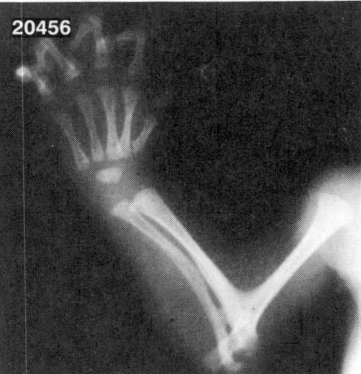

**2125-20455:** Craniosynostosis, proptosis and midface hypoplasia. **20456:** Radiohumeral synostosis and finger contractures.

may be complicated by upper respiratory obstruction secondary to choanal stenosis/atresia. Intellectual performance has been variable. The etiology of developmental delays is not known. Motor performance is adversely affected by synostoses and joint contractures. The altered craniofacial appearance is thought to be secondary to a shortened cranial base. Auditory dysfunction may be conductive or neurosensory. Upper airway congestion is not permanent but is of variable duration. Nasal stenting may be required in early infancy. Radiohumeral synostosis (RHS) has been observed prenatally. In one patient on whom the RHS was released, bony fusion recurred. Carpal fusion also limits motion. Flexion contractures at the fingers have been associated with shortened tendons. These improve with time and physical therapy. Contractures at the hips limit movement and may predispose to femoral fractures during birth. All patients followed beyond infancy have been ambulatory.

**Complications:** Respiratory distress secondary to choanal stenosis/atresia; Femoral fractures secondary to hip contractures, femoral bowing, and trauma of delivery; limited range of motion at elbow secondary to radiohumeral synostosis, and secondary to digital contractures.

**Associated Findings:** **Atrial septal defects** (3 of 9 cases), and carpal fusion.

**Etiology:** Autosomal recessive inheritance is suggested by the fact that affected siblings have been born to unaffected parents.

**Pathogenesis:** Unknown.

**MIM No.:** 20741

**POS No.:** 3570

**Sex Ratio:** M2:F7 (Observed).

**Occurrence:** Undetermined but presumed rare. About a dozen cases have been documented, including one case from Japan.

**Risk of Recurrence for Patient's Sib:**
    See Part I, *Mendelian Inheritance.*

**Risk of Recurrence for Patient's Child:**
    See Part I, *Mendelian Inheritance.*

**Age of Detectability:** At birth. Prenatal diagnosis with ultrasound has detected this disorder in an at-risk pregnancy.

**Gene Mapping and Linkage:** Unknown.

**Prevention:** None known. Genetic counseling indicated.

**Treatment:** Choanal stenting decreases airway obstruction. Casting for femoral fractures appears indicated. Physical therapy for improved range of motion at joint contractures should be undertaken.

**Prognosis:** Guarded. Based upon nine reported cases, three patients have died in infancy of unexplained causes. Of the three individuals who have survived past infancy, and on whom data are available, two have had normal development and one has had developmental delay with IQ approximately 60 at age 10 years.

**Detection of Carrier:** Unknown.

**References:**

Antley R, Bixler D: Trapezoidocephaly, midfacial hypoplasia and cartilage abnormalities with multiple synostoses and skeletal fractures. BD:OAS XI(2). New York: March of Dimes Birth Defects Foundation, 1974:397–401.

Lacheretz M, et al.: L'acrocephalo-synankie: a propos d'une observation avec synostoses multiples. Pediatrie 1974; 29:169–177.

DeLozier CD, et al.: The syndrome of multisynostotic osteodysgenesis with long bone fractures. Am J Med Genet 1980; 7:391–403.

Robinson LK, et al.: The Antley-Bixler syndrome. J Pediatr 1982; 101:201–205.

Schinzel A, et al.: The Antley-Bixler syndrome in sisters: a term newborn and a prenatally diagnosed fetus. Am J Med Genet 1983; 14:1139–147.

Robert E, et al.: Le syndrome D'Antley-Bixler: revue de la literature, a propos d'une observation personnelle. J Genet Hum 1984; 32:291–298.

R0007                                 **Luther K. Robinson**

**Antral atresia**
*See STOMACH, PYLORIC ATRESIA*
**Antral G-cell hyperfunction DU**
*See PEPTIC ULCER DISEASES, NON-SYNDROMIC*
**Antral web**
*See STOMACH, PYLORIC ATRESIA*
**Anus, imperforate-hand, foot, and ear anomalies**
*See ANUS-HAND-EAR SYNDROME*

---

## ANUS-HAND-EAR SYNDROME                           0072

**Includes:**
Anus, imperforate-hand, foot, and ear anomalies
Deafness (sensorineural)-imperforate anus-hypoplastic
thumbs
REAR syndrome
Townes-Brocks syndrome

**Excludes:**
**Branchio-oto-renal dysplasia** (2224)
**Deafness-onycho-osteo-dystrophy-retardation-seizures (doors)**
(0262)
**Deafness-triphalangeal thumbs-onychodystrophy** (2151)
**FG syndrome, Opitz-Kaveggia type** (0754)
**Heart-hand syndrome** (0455)
**Vater association** (0987)
Nonsyndromic anorectal, hand, or ear malformation

**Major Diagnostic Criteria:** Two or more of the following: 1)
anorectal malformation (imperforate anus, anteriorly placed anus,
anal stenosis); 2) hand malformation (preaxial polydactyly, broad
or bifid thumb, triphalangeal thumb); 3) external ear malformation
(microtia, "satyr" or "lop" ear, preauricular tags or pits) with
sensorineural hearing loss; 4) a relative with the syndrome.

**Clinical Findings:** Of the patients described by Townes and
Brocks (1972), Kurnit et al. (1978), and Walpole and Hockey
(1982), ten were male, nine were female, all had anorectal malformation, (9/16) had hand malformation, and (15/16) had ear malformation. In the family described by Reid and Turner (1976) there
were 12 males and 7 females: all had an anorectal malformation
(skin covered anus), five males had broad or bifid thumbs (none
had triphalangeal thumbs), and five males had preauricular tags
(none with pinna malformation or deafness).

**Complications:** Developmental delays may occur if hearing loss
is not diagnosed early, and patients with urinary tract anomalies
may be predisposed to pyelonephritis.

**Associated Findings:** Urinary tract malformation (unilateral renal hypoplasia, meatal stenosis, posterior urethral valves), absent
or hypoplastic toes, clinodactyly of 5th toes, pes planus, abnormal

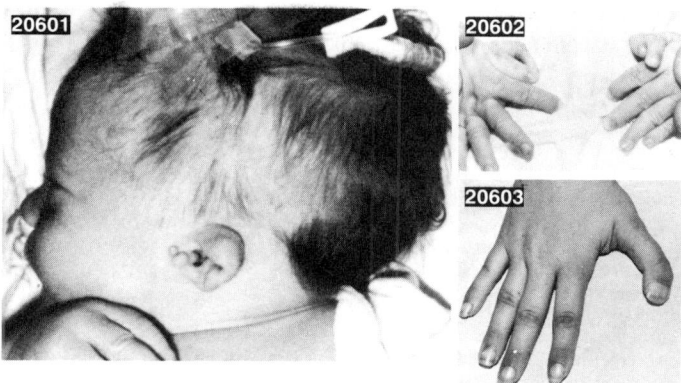

**0072-20601:** Anus-hand-ear syndrome; note small, lop ear from
deficient cartilage and pre-auricular ear tags. **20602:** Bilateral
bifid thumbs. **20603:** Triphalangeal thumb is bilateral in this
subject.

toes with bony exostoses, fused metatarsals, pseudoepiphyses of
second metacarpals, absent triquetrals, fusion of triquetrum and
hamate, cone-shaped epiphyses, cleft lip and palate, hypoplastic
mandible, incomplete closure of left side of mouth, widely spaced
incisors.

**Etiology:** Autosomal dominant inheritance.

**Pathogenesis:** Unknown.

**MIM No.:** *10748

**POS No.:** 3026

**Sex Ratio:** Generally M1:F1 (some syndromes may have sex-
influenced expression).

**Occurrence:** About 75 cases documented.

**Risk of Recurrence for Patient's Sib:**
See Part I, *Mendelian Inheritance.*

**Risk of Recurrence for Patient's Child:**
See Part I, *Mendelian Inheritance.*

**Age of Detectability:** At Birth.

**Gene Mapping and Linkage:** Unknown.

**Prevention:** None known. Genetic counseling indicated.

**Treatment:** Surgical repair of thumb and anal anomalies; early
hearing evaluation with close follow-up for speech development;
early urinary tract evaluation and treatment.

**Prognosis:** Depends on severity of malformations; probably
good for normal life span.

**Detection of Carrier:** By physical examination; penetrance unknown.

**Special Considerations:** There may be a spectrum of anus-hand-
ear syndromes that are autosomal dominant with variable expressivity. This community of syndromes may include a number of
"private" syndromes with similar but distinct features that occur
consistently within single families. The patients reported by
Townes and Brocks (1972) and Walpole and Hockey (1982) appear
to have a specific, recognizable, autosomal dominant malformation syndrome. The patients reported by Reid and Turner (1976)
have a similar but distinct syndrome that is autosomal dominant
with sex-influenced expression. The patients reported by Kurnit et
al. (1978) have anorectal malformations similar to those reported
by Reid and Turner but other clinical features similar to the
Townes-Brocks patients. Their observations suggest that urinary
tract malformation may be an important feature of these syndromes. The single patient reported by Monteiro de Pina-Neto
(1984) had anomalies typical of **Vater association**. On the other
hand, the nonfamilial case reported by Hersh et al. (1986) had
anomalies more typical of the Townes-Brocks syndrome.

Counseling and clinical management of a patient or family
should emphasize the manifestations exhibited in that particular
family but take into account features described for the entire
community of syndromes. Pinsky (1978) has provided a review of
syndromes that includes anorectal malformation.

**References:**
Townes PL, Brocks E: Hereditary syndrome of imperforate anus with
hand, foot and ear anomalies. J Pediatr 1972; 81:321–326. *
Reid IS, Turner G: Familial anal abnormality. J Pediatr 1976; 88:992–
994.
Kurnit DM, et al.: Autosomal dominant transmission of a syndrome of
anal, ear, renal, and radial congenital malformations. J Pediatr 1978;
93:270–273.
Pinsky L: The syndromology of anorectal malformation (atresia,
stenosis, ectopia). Am J Med Genet 1978; 1:461–474.
Walpole IR, Hockey A: Syndrome of imperforate anus, abnormalities
of hands and feet, satyr ears, and sensorineural defects. J Pediatr
1982; 100:250–252.*
Monteiro de Pina-Neto J: Phenotypic variability in Townes-Brocks
syndrome. Am J Med Genet 1984; 18:147–152.
Hersh JH, et al.: Townes syndrome. A distinct multiple malformation
syndrome resembling VACTERL association. Clin Pediatr 1986;
25:100–102.

AY000                                            **Arthur S. Aylsworth**

## AORTA, COARCTATION                                    0073

**Includes:**
> Aorta, coarctation of abdominal
> Coarctation, postductal
> Coarctation, preductal
> Thoracic aorta, coarctation of lower

**Excludes:**
> Aorta, coarctation, infantile type (2909)
> Aortic arch, absence of
> Aortic arch, hypoplasia of
> Aortic arch interruption (0076)
> Aortic hypoplasia
> Pseudocoarctation cervical arch

**Major Diagnostic Criteria:** A blood pressure difference between the upper and lower limbs is diagnostic. Typical X-ray findings, aortography, and suprasternal notch echocardiogram are confirmatory.

**Clinical Findings:** The typical thoracic coarctation consists of a localized area of narrowing just distal to the left subclavian artery and situated just proximal to, opposite, or distal to the insertion of the ductus arteriosus. Collateral circulation arises primarily from the subclavian artery and its branches and includes: upper intercostal, internal mammary, scapular, lateral thoracic, transverse cervical, and anterior spinal arteries. Associated cardiovascular malformations may include: patent ductus arteriosus (40% of preductal coarctations), bicuspid aortic valve (up to 85% of the cases), ventricular septal defect, anomalous origin of the right subclavian artery above or below the coarctation, stenosis or atresia of the left subclavian artery.

Approximately 2% of aortic coarctations are situated in atypical locations in the thoracic or abdominal aorta and may be localized or involve a larger segment of the aorta. Coarctation of the abdominal aorta is more frequently located above or at the level of the renal arteries and may involve these vessels as well as the celiac and superior mesenteric vessels. Significant collateral circulation may be present through anastomoses of the middle colic branch of the inferior mesenteric artery. Associated cardiovascular lesions occur infrequently.

The infant with coarctation of the aorta often develops congestive heart failure between 2 and 6 weeks of age. An additional cardiovascular lesion such as patent ductus arteriosus or ventricular septal defect may frequently be present. The older child with coarctation usually presents with findings of a heart murmur, absent or diminished and delayed femoral pulses together with a significant pressure gradient between the upper and lower limbs, and frequently a systolic suprasternal notch thrill. A mid-to-late systolic murmur is best heard along the left sternal border. Posteriorly, between the scapulae, this systolic murmur may extend past the second sound. In older children, systolic or continuous bruits are related to the presence of collateral circulation. A high-pitched decrescendo diastolic murmur at the third left intracostal space suggests the association of aortic insufficiency due to a bicuspid valve. An aortic systolic click may be encountered, especially in the presence of a bicuspid aortic valve. A murmur in the epigastric and lumbar areas suggests a lower thoracic or abdominal coarctation.

The EKG frequently demonstrates right ventricular hypertrophy in the infant, especially in the presence of an associated lesion. In the absence of associated lesions, most children over 6 months of age demonstrate left ventricular hypertrophy. Thoracic X-rays are usually diagnostic once the patient is beyond the infant age range. There are two primary signs. Notching of the inferior margin of the ribs (usually the third rib through the eighth) is the first indication. This finding, not commonly seen in children less than 4 years of age, is not always present, and is usually confined to the posterior aspect of the ribs. Secondly, some distortion or disfigurement of the aortic knob is present in the vast majority of cases. This distortion may cause densities in this region which resemble a "figure of three." The remainder of findings involving the heart and great vessels may be identical to any condition which places the left ventricle under an obstructive stress. When

this occurs, the heart assumes a left ventricular configuration. If the left ventricle maintains compensation, the vasculature is normal and the heart is normal sized. With left ventricular failure, there are signs of pulmonary venous obstruction and left atrial enlargement. The ascending aorta is prominent in nearly all cases. In an atypical coarctation, thoracic X-rays fail to demonstrate indentation of the aortic isthmus. Rib-notching is absent or confined to the lower ribs. Cardiac catheterization generally demonstrates hypertension above the site of the coarctation, while below the lesion, aortic pressure is decreased and the pressure curve reveals a narrow pulse pressure, slow rise and delay of peak pressure. Aortography demonstrates the site, severity and extent of the coarctation, together with the degree of collateral circulation. Injection of contrast material in the ascending aorta demonstrates the presence or absence of a bicuspid aortic valve. When aortography demonstrates that an abdominal coarctation involves one or both renal arteries, individual renal function studies are indicated.

Echocardiographically detectable abnormalities associated with coarctation of the aorta such as bicuspid aortic valve, parachute deformity of the mitral valve or the presence of left ventricular hypertrophy can aid in the serial follow-up of these patients. Infants with clinical findings of coarctation should be screened for hypoplastic left heart syndrome. The area of coarctation is revealed only by invasive techniques.

**Complications:** Congestive heart failure is common in infancy (2–4 weeks), especially when a patent ductus arteriosus, ventricular septal defect or other cardiovascular lesion is present.

**Associated Findings:** The most common cardiovascular anomaly in patients with gonadal dysgenesis is coarctation of the aorta. Aneurysms of the cerebral vasculature may be present and may rupture at some time in life.

**Etiology:** Multifactorial inheritance.

**Pathogenesis:** Has been related to the presence of ductal tissue in the wall of the aorta at the site of the coarctation. May be caused by exaggeration of the normal infolding of the wall of the aorta distal to the left subclavian artery producing a "subclavian shelf." Coarctation may be present at birth or occasionally may develop postnatally. Abdominal coarctation may be congenital or acquired, and has been reported in patients with neurofibromatosis, pulseless disease, and certain infectious diseases.

**MIM No.:** 12000

**CDC No.:** 747.1

**Sex Ratio:** M2:F1

**Occurrence:** Incidence 1:1600 live births. Prevalence less than 1:2000 in the pediatric population.

**Risk of Recurrence for Patient's Sib:** About 2%.

**Risk of Recurrence for Patient's Child:** If mother is affected: 4%. If father is affected: 2%.

**Age of Detectability:** From birth by selective angiography.

**Gene Mapping and Linkage:** Unknown.

**Prevention:** None known. Genetic counseling indicated.

**Treatment:** Thoracic coarctation: resection and end-to-end anastomosis or graft (preferable after 3 years of age). Abdominal coarctation, resection or bypass graft. Correction of associated renal vascular abnormality by bypass graft or resection. In infants, subclavian flap operation. A recent advance in the treatment of coarctation is the use of non-surgical balloon angioplasty. Originally most useful in recurrent coarctations, this procedure has recently been successfully used as an initial approach to the treatment of aortic coarctation.

Symptomatic therapy for hypertension and congestive heart failure. The infant with congestive heart failure and isolated coarctation usually responds to medical management and does not require immediate operation. When heart failure is unresponsive to medical management in complicated coarctation, operation is indicated.

**Prognosis:** The average age of death in untreated coarctation is 35 years, due to cerebral hemorrhage, aortic rupture, progressive aortic insufficiency with congestive heart failure or subacute bacterial endocarditis. Prognosis is much improved in surgically treated coarctation with decrease in hypertension often to normal levels. Surgical correction in infancy may provide initial improvement, but can result in later development of obstruction as the anastomotic site fails to keep up with growth of the aorta.

**Detection of Carrier:** Unknown.

**Special Considerations:** Postoperative complications: hemorrhage from anastomotic site, pulmonary infection, paradoxical hypertension, necrotizing arteritis of the GI tract blood vessels. Paradoxical hypertension occurring in the first 24 to 36 hours postoperatively usually does not require treatment. Delayed hypertension may occur 48 hours after surgery and last for 7 to 14 days. Necrotizing arteritis of the GI tract blood vessels may occur in up to 19% of patients undergoing repair of coarctation. On about the 4th postoperative day there is onset of abdominal pain and distention, fever, vomiting, and melena associated with leukocytosis. Conservative management is usually recommended with sympatholytics, intestinal antibiotics and decompression. The hypertension occurring with coarctation of the aorta has been attributed to mechanical obstruction and to the development of humoral factors. More recent reports have implicated the renin-angiotensin-aldosterone mechanism as the basis of a humoral involvement, or to increased sympathetic nerve activity. Prognosis in coarctation of the aorta is also affected by the presence of the associated defects, particularly by a bicuspid aortic valve. This, in later life, may become insufficient or stenotic.

**References:**

Riemenschneider TA, et al.: Coarctation of the abdominal aorta in children: report of three cases and review of the literature. Pediatrics 1969; 44:716.

Liberthson RR, et al.: Coarctation of the aorta: review of 234 patients and clarification of management problems. Am J Cardiol 1979; 43:835–840.

Berman LB, et al.: Coarctation of the aorta in children: late results after surgery. Am J Dis Child 1980; 134:464–468.

Gersony WM: Coarctation of the aorta. In Adams FH, Emmanualdes GC, eds, Heart disease in infants, children and adolescents. Baltimore: Williams & Wilkins, 1983:188–198. *

Nora JJ, Nora AH: Maternal transmission of congenital heart disease. Am J Cardiol 1987; 59:459–463. *

RI007
LI011

**Thomas A. Riemenschneider**
**Leonard M. Linde**

**Aorta, coarctation of abdominal**
*See AORTA, COARCTATION*

---

**AORTA, COARCTATION, INFANTILE TYPE**　　2909

**Includes:**
　　Coarctation of the aortic isthmus
　　Preductal aortic coarctation
　　Short-segment coarctation

**Excludes:**
　　**Aorta, coarctation** (0073)
　　Coarctation of the abdominal aorta
　　Coarctation of the thoracic aorta
　　Long-segment coarctation (tubular aortic hypoplasia)
　　Physiologic aortic coarctation
　　Short-segment supravalvular aortic stenosis

**Major Diagnostic Criteria:** An abrupt constriction of the aortic lumen situated in the isthmus region between the origin of the left subclavian artery proximally and the aortic-ductus arteriosus junction distally. Significant narrowing (40% reduction in lumen or more) of the aortic lumen in the isthmus (preductal) region of the aortic arch is demonstrated by direct morphometry at surgery or at necropsy. The lesion can be suspected by demonstrating lumen narrowing in the isthmus region by angiography or by demonstrating abnormal blood flow by magnetic resonance (MR) projection angiography. The degree of coarctation has been classified as *physiologic* (normal narrowing of the aorta isthmus in the

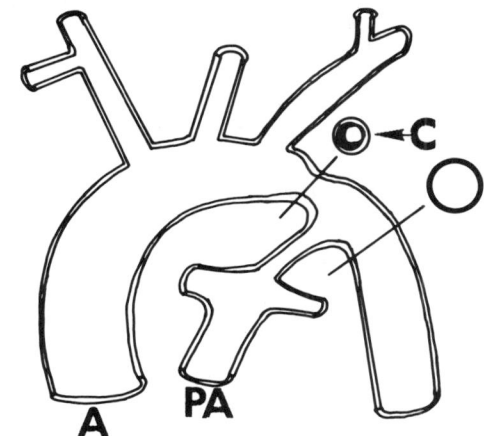

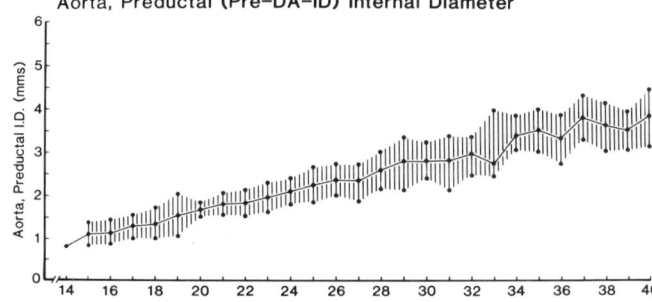

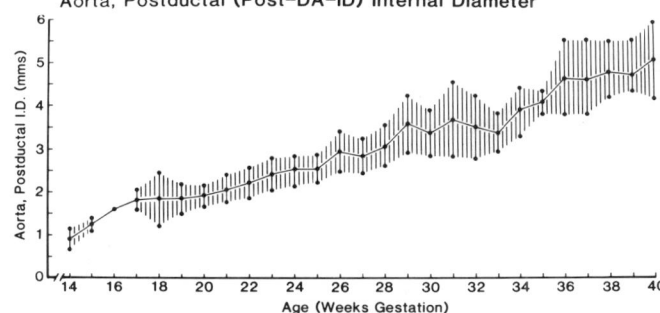

**2909-20237:** Schematic drawing of coarctation of the isthmus region of the aorta. A-aorta; PA-pulmonary artery; C-coarctation site. **20238:** Normal aorta lumen internal diameters in the preductal (isthmus) and postductal regions at various gestational ages (14–40) weeks. Measurements in millimeters.

---

fetua), 0–39% lumen reduction as compared with the postductal aortic lumen; *mild*, 40–44% reduction; *moderate*, 45–49% reduction; and *severe*, 50% or more reduction.

**Clinical Findings:** Coarctation may be an isolated anomaly (32%), usually of a mild degree. Additional anomalies are present in 68% of patients and involve the cardiovascular (24%), genitourinary (20%), CNS (12%), and skeletal systems (6%). Hypertension develops in the proximal arterial circuit, and, in time, collateral circulation develops from the subclavian and intercostal arteries. Reduced pulsation, blood flow, and pressure develop in the distal arterial circulation (e.g., lower extremities). Hypertension in one or both arms is usually present. Blood pressure in the upper extremities of 20 mm Hg or more as compared with that in the legs is indicative of coarctation.

**Complications:** Hypertension, increased pulses, and accelerated atherosclerosis in upper segments. Alterations (pulmonary hypertension) in the pulmonary vascular bed may or may not develop, depending on patency of ductus arteriosus (see **Ductus arteriosus, patent**).

**Associated Findings:** Coarctation is accompanied by additional anomalies in 68% of patients and represents 37% of all aortic arch anomalies. Associated heart anomalies include **Ventricular septal defect**, **Aortic valve, bicuspid**, and **Atrial septal defects**. Preductal coarctation is closely associated with a variety of syndromes including **Turner syndrome** (XO), **Acrocephalosyndactyly type I** (18%), **Umbilical cord, short umbilical cord syndrome**, **Chondrodysplasia punctata**, **Achondroplasia**, **Thanatophoric dysplasia**, **Chromosome 9, trisomy 9** (mosiac), **Chromosome 13, trisomy 13**, **Chromosome 18, trisomy 18**, **Chromosome 21, trisomy 21**, **Fetal rubella syndrome**, **Fetal hydantoin syndrome**, **De Lange syndrome**, **Anencephaly**, renal agenesis-polycystic renal disease, and **Poland syndrome**. Often the fifth aortic arch is persistent.

**Etiology:** Both sporadic and heritable influences have been noted. Infantile coarctation has been reported in families and in sibs.

**Pathogenesis:** The lesion may represent a regional zone of hypoplasia as demonstrated by marked thinning of the muscularis zone. Intramural narrowing has also been attributed to constriction of ductus arteriosus tissues present in this region. In fetuses with **Turner syndrome**, lymphedema and lymphstasis in the aortic adventitial tissues have been postulated to play a role.

**MIM No.:** 12000

**CDC No.:** 747.1

**Sex Ratio:** M2:F1, clinical; M1:F1 on necropsy.

**Occurrence:** 2–3:10,000 live births. Reported in 1.3 Black infants for every one white infant.

**Risk of Recurrence for Patient's Sib:** Estimated at 2%.

**Risk of Recurrence for Patient's Child:** Estimated at about 4% if the mother is affected; about 2% if the father is affected.

**Age of Detectability:** In the infant by angiography and MR projection angiography. All infants should be screened with blood pressure determinations in the upper and lower extremities before age 12 months. Simultaneous pulse comparisons between the upper and lower extremities are also valuable.

**Gene Mapping and Linkage:** Unknown.

**Prevention:** None known. Genetic counseling indicated.

**Treatment:** Surgical repair before age one year is recommended. Left subclavian artery "patch" technique prevents "recoarctation."

**Prognosis:** Guarded but improved if repair is made early. Long-term follow-up shows a high incidence of premature cardiovascular disease and a high premature death rate (12%). Average age of death is 34 years. Approximately 31% ultimately develop systemic hypertension.

**Detection of Carrier:** Unknown.

**References:**

Maron BJ, et al.: Prognosis of surgically corrected coarctation of the aorta: a 20 year postoperative appraisal. Circulation 1973; 47:119–126.
Boon AR, Roberts DF: A family study of coarctation of the aorta. J Med Genet 1976; 13:420–433.
Hamilton DI, et al.: Early and late results of aortoplasty with a left subclavian flap for coarctation of the aorta in infancy. J Thorac Cardiovasc Surg 1978; 75:699–704.
Blackburn WR: Vascular pathology in hypertensive children. In: Loggie JMH, et al., eds: NHLBI workshop on juvenile hypertension. New York: Biomedical Information, 1983:335–364.
Moss AJ: Coarctation of the aorta: current status. J Pediatr 1983; 102:253–255.
Clark EB: Cardiac embryology: its relevance to congenital heart disease. Am J Dis Child 1986; 140:41–44.
Nora JJ, Nora AH: Maternal transmission of congenital heart disease: new recurrence risk figures and the question of cytoplasmic inheritance and vulnerability to teratogens. Am J Cardiol 1987; 59:329–334.
Cohen M, et al.: Coarctation of the aorta: long-term follow-up and prediction of outcome after surgical correction. Circulation 1989; 80:840–845.

BL002                                                    **Will Blackburn**

**Aorta, idiopathic calcification**
*See SINGLETON-MERTEN SYNDROME*

## AORTA, ISOLATION OF SUBCLAVIAN ARTERY FROM AORTA                                                          0546

**Includes:**
    Bilateral subclavian steal syndrome, congenital
    Contralateral subclavian steal syndrome
    Extracardiac shunt to proximal pulmonary artery
    Pulmonary artery subclavian steal
    Subclavian artery, isolation from aorta

**Excludes:**
    Acquired occlusion at the origin of subclavian artery
    Retroesophageal subclavian artery
    Subclavian artery connected to the aorta or its major
        branches
    Subclavian ostial stenosis
    Subclavian steal due to stenotic origin of the subclavian
        artery
    Subclavian steal syndrome with origin distal to the
        coarctation
    Surgical division of subclavian artery (Blalock-Taussig
        operation)

**Major Diagnostic Criteria:** There is a lack of agreement about what to include in this category. Several reports have included cases with an atretic portion of subclavian artery attached to the aorta as congenital isolation of the subclavian artery. Isolation should indicate subclavian connection to the pulmonary artery by a ductus arteriosus (either closed or patent). Either a right or a left aortic arch may be present. The subclavian artery that is isolated is contralateral to the arch (e.g., isolated left subclavian with right arch). In some instances the carotid and subclavian arteries may both be isolated from the aortic arch.

**Clinical Findings:** This defect should be suspected in any patient with diminished pulse in either arm. Many cases, however, have had a normal pulse. The limb on the affected side may be short. This defect may be recognized at the time of angiographic studies for an associated cardiovascular defect. Recognition has occurred at the time of attempted surgical palliation or surgical correction of an associated defect. Symptomatic basilar artery insufficiency (subclavian steal syndrome) may occur in cases in which the ductus is closed and extensive vertebral collateral circulation exists. This is manifested by weakness, light-headedness, and numbness or fatigue of the affected arm. Patency of the ductus arteriosus may result in a left-to-right shunt at the level of the pulmonary artery. A right-to-left shunt from the pulmonary artery to the subclavian artery with greater cyanosis and hypoxemia in the affected arm was documented in one case. Clinical findings may be due to associated cardiac anomalies (usually **Heart, tetralogy of Fallot**) or associated extracardiac abnormalities.

Definitive diagnosis during life is by angiography. Aortic angiograms with special attention paid to delayed films (in cases with ductal atresia) or pulmonary angiography (in cases with ductal patency) will confirm the diagnosis. These studies may become unnecessary for diagnosis as additional experience with identification of thoracic vessels by 2-dimensional echocardiography, computerized axial tomography, and digital-enhanced angiography is accumulated. Because of the importance of recognition of this anomaly prior to attempted Blalock-Taussig anastomosis, it has been suggested that this defect be specifically excluded preoperatively.

**Complications:** Subclavian steal syndrome may develop. Bla-lock-Taussig shunt (subclavian-to-pulmonary anastomosis) on the affected side is unsuccessful because the subclavian artery, which is isolated from the aorta, does not provide an adequate source of pulmonary blood flow.

**Associated Findings:** Associated cardiovascular defects are common. Approximately 60% of cases have tetralogy of Fallot. Left, right, or bilateral ductus arteriosi may be present. Other reported cardiovascular defects include ventricular septal defect, atrial septal defect, interrupted aortic arch, aortic atresia, subvalvular aortic stenosis, mitral atresia, valvular pulmonary stenosis, infundibular pulmonary stenosis, pulmonary artery branch stenosis, complete atrio-ventricular canal defect, isolation of the carotid artery from the aorta, left superior vena cava, dextrocardia, transposition of the great vessels, double-outlet right ventricle, scimitar syndrome, truncus arteriosus, and pulmonary vascular obstructive disease. About 20% of cases have no associated cardiovascular abnormality.

Associated extracardiac abnormalities have included **Mandibulo-facial dysostosis**, Goldenhar syndrome, **Chromosome 21, trisomy 21, Cardiofacial syndrome-assymetric facies**, polysplenia, myelomeningocele, tracheoesophageal fistula, malformation of the hand ipsilateral to the isolation, small arm ipsilateral to the isolation, clinodactyly, scoliosis, clubfeet, and cleft palate. Associated extracardiac defects are uncommon with this entity.

**Etiology:** Unknown.

**Pathogenesis:** It is hypothesized that the embryonic double aortic arch undergoes resorption both distally and proximally to the isolated subclavian on the side of the isolation in the usual case of this type of defect. Normally the distal portion of that arch only is resorbed. The portion that is abnormally resorbed is a remnant of the IVth aortic arch. Thus the isolated segment is left with connection only to the pulmonary artery via a ductus arteriosus. The arch contralateral to the isolation develops normally.

**Sex Ratio:** M1:F1

**Occurrence:** Many asymptomatic cases may be undiagnosed. Although once believed to be extremely rare, there are over 50 well-documented cases in the literature. This defect was found in 1.2% of specimens with right aortic arch in one large study and 1.7% of cases with right aortic arch in another. The prevalence among individuals with left aortic arch is extremely low. One series recognized this defect four times in approximately 60,000 patients referred for suspected heart disease.

**Risk of Recurrence for Patient's Sib:** Unknown. No case found of affected siblings.

**Risk of Recurrence for Patient's Child:** Unknown.

**Age of Detectability:** From birth by aortography. A number of cases have been detected in early infancy.

**Gene Mapping and Linkage:** Unknown.

**Prevention:** None known. Genetic counseling indicated.

**Treatment:** Many cases are asymptomatic and require no intervention. Symptomatic treatment of vertebrobasilar insufficiency may be necessary. Aorta-to-subclavian artery graft or vertebral artery ligation may be required to alleviate symptomatic subclavian steal. The associated cardiovascular defects may require treatment. In such a case, a Blalock-Taussig operation should not be performed on the side of the isolated subclavian artery.

**Prognosis:** Good. Symptomatic subclavian steal syndrome may subsequently develop in asymptomatic individuals. Associated cardiovascular defects may influence prognosis.

**Detection of Carrier:** Unknown.

**References:**
Stewart JR, et al.: An atlas of vascular rings and related malformations of the aortic arch system. Springfield, Illinois: Charles C Thomas, 1964.
Knight L, Edwards JE: Right aortic arch: types and associated cardiac anomalies. Circulation 1974; 50:1047–1051.
Rodriquez L, et al.: Surgical implications of right aortic arch with isolation of left subclavian artery. Br Heart J 1975; 37:931–936. *
Crump WD, et al.: Right aortic arch, isolated left common carotid and left subclavian arteries, and subclavian steal syndrome: a variant of polysplenia syndrome. Hum Pathol 1981; 12:936–938.
Nath, et al.: Isolation of a subclavian artery. Am J Radiol 1981; 137:683–688.
Bricker JT, et al.: Tetralogy of Fallot and congenital connection between the left subclavian artery and the pulmonary artery: possible relationship to a congenital left-hand deformity. Texas Heart Inst J 1984; 11:84–88.

BR014
MC028

**J. Timothy Bricker
Dan G. McNamara**

## AORTIC ARCH INTERRUPTION　　0076

**Includes:** Aortic fourth arches, absence of left or both

**Excludes:**
　Aorta, coarctation (0073)
　Immunodeficiency, thymic agenesis (0943)

**Major Diagnostic Criteria:** Selective ascending aortography is diagnostic, but in some cases even this may fail to differentiate interruption of the aortic arch from the most extreme form of coarctation of the aorta in the living patient. Two-dimensional echocardiography is often diagnostic.

**Clinical Findings:** The interruption may occur distal to the left subclavian artery (type A - 40%), between the left subclavian and left carotid artery (type B - 57%) or distal to the right innominate artery (type C - 4%). Both subclavian arteries may arise from the descending aorta just beyond the entrance of a very large ductus arteriosus which connects the pulmonary trunk with the descending aorta and forms its only blood supply.

Only 4% of patients have no additional cardiac anomaly other than the obligatory patent ductus arteriosus. In 60% of the cases a ventricular septal defect is the only associated lesion, but other cardiovascular anomalies, such as transposition of the great arteries, aortic valve stenosis and truncus arteriosus, are not uncommon. In the few cases where the interrupted arch is the only malformation, the symptoms and signs are similar to those seen in severe preductal coarctation of the aorta, and differential cyanosis of only the lower body and lower limbs, may be present. In cases with associated ventricular septal defect, the signs and symptoms are those seen in any patient with a large left-to-right shunt at the ventricular or great arterial level. In such cases differential cyanosis is not usually apparent because of the relatively high oxygen content of the right ventricular blood.

In most patients the pressures in ascending and descending aorta are approximately equal. In others, the patent ductus arteriosus may become small enough so that diminished pulses and lower arterial pressure in the lower limbs may lead to the erroneous diagnosis of coarctation of the aorta.

Thoracic X-ray usually show hypervascular lungs, cardiomegaly and left atrial enlargement. The linear density formed by the upper descending thoracic aorta is almost invariably absent. The EKG may be normal but usually shows right, left or combined ventricular hypertrophy. Two-dimensional echocardiography can usually identify the site of interruption, the size of the ductus, and other associated anomalies. The diagnosis of interrupted aortic arch and clarification of any associated cardiovascular malformations necessitate cardiac catheterization and angiocardiography.

**Complications:** Dyspnea and pulmonary edema as seen in other types of congenital heart disease with large left-to-right shunt associated with left ventricular outflow obstruction. Constriction of the ductus produces right heart failure and renal ischemia.

**Associated Findings:** Other cardiovascular anomalies such as ventricular septal defect, persistent truncus arteriosis and aortopulmonary window commonly occur with types A and C interruption. Rarely the ductus may be absent with distal body flow via the vertebral-subclavian artery pathway. Sixty-eight percent of patients with type B interruption have been found to be associated with **Immunodeficiency, thymic agenesis**, while this is rare in types A and C interruption.

Facial palsy and retinal coloboma have been reported.

**Etiology:** Teratogenic exposure documented in some cases, compatible with multifactorial inheritance in most.

**Pathogenesis:** Type B interruption may be a manifestation of a more generalized defect in the mesencephalic and rhomebencephalic neural crest, while types A and C interruption are pathogenically related to **Aorta, coarctation.**

**MIM No.:** 10755

**CDC No.:** 747.215

**Sex Ratio:** M1:F1

**Occurrence:** Accounts for < 1% of all congenital heart defects; < 1:10,000 live births. Very rare in general population because of high infant mortality.

**Risk of Recurrence for Patient's Sib:** Unknown.

**Risk of Recurrence for Patient's Child:** Unknown.

**Age of Detectability:** From birth.

**Gene Mapping and Linkage:** Unknown.

**Prevention:** None known. Genetic counseling indicated.

**Treatment:** Initial treatment of pulmonary edema, together with prostaglandins, if signs of a restrictive ductus arteriosus at birth. Surgery is indicated in virtually all cases. An attempt is made to reestablish continuity between the ascending aorta and the descending aorta with division of the patent ductus arteriosus. Since most cases are associated with ventricular septal defect, it is probably initially advisable to also carry out pulmonary arterial banding. Complete repair of all defects is possible in many infants. If thymus is absent, aggressive treatment of all infections is recommended.

**Prognosis:** The prognosis without surgical treatment is extremely poor. Approximately 90% of patients die within the first year of life, and of these the great majority die within the first 20 days.

**Detection of Carrier:** Unknown.

**References:**

Stewart JR, et al.: An atlas of vascular rings and related malformations of the aortic arch system. Springfield: Charles C Thomas, 1964:147–155.

McNamara DG, Rosenberg HS: Interruption of the aortic arch. In: Watson H, ed: Paediatric cardiology. St. Louis: CV Mosby Co, 1968:224–232.

Reardon MJ, et al.: Interrupted aortic arch: brief review and summary of an 18-year experience. Texas Heart Inst J 1984; 11:250–259. *

Van Mierop LHS, Kutsche LM: Interruption of the aortic arch and coarctation: pathogenic relations. Am J Cardiol 1984; 54:829–834.

Van Mierop LHS, Kutsche LM: Cardiovascular anomalies in DiGeorge syndrome and importance of neural crest as a possible pathogenic factor. An J Cardiol 1986; 58:133–137. *

NI006         **Michael R. Nihill**

**Aortic arch, bilateral, with left or right descending aorta**
*See AORTIC ARCH, DOUBLE*

---

## AORTIC ARCH, CERVICAL        0074

**Includes:**
Aortic arch, persistence of third
Cervical aortic arch

**Excludes:**
Aneurysms of individual brachiocephalic vessels
Aorta, congenitally unwound
Pathologic elongation of individual brachiocephalic vessels
Pseudocoarctation

**Major Diagnostic Criteria:** A pulsating mass in the supraclavicular area, compression of which will diminish the femoral pulses. The mass may be on either side.

**Clinical Findings:** What appears to be the aortic arch is located much higher than the normal aortic arch in the lower neck. The striking clinical feature of this anomaly is the presence of a large pulsating mass in either the right or left supraclavicular region. This mass may extend as high as the hyoid bone, the fifth or sixth cervical vertebra. The mass may be associated with symptoms of a vascular ring, ie dysphagia or airway obstruction, or it may be completely asymptomatic. Several affected individuals have shown discrepancies in the pulses and blood pressures in the upper limbs. The diminution of the femoral pulses by compression of the pulsating mass against the adjacent vertebra provides a pathognomonic clinical maneuver. On PA chest roentgenogram, there is an asymmetric widening of the superior mediastinal shadow; the aortic arch is inconspicuous. On barium swallow there is a large posterior indentation of the esophagus at the level of the usual position of the aortic arch. This is a result of the retroesophageal passage of the descending limb of the cervical aorta. Definitive diagnosis made from thoracic aortography.

**Complications:** Symptoms of vascular ring (in 3/8) may occur. The long-term effects of the vascular aging process on the tortuous aorta are unknown.

**Associated Findings:** None known.

**Etiology:** Unknown.

**Pathogenesis:** It most likely represents a persistence of the third aortic arch, instead of the usual fourth, and the ductus caroticus, the segment of the dorsal aorta between the third and fourth arches. A similar anomaly may involve the contralateral subclavian artery which then arises from the innominate artery at a much higher level than normal.

**Sex Ratio:** M1:F1

**Occurrence:** About 40 cases recorded in the literature.

**Risk of Recurrence for Patient's Sib:** Unknown.

**Risk of Recurrence for Patient's Child:** Unknown.

**Age of Detectability:** From birth.

**Gene Mapping and Linkage:** Unknown.

**Prevention:** None known. Genetic counseling indicated.

**Treatment:** Surgical relief of encircling structures such as contralateral ductus or ligamentum arteriosus may be necessary when symptoms of vascular ring are present.

**Prognosis:** Undetermined. Probably benign

**Detection of Carrier:** Unknown.

**References:**

Wei C, et al.: Cervical aortic arch associated with aortic kinking and aneurysm. Nippon Kyobu Geka Gakkai Zasshi 1983; 31:2202–2208. *

Alvarez-Coca J, et al.: Right cervical aortic arch: report of 2 cases, one associated with aortic coarctation. An Esp Pediatr 1984; 21:157–162.

Yeager SB, et al.: Cervical aortic arch: an unusual cause of a suprasternal notch thrill and deminished left arm pulse. W Va Med J 1984; 80:141–142.

Hagel KJ, et al.: Cervical aortic arch: symptoms and diagnosis in 2 children. Z Kardiol 1986; 75:182–185.

Van Nooten G., et al.: Left-sided cervical aortic arch. Acta Chir Beig 1986; 86:248–250.

MC028         **Dan G. McNamara**
MU008         **Charles E. Mullins**

---

## AORTIC ARCH, DOUBLE        0075

**Includes:** Aortic arch, bilateral, with left or right descending aorta

**Excludes:** Aortic arch anomalies causing vascular ring syndrome

**Major Diagnostic Criteria:** Demonstration of characteristic indentations of the barium-filled esophagus and air-filled trachea in infants with symptoms and signs of upper airway obstruction. Aortography is confirmatory.

**Clinical Findings:** An aortic arch is present on each side of the trachea and esophagus. Both arise anteriorly from the ascending aorta, encircle the trachea and esophagus and join posteriorly to continue as the descending aorta. The descending aorta is usually located on the left side but is on the right in some cases. The right posterior aortic arch is generally (80%) the larger, but in 20% of the cases, it may be the smaller of the 2, or the 2 arches are of approximately equal size. Each of the 2 arches gives rise to the ipsilateral common carotid and subclavian arteries.

In the great majority of patients the encirclement of the trachea and esophagus by the two arches causes significant symptoms, usually appearing in infancy. Occasionally, symptoms do not occur until later in childhood, or, rarely, in adult life. The severity of the symptoms is directly related to the degree of obstruction to the trachea and esophagus. In infants, the most obvious and sometimes alarming symptom is severe inspiratory stridor associated with wheezing and a hacking cough. Respiratory tract infections are common, not only due to airway obstruction, but also to obstruction of the esophagus leading to aspiration. Hyperextension of the head alleviates the respiratory symptoms more or less successfully and this position is usually assumed by the child as the most comfortable. In older children or adults, the only symptom may be dysphagia.

Cardiac murmurs are not present unless there are associated cardiovascular anomalies. The findings on physical examination are dominated by those caused by upper airway obstruction. Unless other cardiovascular anomalies are present, the EKG is normal. X-rays of the chest may show a widened upper mediastinum and direct or indirect evidence of airway obstruction such as hyperaeration, atelectasis and pneumonic infiltrates. In the most common type of double aortic arch in which the right posterior arch is the larger of the 2, this arch will cause a large indentation in the right lateral wall of the barium-filled esophagus. A similar but smaller indentation may be visible on the left side. The air-filled trachea almost invariably shows an anterior indentation from the anterior arch. Aortography will confirm the diagnosis and reveal the precise anatomy and relative size of the 2 arches.

**Complications:** Hyperaeration of the lungs, atelectasis, pneumonia and dysphagia.

**Associated Findings:** None known.

**Etiology:** Unknown.

**Pathogenesis:** In cases of double aortic arch, both dorsal aortae persist rather than only the usual left.

**CDC No.:** 747.250

**Sex Ratio:** M1:F1

**Occurrence:** Incidence approximately 1:20,000 live births.

**Risk of Recurrence for Patient's Sib:** Unknown.

**Risk of Recurrence for Patient's Child:** Predicted risk 1:100; empiric risk: Undetermined.

**Age of Detectability:** Neonatal period.

**Gene Mapping and Linkage:** Unknown.

**Prevention:** None known. Genetic counseling indicated.

**Treatment:** The treatment is surgical when the presence of a double aortic arch causes symptoms. The surgery consists of a division of the smaller of the two arches.

**Prognosis:** In symptomatic patients, particularly infants, the prognosis without surgical treatment is poor.

**Detection of Carrier:** Unknown.

**References:**
Stewart JR, et al.: An atlas of vascular rings and related malformations of the aortic arch system Springfield: Charles C Thomas, 1964. *
Nora JJ, McNamara DG: Vascular rings and related anomalies. In: Watson H, ed: Paediatric cardiology. St. Louis: CV Mosby Co. 1968:233–242. *
Netter FH, ed: Ciba collection of medical illustrations: the heart. Summit, NJ: Ciba 1969: vol 5.

N0003                                          **James J. Nora**

**Aortic arch, persistence of third**
*See AORTIC ARCH, CERVICAL*

**AORTIC ARCH, RIGHT                               0077**

**Includes:**
    Right aortic arch types I, II and III
    Right aortic arch-retroesophageal anomalous subclavian artery

**Excludes:**
    **Aortic arch, double** (0075)
    **Aorta, isolation of subclavian artery from aorta** (0546)

**Major Diagnostic Criteria:** Right aortic arch is easily distinguishable on plain films. A barium esophagram is necessary to distinguish Types I and II arches. Type III arch (isolation of the left subclavian) is recognizable by the combination of X-ray signs of right arch plus decreased amplitude of the arterial pulses of the left arm. Thoracic aortography is definitive.

**Clinical Findings:** Right aortic arch is defined as the transverse aortic arch coursing to the right of the trachea. This anomaly is usually asymptomatic and therefore diagnosed incidentally on chest X-ray. The most reliable X-ray sign is a concave deformity on the right side of the trachea. Additional signs are an aortic knob on the right side of the dorsal spine, a clear space on the left side of the dorsal spine, the superior vena cava deviated to the right, the descending thoracic aorta coursing inferiorly along the right side of the spine and signs on the esophagram of an aberrant left subclavian artery if present. When the right arch is present it has 1 of 2 relationships to the esophagus. In one form the arch occupies a retroesophageal position. In the other form it does not pass behind the esophagus but remains to the right of it. By far, the most common form is the right aortic arch without a retroesophageal aortic segment.

For practical purposes, there are three main types of right aortic arch without a retroesophageal segment:

Type I: Mirror Image Branching: In this type the aortic arch passes over the right main stem bronchus and connects with a right-sided proximal aorta. This form demonstrates mirror image branching of the major arteries from that observed in the normal left aortic arch. The first branch of the arch is the left innominate artery and is followed by the right carotid and the right subclavian arteries, in that order. It is the most common right-sided arch and has a very high incidence of congenital heart disease with tetralogy of Fallot being the most common.

Type II: Aberrant Left Subclavian Artery: The aortic arch in this type has a similar course to type I with the same reversal of branches. In this type, however, the left subclavian, instead of coming off the left innominate, comes off distal to the right subclavian. It courses toward the left arm by crossing the midline behind the esophagus, and subsequently causes an indentation in the posterior esophagus. In contrast to what formerly was suspected, this type may be associated with a high incidence of cardiac anomalies. When there is a left-sided ductus arteriosus (or ligamentum arteriosum) present there may be significant compression of the trachea and the esophagus. In elderly adults, the bulbous origin of the left subclavian may project to the left of the spine and be misinterpreted as a nonvascular mass.

Both types I and II right aortic arches are easily recognizable and distinguishable on chest X-rays with barium in the esophagus. In the type II aortic arch, if the ductus arteriosus is on the left, the retroesophageal component produces a wide, concave compression on the esophagus. Uncommonly, when the ductus arteriosus is on the right, the retroesophageal compression is smaller, shallower and angles upward from right to left at approximately 70° from the horizontal. These findings are caused by the anomalous left subclavian arising directly from the aortic arch below the right subclavian.

Type III: Isolation of the Left Subclavian Artery: In this type of right aortic arch the configuration of the arch and descending aorta is similar to types I and II. As before, the 3 branches from the arch are reversed with the left common carotid coming off first, then the right carotid and then the right subclavian. The left subclavian artery is not attached to the aorta but is connected to the left pulmonary artery through a ductus arteriosus or ligamentum arteriosum. In the latter, the left subclavian and brachial artery are perfused by the left vertebral artery; so-called "subclavian steal." The pulses in the left arm are diminished when compared with the right. This type of right aortic arch is extremely rare.

Right arch with retroesophageal aortic segment is an uncommon form of right aortic arch. In this type, the aortic arch occupies a retroesophageal position. The solitary arch passes over the right main bronchus to the right of the trachea and esophagus. It then turns abruptly toward the left behind the esophagus and upon reaching the left side of the esophagus it joins the proximal end of a left-sided descending aorta. A left-sided ductus arteriosus commonly attaches to a diverticula at the junction of the arch and the descending aorta and thus creates a vascular ring. The ring is comprised of the right arch to the right, its retroesophageal segment posteriorly, the PA to the left and the pulmonary arterial bifurcation anteriorly.

In a case of congenital heart disease having a right aortic arch, a number of conditions should be considered as they frequently occur together. The approximate incidence of right aortic arch occurring in each condition is:

Tetralogy of Fallot - 25%: The more severe the degree of obstruction to pulmonary flow, the higher the incidence of right arch. End-stage tetralogy has an incidence of right arch of nearly 50%.

Persistent truncus arteriosus - 35%

Complete transposition with ventricular septal defect and pulmonary stenosis - 25%

Tricuspid atresia - 8%

Isolated ventricular septal defect, usually Eisenmenger anatomy in type - 2%

**Complications:** A vascular ring may be created with either a left posterior ligamentum arteriosum or an aberrant left subclavian artery.

**Associated Findings:** None known.

**Etiology:** Presumably multifactorial inheritance.

**Pathogenesis:** A right aortic arch in situs solitus is due to retention of the right dorsal aorta rather than the left.

**CDC No.:** 747.230

**Sex Ratio:** M1:F1

**Occurrence:** 1:2500.

**Risk of Recurrence for Patient's Sib:** Unknown.

**Risk of Recurrence for Patient's Child:** Unknown.

**Age of Detectability:** From birth.

**Gene Mapping and Linkage:** Unknown.

**Prevention:** None known. Genetic counseling indicated.

**Treatment:** When a retroesophageal component creates a vascular ring, surgical intervention may be necessary to alleviate the obstruction. The left ligamentum or ductus may be divided. Occasionally, division of the left subclavian is necessary.

**Prognosis:** Without associated cardiac defects or retroesophageal component, the prognosis is normal. With an associated cardiac defect, the prognosis would be dependent only on the cardiac defect. When there is a retroesophageal component, a vascular ring may occur which may be relieved by surgical intervention.

**Detection of Carrier:** Unknown.

**References:**

Nora JJ, McNamara DG: Vascular rings and related anomalies. In: Watson H, ed: Paediatric cardiology. St. Louis: CV Mosby Co. 1968:233–242.

Matthew R, et al.: The significance of right aortic arch in D-transposition of the great arteries. Am J Cardiol 1974; 87(3):314–320.

Sissman NJ: Anomalies of the aortic arch complex. In: Moss AJ, Adams FH, eds: Heart disease in infants, children, and adolescents, 3rd ed. Baltimore: Williams and Wilkins. 1983:199–214. *

N0004         **Audrey H. Nora**
N0003         **James J. Nora**

**Aortic atresia**
  *See AORTIC VALVE ATRESIA*
**Aortic fourth arches, absence of left or both**
  *See AORTIC ARCH INTERRUPTION*
**Aortic pulmonary lobe**
  *See LUNG, LOBE SEQUESTRATION*
**Aortic septal defect**
  *See AORTICO-PULMONARY SEPTAL DEFECT*
**Aortic sinus aneurysm with or without rupture, congenital**
  *See AORTIC SINUS OF VALSALVA, ANEURYSM*

---

## AORTIC SINUS OF VALSALVA, ANEURYSM      0053

**Includes:**

Aneurysm of aortic sinus of Valsalva
Aortic sinus aneurysm with or without rupture, congenital

**Excludes:**

Acquired aortic sinus aneurysm
Aorticocardiac fistula, congenital
Cystic medial necrosis-aneurysmal dilatation of aortic root

**Major Diagnostic Criteria:** The diagnosis is strongly suspected in a previously healthy individual with a loud, continuous murmur at the lower precordial area and a dilated aortic root in the echocardiogram. Cardiac catheterization reveals left-to-right shunting at the ventricular or atrial level. The diagnosis is confirmed by retrograde aortography with contrast injection into the ascending aorta. This outlines the aortic sinus aneurysm, the fistulous communication into the right heart chamber, and normal coronary arteries.

**Clinical Findings:** The aneurysm is present since birth and, generally speaking, involves one sinus only; the right coronary sinus in about 70%, the noncoronary sinus in 22%, and the left coronary sinus in about 4%. Congenital aneurysm of more than 1 aortic sinus is observed only in about 3%. The aneurysm grows insidiously and bulges into the adjacent low-pressure right heart chambers. Eventually, its protruding weakest point ruptures, resulting in an aorticocardiac fistula. The usual receiving chamber is either the right ventricle or the right atrium. Right coronary sinus aneurysms rupture into the right ventricle in more than 70%, and into the right atrium in about 25%. Noncoronary sinus aneurysms rupture into the right atrium in 85%, and into the right ventricle in 11%. The rare left coronary sinus aneurysms may rupture into the right atrium or left atrium.

In more than one-third of the cases, an associated ventricular septal defect is present. It is especially common (80%) in aneurysms of the right coronary sinus. The septal defect tends to be located immediately beneath the pulmonary valve. Congenital aortic sinus aneurysms may sometimes accompany coarctation of the aorta.

The unruptured aneurysm is generally not large enough to cause significant hemodynamic effects. It is, therefore, a clinically silent lesion. Occasionally, it may cause some right ventricular outflow obstruction as it protrudes into the subpulmonary conus. An ejection systolic murmur at the upper left sternal border and wide splitting of the second sound may then be observed, simulating the findings of mild pulmonary stenosis. If a ventricular septal defect is present, a typical harsh pansystolic murmur at the left lower sternal border, due to the septal defect, is observed.

Following rupture of the aortic sinus aneurysm, an aorticocardiac fistula develops, with continuous runoff of blood from the aorta to the receiving chamber during systole and diastole. Acute symptoms may accompany this episode, such as severe chest or right upper abdominal pain, weakness, nausea, or shortness of breath. These symptoms may last several minutes to an hour. An intervening period lasting for several weeks or months then follows, during which time exertional dyspnea, palpitation, fatigability, and angina are common. Eventually, death from cardiac failure occurs within a year. Rarely, death may occur immediately following the rupture or after an intervening period lasting for several years.

The striking clinical finding is a loud, continuous, machinery-like murmur along the left or right sternal border. Unlike the continuous murmur of patent ductus arteriosus which is maximally heard at the left infraclavicular area, the murmur is loudest at the lower left or right sternal border where a thrill is often present. The arterial pulses are bounding and the apical impulse as well as precordium are hyperactive due to combined ventricular volume overload.

The chest X-rays are normal in isolated unruptured sinus aneurysms as long as the aortic valve remains competent. The aneurysm is intracardiac and not sufficiently large to cause distortion of the cardiac silhouette. If a ventricular septal defect is also present, shunt vascularity and cardiac enlargement may be observed. Following rupture of the aneurysm, enlargement of all cardiac chambers and increase of pulmonary vascularity occur depending upon the size of the fistulous communication.

The EKG in unruptured aneurysms is normal. Following rupture, combined ventricular hypertrophy, usually with left ventricular preponderance, appears. Disturbances in conduction, including varying forms of A-V block and right bundle branch block, may occur when the aneurysm projects immediately above or below the tricuspid valve in the area of the A-V node or bundle of His. This is likely to be observed in aneurysms arising from the posterior portion of the right coronary sinus or from the noncoronary sinus where rupture tends to occur into the right atrium.

Cross-sectional echocardiography may strongly suggest the diagnosis. It demonstrates an asymmetric aortic root with a somewhat elongated and enlarged right anterior or non-coronary sinus extending distalwards into adjacent structures. Consistent discontinuity of the aortic sinus wall may indicate the fistula. Doppler flow analysis shows an abnormal pattern consisting of high velocity flow throughout systole and diastole, localized at or distal to the site of fistula but not in the aorta or aortic root. A ventricular septal defect, if present, may also be identified.

Cardiac catheterization demonstrates a left-to-right shunt of varying magnitude at the ventricular or atrial level. Pulmonary hypertension is uncommon and pulmonary vascular resistance is usually normal. A pressure gradient across the right ventricular outflow tract may sometimes be present. Aortography with selective injection of contrast material close to the aortic root outlines the aneurysm and its fistulous communication into the right heart chamber. Unlike in coronary-camaral fistulae, the coronary arteries are of normal caliber and distribution.

**Complications:** Aortic insufficiency is common, particularly in those where there is associated ventricular septal defect. Bacterial endocarditis is not uncommon. Congestive heart failure terminating in death develops usually within a period of 1 year following rupture. Hemorrhage into extracardiac tissues, resulting in hemopericardium or hemothorax does not occur.

**Associated Findings:** Ventricular septal defect, coarctation of aorta.

**Etiology:** Sporadic and syndrome-associated cases (See, for example, **Marfan syndrome**).

**Pathogenesis:** The aneurysm is presumed to be due to the presence of a weak point in the aortic root resulting in congenital separation or discontinuity of the aortic media and annulus fibrosus. Inadequate fusion of the bulbar septum has also been incriminated. The weak aortic root segment gradually bulges toward the low-pressure right heart chambers, becoming aneurysmal as it increases in size and finally rupturing at its weakest point. If a high ventricular septal defect is present, the aneurysm may protrude across the defect into the right ventricular outflow tract resulting in functional diminution of the septal defect, aortic insufficiency, and some right ventricular outflow obstruction. Fibrosis with focal or diffuse chronic inflammatory reaction may also be noted in the wall of the aneurysm as well as in the adjoining myocardium. Following rupture, continuous runoff of blood from aorta to the receiving right heart chamber occurs, with consequent volume overloading of both ventricular chambers.

**CDC No.:** 747.240

**Sex Ratio:** M3:F1

**Occurrence:** Less than 1:20,000 (less than 0.5% of CHD).

**Risk of Recurrence for Patient's Sib:** Unknown; may vary with associated syndromes.

**Risk of Recurrence for Patient's Child:** Unknown; may vary with associated syndromes.

**Age of Detectability:** From infancy on, if ruptured, by aortography or selective angiography. In unruptured aneurysms, the diagnosis is incidental during echocardiography or following angiocardiography for other suspected congenital heart defects (eg, ventricular septal defect, coarctation of the aorta).

**Gene Mapping and Linkage:** Unknown.

**Prevention:** None known. Genetic counseling indicated.

**Treatment:** Once a diagnosis of ruptured aneurysm is made, surgical occlusion of the fistula and reconstruction of the aortic root are indicated. This is accomplished with the aid of cardiopulmonary bypass, alone or with additional hypothermia. Surgical treatment for isolated, unruptured aortic sinus aneurysm is still debatable.

In unruptured aneurysms not surgically corrected, chemoprophylaxis for infective endocarditis is important. In ruptured aneurysms with heart failure, the usual medical therapy, consisting of digitalis, diuretics, oxygen, etc., is indicated. Relief from these measures is only temporary.

**Prognosis:** Although hemodynamically benign, the solitary aneurysm is a serious condition due to its tendency to rupture. Following the latter complication, death from congestive heart failure generally occurs within a year. The time of rupture varies but is uncommon during childhood, and occurs more frequently during the 4th decade. The risk of bacterial endocarditis is also higher in this condition than in most other congenital heart defects.

**Detection of Carrier:** Unknown.

**References:**

Sakakibara S, Konno S: Congenital aneurysm of the sinus of Valsalva: anatomy and classification. Am Heart J 1962; 63:405–424. *

Morch JE, Greenwood WF: Rupture of the sinus of Valsalva: a study of eight cases with discussion on the differential diagnosis of continuous murmurs. Am J Cardiol 1966; 18:827–836.

Howard RJ, et al.: Surgical correction of sinus of Valsalva aneurysm. J Thorac Cardiovasc Surg 1973; 66:420–427. *

Mayer JH, et al.: Isolated, unruptured sinus of Valsalva aneurysm. Serendipitous detection and correction. J Thorac Cardiovasc Surg 1975; 69:429–432.

AR001                                                    **René A. Arcilla**

---

## AORTIC STENOSIS-CORNEAL CLOUDING-GROWTH AND MENTAL RETARDATION                           **2819**

**Includes:** Peters anomaly-aortic stenosis-growth and mental retardation

**Excludes:**
Cornea, isolated dysgenesis mesodermalis of
**Dwarfism (short limbed)-Peters anomaly of the eye** (2812)
**Eye, anterior segment dysgenesis** (0439)
**Mietens-Weber syndrome** (2013)
**Roberts syndrome** (0875)

**Major Diagnostic Criteria:** Peters anomaly, i.e., dysgenesis mesodermalis of the cornea; midfacial hypoplasia; subvalvular aortic stenosis; short hands and feet; mental retardation; and growth retardation.

**Clinical Findings:** The ocular symptoms present as Peters anomaly. One child was severely affected in both eyes with concomitant microphthalmia and glaucoma. Only the right eye of her younger brother was affected with a corneal opacity, a deficit of the Descemet membrane, and narrowing of the iridocorneal angle. In both, there was evident midfacial hypoplasia with round flat face, broad nasal bridge, bilateral epicanthus, small maxillae, upturned nose, short upper lip, and microstomia. In both patients, subvalvular aortic stenosis was detected during infancy; it was shown to

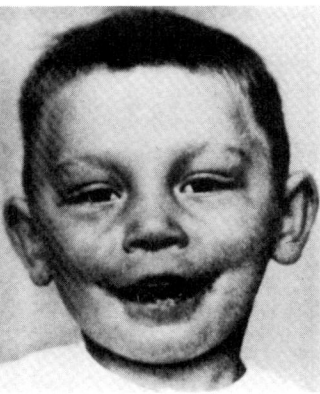

**2819-20081:** Note the typical midface hypoplasia and variable ocular changes in this sister (left) and brother (right).

be of the membranous type in the brother. Hands and feet were short and stubby. In the sister, mental retardation was moderate and growth retardation pronounced; in the brother, growth was borderline and mental retardation only slight.

**Complications:**  Unknown.

**Associated Findings:**  Additional skeletal abnormalities were present in one patient: cubiti valgi with limited extension, equinovarus deformity of both feet, overriding of the first and second toes, and broad halluces in a valgus position.

**Etiology:**  Presumably autosomal recessive inheritance. Variability seems to exist in the severity of ocular changes and in the degree of growth and mental deficiency.

**Pathogenesis:**  Unknown.

**Sex Ratio:**  M1:F1

**Occurrence:**  The delineation of this syndrome is based on the findings in two mentally retarded sibs; brother and sister. At least one other patient has been diagnosed with the same syndrome (A. Schinzel, personal communication).

**Risk of Recurrence for Patient's Sib:**
See Part I, *Mendelian Inheritance.*

**Risk of Recurrence for Patient's Child:**
See Part I, *Mendelian Inheritance.* Mental retardation makes reproduction highly unlikely.

**Age of Detectability:**  At birth.

**Gene Mapping and Linkage:**  Unknown.

**Prevention:**  None known. Genetic counseling indicated.

**Treatment:**  Surgical correction of the subvalvular aortic membrane is indicated.

**Prognosis:**  Life span is variable. Blindness is present in the most affected patients. Growth and mental retardation may vary in severity.

**Detection of Carrier:**  Unknown.

**References:**
Fryns JP, Van den Berghe H: Corneal clouding, subvalvular aortic stenosis, and midfacial hypoplasia associated with mental deficiency and growth retardation: a new syndrome? Eur J Pediatr 1979; 131:179–183.

**Jean-Pierre Fryns**

## AORTIC STENOSIS, SUPRAVALVAR 0078

**Includes:**
Eisenberg supravalvar aortic stenosis
Supraaortic stenosis
Supravalvar aortic stenosis

**Excludes:**
**Aorta, coarctation** (0073)
Aortic hypoplasia
**Aortic valve stenosis** (0080)
**Williams syndrome** (0999)

**Major Diagnostic Criteria:**  Patient may be asymptomatic except in cases of severe stenosis when dyspnea, fatigue, syncope, or angina may be present. Generally, a harsh systolic murmur, thrill, and normal heart size are present. However, definitive localization of the site of left ventricular outflow obstruction requires the demonstration of a pressure gradient a short distance beyond the aortic valve via echocardiography and Doppler ultrasound examination and/or left heart catheterization.

**Clinical Findings:**  Supravalvar aortic stenosis is a congenital narrowing of the ascending aorta, either localized or diffuse, originating at the superior margin of the sinuses of Valsalva just above the level of the coronary arteries. It may be separated anatomically into 3 categories, although any specific patient may demonstrate pathologic findings characteristic of more than 1 type. Most common is the hour-glass type, in which a constricting annular ridge at the superior margin of the sinuses of Valsalva is produced by extreme thickening and disorganization of the aortic media. Although the lumen of the aorta is reduced, the constriction may not be evident on gross inspection of the external surface of the vessel. It has been suggested that this lesion results from a developmental exaggeration of the normal transverse supravalvar aortic plica. The membranous type is produced by a fibrous or fibromuscular diaphragm with a small central opening stretched across the lumen of the aorta. The hypoplastic type is characterized by uniform hypoplasia of the ascending aorta. In the older cardiovascular literature, a fourth anomaly, consisting of a nonobstructing band or cord stretched across the lumen of the aorta at the level of the aortic leaflets, was designated supravalvar aortic stenosis, although it most likely has no functional significance. Rarely, supravalvar aortic stenosis occurs in individuals homozygous for familial hypercholesterolemia due to accumulation of atherosclerotic plaque.

In contrast to other forms of aortic stenosis, in the supravalvar variety the coronary arteries arise proximal to the site of outflow obstruction and are subjected to the elevated pressure that exists within the left ventricle. These vessels are often dilated and tortuous and coronary arteriosclerosis has been observed, even in children. In addition, if the free edges of some or all of the aortic cusps are adherent to the site of supravalvar stenosis, there may be interference with coronary arterial flow. The clinical picture of supravalvar aortic stenosis differs from that observed in other forms of left ventricular outflow obstruction. Chief among these differences is the association of supravalvar aortic stenosis with idiopathic infantile hypercalcemia. The designation **Williams syndrome** has been applied to the distinctive clinical picture produced by coexistence of the cardiac and metabolic disorder. Patients with **Williams syndrome** have, in addition, mental retardation, characteristic facial features, and anomalies in dentition. They may also have strabismus, hernias, sensitivity to sound and noise, and renal dysfunction. Most commonly, supravalvar aortic stenosis is a feature of the distinctive syndrome described above. However, the aortic anomaly and peripheral pulmonary arterial stenosis are also seen in familial and sporadic forms unassociated with the other features of the syndrome. Occasionally, there is moderate thickening of the aortic cusps, and valvar pulmonary stenosis may occur in association with the narrowing of peripheral pulmonary arteries. Rare patients may have mitral valve abnormalities with prolapse and mitral regurgitation and narrowing of other systemic arteries.

A positive family history in a patient with a normal appearance and clinical signs suggesting left ventricular outflow obstruction should alert the physician to a diagnosis of either supravalvar aortic stenosis or muscular subaortic stenosis.

With a few exceptions, the major physical findings resemble those observed in patients with **Aortic valve stenosis**. Among these exceptions are the frequent accentuations of the sound of aortic valve closure due to the elevated pressure in the aorta proximal to the stenosis, the infrequency of an ejection sound, and the more prominent transmission of the thrill and murmur into the jugular notch and along the carotid vessels. Occasionally, there is an early diastolic decrescendo blowing murmur of aortic regurgitation, due to the fusion of 1 or more cusps to the area of stenosis. The narrowing of the peripheral pulmonary arteries that frequently coexists in these patients may produce a continuous murmur that may help distinguish this anomaly from stenosis of the aortic valve. The latter distinction is reinforced by the frequent finding of a significant disparity between the arterial pressures in the upper limbs in supravalvar aortic stenosis; the systolic pressure in the right arm tends to be the higher of the two and may even exceed that in the femoral arteries. When obstruction is severe, the EKG reveals left ventricular hypertrophy. However, biventricular, or even right ventricular hypertrophy may be observed if significant narrowing of the peripheral pulmonary arteries coexists. On X-ray, in contrast to valvar and discrete subvalvar aortic stenosis, poststenotic dilatation of the ascending aorta is rarely seen. Most often the sinuses of Valsalva are dilated and the ascending aorta and the aortic arch are of normal size or appear small. Echocardiography, Doppler ultrasound, and retrograde arterial catheterization are the most valuable techniques for localizing the site of obstruction to the supravalvar area and to assess the degree of hemodynamic abnormality. The diagnosis is confirmed by the demonstration of a pressure gradient just above the aortic valve and a constriction at this level by aortography. The angiogram may also permit visualization of narrowed segments of the aorta or great vessels distal to the obstruction. At right heart catheterization the presence of stenosis of peripheral pulmonary arteries may be detected by continually recording pressure as a catheter is withdrawn from a peripheral artery to the main pulmonary artery and by right ventricular or pulmonary artery angiocardiography.

The level of narrowing of the outflow tract may be observed clearly by two-dimensional echocardiography, digital subtraction angiography, and magnetic resonance imaging.

**Complications:** Syncope, aortic regurgitation, congestive heart failure, bacterial endocarditis, premature coronary arteriosclerosis, sudden unexpected death.

**Associated Findings:** A high incidence of narrowing of peripheral pulmonary arteries is seen (80%). Commonly, there is narrowing of the peripheral systemic arteries, including renal and carotid arteries. Mild degrees of pulmonary and aortic valvular stenosis, as well as coarctation of the aorta, and mitral valve prolapse may also be observed.

**Etiology:** When familial, by autosomal dominant inheritance with variable expression. Some family members may have supravalvar pulmonic stenosis either as an isolated lesion or in combination with supravalvar aortic stenosis.

**Pathogenesis:** The multiple system involvement observed when supravalvar aortic stenosis is associated with **Williams syndrome** may be related to a derangement of vitamin D metabolism in the mother or fetus during pregnancy. The creation of hypervitaminosis D in the pregnant rabbit has resulted in cardiovascular and craniofacial malformations in the offspring resembling those observed in this syndrome.

**MIM No.:** *18550

**CDC No.:** 747.220

**Sex Ratio:** M1:F1

**Occurrence:** Several dozen cases reported in the literature.

**Risk of Recurrence for Patient's Sib:**
See Part I, *Mendelian Inheritance.*

**Risk of Recurrence for Patient's Child:**
See Part I, *Mendelian Inheritance.*

**Age of Detectability:** From birth by typical clinical features and echocardiograph, left heart catheterization, and selective left ventricular or aortic angiocardiography.

**Gene Mapping and Linkage:** Unknown.

**Prevention:** None known. Genetic counseling indicated.

**Treatment:** Early recognition may prove to be a prerequisite to successful medical management, insofar as prompt diagnosis and treatment of the idiopathic hypercalcemia in infancy. Supravalvar aortic stenosis is often amenable to operative treatment. The lumen of the aorta at the supravalvar level may be widened effectively by the insertion of an oval or diamond-shaped fabric prosthesis only in those patients with a normal ascending aorta. If the aorta is hypoplastic, this procedure merely displaces the pressure gradient distally, without abolishing the obstruction. Under these circumstances, totally effective surgical treatment may necessitate replacement or widening of the entire hypoplastic aorta with an appropriate prosthesis.

**Prognosis:** The prognosis depends upon the severity of obstruction, the extent of the aortic wall and other great vessels involved by the pathologic process, the degree of coronary arteriosclerosis and the severity of the associated peripheral pulmonary or peripheral arterial stenoses.

**Detection of Carrier:** Unknown.

**References:**

Kahler RL, et al.: Familial congenital heart disease; familial occurrence of atrial septal defect with a-v conduction abnormalities; supravalvular aortic and pulmonic stenosis, and ventricular septal defect. Am J Med 1966; 40:384–399.

Friedman WF: Vitamin D and the supravalvular aortic stenosis syndrome. In: Woollam DHM, ed: Advances in teratology. New York: Academic Press, 1968:85–96.

Friedman WF, Mills LF: The relationship between vitamin D and the craniofacial and dental anomalies of the supravalvular aortic stenosis syndrome. Pediatrics 1969; 43:12–18. *

Williams DE, et al.: Cross-sectional echocardiographic localization of the sites of left ventricular outflow tract obstructions. Am J Cardiol 1976; 37(2):250–255. *

Usher BW, et al.: Echocardiographic detection of supravalvular aortic stenosis. Circulation 1979; 49:1257–1259.

Taylor AB, et al.: Abnormal regulation of circulating 25-hydroxyvitamin D in the Williams syndrome. N Engl J Med 1982; 306:972–975.

O'Connor WN, et al.: Supravalvular aortic stenosis: clinical and pathologic observations in six patients. Arch Path Lab Med 1985; 109:179–185.

Schmidt MA, et al.: Autosomal dominant supravalvular aortic stenosis: large three-generation family. Am J Med Genet 1989; 32:384–389.

FR019

**William F. Friedman**

## AORTIC VALVE ATRESIA                    0079

**Includes:**  Aortic atresia

**Excludes:**
   **Aortic valve stenosis** (0080)
   **Aorta, coarctation** (0073)
   Hypoplastic left heart if aortic valve is patent

**Major Diagnostic Criteria:** Cardiomegaly and congestive heart failure during the 1st week of life in a mildly to moderately cyanotic infant with weak or absent pulses and marked right ventricular hypertrophy on the EKG strongly suggest the diagnosis. 2-dimensional echocardiograph shows no aortic orifice with a small ascending aorta, underdeveloped left ventricle, and mitral stenosis or atresia. If cardiac catheterization is done, angiocardiography will demonstrate retrograde filling of the hypoplastic proximal aorta by way of a patent ductus.

**Clinical Findings:** Aortic valve maldevelopment varies from complete absence of identifiable valve tissue, to the appearance of definite raphae, to the formation of an imperforate dome. The coronary arteries arise from the base of the aorta, which is hypoplastic in the ascending portion and the arch. Many have a coarctation proximal to or at the level of the ductus arteriosus. The left atrium and ventricle are hypoplastic and may exhibit endocardial fibroelastosis; the mitral valve may be hypoplastic or atretic. An interatrial opening is usually present. The right atrium, right ventricle, and pulmonary arteries are enlarged, and there is always a large patent ductus. Only 5–10% have a ventricular septal defect with an adequate left ventricle. Complete transposition of the great arteries is quite rare.

The pulmonary venous blood does not enter the left ventricle from the left atrium, but passes to the right atrium, right ventricle, pulmonary artery, and then not only to the lungs, but also via the patent ductus to both the ascending and descending aortas. The pressure in the pulmonary arteries is at systemic level.

Aortic atresia is the most common cause of heart failure in the 1st week of life. Failure tends to occur early and to progress rapidly. Cyanosis occurs in nearly all cases, with an average age of onset at 2 days, but may be delayed in appearance. The peripheral pulses may be weak or absent and blood pressures, when obtained, are lower than normal. More than half the patients have grade 1–4/6 systolic murmurs along the sternal border, probably due to increased pulmonary valve flow or to tricuspid insufficiency. Systolic ejection clicks and mid-diastolic murmurs may occur, but thrills are rare.

Thoracic X-rays show prominent pulmonary vasculature in nearly all cases. In most cases, vasculature is of the shunt type, whereas the remainder show severe pulmonary venous obstruction. A prominent main pulmonary artery helps distinguish this defect from transposition of the great arteries. The heart is usually moderately enlarged. The "ductus infundibulum" is evident in the aortic knob region in at least half the cases. The EKG usually shows right axis deviation, but left axis deviation has been reported. Two-thirds show right atrial hypertrophy, and most show right ventricular hypertrophy, often with a qR pattern or upright T waves in the right precordial leads. In the left precordial leads, ST-T abnormalities are frequent, and the q wave is often absent.

The echocardiogram in aortic valve atresia shows little or no motion in the area of the aortic valve. The aorta is hypoplastic as viewed in both the anterior-posterior and superior-inferior axes. The mitral valve echo is usually absent, and the left ventricular cavity is usually slit-like. The left atrium may be dilated. The right ventricle is dilated, as is the pulmonary artery (suprasternal), and tricuspid motion is excessive.

Cardiac catheterization shows reduced oxygen saturation in the venae cavae, with a rise in the right atrium. The oxygen saturation and systolic pressure in the right ventricle is similar to those in the aorta and systemic arteries. A right-sided angiocardiogram can show the right-to-left flow through the patent ductus with retrograde filling of the hypoplastic descending aorta. These structures may also be shown by thoracic aortography.

**Complications:** Death from congestive heart failure or hypoxia. Myocardial infarction has been reported.

**Associated Findings:** Extracardiac anomalies (mostly minor GU malformations) occur in approximately 25% of the cases.

**Etiology:** Unknown.

**Pathogenesis:** Possibly faulty early development of the outflow portion of the left ventricle, probably between the 5th and 8th weeks of fetal life.

**CDC No.:** 746.480

**Sex Ratio:** Estimated to be M2:F1. The sex ratio seems more equal in those patients with associated mitral atresia.

**Occurrence:** 1:10,000 live births. Pobably <1:100 cases of congenital heart disease.

**Risk of Recurrence for Patient's Sib:** Unknown.

**Risk of Recurrence for Patient's Child:** No record of an affected individual reaching reproductive age.

**Age of Detectability:** From mid-pregnancy, by fetal 2-dimensional echocardiography.

**Gene Mapping and Linkage:** Unknown.

**Prevention:** None known. Genetic counseling indicated.

**Treatment:** Prostaglandin E₁ is useful to maintain patency of the ductus arteriosus. There is growing surgical experience with staged repair. In the first stage a broad anastomosis is made between the main pulmonary artery and the ascending aorta and/or aortic arch; and the pulmonary artery bifurcation and branches are separated from the proximal main pulmonary artery and reconnected to the systemic circulation, usually by a tubular shunt. Only a few patients have survived the second stage, which is a modified Fontan procedure with partitioning of the right atrium. Heart transplant is another surgical approach that has been tried.

**Prognosis:** Without cardiac repair or replacement, this condition is fatal, usually within the 1st week of life.

**Detection of Carrier:** Unknown.

**References:**
Watson DG, Rowe RD: Aortic-valve atresia: report of 43 cases. JAMA 1962; 179:14–18. *
Deely WJ, et al.: Hypoplastic left heart syndrome. Am J Dis Child 1971; 121:168–175.
Meyer RA, Kaplan S: Echocardiography in the diagnosis of hypoplasia of the left or right ventricle in the neonate. Circulation 1972; 46:55–64.
Moodie DS, et al.: Congenital aortic atresia: report of long survival and some speculations about surgical approaches. J Thorac Cardiovasc Surg 1972; 63:726–731.
Norwood WI, et al.: Experience with operations for hypoplastic left heart syndrome. J Thorac Cardiovasc Surg 1981; 82:511–519.
Norwood WI, et al.: Physiologic repair of aortic atresia-hypoplastic left heart syndrome. N Engl J Med 1983; 308:23–26. *

WA040                                                              **David G. Watson**

## AORTIC VALVE STENOSIS                                          **0080**

**Includes:**
  Aortic valve, incomplete tricuspid
  Aortic valve, stenotic bicuspid
  Aortic valve stenosis, unicommissural
  Valvar aortic stenosis

**Excludes:**
  Aortic hypoplasia
  **Aortic stenosis, supravalvar** (0078)
  **Aortic valve atresia** (0079)
  **Heart, subaortic stenosis, fibrous** (0916)
  Hypoplastic left heart syndrome

**Major Diagnostic Criteria:** Left heart catheterization establishes the site and severity of obstruction. The essential hemodynamic abnormality produced by the obstruction to left ventricular outflow is the pressure gradient between the left ventricle and aorta during the systolic ejection period localized to the level of the aortic valve.

**Clinical Findings:** In approximately 65% of patients the aortic valve is bicuspid with a single, fused commissure and an eccentrically placed orifice; a 3rd incomplete or rudimentary commissure may sometimes be apparent. About 15% of patients have an aortic valve in which each of the commissures is partially fused. In 10–20% of patients, especially symptomatic infants, the stenotic aortic valve is unicommissural, possesses only a single leaflet, and is dome-shaped. The aortic valve ring may be relatively underdeveloped in infants and young children with severe stenosis of the aortic valve, a lesion which represents a segment of the spectrum extending to the hypoplastic left heart syndrome and the aortic hypoplasia and atresia complexes. The dynamics of blood flow associated with a congenitally deformed aortic valve commonly lead to thickening of the cusps and ultimately to calcification in later life. Secondary calcification of the valve is extremely rare in childhood. When the obstruction is hemodynamically significant, concentric hypertrophy of the left ventricular wall and dilatation of the ascending aorta occur.

Congenital aortic stenosis may be responsible for severe obstruction to left ventricular outflow without the clinical symptoms of diminished cardiac reserve that are so frequent in other forms of congenital heart disease. Conversely, in an occasional patient with mild obstruction, the clinical findings may be striking. Most children with congenital aortic stenosis are asymptomatic and grow and develop normally. Initial attention is usually called to these children only when a murmur is detected on a routine examination. When symptoms do occur, those most commonly noted are fatigability, exertional dyspnea, angina and syncope. Rarely described are abdominal pain, profuse sweating and epistaxis. The obstruction is at least moderately severe if there is a definite history of fatigability and exertional dyspnea. Exertional syncope occurs usually only in patients with gradients exceeding 50 mmHg and is related to inability of the left ventricle to increase its output and to maintain cerebral flow during exercise. The disparity between the oxygen supply to the left ventricle and myocardial oxygen requirements is responsible for anginal pain. The diminished coronary perfusion pressure and the increased duration of left ventricular systole limit coronary blood flow, while the elevated systolic wall tension developed by myocardial fibers and the increased left ventricular mass increase the oxygen requirements of the heart.

When the degree of aortic stenosis is significant, a left ventricular lift is usually palpable. If the systolic pressure gradient across the aortic valve exceeds approximately 25 mmHg, a precordial systolic thrill is often palpated over the base of the heart with transmission to the jugular notch and along the carotid arteries. Ordinarily, the obstruction is mild if neither a left ventricular lift nor a thrill is present. The increased force of left atrial contraction in the presence of left ventricular hypertrophy results in a palpable presystolic expansion. The latter sign is almost always associated with a severe degree of obstruction and an elevated left ventricular end diastolic pressure.

A systolic aortic ejection sound (click) may be heard at the cardiac apex when the valve is mobile; and it is more often heard in patients with mild or moderate stenosis than in those with severe stenosis. In most instances the opening of the aortic valves is responsible for the ejection sound. Disappearance of the ejection sound suggests that progression has occurred. Prolongation of left ventricular emptying and delayed closure of the aortic valve may lead to a single or a closely split second heart sound. With increasingly more severe degrees of obstruction the aortic closure sound may follow the pulmonic sound during expiration; ie, paradoxical splitting is present. The systolic murmur which is characteristic of valvar aortic stenosis starts after the completion of left ventricular isometric contraction or with the ejection sound, and is diamond-shaped, loud, harsh, and best heard at the base of the heart. The murmur, like the thrill, radiates to the jugular notch and carotid vessels as well as to the apex. In approximately 1/4th of the patients with stenosis of the aortic valve an early diastolic blowing murmur of aortic regurgitation is present. Since the degree of regurgitation is usually not hemodynamically significant, the diastolic murmur is faint and the arterial pulse pressure is normal or decreased.

Although it is true that the EKG findings in congenital aortic stenosis often vary with the severity of obstruction, a normal or near normal EKG does not exclude severe stenosis. In patients under 10 years of age the electrocardiogram appears to be a more reliable guide in indicating the severity of the stenosis than in older patients. The findings in the younger age group that tend to accompany severe obstruction are T wave vectors in the frontal plane to the left of -40°, widening of the angle between the mean QRS and T forces in the frontal plane in excess of 100°, an S wave in $V_1$ greater than 20 mm and an R wave in $V_6$ exceeding 30 mm. Perhaps the most reliable index of the severity of obstruction in patients not receiving digitalis is the left ventricular "strain pattern" which consists of the findings of left ventricular hypertrophy combined with ST segment depressions and T wave flattening or inversion in the left precordial leads. This pattern generally, but not always, indicates that severe aortic stenosis is present.

A good relationship appears to exist between exercise induced EKG changes and the severity of obstruction. Thus, the development during exercise of ischemic ST-segment changes has been observed in patients with normal resting cardiac indices and transvalvar pressure differences in excess of 50 mmHg.

On chest X-rays the overall heart size is usually normal or the degree of enlargement is minimal. However, concentric left ventricular hypertrophy accompanies moderate or severe obstruction and is manifested by rounding of the cardiac apex in the frontal projection. More striking left ventricular enlargement may exist in the presence of severe obstruction. Left atrial enlargement and evidence of pulmonary venous obstruction strongly suggest that a severe degree of stenosis exists. Poststenotic dilatation of the ascending aorta is a common finding in patients with valvar aortic stenosis. Roentgenographic evidence of calcification of the valve does not usually occur in the pediatric age group but is a relatively common finding in adults with congenital aortic stenosis.

Real-time cross-sectional echocardiography reveals impaired mobility of cusp tissue, an alteration in the phasic movement of the aortic valve with reduced lateral and increased superior excursions of valve echoes, and an increase in the internal aortic root dimension beyond the level of the valve annulus. Two-dimensional echocardiographic long axis views of the left ventricular outflow tract demonstrate doming of the aortic valve. The parasternal short axis view bisects the face of the valve demonstrating the anatomy of the commisures. Pulse-Doppler echocardiography allows inspection of the pattern flow velocity within the circulation. The technique detects the altered and disturbed turbulence of flow in patients with aortic stenosis. The most accurate noninvasive approach to quantify the severity of obstruction combines continuous wave Doppler flow analysis with cross-sectional echocardiographic determination of the area of the orifice. A simplified Bernoulli equation utilizes the measurement of the maximum velocity of the aortic jet, and time averaged pressure drop obtained from planimetry of the maximal velocity spectral recording. A simple estimate of the transvalvular gradient (in mm Hg) may be calculated as four times the square of the peak of Doppler velocity (meters/sec.).

The malformation may create unique problems in infants, and the clinical picture in this group therefore deserves special comment. Although isolated stenosis of the aortic valve seldom causes symptoms in infancy, occasionally the lesion is responsible for profound and intractable congestive heart failure. In spite of apparently normal coronary arteries, infarction of the left ventricular papillary muscles may occur in some of these infants, resulting in an acquired form of mitral valvar regurgitation, which intensifies the heart failure state. Moreover, endocardial fibroelastosis often results from reduced subendocardial oxygen delivery and myocardial degeneration may be prominent. The symptomatic infant with isolated valvar aortic stenosis is irritable, pale and hypotensive. Presenting manifestations include tachycardia, cardiomegaly and pulmonary venous congestion, manifested by dyspnea, tachypnea, subcostal retractions and diffuse rales. Cyanosis secondary to pulmonary venous unsaturation may be observed. The systolic murmur is often atypical, particularly when the infant is suffering from heart failure. The murmur is frequently best heard at the apex or along the lower left sternal border and may be confused with that caused by a ventricular septal defect. In some infants with heart failure, the murmur may be absent or extremely soft, but it becomes louder when myocardial contractility is improved with digitalis therapy and other medical measures. Often, however, the response to medical management of the infant with congestive heart failure is poor.

The EKG findings in infants may not be characteristic; left ventricular hypertrophy with strain as well as right atrial enlargement and right ventricular hypertrophy may be detected shortly after birth. The EKG signs of right heart involvement result from pulmonary hypertension secondary to elevated left ventricular diastolic and left atrial pressures and volume loading of the right ventricle due to left-to-right shunting across the foramen ovale.

**Complications:** Left ventricular failure, aortic regurgitation (25%), and sudden death (the world's literature yields values ranging from 1–18%. Clearly, a large number of factors regarding selection are operative in providing this range of numbers). Bacterial endocarditis (4%).

**Associated Findings:** As many as 20% of patients may have associated cardiovascular anomalies. Patent ductus arteriosus and coarctation of the aorta occur most frequently, and all 3 lesions may coexist in the same patient. Less often, a ventricular septal defect and pulmonic stenosis are associated malformations.

**Etiology:** Multifactorial inheritance.

**Pathogenesis:** In a true bicuspid valve, 1 of the valve anlagen presumably has never formed. In other cases, 2 of the cusps have fused, forming a functional, single cusp containing a raphe (incomplete tricuspid valve). If 2 commissures have fused completely, a so-called unicuspid valve is formed. Rarely, there is partial fusion of all 3 commissures, resulting in a stenotic tricuspid valve.

**CDC No.:** 746.300

**Sex Ratio:** M4:F1

**Occurrence:** 1:2000 (5% of patients with congenital heart disease).

**Risk of Recurrence for Patient's Sib:** About 2%.

**Risk of Recurrence for Patient's Child:** If mother is affected, risk is 13 - 18%. If father is affected, risk is about 3%.

**Age of Detectability:** From birth by left echocardiography, heart catheterization, and angiography.

**Gene Mapping and Linkage:** Unknown.

**Prevention:** None known. Genetic counseling indicated.

**Treatment:** Since the malformed aortic valve is a potential site of bacterial infection, careful prophylaxis against this complication should be followed in all patients, regardless of the severity of obstruction. Strict avoidance of strenuous physical activity is advised even when the patient is asymptomatic if severe aortic stenosis is present. Participation in competitive sports should probably also be restricted in patients with milder degrees of obstruction. Digitalis should be administered to patients with symptoms of diminished cardiac reserve.

The most critical decision concerns the advisability of surgical treatment. Among the factors influencing the indications, techniques, and results of operation are the patient's age, the nature of the valvar deformity, and the experience of the surgical team. The decision to advise operation depends primarily on the presence of severe obstruction rather than on the symptoms described by the patient. At the present time, operation is recommended for any child with critical stenosis, ie, peak systolic pressure gradient exceeding 75 mmHg, measured in the basal state when the cardiac output is normal, or calculated effective orifice less than 0.5 cm$^2$ per M$^2$ of body surface area. At operation, the fused commissures are opened. When this is done precisely and judiciously, the commissural incision enlarges the valvar orifice appreciably and does not result in significant aortic regurgitation. Complete or almost complete relief of obstruction occurs in the majority of patients unless the valve ring is hypoplastic.

Following commissurotomy, the valve leaflets remain somewhat deformed, and it is possible that further degenerative changes, including calcification, will lead to significant stenosis in later years. Because the valves are not rendered normal anatomically, antibiotic prophylaxis is indicated in the postoperative patient, even if the systolic pressure gradient has been completely abolished.

Special mention of the treatment of aortic stenosis in infancy is important. The seriously ill newborn with congenital aortic stenosis must be considered to be a medical emergency. Because imminent death may be anticipated unless surgical treatment is undertaken promptly, definitive establishment of the diagnosis and valvotomy are usually justified, despite the high risk.

**Prognosis:** The prognosis varies with the degree of obstruction. Mild aortic stenosis is compatible with a nearly normal life span. However, even when the obstruction is mild, the potential hazard of bacterial endocarditis remains and there is a tendency for sclerosis and calcification of the aortic valve to develop in later life so that a note of caution regarding prognosis is necessary. Not only may sclerosis lead to further diminution of the valve orifice with age, but the increase in the cardiac output and participation in strenuous athletic activities accompanying adolescence may also lead to a markedly elevated left ventricular systolic pressure. Moreover, although sudden death usually occurs in patients with the clinical signs of severe obstruction, this type of demise rarely occurs unexpectedly even in patients who are relatively asymptomatic.

The worst prognosis is encountered in infants in congestive heart failure whose clinical course can usually be improved only if operative relief of the obstruction is accomplished. With the exception of infants, death is rarely due to congestive heart failure in the pediatric age group. Rather, ventricular arrhythmias are probably the most common cause of fatal outcome.

**Detection of Carrier:** Unknown.

**References:**

Friedman WF, Pappelbaum SJ: Indications for hemodynamic evaluation and surgery in congenital aortic stenosis. Pediatr Clin North Am 1971; 18:1207.

Friedman WF: Congenital aortic stenosis. In: Moss AJ, Adams FH, eds: Heart disease in infants, children and adolescents. Baltimore: Williams & Wilkins Co, 1983:171. *

Huhta JC, et al.: Echocardiography in the diagnosis and management of symptomatic aortic valve stenosis in infants. Circulation 1984; 70:438.

Sink JD, et al.: Management of critical aortic stenosis in infancy. J Thorac Cardiovasc Surg 1984; 87:82.

Nora JJ, Nora AH: Maternal transmission of congenital heart defects. Am J Cardiol 1987; 59:459–463.

FR019                                                    **William F. Friedman**

**Aortic valve stenosis, unicommissural**
*See AORTIC VALVE STENOSIS*

---

**AORTIC VALVE, BICUSPID**                                              **0108**

**Includes:** Bicuspid aortic valve

**Excludes:**
    Aortic valve incompetence
    **Aortic valve stenosis** (0080)
    Bicuspid aortic valve, acquired

**Major Diagnostic Criteria:** No reliable clinical criteria exist to establish a diagnosis of a bicuspid aortic valve in the absence of left ventricular outflow obstruction or aortic valve incompetence. If selective left ventriculography or thoracic aortography is performed during cardiac catheterization for other cardiovascular anomalies, the bicuspid aortic valve may be an incidental finding; the same is true of 2-dimensional echocardiography.

**Clinical Findings:** The uncomplicated bicuspid aortic valve may be undetected in early life and produce no hemodynamic abnormality until it becomes stenotic and of clinical significance in adult life. When stenosis occurs in childhood, there is usually an aortic systolic ejection murmur, often preceded by an ejection click. A congenital bicuspid aortic valve should be suspected when bacterial endocarditis occurs in a child previously thought to be normal. An increased incidence of bacterial endocarditis occurs in patients with a bicuspid aortic valve, even in the absence of stenosis. Among cases of isolated, calcified aortic stenosis in adults, the congenital bicuspid aortic valve is often the underlying lesion. Rarely, at any age, prolapse of one cusp may result in valve incompetence. Chest X-ray may show a prominent ascending aorta or poststenotic dilatation. The aortic valve is calcified in a majority of adults over the age of 30.

By single crystal echocardiography, bicuspid aortic valves can sometimes be identified by the asymmetric placement of the diastolic closure line within the aortic root. Aortic root enlargement is often seen in such patients. Great variability often exists in the position of diastolic aortic closure, even in normals. Nevertheless, if multiple redundant echoes are consistently asymmetrically placed within the aortic root, the diagnosis of bicuspid aortic valve stenosis can be made. The severity of aortic stenosis is most easily judged by the detection and serial follow-up of left ventricular hypertrophy on the echocardiogram and the ratio of left ventricular systolic dimension to systolic wall thickness. Suprasternal notch echo demonstration of a dilated aortic arch can often be achieved. Cross-sectional echo studies delineating a bi-leaflet aortic valve, abnormal leaflet motion (doming) or the presence of poststenotic dilation are of assistance in making this diagnosis. The presence of fluttering of the mitral valve in patients suspected of having a bicuspid aortic valve is usually confirmatory of aortic insufficiency.

**Complications:** Aortic incompetence secondary to cusp prolapse; sclerosis and calcification resulting in aortic stenosis; bacterial endocarditis.

**Associated Findings:** Coarctation of the aorta (20%).

**Etiology:** Presumably multifactorial inheritance.

**Pathogenesis:** The pathologic anatomy is the presence of 2, rather than 3, aortic valve cusps. The cusps may be equal in size but, more commonly, are unequal. Usually, 1 of the 2 cusps is divided by a vertical raphe into 2 segments. Progressive trauma to the valve may lead to the typical appearance of calcific aortic stenosis in adulthood.

**MIM No.:** 10973

**CDC No.:** 746.400

**Sex Ratio:** M4:F1

**Occurrence:** Still controversial. Some authorities believe it may be as high as 1:250.

**Risk of Recurrence for Patient's Sib:** Unknown.

**Risk of Recurrence for Patient's Child:** Unknown.

**Age of Detectability:** Beyond the third decade by clinical findings of aortic stenosis or aortic incompetence. Definitive diagnosis may be made by echocardiograph or ascending aorta angiography at any age.

**Gene Mapping and Linkage:** Unknown.

**Prevention:** None known. Genetic counseling indicated.

**Treatment:** Institution of appropriate prophylaxis for bacterial endocarditis. Other therapy, as indicated, for complications of aortic stenosis and aortic incompetence.

**Prognosis:** The prognosis is directly related to the nature and severity of the complications. These include aortic stenosis, aortic incompetence, and bacterial endocarditis. By the fifth decade, sclerotic and calcific changes almost always occur in the bicuspid valve.

**Detection of Carrier:** Unknown.

**Special Considerations:** This defect may represent the most common congenital cardiovascular malformation. In the past, even in the absence of a history of rheumatic fever, when isolated aortic stenosis was first detected after age 15 years, the lesion was considered to be of rheumatic etiology. It is now apparent that as many as 70% of these patients have congenital bicuspid aortic valve.

**References:**
Edwards JE: The congenital bicuspid aortic valve. Circulation 1961; 23:485–488.
Gould SE: Pathology of the heart and blood vessels, ed 3. Springfield: Charles C Thomas, 1968.
Roberts WE: The congenitally bicuspid aortic valve. A study of 85 autopsy cases. Am J Cardiol 1970; 26:72–83.
Nanda NC, et al.: Echocardiographic recognition of the congenital bicuspid aortic valve. Circulation 1974; 48:870–875.
Emanuel R, et al.: Congenitally bicuspid aortic valves: clinicogenetic study of 41 families. Brit Heart J 1978; 40:1402–1407.
Friedman WF, Johnson AD: Congenital aortic stenosis in adult congenital heart diseases. In Robert WC, ed: Cardiovascular clinics, 2nd ed. Philadelphia: FA Davis Co., 1987:357–374. *

FR019                                    **William F. Friedman**

**Aortic valve, four-cusped**
*See AORTIC VALVE, TETRACUSPID*
**Aortic valve, incomplete tricuspid**
*See AORTIC VALVE STENOSIS*

**Aortic valve, quadricuspid**
*See AORTIC VALVE, TETRACUSPID*
**Aortic valve, stenotic bicuspid**
*See AORTIC VALVE STENOSIS*

## AORTIC VALVE, TETRACUSPID                    0081

**Includes:**
   Aortic valve, four-cusped
   Aortic valve, quadricuspid

**Excludes:**
   Aortic valve incompetence
   Four-cusped truncal valve-persistent truncus arteriosus

**Major Diagnostic Criteria:** Four distinct aortic valve cusps may be noted at cardiac operation. Angiographic visualization, although possible, is difficult.

**Clinical Findings:** Usually, the tetracuspid aortic valve is a random finding at autopsy. Rarely, symptoms and signs of aortic incompetence may occur.

**Complications:** Aortic insufficiency (20%).

**Associated Findings:** Displacement of the coronary orifice above the aortic ring.

**Etiology:** Unknown.

**Pathogenesis:** Probably results from the formation of an additional intercalated valve swelling.

**Sex Ratio:** Presumably M1:Fl

**Occurrence:** About a dozen cases reported.

**Risk of Recurrence for Patient's Sib:** Unknown.

**Risk of Recurrence for Patient's Child:** Unknown.

**Age of Detectability:** From birth by aortography in cases with insufficiency.

**Gene Mapping and Linkage:** Unknown.

**Prevention:** None known. Genetic counseling indicated.

**Treatment:** Antibiotic prophylaxis for dental procedure if clinical diagnosis is established.

**Prognosis:** Excellent, unless complicated by development of aortic incompetence.

**Detection of Carrier:** Unknown.

**References:**
McRonald RE, Dean DC: Congenital quadricuspid aortic valve. Am J Cardiol 1966; 18:761–763. *
Peretz DI, et al.: Four-cusped aortic valve with significant hemodynamic abnormality. Am J Cardiol 1969; 23:291–293.
Robicsek F, et al.: Congenital quadricuspid aortic valve with displacement of the left coronary orifice. Am J Cardiol 1969; 23:288–290.

FR019                                    **William F. Friedman**

## AORTICO-LEFT VENTRICULAR TUNNEL              0082

**Includes:** Aorticocardiac fistula

**Excludes:**
   Acquired aneurysms
   **Aortic sinus of valsalva, aneurysm** (0053)
   Coronary artery anomalies
   Other forms of aortic valvular incompetence

**Major Diagnostic Criteria:** In individuals with a general state of aortic regurgitation, aortography reveals the tunnel itself arising from the anterior aspect of the ascending aorta, beginning above the level of the origin of the right coronary artery and associated with early opacification of the left ventricle.

**Clinical Findings:** Clinical findings are those of aortic insufficiency with left ventricular strain. This condition also may be seen in the newborn period. Left ventricular enlargement is present and prominent pericardial bulge is commmon, as is a systolic thrill over "aortic area" and a diastolic thrill maximal along the left

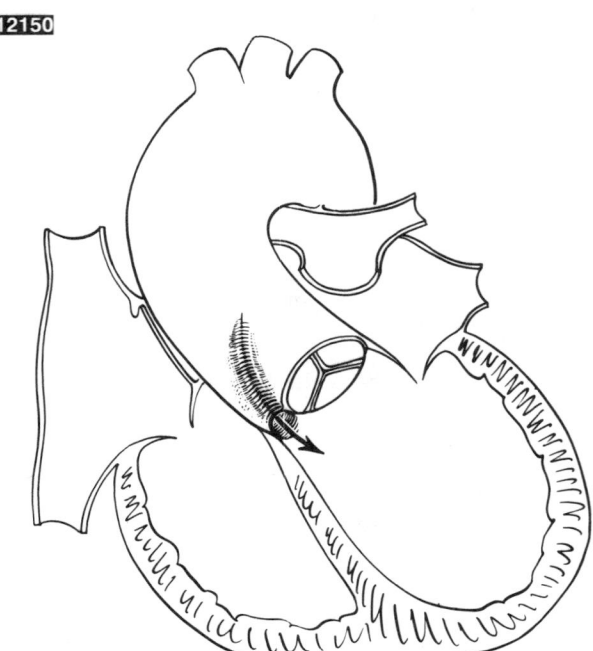

12150

**0082**-12150:  Drawing of aortico-left ventricular tunnel.

sternal border. Loud, harsh systolic and blowing diastolic murmurs are present in areas corresponding to those of thrills. Murmurs are separate, and do not resemble the continuous murmur of patent ductus arteriosus. Wide pulse pressure is a feature. There are EKG signs of left ventricular hypertrophy and strain. Radiologically, if the left ventricle fails, the pulmonary vascularity shows pulmonary congestion. The left ventricle is almost invariably enlarged with a prominent ascending aorta. Aortography shows enlargement of aorta with early opacification of left ventricle. In frontal projections, a tubular-like density, which represents the tunnel, projects from the anterior aspect of the ascending aorta in the region of the pulmonary trunk without opacification of the latter. In lateral views the tunnel projects anteriorly above the level of the right coronary arterial origin, and terminates in the left ventricle. The latter becomes densely opacified. The coronary arteries are normal. The aortic valve may appear stenotic.

**Complications:**  Left ventricular failure. Bacterial endocarditis in the tract is a theoretical possibility.

**Associated Findings:**  None known.

**Etiology:**  Unknown.

**Pathogenesis:**  Undetermined. The tract beginning in the aorta may be an accessory coronary artery which, in the ventricular septum, has direct communication with myocardial sinusoids.

**CDC No.:**  747.290

**Sex Ratio:**  M>1:F1

**Occurrence:**  1 in 1000 cases of congenital heart disease.

**Risk of Recurrence for Patient's Sib:**  Unknown.

**Risk of Recurrence for Patient's Child:**  Unknown.

**Age of Detectability:**  From birth.

**Gene Mapping and Linkage:**  Unknown.

**Prevention:**  None known. Genetic counseling indicated.

**Treatment:**  Surgical obliteration of fistula. Early operation advisable.

**Prognosis:**  In general, good to excellent. Aortic valvular insufficiency may be observed postoperatively in some cases.

**Detection of Carrier:**  Unknown.

**References:**
Levy MJ, et al.: Aortico-left ventricular tunnel. Circulation 1963; 27:841–852.
Somerville J, et al.: Aortico-left ventricular tunnel: clinical features and surgical management. Br Heart J 1974; 36:321–328.

N0003                                          **James J. Nora**

---

## AORTICO-PULMONARY SEPTAL DEFECT                    0083

**Includes:**
　　Aortic septal defect
　　Aorticopulmonary fenestration
　　Aorticopulmonary fistula
　　Aorticopulmonary window
　　Aortopulmonary defect
　　A-P window

**Excludes:**
　　**Heart, truncus arteriosus** (0972)
　　Patent ductus arteriosus simulating aorticopulmonary
　　　　window
　　Pulmonary artery, isolated right, arising from aorta

**Major Diagnostic Criteria:**  Root of aorta aortography best delineates the abnormal communication between the ascending aorta and the main pulmonary artery, and is the diagnostic procedure of choice. Right ventriculography will reveal a normally formed infundibulum, a finding not present in truncus arteriosus.

**Clinical Findings:**  The pathologic anatomy of aorticopulmonary septal defect consists of a window-like communication between the ascending aorta and main pulmonary artery. The defect is usually large and oval shaped with its lower margin lying at, or a few millimeters above, the normal pulmonary and aortic valve rings. The defect is rarely small. Approximately 25% of patients will have additional cardiovascular anomalies, the most common of which are patent ductus arteriosus, coarctation of the aorta, right aortic arch and ventricular septal defect.

The hemodynamic abnormalities in patients with aorticopulmonary window result from a large left-to-right shunt at the level of the great vessels. Because of the large size of the defect, the magnitude of the shunt and the clinical presentation depend almost entirely upon the relationship between pulmonary and systemic vascular resistances. The usual auscultatory findings consist of a loud systolic ejection murmur along the upper left sternal border that ends before the second sound. In less than 20% of patients there is a continuous murmur similar to a patent ductus arteriosus. When a continuous murmur is present, one can be sure that the defect is relatively small. Approximately 45% of patients will also have a low-pitched mid and late diastolic mitral flow murmur over the midprecordium and apex. As pulmonary vascular resistance increases, the systolic murmur may eventually disappear. Under such circumstances a loud, narrowly split second sound becomes the most prominent auscultatory finding with an increased intensity of the pulmonic component followed by a high-pitched diastolic murmur of pulmonic valve insufficiency. At this stage with pulmonary vascular hyperresistance, mild cyanosis is common secondary to some right-to-left shunting at the site of the defect (Eisenmenger physiology). Differential cyanosis of upper and lower limbs is not seen with right-to-left shunting in this lesion, as might be seen with a reversing ductus arteriosus and pulmonary hyperresistance, since with an A-P window desaturated blood flows directly into the ascending aorta, and is distributed to the entire body.

Thoracic X-ray findings are nonspecific and are consistent with any number of lesions that produce left-to-right shunting at the level of the ventricles or great vessels. Prominence of the main pulmonary arteries, increased pulmonary arterial vascularity, biventricular enlargement and left atrial enlargement are usually present. EKG findings vary and are directly related to the presence and severity of pulmonary hypertension and pulmonary vascular resistance. The majority of patients will present with a combination of right ventricular hypertrophy of the pressure overload variety and left ventricular hypertrophy of the volume overload type. Right ventricular hypertrophy alone is detected when the "Eisenmenger physiology" is present. Cardiac catheterization reveals a large shunt at the level of the great vessels just above the aortic valve. At times the catheter can be passed through the defect between the great vessels.

**Complications:** Frequent development of marked pulmonary vascular obstructive disease (Eisenmenger physiology). Death from congestive heart failure or bacterial endocarditis.

**Associated Findings:** None known.

**Etiology:** Presumably multifactorial inheritance.

**Pathogenesis:** Aorticopulmonary septal defect appears to result from a failure of fusion of the embryonic aorticopulmonary septum and truncus septum. This would account for the persistent communication between the ascending aorta and pulmonary trunk in the presence of normally developed arterial roots. In cases where the defect is large, the aorticopulmonary septum is probably hypoplastic as well.

**CDC No.:** 745.010

**Sex Ratio:** M1.5:F1

**Occurrence:** Less than 125 cases reported in the English and European literature.

**Risk of Recurrence for Patient's Sib:** Unknown.

**Risk of Recurrence for Patient's Child:** Unknown.

**Age of Detectability:** From birth by selective angiocardiography.

**Gene Mapping and Linkage:** Unknown.

**Prevention:** None known. Genetic counseling indicated.

**Treatment:** Repair of the defect utilizing total cardiopulmonary bypass; treatment for congestive heart failure or bacterial endocarditis.

**Prognosis:** In the presence of a large defect, the prognosis is poor unless repair of the defect is accomplished early in childhood. Many patients will die in the neonatal period and virtually all by the 4th or 5th decade. With early repair, patients should have restoration of normal hemodynamics with minimal risk of residual pulmonary hypertension.

**Detection of Carrier:** Unknown.

**References:**
Morrow AG, et al.: Congenital aortopulmonary septal defect: clinical and hemodynamic findings, surgical technique, and results of operative correction. Circulation 1962; 25:463–476.
Neufeld HN, et al.: Aorticopulmonary septal defect. Am J Cardiol 1962; 9:12–25.
Wright JG, et al.: Aortopulmonary fenestration. A technique of surgical management. J Thorac Cardiovasc Surg 1968; 55:280–283.
Perloff JK: The Clinical recognition of congenital heart disease, 3rd ed. Philadelphia: W.B. Saunders Co, 1986:442–493.

BU001
SC013

**Richard L. Bucciarelli**
**Gerold L. Schiebler**

**Aorticocardiac fistula**
*See AORTICO-LEFT VENTRICULAR TUNNEL*
**Aorticopulmonary fenestration**
*See AORTICO-PULMONARY SEPTAL DEFECT*
**Aorticopulmonary fistula**
*See AORTICO-PULMONARY SEPTAL DEFECT*
**Aorticopulmonary window**
*See AORTICO-PULMONARY SEPTAL DEFECT*
**Aortopulmonary defect**
*See AORTICO-PULMONARY SEPTAL DEFECT*
**Aparoschisis**
*See GASTROSCHISIS*
**Apert syndrome**
*See ACROCEPHALOSYNDACTYLY TYPE I*

**Apert-Crouzon disease (Acrocephalosyndactyly type II)**
*See ACROCEPHALOSYNDACTYLY TYPE I*
**Aphakia**
*See LENS, APHAKIA*
**Apical dystrophy**
*See MACULAR COLOBOMA-BRACHYDACTYLY*
**Aplasia and hypoplasia of the radius**
*See HAND, RADIAL CLUB HAND*
**Aplasia cutis congenita**
*See SKIN, LOCALIZED ABSENCE OF*

## APLASIA CUTIS CONGENITA-GASTROINTESTINAL ATRESIA 2403

**Includes:**
   Carmi syndrome
   Epidermal dysplasia, type I, late fetal
   Gastrointestinal atresia-aplasia cutis congenita

**Excludes:**
   **Epidermolysis bullosum, type II** (2561)
   **Restrictive dermatopathy** (2757)

**Major Diagnostic Criteria:** The combination of extensive aplasia cutis congenita with or without skin slippage suggestive of epidermolysis bullosa, and gastrointestinal atresias.

**Clinical Findings:** All affected infants have had extensive congenital skin defects, preferentially involving the lower part of the limbs, genital area, and head and neck. In some infants the skin defect resembled aplasia cutis congenita, in that denuded areas were next to normal skin; in other infants, it more closely resembled epidermolysis bullosa with positive "Nikolsky sign." Gastrointestinal atresias are common, although not consistent, and can involve the esophagus, pylorus, and/or duodenum. The ears appear low-set in many cases. X-rays of affected areas have shown underlying hypoplasia of soft tissue and bone. Histologic investigation showed absence of epidermis and skin appendages. Where skin separation occurred, it was between the basement membrane and dermis.

**Complications:** Infection is common.

**Associated Findings:** Findings present in one case only include ectropion, axillary pterygia, hypoplastic fingernails, **Syndactyly** of toes 2 and 3, absent testes, and hydroureter.

**Etiology:** Autosomal recessive inheritance.

**Pathogenesis:** Unknown.

**MIM No.:** *20773

**POS No.:** 3897

**Sex Ratio:** M1:F1

**Occurrence:** Undetermined but presumed rare. Cases have been reported from different parts of the world, including North America, Italy, Israel, and the Netherlands.

**Risk of Recurrence for Patient's Sib:**
   See Part I, *Mendelian Inheritance.*

**Risk of Recurrence for Patient's Child:**
   See Part I, *Mendelian Inheritance.*

**Age of Detectability:** At birth, by the presence of skin defects. Prenatal diagnosis may be possible in that elevated amniotic fluid AFP was present in one case.

**Gene Mapping and Linkage:** Unknown.

**Prevention:** None known. Genetic counseling indicated.

**Treatment:** Unknown.

**Prognosis:** All infants have died before or soon after birth.

**Detection of Carrier:** Unknown.

**References:**
Leschot NJ, et al.: Severe congenital skin defects in a newborn. Europ J Obstet Gynecol Reprod Biol 1980; 10:381–388.
Carmi R, et al.: Aplasia cutis congenita in two sibs discordant for pyloric dysplasia. Am J Med Genet 1982; 11:319–328. *
Carey JC, et al.: Aplasia cutis-congenita - the Carmi syndrome:

confirmation of a new neonatal generalized skin disorder. Proc Greenwood Genet Center 1983; 2:116–117.

Vivona G, et al.: Aplasia cutis congenita and/or epidermolysis bullosa. (Letter) Am J Med Genet 1987; 26:497–502. †

T0007                                              **Helga V. Toriello**

**Aplasia cutis congenita-terminal, transverse defects of limbs**
  *See LIMB AND SCALP DEFECTS, ADAMS-OLIVER TYPE*
**Aplasia of pylorus, congenital**
  *See STOMACH, PYLORIC ATRESIA*

## APO B-100, DEFECTIVE, FAMILIAL                    3227

**Includes:**  Apolipoprotein B100, familial defective

**Excludes:**  Apo-B100 mutations not impairing LDL receptor interaction

**Major Diagnostic Criteria:**  Hypercholesterolemia; defective binding of plasma LDL to LDL receptors; retarded clearance of plasma LDL from the circulation.

*Specific Diagnostic Criteria for Apo-B100(Arg$_{3500}$→Gln):* occurrence of glutamine substitution for the normally occurring arginine at amino acid residue 3500 of apo-B100; enhanced binding of monoclonal antibody MB47 (an antibody to apo-B100 that blocks LDL interaction with the LDL receptor).

**Clinical Findings:**  There has only been one documented mutation of apo-B100 responsible for familial defective apo-B100 thus far, i.e., apo-B100(Arg$_{3500}$→Gln). All patients identified to date are heterozygous for this defect. The clinical findings for these individuals include moderate hypercholesterolemia (adults usually have plasma cholesterol levels of 250 to 350 mg/dl; plasma cholesterol levels are usually greater than the 90th percentile for age- and sex-matched controls). The increased plasma cholesterol is manifested as a pure elevation of plasma LDL. Plasma triglyceride levels are normal.

Diagnosis requires determination of the ability of plasma LDL to bind to LDL receptors expressed on cultured skin fibroblasts. The defective LDL bind poorly to the receptor as compared with normal LDL. Identification of the mutation at residue 3500 is accomplished using polymerase chain reaction DNA amplification followed by annealing with allele-specific oligonucleotide probes. A solid-phase radioimmunoassay comparing the binding of normal and defective LDL to the MB47 antibody can also be used to diagnose the apo-B100(Arg$_{3500}$→Gln) mutation.

The elevation of plasma cholesterol and LDL levels is likely to predispose affected individuals to accelerated atherosclerosis. However, studies to date have not been extensive enough to prove or disprove this postulate.

**Complications:**  Possibly accelerated atherosclerosis.

**Associated Findings:**  Possible premature coronary artery disease, angina, stroke, and/or intermittent claudication.

**Etiology:**  Autosomal dominant inheritance.

**Pathogenesis:**  Mutation of apo-B100 results in defective binding of LDL to the LDL receptor. To date, the only documented mutation is a glutamine-for-arginine substitution at amino acid residue 3500 in apo-B100. Defective binding of LDL to the LDL receptor results in impaired plasma clearance of LDL. This causes an elevation of total plasma cholesterol and LDL, both of which have been associated with an increased risk of developing accelerated atherosclerosis.

**MIM No.:**  *10773

**Sex Ratio:**  M1:F1

**Occurrence:**  Prevalence of the apo-B100(Arg$_{3500}$→Gln) mutation has not been determined; however, it does not appear to be rare. The mutation at residue 3500 has been reported in the United States, Canada, Austria, and Italy.

**Risk of Recurrence for Patient's Sib:**
  See Part I, *Mendelian Inheritance.*

**Risk of Recurrence for Patient's Child:**
  See Part I, *Mendelian Inheritance.*

**Age of Detectability:**  At birth.

**Gene Mapping and Linkage:**  APOB (apolipoprotein B (including Ag(x) antigen)) has been mapped to 2p24-p23.

**Prevention:**  None known. Genetic counseling indicated.

**Treatment:**  Reduction of total plasma cholesterol and LDL; diet low in saturated fat and cholesterol, plus use of hypolipidemic drugs if diet fails. Patients should be counseled to eliminate other risk factors for premature atherosclerosis such as smoking and hypertension.

**Prognosis:**  Unknown.

**Detection of Carrier:**  Polymerase chain reaction DNA amplification, LDL receptor binding studies, or MB47 binding studies can detect the apo-B100(Arg$_{3500}$→Gln) mutation.

**Special Considerations:**  The use of the term familial defective apolipoprotein B100 should be restricted to apo-B100 mutations that impair binding of LDL to LDL receptors and result in an elevation of plasma cholesterol and LDL concentrations. Despite the fact that only one mutation [apo-B100(Arg$_{3500}$→Gln)] has thus far been documented, it is predictable that additional mutations will cause impaired LDL receptor interaction.

**References:**
Vega GL, Grundy SM: In vivo evidence for reduced binding of low density lipoproteins to receptors as a cause of primary moderate hypercholesterolemia. J Clin Invest 1986; 78:1410–1414.

Innerarity TL, et al.: Familial defective apolipoprotein B-100: low density lipoproteins with abnormal receptor binding. Proc Natl Acad Sci USA 1987; 84:6919–6923.

Weisgraber KH, et al.: Familial defective apolipoprotein B-100: enhanced binding of monoclonal antibody MB47 to abnormal low density lipoproteins. Proc Natl Acad Sci USA 1988; 85:9758–9762.

Soria LF, et al.: Association between a specific apolipoprotein B mutation and familial defective apolipoprotein B-100. Proc Natl Acad Sci USA 1989; 86:587–591.

MA093                                              **Robert W. Mahley**

**Apolipoprolipoprotein A-I variants (3A, 3B, 3C)**
  *See HYPOALPHALIPOPROTEINEMIA*
**Apolipoprotein A deficiency**
  *See ANALPHALIPOPROTEINEMIA*
**Apolipoprotein A-I absence**
  *See APOLIPOPROTEIN A-I AND C-III DEFICIENCY STATES*

## APOLIPOPROTEIN A-I AND C-III DEFICIENCY STATES     3165

**Includes:**
  Apoliprotein A-I and C-III deficiency
  Apolipoprotein A-I absence
  Apolipoprotein A-I, C-III, and A-IV deficiency
  Apolipoprotein A-I and C-III deficiency, variant II
  Plasma high density lipoprotein deficiency-planar
    xanthomas

**Excludes:**
  Analphalipoproteinemia (0048)
  Hypoalphalipoproteinemia (3096)
  Lecithin-cholesterol acyl transferase deficiency (0580)

**Major Diagnostic Criteria:**  Plasma high density lipoprotein (HDL) cholesterol levels between 0–5 mg/dl and undetectable or trace amounts of plasma apolipoprotein A-I and C-III in homozygotes, and values for these constituents of approximately 50% of normal in heterozygotes.

In Apolipoprotein A-I, C-III, and A-IV, deficiency apoA-IV values are also decreased. Plasma concentrations of low density lipoprotein (LDL) cholesterol are generally normal, and triglyceride levels are usually decreased. In contrast to homozygous **Analphalipoproteinemia**, plasma apoA-I levels are 1–2 mg/dl, apoC-III values are normal or increased, LDL cholesterol levels are about 50% of normal, and triglyceride levels are usually increased. Moreover, for Apolipoprotein A-I and C-III Deficiency, restriction site polymorphisms will be present following restriction with such enzymes as EcoRI and PstI and genomic blotting with a probe which spans the apoA-I gene. For Apolipoprotein A-I, C-III, and A-IV deficiency, restriction site polymorphisms will be present following restriction with a variety of enzymes (XbaI, Xmn, PstI) and genomic blotting with a probe which spans a region 2 kb 5' to the apoA-I gene. These findings are not present in homozygous **Analphalipoproteinemia.**

**Clinical Findings:** Homozygotes with these disorders develop markedly premature coronary artery disease (CAD) prior to age 40 years, while heterozygotes appear to be at increased risk for CAD prior to age 60 years. In addition, homozygotes have mild diffuse corneal opacification visible on slit examination of the eye. In homozygous Apolipoprotein A-I and C-III deficiency, yellow-orange indurated plaques are noted on the skin over the trunk, neck, eyelids, chest, arms, and back, while these findings were not noted in Apolipoprotein A-I, C-III, and A-IV deficiency. In contrast, in the latter disorder, plasma deficiency of alpha-tocopherol and essential fatty acids is noted; a finding not reported to be present in the former disorder. The cholesterol-ester laden macrophages reported for homozygous **Analphalipoproteinemia** in the lymph nodes, skin, spleen, and liver do not appear to be present in these disorders.

**Complications:** Premature vascular disease.

**Associated Findings:** Yellow-orange skin plaques in homozygous familial Apolipoprotein A-I and C-III deficiency.

**Etiology:** Autosomal codominant inheritance in which the full-blown clinical and biochemical picture is only observed in homozygotes.

**Pathogenesis:** An inability to synthesize normal apoA-I and apoC-III in the case of Apolipoprotein A-I and C-III deficiency, due to a DNA inversion affecting the adjacent apoA-I and apoC-III genes. The breakpoints of this inversion are located within the fourth exon of the apoA-I gene and the first intron of the apoC-III gene, resulting in reciprocal fusion of the apoA-I and apoC-III transcriptional units. In contrast, in familial Apolipoprotein A-I, C-III, and A-IV deficiency there is complete deletion of the entire apoA-I, apoC-III, and apoA-IV gene complex on the long arm of chromosome 11, resulting in an inability to synthesize these apolipoproteins.

**MIM No.:** *10768

**Sex Ratio:** M1:F1

**Occurrence:** These disorders appear to be rare, with each disorder having been described in one kindred only.

**Risk of Recurrence for Patient's Sib:**
See Part I, *Mendelian Inheritance.*

**Risk of Recurrence for Patient's Child:**
See Part I, *Mendelian Inheritance.*

**Age of Detectability:** At birth by measurement of plasma HDL cholesterol and apoA-I concentrations, and by genomic blotting.

**Gene Mapping and Linkage:** APOA1 (apolipoprotein A-I) has been mapped to 11q23-q24.
APR (apolipoprotein receptor) has been provisionally mapped to 12q13-q14.
The defects in these disorders are due to inversions or deletions of DNA within the apoA-I, apoC-III, apoA-IV gene complex on the long arm of chromosome 11.

**Prevention:** None known. Genetic counseling indicated.

**Treatment:** Measures to prevent premature atherosclerosis are indicated in these disorders, especially in the homozygous state. Treatment of hypertension, obesity, diabetes, cigarette smoking, and elevated LDL cholesterol, if present, are indicated. A prudent low saturated fat, low cholesterol diet is also indicated, as is a regular exercise program and maintenance of ideal body weight. Medication which may be useful for raising HDL levels in the heterozygous state include niacin and gemfibrozil. Treatment with dietary essential fatty acids and alpha-tocopherol are indicated if deficiency exists.

**Prognosis:** Good. Incidence of premature atherosclerosis is high prior to age 40 years in homozygotes, and prior to age 60 years in heterozygotes.

**Detection of Carrier:** Heterozygotes have HDL cholesterol, apoA-I, and apoC-III levels which are approximately 50% of normal. Moreover the heterozygous state for these disorders can be diagnosed with certainty by genomic blotting analysis.

**References:**
Norum RA, et al: Familial deficiency of apolipoprotein A-I and C-III and precocious coronary artery disease. New Engl J Med 1982; 306:1513–1519.
Schaefer EJ, et al: Plasma apolipoprotein A-I absence associated with a marked reduction of plasma high density lipoproteins and premature coronary artery disease. Arteriosclerosis 1982; 2:16–26.
Schaefer EJ: Clinical, biochemical, and genetic features in familial disorders of high density lipoprotein deficiency. Arteriosclerosis 1984; 4:303–322.
Schaefer EJ, et al: Familial apolipoprotein A-I and C-III deficiency, variant II. J Lipid Red 1985; 26:1089–1101.
Karathanasis SK, et al: DNA inversion within the apolipoproteins AI/CIII/AIV-encoding gene cluster of certain patients with premature atherosclerosis. Proc Natl Acad Sci USA 1987; 84:7198–7202.

SC065                   **Ernst J. Schaefer**
0R006                  **Jose M. Ordovas**

**Apolipoprotein A-I and C-III deficiency, variant II**
*See APOLIPOPROTEIN A-I AND C-III DEFICIENCY STATES*
**Apolipoprotein A-I, C-III, and A-IV deficiency**
*See APOLIPOPROTEIN A-I AND C-III DEFICIENCY STATES*
**Apolipoprotein B deficiency**
*See ANEMIA, HEMOLYTIC, RED CELL MEMBRANE DEFECTS*
*also ABETALIPOPROTEINEMIA*
**Apolipoprotein B100, familial defective**
*See APO B-100, DEFECTIVE, FAMILIAL*
**Apolipoprotein E, deficiency or defect of**
*See HYPERLIPOPROTEINEMIA, BROAD BETA TYPE*
**Apoliprotein A-I and C-III deficiency**
*See APOLIPOPROTEIN A-I AND C-III DEFICIENCY STATES*
**Apoprotein in intestinal cells-hypobetalipoproteinemia**
*See LIPID TRANSPORT DEFECT OF INTESTINE*
**Appalachian amyloid polyneuropathy, familial**
*See AMYLOIDOSIS, APPALACHIAN TYPE*
**Appelt-Gerken-Lenz syndrome**
*See ROBERTS SYNDROME*
**Apple peel syndrome**
*See JEJUNAL ATRESIA*
**Apraxia, oculomotor-contractures-muscle atrophy**
*See CONTRACTURES-MUSCLE ATROPHY-OCULOMOTOR APRAXIA*
**Apraxia-mental retardation, X-linked-muscle atrophy-contractures**
*See X-LINKED MENTAL RETARDATION-MUSCLE ATROPHY-CONTRACTURES-APRAXIA*

---

**APROSOPIA**                            **2487**

**Includes:** Face, absence of facial structures

**Excludes:**
    **Agnathia-microstomia-synotia** (0028)
    **Anencephaly** (0052)

**Major Diagnostic Criteria:** Absence of facial structures.

**Clinical Findings:** The mouth and nose are completely absent, while a rudimentary eye may be present. The ears are present and fused at the anterior midline (synotia). The tongue, epiglottis, thyroid gland, and hyoid bones are absent.

**Complications:** The flat, membranous bones of the skull may be hypoplastic and incompletely fused.

**Associated Findings:** Patent foramen ovale, **Ductus arteriosus, patent, Anencephaly.**

**Etiology:** Unknown.

**Pathogenesis:** Unknown.

**Sex Ratio:** Undetermined but presumed M1:F1.

**Occurrence:** Undetermined but presumed rare.

**Risk of Recurrence for Patient's Sib:** Unknown. Few if any reported instances of sibling recurrence.

**Risk of Recurrence for Patient's Child:** No affected individuals have survived to reproduce.

**Age of Detectability:** At birth.

**Gene Mapping and Linkage:** Unknown.

**Prevention:** None known. Genetic counseling indicated.

**Treatment:** Unknown.

**Prognosis:** Invariably fatal in the first few minutes of life.

**Detection of Carrier:** Unknown.

**Special Considerations:** Aprosopia may represent the extreme of a spectrum of defects involving the absence of craniofacial structures.

**References:**
Leary M: A case of aprosopia associated with anencephaly. S Afr Med J 1965; 39:657–658.

J0027                                                    **Ronald J. Jorgenson**

**Aqueductal stenosis**
*See HYDROCEPHALY*

---

## ARACHNODACTYLY, CONTRACTURAL BEALS TYPE     0085

**Includes:**
   Beals syndrome
   Beals-Hecht syndrome
   Contractural arachnodactyly, congenital
   Contractures, multiple with arachnodactyly
   Ear anomalies-contractures-dysplasia of bone with
      kyphoscoliosis

**Excludes:**
   Achard syndrome
   Arachnodactyly-cataracts-mental retardation
   **Arthrogryposis, distal types** (2280)
   **Contracture, dupuytren** (0301)
   **Homocystinuria** (0474)
   **Marfan syndrome** (0630)

**Major Diagnostic Criteria:** Arachnodactyly with multiple congenital contractures of limbs, "crumpled" ears.

**Clinical Findings:** Multiple congenital joint contractures of fingers, knees, hips, elbows, and ankles. There may be limitation of elbow extension. Fingers are usually long and narrow at birth, with flexion contractures of the proximal interphalangeal joints. Thumb tends to be adducted onto palm at birth. Ankles, usually mildly valgus, have excessive dorsiflexion. Toes are long and often slightly incurving. Contractures improve spontaneously. Arachnodactyly is present with particularly long, thin feet and elongation of proximal phalanges of digits. Most affected individuals are taller than average. Pectus excavatum and carinatum are seen. "Crumpled" ears are almost always present with flattened top of helix, "crumpled" anthelix, with prominent crura and partial obliteration of the concha. Kyphoscoliosis and osteopenia are inconstant features. They may be present in infancy or progress with age, becoming quite severe in older affected individuals. Intelligence is normal. Keratoconus and myopia has been described. Floppy mitral valve and mitral regurgitation have been reported.

**Complications:** Knee and hand contractures may persist but are responsive to physical therapy. Scoliosis may become worse with age.

**Associated Findings:** Affected individuals are frequently breech deliveries. They may have delayed motor development because of contractures and hypotonia. Congenital heart anomalies have been reported in a few cases.

**Etiology:** Autosomal dominant inheritance with variable expression, even within a given family.

**Pathogenesis:** This condition would appear to be a generalized connective tissue disorder which affects connective tissue in utero and improves with age in most cases.

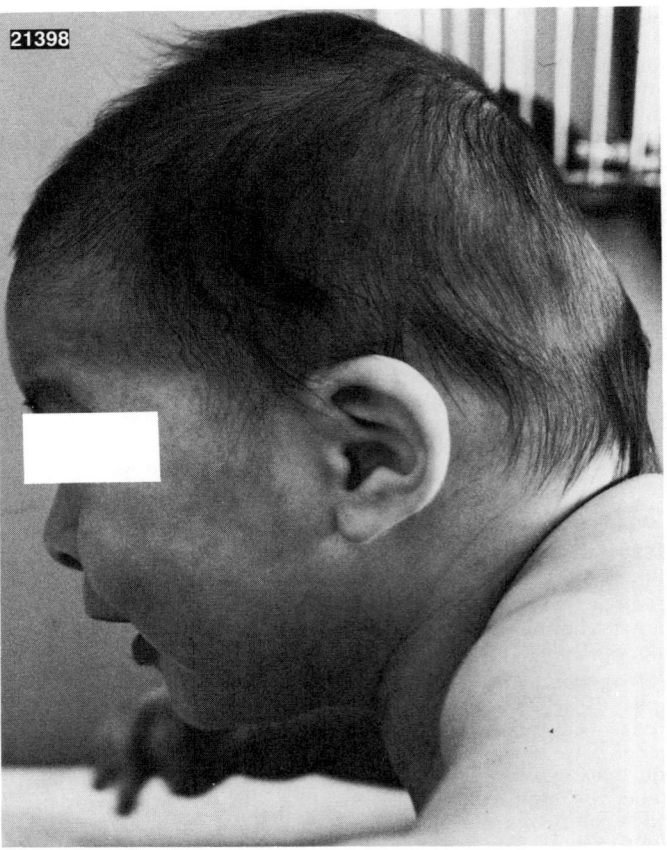

21398

**0085A-21398:** Note flattened helix, prominent crura and shallow concha.

---

**MIM No.:** *12105

**POS No.:** 3027

**Sex Ratio:** M1:F1

**Occurrence:** Twenty affected families and over 13 isolated cases have been reported.

**Risk of Recurrence for Patient's Sib:**
   See Part I, *Mendelian Inheritance.*

**Risk of Recurrence for Patient's Child:**
   See Part I, *Mendelian Inheritance.*

**Age of Detectability:** At birth.

**Gene Mapping and Linkage:** CCA (congenital contractual arachnodactyly) is unassigned.

**Prevention:** None known. Genetic counseling indicated.

**Treatment:** Physical therapy. Surgery rarely needed. Cardiovascular and ophthalmologic evaluation required. Plastic surgery to repair ear, if necessary.

**Prognosis:** Normal life span, with improvement of contractures by adulthood.

**Detection of Carrier:** Adults may appear almost normal with regard to contractures, but abnormal ear shape may help identify affected adults.

**Special Considerations:** Marfan's original patient may have had this condition rather than what we now recognize as **Marfan syndrome**.

**References:**
Beals RK, et al: Congenital contractural arachnodactyly. J Bone Joint Surg [Am] 1971; 53:987–993.

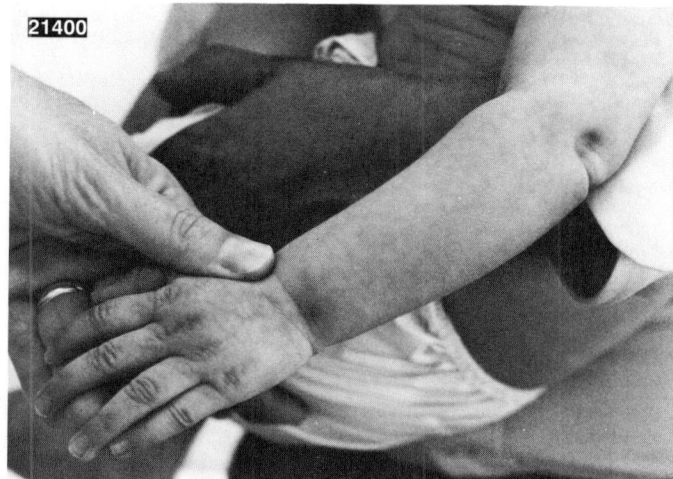

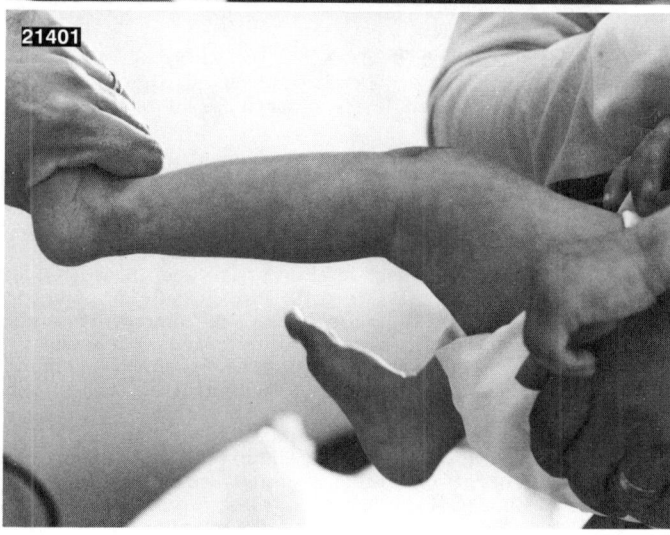

**0085B**-21400: Arachnodactyly and elbow contracture. 21401: Left knee contracture in this infant resolved by age three years.

Lipson EH, et al: The clinical spectrum of congenital contractural arachnodactyly. Z Kinderheilkd 1974; 118:1–8.

Bass HN, et al: Congenital contractural arachnodactyly, karatoconus, and probable Marfan syndrome in the same pedigree. J Pediatr 1981; 98:591–593.

Anderson RA, et al.: Cardiovascular findings in congenital contractual arachnodactyly: report of an affected kindred. Am J Med Genet 1984; 18:265–271.

Ramos Arroyo MA, et al.: Congenital contractural arachnodactyly: report of four additional families and review of the literature. Clin Genet 1985; 27:570–581.

HA014                                                        **Judith G. Hall**

**Arachnodactyly-craniosynostosis-hernia**
 *See CRANIOSYNOSTOSIS-ARACHNODACTYLY-HERNIA*
**Aran-Duchenne disease**
 *See AMYOTROPHIC LATERAL SCLEROSIS*
 *also AMYOTROPHIC LATERAL SCLEROSIS, FAMILIAL ADULT AND JUVENILE TYPES*
**Arcuate uterus**
 *See MULLERIAN FUSION, INCOMPLETE*

## AREDYLD SYNDROME                                        2785

**Includes:**
 Acrorenal field defect-ectodermal dysplasia-lipoatrophic diabetes
 Diabetes, lipoatrophic-acrorenal field defect-ectodermal dysplasia
 Ectodermal dysplasia-acrorenal field defect-lipoatrophic diabetes

**Excludes:**
 **Acro-renal-mandibular syndrome** (2778)
 **Radial-renal-ocular syndrome** (2643)

**Major Diagnostic Criteria:** Lipoatrophic diabetes, limb and kidney abnormalities, dental alterations, trichodysplasia.

**Clinical Findings:** Low birth weight, natal teeth, generalized lipoatrophy, typical nonketotic diabetes, marked resistance to insulin, hepatosplenomegaly, generalized hypotrichosis, short stature, enamel hypoplasia, dysplastic deciduous teeth, anodontia of permanent dentition, lumbar scoliosis, renal alterations, aplasia and hypoplasia of breasts, hypoplastic and hypopigmented areolae with diffuse limits, hyperostosis of the cranial vault, metacarpal hypoplasias, difficulty of grasping with left hand, exertional dyspnea, absent DIP extension and flexion creases, dermatoglyphic alterations, unusual facial appearance, abnormal auricles.

**Complications:** Those due to diabetes. Psychologic problems due to hair, dental, and breast alterations.

**Associated Findings:** None known.

**Etiology:** Probable autosomal recessive inheritance. Parental consanguinity was present in the only family described.

**Pathogenesis:** Unknown.

**MIM No.:** 20778

**POS No.:** 3529

**Sex Ratio:** Presumably M1:F1.

**Occurrence:** One Caucasian Brazilian sibship was described to have two affected sisters among nine sibs. The parents were normal and were second cousins. The proposita's sister, who died at age 1.5 years, was born after a normal pregnancy at term with low birth weight. She had thin and sparse hair and never walked or talked.

**Risk of Recurrence for Patient's Sib:**
 See Part I, *Mendelian Inheritance.*

**Risk of Recurrence for Patient's Child:**
 See Part I, *Mendelian Inheritance.*

**Age of Detectability:** During childhood, by physical examination.

**Gene Mapping and Linkage:** Unknown.

**Prevention:** None known. Genetic counseling indicated.

**Treatment:** Specific for lipoatrophic diabetes. Breast plastic surgery, wigs, and dentures are cosmetically and psychologically helpful.

**Prognosis:** Determined by the progression of the diabetes.

**Detection of Carrier:** Unknown.

**Special Considerations:** The possibility that the proposita presents a concurrence (or syntropy) of two different recessive genes (one for the lipoatrophic diabetes and the other for an ectodermal dysplasia syndrome) was considered by Pinheiro et al. (1983); the conclusion was reached that the probability of this event is extremely low.
 AREDYLD is an acronym derived from the main features of the syndrome.

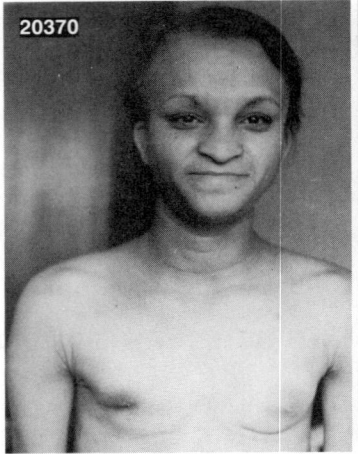
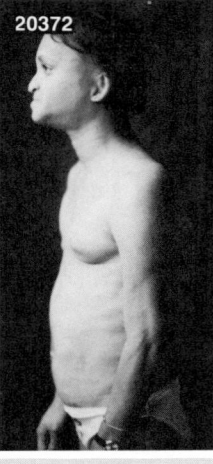
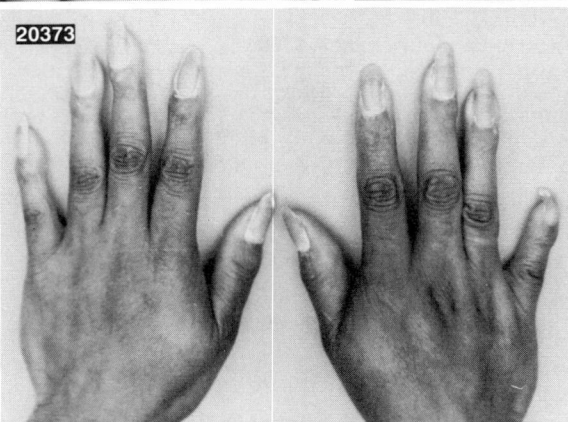
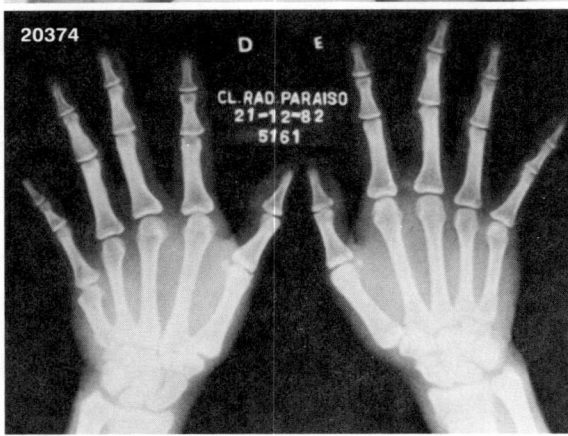

**2785-20370:** Affected 22-year-old woman; note hypotrichosis, mandibular prognathism, abnormal auricle, right amastia, left hypomastia, and abnormal areolae. **20372:** Note facial profile and body habitus; the lateral face shows the short nasal septum, flattened nasal tip and prominent chin. **20373:** Note fifth right fingernail angling downward, absence of DIP extension creases and lower positioning of the right fourth and fifth fingers. **20374:** Note shorter right (D) fourth and fifth metacarpals.

**References:**
Pinheiro M, et al.: AREDYLD: a syndrome combining an acrorenal field defect, ectodermal dysplasia, lipoatrophic diabetes, and other manifestations. Am J Med Genet 1983; 16:29–33.

Araujo LMB, et al.: Diabetes lipoatrófico associado a displasia ecto-dérmica: estudo metabólico. Canela, RS, Brasil: XVI Congr Brasil Endocrinol Metab, October 27–31, 1984.
Freire-Maia N, Pinheiro M: Ectodermal dysplasias: a clinical and genetic study. New York: Alan R. Liss, 1984.

FR033                                                    **Newton Freire-Maia**

**Aregenerative anemia, chronic congenital**
 *See* ANEMIA, HYPOPLASTIC CONGENITAL
**Arginase deficiency**
 *See* ARGININEMIA

## ARGININEMIA                                           0086

**Includes:**
 Arginase deficiency
 Cystinuria, some forms of atypical
 Hyperargininemia

**Excludes:**
 **Aciduria, argininosuccinic** (0087)
 **Hyperammonemia** (1519)
 **Hyperdibasic aminoaciduria** (0491)

**Major Diagnostic Criteria:** Elevated levels of arginine in the blood; absent or reduced levels of arginase in red blood cell lysates.

**Clinical Findings:** The onset may be delayed in some patients who appear normal for the first 2–3 years of life. Other patients were considered to be retarded and to have had neurologic impairment in the first 6 months of life. Increasing clumsiness, spastic quadriplegia (lower limbs more than upper limbs), and loss of language and intellectual ability have been noted. Older patients have lost the ability to walk and virtually all ability to speak. Seizures and EEG abnormalities are common. Periodic lethargy, irritability, and coma are present in most patients.

Blood arginine level is elevated in all cases, usually to >10 mg/dl (1$\mu$M). Other blood amino acid levels are usually normal. Urea is at the lower end of the normal range. Urinary amino acid excretion may be normal on a low or moderate protein intake, but an atypical cystinuric pattern with arginine predominating can be seen in all patients at some time. Arginine also is elevated in the cerebrospinal fluid (CSF). Intermittent elevation of blood ammonia occurs with lethargy, irritability, and sometimes vomiting.

**Complications:** Progressively more severe mental retardation and neurologic impairment.

**Associated Findings:** None known.

**Etiology:** Autosomal recessive inheritance.

**Pathogenesis:** The diminution of arginase in liver is the cause of arginine accumulation in the blood, CSF, and usually the urine. Impairment of urea synthesis is suggested by the persistently low blood levels and the intermittent hyperammonemia, which may result from increased protein intake, intercurrent infection, or other stress.

**MIM No.:** *20780

**Sex Ratio:** M1:F1

**Occurrence:** About 25 cases reported in the literature.

**Risk of Recurrence for Patient's Sib:**
 See Part I, *Mendelian Inheritance.*

**Risk of Recurrence for Patient's Child:**
 See Part I, *Mendelian Inheritance.* None of the known affected individuals has reached reproductive age. Risk is likely to be low.

**Age of Detectability:** At birth with assay of red cell arginase levels in cord blood. Condition likely to be detectable in fetal red blood cells and fetal liver.

**Gene Mapping and Linkage:** ARG1 (arginase, liver) has been provisionally mapped to 6q23.

**Prevention:** None known. Genetic counseling indicated. Decreased protein intake and semisynthetic diets including essential amino acids as the sole nitrogen source diminish the ammonia load to the impaired urea cycle and has been shown to lower blood ammonia and blood arginine. Significant prevention and regression of symptoms has occurred with such regimens.

**Treatment:** Physical therapy to mitigate the impact of increasing spasticity; nonprotein, high-carbohydrate fluids to treat the signs and symptoms of hyperammonemia. Sodium benzoate with or without phenylacetate appears to reduce plasma ammonia and arginine on both an acute and long-term basis.

**Prognosis:** The oldest known patient is aged 26 years. Clinical deterioration in this and other patients had been continuous. Therapy as outlined above appears to arrest deterioration and may result in the regression of some symptoms.

**Detection of Carrier:** Red blood cell arginase levels in five carriers were at least 2.5 SD below the mean.

**Special Considerations:** Abnormal urinary amino acid excretion pattern is seen at some time in all patients. The abnormal urinary amino acid pattern might be considered to be coincidental cystinuria.

**References:**
Snyderman SE, et al.: Argininemia. J Pediatr 1977; 90:563–568.
Cederbaum SD, et al.: Hyperargininemia with arginase deficiency. Pediatr Res 1979; 13:827–833.
Snyderman SE, et al.: Argininemia treated from birth. J Pediatr 1979; 95:61–63.
Cederbaum SD, et al.: Treatment of hyperargininemia due to arginase deficiency with a chemically defined diet. J Inherited Metab Dis 1982; 5:95–99.
Dizikes GJ, et al.: Isolation of human arginase cDNA and absence of homology between the two human arginase genes. Biochem Biophys Res Commun 1986; 141:53–59.

CE001                                   **Stephen D. Cederbaum**

**Argininosuccinate synthetase deficiency**
*See CITRULLINEMIA*
**Argininosuccinic aciduria**
*See ACIDURIA, ARGININOSUCCINIC*
**Argyrophil myenteric plexus, deficiency of**
*See INTESTINAL PSEUDO-OBSTRUCTION SYNDROMES*
**Arhinencephaly**
*See HOLOPROSENCEPHALY*
**Arias hyperbilirubinemia**
*See HYPERBILIRUBINEMIA, UNCONJUGATED*
**Arnold-Chiari malformation**
*See ANENCEPHALY*
*also BRAIN, ARNOLD-CHIARI MALFORMATION*
**Aromatase**
*See GYNECOMASTIA DUE TO INCREASED AROMATASE ACTIVITY, FAMILIAL*
**Arrhinencephalia unilateralis**
*See NOSE, PROBOSCIS LATERALIS*

## ARRHYTHMIA, CARDIAC CONDUCTION DEFECTS, NEONATAL                                         2401

**Includes:**
Cardiac conduction defects, neonatal
Perinatal conduction system defects
Perinatal/neonatal cardiac conduction system defects-arrhythmia

**Excludes:**
Conducting tissue disturbance-atrio ventriculat block
Congenital heart disease-disturbance of conducting tissues

**Major Diagnostic Criteria:** Hypoplasia of sinoatrial node, atrioventricular node, or bundles; associated with intrauterine fetal arrhythmia or intractable neonatal arrhythmia; in the absence of major structural malformation of the heart.

**Clinical Findings:** Range from hydrops fetalis and stillbirth to full term delivery with postpartum development of cardiac arrhythmia. Diagnosis is confirmed clinically by EKG, and should be considered in cases of suspected congenital heart disease. Ar-

rhythmias recorded include tachycardia, supraventricular extrasystoles, and bradycardia.

**Complications:** Cardiac failure; hydrops fetalis/ascites; hydramnios.

**Associated Findings:** None known.

**Etiology:** Unknown.

**Pathogenesis:** The arrhythmias noted in cases so far reported have been associated with hypoplasia of SA and AV nodes and of the atrioventricular conducting tissue, with deficiency of collagen within the nodes. The nodal collagen appears to play a role in stabilizing the sinus node, and its deficiency could lead to electrical instability, even in normal infants. It is also probable that the sinus node hypoplasia could itself affect heart rhythm.

**MIM No.:**  23470

**CDC No.:**  746.880

**Sex Ratio:**  M4:F0 (observed).

**Occurrence:**  Four cases have been reported in the literature.

**Risk of Recurrence for Patient's Sib:**  Unknown.

**Risk of Recurrence for Patient's Child:**  Unknown.

**Age of Detectability:**  Antenatal or neonatal

**Gene Mapping and Linkage:**  Unknown.

**Prevention:**  None known. Genetic counseling indicated.

**Treatment:**  Resuscitation as appropriate.

**Prognosis:**  Cases examined to date suggest that the condition is invariably fatal.

**Detection of Carrier:**  Unknown.

**Special Considerations:**  Detailed examination of the cardiac conducting tissue in normal and abnormal neonates has not been widely reported, so that the significance of the few reported abnormal cases is not established. Greater awareness of the possibility that fatal perinatal arrhythmia (particularly supraventricular tachycardia) may be due to hypoplasia of the conducting tissues is required to settle this dilemma, through detailed pathological assessment at necropsy of normal and abnormal hearts.

**Support Groups:**  Dallas; American Heart Association

**References:**
Fox KM, et al.: Hypoplastic and fibrotic sinus node associated with intractable tachycardia in a neonate. Circulation 1980; 61:1048–1052. †
Ho SY, et al.: Conduction system defects in three perinatal patients with arrhythmia. Br Heart J 1985; 53:158–163. * †

M0036                                   **Gabriel Mortimer**

## ARRHYTHMIA, FROM MATERNAL AUTOIMMUNE DISEASE, CONGENITAL                              2112

**Includes:**
Autoimmune disease, congenital arrhythmia
Heart block with maternal systemic lupus erythematosis
Heart block with other maternal connective tissue diseases
Lupus erythematosis, neonatal, arrhythmia from

**Excludes:**
Heart block without maternal autoimmune disease
**Lupus erythematosis, systemic** (2515)

**Major Diagnostic Criteria:** Clinical and laboratory evidence of maternal autoimmune disease. Slow fetal heart rate may be detected in utero. Complete heart block in the the newborn. Skin lesions of lupus may appear in the newborn, at birth or during the first weeks of life.

**Clinical Findings:** It is essential to monitor all maternal connective tissue disease pregnancies for the presence of fetal bradycardia. Be prepared at the time of delivery for resuscitation and the maintenance of adequate cardiac output in the newborn until his/her condition is stabilized. Once stability is achieved, the infant with complete heart block can usually be maintained without medication or a pacemaker. The heart rate, as is so often

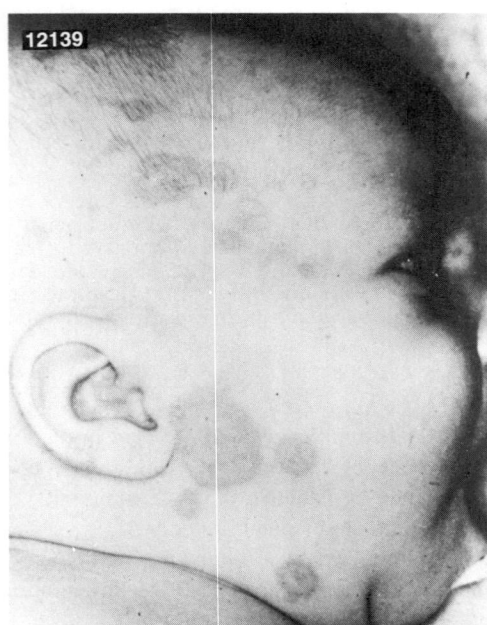

**2112-12139:** Discoid lupus rash on newborn whose mother has lupus erythematosis.

the case in congenital complete heart block, is responsive to exercise. A pacemaker may be required eventually in later childhood or adult life. If attention is not directed aggressively in the immediate newborn period towards maintenance of cardiac output, death may result.

Other clinical findings include the development in the infant of a discoid lupus rash in the presence of **Lupus erythematosis, systemic** in the mother.

The mother may have asymptomatic autoimmune disease, but symptoms can still occur in the offspring. In fact, if bradycardia is detected in the fetus, the mother should be evaluated for potential autoimmune disease, if such a diagnosis has not been previously made.

**Complications:** Congestive heart failure, edema, anasarca, thrombocytopenia, respiratory distress, pericardial effusion, and death.

**Associated Findings:** Cardiomegaly and increased pulmonary vascularity are present on chest X-ray. Electrocardiogram reveals complete heart block, atrioventricular dissociation, right atrial enlargement, and right ventricular hypertrophy. Immunologic studies may or may not be positive.

**Etiology:** Maternal autoimmune disease with transplacental transfer of antibody.

**Pathogenesis:** Maternal IgE antibodies to Ro (a soluble tissue ribonucleoprotein) damang the conducting system of the developing heart with evidence of selective calcification within the ventricular septum in an autopsied case.

**MIM No.:** 15270

**CDC No.:** 746.880

**Sex Ratio:** Presumably M1:F1.

**Occurrence:** May be as high as 40% in mothers with autoimmune disease. Fetal loss is approximately 30% in mothers with **Lupus erythematosis, systemic.**

**Risk of Recurrence for Patient's Sib:** In the range of 20–40%. No apparent relationship to clinical status of maternal disease.

**Risk of Recurrence for Patient's Child:** Unknown.

**Age of Detectability:** May be suspected in utero by detecting total bradycardia. Diagnosis is usual at birth but may occur as late as three months to eight years.

**Gene Mapping and Linkage:** Unknown.

**Prevention:** None known. Genetic counseling indicated.

**Treatment:** Be prepared for resuscitation and treatment of congestive heart failure at birth. Monitoring for complete heart block with treatment as indicated is recommended. A pacemaker may be required in late childhood or during adult life.

**Prognosis:** The rash usually resolves completely. The congenital complete heart block is permanent in most cases.

**Detection of Carrier:** Same as for identification of maternal autoimmune disease.

**Support Groups:** Dallas; American Heart Association

**References:**

McCue CM, et al.: Congenital heart block in newborns of mothers with connective tissue disease. Circulation 1977; 56:82–90.
Winkler RB, et al.: Familial complete heart block and maternal systemic lupus erythematosus. Circulation 1977; 56:1103–1107.
Lee L, et al.: Immunogenetics of maternal lupus syndrome. Ann Intern Med 1983; 99:592–596. *

N0004
N0003

**Audrey H. Nora**
**James J. Nora**

---

## ARRHYTHMIA, HEART BLOCK, CONGENITAL COMPLETE                                    0454

**Includes:**

Atrioventricular block, congenital complete
Atrioventricular block, congenital third degree
Heart block, congenital complete
Sinoatrial block, congenital complete

**Excludes:**

Atrioventricular dissociation due to AV junctional pacemaker
Atrioventricular dissociation due to sinus bradycardia
Heart block, acquired post-natal complete

**Major Diagnostic Criteria:** An abnormally slow heart rate at an early age. Dissociation between atrial and ventricular excitation in AV block, or absence of normal atrial excitation in SA block. The absence of other causes, e.g. diphtheritic or viral myocarditis. A slow heart rate, changing intensity of the first heart sound, and "cannon waves" in the jugular venous pulse should suggest the diagnosis of CHB. Diagnosis is established, however, by EKG.

**Clinical Findings:** Congenital CHB is diagnosed "in utero" in approximately 30% of all cases by the persistently slow fetal heart beat noted in heart tones, EKG, or echocardiogram. In some instances this dysrhythmia must be distinguished from the bradycardia of fetal distress in which the rate is more variable. An additional 15% of CHB cases are recognized between birth and the first year. Therefore, in the majority, the diagnosis is not made until infancy or childhood. CHB occurs as a single anomaly in 70% of cases. Most children with isolated CHB are asymptomatic even at exercise but a few develop mild dyspnea and fatigue on exertion. A slow heart rate, between 30 and 80 beats per minute at rest, is the most striking sign of CHB. Bounding arterial pulses are characteristic and the pulse pressure ranges from 35 to 100 mm Hg. "Cannon waves", large venous pulses in the neck veins, are caused by atrial contraction against closed AV valves during ventricular systole and are often noted in older children. Upon auscultation, variation in intensity of the first heart sound is almost always present. The second sound is usually normal. A third heart sound is often heard with an intermittent accentuation or a third sound may be audible only intermittently, occurring when atrial contraction is coincident with the rapid ventricular filling phase of the cardiac cycle. A systolic ejection murmur, grade II-III/VI, over the left midsternal border is the rule and an apical diatolic flow murmur is often present. These murmurs are due to the large stroke volume compensatory for the slow rate.

Cases without any murmur have also been reported. The coincidence of CHB with another congenital heart defect jeopardizes the hemodynamic compensation, and the clinical symptoms and signs are modified by and may be predominantly those of the structural defect (cyanosis, signs of large shunts and/or cardiac failure). The presence or absence of cardiac malformations in addition to the CHB often requires further diagnostic studies: X-ray, echocardiography, and in many cases cardiac catheterization and angiocardiography.

The EKG in complete AV block shows dissociated atrial and ventricular rhythms with a slower ventricular rate. Both rhythms are usually stable. The atria under the control of the sinus node beat at a normal rate for age (85 beats per minute in the older child and 100 to 150 beats per minute in the infant at rest) with sinus arrhythmia commonly present. The ventricles beat at 30–80 beats per minute, often approximately half the atrial rate at the time. In most cases the ventricular rate increases considerably in response to physical exertion (average of 150% of the resting rate). Atrial fibrillation occurs rarely. The QRS complex is usually of normal duration indicating an origin of excitation of the ventricular escape rhythm proximal to the bifurcation of the bundle of His, i.e. junctional. Prolongation of the QRS complex (more than 0.10 sec.) suggests a lower level of block and ventricular escape rhythm. Right and left bundle branch block patterns have been described; signs of left or biventricular hypertrophy are common. In cases with structural heart defects and CHB, the QRS may be modified according to the type of malformation; however, CHB is associated with an abnormal sequence of activation and the EKG contours are not truly representative. Complete SA block, a rare form of CHB, may be suspected when there is no evidence of atrial activity on the EKG and the ventricular rate is slow. Exercise EKG testing can be done from 3 years of age for heart rate response and exercise-induced ventricular ectopy. Those who are able to increase their heart rate most on exercise have been shown on electrophysiologic testing to be more likely to have the A-V block situated at the level of the A-V node rather than in the bundle of His or below. In one study of CHB 68% developed ventricular ectopy during exercise with a trend towards more frequent severe ectopy in the older children who had a prolonged QRS at rest. There is early evidence that CHB patients with ventricular dysrhythmia on exercise are at increased risk for sudden death. Ambulatory EKG (Holter) monitoring can provide additional rhythm information, specifically sleeping phenomena, which are, in some cases, runs of marked ventricular slowing (less than 20 beats per minute) and/or superimposed dysrhythmias.

In isolated CHB the X-ray shows mild cardiomegaly with left ventricular enlargement and a minor degree of pulmonary venous obstruction. In cases with an associated malformation, the X-ray varies with the hemodynamics of that particular lesion. The echocardiogram in AV block shows varying amplitudes and timing of the A wave (which follows atrial systole) on the mitral valve, and at times on the pulmonic valve, depending upon the relationship of the atrial and ventricular contractions. The cardiac cavity dimensions exceed normal and may vary in size from beat-to-beat. Associated cardiac malformations add their specific features. Cardiac catheterization in CHB without associated heart disease usually reveals mild elevation of pulmonary arterial systolic, left atrial mean, and left ventricular and aortic systolic pressures. Cardiac output is usually normal in spite of the slow heart rate; this is accomplished by an increase in the stroke volume. When there is an associated heart defect, the hemodynamic and angiocardiographic findings reflect both disorders. An electrophysiologic study recording the His bundle potential with an electrode catheter can demonstrate the level of A-V block, whether at the head of the AV node, in the bundle of His, or lower within the ventricles. Atrial pacing confirms a presumptive diagnosis of SA block by showing atrial capture and AV conduction. Overdrive ventricular pacing assesses subsidiary ventricular pacemaker function.

**Complications:** Adams-Stokes attacks (ventricular asystole or fibrillation with cerebral ischemia) are the most serious complications. Depending on the duration of the ventricular standstill and interruption of circulation, the attacks may be lethal (if the heart does not start to beat again) or may result in dizziness, unconsciousness and convulsions. In a large series, the incidence of this complication in all cases (with and without associated congenital heart disease) is about 15% in the first weeks of life and progressively diminishes to less than 5% per 5 years follow-up in the first decade and even lower thereafter. Heart failure is a major problem in the neonate with a slow ventricular rate or when associated heart defects are present.

**Associated Findings:** The overall incidence of associated heart defects is 30%. Most common, making up 80% of those CHB cases with associated congenital heart defects, is inversion of the ventricles with transposition (corrected transposition of the great arteries) with or without other defects, the most frequent being ventricular septal defect. Other abnormalities may include: ASD, VSD, PDA, single ventricle, endocardial fibroelastosis, or cardiomyopathy.

**Etiology:** In the familial form, most often through autosomal recessive inheritance. However, autosomal dominant inheritance with variable penetrance is reported in families, but this appears to be more common in mixed conduction system disease with SA and AV nodal involvement. Multifactoral inheritance and "in utero" myocarditis may also be considered. There is an association with maternal connective tissue disease, primarily lupus erythematosus, with definite evidence in some recent cases for transplacental transmission of maternal antibodies which react with fetal cardiac antigens.

**Pathogenesis:** Discontinuity of the AV conduction system may result from under-development (or abnormal resorption) of its components or from abnormal development of the central fibrous body. In cases where there is no anatomic interruption of the conduction pathway, functional blockage of the electrical excitation is presumed.

**MIM No.:** *14040, 23470

**CDC No.:** 746.870

**Sex Ratio:** M1.8:F1

**Occurrence:** 1:20,000 live births.

**Risk of Recurrence for Patient's Sib:**
See Part I, *Mendelian Inheritance.*

**Risk of Recurrence for Patient's Child:**
See Part I, *Mendelian Inheritance.* 2.5% sporadic.

**Age of Detectability:** Before birth.

**Gene Mapping and Linkage:** Unknown.

**Prevention:** None known. Genetic counseling indicated.

**Treatment:** Medication, pacemaker and operative palliation or correction of associated cardiac defects are options. Implantation of a permanent artificial electronic pacemaker should be seriously considered in these cases: 1) with the first definite Adams-Stokes attack, even mild, e.g. dizziness; 2) in a neonate with a slow ventricular rate (less than 55, often with a fast atrial rate, 140 or greater) or with significant cardiomegaly or signs of congestive failure; 3) for intractable congestive heart failure, more likely when there is an associated cardiac defect. Temporary pacemaker therapy is advisable for patients with CHB who are to undergo general anesthesia for any operative procedure including implantation of a pacemaker, and should be considered for a distressed neonate, e.g., with hyaline membrane disease. Isoproterenol may be used intravenously in the interim preparatory to establishing pacemaker control. Long-term therapy with isoproterenol is rarely efficacious. Digitalis is indicated in congestive heart failure, in spite of the slow heart rate inherent in the condition.

**Prognosis:** In an international study of 599 cases of CHB the outlook for the majority (those without associated congenital heart disease and presenting after the first week of life) was good, with a long-term mortality of 8%. When other congenital heart defects were associated, the mortality increased to 29%. The highest risk period is in early infancy for all patients with CHB with and without associated structural defects. Most of these deaths occur during the first week of life and are due to congestive heart failure. CHB diagnosed "in utero" is usually well tolerated during the third trimester. However, severe congestive heart failure may develop if the ventricular rate is extremely slow, or if associated cardiac defects result in AV valve regurgitation, and may lead to hydrops fetalis which has an extremely high risk of death "in utero" or in the perinatal period.

The first Adams-Stokes attack may be fatal in individuals with CHB. Predictors of a higher risk status in CHB are: a persistently slow ventricular rate at rest (less than 50 at any age including the neonate), widening of the QRS complex (100 msec. or greater), or significant cardiac enlargement. Additional predictors of higher risk are a low work capacity, a slower heart rate response or emergence of ventricular ectopy on exercise testing, a slow recovery of the subsidiary ventricular pacemaker (greater than 3.0 sec.) on overdrive pacing, or ambulatory monitoring which shows additional dysrhythmias. Unfortunately none of these are entirely reliable as indicators. The familial occurrence of congenital complete AV block is associated with a greater likelihood of Adams-Stokes attacks and a higher mortality.

In the absence of clinical or noninvasive criteria for permanent pacemaker therapy, intra-cardiac electrophysiologic studies can separate the higher risk individuals with intra or infra-Hisian block from those with block at the head of the AV node. The wider application of pacemaker therapy has improved the outlook; but, in spite of technical advances, long-term artificial pacemaker therapy continues to have its own morbidity and mortality (greatest in the neonate, where the need for pacing is frequent) which must be weighed against that of nonintervention.

**Detection of Carrier:** Unknown.

**Support Groups:** Dallas; American Heart Association

**References:**

Michaelson M, Engle MA: Congenital complete heart block: an international study of the natural history. Cardiovasc Clin 1972;4:85–101. *

Schneider MD, et al: The syndrome of familial atrioventricular block with sinus bradycardia: prognostic indices, electrophysiologic and histopathologic correlates. Eur J Cardiol 1978; 7:337–351.

Pinsky W, et al: Diagnosis, management, and long-term results of patients with congenital complete atrioventricular block. Pediatrics 1982; 69:728–733. *

Simon AB, et al: Ventricular pacing in children. PACE 1982; 5:836–844.

Kleinman CS, Donnerstein RL: Ultrasonic assessment of cardiac function in the intact human fetus. JACC 1985; 5:84S-93S.

Ho SY, et al: Anatomy of congenital complete heart block and relation to maternal anti-Ro antibodies. Am J Cardiol 1986; 58:291–294.

Reichli M, et al.: Complete congenital heart block followed by anti-Ro/SSA in adult life. Am J Med 1988; 84:339–344.

MI020                                            **B. Lynn Miller**

## ARRHYTHMIA, SUPRAVENTRICULAR TACHYCARDIAS, CONGENITAL                                                 0922

**Includes:**

> Atrial fibrillation
> Atrial flutter, persistent and paroxysmal
> Atrial tachyarrhythmia
> Supraventricular tachycardia paroxysmal
> Supraventricular tachycardias, congenital
> Tachycardia, junctional

**Excludes:**

> **Arrhythmia, Wolff-Parkinson-White type** (1002)
> Supraventricular tachyarrhythmias, acquired

**Major Diagnostic Criteria:** Fast heart rate over 180/min. Irregularity of the heart rhythm with grouped beats is strongly suggestive even when the minute rate is normal. The EKG confirms the diagnosis.

**Clinical Findings:** Three forms of atrial tachyarrhythmias are described together because they are closely related. All three "entities" are rare as congenital manifestations. The congenital nature of these has been confirmed by fetal monitoring during pregnancy or labor, or recording the infant's EKG immediately after birth. In practice, tachyarrhythmias detected during the first four weeks of life are regarded as congenital.

*Supraventricular paroxysmal tachycardia* is defined as a rapid, regular atrial rate of 180–320 beats per minute originating from an ectopic atrial focus. The P waves are often not seen because they are merged in the preceding T waves. It is usually impossible to distinguish between atrial and atrioventricular junctional (nodal) tachycardia. Paroxysms usually begin suddenly and end as abruptly. T wave abnormalities may persist for several days following a paroxysm. Atrioventricular (A-V) conduction may allow each atrial beat to activate the ventricles 1:1 or block some impulses (see atrial flutter).

*Atrial flutter* implies atrial ectopic activity of 250–480 beats per minute. The EKG shows flutter waves, which produce a "saw-tooth pattern" in some leads. A-V conduction ratio varies: most common is a 2:1 ratio leading to a ventricular rate half of the atrial rate. In the case of 3:1 (rare), or 4:1 (second most common), and mixed ratios with up to 8:1 A-V block, the ventricular rate may be within normal limits. A-V conduction may also be of the Wenckebach type (progressive prolongation of the PR interval followed by a dropped beat which produces an irregularity of ventricular rhythm with grouped beating).

In *atrial fibrillation* the ectopic atrial impulse is excessively rapid and variable. This leads to uneven and irregular deviations of low amplitude in the EKG. The ventricular rate is also irregular. QRS complexes are usually normal, but sometimes vary in amplitude.

The distinction between these three forms of supraventricular tachycardias according to atrial rate is somewhat arbitrary. There are transitions from one form to another in one patient, or a mixture of two as seen in flutter-fibrillation. The attacks of tachycardia as well as atrial flutter may continue for longer periods (at times, months after birth). The EKG of the arrhythmia in the fetus has been described as rapid, irregular, or both, revealing atrial paroxysmal tachycardia, atrial flutter or fibrillation (which is rare without congenital heart disease).

In the fetus, paroxysms of tachycardia without other congenital heart disease, even if they last several months, usually do not affect growth or development. It has been noticed that these children appear to have a larger birthweight than the average. The condition of the child during labor is good in most cases. Rarely, intrauterine congestive heart failure can be severe enough to produce hydrops fetalis. In such cases fetal distress may be severe enough to warrant emergency cesarean section. Perinatal diagnosis and treatment of congestive heart failure is a medical emergency.

The echocardiogram in atrial fibrillation shows absence of mitral A waves, whereas those waves are present in atrial tachycardia. Left atrial dimension is increased and left ventricular dimension is decreased. After cardioversion these return toward normal, indicating improvement in cardiac function. In atrial flutter, anterior peaking of the mitral valve has been noted just after the flutter wave.

The clinical picture of supraventricular tachycardia varies considerably. The minority (about 10%) have no symptoms, whereas the majority are obviously ill with slight cyanosis and ashen grey skin, which is cold and moist. The infants are restless and dyspneic. Cardiac failure is relatively common (in contrast to adults) and mainly dependent on the duration of the tachycardia, less on its frequency. Usually, there is no heart failure in the first 24 hours of life, or in the first 24 hours of a paroxysm, but it develops in at least 50% if the tachycardia lasts 48 hours. The younger the child, the more likely is the development of cardiac failure. Transient functional murmurs may appear. The X-ray frequently reveals signs of pulmonary venous congestion and cardiac enlargement. In the presence of congenital heart defects, the clinical picture will be influenced by the underlying malformation.

**Complications:** Dyspnea, mild cyanosis, and eventually signs of congestive heart failure with enlargement of the liver, vomiting, peripheral edema, and oliguria.

**Associated Findings:** **Arrhythmia, Wolff-Parkinson-White type** in approximately 12% of infants with paroxysmal supraventricular tachycardia, **Atrial septal defects**, **Pulmonary valve, atresia**, **Tricuspid**

valve, **Ebstein anomaly**, **Heart, transposition of great vessels**, idiopathic myocardial hypertrophy, endocardial fibroelastosis, and heart tumors may be present.

**Etiology:** Unknown. Transient immaturity of the conduction system and inflammatory disease (myocarditis) have been suggested. In the presence of congenital heart disease, dilatation of the atria, vagal and sympathetic effects, toxic agents, hypoxemia, and electrolyte disturbances are possible causes. Heart tumors, especially in the region of the sinoatrial and the A-V nodes, may lead to anatomic defects of the conduction system.

**Pathogenesis:** Two theories for the mechanism of supraventricular arrhythmias are 1) increased automaticity with origin of the beats from one or more ectopic atrial foci outside the sinoatrial node, and 2) reentry as a large circus movement of the impulse within the atria, a circuit within the A-V junction or multiple small uncoordinated areas of atrial activation. Reentry can be initiated by a premature beat which encounters an area only partially recovered from the preceding beat. This has been thought to be the mechanism of atrial flutter and fibrillation, but the best demonstration is found in the tachycardia associated with **Arrhythmia, Wolff-Parkinson-White type**. As the mechanism for atrial fibrillation, it is consistent with the rarity of the problem in infants since the available length of atrial muscle would generally be insufficient for perpetuation of multiple reentry circuits in the absence of ischemia or other cause of depressed conduction. The first theory, i.e. increased automaticity, is more widely accepted as the mechanism of most supraventricular tachycardias in the young.

**CDC No.:** 427.900

**Sex Ratio:** M3:F1

**Occurrence:** Estimated at 1:25,000.

**Risk of Recurrence for Patient's Sib:** Unknown.

**Risk of Recurrence for Patient's Child:** Unknown.

**Age of Detectability:** Prenatal, from the eleventh week of gestation, by fetal EKG or ultrasonography.

**Gene Mapping and Linkage:** Unknown.

**Prevention:** None known. Genetic counseling indicated.

**Treatment:** Digitalis is the drug of choice. Within the past few years, primary conversion of supraventricular tachycardia with *verapamil* has gained popularity. However, more experience is needed before the use of calcium blockers can be recommended as the drug of choice in infants. Electrical cardioversion is an additional alternate therapy, and low energy levels often suffice. In atrial fibrillation, digitalis provides control of the ventricular rate. In refractory paroxysmal atrial tachyarrhythmia, long-term artificial pacemaker therapy has been used. It has been shown, in a few cases with **Arrhythmia, Wolff-Parkinson-White type** (WPW) syndrome and incapacitating tachycardia, that surgical transection of a previously well-identified anomalous pathway of conduction from atria to ventricles may abolish signs of WPW syndrome and prevent further episodes of tachycardia. Unfortunately, the abnormal conduction pathway often cannot be identified with certainty, and this form of therapy is far from established.

Procainamide, quinidine, or other antiarrhythmic agents, may be successful in preventing recurrences.

**Prognosis:** In paroxysmal atrial tachycardia, the prognosis is usually good in young infants. The best prognosis is in males with the first attack occurring prior to three months of age. Recurrences are rare beyond one year after the first attack. The prognosis is guarded if the paroxysm is prolonged or if attacks recur repeatedly in spite of therapy. In atrial flutter, prognosis is equally favorable. Atrial fibrillation is a serious complication. It usually occurs in association with severe congenital heart disease and is often fatal. The combination of a congenital heart defect with a supraventricular tachycardia worsens the prognosis.

**Detection of Carrier:** Unknown.

**Support Groups:** Dallas; American Heart Association

**References:**

Ferrer P: Arrhythmias in the neonate. In: Roberts N, Gelband H, eds: Cardiac arrhythmi in the neonate, infant and child. New York: Appleton-Century Crofts, 1977:265–316. *

Shahar E, et al.: Verapamil in the treatment of paroxysmal supraventricular tachycardia in infants and children. J Pediatr 1981; 98:323–326.

Garson A, et al.: Supraventricular tachycardia in children: clinical features, response to treatment, and long-term follow-up in 217 patients. J Pediatr 1981; 98:875–882. *

BU001                                               **Richard L. Bucciarelli**

---

## ARRHYTHMIA, WITH LONG QT INTERVAL WITHOUT DEAFNESS      0610

**Includes:**

Long QT syndrome without deafness
Romano-Ward syndrome
Syncope and QT prolongation without deafness
Ventricular fibrillation with prolonged Q-T interval
Ward-Romano syndrome

**Excludes:** Cardio-auditory syndrome (0123)

**Major Diagnostic Criteria:** Syncopal attacks in individuals with prolonged QT interval and with normal hearing.

**Clinical Findings:** Syncopal episodes commonly begin in early childhood. These may be mild and transient, or severe leading to several minutes of unconsciousness or even to sudden death. Early mortality among reported cases is high. Most commonly the syncopal episodes are provoked by violent emotions or physical exercise. The frequency of the syncopal attacks varies from several per month in some individuals to only 1 or 2 episodes in a lifetime in others. In those who survive to early adulthood there appears to be a lessening of the episodes.

The EKG shows a long QT interval. Although this superficially appears to be a QT interval, in some cases there clearly is a Q-U interval with a low amplitude T wave and a large U wave. Episodes of spontaneous T wave alternation (from positive to negative in a given EKG lead) have been observed; and in 1 reported case this was followed in a few seconds by ventricular fibrillation. The QT interval may vary in the same individual. The basic sinus rhythm commonly shows a slow rate at rest. In the face of exercise, the sinus rate may show less acceleration than is appropriate for the amount of work performed, ie a relative sinus bradycardia.

**Complications:** Syncope and sudden death.

**Associated Findings:** None known.

**Etiology:** Autosomal dominant inheritance.

**Pathogenesis:** Syncope and sudden death in this syndrome are consistent with either asystole or fibrillation. Postmortem examinations have shown damage to the SA node's arterial blood supply as well as to the Purkinje system. In addition, the clinical prolongation of the QT interval may be produced experimentally by causing imbalances of the sympathetic innervation to the heart (right stellate ganglion vs left stellate ganglion). The long QT interval increases the duration of the vulnerable period and would lower the fibrillation threshold. Patients with this syndrome exhibit abnormally low heart rates and an inability to increase their rate with exercise or atropine. It is possible that in the younger patients with smaller hearts, which would be resistant to fibrillation, the cause of death is asystole due to default of the SA node and failure of any secondary pacemaker to take over. In older patients with larger hearts, the cause of death is probably fibrillation initiated by an R on T phenomenon. This dual mechanism would explain the incomplete success of various rational therapeutic measures. Propranolol and sympathectomy prevent the fibrillation by raising fibrillation thresholds but suppress pacemaker function, whereas artificial electronic pacemakers prevent asystole but leave the patient vulnerable to fibrillation.

**MIM No.:** *19250

**CDC No.:** 427.900

**Sex Ratio:** M1:F1

**Occurrence:** Approximately 200 cases reported in the literature, most within the last eight years with increased recognition of the syndrome. Prevalence low, and falls with age due to nonsurvival of some affected individuals.

**Risk of Recurrence for Patient's Sib:**
See Part I, *Mendelian Inheritance.*

**Risk of Recurrence for Patient's Child:**
See Part I, *Mendelian Inheritance.*

**Age of Detectability:** At birth by EKG and theoretically in utero by fetal EKG with improved resolution for T wave analysis.

**Gene Mapping and Linkage:** LQT (long QT (Romano-Ward) syndrome) has been DISCONTINUED.

**Prevention:** None known. Genetic counseling indicated.

**Treatment:** Propranolol which shortens the QT interval and increases the threshold for ventricular fibrillation is the recommended therapy. Artificial pacemaker therapy and beta blockade are advised for those patients who have a significant degree of abnormality of the cardiac conduction system as an associated defect. In these patients, ventricular pacing both controls the bradycardia and has the direct beneficial effect of shortening the QT interval. Surgical ablation of the left stellate ganglion shortens the QT interval and has been employed with success in patients who have not responded to medical therapy. The recently introduced automatic implantable cardioverter defibrillator offers another option for those long QT interval patients who suffer recurrent ventricular tachycardia or ventricular fibrillation.

**Prognosis:** Poor: One-half of the cases reportedly died before adolescence. However, this figure is influenced by the fact that often only the more severe forms of the syndrome have been reported; also, most of these were in the period of time preceding the therapy listed above. The prognosis should be improved by earlier recognition and application of current therapy.

**Detection of Carrier:** QT interval on EKG is normal or long, but may be increased by exercising the subject.

**Special Considerations:** There are similarities between the findings in this syndrome, and the cardiac aspects of the **Cardio-auditory syndrome**. The syndrome of familial paroxysmal ventricular fibrillation, although excluded by the absence of a long QT interval, does have several features in common, including prominent U waves and prolongation of the QT interval with exercise.

**Support Groups:** Dallas; American Heart Association

**References:**
Romano C, et al.: Aritmic cardiache rare dell 'eta pediatrica. Clin Pediatr (Bologna) 1963; 45:656–683.
Ward OC: New familial cardiac syndrome in children. J Irish Med Assoc 1964; 54:103–106. *
Garza LA, et al.: Heritable Q-T prolongation without deafness. Circulation 1970; 41:39–48. *
Tye K-H, et al.: Survival following spontaneous ventricular flutter-fibrillation associated with QT syndrome. Arch Intern Med 1980; 140:255–256.
Mitsutake A, et al.: Usefulness of the valsalva maneuver in management of the long QT syndrome. Circulation 1981; 63:1029–1035.
Milne JR, et al.: The long QT syndrome: effects of drugs and left stellate ganglion block. Am Heart J 1982; 104:194–198.
Bhandari AK, Scheinman M: The long QT syndrome. Mod Concepts Cardiovasc Dis 1985; 54:45–50.
Vincent GM: The heart rate of Romano-Ward syndrome patients. Am Heart J 1986; 112:61–64.

**B. Lynn Miller**

---

**ARRHYTHMIA, WOLFF-PARKINSON-WHITE TYPE**      **1002**

**Includes:**
   Accelerated AV conduction
   Anomalous atrioventricular (AV) conduction
   Atrioventricular pathways, accessory
   Preexcitation syndromes
   Ventricular preexcitation
   Wolff-Parkinson-White syndrome

**Excludes:**
   **Arrhythmia, supraventricular tachycardias, congenital** (0922)
   Lown-Ganong-Levine syndrome
   Short PR interval-normal QRS syndrome

**Major Diagnostic Criteria:** Diagnosis is by EKG which, during sinus rhythm, shows ventricular preexcitation by a short PR interval and a prolonged QRS complex (both compared to normal limits for age) with the QRS widened in its initial portion by a slurred onset, termed a delta wave. When the EKG is recorded frequently, the Wolff-Parkinson-White (WPW) pattern is found to be present only intermittently in approximately 40% of cases. Comparison of the EKG during normal AV conduction with that during preexcitation reveals a constant P-J interval (the J point is the junction of the end of the QRS complex with the beginning of the ST segment), but a shorter PR interval and a longer QRS complex during preexcitation. Rarely, preexcitation presents with a normal PR interval when there is associated first degree heart block.
The Wolff-Parkinson-White (WPW) syndrome has been classified by EKG as WPW type A when an R wave is the sole or dominant QRS deflection in lead V1, and WPW type B when the dominant QRS deflection in lead V1 is negative. The delta wave is positive in lead V1 in type A, but may be either negative or biphasic in type B. Cases which fulfill the criteria of neither type A nor type B are best termed atypical. With the use of vectorcardiographic tracings the WPW syndrome has been classified according to the direction of the initial slow portion of the QRS which corresponds to the delta wave: type A when the mean delta is anterior, type B when it is directly to the left or leftward and posterior. The delta wave is directed leftward in almost all cases, regardless of whether anterior or posterior, and is therefore positive in lead V6. WPW is further subdivided into ten types by using all 12 leads of the EKG and more subtle differences in the direction of the delta wave by those who plan to proceed to electrophysiologic studies.
Ventricular preexcitation may either simulate or obscure bundle branch block, ventricular hypertrophy or myocardial infarction EKG patterns. In the presence of WPW conduction any additional EKG diagnosis must be made with reservation. Drugs that mimic or block the effects of the autonomic nervous system have been shown to influence the degree of preexcitation. An atropine test is sometimes used to abolish the WPW pattern transiently, permitting the EKG to be of more assistance in diagnosis of associated cardiopathy.

**Clinical Findings:** Originally described as a specific EKG pattern in individuals with otherwise normal hearts but subject to paroxysms of tachycardia, WPW syndrome has since been employed to denote the EKG abnormality with or without paroxysmal tachycardia. There may be no clinical findings in the absence of paroxysmal tachycardia or between bouts. However, an increased intensity of S1 or abnormal splitting of the first and second heart sounds may be heard. The frequent association of congenital heart disease has been confirmed since the original description. Approximately 30–50% of the affected individuals with WPW syndrome seen in hospital practice have some type of structural heart disease; approximately 40% of those affected have **Tricuspid valve, Ebstein anomaly** (usually associated with WPW type B).
Paroxysmal tachycardia is present in approximately one-half of the WPW cases of most hospital practices. Some 22% of infants with the first episode of supraventricular tachycardia will have WPW which, in a few, is seen during the tachycardia, but much more commonly is not apparent until the follow-up EKG. The incidence of tachycardia with WPW has been reported from 4% to

90%, an inconsistency largely accounted for by the selection of subjects and the method of study. In a healthy population with WPW first detected in adulthood, 13% developed tachycardia during long term follow-up. The type of paroxysmal tachycardia is in part age dependent. Although reciprocating tachycardia is seen at all ages, as is the least common form of tachycardia, atrial flutter, atrial fibrillation is extremely rare in the first decade of life but has a gradually increasing risk of occurrence thereafter. In one study of tachycardia with WPW, atrial fibrillation was present in 32%. Atrial fibrillation in WPW often causes an unusually rapid ventricular rate with broad QRS complexes, "pseudoventricular tachycardia," and may degenerate to ventricular fibrillation.

Exercise testing and ambulatory EKG monitoring allow for more comprehensive non-invasive rhythm analysis. Echocardiogram in WPW type A shows early left ventricular posterior wall systolic motion. In type B WPW the septal systolic contraction pattern can have a double notch, in contrast to the normal single notch. Recently, continous loop 2-D echocardiography has been shown to provide accurate localization of the initial ventricular activation. Cardiac catheterization and angiocardiography are undertaken to define associated cardiac abnormalities. Electrophysiologic studies are done with specialized catheterization techniques to localize and characterize the anomalous AV connection and demonstrate the propensity to and behavior of ectopic tachycardia both before and after the administration of various antiarrhythmic medications. Intraoperative mapping of earliest ventricular activation which further details the position of the anomalous AV connection has recently been done with simultaneous computer analysis with a considerable reduction in the time involved.

**Complications:**  In some cases of WPW syndrome, paroxysmal tachycardia is of major significance. The decrease in cardiac output may cause acute heart failure or hemodynamic collapse, especially in infants or patients with significant associated cardiopathy. Tachycardia may lead to angina or cerebral insufficiency with faintness and even death. Atrial fibrillation presents a particular threat due to the risk of precipitation of ventricular fibrillation by the rapid transmission of impulses from atria to ventricles without the normal AV delay.

**Associated Findings:**  Although WPW occurs more commonly as an isolated defect, it has been found in association with many types of cardiac defects. In addition to **Tricuspid valve, Ebstein anomaly**, these include: prolapsing mitral valve leaflet (usually with WPW type A); **Aorta, coarctation**; aortic valvar or subvalvar stenosis; hypoplastic left heart syndrome; primary myocardial disease; inversion of the ventricles with transposition and "left-sided" Ebstein's anomaly; double-inlet left ventricle; **Heart, tetralogy of Fallot; Tricuspid valve, atresia; Ventricular septal defect; Atrial septal defects**; and **Ductus arteriosus, patent**. Acquired heart disease is rare in infants and children, but increases in adults in whom 30% have acquired disorders, predominantly myocardial and ischemic. The only known associated extra-cardiac abnormalities are those of the CNS; these include microcephaly with mental retardation and seizures, and **Ataxia, Friedreich type**.

**Etiology:**  Autosomal dominant inheritance has been suggested. A congenital etiology is supported by the fact that the WPW pattern is often detected in infancy, commonly associated with congenital heart disease and is occasionally familial. A congenital defect with delayed manifestation or an intermittent form of WPW seems likely when WPW is detected later in life and in association with acquired heart disease.

**Pathogenesis:**  The anatomic substrate of WPW syndrome is a small strand of muscle fibers, the bundle of Kent, which crosses from atrium to ventricle and forms an accessory pathway (AP) of A-V conduction. An AP may be situated in the right ventricular free wall, left ventricular free wall, anterior septum or posterior septum. Multiple AP are found in 5–30% of cases. The functional characteristics of the AP permit rapid conduction of an atrial impulses to the ventricles relative to that through the specialized AV conduction system with its inherent physiologic delay at the AV node. This results in premature excitation of common ventricular myocardium near the AV groove which causes the delta wave of the QRS complex. In most instances the remainder of the

ventricles undergo a dual activation and the QRS is strongly influenced by the normal activation.

The atrioventricular reciprocating tachycardia of WPW syndrome is most often initiated by a premature beat (atrial, junctional or ventricular), which dissociates the near-parallel conduction of AP and normal AV system that is present during sinus rhythm. The more common narrow QRS tachycardia results from an atrial impulse passing anterograde over the normal AV system to activate the ventricles, and then retrograde to the atria via the AP to complete the circuit. Tachycardia with the broad QRS complex of WPW is due to anterograde conduction of the AP. Electrophysiologic studies of supraventricular tachycardia unresponsive to medical treatment have, in many instances, revealed a previously unsuspected AP capable only of retrograde conduction, a state termed "concealed" WPW syndrome.

**MIM No.:**  19420

**CDC No.:**  426.705

**Sex Ratio:**  M1.8:F1

**Occurrence:**  1:2500 live births, with no known predilection for any specific group. 1:200 cases of congenital heart disease.

**Risk of Recurrence for Patient's Sib:**  Undetermined, except in the rare autosomal dominant family.

**Risk of Recurrence for Patient's Child:**  Undetermined, except in the rare autosomal dominant family.

**Age of Detectability:**  From birth, by EKG.

**Gene Mapping and Linkage:**  Unknown.

**Prevention:**  None known. Genetic counseling indicated.

**Treatment:**  Preexcitation per se does not produce symptoms and does not require treatment as long as the heart rate is normal. However, when supraventricular tachycardia complicates the WPW syndrome, it is commonly severe. The acute episode of tachycardia may constitute a medical emergency in the case of infants or a severely symptomatic patient of any age. Cardioversion is indicated in any patient with hemodynamic instability. Cardioversion and digitalis are each approximately 80% effective in converting the narrow QRS tachycardia to sinus rhythm in infants. However, digitalis should be avoided in the adult because of the tendency for either atrial fibrillation or reciprocating tachycardia to deteriorate into ventricular fibrillation in WPW is even greater in the presence of digitalis. Atrial pacing to overdrive the reciprocating tachycardia also has a risk of ventricular fibrillation. In tachycardia with wide QRS complexes cardioversion is usually best, but intravenous procainamide may be used. Otherwise, the usual antiarrhythmic measures may be used.

For long-term management, i.e., prevention of paroxysmal tachycardia, digitalis is effective for the majority of infants and children but is contraindicated in the adult, for whom the combination of quinidine and propranolol are generally best. Neither these agents nor alternatives (amiodarone, disopyramide, procainamide) are always effective; and amiodarone, though usually effective, has severe adverse reactions. Artificial pacemaker therapy has been used successfully to interrupt the paroxysmal tachycardia in a few appropriately selected cases.

Surgical transsection of a previously well-identified AP or multiple pathways (which are more common in patients who are symptomatic from recurrent tachycardia) has been done in selected cases since 1968. Ablation of the AP is effective in preventing further episodes of tachycardia and usually, but not always, abolishes the signs of WPW. This therapeutic approach has been a boon to those patients with life-threatening or incapacitating tachycardia that was refractory to medical therapy. In a few special circumstances it has been elected to ablate the AV node and insert a permanent artificial pacemaker. In a recent series of 118 patients, the success rate of surgical ablation of the AP in the last 108 was 99%, with morbidity and mortality totaling 1.6%. However, this approach involves open heart surgery and requires highly specialized, and generally prolonged, preoperative and intraoperative procedures. Although operative correction of WPW offers an alternative to life-long drug therapy, the risks and benefits should be balanced carefully. Surgical treatment by ablation of the AP tracts is usually reserved for high risk or severely symptomatic cases.

**Prognosis:** In the absence of associated cardiac defects and paroxysmal tachycardia, the WPW syndrome is compatible with a normal life span. In a series of 90 children in whom tachycardia started before four months of age, 33% had recurrence after 18 months of age. Reciprocating tachycardia in infants or when associated with other cardiac defects may be fatal, and the long-term mortality in the above series was 4.4%. Therefore the majority follow a benign course. When the initial episode is in childhood or adulthood, tachycardia recurrences are more common. Patients who have atrial fibrillation with rapid ventricular response (shortest R-to R of preexcited beats less than 200 msec) patients are a high risk sub-group. Any episode of ventricular fibrillation reveals the life-threatening potential of WPW. A few cases have been recorded to expire with the first episode of ventricular fibrillation, whereas other cases of sudden death can only be suspected of this mechanism by previously having had atrial fibrillation. Less substantiated are the few cases of sudden infant death syndrome in which an autopsy has shown the presence of an AP. Any patient with WPW who has an episode of cardiac arrest, atrial fibrillation, or uncontrolled paroxysmal tachycardia should be seriously considered for electrophysiologic evaluation for determination of best therapy, whether medical or surgical.

**Detection of Carrier:** Unknown.

**Support Groups:** Dallas; American Heart Association

**References:**
Gallagher JJ, et al: The preexcitation syndromes. Prog Cardiovasc Dis 1978; 20:285–327. *

Becker AE, Anderson RH: The Wolff-Parkinson-White syndrome and its anatomical substrates. The Anatomical Record 1981; 201:169–177.

Cox JL, et al: Experience with 118 consecutive patients undergoing operation for the Wolff-Parkinson-White syndrome. J Thorac Cardiovasc Surg 1985; 90:490–501.

Deal BJ, et al: Wolff-Parkinson-White syndrome and supraventricular tachycardia during infancy: management and follow-up. J Am Coll Cardiol 1985; 1:30–35.

Vidaillet HJ, et al: Computer-assisted intraoperative mapping of the entire ventricular epicardium in the Wolff-Parkinson-White syndrome. Am J Cardiol 1986; 58:940–948.

Winters SL, Gomes JA: Intracardiac electrode catheter recordings of atrioventricular bypass tracts in Wolff-Parkinson-White syndrome: techniques, electrophysiologic characteristics and demonstration of concealed and decremental propagation. J Am Coll Cardiol 1986; 7:1392–1403.

Fischell TA, et al: Long-term follow-up after surgical correction of Wolff-Parkinson-White syndrome. J Am Coll Cardiol 1987; 9:283–287.

MI020                                                      **B. Lynn Miller**

**Arsacerebroside sulfatase deficiency**
*See METACHROMATIC LEUKODYSTROPHIES*
**Arterial calcification, generalized, of infancy**
*See ARTERY, CORONARY CALCINOSIS*
**Arterial type Ehlers-Danlos syndrome**
*See EHLERS-DANLOS SYNDROME*

---

## ARTERIO-HEPATIC DYSPLASIA                          2084

**Includes:**
    Alagille syndrome
    Arteriohepatic Dysplasia
    Cholestasis-congenital heart disease
    Cholestasis-peripheral pulmonary stenosis
    Dysplasia, arterio-hepatic
    Hepatic ductular hypoplasia, syndromatic
    Hepato-skeleto-cardiac syndrome
    Pulmonary arterial stenosis-neonatal liver disease

**Excludes:**
    Acidemia, Trihydroxycoprostanic (3275)

    Bile ducts, interlobular, nonsyndromic paucity (3277)
    Cat eye syndrome (0544)
    Cerebro-hepato-renal syndrome (0139)
    Cholestasis-lymphedema, Aagenaes type (3118)
    Chromosome 18, trisomy 18 (0160)
    Fetal rubella syndrome (0384)
    Jaundice, intrahepatic cholestatic, Byler type (2371)
    Noonan syndrome (0720)
    Williams syndrome (0999)

**Major Diagnostic Criteria:** Hepatic disease secondary to hepatic ductular hypoplasia. Congenital heart disease, particularly pulmonary artery stenosis or hypoplasia.

**Clinical Findings:** The most crucial organs involved are the liver and the heart, although there may be multisystem involvement. Perhaps 50% of affected individuals present during the neonatal period with prolonged jaundice. Liver disease of varying severity is due to intrahepatic cholestasis. Hepatomegaly may be present with or without splenomegaly. The most characteristic and frequent cardiac anomaly is peripheral pulmonary artery stenosis, present in 88% of patients studied by cardiac catheterization. Approximately 50% of patients have additional cardiac malformations, including atrial and ventricular defects and others. Facial features described as being typical for the condition include a triangular-shaped facies with a prominent forehead and appearance of deeply set eyes. Anomalies of the anterior chamber of the eye also occur, including posterior embryotoxon. The digits may be short, particularly the distal phalanges, and there may be abnormal placement of the thumbs.

X-rays reveal abnormalities of shape and segmentation of the vertebral column. Butterfly vertebrae are typical for the condition and are due to failure of anterior vertebral arch fusion. Liver biopsies usually show hypoplasia of intrahepatic bile ducts and signs of cholestasis.

**Complications:** Mild short stature, hypersplenism, fat malabsorption during infancy, rickets, pruritus, hypercholesterolemia, hyperlipidemia, hypogonadism, and hepatic failure.

**Associated Findings:** Retinal pigmentary changes, hepatocarcinoma, hypoflexia or arreflexia, vocal cord nodules, renal abnormalities, mild to moderate mental retardation, poor school performance, xanthomata, extrahepatic biliary atresia, ascites.

**Etiology:** Autosomal dominant inheritance with considerable variability in clinical expression. Sporadic cases have been reported. Affected siblings born to apparently normal parents in a few families could be due to decreased penetrance, but also raises the possibility of recessive transmission.

**Pathogenesis:** Undetermined. Possibly a connective tissue defect. A chromosome deletion (20 p) was reported in one case.

**MIM No.:** *11845

**POS No.:** 3019

**Sex Ratio:** M1:F1

**Occurrence:** Over 100 cases have been reported in the literature.

**Risk of Recurrence for Patient's Sib:**
    See Part I, *Mendelian Inheritance.*

**Risk of Recurrence for Patient's Child:**
    See Part I, *Mendelian Inheritance.*

**Age of Detectability:** In the first three months for neonatal liver disease. Cardiac defect may cause problems in infancy, but if mild, patient may be asymptomatic.

**Gene Mapping and Linkage:** AGS (Alagille syndrome) has been provisionally mapped to 20p12-p11.

**Prevention:** None known. Genetic counseling indicated.

**Treatment:** No specific therapy can be recommended for all patients. Cholestyramine and fat-soluble vitamins when indicated.

**Prognosis:** The serum bilirubin falls to normal with increasing age. Cholestasis tends to improve as the children approach adulthood. This syndrome has been considered to be generally benign, but several patients have died during childhood of cardiovascular or hepatic complications, and a few have died of unexplained sepsis.

**Detection of Carrier:** For apparently sporadic cases, the parents should be examined carefully for unusual facial appearance and other physical signs of the condition. X-rays should also be taken to look for butterfly vertebrae, and liver function tests should be performed, since the SGOT and 5'-nucleotidase may remain elevated in adults.

**Special Considerations:** In one series, intelligence was thought to be normal whereas mild mental retardation was considered common in another.

No unifying hypothesis for the varied constellation of features of this syndrome has been suggested. An inborn error of synthesis, secretion, or transport of bile acids could cause cholestasis with secondary hypoplasia of the intrahepatic biliary tree. However, this type of metabolic error could not produce the cardiovascular or skeletal abnormalities. Theoretically, a defect of a specific connective tissue component present in bile ducts, vasculature, and bone could account for many of the clinical features.

**References:**
Alagille D, et al.: Hepatic ductular hypoplasia associated with characteristic facies, vertebral malformations, retarded physical, mental, and sexual development, and cardiac murmur. J Pediatr 1975; 86:63–71.
Reily CA, et al.: Arteriohepatic dysplasia: a benign syndrome of intrahepatic cholestasis with multiple organ involvement. Ann Int Med 1979; 91:520–527.
Levin SE, et al.: Arteriohepatic dysplasia: association of liver disease with pulmonary artery stenosis as well as facial and skeletal abnormalities. Pediatrics 1980; 66:876–883.
Romanchuk KG, et al.: Ocular findings in arteriohepatic dysplasia. Canad J Ophthal 1981; 16:94–99.
Shulman SA, et al.: Arteriohepatic dysplasia: extreme variability among affected family members. Am J Med Genet 1984; 19:325–332.
Byrne JLB, et al.: Del(20p) with manifestations of arteriohepatic dysplasia. Am J Med Genet 1986; 24:673–678.
Alagille D, et al.: Syndromatic paucity of interlobular bile ducts: review of 80 cases. J Pediatr 1987; 110:195–200 *
Mueller RF: The Alagille syndrome. J Med Genet 1987; 24:621–626. *

AB004                                      **Dianne N. Abuelo**

**Arteriohepatic Dysplasia**
  *See ARTERIO-HEPATIC DYSPLASIA*
**Arteriopathy, occlusive infantile**
  *See ARTERY, CORONARY CALCINOSIS*
**Arteriovenous aneurysm of external ear**
  *See EAR, ARTERIOVENOUS FISTULA*
**Arteriovenous hemangioma/malformation**
  *See HEMANGIOMAS OF THE HEAD AND NECK*
**Arteriovenous malformations: spinal, cortical, and cerebellar**
  *See CNS ARTERIOVENOUS MALFORMATION*
**Arteritis-arthritis syndrome**
  *See ARTHRITIS-ARTERITIS SYNDROME*

## ARTERY, ANOMALOUS ORIGIN OF CONTRALATERAL
## SUBCLAVIAN                                    0063

**Includes:** Subclavian artery, anomalous origin of contralateral
**Excludes:**
  Carotid and subclavian artery, common
  Ipsilateral common origin to arch
  **Aorta, isolation of subclavian artery from aorta** (0546)

**Major Diagnostic Criteria:** An esophagram in the PA, lateral and both oblique views is necessary to suspect the anomalous vessel. However, an aortic root aortogram may be necessary to demonstrate associated anomalies in the symptomatic case.

**Clinical Findings:** The anomaly, regardless of side, is usually an incidental finding on barium esophagram, on angiocardiography, during cardiac surgery for other anomalies or at autopsy. Occasionally, the anomalous vessel will be related to dysphagia. In the case of the anomalous left subclavian artery with a right aortic arch, this is commonly associated with a left ductus arteriosus or

ligamentum arteriosus which completes a true vascular ring. In the case of anomalous right subclavian artery with a left aortic arch, recent evidence has related the symptomatic cases to associated anomalous origin of the carotid vessels. This is either an unusual closeness of their origins from the arch, or even a true common origin. This anomalous origin of the carotids creates an anterior sling which prevents the trachea and esophagus from bending away from the posterior compression of the anomalous right subclavian artery. This combined anomaly occasionally also causes tracheal compression and resultant respiratory symptoms.

For either the anomalous right or left subclavian artery, barium esophagram demonstrates a posterior and sharp oblique (running cephalad to the side contralateral to the arch) indentation in the esophagus. An aortic root angiocardiogram will confirm this anomaly.

**Complications:** Rarely, dysphagia will occur. Minimal dysphagia or stridor occurs more often, but considering the frequency of the defect, this is still a rare occurrence.

**Associated Findings:** Contralateral origin of the right subclavian artery is frequently found with other congenital heart defects, especially **Heart, tetralogy of Fallot** and **Aorta, coarctation.** It is also found quite often in **Chromosome 21, trisomy 21.**

**Etiology:** Unknown.

**Pathogenesis:** The contralateral origin of the subclavian artery results from the early obliteration of the contralateral embryonic 4th arch and the corresponding distal dorsal aorta is retained to form the 1st part of the anomalous vessel. This explains why such a subclavian artery passes behind the esophagus.

**Sex Ratio:** M1:F1

**Occurrence:** Incidence of anomalous origin of contralateral right subclavian artery approximately 1:200 live births. Anomalous origin of contralateral left subclavian artery occurs in approximately 1:5000 to 1:6000 live births. Right aortic arch occurs in approximately 1:2500 live births.

Prevalence of anomalous origin of right subclavian artery with left aortic arch < 1:2000 persons of all studied populations. Isolated right arch is probably < 1:2500 persons. However, most of these without heart defects have contralateral origin of left subclavian artery, ie 40–50%. Anomalous origin of left subclavian with right aortic arch in approximately 1:5000 to 1:6000.

**Risk of Recurrence for Patient's Sib:** Unknown.

**Risk of Recurrence for Patient's Child:** Unknown.

**Age of Detectability:** If symptomatic, usually found during infancy, otherwise detectable at any age or at necropsy.

**Gene Mapping and Linkage:** Unknown.

**Prevention:** None known. Genetic counseling indicated.

**Treatment:** Usually none required. Rarely, a division of the right subclavian or of the left ligamentum with anomalous left subclavian will be necessary to relieve dysphagia. It is important to note the presence of the contralateral origin of the subclavian prior to cardiac catheterization or when associated with other congenital heart lesions, particularly when a subclavian to pulmonary artery shunt is under consideration. Use of such an anomalous left subclavian artery to left pulmonary artery anastomosis with a right aortic arch would produce a vascular ring.

**Prognosis:** The anomaly is compatible with normal life expectancy in the great majority of cases. Death, when it occurs, is either nonrelated or secondary to associated congenital heart disease.

**Detection of Carrier:** Unknown.

**Special Considerations:** Right aortic arch has high correlation with certain congenital heart defects, especially **Heart, tetralogy of Fallot, Heart, truncus arteriosus** and, less frequently, **Tricuspid valve, atresia.** On the other hand, many patients with a right aortic arch and anomalous origin of left subclavian artery do not have other congenital heart defects.

**References:**
Kienast W, et al.: Clinical relevance of the so-called arteria lusoria in childhood. Z Kardiol 1984; 73:354–360.

Austin EH, Wolfe WG: Aneurysm of aberrant subclavian artery with a review of the literature. J Vasc Surg 1985; 2:571–577. *

Seres-Sturm M, et al.: The aberrant retroesophageal right subclavian artery. Morphol Embryol 1985; 31:183–186.

Motta R, et al.: Aneurysm of right retroesophageal subclavian artery. Ital J Surg Sci 1986; 16:211–215.

Nathan H: Association of retroesophageal right subclavian arteries with thoracic ducts terminating in the right venous angle. J Thorac Cardiovasc Surg 1987; 93:148–149.

MC028                                            **Dan G. McNamara**

---

## ARTERY, BRACHIOCEPHALIC AND CONTRALATERAL CAROTID, COMMON ORIGIN                    0200

**Includes:**
  Brachiocephalic and contralateral corotid artery, common origin of
  Carotid artery, common origin of brachiocephalic and contralateral
  Left common carotid artery arising from innominate artery

**Excludes:**  N/A

**Major Diagnostic Criteria:**  Arch aortography is definitive. Includes right common carotid artery from left innominate artery with a right-sided aortic arch, but excludes abnormalities in which all branches arise from a common stem which in turn originates from the aortic arch.

**Clinical Findings:**  The brachiocephalic and contralateral common carotid arteries arise from the aortic arch with a common stem. The abnormally originating carotid artery crosses in front of the trachea as it courses to the opposite side and may compress the trachea. When the contralateral common carotid artery originates as a branch of the brachiocephalic (innominate) artery it crosses the trachea anteriorly.

The clinical manifestations vary with the degree of tracheal compression. Most patients are asymptomatic, but there may be respiratory distress with stridor or crowing during inspiration and a predisposition to respiratory infections. Dysphagia is not present. The esophagram is usually normal. In the rare case associated with tracheal compression, plain films show indentation or grooving in the anterior tracheal surface. This is best seen in the lateral projection.

**Complications:**  Unknown.

**Associated Findings:**  None known.

**Etiology:**  Unknown.

**Pathogenesis:**  Unknown.

**Sex Ratio:**  Presumably M1:F1

**Occurrence:**  Undetermined but presumed rare.

**Risk of Recurrence for Patient's Sib:**  Unknown.

**Risk of Recurrence for Patient's Child:**  Unknown.

**Age of Detectability:**  At any age by arch aortography.

**Gene Mapping and Linkage:**  Unknown.

**Prevention:**  None known. Genetic counseling indicated.

**Treatment:**  In symptomatic cases, the anomalous vessel may be sutured to the posterior aspect of the sternum.

**Prognosis:**  Excellent. In asymptomatic patients it has no effect on life expectancy. In those with tracheal compression, once surgically relieved, patient should have a normal life expectancy.

**Detection of Carrier:**  Unknown.

**References:**
Gross RE: Arterial malformations which cause compression of trachea and esophagus. Circulation 1955; 11:124.

Liechty JD, et al.: Variations pertaining to the aortic arches and their branches. Q Bull NW Univ Med Sch 1957; 31:136.

Bosniak MA: An analysis of some anatomic-roentgenologic aspects of the brachiocephalic vessels. Am J Roentgenol Radium Ther Nucl Med 1964; 91:1222.

Yeh HC, et al.: Ultrasonography of the brachiocephalic arteries. Radiology 1979; 132:403–408. *

Pokrovskii AV, et al.: Ultrasonic angiography in the diagnosis of lesions of the brachiocephalic branches of the aorta. Kardiologiia 1985; 25:82–86.

MU008                                            **Charles E. Mullins**
MC028                                            **Dan G. McNamara**

---

## ARTERY, CORONARY CALCINOSIS                    0217

**Includes:**
  Arterial calcification, generalized, of infancy
  Arteriopathy, occlusive infantile
  Coronary arterial calcinosis
  Coronary arteries, congenital medial sclerosis of
  Coronary artery sclerosis
  Coronary calcification of infancy
  Coronary sclerosis, juvenile or infantile
  Medial coronary sclerosis of infancy

**Excludes:**  Coronary atherosclerosis of infancy or childhood

**Major Diagnostic Criteria:**  This syndrome cannot at present be diagnosed antemortem. The typical clinical picture, plus X-ray proof of arterial calcification, would be highly suggestive.

**Clinical Findings:**  Coronary calcinosis undoubtedly encompasses a number of conditions with varying etiologies. The common finding is one of interruption of normal myocardial blood flow by extensive generalized narrowing of coronary arteries with calcification. Both the intima and media are involved without atheroma. This is a disease of infancy with the majority of patients dying before age 6 months.

The classic clinical presentation is that of an infant with acute onset of pallor, dyspnea, and signs of congestive heart failure which rapidly progress to death in several hours to several days. There may be a recent history of viral infection or even an intercurrent viral illness. There is also a less fulminant form of the disease characterized by more gradual onset of congestive failure with death in a period of weeks or months. There are no heart murmurs.

The EKG in the few patients in whom it has been obtained has shown ischemia or infarction. Progressive heart block also has been reported. Chest X-rays show cardiomegaly and pulmonary venous congestion. Some patients will have generalized arterial calcification, and films of the neck may prove useful in delineating thyroid artery or carotid artery calcification.

**Complications:**  Myocardial infarction, arrhythmias, hypertension, congestive heart failure and death.

**Associated Findings:**  Some patients may have generalized arterial calcification.

**Etiology:**  Autosomal recessive inheritance presumably involving a defect of elastic fibers. Possibly an associated environmental component.

**Pathogenesis:**  It is not known whether the infants involved with this syndrome are affected pre- or postnatally. Intrauterine insults such as rubella and other viremias may play a role in some patients. Altered calcium metabolism also may play a role in certain patients. Extrauterine infections, as well as anoxia, may be capable of producing coronary arterial medial necrosis with subsequent fibrous proliferation accounting for the pathologic findings.

**MIM No.:**  *20800

**Sex Ratio:**  M1:Fl

**Occurrence:**  Undetermined. Less than 1:1000 cases of congenital heart disease.

**Risk of Recurrence for Patient's Sib:**  Undetermined. Two of 44 reported cases occurred in sibs.

**Risk of Recurrence for Patient's Child:**  Affected individuals are not expected to survive to reproduce.

**Age of Detectability:**  Antemortem diagnosis is not possible.

**Gene Mapping and Linkage:** Unknown.

**Prevention:** None known. Genetic counseling indicated.

**Treatment:** Supportive.

**Prognosis:** Usually fatal, although an instance of spontaneous regression and survival at 7 years of age has been reported.

**Detection of Carrier:** Unknown.

**References:**

Moran JJ, Becker SM: Idiopathic arterial calcification of infancy. Am J Clin Pathol 1959; 31:517–529.

Nora JJ, McNamara DG: Coronary artery sclerosis. In: Watson H, ed: Paediatric Cardiology. St. Louis: C.V. Mosby Co., 1968:311.

Bird T: Idiopathic arterial calcification in infancy. Arch Dis Child 1974; 49:82–89. *

Maayan C, et al.: Idiopathic infantile arterial calcification: a case report and review of the literature. Europ J Pediat 1984; 142:211–215.

Anderson KA, et al.: Idiopathic arterial calcification of infancy in newborn siblings with unusual light and electron microscope findings. Arch Path Lab Med 1985; 109:838–842.

GR002 **Thomas P. Graham, Jr.**

## ARTERY, CORONARY, ANOMALOUS ORIGIN FROM PULMONARY ARTERY                                    0064

**Includes:**

Coronary arteries, anomalous origin from pulmonary artery
Left coronary artery, anomalous origin from pulmonary artery
Right coronary artery, anomalous origin from pulmonary artery

**Excludes:**

**Artery, coronary, arteriovenous fistula (0218)**
**Artery, single coronary (0219)**

**Major Diagnostic Criteria:** Aortic root angiography confirms the diagnosis. This procedure also differentiates anomalous left coronary artery from endocardial fibroelastosis, myocarditis, glycogen storage disease, congenital mitral insufficiency, and cardiomyopathy of unknown cause. Cross-sectional echocardiography can be useful to diagnose this anomaly, but specificity and diagnostic accuracy for this technique have not been established.

**Clinical Findings:** *Anomalous origin of the left coronary artery from the pulmonary artery:* this lesion is characterized by a normal right coronary artery arising from the aorta, while the left coronary artery arises wholly from the pulmonary trunk. There is no intrauterine disturbance of myocardial blood supply since pulmonary artery and aortic pressures, as well as oxygen contents, are similar. With the normal drop in pulmonary vascular resistance after birth, however, perfusion pressure in the left coronary artery will become insufficient for antegrade flow. As a consequence of this decrease in pulmonary artery pressure, perfusion of the myocardium supplied by the left coronary artery will be dependent on adequate anastomoses between the right and left coronary arteries. Thus the left coronary artery can be filled retrogradely and the direction of the blood flow will then be out into the pulmonary artery. The presence or absence of symptoms or signs of this defect then will be related to the adequacy of myocardial perfusion which in turn will be related to intercoronary anastomoses, intracoronary vascular resistance, aortic pressure, pulmonary pressure and cardiac metabolic demands.

The majority of patients will present with symptoms during the first 6 months of life. The typical history is one of gradually increasing irritability, sweating, tachypnea, dyspnea and excessive crying as if in pain. The onset of these symptoms has been reported as early as the 1st month of life. A small number of children will present after infancy with only mild symptoms of exercise intolerance. Asymptomatic adults have been reported and may comprise 10–15% of patients with this lesion.

Physical examination in the sick infant will reveal signs of congestive heart failure. Cardiac examination generally reveals cardiomegaly and a prominent third sound. Mitral insufficiency is a common finding in infants as well as older children. Older children and adults may have diastolic or continuous murmurs.

Cardiac X-rays usually show severe left ventricular enlargement with a small aorta. The left atrium may be normal in size unless there is mitral insufficiency. Signs of pulmonary venous congestion of the lungs are almost invariably present. The EKG is the key to the diagnosis and classically shows signs of anterolateral myocardial infarction with broad deep Q waves in I, aVL and left precordial leads. In addition there may be decreased anterior-lateral QRS forces with poor progression of R wave with ST elevation or T wave inversion over the left precordium. The pattern of anteroseptal infarction with Q in $V_5$ greater than Q in $V_6$ has also been reported as well as a reversed Q loop. In addition, criteria for left ventricular hypertrophy generally are present. Thallium imaging of the heart may reveal anterio-lateral perfusion abnormalities of the left ventricle and can be useful.

Cardiac catheterization usually fails to reveal oximetry evidence of a left-to-right shunt in infants but may do so in adults. Left ventricular end diastolic pressure is elevated and left ventricular angiocardiography reveals a poorly contracting ventricle. Mitral insufficiency will be evident in many patients. Pulmonary artery angiography may reveal transient filling of the proximal part of the anomalous vessel. Aortic root angiography is diagnostic and reveals a single right coronary artery arising from the aorta and usually sequential retrograde filling of the left coronary and pulmonary artery. Rarely, patients with sparse collaterals fail to show this retrograde filling, and these infants generally have the most severe symptoms.

*Anomalous origin of the right coronary artery from the pulmonary artery:* this lesion has been discovered as an incidental finding at surgery or autopsy, and there have been no cases reported with symptoms related to its presence. The vessel frequently is thin walled and suggestive evidence of retrograde flow has been shown in one case at surgery. Physical examination, X-ray and EKG are generally normal.

*Anomalous origin of both coronary arteries from the pulmonary artery:* this lesion is felt to be incompatible with life after pulmonary artery pressure declines postnatally. Eight patients have been reported with age at death ranging from 8 hours-10 days.

Echocardiographic findings include dilatation of the left ventricle with areas of akinesis or dyskinesis. Since the problem is frequently a segmental one, two-dimensional high resolution examination is required in most instances to image these abnormalities.

Symptoms include early onset of congestive failure of increasing severity with marked cardiomegaly. Murmurs have not been reported and an EKG has not been recorded in an infant with this lesion.

**Complications:** Anomalous left coronary artery--myocardial ischemia and infarction, papillary muscle dysfunction, mitral insufficiency and congestive heart failure. Anomalous right coronary artery--none known. Anomalous origin of both coronaries--progressive myocardial ischemia, congestive heart failure and death.

**Associated Findings:** None known.

**Etiology:** Unknown.

**Pathogenesis:** Two theories have been proposed. The first states that either the truncus arteriosus is abnormally divided so that one or both coronary anlagen are included in the pulmonary artery or that a coronary bud arises in an anomalous position from a part of the truncus which will become the pulmonary artery. An alternate theory proposes that there are six coronary anlagen from the truncus, each of which is related to a portion which will become an aortic or pulmonary sinus of Valsalva. Normally all but two anlagen involute but variations in involution and persistence of such anlagen could explain the known anomalous origins of coronary arteries.

**Sex Ratio:** Presumably M1:F1

**Occurrence:** Anomalous left coronary artery <3:1000 cases of congenital heart disease.

Anomalous right coronary artery undetermined.

Anomalous origin both coronaries is rare.

**Risk of Recurrence for Patient's Sib:**  Unknown.

**Risk of Recurrence for Patient's Child:**  Unknown.

**Age of Detectability:**  Anomalous left coronary is detectable from birth by aortic root angiography: as soon as pulmonary vascular resistance falls, retrograde filling of the left coronary may be evident (normally by 1–3 months).

Anomalous right coronary artery detectable from birth by proximal aortography.

Anomalous origin of both coronaries detectable from birth by selective pulmonary arteriogram.

**Gene Mapping and Linkage:**  Unknown.

**Prevention:**  None known. Genetic counseling indicated.

**Treatment:**  Anomalous left coronary artery—most groups advocate surgical reconstruction of a two-coronary system when catheterization data indicate coronary flow into the pulmonary artery. Surgical ligation of the anomalous coronary may be preferable in very small, critically ill infants. Anomalous right coronary artery—surgery not indicated in asymptomatic infants. In older patients, reconstruction of a two-coronary system may be indicated. Anomalous origin of both coronaries—surgery has not been attempted. Theoretic considerations include prosthetic or venous graft for anastomosis of one or both vessels to the aorta in early infancy.

**Prognosis:**  Prognosis, in general, is poor in infants with anomalous left coronary artery and severe congestive heart failure. When reconstruction of a 2-coronary artery system can be accomplished, prognosis has been good with amelioration of symptomatology.

The long-term prognosis of associated mitral insufficiency is unknown. In older children and adults with minimal symptoms, prognosis is excellent. Prognosis for anomalous right coronary artery is excellent. Anomalous origin of both coronaries is uniformly fatal in infancy.

**Detection of Carrier:**  Unknown.

**References:**

Sabiston DC Jr, et al.: The direction of blood flow in anomalous left coronary artery arising from the pulmonary artery. Circulation 1960; 22:591–597.
Roberts WC: Anomalous origin of both coronary arteries from the pulmonary artery. Am J Cardiol 1962; 10:595–600.
Nora JJ, McNamara DC: Anomalies of the coronary arteries and coronary artery fistula. In: Watson H, ed: Paediatric cardiology. St. Louis: CV Mosby, 1968:295–310. *
Wesselhoeft H, et al.: Anomalous origin of the left coronary artery from the pulmonary trunk. Circulation 1968; 38:403–425. *

GR002                                    **Thomas P. Graham, Jr.**

---

## ARTERY, CORONARY, ARTERIOVENOUS FISTULA          0218

**Includes:**

Coronary arteriovenous fistula
Coronary artery-cameral shunt

**Excludes:**  Artery, coronary, anomalous origin from pulmonary artery (0064)

**Major Diagnostic Criteria:**  Aortic root angiography confirms the diagnosis of coronary arteriovenous fistula.

**Clinical Findings:**  A coronary arteriovenous fistula is characterized by a single or multiple channel communicating between one or both coronary arteries and a cardiac chamber or pulmonary artery. The most common site of communication is the right heart (90%). This includes the right ventricle (45%), followed in order by the right atrium (including coronary sinus) (30%), and the pulmonary artery (15%). In less than 10% of the cases, the communication is into the left atrium or the left ventricle. The right coronary artery alone is most commonly involved (60%), but the anomaly may occur in both right and left coronary arteries. Rarely, an extra coronary artery may be involved. The hemodynamic findings are related to the magnitude of flow through the fistula. Congestive

heart failure has been reported in 21 of 150 patients (14%), usually in infancy or in late adult life.

Physical examination is variable, depending upon the magnitude and point of egress of the shunt. In the common variety (ie into the right heart) there is usually a continuous murmur and thrill maximally along the lower sternal border, either on the right or left side. The murmur may be loud, harsh and machinery-like with a superficial high-pitched quality. The continuous murmur may be differentiated from a patent ductus arteriosus by its location. In addition, it usually peaks near the first heart sound, the diastolic component may be louder than the systolic component. Atrioventricular valve flow murmurs are usually obscured by the continuous murmur. With a large shunt causing considerable aortic run-off, the increased pulse pressure manifests itself as bounding peripheral arterial pulses.

The thoracic X-ray generally reveals increased shunt vascularity and cardiomegaly in patients with large shunts to the right heart or pulmonary artery. In patients with small left-to-right shunts, the roentgen findings are normal. The EKG is usually normal. With large left-to-right shunts, left or biventricular hypertrophy is present.

Cardiac catheterization will reveal a left-to-right shunt when a large communication enters the right heart. Right pressures may be elevated. Aortic root angiography will reveal a dilated coronary vessel(s) communicating with a cardiac chamber or vessel.

**Complications:**  Congestive heart failure, subacute bacterial endocarditis, development of a coronary artery aneurysm, formation of mural thrombi within tortuous coronary artery.

**Associated Findings:**  None known.

**Etiology:**  Probably multifactorial inheritance.

**Pathogenesis:**  In normal embryologic development of the coronary arteries, angioblastic buds arise from the truncus arteriosus, acquire lumens, and proliferate through the myocardium connecting through capillary beds with the coronary veins. The veins form also as buds from the caudal end of the primitive cardiac tube at a slightly earlier stage of development. During early development of the coronary arteries, there are communications with muscular intratrabecular spaces which may become lined with endothelium. Persistence of such channels provides a plausible explanation for intracardiac arteriovenous fistula.

**CDC No.:**  746.885

**Sex Ratio:**  Presumably M1:F1

**Occurrence:**  Less than 4:1000 cases of congenital heart disease.

**Risk of Recurrence for Patient's Sib:**  Unknown.

**Risk of Recurrence for Patient's Child:**  Unknown.

**Age of Detectability:**  From birth by selective angiography.

**Gene Mapping and Linkage:**  Unknown.

**Prevention:**  None known. Genetic counseling indicated.

**Treatment:**  Surgery on fistula obliterating left-to-right shunt. Symptomatic for congestive heart failure, appropriate antibiotic prophylaxis to prevent subacute bacterial endocarditis.

**Prognosis:**  The prognosis is excellent for patients who are detected and have surgical correction. Patients with congestive failure require digitalis followed by surgical therapy. Asymptomatic patients should in most cases have ligation unless the fistula is quite small or other considerations supervene.

**Detection of Carrier:**  Unknown.

**References:**

Sabiston DC Jr, et al.: Surgical management of congenital lesions of the coronary circulation. Ann Surg 1963; 157:908.
Gasul BM, et al.: Systemic arteriovenous fistula. In: Gasul BM, et al., eds: Heart disease in children: diagnosis and treatment. Philadelphia: J.B. Lippincott, 1966:442.
Nora JJ, McNamara DG: Anomalies of the coronary arteries and coronary artery fistula. In: Watson H, ed: Paediatric cardiology. London: Lloyd-Luke, 1968:295. *

GR002                                    **Thomas P. Graham, Jr.**

## ARTERY, INDEPENDENT ORIGIN OF IPSILATERAL VERTEBRAL     0527

**Includes:** Ipsilateral vertebral artery from aortic arch

**Excludes:** Vertebral artery, other abnormal origin of

**Major Diagnostic Criteria:** The vertebral artery ipsilateral to the aortic arch usually arises as the first branch of the subclavian artery. In this variant with a normal left aortic arch, the left vertebral artery arises from the aortic arch, the left common carotid and the left subclavian artery. Most cases are found incidentally at autopsy. Selective aortic arch angiography is diagnostic.

**Clinical Findings:** This variant is asymptomatic and may be found incidentally in about 6% of normal individuals. Origin of the vertebral artery directly from the aorta may be of diagnostic importance during angiography since its presence rules out the possibility of a pathologic occlusion if there is an absence of filling of the left vertebral artery from the left subclavian artery. Patients with occlusion of the proximal part of the left subclavian artery and with the artery originating in the left vertebral artery directly from the aorta have been reported without symptoms of subclavian steal syndrome.

**Complications:** When this anatomic variant is associated with other aortic arch abnormalities (such as coarctation of the aorta or hypoplastic aortic arch), resection of the vertebral artery origin with the involved portion of the aortic arch may occur at the time of surgical repair.

**Associated Findings:** None known.

**Etiology:** Unknown.

**Pathogenesis:** The vertebral arteries develop embryologically from longitudinal anastomoses between the paired cervical intersegmental arteries. Although most of these intersegmental arteries involute, the left 6th persists as the eventual left subclavian artery and proximal portion of the left vertebral artery. The 4th or 5th left intersegmental artery may persist as the direct attachment of the vertebral artery to the aorta.

**Sex Ratio:** Presumably M1:F1

**Occurrence:** Between 2.6% and 7.0% prevalence has been found in autopsy series. Several large autopsy and angiography series have shown a prevalence of 6.0%

**Risk of Recurrence for Patient's Sib:** Unknown.

**Risk of Recurrence for Patient's Child:** Unknown.

**Age of Detectability:** At birth by aortic arch angiography.

**Gene Mapping and Linkage:** Unknown.

**Prevention:** None known. Genetic counseling indicated.

**Treatment:** Unknown.

**Prognosis:** Excellent; should have a normal life span.

**Detection of Carrier:** Unknown.

**References:**
Helenon CH, et al.: Left subclavian steal syndrome associated with separate origin of left vertebral artery from the aorta. Sem Hop Paris 1974; 50:2673–2677.
Kuwabara Y, et al.: Anomalous origin of left vertebral artery. Nippon Igaku Hoshasen Gakkai Zasshi 1978; 38:521–527.
Denkhaus H, et al.: Variant of the subclavian steal syndrome associated with an anomalous origin of the left vertebral artery. Radiologe 1981; 21:77–80.
Holder J, et al.: Ipsilateral subclavian steal in association with aberrant origin of left vertebral artery from the aortic arch. A.J.N.R. 1981; 2:411–413.
Nathan H, Seidel MR: The association of a retroesophageal right subclavian artery, a right-sided terminating thoracic duct, and a left vetebral artery of aortic origin: anatomical and clinical considerations. Acta Anat 1983; 117:362–373.

MU008
MC028

**Charles E. Mullins**
**Dan G. McNamara**

## ARTERY, RENAL FIBROMUSCULAR DYSPLASIA     2307

**Includes:**
  Fibrodysplasia of arteries
  Fibromuscular dysplasia of arteries
  Fibromuscular dysplasia with medial fibroplasia
  Fibromuscular hyperplasia
  Fibroplastic renal artery disease
  Intimal fibrosis with fibromuscular dysplasia
  Medial fibroplasia
  Renal artery stenosis, congenital

**Excludes:**
  Atherosclerotic renal artery disease
  Diabetic renovascular changes
  Embolic renal disease
  Inflammatory renal artery disease
  Middle aortic syndrome
  **Neurofibromatosis** (0712)
  Renal artery disease in transplanted kidneys due to rejection
  Renal artery disease due to anastomotic obstruction
  Secondary fibrotic renal disease
  Takayasu artesitis

**Major Diagnostic Criteria:** The diagnosis is made by renal arteriography. The renal arteries have a typical "beaded" appearance. Children with fibromuscular dysplasia are said to be less likely than adults to have the typical angiographic features. Renal vein renin levels and renal vein to peripheral blood renin ratios may be used to confirm the renovascular origin of the hypertension. Abnormal findings on intravenous pyelography may be found in between 30% and 87% of individuals with renovascular hypertension, depending upon criteria for diagnosis, and a false positive intravenous pyelogram will be found in 11.4% of hypertensives without renovascular hypertension.

Appropriate studies should be performed to rule out an arteritis due to a diffuse, systemic inflammatory disorder. Investigation to rule out **Neurofibromatosis** is also recommended.

**Clinical Findings:** Fibromuscular dysplasia of the renal arteries will present with findings and symptoms of renovascular hypertension. Features suggestive of renovascular hypertension include the finding of an abdominal bruit (particulary if the bruit is continuous and radiates to the flanks), onset of hypertension at a young age, sudden onset of hypertension, hypertension that is particularly severe or difficult to control, and hypertension associated with deteriorating renal function. Rapidly accelerating hypertension associated with severe retinopathy has an increased likelihood of being renovascular in origin. Renovascular hypertension may present with epistaxis, anorexia, poor weight gain in infancy, headaches, or be found on routine examination in an asymptomatic individual.

**Complications:** Unrecognized and untreated renovascular hypertension from fibromuscular dysplasia can lead to the sequelae of severe systemic arterial hypertension including hypertensive encephalopathy, cerebral hemorrhage, severe hypertensive retinopathy with blindness, left ventricular dilation, left ventricular hypertrophy, congestive heart failure, myocardial infarction, progressive renal insufficiency, and death. Unilateral renovascular hypertension may result in nephrosclerosis in the contralateral normal kidney. Complications from surgical procedures to revascularize the kidney, from balloon angioplasty for renal artery stenosis, and from pharmacologic therapy of renovascular hypertension may occur as well.

**Associated Findings:** **Neurofibromatosis** is associated with renal artery stenosis which is similar to fibromuscular dysplasia histologically. Characteristically, the renal artery lesion with neurofibromatosis is closer to the aortic orifice of the renal artery and is less diffuse than that found with isolated fibromuscular dysplasia. Investigation to rule out neurofibromatosis with the diagnosis of fibromuscular dysplasia, and to rule out renal artery disease in individuals with neurofibromatosis who become hypertensive, is appropriate.

An association between right renal artery fibroplastic disease and nephroptosis of that kidney has been reported.

**Etiology:** Some cases found in young children have been presumed to be congenital in origin. Possibly autosomal dominant inheritance with variable and often no clinical effects.

**Pathogenesis:** The renal artery lesions may be unilateral or bilateral. Focal, multifocal, or tubular stenosis may be present. Poststenotic dilation with multifocal stenosis give rise to the typical "beaded" appearance of the renal artery angiographically. Intimal fibrosis, medial smooth muscle hyperplasia, perimedial and external elastic membrane fibrosis, or adventitial changes may predominate on histologic examination. It has been speculated that trauma could be related to some cases, particularly those with intimal or adventitial fibrosis. The pathogenesis is unknown and, although these lesions are generally grouped together, it may be that pathogenesis and etiologies for the various histologic types of fibromuscular dysplasia are different.

**MIM No.:** 13558

**CDC No.:** 747.610

**Sex Ratio:** M1:F1 in pediatric cases. Reportedly more frequent among females adults.

**Occurrence:** Represented 12% (2/17) of cases of renovascular hypertension in childhood found in a 10 year period at the Hospital for Sick Children in Toronto. In adults, renovascular hypertension is estimated to account for less than 2% of hypertension and, of these, the majority are atherosclerotic renal artery disease. An incidence and prevalence of less than 1:100,000 is likely.

**Risk of Recurrence for Patient's Sib:**
See Part I, *Mendelian Inheritance.*

**Risk of Recurrence for Patient's Child:**
See Part I, *Mendelian Inheritance.*

**Age of Detectability:** Usually detected in childhood or as a young adult after onset of hypertension.

**Gene Mapping and Linkage:** Unknown.

**Prevention:** None known. Genetic counseling indicated.

**Treatment:** Pharmacologic treatment may be successful in some cases. Surgical treatment may include nephrectomy, partial nephrectomy with ligation of stenosed vessels, auto-transplantation, angioplasty, or bypass of an obstructed segment of artery. Preservation of renal parenchyma as well as cure of hypertension should be the goal of surgical treatment. Transluminal balloon angioplasty has been used successfully in adult and pediatric patients with fibromuscular dysplasia of the renal arteries.

**Prognosis:** Untreated cases would be expected to develop complications of systemic arterial hypertension and, in some cases, progressive renal insufficiency which would shorten survival to varying degrees depending upon the severity of hypertension and uremia. Successfully treated cases should have a normal life span.

**Detection of Carrier:** Unknown.

**References:**
Harrison EG Jr, McCormack LJ: Pathologic classification of renal artery disease in renovascular hypertension. Mayo Clin Proc 1971; 46:161–167.
de Zeeuw D, et al.: Nephroptosis and hypertension. Lancet 1977; 1:213–215.
Makker SP, Moorthy B: Fibromuscular dysplasia of the renal arteries: an important cause of renovascular hypertension in children. J Pediatr 1979; 95:940–945.
Inglefinger J: Renovascular hypertension. In: Pediatric Hypertension. Chap 11. W.B. Saunders, 1982:150–167.
Watson AR, et al.: Renovascular hypertension in childhood: a changing perspective in management. J Pediatr 1985; 106:366–372.

ST050
BR014

**Fernando Stein**
**J. Timothy Bricker**

## ARTERY, SINGLE CORONARY 0219

**Includes:** Coronary artery, single left or right

**Excludes:** Artery, coronary, anomalous origin from pulmonary artery (0064)

**Major Diagnostic Criteria:** No symptoms or signs are evident unless accompanied by other major cardiac abnormalities. Diagnosis can be made with aortic root angiography or cineangiography at the time of cardiac catheterization.

**Clinical Findings:** This is a single coronary artery arising from the aorta by a single ostium. In 22 of 37 cases, with data available, the single artery had the origin of a left coronary artery, while the remaining 15 had the origin of a right coronary artery.

Three anatomic types have been described with approximately one-third of patients falling into each category. Type I includes cases in which the single vessel follows the course of either the normal right or left coronary and supplies the remainder of the heart by extension of those branches. Type II includes cases in which the single artery branches into 2 vessels shortly after its origin, and these 2 vessels then follow the normal right and left artery distributions. Type III includes all cases in which the coronary distribution is atypical of either a normal right or left coronary pattern.

This anomaly causes no hemodynamic abnormalities when it occurs as an isolated cardiac defect. Because of the few reported cases, it is not known whether the patient is more vulnerable to coronary occlusive disease in later life.

The EKG and X-rays are normal in isolated, uncomplicated single coronary artery.

**Complications:** In 4 of 27 adults with single coronary artery examined at necropsy, myocardial infarction was found. These 4 patients were ages 38, 46, 46 and 62. The relationship of the single coronary artery to the myocardial infarcts in these patients is unknown. There is an increase in the incidence of myocardial ischemia and infarction when the main left coronary artery or the anterior descending coronary artery runs between the aorta and the pulmonary trunk even in the absence of atherosclerotic disease. The reason for this complication remains unknown at the present time.

**Associated Findings:** There is a high percentage of associated cardiac defects in children with proven single coronary arteries. In 16 of 20 such patients, there were symptoms referable to the associated lesions. These associated defects include common ventricle (4), bicuspid aortic valve (3), fistulous communication with the right ventricle (2) and truncus arteriosus (2).

**Etiology:** Probably multifactorial inheritance.

**Pathogenesis:** Several possibilities seem reasonable. First, there could be an absence of 1 coronary anlage or a development and subsequent involution of 1 anlage. The single artery which develops then would supply the entire myocardium by extension of and addition to its normal branches. Another possibility would be the development of 2 coronary artery anlagen in close proximity.

**Sex Ratio:** Presumably M1:F1

**Occurrence:** Probably less than 1:200 cases of congenital heart disease.

**Risk of Recurrence for Patient's Sib:** Unknown.

**Risk of Recurrence for Patient's Child:** Unknown.

**Age of Detectability:** From birth by aortic root angiography.

**Gene Mapping and Linkage:** Unknown.

**Prevention:** None known. Genetic counseling indicated.

**Treatment:** None indicated for isolated condition.

**Prognosis:** Excellent for the isolated condition. Prognosis for patients with associated cardiac defects is entirely related to the severity of these defects. Relationship to development of coronary atherosclerosis is undetermined.

**Detection of Carrier:** Unknown.

**References:**
Smith JC: Review of a single coronary artery with report of two cases. Circulation 1950; 1:1168.
Nora JJ, McNamara DG: Anomalies of the coronary arteries and coronary artery fistula. In: Watson H, ed: Paediatric cardiology. London: Lloyd-Luke, 1968:295.
Chaitman BR, et al.: Clinical, angiographic and hemodynamic findings in patients with anomalous origin of the coronary arteries. Circulation 1976; 53:122. *

GR002                                          **Thomas P. Graham, Jr.**

**Artery, umbilical cord, single**
  *See UMBILICAL CORD, SINGLE ARTERY*
**Arthritis, E family**
  *See SYNOVITIS, FAMILIAL HYPERTROPHIC*

## ARTHRITIS, RHEUMATOID                             2517

**Includes:**   Rheumatoid arthritis
**Excludes:**
   Ankylosing spondylitis (2516)
   Inflammatory osteoarthritis
   Juvenile rheumatoid arthritis

**Major Diagnostic Criteria:**   Morning stiffness, joint pain with swelling (arthritis), and subcutaneous nodules. The swelling involves one or more joints and is often symmetrical and polyarticular. Other common features include elevated erythrocyte sedimentation rate, inflammatory synovial fluid, positive test for rheumatoid factor, X-ray changes of joint space narrowing and erosions, and characteristic histopathologic changes of the synovium and rheumatoid nodule. These features are grouped into seven diagnostic criteria, and rheumatoid arthritis is diagnosed at three levels of certainty (classic, definite, probable) based on the number of criteria present (Arnett et al, 1988).

**Clinical Findings:**   Rheumatoid arthritis (RA) is a chronic systemic inflammatory disease, with the cardinal feature of arthritis involving the synovial joints as well as the surrounding tendons, ligaments, fascia, muscle, and bone. Inflammation of the synovium results in swelling, pain, stiffness, limitation of motion of the affected joints. Any synovial joint may be involved, but there is a predilection for the small joints of the hand and foot, with the exception of the distal interphalangeal joints, and the wrist. Extra-articular features are an integral part of the systemic nature of the disease and include rheumatoid nodules, vasculitis, hematologic abnormalities, and involvement of the heart, lungs, pleura, eyes, peripheral nerves, lymph nodes, and spleen. X-ray changes include periarticular osteoporosis, narrowing of the joint space secondary to loss of articular cartilage, and bony erosions. Rheumatoid factors are present in 70–90% of cases.

**Complications:**   Vary depending on the organ systems involved. For example, scleritis may lead to perforation of the eyeball. Presence of rheumatoid vasculitis leads to more serious complications such as cerebrovascular accident and bowel perforation. Cervical spine involvement may lead to spinal cord compression. Drugs used in the treatment of RA may also lead to specific complications (e.g. nephropathy due to gold, and hepatotoxicity due to methotrexate).

**Associated Findings:**   None known.

**Etiology:**   RA is a disease characterized by immunologic hyperreactivity and defective immunoregulation. Available data suggest that RA is a heterogenous disease with multiple genetic and environmental components involved in its development and expression. The responsible environmental agents have not been identified.
Evidence for a genetic component in RA is the familial clustering, with a one-to-five-fold increased risk for RA in first-degree relatives of an affected individual and the increased concordance among monozygotic twins when compared with dizygotic twins. Population studies show a positive association between seropositive RA and HLA-DR4 (relative risk of 3–6) and a weaker association with HLA-DR1. The HLA-Dw4 and HLA-Dw14 sub-

sets of HLA-DR4 appear to be important in the association. HLA-DR4 is the most common DR allele found with RA in family studies, but other DR alleles are found in some families. However, the association between DR4 and the disease susceptibility is not absolute. Recent studies using molecular probes suggest that the DR4 positive populations consist of several distinct subtypes.
Family studies show that affected sibs share their HLA haplotypes more often than expected, and linkage studies demonstrate significant linkage between RA and HLA, suggesting the presence of an RA susceptibility gene (or genes) in the HLA-DR region on chromosome 6. Immunoglobulin G (Gm) allotypes (specifically Gm2) are associated with RA, particularly when the HLA type of the affected individual is considered, suggesting the presence of a separate RA susceptibility gene (or genes) on chromosome 14, which interacts with the susceptibility gene or genes in the HLA region.
The concept of genetic heterogeneity of RA is supported by the differences in seropositive and seronegative RA. Seropositive RA is more severe and is associated with HLA-DR4, while seronegative RA is associated with HLA-DR1. The frequency of RA in first-degree relatives is 2–16% for seropositive probands and 1–6% for seronegative probands. Immunoglobulin G (Gm) allotypes are associated with HLA-DR4 and seropositive RA, and not with seronegative RA. Further genetic heterogeneity of RA is suggested in a subgroup of seropositive individuals who have circulating antibodies to native type II collagen, and an increased frequency of HLA-DR3 or HLA-DR7 rather than HLA-DR4.
The current view is that the immunoglobulin supergene family is involved in the predisposition to many rheumatic diseases.

**Pathogenesis:**   The cellular pathology of rheumatoid synovium is characterized by synovial lining cell hyperplasia, proliferation of vasculature with inflammation of the vessel walls, formation of villi infiltrated with lymphocytes and plasma cells and pannus infiltrating and destroying the articular cartilage. Based on these observations, RA may be considered a disease mediated by immune complexes, altered cellular immunity, or both.

**MIM No.:**   18030

**Sex Ratio:**   Variable, depending on age of onset. Ranges betwee M1:F1.3 to M1:F6.8.

**Occurrence:**   RA is found in all parts of the world and in all ethnic groups. The prevalence in approximately 0.5–3.0%, depending on the population and the diagnostic criteria used.

**Risk of Recurrence for Patient's Sib:**   Risk for first-degree relatives is increased by a factor of 1–5.

**Risk of Recurrence for Patient's Child:**   Risk for first-degree relatives is increased by a factor of 1–5.

**Age of Detectability:**   Onset may be at any age, but is usually between the ages of 35 and 60 years. The frequency increases with age.

**Gene Mapping and Linkage:**   Unknown.

**Prevention:**   None known. Genetic counseling indicated.

**Treatment:**   Same as for nonfamilial RA; nonsteroidal antiinflammatory agents and slow-acting antirheumatic drugs (e.g., gold). Other treatment modalities in use include corticosteroids and methotrexate. The presence of HLA-DR3 may improve the response and increase the risk of developing proteinuria or thrombocytopenia with gold therapy.

**Prognosis:**   The course of RA is unpredictable. The severity of RA is increased by the presence of rheumatoid factor (seropositive RA), erosions present at the time of diagnosis, and extra-articular manifestations, including rheumatoid nodules and vasculitis. Mortality is increased in RA, in part due to complications of treatment. Genetic studies do not identify an inherited component of prognosis, except for the association of HLA-DR4 with seropositive RA.

**Detection of Carrier:**   Unknown. HLA studies of family members are not useful for genetic counseling at the present time.

**Special Considerations:**   The phenotypic expression of RA should be viewed as a multifactorial process. The genetic components include HLA-DR (and Gm)-linked susceptibility genes. The environmental components have not been identified. Experimental animal models of arthritis include streptococcal cell-wall induced and collagen induced arthritis in rats.

**Support Groups:** Atlanta; Arthritis Foundation

**References:**
Lawrence JS: Rheumatoid arthritis-native or nurture. Ann Rheum Dis 1970; 29:357–379.
Harris ED, Jr.: Rheumatoid arthritis: the clinical spectrum. In: Kelly WN, et al, eds: Textbook of rheumatology. Philadelphia: W.B. Saunders, 1985:915–950.
Jaraquemada D, et al.: HLA and rheumatoid arthritis: a combined analysis of 440 British patients. Ann Rheum Dis 1986; 45:627–636.
Nepom GT, et al.: Identification of HLA-Dw4 genes in DR4 + rheumatoid arthritis. Lancet 1986; II:1002–1005.
Woodrow JL: Analysis of the HLA association with rheumatoid arthritis. Dis Marker 1986; 4:7–12.
van Kercklove C, Glass DN: The immunoglobulin supergene family and the polygenic nature of inherited predisposition to rheumatic disease. Arth Rheum 1987; 30:951–953.
Walker DJ, et al.: Linkage studies of HLA and rheumatoid arthritis in multicase families. Arthritis Rheum 1987; 30:31–35.
Arnett FC, et al.: The ARA 1987 revised criteria for classification of rheumatoid arthritis. Arthritis Rheum 1988; 31:315–324.
Bull BS, et al.: Efficacy of tests used to monitor rheumatoid arthritis. Lancet 1989; II:965–967.
Riskin WG, et al.: Amiprilose hydrochloride for rheumatoid arthritis. Ann Intern Med 1989; 111:455–465.

KI007      **Richard A. King**

---

## ARTHRITIS-ARTERITIS SYNDROME    2122

**Includes:**
Arteritis-arthritis syndrome
Granulomatous arteritis-polyarthritis of juvenile onset
Tenosynovitis, progressive-contractures-systemic involvement

**Excludes:**
**Arthritis, rheumatoid** (2517)
Churg-Strauss vasculitis
**Immunodeficiency, hyper IgE type** (2211)
Polyarteritis nodosa
Takayasu arteritis
Temporal arteritis

**Major Diagnostic Criteria:** Juvenile-onset polyarthritis and granulomatous arteritis.

**Clinical Findings:** Polyarthritis (100%), with or without symptomatic inflammation, begins in childhood; sometimes as early as the second year of life. The hands, ankles, elbows, and knees seem to be most involved, in that order. Relapsing fever may accompany the arthritis, but is not always evident. Granulomatous arteritis has been found in all studied cases but does not always produce obvious signs and symptoms. Mononuclear and eosinophilic giant cells are found in many tissues, particularly heart, kidney, and aorta. Iritis was present in at least 33% of cases, with formation of synechiae and significant visual impairment in some. A nonspecific skin rash has been observed occasionally. No specific laboratory tests have been identified, and the usual serologic tests for collagen vascular disease are uniformly negative.

**Complications:** Joint contractures, periarticular osteoporosis, hypertension, and synechiae.

**Associated Findings:** None known.

**Etiology:** Possibly autosomal dominant inheritance.

**Pathogenesis:** Unknown.

**MIM No.:** 10805

**Sex Ratio:** Presumably M1:F1

**Occurrence:** Less than a dozen cases have been documented.

**Risk of Recurrence for Patient's Sib:**
See Part I, *Mendelian Inheritance.*

**Risk of Recurrence for Patient's Child:**
See Part I, *Mendelian Inheritance.*

**Age of Detectability:** Early to mid-childhood, in most cases.

**Gene Mapping and Linkage:** Unknown.

**Prevention:** None known. Genetic counseling indicated.

**Treatment:** One patient appeared to improve following corticosteroid and cyclophosphamide therapy.

**Prognosis:** Variable. One affected case survived into the seventh decade, but death within the first five years of life has occurred, apparently secondary to severe coronary arteritis. The extent of disability from arthritis varies from minimal to severe; vasculitis is often asymptomatic but can produce life-threatening hypertension.

**Detection of Carrier:** Unknown.

**Special Considerations:** This disorder does not seem to have any associations with specific HLA types, and the complement system does not demonstrate significant derangement.

**Support Groups:** Atlanta; Arthritis Foundation

**References:**
Di Liberti JH, et al.: Progressive tenosynovitis with contractures and possible systemic involvement--a new heritable disorder of connective tissue? BD:OAS XI(6). New York: March of Dimes birth Defects Foundation, 1975:81–82.
Rotenstein D, et al.: Familial granulomatous arteritis with polyarthritis of juvenile onset. New Engl J Med 1982; 306:86–90.
Di Liberti JH: Granulomatous vasculitis. (Letter) New Engl J Med 1982; 306:1365 only.

DI001      **John H. Di Liberti**

**'Arthritis-like' condition-short stature**
  *See WINCHESTER SYNDROME*
**Arthritis-pericarditis-camptodactyly**
  *See PERICARDITIS-ARTHRITIS-CAMPTODACTYLY*
**Arthro-dento-osteodysplasia**
  *See HAJDU-CHENEY SYNDROME*

---

## ARTHRO-OPHTHALMOPATHY, HEREDITARY, PROGRESSIVE, STICKLER TYPE    0090

**Includes:**
Epiphyseal changes and high myopia
Ophthalmoarthropathy
Progressive arthro-ophthalmopathy
Robin anomaly (some)
Stickler syndrome

**Excludes:**
**Arthro-ophthalmopathy, Weissenbacher-Zweymuller variant** (2424)
**Ehlers-Danlos syndrome** (0338)
**Epiphyseal dysplasia, multiple** (0358)
**Kniest dysplasia** (0557)
**Marfan syndrome** (0630)
**Oto-spondylo-megaepiphyseal dysplasia** (2304)
**Spondyloepiphyseal dysplasia congenita** (0897)
**Spondyloepiphyseal dysplasia, late** (0898)
**Retina, hyaloideoretinal degeneration of Wagner** (0479)

**Major Diagnostic Criteria:** Congenital myopia with vitreoretinal changes in combination with epiphyseal changes on X-rays.

**Clinical Findings:** The primary ocular features are moderate-to-high myopia, radial perivascular lattice, and fluid vitreous with peripheral condensations manifesting as circular bands. Total retinal detachments occur in more than one-half of the patients spontaneously, often in the first two decades of life or after extraction of presenile cataracts. Intractable glaucoma may be an associated finding.

The joint manifestations may be recognizable at birth by bony enlargement of certain joints, especially ankles, knees, and wrists. Often these changes are subtle and seen only on X-ray examination. During childhood, stiffness and soreness occur after overuse;

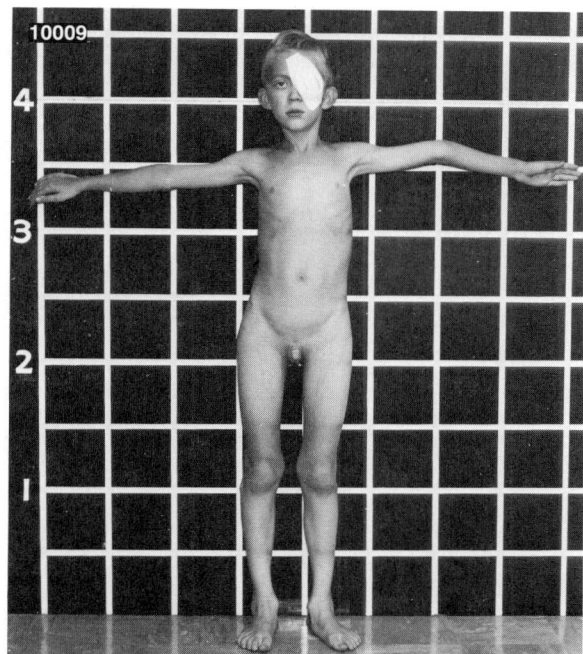

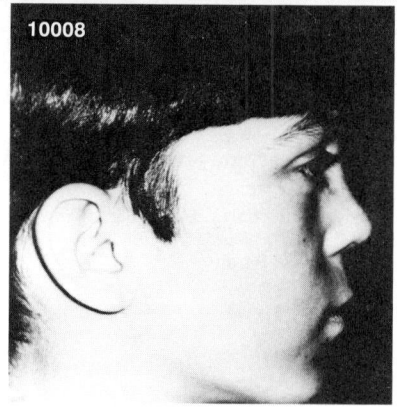

**0090**-10009: Affected male has characteristic slender body conformation, joint hyperextensibility, genu valgum and flat feet; a left retinal detachment is bandaged postoperatively. 10008: Lateral view of facies shows the flat mid-face.

swelling, redness, and heat occur occasionally, leading to crepitation and temporary locking of the joints. The most severely involved joints are hips, ankles, and wrists. Hypermobility is observed in some of the affected individuals. They may have a marfanoid habitus. Other individuals may appear short and stocky, and often have unusual facies with flattening of the nasal bridge. There is an increased incidence of sensorineural hearing loss. **Cleft palate-micrognathia-glossoptosis** (Robin anomaly) are common. The skin is normal clinically and histologically. Laboratory findings are within normal limits. On X-ray evaluation flattening of the epiphyseal ossification centers is seen.

**Complications:** Total blindness after the first decade and progressive mild to severe arthropathy.

**Associated Findings:** None known.

**Etiology:** Autosomal dominant inheritance with variable expressivity.

**Pathogenesis:** Probably part of a heterogeneous disease group involving collagen abnormalities.

**MIM No.:** *10830

**POS No.:** 3030

**CDC No.:** 759.860

**Sex Ratio:** M1:F1

**Occurrence:** Estimated 1:20,000 people.

**Risk of Recurrence for Patient's Sib:**
See Part I, *Mendelian Inheritance*.

**Risk of Recurrence for Patient's Child:**
See Part I, *Mendelian Inheritance*.

**Age of Detectability:** Shortly after birth in case of positive family history or Robin anomaly.

**Gene Mapping and Linkage:** AOM (arthroophthalmopathy, progressive (Stickler syndrome)) has been mapped to 12q14.

**Prevention:** None known. Genetic counseling indicated.

**Treatment:** Avoidance of excessive exertion including contact sports. Repeat examination for early detection of retinal detachments. Management of cataracts and glaucoma as required. For neonatal management of micrognathia and cleft palate (Robin Anomaly), see **Cleft palate-Micrognathia-Glossoptosis** If sensorineural hearing loss is present special training and amplification should be considered.

**Prognosis:** Normal for life span and intelligence. Visual disability exists in the majority of cases after age 10 years. Joint mobility and ambulation are preserved throughout life.

**Detection of Carrier:** Mild vitreous liquefaction in positive families.

**Special Considerations:** Opitz (1972) has postulated that Stickler syndrome is a common cause of severe myopia and Robin anomaly and may be more common than the **Marfan syndrome**.
It has been suggested Stickler syndrome is expressed in the neonate as **Arthro-ophthalmopathy, Weissenbacher-Zweymuller variant**, and McKusick's *Mendelian Inheritance in Man* assigns the two conditions to the same number. Other authors maintain that these are distinct conditions.
Herrmann, et al. (1975) have suggested that the Stickler syndrome may have affected Abraham Lincoln and his son, Tad, although others have felt that the Lincoln appearance was attributable to **Marfan syndrome**.

**References:**
Stickler GB, et al.: Hereditary progressive arthroophthalmopathy. Mayo Clin Proc 1965; 40:433–455.
Stickler GB, Pugh DG: Hereditary progressive arthro-ophthalmopathy: additional observations on vertebral abnormalities, a hearing defect, and a report of a similar case. Mayo Clin Proc 1967; 42:495–500.
Knobloch WH, Layer JM: Clefting syndromes associated with retinal detachment. Am J Ophthalmol 1972; 73:517.
Opitz JM, et al.: The Stickler syndrome. New Engl J Med 1972; 286:546–547.
Herrmann J, et al.: The Stickler syndrome (hereditary arthro-ophthalmopathy). BD:OAS XI(2). New York: March of Dimes Birth Defects Foundation, 1975:76–103.
Maumenee, IH: Vitreoretinal degeneration: a sign of generalized connective tissue diseases. Am J Ophthalmol 1979; 88:432–439.
Ayme S, Preus M: The Marshall and Stickler syndromes: objective rejection of lumping. J Med Genet 1984; 21:34–38.
Spallone A: Stickler's syndrome: a study of 12 families. Brit J Opthal 1987; 71:504–509.
Beighton P, et al.: International nosology of heritable disorders of connective tissue, Berlin, 1986. Am J Med Genet 1988; 29:581–594.

MA054                                          **Irene H. Maumenee**

## ARTHRO-OPHTHALMOPATHY, WEISSENBACHER-ZWEYMULLER VARIANT      2424

**Includes:** Weissenbacher-Zweymuller variant of arthro-ophthalmopathy

**Excludes:**
    **Arthro-ophthalmopathy, hereditary, progressive, Stickler type** (0090)
    **Deafness-myopia-cataract-saddle nose, Marshall type** (0261)
    Ophthalmopathy, other forms of hereditary
    **Oto-spondylo-megaepiphyseal dysplasia** (2304)

**Major Diagnostic Criteria:** Rhizomelic chrondrodysplasia with dumbbell-shaped femora and humeri; ophthalmopathy; hypoplasia of the maxilla. Clinical signs are evident during the newborn period. Regression of bone changes and normal growth occur in later years.

**Clinical Findings:** Rhizomelic chondrodysplasia and ophthalmopathy consisting of high myopia, with or without glaucoma and corneal clouding, may be the first presenting features. Other findings are hypoplasia of the maxilla; micrognathia, sometimes associated with **Cleft palate**; depressed nasal bridge and large anterior fontanelle; flattened occiput and short neck.

X-ray skeletal survey may reveal dumbbell-shaped long bones, flattened acetabular roofs, posterior defects in the vertebral bodies in the thoracic region, and platyspondyly. Mild muscle weakness, hyperextensible joints, moderate delay in development may be present in infancy.

Regression of bone changes and normal growth in later years has been described as part of the natural history of this disorder. Detailed family history and careful examination of all family members are essential.

**Complications:** Retinal detachment, glaucoma.

**Associated Findings:** Hypotonia, hyperextensible joints, moderate developmental delay, and hearing loss (in the patients who developed the Marshall phenotype).

**Etiology:** Autosomal dominant inheritance with variable expression.

**Pathogenesis:** Unknown.

**MIM No.:** *10830

**POS No.:** 3030

**Sex Ratio:** M1:F1

**Occurrence:** Undetermined but presumed rare. Several kindreds have been reported.

**Risk of Recurrence for Patient's Sib:**
See Part I, *Mendelian Inheritance.*

**Risk of Recurrence for Patient's Child:**
See Part I, *Mendelian Inheritance.*

**Age of Detectability:** Newborn period or early infancy. Prenatal diagnosis by ultrasonography may be possible.

**Gene Mapping and Linkage:** AOM (arthroophthalmopathy, progressive (Stickler syndrome)) has been mapped to 12q14.

**Prevention:** None known. Genetic counseling indicated.

**Treatment:** Management of the ophthalmopathy and its complications. Appropriate therapy programs in cases of developmental delay.

**Prognosis:** Normal life span. Potential visual impairment because of the ophthalmopathy and its complications.

**Detection of Carrier:** Careful clinical/ophthalmologic examination and history of all first degree relatives will help indicate those who are minimally affected.

**Special Considerations:** It has been suggested that the Weissenbacher-Zweymuller form is a neonatal expression of **Arthro-ophthalmopathy, hereditary, progressive, Stickler type** based on the findings characteristic for this syndrome in an infant from a family segregating for the Stickler phenotype. Also, the findings of the Weissenbacher-Zweymuller phenotype in three infants who subsequently developed **Deafness-myopia-cataract-saddle nose, Mar-**shall type support the suggestion that these conditions represent variable manifestations of the same gene. Other authors concluded that the Stickler, Marshall, and Weissenbacher-Zweymuller syndromes are separate entities.

**References:**
Weissenbacher G, Zweymuller E: Gleichzeitiges Vorkommen eines Syndroms von Pierre Robin und einer fetalen Chrondrodysplasie. Monatsschr Kinderheilkd 1964; 112:315–317.
Kelly TE, et al.: The Weissenbacher-Zweymuller syndrome: possible neonatal expression of the Stickler syndrome. Am J Med Genet 1982; 11:113–119. *
Winter RM, et al.: The Weissenbacher-Zweymuller, Stickler, and Marshall syndromes: further evidence for their identity. Am J Med Genet 1983; 16:189–199.
Ayme S, Preus M: The Marshall and Stickler syndromes: objective rejection of lumping. J Med Genet 1984; 21:34–38.
Scribanu N, et al.: Weissenbacher-Zweymuller phenotype in the neonatal period as an expression in the continuum of manifestations of the hereditary arthroophthalmopathies. Ophthalmol Paediatr Genet (Lond) 1987; 8:159–163.

SC052      **Nina Scribanu**

**Arthrochalasis multiplex congenita**
  *See EHLERS-DANLOS SYNDROME*
**Arthrodentoosteodysplasia**
  *See OSTEOLYSIS, ESSENTIAL*

## ARTHROGRYPOSES      0088

**Includes:**
    Arthrogryposes multiplex congenita
    Contractures, congenital arthrogrypotic type
    Guerin-Stern syndrome
    Joints, multiple congenital articular rigidities

**Excludes:**
    **Arachnodactyly, contractural Beals type** (0085)
    **Arthrogryposis, amyoplasia type** (2281)
    **Arthrogryposis, distal types** (2280)
    **Camptodactyly-trismus syndrome** (0882)
    **Cerebro-oculo-facio-skeletal syndrome** (0140)
    **Chromosome 18, trisomy 18** (0160)
    **Diastrophic dysplasia** (0293)
    Distal arthrogryposis
    **Kuskokwin syndrome** (0560)
    **Pena-Shokeir syndrome** (2080)
    **Pterygium** syndromes

**Major Diagnostic Criteria:** Congenital, usually nonprogressive limitation of joint movement in multiple sites.

**Clinical Findings:** Heterogeneous group of conditions, all with congenital nonprogressive limitation of movement in two or more joints in two or more body areas. Multiple congenital contractures are also seen in a number of etiologically distinguishable conditions (**Chromosome 18, trisomy 18, Renal agenesis, bilateral, Myotonic dystrophy, Meningomyelocele,** and so on). All combinations of flexion and extension deformities of joints can be found. Absence of normal skin creases and the presence of dimpling and webs over joints are commonly seen.

Three categories of arthrogryposis not secondary to recognizable syndromes can be distinguished: 1) primarily limb involvement; 2) limb joint limitation plus scoliosis, ptosis, cleft palate, generalized weakness, or other anomalies and malformations; and 3) limitation of joint movement associated with severe CNS disturbance. All three categories are heterogeneous.

**Complications:** Skeletal changes secondary to the original deformities, i.e. scoliosis and changes in shapes of carpal and tarsal bones. Delayed developmental landmarks because of limitation of movement. Breech presentation at birth. External genitalia may be abnormal depending on hip position (i.e. cryptorchid, or absent labia major). Limbs with long-standing contractures have undergrowth.

**Associated Findings:** Non-limb anomalies are seen almost entirely in categories 2 and 3.

**Etiology:** Possibly autosomal dominant inheritance.

**Pathogenesis:** Apparently anything causing decreased or absent limb movement in utero (neurogenic, myogenic, connective tissue, infection, space limitation, drugs) can lead to congenital contractures of the limbs. Generalized fetal akinesia also leads to polyhydramnios, pulmonary hypoplasia, micrognathia, ocular hypertelorism, and short umbilical cord.

**MIM No.:**  10811

**CDC No.:**  755.800

**Sex Ratio:**  M1:F1

**Occurrence:**  1–3:10,000.

**Risk of Recurrence for Patient's Sib:** If no specific diagnosis can be made the empiric risk is for category 1, 3–5%; category 2, 1–3%; category 3, 7–15%.

**Risk of Recurrence for Patient's Child:** If no specific diagnosis can be made, the empiric risk is about 4%.

**Age of Detectability:** At birth, or in utero by real-time ultrasound.

**Gene Mapping and Linkage:** Heterogeneous disorder, no known linkage.

**Prevention:** None known. Genetic counseling indicated.

**Treatment:** Aggressive physical therapy and multiple orthopedic procedures are often necessary.

**Prognosis:** Life span may be normal, but it is probably related to the degree of severity of involvement and the number of other malformations. In category 3, 50% die in the first year of life. Scoliosis may compromise respiratory function. Functional prognosis depends on persistence and emotional support by family and physician. Patients can do surprisingly well and live independently.

**Detection of Carrier:** Unknown.

**Special Considerations:** Arthrogryposis is term that has been used loosely in the past to refer to any congenital contracture. Etiologic heterogeneity is definitely present. It is most important to make an attempt to recognize and distinguish known syndromes for prognosis and genetic counseling.

**Support Groups:**
NY; North Bellemore; Arthrogryposis Multiplex Congenita Association
CA; Sonora (Box 5192); National Support Group for Arthrogryposis Multiplex Congenita (AVENUES)

**References:**
Hall JG: Arthrogryposes. In: Emery, Limoin, eds: Principles and practice of medical genetics. Edinburgh: Churchill Livingstone, 1983:781–811.
Hall JG: Genetic aspects of arthrogryposis. In: Thompson G, ed: Clinical orthopedics. Philadelphia: J.B. Lippincott, 1985:44–53.

HA014                                    **Judith G. Hall**

**Arthrogryposes multiplex congenita**
*See ARTHROGRYPOSES*
**Arthrogryposis multiplex congenita (AMC)**
*See ARTHROGRYPOSIS, AMYOPLASIA TYPE*
**Arthrogryposis multiplex congenita, distal type I**
*See ARTHROGRYPOSIS, DISTAL TYPES*
**Arthrogryposis multiplex congenita, distal type II**
*See ARTHROGRYPOSIS, DISTAL TYPES*
**Arthrogryposis multiplex congenita, distal, type IIA**
*See CAMPTODACTYLY-CLEFT PALATE-CLUB FOOT, GORDON TYPE*
**Arthrogryposis multiplex congenita-muscle involvement**
*See MUSCULAR DYSTROPHY, CONGENITAL WITH ARTHROGRYPOSIS*
**Arthrogryposis multiplex congenita-pulmonary hypoplasia**
*See PENA-SHOKEIR SYNDROME*

## ARTHROGRYPOSIS, AMYOPLASIA TYPE  2281

**Includes:** Arthrogryposis multiplex congenita (AMC)

**Excludes:** Arthrogryposis (other)

**Major Diagnostic Criteria:** Bilateral internally rotated shoulders, fixed extended elbows, and fixed wrists if arms involved; bilateral equinovarus position of feet if lower limbs involved. Marked hypoplasia of limb muscles replaced by fibrous and fatty tissue.

**Clinical Findings:** Appearance of bilaterally symmetric involvement with decreased muscle mass; lack of creases at either the elbows or knees, or both; a relative increase in subcutaneous fat in infancy; and rigidity of joints. There is a characteristic positioning of the limbs, internally rotated arms with downward-sloping shoulders, elbows extended straight in infancy but tending to become flexed with growth, a flexed wrist and cupped hands, short feet with severe equinovarus deformities, and other deformities such as dimpling over joints. Sixty-three percent of patients had this type of involvement with all four limbs involved; 24% had mainly upper limb involvement; and 13% had mainly lower limb involvement. The positions of the other major joints are more variable. Midface capillary hemangiomas are seen in at least 90% of the patients with all four limbs involved, 70% of those with upper limb involvement, and 10% with lower limb involvement. The face appears round with short anteverted nostrils and mild micrognathia. Other abnormalities include facial asymmetry, hypoplastic labia/scrotum, cryptorchidism. Hernias, scoliosis, and gastroschisis; bowel atresia or abdominal wall defect (about 10% of cases).

**Complications:** Breech presentation (30%); fractures at birth (10%).

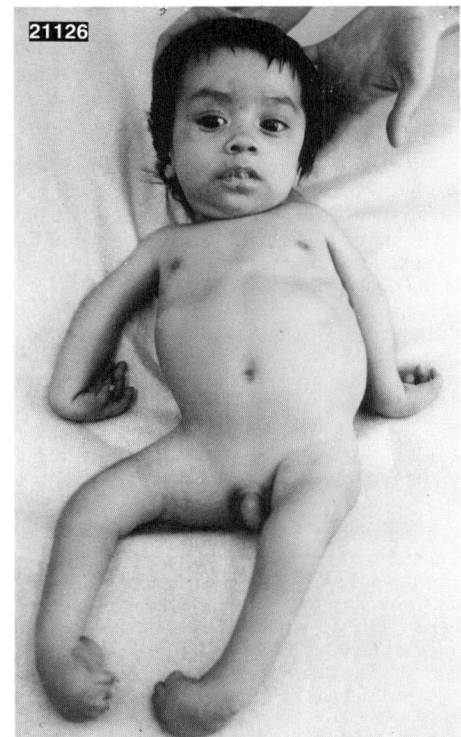

**2281-21126:** This child has typical amyoplasia. Note the symmetric involvement with internally rotated shoulders, extended elbows and flexed wrists as well as severe equinovarus deformity of the foot. The child also has a hemangioma over the glabella area.

**Associated Findings:** Five percent of reported patients were discordant monozygotic twins.

**Etiology:** A sporadic condition. There has been no recurrence of amyoplasia in the families of the 220 patients with amyoplasia studied; 11 discordantly affected monozygotic twins have been reported.

**Pathogenesis:** The presence of contractures at birth is undoubtedly related to decreased use or lack of limb movements in utero. In addition, amyoplasia is associated with muscle tissue loss at some point in development, probably early in the second trimester after the limb nerve and muscle tissues have already been formed.

**MIM No.:** 10811

**POS No.:** 3664

**CDC No.:** 755.800

**Sex Ratio:** M1:F1

**Occurrence:** Most common type of arthrogryposis; approximately 1:10,000 births.

**Risk of Recurrence for Patient's Sib:** Minimal.

**Risk of Recurrence for Patient's Child:** Minimal.

**Age of Detectability:** At birth, or prenatally by real-time ultrasound.

**Gene Mapping and Linkage:** Unknown.

**Prevention:** None known. Genetic counseling indicated.

**Treatment:** Therapy for and treatment of abdominal problems. Mobilize limbs early so that atrophy in the remaining muscles will be minimized. Aggressive physical and occupational therapy. Casting and immobilization may lead to greater muscle atrophy.

**Prognosis:** The limb deformities seen at birth undergo predictable, characteristic changes with growth. With decreased movement, bone growth is diminished, and the affected limbs of adults are shorter than is normal. Thus, if the limbs are not mobilized at birth, there will be less bone growth and less calcium deposited in bone than is normal.

**Detection of Carrier:** Unknown.

**Support Groups:**
NY; North Bellemore; Arthrogryposis Multiplex Congenita Association
CA; Sonora; National Support Group for Arthrogryposis Multiplex Congenita (AVENUES, P.O. Box 5192

**References:**
Hall JG, et al.: Amyoplasia: a common sporadic condition with congenital contractures. Am J Med Genet 1983; 15:571–590.
Hall JG, et al.: Amyoplasia: twinning in amyoplasia: a specific type of arthrogryposis with an apparent excess of discordant identical twins. Am J Med Genet 1983; 15:591–599.
Reid COMV, et al.: The association of amyoplasia with gastroschisis: bowel atresia and defects of the muscular layer of the trunk. Am J Med Genet 1986; 24:701–710.

HA014                                                    **Judith G. Hall**

**Arthrogryposis, digito-talar dysmorphism**
*See DIGITO-TALAR DYSMORPHISM*

---

## ARTHROGRYPOSIS, DISTAL TYPES                          **2280**

**Includes:**
Arthrogryposis multiplex congenita, distal type I
Arthrogryposis multiplex congenita, distal type II
Distal arthrogryposis

**Excludes:**
**Arthrogryposis, amyoplasia type** (2281)
**Arachnodactyly, contractural Beals type** (0085)
**Camptodactyly-cleft palate-club foot, Gordon type** (2396)
**Cranio-carpo-tarsal dysplasia, whistling face type** (0223)

**Major Diagnostic Criteria:** *Type I:* Tightly clenched fists at birth, with medially overlapping fingers; ulnar deviation and camptodactyly in adults, and positional foot deformities.
*Type II:* The association of congenital distal joint contractures with various additional manifestations in particular combinations.

**Clinical Findings:** *Type I:* The hand of the infant is characteristic. Typically, the hand is held in a tight fist with medial overlapping of the fingers, and the thumb is held tightly in adduction, usually across the palm. The position of the fingers is often similar to that seen in **Chromosome 18, trisomy 18**. The hands are involved in 98% of reported patients. The feet are often involved (88%), with about one-half of the patients having an equinovarus or calcaneovalgus deformity of one or both feet at birth. There may be varying degrees of congenital flexion contractures at elbows, knees, and hips.
*Type II:* This heterogeneous group of patients has been sorted into five groups on a phenotypic basis:
*Type IIA:* Gordon syndrome (see **Camptodactyly-cleft palate-club foot, Gordon type**). Almost all affected individuals have **Cleft palate**, short necks, submucous cleft or bifid uvula, **Camptodactyly**, and epicanthal folds. **Eyelid, ptosis, congenital** have also been reported.
*Type IIB:* The most distinctive manifestations are short stature, short neck, **Eyelid, ptosis, congenital**, a somewhat immobile facies

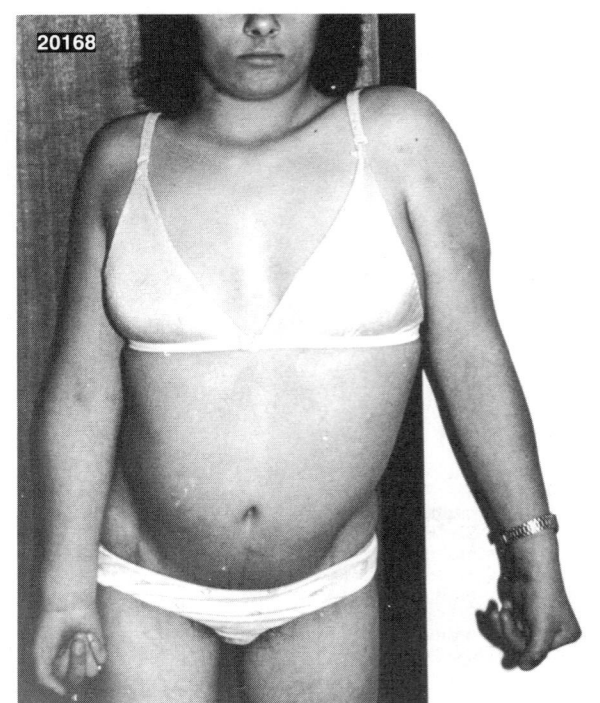

**2280A-20168:** Type II distal arthrogryposis; note scoliosis, short neck and hand contractures. The patient also had trismus, lower limb involvement and a VSD.

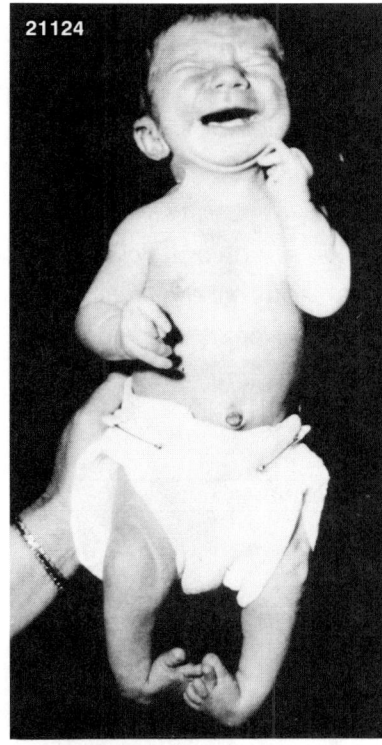

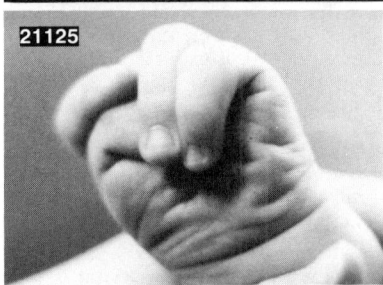

**2280B**-21124:  A child with typical distal arthrogryposis; note overlapping fingers which open ulnarly and primarily involved hands and feet.    21125:  A typical hand of distal arthrogryposis in the newborn period which is flexed with overlapping fingers. With time the hand opens out and deviates laterally.

with or without keratoconus, decreased range of ocular motion, and very smooth, shiny, tapering fingers with mild **Camptodactyly**.

*Type IIC:* Ch017arcterized by a combination of distal contractures and cleft lip and/or palate. The most notable contractures affect the feet with equinovarus deformity of the feet. The presence of cleft lip and lack of short stature seem to separate this from the other type II groups.

*Type IID:* Characterized by congenital contractures with scoliosis and without shortness of stature, **Cerebral palsy, Eyelid, ptosis, congenital**, epicanthal folds, keratoconus, immobile face, or **Cleft lip**.

*Type IIE:* May be identified by an unusual hand configuration of **Camptodactyly** with hyperextension of the metacarpo-phalangeal joint, distal flexion contractures, and limited jaw movement. Contractures of the feet are also seen in all affected patients. In addition, there may be developmentally delayed when compared to other family members.

**Complications:**  Without physical therapy, contractures may progress. The patient should be monitored for scoliosis.

**Associated Findings:**   A variety of other anomalies can be seen in the type II form.

**Etiology:**  *Type I and Type IIA*: Probably autosomal dominant inheritance with variable expressivity.

*Type II*: Depends on the subtype, but most are also thought to be autosomal dominant. Sporadic cases have been reported, particularly in association with increased paternal age. The Trismus seen in Type IIE is a sporadic condition.

**Pathogenesis:**  In theory, anything that leads to decreased limb movements *in utero* can result in congenital joint contractures. The contractures in distal arthrogryposis Type I appear to be due to misplaced, hypoplastic, or absent tendons. Scoliosis could be due to a weakness in musculature supporting the spine, or misplaced muscle attachments. An imbalance of misplaced tendons, and fibrosis and atrophy of muscles, play an important role in producing *in utero* contractures. There is heterogeneity in the etiology and pathogenesis of these disorders.

**MIM No.:**  10812, 10813

**POS No.:**  3166, 3388

**CDC No.:**  755.800

**Sex Ratio:**  M1:F1

**Occurrence:**  Some 35 kinships, with over 150 individuals, have been reported.

**Risk of Recurrence for Patient's Sib:**
See Part I, *Mendelian Inheritance.*

**Risk of Recurrence for Patient's Child:**
See Part I, *Mendelian Inheritance.*

**Age of Detectability:**  At birth. Prenatal diagnosis using real-time ultrasound has been successful.

**Gene Mapping and Linkage:**  Unknown.

**Prevention:**  None known. Genetic counseling indicated.

**Treatment:**  Physical and occupational therapy, with surgery where indicated.

**Prognosis:**  Good if proper management is followed from birth. Stretching exercises should be started on hands and feet at birth, before disuse atrophy occurs. Surgery may be indicated for clefting, cord releases, tendon tansfers, and club feet.

**Detection of Carrier:**  Unknown.

**Support Groups:**
NY; North Bellemore; Arthrogryposis Multiplex Congenita Association
CA; Sonora; National Support Group for Arthrogryposis Multiplex Congenita (AVENUES, P.O. Box 5192

**References:**
Hall JG et al.: The distal arthrogryposis: delineation of new entities - review and nosologic discussion. Am J Med Genet 1982; 11:185–239. * †
Kawira EL, Bender HA: An unusual distal arthrogryposis. Am J Med Genet 1985; 20:425–429.
Reiss JA, Sheffield LJ: Distal arthrogryposis type II: a family with varying congenital abnormalities. Am J Med Genet 1986; 24:255–267. * †

HA014                                                            **Judith G. Hall**

**Arthrogryposis-like disorder**
*See KUSKOKWIN SYNDROME*
**Arthrogryposis-like hand anomaly-sensorineural deafness**
*See MUSCLE WASTING OF HANDS-SENSORINEURAL DEAFNESS*
**Arthroosteoonychodysplasia**
*See NAIL-PATELLA SYNDROME*
**Arthropathies of ulcerative colitis**
*See ANKYLOSING SPONDYLITIS*
**Arthropathy-camptodactyly syndrome**
*See SYNOVITIS, FAMILIAL HYPERTROPHIC*
**Arthropathy-rash-uveitis-mental retardation**
*See INFLAMMATORY DISEASE, NEONATAL BATES-LORBER TYPE*

## ARTICULAR HYPERMOBILITY, FAMILIAL 3220

**Includes:**
Ehlers-Danlos syndrome XI (obsolete)
Familial articular hypermobility, uncomplicated type
Familial articular hypermobility, dislocating type
Joint instability, familial
Joint laxity, familial

**Excludes:**
**Ehlers-Danlos syndrome** (0338)
**Larsen syndrome** (0570)

**Major Diagnostic Criteria:** Abnormal range of movements in the joints without skin involvement. Two major groups of Familial Articular Hypermobility Syndrome (FAHS) are recognised: (a) Familial articular hypermobility, uncomplicated type, and (b) Familial articular hypermobility, dislocating type.

**Clinical Findings:** The hallmark of this heterogeneous group of disorders is hypermobility of joints in the absence of skin hyperextensibility or connective tissue fragility. The mildest forms overlap with normal limits, while at the severe end of the spectrum variable orthopaedic complications include subluxations and dislocation of joints. Malalignment of the spine may occur.

FAHS was initially designated "Ehlers-Danlos syndrome XI". The absence of skin fragility or hyperextensibility resulted in this designation being removed at the Symposium for Heritable Diseases of Connective Tissue in Berlin in 1986 (Beighton et al, 1988); the category EDS XI now remains vacant and the Familial Articular Hypermobility Syndromes are now accepted in their own right. The basic defect is unknown, and no diagnostic tests are available.

**Complications:** Complications of joint laxity: recurrent dislocations, subluxation, spinal malalignment, pes planus, sprains, and effusions.

**Associated Findings:** An association between FAHS and **Mitral valve prolapse** has been recognised.

**Etiology:** Autosomal dominant inheritance. An autosomal recessive variant of the uncomplicated form has been suggested.

**Pathogenesis:** Probable collagen abnormality.

**MIM No.:** *14790

**Sex Ratio:** M1:F1

**Occurrence:** Since the condition overlaps with the normal range of joint mobility, its occurrence remains undetermined but presumed common.

**Risk of Recurrence for Patient's Sib:**
See Part I, *Mendelian Inheritance.*

**Risk of Recurrence for Patient's Child:**
See Part I, *Mendelian Inheritance.*

**Age of Detectability:** During infancy.

**Gene Mapping and Linkage:** Unknown.

**Prevention:** None known. Genetic counseling indicated.

**Treatment:** Orthopedic management.

**Prognosis:** Life span not reduced.

**Detection of Carrier:** Unknown.

**References:**
Hass J, Hass R: Arthrochalasis multiplex congenita. J Bone Joint Surg 1958; 40:663–674.
Carter C, Sweetnam R: Recurrent dislocation of the patella and of the shoulder, their association with familial joint laxity. J Bone Joint Surg 1960; 42:721–727.
Beighton P, Horan FT: Dominant inheritance in familial generalized articular hypermobility. J Bone Joint Surg 1970; 52B:145–147.
Horan FT, Beighton P: Recessive inheritance of generalized joint hypermobility. Rhumatol and Rehab, 1973; 12:47–49.
Horton WA, et al.: Familial joint instability syndrome. Am J Med Genet 1980; 6:221–228.
Beighton P, et al.: Hypermobility of joints, 2nd ed. Heidelberg: Springer-Verlag, 1983.
Beighton P, et al.: International Nosology of Heritable Disorders of connective Tissue, Berlin, 1986. Am J Med Genet 1988; 29:581–594.

WI055 **Ingrid M. Winship**

**Aryl hydrocarbon hydroxylase**
*See CANCER, LUNG, FAMILIAL*
**Arylsulfatase A deficiency**
*See METACHROMATIC LEUKODYSTROPHIES*
**Arylsulfatase B deficiency**
*See MUCOPOLYSACCHARIDOSIS VI*
**Ascending aorta, origin of pulmonary artery**
*See PULMONARY ARTERY, ORIGIN FROM ASCENDING AORTA*
**Ascher syndrome**
*See BLEPHAROCHALASIS-DOUBLE LIP-NONTOXIC GOITER*
**Aseptic necrosis**
*See JOINTS, OSTEOCHONDRITIS DISSECANS*
**Asexual ateleotic dwarfism**
*See DWARFISM, PANHYPOPITUITARY*
**Askin tumor**
*See CANCER, EWING SARCOMA*

## ASPARTYLGLUCOSAMINURIA 2042

**Includes:** Aspartylglycosaminuria

**Excludes:**
**Mannosidosis** (2079)
**Mucolipidosis I** (0671)
**Mucolipidosis II** (0672)
**Mucolipidosis III** (0673)
**Mucopolysaccharidosis**
**Salla disease** (2041)

**Major Diagnostic Criteria:** As indicated by the name, aspartylglucosaminuria patients excrete abnormal amounts of aspartylglucosamine (2-acetamido-1-β-L-aspartamido-1,2-dideoxy-β-D-glucose). Several urinary tests have been developed to detect the presence or absence of increased amounts of this compound as a means of screening for the disorder. The definitive diagnosis of aspartylglucosaminuria is based on the demonstration of a deficiency of the lysosomal enzyme aspartylglucosaminidase (AGA) in any of several tissues or fluids, i.e., blood lymphocytes, plasma, cultured skin fibroblasts, cultured amniocytes, or chorionic villus sample.

**Clinical Findings:** Pregnancy and neonatal courses are, in general, uneventful. During childhood, enlargement of the pharyngeal tonsils and umbilical and inguinal hernias are frequently found. Facial features and psychomotor development are usually within normal limits during the first 1–2 years. Delayed speech formation is often the first sign of mental retardation. Motor clumsiness and behavioral changes may also be early manifestations of the disease. By ages six to eight years, all patients are mildly to moderately retarded. The facial features coarsen slowly during the next 5–10 years. In older patients, the nasal bridge is low; the mouth and the tongue are large; and the lips are often thick. The eyes are normal; hepatomegaly and splenomegaly usually do not occur. Although the mental and somatic deterioration in aspartylglucosaminuria is rather slow, life span appears to be shortened. A generalized bone dysplasia, which resembles mild forms of mucopolysaccharidosis and is most prominent in the long bones, becomes evident simultaneously with the appearance of the characteristic facial features. Approximately 5 to 10% of the peripheral blood lymphocytes show vacuolation, and enlarged lysosomes can be seen in the various cells of the skin, liver, kidney, and central nervous system. All patients appear to excrete increased amounts of aspartylglucosamine in the urine. Aspartylglucosamine is also the main material accumulating in various tissues in this disease.

**Complications:** Respiratory infections are common during infancy and early childhood. Death is usually caused by bacterial or viral infections before age 50 years.

**Associated Findings:** None known.

**Etiology:** Autosomal recessive inheritance.

**Pathogenesis:** The lysosomal enzyme 1-aspartamido-$\beta$-N-acetyl-glucosamine aminohydrolase (AGA), E.C. 3.5.1.26, is deficient. This enzyme is responsible for splitting the N-acetylglucosaminyl-asparagine linkage, which is a common structure in several glycoproteins. Defective degradation leads to lysosomal accumulation of aspartylglucosamine in the central nervous system and visceral organs.

**MIM No.:** *20840

**Sex Ratio:** M1:F1

**Occurrence:** The gene frequency for this disorder is relatively high in the Finnish population (1:100 to 1:200). About 200 patients are known in Finland (population, 4.9 million), seven in Norway (of Finnish origin), and at least 11 elsewhere, including one American black and one Native American.

**Risk of Recurrence for Patient's Sib:**
See Part I, *Mendelian Inheritance.*

**Risk of Recurrence for Patient's Child:**
See Part I, *Mendelian Inheritance.*

**Age of Detectability:** Clinical signs usually appear after the second year of life. Onset of urinary aspartylglucosamine excretion precedes clinical manifestations. The enzyme defect is identifiable in utero in cultured amniotic fluid cells. First trimester prenatal diagnosis is possible.

**Gene Mapping and Linkage:** AGA (aspartylglucosaminidase) has been mapped to 4q21-qter.

**Prevention:** None known. Genetic counseling indicated.

**Treatment:** No specific therapy is available. Supportive therapy should be similar to that given any child with a progressive CNS disease.

**Prognosis:** Life span is shortened, usually to ages 30–40 years. Death is usually caused by infection.

**Detection of Carrier:** The AGA assay in peripheral blood lymphocytes (but not in plasma or unfractionated leukocytes) separates heterozygotes from normal individuals.

**References:**
Aula P, et al.: Enzymatic diagnosis and carrier detection of aspartyl-glucosaminuria using blood samples. Pediatr Res 1976; 10:625–629.
Isenberg JN, Sharp HL: Aspartylglucosaminuria-psychomotor retardation masquerading as a mucopolysaccharidosis. J Pediatr 1975; 86:713–717.
Maury P: Accumulation of two glycoasparagines in the liver in aspartylglycosaminuria. J Biol Chem 1979; 254:1513–1515.
Palo J, et al.: Glycoasparagine metabolites in patients with aspartyl-glycosaminuria: comparison between English and Finnish patients with special reference to storage materials. Clin Chim Acta 1973; 47:69–74.
Pollitt RJ, et al.: Aspartylglycosaminuria: an inborn error of metabolism associated with mental defect. Lancet 1968; II:253–255.
Hreidarsson S, et al.: Aspartylglucosaminuria in the United States. Clin Genet 1983; 23:427–435.
Aula P, et al.: Prenatal diagnosis and fetal pathology of aspartylglu-cosaminuria. Am J Med Genet 1984; 19:359–367.
Chitayat D, et al.: Aspartylglucosaminuria in a Puerto Rican family: additional features of a panethnic disorder. Am J Med Genet 1988; 31:527–532.

AU001
TH021
RE016
SI016

**Pertti Aula**
**George H. Thomas**
**Martin Renlund**
**Olli G. Simell**

**Aspartylglycosaminuria**
*See ASPARTYLGLYCOSAMINURIA*

## ASPHYXIATING THORACIC DYSPLASIA 0091

**Includes:**
Asphyxiating thoracic dystrophy
Jeune syndrome
Thoracic dysplasia, asphyxiating
Thoracic-pelvic-phalangeal dystrophy

**Excludes:**
**Chondroectodermal dysplasia** (0156)
**Metatropic dysplasia** (0656)
**Mucolipidosis II** (0672)
**Thanatophoric dysplasia** (0940)

**Major Diagnostic Criteria:** The narrow thorax and short limbs are present at birth. Respiratory distress is a clue to the diagnosis, which can be made only by careful X-ray study of the thorax, pelvis, and long bones. Although involvement of the pelvis may not be a consistent finding, its absence must cast some doubt upon the diagnosis. Key X-ray findings are short horizontal ribs, square iliac wings, and horizontal acetabular roof with a medial

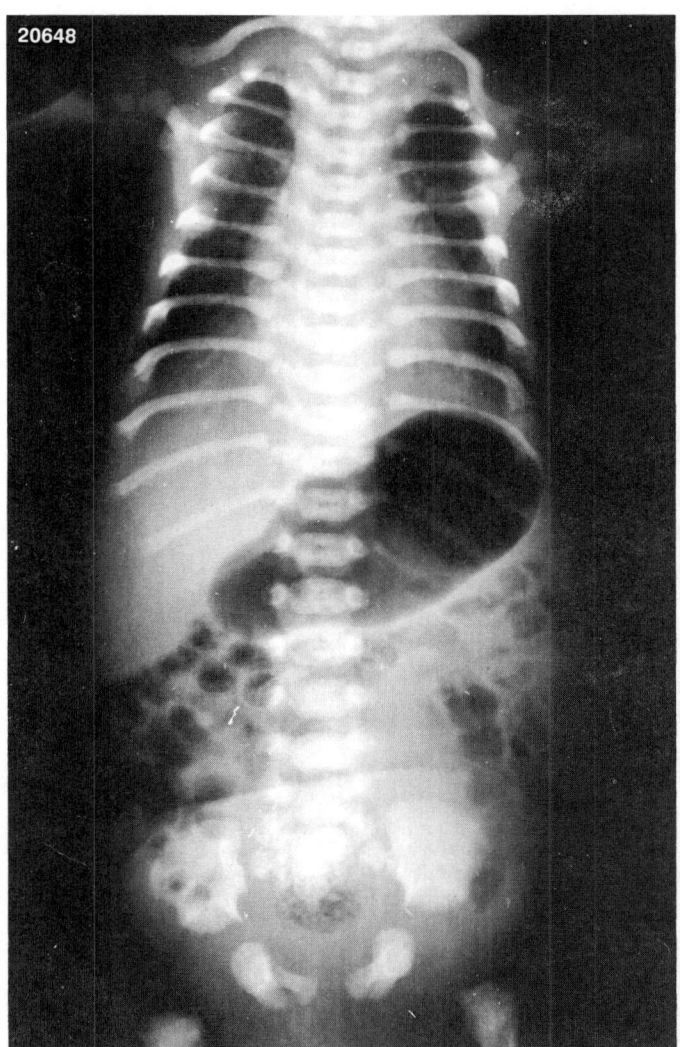

**0091A-20648:** Asphyxiating thoracic dysplasia in a newborn; note small thoracic cage, and trident appearance of the acetabular margin.

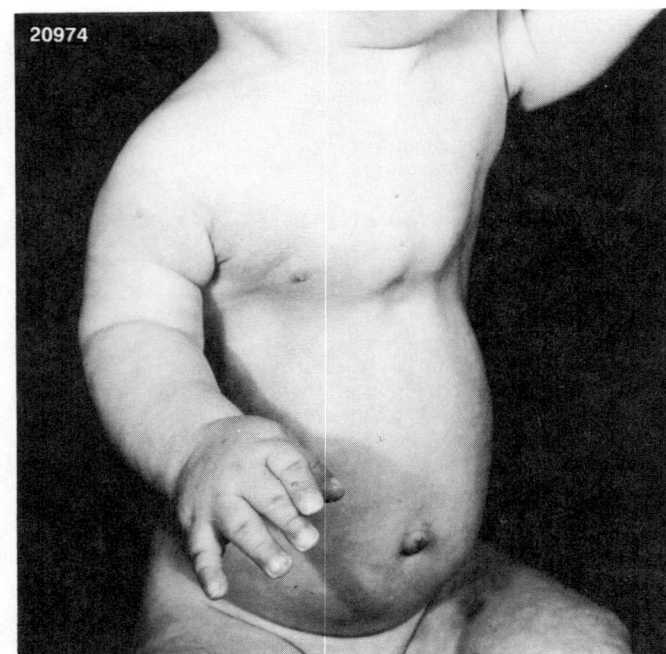

**0091B-20974**: Small, narrow chest with short ribs and pectus carinatum.

spur-shaped projection. The long bones are short and stubby with some irregular metaphyses.

**Clinical Findings:** Asphyxiating thoracic dysplasia can be diagnosed at birth by a careful physical examination and a high index of suspicion. Findings include a narrow thorax, in contrast to the shortness of the limbs. However, diagnosis of the condition is more often not made until the onset of respiratory distress, which usually occurs in the early months of life in association with an upper respiratory infection. The narrowness and immobility of the thorax leads to tachypnea and cyanosis. Expandability of the thorax is so severely limited that respiration is diaphragmatic. The limbs appear short in comparison to the trunk, but the morphology of the limbs is not otherwise altered. The craniofacial morphology is also normal. In occasional cases, some polydactyly may be observed.

Asphyxiating thoracic dysplasia is often rapidly fatal in spite of intensive therapeutic measures. Some less severe cases survive, and some rare cases are latent (Sandomenico et al., 1981). Functional respiratory problems do not always occur. In such cases, the diagnosis is possible only upon X-ray examination. The X-rays show shortening of the ribs, which is particularly evident on the lateral view of the thorax. The ribs are horizontal, short, and stubby, and the anterior portions of the ribs are widened.

The characteristic appearance of the pelvis aids in confirmation of the diagnosis of asphyxiating thoracic dysplasia. The iliac wings are square, the roof of the acetabulum is horizontal, and its medial portion is deformed by a rounded protuberance limited on each side by a spur-shaped projection.

The long bones are in some cases somewhat short and stubby, and the metaphyseal ends may be irregular. Often X-rays reveal a small spine on the distal metaphysis of the humerus or on the proximal end of the tibia. The bones of the hands and feet are minimally involved; however, cone-shaped epiphyses may be observed. In patients who survive, the metaphyseal lesions of the long bones usually become more apparent, especially at the proximal end of the femur. On the other hand, asymmetry of the tibial plateau and fusion of the carpal bones are not observed as they are in **Chondroectodermal dysplasia** (Cortina et al., 1979).

**Complications:** In addition to the severe respiratory problems that are characteristic of the condition, Herdman and Langer (1968) have noted the occurrence of complicating renal insufficiency with proteinuria and hypertension in surviving patients.

**Associated Findings:** None known.

**Etiology:** Autosomal recessive inheritance.

**Pathogenesis:** Undetermined. The functional respiratory problems are the result of a structural defect involving narrowness and immobility of the thoracic cage. Histologic study of the costochondral junctions reveals an oblique growth line with alteration of the cartilaginous portion. These alterations allow the condition to be classed as a form of chondrodysplasia. The lesions of the kidney are variable. In some cases the picture is not unlike that seen in nephronophtisia. In other cases, polycystic disease of the kidney is present.

**MIM No.:** *20850

**POS No.:** 3032

**CDC No.:** 756.400

**Sex Ratio:** M1:F1

**Occurrence:** Undetermined. Limited primarily to Caucasians.

**Risk of Recurrence for Patient's Sib:**
See Part I, *Mendelian Inheritance.*

**Risk of Recurrence for Patient's Child:**
See Part I, *Mendelian Inheritance.*

**Age of Detectability:** The condition may be recognized in the newborn period through clinical ultrasound.

**Gene Mapping and Linkage:** Unknown.

**Prevention:** None known. Genetic counseling indicated.

**Treatment:** Respiratory infections should be treated promptly and vigorously. Affected infants should be immunized early against such diseases as influenza, measles, and pertussis.

**Prognosis:** Some cases are lethal in the newborn and similar to the **Short rib-polydactyly syndrome** but without polydactyly. Most affected infants do not survive early infancy. If the patient does survive the first months of life, death may later result from renal involvement. There is no effect upon intelligence in surviving patients, but the growth of long bones is moderately altered. Respiratory problems become less severe, but the thoracic malformation persists. Impaired renal function may sometimes occur after the twentieth year of life.

**Detection of Carrier:** Unknown.

**Special Considerations:** The relationship of asphyxiating thoracic dysplasia to **Chondroectodermal dysplasia** has been a point of discussion for several years. Indeed, the X-ray features of the two conditions are very similar, particularly those of the pelvis. Narrowness of the thorax, at times very pronounced, is not rare in chondroectodermal dysplasia. Moreover, the presence of polydactyly and dental anomalies has been observed in asphyxiating thoracic dysplasia, further illustrating its resemblance to chondroectodermal dysplasia. Despite these similarities, the two conditions are probably due to two different gene mutations, the modes of action and end results of which are similar.

**References:**
Maroteaux P, Savart P: La dystrophie thoracique asphyxiante. Etude radiologique et rapports avec le syndrome d'Ellis et van Creveld. Ann Radiol (Paris) 1964; 7:332–338.
Herdman RC, Langer LO: The thoracic asphyxiant dystrophy and renal disease. Am J Dis Child 1968; 116:192–201.
Burkle FM Jr, Bravo AJ: Asphyxiating thoracic dystrophy: malformation of the newborn. Clin Pediatr (Phila) 1969; 8:165.
Tahernia AC, Stamps P: Jeune syndrome (asphyxiating thoracic dystrophy). Clin Pediatr (Phila) 1977; 16:903–908.
Cortina H, et al.: The wide spectrum of the asphyxiating thoracic dysplasia. Pediatr Radiol 1979; 8:93–99. *
Sandomenico C, et al.: Dysplasie thoraco-pelvi-phalangienne ou "forme latente" de la dysplasie thoracique asphyxiante. Un cas clinique. Ann Radiol (Paris) 1981; 24:589–593.

Wilson DJ, et al.: Retinal dystrophy in Jeune's syndrome. Arch Ophthal 1987; 105:651–657.

MA034                                    **Pierre Maroteaux**

**Asphyxiating thoracic dystrophy**
*See ASPHYXIATING THORACIC DYSPLASIA*

## ASPLENIA SYNDROME                                    0092

**Includes:**
    Asplenia-cardiovascular anomalies
    Ivemark syndrome
    Polysplenia syndrome
    Splenic agenesis
    Teratologic syndrome of visceral heterotaxy

**Excludes:**
    Asplenia with cystic liver, kidney and pancreas
    Splenic agenesis, isolated congenital

**Major Diagnostic Criteria:** Evidence for partial visceral situs inversus and presence of Howell-Jolly and Heinz bodies in the blood smear in an infant with (cyanotic) congenital heart disease. Radiographically, dextrocardia in combination with signs of severe pulmonary venous hypertension is virtually pathognomonic.

**Clinical Findings:** Asplenia rarely occurs as an isolated defect. Asplenia syndrome indicates a characteristic constellation of visceral anomalies of which the outstanding feature, in addition to the splenic agenesis, is a strong tendency for normally asymmetric

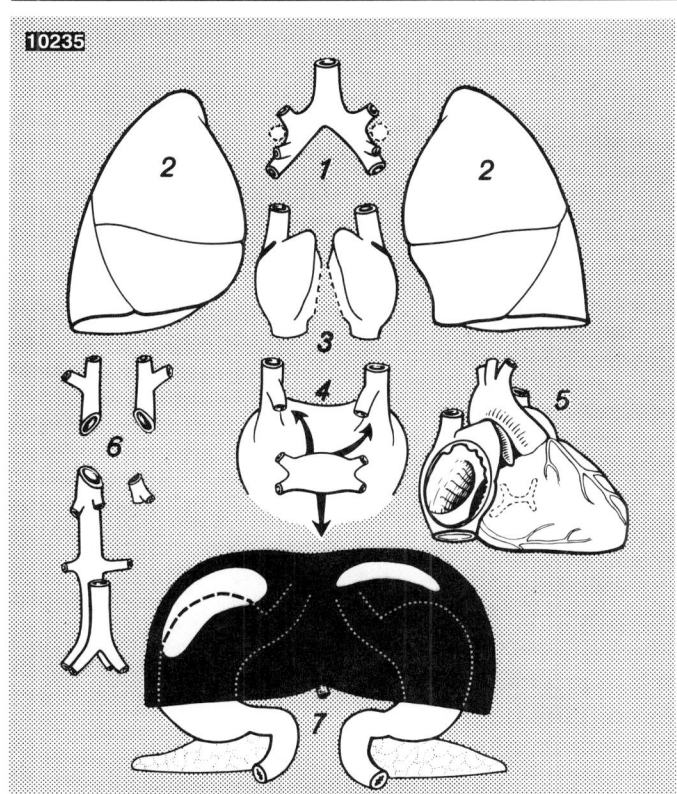

**0092A-**10235: Note partial or complete failure of bowel rotation. Asplenia: 1) bilateral eparterial bronchi; 2) bilateral trilobed lungs; 3) bilateral morphologic right atria; 4) pulmonary venous anomalies; 5) cardiac malformations; 6) systemic venous anomalies; 7) symmetric liver and right- or left-sided stomach.

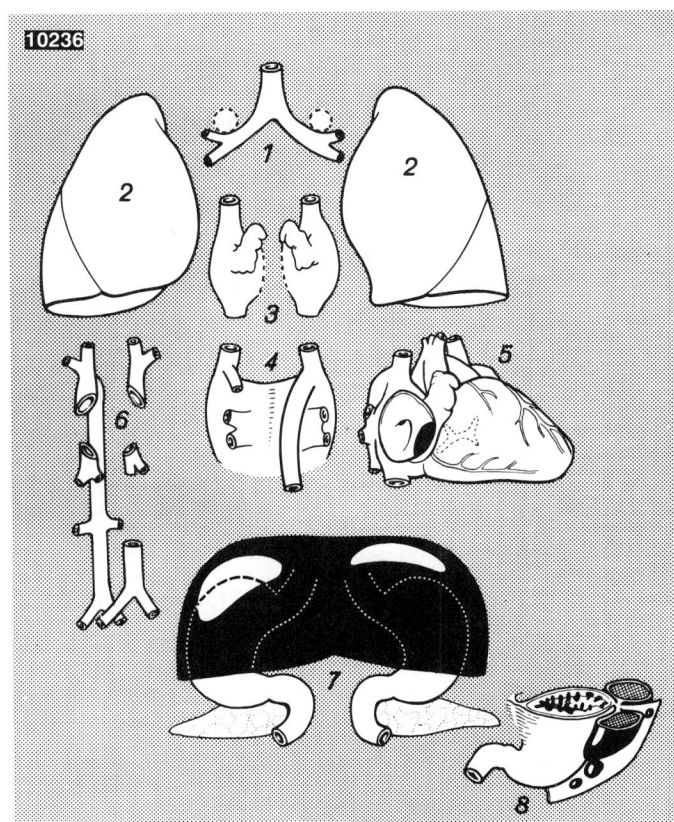

**0092B-**10236: Partial or complete failure of bowel rotation. Polysplenia: 1) bilateral hyparterial bronchi; 2) bilateral bilobed lungs; 3) bilateral morphologic left aorta; 4) pulmonary venous anomalies; 5) cardiac malformations; 6) systemic venous anomalies; 7) symmetric liver and right- or left-sided stomach; 8) stomach and double spleen.

organs or pairs of organs to develop more or less symmetrically. The left-sided organs or members of pairs of organs assume the morphologic characteristics of their right-sided counterparts, but in mirror image (isomerism). In at least 90% of cases an eparterial bronchus is present bilaterally, and the lobation of both lungs resembles that of a normal trilobed right lung. Accessory pulmonary fissures are common. The right and left lobes of the liver are about equal in size in 40% of cases and the lower edge of the liver is essentially horizontal. The stomach is located on the right side in about half the cases. Occasionally the stomach has retained a midline position with a proximal portion located in the posterior mediastinum. Usually the intestinal tract has failed to rotate in which case the colon lies behind and below the small bowel and the mesentery is free with its root located in the midline. In rare cases a hypoplastic spleen may be present.

The echocardiographic findings are directly related to the specific associated lesions. Bilateral superior vena cava will not be appreciated by echocardiography. A total anomalous pulmonary venous connection may be found if the collecting chamber is posterior to the left atrium (see **Pulmonary venous connection, total anomalous**).

Absence of the coronary sinus has not been appreciated by M-mode echocardiography. If an endocardial cushion defect is present, it will be associated with the usual findings (see **Heart, endocardial cushion defects**).

Right ventricular outflow tract obstruction and transposition of the great arteries, usually present, will demonstrate their usual echocardiographic characteristics.

Complex cardiovascular anomalies are almost always present. Bilateral superior venae cavae are common, as is a common hepatic vein, contralateral to the inferior vena cava, draining the corresponding liver lobe. Some form of total anomalous pulmonary venous connection is found in almost all cases; at least 10% of these are of the infradiaphragmatic type. There is isomerism of the atria, ie both atria morphologically resemble right atria. The atrial septum in most cases is absent except for a peculiar triangularly shaped band of muscle which crosses the atrial cavity. The coronary sinus is absent. Some form of endocardial cushion defect, usually of the complete type, is present in the great majority of cases and generally there is only one functioning ventricle. Partial or complete obstruction to pulmonary arterial blood flow is found in at least 70% of the cases and the great arteries, as a rule, are transposed. The cardiac apex may be directed to either side.

Clinically children with asplenia syndrome generally present themselves within days or weeks after birth with marked cyanosis, respiratory distress, feeding difficulties and congestive heart failure. Early death is common and infants who survive for any length of time often fail to thrive and tend to suffer from cutaneous, respiratory, and other infections. The P vector may be abnormal, or change from time to time. Left axis deviation is common as might be expected, considering the high incidence of endocardial cushion defects; otherwise, the EKG varies so much from case to case as to be of little help. X-rays commonly demonstrate partial visceral heterotaxy and the liver shadow may be evenly distributed bilaterally. There is a high incidence of dextrocardia. Because severe pulmonary stenosis or atresia is almost invariably present, the pulmonary vascularity is usually diminished. Occasionally, the air filled tracheobronchial tree may be seen to be symmetric. Cardiac catheterization is of limited value, but angiocardiography will show the complexity of the cardiovascular lesions. Probably the most important angiographic finding is the disclosure that the abdominal aorta and inferior vena cava are found together on the same side of the spine.

The peripheral blood usually shows the presence of polycythemia, Howell-Jolly bodies, Heinz bodies, siderocytes, target cells and normoblasts.

**Complications:** Persistent or recurrent infections which respond poorly to treatment. Volvulus has been reported.

**Associated Findings:** None known.

**Etiology:** The great majority of cases appear to be sporadic but studies have revealed consanguinity in families in which there were multiple affected sibs, suggesting autosomal recessive inheritance.

**Pathogenesis:** The spleen first appears in human embryos of 10 mm C-R length, ie about 36–37 days of gestation. Splenic agenesis must therefore be determined by the 34th-36th day. The conotruncal structures of the heart, abnormalities of which are so constantly associated with splenic agenesis, develop a day or two later and, therefore, some common factors acting at this period in gestation may be responsible for both anomalies. It has also been proposed that splenic agenesis and symmetric liver may be produced by vascular changes associated with partial situs inversus. The cause of the latter is unknown.

**MIM No.:** 20853

**CDC No.:** 759.000

**Sex Ratio:** M2:F1. In some series, male predominance has been much more pronounced.

**Occurrence:** Exact incidence figures are not available, but a growing established literature indicates that the syndrome is being recognized with increasing frequency. Very low prevalence due to extremely high, early mortality.

**Risk of Recurrence for Patient's Sib:** Small, but possible recessive inheritance.

**Risk of Recurrence for Patient's Child:** Affected individuals are not expected to survive to reproduce.

**Age of Detectability:** Prenatal ultrasonography shows bradycardia, single ventricle, edema, ascites, and displaced intestinal loops. Shortly after birth, by examination of peripheral blood smear.

**Gene Mapping and Linkage:** Unknown.

**Prevention:** None known. Genetic counseling indicated.

**Treatment:** Because of the extreme complexity of the malformations and the poor prognosis, therapy including palliative surgery is of little value.

**Prognosis:** Extremely poor, more than 90% of infants die during the first year of life from associated defects or infection.

**Detection of Carrier:** Unknown.

**Special Considerations:** Families in which one sib has asplenia syndrome and another polysplenia syndrome suggest that these are a single entity.

**Support Groups:** Dallas; American Heart Association

**References:**

Ivemark BI: Implications of agenesis of the spleen on the pathogenesis of cono-truncus anomalies in childhood; analysis of heart malformations in splenic agenesis syndrome with 14 new cases. Acta Paediatr (Uppsala) 1955; 44(Suppl. 104):1–110.

Van Mierop LHS, et al.: Asplenia and polysplenia syndrome. In: Bergsma D, Blumenthal S, eds: BD:OAS vol VIII(1). Baltimore: Williams & Wilkins Co, for The National Foundation-March of Dimes, 1972:74. *

Simpson J: Familial occurence of Ivemark syndrome. J Med Genet 1973; 10:303–304.

Rose V, Izukawa T, Moes CAF: Syndromes of asplenia and polysplenia: a review of cardiac and non-cardiac malformation in 60 cases with special reference to diagnosis and prognosis. Brit Heart J 1975; 37:840–852.

Silverman NH, Snider AR: Two-dimensional echocardiography in congenital heart disease. East Norwalk, CT: Appleton-Century-Crofts, 1982.

Niikawa N, et al.: Familial clustering of situs inversus totalis, and asplenia and polysplenia syndromes. Am J Med Genet 1983; 16:43–47.

de la Monte SM, Hutchins GM: Sisters with polysplenia. Am J Med Genet 1985; 21:171–173.

N0003                                              **James J. Nora**

**Asplenia-cardiovascular anomalies**
*See ASPLENIA SYNDROME*
**Asthma, inherited**
*See SKIN, ATOPY, FAMILIAL*
**Asthma, ragweed pollen-induced**
*See RAGWEED POLLEN SENSITIVITY*
**Astrocytoma including optic nerve glioma**
*See CNS NEOPLASMS*
**Astrocytoma types 3 & 4**
*See CANCER, GLIOMA, FAMILIAL*
**Asucrosia**
*See SUCRASE-ISOMALTASE DEFICIENCY*
**Asymmetrical crying facies (ACF)**
*See CARDIOFACIAL SYNDROME-ASSYMETRIC FACIES*
**Asymmetry, congenital**
*See HEMIHYPERTROPHY*
**Asymmetry, congenital-short stature-sexual development variations**
*See SILVER SYNDROME*
**AT III deficiencies**
*See ANTITHROMBIN III DEFICIENCY*
**Ataxia with lactic acidosis**
*See PYRUVATE DEHYDROGENASE DEFICIENCY*
**Ataxia with lactic acidosis II**
*See PYRUVATE CARBOXYLASE DEFICIENCY WITH LACTIC ACIDEMIA*

## ATAXIA, FRIEDREICH TYPE                    2714

**Includes:**
> Friedreich ataxia (FA)
> Friedreich disease
> Spinal ataxia, hereditofamilial
> Tabes of Friedreich

**Excludes:**
> **Abetalipoproteinemia** (0002)
> **Aciduria**
> **Anemia, pernicious congenital** (2656)
> **Ataxia-telangiectasia** (0094)
> Cerebellar ataxia, congenital
> **Cockayne syndrome** (0189)
> **G(M2)-gangliosidosis with hexosaminidase A deficiency** (0434)
> **Metachromatic leukodystrophies** (0651)
> **Neuropathy, hereditary motor and sensory, type I** (2104)
> **Paraplegia, familial spastic** (0295)
> Taboparetic syphilis
> **Xeroderma pigmentosum** (1005)

**Major Diagnostic Criteria:** Ataxia (unsteadiness of gait), dysarthria (of the cerebellar type), weakness (lower extremities are more severely affected than the upper), and areflexia (especially of the lower extremities). The disease may be confidently diagnosed when these features are combined with plantar extension reflexes, cardiomyopathy, and the age of onset less than 25 years.

**Clinical Findings:** Relentlessly progressive truncal ataxia, and to a lesser extent, limb (appendicular) ataxia, are the most striking findings. Cerebellar dysarthria may preclude intelligible speech; although it is not a prominent finding early in the disease, it is invariably present within 10 years of onset. Extremity weakness may also take years to develop; it is much more marked in the legs than in the arms and is usually associated with normal or reduced tone. Lack of knee and ankle jerks is an early, universal finding. Upper limb areflexia is less common. The plantar response is extensor.

Ninety percent of patients demonstrate a sensory deficit, usually defective joint position sense in the lower extremities. Vibratory sense appreciation is also commonly impaired, but pain and temperature senses are normal. Lateral gaze nystagmus or other disturbance of eye movement is present in approximately one half of established cases; optic atrophy is noted in one-fourth. Other less common neurologic abnormalities include deafness, tremor, and vertigo. Nonneurologic findings include pes cavus, scoliosis, and cardiomyopathy; all present in more than 90% of established cases. The cardiomyopathy results in dyspnea and palpitations; the characteristic EKG abnormalities are described below. Twenty percent of patients develop diabetes, and this seems to cluster in families.

CT scans show nonspecific atrophy. There is some evidence that this is most marked in patients with disease of early onset. Most (>90%) patients have delayed sensory nerve conduction velocities and absent sensory nerve action potentials, although these may be late findings. Somatosensory evoked potential studies are usually abnormal, with reduction of the Erb point potential and cortical waveform dispersal. Electroretinography may disclose a nonspecific abnormality; visual evoked potentials reveal P100 prolongation in about one half of established cases. An electrocardiogram should be obtained in all (even nonsymptomatic) cases. Investigators have reported abnormalities in up to 90% of cases; T-wave inversion is most common and is usually best seen in the inferior and precordial leads. Other changes include left ventricular hypertrophy and axis deviation. Cardiomegaly may be seen on chest X-ray. Echocardiography may show ventricular outflow obstruction and, occasionally, asymmetric septal hypertrophy. Periodic investigation for insulin-dependent diabetes is similarly warranted. Glycosuria, hyperglycemia, and abnormal glucose tolerance curves have been reported. Finally, X-ray films of the feet and spine may document the bony abnormalities described above; although the abnormalities are usually clinically apparent, serial films may be useful for monitoring progression.

Postmortem studies have disclosed spinal cord atrophy and degeneration of the posterior columns, dorsal root ganglion cells, and pyramidal and spinocerebellar tracts. Less marked changes are seen in the anterior horns; peripheral nerves show a loss of large, myelinated fibers. There may be loss of Purkinje and Betz cells and loss of the cells in cranial nerve nuclei. Cardiac histology may demonstrate interstitial fibrosis and occasional inflammatory changes.

**Complications:** Cardiac disease, diabetes, and progressive skeletal disease. Patients have succumbed to heart failure or ketoacidosis.

**Associated Findings:** Vertigo, peripheral vascular insufficiency, and pain. Glaucoma was reported in an inbred Spanish family (Combarros et al, 1988).

**Etiology:** Autosomal recessive inheritance.

**Pathogenesis:** Several theories have been advanced, but not proven, since Friedreich postulated that the disease was due to alcohol excess. Abnormalities of purine and amino acid metabolism have been reported but not confirmed. Other investigators have suggested lipoprotein, organic acid, or mitochondrial defects. Most recently, attention has focused on the pyruvate dehydrogenase complex and on lipoamide dehydrogenase activity. The original concept of the disease as a metabolically induced, progressive "dying back" degeneration also remains viable.

**MIM No.:** *22930, 22931

**POS No.:** 3797

**Sex Ratio:** M1:F1

**Occurrence:** Considered to be the most common of the hereditary ataxias. Harding (1984) reported a prevalence of 1:48,000 in England, in keeping with the estimates of other investigators of 1:46,000–52,000.

**Risk of Recurrence for Patient's Sib:**
See Part I, *Mendelian Inheritance.*

**Risk of Recurrence for Patient's Child:**
See Part I, *Mendelian Inheritance.*

**Age of Detectability:** Usually during puberty. Harding (1984) reported a mean of 10.52 ± 7.4 years of age. A diagnosis of Friedreich ataxia in an individual whose symptoms began after age 25 years is untenable.

Prenatal diagnosis was accomplished in a family in which there was a prior affected child and in which both parents were heterozygous for a closely-linked DNA marker.

**Gene Mapping and Linkage:** FRDA (Friedreich ataxia) has been mapped to 9q13-q21.1.

**Prevention:** None known. Genetic counseling indicated.

**Treatment:** No reports have appeared of unequivocal benefit from any of the various agents tried. Cholinergic agonists and precursors (lecithin and choline), gamma-vinyl GABA, 5-hydroxy-tryptophan, and benserazide have been used without clear-cut success. Cardiac disease may require propranolol and digoxin; insulin may be required in those patients who are diabetic, though there are reports of success with oral hypoglycemic agents. Many authors have commented on their patient's observation that bedrest seems to aggravate the condition, and this must be considered when surgery is contemplated. The need for and the timing of surgical intervention to correct the bony deformities are not clear, although work is currently in progress on this issue. Respiratory insufficiency and inability to ambulate are the most common indications.

**Prognosis:** There is steady progression of the disease, which may be exacerbated by intercurrent illness. Life span estimates for individual patients are difficult because of the considerable variability in rate of progression. Patients have lived from 18 months to 50 years after the onset of symptoms, although the disease does seem to be similar among patients in individual families. Patients with cardiac disease with or without diabetes do less well; these features also tend to cluster within a given kindred. The average patient with Friedreich ataxia dies of intercurrent infection or heart failure within 30 years of onset of symptoms.

**Detection of Carrier:** Unknown.

**Special Considerations:** The hereditary ataxias constitute a heterogeneous group of disorders with overlapping features. Recent work by Harding and others in defining uniform diagnostic criteria allows more specific patient classification than has been possible previously. The varied and inconsistent biochemical abnormalities reported in the past may in part be a reflection of the heterogeneity of the populations studied. Current work with homogeneous groups of patients with "true" Friedreich ataxia may demonstrate more specific and reproducible findings. Finally, improvements in supportive care have resulted in greater patient longevity, and investigations into such issues as the timeliness of surgical intervention are underway.

Roussy-Levy hereditary dystasia, a dominant condition (see **Neuropathy, hereditary motor and sensory, type I**), has been called "an abortive type of Friedreich disease" (Yudell et al, 1965).

**Support Groups:**
CA; Oakland; Friedreich's Ataxia Group in America, Inc.
MN; Wayzata; National Ataxia Foundation

**References:**
Yudell A, et al.: A kinship with the Roussy-Levy syndrome. Arch Neurol 1965; 13:432–440.
Tyrer J: Friedreich's ataxia. In: Handbook of clinical neurology. Amsterdam: North Holland, 1974:14:319–364.
Harding A: Friedreich's ataxia. In: The hereditary ataxias and related disorders. Edinburgh: Churchill Livingstone, 1984:57–103. * †
Chamberlain S, et al.: Mapping of mutation causing Friedreich's ataxia to human chromosome 9. Nature 1988; 334:248–250.
Combarros O, et al.: Association of an ataxia indistinguishable from Friedreich's ataxia and congenital glaucoma in a family: a new syndrome. J Med Genet 1988; 25:44–46.
Keats BJB, et al.: "Acadian" and "classical" forms of Friedreich ataxia are most probably caused by mutations at the same locus. Am J Med Genet 1989; 33:266–268.

H0057
KA008

**John H. Holtkamp**
**Raymond S. Kandt**

**Ataxia, hereditary cerebellar-childhood cataracts**
*See MARINESCO-SJOGREN SYNDROME*
**Ataxia, intermittent-pyruvate decarboxylase deficiency**
*See PYRUVATE DEHYDROGENASE DEFICIENCY*
**Ataxia, intermittent-pyruvate dehydrogenase deficiency**
*See PYRUVATE DEHYDROGENASE DEFICIENCY*
**Ataxia-deafness (sensorineural)-hyperuricemia**
*See PHOSPHORIBOSYL PYROPHOSPHATE (PRPP) SYNTHETASE ABNORMALITY*

---

## ATAXIA-DYSMORPHIC FACIES-TRICHODYSPLASIA　　　2341

**Includes:**
Dysmorphic facies-ataxia-trichodysplasia
Spinocerebella ataxia with dysmorphism
Trichodysplasia-dysmorphic facies-ataxia

**Excludes:**
**Ataxia, Friedreich type** (2714)
Spinocerebellar ataxia (others)

**Major Diagnostic Criteria:** Unusual facial appearance, delayed psychomotor development, and limb and gait ataxia. Cerebellar atrophy with cortical and subcortical involvement, and hair configuration, as seen by the scanning electron microscopy, characterized by large cuticular scales.

**Clinical Findings:** The unusual facies is characterized by thick, rough, and abundant hair; wide forehead; mild palpebral ptosis; small nose; anteverted nostrils; thick lips; and downslanting corners of the mouth. Other findings are cubitus valgus, genu recurvatum, plano varus/valgus foot deformity, first hammertoe, scoliosis, unstable gait, upper and lower limb ataxia, dysarthria, diminished deep tendon reflexes, and Babinski and Romberg signs. The delayed psychomotor development (IQ: 60–65) is of early onset and apparent mainly in speech and locomotion.
The EEG shows diffuse abnormalities and maturation deficit.

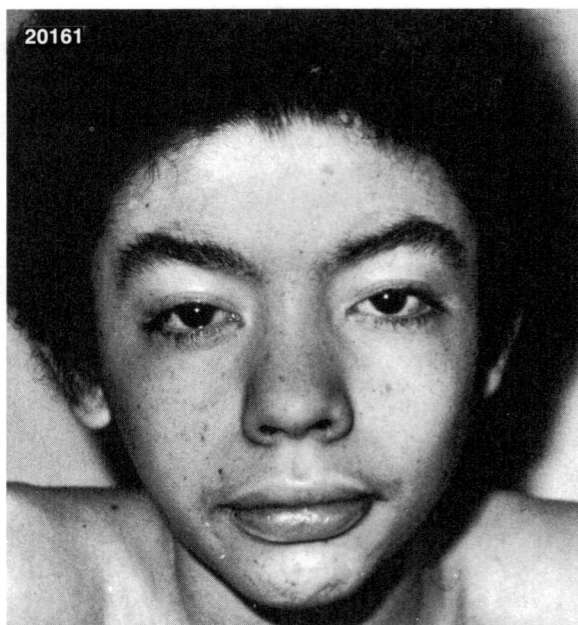

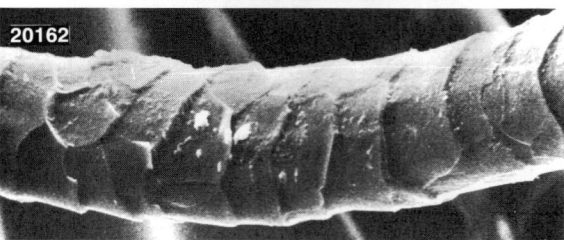

2341-20161: Abundant coarse hair, broad forehead, mild ptosis, thick lips, and downward slanting of the corners of the lips. 20162: Scanning electron microscopic study of the clinically abnormal hair shows the unusual configuration with large cuticular scales.

---

Cranial CT scan reveals cerebellar atrophy with cortical and subcortical involvement. A denervation pattern predominantly in distal limbs is confirmed by electromyographic studies. The X-ray findings are dolichocephaly, scoliosis, slender long bones, generalized osteopenia, and delayed bone age. Two of three patients had spina bifida occulta at L-5. Light microscopy of the hair is normal, but scanning electron microscopy reveals a peculiar hair configuration characterized by large cuticular scales.

**Complications:** Skeletal deformities, mainly scoliosis and foot deformities, occur primarily as a consequence of muscle wasting and weakness.

**Associated Findings:** Mild optic atrophy.

**Etiology:** Autosomal recessive inheritance.

**Pathogenesis:** Unknown.

**MIM No.:** 27127

**Sex Ratio:** M2:F1 (observed).

**Occurrence:** Reported in two brothers and one sister in a single family.

**Risk of Recurrence for Patient's Sib:**
See Part I, *Mendelian Inheritance.*

**Risk of Recurrence for Patient's Child:**
See Part I, *Mendelian Inheritance.*

**Age of Detectability:** At birth, by facial appearance. The neurologic signs are apparent at 3–4 years of age.

**Gene Mapping and Linkage:** Unknown.

**Prevention:** None known. Genetic counseling indicated.

**Treatment:** Physical therapy and other symptomatic treatments.

**Prognosis:** Poor, due to neurologic incapacitation.

**Detection of Carrier:** Unknown.

**Support Groups:** MN; Wayzata; National Ataxia Foundation

**References:**

Becker PE, et al.: Dominant erblicher Typ von cerebellarer ataxia. Z Neurol 1971; 199:116–139.

Sánchez-Corona J, et al.: A distinct dysmorphic syndrome with spinocerebellar ataxia and probable autosomal recessive inheritance. Hum Genet 1985; 69:243–245. *

C0064
CA011

José Sánchez-Corona<br>José María Cantú

**Ataxia-erythrokeratodermia**
*See GIROUX-BARBEAU SYNDROME*

## ATAXIA-HYPOGONADISM SYNDROME 0093

**Includes:**
 Boucher-Neuhauser syndrome
 Cerebellar ataxia-hypogonadotropic hypogonadism
 Luteinizing hormone-releasing hormone (LHRH) deficiency-ataxia

**Excludes:** Nonhypogonadism in other hereditary ataxias

**Major Diagnostic Criteria:** Cerebellar ataxia and hypogonadotropic hypogonadism.

**Clinical Findings:** Cerebellar ataxia, predominantly truncal type, occurs in adolescence or early adulthood, usually accompanied by nystagmus, hypotonia, rebound phenomenon, dysdiadochokinesia, and/or tremor. CT may reveal cerebellar and brainstem atrophy. Incoordination and dysarthric speech become more pronounced with advancing age. Signs of peripheral neuropathy may be present. External and internal genitalia are hypoplastic. There is no breast development or menses in affected females. Eunuchoid body habitus, gynecomastia, and infertility are features in affected males. Emotional disturbance and personality disorders may occur. Endocrine studies reveal the hypogonadism to be of hypogonadotropic origin. Hypothalamic luteinizing hormone-releasing hormone (LHRH) deficiency has been shown.

**Complications:** Physical handicap because of difficulties in walking and coordination; speech disorder; infertility.

**Associated Findings:** Macular degeneration, mental deterioration, and anomalies of amino acid distribution have been observed in some.

**Etiology:** One form appears to be either an autosomal dominant male sex-limited or an X-linked recessive inherited trait. Autosomal recessive transmission postulated because of occurrence in both sexes, and parental consanguinity is reported in at least one family.

**Pathogenesis:** Unknown.

**MIM No.:** *21284, 30740

**POS No.:** 3999

**Sex Ratio:** Unknown.

**Occurrence:** Rare; About ten cases described in the literature.

**Risk of Recurrence for Patient's Sib:**
See Part I, *Mendelian Inheritance.*

**Risk of Recurrence for Patient's Child:**
See Part I, *Mendelian Inheritance.* No affected individuals are known to have reproduced.

**Age of Detectability:** Hypogonadism can be detected at puberty. Ataxia at adolescence or early adulthood (20–30 years).

**Gene Mapping and Linkage:** Unknown.

**Prevention:** None known. Genetic counseling indicated.

**Treatment:** Physiotherapy; hormone therapy may be helpful.

**Prognosis:** Ataxia is slowly progressive in most patients; life expectancy may be reduced.

**Detection of Carrier:** Unknown.

**Special Considerations:** Sporadic and familial cases of hypogonadotropic hypogonadism and cerebellar ataxia were described predominantly in male patients; in a small number of sibships both sexes were affected, suggesting autosomal recessive inheritance. The ataxia syndrome is not fully comparable with other forms of hereditary ataxia, but this suggestion deserves further study. Endocrine dysfunctions may occur in patients with hereditary ataxias or ataxia syndromes; however, hypergonadotropic hypogonadism usually is found. Extensive endocrinologic studies in such patients are necessary for clarification. Hypogonadism may be caused by the CNS defect, but more likely it is an expression of pleiotropic gene effects.

**Support Groups:** MN; Wayzata; National Ataxia Foundation

**References:**

Rimoin DL, Schimke RN: Genetic disorders of the endocrine glands. St. Louis: C.V. Mosby, 1971.

Neuhäuser G, Opitz JM: Autosomal recessive syndrome of cerebellar ataxia and hypogonadotropic hypogonadism. Clin Genet 1975; 7:426–434. *

Skre H, et al.: Cerebellar ataxia and hypergonadotropic hypogonadism in two kindreds. Chance concurrence, pleiotropism or linkage? Clin Genet 1976; 9:234–244.

Lowenthal A, et al.: Familial cerebellar ataxia with hypogonadism. J Neurol 1979; 222:75–80.

Berciano J, et al.: Familial cerebellar ataxia and hypogonadotropic hypogonadism: evidence for hypothalamic LHRH deficiency. J Neurol Neurosurg Psychiatry 1982; 45:747–751. *

Limber ER, et al.: Spinocerebellar ataxia, hypogonadotropic hypogonadism, and choroidal dystrophy (Boucher-Neuhäuser syndrome). Am J Med Genet 1989; 33:409–414.

NE012

Gerhard Neuhäuser

## ATAXIA-TELANGIECTASIA 0094

**Includes:**
 Ataxia-telangiectasia (AT) variants
 Boder-Sedgwick syndrome
 Louis-Barr syndrome

**Excludes:**
 Ataxia without immunodeficiency
 **Ataxia, Friedreich type** (2714)
 "AT-like" syndromes
 **Bloom syndrome** (0112)
 Cerebellitis

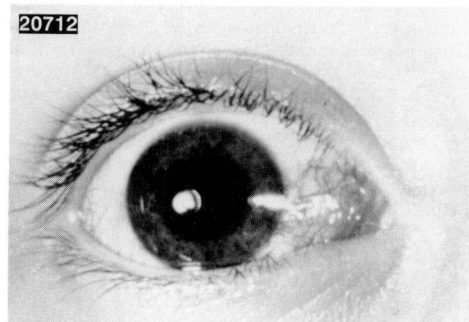

0094-20712: Telangiectasia in bulbar conjunctiva.

Cerebral palsy (2931)
Chromosome instability, Nijmegen type (2551)
G(m2)-gangliosidosis with hexosaminidase A and B deficiency (0433)
G(m2)-gangliosidosis with hexosaminidase A deficiency (0434)
Immunoglobulin A deficiency (0525)
Marinesco-Sjogren syndrome (2031)

**Major Diagnostic Criteria:** Cerebellar ataxia, dysarthric speech, oculocutaneous telangiectasia, immunodeficiency, radioresistant DNA synthesis. Other diagnostic criteria includes elevated alpha-fetoprotein, sinopulmonary infections, and characteristic chromosomal aberrations.

**Clinical Findings:** Cerebellar ataxia becomes evident when the child begins to walk. Commencing as a truncal ataxia manifested by swaying of the head and trunk, slow progression subsequently involves the gait, with later development of intention tremor and choreoathetosis. Speech becomes slurred or dysarthric. Characteristic oculomotor signs are apraxia of eye movements, fixation nystagmus, and strabismus. Telangiectasia of the bulbar conjunctiva may not become apparent until later. Faint telangiectasia may also appear on other exposed skin areas, such as the pinnae. Cerebellar histology reveals grossly depleted numbers of Purkinje cells; however, Bielschowsky-silver staining reveals near-normal numbers of basket cells, indicating that at birth Purkinje cell numbers are near normal and deteriorate with time. This finding correlates with the unrelenting progress of the cerebellar ataxia. A striking histopathologic finding has been extensive nucleomegaly, involving most organs, especially the liver.

Sinopulmonary infections of viral or bacterial etiology are common in ataxia-telangiectasia (AT) patients and are indicative of underlying immunodeficiencies. The type and degree of immunodeficiency can vary, even among affected sibs. Decreased or absent levels of IgG2, IgA, and IgE have been noted in most patients. Cellular immune functions are also impaired, as evidenced by skin anergy and poor lymphocyte responses to *in vitro* stimulation with mitogens and allogeneic cells. T/B-cell proportions in the peripheral blood are usually within normal ranges. Peripheral lymph nodes show depletion of lymphocytes but increased numbers of reticulum cells. Proliferation of reticular-epithelial stromal cells also predominates in thymic tissue. Hassal corpuscles are rare or absent, and the entire thymus appears embryonic or atrophic. Serum alpha-fetoprotein (AFP) levels are elevated in almost all patients, making the diagnosis of AT questionable (but still possible) if AFP is normal. This elevated AFP is thought to originate in the liver.

Cytogenetic abnormalities are characteristic of AT, although poor lymphocyte responses to phytohemagglutinin often impede these studies. Aberrations involve approximately 10% of mitoses, the most common breakpoints being: 7p14, 7q35, 14q11, 14q32, 2p11, and 22q11. The latter constitute about 80% of aberrations and correspond to the sites of gene complexes for T- and B-cell receptors. Clonal patterns are commonly observed and occasionally are associated with leukemia.

Radioresistant DNA synthesis measures the effects of ionizing radiation on fibroblasts or lymphocytes. Although this test is not generally available, it is at present considered the *sine qua non* by most clinical investigators, since without this abnormality, complementation studies are impossible. The latter presently form the basis for inclusion or exclusion of some "AT-like" syndromes. For example, **Chromosome instability, Nijmegen type** manifests the chromosomal aberrations and radioresistant DNA synthesis that are characteristic of AT, but the patients do not have ataxia or telangiectasia. Most important, the fibroblasts of **Chromosome instability, Nijmegen type** patients complement fibroblasts of AT patients of complementation group V1. In limited testing, complementation groups (excluding V1) distribute worldwide approximately as follows: Group A, 55%; Group C, 28%; Group D, 14%; Group E, 3%; and Group V1, rare. Groups A, C, D and E are indistinguishable except by complementation assays. Patients in Group V1 have **Microcephaly** and mental retardation in addition to all other signs and symptoms of AT; the AFP level is not elevated.

Progeric changes in AT patients include gray strands of hair in young children, neurofibrillary tangles and lipofuchsin deposits in the brain at postmortem examination, and precocious onset of certain malignancies, such as basal cell carcinomas and uterine tumors in the 20s. Approximately one-third of all AT patients develop a malignancy during their shortened life. Eighty percent of these malignancies involve lymphoreticular tissue. Heterozygotes also develop malignancies, with approximately a 5-fold increase over the general population; these are primarily nonlymphoid, such as breast, pancreas, and liver. Infections and malignancy are the most frequent causes of death in AT patients. Endocrinopathy in some patients includes decreased 17-ketosteroid excretion consistent with gonadal dysgenesis, abnormal glucose metabolism associated with elevated plasma insulin levels and diabetes mellitus (often without ketosis or glycosuria), and growth retardation. Ovarian agenesis or hypoplasia has been found at autopsy. Most patients have normal pubertal development.

**Complications:** Ataxia, 100%; choreoathetosis, 90–100%; nystagmus, 90–100%; ocular apraxia, 80–90%; dysarthria, 90–100%; recurrent sinopulmonary infections, 50–70%; malignancy (mainly lymphoreticular), 35%. Severe radiation fibrosis follows radiation whenever conventional therapeutic dosage is used to treat cancer, 100%. To a lesser degree, AT carriers are also radiation hypersensitive.

**Associated Findings:** Ovarian dysgenesis, uterine tumors, growth retardation, testicular atrophy, abnormal carbohydrate metabolism, and hepatic dysfunction.

Carriers of one mutant gene are estimated to have a 6.8 relative risk of breast cancer, and, assuming a frequency of 1.4% of such heterozygotes in the United States population, about 9% of breast cancer may occur in association with the ataxia telagiectasia gene (see **Cancer, breast, familial**).

**Etiology:** Autosomal recessive inheritance with genetic heterogeneity, as evidenced by the existence of at least five different complementation groups.

**Pathogenesis:** Evidence exists that some Purkinje cells overmigrate into ectopic positions during the third trimester *in utero*. Normal numbers of Purkinje cells are present at birth but begin to degenerate thereafter. It is unclear at present whether this occurs through disuse atrophy secondary to faulty neuronal connections or secondary to an enzymatic deficiency that plays a key role in normal Purkinje cell function. At a more basic level, DNA maintenance or processing or both is abnormal and may involve a defective DNA-binding protein or enzyme that is important to gene expression and DNA repair, such as a recombinase, topoisomerase, ligase, endonuclease, resolvase or terminal transferase.

**MIM No.:** *20890, 20891

**POS No.:** 3033

**Sex Ratio:** M1:F1

**Occurrence:** 1:30,000–100,000 live births. More common in countries where the incidence of consanguinity is high, such as Turkey. Prevalence equals incidence up to adolescence, then declines as patients die. Longest known survival is 49 years.

### Risk of Recurrence for Patient's Sib:

See Part I, *Mendelian Inheritance*. Sixty-six percent of unaffected sibs will be carriers; 25% of their offspring will be affected if their spouse carries the same complementation group for the defective AT gene. The frequency of the gene in the general population has been roughly estimated at 0.5–5.0%.

### Risk of Recurrence for Patient's Child:

See Part I, *Mendelian Inheritance*. Affected individuals are not known to have reproduced.

**Age of Detectability:** One to six years of age. Earlier diagnosis is possible by measuring radioresistant DNA synthesis and performing extensive karyotyping. Measuring AFP level may also help. Attempts at prenatal diagnosis should be followed up by postmortem studies whenever possible, with special attention to establishing fibroblast cultures for evaluating radioresistant DNA synthesis and examining thymus and other lymphoid organs.

**Gene Mapping and Linkage:** ATA (ataxia telangiectasia (complementation group A)) has been provisionally mapped to 11q22-q23.

**Prevention:** None known. Genetic counseling indicated.

**Treatment:** Patients should avoid hospital visits and contact with respiratory pathogens; patients should be immunized with killed vaccines only; physical therapy appropriate to neurologic dysfunction (swimming is often well tolerated by AT patients); aggressive pulmonary toilet; microbiologic cultures followed by appropriate and timely antibiotic therapy of infections; aggressive diagnostic studies of chronic low-grade fevers for evidence of malignancy or infection. Early use of a typewriter keyboard, fitted with a special guard to minimize striking the wrong keys by accident, is often helpful with schooling in later years, after the handwriting has deteriorated to illegible.

While no specific therapy is available to halt the progress of the disease, antispasmodics and antidepressants sometimes provide subjective relief of symptoms. Use of radiotherapy or radiomimetic agents in the treatment of associated malignancies should proceed with caution in view of reports of untoward reactions to conventional doses in AT patients. Known AT carriers should also be treated cautiously. Treatment of IgA-deficient AT patients with gamma globulin is generally ineffective and incurs the risk of severe hypersensitivity reactions. However, IgA-free intravenous gamma globulin preparations may be used for replacement of any IgG or IgG subclass deficiencies. Ineffective immunotherapeutic trials have included thymosin, thymus implants, transfer factor, levamisol, fresh frozen plasma, and fresh bovine colostrum.

**Prognosis:** Most patients are confined to a wheelchair by age 10 years; however, in some families this is delayed by 3–4 years. Infections and malignancy account for over 90% of deaths. Most North American patients are living into their 30s in facilities for the handicapped. Several have married.

**Detection of Carrier:** This is an area of intense investigation. Most carrier-detection assays depend on the hypersensitivity of fibroblasts or lymphocytes to ionizing radiation. With *extensive* testing of an individual, carrier detection is about 80–90% accurate; still impractical for routine clinical use or for screening populations. Carrier detection is now possible for Group A families by genotyping with linked DNA markers, if DNA is available on at least one affected family member. It is estimated that this testing is 95% accurate.

**Special Considerations:** There is a Ataxia-Telangiectasia Medical Research Foundation in Los Angeles, CA, which both conducts scientific research and provides support group services.

**Support Groups:** MN; Wayzata; National Ataxia Foundation

**References:**

Boder E, Sedgwick RP: Ataxia-telangiectasia: a familial syndrome of progressive cerebellar ataxia, oculocutaneous telangiectasia and frequent pulmonary infection. Pediatrics 1958; 21:526–554.

Gatti RA: Immune dysfunction is one of many defects. Immunol Today 1984; 5:121–123. *

Boder E: Ataxia-telangiectasia: an overview. In: Gatti RA, Swift M, eds: Ataxia-telangiectasia: genetics, neuropathology, and immunology of a degenerative disease of childhood. New York: Alan R. Liss, 1985:1–63. *

Bridges BA, et al.: Workshop on ataxia-telangiectasia heterozygotes and cancer. Cancer Res 1985; 45:3979–3980.

Gatti RA, et al.: Translocations involving chromosomes 2p and 22q in ataxia-telangiectasia. Dis Markers 1985; 3:169.

Jaspers NGJ, et al.: Complementation analysis of ataxia-telangiectasia. In: Gatti RA, Swift M, eds: Ataxia-telangiectasia: genetics, neuropathology, and immunology of a degenerative disease of childhood. New York: Alan R. Liss, 1985: 147–162.

Paterson MC, et al.: Cellular hypersensitivity to chronic gamma-radiation in cultured fibroblasts from ataxia-telangiectasia heterozygotes. In: Gatti RA, Swift M, eds: Ataxia-telangiectasia: genetics, neuropathology, and immunology of a degenerative disease of childhood. New York: Alan R. Liss, 1985: 73–87.

Vinters HV, et al.: Sequence of cellular events in cerebellar ontogeny relevant to expression of neuronal abnormalities in ataxia-telangiectasia. In: Gatti RA, Swift M, eds: Ataxia-telangietasia: genetics,

neuropathology, and immunology of a degenerative disease of childhood. New York: Alan R. Liss, 1985: 233–255.

Swift M, et al.: The incidence and gene frequency of ataxia-telangiectasia in the United States. Am J Hum Genet 1986; 39:573–583. *

Swift M, et al.: Breast and other cancers in families with ataxia-telangiectasis. N Eng J Med 1987; 316:1289–1294.

Taylor A, et al.: Variant forms of ataxia telangiectasia. J Med Genet 1987; 24:669–677.

Norman A, et al.: The importance of genetics for the optimization of radiation therapy. Am J Clin Oncol 1988; 11:84–88.

Gatti RA, et al.: Localization of an ataxia-telangiectasia gene to chromosome 11q22–23. Nature 1988; 336:577–580. *

Curry CJR, et al.: AT: a phenotype linking ataxia-telangiectasia with the Nijmegen breakage syndrome. Am J Hum Genet 1989; 45:270–275.

Jaspers NGJ, et al.: Genetic complementation analysis of ataxia-telangiectasia and the Nijmegen breakdown syndrome: a survey of 50 patients. Cytogenet Cell Genet 1989; 49:259–263.

Carbonari M, et al.: Relative increase of T cell expressing the gamma/delta rather than the alpha/beta receptor in ataxia-telangiectasia. New Engl J Med 1990; 322:73–76.

GA020                                                        **Richard A. Gatti**

**Ataxia-telangiectasia (AT) variants**
  *See ATAXIA-TELANGIECTASIA*
**Ateliotic dwarfism**
  *See DWARFISM, PANHYPOPITUITARY*

---

## ATELOSTEOGENESIS                                               2521

**Includes:**

  Chondrodysplasia
  Giant cell chondrodysplasia
  Spondylohumerofemoral hypoplasia, giant cell

**Excludes:** Skeletal dysplasia, De La Chapelle type (2631)

**Major Diagnostic Criteria:** Lethal neonatal dwarfism with diagnostic X-ray and characteristic clinical and histopathologic features.

**Clinical Findings:** This disorder is a form of neonatal micromelic dwarfism associated with death *in utero* or shortly thereafter. The proximal limb segments are most severely affected. The lower extremities are bowed with equinovarous deformity of the feet. There is a depressed nasal bridge and small mouth. X-rays show hypertrophy of the proximal humeri and femora with club foot deformity. There is distal humeral and, to a much lesser degree, distal femoral hypoplasia. The fibulae are hypoplastic or absent. There are dislocations at the elbow joint, and hypoplasia of the vertebral bodies with coronal clefts. The ossification of the short tubular bones is anarchic, with slightly abnormal ossification of some of the tubular bones and severe hypoplasia or no ossification of the others. The pelvis and the skull show no gross abnormality.

**Complications:** Intrauterine or neonatal death.

**Associated Findings:** None known.

**Etiology:** Unknown. Possibly autosomal recessive inheritance.

**Pathogenesis:** Pathologic examination of cartilage shows that reserve zone cartilage is relatively intact but shows hypocellular areas interspersed with areas of normal cellularity. Sometimes multinucleate giant cells are found in the areas of hypocellularity. These giant chondrocytes are not specific to any single lethal skeletal dysplasia.

**MIM No.:** 10872

**POS No.:** 3552

**Sex Ratio:** Presumably M1:F1

**Occurrence:** About a dozen cases have been documented.

**Risk of Recurrence for Patient's Sib:**
  See Part I, *Mendelian Inheritance.*

**Risk of Recurrence for Patient's Child:** Affected individuals are not expected to survive to reproduce.

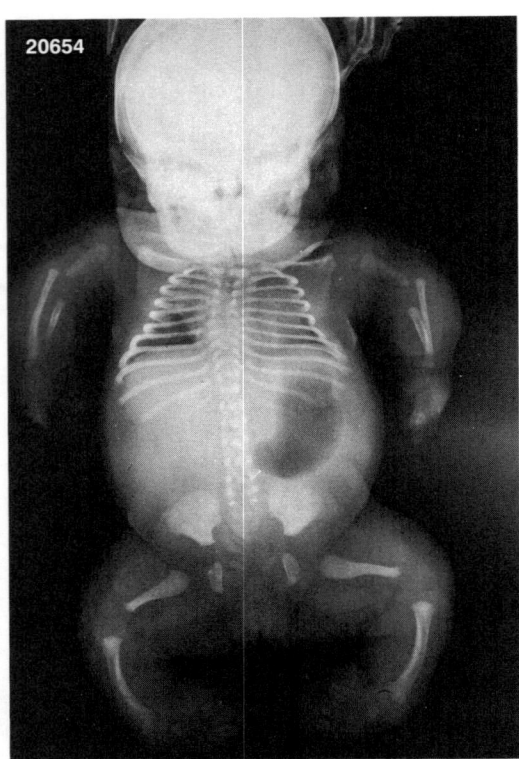

2521-20654: Atelosteogenesis in a newborn; note the club-shape of the humerus and femur, absence of the fibula and short cubitus.

**Age of Detectability:** At birth. Prenatal diagnosis by ultrasound in the second trimester is possible.

**Gene Mapping and Linkage:** Unknown.

**Prevention:** None known. Genetic counseling indicated.

**Treatment:** Unknown.

**Prognosis:** Usually fatal in the neonatal period.

**Detection of Carrier:** Unknown.

**References:**
Kozlowski K, et al.: New forms of neonatal death dwarfism: report of 3 cases. Pediatr Radiol 1981; 10:155–160.
Maroteaux P, et al.: Atelosteogenesis. Am J Med Genetics 1982; 13:15–25.
Silence D, Kozlowski K: "Giant cell" chondrodysplasia. (Letter) Am J Med Genet 1983; 15:627 only.
Stevenson RE, Wilkes G: Atelosteogenesis with survival beyond the neonatal period. Proc Greenwood Genet Center 1983; 2:32–38.
Kozlowski K, Bateson E: Atelosteogenesis. Fortschr Röntgenstr 1984; 140:224–225.

K0021                                              **K.S. Kozlowski**

**Athelia**
*See BREAST, AMASTIA*
**Athetosis-gingival fibromatosis-depigmentation-microphthalmia**
*See GINGIVAL FIBROMATOSIS-DEPIGMENTATION-MICROPHTHALMIA*
**Athyreotic hypothyroidism**
*See THYROID, DYSGENESIS*
**Athyrosis**
*See THYROID, DYSGENESIS*
**Ativan∧, fetal effects**
*See FETAL BENZODIAZEPINE EFFECTS*
**Atkin-Flaitz X-linked mental retardation**
*See X-LINKED MENTAL RETARDATION, ATKIN TYPE*

**Atonic sclerotic muscular dystrophy, Ullrich type**
*See MUSCULAR DYSTROPHY, CONGENITAL WITH ARTHROGRYPOSIS*
**Atopic dermatitis**
*See SKIN, ATOPY, FAMILIAL*
**Atopic dermatitis and (sensorineural) hearing loss**
*See DEAFNESS-ATOPIC DERMATITIS*
**Atopic diathesis with asthma and hayfever**
*See SKIN, ATOPY, FAMILIAL*
**Atopic hypersensitivity**
*See SKIN, ATOPY, FAMILIAL*
**ATPase deficiency**
*See ANEMIA, HEMOLYTIC, RED CELL MEMBRANE DEFECTS*

---

## ATRANSFERRINEMIA                                    0095

**Includes:**
> Iron-binding globulin deficiency
> Siderophilin deficiency

**Excludes:**
> Ferridoxin abnormalities
> Ferritin abnormalities

**Major Diagnostic Criteria:** Demonstration of markedly decreased levels of transferrin or serum iron-binding capacity. Serum iron of 9–30 $\mu$g/dl, total iron-binding capacity of 30–81 $\mu$g/dl, and transferrin levels of 0–39 mg/dl have been noted.

**Clinical Findings:** The first patient with hereditary atransferrinemia was a young girl who had severe hypochromic, microcytic anemia (Heilmeyer et al., 1961). Death resulted from cardiac failure at age 7 years. Hemosiderosis of the heart and liver was seen at autopsy. Low transferrin (Tf) levels were found in both parents. Similar patients have been reported in Japan and Mexico. Acquired atransferrinemia may result from the presence of anti-Tf antibodies following multiple transfusions.

**Complications:** Severe anemia and hemosiderosis with their consequences.

**Associated Findings:** None known.

**Etiology:** Possibly autosomal recessive inheritance.

**Pathogenesis:** Atransferrinemia presumably results from homozygosity for an allele, probably at the structural locus for transferrin, that cannot produce translatable transferrin messenger RNA. In the family reported by Goya et al. (1972), transferrin absence was demonstrated by immunodiffusion, indicating absence of normal levels of cross-reactive material.

**MIM No.:** 20930

**Sex Ratio:** M1:F1

**Occurrence:** Rare, but cases reported in the United States, Europe, Japan and Mexico.

**Risk of Recurrence for Patient's Sib:**
> See Part I, *Mendelian Inheritance.*

**Risk of Recurrence for Patient's Child:**
> See Part I, *Mendelian Inheritance.*

**Age of Detectability:** Presumably at birth.

**Gene Mapping and Linkage:** Unknown.

**Prevention:** None known. Genetic counseling indicated.

**Treatment:** Transfusion has been tried, but only modest increases in plasma transferrin levels can be achieved and clinical improvement is questionable. Goya et al. (1972) administered 1 g of purified human iron-free transferrin to their patient on several occasions and each time produced a marked increased in red cell and hemoglobin levels. The injected transferrin was detectable only for about 1 week, and the red cell and hemoglobin levels returned to pretreatment values after 3 to 6 months.

**Prognosis:** Shortened life span because of hemosiderosis and increased susceptibility to infections.

**Detection of Carrier:** Heterozygotes for atransferrinemia have plasma transferrin levels in the low to normal range and would not be readily identified except by relationship to a known homozygote.

**Special Considerations:** Transferrin Tf C is the electrophoretic type most common, but some 20 codominantly inherited electrophoretic variants are known. Variants more negatively charged than transferrin C are designated *Tf B*, and those more positively charged are *Tf D*, but all have similar iron-binding abilities. Each variant corresponds to a separate Tf allele, all apparently at the same locus and provide a useful genetic marker for population studies. A hypochromic microcytic anemia resulting from an abnormality of transferrin-receptor interaction or in the mechanism of iron release may also be a hereditary defect of the transferrin system. (Morgan, 1981). The transferrin gene has been cloned and sequenced (Park et al., 1985), and the regulatory binding sites for metals, progesterone, glucocorticoids, cAMP, and cis-acting DNA enhancers have been identified (Lucerno et al., 1986).

**References:**

Heilmeyer L, et al.: Kongenitale Atransferrinaemia bei einem sieben Jahre alten Kind. Dtsch Med Wochenschr 1961; 86:1745–1751.

Goya N, et al.: A family of congenital atransferrinemia. Blood 1972; 40:239–245. *

Sutton HE, Jamieson BA: Plasma glycoproteins: transferrins, haptoglobin, and ceruloplasmin. In: Gottschalk A, ed: The glycoproteins, ed. 2. Amsterdam: Elsevier, 1972:653–689.

Chautard-Freire-Maia EA: Probable assignment of the serum cholinesterase (E1) and transferrin (Tf) loci to chromosome 1 in man. Hum Hered 1977; 27:134–142.

Morgan EH: Transferrin, biochemistry, physiology, and clinical significance. Mol Aspects Med 1981; 4:1–123.*

Park I, et al.: Organization of the human transferrin gene: direct evidence that it originated by gene duplication. Proc Natl Acad Sci USA 1985; 82:3149–3153.

Lucerno MA, et al.: The 5' region of the human transferrin gene: structure and potential regulatory sites. Nucleic Acids Res 1986; 14:86–92.

GR035

**Alice A. Greene**

**Atresia choanal posterior**
*See NOSE, POSTERIOR ATRESIA*
**Atresia choanal posterior-lymphedema**
*See NOSE, CHOANAL ATRESIA-LYMPHEDEMA*
**Atresia of anterior nares**
*See NOSE, ANTERIOR ATRESIA*
**Atresia of esophagus with or without tracheoesophageal atresia**
*See ESOPHAGUS, ATRESIA AND TRACHEOESOPHAGEAL FISTULA*
**Atresia of foramina of Luschka and Magendie**
*See HYDROCEPHALY*
**Atresia of larynx, types I, II and III**
*See LARYNX, ATRESIA*
**Atresia of nasopharynx, congenital**
*See CLEFT PALATE-PERSISTENCE OF BUCCOPHARYNGEAL MEMBRANE*
**Atresia of posterior nares**
*See NOSE, POSTERIOR ATRESIA*
**Atresia of posterior nares-lymphedema**
*See NOSE, CHOANAL ATRESIA-LYMPHEDEMA*
**Atresia of pulmonary valve**
*See PULMONARY VALVE, ATRESIA*
**Atresia of tricuspid valve**
*See TRICUSPID VALVE, ATRESIA*
**Atresia, bronchial**
*See BRONCHIAL ATRESIA*
**Atresia, esophageal**
*See ESOPHAGUS, ATRESIA*
**Atresia, mitral valve**
*See MITRAL VALVE ATRESIA*
**Atresia, nasal anterior**
*See NOSE, ANTERIOR ATRESIA*
**Atretic atrioventricular (AV) valve of the right atrium**
*See TRICUSPID VALVE, ATRESIA*
**Atrial fibrillation**
*See ARRHYTHMIA, SUPRAVENTRICULAR TACHYCARDIAS, CONGENITAL*
**Atrial flutter, persistent and paroxysmal**
*See ARRHYTHMIA, SUPRAVENTRICULAR TACHYCARDIAS, CONGENITAL*
**Atrial septal defect at fossa ovalis**
*See ATRIAL SEPTAL DEFECTS*

## ATRIAL SEPTAL DEFECTS 0096

**Includes:**
> Atrial septum, absent
> Atrial septal defect at fossa ovalis
> Common atrium
> Communication interauriculaire
> High sinus venosus with partial pulmonary venous connection
> High sinus venosus without partial pulmonary venous connection
> Low sinus venosus type defect

**Excludes:**
> Atrial septal defect, primum type
> **Heart, endocardial cushion defects** (0347)
> **Pulmonary venous connection, total anomalous** (0842)

**Major Diagnostic Criteria:** The clinical findings of a pulmonary ejection systolic murmur, tricuspid inflow diastolic murmur, widely split and relatively fixed second sound with an accentuated pulmonic component when combined with confirmatory echocardiogram, EKG, vectorcardiogram, and X-rays are diagnostic of an atrial septal defect and may allow surgical intervention without further testing by catheterization and angiocardiography.

**Clinical Findings:** Atrial septal defect (ASD) as an independent lesion comprises 10% of all congenital heart anomalies. Although the size of the defect affects the amount of shunting, the defect is usually large and the shunt therefore depends on the relative compliance of the left and right ventricles. The most common anatomic type is the large, central fossa ovalis variety, but ASD may also occur at the entrance of the superior vena cava and more rarely at the inferior vena cava entrance. In the former, partial anomalous right pulmonary venous connection may be an associated abnormality. In the early weeks of life, the persistence of increased pulmonary vascular resistance and the thick-walled, relatively noncompliant right ventricle limit left-to-right shunting. With increasing age, pulmonary vascular resistance and the right ventricular thickness decrease and the left-to-right shunt increases. It is at this time that the murmurs and the clinical and laboratory consequences of increased right heart flow become evident and the diagnosis is made.

Although the left atrial pressure is only slightly higher than the right atrial pressure, a left-to-right shunt is present and the pulmonary blood flow may exceed the systemic blood flow by 3–4 times. This flow produces the characteristic systolic ejection murmur of relative pulmonary stenosis. The usual absence of a thrill is a helpful clinical finding. Right ventricular systolic pressure is seldom more than 50 mm Hg in an uncomplicated case of ASD, and a systolic gradient as high as 20 mm Hg may be present across the pulmonary valve related to excessive flow across a normal outflow tract. With large flow (eg exceeding 2:1 ratio of pulmonary:systemic blood flow) a diastolic inflow murmur is heard from relative tricuspid stenosis. Wide and relatively fixed splitting of the second sound with a late loud pulmonary component is the most valuable and consistent diagnostic finding. A precordial bulge and right ventricular hyperactivity may be observed and palpated. The presence of partial anomalous pulmonary venous connection as an associated defect does not significantly alter the clinical picture.

X-ray findings include increased pulmonary blood flow and enlargement of the right atrium, right ventricle and main pulmonary artery. In contrast to lesions with left-to-right shunting at the ventricular and the great vessel level, left atrial enlargement is absent. The EKG commonly shows moderate right ventricular enlargement in the form of the rSR[1] pattern. Some cardiographic evidence of right atrial enlargement is seen in about 25% of cases. The PR interval is at the upper limits of normal except in sinus venosus defects which are often accompanied by first degree heart block. Axis is normal or rightward, and rarely may be leftward. In these latter cases, it is necessary to differentiate an ostium secundum atrial defect from the ostium primum variety in which left axis deviation and first degree heart block are characteristic. The vectorcardiogram shows right ventricular hypertrophy consistently with increased terminal rightward and anterior QRS forces.

The atrial septal defect itself usually cannot be imaged by conventional M-mode echocardiographic technique, but changes in blood flow which result from the defect can be observed. The right ventricular cavity is enlarged with respect to normal and the septum may exhibit paradoxical motion. Valvular motions are usually normal. The size and location of the defect can be seen with two dimensional echocardiography.

Right ventricular anterior wall thickness is usually normal. These individual findings are not exclusive for ASD but, when all are combined, a right ventricular volume overload is suggested. Contrast echocardiography is very helpful in non-invasive diagnosis.

Cardiac catheterization data show an increase in oxygen saturation at the right atrial level. Right ventricular systolic pressure is usually mildly elevated. Tiny defects requiring detection by more sensitive methods (eg hydrogen electrode) are rare. Angiocardiographic demonstration can be accomplished by injection into the main pulmonary artery with the shunt into the right atrium seen in the anterior-posterior view right after pulmonary venous return into the left atrium. The ASD can be more precisely delineated with left atrial injection with the patient in the LAO position. The diagnosis of partial anomalous pulmonary venous connection as an alternate or accompanying cause of increased oxygen saturation of the right atrium can be made by selective pulmonary artery angiocardiography or indicator dilution techniques.

**Complications:** Congestive heart failure, when present, develops only with large shunts, usually in infancy or in adult life. Pneumonia may occur. Bacterial endocarditis is very rare in unoperated ostium secundum defects. Pulmonary hypertension with later development of the Eisenmenger physiology usually does not occur until after the second decade.

**Associated Findings:** None known.

**Etiology:** Multifactorial inheritance accounts for the majority of cases. The condition is also associated with certain single mutant gene syndromes such as **Heart-hand syndrome** and **Chondroectodermal dysplasia** which are clearly Mendelian in some families. ASD is a frequent lesion in pregnancies complicated by drug ingestion in first trimester (alcohol, amphetamines, chemotherapy, thalidomide, lithium, etc).

**Pathogenesis:** Defects at the fossa ovalis may be due to overabsorption of septum primum or hypoplasia of the septum secundum, or both. The pathogenesis of the sinus venosus defect is unknown.

**MIM No.:** *10880

**CDC No.:** 745.5

**Sex Ratio:** M1:F2

**Occurrence:** Approximately 1:1000 in the pediatric population.

**Risk of Recurrence for Patient's Sib:**
See Part I, *Mendelian Inheritance.* Empiric risk is 2.5:100.

**Risk of Recurrence for Patient's Child:**
See Part I, *Mendelian Inheritance.* Empiric risk if mother is affected is 4.5%. If father is affected, risk is 1.5%.

**Age of Detectability:** The ASD may be diagnosed in early infancy but more typically becomes apparent between 6 months and 3 years.

**Gene Mapping and Linkage:** Unknown.

**Prevention:** None known. Genetic counseling indicated.

**Treatment:** Open heart surgery is performed with the heart-lung machine and cardiopulmonary bypass. The operation can be performed whenever the child is of sufficient size (usually 30 pounds is quite safe), and is done if the pulmonary blood flow is >1.5 times that of the systemic flow. Usually direct suture closure is feasible, but occasionally a prosthetic patch may be needed. Septal repositioning may be necessary with partial anomalous pulmonary venous connection and with sinus venosus type defects.

Medical management is usual until age 3 years. Usually this consists of observation alone, but rarely, treatment for congestive heart failure or earlier surgical intervention may be necessary.

Closure of small atrial septal defects has recently been accomplished by threading an umbrella-like device into the heart by catheter technique. This method has been used successfully and safely in a few patients and may eliminate the need for thoracotomy in ASD repair in selected individuals.

**Prognosis:** Small secundum type atrial septal defects are compatible with a long life. Spontaneous closure of secundum atrial septal defects may rarely occur, particularly early in life.

Death in early infancy is rare but it has been reported, usually from congestive failure. Pneumonia is also a rare cause of mortality, but death from all causes is rare before the 4th decade. In later life, patients with an ASD have a higher incidence of arrhythmias and unoperated cases may die from progressive pulmonary vascular disease.

**Detection of Carrier:** Unknown.

**Special Considerations:** Larger defects with cardiomegaly and clinical symptoms require operative closure. Closure should be accomplished before pulmonary hypertension occurs. This usually does not occur until early adult life and the occurrence then of cyanosis with right-to-left shunting implies inoperability. Patients with small defects without clinical symptoms, without cardiomegaly and without pulmonary vascular disease can probably live a full lifetime without operation. On the other hand, operation in the pediatric age group carries a mortality which is less than 0.5%, so that some cardiologists advise operation more freely in milder cases.

**Support Groups:** Dallas; American Heart Association

**References:**
Keith JD, et al.: Atrial septal defect. In: Heart disease in infancy and childhood, 2nd ed. New York: Macmillan Co., 1967: 392–431.
Diamond MA, et al.: Echocardiographic features of atrial septal defect. Circulation 1971; 43:129–135.
Goldberg SJ, et al.: Pediatric and adolescent echocardiography. Chicago: Year Book Medical Publishers, 1975:71–76.
Krovetz LJ, et al.: Atrial septal defect: ostium secundum. In: Handbook of pediatric cardiology, 2nd ed. New York: Harper and Row, 1980:167–175.
Feldt RH, et al.: Atrial septal defects and atrioventricular canal. In: Adams FH, Emmanouilides GC, eds. Heart disease in infants, children and adolescents. Baltimore: Williams and Wilkins, 1983: 118–128. *
Nora JJ, Nora AH: Maternal transmission of congenital heart disease. Am J Cardiol 1987; 59:459–463.

LI011                                                    **Leonard M. Linde**

**Atrial septum, absent**
  *See ATRIAL SEPTAL DEFECTS*
**Atrial tachyarrhythmia**
  *See ARRHYTHMIA, SUPRAVENTRICULAR TACHYCARDIAS, CONGENITAL*
**Atrial, myxoma**
  *See MYXOMA, INTRACARDIAC*
**Atriodigital dysplasia**
  *See HEART-HAND SYNDROME*
**Atrioventricular block, congenital complete**
  *See ARRHYTHMIA, HEART BLOCK, CONGENITAL COMPLETE*
**Atrioventricular block, congenital third degree**
  *See ARRHYTHMIA, HEART BLOCK, CONGENITAL COMPLETE*
**Atrioventricular canal, persistent common**
  *See HEART, ENDOCARDIAL CUSHION DEFECTS*
**Atrioventricular discordance with ventriculoarterial discordance**
  *See VENTRICLES, INVERTED WITH TRANSPOSITION OF GREAT ARTERIES*
**Atrioventricular pathways, accessory**
  *See ARRHYTHMIA, WOLFF-PARKINSON-WHITE TYPE*
**Atrioventricularis communis**
  *See HEART, ENDOCARDIAL CUSHION DEFECTS*
**Atrophia bulborum hereditaria**
  *See NORRIE DISEASE*
**Atrophy, optic**
  *See OPTIC ATROPHY, INFANTILE HEREDOFAMILIAL*
**Attention deficit disorder**
  *See ATTENTION-DEFICIT HYPERACTIVITY DISORDER (ADHD)*

## ATTENTION-DEFICIT HYPERACTIVITY DISORDER (ADHD)      3240

**Includes:**
    Attention deficit disorder
    Hyperactive child syndrome
    Hyperkinetic-impulse disorder
    Hyperkinetic syndrome

**Excludes:**
    **Autism, infantile** (2128)
    Pervasive developmental disorders

**Major Diagnostic Criteria:** Age-inappropriate levels of inattention, impulsivity, and motor hyperactivity. The *Diagnostic and statistical manual of mental disorders* (DSM-III-R) lists diagnostic criteria for ADHD (DSM-III-R code 314.01) (American Psychiatric Association, 1987), and describes clinical and epidemiological findings.

**Clinical Findings:** Onset is before seven years of age. The most prominent feature of ADHD in preschool children is gross motor overactivity, with inattention and impulsivity manifested as frequent shifting among activities. In later childhood and adolescence, excessive restlessness and fidgeting are more prominent than gross overactivity, and inattention and impulsivity substantially impair academic performance. Symptoms may be exacerbated by increasing attentional demands, and may be ameliorated by behavioral reinforcement or increased environmental salience (DSM-III-R).

Frequently present are symptoms of specific developmental disorders (DSM-III-R diagnostic code 315), conduct disorder (DSM 312), and oppositional defiant disorder (DSM 313.81). Patients sometimes have functional enuresis (DSM 307.60) and encopresis (DSM 307.70). Overrepresentation of nonlocalized, neurological ("soft-") signs is found in this disorder. ADHD symptomatology may be present in mentally retarded individuals due to a general, intellectual developmental delay; the diagnosis of ADHD is made if symptoms are extreme for the patient's mental age.

Abnormalities have been reported in cortical evoked potentials, cerebral blood flow, neurotransmitter metabolites, and neuroendocrine measures.

**Complications:** School difficulties.

**Associated Findings:** Several laboratories have reported an excess of minor physical anomalies in children with ADHD. These studies have relied almost exclusively on a protocol developed by Waldrop and Halverson (1971), which yields a full-scale score equal to the weighted sum of individual minor physical anomalies, e.g., epicanthus, hypertelorism, low-set ears, and single transverse palmar crease.

The full-scale Waldrop and Halverson score is continuously distributed in the general population, and cut-off points are sometimes used to operationally define dysmorphology. The range of full-scale scores reported for ADHD patients in the literature is 2.2 - 5.6 (median 3.5), compared to 0.8 - 3.5 (median 2.5) in normal controls. Using a cut-off point > 5 to indicate dysmorphology, 18.0 - 31.0% (median 29.8%) of ADHD cases meet this criterion, compared to 8.3 - 12.6% (median 10.4%) of normal controls.

There is also a statistical overrepresentation of non-relative adoptive status in children with ADHD (12 - 20%, compared to a population base rate of approximately 2%).

**Etiology:** Considered to be etiologically heterogeneous. Most firmly supported by the literature are genetic influences, which may be varied and interact with environmental factors. The mode of inheritance, presently unclear, is dependent on assumptions made in quantitative models of transmission. ADHD appears to be overrepresented in normally intelligent children with specific genetic syndromes, including **Tourette syndrome**, **Neurofibromatosis**, and **Phenylketonuria** treated with a strict low phenylalanine diet.

Several prenatal environmental etiologies have been suggested, including: (1) damage resulting in CNS insult (e.g., physical disruption, anoxia), (2) infection (e.g., viral encephalopathies), (3) malnourishment, and (4) exposure to teratogens (e.g., ethanol). The role that factors (1)-(3) play in the etiology of ADHD is conjectural and narrowly-based. There is more evidence that factor (4) plays a role in the genesis of ADHD, specifically in **Fetal alcohol syndrome** (Shaywitz et al., 1980). Recent epidemiological studies implicate body lead burden and early childhood malnourishment as potential factors in the development of ADHD symptomatology.

**Pathogenesis:** Unknown. Neuropsychological and brain imaging studies point to frontal lobe dysfunction in ADHD (Zametkin and Rapoport, 1987).

**Sex Ratio:** M6:F1 to M9:F1 in clinical samples; M3:F1 in community samples.

**Occurrence:** Estimates depend on the severity of symptomatology required for a diagnosis. The prevalence of ADHD may be as high as 3% in school-aged children.

**Risk of Recurrence for Patient's Sib:** For the sibs of male probands, estimates for brothers is 26–42%, and for sisters 9–24%.

**Risk of Recurrence for Patient's Child:** Unknown.

**Age of Detectability:** Before age four in approximately one-half of cases (DSM-III-R); some parents note ADHD symptoms earlier (Jellinek and Herzog, 1988). Often the condition is not recognized until the child enters school.

**Gene Mapping and Linkage:** Unknown.

**Prevention:** Pregnant women should be informed of the risk of ADHD associated with teratogens (e.g., ethanol), and body lead burden should be minimized.

**Treatment:** Stimulant medication (e.g., methylphenidate) and behavior modification are commonly used (Barkley, 1981; Zametkin & Rapoport, 1987; Jellinek & Herzog, 1988).

**Prognosis:** Usually persists throughout childhood, and approximately one-third of cases have residual ADHD symptomatology in adulthood (DSM-III-R).

**Detection of Carrier:** Possibly by clinical assessment.

**Support Groups:** FL; Plantation; Children with Attention Deficit Disorders (CH.A.D.D.)

**References:**
Waldrop M, Halverson CF: Minor physical anomalies and hyperactive behavior in young children. In: Hellmuth J, ed: The exceptional infant. New York: Brunner & Mazel, 1971:343–380.
Shaywitz SE, et al.: Behavior and learning difficulties in children of normal intelligence born to alcoholic mothers. J Pediat 1980; 96:978–982.
Barkley RA: Hyperactive children: a handbook for diagnosis and treatment. New York: Guilford, 1981.
Vandenberg SG, et al.: The heredity of behavior disorders in adults and children. New York: Plenum, 1986.
American Psychiatric Association: Diagnostic and Statistical Manual of Mental Disorders, ed. 3, Revised (DSM-III-R). Washington, APA, 1987.
Zametkin AJ, Rapoport JL: Neurobiology of Attention Deficit Disorder with hyperactivity: where have we come in 50 years? J Am Acad Child Adol Psychiat 1987; 26:676–686.
Jellinek MS, Herzog DB: Special populations: the child. In: Nicholi AM, ed: The new Harvard guide to psychiatry. Cambridge: Harvard University Press, 1988.
Deutsch CK, et al.: Genetic latent structure analysis of dysmorphology in attention deficit disorder. Special issue on psychiatric genetics (Leckman J, Pauls D, eds). J Am Acad Child Adol Psychiat 1990; 29:189–194.
Lou HC, et al.: Focal cerebral dysfunction in developmental learning disabilities. Lancet 1990; 335:8–11.

DE027        **Curtis K. Deutsch**

**Auditory canal, atresia of**
*See EAR, AUDITORY CANAL ATRESIA*

## AURAL ATRESIA-DYSMORPHIC FACIES-SKELETAL DEFECTS 3130

**Includes:**
Aural atresia-multiple congenital anomalies-mental retardation
Cooper-Jabs syndrome
Face, dysmorphic-skeletal defects-aural atresia
Skeletal defects-dysmorphic facies-aural atresia

**Excludes:**
**Johanson-Blizzard syndrome** (2026)
**Velo-cardio-facial syndrome** (2129)

**Major Diagnostic Criteria:** The combination of aural atresia, abnormal facial appearance, skeletal anomalies, and mental retardation.

**Clinical Findings:** Present in the two reported sibs were brachycephaly, esotropia, midface hypoplasia, anteverted nares, low-set and posteriorly rotated ears, atretic ear canals, long fifth fingers, proximally placed thumbs, positional defects of feet (calcaneus in one, equinovarus in the other), anteriorly displaced anus, hypotonia, growth failure, normal head circumference, and mental retardation.

**Complications:** Deafness secondary to the aural atresia.

**Associated Findings:** One sib also had **Hernia, umbilical, Camptodactyly**, dislocated left hip, osteoporosis, 13 ribs, scoliosis, and arrested **Hydrocephaly**. The other sib had hyperextensible joints.

**Etiology:** Possibly autosomal recessive inheritance.

**Pathogenesis:** Unknown.

**MIM No.:** 20977

**Sex Ratio:** M0:F2 (observed).

**Occurrence:** Reported in a pair of sibs from the United States.

**Risk of Recurrence for Patient's Sib:**
See Part I, *Mendelian Inheritance.*

**Risk of Recurrence for Patient's Child:**
See Part I, *Mendelian Inheritance.*

**Age of Detectability:** At birth, by physical examination.

**Gene Mapping and Linkage:** Unknown.

**Prevention:** None known. Genetic counseling indicated.

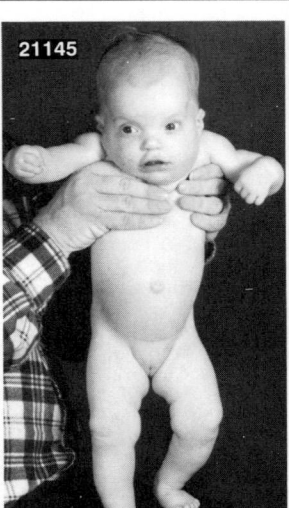
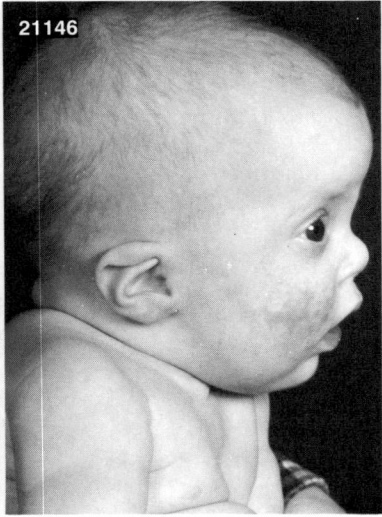

**3130-21145:** Five-month-old infant with aural atresia, multiple congenital anomalies and mental retardation. 21146: Lateral view of the face shows low-set and posteriorly rotated ear with overlap of the upper helix.

**Treatment:** Orthopedic treatment for positional anomalies of the feet and hip dislocation; hearing aids for deafness.

**Prognosis:** Mental retardation is moderately severe, with a measured IQ in one sib of 30–40. Life span is undetermined.

**Detection of Carrier:** Unknown.

**References:**
Cooper LF, Jabs EW: Aural atresia associated with multiple congenital anomalies and mental retardation: a new syndrome. J Pediatr 1987; 110:747–750.

T0007      Helga V. Toriello
C0072      Linda F. Cooper
JA015      Ethylin Wang Jabs

**Aural atresia-multiple congenital anomalies-mental retardation**
*See AURAL ATRESIA-DYSMORPHIC FACIES-SKELETAL DEFECTS*
**Aural exostoses**
*See EAR, EXOSTOSES*

## AURICULO-OSTEODYSPLASIA 0098

**Includes:**
Beals auriculo-osteodysplasia syndrome
Ear abnormalities-short stature-elbow/hip dislocation
Elbow/hip dislocation-ear abnormalities-short stature
Osteodysplasia, auricular
Short stature-ear abnormalities-elbow/hip dislocation

**Excludes:**
Coxoauricular syndrome
**Mesomelic dysplasia, Reinhardt-Pfeiffer type** (0648)
**Nail-patella syndrome** (0704)
Oculo-palato-digital syndrome

**Major Diagnostic Criteria:** Unusual ear lobe and ear lobe attachment; dislocation of the elbows and hips.

**Clinical Findings:** Height is between the 3rd and 50th percentiles in all affected individuals. Malformed external ears characterized by elongated lobes with cone-shaped attachment to the head, prominent antihelix and overfolded helix are usually present. In addition, the ears in some individuals are small and superiorly flattened. Skeletal abnormalities include dysplasia of the capitellum, with or without bilateral radial-head dislocation; hypoplasia of the distal radial epiphyses; horizontal position of the clavicles, changes in the shape of the scapulas; and in some affected females, dysplasia or dislocation of the hips. Muscular appearing neck with broad shoulders is also present. Ectodermally derived structures are normal. Mental retardation is not associated with this condition.

**Complications:** Degenerative joint disease may occur in the hips. Variable limitations of elbow and hip mobility are frequently present.

**Associated Findings:** None known.

**Etiology:** Autosomal dominant inheritance with full penetrance, but variability of expression.

**Pathogenesis:** Unknown.

**MIM No.:** *10900

**POS No.:** 3035

**Sex Ratio:** M1:F1

**Occurrence:** Rare. Two kindreds have been reported in the American literature and one isolated case in the Czechoslovakian literature.

**Risk of Recurrence for Patient's Sib:**
See Part I, *Mendelian Inheritance.*

**Risk of Recurrence for Patient's Child:**
See Part I, *Mendelian Inheritance.*

**Age of Detectability:** At birth by physical examination. At this time the characteristic ear changes are present while mild limitation to elbow motion may be evident. Elbow dislocation may develop later.

**Gene Mapping and Linkage:** Unknown.

**Prevention:** None known. Genetic counseling indicated.

**Treatment:** Early detection and treatment of hip dislocation.

**Prognosis:** Independent life and normal intelligence is expected in all cases. Limb function is variable; there may be significant disability from the hip dislocation/dysplasia.

**Detection of Carrier:** Unknown.

**References:**

Beals RK: Auriculo-osteodysplasia: a syndrome of multiple osseous dysplasia, ear anomaly, and short stature. J Bone Joint Surg 1967; 49A:1541–1550. *
Duca D, et al.: A previously unreported, dominantly inherited syndrome of shortness of stature, ear malformations, and hip dislocation: the coxoauricular syndrome-autosomal or X-linked male-lethal. Am J Med Genet 1981; 8:173–180.
Vanek J: Aurikulo-osteodysplazie. Cas Lek Cesk 1981; 120:452–453. †

ES004                                                                **Luis F. Escobar**
WE005                                                             **David D. Weaver**

**Auriculotemporal syndrome**
*See SWEATING, GUSTATORY*

---

## AUTISM, INFANTILE                                                                2128

**Includes:**

    Infantile psychosis
    Kanner disease

**Excludes:**

    Depression, infant
    Deprivation syndromes
    Ego development, atypical
    Mental retardation syndromes with autistic features
    **Mood and thought disorders** (1532)
    **Rett syndrome** (2226)
    Sensory deprivation syndromes with autistic features
    Symbiotic psychosis

**Major Diagnostic Criteria:** A combination of most of the following features should be present for this diagnosis to be strongly suspected: 1) impaired social development, which includes a profound inability to relate to other people; Kanner's "extreme autistic aloneness" or Chess's "lack of effective human contact," 2) onset before the age of 30 months, 3) delayed and deviant communication abilities, particularly manifest in language development, including impaired comprehension appropriate for age and unusual use of language, 4) ritualistic and compulsive behavior, including an "insistence on sameness," 5) disturbances of motility, particularly hand flapping and stereotypies, 6) abnormal perceptual responses to sensory stimuli, particularly in auditory, visual, and tactile modalities, and, in a smaller percentage of cases, 7) an "area of excellence," that is, isolated normal or superior level of mental functioning in a child functioning at a much lower level in most other areas; also called "splinter skills."

**Clinical Findings:** The onset of clinical symptoms varies from the neonatal period to as late as 30 months of age. The three physical stigmata that occur in some cases are hypertelorism, low-set ears, and partial syndactyly of the second and third toes. In patients with neonatal onset, irritability, failure to mold in the mother's arms, arching of the back (or actual opisthotonos), tactile, auditory, and visual hypersensitivity may be present. Failure of eye contact often is striking. Seizure disorders occur in some patients past adolescence. Laboratory findings include abnormalities in whole blood serotonin which is elevated in the majority of patients and below normal limits in less than 10% of the patients. Hyperuricosuria is seen in 22% of patients and hypocalciuria in 21% of the patients. Other laboratory findings show the fragile X syndrome in a small percentage of patients, usually males. Rare cases have positive laboratory tests for gestational rubella, phenylketonuria, or pyruvic acidosis (see **Fetal rubella syndrome** and **Fetal effects from maternal PKU**).

**Complications:** Self-stimulatory behaviors, apparently unprovoked explosive rages, cyclic diarrhea, or constipation.

**Associated Findings:** EEG and CT often are within normal limits, but not always. MRI are also usually within limits (the occasional finding of vermal cerebellar atrophy is not specific to this syndrome).

**Etiology:** About ten percent of the patients show a familial pattern usually suggesting autosomal recessive inheritance. Other etiologies include **X-linked mental retardation, Fragile X syndrome, Adenylosuccinate monophosphate lyase deficiency**, phenylketonuria (see **Fetal effects from maternal PKU**), **Fetal rubella syndrome**, one of the **Hydrocephaly** syndromes, and sequelae of the infantile spasms syndrome. The majority of patients do not have a definitive etiology. No relationship has been found to parental education or occupation, or to religion or racial origin.

**Pathogenesis:** "Perceptual inconstancy" suggests that affected individuals have much difficulty handling sensory input. The slowness of language development in almost all of the patients suggests that the auditory pathways may be one area primarily affected in many children.

**MIM No.:** 20985

**Sex Ratio:** M4:F1

**Occurrence:** 1:2,500 live births

**Risk of Recurrence for Patient's Sib:** The overall recurrence rate is 8.6% (if the first autistic child is male, 7%; if the first autistic child is female, 14.5%).

**Risk of Recurrence for Patient's Child:** No report exists of a patient having reproduced.

**Age of Detectability:** Any time between birth and 30 months of age.

**Gene Mapping and Linkage:** Unknown.

**Prevention:** Vaccine for rubella in females prior to childbearing age, PKU screening of neonates. Genetic counseling is indicated.

**Treatment:** Treatment is of two types. First is educational programming which primarily should be some type of behavior conditioning or behavior modifying techniques. Second, there is medical management of any documented biochemical abnormality.

**Prognosis:** Most patients live into the adult age group. Few are self-sufficient as adults.

**Detection of Carrier:** Undetermined, except in the fragile X subgroup (see **X-linked mental retardation, Fragile X syndrome**).

**Special Considerations:** This syndrome was first identified by Kanner in 1943 when he described a group of children having "autistic disturbances of affective contact." In 1944 he adopted the term "early infantile autism." The fact that the syndrome has multiple etiologies has only recently been documented.

**Support Groups:**

    NY; Albany; National Society for Autistic Children
    DC; Washington; National Society for Children and Adults with Autism

**References:**

Kanner L: Autistic disturbances of affective contact. New Child 1943; 2:207–250.
Folstein S, Rutter M: Infantile autism: a genetic study of 21 twin pairs. J Child Psychol Psychiatr 1977; 18:297–321.
Rutter M, Schopler E, eds: Autism: a reappraisal of concepts and treatment. New York: Plenum Press, 1978.
Blomquist HK, et al.: Frequency of the fragile X syndrome in infantile autism: a Swedish multicenter study. Clin Genet 1985; 27:113–117.
Coleman M, Gillberg C: The biology of the autistic syndromes. New York: Praeger Scientific, 1985. *
Ritvo E, et al.: The UCLA-University of Utah epidemiologic survey of autism: prevalence. Am J Psychiatry 1989; 146:194–199.
Ritvo E, et al.: The UCLA-University of Utah epidemiologic survey of autism: recurrence risk estimates and genetic counseling. Am J Psychiatry 1989; 146:1032–1036.

Gillberg C, ed: Diagnosis and treatment of Autism. New York: Plenum Press, 1990.

C0018                                    **Mary Coleman**

**Autism, succinylpurinemic type**
  *See ADENYLOSUCCINATE MONOPHOSPHATE LYASE DEFICIENCY*
**Autism-dementia-ataxia-loss of purposeful hand use**
  *See RETT SYNDROME*
**Autoimmune disease, congenital arrhythmia**
  *See ARRHYTHMIA, FROM MATERNAL AUTOIMMUNE DISEASE,
    CONGENITAL*
**Autoimmune disease, deficiency of C2**
  *See COMPLEMENT COMPONENT 2, DEFICIENCY OF*
**Autoimmune disease, deficiency of C4**
  *See COMPLEMENT COMPONENT 4, DEFICIENCY OF*
**Autoimmune disease, deficiency of regulatory component C1**
  *See ANGIOEDEMA, HEREDITARY*
**Autoimmune polyendocrinopathy-candidiasis-ectodermal dystrophy**
  *See POLYGLANDULAR AUTOIMMUNE SYNDROME*
**Autonomic control, congenital failure of**
  *See HYPOVENTILATION, CONGENITAL CENTRAL ALVEOLAR TYPE*
**Autonomic nervous system dysfunction (congenital)**
  *See HYPOVENTILATION, CONGENITAL CENTRAL ALVEOLAR TYPE*
**Autonomic noradrenergic and adrenomedullary failure (some)**
  *See DOPAMINE BETA-HYDROXYLASE DEFICIENCY, CONGENITAL*
**Autosomal recessive spastic ataxia of Charlevoix-Saguenay
    (ARSACS)**
  *See SPASTIC ATAXIA, CHARLEVOIX-SAGUENAY TYPE*
**Autosomal recessive vitamin D dependency (ARVD)**
  *See RESISTANCE TO 1,25 DIHYDROXY VITAMIN D*
**Autosomal recessive vitamin D-dependency (ARVDD)**
  *See RICKETS, VITAMIN D-DEPENDENT, TYPE I*
**Axial osteosclerosis**
  *See OSTEOMESOPYKNOSIS*
**Axonal type Charcot-Marie-Tooth disease**
  *See NEUROPATHY, HEREDITARY MOTOR AND SENSORY, TYPE II*
**Azorean neurologic disease (pejorative)**
  *See MACHADO-JOSEPH DISEASE*
**Azygos continuation of inferior vena cava**
  *See VENA CAVA, ABSENT HEPATIC SEGMENT*

# ❖ B ❖

B responsive homocystinuria without methylmalonic aciduria
See *METHYLCOBALAMIN DEFICIENCY*
B-cell chronic lymphocytic leukemia
See *LEUKEMIA/LYMPHOMA, B-CELL*
B-cell prolymphocytic leukemia
See *LEUKEMIA/LYMPHOMA, B-CELL*
B-K mole syndrome
See *CANCER, MALIGNANT MELANOMA, FAMILIAL*
B-responsive forms of methylmalonic acidemia
See *ACIDEMIA, METHYLMALONIC*
B2M amyloidosis
See *AMYLOIDOSIS, HEMODIALYSIS-RELATED*
BADS syndrome
See *ALBINISM-BLACK LOCKS-DEAFNESS*
Baelz syndrome
See *LIP, CHEILITIS GLANDULARIS*
Baller-Gerold syndrome
See *CRANIOSYNOSTOSIS-RADIAL APLASIA SYNDROME*
Balloon or billowing mitral valve
See *MITRAL VALVE PROLAPSE*
Baltic myoclonus epilepsy
See *SEIZURES, PROGRESSIVE MYOCLONIC, UNVERRICHT-LUNDBORG TYPE*
Bamatter Syndrome
See *OSTEODYSPLASTICA GERODERMIA, BAMATTER TYPE*
Bamboo hair
See *ICHTHYOSIS, LINEARIS CIRCUMFLEXA*
Band keratitis
See *EYE, KERATOPATHY, BAND-SHAPED*
Band-shaped keratopathy
See *EYE, KERATOPATHY, BAND-SHAPED*
Bannayan-Zonana syndrome
See *OVERGROWTH, BANNAYAN TYPE*
Bannworth syndrome
See *FETAL EFFECTS FROM LYME DISEASE*
Barakat syndrome
See *NEPHROSIS-NERVE DEAFNESS-HYPOPARATHYROIDISM, BARAKAT TYPE*
Barbiturate effects, fetal
See *FETAL BARBITURATE EFFECTS*

## BARDET-BIEDL SYNDROME                                    2363

**Includes:**
Biedl-Bardet syndrome
Laurence-Moon-Bardet-Biedl syndrome (some)

**Excludes:**
Acrocephalopolysyndactyly (0013)
Alstrom syndrome (0041)
Biemond II syndrome (2169)
Cohen syndrome (2023)
Laurence-Moon syndrome (0578)
Prader-Willi syndrome (0823)
X-linked mental retardation-growth-hearing and genital defects (2480)

**Major Diagnostic Criteria:** Polydactyly, genital hypoplasia, pigmentary retinopathy, obesity, mental retardation.

**Clinical Findings:** Postaxial polydactyly and hypoplastic genitalia are present at birth. The extra digits are often also syndactylic. Most cases have some degree of hypogonadotrophism but primary gonadal hypoplasia is also present. Pale optic discs may be present at birth. Visual acuity is poor and worsens slowly. A combined rod and cone retinal dystrophy produces pigmentary mottling of the retina, most noticeable around the macula. The dystrophy has variable rates of progression. Some cases develop pigment changes such as **Retinitis pigmentosa**. Obesity develops during infancy and mental retardation becomes evident during childhood. Height growth is poor; most patients are small at birth and become short adults.

**Complications:** Many are classified as legally blind. The mental defect is quite limiting.

**Associated Findings:** Several cases have had progressive nephropathy.

**Etiology:** Autosomal recessive inheritance.

**Pathogenesis:** Failure of normal embryologic development.

**MIM No.:** *20990

**POS No.:** 3276

**CDC No.:** 759.820

**Sex Ratio:** M1:F1

**Occurrence:** Over 60 cases have been documented. Reportedly increased in the Arab population of Kuwait.

**Risk of Recurrence for Patient's Sib:**
See Part I, *Mendelian Inheritance*.

**Risk of Recurrence for Patient's Child:**
See Part I, *Mendelian Inheritance*. Most affected individuals are infertile.

**Age of Detectability:** Evident at birth, although definitive diagnosis is difficult until the obesity develops and mental retardation becomes evident.

**Gene Mapping and Linkage:** Unknown.

**Prevention:** None known. Genetic counseling indicated.

**Treatment:** Careful nutritional management controls the obesity but does not abolish it. Severe calorie restriction may cause malnutrition.

**Prognosis:** A chronic handicapping condition due mainly to the visual defect and mental retardation.

**Detection of Carrier:** If genealogic studies identify the underlying cause as parental consanguinity stemming from membership in a small genetic isolate, normal relatives have as high as 50% chance of heterozygosity.

**Special Considerations:** Bardet and Biedl described a familial syndrome in which **Polydactyly** was present but spastic paraplegia was absent. Laurence and Moon described a familial syndrome in which spastic paraplegia was present but polydactyly was absent. Shortly after Biedl's report, the medical literature became confused, grouping many different disorders under the terms *Laurence-Moon-Biedl syndrome* or *Laurence-Moon-Bardet-Biedl syndrome*.

Very few case descriptions truly fit into either the syndrome described by Bardet and Biedl or the syndrome described by Laurence and Moon. Most published case descriptions appear to represent either familial or isolated cases of quite distinct syndromes, rather than variants of either of the two classic syndromes.

**Support Groups:** MD; Lexington Park; Laurence-Moon-Biedl Syndrome (LMBS) Support Network

**References:**
Bardet G: Sur un syndrome d'obésité infantile avec polydactylie et retinite pigmentaire. (Contribution a l'étude des formes cliniques de l'obésité hypophysaire). Ph.D. Thesis, No. 479, 1920; Paris.
Biedl A: Ein geschwisterpaar mit adiposo-genitaler dystrophie. Dtsch Med Wochenschr 1922; 48:1630 only.
Campor RV, Aaberg TM: Ocular and systemic manifestations of the Bardet-Biedl syndrome. Am J Ophthalmol 1982; 94:750–756.
Schachat AP, Maumenee IH: The Bardet-Biedl syndrome and related disorders. Arch Ophthalmol 1982; 100:285–288.
Pagon RA, et al.: Hepatic involvement in the Bardet-Biedl syndrome. Am J Med Genet 1982; 13:373–381.
Farag TI, Teebi AS: Bardet-Biedl and Laurence-Moon syndromes in a mixed Arab population. Clin Genet 1988; 33:78–82.

TH017  
UR001

**T.F. Thurmon**  
**S.A. Ursin**

**Bare lymphocyte syndrome**
*See IMMUNODEFICIENCY, SEVERE COMBINED*
**Barlow syndrome**
*See MITRAL VALVE PROLAPSE*
**Barnes syndrome**
*See THORACOPELVIC DYSOSTOSIS*
**Bart syndrome**
*See EPIDERMOLYSIS BULLOSUM, TYPE III*
**Bart-Pumphrey syndrome**
*See KNUCKLE PADS-LEUKONYCHIA-DEAFNESS*
**Bartsocas-Papas syndrome**
*See PTERYGIUM SYNDROME, POPLITEAL, LETHAL*

## BARTTER SYNDROME 0100

**Includes:**
Hypokalemic alkalosis
Pseudohypoadrenocorticism

**Excludes:**
Secondary hyperaldosteronism due to chronic diuretic abuse
Secondary hyperaldosteronism due to chronic laxative abuse
Secondary hyperaldosteronism due to juvenile nephrophthisis
Secondary hyperaldosteronism due to medullary cystic disease of kidney

**Major Diagnostic Criteria:** Growth retardation, muscle weakness, mental retardation, and polyuria with inability to concentrate urine, most frequently presenting in infancy or early childhood. The term "Bartter syndrome" should be restricted to those patients having hypokalemic alkalosis, normotension, hyperaldosteronism, and juxtaglomerular hyperplasia without a primary renal, GI, or drug-induced cause.

**Clinical Findings:** This syndrome most commonly presents in late infancy or early childhood and is characterized by hypokalemia, hypochloremia, alkalosis, normal blood pressure, hyperaldosteronism, and hyperplasia of the juxtaglomerular apparatus. Other features include growth retardation, muscle weakness, mental retardation, and polyuria with inability to concentrate urine. Edema is not present. Plasma renin and angiotensin levels are elevated. The pressor response to infused angiotensin is diminished, as is the rise in aldosterone following infusion of renin. Urinary excretion of prostaglandin E and its derivatives is markedly increased.

Adolescents and young adults also have been reported with this syndrome. In these cases intellect and stature have been normal,

periods of severe weakness have even been diagnosed as periodic paralysis, and weight loss with vomiting has been ascribed to psychologic disturbances, including anorexia nervosa.

Chronic abuse of diuretics and purgatives may mimic this condition. Indeed, chronic sodium depletion of various etiologies may mimic the findings by its effect of stimulating the renin-angiotensin-aldosterone system and the juxtaglomerular renal apparatus. Consequently, renal diseases such as medullary cystic disease and juvenile nephronophthisis may simulate the Bartter syndrome.

**Complications:** The complications are predominantly due to the effects of hypokalemia.

**Associated Findings:** Erythropoietin overproduction and erythrocytosis have been described. Also, capillary basement membrane thickening has been described in the renal glomeruli.

**Etiology:** Presumably autosomal recessive inheritance.

**Pathogenesis:** Possibly a defect in renal tubular reabsorption of sodium or a defect in the conversion of angiotensin I to angiotensin II, as a result of deficiency in renin substrate. Expansion of the plasma volume by sodium loading does not lower aldosterone excretion in Bartter syndrome, whereas expansion of plasma volume will lower aldosterone secretion when the syndrome is simulated by renal, GI, or drug-induced causes. More recent observations on this syndrome strongly suggest that renal overproduction of prostaglandin substantially contributes to the pathogenesis and clinical features of this condition. Excessive urinary excretion of prostacyclin has been documented. Excessive renal production of prostaglandin E may also be responsible for the high plasma bradykinin and low urinary kinins. Although the primary role of prostaglandin overproduction has been questioned, dramatic improvement in biochemical and clinical abnormalities has resulted in the use of prostaglandin synthetase inhibitors such as indomethacin, aspirin, or ibuprofen in some cases.

**MIM No.:** *24120

**Sex Ratio:** M1:F1

**Occurrence:** Rare, but reported in a wide range of populations.

**Risk of Recurrence for Patient's Sib:**
See Part I, *Mendelian Inheritance.*

**Risk of Recurrence for Patient's Child:**
See Part I, *Mendelian Inheritance.*

**Age of Detectability:** May be detected in infancy through adulthood, but most commonly in early childhood.

**Gene Mapping and Linkage:** Unknown.

**Prevention:** None known. Genetic counseling indicated.

**Treatment:** Aldosterone antagonists such as spironolactone or triamterene in association with supplementation by large doses of potassium have tended to correct the hypokalemia in some patients. The beta-adrenergic blocking agent propranolol, which can inhibit the production of renin when given in conjunction with spironolactone, has also proven efficacious. While the safety of long-term use of aspirin, indomethacin, or ibuprofen is yet to be determined in this condition, these are now the therapies of choice with documented effectiveness in Bartter syndrome. Secondary causes such as diuretic abuse should be eliminated.

**Prognosis:** Guarded for normal life span.

**Detection of Carrier:** Unknown.

**References:**
Bartter FC, et al.: Hyperplasia of the juxtaglomerular complex with hyperaldosteronism and hypokalemic alkalosis: a new syndrome. Am J Med 1962; 33:811–828.
Goodman AD, et al.: Pathogenesis of Bartter's syndrome. N Engl J Med 1969; 281:1435.
Gardner JD, et al.: Altered membrane sodium transport in Bartter's syndrome. J Clin Invest 1972; 51:1565.
Modlinger RS, et al.: Some observations on the pathogenesis of Bartter's syndrome. N Engl J Med 1973; 289:1022.
Tarm F, et al.: Bartter's syndrome: an unusual presentation. Mayo Clin Proc 1973; 48:280–283.

Bartter's syndrome. Editorial. Lancet 1976; II:721.

Fichman MP, et al.: Role of prostaglandins in the pathogenesis of Bartter's syndrome. Am J Med 1976; 60:785.

Vinci JM, et al.: The kallikrein-kinin system in Bartter's syndrome and its response to prostaglandin synthetase inhibition. J Clin Invest 1978; 61:1671.

Güllner HG, et al.: Prostacyclin overproduction in Bartter's syndrome. Lancet 1979; II:767.

Etzioni A, et al.: Effect of indomethacin in a patient with Bartter's syndrome: evidence against a primary role of prostaglandins in this disorder. Pediatr Res 1980; 14:1395.

Garin EH, et al.: Treatment of Bartter's syndrome with indomethacin. Am J Dis Child 1980; 134:258.

Güllner HG, et al.: Correction of increased sympathoadrenal activity in Bartter's syndrome by inhibition of prostaglandin synthesis. J Clin Endocrinol Metab 1980; 50:857.

Shimoyama R: Reversal of altered vascular responsiveness in Bartter's syndrome by indomethacin treatment. J Clin Endocrinol Metab 1980; 51:908.

Cole CH, et al.: Effect of treatment with prostaglandin synthetase inhibitors on the erythrocyte sodium transport abnormality of Bartter's syndrome. Pediatr Res 1981; 15:926.

Rodrigues-Pereira R, van Wersch J: Inheritance of Bartter syndrome. Am J Med Genet 1983; 15:79–84.

Watson ML et al.: Systematic prostaglandin I2 synthesis is normal in patients with Bartter syndrome. Lancet 1983; II:368.

SP004                                   **Mark A. Sperling**

**Basal cell epithelioma, multiple benign nodular intraepidermal**
*See SCALP, CYLINDROMAS*

**Basal cell nevi**
*See NEVOID BASAL CELL CARCINOMA SYNDROME*

**Basal cell nevus syndrome**
*See NEVOID BASAL CELL CARCINOMA SYNDROME*

**Basal ganglion disorder-mental retardation**
*See X-LINKED MENTAL RETARDATION-BASAL GANGLION DISORDER*

**Basan syndrome**
*See ECTODERMAL DYSPLASIA, BASAN TYPE*

## BASILAR IMPRESSION, PRIMARY               0103

**Includes:** Primary basilar impression

**Excludes:** Secondary basilar impression

**Major Diagnostic Criteria:** Demonstrated congenital bony abnormality in the occipitocervical region associated with limitation of movement of the neck and progressive neurologic signs such as sensory disturbances, dysphagia, aphonia, and diplopia due to compression of the pons, medulla, cerebellum, and spinal cord.

**Clinical Findings:** Symptoms usually begin insidiously in the third or fourth decade. The patient may complain of occipital headaches, neck stiffness, dysphagia, aphonia, diplopia, trigeminal pain, mental deterioration, unsteady gait, and various sensory disturbances. Examination may reveal a short neck with restricted movements. Dorsal kyphosis with increased cervical lordosis is common. The neurologic findings may include increased intracranial pressure, signs of compression of the medulla and pons, cerebellar signs, as well as evidence of spinal cord compression producing long tract and sensory disturbances. Examination of the cerebrospinal fluid (CSF) reveals, in most cases, a modest elevation of protein. Occasionally, a block is demonstrated by the Queckenstedt test or by myelography. The X-ray criteria for diagnosis are debatable but commonly include abnormalities in position of the atlas and odontoid process in relation to the Chamberlain line, (drawn from the posterior edge of the foramen magnum to the hard palate).

**Complications:** Directly related to the bony deformities at the base of the skull in which there is upward displacement of the floor of the posterior fossa, producing combinations of the following: 1) pressure on cranial nerves, brainstem, cerebellum, or cervical spinal cord; 2) altered blood supply to these structures because of direct pressure or adhesions; and 3) interference with CSF flow, producing hydrocephalus.

**Associated Findings:** Abnormally small foramen magnum, defects of the atlas, **Klippel-Feil anomaly, Brain, Arnold-Chiari malformation,** and vascular anomalies, particularly of the vertebral artery, which may explain some of the symptoms and signs.

**Etiology:** Possibly autosomal dominant inheritance.

**Pathogenesis:** There is evidence to suggest that primary basilar impression is the result of a defect in embryogenesis of the occipital bone.

**MIM No.:** 10950

**Sex Ratio:** M1:F1

**Occurrence:** 1:3,300. Russell (1900) reported a high incidence of basilar impression in Eskimos; others, in poorly documented studies, have noticed an increased prevalence in The Netherlands and northern Brazil.

**Risk of Recurrence for Patient's Sib:**
See Part I, *Mendelian Inheritance.*

**Risk of Recurrence for Patient's Child:**
See Part I, *Mendelian Inheritance.*

**Age of Detectability:** First decade by means of X-rays; third or fourth decade by onset of neurologic signs.

**Gene Mapping and Linkage:** Unknown.

**Prevention:** None known. Genetic counseling indicated.

**Treatment:** Most patients are asymptomatic. Immobilization is of limited use. Surgical decompression should be approached with considerable caution. Ventricular shunting procedures are indicated for those with progressive hydrocephalus.

**Prognosis:** Death may occur in fourth or fifth decades or patient may be totally asymptomatic.

**Detection of Carrier:** Skull X-rays for parents of an affected individual.

**Special Considerations:** Secondary basilar impression may be the result of bone diseases, such as Paget disease, rickets, **Osteogenesis imperfecta,** osteomalacia, osteoporosis, cleidocranial dysostosis, Morquio disease, syphilis, and tuberculosis, or possibly from carrying heavy loads upon the head.

**References:**
Russell F: Studies in cranial variation. Am Natural 1900; 34:737.

List CF: Neurologic syndromes accompanying developmental anomalies of occipital bone, atlas and axis. Arch Neurol Psychiatr 1941; 45:577.

Bull JWD, et al.: Radiological criteria and familial occurrence of primary basilar impression. Brain 1955; 78:229–247. *

HA053                                **Robert H.A. Haslam**

**Basilar migraine**
*See MIGRAINE*

**Bassen-Kornzweig syndrome**
*See ABETALIPOPROTEINEMIA*
*also ANEMIA, HEMOLYTIC, RED CELL MEMBRANE DEFECTS*

**Bat ear**
*See EAR, LOP*

**Bates syndrome**
*See INFLAMMATORY DISEASE, NEONATAL BATES-LORBER TYPE*

**Batten disease**
*See NEURONAL CEROID-LIPOFUSCINOSES (NCL)*

**Batten-Mayou disease**
*See NEURONAL CEROID-LIPOFUSCINOSES (NCL)*

**Batten-Vogt syndrome**
*See NEURONAL CEROID-LIPOFUSCINOSES (NCL)*

**BBB syndrome**
*See HYPERTELORISM-HYPOSPADIAS SYNDROME*

**Beals auriculo-osteodysplasia syndrome**
*See AURICULO-OSTEODYSPLASIA*

**Beals syndrome**
*See ARACHNODACTYLY, CONTRACTURAL BEALS TYPE*

**Beals-Hecht syndrome**
*See ARACHNODACTYLY, CONTRACTURAL BEALS TYPE*

**Bean syndrome**
*See NEVUS, BLUE RUBBER BLEB NEVUS SYNDROME*

**Bear tracks**
  See *RETINA, GROUPED HYPERTROPHY OF RETINAL PIGMENT*
    *EPITHELIUM*
**Bechterew syndrome**
  See *ANKYLOSING SPONDYLITIS*
**Becker generalized myotonia**
  See *MYOTONIA CONGENITA*
**Becker muscular dystrophy**
  See *MUSCULAR DYSTROPHY, ADULT PSEUDOHYPERTROPHIC*
**Beckwith syndrome**
  See *BECKWITH-WIEDEMANN SYNDROME*

## BECKWITH-WIEDEMANN SYNDROME                    0104

**Includes:**
  Beckwith syndrome
  EMG syndrome
  Exomphalos-macroglossia-gigantism syndrome
  Macroglossia-omphalocele-visceromegaly syndrome
  Omphalocele-visceromegaly-macroglossia syndrome
  Visceromegaly-umbilical hernia-macroglossia
  Wiedmann-Beckwith syndrome

**Excludes:**
  **Chromosome 11, trisomy 11p** (2459)
  **Hypoglycemia, familial neonatal** (0512)
  **Macroglossia** (0618)
  **Omphalocele** (0748)
  **Thyroid, iodide transport defect** (0542)

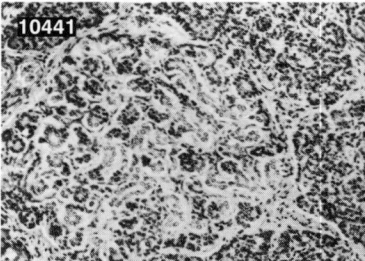

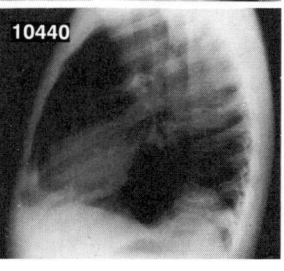

**0104**-10435: Macroglossia.  10436: Anterior open bite.  10439: Omphalocele.  10437: Ear lobe groove.  10438: Circular depression on posterior rim of helix.  10441: Hyperplasia of the ducts and acini in pancreas.  10440: Diaphragmatic eventration.

**Thyroid, iodotyrosine deiodinase deficiency** (0543)
**Thyroid, peroxidase defect** (0947)
**Thyrotropin unresponsiveness** (0948)

**Major Diagnostic Criteria:**  Clinical findings may be quite variable, but the diagnosis should be considered in an infant with **Macroglossia** and **Omphalocele** or umbilical anomaly. **Hypoglycemia, familial neonatal** may be present and ear lobe grooves or circular depressions on the posterior helices, when present, are especially significant for diagnosis.

**Clinical Findings:**  The frequency of clinical features in 248 Beckwith-Wiedemann syndrome patients from the literature was recently summarized by Pettenati et al. (1986). These findings include macroglossia (98%), visceromegaly [nephromegaly (97%), splenomegaly (82%), heptomegaly (73%)], somatic gigantism (average birth weight and birth length for both sexes greater than the 90th percentile), midface hypoplasia (81%), cryptorchidism (81%), omphalocele (76%), prominent occiput (72%), ear anomalies (pits and/or creases - 66%), facial nevus flammeus (62%), neonatal hypoglycemia (61%), polyhydramnios (51%), **Hernia, umbilical** (49%), cardiac defects (34%), hemihypertrophy (33%), diastasis recti (33%), clitoromegaly (16%), and malignant tumors (e.g., Wilms) in approximately 5% of the patients. Other reported findings include microcephaly, polycythemia, advanced bone age, prematurity, mental retardation, diaphragmatic eventration (occasionally diaphragmatic hernia), **Hypospadias**, bicornuate uterus, intestinal malrotation, enlarged labia, hypercalcemia, hyperlipemia, hypercholesterolemia, and hypocalcemia.

Neonatal hypoglycemia occurs in about 60% or more of the infants. This hypoglycemia is due to relative hyperinsulinemia (leucine sensitive) associated with pancreatic islet hyperplasia (nesidioblastosis) and is most common in Beckwith-Wiedemann infants with high birth weight (> 4000 g). The hypoglycemia tends to be severe and resists simple treatment (frequent feedings, intravenous glucose). A nonketogenic diet high in calories and low in protein (leucine) may be helpful. Diazoxide, long-acting epinephrine, corticosteroids, ACTH, or a partial pancreatectomy may be necessary.

**Complications:**  Mental retardation may result from undetected or untreated neonatal hypoglycemia. In light of the recently reported chromosome 11p abnormalities in patients with this syndrome, high-resolution chromosome studies should be carried out on any child with this syndrome, particularly with unexplained mental retardation.

**Associated Findings:**  Wilms tumor and adrenal cortical carcinoma occur in about 5% of reported cases. Hepatoblastoma, glioma, embryonal rhabdomyosarcoma, carcinoid tumor, myxoma, and fibroma have been noted rarely. There also appears to be an increased risk of malignancies in those patients with hemihypertrophy. Gonadal interstitial cell hyperplasia occurs in males and may be due to elevated serum gonadotropin levels. Seizures can also occur in children with this syndrome.

**Etiology:**  Although most cases (85%) are sporadic, familial cases have been reported. Affected sibs appear occasionally, and consanguinity has been reported. Based on familial cases, autosomal recessive, autosomal dominant, multifactorial, and autosomal dominant sex-dependent inheritance have been proposed. Recent segregation analysis is most consistent with autosomal dominant inheritance with incomplete penetrance. Etiologic heterogeneity is possible with recent reports of patients with features of Beckwith-Wiedemann syndrome and a chromosome 11p abnormality, usually a duplication.

**Pathogenesis:**  Altered placental endocrine physiology may play a role in producing many of the features found during the neonatal period. Omphalocele, anomalies of intestinal rotation and fixation, and diaphragmatic eventration may be secondary to early visceromegaly. A possible reason for somatic gigantism may be due to increased levels of growth hormone, including insulin and/or insulin-like growth factors.

**MIM No.:**  *13065
**POS No.:**  3036
**CDC No.:**  759.870

**Sex Ratio:** M1:F1

**Occurrence:** Undetermined; 1:13,700 live births in the West Indies.

**Risk of Recurrence for Patient's Sib:**
See Part I, *Mendelian Inheritance*. Recurrence risk low, but not negligible in sporadic instances.

**Risk of Recurrence for Patient's Child:**
See Part I, *Mendelian Inheritance*.

**Age of Detectability:** At birth by clinical evaluation.

**Gene Mapping and Linkage:** BWS (Beckwith-Wiedemann syndrome) has been mapped to 11pter-p15.4.

**Prevention:** None known. Genetic counseling indicated.

**Treatment:** Omphalocele repair, treatment of neonatal hypoglycemia. Partial glossectomy may be indicated if macroglossia persists. Orthognathic surgery, orthodontic and speech therapy.

**Prognosis:** Fair. A number of patients have died during infancy from complications of the syndrome.

**Detection of Carrier:** Unknown.

**References:**

Beckwith JB: Macroglossia, omphalocele, adrenal cytomegaly, gigantism and hyperplastic visceromegaly. BD:OAS(V). New York: March of Dimes Birth Defects Foundation, 1969:188–196. *

Wiedemann HR: Tumors and hemihypertrophy associated with Wiedemann-Beckwith syndrome. Eur J Pediatr 1983; 141:129.

Hecht F, Sandberg AA: Wiedermann-Beckwith syndrom: cancer predisposition and chromosome 11 (Editorial) Cancer Genet Cytogenet 1986; 23:159–161.

Pettenati MJ, et al.: Wiedemann-Beckwith syndrome: presentation of clinical and cytogenetic data on 22 new cases and review of literature. Hum Genet 1986; 74:143–154. *

Aleck KA, Hadro T: Dominant inheritance of Weidemann-Beckwith syndrome: further evidence for transmission of "unstable premutation" through carrier women. Am J Med Genet 1989; 33:155–160. †

BU040                                                   **Merlin G. Butler**

**Beckwith-Wiedemann syndrome with 11p15 duplication**
*See CHROMOSOME 11, TRISOMY 11p*

**Beemer lethal malformations syndrome**
*See HYDROCEPHALUS-HEART DEFECT-DENSE BONES, BEEMER TYPE*

**Beguez Cesar-Steinbrinck-Chediak-Higashi syndrome**
*See CHEDIAK-HIGASHI SYNDROME*

**Behavioral disturbance, reversible**
*See HARTNUP DISORDER*

**Behr syndrome (complicated optic atrophy)**
*See OPTIC ATROPHY, INFANTILE HEREDOFAMILIAL*

**Bell palsy, single or recurrent episodes of**
*See PALSY, LATE-ONSET FACIAL, FAMILIAL*

**Bencze syndrome**
*See OCULO-FACIAL SYNDROME, BENCZE TYPE*

**Benign cystinosis**
*See CYSTINOSIS*

**Benign exertional headache**
*See MIGRAINE*

**Benign intraepithelial dyskeratosis**
*See MUCOSA (ORAL/EYE), INTRAEPITHELIAL DYSKERATOSIS, BENIGN*

**Benign mellituria**
*See RENAL GLYCOSURIA*

**Benign recurrent intrahepatic cholestasis (BRIC)**
*See CHOLESTASIS, INTRAHEPATIC, RECURRENT BEGIGN*

**Benign sexual headache**
*See MIGRAINE*

**Benign tertian malaria**
*See MALARIA, VIVAX, SUSCEPTIBILITY TO*

**Benzodiazepine, fetal effects**
*See FETAL BENZODIAZEPINE EFFECTS*

**Berardinelli-Seip syndrome**
*See LIPODYSTROPHY SYNDROME, BERARDINELLI TYPE*

**Berdon syndrome**
*See INTESTINAL HYPOPERISTALSIS, MEGACYSTIS-MICROCOLON TYPE*

**Berg syndrome**
*See EYE, ANISOMETROPIA*

---

## BERLIN SYNDROME                                                   0105

**Includes:**
Ectodermal dysplasia, Berlin type
Leukomelanoderma-hypodontia-hypotrichosis-retardation
Leukomelanoderma-infantilism-retardation-hypodontia-hypotrichosis
Melanoleucoderma

**Excludes:**
**Dyskeratosis congenita** (2024)
**Ectodermal dysplasia, Naegeli type** (0703)
**Ectodermal dysplasia** without pigmentary changes
**Incontinentia pigmenti** (0526)
**Rothmund-Thomson syndrome** (2037)
**Werner syndrome** (0998)

**Major Diagnostic Criteria:** 1) Melanoleucoderma: Generalized mottled dyschromia with various shades of hyper- and hypopigmentation involving the trunk and extremities but sparing the scalp; 2) Hyperkeratosis, hyperhidiosis of the palms and soles; 3) Absence of lanugo hair, sparse eyebrows with normal scalp hair, nails, eyelashes, and sweating; 4) Delayed dentition with hypodontia; 5) Hypogonadism in males; 6) Mental and growth retardation. Clinically characterized by short stature, slender build with "bird-like" legs, moderate hyperflexibility of fingers, sparse eyebrows with absence of the lateral portions, flat saddle-shaped nose, deep furrows about the eyes and mouth and generalized melanoleukoderma (leopard skin).

**Clinical Findings:** One family reported to date with this condition. Based on the two males and two females affected, the clinical findings include A. Postnatal proportionate short stature; mild to moderate mental retardation. B. Generalized mottled dyschromia with shades of hyper- and hypopigmentation beginning by one year of age, completed by 3 years of age; telangiectasias on the lips and poikiloderma-like lesions on elbows, knees, and proximal phalangeal joints; hyperkeratosis, hyperhidiosis of the palms and soles; normal sweating, hypofunction of the sebaceous glands. C. Hair of scalp abundant with premature graying; absence of lanugo hair; sparse eyebrows, laterally absent; normal nails. D. Delayed eruption of primary and secondary dentition; hypodontia (incisors, canines, premolars, molars variably involved); teeth which are present are normal. E. Hypogonadism in the 2 males, including hypospadias, small genitalia, and lack of pubertal changes; normal pubertal changes and fertility in the female.

Routine laboratory tests including "Thorn test" after 25 mg corticotropin, urinary 24 hr. 17-ketosteroids and X-rays were normal.

The glucose tolerance curve was flat.

Skin biopsy findings include malpighian layer reduced in thickness; basal layer contained a pathologic amount of pigment; pigment was also found in the upper portion of the epidermis; there were areas totally devoid of pigment; no inflammatory changes; no hair follicles or sebaceous glands; sweat glands were present.

**Complications:** Impotence and minimal libido in the male; renal calculus in one-half of males resulting in urinary tract infections.

**Associated Findings:** None known.

**Etiology:** Possibly autosomal recessive inheritance. In the only known family, the affected children are the product of a marriage between cousins.

**Pathogenesis:** Unknown.

**MIM No.:** 24650

**POS No.:** 3827

**CDC No.:** 757.340

**Sex Ratio:** M1:F1

**Occurrence:** Rare; only one family known (Iranians living in Israel), two males and two females were affected out of 12 offspring.

**Risk of Recurrence for Patient's Sib:**
See Part I, *Mendelian Inheritance*.

**Risk of Recurrence for Patient's Child:**
See Part I, *Mendelian Inheritance.*

**Age of Detectability:** At one year of age when skin changes begin.

**Gene Mapping and Linkage:** Unknown.

**Prevention:** None known. Genetic counseling indicated.

**Treatment:** No specific measures. Educational services should be made available. Complete endocrinology studies were not performed. Therefore, these should be evaluated, including studies of growth hormone.

**Prognosis:** Life expectancy appears normal. Oldest male was 29 years. Mental retardation is present, but degree has not been established. Females are sexually functional, males are not.

**Detection of Carrier:** Unknown.

**Special Considerations:** This syndrome is probably best classified as an ectodermal dysplasia with endocrine and neurological involvement. The endocrine involvement in this family was not fully evaluated, as growth hormone studies were not clinically available. Other reported females with similar but additional findings include those reported by Pinheiro et al. (1981), and the patient described by Alves et al. (1981).

**Support Groups:** IL; Mascoutah; National Foundation for Ectodermal Dysplasias (NFED)

**References:**
Berlin CI: Congenital generalized melanoleucoderma associated with hypodontia, hypotrichosis, stunted growth, and mental retardation occurring in two brothers and two sisters. Dermatologica 1961; 123:227–243. *
Kristensen DK: Poikilodermal congenitale: an early case of Rothmund-Thompson's syndrome. Acta Dermato-Venerol 1975; 55:316.
Sparrow GP, et al.: Hypopigmentation and hypohidosis (The Naegeli-Franceschetti-Tadassohn syndrome): report of a family and review of the literature. Clin Exp Dermatol 1976; 1:127–140.
Alves AFP, et al.: An autosomal recessive ectodermal dysplasia syndrome of hypohidiosis, onchodysplasia, hyperkeratosis, kyphoscoliosis, cataract, and other manifestations. Am J Med Genet 1981; 10:213–218.
Pinheiro M, et al.: A previously undescribed condition: tricho-odonto-onchyo-dermal syndrome. A review of the tricho-odonto-onchyial subgroup of ectodermal dysplasias. Br J Dermatol 1981; 105:371–382.

GR021
TR008

**Arthur W. Grix**
**Carlos J. Trujillo-Botero**

**Bertrand spongy degeneration of the CNS**
*See BRAIN, SPONGY DEGENERATION*
**Besnier-Boek-Schaumann disease**
*See SARCOIDOSIS*
**Best disease**
*See RETINA, MACULAR DEGENERATION, VITELLIRUPTIVE*
**Beta-2-microglobulin**
*See AMYLOIDOSIS, HEMODIALYSIS-RELATED*
**Beta-galactosidase-1 deficiency**
*See G(M1)-GANGLIOSIDOSIS, TYPE 1*
**Beta-glucuronidase deficiency**
*See MUCOPOLYSACCHARIDOSIS VII*
**Beta-hydroxyisovaleric acidemia**
*See ACIDURIA, BETA-METHYL-CROTONYL-GLYCINURIA*
**Beta-interferon deficiency**
*See INTERFERON DEFICIENCY*
**Beta-ketothiolase deficiency**
*See ACIDEMIA, 3-KETOTHIOLASE DEFICIENCY*
**Beta-LCAT deficiency**
*See ANEMIA, HEMOLYTIC, RED CELL MEMBRANE DEFECTS*
**Beta-lipoprotein deficiency, congenital**
*See HYPOBETALIPOPROTEINEMIA*
**Beta-mercaptolactate-cysteine disulfiduria**
*See ACIDURIA, BETA-MERCAPTOLACTATE-CYSTEINE DISULFIDURIA*
**Beta-methylcrotonylglycinurie**
*See ACIDURIA, BETA-METHYL-CROTONYL-GLYCINURIA*
**Betalipoprotein deficiency**
*See ABETALIPOPROTEINEMIA*
**Bianchine-Lewis syndrome**
*See X-LINKED MENTAL RETARDATION-CLASPED THUMB*

**Biatrial myxoma with atrial septal defect**
*See MYXOMA, INTRACARDIAC*
**Biber-Haab-Dimmer degeneration**
*See CORNEAL DYSTROPHY, LATTICE TYPE*
**Bicornuate uterus**
*See MULLERIAN FUSION, INCOMPLETE*
**Bicuspid aortic valve**
*See AORTIC VALVE, BICUSPID*
**Bicuspid pulmonary valve with or without a raphe**
*See PULMONARY VALVE, BICUSPID*
**Bidermoma of head or neck**
*See NECK/HEAD, DERMOID CYST OR TERATOMA*
**Biedl-Bardet syndrome**
*See BARDET-BIEDL SYNDROME*

## BIEMOND I SYNDROME   3034

**Includes:**

Brachydactyly-nystagmus-cerebellar ataxia syndrome
Cerebellar ataxia-brachydactyly-nystagmus syndrome
Nystagmus-brachydactyly-cerebellar ataxia syndrome

**Excludes:** Biemond II syndrome (2169)

**Major Diagnostic Criteria:** Brachydactyly, cerebellar ataxia, and nystagmus. One or two of these findings with positive family history also suggest the diagnosis.

**Clinical Findings:** This condition has only been described in a single family. The full expression consists of short metacarpals and sometimes metatarsals, cerebellar ataxia, nystagmus, strabismus, and mental deficiency; however, most affected individuals did not have full expression of the syndrome.

**Complications:** Unknown.

**Associated Findings:** None known.

**Etiology:** Possibly autosomal dominant inheritance with variable expressivity and reduced penetrance.

**Pathogenesis:** Unknown.

**MIM No.:** 11340

**POS No.:** 3816

**Sex Ratio:** M1:F1

**Occurrence:** Documented in four generations of one family.

**Risk of Recurrence for Patient's Sib:**
See Part I, *Mendelian Inheritance.*

**Risk of Recurrence for Patient's Child:**
See Part I, *Mendelian Inheritance.*

**Age of Detectability:** Presumably at birth by the presence of brachydactyly.

**Gene Mapping and Linkage:** Unknown.

**Prevention:** None known. Genetic counseling indicated.

**Treatment:** Unknown.

**Prognosis:** Mental deficiency is not always present; life span may not be affected.

**Detection of Carrier:** Unknown.

**Special Considerations:** It has been questioned whether this entity is actually a syndrome or the occurrence of two or more independently segregating traits within a single family.

**References:**
Biemond A: Brachydactylie, Nystagmus en cerebellaire Ataxie als familiair Syndroom. Ned Tijdschr Geneeskd 1934; 78:1423–1431.
Temtamy S, McKusick VA: The genetics of hand malformations. New York: Alan R. Liss, 1978:259.

T0007

**Helga V. Toriello**

## BIEMOND II SYNDROME                                      2169

**Includes:**
Coloboma-obesity-polydactyly-hypogenitalism
Polydactyly-obesity-hypogenitalism-iris coloboma

**Excludes:**
**Bardet-Biedl syndrome** (2363)
**Biemond I syndrome** (3034)
**Eye, microphthalmia/coloboma** (0661)
**Laurence-Moon syndrome** (0578)
**Prader-Willi syndrome** (0823)

**Major Diagnostic Criteria:**  The combination of iris coloboma, mental retardation, obesity, hypogenitalism, and postaxial polydactyly.

**Clinical Findings:**  Iris coloboma, **Polydactyly**, and hypogenitalism are noticed at birth. The baby is usually hypotonic at birth and may have periods of apnea. Slow development is apparent in the first year of life, and mental retardation follows. Several patients have had short stature. Obesity has its onset after the first year of life. **Hydrocephaly** or **Craniofacial dysostosis** is discovered shortly after birth in those patients so afflicted.

**Complications:**  Most of the patients with hydrocephaly died of its complications in the first year of life.

**Associated Findings:**  **Hypospadias** has been noted in some patients.

**Etiology:**  Presumed autosomal recessive inheritance. In one family, iris coloboma, and in another, postaxial polydactyly were found in family members who did not have the other findings of the Biemond II syndrome.

**Pathogenesis:**  Unknown.

**MIM No.:**  21035

**POS No.:**  3701

**Sex Ratio:**  Presumably M1:F1.

**Occurrence:**  About ten cases have been documented.

**Risk of Recurrence for Patient's Sib:**
See Part I, *Mendelian Inheritance.*

**Risk of Recurrence for Patient's Child:**
See Part I, *Mendelian Inheritance.* The hypogenitalism of the full syndrome precludes reproduction in most cases.

**Age of Detectability:**  At birth.

**Gene Mapping and Linkage:**  Unknown.

**Prevention:**  None known. Genetic counseling indicated.

**Treatment:**  Unknown.

**Prognosis:**  Those affected with hydrocephaly fare poorly and usually die at an early age.

**Detection of Carrier:**  Unknown.

**Special Considerations:**  Most cases have been reported as **Laurence-Moon syndrome.** Some of the cases reported long ago might now be diagnosed as other syndromes; many of the findings of this syndrome are typical of chromosomal disorders.

**References:**
Grebe H: Contribution au diagnostic differentiel du syndrome de Bardet-Biedl. J Genet Hum 1953; 2:127–144.
Blumel J, Kniker WT: Laurence-Moon-Biedl syndrome: review of the literature and a report of five cases including a family group with three affected males. Texas Rep Biol Med 1959; 17:391–410.
Klein N, Amman F: The syndrome of Laurence-Moon-Biedl and allied disease in Switzerland: clinical, genetic and epidemiological studies. J Neurol Sci 1969; 9:479–494.

TH017                                                **T.F. Thurmon**
UR001                                                **S.A. Ursin**

**Bifid nose**
*See NOSE, BIFID*
**Bifid uvula**
*See UVULA, CLEFT*

**Bilateral acoustic neuromas**
*See ACOUSTIC NEUROMATA*
**Bilateral hilar involvement**
*See SARCOIDOSIS*
**Bilateral subclavian steal syndrome, congenital**
*See AORTA, ISOLATION OF SUBCLAVIAN ARTERY FROM AORTA*

## BILE DUCT CHOLEDOCHAL CYST                             0149

**Includes:**
Bile duct, diverticulum of common
Bile ducts, intrahepatic cystic dilatation of
Choledochal cyst
Choledochocele
Cystic dilation of common duct, congenital

**Excludes:**
**Gallbladder, anomalies** (0404)
**Liver, cyst, solitary** (0465)
**Liver, hamartoma** (0604)
**Liver, hepatic fibrosis, congenital** (0605)
**Mesenteric cysts** (0645)
Pancreatic pseudocyst
Parasitic hepatic cyst

**Major Diagnostic Criteria:**  An right upper quadrant mass in a female child or young adult with a history of recurrent intermittent pain and jaundice.

**Clinical Findings:**  A right upper quadrant mass (80%), jaundice (75%), and pain (60%) are common findings, with the entire triad present in 60% of cases. Intermittent episodes of pain and jaundice associated with chills and fever may occur repeatedly. Leukocytosis, elevated bilirubin and alkaline phosphatase, acholic stools, and dark urine may be observed during such episodes. In the absence of jaundice, intravenous cholangiography may be diagnostic. Barium swallow may be helpful in delineating a mass or displacement of the duodenum (anteriorly or to the left), the colon, or stomach. Percutaneous transhepatic cholangiography, ultrasound, CAT scan, and $99_m$ $T_c$-HIDA biliary scintiscan may also be useful in achieving a diagnosis, whereas oral cholecystograms rarely show the dilatation since the dye fails to concentrate.

**Complications:**  Cholangitis, biliary cirrhosis, portal hypertension and varices. Obstruction of adjacent structures (e.g. duodenum) by enlarging cysts, pancreatitis, and malignant degeneration to carcinoma.

**Associated Findings:**  None known.

**Etiology:**  The exact cause is obscure. However, the cyst appears to be of congenital origin, most likely representing an embryologic weakness in the bile duct wall. Some investigators believe cystic dilation of the common duct is related to a variant of biliary atresia and hypoplasia, possibly due to inflammation.

**Pathogenesis:**  The wall of the cyst is composed of fibrous tissue, with occasional smooth muscle or elastic fibers noted. The inner lining is often devoid of epithelium. The common duct proximal to the cyst may be dilated, whereas distally the common bile duct is narrow. Stasis and intermittent obstruction result in cholangitis and biliary cirrhosis.

**CDC No.:**  751.660

**Sex Ratio:**  M1:F4

**Occurrence:**  Over 500 cases reported; 1:13,500 hospital admissions. Appears more common in Japanese patients.

**Risk of Recurrence for Patient's Sib:**  Not increased.

**Risk of Recurrence for Patient's Child:**  Not increased.

**Age of Detectability:**  22% in first year, 33% between 1–10 years, with 80% of all patients being diagnosed in the first 30 years of life.

**Gene Mapping and Linkage:**  Unknown.

**Prevention:**  None known. Genetic counseling indicated.

**Treatment:**  Surgical procedures include biliary-intestinal drainage procedure (cyst-duodenostomy, cyst Roux-Y jejunostomy, or cyst resection and anastomosis), with the latter operation currently the procedure of choice. Close follow-up is required after initial operation for anastomotic stricture, cholangitis, and calculus formation. Antibiotics for cholangitis may be suggested.

**Prognosis:** If untreated, this defect is lethal with eventual death due to cholangitis and biliary cirrhosis (29 of 30 dead by age 32).

Life expectancy of many of these children (25–35%) is adversely affected by this anomaly. Drainage procedures carried out in childhood may be followed by a protracted life-limiting chronic hepatobiliary disease process. Improved results may be expected with early diagnosis, cyst resection, and subsequent hepatojejunostomy or cystojejunostomy (Roux-Y type) as the initial procedure.

**Detection of Carrier:** Unknown.

**Special Considerations:** The diagnosis of choledochal cyst should be entertained whenever the triad of pain, jaundice, and right upper quadrant mass present in a girl; repeated episodes of chills and fever occur as well. In many instances only one of the major triad components exists. The treatment of choice is surgical. At the time of operation, cholangiography is a very helpful diagnostic adjunct. The procedure of choice in most centers is biliary-intestinal drainage. In past years cyst duodenostomy was the most popular operation employed. Recent reports, however, stress that after this procedure, the occurrence of postoperative complications requires revision to a cyst Roux-Y jejunostomy. A few centers in Japan, Switzerland, and the United States regard complete cyst excision (when possible) and hepatoenterostomy to be the therapy of choice. Residual cyst is reported to accompany an increased risk of cancer. This is the procedure currently performed most commonly at most major centers. The cyst has little or no epithelial lining, with disruption of elastic fibers in the wall, it is fibrotic; its poor motility may cause stasis. Stasis and inappropriate cyst-duodenostomy are probably why, in the past, chronic hepatobiliary disease in children with choledochal cysts was observed even after drainage operations. Many of these former cases developed biliary calculi and evidence of permanent hepatic damage from instances of recurrent cholangitis and biliary cirrhosis, which adversely affected the life expectancy of these children. It is obvious that early intervention and long-term follow-up in these cases is most essential.

**References:**

Fonkalsrud EW, Boles ET, Jr: Choledochal cysts in infancy and childhood. Surg Gynecol Obstet 1965; 121:733.

Hays DM, et al.: Congenital cystic dilatation of the common bile duct. Arch Surg 1969; 98:457.

Mahour GH, Lynn HB: Choledochal cyst in children. Surgery 1969; 65:967.

Saito S, Ishida M: Congenital choledochal cyst (cystic dilatation of common bile duct). Prog Pediatr Surg 1974; 6:63.

Reuter K, et al.: The diagnosis of choledochal cyst by ultrasonography. Radiology 1980; 136(2);437–438.

Yamaguchi M, et al.: Observation of cystic dilatation of the common bile duct by ultrasonography. J Pediatr Surg 1980; 15(2):207–210.

Wong KC, et al.: Human fetal development of the hepato-pancreatic duct junction - a possible explanation of congenital dilatation of the biliary tract. J Pediatr Surg 1981; 16(2):139–145.

GR022
CL007

**Jay L. Grosfeld**
**H. William Clatworthy, Jr.**

**Bile duct, diverticulum of common**
*See BILE DUCT CHOLEDOCHAL CYST*
**Bile ducts, atresia of intrahepatic**
*See BILE DUCTS, INTERLOBULAR, NONSYNDROMIC PAUCITY*
**Bile ducts, hypoplasia of terminal**
*See BILE DUCTS, INTERLOBULAR, NONSYNDROMIC PAUCITY*

## BILE DUCTS, INTERLOBULAR, NONSYNDROMIC PAUCITY

**Includes:**
>    Bile ducts, atresia of intrahepatic
>    Bile ducts, hypoplasia of terminal

**Excludes:**
>    **Alpha(1)-antitrypsin deficiency** (0039)
>    **Arterio-hepatic dysplasia** (2084)
>    **Chromosome 21, trisomy 21** (0171)
>    **Jaundice, intrahepatic cholestatic, Byler type** (2371)

**Major Diagnostic Criteria:** Demonstration of hepatocellular cholestasis associated with a paucity of interlobular bile ducts as defined by a ratio of intrahepatic bile ducts to portal spaces of 0.6 before 90 days of age.

**Clinical Findings:** Patients typically present with cholestasis in the neonatal period. Liver function other than excretion remains normal during the early phases of this disease. Examination of the extrahepatic biliary tree reveals small but patent common duct and gallbladder. Liver biopsy reveals paucity of intrahepatic bile ducts, hepatocellular cholestasis and a variable degree of portal fibrosis and or inflammation. In some patients clinical signs of cholestasis resolve spontaneously and in others symptoms persist. Many patients develop intractable pruritus even in the absence of jaundice. Elevated serum lipids are common in this group frequently resulting in xanthomata as early as 18 months of age. In patients with a chronic course, rickets and other complications associated with malabsorption of fat soluble vitamins are likely to occur. Growth failure and malnutrition secondary to fat malabsorption are also seen.

Documentation of this disease is limited. Since paucity of bile ducts is a feature of several other disorders, it has been speculated that patients with a familial history or rapidly progressive course may represent a different disease entity.

**Complications:** All of the complications of chronic cholestatic liver disease, including malabsorption of fat and fat-soluble vitamins, pruritus, hypercholesterolemia, xanthomatosis, growth failure, and cirrhosis, including portal hypertension, hypersplenism, ascites, porto-systemic encephalopathy, esophageal varices, and related conditions.

**Associated Findings:** None known.

**Etiology:** Presumably sporadic, but one report describes two affected siblings.

**Pathogenesis:** Electron microscopic evidence of breaks in bile duct basal lamina and lymphocytic infiltration of duct epithelium suggests that paucity results from duct destruction, but the exact pathogenesis is unknown.

**Sex Ratio:** Presumably M1:F1.

**Occurrence:** Fewer than 50 cases have been documented in the literature.

**Risk of Recurrence for Patient's Sib:** Unknown.

**Risk of Recurrence for Patient's Child:** Unknown.

**Age of Detectability:** At 2–4 weeks, by liver biopsy.

**Gene Mapping and Linkage:** Unknown.

**Prevention:** None known. Genetic counseling indicated.

**Treatment:** Treatment as for other forms of chronic cholestasis. Pruritus may respond to phenobarbital or cholestyramine. Supplementation of fat soluble vitamins is required.

**Prognosis:** Highly variable, ranging from complete resolution of symptoms to cirrhosis in as many as 55%.

**Detection of Carrier:** Unknown.

**References:**

Gherardi GJ, MacMahon HE: Hypoplasia of terminal bile ducts. Amer J Dis Child 1970; 120:151–153.

Odievre M, et al.: Long-term prognosis for infants with intrahepatic cholestasis and patent extrahepatic biliary tract. Arch Dis Child 1981; 56:373–376.

Kahn E, et al.: Nonsyndromic paucity of interlobular bile ducts: light and electron microscopic evaluation of sequential liver biopsies in early childhood. Hepatology 1986; 6:890–901.

Sacher M, Thaler H: Prognosis of nonsyndromic paucity of intrahepatic bile ducts. J Pediatr Gastroenterol Nutr 1988; 7:303 only.

AL037                      **Estella M. Alonso**
FI035                      **Mark Fishbein**

**Bile ducts, intrahepatic cystic dilatation of**
*See BILE DUCT CHOLEDOCHAL CYST*

## BILIARY ATRESIA                     0110

**Includes:**
> Biliary atresia, complete extrahepatic
> Cholestatic jaundice-renal tubular insufficiency
> Extrahepatic biliary atresia-discontinuity of bile duct
> Idiopathic extrahepatic biliary atresia (EHBA)
> Renal tubular insufficiency-biliary malformation

**Excludes:**
> **Arterio-hepatic dysplasia** (2084)
> Bile ducts, mechanical obstruction of
> Choledochal cyst
> Ductal paucity syndromes
> Intrahepatic cholestasis

**Major Diagnostic Criteria:** Any infant in the first three months of life with cholestasis should be evaluated for biliary atresia.

**Clinical Findings:** Because the disease is a progressive obliterative cholangiopathy, it is not apparent at birth. Affected infants are sometimes jaundiced during the perinatal period, but the cause, mechanism, and severity of their jaundice has not been shown to differ from that of normal newborns. Patients often present at 1–2 months with jaundice, hypopigmented stools, and dark urine. The serum bilirubin level is usually 6–10 mg% and predominantly conjugated. Hepatosplenomegaly is usually evident, increases as biliary cirrhosis develops, and is not as prominent early, as in patients with neonatal hepatitis. Although the majority of affected infants are otherwise normal, finding other anatomic anomalies, particularly situs abnormalities, suggests the diagnosis.

Early diagnosis is important and affects the outcome. Evaluation should include a search for other causes of cholestasis (including alpha-1-antitrypsin level, CMV culture and serology, urine metabolic screen, and so forth), which, if found, preclude the need for further evaluation. Ultrasound of the liver will exclude choledochal cyst and may help to exclude biliary atresia if normal ducts are visualized. Excretory biliary scan with $^{99m}$Tc-HIDA (or analogues thereof) is useful to exclude biliary atresia. Apparent complete obstruction in the absence of biliary atresia (false-positive test) is relatively common, but error can be reduced by pretreatment with 1 week of oral phenobarbital at 5 mg/kg/day. A normal scan in the presence of biliary atresia (false-negative test) is uncommon. Percutaneous liver biopsy is most useful. Finding expanded portal areas with characteristic proliferation of ductular elements and bile plugs suggests biliary atresia with 95% confidence. Operative exploration with cholangiogram is the most definitive study and should be undertaken if there is any question regarding the diagnosis.

**Complications:** Biliary cirrhosis with all of its complications. Deficiency of fat-soluble vitamins and fat malabsorption secondary to bile salt deficiency in the intestinal lumen. Hyperlipidemia and pruritus secondary to retention of bile.

**Associated Findings:** 1) Situs abnormalities, particularly polysplenia/asplenia. 2) Abnormal cilia syndrome.

**Etiology:** Possibly autosomal recessive inheritance.

**Pathogenesis:** Biliary atresia is thought to represent the end stage of a process of obliterative cholangiopathy. Several patients have been studied as their disease progressed from what is reminiscent of neonatal hepatitis into biliary atresia. Moreover, newborns who have died of other causes have not been found to have biliary atresia with nearly the frequency predicted by the incidence of the disease. These findings suggest that it is an acquired disease, being contracted intrauterinely. Several instances of time and space clustering have been observed, which suggest that infectious or environmental toxic factors cause or promote the disease. Although not a uniform finding, serologic and culture evidence suggests that reovirus type 3 might be the causitive agent in biliary atresia.

**MIM No.:** 21050, 21055

**CDC No.:** 751.650

**Sex Ratio:** M1:F1–2

**Occurrence:** 1:8–10,000. There are time and space clusters, and there is an increased incidence in Hawaii, Japan, and China.

**Risk of Recurrence for Patient's Sib:** Not known to be greater than that for the general population. Several sets of monozygotic twins have been reported to be discordant for biliary atresia.

**Risk of Recurrence for Patient's Child:** Unknown.

**Age of Detectability:** In Infancy.

**Gene Mapping and Linkage:** Unknown.

**Prevention:** None known. Genetic counseling indicated.

**Treatment:** Special attention to the nutritional needs of these patients is imperative. If biliary atresia is diagnosed and confirmed by surgical exploration and cholangiography, an attempt to obtain bile drainage by hepatic portoenterostomy can be made. The several variants of the procedure described by Kasai rely on ductal remnants in the portahepatis to provide drainage. If the duct remnant is examined by frozen section and contains duct elements of >70–100μm diameter, the procedure can successfully be completed and expected to provide temporary drainage. The long-term prognosis is poor; most patients progress to end-stage cirrhosis within the first decade despite successful surgery.

Orthotopic hepatic transplantation at present plays a prominent role in the long-term treatment of patients with biliary atresia. Repeated abdominal surgery in an attempt to "re-do" a nonfunctioning portoenterostomy is to be avoided, because it complicates transplantation and reduces overall survival.

**Prognosis:** Determined by the effectiveness of surgical therapy. Although about one-third of patients experience prolonged improvement after Kasai procedure, most progress to end-stage cirrhosis within the first decade. Orthotopic liver transplantation is the only effective therapy for such patients. The current survival rates vary from 40% for critically ill infants of less than 8 kg body weight to 80% for school aged children transplanted electively.

**Detection of Carrier:** Unknown.

**Special Considerations:** Early diagnosis and portoenterostomy improve outcome. Portoenterostomy performed after age three months is usually unsuccessful.

**Support Groups:**
> NJ; Maplewood; The Children's Liver Foundation, Inc.
> NJ; Cedar Grove; American Liver Foundation

**References:**
Moreki R, et al.: Biliary atresia and reovirus type 3 infection. N Engl J Med 1982; 307:481–484.

Strickland AD, Shannon K: Studies in the etiology of extrahepatic biliary atresia: time-space clustering. J Pediatr 1982; 100:749–753.

Glaser JH, et al.: Role of reovirus type 3 in persistent infantile cholestasis. J Pediatr 1984; 105:912–915.

Iwatsuki S, et al.: Liver transplantation for biliary atresia. World J Surg 1984; 8:51–56.

Kobayashi A, et al.: Long-term prognosis in biliary atresia after hepatic portoenterostomy: analysis of 35 patients who survived beyond 5 years of age. J Pediatr 1984; 105:243–264.

Strickland AD, et al.: Biliary atresia in two sets of twins. J Pediatr 1985; 107:418–420.

Kaufman SS, et al.: Nutritional support for the infant with extrahepatic biliary atresia. J Pediatr 1987; 110:679–686.

Cunningham ML, Sybert VP: Idiopathic extrahepatic biliary atresia. Am J Med Genet 1988; 31:421–426.

Grosfeld JL, et al.: The efficacy of hepatoportoenterostomy in biliary atresia. Surgery 1989; 106:692–701.

Lilly JR, et al.: The surgery of biliary atresia. Ann Surg 1989; 210: 289–296. *

WH007                                    Peter F. Whitington

**Bicarbonate-wasting renal tubular acidosis**
    See *RENAL BICARBONATE REABSORPTIVE DEFECT*
**Biliary atresia, complete extrahepatic**
    See *BILIARY ATRESIA*
**Binder syndrome**
    See *MAXILLONASAL DYSPLASIA, BINDER TYPE*
**Bing-Siebenmann dysplasia**
    See *EAR, INNER DYSPLASIAS*

---

## BIOPTERIN SYNTHESIS DEFICIENCY                2002

**Includes:**
    Dihydrobiopterin synthetase deficiency
    Hyperphenylalaninemia due to abnormal biopterin
        metabolism
    Pee deficiency
    Phenylketonuria III
    Phenylketonuria VI
    Phosphate-eliminating enzyme, deficiency of
    Six-pyruvoyl tetrahydropterin synthase deficiency

**Excludes:**
    **Dihydropteridine reductase deficiency** (2001)
    Hyperphenylalaninemia, transient
    Hyperphenylalaninemias, other
    **Phenylketonuria** (0808)

**Major Diagnostic Criteria:** Progressive cerebral deterioration occurs despite excellent dietary control of concentrations of phenylalanine in the blood. The diagnosis is most readily confirmed by the prompt fall in the elevated serum concentration of phenylalanine following the administration of synthetic tetrahydrobiopterin; this characteristic readily distinguishes biopterin synthesis deficiency from classic phenylketonuria (PKU).

**Clinical Findings:** Affected individuals are first noticed when hyperphenylalaninemia is detected in neonatal screening. Tetrahydrobiopterin, an obligatory cofactor for phenylalanine hydroxylase, is also the cofactor for the hydroxylation of tryptophan and tyrosine which are both essential for the synthesis of serotonin, norepinephrine, and dopamine.

The diagnosis, confirmed by an assay of the pattern of excretion of pterins in the urine, can also be made by quantitative measurement of the concentration of tetrahydrobiopterin in plasma, especially after the administration of phenylalanine. In normal individuals and in those with PKU or dihydropteridine reductase deficiency, phenylalanine dramatically increases the level of tetrahydrobiopterin; in patients with defective biopterin synthesis there is no change. The pattern of biopterin excretion may be studied using a variety of chromatographic techniques. The total excretion is low, although there is specific reduction in 7,8-dihydrobiopterin while concentrations of neopterin are normal.

**Complications:** Severe mental retardation; seizures.

**Associated Findings:** None known.

**Etiology:** Autosomal recessive inheritance.

**Pathogenesis:** The defective synthesis of tetrahydrobiopterin interferes with the conversion of phenylalanine to tyrosine, and produces a metabolic milieu identical to that of the patient with PKU. In addition, defective hydroxylation of tryptophan and tyrosine interferes with the synthesis of the neurotransmitters which are essential to the functioning of the nervous system.

**MIM No.:** *26164

**Sex Ratio:** M1:F1

**Occurrence:** Undetermined but presumed rare.

**Risk of Recurrence for Patient's Sib:**
    See Part I, *Mendelian Inheritance.*

**Risk of Recurrence for Patient's Child:**
    See Part I, *Mendelian Inheritance.*

**Age of Detectability:** As in PKU, usually within 48 hours if protein intake is normal; by six days virtually all cases should be detectable. Prenatal diagnosis is possible.

**Gene Mapping and Linkage:** PTS (6-pyruvyltetrahydropterin synthase) is unassigned.

**Prevention:** None known. Genetic counseling indicated.

**Treatment:** Synthetic tetrahydrobiopterin or a low phenylalanine diet should prevent the consequences of hyperphenylalaninemia. It is recommended that the patient also be given 5-hydroxytryptophan and dihydroxyphenylalanine along with a peripheral decarboxylase inhibitor such as carbidopa.

**Prognosis:** Usually grave. In those patients detected before the onset of symptoms, treatment should be effective.

**Detection of Carrier:** Unknown.

**References:**
Bartholome K: A new molecular defect in phenylketonuria. Lancet 1974; II:1580.
Bartholome K, Byrd DJ: L-dopa and 5-hydroxytryptophan therapy in phenylketonuria with normal phenylalanine hydroxylase activity. Lancet 1975; II:1042–1043.
Kaufman S, et al.: Phenylketonuria due to a deficiency of dihydropteridine reductase. New Engl J Med 1975; 293:785–790. *
Schaub J, et al.: Tetrahydrobiopterin therapy of atypical phenylketonuria due to defective dihydrobiopterin biosynthesis. Arch Dis Child 1978; 53:674–676.
Butter I-J, et al.: Neurotransmitter defects and treatment of disorders of hyperphenylalaninemia. J Pediatr 1981; 98:729–733.
Nyhan WL: Hyperphenylalaninemia and defective metabolism of tetrahydrobiopterin. In: Nyan WL, ed: Diagnostic recognition of genetic disease. Philadelphia: Lea & Febiger, 1987:107–112.
Scriver CR, et al.: Hyperphenylalaninemia due to deficiency of 6-pyruvoyl tetrahydropterin synthase: unusual gene dosage effect in heterozygotes. Hum Genet 1987; 77:168–171.
Blaskovics M, Giudici TA: A new variant of biopterin deficiency. New Engl J Med 1988; 319:1611–1612.

NY000                                    William L. Nyhan

**Biotin-responsive 3-beta-methylcrotonylglycinuria (some)**
    See *CARBOXYLASE DEFICIENCY, HOLOCARBOXYLASE DEFICIENCY TYPE*

---

## BIOTINIDASE DEFICIENCY                    2591

**Includes:**
    Combined carboxylase deficiency, late-onset
    Multiple carboxylase deficiency, infantile
    Multiple carboxylase deficiency, juvenile-onset
    Multiple carboxylase deficiency, late-onset

**Excludes:**
    Biotin deficiency
    **Carboxylase deficiency, holocarboxylase deficiency type** (2006)

**Major Diagnostic Criteria:** Any or all of the following common clinical features may be present: seizures, hypotonia, ataxia, skin rash, and alopecia. There is usually metabolic ketolactic acidosis and organic aciduria with metabolites suggestive of multiple carboxylase deficiency. Deficient biotinidase activity in serum or other tissues definitively establishes the diagnosis. Biotinidase activity is readily determined using a colorimetric procedure that measures the liberation of p-aminobenzoate from biotinyl-p-aminobenzoate, an analogue of the natural substrate of biotinidase, biocytin.

**Clinical Findings:** The age of onset varies from two weeks to two years, with a mean age of six months. The most frequent initial neurologic symptoms are myoclonic seizures and hypotonia. Several patients exhibited ataxia, hyperventilation, apnea, stridor or developmental delay. Common nonneurologic initial symptoms included eczematoid or seborrheic skin rash, partial or complete alopecia, and conjunctivitis. Some affected individuals had combinations of these neurologic and cutaneous findings. More than 70% of the patients had seizures, hypotonia, skin rash, or alopecia at some time prior to diagnosis and treatment. About one-half of the children had ataxia, developmental delay, conjunctivitis, and visual problems, including optic atrophy. Hearing loss was found in about 50%. The hearing loss, which was usually high-frequency sensorineural, was often demonstrated in patients before the initiation of biotin treatment.

Several affected children died while in metabolic coma. Patients have exhibited fungal infections, such as candidiasis, which has been attributed to immunoregulatory dysfunction. Over 80% of the patients had episodes of ketolactic acidosis and organic aciduria. The most frequently observed abnormal urinary metabolite has been 3-hydroxyisovaleric acid. Other commonly observed metabolites included 3-ethylcrotonylglycine, 3-hydroxypropionate, and methylcitrate. Mild hyperammonemia may be present. If affected individuals are not treated with pharmacological doses of biotin, they may suffer irreversible neurologic damage, become comatose, or die.

All children with the disorder who were treated with biotin have improved clinically. The cutaneous manifestations usually resolve quickly, and the seizures and ataxia usually stop; the hearing loss and optic atrophy appear to be less reversible than the other symptoms. Depending on the severity and frequency of the episodes of metabolic and neurologic compromise, many children with developmental delay achieve or regain milestones.

**Complications:** Numerous or severe neurologic or metabolic exacerbations may result in optic atrophy, neurosensory hearing loss or other neurologic and mental abnormalities that are not reversible by biotin treatment.

**Associated Findings:** Unknown.

**Etiology:** Autosomal recessive inheritance.

**Pathogenesis:** There are four biotin-dependent enzymes in humans; propionyl CoA carboxylase, pyruvate carboxylase, β-methylcrotonyl-CoA carboxylase, and acetyl-CoA carboxylase, which have important roles in amino acid catabolism, fatty acid synthesis and gluconeogenesis. Biotin is bound covalently to the various apocarboxylases by one or more holocarboxylase synthetases to form active holoenzymes. During the proteolytic degradation of these carboxylases, biotin is cleaved from small biotinylpeptides or biocytin (ε-N-biotinyl-lysine) by biotinidase, thereby recycling the vitamin. Free dietary biotin can be absorbed in the intestines, whereas protein-bound biotin in the diet may have to be processed by biotinidase from pancreatic juice or in the intestinal mucosa to become bioavailable.

Children with biotinidase deficiency cannot recycle the vitamin and probably cannot process protein-bound dietary biotin. Therefore, affected individuals become biotin deficient during infancy or early childhood. The symptoms are apparently caused, in part, by the effects of accumulating abnormal metabolites formed by the secondary carboxylase deficiencies. The biochemical abnormalities attributed to biotinidase deficiency are often life threatening and appear to represent relatively late effects of the disorder. The cutaneous symptoms and some of the neurologic findings are similar to those seen in biotin deficiency states and may result from depletion of biotin when the residual carboxylase activities are still adequate. Ketoacidosis and organic aciduria usually occur only after protracted biotin deficiency.

**MIM No.:** *25326

**Sex Ratio:** M1:F1

**Occurrence:** 1:70,000–80,000 live births (based on the results of newborn screening in the United States and other countries). No oriental children with biotinidase deficiency have been reported.

**Risk of Recurrence for Patient's Sib:**
See Part I, *Mendelian Inheritance.*

**Risk of Recurrence for Patient's Child:**
See Part I, *Mendelian Inheritance.*

**Age of Detectability:** Biotinidase deficiency can be diagnosed at birth by demonstrating enzyme deficiency in serum or in blood soaked filter paper samples used in newborn screening. A potential exists for prenatal diagnosis by determining biotinidase activity in amniotic fluid cells using a sensitive radioassay.

**Gene Mapping and Linkage:** Unknown.

**Prevention:** Neonatal screening for the enzyme deficiency is being conducted in several states and countries. Symptoms can be prevented in a biotinidase-deficient child by treatment with oral biotin, 5–10 mg/day.

**Treatment:** Currently, the empiric dose of 5–10 mg of biotin per day for life is recommended. Lower doses of biotin may be found to be adequate, but the appropriate dose will depend on the determination of the rates of metabolic turnover of the biotin-dependent carboxylases.

**Prognosis:** Several teenage children with biotinidase deficiency, who were treated with biotin since early childhood, have remained asymptomatic. Their physical and mental development has been normal. The oldest child detected on newborn screening for biotinidase deficiency is two years old and is asymptomatic. All biotinidase-deficient children are expected to respond to therapy because biotin treatment circumvents the enzymatic defect.

**Detection of Carrier:** Biotinidase activity in serum is 35–60% of mean normal activity, as determined by the colorimetric enzyme assay. This method is about 95% accurate.

**Special Considerations:** Infants with 15–30% of mean normal activity have been detected through screening. Recently, several teenagers with partial biotinidase deficiency in this enzyme range have been described; they have had intractable seborrheic dermatitis since infancy.

**References:**
Wolf B, et al.: Biotinidase deficiency: the enzymatic defect in late-onset multiple carboxylase deficiency. Clin Chim Acta 1983; 131: 273–281.
Wolf B, et al.: Phenotypic variation in biotinidase deficiency. J Pediatr 1983; 103:233–237.
Wolf B, et al.: Biotinidase deficiency: a novel vitamin recycling defect. J Inher Metab Dis 1985; 8(Suppl 2):53–58.
Wolf B, et al.: Biotinidase deficiency: initial clinical features and rapid diagnosis. Ann Neurol 1985; 18:614–617.
Wolf B, et al.: Clinical findings in four children with biotinidase deficiency detected through a statewide neonatal screening program. New Engl J Med 1985; 313:16–19.
Heard GS, et al.: Newborn screening for biotinidase deficiency: results of a one year pilot study. J Pediatr 1986; 108:40–46. *
Sweetman L, Nyhan WL: Inheritable biotin-treatable disorders and associated phenomena. Ann Rev Nutr 1986; 6:317–343.
Wolf B, Heard GS: Disorders of biotin metabolism. In: Scriver CR, et al, eds: The metabolic basis of inherited disease, 6th ed. New York: McGraw-Hill, 1989:2083–2105.

W0002                                   **Barry Wolf**
HE041                          **Gregory S. Heard**

**Bipolar affective disorder**
*See MOOD AND THOUGHT DISORDERS*
**Bird-headed dwarf (obsolete/pejorative)**
*See SECKEL SYNDROME*
**Bird-headed dwarf, Montreal type**
*See SECKEL SYNDROME*
**Bird-headed dwarfism, osteodysplastic, type I**
*See DWARFISM, OSTEODYSPLASTIC PRIMORDIAL, MAJEWSKI-WINTER TYPE*
**Bird-headed dwarfism, osteodysplastic, type III**
*See DWARFISM, OSTEODYSPLASTIC PRIMORDIAL, MAJEWSKI-RANKE TYPE*
*also DWARFISM, OSTEODYSPLASTIC PRIMORDIAL, MAJEWSKI-WINTER TYPE*
**Bird-headed dwarfism, Virchow type**
*See SECKEL SYNDROME*
**'Birthmark' (obsolete)**
*See NEVUS FLAMMEUS*
**Bisphosphoglycerate mutase, (E.C.2.7.5.4) deficiency**
*See ERYTHROCYTE, DIPHOSPHOGLYCERATE MUTASE (2,3) DEFICIENCY*
**Bitemporal aplasia cutis congenita**
*See ECTODERMAL DYSPLASIA, CONGENITAL FACIAL, SETLEIS TYPE*

**Bixler syndrome**
  See *HYPERTELORISM-MICROTIA-FACIAL CLEFT-CONDUCTIVE DEAFNESS*
**Bjornstad syndrome**
  See *DEAFNESS-PILI TORTI, BJORNSTAD TYPE*
**Blackfan-Diamond syndrome**
  See *ANEMIA, HYPOPLASTIC CONGENITAL*
**Bladder (dysplastic)-hydronephrosis-hydroureter-grimacing facies**
  See *UROFACIAL SYNDROME*
**Bladder diverticulum, superior**
  See *URACHAL ANOMALIES*

---

## BLADDER EXSTROPHY                                          3015

**Includes:**

  Epispadias-exstrophy complex (one component)
  Exstrophy of the bladder
  Vesical exstrophy

**Excludes:**
  Cloacal anomalies, other
  **Epispadias** (2008)
  **Exstrophy of cloaca sequence** (3193)
  Exstrophy variants, other

**Major Diagnostic Criteria:**  Physical examination establishes the diagnosis: The urinary tract is open anteriorly from the urethral meatus to the umbilicus. Wide separation of the pubic symphysis and the rectus muscles is invariably present.

**Clinical Findings:**  Apparent eversion of the posterior bladder wall, with the bladder mucosa, ureteral orifices, posterior bladder neck, and urethra exposed. The pubic bones are separated. The anus is anteriorly displaced and may be slightly patulous.
*In males*: the scrotum is broad and the testes are retractile. The penis is attached to the inferior ramus of the pubis, leading to a short, stubby penis with dorsal chordee. The glans penis is spade-like in form, with no tubularization. Hernias are usually noted sometime during the first year of life.
*In females*: the halves of the clitoris and labia are widely separated. The vaginal opening is anteriorly placed and often stenotic. There is occasional duplication of the müllerian structures. Uterine prolapse, especially in later years, may be troublesome.

**Complications:**  Initially, there are no major medical complications. After surgical intervention and bladder closure, vesicoureteral reflux is invariably present. The upper tracts are almost always normal at first, and hydronephrosis occurs mainly if there are problems after reconstructive procedures. Long-term difficulties with urinary incontinence and inadequate genitalia may persist despite surgery.

**Associated Findings:**  Lateral rotation of the acetabulum and femurs is present in association with the diastasis pubis. This may lead to a slightly broad-based gait.

**Etiology:**  Unknown.

**Pathogenesis:**  It is postulated on the basis of embryologic studies and experimental work that there is a defect with overdevelopment of the cloacal membrane, preventing medial migration of the mesenchyme. This is thought by some to be due to a caudal displacement of the primorida of the genital tubercle.

**CDC No.:**  753.500

**Sex Ratio:**  M3:F1

**Occurrence:**  1:30,000 deliveries.

**Risk of Recurrence for Patient's Sib:**  Unknown. There have been only isolated occurrences of bladder exstrophy in sibs or twins.

**Risk of Recurrence for Patient's Child:**  None known, although overall fertility rates for males with exstrophy are reduced.

**Age of Detectability:**  At birth.

**Gene Mapping and Linkage:**  Unknown.

**Prevention:**  None known. Genetic counseling indicated.

**Treatment:**  The accepted treatment plan for most neonates with bladder exstrophy is initial (within 72 hours) closure of the bladder, with supplementary procedures to achieve continence (bladder neck reconstruction with ureteral reimplantation) and external genitalia reconstruction (epispadias repair with further penile straightening). These operations are technically difficult and not universally successful. If these procedures fail or the bladder is too small or fibrotic to close, then delayed elective diversion of the urine by an intestinal conduit and genital reconstruction is an alternative. Antirefluxing, continent diversion has also been successfully performed. Long-term problems with upper tract deterioration, stones, and infections have not been entirely eliminated with these techniques.

Ureterosigmoidostomy, once the preferred method of reconstruction, has lost advocacy due to the increased risk of carcinoma of the colon at the site of the uretercolonic anastomosis. If a patient has this type of ''internal diversion'', yearly follow-up with ultrasound and sigmoidoscopy is mandatory.

**Prognosis:**  The risk of adenocarcinoma in the bladder of untreated exstrophy is significant and probably related to the length of time that the bladder is left exposed. The other main cancer risk is with ureterosigmoidostomy.

The results from modern day surgery can achieve a success rate of continence with an intact bladder and healthy upper tracts in about 60–70% of cases. With tenacity in reconstructing the genitalia in the male, who often requires additional surgery after puberty, an adequate phallus can result. Females are fertile but may have problems with carrying to term and with delivery due to lax pelvic structure support.

**Detection of Carrier:**  Unknown.

**Special Considerations:**  Exstrophy is the most commonly seen anomaly in the so-called *Epispadias-exstrophy complex*. The long-term prognosis for life span is good. The major challenge is the quality of life. In previous years, suicide during the adolescent and young adult years, especially in males, was very high. It requires a commitment on the part of the physicians and family to achieve the best possible result with these difficult problems.

**Support Groups:**   OH; Solon; National Support Group for Exstrophy

**References:**

Marshall VF, Muecke EC: Variations in exstrophy of the bladder. J Urol 1962; 88:766–796.
Allen TD, et al.: Reconstruction of the external genitalia in exstrophy of the bladder. J Urol 1974; 111:830–834.
Erakalis A, Folkman J: Adenocarcinoma at the site of ureterosigmoidostomy for exstrophy of the bladder. J Pediatr Surg 1978; 13:730–734.
Jeffs RD: Exstrophy and cloacal exstrophy. Urol Clin North Am 1978; 5:127–140.
Mesrobian HJ, et al.: Longterm follow-up of 103 patients with bladder exstropy. J Urol 1988; 140:719–722.

MA074                                          **James Mandell**

**Bleomycin induced scleroderma**
  See *SCLERODERMA, FAMILIAL PROGRESSIVE*

---

## BLEPHARO-NASO-FACIAL SYNDROME                             2088

**Includes:**

  Face (dysmorphic)-skeletal defects-torsion dystonia
  Naso-blepharo-facial syndrome
  Skeletal defects-dysmorphic facies-torsion dystonia
  Torsion dystonia-skeletal and facial defects

**Excludes:**  **Blepharoptosis-blepharophimosis-epicanthus inversus-telecanthus** (2103)

**Major Diagnostic Criteria:**  Mental retardation and characteristic craniofacial findings are the significant features. A movement disorder described in this family may represent an important diagnostic sign.

**Clinical Findings:**  The facial appearance is distinctive. Telecanthus, redundant nasal eyelid tissue, lateral displacement of the lacrimal puncta, with nasolacrimal duct obstruction and secondary epiphora, blepharophimosis, and downslanting palpebral fissures are the characteristic ophthalmologic features. There are projections of the hairline laterally onto the forehead, bushy eyebrows, prominent nasal bridge, thick alae with wide nasal tip, midfacial hypoplasia, trapezoidal mouth with protruding lower lip, longitudinal furrow of the cheeks, and coarse skin of the face with decreased expression. Extracranial features include joint laxity and mild interdigital webbing. The neurologic examination is abnormal, with Babinski signs present and impaired fine and gross motor coordination. Constant writhing, restless, purposeless movements were observed in the four affected members of one family.

**Complications:** Affected individuals are retarded, with intelligence quotients of 35–68.

**Associated Findings:** The **Torsion dystonia** may have been a secondary feature in one family described.

**Etiology:** In the reported family, the syndrome appears to have been transmitted as an autosomal dominant trait. X-linked inheritance or multifactorial inheritance are also compatible with the pedigree. Karyotypes were unremarkable.

**Pathogenesis:** Unknown.

**MIM No.:** 11005

**POS No.:** 3039

**Sex Ratio:** M2:F1 (observed).

**Occurrence:** One family has been reported.

**Risk of Recurrence for Patient's Sib:**
See Part I, *Mendelian Inheritance.*

**Risk of Recurrence for Patient's Child:**
See Part I, *Mendelian Inheritance.*

**Age of Detectability:** The craniofacial features are present at birth. Psychomotor retardation and torsion dystonia develop in the first year.

**Gene Mapping and Linkage:** Unknown.

**Prevention:** None known. Genetic counseling indicated.

**Treatment:** Unknown.

**Prognosis:** The mental retardation appears to be nonprogressive, static, and prenatal in origin. The disability appears to be only moderate in the reported family.

**Detection of Carrier:** By clinical evaluation.

**Special Considerations:** An individual with a striking resemblance in facial features to affected members of the index family was reported by John P. Johnson and John C. Carey in August 1981 at the David Smith meeting on Malformations and Morphogenesis at Dartmouth, NH. This patient had disproportionate short stature with mesomelic shortening, deafness, and profound mental retardation (IQ 6) with seizures and unusual movements in addition to the characteristic facial findings. The family history is unremarkable, and it is unclear whether this female has the same syndrome.

**References:**
Pashayan H, et al.: A family with blepharo-naso-facial malformations. Am J Dis Child 1973; 125:389–393. * †
Putterman AM, et al.: Eye findings in the blepharo-naso-facial malformation syndrome. Am J Ophthalmol 1973; 76:825–831. * †

**John P. Johnson**

## BLEPHAROCHALASIS-DOUBLE LIP-NONTOXIC GOITER 0111

**Includes:**
Ascher syndrome
Goiter-double lip-blepharochalasis
Lip, double-blepharochalasis-goiter

**Excludes:**
Blepharochalasis superior
**Cheilitis granulomatosa, Melkersson-Rosenthal type** (2083)
**Lip, double** (0594)
Vascular hemangiomas

**Major Diagnostic Criteria:** Sagging eyelids and a double upper lip on smiling are apparent clinically. Thyroid enlargement may occur in the second decade.

**Clinical Findings:** Sagging eyelids and abnormality involving the lips usually results in horizontal duplication of the upper lip between the inner and outer parts. This manifestation may be seen in childhood. The swelling of the eyelids, usually the upper, begins between childhood and puberty and results in relaxation of the supratarsal fold with the lid hanging slack over the palpebral fissure. Thyroid enlargement is more variable and is nontoxic. Its onset is usually after swelling or drooping of the upper lid is noticed, usually during the second decade.

The abnormality of the lips cannot be seen with the mouth closed, but it is noted when the patient talks or smiles. Angioneurotic edema is reported in some patients prior to the onset of the drooping of the lids. Rarely the lower lip can be involved as well.

Pathologic examination of the lids has shown prolapsed orbital fat and hyperplastic lacrimal gland tissue. Histopathologic examination of the lips reveals loose areolar tissue with hyperplastic mucous glands, numerous blood-filled capillaries, and perivascular infiltration with plasma cells and lymphocytes.

**Complications:** Unknown.

**Associated Findings:** None known.

**Etiology:** Possible autosomal dominant inheritance with variability in expression.

**Pathogenesis:** Unknown.

**MIM No.:** 10990

**POS No.:** 3031

**Sex Ratio:** M1:F1

**Occurrence:** Rare; less than a half-dozen cases reported.

**Risk of Recurrence for Patient's Sib:**
See Part I, *Mendelian Inheritance.*

**Risk of Recurrence for Patient's Child:**
See Part I, *Mendelian Inheritance.*

**Age of Detectability:** Childhood to early adolescence.

**Gene Mapping and Linkage:** Unknown.

**Prevention:** None known. Genetic counseling indicated.

**Treatment:** Unknown.

**Prognosis:** Surgical correction of the eyelids and lips is possible for cosmetic reasons. The thyroid abnormalities are nonfunctional, and therefore no specific treatment is necessary.

**Detection of Carrier:** Examination of relatives for evidence of the trait.

**References:**
Ascher KW: Blepharochalasis mit Struma und Doppellippe, Klin Monatsbl Augenheikd 1920; 65:86–97.
Findlay, GH: Idiopathic enlargements of the lips: cheilitis granulomatosa, Ascher's syndrome and double lip. Br J Dermatol 1954; 66:129–138.
Franceschetti A: Manifestation de blépharochalasis chez le père associé à des doubles lèvres apparaissant également chez sa filette âgée d'un mois. J Génét Hum 1955; 4:181–182.
Barnett ML, et al.: Double lip and double lip with blepharochalasis (Ascher's syndrome). Oral Surg 1972; 34:727–733.

**Raymond C. Lewandowski**

**Blepharophimosis**
*See BLEPHAROPTOSIS-BLEPHAROPHIMOSIS-EPICANTHUS
INVERSUS-TELECANTHUS*
**Blepharophimosis syndrome (tetrad)**
*See BLEPHAROPTOSIS-BLEPHAROPHIMOSIS-EPICANTHUS
INVERSUS-TELECANTHUS*
**Blepharophimosis-blepharoptosis-heart defects-mental retardation**
*See MENTAL RETARDATION-HEART DEFECTS-
BLEPHAROPHIMOSIS*
**Blepharoptosis**
*See BLEPHAROPTOSIS-BLEPHAROPHIMOSIS-EPICANTHUS
INVERSUS-TELECANTHUS*
**Blepharoptosis, congenital**
*See EYELID, PTOSIS, CONGENITAL*
**Blepharoptosis-absent eye movements**
*See EYE, FIBROSIS OF THE EXTRAOCULAR MUSCLES,
GENERALIZED*

## BLEPHAROPTOSIS-BLEPHAROPHIMOSIS-EPICANTHUS INVERSUS-TELECANTHUS                    2103

**Includes:**
Blepharophimosis
Blepharophimosis syndrome (tetrad)
Blepharoptosis
Epicanthus inversus
Eyelid, blepharophimosis tetrad
Kohn-Romano syndrome
Telecanthus

**Excludes:**
**Cranio-carpo-tarsal dysplasia, whistling face type** (0223)
Epicanthus palpebralis
Epicanthus supraciliaris
Epicanthus tarsalis

**Major Diagnostic Criteria:** The external appearance of the eyes and mid-face is characteristic, with vertical and horizontal shortening of the palpebral fissures (blepharophimosis), congenial drooping of the eyelids (blepharoptosis) with attenuation of the horizontal lid folds, a fold of skin running upwards from the inner aspect of the lower eyelid onto the medial canthus (epicanthus inversus), and increased distance between the medial canthi (telecanthus). Clinical variability is common; however all four primary features of this tetrad are present to some degree in all cases.

**Clinical Findings:** Blepharoptosis is usually severe, with the levator palpebrae superiors hypoactive and fibrotic. These patients have hypoplasia of the tarsal plate with absence of the eyelid fold and smooth overlying skin which correlates with poor levator function commonly found. Vertical brow width is increased from constant utilization of the frontalis muscle for eyelid lifting. To compensante for the severe blepharoptosis, the head may assume a backward tilt while the chin arches upward.

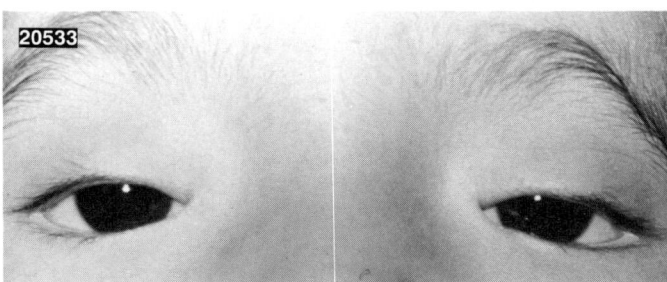

**2103-20533:** Typical appearance of patient with blepharophimosis syndrome. Note shortened horizontal and vertical palpebral apertures and bilateral ptosis with absent horizontal lid folds. Note brow elevation as patient is using frontalis muscle to lift upper lids. There is telecanthus and mild epicanthus inversus.

Blepharophimosis denotes a diminution of horizontal palpebral fissure length from a normal 25 - 30 mm to 18 - 22 mm in this condition.

Epicanthus inversus is an epicanthal fold that arises in the lower eyelid, extending upward to partially obscure the inner canthus. It is seen almost exclusively as part of this congenital syndrome in conjunction with blepharoptosis, blepharophimosis, and telecanthus (*Kohn-Romano syndrome*). The epicanthus inversus fold may diminish the normal depression at the medial canthus. Both the caruncle and plica semilunaris may be hypoplastic and secluded beneath the epicanthal fold.

Telecanthus denotes increased distance between the internal canthi. This is subdivided into primary and secondary forms based upon radiologic evidence of hypertelorism. In this syndrome the length of the medial canthal tendon is increased from a normal 8 - 9mm to 13mm.

**Complications:** This condition represents both a reconstructive and cosmetic handicap. The reconstructive element relates to the severe blepharoptosis with resultant diminution of the upper portion of the visual field.

**Associated Findings:** Additional eyelid features include the upper eyelid margin characteristically S-shaped and the lower eyelid margin with a downward concavity, particularly laterally, which may result in ectropion. Trichiasis was additionally present in several reports. The lacrimal system is often affected. The lower punctum is uniformly laterally displaced, while the upper punctum is medially displaced. Posterior ectopia of the lower punctum and aplasia of the upper punctum were recently described. Other variations may include stenosis of all canaliculi, elongation of the horizontal canaliculi, and punctal reduplication.

Additional ophthalmic features may occasionally include microphthalmos, exotropia, esotropia, underaction of the superior rectus muscle with limitation of upgaze, underaction of the inferior rectus muscle with limitation of downgaze, nystagmus, and optic disc colobomas.

Additional facial features include a broad and flat nasal bridge with a bony deficiency at the supraorbital rim and brow. The palate may be high arched and the ears may be low set and cupped with an overhanging helix. Despite their appearance, mental status is normal, although some patients have developed secondary psychological problems from their cosmetic handicap. This condition is quite stable over time.

**Etiology:** Autosomal dominant inheritance with essentially 100% penetrance, occurence more commonly in males, and expression more commonly through male lineage. The syndrome is associated with an increased incidence of amenorrhea. Anomalies of male reproduction have not been reported. Two subcategories of this syndrome have recently been postulated. Type I is said to be an autosomal dominant trait transmitted by males (due to female infertility). Type II is said to be an autosomal dominant trait without associated female infertility. Approximately one-half of cases are due to new mutations, and sporadic cases are occasionally found. All chromosomal studies have been normal.

**Pathogenesis:** Unknown.

**MIM No.:** *11010

**POS No.:** 3230

**CDC No.:** 743.635, 743.600

**Sex Ratio:** M1:F<1

**Occurrence:** Over 40 cases have been documented in a literature extending back 100 years.

**Risk of Recurrence for Patient's Sib:**
See Part I, *Mendelian Inheritance.*

**Risk of Recurrence for Patient's Child:**
See Part I, *Mendelian Inheritance.*

**Age of Detectability:** At birth.

**Gene Mapping and Linkage:** Unknown.

**Prevention:** None known. Genetic counseling indicated.

**Treatment:** Management is often deferred until the preschool years when the anatomy becomes larger and easier to work with.

The surgery is based upon a medial canthoplasty which eliminates the epicanthus inversus, while reducing the blepharophimosis and telecanthus. Blepharoptosis is corrected as the final stage or the first procedure or at a second operation. Usually frontalis suspension is required due to the very poor levator function present in these cases. In selected patients, though, with less blepharoptosis and domonstrable levator function, a maximum levator resection may prove adequate.

**Prognosis:** Good, when surgically corrected.

**Detection of Carrier:** Careful clinical examination of relatives for evidence of this syndrome.

**Special Considerations:** It should be emphasized that epicanthus supraciliaris, palpebralis, and tarsalis are variations of normal and not part of this condition. To establish the diagnosis of this syndrome all features of the tetrad (blepharoptosis, blepharophimosis, epicanthus inversus, and telecanthus) must be evident.

**References:**

Kohn R, Romano P: Blepharoptosis, blepharophimosis, epicanthus inversus, and telecanthus: a syndrome with no name. Am J Ophthalmol 1971; 72:625–632.

Geeraets W: Ocular syndromes (Kohn - Romano syndromes). Philadelphia: Lea and Febiger, 1976.

Johnson C: Epicanthus and epiblepharon. Arch Opththalmol 1978; 96:1030.

Townes P, Muechler E: Blepharophimosis, ptosis, epicanthus inversus, and primary amenorrhea: a dominant trait. Arch Ophthalmol 1979; 97:1664–1666.

Kohn R: Additional lacrimal findings in the syndrome of blepharoptosis, blepharophimosis, epicanthus inversus, and telecanthus. J Ped Ophthalmol and Strabismus 1983; 20:98.

Zlotogora J, et al.: The blepharophimosis, ptosis, and epicanthus inversus syndrome: delineation of two types. Am J Hum Genet 1983; 35:1020–1027.

Jones C, Collin J: Blepharophimosis and its association with female infertility. Br J Ophthalmol 1984; 68:533–534.

Roy F: Ocular syndromes and systemic diseases. (Kohn-Romano Syndrome). New York, Grune and Stratton, 1985.

Ohdo S, et al.: Mental retardation associated with congenital heart disease, blepharophimosis, blepharoptosis and hypoplastic teeth. J Med Genet 1986; 23:242–244.

Elliot D, Wallace A: Ptosis with blepharophimosis and epicanthus inversus. Br J Plast Surg 1986; 39:3–17.

Kohn R: Congenital Anomalies of the Eyelids, Socket, and Orbit. In: Hornblass A, ed: Ophthalmic and Orbital Plastic and Reconstructive Surgery, vol I. Baltimore, Williams and Wilkins, 1988.

Kohn R: Textbook of Ophthalmic Plastic and Reconstructive Surgery. Philadelphia: Lea and Febiger, 1988.

K0025
MA080
RE023

**Roger Kohn**
**Bartholomew Martyak**
**Philip R. Reilly**

## BLINDNESS (CORTICAL)-RETARDATION-POSTAXIAL POLYDACTYLY                    2789

**Includes:**
Growth retardation-cortical blindness-postaxial polydactyly
Polydactyly (postaxial)-cortical blindness-growth retardation

**Excludes:**
**Bardet-Biedl syndrome** (2363)
Cortical blindness, other
Hamartoblastoma, congenital
**Oro-facio-digital syndrome I** (0770)

**Major Diagnostic Criteria:** Congenital cortical blindness, growth and psychomotor retardation, postaxial **Polydactyly**.

**Clinical Findings:** Polydactyly in both hands and feet. Cortical blindness and psychomotor retardation are noted early. Prominent forehead, short nose, long philtrum, high-arched palate, microretrognathia. Normal ophthalmologic data indicate a cortical origin of the blindness.

X-rays show an unarticulated postaxial extra digit in each hand

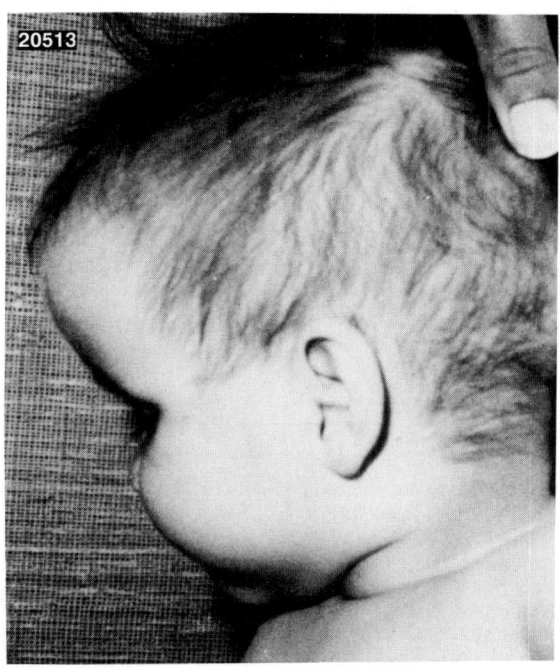

**2789-20513:** Note prominent forehead, short nose and microretrognathia.

and a well-formed supernumerary sixth digit joined to the fifth metatarsal bone in the feet.

**Complications:** Recurrent respiratory and intestinal infections.

**Associated Findings:** None known.

**Etiology:** Possibly autosomal recessive inheritance.

**Pathogenesis:** Unknown.

**MIM No.:** 21801

**Sex Ratio:** Presumably M1:F1.

**Occurrence:** Documented in three children of first cousin parents.

**Risk of Recurrence for Patient's Sib:**
See Part I, *Mendelian Inheritance.*

**Risk of Recurrence for Patient's Child:**
See Part I, *Mendelian Inheritance.*

**Age of Detectability:** At birth.

**Gene Mapping and Linkage:** Unknown.

**Prevention:** None known. Genetic counseling indicated.

**Treatment:** Cosmetic surgery for polydactyly.

**Prognosis:** Uncertain, due to recurrent respiratory and intestinal infections. Two of the three known cases died at five and 20 months of age respectively.

**Detection of Carrier:** Unknown.

**References:**

Hernández A, et al.: Cortical blindness, growth and psychomotor retardation and postaxial polydactyly: a probably distinct autosomal recessive syndrome. Clin Genet 1985; 28:251–254.

HE039
CA011

**Alejandro Hernández**
**José María Cantú**

**Blindness (pseudogliomatous)-osteoporosis-mild mental retardation**
*See OSTEOPOROSIS-PSEUDOGLIOMA SYNDROME*
**Blindness-polycystic kidney disease-cataract**
*See KIDNEY, POLYCYSTIC DISEASE-CATARACT-BLINDNESS*

**Bloch-Miescher syndrome**
See LIPODYSTROPHY-COARSE FACIES-ACANTHOSIS NIGRICANS, MIESCHER TYPE
**Bloch-Siemens incontinentia pigmenti**
See INCONTINENTIA PIGMENTI
**Bloch-Sulzberger syndrome**
See INCONTINENTIA PIGMENTI
**Blood group, Rhesus system (Rh)**
See ERYTHROBLASTOSIS FETALIS
**Blood pressure, fetal effects of maternal hypertension medication**
See FETAL EFFECTS FROM MATERNAL VASODILATOR
**Blood, diphosphoglycerate mutase (2,3) deficiency**
See ERYTHROCYTE, DIPHOSPHOGLYCERATE MUTASE (2,3) DEFICIENCY
**Blood, red cell membrane defects**
See ANEMIA, HEMOLYTIC, RED CELL MEMBRANE DEFECTS
**Blood-limb syndrome**
See WT SYNDROME

## BLOOM SYNDROME                                    0112

**Includes:**  Growth deficiency-facial erythema-chromosome instability

**Excludes:**
   **Chromosome instability, Nijmegen type** (2551)
   Primordial (idiopathic) dwarfism
   **Rothmund-Thomson syndrome** (2037)
   **Silver syndrome, X-linked** (2829)

**Major Diagnostic Criteria:**  1) Growth deficiency with normal body proportions; 2) an erythematous, sun-sensitive facial erythema; and 3) chromosome instability of a specific type, i.e., a tendency to chromatid exchange. Demonstration of a greatly increased frequency of sister-chromatid exchange (SCE) is diagnostic.

**Clinical Findings:**  The cardinal clinical features are 1) growth deficiency, both intra- and extrauterine, proportionate except for slight relative microcephaly, and 2) a sun-sensitive facial erythema. The facies is characteristic: malar hypoplasia, nasal

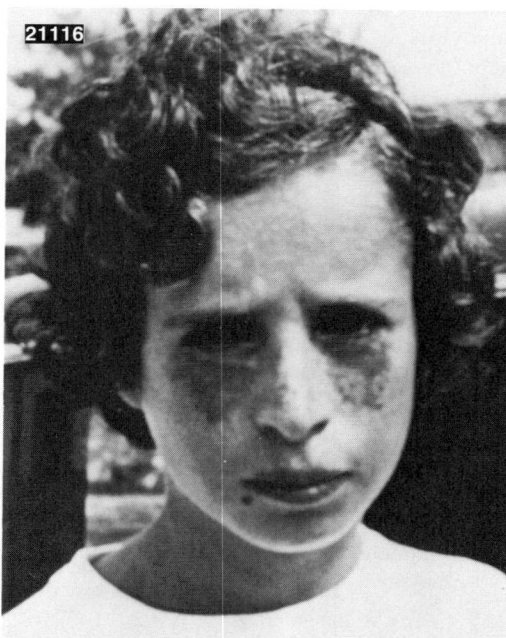

**0112-21116:**  Note telangiectatic erythema in the butterfly area of the face along with prominent nose and narrow facies with malar hypoplasia.

prominence, small mandible, and narrow dolichocephalic skull and face. The skin of the dorsa of the hands and forearms and occasionally of the ears and neck may be affected by the erythematous, often telangiectatic, lesion, but such lesions in other areas speak against the diagnosis. The skin lesion varies in severity, is milder in females than in males, and is occasionally absent.

**Complications:**  Malignant neoplasia, often multiple, occurs at an increased frequency at all ages. Acute leukemia and lymphoid neoplasms predominate before age 25 years, and after age 20 years carcinomas (tongue, larynx, lung, esophagus, colon, skin, breast, cervix) predominate, that of any given site appearing several decades earlier than expected in the general population. Chronic bronchitis and bronchiectasis, probably the consequence of inadequately treated acute respiratory infections early in life, can be severe and disabling. Diabetes mellitus occurs with increased frequency.

**Associated Findings:**  *Characteristic:* infantile diarrhea and vomiting, café-au-lait with or without hypopigmented spots, high-pitched voice of characteristic timbre, azoospermia, sun-tolerance except of the face. *Frequent:* minor developmental defects, benign neoplasia, learning disability, low average intellectual ability. *Occasional:* mild mental deficiency.

**Etiology:**  Autosomal recessive inheritance.

**Pathogenesis:**  The growth deficiency is unexplained. The proneness to infection is the consequence of a widespread immunodeficiency. The proneness to neoplasia probably is the consequence of the increased genomic instability, enhanced possibly by the immunodeficiency. Decreased activity of DNA ligase I appears to be the explanation for the genomic instability.

**MIM No.:**  *21090

**POS No.:**  3040

**Sex Ratio:**  M4:F3

**Occurrence:**  Recognized in many ethnic groups but relatively more common in Ashkenazi Jews whose ancestors were from Poland or the Ukraine. Patients diagnosed throughout the world (approximately 130) are tabulated in progress reports from the *Bloom's Syndrome Registry* (German et al., 1984).

**Risk of Recurrence for Patient's Sib:**
   See Part I, *Mendelian Inheritance.*

**Risk of Recurrence for Patient's Child:**
   See Part I, *Mendelian Inheritance.*

**Age of Detectability:**  Any time after birth. Prenatal diagnosis is theoretically possible.

**Gene Mapping and Linkage:**  Unknown.

**Prevention:**  None known. Genetic counseling indicated.

**Treatment:**  Prompt antibiotic therapy for infections. Increased surveillance for carcinomas after age 20 years.

**Prognosis:**  Good general health, but with the serious complications mentioned above. Improved resistance to infections and decreasingly severe skin lesions with advancing age.

**Detection of Carrier:**  Unknown.

**Special Considerations:**  The *Bloom's Syndrome Registry* serves as a repository for clinical and genetic information about the syndrome. For information, or to report a newly recognized patient, contact Laboratory of Human Genetics, The New York Blood Center, New York, NY 10021.

**References:**
German J: Bloom's syndrome I: genetical and clinical observations in the first twenty-seven patients. Am J Hum Genet 1969; 21:196–227. †
German J: Bloom's syndrome VIII: review of clinical and genetic aspects. In: Goodman RM, Motulsky AG, eds: Genetic diseases among Ashkenazi Jews. New York: Raven, 1979:121–139.
German J: Patterns of neoplasia associated with the chromosome-breakage syndromes. In: German J, ed: Chromosome mutation and neoplasia. New York: Alan R. Liss, 1983:97–134.
Ray JH, German J: The cytogenetics of the "chromosome-breakage syndromes." In: German J, ed: Chromosome mutation and neoplasia. New York: Alan R. Liss, 1983:135–167.

German J: The significance of identifying a cancer-predisposed person
- lessons from the chromosome-breakage syndromes. In: Chaganti
RSK, German J, eds: Genetics in clinical oncology. New York:
Oxford University Press, 1985:211–221.
Chan JHY, et al.: Altered DNA ligase in Bloom's syndrome. Nature
1987; 325:357–359.
German J, Passarge E: Bloom's syndrome XII: Report from the
Registry for 1987. Clin Genet 1987; 35:57–69.

GE009 **James German**

**Blue colorblindness**
See COLOR BLINDNESS, YELLOW-BLUE TRITAN
**Blue diaper syndrome**
See TRYPTOPHAN MALABSORPTION
**Blue monocone-monochromatic, color blindness**
See COLOR BLINDNESS, BLUE MONOCONE-MONOCHROMATIC
**Blue rubber bleb nevus of skin and gastrointestinal tract**
See NEVUS, BLUE RUBBER BLEB NEVUS SYNDROME
**Blueberry muffin rash**
See TEETH, ENAMEL AND DENTIN DEFECTS FROM
ERYTHROBLASTOSIS FETALIS
**Bochdalek hernia**
See DIAPHRAGMATIC HERNIA
**Boder-Sedgwick syndrome**
See ATAXIA-TELANGIECTASIA
**Bohn nodules**
See MUCOSA, ORAL INCLUSION CYSTS OF THE NEWBORN
**Bone aplasias-hypoplasias of the upper extremities**
See LIMB, REDUCTION DEFORMITIES OF UPPER LIMBS
**Bone atrophy, deffuse**
See TEETH, PERIODONTITIS, JUVENILE
**Bone density (increased)-syndactyly**
See CRANIODIAPHYSEAL DYSPLASIA, LENZ-MAJEWSKI TYPE
**Bone disease, hypophosphatemic (HBD)**
See HYPOPHOSPHATEMIA, NON X-LINKED
**Bone dysplasia, Worth type hyperostosis**
See HYPEROSTOSIS, WORTH TYPE
**Bone fragility-skeletal bowing-cortical thickening-ichthyosis**
See SKELETAL BOWING-CORTICAL THICKENING-BONE FRAGILITY-
ICTHYOSIS
**Bone marrow dysfunction-pancreatic insufficiency-short stature**
See SHWACHMAN SYNDROME
**Bone, absence deformities of long-cleft lip/palate**
See ROBERTS SYNDROME
**Bone, excessive turnover**
See OSTEOECTASIA

## BONE, PAGET DISEASE  3081

**Includes:**
Osteitis deformans
Paget disease
**Excludes:**
Hyperphosphatasia
Osteitis fibrosa cystica
**Osteoectasia** (0776)

**Major Diagnostic Criteria:** Slowly progressive asymmetric expansion of bones, especially in the skull and shins. On X-ray there are characteristic areas of bone lucency and sclerosis.

**Clinical Findings:** The prevalence increases with advancing age and Paget disease is seldom encountered before middle life (see **Osteoectasia** for a juvenile form). The skull, axial skeleton, and proximal long bones are the sites of predilection. Bone pain is sometimes intractable. The serum alkaline phosphatase level is consistently raised.

On X-ray, bone involvement may be localized or widespread. Radiolucent areas appear in the early stages of the disease, followed by sclerosis, expansion, and distortion of the bones. These changes sometimes mimic neoplastic metastases. Individuals with the characteristic X-ray bone changes may remain totally asymptomatic.

**Complications:** Deafness, skeletal deformity, spontaneous fractures, and osteosarcomatous changes are late complications. In severe cases the vascular component acts as an arteriovenous shunt, and cardiac failure may supervene.

**Associated Findings:** None known.

**Etiology:** Possibly autosomal dominant inheritance with varying clinical expression. Slow virus infection has also been suggested as a possible etiology.

**Pathogenesis:** Unknown.

**MIM No.:** 16725

**Sex Ratio:** Presumably M1:F1.

**Occurrence:** Paget disease has a worldwide distribution, but it seems to be unusually common in Lancashire, England, and in British immigrants in Australia. About 40 pedigrees are well documented.

**Risk of Recurrence for Patient's Sib:**
See Part I, Mendelian Inheritance.

**Risk of Recurrence for Patient's Child:**
See Part I, Mendelian Inheritance.

**Age of Detectability:** Onset before middle age is unusual.

**Gene Mapping and Linkage:** Unknown.

**Prevention:** None known. Genetic counseling indicated.

**Treatment:** The management of Paget disease has been improved by the introduction of calcitonin therapy, and, in adequately treated patients, symptomatic remission can be induced.

**Prognosis:** Slow progression in untreated cases. Late complications may eventually be lethal.

**Detection of Carrier:** Unknown.

**Special Considerations:** Characteristic cytoplasmic inclusions are present in the osteoclasts. These bodies resemble virus particles, and their frequency corresponds to the severity of the disorder. Familial clustering may reflect exposure or propensity to infection by the causative agent rather than mendelian inheritance.

**Support Groups:** NY; Brooklyn; Paget's Disease Foundation

**References:**
McKusick VA: Paget's disease of the bone. In: Heritable disorders of
connective tissue, ed 4. St. Louis: C.V. Mosby, Co. 1972:718–723.
Gardner MJ, et al.: Radiological prevalence of Paget's disease of bone
in British migrants to Australia. Br Med J 1978; I:1655–1657.
Barker DJP, et al.: Paget's disease of bone: the Lancashire focus. Br
Med J 1980; 280:1105–1107.
Harvey L, et al.: Ultrastructural features of the osteoclasts from Paget's
disease of bone in relation to a viral aetiology. J Clin Pathol 1982;
35:771–779.
Sofaer JA, et al.: A family study of Paget's disease of bone. J Epidemiol
Community Health 1983; 37:226–231.

BE008 **Peter Beighton**

**Bone-hair-nail-tooth dysplasia**
See TRICHO-DENTO-OSSEOUS SYNDROME
**Bones, dense-heart defects-hydrocephalus**
See HYDROCEPHALUS-HEART DEFECT-DENSE BONES, BEEMER
TYPE
**Bony choanal atresia, anterior**
See NOSE, ANTERIOR ATRESIA
**Bony choanal atresia, posterior**
See NOSE, POSTERIOR ATRESIA
**Bony choanal atresia, posterior-lymphedema**
See NOSE, CHOANAL ATRESIA-LYMPHEDEMA
**Book syndrome**
See HYPERHIDROSIS-PREMATURE GREYING-PREMOLAR APLASIA
**Boomerang skeletal dysplasia**
See SKELETAL DYSPLASIA, BOOMERANG DYSPLASIA
**BOR syndrome**
See BRANCHIO-OTO-RENAL DYSPLASIA
**Borjeson syndrome**
See BORJESON-FORSSMAN-LEHMANN SYNDROME

## BORJESON-FORSSMAN-LEHMANN SYNDROME     2272

**Includes:**
Borjeson syndrome
Endocrine disorders-epilepsy-mental deficiency
Mental deficiency-epilepsy-endocrine disorders

**Excludes:**
**Bardet-Biedl syndrome** (2363)
**Coffin-Lowry syndrome** (0190)
**Prader-Willi syndrome** (0823)

**Major Diagnostic Criteria:** Characteristic craniofacial appearance, hypotonia, severe mental retardation, hypogonadism, and ophthalmologic, EEG, and skeletal abnormalities in males. Manifestations are less severe and more variable in females.

**Clinical Findings:** Craniofacial characteristics include **Microcephaly** in some, prominent supraorbital ridge, deep-set eyes, ptosis, large ears, and coarse, fleshy facial features. The skin has a soft doughy consistency. Nearly all affected individuals have been shorter than average and obese at some point in their lives. Supraspinal hypotonia is present.

Most affected males have had severe mental retardation with an IQ less than 60, although males with this disorder with mild to moderate retardation have recently been identified. Affected females have mild-to-moderate mental retardation; some obligate carrier females have had normal to above average intelligence.

Hypogonadism in the form of small penis and small and/or undescended testes has been seen in all males. The hypogonadism has elements of both central and end-organ dysfunction, with a lag in the expected increase in gonadotropins, delayed puberty, and abnormal testicular function with elevated FSH levels once pubertal changes have begun. Females may have a delay in development of secondary sexual characteristics.

Ophthalmologic abnormalities include nystagmus, decreased visual acuity, optic nerve abnormalities, decreased retinal function on electroretinogram (ERG) and corneal or lenticular changes. EEG abnormalities have included markedly decreased alpha rhythms, excessive theta slow waves, or excessive beta waves.

Various skeletal abnormalities have been observed including abnormally steep radiocarpal angle, narrow cervical spinal canal, Scheuermann-like vertebral changes, kyphoscoliosis, mild epiphyseal dysplasia, delayed closure of the radial and ulnar epiphyses, short distal phalanges, small heads of the proximal long bones, and thickened calvaria.

**Complications:** About one-half of the reported males have developed convulsions.

**Associated Findings:** None known.

**Etiology:** X-linked inheritance with variable expression in female heterozygotes.

**Pathogenesis:** Autopsy findings have suggested that the CNS anomalies are due to a primary disturbance of neuronal migration.

**MIM No.:** 30190

**POS No.:** 3502

**Sex Ratio:** M1:F1

**Occurrence:** Some six kinships have been reported.

**Risk of Recurrence for Patient's Sib:**
See Part I, *Mendelian Inheritance.*

**Risk of Recurrence for Patient's Child:**
See Part I, *Mendelian Inheritance.* No affected males are known to have reproduced.

**Age of Detectability:** In early childhood.

**Gene Mapping and Linkage:** BFLS (Borjeson-Forssman-Lehmann syndrome) has been mapped to Xq26-q27.

**Prevention:** None known. Genetic counseling indicated.

**Treatment:** A sheltered environment is generally necessary because of severe limitations of nervous system performance in affected males. Affected females may benefit from early special education programs.

**Prognosis:** Life span is presumably normal in both males and females, although two institutionalized males of the original report died of pneumonia at ages 20 and 44 years. Males have severe mental retardation with additional limitations due to their hypotonia and poor vision. Carrier females range from those with no observable abnormalities to those with mild-to-moderate visual and intellectual limitations.

**Detection of Carrier:** Unknown. May become possible by linkage studies.

*The author wishes to thank James W. Hanson for his help in the preparation of this article.*

**References:**
Börjeson M, et al.: An X-linked recessively inherited syndrome characterized by grave mental deficiency, epilepsy, and endocrine disorder. Acta Med Scand 1962; 171:13–21.
Brun A, et al.: An inherited syndrome with mental deficiency and endocrine disorder: a pathoanatomical study. J Ment Defic Res 1974; 18:317–325.
Robinson LK, et al.: The Börjeson-Forssman-Lehmann syndrome. Am J Med Genet 1983; 15:457–468.
Ardinger HH, et al.: Börjeson-Forssman-Lehmann syndrome: further delineation in five cases. Am J Med Genet 1984; 19:653–664. *

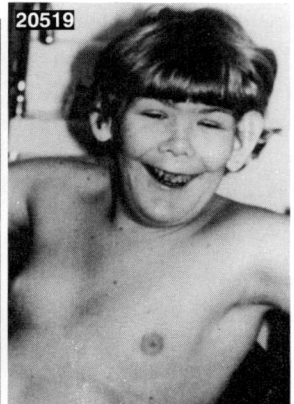
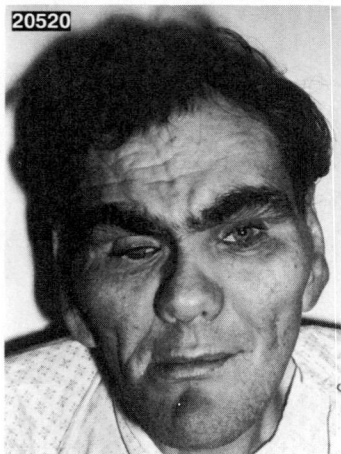
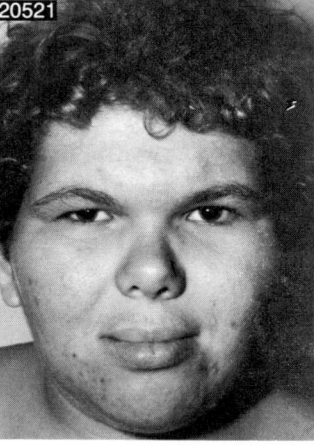

**2272**-20518: Borjeson-Forssman-Lehman syndrome; note 10-month-old male infant with large ears and ptosis.   20519: 21-year-old male subject; ptosis and large ears are still apparent. 20520:   40-year-old male subject; note ptosis, prominent supraorbital ridges, and coarse, fleshy facial features.   20521: 23-year-old female subject; note characteristic facies with deep-set eyes, prominent supraorbital ridges, and coarse, fleshy facial features.

Flannery DB, et al.: Dermatoglyphics in Börjeson-Forssman-Lehmann syndrome. (Letter) Am J Med Genet 1985; 21:401–404.
Mathews K, et al.: Börjeson-Forssman-Lehmann syndrome localization. (Letter) Am J Med Genet 1989; 34:475.

AR009                                          **Holly H. Ardinger**

**Borrelia burgdorferi infection**
  *See FETAL EFFECTS FROM LYME DISEASE*
**Boucher-Neuhauser syndrome**
  *See ATAXIA-HYPOGONADISM SYNDROME*
**Bourneville syndrome**
  *See TUBEROUS SCLEROSIS*
**Bowen-Conradi Hutterite syndrome**
  *See HUTTERITE SYNDROME, BOWEN-CONRADI TYPE*
**Bowing of legs, anterior, with dwarfism**
  *See SKELETAL DYSPLASIA, WEISMANN-NETTER-STUHL TYPE*
**Bowing of the limbs, congenital**
  *See CAMPOMELIC DYSPLASIA*
**Bowing, congenital, with short bones**
  *See KYPHOMELIC DYSPLASIA*
**Brachial neuritis, recurrent familial**
  *See NEUROPATHY, HEREDITARY RECURRENT BRACHIAL*
**Brachial neuropathy, familial**
  *See NEUROPATHY, HEREDITARY RECURRENT BRACHIAL*
**Brachial plexopathy, hereditary**
  *See NEUROPATHY, HEREDITARY RECURRENT BRACHIAL*
**Brachial plexus neuropathy, heredo-familial**
  *See NEUROPATHY, HEREDITARY RECURRENT BRACHIAL*
**Brachiocephalic and contralateral corotid artery, common origin of**
  *See ARTERY, BRACHIOCEPHALIC AND CONTRALATERAL CAROTID, COMMON ORIGIN*
**Brachmann-de Lange syndrome**
  *See DE LANGE SYNDROME*
**Brachycephaly**
  *See CRANIOSYNOSTOSIS*

## BRACHYDACTYLY                                    0114

**Includes:**
  Brachydactyly types A1, A2, A3, B, C, D and E
  Brachymesophalangy-brachymetapody
  Brachymesophalangy II, Mohr-Wriedt type
  Brachymesophalangy V, clinodactyly
  Digits, short
  Farabee brachydactyly
  "Stub thumb"

**Excludes:**
  **Chromosome 21, trisomy 21** (0171)
  **Macular coloboma-brachydactyly** (0621)
  **Parathormone resistance** (0830)
  **Poland syndrome** (0813)
  **Rubinstein-Taybi broad thumb-hallux syndrome** (0119)
  Tabatznik syndrome
  **Turner syndrome** (0977)
  Brachydactyly in other syndromes

**Major Diagnostic Criteria:** Short digits. Genetic types may be separated from others by determining if they fit into one of the characteristic patterns and identifying similarly affected relatives.

**Clinical Findings:** Brachydactyly is shortening of the digits due to shortening of any of its components, the metacarpals or phalanges. Brachydactyly has been classified into seven genetic types according to the inheritance of selective and specific shortening of certain parts of the digits consistently within families. In brachydactyly types $A_1$, $A_2$, and $A_3$ brachydactyly, shortening is confined to the middle phalanges.

In type $A_1$ (Farabee type) it affects all the middle phalanges, which are rudimentary and sometimes fused with the terminal phalanges. The proximal phalanges of the thumbs and big toes are short. The subjects are short in stature.

In type $A_2$ shortening of the middle phalanges is confined to the index finger and the second toe with the other digits being more or less normal. Because of a rhomboid or triangular shape of the affected middle phalanx, the end of the second finger usually deviates radially.

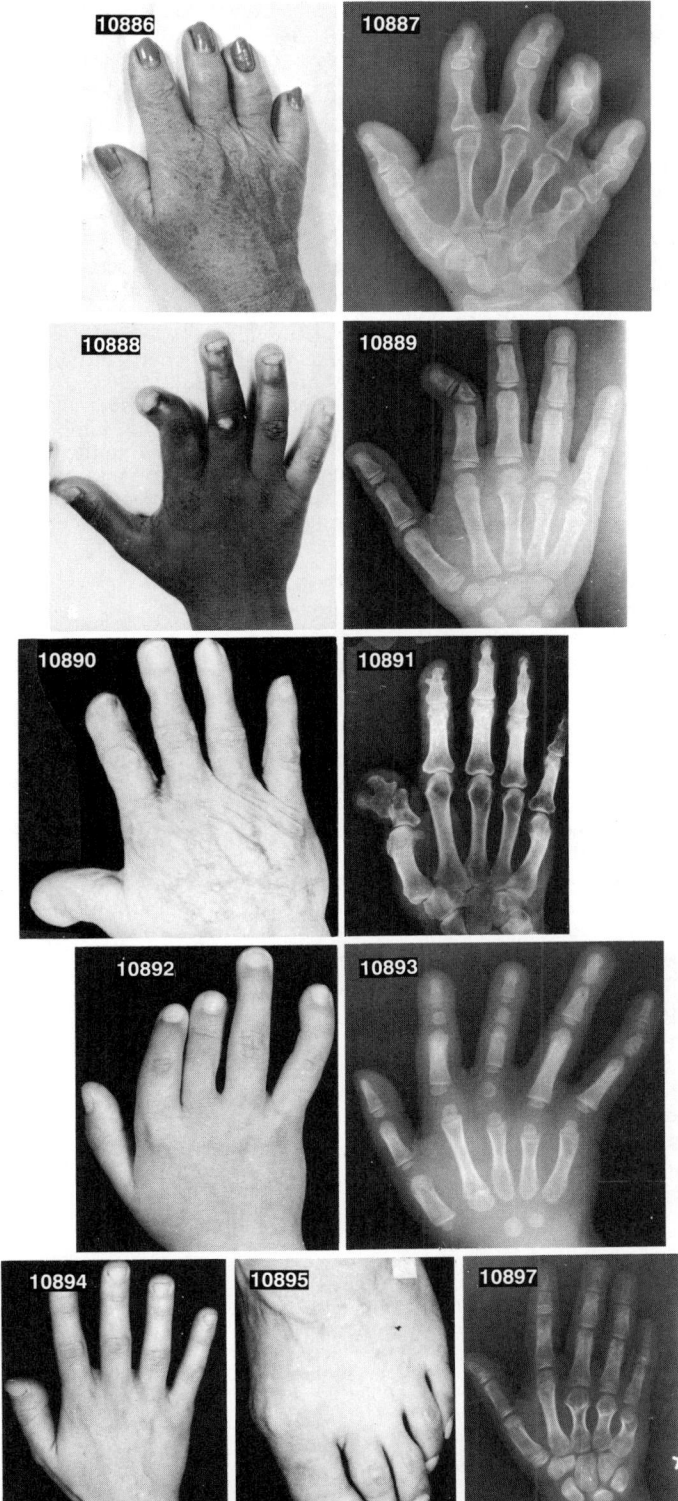

**0114**-10886–10887: Type A1 brachydactyly. 10888–10889: Type A2 brachydactyly. 10890–10891: Type B brachydactyly. 10892–10893: Type C brachydactyly. 10894–10895: Type D brachydactyly. 10897: Type E brachydactyly.

In type $A_3$ shortening affects the middle phalanx of the fifth digit.

In type B brachydactyly, the middle phalanges are also short but in addition, the terminal phalanges are rudimentary or absent. Thumbs and big toes are usually deformed. Symphalangism is also a feature. The absence of distal phalanges has led some authors to define this malformation as ectrodactyly and as apical dystrophy. The association with syndactyly has led some authors to describe it as symbrachydactyly.

In type C brachydactyly, the middle phalanges as well as some metacarpals are shortened. The characteristic change is a deformity of the middle and proximal phalanges of the second and third digits (index and middle fingers), sometimes with hypersegmentation of the proximal phalanx. The ring finger may be essentially normal and, therefore, is the longest digit.

Type D brachydactyly is characterized by short and broad terminal phalanges of the thumbs and big toes.

Type E brachydactyly is due mainly to shortening of the metacarpals and metatarsals. Wide variability in the number of digits affected occurs from person to person even within the same family. The patients are moderately short in stature and have a round face but do not have ectopic calcification, mental retardation, or cataract as occurs in **Parathormone resistance**.

**Complications:** Unknown.

**Associated Findings:** None known.

**Etiology:** Autosomal dominant inheritance.

**Pathogenesis:** Unknown.

**MIM No.:** *11250, *11260, *11270, *11300, *11310, *11320, *11330

**POS No.:** 3042

**Sex Ratio:** M1:F1

**Occurrence:** While types $A_1$, $A_2$, B, C, and E are rather rare, types $A_3$ (fifth finger clinodactyly) and D ("stub thumb") are common and can be considered as normal variations.

**Risk of Recurrence for Patient's Sib:**
See Part I, *Mendelian Inheritance*.

**Risk of Recurrence for Patient's Child:**
See Part I, *Mendelian Inheritance*. (Extreme variability in lesion from very mild to very severe should be considered).

**Age of Detectability:** From birth to late in childhood.

**Gene Mapping and Linkage:** Unknown.

**Prevention:** None known. Genetic counseling indicated.

**Treatment:** Surgical intervention is recommended in type $A_2$, when syndactyly is an associated malformation, and in some cases with type C brachydactyly when talipes is an associated malformation.

**Prognosis:** Brachydactyly as an isolated malformation does not affect life span.

**Detection of Carrier:** Unknown.

**References:**
Haws DV, McKusick VA: Farabee's brachydactylous kindred revisited. Bull Johns Hopkins Hosp 1963; 113:20–30.
McKusick VA, Milch RA: The clinical behavior of genetic diseases: selected aspects. Clin Orthop 1964; 33:22.
Temtamy SA: Genetic factors in hand malformations. Unpublished doctoral dissertation. Baltimre: Johns Hopkins University, 1966.
Temtamy SA, McKusick VA: The genetics of hand malformations. New York: Alan Liss, 1978. *
Baraitser M, Burn J: Recessively inherited brachydactyly type C. J Med Genet 1983; 20:128–129.
Gray E, Hurt VK: Inheritance of brachydactyly type D. J Hered 1984; 75:297–299.

TE004

**Samia A. Temtamy**

**Brachydactyly and macular coloboma**
*See MACULAR COLOBOMA-BRACHYDACTYLY*
**Brachydactyly due to absence of distal phalanges**
*See DIGITO-RENO-CEREBRAL SYNDROME*
**Brachydactyly type E-Anetodermia-exostoses**
*See EXOSTOSES-ANETODERMIA-BRACHYDACTYLY TYPE E*

**Brachydactyly types A1, A2, A3, B, C, D and E**
*See BRACHYDACTYLY*
**Brachydactyly, long thumb type**
*See BRACHYDACTYLY-LONG THUMB SYNDROME*
**Brachydactyly-corneal dystrophy-hyperkeratosis-short stature**
*See CORNEO-DERMATO-OSSEOUS SYNDROME*
**Brachydactyly-growth deficiency-dysmorphic faces**
*See GROWTH DEFICIENCY-FACIAL DEFECTS-BRACHYDACTYLY*

## BRACHYDACTYLY-LONG THUMB SYNDROME     3035

**Includes:**
Brachydactyly, long thumb type
Thumb, long-brachydactyly syndrome

**Excludes:**
Cryptodontic brachymetacarpalia
**Heart-hand syndrome II** (3265)

**Major Diagnostic Criteria:** This condition is characterized by a combination of **Brachydactyly**, clinodactyly, and other skeletal and cardiac defects.

**Clinical Findings:** Four affected individuals have been reported. All affected individuals had brachydactyly with relatively long thumbs, clinodactyly, narrow shoulders, **Pectus excavatum**, short upper and lower limbs, and cardiac defects, including mild pulmonic stenosis, apparent cardiac conduction defects, and cardiomegaly. Small feet were described in three individuals.

X-rays on three persons demonstrated short, broad clavicles and short humeri in all. The brachydactyly was characterized by severe shortening of the middle phalanges, moderate shortness of the proximal phalanges, and mild shortness of the distal phalanges. The metacarpals were normal.

**Complications:** Shoulder and metacarpophalangeal joint limitation occur, likely secondary to the skeletal anomalies; the cardiac anomalies are likely secondary to the pectus excavatum.

**Associated Findings:** None known.

**Etiology:** Probably autosomal dominant inheritance.

**Pathogenesis:** Unknown. Probably related to skeletal tissue.

**MIM No.:** 11243

**POS No.:** 3508

**Sex Ratio:** M1:F1

**Occurrence:** Documented in four members from three generations of one family.

**Risk of Recurrence for Patient's Sib:**
See Part I, *Mendelian Inheritance*.

**Risk of Recurrence for Patient's Child:**
See Part I, *Mendelian Inheritance*.

**Age of Detectability:** Probably at birth by the presence of the hand anomalies.

**Gene Mapping and Linkage:** Unknown.

**Prevention:** None known. Genetic counseling indicated.

**Treatment:** Orthopedic intervention may be indicated; treatment of the cardiac defect was not necessary in the reported cases.

**Prognosis:** Apparently normal intellectual development and near-normal life span. One affected person died at age 66 years of unrelated causes.

**Detection of Carrier:** Unknown.

**References:**
Hollister DW, Hollister WG: The "long-thumb" brachydactyly syndrome. Am J Med Genet 1981; 8:5–16.

T0007

**Helga V. Toriello**

**Brachydactyly-maxillary hypoplasia-metaphyseal dysplasia**
*See METAPHYSEAL DYSPLASIA-MAXILLARY HYPOPLASIA-BRACHYDACTYLY*
**Brachydactyly-nystagmus-cerebellar ataxia syndrome**
*See BIEMOND I SYNDROME*

**Brachydactyly-oto-dental-cataract defects**
*See CATARACTS-OTO-DENTAL DEFECTS*
**Brachydactyly-peculiar facies-mental retardation syndrome**
*See RUBINSTEIN-TAYBI BROAD THUMB-HALLUX SYNDROME*
**Brachyectrodactyly-triphalangeal thumb**
*See THUMB, TRIPHALANGEAL-BRACHYECTRODACTYLY*
**Brachymelic primordial dwarfism**
*See DWARFISM, OSTEODYSPLASTIC PRIMORDIAL, MAJEWSKI-WINTER TYPE*
**Brachymesophalangy II, Mohr-Wriedt type**
*See BRACHYDACTYLY*
**Brachymesophalangy V, clinodactyly**
*See BRACHYDACTYLY*
**Brachymesophalangy-brachymetapody**
*See BRACHYDACTYLY*
**Brachymetapody-anodontia-hypotrichosis-albinoidism**
*See OCULO-OSTEO-CUTANEOUS SYNDROME, TOUMAALA-HAAPANEN TYPE*

---

## BRACHYOLMELIA, DOMINANT TYPE     3144

**Includes:** Spondylodysplasia, dominant type

**Excludes:**
    **Brachyolmelia, Hobaek type** (3036)
    **Brachyolmelia, Maroteaux type** (3143)
    **Spondyloepimetaphyseal dysplasia** (2313)
    **Spondyloepiphyseal dysplasia**

**Major Diagnostic Criteria:** Short trunk dwarfism characterized on X-ray by generalized platyspondyly without significant epiphyseal or metaphyseal changes in the long bones.

**Clinical Findings:** Childhood onset short trunk dwarfism. Universal platyspondyly without significant changes in the epiphyses, diaphyses and metaphyses of the long bones. The vertebral changes of this type are similar to those seen in **Brachyolmelia, Maroteaux type**, but may be more severe. Most patients have scoliosis and or kyphosis. Marked cervical vetebral flattening and irregularity were noted in one family (Shohat et al, 1987). In a few cases (Brown & MacDonald, 1933; Lomas & Boyle, 1959) metaphyseal irregularities were found in the femur and humerus, which lead one team (Kozlowski et al, 1982) to conclude that pure brachyolmia does not exist and that metaphyseal involvement may be minimal and scattered but always is present.

**Complications:** Final height <150 cm. Scoliosis. Neck stability by extension/flexion films may be indicated when severe cervical vertebral flattening exist. Osteoarthritis of the large joints has been reported in a few older patients.

**Associated Findings:** Clinodactyly and hyperopia.

**Etiology:** Autosomal dominant inheritance. Reported families differ in regard to the severity of the skeletal changes as well as the existance of femoral metaphyseal irregularities, and may represent heterogenous groups within the dominantly inherited spondylodysplasias.

**Pathogenesis:** Unknown.

**MIM No.:** 11350

**POS No.:** 3679

**Sex Ratio:** M1:F1

**Occurrence:** Several families have been documented.

**Risk of Recurrence for Patient's Sib:**
See Part I, *Mendelian Inheritance.*

**Risk of Recurrence for Patient's Child:**
See Part I, *Mendelian Inheritance.*

**Age of Detectability:** Most cases were found to be short in early childhood (2–6 years of age). It is possible that X-ray changes can be detected earlier.

**Gene Mapping and Linkage:** Unknown.

**Prevention:** None known. Genetic counseling indicated.

**Treatment:** As needed to correct scoliosis.

**Prognosis:** Depends on the severity of the scoliosis.

**Detection of Carrier:** Unknown.

**Special Considerations:** This brachyolmia which is inherited autosomal dominantly may be more severe than **Brachyolmelia, Hobaek type**. Since this entity was not classified until recently, it is possible that milder cases exist but have not been diagnosed.

**References:**
Brown DO, MacDonald C: Three cases of familial osseous dystrophy. Aust New Zeal J Surg 1933; 3:78–88.
Lomas JJP, Boyle AC: Osteo-chondrodystrophy (Morquio's disease) in three generations. Lancet 1959; II:430–432.
Kozlowski K, et al: Spondylo-metaphyseal dysplasia: report of 7 cases and essays of classification. In, Papadatos, CJ & Bartsocas CS, eds: Skeletal Dysplasias. New York: Alan R. Liss, 1982:89–101.
Shohat M, et al: Brachyolimia; genetic, clinical and radiographic heterogenity. Am J Hum Genetic 1987; 41:A84.
Shohat M, et al: Brachyolmia: radiographic and genetic evidence of heterogeneity. Am J Med Genet 1989; 33:209–219. †

SH053        **Mordechai Shohat**

---

## BRACHYOLMELIA, HOBAEK TYPE     3036

**Includes:**
    Brachyolmelia, Toledo type
    Spondylodysplasia with pure brachyolmia

**Excludes:**
    **Brachyolmelia, dominant type** (3144)
    **Brachyolmelia, Maroteaux type** (3143)
    **Dyggve-Melchior-Clausen syndrome** (0306)
    **Spondylometaphyseal chondrodysplasia, Kozlowski type** (0899)

**Major Diagnostic Criteria:** Short stature of late childhood or early teen onset, X-ray abnormalities of the spine, and lack of nonskeletal anomalies.

**Clinical Findings:** This condition is limited to the skeletal system, particularly to vertebral involvement. Clinically, affected individuals manifest short stature between childhood and teen years. The shortness is mainly limited to the trunk, although limbs are also somewhat short. The diagnosis of brachyolmia is confirmed on X-ray, with platyspondyly of cervical, thoracic, and lumbar bodies a consistent finding. Additional findings include mild scoliosis, short iliac bones, and slightly short tubular bones. Dense phalangeal epiphyses were described in one patient.

**Complications:** Back stiffness and pain; hip and other joint pain also occur.

**Associated Findings:** None known.

**Etiology:** Autosomal recessive inheritance.

**Pathogenesis:** Unknown.

**MIM No.:** 27153

**POS No.:** 3679

**Sex Ratio:** Presumably M1:F1.

**Occurrence:** Fewer than a dozen cases have been documented in the literature.

**Risk of Recurrence for Patient's Sib:**
See Part I, *Mendelian Inheritance.*

**Risk of Recurrence for Patient's Child:**
See Part I, *Mendelian Inheritance.*

**Age of Detectability:** Short stature becomes evident in late childhood or early teen years; however, X-ray changes were present in one child at age 3 1/2 years, so X-ray findings may precede the onset of short stature.

**Gene Mapping and Linkage:** Unknown.

**Prevention:** None known. Genetic counseling indicated.

**Treatment:** Symptomatic.

**Prognosis:** Intellectual development is normal; life span is unlikely to be affected.

**Detection of Carrier:** Unknown.

**Special Considerations:** The term brachyolmia is Greek for "short trunk". *Brachyolmia, Toledo type*, reported in four sibs by

Toledo et al (1978), may also be the same condition; however, three of four had corneal opacities visible on slit-lamp examination. Qualitative urinary mucopolysaccharide abnormalities were also found in these sibs. However, chondroosseous morphology in patients with Hobaek type brachyolmia was identical to that in a patient with the Toledo type.

**References:**
Hobaek A: Problems of hereditary chondrodysplasia. Oslo: University Press, 1961:82–95.
Toledo SP, et al.: Recessively inherited late onset spondylar dysplasia and peripheral corneal opacity with anomalies in urinary mucopolysaccharides: a possible error of chondroitin-6-sulfate synthesis. Am J Med Genet 1978; 2:385–396.
Horton WA, et al.: Brachyolmia, recessive type (Hobaek): a clinical, radiographic, and histochemical study. Am J Med Genet 1983; 16:201–211.
Shohat M, et al.: Brachyolmia: radiographic and genetic evidence of heterogeneity. Am J Med Genet 1989; 33:209–219. * †

T0007                                            **Helga V. Toriello**

---

## BRACHYOLMELIA, MAROTEAUX TYPE                           3143

**Includes:**
 Brachyolmia, Maroteaux type
 Spondylodysplasia, Maroteaux type

**Excludes:**
 **Brachyolmelia, dominant type** (3144)
 **Brachyolmelia, Hobaek type** (3036)
 **Spondyloepimetaphyseal dysplasia** (2313)
 **Spondyloepiphyseal dysplasia**

**Major Diagnostic Criteria:**  Short trunk dwarfism characterized on X-ray by generalized platyspondyly without significant epiphyseal or metaphyseal changes in the long bones. Rounding of the anterior and posterior vertebral borders on lateral spine films differentiates this condition from **Brachyolmelia, Hobaek type**.

**Clinical Findings:**  Childhood onset short trunk dwarfism. On X-ray, universal platyspondyly, irregular and reduced intervertebral spaces, and marked extension of the lateral margins of the vertebrae. Characteristically, rounding of the anterior and posterior vertebral borders is seen on the lateral aspect of the spine. No significant metaphyseal, diaphyseal, or epiphyseal changes in the long bones exist.

**Complications:**  Final height between 125 and 156 cm. Scoliosis.

**Associated Findings:**  A few cases have shown precocious calcification of falx cerebri. Short, stubby fingers and hyperlaxity of joints have also been reported, along with a few reports of slightly dysmorphic features, with flat nose and thick lips.

**Etiology:**  Presumably autosomal recessive inheritance.

**Pathogenesis:**  Unknown.

**POS No.:**  3679

**Sex Ratio:**  M1:F1

**Occurrence:**  Six families have been documented.

**Risk of Recurrence for Patient's Sib:**
 See Part I, *Mendelian Inheritance*.

**Risk of Recurrence for Patient's Child:**
 See Part I, *Mendelian Inheritance*.

**Age of Detectability:**  Early childhood (ages 2–6 years).

**Gene Mapping and Linkage:**  Unknown.

**Prevention:**  None known. Genetic counseling indicated.

**Treatment:**  As needed to correct scoliosis.

**Prognosis:**  Good. Final height between 125 and 156 cm. Normal life span.

**Detection of Carrier:**  Unknown.

**Special Considerations:**  The term *brachyolmia* was originally proposed to describe the short trunk of these patients. Since clinically

there is also shortening of the extremities, it is suggested that the term *spondylodysplasia* be used.

**References:**
Fontaine G, et al.: La dysplasie spondyloaire pure oun brachyolmie. Arch Fr Pediatr 1975; 32:695–708.
Shohat M, et al.: Brachyolmia-genetic, clinical and radiographic heterogeneity. Am J Hum Genet 1987; 41:A84.
Shohat M, et al.: Brachyolmia: radiographic and genetic evidence of heterogeneity. Am J Med Genet 1989; 33:209–219. †

SH053                                            **Mordechai Shohat**

**Brachyolmia, Maroteaux type**
 *See BRACHYOLMELIA, MAROTEAUX TYPE*
**Brachyolmia, Toledo type**
 *See BRACHYOLMELIA, HOBAEK TYPE*
**Brachytelephalangy-peripheral pulmonary stenoses-deafness**
 *See KEUTEL SYNDROME*
**Brailsford syndrome**
 *See MUCOPOLYSACCHARIDOSIS IV*
**Brain (fetal) disruption sequence**
 *See FETAL BRAIN DISRUPTION SEQUENCE*
**Brain anomalies-frontal bone protuberance**
 *See CRANIOTELENCEPHALIC DYSPLASIA*
**Brain tumor, neuroepithelial and meningeal**
 *See CANCER, NEUROEPITHELIAL AND MENINGEAL*
**Brain tumor-adenomatous polyposis syndrome**
 *See TURCOT SYNDROME*

---

## BRAIN, ARACHNOID CYSTS                           3002

**Includes:**
 Agenesis of the temporal lobe
 Temporal lobe, agenesis

**Excludes:**
 **Brain, midline caves** (3000)
 Choroid plexus cyst
 Dandy-Walker cyst

**Major Diagnostic Criteria:**  Demonstration by CT or MRI scan of a fluid filled cyst in the subarachnoid space, confined to the surface of the central nervous system. The cyst does not communicate with the ventricles.

**Clinical Findings:**  Small subarachnoid cysts are often found incidentally when the patient's head is scanned for some unrelated neurologic problem. Such cysts may remain asymptomatic throughout the patient's life. Some arachnoid cysts will increase in size, either in infancy or childhood or even in adulthood. The patient then presents with symptoms and signs of increased pressure plus signs of compression of neighboring neural tissue. Some subarachnoid cysts may fill half or more of the intracranial space. Since the cysts may occur at any site within the craniovertebral space, the accompanying neurologic signs will depend on the location of the cyst.

**Complications:**  Enlarging cysts compress the adjacent neural tissue and cause increased intracranial pressure. Cysts in the Sylvian fissure may compress the temporal lobe, a condition erroneously called temporal lobe agenesis. Free blood vessels may cross the lumen of the cyst and may rupture after head trauma. Posterior fossa arachnoid cysts are difficult to distinguish from a large cisterna magna cerebelli.

**Associated Findings:**  None known. Intra- or extracranial lesions are not usually found.

**Etiology:**  Unknown.

**Pathogenesis:**  Arachnoid cysts are thought to represent a cleft in the arachnoid. They may arise as a developmental disturbance in the splitting of the primitive mesenchyme which surrounds the CNS and produces its meninges, or possibly in response to an intrauterine inflammatory process of the meninges.

**CDC No.:**  742.420

**Sex Ratio:**  M1:F1

**Occurrence:** Undetermined but not uncommon; no geographic or racial predominance.

**Risk of Recurrence for Patient's Sib:** Minimal if any increase.

**Risk of Recurrence for Patient's Child:** Not increased.

**Age of Detectability:** From birth to senility.

**Gene Mapping and Linkage:** Unknown.

**Prevention:** None known. Genetic counseling indicated.

**Treatment:** Surgical drainage, removal, or shunting if the lesion is considered symptomatic. Small, asymptomatic cysts require no treatment.

**Prognosis:** Cysts may remain static or asymptomatic throughout life, but can enlarge at any age, or bleed.

**Detection of Carrier:** Unknown.

**References:**

Menezes AH, et al: Arachnoid cysts in children. Arch Neurol 1980; 37:168–172.

Varma TRK, et al: Post-traumatic complications of arachnoid cysts and temporal lobe agenesis. J Neurol Neurosurg Psychiatr 1981; 44:29–34.

Braakman R, et al: Arachnoidal cysts in the middle cranial fossa: cause and treatment of progressive and non-progressive symptoms. J Neurol Neurosurg Psychiatr 1983; 46:1102–1106.

DeMyer W: Arachnoid and porencephalic cysts. In: Johnson RT, ed: Current Therapy in Neurologic Disease. Philadelphia: B.C. Decker, 1985; 98:101.

DE007                                                **William DeMyer**

## BRAIN, ARNOLD-CHIARI MALFORMATION                    2944

**Includes:**

   Anencephaly-spina bifida
   Arnold-Chiari malformation
   Spina bifida-anencephaly

**Excludes:** Dandy-Walker malformation

**Major Diagnostic Criteria:** Caudal displacement of the brainstem and cerebellum through the foramen magnum into the upper cervical areas with or without associated **Meningomyelocele**.

**Clinical Findings:** *Type I:* Tongue-like lowered inferior pole of the cerebellum. The tonsils are lowered but the fourth ventricle is entirely in the posterior fossa. *Type II:* Short neck, epilepsy, possible **Hydrocephaly** and possible **Meningomyelocele**. The fourth ventricle is also lowered and communicates directly with the ependymal canal. Supratentorial **Hydrocephaly**. Eventual lumbar spina bifida (see **Meningocele**). *Type III:* **Hydrocephaly** with spina bifida, cervical or lumbar **Meningomyelocele**, severe neurologic deficits, and epilepsy. An important part of the cerebellum and brainstem are located in the enlarged cervical canal. Cervical or lumbar meningomyelocele. Associated malformations of the bones and nervous system.

**Complications:** Infections, compressions.

**Associated Findings:** Basilar invagination, Lüeckenschäedel, obstructed foramen of Magendie, syringomyelia, diastematomyelia.

**Etiology:** A sporadic malformation. Various teratogenic agents have been postulated. Lindenberg and Walker (1971) described a family with two affected sisters.

**Pathogenesis:** Possibly a dissociation between the development of the craniodural posterior fossa container with regard to the nervous structures and too rapid growth.

**MIM No.:** 20795

**CDC No.:** 742.480

**Sex Ratio:** Presumably M1:F1.

**Occurrence:** Undetermined but presumed rare. No geographic or racial predominance has been identified.

**Risk of Recurrence for Patient's Sib:** Unknown.

**Risk of Recurrence for Patient's Child:** Unknown.

**Age of Detectability:** At birth for severe cases or cases with **Meningomyelocele**. Type I is often undetected.

**Gene Mapping and Linkage:** Unknown.

**Prevention:** None known. Genetic counseling indicated.

**Treatment:** Neurosurgical as needed.

**Prognosis:** Type I is tolerated well. Types II and III are associated with life spans related to infection and the results of surgical treatment.

**Detection of Carrier:** Possibly by computed tomography scanning and nuclear magnetic resonance imaging.

**References:**

Chiari H: Uber Veräenderungen des Kleinhirns, des Pons und der Medulla oblongata in Folge von congenitaler Hydrocephalie des Grosshirns. Dtsch Med Wochenschr 1891; 27:1172–1175.

Arnold J: Myelocyste, Transposition von Gewebskeimen und Sympodie. Beitr Pathol Anat 1894; 16:1–28.

Chiari H: Uber Veränderungen des Kleinhirns, des Pons und der Medulla oblongata in Folge von congenitaler Hydrocephalie des Grosshirns. Dtsch Akad Wiss Wien 1895; 63:71–116.

Lindenberg R, Walker BA: Arnold-Chiari malformation. BD:OAS VII(1). New York: March of Dimes Birth Defects Foundation, 1971:234–236.

Naidich TP, et al.: The Chiari II malformation: part IV. The hindbrain deformity. Neuroradiology 1983; 25:179–197.

WA050                                                **A. Wackenheim**

**Brain, glioma of**
   *See CANCER, GLIOMA, FAMILIAL*
**Brain, lobar atrophy of**
   *See PICK DISEASE OF THE BRAIN*

## BRAIN, MICROPOLYGYRIA                                2999

**Includes:**

   Microgyria
   Micropolygyria
   Polymicrogyria

**Excludes:**

   Brain warts
   **Muscular dystrophy, congenital with mental retardation** (2705)
   Nodular cortical dysplasia
   Pachygyria
   Status verrucosus
   Stenogyria
   Ulegyria

**Major Diagnostic Criteria:** Spastic **Cerebral palsy** (quadriplegia or hemiplegia), mental retardation, **Microcephaly**, and seizures.

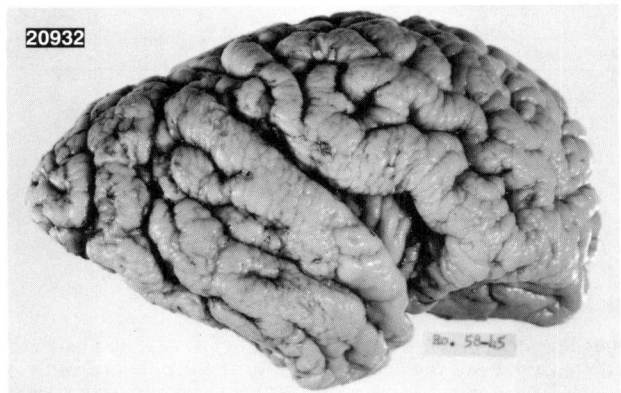

**2999-20932:** Lateral view of the right cerebral hemisphere; polymicrogyria affects the entire cerebral cortex.

**Clinical Findings:** Vary depending on the extent and localization of the lesions. Small lesions are an occasional, incidental finding at autopsy. Most patients are born with **Microcephaly** and spastic. Quadriplegia is the most common motor deficit; hemiplegia is much less frequent. Generalized seizures and mental retardation are almost invariably present. Chorioretinitis is observed in 15% of cases. Less frequent findings include blindness, deafness, ophthalmoplegia, nystagmus, and microphthalmia.

**Complications:** Deformities due to motor deficits (hypotrophy of extremities, scoliosis, kyphosis, talipes calcaneovalgus, **Foot, talipes equinovarus (TEV)**, and **Arthrogryposes.**

**Associated Findings:** **Muscular dystrophy, congenital with mental retardation.**

**Etiology:** Thought to be related to a damaging event occurring about the fifth to sixth month of fetal life.

**Pathogenesis:** Possibly a disturbance of neuronal migration. Nevertheless, most investigators favor the concept that the malformation results from a "hypoxic" event with selective destruction of the medial cortical layers. A few cases have been reported that were associated with intrauterine infection with toxoplasma or cytomegalovirus.

**CDC No.:** 742.280

**Sex Ratio:** M1:F1

**Occurrence:** Undetermined but presumed rare.

**Risk of Recurrence for Patient's Sib:** Unknown.

**Risk of Recurrence for Patient's Child:** Unknown.

**Age of Detectability:** Varies with extent and localization of the lesions.

**Gene Mapping and Linkage:** Unknown.

**Prevention:** None known. Genetic counseling indicated.

**Treatment:** Physical therapy to avoid deformities. Treatment of epilepsy.

**Prognosis:** Patients who survive their first year of life have markedly retarded psychomotor development.

**Detection of Carrier:** Unknown.

**References:**
Crome L: Microgyria. J Pathol Bacteriol 1952; 64:479–495.
Crome L, France NE: Microgyria and cytomegalic inclusion disease in infancy. J Clin Pathol 1959; 12:427–434.
DeLeon GA: Observations on cerebral and cerebellar microgyria. Acta Neuropathol 1972; 20:278–287.
Richman DP, Stewart RM: Cerebral microgyria in a 27-week fetus: an architectonic and topographic analysis. J Neuropathol Exp Neurol 1974; 33:374–384.
Larroche JC: Cytoarchitectonic abnormalities (abnormalities of cell migration). In: Vinken PJ, Bruyn, eds: Congenital malformations of the brain and skull, Vol 30, Part I. New York: Elsevier/North-Holland Biomedical, 1977:479–485.

AZ001                                                       **Biagio Azzarelli**

## BRAIN, MIDLINE CAVES                                      3000

**Includes:**
   Cavum septi pellucidi
   Cavum velli interpositi
   Cavum vergae
   Cyst of septum pellucidum
   Dorsal cyst or sac
   Suprapineal recess

**Excludes:**
   **Brain, arachnoid cysts** (3002)
   Choroid plexus cysts

**Major Diagnostic Criteria:** CT or MRI scans readily visualize the midline cavities of the brain related to the fornix and ventricular system. These cavities are normally present but vary greatly in size, resembling in this respect the cisterna magna cerebelli.

The cavum septi pellucidi is between the two layers of the septum pellucidum, which stretches between the undersurface of the corpus callosum and the anterior pillars of the fornix. The cavum Vergae is simply a posterior extension of the cavum septi pellucidi, separating the midportion of the fornix from the undersurface of the corpus callosum.

The cavum velli interpositi is between the roof of the third ventricle and the undersurface of the fornix and hippocampal commissure. It is part of the subarachnoid space and communicates with the cistern of the vein of Galen and the quadrigeminal and ambient cisterns.

A suprapineal recess occurs in normal individuals when the roof of the third ventricle balloons upward and backward between the pineal body and the splenium of the corpus callosum. This sac contains ventricular fluid, and its ostium generally communicates with the third ventricle.

**Clinical Findings:** Since these caves and the suprapineal recess are normal spaces, they do not of themselves produce symptoms, but alterations in their size or contour may reflect other brain lesions. The cavum septi pellucidi is almost always present at birth, but undergoes obliteration in the first several months. Its persistence is sometimes spoken of as a cyst of the septum pellucidum, but by itself it is asymptomatic. A large cavum septi pellucidi and cavum Vergae are associated with mental retardation and **Megalencephaly.** The cavum septi pellucidi is completely absent in opticoseptal dysplasia. The leaves of the septum pellucidum may rupture as a result of trauma, resulting in fenestration, which may also occur as a congenital malformation.

The cavum veli interpositi is absent in agenesis of the corpus callosum, since the backward growth of the corpus callosum over the third ventricle and thalamus forms its roof. The roof of the third ventricle is the floor of the cavum velli interpositi. In atrophic brains the cavum is enlarged. Its space may be encroached on by a dorsal sac, an aneurysm of the vein of Galen, or by pinealomas or teratomas.

In some individuals, the suprapineal recess extends as a dorsal sac, often erroneously called a cyst, into the interhemispheric fissure, where it acts as a mass lesion. In patients lacking a corpus callosum, the third ventricular roof is always elevated to some degree, and in some the roof extends as a dorsal sac toward and sometimes reaching the vertex or posterior circumference of the calvarium.

**Complications:** Unknown.

**Associated Findings:** None known.

**Etiology:** Unknown.

**Pathogenesis:** Unknown.

**CDC No.:** 742.280

**Sex Ratio:** M1:F1

**Occurrence:** Undetermined. A cavum septi pellucidi remains in a small percentage of mature normal brains. Absence of the septum pellucidum occurs rarely.

**Risk of Recurrence for Patient's Sib:** Presumably not increased.

**Risk of Recurrence for Patient's Child:** Presumably not increased.

**Age of Detectability:** At any age.

**Gene Mapping and Linkage:** Unknown.

**Prevention:** None known. Genetic counseling indicated.

**Treatment:** Unknown.

**Prognosis:** Unknown.

**Detection of Carrier:** Unknown.

**References:**
Larroche JC, et al: Cavum septi lucidi, cavum Vergae, Cavum veli interpositi: Cavites de la lignemediane. Biol Neonat 1961; 3:193–236.
Bergleiter R, et al: Das Cavum septi pellucidi und Cavum Vergae in Klinik und Röntgenbild. Fortschritte der Neurologie Psychiatrie und Ihrer Grenzgebiete 1964; 32:361–399.
Miller ME, et al: Cavum Vergae. Arch Neurol 1986; 43:821–823.

DE007                                                       **William DeMyer**

## BRAIN, PORENCEPHALY                                                 2998

**Includes:**
    Hemiplegia, infantile-porencephaly
    Porencephaly, prenatal

**Excludes:**
    **Brain, arachnoid cysts** (3002)
    **Brain, midline caves** (3000)
    **Brain, schizencephaly** (3001)
    Central porencephaly
    Cystic degeneration of the brain
    Encephaloclastic porencephaly
    False porencephaly
    **Hydranencephaly** (0480)
    Internal porencephaly
    Multiocular cystic encephalopathy
    Polyporencephaly
    Porencephaly, "mark" or medullary
    Pseudoporencephaly

**Major Diagnostic Criteria:** Porencephaly (cystic structures or cavitations within the brain) is a major malformation of the brain. The association of mental retardation, spastic paralysis, ophthalmoplegia, and epilepsy suggest the diagnosis. Porus can be demonstrated by pneumoencephalogram or CT scan.

**Clinical Findings:** In a series of 22 cases described by Gross and Simanyi (1977), moderate to severe mental retardation was present in almost all cases. In addition, there was spastic tetraplegia in 95.4%, paresis of cranial nerves (ophthalmoplegia) in 68.2%, dysphagia in 18.2%, nystagmus in 18.2%, optic atrophy in 22%, and facial paralysis in 9.1%. Development of speech is absent or poor. Epilepsy is common. Porencephaly is readily recognizable on CT examination.

**Complications:** **Hydrocephaly**, epileptic seizures, spastic contractures, and mental retardation.

**Associated Findings:** Often seen with congenital heart malformations.

**Etiology:** Unknown. A familial form has been described but is apparently rare.

**Pathogenesis:** Speculative interpretations are that porencephaly 1) is a primary malformation due to focal agenesis of the cerebral wall, 2) results from encephaloclastic process in early gestational period due to an infectious process or circulatory disturbance, and 3) is caused by anoxia.

    The prenatal origin of the process is suggested by the radial arrangement of the marginal gyri and more convincingly by the presence in many cases of micropolygyria around the porus. In the majority of cases it seems reasonable to ascribe both the porus and micropolygyria to the action of a single pathologic process occurring about the fourth or fifth fetal month.

**MIM No.:** 17578

**CDC No.:** 742.410

**Sex Ratio:** M1:F1

**Occurrence:** About 50 cases have been documented, of which some 15 cases in at least four families appear to reflect an autosomal dominant form of inheritance.

**Risk of Recurrence for Patient's Sib:** Unknown.

**Risk of Recurrence for Patient's Child:** Unknown.

**Age of Detectability:** When symptomatic, any age from birth on.

**Gene Mapping and Linkage:** Unknown.

**Prevention:** None known. Genetic counseling indicated.

**Treatment:** Physical therapy, treatment of seizure disorder, and shunt procedures in cases complicated by **Hydrocephaly**.

**Prognosis:** Depends on the site and extent of the lesion. Many patients are institutionalized. Others die before the second decade of life. In a few reported cases patients survived up to the sixth decade with minimal or no neurologic improvement.

**Detection of Carrier:** By CT scan in familial cases.

**References:**
Dekaban A: Large defects in cerebral hemisphere associated with cortical dysgenesis. J Neuropathol Exp Neurol 1965; 24:512–530.
Gross H, Simanyi: Porencephaly. In: Handbook of clinical neurology, Vol 30. New York: Elsevier/North-Holland, 1977:27:681–692.
Ramsey RG, Huckman MS: Computed tomography of porencephaly and other cerebrospinal fluid containing lesions. Radiology 1977; 123:73–77.
Berg RA, et al.: Familial porencephaly. Arch Neurol 1983; 44:567–569.
Zonana J, et al.: Familial porencephaly and congenital hemipgia. J Pediatr 1986; 109:671–674.

AZ001                                                    **Biagio Azzarelli**

**2998-20929:** Brain, porencephaly; external aspect of right cerebral hemisphere. Large cortical defect which communicates with the lateral ventricle (porus).

## BRAIN, SCHIZENCEPHALY                                              3001

**Includes:** Cerebral clefts symmetrical

**Excludes:**
    **Brain, porencephaly** (2998)
    **Lissencephaly syndrome** (0603)

**Major Diagnostic Criteria:** The cerebrum shows bilaterally symmetric clefts, which follow the line of a major sulcus, usually the central sulcus. A thick, richly cellular cortex persists in the cleft wall. The marginal layers of the cortex covering the lips of the cleft fuse into a solid cellular seam, and the seam retains continuity with the subependymal cell plate around the ventricle or with the striatum. A second type of schizencephaly, with the lips of the cleft separated, is also recognized.

**Clinical Findings:** The patients have varying degrees of **Microcephaly**, mental retardation, and hemiparesis or quadriparesis, but many are hypotonic. Most have seizures.

**Complications:** Some patients have **Hydrocephaly** which may require shunting.

**Associated Findings:** None known. Extracephalic malformations do not usually occur.

**Etiology:** Unknown.

**Pathogenesis:** Whether schizencephaly exists as a separate entity from **Brain, porencephaly** is uncertain. Yakovlev et al (1946) initially separated it as a malformation in contradistinction to the encephaloclastic porencephalies, which they regarded as destructive in origin.

**CDC No.:** 742.280

**Sex Ratio:** M1:F<1

**Occurrence:** Undetermined but presumed rare.

**Risk of Recurrence for Patient's Sib:** Unknown.

**Risk of Recurrence for Patient's Child:** Unknown.

**Age of Detectability:** At birth.

**Gene Mapping and Linkage:** Unknown.

**Prevention:** None known. Genetic counseling indicated.

**Treatment:** Unknown.

**Prognosis:** Depends on the degree of neurologic deficit.

**Detection of Carrier:** Unknown.

**Special Considerations:** Neuropathologists differ in separating schizencephaly from **Brain, porencephaly**. Schizencephaly may represent a form or degree of the latter rather than a disease sui generis. Patients with **Lissencephaly syndrome** often demonstrate bilateral clefts in the midportion of the hemispheres, approximately along the line of the central sulcus. Although some authors describe these patients as having schizencephaly, the cleft may represent an upper extension of the Sylvian fissure rather than the central sulcus. A pathogenetic relation between the schizencephaly of Yakovlev et al (1946) and lissencephaly is not established.

**References:**
Yakovlev PI, et al: Schizencephalies: a study of the congenital clefts in the cerebral mantle. J Neuropath Exp Neurol 1946; 5:116–130.
Zimmerman RA, et al: Computed tomography in migratory disorders of human brain development. Neuroradiology 1983; 25:257–263.
Miller GM, et al: Schizencephaly: a clinical and CT study. Neurology 1984; 34:997–1001.

DE007                                                    **William DeMyer**

---

## BRAIN, SPONGY DEGENERATION                          0115

**Includes:**
Bertrand spongy degeneration of the CNS
Canavan disease
Van Bogaert spongy degeneration of the CNS

**Excludes:**
**Adrenoleukodystrophy, X-linked** (2533)
**Alexander disease** (2712)
Amino acid metabolism, inborn errors of
Creutzfeldt-Jacob disease
**G(m1)-gangliosidosis, type 1** (0431)
**G(m2)-gangliosidosis with hexosaminidase A deficiency** (0434)
**Leukodystrophy, globoid cell type** (0415)
**Metachromatic leukodystrophies** (0651)
**Phytanic acid oxidase deficiency, infantile type** (2278)

**Major Diagnostic Criteria:** Normal development in the first few weeks of life followed by onset of apathy, sluggishness, megalencephaly, spasticity, optic atrophy and blindness. Pathologically there is widespread vacuolation in the brain, characteristically involving the deeper layers of the cortex and the subcortical white matter. It is not so much the presence but rather the topography of the vacuolation which is characteristic. There are no diagnostic laboratory tests short of examination of brain tissue.

**Clinical Findings:** Most commonly the infant is the product of a normal pregnancy and delivery, feeds well, thrives and achieves normal developmental milestones in the first few weeks of life. In the majority of patients, the onset of the disease is between two and six months of age. There are rare instances of the clinical onset of the disease in the neonatal period or after the age of five years.

Loss of head control, reduced motor activity, deterioration in alertness and a decrease in appetite are the earliest features of the disease, becoming apparent in the second and third months of life. Generalized hypotonia is considered to be an important early feature but some patients may never develop hypotonia and be spastic from onset. Hypotonia is invariably followed by spasticity manifested by abnormal posturing of extremities, hyperreflexia,

clonus and Babinski's sign. Ultimately they develop pseudobulbar palsy and decerebrate and decorticate posturing.

Bilateral optic atrophy is evident at two months and is associated with attenuation of retinal vessels.

Pigmentary retinal degeneration and cherry-red spot as seen in the lipid storage diseases are not a feature of this disease. Marked visual impairment and blindness associated with roving eye movements and nystagmus are important components of this disease. Strabismus has also been described in some cases. Pupillary light reflex is sluggish.

Enlargement of the head is frequent, gradual, symmetric and becomes evident between four and six months of life. It is associated with a delay in closure of the anterior fontanel. The head circumference crosses percentiles on the head circumference chart and the head is enlarged relative to body size but does not reach extreme proportions. The enlargement is due to increased size of the brain.

Autonomic dysfunction is associated with the onset of spasticity and characterized by marked thirst, abnormal diuresis, constipation, pallor, episodic sweating, temperature instability and occasionally projectile vomiting. These disturbances have a grave prognosis and may be signs of impending coma and death.

Seizures occur in about half the patients and may be partial or generalized tonic clonic in type. Recognition of seizures may be difficult because these patients also are prone to excessive startle response and choreoathetoid movements.

Clinical findings in 26 cases (Buchanan & Davis, 1965): Onset before ten months (26/26); eventual spasticity (22/26); visual impairment (22/26); initial hypotonia (17/26); Jewish extraction (14/26); optic disc pallor (13/26); seizures (9/26); involuntary movements (8/26).

The juvenile-onset spongy degeneration is characterized by cerebellar signs, mental deterioration, optic atrophy, visual loss, spasticity and a protracted course. Megalencephaly has not been observed. In addition to the typical spongy changes, neuroaxonal dystrophy is also seen mainly in the pallido-nigral system.

Laboratory investigations do not reveal any distinct abnormalities. Blood counts, chemistries and urinalysis are normal. Cerebrospinal-fluid (CSF) examination is almost always normal with occasional reports of slight increase in the protein concentration. EEG has been diffusely abnormal in those cases in whom it was obtained. Urine amino acid chromatography is normal. Brain computerized tomography shows *diffuse* low attenuation of the white matter in contrast to Alexander's disease in which the *frontal regions* of the cerebral hemispheres show more prominent low attenuation of white matter and Adrenoleukodystrophy in which white matter in the *occipital lobes* seems to be preferentially affected.

**Complications:** Aspiration pneumonia, failure to thrive, hyperpyrexia, hypothermia, pressure sores and contractures are possible complications. None of these complications is peculiar to spongy degeneration of the brain.

**Associated Findings:** In one study it was noted that affected children, all of Jewish extraction of eastern European origin, had fair complexion, blond or red hair and commonly blue eyes. Dark hair or dark complexion were the dominant characteristics in the non-affected members of their families.

**Etiology:** Autosomal recessive inheritance.

**Pathogenesis:** Matalone et al (1988) reported two patients with Canavan disease who had aspartoacylase deficiency in skin fibroblasts and N-acetylaspartic aciduria. Synthesis of N-acetylaspartic acid is not known to occur elsewhere than the CNS. Abnormal metabolism of N-acetylaspartic acid in the brain may cause abnormalities of myelin formation or myelin breakdown, or a defect in hydrolysis may affect neurotransmitter balance. In other cases, electron microscopic studies indicate accumulation of excess fluid within the astrocytic cytoplasm and myelin lamellae. In the first reported cases, it was postulated that the spongy change was a result of excessive absorption of fluid causing chronic edema which in turn interfered with myelination or caused demyelination in previously myelinated areas. Excessive absorption of fluid was thought to be secondary to abnormal permeability of blood-brain barrier. Other studies have considered arrest of myelination in fetal life, breakdown of myelin with accumulation of low-molecular-weight products and subsequent absorption of fluid by osmotic gradient and abnormality of sodium- and potassium-activated ATPase and cytochrome oxidase in cerebral tissue. At least one study has raised the question that the spongy changes are an artifact resulting from postmortem glycogenolysis with release of $CO_2$. Ultrastructural and histochemical studies are suggestive of a metabolic disturbance in the abnormal astrocytic mitochondria.

**MIM No.:** *27190

**Sex Ratio:** M1:F1

**Occurrence:** As of 1973, there were 94 cases of spongy degeneration reported in the literature, 72 of which were verified by histologic examination. Although original reports indicated that the disease occurred in children of Jewish extraction of eastern European origin, subsequently it has been reported in a variety of ethnic groups including Irish, Italian, Chinese and Iranian.

**Risk of Recurrence for Patient's Sib:**
See Part I, *Mendelian Inheritance.*

**Risk of Recurrence for Patient's Child:**
See Part I, *Mendelian Inheritance.*

**Age of Detectability:** Second and third month of life.

**Gene Mapping and Linkage:** Unknown.

**Prevention:** None known. Genetic counseling indicated.

**Treatment:** Care to prevent malnutrition, contractures, pressure sores and aspiration pneumonia may increase comfort and prolong life. Anti-seizure medications may be required.

**Prognosis:** Clinical course is progressively downhill with wide variations in survival time, ranging from a few days to as long as seven and half years in the infantile type. Average life expectancy from onset of the disease in this type is nineteen months. Juvenile-onset disease has a much more protracted course and a patient has been reported to live for fifteen and a half years from the onset of his disease at age five years.

**Detection of Carrier:** Unknown.

**Special Considerations:** The eponym Canavan's disease is considered by many to be unjustified because this author did not seem to appreciate that the spongy degeneration in her patient was a unique pathologic alteration and one which distinguished her patient from that described by Schilder. Pathologically there is increase in size and weight of the brain in most cases. White matter appears soft, gelatinous and retracts from the cut surface. Microscopically, in addition to the characteristic vacuolation alluded to earlier, there is widespread disintegration of white matter both in the areas of spongy change and elsewhere. Despite the severe degree of myelin loss there is conspicous absence of myelin breakdown products. Oligodendroglia are preserved and there is an increase in the size and numbere of protoplasmic astrocytes.

**References:**
Banker BQ, et al.: Spongy degeneration of the CNS in infancy. Neurology 1964; 14:981–1001.
Buchanan DS, Davis RL: Spongy degeneration of the nervous system. Neurology 1965; 15:207–222.
Jellinger K, Seitelberger F: Juvenile form of spongy degeneration of the CNS. Acta Neuropath 1969; 13:276–281.
Van Bogaert: Spongy degeneration of the brain. In: Handbook of Neurology North Holland Publishing Company 1970; 10:203–211.
Adachi M, et al.: Spongy degeneration of the CNS. Human Pathology 1973; 4:331–347.
Rushton AR, et al.: Computed Tomography in the Diagnosis of Canavan's disease. Ann Neurol 1981; 10:57–60.
Matalon R, et al.: Aspartoacylase deficiency and N-acetylaspartic aciduria in patients with Canavan disease. Am J Med Genet 1988; 29:463–471.

**I. Hussain Bangash**
**Raymond S. Kandt**

**Brain-bone-fat disease**
See OSTEODYSPLASIA, LIPOMEMBRANOUS POLYCYSTIC-DEMENTIA
**Brain-muscle-eye syndrome**
See MUSCLE-EYE-BRAIN SYNDROME
**Bran ear wax**
See EAR, CERUMEN VARIATIONS
**Branched-chain alpha-keto acid dehydrogenase deficiency**
See MAPLE SYRUP URINE DISEASE
**Branched-chain ketoaciduria**
See MAPLE SYRUP URINE DISEASE
**Branched-chain ketonuria**
See MAPLE SYRUP URINE DISEASE
**Brancher deficiency**
See GLYCOGENOSIS, TYPE IV

## BRANCHIAL ARCH SYNDROME, X-LINKED      2825

**Includes:** Microcephaly-brachial arch, X-linked

**Excludes:**
    Branchio-oto-renal dysplasia (2224)
    Branchio-skeleto-genital syndrome (0118)
    Mandibulofacial dysostosis (0627)
    Noonan syndrome (0720)

**Major Diagnostic Criteria:** The combination of **Microcephaly**, branchial arch defects, and short stature in a male.

**Clinical Findings:** Of three known affected boys, **Microcephaly**, sparse lateral eyebrows, epicanthal folds, downslanting palpebral fissures, malar hypoplasia, high-arched palate, micrognathia, apparently low-set ears, protruding ears, slight neck webbing, short stature, and mixed-type hearing loss were present in all three. Additional findings include ptosis (1/3), preauricular pit (1/3), subvalvar pulmonic stenosis (1/3), cryptorchidism (2/3), and asymmetry (1/3). Mild developmental delay or learning disability was also present.

**Complications:** Unknown.

**Associated Findings:** None known.

**Etiology:** Presumably X-linked inheritance based on the presence of the condition in two male sibs and their maternal cousin.

**Pathogenesis:** The basic genetic defect is unknown, although abnormal neural crest cell migration is likely a pleiotropic effect of the mutant gene.

**MIM No.:** 30195

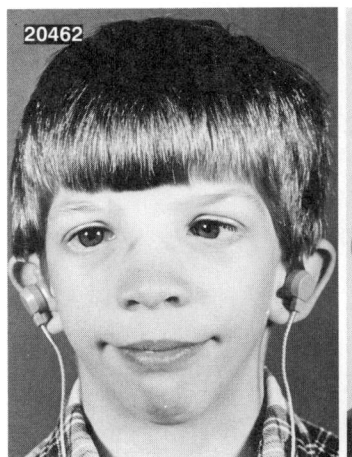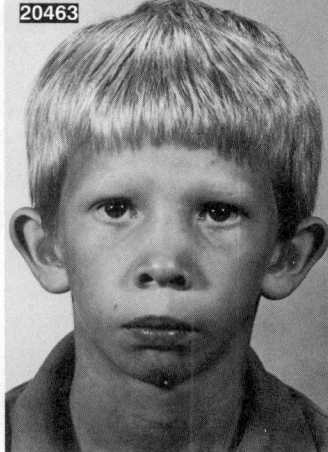

2825-20462: Micrognathia, malar hypoplasia, downward slanting palpebral fissures, low-set ears and hearing loss. 20463: Sparse eyebrows, malar hypoplasia, and micrognathia.

**POS No.:** 3623

**Sex Ratio:** M3:F0 (observed).

**Occurrence:** Two brothers and a cousin from Michigan have been documented.

**Risk of Recurrence for Patient's Sib:**
See Part I, *Mendelian Inheritance.*

**Risk of Recurrence for Patient's Child:**
See Part I, *Mendelian Inheritance.*

**Age of Detectability:** At birth by physical examination.

**Gene Mapping and Linkage:** Unknown.

**Prevention:** None known. Genetic counseling indicated.

**Treatment:** Hearing aids are indicated for the hearing defect.

**Prognosis:** Mild developmental delay or learning disability was present in all three boys; life span is presumably normal.

**Detection of Carrier:** Carrier females may exhibit partial expression of the defect, although this was not observed in the reported family.

**Special Considerations:** A mother and son with deafness, malformed ears, mental retardation and "peculiar facies" described by Kawashima & Tsuji (1987) may have the same condition.

**References:**
Toriello HV, et al.: X-linked syndrome of branchial arch and other defects. Am J Med Genet 1985; 21:137–142. †
Kawashima H, Ksuji N: Syndrome of microcephaly, deafness, malformed ears, mental retardation and peculiar facies in a mother and son. Clin Genet 1987; 31:303–307.

T0007 **Helga V. Toriello**

**Branchial arch-premature aging syndrome**
*See BRANCHIO-OCULO-FACIAL SYNDROME*

## BRANCHIAL CLEFT CYSTS 2723

**Includes:**
Branchial cleft cysts type I
Branchial cleft cysts type II
Parotid gland, swelling of
Salivary gland, branchial cleft cysts

**Excludes:**
Cysts of parotid gland, acquired
**Salivary gland, dermoid cyst** (2724)
**Salivary gland, ductal cyst** (2725)

**Major Diagnostic Criteria:** Painless unilateral swelling of the parotid gland. Bilateral swelling is rare.

**Clinical Findings:** Classified by Work into Type I and Type II:
*Type I:* is located within the periauricular soft tissue and parotid gland. Presents as sinus tract or localized swelling near the postauricular sulcus, concha, or anterior to the tragus. Rarely involves the tympanic membrane or middle ear.
*Type II:* may form an anomalous external auditory canal and rudimentary pinna. Presents in upper neck with possible extension to middle ear or tympanic cavity.

**Complications:** Type I may result in abscess formation which may make diagnosis difficult.
Type II may be complicated by infection with abscess formation.

**Associated Findings:** None known.

**Etiology:** Unknown.

**Pathogenesis:** *Type I:* Duplication anomaly of the external auditory canal (membranous and bony), which histologically contains squamous epithelium without skin appendages.
*Type II:* Duplication anomaly forming an anomalous external auditory canal and pinna. Formed of two germinal layers; ectoderm and mesoderm.

**CDC No.:** 744.400

**Sex Ratio:** Undetermined but presumably M1:F1.

**Occurrence:** Undetermined. Type I occurs more frequently than Type II.

**Risk of Recurrence for Patient's Sib:** Unknown.

**Risk of Recurrence for Patient's Child:** Unknown.

**Age of Detectability:** Variable.

**Gene Mapping and Linkage:** Unknown.

**Prevention:** None known. Genetic counseling indicated.

**Treatment:** For both *Type I and II* complete surgical excision with preservation of the facial nerve. *Type II* may have scar tissue in close proximity to the facial nerve; therefore, identification of the facial nerve during dissection is essential.

**Prognosis:** Good for life span, intelligence, and function. Otherwise dependent on concomitant defects.

**Detection of Carrier:** Unknown.

**References:**
Batsakis JG, Regezi JA: Selected controversial lesions of salivary tissues. Otolaryngol Clin North Am 1977; 10:309–328.
Work WP: Cysts and congenital lesions of the parotid glands. Otolaryngol Clin North Am 1977; 10:339–344.
Work WP: Non-neoplastic disorders of the parotid gland. J Otolaryngol 1981; 10:35–40.
Sucupira MS, et al.: Salivary gland imaging and radionuclide dacryocystography in agenesis of salivary glands. Arch Otolaryngol 1983; 109:197–198.

MY003 **Charles M. Myer III**
OR005 **Peter Orobello**

**Branchial cleft cysts type I**
*See BRANCHIAL CLEFT CYSTS*
**Branchial cleft cysts type II**
*See BRANCHIAL CLEFT CYSTS*
**Branchial cleft cysts, Bailey type IV**
*See NASOPHARYNGEAL CYSTS*
**Branchial cleft fistula**
*See NECK, BRANCHIAL CLEFT, CYSTS OR SINUSES*
**Branchial clefts, hemangiomatous-lip pseudoclefts-unusual facies**
*See BRANCHIO-OCULO-FACIAL SYNDROME*

## BRANCHIO-OCULO-FACIAL SYNDROME 2563

**Includes:**
Branchial arch-premature aging syndrome
Branchial clefts, hemangiomatous-lip pseudoclefts-unusual facies

**Excludes:**
Branchial cleft syndromes, other
Chromosomal disorders.

**Major Diagnostic Criteria:** Prominent vertical ridges on the upper lip resembling a poorly repaired **Cleft lip**, branchial cleft consisting of a sinus and/or hemangiomatous or atrophic skin lesion in post-auricular area, lacrimal duct obstruction, and broad misshapen nose.

**Clinical Findings:** Subcutaneous cysts of scalp (3/7); premature graying of hair (4/4); lacrimal duct obstruction (11/11); coloboma (5/9); microphthalmia (3/11); cataract (3/8); myopia (3/3); strabismus (2/11); malformed ears (10/11); auricular pits (3/11); conductive hearing deficit (5/6); misshapen nose (11/11); lip pseudoclefts (11/11); lip pits (2/11); dental abnormality (5/8); high-arched palate (4/7); branchial clefts (branchial sinus, atrophic skin, and/or hemangioma) (6/10); prenatal growth deficiency (6/10); postnatal growth deficiency (2/11); mental retardation (2/11); hand anomalies (clinodactyly, single transverse palmar crease, **Polydactyly**) (5/9).

**Complications:** Chronic dacryocystitis, myopia, and hearing loss. Psychological adjustment may pose a problem because of the unusual facial appearance.

**Associated Findings:** One patient had right facial palsy, an accessory nipple, absence of the right kidney, and **Hypospadias**.

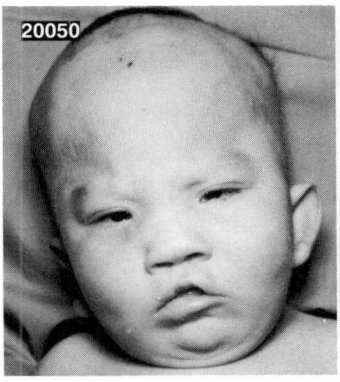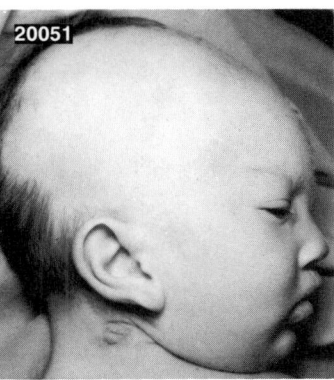

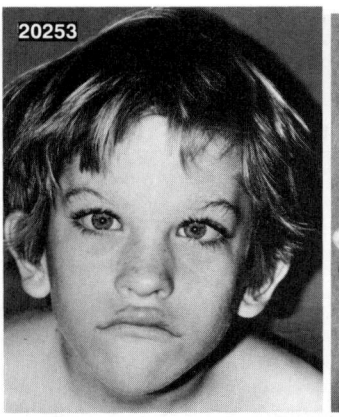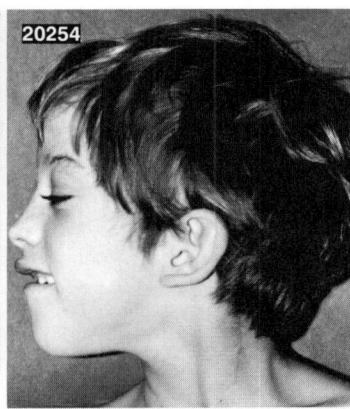

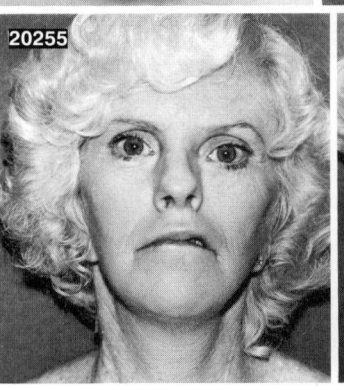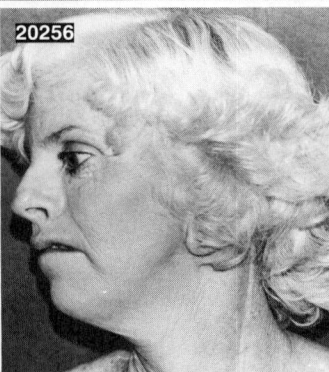

**2563A-20050:** Note the prominent vertical ridges on the upper lip which resemble a poorly repaired cleft lip. **20051:** Lateral view demonstrates the hemangiomatous lesion and the branchial cleft.

**Etiology:** Autosomal dominant inheritance. Seventy percent of cases have been sporadic.

**Pathogenesis:** Possibly ectodermal and mesodermal dysplasia including but not limited to the second branchial arch.

**MIM No.:** 11362

**POS No.:** 3618

**CDC No.:** 758.990

**Sex Ratio:** Presumably M1:F1; M8:F5 observed.

**Occurrence:** More than a dozen cases have been documented.

**Risk of Recurrence for Patient's Sib:**
See Part I, *Mendelian Inheritance.*

**Risk of Recurrence for Patient's Child:**
See Part I, *Mendelian Inheritance.*

**Age of Detectability:** At birth.

**Gene Mapping and Linkage:** Unknown.

**Prevention:** None known. Genetic counseling indicated.

**Treatment:** Chronic dacryocystitis requires almost continuous antibiotic treatment during infancy, and surgical probing of the ducts in some. Removal of subcutaneous cysts and branchial sinuses and cosmetic surgeries as indicated.

**Prognosis:** Probably normal life expectancy even though premature graying of hair occurs in adults. Intelligence is normal in the majority, and mental retardation, if present, is mild. A decrease in reproductive fitness is implied by family pedigrees.

**Detection of Carrier:** Clinical examination.

**References:**

Lee WK, et al.: Bilateral branchial cleft sinuses associated with intrauterine and postnatal growth retardation, premature aging, and unusual facial appearance: a new syndrome with dominant transmission. Am J Med Genet 1982; 11:345–352.

Root JD, Tedesco TA: Growth characteristics of fibroblasts from patients with the syndrome of intrauterine growth retardation, branchial cleft sinuses, and premature aging. Pediatr Res 1982; 16:272A.

Hall BD, et al.: A new syndrome of hemangiomatous branchial clefts, lip pseudoclefts, and unusual facial appearance. Am J Med Genet 1983; 14:135–138.

Fujimoto A, et al.: A new autosomal dominant branchio-oculo-facial syndrome. Am J Med Genet 1987; 27:943–951. * †

FU003
R0047
LE045

**Atsuko Fujimoto**
**Allen W. Root**
**Woon K. Lee**

**2563B-20253:** Branchio-oculo-facial syndrome; note characteristic facies in the 12-year-old proband including arched eyebrows, upward slanting palpebral fissures, short upper lip, downturned corners of the mouth and prominent ears. **20254:** Lateral view of proband's face shows short upper lip, low-set ear and ear conformation. **20255:** Mother of the proband at age 42 years; note premature aging. **20256:** Lateral view of affected mother.

**Branchio-oto dysplasia**
*See BRANCHIO-OTO-RENAL DYSPLASIA*

## BRANCHIO-OTO-RENAL DYSPLASIA      2224

**Includes:**
> BOR syndrome
> Branchio-oto dysplasia
> Ear malformations-cervical fistulas/nodules-mixed hearing loss
> Ear pit-deafness syndrome
> Melnick-Fraser syndrome
> Oto-branchio-renal dysplasia
> Oto-facio-cervical syndrome
> Preauricular pit-cervical fistula-hearing loss syndrome
> Renal-branchio-oto dysplasia

**Excludes:**
> **Branchio-oto-ureteral syndrome** (3037)
> **Deafness-malformed, low-set ears** (0254)

**Major Diagnostic Criteria:** Preauricular pits or ear tags, branchial cysts or fistulas, sensory or mixed hearing loss, and renal hypoplasia.

**Clinical Findings:** *Otologic findings:* preauricular pit; typically a shallow, pinhead-sized blind depression in the helix of the upper ear or the skin just anterior to the upper attachment or preauricular cartilaginous tags. The external ear may be cupped ("lop," "bat") or hypoplastic (microtia). The external canal may be narrow or slanted upward. Hearing loss is most frequently mixed but may be sensorineural or, rarely, conductive. Onset varies from early childhood to young adulthood. Sudden hearing loss may be associated with intense effort; periods of rapid deterioration have also been described. The middle ear, vestibular system, and cochlea may be malformed; the ossicles may be displaced or malformed; and the stapes and incus may be fused or unconnected.

*Branchial findings*: branchial cleft fistulas that open externally in the lower one-third of the neck, usually on the median border of the sternomastoid muscle. There may be an internal opening in the tonsillar fossa, or a cyst or cartilaginous mass without any opening.

*Renal anomalies* may range from none, through sharply tapered superior poles with blunting of calyces, to marked hypoplasia or agenesis. Polycystic kidneys have been reported occasionally. Renal histology in severe cases may show oligomeganephronic, hypoplastic, or multicystic dysplasia.

**Complications:**  Cysts or fistulas may become infected and require surgical removal. Renal failure may intervene in cases with severe hypoplasia. Other patients may show diminished glomerular filtration rate. The milder renal abnormalities do not seem to be progressive.

**Associated Findings:**  Lacrimal duct stenosis (8%); long narrow face, constricted palate with deep overbite, and cleft palate (2%); paralysis of certain facial muscles (4%). Possible hemifacial microsomia may be a component in some families (Rollnick & Kaye, 1985).

**Etiology:**  Autosomal dominant inheritance with high penetrance.

**Pathogenesis:**  The external ear anomalies presumably result from abnormal differentiation of the first and second branchial arches, from which they arise, as do the abnormalities of cochlea and otic capsule (ossicles). Incomplete epithelial fusion of the first branchial cleft leads to the ear pits, and of the second branchial cleft to the sinuses and cysts.

The renal anomalies presumably result from abnormal differentiation of the ureteral bud and its inductive interactions with the metanephrogenic mesenchyme. Presumably there is some molecule common to these processes, like a membrane component, whose alteration affects these but not other developmental processes. Such tautologic speculations do not "explain" the pathogenesis, but it is interesting that the embryonic kidney and ear have antigens in common.

**MIM No.:**  *11365

**POS No.:**  3133

**Sex Ratio:**  M1:F1

**Occurrence:**  Estimated 1:40,000 (assuming 1:1,000 children has profound hearing loss, 1:20 of these has branchial anomalies, and 1:2 of these has the BOR syndrome.

**Risk of Recurrence for Patient's Sib:**
See Part I, *Mendelian Inheritance*.

**Risk of Recurrence for Patient's Child:**
See Part I, *Mendelian Inheritance*.

**Age of Detectability:**  At birth. Prenatal diagnosis can be done for renal agenesis or severe hypoplasia.

**Gene Mapping and Linkage:**  Unknown.

**Prevention:**  None known. Genetic counseling indicated.

**Treatment:**  Hearing aid may be indicated. Surgery for external ear defects and branchial sinuses or cysts. Exploratory tympanotomy has had disappointing results. Renal transplant if indicated.

**Prognosis:**  Summaries from the literature are biased by uncertainty about whether certain traits were present but not recorded by the observer. In carriers of the gene, about one-half will have pits, branchial clefts, and deafness; 1/10 will have clefts and deafness; 1/10 will have deafness without pits or clefts; and 1/20 will have pits and deafness. Only 1% will have none of these. The frequency of renal anomalies is about 1/2, and of severe anomalies

between 1/10 to 1/4. For counseling, these figures provide the following answers: 1) a newborn child with ear pits only and a negative family history has about a 1/200 chance of having severe hearing loss; the pits are probably nongenetic or (occasionally) a fresh mutation for the gene for preauricular pits only; 2) offspring of carriers who have pits and/or clefts have about a 4/5 chance of hearing loss; 3) offspring of carriers who do not have pits or clefts may nevertheless be carriers, with about a 1/20 chance of developing hearing loss; much higher if they have anomalies of the external ear, lacrimal ducts, or kidneys, and lower if they do not; 4) prenatal diagnosis can be offered for detection of severe renal anomalies.

**Detection of Carrier:**  Unknown.

**Special Considerations:**  Ear pits, branchial sinuses, and deafness associated with duplicated ureters, bifid renal pelvis, or both, may be a separate entity which has been termed the **Branchio-oto-ureteral syndrome** (BOU syndrome), although further family studies are needed to confirm this delineation.

**References:**
Melnick M, et al.: Familial branchio-oto-renal dysplasia: a new addition to the branchial arch syndromes. Clin Genet 1976; 9:25–34.
Fraser FC, et al.: Genetic aspects of the BOR syndrome: branchial fistulas, ear pits, hearing loss, and renal anomalies. Am J Med Genet 1978; 2:241–252. * †
Cremers CWRJ, et al.: The earpits-deafness syndrome: clinical and genetic aspects. Int J Pediatr Otolaryngol 1980; 2:309–322.
Fraser FC, et al.: Frequency of the branchio-oto-renal (BOR) syndrome in children with profound hearing loss. Am J Med Genet 1980; 7:341–349.
Widdershoven J, et al.: Renal disorders in the branchio-oto-renal syndrome. Helv Paediatr Acta 1983; 38:513–522. *
Rollnick BR, Kaye CI: Hemifacial microsomia and the branchio-oto-renal syndrome. J Craniofac Genet Devel Biol 1985; 1:287–295.
Heimler A, Lieber E: Branchio-oto-renal syndrome: reduced penetrance and variable expressivity in four generations of a large kindred. Am J Med Genet 1986; 25:15–27.
Joseph MP, et al.: Heterotopic cervical salivary gland tissue in a family with probable branchio-oto-renal syndrome. Head & Neck Surg 1986; 8:456–462.

FR009                                                    **F. Clarke Fraser**

---

## BRANCHIO-OTO-URETERAL SYNDROME          3037

**Includes:**
   Fraser-Ayme-Hall syndrome
   Oto-branchio-ureteral syndrome
   Renal duplication-hearing loss-external ear anomalies

**Excludes:**  **Branchio-oto-renal dysplasia** (2224)

**Major Diagnostic Criteria:**  The combination of hearing loss with or without preauricular pits or tags and bifid renal collecting system should suggest the diagnosis in an isolated case. One of the above findings plus a family history of the other findings should suggest the diagnosis.

**Clinical Findings:**  Branchial anomalies included preauricular tags or pits, cone-shaped pinnae, and microtia. Deafness ranged from mild to severe, and sensorineural, conductive, and mixed deafness all occurred. Ureteral anomalies ranged from duplicated ureters with ureterocele to bifid renal pelves. Expression of the condition was variable in that only 2/14 individuals had all three findings; 4/14 had two findings; and 8/14 had only one finding. In addition, five individuals had spina bifida occulta at L-5 or S-1.

**Complications:**  Those associated with duplicated ureters.

**Associated Findings:**  None known.

**Etiology:**  Presumably autosomal dominant inheritance with variable expression and reduced penetrance.

**Pathogenesis:**  Unknown.

**POS No.:**  3588

**Sex Ratio:**  Presumably M1:F1.

**Occurrence:** Two families, with a total of 14 affected members, have been reported.

**Risk of Recurrence for Patient's Sib:**
See Part I, *Mendelian Inheritance.*

**Risk of Recurrence for Patient's Child:**
See Part I, *Mendelian Inheritance.*

**Age of Detectability:** Potentially at birth if the ureteral or branchial anomaly is present; otherwise, during childhood.

**Gene Mapping and Linkage:** Unknown.

**Prevention:** None known. Genetic counseling indicated.

**Treatment:** Hearing aids for deafness and surgery for the ureteral defect may be indicated.

**Prognosis:** Intellect and life span are apparently unimpaired.

**Detection of Carrier:** Unknown.

**References:**
Fraser FC, et al.: Autosomal dominant duplication of the renal collecting system, hearing loss, and external ear anomalies: a new syndrome? Am J Med Genet 1983; 14:473–478.

T0007                                    **Helga V. Toriello**

---

## BRANCHIO-SKELETO-GENITAL SYNDROME          0118

**Includes:**
>  Craniofacial-genital-dental syndrome (CFGD)
>  Elsahy syndrome
>  Elsahy-Waters syndrome
>  Genito-branchio-skeletal syndrome
>  Genito-oculo-oligophrenic-dento-skeleto syndrome
>  (GOODS)
>  Skeleto-branchio-genital syndromes

**Excludes:**
**Oculo-mandibulo-facial syndrome** (0738)
**Spherophakia-brachymorphia syndrome** (0893)

**Major Diagnostic Criteria:** Hypoplasia of the maxilla and relative prognathism, cleft palate or uvula, hypertelorism, brachycephaly, dentine dysplasia, pectus excavatum, hypospadias.

**Clinical Findings:** *Branchial arch (first and second) anomalies:* Maxilla: hypoplasia, multiple dentigerous cysts, and unerupted teeth. Mandible: relative prognathism, multiple dentigerous cysts, unerupted teeth, dentin dysplasia (radicular type), teeth with demilune or obliterated chambers with abnormal short roots. Palate: bifid uvula; high-arched, cleft palate; and submucous palatal cleft causing nasal speech with articulation defects. Mastoid bone: undeveloped. Nose: broad and flat with wide nasal tip and flared alar cartilages. Eyes: hypertelorism, strabismus, ptosis, nystagmus.

*Skeletal anomalies:* Skull: brachycephaly. Vertebral column: fusion of second and third cervical spinous processes, Schmorl nodes in lumbar vertebrae. Sternum: pectus excavatum.
*Genital anomalies:* penoscrotal hypospadias.

**Complications:** Mental retardation, convulsions, nasal speech, destruction of mandible and maxilla from cyst expansion.

**Associated Findings:** None known.

**Etiology:** Probably autosomal recessive inheritance. In the one reported kinship, unaffected parents were first cousins.

**Pathogenesis:** Defect appears to be a midline clefting syndrome, i.e., hypertelorism, cleft palate, pectus excavatum, and hypospadias, probably indicating an embryonic somite fusion defect involving the embryologic origin of the head and neck (namely, the first and second branchial arch derivatives, the forebrain, skull, and cervical vertebrae) and the rest of the body. Histologic changes in teeth are identical with those of radicular dentin dysplasia.

**MIM No.:** 21138

**POS No.:** 3046

**Sex Ratio:** Presumably M1:F1 (M3:F0 observed).

**Occurrence:** Rare. One kinship with three affected sibs has been reported.

**Risk of Recurrence for Patient's Sib:**
See Part I, *Mendelian Inheritance.*

**Risk of Recurrence for Patient's Child:**
See Part I, *Mendelian Inheritance.*

**Age of Detectability:** At birth by clinical and X-ray examination.

**Gene Mapping and Linkage:** Unknown.

**Prevention:** None known. Genetic counseling indicated.

**Treatment:** Surgical repair of anatomic defects of palate and teeth; correction of hypertelorism with either subcranial or transcranial approaches at age 5 years; hypospadias repair; dental care; speech therapy; medical therapy for seizures.

**Prognosis:** Not a life-threatening disorder; affected individuals have survived to adulthood but are psychosocially retarded.

**Detection of Carrier:** Unknown.

**Special Considerations:** This syndrome was originally described by Elsahy and Waters in 1971 in a family as the branchio-skeleto-genital syndrome. The same family was subsequently inadvertently designated Unger-Trott syndrome by Witkop (1972, 1975). The histologic pictures of the tooth defect in the paper by Elsahy and Waters (1971) had been erroneously replaced by a picture of Witkop's patient with fibrous dysplasia of dentin.

**References:**
Elsahy NI, Waters WR: The branchio-skeleto-genital syndrome: a new hereditary syndrome. Plast Reconstr Surg 1971; 58:542–550.
Witkop CJ Jr, Rao S: Inherited defects in tooth structure. BD:OAS VII(7), 1971:153.
Elsahy NI, Vistnes LM: Anomalies of the head and neck: an attempt at classification. Acta Chir Plast (Prague) 1972; 14:1.
Witkop CJ Jr: Genetics. Schweiz Monatsschr Zahnheilkd 1972; 82:917.
Witkop CJ Jr: Hereditary defects of dentin. Dent Clin North Am 1975; 19:25.
Converse JM: Plastic and reconstructive surgery, vol 4. Philadelphia: W.B. Saunders, 1977:2116–2161.
Goodman RM, Gorlin RJ: Atlas of the face in genetic disorders. St. Louis: C.V. Mosby Co., 1977:226.
Wedgwood DL, et al.: Cranio-facial and dental anomalies in the branchio-skeleto-genital syndrome with suggestions for more appropriate nomenclature. Br J Oral Surg 1983; 21:94.
Serafin G: Pediatric plasic surgery. St. Louis: C.V. Mosby, 1984:467.

EL008                                    **Nabil I. Elsahy**
WI043                                    **Carl J. Witkop, Jr.**

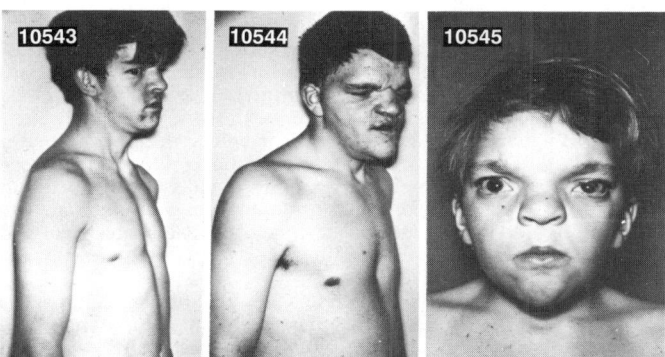

**0118**-10543–45: Affected male sibs show hypertelorism, flat nose with wide nasal tip and prognathism.

**Brandt syndrome**
*See ACRODERMATITIS ENTEROPATHICA*
**Brauer keratoderma palmoplantar**
*See SKIN, PAINFUL PLANTAR CALLOSITIES*

**Braun-Bayer syndrome**
  *See NEPHROSIS-DEAFNESS-URINARY TRACT AND DIGITAL DEFECTS*
**Brazilian achondrogenesis**
  *See GREBE SYNDROME*
**Brazilian type acheiropody**
  *See ACHEIROPODY*
**Breakpoint cluster region-1**
  *See LEUKEMIA, CHRONIC MYELOID (CML)*
**Breast cancer, familial, site-specific**
  *See CANCER, BREAST, FAMILIAL*
**Breast fibroadenomas-hypertrichosis-gingival fibromatosis**
  *See GINGIVAL MULTIPLE HAMARTOMA SYNDROME*
**Breast tissue, congenital absence**
  *See BREAST, AMASTIA*

---

## BREAST, AMASTIA                                    0042

**Includes:**

  Amastia, breast
  Athelia
  Breast tissue, congenital absence
  Nipple, congenital absence

**Excludes:**

  **Ectodermal dysplasia, Christ-Siemens-Touraine type** (0333)
  **Poland syndrome** (0813)
  Tricho-Odonto-Onycho-Dermal Syndrome

**Major Diagnostic Criteria:** Absence of at least one mamma with or without underlying muscle abnormality.

**Clinical Findings:** Absence of nipples, unilateral or bilateral, from birth; lack of breast development at puberty or during pregnancy; no abnormality of other secondary sexual characters and normal fertility.

**Complications:** Lack of lactation.

**Associated Findings:** Unilateral amastia is frequently associated with absence of corresponding pectoral muscles. Nearly 40% of cases of bilateral amastia have multiple congenital anomalies: skeletal anomalies, cleft or high-arched palate, hypertelorism.

**Etiology:** Pedigrees consistent with both autosomal dominant and autosomal recessive inheritance have been reported.

**Pathogenesis:** Absence of breast results from failure of the pectoral portions of the mammary ridge to develop. There is lack of breast enlargement in affected female at puberty and during pregnancy.

**MIM No.:** 11370

**CDC No.:** 757.600

**Sex Ratio:** M1:F5 in one series.

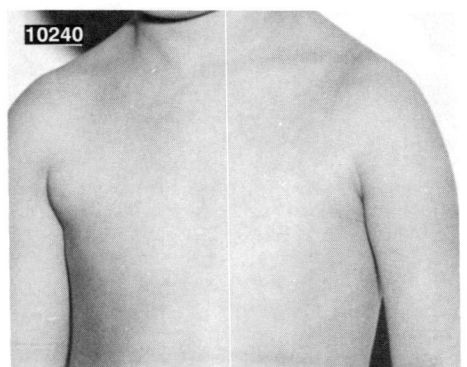

**0042-10240:** Absence of nipples (amastia).

**Occurrence:** Rare, although several pedigrees have been documented, and a report of the condition appears in the Bible (Song of Solomon VIII:8).

**Risk of Recurrence for Patient's Sib:**
  See Part I, *Mendelian Inheritance.*

**Risk of Recurrence for Patient's Child:**
  See Part I, *Mendelian Inheritance.*

**Age of Detectability:** At birth.

**Gene Mapping and Linkage:** Unknown.

**Prevention:** None known. Genetic counseling indicated.

**Treatment:** Tattoing of the nipples or grafting of the skin from labia minora or scrotum to simulate the nipple. Injection of plastic materials (silastic gel or equivalent) to produce protuberance of the breast in pubertal female.

**Prognosis:** Normal life span and reproductive fitness.

**Detection of Carrier:** Unknown.

**References:**

Trier WC: Complete breast absence: case report and review of the literature. Plast Reconstr Surg 1965; 36:431–439. *
Kowlessar M, Orti E: Complete breast absence in siblings. Am J Dis Child 1968; 115:91–92. †
Tawil HM, Najjar SS: Congenital absence of the breasts. J Pediatr 1968; 73:751–753.
Wilson MG, et al.: Dominant inheritance of absence of the breast. Humangenetik 1972; 15:268 only.
Goldberg F: Choanal atresia and athelia: methimazole teratogenicity or a new syndrome? Am J Med Genet 1987; 28:931–934.

QA000                                      **Qutub H. Qazi**
                                           *Eduardo Orti*

---

## BREAST, POLYTHELIA                              0815

**Includes:**

  Mammary gland tissue without nipple or areola
  Mammary glands, complete supernumerary
  Nipples, accessory
  Nipples, supernumerary nipples
  Polymastia (polymastie)

**Excludes:**

  Nipples, supernumerary associated with malformation syndromes
  Polythelia, intra-areolar

**Major Diagnostic Criteria:** A supernumerary nipple or breast with histologic presence of breast tissue situated anywhere along the mammary line. Supernumerary nipple must be distinguished from congenital moles, macules, plane warts, papilloma, and the like.

**Clinical Findings:** Complete supernumerary mammary glands are very rare. Supernumerary nipple (polythelia), commonly regarded as a benign congenital anomaly, is by far the most frequent. A vast majority occur along the so-called "milk-line" (mammary line) extending from the axilla to the groin, and most are observed in the thoracic region. In rare instances the accessory breasts have occurred outside the mammary line, in such locations as the face, neck, arm, shoulder, thigh, buttock, and back. They may be unilateral or bilateral, above or below the normal mammae, and more frequently on the left side than on the right. Those situated above the normal mammae are usually lateral to them, whereas those placed below the normal mammae are medial. The laterally situated glands are well-formed, of considerable size, and can lactate; medial ones are usually small, imperfectly developed, and incapable of lactation.

  In the majority of cases a single accessory nipple or breast is present; about one-third of the affected have two. The incidence decreases inversely to the number of mammae. Patients with eight or nine supernumerary breasts have been described. Complete supernumerary breasts have all complements, of normal breast, including well-formed nipple, areola, and ductal system. Polymastia will have a ductal system but may lack nipple and areola. Supernumerary nipple may appear like a mole or wart, and may or may not have breast tissue or areola. Histologically, a supernumerary nipple shows all the components of a normal nipple, including epidermal thickening, pilosebaceous structures, smooth muscle, and remnant of duct system.

Supernumerary breasts undergo cyclic changes in size and density of the normal breast and are subject to the same diseases, including cancer. They generally attract attention at the time of puberty or in association with pregnancy and lactation. However, they may remain unnoticed and quiescent. In Caucasians more than 90% of the accessory breasts are found below the normally situated mammae, while in Japanese 88% are above the normal mammae.

**Complications:** Pain and swelling during menstruation and pregnancy and pain and/or dribbling of milk during lactation, causing esthetic and psychologic embarrassment. Bacterial and mycoplasma infections can occur. Fibroadenoma, chronic cystic disease, and malignant change (such as infiltrating ductal carcinoma) have been reported. It is, however, not established that the tumors arise with greater frequency in accessory mammary glands or that the prognosis of cancer of such glands is worse than that of the normal breast.

**Associated Findings:** Association with multiple births, tuberculosis, and left handedness has been reported in the earlier literature, but more careful evaluation of the data failed to bear any such relationship. Recent reports point to association with cardioarterial disease, obstructive urinary tract anomalies (purportedly in Caucasians), renal adenocarcinoma, unilateral renal agenesis, testicular cancer, and congenital pyloric stenosis.

**Etiology:** A small proportion of cases (about 6%) are familial. Autosomal dominant inheritance has been postulated. Hereditary transmission through four generations has been reported.

**Pathogenesis:** Those occurring along the mammary line are thought to result when the embryonic mammary crest fails to undergo normal regression. Lateral, cephalad, or caudal displacement of the mammary crest could explain locations outside the ventral surface of the body.

**MIM No.:** *16370

**CDC No.:** 757.650

**Sex Ratio:** M1:F<1 Caucasians, M1:F>1 in Japanese.

**Occurrence:** Approximately 1–2% (0.22 - 2.5%). Racial and geographic differences have been noted.

**Risk of Recurrence for Patient's Sib:**
See Part I, *Mendelian Inheritance.*

**Risk of Recurrence for Patient's Child:**
See Part I, *Mendelian Inheritance.*

**Age of Detectability:** Neonatal period. May remain unnoticed in males, and until after puberty or pregnancy in females.

**Gene Mapping and Linkage:** Unknown.

**Prevention:** None known. Genetic counseling indicated.

**Treatment:** Excision for cosmetic reasons. Supernumerary breasts should be examined with the same care and frequency as the normal breasts for detection of breast disease, namely tumors.

**Prognosis:** Normal for life span, intelligence, and function. Normal reproductive fitness.

**Detection of Carrier:** Unknown.

**References:**
De Cholnoky T: Supernumerary breast. Arch Surg 1939; 39:926–941. *
Weinberg SK, Motulsky AG: Aberrant axillary breast tissue: a report of a family with six affected women in two generations. Clin Genet 1976; 10:326–328.
Mehes K: Association of supernumerary nipples with other anomalies. J Pediatr 1979; 95:274–275.
Smith GMR, Greening WP: Carcinoma of aberrant tissue. Obstet Gynecol 1980; 55:845–847.
Mehergan AH: Supernumerary nipple: a histologic study. J Cutan Pathol 1981; 8:96–104.
Johnson CA, et al.: Polythelia (supernumerary nipple): an update. South Med J 1986; 79:1106–1108. * †

QA000
**Qutub H. Qazi**
*Eduardo Orti*

**Brevicollis, congenital**
See *KLIPPEL-FEIL ANOMALY*
**'Broad beta' disease**
See *HYPERLIPOPROTEINEMIA, BROAD BETA TYPE*
**Broad thumb-hallux-syndrome**
See *RUBINSTEIN-TAYBI BROAD THUMB-HALLUX SYNDROME*

## BRONCHIAL ATRESIA                                     0120

**Includes:** Atresia, bronchial

**Excludes:** Emphysema, lobar, congenital

**Major Diagnostic Criteria:** Atresia of a segmental bronchus with associated emphysema demonstrated by X-ray, computed tomography, and bronchoscopy.

**Clinical Findings:** Most cases have been discovered on routine chest X-ray, and are not clinically symptomatic. Mild shortness of breath and recurrent pulmonary infections have been reported. Physical examination findings include diminished or absent breath sounds over the emphysematous area. Evidence of cardiac displacement, as in congenital lobar emphysema, may be found. On X-ray there is a localized radiolucent area of emphysema with an adjacent perihilar density. The latter finding is caused by mucous-filled bronchus or mucocele beyond the point of the atretic segment. Most cases, 23 of 32 in the largest literature review, have involved the apical-posterior segment of the left upper lobe. In all, there were 28 cases involving the upper lobes.

**Complications:** A mild obstructive ventilation defect was demonstrated in one case. Reported patients have usually not had physiologic assessments of function. Pulmonary infection occurs in some patients.

**Associated Findings:** One case report of associated pericardial defect and lung sequestration. Atrial septal defect with left-sided inferior vena cava, unilateral renal agenesis, anomalous venous drainage of the left upper lobe, congenital cystic adenomatoid malformation, and fusion of C2-C3 apophyseal joints have been reported.

**Etiology:** Unknown.

**Pathogenesis:** An interruption of a bronchial artery branch to the involved bronchus after branching is complete has been postulated. Distal branches of the pulmonary artery supplying the involved segment are hypoplastic. The nature of the defect appears to parallel intestinal atresias for which a vascular origin has been postulated and demonstrated in animal models.

**CDC No.:** 748.350

**Sex Ratio:** M17:F11 (observed).

**Occurrence:** Rare; twenty-eight cases have been reported.

**Risk of Recurrence for Patient's Sib:** Unknown.

**Risk of Recurrence for Patient's Child:** Unknown.

**Age of Detectability:** From birth. Most cases discovered during adulthood.

**Gene Mapping and Linkage:** Unknown.

**Prevention:** None known. Genetic counseling indicated.

**Treatment:** Depends on age at presentation and presence of symptoms. The presence of an emphysematous segment may impede normal alveolar development in adjacent lung segments. Surgical approach with lobectomy or segmental resection is indicated. In asymptomatic adults conservative management may be indicated.

**Prognosis:** Excellent. No limitation in function.

**Detection of Carrier:** Unknown.

**Special Considerations:** Computed tomography has improved the accuracy of noninvasive diagnosis of this disorder.

**References:**
Montague NT, Shaw RR: Bronchial atresia. Ann Thorac Surg 1974; 18:337–345.
Oh KS, et al.: The syndrome of bronchial atresia or stenosis with mucocele and focal hyperinflation of the lung. Johns Hopkins Med J 1976; 138:48–53.
Haller JA Jr, et al.: The natural history of bronchial atresia. J Thorac Cardiovasc Surg 1980; 79:868–872.
Robotham JL, et al.: A physiologic assessment of segmental bronchial atresia. Am Rev Respir Dis 1980; 121:533–540.
Pugatch RD, Gale ME: Obscure pulmonary masses: bronchial impaction revealed by CT. Am J Radiol 1983; 141:909–914.

BI009                                    **Robert M. Bilenker**

**Bronchiectasis, sinusitis, and dextrocardia**
 *See DEXTROCARDIA-BRONCHIECTASIS-SINUSITIS SYNDROME*
**Bronchiectasis-dextrocardia-sinusitis syndrome**
 *See DEXTROCARDIA-BRONCHIECTASIS-SINUSITIS SYNDROME*
**Bronchogenic cyst**
 *See LUNG, BRONCHOGENIC CYST*

---

# BRONCHOMALACIA                          2995

**Includes:**
 Central bronchomalacia
 Diffuse segmental bronchomalacia
 Williams-Campbell syndrome

**Excludes:**
 **Alpha(1)-antitrypsin deficiency** (0039)
 Bronchial stenosis
 **Cystic fibrosis** (0237)
 **Dextrocardia-bronchiectasis-sinusitis syndrome** (0285)
 **Immunodeficiency**
 **Lung, emphysema congenital lobar** (2703)
 **Tracheomalacia** (2505)
 Tuberculosis

**Major Diagnostic Criteria:** For central bronchomalacia, ipsilateral air trapping or atelectasis may be seen on chest X-rays and excessive expiratory collapse of central bronchi may be visualized by fluoroscopy. The diagnosis must be confirmed with bronchoscopy, which demonstrates excessive (i.e., >75%) anterior-posterior apposition of the bronchial walls during expiration. Since the airways may be artificially stented open with positive pressure ventilation and a rigid bronchoscope, flexible bronchoscopy is the procedure of choice. A concomitant bronchogram may be needed to determine the axial extent of the lesion. The left mainstem bronchus is the most frequent site of involvement, but the lesion may be right-sided or bilateral.

Diffuse bronchiectasis is seen in routine chest X-rays. Since the defect in this disorder is more distal, characteristically involving the fourth to eighth generation bronchi, bronchoscopic findings are normal or nonspecific (i.e., demonstrating airway inflammation or mucopurulent secretions). Diagnosis depends on bronchography, which demonstrates alternating inspiratory ballooning and expiratory collapse of the segmental bronchi and no bronchiolar dye filling, and the exclusion of other etiologies of bronchiectasis.

**Clinical Findings:** Clinical features and age of onset depend on the location, length, and degree of airway collapse. Patients with less severe and focal involvement may present in the first year of life with chronic cough, harsh expiratory wheezing often unresponsive to bronchodilators, recurrent pneumonia, lobar emphysema, or atelectasis. With more severe involvement, wheezes, retractions, cyanotic episodes, and progressive respiratory distress may begin at birth. Symptoms are typically exacerbated by agitation and respiratory tract infections.

Initial symptoms usually develop following an upper respiratory tract infection in the first year of life, and consist of a persistent and frequently productive cough, variable wheezing, recurrent pneumonia, and dyspnea on exertion. With time, affected patients manifest growth failure, persistent pulmonary

hyperinflation resulting in barrel-shaped chests, and digital clubbing.

**Complications:** Recurrent pneumonia; focal or diffuse air trapping and/or atelectasis; bronchiectasis; dyspnea; hypoxemia; respiratory failure; and respiratory arrest.

**Associated Findings:** Approximately 50% of patients with **Tracheomalacia** will also have unilateral or bilateral bronchomalacia.

Other associated findings include **Pectus excavatum**; congenital heart disease (e.g., **Heart, tetralogy of Fallot**; gastro-esophageal reflux; bronchopulmonary dysplasia; **Ehlers-Danlos syndrome**; and **Chondroectodermal dysplasia**.

**Etiology:** Possibly autosomal recessive inheritance.

**Pathogenesis:** Congenital bronchomalacia results from a defect in bronchial cartilage formation, wherein the latter may be entirely absent or present as irregularly shaped and distributed islands rather than rings. It may be primary (i.e., idiopathic) or secondary, with bronchial maldevelopment associated with an external compression (e.g., from a dilated pulmonary artery). More commonly, however, bronchomalacia is acquired, usually with **Tracheomalacia**, in children with chronic airways inflammation resulting from prolonged endotracheal intubation, bronchopulmonary dysplasia, and gastroesophageal reflux.

*Williams-Campbell syndrome* is generally attributed to a congenital absence of cartilage in the third to fourth through the eighth generation bronchi, although the latter syndrome has also been ascribed to obliterative bronchiolitis in infancy.

**MIM No.:** 21145

**Sex Ratio:** M2:F1 for central bronchomalacia; M1:F1 in *Williams-Campbell syndrome*.

**Occurrence:** Undetermined but presumed rare. All primary forms are less common than **Tracheomalacia** or acquired tracheobronchomalacia Fewer than a dozen cases have been documented in the literature.

**Risk of Recurrence for Patient's Sib:**
 See Part I, *Mendelian Inheritance.*

**Risk of Recurrence for Patient's Child:**
 See Part I, *Mendelian Inheritance.*

**Age of Detectability:** From the first days of life to several months of age.

**Gene Mapping and Linkage:** Unknown.

**Prevention:** None known. Genetic counseling indicated.

**Treatment:** For severe central bronchomalacia, prolonged administration of continuous positive airway pressure (CPAP) or possibly intermittent positive pressure ventilation (IPPV) may be necessary for an extended period. If vascular compression (e.g., pulmonary artery) is noted on bronchoscopy, arteriopexy may relieve the obstruction. Refractory cases may require pneumonectomy or bronchoplasty. Bronchial stenting is usually unsuccessful in congenital lobar emphysema. Patients with *Williams-Campbell syndrome* benefit from chest percussion and the use of antibiotics to control secondary infection.

**Prognosis:** Excellent for mild cases of central bronchomalacia, with spontaneous resolution by 12–18 months of age; fair to good for severe cases requiring surgery or extended CPAP. Fair for *Williams-Campbell syndrome*, with ~75% survival beyond five years and 50% survival beyond 15 years of age.

**Detection of Carrier:** Unknown.

**Special Considerations:** Although *Williams-Campbell syndrome* is generally considered to be a form of congenital bronchiectasis, its pathophysiology more accurately classifies it as *diffuse segmental bronchomalacia*.

The variations in tracheal and bronchial luminal area that occur with changes in intrathoracic pressure during the respiratory cycle are normally more pronounced in infants because of the smaller initial diameters and more compliant walls of infant airways. If an airway's cartilaginous framework is deficient or absent, transmural forces during expiration may exceed the intrinsic rigidity of the airway, resulting in its collapse. Factors that increase transmural pressure (e.g., coughing, agitation, peripheral obstructive airway disease) or decrease initial luminal area (e.g., inflammation) will exacerbate this dynamic collapse.

**Support Groups:** New York; American Lung Association

**References:**

Williams HE, et al.: Generalized bronchiectasis due to extensive deficiency of bronchial cartilage. Arch Dis Child 1972; 47:423–428. *

Neijens HJ, et al. Successful treatment with CPAP of two infants with bronchomalacia. Acta Paediatr Scand 1978; 67:293–296. †

Denneny JC III: Bronchomalacia in the neonate. Ann Otol Rhinol Laryngol 1985; 94:466–469. *

Sotomayor JL, et al.: Large-airway collapse due to acquired tracheo-bronchomalacia in infancy. Am J Dis Child 1986; 140:367–371.

Vinograd I, et al.: Long-term functional results of prosthetic airway splinting in tracheomalacia and bronchomalacia. J Pediatr Surg 1987; 22:38–41.

SC066                        **Craig M. Schramm**
SC064                        **Thomas F. Scanlin**

**Bronchus, aberrant**
*See LUNG, ABERRANT LOBE*
**Bronze diabetes**
*See HEMOCHROMATOSIS, IDIOPATHIC*
**Bronze Schilder disease**
*See ADRENOLEUKODYSTROPHY, X-LINKED*
**Brooke tumor**
*See EPITHELIOMAS, HEREDITARY MULTIPLE CYSTIC*
**Brooke-Fordyce trichoepithelioma**
*See EPITHELIOMAS, HEREDITARY MULTIPLE CYSTIC*
**Brown albino**
*See ALBINISM, OCULOCUTANEOUS, BROWN TYPE*

---

## BROWN SYNDROME                             3179

**Includes:**
Eye movement disorder
Eye, superior oblique tendon sheath syndrome of Brown
Eye, superior orbital click syndrome

**Excludes:** Eye, inferior oblique paresis

**Major Diagnostic Criteria:** An eye movement disorder characterized by a lack of elevation in adduction. Other diagnostic features include a positive forced duction test and minimal or no overaction of the ipsilateral superior oblique.

**Clinical Findings:** Brown syndrome can be congenital or acquired, and its motility defect can be permanent, transient, or intermittent. Its clinical findings include: 1) limitation of elevation in adduction, occasionally with depression of the globe on adduction; 2) a positive forced duction test to elevation in adduction indicating a mechanical restriction; 3) minimal or no overaction of the contralateral superior oblique; and 4) divergence of the eyes on straight elevation. There may be a widening of the lid fissure on adduction. Occasionally, there is an associated chin-up head position or a head turn to the side opposite the impaired muscle in an effort to maintain single binocular vision. The involved eye may be hypotropic in the primary position.

A variant of this motility disorder is the *superior orbital click syndrome*. Affected patients have a clinical motility pattern identical to that of Brown syndrome with the exception of an audible (and palpable) click that occurs on successful elevation in adduction. There may also be a palpable mass or subjective tenderness in the trochlear region.

**Complications:** Anomalous head position to maintain binocular vision.

**Associated Findings:** None known.

**Etiology:** The majority of cases are isolated, but there have been several reports of familial Brown syndrome with autosomal dominant inheritance. Katz et al (1981) and Wortham & Crawford (1988) reported Brown syndrome in monozygotic twins.

**Pathogenesis:** The cause is felt to be a tight, short, or mechanically restricted superior oblique tendon. The acquired form may result from inflammation restricting the passage of the superior

oblique tendon through the trochlea. This may be associated with systemic inflammatory disorders such as adult or juvenile rheumatoid arthritis or may be secondary to local inflammatory processes such as infection in an adjacent sinus. Brown syndrome may appear post-operatively after tucking a palsied superior oblique tendon or after frontal sinus window surgery if the sinus is entered through the supero-nasal quadrant of the orbit.

**Sex Ratio:** Presumably M1:F1, but in 126 patients reported by Brown (1973), the ratio was M1:F1.4.

**Occurrence:** Incidence in patients with strabismus is 1:450. Ten percent of cases are bilateral. Of the 126 patients reported by Brown (1973), 114 were under 13 years at age of detection.

**Risk of Recurrence for Patient's Sib:** Most cases are isolated.

**Risk of Recurrence for Patient's Child:** Most cases are isolated.

**Age of Detectability:** The congenital form is present at birth, but usually not recognized until early childhood.

**Gene Mapping and Linkage:** Unknown.

**Prevention:** None known. Genetic counseling indicated.

**Treatment:** Anti-inflammatory agents are used to treat Brown syndrome associated with inflammation such as juvenile rheumatoid arthritis. The congenital form may require surgery if the involved eye is hypotropic in the primary position or in the presence of an anomalous head posture which is cosmetically embarrassing. Tenotomy or tenectomy of the superior oblique tendon is the treatment of choice. This often results in a superior oblique palsy which may require further surgery. Some authors have suggested combining the tenotomy of the superior oblique tendon with a weakening procedure of the ipsilateral inferior oblique.

**Prognosis:** The acquired form may be transient, or responds to systemic anti-inflammatory agents.

**Detection of Carrier:** Unknown.

**References:**

Brown HW: Congenital structural muscle anomalies. In: Allen JH, ed: Strabismus ophthalmic symposium I. St Louis: C.V. Mosby, 1950: 205–36.

Brown HW: True and simulated superior oblique tendon sheath syndromes. Doc Ophthalmol 1973; 34:123–136.

Parks MM: Ocular motility and strabismus. Hagerstown, MD: Harper & Row, 1975:167–169. †

Katz NNK, et al.: Brown's syndrome in twins. J Pediatr Ophthalmol Strabismus 1981; 18:32–34.

Von Noorden GK: Binocular vision and ocular motility, 3rd ed. St Louis: C.V. Mosby, 1985:377–380. *

Magli A, et al: Inheritance in Brown syndrome. Ophthalmologica 1986; 192:82–87.

Wortham EV, Crawford JS: Brown's syndrome in twins. Am J Ophthalmol 1988; 105:562–563.

SC067                        **Bruce M. Schnall**
JA016                        **Mohammad S. Jaafar**

**Brown teeth**
*See TEETH, DEFECTS FROM TETRACYCLINE*
**Brown-Vialetto-Van Leare syndrome**
*See PALSY, PROGRESSIVE BULBAR OF CHILDHOOD*
**Brush border, congenital disorganization of**
*See MICROVILLUS INCLUSION DISEASE*
**Bruton agammaglobulinemia**
*See IMMUNODEFICIENCY, AGAMMAGLOBULINEMIA, X-LINKED, INFANTILE*
**Bulbar palsy, progressive**
*See AMYOTROPHIC LATERAL SCLEROSIS*
*also AMYOTROPHIC LATERAL SCLEROSIS, FAMILIAL ADULT AND JUVENILE TYPES*
**Bulbopontine paralysis, chronic-deafness**
*See PALSY, PROGRESSIVE BULBAR OF CHILDHOOD*
**Bulbospinal muscular atrophy, X-linked**
*See MUSCULAR ATROPHY, SPINAL AND BULBAR, X-LINKED KENNEDY TYPE*
*also SPINAL MUSCULAR ATROPHY*
**Bull teeth**
*See TEETH, TAURODONTISM*

**Bulldog syndrome**
See *SIMPSON-GOLABI-BEHMEL SYNDROME*
**Bullous acrokeratotic poikiloderma of Kindler and Weary**
See *POIKILODERMA, HEREDITARY ACROKERATOTIC, KINDLER-WEARY TYPE*
**Bullous congenital ichthyosiform erythroderma**
See *ICHTHYOSIFORM HYPERKERATOSIS, BULLOUS CONGENITAL*
**Bullous erythroderma ichthyosiformis congenita of Brocq**
See *ICHTHYOSIFORM HYPERKERATOSIS, BULLOUS CONGENITAL*
**Bullous ichthyosis**
See *ICHTHYOSIFORM HYPERKERATOSIS, BULLOUS CONGENITAL*
**Buphthalmos, congenital**
See *GLAUCOMA, CONGENITAL*
**Burger-Grutz syndrome**
See *HYPERCHYLOMICRONEMIA*
**Burkitt-like lymphoma**
See *LYMPHOMA, BURKITT TYPE*
**Burns syndrome**
See *ICHTHYOSIFORM ERYTHROKERATODERMA, ATYPICAL WITH DEAFNESS*
**Buschke-Fischer keratoderma palmoplantar**
See *SKIN, PAINFUL PLANTAR CALLOSITIES*
**Buscke-Ollendorf syndrome**
See *OSTEOPOIKILOSIS*
**Butyryl-CoA dehydrogenase deficiency**
See *ACYL-CoA DEHYDROGENASE DEFICIENCY, SHORT CHAIN TYPE*
**Byler disease (Amish kindred)**
See *JAUNDICE, INTRAHEPATIC CHOLESTATIC, BYLER TYPE*

# ❖ C ❖

## C SYNDROME                                                          0121

**Includes:**
    Opitz trigonocephaly syndrome
    Trigonocephaly "C" syndrome

**Excludes:   Trigonencephaly, autosomal dominant type** (3030)

**Major Diagnostic Criteria:**   C syndrome should be considered in all patients with trigonocephaly without an extra chromosome. Trigonocephaly, hypoplastic nasal root, abnormal external ears, strabismus, joint deformities, contractures or dislocations, and loose skin are the most consistent features found. The characteristic deeply furrowed palate is a common and distinctive anomaly in this syndrome but is otherwise rare. The palate is the best cranial sign after trigonocephaly.

**Clinical Findings:**   Based on data from 11 published cases, the C syndrome is a sublethal condition. The pattern of findings includes an anomaly of the anterior cranium and frontal cortex (trigonocephaly), the root of the nose (broad nasal bridge, epicanthus, and short nose), and palate (thick anterior alveolar ridges); abnormalities of the limbs (polysyndactyly, bridged palmar creases, short limbs, and joint dislocations with or without contractures); visceral defects (congenital heart defects, cryptorchid-

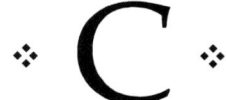

**0121**-10705–06:  Note short nose, prominent maxilla and slightly receding chin.

ism, and abnormal lobulations of the lungs and kidneys). Auricular, mandibular, skin, and genital abnormalities also occur. Consistent neurologic findings are hypotonia, strabismus, and psychomotor retardation; seizures have been reported.

*General findings*  Observations on the first 11 cases of C syndrome support the original associations of trigonocephaly (11/11); hypoplasia of the nasal root (11/11); abnormalities of external ears (11/11), which are posteriorly angulated, appear low-set, and sometimes have an abnormal helix; upward-slanting palpebral fissures (9/10); strabismus (7/10); joint deformities: contractures or dislocations (9/11); and loose skin (8/9). These anomalies are present in over 70% of cases. The characteristic palate has been positively identified in seven patients and probably was present in two; the palate is of uncertain configuration in two other patients. When present, this is an important diagnostic sign (Oberklaid and Danks, 1975). At the moment, the presence of trigonocephaly with wide alveolar ridges meeting in a deep midline furrow is still unique to this syndrome.

Besides the above-mentioned ear findings, most patients have some abnormality of the helix, apparently decreased cartilage, and incomplete or abnormal formation of the helix. The least auricular finding may be the single report of helical pits in one patient. Attached frenula is a useful, associated finding, which is easy to miss and may be under-reported. Combined abnormalities of the sternum (pectus excavatum, short and keel-shaped sternum) are seen in about one-half of reported cases.

Other anomalies are more variable, and there is a suggestion that the age of the patient may have a significant influence on the frequency of specific anomalies. For example, head size seems to be within a normal range at birth, but measurements over time suggest an increasing tendency toward microcephaly. Girls examined at birth have tended to have clitoral enlargement, which apparently does not persist. Also, micrognathia is not present in the two older children but is consistent among infants. These observations suggest that the apparent micrognathia may be a relative accentuation of the small jaw of normal infants. Findings at autopsy included trigonocephaly with shallow anterior fossa, and deep, funnel-shaped posterior fossa platybasia; bone defects over the cribriform plate, ridging of cranial sutures with fused posterior fontanelle, ethmoid sinuses, and absence of bone between the superior portions of the orbits; short sternum with reduced number of ossification centers but long xiphisternum, deformity of ribs; severe shortness of all metacarpals; bilateral postaxial hexadactyly. The patient of Oberklaid and Danks (1975) had bilateral dislocation of head of radius.

*Visceral and cardiovascular anomalies*:  Complete atrioventricular canal, hepatomegaly, free-floating cecum, and ascending colon combined within the mesentery of the ileum (leading to cecal volvulus in patient 1 of Preus et al., 1975); renal agenesis, prominent fetal lobulations of the kidneys, histologic immaturity of lung and kidneys, abnormal lobulation of the lungs, extensive fibrosis of the pancreas, and heterotopic pancreas. Patent ductus arteriosus, separate origin of left internal and external carotids from the aorta, thin-walled pulmonary arteries, and congenital heart disease of unspecified type in both patients of Preus et al (1975).

*Central nervous system findings.* Incomplete development of tentorium, many foci of cerebral, cerebellar, and meningeal hemorrhage, poor myelinization of the brain.

**Complications:** The patient of Oberklaid and Danks (1975) had a macroscopically normal brain, persistent pupillary membranes, central hyaloid arteries, and a coloboma of the optic disks. Patient 1 of Preus et al. (1975) had glaucoma requiring goniotomy. Patient 3 of Antley et al. (1981) had microcephaly.

**Associated Findings:** The neurologic findings in C syndrome include severe mental retardation. A single patient has moderate mental retardation and represents the best prognosis known to date. Other consistent neurologic findings are hypotonia and poor suck. Feeding is often so poor that gavage supplementation is required. The extensive joint dislocations found in some of the patients may represent neurologic deficiencies and hypotonia or a connective tissue problem related to the cutis hyperelastica. In addition, seizures, facial palsy, and depressed deep tendon reflexes have been noted.

**Etiology:** Probably homozygous state of autosomal recessive mutant gene.

**Pathogenesis:** Unknown.

**MIM No.:** *21175

**POS No.:** 3048

**Sex Ratio:** Presumably M1:F1

**Occurrence:** Less than twenty-five reported cases.

**Risk of Recurrence for Patient's Sib:**
See Part I, *Mendelian Inheritance.*

**Risk of Recurrence for Patient's Child:**
See Part I, *Mendelian Inheritance.*

**Age of Detectability:** At birth, by physical examination.

**Gene Mapping and Linkage:** Unknown.

**Prevention:** None known. Genetic counseling indicated.

**Treatment:** As may be indicated.

**Prognosis:** Lethal in infancy in 5/11 cases. Mental retardation among the survivors is a consistent finding.

**Detection of Carrier:** Unknown.

**References:**
Opitz JM, et al: The C syndrome of multiple congenital anomalies. In: BD:OAS 1969; V(2):161–166.
Oberklaid F, Danks DM: The Opitz trigonocephaly syndrome; a case report. Am J Dis Child 1975; 129:1348–1349.
Preus M, et al.: The C syndrome. In: BD:OAS 1975; XI(2):58–62.
Antley RM, et al.: Further delineation of the C (trigonocephaly) syndrome. Am J Med Genet 1981; 9:147–163.
Flatz SD, et al.: Opitz trigonocephaly syndrome: report of two cases. Eur J Pediatr 1984; 141:183–185.
Sargent C, et al.: Trigonocephaly and the Opitz C syndrome. J Med Genet 1985; 22:39–45.

AN014                                               **Ray M. Antley**

C2 deficiency
*See COMPLEMENT COMPONENT 2, DEFICIENCY OF*
C3b inactivator deficiency (Factor I)
*See COMPLEMENT COMPONENT 3, DEFICIENCY OF*
Cafe-au-lait spots-pulmonary stenosis
*See PULMONIC STENOSIS-CAFE-AU-LAIT SPOTS, WATSON TYPE*
Cafe-au-lait-ulcer, peptic/hiatal hernia-hypertelorism-myopia
*See GASTROCUTANEOUS SYNDROME*
Caffey disease
*See CORTICAL HYPEROSTOSIS, INFANTILE*
Calcification of cartilages-brachytelephalangy-pulmonary stenosis
*See KEUTEL SYNDROME*
Calcifying epithelioma of Malherbe
*See PILOMATRIXOMA*
Callosities, painful plantar
*See SKIN, PAINFUL PLANTAR CALLOSITIES*

Calves, hypertrophy of-spinal muscular atrophy
*See MUSCULAR ATROPHY, SPINAL AND BULBAR, X-LINKED KENNEDY TYPE*
CAMFAK syndrome
*See CATARACT, CORTICAL AND NUCLEAR*
Campailla-Martinelli acromesomelic dysplasia
*See ACROMESOMELIC DYSPLASIA, CAMPAILLA-MARTINELLI TYPE*
Campomelia-wormian bones-blue sclerae-mandibular hypoplasia
*See SHORT STATURE-WORMIAN BONES-JOINT DISLOCATIONS*

---

## CAMPOMELIC DYSPLASIA                            0122

**Includes:**
   Bowing of the limbs, congenital
   Campomelic syndrome
   Dwarfism, campomelic

**Excludes:**
   Short limb varieties of campomelia
   Other forms of congenital bowing of the limbs

**Major Diagnostic Criteria:** Congenital bowing of the long bones in a short-limbed dwarf in whom the bent femur is relatively long and slender.

**Clinical Findings:** The typical campomelic syndrome is associated with short-limbed dwarfism selectively affecting the lower limbs with anterior bending of the femur and tibia over which there are pretibial skin dimples. The calvarium is large with disproportionately small facies. The ears are low-set, and there is micrognathia and hypertelorism. The facies appear flat with a depressed nasal root, and a posterior cleft palate is usually present. Hypotonia and absence of olfactory nerves are found, and death usually occurs in the neonatal period as a result of respiratory distress. In the classic form of campomelic syndrome, on X-ray the bent long bones are fairly long and slender. There is femoral and tibial bowing and hypoplastic fibulae. Eleven pairs of ribs have been described in these patients, with hypoplasia of the scapulae. The ribs are narrow and wavy, and the clavicles are

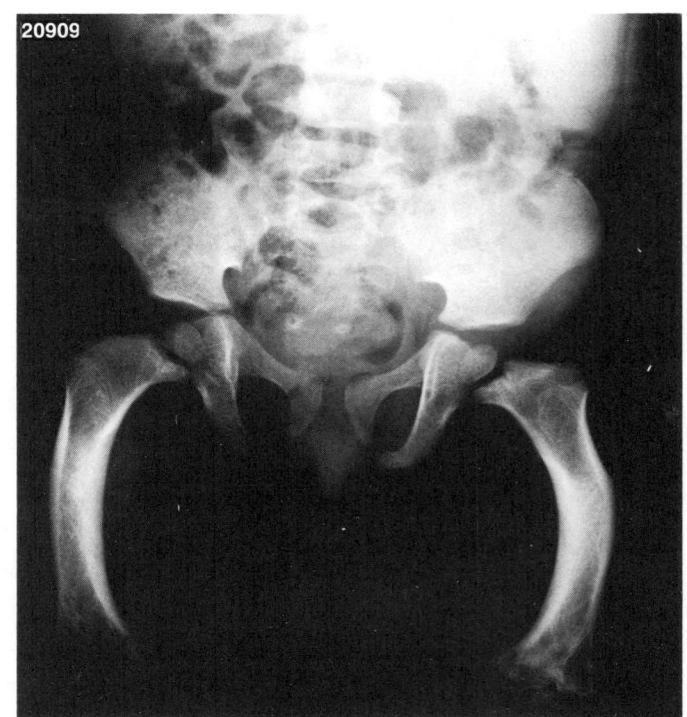

**0122A-20909:** Femoral bowing in campomelic dysplasia.

slender. There is scoliosis or kyphoscoliosis. The pelvis is high and narrow with hypoplasia of the ischiopubic rami. The ischia appear vertical in their orientation.

**Complications:** Respiratory distress is secondary to decreased rib cage size and tracheal cartilage abnormalities.

**Associated Findings:** Sex reversal in some karyotypic males with reported absence of H-Y antigen. CNS, cardiac, and renal abnormalities reported in some cases.

**Etiology:** Autosomal recessive inheritance. Seven instances of affected sibs with the typical form of the disease have been described.

**Pathogenesis:** Histologic examination of the site of bowing of the long bones shows parallel masses of periosteal new bone extending into the medullary cavity at right angles to the axis of the bone. This is probably secondary to the stress that produced the bending of the bone. While cartilage appears normal, temporal bone histology suggests a disturbance in cartilage growth.

**MIM No.:** *21197

**POS No.:** 3049

**Sex Ratio:** Phenotypic sex ratio: approximately M1:F2.3; karyotypic sex ratio: approximately M2:F1

**Occurrence:** Unknown. Extensive literature.

**Risk of Recurrence for Patient's Sib:**
See Part I, *Mendelian Inheritance.*

**Risk of Recurrence for Patient's Child:** Affected individuals are not expected to survive to reproduce.

**Age of Detectability:** Newborn. Has been diagnosed prenatally by ultrasound.

**Gene Mapping and Linkage:** Unknown.

**Prevention:** None known. Genetic counseling indicated.

**Treatment:** Support of respiratory function in the newborn.

**Prognosis:** Almost all result in neonatal or infant death.

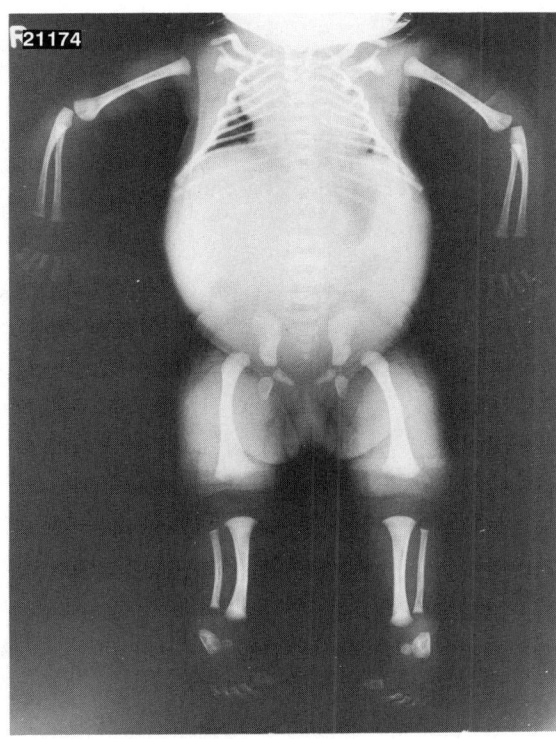

0122B-21174:  Skeletal findings in campomelic dysplasia.

**Detection of Carrier:**  Unknown.

**Special Considerations:**  Campomelia, or bending of the long bones, can be produced by a heterogeneous group of disorders. This classic or long-bone variety of campomelic dwarfism must be distinguished from various generalized bone dysplasias that can produce bending of the long bones, such as osteogenesis imperfecta and hypophosphatasia, as well as several recently described rare conditions. Thus, the campomelic syndrome appears to be a well-defined, distinct disorder that can be delineated by a variety of X-ray findings, including the long, slender, bent bones. Two apparently distinct syndromes which have been termed "short-bone varieties" of campomelic dwarfism, have been described.

The short bone craniostenotic type is characterized by campomelic limbs with short, bent bones and normal metaphyses; gross skull deformities with craniostenosis and hydrocephalus (Kleeblattschädel) and facial hypoplasia with micrognathia; slender ribs and hypoplastic scapulae; and radioulnar synostosis and precocious ossification of the carpal bones. The vertebral bodies appear square with stellate fissured centers, and there is an abnormal pelvis. The etiology of this syndrome is supportive of autosomal recessive.

In the short-bone normocephalic type, the campomelic limbs are also short and broad, but there is metaphyseal flaring or irregularity. The upper limbs are frequently bowed as well and there are 11 pairs of ribs. One pair of sibs has been reported with this syndrome, suggesting autosomal recessive inheritance. Both of these short bone varieties also result in neonatal death. Several cases of classic campomelic dsysplasia without campomelia (bent extremities) have been seen.

**References:**

Khajavi A, et al.: Heterogeneity in the campomelic syndromes. Long and short bone varieties. Radiology 1976; 120:641–647. *
Kozlowski K, et al.: Syndromes of congenital bowing of the long bones. Pediatr Radiol 1978; 7:40–48.
Tokita N, et al.: The campomelic syndrome. Temporal bone histopathalogic features and otolargngolic manifestations. Arch Otolargngol 1979; 105:449–454.
Hall BD, Spranger JW: Campomelic dysplasia. Am J Dis Child 1980; 124:285–289.
Puck SM, et al.: Absence of H-Y antigen in an XY female with campomelic dysplasia. Hum Genet 1981; 57:23–27.
Houston SC et al.: The campomelic syndrome: review, report of 17 cases, and follow-up on the current 17-year-old boy first reported by Maroteaux et al in 1971. Am J Med Genet 1983; 15:3–28. *

B0025                                                    **Zvi Borochowitz**
LA006                                                    **Ralph S. Lachman**
                                                         *David L. Rimoin*

**Campomelic syndrome**
*See CAMPOMELIC DYSPLASIA*

---

## CAMPTODACTYLY                                          2255

**Includes:**
  Dupuytren contracture, congenital
  Fingers, congenital contracture of
  Fingers, flexed
  Fingers, hammer
  Palmar clinodactyly
  Streblodactyly
  Streblomicrodactyly

**Excludes:**
  **Camptodactyly syndrome, Guadalajara type I** (2257)
  **Camptodactyly syndrome, guadalajara type ii** (2191)
  **Camptodactyly syndrome, Tel Hashomer type** (2256)
  **Contracture, dupuytren** (0301)
  Digital malformations, all other

**Major Diagnostic Criteria:**  Flexion contractures of the digits are usually present at birth, although they may not be noticed until early childhood or later. There is usally no or minimal progression of the contracture at the proximal interphalangeal joints. In most

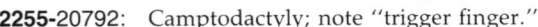

**2255-20792:** Camptodactyly; note "trigger finger."

instances, camptodactyly involves the little finger and commonly affects other fingers except the thumb. Malformation is usually bilateral. The flexed fingers are usually slender with tight skin. Contracture bands are frequently palpated beneath the skin on the volar surface of the affected joint, and the transverse skin creases in this location are lost. Dermatoglyphics are commonly abnormal.

**Clinical Findings:** Finger involvement in decreasing order of severity is as follows: fifth, fourth, third and second digits, with the thumb rarely affected. Involvement is usually bilateral and symmetrical, and may vary from mild to severe. The toes may also be involved. X-ray findings merely confirm the degree of flexion contracture.

*Streblodactyly*, from the Greek, is a related condition characterized by twisted or crooked fingers (Donofrio and Ayala, 1983).

**Complications:** Alteration in hand function depends upon the degree of involvement, but in the most cases there is little loss of function.

**Associated Findings:** Camptodactyly can occur as an isolated malformation, and is also commonly found in a number of syndromes.

**Etiology:** Isolated camptodactyly by autosomal dominant inheritance. When associated with a syndrome, the mode of transmission will depend on the etiology of the syndrome.

**Pathogenesis:** Unknown.

**MIM No.:** *11420

**CDC No.:** 755.500

**Sex Ratio:** Theoretically M1:F1, but some reports suggest females are more affected.

**Occurrence:** Undetermined but presumably relatively common.

**Risk of Recurrence for Patient's Sib:**
See Part I, *Mendelian Inheritance.*

**Risk of Recurrence for Patient's Child:**
See Part I, *Mendelian Inheritance.*

**Age of Detectability:** Possible at birth, but probably more common during childhood.

**Gene Mapping and Linkage:** Unknown.

**Prevention:** None known. Genetic counseling indicated.

**Treatment:** Nonoperative measures include physiotherapy, casts, and splints. Surgical procedures have shown discouraging results with only 35% improvement. It may be best to guide the patient to accepting the deformity, particularly if there is no severe functional disturbance.

**Prognosis:** As an isolated malformation, camptodactyly does not influence life span. Functional impairment is usually mild to moderate.

**Detection of Carrier:** Unknown.

**References:**
Goodman RM, et al.: Camptodactyly: occurrence in two new genetic syndromes and its relationship to other syndromes. J Med Genet 1972; 9:203–212.
Engber WD, Flatt AE: Camptodactyly: an analysis of sixty-six patients and twenty-four operations. J Hand Surg 1977; 2:216–224.
Temtamy, SA, McKusick VA: The genetics of hand malformations. New York: Alan R. Liss, 1978.
Hall JG, et al.: The distal anrthrogryposes: delineation of new entities: review and nosologic discussion. Am J Med Genet 1982; 11:185–239.
Donofrio P, Ayala F: Familial streblodactyly. Acta Derm Venereol 1983; 63:361–363.
Rozin MM, et al.: A new syndrome with camptodactyly, joint contractures, facial anomalies, and skeletal defects: a case report and review of syndromes with camptodactyly. Clin Genet 1984; 26:342–355.

G0026                                                                    **Richard M. Goodman**

## CAMPTODACTYLY SYNDROME, GUADALAJARA TYPE I                                    2257

**Includes:** Guadalajara camptodactyly, type I

**Excludes:**
**Camptodactyly syndrome, Guadalajara type II** (2191)
**Camptodactyly syndrome, Tel Hashomer type** (2256)
**Camptodactyly** (in other syndromes)

**Major Diagnostic Criteria:** Intrauterine growth retardation, short stature, typical facial features, camptodactyly of fingers, hallux valgus, and other skeletal anomalies.

**Clinical Findings:** Low birth weight, short stature, flat facies with ample forehead, epicanthal folds, telecanthus, microcornea, short nose with anteverted nostrils, long philtrum, microstomia, abnormal dental eruption and malocclusion, small low-set ears, **Pectus excavatum**, small pelvis, cubitus valgus, **Syndactyly, Camptodactyly** of fingers 2–5, short feet with an increased space between toes 1 and 2, bilateral hallux valgus, pigmented nevi, normal intelligence.

X-ray findings are frontal and ethmoidal sinus agenesis, prognathism, cuboid vertebral bodies, spina bifida occulta, gynecoanthropoid pelvis, hypoplastic iliac bones, tubular-shaped metacarpal bones, hypoplasia of metacarpal bones, hypoplasia of the second phalanx, fibular hypoplasia, mild metaphyseal broadening, interphalangeal subluxation of the first toe, bilateral hallux valgus.

**Complications:** Unknown.

**Associated Findings:** Microphthalmia, **Myopia, congenital**, decreased visual acuity.

**Etiology:** Possibly autosomal recessive inheritance.

**Pathogenesis:** Unknown.

**MIM No.:** 21191

**POS No.:** 4313

**Sex Ratio:** Presumably M1:F1 (two female sibs were originally reported).

**Occurrence:** Undetermined but presumed rare. Reported in two sister of a Mexican family.

**Risk of Recurrence for Patient's Sib:**
See Part I, *Mendelian Inheritance.*

**Risk of Recurrence for Patient's Child:**
See Part I, *Mendelian Inheritance.*

**Age of Detectability:** At birth.

**Gene Mapping and Linkage:** Unknown.

**Prevention:** None known. Genetic counseling indicated.

**Treatment:** Plastic surgery for the camptodactyly.

**Prognosis:** Apparently normal life span.

**Detection of Carrier:** Unknown.

**References:**

Cantú JM, et al.: Guadalajara camptodactyly syndrome: a distinct probably autosomal recessive disorder. Clin Genet 1980; 18:153–159.

Cantú JM, et al.: Guadalajara camptodactyly syndrome. (Abstract) Jerusalem: Sixth Int Cong Hum Genet, 1981:263.

Rozin MM, et al.: A new syndrome with camptodactyly, joint contractures, facial anomalies, and skeletal defects: a case report and review of syndromes with camptodactyly. Clin Genet 1984; 26:342–355.

CR019                       **Diana García-Cruz**
CA011                       **José María Cantú**

## CAMPTODACTYLY SYNDROME, GUADALAJARA TYPE II     2191

**Includes:** Guadalajara camptodactyly

**Excludes:** Camptodactyly syndrome, Guadalajara type I (2257)

**Major Diagnostic Criteria:** Prenatal onset of short stature, **Microcephaly**, hypotelorism, unusual facies, and multiple skeletal defects including **Camptodactyly** of all fingers and hypoplasia of genitalia and gluteal areas.

**Clinical Findings:** Based on two known sibs and one sporadic case with histories of intrauterine growth retardation, and dwarfism: microcephaly, unusual facies with ocular hypotelorism, long philtrum, micrognathia and short neck, large and low-set ears, **Pectus excavatum**, and widely spaced nipples. Limb defects include hypotrophic limbs, camptodactyly of all fingers, simian creases, altered dermatoglyphics, limited pronation and supination movements, **Foot, talipes equinovarus (TEV)**, prominent tallus, bilateral hallux valgus, **Brachydactyly** of second, fourth and fifth toes, and patellar hypoplasia; and hypoplasia of the pubic region involving labia minora and majora and hypoplasia of gluteal area.

X-ray findings include microcephaly, cuboid vertebral bodies, hypoplasia of iliac and ischiopubic bones, slender long bones with growth delay bands, patellar hypoplasia, generalized osteopenia, delayed bone age and brachydactyly of digits of toes and second metatarsal.

**Complications:** Unknown.

**Associated Findings:** None known.

**Etiology:** Possibly autosomal recessive inheritance.

**Pathogenesis:** Unknown.

**MIM No.:** 21192

**POS No.:** 4412

**Sex Ratio:** Presumably M1:F1; in the reported family two female sibs were affected.

**Occurrence:** One family, of Mexican origin, with two affected daughters has been reported.

**Risk of Recurrence for Patient's Sib:**
See Part I, *Mendelian Inheritance.*

**Risk of Recurrence for Patient's Child:**
See Part I, *Mendelian Inheritance.* Very unlikely in the absence of consanguinity.

**Age of Detectability:** Theoretically at birth, but more likely during early childhood.

**Gene Mapping and Linkage:** Unknown.

**Prevention:** None known. Genetic counseling indicated.

**Treatment:** Symptomatic care.

**Prognosis:** Unknown.

**Detection of Carrier:** Unknown.

**References:**

Cantú JM, et al.: Guadalajara camptodactyly syndrome. Clin Genet 1980; 18:153–159.

Rozin MM, et al.: A new syndrome with camtodactyly, joint contrac-

tures, facial anomalies, and skeletal defects: a case report and review of syndromes with camptodactyly. Clin Genet 1984; 26:342–355.

Cantú JM, et al.: Guadalajara camptodactyly syndrome type II. Clin Genet 1985; 28:54–60.

G0026                       **Richard M. Goodman**

## CAMPTODACTYLY SYNDROME, TEL HASHOMER TYPE     2256

**Includes:**
Camptodactyly-muscular hypoplasia-skeletal and palmar anomalies
Tel-Hashomer camptodactyly syndrome

**Excludes:**
Camptodactyly (2255)
Camptodactyly syndrome, Guadalajara type I (2257)
Camptodactyly syndrome, guadalajara type ii (2191)
Camptodactyly (in any other syndrome)

**Major Diagnostic Criteria:** Camptodactyly involving mainly the fingers, distinct facial features with multiple musculoskeletal defects, characteristic dermatoglyphic changes.

**Clinical Findings:** *Stature*: short. *Skull*: brachycephaly, prominent forehead. *Facies*: asymmetry, ocular hypertelorism, small mouth, high-arched palate, increased philtrum length, dental crowding. *Chest*: thoracic scoliosis, winging of scapulae. *Extremities*: **Camptodactyly**, **Syndactyly**, clinodactyly, **Brachydactyly** of thumbs, spindle-shaped fingers, abnormal handprints, dislocated radii, clubbed feet, pes planus, malformed toes. *Muscular system*: hypoplasia of chest, pelvis, and limb and hand muscles.

The dermatoglyphic changes have tended to be characteristic, showing an increase in whorls that extend beyond the borders of the terminal phalanges; a low mainline index resulting from a vertical orientation of the A-D radiants; and numerous palmar creases obliterating the normal structure of the ridges and openings of the sweat pores.

**Complications:** Various musculoskeletal problems involving mainly the feet and spine.

**Associated Findings:** None known.

**Etiology:** Autosomal recessive inheritance. In most reported cases, the parents have been consanguineous.

**Pathogenesis:** Probably a myopathy. A raised creatine kinase level, an abnormal electromyogram, and an abnormal muscle biopsy specimen were noted in one patient. The histology of the muscle biopsy specimen showed fiber diameter in type 1 and type 2 range, with a relative deficiency of type 2b fibers.

**MIM No.:** *21196

**POS No.:** 3051

**Sex Ratio:** M1:F1

**Occurrence:** Undetermined but presumed rare. Less than a dozen cases from six families have been reported in the literature.

**Risk of Recurrence for Patient's Sib:**
See Part I, *Mendelian Inheritance.*

**Risk of Recurrence for Patient's Child:**
See Part I, *Mendelian Inheritance.*

**Age of Detectability:** At birth. Prenatal diagnosis is possible using ultrasound.

**Gene Mapping and Linkage:** Unknown.

**Prevention:** None known. Genetic counseling indicated.

**Treatment:** Surgical correction of skeletal problems.

**Prognosis:** Life span does not appear to be reduced.

**Detection of Carrier:** Unknown.

**References:**

Goodman RM, et al.: Camptodactyly occurrence in two new genetic syndromes and its relationship to other syndromes. J Med Genet 1972; 9:203–212.

Goodman RM, et al.: Camptodactyly with muscular hypoplasia,

skeletal dysplasia and abnormal palmar creases: Tel-Hashomer camptodactyly syndrome. J Med Genet 1976; 13:136–141.

Gollop TR, Colletto SMDD: The Tel Hashomer camptodactyly syndrome in a consanguineous Brazilian family. Am J Med Genet 1984; 17:399–406.

Patton MA, et al.: Tel-Hashomer camptodactyly syndrome: report of a case with myopathic features. J Med Genet 1986; 23:268–270.

Tylki-Szymanska A: Three new cases of Tel-Hashomer camptodactyly syndrome in one Arabic family. Am J Med Genet 1986; 23:759–763.

Pagnan NAB, et al.: The Tel Hashomer camptodactyly syndrome: report of a new case and review of the literature. Am J Med Genet 1988; 29:411–417.

G0026

**Richard M. Goodman**

**Camptodactyly, facultative type**
 *See* CAMPTODACTYLY-TRISMUS SYNDROME
**Camptodactyly-arthropathy syndrome**
 *See* SYNOVITIS, FAMILIAL HYPERTROPHIC

---

## CAMPTODACTYLY-CLEFT PALATE-CLUB FOOT, GORDON TYPE     2396

**Includes:**
 Arthrogryposis multiplex congenita, distal, type IIA
 Distal arthrogryposis, type IIA
 Gordon syndrome

**Excludes:**
 **Arthrogryposis, distal types** (2280)
 **Arachnodactyly, contractural Beals type** (0085)
 Camptodactyly and cleft palate syndromes, other

**Major Diagnostic Criteria:** Camptodactyly and clubfeet, frequently associated with cleft palate.

**Clinical Findings:** Varying combinations of **Camptodactyly** (90%), clubfeet (75%), and **Cleft palate** (30%).

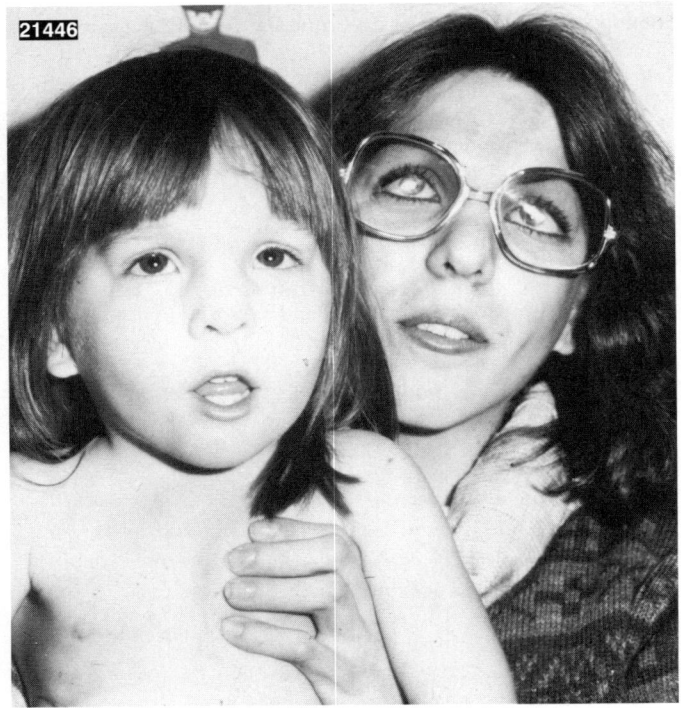

**2396A-**21446: Striking facial resemblance in this affected mother and daughter.

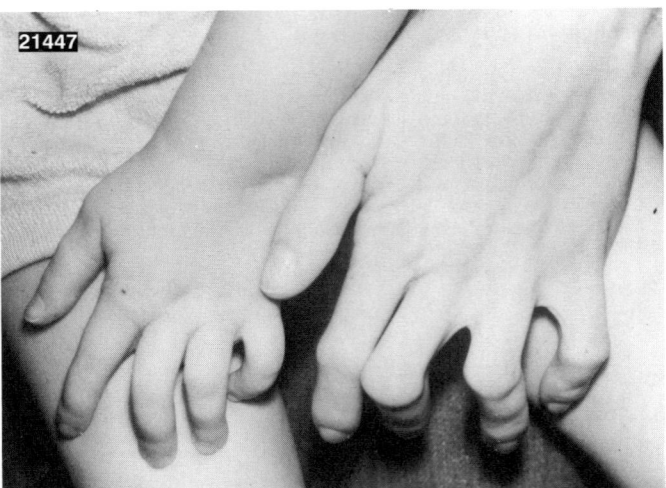

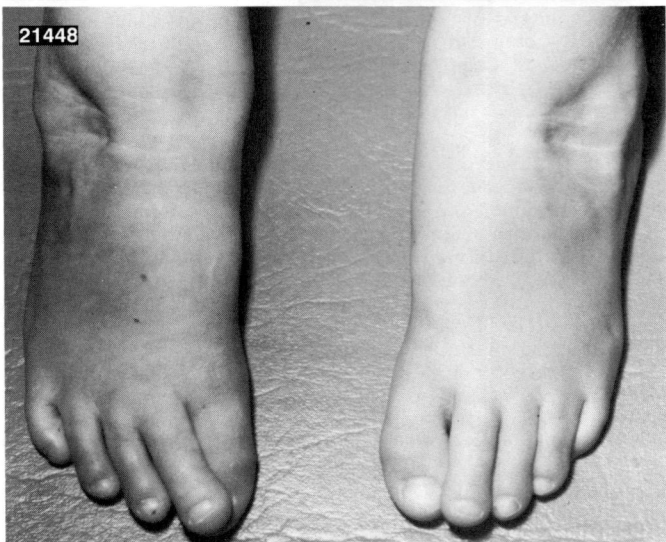

**2396B-**21447: Camptodactyly of the hands in a mother and daughter. 21448: Clubfeet of the mother after several operations.

---

**Complications:** Usually orthopedic in nature. In some of the reported cases, camptodactyly and clubfeet were quite severe, requiring casting of long duration and multiple surgical corrections.

**Associated Findings:** Short stature, **Syndactyly**, dermatoglyphic abnormalities, undescended testes, stenosis of spinal canal, and narrowed intervertebral spaces.

**Etiology:** Autosomal dominant inheritance with incomplete penetrance and variable expressivity.

**Pathogenesis:** Unknown.

**MIM No.:** *11430

**POS No.:** 3166

**Sex Ratio:** M1:F1

**Occurrence:** Five families with 38 affected members have been reported.

**Risk of Recurrence for Patient's Sib:**
 See Part I, *Mendelian Inheritance.*

**Risk of Recurrence for Patient's Child:**
 See Part I, *Mendelian Inheritance.*

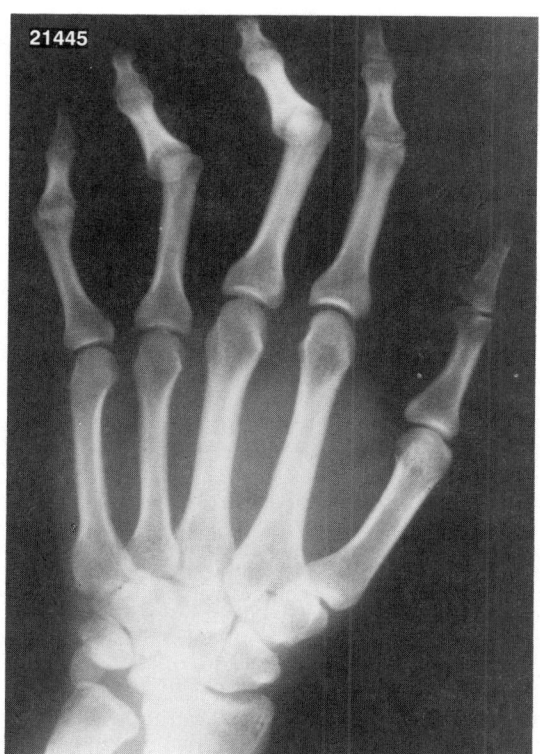

**2396C-21445:** X-ray of the hand shows joint deformities.

Camptodactyly-limited jaw excursion
*See CAMPTODACTYLY-TRISMUS SYNDROME*
Camptodactyly-muscular hypoplasia-skeletal and palmar anomalies
*See CAMPTODACTYLY SYNDROME, TEL HASHOMER TYPE*
Camptodactyly-pericarditis-arthritis
*See PERICARDITIS-ARTHRITIS-CAMPTODACTYLY*

## CAMPTODACTYLY-TRISMUS SYNDROME    0882

**Includes:**
>Camptodactyly-limited jaw excursion
>Camptodactyly, facultative type
>Finger flexor tendons, short
>Hecht syndrome
>Jaw excursion, limitation of
>Mouth, inability to open completely-camptodactyly
>Trismus-pseudocamptodactyly

**Excludes:**
>**Camptodactyly** (see others)
>**Cranio-carpo-tarsal dysplasia, whistling face type** (0223)

**Major Diagnostic Criteria:** Shortening of the flexor tendons of the wrist or deformity of the feet, with inability to open the mouth fully.

**Clinical Findings:** Characterized by inability to open the mouth fully, and curved fingers (camptodactyly) that occur at all the interphalangeal joints on dorsiflexion of the wrist. Volar flexion of the wrist allows complete extension of the fingers; forearm flexor tendons are short. Deformities of the feet also occur, including combinations of talipes equinovarus, pes planus, metatarsus varus, and calcaneovalgus. The gastrocnemii and hamstrings are often short. The latter cause a pelvic tilt. The affected individuals

**Age of Detectability:** At birth.

**Gene Mapping and Linkage:** Unknown.

**Prevention:** None known. Genetic counseling indicated.

**Treatment:** Mainly surgical for skeletal abnormalities and cleft palate. Psychotherapeutic intervention may be required during childhood for patients with severe malformations and deformations. Speech therapy may also be needed.

**Prognosis:** Rehabilitation varies depending on the severity of the limb deficiencies. Prognosis appears to be good for mental development and life span.

**Detection of Carrier:** Unknown.

**Special Considerations:** Hall et al (1982) has designated this condition *Distal arthrogryposis, type IIA* (see **Arthrogryposis, distal types**), and suggested that the first case was reported by Moldenhauer (1964), and that the disorder was also present in the case reported by Krieger and Espiritu (1972).

**References:**
Moldenhauer E: Zur klinik des Nielson-syndromes. Derm Wschr 1964; 150:594–601.
Gordon H, et al.: Camptodactyly, cleft palate, and club feet. J Med Genet 1969; 6:266–274.
Krieger I, Espiritu CE: Athrogryposis multiplex congenita and the Turner phenotype. Am J Dis Child 1972; 123:141–144.
Halal F, Fraser C: Camptodactyly, cleft palate and clubfoot (the Gordon syndrome). J Med Genet 1977; 16:149–150.
Say B, et al.: The Gordon syndrome. J Med Genet 1980; 17:405. *
Robinow M, Johnson, GF: The Gordon syndrome: autosomal dominant cleft palate, camptodactyly and clubfeet. Am J Med Genet 1981; 9:139–146. *
Hall JG, et al.: The distal arthrogryposis: delineation of new entities. Am J Med Genet 1982; 11:185–239.

SA033                                    **Burhan Say**

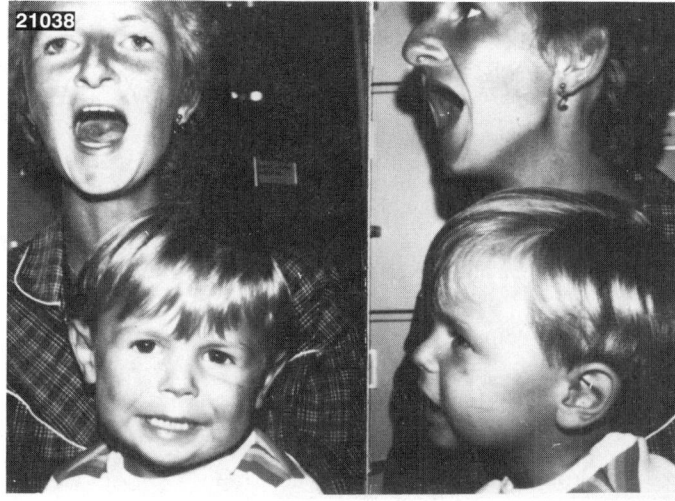
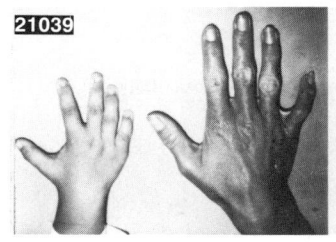
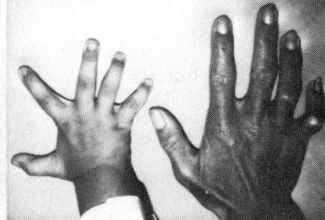

**0882-21038:** Camptodactyly-trismus syndrome in an affected mother and son; note the maximal opening of their mouths. **21039:** Pseudocamptodactyly; dorsiflexion of the hands on the right shows flexion of the fingers.

are all below the third percentile in height. Intelligence is normal. Mild torticollis is described.

**Complications:**  Difficulty with eating and locomotion.

**Associated Findings:**  One 13-day-old died of intestinal obstruction.

**Etiology:**  Autosomal dominant inheritance.

**Pathogenesis:**  Unknown.

**MIM No.:**  *15830

**POS No.:**  3017

**Sex Ratio:**  M1:F1

**Occurrence:**  At least 35 cases described in the literature. Described in at least two kindreds and through four generations. Many of the cases are of Dutch ancestry, including United States cases which trace back to a Dutch girl who migrated to Tennessee soon after the American Revolution.

**Risk of Recurrence for Patient's Sib:**
See Part I, *Mendelian Inheritance.*

**Risk of Recurrence for Patient's Child:**
See Part I, *Mendelian Inheritance.*

**Age of Detectability:**  In infancy.

**Gene Mapping and Linkage:**  Unknown.

**Prevention:**  None known. Genetic counseling indicated.

**Treatment:**  Orthopedic care for the foot deformities. Surgery has not been required for the flexor tendon shortening of the wrist.

**Prognosis:**  Good for normal life span and intelligence. Variable for function.

**Detection of Carrier:**  Unknown.

**Special Considerations:**  The cause of the inability to fully open the mouth has not been established.

**References:**
Hecht F, Beals RK: Inability to open the mouth fully: an autosomal dominant phenotype with facultative campylodactyly and short stature (preliminary note). BD:OAS V(3). New York: National Foundation-March of Dimes, 1969:96–98.
Wilson RV, et al.: Autosomal dominant inheritance of shortening of the flexor profundus muscle-tendon unit with limitation of jaw excursion. BD:OAS V(3). New York: The National Foundation-March of Dimes, 1969:99–102.
De Jong, JGY: A family showing strongly reduced ability to open mouth and limitation of some movements of the extremities. Humangenetik 1971; 13:210–217.
Mabry CC, et al.: Trismus pseudocamptodactyly syndrome: Dutch-Kentucky syndrome. J Pediat 1974; 85:503–508.
Hall JG, et al.: The distal arthrogryposes: delineation of new entries: review and nosologic discussion. Am J Med Genet 1982; 11:185–239.
Tsukahara M, et al.: Trismus-pseudocamptodactyly syndrome in a Japanese family. Clin Genet 1985; 28:247–250.

OS001                                                         **A. Lee Osterman**

**Camurati-Engelmann syndrome**
  *See DIAPHYSEAL DYSPLASIA*
**Canavan disease**
  *See BRAIN, SPONGY DEGENERATION*
**Cancer (lymphoreticular)-immunodeficiency-microcephaly**
  *See CHROMOSOME INSTABILITY, NIJMEGEN TYPE*
**Cancer family syndrome**
  *See CANCER, SEBACEOUS GLAND TUMOR-MULTIPLE VISCERAL CARCINOMA*
**Cancer family syndrome (some cases)**
  *See CANCER, BREAST, FAMILIAL*
**Cancer family syndrome, Lynch syndrome II**
  *See CANCER, COLORECTAL*
**Cancer of the colon**
  *See CANCER, COLORECTAL*
**Cancer of the esophagus-palmo-plantar keratoderma**
  *See HOWEL EVANS SYNDROME*

**Includes:**
  Breast cancer, familial, site-specific
  Cancer family syndrome (some cases)
  Li-Fraumeni syndrome (some cases)
  Lynch syndrome II (some cases)
  Sarcoma family syndrome of Li and Fraumeni (some cases)
  SBLA syndrome (some cases)

**Excludes:**
  Cancer, familial (1505)
  Gingival multiple hamartoma syndrome (0412)
  Klinefelter syndrome (0556)

**Major Diagnostic Criteria:**  Presence of three first-degree relatives with breast cancer, usually adenocarcinoma of the female breast, without an alternate explanation and generally without other relatives with dissimilar cell types. Age at diagnosis is an important element in making a diagnosis that, ultimately, is largely based on intuition.

**Clinical Findings:**  Since one of every 10 of American women gets breast cancer in their lifetime, many family members may, by chance, have breast cancer. Making a diagnosis depends, in part, on criteria that have derived from studying Mendelian traits that predispose to cancer, such at retinoblastoma, early age at diagnosis, affected male relatives, bilaterality, and members with multiple primary cancers. Two elderly sisters with breast cancer may well represent a chance occurrence, whereas three middle-aged sisters are notable, and two brothers affected in their thirties would be rare indeed.

**Complications:**  Most series suggest that the types of breast cancers do not differ from sporadic tumors in clinical presentation, response to therapy, histologic pattern, and prognosis. One series suggested that lobular carcinoma occurs in slight excess compared with other cell types; but lobular cancers generally do occur at a young age.

**Associated Findings:**  None known.

**Etiology:**  Mathematical modeling shows that some families fit the single gene inheritance of the dominant trait, whereas others are multifactorial.
  Familial breast cancer may be passed by unaffected males just as by affected females. In other words, a positive paternal family history is as relevant as a positive maternal history.

**Pathogenesis:**  Among adult cancers, breast cancer is the tumor with the greatest familial aggregation, which of course could arise from shared environmental determinants, the action of major or minor genes, or, most likely, the interaction of environmental and genetic influences (ecogenetics). Great etiologic and genetic heterogeneity has been recognized, and so the differential diagnosis would include **Klinefelter syndrome**, the *Cancer family syndrome* or *Lynch syndrome II* (Abusamra et al, 1987), the *Li-Fraumeni* or *SBLA syndrome* (Lynch et al, 1985), and the **Gingival multiple hamartoma syndrome**.
  Elevated risk for breast cancer is associated with early menarche and late age at first full-time pregnancy and natural menopause; it is reduced in women with early loss of an ovarian function due to surgery. Hence, *endogenous* female sex hormones seem to increase the breast cancer risk, whereas the association of *exogenous* estogen use (for example, for menopausal symptoms) is controversially related to breast cancer risk.
  Early metabolic studies suggested that an elevated estriol-to-estrone ratio and estradiol urinary fractions were important metabolic determinants of breast cancer risk that might have a genetic basis. *In vitro* studies of cultured skin biopsy material showed an excess of tetraploidy in endothelial outgrowths and fetal-like behavior of fibroblasts from women with or at high risk of hereditary breast cancer compared with biopsy material from healthy controls. Some premenopausal breast cancers have lost molecular heterogeneity, indicating a role of recessive mutation on chromosome 13.

**MIM No.:**  *11371, *11440, 11448

**Sex Ratio:** Largely females, but some males, especially with **Klinefelter syndrome**, are affected.

**Occurrence:** Genetic determinants are important in a substantial but unclear fraction of the estimated 100,000 new cases of breast cancer in the United States each year. In one oncology clinic, 5% of breast cancer patients had two or more relatives within the nuclear family who also had breast cancer.

**Risk of Recurrence for Patient's Sib:** Varies with etiology, but may be as high as 1:2 among sisters of an affected person. Since autosomal dominant inheritance has not been proved, it is best to counsel using empiric risk estimates, which vary with age of onset and family pattern; the highest risk is 39-fold when a sister had breast cancer under age 40 years and their mother also had breast cancer. Additional factors, not necessarily of genetic origin, may further increase the risk, for example, proliferative fibrocystic disease and nulliparity.

A strategy for calculating the absolute risk has been developed (Mulvihill et al, 1982), which advises multiplying the individual relative risks together, along with age-specific annual incidence in the general population. Experience and empiric data have shown that multiplying risk factors usually produces an overestimate of the relative risk, so the individual risk elements should be added together *before* multiplying by the incidence. The risk estimate is best done in five-year intervals, because the age-specific incidence increases with age, whereas the relative risk for family history decreases.

**Risk of Recurrence for Patient's Child:** Varies with etiology, but may be as high as 1:2 among daughters of an affected woman. As for sibs, empiric recurrence risk estimates for children vary, reaching as much as tenfold.

**Age of Detectability:** Twenty percent of all sporadic breast cancers are diagnosed under age 50 years. In general, familial breast cancer occurs at a younger-than-average age, and is more often bilateral.

**Gene Mapping and Linkage:** BCEI (breast cancer, estrogen-inducible sequence expressed in) has been mapped to 21q22.3.

**Prevention:** Persons at high risk are advised to minimize their other risk factors and to participate in reasonable screening efforts (monthly self-examination, semiannual examination by a breast cancer surgeon, a baseline mammogram by age 30 years, and then annually thereafter.) Prophylactic mastectomy (simple or subcutaneous procedures with reconstruction) may be considered by women at highest risk because of prior breast cancer, severe proliferative fibrocystic disease, or cancer phobia often arising from a strong family history.

**Treatment:** Treatment of familial breast cancer should be identical to that of sporadic breast cancer.

**Prognosis:** Despite one report that familial breast cancer patients have a better prognosis, it is likely to be a small advantage, not sufficient to alter therapy.

**Detection of Carrier:** No clinically useful bioassays are available.

**Special Considerations:** Mothers of children with sarcomas have a threefold risk of breast cancer, probably as part of the *Li-Fraumeni cancer family syndrome*. Carriers of one mutant gene for **Ataxia-telangiectasia** are estimated to have a 6.8 relative risk of breast cancer, and, given a frequency of 1.4% of such heterozygotes in the United States population, about 9% of breast cancer may occur in association with the ataxia telangiectasia gene.

Updated versions of the individualized probabilities for breast cancer can be obtained from Dr. John J. Mulvihill at the National Cancer Institute of the United States National Institutes of Health in Bethesda, MD.

**Support Groups:** Atlanta; American Cancer Society

**References:**

Lynch HT, ed: Genetics and breast cancer. New York: Van Nostrand Reinhold, 1981. *

Mulvihill JJ, et al.: Prevention in familial breast cancer: counseling and prophylactic mastectomy. Prev Med 1982; 11:500–511. *

Ottman R, et al.: Practical guide for estimating risk for familial breast cancer. Lancet 1983; II:556–558.

Brinton LA: The relationship of exogenous estrogens to cancer risk. Cancer Detect Prevent 1984; 7:159–171.

Lynch HT, et al.: The sarcoma, breast cancer, lung cancer, and adrenocortical carcinoma syndrome revisited. Am J Dis Child 1985; 139:134–136.

Bailey-Wilson JE, et al.: Genetic analysis of human breast cancer: a synthesis of contributions to GAW IV. Genet Epidemiol (suppl) 1986; 1:15–35.

Hartley AL, et al.: Breast cancer risk in mothers of children with osteosarcoma and chondrosarcoma. Br J Cancer 1986; 54:819–823.

Abusamra H, et al.: Cancer family syndrome of Lynch. Am J Med 1987; 83:981–983.

Haggie JA, et al.: Fibroblasts from relatives of patients with hereditary breast cancer show fetal-like behaviour in vitro. Lancet 1987; I:1455–1457.

Lundberg C, et al.: Loss of heterozygosity in human ductal breast tumors indicates a recessive mutation on chromosome 13. Proc Natl Acad Sci USA 1987; 84:2372–2376.

O'Malley MS, Fletcher SW: Screening for breast cancer with breast self-examination: a critical review. J Am Med Asso 1987; 257:2197–2208.

Swift M, et al.: Breast and other cancers in families with ataxia-telangiectasia. New Engl J Med 1987; 316:1289–1294.

Hall JM, et al.: Oncogenes and human breast cancer. Am J Hum Genet 1989; 44:577–584.

Slamon DJ, et al.: Studies of the HER-2/neu proto-oncogene in human breast and ovarian cancer. Science 1989; 244:707–712.

MU009                                                    **John J. Mulvihill**

---

**CANCER, COLORECTAL**                                          **2343**

**Includes:**

Cancer family syndrome, Lynch syndrome II
Cancer of the colon
Colorectal cancer
Hereditary nonpolyposis colorectal cancer (HNPCC)
Nonpolyposis colerectal cancer, hereditary Lynch sydromes
Site-specific colorectal cancer, Lynch syndrome I
Solitary polyp syndrome

**Excludes:**

Intestinal polyposis, juvenile type (2259)
Intestinal polyposis, type I (0535)
Intestinal polyposis, type II (2344)
Intestinal polyposis, type III (0536)

**Major Diagnostic Criteria:** Colorectal cancer is a histologic diagnosis. Although the findings on barium enema and colonoscopy may be strongly suggestive, confirmatory histology of tissue obtained endoscopically or surgically is mandatory.

Hereditary nonpolyposis colorectal cancer (HNPCC) is an inherited subtype of colorectal cancer. It is defined as the occurrence of highly penetrant, autosomally dominant inherited colorectal cancer without the adenomatous polyposis trait. HNPCC is divided into hereditary site-specific colorectal cancer (*Lynch syndrome I*), and cancer family syndrome (*Lynch syndrome II*). Lynch syndrome I consists of the inherited colon cancer phenotype, while Lynch syndrome II includes this phenotype and certain extracolonic cancers, particularly carcinoma of the endometrium and ovary. Gastric, small bowel, pancreatic, urologic and laryngeal malignancies have also been noted to occur in certain pedigrees.

**Clinical Findings:** Colorectal cancer is a disease of later life. Ninety-three percent of cases occur after age 50 years. The average age of diagnosis is 62–65 years.

Early stage colorectal cancer is usually asymptomatic. More advanced tumors are characterized by changes in bowel habit, rectal bleeding, abdominal pain, anemia, anorexia, weight loss, and malaise. Changes in bowel habits, abdominal pain, and visible rectal bleeding are more characteristic of distal or "left-sided" colonic cancer, while anemia without visible rectal bleeding favors a diagnosis of proximal colonic cancer. Generalized symptoms such as anorexia, weight loss, and malaise often portend advanced tumors. The anatomic distribution of colorectal cancer is: rectum, 22%; rectosigmoid, 10%; sigmoid, 25%; descending colon, 6%; transverse colon, 13%; ascending colon, 8%; cecum, 15%; and appendix, 1%.

HNPCC, both Lynch syndromes I and II, differs from other colon cancers in that the average age of diagnosis is 44 years. HNPCC also exhibits a predilection to cancers of the proximal colon, and an increase in synchronous and metachronous colon cancers. Although adenomatous polyposis is not present in HNPCC, one or several adenomatous polyps are often observed in affected individuals.

**Complications:** Colonic obstruction, perforation, volvulus, and intussusception may all occur. Fistulas sometimes develop between the colon and other abdominal organs. Colonic tumors may compress or invade adjacent organs, and distant metastases are most frequently found in the liver, lungs, bones, and brain. Complications referable to the extracolonic malignancies of Lynch syndrome II also occur in that syndrome.

**Associated Findings:** Elevated serum carcinoembryonic antigen (CEA) is found in many patients with colorectal cancer, and has a role in detecting early recurrences. However, the test is not useful diagnostically, because it is insensitive, particularly to early-stage tumors, and because it is nonspecific.

**Etiology:** Most if not all colorectal cancers arise from adenomatous polyps. Clinically detectable polyps are present in 10–15% of adults over 40 years of age in the United States.

Population and migration studies suggest that environmental factors are important to the etiology of colorectal cancer. Diets high in fat and low in fiber are correlated with an increased incidence of colon cancer.

Hereditary factors likewise appear to be etiologically important. There are inherited syndromes of colon cancer and familial clustering of colon cancer cases in general. The inherited syndromes include the colonic adenomatous polyposis conditions, familial adenomatous polyposis and Gardner syndrome, and the HNPCC syndromes, Lynch Syndromes I and II. The polyposis syndromes are reviewed in other chapters. They account for less than 1% of colon cancer cases. The HNPCC syndromes account for approximately 6% of colon cancers. The importance of environmental factors in these inherited syndromes remains to be determined.

Population genetic studies demonstrate that first-degree relatives of those with colon cancer exhibit a two to three-fold increased risk for colon malignancy in general. A similar risk is observed in first-degree relatives of individuals with colonic adenomatous polyps, the precursor lesions of colon cancer. Genetic epidemiologic studies in pedigrees suggest that this common familial clustering probably occurs on the basis of partially penetrant inherited susceptibility factors. The responsible gene (or genes) appears to be common (estimated gene frequency of 19%) and accounts for a significant fraction of clinically observed adenomas. Environmental factors likely interact with inherited susceptibility factors to allow expression of polyps and cancer.

A small number of colon cancer cases arise from inflammatory bowel disease, which also exhibits some familial clustering.

**Pathogenesis:** Adenomatous polyps and colon cancers arise as a clone of cells in which mutational events take place. Adenoma cells exhibit hypomethylation of DNA, which may contribute to nondisjunction and chromosomal aberrations in some cases. As the polyps grow and undergo malignant change, DNA sequence deletions are often found in consistent locations on chromosomes 5, 17, and 18. Expression of the ras oncogenes is also frequently observed. The chromosome 5 deletion is at or near the 5q locus of adenomatous polyposis, which is thought to regulate expression of the c-myc oncogene. The deletion on chromosome 17 is thought to represent mutations of the gene for the transformation-associated protein, p53.

**MIM No.:** 11450, 10558

**Sex Ratio:** M3:F2; M1:F1 if colon and rectal cancers are combined.

**Occurrence:** 58.2:100,000 cases per year for males; 42.6:100,000 cases per year for females.

**Risk of Recurrence for Patient's Sib:**
See Part I, *Mendelian Inheritance*. In general, a three-fold increased risk over that expected by chance is observed among sibs of colon cancer patients. In HNPCC, the risk approaches 50%.

**Risk of Recurrence for Patient's Child:**
See Part I, *Mendelian Inheritance*. In general, a three-fold increased risk over that expected by chance is observed among first-degree relatives of colon cancer patients. In HNPCC the risk approaches 50%.

**Age of Detectability:** Ninety-three percent of colorectal cancer cases are diagnosed after 40 years of age. The age of diagnosis in well defined inherited syndromes is 10–20 years younger than expected in the general population.

**Gene Mapping and Linkage:** The inherited polyposis conditions have been mapped to 5q21–22. Lynch syndrome II exhibits linkage to JK blood group on chromosome 18. The molecular results of these mutations are not known. The purported susceptibility gene (or genes) for common inherited susceptibility has not been mapped.

**Prevention:** A high-fiber, low-fat diet has been recommended as possibly preventative in nonsyndromic colon cancer. Screening is also advocated by many because asymptomatic cancers are usually curable, while symptomatic tumors are often metastatic and not curable. The purpose of screening is both to detect malignancies while they are still curable, and to detect and remove adenomatous polyps before they undergo maligant change.

If one first-degree relative is affected with colon cancer, screening should begin by 35–40 years of age and include an annual digital rectal exam and fecal occult blood test, and proctosigmoidoscopy every three to five years. If two first-degree relatives are affected, screening should consist of an annual fecal occult blood test and colonoscopy every three to five years beginning by age 35–40 years, or at an age five years younger than the age of the earliest colon cancer in relatives, whichever comes first. If three or more first-degree relatives are affected but do not have polyposis coli, HNPCC should be the presumed diagnosis. An inherited syndrome should be suspected if colon cancer is diagnosed at an age younger than 30 years.

Those at risk for HNPCC should have a fecal occult blood test annually and full colonoscopy every two years beginning at age 25, or beginning at an age five years younger than the age of the earliest colon cancer diagnosis in the family. Colonoscopy should be done annually after age 35.

**Treatment:** Surgical resection is the primary treatment. When the cancer is unresectable, chemotherapy and radiation protocols are of limited benefit. Subtotal colectomy is the surgical procedure of choice for individuals with HNPCC.

**Prognosis:** If cancer is confined to the bowel wall, the five-year survival is 95%. If cancer involves serosa and mesenteric fat, the five-year survival is 80%. If lymph node metastases are present, the five-year survival is 40%. If distant metastases are present, the five-year survival is negligible. The presence of chromosome 17 and 18 deletions in cancer tissues have been associated with distant metastasis.

**Detection of Carrier:** Unknown. DNA markers may soon be available for adenomatous polyposis.

**Special Considerations:** The etiology of adenomatous polyps, the precursor of colorectal cancer, is not understood. Five to ten percent of United States adults harbor polyps large enough to have some cancer risk. Studies addressing cancer and polyp etiology should clarify environmental and genetic risk. More specific guidelines for polyp and cancer detection in those with a family history of colonic cancer or polyps will then evolve.

**Support Groups:** Atlanta; American Cancer Society

**References:**
Winawer SJ, et al.: Surveillance and early diagnosis of colorectal cancer. Cancer Detect Prevent 1985: 8:373–392.
Fearon ER, et al.: Clonal analysis of human colorectal tumors. Science 1987; 238:193–197.
Cannon-Albright LA, et al.: Common inheritance of susceptibility to

colonic adenomatous polyps and associated colorectal cancers. New Engl J Med 1988; 319:533–537. *

Lynch HT, et al.: Natural history of colorectal cancer in hereditary nonpolyposis colorectal cancer (Lynch syndromes I and II). Dis Colon Rectum 1988; 31:439–444. *

Vogelstein B, et al.: Genetic alterations during colorectal tumor development. New Engl J Med 1988; 319:525–532. *

Baker SJ, et al.: Chromosome 17 deletions and p53 gene mutations in colorectal carcinomas. Science 1989; 244:217–221.

Bresalier RS, Kim YS: Malignant neoplasms of the large and small intestine. In: Sleisenger MH, Fordtran JS, eds: Gastrointestinal disease, Philadelphia, W.B. Saunders, 1989:1519–1560. * †

Erisman MD, et al.: Evidence that the familial adenomatous polyposis gene is involved in a subset of colon cancers with a complementable defect in c-myc regulation. Proc Natl Sci 1989; 86:4264–4268.

Fleischer DE, et al.: Detection and surveillance of colorectal cancer. J Am Med Asso 1989; 261:580–609.

Vogelstein B, et al.: Allelotype of colorectal carcinomas. Science 1989; 244:207–211.

Fearon ER, et al.: Identification of a chromosome 18q gene that is altered in colorectal cancers. Science 1990; 247:49–56.

BU036
LY000

**Randall W. Burt**
**Henry T. Lynch**

## CANCER, EWING SARCOMA                                      3112

**Includes:**

    Askin tumor
    Ewing sarcoma of bone
    Neuroblastoma, adult
    Neuroepithelioma
    Peripheral neuroblastoma

**Excludes:**

    **Cancer, neuroblastoma** (2736)
    **Cancer, soft tissue sarcoma** (2749)
    **Osteosarcoma** (3101)

**Major Diagnostic Criteria:**  Ewing sarcoma is the second most common tumor of bone primarily afflicting children and young adults. This tumor can involve any bone in the body but is most frequently found either in an extremity (60%), the pelvis (18%), or a rib (8%). Diagnosis is routinely made by clinical presentation and histologic examination. Because of its lack of definitive histologic features, one diagnostic criteria is a karyotype of the tumor, since almost all Ewing sarcomas studied have shown a characteristic rearrangement: t(11;22)(q24;q12). Several other tumors have been described that contain this characteristic translocation as well as many clinical and biochemical similarities, hence they are included here.

**Clinical Findings:**  Ewing sarcoma is a tumor that occurs in children and young adults. Approximately 80% of the cases are diagnosed in the first two decades of life. The tumor first manifests as an area of painful swelling located most often in an extremity. The single most frequent primary site is the femur, which accounts for approximately 20% of all cases. On X-ray, the tumor usually appears as an area of bone destruction that is typically associated with a soft tissue mass. The diagnosis of Ewing sarcoma requires a biopsy for pathologic evaluation of the tissue. Histologically, the tumor consists of uniform, small, undifferentiated cells. Because of its lack of distinguishing cytologic features, it has been difficult to diagnose this tumor. The finding that almost all Ewing sarcomas have a characteristic chromosome rearrangement: (t[11;22][q24,q12]), has provided a diagnostic tool for the tumor as well as suggested a possible etiology. This finding has allowed reevaluation of this group of tumors. Two tumors that had been thought to be distinct from Ewing sarcoma have been shown to have the 11;22 translocation: *Askin tumor* of the chest wall and *neuroepithelioma*. Both of these tumors differ from classic Ewing sarcoma because they have primitive neuronal features that can be seen by electron microscopy. Recently, several groups have demonstrated the presence of neuron-specific proteins in morphologically undifferentiated Ewing sarcoma. This finding may establish an ontologic link between these tumors.

Even though Ewing sarcoma is a radiosensitive tumor, patients have had a poor prognosis because of the high frequency of metastasis. Because of the subtle symptoms, there is often a long interval between the first appearance of symptoms and medical intervention. As a result, between 10 and 30% of all patients present with metastases. Even 25–42% of those patients who are apparently rendered free of disease by treatment will develop metastasis. Frequent sites of metastasis include such diffuse locations as the lungs, other bones (including the skull), bone marrow, and lymph nodes. Clearly, surgical removal of the tumor and local irradiation are inadequate means of achieving a cure in most patients. Recently, an aggressive multimodal therapy, including surgical intervention, multidrug chemotherapy, and high-dose radiation, has dramatically improved survival, with over 50% of patients free of disease two years after diagnosis.

**Complications:**  Aside from pathologic bone fractures at the site of the primary tumor, the major complications for these patients are problems associated with their treatment. Myelosuppression is often a consequence of both chemotherapy and radiotherapy. The resulting immunosuppression can contribute to the development of life-threatening infections that require immediate treatment. Skeletal disabilities can also result from treatment of the primary tumor due to local bone erosion.

**Associated Findings:**  One study has reported an increased incidence of congenital urogenital malformations in 12% of these patients.

**Etiology:**  Ewing sarcoma is a sporadic condition whose etiology is unknown. Autosomal dominant inheritance has been suggested. The finding that Ewing sarcoma is virtually absent in Blacks has prompted investigators to look for genetic factors that may predispose certain individuals to develop the cytogenetic translocation that is closely associated with this tumor. The demonstration of a spontaneous fragile site, fra(11)(q23), in one patient's constitutional cells has identified one such predisposing factor. In addition, several studies have shown a higher incidence of Ewing sarcoma in rural communities. These studies have suggested that exposure to either an animal virus or an insecticide might be involved in the etiology of this tumor.

**Pathogenesis:**  The finding of an invariant t(11;22)(q24,q12) in this tumor indicates that altered regulation of a gene residing in this location may be responsible for the malignant transformation. Two known oncogenes reside near the translocation breakpoints: c-sis on 22q13 and c-ets-1 on 11q23.3. Rearrangement and expression of these genes have been studied. Although the oncogene c-sis has been shown to be translocated to chromosome 11, no expression of its mRNA could be detected in this tumor. The oncogene c-ets-1 remains on chromosome 11 and its expression in tumor tissue is quite variable. This suggests that its regulation may be disrupted by the translocation.

**MIM No.:**  13345

**CDC No.:**  171.800

**Sex Ratio:**  M1.5:F1

**Occurrence:**  Varies with racial origin, with over 95% of the cases occuring in the white population where its incidence is 1.7: 1,000,000. The occurrence in both American and African Blacks, as well as Orientals, is exceptionally rare.

**Risk of Recurrence for Patient's Sib:**  Unknown. Only four cases of families with two affected sibs have been reported in the literature.

**Risk of Recurrence for Patient's Child:**  Unknown. No instance of recurrence in offspring has been reported. However, in the past, most patients with this condition died in adolescence.

**Age of Detectability:**  From birth to age 30 years.

**Gene Mapping and Linkage:**  The genes responsible remain unknown; however, the linkage will presumably be to 11q24 and/or 22q12.

**Prevention:**  None known. Genetic counseling indicated.

**Treatment:**  Patients are treated with multimodal therapy, including surgery, radiation, and chemotherapy.

**Prognosis:** The prognosis for patients with these tumors has improved dramatically in recent years. For each patient, the prognosis will vary depending on the site of the primary tumor and if there is metastatic disease. With current aggressive treatment, over 95% of all patients achieve complete clinical remission, and over 50% of the patients presenting without metastasis will survive the first five years.

**Detection of Carrier:** Unknown.

**Special Considerations:** It is essential for proper patient care and treatment that Ewing sarcoma be differentiated from other small, round cell tumors of childhood, especially **Cancer, neuroblastoma**. The prognosis for neuroblastoma is poor, with only 2% of late-stage neuroblastoma patients surviving five years. Although neuroblastoma can be differentiated from classic Ewing sarcoma by its primitive neuronal features on histology, the more differentiated subtypes such as neuroepithelioma are histologically indistinguishable. Although the diagnosis of Ewing sarcoma should be suspected when the tumor occurs in a child older than five years, prior to that time both tumors can occur. A karyotype of the tumor is one definitive way to distinguish these tumors.

A study of proto-oncogenes revealed another difference that may be useful for diagnosis. High levels of the mRNA for the oncogene c-*myc* were detected in Ewing sarcoma but not in neuroblastoma. Instead, neuroblastoma had high levels of the mRNA for the proto-oncogene N-*myc*, which was also amplified in many late-stage tumors. Another distinguishing feature of every Ewing sarcoma is the presence of the neurotransmitter synthetic enzyme choline acetyltransferase. In contrast, neuroblastoma has high levels of the adrenergic synthetic enzyme dopamine-β-hydroxylase.

The finding of a neurotransmitter synthetic enzyme in all Ewing sarcomas also addresses another major controversy: the cell of origin of this tumor. Because Ewing sarcoma is found in and around bone, it was originally thought to have a mesenchymal origin. Even though Ewing sarcoma shows no neuronal features by electron microscopy and is negative when stained with neuron-specific enolase, several investigators have now shown the presence of neuron-specific proteins. In addition, some Ewing sarcoma cell lines have been induced toward neuronal differentiation in culture. The cholinergic phenotype and the location of this tumor near efferent nerves has prompted the hypothesis that the cell of origin may be a postganglionic parasympathetic neuron.

**Support Groups:** Atlanta; American Cancer Society

**References:**
Ewing J: Diffuse endothelioma of bone. Proc NY Pathol Soc 1921; 21:17–24.
Turc-Carel C, et al.: Chromosomal translocations in Ewing's sarcoma. New Engl J Med 1983; 309:497–498.
Gollin SM, et al.: Spontaneous expression of fra(11)(q23) in a patient with Ewing's sarcoma and t(11;22)(q23:q11). Cancer Genet Cytogenet 1986; 20:331–339.
Griffin CA, et al.: Comparison of constitutional and tumor-associated 11;22 translocations: nonidentical breakpoints on chromosome 11 and 22. Proc Natl Acad Sci 1986; 83:6122–6126.
Triche TJ, et al.: Neuroblastoma, Ewing's sarcoma, and the differential diagnosis of small-, round-, blue-cell tumors. Major Prob Pathol 1986; 18:145–195. * †
Zamora P, et al.: Ewing's tumor in brothers. Am J Clin Oncol 1986; 9:358–360.
McKeon C, et al.: Indistinguishable patterns of protooncogene expression in the two distinct but closely related tumors: Ewing's sarcoma and neuroepithelioma. Can Res 1988; 48:4307–4311.

MC038                                            **Catherine McKeon**

---

**Includes:** Cancer; nonspecific aggregation in a family

**Excludes:**
    Cancer family patterns, site-specific
    Cancer family syndrome of Li-Fraumeni (SBLA syndrome)
    Cancer family syndrome of Lynch

**Major Diagnostic Criteria:** In general, three or more first degree relatives with malignant neoplasms.

**Clinical Findings:** Because one in four Americans develops cancer in his lifetime, everyone will have some relatives with cancer, and, by chance, some will have many affected family members.

The definition of a "cancer family" is not statistically precise, but somewhat a matter of intuition. An excessive aggregation of cancer within a family can be suspected when malignant neoplasms occur in the following circumstances: in members of more than one generation, in a number of sibs, at an unusual age, with an atypical tumor type or site, in an atypical sex, or in association with other primary tumors or birth defects in the same individuals or relatives.

The best documentation of a true excess of cancer in a family is made by following the same family for years and comparing the observed numbers of cancers with those expected in the general population. The tumor type that has shown greatest familiality in the genealogic survey of Mormons in Utah has been prostate cancer, contrary to the impression gained from case reports and clinical observations.

**Complications:** Cancer kills by metastases, local invasion, or metabolic disturbances. Modern multiple modality therapy has improved survival for some tumor types, in children more than in adults and in rare cancers more than in common ones. As survival improves, questions are raised about empiric recurrence risk and the possible genetic consequences to offspring from mutagenicity among survivors of intensive chemotherapy and radiotherapy.

**Associated Findings:** The psychological impact of being in a cancer family is variable. Certain families become quiet and secretive. Medical attention is shunned by some who fear discovery of cancer and is abused by others who hope to find the earliest possible tumor. Some families go public, using the media as a source of attention and funds to meet large expenses. Some try to make the best of an unfortunate situation by volunteering for biomedical research.

**Etiology:** Often no single cause can be detected. Shared environmental factors have been identified in familial aggregations of asbestos-associated lung and pleural tumors and benzene-associated leukemia. Some 394 single gene traits are known to predispose to neoplasia, such as the multiple endocrine neoplasia syndromes or neurofibromatosis; these could explain some familial aggregation.

**Pathogenesis:** Not specifically known; in general, however, each cancer probably arises from a complex interaction of host susceptibility and diverse environmental influences through a series of steps, some of which are mutations. The step of initiation is likely a single locus or chromosome mutation; subsequent steps, called *promotion*, enable the cells to achieve independent unregulated growth, manifested as a clinical cancer.

**MIM No.:** *11440

**Sex Ratio:** M1:F1

**Occurrence:** In surveys of adult medical oncology clinics 6% of persons with cancer had three or more first degree relatives with cancer, 12% had two, and 30% had one.

**Risk of Recurrence for Patient's Sib:**
    See Part I, *Mendelian Inheritance*.

**Risk of Recurrence for Patient's Child:**
    See Part I, *Mendelian Inheritance*.

**Age of Detectability:** Lifelong, depending on tumor types and age of onset in the family.

**Gene Mapping and Linkage:** LCO (liver cancer oncogene) has been mapped to 2q14-q21.

**Prevention:** Counseling about the guidelines of the American Cancer Society and National Cancer Institute for cancer prevention and early screening and detection, according to the cell types occurring in the family. Very occasionally, prophylactic surgery could be considered, e.g., thyroidectomy in the multiple mucosal neuroma syndrome and colectomy in familial polyposis coli.

**Treatment:** As cancers arise they should be handled by standard means. Family members first affected may have had less than ideal cancer therapy; so, as additional relatives develop cancer, early referral to a comprehensive cancer center may be useful.

**Prognosis:** Familial cancers seem to have the same natural history as sporadic cancers of the same type and stage.

**Detection of Carrier:** Examination of relatives and standard screening tests.

**Support Groups:**
Atlanta; American Cancer Society
AUSTRALIA: NSW; Sydney; Australian Cancer Society
ENGLAND: London; World Federation for Cancer Care
SWITZERLAND: Geneva; International Union Against Cancer

**References:**

Albert S, Child M: Familial cancer in the general population. Cancer 1977; 40:1674–1679.
Mulvihill JJ, et al., eds: Genetics of human cancer. New York: Raven, 1977.
Lynch HT, et al.: Family history in an oncology clinic: implications for cancer genetics. J Am Med Asso 1979; 242:1268–1272.
Knudson AG, Jr., Kelly PT: Genetic counseling with the cancer patient's family. In: Hickey RC, Clark RL, eds: Current problems in cancer. Chicago: Yearbook Medical, 1983:15–41.
Schneider NR, et al.: Familial predispostion to cancer and age at onset of disease in randomly selected cancer patients. Am J Hum Genet 1983; 35:454–467.
Chaganti RSK, German J, eds: Genetics in clinical oncology. New York: Oxford University, 1985.
Muller H-J, Weber W, eds: Familial cancer. Basel: Karger, 1985.*
Parry DM, et al.: Strategies for controlling cancer through genetics: report of a workshop. Am J Hum Genet 1987; 41:63–69.

MU009                                                  **John J. Mulvihill**

## CANCER, GASTRIC FAMILIAL                                     2746

**Includes:**
Gastric cancer
Lynch syndrome II (some)
Stomach cancer

**Excludes:**
Leiomyosarcoma of stomach
Lymphoma of stomach

**Major Diagnostic Criteria:** The presence of two or more first degree relatives with gastric cancer. Barium upper GI series is a standard diagnostic approach. However, the advent of flexible fiberoptic gastroscopy, which while providing excellent visualization also enables the physician to obtain tissue biopsy or exfolitative cytology, has made this procedure the preferred method. Other methods include CT scanning, ultrasound, and plasma tumor markers.

**Clinical Findings:** There has been a significant decrease in age-adjusted mortality in the United States due to decreased incidence in rates of stomach cancer. No adequate explanation for this decline in incidence has been identified. Premalignant lesions of the stomach are important, and these include atrophic gastritis, particularly when associated with intestinal metaplasia (80% of patients with resection for gastric cancer in Japan showed intestinal metaplasia). Symptoms in the early and potentially curable phase are usually minimal or nonexistent. Presentation may be vague and nonspecific. Dysphagia and obstruction may present, depending on location of the lesion. When physical signs are present, patients are usually incurable.

**Complications:** Malnutrition, weight loss, and abdominal pain. In addition to mechanical obstruction, pseudo-obstruction can occur from neurovascular involvement of the mesentery root. Significant upper GI bleeding is rare. However, chronic anemia from slow GI blood loss is not unusual. Further complications depend on the site of metastases. The most common local organ is the liver. Metastases to the liver can cause jaundice and pain. Metastases to the omentum and peritoneum are also common local sites. Splenic involvement is infrequent. Distant organs most commonly involved are the lung and, secondly, the adrenals. Complications can include ascites, pleural effusion, adrenal insufficiency, chyloascites, and chylothorax. These can also be presenting manifestations of gastric adenocarcinoma.

Syndromes of remote effects of carcinoma are rare in gastric adenocarcinoma. It is the most common abdominal cancer associated with acanthosis nigricans. Both glucose intolerance and hypoglycemia have been reported as have neuromyopathy, nephrotic syndrome, migrating thrombophlebitis, and thrombotic nonbacterial endocarditis. Proximal gastric cancer can present with symptoms and X-ray findings classic for **Esophagus, achalasia**.

**Associated Findings:** Certain distant lymph node metastases involve lymph nodes in the left supraclavicular area (verchaus nodes), and periumbilical lymph node involvement (Sister Mary Joseph nodes), and should be actively sought during the initial presentation.

**Etiology:** High incidence rates in Japan and Chile, although in migrant populations going from high-to-low incidence countries with significant decrease in gastric cancer occurrence, suggest that this disease must have strong environmental perturbation. Environmental factors considered important include consumption of smoked and salted foods and aflatoxin contamination. Gastric cancer twice as frequent in the *lower* as opposed to the higher socioeconomic groups in the United States and western Europe. High-risk occupational groups include farmers (in Japan), nickel refinery workers, coal miners, rubber workers, and those who process timber. High rates are also found in asbestos workers. Studies from Japan have shown that nitro-N-nitrosoguanidines are gastric carcinogens, which induce gastrointestinal metaplasia that is followed by gastric cancer.

Patients with pernicious anemia have a 5–10% incidence of gastric cancer (gastric cancer is 20 times more common in patients with PA than in age-matched control population). Gastric resection for peptic ulcer disease is also associated with increased gastric cancer risk. Villous adenomatous polyps of the stomach appear to be premalignant. Hyperplastic polyps, while significantly more common, are very infrequently associated with gastric cancer. There is controversy relevant to gastric ulcer and malignancy wherein data from the United States fail to support association while in Japan a high correlation between chronic gastric ulcer and cancer has been observed.

The risk for gastric cancer in patients with blood group A has been thought to be significant, but recent data show only a moderate (1.2%) increased risk, while extensive investigations in Scandanavia have failed to identify a relationship between gastric cancer and blood group A. There is a strong association between atrophic gastritis and gastric cancer, but this does not mean that atrophic gastritis is a precursor to gastric cancer. Atrophic gastritis appears in approximately 80–95% of individuals of older ages. Familial clustering has been observed in families, as in the family of Napoleon Bonaparte, with vertical transmission through three generations and in Lynch syndrome II (Cristofaro et al, 1987; Lynch, 1976). The condition is found in patients with **Ataxia-telangiectasia**, and heterozygous carriers of this deleterious gene. There is a weak concordance in monozygous as opposed to dizygous twins. The condition is common in Japan, Central and South America, Iceland, and Scandanavia, and is associated with the consumption of hypertonic, salted, pickled, or smoked foods (particularly fish in Japan). May be related to conversion of nitrates to nitrites through formation of N-nitroso compounds through interaction with secondary or tertiary amines in the stomach.

**Pathogenesis:** Ninety-five percent of gastric cancers are adenocarcinomas, but adenoacanthanomas, squamous cell carcinomas, and carcinoids account for about 1% of gastric cancer, while leiomyosarcomas may account for 1–3% of malignant gastric lesions. Environmental factors have been considered, particularly dietary, as in areas of low consumption of green vegetables and citrus fruits. There is an increased incidence in countries where nitrates are used as preservatives, and where charcoal is used for cooking. There are increased rates in certain occupational groups, such as coal miners, farmers, nickle refinery workers, rubber workers, rubber workers, and asbestos workers, but it is also necessary to control for socioeconomic background as a factor in these groups.

**MIM No.:** *11440

**Sex Ratio:** M1.6:F1

**Occurrence:** The sixth most common cause of cancer death in the United States. There were 24,600 new cases in 1987 (15,000 male, 9,600 female).

**Risk of Recurrence for Patient's Sib:** About three-fold increased risk over general population; may approach 50% in selected hereditary cancer-prone syndromes, including some kindreds with *Lynch syndrome II.*

**Risk of Recurrence for Patient's Child:** About three fold increased risk over general population; may approach 50% in selected hereditary cancer-prone syndromes, including some kindreds with *Lynch syndrome II.*

**Age of Detectability:** About 60 years of age, with less than 5% under the age of 40 years. The age of onset is ten to 15 years earlier in hereditary cases, including *Lynch syndrome II.*

**Gene Mapping and Linkage:** Unknown.

**Prevention:** None known. Genetic counseling indicated. No surveillance strategies of proven sensitivity and specificity are available in the United States. In Japan, experience has been excellent with combined endoscopy and cytology.

**Treatment:** Surgical treatment of resectable candidates (first search for evidence of distant metastases to avoid unnecessary surgery). Chemotherapy with 5- fluorouracil (5-FU) causes remission in 10% of cases. Combination chemotherapy with 5-FU, doxorubicin, and mitomycin-C provides a better statistical response rate, but only a nonsignificant gain in overall median survival (less than one year). Adjuvant radiotherapy or chemotherapy is experimental and of unproven efficacy.

**Prognosis:** Related to the status at initial presentation; gross appearance, site, extent of local invasion, and histology. Less than 15% survive five years.

**Detection of Carrier:** Unknown.

**Support Groups:** Atlanta; American Cancer Society

**References:**
Lynch HT: Cancer genetics. Springfield, IL: C.C. Thomas, 1976.
Cristofaro G, et al.: New phenotypic aspects in a family with Lynch syndrome II. Cancer 1987; 60:51–58.

LY000
LA042

**Henry T. Lynch**
**Stephen J. Lanspa**

Cancer, glioblastoma, familial
*See CANCER, GLIOMA, FAMILIAL*

**Includes:**
   Astrocytoma types 3 & 4
   Brain, glioma of
   Cancer, glioblastoma, familial
   GLI gene
   Glioblastoma multiforme, familial
   Glioma oncogene
   Gliomas, familial aggregation
   Spongioblastoma multiforme

**Excludes:**
   **Cancer, familial** (1505)
   **Cancer, neuroepithelial and meningeal** (2748)
   **Chromosome instability, Nijmegen type** (2551)

**Major Diagnostic Criteria:** Two or more first-degree relatives with glioma. The diagnosis of glioma is based on the development of a seizure disorder and progressive weakness, gait, speech and/or visual disturbances, and is confirmed by computed tomography of the brain and histology following excision of the tumor. Since gliomas are not rare, especially in young people, some instances of familial aggregation will occur by chance.

**Clinical Findings:** The most frequent site of glioblastoma multiforme is the frontal lobe, followed by the temporal lobe and the corpus callosum, also with multiple foci (multifocal glioblastoma multiforme). The cerebellum is only rarely affected. Clinical signs can develop early in infancy and childhood or as late at the fourth, fifth or even the sixth decade. There is striking clinical and anatomical similarity in familial cases. Sibs tend to have common features with regard to localization of the tumor and initial symptomatology, and also a similar age of onset.
   Skull X-rays may be normal. Electroencephalogram, computed tomography of the brain and angiography reveal the intracerebral mass. The final diagnosis can only be made by histopathology. The histology and the localization of the familial glioblastoma multiforme does not differ from that of the tumor associated with neurocutaneous syndromes: polymorphic astrocytes, often of the bipolar type, scattered giant cells with a high frequency of mitoses, representing dedifferentiation of astrocytes. Central necrosis is a constant finding. Metastatic spread is mainly intrathecal, to the spinal cord and less frequently to the liver.

**Complications:** Derived from the original tumor, localization in the brain or the spinal cord, number of tumors, metastases, and associated tumors. Like sporadic glioma, familial glioma kills by local invasion and expansion and endocrinologic and metabolic derangements.

**Associated Findings:** Glioma may occur in families because of a predisposing disease that is genetic or familial, such as **Neurofibromatosis, Tuberous sclerosis,** and **Turcot syndrome.** Cancers of various organs have also been described in these families, as well as skeletal abnormalities, osteochondrodysplasia, multiple exostoses, and vascular malformations. Because of the frequent association of **Neurofibromatosis** and gliomatous tumors of the central nervous system, it is important to rule out neurocutaneous syndromes in families with these tumors.

**Etiology:** Of all brain tumor types, glioma was the one common variety that showed the greatest numbers of case reports in a global literature review that served to launch an International Registry of Familial Brain Tumors. Apart from medulloblastoma, there were five reported concordant twins (all monozygotic), 50 sib-pairs, and 34 reports of multiple generations with neuroepithelial tissue tumor. Familial glioma could, in theory, be explained by shared environmental determinants. Case-control studies have associated brain tumors with many environmental factors, including paternal exposure to hydrocarbons, maternal exposures to N-nitrose compounds, and personal exposure in childhood to ionizing radiation and insecticides, and in adults to the manufacture and maintenance of electronic equipment. Features that suggest excessive familial aggregation are extrapolated from the characteristics of classic examples of single genes that cause cancer, like retinoblastoma: early age of onset, multifocality, presence of multiple primary malignant neoplasms, and of course familial aggregation.

Glioblastoma multiforme is an extreme manifestation of anaplasia and dedifferentiation of mature astrocytes. Familial glioblastoma multiforme is only rarely found as an isolated tumor, not associated with one of the neurocutaneous syndromes. Specific genetic or predisposing factors that may be found in particular families are not necessarily common to all families. In some of the reported families, affected individuals are found among siblings only, whereas in others there is parent to offspring transmission. In some families only males are affected suggesting X-linked inheritance or at least sex-limited factors.

**Pathogenesis:** A gene termed "GLI" has been identified, that is expressed more than 50-fold in a malignant glioma cell line. This gene is mapped to chromosome 12 (q13-q14.3). The tumor derived DNA was obtained from a 46-year-old male with a normal constitutional karyotype. Chromosomes of the original tumor and the established cell lines revealed numerous double minute chromosomes. Molecular evidence for amplification suggested a highly amplified sequence which, when screened to 22 known oncogene sequences, failed to show homology to any previously described gene sequence.

Polysomy of chromosome 7 in human glioblastoma cell lines has been shown, and a correlation with an increased expression of the erbB oncogene was observed. This oncogene has been mapped to chromosome 7pter-q22. Other cytogenetic findings include loss of chromosome 10, structural anomalies of chromosomes 9p and 19q and double minute chromosomes (suggesting the presence of gene amplification). In all, about 22% of human malignant gliomas have chromosomal abnormalities. Peripheral blood constitutional karyotypes of patients have consistently been normal.

Polymorphic markers on chromosome 10 in 13 patients with glioblastoma multiforme, using tumor and lymphocyte DNA, suggest that the expression of a recessive mutant gene on chromosome 10 leads to the formation of the tumor. This observation fits well the "two hit" theory, where the first mutational event may be related to the expression of an oncogene.

**MIM No.:** *13780

**CDC No.:** 191.000

**Sex Ratio:** Usually M1:F1. In some families, only males have been affected.

**Occurrence:** With the assumption that 60% of all primary central nervous system tumors are gliomas, some 8,800 persons were estimated to develop glioma in 1987. Only a small fraction would be expected to be familial. At least 25 families have been reported, but the description of clinical findings is frequently insufficient to rule out a neurocutaneous syndrome. In at least 10 families with the "family cancer syndrome" (see **Cancer, familial**) glioblastoma multiforme was one of the malignant tumors.

**Risk of Recurrence for Patient's Sib:** Depends on etiology, but in general very low. Analysis of death certificates from overall childhood brain tumors in the U. S. indicated a ten-fold excess of brain tumors and bone cancer in siblings. A similar study found 30 sib pairs with at least one brain tumor compared to 11 pairs expected by chance. The frequency in the general population is unknown.

**Risk of Recurrence for Patient's Child:** Undetermined but low, in the absence of a dominant trait predisposing to glioma.

**Age of Detectability:** The age of diagnosis of sporadic glioma has two peaks and tends to be in the same range within a family: one in childhood, the other basically in early and middle adult life. The youngest age of detection has been six months, the oldest in the sixth decade. Data are insufficient to document the generalization that familial glioma occurs at an earlier age than sporadic glioma.

**Gene Mapping and Linkage:** GLI (glioma-associated oncogene homolog) has been provisionally mapped to 12q13-q14.3.

**Prevention:** None known. Genetic counseling is indicated in families in which the history of familial aggregation may point to individuals at potential risk.

**Treatment:** Surgical excision of the tumor(s), with additional radiotherapy and chemotherapy.

**Prognosis:** Poor. Survival is determined by age at diagnosis, histologic grade, localization and treatment. The half-time survival of 50% of the patients is six months. Average five-year survival for all types of brain tumors in the United States is 24%.

**Detection of Carrier:** Unknown.

**Support Groups:** Atlanta; American Cancer Society

**Special Considerations:** An attempt has been made to classify familial gliomas into four groups (Vieregge, 1987): 1) familial brain gliomas associated with neurocutaneous and phakomatosis syndromes; 2) familial brain tumors not associated with the above; 3) brain gliomas within the familial cancer syndrome; and 4) brain gliomas as congenital tumors. The present discussion would include only glioblastoma multiforme of the second group, but it is difficult to follow a rigid classification, since many reports lack complete clinical descriptions and there is much overlap among these groups. The main unique characteristic of familial glioblastoma multiforme is the occurrence of these tumors in families without neurocutaneous syndromes.

Chromosomal abnormalities in tumors may be specific and may help investigate genetic alterations that play a role in tumor development. This should not be considered a useful technique to establish risks for tumor development. The GLI oncogene is an important development in understanding the genetic mechanisms of tumor development. Several other genes have been found to be abnormal in human primary tumors. The GLI1 oncogene has been extensively studied, but it should be clear that this gene was identified from the malignant glioma of one single patient. Similar studies on other clinically and pathologically diagnosed tumors of this type have not yet been reported.

**References:**

Miller RW: Deaths from childhood leukemia and solid tumors among twins and other sibs in the United States. J Natl Cancer Inst 1971; 46:203–209.

Draper GJ, et al: Occurence of childhood cancers among sibs and estimation of familial risks. J Med Genet 1977; 14:81–90.

Von Motz IP, et al.: Astrocytoma in three sisters. Neurology 1977; 27:1039–1041.

Chemke J, et al.: Familial glioblastoma multiforme without neurofibromatosis. Am J Med Genet 1985; 21:731–735.

Tijssen CC: Genetic aspects of brain tumors; tumors of neuroepithelial and meningeal tissue. In: Muller HJ, Weber A, eds: Familial Cancer. Basel: Karger, 1985:98–102.

Henn W, et al.: Polysomy of chromosome 7 is correlated with overexpression of the erbB oncogene in human glioblastoma cell lines. Hum Genet 1986; 74:104–106.

Heuch I, Blom GP: Glioblastoma multiforme in three family members, including a case of true multicentricity. J Neurol 1986; 233:142–144.

Kinzler KW, et al.: Identification of an amplified, highly expressed gene in a human glioma. Science 1987; 236:70–73.

Vieregge P, et al.: Familial glioma: occurrence within the "familial cancer syndrome" and systemic malformations. J Neurol 1987; 234:220–232.

Bigner SH, et al.: Specific chromosomal abnormalities in malignant human gliomas. Cancer Res 1988; 48:405–411.

Fujimoto M, et al.: Loss of heterozygosity on chromosome 10 in human glioblastoma multiforme. Genomics 1989; 4:210–214.

CH013

MU009

TR010

**Juan Chemke**
**John J. Mulvihill**
**Jeffrey M. Trent**

## CANCER, HODGKIN DISEASE, FAMILIAL                2352

**Includes:**

Hodgkin disease, site-specific aggregations
Hodgkin's disease

**Excludes:  Ataxia-telangiectasia** (0094)

**Major Diagnostic Criteria:** In general, two or more relatives also with Hodgkin disease.

**Clinical Findings:** Familial Hodgkin disease is a well recognized rare clinical entity which has been of interest for several decades. Since Hodgkin disease is relatively rare, two or more individuals in one family are unlikely to develop Hodgkin disease by random chance alone. Accruing sufficient numbers of multiplex families in any one institution has been a major problem in studying the genetics of this disease. In most of the reported kindreds, the affected individuals have tended to fall within the early age peak of Hodgkin disease, and the most common histology has been nodular sclerosing. On the basis of fairly limited data, familial Hodgkin disease does not differ in clinical presentation, response to therapy, or prognosis from sporadic disease.

**Complications:** Whether or not individuals with familial Hodgkin disease have more extensive immunosuppression at the initiation or completion of therapy compared to individuals with sporadic disease has not been well studied. Individuals treated for Hodgkin disease are at increased risk of second primary cancers.

**Associated Findings:** None known.

**Etiology:** One of the major hypotheses is that Hodgkin disease develops as an uncommon response to a common environmental exposure (possibly a virus) in a susceptible host. The nature of the host susceptibility has been investigated by assessing the relationship between the immune response genes near and within the HLA complex and Hodgkin disease. Current evidence suggests that there is heterogeneity within the families, with approximately 60% of the cases in families being associated with a recessive host susceptibility gene tightly linked to the HLA complex, and the other 40% being due to other familial or environmental exposures.

**Pathogenesis:** Associations with multiple viruses have been extensively investigated, especially Epstein-Barr virus, and most recently HBLV. No causative associations have been demonstrated, however. The etiology of the persistent T-cell immunodeficiency associated with Hodgkin disease is also not well established.

**MIM No.:** 23600

**Sex Ratio:** M3:F2; similar to sporadic Hodgkin disease.

**Occurrence:** Genetic determinants are important in a small, but not quantified, proportion of the 7,400 new cases in United States each year.

**Risk of Recurrence for Patient's Sib:** Differs by etiology, but various estimates have been in the range of 10-fold compared to population controls.

**Risk of Recurrence for Patient's Child:** Undetermined, but multiple kindreds with an affected parent and child have been reported.

**Age of Detectability:** Familial Hodgkin disease frequently, but not invariably, occurs within the young age peak (age 15–30).

**Gene Mapping and Linkage:** Complex segregation analysis has suggested that the genetic model is perhaps intermediate to a recessive and dominant one. As above, there appears to be a recessive gene that is tightly linked to the HLA complex. Other familial factors, possibly polygenic and/or environmental, also appear to be involved in etiology.

**Prevention:** None known. Genetic counseling indicated.

**Treatment:** Treatment of familial Hodgkin disease should be identical to that of sporadic Hodgkin disease.

**Prognosis:** There is no difference in prognosis between familial and sporadic Hodgkin disease.

**Detection of Carrier:** No clinically useful bioassays are available. HLA typing of first degree relatives may be somewhat useful in detecting relatives at possible increased risk.

**Support Groups:** Atlanta; American Cancer Society

**References:**

Gutensohn N, Cole P: Childhood social environment and Hodgkin's disease. New Engl J Med 1981; 296:248–253.
Gutensohn NM: Social class and age at diagnosis of Hodgkin's disease: new epidemiologic evidence for "two-disease hypothesis." Cancer Treat Rep 1982; 66:689–695.
Grufferman S: Hodgkin's disease. In: Schottenfeld D, Fraumeni JF Jr., eds: Cancer Epidemiology and Prevention. Philadelphia, W.B. Saunders 1982:739–753.
Hors J, Dausset J: HLA and susceptibility to Hodgkin's disease. Immunol Rev 1983; 70:167–192.
Harris EL, et al: Complex segregation analysis of multiple case Hodgkin's disease families. Am J Hum Genet 1985; 37:A197.
Chakravarti A, et al: Etiologic heterogeneity in Hodgkin's disease: HLA linked and unlinked determinants of susceptibility independent of histologic concordance. Genet Epidem 1986; 3:407–415.
Tucker MA, et al.: Risk of second cancers after treatment for Hodgkin's disease. New Engl J Med 1988; 318:76–81.
Kaldor JM, et al.: Leukemia following Hodgkin's disease. New Engl J Med 1990; 322:7–13.

TU014                                        **Margaret A. Tucker**

**Cancer, intestinal polyposis I**
*See INTESTINAL POLYPOSIS, TYPE I*

## CANCER, LUNG, FAMILIAL                      2747

**Includes:**

Aryl hydrocarbon hydroxylase
Cytochrome P450, subfamily I (aromatic compound-
   inducible)
Larynx cancer
Lung cancer
Pharynx cancer

**Excludes:**

**Cancer, soft tissue sarcoma** (2749)
**Cancer, familial** (1505)

**Major Diagnostic Criteria:** Two or more first-degree relatives with respiratory tract cancer.

**Clinical Findings:** The definition of familial lung cancer is arbitrary, and making a diagnosis is somewhat a matter of intuition. Since lung cancer is common in men and now in women, many persons will have affected relatives, and, by chance, some will have two or more. Familial lung cancer could, of course, be explained by shared environmental determinants, most often smoking tobacco alone or together with an occupational exposure, such as to asbestos. Features that suggest an excessive familial aggregation are extrapolated from the characteristics of classic examples of single genes that cause cancer, like **Retinoblastoma**: early age of onset, bilaterality, presence of multiple primary malignant neoplasms, and, of course, familial aggregation.

The presenting clinical findings do not differ from those of sporadic lung cancer: cough, hemoptysis, chest pain, recurring bronchitis or pneumonia, and mass on chest X-ray.

**Complications:** Like sporadic lung cancer, familial lung cancer kills by metastasis, local invasion, and endocrinologic and metabolic derangements.

**Associated Findings:** Lung cancer may occur in families because of a predisposing disease that is familial: **Scleroderma, familial progressive, Tuberous sclerosis**, and interstitial pulmonary fibrosis. The patients may have signs of tobacco abuse in the skin, lungs, and vascular system.

**Etiology:** Diverse etiologies are possible. As with sporadic lung cancer, tobacco abuse is likely the single major cause of familial lung cancer. The Carney triad of unknown etiology has pulmonary chondroma as one feature, the others being gastric leiomyosarcoma and paraganglioma. There have been asbestos-associated familial chest tumors, including mesothelioma and lung cancer. Early reports linked a high risk of lung cancer among smokers to hereditary variations in the inducible levels of the enzyme system, called *aryl hydrocarbon hydroxylase;* subsequently the work was shown to be controversial, if not wrong, in detail but doubtlessly correct in principle. Specific P-450 genes surely produce human variation in the metabolism of xenobiotics, including carcinogens. Another pharmacogenetic trait that seems to be related to lung cancer risk involves the hydroxylation of the test drug debrisoquine.

**Pathogenesis:** Regardless of specific primary etiology, cytogenetic and single-gene abnormalities are probably a common pathway in the progression to clinical lung cancer, whether familial or sporadic. Specifically, a chromosome 3 deletion (3p14–23) is seen in almost all small cell carcinomas of the lung. The presence of homogenously staining regions and double minutes in small cell carcinoma of the lung seems to represent specific amplification of a gene in the *myc* family, and H-*ras* oncogene activation has been documented by transfection assays.

**MIM No.:** *10833, 21198

**Sex Ratio:** M2:F1. There is no reason to think that familial lung cancer has a different sex ratio than sporadic lung cancer.

**Occurrence:** Of the estimated 150,000 new cases of lung cancer in 1987, just a small fraction was familial.

**Risk of Recurrence for Patient's Sib:** Depends on etiology, but in general, very low. Population surveys have shown a 2.4 increase in risk of lung cancer among relatives of lung cancer patients, even after adjusting for smoking behavior.

**Risk of Recurrence for Patient's Child:** Undetermined, but prabably a relative risk of 3, which could be multiplied by the age, sex, and race-specific incidence rate to estimate absolute risk. For example, a 50-year-old white male whose parents had lung cancer has an annual risk of 3 times 115:100,000 per year, or 1.7% over a five year period.

**Age of Detectability:** The median age of diagnosis of sporadic lung cancer is 65 years. Data are insufficient to document the generalization that familial lung cancer occurs at an earlier age than sporadic.

**Gene Mapping and Linkage:** AHH (aryl hydrocarbon hydroxylase) has been mapped to 2pter-q31.
  CYP1 (cytochrome P450, subfamily I (aromatic compound-inducible)) has been mapped to 15q22-q24.

**Prevention:** Primary prevention of lung cancer in the population depends on achieving a smoke-free environment. Genetic counseling may be offered to persons at highest risk. Secondary prevention of lung cancer deaths through early screening has not been successful with the classic tools of sputum cytology and chest X-ray.

**Treatment:** Small cell carcinoma, with 3p-, seems to be the one type of lung cancer with improved survival due to combined chemotherapy and radiotherapy.

**Prognosis:** It has been shown that increased amplification of the activated *myc* oncogenes is associated with a less favorable prognosis.

**Detection of Carrier:** Unknown.

**Support Groups:** Atlanta; American Cancer Society

**References:**
Tokuhata DK, Lilienfeld AM: Familial aggregation of lung cancer among hospital patients. Public Health Rep 1963; 78:277–283.
Goffman TE, et al.: Familial respiratory tract cancer: opportunities for research and prevention. J Am Med Asso 1982; 247:1020–1023.
Ayesh R, et al.: Metabolic oxidation phenotypes as markers for susceptibility to lung cancer. Nature 1984; 312:169–170.
Mulvihill JJ, Bale AE: Ecogenetics of lung cancer: genetic susceptibility in the etiology of lung cancer. In Mizell M, Correa P (eds): Lung cancer: causes and prevention. Deerfield Beach: Verlag Chennie International, 1984; 141–152. *

Lynch HT, et al.: Genetics and smoking-associated cancers. a study of 485 families. Cancer 1986; 57:1640–1646.
Ooi WL, et al.: Increased familial risk for lung cancer. J Nat Cancer Inst 1986; 76:217–222.
Caporaso N, et al.: Debrisoquine metabolic phenotype (MP), asbestos exposure, and lung cancer. Proc ASCO 1987; 6:229 only.

MU009                                                      **John J. Mulvihill**

## CANCER, MALIGNANT MELANOMA, FAMILIAL          2318

**Includes:**
  B-K mole syndrome
  Cutaneous malignant melanoma, hereditary
  Dysplastic nevus syndrome
  Familial atypical mole-malignant melanoma (FAMMM)
  FAMMM syndrome of Lynch
  Hereditary cutaneous malignant melanoma (HCMM)
  Malignant melanoma
  Malignant melanoma, site-specific aggregation of

**Excludes: Xeroderma pigmentosum** (1005)

**Major Diagnostic Criteria:** Two or more relatives with malignant melanoma.

**Clinical Findings:** The definition of familial malignant melanoma is straightforward. Although cutaneous malignant melanoma is one of the most rapidly increasing cancers, it is still relatively rare, and the chance occurrence of two or more members of a family developing melanoma is unlikely. Melanoma-prone families have distinctive cutaneous precursor lesions, dysplastic nevi, which identify family members at increased risk of melanoma.
  Individuals with these nevi have a 148-fold increased risk of developing melanoma compared to individuals in the general population, and over a lifetime, have approximately 100% cumulative risk of developing malignant melanoma. The melanomas which occur in this familial setting have the characteristics of other hereditary cancers, such as retinoblastoma. The melanomas occur at an early age and affected individuals develop multiple primary melanomas. The presenting clinical findings do not differ from those of sporadic cutaneous melanoma. The back is the most common site for melanomas to develop in males, whereas the lower leg and back are the most common locations for the females. The histology is most frequently superficial spreading melanoma, followed by nodular melanoma. Acral lentiginous and lentigo maligna melanomas are rare in these families. Once the families are identified as being at increased risk of melanoma, the melanomas tend to be diagnosed at earlier stages, when they are more easily cured by relatively simple surgery.

**Complications:** Familial malignant melanoma, if not diagnosed at an early stage, kills by metastases. If the melanoma is relatively thick when initially diagnosed, surgical resection to adequate margins leads to a large soft tissue defect.

**Associated Findings:** Affected family members have large, variably pigmented, irregularly shaped, flat nevi which occur in an unusual distribution, including non-sun-exposed skin surfaces.

**Etiology:** Autosomal dominant inheritance with about 90% penetrance.

**Pathogenesis:** Virtually all of the familial melanomas arise in precursor dysplastic nevi. The events triggering the transformation of a dysplastic nevus to melanoma are unknown, but similar to individuals who develop sporadic melanoma, family members with melanoma are more likely to have had multiple blistering sunburns. This observation is consistent with the laboratory findings of enhanced mutagenesis in lymphocytes of affected family members following exposure to ultraviolet light. Fibroblasts from affected individuals also show enhanced cell killing when exposed to ultraviolet light.

**MIM No.:** *15560

**Sex Ratio:** M1:F1

**Occurrence:** Approximately 8–10% of the 27,000 new cutaneous melanomas per year in the United States are familial.

**Risk of Recurrence for Patient's Sib:**
See Part I, *Mendelian Inheritance.* May be as high as 100% in sibling with dysplastic nevi. This risk may be significantly modified by surveillance and early biopsy of changing nevi. Among clinically unaffected siblings (without dysplastic nevi) there is a < 5% chance (based on estimations of penetrance).

**Risk of Recurrence for Patient's Child:**
See Part I, *Mendelian Inheritance.*

**Age of Detectability:** Dysplastic nevi are usually apparent by the age of puberty. These nevi detect those individuals at increased risk of melanoma. The average age at first diagnosis of familial malignant melanoma is approximately 30 years of age, but may be as young as 10 years old.

**Gene Mapping and Linkage:** CMM (cutaneous malignant melanoma/dysplastic nevus) has been provisionally mapped to 1p36.

**Prevention:** Persons at high risk can be detected fairly reliably by the presence of dysplastic nevi. These individuals should minimize sun exposure, avoiding sunburns in particular. They should also examine their own skin monthly, and be examined by a health care practitioner every 3–6 months. Nevi should be biopsied if there is any suspicion of melanoma (large size, usually greater than 5mm; multiple colors, especially black, in a nevus; irregular border; abnormal surface, such as scaly, flaky, oozing, or bleeding; unusual sensation, particularly itching or tenderness; or abnormal skin adjacent to the nevus). Individuals with dysplastic nevi should be watched particularly closely during times of hormonal change such as pregnancy or puberty. Early biopsy of changing nevi can lead to earlier diagnosis of melanoma when it is easily cured by minimal surgery.

**Treatment:** Familial melanoma should be treated using the same procedures as those used in the treatment of sporadic melanoma (Balch et al, 1989).

**Prognosis:** Members of melanoma-prone families who develop melanoma have no different prognosis than individuals with sporadic melanoma. Melanomas in these family members, however, tend to be found at earlier stages because of close surveillance.

**Detection of Carrier:** Dysplastic nevi identify the individuals at increased risk of melanoma. There are infrequent obligate gene carriers who do not have dysplastic nevi.

**Support Groups:** Atlanta; American Cancer Society

**References:**
Greene MH, et al: Familial cutaneous malignant melanoma: autosomal dominant trait possibly linked to the Rh locus. Proc Nat Acad Sci 1983; 80:6071–6075.
Greene MH, et al: High risk of malignant melanoma in melanoma-prone families with dysplastic nevi. Ann Int Med 1985; 102:458–465.
Greene MH, et al: Acquired precursors of cutaneous malignant melanoma: the familial dysplastic nevus syndrome. New Engl J Med 1985; 312:91–97.
Bale SJ, et al: Cutaneous malignant melanoma and familial dysplastic nevi: evidence for autosomal dominance and pleiotropy. Am J Hum Genet 1986; 38:188–196.
Greene MH, Bale SJ: Genetic Aspects of cutaneous malignant melanoma. In: Gallagher RP, ed: Recent Results in Cancer Research, vol 102, Epidemiology of Malignant Melanoma. Philadelphia: Springer Verlag, 1986:144–153.
Greene MH, et al: Hereditary melanoma and the dysplastic nevus syndrome: the risk of cancers other than melanoma. J Amer Acad Dermatol 1987; 16:792–797.
Greene MH: Laboratory studies in patients with hereditary cutaneous malignant melanoma and dysplastic nevus syndrome. In: MacKie RM, ed: Pigment Cell, vol 8. Berlin: S Karger, 1987:29–50.
Dracopoli NC, Bale SJ: Genetic aspects of familial cutaneous malignant melanoma. Semin Oncol 1988; 15:541–548.
Balch CM, et al.: Cutaneous melanoma. In: DeVita VT, et al, eds: Cancer: principles and practice of oncology, 3rd ed. Piladelphia: J.B. Lippincott, 1989:1499–1542.
Bale SJ, et al.: Mapping the gene for hereditary cutaneous malignant melanoma-dysplastic nevus to chromosome 1p. New Engl J Med 1989; 320:1367–1372.

TU014                                      **Margaret A. Tucker**

## CANCER, MULTIPLE MYELOMA                                2744

**Includes:**
    Kahler disease
    Myeloma, multiple
    Myelomatosis
    Multiple myeloma
    Plasma cell myeloma

**Excludes:**
    Alpha-heavy-chain disease
    **Amyloidosis**
    Heavy-chain diseases, such as gamma-heavy-chain disease
    Mu-heavy-chain disease
    Plasma cell leukemia

**Major Diagnostic Criteria:** Diagnostic triad of marrow plasmacytosis, lytic bone lesions (characteristically "punched out") and a serum and/or urine M component. Serum M component will show IgG (53%), IgA (25%), or IgD (1%), while 20% will have only light chains in serum and urine.

**Clinical Findings:** Two-thirds of myeloma patients will present with bone pain, often involving the back and ribs, and occasionally the extremities, with pain accentuated by movement, and does not occur at night except with positional change. This is in contrast to bone pain in metastatic carcinoma, which is often more pronounced at night. Persistence of localized pain may indicate a pathologic fracture. There is an increased susceptibility to infection. Hematologic findings include anemia and rouleaux formation. Renal findings include proteinuria and may progress to renal failure. Anemia, abnormal bleeding tendency, occasional macroglossia, carpal tunnel syndrome, and gastrointestinal symptoms, particularly diarrhea, which may be secondary to amyloid disease, may occur. Central nervous system (CNS) signs and symptoms may be secondary to hyperviscosity syndromes. Acute or chronic advanced disease may be heralded by weight loss, weakness, intermittent or sustained fever in the absence of infection, and dehydration.

**Complications:** Hyperuricemia, hypercalcemia, hyperviscosity with neurologic sequelae, and metastatic complications including nerve compression.

**Associated Findings:** Amyloid disease, hyperviscosity syndrome, uremia.

**Etiology:** Undetermined. Occurs rarely in two or more primary relatives. Nevertheless, an unknown fraction of patients will show excess in their families, with 43 such familial occurrences (most in sibs) having been reported (Grosbois et al, 1986). Investigation of tumor associations (all sites) will be essential in family studies (Bourguet et al, 1985).

**Pathogenesis:** Myeloma occurs when a cell of the B-lymphocyte lineage proliferates, giving rise to a population of similar cells, believed to be monoclonal due to production of a homogeneous immunoglobulin (M protein). This immunoglobulin is comprised of a single class of heavy chain and a single type of light chain, with each clone producing a unique protein with an idiotypic marker distinguishing it from all other immunoglobulins. Viral etiology has been pursued in mouse plasmacytomas, but status remains unclear. Chromosome rearrangements have been studied in murine plasmacytomas. Aleutian disease of mink has been investigated wherein the Aleutian disease virus (ADV) appears to be transmissible to humans. ADV has been characterized by hyperglobulinemia and plasmacytosis. However, links of myeloma to humans are not established.

Chronic antigenic stimulation has been considered, since such disorders as rheumatoid arthritis, hereditary spherocytosis, osteomyelitis, and cholecystitis, among others, have been shown to have variable statistical association with development of plasma cell tumors. Radiation and asbestos exposure have also been suspect. Genetic factors appear to be important (Grosbois et al., 1986). Myeloma-prone families provide invaluable models for systematic immunochemical and immunogenetic investigations in concert with environmental factors.

**MIM No.:**  25450

**Sex Ratio:**  M1:F<1 (slight male excess).

**Occurrence:**  Approximately 3:100,000. Black/white ratio approximately 2:1. Increases progressively with age, with the highest rates in women over 70 and males over 80 years of age.

**Risk of Recurrence for Patient's Sib:**  Unknown.

**Risk of Recurrence for Patient's Child:**  Unknown.

**Age of Detectability:**  Average age of onset is 64 years. Fewer than 20% of patients are younger than age 40 years. There have been rare reports in children and youth.

**Gene Mapping and Linkage:**  Unknown.

**Prevention:**  None known. Genetic counseling indicated.

**Treatment:**  Alkylating agents, particularly Melphalan and cyclophosphamide, in association with adrenocorticosteroids have been shown to be effective and have resulted in remissions. However, patients may eventually go into acute phase with marked pancytopenia, a cellular marrow with immature plasma cells, and an increased risk of a terminal acute leukemia. Combination chemotherapy has been tried, but remains experimental.

**Prognosis:**  About 10% of patients will have an indolent course, demonstrating only very slow progression of disease over many years, and will rarely require antitumor therapy. About 15% of patients will die within the first three months following diagnosis. Subsequently, the death rate is about 15% per year. The disease usually follows a chronic course for 2–5 years before developing into an acute terminal phase marked by pancytopenia with a cellular marrow that is refractory to treatment. Patients with solitary bone plasmacytomas and extramedullary plasmacytomas (a fraction of whom will develop multile myeloma) may be expected to enjoy prolonged disease-free survival after local radiation therapy. Chronic phase may last for several years, but acute phase is often fulminant. There is no known cure.

**Detection of Carrier:**  Benign monoclonal gammopathy (BMG) may precede clinical evidence of multiple myeloma. BMG appears to be a preneoplastic setting in that in studies at the Mayo Clinic, ongoing for more than a decade, approximately 18% of patients with BMG developed a B-cell neoplasm, and an additional 9% manifested an increase in the M protein.

**Special Considerations:**  Plasma cell tumors have been extensively investigated in inbred mouse strains, a model that has been useful for human considerations, but to date the identification of an etiologic agent remains elusive. Genetic factors may be important in that the induction of plasmacytomas through pristane is restricted to BALB/C or NZB mice. Familial myeloma has been reported in humans, and, in one study from the Mayo Clinic, myeloma was observed in the sibs of eight of 440 myeloma patients. While the Mendelian inheritance pattern has not been identified, evidence in support of genetic factors for myeloma susceptibility in humans has been gleaned from identification of familial association of myeloma, macroglobulinemia, and BMG as well as the increased incidence in blacks. High-dose radiation exposure has been attributed to plasma cell myeloma etiology among controls and survivors of the Hiroshima and Nagasaki atomic bombs. Risk in the high-exposure group was recognized approximately 20 years following exposure. Asbestos exposure has also been suggested as an etiologic link, but more investigation is required.

**Support Groups:**  Atlanta; American Cancer Society

**References:**
Bourguet CC, et al.: Multiple myeloma and family history of cancer: a case-control study. Cancer 1985; 56:2133–2139.
Horwitz L, et al.: Multiple myeloma in three siblings. Arch Intern Med 1985; 145:1449–1459.
Grosbois B, et al.: Multiple myeloma in two brothers: an immuno-chemical and immunogenetic familial study. Cancer 1986; 58:2417–2421.
Comotti B, et al.: Multiple myeloma in a pair of twins. Brit J Haemat 1987; 65:123–124.

LY000                                    **Henry T. Lynch**

## CANCER, NEUROBLASTOMA                              2736

**Includes:**  Neuroblastoma and related lesions (all types)
**Excludes:**
  **Cancer, Ewing sarcoma** (3112)
  Central (cerebral and cerebellar) neuroblastoma
  Esthesioneuroblastoma
  **Jaw, neuroectodermal pigmented tumor** (0711)
  Malignant ectomesenchymoma
  Melanotic neuroectodermal tumor of infancy
  Neuroectodermal tumor, primitive
  Olfactory neuroblastoma

**Major Diagnostic Criteria:**  Elevated urine or blood dihydroxyphenylalnine (DOPA) and catecholamine metabolite levels. Elevated urinary vanillylmandelic acid (VMA), homovanillic acid (HVA), or both is seen in 95% of patients. X-ray demonstration of a suprarenal or posteromediastinal mass with calcifications.

**Clinical Findings:**  Neuroblastoma has a unique biology. Despite its very malignant and invasive capabilities, its in situ (microscopic aggregate of neuroblasts confined to the adrenal medulla, and incidently found in perinatal autopsies), and IV-S (hepatic, bone marrow, and skin involvement without radiologic bony lesions) forms may regress spontaneously. Neuroblastoma may also mature into a benign tumor, the ganglioneuroma, after going through an intermediate stage of ganglioneuroblastoma.

About 50–75% are retroperitoneal, arising in the adrenal medulla or a sympathetic ganglion, and 10–15% are mediastinal. Other sites are rare.

Some clinical findings lack specificity: irritability, tiredness, anorexia and weight loss, irregular fever, sweating, and pallor. They are the presenting signs in nearly one-half of the abdominal tumors. Other possible findings are abdominal pain; hypertension; diarrhea; bone pain; and subcutaneous nodules, sometimes affecting the scalp. Less common findings are polymyoclonus-opsoclonia syndrome, diabetes insipidus, hyperthyroidism, agranulocytosis, and myasthenia gravis. Polymyoclonus-opsoclonia-associated neuroblastoma is usually not accompanied by VMA elevation.

Some findings are directly determined by the site of the tumor. Signs of cord compression can be seen with dumbbell-shaped paravertebral tumors arising from sympathetic ganglia (weakness of an extremity, paralysis, and incontinence). Coughing, dyspnea, pulmonary infection, and paraplegia may accompany a mediastinal tumor. **Horner syndrome** and heterochromia iridis may be seen when the cervical sympathetic trunk is affected. Tumors of the pelvic region may present with difficulties at micturition or defecation, simulating presacral teratomas. Intrapelvic tumors may mimic embryonal rhabdomyosarcomas.

Congenital and neonatal neuroblastomas often present in stage IV-S. Skin lesions (32% of cases) consist of bluish nodules likened to a blueberry muffin; they become erythematous for a couple of minutes after palpation, then blanch, presumably as a result of catecholamine-induced vasoconstriction, a helpful diagnostic sign.

Cases of congenital neuroblastoma have manifested in utero. The fetal tumor may produce signs and symptoms of hypersecretion of catecholamine metabolites in the mother. These disappear after delivery. Neuroblastomas have been found in abortuses and stillborn fetuses.

**Complications:**  Metastatic dissemination develops rapidly and widely: local invasion, lymphatic dissemination, and hematogenous spread predominantly to the liver and bones. Metastases to the lungs occur in late stages. Three-fourths of the cases have metastases at the time of diagnosis. Pathologic fractures may occur. Profuse bony metastases, particularly to the skull and orbit with periorbital ecchymoses and exophthalmus, are sometimes seen. Widespread dissemination throughout the bone marrow is a distinctive and common pattern of spread. This may lead to thrombocytopenia and anemia. Anemia may also result from bleeding into the tumor mass or from consumption coagulopathy.

Subsequent development of a second malignancy (neurogenic tumors, acute lymphoblastic leukemia) is possible.

**Associated Findings:** There may be a higher incidence of skull and brain defects than expected for the general childhood population. The association with **Colon, aganglionosis** and **Neurofibromatosis** seems to be more than coincidental. The significance of heterochromia iridis is controversial.

**Etiology:** The mode of inheritance of the predisposition to the tumor is not established, but a hypothesized autosomal dominant mechanism with decreased penetrance (63%) is gaining acceptance over an autosomal recessive mode. Several children with the **Fetal hydantoin syndrome** have had neuroblastomas. The role of alcohol during pregnancy is not clear. There are sporadic and familial cases, and as much as 22% of neuroblastomas may have a heritable component. Both vertical and lateral transmissions have been observed.

**Pathogenesis:** Knudson and Strong (1972) have suggested a two-mutation model for familial neuroblastoma, the first mutation being prezygotic. In sporadic neuroblastoma, both mutations are postzygotic. *In situ* and IV-S neuroblastomas may represent a manifestation of the first (prezygotic) mutation. It has been suggested that neuroblastoma IV-S represents nonmalignant cells bearing a mutation preventing them from differentiating normally. Systemic chromosomal anomalies are rarely reported in patients with neuroblastoma. Double minute chromosomes and homogeneously staining regions are associated with N-*myc* amplification and are commonly seen in neuroblastoma tumor cells. N-*myc* amplification seems to correlate with advanced disease and poor prognosis, being usually absent from IV-S neuroblastoma and always from ganglioneuroma cells.

**MIM No.:** 25670

**CDC No.:** 194.000

**Sex Ratio:** M1:F1 in some series. In other series, it seems that both sporadic and familial neuroblastomas show a preponderance of affected males. This has been attributed to the more frequent maturation of neuroblastoma into ganglioneuroma in females.

**Occurrence:** The second most common malignant solid tumor in childhood, preceded only by brain tumors. There are some geographic, racial, and possibly seasonal variations. For unclear reasons, the incidence is much lower in certain parts of Africa and Asia than in Western Europe and the United States, where the annual incidence is approximately 9.6:1 million in white children and 7.0:1 million in black children. The proportion of sporadic and familial cases does seem to be similar from one country to another.

**Risk of Recurrence for Patient's Sib:** Unknown.

**Risk of Recurrence for Patient's Child:** Estimated at around 7%.

**Age of Detectability:** Only the tumor (and not the predisposition) can be detected. One-half of the cases occur in children less than two years of age, and about three-fourths of all cases are encountered during the first four years of life. Some investigators are attempting very early detection of the tumor by systematic and repeated evaluation of catecholamine metabolites in the urine from the time of birth. Ganglioneuromas can be detected incidentally and at any age.

**Gene Mapping and Linkage:** Unknown. The relationship between N-*myc* amplification, the deletion affecting the short arm of chromosome 1 and observed in as many as 70% of neuroblastoma cells, and the reported activation of N-*ras*, which also resides on chromosome 1, is not clear.

**Prevention:** None known. Genetic counseling indicated. A family history of neuroblastoma should alert the clinician for the need to follow up the child, his sibs, and eventually his offspring closely. Close follow-up is also indicated for sibs and offspring of patients with congenital and IV-S neuroblastomas.

**Treatment:** Various modalities consisting of surgical excision, radiation, and chemotherapy, are possible. Total body irradiation followed by bone marrow transplantation is sometimes attempted. Ganglioneuromas require surgical excision only. Congenital, neonatal, and infantile neuroblastomas, including stage IV-S, are often treated with chemotherapy alone.

**Prognosis:** The most valuable prognostic factors are the age of the patient, histology, and stage and location of the tumor. Disease-free two-year survival for treated infants, including the IV-S group and patients under age two years in stages I and II, is consistently reported to be over 90%. In patients in stages III and IV and who are generally older, the two-year disease-free survival rate nears 20–35%. Paraspinal dumbbell tumors have a better prognosis and a more pronounced tendency toward maturation into ganglioneuroma. Neuroblastomas associated with polymyoclonus-opsoclonia seem to have an excellent prognosis. This symptomatology has been attributed to a possible autoimmune factor directed against the tumor, and may be cross-reacting with cerebellar cells.

Determination of serum levels of ferritin, serum neuron-specific enolase (NSE), degree of N-*myc* amplification in the tumor cells, E-rosette inhibition, and nuclear DNA content of tumor cells are emerging as additional tools helpful in predicting the outcome. High VMA/HVA ratios also seem to predict a better prognosis. Determination of carcinoembryonic antigen (CEA) levels is useful in monitoring response to therapy and recurrence of the disease.

**Detection of Carrier:** None known for the predisposition to develop neuroblastoma.

**Special Considerations:** Tumors not clearly established as being directly related to the usual adrenal neuroblastoma have been excluded from this article. The most important diagnostic criterion is the pathologic diagnosis, as catecholamine metabolite levels are not always increased and, albeit rarely, may be increased in the absence of neuroblastoma. Determination of hereditary versus sporadic forms is rarely possible histologically, as multifocality and precursor lesions (i.e., *in situ* neuroblastoma) can no longer be recognized once the tumor is fully developed. The actual incidence of neuroblastoma may be higher than the clinically observed incidence, which does not take into consideration instances of *in situ* neuroblastoma or tumors developing in abortuses. Also, when investigated, parents and sibs of patients with neuroblastoma have been discovered to have elevated VMA levels or incidental ganglioneuromas. Thus, the estimated penetrance of 63%, implying a risk of about 7% to each offspring of an affected individual, cannot be considered as established.

**Support Groups:** Atlanta; American Cancer Society

**References:**

Knudson AG, Jr., Strong LC: Mutation and cancer: neuroblastoma and pheochromocytoma. Am J Hum Genet 1972; 24:514–532.

Knudson AG, Jr., Meadows AT: Regression of neuroblastoma IV-S: a genetic hypothesis. New Engl J Med 1980; 302:1254–1256.

Hecht F, et al.: Genetics of familial neuroblastoma: long-range studies. Cancer Genet Cytogenet 1982; 7:227–230.

Pochedly C, ed: Neuroblastoma: clinical and biological manifestations. New York: Elsevier Science, 1982. * †

Seeger RC, et al.: Association of multiple copies of the N-*myc* oncogene with rapid progression of neuroblastomas. New Engl J Med 1985; 313:1111–1116.

Evans AE, et al.: Prognostic factors in neuroblastoma. Cancer 1987; 59:1853–1859.

Nishi M, et al.: Effects of the mass screening of neuroblastoma in Sapporo City. Cancer 1987; 60:433–436.

Tsuda T, et al.: Analysis of N-myc amplification in relation to disease stage and histologic types in human neuroblastomas. Cancer 1987; 60:820–826.

Hayashi Y, et al.: Cytogenetic findings and prognosis in neuroblastoma with emphasis on marker chromosome 1. Cancer 1989; 63:126–132.

DE037                                           **Jean-Pierre de Chadarévian**

## CANCER, NEUROEPITHELIAL AND MENINGEAL  **2748**

**Includes:**
Central nervous system tumors
Tumors of the central nervous system, site-specific
aggregation
Brain tumor, neuroepithelial and meningeal

**Excludes:**
**Cancer, familial** (1505)
**Cancer, glioma, familial** (2839)
Mendelian disorders that predispose to brain tumors
(other)

**Major Diagnostic Criteria:** Two or more first-degree relatives also with central nervous system tumors other than glioma.

**Clinical Findings:** The definition of familial brain tumors is arbitrary and making a diagnosis is somewhat a matter of intuition. Since brain tumors are not rare, especially in young people, some instances of familial aggregation could occur by chance. Familial brain tumors could, in theory, be explained by shared environmental determinants. Case-control studies have associated brain tumors with many environmental agents including paternal exposure to N-nitroso compounds and personal exposure to ionizing radiation and insecticides in childhood and, in adults, to the manufacture and maintenance of electronic equipment. Features that suggest an excessive familial aggregation are extrapolated from the characteristics of classic examples of single genes that cause cancer, like **Retinoblastoma**: early age of onset, bilaterality, presence of multiple primary malignant neoplasms, and of course familial aggregation. The presenting clinical findings do not differ from those of sporadic brain tumors: seizures, headache, mental and visual changes, and lateralizing weakness.

**Complications:** Like sporadic brain tumors, familial brain tumors kill by local invasion and expansion, and endocrinologic and metabolic derangements.

**Associated Findings:** Brain tumors may occur in families because of a predisposing disease that is genetic or familial; such as, **Neurofibromatosis, Tuberous sclerosis**, and **Nevoid basal cell carcinoma syndrome**.

**Etiology:** Diverse etiologies are likely, as might be expected for this heterogeneous grouping of tumor types. Medulloblastoma has been seen as the first manifestation of the **Nevoid basal cell carcinoma syndrome** and, on occasion, in patients with **Turcot syndrome** and **Ataxia-telangiectasia**. In the tissue of sporadic meningioma, one chromosome 22 is almost always missing, even when the constitutional karyotype is normal. In an informative but thus far unique family with four members in two generations with meningioma, a heritable translocation was seen (t(14;22)). A pathogenetic role for genes on chromosome 22 is likely in the origins of meningioma as supported by the loss in genetic heterogeneity seen in meningiomas arising in persons with **Acoustic neuromata**, mapped to chromosome 22 by family studies. Meningioma has also been reported in **Werner syndrome** and **Gingival multiple hamartoma syndrome**. Pinealblastoma is a pleiotropic effect of the hereditary retinoblastoma gene. It sometimes occurs even before retinoblastoma is diagnosed, and sometimes at an ectopic site, such as the cheek. The term "trilateral retinoblastoma" for pinealoblastoma recalls the facts that the pineal gland is the third eye of amphibions and that the human pineal body has some photoreceptor cells. Childhood pinealomas seem to occur to excess in Japan. Central nervous system lymphomas are rare but occur at vast excess in persons with hereditary or acquired immunodeficiencies, such as **Immunodeficiency, Wiskott-Aldrich type** and renal transplant recipients.

**Pathogenesis:** Regardless of specific primary etiology, cytogenetic and single gene abnormalities are probably a common pathway in the progression from normal brain tissue to clinical brain tumor, whether familial or sporadic. Specifically, chromosome 22 has been implicated in meningiomas as seen by direct tumor studies, by its association with **Acoustic neuromata**, and by reports of isolated patients and families with meningiomas and constitutional defects involving chromosome 22. Likewise, chromosome 13 seems involved with pinealoblastoma, at least when it complicated **Retinoblastoma**.

**MIM No.:**  13345

**Sex Ratio:**  M1:F1. There is no reason to think that familial brain tumors have different sex ratios than sporadic ones.

**Occurrence:**  With the assumption that 60% of all primary central nervous system tumors are gliomas, some 6,000 persons were estimated to develop brain tumors other than gliomas in 1987. Only a small fraction would be expected to be a familial.

**Risk of Recurrence for Patient's Sib:**  Depends on etiology, but in general low. Analysis of death certificates from childhood brain tumor in the United States (including some gliomas) indicated a ten-fold excess of brain tumors and bone cancer in siblings. A similar study found 30 sib pairs with at least one brain tumor, compared to 11 pairs expected by chance.

**Risk of Recurrence for Patient's Child:**  Undetermined but low, in the absence of a dominant trait predisposing to brain tumors.

**Age of Detectability:**  Primary brain tumors may present at any age. Data are insufficient to document the generalization that familial brain tumors occur at earlier ages than sporadic ones.

**Gene Mapping and Linkage:**  Several gene that predispose to brain tumor have been mapped. See **Neurofibromatosis, Acoustic neuromata, Tuberous sclerosis**, and **Von Hippel-Lindau syndrome**.

**Prevention:**  None known. Genetic counseling indicated.

**Treatment:**  As for sporadic cases; surgery with additional chemotherapy and radiotherapy as indicated.

**Prognosis:**  As for sporadic brain tumors, survival is determined by age at diagnosis, histologic grade, localization, and treatment. Average five-year survival for all types of brain tumors in the United States is 24%.

**Detection of Carrier:**  Unknown.

**Support Groups:**
Atlanta; American Cancer Society
Chicago; Association for Brain Tumor Research

**References:**
Miller RW: Deaths from childhood leukemia and solid tumors among twins and other sibs in the United States. J Natl Cancer Inst 1971; 46:203–209.
Draper GJ, et al: Occurrence of childhood cancers among sibs and estimation of familial risks. J Med Genet 1977; 14:81–90.
Tijssen CC, et al: Familial brain tumors. Developments in Oncology, vol 9. The Hague: Nijhoff, 1982:469. *
Farwell J, Flannery JT: Cancer in relatives of children with central-nervous-system neoplasms. New Engl J Med 1984; 311:749–753.
Arinami T, et al: Multifocal meningiomas in a patient with a constitutional ring chromosome 22. J Med Genet 1985; 22:178–180.
Bolger GB, et al: Chromosome translocation t(14;22) and oncogene (c-sis) variant in a pedigree with familial meningioma. New Engl J Med 1985; 312:564–567.
Lesnick JE, et al: Familial pineoblastoma. J Neurosurg 1985; 62:930–932.
Tijssen CC: Genetics aspects of brain tumors: tumors of neuroepithelial and meningeal tissue. In: Muller HJ, Weber, eds: Familial Cancer. Basel: Karger, 1985:98–102.

MU009                                                      **John J. Mulvihill**

**Cancer, osteosarcoma**
*See OSTEOSARCOMA*

## CANCER, PANCREAS, FAMILIAL ADENOCARCINOMA OF 2374

**Includes:**
  Adenocarcinoma of the pancreas
  Carcinoma of the pancreas
  Pancreatic acinar carcinoma
  Pancreatic cancer

**Excludes:**
  Carcinoma of the ampulla of Vater
  Glucagonoma
  Insulinoma
  Pancreatic adenoma
  **Pancreatitis, hereditary** (0793)

**Major Diagnostic Criteria:** The diagnosis is established by histopathologic demonstration of adenocarcinoma of the exocrine pancreas.

**Clinical Findings:** Typical presenting features include abdominal pain, jaundice, anorexia, and weight loss.
  Sonography, computerized axial tomography, endoscopic retrograde choledochopancreatography, and selective angiography are useful means of visualizing pancreatic carcinoma.

**Complications:** Diabetes mellitus occurs in 10–20% of patients with pancreatic carcinoma. Pancreatitis is sometimes seen.

**Associated Findings:** Carcinoma of the pancreas has been reported in association with **Pancreatitis, hereditary**, multiple endocrine adenomatosis type I, **Ataxia-telangiectasia**, familial pancreatic and colon cancer syndrome, and **Intestinal polyposis, type III**. In families with these conditions, the recurrence risk and genetic counselling depend on the underlying diagnosis.

**Etiology:** Most cases are sporadic, but rare familial instances have been reported. Cigarette smoking, coffee drinking, and environmental chemicals have been suggested as possible predisposing factors, but these associations appear to be weak.

**Pathogenesis:** Unknown.

**MIM No.:** 26035

**Sex Ratio:** M1.5:F1

**Occurrence:** 1–12:100,000

**Risk of Recurrence for Patient's Sib:** Presumably small.

**Risk of Recurrence for Patient's Child:** Presumably small.

**Age of Detectability:** Any age, but usually late adulthood. Mean age at diagnosis is about 57 years.

**Gene Mapping and Linkage:** Unknown.

**Prevention:** Avoidance of cigarettte smoking and other environmental hazards. Genetic counseling is indicated.

**Treatment:** Surgical, radiation, and medical therapy in various combinations have been used.

**Prognosis:** Ninty percent of patients with carcinoma of the pancreas die within five years of diagnosis, even with the best available treatment.

**Detection of Carrier:** Unknown.

**Support Groups:** Atlanta; American Cancer Society

**References:**
MacDermott RP, Kramer P: Adenocarcinoma of the pancreas in four siblings. Gastroenterology 1973; 65:137–139.
Friedman JM, Fialkow PJ: Familial carcinoma of the pancreas. Clin Genet 1976; 9:463–469. *
Reimer RR, et al.: Pancreatic cancer in father and son. Lancet 1977; 1:911.
Danes BS, Lynch HT: A familial aggregation of pancreatic cancer: an in vitro study. J Am Med Asso JAMA 1982; 247:2798–2802.
Dat NM, Sontag SJ: Pancreatic carcinoma in brothers. Ann Intern Med 1982; 97:282.
Higginson J, Muir CS: Epidemiology of cancer. In: Holland JF, Frei E, eds: Cancer medicine, 2nd ed. Philadelphia: Lea & Febiger, 1982: 257–327.
Macdonald JS, et al.: Cancer of the pancreas. In: DeVita VT, et al., eds: Cancer: principles and practice of oncology. Philadelphia: J.B. Lippincott Company, 1982:563–589. *
Moertel CG: Exocrine pancreas. In: Holland JF, Frei E, eds: Cancer medicine, 2nd ed., Philadelphia: Lea & Febiger, 1982:1792–1804.
Grajower MM: Familial pancreatic cancer. Ann Intern Med 1983; 97:111.
Moossa AR, et al.: Tumors of the pancreas. In: Moossa AR, eds: Comprehensive textbook of oncology. Baltimore: Williams & Wilkins, 1986:1105–1132.

FR017                                                    **J.M. Friedman**

## CANCER, RENAL CELL CARCINOMA 2689

**Includes:**
  Adenocarcinoma of the kidney
  Clear cell carcinoma of the kidney
  Hypernephroma
  Kidney, renal cell carcinoma
  Renal cell carcinoma

**Excludes:** Cancer, Wilms tumor (2742)

**Major Diagnostic Criteria:** Diagnosis is based on microscopic examination of tumor tissue obtained at biopsy or nephrectomy.

**Clinical Findings:** Classically presents with triad of flank mass, pain with fever, and hematuria. Other constitutional symptoms may also be present. Diagnosis often suspected from sonography, intravenous pyelogram, and angiography studies, but definitive diagnosis requires tumor tissue.

**Complications:** Propensity of tumor for hematogenous spread, particularly to bones and lungs. Death can result from renal failure, metastatic disease, or both.

**Associated Findings:** None known.

**Etiology:** Possibly autosomal dominant inheritance. A weak association has been reported with cigarette smoking. Increased in **Von Hippel-Lindau syndrome**.

**Pathogenesis:** Unknown.

**MIM No.:** 14470

**Sex Ratio:** M2:F1

**Occurrence:** Rate increases with age. About ten affected kinships have been reported.

**Risk of Recurrence for Patient's Sib:** Very small.

**Risk of Recurrence for Patient's Child:** Very small.

**Age of Detectability:** Median age at diagnosis is around age 65 years. The cancer is rare before age 40 years.

**Gene Mapping and Linkage:** Chromosome and molecular analysis of renal cancer cells shows changes in chromosome 3 to be most common, usually deletion of 3p (del 3p14–21).

**Prevention:** Avoidance of heavy smoking.

**Treatment:** Cure of local disease can be attained by nephrectomy. Radiotherapy and chemohumoral therapy have little effect. Recently, responses have been reported with interleukin-2 with lymphokine-activated killer cells.

**Prognosis:** Almost always fatal unless a surgical cure is achieved. Recurrences can occur years after initial total tumor excision.

**Detection of Carrier:** Unknown.

**Special Considerations:** Familial renal cancer has been reported in appoximately ten families without **Von Hippel-Lindau syndrome** which is a known risk factor. Of note is a family with ten affected persons and a 3;8 chromosome translocation that is constitutional and dominantly transmitted. The breakpoint on chromosome 3 is at 3p14, the most common site of chromosomal change among all renal cancers.

**Support Groups:** Atlanta; American Cancer Society

**References:**
Cohen AJ, et al.: Hereditary renal-cell carcinoma associated with a chromosomal translocation. New Engl J Med 1979; 301:592–595.

Li FP, et al.: Familial renal carcinoma. Cancer Genet Cytogenet 1982; 7:271–275.
Outzen HC, Maguire HC, Jr: The etiology of renal-cell carcinoma. Semin Oncol 1983; 10:378–384.
Drabkin HA, et al.: Translocation of *c-myc* in the hereditary renal cell carcinoma associated with a t(3;8)(p14.2;q24.13)chromosomal translocation. Proc Natl Acad Sci USA 1985; 82:6980–6985.
Zbar B, et al.: Loss of alleles of loci on the short arm of chromosome 3 in renal cell carcinoma. Nature 1987; 327:721–724.

LI028                                  **Frederick P. Li**

**Cancer, reticulosis, familial histiocytic, Omenn type**
*See IMMUNODEFICIENCY, RETICULOENDOTHELIOSIS WITH EOSINOPHILIA*
**Cancer, retinoblastoma**
*See RETINOBLASTOMA*

## CANCER, SEBACEOUS GLAND TUMOR-MULTIPLE VISCERAL CARCINOMA        2743

**Includes:**
> Cancer family syndrome
> Cutaneous sebaceous neoplasms-keracanthomas-GI and other cancers
> Hereditary nonpolyposis colorectal cancer (HNPCC)
> Keratocanthomas-cutaneous sebaceous tumors-other cancers
> Lynch syndromes I and II
> Muir-Torre (MT) syndrome

**Excludes:**
> **Cancer** (other)
> **Intestinal polyposis, type III** (0536)

**Major Diagnostic Criteria:** The cutaneous findings of sebaceous hyperplasia, sebaceous adenoma, sebaceous carcinoma, basal cell carcinoma with sebaceous differentiation, or multiple keratoacanthoma are essential components. These skin signs may occur singly or in combination with multiple primary visceral cancer and a rather extraordinary increased survival, even in the presence of distant metastases. Thus, the combination of these cutaneous findings and visceral cancer comprise the full complement of the syndrome.

**Clinical Findings:** Cutaneous signs of sebaceous hyperplasia, adenoma and carcinoma, basal cell carcinoma with sebaceous differentiation, and keratoacanthoma in association with visceral cancer (often multiple), including tumors of the gastrointestinal tract, ovary, endometrium, and, more rarely, the hematopoietic system comprise the syndrome. There is often an extraordinarily improved cancer survival even in the presence of distant metastases. Lynch et al (1981, 1985) have linked these cutaneous features with the Lynch syndromes I and II.

**Complications:** All of the sequelae accompanying each anatomic site of cancer predilection in the HNPCC syndromes.

**Associated Findings:** The distinctive cutaneous stigmata are reported in only a small number of patients within Lynch syndrome kindreds.

**Etiology:** Autosomal dominant inheritance.

**Pathogenesis:** Unknown.

**MIM No.:** 15832, *11440

**Sex Ratio:** M1:F1

**Occurrence:** Undetermined in the general population, but occurs in about one-fifth of hereditary nonpolyposis colorectal cancer (HNPCC) kindreds (Lynch syndromes I and II).

**Risk of Recurrence for Patient's Sib:**
> See Part I, *Mendelian Inheritance.*

**Risk of Recurrence for Patient's Child:**
> See Part I, *Mendelian Inheritance.*

**Age of Detectability:** Age of onset of cutaneous findings is not well defined. Sebaceous tumors occur around puberty in the general population. Average age of cancer onset is early (about age 44 years) in the Lynch syndromes.

**Gene Mapping and Linkage:** Unknown.

**Prevention:** None known. Genetic counseling indicated. Highly targeted cancer surveillance with colonoscopy (or double air contrast barium enema if expertise for colonoscopy is unavailable) is essential, since there is a proximal colon cancer excess in Lynch syndromes. Colonoscopy should be initiated at age 25 and performed annually thereafter. Other measures appropriate for cancer sites of predilection in specific families.

**Treatment:** That which is appropriate for each particular form of cancer.

**Prognosis:** Cancer is often indolent with occasional extraordinary survival in the presence of metastases.

**Detection of Carrier:** Unknown.

**Special Considerations:** Over 50 disorders are characterized by distinguishing cutaneous signs that are associated with hereditary cancer-prone syndromes (Lynch and Fusaro, 1982), and this syndrome joins the list of these cancer-associated genodermatoses (Lynch et al, 1985). Recognition of the hereditary component, with particular relevance to the Lynch syndromes, has only recently been appreciated mainly due to the fact that in early reports linking the cutaneous manifestations with visceral cancer, this family history was often ignored. Syndrome recognition requires meticulous documentation of cutaneous findings in concert with visceral cancer (all sites), including attention to the pattern of multiple primary cancer. Particular attention must be given to a search for nonpolyposis colonic cancer with proximal predominance, carcinoma of the endometrium, ovary, breast, and other anatomic sites, including, on occasion, the hematopoietic system. Cutaneous manifestations require biopsy, since histologic interpretation is essential for diagnosis. Characteristic cutaneous signs have been observed in only a small fraction of the total membership of our Lynch syndrome kindreds. This phenomenon is not unlike that which occurs in such hereditary cancer-prone disorders as Gardner syndrome (see **Intestinal polyposis, type III** in which it is rare to encounter a patient in a given family who manifests *all* components that are consonant with the so-called classic definition of the syndrome.

**Support Groups:** Atlanta; American Cancer Society

**References:**
Lynch HT, et al.: The cancer family syndrome: rare cutaneous phenotypic linkage of Torre's syndrome. Arch Intern Med 1981; 141:607–611.
Lynch HT, Fusaro RM: Cancer-associated genodermatoses. New York: Van Nostrand Reinhold, 1982.
Lynch HT, et al.: Muir-Torre syndrome in several members of a family with a variant of the cancer family syndrome. Br J Dermatol 1985; 113:295–301.
Lynch HT, et al.: Hereditary nonpolyposis colorectal cancer: Lynch syndromes I and II. Gastroenterol Clinics North Am 1988; 17:679–712.

LY000                                  **Henry T. Lynch**

## CANCER, SOFT TISSUE SARCOMA        2749

**Includes:**
> Fibrosarcoma
> Leiomyosarcoma
> Liposarcoma
> Malignant fibrous histiocytoma
> Rhabdomyosarcoma

**Excludes:**
> **Cancer, Ewing sarcoma** (3112)
> Connective tissue disorders, benign
> **Osteosarcoma** (3101)

**Major Diagnostic Criteria:** Diagnosis is established by light microscopy of biopsy specimen.

**Clinical Findings:** May arise at any age and in diverse primary sites. Congenital lesions are rare, but reported. Usually presents as a tumor mass that is palpable or that impinges on adjacent tissues to produce symptoms. Occasionally, disease detected at metastatic site, such as lung. X-ray studies, including CT scanning are used in determining the extent of the disease.

**Complications:** Death from disease progression at the primary site or a metastatic site.

**Associated Findings:** None known.

**Etiology:** Undetermined, except for rare cases induced by high doses of radiation. Possibly through autosomal dominant inheritance in some families.

**Pathogenesis:** Chromosomal translocations and deletions t(x;18) in synovial sarcoma, t(12;16) in some myxoid liposarcomas, and del 3 in some rhabdomyosarcomas) are reported for several forms of sarcoma.

**MIM No.:** *11440

**Sex Ratio:** M5:F4

**Occurrence:** Incidence: 1–10:10⁶ persons per year.

**Risk of Recurrence for Patient's Sib:** Very small except in rare families.

**Risk of Recurrence for Patient's Child:** Very small except in rare families.

**Age of Detectability:** All ages, with slightly higher rates after age 40 years of age.

**Gene Mapping and Linkage:** Unknown.

**Prevention:** None known. Genetic counseling indicated. Avoidance of high-dose radiation.

**Treatment:** Surgery, radiation therapy, and chemotherapy.

**Prognosis:** Depends on the extent of the disease (stage) and tumor differentiation (histologic grade).

**Detection of Carrier:** Unknown.

**Special Considerations:** Approximately 30 families have been reported with an autosomal dominant pattern of sarcomas in children associated with breast cancer, brain tumors, acute leukemia, and adrenocortical carcinoma in young relatives (hence the occasional designation *SBLA cancer family syndrome*, see **Cancer, breast, familial**). Pathogenesis of this familial condition is undetermined.

**Support Groups:** Atlanta; American Cancer Society

**References:**

Li FP, Fraumeni JF: Prospective study of a family cancer syndrome. J Am Med Asso 1982; 247:2692–2694.
Birch JM, et al.: Excess risk of breast cancer in the mothers of children with soft tissue sarcomas. Br J Cancer 1984; 49:325–331.
Turc-Carel C, et al.: Involvement of chromosome X in primary cytogenetic change in human neoplasia. nonrandom translocation in synovial sarcoma. Proc Natl Acad Sci USA 1987; 84:1981–1985.

LI028                                          **Frederick P. Li**

## CANCER, THYMOMA                              2745

**Includes:**
    Epithelial thymomas, pseudorosette type
    Superior vena cava syndrome
    Thymoma, familial

**Excludes:**
    Carcinoids
    Germ cell tumors
    **Lymphoma**
    Thymolipomas involving the thymic gland

**Major Diagnostic Criteria:** The epithelial component of the thymus gland must be neoplastic for diagnosis of thymoma.

**Clinical Findings:** May be identified fortuitously through its discovery on a chest X-ray obtained for reasons unrelated to this lesion. Onset is often between 40 and 60 years of age. Symptoms are vague and often pulmonary, including dyspnea, tightness of the chest, pain in the chest, and cough. Dysphagia may also occur. In the advanced stage, one may encounter the *superior vena cava syndrome*. This is characterized by dilation of veins of the upper neck and thorax with associated headache, reduced cognition and consciousness, edema of the head and neck, and plethora, secondary to tumor compression of vessels. Thymomas are slow growing, with some having been reported to remain the same size for as long as 15 years. Distinction between "benign" and "malignant" thymomas is artificial, and all thymomas must be considered malignant and thereby capable of infiltrating surrounding tissue. Metastases to regional or distant nodes is uncommon and, when observed, the most common blood-borne metastatic sites have been liver, bone, brain, spleen, colon, and kidney.

Thymomas are rare in children, with fewer than 10% being found in individuals below age 20 years. They appear to have a more malignant outcome in children as opposed to thymomas in adults. Thymomas are located primarily in the anterior mediastinum (75% of cases). Fifteen percent may occur in both the anterior and superior mediastinum, while 6% are primarily in the superior mediastinum, with no more than 5–10% in other locations (neck, middle and posterior mediastinum). The tumors are round or oval and have smooth or lobulated margins, with calcifications in about 20% of thymomas. CT scan is helpful in defining the extent and involvement of lesions suspected as being thymoma.

**Complications:** Malignant potential correlates with invasive characteristics as opposed to its microscopic appearance.

**Associated Findings:** Most common are myasthenia gravis, hypogammaglobulinemia (5–10% of patients with thymoma), and red cell aplasia, considered an autoimmune disorder (5% of patients with thymoma). Other associated conditions include polymyositis, **Lupus erythematosus, systemic, Arthritis, rheumatoid,** thyroiditis, **Scleroderma, familial progressive,** dermatomyositis, sarcoid, rheumatic endocarditis, chronic ulcerative colitis (see **Inflammatory bowel disease**), and **Sjogren syndrome,** in addition to endocrine disorders. The most common association is with myasthenia gravis. About 40–50% of patients with associated syndromes will show this particular combination. Fifteen to 50% of patients with myasthenia gravis will have gross or microscopic evidence of thymomas. In some circumstances, more than one disease may occur in association with thymoma, e.g., myasthenia gravis and thrombocytopenia. Severe inflammations such as myocarditis may also be associated with thymoma.

**Etiology:** There are rare reports of affected sibs, the significance of which remains elusive.

**Pathogenesis:** Epithelium of the thymus gland is derived from the third pharyngeal pouches. For a neoplasm to be considered a thymoma, the epithelial component must form a neoplastic component. **Cancer, Hodgkin disease, familial** and **Lymphoma, non-Hodgkin,** when involving the thymus gland, are essentially the same as their occurrence in any other tissue, and they must not be considered as thymomas. Epithelial thymomas have a more extensive and aggressive course than in patients with spindle cell or predominantly lymphocytic types of involvement of the thymus. There does not appear to be any correlation between the histology of a thymoma and its coexistence with other associated disorders or between histology and prognosis. Two reports show thymic neoplasia in sibs (Wick et al, 1982; Matani and Dritsas, 1973). The first report of familial involvement showed two middle-aged brothers affected, one with histologically verified thymic carcinoma and the other with histologically verified, invasive, spindle cell thymoma with associated hypogammaglobulinemia. In the second familial occurrence (Matani and Dritsas, 1973), a 27-month-old girl manifested a large tumor of the thymus gland, which histologically was predominantly of the lymphocytic type. Her brother died of a similar lesion at age 9 months. Thymic tumors have also occurred in multiple endocrine neoplasia wherein the histology has consistently been that of thymic carcinoid tumors (Rosai et al, 1972; Manes and Taylor, 1973).

**MIM No.:** 27423

**Sex Ratio:** M1:F1

**Occurrence:**   Unknown.

**Risk of Recurrence for Patient's Sib:**   Unknown.

**Risk of Recurrence for Patient's Child:**   Unknown.

**Age of Detectability:**   Usually between ages 40 and 60 years, with about 10% in patients under age 20 years, and rare in children.

**Gene Mapping and Linkage:**   Unknown.

**Prevention:**   None known. Genetic counseling indicated.

**Treatment:**   Complete surgical extirpation is the most effective treatment, with virtually 100% cure when the entire thymus is removed without disturbing the capsule. Invasiveness of the tumor or association with myasthenia gravis renders a poor outcome. Thymomas are relatively radiosensitive; therefore, radiation therapy is excellent for adjuvant use and is mandatory for patients with invasive thymomas, regardless of whether complete resection has been obtained. Preoperative radiation therapy has been used by some, but its benefit has not been proven. Regression of resectable thymomas has been reported to result from administration of corticosteroids. Single drug chemotherapy agents have included doxorubicin, cis-diamminedichlorplatinum, and alkylating agents. Combination therapy has included vincristine, cyclophosphamide, lomustine, and prednisone, with which response rates have been as high as 56%.

**Prognosis:**   Good in general. Poorer survivals are associated with tumor invasiveness and presence of myasthenia gravis.

**Detection of Carrier:**   Unknown.

**Support Groups:**   Atlanta; American Cancer Society

**References:**

Rosai J, et al.: Mediastinal endocrine neoplasia in patients with multiple endocrine adenomatosis: a previously unrecognized association. Cancer 1972; 29:1075–1083.

Manes JL, Taylor HB: Thymic carcinoid in familial multiple endocrine adenomatosis. Arch Pathol 1973; 95:252–255.

Matani A, Dritsas C: Familial occurrence of thymoma. Arch Pathol 1973; 95:90–91.

Rosai J: Tumors of the thymus. In: Atlas of tumor pathology, Ser 2, Fasc 13. Washington, D.C.: Armed Forces Institute of Pathology, 1976.

Wick MR, et al.: Thymic neoplasia in two male siblings. Mayo Clin Proc 1982; 57:653–656.

LY000                                           **Henry T. Lynch**

## CANCER, THYROID, FAMILIAL PAPILLARY CARCINOMA OF                                          2641

**Includes:**
> Differentiated carcinoma of the papillary type
> Follicular variant of papillary carcinoma
> Papillary carcinoma with follicular elements
> Papillary cystadenocarcinoma
> Thyroid, familial papillary carcinoma
> Thyroid 1, transforming sequence

**Excludes:**
> Carcinoma, familial medullary
> **Intestinal polyposis, type I** (0535)
> **Intestinal polyposis, type III** (0536)
> Neoplasia, multiple endocrine

**Major Diagnostic Criteria:**   Two or more cases of papillary carcinoma of the thyroid gland within a family. The diagnosis is based on characteristic histology, which includes papillae. Frequently a follicular pattern is also observed. The nuclei have a characteristic clear watery appearance. Forty percent of papillary carcinomas contain laminated calcific spherules, called psammoma bodies. Lymphatic, capsular, and occasional vascular invasion may be identified.

**Clinical Findings:**   Thyroid nodule(s) and occasionally palpable lymph nodes identified by careful palpation of the neck by an experienced examiner. Confirmation by appropriate studies, which currently include outpatient needle biopsy. Benign thyroid diseases appear to be common in these families.

**Complications:**   The tumor usually remains localized and may remain indolent for decades, but may metastasize locally or spread to more distant cervical or upper mediastinal lymph nodes or, rarely, to bone or lung.

**Associated Findings:**   Several parents of papillary carcinoma patients in papillary carcinoma families have had **Cancer, colorectal**. Thus it is possible that colon carcinoma is one manifestation of the gene.

**Etiology:**   Possibly autosomal dominant inheritance with reduced penetrance. Expressivity appears to be variable, ranging from benign thyroid disease to papillary carcinoma of the thyroid and, possibly, colon cancer. Familial exposure to radiation, e.g., for enlarged thymus or tonsillar disease, could, in theory, account for some familial aggregation. At least one set of monozygotic twins, concordant for papillary carcinoma of the thyroid gland, has been reported (Austoni, 1988). Their mother had a nodular goiter.

**Pathogenesis:**   The pathogenesis of papillary thyroid carcinoma may follow Knudson's two-hit theory for the initiation of carcinogenesis. Thus, in the papillary carcinoma family, the first hit is the inherited mutation, and a second mutation (hit) in a susceptible cell is sufficient to cause carcinogenesis. In these families, the susceptible cells may include cells in the colon as well as in the thyroid gland. The benign thyroid disease may be a more direct effect of the mutation and may increase the likelihood of carcinogenesis by increasing the number of susceptible cells through cellular hyperplasia. Radiation to the head or neck may be a predisposing environmental variable. The high-resolution karyotype is normal, and there is no evidence of increased chromosome instability. It is possible that in some cases papillary carcinoma is caused by the same mutant gene that causes familial polyposis.

**MIM No.:**   18855

**Sex Ratio:**   M1:F2–3

**Occurrence:**   Discovered in 1:1,000 routine autopsies. Papillary carcinoma of the thyroid is usually sporadic, but at least 3.5%, probably more, of new patients will be members of a papillary carcinoma family. Occasionally it is associated with **Intestinal polyposis, type III** and **Intestinal polyposis, type I**. Papillary carcinoma was diagnosed in about 7,000 patients in the United States during 1986.

**Risk of Recurrence for Patient's Sib:**
> See Part I, *Mendelian Inheritance*.

**Risk of Recurrence for Patient's Child:**
> See Part I, *Mendelian Inheritance*.

**Age of Detectability:**   Age of onset varies, with thyroid disease occurring in younger individuals and colon cancer in older individuals.

The peak incidence of papillary carcinoma is in the third and fourth decades of life; age range is five to 90 years. The youngest papillary carcinoma family member diagnosed thus far was 16 years old, but the carcinoma can be diagnosed in childhood. The mean age of diagnosis of the confirmed familial cases of papillary carcinoma is 37.8 ± 14.2 years.

**Gene Mapping and Linkage:**   TST1 (transforming sequence, thyroid 1) has been provisionally mapped to 10q11.2.

**Prevention:**   None known. Genetic counseling indicated.

**Treatment:**   Surgical excision. The extent of surgical treatment depends on the extent of the tumor. Iodine-131 ablation is sometimes helpful following surgery. Replacement therapy with levothyroxine is important to prevent recurrence.

**Prognosis:**   For tumors less than 4 cm in size with either no metastatic disease or only metastatic cervical nodes: excellent; distal metastatic disease involving lung or bone: 53% five-year survival, 38% ten-year survival, and 30% 15-year survival. The prognosis tends to be least favorable when onset of treatment begins beyond age 50 years.

**Detection of Carrier:** Palpation of the neck by an experienced examiner or, for a less experienced examiner, ultrasound or nuclear medicine imaging procedures.

**Special Considerations:** About 70% of all thyroid carcinoma is papillary. About two-thirds of patients have unifocal disease, and one-third multifocal or with lymph node metastasis. There may be a disproportionate risk to irradiated subjects who are Jewish. When two or more persons in a family have papillary carcinoma of the thyroid, all first and second degree relatives should have their necks palpated by an experienced examiner and perhaps tested for possible colon cancer.

**Support Groups:** Atlanta; American Cancer Society

**References:**
Lote K, et al.: Familial occurrence of papillary thyroid carcinoma. Cancer 1980; 46:1291–1297.
Mazzaferi EL, Young RL: Papillary thyroid carcinoma: a 10 year follow-up report of the impact of therapy in 576 patients. Am J Med 1981; 70:511–518.
Phade VR, et al.: Familial papillary carcinoma of the thyroid. Arch Surg 1981; 116:836–837.
McConahey WM, et al.: Papillary thyroid cancer treated at the Mayo Clinic, 1946 through 1970: initial manifestations, pathologic findings, therapy, and outcome. Mayo Clin Proc 1986; 61:978–996.
Schlumberger M, et al.: Long-term results of treatment of 283 patients with lung and bone metastases from differentiated thyroid carcinoma. J Clin Endocrinol Metabol 1986; 63:960–967.
Stoffer SS, et al.: Familial papillary carcinoma of the thyroid. Am J Med Genet 1986; 25:775–782.
Austoni M: Thyroid papillary carcinoma in identical twins. Lancet 1988; I:1115 only.

ST051
VA004

**Sheldon S. Stoffer**
**Daniel L. Van Dyke**

**Cancer, trichomatrical**
*See PILOMATRIXOMA*

## CANCER, WILMS TUMOR                          2742

**Includes:**
    Clear cell sarcoma of the kidney (CCSK)
    Kidney, clear cell sarcoma
    Malignant rhabdoid tumor of the kidney (MRTK)
    Nephroblastoma
    Nephroblastomatosis
    Renal blastema, nodular or persistent
    Wilms tumor

**Excludes:**
    **Chromosome 11, partial monosomy 11p** (2245)
    Juxtaglomerular cell tumor
    Mesoblastic nephroma, congenital
    Wilms tumor of the adult
    Wilms tumor, extrarenal

**Major Diagnostic Criteria:** Tissue diagnosis is essential. A non-mobile mass in an upper quadrant is found in nearly 95% of the cases of Wilms tumor. In more than one-half of the cases, this mass is the only sign.

**Clinical Findings:** In nearly 85% of the cases, the mass is discovered by the family. It may be associated with abdominal pain (33%), microscopic hematuria (25%), macroscopic hematuria (20%), hypertension (12–50%), or fever.

Nephroblastomatosis presents as bilateral nephromegaly. It may be one element of more complex syndromes (**Hemihypertrophy, Beckwith-Wiedemann syndrome, Overgrowth-renal hamartoma, Perlman type, Wilms tumor-pseudohermaphroditism-glomerulopathy, Denys-Drash type**). Even when not complicated by conventional Wilms tumor, it may be associated with hypertension, but usually not with hematuria.

Wilms tumor may be bilateral (1.4–14% of cases) and familial. Bilateral tumors may be synchronous (55–75%). When metachronous, the contralateral tumor is discovered six months to two years after the initial diagnosis, but may take as long as 19 years to manifest. Hypertension and hematuria are more commonly seen with bilateral tumors. About 20% of the familial and 3% of the seemingly sporadic cases are bilateral. Familial cases are thought to represent 1% of the total. Some studies suggest that 32% of tumors have a hereditary component, and that all bilateral tumors may be familial.

**Complications:** Acute hemorrhage into the tumor with fever and anemia; venous thrombosis and disseminated intravascular coagulation; intratumoral arteriovenous shunting; metastatic dissemination, usually hematogenous, and relapses; complications of the therapy itself.

About one-half of the cases have metastases at the time of diagnosis. The most common sites for metastases and relapses are the lungs (80%), liver (19%), and other abdominal sites (33%). The brain, lymph nodes, and bones are sometimes involved, but rarely the bone marrow. The emergence of a second malignant neoplasm is possible (3–4%).

**Associated Findings:** Hyperreninism, increased erythropoietic stimulating factor (ESF), and erythropoietin production with or without polycythemia (it is possible to detect high ESF in the absence of polycythemia), hypercalcemia with (one case) or without increased production of parathyroid hormone, hyaluronic acidemia and aciduria, tumor-associated antigenemia, and coagulopathy similar to that in **Von Willebrand disease** have been observed.

Nodular renal blastema, nephroblastomatosis, and 13–15% of Wilms tumors may be associated with congenital anomalies. Anomalies of the genitourinary tract account for nearly 28% of congenital anomalies and are seen in as many as 5% of children with the tumor. Cryptorchidism is seen in 1.3%, hypospadias in 0.8%, double collecting system in 1.5%, and fused kidneys in 0.4%. Male pseudohermaphroditism, renal dysplasia, and various forms of intersexual disorders and nephropathies may be also seen (*Drash syndrome*). Associated congenital anomalies are common in bilateral tumors (55–65% versus 4% in unilateral tumors).

**Hemihypertrophy** is present in 1–3% of patients with Wilms tumor and accounts for nearly 18% of all associated congenital anomalies. Its occurrence is sporadic, although it may be present in a parent or a sib who does not have the tumor; therefore, some forms could be inherited. The **Beckwith-Wiedemann syndrome** (BW) is present in 0.2% of cases of Wilms' tumor. The incidence of Wilms tumor in the BW syndrome is 6–8%. When the BW syndrome includes hemihypertrophy, the incidence may rise to 33%. In this syndrome and in hemihypertrophy, in addition to Wilms tumor there is a predisposition to develop other neoplasms, primarily hepatoblastoma and adrenal cortical carcinoma. **Overgrowth-renal hamartoma, Perlman type**, familial syndrome of fetal gigantism, renal hamartomas, and nephroblastomatosis, shares many features with the BW syndrome, but does not include hemihypertrophy, omphalocele, or umbilical abnormalities.

About 1–1.6% of patients with Wilms tumor have aniridia, which is almost always sporadic in type. Deletion of chromosome 11p13 has been detected in (and only in) such patients. About 33–40% of them develop Wilms tumor, which is bilateral in about 40% of the cases. This syndrome also includes ambiguous genitalia, gonadoblastoma, and mental retardation (WAGR complex). Other ocular and genitourinary anomalies sometimes seen are cataract, glaucoma, cryptorchidism, and hypospadias. There is one documented case of hemihypertrophy in a patient with sporadic aniridia.

**Neurofibromatosis** is seen in 0.87% of patients with the tumor (the incidence in the general population is 0.03%). On rare occasions, the tumor has been reported in association with pigmented nevi, **Angio-osteohypertrophy syndrome, Dwarfism, Mulibrey type, Chromosome 8, trisomy 8, Chromosome 18, trisomy 18,** B-C translocation, **Turner syndrome**, XX/XY mosaicism, **Marfan syndrome**, familial distal tubular acidosis, **Pancytopenia syndrome, Fanconi type**, and **Cerebral gigantism**. The significance of these associations is not clear.

In patients with nephroblastomatosis, the incidence of congenital malformations has been estimated at 32%. The malformations include hemihypertrophy, elements of the BW syndrome, and genitourinary malformations. The **Angio-osteohypertrophy syndrome**, asplenia, and enophthalmos have also been seen.

**Etiology:** The nature of the event leading to the development of the tumor is not known. In familial cases, a predisposition to the tumor, is inherited. Thus, mutation is thought to be autosomal dominant.

**Pathogenesis:** According to the hypothesis of Knudson and Strong, Wilms tumor results from two sequential events. In the hereditary cases, the first event (or "hit," or mutation) occurs prezygotically, and may be responsible for the development of premalignant lesions such as nodular renal blastema and nephroblastomatosis. The second hit is always postzygotic. Nonhereditary tumors are the result of two somatic hits.

Tumor predisposition, the first mutation in the hereditary forms, affects all cells but requires a second mutation to develop a tumor. This second event can occur in many cells, leading, at an earlier age, to a higher incidence of multiple or multifocal tumors in which study of the renal tissue unaffected by the tumor often reveals morphologic evidence of the first hit in the form of residual nodular renal blastema and sometimes also nephroblastomatosis. When the mutation is transmitted, this follows an autosomal dominant mode with variable penetrance (60–70%) and expressivity (unilateral, bilateral). However, the high frequency of unaffected parents with two or more affected sibs cannot be explained simply by incomplete penetrance. Gonadal mosaicism, unequal inheritance of parental balanced translocation, delayed mutations, multiple allelism, and host resistance may explain some of these cases.

The host resistance hypothesis suggests that expression of a tumor predisposition gene, the second event, is determined by an inherited host resistance to tumor development.

In patients with sporadic **Aniridia**, the 11p13 deletion may represent the first event. This deletion has also been transmitted from an unaffected parent who had a balanced chromosomal translocation. Occasional reports of BW syndrome describing abnormalities different from the 11p13 deletion have also appeared. In some of the cases, an 11p15 deletion was detected, but the significance of these observations is not yet determined.

Studies of Wilms tumor cells indicate that the malignant cells may have the 11p13 deletion in the absence of a cytogenetically detectable systemic deletion, that the tumor cells are homozygous for the deletion, and that introduction of a normal chromosome 11 into a Wilms tumor cell line may control its tumorigenic expression. Furthermore, it appears that the lost chromosome allele is of maternal origin. About 18–20% of Wilms tumors are thought to follow a germinal mutation with no detectable cytogenetic abnormality.

Recent investigation of several families segregating for Wilms tumor found that, in the families studied, the location of the predisposing gene was not the 11p13 locus involved in WAGR and tumorigenesis, nor the 11p15 locus involved in the **Beckwith-Wiedemann syndrome**. A possible similarity with **Endocrine neoplasia, multiple type II**, in which the predisposing gene is believed to be at a different location from the tumorigenesis gene, was suggested.

**MIM No.:** *19407

**CDC No.:** 189.000

**Sex Ratio:** M1:F1. There may be a slight preponderance of males, although this does not appear to be true for nephroblastomatosis and for Wilms tumor associated with hemihypertrophy.

**Occurrence:** Wilms tumor accounts for 8% of pediatric solid malignancies. It occurs less frequently than central nervous system tumors, lymphomas, neuroblastomas, and soft tissue sarcomas, but it is the most frequent intra-abdominal tumor in children. The random risk of developing the tumor is 1:10,000 live births. Congenital Wilms tumors are extremely rare.

The tumor has no significant racial predilection. It has a uniform worldwide incidence of 7–8:1,000,000 per year, for persons less than age 15 years. No data are available regarding incidence and racial predilection in isolated nephroblastomatosis, as the number of cases documented is still extremely limited. Thus far, all

reported cases in which the race was recorded occurred in white children. Familial nephroblastomatosis has been described in a Yemenite-Jewish family.

**Risk of Recurrence for Patient's Sib:** In the absence of a family history or predisposing anomalies, 1% if the tumor is unilateral and unifocal; at least 1% if it is multifocal; and 1–2% if it is bilateral. When two sibs are affected, the chance of another sib having the tumor is 20%. The risk for a monozygotic twin of a patient with a hereditary tumor is 63%; 24% if the tumor is sporadic.

**Risk of Recurrence for Patient's Child:** If a parent has a unilateral tumor and there is no family history or predisposing anomalies, the risk for each child to have Wilms tumor may be as high as 5–9%. This risk could be 30–32% if the parental tumor is considered hereditary. One study found one offspring with Wilms tumor born to 218 survivors.

**Age of Detectability:** Seventy-seven percent occur in children under age five years, and 90% occur under age seven. The mean age of onset of the tumor, based on nearly 2,000 patients followed by three National Wilms Tumor Studies, is 45.1 months for unilateral unicentric tumors and 44.6 months for unilateral multicentric tumors. The mean age of onset for bilateral tumors is 30.5 months. The age distribution seems to be sex-dependent: the male incidence peaks in the second to third year of life, while the female peak remains high into the fourth year.

**Gene Mapping and Linkage:** WAGR (Wilms tumor, aniridia, genitourinary abnormalities, and MR) has been mapped to 11p13.
WT1 (Wilms tumor 1) has been mapped to 11p13.
WT2 (Wilms tumor 2) is unassigned.
GUD (genitourinary dysplasia component of WAGR) is 11p13.
E7-associated cell surface antigen has been detected in cases of WAGR. The level of expression of the insulin-like growth factor 2 (IGF2) gene seems to correlate with the stage of tissue differentiation, and it has been suggested that this gene may be involved in the neoplastic transformation process. Similarly, enhanced expression of the N-*myc* gene, without amplification, has been shown in these tumors.

**Prevention:** None known. Genetic counseling indicated.

**Treatment:** Surgery, chemotherapy, and radiotherapy. Choice of a single modality or various combinations is dictated by the stage and histology (favorable, unfavorable) of the process.

There is no widely accepted therapeutic modality for either nephroblastomatosis or bilateral tumors, which creates therapeutic dilemmas. Some cases of nephroblastomatosis have regressed with chemotherapy alone. Nodular renal blastema may regress spontaneously, as documented by autopsy studies comparing its incidence in infants younger than age four months with the incidence in older children.

**Prognosis:** Numerous factors adversely affect the prognosis: advanced patient age and disease stage, "unfavorable" histology of the tumor, inadequacy of treatment, recurrences, and complications of therapy. Heredity and associated features predisposing to tumor development do not seem to affect the prognosis adversely. Large tumors have been associated with increased risk of recurrence, but it is not established whether tumor size or even rupture otherwise have a prognostic significance. This is probably also true for the presence of hematuria, elevated levels of ESF, and erythrocytosis.

Nearly 57% of patients with "unfavorable" histology die of the tumor compared with 6.9% of patients with "favorable" histology. Tumors with "unfavorable" histology usually are not associated with congenital anomalies and hereditary features, but often metastasize to lymph nodes. CCSK metastasizes to bones.

It is debatable whether age and histology correlate. However, the incidence of "unfavorable" histology is 7.4% in children under age two years and 13% in older children. Correlation between age and stage seems to exist; the median age for stage I is 1.3 years and for stage IV is 4.3 years.

The overall mortality rate for children under age two years with "favorable" histology, is 2.7%, but is 8.7% for older children. When the histology is "unfavorable," the mortality rates become, respectively, 78 and 52%. When anaplasia is seen in a relapsing tumor, the mortality rate is 85%. Results of the Third National Wilms Tumor Study (NWTS-3) show that the disease-free survival rate, at two years, for "favorable" histology tumors in stages I to III are, respectively, 90, 88, and 80%; the worst results are seen in patients in stage IV with "unfavorable" histology, with a 62% disease-free survival rate at two years.

Factors valuable in evaluating the prognosis in unilateral tumors are also operative in bilateral tumors. The survival rates after two years are 87%, but, probably because of a relatively high incidence of late recurrence and metastases, this rate is often reported as being closer to 50%. "Unfavorable" histology is unusual in bilateral tumors.

Survival after congenital Wilms tumor is exceptional. Congenital, neonatal, and familial nephroblastomatosis are also usually fatal. Nephroblastomatosis, when not associated with Wilms tumor or congenital malformations, and seen in older children but under age two years, seems to be amenable to cure with chemotherapy.

**Detection of Carrier:** Examination of patient and relatives for evidence of the trait, i.e., a family history of Wilms tumor, congenital anomalies. In the presence of sporadic aniridia, detection of a constitutional chromosomal abnormality involving chromosome 11p13 and determination of decreased catalase activity.

**Special Considerations:** The concept of Wilms tumor has evolved drastically. Several entities have been delineated, and some were shown not to be related to Wilms tumor (i.e., congenital mesoblastic nephroma); the place of others is still unclear, and some were demonstrated to be part of a well-delineated syndrome in which a specific constitutional chromosomal abnormality has been established (WAGR). At present, CCSA, and MRTK are emerging as candidates for exclusions from the Wilms family. CCSK and MRTK, however, account respectively for six and 2% of all tumors in the NWTS-3, and CCSK makes up 50% of the "unfavorable" histology cases. Similarly, the concept of a nodular renal blastema - nephroblastomatosis complex is being refined, and several entities probably differing in pathologic, pathogenetic, and clinical aspects are being recognized: perilobar, intralobar, combined, and diffuse panlobar nephroblastomatosis. However, most data used as the basis for the present review do not take these aspects into consideration. Therefore, although the figures provided are useful, they should be considered as relatively rough estimates. This word of caution also applies to the results of cytogenetic, gene mapping, and linkage studies on patients and tumor cells. Such studies are still in their infancy, and a very limited number of cases has been evaluated.

**Support Groups:** Atlanta; American Cancer Society

**References:**
Pochedly C, Baum ES, eds: Wilms' tumor. New York: Elsevier Science, 1984. * †
Koufos A, et al.: Loss of heterozygosity in three embryonal tumors suggests a common pathogenetic mechanism. Nature 1985; 316:330–334.
Scoggin CH, et al.: The E7-associated cell-surface antigen: a marker for the 11p13 chromosomal deletion associated with aniridia-Wilms tumor. Am J Hum Genet 1985; 37:883–889.
Glaser T, et al.: The β-subunit of follicle-stimulating hormone is deleted in patients with aniridia and Wilms' tumor, allowing further definition of the WAGR locus. Nature 1986; 321:882–887.
Nisen PD, et al.: Enhanced expression of the N-myc gene in Wilms' tumors. Cancer Res 1986; 46:6217–6222.
Shroeder WT, et al.: Nonrandom loss of maternal chromosome 11 alleles in Wilms tumors. Am J Hum Genet 1987; 40:413–420.
Weissman BE, et al.: Introduction of a normal human chromosome 11 into a Wilms' tumor cell line controls its tumorigenic expression. Science 1987; 236:175–180.
Greenberg F, et al.: Expanding the spectrum of the Perlman syndrome. Am J Hum Genet 1988; 29:773–776.
Grundy P, et al.: Familial predisposition to Wilms' tumor does not map to the short arm of chromosome 11. Nature 1988; 336:374–376.
Huff V, et al.: Lack of linkage of familial Wilms' tumor to chromosomal band 11p13. Nature 1988; 336:377–378.
Hoffman M: One Wilms' tumor gene is cloned; are there more? Science 1989; 246:1387.

DE037                    **Jean-Pierre de Chadarévian**

**Cancer; nonspecific aggregation in a family**
See CANCER, FAMILIAL
**Candida albicans infection, chronic, median rhomboid glossitis**
See GLOSSITIS, MEDIAN RHOMBOID

---

## CANDIDIASIS, FAMILIAL CHRONIC MUCOCUTANEOUS    2117

**Includes:** Familial chronic mucocutaneous candidiasis (FCMC)

**Excludes:**
Candidiasis, other
**Polyglandular autoimmune syndrome** (2623)

**Major Diagnostic Criteria:** Familial chronic oral candidiasis, usually from early childhood, with frequent involvement of nails and of skin and other sites to a mild degree; no significant endocrinopathy but generally consistent defects in delayed hypersensitivity.

**Clinical Findings:** All of the patients develop chronic oral candidiasis early in life, often by the age of two years, and this is usually the patient's chief complaint at presentation. Typically, the tongue exhibits white candidal plaques, is enlarged, fissured, and crenated by the teeth. The buccal mucosa may also be covered by a thick white membrane and may also exhibit hyperkeratosis. White candidal plaques can be scraped off (although sometimes with difficulty) leaving a raw, red, shiny surface. Bilateral angular cheilitis is present in most patients, usually symmetrical and often very painful. Approximately half the patients exhibit chronic candidal paronychia with some associated onychomycosis. Those most affected are often chronic nail biters.

Some patients relate a history of chronic blepharitis, although this has not been proven to be caused by candida. Mild cutaneous candidiasis is sometimes seen, most often involving the scalp, face, hands, and groin. Occasional patients exhibit chronic hoarseness due to candidal laryngitis and a few females have presented with proven chronic candidal vaginitis. Patients are typically in generally good health and none exhibit hypoparathyroidism, hypoadrenocorticism, or diabetes mellitus. Immunologically, although neutrophil function is normal, many patients appear unable to produce migration inhibition factor (MIF) from their lymphocytes. This defect is usually accompanied by absent delayed skin hypersensitivity to candida antigen and sometimes also with inability to be sensitized to dinitrochlorobenzene. Blood group O is presently associated with H substance in many patients. Many exhibit latent iron deficiency and some present with frank iron deficiency anemia. Some patients also have low levels of serum Vitamin A.

**Complications:** Painful angular cheilitis, glossitis, onychomycosis, and hoarseness.

**Associated Findings:** None known.

**Etiology:** Autosomal recessive inheritance in most cases, although examples of possible autosomal dominant transmission have been reported. Consanguinity is common.

**Pathogenesis:** There is no evidence that organisms involved differ from Candida found in environment or in unaffected patients. Postulations include 1.) inherited deficiency in cell-mediated immunity to Candida or general deficiency in cell-mediated immunity; 2.) iron deficiency leading to defective epithelium formation in turn predisposing to chronic superimposed candidal infection leading over a prolonged period of time to an altered immune response.

**MIM No.:** *21205

**Sex Ratio:** M1:F1

**Occurrence:** A few dozen cases have been documented.

**Risk of Recurrence for Patient's Sib:**
See Part I, *Mendelian Inheritance.*

**Risk of Recurrence for Patient's Child:**
See Part I, *Mendelian Inheritance*.

**Age of Detectability:** In early childhood.

**Gene Mapping and Linkage:** Unknown.

**Prevention:** None known. Genetic counseling indicated.

**Treatment:** Oral ketoconzaole, clotrimazole or topical nystatin; 5 fluorocytosine, oral or parenteral iron.

**Prognosis:** Good. Skin and mucosal lesions often substantially improve or disappear with antimycotic therapy. Recurrences occur but can be successfully treated by reinstituting therapy.

**Detection of Carrier:** Unknown.

**Special Considerations:** Okamoto et al (1977) described a mother and two daughters suffering from a syndrome of chronic mucocutaneous candidiasis, alopecia universalis, progressive keratoconjuctivitis with corneal vascularization and B cell as well as T cell abnormalities. This syndrome, apparently autosomal or X-linked dominant, differs in many aspects from the condition described above. The role of the candidal infection in this condition is unclear. In addition, Sams et al (1979) have described a family comprising eight unaffected relatives. The affected patients in this family greatly resembled those with FCMC but the genetic transmission appeared to be autosomal dominant. The affected patients were also said to exhibit a high incidence of dermatophytosis as well as ''enamel dysplasia'' (not well documented).

**References:**
Wells RS, et al.: Familial chronic muco-cutaneous candidiasis. J Med Genet 1972; 9:302–310. *
Kroll JJ, et al.: Mucocutaneous candidiasis in a mother and son. Arch Dermatol 1973; 108:259–262.
Rothschild J, et al.: An immunological investigation of a family with chronic mucocutaneous candidiasis. Int Archs Allergy Appl Immunol 1976; 52:291–296.
Okamoto GA, et al.: New syndrome of chronic mucocutaneous candidiasis. BD:OAS XXIII(3B). New York: March of Dimes Birth Defects Foundation, 1977:117–125.
Sams WM Jr, et al.: Chronic mucocutaneous candidiasis: immunologic studies of three generations of a single family. Am J Med 1979; 67:948–959.
Morrison JGL, Anderson R: Familial chronic mucocutaneous candidiasis successfully treated with oral ketoconazole. South Afr Med J 1981; 59:237–239.

G0009                                    **Lawrence I. Goldblatt**

**Candidiasis-endocrinopathy syndrome**
  *See POLYGLANDULAR AUTOIMMUNE SYNDROME*
**Cantrell pentalogy**
  *See PENTALOGY OF CANTRELL*
**Cantrell-Haller-Ravitch syndrome**
  *See PENTALOGY OF CANTRELL*
**Cantu syndrome**
  *See DERMO-FACIO-CARDIO-SKELETAL SYNDROME*
**Capillary hemangioma**
  *See NEVUS FLAMMEUS*
  *also HEMANGIOMAS OF THE HEAD AND NECK*
**Capillary lymphangiomas of orbit**
  *See ORBITAL AND PERIORBITAL LYMPHANGIOMA*
**Capillary nevus**
  *See NEVUS FLAMMEUS*
**Capoten⌃, fetal effects**
  *See FETAL ANGIOTENSIN CONVERTING ENZYME (ACE) INHIBITION RENAL FAILURE*
**Capsular and polar cataracts**
  *See CATARACT, POLAR AND CAPSULAR*
**Capsulolenticular cataract**
  *See CATARACT, POLAR AND CAPSULAR*
**Captopril, fetal effects**
  *See FETAL ANGIOTENSIN CONVERTING ENZYME (ACE) INHIBITION RENAL FAILURE*
**Carbamazepine exposure, fetal effects**
  *See FETAL CARBAMAZEPINE EXPOSURE*

## CARBAMOYL PHOSPHATE SYNTHETASE DEFICIENCY 3022

**Includes:**
  Carbamoyl phosphate synthetase I deficiency
  Hyperammonemia, congenital (some)

**Excludes:**
  **Aciduria, argininosuccinic** (0087)
  **Argininemia** (0086)
  **Citrullinemia** (0174)
  **Hyperdibasic aminoaciduria** (0491)
  **Hyperornithinemia-hyperammonemia-homocitrullinuria** (3169)
  Lactic acidosis, congenital
  **N-acetylglutamate synthetase deficiency** (3170)
  Organic acidemias
  **Ornithine transcarbamoylase deficiency** (3023)
  Reye syndrome
  Transient hyperammonemia of the newborn

**Major Diagnostic Criteria:** In complete deficiencies, coma associated with hyperammonemia (plasma ammonium >500 $\mu$M, normal <50 $\mu$M) occurs in the first week of life. In partial deficiencies, recurrent episodes of ataxia, vomiting, lethargy, and coma with elevated plasma ammonium levels (>100 $\mu$M) and low serum urea nitrogen levels occur. Plasma amino acids show low levels of citrulline (absent to trace levels in the neonatal onset form of the disorder), distinguishing it from citrullinemia and argininosuccinic aciduria, in which citrulline levels are high. Plasma arginine level is low, in contrast to that in argininemia, in which the arginine level is elevated. Plasma glutamine and alanine levels are elevated. Urinary orotic acid excretion is low, distinguishing this disorder from ornithine transcarbamoylase deficiency, in which urinary orotic acid excretion is high. Organic acids and dibasic amino acids are not found in the urine. A definitive diagnosis can be made by measuring activity of carbamoyl phosphate synthetase in liver, duodenal, or rectal tissue. The enzyme is not expressed in fibroblasts or leukocytes.

**Clinical Findings:** Fourteen infants have been reported with a complete deficiency of carbamoyl phosphate synthetase. They presented with respiratory distress, poor feeding, hypotonia, progressive lethargy, and coma in the first week of life. Untreated, there was universal mortality. Approximately one-half survived following treatment with hemodialysis/peritoneal dialysis. Pulmonary and gastrointestinal hemorrhages have been reported. Seven patients have had partial deficiencies with recurrent episodes of vomiting, hyperactivity, lethargy, and coma, occurring from early childhood and often associated with protein intolerance or intercurrent infections.

**Complications:** In children with neonatal-onset hyperammonemic coma lasting longer than 48 hours, there is a high incidence of cortical atrophy associated with mental retardation and other developmental disabilities. Despite treatment, affected children are at risk for future episodes of hyperammonemic coma, which may cause further brain damage or death.

**Associated Findings:** Chronic anorexia, food avoidance.

**Etiology:** Autosomal recessive inheritance.

**Pathogenesis:** CPS deficiency is caused by a partial or complete deficiency of the mitochondrial urea cycle enzyme carbamoyl phosphate synthetase. Carbamoyl phosphate synthetase is the first enzyme in the urea cycle. Deficient activity leads to an accumulation of ammonium in blood and brain, especially following a protein load or intercurrent infection. Ammonia is a neurotoxin. Additionally, there may be alterations in brain energy and neurotransmitter metabolism induced by prolonged hyperammonemic coma that result in brain damage. Alzheimer type II cells are found in the brain.

**MIM No.:** *23730

**Sex Ratio:** M1:F1

**Occurrence:** Estimated at <1:60,000.

**Risk of Recurrence for Patient's Sib:**
See Part I, *Mendelian Inheritance*.

**Risk of Recurrence for Patient's Child:**
See Part I, *Mendelian Inheritance.*

**Age of Detectability:** In complete deficiencies, symptoms are evident by one week of age. In partial defects, detection may be delayed to early childhood or later. Prenatal detection by RFLP is possible in about 85% of affected families. Prospective treatment of at-risk infants is possible from birth.

**Gene Mapping and Linkage:** CPS1 (carbamoyl phosphate synthetase 1, mitochondrial) has been provisionally mapped to 2p.

**Prevention:** None known. Genetic counseling indicated.

**Treatment:** Treatment involves combining protein restriction with the induction of alternate pathways of waste nitrogen excretion. This is accomplished using a protein-restricted diet supplemented with essential amino acids (including citrulline) and providing sodium benzoate and sodium phenylacetate.

**Prognosis:** The few affected children who have been treated prospectively from birth, because of a previously affected sib, have done well. However, the majority of children who have suffered neonatal hyperammonemic coma are mentally retarded. Results in partial deficiencies have depended on maintaining adequate control of plasma ammonium levels. Life span is uncertain because of the risk of intercurrent hyperammonemic episodes.

**Detection of Carrier:** Carrier detection has been attempted using protein tolerance tests, but false-negative results have been obtained. RFLP has been useful in carrier detection of informed families.

**References:**

Batshaw M, et al.: Treatment of carbamoyl-phosphate-synthetase deficiency with keto analogues of essential amino acids. New Engl J Med 1975; 292:1085–1090.

Montagos S, et al.: Neonatal hyperammonemia with complete absence of liver carbamoyl phosphate synthetase activity. Arch Dis Child 1978; 53:230–234.

Zimmermann A, et al.: Ultrastructural pathology in congenital defects of the urea cycle: ornithine transcarbamylase and carbamoyl phosphate synthetase deficiency. Virchows Arch Pathol 1981; 393:321.

Batshaw ML, et al.: Treatment of inborn errors of urea synthesis: activation of alternative pathways of waste nitrogen synthesis and excretion. New Engl J Med 1982; 306:1387–1392.

Batshaw ML: Hyperammonemia. Curr Prob Pediatr 1984; 14:1–69.

Msall M, et al.: Neurologic outcome of children with inborn errors of urea synthesis. New Engl J Med 1984; 310:1500–1505.

Fearon ER, et al.: Genetic analysis of carbamoyl phosphate synthetase I deficiency. Hum Genet 1985; 70:207–210.

Brusilow SW: Urea cycle disorders and other hereditary hyperammonemic syndromes. In: Scriver CR, et al, eds: The metabolic basis of inherited disease, 6th ed. New York: McGraw-Hill, 1989:629–664.

BA066                                    **Mark L. Batshaw**

**Carbamoyl phosphate synthetase I deficiency**
  *See CARBAMOYL PHOSPHATE SYNTHETASE DEFICIENCY*
**Carbimazole fetal effects, scalp and urachal**
  *See FETAL EFFECTS FROM METHIMAZOLE AND CARBIMAZOLE*
**Carbohydrate-induced hyperlipemia**
  *See HYPERLIPOPROTEINEMIA, BROAD BETA TYPE*
  *also HYPERTRIGLYCERIDEMIA*
**'Carbon baby'**
  *See SKIN, HYPERPIGMENTATION, FAMILIAL*
**Carbon monoxide, fetal effects of**
  *See FETAL EFFECTS FROM MATERNAL CARBON MONOXIDE EXPOSURE*
**Carbonic anhydrase B**
  *See RENAL TUBULAR ACIDOSIS-OSTEOPETROSIS SYNDROME*
**Carbonic anhydrase B deficiency**
  *See RENAL TUBULAR ACIDOSIS-SENSORINEURAL DEAFNESS*
**Carbonic anhydrase II deficiency**
  *See OSTEOPETROSIS, MALIGNANT RECESSIVE*
  *also RENAL TUBULAR ACIDOSIS-OSTEOPETROSIS SYNDROME*
**Carbonic anhydrase II, erythrocyte, electrophoretic variant**
  *See RENAL TUBULAR ACIDOSIS-OSTEOPETROSIS SYNDROME*

## CARBOXYLASE DEFICIENCY, HOLOCARBOXYLASE DEFICIENCY TYPE 2006

**Includes:**
  Biotin-responsive 3-beta-methylcrotonylglycinuria (some)
  Carboxylase deficiency, multiple, biotin-responsive
  Holocarboxylase synthetase deficiency
  Multiple carboxylase deficiency, neonatal or early onset form

**Excludes:**
  **Biotinidase deficiency** (2591)
  Biotin-unresponsive 3-beta-methylcrotonylglycinuria
  Multiple carboxylase deficiency, late-onset form

**Major Diagnostic Criteria:** Before biotin treatment, urinary organic acids include highly elevated 3-hydroxyisovaleric acid, variably elevated 3-methylcrotonylglycine, variably elevated lactic acid, and modest elevations of 2-methylcitric acid and 3-hydroxypropionic acid. The elevated acids decrease or normalize with biotin treatment. The activities of 3-methylcrotonyl-CoA, propionyl-CoA, and pyruvate carboxylases are low in white cells before biotin treatment and in fibroblasts cultured without added biotin, and the activities increase in white cells after treatment of the patient with biotin and increase in fibroblasts cultured with 1 $\mu$mol/liter biotin. Biotinidase activity is normal in serum. Activity of holocarboxylase synthetase is deficient (or the Km for biotin is elevated) in white cells or cultured fibroblasts.

**Clinical Findings:** The presentation may be acute in the first few days or months of life or may be chronic during the first year. Typical acute findings are severe metabolic acidosis, ketosis, lactic acidosis, moderate hyperammonemia, and organic aciduria. Hypotonia may occur, progressing to coma and death. Chronic symptoms may include vomiting, developmental delay or regression, an erythematous skin rash, and alopecia. Without treatment with biotin, this can be a fatal disorder. Upon treatment with large doses of biotin (10 mg/day or more) patients respond dramatically with normalization of clinical symptoms and most biochemical abnormalities, although some patients are not fully responsive and continue to have a moderate organic aciduria and continuing rash. Clinical features overlap many of those of **Biotinidase deficiency.**

**Complications:** None, except that if not fully responsive to biotin the skin rash may be subject to *candida* infections. Unlike biotinidase deficiency, there are no complications of nerve deafness or optic nerve atrophy.

**Associated Findings:** None known.

**Etiology:** Autosomal recessive inheritance.

**Pathogenesis:** There is deficient activity of holocarboxylase synthetase, the enzyme which attaches the vitamin biotin as a covalently bound cofactor to the four inactive apocarboxylases to form the enzymatically active holocarboxylases. The clinical and biochemical abnormalities are believed to be due to the deficient activity of 3-methylcrotonyl-CoA carboxylase required for the catabolism of leucine, propionyl-CoA carboxylase required for the catabolism of propionate derived from five amino acids and other sources, pyruvate carboxylase required for gluconeogenesis, and acetyl-CoA carboxylase required for fatty acid synthesis. In addition to having a low maximum velocity, most of the abnormal holocarboxylase synthetases have an elevated Km for biotin. The response to pharmacologic doses of biotin can be explained as due to raising the intracellular concentrations of biotin above the elevated Km of the holocarboxylase synthetase, resulting in increased or even normal activity of all four biotin-containing carboxylases.

**MIM No.:** *25327

**Sex Ratio:** M1:F1

**Occurrence:** Undetermined; perhaps one in several hundred thousand.

**Risk of Recurrence for Patient's Sib:**
See Part I, *Mendelian Inheritance.*

**Risk of Recurrence for Patient's Child:**
See Part I, *Mendelian Inheritance.*

**Age of Detectability:** Postnatally on first day of life from urinary organic acids or white cell carboxylases. Prenatal diagnosis can be done by amniocentesis at 16–18 weeks, by measurement of elevated 3-hydroxyisovaleric acid in amniotic fluid and biotin-responsive deficiencies of carboxylases in cultured amniocytes.

**Gene Mapping and Linkage:** Unknown.

**Prevention:** None known. Genetic counseling indicated.

**Treatment:** Treatment with biotin is essential. A typical dose of 10 mg/day orally is effective for many patients. Some patients are less responsive, and the dose should be increased to as much as 60 mg/day to minimize excretion of organic acids. The most reliable indicator of response is the urinary 3-hydroxyisovaleric acid levels. Dietary protein restriction has not been necessary. Biotin treatment must continue the entire life. Prenatal treatment of the pregnant mother with biotin and postnatal treatment of the infant has prevented symptoms at birth and postnatally.

**Prognosis:** With optimal biotin therapy the prognosis is excellent, with normal growth and development, provided that there is no neurological damage from any acute acidotic episode. A normal life span is expected.

**Detection of Carrier:** Carriers cannot be detected since they have normal urinary organic acids, normal white cell and fibroblast carboxylases, and the assay of holocarboxylase synthetase is not currently accurate enough to distinguish carriers from normal subjects.

**References:**

Gompertz D, et al.: Biotin-responsive beta-methylcrotonylglycinuria. Lancet 1971; II:22–24.
Burri BJ, et al.: Mutant holocarboxylase synthetase: evidence for the enzyme defect in early infantile biotin-responsive multiple carboxylase deficiency. J Clin Invest 1981; 68:1491–1495.
Packman S, et al.: Prenatal treatment of biotin-responsive multiple carboxylase deficiency. Lancet 1982; I:1435–1439.
Burri BJ, et al.: Heterogeneity of holocarboxylase synthetase in patients with biotin-responsive multiple carboxylase deficiency. Am J Hum Genet 1985; 37:326–337.
Sweetman L, Nyhan WL: Inheritable biotin-treatable disorders and associated phenomena. Ann Rev Nutr 1986; 6:317–343.

SW002            **Lawrence Sweetman**

**Carboxylase deficiency, multiple, biotin-responsive**
*See CARBOXYLASE DEFICIENCY, HOLOCARBOXYLASE DEFICIENCY TYPE*
**Carcinoma of the pancreas**
*See CANCER, PANCREAS, FAMILIAL ADENOCARCINOMA OF*
**Carcinoma, nevoid basal cell syndrome**
*See NEVOID BASAL CELL CARCINOMA SYNDROME*
**Cardiac conduction defects, neonatal**
*See ARRHYTHMIA, CARDIAC CONDUCTION DEFECTS, NEONATAL*
**Cardiac form of generalized glycogenosis**
*See GLYCOGENOSIS, TYPE IIa*
**Cardiac limb syndrome**
*See HEART-HAND SYNDROME*
**Cardiac type amyloidosis**
*See AMYLOIDOSIS, DANISH CARDIAC TYPE*
**Cardiac-limb-oto syndrome**
*See LIMB-OTO-CARDIAC SYNDROME*

## CARDIO-AUDITORY SYNDROME        0123

**Includes:**
Deafness-functional heart disease
EKG, prolonged QT interval-deafness-sudden death
Jervell syndrome
Lange-Nielsen syndrome
Long QT syndrome (one form)
Surdocardiac syndrome

**Excludes:** Arrhythmia, with long QT interval without deafness (0610)

**Major Diagnostic Criteria:** Sensorineural deafness and EKG prolongation of the QT interval.

**Clinical Findings:** Deafness, prolongation of the QT interval, syncope, and, possibly, sudden death.

The deafness is congenital or at least of very early onset and probably not progressive. It is sensorineural and of profound degree; the hearing loss is symmetric. There is variable preservation of hearing in the low tones but this is insufficient for the normal learning of speech, and special education is often necessary. No results of tests of vestibular function are available.

The syncopal attacks commonly occur in childhood although rarely they may be delayed into the adult years. They are usually precipitated by fear, excitement, exercise or loud noises. The attacks may be infrequent or may occur several times per day and range from mild to so severe as to cause loss of consciousness for several minutes. Seizure activity and urinary incontinence have been observed with the resultant misdiagnosis of epilepsy.

Commonly there is a resting bradycardia and the heart rate may fail to accelerate normally with exercise. The T waves may be normal, inverted, diphasic, broad or variably fused with a prominent U wave. QT prolongation varies greatly both between patients and from day to day in the same patient. A normal QT interval may become prolonged with an exercise stress test.

In patients with EKG recordings during syncope the commonest finding has been rapid ventricular fibrillation. Death may occur with one of the syncopal attacks and is probably due to ventricular fibrillation, ventricular tachycardia or asystole.

It is said that attacks become less frequent with increasing age.

**Complications:** Sudden death.

**Associated Findings:** None known.

**Etiology:** Autosomal recessive inheritance.

**Pathogenesis:** The cardiac abnormality appears to be the result of an imbalance between various components of the cardiac sympathetic innervation. Dominance of the left side secondary to a decreased activity through the right cardiac sympathetic nerves seems to be the more likely pathogenetic mechanism for the majority of cases.

Inner ear abnormalities on autopsy show disorganization of the organ of Corti. Widespread presence of Periodic Acid-Schiff (PAS)-positive deposits throughout the membranous labyrinth, spiral prominence and into the region of the organ of Corti as well as the crista of the horizontal canal are most striking.

**MIM No.:** *22040

**POS No.:** 3660

**Sex Ratio:** M1:F1

**Occurrence:** Approximately 0.25% of deaf children.

**Risk of Recurrence for Patient's Sib:**
See Part I, *Mendelian Inheritance.*

**Risk of Recurrence for Patient's Child:**
See Part I, *Mendelian Inheritance.*

**Age of Detectability:** EKG abnormalities have been detected prenatally. Deafness can be detected in the first year of life.

**Gene Mapping and Linkage:** Unknown.

**Prevention:** None known. Genetic counseling indicated.

**Treatment:** Adrenergic β-blockage, i.e. propranolol in full doses. If symptoms persist, a left stellate ganglionectomy with continuation of propranolol in lower doses. If cardiac events persist after both treatments, an implanted automatic defibrillator may be of use although there are no reported cases as yet in the literature of such a device being used in a patient with the Cardio-auditory syndrome.

**Prognosis:** High mortality if untreated. Significant improvement of mortality with the treatment outlined above. A prospective study began in 1979, by, Moss includes cases with a prolonged QT interval with and without deafness (**Arrhythmia, with long QT interval without deafness**). The present prospective registry mortality rate is 1.3% per year with the average age of the affected population being 24 years. Congenital deafness was present in only 6% of the registry population and was the most potent risk factor with regards to having a cardiac event, i.e. syncope/cardiac death.

**Detection of Carrier:** It has been postulated that there are heterozygote carriers of the trait because of moderate prolongation of the QT interval in otherwise unaffected members of the family.

**Special Considerations:** Many reports in the literature include the Cardio-auditory syndrome and **Arrhythmia, with long QT interval without deafness** together as the Long QT Syndrome (LQTS).

A mild form of the long QT syndrome has been established with some patients having one or two attacks in the course of a lifetime. As adults, they are likely to have normal lives.

A normal EKG does not eliminate the possibility of the syndrome because the QT changes can be intermittent.

**Support Groups:** Dallas; American Heart Association

**References:**
Schwartz PJ.: The long Q-T syndrome. Am Heart J 1975; 89(3):378–390.
Fraser GR: The causes of profound deafness in childhood, Baltimore: The Johns Hopkins University Press, 1976.
Mirowski M, et al.: Termination of malignant ventricular arrhythmias with an implanted automatic defibrillator in human beings. N Engl J Med 1980; 303(6):322–324.
Smith W: The Long Q-T syndrome. Aust NZ Med 1984; 14:700- 704.
Jervell A: The pseudo-cadiac syndrome. Europ Heart J 1985; 6(suppl. D):97–102.
Moss AJ, et al.: The long QT syndrome: a prospective international study. Circulation 1985; 71:17–21. *
Schwartz PJ: Idiopathic long QT syndrome: progress and questions. Am Heart J 1985; 109:399–411.

K0023                                                    **Frederick K. Kozak**

**Cardio-dermo-facio-skeletal syndrome**
*See DERMO-FACIO-CARDIO-SKELETAL SYNDROME*

---

## CARDIO-FACIAL-CUTANEOUS SYNDROME            2587

**Includes:**
>   Cardio-facio-cutaneous syndrome
>   CFC syndrome
>   Facio-cardio-cutaneous syndrome
>   Skin changes-typical facies-heart defect

**Excludes:**
>   **Ichthyosis**
>   **Noonan syndrome** (0720)
>   Trimethylaminuria

**Major Diagnostic Criteria:** Typical facies, skin changes (hyperkeratosis), sparse and curly hair, heart defect, and mental retardation.

---

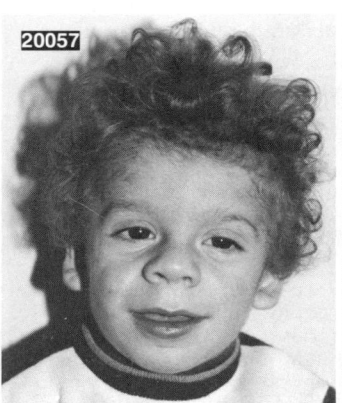 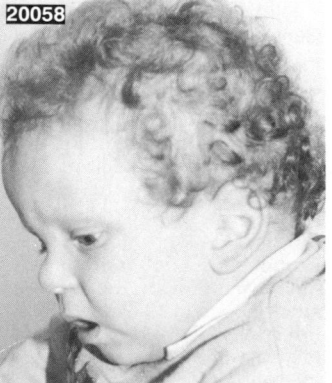

**2587-20057–58:** Cardio-facio-cutaneous syndrome; note these 2 unrelated boys ages 18 months and 22 months respectively with sparse, curly hair, hypoplastic supraorbital ridges, downward slanting palpebral fissures and abnormal ears.

**Clinical Findings:** Relative **Megalencephaly**; typical facial characteristics, with high forehead, bitemporal constriction, hypoplasia of supraorbital ridges, downward slant of palpebral fissures, depressed bridge of nose, posteriorly angulated ears with prominent helices; sparse and friable hair; skin changes, varying from patchy hyperkeratosis to generalized **Ichthyosis**; hemangiomatosis; variable cardiac defects, the most common being **Pulmonary valve, stenosis** and **Atrial septal defects**; and splenomegaly.

**Complications:** Developmental delay, characterized by growth and psychomotor retardation, usually moderate; **Hydrocephaly**.

**Associated Findings:** None known.

**Etiology:** All reported cases have been sporadic. Parents have been healthy and non related. Possibly autosomal dominant inheritance or a presently undetectable chromosome abnormality. Mitochondrial inheritance also can not be ruled out.

**Pathogenesis:** Unknown.

**MIM No.:** 11515

**POS No.:** 3627

**Sex Ratio:** Presumably M1:F1.

**Occurrence:** Sixteen cases have been reported; from the United States, Europe, and Australia.

**Risk of Recurrence for Patient's Sib:**
See Part I, *Mendelian Inheritance.* Probably not increased.

**Risk of Recurrence for Patient's Child:**
See Part I, *Mendelian Inheritance.* No affected individuals are known to have reproduced.

**Age of Detectability:** In infancy; probably even at birth.

**Gene Mapping and Linkage:** Unknown.

**Prevention:** None known. Genetic counseling indicated.

**Treatment:** Symptomatic treatment of skin lesions; surgical treatment of heart defect and hydrocephalus, as indicated.

**Prognosis:** Developmental delay, with mental retardation varying from mild to severe, usually moderate. Life span is presumed to be normal.

**Detection of Carrier:** Unknown.

**Special Considerations:** The condition can be distinguished from the inborn error of oxidative metabolism *trimethylaminuria* (Al-Waiz et al, 1987) by the lack of fish odor.

**Support Groups:** Dallas; American Heart Association

**References:**
Reynolds JF, et al.: New multiple congenital anomalies/mental retardation syndrome with cardio-facio-cutaneous involvement: the CFC syndrome. Am J Med Genet 1986; 25:413–427.
Neri G, et al.: The CFC syndrome: report of the first two cases outside the United States. Am J Med Genet 1987; 27:767–771.
Chrzanowska K, et al.: Cardio-facio-cutaneous (CFC) syndrome: report of a new patient. Am J Med Genet 1989; 33:471–473 †
Mucklow ES: A case of cardio-facio-cutaneous syndrome. Am J Med Genet 1989; 33:474–475 †
Sorge G: CFC syndrome: report on three additional cases. Am J Med Genet 1989; 33:476–478. †

NE019                                                    **Giovanni Neri**

**Cardio-facio-cutaneous syndrome**
*See CARDIO-FACIAL-CUTANEOUS SYNDROME*
**Cardiocutaneous syndrome**
*See LENTIGINES SYNDROME, MULTIPLE*
**Cardioduodenal duct**
*See STOMACH, DUPLICATION*

## CARDIOFACIAL SYNDROME-ASSYMETRIC FACIES          2035

**Includes:**
  Asymmetrical crying facies (ACF)
  Cayler syndrome
  Depressor anguli oris muscle, hypoplasia of
  Facial paresis, partial, unilateral

**Excludes:**
  Facial nerve dysfunction
  **Hemihypertrophy** (0458)
  **Oculo-auriculo-vertebral anomaly** (0735)
  Wilms association

**Major Diagnostic Criteria:**   Facial asymmetry on crying (ACF); no evidence of asymmetry when not crying. Electrodiagnostic studies conclusive of hypoplasia of anguli oris depressor muscle (HAODM), but ACF due to HAODM may be differentiated from ACF due to facial nerve palsy by clinical presentation. A history of obstetric trauma or signs of upper and lower facial weakness may indicate facial nerve palsy. In ACF due to HAODM, there is no history of birth trauma, abnormal eye closure, or forehead wrinkling. The baby feeds normally and usual drooling occurs. Other associated congenital anomalies (cardiac, respiratory, vertebral, renal, and anal defects) may be present.

**Clinical Findings:**   Various congenital anomalies have been found in association with ACF-cardiofacial syndrome. Cardiac defects, most commonly **Ventricular septal defect**, but also **Atrial septal defects**, AV canal, **Aorta, coarctation, Pulmonary valve, stenosis,** and **Heart, tetralogy of Fallot,** have been reported. Other major malformations include those seen in **Vater association,** i.e. vertebral, gastrointestinal, renal and limb anomalies. Minor malformations have also been reported, including unusual facies with small head, small and low-set ears, micrognathia, and microphthalmia.

**Complications:**   Those related to the associated cardiac and other malformations.

**Associated Findings:**   Depends upon other associated anomalies.

**Etiology:**   Autosomal dominant inheritance in some families, although multifactorial inheritance with teratogenic exposure has also been postulated.

**Pathogenesis:**   Partial agenesis of the anguli oris depressor muscle, rather than a facial nerve palsy.

**MIM No.:**   *12552

**POS No.:**   3614

**Sex Ratio:**   Presumably M1:F1.

**Occurrence:**   6–8:1,000. The reported incidence of associated anomalies varies greatly.

**Risk of Recurrence for Patient's Sib:**
  See Part I, *Mendelian Inheritance.*

**Risk of Recurrence for Patient's Child:**
  See Part I, *Mendelian Inheritance.*

**Age of Detectability:**   At birth.

**Gene Mapping and Linkage:**   Unknown.

**Prevention:**   None known. Genetic counseling indicated.

**Treatment:**   No known treatment for face asymmetry on crying; correction of associated anomalies.

**Prognosis:**   Depends on severity of associated anomalies.

**Detection of Carrier:**   Clinical examination of first degree relatives.

**Special Considerations:**   It has been recommended that an infant with congenital ACF should undergo a thorough clinical examination for other associated anomalies. Right-sided facial asymmetry has been reported to be more commonly associated with other defects than left-sided asymmetry.

**Support Groups:**   Dallas; American Heart Association

**References:**
Cayler GC: Cardiofacial syndrome: congenital heart disease and facial weakness. Arch Dis Child 1969; 44:69–75.

Miller M, Hall JG: familial asymmetric crying facies. Am J Dis Child 1979; 133:743–746.
Singhi S, et al.: Congenital asymmetrical crying facies. Clin Pediatr 1980; 19:673–678. *
Silengo MC, et al.: Asymmetric crying facies with microcephaly and mental retardation: an autosomal dominant syndrome with variable expressivity. Clin Genet 1986; 30:481–484.

N0003                                                    **James J. Nora**

**Cardiogenital syndrome**
  *See CARDIOMYOPATHY-GENITAL DEFECTS*
**Cardiomegalia glycogenica diffusa**
  *See GLYCOGENOSIS, TYPE IIa*
**Cardiomelic dysplasia-mesoaxial hexadactyly**
  *See HEART-HAND SYNDROME IV*
**Cardiomelic syndrome**
  *See HEART-HAND SYNDROME*
**Cardiomelic-facio dysplasia, lethal**
  *See FACIO-CARDIOMELIC DYSPLASIA, LETHAL*
**Cardiomyopathic lentiginosis**
  *See LENTIGINES SYNDROME, MULTIPLE*
**Cardiomyopathy due to desmin defect**
  *See MYOPATHY OR CARDIOMYOPATHY DUE TO DESMIN DEFECT*
**Cardiomyopathy due to lysosomal glycogen storage**
  *See GLYCOGENOSIS, TYPE IIc*
**Cardiomyopathy, congestive-hypergonadotropic hypogonadism**
  *See HYPERGONADOTROPIC HYPOGONADISM WITH CARDIOMYOPATHY*

## CARDIOMYOPATHY, FAMILIAL DILATED          3234

**Includes:**
  Cardiomyopathy, familial idiopathic
  Congestive cardiomyopathy, familial
  Peripartum cardiomyopathy (some cases)

**Excludes:**
  Cardiomyopathies, dilated, secondary
  Cardiomyopathy, restrictive
  **Heart, subaortic stenosis, muscular** (0917)
  Myocarditis
  **Ventricle, endocardial fibroelastosis**

**Major Diagnostic Criteria:**   Based on echocardiographic or cardiac catheterization determination of ventricular internal dimension in diastole above the normal limits for the patient's age and body surface area, plus reduced ventricular systolic function (ejection fraction of less than 50%). Since these abnormalities are nonspecific and can be due to other diseases such as atherosclerosis, the diagnosis of idiopathic dilated cardiomyopathy is one of exclusion that requires careful history, physical examination and appropriate laboratory studies. In some cases it may be made only after investigations such as coronary angiograms or cardiac biopsy. By definition, familial idiopathic dilated cardiomyopathy can only be diagnosed when two or more relatives are affected.

**Clinical Findings:**   Clinical signs may develop at any age, but most frequently they appear in adolescence or adulthood. There is great variability of age of onset even within families. Initial symptoms may be due to cardiac arrhythmias or congestive heart failure. Some patients first become symptomatic during periods of physiologic stress, such as during pregnancy or during an intercurrent illness such as a viral infection or pneumonia. In these cases the disease may be erroneously attributed to the precipitating factor and the familial nature of the disease may be missed without a careful review of the family history or family investigations.

In some patients clinical onset of the disease may be precipitous and the first sign may be sudden death. In other patients within the same family, the condition may be detected only because of echocardiographic screening; these patients may do well for many years and may have slowly progressive disease.

In a population-based study of idiopathic dilated cardiomyopathy patients (not specifically investigated for familial disease), the relative one-year survival was 95% and the five-year survival was 94%. This is considerably better than survival rates of 69% at one year and 40% at five years based on patients referred to tertiary medical centers. However, the natural history of familial dilated cardiomyopathy has not been well defined; it is likely that some persons who have acute onset of symptoms may have had presymptomatic disease for many years.

Non-penetrance has been shown to occur infrequently but precise age-dependent penetrance data are not available. Some patients with familial dilated cardiomyopathy will not be determined to have familial disease based on review of their family history. Therefore, screening of first degree relatives for occult disease by echocardiogram is indicated in some cases.

Familial dilated cardiomyopathy is a heterogeneous group of disorders. Although most cases involve left ventricular dysfunction which may progress to involve the right ventricle, some families primarily have right ventricular involvement. Some families with primarily right ventricular involvement have right ventricular dysplasia which may be a less severe form of Uhl anomaly. Other families with right ventricular cardiomyopathy do not have the typical histologic abnormalities of fibrous and fatty replacement of the right ventricular free wall that is seen in right ventricular dysplasia. Furthermore, some family members may have early left ventricular involvement that is indistinguishable from the more common familial idiopathic dilated cardiomyopathy that affects primarily the left ventricle. The histology of left ventricular idiopathic dilated cardiomyopathy is not specific and shows variable interstitial fibrosis and cellular hypertrophy. Electron microscopic studies may show abnormal mitochondria in some cases.

**Complications:** Cardiac arrhythmia may result in syncope, anoxic spells with seizures, angina, or sudden death. Progressive congestive heart failure may lead to death. Since this disease may afflict otherwise young and healthy persons, cardiac transplantation should be considered.

**Associated Findings:** None known.

**Etiology:** Heterogeneous. Most families are compatible with autosomal dominant inheritance, although autosomal recessive and X-linked inheritance have been observed. In cases with only a few affected family members and without an obvious inheritance pattern, multifactorial etiology or a mixed model (e.g., autosomal dominant gene effect plus multifactorial or polygenic factors) has not been excluded. Most cases of idiopathic dilated cardiomyopathy are sporadic.

**Pathogenesis:** Unknown.

**MIM No.:** *11520, 21211

**Sex Ratio:** M1:F1, with the exception of possible X-linked cases.

**Occurrence:** The prevalence of idiopathic dilated cardiomyopathy in persons <55 years is 1:5,000. In series of patients with idiopathic dilated cardiomyopathy, approximately 9–33% are familial.

**Risk of Recurrence for Patient's Sib:**
See Part I, *Mendelian Inheritance.* In sporadic cases of idiopathic dilated cardiomyopathy, the empiric recurrence risk is probably less than 5–10%.

**Risk of Recurrence for Patient's Child:**
See Part I, *Mendelian Inheritance.*

**Age of Detectability:** Patients as young as 15 months have been detected, but the disease can become manifest at any age. There are no biochemical or physiologic markers. Presymptomatic detection by echocardiography is sometimes possible, but normal findings do not preclude later development of the disease.

**Gene Mapping and Linkage:** Unknown.

**Prevention:** None known. Genetic counseling indicated. For persons at significant risk, cigarette smoking and excessive alcohol ingestion should be avoided, since these may aggravate the disease. However, avoidance of these agents may or may not reduce the likelihood of developing disease in genetically predisposed persons.

**Treatment:** Medications to control cardiac arrhythmias and/or congestive heart failure are indicated for some patients. Heart transplantation should be considered. Whether or not treatment

of asymptomatic patients detected by screening will slow progression of the disease or improve longevity is undetermined.

**Prognosis:** In some patients, cardiac function deteriorates inexorably in spite of medications and results in terminal heart failure or need for cardiac transplant. The course of illness from the time symptoms develop to death may be less than one month. Other patients have remained stable for over 12 years. The course of illness in asymptomatic relatives detected by screening is undetermined.

**Detection of Carrier:** Unknown. Presymptomatic detection by echocardiography is sometimes possible.

**Special Considerations:** There is marked heterogeneity of idiopathic dilated cardiomyopathy, and it is likely that there are both genetic and non-genetic forms of the disease. It is probable that there is significant heterogeneity of the genetic forms of the disease, since autosomal dominant, autosomal recessive, and X-linked inheritance have been reported. Delineation of distinct forms of the disease based on clinical signs and symptoms is hampered by the marked variability of age of onset, clinical symptoms, and course of the disease within a given family. Careful histologic and/or genetic linkage studies may be helpful in delineating this group of diseases.

**References:**
Michels VV, et al.: Familial aggregation of idiopathic dilated cardiomyopathy. Am J Cardiol 1985; 55:1232–1233. *
Berko BA, Swift M: X-linked dilated cardiomyopathy. New Engl J Med 1987; 316:1186–1191.
Fragola PV, et al.: Familial idiopathic dilated cardiomyopathy. Am Heart J 1988; 115:912–914.
Klein LW, Horowitz LN: Familial right ventricular dilated cardiomyopathy associated with supraventricular arrhythmias. Am J Cardiol 1988; 62:482–483.
Schmidt MA, et al.: Familial dilated cardiomyopathy. Am J Med Genet 1988; 31:135–143. *
Michels VV, et al.: Frequency of familial dilated cardiomyopathy in an unselected series of patients with idiopathic dilated cardiomyopathy. (Abstract) Am J Hum Genet 1989; 45 (Suppl 4):A55. *
Valantine HA, et al.: Frequency of familial nature of dilated cardiomyopathy and usefulness of cardiac transplantation in this subset. Am J Cardiol 1989; 63:959–963. *

MI002                                           **Virginia V. Michels**

**Cardiomyopathy, familial idiopathic**
  *See CARDIOMYOPATHY, FAMILIAL DILATED*
**Cardiomyopathy, hypertrophic obstructive**
  *See HEART, SUBAORTIC STENOSIS, MUSCULAR*

---

## CARDIOMYOPATHY-GENITAL DEFECTS                2246

**Includes:**
  Cardiogenital syndrome
  Genital anomaly-cardiomyopathy

**Excludes:**
  **Collagenoma, multiple cutaneous, familial** (3166)
  **Hypergonadotropic hypogonadism with cardiomyopathy** (3195)

**Major Diagnostic Criteria:** Genital anomaly, cardiomyopathy, and mental retardation.

**Clinical Findings:** The abnormality of the external genitalia consists of a very small phallus, poor development of the scrotal sac, and, in some patients, persistence of the urogenital sinus with a vestigeal vaginal pouch. There is lack of response to the administration of human chorionic gonadotropin, and elevated concentration of follicle-stimulating hormone, strongly suggesting primary testicular failure. The karyotype has been normal 46, XY in the reported male patients.

Mental retardation is moderate and is not apparent in early infancy. It is associated with delayed and defective speech, but normal motor development.

The cardiomyopathy is documented by auscultation, electrocardiography and X-rays. The heart sounds are muffled. S₃ is

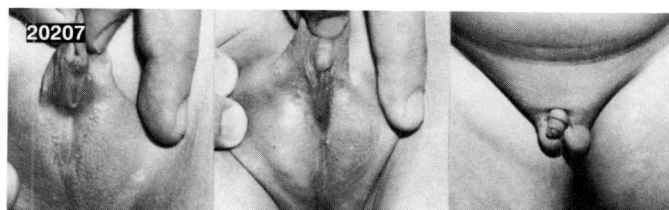

**2246-20207:** Note the varying degrees of partial virilization of the external genitalia of three brothers with cardiomyopathy and genital defects.

accentuated at the apex. No significant murmurs are heard. The electrocardiogram reveals nodal tachycardia, premature ventricular contraction, QRS complexes of small amplitude, inverted T waves in leads I, V5, and V6, and a prolonged Q-T interval. These may lead to congestive heart failure, pericardial effusion, and death by the age of 14 years.

**Complications:** Congestive heart failure.

**Associated Findings:** None known.

**Etiology:** Probably autosomal recessive inheritance.

**Pathogenesis:** Unknown.

**MIM No.:** 21212

**POS No.:** 3732

**Sex Ratio:** M1:F0. All reported patients have been chromosomally male.

**Occurrence:** Five patients have been reported from two Lebanese families.

**Risk of Recurrence for Patient's Sib:**
See Part I, *Mendelian Inheritance.*

**Risk of Recurrence for Patient's Child:**
See Part I, *Mendelian Inheritance.* No report exists of a patient having reproduced.

**Age of Detectability:** The anomalies of the genitalia are apparent at the time of birth. Mental retardation and speech impairment do not manifest until the age of five years. The cardiac findings may appear as early as two months of age.

**Gene Mapping and Linkage:** Unknown.

**Prevention:** None known. Genetic counseling indicated.

**Treatment:** Undetermined except the symptomatic therapeutic modalities for the complications of the cardiomyopathy. Sex of rearing should be guided by the degree of genital anomaly.

**Prognosis:** In general, life expectancy is shortened and death may occur by the age of 14 years.

**Detection of Carrier:** Unknown.

**Support Groups:** Dallas; American Heart Association

**References:**
Najjar SS, et al.: Genital anomaly, mental retardation, and cardiomyopathy: a new syndrome? J Pediatr 1973; 83:286–288.
Najjar SS, et al.: Genital anomaly and cardiomyopathy: a new syndrome. Clin Genet 1984; 26:371–373.
Malouf J, et al.: Hypergonadotropic hypogonadism with congestive cardiomyopathy: an autosomal recessive disorder? Am J Med Genet 1985; 20:483–489.

NA009
DE030

**Samir S. Najjar**
**Vazken M. Der Kaloustian**

**Cardiomyopathy-hypogonadism-collagenoma syndrome**
*See COLLAGENOMA, MULTIPLE CUTANEOUS, FAMILIAL*
**Cardiopathy, constrictive**
*See VENTRICLE, ENDOMYOCARDIAL FIBROSIS OF RIGHT*
*also VENTRICLE, ENDOMYOCARDIAL FIBROSIS OF LEFT*
**Cardiospasm**
*See ESOPHAGUS, ACHALASIA*

**Carmi syndrome**
*See SKIN, LOCALIZED ABSENCE OF*
*also APLASIA CUTIS CONGENITA-GASTROINTESTINAL ATRESIA*
**Carney complex**
*See NEVI-ATRIAL MYXOMA-MYXOID NEUROFIBROMAS-EPHELIDES*
**Carney syndrome**
*See NEVI-ATRIAL MYXOMA-MYXOID NEUROFIBROMAS-EPHELIDES*
**Carnitine deficiency, myopathic**
*See MYOPATHY-METABOLIC, CARNITINE DEFICIENCY, PRIMARY AND SECONDARY*
**Carnitine deficiency, primary**
*See MYOPATHY-METABOLIC, CARNITINE DEFICIENCY, PRIMARY AND SECONDARY*
**Carnitine deficiency, primary systemic (some)**
*See VISCERA, FATTY METAMORPHOSIS*
**Carnitine deficiency, secondary**
*See MYOPATHY-METABOLIC, CARNITINE DEFICIENCY, PRIMARY AND SECONDARY*
**Carnitine deficiency, systemic**
*See MYOPATHY-METABOLIC, CARNITINE DEFICIENCY, PRIMARY AND SECONDARY*
**Carnitine palmityl-transferase-A(I) deficiency**
*See MYOPATHY-METABOLIC, CARNITINE PALMITYL TRANSFERASE DEFICIENCY*
**Carnitine palmityl-transferase-B(II) deficiency**
*See MYOPATHY-METABOLIC, CARNITINE PALMITYL TRANSFERASE DEFICIENCY*
**Carnosinase deficiency**
*See CARNOSINEMIA*

## CARNOSINEMIA    0126

**Includes:**
Carnosinuria
Carnosinase deficiency
Hyper-beta-carnosinemia
Serum carnosinase deficiency, disorders of

**Excludes:**
Dietary carnosinuria
Homocarnosinosis
Imidazole aminoaciduria

**Major Diagnostic Criteria:** Increased excretion of carnosine in the urine despite a meat-free diet for 3 days. Decreased serum carnosinase activity ranging from 0 to 30% of normal. Eating meat or fowl causes individuals with serum carnosinase deficiency to excrete anserine but not 1-methylhistidine. Individuals with normal carnosinase after exposure to meat or fowl excrete both 1-methylhistidine and large amounts of anserine. Serum carnosine level may also be elevated, but this is not a consistent finding even when carnosine is being excreted in the urine. Tissue carnosinase activity in carnosinemia has been normal in spite of low serum carnosinase levels, and this has led to the proposal that tissue carnosinase may be a different enzyme than the serum enzyme.

**Clinical Findings:** Twenty-three patients have been described with the serum carnosinase deficiency. Their serum carnosinase activity ranged from 0 to 30% of normal, and they all excreted increased amounts of carnosine after a meat-free diet for 3 days. The clinical symptoms noted in the patients did not correlate with either serum carnosinase activity or amount of excreted carnosine. The symptoms included attention deficit disorder in four patients, a nonprogressive developmental delay in one, neurofibromatosis in one, absences seizures in one, childhood dementia in one, and neurosensory hearing loss in one. One of the patients in the study was considered to be clinically normal. There has not yet been correlation between severity of the neurologic symptoms or the type of symptoms and serum carnosinase activity. This has suggested that serum carnosinase deficiency is not directly related to the neurologic symptoms but may be an associated predisposition or a marker for another genetic problem.

**Complications:** At present, a direct relationship between the biochemical abnormalities and the clinical findings has not been established.

**Associated Findings:** None known.

**Etiology:** Probably autosomal recessive inheritance, although X-linked recessive inheritance has not been rules out.

**Pathogenesis:** Deficiency of serum carnosinase activity.

**MIM No.:** *21220

**Sex Ratio:** Presumably M1:F1

**Occurrence:** Twenty-three cases have been reported, but the condition is thought to be under-reported because of a long-standing assumption that it is a "non-disease".

**Risk of Recurrence for Patient's Sib:**
See Part I, *Mendelian Inheritance.*

**Risk of Recurrence for Patient's Child:**
See Part I, *Mendelian Inheritance.*

**Age of Detectability:** Early infancy.

**Gene Mapping and Linkage:** Unknown.

**Prevention:** None known. Genetic counseling indicated.

**Treatment:** Decreased intake of meat and fowl would decrease exogenous carnosine, but since symptomatology does not correlate with levels, dietary therapy it is not recommended.

**Prognosis:** Difficult to determine since there have been severely affected individuals and clinically normal individuals with established serum carnosinase deficiency.

**Detection of Carrier:** Not established, but serum carnosinase activity has been intermediate in three of the mothers and both parents in two pedigrees.

**Special Considerations:** It remains unproven whether the presence of serum carnosinase deficiency is in anyway related to the various outcomes that have been reported. Since there has been a wide spectrum of neurologic involvement, including clinically normal, it is difficult to prove that carnosinase deficiency is clinically relevant. It is possible this is an association or merely a bias of ascertainment, since many of the patients have been studied due to their neurologic involvement. To date, no random studies have been done to look at the presence of carnosinase deficiency in the general population.

In one patient studied, homocarnosine, which is a product of GABA metabolism, was normal, thus suggesting that carnosinase deficiency may have no neurologic effects. Finally, tissue carnosinase deficiency has been normal in those individuals with serum carnosinase deficiency, and it is difficult to propose a mechanism by which the serum deficiency would cause brain symptomatology.

**References:**
Perry TL, et al.: Carnosinemia: a metabolic disorder with neurologic disease and mental defect. N Engl J Med 1967; 277:1219–1227.
Fleisher LD, et al.: Carnosinase deficiency: a new variant with high residual activity. Pediatr Res 1980; 14:269–271.
Stanbury JB, et al.: Serum carnosinase deficiency. In Stanbury JB, ed: The metabolic basis of inherited disease, ed 5. New York: McGraw Hill, 1983:579–583.
Cohen M, et al.: Serum carnosinase deficiency: a non-disabling phenotype? J Ment Defic Res 1985; 29:383–389.

BU007                                              **Bruce A. Buehler**

**Carnosinuria**
*See CARNOSINEMIA*
**Caroli disease**
*See LIVER, CONGENITAL CYSTIC DILATATION OF INTRAHEPATIC DUCTS*
**Carotid artery aneurysm**
*See EAR, ANEURYSM OF INTERNAL CAROTID ARTERY*
**Carotid artery, common origin of brachiocephalic and contralateral**
*See ARTERY, BRACHIOCEPHALIC AND CONTRALATERAL CAROTID, COMMON ORIGIN*

## CAROTID BODY TUMOR                              0127

**Includes:**
Chemodectoma of neck
Ganglion nodosum tumor
Glomus jugulare tumors
Paragangliomata
Tumor, juxtavagal

**Excludes:**
Aortic body tumor
Chemodectoma located elsewhere in the body
**Ear, chemodectoma of middle ear** (0145)

**Major Diagnostic Criteria:** Presence of a mass in the region of the carotid bifurcation and a positive tumor flush by arteriography. Biopsy should be avoided if possible, but if tissue is obtained the findings are characteristic.

**Clinical Findings:** A painless neck mass is found, which may or may not be associated with a bruit. The mass can be moved laterally (side to side) but not vertically. Dysphagia, hoarseness or cough, syncope with carotid sinus syndrome, headache, and occasionally pain or tenderness may be seen. Tumors may present in the lateral pharyngeal wall. Also paralysis of one or more of the 9th, 10th, 11th and 12th cranial nerves may occur. If these tumors are of a secreting nature, laboratory findings would be similar to those of a pheochromocytoma; namely, elevated catecholamines in the blood and urine. However, the incidence of secreting chemodectomas of the neck is only about 1 or 2%. Arteriography provides significant information. A typical tumor blush is seen, and venous studies may show obstruction of the internal jugular vein or the jugular bulb. It is possible to have multiple tumors which could be bilateral and involve other areas.

**Complications:** Local mass or pressure effects, including obstruction of the carotid vessel or internal jugular vein. Present 15% of the time are cranial nerve paralysis, 10th nerve first, then 11th and 12th nerves followed by the 9th nerve. Rare tumors secrete norepinephrine and are associated with hypertension, and some tumors are malignant, with multiple metastatic lesions.

**Associated Findings:** Chemodectomas may be multiple, occurring in the neck, ear, thorax, or abdomen.

**Etiology:** Presumably autosomal dominant inheritance.

**Pathogenesis:** Tumor growth by one or more elements of chemoreceptor tissue. Primarily these are locally invasive tumors. Incidence of malignancy is undetermined. Probably 3–4% develop metastases. Multicentric location is at least 5%, going up to 26% in familial cases.

**MIM No.:** *16800

**Sex Ratio:** M1:F1

**Occurrence:** Unknown. Over 500 cases of carotid body tumors have been reported. It is the most frequent type of paraganglioma of the head and neck.

**Risk of Recurrence for Patient's Sib:**
See Part I, *Mendelian Inheritance.* Incidence of multiple chemodectomas is highest in carotid body tumors and approaches 5%. When there is a positive family history, the incidence of multiple tumors as distinct from a single carotid body tumor increases to 26%.

**Risk of Recurrence for Patient's Child:**
See Part I, *Mendelian Inheritance.*

**Age of Detectability:** Most commonly noted in the third and fourth decades; however, one case has been reported at birth. Somewhat younger average age of detection in families with positive history.

**Gene Mapping and Linkage:** Unknown.

**Prevention:** None known. Genetic counseling indicated.

**Treatment:** Early diagnosis and surgical excision whenever possible, which leaves a low incidence of local recurrence. Careful arteriography may lead to the discovery of multiple tumors.

For large, unresectable lesions or poor surgical risks, radiation therapy in the range of 4,000 to 6,000 rads.

**Prognosis:** Fortunately the majority of patients have a slow-growing tumor. The incidence of metastases is low. Small tumors have a very good prognosis with surgical excision. Large tumors carry a fair to poor prognosis over a long duration. Because of the slow growth of these tumors, survival is usually of long duration.

**Detection of Carrier:** Unknown.

**References:**
Berman SO: Chemoreceptor system and its tumor - the chemodectoma. Int Abstr Surg 1956; 102:330.
Rush BF Jr: Familial bilateral carotid body tumors. Ann Surg 1963; 157:633.
Akkary S: Malignant carotid body tumor in the neck of a newborn infant. Arch Dis Child 1964; 39:194.
Resler DR, et al.: Multiplicity and familial incidence of carotid body and glomus jugulare tumors. Ann Otol Rhinol Laryngol 1966; 75:114.
Grimley PM, Glenner GG: Ultrastructure of the human carotid body: a perspective on the mode of chemoreception. Circulation 1968; 37:648.
Glenner G, Grimley P: Tumors of the extra-adrenal paraganglion system. Washington DC: Armed forces Institute of Pathology, 1974: (II)9.
McGuirt WF, Harker LA: Carotid body tumors. Arch Otolaryngol 1975; 101:58–62.
Batsakis JG: Paragangliomas of the head and neck. In: Batsakis JG, ed: Tumors of the head and neck: clinical and pathologic considerations, ed. 2. Baltimore: Williams & Wilkins, 1979:369–380.
Parry DM, et al.: Carotid body tumors in humans: genetics and epidemiology. J Nat Cancer Inst 1982; 68:573–578.

AU005                                                    **Thomas Aufdemorte**

**Carpal osteochondroma**
*See DYSPLASIA EPIPHYSEALIS HEMIMELICA*
**Carpal tunnel amyloid of chronic hemodialysis**
*See AMYLOIDOSIS, HEMODIALYSIS-RELATED*
**Carpal-tarsal osteolysis, recessive**
*See OSTEOLYSIS, RECESSIVE CARPAL-TARSAL*
**Carpal-tarsal osteolysis-chronic progressive glomerulopathy**
*See OSTEOLYSIS, CARPAL-TARSAL AND CHRONIC PROGRESSIVE GLOMERULOPATHY*
**Carpenter syndrome**
*See ACROCEPHALOPOLYSYNDACTYLY*
**Carpo-tarsal and cranial dystrophy**
*See CRANIO-CARPO-TARSAL DYSPLASIA, WHISTLING FACE TYPE*
**Cartilage-hair hypoplasia**
*See METAPHYSEAL CHONDRODYSPLASIA, TYPE McKUSICK*
**Caruncle aberrations**
*See EYE, CARUNCLE ABERRATIONS*
**Caruncle, absence of**
*See EYE, CARUNCLE ABERRATIONS*
**Caruncle, hyperplasia of**
*See EYE, CARUNCLE ABERRATIONS*
**Caruncle, hypoplasia of**
*See EYE, CARUNCLE ABERRATIONS*
**Caruncle, notch or cleavage of**
*See EYE, CARUNCLE ABERRATIONS*
**Caruncle, supernumerary**
*See EYE, CARUNCLE ABERRATIONS*
**Cat cry syndrome**
*See CHROMOSOME 5, MONOSOMY 5p*
**Cat ear wax**
*See EAR, CERUMEN VARIATIONS*

## CAT EYE SYNDROME                                      0544

**Includes:**
    Anal atresia-iris coloboma
    Chromosome 22, partial trisomy 22
    Iris coloboma-anal atresia
    Ocular coloboma, imperforated anus, preauricular
      appendages
    Schmid-Fraccaro syndrome

**Excludes:** coloboma or anal atresia without chromosomal abnormality

**Major Diagnostic Criteria:** Colobomatous anomalies of the eye, preauricular appendages or fistulae, anal atresia.

**Clinical Findings:** Colobomatous anomalies of the eye, mostly of the iris but also of the choroid and retina, sometimes associated with microphthalmos, usually bilateral. The patients may exhibit a peculiar facies with depressed nose, hypertelorism, downward-slanting palpebral fissures, and micrognathia. Important features are preauricular cutaneous tags, pits, or fistulae frequently associated with deformity of the ear, even microtia. The secondary palate may also have a cleft. Anal atresia and/or rectal stenosis with rectoperineal or rectovaginal fistula is common. Hypospadias was noted in some patients, vaginal atresia in one patient. Abnormalities of the kidneys, mostly hypoplasia or agenesis and hydronephrosis and cystoureteral reflux, were shown. Anomalies of the ribs and vertebrae, e.g. hemivertebrae, and dislocation of the hips may be associated. Single or complex malformations of the heart, such as septum defects, pulmonic stenosis, or **Heart, tetralogy of Fallot**, and gross abnormalities of the great vessels, namely **Pulmonary venous connection, total anomalous**, were noted. Dermatoglyphics may be unusual. At least two-thirds of the patients are moderately mentally retarded. Short stature seems to be common.

**Complications:** Cardiovascular failure, infections of the urinary tract, hydronephrosis, glaucoma, cataract, moderate conductive hearing loss.

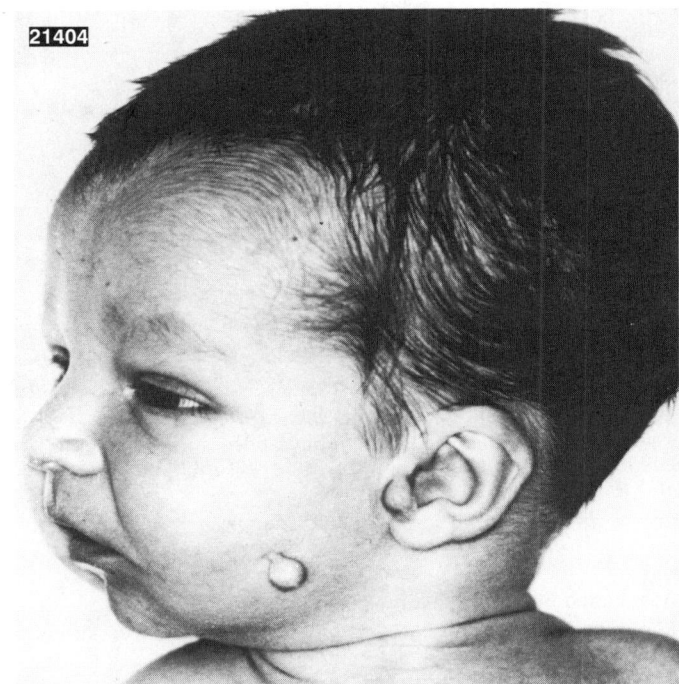

**0544A-**21404: Note skin tags and low-set ear.

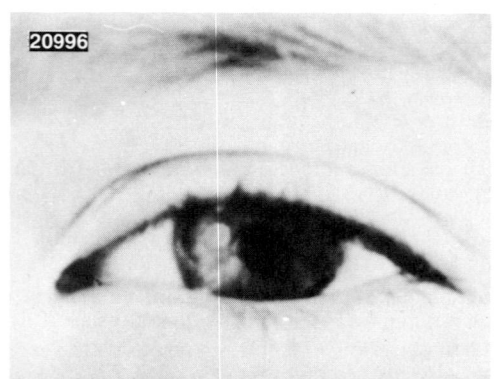

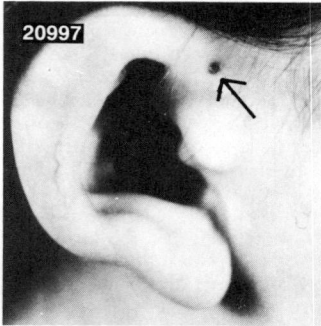
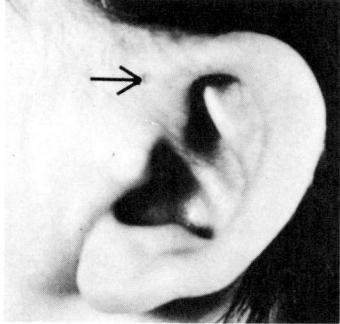

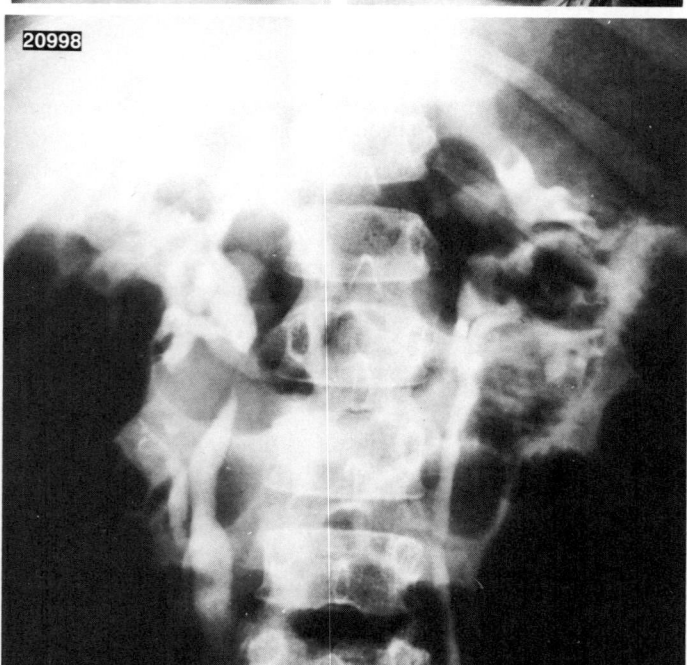

**0544B-20996:** Left-sided coloboma of the iris. **20997:** Preauricular pits; the preauricular tags have been surgically removed. **20998:** Intravenous pyelography shows doubling of the ureter and renal pelvis bilaterally.

---

**Associated Findings:** None known.

**Etiology:** Probably due to chromosomal imbalance, although Mendelian factors may also be important.

**Pathogenesis:** An additional small extra chromosome, sometimes with mosaicism, with a minority of euploid cells, has been

found in more than 50 cases; some familial. After the introduction of the banding techniques, different authors identified the extra-chromosomes as a bisatellited dicentric chromosome, most likely of the chromosome 22 origin. The chromosome 22 derivation of the marker was recently confirmed by the use of a chromosome 22-derived single sequence probe, p22/34, which identifies locus D22S9 which was shown to anneal to 22q11 by *in situ* hybridisation. High-resolution quinacrine-stained chromosomes from parents and patients further showed that the extra chromosomes have different short arm/satellite regions on each end, and that these match both chromosome 22 heteromorphism of the mothers, i.e.; the abnormal extra chromosome is the result of a first meiotic structural error in the mother, as well as of a segregation error involving both chromosomes 22.

**MIM No.:** 11547

**POS No.:** 3267

**Sex Ratio:** About F1:F2 obsered in patients with a non-familial marker chromosome (21/33).

**Occurrence:** Over sixty cases have been documented.

**Risk of Recurrence for Patient's Sib:** Unknown. Increased.

**Risk of Recurrence for Patient's Child:** Unknown. Increased.

**Age of Detectability:** At birth.

**Gene Mapping and Linkage:** CECR (cat eye syndrome chromosome region) has been mapped to 22pter-q11.

**Prevention:** None known. Genetic counseling indicated.

**Treatment:** Corrective surgery.

**Prognosis:** Life span depends upon cardiovascular and renal functions. Various degrees of mental deficiency.

**Detection of Carrier:** By cytogenetic studies.

**Special Considerations:** The association of coloboma of the eye with anal atresia and cystic dysplasia of one kidney was first observed in 1878. What has been considered the typical (cat eye) syndrome should therefore comprise not only colobomatous anomalies, anal atresia and preauricular dysmorphism but an additional extra chromosome as well. There are associations of coloboma and anal atresia (and genitourinary abnormalities) without any chromosomal aberration, and some cases with the typical syndrome including cardiac malformations. Observations of two sisters, and in a male infant of related parents, suggesting homozygosity of a rare mutation, have been inconclusive. However, the association of coloboma and anal atresia in otherwise healthy individuals without a chromosomal aberration could be coincidental.

**References:**
Schachenmann G, et al.: Chromosomes in coloboma and anal atresia. Lancet 1965; II:290 only.
Weleber RB, et al.: Cytogenetic investigation of cat-eye syndrome. Am J Ophthalmol 1977; 84:477.
Schinzel A, et al.: The "Cat Eye syndrome". dicentric small marker chromosome probably derived from a no.22 (tetrasomy 22pter-q11) associated with a characteristic phenotype. Hum Genet 1981; 57: 148–158.
McDermid HE, et al.: Characterization of the supernumerary chromosome in Cat Eye syndrome. Science 1986; 232:646–648.
Magenis RE, et al.: Parental origin of the extra chromosome in the Cat Eye Syndrome: evidence from heteromorphism and in situ hybridisation analysis. Am J Med Genet 1988; 29:9–19.

PF001
FR030

**Rudolf A. Pfeiffer**
**Jean-Pierre Fryns**

**Cataplexy**
*See NARCOLEPSY*
**Cataract, anterior polar (CAP)**
*See CATARACT, POLAR AND CAPSULAR*

## CATARACT, AUTOSOMAL DOMINANT CONGENITAL 2342

**Includes:**
> Coralliform cataract
> Cortical cataract
> Crystalline aculeiform or frosted cataract
> Floriform cataract
> Lamellar cataract
> Lenticular cataract
> Membranous cataract
> Nuclear cataract
> Perinuclear cataract
> Polar cataract
> Posterior polar
> Pulverulent zonular cataract
> Sutural cataract
> Total cataract
> Zonular cataract

**Excludes:**
> **Cataract, cortical and nuclear** (0132)
> **Cataract, polar and capsular** (0133)
> **Cataract** (other)

**Major Diagnostic Criteria:** Opacities in the lens. Slit lamp examination may be required for identification.

**Clinical Findings:** The clinical picture varies from visually insignificant opacities to severe visual impairment. The morphologic characteristics of the opacities exhibit intra- and interfamilial variability in the location (embryonal, anterior and posterior polar, or cortical regions), shape (coralliform or star-like), and density. In general, the intrafamilial variable expressivity includes asymmetry as well as variable density and morphology. Differences in the morphology of the cataracts are more impressive among than within families, suggesting genetic variability. Penetrance is usually high.

**Complications:** Visual deprivation amblyopia, which is associated with nystagmus, strabismus, and absent or diminished binocularity, may be associated with bilateral congenital cataracts.

**Associated Findings:** Microphthalmia was reported in two families (Capella et al, 1963).

**Etiology:** Autosomal dominant inheritance.

**Pathogenesis:** Unknown.

**MIM No.:** *11570, *11580, *11590, 11610, *11620, *11630, *11640, *11660, 11670, *11680, *15685

**CDC No.:** 743.326

**Sex Ratio:** M1:F1

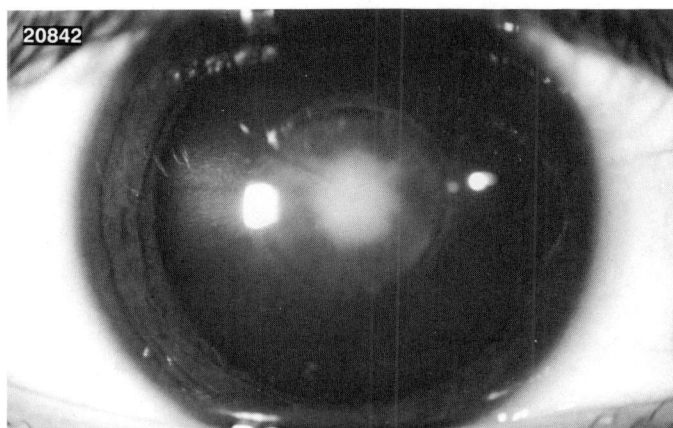

2342-20842: Cataract, congenital autosomal dominant.

**Occurrence:** Undetermined, but autosomal dominant nuclear cataract is one of the most frequent types of congenital cataract.

**Risk of Recurrence for Patient's Sib:**
See Part I, *Mendelian Inheritance.*

**Risk of Recurrence for Patient's Child:**
See Part I, *Mendelian Inheritance.*

**Age of Detectability:** Usually evident at birth if eyes are dilated and examined with a slit lamp.

**Gene Mapping and Linkage:** CAE (cataract, zonular pulverulent (FY-linked)) has been mapped to 1q21-q25.
CTM (cataract, Marner) has been provisionally mapped to 16.
Several Japanese investigators have reported the association of blood phenotype i, rare in all populations studied, and congenital cataracts. A three-generation family with autosomal dominant anterior polar cataracts which segregated with an apparently balanced 2;14 reciprocal chromosome translocation has been reported.

**Prevention:** None known. Genetic counseling indicated.

**Treatment:** Cataract extraction.

**Prognosis:** Ultimate visual acuity is a function of density and morphology of the cataract and the age at which surgery is performed.

**Detection of Carrier:** Slit lamp examination may help identify some mildly affected individuals.

**Support Groups:** PA; Devon; Parents of Cataract Kids (PACK)

**References:**

Capella JA, et al.: Hereditary cataracts and microphthalmia. Am J Ophthal 1963; 56:454-458.
Conneally PM, et al.: Confirmation of genetic heterogeneity in autosomal dominant forms of congenital cataracts from linkage studies. Cytogenet Cell Genet 1978; 22:295-297. *
Maumenee IH: Classification of hereditary cataracts in children by linkage analysis. Trans Am Acad Ophthalmol Otolaryngol 1979; 86:1554-1558. *
Jaafar MS, Robb RM: Congenital anterior polar cataract: a review of 63 cases. Ophthalmology 1984; 91:249-252. *
Ogata H, et al.: Phenotype i associated with congenital cataract in Japanese. Transfusion 1984; 19:166-168.
Moross T, et al.: Autosomal dominant anterior polar cataracts associated with a familial 2;14 translocation. J Med Genet 1984; 21:52-53.
Bateman JB, et al.: Genetic linkage analysis of autosomal dominant congenital cataracts. Am J Ophthalmol 1986; 101:218-225.

BA042                                    **J. Bronwyn Bateman**

**Cataract, congenital-microcornea or slight microphthalmia**
*See CATARACT, CORTICAL AND NUCLEAR*

## CATARACT, COPPOCK 3174

**Includes:**
> Cataract, discoid
> Cataract, pulverulent nuclear
> Cataract, pulverulent zonular
> Discoid cataract
> Doyne discoid cataract
> Nuclear cataract
> Pulverulent nuclear cataract
> Pulverulent zonular cataract

**Excludes:** **Cataract** (other)

**Major Diagnostic Criteria:** Congenital, bilateral, nuclear cataracts in a person derived from the original pedigree first studied by Doyne, with subsequent elaboration and publication by Nettleship & Ogilvie (1906). These cataracts are usually mild, often asymptomatic, or minimally symptomatic for glare in bright light; occasional exceptions with more opacity may occur. First described without the aid of the slit lamp as a sharply defined disc placed deep in the lens between the nucleus and the posterior pole. In a slit lamp study of one member of this pedigree by

Adams (1942), the cataract was redescribed to involve the embryonal nucleus only.

**Clinical Findings:** The cataracts are bilateral, congenital, and generally stationary. Vision is usually normal, and seldom reduced to less than 20/40. Symmetry between the eyes is the rule. The patient is usually unaware of the ocular defect at the time of diagnosis. Lenticular opacification may progress later in life, and cataract extraction may be required.

**Complications:** Unknown.

**Associated Findings:** None known.

**Etiology:** Autosomal dominant inheritance.

**Pathogenesis:** Unknown.

**MIM No.:** *11620

**Sex Ratio:** M1:F1

**Occurrence:** Undetermined but presumed rare.

**Risk of Recurrence for Patient's Sib:**
See Part I, *Mendelian Inheritance.*

**Risk of Recurrence for Patient's Child:**
See Part I, *Mendelian Inheritance.*

**Age of Detectability:** During the newborn period, but since cataract is mild, detection usually occurs much later.

**Gene Mapping and Linkage:** CAE (cataract, zonular pulverulent (FY-linked)) has been mapped to 1q21-q25.
A family with Coppock-like cataracts had linkage established to the Duffy blood group by Renwick and Lawler (1968). The Duffy blodd group has since been assigned to chromosome 1. Similar appearing cataracts in other pedigrees have not had this linkage. Another Coppock-like cataract has been linked to the gamma crystallin gene cluster on chromosome 2 by Lubsen et al (1987).

**Prevention:** None known. Genetic counseling indicated.

**Treatment:** Cataract extraction may be required if vision is severely reduced.

**Prognosis:** Good. Cataract is stationary in most cases.

**Detection of Carrier:** By slit lamp examination of relatives, and evaluation of pedigree.

**Special Considerations:** Many families have been reported with dominant congenital cataract as the only known defect. Some of these are similar in appearance to the Coppock type. These are summarized by Bateman et al (1986).

**References:**
Nettleship E, Ogilvie FM: A peculiar form of hereditary congenital cataract. Trans Ophthalmol Soc UK 1906; 26:191–207.
Adams PH: Doyne's discoid cataract (Coppock). Br J Ophthalmol 1942; 26:152–153.
Renwick JH, Lawler SD: Probable linkage between a congenital cataract locus and the Duffy blood group locus. Ann Hum Genet 1963; 27:67–84.
Bateman JB, et al: Genetic linkage analysis of autosomal dominant congenital cataracts. Am J Ophthalmol 1986; 101:218–225.
Lubsen NH, et al: A locus for a human hereditary cataract is closely linked to the gamma crystallin gene family. Proc Natl Acad Sci USA 1987; 84:489–492.

HU016
JA016

**Lee R. Hunter**
**Mohammad S. Jaafar**

**Cataract, coralliform-uncombable hair (misnomer)**
*See HAIR, UNCOMBABLE-CRYSTALLINE CATARACT*
**Cataract, cortical**
*See CATARACT, CORTICAL AND NUCLEAR*

## CATARACT, CORTICAL AND NUCLEAR     0132

**Includes:**
 CAMFAK syndrome
 Cataract, congenital-microcornea or slight microphthalmia
 Cataract, total congenital
 Cataract, total-posterior sutural opacities in heterozygotes
 Cataract, cortical
 Cataract, crystalline coralliform
 Cataract, crystalline aculeiform or frosted
 Cataract, floriform
 Cataract, lamellar
 Cataract, lenticular
 Cataract, Marner
 Cataract, membranous
 Cataract, nuclear
 Cataract, nuclear diffuse nonprogressive
 Cataract, nuclear total
 Cataract, perinuclear
 Cataract, sutural
 Cataract, total
 Cataract, zonular
 Cataract-microcephaly-failure to thrive-kyphoscoliosis
 Cataract-microphthalmia-nystagmus

**Excludes:** Cataracts (all others)

**Major Diagnostic Criteria:** Opacities in the lens may be so small that they can be detected only by slit-lamp examination with pupil dilated. Large opaque cataracts are easily seen.

**Clinical Findings:** The clinical picture varies from functionally insignificant, minute opacities to a variety of rarer and sometimes vision-affecting opacifications to the totally opacified lens. Duke-Elder divides these into cataracts affecting a particular zone, those not so limited, and those affecting most of the lens. Combinations of types occur. In a central pulverulent (fine powdery) cataract the embryonic nucleus has many small white dots. Vision is rarely disturbed and the condition is usually bilateral and nonprogressive. Total nuclear cataract accounts for about 25% of all congenital cataracts and appears as a large white opacity of the embryonic and infantile nuclei. It occurs bilaterally and affects vision, sometimes seriously. Zones of opacity between the embryonic nucleus and cortex are called lamellar cataracts. The more central the affected concentric zone, the earlier the insult in embryogenesis. The condition is usually bilateral and the visual disability is variable, depending upon the degree of opacification. This form of congenital cataract is said to account for 40% of all types. It may be slowly progressive and quite disabling. Cataracts may affect just the Y sutures. Others form discrete opacities particularly in the axial region of the lens affecting several layers. They are usually bilateral, nonprogressive and do not affect vision. Morphologic types include anterior axial embryonic cataract, floriform cataract (resemble flower petals), dilacerated cataract (mossy) or punctate or blue dot cataract (affects fetal nucleus). Crystalline forms include coralliform cataract (resemble coral) and spear-shaped cataract (resemble grains of wheat). Much or all of the lens is

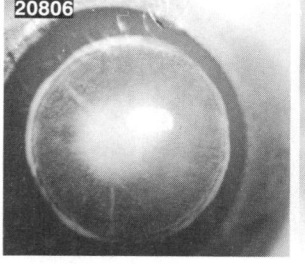
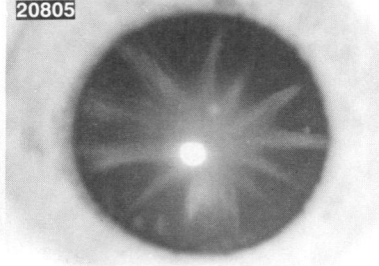

**0132-20806:** Zonular cataract. **20805:** Cortical cataract.

affected in total cataract. In disk- shaped cataract the nucleus is missing, and in membranous cataract the lens is mostly resorbed. Vision is severely impaired in these forms.

**Complications:** Nystagmus and strabismus in about 30% of cases if visual impairment is present.

**Associated Findings:** Combinations of the above occur especially with lamellar cataract. In axial fusiform cataract, opacities of the nucleus may combine with polar cataracts. In membranous cataract, other sequelae of intrauterine inflammation may be present. Almost all other ocular anomalies can be found in conjunction with congenital cataract, particularly the more severe lens afflictions. Microphthalmia is said to occur in about 25% of unilateral and 11% of bilateral cases of congenital cataract. Colobomata, aniridia, ectopia lentis, persistent hyperplastic primary vitreous and vasculosa lentis are not uncommon. Possibly one-half the cases of congenital cataract have other ocular defects. Many syndromes include congenital cataract, i.e. rubella embryopathy, galactosemia, etc. Recently, patients with **Acoustic neuromata** have been described with presenile posterior subcapsular and nuclear cataracts. In one family (Scott-Emuakpor et al, 1977) cataracts were associated with microcephaly and a variety of other malformations known as "CAMFAK".

**Etiology:** This condition includes a large and heterogeneous group of lens opacities, often indistinguishable. About 25% of cases are due to heritable traits. Most of these appear to be autosomal dominant. Recessive pedigrees are uncommon. X-linked inheritance has been suggested in some pedigrees but has been convincingly shown in very few; such as the pedigree described by Krill et al (1969). Cataracts which occur as part of a complex malformation syndrome are transmitted in the same manner as the syndrome. Well documented dominant pedigrees are noted for central pulverulent cataract, total nuclear cataract, lamellar cataract and coralliform cataract. Total cataract may be inherited in a number of ways. A few dominant pedigrees are documented for the axial type cataracts. Sporadic cases, possibly due to environmental causes, have been seen in all forms of cataract but are prevalent in total cataract, disk-shaped cataract and membranous cataract. In sporadic cases of lamellar cataract, biochemical disturbances have been implicated. Thus exogenous factors, both constitutional and local, either hereditary or not, play a role in the majority of congenital cataracts.

**Pathogenesis:** This is a heterogeneous group of disorders of which some are heritable and others environmentally induced. Little is known about the pathogenesis of congenital cataracts. Discrete opacities may consist of poorly formed lens fibers which have degenerated as in the punctate cataract. Some crystalline opacities have been found to be composed of cysteine, tyrosine, and calcium. Disk-shaped cataracts may result from interferences with development about the fifth fetal month. Total cataract could relate to persistence of the hyaloid artery, faulty lens vesicle separation or intrauterine inflammation. Genetic influences on embryogenesis may play a role. Environmental factors such as toxins and their direct effect or their effect on induction are exemplified by viral infections such as rubella. Metabolic factors include a potential defect in calcium metabolism, as suggested in lamellar cataracts where hypocalcemia and tetany are known to be deleterious, and carbohydrate metabolism such as in galactosemia and galactokinase deficiency. These have a hereditary basis. Finally local changes induced by intrauterine inflammation could produce sporadic abnormalities.

**MIM No.:** *11570, *11580, *11590, 11610, *11630, *11640, 11670, *11680, 21260, 21270, *30220, 30230

**CDC No.:** 743.326

**Sex Ratio:** M1:F1, although lamellar cataracts M>1:F1.

**Occurrence:** Dependent upon type of lens opacity. Minute opacities in the lens present in over 90% of children. Anterior axial embryonic cataract occurs in 20–30% of children as does blue-dot cataract.

**Risk of Recurrence for Patient's Sib:**
See Part I, *Mendelian Inheritance.*

**Risk of Recurrence for Patient's Child:**
See Part I, *Mendelian Inheritance.*

**Age of Detectability:** Variable, depending on cataract size; at birth by slit lamp examination.

**Gene Mapping and Linkage:** CTM (cataract, Marner) has been provisionally mapped to 16.
CCT (cataract, congenital, total) has been mapped to X.

**Prevention:** See **Galactosemia, Galactose epimerase deficiency,** and **Galactokinase deficiency** for prevention of cataract in those disorders. There is no known prevention for other types. Genetic counseling is recommended.

**Treatment:** Cataract extraction where indicated.

**Prognosis:** Normal life span; ocular prognosis is generally good unless associated defects are present or dense opacities are present at birth or infancy.

**Detection of Carrier:** By slit lamp examination.

**Support Groups:** PA; Devon; Parents of Cataract Kids (PACK)

**References:**
Francois J: Congenital cataracts. Netherlands: C.C. Thomas, 1963.
Krill AE, et al.: X-chromosomal-linked sutural cataracts. Am J Ophthal 1969; 68:867–872.
Scott-Emuakpor AB, et al.: A syndrome of microcephaly and cataracts in four siblings. Am J Dis Child 1977; 131:167–169.
Conneally PM, et al.: Confirmation of genetic heterogeneity in autosomal dominant forms of cataract from linkage studies. Cytogenet Cell Genet 1978; 22:295–297.
Francois J: Genetics of cataract. Opthalmolopia 1982; 184:61–71.
Pearson-Webb M, et al.: Eye findings in bilateral acoustic (rential) neurofibromatosis. N Eng J Med 1986; 315:1553–1554.
Reese PD, et al.: Autosomal dominant congenital cataracts associated with chromosomal translocations [t(3;4)(p26.2;p15)] Arch Ophthalmol 1987; 105:1382–1384.

CR012 **Harold E. Cross**

**Cataract, crystalline aculeiform or frosted**
*See CATARACT, CORTICAL AND NUCLEAR*
**Cataract, crystalline coralliform**
*See CATARACT, CORTICAL AND NUCLEAR*
**Cataract, crystalline-uncombable hair**
*See HAIR, UNCOMBABLE-CRYSTALLINE CATARACT*
**Cataract, discoid**
*See CATARACT, COPPOCK*
**Cataract, floriform**
*See CATARACT, CORTICAL AND NUCLEAR*

## CATARACT, HUTTERITE 3173

**Includes:** Hutterite cataract

**Excludes:**
Cataract (others)
Cataract, in other populations
Cataract, with known metabolic cause

**Major Diagnostic Criteria:** Bilateral (can occur asynchronously) anterior or posterior polar, or total cortical cataracts in the absence of other systemic disease.

**Clinical Findings:** These developmental cataracts (possibly with congenital features) are usually diagnosed between the ages of 3–6 years. Often the lens of the fellow eye will show minimal or no cataract at the time of diagnosis, but will progress to cataract formation within months. The cataract is often of a white cortical type when discovered, but anterior and posterior subcapsular opacities with less marked cortical involvement have been found; these may progress to the mature type. The distinguishing feature of this disorder is that the cataracts occur alone, separating it from recessive genetic syndromes that may present with cataracts within a constellation of other findings. No underlying metabolic abnormality has been discovered.

**Complications:** Amblyopia may occur.

**Associated Findings:** None known.

**Etiology:** Autosomal recessive inheritance.

**Pathogenesis:** Unknown.

**MIM No.:** *21250

**Sex Ratio:** M1:F1

**Occurrence:** Nine cases have been documented in four sibships of an inbred Lehrerleut Hutterite group.

**Risk of Recurrence for Patient's Sib:**
See Part I, *Mendelian Inheritance.*

**Risk of Recurrence for Patient's Child:**
See Part I, *Mendelian Inheritance.*

**Age of Detectability:** Usually ages 3–6 years, possibly during infancy in some cases.

**Gene Mapping and Linkage:** CCAT (cataract, congenital) is ULG3.

**Prevention:** None known. Genetic counseling indicated.

**Treatment:** Cataract aspiration with amblyopia therapy as required.

**Prognosis:** Good for vision following treatment.

**Detection of Carrier:** Unknown.

**References:**
Shokeir MHK, Lowry RB: Juvenile cataract in Hutterites. Am J Med Genet 1985; 22:495–500.

HU016
JA016

Lee R. Hunter
Mohammad S. Jaafar

**Cataract, lamellar**
*See CATARACT, CORTICAL AND NUCLEAR*
**Cataract, lenticular**
*See CATARACT, CORTICAL AND NUCLEAR*
**Cataract, Marner**
*See CATARACT, CORTICAL AND NUCLEAR*
**Cataract, membranous**
*See CATARACT, CORTICAL AND NUCLEAR*
**Cataract, nuclear**
*See CATARACT, CORTICAL AND NUCLEAR*
**Cataract, nuclear diffuse nonprogressive**
*See CATARACT, CORTICAL AND NUCLEAR*
**Cataract, nuclear total**
*See CATARACT, CORTICAL AND NUCLEAR*
**Cataract, perinuclear**
*See CATARACT, CORTICAL AND NUCLEAR*

## CATARACT, POLAR AND CAPSULAR 0133

**Includes:**
Capsular and polar cataracts
Capsulolenticular cataract
Cataract, anterior polar (CAP)
Cataract, posterior polar
Microphthalmia-cataract
Polar and capsular cataracts

**Excludes:**
**Cataract** (all others)
**Eye, pupillary membrane persistence** (0845)

**Major Diagnostic Criteria:** Pinpoint lens opacities detectable by slit-lamp examination.

**Clinical Findings:** Capsular cataracts, anterior and posterior, are small discrete flecks of opacity and pigmented satellite formations in the lens epithelium and capsule, usually less than 1 mm and which do not interfere with vision.

Polar cataracts involve the lens capsule, epithelium and underlying lens fibers. The anterior variety assumes a multitude of shapes and sizes (most 0.5 to 1.5 mm in size). Anterior protrusion leads to the pyramidal form. After formation, normal lens fibers may develop between the cortical and capsular opacities (reduplication). The changes are usually bilateral, stationary and functionally insignificant, but progression on to complete lens opacification may occur.

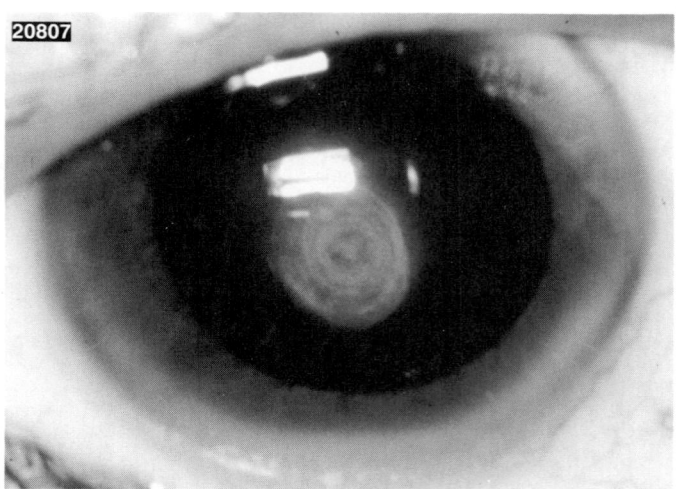

0133-20807: Cataract, polar.

Posterior polar cataracts occur as described above in a stationary form present at birth with a variety of opaque bodies in the posterior pole of the lens, and also as a progressive variety in which radiating opacities form in the posterior lens cortex resulting in progressive decrease of vision.

**Complications:** Visual impairment.

**Associated Findings:** Microphthalmia, persistence of the pupillary membrane and hyaloid vascular system, corneal opacities, anterior lenticonus, axial fusiform cataract (whereby a central nuclear cataract connects to one or both poles). Amblyopia and strabismus may occur in up to one-third of patients.

**Etiology:** In cases of polar cataracts, autosomal dominant inheritance of a defect in embryogenesis. But there is no doubt that this a heterogeneous group of disorders with various etiologies. Intrauterine inflammation is a possibility in other cases, especially those with corneal opacities.

**Pathogenesis:** Intrauterine inflammation produced by a corneal perforation or adhesion to the lens could lead to anterior polar lens changes. Adhesions of the tunica vasculosa lentis or pupillary membrane to the lens in the anterior polar cataracts, and adhesion or invasion of the posterior lens by the fetal vascular system in the posterior polar cataracts are the explanations usually given.

**MIM No.:** *11565, *11660, *15685

**CDC No.:** 743.325

**Sex Ratio:** M1:Fl

**Occurrence:** Undetermined. Pedigrees reported as early as 1909.

**Risk of Recurrence for Patient's Sib:**
See Part I, *Mendelian Inheritance.*

**Risk of Recurrence for Patient's Child:**
See Part I, *Mendelian Inheritance.*

**Age of Detectability:** At birth.

**Gene Mapping and Linkage:** Unknown.

**Prevention:** None known. Genetic counseling indicated.

**Treatment:** Cataract extraction and visual rehabilitation when indicated.

**Prognosis:** Normal life span with ocular prognosis is variable according to the degree of the defect.

**Detection of Carrier:** By split lamp examination.

**Support Groups:**  PA; Devon; Parents of Cataract Kids (PACK)

**References:**

Harman NB: Hereditary anterior polar cataract and microphthalmia. Trans Ophthalmol Soc UK 1909; 29:101–108.

Tulloh CG: Heredity of posterior polar cataract with report of a pedigree. Brit J Ophthal 1955; 39:374–379.

Capella JA: Hereditary cataract and microphthalmia. Am J Ophthal 1963; 56:454–458.

Francois J: Congenital cataracts. Netherlands: C.C. Thomas, 1963.

Jaafar MS, Robb RM: Congenital anterior polar cataract. Ophthal 1984; 91:249–254.

CR012                                                   **Harold E. Cross**

**Cataract, posterior polar**
  *See CATARACT, POLAR AND CAPSULAR*
**Cataract, pulverulent nuclear**
  *See CATARACT, COPPOCK*
**Cataract, pulverulent zonular**
  *See CATARACT, COPPOCK*
**Cataract, sutural**
  *See CATARACT, CORTICAL AND NUCLEAR*
**Cataract, total**
  *See CATARACT, CORTICAL AND NUCLEAR*
**Cataract, total congenital**
  *See CATARACT, CORTICAL AND NUCLEAR*
**Cataract, total-posterior sutural opacities in heterozygotes**
  *See CATARACT, CORTICAL AND NUCLEAR*
**Cataract, X-linked with Hutchinsonian teeth**
  *See CATARACTS-OTO-DENTAL DEFECTS*
**Cataract, zonular**
  *See CATARACT, CORTICAL AND NUCLEAR*
**Cataract-deafness-myopia-saddle nose**
  *See DEAFNESS-MYOPIA-CATARACT-SADDLE NOSE, MARSHALL TYPE*
**Cataract-dental syndrome**
  *See CATARACTS-OTO-DENTAL DEFECTS*

## CATARACT-ICHTHYOSIS                                        0131

**Includes:**  Ichthyosis-cataract

**Excludes:**
  **Chondrodysplasia punctata, X-linked dominant type** (2730)
  **Ichthyosiform hyperkeratosis, bullous congenital** (2852)
  **Ichthyosis vulgaris** (2534)
  **Ichthyosis, X-linked with steroid sulfatase deficiency** (2532)
  **Phytanic acid storage disease** (0810)
  **Sjogren-Larsson syndrome** (2030)
  **Trichothiodystrophy** (2559)

**Major Diagnostic Criteria:**  The clinical picture is characterized by congenital ichthyosis and lens opacities. A dermal biopsy confirms the diagnosis of ichthyosis.

**Clinical Findings:**  Congenital ichthyosis associated with cortical opacities of the lens, which were identified by age 5 years in the male sibs reported by Pinkerton (1958). Although ectropion of the lids, conjunctivitis, and deep stromal corneal opacities may be seen in some forms of ichthyoses, these brothers were not so affected. Jancke (1950) reported three affected sisters.

**Complications:**  Unknown.

**Associated Findings:**  None known.

**Etiology:**  Autosomal recessive inheritance.

**Pathogenesis:**  Unknown.

**MIM No.:**  *21240

**POS No.:**  4061

**Sex Ratio:**  Presumably M1:F1

**Occurrence:**  Documented in two families; one Japanese.

**Risk of Recurrence for Patient's Sib:**
  See Part I, *Mendelian Inheritance.*

**Risk of Recurrence for Patient's Child:**
  See Part I, *Mendelian Inheritance.*

**Age of Detectability:**  In the neonate.

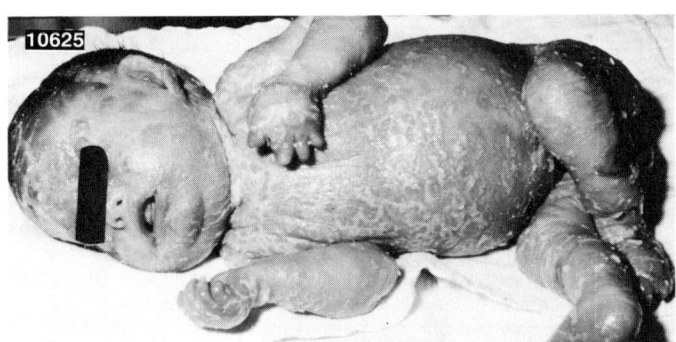

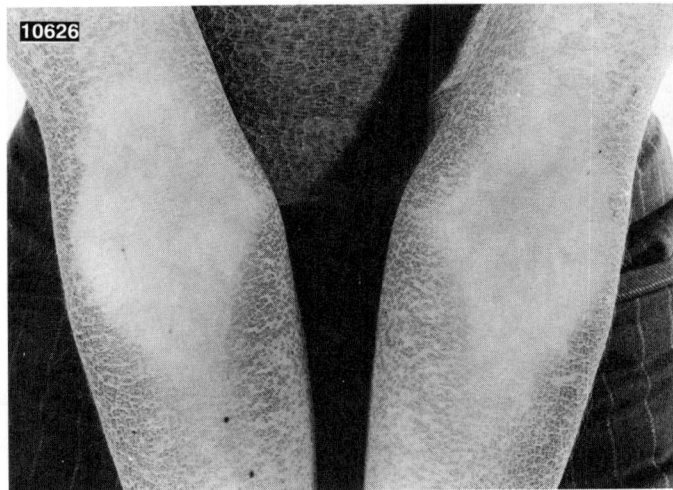

0131-10625:  Congenital ichthyosis.  10626:  Skin changes of ichthyosis in the antecubital fossa.

**Gene Mapping and Linkage:**  Unknown.

**Prevention:**  None known. Genetic counseling indicated.

**Treatment:**  Local amelioration of ichthyosis and surgery for cataract if vision is impaired.

**Prognosis:**  Unknown.

**Detection of Carrier:**  Unknown.

**Support Groups:**  PA; Devon; Parents of Cataract Kids (PACK)

**References:**

Jancke G: Cataracta syndermatotica und ichthyosis congenita. Klin Mbl Augenheilk 1950; 117:286–290.

Pinkerton OD: Cataract associated with congenital ichthyosis. Arch Ophthalmol 1958; 60:393–396.

Jay B, et al.: Ocular manifestations of ichthyosis. Br J Ophthalmol 1968; 52:217–226.

BA042                                               **J. Bronwyn Bateman**

**Cataract-mental retardation-hypogonadism-microcephaly**
  *See MARTSOLF SYNDROME*
**Cataract-microcephaly-failure to thrive-kyphoscoliosis**
  *See CATARACT, CORTICAL AND NUCLEAR*

## CATARACT-MICROCORNEA SYNDROME 2758

**Includes:**
Cataract-myopia
Microcornea-cataract

**Excludes:**
**Cataract** (other)
**Eye, anterior segment dysgenesis** (0439)
Microcornea, isolated

**Major Diagnostic Criteria:** Cataracts and microcornea with or without myopia occurring in an autosomal dominant pattern. In some individuals the gene expression may take the form of Peter anomaly (see **Eye, anterior segment dysgenesis**).

**Clinical Findings:** Microcornea occurred in all examined individuals, with cataracts present in the majority. Myopia was also noted in several cases. Two individuals had iridal colobomas and several had Peter anomaly. Axial length and globe size are normal, although cornea, in addition to being small, had steeper curvatures than normal.

**Complications:** Retinal detachment and glaucoma may be rare complications. Amblyopia is uncommon.

**Associated Findings:** None known.

**Etiology:** Autosomal dominant inheritance.

**Pathogenesis:** An abnormality of growth of optic cup ectoderm occurring around the fifth month of gestation had been postulated, although more recent work suggests that a defect in neural crest cell migration occurring around the eighth week may be responsible for the ocular anomalies.

**MIM No.:** *11615

**POS No.:** 3723

**Sex Ratio:** M1:F1

**Occurrence:** Over 100 affected individuals from five families from different parts of the world have been documented.

**Risk of Recurrence for Patient's Sib:**
See Part I, *Mendelian Inheritance.*

**Risk of Recurrence for Patient's Child:**
See Part I, *Mendelian Inheritance.*

**Age of Detectability:** The microcorneae are congenital, although lens opacities may not occur until later. The rarity of ambylopia suggests that significant cataracts are not usually congenital, but that they do appear before the third decade of life.

**Gene Mapping and Linkage:** Unknown.

**Prevention:** None known. Genetic counseling indicated.

**Treatment:** Surgical removal of cataracts is indicated; eyeglasses for myopia. All offspring of affected parents should be examined for cataracts at birth and annually thereafter until adulthood.

**Prognosis:** Intellectual development and life span are normal. With early surgery and visual rehabilitation, blindness should not occur.

**Detection of Carrier:** By slit lamp examination.

**Support Groups:** PA; Devon; Parents of Cataract Kids (PACK)

**References:**
Friedmann MW, Wright ES: Hereditary microcornea and cataract in 5 generations. Am J Ophthalmol 1952; 35:1017–1021.
Polomeno RC, Cummings C: Autosomal dominant cataracts and microcornea. Can J Ophthalmol 1979; 14:227–229.
Mollica F, et al.: Autosomal dominant cataract and microcornea associated with myopia in a Sicilian family. Clin Genet 1985; 28:42–46.
Green JS, Johnson GJ: Congenital cataract with microcornea and Peters anomaly as expression of one autosomal dominant gene. Ophthalm Paediatr Genet 1986; 7:187–194.
Salmon JF, et al.: Variable expressivity of autosomal dominant microcornea with cataract. Arch Ophthalmol 1988; 106:505–510.

T0007
CR012

**Helga V. Toriello**
**Harold E. Cross**

---

**Cataract-microphthalmia-nystagmus**
*See CATARACT, CORTICAL AND NUCLEAR*
**Cataract-myopia**
*See CATARACT-MICROCORNEA SYNDROME*
**Cataract-poikiloderma atrophicans**
*See ROTHMUND-THOMSON SYNDROME*
**Cataract-polycystic kidney disease-blindness**
*See KIDNEY, POLYCYSTIC DISEASE-CATARACT-BLINDNESS*

---

## CATARACT-RENAL TUBULAR NECROSIS-ENCEPHALOPATHY, CROME TYPE 2162

**Includes:**
Crome syndrome
Encephalopathy-cataract-renal tubular necrosis
Renal tubular necrosis-cataract-encephalopathy

**Excludes:**
**Brain, spongy degeneration** (0115)
**Galactosemia** (0403)
**Kidney, polycystic disease-cataract-blindness** (3288)
**Marinesco-Sjogren syndrome** (2031)
**Oculo-cerebro-renal syndrome** (0736)
**Phytanic acid oxidase deficiency, infantile type** (2278)

**Major Diagnostic Criteria:** 1) Cataracts in the newborn; 2) infantile seizures, with developmental delay; 3) spongy degeneration of the gray and white matter, uneven neuronal degeneration and cerebellar dysplasia; and 4) renal tubular necrosis.

**Clinical Findings:** Crome (1963) first described two female siblings who had cataracts and nystagmus, a generalized seizure disorder beginning in the second month, which responded poorly to medication, and developmental delay. The first child had trace albumin with a few red blood cells, some white cells and casts in her urine at eight months of age, three days before her death. Urinalysis and urinary amino acid studies on the second child were normal with no galactose being found. The second child died of pneumonia at 4 months of age.

Laboratory studies included: CSF protein was 120 - 70 mg/100 ml CSF glucose was 85 mg/100 ml; Wasserman was negative; blood sugar was 116 mg/199 ml; BUN 68 mg/100 ml; serum calcium 11.4 mg/100 ml; serum potassium 6 mg/100 ml; EEG showed abnormally slow record with random bilateral epileptic discharges; skull X-rays were normal.

Post mortem studies in both sisters were similar: the eyes had irregular nucleus/cortex lenticular opacities and gliosis of the optic nerve. The liver had fatty changes; cellular vacuolation. The brain showed generalized decreased myelinization with spongy degeneration of gray and white matter. The brain stem had decreased myelinization of the corticopontine and corticospinal tracts. The cerebellum had total loss of Purkinje cells; proliferation of Bergmann glia; and spongy degeneration of the white matter. The basal ganglia and inferior olive were normal. The spinal cord had decreased myelinization of lateral and anterior columns. The kidney had necrotic foci in the boundary zone of the medulla. The central parts of the lesions showed coagulative necrosis, which when cut tangentially, displayed densely arranged lymphocytes and histiocytes. Arteries were often surrounded by a sleeve or lymphocytes with some showing thickening of their adventitia and intima.

**Complications:** Unknown.

**Associated Findings:** None known.

**Etiology:** Possibly autosomal recessive inheritance.

**Pathogenesis:** Unknown.

**MIM No.:** *21890

**POS No.:** 3956

**Sex Ratio:** M0:F2 (observed)

**Occurrence:** Two affected sisters have been documented.

**Risk of Recurrence for Patient's Sib:**
See Part I, *Mendelian Inheritance.*

**Risk of Recurrence for Patient's Child:**
See Part I, *Mendelian Inheritance.*

**Age of Detectability:** At birth.

**Gene Mapping and Linkage:** Unknown.

**Prevention:** None known. Genetic counseling indicated.

**Treatment:** Treatment of the seizures appeared ineffective, but newer therapies are now available.

**Prognosis:** Poor. Death occurred at ages four and eight months.

**Detection of Carrier:** Unknown.

**Support Groups:** PA; Devon; Parents of Cataract Kids (PACK)

**References:**
Crome L, et al.: Congenital cataracts, renal tubular necrosis and encephalopathy in two sisters. Arch Dis Child 1963; 38:505–515.
Richards W, et al.: The oculo-cerebro-renal syndrome of Lowe. Am J Dis Child 1965; 109:2–20.

GR021                                            **Arthur W. Grix**

---

## CATARACTS                                    1514

**Includes:**

Eye, cataracts
Lens opacities

**Major Diagnostic Criteria:** A cataract results from any alteration, focal or general, in the transparency of the crystalline lens, although some investigators suggest that only clinically significant opacification should be so designated. Nonprogressive and isolated micro-opacities with no effect on vision are so common that they should probably not be called cataracts, except those of known association with various metabolic (systemic) or genetic disorders.

**Clinical Findings:** The human crystalline lens is a transparent structure that contributes approximately 30% of the dioptic power of the eye. It is located between the anterior hyaloid face of the vitreous and the posterior surface of the iris, thus anatomically dividing the eye into anterior and posterior chambers. The lens is suspended in place by zonules or capsular ligaments that stretch between the ciliary processes and the lens capsule near its equator.

The lens is derived from surface ectoderm beginning at about the 4.5-mm stage of embryogenesis and continues to develop through the eighth month of gestation. In fact, new cortical fibers are added throughout adulthood, making the lens the only human tissue that continuously enlarges throughout life. The original ectodermal cells that form the lens plate (placode) subsequently obliterate the lens vesicle with primitive lens epithelial "fibers" to form the embryonic nucleus (by 3 months of gestation); then new layers are added to form the fetal nucleus (third to eighth months), and finally the infantile nucleus that develops from late fetal life through puberty. The adult nucleus develops during early adult life and is continuously covered by the layers of cortical fibers to produce the lens cortex. Addition of more lens fibers increases the mass of the neonatal lens by a factor of two at puberty and triples it by the 70th year.

Optical transparency results from both composition and organization of lens fibers, and any metabolic and morphologic changes can result in some opacification. The pattern of continuous development and the ability to visualize directly the entire lens sometimes allow one to identify the stage of developmental insults. Opacifications of the embryonic nucleus are seldom purely metabolic in origin and suggest a maternal infection instead as the nucleus develops during the first three months of gestation.

Zonular cataracts involving the fetal nucleus, on the other hand, are usually hereditary and appear to involve almost the entire lens at birth, although postnatal cortical fibers may be clear. Opacification of the infantile nucleus and cortex occuring postnatally suggests an exogenous or metabolic cause with frequent progression throughout the first two decades of life.

The developing embryonic lens is surrounded and nourished by a capillary network known as the *tunica vasculosa lentis,* which usually disappears by 8.5 months gestation. Failure of complete regression can result in axial opacities at the anterior and posterior poles. These are apparent at birth, are usually unilateral, rarely progress, and usually do not interfere with vision. Anterior polar cataracts seldom meet a critical 3-mm size to interfere with fixation (due to visual loss) but need to be watched as their size may increase postnatally. Posterior polar opacities, particularly of the type known as *posterior lenticonus,* are often associated with some persistence of the embryonic hyaloid vascular system and are more likely to progress to visual significance than are anterior opacities.

While any degree or type of opacification can be called a cataract, the nomenclature can be confusing since cataracts can be classified according to presumed etiology (traumatic, metabolic, genetic or inflammatory), time of onset (congenital or senile), location (nuclear, cortical, or subcapsular), morphology (crystalline, shield, or coralliform), or degree (incipient, immature, or morgagmian).

New opacities may be reversible, as exemplified by the transient lens vacuoles sometimes seen in the first week of life or by the early galactosemic cataracts prior to therapy. Cataracts can, of course, occur as isolated abnormalities or in association with other malformations as part of a syndrome. Recognition and classification often require examination of other relatives.

**Complications:** Isolated, small lens opacities create no symptoms and are usually of no clinical significance in adolescents or adults. In children, they should be periodically evaluated to ensure they are not progressive.

In infants and children, deprivation amblyopia is by far the most frequent and significant complication of cataracts. The ocular media must be sufficiently clear during the first 10–12 weeks of life to stimulate the development of the visual pathways and acquire the fixation reflex. The onset and degree of amblyopia is influenced by the location, size, and density of the lens opacity, although fixation can be blocked by central opacification of 3 mm or more (as the image pathway through the normal pupil is blocked). Cataracts need not be congenital to cause amblyopia, since interruption of fixation for as little as a 1-month duration during the first 7–8 years of life can result in a "lazy eye."

After the first decade of life, the major complication is loss of vision proportionate to the density of the opacification in the visual axis. Rarely, cataracts may progress to maturity and intumescence producing intraocular inflammation and secondary glaucoma, which require immediate surgical attention.

Complications of cataract surgery such as glaucoma, retinal detachments, and corneal decompensation as well as inadequate visual rehabilitation may also result in permanent visual impairment.

**Associated Findings:** The majority of congenital cataracts are associated with systemic and other ocular abnormalities. Glaucoma and retinal detachments are among the more serious, but malformations of the globes, uveal colobomas, corneal opacities, ametropia, strabismus, and nystagmus (suggesting severe visual deprivation) are also frequently found.

Cataracts are also found in numerous metabolic disorders, including **Diabetes mellitus**, **Hepatolenticular degeneration**, **Oculo-cerebro-renal syndrome**, **Fabry disease**, **Nephritis-deafness (sensorineural), hereditary type**, and **Galactosemia**. Lens opacification occurs frequently in patients with chromosomal disorders, including **Chromosome 21, trisomy 21; Chromosome 13, trisomy 13**; and **Chromosome 18, trisomy 18**. Dermatologic disorders such as **Ichthyoses**, atopic dermatitis (see **Skin, atopy, familial**), **Poikiloderma** and **Ectodermal dysplasias** may also be associated with cataracts.

**Occurrence:** Minor sutural and discrete dot opacities are found in over 50% of the population. Clinically significant opacities are seen in about 1:250 live births, and a genetic etiology can be found in up to 25% of these cases. Surveys of children at schools for the visually impaired reveal that 18–25% have or have had cataracts.

**Prevention:** Identification of specific genetic or familial features. Genetic counseling is indicated.

**Treatment:** Surgical removal is the only known effective treatment for visually significant cataracts. Among children under age eight years of age, early intervention and visual rehabilitation are absolutely essential to treat or to prevent amblyopia, including correction of the aphakic refractive error with glasses or contact lenses, followed by patching and other orthoptic therapy throughout the first decade. In adults, replacement of the crystalline lens with a plastic implant has been one of the most beneficial of recent technical advances in visual restoration.

**Prognosis:** Excellent after surgery.

**Detection of Carrier:** Slit-lamp examination.

**Support Groups:** PA; Devon; Parents of Cataract Kids (PACK)

CR012                                                    **Harold E. Cross**

**Cataracts, due to galactokinase deficiency**
   *See GALACTOKINASE DEFICIENCY*
**Cataracts-gonadal dysgenesis-myopathy, family congenital type**
   *See MYOPATHY-CATARACT-GONADAL DYSGENESIS*
**Cataracts-microcephaly-kyphosis-limited joint movement (Lowry)**
   *See CEREBRO-OCULO-FACIO-SKELETAL SYNDROME*

---

## CATARACTS-OTO-DENTAL DEFECTS                          2119

**Includes:**
   Brachydactyly-oto-dental-cataract defects
   Cataract-dental syndrome
   Cataract, X-linked with Hutchinsonian teeth
   Dental-cataract-oto-brachydactyly defects
   Mesiodens-cataract syndrome
   Nance-Horan syndrome

**Excludes:**
   **Cataracts**
   **Lenz microphthalmia syndrome** (3171)
   **Oculo-cerebro-renal syndrome** (0736)
   **Parathyroid hormone resistance** (0830)

**Major Diagnostic Criteria:** The association of congenital cataracts, microcornea, and aural and dental anomalies in affected males with an X-linked pattern of inheritance is diagnostic, although there may be various combinations of symptoms with differing intra- and inter-familial expression.

**Clinical Findings:** The main components of this syndrome include X-linked congenital cataract, microcornea, aural and dental anomalies, and shortened fourth metacarpals. Affected males frequently undergo cataract surgery in infancy but usually show minimal improvement in vision. They have a pendular nystagmus and corneal diameters ranging between 8 and 10 mm. The ears are anteverted. The teeth are widely spaced and supernumerary cone-shaped incisors with short roots may be present. Typically, the cervical width of the teeth is larger than the incisal width.

**Complications:** Decreased visual acuity, nystagmus, and possibility of total cataracts in carrier females of advanced age. Supernumerary incisors may disrupt the eruption of permanent incisors.

**Associated Findings:** Microphthalmia, ptosis, and mental retardation in at least two individuals.

**Etiology:** X-linked recessive inheritance.

**Pathogenesis:** The disease state is presumably caused by a mutation on the X-chromosome which affects multiple systems. A single basic defect which will explain all the features of the syndrome is unknown.

**MIM No.:** *30235

**POS No.:** 3464

**Sex Ratio:** M1:F0

**Occurrence:** About one-half dozen kindreds have been documented.

**Risk of Recurrence for Patient's Sib:**
   See Part I, *Mendelian Inheritance.*

**Risk of Recurrence for Patient's Child:**
   See Part I, *Mendelian Inheritance.*

**Age of Detectability:** At birth.

**Gene Mapping and Linkage:** NHS (Nance-Horan syndrome (congenital cataracts and dental anomalies)) has been provisionally mapped to Xp22.3-p21.1.

**Prevention:** None known. Genetic counseling indicated.

**Treatment:** Cataract extraction and vision correction as indicated. Removal of supernumerary teeth.

**Prognosis:** Normal life span, but poor visual prognosis.

**Detection of Carrier:** Carrier females show posterior Y-sutural opacification of the lens which may develop into total cataracts, slightly smaller corneal diameters, aural anomalies, and widely spaced teeth. Intra- and inter-familiar variation in expression of the signs may exist between the carrier females due to random inactivation of the X-chromosomes early in embryogenesis.

**Special Considerations:** It has been suggested that the various disease states involving X-linked cataracts may represent allelic or pseudoallelic mutations on the X-chromosome. The alternative hypothesis is that the several clinical syndromes may be determined by separate loci on the X-chromosome. Additional linkage studies or precise localization of the genes, using recombinant DNA techniques, might serve to discriminate these two possibilities. The family reported by Walsh and Wegman (1937) may represent an instance in which the ocular anomalies have occurred without the systemic abnormalities.

Considering the phenotypic heterogeneity within this group of clinical syndromes, it has further been suggested that families with X-linked cataract and X-linked microphthalmia, be examined more closely for anomalies of the ears and teeth.

**Support Groups:** PA; Devon; Parents of Cataract Kids (PACK)

**References:**
Walsh FB, Wegman ME: A pedigree of hereditary cataract, illustrating sex- limited type. Bull Johns Hopkins Hosp 1937; 61:125.
Horan MB, Billson FA: X-linked cataract and Hutchinsonian teeth. Aust Paediat J. 1974; 10:98–102.
Nance WE, et al.: Congenital X-linked cataract, dental anomalies and brachymetacarpalia. BD:OAS X(4). New York: March of Dimes Birth Defects Foundation, 1974:285–291.
van Dorp DB, Delleman JW: A family with X-chromosomal recessive congenital cataract, microphthalmia, a peculiar form of the ear and dental anomalies. J Ped Ophthal Strab 1979; 16:166–171.
Bixler D, et al.: The Nance-Horan syndrome. Clin Genet 1984; 26:30–35. *

AW000                                                  **Paula D. Awrich**
NA007                                                   **Walter E. Nance**

**Catel-Hempel dysostosis enchondralis metaepiphysaria**
   *See CHONDRODYSTROPHIC MYOTONIA, SCHWARTZ-JAMPEL TYPE*
**Catel-Manzke syndrome**
   *See DIGITO-PALATAL SYNDROME, STEVENSON TYPE*
**Cauda equina lipoma**
   *See LIPOMENINGOCELE*
**Caudal dysplasia**
   *See CAUDAL REGRESSION SYNDROME*

---

## CAUDAL REGRESSION SYNDROME                           3211

**Includes:**
   Caudal dysplasia
   Sacral agenesis, congenital
   Sacral regression

**Excludes:**
   Cloacal dysgenesis
   Hemisacral dysplasia, types I and II
   **Mullerian aplasia** (0682)
   **Sirenomelia sequence** (3191)
   **Urorectal septum malformation sequence** (3161)
   **Vater association** (0987)

**Major Diagnostic Criteria:** The caudal regression syndrome (CRS) originally consisted of anomalies of the lower areas of the neural tube, primarily represented by sacral agenesis and anomalies of all or several lumbar vertebrae. Subsequently, anomalies of the lower extremities, gastrointestinal and genitourinary tracts also have been included in this condition.

**Clinical Findings:** The CRS differs from other caudal developmental defects by agenesis or hypoplasia of caudal structures particularly, those of the lower spine. The spectrum of the disorder extends from agenesis of the coccyx with few or no symptoms to extensive deletion of the lumbosacral spine with severe physical dysfunction and shortened survival. The clinical findings can be divided according to: 1) vertebral defects; absent or malformed lumbar vertebrae, sacrum and coccyx, and spina bifida cystica or spina bifida occulta; 2) neurological defects; paralysis, paresthesias and weakness of the legs, neurogenic bladder, and loss of control of the anal sphincter with urinary and fecal incontinence and anesthesia of the sacral region; 3) pelvic defects; fusion or hypoplasia of the pelvis, and hip dislocation, 4) lower extremity defects; **Arthrogryposes**, muscle hypoplasia, femoral aplasia, and clubfoot deformities; 5) gastrointestinal defects; imperforate anus, and gut malrotation; 6) genitourinary defects; **Kidney, horseshoe**, renal adysplasia, **Kidney, polycystic**, hydronephrosis, partial uteropelvic junction obstruction and urachal remnant, and 7) genital defects; hypospadias and displacement of the external genitalia.

**Complications:** Unknown.

**Associated Findings:** Marked growth retardation, agenesis of the pituitary gland, **Hydrocephaly**, Robin sequence, **Cleft lip**, **Cleft palate**, micrognathia, congenital heart defects, radial clubhand deformity, **Polydactyly**, radial aplasia, **Meningomyelocele**, **Bladder exstrophy**, and rectovaginal fistula.

**Etiology:** The majority of the cases are sporadic and of unknown etiology. Approximately 16% of affected individuals are born to latent, pre- or diabetic mothers. Autosomal and X-linked dominant inheritance have been suggested, in some families.

**Pathogenesis:** It has been suggested that failure of the inductive tissue-tissue mechanism can lead to such type of abnormalities. Vascular abberations also have been suggested. Chick embryos injected with insulin during the first two days of incubation result in caudal neural tube defects similar to those seen in CRS. How insulin affects these embryos is still unknown.

**MIM No.:** 18294

**POS No.:** 3399

**Sex Ratio:** Presumably M1:F1.

**Occurrence:** From 1–5:100,000 live births.

**Risk of Recurrence for Patient's Sib:** Unknown.

**Risk of Recurrence for Patient's Child:** Usually less than one percent in sporadic case.

**Age of Detectability:** Prenatal diagnosis by ultrasound has been accomplished during the second trimester by detecting sacral agenesis and absence of multiple lumbar vertebrae.

**Gene Mapping and Linkage:** Unknown.

**Prevention:** Genetic counseling in the familial cases and adequate early control of maternal diabetes.

**Treatment:** Appropriate colonic diversion and/or correction should be done if imperforate anus is present. Orthopedic management should be undertaken for any problems of the back hips and lower extremities.

**Prognosis:** Mild cases may be asymptomatic and can go undetected throughout life. On the other hand there may be significant neurologic deficiency leading to neurogenic bladder, paralysis of the lower extremities, and associated orthopedic problems. Parents of affected children should have X-ray evaluation of the pelvis in order to rule out familial occurrence.

**Detection of Carrier:** Unknown.

**Special Considerations:** The caudal regression syndrome is probably a part of a spectrum of anomalies belonging to the caudal developmental field.

**References:**
Stewart JM, Stoll S: Familial caudal regression anomalad and maternal diabetes. J Med Genet 1979; 16:17–20.
Welch JP, Aterman K: The syndrome of caudal dysplasia: a review, including considerations and evidence of heterogeneity. Ped Path 1984; 2:313–327. *

ES004      **Luis F. Escobar**
WE005      **David D. Weaver**

**Cavernoma multiplex**
See RETINA, CAVERNOUS HEMANGIOMA
**Cavernous hemangioma**
See HEMANGIOMAS OF THE HEAD AND NECK
**Cavernous lymphangiomas of orbit**
See ORBITAL AND PERIORBITAL LYMPHANGIOMA
**Cavernous transformation of portal vein**
See LIVER, VENOUS ANOMALIES
**Cavum septi pellucidi**
See BRAIN, MIDLINE CAVES
**Cavum velli interpositi**
See BRAIN, MIDLINE CAVES
**Cavum vergae**
See BRAIN, MIDLINE CAVES
**Cayler syndrome**
See CARDIOFACIAL SYNDROME-ASSYMETRIC FACIES
**CBG-transcortin abnormalities**
See STEROID, BINDING GLOBULIN ABNORMALITIES
**CD11/CD18 leukocyte glycoprotein deficiency syndrome**
See GRANULOCYTE GLYCOPROTEIN CD11/CD18 DEFICIENCY
**CDA (congenital dyserythropoietic anemia) I**
See ANEMIA, DYSERYTHROPOIETIC, TYPE I
**CDA (congenital dyserythropoietic anemia) II**
See ANEMIA, DYSERYTHROPOIETIC, TYPE II
**CDA (congenital dyserythropoietic anemia) III**
See ANEMIA, DYSERYTHROPOIETIC, TYPE III
**Cebocephaly**
See HOLOPROSENCEPHALY
also CYCLOPIA
**Celiac disease**
See GLUTEN-SENSITIVE ENTEROPATHY
**Celiac sprue**
See GLUTEN-SENSITIVE ENTEROPATHY
**Cellular hemangioma of infancy**
See ORBITAL HEMANGIOMA
**Celosomia**
See OMPHALOCELE
**Cementopathia, deep**
See TEETH, PERIODONTITIS, JUVENILE
**Cementum, environmental defects in**
See TEETH, ROOT CONCRESCENCE
**Cenani syndactylism**
See SYNDACTYLY, CENANI TYPE
**Cenani-Lenz syndactyly**
See SYNDACTYLY, CENANI TYPE
**Central bronchomalacia**
See BRONCHOMALACIA
**Central cloudy corneal dystrophy of Francois**
See CORNEA, CENTRAL CLOUDY DYSTROPHY OF FRANCOIS
**Central core disease of muscle (CCD)**
See MYOPATHY, CENTRAL CORE DISEASE TYPE
**Central crystalline corneal dystrophy**
See CORNEAL DYSTROPHY, SCHNYDER CRYSTALLINE
**Central cystoid dystrophy**
See RETINA, MACULAR DEGENERATION, VITELLIRUPTIVE
**Central nervous system arteriovenous malformation**
See CNS ARTERIOVENOUS MALFORMATION
**Central nervous system neoplasms**
See CNS NEOPLASMS
**Central nervous system tumors**
See CANCER, NEUROEPITHELIAL AND MENINGEAL
**Central nervous system tumors-polyposis of colon**
See TURCOT SYNDROME
**Central neurofibromatosis**
See ACOUSTIC NEUROMATA
**Central ray defects**
See LIMB REDUCTION DEFECTS

**Centralopathic epilepsy**
*See SEIZURES, CENTRALOPATHIC*
**Centromere abnormalities-chromatid apposition-Roberts spectrum**
*See ROBERTS SYNDROME*
**Centromere separation, premature**
*See ROBERTS SYNDROME*
**Centromere spreading**
*See ROBERTS SYNDROME*
**Centromeric instability-immunodeficiency**
*See IMMUNODEFICIENCY WITH CENTROMERIC INSTABILITY*
**Centronuclear myopathy**
*See MYOPATHY, MYOTUBULAR*
**Cephalopolysyndactyly syndrome, Greig type**
*See POLYSYNDACTYLY-DYSMORPHIC CRANIOFACIES, GREIG TYPE*
**Ceramidase deficiency**
*See LIPOGRANULOMATOSIS*
**Ceramide deficiency**
*See LIPOGRANULOMATOSIS*
**Ceramide trihexosidase deficiency**
*See FABRY DISEASE*

---

## CEREBELLAR AGENESIS                                   2011

**Includes:**
> Cerebellar aplasia
> Cerebellar hemiagenesis
> Cerebellar hypoplasia

**Excludes:**
> **Brain, Arnold-Chiari malformation** (2944)
> **Hydrocephaly** (0481)
> **Vermis agenesis** (2106)

**Major Diagnostic Criteria:** The presence of cerebellar signs suggests the diagnosis. Pneumoencephalographic and CT findings show an enlarged fourth ventricle and large cisterna magna.

**Clinical Findings:** Partial or incomplete agenesis of the cerebellum may be asymptomatic. Complete agenesis is more likely to show signs of cerebellar deficiency like hypotonia, ataxia, tremor and nystagmus.

**Complications:** Muscle stretch reflexes may be normal or depressed. Mental deficiency as a result of concomitant cerebral malformations may be present but is not necessary.

**Associated Findings:** Atrophy or maldevelopment of the inferior olivary nucleus, the nuclei of the pontine basis and the red nucleus is frequently present. Other anomalies of the brain may be present and responsible for mental retardation.

**Etiology:** Possibly autosomal recessive inheritance.

**Pathogenesis:** Agenesis of the cerebellum is generally considered to be due to defective neuronal proliferation or migration during the development of the rhombic lips. Cerebellar atrophy occurs following destruction of the contralateral cerebral hemisphere and is often difficult to distinguish from primary cerebellar hemihypoplasia.

**MIM No.:** *21300

**Sex Ratio:** Presumably M1:F1.

**Occurrence:** About seven families have been documented.

**Risk of Recurrence for Patient's Sib:**
See Part I, *Mendelian Inheritance.*

**Risk of Recurrence for Patient's Child:**
See Part I, *Mendelian Inheritance.*

**Age of Detectability:** Variable.

**Gene Mapping and Linkage:** Unknown.

**Prevention:** None known. Genetic counseling indicated.

**Treatment:** Unknown.

**Prognosis:** Varies from poor to excellent.

**Detection of Carrier:** Unknown.

**Special Considerations:** Complete absence of the cerebellum is rare. Hypoplasia or agenesis of one cerebellar hemisphere is more common. Agenesis almost always results in clinical dysfunction; partial aplasia may be asymptomatic.

**References:**
Rubinstein HS, Freeman W: Cerebellar agenesis. J Nerv Ment Dis 1940; 92:489–502. *
Dow R, Moruzzi G: The physiology and pathology of the cerebellum. Minneapolis: Minneapolis: University of Minnesota Press, 1958:424–441.
Urich H: Malformations of the nervous system. In: Blackwood W, Corsellis J, eds: Greenfield's neuropathology. London: Edward Arnold, 1976:401–409.
Macchi G, Bentivoglio M: Agenesis or hypoplasia of cerebellar structures. In: Vinken PJ, Bruyn GW, eds: Congenital malformations of the brain and skull, part 1, Handbook of clinical neurology. Amsterdam: North Holland Publishing, 1977:367–393.

GA018                                                **Bhuwan P. Garg**

**Cerebellar aplasia**
*See CEREBELLAR AGENESIS*
**Cerebellar ataxia-brachydactyly-nystagmus syndrome**
*See BIEMOND I SYNDROME*
**Cerebellar ataxia-hypogonadotropic hypogonadism**
*See ATAXIA-HYPOGONADISM SYNDROME*
**Cerebellar ataxia-progressive dementia-amyloid deposits in CNS**
*See GERSTMANN-STRAUSSLER SYNDROME*
**Cerebellar atrophy**
*See DYSEQUILIBRIUM SYNDROME*
**Cerebellar disorder (nonprogressive)-mental retardation**
*See DYSEQUILIBRIUM SYNDROME*
**Cerebellar hemiagenesis**
*See CEREBELLAR AGENESIS*
**Cerebellar hypoplasia**
*See CEREBELLAR AGENESIS*
*also DYSEQUILIBRIUM SYNDROME*
**Cerebellar parenchymal disorder, type IV**
*See JOUBERT SYNDROME*
**Cerebellar vermis agenesis**
*See VERMIS AGENESIS*
**Cerebellar vermis agenesis, familial**
*See JOUBERT SYNDROME*
**Cerebellar vermis agenesis-neurologic abnormalities**
*See JOUBERT SYNDROME*
**Cerebellar-macular abiotrophy**
*See OLIVOPONTOCEREBELLAR ATROPHY, DOMINANT WITH RETINAL DEGENERATION*
**Cerebellar-oculo-renal syndrome**
*See OCULO-RENO-CEREBELLAR SYNDROME*
**Cerebello-lental degeneration with mental retardation**
*See MARINESCO-SJOGREN SYNDROME*
**Cerebello-parenchymal disorder IV**
*See VERMIS AGENESIS*

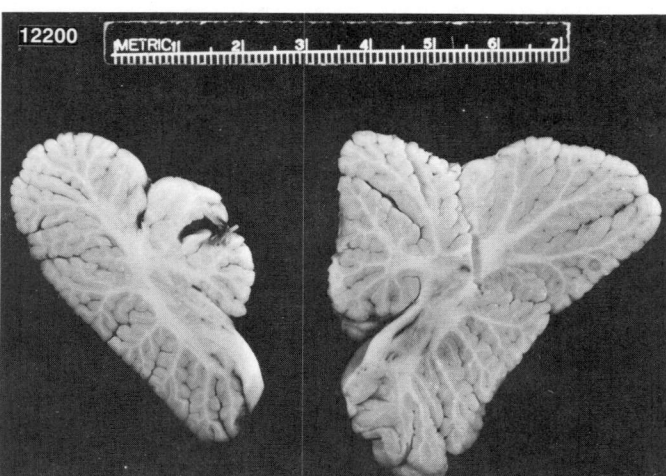

**2011-12200:** Cerebellar agenesis.

Cerebelloolivary degeneration-rigidity and dementia
  See OLIVOPONTOCEREBELLAR ATROPHY, DOMINANT WITH
    OPHTHALMOPLEGIA
Cerebelloparenchymal disorder IV
  See JOUBERT SYNDROME
Cerebral amyloid angiopathy, familial
  See AMYLOIDOSIS, ICELANDIC TYPE
Cerebral arterial amyloidosis
  See AMYLOIDOSIS, ICELANDIC TYPE
Cerebral atrophy-keratosis follicularis-short stature, X-linked
  See SHORT STATURE-CEREBRAL ATROPHY-KERATOSIS
    FOLLICULARIS, X-LINKED
Cerebral cholesterinosis
  See XANTHOMATOSIS, CEREBROTENDINOUS
Cerebral clefts symmetrical
  See BRAIN, SCHIZENCEPHALY

## CEREBRAL GIGANTISM 0137

Includes:
  Gigantism, cerebral
  Sotos syndrome
Excludes:
  Beckwith-Wiedemann syndrome (0104)
  Chromosome XYY (2552)
  Constitutional tall stature
  Excessive growth hormone secretion (pituitary gigantism)
  Fibrous dysplasia, polyostotic (0391)
  Gigantism secondary to a pinealoma or teratoma

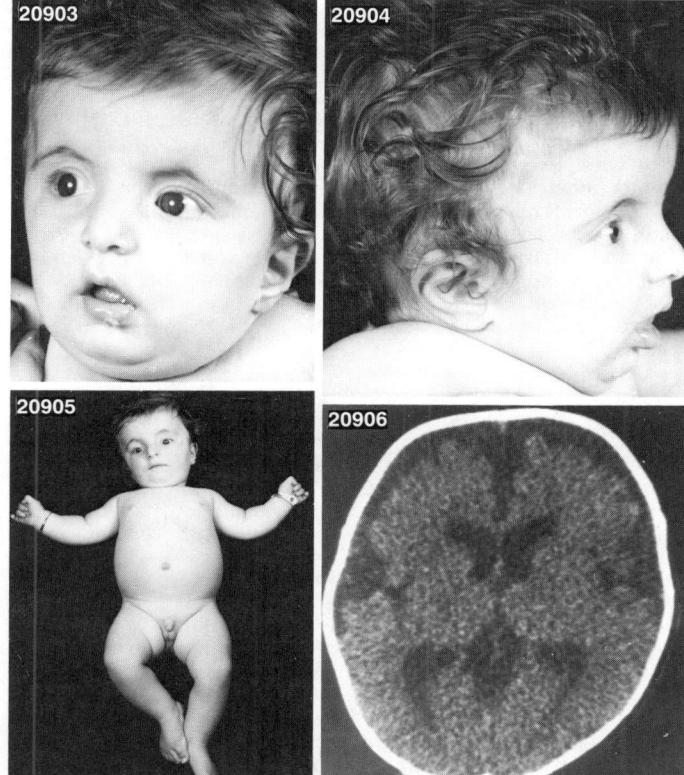

**0137A-20903:** Cerebral gigantism; facies show a prominent fore-head, downward slanting palpebral fissures and low-set ears. 20904: Lateral view of the face. 20905: Full body view shows prominent forehead and relatively large hands and feet. 20906: CAT scan of the head shows enlarged subarachnoid space and mild ventricular enlargement typical of cerebral gigantism. This may be misdiagnosed as cerebral atrophy.

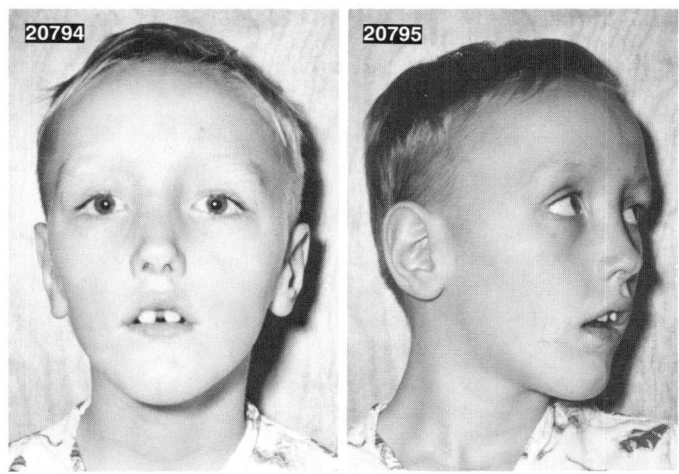

**0137B-20794–95:** Cerebral gigantism: note prominent forehead and supraorbital ridges, receding anterior hairline, downward slant of the palpebral fissures, prognathism and flat facies in this subject with excessive growth.

Lipodystrophy-gigantism-associated endocrine
    manifestations
  Marfan syndrome (0630)
  Neurofibromatosis (0712)
  Nevo syndrome (3273)
  Overgrowth, Ruvalcaba-Myhre-Smith type (2120)
  Steroid 21-hydroxylase deficiency (0908)
  Thyrotoxicosis
  X-linked mental retardation, Fragile X syndrome (2073)

**Major Diagnostic Criteria:** Gigantism, prominent forehead, high arched palate, hypertelorism, long arm span, dolichocephaly, mental retardation, enlarged ventricles or subarachnoid space on pneumoencephalogram or computerized tomographic (CT) scan, normal growth hormone secretion. There is no biochemical marker.

**Clinical Findings:** Clinical findings based on the sample of 80 of Jaeken et al. (1972) include the following: gigantism (100%); prominent forehead (96%); high-arched palate (96%); hypertelorism (91%); arm span greater than height (91%); dolichocephaly (84%); developmental retardation (median IQ 72) (83%); large hands and feet (83%); pointed chin (83%); downslanting palpebral fissures (77%); lack of fine motor control (67%); premature eruption of teeth (57%); neonatal adaptation with or without feeding difficulties (44%); abnormal dermatoglyphics (nonspecific) (33%); other eye abnormalities, mainly strabismus (17%); seizures, and large ears (frequency undetermined).

Mean birth weight = 3.9 kg. Mean birth length = 55.2 cm.

Laboratory findings include enlarged ventricles on pneumoencephalogram (thought to occur in most cases); Abnormal electroencephalogram, usually nonspecific and diffusely abnormal (45%); abnormal glucose tolerance test, diabetic profile (14%); and enlarged ventricles or subarachnoid space on CT scan (undetermined frequency).

**Complications:** Unknown.

**Associated Findings:** Hyperthyroidism in three cases; hypothyroidism in three cases; abnormal plasma amino acids in four cases; Wilms tumor in two cases. The following findings may or may not be important (i.e., single case reports): syndactyly, anterior fontanel bones, functional megacolon, vertebra plana, kyphoscoliosis, unequal leg length, peripheral dysostosis, autonomic failure with persistent fever, Kocher-Debré-Semelaigne syndrome (familial nongoiterous cretinism accompanied by muscular hypertrophy), hepatocarcinoma, cataracts, juvenile macular degeneration.

**Etiology:** Autosomal dominant inheritance has been suggested by the occurrence of cerebral gigantism in successive generations in six families, but most cases are isolated. Cerebral gigantism in sibs has raised the possibility of recessive inheritance.

**Pathogenesis:** Undetermined. Speculations exist concerning a biologically active but immunologically inactive growth-stimulating material (as yet unidentified), possible excessive growth hormone secretion in early life, and possible excessive growth hormone secretion over a 24-hour period. Studies of growth hormone secretion almost always show normal results. Unusual dermatoglyphics suggest a prenatal abnormality.

**MIM No.:** *11755

**POS No.:** 3055

**Sex Ratio:** M1:F1

**Occurrence:** 150 cases since 1964 (Dodge et al., 1983).

**Risk of Recurrence for Patient's Sib:**
See Part I, *Mendelian Inheritance.*

**Risk of Recurrence for Patient's Child:**
See Part I, *Mendelian Inheritance.*

**Age of Detectability:** Large size at birth may raise suspicion; usually can be diagnosed by 2–3 years of age. Median age at first examination for gigantism and retardation is 5 years (Jaeken et al., 1972).

**Gene Mapping and Linkage:** Unknown.

**Prevention:** None known. Genetic counseling indicated.

**Treatment:** Special education; possible estrogen treatment to decrease excessive linear growth; treatment of scoliosis.

**Prognosis:** Appears good within limits of the mental retardation.

**Detection of Carrier:** Unknown.

**Special Considerations:** Numerous investigations of endocrine status have been normal with the exceptions of three cases of hyperthyroidism, three cases of hypothyroidism, one case of the Kocher-Debré-Semelaigne syndrome, one case with a paradoxical rise in his serum growth hormone level following hyperglycemia (rather than hypoglycemia), and 11 out of 80 cases (14%) with glucose tolerance curves of diabetic type.

Total 24-hour growth hormone secretion studies have not been reported. With routine methods, growth hormone levels have not been elevated. Elevations of urinary steroids and early sexual development have been reported but are thought to be due to advanced biologic age rather than endocrine abnormality. Other studies have suggested normal peripheral sensitivity to growth hormone and no conclusive abnormalities of somatomedin.

The brain was without structural abnormalities or ventricular enlargement in the sole reported autopsy case (Sugarman et al., 1977).

The review of Jaeken (1972) of data from 21 boys shows rapid growth of height during the first 4–5 years, and then the height values remain above but parallel to the normal growth curve. In contrast, the growth of height in 24 girls is only slightly above the 97th percentile until approximately age five years at which point the growth rate gradually increases (height data is plotted only until age 10 years).

**References:**
Jaeken J, et al.: Cerebral gigantism syndrome: a report of four cases and review of the literature. Z Kinderheilk 1972; 112:332–346. *
Sugarman GI, et al.: A case of cerebral gigantism and hepatocarcinoma. Am J Dis Child 1977; 131:631–633.
Dodge PR, et al.: Cerebral gigantism. Dev Med Child Neurol 1983; 25:248–252. *
Maldonado V, et al.: Cerebral gigantism associated with Wilms' tumor. Am J Dis Child 1984; 138:486–488.

KA008
DS000

**Raymond S. Kandt**
**Bernard D'Souza**

**Cerebral G(M1)-gangliosidosis**
*See G(M1)-GANGLIOSIDOSIS, TYPE 1*

**Cerebral hemorrhage, familial**
*See AMYLOIDOSIS, ICELANDIC TYPE*

## CEREBRAL PALSY                                    2931

**Includes:**
Paralysis (cerebral), congenital spastic
Spastic infantile paralysis (cerebral)

**Excludes:**
Brachial plexus (Erb) palsy motor deficit, acquired
**Meningomyelocele** (0693)
Motor deficit secondary to hereditary, degenerative disease
Motor deficit secondary to spinal injury
Motor deficit secondary to disorder of nerve or muscle
**Paraplegia, familial spastic** (0295)

**Major Diagnostic Criteria:** Abnormality of movement or posture, present since early in life and not the result of recognized progressive disease.

**Clinical Findings:** Except for the 10–12% of cerebral palsy cases acquired through known infection or injury after the first month of life, this condition does not have a definable onset but is generally assumed to be congenital or, in a small percentage of cases, acquired during the perinatal period. Many but not most children with cerebral palsy demonstrate abnormal neurologic signs during the neonatal period. Usually the presenting complaint is failure to meet early developmental milestones. The child may manifest early abnormality of muscle tone, with hypertonus, hypotonus, hypertonus and pathologic reflexes in the extremities, or hypotonus of neck and trunk, combined with absence of age-appropriate postural reflexes.

The major forms of cerebral palsy are spastic, with hypertonus of the claspknife type (anatomic subtypes are hemiplegia, with involvement of both limbs of one side; diplegia, with involvement of legs more than arms; and quadriplegia, with involvement of all extremities, the arms more markedly than the legs); extrapyramidal, with hypertonus tending to be of the rigid or leadpipe variety and with defects of posture and often with involuntary movements (athetosis, dystonia, or ataxia); and mixed types.

The deficit may be manifested somewhat differently at different ages, but there is not, overall, a progression of the disorder. Physical therapy can prevent contractures and secondary complications of imbalance of tonus around such joints as the hip. Depending on severity of the motor deficit and the presence and degree of associated disabilities, the handicap may be major or minor.

Other neurologic and sensory disabilities often coexist with motor abnormalities in cerebral palsy. Mental retardation is a relatively common concomitant, present in about one-half of the children with cerebral palsy. Persons with spastic quadriplegia are especially likely to have associated severe intellectual deficits. One-fourth to one-third of persons with cerebral palsy have some type of seizure disorder. Visual and visual-motor abnormalities affect approximately one-half of persons with cerebral palsy. Abnormalities in the control of ocular muscles, with resulting strabismus, are frequent, and refractive errors are also common. Abnormalities of hearing are found in 10–15% of affected persons. Somatic sensory abnormalities may be present in hemiplegia, and dental defects are common. Speech and learning defects are major handicaps in persons with cerebral palsy and may stem from an interaction of factors including motor, intellectual, and experiential elements. Social and emotional maladjustment and depression, especially in adolescence, are common.

There is usually not a family history of similar involvement, and there are no specific laboratory findings.

**Complications:** Subluxation or dislocation of the hip at the acetabulum in spastic varieties, and aspiration pneumonia, particularly in those with quadriplegia and severe mental retardation.

**Associated Findings:** Congenital malformations are more common in persons with cerebral palsy than in comparison populations.

**Etiology:** No known mode of inheritance in most cases. Intrauterine infection and postnatal injury or infection are among potential causes. Some, probably a relatively small minority, may be related to birth asphyxia. Maldevelopment of the nervous system is likely in some cases. In most cases, the cause is unknown.

**Pathogenesis:** Unknown.

**Sex Ratio:** About M1:F1. A slight excess of males has been noted.

**Occurrence:** Approximately 2–2.5:1,000 live births.

**Risk of Recurrence for Patient's Sib:** Undetermined, but low. Estimated at 10% in the ataxic and dystonic forms.

**Risk of Recurrence for Patient's Child:** Undetermined, but presumably low.

**Age of Detectability:** Severe cases in term babies may be suspected in the early months of life, but, because there is apparent resolution of mild or moderate cases, and further identification of other mild or moderate cases in the early years, confident diagnosis should wait until about age three years.

**Gene Mapping and Linkage:** Unknown.

**Prevention:** Avoidance of isoimmunization for rH factors is among the only known means of prevention. Avoidance of obstetric trauma is obviously desirable, but improvements in obstetric and neonatal care have not been followed by a decrease in incidence of cerebral palsy.

**Treatment:** Recognition and remediation of associated handicaps is important. Physical therapy can avoid complications such as contractures, and physical therapy and occupational and speech therapy can help affected persons to maximize their use of remaining capabilities. Braces and other assistive devices can be of marked benefit. Drug therapies have been of limited benefit. Surgical treatment can minimize limitations of range of joint movement. Family counseling and psychologic therapy may be appropriate.

**Prognosis:** Life span depends on type and severity of involvement and, most critically, on level of intelligence. Severe quadriplegia and profound mental retardation are associated with the most marked limitation of life span. Level of care is also relevant.

**Detection of Carrier:** Unknown.

**Support Groups:**
New York; United Cerebral Palsy Associations (UCPA)
CANADA: Ontario; Toronto; The Canadian Cerebral Palsy Association
ENGLAND: London; The Spastics Society

**References:**
Freud S: Infantile cerebral palsy. Coral Gables, FL: University of Miami Press, 1968 (L.A. Russin, translator).
Stanley A, Alberman E, eds: The epidemiology of the cerebral palsies. Philadelphia: J.B. Lippincott, 1984.
Nelson KB, Ellenberg JH: Antecedents of cerebral palsies: multivariate analysis of risk. New Engl J Med 1986; 315:81–86.
Kitchen WH, et al.: Cerebral palsy in very low birthweight infants surviving to 2 years with modern perinatal intensive care. Am J Perinatol 1987; 4:29–35.
Freeman JM, Nelson KB: Intrapartum asphyxia and cerebral palsy. Pediatrics 1988; 82:240–249.
Nelson KB: What proportion of cerebral palsy is related to birth asphyxia? J Pediatr 1988; 112:572–574.
Emond A, et al.: Cerebral palsy in two national cohort studies. Arch Dis Childhd 1989; 64:848–852.
Pharoah POD, et al.: Acquired cerebral palsy. Arch Dis Childhd 1989; 64:1013–1016.

NE021

**Karin B. Nelson**

**Cerebral sclerosis, degenerative diffuse-Scholz type**
*See METACHROMATIC LEUKODYSTROPHIES*
**Cerebral sclerosis, diffuse chronic infantile**
*See PELIZAEUS-MERZBACHER SYNDROME*
**Cerebral vascular amyloid peptide**
*See ALZHEIMER DISEASE, FAMILIAL*

**Cerebral-digito-reno syndrome**
*See DIGITO-RENO-CEREBRAL SYNDROME*

---

## CEREBRO-COSTO-MANDIBULAR SYNDROME 0138

**Includes:** Rib gap defects-micrognathia

**Excludes:**
Micrognathia, other conditions with severe
Pierre Robin anomaly, other syndromes with

**Major Diagnostic Criteria:** Combination of microcephaly, micrognathia and posterior rib gap defects.

**Clinical Findings:** Severe micrognathia, glossoptosis, cleft palate, posterior rib gap defects, microcephaly and mental retardation in some patients; others have normal intelligence. The rib defects consist of replacement of bone by fibroconnective tissue in the posterior paravertebral portions of the ribs. The lesions are bilateral, but not necessarily symmetric, and may involve all or only some ribs, particularly the fourth and fifth pairs. Cartilage or bone may be abnormal in other areas (trachea, hip, elbow). Pterygium colli has been found in four patients. The combination of micrognathia, glossoptosis and "flat chest" causes severe respiratory distress. Mortality in early infancy is high.

**Complications:** Respiratory distress, respiratory infection, feeding difficulties, failure to thrive, mental retardation possibly secondary to neonatal hypoxia, speech delay, high infant mortality, conductive hearing loss, round and oval window abnormalities.

**Associated Findings:** **Ventricular septal defect, Kidney, polycystic adult type, Meningocele** and **Meningomyelocele.**

**Etiology:** Possibly autosomal dominant inheritance.

**Pathogenesis:** Unknown.

**MIM No.:** 11765

**POS No.:** 3056

**CDC No.:** 759.870

**Sex Ratio:** Presumably M1:F1

**Occurrence:** Two dozen cases have been observed in different (Caucasian) populations.

**Risk of Recurrence for Patient's Sib:**
See Part I, *Mendelian Inheritance.*

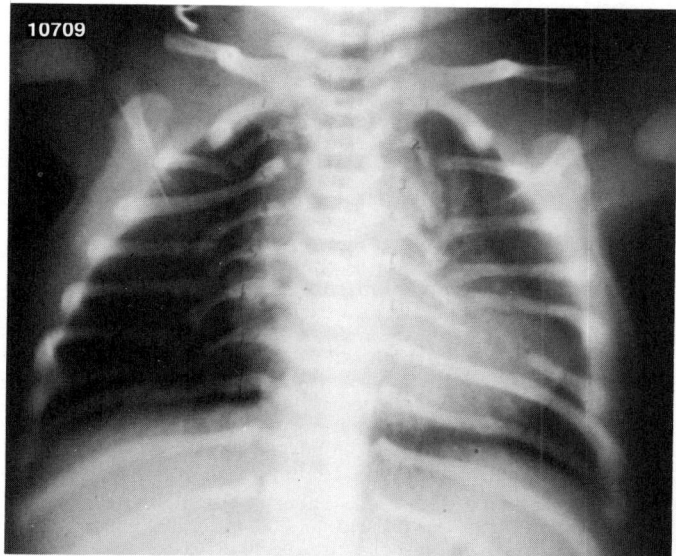

0138-10709: Bilateral posterior rib gap defects.

**Risk of Recurrence for Patient's Child:**
See Part I, *Mendelian Inheritance.*

**Age of Detectability:** At birth; prenatal diagnosis by ultrasound.

**Gene Mapping and Linkage:** Unknown.

**Prevention:** None known. Genetic counseling indicated.

**Treatment:** Intensive care for respiratory distress, feeding difficulty and infection. Cleft palate repair. Special education for hearing loss. Hearing aids.

**Prognosis:** Of 24 reported patients, ten died before 3 months of age. Survival has extended to adulthood. All survivors showed growth disturbances.

**Detection of Carrier:** Unknown.

**References:**

McNicholl B, et al.: Cerebro-costo-mandibular syndrome. Arch Dis Child 1970; 45:521.

Miller KE, et al.: Rib gap defects with micrognathia. Am J Roentgen 1972; 114:253–256.

Langer LO Jr, Herrmann J: The cerebrocostomandibular syndrome. Malformation Syndromes BD:OAS 1974; X(7):167.

Silverman FN, et al.: Cerebro-costo-mandibular syndrome. J Pediatr 1980; 97:406–416.

Tachibana K, et al.: Cerebro-costo-mandibular syndrome. A case report and review of the literature. Hum Genet 1980; 54:283–286.

LeRoy JG, et al.: Cerebro-costo-mandibular syndrome with autosomal dominant inheritance. J Pediatr 1981; 99:441–443.

Schroer RJ, Meyer LC: Cerebro-costo-mandibular syndrome. Proc Greenwood Genet Center 1985; 4:55–59.

Merlob P, et al.: Autosomal dominant cerebro-costo-mandibular syndrome: ultrasonographic and clinical findings. Am J Med Genet 1987; 26:195–202.

*Frederic N. Silverman*

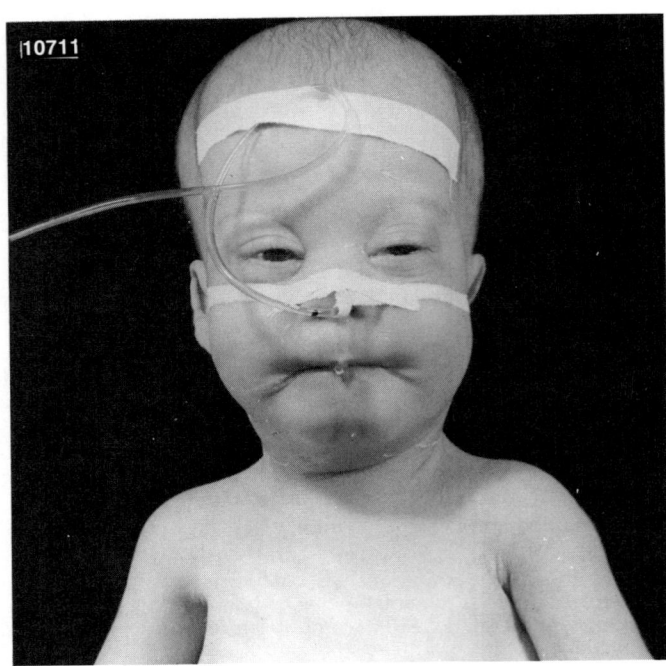

**0139-10711:** Note high forehead, epicanthal folds, ptosis, and rounded face.

---

## CEREBRO-HEPATO-RENAL SYNDROME      0139

**Includes:**

Acidemia, hyperpipecolic
Adrenoleukodystrophy, neonatal
Peroxisomal biogenesis, disorders of
Peroxisome deficiency
Pipecolic acidemia
Refsum disease (some neonatal or infantile forms)
Zellweger syndrome

**Excludes:**

**Acidemia, glutaric acidemia II, neonatal onset** (2289)
**Acidemia, Trihydroxycoprostanic** (3275)
Beta-hydroxylisobutyryl CoA deacylase deficiency
**Chondrodysplasia punctata, rhizomelic type** (0154)
Floppy infant, other types of
Iron storage disease, idiopathic neonatal
Hyperoxaluria, type I
**Phytanic acid oxidase deficiency, infantile type** (2278)
**Phytanic acid storage disease** (0810)

**Major Diagnostic Criteria:** Profound muscular hypotonia with areflexia, cerebral depression, non-responsiveness, absent psychomotor development, severe feeding difficulties, convulsions, attacks of apnea, dysmorphic craniofacial features, glaucoma, cataracts, thymus hypoplasia, congenital heart lesions, hepatomegaly, stippling of patella and triradiate cartilage of hip socket, elevated serum iron, high normal or elevated iron binding capacity, elevated very long chain fatty acids in plasma and cultured fibroblasts, elevated phytanic acid, decreased particulate (peroxisomal) catalase, high pipecolic acid and increased di- and trihydroxycoprostanic acid in bile, serum and urine, absence or decrease of peroxisomes in liver biopsy.

**Clinical Findings:** Prenatal history is unrevealing, though fetal movements may be decreased. There is prenatal growth failure with full term birthweights below 3,000 and 2,500 grams in 50% and 25%, respectively. Patients are cerebrally depressed, motionless, non-responsive with weak or absent Moro response. Sucking and swallowing reflexes are absent and feeding by gavage or through gastrostomy may be necessary throughout life. There is extreme muscular hypotonia in all cases, withdrawal and tendon reflexes cannot be elicited. The hypotonia is of supranuclear origin, though a mitochondrial myopathy may contribute to the hypotonia. Patients display craniofacial dysmorphic features with a high bulging and receding forehead, dolichoturricephaly, wide open fontanels and sutures including the metopic suture, puffy eyelids, mongoloid slant, poorly developed supraorbital ridges, ocular hypertelorism, epicanthic folds, Brushfield spots, corneal cloudiness, glaucoma, buphthalmos, cataracts, pigmentary retinopathy, optic nerve dysplasia, low set ears, abnormal helices, high arched palate with cleft of the soft palate, micrognathia and somewhat rounded face. The thymus is small and some immunodeficiency may be present. Congenital heart lesions are rare, but septal defects, delayed closure of ductus arteriosus, and foramen ovale occur. Hepatomegaly may develop soon after birth and is then a nearly constant finding and jaundice and melena are often encountered in the first two months of life. Boys are frequently cryptorchid while clitoromegaly is found in girls. Some patients have difficulties in regulating their body temperature. Limb anomalies include cubitus valgus, camptodactyly, transverse palmar crease, metatarsus adductus, and talipes equinovarus. Dermatoglyphics are non-specific, ridge counts are often low, ulnar loops prevail in some, whorls in other patients. Failure to thrive is conspicuous. Most children show no psychomotor development. Therapy-resistant convulsions often beginning in the neonatal period are frequent. Life expectancy is severely curtailed; 70% of the children die within the first 3 months and most die within the first year. The longest recorded survival has been 2 1/2 years. There are, however, rare variants of the condition which show initially some development, but which regress subsequently. The pace of deterrioration varies. These individuals survive longer, and exceptional patients may even reach the second decade.

A special variant with longer survival has been described by Versmold et al. It is characterized by muscular hypertonia, decreased liver catalase, with a respiratory chain deficiency at the cytochrome b level, while the electron chain defect in the classic condition is at levels preceding the cytochrome steps. In all other respects the Versmold variant is identical.

Impaired liver functions include elevated serum bilirubin, elevated liver enzymes such as SGOT, SGPT, hypoprothombinemia, altered catabolism of bile acids with elevated di- and trihydroxy-coprostanic acid in bile, serum, and urine. Serum iron is frequently increased, iron binding capacity is high normal or elevated. Breakdown of lysine is altered as evidenced by elevated pipecolic acid in serum and urine which, however, appears only after a few weeks of postnatal life. The beta-oxidation of very long chain fatty acids is impaired, hence, elevated levels of saturated and monounsaturated $C_{26}$ fatty acids in plasma and fibroblasts. Recently, a deficiency of a membrane-bound phospholipid, plasmalogen, was discovered in various organs, which is presumably due to deficiency of Acyl CoA dihydroxyacetone phosphate acyltransferase; a peroxisomal enzyme catalyzing the initial step of glycerol ether lipid biosynthesis. Phytanic acid oxidase is deficient and phytanic acid is increased. The particulate (peroxisomal) catalase is absent or decreased, although the cytosolic catalase is present. Urinary excretion of dicarboxylic acid is increased. EEG is abnormal and ERG (electroretinogram) may be extinguished. X-rays show stippling (sometimes scimitar shaped calcifications) of patella, triradiate cartilage of the hip sockets, and various epiphyses. There are essential alterations in the electron transport respiratory chain between succinic dehydrogenase flavoprotein and coenzyme Q at the level of succinate-ubiquinone oxidoreductase, as evidenced by the abnormal oxidation of succinate, glutamate, pyruvate, malate, and alpha-keto-glutarate.

Neuropathological studies indicate that the early differentiation of the neuraxis, closure of the neural groove, diverticulation of the major brain vesicles, and prosencephalic cleavage are essentially undisturbed. The developmental abnormalities involve the finer differentiation of the CNS structures which takes place during the 4th to 6th week of gestation and includes pachygyria, micropolygyria, hypoplastic commissural structures such as hypoplasia of the corpus callosum, deep furrows between the gyri, dysplasia of the inferior olives and paraventricular cysts. The histoarchitecture of the CNS is distorted to a degree varying from case to case. The cortical layers are poorly organized. There are heterotopias due to incomplete migration of the subependymal neurons to the cortex. Heterotopias of Purkinje cells are found in the cerebellum. Sudanophilic deposits are found in neuronal and glial cells and large multinucleated "globoid" cells are scattered throughout the cortex. Glygcogen deposits are found in some instances. Gliosis dys- and demyelination are likewise encountered.

Histological findings in the liver vary between minor abnormalities in the beginning and micronodular cirrhosis, notably in children who survive the first six months. Abnormal liver lobules, dysgenesis of the biliary duct system, intralobular and periportal fibrosis, and hemosiderosis are often found. Hemosiderosis is also found in other organs, notably bone marrow, and is due to alterations of iron transfer, not to increased hemolysis. The kidneys show dysgenesis of the parenchyma and small subcortical cysts which are almost pathognomonic and can sometimes be discovered in vivo by CT scan. Hypoplasia of lungs, thymus, and hypertrophic islets in the pancreas are frequently found.

Most important is the absence of perixomes in liver and proximal kidney tubules and mitochondrial abnormalities in various organs, notably brain, liver, and muscle. The mitochondria show abnormal size and abnormal structure, such as dilated and concentric cristae. The mitochondrial abnormalities are presumably secondary to the absence of the peroxisomes.

**Complications:** Jaundice and hypoprothrombinemic hemorrhages may occur during the first two months. Attacks of respiratory arrest are occasionally observed. Aspiration due to feeding difficulties and repeated infections of the respiratory tract occur. A certain immunodeficiency connected with the small thymus may influence the outcome of the infections.

**Associated Findings:** None known.

**Etiology:** Autosomal recessive inheritance. Occurrence in more than one sibling is frequently encountered and parental consanguinity has been reported several times. Clinical, anatomical, and biochemical findings vary more than is usually seen in autosomal recessive conditions, and genetic heterogeneity has been proven by cell fusion and complementation of the heterokaryon.

**Pathogenesis:** Due to the absence or marked diminution of peroxisomes. Peroxisomes are small intracellular organelles which perform a multitude of metabolic functions. Absence of peroxisomes has, therefore, a profound and complex impact on the metabolism which is barely compatible with a longer postnatal survival. The basic defect consists in a defective import of the matrix proteins into the peroxisomes. Peroxisomal matrix proteins are encoded by nuclear genes and originate in free polyribosomes. They are then directed from the cytosol to pre-existing peroxisomes by a not fully understood but probably complex mechanism. The pre-existing peroxisomes which come from the germ cells grow after the matrix proteins have been imported, and then multiply by division or budding. If the matrix proteins fail to reach the peroxisomes, no further peroxisomes are formed and a state of absent or diminished peroxisomes ensues.

Peroxisomes also have an effect on the mitochondria; mitochondrial abnormalities found in the present syndrome are secondary to the absence of peroxisomes.

The present syndrome is among the first in which dysmorphic signs and malformations could be causally related to a metabolic error.

Several other peroxisomal disorders have been described (See **Chondrodysplasia punctata, rhizomelic type** and **Phytanic acid oxidase deficiency, infantile type**). Through cell fusion and complementation studies of the heterokarya, it was recognized that these conditions compliment each other in some, but not in all instances; which suggests that they can be encoded by the same gene, but different genes can encode for the same phenotype. Six complementation groups have been identified. One of them complements for this condition as well as **Phytanic acid oxidase deficiency, infantile type** (Roscher et al, 1989).

Besides the heterogeneous disorders of peroxisomal biogenesis, there exists a second class of peroxisomal disorders which are due to the deficiency of one or several peroxisomal enzyme(s). The so-called *Pseudo-Zellweger syndrome(s)* display phenotypic similarities to the disorders of peroxisomal biogenesis, while other single peroxisomal enzyme deficiencies cause different disease conditions (for example **Phytanic acid storage disease**).

**MIM No.:** *21410

**POS No.:** 3057

**CDC No.:** 759.870

**Sex Ratio:** M1:F1

**Occurrence:** 1:25,000–50,000 live births. Many cases die before the correct diagnosis is made. About 200 cases have been reported.

**Risk of Recurrence for Patient's Sib:**
See Part I, *Mendelian Inheritance.*

**Risk of Recurrence for Patient's Child:** Affected individuals are not expected to survive to reproduce.

**Age of Detectability:** At birth or soon thereafter.

**Gene Mapping and Linkage:** ZWS (Zellweger syndrome) has been tentatively mapped to 7q11.

**Prevention:** Prenatal diagnosis possible by determining long-chain fatty acids and possibly by the absence of dihydroxyacetone phosphate acyltransferase in cultured amniocytes.

**Treatment:** None, except symptomatic. Attempts to treat with Clofibrate (to stimulate formation of peroxisomes) and glycerol-ether-lipid preparations have not been successful.

**Prognosis:** Death in infancy or early childhood.

**Detection of Carrier:** Lenticular opacities can be found in some carriers by biomicroscopy after maximal dilatation of the pupils.

**References:**
Moser HW: Peroxisomal disorders. J Pediatr 1986; 108:398–400.
Schutgens RBH et al.: Review: peroxisomal disorders: a newly recognized group of genetic diseases. Europ J Pediatr 1986; 144:430–440.
Vamecq J, et al.: Multiple peroxisomal enzymatic deficiency disorders:

A comparative biochemical and morphological study of Zellweger cerebrohepatorenal syndrome and neonatal adrenoleukodystrophy. Am J Pathol 1986; 125:524–535.

Wanders RJA, et al.: Infantile Refsum disease. Eur J Pediat 1986; 145:172–175.

Wilson GN et al.: The Zellweger syndrome: Diagnostic assays, syndrome delineation and potential therapy. Am J Med Genet 1986; 24:69–82.

Wanders RJA, et al.: Neonatal adrenoleukodystrophy. J Neurol Sci 1987; 77:331–340.

Zellweger H: The Zellweger syndrome and related peroxisomal disorders. Devel Med Child Neurol 1987; 29:821–829. *

Singh I, et al.: Peroxisomal disorders: biochemical and clinical diagnostic considerations. Am J Dis Child 1988; 142:1297–1301.

Lazarow PB, Moser HW: Disorders of peroxisome biogenesis. In: Scriver CR, et al, eds: The metabolic basis of inherited disease, 6th ed. New York: McGraw-Hill, 1989:1479–1510.

ZE001                                                     **Hans Zellweger**

## CEREBRO-NEPHRO-OSTEODYSPLASIA, HUTTERITE TYPE                                                              2795

**Includes:**  Hutterite cerebro-osteo-nephrodysplasia

**Excludes:**
  **Adrenoleukodystrophy, X-linked** (2533)
  **Cerebro-hepato-renal syndrome** (0139)
  **Leukodystrophy, globoid cell type** (0415)
  **Metachromatic leukodystrophies** (0651)
  **Rett syndrome** (2226)

**Major Diagnostic Criteria:**  The combination of rhizomelic, short trunk dwarfism, development of **Microcephaly**, subsequent failure to thrive, and renal involvement; particularly in a child of Hutterite background.

**Clinical Findings:**  This condition has been documented in two Hutterite sisters. Both had congenital short stature and a neonatal period characterized by jaundice, feeding difficulties, and seizure-like activity. One also had nystagmus. Brachycephaly was present in both, whereas only one had a large anterior fontanelle. The facial features present in one or both included flat facial profile, sixth nerve palsy, anteverted nares, long upper lip, flat philtrum, thin upper vermilion, large tongue, and posteriorly rotated ears. The liver and spleen were palpable in both; one sister also had a **Hernia, umbilical**, whereas the other had diastasis recti. The trunk and limbs were short, with rhizomelic shortness of the limbs more pronounced than mesomelic or acromelic shortness.

Although early developmental milestones were achieved, developmental progress slowed or stopped in later infancy; head growth also slowed, so that microcephaly was present by age one year. Failure to thrive also occurred by this age. The older girl died at age three years because of an apparent nephrotic syndrome.

X-ray examination demonstrated brachycephaly with a small midface, six cervical vertebrae, vertebral platyspondyly with coronal clefting, mild iliac hypoplasia, and flared femoral metaphyses. CT scan showed diffuse cerebral atrophy at age one year. Numerous biochemical investigations were normal, with the exception of slight elevations of creatine kinase, lactate dehydrogenase, and ASOT levels on liver function tests.

**Complications:**  Failure of growth is likely as a result of by CNS-based feeding difficulties.

**Associated Findings:**  None known.

**Etiology:**  Possibly autosomal recessive inheritance.

**Pathogenesis:**  Unknown. Tissues of both ectodermal and mesodermal origin seem affected.

**MIM No.:**  23645

**POS No.:**  3717

**Sex Ratio:**  M0:F2 (observed).

**Occurrence:**  One Lehrerleut Hutterite sibship has been reported.

**Risk of Recurrence for Patient's Sib:**
  See Part I, *Mendelian Inheritance.*

**Risk of Recurrence for Patient's Child:**
  See Part I, *Mendelian Inheritance.*

**Age of Detectability:**  At birth, by the presence of short-limbed, short trunk dwarfism. Prenatal diagnosis by ultrasound is possible.

**Gene Mapping and Linkage:**  Unknown.

**Prevention:**  None known. Genetic counseling indicated.

**Treatment:**  Supportive.

**Prognosis:**  The older of the two sisters died by age three years. Mental retardation appears to become severe.

**Detection of Carrier:**  Unknown.

**References:**
Opitz JM, et al.: Hutterite cerebro-osteo-nephrodysplasia: autosomal recessive trait in a Lehrerleut Hutterite family from Montana. Am J Med Genet 1985; 22:521–529.

T0007                                                  **Helga V. Toriello**

**Cerebro-oculo-facial syndrome**
  *See OCULO-CEREBRO-FACIAL SYNDROME, KAUFMAN TYPE*

## CEREBRO-OCULO-FACIO-SKELETAL SYNDROME                                                          0140

**Includes:**
  Cataracts-microcephaly-kyphosis-limited joint movement (Lowry)
  COFS syndrome
  Microcephaly-multiple congenital anomalies
  Pena-Shokeir II syndrome

**Excludes:**
  **Arthrogryposes** (0088)
  **Cerebro-costo-mandibular syndrome** (0138)
  **Cerebro-hepato-renal syndrome** (0139)
  **Chromosome** anomalies (all other)
  **Cockayne syndrome** (0189)
  **Fetal rubella syndrome** (0384)
  **Hutterite syndrome, Bowen-Conradi type** (2422)
  **Oculo-auriculo-vertebral anomaly** (0735)
  **Oculo-cerebro-renal syndrome** (0736)
  **Oculo-mandibulo-facial syndrome** (0738)
  **Pena-Shokeir syndrome** (2080)
  Viral infections

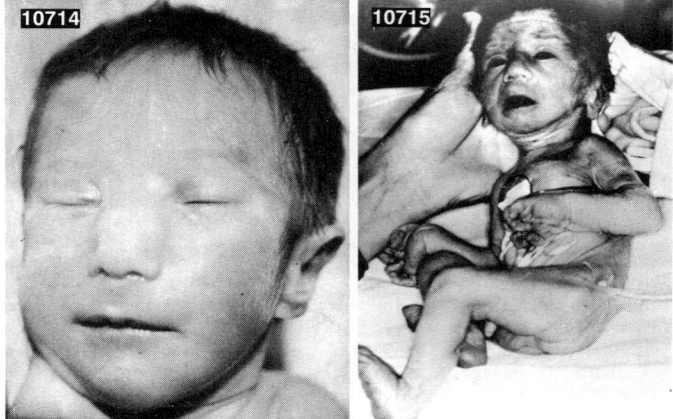

0140-10714: Facies shows sloping forehead, microphthalmia and a high nasal bridge. 10715: Affected infant with prominent nose; small, receding chin; large, low-set ears and contractures.

**Major Diagnostic Criteria:** Craniofacial anomalies in this condition include microcephaly, ocular anomalies such as cataract and microphthalmia, dysmorphic facies with prominent nasal bridge, large ears, overhanging upper lip, and small chin. The skeletal defects include a variety of problems such as scoliosis, hip and pelvis defects, and flexion contractures of limbs. The diagnosis should be considered in patients with some combination of these problems.

**Clinical Findings:** The cerebral feature is microcephaly, sometimes with a sloping forehead; the ocular features are cataract, microphthalmia, and narrow palpebral fissures; the facial features are high nasal bridge with a prominent saddle-like bony ridge, large ears, upper lip overhanging the lower, and micro- or retrognathia; and the skeletal features are kyphosis, scoliosis, hip dislocation or acetabular dysplasia, narrow pelvis, coxa valga, flexion contractures of the limbs and digits, rocker bottom feet, and osteoporosis. In addition, affected infants are usually small for dates, and they may have renal anomalies, short neck, widely spaced nipples, simian creases, a longitudinal foot groove, and hypotonia.

**Complications:** Feeding difficulty, respiratory distress, repeated lower respiratory infections.

**Associated Findings:** Osteopetrosis and severe degeneration of skeletal muscles have been reported (Lerman-Sagie et al, 1987).

**Etiology:** Autosomal recessive inheritance strongly suggested by pedigree analysis and by consanguinity in parents.

**Pathogenesis:** Unknown.

**MIM No.:** 21415

**POS No.:** 3136

**Sex Ratio:** M1:F1

**Occurrence:** Probably rare. Wide geographic and ethnic range, including Black and Italian cases.

**Risk of Recurrence for Patient's Sib:**
See Part I, *Mendelian Inheritance.*

**Risk of Recurrence for Patient's Child:** Affected individuals are not expected to survive to reproduce.

**Age of Detectability:** At birth.

**Gene Mapping and Linkage:** Unknown.

**Prevention:** None known. Genetic counseling indicated.

**Treatment:** Unknown.

**Prognosis:** Most patients die within the first 3 years of life. The cause of death has been respiratory failure, in some instances due to repeated lower respiratory infections.

**Detection of Carrier:** Unknown.

**Special Considerations:** Detailed gross and microscopic examination of the eyes in 1 patient revealed microphthalmia, incomplete cleavage of the chamber angle, persistent pupillary membrane, partial detachment and absence of the corneal endothelium and corneal edema, and cataract. Ganglion cell and nerve fiber layers of the retina were absent and there were intraretinal hemorrhages with decreased presence of retinal blood vessels, exudates in the anterior and posterior chambers, vitreous cavity and subretinal space, and optic atrophy.

There may be two types (Pena et al, 1978); both with autosomal recessive inheritance. The first may be a primary degenerative disorder and includes the patients of Lowry et al, 1971; Pena and Shokeir, 1974; and Scott-Emuakpor et al, 1977. The onset may be congenital or by early infancy, and it is progressive. This condition is similar to **Cockayne syndrome.** The second may be more severe and have major visceral anomalies, such as renal or heart malformations. This type includes the patients of Preus et al, 1977 and Lurie, 1976. These 3 patients were all severely affected and died within the first month of life. It is not always clear in which category a patient belongs. For example, the patient of Preus and Fraser, 1974, had congenital onset and died after 6 days of life, but had no apparent visceral malformations.

**References:**

Lowry RB, et al.: Cataracts, microcephaly, kyphosis, and limited joint movement in two siblings: a new syndrome. J Pediatr 1971; 79:282–284. †

Preus M, Fraser FC: The cerebro-oculo-facio-skeletal syndrome. Clin Genet 1974; 5:294–297. †

Lurie IW, et al.: Further evidence for the autosomal-recessive inheritance of the COFS syndrome. Clin Genet 1976; 10:343–346. †

Preus M, et al.: Renal anomalies and oligohydramnios in the cerebro-oculo-facio-skeletal syndrome. Am J Dis Child 1977; 131:62–64. †

Scott-Emuakpor AB, et al.: A syndrome of microcephaly and cataracts in 4 siblings. Am J Dis Child 1977; 131:167–169. †

Pena SDJ, et al.: COFS syndrome revisited. BD:OAS 1978:XIV(6B): 205–213. * †

Lerman-Sagie T, et al.: Syndrome of osteopetrosis and muscular degeneration associated with cerebro-oculo-facio-skeletal changes. Am J Med Genet 1987; 28:137–142.

PR004 **Marilyn Preus**

**Cerebro-oculo-muscular syndrome**
*See WALKER-WARBURG SYNDROME*
**Cerebro-oculo-renal syndrome**
*See OCULO-CEREBRO-RENAL SYNDROME*
**Cerebromacular degeneration, familial**
*See NEURONAL CEROID-LIPOFUSCINOSES (NCL)*
**Cerebromuscular dystrophy, Fukuyama type**
*See MUSCULAR DYSTROPHY, CONGENITAL WITH MENTAL RETARDATION*
**Cerebrooocular dysgenesis**
*See WALKER-WARBURG SYNDROME*
**Cerebroocular dysplasia-muscular dystrophy**
*See WALKER-WARBURG SYNDROME*
**Cerebroside lipidosis**
*See GAUCHER DISEASE*
**Cerebroside sulfatidosis**
*See METACHROMATIC LEUKODYSTROPHIES*
**Cerebrosidosis**
*See GAUCHER DISEASE*
**Cerebrotendinous xanthomatosis**
*See XANTHOMATOSIS, CEREBROTENDINOUS*
**Ceruloplasmin deficiency**
*See HEPATOLENTICULAR DEGENERATION*
**Cerumen variation**
*See EAR, CERUMEN VARIATIONS*
**Cervical aortic arch**
*See AORTIC ARCH, CERVICAL*
**Cervical cyst or sinus**
*See NECK, BRANCHIAL CLEFT, CYSTS OR SINUSES*
**Cervical lipomatosis, familial benign**
*See NECK/FACE, LIPOMATOSIS*
**Cervical teratomas**
*See NECK/HEAD, DERMOID CYST OR TERATOMA*
**Cervical tracheoesophageal fistula, congenital isolated H-type**
*See TRACHEOESOPHAGEAL FISTULA*
**Cervical vertebral fusion, congenital**
*See KLIPPEL-FEIL ANOMALY*
**Cervical, thoracic-thoracoabdominal ectopia cordis**
*See HEART, CORDIS ECTOPIA*

---

**CERVICO-DERMO-GU SYNDROME, GOEMINNE TYPE** **2174**

**Includes:**
  Cervico-dermo-reno-genital dysplasia
  Dermo-gu-cervico syndrome
  Goeminne syndrome
  Gu-dermo-cervico syndrome
  TKCR syndrome
  Torticollis-keloids-cryptorchidism-renal dysplasia

**Excludes:**
  Keloids
  **Klinefelter syndrome** (0556)

**Major Diagnostic Criteria:** The combination of torticollis, keloids, cryptorchidism, and renal "dysplasia" in a male should suggest the diagnosis.

**Clinical Findings:** In five affected males, the clinical findings were as follows: facial asymmetry (1); plagiocephaly (1); periocular skin pigmentation (1); congenital **Torticollis** (5); duodenal ulcer/gastric complaints (2); progressive pyelonephritis (2); infertility (1); cryptorchidism (3); varicose veins (2); keloids and/or nevi (2).

In five carrier females, the findings were as follows: slight facial asymmetry (1); pigmented eyelids (1); **Torticollis** (1); pyelonephritis (1); nephrolithiasis (1); hypertension (2); nevi (2).

The muscular **Torticollis** is congenital; the facial asymmetry and plagiocephaly may be secondary deformation. The other findings appear with age. The keloids appear at puberty. Renal disease occurred in the first decade in one patient and age 19 in another. In female carriers, renal disease was diagnosed in the third decade. Infertility in males is secondary to decreased sperm count and sperm immotility. Intelligence is normal to above average.

Laboratory findings have included normal metabolic studies, karyotype, and gonadotropins. IVPs have generally been normal. Biopsies of keloids have been histologically typical of keloids.

**Complications:** Hypertension and renal failure.

**Associated Findings:** A long second toe was found in one affected male and one female carrier. Dental caries, asthma, clinodactyly, and low birth weight were each described in only one individual.

**Etiology:** Presumably X-linked recessive inheritance, with some expression in carrier females likely.

**Pathogenesis:** Unknown.

**MIM No.:** *31430

**POS No.:** 3890

**Sex Ratio:** M5:F2 (observed).

**Occurrence:** One family has been reported.

**Risk of Recurrence for Patient's Sib:**
See Part I, *Mendelian Inheritance*.

**Risk of Recurrence for Patient's Child:**
See Part I, *Mendelian Inheritance*.

**Age of Detectability:** At birth, if torticollis is present. Otherwise in late childhood or early teens.

**Gene Mapping and Linkage:** TKC (torticollis, keloids, cryptorchidism and renal dysplasia) has been provisionally mapped to Xq28-qter.

**Prevention:** None known. Genetic counseling indicated.

**Treatment:** If indicated, treatment for renal disease. Radiation for keloids has not proven effective.

**Prognosis:** If renal disease is not present, life span is not impaired. Intelligence has been normal to above average. Males are infertile, whereas female carriers appear to have normal fertility.

**Detection of Carrier:** In four of five female carriers, some manifestations of the syndrome were present.

**References:**
Goeminne L: A new probably X-linked inheritance syndrome: congenital muscular torticollis, multiple keloids, cryptorchidism and renal dysplasia. Acta Genet Med Gemellol (Rome) 1968; 17:439–467. * †

Zuffardi A, Fraccaro M: Gene mapping and serendipity: the locus for torticollis, keloids, cryptorchidism and renal dysplasia (31430, McKusick) is at Xq28, distal to the G6PD locus. Hum Genet 1982; 62:280–281.

Schinzel A: Catalogue of unbalanced chromosomal aberrations in Man. New York, Walter de Gruyter, 1984:397.

T0007                      **Helga V. Toriello**

**Cervico-dermo-reno-genital dysplasia**
*See CERVICO-DERMO-GU SYNDROME, GOEMINNE TYPE*

---

# CERVICO-OCULO-ACOUSTIC SYNDROME      **0142**

**Includes:**
Acoustic-cervico-oculo syndrome
Cervicooculofacial dysplasia
Oculo-cervico-acoustic syndrome
Klippel-Feil anomaly-deafness-abducens palsy
Wildervanck syndrome

**Excludes:** Oculo-auriculo-vertebral anomaly (0735)

**Major Diagnostic Criteria:** Klippel-Feil anomaly (KF), unilateral or bilateral congenital sensorineural hearing loss and abducens palsy with retractio bulbi (Duane syndrome). Some authors feel that the triad need not always be complete, as in many syndromes.

**Clinical Findings:** Clinical features of the KF anomaly are limitation of movements of the head, a low hairline, and absence of the neck making the head appear to be attached to the trunk. Three subtypes are described: 1) fusion of most of the cervical vertebrae sometimes including the upper thoracic vertebrae, 2) fusion at one or two cervical or thoracic vertebrae associated with hemivertebrae and other abnormalities of the cervical spine, and 3) fusion of two or more cervical vertebrae and possibly fusion of lumbar or lower thoracic vertebrae.

The congenital hearing loss is sensorineural although a few cases of mixed hearing loss have been described. X-ray findings may include absence of the semicircular canals, a short internal auditory meatus, and incomplete cochlear and vestibular systems.

The main eye abnormality is abducens palsy with retractio bulbi of one or both eyes (Duane syndrome), i.e., an inward retraction of the orbit when looking with the affected eye in the direction of the nose.

This disorder is congenital and not progressive.

**Complications:** Cervical osteoarthritis appears at an early age. Kyphoscoliosis and the usual difficulties associated with hearing loss such as communication and speech in the hearing world.

**Associated Findings:** Other anomalies described are preauricular appendages and fistulae, auricular malformations, epibulbar dermoids and lipodermoids, cleft palate, occipital meningocoele, pseudopapilloedema, facial paralysis, bilateral subluxation of the lens, **Torticollis**, high scapula **Sprengel deformity**, kyphoscoliosis, and spina bifida.

**Etiology:** Polygenic or multifactorial inheritance with limitation to females. Sex-linked dominance with lethality in the hemizygous male is also possible.

**Pathogenesis:** Unknown.

**MIM No.:** 31460

**POS No.:** 3059

**Sex Ratio:** M7:F75

**Occurrence:** Frequency among hearing loss children has been estimated to be around 1% in England and the Netherlands.

**Risk of Recurrence for Patient's Sib:**
See Part I, *Mendelian Inheritance*.

**Risk of Recurrence for Patient's Child:**
See Part I, *Mendelian Inheritance*.

**Age of Detectability:** Within the first year of life.

**Gene Mapping and Linkage:** Unknown.

**Prevention:** None known. Genetic counseling indicated.

**Treatment:** Special education. Middle ear surgery for cases with conductive hearing loss. Eye surgery for restriction of abduction of the eye can be partly or completely corrective.

**Prognosis:** Most patients have normal intelligence, but mental retardation or "dullness" has been reported. The three main anomalies remain stationary throughout life in most cases. Life expectancy is normal.

**Detection of Carrier:** Unknown.

References:
Konigsmark BW, Gorlin RJ: Genetic and metabolic deafness, Philadelphia: W.B. Saunders, 1976.
Wildervanck LS: The cervico-oculo-acusticus syndrome. In: Vinken PJ, Bruyn GW, eds: Congenital malformations of the spine and spinal cord, handbook of clinical neurology. New York: Elsevier North-Holland, 1978; 32:123–130. *
Wilkinson M: The Klippel-Feil syndrome. In: Vinken PJ, Bruyn GW, eds: Congenital malformations of the spine and spinal cord, handbook of clinical neurology. New York: Elsevier North-Holland, 1978:111–122.
Cremers WRJ, et al.: Hearing loss in the cervico-oculo-acoustic (Wildervanck) syndrome. Arch Otolaryngol 1984; 110:54–57. *

K0023                                     **Frederick K. Kozak**

**Cervicooculofacial dysplasia**
*See CERVICO-OCULO-ACOUSTIC SYNDROME*
**CFC syndrome**
*See CARDIO-FACIAL-CUTANEOUS SYNDROME*
**Chalastoderma**
*See CUTIS LAXA*
**Chalastoderma with exposure to D-penicillamine**
*See FETAL D-PENICILLAMINE SYNDROME*
**Chanarin syndrome**
*See STORAGE DISEASE, NEUTRAL LIPID TYPE*
**Chanarin-Dorfman syndrome**
*See STORAGE DISEASE, NEUTRAL LIPID TYPE*

## CHANDS                                                      3039

**Includes:**
> Ankyloblepharon-curly hair-nail dysplasia syndrome
> Curly hair-ankyloblepharon-nail dysplasia syndrome (CHANDS)
> Hair(curly)-ankyloblepharon-nail dysplasia syndrome
> Nail dysplasia-curly hair-ankyloblepharon syndrome

**Excludes:**
> **Cleft lip/palate-filiform fusion of eyelids** (0176)
> **Ectodermal dysplasia**

**Major Diagnostic Criteria:** The presence of curly hair, ankyloblepharon, and nail dysplasia, but without other ectodermal defects, should suggest the diagnosis.

**Clinical Findings:** All affected individuals in the reported family had curly hair that did not grow past shoulder length, short and dysplastic nails, and ankyloblepharon at birth.

**Complications:** Unknown.

**Associated Findings:** None known.

**Etiology:** Probably autosomal recessive inheritance, although in the reported family, extensive inbreeding led to quasidominant transmission, with the mother and three of her eight children affected.

**Pathogenesis:** Unknown. Probably an ectodermal defect.

**MIM No.:** 21435

**POS No.:** 3845

**Sex Ratio:** M1:F1

**Occurrence:** Only one family of Dutch ethnic origin has been documented.

**Risk of Recurrence for Patient's Sib:**
> See Part I, *Mendelian Inheritance.*

**Risk of Recurrence for Patient's Child:**
> See Part I, *Mendelian Inheritance.*

**Age of Detectability:** At birth by the presence of ankyloblepharon.

**Gene Mapping and Linkage:** Unknown.

**Prevention:** None known. Genetic counseling indicated.

**Treatment:** Surgical correction of the ankyloblepharon

**Prognosis:** Normal life span and intellectual development.

**Detection of Carrier:** Unknown.

References:
Baughman FA: CHANDS: the curly hair-ankyloblepharon-nail dysplasia syndrome. BD:OAS VII(8). New York: March of Dimes Birth Defects Foundation, 1971:100–102.
Valdmanis H, et al.: Re-evaluation of CHANDS. J Med Genet 1979; 16:316–317.

T0007                                     **Helga V. Toriello**

## CHARCOT MARIE TOOTH DISEASE-DEAFNESS          2419

**Includes:**
> Charcot-Marie-Tooth disease-nephritis
> Deafness-Charcot-Marie-Tooth disease
> Friedreich ataxia-Charcot-Marie-Tooth disease-deafness

**Excludes:**
> **Neuropathy, hereditary motor and sensory, type I** (2104)
> **Neuropathy, hereditary motor and sensory, type II** (2105)
> Peripheral neuropathies (other inherited)

**Major Diagnostic Criteria:** Slowly progressive muscular weakness and atrophy that starts in the feet and peroneal muscles and is secondary to hereditary motor and sensory neuropathy. Slowly progressive sensorineural hearing loss becomes evident, usually in the second decade of life. Occasionally evidence of chronic nephritis is found. Nerve conduction velocity studies, electromyograms and audiometries are necessary for the diagnosis. Sural nerve biopsy is indicated for isolated cases.

**Clinical Findings:** Clinical signs may manifest any time in the first decade of life. Peroneal and foot weakness are the earliest signs; they cause a foot drop. As the muscle weakness progresses, pes equinovarus and pes cavus appear, in addition to obvious muscle wasting and clawing of fingers and toes. Diminished vibratory sense appears to be the first sign of sensory involvement. Intention tremor and ataxia are relatively infrequent and late signs. The patient usually becomes aware of hearing loss during the second decade of life. By the fifth decade, the hearing loss is severe.

The renal symptomatology in the few reported patients occurred during the third decade of life. Since renal involvement was not found in a large kindred, it is not clear whether the chronic interstitial nephritis reported in a small sibship is a salient clinical feature.

There is variable expressivity both within and between families. Intrafamilial variability and clinical expression of the trait is encountered. Penetrance appears to be complete. In a few patients studies, the trait was classified with the hypertrophic types of Charcot-Marie-Tooth disease through nerve biopsy findings.

**Complications:** Increasing limitations in mobility lead to wheelchair-bound existence in scores of patients. The hearing impairment is considerable and represents a handicap of long standing.

**Associated Findings:** Tonic pupils, frequently misdiagnosed as Adie syndrome (Adie, 1932). **Ataxia, Friedreich type** was reported in one family (Van Bogaert and Moreau, 1939–1940).

**Etiology:** Autosomal dominant inheritance with variable expression and complete penetrance. A large kindred with 72 affected members, 61 with hearing loss, showed male-to-male transmission on 13 occasions; on six occasions the gene was transmitted exclusively by males through three generations.

**Pathogenesis:** Segmental demyelination and onion-bulb-type hypertrophy of peripheral nerves have been documented in the studied patients.

**MIM No.:** *11830, 30290

**POS No.:** 4384

**Sex Ratio:** M1:F1

**Occurrence:** Undetermined. Probably less frequent than the other types of Charcot-Marie-Tooth disease.

**Risk of Recurrence for Patient's Sib:**
> See Part I, *Mendelian Inheritance.*

**Risk of Recurrence for Patient's Child:**
See Part I, *Mendelian Inheritance.*

**Age of Detectability:** Usually clinically evident by 10–20 years of age; earlier onset of clinical signs and symptoms occurs. Clinically, the hearing loss appears to lag behind the signs of neuropathy by 5–10 years.

**Gene Mapping and Linkage:** Unknown.

**Prevention:** None known. Genetic counseling indicated.

**Treatment:** Palliative. Orthopedic procedures and devices and hearing aids prolong the duration of an independent life-style.

**Prognosis:** Life-span does not appear to be shortened. Due to the physical handicaps, change of life-style occurs in most patients. Intelligence is normal.

**Detection of Carrier:** Detailed diagnostic evaluation, including skeletal survey and a test for color blindness, of the first-degree relatives should detect those who are minimally affected.

**References:**
Taylor J: Peroneal atrophy. Proc Roy Soc Med 1912; 642:50–51.
Adie WJ: Tonic pupils and absent tendon reflexes. Brain 1932; 55:98–113.
Van Bogaert L, Moreau M: Combinaison de l'amyotrophie de Charcot-Marie-Tooth et de la maladie de Friedreich chez plusieurs membres d'une meme famille. Encephale 1939–1940; 34:312–320.
Lemieux G, Neemeh JA: Charcot-Marie-Tooth disease and nephritis. Can Med Assoc J 1967; 97:1193–1198.
Hanson PA, et al.: Distal muscle wasting, nephritis and deafness. Neurology 1970; 20:426–434.
Kousseff BG, et al.: Charcot-Marie-Tooth disease with sensorineural hearing loss-an autosomal dominant trait. BD:OAS XVIII(3B). New York: March of Dimes Birth Defects Foundation, 1982:223–228. *

K0018            **Boris G. Kousseff**

**Charcot-Marie-Tooth disease with optico-acoustic degeneration**
*See DEAFNESS-POLYNEUROPATHY-OPTIC ATROPHY*
**Charcot-Marie-Tooth disease with skeletal and laryngeal anomalies**
*See NEUROPATHY, CONGENITAL MOTOR & SENSORY-SKELETAL-LARYNGEAL DEFECTS*
**Charcot-Marie-Tooth disease, hypertrophic (some cases)**
*See NEUROPATHY, HEREDITARY MOTOR AND SENSORY, TYPE I*
**Charcot-Marie-Tooth disease, neuronal (some cases)**
*See NEUROPATHY, HEREDITARY MOTOR AND SENSORY, TYPE II*
**Charcot-Marie-Tooth disease, slow nerve conduction type**
*See NEUROPATHY, HEREDITARY MOTOR AND SENSORY, TYPE I*
**Charcot-Marie-Tooth disease-nephritis**
*See CHARCOT MARIE TOOTH DISEASE-DEAFNESS*
**Charcot-Marie-Tooth peroneal muscular atrophy**
*See NEUROPATHY, HEREDITARY MOTOR AND SENSORY, TYPE I*

---

**CHARGE ASSOCIATION**           **2124**

**Includes:**
    CHARGE syndrome
    Choanal atresia, posterior

**Excludes:**
    **Antley-Bixler syndrome** (2125)
    **Cat eye syndrome** (0544)
    **Chromosome 4, monosomy 4p** (0164)
    **Eye, microphthalmia/coloboma** (0661)
    **Nose, choanal atresia-lymphedema** (2597)
    **Nose, posterior atresia** (0727)

**Major Diagnostic Criteria:** The acronym CHARGE has been used to represent the major features of this condition: *c*oloboma of the eye or eye defects, *h*eart disease, choanal *a*tresia, *r*etarded growth and development with or without CNS anomalies, *g*enital hypoplasia, and *e*ar anomalies with or without deafness (Pagon et al., 1981). To be classified as having CHARGE association, the patient must have two or more of the defects.

**Clinical Findings:** The association of certain defects with choanal atresia was first reported by Hall (1979). Subsequently, Pagon et al. (1981) suggested CHARGE as an acronym for this association. More recently, Davenport et al. (1986) postulated that the condi-

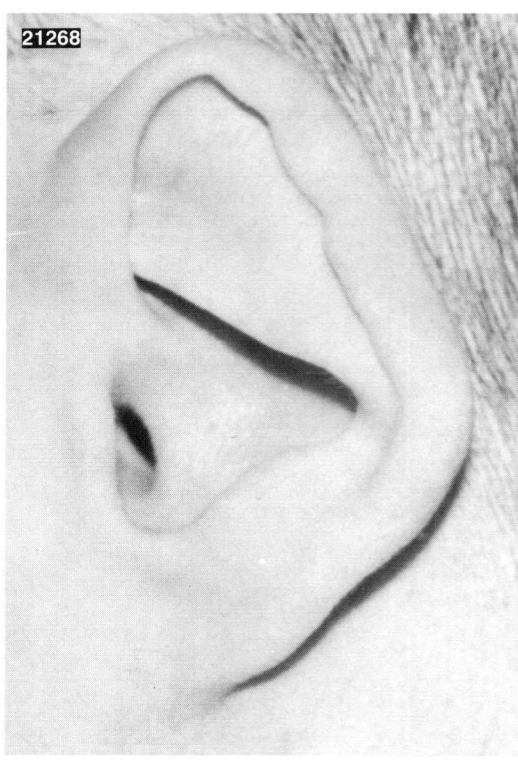

2124-21268: The ear of a patient with CHARGE association demonstrating the characteristic triangular shape of the concha.

---

tion constitutes a syndrome rather than a nonrandom association of defects.

At birth, choanal atresia can represent a life-threatening anomaly if not recognized immediately and treated promptly. This defect may be either bilateral or unilateral, with membranous and sometimes bony obstruction of the posterior choanae. Anomalies of the heart include patent ductus arteriosus, double outlet right ventricle with atrioventricular canal, tetralogy of Fallot, ventricular septal defect, atrial septal defect, and right-sided aortic arch with a vascular ring. A careful assessment of the heart is needed in any neonate with recognized choanal atresia.

Approximately 80% of cases have ocular colobomas. These defects vary from unilateral or bilateral typical colobomas of the iris, choroid, retina, or disk and optic nerve to clinical anophthalmia. Due to the colobomatous malformations, visual impairment and retinal detachments can occur.

Mental retardation is present in most patients with CHARGE association and ranges in severity from mild to severe (IQ range, 30–80).

Newborns with this condition are usually normal in length and weight at birth. By age six months, however, 80% of patients show linear growth at or below the 3rd percentile. In addition, partial growth hormone deficiency may contribute to the short stature and retarded bone age.

Other consistent findings in CHARGE association are hypoplastic genitalia and cryptochidism in male patients. In these males, one-half have microphallus. Three patients with anosmia-hypogonadotrophic hypogonadism or Kallmann syndrome have been reported.

Ear abnormalities have also been noted. The spectrum of external ear abnormalities includes reduction in size to cup-shaped hypoplastic ear. Hearing loss also occurs. It may be either conductive or sensorineural, and varies from mild to profound.

Other anomalies reported include micrognathia, cleft lip, cleft palate or bifid uvula, Robin sequence, unilateral facial palsy or facial asymmetry, velopharyngeal incompetency, the DiGeorge sequence with its associated problems, and **Vater association**.

**Complications:** Decreased visual acuity, limited visual fields, myopia, retinal detachment, and optic atrophy are secondary to the colobomatous defects. Respiratory failure during the newborn period most frequently results from the choanal atresia. However, if Robin sequence (micrognathia, posterior placement of the tongue, and cleft palate) is present, airway obstruction may occur from glossoptosis. Congestive heart failure may develop as the result of a congenital heart defect.

**Associated Findings:** Dysmorphic findings of the face include flattened, squared, and asymmetric face; asymmetry of the ears; malar hypoplasia; long philtrum; and lower lip frenula. Urinary tract defects include bilateral ureteral reflux, urethral atresia, hydronephrosis, urethroperitoneal fistulae, and posterior urethral valves. Imperforate anus and **Pectus carinatum** have also been reported.

**Etiology:** In most situations the case is an isolated one, and the etiology is undetermined. However, autosomal dominant and recessive inheritance have been reported; thus, a family history is essential. Multiple inheritance patterns also suggest that the condition is heterogeneous.

**Pathogenesis:** Unknown.

**MIM No.:** 21480

**POS No.:** 3480

**Sex Ratio:** M2:F1

**Occurrence:** Over 50 cases have been reported.

**Risk of Recurrence for Patient's Sib:**
See Part I, *Mendelian Inheritance*. If of nongenetic etiology, probably less than 1%.

**Risk of Recurrence for Patient's Child:**
See Part I, *Mendelian Inheritance*. There have been no reports of reproduction in affected individuals.

**Age of Detectability:** Usually at birth.

**Gene Mapping and Linkage:** Unknown.

**Prevention:** None known. Genetic counseling indicated.

**Treatment:** Surgical treatment is usually required for the choanal atresia and may be required for palliation or correction of any heart defect that is present. Because of the frequency of intellectual impairment, all patients should have developmental and intelligence testing done at appropriate times. Hearing aids and intensive speech and language therapy should be instituted for children with hearing deficiencies. Visual correction, if needed, should be done during early childhood. If a growth hormone deficiency is present, replacement therapy should be considered. In addition, testosterone therapy may be used effectively for achieving phallic enlargement in patients with microphallus. Testosterone supplementation for males also has been suggested if inadequate development occurs at puberty.

**Prognosis:** Variable, depending on the extent of the defects and severity of the retardation. If the choanal atresia and congenital heart defects are successfully treated, normal life span is expected.

**Detection of Carrier:** Clinical examination and family history.

**References:**
Hall BD: Choanal atresia and associated multiple anomalies. J Pediatr 1979; 95:395–398.
Pagon RA, et al.: Coloboma, congenital heart disease, and choanal atresia with multiple anomalies: CHARGE association. J Pediatr 1981; 99:223–227. *
Koletzko B, Majewski F: Congenital anomalies in patients with choanal atresia: CHARGE association. Europ J Pediatr 1984; 142:271–275.
Davenport SL, et al.: The spectrum of clinical features in CHARGE syndrome. Clin Genet 1986; 29:298–310. †
Goldson E, et al.: The CHARGE association: how well can they do? Am J Dis Child 1986; 140:918–921.
Metlay LA, et al.: Familial CHARGE syndrome: clinical report with autopsy findings. Am J Med Genet 1987; 26:577–581.

Meinecke P, et al.: Limb anomalies in the CHARGE association. J Med Genet 1989; 26:202–203. †

ES004
WE005

**Luis F. Escobar**
**David D. Weaver**

**CHARGE syndrome**
*See CHARGE ASSOCIATION*
**Charlevoix disease (one type)**
*See CORPUS CALLOSUM AGENESIS-SENSORIMOTOR NEUROPATHY, FAMILIAL*
**Charlevoix-Saguenay spastic ataxia**
*See SPASTIC ATAXIA, CHARLEVOIX-SAGUENAY TYPE*

## CHARLIE M SYNDROME 2170

**Includes:**
Face-limb syndrome (one form)
Limb-face syndrome (one form)

**Excludes:**
**Amniotic bands syndrome** (0874)
**Diplegia, congenital facial** (0376)
**Hypoglossia-hypodactylia** (0451)

**Major Diagnostic Criteria:** Differentiating between Charlie M patients and those with other disorders within the face-limb syndrome community is controversial and requires a typical facies with hypertelorism, small mouth, cleft palate, dental anomalies, and digital anomalies.

**Clinical Findings:** These are manifest at birth and include distal, asymmetric, amputation-like defects of the limbs, cleft hard or soft palate without cleft lip, and dental abnormalities including absent or hypoplastic incisors, which may be in a conical crown form. There is midface hypoplasia with broad nose, hypertelorism, small mouth and philtrum, micrognathia, and variable degrees of facial nerve paralysis. Cone-shaped or ivory epiphyses may be seen on hand X-rays.

**Complications:** Nasal speech due to cleft palate, and a mild conductive hearing loss, were documented in one patient. Intelligence is unaffected.

**Associated Findings:** Until definitive evidence is available for separating Charlie M from other face-limb syndromes, several malformations typical of this patient community must be considered. These include aglossia or **Tongue, cleft**, **Poland syndrome**, and congenital contractures such as clubfoot. A patient of R. Hoehn, cited by Kaplan et al. (1976), had cleft lower eyelid and **Nose, bifid**.

**Etiology:** There is no evidence of genetic transmission, partial manifestations in relatives, or consanguinity in the five reported families. The male predominance may suggest polygenic or X-linked inheritance.

**Pathogenesis:** The limb anomalies in conjunction with facial clefts suggest amniotic bands or vascular hemorrhage with necrosis as pathogenetic factors.

**POS No.:** 3182

**Sex Ratio:** M1:F0

**Occurrence:** About five families have been reported.

**Risk of Recurrence for Patient's Sib:** Minimal, based on current data.

**Risk of Recurrence for Patient's Child:** Minimal, although there is no documented instance of reproduction.

**Age of Detectability:** The disorder is obvious at birth, with potential prenatal detection by ultrasound imaging of limb and facial defects.

**Gene Mapping and Linkage:** Unknown.

**Prevention:** None known. Genetic counseling indicated.

**Treatment:** Orthopedic therapy, plastic surgery, and physical therapy are required for limb and facial defects. Patients with oral clefts will need surveillance for otitis, conductive hearing loss, and speech problems.

**Prognosis:** Normal life span and intelligence can be anticipated, although long-term follow-up of reported cases is not available.

**Detection of Carrier:** Unknown.

**Special Considerations:** Further delineation of the face-limb malformation community will be required before Charlie M syndrome can be considered a definite entity. The distinctive facies of at least two patients affords preliminary support for its recognition as a discrete syndrome.

**Hypoglossia-hypodactylia**, Hanhart syndrome, Glossopalatine ankylosis syndrome, **Charlie M syndrome**, and Moebius syndrome are grouped together under the category of *Oromandibular-Limb Hypogenesis syndrome*. These are clearly overlapping conditions of unknown etiology. While we recognize that these may be variants of an environmentally (or other) induced spectrum of anomalies, the *Encyclopedia* has placed Hanhart syndrome and Glossopalatine ankylosis under the title **Hypoglossia-hypodactylia** and has separate articles on Moebius syndrome (**Diplegia, congenital facial**) and **Charlie M syndrome**.

**References:**
Gorlin RJ: Some facial syndromes. BD:OAS V(2). New York: March of Dimes Birth Defects Foundation, 1969:66–76.
Kaplan P, et al.: A "community" of face-limb malformation syndromes. J Pediatr 1976; 89:241–247.†
Bonioli E, et al.: The "Charlie M" syndrome: a new clinical entity? Description of a case. Minerva Pediatr 1980; 32:699–702. *

WI024                                                    **Golder N. Wilson**

**Chediak (anomaly, syndrome, or disease)**
*See CHEDIAK-HIGASHI SYNDROME*

---

## CHEDIAK-HIGASHI SYNDROME                              0143

**Includes:**
Albinism, incomplete oculocutaneous
Beguez Cesar-Steinbrinck-Chediak-Higashi syndrome
Chediak (anomaly, syndrome, or disease)
Chediak-Steinbrinck syndrome
Constitutional giant granulations of leukocytes, hereditary
Constitutional granular gigantism
Gigantism of cytoplasmic organelles, hereditary
Gigantism of peroxidase granules, congenital
Leukocytes, granulation anomaly of
Lymphocytes, natural killer, defect in
Panleukocytic granulation, anomalous

**Excludes:**
Alder-Reilly anomaly
Dohle bodies
May-Hegglin anomaly
Riley bodies

**Major Diagnostic Criteria:** The pathognomonic feature of this syndrome is the presence of giant lysosomal granules in the granulocytes of the peripheral blood. The examination for these granules should be prompted by a combination of fevers of unknown origin, recurrent bacterial infections, and the pigmentation abnormalities described below. Less commonly, the neurologic features or the accelerated phase of this C-H syndrome may bring the patient to medical attention.

**Clinical Findings:** The principal clinical features of this disorder are a pseudoalbinism or pigmentary dilution, frequent bacterial infections, and hematologic abnormalities. The skin is light cream to slate gray and may approach albinism in offspring of pale individuals. After exposure to sunlight, the skin may develop papillary or hyperpigmented lesions. The decreased hair pigmentation may cause color variations from light blond to brunette, often with a prominent silver-gray sheen. The hypopigmentation of hair and skin may only be evident on comparison with other family members. The eyes usually have decreased or absent uveal pigment and resultant photophobia and nystagmus in the majority of patients. The hair may be examined microscopically to reveal the giant melanin granules. Frequent bacterial infections, which

are the characteristic that usually brings the patient to the attention of a physician, are a complication of the disorder and are described below.

Hematologic abnormalities are reflected in each of the cellular elements of blood. Granulocytes of all types display one or more characteristic giant granules. Not every cell will contain giant granules, and most that do also contain some normal-appearing granules as well. Lymphocytes and monocytes may also contain one or more enlarged azurophilic granules. Other morphologic features of the leukocytes are unaltered. Giant granulation of platelets has been reported less frequently and may be absent or may vary from 1 in 1,000 platelets to as high as 5% of platelets. Erythrocytes are of normal microscopic appearance unless influenced secondarily. However, anemias occur in over 80% of cases, most often in association with the accelerated phase. Leukopenia is present at times in the majority of cases, but even in the face of a normal total leukocyte count most patients will have chronic or intermittent depressions of absolute granulocyte counts and diminished granulocyte responses to infection or steroid challenge. Bone marrows are usually normocellular to hypercellular. Giant granulations are found in myeloid precursors and mature forms and in some erythroid precursors. Extensive vacuolization of bone marrow neutrophils and their precursors has been described in several cases and is attributed to ineffective myelopoiesis with intramedullary granulocyte destruction. Serum lysozyme (muramidase) levels were consistently and markedly elevated in these cases.

Functional studies of C-H neutrophils and mononuclear phagocytosis reveal several abnormalities. Skin window cell mobilization may be decreased. Chemotactic responses of neutrophils and monocytes are depressed, probably on the basis of an effector defect rather than a deficient receptor mechanism. Phagocytic indices in vitro are normal to increased, but degranulation and bactericidal functions are depressed, especially early or when encountering a large bacterial challenge. C-H neutrophils have a resting metabolic rate above normal and respond to challenge with a normal metabolic burst. In vitro surface adherence of C-H neutrophils may be depressed.

Parameters of specific immunity as reflected in lymphocyte numbers, immunoglobulin levels, capacities for delayed hypersensitivity, and antibody formation have routinely been normal in the absence of the accelerated phase. Where studied, patients have shown deficiencies in both natural killer (NK) cell function and antibody-dependent cell-mediated cytolysis (ADCC). NK cells, as reflected in the large granular lymphocyte population, are present in normal numbers but demonstrate the giant granular abnormality. While the exact mechanisms of NK cell dysfunction remain in doubt, these cells in the C-H syndrome appear to posseess the basic cellular systems necessary to function as lytic effector cells.

A large minority of patients have had easy bruising, epistaxis, or intestinal bleeding. These bleeding diatheses are not always accompanied by thrombocytopenia, although the latter is present in about one-half of the C-H cases, especially during the accelerated phase. The platelets from many patients, with or without bleeding, have a storage pool deficiency of nucleotides, serotonin, and releasable divalent cations detectable by platelet aggregometry. The patients may show a prolonged bleeding time. Coagulation studies are usually normal in the absence of the accelerated phase.

Many patients have neurologic dysfunctions that may take the form of ataxia, muscle weakness, decreased deep tendon reflexes, sensory loss, diffusely abnormal electroencephalogram, abnormal electromyogram, decreased motor nerve conduction velocity, or, rarely, convulsions. Hypotonia of the upper and lower gastrointestinal tract has been reported. Patients may have defective stereovision, abnormal visually evoked potentials, or asymmetric auditory brainstem responses; all findings similar to those seen in true oculocutaneous albinism. Mental retardation has been reported in 10–15% of cases; about two-thirds of those with mental retardation have come from consanguineous parentage.

Giant granules have also been observed in melanocytes, plasma cells, histiocytes, liver parenchymal and Kupffer cells, adrenal cortex, anterior pituitary, vascular endothelium and pericytes, neurons, Schwann cells, renal tubules, gut epithelium, thyroid, osteoclasts, and fibroblasts in cell cultures.

There are no characteristic X-ray findings in this disorder.

**Complications:** The major complications of the C-H syndrome are recurrent bacterial infections. Reported cases have most often had infections of the upper and lower respiratory tract and skin (50–90%). Infections of the gastrointestinal tract, ears, and urinary tract are a less frequent but significant part of the infectious complications. Periodontal disease may be especially pronounced with secondary loss of teeth at an early age. Among the numerous bacterial pathogens encountered in this syndrome, only *Staphylococcus* has been reported with any notable dominance. Infections may be occult and suggested only by fevers of unknown origin. The infections accompanying the C-H syndrome are usually not as severe as those seen in children with agammaglobulinemia or chronic granulomatous disease. Fungal infections do not occur with an appreciably greater frequency than in the general population. C-H syndrome patients do not appear to be at any increased risk for viral infections.

The accelerated phase of the disorder is a lymphohistiocytic proliferation of unknown origin that occurs in the great majority of cases. It is characterized by hepatosplenomegaly, lymphadenopathy, and accentuations of the anemia, neutropenia, and thrombocytopenia. Coombs-negative hemolysis is frequent. Neurologic findings may become worse or may arise anew during the accelerated phase. Previously normal tests of liver function, coagulation, immunoglobulins, and cellular immunity may become abnormal. Histologically, the accelerated phase is characterized by infiltrates of mature-appearing lymphocytes and monocytes or histiocytes without significant numbers of plasma cells, eosinophils, or neutrophils. The infiltrates are often perivascular, and usually there is little destruction of normal tissue architecture. Erythrophagocytosis is seen in about one-third of the cases with the accelerated phase.

There have been reports of very high titers of some Epstein-Barr virus-induced antibodies in some patients before any evidence of accelerated phase development. Titers as high as those reported are usually seen only with Burkitt lymphoma, and the reporting authors speculate that the accelerated phase may be due to a population of Epstein-Barr virus-transformed cells that are not suppressed because of the defective NK and ADCC activity. The cellular infiltrate in the accelerated phase has been identified as being due to T lymphocytes in at least one patient.

**Associated Findings:** A few patients have been reported with varieties of hyperlipidemia. In one patient there was also a glucose-6-phosphate dehydrogenase deficiency. The rather high incidence of consanguinity in these families suggests that the above findings may occur by chance association.

**Etiology:** Autosomal recessive inheritance of a single defective gene. The primary lesion of this syndrome appears to reside in the formation of defective giant cytoplasmic granulations of numerous cell types. The biochemical basis of this lesion is unknown.

**Pathogenesis:** Giant cytoplasmic granulations appear in infancy in a variety of cell types. In general, the giant granulations resemble the normal granules of the specific cell type in both fine structure and cytochemical reactions. The best studied of the cells with giant granules are the neutrophils. Enlarged granules are found in neutrophil precursors of the bone marrow at a stage shortly after granule formation has begun. The giant granules are the product of abnormal fusion of normal-sized granules, initially involving azurophilic granules. Later the specific granules of the neutrophil participate, resulting in giant granules taking the character of secondary lysosomes. This process continues after cell maturation and during circulation in the peripheral blood. One consequence of the fusion of both azurophilic and specific granules appears to be a labilization and loss of some lysosomal enzyme activity. The giant granules fail to participate significantly in the degranulation process. Depletion of normal granules and the failure of the giant granules to fuse with phagosomes may largely explain the bacterial defect noted above. Present evidence indicates that the underlying fault in C-H neutrophils lies in a

membrane abnormality that fosters the giant granule formation. This membrane fault may be linked in some way to microtubule assembly, which some authors have found defective.

The pigmentary dilution appears to be due to a similar process of melanosome fusion that results in giant melanin granules. These granules are improperly distributed in tissues, leading to the clinically noted pigmentation abnormalities.

The mechanism whereby the genetic fault in this syndrome leads to the neurologic dysfunctions and the accelerated phase of the disease remains unknown.

**MIM No.:** *21450

**POS No.:** 3060

**Sex Ratio:** M1:F1

**Occurrence:** Very rare; less than 100 cases reported. Cases have come from over 15 countries on four continents and have involved several races, including Orientals and blacks.

**Risk of Recurrence for Patient's Sib:**
See Part I, *Mendelian Inheritance.*

**Risk of Recurrence for Patient's Child:**
See Part I, *Mendelian Inheritance.* Two-thirds of unaffected sibs of a patient will be heterozygous carriers of the C-H gene.

**Age of Detectability:** Birth to a few months of age.

**Gene Mapping and Linkage:** Unknown.

**Prevention:** None known. Genetic counseling indicated.

**Treatment:** Primary disorder: high-dose vitamin C (ascorbic acid), 200 mg in infants to as high as 6 g per day in adults orally, has been advocated for long-term treatment of patients with this syndrome. The rationale for this therapy is derived from the observed potentiation by ascorbic acid of directed cell movement of normal monocytes and neutrophils. Where tested, there has been a partial restoration of neutrophil chemotaxis and normalization of bactericidal function. NK cell function remains abnormal after vitimin C therapy. The ultimate efficacy of vitamin C in preventing the neurological features or the accelerated phase of the disorder is unevaluated. However, one patient is reported to have developed the accelerated phase while taking vitamin C. Parenteral lithium chloride has been shown in a single study to improve the bactericidal function of neutrophils from beige mice, an animal analog of the C-H syndrome. The latter form of treatment has not been tried in human C-H patients. Bone marrow transplantation successfully converted the neutrophil and NK cell abnormalities in one patient.

The infectious episodes require vigorous specific and supportive therapy as indicated by the site of infection, the pathogen, and complications.

The accelerated phase has usually been treated as a form of lymphoid malignancy. Vinca alkaloids in conjunction with steroids have been effective in causing remissions; however, these have most often been temporary, and death has occurred within months. Splenectomy has produced a transient effect in patients with evidence of hypersplenism, but this has not demonstrably altered the lethal course of the disease.

**Prognosis:** Of reported cases, about 60% have died (average age at death, 4 years), and less than 10% have survived beyond age 20 years.

**Detection of Carrier:** Heterozygous carriers can occasionally be detected by finding rare giant granules in leukocytes during microscopic examination, but this is not sensitive enough to be useful as a carrier test. The carriers do not demonstrate functional abnormalities or clinical findings. One author has reported an abnormal enzyme pattern in the leukocytes of probable carriers that may serve to identify the carrier state.

**Special Considerations:** An analogous anomaly has been described in beige mice, Aleutian mink, Hereford cattle, cats, and a killer whale. There have been a few reports of individual patients with a giant granule anomaly of their leukocytes but who lack some of the more typical findings of this syndrome. Therefore, these patients have been presented as possible newly described entities. None of these patients has been evaluated completely enough to know whether or not they are unusual examples of the C-H syndrome.

**References:**
Blume RS, Wolff SM: The Chédiak-Higashi syndrome: studies in four patients and a review of the literature. Medicine 1972; 51:247–280. *
Boxer LA, et al.: Correction of leukocyte function in Chédiak-Higashi syndrome by ascorbate. N Engl J Med 1976; 295:1041–1045.
Clawson CC, et al.: The Chédiak-Higashi syndrome: quantitation of a deficiency in maximal bactericidal capacity. Am J Pathol 1979; 94:539–548.
Tanaka T: Chediak-Higashi syndrome: abnormal lysosomal enzyme levels in granulocytes of patients and family members. Pediatr Res 1980; 14:901–904.
White JG, Clawson CC: The Chédiak-Higashi syndrome: the nature of the giant neutrophil granules and their interactions with cytoplasm and foreign particulates. Am J Pathol 1980; 98:151–196.
Weening RS, et al.: Effects of ascorbate on abnormal neutrophil, platelet, and lymphocyte function in a patient with the Chediak-Higashi syndrome. Blood 1981; 57:856–865.
Roder JC, et al.: The Chediak-Higashi gene in humans. III. Studies on the mechanisms of NK impairment. Clin Exp Immunol 1983; 51:359–368.
Penner JD, Prieur DJ: Interspecific genetic complementation analysis with fibroblasts from humans and four species of animals with Chediak-Hagashi syndrome. Am J Med Genet 1987; 28:455–470.

CL008                                                      **C.C. Clawson**

**Chediak-Higashi-like syndrome**
*See HYPOPIGMENTATION-IMMUNE DEFECT, GRISCELLI TYPE*
**Chediak-Steinbrinck syndrome**
*See CHEDIAK-HIGASHI SYNDROME*
**Cheek-eyebrow-ichthyosis syndrome**
*See ICHTHYOSIS-CHEEK-EYEBROW SYNDROME*
**Cheilitis glandularis apostematosa**
*See LIP, CHEILITIS GLANDULARIS*
**Cheilitis granulomatosa (oligosymptomatic forms)**
*See CHEILITIS GRANULOMATOSA, MELKERSSON-ROSENTHAL TYPE*

## CHEILITIS GRANULOMATOSA, MELKERSSON-ROSENTHAL TYPE                                          2083

**Includes:**
  Cheilitis granulomatosa (oligosymptomatic forms)
  Meischer cheilitis (oligosymptomatic forms)
  Melkersson-Rosenthal syndrome

**Excludes:**
  Abscess
  **Amyloidosis, Finnish type** (2145)
  **Angioedema, hereditary** (0054)
  **Ankylosing spondylitis** (2516)
  **Blepharochalasis-double lip-nontoxic goiter** (0111)
  Cellulitis
  Erysipelis
  Herpes labialis
  **Lip, cheilitis glandularis** (0144)
  Lymphangioma
  Oro-facial granulomatosis
  **Palsy, late-onset facial, familial** (0378)
  **Sarcoidosis** (2966)
  Tuberculosis
  Uveoparotid fever

**Major Diagnostic Criteria:** Facial swelling, facial paralysis and fissured tongue.

**Clinical Findings:** Sudden onset of unilateral or bilateral non-pitting asymptomatic swelling of one or both lips, usually the upper, sometimes producing a reddish brown appearance and which may become recurrent and then permanent. Swelling may also involve the eyelids, nose, chin and forehead. Usually following this swelling, but sometimes preceding it or occurring simultaneously, is a peripheral facial nerve paralysis (Bell's palsy, see **Palsy, late-onset facial, familial**) either complete or incomplete,

unilateral or bilateral, and usually but not always ipsilateral with the swelling. Accompanying the swelling and/or paralysis may be a fissured tongue. Histologically the swollen tissues exhibit most commonly a perivascular chronic granulomatous inflammation of lymphohistiocytic, sarcoidal or tuberculoid type located in the lamina propria and sometimes in the muscle and/or accessory salivary gland; in other cases only a lymphedematous reaction is seen.

**Complications:** Chapping and fissuring of lip, taste deficit along anterior two-thirds of tongue, occasional permanent facial paralysis, corneal drying, and migraine headache.

**Associated Findings:** Herpes labialis, hyperpyrexia, chills, auditory and visual disturbances, swelling of hands, chest and buttocks, acroparesthesia, hyperhidrosis, hyposialosis, blepharospasm, epiphora, hypacusia, megacolon, **Cancer, Hodgkin disease, familial**, Anderson-Fabry disease, hairy cell leukemia.

**Etiology:** Presumabbly autosomal dominant inheritance. Postulated causes include genetically determined defects in autonomic nervous system, exposure to cold, sarcoidosis, tuberculosis, or herpes virus.

**Pathogenesis:** Undetermined. Postulations include allergy, local immune response angioneurotic edema, and vasomotor disturbance in vasa vasorum of vessels supplying facial nerve and neighboring subcutaneous tissue produces edema of both nerve and face, and endovasal granulomatous lymphangitis.

**MIM No.:** *15590

**POS No.:** 3491

**Sex Ratio:** M1:F1

**Occurrence:** About one-half dozen kindreds have been documented in the literature, including one Greek kindred.

**Risk of Recurrence for Patient's Sib:**
  See Part I, *Mendelian Inheritance.*

**Risk of Recurrence for Patient's Child:**
  See Part I, *Mendelian Inheritance.*

**Age of Detectability:** Swelling usually begins during childhood; paralysis may be observed in childhood or young adulthood.

**Gene Mapping and Linkage:** Unknown.

**Prevention:** None known. Genetic counseling indicated.

**Treatment:** For swelling: intralesional steroid injections, cold packs and skin care during acute phase, cosmetic surgical reduction if swelling becomes permanent. For paralysis: protection of cornea, decompression of facial nerve, prednisone.

**Prognosis:** Both swelling and paralysis may be self-limiting but commonly become recurrent.

**Detection of Carrier:** Unknown.

**References:**
Carr RD: Is the Melkersson-Rosenthal syndrome hereditary? Arch Dermatol 1966; 93:426–427.
Vistness LM, Kernahan DA: The Melkersson-Rosenthal syndrome. Plast Reconstr Surg 1971; 48:126–132.
Lygidakis C, et al.: Melkersson-Rosenthal's syndrome in four generations. Clin Genet 1979; 15:189–192.
Graff-Radford SB: Melkersson-Rosenthal syndrome: a review of the literature and a case report. S Afr Med J 1981; 60:71–74.
Worsaae N, et al.: Melkersson-Rosenthal syndrome and cheilitis granulomatosa: a clinicopathologic study of 33 patients with special reference to their oral lesions. Oral Surg 1982; 54:404–413. * †
Hernandez G, et al.: Miescher's granulomatous cheilitis: Surg 1986; 44:474–478. *

G0009                                                **Lawrence I. Goldblatt**

**Cheilopalatoschisis**
  *See CLEFT LIP*
**Cheiloschisis**
  *See CLEFT LIP*
**Cheirolumbar dysostosis**
  *See DYSOSTOSIS, CHEIROLUMBAR*
**Chemke syndrome**
  *See WALKER-WARBURG SYNDROME*

**Chemodectoma of neck**
  See CAROTID BODY TUMOR
**Cheney syndrome**
  See OSTEOLYSIS, ESSENTIAL
  also HAJDU-CHENEY SYNDROME
**Cherry-red spot-myoclonus syndrome**
  See MUCOLIPIDOSIS I
**Cherry-red spot-myoclonus with dementia**
  See GALACTOSIALIDOSIS

---

## CHERUBISM                                         0539

**Includes:** Jaws, intraosseous fibrous swelling

**Excludes:**
  Dentigerous keratocysts
  Fibrous dysplasia of jaws
  Giant cell (reparative) granuloma of jaws
  Giant cell tumor of jaws
  Infantile cortical hyperostosis of jaws
  **Nevoid basal cell carcinoma syndrome** (0101)
  Odontogenic keratocysts
  Pseudohypoparathyroidism

**Major Diagnostic Criteria:** Clinical swellings occur at angles of mandible, with X-ray evidence of bilateral, radiolucent lesions in molar-angle region. Biopsy should be performed to establish diagnosis.

**Clinical Findings:** Exaggerated chubbiness of face, especially over angles of mandible. In more severe cases, there may be extensive maxillary swelling with involvement of orbital floor causing upward displacement of globe and exposure of scleral rims. In extreme cases, the swellings may result in a grotesque facial deformity. Swellings are due to expansion of mandible and maxilla. On X-ray, the lesions are bilaterally symmetric, radiolucent, and usually multilocular in character. Alkaline phosphatase may be slightly elevated. Other laboratory studies are generally within normal limits. In several reports, lesions have been noted in other bones (rib, humerus, femur). These appear to be incidental findings and may not be related to cherubism. In some cases, the submandibular and cervical lymph nodes have been enlarged by 50%.

Bilateral symmetric involvement of mandibular molar region, angle of mandible, or ascending ramus of mandible is 100%. The frequency of involvement of the entire mandible is unknown; it is probably less than 25%. Bilateral symmetric involvement of the posterior maxillary (tuberosity) area is 60%. The frequency of involvement of the entire maxilla is unknown; it is probably less than 20%. There is apparently a considerable range of involvement in cherubism. While bilateral lesions at the angles of the mandible are necessary for the diagnosis and represent the consistent feature of the disease, cases are known where children first presented with unilateral swellings but developed bilateral involvement while under observation. Expansion of the posterior maxillary region (tuberosity) represents the mildest maxillary involvement and is present in about 2/3 of cases. In the more severe examples, the entire maxilla and mandible may be involved. The affected child is normal at birth, and swellings may become apparent between one and eight years of age.

The natural history of this disease is not well understood, and treatment is not standardized. Some instances regress without treatment in early adult life, while in others, the deformity remains or is slowly progressive. No instances of malignant change are known.

**Complications:** In severe cases, there may be severe deformity and difficulty with mastication, swallowing, respiration, or speech, and visual distortions such as diplopia. Tumor may displace teeth.

**Associated Findings:** There are several reports of asymptomatic, isolated lesions in other bones. In most cases, these have not been studied histologically, and the relation of such lesions to cherubism is uncertain. Several cases have had multiple warty nevi or multiple café-au-lait spots.

**Etiology:** Autosomal dominant inheritance with variable expressivity and possibly reduced penetrance in females (50–70%). Isolated cases may be due to new mutations. In many instances, one parent will have only a history of prominent facial swellings or X-ray evidence of abnormal bone pattern in the mandible, but is not overtly affected at the time of examination. Some lesions may heal spontaneously.

**Pathogenesis:** Grossly, the lesion is soft to fibrous in character and appears whitish to reddish in color. Microscopically, it is composed of fibroblasts, polyhedral mononuclear cells, and varying numbers of multinucleated giant cells. The tissue closely resembles that of the giant cell granuloma (benign giant cell tumor) of the jaws. Some authorities consider that cherubism is microscopically indistinguishable from giant cell granuloma, while others believe the microscopic features of cherubism are distinctive and diagnostic. (This contributor subscribes to the former view.) Lesions continue to enlarge until about puberty when they often, but not always, regress. In some patients, small lesions completely heal, with only slight enlargement of bones as the end result.

**MIM No.:** *11840

**POS No.:** 3266

**Sex Ratio:** Presumably M1:F1. Reported cases show male predominance (actual M2:F1), but male-to-male transmission rules out X-linkage.

**Occurrence:** About 150 have been reported.

**Risk of Recurrence for Patient's Sib:**
  See Part I, *Mendelian Inheritance.*

**Risk of Recurrence for Patient's Child:**
  See Part I, *Mendelian Inheritance.*

**Age of Detectability:** Facial swelling usually becomes noticeable between ages 2–4 years. In less severe cases, swelling may not be apparent until ages 6 or 7 years. In a few instances, swellings have been apparent by one year of age.

**Gene Mapping and Linkage:** Unknown.

**Prevention:** None known. Genetic counseling indicated.

**Treatment:** Management is not standardized. Some cases have shown regression and considerable improvement in early adult life. In others, the deformity has continued and even slowly progressed. Conservative surgical curettage performed early has given good results in some cases and poor results in others. A more radical surgical approach has been advocated for extensive lesions. Others have suggested delay of therapy until late adolescence or early adult life and then operative reduction of the expanded bone. Radiation therapy has given poor results and is contraindicated due to the possible sequelae of osteoradionecrosis and induction of sarcoma. Prosthetic replacement of teeth may be helpful.

**Prognosis:** Good. Life span not affected. Facial swellings may cause varying degrees of cosmetic and psychologic disability.

**Detection of Carrier:** X-ray study of the mandible in two clinically normal fathers who had multiple affected offspring with cherubism revealed changes in the gonial angle which appeared to be the net result of the disease process acting on bony recontouring (Bixler & Garner, 1971).

**References:**
Anderson DE, McClendon JL: Cherubism-hereditary fibrous dysplasia of the jaws. I. Genetic considerations. Oral Surg Oral Med Oral Pathol 1962; 15(Suppl. 2):5–16. * †
Hamner JE III, Ketcham AS: Cherubism: an analysis of treatment. Cancer 1969; 23:1133–1143. †
Bixler D, Garner L: Cherubism: a family study to delineate gene action on mandibular growth and development. BD:OAS;VII(7). New York: March of Dimes Birth Defects, 1971:222–225.
Peters WJN: Cherubism: a study of twenty cases from one family. Oral Surg Oral Med Oral Pathol 1979; 47:307–311. * †

WA008                                    **Charles A. Waldron**

**Cherubism-gingival fibromatosis-epilepsy-hypertrichosis**
*See GINGIVAL FIBROMATOSIS-CHERUBISM-SEIZURES, RAMON TYPE*
**Chest, funnel**
*See PECTUS EXCAVATUM*
**Chicken breast**
*See PECTUS CARINATUM*
**Chickenpox, fetal effects**
*See FETAL EFFECTS FROM VARICELLA-ZOSTER*
**Child spot**
*See SKIN, CUTANEOUS MELANOSIS: MONGOLIAN SPOT*
**CHILD syndrome**
*See LIMB REDUCTION-ICHTHYOSIS*
**Childhood migraine**
*See MIGRAINE*
**Childhood pseudohypertrophic muscular dystrophy**
*See MUSCULAR DYSTROPHY, CHILDHOOD PSEUDOHYPERTROPHIC*
**CHIME syndrome**
*See ICHTHYOSIS-COLOBOMA-HEART DEFECT-DEAFNESS-MENTAL RETARDATION*
**Chin cleft**
*See FACE, CHIN FISSURE*
**Chin dimple**
*See FACE, CHIN FISSURE*
**Chin fissure**
*See FACE, CHIN FISSURE*
**Chin groove or furrow**
*See FACE, CHIN FISSURE*
**Chin, quivering**
*See CHIN, TREMBLING*

---

## CHIN, TREMBLING                                              0147

**Includes:**
    Chin, quivering
    Quivering of chin, hereditary

**Excludes:**
    Facial myokymia
    Facial tics

**Major Diagnostic Criteria:**   The presence of a trembling chin in a person with similarly affected relatives.

**Clinical Findings:**   Trembling of the chin may last for a few seconds or for several minutes. The tremor consists of either fine or coarse movements and is not particularly related to the precipitating cause. The chin trembling occurs in a perpendicular direction and at a rate of two or three times per second. In most cases an emotional stimulus is the trigger mechanism, but it may also occur during sleep. EEG studies have yielded no unusual findings.

**Complications:**   None, other than possible social discomfort.

**Associated Findings:**   Horizontal nystagmus.

**Etiology:**   Autosomal dominant inheritance.

**Pathogenesis:**   Electromyographic studies suggest that the chin movement is due to a rapid rhythmic simultaneous discharge of a number of motor units, producing virtually a tetanic twitch.

**MIM No.:**   *19010

**Sex Ratio:**   M1:F1

**Occurrence:**   Undetermined but rare.

**Risk of Recurrence for Patient's Sib:**
    See Part I, *Mendelian Inheritance.*

**Risk of Recurrence for Patient's Child:**
    See Part I, *Mendelian Inheritance.*

**Age of Detectability:**   Noted frequently in the first few weeks of life.

**Gene Mapping and Linkage:**   Unknown.

**Prevention:**   None known. Genetic counseling indicated.

**Treatment:**   Avoidance of known precipitating factors (anger, rapid eye movement, and so forth). The occasional intermittent use of tranquilizing drugs may be justified in patients in whom anxiety and tension are the sole precipitating factors. Long-term drug therapy is not indicated for this benign condition.

**Prognosis:**   Excellent. There is usually a lessening severity of the trembling with increasing age. One patient is reported to have stopped quivering spontaneously. Another reported patient was "cured" by a blow on the chin.

**Detection of Carrier:**   Unknown.

**References:**
Frey E: Ein streng dominant erbliches Kinnmuskelzittern (Beitrag zur Erforschung der menschlichen Affektäusserungen). Dtsch Z Nervenheilk 1930; 115:9–26.
Wadlington WB: Familial trembling of the chin. J Pediatr 1958; 53:316–321.
Laurance BM, et al.: Hereditary quivering of the chin. Arch Dis Child 1968; 43:249–251.

WA003                                              **William B. Wadlington**

**Chlomaphen, ovulation induction trisomy**
*See OVULATION INDUCTION TRISOMY*
**Chlordiazepoxide, fetal effects**
*See FETAL BENZODIAZEPINE EFFECTS*
**Chloride diarrhea, congenital**
*See DIARRHEA, CONGENITAL CHLORIDE*
**Choanal atresia, anterior**
*See NOSE, ANTERIOR ATRESIA*
**Choanal atresia, posterior**
*See NOSE, POSTERIOR ATRESIA*
*also CHARGE ASSOCIATION*
**Choanal atresia, posterior-lymphedema**
*See NOSE, CHOANAL ATRESIA-LYMPHEDEMA*
**Choanalatresie-lymphedema**
*See NOSE, CHOANAL ATRESIA-LYMPHEDEMA*
**Choledochal cyst**
*See BILE DUCT CHOLEDOCHAL CYST*
**Choledochocele**
*See BILE DUCT CHOLEDOCHAL CYST*
**Cholestanalosis**
*See XANTHOMATOSIS, CEREBROTENDINOUS*
**Cholestasis associated with oral contraceptive therapy**
*See INTRAHEPATIC CHOLESTASIS OF PREGNANCY (ICP)*
**Cholestasis, intrahepatic, of pregnancy**
*See INTRAHEPATIC CHOLESTASIS OF PREGNANCY (ICP)*

---

## CHOLESTASIS, INTRAHEPATIC, RECURRENT BENIGN      3276

**Includes:**
    Benign recurrent intrahepatic cholestasis (BRIC)
    Summerskill disease
    Summerskill-Tygstrup disease

**Excludes:**
    Cholestasis, benign, of pregnancy
    **Intrahepatic cholestasis of Pregnancy (ICP)** (3278)
    Intrahepatic cholestasis, secondary
    **Jaundice, intrahepatic cholestatic, Byler type** (2371)

**Major Diagnostic Criteria:**   Episodes of jaundice and pruritus lasting for days to months separated by symptom free intervals of months to years.

**Clinical Findings:**   The first episode of cholestasis can occur between eight months to 60 years of age, with a majority of patients experiencing the first episode before 20 years of age. Episodes last from two days to 24 months. Asymptomatic intervals vary from one month to twenty years. The attacks are associated with itching, fatigue, loss of appetite, steatorrhea, nausea and vomiting followed by jaundice. Hepatomegaly is moderate. Cholestasis results in elevations of total bilirubin, conjugated bilirubin, alkaline phosphatase, and serum bile salts. Fat malabsorption results in raised fecal fat and fat-soluble vitamin deficiency. During symptomatic periods, the hepatic excretion of organic anions is defective, cholangiogram demonstrates no extrahepatic obstruction and liver histology shows accumulation of bile pigment in hepatocytes, and bile canaliculi. A mild fibrosis is frequently present in the periportal or centrilobular zones and, in some cases, focal areas of hepatocellular necrosis are seen. Between attacks liver functions and histology return to normal.

**Complications:**  Pruritus, fat malabsorption, fat-soluble vitamin deficiency.

**Associated Findings:**  None known.

**Etiology:**  Presumably autosomal recessive inheritance.

**Pathogenesis:**  A primary defect in hepatic bile formation is suspected. This results in an inconstant defect in the excretion of bile salts, conjugated bilirubin, and other substances at the hepatocyte or canalicular level, resulting in clinical cholestasis. Spontaneous recovery occurs after a variable time.

**MIM No.:**  24330

**Sex Ratio:**  M1:F<1 (predominantly male).

**Occurrence:**  Thirty-nine known cases have been identified, of which one-third are familial.

**Risk of Recurrence for Patient's Sib:**
See Part I, *Mendelian Inheritance.*

**Risk of Recurrence for Patient's Child:**
See Part I, *Mendelian Inheritance.*

**Age of Detectability:**  From infancy to adulthood.

**Gene Mapping and Linkage:**  Unknown.

**Prevention:**  None known. Genetic counseling indicated.

**Treatment:**  Therapy is symptomatic. Cholestyramine may be administered to help treat itching. Supplementation of fat soluble vitamins including A, D, E and K is necessary during prolonged bouts of cholestasis.

**Prognosis:**  Good. Progression of hepatocellular failure or cirrhosis has not been reported.

**Detection of Carrier:**  Unknown.

**References:**
Summerskill WHJ, Walsh JM: Benign recurrent intrahepatic "obstructive" jaundice. Lancet 1959; 2:686 only.
Tygstrup N: Intermittent, possible familial, intrahepatic cholestatic jaundice. Lancet 1960; 1:1171–1172.
Beaudoin M, et al.: Benign recurrent cholestasis. Digestion 1973; 9:49–65.
Lesser P: Benign familial recurrent intrahepatic cholestasis. Amer J Dig Dis 1973; 18:259–264.
Summerfield JA, et al.: Benign recurrent intrahepatic cholestasis: studies of bilirubin, kinetics, bile acids and cholangiography. Gut 1980; 21:154–160.
Schiff L: Idiopathic benign recurrent cholestasis. In: Schiff L, Schiff ER, eds: Diseases of the liver. Philadelphia: Lippincott, 1987:1473–1477.

FI035                                                      **Mark Fishbein**
AL037                                                **Estella M. Alonso**

**Cholestasis, neonatal**
*See ALPHA(1)-ANTITRYPSIN DEFICIENCY*
**Cholestasis, progressive idiopathic**
*See JAUNDICE, INTRAHEPATIC CHOLESTATIC, BYLER TYPE*
**Cholestasis-congenital heart disease**
*See ARTERIO-HEPATIC DYSPLASIA*

---

# CHOLESTASIS-LYMPHEDEMA, AAGENAES TYPE          3118

**Includes:**
Aagenaes syndrome
Lymphedema-cholestasis, Aagenaes type

**Excludes:**
**Alpha(1)-antitrypsin deficiency** (0039)
**Arterio-hepatic dysplasia** (2084)
**Cholestasis, intrahepatic, recurrent benign** (3276)
Disorders of bile acid metabolism
**Jaundice, intrahepatic cholestatic, Byler type** (2371)
**Lymphedema I** (0614)
**Liver, hemangiomatosis** (0466)

**Major Diagnostic Criteria:**  Occurrence of intrahepatic cholestasis in association with chronic lymphedema of lower extremities.

**Clinical Findings:**  The onset of cholestasis occurs between ages 1–16 weeks. Jaundice with light stools and dark urine are usual presenting features. Hepatomegaly is moderate. Hyperbilirubinemia, mostly conjugated, ranges from 4–12 mg/dl. Hyperlipidemia with cholesterol levels of 200–400 mg/dl is a constant finding. Elevated serum bile salt concentration is sometimes associated with severe itching. The cholestasis tends to lessen as the child grows older and sometimes subsides by age ten years. Liver histology demonstrating marked giant-cell transformation becomes less evident and portal fibrosis becomes more prominent. Sometimes fibrosis is severe, and one patient has developed cirrhosis. The extrahepatic biliary tree is normal, but often contains thick, sticky bile at the time of operative cholangiogram. Interlobular bile duct radicles are normal in number. Portal and central venules and hepatic arterioles are normal. No abnormality of hepatic lymphatics has been demonstrated.

Edema of the lower extremities has its onset usually in the third to sixth years. The edema is pitting and is not associated with hypoalbuminemia. It is bilaterally symmetric and usually involves the entire leg and sometimes the genitalia. Lymphangiogram and histology demonstrate hypoplasia of lymph vessels. The lymphedema persists after the cholestasis remits.

**Complications:**  *Hepatic:* fibrosis with portal hypertension, cirrhosis with attendant complications, malabsorption, growth failure, fat-soluble vitamin deficiency.
*Lymphedema:* infection of skin and subcutaneous tissues, tissue necrosis, immobility.

**Associated Findings:**  Defects of dental enamel, discoloration of the teeth.

**Etiology:**  Autosomal recessive inheritance.

**Pathogenesis:**  Experimental data suggest that occlusion of hepatic lymphatics can produce transient cholestasis. Thus, it has been proposed that hepatic lymphatics are underdeveloped in this disease. However, because hepatic lymphatics are very difficult to demonstrate in histologic preparations, their hypoplasia cannot be documented. Hypoplasia of the lymphatics of the legs is thought to be a developmental defect that becomes clinically apparent when hydrostatic pressure overcomes the limited capacity for lymph drainage.

**MIM No.:**  *21490

**POS No.:**  3768

**Sex Ratio:**  M1:F1

**Occurrence:**  Six families with 37 affected members have been reported. All but one have been of Norwegian descent.

**Risk of Recurrence for Patient's Sib:**
See Part I, *Mendelian Inheritance.*

**Risk of Recurrence for Patient's Child:**
See Part I, *Mendelian Inheritance.*

**Age of Detectability:**  *Cholestasis:* from birth to 16 weeks.
*Lymphedema:* from ages 3–10 years.

**Gene Mapping and Linkage:**  Unknown.

**Prevention:**  None known. Genetic counseling indicated.

**Treatment:**  Conservative management of liver disease with attention to maintaining nutritional status. Treatment with phenobarbital as a choleretic and cholestyramine as a bile salt-binding agent is suggested. In patients with cirrhosis, liver transplantation is considered. Conservative treatment of lymphedemia is also recommended. Positional therapy and orthopedic stockings may reduce disability.

**Prognosis:**  *Hepatic:* The majority have no long-term disability. Few will have fibrosis or cirrhosis.
*Lymphedema:* Chronic disability is expected.

**Detection of Carrier:**  Clinical and laboratory examinations.

**References:**
Aagenaes Ø, et al.: Hereditary recurrent intrahepatic cholestasis from birth. Arch Dis Child 1968; 43:646–657.

Aagenaes Ø, et al.: Lymphoedema in hereditary recurrent cholestasis from birth. Arch Dis Child 1970; 45:690–695.

Sigstad H, et al.: Primary lymphoedema combined with hereditary recurrent intrahepatic cholestasis. Acta Med Scand 1970; 188:213–219.

Sharp HL, Krivit W: Hereditary lymphedema and obstructive jaundice. J Pediatr 1971; 78:491–496.

Aagenes Ø: Hereditary recurrent cholestasis with lymphoedema-two new families. Acta Paediatr Scand 1974; 63:465–471.

Vajro P, et al.: Aagenaes's syndrome in an Italian child. Acta Paediatr Scand 1984; 73:695–696.

WH007                                         **Peter F. Whitington**

**Cholestasis-peripheral pulmonary stenosis**
  *See ARTERIO-HEPATIC DYSPLASIA*
**Cholestatic jaundice-renal tubular insufficiency**
  *See BILIARY ATRESIA*
**Cholesteatoma of temporal bone**
  *See EAR, CHOLESTEATOMA OF TEMPORAL BONE*
**Cholesteatoma, congenital**
  *See EAR, CHOLESTEATOMA OF TEMPORAL BONE*
**Cholesteatoma, primary**
  *See EAR, CHOLESTEATOMA OF TEMPORAL BONE*
**Cholesteatoma, true**
  *See EAR, CHOLESTEATOMA OF TEMPORAL BONE*
**Cholesterol ester storage disease**
  *See CHOLESTERYL ESTER STORAGE DISEASE*
**Cholesterol, familial elevated**
  *See HYPERCHOLESTEREMIA*

## CHOLESTERYL ESTER STORAGE DISEASE          0151

**Includes:**
  Acid cholesteryl ester hydrolase deficiency, type 2
  Cholesterol ester storage disease
  Hepatic cholesteryl ester storage disease
  Histiocytosis, sea-blue
  LIPA deficiency
  Liver cholesteryl ester storage
  Lysosomal acid lipase deficiency

**Excludes:**
  **Analphalipoproteinemia** (0048)
  **Wolman disease** (1003)

**Major Diagnostic Criteria:**  Acid lipase deficiency in leukocytes, cultured skin fibroblasts, or body tissues. The generally mild phenotype in cholesteryl ester storage disease is distinguished from the rapidly progressive fatal phenotype in **Wolman disease**, which also results from acid lipase deficiency.

**Clinical Findings:**  Massive hepatomegaly is constant, and splenomegaly occurs in many patients. The cholesteryl ester content of liver is markedly increased. Plasma cholesterol and triglycerides are usually moderately elevated (a type 2b pattern in the Fredrickson classification of hyperlipoproteinemia), and HDL cholesterol is very low. Hepatic fibrosis and esophageal varices are frequent. Foam cells are found in the bone marrow and in the lamina propria of the intestine.

**Complications:**  Evidence of premature atherosclerosis was found at autopsy in at least three cases. In one sibship, possibly representing a more severe phenotype, three sisters died with acute hepatic failure at the ages of 7, 9, and 17 years.

**Associated Findings:**  None known.

**Etiology:**  Presumably autosomal recessive inheritance. All patients adequately studied are deficient in both lysosomal cholesteryl ester hydrolase and triglyceride lipase activities. These activities may be attributable to a single enzyme; acid lipase.

**Pathogenesis:**  Acid lipase deficiency in tissues results in accumulation of cholesteryl esters and, to a lesser extent, triglycerides. This lysosomal enzyme is an essential component of the LDL pathway for the feedback regulation of cholesterol metabolism and biosynthesis. Disturbance of the LDL pathway may explain the hyperlipidemia in these patients.

**MIM No.:**  21500

**Sex Ratio:**  M1:F1

**Occurrence:**  At least 20 cases known, including one black and two Mexican families, and at least one case from Ireland.

**Risk of Recurrence for Patient's Sib:**
  See Part I, *Mendelian Inheritance.*

**Risk of Recurrence for Patient's Child:**
  See Part I, *Mendelian Inheritance.*

**Age of Detectability:**  Enzyme assay can be performed at birth, and prenatal diagnosis has been performed. Hepatomegaly probably is detectable during the first two years of life.

**Gene Mapping and Linkage:**  LIPA (lipase A, lysosomal acid (Wolman disease)) has been mapped to 10.

**Prevention:**  None known. Genetic counseling indicated.

**Treatment:**  Treatment is symptomatic for most patients; the disease is often relatively benign. Iron deficiency anemia may require treatment because of intestinal involvement and esophageal varices. Bile acid-binding resins may be used to treat the hyperlipidemia. Enzyme replacement therapy, liver transplantation, or somatic gene replacement are all theoretically possible, but have not been reported for this disease.

**Prognosis:**  Some patients have survived in good health into adult life. One patient died at age 21 years because of aortic stenosis, perhaps on an unrelated basis. Childhood death because of acute liver failure has occurred in one sibship. The frequent occurrence of premature atherosclerosis, hepatic fibrosis, and esophageal varices make the long-term prognosis guarded.

**Detection of Carrier:**  Reduced levels of acid lipase activity have been reported in leukocytes and cultured skin fibroblasts from heterozygotes. Heterozygotes are asymptomatic, although some have been found to have plasma lipoprotein abnormalities.

**Special Considerations:**  Cholesteryl ester storage disease and **Wolman disease** may be allelic disorders. A spectrum of clinical disease is associated with acid lipase deficiency.

**References:**
Beaudet AL, et al.: Cholesterol ester storage disease: clinical, biochemical and pathological studies. J Pediatr 1977; 90:910–914.

Besley, GTN, et al.: Cholesteryl ester storage disease in an adult presenting with sea-blue histiocytosis. Clin Genet 1984; 26:195–203.

Hoeg JM, et al.: Cholesteryl ester storage disease and Wolman disease: phenotypic variants of lysosomal acid cholesteryl ester hydrolase deficiency. Am J Hum Genet 1984; 36:1190–1203.

Cagle PT, et al.: Clinicopathologic conference: Pulmonary hypertension in an 18-year-old girl with cholesteryl ester storage disease (CESD). Am J Med Genet 1986; 24:711–722.

Desai PK, et al.: Cholesteryl ester storage disease: pathologic changes in an affected fetus. Am J Med Genet 1987; 26:689–698.

Schmitz G, Assmann G: Acid lipase deficiency: Wolman's disease and cholesteryl ester storage disease. In: Scriver CR, et al, eds: The metabolic basis of inherited disease, 6th ed. New York: McGraw-Hill, 1989:1623–1644. *

C0063                                          **Paul M. Coates**

## CHOLINESTERASE, ATYPICAL                    0152

**Includes:**
  Acylcholine acyl-hydrolase EC 3.1.1.8
  Anectine apnea
  Dibucaine resistant variant E1a
  Plasma cholinesterase, atypical
  Post-anesthesia apnea
  Pseudocholinesterase deficiency
  Pseudocholinesterase, E(1)
  Pseudocholinesterase types E(2) variants
  Succinylcholine apnea
  Suxamethonium sensitivity

**Excludes:**  Succinylcholine apnea-normal plasma cholinesterase

**Major Diagnostic Criteria:**  No physical findings prior to apnea. Occurrence of prolonged apnea after succinylcholine administration. Detecting the occurrence of prolonged apnea is dependent upon the amount and anticipated duration of the drug in relation to the total anesthesia procedure. Apnea lasting longer than 10 minutes is considered abnormal. A peripheral nerve stimulator may aid confirmation of diagnosis by demonstrating flaccidity of hand muscles. Confirmation of clinical diagnosis by laboratory tests.

**Clinical Findings:** Prolonged apnea occurs after succinylcholine administration (1–3 mg/kg). Apnea lasts longer than 10 minutes in the absence of significant amounts of depressant premedication, anesthetic agent or neurologic defect. The recovery of adequate spontaneous ventilation is prolonged with obvious persistent weakness of intercostal and cervical musculature, e.g. inability to raise head while supine.

**Complications:** Complications may include hypoxia (may lead to cardiac arrest), hypercarbia (acidosis--both respiratory and metabolic), dehydration, and postoperative psychologic disturbances (failure to keep patient asleep during apnea).

**Associated Findings:** None known.

**Etiology:** Autosomal dominant inheritance.

**Pathogenesis:** Succinylcholine is a skeletal muscle relaxant that acts at the neuromuscular junction to provide alteration in sensitivity to acetylcholine, the transmitter substance. The circulating drug molecules have a short route from the blood to their site of action, and onset of paralysis after intravenous injection of the drug is rapid. The high concentration of drug in plasma immediately after intravenous injection falls very quickly in the normal individual because of the rapid action of plasma cholinesterase. The prolonged effect of succinylcholine in persons with atypical plasma cholinesterase is considered to be due to an excessive amount of the drug reaching the endplate. Not all cases of prolonged apnea during anesthesia are associated with atypical cholinesterase, but it should be recognized that the atypical homozygote is always at risk of a prolonged effect of succinylcholine.

**MIM No.:** *17740, *17750

**CDC No.:** 277.630

**Sex Ratio:** M1:F1

**Occurrence:** The occurrence of atypical homozygotes for the dibucaine-resistant form has been estimated to be from 1:2000 to 1:4000 in various populations. The fluoride-resistant $E_1{}^f$, the silent gene, $E_1{}^s$ and $E_1$ Newfoundland variants are much rarer.

The gene for dibucaine-resistant atypical cholinesterase appears to be widely distributed. An unusually high rate has been reported among Jews from Iran and Iraq, but a low incidence in Jews from North Africa. Low carrier rates have been found in Orientals and blacks. An unusually high rate of occurrence of the silent gene has been described in southern Eskimos.

**Risk of Recurrence for Patient's Sib:**
See Part I, *Mendelian Inheritance.*

**Risk of Recurrence for Patient's Child:**
See Part I, *Mendelian Inheritance.*

**Age of Detectability:** It is not possible to detect atypical homozygous individuals by inhibition studies at any age. The relatively low plasma cholinesterase activity in the neonate may prejudice screening tests dependent only on enzyme activity measurement.

**Gene Mapping and Linkage:** CHE1 (cholinesterase (serum) 1) has been mapped to 3q26-qter.
CHE2 (cholinesterase (serum) 2) has been provisionally mapped to 2q.

**Prevention:** None known. Genetic counseling indicated.

**Treatment:** It is essential in taking the history to elicit information concerning a previous occurrence of apnea in the patient or in the family and, pending biochemical evaluation, to avoid the use of succinylcholine with an individual possibly at risk. The essential therapy is assisted respiration and associated care during the period of apnea. Because of the risk of psychic trauma associated with consciousness of the patient during a part of the period of paralysis, it is advisable to administer an agent such as nitrous oxide as soon as the fact of the existence of apnea is recognized. The infusion of normal plasma as a source of normal cholinesterase has been advocated as a means of shortening the period of paralysis, but this treatment has not come into general use. Injection of normal purified plasma cholinesterase before and after injection of succinylcholine has been advocated for control of apnea.

**Prognosis:** Good, providing the apnea is recognized early and appropriate therapy is given.

**Detection of Carrier:** Identification of the heterozygous state on clinical grounds is uncertain. Some individuals experiencing apnea of short duration have been shown to be heterozygotes by biochemical studies. Detection of the heterozygote state by biochemical means requires study of the inhibition of plasma cholinesterase activity.

**Special Considerations:** Women of childbearing age using oral contraceptives have reduced plasma cholinesterase levels.

Biochemical abnormalities are indicated by the presence of atypical enzymes that have different properties with respect to substrates than the normal form of plasma cholinesterase. Atypical plasma cholinesterase can be detected by inhibition studies with compounds such as dibucaine and sodium fluoride.

Electrophoresis: Migration in starch gels of plasma cholinesterase in four or more separate activity bands can be demonstrated. Evidence for structural differences has been reported between normal and atypical cholinesterase. Separation of normal and atypical forms of plasma cholinesterase has been demonstrated on chromatographic columns.

**References:**
Harris H, Whittaker M: The genetics of drug sensitivity with special reference to suxamethonium. In: Mongar JL, de Reuck AVS, eds: Ciba Foundation symposium on enzymes and drug action. Boston: Little Brown, 1962.
Rubinstein HM: Silent cholinesterase gene: variations in the properties of serum enzyme in apparent homozygotes. J Clin Invest 1970; 49:479–486.
Scott EM, et al.: Discrimination of phenotypes in human serum cholinesterase deficiency. Am J Hum Genet 1970; 22:363–369.
Simpson NE, Elliott CR: Cholinesterase Newfoundland: a new succinylcholine-sensitive variant of cholinesterase at locus 1. Am J Hum Genet 1981; 33:366.
Lockridge O, et al.: Complete amino acid sequence of human serum cholineesterase. J Biol Chem 1987; 262:549–557.
Muensch H, et al.: Structural difference at the active site of dibucaine resistant variant of human plasma cholinesterase. Am J Hum Genet 1987; 30:302–307.

D0009                                              **George N. Donnell**

**Chondro-dermo-corneal dystrophy of Francois**
*See DERMO-CHONDRO-CORNEAL DYSTROPHY, FRANCOIS TYPE*
**Chondro-osteodystrophy**
*See SPONDYLOEPIPHYSEAL DYSPLASIA, LATE*
**Chondrodysplasia**
*See ATELOSTEOGENESIS*
**Chondrodysplasia punctata, Conradi-Hunermann type**
*See CHONDRODYSPLASIA PUNCTATA, MILD SYMMETRIC TYPE*

---

**CHONDRODYSPLASIA PUNCTATA, MILD SYMMETRIC TYPE**                    **0153**

**Includes:**
Chondrodysplasia punctata, Conradi-Hunermann type
Chondrodystrophia calcificans congenita
Conradi-Hunermann disease
"Koala bear" faces
Nose, flattened tip and depressed bridge (some)

**Excludes:**
Chondrodysplasia punctata, rhizomelic type (0154)
Chondrodysplasia punctata, X-linked dominant type (2730)
Fetal warfarin syndrome (0389)
Symptomatic stippling associated with other syndromes

**Major Diagnostic Criteria:** The characteristic facial features of the newborn and young child are flattened tip and depressed bridge of the nose. Mild, symmetric calcific stippling, most notably of the tarsal bones, also occurs.

**Clinical Findings:** The most consistent physical feature is the unusual shape of the nose, with a shortened columella resulting in a flattened nasal tip. The nasal bridge is frequently depressed. Respiratory and feeding problems may occur after birth. The morphologic anomalies lessen with age. X-rays show comparatively mild, symmetric calcific stippling most commonly in the tarsus, less constantly in the vertebrae and carpal bones. Since the calcifications disappear with age, the disorder may be impossible to detect in an older individual. Cataracts and skin changes are not found in this form of chondrodysplasia punctata.

**Complications:** Respiratory and feeding problems secondary to nasal obstructions have been observed in infants.

**Associated Findings:** Mild mental retardation and postaxial polydactyly has been rarely described.

**Etiology:** Autosomal dominant inheritance.

**Pathogenesis:** Unknown.

**MIM No.:** *11865

**POS No.:** 3065

**CDC No.:** 756.575

**Sex Ratio:** M3:F1

**Occurrence:** Over 100 cases reported. Dr. L.J. Sheffield has reported seeing 120 cases chondrodysplasia punctata in Australia, of which 90 were of a "mild" type.

**Risk of Recurrence for Patient's Sib:**
See Part I, *Mendelian Inheritance*.

**Risk of Recurrence for Patient's Child:**
See Part I, *Mendelian Inheritance*.

**Age of Detectability:** At birth.

**Gene Mapping and Linkage:** Unknown.

**Prevention:** None known. Genetic counseling indicated.

**Treatment:** Symptomatic. Plastic surgery for nasal dysplasia has been performed.

**Prognosis:** Excellent for function and lifespan.

**Detection of Carrier:** Nasal abnormality may persist into adulthood and this may be the only marker of the condition. On the other hand, regression of the morphologic changes with age makes identification of hypothetically affected parents very difficult.

Extrinsic factors such as intrauterine exposure to alcohol or warfarin produce similar facial and bone changes, and these factors must be ruled out before genetic causes are assumed in an individual patient. Bone changes produced by warfarin tend to be more severe than in the typical case with mild chondrodysplasia punctata.

Symptomatic symmetric stippling has been observed in a range of other genetic disorders which must be delineated from the present condition.

**References:**
Silverman FN: Discussion on the relation between stippled epiphyses and the multiplex form of epiphyseal dysplasia. In: BD:OAS 1969; V(4):68–71.
Spranger J, et al.: Heterogeneity of chondrodysplasia punctata. Humangenetik 1971; 11:190–212.
Sheffield LJ, et al.: Chondrodysplasia punctata: 23 cases of a mild and relatively common variety. J Pediatr 1976; 89:916–923.
Silengo MC, et al.: Clinical and genetic aspects of Conradi-Hunermann disease: a report of three familial cases and a review of the literature. J Pediat 1980; 97:911–917.
Whitfield MF: Chondrodysplasia punctata after warfarin in early pregnancy: case report and a summary of the literature. Arch Dis Child 1980; 55:139–142.
Trowitzsch E, et al.: Severe pulmonary arterial stenoses in Conradi-Hunermann disease. Europ J Pediat 1986; 145:116–118.

SP007                                                       **Jürgen W. Spranger**

## CHONDRODYSPLASIA PUNCTATA, RHIZOMELIC TYPE     0154

**Includes:**
> Chondrodystrophia calcificans congenita
> Peroxisomal disorder (one form)
> Rhizomelic chondrodysplasia punctata

**Excludes:**
**Cerebro-hepato-renal syndrome** (0139)
**Chondrodysplasia punctata, X-linked dominant type** (2730)
**Fetal warfarin syndrome** (0389)
**Phytanic acid oxidase deficiency, infantile type** (2278)
**Rhizomelic syndrome, Urbach type** (2816)
Stippling, calcificic, other forms

**Major Diagnostic Criteria:** Coronal clefts in lateral X-ray views of the vertebral bodies and shortening of the humeri or femora. The coronal clefts affect all or most of the vertebral bodies.

**Clinical Findings:** Disproportionate shortness of stature affecting primarily the proximal parts of the limbs; **Microcephaly** in most cases; flat face with upward-slanting palpebral fissures; lymphedema of the cheeks ("chipmunk" appearance) in the newborn; bilateral cataracts (approximately 80% of cases); ichthyosiform skin changes; alopecia (27%); contractures of multiple joints (60%).

X-rays show dorsal and ventral ossification centers of the vertebral bodies in lateral views of the spine; symmetric shortening and metaphyseal irregularities of the humeri or femora; extracartilaginous and epiphyseal stippling in most cases; a trapezoid shape of the iliac bones in anteroposterior projections of the pelvis. Stippling is not a condition sine qua non. It disappears during the first year of life. The ossification centers of the vertebral bodies fuse during later infancy.

**Complications:** Cerebral hypoplasia; severe mental deficiency; spastic quadriplegia in survivors with the syndrome.

**Associated Findings:** Congenital heart disease; optic atrophy.

**Etiology:** Autosomal recessive inheritance.

**Pathogenesis:** Pathohistologic examination of the long bones shows disruption of the growth plates, foci of calcification, ossification, cyst formation, and zones of inflammation. The changes possibly reflect some damage during development with subsequent healing of the cartilage by fibrosis, calcification, and ossification. The clefts of the vertebral bodies are due to an embryonic arrest of development. The microcephaly is related to a decrease in the number of nerve cells found in neurohistologic examinations.

Rhizomelic chondrodysplasia punctata has recently been shown to be a peroxisomal disorder with severe deficiency of plasmalogens and deficient activity of the peroxisomal enzyme acyl-CoA: dihydroxy-acetone-phosphate acyltransferase in thrombocytes and cultured cell fibroblasts. Plasma phytanic acid levels are elevated. It is similar clinically and biochemically to **Cerebro-hepato-renal syndrome** but somatic cell studies indicate that it is genetically distinct from both **Cerebro-hepato-renal syndrome** and **Phytanic acid oxidase deficiency, infantile type**.

**MIM No.:** *21510

**POS No.:** 3064

**CDC No.:** 756.575

**Sex Ratio:** M1:F1

**Occurrence:** Undetermined but rare.

**Risk of Recurrence for Patient's Sib:**
See Part I, *Mendelian Inheritance*.

**Risk of Recurrence for Patient's Child:**
See Part I, *Mendelian Inheritance*.

**Age of Detectability:** Prenatal detection of peroxisomal dysfunction is possible in amniotic fluid cells or through chorionic villus biopsy.

**Gene Mapping and Linkage:** Unknown.

**Prevention:** None known. Genetic counseling indicated.

**Treatment:** Supportive.

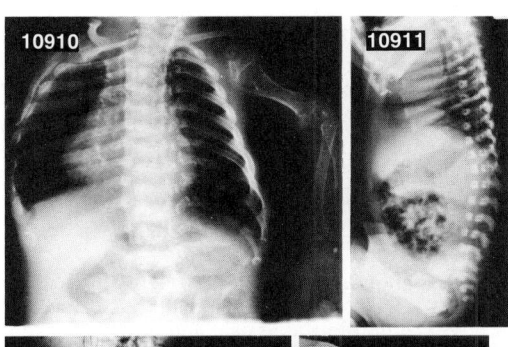

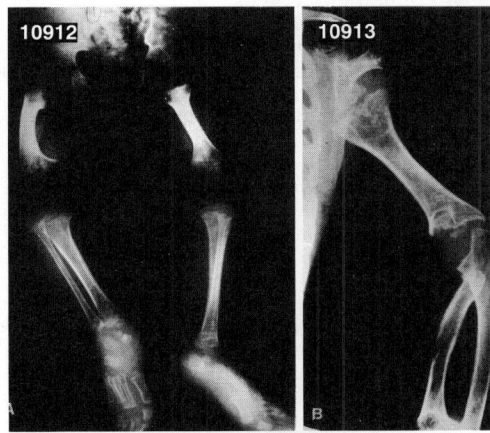

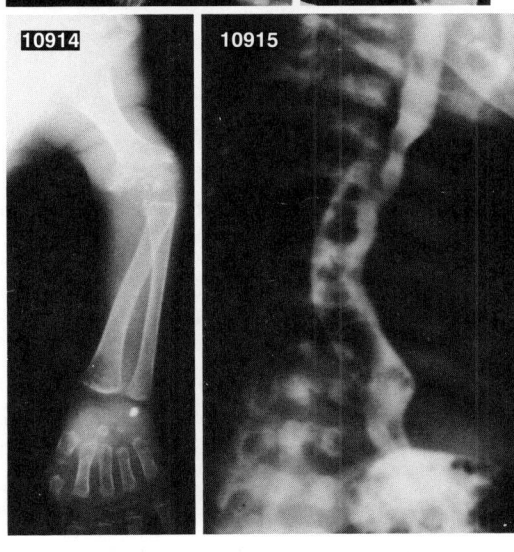

**0154-10910:** Stippled calcifications at base of ribs, sternum and elbow; short humerus with widened metaphysis. **10911:** Thoracic and lumbar vertebral bodies in newborn are divided into dorsal and ventral segments by radiolucent bars of cartilage. **10912:** At age 1 year, the femora are short and deformed. **10913:** At age 4 years there is severe shortening with metaphyseal widening of the humerus. **10914:** Single dense calcific focus in the wrist, shortened humerus with widened metaphysis and stippled calcifications. **10915:** Stippled calcifications at periphery of cartilagenous structure of vertebral bodies.

**Prognosis:** Lethal condition. Affected infants fail to thrive and usually die in the first weeks of life from recurrent infections. Patients who survive their first year of life are severely retarded in psychomotor development. They usually die before age 10 years.

**Detection of Carrier:** Unknown.

**References:**

Spranger J, et al.: Heterogeneity of chondrodysplasia punctata. Humangenetik 1970; 11:190–212.
Visekul C, et al.: Pathology of chondrodysplasia punctata, rhizomelic type. In Bergsma, D ed: Skeletal dysplasias. Amsterdam: Excerpta Medica. 1974:327–333.
Heymans HSA, et al.: Rizomelic chondrodysplasia punctata: another peroxisomal disorder. New Engl J Med 1985; 313:187–188.
Schutgens RBH, et al.: Peroxisomal disorders. Eur J Pediatr 1986; 144:430–440.
Wanders RJA, et al.: Genetic relation between the Zellweger syndrome, infantile Refsum's disease, and rhyizomelic chondrodysplasia punctata. New Engl J Med 1986; 314:787–788.

SP007                                                    **Jürgen W. Spranger**

## CHONDRODYSPLASIA PUNCTATA, X-LINKED DOMINANT TYPE                                           2730

**Includes:**

    Chondrodysplasia calcificans congenita
    Chondrodysplasia punctata, X-linked recessive type
    Dysplasia epiphysealis punctata
    Stippled epiphyses

**Excludes:**

**Chondrodysplasia punctata**
**Fetal warfarin syndrome** (0389)
Stippling, symptomatic

**Major Diagnostic Criteria:** Flat face with depressed nasal bridge, cataracts, ichthyosiform skin changes, asymmetric calcific stippling in the newborn, and asymmetric epiphyseal and vertebral changes in the older child.

**Clinical Findings:** The newborn is short and has a saddle nose. In severe cases, the tip of the nose shows a bilateral groove. Ichthyosiform skin changes, cataracts, and foot deformities are frequently present. Older children are short, with asymmetric shortening of limbs and/or fingers; kyphoscoliosis; joint contractures; asymmetric and often unilateral cataracts; partial alopecia; and irregularly distributed, linear or whorly areas of ichthyosiform erythroderma or follicular atrophoderma. Skin and hair lesions may be discrete. X-rays show irregularly distributed, asymmetric punctate calcifications affecting primarily the ends of the long bones, carpal and tarsal regions, vertebrae, and ischiopubic bones of the newborn. During infancy the calcifications disappear, but ossification remains defective in areas of prominent stippling. This results in a characteristically asymmetric bone dysplasia with irregular vertebral and epiphyseal defects. Mental development has been normal.

**Complications:** Patients with severe chondrodysplasia punctata may die before or shortly after birth. In survivors, orthopedic complications are common, depending on the degree and severity of bone lesions.

**Associated Findings:** There have been isolated reports of **Polydactyly.**

**Etiology:** X-linked dominant inheritance, with possible lethality in the hemizygous male. X-linked recessive cases have also been reported.

**Pathogenesis:** Peroxisomal enzyme deficiency has been reported in a single patient.

**MIM No.:** *30295, 30296

**POS No.:** 4299

**Sex Ratio:** M0:F1

**Occurrence:** About 50 cases have been reported in the literature.

**Risk of Recurrence for Patient's Sib:**
    See Part I, *Mendelian Inheritance.*

**Risk of Recurrence for Patient's Child:**
    See Part I, *Mendelian Inheritance.*

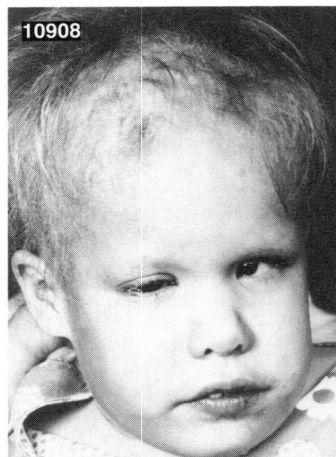

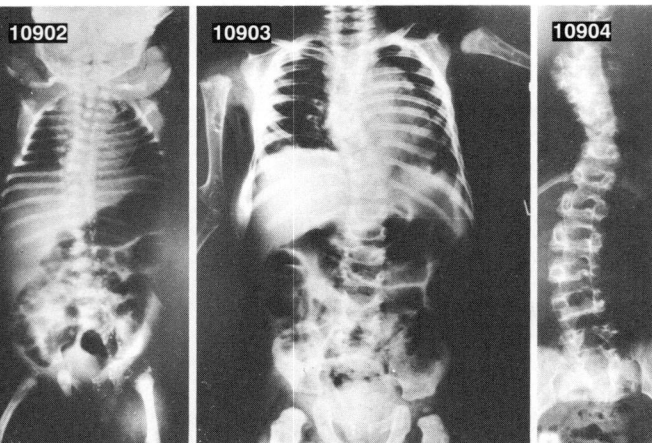

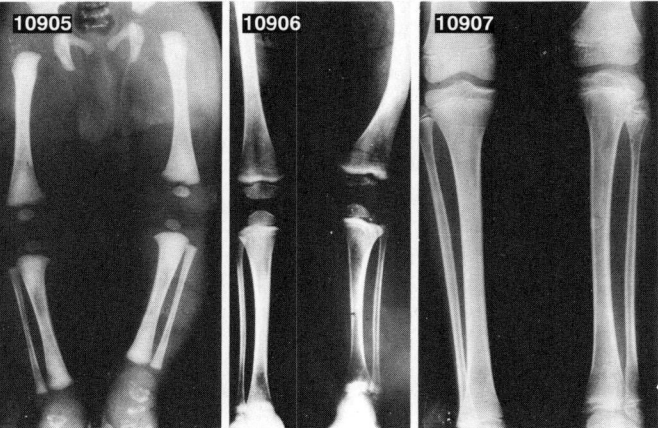

**Age of Detectability:** During the prenatal period.

**Gene Mapping and Linkage:** CDPX (chondrodysplasia punctata) has been mapped to Xp22.32.

**Prevention:** None known. Genetic counseling indicated.

**Treatment:** Symptomatic.

**Prognosis:** Extremely variable, from neonatal death to bare detectability of the disorder in the adult.

**Detection of Carrier:** Discrete skin changes or alopecia may be the only signs in an adult carrier.

**Special Considerations:** The genetics of this type of chondrodysplasia punctata are not entirely clear. X-linked dominant inheritance with lyonization in the female and lethality in the hemizygous male is suggested by the asymmetric distribution of skin, eye, and bone changes, female preponderance, and paucity of male offspring in some families. In some patients, the disorder is very mild and limited to minimal skin, hair, and eye changes. Lethal cases may present the severe end of a phenotypic spectrum. A number of males with lethal chondrodysplasia punctata have been observed.

X-linked recessive inheritance has been demonstrated in two families with a chromosomal deletion at Xp22.32. The phenotype differed from X-linked dominant chondrodysplasia punctata by the symmetric distribution of calcifications, hypoplasia of the distal phalanges, and the presence of mental retardation in affected males.

Unilateral stippling may be present in newborns with congenital hemidysplasia with ichthyosiform erythroderma and limb defects (CHILD syndrome; see **Limb reduction-ichthyosis**). Mild, symmetric calcifications are seen in a number of other conditions (see **Chondrodysplasia punctata, mild symmetric type**).

**References:**

Spranger JW, et al.: Heterogeneity of chondrodysplasia punctata. Humangenetik 1971; 11:190–212.

Happle R, et al.: Sex-linked chondrodyspasia punctata? Clin Genet 1977; 11:73–76.

Manzke H, et al.: Dominant sex-linked inherited chondrodysplasia punctata: a distinct type of chondrodysplasia punctata. Clin Genet 1980; 14:97–107.

Curry CJR, et al.: Inherited chondrodysplasia punctata due to a deletion of the terminal short arm of an X chromosome. New Engl J Med 1984; 311:1010–1015.

Mueller RF, et al.: X-linked dominant chondrodysplasia punctata: a case report and family studies. Am J Med Genet 1985; 20:137–144.

Holmes RD, et al.: Peroxisomal enzyme deficiency in the Conradi-Hunermann form of chondrodysplasia punctata. New Engl J Med 1987; 316:1608.

Bick D, et al.: Male infant with ichthyosis, Kallmann syndrome, chondrodysplasia punctata, and an Xp chromosome deletion. Am J Med Genet 1989; 33:100–107.

Maroteaux P: Brachytelephalangic chondrodysplasia punctata: a possible X-linked recessive form. Hum Genet 1989; 82:167–170.

SP007                                    **Jürgen W. Spranger**

**Chondrodysplasia punctata, X-linked recessive type**
  *See CHONDRODYSPLASIA PUNCTATA, X-LINKED DOMINANT TYPE*
**Chondrodysplasia secondary to chondroosseous transformation defect**
  *See OPSISMODYSPLASIA*
**Chondrodysplasia, Kniest-like**
  *See KNIEST-LIKE DYSPLASIA*
**Chondrodysplasia, lethal neonatal with snail-like pelvis**
  *See SKELETAL DYSPLASIA, SCHNECKENBECKEN TYPE*
**Chondrodysplasia, micromelic (misnomer)**
  *See KNIEST-LIKE DYSPLASIA*
**Chondrodysplasia, spondylometaphseal, Kozlowski type**
  *See SPONDYLOMETAPHYSEAL CHONDRODYSPLASIA, KOZLOWSKI TYPE*
**Chondrodysplasias**
  *See DWARFISM*
**Chondrodystrophia**
  *See ACHONDROPLASIA*
**Chondrodystrophia calcificans congenita**
  *See CHONDRODYSPLASIA PUNCTATA, MILD SYMMETRIC TYPE*
  *also CHONDRODYSPLASIA PUNCTATA, RHIZOMELIC TYPE*

**2730**-10908: Affected child has dry, lusterless hair, which is sparse with areas of alopecia. 10902: X-ray of the newborn shows widespread stippling. 10903: At age 9 months, the stippling is no longer seen; the humerus is short and deformed. 10904: Spine at age 11 years has marked scoliosis; there are irregular endplates of the lumbar vertebrae. 10905: X-ray of lower limbs in the newborn shows discrete stippling in the sacral spine, greater trochanters, and tarsal bones. 10906: At age 2 years the left leg is shorter than the right; there is external bowing of the small and deformed left femur. 10907: Short left tibia and fibula at age 11 years.

## CHONDRODYSTROPHIC MYOTONIA, SCHWARTZ-JAMPEL TYPE

**0155**

**Includes:**
- Aberfeld syndrome
- Catel-Hempel dysostosis enchondralis metaepiphysaria
- Dysostosis enchondralis metaepiphysaria, Catel-Hempel type
- Myotonic myopathy-dwarfism-chondrodystrophy-eye/face anomalies
- Schwartz-Jampel syndrome

**Excludes:**
- **Arthrogryposes** (0088)
- **Cranio-carpo-tarsal dysplasia, whistling face type** (0223)
- Mandibular arch syndrome-dwarfism
- **Mucopolysaccharidosis** (all)
- **Muscular dystrophy, congenital with arthrogryposis** (2706)
- **Myotonia congenita** (0701)
- **Myotonic dystrophy** (0702)
- **Seckel syndrome** (0881)

**Major Diagnostic Criteria:** The diagnosis is primarily clinical. It is based on the association between muscle disease with clinical myotonia, which must be confirmed electromyographically, facial and ocular abnormalities of variable severity, and skeletal deformities of the type indicative of abnormal bone formation with corresponding X-ray changes. All but three reported patients had short stature. One of the originally studied patients grew from 115.6 cm at age 10 years to 162.6 cm at age 17 years (unpublished, personal observation). Short stature cannot be considered to be an obligatory feature of chondrodystrophic myotonia.

**Clinical Findings:** The birth weight is normal or low. Symptoms begin to appear at the end of the first year or during the second year of life. Motor development is abnormally slow, growth falls

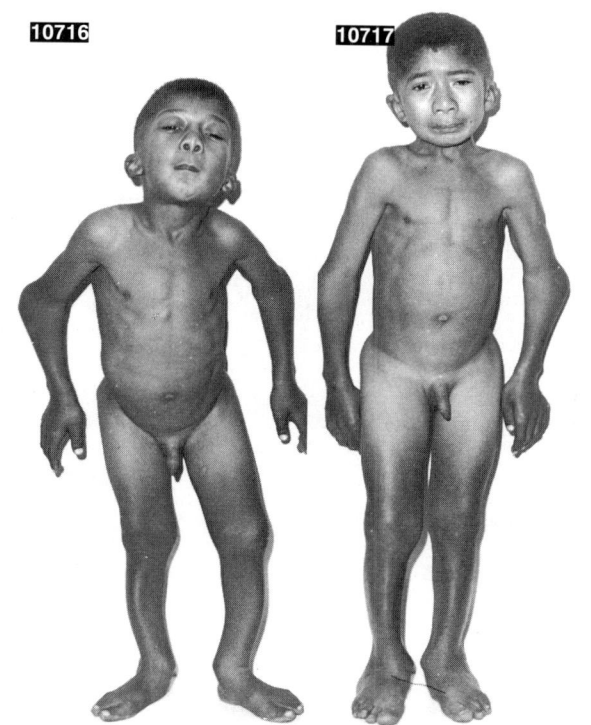

**0155**-10716–17:  Note short neck, joint contractures, fixed facial expression, small mouth and ptosis.

below the normal range, skeletal deformities become apparent, the facial features change, and myotonia is diagnosed after age 2 years. After the second year motor function improves: In one of the originally studied patients, clinical myotonia gradually subsided, and height reached the normal range.

At least 25 patients with this syndrome have been reported. All had myotonia, ocular and facial abnormalities, and bone disease. Three patients, one of them studied by the author, reached normal height, while the remaining two had abnormally short stature. Persistent muscle fiber activity during rest was present in some patients.

The clinical findings also include skeletal deformities: short neck, pigeon breast deformity, kyphoscoliosis, hip dysplasia and joint contractures; anomalies of the face: flattened face - relatively small in relation to the size of the skull, small mouth, small chin, and fixed facial expression; anomalies of the eyes: short and narrow palpebral fissures, shortening of the distance between the outer angles of the eyes in relation to the distance between the inner angles, increased distance between the inner angles of the eyes, intermittent unilateral ptosis; microcornea; probable microphthalmos and bilateral pseudoptosis, severe myopia, juvenile cataract, eyelashes inserted in two or more rows; abnormalities of the skeletal muscles: increased muscle consistency, small muscles, generalized muscular hypertrophy, and suspected muscular hypertrophy.

Other abnormalities include transient lactosuria; umbilical and inguinal hernia; abnormally small testes; patency of the anal sphincter; and indistinct speech and drooling.

**Complications:** Inability to ambulate independently because of hip dysplasia. Limitation of movement because of joint contractures and myotonia. Impaired vision because of narrowing of the palpebral fissures, myopia, or juvenile cataract. Psychologic abnormalities related to crippling by the disease and to repeated or prolonged hospitalization.

**Associated Findings:** Bilateral carpal tunnel has been reported.

**Etiology:** Autosomal recessive inheritance.

**Pathogenesis:** The primary effect of the mutant autosomal gene is not known and is apparently confined to tissues derived from the mesoderm. Bone biopsy was performed in one patient and revealed changes suggestive of abnormal ossification of the proximal epiphyseal cartilage plate of the femur. A generalized defect of enchondral ossification is perhaps responsible for the retarded growth rate and the anomalies of the facial and body skeleton. Light microscopy of muscle biopsies in four cases have revealed diffuse atrophy in two, and were normal in two. Electron microscopy in two cases revealed vacuolation of muscle fibers.

**MIM No.:** *25580

**POS No.:** 3403

**Sex Ratio:** M11:F12 (observed)

**Occurrence:** Several dozen cases reported. Two reported pairs were affected sibs. Caucasian patients were of Italian, Irish, Dutch, German, and Portuguese descent. One patient was reported from Brazil and two sibs belonged to the Cape black community, South Africa.

**Risk of Recurrence for Patient's Sib:**
See Part I, *Mendelian Inheritance.*

**Risk of Recurrence for Patient's Child:**
See Part I, *Mendelian Inheritance.* (None of the described patients has yet reached reproductive age.)

**Age of Detectability:** Ordinarily in the second year of life.

**Gene Mapping and Linkage:** Unknown.

**Prevention:** None known. Genetic counseling indicated.

**Treatment:** Surgical widening of the palpebral fissures; orthopedic treatment for joint contractures and hip dysplasia; correction of refractive errors with glasses.

**Prognosis:** There is no evidence that life span is shortened. All but one patient, who died accidentally, are still alive. All patients have had normal intelligence. Satisfactory functioning can be anticipated, provided that adequate corrective measures are taken for the ocular and orthopedic abnormalities.

**Detection of Carrier:** Unknown.

**Special Considerations:** The diagnosis of this syndrome is necessarily clinical since there are no specific biochemical, cytogenetic, or histopathologic changes. Muscle disease with myotonia is an essential feature, which can be easily overlooked because skeletal and oculofacial abnormalities dominate the clinical picture.

**References:**
Aberfeld DC, et al.: Myotonia, dwarfism, diffuse bone disease and unusual ocular and facial abnormalities (a new syndrome). Brain 1965; 88:313–322.
Huttenlocher PR, et al.: Osteo-chondro-muscular dystrophy: a disorder manifested by multiple skeletal deformities, myotonia and dystrophic changes in muscle. Pediatrics 1969; 44:945–958.
Aberfeld DC, et al.: Chondrodystrophic myotonia: report of two new cases; myotonia, dwarfism, diffuse bone disease and unusual ocular and facial abnormalities. Arch Neurol 1970; 22:455–462.
Fowler WM Jr, et al.: The Schwartz-Jampel syndrome: its clinical, physiological and histological expressions. J Neurol Sci 1974; 22:127–146. *
van Huffelen AC, et al.: Chondrodystrophic myotonia. A report of two unrelated Dutch patients. Neuropadiatrie 1974; 5:71–90.
Scaff M, et al.: Chondrodystrophic myotonia: electromyographic and cardiac features of a case. Acta Neurol Scand 1979; 60:243–249.
Farrel SA, et al.: Neonatal manifestations of Schwartz-Jampel syndrome. Am J Med Genet 1987; 27:799–805.

AB002                                    **Donald C. Aberfeld**

**Chondrodystrophy**
*See ACHONDROPLASIA*
**Chondrodystrophy, hyperplastic form**
*See METATROPIC DYSPLASIA*
**Chondrodystrophy-sensorineural deafness**
*See OTO-SPONDYLO-MEGAEPIPHYSEAL DYSPLASIA*
*also CHONDRODYSTROPHY-SENSORINEURAL DEAFNESS, NANCE-INSLEY TYPE*

## CHONDRODYSTROPHY-SENSORINEURAL DEAFNESS, NANCE-INSLEY TYPE                              2366

**Includes:**
Chondrodystrophy-sensorineural deafness
Nance-Insley syndrome
Nance-Sweeney syndrome
Oto-spondylo-megaepiphyseal dysplasia
Sensorineural deafness-chondrodystrophy

**Excludes:**
Achondroplasia (0010)
Arthro-ophthalmopathy, hereditary, progressive, Stickler type (0090)
Arthro-ophthalmopathy, Weissenbacher-Zweymuller variant (2424)
Deafness-myopia-cataract-saddle nose, Marshall type (0261)
Kniest dysplasia (0557)

**Major Diagnostic Criteria:** Flat facial profile, deafness, and skeletal dysplasia.

**Clinical Findings:** A characteristic facial appearance, including a depressed nasal bridge; a short nose with anteverted nares; flat facial profile; midfacial hemangioma; and either cleft hard or soft palate, or both. The limbs are short, and stature is below the 25th centile in all cases. Joint mobility is limited: metacarpophalangeal in young patients and elbow in older patients. X-ray examination has shown short, broad tubular bones with metaphyseal flaring, and vertebral anomalies. The vertebral anomalies tend to be progressive, being described as defects of the upper anterior angle in younger patients and progressing to widespread vertebral flattening, irregularity of vertebral surfaces, and disk space narrowing in older patients. In the oldest reported patient, cartilage

calcification was also noted in several areas. Strabismus and recurrent infection each occurred in two cases.

**Complications:** Scoliosis and/or kyphosis often develop, likely secondary to the vertebral anomalies. Conductive deafness may occur as a result of frequent otitis media.

**Associated Findings:** Lacrimal duct stenosis, **Ventricular septal defect**, hyperopia, and fused carpal bones were each reported in one patient.

**Etiology:** Autosomal recessive inheritance.

**Pathogenesis:** Unknown.

**MIM No.:** *21515

**POS No.:** 3062

**Sex Ratio:** M1:F1

**Occurrence:** Eight cases from North and South America and Europe have been reported.

**Risk of Recurrence for Patient's Sib:**
See Part I, *Mendelian Inheritance.*

**Risk of Recurrence for Patient's Child:**
See Part I, *Mendelian Inheritance.*

**Age of Detectability:** At birth by the facial appearance and presence of **Cleft palate**.

**Gene Mapping and Linkage:** Unknown.

**Prevention:** None known. Genetic counseling indicated.

**Treatment:** Treatment of infections and orthopedic management are indicated.

**Prognosis:** Life span and intelligence appear to be unimpaired.

**Detection of Carrier:** Unknown.

**References:**
Nance WE, Sweeney A: A recessively inherited chondrodystrophy. BD:OAS VI(4). New York: March of Dimes Birth Defects Foundation, 1970:25–27.
Insley J, Astley R: A bone dysplasia with deafness. Br J Radiol 1974; 47:244–251.
Miny P, Lenz W: Autosomal recessive deafness with skeletal dysplasia and facial appearance of Marshall syndrome. Am J Med Genet 1985; 21:317–324. * †
Salinas CF, et al.: Bone dysplasia, deafness and cleft palate syndrome. (Abstract) 7th Int Cong Hum Genet. Berlin, 1986:259.

T0007                                    **Helga V. Toriello**

## CHONDROECTODERMAL DYSPLASIA                              0156

**Includes:**
Dwarfism-polydactyly-dysplastic nails
Dwarfism, six-fingered
Ellis-van Creveld syndrome
Mesoectodermal dysplasia
Polydactyly-chondrodystrophy

**Excludes:**
Asphyxiating thoracic dysplasia (0091)
Heart-Hand syndrome IV (3272)
Oculo-cerebro-facial syndrome, Kaufman type (2179)
Other short-limb dwarfism detectable at birth

**Major Diagnostic Criteria:** Postaxial polydactyly of the hands with short-limbed dwarfism and dysplastic fingernails.

**Clinical Findings:** Short-limb dwarfism and postaxial polydactyly permit recognition at birth. All cases have postaxial polydactyly of the hands. Polydactyly of the feet occurs in a minority of cases, perhaps 10%. The extra fingers are rather well developed. All cases have dysplasia of the fingernails, which are underdeveloped. So-called partial harelip is usual and consists of a midline puckering of the upper lip with prominent frenulum. This condition is associated with natal teeth that erupt and exfoliate very early.
The shortening of the limbs is more striking in the distal portion; in the fingers the proximal phalanges are longer than the

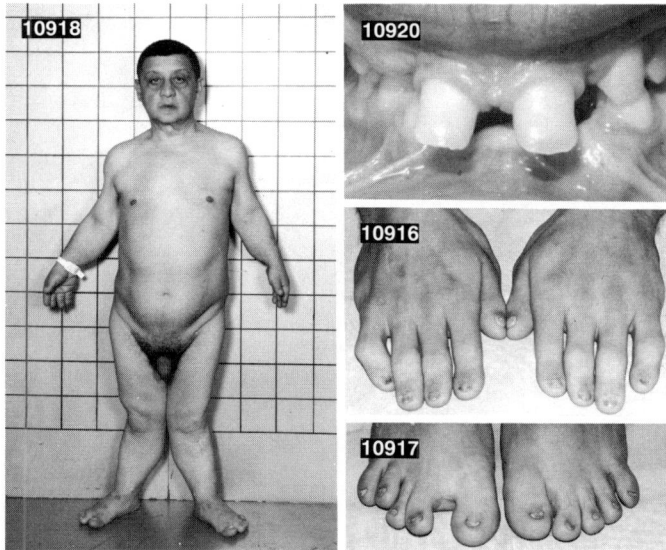

**0156-10918:** Short stature with short limbs especially in the distal segments; genu valgum. **10920:** Hypertrophied frenula and barrel-shaped incisors. **10916:** Brachydactyly, clinodactyly and hypoplastic nails. **10917:** Hypoplastic nails and wide space between 1st and 2nd toes on the left.

middle and distal phalanges so that the patient cannot make a tight fist.

Genu valgum is always present, and by age 5 or 6 years typical X-ray changes consist of erosion of the lateral aspect of the proximal tibial metaphysis. X-ray views of the pelvis show a trident configuration over the acetabulum rather like that of asphyxiating thoracic dysplasia. A characteristic X-ray finding in the wrist is fusion of the hamate and capitate bones.

Over one half of the patients have congenital malformation of the heart and usually a large atrial septal defect of either ostium primum or ostium secundum type, more often the former. **Hydrocephaly** due to Dandy-Walker malformation has been found in some patients.

**Complications:** Heart failure; respiratory failure from thoracic and tracheobronchial abnormalities; severe leg deformity, especially knock-knees.

**Associated Findings:** Natal teeth, precocious exfoliation of teeth, epispadias.

**Etiology:** Autosomal recessive inheritance.

**Pathogenesis:** Unknown.

**MIM No.:** *22550

**POS No.:** 3066

**CDC No.:** 756.525, 756.520

**Sex Ratio:** M1:F1

**Occurrence:** Ordinarily rare. No racial predilection. Very frequent in one Amish group.

**Risk of Recurrence for Patient's Sib:**
See Part I, *Mendelian Inheritance.*

**Risk of Recurrence for Patient's Child:**
See Part I, *Mendelian Inheritance.*

**Age of Detectability:** At birth. Prenatal diagnosis may be possible with ultrasound or fetoscopy.

**Gene Mapping and Linkage:** Unknown.

**Prevention:** None known. Genetic counseling indicated.

**Treatment:** Orthopedic correction of genu valgum, amputation of extra digits, and surgical repair of cardiac malformation.

**Prognosis:** In about one-third of cases death occurs before age six months. Survival to adulthood occurs, especially in those patients who are free of cardiac malformation.

**Detection of Carrier:** Unknown.

**Special Considerations:** Among the Old Order Amish of Lancaster County, Pennsylvania, over 100 cases in almost 50 sibships have been observed. Founder effect, endogamy, consanguinity, and perhaps random genetic drift are factors responsible for the high frequency of the condition in this group. It has been reported rarely in many other ethnic groups.

**References:**

McKusick FA, et al.: Dwarfism in the Amish. I. The Ellis-van Creveld syndrome. Bull Johns Hopkins Hosp 1964; 115:306.

Murdoch JL, Walker BA: Ellis-van Creveld syndrome. In: BD:OAS 1969; V:279. New York: The National Foundation - March of Dimes.

Mahoney MJ, Hobbins JC: Prenatal diagnosis of chondroectodermal dysplasia (Ellis-van Creveld syndrome) with fetoscopy and ultrasound. N Engl J Med 1977; 297:258–260.

Christian JC, et al.: A family with three recessive traits and homozygosity for a long 9qh+ chromosome segment. Am J Med Genet 1980; 6:301–308.

Da Silva EO, et al.: Ellis-van Creveld syndrome: A report of 15 cases in an inbred kindred. Am J Med Genet 1980; 17:349–356.

Rosenberg S, et al.: Chondroectodermal dysplasia (Ellis-van Creveld) with anomalies of CNS and urinary tract. Am J Med Genet 1983; 15:291–295.

Taylor GA, et al.: Polycarpaly and other abnormalities of the wrist in chonodroectodermal dysplasia: the Ellis-van Creveld syndrome. Radiology 1984; 151:393–396.

MC023                                          **Victor A. McKusick**

**Chondrogenesis imprefecta**
*See ACHONDROGENESIS, LANGER-SALDINO TYPE*
**Chondroitin sulfate sulfotransferase deficiency**
*See SPONDYLOEPIPHYSEAL DYSPLASIA, LATE*
**Chondroosteodystrophy**
*See MUCOPOLYSACCHARIDOSIS IV*
**Chondrosternal prominence, congenital**
*See PECTUS CARINATUM*
**Chonechondrosternon**
*See PECTUS EXCAVATUM*
**Chordae tendineae, anomalous shortened**
*See MITRAL VALVE INSUFFICIENCY*

---

**CHOREA, BENIGN FAMILIAL**          **2306**

**Includes:** Choreoathetosis, autosomal dominant

**Excludes:**
**Acanthocytosis-neurologic defects** (2398)
**Huntington disease** (0478)
Hypoxic encephalopathy, neonatal
Kernicterus
Paroxysmal choreoathetosis
Rheumatic ("Sydenham") chorea

**Major Diagnostic Criteria:** Nonprogressive chorea beginning in infancy, in the absence of other neurologic signs, and the absence of dementia.

**Clinical Findings:** Onset of chorea (and athetosis in some cases) occurs in early childhood, often interfering with the development of motor milestones. The chorea is nonprogressive. Intellect is normal. There is no dementia. Poor coordination of the movements of the upper and lower extremities occurs, including gait ataxia.

**Complications:** The condition is more of an inconvenience than disabling.

**Associated Findings:** Dysarthria or anarthria.

**Etiology:** Autosomal dominant inheritance, with incomplete penetrance in a few cases.

**Pathogenesis:** Chorea has been postulated to arise from an excess of dopamine, probably acting via D1 receptors.

**MIM No.:** *11870

**Sex Ratio:** M1:F1

**Occurrence:** Incidence estimated at 1:500,000.

**Risk of Recurrence for Patient's Sib:**
See Part I, *Mendelian Inheritance.*

**Risk of Recurrence for Patient's Child:**
See Part I, *Mendelian Inheritance.*

**Age of Detectability:** Usually at birth, or in the first year of life.

**Gene Mapping and Linkage:** BCH (benign chorea) is unassigned.

**Prevention:** None known. Genetic counseling indicated.

**Treatment:** Use of aids for writing and school work (typewriters, word processors). Research treatments include steroids and copper.

**Prognosis:** Life span is not impaired.

**Detection of Carrier:** Unknown.

**References:**
Haerer AF, et al.: Hereditary nonprogressive chorea of early onset. New Engl J Med 1967; 276:1220–1224.
Harper PS: Benign hereditary chorea: clinical and genetic aspects. Clin Genet 1978; 13:85–95.
Robinson RO, Thornett CEE: Benign hereditary chorea: response to steroids. Dev Med Child Neurol 1985; 27:814–821.
Stapert JLRH, et al.: Benign (nonparoxysmal) familial chorea of early onset: an electroneurophysiological examination of two families. Brain Dev 1985; 7:38–42.

C0018                           **Mary Coleman**

**Choreoacanthocytosis**
   *See ACANTHOCYTOSIS-NEUROLOGIC DEFECTS*
**Choreoathetosis, autosomal dominant**
   *See CHOREA, BENIGN FAMILIAL*
**Choreoathetosis-mental retardation, X-linked**
   *See X-LINKED MENTAL RETARDATION-CHOREOATHETOSIS*
**Chorioretinal coloboma-Joubert syndrome**
   *See JOUBERT SYNDROME*
**Chorioretinitis, toxoplasmic**
   *See FETAL TOXOPLASMOSIS SYNDROME*
**Chorioretinopathy-congenital microcephaly**
   *See MICROCEPHALY WITH CHORIORETINOPATHY*
**Choroid, coloboma**
   *See EYE, MICROPHTHALMIA/COLOBOMA*
**Choroid, gyrate atrophy**
   *See GYRATE ATROPHY OF THE CHOROID AND RETINA*
**Choroidal sclerosis**
   *See CHOROIDEREMIA*

## CHOROIDEREMIA                  0925

**Includes:**
   Choroidal sclerosis
   Choroidoretinal degeneration
   Retina, tapetochoroidal dystrophy
   Tapetochoroidal dystrophy, progressive

**Excludes:**
   **Gyrate atrophy of the choroid and retina** (0449)
   **Retinitis pigmentosa** (0869)

**Major Diagnostic Criteria:** A bilateral X-linked progressive dystrophic disease of the choroid and retina characterized by night blindness and visual field constriction in affected males, with a characteristic fundus appearance. Female carriers have a mosaic of hypopigmented and hyperpigmented changes at the level of the retinal pigment epithelium, accentuated in the peripheral retina.

**Clinical Findings:** Early in the disease, there is hypopigmentation of the retinal pigment epithelium (RPE) with prominent choroidal vessels throughout the fundus. Atrophy of the choroid and pigment epithelium progresses during the first two decades with attendant night blindness and peripheral visual field constriction. Changes occur diffusely throughout the retina but progress towards the macular area, which is usually affected last in the third or fourth decades of life, thus leaving hemizygous males

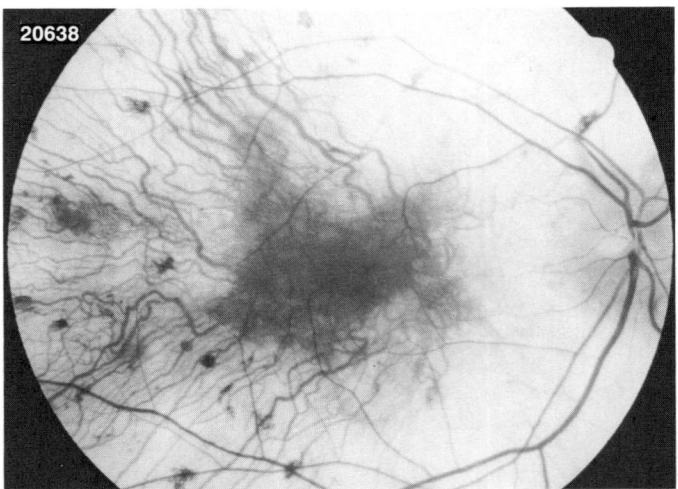

**0925A-20638:** Choroideremia in a male in his third decade; the retinal vessels and optic nerve are well preserved but there has been a circumferential loss of the retinal pigment epithelium, choriocapillaris, and some large choroidal vessels, sparing only the central macular region.

with reasonable central acuity until late in the disease. Occasional islands of reactive hyperpigmentation can be seen in or near large areas of atrophy of choriocapillaris and choroid. Both electrophysiology and dark adaptation are abnormal. Carriers are usually asymptomatic, although some in the sixth and seventh decades will complain of moderate night blindness and show peripheral coarse pigment clumping.

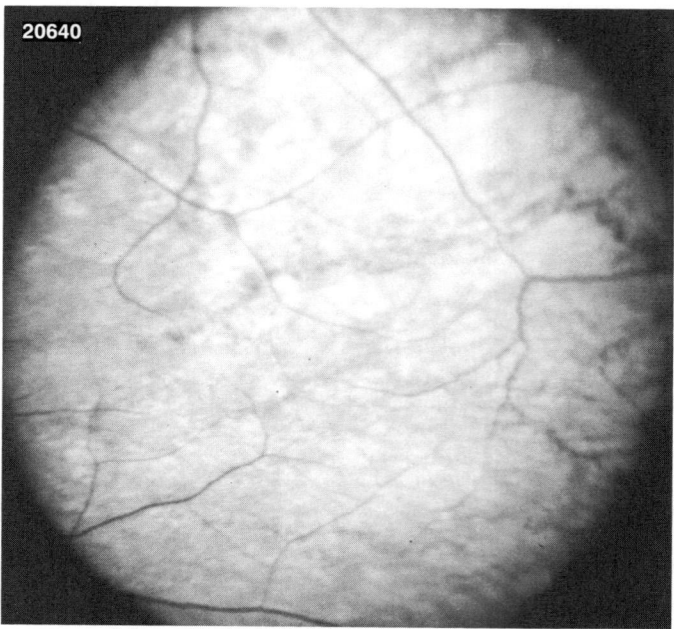

**0925B-20640:** Note the reticulated curvilinear clumping of the retinal pigment epithelium in the midperiphery of an obligate carrier of choroideremia.

**Complications:** Progressive visual impairment with eventual blindness in middle thirties to forties. One 14 year-old patient has been reported with disciform macular degeneration.

**Associated Findings: Van Den Bosch syndrome** includes choroideremia as a main feature. Ayazi (1981) reported a family with X-linked choroideremia, obesity, mental retardation, and deafness. Several other cases and families with overlapping features have been reported. In the majority of cases, however, choroideremia is an isolated ophthalmic finding.

**Etiology:** X-linked inheritance.

**Pathogenesis:** Unknown.

**MIM No.:** *30310, 30311, 30320

**Sex Ratio:** M1:F0

**Occurrence:** Probably less than 1:60,000.

**Risk of Recurrence for Patient's Sib:**
See Part I, *Mendelian Inheritance.*

**Risk of Recurrence for Patient's Child:**
See Part I, *Mendelian Inheritance.*

**Age of Detectability:** Fundus changes are identifiable in first decade by a skilled observer. Hypopigmentation and hyperpigmentation of the RPE have been observed in the second year of life. Prenatal diagnosis is possible in cases where choroideremia is associated with a detectable deletion (Hodgson, 1987) and, theoretically, using RFLP techniques.

**Gene Mapping and Linkage:** TCD (tapeto-choroidal dystrophy, progressive choroidemia) has been mapped to Xq21.1-q21.2.
CRD (choroidoretinal degeneration) has been mapped to X.

**Prevention:** None known. Genetic counseling indicated.

**Treatment:** Unknown.

**Prognosis:** Blindness by middle to late adulthood.

**Detection of Carrier:** Possible by retinal examination in more than 90% of cases. Retinal electrophysiologic studies are normal in 90% of carriers.

**References:**
McCulloch Jc, McCulloch RFP: Hereditary and clinical study of choroideremia. Trans Am Acad Ophthalmol Otolaryngol 1948; 52:160–168.
Ayazi S: Choroideremia, obesity, and congenital deafness. Am J Ophthalmol 1981; 92:63–69.
Rodrigues MM, et al: Choroideremia: a clinical, electron microscopic, and biochemical report. Ophthalmol 1984; 91:873–883.
Sieving PA, et al: Electroretinographic findings in selected pedigrees with choroideremia. Am J Ophthalmol 1986; 101:361–367.
Hodgson SV, et al.: Prenatal diagnosis of X-linked choroideremia with mental retardation, associated with a cytologically detectable X-chromosome deletion. Hum Genet 1987; 75:286–290.
Sankila E-M, et al.: Haplotyping Finnish choroideremia patients. (Abstract) Cytogenet Cell Genet 1987; HGM9.

TR009                                                    **Elias I. Traboulsi**

**Choroidoretinal degeneration**
*See CHOROIDEREMIA*
**Chotzen syndrome**
*See ACROCEPHALOSYNDACTYLY TYPE III*
**Christ-Siemens-Touraine syndrome**
*See ECTODERMAL DYSPLASIA, CHRIST-SIEMENS-TOURAINE TYPE*
**Christensen Krabbe disease**
*See ALPERS DISEASE*
**Christian syndrome**
*See X-LINKED MENTAL RETARDATION-SKELETAL DYSPLASIA*
**Christmas disease**
*See HEMOPHILIA B*
**Christmas tree syndrome**
*See JEJUNAL ATRESIA*
**Chromatophore nevus of Naegeli**
*See ECTODERMAL DYSPLASIA, NAEGELI TYPE*
**Chromosome 1, 45,XY,-1/46,XY/47,XY+1**
*See CHROMOSOME 1, TRISOMY-MONOSOMY 1 MOSAIC*
**Chromosome 1, centromeric instability-immunodeficiency**
*See IMMUNODEFICIENCY WITH CENTROMERIC INSTABILITY*

**Chromosome 1, deletion (1)(q42) syndrome**
*See CHROMOSOME 1, MONOSOMY 1q4*
**Chromosome 1, deletion (1)(q43) syndrome**
*See CHROMOSOME 1, MONOSOMY 1q4*
**Chromosome 1, deletion of chromosome 1q (42 or 43-ter)**
*See CHROMOSOME 1, MONOSOMY 1q*
**Chromosome 1, duplication 1q25-1q32**
*See CHROMOSOME 1, TRISOMY 1q25-1q32*
**Chromosome 1, duplication 1q32-qter**
*See CHROMOSOME 1, TRISOMY 1q32-qter*

## CHROMOSOME 1, MONOSOMY 1Q                      2325

**Includes:** Chromosome 1, deletion of chromosome 1q (42 or 43-ter)

**Excludes: Chromosome** (other defects)

**Major Diagnostic Criteria:** The diagnosis is suspected on the basis of **Microcephaly** from birth, brachycephaly, fine and scant hair, round face, heavy cheeks and a characteristic mouth which is carp-shaped with a pulled-in lower lip giving the appearance of chewing on the lower lip. Diagnosis is confirmed by chromosome analysis.

**Clinical Findings:** The most common features and their approximate frequencies are based on 28 cases:
*General:* full term or postmature (13/20); generalized hypotonia (13/16); marked growth delay (22/25); severe psychomotor delay (24/25); shrill cry (9/10); and seizures (12/21).
*Craniofacial:* severe **Microcephaly** from birth (23/28); brachycephaly (17/23); fine scant hair (11/11); round face (12/17); short broad nose (24/28); prominent philtrum (12/17); oblique palpebral fissures (16/22); epicanthus (20/24); pseudohypertelorism (16/20); strabismus (10/10); bilateral microphthalmia (2/28); carp shaped mouth (24/28); pulled in lower lip (8/11); appearance of chewing on lower lip (8/11); **Cleft palate** (7/24); micrognathia or retrognathia (21/28); abnormal ears (21/28).
*Heart:* predominantly **Ventricular septal defect** (12/26).
*Genitourinary:* hypospadias/cryptorchidism (13/13 males); vaginal stenosis (1/15 females); single kidney (1/28); hydronephrosis (2/24).
*Extremities:* hands, including clinodactyly, abnormal length or tapering of fingers, or hypoplastic nails (18/26); feet, including talipes deformity, **Syndactyly**, or hypoplastic nails (11/24).
*Central nervous system:* cortical atrophy (4/17); **Hydrocephaly** (5/17); partial or complete agenesis of the corpus callosum (7/26); occipital encephalocele (3/27); and spina bifida (2/28).
*Other:* short neck (21/23); vertebral anomalies; skin aplasia of scalp (1/28); sclerocornea (1/28).
*Dermatoglyphics:* case reports are too fragmentary to draw any firm conclusions. Hallucal arches may be specific to this group.

**Complications:** Cardiac failure and problems with cleft palate.

**Associated Findings:** Seizures may be difficult to control.

**Etiology:** Usually the result of the deletion of some of the genetic material from the terminal portion of the long arm of chromosome 1 during gametogenesis. This particular segment which is lost is distal to band q42 or q43. Four of the cases resulted from maternal balanced translocations involving chromosomes 2, 10 and 16, of which two were from the same mother. The remainder proved to be *de novo.*

**Pathogenesis:** Unknown.

**POS No.:** 3112, 3684

**CDC No.:** 758.990

**Sex Ratio:** M1:F1

**Occurrence:** Twenty-eight cases have been reported in the literature.

**Risk of Recurrence for Patient's Sib:** Varies depending upon the specific balanced translocation if present in the parents.

**Risk of Recurrence for Patient's Child:** Unknown.

**Age of Detectability:** At birth or prenatally by chromosome analysis.

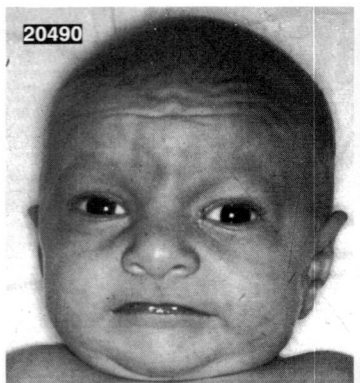
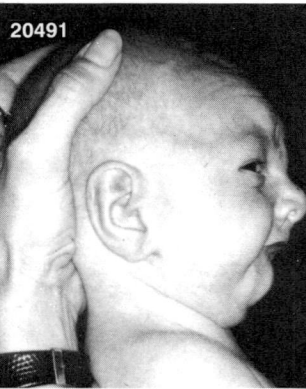

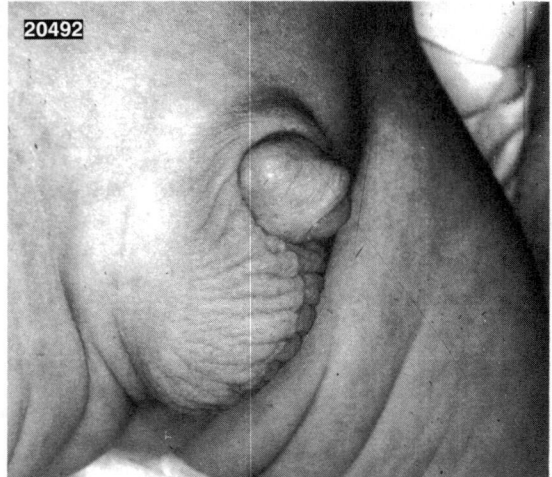

**2325-20490:** Chromosome 1, monosomy 1q; note round face; short, broad nose; oblique palpebral fissures; long smooth philtrum; and carp-shaped mouth. **20491:** Lateral view of face; note micrognathia, pulled-in lower lip and the appearance of chewing on the lower lip. **20492:** Hypospadias and small phallus.

**Gene Mapping and Linkage:** See *Gene Map.*

**Prevention:** None known. Genetic counseling indicated.

**Treatment:** As may be indicated for any congenital anomalies.

**Prognosis:** The average life span is unknown. Five of the 28 affected patients died in infancy. The oldest surviving patient is now 30 years of age. The children, if they survive infancy, remain severely delayed in growth and development.

**Detection of Carrier:** By chromosomal analysis.

**References:**

Mankinen CB, et al.: Terminal (1)(q43) long arm deletion of chromosome no. 1 in a three-year-old female. BD:OAS (XII). New York: March of Dimes Birth Defects Foundation, 1976:131–136.

Juberg RC, et al.: New deletion syndrome: 1q43. Am J Hum Genet 1981; 33:455–463.

Johnson VP, et al.: Deletion of the distal long arm of chromosome 1: a definable syndrome. Am J Med Genet 1985; 22:685–694. * †

Watson MS, et al.: Chromosome deletion 1q42–43. Am J Med Genet 1986; 24:1–6. *

Meinecke P, Vogtel D: A specific syndrome due to the deletion of the distal long arm of chromosome 1. Am J Med Genet 1987; 28:371–376. *

Reed T, Milatovich A: Dermatoglyphic findings in chromosome 1 long arm deletions. Am J Med Genet 1988; 29:685–689.

LA008                                                        **Charlotte Z. Lafer**

---

## CHROMOSOME 1, MONOSOMY 1Q4                                            2429

**Includes:**
    Chromosome 1, deletion (1)(q42) syndrome
    Chromosome 1, deletion (1)(q43) syndrome

**Excludes:** N/A

**Major Diagnostic Criteria:** Demonstration of deletion of the distal bands of the long arm of chromosome 1 from q42 or q43 to q terminal.

**Clinical Findings:** Based on the 15 reported cases as of 1985 (Johnson et al., 1985): **Microcephaly** (15/15); brachycephaly (7/8); small fontanelle (4/4); oblique palpebral fissures (8/10); epicanthal folds (11/12); impression of hypertelorism (8/9); strabismus (6/11); short, broad nose (13/14); smooth, long philtrum (7/9); thin vermilion border and downturned corners of the mouth (13/13); micro- or retrognathia (12/15); apparently low-set anomalous ears (12/13); abnormal palate (7/8); short neck (11/12); cardiac anomaly (5/13); genital anomaly (11/14); abnormal hands (13/14); abnormal feet (10/10); psychomotor retardation (13/13); and growth retardation (9/10).

The craniofacial characteristics are microbrachycephaly, round face, short and broad nose with a tendency to anteverted nares, mild-to-moderate epicanthal folds, upslanting palpebral fissures, long upper lip with smooth philtrum, thin vermillion border of lips with well-formed cupid's bow and downturned corners, micrognathia or retrognathia, apparently low-set ears, palatal defect, narrow high-arched palate, absent uvula, and **Cleft palate.**

Congenital heart defect reported consists of **Ventricular septal defect** (VSD), valvular pulmonary stenosis, pseudotruncus arteriosus, and **Pulmonary valve, atresia.** The genital abnormalities vary, such as ambiguous genitalia with perineal urethra and bifid scrotum, small genitalia, hypospadias, cryptorchidism, vaginal stenosis, and prominent labia minora.

CNS abnormalities include **Corpus callosum agenesis** in three cases, cortical atrophy, **Hydranencephaly,** and various grades of neural tube defect. Postnatal growth retardation, failure to thrive, and profound-to-severe mental retardation were present in all cases.

**Complications:** Unknown.

**Associated Findings:** Respiratory problems include apneic episodes, bronchospasm and repeated infections. Heart problems include arrhythmia and congestive failure from heart malformations. Urinary tract problems include urethral reflux and recurrent infections.

**Etiology:** The majority of cases had *de novo* deletions with breakpoints at 1q42 or 1q43. Three had a derived deletion from a parental translocation.

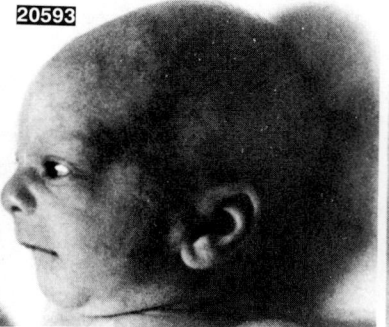
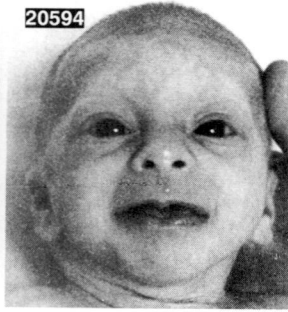

**2429A-20593–94:** Chromosome 1, monosomy 1q4; note microbrachycephaly; epicanthal folds; short, broad nose; long, smooth philtrum; and thin vermilion border. Lateral view shows micrognathia and low-set ear.

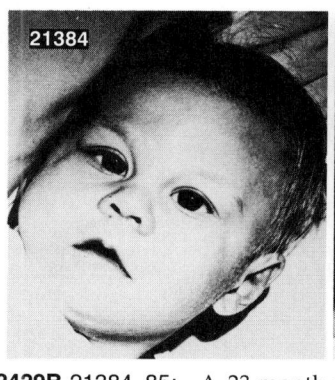
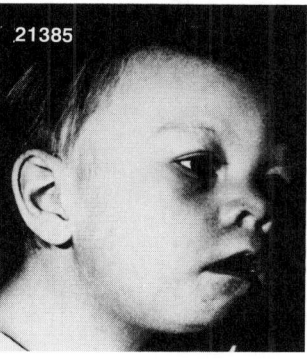

**2429B-21384–85:** A 23-month-old male with epicanthal folds, flat nasal bridge, and downturned mouth; he had a terminal deletion of the long arm of chromosome one.

**Pathogenesis:** Chromosomal imbalance leads to multiple malformations, mental retardation, and growth retardation.

**POS No.:** 3118

**CDC No.:** 758.990

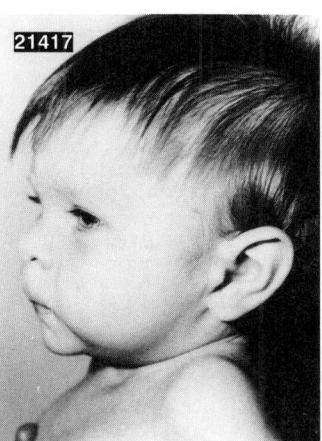
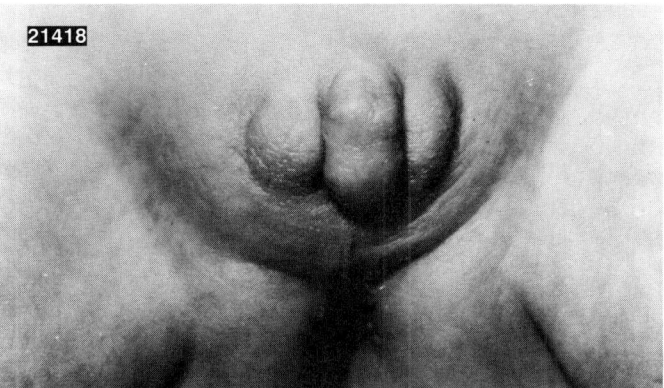

**2429C-21416:** Affected 11-month-old male with dysmorphic facies, flattened nasal bridge, bulbous nose and abnormal eyelids. **21417:** Lateral view of the face shows brachycephaly, micrognathia, short neck, sparse fine hair, and large ears. **21418:** Abnormal scrotum and hypospadias.

**Sex Ratio:** M7:F8 (observed).

**Occurrence:** At least 23 cases have been documented.

**Risk of Recurrence for Patient's Sib:** Very small unless parent is a translocation carrier. Parental karyotyping should be done in all cases.

**Risk of Recurrence for Patient's Child:** Affected individuals are not expected to survive to reproduce.

**Age of Detectability:** Midtrimester by amniocentesis and karyotyping of amniocytes, or at birth.

**Gene Mapping and Linkage:** See *Gene Map*.

**Prevention:** None known. Genetic counseling indicated.

**Treatment:** As indicated.

**Prognosis:** A shortened life span appears to be the rule. Retardation is profound to severe.

**Detection of Carrier:** Parental karyotyping is indicated in all cases with translocations between 1 and 16 and between 1 and 12.

**References:**

Juberg RC, et al.: New deletion syndrome: del 1q43. Am J Hum Genet 1981; 33:455–463.

Johnson VP, et al.: Deletion of the distal long arm of chromosome I: a definable syndrome. Am J Med Genet 1985; 22:685–694.

Meinecke P, Vögtel D: A specific syndrome due to deletion of the distal long arm of chromosome 1. Am J Med Genet 1987; 28:371–376.

Yamamoto Y, et al.: Deletion of the distal long arm of chromosome 1: an analytical approach may contribute to the diagnosis. Acta Pediatr Jpn 1988; 30:696–702.

J0010                                        **Virginia P. Johnson**

---

### CHROMOSOME 1, TRISOMY 1Q25–1Q32          **2428**

**Includes:** Chromosome 1, duplication 1q25–1q32

**Excludes:** Chromosome 1, trisomies of other portions

**Major Diagnostic Criteria:** Multiple congenital anomalies including facial dysmorphism, developmental delay or mental retardation, and congenital heart disease. The diagnosis is made by chromosome evaluation looking for either a duplication of 1q25→1q32 or an unbalanced translocation involving translocation of 1q25→1q32 to another chromosome, and confirming the translocation by demonstration of a parental balanced translocation.

**Clinical Findings:** Birth weight is normal. Head circumference is normal to megalencephalic. There is facial dysmorphism with deep-set eyes, broad nasal bridge, small mouth, retrognathia, and low-set posteriorly rotated ears. There is **Camptodactyly** with overlapping fingers. Congenital heart defects have been described (4/7). Eye malformations have been reported, including colobomas (1/7) and microphthalmia (2/7). Pectus deformities may be seen.

Outcome is quite variable, with intellect in survivors ranging from normal (3/6) to mild-to-moderate mental retardation (1/6).

**Complications:** Respiratory distress may be seen secondary to glossoptosis, which is related to the retrognathia. Severe hypoglycemia has been reported in one patient.

**Associated Findings:** Retinal colobomas have been described in one child.

**Etiology:** May arise as a result of an inherited unbalanced translocation from a parent with a balanced chromosome translocation. *De novo* cases have been described.

**Pathogenesis:** Unknown.

**POS No.:** 3683

**CDC No.:** 758.990

**Sex Ratio:** M0:F7 (observed).

**Occurrence:** Seven cases have been reported in the literature.

**Risk of Recurrence for Patient's Sib:** Relatively high if one parent is a carrier of a balanced chromosomal translocation. Very low

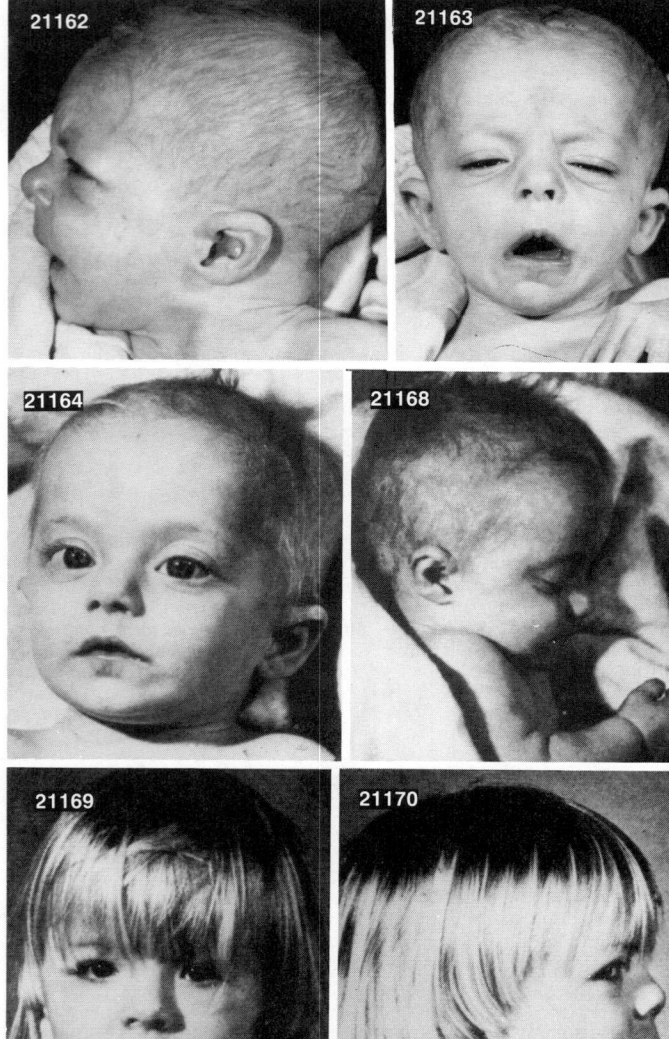

**2428**-21162–63: Affected 3-month-old sib showing unusual facial features including prominent eyes, low-set ears, prominent lower eyelid folds, long philtrum, and micrognathia. 21164–68: Affected 17-month-old sib with prominent eyes, micrognathia and low-set ears. 21169–70: Affected 4-year-old sib also shows low-set ears, short nose, and long philtrum.

recurrence risk for sib if proband is carrier of a *de novo* duplication or translocation.

**Risk of Recurrence for Patient's Child:** High recurrence risk for patients with a duplication; theoretically 50%. No cases of reproduction in affected individuals have been reported.

**Age of Detectability:** At birth, by karyotype. Prenatal diagnosis with either chorionic villus sampling or amniocentesis.

**Gene Mapping and Linkage:** See *Gene Map*.

**Prevention:** None known. Genetic counseling indicated.

**Treatment:** Unknown.

**Prognosis:** Variable. Individuals with normal intellect have been described, as well as individuals with moderate-to-severe mental retardation. Congenital heart defects have been seen in 4/7 individuals and may be a cause of morbidity and mortality.

**Detection of Carrier:** The balanced translocation carrier is recognizable by karyotype analysis.

**References:**
Palmer CG, et al.: Partial trisomy 1 due to a "shift" and probable location of Duffy (Fy) locus. Am J Hum Genet 1977; 29:371–377.
Pan SF, et al.: Meiotic consequences of an intrachromosomal insertion of chromosome No 1: a family pedigree. Clin Genet 1977; 12:303–313.
Schinzel A: Possible trisomy 1q25→1q32 in a malformed girl with a de novo insertion in 1q. Hum Genet 1979; 49:167–173.

SA001 **Howard M. Saal**

---

**CHROMOSOME 1, TRISOMY 1Q32-QTER** 2426

**Includes:** Chromosome 1, duplication 1q32→qter

**Excludes:** Chromosome 1, trisomies of other portions

**Major Diagnostic Criteria:** Multiple congenital anomalies including facial dysmorphism, severe developmental delay or mental retardation, and growth retardation. The diagnosis is made by chromosome evaluation looking for either a duplication of 1q32→qter or an unbalanced translocation involving translocation of 1q32→qter to another chromosome and confirming the translocation by demonstration of a parental balanced translocation.

**Clinical Findings:** There is mild intrauterine growth retardation, with mean birth weight being about 2,500 g. Severe malformations are present at birth, and most affected infants die within the first days of life. There is relative **Megalencephaly**, with prominent forehead, large anterior fontenelle, and metopic suture. The palpebral fissures are downslanting, and hypertelorism is often present. The nose is small, and the nasal bridge is flat. The ears are small, malformed, and low set. Micrognathia is a common feature. Redundant nuchal skin may be seen. The fingers are long and often overlap. Simian lines are often seen. Congenital heart disease is common and is often a cause for morbidity and mortality. The most common congenital heart defect is **Heart, truncus arteriosus**.

Perinatal death is common, especially in the presence of congenital heart disease. Individuals who survive have moderate-to-severe mental retardation.

**Complications:** Feeding difficulties and sensorineural hearing loss have been described.

**Associated Findings:** **Hernia, inguinal** has been seen in one patient, and kyphoscoliosis has been seen in one patient.

**Etiology:** May arise as an inherited unbalanced translocation from a parent with a balanced chromosomal translocation. *De novo* cases have been described.

**Pathogenesis:** Unknown.

**POS No.:** 3126

**CDC No.:** 758.990

**Sex Ratio:** M4:F3

**Occurrence:** Seven cases have been described in the literature.

**Risk of Recurrence for Patient's Sib:** Relatively high if one parent is a carrier of a balanced chromosomal translocation. Very low recurrence risk for sib if proband is a carrier of a *de novo* duplication or translocation.

**Risk of Recurrence for Patient's Child:** Reproduction of survivors has not been reported.

**Age of Detectability:** At birth, by karyotype. Prenatal diagnosis with either chorionic villus sampling or amniocentesis.

**Gene Mapping and Linkage:** See *Gene Map*.

**Prevention:** None known. Genetic counseling indicated.

**Treatment:** Unknown.

**Prognosis:** Moderate-to-severe mental retardation.

**Detection of Carrier:** The balanced translocation carrier is recognizable by karoytype analysis.

**References:**
van den Berghe H, et al.: Partial trisomy 1: karyotype 46,XY, 12-, t(1q, 12p)+. Humangenetik 1973; 18:225–230.
Rehder H, Friedrich U: Partial trisomy 1q syndrome. Clin Genet 1979; 15:534–540.
de Grouchy J, Turleau C: Clinical atlas of human chromosomes, ed 2. New York: John Wiley & Sons, 1984.
Michels VV, et al.: Duplication of part of chromosome 19: clinical report and review of the literature. Am J Med Genet 1984; 18:125–134. *

SA001                                          **Howard M. Saal**

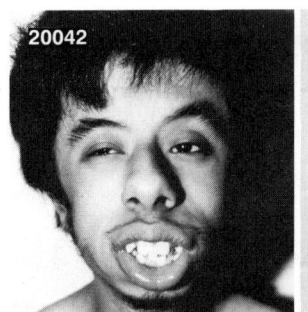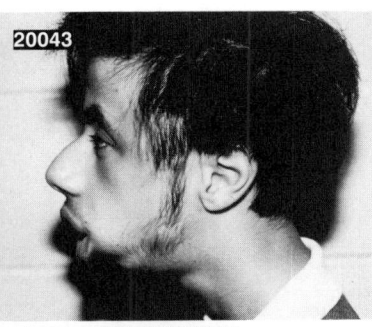
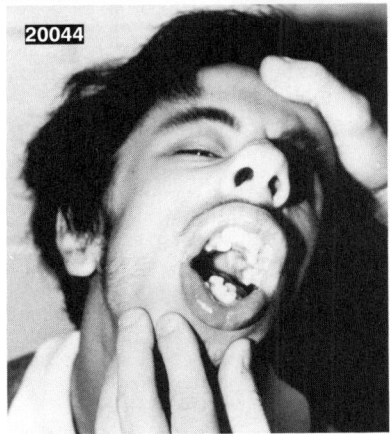

## CHROMOSOME 1, TRISOMY-MONOSOMY 1 MOSAIC    2536

**Includes:** Chromosome 1, 45,XY,-1/46,XY/47,XY+1

**Excludes:**
  Chromosome 1, inversions of
  Chromosome 1, partial monosomies of
  Chromosome 1, partial trisomies of
  Ghromosome 1, other anomalies

**Major Diagnostic Criteria:** Since only one patient with this cytogenetic entity has been encountered, it is premature to consider the major diagnostic criteria of this condition. In addition, variations in the ratio of the different cell lines should be expected to lead to considerable phenotypic changes. A constellation of congenital anomalies, however, should be present. Thus, cytogenetic studies of patients with multiple congenital anomalies may detect more individuals with this entity.

**Clinical Findings:** Postnatal slow physical and psychomotor development results in severe proportionate short stature with **Microcephaly** and mental retardation. Congenital cataracts, microcornea, mild microphthalmia, optic atrophy, facial dysmorphy and premature graying define further the phenotype. The latter, however, is expected to show considerable pleiotrophy secondary to variations of the cell ratio.

**Complications:** Failure to thrive, with spitting up in infancy.

**Associated Findings:** None known.

**Etiology:** Unequal division of the chromosomes.

**Pathogenesis:** Unknown.

**Sex Ratio:** M1:F0 (the only known case was male).

**Occurrence:** One case has been documented. Since chromosome 1 represents almost 10% of the haploid genome, trisomy or monosomy 1 is expected to be incompatible with life. It may be presumed that only low percentage mosaicism, just as in this patient, will be seen in individuals with aberrant phenotypes.

**Risk of Recurrence for Patient's Sib:** Expected to be low; probably lower than that for any other mosaicism involving smaller size chromosomes.

**Risk of Recurrence for Patient's Child:** Unknown. May not be compatible with reproduction.

**Age of Detectability:** Whenever a karyotype is performed. Prenatal diagnosis is possible.

**Gene Mapping and Linkage:** See *Gene Map.*

**Prevention:** None known. Genetic counseling indicated.

**Treatment:** Palliative, addressing specific clinical features. Home rearing with early intensive stimulation could be beneficial.

**Prognosis:** Life span is expected to be shortened.

**Detection of Carrier:** By cytogenetic study.

**Special Considerations:** The phenotype of the patient showed bilateral microcornea (7mm). By definition, microcornea implies microphthalmia. On CT orbital scan, however, the total axial length was only minimally reduced to 21.7 mm (borderline

**2536-20042:** Note dysmorphic facies, microphthalmia, prominent nose and full lips. **20043:** Lateral facies; note beaked nose and short upper lip with microretrognathia. **20044:** Constricted dental arches lead to a double row of teeth.

microphthalmia). This suggests that total axial length measurements are necessary whenever microcornea is encountered.

Cytogenetically, 39 (8.5%) of the 458 metaphases examined in peripheral lymphocyte and skin fibroblast cultures had an abnormality involving chromosome 1. On three occasions, months apart, lymphocyte studies showed ratios 1:96:7,3:46:3 and 6:91:3, respectively. Two skin fibroblast cultures, six months apart, showed 45,XY,-1/46,XY with ratios of 1:94 and 5:92. In addition, there were metaphases with isochromosomes 1p and 1q, as well as del (1p), del (1q) and translocations involving chromosome 1. These structural abnormalities were found only in one of the two flasks initiated from each skin specimen. This suggested an *in vitro* phenomenon. In 571 bone marrow metaphases, only one 47,XY,+1 cell was found. This corroborated reported observations of chromosome abnormality present in lymphocytes and not in the bone marrow cultures. In 2% of the examined lymphocyte, fibroblast and bone marrow metaphases of this patient, there were two fragile sites at 1p11 and 1p22, respectively. Folic acid deficient and BrdU-containing media did not increase the number of metaphases with fragile 1p sites. Only the fra(1) (p11) site appeared to be the break point for one of the structural anomalies, t(1p;8q). Therefore, it might have played a role in the genesis of the structural abnormalities and the non-disjunction. This also suggests chromosome instability.

**References:**
Reyes PG, et al.: Trisomy 8 mosaicism syndrome: report of monozygotic twins. Clin Genet 1978; 14:90–97.
Hustinx TWJ, et al.: Karyotype instability with multiple 7/14 and 7/7 rearrangements. Hum Genet 1979; 49:199–208.
Garcia-Sagredo JM, et al.: Fragile chromosome 16(q22) causes a balanced translocation at the same point. Hum Genet 1983; 65:211–213.

Defendi G, et al.: New chromosome rearrangements in human amniotic fluid cells in respect to heritable fragile sites. (Abstract) Atlanta, GA: The 11th Annual Meeting Association of Cytogenetic Technologists, 1986.

Neu RL, et al.: Monosomy, trisomy, fragile site and rearrangements of chromosome 1 in a mentally retarded male with MCA. Clin Genet 1988; 33:73–77. *

K0018 **Boris G. Kousseff**

## CHROMOSOME 2, MONOSOMY OF MEDIAL 2Q    2349

**Includes:** N/A

**Excludes:** N/A

**Major Diagnostic Criteria:** Multiple congenital anomalies, failure to thrive, developmental delay, and cytogenetic demonstration of monosomy of 2q (interstitial deletion).

**Clinical Findings:** Over 50% of the patients exhibit low birthweight (approximate mean 2,400 g), failure to thrive, severe psychomotor retardation, no speech development, **Microcephaly**, micrognathia, low-set ears, clenched hands, large cleft between first and second toes, and clubfoot. Findings with a frequency of 10–45% are: microphthalmia, cataracts, corneal opacity, downward-slanting palpebral fissures, prominent/beaked nose, maxillary hypoplasia, **Cleft palate**, defective dentition, feet brachy/syndactyly, joint hyperextensibility, CNS defect (internal hydrocephalus, meningomyelocele) and cardiac malformation (patent ductus Botallo, pulmonary artery stenosis, **Aorta, coarctation**, **Atrial septal defects**, or **Ventricular septal defect**).

**Complications:** Unknown.

**Associated Findings:** Plagiocephaly, iris coloboma, hypertelorism, **Cleft lip**, preauricular sinus, pilonidal dimple, feet ectrodactyly, postaxial polydactyly, absent 12th ribs, faulty lung segmentation, renal hypoplasia.

**Etiology:** The monosomy had a (definite or presumed) *de novo* origin in 11 of 16 cases. It resulted from familial insertions (1 intra- and 1 interchromosome) in the remaining five patients.

**Pathogenesis:** Unknown.

**POS No.:** 3685

**CDC No.:** 758.990

**Sex Ratio:** M4:F12.

**Occurrence:** More than 16 cases have been reported in the literature.

**Risk of Recurrence for Patient's Sib:** Significant if a parent carries a balanced rearrangement; otherwise not increased.

**Risk of Recurrence for Patient's Child:** No patient is known to have reproduced.

**Age of Detectability:** At birth, or through prenatal diagnosis.

**Gene Mapping and Linkage:** See *Gene Map.*

**Prevention:** None known. Genetic counseling indicated.

**Treatment:** Symptomatic for congenital defects; special education.

**Prognosis:** Seven of 16 patients are known to have died, most within the first year of life. Severe mental retardation should be expected.

**Detection of Carrier:** By chromosome analysis.

**References:**

Taysi K, et al.: Interstitial deletion of the long arm of chromosome 2: case report and review of literature. Ann Genet 1981; 24:245–247.

Shabtai F, et al.: Partial monosomy of chromosome 2: delineable syndrome of deletion 2(q23→q32). Ann Genet 1982; 25:156–158.

Buchanan PD, et al.: Interstitial deletion 2q31→q33. Am J Med Genet 1983; 15:121–126.

Pai GS, et al.: Identical multiple congenital anomalies mental retardation (MCA/MR) syndrome due to del(2)(q32) in two sisters with intrachromosomal insertional translocations in their father. Am J Med Genet 1983; 14:189–195. * †

Moller M, et al.: Pure monosomy and trisomy 2q24.2→q3105 due to an inv ins(7;2) (q21.2;q3105q24.4) segregating in four generations. Hum Genet 1984; 68:77–86. †

Bernar J, et al.: Interstitial deletion 2q24.3: case report with high resolution banding. J Med Genet 1985; 22:226–228. *

Ramer JC, et al.: A review of phenotype-karyotype correlations in individuals with interstitial deletions of the long arm of chromosome 2. Am J Med Genet 1989; 32:359–363.

RI014 **Horacio Rivera**
CA011 **José María Cantú**

**Chromosome 2, partial trisomy**
*See CHROMOSOME 2, PARTIAL TRISOMY 2p*

## CHROMOSOME 2, PARTIAL TRISOMY 2P    2132

**Includes:** Chromosome 2, partial trisomy

**Excludes:** Chromosome 2 (other)

**Major Diagnostic Criteria:** Prenatal and postnatal growth retardation, severe mental handicap, and peculiar facial dysmorphism.

**Clinical Findings:** Facial features include **Microcephaly**, prominent forehead, ocular hypertelorism, epicanthus, ptosis of eyelids, lacrimal duct stenosis, wide and flat nasal bridge, low-set posteriorly rotated and malformed ears, small triangular mouth, microglossia, and micro-retrognathia. Long and slender extremities with arachnodactyly, hypoplastic genitalia with shawl scrotum and/or cryptorchidism, and hirsutism are also observed.

**Complications:** Unknown.

**Associated Findings:** Cardiopulmonary malformations with agenesis or faulty lobulation of lungs, neural tube defects, cleft palate, neuroblastoma, megacolon, and scoliosis and/or kyphosis.

**Etiology:** In the majority of patients the 2p duplication was the unbalanced product of a parental translocation involving 2p and another autosome. The concomitant partial monosomies of the other autosomes involved in the translocation may influence the phenotypic expression. In one patient a direct duplication (dir dup 2(p14→p23)) was documented.

**Pathogenesis:** Unknown.

**POS No.:** 3693

**CDC No.:** 758.990

**Sex Ratio:** M2:F1

**Occurrence:** About two dozen cases have been reported in the literature.

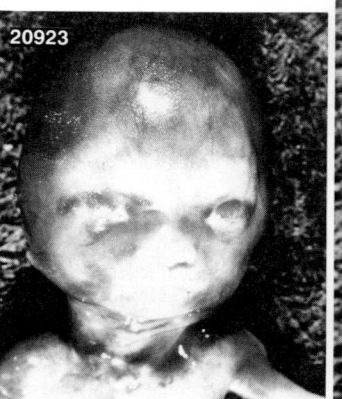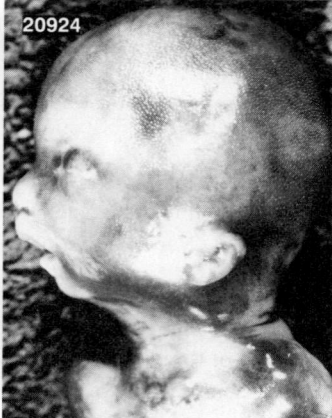

**2132A-20923–24:** Chromosome 2, partial duplication of 2p; note severe micrognathia and low-set ears in this affected fetus.

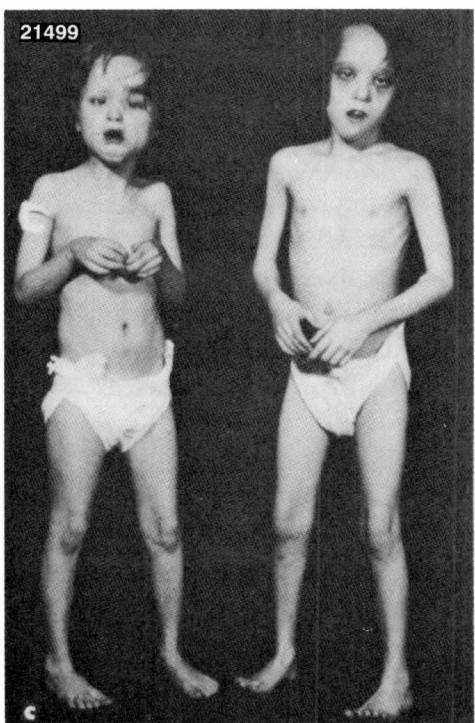

**2132B-21499:** Chromosome 2, trisomy 2p; note prominent forehead, hypertelorism, short nose with prominent tip, pointed chin, and long, narrow trunk.

**Risk of Recurrence for Patient's Sib:** Negligible if parental chromosomes are normal. Considerably increased (to an estimated 5–10%) if reciprocal translocation involving chromosome 2 and another autosome is found in one of the parents.

**Risk of Recurrence for Patient's Child:** Severe mental retardation in surviving patients makes reproduction unlikely.

**Age of Detectability:** At birth. Prenatal diagnosis by amniocenthesis or CVS is possible.

**Gene Mapping and Linkage:** See *Gene Map.*

**Prevention:** None known. Genetic counseling indicated.

**Treatment:** As indicated for specific symptoms and malformations.

**Prognosis:** Limited survival mainly due to the severe autosomal translocations involving 2p.

**Detection of Carrier:** Cytogenetic examination of the parents to exclude autosomal translocations involving 2p.

**References:**
Yunis E, et al: Direct duplication 2p14→2p23. Hum Genet 1979; 48:241–244.
Fryns JP, et al: The fetal phenotype in 2p trisomy. Ann Génét 1986; 29:269–271. *
Pueschel SM, et al: Partial trisomy 2p. J Ment Defic Res 1987; 31:293–298.

FR030
KL007

**Jean-Pierre Fryns**
**Alice Kleczkowska**

## CHROMOSOME 2, TRISOMY DISTAL 2Q 2348

**Includes:** N/A

**Excludes:** N/A

**Major Diagnostic Criteria:** Growth and developmental delay, characteristic facies, and demonstration of cytogenetic defect.

**Clinical Findings:** In over 50% of cases there is low birthweight (approximate average 2,750 g) with normal gestation, muscular hypotonia and/or hypotrophy, feeding difficulties (during infancy), moderate to severe mental deficiency, growth retardation, microcephaly, square facies, prominent glabella and/or forehead, hypertelorism, downward-slanting palpebral fissures, depressed nasal bridge, hypoplastic nasal bones, upturned nostrils, long and well-developed philtrum, "Cupid's-bow" mouth, thin upper lip, short neck, short stubby hands, clinodactyly and brachymesophalangy V, hypoplastic nails, abnormal dermatoglyphics (predominantly t' or t" placed axial triradii, hypothenar patterns, and high ridge count), and dry, wrinkled skin. Ten to fifty percent of patients have epicanthal folds, nystagmus, strabismus, micrognathia, cleft palate, congenital heart defect (aortic stenosis, ventricular septal defect), kyphosis, scoliosis, urinary tract and genital anomalies, and clubfoot.

**Complications:** Variable and related to primary defects.

**Associated Findings:** Uveal coloboma, congenital glaucoma, aniridia, corneal opacification, thumb duplication, camptodactyly, persistence of archaic muscles, and sacrococcygeal fistula.

**Etiology:** Partial trisomy (duplication) for all or a part of the region 2q3. Usually the abnormality results from a balanced translocation or insertion in either parent. In two sibs the imbalance was secondary to a pericentric inversion, and in only two of 35 cases was there a *de novo* tandem duplication.

**Pathogenesis:** Unknown.

**POS No.:** 3686

**CDC No.:** 758.990

**Sex Ratio:** M1:F1

**Occurrence:** Undetermined, but appears to have world-wide distribution. Some 35 cases have been documented.

**Risk of Recurrence for Patient's Sib:** Moderate to high if a parent is a balanced translocation, insertion, or inversion carrier; otherwise probably negligible.

**Risk of Recurrence for Patient's Child:** Theoretical 50% risk.

**Age of Detectability:** At birth or prenatally, by first or second trimester karyotyping. Prenatal chromosome analysis is indicated if a parent has a balanced rearrangement.

**Gene Mapping and Linkage:** See *Gene Map.*

**Prevention:** None known. Genetic counseling indicated.

**Treatment:** Symptomatic for congenital defects; special education.

**Prognosis:** About 20% of the 35 known patients died during the first three months of life. Survival to 28 years of age has been recorded. Mental retardation ranges from moderate to severe.

**Detection of Carrier:** By chromosome analysis; at present, high-risk carriers are only identifiable after the birth of an affected child. Careful pedigree studies may also be useful.

**Special Considerations:** In addition to the 2q3 trisomy syndrome, there would be other distinct 2q trisomy entities. For instance, two sibs (aged 45 and 26 years) with trisomy 2q24.2→q3105 appeared to have a separate syndrome, including upward slanting palpebral fissures and malar hypoplasia as distinctive features.

**References:**
Francke U: Clinical syndromes associated with partial duplications of chromosome 2 and 3: dup(2p), dup(2q), dup(3p), dup(3q). BD:OAS XIV(6C). New York: March of Dimes Birth Defects Foundation, 1978:191–217.
Zankl M, et al.: Distal 2q duplication: Report of two familial cases and an attempt to define a syndrome. Am J Med Genet 1979; 4:5–16. *

Yu CW, Chen H: De novo inverted tandem duplication of the long arm of chromosome 2(q34→q37). BD:OAS XVIII(3B). New York: March of Dimes Birth Defects Foundation, 1982:311–320.

Kyllerman M, et al.: Delineation of a characteristic phenotype in distal trisomy 2q. Helv Paediat Acta 1984; 39:499–508. *

Moller M, et al.: Pure monosomy and trisomy 2q24.2→q3105 due to an inv ins(7;2) (q21.2;q3105q24.2) segregating in four generations. Hum Genet 1984; 68:77–86. *

RI014
CA011

**Horacio Rivera**
**José María Cantú**

**Chromosome 3, deletion of distal 3p**
*See CHROMOSOME 3, MONOSOMY 3p2*
**Chromosome 3, distal 3p monosomy**
*See CHROMOSOME 3, MONOSOMY 3p2*
**Chromosome 3, distal 3p trisomy/duplication**
*See CHROMOSOME 3, TRISOMY 3p2*
**Chromosome 3, distal 3q2 trisomy/duplication**
*See CHROMOSOME 3, TRISOMY 3q2*

## CHROMOSOME 3, MONOSOMY 3P2      2431

**Includes:**
Chromosome 3, distal 3p monosomy
Chromosome 3, deletion of distal 3p

**Excludes:** Chromosome 3, proximal 3p monosomy

**Major Diagnostic Criteria:** Multiple congenital anomalies syndrome with mental retardation, severe-to-profound developmental delay, marked pre- and postnatal growth retardation, and typical craniofacial dysmorphism in most patients. Although the number of reported patients is too small to delineate a typical 3p monosomy syndrome, marked **Microcephaly**, hypertrichosis, and synophrys seem to be the most constant findings.

**Clinical Findings:** The craniofacial dysmorphism is further characterized by dolichocephaly, triangular face, frontal bossing, palpebral ptosis and upturned palpebral fissures, hypertelorism and epicanthus, short and thick nose, micrognathia, and low-set, malformed ears. Thoracic abnormalities include **Pectus excavatum** and scoliosis. Hypogenitalia is present in male patients, and minor limb anomalies include clinodactyly of the 5th finger, **Syndactyly**, and postaxial polydactyly.

**Complications:** Early death.

**Associated Findings:** Several congenital malformations have been sporadically reported, i.e., cardiac defects, **Hernia, hiatal**, optic atrophy, fetal lobulation of kidneys, polycystic renal dysplasia, and hypoplastic clavicles.

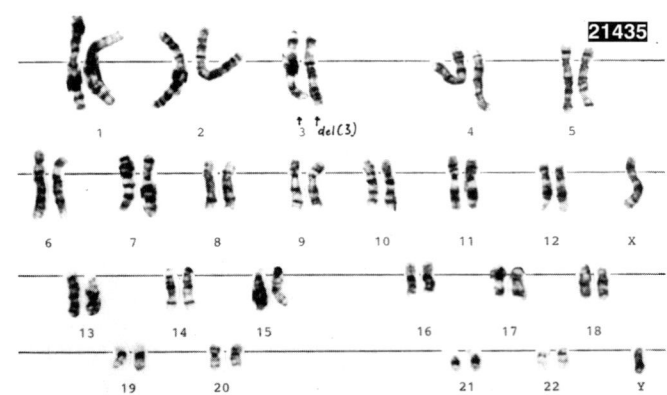

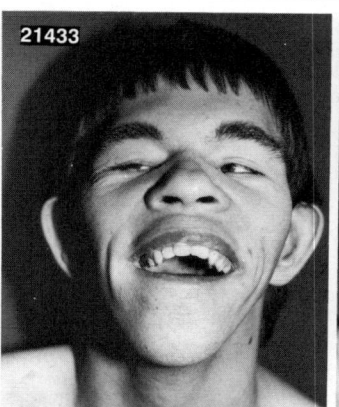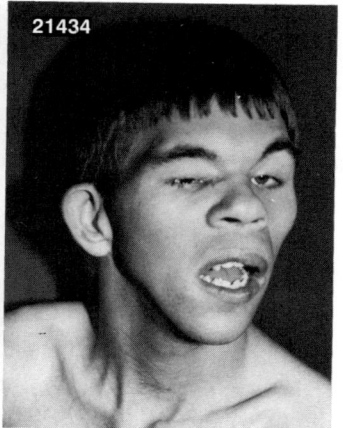

**2431A-21433–34:** Adult male with terminal deletion of chromosome 3p; note coarse facies.

**2431B-21435:** Karyogram showing terminal deletion of 3p: 46,XY,del(3) (p25).

**Etiology:** In the majority of patients the unbalanced karyotype is the product of a duplication/deficiency rearrangement in a parental inverted chromosome 3. A *de novo* deletion was reported in one patient.

**Pathogenesis:** Unknown.

**POS No.:** 3687

**CDC No.:** 758.990

**Sex Ratio:** M1:F1

**Occurrence:** About a dozen patients have been reported.

**Risk of Recurrence for Patient's Sib:** Very low if parental chromosomes are normal. Considerably increased (possibly 5–10%) if a pericentric inversion of chromosome 3 is present in one of the parents.

**Risk of Recurrence for Patient's Child:** Reproduction in affected patients is highly unlikely.

**Age of Detectability:** In the first years of life, by the presence of developmental delay and craniofacial stigmata. Prenatal diagnosis by chorionic villus sampling or amniocentesis is possible.

**Gene Mapping and Linkage:** Unknown.

**Prevention:** None known. Genetic counseling indicated.

**Treatment:** Unknown.

**Prognosis:** Life span seems to be considerably limited by the presence of internal malformations.

**Detection of Carrier:** By cytogenetic examination.

**References:**
de Grouchy J, Turleau C: Clinical atlas of human chromosomes. New York: John Wiley & Sons, 1984:42–43. *

Schinzel A: Catalogue of unbalanced chromosome aberrations in man. Berlin: Walter De Gruyter, 1984:130–139.†

Preus M, et al.: Diagnosis of chromosome 3 duplication q23 → qter, deletion q25 → qter in a patient with the C (trigonocephaly) syndrome. Am J Med Genet 1986; 23:935–943.†

Narahara K, et al.: Loss of the 3p25.3 band is critical in the manifestation of del(3p) syndrome. Am J Med Genet 1990; 35:269–273.†

FR030

**Jean-Pierre Fryns**

## CHROMOSOME 3, TRISOMY 3P2     2432

**Includes:** Chromosome 3, distal 3p trisomy/duplication

**Excludes:**
Chromosome 3, proximal 3p trisomy/duplication
**Chromosome 3, trisomy 3q2** (2430)

**Major Diagnostic Criteria:** Multiple congenital anomalies syndrome with severe mental retardation, characteristic craniofacial changes, and absence of other gross external abnormalities. The craniofacial dysmorphism includes frontal bossing and temporal indentation, square face, marked hypertelorism with or without epicanthus, thick and short nose, full lips, and a large mouth with downturned corners. Most patients have striking micrognathia, but ears are well-shaped and in normal position.

**Clinical Findings:** In addition to the severe mental retardation and the typical facial changes, the neck is short with redundant skin. Thoracic abnormalities include widely spaced nipples, pectus excavatum, and short sternum. Microgenitalia and testicular ectopy is present in male patients. Minor limb abnormalities include **Camptodactyly**, cutaneous **Syndactyly**, and deep plantar creases between toes 1 and 2.In most patients, postnatal growth retardation is severe.

**Complications:** Early death.

**Associated Findings:** Congenital heart defects, most frequently **Atrial septal defects** and **Ventricular septal defect**, are found in most patients. A holoprosencephaly sequence was present in several patients and this, together with the cardiac malformation, seems to be the most pathognomonic internal malformation in this chromosomal syndrome. Several other congenital malformations have been sporadically reported, i.e., cleft lip, cleft palate, muscular hypoplasia, retinal myopic degeneration, absence of gallbladder, renal anomalies, and clubfeet.

**Etiology:** In the majority of patients the 3p2 duplication is the unbalanced product of a parental autosomal translocation involving 3p2 and another autosome.

**Pathogenesis:** Unknown.

**POS No.:** 3067

**CDC No.:** 758.990

**Sex Ratio:** M1:F1

**Occurrence:** About 40 cases have been reported in the literature.

**Risk of Recurrence for Patient's Sib:** Not increased if parental chromosomes are normal. Considerably increased (possibly 5–10%) if one of the parents is a carrier of an autosomal balanced translocation involving 3p2.

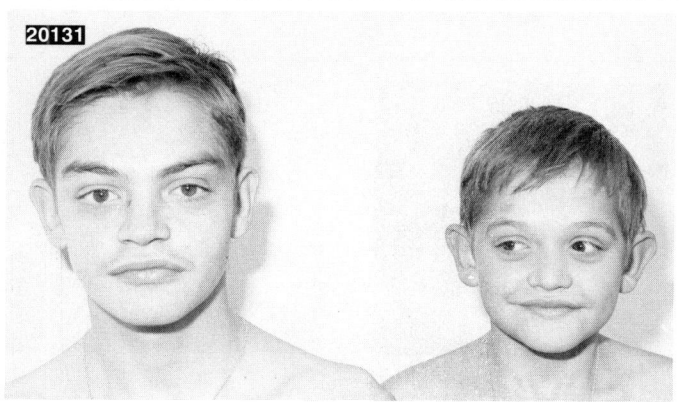

**2432-20134:** Note square facies, hypertelorism, thick, short nose, full lips and a large mouth with downturned corners in these two brothers.

**Risk of Recurrence for Patient's Child:** Reproduction in affected patients is highly unlikely.

**Age of Detectability:** In the first years of life by clinical examination. Prenatal diagnosis by chronic villus sampling or amniocentesis is possible.

**Gene Mapping and Linkage:** See *Gene Map*.

**Prevention:** None known. Genetic counseling indicated.

**Treatment:** Unknown.

**Prognosis:** Life span seems to be considerably limited in the majority of patients by the presence of CNS and cardiac malformations.

**Detection of Carrier:** By cytogenetic examination.

**References:**
Aula P, et al.: Distribution of spontaneous chromosome breaks in human chromosomes. Hum Genet 1976; 32:142–148.
Kleczkowska A, et al.: Partial trisomy of chromosome 3 (p14→p22) due to maternal insertional translocation. Ann Genet 1984; 27:180–183.
Schwanitz G, Zerres K: Signes phénotypiques à différents âges d'une trisomie partiëlle 3p par translocation familiale 3/5. Ann Genet (Paris) 1984; 27:167–172. *
Gimelli G, et al.: Dup(3) (p2→ pter) in two families, including one infant with cyclopia. Am J Med Genet 1985; 20:341–348.
Gillerot Y, et al.: Brief clinical report: prenatal diagnosis of a dup(3p) with holoprosencephaly. Am J Med Genet 1987; 26:225–227.

FR030      **Jean-Pierre Fryns**

## CHROMOSOME 3, TRISOMY 3Q2     2430

**Includes:** Chromosome 3, distal 3q2 trisomy/duplication

**Excludes:**
**Chromosome 3, monosomy 3p2** (2431)
Chromosome 3, proximal 3q trisomy/duplication
**Chromosome 3, trisomy 3p2** (2432)
**De Lange syndrome** (0242)

**Major Diagnostic Criteria:** Multiple congenital anomalies syndrome with mental retardation, moderate-to-severe developmental delay, and clinical findings strikingly similar to those in **De Lange syndrome**, i.e., brachycephaly, synophrys, and hirsutism.

**Clinical Findings:** Characteristic craniofacial dysmorphism with acro- and brachycephaly, low hair implantation, hirsutism, synophrys, long eyelashes, hypertelorism, epicanthus, and up-slanted palpebral fissures. Ocular malformations are frequent and vary from strabismus, nystagmus, cataract, corneal opacities, and colobomas of the iris to anophthalmia. Other findings reminiscent of the **De Lange syndrome** are a small nose with upturned nares, prominent philtrum, fine upper lip, downslanting mouth corners, microretrognathia, and high-arched palate. In addition to generalized hirsutism, the neck is short with redundant skin and the thorax is small with sloping shoulders. Hypogenitalism with cryptorchidism in the male and malformations of the internal genital organs in females are frequently documented. Limb anomalies include hypoplasia of the terminal phalanges of fingers, **Camptodactyly**, and clinodactyly.

**Complications:** Unknown.

**Associated Findings:** Cardiac malformations are noted in one-third of the patients, especially in those with a proximal 3q2 duplication. Renal malformations, i.e., polycystic kidneys or dysplasia, are equally frequently observed. Occasional malformations include brain abnormalities with micropolygyria, cerebellar hypoplasia, arrhinencephaly, and intestinal malrotation.

**Etiology:** Most frequently the 3q2 duplication in the patient is the unbalanced product of a parental autosomal translocation involving 3q2 and another autosome. In other patients a *de novo* 3q2 duplication is observed, and in others the chromosomal anomaly is the product of a duplication/deficiency rearrangement in a parental inverted chromosome 3.

**Pathogenesis:** Unknown.

**POS No.:** 3688

**CDC No.:** 758.990

**Sex Ratio:** M1:F1

**Occurrence:** At least 30 patients have been reported in the literature.

**Risk of Recurrence for Patient's Sib:** Very low if parental chromosomes are normal. Considerably increased (possibly 5–10%) if one of the patients is a carrier of a pericentric inversion in chromosome 3 or has an autosomal balanced translocation involving 3q2.

**Risk of Recurrence for Patient's Child:** Reproduction in affected patients is highly unlikely.

**Age of Detectability:** In infancy by clinical examination. Prenatal diagnosis by chorionic villus sampling or amniocentesisis is possible.

**Gene Mapping and Linkage:** See *Gene Map.*

**Prevention:** None known. Genetic counseling indicated.

**Treatment:** Unknown.

**Prognosis:** Life span is variable and depends on the presence of associated internal malformations.

**Detection of Carrier:** By cytogenetic examination.

**References:**
Steinbach P, et al.: The dup(3q) syndrome: report of eight cases and review of the literature. Am J Med Genet 1981; 10:159–177.
Schinzel A: Catalogue of unbalanced chromosome aberrations in man. Berlin: Walter De Gruyter, 1984:140–147.
Wilson GN, et al.: Further delineation of the dup(3q) syndrome. Am J Med Genet 1985; 22:117–123.
Preus M, et al.: Diagnosis of chromosome 3 duplication q23 → qter deletion p25 → pter in a patient with the C (trigonocephaly) syndrome. Am J Med Genet 1986; 23:935–943.

FR030                                              **Jean-Pierre Fryns**

**Chromosome 4, 4q terminal deletion syndrome**
    *See CHROMOSOME 4, MONOSOMY DISTAL 4q*
**Chromosome 4, deletion 4q31-qter syndrome**
    *See CHROMOSOME 4, MONOSOMY DISTAL 4q*
**Chromosome 4, deletion 4q32-qter syndrome**
    *See CHROMOSOME 4, MONOSOMY DISTAL 4q*
**Chromosome 4, deletion 4q33-qter syndrome**
    *See CHROMOSOME 4, MONOSOMY DISTAL 4q*
**Chromosome 4, distal 4q-syndrome**
    *See CHROMOSOME 4, MONOSOMY DISTAL 4q*
**Chromosome 4, dup(4) (q25-qter)**
    *See CHROMOSOME 4, TRISOMY DISTAL 4q*
**Chromosome 4, dup(4) (q26 or 27-qter)**
    *See CHROMOSOME 4, TRISOMY DISTAL 4q*
**Chromosome 4, dup(4) (q31 or 32-qter)**
    *See CHROMOSOME 4, TRISOMY DISTAL 4q*

---

**CHROMOSOME 4, MONOSOMY 4P**                        **0164**

**Includes:**
    Chromosome 4, partial chromosome 4 deletion syndrome
    Wolf-Hirschhorn syndrome
    Wolf syndrome

**Excludes:**
    **Chromosome 5, monosomy 5p** (0163)
    **Chromosome 13, trisomy 13** (0168)

**Major Diagnostic Criteria:** The presence in a profoundly retarded individual of low birthweight, microcephaly, hypertelorism and downward slanting palpebral fissures is suggestive of a short arm deletion of chromosome 4 and clinical signs include a weak cry in early infancy, and the presence of cleft palate, beaked nose, carp-like mouth, preauricular dimples, underdeveloped dermal ridges, hypospadias and delayed ossification of the carpals and pelvis. Chromosomal identification of the deleted chromosome as a number 4 confirm the diagnosis.

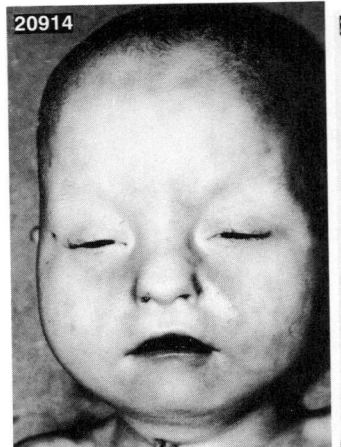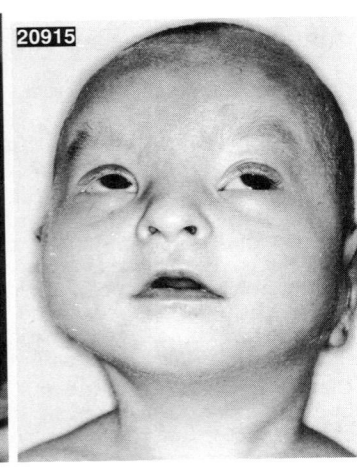

**0164A**-20914–15: Chromosome 4, monosomy 4p; note high forehead, wide glabella, hypertelorism, prominent philtrum and carp-shaped mouth.

**Clinical Findings:** In most cases there is low birthweight with normal or prolonged gestation (mean birthweight of 25 cases was 2015 gm), severe psychomotor retardation, postnatal growth retardation, microcephaly, hypertelorism, broad or beaked nose, low-set simple ears, micrognathia, hypoplastic dermal ridges, ridge disassociation, seizures and hypospadias in males and hypoplastic mullerian derivitives in females. More than half of all cases have epicanthus, antimongoloid slant to the eyes, colobomata, strabismus, cleft lip, palate or uvula, preauricular sinus, midline scalp defect, hemangioma of the forehead, low ridge count on the fingers (< 100), delayed bone age, heart defect and orthopedic deformities.

When midline scalp defect, cleft lip and palate and coloboma are present, the 4p- syndrome may be confused with the 13 trisomy syndrome clinically, although (in 4p- syndrome) polydactyly has been reported in only 1 case and colobomata are limited to the iris.

**Complications:** Seizures; present in most individuals surviving infancy and difficult to control.

**Associated Findings:** CNS defects (1/3) and renal anomalies seen frequently at autopsy.

**Etiology:** The syndrome is the result of the deletion of some of the genetic material of the short arm of chromosome number 4. Chromosome breakage during gametogenesis leads to a reciprocal translocation and subsequent segregation of the chromosomes at

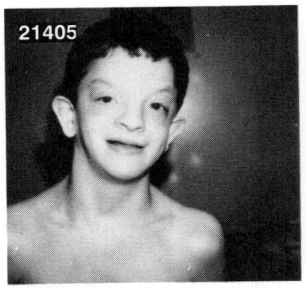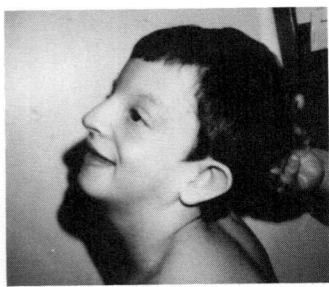

**0164B**-21405: A 15-year-old male with monosomy 4p (46, XY del(4) (p16.1)). In addition to severe psychomotor retardation and hypotonia, he has microcephaly, hypertelorism, epicanthal folds, the "Greek helmet" appearance of the nose, and short and deep philtrum.

meiosis gives rise to a gamete with a deletion. A balanced translocation carrier may also be produced in this way; he or she can then have offspring who are balanced carriers, or have a deletion (thus the 4p- syndrome), or have a duplication of chromosome material. Chromosome deletion may also occur without translocation, with loss of the deleted segment, either from the end of the chromosome or interstitially.

It appears that deletion of band 4p16 is necessary for full expression of this phenotype. Families with reciprocal translocations involving the short arm of cromosome 4 have been shown to be at high risk for offspring with unbalanced chomosomes under some circumstances.

Most cases are sporadic. Approximately 13% of reported cases result from segregations of parental chromosomal aberrations, primarily translocations.

**Pathogenesis:** Although many factors such as chemicals and radiation are known to be capable of breaking chromosomes, factors which influence breakage in the human in vivo are unknown. Maternal and paternal ages do not seem to be a factor.

**POS No.:** 3069

**CDC No.:** 758.320

**Sex Ratio:** Female predominance observed.

**Occurrence:** About 120 cases have been reported.

**Risk of Recurrence for Patient's Sib:** Negligible unless a parent is a translocation carrier.

**Risk of Recurrence for Patient's Child:** No affected individual is known to have reproduced.

**Age of Detectability:** At birth or in second trimester by analysis of cultured fetal fibroblasts.

**Gene Mapping and Linkage:** See *Gene Map.*

**Prevention:** None known. Genetic counseling indicated.

**Treatment:** Unknown.

**Prognosis:** Several stillbirths and perinatal deaths have been reported. Most reported deaths have occured in the first year. The average lifespan for those who survive is unknown, but affected adults have been reported.

**Detection of Carrier:** Balanced translocation carriers may be recognized by chromosomal studies.

**References:**
Centerwall WR, et al.: Translocation 4p- syndrome. Am J Dis Child 1975; 129:366–370.
Johnson VP, et al.: The Wolf-Hirschhorn (4p-) syndrome. Clinical Genetics 1976:10:104–112.
Lazjuk GI, et al.: The Wolf-Hirschhorn syndrome. Clinical Genetics 1980; 18:6–12.
Lurie IW, et al.: The Wolf-Hirschhorn syndrome. Clinical Genetics 1980; 17:375–384.
Wilson MG, et al.: Genetic and clinical studies in 13 patients with the Wolf-Hirschhorn syndrome. Human Genetics 1981; 59:297–307. *
Stengel-Rutkowski S, et al.: Familial Wolf's syndrome with a hidden 4p deletion by translocation of an 8p segment: Case report, review and risk estimates. Clinical Genetics 1984; 25:500–521. *

BU011
                                          **Marilyn J. Bull**
                                          *Dorothy Warburton*

---

## CHROMOSOME 4, MONOSOMY DISTAL 4Q     2435

**Includes:**
   Chromosome 4, deletion 4q31-qter syndrome
   Chromosome 4, deletion 4q32-qter syndrome
   Chromosome 4, deletion 4q33-qter syndrome
   Chromosome 4, distal 4q-syndrome
   Chromosome 4, partial monosomy of distal 4q
   Chromosome 4, 4q terminal deletion syndrome

**Excludes:**
   Chromosome 4, partial monosomy for proximal 4q
   Chromosome 4, proximal 4q- syndrome

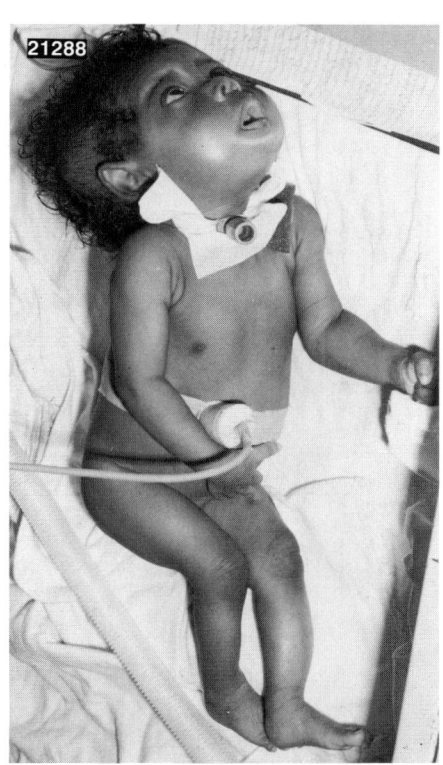

2435-21288: Note unusual facies with short snub nose and micrognathia, and large pointed ears.

---

**Major Diagnostic Criteria:** Normal birth weight, dysmorphic features (including the Robin malformation sequence), and mental retardation. Limb anomalies and cardiac defects are usually present. Karyotype analysis is needed to confirm the diagnosis.

**Clinical Findings:** *Development*: normal birth weight, 24/28; postnatal growth retardation, 17/22; developmental delay, 21/22; *Craniofacial*: Robin malformation: micro-, retrognathia, 26/28; **Cleft palate**, 23/28; **Cleft lip**, 8/28; Cranial shape abnormality, 19/28; hypertelorism, 14/28; oblique palpebral fissures, 7/28; short nose with depressed nasal bridge, 20/28; low-set ears with pointed helices, 18/28; *Limb*: abnormal implantation of thumbs, 12/28; absent flexion creases of fifth finger, 14/28; Cardiac defects, 16/28.

**Complications:** Respiratory and feeding problems, cardiac failure, seizures.

**Associated Findings:** In some cases, renal, **Microcephaly**, skeletal, and genital anomalies were reported. Esophageal atresia with tracheoesophageal fistula and ectopic anus were seen in one patient.

**Etiology:** Familial translocations were only observed in 3/21 cases. The majority of cases occur *de novo.*

**Pathogenesis:** Unknown.

**POS No.:** 3072

**CDC No.:** 758.990

**Sex Ratio:** M1:F1

**Occurrence:** Eighteen cases of 4q31→qter deletions, four cases of 4q32→qter deletions, and six cases of 4q33→qter deletions have been reported in the literature.

**Risk of Recurrence for Patient's Sib:** Appears to be low unless a parent carries a balanced translocation.

**Risk of Recurrence for Patient's Child:** No known case of reproduction.

**Age of Detectability:** At birth, or prenatal diagnosis by chorionic villus sampling, amniocentesis, or percutaneous umbilical blood sampling.

**Gene Mapping and Linkage:** See *Gene Map.*

**Prevention:** None known. Genetic counseling indicated.

**Treatment:** Symptomatic for congenital defects, special education.

**Prognosis:** Patients are thought to have a diminished life span. Ten of 22 patients died within the first 15 months of life from either complications of cardiac defects or oropharyngeal incoordination. The oldest reported living patient with distal 4q- was 14 years old.

**Detection of Carrier:** By chromosomal analysis.

**Special Considerations:** There have been three cases of monosomy distal 4q occurring with another chromosomal abnormality.

The more terminal deletions seem to be associated with a milder phenotype and less severe complications. One case report describes a patient who has a 4q33→qter deletion and phenotypic features of the **Williams syndrome.**

**References:**

Ockey CH, et al.: A large deletion of the long arm of chromosome No. 4 in a child with limb abnormalities. Arch Dis Child 1967; 42:428–434.

Townes PL, et al.: 4q-syndrome. Am J Dis Child 1979; 133:383–385.

Davis JM, et al.: The del(4)(q31) syndrome-a recognizable disorder with atypical Robin malformation sequence. Am J Med Genet 1981; 9:113–117.

Mitchell JA, et al.: Deletion of different segments of the long arm of chromosome 4. Am J Med Genet 1981; 8:73–89.

Stamberg J, et al.: Terminal deletion (4)(q33) in a male infant. Clin Genet 1982; 21:125–129.

Jefferson RD, et al.: A terminal deletion of the long arm of chromosome 4 (46,XX,del[4][q33]) in an infant with phenotypic features of the Williams syndrome. J Med Genet 1986; 23:474–480.

Lin AE, et al.: Interstitial and terminal deletions of the long arm of chromosome 4: further delineation of phenotypes. Am J Med Genet 1988; 31:533–548.

C0072
JA014

**Linda F. Cooper**
**Ethylin Wang Jabs**

**Chromosome 4, partial chromosome 4 deletion syndrome**
*See CHROMOSOME 4, MONOSOMY 4p*
**Chromosome 4, partial monosomy of distal 4q**
*See CHROMOSOME 4, MONOSOMY DISTAL 4q*
**Chromosome 4, partial trisomy 4p**
*See CHROMOSOME 4, TRISOMY 4p*
**Chromosome 4, partial trisomy 4q syndrome**
*See CHROMOSOME 4, TRISOMY DISTAL 4q*
**Chromosome 4, r(4)(p16q35)**
*See CHROMOSOME 4, RING 4*

## CHROMOSOME 4, RING 4                    2554

**Includes:**
Chromosome 4, terminal deletion of short (p) and long (q) arms of
Chromosome 4, r(4)(p16q35)

**Excludes:**
Chromosome 4, monosomy 4p (0164)
Chromosome 4, trisomy 4p (2433)

**Major Diagnostic Criteria:** Low birth weight, retardation in growth and development, **Microcephaly**, and beaked nose.

**Clinical Findings:** Affected infants who are of low birth weight feed poorly and are slow to gain weight. They have some features in common with **Chromosome 4, monosomy 4p.** Physical findings are **Microcephaly**, micrognathia, rounded broad nose, malformed ears, and a cleft of the soft palate. Other findings may include ptosis, clinodactyly, abnormal palmar creases, and hypospadias.

The clinical course shows failure to gain weight and to reach developmental milestones. There is speech delay. Laboratory

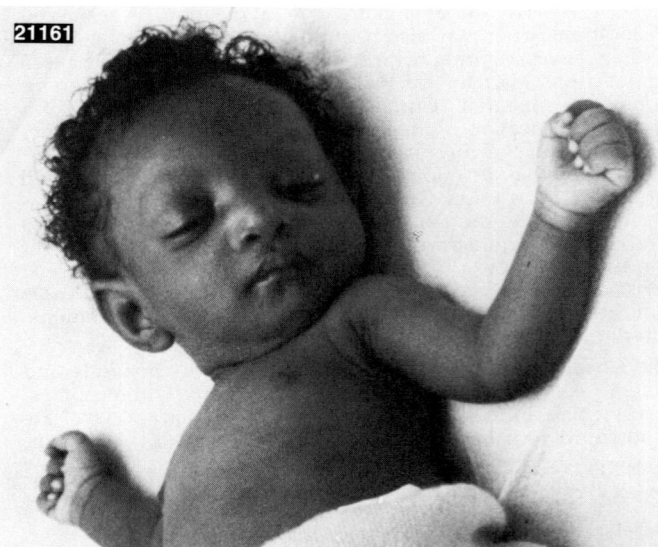

2554-21161: Microcephaly, micrognathia, rounded broad nose and malformed ears.

findings show a deletion of the terminal bands on both the short and long arms of chromosome 4. Parents have normal karyotypes.

Patients seem to differ from **Chromosome 4, monosomy 4p** patients by not having hypertelorism, prominent glabella, coloboma, beaked lip, short philtrum, downturned mouth, large ears, and heart malformations. Patients missing both 4p15 and 4p16 more closely resemble those with **Chromosome 4, monosomy 4p** than do those missing only 4p16.

**Complications:** Multiple congenital malformations as characteristic of chromosomal aberration syndromes.

**Associated Findings:** Retarded bone age.

**Etiology:** Patients with the deletion of 4p16 and 4q35 are similar to those with a deletion of 4p16 and 4q33. The deletion of more genetic material in the latter cases does not seem to modify the phenotype; thus 4p16 is crucial.

**Pathogenesis:** Unknown.

**CDC No.:** 758.990

**Sex Ratio:** Presumably M1:F1

**Occurrence:** Undetermined but presumed rare.

**Risk of Recurrence for Patient's Sib:** Presumably not increased.

**Risk of Recurrence for Patient's Child:** Presumably not increased.

**Age of Detectability:** During the newborn period.

**Gene Mapping and Linkage:** See *Gene Map.*

**Prevention:** None known. Genetic counseling indicated.

**Treatment:** Unknown.

**Prognosis:** Unknown.

**Detection of Carrier:** Unknown.

**References:**

Niss R, Passarge E: Derivative chromosome structure from a ring chromosome 4. Humangenetik 1975; 28:9–23.

Chavin-Colvin F, et al.: Anneau du chromosome 4 II: sans dysmorphie faciale. Ann Genet 1977; 20:105–109.

Fraisse J, et al.: Anneau de chromosome 4 I: avec phenotype 4p-. Ann Genet 1977; 20:101–104.

McDermott A, et al.: Ring chromosome 4. J Med Genet 1977; 14:228–232.

Perez-Castillo A, Abrisqueta J: Ring chromosome 4 and Wolf syndrome. Hum Genet 1977; 37:87–91.

Finley WH, et al.: Ring 4 chromosome with terminal p and q deletions. Am J Dis Child 1981; 135:729–731.

FI007                                                           **Wayne H. Finley**

**Chromosome 4, terminal deletion of short (p) and long (q) arms of**
  *See* CHROMOSOME 4, RING 4
**Chromosome 4, trisomies 4q2 and 4q3**
  *See* CHROMOSOME 4, TRISOMY DISTAL 4q

## CHROMOSOME 4, TRISOMY 4P                               2433

**Includes:**  Chromosome 4, partial trisomy 4p

**Excludes:**
  Chromosome 4, trisomy 4p occurring with another
    abnormality
  Chromosome 4, trisomy 4q

**Major Diagnostic Criteria:**  Dysmorphic facial features, malformed ears, short neck, skeletal anomalies, mental retardation. Karyotype analysis is needed to confirm diagnosis.

**Clinical Findings:**  *Development*: full-term gestation, 24/32; postnatal growth retardation, 21/34; psychomotor retardation, 34/34. *Craniofacial*: **Microcephaly**, 20/34; prominent glabella or supraorbital ridge, 21/34; hypertelorism, 14/34; bulbous nose, 26/34; depressed nasal bridge, 21/34; ear abnormalities, 29/34; short neck, 26/34; prominent chin, 16/34; widely spaced nipples, 16/33. *Skeletal*: limb deformities and contractures, 30/34; scoliosis, 14/34. Abnormal genitalia in males, 14/16; abnormalities of fingers and hands, 21/34; clinodactyly, 10/33; and abnormalities of toes and feet, 22/34.

**Complications:**  Respiratory and feeding problems, seizures.

**Associated Findings:**  Some cases have been reported with congenital heart disease, kidney malformations, **Hernia, inguinal**, and ocular anomalies.

**Etiology:**  In each of 16 families, one parent was found to carry a balanced translocation; t(4;22) was the most common. Pericentric inversions were found in three families, and a maternal centric fission was detected in another. In three cases, the patients had a *de novo* duplication of 4p.

**Pathogenesis:**  Unknown.

**POS No.:**  3070

**CDC No.:**  758.990

**Sex Ratio:**  M1:F1

**Occurrence:**  Thirty-four cases have been reported from 22 different kindreds.

**Risk of Recurrence for Patient's Sib:**  Appears to be low unless a parent carries a balanced translocation. Based on segregation analysis, the risk for either male or female reciprocal translocation carriers is approximately 14%. The spontaneous abortion rate for these individuals is not increased over the general population, but a sevenfold increase in the frequency of stillborns has been observed.

**Risk of Recurrence for Patient's Child:**  No known case of reproduction.

**Age of Detectability:**  At birth, or prenatal diagnosis by chorionic villus sampling, amniocentesis, or percutaneous umbilical blood sampling.

**Gene Mapping and Linkage:**  *See Gene Map.*

**Prevention:**  None known. Genetic counseling indicated.

**Treatment:**  Symptomatic for congenital defects, special education.

**Prognosis:**  Shortened life span may occur secondary to cardiac and respiratory complications or status epilepticus. More than one-third of the patients die in childhood as a result of pneumopathies. Patients have an average IQ of 50.

**Detection of Carrier:**  By chromosomal analysis.

**Special Considerations:**  Because most cases of trisomy 4p are due to parental translocations, patients may also have cytogenetically undetectable deletions or duplications of another chromosome. It has been suggested that these additional chromosomal abnormalities may account for the variability of the trisomy 4p phenotype.

**References:**

Gustavson KH, et al.: A 4–5/21–22 chromosomal translocation associated with multiple congenital anomalies. Acta Paediatr 1964; 53:172–181.

Wilson MG, et al.: Inherited pericentric inversion of chromosome No. 4. Am J Hum Genet 1970; 22:679–690.

Dallapiccola B, et al.: Centric fission of chromosome No. 4 in the mother of two patients with trisomy 4p. Hum Genet 1976; 31:121–125.

Gonzalez CH, et al.: The trisomy 4p syndrome: case report and review. Am J Hum Genet 1977; 1:137–156.

Crane J, et al.: 4p trisomy syndrome: report of 4 additional cases and segregation analysis of 21 families with different translocations. Am J Med Genet 1979; 4:219–229.

C0072                                                        **Linda F. Cooper**
JA014                                                     **Ethylin Wang Jabs**

## CHROMOSOME 4, TRISOMY DISTAL 4Q                        2434

**Includes:**

  Chromosome 4, dup(4) (q25-qter)
  Chromosome 4, dup(4) (q26 or 27-qter)
  Chromosome 4, dup(4) (q31 or 32-qter)
  Chromosome 4, partial trisomy 4q syndrome
  Chromosome 4, trisomies 4q2 and 4q3

**Excludes:**
  Chromosome 4, trisomy 4p (2433)
  Chromosome 4, trisomy distal 4q with another abnormality

**Major Diagnostic Criteria:**  Dysmorphic facial features, **Microcephaly**, low-set or malformed ears, short neck, limb anomalies, and mental retardation. Karyotype analysis is needed to confirm diagnosis.

**Clinical Findings:**  *Developmental*: psychomotor retardation, 21/30; hypotonia, 12/27; low birth weight, 11/30. *Craniofacial*: **Microcephaly**, 22/30; sloping forehead, 12/29; antimongoloid slant, 17/30; epicanthal folds, 15/28; malformed or low-set ears, 28/30; depressed or wide nasal bridge, 13/30; short philtrum with downturned corners of mouth, 12/30; micrognathia, 15/30; short neck, 19/30. *Limb*: malformed hands and feet, thumb anomalies, **Syndactyly** of toes, and talipes valgus, 23/30. Heart defects and vascular anomalies, 14/30; urinary tract anomalies, 11/29; and cryptorchidism, 11/14.

**Complications:**  Cardiac failure, seizures.

**Associated Findings:**  Hernias and ocular anomalies, including blepharophimosis, epicanthus, ptosis, and microphthalmos, have been reported in a few cases.

**Etiology:**  Usually the result of parental translocation, most frequently involving chromosome 18. Only 2/29 cases of partial trisomy 4q have occurred *de novo*.

**Pathogenesis:**  Unknown.

**POS No.:**  3071

**CDC No.:**  758.990

**Sex Ratio:**  M1:F1

**Occurrence:**  Of the 30 reported cases, trisomy 4q26 or 27→qter was diagnosed in ten cases, 4q25→qter in seven cases, and 4q31 or 32→qter in six cases.

**Risk of Recurrence for Patient's Sib:**  Appears to be low unless a parent carries a balanced translocation.

**Risk of Recurrence for Patient's Child:**  No known case of reproduction.

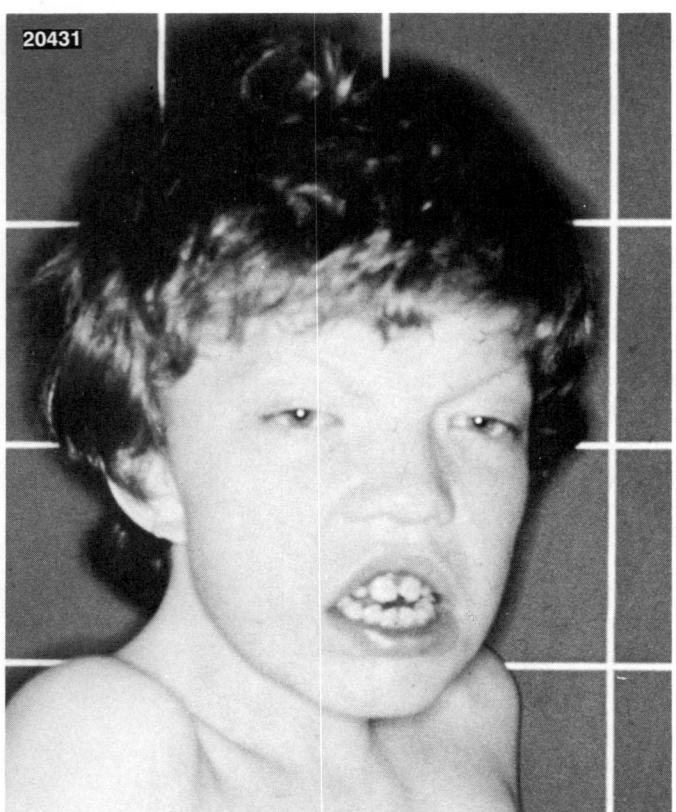

2434-20431: Chromosome 4, trisomy distal 4q; note ptosis, and downcurved mouth with short upper lip.

**Age of Detectability:** At birth, or prenatal diagnosis by chorionic villus sampling, amniocentesis, or percutaneous umbilical blood sampling.

**Gene Mapping and Linkage:** See *Gene Map*.

**Prevention:** None known. Genetic counseling indicated.

**Treatment:** Symptomatic for congenital defects, special education.

**Prognosis:** Patients may have a shortened life span due to complications of congenital malformations. Mental retardation is severe, with an IQ of less than 50. The oldest reported living patient with dup(4)q26 or q27→ter was 42 years of age.

**Detection of Carrier:** By chromosomal analysis.

**Special Considerations:** The severity of this syndrome does not directly correlate to the size of the trisomy (4q2→qter or 4q3→qter). The phenotype seems to be determined mainly by trisomy for the 4q3 region. Because most cases of trisomy 4q are the result of parental translocations, patients may also have cytogenetically undetectable deletions or duplications of another chromosome.

**References:**
Dutrillaux B, et al.: La trisomie 4q partielle a propos de trois observations. Ann Genet 1975; 18:21–27.
Yunis E, et al.: Partial trisomy 4q. Ann Genet 1977; 20:243–248.
Bonfante A, et al.: Partial trisomy 4q: two cases resulting from a familial translocation t(4;18)(q27;p11). Hum Genet 1979; 52:85–90.

**Linda F. Cooper**
**Ethylin Wang Jabs**

C0072
JA014

---

**Chromosome 5, 46,XX or 46,XY, 5q**
 *See CHROMOSOME 5, MONOSOMY 5q INTERSTITIAL*
**Chromosome 5, 5q- syndrome**
 *See CHROMOSOME 5, MONOSOMY 5q INTERSTITIAL*
**Chromosome 5, complete trisomy 5p syndrome (5p11-pter)**
 *See CHROMOSOME 5, TRISOMY 5p*
**Chromosome 5, deletion 5q**
 *See CHROMOSOME 5, MONOSOMY 5q INTERSTITIAL*
**Chromosome 5, interstitial deletion 5q**
 *See CHROMOSOME 5, MONOSOMY 5q INTERSTITIAL*

---

## CHROMOSOME 5, MONOSOMY 5P 0163

**Includes:**
  Cat cry syndrome
  Cri du chat syndrome

**Excludes:** Chromosome 4, monosomy 4p (0164)

**Major Diagnostic Criteria:** The diagnosis is suspected on the basis of the more common features noted below. Although none is diagnostic, the characteristic cry in the younger patients is the most important feature. Confirmation is made by demonstrating a deletion involving the short arm of chromosome 5.

**Clinical Findings:** The most common, and, therefore, characteristic, features are the cat-like, weak, or high-pitched cry in infancy; growth failure; microcephaly; facial abnormalities including hypertelorism, downward slanting palpebral fissures, and micrognathia; and severe mental retardation.

The more common features and their approximate frequencies are mental retardation-usually profound, IQ rarely above 35 (100%); low birthweight-<2,600 g (50%); slow growth, height-<3rd percentile (85%); feeding difficulties in infancy (>50%); abnormal cry, usually cat-like, occasionally weak or high-pitched, in

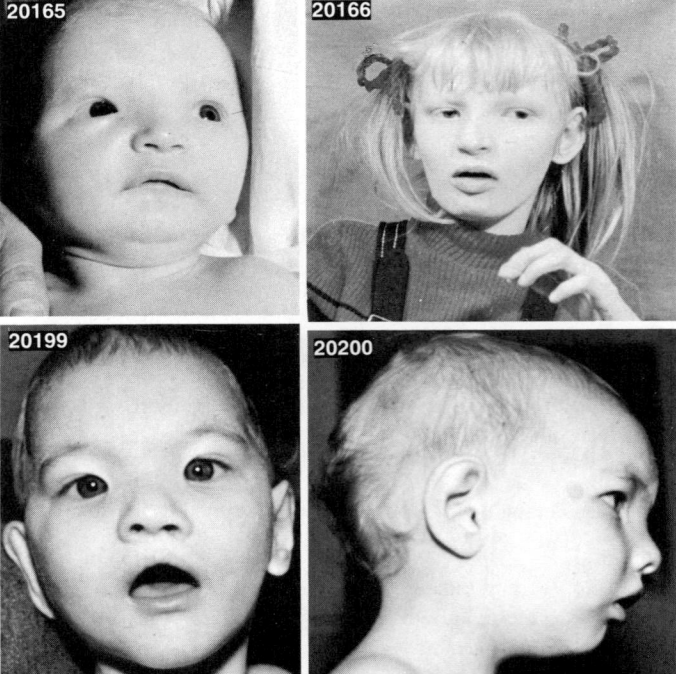

0163-20165: Note subject's features in infancy: hypertelorism, round face and downturned lips. 20166: At 9 years of age, the face has lengthened but hypertelorism persists. 20199: Facial features include hypertelorism, round facies and low-set ears. 20200: Note micrognathia on lateral view.

infancy-normalizes with age (98%); abnormal larynx (55–65%); and hypotonia in infancy, or poor muscular development in older patients (60–80%).

Craniofacial abnormalities include: **Microcephaly** (98%); face-round in infants, thin in adults (70%); facial asymmetry, older patients (25%); broad base of nose in infancy, less frequent in adults (85%); ears low-set or poorly formed (85%); preauricular tags (40%); micrognathia in infancy, less common in adults (75–85%); occasional prognathism in adults; malocclusion in older patients (70–80%); abnormal palate, either high and narrow or broad and flat (50–75%), and large frontal sinuses, in adults (85-90%).

Eye characteristics include: hypertelorism in young patients, less frequent in adults (90–95%); **Eye, hypotelorism**, occasional; epicanthal folds in young patients, less frequent in adults (85–90%); oblique palpebral fissures, usually downward-slanting, occasionally upward (75–85%); strabismus, usually divergent, after infancy (60–70%); deficient tears, Schirmer test-in adults (6/6); increased sensitivity of pupil to methacholine, adults (5/5); tortuous retinal vessels, adults (6/6); and optic atrophy, adults (2/6).

Congenital heart defects are found in 15–30% of observed cases. Types vary, but patent ductus arteriosus is most common. Abdominal features include: **Hernia, inguinal** (25–30%), diastasis recti (30–35%), and occasional renal anomalies. Limb abnormalities include: short metacarpals or metatarsals-adult (65–75%); simian crease (80–90%); distal axial triradius-t' or t″ (80–90%); partial syndactyly (25–30%); pes planus-older individuals (65–75%); and occasional clinodactyly.

Skeletal abnormalities include small wings of the ilia or increased iliac angle (70–80%) and scoliosis in adults (55–65%). Other characteristics include short neck (45–65%), premature graying of hair in adults (30–35%), and occasional cryptorchidism.

**Complications:** Severe respiratory and feeding problems soon after birth.

**Associated Findings:** None known.

**Etiology:** In most cases, there is simple deletion of the short arm of chromosome 5, which presumably occurs during gametogenesis. The particular segment, loss of which results in the characteristic features, appears to be the distal portion of band p14 or proximal part of band p15. A 5p- chromosome is usually present in every cell, although there have been infrequent reports of patients with mosaicism in whom normal cells are also found. Occasionally the deletion results from ring formation or a *de novo* translocation (unbalanced).

The etiology of the chromosomal abnormality is usually not known; average parental age is not increased. However, between 10–15% of cases have inherited the 5p- chromosome from a parent who is heterozygous for a reciprocal translocation involving the short arm of chromosome 5. Infrequently the deleted chromosome may be attributed to a pericentric inversion of chromosome 5 or mosaicism with normal and 5p- cells in a parent.

**Pathogenesis:** Unknown.

**POS No.:** 3073

**CDC No.:** 758.310

**Sex Ratio:** There has been a preponderance of females among infants and young children. The sex ratio is more nearly equal in the patients identified in later life. These differences may reflect differences in diagnostic methodology.

**Occurrence:** Of 59,452 unselected newborns studied cytogenetically, 3 (or 1:20,000) had deletion of the short arm of chromosome 5. One of these cases was a mosaic with normal and 5p-cells.

Prevalence in the general population is unknown. Up to 1% of profoundly retarded (IQ < 20) individuals have this syndrome.

**Risk of Recurrence for Patient's Sib:** Appears to be low (exact figure not available) unless a parent is a carrier of a reciprocal translocation of an inversion involving chromosome 5 or is a mosaic with normal or 5p-cells. In cases with a parental translocation, the risk appears to be between 15–25%. Because of the rarity of cases with parental inversion or mosaicism, the risk is unknown, but is presumed to be increased.

**Risk of Recurrence for Patient's Child:** No affected individuals are known to have reproduced. If reproduction were to occur, risk could be up to 50%.

**Age of Detectability:** At birth or prenatal diagnosis when a parent is a translocation or inversion carrier, or is a mosaic.

**Gene Mapping and Linkage:** See *Gene Map*.

**Prevention:** None known. Genetic counseling indicated.

**Treatment:** Symptomatic only; home rearing with comprehensive, early stimulation appears beneficial.

**Prognosis:** Diminished life span, but many of these patients survive into adulthood. Survival to 56 years of age is recorded.

**Detection of Carrier:** Karyotype studies of the parents.

**References:**

Breg WR, et al.: The cri du chat syndrome in adolescents and adults: clinical findings in 13 older patients with partial deletion of the short arm of chromosome No. 5(5p-). J Pediatr 1970; 77:782–791.
Howard RO: Ocular abnormalities in the cri du chat syndrome. Am J Ophthalmol 1972; 73:949–954. * †
Niebuhr E: The cri du chat syndrome: epidemiology, cytogenetics, and clinical features. Hum Genet 1978; 44:227–275. * †
Kousseff BG, et al.: Aberrations of chromosome no. 5 and phenotypic expression. Clin Res 1982; 30:890A.
Wilkins LE, et al.: Clinical heterogeneity in 80 home-reared children with cri du chat syndrome. J Pediatr 1983; 102:528–533. * †

K0018                                              **Boris G. Kousseff**

**Chromosome 5, monosomy 5q**
*See CHROMOSOME 5, MONOSOMY 5q INTERSTITIAL*

## CHROMOSOME 5, MONOSOMY 5Q INTERSTITIAL    2544

**Includes:**
   Chromosome 5, 5q-syndrome
   Chromosome 5, 46,XX or 46,XY, 5q
   Chromosome 5, deletion 5q
   Chromosome 5, interstitial deletion 5q
   Chromosome 5, monosomy 5q

**Excludes:** Chromosome 5, other anomalies

**Major Diagnostic Criteria:** Frontal bossing, anteverted nostrils, and severe mental retardation. The diagnosis is confirmed by karyotype.

**Clinical Findings:** *5q-syndrome (5q-):* Constitutional interstitial deletion of the long arm of chromosome 5 is rare. Seventeen cases are known, ten of which were reported in detail. Facial dysmorphia is noticeable at birth in one-half of the cases. In the other one-half of the cases the facial features or the mental retardation become apparent after age six months. The oldest patient was diagnosed at age 42 years. Birth weight is normal or subnormal (3/8). The facial dysmorphology is mild in all patients. Brachycephaly, a narrow forehead, and frontal bossing are the main features. The face is round. Palpebral fissures may slant horizontally or upward, but more often downward. Hypertelorism is not always present (2/9). Depressed nasal bridge, anteverted nostrils, and large philtrum with a deep groove are constant signs. Ears are low-set. The neck is short. Some patients have a **Cleft palate** with or without a heart murmur (2/8), dislocated hips (5/8), clubfoot (5/8), kidney abnormalities (**Kidney, horseshoe**) (3/8), or a heart malformation (bundle branch block), **Aorta, coarctation**, persistent ductus arteriosus, rounded heart).

One patient had **Intestinal polyposis, type III**, and a missing right lobe of the liver and agenesis of the gallbladder. Hypertonia is present in the newborn and in the adult. Hypotonia is present only in the infant. Mental retardation has been severe in all but one case in which it was moderate. Clinical variability is common. Parent and sibs are normal. Dermatoglyphics shows the finger patterns to consist of seven or eight whorls. Chromosome analysis demonstrates a deletion of band q13 to q15 or 22 or 31. Parents' karyotypes are normal.

One case has to be considered apart from the others. The

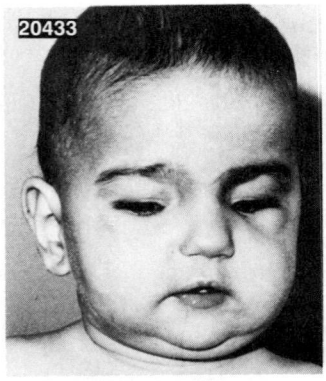
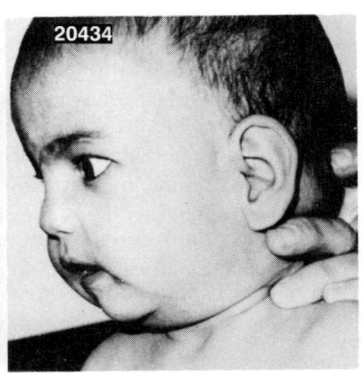
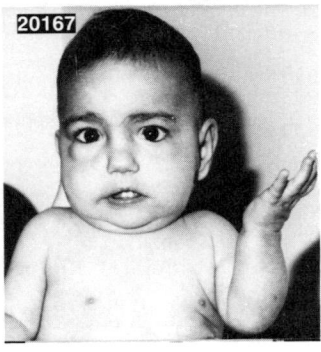
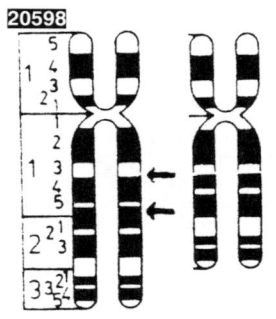

**2544**-20433–34, 20167: Note round facies, narrow forehead, large philtrum and short neck. 20598: The critical segment which is deleted in the chromosome 5, monosomy interstitial. Arrows indicate where breakages occur.

---

patient of Dudin et al (1984) who was a six-month-old girl with psychomotor retardation and multiple congenital malformations also had low-set ears, thick eyelashes, epicanthal folds, dolichocephaly, and spade-like hands. This patient had a deletion of band q12 of chromosome 5.

**Complications:** Kyphoscoliosis and pes adductus are sometimes seen.

**Associated Findings:** Weight gain is greatly retarded. An interstitial deletion of 5q13→q15 or 5q15→q22 was observed in two intellectually handicapped brothers with **Intestinal polyposis, type I**.

**Etiology:** All reported cases of 5q- have been *de novo*.

**Pathogenesis:** Unknown.

**CDC No.:** 758.990

**Sex Ratio:** M1:F1

**Occurrence:** Undetermined but presumed rare.

**Risk of Recurrence for Patient's Sib:** Probably not increased.

**Risk of Recurrence for Patient's Child:** Theoretically 1:2, but severe mental retardation usually prevents reproduction.

**Age of Detectability:** At birth or during the first months of life, or by prenatal diagnosis.

**Gene Mapping and Linkage:** See *Gene Map*.

**Prevention:** None known. Genetic counseling indicated.

**Treatment:** Physical therapy to prevent kyphoscoliosis or pes adductus. Infant stimulation.

**Prognosis:** Severe mental retardation. The oldest patient died from an abdominopelvic neoplasm at age 42 years.

**Detection of Carrier:** By chromosomal examination.

**Special Considerations:** The term *5q- syndrome* should only be used for patients who have all the clinical features of the syn-

drome and an interstitial deletion of the long arm of chromosome 5, including all or part of 5q13 to 5q31.

**References:**

Stoll C, et al.: Interstitial deletion of the long arm of chromosome 5 in a deformed boy: 46,XY,del(5)(q13q15). J Med Genet 1980; 17:486–487.

Harprecht-Beato W, et al.: Interstitial deletion of the long arm of chromosome No. 5. Clin Genet 1983; 23:167–171.

Dudin G, et al.: Interstitial deletion of band q12 of chromosome 5. Clin Genet 1984; 25:455–458.

Borgaonkar DS, et al.: Repository of chromosomal variants and anomalies in man. Twelveth Listing, Medical Center of Delaware, Newark, Delaware, 1987.

Rivera H, et al.: Constitutional del (5) (q23;3q31.1). Ann Genet 1987; 30:91–93.

Hockey KA, et al.: Deletion of chromosome 5q and familial adenomatous polyposis. J Med Genet 1989; 26:61–68.

ST029 **Claude Stoll**

**Chromosome 5, partial trisomy 5p syndrome 5p13 or 14-pter**
*See CHROMOSOME 5, TRISOMY 5p*
**Chromosome 5, partial trisomy 5q3**
*See CHROMOSOME 5, TRISOMY 5q3*

---

### CHROMOSOME 5, TRISOMY 5P        2436

**Includes:**
> Chromosome 5, "complete" trisomy 5p syndrome (5p11-pter)
> Chromosome 5, partial trisomy 5p syndrome 5p13 or 14-pter

**Excludes:** Chromosome 5, trisomy 5q3 (2437)

**Major Diagnostic Criteria:** Normal birth weight, **Microcephaly**, facial dysmorphism, hypotonia, and psychomotor retardation. Karyotype analysis is required for confirmation.

**Clinical Findings:** *General*: normal birth weight, 13/13; hypotonia, 10/10; postnatal growth failure, 6/6; psychomotor retardation, 16/18. *Craniofacial*: **Microcephaly** (macrodolichoscaphocephaly), 14/16; hypertelorism, 9/19; mongoloid slant of eye, 11/14; epicanthus, 9/12; low-set ears, 15/16; depressed nasal bridge, 13/15; macroglossia, 8/11; micrognathia, 7/11. *Eye abnormalities*: coloboma of iris, 2/13; microphthalmia, 4/13; strabismus, 4/13. Congenital heart disease, 6/11. *Skeletal*: long fingers, 10/13; short first toe, 7/14; clubfeet, 7/12. *CNS*: seizures, 9/13.

**Complications:** Recurrent respiratory infections and feeding problems are sometimes seen.

**Associated Findings:** There are one or two reported cases of obesity, diaphragmatic and umbilical hernias, hydronephrosis, and **Pectus excavatum**.

**Etiology:** Three cases of complete trisomy (5p11→pter) have been reported. They were all *de novo* unbalanced translocations. One case was associated with a maternal pericentric inversion of chromosome 2.

Most cases of partial trisomy of chromosome 5 are duplications of the region of the short arm (5p13 or 14→pter). The partial trisomy 5p appears to be a consequence of an error during gametogenesis if a parent has a balanced translocation.

**Pathogenesis:** Unknown.

**CDC No.:** 758.990

**Sex Ratio:** M1:F2

**Occurrence:** Three reported cases of "complete" trisomy 5p11→pter; 21 reported cases of partial trisomy 5p.

**Risk of Recurrence for Patient's Sib:** In all reported kindreds with balanced translocations, 100 pregnancies resulted from 26 heterozygous parents. The distribution of the outcome of 76 pregnancies with the 24 probands eliminated to reduce bias of ascertainment is 32% normal; 26% carrier-balanced translocations; 20% unbalanced translocations; 12% stillbirths, spontaneous abortions, or children with multiple congenital abnormalities; and 6% unknown.

**Risk of Recurrence for Patient's Child:**  No reported reproduction by patient. Two adult cases reported with normal menses and puberty.

**Age of Detectability:**  At birth, or prenatal diagnosis by chorionic villus sampling, amniocentesis, or percutaneous umbilical blood sampling.

**Gene Mapping and Linkage:**  See *Gene Map.*

**Prevention:**  None known. Genetic counseling indicated.

**Treatment:**  Symptomatic therapy for congenital defects, special education.

**Prognosis:**  Psychomotor retardation with postnatal growth failure has been reported. Life span in those with the terminal duplication appears to be longer than those with the complete duplication. The oldest known living patient is 31 years old. Early death from respiratory complications has been reported.

**Detection of Carrier:**  By chromosomal analysis.

**Special Considerations:**  The severity of clinical findings and presentation in the reported cases correlate to the length of the duplicated portion. The larger duplication 5p11→pter has more severe clinical signs. Duplication of 5p14→pter results in mental retardation with few clinical findings.

**References:**
Lejeune J, et al.: Maladie du cri du chat et sa reciproque. Ann Genet 1965; 8:11–15.
Leschot NJ, Lim KS: "Complete" trisomy 5p de novo translocation t(2;5)(q36;p11) with isochromosome 5p. Hum Genet 1979; 46,271–278.
Carnevale A, et al.: A clinical syndrome associated with dup(5p). Am J Med Genet 1982; 13:277–283.
Khodr GS, et al.: Duplication of (5p13→pter): prenatal diagnosis and review of literature. Am J Med Genet 1982; 12:43–49.

MA078
JA014

**Laura S. Martin**
**Ethylin Wang Jabs**

## CHROMOSOME 5, TRISOMY 5Q3     2437

**Includes:**
    Chromosome 5, partial trisomy 5q3
    Chromosome 5, Trisomy 5q31-qter
    Chromosome 5, trisomy 5q33-qter
    Chromosome 5, trisomy 5q34-qter

**Excludes:**
    Chromosome 5, more proximal trisomies
    Chromosome 5, trisomy 5q13–22
    Chromosome 5, trisomy 5q13–31
    Chromosome 5, trisomy 5q15-q31
    Chromosome 5, trisomy 5q22-qter

**Major Diagnostic Criteria:**  Characteristic clinical signs and symptoms include normal birth weight with growth failure, **Microcephaly**, dysmorphic facies, congenital heart defects, and digital abnormalities. Karyotype confirmation is required.

**Clinical Findings:**  *General*: psychomotor retardation, 21/21; growth retardation, 21/21. *Craniofacial*: **Microcephaly**, 21/23; receding forehead, 5/13; hypertelorism, 12/20; antimongoloid slant of eyes, 8/19; epicanthus, 5/19; dysplastic ears, 15/20; long upper lip, 5/17; microstomia, 9/15; carp mouth, 6/15; micrognathia, 9/16. *Eye*: strabismus, 9/15. *Heart*: congenital heart defects, 15/20. *Abdomen*: umbilical and inguinal hernias, 8/23; diaphragmatic hernia, 2/22; accessory spleen, 2/2. *Limbs*: brachydactyly, 8/15; preaxial polydactyly, 3/23.

**Complications:**  Feeding problems and subsequent failure to thrive usually occur.

**Associated Findings:**  Arhinencephaly, double uterus and vagina, hip dislocations, and dysplasias have been reported. Eczema, delayed puberty, and cardiac conduction defects were reported in three cases with trisomy 5q34→qter in one family.

**Etiology:**  Partial trisomy 5q31→qter is transmitted during gametogenesis via parental translocations. A single case of a parental pericentric inversion of chromosome 5 has been associated with a partial trisomy. No *de novo* cases have been reported.

**Pathogenesis:**  Unknown.

**CDC No.:**  758.990

**Sex Ratio:**  M1:F2

**Occurrence:**  Eleven cases of trisomy 5q31→qter, seven cases of trisomy 5q33→qter, and five cases of trisomy 5q34→qter have been reported.

**Risk of Recurrence for Patient's Sib:**  Low except when one of the parents has a balanced translocation.

**Risk of Recurrence for Patient's Child:**  No reported reproduction by a patient.

**Age of Detectability:**  At birth, or prenatal diagnosis by chorionic villus sampling, amniocentesis, or percutaneous umbilical blood sampling.

**Gene Mapping and Linkage:**  See *Gene Map.*

**Prevention:**  None known. Genetic counseling indicated.

**Treatment:**  Symptomatic therapy for congenital defects, special education.

**Prognosis:**  All patients described have mental, developmental, and growth retardation. Life span may be shortened by complications of major malformations. Patients in their 20s have been reported.

**Detection of Carrier:**  By chromosomal analysis.

**Special Considerations:**  Mental retardation is universal in this syndrome. The facial features are more prominent as the trisomic duplication increases in size. Trisomy 5q34→qter lack characteristic eye and mouth features. The few reported cases of duplications that are more proximal than 5q31 share some of the same clinical features, such as psychomotor retardation, facial dysmorphism, musculoskeletal abnormalities, and growth retardation.

**References:**
Ferguson-Smith MA, et al.: Assignment by deletion of human red cell acid phosphatase gene locus to the short arm of chromosome 2. Nature 1973; 243:271–273.
Curry CJR, et al.: Partial trisomy for the distal long arm of chromosome 5 (region q34→qter). A new clinically recognizable syndrome. Clin Genet 1979; 15:454–461.
Bremer FA, et al.: Familial partial monosomy 5p and trisomy 5q: three cases due to parental pericentric inversion 5 (p15 q33). Clin Genet 1984; 26:209–215.
Lazjuk GI, et al.: Partial trisomy 5q and partial monosomy 5p within the same family. Clin Genet 1985; 28:122–129.
Kumar D, et al.: Clinical manifestations of trisomy 5q. J Med Genet 1987; 24(3):180–184.

MA078
JA014

**Laura S. Martin**
**Ethylin Wang Jabs**

**Chromosome 5, Trisomy 5q31-qter**
  *See CHROMOSOME 5, TRISOMY 5q3*
**Chromosome 5, trisomy 5q33-qter**
  *See CHROMOSOME 5, TRISOMY 5q3*
**Chromosome 5, trisomy 5q34-qter**
  *See CHROMOSOME 5, TRISOMY 5q3*
**Chromosome 6, del(6)(q13q15),(q12q14) or (q14q16)**
  *See CHROMOSOME 6, MONOSOMY PROXIMAL 6q*
**Chromosome 6, deletion of proximal 6q**
  *See CHROMOSOME 6, MONOSOMY PROXIMAL 6q*
**Chromosome 6, distal 6p trisomy (duplication)**
  *See CHROMOSOME 6, TRISOMY 6p2*
**Chromosome 6, interstitial deletion of proximal 6q**
  *See CHROMOSOME 6, MONOSOMY PROXIMAL 6q*

## CHROMOSOME 6, MONOSOMY DISTAL 6Q                2518

**Includes:**  Chromosome 6, terminal 6q deletion [del(6)(q23qter)]

**Excludes:**  Chromosome 6, proximal/interstitial 6q deletions [del(6)(q3q15)]

**Major Diagnostic Criteria:**  1) Neonatal hypotonia. 2) Characteristic craniofacial findings: small and high forehead, narrow palpebral fissures, flat nasal bridge, small nose, long philtrum, small triangular mouth, and short neck. 3) Long thorax, truncal obesity, relative small hands and feet. 4) Moderate developmental retardation.

**Clinical Findings:**  Neonatal hypotonia; characteristic craniofacial findings: small and high forehead, narrow palpebral fissures, flat nasal bridge, small nose, long philtrum, small triangular mouth, and short neck; long thorax, truncal obesity, relative small hands and feet; and moderate developmental retardation. Internal malformations are apparently rare.

**Complications:**  Unknown.

**Associated Findings:**  None known.

**Etiology:**  Interstitial 6q23(?) deletion in one patient, *de novo* der(6),t(5;6)(q22;q23.3) translocation in the second patient. The clinical findings are related to deletion of band 6q23. The 6q deletion occured *de novo*, as parental karyotypes were normal.

**Pathogenesis:**  Unknown.

**CDC No.:**  758.990

**Sex Ratio:**  Undetermined but presumably M1:F1.

**Occurrence:**  Two cases have been documented.

**Risk of Recurrence for Patient's Sib:**  Not increased if parental chromosomes are normal.

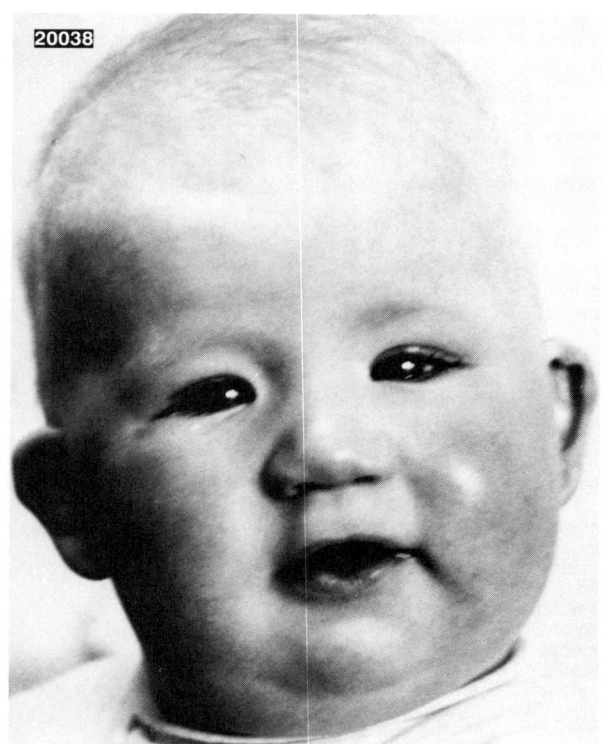

**2518-20038:**  Note high forehead, small nose, long philtrum, and short neck.

**Risk of Recurrence for Patient's Child:**  Theoretically 1:2 (50%). Fertility status is undetermined. Reproduction is unlikely in surviving patient due to mental retardation.

**Age of Detectability:**  At birth, or by prenatal diagnosis by CVS or amniocentesis.

**Gene Mapping and Linkage:**  See *Gene Map.*

**Prevention:**  None known. Genetic counseling indicated.

**Treatment:**  Unknown.

**Prognosis:**  Long-term prognosis is good, by the absence of severe internal malformations, in the two reported patients.

**Detection of Carrier:**  Cytogenetic examination for autosomal translocation involving 6q.

**References:**
Young RS, et al.: Deletions of the long arm of chromosome 6: two new cases and review of the literature. Am J Med Genet 1985; 20:21–29.
Fryns JP, et al.: Distal deletion of the long arm of chromosome 6: a specific phenotype? Am J Med Genet 1986; 24:175–178.

FR030                                        **Jean-Pierre Fryns**

## CHROMOSOME 6, MONOSOMY PROXIMAL 6Q              2543

**Includes:**
Chromosome 6, deletion of proximal 6q
Chromosome 6, del(6)(q13q15),(q12q14) or (q14q16)
Chromosome 6, interstitial deletion of proximal 6q

**Excludes:**
Chromosome 6, distal 6q and other interstitial deletion
**Vater association** (0987)

**Major Diagnostic Criteria:**  Facial dysmorphia, generalized retardation of growth and development, minor skeletal abnormalities, excessive whorls, and a demonstration of the deletion of 6q13–15.

**Clinical Findings:**  Short stature (3rd to 25th percentile); motor and mental retardation (DQ-IQ 23–44); facial dysmorphia, including full cheeks (6/6) upslanting palpebral fissures (5/6), long philtrum (4/6), dolichocephaly (2/6), facial asymmetry (2/6), epicanthus (4/6), and thin upper lip (3/6); short neck (4/6), various vertebral anomalies (3/5), congenital heart disease (PDA, VSD) (3/6), **Hernia, umbilical** (5/6), excessive whorls (5/5), and simian crease (3/6).

**Complications:**  Unknown.

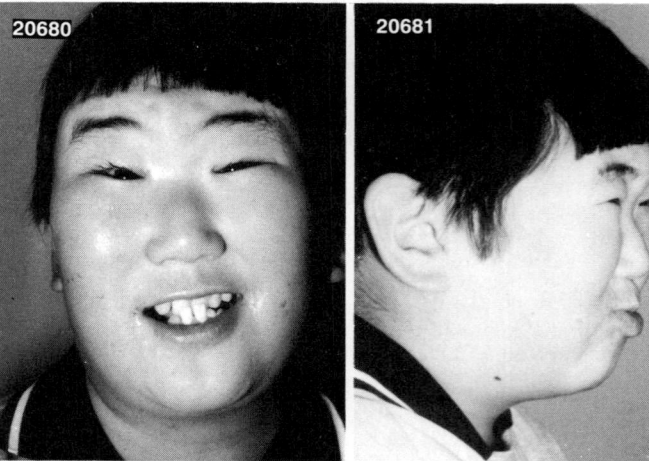

**2543-20680–81:**  Chromosome 6, monosomy proximal 6q; note facial asymmetry, upward slanting palpebral fissures, epicanthi, flat nasal root, and protrusion of the glabella.

**Associated Findings:** Tracheoesophageal fistula, **Hernia, hiatal, Hernia, inguinal, Cleft palate,** and ectopic kidney.

**Etiology:** Interstitial deletion of the proximal part of the long arm of chromosome 6 (6q13–15), (q12q14), or (q14q16).

**Pathogenesis:** Unknown.

**POS No.:** 3678

**CDC No.:** 758.990

**Sex Ratio:** M1:F5 (observed).

**Occurrence:** Undetermined but presumed rare.

**Risk of Recurrence for Patient's Sib:** Not increased unless a parent has a balanced insertional translocation (such a case has not been reported to date).

**Risk of Recurrence for Patient's Child:** Unknown.

**Age of Detectability:** At birth, or prenatally by chromosome analysis.

**Gene Mapping and Linkage:** See *Gene Map.*

**Prevention:** None known. Genetic counseling indicated.

**Treatment:** Symptomatic.

**Prognosis:** Moderate-to-severe mental retardation. The oldest patient was last seen at 14 years of age.

**Detection of Carrier:** By cytogenetic analysis.

**References:**
McNeal RM, et al.: Congenital anomalies including the VATER association in a patient with a del(6)q deletion. J Pediatr 1977; 91:957–960.
Young RS, et al.: Deletions of the long arm of chromosome 6: two new cases and review of the literature. Am J Med Genet 1985; 20:21–29.
Yamamoto Y, et al.: Deletion of proximal 6q: a clinical report and review of the literature. Am J Med Genet 1986; 25:467–471.
Lonardo F, et al.: A malformed girl with a de novo proximal 6q deletion. Ann Genet 1988; 31:57–59.
Turleau C, et al.: 6q1 monosomy: a distinctive syndrome. Clin Genet 1988; 34:38–42.

YA001                                    **Yoshifumi Yamamoto**

**Chromosome 6, partial trisomies 6q between 6q21 and 6q26**
*See CHROMOSOME 6, TRISOMY 6q2*

## CHROMOSOME 6, RING 6                     2440

**Includes:** Ring 6

**Excludes:**
Mental-motor-growth retardation due to other causes
Multiple minor anomalies-CNS/ocular defects due to other causes

**Major Diagnostic Criteria:** Growth and psychomotor retardation and a cytogenetic demonstration of the ring 6 chromosome.

**Clinical Findings:** The phenotypic spectrum is very broad. Among a total of 17 patients: growth retardation (94%); psychomotor retardation (82%); malformed or low-set ears (71%); **Microcephaly** (76%); micrognathia (71%); eye abnormalities (63%); flat nasal bridge (53%); **Eye, hypertelorism** (53%); high-arched palate (53%); epicanthal folds (47%); **Foot, talipes equinovarus (TEV)** (35%); low birth weight (65%); CNS malformations, including **Hydrocephaly** (41%); short neck, webbed or with redundant skin (31%); convulsions (29%); downward slanting palpebral fissures (29%); congenital heart disease (19%); hip dislocation (24%); and wide-spaced nipples (18%).

The degree of psychomotor retardation may be severe to mild. Children with minimal physical abnormalities and normal intelligence have been reported. Ocular abnormalities are relatively frequent, including microphthalmia, iris coloboma, megalocornea, posterior embryotoxon, glaucoma, ptosis, strabismus, nystagmus, optic atrophy, and albinoid fundi. Talipes equinovalgus or ankle contracture and CNS malformations, including **Hydrocephaly** and agenesis of corpus callosum and olfactory bulbs, are noteworthy.

**Complications:** Unknown.

**Associated Findings:** Imperforate anus, **Hernia, umbilical,** undescended testis, arachnodactyly, blue sclerae, nail hypoplasia, clinodactyly of the 5th finger, nevus pigmentosus, hyperkeratosis of the soles, hemivertebrae, sacral dimple, bird-headed face.

**Etiology:** Monosomic state of the short and long arms of chromosome 6 of variable degree resulting from ring formation. The existence of dicentric rings, monosomic cells for chromosome 6, and so forth, may contribute to phenotypic variability.

**Pathogenesis:** Unknown.

**CDC No.:** 758.990

**Sex Ratio:** M10:F7 (observed).

**Occurrence:** Some 17 cases have been documented.

**Risk of Recurrence for Patient's Sib:** Presumably not significantly increased.

**Risk of Recurrence for Patient's Child:** Unknown.

**Age of Detectability:** At birth, or prenatally by cytogenetic analysis.

**Gene Mapping and Linkage:** See *Gene Map.* Low leukocyte SOD2 in a patient with a ring chromosome 6 has been reported.

**Prevention:** None known. Genetic counseling indicated.

**Treatment:** Symptomatic.

**Prognosis:** Near-normal (up to IQ 92) to severe mental retardation. The oldest patient was six years of age when last seen.

**Detection of Carrier:** By cytogenetic analysis.

**Special Considerations:** In many cases it has been difficult to identify precisely the break points of the ring. The clinical severity of r(6) patients depends not only on the amount of chromosome material lost but also on the stability of the ring and its proportion of mosaicism *in vivo.*

**References:**
Moore CM, et al.: Developmental abnormalities associated with a ring chromosome 6. J Med Genet 1973; 10:299–303.
Peeden JN, et al.: Ring chromosome 6: variability in phenotypic expression. Am J Med Genet 1983; 16:563–573.
Levin H, et al.: Aniridia, congenital glaucoma, and hydrocephalus in a male infant with ring chromosome 6. Am J Med Genet 1986; 25:281–287.
Chitayat D, et al.: Ring chromosome 6: report of a patient and literature review. Am J Med Genet 1987; 26:145–151.
Yoshimitsu K, et al.: Decreased superoxide dismutase-2 activity in a patient with ring chromosome 6. Am J Med Genet 1987; 28:211–214.

YA001                                    **Yoshifumi Yamamoto**

**Chromosome 6, terminal 6p trisomy (duplication)**
*See CHROMOSOME 6, TRISOMY 6p2*
**Chromosome 6, terminal 6q deletion [del(6)(q23qter)]**
*See CHROMOSOME 6, MONOSOMY DISTAL 6q*

## CHROMOSOME 6, TRISOMY 6P2                 2438

**Includes:**
Chromosome 6, distal 6p trisomy (duplication)
Chromosome 6, terminal 6p trisomy (duplication)

**Excludes:**
Chromosome 6, complete 6p trisomy (duplication)
Chromosome 6, proximal 6p1 trisomy (duplication)

**Major Diagnostic Criteria:** Characteristic craniofacial dysmorphism: dolichocephaly with high forehead, hypertelorism, long eye lashes, blepharophimosis and blepharoptosis, high and broad nasal bridge and bulbous nose with hyperplastic nares, short philtrum, small mouth, thin lips and micrognathia.

**Clinical Findings:** Multiple congenital anomalies syndrome with pre- and postnatal growth retardation, characteristic face, short neck, broad thorax with widely-set nipples, long fingers and toes, and severe mental retardation in surviving patients.

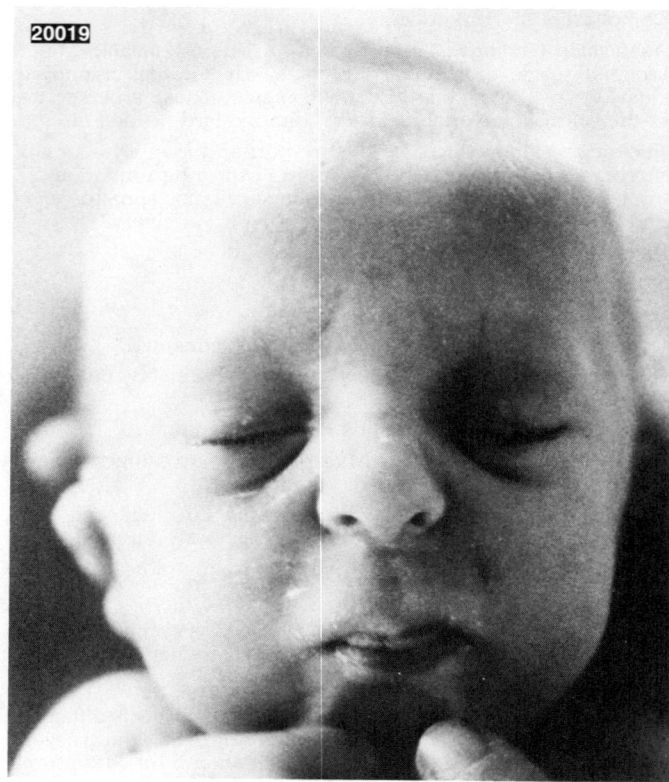

**2438-20019:** Note characteristic facies: close-set eyes with narrow palpebral fissures; closed eyes, high forehead, short nose and long philtrum.

**Complications:** Unknown.

**Associated Findings:** Ocular malformations including microphthalmia, iris and/or pupilla colobomata, optic nerve atrophy, and strabismus convergens are reported in more than one-third of the patients. In addition to the characteristic morphology of the nose, choanal atresia and absence of bulbi olfactorii were noted in some patients. Clinodactyly of the 5th fingers, **Camptodactyly**, **Syndactyly**, and abnormal palmar and solar creases are regularly observed. A variety of internal malformations were noted, of which the genito-urinary malformations are the most constant. In a post-pubertal female patient, hypoplasia of internal and external genitalia and lack of secondary sexual development was observed.

**Etiology:** In all patients a 6p2 trisomy is present. In the majority of cases the 6p2 trisomy is the unbalanced product of a parental reciprocal autosomal translocation involving 6p2 and another autosome. In one patient the 6p trisomy resulted from a *de novo* t(6;9) (p21.2;p22), and in two other patients the 6p trisomy resulted from a paternal inversion in chromosome 6.

**Pathogenesis:** Unknown.

**POS No.:** 3075

**CDC No.:** 758.990

**Sex Ratio:** M1:F1

**Occurrence:** About two dozen cases have been reported in the literature.

**Risk of Recurrence for Patient's Sib:** Not increased if parental chromosomes are normal. Considerably increased (possibly 5–10%) if one of the parents is a carrier of an autosomal balanced translocation involving 6p2.

**Risk of Recurrence for Patient's Child:** Reproduction in affected patients is highly unlikely.

**Age of Detectability:** At birth by clinical examination, or prenatal diagnosis by CVS or amniocenthesis.

**Gene Mapping and Linkage:** See *Gene Map*.

**Prevention:** None known. Genetic counseling indicated.

**Treatment:** Unknown.

**Prognosis:** Long-term prognosis is poor, and most patients do not survive the neonatal period due to the presence of severe internal anomalies. Only three out of 22 reported cases have been adults.

**Detection of Carrier:** Cytogenetic examination.

**References:**

Pearson G, et al.: Inversion duplication of chromosome 6 with trisomic codominant expression of HLA antigens. Am J Hum Genet 1979; 31:29–34.

Grouchy J de, Turleau C: Clinical atlas of human chromosomes, 2nd ed. New York: John Wiley and Sons, 1984.

Smith BS, Peterssen JC: An anatomical study of a duplication 6p based on two sibs. Am J Med Genet 1985; 20:649–663.

Fryns JP, et al.: Partial distal 6p trisomy in a malformed fetus. Ann Génét 1986; 29:53–54.

FR030                                                    **Jean-Pierre Fryns**

---

## CHROMOSOME 6, TRISOMY 6Q2                        2439

**Includes:** Chromosome 6, partial trisomies 6q between 6q21 and 6q26

**Excludes:** N/A

**Major Diagnostic Criteria:** Karyotype showing trisomy for part or all of 6q2. Mental retardation, dysmorphic features, webbing of the neck, joint flexion contractures.

**Clinical Findings:** Dysmorphism is relatively minor in infancy and becomes very striking in childhood. The cranium is often abnormal in shape, with turricephaly and prominent forehead with or without **Microcephaly**. The face is flat, and the features seem to be pulled downward. The palpebral fissures slant downward, with thin, arched eyebrows. There is hypertelorism. The nose is enlarged. The lips are thin, and the mouth has a peculiar shape, the median part of the upper lip seeming to be pulled upward and the lower lip being slightly everted.

The most characteristic feature of the syndrome is the neck deformity: the neck is very broad, short, and has an anterior webbing that is entirely different from the pterygium colli observed in **Turner syndrome**. The angles of the jaw may be com-

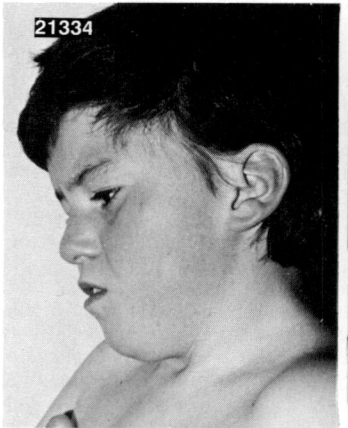
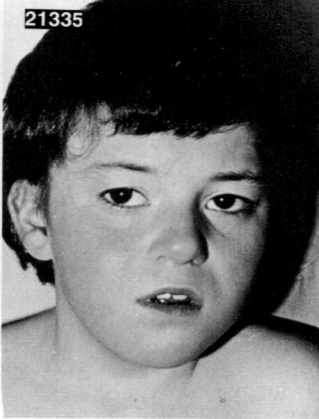

**2439-21334–35:** Chromosome 6, trisomy 6q2; note downturned corners of the mouth and anterior webbing of the neck.

pletely effaced by this webbing. The hair line is low-set on the nape.

There may be deformity of the chest, possibly severe. The nipples are widely spaced. Deformities of the spine are regularly found in older children.

Flexion contractures are a major sign of the syndrome. They involve the fingers and major articulations as well, leading to faulty posture. There is hypospadias and cryptorchidism.

Inner organ malformations are various. They are more frequent when the breakpoint is more proximal (q21-q23). Likewise, the clinical features, in particular the contractures, are less severe when the breakpoint is distal (q26). Mental retardation is severe to profound. Growth retardation may be pronounced.

**Complications:** Those due to inner organ malformations and contractures.

**Associated Findings:** None known.

**Etiology:** Trisomy for part or all of 6q2 due to malsegregation of a parental rearrangement in all known cases but one. The rearrangement is a reciprocal translocation in most cases, a pericentric inversion in one, and an insertion in two. In practically all instances the rearrangement is of maternal origin.

**Pathogenesis:** Unknown.

**POS No.:** 3689

**CDC No.:** 758.990

**Sex Ratio:** M7:F10

**Occurrence:** Seventeen cases have been documented in the literature.

**Risk of Recurrence for Patient's Sib:** Depends on the presence of a parental rearrangement and of its type. Recurrence risk seems to be high, since several examples of familial occurrence are known. Furthermore, numerous spontaneous abortions and stillbirths are known in families at risk.

**Risk of Recurrence for Patient's Child:** There is no known instance of reproduction in patients.

**Age of Detectability:** Theoretically at birth or even prenatally by karyotype analysis. In the neonate, psychomotor retardation, **Microcephaly**, facial dysmorphism, joint contractures, and fingers anomalies are evocative.

**Gene Mapping and Linkage:** See *Gene Map*.

**Prevention:** None known. Genetic counseling indicated.

**Treatment:** Symptomatic care as indicated.

**Prognosis:** Inner organ malformations being rare, survival is the rule. The oldest patient was seen at age 33 years. Growth and mental retardation is severe.

**Detection of Carrier:** By karyotype.

**References:**
Chen H, et al.: Familial partial trisomy 6q syndromes resulting from inherited ins(5;6) (q33;q15q27). Clin Genet 1976; 9:631–637.
Tipton RE, et al.: Duplication 6q syndrome. Am J Med Genet 1979; 3:325–330.
Clark CE, et al.: Trisomy 6q25→6qter in two sisters resulting from maternal 6;11 translocation. Am J Med Genet 1980; 5:171–178.
Turleau C, de Grouchy J: Trisomy 6q2. Clin Genet 1981; 19:202–206.
de Grouchy J, Turleau C: Clinical atlas of human chromosomes, 2nd ed. New York: John Wiley Medical, 1984:487.

DE029
TU013

**Jean de Grouchy
Catherine Turleau**

**Chromosome 7, distal deletion of 7q3**
See CHROMOSOME 7, MONOSOMY 7q3
**Chromosome 7, intersititial deletion of 7q2**
See CHROMOSOME 7, MONOSOMY 7q2
**Chromosome 7, interstitial deletion of 7q1**
See CHROMOSOME 7, MONOSOMY 7q1

## CHROMOSOME 7, MONOSOMY 7P2     2447

**Includes:** Chromosome 7, terminal 7p deletion [del(7) (p21p22)]

**Excludes:**
Chromosome 7, interstitial 7p deletions [del(7) (p11p15)]
**Chromosome 7, monosomy 7** (other)

**Major Diagnostic Criteria:** Severe developmental delay and characteristic craniofacial findings including premature craniosynostosis with scaphocephaly and trigonocephaly. Cytogenetic analysis confirms the diagnosis.

**Clinical Findings:** Severe developmental delay and characteristic craniofacial findings including premature craniosynostosis with scaphocephaly and trigonocephaly. Limitation of joint movements and **Camptodactyly** have been present in one-half of the cases seen.

**Complications:** Unknown.

**Associated Findings:** Skeletal deformities with talipes calcaneovalgus, hypoplastic external genitalia, heart defects (**Ventricular septal defect**, left heart hypoplasia), glossoptosis, microcolon and renal hypoplasia.

**Etiology:** In all reported patients, a terminal 7p deletion [7p22 or 7p22p21] was found. The characteristic clinical findings are due to a deletion of the terminal 7p22 band. In the majority of patients the 7p terminal deletion occurred *de novo*.

**Pathogenesis:** Unknown.

**POS No.:** 4369

**CDC No.:** 758.990

**Sex Ratio:** M4:F3 (observed).

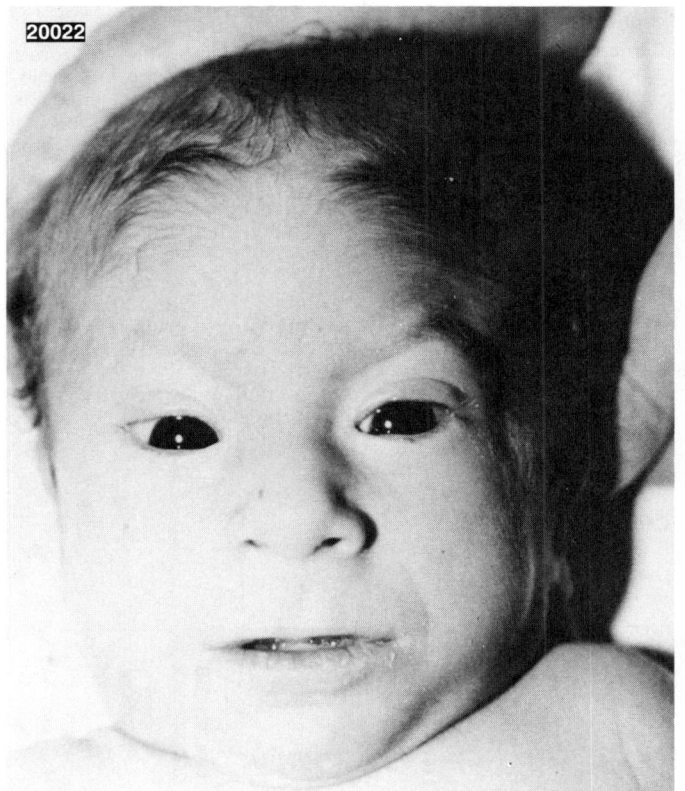

**2447-20022:** Note craniofacies with high narrow forehead, hypotelorism and prominent eyes. These features occur with craniosynostosis which is often present.

**Occurrence:** Less than a dozen cases have been reported.

**Risk of Recurrence for Patient's Sib:** Not increased if parental chromosomes are normal.

**Risk of Recurrence for Patient's Child:** Mental retardation in surviving patients makes reproduction unlikely.

**Age of Detectability:** At birth clinically, or by prenatal diagnosis through CVS or amniocentesis.

**Gene Mapping and Linkage:** See *Gene Map.*

**Prevention:** None known. Genetic counseling indicated.

**Treatment:** Unknown.

**Prognosis:** Long-term prognosis is unknown. At least one-half of the patients died within the first years of life from severe growth failure and the associated internal malformations.

**Detection of Carrier:** Cytogenetic or clinical examination.

**References:**
Friedrich U, et al.: A girl with karyotype 46,XX, del(7) (qter→p15:). Hum Genet 1975; 26:161–165.
Fryns JP, et al.: De Novo partial 2q3 trisomy/distal 7p22 monosomy in a malformed newborn with 7p deletion phenotype and craniosynostosis. Ann Génét 1985; 28/1:45–48.

FR030                                    **Jean-Pierre Fryns**

---

## CHROMOSOME 7, MONOSOMY 7Q1            **2445**

**Includes:** Chromosome 7, interstitial deletion of 7q1

**Excludes:**
    Chromosome 7, monosomy 7q2 (2444)
    Chromosome 7, monosomy 7q3 (2443)

**Major Diagnostic Criteria:** Severe mental retardation and growth failure. No specific dysmorphic syndrome has been delineated in the reported patients. Cytogenetic findings are necessary to confirm the diagnosis.

**Clinical Findings:** Although no distinct dysmorphic syndrome is associated, most patients share a number of clinical findings stigmata in common including **Microcephaly**, flat face, flat nasal bridge, broad nose, hypertelorism, low-set and malformed ears, long upper lip, webbed neck, short extremities, and genital hypoplasia; especially in males.

**Complications:** Unknown.

**Associated Findings:** Severe internal malformation (cardiac anomalies with preductal type of coarctatio aortae, absence of adrenal gland).

**Etiology:** Interstitial deletion of band 7q1, either occurring *de novo*, or as the unbalanced product of a rearranged parental chromosome. Two male siblings with 7q1 interstitial deletion were reported born from a mother with karyotype 47,XX, del (7) (pter→cen::q21→qter), +fr. The interstitial 7q deletion in the mother included centromeric fission, break at 7q21 and preservation of the proximal q arm fragment.

**Pathogenesis:** Unknown.

**POS No.:** 3122

**CDC No.:** 758.990

**2445-21046:** Chromosome 7 of a child with multiple congenital anomalies and a schematic representation of the rearrangement of chromosome 7 in the mother.

---

**Sex Ratio:** Undetermined but presumably M1:F1.

**Occurrence:** Less than 15 cases have been reported.

**Risk of Recurrence for Patient's Sib:** Not increased if parental chromosomes are normal. The risk of recurrence is considerably increased if one parent is carrier of a rearranged chromosome 7.

**Risk of Recurrence for Patient's Child:** Reproduction in affected patients is unlikely.

**Age of Detectability:** At birth clinically, or by prenatal diagnosis through CVS or amniocentesis.

**Gene Mapping and Linkage:** See *Gene Map.*

**Prevention:** None known. Genetic counseling indicated.

**Treatment:** Unknown.

**Prognosis:** Poor long term prognosis due to the severe internal malformations.

**Detection of Carrier:** Cytogenetic and clinical examination.

**References:**
Pfeiffer RA: Interstitial deletion of a chromosome 7 (q11.2q22.1) in a child with splithand/splitfoot malformation. Ann Génét 1984; 27:45–48.
Fryns JP, et al.: Centric fission of chromosome 7 with 47,XX,del(7) (pter→cen: q21→qter) + cen fr karyotype in a mother and proximal 7q deletion in two malformed newborns. Ann Génét 1985; 28/4:248–250.

FR030                                    **Jean-Pierre Fryns**

---

## CHROMOSOME 7, MONOSOMY 7Q2            **2444**

**Includes:** Chromosome 7, intersititial deletion of 7q2

**Excludes:**
    Chromosome 7, monosomy 7q1 (2445)
    Chromosome 7, monosomy 7q3 (2443)
    Chromosome 7, trisomy 7q2–3 (2442)

**Major Diagnostic Criteria:** Multiple congenital anomalies syndrome with moderate to severe mental retardation, but absence of growth retardation in some patients. No specific dysmorphic syndrome was delineated in the reported patients. Cytogenetic confirmation is required to confirm the diagnosis.

**Clinical Findings:** Most patients share a number of general findings in common: mild facial hypoplasia, hypertelorism, epicanthus, short and upslanting palpebral fissures, broad nasal bridge with stubby nose, large mouth with everted lower lip and downturned corners, low-set and malformed ears, and broad short hands and feet.

**Complications:** Unknown.

**Associated Findings:** Central nervous system anomalies with generalized cortical atrophy and severe convulsive disorders. Skeletal anomalies include clubfeet and lobster-claw deformities.

**Etiology:** Interstitial deletion of band 7q2, either occurring *de novo*, or as the unbalanced product of a rearranged parental chromosome 7.

**Pathogenesis:** Unknown.

**CDC No.:** 758.990

**Sex Ratio:** Undetermined but presumably M1:F1.

**Occurrence:** Less than 15 cases have been documented.

**Risk of Recurrence for Patient's Sib:** Not increased if parental chromosomes are normal. Considerably increased if one parent is the carrier of a rearranged chromosome 7.

**Risk of Recurrence for Patient's Child:** Reproduction in affected patients is unlikely.

**Age of Detectability:** At birth clinically, or by prenatal diagnosis through CVS or amniocentesis.

**Gene Mapping and Linkage:** See *Gene Map.*

**Prevention:** None known. Genetic counseling indicated.

**Treatment:** Unknown.

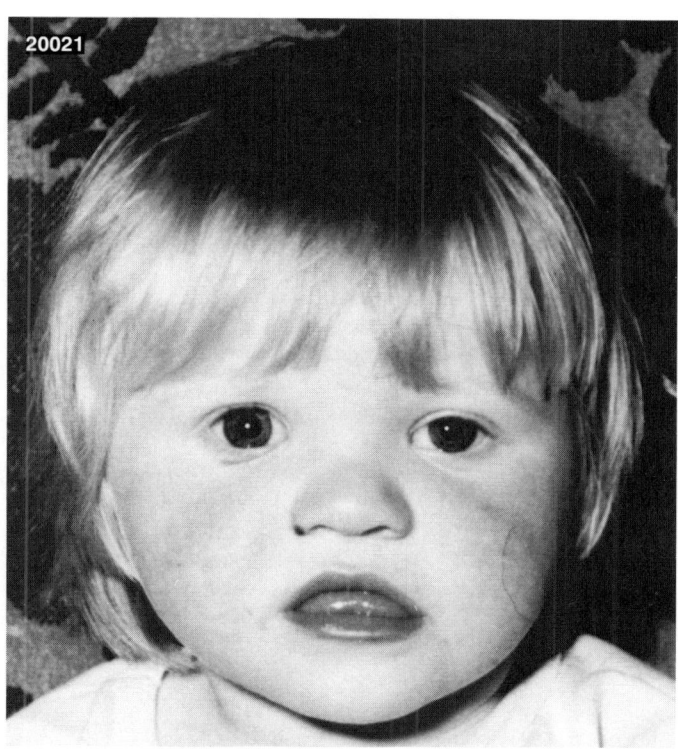

2444-20021: Note characteristic facies: widely set eyes, short palpebral fissures, epicanthal folds, wide nasal bridge with down-turned corners of the mouth.

**Prognosis:** Life span prognosis seems to be better than in proximal and distal 7q deletions.

**Detection of Carrier:** Cytogenetic and clinical examination.

**References:**
Young RS, et al.: Terminal and interstitial deletions of the long arm of chromosome 7: a review with five new cases. Am J Med Genet 1984; 17:437–450.

FR030 **Jean-Pierre Fryns**

---

### CHROMOSOME 7, MONOSOMY 7Q3      2443

**Includes:** Chromosome 7, distal deletion of 7q3

**Excludes:**
**Chromosome 7, monosomy 7q1 (2445)**
**Chromosome 7, monosomy 7q2 (2444)**

**Major Diagnostic Criteria:** Multiple congenital anomalies syndrome with severe mental retardation and growth failure. No specific clinical syndrome has yet been delineated in the reported patients. Cytogenetic confirmation is required.

**Clinical Findings:** Most patients share a number of congenital features in common: micro- and brachycephaly, upslanted palpebral fissures, bulbous nose, short neck, broad and short fingers, hypospadias, hyperlaxity of skin, and hypertonia.

**Complications:** Unknown.

**Associated Findings:** Skeletal anomalies include scoliosis and **Foot, talipes equinovarus (TEV)**. Central nervous system anomalies and retinal coloboma have also been reported.

**Etiology:** Terminal deletion of band 7q3, either occurring *de novo*, or as the unbalanced product of a parental autosomal translocation involving 7q3.

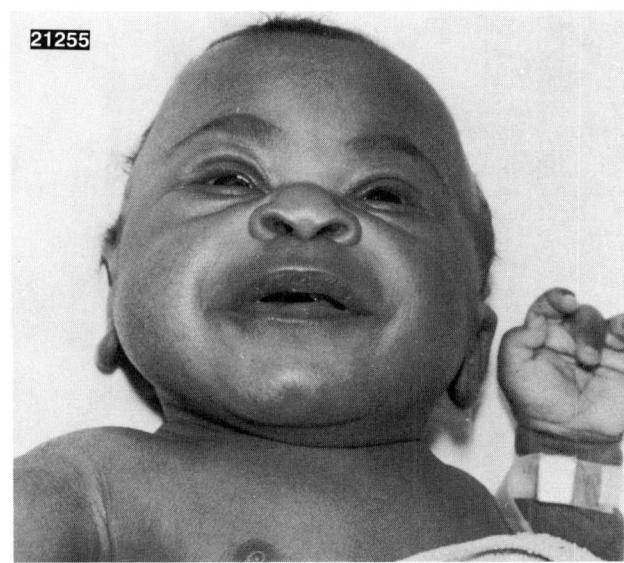

2443A-21255: Note microcephaly and short neck.

**Pathogenesis:** Unknown.

**CDC No.:** 758.990

**Sex Ratio:** Undetermined but presumably M1:F1.

**Occurrence:** Less than a dozen cases have been reported.

**Risk of Recurrence for Patient's Sib:** Not increased if parental chromosomes are normal. Increased if one parent is carrier of an autosomal translocation involving 7q3.

**Risk of Recurrence for Patient's Child:** Reproduction in affected patients is unlikely.

**Age of Detectability:** At birth clinically, or by prenatal diagnosis through CVS or amniocentesis.

**Gene Mapping and Linkage:** See *Gene Map*.

**Prevention:** None known. Genetic counseling indicated.

**Treatment:** Unknown.

**Prognosis:** Poor life prognosis and severe developmental retardation.

**Detection of Carrier:** Cytogenetic and clinical examination.

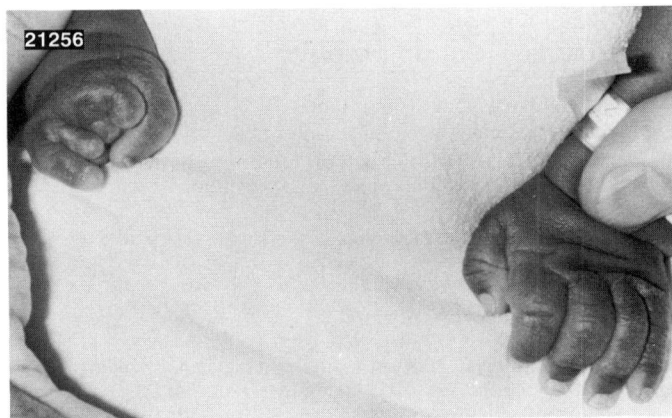

2443B-21256: Symbrachydactyly of the right hand.

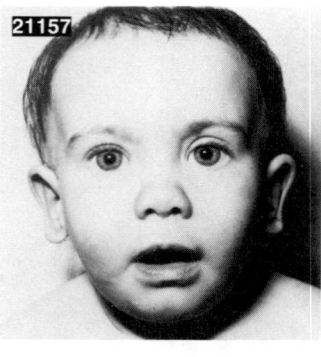
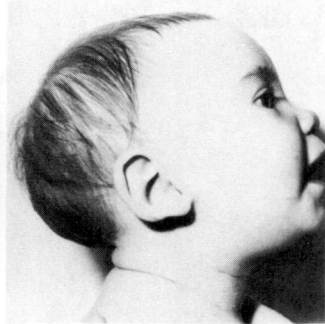
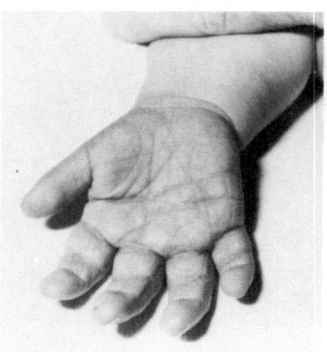
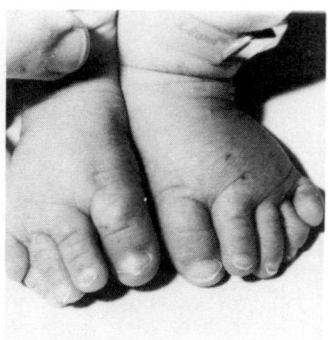

**2443C-21157:** Proband at 1 year. *Upper left*, low set ears; anteverted nares; thin upper lip; downturned mouth. *Upper right*, prominent antitragus with nearby helical prominence; preauricular prominence. *Lower left*, right hand with digitalized thumb and Sydney-type flexion crease. *Lower right*, feet showing tibially turned 5th toes.

**References:**
Koussef BG, et al.: A partial long arm deletion of 7:46,XY, del(7) (q32). J Med Genet 1977; 14:144–147.
Nielsen KB, et al.: Familial partial 7q monosomy resulting from segregation of an insertional chromosome rearrangement. J Med Genet 1979; 16:461–466.
Turleau C, et al.: Monosomie 7qter. Ann Génét 1979; 22:242–244.
Nistrup-Madsen H, et al.: A case of partial deletion of the long arm of chromosome 7 (7q34→qter). Danish Med Bull 1983; 30:14–16.
Stallard R, Juberg RC: Partial monosomy 7q syndrome due to distal interstitial deletion. Hum Genet 1981; 57:210–213.

FR030                                                    **Jean-Pierre Fryns**

## CHROMOSOME 7, MOSAIC TRISOMY 7                          2553

**Includes:** N/A

**Excludes:** Chromosome 7, other anomalies

**Major Diagnostic Criteria:** A lethal condition with characteristic craniofacial findings. Diagnosis is confirmed by chromosome analysis.

**Clinical Findings:** Flat face with low nasal bridge and pug nose, low-set, posteriorly rotated ears with deficient cartilage and short neck with redundant skin. Positional deformities of the extremities.

**Complications:** Unknown.

**Associated Findings:** Potter sequence (see **Renal agenesis, bilateral**) with concomitant lung hypoplasia, unilateral or bilateral renal agenesis, hyaline membranes, cardiac defects, spina bifida occulta, thoracic kyphosis, and rocker bottom feet.

**Etiology:** As with mosaicism of other autosomes, apparently of postzygotic origin. The phenotypic features of mosaic trisomy 7 and, more specifically, the Potter sequence are almost exclusively related to the 7q duplication.

**Pathogenesis:** Unknown.

**CDC No.:** 758.990

**Sex Ratio:** M2:F4 (observed).

**Occurrence:** Undetermined but presumed rare.

**Risk of Recurrence for Patient's Sib:** Probably not increased.

**Risk of Recurrence for Patient's Child:** Affected individuals are not expected to survive to reproduce.

**Age of Detectability:** At birth, or by prenatal diagnosis by amniocenthesis or fetal blood sampling.

**Gene Mapping and Linkage:** See *Gene Map*.

**Prevention:** None known. Genetic counseling indicated.

**Treatment:** Symptomatic.

**Prognosis:** Mosaic trisomy 7 is, as full trisomy 7, a lethal condition. Severe renal and other internal malformations.

**Detection of Carrier:** Unknown.

**References:**
Pflueger SMV, et al: Trisomy 7 and Potter sequence. Clin Genet 1984; 25:543–548. *
Verp MS, et al: Mosaic trisomy 7 and renal dysplasia. Am J Med Genet 1987; 26:139–143.

FR030                                                    **Jean-Pierre Fryns**

**Chromosome 7, rearrangements**
  *See CHROMOSOME INSTABILITY, NIJMEGEN TYPE*
**Chromosome 7, Terminal 7p deletion [del(7) (p21p22)]**
  *See CHROMOSOME 7, MONOSOMY 7p2*
**Chromosome 7, Terminal 7p2 trisomy**
  *See CHROMOSOME 7, TRISOMY 7p2*

## CHROMOSOME 7, TRISOMY 7P2                               2446

**Includes:** Chromosome 7, terminal 7p2 trisomy

**Excludes:**
   Chromosome 7, interstitial 7p duplication
   Chromosome 7, trisomy 7p1

**Major Diagnostic Criteria:** Severe developmental retardation, growth failure and typical craniofacial findings including sloping forehead, with large anterior fontanelle and wide metopic and sagittal sutures, hypertelorism, short palpebral fissures, full cheeks, short nose, small mouth with down-turned corners, micrognathia and short neck. Cytogenetic findings confirm the diagnosis.

**Clinical Findings:** Severe developmental retardation, growth failure and typical craniofacial findings including sloping forehead, with large anterior fontanelle and wide metopic and sagittal sutures, hypertelorism, short palpebral fissures, full cheeks, short nose, small mouth with down-turned corners, micrognathia and short neck. craniofacial anomalies are "en contretype" with the craniosynostosis present in 7p2 deletion.

**Complications:** Unknown.

**Associated Findings:** Skeletal anomalies (**Camptodactyly**, hip luxation, rocker-bottom feet), anal atresia, genital hypoplasia, cardiac, renal and cerebral malformations were reported in one or more patients.

**Etiology:** In all reported patients a duplication of 7p2 was described. Duplication of the sole 7p22 band seems to be responsible for the typical clinical findings. In all cases, the 7p2 duplication was the unbalanced product of a parental autosomal translocation involving 7p2 and another autosome.

**Pathogenesis:** Unknown.

**CDC No.:** 758.990

**Sex Ratio:** Undetermined but presumably M1:F1.

**Occurrence:** Less than a dozen cases have been reported.

**Risk of Recurrence for Patient's Sib:** Not increased if parental chromosomes are normal. Considerably increased (possibly 5–10%) if one of the parents is the carrier of an autosomal balanced translocation involving 7p2.

**Risk of Recurrence for Patient's Child:** Reproduction in affected patients is unlikely.

**Age of Detectability:** At birth clinically or by prenatal diagnosis through CVS or amniocentesis.

**Gene Mapping and Linkage:** See *Gene Map.*

**Prevention:** None known. Genetic counseling indicated.

**Treatment:** Unknown.

**Prognosis:** Long-term prognosis is poor, and most patients do not survive the neonatal period due to the presence of severe internal anomalies.

**Detection of Carrier:** Cytogenetic and clinical examination.

**References:**

Berry C, et al.: Two children with partial trisomy for 7p. J Med Genet 1979; 16:320–321. †

Milunsky J, et al.: Emerging phenotype of duplication (7p): a report of three cases and a review of the literature. Am J Med Genet 1989; 33:364–368. * †

FR030                                                         **Jean-Pierre Fryns**

## CHROMOSOME 7, TRISOMY 7Q2–3                          2442

**Includes:** Chromosome 7, trisomy/duplication of region 7q3

**Excludes:** Chromosome 7, other anomalies

**Major Diagnostic Criteria:** In patients with parental balanced rearrangements, the diagnosis is based on demonstration of both the balanced rearrangement in the parent and the unbalanced leading to partial trisomy in the proband. In *de novo* rearrangements, it is based on the banding pattern of the additional chromosome segment, the phenotype of the patient, and, in the future, of the results of in situ hybridization with cloned DNA segments localized on distal 7q.

**Clinical Findings:** Duplication of region 7q3 with or without 7q2 goes along with a rather distinct pattern of minor and, more facultative, major anomalies. There is some clinical variability in carriers of identical unbalanced rearrangements, however, the individual pattern mostly depends on the size of the duplicated segment and on additional duplication or deletion of a second chromosome involved in a rearrangement.

*Growth, performance, nervous system:* pre- and postnatal growth retardation, delayed skeletal maturation and closure of fontanelles, severe to profound mental deficiency, all of the above-mentioned correlating in extent with the size of the duplicated segment. Severe neonatal adaptation problems in patients with duplications of at least the distal one-half of 7q, often leading to early postnatal death; muscular hypotonia; occasionally seizures. Cerebral malformations may include **Hydrocephaly**; hypoplasia of the corpus callosum, cortical, cerebral, and cerebellar atrophy and cerebellar vermis hypoplasia.

*Facies:* a pattern of minor anomalies including frontal bossing, prominent eyes, downslanting palpebral fissures, short nose with a depressed bridge and upturned nares, long philtrum, **Cleft palate**, small mandible, dysplastic ears, and short neck. Occasionally, coloboma of iris, microphthalmia, short palpebral fissures, strabismus, microstomia, and preauricular pits are seen.

*Trunk and genitalia:* anomalies are mostly found in skeleton and male genitalia. Skeletal findings include scoliosis, hemivertebrae, other vertebral anomalies and absence of 12th ribs. Male genitalia may show cryptorchidism, a small penis with hypospadias, and scrotum bifidum. Further, occasional findings include congenital heart defects, intestinal malrotation, anterior placement of anus.

*Extremities:* characteristic findings are either joint laxity or stiffness, the latter with foot position anomalies, hip dislocation, **Camptodactyly** and stiffness in a flexion position of fingers. Midhands are short with single transverse palmar creases, but fingers and toes tend to be long and may exhibit additional flexion creases.

**Complications:** Shortened life span in many cases, particularly with larger duplicated segments.

**Associated Findings:** None known.

**Etiology:** Cases with a balanced parental rearrangement follow unbalanced meiotic segregation. Non-familial cases may arise through a *de novo* unbalanced rearrangement, or a direct or tandem duplication in a germ cell.

**Pathogenesis:** Unknown.

**CDC No.:** 758.990

**Sex Ratio:** Presumably M1:F1 (M19:F13 observed).

**Occurrence:** A few dozen cases have been documented.

**Risk of Recurrence for Patient's Sib:** Parents carrying a balanced rearrangement: the risk of unbalanced segregation in offspring of balanced rearrangement carriers is theoretically 50%; empirically about 5–10% in addition to increased reproductive vastage.

Parents not carrying a balanced rearrangement: mildly increased (at best to 1%) for the parents of a case with *de novo* unbalanced rearrangement. Not increased for any other relatives.

**Risk of Recurrence for Patient's Child:** Theoretically 50%; in practice much lower because of increased abortion rates of unbalanced products. Unbalanced carriers will almost invariably not reproduce because of their mental handicap.

**Age of Detectability:** Prenatally through chorionic villus chromosome studies at about 10 weeks gestation or through chromosome examination from cultured amniotic fluid cells during about 18–19 weeks gestation. Many unbalanced products wil show abnormal ultrasound findings which may prompt prenatal chromosome examination in cases with no previous affected child. At birth or after through regular blood chromosome examination prompted by the clinical features.

**Gene Mapping and Linkage:** See *Gene Map.*

**Prevention:** None known. Genetic counseling indicated. If the father is a balanced carrier, possibly through heterologous insemination.

**Treatment:** Symptomatic treatment of orthopedic, cardiac, or renal problems, and of seizures. Antibiotic therapy for recurrent infections to which many patients are prone during the first postnatal years.

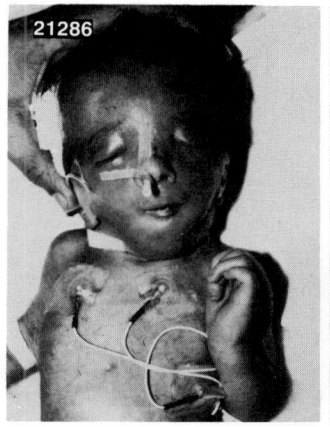 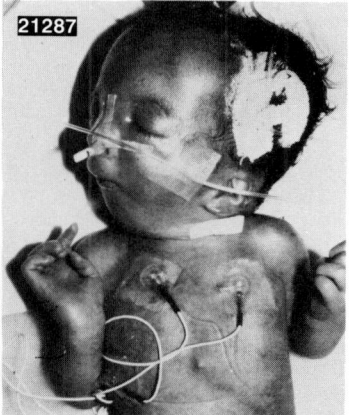

**2442-21286–87:** Facies of an infant with duplication of 7q22-qter at 2 days of age; note frontal bossing, downslanting palpebral fissures, long philtrum, and small mandible.

**Prognosis:** For life: survival greatly depends on the size of the duplicated segment; the larger the latter, the shorter is life expectancy. Patients with duplications of 7q21 or q22→qter usually do not survive. Most patients with duplications of 7q32→qter and almost all with smaller duplications survive at least the first decades. For intelligence: similar negative correlation with the size of the duplicated segment. Patients with duplication of the distal one-half (appr. 7q31→qter) to 2/3 (appr. 7q21→qter) of 7q are profoundly mentally retarded, patients with duplication of the distal one-third (7q32→qter) usually are severely retarded, and retardation in patients with even smaller duplications may range from moderate to severe. For growth: shortness of stature is very common in this condition.

**Detection of Carrier:** By clinical and cytogenetic examination.

**Special Considerations:** Duplication of distal 7q shows a clear-cut positive correlation between size of the duplicated segment, presence and severity of major malformations, extent of growth and mental retardation, and a negative relationship to life span. Patients with larger duplications (7q21→qter) are profoundly retarded, small for dates, face severe neonatal adaptation problems and profound mental retardation, are born with a variety of often severe congenital defects, and often do not survive. Segments longer than the former have not been found in familial and/or non-mosaic cases, and thus might be incompatible with intra-uterine survival. Duplication of 7q22→qter is associated with a distinct dysmorphic pattern and severe mental retardation. Dysmorphic features are very similar in patients whose duplicated segments range from the distal one-third (q32→qter) to two-thirds (q22→qter) of 7q. On the milder side of the spectrum is duplication of only 7q36→qter which is associated with mental retardation in absence of major malformations, and distinct dysmorphisms. If there is additional autosomal deletion (e.g. duplication-deletion due to unbalanced segregation of reciprocal translocations), the latter has its influence on the phenotype, and its associated clinical features may even overshadow those of 7q duplication.

Interstitial duplications of 7q (mostly through unbalanced segregation of interstitial translocations/insertions) are associated with a clinical picture different from that discussed in this article.

**References:**
Schinzel A, Tönz O: Partial trisomy 7q and probable partial monosomy of 5p in the son of a mother with a reciprocal translocation between 5p and 7q. Hum Genet 1979; 53:121–124.

Johnson DC: Duplication of 7q31.2→7qter and deficiency of 18qter: report of two patients and literature review. Am J Med Genet 1986; 25:477–488.

Forabosco A, et al.: The phenotype of partial dup (7q) reconsidered: a report of five new cases. Clin Genet 1988; 34:48–59.

SC017                              **Albert A.G.L. Schinzel**

**Chromosome 7, trisomy/duplication of region 7q3**
  *See CHROMOSOME 7, TRISOMY 7q2-3*
**Chromosome 8, 46, +8p**
  *See CHROMOSOME 8, TRISOMY 8p*

## CHROMOSOME 8, MONOSOMY 8P2                     2450

**Includes:** Chromosome 8, partial monosomy 8p2

**Excludes:** Chromosome 8, other anomalies

**Major Diagnostic Criteria:** The deletion of all or part of the short arm of chromosome 8.

**Clinical Findings:** The first case of monosomy 8p2 was described by Lubs and Lubs in 1973. Since that time an additional ten cases have been reported. Patients with monosomy 8p2 are mentally retarded, with physical features during infancy that may diminish with time. At birth the child usually presents with **Microcephaly**; a distinctive, narrow head with high forehead; protruding occiput; epicanthal folds; a flat nasal bridge with a short, stubby nose; short neck; micrognathia; and a broad chest with wide-set, hypoplastic nipples. Heart defects are often present and include

pulmonary stenosis, **Ventricular septal defect**, or more complicated malformations. Complications due to heart defects are among the leading causes of early death. Failure to thrive and growth retardation are typical findings. Varying degrees of mental retardation and speech difficulties are consistently found. Glandular hypospadias and cryptorchidism have been noted in males, and testicular hypoplasia is sometimes found in adolescents.

**Complications:** Failure to thrive and growth retardation may be related to heart failure caused by the congenital heart defect.

**Associated Findings:** None known.

**Etiology:** In the majority of cases, the deletions are *de novo*, with the break point located at 8p21 or 8p22.

**Pathogenesis:** Chromosomal deletions can occur as errors in gametogenesis or during mitotic cell division in the embryo. The deletion may arise from one parent carrying a balanced translocation involving chromosome 8, in which case the deleted chromosome 8 is passed on to the child.

**POS No.:** 3691

**CDC No.:** 758.990

**Sex Ratio:** M1:F1

**Occurrence:** Eleven cases have been reported.

**Risk of Recurrence for Patient's Sib:** No increase or background risk if deletion is *de novo*. If a familial translocation is present, risk will be increased.

**Risk of Recurrence for Patient's Child:** No reports of patients reproducing.

**Age of Detectability:** At birth, infants may present with **Microcephaly**, narrow cranium, short and stubby nose, and heart defects. Facial features tend to diminish with age. Therefore, older individuals may present with mental retardation but without the features seen during infancy. Prenatal diagnosis is possible.

**Gene Mapping and Linkage:** See *Gene Map*.

**Prevention:** None known. Genetic counseling indicated.

**Treatment:** Medical and surgical management of heart defects. Appropriate educational or training programs to match the ability of the child should be arranged.

**Prognosis:** Children have been observed in infancy and adolescence. Life span may depend on the severity of the heart malformations. Mental retardations is variable, but consistently present.

**Detection of Carrier:** By karyotyping and clinical examination.

**Special Considerations:** The phenotype in this syndrome is not distinctive. Children who are dysmorphic and mentally retarded should be karyotyped to rule out chromosomal abnormalities and concomitant familial balanced translocations, if present.

**References:**
Lubs HA, Lubs ML: New cytogenetic techniques applied to a series of children with mental retardation. In: Casperson T, Zech L, eds: Nobel symposia 23. Chromosome identification-technique and applications in biology and medicine. New York: Academic, 1973:241–250.

Orye E, Craen M: A new chromosome deletion syndrome. Report of a patient with 46,XY,8p-chromosome constitution. Clin Genet 1976; 9:289–301. †

Magenis RE, et al.: Exclusion of glutathione reductase from 8pter→8p22 and localization to 8p21. Cytogenet Cell Genet 1978; 22:446–448.

Reiss JA, et al.: The 8p-syndrome. Hum Genet 1979; 47:135–140. *

Brocker-Vriends AHJT, et al.: Monosomy 8p: an easily overlooked syndrome. J Med Genet 1986; 23:153–154.

DA029                              **Margaret A. Davee**
WE005                              **David D. Weaver**

**Chromosome 8, partial monosomy 8p2**
  *See CHROMOSOME 8, MONOSOMY 8p2*
**Chromosome 8, partial trisomy 8p**
  *See CHROMOSOME 8, TRISOMY 8p*

## CHROMOSOME 8, TRISOMY 8                    0157

**Includes:**
  Chromosome 8, trisomy 8, normal diploid mosaicism
  Warkany Syndrome

**Excludes:**
  Chromosome 8, partial 8 trisomies
  Other C trisomies not involving 8

**Major Diagnostic Criteria:** Multiple congenital abnormalities include dysmorphic facies with everted lip, large ears, and prominent forehead. Skeletal features include a long, thin trunk, rib and vertebral anomalies with multiple joint contractures, absent or dysplastic patellae, camptodactyly and clinodactyly. Deep palmar and plantar furrows are characteristic. Mosaicism for trisomy of chromosome 8 is demonstrated by banding techniques in peripheral leukocytes and/or skin fibroblasts.

**Clinical Findings:** *Growth:* Birth weight and length are normal. Growth is generally normal, but may be delayed.

*Psychomotor development:* Mild to moderate retardation, often with delayed and poorly articulated speech. A proportion of patients have normal IQ, but may display personality disorders and/or psychosis. Average IQ is about 60 (range 12 to normal). Autistic features in a four-year-old male have been described.

*Facies:* Characteristic, with prominent forehead, down-slanting palpebral fissures, broad-based upturned nose, everted lower lip, high-arched or cleft palate, stretched lingual frenulum, micrognathia, and large, dysplastic ears often with a prominent antihelix which is fused to the descending portion of the helix, and a large, rotated, sometimes low-set lobule. Ocular abnormalities may include microphthalmia and convergent strabismus, as well as unilateral corneal opacity, congenital cataract, or heterochromia of the iris.

*Musculoskeletal:* The trunk is long and thin with narrow shoulders, chest, and pelvis. The neck is short and broad and occasionally webbed. There are abnormalities in number and shape of vertebrae (hemivertebrae, fusion of vertebrae, spina bifida) and broad dorsal ribs. Kyphoscoliosis, pectus carinatum, and hip

**0157-20710:** Chromosome 8, trisomy; note bilateral ptosis.
**20711:** Very deep plantar creases.

abnormalities (coxa valga) are common. Flaring of the metaphysis and proximal diaphysis of the femur, humerus, and distal radius has been noted. Joint flexion contractures are present at birth and progress. Digits are long and thin with camptodactyly and clinodactyly. Metacarpal and metatarsal bones may be shortened and irregular in form. Absence or hypoplasia of the patellae is frequent. Nail hypoplasia is common.

*Visceral anomalies:* Renal and ureteral anomalies are frequent, most often hydronephrosis and ureteral reflux. Cryptorchidism is common, as is congenital heart defect, particularly septal defects and great vessel anomalies. Rarer malformations include diaphragmatic hernia, esophageal atresia, and malrotation or absence of the gallbladder.

*Central nervous system malformations:* Agenesis of the corpus callosum is present in a small proportion of cases. A single case with **Hydrocephaly** and bilateral cystic nephroblastomas has been reported.

*Dermatoglyphics:* Deep plantar and palmar furrows are particularly striking in infancy and are characterized by a low ridge count, excessive number of arches or the unusual association of both arches and whorls on the fingertips, and high palmar and plantar pattern intensity.

*Laboratory and X-ray findings:* Banded cytogenetic studies reveal trisomy 8 in a proportion of cells in peripheral blood lymphocytes and in cultured skin fibroblasts, generally with euploid mosaicism. The proportion is usually greater in skin fibroblasts. The percentage of trisomic cells in lymphocytes often decreases with time, and there are reported cases of normal blood chromosome studies in patients with trisomy 8 demonstrable in skin fibroblasts. Most patients with trisomy 8 have mosaicism with a euploid cell line. There is a single description of a living individual with non-mosaic trisomy 8 demonstrated in several tissues; however, this patient may represent mosaicism in other, unexamined tissues.

Partial deficit of coagulation factor VII has been found in several patients. X-rays demonstrate the skeletal anomalies and contractures, most commonly spina bifida occulta and supernumerary vertebrae and ribs as well as hip dysplasia and coxa valga and vara. The rib index, which is the ratio of the narrowest medial height to the broadest height of the dorsal aspect of ribs 4, 6, and 8, is significantly lower than the mean of 0.83 for normals. This may be a helpful diagnostic sign. Focal EEG abnormalities are seen in half of the individuals. CT scan will demonstrate absence of corpus callosum, if present.

**Complications:** Major consequences may result from musculoskeletal or visceral anomalies. Renal insufficiency, significant cardiac dysfunction, restricted mobility, and developmental and learning problems are common. Speech delay and articulation problems are frequent. Feeding problems may occur due to the stretched lingual frenulum.

**Associated Findings:** Malignancy has been noted in 3 of 74 reported patients with trisomy 8 (4%), and trisomy 8 is a common finding in bone marrow chromosomes in various hematologic disorders. The significance of this is unknown.

High incidence of advanced paternal age has been reported.

**Etiology:** Chromosome non-disjunction, due to unknown factors.

**Pathogenesis:** The phenotypic features of trisomy 8 mosaicism are most probably due to gene overdose interfering with the normal ontogenic process. The details are unknown.

**POS No.:** 3077

**CDC No.:** 758.500

**Sex Ratio:** M2–3:F1 (observed)

**Occurrence:** Some 75 reported cases. Has not been detected in the large number of infants reported in newborn karyotyping surveys. The estimated incidence in conceptuses may be as high as 0.45 per 1000, based on incidence in abortuses and assuming 15% of conceptuses spontaneously abort. Full trisomy 8 without mosaicism is probably the most frequent one of the C group trisomies in spontaneous first trimester abortions. Surveys involving a total of 800 perinatal deaths showed only 1 case of trisomy 8. Many cases may be unrecognized.

**Risk of Recurrence for Patient's Sib:** Unknown.

**Risk of Recurrence for Patient's Child:** Unknown.

**Age of Detectability:** Has been observed clinically in the neonatal period. Can be detected in amniotic fluid cell culture in midtrimester. Clinically, trisomy 8 may fail to be recognized until later in life.

**Gene Mapping and Linkage:** See *Gene Map*.

**Prevention:** None known. Genetic counseling indicated.

**Treatment:** Symptomatic therapy can attempt to correct or compensate for anatomic defects, including surgery and/or physical and occupational therapy for skeletal defects, early treatment for renal anomalies to prevent progression of obstruction to renal insufficiency, and medical or surgical treatment of cardiac defects. Speech therapy and remedial education may be beneficial. Surgical correction of stretched lingual frenulum may facilitate feeding and more normal speech.

**Prognosis:** Life span is unknown, but relatively healthy adult patients have been reported. Survival is less reduced than in most other chromosome abnormalities. Cardiac and renal problems may interfere with normal life expectancy. Physical restrictions and psychomotor retardation may be significant factors in altering quality of life.

**Detection of Carrier:** Unknown.

**Special Considerations:** Trisomy 8 cells are more stable in skin fibroblasts than in lymphocytes, and in many individuals, the trisomy 8 cells are found in higher proportion in skin than in blood. If the diagnosis of trisomy 8 syndrome is suspected clinically and the blood karyotype is normal, skin fibroblast karyotype is indicated. A few patients with mosaic trisomy 8 do not exhibit the characteristic phenotype.

**References:**

Riccardi VM: Trisomy 8: an international study of 70 patients. BD:OAS 1977:XIII(3C):171–184.

Anneren G, et al.: Trisomy 8 syndrome. Helv Paediat Acta 1981; 36:465–472. *

Frangoulis M, Taylor D: Corneal opacities: a diagnostic feature of the trisomy 8 mosaic syndrome. Br J Ophthalmol 1983; 67:619–622.

Schinzel A: Trisomy 8 mosaicism. in Catalogue of Unbalanced Chromosome aberrations in man. Berlin: Walter de Gruyter and Co., 1983:325–328.

Burd L, et al,: A case of autism and mosaic of trisomy 8. J Autism Develop Disorders 1985; 15:351–352.

NaKamura Y, et al.: Bilateral cystic nephroblastomas and multiple malformations with trisomy 8 mosaicism. Hum Pathol 1985; 16:754–756.

R0057                         **Sally Shulman Rosengren**
CA032                         **Suzanne B. Cassidy**

**Chromosome 8, trisomy 8, normal diploid mosaicism**
*See CHROMOSOME 8, TRISOMY 8*

---

## CHROMOSOME 8, TRISOMY 8P             2449

**Includes:**

Chromosome 8, partial trisomy 8p

**Excludes:** Chromosome 8, trisomy 8 (0157)

**Major Diagnostic Criteria:** High prominent forehead; wide face during infancy; fleshy, everted lower lip; poorly defined philtrum; marked macrostomia with gingival hypertrophy; low nasal bridge and anteverted nostrils; large, abnormally soft ears with excess folds and elongated conchae. Definitive diagnosis is made cytogenetically when partial trisomy of the short arm of chromosome 8 can be demonstrated by a translocation to another chromosome, or because of an interstitial or terminal duplication.

The gene for glutathione reductase has been mapped to 8p21. A gene dosage effect is seen in trisomies involving this band.

**Clinical Findings:** Infants may be rather large and long-limbed at birth, although growth retardation is usually observed later. Moderate-to-severe hypotonia is frequently noted. Observed

anomalies are relatively minor and generally involve the craniofacial region. The most striking features include macrostomia with a long and poorly defined philtrum, a fleshy and everted lower lip, and large, abnormally soft ears that tend to be posteriorly rotated. The palpebral fissures are downslanting. In addition, the neck is often short, with an excess of skin. The thorax may appear long in comparison to the rest of the body, and kyphoscoliosis may eventually occur. In males, the penis is usually small, and cryptorchidism may be present.

There may be flexion contractures of the hands and legs, coxa valga, and clubfeet deformities. Hyperextensibility of the finger joints, clinodactyly of the fifth digits, short fingers, and hypoplastic nails have been noted. Dermatoglyphics show an increased frequency of a single median palmar crease (simian crease), absence of digital flexion creases, and an excess of arches on the fingertips. Deep plantar furrows may be observed in infants.

Cardiac malformations have been observed in about one-third of the cases. Cerebral malformations may also be present, the most common being agenesis of the corpus callosum. Spina bifida occulta, ureteral stenosis, absence of the bladder, or a single umbilical artery have occasionally been noted. Delayed bone age, various osseous findings, such as supernumerary ribs, and anomalies of the phalanges have been found. Mental retardation is more severe in these children than in those with trisomy 8 mosaicism. Affected individuals may be unable to walk, and may move about on the floor by bracing themselves on their arms.

**Complications:** Additional complications can arise if there are malformations of the heart, nervous system, or urogenital system.

**Associated Findings:** Translocation of the short arm of chromosome 8 may result in deletions in the chromosome to which it has been translocated. These deletions may cause additional physical and behavioral problems in the patient, depending on the size of the deletion and the particular chromosome involved.

**Etiology:** A number of cases have been due to a parental balanced translocation to an acrocentric chromosome. In these cases translocations have involved all of 8p. In nearly one-half of the cases, a *de novo* duplication of nearly all of 8p is found, resulting in an interstitial or terminal duplication of the chromosome or in a pericentric inversion. In a few cases, the trisomy included the most proximal portion of 8q.

**Pathogenesis:** Partial trisomy of the short arm of chromosome 8 can occur as a result of duplications of chromatin within the chromosome or as the result of a translocation.

**POS No.:** 3078

**CDC No.:** 758.990

**Sex Ratio:** M1:F1

**Occurrence:** Fewer than 50 cases have been reported since the first case was published in 1971.

**Risk of Recurrence for Patient's Sib:** If the translocation is *de novo*, the risk is probably less than 1%. If a balanced translocation is present in one of the parents, the recurrence risk is 5–20%.

**Risk of Recurrence for Patient's Child:** There have been no reports of affected individuals reproducing. However, if they should, there would be an increased risk of producing abnormal offspring.

**Age of Detectability:** Children who present at birth with the major diagnostic findings may be suspected to have trisomy 8p and can diagnosed by cytogenetic investigation. Older individuals who are significantly mentally and physically delayed and who retain the major physical findings should be suspected to have trisomy 8p. Prenatal diagnosis is possible.

**Gene Mapping and Linkage:** See *Gene Map*.

**Prevention:** None known. Genetic counseling indicated.

**Treatment:** Treatment of cardiac disease or other problems arising from malformations, if present.

**Prognosis:** Patients have been observed at various ages. Severe mental retardation is usual. A reduced life span may be expected with early death if severe heart defects or other malformations are present.

**Detection of Carrier:** By karyotyping and clinical examination.

**Special Considerations:** Because of the heterogeneous nature and relatively unremarkable physical manifestations of this condition, the possibility that a chromosomal abnormality exists may be overlooked. In addition, it is possible that there is a deletion in another chromosome along with the +8p, which could mask the clinical features of trisomy 8p. Because a familial balanced translocation may exist, it is critical to rule out a chromosomal abnormality in any case of mental retardation and malformations of unknown etiology.

**References:**
Yanagisawa S, Hiraoka K: Familial G/C translocation in three relatives associated with severe mental retardation, short stature, unusual dermatoglyphics and other malformations. J Ment Defic Res 1971; 15:136–146.

de la Chapelle A, et al.: Mapping of the gene for glutathione reductase on chromosome 8. Ann Genet 1976; 19:253–256.

Clark CE, et al.: A case of partial trisomy 8p resulting from a maternal balanced translocation. Am J Med Genet 1980; 7:21–25.

Mattei JF, et al.: Clinical, enzyme, and cytogenetic investigations in three new cases of trisomy 8p. Hum Genet 1980; 53:315–321. * †

Stengel-Rutkowski S, et al.: Familial Wolf's syndrome with a hidden 4p deletion by translocation of an 8p segment. Unbalanced inheritance from a maternal translocation (4;8)(p15.3;p22): case report, review and risk estimates. Clin Genet 1984; 25:500–521.

Fryns JP, et al.: Partial 8p trisomy due to interstitial duplication: karyotype: 46,XX, inv dup(8) (p21.1→p22). Clin Genet 1985; 28:546–549. * †

DA029
WE005

**Margaret A. Davee**
**David D. Weaver**

**Chromosome 9, centromeric instability-immunodeficiency**
*See IMMUNODEFICIENCY WITH CENTROMERIC INSTABILITY*
**Chromosome 9, duplication 9q3**
*See CHROMOSOME 9, TRISOMY 9q3*

---

**CHROMOSOME 9, PARTIAL MONOSOMY 9P          2231**

**Includes:** N/A

**Excludes:** Chromosome 9, monosomy 9p

**Major Diagnostic Criteria:** Mental retardation and dysmorphic facies consisting of trigonocephaly, midface hypoplasia, upward slanting palpebral fissures, and long philtrum. The diagnosis is confirmed by cytogenetic studies revealing deletion of the short (p) arm of the chromosome 9 distal to band p22.

**Clinical Findings:** The majority of patients have the following features: normal birth weight and length, trigonocephaly, upward-slanting palpebral fissures, arched eyebrows, bilateral epicanthal folds, flattened nasal bridge, short nose, anteverted nares, long philtrum, small mouth, high-arched palate, micrognathia, low-set ears with aplastic lobes and poorly folded helices, short neck, increased internipple distance, apparently long digits due to relative shortness of metacarpals with respect to phalanges, and square hypLECTUREERconvex nails. Dermatoglyphics reveal an excess of whorls, an elevated total ridge count, and accessory finger flexion creases, particularly on the middle phalanx. In females, genital abnormalities include hypoplasia of the labia majora and hyperplasia of the labia minora. Males are likely to have hypospadias. The mental retardation is moderate, with IQ ranging between 30 and 60. The typical personality is described as friendly, affectionate, and sociable.

**Complications:** Advanced osseous maturation, precocious puberty, kyphosis, autism, and seizures.

**Associated Findings:** Cardiac malformations, omphalocoele, and hernias.

**Etiology:** Deletion of genetic material from chromosome 9p. In the majority of cases, the breakpoint is in band p22. The deletion is *de novo* in two-thirds of cases. Mean paternal and maternal ages (*de novo* cases): P= 31.2 years, M= 29 years.

**Pathogenesis:** Unknown.

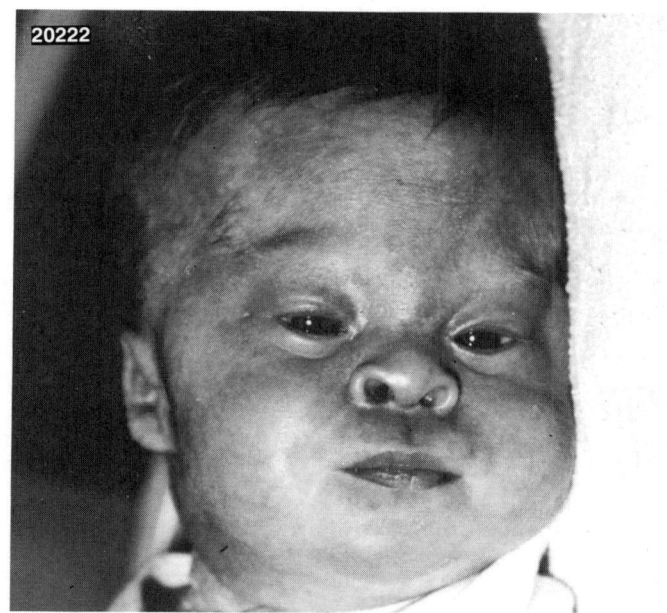

**2231-20222:** Note upward slanting palpebral fissures, epicanthi, trigonencephaly, mid-face hypoplasia, anteverted nares and long philtrum.

---

**POS No.:** 3081

**CDC No.:** 758.990

**Sex Ratio:** M7:F20

**Occurrence:** About 100 cases have been reported in the literature.

**Risk of Recurrence for Patient's Sib:** If the parent is a translocation carrier, the risk is high. If the parental karyotypes are normal, exact risk figures are unknown but presumed to be low.

**Risk of Recurrence for Patient's Child:** There has been no known reproduction by an affected patient.

**Age of Detectability:** At birth. Prenatal diagnosis is possible by chromosome studies of chorionic villus or amniotic fluid cells.

**Gene Mapping and Linkage:** See *Gene Map.*

**Prevention:** None known. Genetic counseling indicated.

**Treatment:** Surgical repair of congenital heart lesions, omphalocoele, and hernia.

**Prognosis:** Depends on the severity of associated malformations. If there are no major congenital heart malformations, life span is normal. A sixty-one year old man with del (9)(p22) has been described.

**Detection of Carrier:** Chromosome analysis.

**References:**
Alfi O, et al: Deletion of the short arm of chromosome #9 (46,9p-): a new deletion syndrome. Ann Genet 1973; 16:17–22.

Nielsen J, et al: The deletion 9p syndrome: a 61 year old man with deletion of short arm 9. Clin Genet 1977; 12:80–84.

Deroover J, et al: Partial monosomy of the short arm of chromosome 9: a distinct clinical entity. Hum Genet 1978; 44:195–200.

Rutten FJ, et al: A case of partial 9p monosomy with some unusual clinical features. Ann Genet 1978; 21:51–55.

Funderburk SJ, et al: The 9p-syndrome. J Med Genet 1979; 16:75–79.

Young RS, et al: The dermatoglyphic and clinical features of the 9p trisomy and partial 9p monosomy syndromes. Hum Genet 1982; 62:31–39.

Young RS, et al: Two children with de novo del(9p). Am J Med Genet 1983; 14:751–757.

De Grouchy J, Turleau C: Clinical Atlas of Human Chromosomes, 2nd ed. New York: John Wiley, 1984:158–163.

Huvet JL, et al: Eleven new cases of del 9p1 and features from 80 cases. J Med Genet 1988; 25:741–749.

BI001                                                    **Diana W. Bianchi**

## CHROMOSOME 9, RING 9                                          2454

**Includes:** Ring (9)

**Excludes:** Chromosome 9, partial monosomy 9p (2231)

**Major Diagnostic Criteria:** Ring chromosome 9 on karyotype. Phenotypic manifestations may be extremely mild, particularly in the newborn period.

**Clinical Findings:** Findings, based on 13 cases, have been similar to del (9) (pter-22) and to **Chromosome 9, trisomy 9**, but are often mild. Craniofacial appearance includes **Microcephaly** and trigonocephaly, a slightly prominent midface with mild exophthalmos and slanting of the palpebral fissures, and an exaggeration of the arch of the eyebrows. The neck may appear short and the chin small, and the antihelix of the ear may protrude. However, some cases do not appear obviously dysmorphic. Heart defects were seen in four of 13, and hypospadias or ambiguous male genitalia in four of ten. Skeletal anomalies of varying sorts and **Cleft palate** have also been seen. Older patients may show growth retardation, and there is typically mental retardation of a moderate to severe degree. Some are agitated and introverted, and difficult to control as they mature. However, cases have had minimal dysmorphology, and only isolated ambiguous genitalia. Intelligence may be in the low normal range, despite some deficits in expressive language.

**Complications:** Unknown.

**Associated Findings:** None known.

**Etiology:** Formation of a ring 9 chromosome with loss of distal short and long arm material.

**Pathogenesis:** Unknown.

**CDC No.:** 785.990

**Sex Ratio:** Undetermined but presumed to be M1:F1.

**Occurrence:** Over a dozen cases have been reported.

**Risk of Recurrence for Patient's Sib:** Low, unless a parent also has a ring.

**Risk of Recurrence for Patient's Child:** Unknown.

**Age of Detectability:** Prenatally by amniocentesis or chorionic villi sampling. Postnatally by karyotype.

**Gene Mapping and Linkage:** See *Gene Map.*

**Prevention:** None known. Genetic counseling indicated.

**Treatment:** Symptomatic for specific anomalies. Special education.

**Prognosis:** The heart defects can be lethal, but long-term survival (minimally, into early adulthood, probably longer) is otherwise expected. Behavioral problems may make management difficult in some cases.

**Detection of Carrier:** By karyotype.

**Special Considerations:** As with other ring chromosomes, findings can be variable. Generally appearances are far less distinctive than with 9p deletion. Findings can also be extremely mild, and caution should be used in predicting final mental function.

**References:**
de Grouchy J, Turleau C: Clinical atlas of human chromosomes. 2nd ed. New York: John Wiley & Sons, 1984.

Schinzel A: Catalogue of unbalanced chromosomal aberrations in man. New York: Walter de Gruyter, 1984.

LU001                                                    **Mark Lubinsky**

## CHROMOSOME 9, TETRASOMY 9P                                   2335

**Includes:** N/A

**Excludes:** Chromosome 9, trisomy 9p (2451)

**Major Diagnostic Criteria:** Moderate to severe psychomotor retardation, normal to mild growth deficiency; **Hydrocephaly**; dysmorphic facial features similar to those seen in **Chromosome 9, trisomy 9p** (microcephaly, enophthalmos, hypertelorism, bulbous nose); congenital heart disease; skeletal; and renal anomalies. Confirmation of i(9p) or idic (9p) in lymphocyte and/or skin cultures.

**Clinical Findings:** Low birthweight (6/10); psychomotor retardation (10/10); microcephaly (9/10); wide open sutures and fontanelles (10/10); hydrocephaly (5/10); hypertelorism (7/10); strabismus (4/10); enophthalmos (4/10); epicanthal folds (5/10); bulbous/beaked nose (8/10); downward slanting mouth (4/10); cleft lip/palate (3/10); microretrognathia (5/10); protruding and malformed ears (5/10); short neck (6/10); widely spaced nipples (3/10); cryptorchidism (3/6); dysplastic fingernails (4/10); clinodactyly of fifth fingers (4/10); single palmar crease (4/10); absence of fusion of C triradius (3/10); congenital heart disease (6/10); renal anomalies (2/10); skeletal anomalies (8/10).

The X-ray studies show: microcephaly, hypertelorism, angulated costal arches, first and 12th hypoplastic vertebral bodies, kyphoscoliosis, clinodactyly and brachymesophalangy of fifth fingers, slender 2–5 metatarsals, delayed ossification of pubic bones and ischiopubic synchondrosis, broad ischiopubic tubera, wide interpubic synchondrosis, delayed ossification of femoral heads, spina bifida occulta, hydrocephalia, and generalized osteopenia.

Tetraplex gene dosage effect for galactose-1-P-uridyltransferase (GALT) has been observed. The majority of patients have i(9p); isodicentric chromosomes and mosaicism are less frequent.

Mean parental age has been about 30 years of age.

**Complications:** Depend on the visceral and the musculo-skeletal involvement.

**Associated Findings:** A few patients have been reported with myopic chorioretinal degeneration. Scanning electron microscopic studies of the hair from one affected female showed notches along the hair fibre, as well as longitudinal gaps.

**Etiology:** Tetrasomy 9p due to an extra isochromosome or isodicentric. All known patients acquired their aneuploidy from a *de novo* event.

**Pathogenesis:** Unknown.

**CDC No.:** 758.990

**Sex Ratio:** M6:F4

**Occurrence:** Over a dozen cases have been reported, with mosaicism found in five.

**Risk of Recurrence for Patient's Sib:** Unknown.

**Risk of Recurrence for Patient's Child:** Unknown.

**Age of Detectability:** At birth or prenatally by chromosome studies.

**Gene Mapping and Linkage:** See *Gene Map.*

**Prevention:** None known. Genetic counseling indicated.

**Treatment:** Special education may be beneficial; skeletal defects may require correction.

**Prognosis:** High mortality rate during the first year of life. Individuals with mosaicism have a better prognosis.

**Detection of Carrier:** Unknown.

**References:**
Eydoux P, et al.: Gene dosage effect for GALT in 9p trisomy and in 9p tetrasomy with an improved technique for GALT determination. Hum Genet 1981; 57:142–144. *

García-Cruz D, et al.: Tetrasomy 9p: clinical aspects and enzymatic gene dosage expression. Ann Genet 1982; 25:237–242. * †

Peters J, et al.: Case report of mosaic partial tetrasomy 9 mimicking

Klinefelter syndrome. BD:OAS XVIII (3B). New York: March of Dimes Birth Defects Foundation, 1982:287–293.

Balestrazzi P, et al.: Tetrasomy 9p confirmed by GALT. J Med Genet 1983; 20:396–399. †

Shapiro SD, et al.: Non-mosaic partial tetrasomy and partial trisomy 9. Am J Med Genet 1985; 20:271–276.

CR019
CA011

**Diana García-Cruz**
**José María Cantú**

## CHROMOSOME 9, TRISOMY 9      2452

**Includes:** Chromosome 9, trisomy 9 mosaicism

**Excludes:**
> Chromosome 9, partial trisomy 9
> **Chromosome 9, trisomy 9p** (2451)
> **Chromosome 9, trisomy 9q3** (2453)

**Major Diagnostic Criteria:** Cytogenetic evidence for trisomy of the entire chromosome 9. Most cases are mosaic with a normal and trisomic cell line in varying ratios, ranging from 2% to 97% trisomic cells.

**Clinical Findings:** Fewer than 30 cases of Trisomy 9 have been reported among livebirths, and only eight are reported to be non-mosaic. Because so few cases are known the clinical description below includes both mosaic and non-mosaic case.

The most constant dysmorphic features of the syndrome are micrognathia (17/24), low-set anomalous ears (16/24), deep-set eyes (13/24), small palpebral fissures (11/24), and broad-based nose with bulbous tip (13/24). The typical major malformations include cardiac defects (13/24), **Microcephaly** (11/24), fixed or dislocated large joints, especially hips and knees (15/24), hypoplastic/aplastic bones (10/24), hand anomalies (11/24), widening of cranial sutures (7/24), genital (11/24) and renal (8/24) anomalies, and intrauterine growth retardation (6/24).

Other findings include: *CNS:* neurologic impairment, brain malformations; *Craniofacial:* microphthalmia (5/24), hypertelorism (6/24), high palate (6/24), cleft palate with or without cleft lip (6/24), downturned mouth (5/24), short neck (7/24), narrow temples (5/24), cranial asymmetry or craniosynostosis (5/24); *Musculoskeletal:* dislocations or limitations of hips, knees, elbows, radius, wrists, fingers; rocker-bottom feet (5/24), abnormalities of hand including hyperconvex nails, overriding of fingers, hypoplastic phalanges; *Cardiovascular:* **Ventricular septal defect** (10/24), **Ductus arteriosus, patent** (6/24), **Atrial septal defects** (5/24), persistent left superior vena cava (4/24), or others; single umbilical artery (5/24); *Renal:* renal cysts (7/24) and other urinary tract anomalies (11/24) such as hypoplasia of kidney, ureter, bladder, and hydronephrosis; *Genital:* cryptorchidism (8/24), small penis (6/24), hypoplastic scrotum (3/24); *Other:* hypoplastic lungs (5/24), malrotation of gut (3/24); *Dermatoglyphics:* deeply furrowed palms and soles (7/24), simian crease (7/24).

Mental retardation is probable although not proven. While the majority of infants die within the first four months of life, one patient with a low percentage of trisomic cells who died at age nine years was described as having severe mental retardation. One female with 58% trisomic cells was evaluated at age 12 months and was developmentally normal. She had major anomalies and dysmorphic facies characteristic of the syndrome.

**Complications:** Early death.

**Associated Findings:** The following have been reported in one or two cases only: **Corpus callosum agenesis**, cloverleaf skull, leukomalacia, torticollis, epibulbar dermoid, coloboma of the iris, corneal opacities, atretic ear canal with absence of ossicles, small mouth, absent nose and nostrils, unilateral renal agenesis, accessory spleen, **Diaphragmatic hernia**, omphalocele, uterine anomaly, small closed lumbar meningocele, sacral dimple, and punctate mineralization in developing cartilage.

**Etiology:** Meiotic or mitotic non-disjunction, felt to be unassociated with parental age. Variations in the size of the 9qh segment and pericentric inversions have been reported in parents of probands. It has been hypothesized that these variations may predispose to non-disjunction, but the limited number of cases precludes conclusions.

**Pathogenesis:** Considering the rarity among live-births and the wide variability of the major and minor malformations, the presence of an extra chromosome 9 can be presumed to present a serious disruption to embryogenesis.

**POS No.:** 3080

**CDC No.:** 758.990

**Sex Ratio:** M1:F1

**Occurrence:** A few dozen cases have been reported, and only eight of these have been without mosaicism.

**Risk of Recurrence for Patient's Sib:** Unknown.

**Risk of Recurrence for Patient's Child:** Affected individuals are not expected to survive to reproduce.

**Age of Detectability:** At birth or prenatally. Pseudomosaicism of Trisomy 9 has been reported on amniocentesis (attributed to extra-embryonic tissue mosaicism); the fetus had normal chromosomes.

**Gene Mapping and Linkage:** See *Gene Map.*

**Prevention:** None known. Genetic counseling indicated.

**Treatment:** Management of major malformations.

**Prognosis:** The majority of infants die shortly after birth, and survival beyond four months is unusual. One child with low percentage mosaicism died at age nine years.

**Detection of Carrier:** Unknown.

**References:**

Feingold M, Atkins L: A case of trisomy 9. J Med Genet 1973; 10:184–187.

Lewandowski RC Jr, Yunis JJ: Trisomy 9 mosaicism. Clin Genet 1977; 11:306–310. †

Carpenter BF, Tomkins DJ: The trisomy 9 syndrome. Perspectives in Pediatric Pathology 1982; 7:109–120. *

Kaminker CP, et al.: Mosaic trisomy 9 syndrome with unusual phenotype. Am J Med Genet 1985; 22:237–241.

Williams T, et al.: Complex cardiac malformations in a case of trisomy 9. J Med Genet 1985; 22:230–233.

Levy I, et al.: Gastrointestinal abnormalities in the syndrome of mosaic trisomy 9. J Med Genet 1989; 26:280–281.

NI001

**Pat Nichols**

**Chromosome 9, trisomy 9 mosaicism**
> See CHROMOSOME 9, TRISOMY 9
**Chromosome 9, trisomy 9(pter-p21 to q32)**
> See CHROMOSOME 9, TRISOMY 9p

## CHROMOSOME 9, TRISOMY 9P      2451

**Includes:**
> Chromosome 9, trisomy 9(pter-p21 to q32)
> Rethore syndrome

**Excludes:**
> **Chromosome 9, trisomy 9** (2452)
> **Chromosome 9, trisomy 9q3** (2453)
> Chromosome 9, trisomy 9 mosaicism

**Major Diagnostic Criteria:** Cytogenetic evidence for trisomy of a portion or all of 9p, with or without trisomy of the proximal portion of 9q. Mental retardation and characteristic facies are virtually constant features.

**Clinical Findings:** The spectrum of physical and developmental features are remarkably consistent despite the varying sizes of the duplicated segments. Phenotypic-cytogenetic correlation has been attempted. In cases secondary to familial reciprocal translocations, partial monosomy or triploidy for other chromosomes may influence phenotype. In general, patients with the trisomic segment extending from 9pter - 9q13 exhibit mental retardation, **Microcephaly**, brachycephaly, delayed bone maturation, bulbous nose, down-turned corners of mouth, anomalous ears, "worried look",

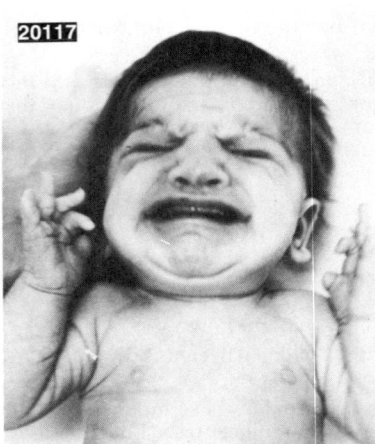
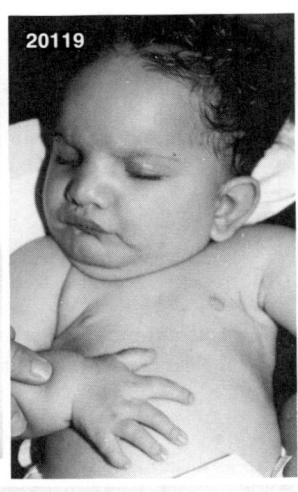
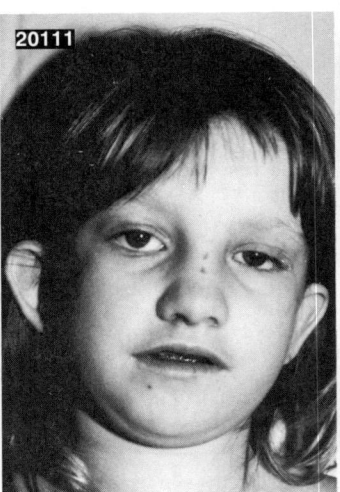
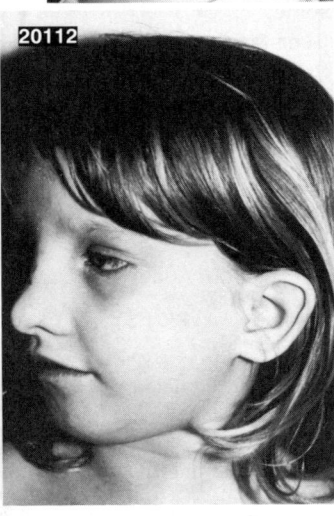

**2451-20117:** Infant with trisomy 9p at one month. Karyotype is 47, XX, +9pter - 9q21 mat. Mother carries a balanced translocation 46, XX, t(9;10) (q21;q13). Note dysmorphic facies with deep-set eyes, hypertelorism, short upper lip and wide, downturned mouth. **20119:** Infant in 20117 shown at 10 months of age. Note short upper lip with prominent philtrum and brachymesophalangy. **20111:** Unrelated girl age 10 years with 46, XX −4, +4pter - 4q35::9p22 - 9pter mat. Mother carries a balanced translocation 46, XX, t(4;9) (q35;p22). Thus this girl is trisomic for 9p22-9pter. Note mild ptosis and simple low-set ears. **20112:** Lateral view of face of girl shown in 20111; note low-set ears and short upper lip.

and those with larger trisomic segments extending through 9q22 or 9q32 have, in addition, intrauterine growth retardation, cleft lip/palate, skeletal anomalies and congenital heart defects.

*Central nervous system anomalies* include mental retardation in virtually all patients, and microcephaly, hypotonia, and growth retardation (60%). The mean I.Q. is 55.

*Craniofacial anomalies* include downturned corners of mouth, bulbous nose (95%); anomalous ears, strabismus, short philtrum, hypertelorism (70–80%); short or webbed neck, low-set ears, enophthalmos, high-arched palate, downslanting palpebral fissures (60–70%); widely spaced nipples, cleft lip and/or palate (40%).

*Congenital heart defects* are reported in approximately 26% of cases (interventricular septal defects).

*Skeletal anomalies* include delayed bone maturation (99%); clino-

dactyly, brachymesophalangy, joint abnormalities (90%); nail hypoplasia, and brachycephaly (70–75%).

*Dermatoglyphics* are unusual and may be helpful from a diagnostic standpoint. Characteristic patterns include fusion or absence of palmar digital triradii, (80–95%); brachymesophalangy, simian crease (80–95%); reduced total finger ridge count, and single flexion crease on fifth finger (30–50%). Axial triradii is usually in the t' position.

**Complications:** Language development may be severely delayed.

**Associated Findings:** Hip dislocation, club foot, **Hydrocephaly, Hernia, umbilical**, and rarely renal anomalies have been noted in case reports.

**Etiology:** In approximately 50% of cases, trisomy 9p arises *de novo*, and the remainder are the result of a familial balanced rearrangement. Average parental age is not increased.

**Pathogenesis:** Unknown.

**POS No.:** 3079

**CDC No.:** 758.990

**Sex Ratio:** M1:F2

**Occurrence:** This is among the most common partial trisomy syndromes. Over 100 cases have been reported.

**Risk of Recurrence for Patient's Sib:** If parent is a carrier of a balanced translocation, the risk is high. For *de novo* index cases, recurrence risk for siblings is not increased.

**Risk of Recurrence for Patient's Child:** No patient is known to have reproduced.

**Age of Detectability:** At birth or by prenatal karyotype.

**Gene Mapping and Linkage:** See *Gene Map*.

**Prevention:** None known. Genetic counseling indicated.

**Treatment:** Infant stimulation and speech therapy should be considered because of language delay.

**Prognosis:** In cases of pure trisomy 9p, major structural malformations are infrequent and life expectancy is not diminished. Major malformations and shortened life span are more likely to occur when trisomy 9p is associated with partial monosomy or trisomy of another chromosome.

**Detection of Carrier:** Chromosome analysis and clinical examination.

**References:**

Rethore MO, et al.: Analyse de la trisomie 9p par denaturation menagee. Hum Genet 1973; 18:129–138.
Young RS, et al.: The dermatoglyphic and clinical features of the 9p trisomy and partial 9P monosomy syndromes. Hum Genet 1982; 62:31–39.
Preus M, Ayme S: Formal analysis of dysmorphism: objective methods of syndrome definition. Clin Genet 1983; 23:1–16. †
Wilson GN, et al.: The phenotypic and cytogenetic spectrum of partial trisomy 9. Am J Med Genet 1985; 20:277–282. *
Smart RD, et al.: Partial trisomy 9: further delineation of the phenotype. Am J Med Genet 1988; 31:947–951.

NI001          **Pat Nichols**

---

| CHROMOSOME 9, TRISOMY 9Q3 | 2453 |
| --- | --- |

**Includes:** Chromosome 9, duplication 9q3

**Excludes:**
> **Arthro-ophthalmopathy, hereditary, progressive, Stickler type** (0090)
> **Chromosome 9, trisomy (other)**
> **Marfan syndrome** (0630)
> **Velo-cardio-facial syndrome** (2129)

**Major Diagnostic Criteria:** Low birth weight with multiple congenital anomalies at birth, including arachnodactyly, dolichocephaly, beaked nose, and micro- and retrognathia. The diagnosis is

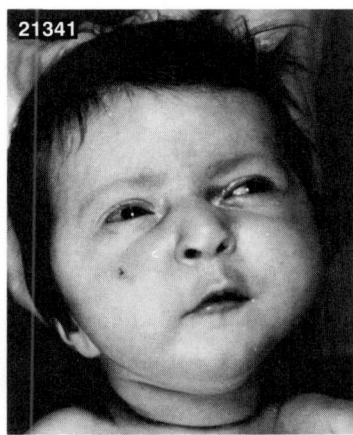
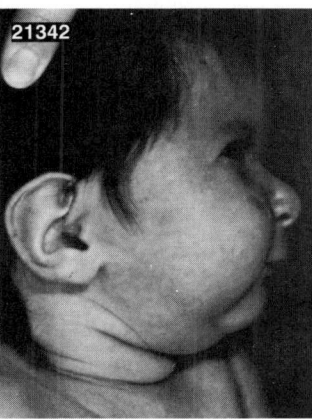

**2453A-21341–42:** Chromosome 9, trisomy 9q3; note deep-set eyes and receding chin.

made by chromosome evaluation looking for either a translocation involving 9q3 or a duplication of 9q3.

**Clinical Findings:** Most affected newborns are of low birth weight with normal birth lengths. There is dolichocephaly with varying degrees of facial asymmetry. The ears are large and malformed. There is a prominent nasal bridge, and the nose is narrow and beaked. There is retrognathia and in some cases micrognathia. Arachnodactyly is present, often associated with **Camptodactyly** and flexion contractures. Cryptorchidism has been described in most affected males (5/6).

Outcome is variable, with most individuals having moderate to severe retardation.

**Complications:** Respiratory obstruction may be associated with glossoptosis secondary to retrognathia. Seizures have been described in some individuals. One patient had hypertonia secondary to brain malformations.

**2453B-21343:** Chromosome 9, trisomy 9q3; note unusual positioning of the fingers.

**Associated Findings:** Pierre-Robin sequence with cleft palate secondary to micrognathia.

**Etiology:** May arise as a result of an inherited unbalanced translocation from a parent with a balanced translocation. *De novo* cases of trisomy 9q3 have been described.

**Pathogenesis:** Unknown.

**CDC No.:** 758.990

**Sex Ratio:** M1:F1

**Occurrence:** Fifteen cases have been reported in the literature, including one large kindred in Newfoundland with seven affected members.

**Risk of Recurrence for Patient's Sib:** Relatively high if patient's mother is a carrier of a balanced translocation (31.5%); risk is high if patient's father is a translocation carrier, but not as high as that associated with a maternal translocation carrier.

**Risk of Recurrence for Patient's Child:** High theoretical recurrence risk, although no affected individuals have reproduced.

**Age of Detectability:** At birth by karyotype or prenatal diagnosis by chorionic villus sampling or amniocentesis.

**Gene Mapping and Linkage:** See *Gene Map.*

**Prevention:** None known. Genetic counseling indicated.

**Treatment:** Unknown.

**Prognosis:** Most affected individuals have moderate-to-severe mental retardation. Life span may be reduced if respiratory difficulties are encountered.

**Detection of Carrier:** By karyotype analysis.

**References:**
Turleau C, et al.: Partial trisomy 9q: a new syndrome. Humangenetik 1975; 29:233–241.
Allerdice PW, et al.: Duplication 9q34 syndrome. Am J Hum Genet 1983; 35:1005–1019. *
de Grouchy J, Turleau C: Clinical atlas of human chromosomes, ed 2. New York: John Wiley & Sons, 1984.
Soltan HC, et al.: Partial trisomy 9q resulting from a familial translocation t(9;16) (q32;q24). Clin Genet 1984; 25:449–454.

SA001                                   **Howard M. Saal**

**Chromosome 10, dup 10p**
*See CHROMOSOME 10, TRISOMY 10p*

---

**CHROMOSOME 10, MONOSOMY 10P**            **2457**

**Includes:** Chromosome 10, partial deletion of the short arm

**Excludes:**
    Chromosome 10, monosomy 10p (2457)
    Immunodeficiency, thymic agenesis (0943)

**Major Diagnostic Criteria:** Terminal deletion of the short arm of chromosome 10.

**Clinical Findings:** Based on at least 15 patients reported: frontal bossing (11/15); downslanted palpebral fissures (11/15); epicanthal folds (9/15); short fissures/ptosis (11/15); low nasal root (12/15); anteverted nares (9/15); cleft lip/palate (1/15); micrognathia (13/15); small, dysplastic ears (14/15); helical pit (3/15); short neck (12/15); wide spaced nipples (8/15); congenital heart defect (7/15); urinary tract defects (6/15); hypoplastic scrotum/cryptorchidism (6/9); **Microcephaly** (7/15); growth delay/short stature (8/11); developmental delay (10/10).

**Complications:** Unknown.

**Associated Findings:** At least three patients have had Di George anomaly (see **Immunodeficiency, thymic agenesis**) with hypoparathyroidism or hypocalcemia and thymic dysplasia or T-cell dysfunction. At least three patients have been reported with arrhinencephaly.

**Etiology:** Deletion of the terminal portion (band p13) of the short arm of chromosome 10. This may be due to a *de novo* deletion or may involve an unbalanced translocation involving 10p and another chromosome, which may be *de novo* or inherited.

**Pathogenesis:** Unknown.

**POS No.:** 3085

**CDC No.:** 758.990

**Sex Ratio:** M8:F5 (observed).

**Occurrence:** At least 15 cases have been reported.

**Risk of Recurrence for Patient's Sib:** Low, unless one parent has a balanced translocation.

**Risk of Recurrence for Patient's Child:** Presumably 1:2 (50%), although no patients have thus far reproduced.

**Age of Detectability:** At birth or by prenatal chromosomal diagnosis.

**Gene Mapping and Linkage:** See *Gene Map.*

**Prevention:** None known. Genetic counseling indicated.

**Treatment:** Supportive care.

**Prognosis:** At least five patients died in the first three months of life. All surviving patients thus far have had developmental delay/psychomotor retardation, with most in moderate to severe range.

**Detection of Carrier:** Chromosome analysis.

**References:**

Elstner CL, et al.: Further delineation of the 10p deletion syndrome. Pediatrics 1984; 73:670–675. * †
Koenig R, et al.: Partial monosomy 10p syndrome. Ann Genet 1985; 28:173–176.
Greenberg F, et al.: Hypoparathyroidism and T cell immune defect in a patient with 10p deletion syndrome. J Pediatr 1986; 109:489–492.

GR011                                    **Frank Greenberg**

---

### CHROMOSOME 10, MONOSOMY 10Q2                    **2458**

**Includes:**

  Chromosome 10, monosomy 10qter
  Chromosome 10, partial deletion 10q
  Chromosome 10, ring chromosome 10
  Chromosome 10, terminal deletion of the long arm

**Excludes:** Chromosome 10, other anomalies

**Major Diagnostic Criteria:** Low birth weight, **Microcephaly**, characteristic facies, and mental retardation. Diagnosis is confirmed by cytogenetic demonstration of a deletion of the long arm of chromosome 10.

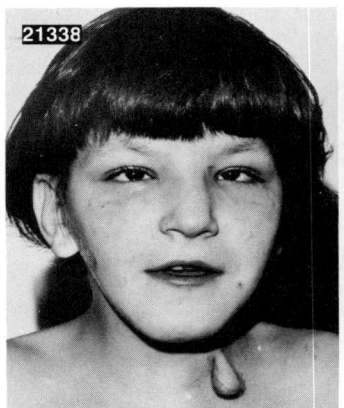 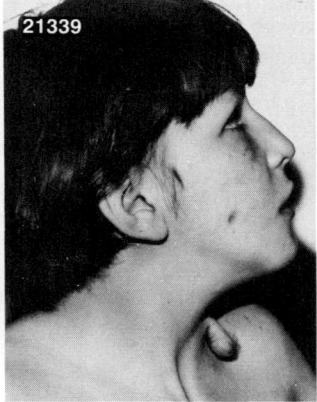

**2458**-21338–39: Chromosome 10, monosomy 10q2; note the long face with effacement of the angles of the jaw.

**Clinical Findings:** Those diagnosed at birth typically have normal gestation, low birth weight, hypotonia, and are microcephalic and possibly brachycephalic. Craniofacial features include **Eye, hypertelorism**, down-slanting short and narrow palpebral fissures, a broad and prominent nasal bridge, a small nose with anteverted nostrils, large and low-set malformed ears, and a prominent upper lip. Other findings include a short neck, abnormal genitalia (small penis and cryptorchidism in males, cloaca in females), and congenital heart malformations (**Ventricular septal defect, Ductus arteriosus, patent**, or **Pulmonary valve, stenosis**).

Those diagnosed in the first year of life or later typically have short stature, hypotonia, mental and psychomotor delay, **Microcephaly**, characteristic facies (triangular facies, strabismus, a prominent nasal bridge, stubby nose, low-set malformed ears), a short neck with a low posterior hairline, abnormal hands (short fingers, clinodactyly of the 5th finger), abnormal dermatoglyphics (abnormal creases, excessive frequency of whorls), abnormal feet (pes equinovarus, **Syndactyly** of the 2nd and 3rd toes), an abnormal chest with widely spaced nipples, a genitourinary abnormality, and delayed bone age.

**Complications:** Respiratory distress, feeding difficulty, cardiac or renal failure (hydronephrosis, recurrent urinary infections).

**Associated Findings:** Ophthalmologic abnormalities (cataract, myopia, macular hypoplasia, choroid atrophy, strabismus, and coloboma); **Cleft lip**, **Cleft palate**, **Uvula, cleft**, micrognathia, webbing of the neck; short neck; male genital hypoplasia; orthopedic deformities (lordosis, **Pectus excavatum**, pes equinovarus); limited elbow extension; **Syndactyly** of the toes; nail hypoplasia; and clinodactyly.

**Etiology:** Partial deletion of the distal portion of the long arm of chromosome 10 (q25-q26). This may result from a ring formation (ten cases) or from a *de novo* deletion (eight cases). Four patients inherited the deleted chromosome from a parent who is heterozygous for a structural rearrangement involving the long arm of chromosome 10. The average paternal age is not increased. No causal association was found with the fragile site on 10q25.

**Pathogenesis:** Unknown.

**CDC No.:** 758.990

**Sex Ratio:** M1:F2

**Occurrence:** A few dozen cases have been reported.

**Risk of Recurrence for Patient's Sib:** Not increased unless there is a parental balanced translocation carrier. The risk of aneuploid offspring for balanced translocation carriers identifed through an affected proband is about 18%.

**Risk of Recurrence for Patient's Child:** Theoretically 1:2 (50%), although there has been no known reproduction by an affected individual.

**Age of Detectability:** Prenatally by CVS or amniotic fluid cell culture, or postnatally by blood cell culture.

**Gene Mapping and Linkage:** See *Gene Map.*

**Prevention:** None known. Genetic counseling indicated.

**Treatment:** Symptomatic for congenital defects, special education.

**Prognosis:** Severe mental retardation.

**Detection of Carrier:** By karyotype analysis and clinical examination.

**References:**

Lewandowski RC, et al.: Partial deletion 10q. Hum Genet 1978; 42:339–343.
Turleau C, et al.: Monosomy 10qter. Hum Genet 1979; 47:233–237.
Michels VV, et al.: Phenotype associated with ring 10 chromosome: report of patient and review of literature. Am J Med Genet 1981; 9:231–237.
Wegner RD, et al.: Monosomy 10qter due to a balanced familial translocation t(10;16)(q25.2;q24). Clin Genet 1981; 19:130–133.
Taysi K, et al.: Terminal deletion of the long arm of chromosome 10:q26 to qter: case report and review of the literature. Ann Genet 1982; 25:141–144.

Chieri P, et al.: Monosomy 10 qter due to a balanced maternal translocation: t(10;8)(q23;q23). Clin Genet 1983; 24:147–150

Zatterale A, et al.: Clinical features of monosomy 10 qter. Ann Genet 1983; 26:106–108.

Shapiro SD, et al.: Deletions of the long arm of chromosome 10. Am J Med Genet 1985; 20:181–196. * †

Mehta L, et al.: Behaviour disorder in monosomy 10qter. J Med Genet 1987; 24:185–187.

Wulfsberg EA, et al.: Chromosome 10 qter deletion syndrome: a review and report of three new cases. Am J Med Genet 1989; 32:364–367.

LE033          **Raymond C. Lewandowski**
VE007            **Michel J.J. Vekemans**

**Chromosome 10, monosomy 10qter**
  See CHROMOSOME 10, MONOSOMY 10q2
**Chromosome 10, partial deletion 10q**
  See CHROMOSOME 10, MONOSOMY 10q2
**Chromosome 10, partial deletion of the short arm**
  See CHROMOSOME 10, MONOSOMY 10p
**Chromosome 10, partial distal 10q trisomy (duplication)**
  See CHROMOSOME 10, TRISOMY 10q2
**Chromosome 10, ring chromosome 10**
  See CHROMOSOME 10, MONOSOMY 10q2
**Chromosome 10, terminal deletion of the long arm**
  See CHROMOSOME 10, MONOSOMY 10q2

## CHROMOSOME 10, TRISOMY 10P                    2456

**Includes:** Chromosome 10, dup 10p

**Excludes:** Chromosome 10, trisomy 10q2 (2455)

**Major Diagnostic Criteria:** Prenatal and postnatal growth retardation; dolichocephaly; narrow face; broad cheeks; high forehead; short bulbous nose; broad nasal root; long philtrum; thin lips; cleft lip and/or cleft palate; highly arched eyebrows; long and curly eyelashes; coloboma; nystagmus; microphthalmia; microcornea; optic nerve atrophy; hypertelorism; usually horizontal or with a mild upward slant of palpebral fissures; fissured tongue; bifid uvula; apparently low-set, large, prominent ears; micrognathia; small rounded chin; congenital heart disease; renal anomalies; cystic kidney, unilateral agenesis; flexion deformities and dermatoglyphic anomalies of flexion creases. Diagnosis is confirmed by karyotype.

**Clinical Findings:** Growth retardation, mental retardation, congenital contractures, hypospadias, and cryptorchidism are found in males; hypoplastic and cystic lungs, additional lung lobes, anal atresia, scoliosis, spina bifida, narrow bones, clubfoot or flatfoot, frontal bossing, hyperflexed upper limbs, **Camptodactyly**, clinodactyly, lower limbs abducted and flexed, hypotonia.

**Complications:** Unknown.

**Associated Findings:** None known.

**Etiology:** A large majority of cases arise due to segregation from a balanced translocation with another autosome and the breakpoint on chromosome 10 is usually proximal to the centromere. A few cases have been found to be duplications of 10p usually from an inversion.

**Pathogenesis:** Unknown.

**POS No.:** 3084

**CDC No.:** 758.990

**Sex Ratio:** Presumably M1:F1.

**Occurrence:** Undetermined but presumed rare.

**Risk of Recurrence for Patient's Sib:** About 20% for this aneuploidy to occur for both male and female balanced carriers.

**Risk of Recurrence for Patient's Child:** Unknown.

**Age of Detectability:** Usually at birth or during infancy by the presence of congenital anomalies. prenatal diagnosis is possible.

**Gene Mapping and Linkage:** See *Gene Map.*

**Prevention:** None known. Genetic counseling indicated.

**Treatment:** Unknown.

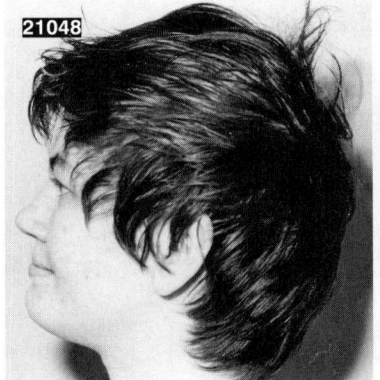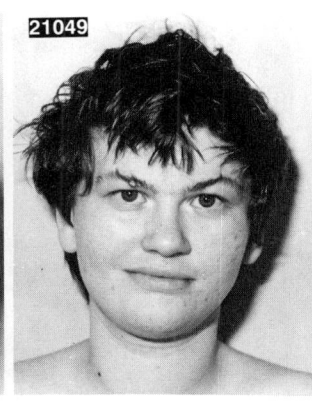

**2456**-21048–49: Chromosome 10, trisomy 10p; note broad cheeks, highly arched eyebrows, bulbous nose and low-set ears.

**Prognosis:** Poor; guarded.

**Detection of Carrier:** By karyotype and clinical examination.

**References:**

Stene J, Stengel-Rutkowski S: Risk for short arm of 10 trisomy: a segregation analysis of eleven families with different translocations. Hum Genet 1977; 39:7–13.

Stene J, Stengel-Rutkowski S: Genetic risks for familial reciprocal translocations with special emphasis on those leading to 9p, 10p and 12p trisomies. Ann Hum Genet 1982; 46:41–74.

Gonzalez CH, et al.: Duplication 10p in a girl due to a maternal translocation t(10:14) (p11;p12). Am J Med Genet 1983; 14:159–167.

Petrosky DL, Borgaonkar DS: Segregation analysis in reciprocal translocation carriers. Am J Med Genet 1984; 19:137–159.

Farge P, et al.: Prenatal diagnosis of trisomy 10p in a twin pregnancy. Prenat Diag 1985; 5:199–203.

Phelan MC, et al.: Trisomy 10p due to a maternal translocation. Proc Greenwood Genet Center 1986; 5:44–48.

B0021                            **Digamber S. Borgaonkar**

## CHROMOSOME 10, TRISOMY 10Q2                    2455

**Includes:** Chromosome 10, partial distal 10q trisomy (duplication)

**Excludes:** Chromosome 10, trisomy 10p (2456)

**Major Diagnostic Criteria:** Craniofacial features including **Microcephaly**, high forehead, small palpebral fissures with blepharophimosis, midfacial hypoplasia with a flat, broad nasal bridge and a small, upturned nose contrasting with prominent philtrum, microstomia, and micrognathia. The diagnosis is confirmed by karyotype.

**Clinical Findings:** Pre- and postnatal growth-retardation, characteristic face, short neck, skeletal anomalies i.e. **Camptodactyly**, large distance between toes I and II, and scoliosis. General hyperlaxity and severe mental retardation.

**Complications:** Unknown.

**Associated Findings:** **Cleft palate** seems to occur in at least 20% of the patients. Various internal malformations, mostly cardiovascular and renal, have been documented in the majority of patients.

**Etiology:** In all reported patients a duplication of 10q2 (most frequently 10q24→10qter) is described. In the majority of cases, the 10q2 duplication is the unbalanced product of a parental autosomal translocation involving 10q2 (most common breakpoint 10q24) and another autosome. Two cases of trisomy 10q2 were the result of a *de novo* reciprocal autosomal translocation. Some

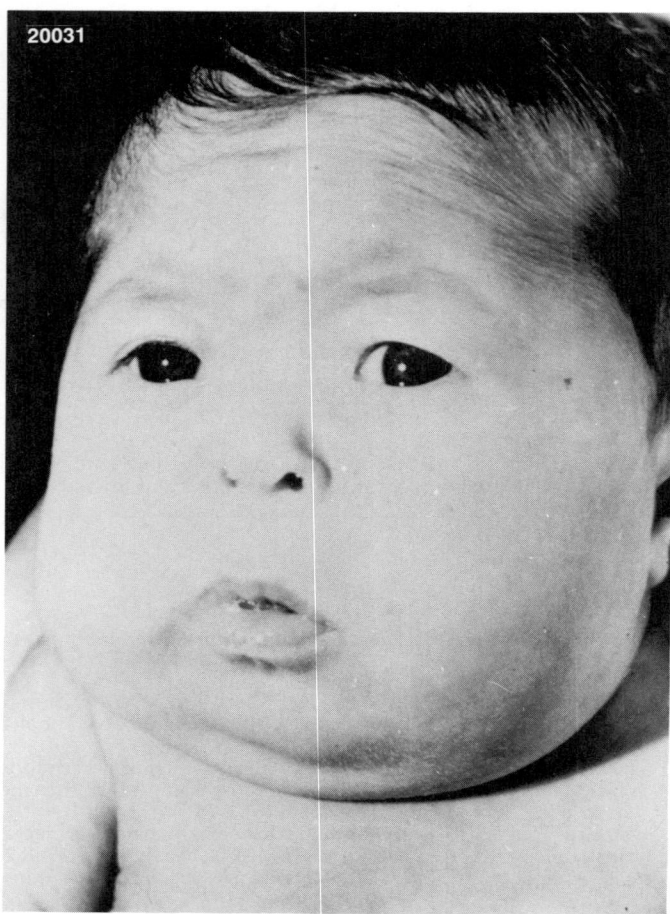

2455-20031: Note the microcephaly, blepharophimosis and small palpebral fissures as well as a flat nasal bridge, small nose, prominent philtrum and microstomia.

patients with 10q2 trisomy due to intrachromosomal duplications or insertional translocations were reported.

**Pathogenesis:** Unknown.

**POS No.:** 3083

**CDC No.:** 758.990

**Sex Ratio:** M1:F1

**Occurrence:** At least 35 cases have been documented.

**Risk of Recurrence for Patient's Sib:** Not increased if parental chromosomes are normal. Considerably increased (5–10%) if one of the parents is carrier of an autosomal balanced translocation involving 10q2.

**Risk of Recurrence for Patient's Child:** Reproduction in affected patients is unlikely.

**Age of Detectability:** At birth clinically or by prenatal diagnosis by CVS or amniocentesis.

**Gene Mapping and Linkage:** See *Gene Map*.

**Prevention:** None known. Genetic counseling indicated.

**Treatment:** Unknown.

**Prognosis:** Long-term prognosis is poor due to the presence of severe internal malformations. These are responsible for death within the first year of life in one third of the patients. In the surviving patients psychomotor retardation is profound.

**Detection of Carrier:** Cytogenetic and clinical examination.

**References:**

Fryns JP, et al.: New chromosomal syndromes: partial trisomy of the distal portion of the long arm of chromosome number 10 (10q24 10qter): a clinical entity. Acta Paediatr Belg 1979; 32:141–143.

de Grouchy J, Turleau C: Clinical atlas of human chromosomes, 2nd ed. New York: J. Wiley and Sons, 1984.

FR030                                                   **Jean-Pierre Fryns**

**Chromosome 11, deletion 11p13**
  *See CHROMOSOME 11, PARTIAL MONOSOMY 11p*
**Chromosome 11, distal 11q- syndrome**
  *See CHROMOSOME 11, MONOSOMY 11q*
**Chromosome 11, duplication of 11p**
  *See CHROMOSOME 11, TRISOMY 11p*
**Chromosome 11, monosomy 11p13**
  *See CHROMOSOME 11, PARTIAL MONOSOMY 11p*

---

## CHROMOSOME 11, MONOSOMY 11Q                    0162

**Includes:**
   Chromosome 11, distal 11q- syndrome
   Chromosome 11, partial monosomy of distal 11q
   Jacobsen syndrome

**Excludes:**
   Chromosome 11, partial monosomy for proximal 11q
   Chromosome 11, proximal 11q- syndrome

**Major Diagnostic Criteria:** Developmental delay, trigonocephaly, demonstration of cytogenetic defect.

**Clinical Findings:** Pre- and postnatal growth retardation is found in more than one-half of all affected individuals. Developmental delay, psychomotor retardation ranging from moderate to profound, and severe speech impairment are constant features. Trigonocephaly (prominent, keel-shaped forehead) is noticeable at birth. Craniofacial dysmorphism includes microencephaly; hypertelorism; a short, broad nose with a wide, depressed nasal bridge; epicanthal folds, a carp-shaped mouth; ptosis; low-set, malformed ears; and micrognathia. Iris coloboma and strabismus are occasionally noted. Congenital heart defects occur in more than 50% of cases and are often the cause of death for individuals with this partial chromosome deletion. Ventricular septal defect is the most frequently encountered cardiac abnormality, but truncus arteriosus and aortic arch defects are also common. Joint contractures, hypoplastic terminal phalanges, simian creases, hammer position of great toes, equinovarus foot deformity, and cutaneous syndactyly are other characteristics of this syndrome. Addition-

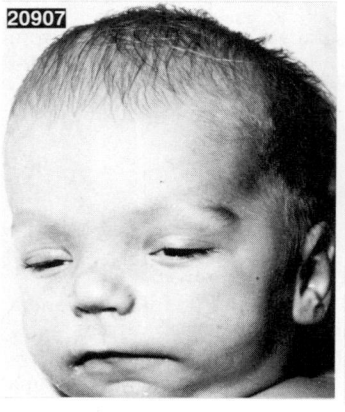 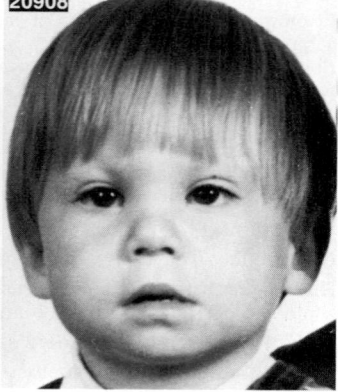

0162A-20907: Chromosome 11, monosomy 11q; note trigonocephaly, broad nasal bridge, short nose, epicanthal fold, thin lips and small chin. 20908: Older affected child shows similar findings.

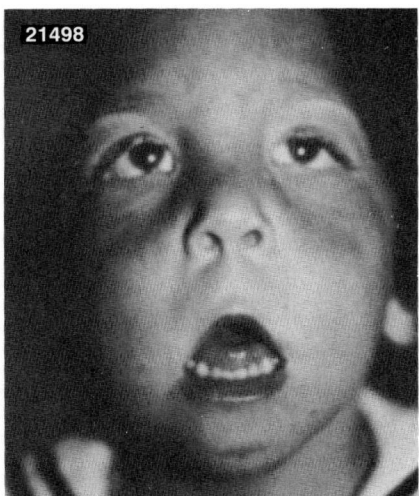

**0162B-21498:** Chromosome 11, partial monosomy 11q; note prominent forehead with scaphocephaly, broad nasal bridge, short nose and poorly defined philtrum with a thin upper lip and downturned angles of the mouth.

ally, thrombocytopenia and pancytopenia have been identified in a significant number of cases. Although most affected individuals are female, males with this syndrome are often noted to have pyloric stenosis and inguinal hernias. These latter two defects have not been identified in females.

**Complications:** Cardiac failure, susceptibility to infection.

**Associated Findings:** Hypospadias, renal duplication, hydronephrosis, adrenal hypoplasia, accessory spleens, polydactyly.

**Etiology:** Partial 11q chromosome deletion, most commonly deletion of 11q23→11qter. Interstitial deletion of 11q23→11q25 has been reported on four occasions in individuals with features typical of the syndrome. Absence of band 11q24.1 appears to be the critical deletion for determining this syndrome. Approximately 85% of cases represent de novo deletions. Five cases involving malsegregation from balanced parental translocations have been reported. Three cases of ring 11 chromosomes with phenotypes compatible with partial monosomy 11q have been reported.

**Pathogenesis:** Unknown.

**POS No.:** 3087

**CDC No.:** 758.990

**Sex Ratio:** M1:F5

**Occurrence:** Over 30 cases have been described in the literature.

**Risk of Recurrence for Patient's Sib:** Negligible if de novo in a patient. Significant if parent is a balanced translocation carrier.

**Risk of Recurrence for Patient's Child:** Theoretically 1:2 (50%). There are no reports of individuals with this chromosome deletion syndrome who have reproduced.

**Age of Detectability:** Prenatal diagnosis by chromosome analysis utilizing chorionic villus sampling or amniocentesis.

**Gene Mapping and Linkage:** See *Gene Map.*

**Prevention:** None known. Genetic counseling indicated.

**Treatment:** Surgical repair of congenital defects, especially heart and craniofacial structures; special education.

**Prognosis:** The majority of deaths in infancy are attributable to severe congenital heart defects. In patients without cardiac disease or in whom treatment is successful, prognosis for survival is fair. The oldest known affected individual is 16 years old. All patients have moderate-to-severe mental deficiency.

**Detection of Carrier:** By cytogenetic analysis.

**References:**
Schinzel A, et al.: Partial deletion of long arm of chromosome 11 [del(11)(q23)]: Jacobsen syndrome. J Med Genet 1977; 14:438–444.
McPherson E, Meissner L: 11q-syndrome: review and report of two cases. In: BD:OAS 1982; XVIII(3B):295–300. *
Monteleone PL, et al.: Brief clinical report: deletion of the long arm of chromosome 11, [del(11)(q23)]. Am J Med Genet 1982; 13:299–304.
Cousineau AJ, et al.: Brief clinical report: ring-11 chromosome: phenotype-karyotype correlation with deletions of 11q. Am J Med Genet 1983; 14:29–35.
O'Hare AE, et al.: Deletion of the long arm of chromosome 11 [46,XX,del(11)(q24.1→qter)]. Clin Genet 1984; 25:373–377.
Fryns JP, et al.: Distal 11q monosomy. The typical 11q monosomy syndrome is due to deletion of subband 11q24.1. Clin Genet 1986; 30:255–260. *
Helmuth RA, et al.: Holoprosencephaly, ear abnormalities, congenital heart defect, and microphallus in a patient with 11q-mosaicism. Am J Med Genet 1989; 32:178–181.

D0025                                          **Alan E. Donnenfeld**
ZA000                                          **Elaine H. Zackai**
EM000                                          **Beverly S. Emanuel**

## CHROMOSOME 11, PARTIAL MONOSOMY 11P     2245

**Includes:**
Aniridia, type II
Aniridia-ambiguous genitalia-mental retardation (AGR triad)
Aniridia-Wilms tumor association (AWTA)
Aniridia-Wilms tumor-gonadoblastoma
Chromosome 11, deletion 11p13
Chromosome 11, monosomy 11p13
Wilms tumor-aniridia
Wilms tumor-aniridia-gonadoblastoma-mental retardation (WAGR)

**Excludes:** Aniridia (0057)

**Major Diagnostic Criteria:** **Aniridia** with a chromosome rearrangement involving a deletion of band 11p13.

**Clinical Findings:** **Aniridia** is, except for one known instance, the only constant clinical feature. In practically all cases, it is accompanied by nystagmus, cataract and/or glaucoma. Nephroblastoma or **Cancer, Wilms tumor** is an important but inconstant feature, occurring in about one-third of the cases. Gonadoblastoma has been observed in two cases with gonadal dysgenesis.

Genital anomalies are practically constant in XY patients. In 75% of the cases, there is cryptorchidism with or without hypospadias, and in 25% of the cases there is more severe ambiguity such as pseudohermaphroditism. Streak gonads have been reported in one girl. Mental retardation is common, but highly variable; some

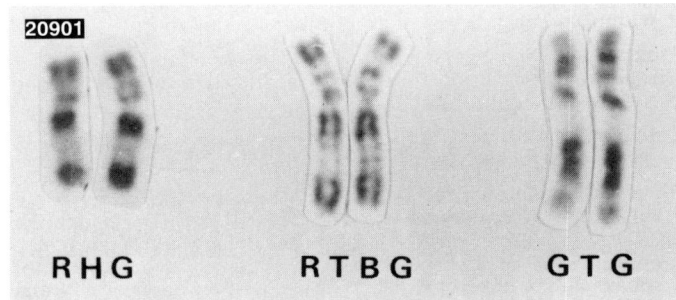

**RHG**          **RTBG**          **GTG**

**2245-20901:** Chromosome 11, monosomy 11p13; note 3 different banding techniques showing the monosomic chromosome on the left.

patients are described as normal or borderline, others as severely retarded. Growth retardation is frequent. There is no specific facial dysmorphism associated with del 11p13. The chromosome rearrangement involves monosomy of all or part of 11p13. The nature and the size of the deletion are variable. *De novo* intercalary deletions are the most frequent. Complex *de novo* rearrangements have also been observed. Balanced parental rearrangements are observed in 10% of the cases. They include insertions in the same or another chromosome. Breakpoints are variable. The smallest region of overlap is the distal part of 11p13. A noteworthy observation is the apparently high frequency, in *de novo* cases, of associated structural rearrangements involving chromosomes other than chromosome 11.

The gene for catalase has been assigned to 11p13. The enzyme shows a gene dosage effect. Reduced catalase activity has been observed in most all tested cases.

**Complications:** Ocular complications of aniridia, Wilms tumor, and more rarely, gonadoblastoma.

**Associated Findings:** Renal malformations, cardiomyopathy, **Heart, tetralogy of Fallot, Microcephaly**, bilateral fibular polydactyly.

**Etiology:** Monosomy of all or part of band 11p13. The deletion may extend on either side of 11p13. Conversely, submicroscopic deletions have been suggested in exceptional aniridia/Wilms tumor associations without visible deletion.

**Pathogenesis:** Moore et al (1986) has suggested that single chromosomal breaks are associated with isolated aniridia, while deletions of 11p13 result in the full WAGR syndrome.

**MIM No.:** *10621

**POS No.:** 3697

**CDC No.:** 758.990

**Sex Ratio:** M24:F13 (observed). Severe genital ambiguity may lead to erroneous sex identification.

**Occurrence:** At least 50 cases of **Aniridia** with del 11p have been documented in the literature.

**Risk of Recurrence for Patient's Sib:** Theoretically negligible in the case of de novo rearrangement. If a parent is a carrier of a balanced rearrangement (insertion), the risk is high (not omitting the risk of trisomy for 11p13).

**Risk of Recurrence for Patient's Child:** If reproduction is possible, the risk is theoretically 50%.

**Age of Detectability:** At birth, for aniridia and high resolution karyotyping, or by prenatal diagnosis if parental balanced rearrangement.

**Gene Mapping and Linkage:** AN2 (aniridia 2 without Wilms' tumor, GU abnormalities, and M.R.) has been mapped to 11p13.
GUD (genitourinary dysplasia component of WAGR) is 11p13.

**Prevention:** None known. Genetic counseling indicated.

**Treatment:** Ophthalmic care for complications of aniridia. Early detection of nephroblastoma. Systematic examination to detect gonadal dysgenesis, and eventually gonadectomy to prevent gonadoblastoma. Management of mental retardation.

**Prognosis:** Depends largely on the degree of mental retardation. Visual prognosis is poor. Prognosis for life span depends on the occurrence of nephroblastoma.

**Detection of Carrier:** High resolution chromosome analysis of first degree relatives.

**Special Considerations:** The identification of constitutional microdeletions in childhood tumors draws attention to specific chromosomal target bands. Molecular biology techniques may then lead to the identification of the genes involved, as for instance Wilms tumor gene(s). The association between aniridia and Wilms tumor was originally discovered by Robert W. Willer at the United States National Cancer Institute, and is an excellent illustration of the association between congenital malformation and malignancy.

**References:**
Riccardi VM, et al.: Chromosomal imbalance in the aniridia-Wilms tumor association: 11p interstitial deletion. Pediatrics 1978; 61:604–610. †
Junien C, et al.: Regional assignment of catalase (CAT) gene to band 11p13: association with the aniridia-Wilms tumor-gonadoblastoma (WAGR) complex. Ann Génét 1980; 23:165–168.
Nakagome Y, et al.: High-resolution studies in patients with aniridia-Wilms tumor association, Wilms tumor or related congenital abnormalities. Hum Genet 1984; 67:245–248.
Narahara K, et al.: Regional mapping of catalase and Wilms tumor-aniridia, genitourinary abnormalities, and mental retardation triad loci to the chromosome segment 11p1305→p1306. Hum Genet 1984; 66:181–185.
Turleau C, et al.: Del 11p/aniridia complex: report of three patients and review of 37 observations from the literature. Clin Genet 1984; 26:256–262. *
Turleau C, et al.: Del 11p13/nephroblastoma without aniridia. Hum Genet 1984; 67:455–456.
Moore JW, et al.: Familial isolated aniridia associated with a translocation involving chromosomes 11 and 22 [t(11;22)(p13;q12.2)]. Hum Genet 1986; 72:297–302.
Davis LM, et al.: Two anonymous DNA segments distinguish thw Wilms' tumor and aniridia loci. Science 1988; 241:840–842.

TU013                                    **Catherine Turleau**

**Chromosome 11, partial monosomy of distal 11q**
*See CHROMOSOME 11, MONOSOMY 11q*

## CHROMOSOME 11, PARTIAL TRISOMY 11Q          0161

**Includes:**
Chromosome 11, partial trisomy 11q13-qter
Chromosome 11, partial trisomy 11q21-qter
Chromosome 11, partial trisomy 11q23-qter

**Excludes:** Chromosome 22, supernumerary der 22, t(11;22) (2043)

**Major Diagnostic Criteria:** Developmental delay, growth retardation, characteristic facies, and cytogenetic demonstration of duplication of distal 11q.

**Clinical Findings:** Sixteen well-documented cases involving 14 families have been reported. Verification by chromosome banding was accomplished in all 16 instances: 11q23→qter (six cases), 11q22→qter (one case), 11q21→qter (three cases), 11q14→qter (one case) and 11q13→qter (five cases).

Growth retardation of prenatal onset, 11/14; moderate-to-severe psychomotor retardation, 16/16; microcephaly, 11/14. Craniofacial dysmorphia includes short nose, 12/13; long philtrum, 12/13; micrognathia, 12/13; low-set ears, 10/13; and high-arched palate, 9/13. Craniofacial abnormalities occurring in <50% of cases include epicanthal folds, hypertelorism, downslanted palpebral fissures, cleft palate, prominent anthelix, and hypoplasia or aplasia of the corpus callosum. An unusual clavicular defect, characterized by fusion between the medial and lateral portions resulting in a bipartite X-ray appearance, has been identified in four cases and is thought by some investigators to be specific for trisomy 11q. Other features of this syndrome are congenital heart disease, 9/12; cutis laxa, 4/12; urinary tract abnormalities, 4/9; dysplastic hip, 4/13; abnormal palmar creases, 8/13; short neck, 3/13; and micropenis, 5/7 males. Craniorachischisis (complete spina bifida and anencephaly) and meningomyelocele have each been reported once. Three newborns suspected of having 11q+ (all born to balanced translocation mothers) have also had neural tube defects. Unfortunately, karyotypes were not performed on these three children.

**Complications:** Cardiac failure, recurrent infections.

**Associated Findings:** Preauricular skin tags, umbilical hernia.

**Etiology:** Duplication of distal 11q (region 11q13, 14, 21, 22, or 23→qter). Derived from a balanced translocation parent (10 maternal, 4 paternal) in 14/16 cases or as a de novo chromosome rearrangement in 2 cases. In all reports, a deleted chromosome segment accompanies the 11q duplication.

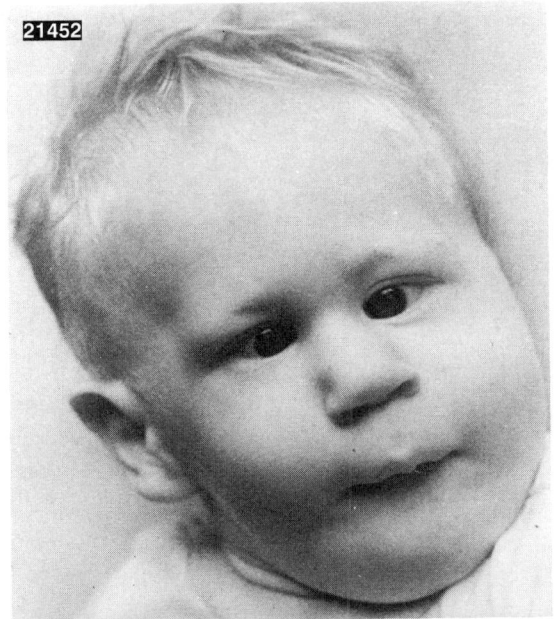

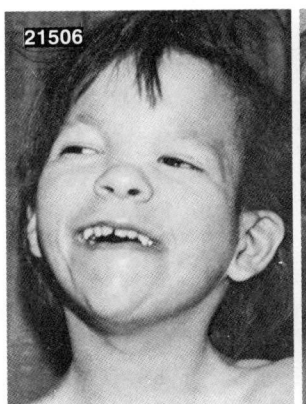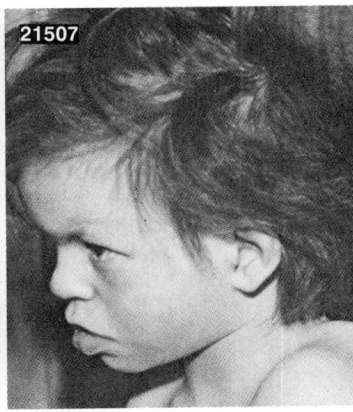

**0161B**-21506–07: Chromosome 11, trisomy 11q; note microcephaly, low-set, posteriorly rotated ears with prominent antihelix and microretrognathia.

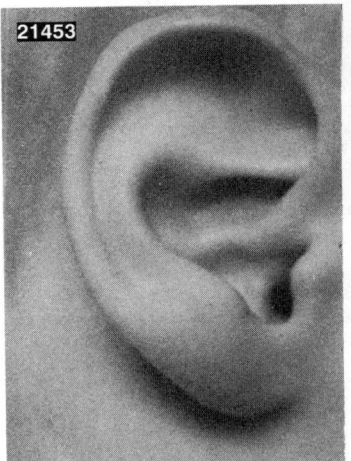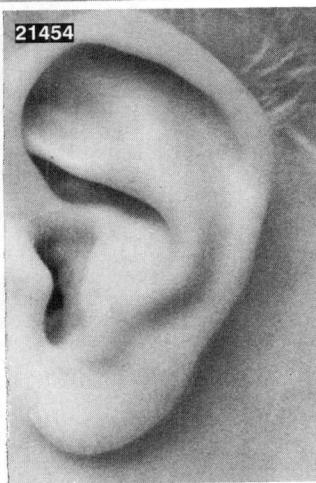

**0161A**-21452: Chromosome 11, partial trisomy 11q; note facial features including short nose and long philtrum, microretrognathia, and retracted lower lip. 21453–54: The auricles differ in shape with prominent anthelix.

Nine families are maternally derived: t(4;11) (q35;q211) mat; t(5;11) (p15;q21) mat; t(3;11) (p26;q21) mat; t(6;11) (q27;q231) mat; t(3;11) (p27;q231) mat (two cases); t(11;17) (q231;p13) mat; t(4;11) (q35;q231) mat; t(11;21) (q23;q22) mat; t(X;11) (q22;q13) mat.

Three families are paternally derived: t(11;13) (q13;q32–34) pat (two cases); t(10;11) (q26;q133) pat; t(11;18) (q142;p1131) pat.

Two families are *de novo* translocations: 46,XX,-2,+der2,t(2;11)(q37;q13); 46,XY,-9,+der9,t(9;11)(q34;q22).

**Pathogenesis:** Unknown.

**CDC No.:** 758.990

**Sex Ratio:** M7:F9 (observed)

**Occurrence:** Sixteen cases documented in 14 families.

**Risk of Recurrence for Patient's Sib:** Significant if parent is a balanced translocation carrier: negligible if de novo in the patient.

**Risk of Recurrence for Patient's Child:** Theoretically as high as 50%, although no reports of reproduction in these patients have been described.

**Age of Detectability:** Prenatal diagnosis by chorionic villus sampling or amniocentesis if a parent has a balanced translocation.

**Gene Mapping and Linkage:** See *Gene Map*.

**Prevention:** None known. Genetic counseling indicated.

**Treatment:** Therapy is symptomatic for congenital defects. Special education is indicated.

**Prognosis:** Nine of 16 were living at the time of their report; six of these were less than 1 year old. Six died within the first year of life. The oldest reported patient died at age 16 years (trisomic for 11q21→qter). Moderate-to-severe mental retardation was present in all.

**Detection of Carrier:** By chromosome analysis.

**Special Considerations:** The severity of manifestations and the prognosis are related to the extent of the duplicated segment of 11q and to the extent of the corresponding deleted derivative chromosome segment. The special case of supernumerary der(22) resulting from a 3:1 meiotic nondisjunction of a balanced 11;22 translocation parent (in most cases) has a separate, distinct phenotype.

**References:**
Barnabei VM, et al.: A possible exception to the critical region hypothesis. Am J Hum Genet 1981; 33:61–66.
Pihko H, et al.: Partial 11q trisomy syndrome. Hum Genet 1981; 58:129–134. *
Bader PI, et al.: Brief clinical report: neural tube defects in dup(11q). Am J Med Genet 1984; 19:5–8.
De France HF, et al.: Partial trisomy 11q due to paternal t(11q;18p); further delineation of the clinical picture. Clin Genet 1984; 25:295–299. †
Greig F, et al.: Duplication 11(q22→qter) in an infant. Ann Genet (Paris) 1985; 28:185–188.

D0025
ZA000
EM000

Alan E. Donnenfeld
Elaine H. Zackai
Beverly S. Emanuel

**Chromosome 11, partial trisomy 11q13-qter**
*See CHROMOSOME 11, PARTIAL TRISOMY 11q*
**Chromosome 11, partial trisomy 11q21-qter**
*See CHROMOSOME 11, PARTIAL TRISOMY 11q*
**Chromosome 11, partial trisomy 11q23-qter**
*See CHROMOSOME 11, PARTIAL TRISOMY 11q*

# CHROMOSOME 11, TRISOMY 11P 2459

**Includes:**
  Beckwith-Wiedemann syndrome with 11p15 duplication
  Chromosome 11, duplication of 11p
**Excludes:**
  **Beckwith-Wiedemann syndrome** (0104)
  Chromosome 11, other anomalies

**Major Diagnostic Criteria:** Mental and growth retardation, prominent frontal bossing, hypertelorism, strabismus, low-set ears, broad flat nasal bridge, cleft lip and palate, macroglossia, umbilical or inguinal **Hernia**, cryptorchidism, hypospadias, broad fingers and toes, and renal and cardiac abnormalities.

**Clinical Findings:** Mental and growth retardation, prominent frontal bossing, hypertelorism, strabismus, low-set ears, broad flat nasal bridge, cleft lip and palate, macroglossia, umbilical or inguinal hernia, cryptorchidism, hypospadias, broad fingers and toes, and renal and cardiac abnormalities.

**Complications:** Unknown.

**Associated Findings:** Macular dysfunction, bilateral absent thumbs and first metacarpals, duodenal ulcers, widely spaced nipples, seizures, ear lobe grooves, **Nevus flammeus**, visceromegaly, spina bifida, hypoglycemia, macrosomia, and cystic hygroma. Six patients with partial duplication of 11p15 were reported as cases of **Beckwith-Wiedemann syndrome**.

**Etiology:** Up to now, no more than 30 patients with trisomy 11p and duplications of different segments of the short arm were described. Twelve of these were the unbalanced product of a parental autosomal balanced translocation involving 11p and another autosome. Four were due to a parental pericentric inversion of chromosome 11, and four were *de novo*.
  The characteristic clinical features of the syndrome correspond to complete trisomy 11p.

**Pathogenesis:** Unknown.

**CDC No.:** 758.990

**Sex Ratio:** M1:F1

**Occurrence:** About 30 cases have been documented.

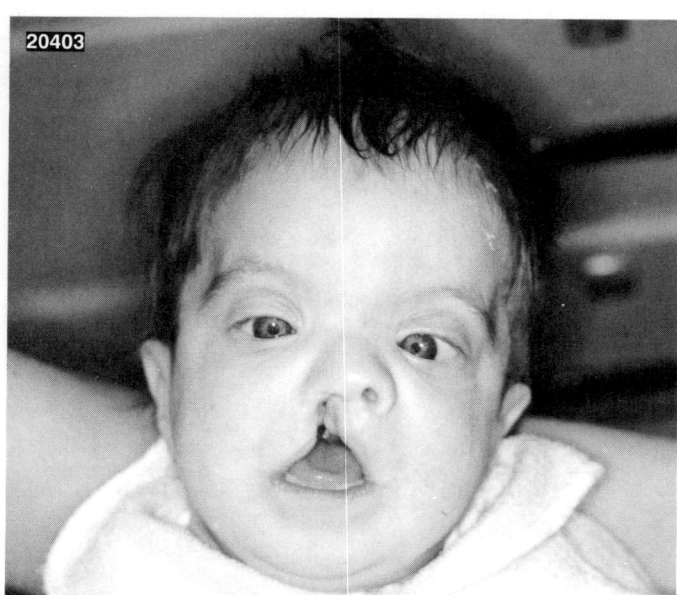

**2459A-20403:** 3-month-old infant with chromosome 11, trisomy 11p; note high forehead, wide nasal bridge, hypertelorism, prominent epicanthi, rounded cheeks and cleft lip.

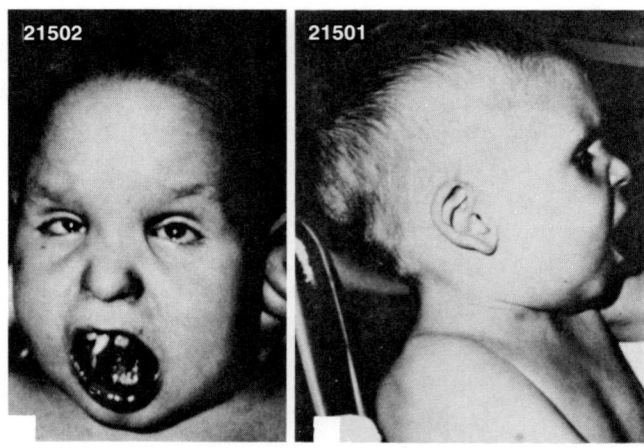

**2459B-21501–02:** Chromosome 11, trisomy 11p; note prominent forehead, downslanting palpebral fissures, epicanthal folds and the wide and flat nasal bridge.

**Risk of Recurrence for Patient's Sib:** Not increased if parental chromosomes are normal. Considerably increased (possibly 5–10%) if reciprocal translocation or pericentric inversion involving chromosome 11 is found in one of the parents.

**Risk of Recurrence for Patient's Child:** Severe mental retardation in surviving patients makes reproduction unlikely.

**Age of Detectability:** At birth, or prenatal by CVS or amniocenthesis.

**Gene Mapping and Linkage:** Further arguments in favor of an association between 11p and **Beckwith-Wiedemann syndrome** come from gene mapping data. Band 11p15 harbours the genes coding for the globins, insulin and the oncogene HRAS1.

**Prevention:** None known. Genetic counseling indicated.

**Treatment:** Symptomatic.

**Prognosis:** Long-term prognosis is poor. At least three patients were stillborn, and four others were born alive but died in the first few hours or weeks of life.

**Detection of Carrier:** Cytogenetic and clinical examination.

**References:**
Falk RE, et al: Partial trisomy of chromosome 11: a case report. Am J Ment Defic 1977; 77:383–388. *
Waziri M, et al: Abnormality of chromosome 11 in patients with features of Beckwith-Wiedemann Syndrome. J Ped 1983; 102:873–876.
Turleau C, et al: Trisomy 11p15 and Beckwith-Wiedemann Syndrome: a report of two cases. Hum Genet 1984; 67:219–221. *
Fryns JP, et al: Cystic Hygroma and Hydrops Fetalis in dup(11p) Syndrome. Am J Med Genet 1985; 22:287–289.
Journel H, et al: Trisomy 11p15 and Beckwith-Wiedemann syndrome. Ann Genet 1985; 28:97–101. *

FR030
CH043

**Jean-Pierre Fryns**
**Krysztyna Chrzanowska**

**Chromosome 12, deletion of 12p**
  *See CHROMOSOME 12, MONOSOMY 12p*
**Chromosome 12, duplication 12p**
  *See CHROMOSOME 12, PARTIAL TRISOMY 12p*
**Chromosome 12, duplication of 12q12**
  *See CHROMOSOME 12, TRISOMY 12q2*
**Chromosome 12, isochromosome 12p mosaicism**
  *See PALLISTER-KILLIAN MOSAIC SYNDROME*

## CHROMOSOME 12, MONOSOMY 12P                2461

**Includes:**  Chromosome 12, deletion of 12p

**Excludes:**  Chromosome 12, other anomalies

**Major Diagnostic Criteria:**  Moderate to severe developmental delay and constant craniofacial abnormalities. The diagnosis is confirmed by cytogenetic analysis.

**Clinical Findings:**  **Microcephaly**, small bitemporal diameter, variable position of the palpebral fissures, long pointed nose, receding chin and micrognathia, large and very low-set ears. The hands are narrow with clinodactyly of the fifth fingers; **Camptodactyly** and brachymetacarpy are rarely observed. In male patients, cryptorchidism and micropenis are frequent findings.

**Complications:**  Unknown.

**Associated Findings:**  Internal malformations are rare: cardiac defects, ureter duplex, and genua valga.

**Etiology:**  In most patients, the 12p deletion occured *de novo*. In a small number, the 12p deletion was the unbalanced product of a parental translocation involving 12p and another chromosome.

**Pathogenesis:**  Unknown.

**CDC No.:**  758.990

**Sex Ratio:**  M1:F1

**Occurrence:**  Less than 20 cases with pure 12p monosomy have been reported.

**Risk of Recurrence for Patient's Sib:**  Not increased if parental chromosomes are normal. Increased (possibly 5–10%) if autosomal translocation involving 12p and another chromosome is found in one of the parents.

**Risk of Recurrence for Patient's Child:**  Mental retardation in surviving patients makes reproduction unlikely.

**Age of Detectability:**  At birth or by prenatal diagnosis by CVS or amniocenthesis.

**Gene Mapping and Linkage:**  See *Gene Map.*

**Prevention:**  None known. Genetic counseling indicated.

**Treatment:**  Symptomatic.

**Prognosis:**  Long-term prognosis seems to be good. Most patients seem to survive the early childhood as severe internal malformations are usually absent. A deterioration of IQ with age is possible.

**Detection of Carrier:**  Cytogenetic and clinical examination.

**References:**
Boilly-Dartigalongue B, et al: Etude d'un nouveau cas de monosomie partielle du chromosome 12, del(12) (p11.01→p12.109) confirmant la localisation du gène de la lacticodéshydrogénase. Ann Génét 1985; 28:55–57.
Romain DR, et al: Partial monosomy 12p13.1→13.3. J Med Genet 1987; 24:434–436. *

FR030                                   **Jean-Pierre Fryns**

---

## CHROMOSOME 12, PARTIAL TRISOMY 12P        2130

**Includes:**
    Chromosome 12, duplication 12p
    Chromosome 12, trisomy 12p

**Excludes:**
    **Chromosome 12, partial trisomy 12p** (2130)
    **Chromosome 12, trisomy 12q2** (2462)

**Major Diagnostic Criteria:**  Severe developmental retardation, hypotonia and, postnatal growth retardation associated with distinct craniofacial dysmorphism.

**Clinical Findings:**  Midfacial hypoplasia is evident with shallow orbits, epicanthus, flat upturned nose with wide bridge, upward slanting of the palpebral fissures, long philtrum. The cheeks are puffy, the lower lip thick and everted, and the tongue large. The

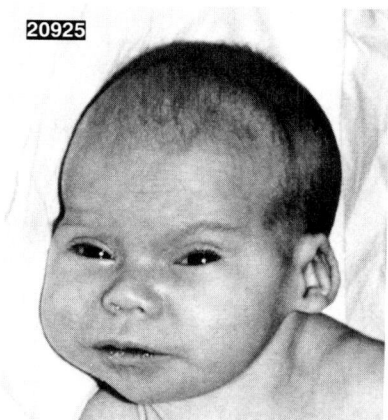

2130-20925:  Chromosome 12, partial duplication of 12p; note broad face with mid-facial hypoplasia, flat, upturned nose, long philtrum and thick, everted lower lip.

---

ears are small but in normal position. The hands are broad and short with clinodactyly of the fifth fingers.

**Complications:**  Unknown.

**Associated Findings:**  Skull deformations (turri-brachycephaly), microphthalmia, micrognathia with high-arched palate, cardiac defects (hypoplastic left heart in three patients), renal malformations, anal atresia, and diastasis recti.

**Etiology:**  In the majority of the patients the 12p duplication was the unbalanced product of a parental translocation involving 12p and another autosome. The breakpoints usually occur at 12p11, 12q11, and 12q12. Centric fission leading to isochromosome 12p formation was reported in one patient.

**Pathogenesis:**  Unknown.

**POS No.:**  3088

**CDC No.:**  758.990

**Sex Ratio:**  M1:F1

**Occurrence:**  About 25 patients have been documented.

**Risk of Recurrence for Patient's Sib:**  Negligible if parental chromosomes are normal. Considerably increased (5–10%) if reciprocal translocation involving chromosome 12p and another chromosome is found in one of the parents.

**Risk of Recurrence for Patient's Child:**  Severe mental retardation in surviving patients makes reproduction unlikely.

**Age of Detectability:**  At birth. Prenatal diagnosis, by amniocenthesis or CVS, is possible.

**Gene Mapping and Linkage:**  See *Gene Map.*

**Prevention:**  None known. Genetic counseling indicated.

**Treatment:**  Governed by extent of internal malformations, which have been severe in a large number of patients.

**Prognosis:**  Unknown.

**Detection of Carrier:**  Cytogenetic examination of the parents to exclude autosomal translocations involving 12p.

**References:**
Ray M, et al: A case of de novo trisomy 12p syndrome. Ann Génét 1985; 28:235–238. *
Rivera H, et al: Centric fission, centromere-telomere fusion and isochromosome formation: a possible origin of a de novo 12p trisomy. Clin Genet 1987; 31:393–398.

FR030                                   **Jean-Pierre Fryns**
KL007                                   **Alice Kleczkowska**

**Chromosome 12, trisomy 12p**
*See CHROMOSOME 12, PARTIAL TRISOMY 12p*

## CHROMOSOME 12, TRISOMY 12Q2     2462

**Includes:** Chromosome 12, duplication of 12q12

**Excludes:** Chromosome 12, other anomalies

**Major Diagnostic Criteria:** Severe mental retardation associated with a similar dysmorphic syndrome of which the craniofacial features are the most typical. Cytogenetic analysis confirms the diagnosis.

**Clinical Findings:** Facial asymmetry, small palpebral fissure, heavy eyebrows, narrow nasal bridge, short upper lip, macrostomia, downturned angles of the mouth, scrotal tongue and large everted ears. Skeletal and limb abnormalities range from proximal implanted thumbs and brachymetatarsy and brachymetacarpy to hip dislocations.

**Complications:** Unknown.

**Associated Findings:** Except for non-life threatening cardiac anomalies, internal malformations were rarely observed.

**Etiology:** In all reported and surviving patients a small distal trisomy 12q i.e. with the breakpoint in 12q24 to qter, is found. In the majority of the patients the 12q12 trisomy is the unbalanced product of a parental translocation involving 12q12 and another autosome. In a minority of patients the 12q12 trisomy originated *de novo*.

**Pathogenesis:** Unknown.

**POS No.:** 3124

**CDC No.:** 758.990

**Sex Ratio:** M1:F1

**Occurrence:** Less than 20 cases have been reported.

**Risk of Recurrence for Patient's Sib:** Not increased if parental chromosomes are normal. Increased risk (2–5%) if autosomal reciprocal translocation involving 12q2 and another autosome is present in one of the parents. The scarcity of duplication 12q in liveborn children is apparently due to a high level of alternate segregation with a low level of interstitial chiasmata.

**Risk of Recurrence for Patient's Child:** Mental retardation in surviving patients makes reproduction unlikely.

**Age of Detectability:** In early childhood. Prenatal diagnosis using CVS or amniocentesis is possible.

**Gene Mapping and Linkage:** See *Gene Map.*

**Prevention:** None known. Genetic counseling indicated.

**Treatment:** Symptomatic.

**Prognosis:** Long term survival is good. In two cases, an early death was caused by infection.

**Detection of Carrier:** Cytogenetic and clinical examination.

**References:**
de Muêlenaere A, et al: Partial distal 12q trisomy. Ann Génét 1980; 23:251–253.
McCorquodale MM, et al: Duplication (12q) syndrome in female cousins, resulting from maternal (11;12) (q15.5;q24.2) translocations. Am J Genet 1986; 24:613–622.

FR030            **Jean-Pierre Fryns**

**Chromosome 13, 13r syndrome**
*See CHROMOSOME 13, MONOSOMY 13q*
**Chromosome 13, deletions of 13ql, 2 and 3**
*See CHROMOSOME 13, TRISOMY DISTAL 13q*
**Chromosome 13, monosomy 13 (q31-qter)**
*See CHROMOSOME 13, MONOSOMY 13q3*
**Chromosome 13, monosomy 13 (q32-qter)**
*See CHROMOSOME 13, MONOSOMY 13q3*
**Chromosome 13, monosomy 13 (q33)**
*See CHROMOSOME 13, MONOSOMY 13q3*
**Chromosome 13, monosomy 13 (q33-qter)**
*See CHROMOSOME 13, MONOSOMY 13q3*
**Chromosome 13, monosomy 13 (q34-qter)**
*See CHROMOSOME 13, MONOSOMY 13q3*

## CHROMOSOME 13, MONOSOMY 13Q     0167

**Includes:** Chromosome 13, 13r syndrome

**Excludes:** Chromosome 13, monosomy 13q3 (2465)

**Major Diagnostic Criteria:** Low birthweight; microcephaly; wide prominent nasal bridge; protruding upper maxilla; eye abnormalities such as microphthalmia, colobomata, retinoblastoma; and large malformed ears. Other clinical findings are listed below. Karyotypic analysis with banded chromosomes is essential to confirm diagnosis and to classify subdivisions of the syndrome accurately.

**Clinical Findings:** Based on an analysis of 72 cases (61% ring chromosome 13; 28% terminal or interstitial deletions), the following frequencies of clinical features: Severe psychomotor retardation 64/68 (94%); microcephaly 55/59 (93%); microphthalmia and/or colobomata 16/62 (25%); retinoblastoma 11/62 (18%); prominent nasal bridge 32/48 (66%); hypertelorism 52/55 (94%); large ears 39/49 (79%); lowset ears 25/47 (53%); hypoplastic or absent thumb 19/71 (27%); congenital heart disease 23/42 (55%); anal atresia 11/66 (16%); and hypospadias (males) 11/29 (38%).

The mean birth weight in these 72 cases was 2220 grams; the mean gestational age was 39 weeks. Necropsy was performed in only 12 cases confirming a ventricular septal defect in 4, atrial septal defect in 4, hypoplastic kidneys in 7, and aplasia of the gallbladder in 4.

About half of all retinoblastoma have interstitial deletion which includes band q14. The retinoblastoma associated with 13q- is usually bilateral and often associated with short stature, microcephaly, moderate to severe mental retardation and minor dysmorphic features, including those reported above. Submicroscopic deletions of 13q14 associated with decreased levels of esterase D activity have been described in some retinblastoma patients. Deletion of bands q14 or 21→qter was found to be associated with significant growth retardation, perinatal mortality and serious internal anomalies including severe forms of holo-

**2462-21047:** Chromosome 12, trisomy 12q2; note rectangular-shaped face, short philtrum and downcurved lips.

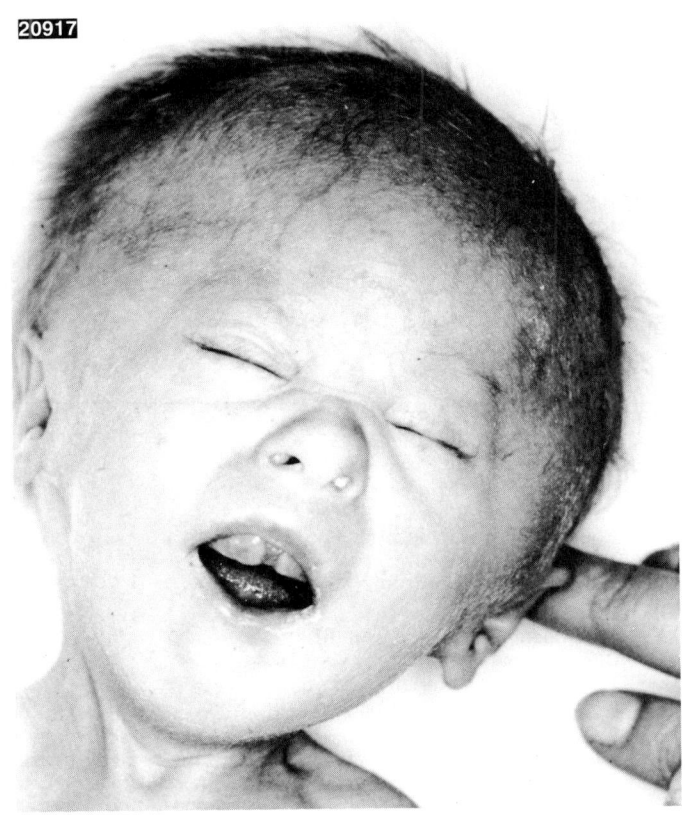

**0167-20917:** Chromosome 13, monosomy 13q; note wide nasal bridge, prominent upper maxilla, and prominent, exposed upper incisors.

**POS No.:** 3125

**CDC No.:** 758.330

**Sex Ratio:** M1:F1.15

**Occurrence:** The birth incidence of ring chromosome 13 has been estimated at 1.72:100,000 in an Anglo-Saxon population.

**Risk of Recurrence for Patient's Sib:** The risk is very small if parental chromosomes are normal with no evidence of submicroscopic deletion. Otherwise, the risk varies depending on the type of parental chromosome abnormality found.

**Risk of Recurrence for Patient's Child:** Individuals with submicroscopic or interstitial deletions of 13q14 have a 1:2 (50%) risk of having a similarly affected child. No individual affected with other deletions is know to have reproduced.

**Age of Detectability:** In utero by karyotyping of cells obtained by amniocentesis or chorionic biopsy; or at birth.

**Gene Mapping and Linkage:** See *Gene Map.*

**Prevention:** None known. Genetic counseling indicated.

**Treatment:** As indicated by complications and clinical features.

**Prognosis:** Overall, 19% of patients die prior to 6 months of age. Fifty percent of patients with deletion of segment q22→qter die by 21 months of age. Survival into adulthood has been described in individuals with terminal and interstitial deletions and with ring chromosomes. The majority of affected individuals are severely mentally retarded, although mild to moderate mental retardation has been observed in some cases, particularly those with smaller deletions.

**Detection of Carrier:** By karyotype of the parents and, if indicated, other family members to allow detection of familial translocations, of inversions, and insertions which may give rise to the 13q- syndrome.

**References:**
Niebuhr E: Partial trisomies and deletions of chromosome 13. In: Yunis JJ, ed: New chromosomal syndromes. New York: Academic Press, 1977:273–299.

Nichols WW, et al.: Interstitial deletion of chromosome 13 and associated anomalies. Hum Genet 1979; 52:169–173.

Sparkes RS, et al.: Assignment of genes for human esterase D and retinoblastoma to chromosome band 13q14. Science 1980; 208:1042–1044.

Martin NJ, et al.: The ring chromosome 13 syndrome. Hum Genet 1982; 61:18–23.

deGrouchy J, et al.: Regional mapping of clotting factors VII and X to 13q34. Expression of factor VII through chromosome 8. Hum Genet 1984; 66:230–233.

Rivera H, et al.: Monosomy 13q32.3→qter: report of two cases. J Med Genet 1985; 22:142–145.

Cowell JK, et al.: The need to screen all retionblastoma patients for esterase D activity: detection of submicroscopic chromosome deletions. Arch Dis Child 1987; 62:8–11.

RU012                                                      **Laura J. Russell**

prosencephaly, renal hypoplasia or agenesis and cleft lip/palate. The majority of conceptuses with deletion of these bands are spontaneously aborted.

Approximately half the individuals with deletion of q22 or 31→qter have colobomata of the iris or choroid, and microphthalmia; other ocular findings include corneal opacities and cataract. Brain malformations, including arrhinencephaly, agenesis of the corpus callosum, meningocele and hydrocephalus are present in half of the patients. Vertebral and rib anomalies, scoliosis, clubfoot deformity and synostosis between metacarpals 4 and 5 have been reported in deletions of these segments and in those of the more distal q32 or q33 qter segments.

The phenotype associated with ring chromosome 13 is a highly variable one in which growth and mental deficiency are associated with clinical features which may be nonspecific and mild, or similar to those described for individuals with deletion q22→qter. The phenotype associated with interstitial deletions is also variable and depends on the size and location of the deleted segments.

**Complications:** Failure to thrive; increased susceptibility to infections; deletion of segment q14 or 21→qter in a conceptus usually results in spontaneous abortion or perinatal death.

**Associated Findings:** None known.

**Etiology:** The 13q-Syndrome results from partial monosomy for a segment of the long arm of one chromosome 13. In the majority of cases, parental chromosomes are normal. However, some cases have resulted from familial translocations, inversions, and insertions or from de novo translocations.

**Pathogenesis:** Unknown.

## CHROMOSOME 13, MONOSOMY 13Q3                    2465

**Includes:**

Chromosome 13, monosomy 13 (q31-qter)
Chromosome 13, monosomy 13 (q32-qter)
Chromosome 13, monosomy 13 (q33)
Chromosome 13, monosomy 13 (q33-qter)
Chromosome 13, monosomy 13 (q34-qter)
Chromosome 13, ring 13 (pter-q31)

**Excludes:**

**Chromosome 13, monosomy 13q** (0167)
Chromosome 13, monosomy 13 (q22-qter)

**Major Diagnostic Criteria:** **Microcephaly,** mental retardation, abnormalities of the nasal bridge giving a "Greek profile," and radial axis abnormalities. Karyotype analysis confirms the diagnosis.

**Clinical Findings:** The most common features of this syndrome and their frequencies are noted below. Only cases with accurate banding were included. Column A refers to cases involving deletion of 13q3. Column B refers to cases of ring 13.

| General: | A | B |
|---|---|---|
| low birth rate (<2500g) | 5/12 | 11/14 |
| growth failure | 6/9 | 11/11 |
| psychomotor retardation | 12/12 | 15/15 |
| Craniofacial: | | |
| microcephaly | 8/12 | 15/15 |
| brachycephaly | 6/8 | - |
| trigonocephaly | 1/5 | 3/14 |
| facial asymmetry | 3/9 | 1/11 |
| hypertelorism | 5/12 | 8/11 |
| upslanting palpebral fissures | 9/12 | 4/10 |
| coloboma | 2/11 | 3/10 |
| broad, abnormal or prominent nasal bridge | 8/10 | 15/15 |
| large or abnormally formed ears | 9/11 | 11/14 |
| short philtrum, protruding maxilla/upper incisors | 5/9 | 5/9 |
| Congenital heart disease | 2/10 | 3/10 |
| Renal abnormalities (agenesis of kidney, hypoplastic kidney) | - | 3/7 |
| Genital abnormalities (cryptorchidism, hypospadius) | 4/9 | 6/9 |
| Anal atresia | - | 1/15 |

**Complications:** Recurrent respiratory infections and otitis media in some patients.

**Associated Findings:** One patient with 13q3 deletion was reported to have no ventricles visible on cranial CT scan; two cases with **Corpus callosum agenesis.**

**Etiology:** Monosomy 13q3 may arise as a result of a *de novo* deletion or may occur as a result of abnormal segregation of a parental translocation. Of the cases in which parental karyotypes are reported, it appears that approximately 60% result from parental translocations. Rings are generally de novo events, however cases have been described in association with translocations.

**Pathogenesis:** Unknown.

**POS No.:** 3091

**CDC No.:** 758.990

**Sex Ratio:** M1:F1

**Occurrence:** While there have been many cases of 13q- reported, and about twice as many cases of ring 13, for the purposes of this article, only recently reported cases with accurate banding techniques are included.

**Risk of Recurrence for Patient's Sib:** Not increased if no parental translocation is present.

**Risk of Recurrence for Patient's Child:** No affected individuals are known to have reproduced.

**Age of Detectability:** Karyotype may be done prenatally by karyotype analysis of fetal cells and/or blood.

**Gene Mapping and Linkage:** See *Gene Map.*

**Prevention:** None known. Genetic counseling indicated. Artificial insemination is possible if the father is a translocation carrier.

**Treatment:** Symptomatic therapy, special education.

**Prognosis:** All show psychomotor retardation, usually moderate to severe. Exact life span is unknown. The oldest patient included in this survey is eight years old.

**Detection of Carrier:** By chromosomal analysis and clinical evaluation.

**Special Considerations:** In the case of ring chromosomes, mitotic instability of the ring may result in mosaic karyotypes and phenotypic modification.

**References:**
Allderdice P, et al: The 13q- deletion syndrome. Am J Hum Genet 1969; 21:499–512.
Niebuhr E: Partial trisomies and deletions of chromosome 13. In: Yunis J ed.: New chromosomal syndromes. New York: Academic Press, 1977:273–299.
Telfer M, et al: Long arm deletion of chromosome 13 with exclusion of esterase D from 13q→13qter. Clin Genet 1980; 17:428–432.
Martin N, et al: The ring chromosome 13 syndrome. Hum Genet 1982; 61:18–23.

HA079
JA014

**Pamela A. Hawks**
**Ethylin Wang Jabs**

**Chromosome 13, ring 13 (pter-q31)**
*See CHROMOSOME 13, MONOSOMY 13q3*

## CHROMOSOME 13, TRISOMY 13     0168

**Includes:**
D Trisomy syndrome
Patau syndrome
Robertsonian translocation
Trisomy D1 syndrome
Trisomy 13–15 syndrome

**Excludes:**
**Chromosome 18, trisomy 18** (0160)
**Chromosome 4, monosomy 4p** (0164)
Partial trisomy 13 syndromes

**Major Diagnostic Criteria:** The 13 trisomy patient may show a triad of microphthalmia, cleft lip and palate, and polydactyly in addition to a number of other abnormalities. One or all of the triad may be absent; however, the syndrome can still be suspected when the patient shows a constellation of other findings mentioned below. Chromosomal study is required.

**Clinical Findings:** Observed clinical findings include: developmental retardation and undescended testes (both 100%); ocular hypertelorism; low-set ears; malformed ears; and distal palmar axial triradius (all > 80%); jitteriness and apneic spells; microcephaly; microphthalmia; cleft lip or palate; polydactyly; congenital heart disease; epicanthal folds; presumptive deafness; micrognathia; extra skin nape of neck; short neck; capillary hemangioma; long narrow hyperconvex nails; retroflexible thumbs; flexion deformity of fingers; single transverse palmar crease; tibial loop hallucal pattern; and prominent calcaneus (all 50–80%).

Additional findings include hypotonia (40–50%); hypertonia (20–30%); seizures (20–30%); and scalp defects (10–50%); absent eyebrows (10–50%); shallow supraorbital ridges; iris colobomata; inguinal or umbilical hernia; single umbilical artery; pilonidal pit;

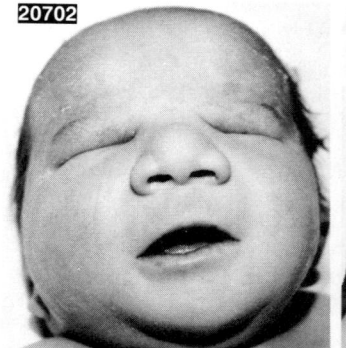
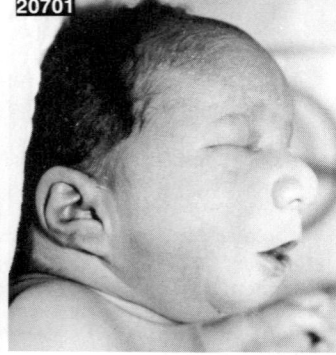

**0168-20701–02:** Chromosome 13, trisomy 13; note microphthalmia, sloping forehead, bulbous nose and low-set ears.

hypoplastic nails; three or more simple arches on digits; fibular S arch hallucal pattern; and short dorsiflexed big toe (all 10–50%).

Less frequent findings (undetermined or under 20%) include omphalocele; limited hip abduction; equinovarus deformity of feet; calcaneovalgus deformity of feet; forehead receding; palpebral fissures horizontal; nose flat and broad; cyclopia; cataracts; retinal dysplasia; retinal detachment; clitoral hypertrophy; scrotal anomalies; muscles hypoplastic or absent; radial loops, especially on thumbs; pear-shaped face; sloping forehead; prominent nasal bridge; and hypoplastic nipples.

Radiologic observations, of undetermined frequency, include cervical rib; absent 12th rib; anomalies of rib number or morphology; and low acetabular angles.

Laboratory findings include elevation of fetal hemoglobin during infancy (100%), as well as undetermined frequencies of persistence of gower-2 embryonic hemoglobin to birth; elevation of hemoglobin Portland$_1$, at birth; delayed rise of hemoglobin A$_2$ to adult levels; increased number of nuclear projections in polymorphonuclear leukocytes; delayed maturation of the I blood group system; and delayed maturation of erythrocyte carbonic anhydrase B.

Autopsy findings include congenital heart defects (> 80%); ventricular septal defect (50–60%); patent ductus arteriosus (50–60%); atrial septal defect (40–50%); dextroposition (20–50%); and coarctation of the aorta (10–20%).

Renal anomalies occur in more than 80% of the cases, and include multiple small renal cortical cysts (40–50%); multiple renal arteries (30–80%); duplication of renal pelvis and/or ureter (10–20%); and hydronephrosis and hydroureter (10–20%).

Brain abnormalities occur in 70–80% of cases and include agenesis of olfactory bulbs (60–70%); and undetermined frequencies of agenesis of corpus callosum; failure of hemispheral cleavage; cerebellar hypoplasia; and hydrocephaly.

Reproductive system abnormalities occur in (50–100%) of cases and include bicornuate uterus (50–80%); bifid vagina, hypoplastic ovaries, and abnormal fallopian tubes of undetermined frequency.

Gastrointestinal system abnormalities occur in 50–80% of cases and include malrotation of the intestine (20–30%); Meckel diverticulum (10–20%); and undetermined frequencies of unattached mesentery; elongated gallbladder; hypoplastic bile ducts; and accessory spleens.

Ear and other abnormalities include, in undetermined frequency, degeneration of cochlea and saccule; organ of Corti absent or replaced by fibrous tissue; tectorial membrane, Peissner membrane and stria vascularis degenerated.

Eye abnormalities include, in undetermined frequency, microphthalmia; colobomata of ciliaxy body, iris and/or optic nerve; persistent primary uitreous; intraocular cartilage; dysplastic retina; cataracts; corneal opacities; and optic nerve hypoplasia.

Muscle abnormalities have been observed in 100% of cases and include absent palmaris longus (100%); absent peroneus tertius (100%); absent palmaris brevis (90%); absent plantaris; absence or variation extensor indicis; and presence of pectorodorsalis muscle (each 80%).

Pathological studies are very important in the recognition of 13 trisomy. Based on autopsy data, 13 trisomy syndrome can be diagnosed with certainty, even in the absence of karyotyping. In addition to the different malformations, histological evidence of organ dysplasia in the central nervous system, eyes, pancreas, kidneys and ovaries are characteristic. Mild cystic renal dysplasia is a constant feature, and foci of persistent nodular renal blastema are found in more than half of the patients. The pancreatic dysplasia appears to be a very specific feature that confirms the diagnosis.

**Complications:** Feeding difficulties (> 80%), failure to thrive (> 80%), jitteriness and apneic spells (50–80%), hypotonia (40–50%), jaundice (40–50%), hypertonia (20–30%) and seizures (20–30%).

**Associated Findings:** None known.

**Etiology:** In the vast majority of cases, a classical free 13 trisomy is found (47,XX or XY,+13), due to a parental meiotic nondisjunction. Mosaic 13 trisomy, in which a normal karyotype is found in a variable percentage of the cells, may account for a less

typical clinical syndrome and longer survival. Much less frequently, 13 trisomy syndrome is due to a translocation trisomy, either occuring de novo or being the result of a meiotic malsegregation in a parent, carrier of a 13/D Robertsonian translocation. Partial trisomies of different parts of chromosome 13 have been reported. These exhibit the more or less typical stigmata of the 13 trisomy syndrome. From these observations, the conclusion can be made that the classical 13 trisomy syndrome, in contrast to the 18 trisomy syndrome, is not due to a trisomy of a specific band or subband of chromosome 13.

**Pathogenesis:** Unknown.

**MIM No.:** 25730

**POS No.:** 3090

**CDC No.:** 758.1

**Sex Ratio:** M1.2:F1

**Occurrence:** About 1:8000 live births. (1:12,000 47+13; 1:24,000 46t (13;D)). There appears to be no preferential occurrence by population or ethnic groups. Prevalence is very low due to high infant mortality.

**Risk of Recurrence for Patient's Sib:** If parent is carrier of 13/14 or 13/15 translocation; about 2% risk.

**Risk of Recurrence for Patient's Child:** No affected individuals are known to have reproduced.

**Age of Detectability:** Prenatally by chorionic villus ampling (CVS) or by amniocentesis and chromosomal analysis of amniotic fluid cells. Ultrasound shows decreased ratio of diameters of fetal head to trunk. Newborn by clinical examination and chromosomal analysis.

**Gene Mapping and Linkage:** See *Gene Map.*

**Prevention:** None known. Genetic counseling indicated.

**Treatment:** As may be clinically indicated.

**Prognosis:** The prognosis is extremely poor. One-half the patients with 47 chromosomes die by 1 month of age, 65% by 3 months, and about 95% by 3 years. Cases with with normal/13 trisomy mosaicism have a somewhat better prognosis. All patients have been profoundly retarded. Adult patients are extremely rare.

**Detection of Carrier:** A small proportion of 13 trisomy patients have been shown to have a translocation; in a few of these a parent, most often a mother, has been shown to be a carrier. Further family studies have revealed members who are also translocation carriers, and who are thus at risk. Risk is reportedly greater in mothers over 35 years of age.

**Special Considerations:** Phenocopies have occurred in this syndrome in which a typical 13 trisomy syndrome picture is associated with apparently normal chromosomes. The cause of these is unknown. There is much overlap of clinical findings with the 18 trisomy syndrome, so that patients with "intermediate" features may be confused. There are also some common findings with the various partial 13 trisomies.

**Support Groups:** UT; West Jordan; Support Organization for Trisomy 18/13 (SOFT)

**References:**
Cogan DG, Kuwababa T: Ocular pathology of the 13–15 trisomy syndrome. Arch Ophthalmol 1964; 72:246–253.
Huehns ER, et al.: Developmental hemoglobin anomalies in a chromosomal duplication: D$_1$ trisomy syndrome. Proc Nat Acad Sci 1964; 51:89.
Huehns ER, et al.: Nuclear abnormalities of the neutrophils in D(13–15) trisomy syndrome. Lancet 1964; 1:589.
Magenis RE, et al.: Trisomy 13(D) syndrome: studies on parental age, sex ratio, and survival. J Pediatr 1968; 73:222–228. *
Taylor AI: Autosomal trisomy syndromes: a detailed study of 27 cases of Edward's syndrome and 27 cases of Patau's syndrome. J Med Genet 1968; 5:227. *
Addor C, et al.: Patau's syndrome: a pathological and cytogenetic study of two cases. J Genet Hum 1975; 23:83.
Hodes ME, et al.: Clinical experience with trisomies 18 and 13. J Med Genet 1978; 15:48.
Pettersen JC, et al.: An examination of the spectrum of anatomic

defects and variations found in eight cases of trisomy 13. Am J Med Genet 1979; 3:183.

MA012
HE007

Ellen Magenis
Frederick Hecht

**Chromosome 13, trisomy 13pter-q12**
*See CHROMOSOME 13, TRISOMY 13q1*
**Chromosome 13, trisomy 13pter-q13**
*See CHROMOSOME 13, TRISOMY 13q1*
**Chromosome 13, trisomy 13pter-q14**
*See CHROMOSOME 13, TRISOMY 13q1*

---

### CHROMOSOME 13, TRISOMY 13Q1       2464

**Includes:**
>Chromosome 13, trisomy 13pter-q12
>Chromosome 13, trisomy 13pter-q13
>Chromosome 13, trisomy 13pter-q14

**Excludes:**
>**Chromosome 13, trisomy 13** (0168)
>**Chromosome 13, trisomy distal 13q** (2463)
>Chromosome 13, trisomy 13pter-q21 or 22

**Major Diagnostic Criteria:** Mental retardation, growth retardation, depressed nasal bridge, cleft lip/palate, clinodactyly, persistence of fetal hemoglobin, increased projections of polymorphonuclear leukocytes. Karyotype analysis confirms the diagnosis.

**Clinical Findings:** *General*: growth retardation, 8/13; psychomotor retardation, 13/13; clinodactyly, 6/13; hemangioma, 2/13. *Craniofacial*: **Microcephaly**, 6/13; frontal bossing, 4/12; low-set, malformed ears, 9/13; broad, bulbous nose, 6/12; depressed nasal bridge, 6/12; long philtrum, 2/12; cleft lip/palate, 5/13; high-arched palate, 2/12; micrognathia, 6/13; epicanthus, 4/13; short neck, 5/12. *Cardiac*: 1/10. *GU*: **Hernia, inguinal**, 1/13; cryptochidism, 4/7. *CNS*: seizures, 2/12; hypotonia, 2/13. *Hematology*: increased polymorphonuclear projections, 6/8; persistence of HgbF, 4/7.

**Complications:** Those resulting from the specific malformations.

**Associated Findings:** One patient was reported with skull and scalp defects, and one patient with **Craniosynostosis, Kleeblattschadel type**, glaucoma, and sacral myelomeningocele.

**Etiology:** Origin of the various trisomic segments occurs secondary to parental translocation in most cases: 11/12 have been maternal in origin, 1/12 paternal in origin. Only one case of *de novo* origin has been reported. No inversions have been reported.

**Pathogenesis:** Unknown.

**POS No.:** 3690

**CDC No.:** 758.990

**Sex Ratio:** M1:F1

**Occurrence:** Twenty-three cases of proximal trisomy 13 syndrome are cited in the literature. Several cases were described prior to accurate banding techniques, and exact break points cannot be defined. Some cases were associated with an abnormality of an additional chromosome. The clinical findings are based only on the 13 cases with break points documented within the 13q1 region.

**Risk of Recurrence for Patient's Sib:** Depends on segregation of parental translocation, if present. There is a low recurrence risk if no parental translocation exists.

**Risk of Recurrence for Patient's Child:** No affected individuals are known to have reproduced.

**Age of Detectability:** At birth, or by prenatal diagnosis by chorionic villus sampling, amniocentesis, or percutaneous umbilical blood sampling.

**Gene Mapping and Linkage:** See *Gene Map*.

**Prevention:** None known. Genetic counseling indicated.

**Treatment:** Symptomatic, special education.

**Prognosis:** All patients show psychomotor retardation. Exact life span is unknown; the oldest reported patient is age 20 years.

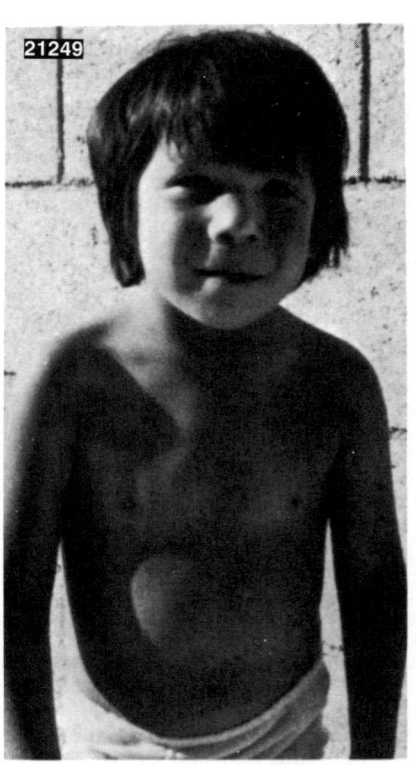

**2464-21249:** Affected male at age 4 years; note the short neck and shield-shaped chest.

---

**Detection of Carrier:** By chromosomal analysis.

**Special Considerations:** The length of the trisomic segment influences clinical features. Increased nuclear projections are associated with trisomy for band 13q12. Persistence of fetal Hgb is associated with trisomy for band 13q14.

**References:**
Escobar J, Yunis J: Trisomy for the proximal segment of the long arm of chromosome 13. Am J Dis Child 1974; 128:221–222.
Moedjono S, Sparkes RS: Partial trisomy of 13(pter→12) due to 47,XY,+der(13),t(13,22)(q12,q13)mat. Hum Genet 1979; 50:241–246.
Tharapel S, et al.: Phenotype-karyotype correlation in patients trisomic for various segments of chromosome 13. J Med Genet 1986; 23:310–315.

HA079
JA014

Pamela A. Hawks
Ethylin Wang Jabs

## CHROMOSOME 13, TRISOMY DISTAL 13Q          2463

**Includes:** Chromosome 13, deletions of 13ql, 2 and 3

**Excludes:** N/A

**Major Diagnostic Criteria:** Psychomotor retardation, frontal bossing, long upwardly curved eyelashes, stubby nose, long philtrum, hemangiomata, ears with a small lobule and anthelix, and post-axial polydactyly.

**Clinical Findings:**

|  | Distal 3/4 13ql | Distal 1/2 13q2 | Distal 1/3 13q3 |
|---|---|---|---|
| Low birth weight | No | Usual | Usual |
| Normal growth | Rare | Usual | Always |
| Psychomotor retardation | Always | Always | Always |
| Microcephaly | Usual | Usual | Rare |
| Frontal bossing | Always | Always | Usual |
| Hypotelorism | Usual | Usual | Usual |
| Epicanthic folds | Usual | Usual | Usual |
| Anti-mongoloid slant | Usual | Usual | Usual |
| Long upwardly curved eyelashes | Always | Always | Always |
| Stubby nose | Usual | Always | Always |
| Long philtrum | Usual | Usual | Always |
| Prominent anthelix with small lobules | Always | Usual | Always |
| Hexadactyly | Usual | Usual | Usual |
| Hemangiomata | Always | Always | Always |
| Anomalies of male external genitalia | Always | Usual | Usual |

**Complications:** Unknown.

**Associated Findings:** Feeding difficulties, respiratory distress and failure to thrive. Many cases who survive the first year are retarded and sometimes have seizures.

**Etiology:** The trisomy 13q syndromes arise usually from parental balanced translocations, sometimes from parental pericentric inversions, and rarely from *de novo* duplications.

**Pathogenesis:** Unknown.

**POS No.:** 3690

**CDC No.:** 758.990

**Sex Ratio:** Presumably M1:F1.

**Occurrence:** Undetermined but presumed rare.

**Risk of Recurrence for Patient's Sib:** Not increased, except when one of the parents is a balanced translocation carrier.

**Risk of Recurrence for Patient's Child:** No patient is known to have reproduced.

**Age of Detectability:** At birth, or by amniocentesis and prenatal diagnosis.

**Gene Mapping and Linkage:** See *Gene Map.*

**Prevention:** None known. Genetic counseling indicated.

**Treatment:** Symptomatic management.

**Prognosis:** Severe mental retardation.

**Detection of Carrier:** By cytogenetic and clinical examination.

**References:**
Bonioli E, et al.: Karyotype-phenotype correlation in partial trisomy 13. Am J Dis Child 1981; 135:115.
Gilsenkrantz S, et al.: Proximal trisomy 13. Hum Genet 1981; 58:436.
Patil SR, Zellweger H: Partial trisomy 13. Clin Pediatr 1981; 20:534.
deGrouchy J, Turlean C: Clinical atlas of human chromosomes. New York: John Wiley & Sons, 1984:232–236.

P0010

Ian H. Porter

**Chromosome 14, duplication of distal 14q**
*See CHROMOSOME 14, PARTIAL TRISOMY 14q*

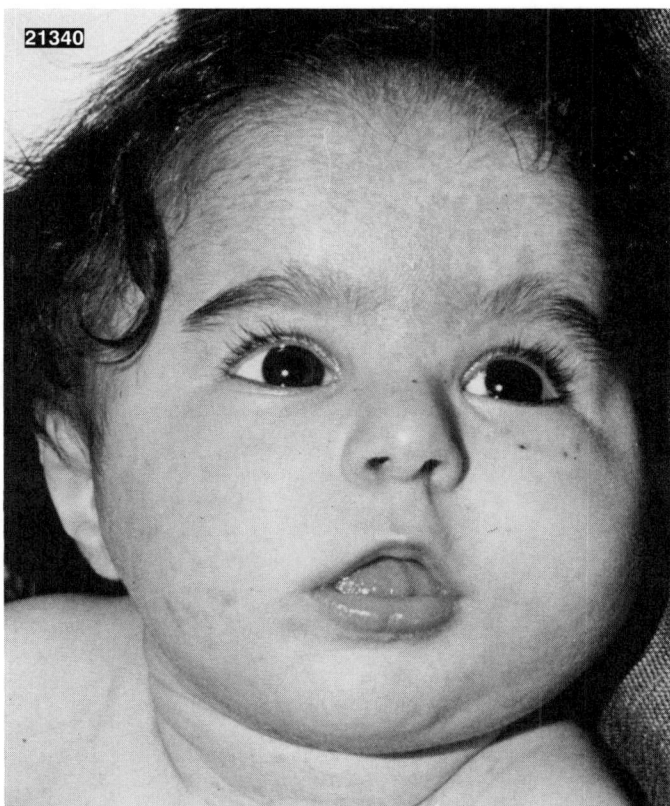

2463-21340: Chromosome 13, trisomy distal 13q; note temporal retraction and bushy converging eyebrows.

**Chromosome 14, duplication of proximal 14q**
*See CHROMOSOME 14, PARTIAL TRISOMY 14q*

## CHROMOSOME 14, MONOSOMY 14Q (Q24.3-Q32.1)          2539

**Includes:** N/A

**Excludes:** Chromosome 14, ring 14 (2467)

**Major Diagnostic Criteria:** Mental retardation. Facial characteristics are round face; horizontal, narrow palpebral fissures; frontal hypertrichosis with thick eyebrows; short bulbous nose with a flat root; long philtrum; and mild micrognathia.

**Clinical Findings:** Dolichocephaly, high-arched palate, brachycephaly, normally set ears with poor helix formation, cleft uvula, micropenis and cryptorchidism, **Atrial septal defects**, and simian line. Most cases are isolated and non-familial.

**Complications:** Respiratory infections, left inguinal hernia, low developmental quotient.

**Associated Findings:** None known.

**Etiology:** Interstitial deletions arising *de novo.*

**Pathogenesis:** Unknown.

**CDC No.:** 758.990

**Sex Ratio:** Undetermined but presumably M1:F1.

**Occurrence:** Undetermined but presumed rare.

**Risk of Recurrence for Patient's Sib:** Not increased if parents have normal karyotypes.

**Risk of Recurrence for Patient's Child:** Unknown.

**Age of Detectability:** During infancy, or prenatally by amniocentesis and karyotyping.

**Gene Mapping and Linkage:** See *Gene Map.*

**Prevention:** None known. Genetic counseling indicated.

**Treatment:** Unknown.

**Prognosis:** One patient in the second decade of life has been reported.

**Detection of Carrier:** Chromosomal analysis to determine translocation state.

**References:**

Hreidarsson SJ, Stamberg J: Distal monosomy 14 not associated with ring formation. J Med Genet 1983; 20:147–149.

Petrosky DL, Borgaonkar DS: Segregation analysis in reciprocal translocation carriers. Am J Med Genet 1984; 19:137–159.

Yamamoto Y, et al.: Deletion 14q(q24.3 to q32.1) syndrome: significance of peculiar facial appearance in its diagnosis and deletion mapping of Pi ($\alpha_1$-antitrypsin). Hum Genet 1986; 74:190–192.

Yen FS, et al.: A terminal deletion (14)(q31.1) in a child with microcephaly, protuberant ears, and mild mental retardation. J Med Genet 1989; 26:130–133.

B0021                                         **Digamber S. Borgaonkar**

---

## CHROMOSOME 14, PARTIAL TRISOMY 14Q          0165

**Includes:**

Chromosome 14, duplication of distal 14q
Chromosome 14, duplication of proximal 14q

**Excludes:**

**Chromosome 14, trisomy 14 mosaic** (2547)
**Chromosome 14, trisomy 14q** (2466)

**Major Diagnostic Criteria:** Dysmorphic features and developmental delay (or mental retardation) together with cytologic demonstration of duplication (partial trisomy) of 14q.

**Clinical Findings:** There are at least 2 distinct syndromes due to partial trisomy of the long arm (q) of chromosome 14. One syndrome is associated with partial trisomy of the proximal portion of 14q. The second syndrome is associated with partial trisomy of the distal portion of 14q.

*Syndrome I results from partial duplication of proximal portion of 14q* Nine of the cases studied to date have shown the following features: low birthweight (1,800–2,600 gm), growth retardation, motor and mental retardation, seizures or hypertonia, microcephaly (and sometimes brachycephaly), low anterior hairline, ocular hyper- or hypotelorism, occasional ptosis of the eyelids with antimongoloid slant of the palpebral fissures, small palpebral fissures, microphthalmia or strabismus. The external ears may be low-set or malformed. The nose is prominent and has a broad base and a prominent tip. The mouth is large with a thin upper lip. The palate is highly arched or cleft. Prominent philtrum and micrognathia may be present. The neck is short. The fingers are long and tapered and clinodactyly or camptodactyly are usually present. Other reported skeletal anomalies include kyphosis, hypoplastic 12th ribs, missing or hypoplastic radius, dislocated or dysplastic hips, and clubfeet. Three of 9 patients had congenital heart malformations, and 2 had mild genital malformations such as cryptorchidism.

*Syndrome II results from partial duplication of distal portion of 14q.* The cases studied have the following features: Development and mental retardation; and hypotonia or spasticity (observed in all cases); growth retardation (90%); abnormally positioned ears; and micrognathia (> 85%); abnormal EEG and/or seizures; microcephaly; ocular hypertelorism; downward-slanting palpebral fissures; hypogonadism; cryptorchidism; and sparse hair (all 50–85%); and widely open sutures and congenital heart disease (both 40–50%).

Other clinical findings include high-arched or cleft palate, protruding upper lip, buccal fat pad, camptodactyly, cyanosis, and hypoplasia of the 12th rib. The growth retardation may be evident at birth or later. The congenital cardiovascular anomaly is usually conotruncal or aortic arch.

**Complications:** Seizures with duplication proximal 14q (syndrome I).

**Associated Findings:** Congenital heart disease.

**Etiology:** Partial trisomy (duplication) of part of the long arm of chromosome 14.

**Pathogenesis:** Unknown.

**CDC No.:** 758.990

**Sex Ratio:** M1:F1

**Occurrence:** Less than 20 cases documented in the literature.

**Risk of Recurrence for Patient's Sib:** Low, except when one of the parents has a balanced translocation.

**Risk of Recurrence for Patient's Child:** Unknown.

**Age of Detectability:** At birth or in second trimester by study of chorionic villus sample (CVS) or cultured amniotic fluid cells.

**Gene Mapping and Linkage:** See *Gene Map.*

**Prevention:** None known. Genetic counseling indicated.

**Treatment:** Unknown.

**Prognosis:** Moderate to severe mental retardation. Patients with duplication of proximal part of 14q (syndrome I) may survive at least into adulthood. As greater amounts of the long arm are involved, the malformations are more pronounced and mental retardation more profound.

**Detection of Carrier:** The balanced translocation carrier or mosaic is recognizable by karyotype analysis. Presently, this has been done only after the birth of an affected child.

**References:**

Pfeiffer RA, et al.: Partial trisomy 14 following a balanced reciprocal translocation t(14q-; 21q+). Humangenetik 1973; 20:187.

Wyandt HE, et al.: Abnormal chromosomes 14 and 15 in abortions, syndromes and malignancy. In: Yunis JJ, ed: New chromosomal syndromes. New York: Academic Press, 1977. *

Atkin JF: Duplication of the distal segment of 14q. Am J Med Genet 1983; 16:357. *

HE007                                              **Frederick Hecht**
WY000                                              **Herman E. Wyandt**

**Chromosome 14, rearrangements**
*See CHROMOSOME INSTABILITY, NIJMEGEN TYPE*

---

## CHROMOSOME 14, RING 14                       2467

**Includes:** Ring 14

**Excludes:** **Tuberous sclerosis** (0975)

**Major Diagnostic Criteria:** Demonstration of the ring 14 chromosome by appropriate cytogenetic studies.

**Clinical Findings:** A characteristic craniofacial dysmorphism consisting of dolicocephaly; **Microcephaly**; high forehead; down slanting palpebral fissures; epicanthic folds; flat nasal bridge; hypertelorism; prominent, bulbous nasal tip; slightly anteverted nares; large, low-set ears; high-arched palate; micrognathia; thin upper lip with down turned corners of the mouth; short neck with redundant skin folds; widely spaced nipples; and simian creases. The clinical course is characterized by growth delay, significant psychomotor retardation, and early onset of difficult-to-control seizures.

**Complications:** Unknown.

**Associated Findings:** Neurologic abnormalities (athetosis, ataxia, intention tremor, and hyperactivity). Abnormalities of skin pigmentation (cafe-au-lait spots, vitiligo, and pigmented nevi). Nonspecific abnormalities of the eye grounds. Orthopedic anomalies (contractures significant enough to interfere with ambulation). Congenital heart disease (stenosis of part of either the pulmonary artery or aorta).

**Etiology:** The formation of the ring chromosome results from breaks in the p and q arm of chromosome 14, obligatory loss of genetic material, and reunion of the p and q arms.

**Pathogenesis:** Unknown.

**CDC No.:** 758.990

**Sex Ratio:** M2:F1

**Occurrence:** At least sixteen cases of ring 14, including seven previously reported cases and nine unpublished cases, are known.

**Risk of Recurrence for Patient's Sib:** Apparently low, unless a parent also has a ring 14 chromosome.

**Risk of Recurrence for Patient's Child:** Unknown.

**Age of Detectability:** Prenatally by chromosome studies, or at birth with cytogenetic studies on cultured peripheral leukocytes.

**Gene Mapping and Linkage:** See *Gene Map.*

**Prevention:** None known. Genetic counseling indicated.

**Treatment:** Physical therapy and/or medical intervention as indicated for secondary complications including contractures, pulmonary infections, and seizures. Corrective surgery for congenital heart lesion.

**Prognosis:** The presence of the ring 14 chromosome does not appear to be incompatible with prolonged survival. The average age of the surviving patients at the time of reporting was 78 months. Two patients died within the first 3 1/2 years of life; one died of complications of pneumonia, the second died suddenly of unexplained causes. Seven patients have been followed into the second decade of life and two other patients are in their twenties.

Follow up clinical evaluations were frequently positive for growth retardation, with several cases reporting feeding difficulties. This was probably a reflection of overall hypotonia and related poor suck. The majority of patients showed significant developmental delay and psychomotor retardation. Seizures, beginning within the first year of life, were noted in all but three cases (in these cases onset was between one and three years). The seizures were usually classified as generalized tonic clonic, myoclonic, or focal. They were not associated with any specific EEG changes. Cerebral atrophy with secondary ventricular enlargement was generally noted on CT scan. The seizures were generally quite difficult to control even on multiple drug regimens. Repeated bouts of upper respiratory or pulmonary infections were noted in many patients; this was thought to be secondary to aspiration during the frequent seizure episodes.

**Detection of Carrier:** Cytogenetic and clinical examination.

**Special Considerations:** Inheritance of various ring chromosomes have been cited in the literature. Though the vast majority of cases of ring 14 chromosome were associated with normal parental karyotypes, Bowser et al (1981) reported the passage of a ring 14 chromosome from a phenotypically normal, slightly retarded mother to her twin daughters and a therapeutically aborted fetus. Therefore, cytogenetic studies of the parents of an affected child are recommended.

The variability noted in various ring chromosome syndromes has been attributed to the difference in the amount of genetic material lost and/or the stability of the ring during mitosis. Review of the cytogenetic findings revealed that the ring 14 appears to be a relatively stable structure. Therefore, the overall consistency of the craniofacial dysmorphism and similar clinical histories were surprising in view of the various breakpoints that were described. Comparison of the ring 14 patients with a patient reported as having simple deletion of 14q, with the breakpoint designated as 14q32.1 identified a very similar facial dysmorphism and psychomotor retardation. Therefore, the major phenotypic features noted in the ring 14 syndrome may be due to loss of only a small amount of genetic material on 14q.

**References:**
Bowser RS, et al.: Inheritance of a ring 14 chromosome. J Med Genet 1981; 8:209–213.
Lippe BM, Sparkes RS: Ring 14 chromosome: an association with seizures. Am J Med Genet 1981; 9:301–305.
Schmidt R, et al.: Ring chromosome 14: a distinct clinical entity. J Med Genet 1981; 18:304–307.
Fryns JP, et al.: Ring chromosome 14 syndrome. Ann Genet 1982; 25:179–180.

SC004                                          **Paula R. Scarbrough**

**Chromosome 14, trisomy 14**
*See CHROMOSOME 14, TRISOMY 14 MOSAIC*

## CHROMOSOME 14, TRISOMY 14 MOSAIC                    2547

**Includes:**
    Chromosome 14, trisomy 14
    Chromosome 14, trisomy 14, normal mosaicism

**Excludes:** N/A

**Major Diagnostic Criteria:** Dysmorphic features, including growth delay, wide nasal bridge, and micrognathia, together with developmental delay (or mental retardation). Diagnosis is confirmed by chromosome analysis.

**Clinical Findings:** One of the more interesting discoveries in clinical cytogenetics has been that in pregnancies with trisomy 14, normal mosaicism can survive beyond chorionic villus sampling and amniocentesis to birth. Ten cases have been summarized by Lipson (1987), and two additional cases have been seen. Growth retardation (100%) is uniform and may be evident by length at birth. Developmental delay and, later, mental retardation are similarly ubiquitous (100%). The forehead tends to be prominent (80%), the eyes widespread (70%), and the nasal bridge wide (100%). The ears usually appear low-set (90%). The palate may be cleft (40%), and there is usually micrognathia (100%). Congenital heart disease (often **Heart, tetralogy of Fallot**) is common (90%). Among the more unusual findings are an evanescent translucent film over the eyes (30%) and body asymmetry (30%).

**Complications:** Polyhydramnios may complicate the pregnancy (30%), and birth may be premature (20%).

**Associated Findings:** Congenital heart disease.

**Etiology:** Trisomy of chromosome 14. This results from nondisjunction in parental meiosis or in fetal mitosis. The zygote has trisomy 14, and then nondisjunction occurs to create a normal cell line, or vice versa. The mean ages of the parents are not increased (fathers, 31.0 years; mothers, 26.1 years of age).

**Pathogenesis:** Unknown.

**POS No.:** 4389

**CDC No.:** 758.990

**Sex Ratio:** M3:F11 (observed).

**Occurrence:** A dozen cases have been documented.

**Risk of Recurrence for Patient's Sib:** Relatively low, except that the total risk for all types of aneuploidy may be elevated to 1–2% at least with the next pregnancy.

**Risk of Recurrence for Patient's Child:** Unknown.

**Age of Detectability:** By prenatal diagnosis with chorionic villus sampling or amniocentesis.

**Gene Mapping and Linkage:** See *Gene Map.*

**Prevention:** None known. Genetic counseling indicated.

**Treatment:** Directed at specific anatomic malformations amenable to surgery, and supportive measures plus early special education.

**Prognosis:** Although all patients recognized to date have been developmentally or mentally retarded, the sample size is small and it is reasonable to expect some patients to be intellectually normal. Some patients have died in infancy, whereas other patients are still alive and in their teens.

**Detection of Carrier:** Unknown.

**Special Considerations:** Because several of the key immunologic genes are on chromosome 14, we suspect that some children with trisomy 14, normal mosaicism may be immune deficient. There may, therefore, be reason to evaluate those children immunologically.

References:
Lipson MH: Trisomy 14 mosaicism syndrome. Am J Med Genet 1987; 26:541.

HE007                                                    Frederick Hecht
HE008                                                    Barbara K. Hecht

**Chromosome 14, trisomy 14, normal mosaicism**
*See CHROMOSOME 14, TRISOMY 14 MOSAIC*

---

## CHROMOSOME 14, TRISOMY 14Q                              2466

**Includes:** Chromosome 14, trisomy mosaic

**Excludes:** Chromosome 14, partial trisomy 14q (0165)

**Major Diagnostic Criteria:** Growth and psychomotor retardation in the presence of trisomic 14q, usually in mosaic with normal cell line. Cytogenetic analysis confirms the diagnosis.

**Clinical Findings:** Growth retardation (11/11); psychomotor retardation (10/10); minor facial abnormalities (11/11); congenital heart disease (11/11); body and/or facial asymmetry (7/11); high-arched or cleft palate (6/9); hypo- and hyper-pigmented skin lesions (5/9).

**Complications:** Unknown.

**Associated Findings:** Three males had a small phallus and cryptorchidism. One female had an anteriorly placed anus. One patient had abnormalities of the neutrophils.

**Etiology:** In ten of eleven patients, trisomy occurred *de novo*; free trisomy in eight and t(14q14q) in two. One patient had t(14;15)(q11;p11) which was inherited from the carrier mother. Cytogenetic investigation with special stainings showed that the normal cell line in this patient was derived from a break of the translocation chromosome and loss of 14q. Mosaicism with normal cell line was found in all eleven. The trisomic cell line ranged from 8–41% in blood and lower percentages in skin. Non-mosaic trisomy 14 is probably lethal since it was found only in abortuses. Maternal and paternal ages do not seem to be factors.

**Pathogenesis:** Unknown.

**CDC No.:** 758.990

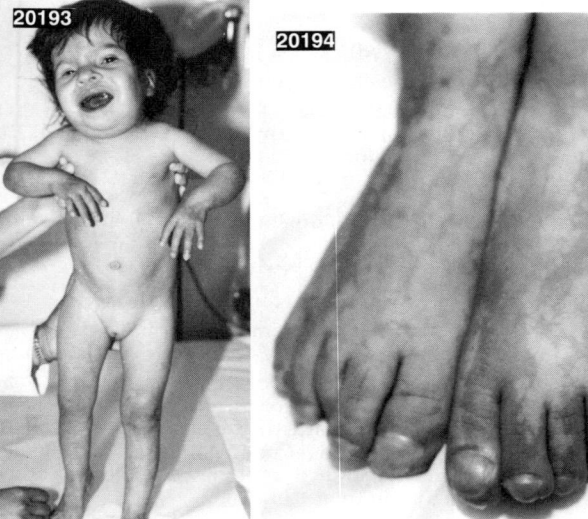

**2466-20193:** This 18-month-old child has asymmetry of the face and body, dysmorphic facies, low-set ears, long fingers and skin pigmentation.    **20194:** Hyperpigmented skin lesions are found bilaterally; note the difference between the size of the right and left feet and the clubbed toes.

**Sex Ratio:** M4:F7 (observed).

**Occurrence:** At least eleven cases have been documented.

**Risk of Recurrence for Patient's Sib:** Very low for *de novo* cases and low even for inherited translocation case since non-mosaic 14 is probably lethal.

**Risk of Recurrence for Patient's Child:** No patient has reached reproductive age.

**Age of Detectability:** At birth, or by prenatal diagnosis.

**Gene Mapping and Linkage:** See *Gene Map.*

**Prevention:** None known. Genetic counseling indicated.

**Treatment:** Treatment of cardiac lesion if indicated. Otherwise, supportive therapy.

**Prognosis:** The average life span is unknown. The oldest reported patient is in the early teens. In one patient with **Heart, tetralogy of Fallot,** Blalock-Taussig procedure resulted in improvement of growth and developmental parameters.

**Detection of Carrier:** Chromosome analysis and clinical evaluation.

**References:**
Rethore MO, et al.: Trisomie 14 en mosaique chez une enfant multimalformee. Ann Genet 1975; 18:71–74.
Martin AO, et al.: 46,XX/47,XX,+14 mosaicism in a liveborn infant. J Med Genet 1977; 14:214–218.
Johnson VP, et al.: Trisomy 14 mosaicism: case report and review. Am J Med Genet 1979; 3:331–339.
Turleau C, et al.: Trisomie 14 en mosaique par isochromosome dicentrique. Ann Genet 1980; 23:238–240.
Jenkins MB, et al.: Trisomy 14 mosaicism in a translocation 14q15q carrier: probable dissociation and isochromosome formation. J Med Genet 1981; 18:68–71.
Fujimoto A, et al.: Trisomy 14 mosaicism with t(14;15)(q11;p11) in offspring of a balanced translocation carrier mother. Am J Med Genet 1985; 22:333–342. * †

FU003                                                    **Atsuko Fujimoto**

**Chromosome 14, trisomy mosaic**
*See CHROMOSOME 14, TRISOMY 14q*
**Chromosome 15, 15 mosaicism**
*See CHROMOSOME 15, RING 15*
**Chromosome 15, duplication of 15q1.**
*See CHROMOSOME 15, TRISOMY 15q1*
**Chromosome 15, partial distal duplication 15q**
*See CHROMOSOME 15, PARTIAL TRISOMY DISTAL 15q*
**Chromosome 15, partial distal trisomy 15q**
*See CHROMOSOME 15, PARTIAL TRISOMY DISTAL 15q*

---

## CHROMOSOME 15, PARTIAL TRISOMY DISTAL 15Q              2131

**Includes:**
    Chromosome 15, partial distal trisomy 15q
    Chromosome 15, partial distal duplication 15q

**Excludes:**
    Chromosome 15, duplication of proximal 15q (15q1)
    **Chromosome 15, trisomy 15q1 (2548)**
    Chromosome 15, trisomy proximal 15q (15q1)

**Major Diagnostic Criteria:** Postnatal growth retardation, failure to thrive due to swallowing difficulties, and severe developmental delay associated with a distinct craniofacial dysmorphism.

**Clinical Findings:** Micro- and microdolichocephaly, prominent occiput, sloping forehead, downward slanting of the palpebral fissures, narrow palpebral fissures and epicanthus, prominent and/or bulbous nose with flattened nasofrontal sulcus, broad nasal bridge, deep and long philtrum, small, triangular mouth with long upper lip, high-arched palate, micro(retro)gnathia, low-set, large ears with marked antihelices, and cryptorchidism and/or hypogenitalism in all male patients. The few patients reported with a very distal 15q duplication (15q24or25→15qter) presented a different phenotype with **Hydrocephaly** rather than **Microcephaly**, and excessive body growth.

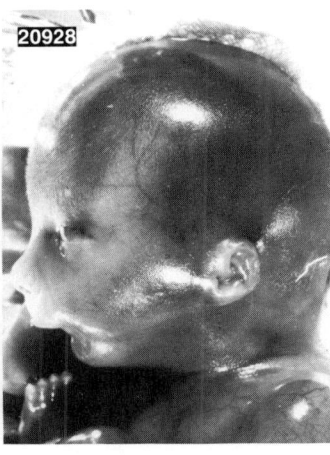

**2131A-20926:** Chromosome 15, partial duplication 15q; cranio-facial findings in an affected fetus include sloping forehead, broad nasal bridge, bulbous nose, and long philtrum. **20928:** Severe micrognathia is evident on the lateral view of the facies.

**Complications:** Unknown.

**Associated Findings:** Cervical vertebral anomalies resulting in short, webbed neck, congenital heart defect, joint deformities and severe general hypertonicity, multiple exostoses, renal agenesis, cortical pseudocysts of the suprarenal glands, and polydactyly/syndactyly.

**Etiology:** In the majority of patients, the 15q2 duplication was the unbalanced product of a parental translocation involving chromosome 15 (breakpoints 15q22, 15q21 or 15q23) and another autosome, most frequently another acrocentric chromosome. Mosaicism with a normal cell line was reported in one patient. In another patient a maternal pericentric inversion (15)(p12q22) resulted in a pure duplication (15)(q22→qter).

**Pathogenesis:** Unknown.

**CDC No.:** 758.990

**Sex Ratio:** M2:F1

**Occurrence:** Some 38 cases have been reported in the literature.

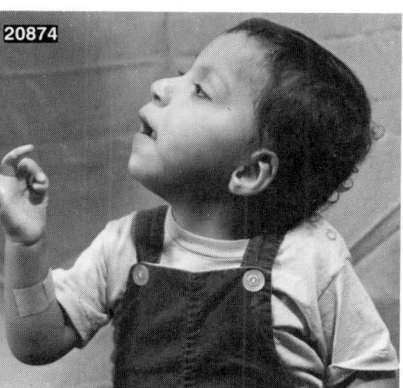

**2131B-20873:** Age 32 months; note microcephaly, asymmetric face, downward slant of the palpebral fissures, prominent nose and long tapering fingers. **20874:** Lateral facies shows low-set ear and micrognathia.

**Risk of Recurrence for Patient's Sib:** Negligible if parental chromosomes are normal. Considerably increased (5–10%) if reciprocal or Robertsonian type translocation involving chromosome 15 and another chromosome is found in one of the parents.

**Risk of Recurrence for Patient's Child:** Severe mental retardation in surviving patients makes reproduction unlikely.

**Age of Detectability:** At birth. Prenatal diagnosis is possible by amniocenthesis or CVS.

**Gene Mapping and Linkage:** See *Gene Map.*

**Prevention:** None known. Genetic counseling indicated.

**Treatment:** As indicated, including prevention of infections and special education.

**Prognosis:** The average life span is undetermined, although at least one survivor has reached age 20. Four infants died before age six months. Survivors have shown profound mental retardation and recurrent infections of the upper respiratory and urinary tracts.

**Detection of Carrier:** Cytogenetic examination of the patients to exclude autosomal translocations involving 15q2.

**Special Considerations:** Phenotypic variation would be expected when a different segment of the distal 15q is duplicated and monosomy of a different second chromosome is present. However, all the patients so far reported as having duplication of the 15q23→qter segment appear to have the common phenotype described for distal 15q trisomy. Three individuals with duplication of 15q25→qter are not included in the above group. Two brothers who had der(6),t(6;15)(p25;q25)mat had mild facial dysmorphism and mild mental retardation. One severely retarded boy with a cloverleaf skull anomaly had der(12),t(12;15)(p13; q25)mat. The different phenotypes seen in these three patients may be due to the involvement of a shorter segment of distal 15q, or the effect of monosomy of the second chromosomes.

**References:**

Fujimoto A, et al.: Inherited partial duplication of chromosome 15. J Med Genet 1974; 11:287–291. * †

Gregoire MJ, et al.: Duplication 15q22→15qter and its phenotypic expression. Hum Genet 1981; 59:429–433.

Sanger WG, et al.: Inherited partial trisomy #15 complicated by neuroblastoma. Cancer Genet Cytogenet 1984; 11:153–159.

Schnatterly P, et al.: Distal 15q trisomy: phenotypic comparison of nine cases in an extended family. Am J Hum Genet 1984; 36:444–451.

FU003
FR030
KL007

**Atsuko Fujimoto**
**Jean-Pierre Fryns**
**Alice Kleczkowska**

---

**CHROMOSOME 15, RING 15**                                   **2468**

**Includes:**
    Chromosome 15, 15 mosaicism
    Ring 15

**Excludes:** Chromosome 15, other anomalies

**Major Diagnostic Criteria:** The diagnosis is suspected based on the more common clinical features, and confirmed by cytogenetic analysis.

**Clinical Findings:** Slow prenatal and/or postnatal physical growth including **Microcephaly** and mental retardation are the most common features. Acromicria, hypertelorism (possibly telecanthus), micrognathia, and gonadal hypoplasia are also common. Varied minor congenital anomalies (informative morphogenetic variants) are frequently present. The approximate frequency of the clinical features are: slow growth [height < 3rd percentile] (31/32); microcephaly (30/32); mental retardation (29/32); hypotonia (27/32); hypertonia (2/32); micrognathia [less common in adults] (21/32); hypertelorism [less frequent in adults] (8/32); bird head profile (2/32); congenital heart defects, varied types (6/32); short phalanges leading to acromicria (13/32); **Syndactyly** (3/32); radial ray hypoplasia (3/32); congenital dislocation of the hip

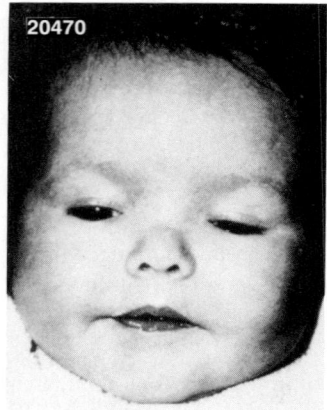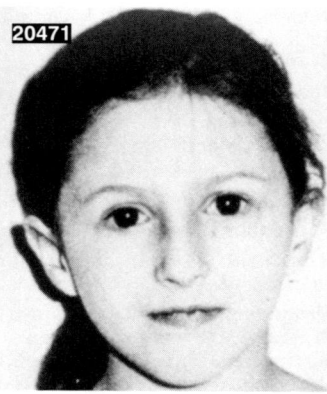

**2468-20470:** Facial features in a 4-month-old male: flat nasal bridge, small, upturned nose, minimal downward slanting of the palpebral fissures, short philtrum, triangular mouth. **20471:** Facial features in a 6-year-old female: somewhat oldish appearance, and triangular-shaped face.

(3/32); scoliosis (3/32); renal anomalies (2/32); seizures (2/32); cafe au lait pigmentations (3/32); and gonadal hypoplasia [apparent in adulthood] (7/32).

**Complications:** Occasional failure to thrive during infancy.

**Associated Findings:** **Camptodactyly,** ectopic anus, eczema, pyloric stenosis, amyotrophy, asymmetric nostrils, and retinal depigmentations (possibly secondary to rod degeneration) have been reported once each.

**Etiology:** Increased parental age may be a factor. Only one patient had the ring secondary to a familial translocation. The rest represented a *de novo* event.

**Pathogenesis:** Unknown.

**CDC No.:** 758.990

**Sex Ratio:** M1:F3

**Occurrence:** Over thirty cases have been reported. Most genetic centers, however, have unreported cases.

**Risk of Recurrence for Patient's Sib:** Appears to be low (exact figure not available) unless a parent is a carrier of a balanced translocation.

**Risk of Recurrence for Patient's Child:** While no affected individuals have reproduced, the risk could be as high as 50%.

**Age of Detectability:** At birth, or prenatally.

**Gene Mapping and Linkage:** See *Gene Map.*

**Prevention:** None known. Genetic counseling indicated.

**Treatment:** Palliative for specific clinical features. Home rearing with comprehensive, early stimulation appears beneficial.

**Prognosis:** Shortened life span; survival to the fifth decade has been reported.

**Detection of Carrier:** Cytogenetic studies and clinical examination.

**Special Considerations:** Varied mosaicism, showing cell lines with monosomy 15, unfolded and double, frequently dicentric, rings implies post-zygotic dynamics with undetermined impact on the phenotype. Extensive cytogenetic studies by Ledbetter et al (1980) report aneuploidy and altered ring morphologies, as well as decondensed and pulverized rings.

**References:**
Jacobsen P: A ring chromosome in the 13–15 group associated with microcephalic dwarfism, mental retardation and emotional immaturity. Hereditas 1966; 55:188–191.

Laszlo J, et al.: Chromosome studies in ovarian hypoplasia. Clin Genet 1976; 9:61–70.
Kousseff BG: Ring chromosome 15 and failure to thrive. Am J Dis Child 1980; 134:798–799.
Ledbetter DH, et al.: Ring chromosome 15, phenotype, Ag-NOR analysis, secondary aneuploidy, and associated chromosome instability. Cytogenet Cell Genet 1980; 27:111–122.
Otto J, et al.: Dysplastic features, growth retardation, malrotation of the gut, and fatal ventricular septal defect in a 4-month old girl with ring chromosome 15. Eur J Ped 1984; 141:229–231.
Butler MG, et al.: Two patients with ring chromosome 15 syndrome. Am J Med Genet 1988; 29:149–154. *

K0018

**Boris G. Kousseff**

---

**CHROMOSOME 15, TRISOMY 15Q1**      **2548**

**Includes:** Chromosome 15, duplication of 15q1.

**Excludes:** Chromosome 15, other anomalies

**Major Diagnostic Criteria:** Severe mental retardation and characteristic craniofacial dysmorphism. The diagnosis is confirmed by chromosome analysis.

**Clinical Findings:** Oval face with deeply-set eyes, prominent supraorbital and zygomatic regions, full cheeks, strabismus, large nose, low-set ears, high-arched and/or **Cleft palate**. Slight **Microcephaly** is present in less than 50% of the patients. Limb anomalies include short, thick fingers and toes, and rocker-bottom deformity of the feet.

**Complications:** Unknown.

**Associated Findings:** Microphthalmia, cardiac defects and **Hernia, inguinal.** Epileptic seizures, hyperactivity and aggressiveness, apparently due to the severe mental retardation, are also frequently observed. Proximal 15q11q12(or 15q12q13) duplication was reported in two patients presenting many manifestations of the **Prader-Willi syndrome:** obesity, compulsive eating, short stature, central hypotonia, hypogonadism, small hands and feet, hypopigmentation, and feeding problems.

**Etiology:** In one-half of the patients, the 15q1 duplication occured *de novo.* In the others, the 15q1 duplication was the unbalanced product of a parental translocation involving chromosome 15 and another autosome, most frequently chromosome 22. Inverted duplication of the 15q1 segment was the cause of the 15q1 trisomy in other patients.

**Pathogenesis:** Unknown.

**CDC No.:** 758.990

**Sex Ratio:** M1:F2 (observed).

**Occurrence:** About 30 cases have been documented.

**Risk of Recurrence for Patient's Sib:** Not increased if parental chromosomes are normal. Considerably increased (5–10%) if reciprocal or Robertsonian type translocation involving chromosome 15 and another chromosome is found in one of the parents.

**Risk of Recurrence for Patient's Child:** Severe mental retardation in surviving patients makes reproduction unlikely.

**Age of Detectability:** At birth, or by prenatal diagnosis by CVS or amniocentesis.

**Gene Mapping and Linkage:** See *Gene Map.*

**Prevention:** None known. Genetic counseling indicated.

**Treatment:** Symptomatic.

**Prognosis:** Death within the first years of life is unlikely, due to the absence of severe growth failure and associated internal malformations.

**Detection of Carrier:** By cytogenetic examination.

**References:**
Hood OJ, et al: Proximal duplications of chromosome 15: clinical dilemmas. Clin Genet 1986; 29:234–240.

Pettigrew AL, et al: Duplication of proximal 15q as a cause of Prader-Willi syndrome. Am J Med Genet 1987; 28:791–802.

FR030                                                    **Jean-Pierre Fryns**

**Chromosome 16, centromeric instability-immunodeficiency**
*See IMMUNODEFICIENCY WITH CENTROMERIC INSTABILITY*
**Chromosome 16, interstitial 16q deletion [del(16)(q13q21 or 22)]**
*See CHROMOSOME 16, MONOSOMY 16q*
**Chromosome 16, interstitial deletions at alpha-globin loci**
*See MENTAL RETARDATION, HEMOGLOBIN H RELATED*

---

## CHROMOSOME 16, MONOSOMY 16Q                2519

**Includes:**
   Chromosome 16, interstitial 16q deletion [del(16)(q13q21 or 22)]
   Chromosome 16, terminal 16q deletion [del(16)(q21q24)]
**Excludes:**
   **Chromosome 16, trisomy 16p** (2469)
   Chromosome 16, other anomalies

**Major Diagnostic Criteria:** Multiple congenital anomalies, with severe problems of growth and development, and malformations mainly confined to the head and the neck. The forehead is high, the anterior fontanel large and bulging with diastasis of the cranial sutures, and prominent metopic suture. All patients had a short neck, upward slanting palpebral fissures, and low-set and/or dysmorphic ears.

**Clinical Findings:** Delayed growth and development, feeble suck, hypotonia, high forehead, prominent metopic suture, large anterior fontanelle, narrow palpebral fissures, low-set folded ears, micrognathia, short neck, narrow thorax, diverse skeletal anomalies, and various internal organ defects.

**Complications:** Unknown.

**Associated Findings:** Intestinal malrotation, ectopic anus, neural deafness, internal hydrocephalus, renal hypoplasia, rhizomelic shortening of the limbs, and **Ventricular septal defect**.

**Etiology:** A monosomy for 16q was found in all patients: three terminal (16q21q24) and four interstitial deletions (16q13q21 or q22). The smallest region of overlap is 16q21. It seems indisputable that band 16q21 is responsible for the distinct clinical findings. In all patients, the 16q deletion occured *de novo*. Parental karyotypes were normal.

**Pathogenesis:** Unknown.

**CDC No.:** 758.990

**Sex Ratio:** M4:F3

**Occurrence:** About 10 patients have been reported in the literature.

**Risk of Recurrence for Patient's Sib:** Not increased if parental chromosomes are normal.

**Risk of Recurrence for Patient's Child:** Severe mental retardation in surviving patients makes reproduction unlikely.

**Age of Detectability:** At birth, or by prenatal diagnosis by CVS or amniocenthesis.

**Gene Mapping and Linkage:** See *Gene Map*.

**Prevention:** None known. Genetic counseling indicated.

**Treatment:** Symptomatic.

**Prognosis:** Two patients died in the neonatal period. Follow-up information on four surviving patients is available. Moderate mental retardation and slight growth retardation was seen in one patient at six years of age. Three other patients were severely mentally retarded, with severe growth failure, and recurrent respiratory infections. One had progressive renal insufficiency.

**Detection of Carrier:** Chromosomal examination for an autosomal translocation involving 16q.

**References:**
Fryns JP, et al.: Partial monosomy of the long arm of chromosome 16: a distinct clinical entity? Hum Genet 1979; 46:115–120.
Coté GB, et al.: Fryns syndrome without deletion 16q. Ann Génét 1980; 23/3:171–172.
Fryns JP, et al.: Interstitial 16q deletion with typical dysmorphic syndrome. Ann Génét 1981; 24/2:124–125.
Rivero H, et al.: Monosomy 16q: a distinct syndrome: apropos of a de novo del(16)(q2100q2300). Clinical Genetics 1985; 28:84–86.

FR030                                                    **Jean-Pierre Fryns**

**Chromosome 16, mosaic trisomy 16q**
*See CHROMOSOME 16, TRISOMY 16q*
**Chromosome 16, partial trisomy 16p**
*See CHROMOSOME 16, TRISOMY 16p*
**Chromosome 16, partial trisomy 16q**
*See CHROMOSOME 16, TRISOMY 16q*
**Chromosome 16, proximal 16p trisomy**
*See CHROMOSOME 16, TRISOMY 16q*
**Chromosome 16, terminal 16q deletion [del(16)(q21q24)]**
*See CHROMOSOME 16, MONOSOMY 16q*

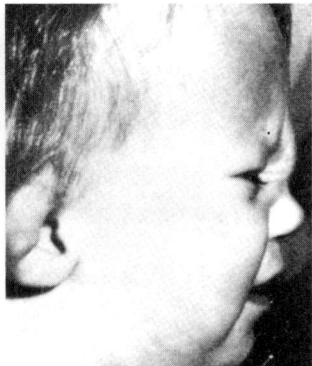

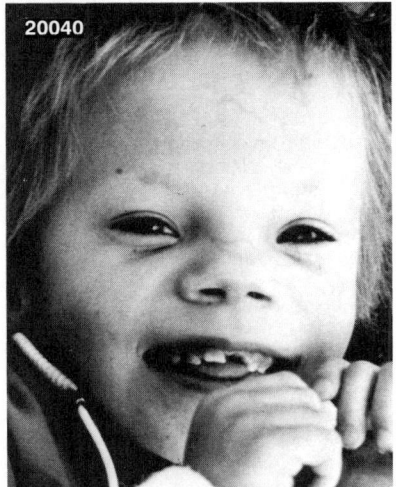

**2519-20039:** Note high forehead, narrow and upslanting palpebral fissures, micrognathia and low-set folded ears at ages 3 months and 1 year.  **20040:** Dysmorphic facies and high forehead at age 6 years.

## CHROMOSOME 16, TRISOMY 16P     2469

**Includes:** Chromosome 16, partial trisomy 16p

**Excludes:** Chromosome 16, trisomy 16q (2470)

**Major Diagnostic Criteria:** Trisomy for all or most of the short arm of chromosome 16, either as the result of reduplication or an unbalanced translocation. Cytogenetic analysis confirms the diagnosis.

**Clinical Findings:** Liveborn patients (7/10) have been small for gestational age. The heads are usually round and small with a flat, round face. Scalp hair is often sparse with sparse eyebrows and lashes. Hypertelorism is usually present along with small palpebral fissures and/or ptosis. **Cleft palate** and micrognathia are also common features. About fifty percent have had contractures involving the fingers, wrist, knees and hips. Each liveborn male has had **Hernia, inguinal** (3/3). Hand abnormalities include absent thumbs, malpositioned thumbs, long tapering fingers, and simian creases. All patients have had severe neurologic impairment. Most have had poorly controlled seizures and/or severe apnea. Only one confirmed child was known to be alive at age eleven. Five died in infancy or early childhood of respiratory infections.

**Complications:** Profound mental retardation or developmental delay. Early death from respiratory infections.

**Associated Findings:** A single umbilical artery was present in 2/5 infants in which the cord was described. Internal defects were uncommon with the exception of cardiac anomalies. Two cases had **Heart, tetralogy of Fallot**, and two had **Atrial septal defects**.

**Etiology:** This condition may arise from an apparent spontaneous reduplication of 16p (2 cases), as the result of an unbalanced translocation involving 16p and another chromosome (8 familial cases and probably the two *de novo* cases of trisomy 16q-).

**Pathogenesis:** Unknown.

**POS No.:** 3696

**CDC No.:** 758.990

**Sex Ratio:** M4:F8 (Two of the males were identified prenatally).

**Occurrence:** About a dozen cases have been documented.

**Risk of Recurrence for Patient's Sib:** If both parents are chromosomally normal, the recurrence risk should be very small. When one parent is a balanced translocation carrier the theoretical risk is 1:3, and in the large pedigree published by Leschot et al (1979) 8:28 at risk pregnancies were affected (five chromosomally documented and three by history).

**Risk of Recurrence for Patient's Child:** No affected individuals are known to have reproduced.

**Age of Detectability:** Prenatally.

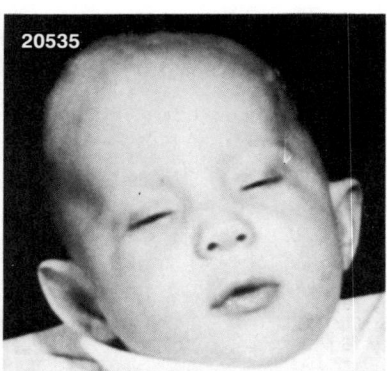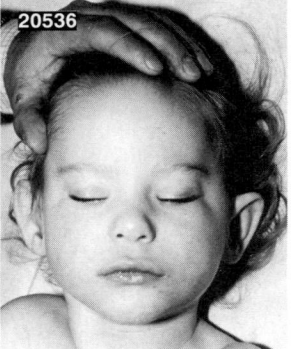

**2469-20535–36:** Chromosome 16, trisomy 16p; subject at 3 months and 2 years respectively, note round facies with scanty eyelashes and brows.

**Gene Mapping and Linkage:** See *Gene Map*.

**Prevention:** None known. Genetic counseling indicated.

**Treatment:** Symptomatic treatment of seizures.

**Prognosis:** Poor. Many cases have died in infancy, and all have been profoundly delayed.

**Detection of Carrier:** Chromosomal analysis.

**References:**
Yunis E, et al.: Partial trisomy 16q-. Hum Genet 1977; 38:347–350. †
Roberts SH, Ducket DP: Trisomy 16p in a liveborn infant and a review of partial and full trisomy 16. J Med Genet 1978; 15:375–381. †"
Dallapiccola B, et al.: De Novo trisomy 16q11→pter. Hum Genet 1979; 49:1–6.
Leschot NJ, et al.: Five familial cases with a trisomy 16p syndrome due to translocation. Clin Genet 1979; 16:205–214. * †
Gabbarron-Llamas J, et al.: Trisomia parcial 16p "de novo". An Esp Pediatr 1981; 15:587–91. †
Golden NL, et al.: Abnormality of chromosome 16 and its phenotypic expression. Clin Genet 1981; 19:41–45. * †
McMorrow LE, et al.: Partial trisomy 16p due to maternal balanced translocation. J Med Genet 1984; 21:315–16.

WA037                         **John R. Waterson**

## CHROMOSOME 16, TRISOMY 16Q     2470

**Includes:**

    Chromosome 16, mosaic trisomy 16q

    Chromosome 16, partial trisomy 16q

    Chromosome 16, proximal 16p trisomy

**Excludes:**

    **Chromosome 16, monosomy 16q** (2519)

    **Chromosome 16, trisomy 16p** (2469)

    Chromosome 16, other anomalies

**Major Diagnostic Criteria:** Postnatal growth failure; pronounced psychomotor retardation; characteristic craniofacial anomalies, including high forehead and enlarged metopic suture; prominent nose with broad tip; diminished upper lip; micrognathia and low-set, poorly formed ears; short neck; imperforate or otherwise abnormally placed anus; **Ductus arteriosus, patent**; and a variety of X-ray and positional abnormalities, particularly in the vertebrae, hands, and feet. Hand X-rays may show absent or hypoplastic phalanges with sclerotic tufts at the tips of the distal phalanges, as well as shortened metacarpals and metatarsals. The presence of three doses of some or all of 16q material on a well-banded karyotype provides definitive evidence.

**Clinical Findings:** All but two of the known cases (one with ring 16; another with partial 16q duplication) are the results of translocations and have another accompanying trisomic and sometimes a monosomic segment. The clinical findings, therefore, most likely represent a composite of findings arising from at least two separate cytogenetic abnormalities.

Parental ages were not elevated, and most infants were full term. Placental abnormalities such as polyhydramnios and falling estriol levels were occasionally noted. Almost all infants had decreased birth measurements, including head circumference. Most had obvious congenital anomalies and were identified cytogenetically in the newborn period, but several were studied during childhood because of retardation or the identification of a familial translocation.

Poor or absent suck and generalized hypotonia were noted in all patients; a few have also developed hypertonia in the lower extremities. Poor myelination has been noted in several patients, and one male had seizures at age 3 1/2 years. All patients showed significant neurologic impairment. One child scored an IQ of 43 at age five months; another was severely retarded at age 3 1/2 years.

The craniofacial findings vary, and they overlap with findings seen in cases of 16p trisomy, 16q monosomy, and phenotypes associated with the accompanying extra or missing chromosomal material. Features in the majority of cases include an asymmetric skull; a high forehead with some bitemporal narrowing and frontal bossing; an open metopic suture; hypertelorism, often with short, downward-slanting palpebral fissures and epicanthal folds; periorbital edema in the newborn period; a short, prominent nose with a high, flattened bridge and a broadened, bulbous tip; a thin upper lip that may not be visible; and retro- and micrognathia and ears that are prominent, low-set, posteriorly rotated, and poorly formed. Several children have had decreased or absent eyelashes, and one had an ectropion of the lower lid. Unequal orbits; deeply set globes, corneas, and pupils; and strabismus have been noted.

All patients have had short necks. Various thoracic configurations are present, such as short, hypoplastic sternum; **Pectus excavatum**; long, narrow thorax; short, narrow ribs; and low-set, widely spaced nipples. Scoliosis with or without kyphosis and gibbus formation occurs in at least 50% of patients, with multiple vertebral anomalies, particularly hemivertebrae and bony fusions, noted on X-ray. Poor ossification and demineralization, especially of cranial bones, is also seen.

Skeletal maturation is delayed in all patients. Contractures, particularly at the elbow, clenched fists with some overlapping of the fingers, and **Camptodactyly** have occurred in more than one-half of patients. The fingers are often short and rounded. Fifth finger clinodactyly is found in all patients, and simian or other unusual palmar creases in 30%. Two had triphalangeal thumbs with poor or absent opposition. The feet often show a hammer toe, with a gap between the first two toes and some metatarsal shortening. In several patients, the middle phalanx is hypoplastic or missing. X-rays also show an unusual sclerosis of the tufts of the distal phalanges of both hands and feet. Some positional deformities such as metatarsus adductus, pes valgus, equinovarus, genu valgus, talus valgus, and calcaneovalgus are encountered in all cases.

More than one-half of the patients have had a heart murmur, with PDA, **Ventricular septal defect**, **Atrial septal defects**, and abnormal branching of the aortic arches noted. Malrotation of the gut has been present in one-third of the patients. Genital anomalies occur in most male patients. These include ambiguous genitalia, hypospadias, small penis, bifid scrotum, and undescended testicles. Female defects are less obvious, but are likely present also. The anus is abnormal in all patients, with anterior displacement and imperforation being the most common defects, followed by an opening into a common cloaca or the presence of an anovesicular fistula.

The skin has been noted to be abnormal in about 50% of patients. Several have shown excess friability; others report dry or excessively wrinkled skin. A temporal scalp defect was present in one patient, a low hairline in another, and hypertrichosis in two. Most patients have a congenital decrease in subcutaneous fat.

**Complications:** Most are secondary to the major malformations, and functional disabilities caused by the extra 16q material, as well as any associated extra or deleted chromosomal material. The inadequate suck and repeated vomiting coupled with major organ anomalies perpetuate growth failure. About 25–50% have prolonged or intractable diarrhea, and some develop a necrotizing enterocolitis. The hypotonia and CNS abnormalities result in developmental retardation and contribute to seizures and repeated bouts of aspiration pneumonia. Frequent apneic episodes occur.

**Associated Findings:** Microphthalmia, sensorineural hearing loss, ectropion, deficient eyelashes, preauricular pit, hypoplastic sternum, pectus, genu valgus, and absent toe have each been noted in only one or two patients. Omphalocele with **Diaphragmatic hernia**, ambiguous genitalia, hypospadias, **Cleft palate**, and thymic hypoplasia have each been reported in one patient. Biliary and liver defects and abnormal lobulation of the liver and lung are occasionally reported. A single umbilical artery has been noted in two patients.

**Etiology:** All cases but two show an unbalanced karyotype resulting from the segregation of a parental translocation. The exceptions involved a ring 16 chromosome with 4% mosaicism for dicentric rings, and a duplication of a portion of 16q. Two more mothers than fathers carried the translocation. 15p was involved

in the translocation in three cases, and 21p and 21q each in two apiece. Chromosomes 9, 11, 18, 20, and 22 have also been involved. Most patients are only trisomic for a portion of the 16q arm, with only two infants showing translocations of most or all of 16q. The patients were either partially trisomic or monosomic for some portion of the other chromosome(s) involved in the translocation. No cases of "pure" complete trisomy 16q exist. The duplicated 16q patient appears to have an isolated partial trisomy for the 16q13-q24 segment.

Trisomy 16 is the most common autosomal trisomy seen in early spontaneous abortions, but it is rarely seen in live births or stillborns and is usually associated with abnormal, disorganized, poorly developed fetuses. Trisomy 16p and 16q have been similarly implicated in early miscarriages. Families with rearrangements involving chromosome 16 frequently show early pregnancy losses. All this supports the current belief that the excess (and possibly also the absence) of some or all of chromosome 16 is usually lethal to the embryo.

**Pathogenesis:** Unknown.

**POS No.:** 3712

**CDC No.:** 758.990

**Sex Ratio:** M8:F10 (observed).

**Occurrence:** Less than 25 cases have been reported in the literature.

**Risk of Recurrence for Patient's Sib:** The presence of a parental rearrangement raises the risk for unbalanced gametes and embryos. Since most fetuses are unlikely to survive past the first trimester, the risk of a liveborn child with an unbalanced karyotype is unknown, but likely to be quite small. There are two families reported in which a second sib with some degree of trisomy 16q has been born. In one family the mother was the balanced carrier, the father in the other. The usual disparity in risks between female and male translocation carriers may be less relevant with this abnormality.

**Risk of Recurrence for Patient's Child:** Affected individuals are not expected to survive to reproduce.

**Age of Detectability:** Prenatally by cytogenetic studies from chorionic villi or amniotic fluid cell culture, should the fetus survive until the second trimester. All reported cases, however, were studied postnatally. The characteristic dysmorphic phenotype and pattern of anomalies is likely to be recognizable at birth.

**Gene Mapping and Linkage:** See *Gene Map.*

**Prevention:** None known. Genetic counseling indicated. It is possible to use artificial insemination or surrogate motherhood for carrier parents.

**Treatment:** The abnormal anal orifice and the gut malrotation usually require neonatal surgical repair. Most infants require gavage feeding, apnea monitoring, and other symptomatic and supportive therapy. The deformities of the spine and extremities may require orthopedic intervention. Developmental stimulation is indicated for those who survive the neonatal period.

**Prognosis:** The congenital anomalies, particularly cardiac defects, significant feeding difficulties, and repeated aspirations, have precipitated early deaths in all but three children. One child survived to age six years, and two others into their fourth year. Prolonged survival seems unlikely. All survivors are severely retarded.

**Detection of Carrier:** Cytogenetic and clinical examination.

**Special Considerations:** Many of the phenotypic features seemingly caused by an excess of 16q material have also been seen in some cases of **Chromosome 16, trisomy 16p** and in many cases of **Chromosome 16, monosomy 16q**. Examples include large forehead; wide metopic suture; hypertelorism; broad, flat nasal bridge; dysmorphic, low-set ears; micrognathia; clinodactyly; overlapping fingers; distal joint contractures and camptodactyly; and abnormal great toe and positional foot deformities. Congenital heart disease, imperforate anus, omphalocele, malrotated gut, umbilical and inguinal hernias, and genital hypoplasia with or without cryptorchidism are also found in both groups. Growth and developmental retardation, hypotonia, and feeding difficulties occur independent of any specific cytogenetic abnormality. It seems possible, therefore, that any perturbation of chromosome 16, although usually incompatible with life, can give rise to a fairly predictable and consistent pattern of dysmorphogenesis. Renal anomalies may be peculiar to 16q monosomy, while cutaneous lesions, vertebral anomalies, absent phalanges or digits, and the presence of a cloaca may be more specific for trisomy 16q.

**References:**

Schmickel R, et al.: 16q trisomy in a family with a balanced 15/16 translocation. BD:OAS XI(5). New York: March of Dimes Birth Defects Foundation, 1975:229–236. †

Balestraszzi P, et al.: Partial trisomy 16q resulting from maternal translocation. Hum Genet 1979; 49:229–235. †

Rethore MO, et al.: Increased activity of adenine phosphoribosyl transferase in a child trisomic for 16q22.2: 16qter due to malsegregation of a t(16;21) (q22.2;q22.2)pat [In French]. Ann Genet (Paris) 1982; 25:36–42. †

Calva P, et al.: Partial trisomy 16q resulting from maternal translocation 11p/16q. Ann Genet (Paris) 1984; 27:122–125. *

de Grouchy J, Turleau C: Clinical atlas of human chromosomes, ed 2. New York: John Wiley & Sons, 1984. *

Hatanaka K, et al.: Trisomy 16q13-qter in a[n] infant from a t(11;16) (q25;q13) translocation-carrier father. Hum Genet 1984; 65:311–315.

CA016        **Mary Esther Carlin**

**Chromosome 17, deletion 17p13**
   *See LISSENCEPHALY SYNDROME*
**Chromosome 17, duplication 17q2**
   *See CHROMOSOME 17, TRISOMY 17q2*
**Chromosome 17, interstitial deletion 17 (p11.2;p11.2)**
   *See CHROMOSOME 17, INTERSTITIAL DELETION 17p*

## CHROMOSOME 17, INTERSTITIAL DELETION 17P    2513

**Includes:**
   Chromosome 17, interstitial deletion 17 (p11.2;p11.2)
   Smith-Magenis syndrome

**Excludes:**
   **Lissencephaly syndrome** (0603)
   **Prader-Willi syndrome** (0823)

**Major Diagnostic Criteria:** Interstitial deletion of chromosome 17p11.

**Clinical Findings:** Brachycephaly (15/15); flat midface (16/16); prominent forehead (15/15); broad face (14/15); broad nasal bridge (13/16); prominent jaw (10/16); delayed dentition (6/13); down-turned upper lip (8/14); nalformed, malpositioned ears (13/16); strabismus (6/12); short, broad hands (10/11); digital anomalies (9/13); congenital heart defects (7/16); genital anomalies (6/15); infantile hypotonia (5/8); seizures (5/10); short stature/growth delay (12/16); **Microcephaly** (6/16); mental retardation (16/16); speech delay (14/15); hearing loss (9/16); and hoarse, deep voice (5/10).

**Complications:** Hyperactivity and self-destructive behavior have been observed in over 75% of patients.

**Associated Findings:** Relative obesity with short stature, craniosynostosis, cleft lip/palate, iris coloboma, scoliosis, hemivertebrae, sacral lipoma, renal anomalies.

**Etiology:** *De novo* interstitial chromosomal deletion in all known cases.

**Pathogenesis:** Unknown.

**CDC No.:** 758.990

**Sex Ratio:** M10:F6 (observed).

**Occurrence:** Twenty cases have been reported, and at least four additional cases have been observed. All racial groups have been represented.

**Risk of Recurrence for Patient's Sib:** Probably not increased.

**Risk of Recurrence for Patient's Child:** Probably 1:2 (50%), if fertile.

**Age of Detectability:** The earliest diagnosis was at three months. Mean age at diagnosis was 15 years of age.

**Gene Mapping and Linkage:** See *Gene Map.*

**Prevention:** None known. Genetic counseling indicated.

**Treatment:** Supportive care.

**Prognosis:** Life expectancy is unknown. However, one patient was diagnosd at age 65 and four patients were over 20 years of age at diagnosis. All reported patients have been moderately to severely retarded, with the greatest delay in speech. All older patients were ambulatory.

**Detection of Carrier:** Chromosome analysis.

**Special Considerations:** Self destructive behavior is a common feature of this condition. For that reason, this syndrome should be considered along with **Lesch-Nyhan syndrome** in children with self-mutilatory behavior.

**References:**

Patil SR, Bartley JA: Interstitial deletion of the short arm of chromosome 17. Hum Genet 1984; 67:237–238.

Smith ACM, et al.: Interstitial deletion of (17) (p11.2p11.2) in nine patients. Am J Med Genet 1986; 34:393–414. * †

Stratton RF, et al.: Interstitial deletion of (17) (p11.2p11.2): report of six additional patients with a new chromosome deletion syndrome. Am J Med Genet 1986; 24:421–432. * †

Lockwood D, et al.: Chromosome subband 17p11.2 deletion: a minute deletion syndrome. J Med Genet 1988; 25:732–737.

GR011        **Frank Greenberg**

**Chromosome 17, monosmy 17p13**
   *See LISSENCEPHALY SYNDROME*
**Chromosome 17, partial trisomy 17**
   *See CHROMOSOME 17, TRISOMY 18*
**Chromosome 17, trisomy 17**
   *See CHROMOSOME 18, TRISOMY 18*

## CHROMOSOME 17, TRISOMY 17Q2    2471

**Includes:** Chromosome 17, duplication 17q2

**Excludes:** **Lissencephaly syndrome** (0603)

**Major Diagnostic Criteria:** Duplication of the distal portion of the long arm of chromosome 17.

**Clinical Findings:** Holoprosencephaly, polymicrogyria, broad forehead, widow's peak, broad midface, narrow palpebral fissures, **Cleft palate**, short neck, scoliosis, wide-spaced nipples, sacral dimple, shortening of proximal limbs, brachydactyly, **Syndactyly**, **Polydactyly**, genital anomalies, renal defects, and congenital heart defects.

**Complications:** Unknown.

**Associated Findings:** Vary according to type of chromosomal defect. Additional findings may be present if there is a partial monosomy of another chromosome due to a translocation or due to a combined deficiency of 17p due to a peri- or paracentric inversion of chromosome 17.

**Etiology:** Trisomy 17q2 due to unbalanced translocation. Duplication 17q2-deficiency 17p1 due to unbalanced peri- or paracentric inversion.
   All cases thus far have been due to parental rearrangement.

**Pathogenesis:** Unknown.

**CDC No.:** 758.990

**Sex Ratio:** M5:F5

**Occurrence:** At least 15 cases have been reported in the literature.

**Risk of Recurrence for Patient's Sib:** Increased if due to a parental balanced translocation of inversion. Low recurrence if due to a *de novo* event with normal parental chromosomes.

**Risk of Recurrence for Patient's Child:** Theoretically a 1:2 risk for fertile survivors.

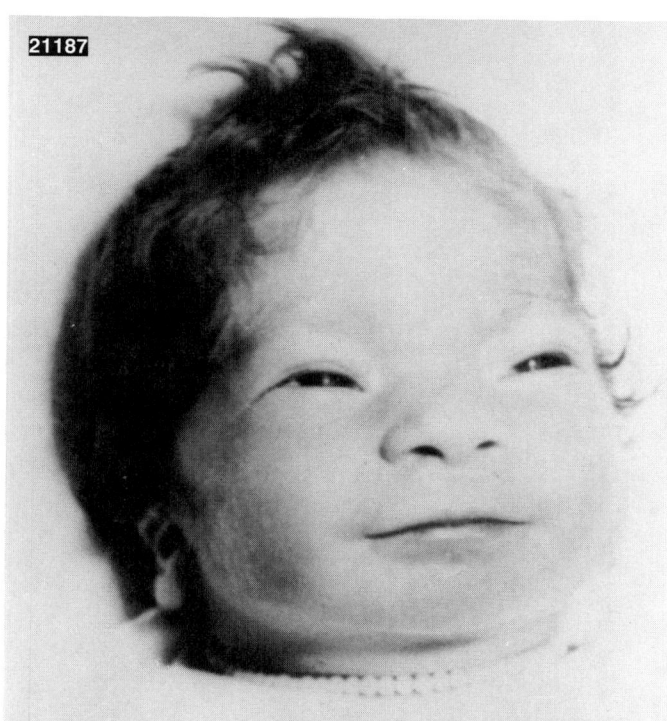

2471A-21187: Affected newborn shows hypertelorism with squinty eyes, long philtrum, and wide mouth.

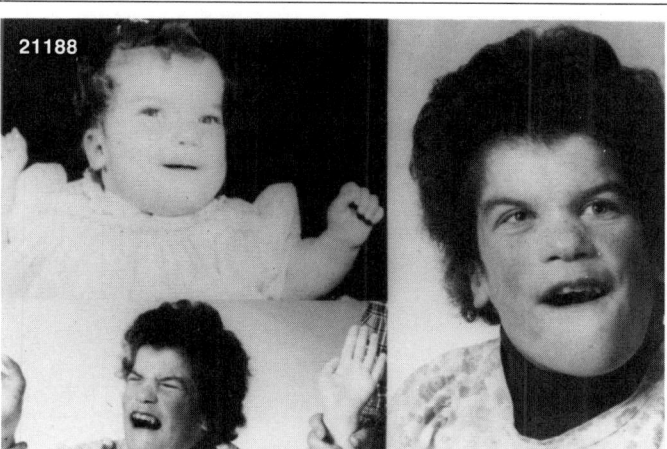

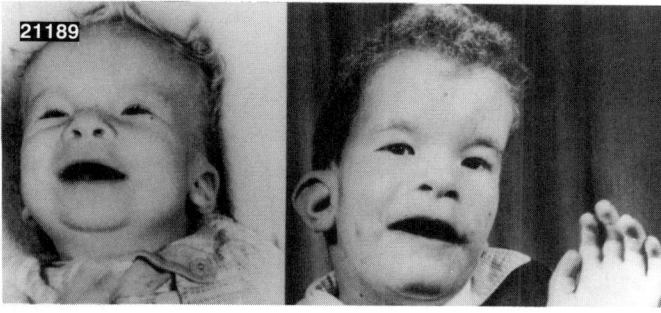

2471B-21188–89: Two individuals with chromosome 17p23 partial trisomy shown in infancy and at 17 years (upper) and 8 years (lower); note high forehead with widow's peak and temporal retraction; narrow palpebral fissures, low-set ears, long philtrum, and wide mouth.

**Age of Detectability:** May be detected prenatally by amniocentesis or chorionic villus sampling, or at birth.

**Gene Mapping and Linkage:** See *Gene Map.*

**Prevention:** None known. Genetic counseling indicated.

**Treatment:** Supportive.

**Prognosis:** Life expectancy unknown. All reported patients are mentally retarded.

**Detection of Carrier:** Chromosome analysis.

**References:**
de Grouchy J, Turleau C: Clinical atlas of human chromosomes, 2nd ed. New York: John Wiley & Sons, 1984:286–289.
Naccache NF, et al.: Duplication of distal 17q. Am J Med Genet 1984; 17:633–639.
Greenberg F, et al.: Familial Miller-Dieker syndrome associated with pericentric inversion of chromosome 17. Am J Med Genet 1986; 23:853–859.
Lenzini E, et al.: Partial duplication of 17 long arm. Ann Genet (Paris) 1988; 31:175–180.

GR011                                                    **Frank Greenberg**

**Chromosome 18, distal 18q trisomy (duplication)**
*See CHROMOSOME 18, TRISOMY 18q2*

---

## CHROMOSOME 18, MONOSOMY 18P                          0158

**Includes:** N/A

**Excludes:**
    **Chromosome 18, monosomy 18q** (0159)
    **Turner syndrome** (0977)

**Major Diagnostic Criteria:** Typical affected individuals have mental retardation, short stature, facial dysmorphism with round facies and prominent pinnae; skeletal abnormalities, and severe dental caries. A deletion involving the short arm of chromosome 18 should be demonstrated in at least a proportion of dividing cells.

**Clinical Findings:** In addition to low birthweight, there may be webbing of the neck, lymphedema, shield chest, and widely spaced nipples. Short stature is very common, as well as an extremely variable degree of mental retardation. Round facies, hypertelorism, epicanthic folds, strabismus, and ptosis are common, and the nasal bridge is generally flattened or broad. Nasal bones were absent in 1 case. The auricles tend to be large, floppy, poorly formed, and may be low-set. A small mandible and severe dental caries are common. Stubby hands with short fingers, high set thumbs, and partial syndactyly of the toes are seen. Less common malformations include microcephaly, cataract, cebocephaly, arhinencephaly, cleft lip and palate, cyclops deformity, and congenital alopecia. Mental retardation, ranging from borderline to profound, is present in virtually all patients. Among the mentally retarded patients, one also finds aphasia or dysphasia.

Negative findings of note are the absence of cardiac, renal or GI malformations, or characteristic dermatoglyphic changes.

**Complications:** Unknown.

**Associated Findings:** Absent or low IgA is reported; as is associated hypothyroidism, diabetes, or other autoimmune disorders. At least two patients have had growth hormone deficiency.

**Etiology:** Deletion of part or all of the short arm of chromosome 18, particularly band p11. Most cases represent de novo deletions.

**Pathogenesis:** Unknown.

**POS No.:** 3095

**CDC No.:** 758.350

**Sex Ratio:** M2:F3 (observed)

**Occurrence:** More than 70 known cases.

**Risk of Recurrence for Patient's Sib:** Very low except when a parent has a balanced translocation--then the recurrence risk may be as high as 1:4--or mosaicism, which has a similar though probably somewhat lower risk.

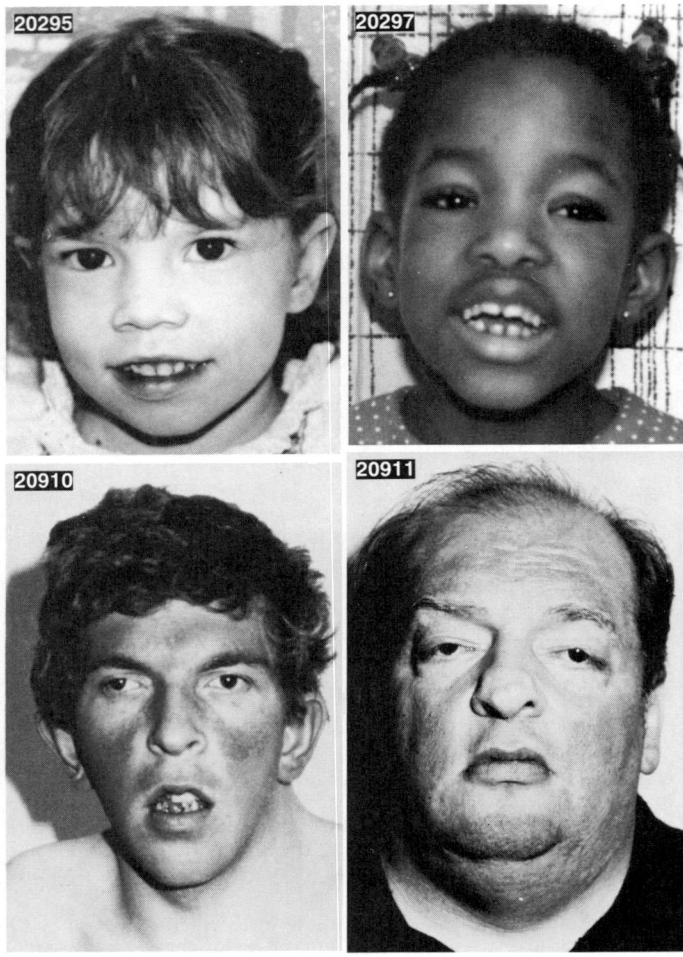

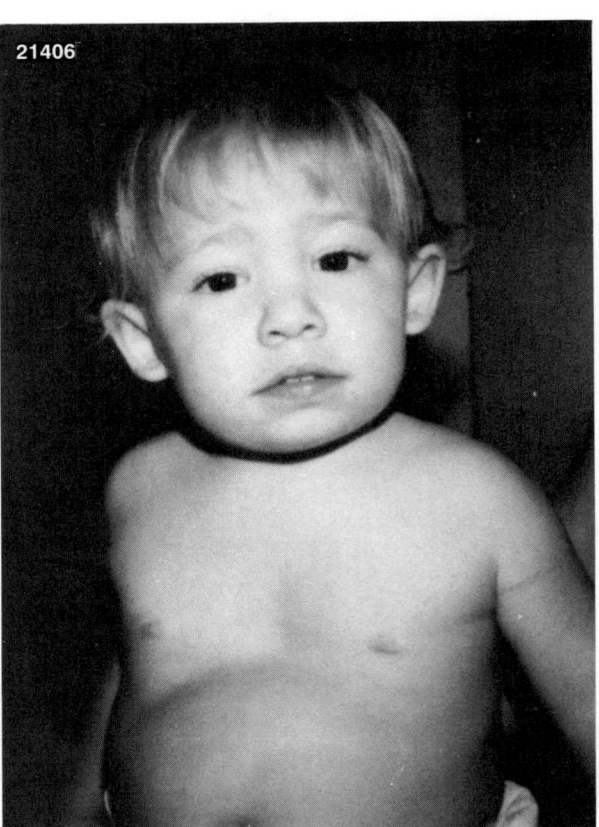

**0158B**-21406: A young girl with monosomy 18p (46,XX, del(18) (p11.1)). In addition to developmental and speech delay, note her rounded face, short upper lip, broad philtrum, everted lower lip and protruding ears.

**0158A**-20295: Girl with chromosome 18, monosomy 18p; note round facies, wide mouth and prominent ears. 20297: Note epicanthal folds, low nasal bridge, rounded facies, wide mouth and prominent ears. 20910–11: Facial stigmata in two affected adults.

Schinzel A, et al.: Structural aberrations of chromosome 18. I. The 18p syndrome. Archiv für Genetik 1974; 47:1–15. *
Wolfsberg EA, et al.: Trisomy 18 phenotype in a patient with iso-pseudodiantric 18 chromosome. J Med Genet 1984; 21:151–153.

GR011                                    **Frank Greenberg**

**Risk of Recurrence for Patient's Child:** Probably 50% if fertile, since occasional patients have produced affected offspring.

**Age of Detectability:** At birth or prenatally by karyotype study of fetal cells.

**Gene Mapping and Linkage:** See *Gene Map.*

**Prevention:** None known. Genetic counseling indicated.

**Treatment:** Unknown.

**Prognosis:** Dependent on severity of associated defects; otherwise life span not decreased.

**Detection of Carrier:** Balanced translocation carrier or mosaic detected only by karyotype analysis. At present, this would be looked for only after the birth of an affected child.

**Special Considerations:** Maternal and paternal ages tend to be advanced in contrast to the findings in other types of structural chromosomal abnormalities.

**References:**
de Grouchy J: The 18p, 18q and 18r syndromes. BD:OAS V. New York: March of Dimes Birth Defects Foundation, 1969: 74–87.
Lurie I, Lazjuk G: Partial monosomies 18. Humangenetik 1972; 15:203–222.

## CHROMOSOME 18, MONOSOMY 18Q                    0159

**Includes:** Chromosome 18, monosomy 18r (most cases)

**Excludes:** Chromosome 18, monosomy 18p (0158)

**Major Diagnostic Criteria:** The characteristic facial dysmorphism includes depressed midface, relative prognathion down-curved lips and folded pinnae; skeletal defects with dimples over limb joints; and ophthalmologic abnormalities should be seen. Demonstration of a deletion (18q or 18r) is confirmatory.

**Clinical Findings:** Characteristic findings include low birthweight, short stature, microcephaly, midface hypoplasia, prominent chin, carp-shaped mouth, prominent anthelix and antitragus, narrow or atretic ear canals, widely spaced nipples, very conspicuous subacromial dimples and dimples on the epitrochlea, the sides of the patellae and on the back of the hands. Long tapering fingertips, clubfoot. Hypotonia and mental retardation (profound) are common. Eye defects include nystagmus, strabismus, glaucoma, tapetoretinal degeneration and bilateral optic atrophy. Congenital heart disease is seen in over 25% of cases. Renal malformations are sometimes seen and genital defects are common. Whorls are frequently found in the dermatoglyphics.

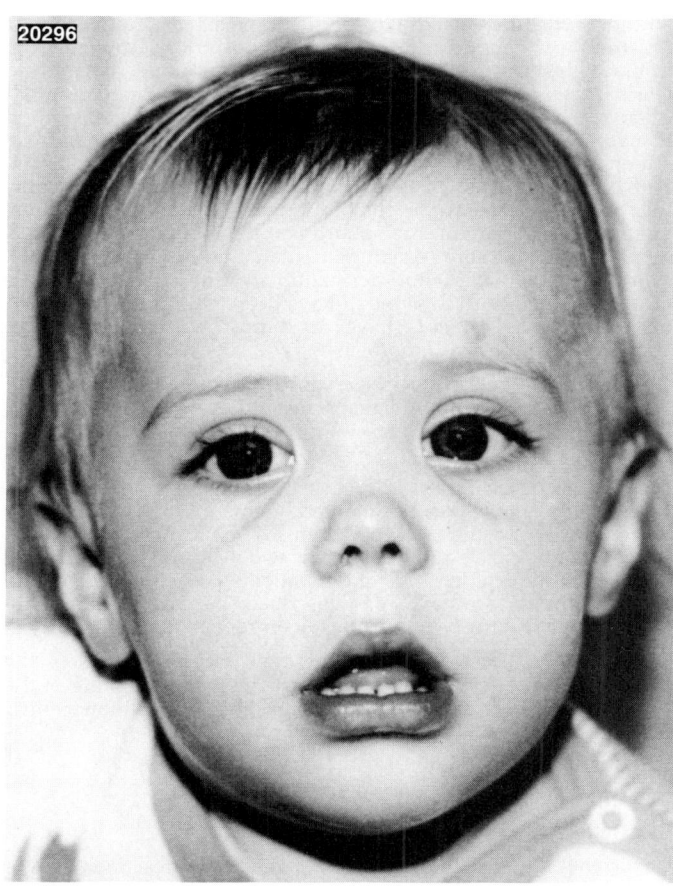

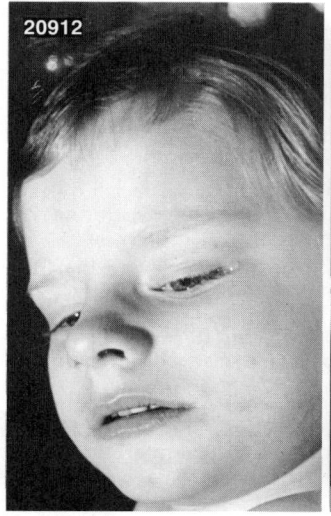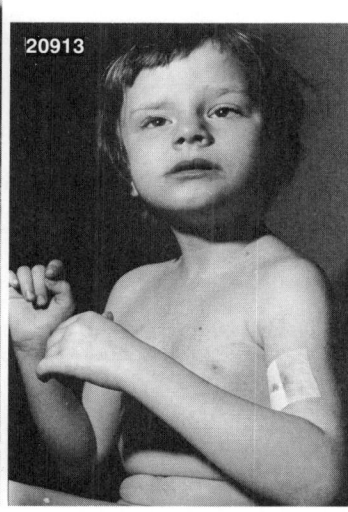

**0159B**-20912–13:  Chromosome 18, monosomy 18q; facial stigmata include deep-set eyes, small mid-face and carp-shaped mouth.

**0159A**-20296:  Girl with chromosome 18, monosomy 18q; note epicanthal folds, deep-set eyes and carp-shaped mouth.

**Prognosis:**  Moderate to severe mental retardation usually observed. Life expectancy is decreased.

**Detection of Carrier:**  Balanced translocation carrier or mosaic detectable by karyotype analysis.

**References:**
de Grouchy J: The 18q, 18q, and 18r syndromes. BD:OAS V. New York: March of Dimes Birth Defects Foundation, 1969:74–87.
Lurie I, Lazjuk G: Partial monosomies 18. Humangenetik 1972; 15:203–222.
Schinzel A, et al.: Structural aberrations of chromosome 18. II. The 18q syndrome: report of three cases. Humangenetik 1975; 26:123–132. *
Wilson MG, et al.: Syndromes associated with deletion of the long arm of chromosome 18 (del(18q)). Am J Med Genet 1979; 3:155–174. * †
Corney MJ, et al.: Early development of an infant with 18q syndrome. J Ment Defic Res 1984; 28:303–307.

GR011                                **Frank Greenberg**

**Chromosome 18, monosomy 18r (most cases)**
*See CHROMOSOME 18, MONOSOMY 18q*
**Chromosome 18, partial trisomy 18(pter q11:)**
*See CHROMOSOME 18, TRISOMY 18p AND q11*

**Complications:**  Seizures occur in a few cases.

**Associated Findings:**  Congenital heart disease and renal malformations. CNS malformations, including holoprosencephaly, are seen occasionally. IgA deficiency is seen in about 1/3 of cases, with increased tendency to infections and eczema. Lymphedema may occasionally occur.

**Etiology:**  Deletion of part of the long arm of chromosome 18, especially band 18q21.3.

**Pathogenesis:**  About 75% de novo deletions. About 10% result from inherited translocations.

**POS No.:**  3096

**CDC No.:**  758.340

**Sex Ratio:**  M1:F1.7

**Occurrence:**  More than fifty cases have been reported.

**Risk of Recurrence for Patient's Sib:**  Low, except when either parent is a balanced translocation carrier (5 of 57 families), where the risk may approach 1:4, or a mosaic (6 of 57 families), where the risk may be somewhat less.

**Risk of Recurrence for Patient's Child:**  Probably 50% if fertile. Transmission to offspring has been reported, although fertility is usually reduced.

**Age of Detectability:**  At birth, or by karyotype analysis of fetal cells.

**Gene Mapping and Linkage:**  See *Gene Map*.

**Prevention:**  None known. Genetic counseling indicated.

**Treatment:**  Symptomatic.

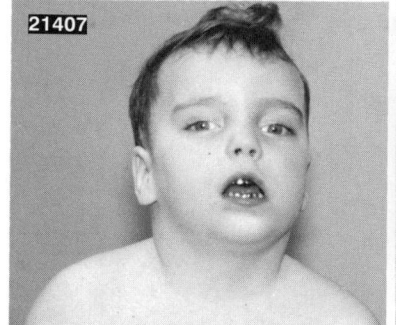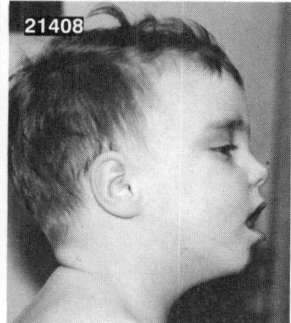

**0159C**-21407–08:  Characteristic facies with microcephaly, deep-set eyes, short nose, low-set ears with prominent anthelix, carp-shaped mouth, and small teeth.

# CHROMOSOME 18, RING 18      **2473**

**Includes:** Ring 18

**Excludes:**
> **Chromosome 18, monosomy 18p** (0158)
> **Chromosome 18, monosomy 18q** (0159)
> Chromosome 18, other anomalies

**Major Diagnostic Criteria:** Mental retardation, facial dysmorphism, **Microcephaly**, and hypotonia. Diagnosis is confirmed by cytogenetic analysis demonstrating a ring 18 chromosome.

**Clinical Findings:** The clinical picture is less severe than that presented by **Chromosome 18, monosomy 18q**, although some clinical features are found in both conditions. There are, however, no clinical features found exclusively in the 18 ring which enable differentiation from either **Chromosome 18, monosomy 18p** or **Chromosome 18, monosomy 18q**.

The clinical course of most patients includes growth retardation, moderate or severe mental deficiency, and increased infections during the first years of life. Normal puberty and fertility occurs. Hypotonia is present in 90% of the patients. **Microcephaly** is demonstrated in 75–90%, and more than two-thirds have epicanthus and/or hypertelorism. Ocular anomalies are found in at least 50% of affected patients, and may include strabismus, nystagmus, ptosis, partial aniridia, and microphthalmia. Malformation of the

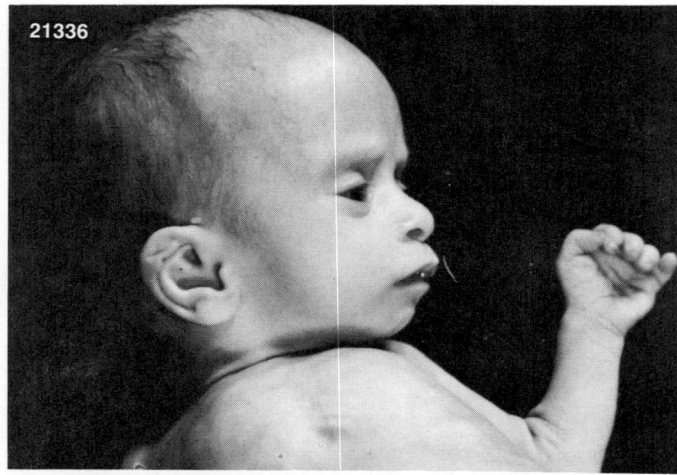

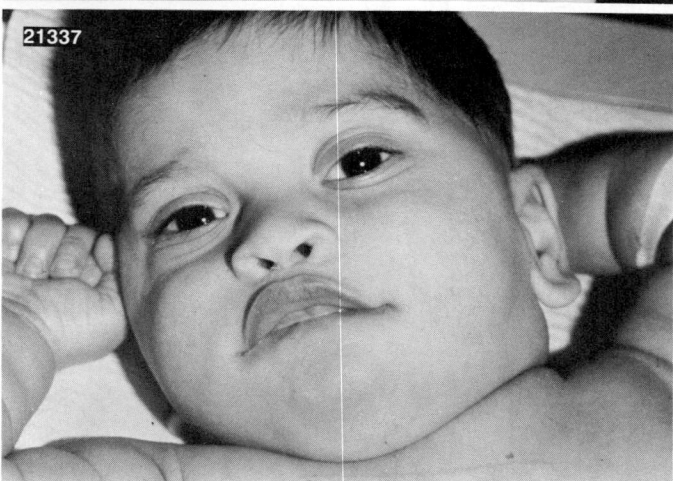

**2473-21336–37:** Chromosome 18, ring 18; note midface retraction, carp-shaped mouth and overfolded ears.

auditory structures include dysplasia of the external ears, stenotic or atretic ear canals, and low-set and posteriorly rotated ears. Midface dysplasia is very common. A short upper lip and an everted lower lip produces a characteristic "carp-shaped mouth". Microglossia is a frequent finding. Highly arched palate is found in over two-thirds of patients. Abnormalities of the mandible, either prognathia or micrognathia, are found in more than one-half of the patients. Skeletal anomalies of the vertebrae, ribs, micromelia, clinodactyly of the fifth finger and overlying toes may be found in more than three-quarters of the affected. Abnormalities of the genitalia are seen in more than one-fifth of the patients. More than 40% have whorl dermal fingerprint patterns in excess of normal. One-third to one-half have decreased or absent IgA. A minority of the patients have an almost normal phenotype, usually presenting with mosaicism.

**Complications:** Deafness is seen as a consequence of stenosis or atresia of the ear canal. Oligospermia was reported in an adult healthy male with mosaicism, who was otherwise normal.

**Associated Findings:** Holoprosencephaly with cebocephaly or cyclopia has been reported in five cases. Congenital heart and renal defects have also been noted. Other notable features reported are pterigyum colli, posterior low hair line implantation, funnel shaped chest, and hypoplastic widely spaced nipples. **Cleft palate** is found in at least 5% of the patients. Hypothyroidism and hypoparathyroidism have been described. Behavioral abnormalities may occur, and psychosis has been repeatedly observed.

**Etiology:** Deletion of part of the small and large arms of the chromosome 18, loss of the acentric fragments and joining of the ends of the short and long arms, forming a ring monocentric chromosome.

**Pathogenesis:** Unknown.

**CDC No.:** 758.990

**Sex Ratio:** M3:F5

**Occurrence:** More than 70 cases have been described in the literature.

**Risk of Recurrence for Patient's Sib:** Low except when either parent has a balanced translocation or mosaicism.

**Risk of Recurrence for Patient's Child:** Inheritance of ring chromosome 18 is uncommon, usually arising *de novo*. Transmission from parent to child has been reported in two families (the mother was affected in both cases).

**Age of Detectability:** Usually at birth, or by prenatal diagnosis.

**Gene Mapping and Linkage:** See *Gene Map*.

**Prevention:** None known. Genetic counseling indicated.

**Treatment:** Symptomatic.

**Prognosis:** Life span is normal.

**Detection of Carrier:** Cytogenetic analysis.

**Special Considerations:** Most authors suspect that the deletion occurs at 18p11 and 18q23. Fukushima et al (1984) reported a predisposition to autoimmune thyroiditis in ring chromosome 18; they found thyroiditis in four of five patients that they studied.

**References:**
Wang HC, et al.: Ring chromosome in human beings. Nature 1962; 195:733–734.
de Grouchy J: The 18p-,18q- and 18r syndromes. BD:OAS V. New York: March of Dimes Birth Defects Foundation, 1969:74–87.
Kunze J, et al.: Ring-chromosom 18. Ein 18p/18q-deletion syndrom. Humangenetik 1972; 15:289–318.
Schinzel A: Catalogue of unbalanced chromosome aberations in man. Berlin, New York: Walter de Gruyter, 1983:616–618.
Fukushima Y, et al.: Predisposition to autoinmune thydoitis in ring chromosome 18 syndrome. Jpn J Hum Genet 1984; 29:127–132.
Donlan MA, Dolan CR: Ring chromosome 18 in a mother and son. Am J Med Genet 1986; 24:171–174.

TR008       **Carlos J. Trujillo-Botero**

## CHROMOSOME 18, TETRASOMY 18P　　　2336

**Includes:** N/A

**Excludes:** N/A

**Major Diagnostic Criteria:** Moderate to severe mental retardation, signs of lesion of the pyramidal system, peculiar craniofacial dysmorphy, and demonstration of the cytogenetic abnormality.

**Clinical Findings:** The following features occur with a frequency of 50% or more in affected infants: subnormal birthweight (average 2,900 g) with normal gestation, moderate to severe mental retardation, signs of lesion of the pyramidal system (increased deep tendon reflexes, Babinski sign, ankle clonus, muscular hypertonia), feeding difficulties and vomiting, asthenic bodily habitus, small skull (sometimes microcephaly), dolichocephaly, delicate facies often referred to as chubby, pinched nose, small triangular mouth, high-arched palate, micrognathia, low-set ears, narrow shoulders and thorax, small iliac wings, absence of distal flexion creases on the fingers, simian creases, renal malformations (malrotation, **Kidney, horseshoe**, double ureter), and temporary immunologic deficiency (low serum IgA). Dermatoglyphics are fairly normal, though increased a-b ridge counts have been reported. Young and adult patients usually exhibit spasticity, abnormal gait, facial asymmetry, severe osteoarticular abnormalities (mainly thoracic kyphoscoliosis), limited speech, irritability, and destructive behavior. Less common findings include flat occiput, epicanthus, faun-like ears, short neck, cryptorchidism, overlapping fingers, **Camptodactyly**, **Syndactyly**, and adducted thumbs.

**Complications:** Unknown.

**Associated Findings:** Motor seizures, hypotelorism, convergent squint, **Cleft palate**, gum hypertrophy, pterygium colli, heart murmur, coxa valga, pes planus.

**Etiology:** This tetrasomy is due to an extra i(18p). The abnormal chromosome usually has a *de novo* origin; however, in 1/19 known cases, it was maternally inherited. The initial defect could be a centromere misdivision occurring during a germinal premeiotic mitosis, whereby a primary gametocyte would have either of the two isochromosomes formed. Then, the faulty pairing at meiosis I between the normal homolog and the isochromosome may determine their non-disjunction; consequently two n+1 and two n-1 gametes will be originated, the extra element being precisely the isochromosome.

**Pathogenesis:** Unknown.

**POS No.:** 3702

**CDC No.:** 758.990

**Sex Ratio:** M11:F8

**Occurrence:** About 20 cases have been documented.

**Risk of Recurrence for Patient's Sib:** Usually negligible.

**Risk of Recurrence for Patient's Child:** No patient has reproduced. If reproduction were to occur, the risk could be as high as 50%.

**Age of Detectability:** At birth or prenatally by chromosome studies.

**Gene Mapping and Linkage:** See *Gene Map.*

**Prevention:** None known. Genetic counseling indicated.

**Treatment:** Physiotherapy, kinesitherapy, special education.

**Prognosis:** Life span appears normal; mental and motor impairment are constant.

**Detection of Carrier:** Chromosome analysis: The only ''carrier'' known is a woman with 47 chromosomes, including a normal 18, a telocentric 18p- and an i(18p).

**References:**
Condron CJ, et al.: The supernumerary isochromosome 18 syndrome (+18pi). BD:OAS 1974; 10:36–42.
Taylor KM, et al.: Origin of a small metacentric chromosome: familial and cytogenetic evidence. Clin Genet 1975; 8:364–369.
Brondum Nielsen K, et al.: Small metacentric nonsatellited extra chromosome: report of five mentally retarded individuals and review of literature. Hum Genet 1978; 44:59–69. †
Batista DAS, et al.: Tetrasomy 18p: tentative delineation of a syndrome. J Med Genet 1983; 20:144–147.
Rivera H, et al.: Tetrasomy 18p: a distinctive syndrome. Ann Genet. 1984; 27:187–189. *
Fryns JP, et al.: 18p tetrasomy: further evidence for a distinctive clinical syndrome. Ann Genet 1985; 28:111–112. *

RI014　　　　　　　　　　　　　**Horacio Rivera**
CA011　　　　　　　　　　　　**José María Cantú**

## CHROMOSOME 18, TRISOMY 18　　　0160

**Includes:**

　　Chromosome E1-trisomy syndrome
　　Chromosome 17, partial trisomy 17
　　Chromosome 17, trisomy 17
　　Chromosome trisomy 17–18 syndrome
　　Edwards syndrome

**Excludes:**

　　**Chromosome 13, trisomy 13** (0168)
　　**Hutterite syndrome, Bowen-Conradi type** (2422)

**Major Diagnostic Criteria:** Should be suspected when an affected person has five or more of the clinical findings with frequency of 50% or greater. Chromosome study is urged in every instance because of serious implications.

**Clinical Findings:** Observed findings include developmental and mental retardation, failure to thrive, and cryptorchidism (each 100%); difficulty feeding with poor suck (> 95%); congenital heart disease [especially ventricular septal defect and patent ductus] (>

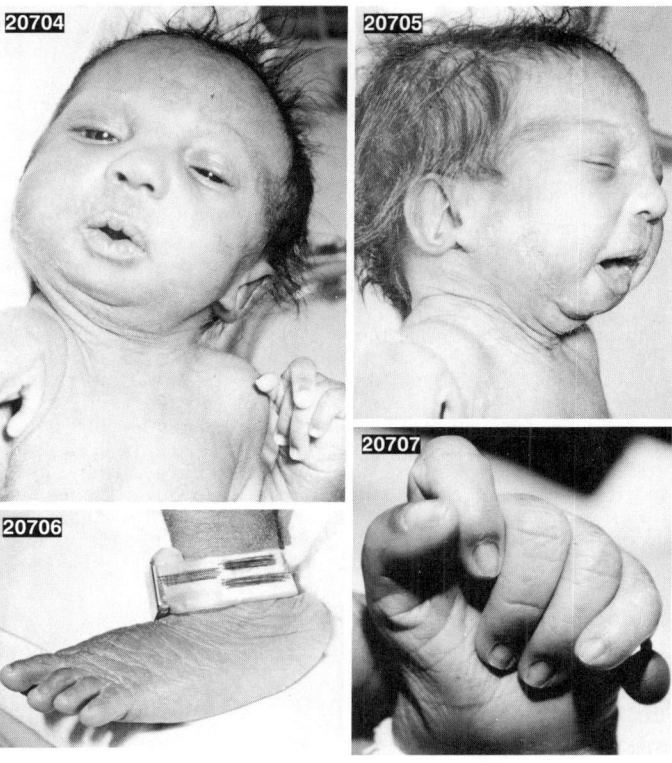

0160-20704: Chromosome 18, trisomy 18; note small mouth and epicanthal folds. 20705: Micrognathia and low-set ears with abnormal pinna. 20706: Rocker-bottom foot. 20707: Closed fist with characteristic overlapping fingers.

95%); fawn-like ears with pointed upper portion; low-set ears; prominent occiput with long skull; small biparietal diameter of skull; narrow palate; small mouth; micrognathia; short sternum; single umbilical artery; flexion deformity of fingers; overlapping fingers; simple arches on 6 or more digits; small, narrow pelvis; and limited hip abduction (all > 80%).

Additional findings include hypotonia followed by hypertonia; short neck; upturned nose; heart murmur; inguinal or umbilical hernia; distally located palmar axial triradius; short, dorsiflexed big toe; and rocker-bottom feet with prominent calcaneus (all 50–80%).

Renal malformations, especially horseshoe kidney and hydronephrosis and hydroureter have been reported in 50–80% of the cases.

Narrow palpebral fissures; retroflexible thumb; distally implanted thumb; extra skin nape of neck; calcaneovalgus feet; and meckel diverticulum have been reported in 40–60% of the cases.

Ten percent to as many as half of the cases have reported diaphragmatic hernia with eventration; ptosis of eyelids; epicanthal folds; corneal opacities; microphthalmos; short upper lip; brain or spinal cord malformation; webbed neck; wide-spaced small nipples; pyloric stenosis; syndactyly; ulnar or radial deviation of hands; single transverse palmar crease; single flexion crease on 5th finger; hypoplastic finger and toenails; and high-pitched cry.

Certain features which occur more frequently in 18 trisomy help to delineate this syndrome: hypertonia, high-pitched cry, prominent occiput, meningomyelocele, webbed neck, short sternum, eventration (thinning) of the diaphragm, pyloric stenosis, horseshoe kidney, hydronephrosis and hydroureter, Meckel diverticulum, limited hip abduction, distally implanted thumb, retroflexible thumb, partial syndactyly, hypoplasia of nails, simple arches on fingertips, short dorsiflexed big toe, talipes equinovalgus, and prominent calcaneus (rocker-bottom feet).

**Complications:** Severe disability and early death usually occur. Other complications are due to the specific defects.

**Associated Findings:** Severe feeding and respiratory (aspiration) problems.

**Etiology:** The cause of 18 trisomy with 47 chromosomes is nondisjunction during meiosis. Cases of 18 trisomy/normal mosaicism involve, in addition, postzygotic nondisjunction or anaphase lag. The causes of meiotic and mitotic nondisjunction involving chromosome 18 are unknown. The factors by which advancing maternal age increases the risk of meiotic nondisjunction are also unknown. Eighteen trisomy syndrome results from triplication of part or all of chromosome 18 in some or all of the patient's cells. This may be due to trisomy/normal mosaicism, or a translocation resulting in partial trisomy. Except in the case of inherited translocations, the parent donating the extra chromosome material has not, in most cases, been identified, although the association between 18 trisomy and increasing maternal age makes it likely that the mother is the more common contributor of the extra chromosome.

The bands of chromsome 18 which all patients with partial duplication 18 and typical 18 trisomy phenotype have in common are 18q11-q12. The finding of a newly specific syndrome in an individual with partial 18q12 trisomy due to intrachromosomal duplication, demonstrated that trisomy of band 18q12 is not accompanied by a full or incomplete trisomy 18 phenotype indicating that this phenotype is due to duplication of the sole 18q11 band.

**Pathogenesis:** Unknown.

**MIM No.:** 25730

**POS No.:** 3094

**CDC No.:** 758.2

**Sex Ratio:** At birth M1:F1.8, after 3 months M1:F2.9

**Occurrence:** Incidence 1:6600 live births in North America and Great Britain. Incidence may be notably higher than 1:6600 live births in series including low birth weight babies. Prevalence very low because of high mortality in infancy.

**Risk of Recurrence for Patient's Sib:** Probably no greater than 1%.

**Risk of Recurrence for Patient's Child:** Affected individuals are not expected to survive to reproduce.

**Age of Detectability:** For suspected cases, in midgestation, by amniotic fluid cell culture with chromosomal analysis. Elevated AFP in amniotic fluid. Ultrasonography shows unusual shaped fetal trunk, small fetal head and chest, and hydramnios.

**Gene Mapping and Linkage:** See *Gene Map*.

**Prevention:** None known. Genetic counseling indicated.

**Treatment:** Unknown.

**Prognosis:** The diagnosis should be carefully confirmed by chromosome analysis since the prognosis is poor: 30% of patients die by 1 month of age, 50% by 2 months, 70% by 3 months, 90% by 1 year, and 99% before age 10. The survivors are profoundly retarded in motor and intellectual development. None has been able to walk, talk or procreate. The usual causes of death are aspiration, apnea or congenital heart disease. The prognosis may, however, be significantly better in patients with mosaicism or "partial trisomy" due to translocation.

**Detection of Carrier:** A parent or sibs of an affected child who has "partial trisomy" due to translocation may have a balanced translocation. High-risk families may also be identifiable by careful pedigree and chromosome studies.

**Special Considerations:** The findings during pregnancy are characteristic with trisomy 18. There is polyhydramnios, small placenta, decreased fetal movement and small biparietal diameter of the fetal head. Postmaturity is the rule with mean duration of pregnancy being 42 weeks. An increasing number of 18 trisomies are diagnosed in the second and third trimesters by echographic examination. Echographic findings include severe symmetrical growth retardation, oligoamnios, and associated congenital malformations; i.e. omphalocoele, cleft lip/cleft palate, and meningomyelocele.

The most helpful diagnostic test on a clinical level after birth is dermatoglyphic inspection of the fingers and especially toes in search of simple digital arch patterns.

The most rapid laboratory test to confirm the diagnosis of trisomy 18 is bone marrow aspiration with direct chromosome analysis.

**Support Groups:** UT; West Jordan (801–882–6635); Support Organization for Trisomy 18/13 (SOFT)

**References:**
Smith DW, et al.: The no. 18 trisomy syndrome. J Pediatr 1962; 60:513.
Hecht F, et al.: The no. 17–18 trisomy syndrome. Studies on cytogenetics, dermatoglyphics, parental age and linkage. J Pediatr 1963; 63:605.
Taylor AI: Autosomal trisomy syndromes: a detailed study of 27 cases of Edwards' syndrome and 27 cases of Patau's syndrome. Am J Med Genet 1968; 5:227.
Nielson J, et al.: Prevalence of Edwards syndrome. Clustering and seasonal variation? Humangenetik 1975; 26:113.
de Grouchy J, Turleau C: Clinical atlas of human chromosomes. New York: John Wiley & Sons, 1977:160–164. *
Turleau C, de Grouchy J: Trisomy 18 qter and trisomy mapping of chromosome 18. Clin Genet 1977; 12:361–371.
Ramirez-Castro JL, et al.: Anatomical analysis of the developmental effects of aneuploidy in man. The 18 trisomy syndrome. Am J Med Genet 1978; 2:285.
Fryns JP, et al.: Partial trisomy 18q12, due to intrachromosomal duplication, is not associated with typical 18 trisomy phenotype. Hum Genet 1979; 46:341–344.

HE007   **Frederick Hecht**
HE008   **Barbara K. Hecht**

## CHROMOSOME 18, TRISOMY 18P AND Q11     2550

**Includes:** Chromosome 18, partial trisomy 18(pter q11:)

**Excludes:** Chromosome 18, other anomalies

**Major Diagnostic Criteria:** Arthrogrypotic and malformative features of the full trisomy 18 phenotype, except for milder visceral damage and longer survival; cytogenetic evidence of trisomy 18pter q11.

**Clinical Findings:** History of polyhydramnios, low birth weight, hypertonia, low-pitched cry, psychomotor retardation, and protracted survival. Malformations include **Microcephaly**, hypotelorism, small and thin nose with a depressed bridge, narrow palate, micrognathia, malformed ears with meatal hypoplasia, short neck with redundant skin folds, narrow shoulders and pelvis, short sternum, wide-spread nipples, chubby and radially deflected hands, distal narrowing of fingers, **Aorta, coarctation**, caput cuadratum, osteopenia, hypoplastic first rib pair, and acetabular dysplasia. Deformations included limited joint mobility, cubitus varus, knuckle dimples, digital flexure contractures and absence of distal flexure creases, pollux varus, and clubfoot. Other manifestations include hyperreflexia, abnormal EEG, and those resulting from unbalanced rearrangements when present. If the trisomy includes regions 18q12.1-q12.2, a full trisomy 18 phenotype may result.

**Complications:** Unknown.

**Associated Findings:** Repeated infections, strabismus, malocclusion, ambiguous external genitalia, cryptorchidism, zygodactyly.

**Etiology:** Trisomy was *de novo* in two cases, and resulted from a parental reciprocal translocation in three.

**Pathogenesis:** Unknown.

**CDC No.:** 758.990

**Sex Ratio:** M2:F3 (observed).

**Occurrence:** Less than ten cases have been reported.

**Risk of Recurrence for Patient's Sib:** Unknown. Increased when a parent carries a balanced rearrangement.

**Risk of Recurrence for Patient's Child:** No affected individuals have survived to reproduce.

**Age of Detectability:** At birth, or prenatally by chromosome analysis.

**Gene Mapping and Linkage:** See *Gene Map*.

**Prevention:** None known. Genetic counseling indicated.

**Treatment:** Surgery and rehabilitation depending on physical and functional effects.

**Prognosis:** Life span is longer than that seen in **Chromosome 18, trisomy 18**. One case has survived more than seven years.

**Detection of Carrier:** By chromosome analysis.

**References:**
Stern LM, et al.: Pseudohermaphroditism with clinical features of trisomy 18 in an infant trisomic for parts of chromosomes 16 and 18: 47,XY,der(18),t(16;18) (p12;q11)mat. J Med Genet 1975; 12:305–307.
Fried K, et al.: Partial 18 trisomy (with 47 chromosomes) resulting from a familial maternal translocation. J Med Genet 1978; 15:76–78.
Hernández A, et al.: De novo partial trisomy of chromosome 18(pter q11). Some observations on the phenotype mapping of chromosome 18 imbalances. Ann Genet 1979; 22:165–167.
Turleau C, et al.: Trisomy 18q-. Trisomy mapping of chromosome 18 revisited. Clin Genet 1980; 18:20–26.

C0073                                 **Enrique Corona-Rivera**
CA011                                 **José María Cantú**

## CHROMOSOME 18, TRISOMY 18Q2     2472

**Includes:** Chromosome 18, distal 18q trisomy (duplication)

**Excludes:**
    Chromosome 18, proximal 18q trisomy (duplication)
    **Chromosome 18, trisomy 18** (0160)
    **Chromosome 18, trisomy 18p and q11** (2550)
    Chromosome 18, other anomalies

**Major Diagnostic Criteria:** In contrast to **Chromosome 18, trisomy 18** and **Chromosome 18, trisomy 18p and q11**, the clinical findings in distal 18q trisomy are much more discrete. The craniofacial dysmorphism is the most constant finding with broad and high forehead, prominent nasal bridge, with absent frontonasal angle,

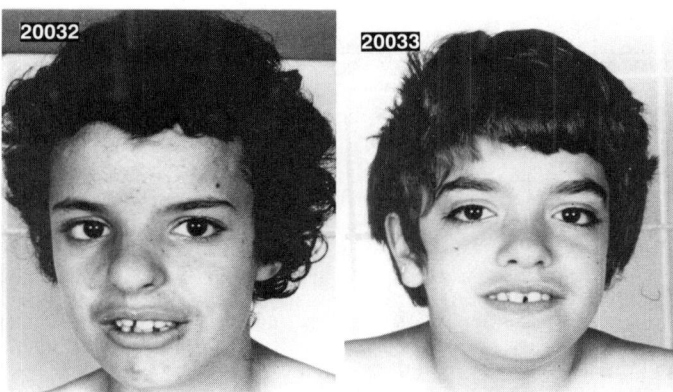

**2472-20032–33:** Similar craniofacial findings in two adults with 18q2 trisomy; note high and broad forehead, prominent nasal bridge, bulbous nasal tip, hypertelorism, and large mouth with full lips.

**2550-20514:** Chromosome 18, trisomy 18p & q1; note dysmorphic facies, short neck and contractures.

bulbous nasal tip, hypertelorism, and large mouth with full lips. Cytogenetic analysis confirms the diagnosis.

**Clinical Findings:**  Moderate pre- and postnatal growth retardation, severe mental retardation, discrete neurological symptoms, absence of evident internal malformations, and discrete dysmorphic features.

**Complications:**  Unknown.

**Associated Findings:**  Severe internal malformations are relatively rare.

**Etiology:**  All patients have shown a distal 18q trisomy involving at least bands 18q22 and 18q23. In the majority of cases the 18q2 duplication was the unbalanced product of a parental autosomal translocation involving 18q2 and another autosome.

**Pathogenesis:**  Unknown.

**POS No.:**  3966

**CDC No.:**  758.990

**Sex Ratio:**  M1:F1

**Occurrence:**  Less than 30 cases have been reported in the literature.

**Risk of Recurrence for Patient's Sib:**  Not increased if parental chromosomes are normal. Considerably increased (5–10%) if one of the parents is carrier of an autosomal balanced translocation involving 18q2.

**Risk of Recurrence for Patient's Child:**  Reproduction in affected patients is unlikely.

**Age of Detectability:**  During the first years of life by the presence of developmental delay and discrete dysmorphic features, or by prenatal diagnosis by CVS or amniocentesis.

**Gene Mapping and Linkage:**  See *Gene Map*.

**Prevention:**  None known. Genetic counseling indicated.

**Treatment:**  Unknown.

**Prognosis:**  Long-term prognosis seems to be good because of the absence of severe internal malformations.

**Detection of Carrier:**  Cytogenetic and clinical examination.

**References:**
Turleau C, de Grouchy J: Trisomy 18qter and trisomy mapping of chromosome 18. Clin Genet 1977; 12:361–371.
Fryns JP, et al.: Partial trisomy 18q12 due to intrachromosomal duplication is not associated with typical 18 trisomy phenotype. Hum Genet 1979; 46:341–344.
De Mûelenaere A, et al.: Familial partial distal 18q (18q22–18q23) trisomy. Clin Genet 1981; 24/3:184–186.

FR030                                                    **Jean-Pierre Fryns**

**Chromosome 19, other anomalies**
*See CHROMOSOME 19, TRISOMY 19q*

## CHROMOSOME 19, TRISOMY 19Q                    2474

**Includes:**  Chromosome 19, other anomalies

**Excludes:**  N/A

**Major Diagnostic Criteria:**  Karyotype showing trisomy for part or all of 19q. Severe mental retardation, facial dysmorphism, and inner organ malformations.

**Clinical Findings:**  Clinical signs may manifest in the neonate as feeding difficulties, seizures, and stridor. Growth is very retarded both pre- and postnatally. Microbrachycephaly is constant. Fontanelles are wide open. The facies is flat, with palpebral fissures slanting downward. There is enophthalmia with hypertelorism and frequent bilateral palpebral ptosis. The nose is small and snubbed with a flat nasal bridge. The philtrum is short and prominent. The mouth is abnormal with downturned corners. The ears are low-set.

The neck is short, and chest deformities are observed in most cases. Various deformities of the hands and feet may be present. In boys, external genitalia are usually abnormal.

Various congenital malformations of the inner organs have been reported: cardiac abnormalities of variable severity and digestive, renal, bronchial, and vertebral malformations. Most patients have neurologic disorders, mainly seizures.

**Complications:**  Complications occur as per inner organ malformations.

**Associated Findings:**  None known.

**Etiology:**  Out of nine known cases, eight are due to a parental translocation, two with a 22, one with a 20, and one with a 17. The breakpoint is in 19q13. The translocation is maternal in all known instances. The smallest common trisomic segment is 19q13.3→qter.

**Pathogenesis:**  Unknown.

**CDC No.:**  758.990

**Sex Ratio:**  M1:F1

**Occurrence:**  Nine cases have been reported, comprising three sib pairs and one nephew-uncle pair.

**Risk of Recurrence for Patient's Sib:**  Depends on the existence of a parental rearrangement. A high risk of recurrence is suggested because eight of nine cases were familial.

**Risk of Recurrence for Patient's Child:**  Reproduction has not been reported in affected individuals.

**Age of Detectability:**  At birth, or by prenatal diagnosis.

**Gene Mapping and Linkage:**  See *Gene Map*.

**Prevention:**  None known. Genetic counseling indicated.

**Treatment:**  Symptomatic care and management of inner organ malformations.

**Prognosis:**  Two sibs died in early infancy. The oldest reported patient was age 25 years. Mental retardation is usually severe.

**Detection of Carrier:**  By karyotyping.

**References:**
Lange M, Alfi OS: Trisomy 19q. Ann Genet 1976; 19:17–21.
de Grouchy J, Turleau C: Clinical atlas of human chromosomes, 2nd ed. New York: Wiley Medical, 1984.
Rivas F, et al.: 19q distal trisomy due to a de novo (19;22) (q13.2;p11) translocation. Ann Genet 1985; 28:113–115.

DE029                                                    **Jean de Grouchy**
TU013                                                    **Catherine Turleau**

## CHROMOSOME 20, PERICENTRIC INVERSION          2540

**Includes:**  N/A

**Excludes:**  Chromosome 20, paracentric inv20p or 20q

**Major Diagnostic Criteria:**  Carriers of pericentric inversions of chromosome 20 are clinically normal.

**Clinical Findings:**  In the two reported families, the index patients were identified after recurrent abortions, and after the birth of a malformed child with recombination aneusomy resulting from a maternal inv(20) (p11.209q1309), respectively.

**Complications:**  Unknown.

**Associated Findings:**  None known.

**Etiology:**  Familial occurence in inv(20) was documented in two reports. *De novo* occurence of inv(20) has not yet been reported.

**Pathogenesis:**  Unknown.

**CDC No.:**  758.990

**Sex Ratio:**  Presumably M1:F1.

**Occurrence:**  Reported in two families. In a total of 51,500 patients seen for constitutional chromosome analyses during the period 1970–1985 at the Leuven Centre, no pericentric inversions of chromosome 20 were detected.

**Risk of Recurrence for Patient's Sib:**  In families, the inversion is probably present in 50% of the family members.

**Risk of Recurrence for Patient's Child:** Of the 11 karyotyped offspring of inv(20) carriers, five had inherited the inversion, five were karyotypically normal, and one boy presented a recombinant chromosome 20.

**Age of Detectability:** Variable. Inv(20) probably remains undetected in a number of carriers in the absence of reproductive problems. Prenatal diagnosis, by (CVS or amniocentesis, can exclude recombination aneusomy in the offspring.

**Gene Mapping and Linkage:** See *Gene Map*.

**Prevention:** None known. Genetic counseling indicated.

**Treatment:** Unknown.

**Prognosis:** Unknown.

**Detection of Carrier:** By cytogenetic examination.

**References:**

Lucas J, et al: Trisomie 20p dérivée d'une inversion péricentrique maternelle et brachymésophalangie de l'index. Génét 1985; 28:167–171.

Groupe de Cytogénéticiens français: Pericentric inversion in man: a French collaborative study. Ann Génét 1986; 29:129–168.

FR030 **Jean-Pierre Fryns**

## CHROMOSOME 20, TRISOMY 20P 2475

**Includes:** N/A

**Excludes:** N/A

**Major Diagnostic Criteria:** Karyotype showing trisomy 20p. Psychomotor retardation and facial dysmorphism.

**Clinical Findings:** Pre- and postnatal development is normal, if not excessive. Mental retardation is moderate with poor motor coordination and speech delay and impediment. Craniofacial dysmorphism is slightly pronounced, but there is a striking likeness in all patients. The face is round with full cheeks. The hair is coarse. Palpebral fissures are slanted upward, with a fold in the upper eyelid and slight enophthalmia. There is usually hypertelorism. The nose is short with a flat bridge and large nares, which are sometimes anteverted. The chin is small. Tooth decay and dental anomalies are frequent. The ears are large, flat, and poorly folded.

Major malformations are not the rule. One can observe vertebral anomalies and nonspecific deformities (clinodactyly of the 5th finger, mild webbing of the toes, and so forth). Hypogonadism and hypospadias may occasionally be seen. Macroorchidism was reported in one case. Heart and kidney anomalies have been described.

**Complications:** Those due to inner organ and skeletal malformations. Two patients died from heart defects in early infancy. Kyphosis was reported in several instances.

**Associated Findings:** Assay of inosine triphosphatase (ITPA) activity shows gene dosage effect.

**Etiology:** In the majority of the cases, trisomy 20p results from a parental translocation with a breakpoint usually in 20p11. In one case, trisomy 20p resulted from recombination of a parental pericentric inversion, and two cases occurred *de novo*.

**Pathogenesis:** Unknown.

**POS No.:** 3099

**CDC No.:** 758.990

**Sex Ratio:** M1:F1

**Occurrence:** Rare or rarely identified due to mild phenotypic manifestations. Twenty cases have been reported.

**Risk of Recurrence for Patient's Sib:** Depends on the existence of a parental rearrangement, if present. In the case of pericentric inversion, the risk is difficult to evaluate. If there is no parental rearrangement, the risk is not increased.

**Risk of Recurrence for Patient's Child:** Reproduction has not been reported in affected individuals.

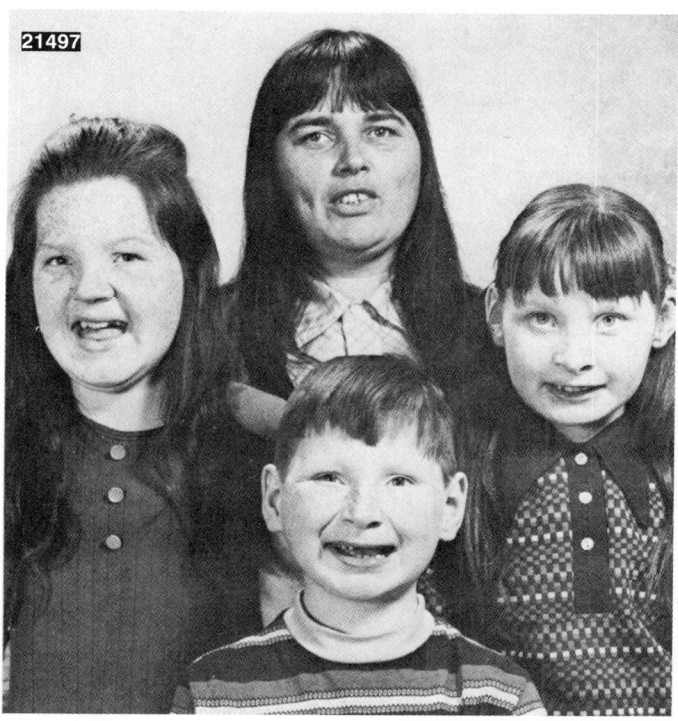

2475-21497: Three affected sibs with chromosome 20, partial trisomy 20p shown with their mother. Facial features of note include round facies with prominent cheeks, short chin, increased innercanthal distances, downward displacement of the medial corner of the palpebral fissures with upward displacement of the lateral part, short nose with broad upturned tip and large nares.

**Age of Detectability:** At birth clinically (or usually later due to mild manifestationsor) or by prenatal diagnosis.

**Gene Mapping and Linkage:** See *Gene Map*.

**Prevention:** None known. Genetic counseling indicated.

**Treatment:** Symptomatic care and management of inner organ malformations.

**Prognosis:** Two patients died from heart defects in early infancy. In the absence of inner organ malformations, the life span prognosis is good. The oldest known patient was aged 45 years at the time of examination. Mental retardation is mild to moderate, with coordination and speech impairment.

**Detection of Carrier:** By karyotyping.

**References:**

Francke U: Abnormalities of chromosomes 11 and 20. In: Yunis JJ, ed: New chromosomal syndromes. New York: Academic, 1977.

Balestrazzi P, et al.: "De novo" trisomy 20p with macroorchidism in a prepubertal boy. Ann Genet 1984; 27:58–59.

Grouchy J de, Turleau C: Clinical atlas of human chromosomes, 2nd ed. New York: Wiley Medical, 1984.

Bown N, et al.: Partial trisomy 20p resulting from a recombination of a familial pericentric inversion. Hum Genet 1986; 74:417–419.

DE029 **Jean de Grouchy**
TU013 **Catherine Turleau**

**Chromosome 21, deletion 21, pter-q21**
*See CHROMOSOME 21, MONOSOMY 21*

## CHROMOSOME 21, MONOSOMY 21      0170

**Includes:**
> Antimongolism
> Chromosome 21, deletion 21, pter-q21
> G deletion syndrome
> Chromosome 21, partial monosomy 21
> Chromosome 21, proximal 21 monosomy

**Excludes:** Chromosome 21 (other anomalies)

**Major Diagnostic Criteria:** Demonstration of a complete or partial deletion of a number twenty-one chromosome. Total monosomy 21 is very rare. Most reported cases have had involved translocations. Major phenotypic effects appear to result from complete or total loss of the number 21 long arm. There is marked clinical variability in reported cases with some unusual clinical features which may aid in establishing the diagnosis.

**Clinical Findings:** Historical features include intrauterine growth retardation, failure to thrive with recurrent respiratory and gastrointestinal illnesses, seizures, severe mental retardation (IQ below 50) and death usually before two years of age. A few infants have died neonatally with the oligohydramnios sequence.

Variable facial features include microcephaly, prominent nose, downslanting palpebral fissures, downturned mouth corners, micrognathia, and cleft lip and/or palate (about 50%). There are several reports of ocular abnormalities including microphthalmia, Peters anomaly of the iris, and cataracts.

Skeletal abnormalities mimicking arthrogryposis have been reported by multiple authors as have joint dislocations. Syndactyly of the fingers and ectrodactyly of the hands and feet have been noted rarely.

Abnormal genitalia have been reported in several male infants with a range of defects from cryptorchidism to frank ambiguity.

At autopsy, renal malformations including unilateral agenesis with contralateral cystic dysplasia has been noted. Variable central nervous system defects have included cortical atrophy, hypoplasia of the cerebellum, and brain stem, agenesis of the corpus callosum, dilated ventricles, and alobar holoprosencephaly.

**Complications:** Unknown.

**Associated Findings:** None known.

**Etiology:** Clinical findings are thought to be due to a deletion of all or part of the long arm of chromosome 21. Cytogenetic findings include complete monosomy, monosomy mosaicism, partial deletion of the long arm, translocations, or **Chromosome 21, ring 21.** The study of enzymatic markers localized to chromosome 21 (i.e. superoxidide dismutase-1 and liver phosphofructokinase) may prove useful in further study.

**Pathogenesis:** Undetermined, except in cases where a parent is a carrier of balanced translocation.

**POS No.:** 3598

**CDC No.:** 758.300

**Sex Ratio:** M1:F<1

**Occurrence:** Undetermined but presumed rare.

**Risk of Recurrence for Patient's Sib:** Probably low, except in cases of parental translocation.

**Risk of Recurrence for Patient's Child:** No affected individuals are known to have reproduced.

**Age of Detectability:** At birth.

**Gene Mapping and Linkage:** See *Gene Map.*

**Prevention:** None known. Genetic counseling indicated.

**Treatment:** Symptomatic.

**Prognosis:** Poor. Longest survivor lived to eleven years with profound mental retardation.

**Detection of Carrier:** By karyotype.

**References:**
Fryns JP, et al.: Full Monosomy 21. A clinically recognizable syndrome? Hum Genet 1977; 37:155–259.
Houston CS, Chudley AE: Separating monosomy-21 from the "arthrogryposis wastebasket" J de l'Assoc Canadienne des Radiologists 1981; 32:220–223.
Rivera J, et al.: "Pure" monosomy 21 pter-q21 in a girl born to a couple 46,XX,t(14;21)(p12;q22) and 46,XY,t(5;8)(q32;q22). Ann Genet 1983; 26:234–237.
Wisniewski K, et al.: Monosomy 21 syndrome: Further delineation including clinical, neuropathological, cytogenetic and biochemical studies. Clin Genet 1983; 23:102–110.
Pellissier MC, et al.: Monosomy 21: a new case confirmed by situ hybridization. Hum Genet 1987; 75:95–96.

CU009      **Cynthia J.R. Curry**

**0170-20920:** Chromosome 21, monosomy 21; infant with the complete monosomy. Findings include prominent nose and wide nasal bridge, large low-set ears, prominent eyes, microcephaly and broad philtrum.

**Chromosome 21, mosaic 21 syndrome**
*See CHROMOSOME 21, TRISOMY 21*
**Chromosome 21, partial monosomy 21**
*See CHROMOSOME 21, MONOSOMY 21*
**Chromosome 21, proximal 21 monosomy**
*See CHROMOSOME 21, MONOSOMY 21*

## CHROMOSOME 21, RING 21      2476

**Includes:** Ring 21

**Excludes:**
    Chromosome 21, monosomy 21 (0170)
    Chromosome 21, trisomy 21 (0171)
    Chromosome 21, other anomalies

**Major Diagnostic Criteria:** Evidence of ring chromosome 21 by cytogenetic analysis.

**Clinical Findings:** The clinical findings can be extremely variable. Some individuals with ring chromosome 21 have been completely normal, with identification by prenatal diagnosis or evaluation of multiple miscarriages. Among the patients with significant clinical findings, many have had features similar to patients with **Chromosome 21, monosomy 21.** Features of **Chromosome 21, trisomy 21** may be present in the mosaic trisomic state.

**Complications:** Variable. Some patients have had profound mental retardation, visceral anomalies, and shortened life span.

**Associated Findings:** Patients have been described with **Eye, anterior segment dysgenesis,** holoprosencephaly, or hemifacial microsomia with lateral clefting of the mouth. Infertility and pregnancy loss may be more common. Acute lymphocytic leukemia occurred in one child.

**Etiology:** Breakage of both the short and the long arms of chromosome 21 with rejoining of the ends to form a ring. Has occurred as a *de novo* event in most cases, although instances of inheritance of the ring have reported.

**Pathogenesis:** Unknown.

**CDC No.:** 758.990

**Sex Ratio:** Presumably M1:F1.

**Occurrence:** Undetermined but presumed rare.

**Risk of Recurrence for Patient's Sib:** Low if *de novo*; theoretically 50% if inherited.

**Risk of Recurrence for Patient's Child:** Theoretically, 50%. There are few cases of parental (mostly maternal) transmission.

**Age of Detectability:** Variable. Has been detected by prenatal diagnosis.

**Gene Mapping and Linkage:** See *Gene Map.*

**Prevention:** None known. Genetic counseling indicated.

**Treatment:** Symptomatic.

**Prognosis:** Variable.

**Detection of Carrier:** Chromosome analysis.

**References:**

Ferrante E, et al.: Partial monosomy for a 21 chromosome: report of a new case of r (21) and review of the literature. Helv Paediatr Acta 1983; 38:73–80. *

Dallapicolla B, et al.: Ring chromosome 21 in healthy persons: different consequences in females and males. Hum Genet 1986; 73:218–220.

Gardner RJM, et al.: Ring 21 chromosome: the mild end of the phenotypic spectrum. Clin Genet 1986; 30:466–470. *

Falchi AM, et al.: Acute lymphoblastic leukemia in a child with constitutional ring chromosome 21. Cancer Genet Cytogenet 1987; 27:219–224.

Hertz JM: Familial transmission of a ring chromosome 21. Clin Genet 1987; 32:35–39.

Hoovers JMN, Janswijer MCE: Holoprosencephaly associated with ring chromosome 21. Clin Genet 1987; 32:207–208.

Miller K, et al.: Tandem duplication chromosome 21 in the offspring of a ring chromosome 21 carrier. Ann Genet 1987; 30:180–182. *

Dalgleish R, et al.: Apparent monosomy 21 owing to a ring 21 chromosome: parental origin revealed by DNA analysis. J Med Genet 1988; 25:851–854. †

Wong C, et al.: Molecular mechanism in the formation of a human ring chromosome 21. Proc Nat Acad Sci 1989; 86:1914–1918. *

B0021
GR011

                                 **Digamber S. Borgaonkar**
                                       **Frank Greenberg**

---

**Chromosome 21, translocation 21 syndrome**
*See CHROMOSOME 21, TRISOMY 21*

## CHROMOSOME 21, TRISOMY 21      0171

**Includes:**
    Chromosome 21, mosaic 21 syndrome
    Chromosome 21, translocation 21 syndrome
    Down syndrome
    Mongolism (obsolete/pejorative)
    Trisomy G syndrome

**Excludes:** Chromosome x, poly x (3007)

**Major Diagnostic Criteria:** Diagnosis usually definite with eight or more of the characteristic clinical findings. In questionable cases, demonstration of one of the characteristic chromosomal abnormalities may be necessary for diagnosis.

**Clinical Findings:** Chromosomal abnormality (99%); twenty-one trisomy (94%); translocation trisomy (3–4%); mosaicism (1–2%); 10 ulnar loops or 8–9 with a radial loop, 4th finger (90%); t'axial triradius (undetermined frequency); flattened facial features (90%); oblique palpebral fissures (80%); flat occiput (78%); and brachycephaly (75%).

    Short limbs (70%); short, broad hands, short fingers, especially the 5th (70%); high-arched, narrow palate (70%); short 5th middle phalanx (62%); hyperextensibility or hyperflexibility (47–77%), and hypotonia (21–77%).

    Depressed nasal bridge (60%); speckled iris (50%); dysplastic ears (50%); incurved 5th finger (50%); and congenital heart defects (40–60%).

    Tibial arch in hallucal area (50%); transverse palmar crease (48%); increased space between 1st and 2nd toes (45%); epicanthic folds (40%); small nose (undetermined frequency); plantar furrow between 1st and 2nd toes (28%); single flexion crease, 5th finger (20%); and small or absent nasal bones (undetermined frequency).

    Additional characteristics useful in the evaluation of newborns or those in early childhood include absent Moro reflex (82%); excess skin at nape of neck (81%); and dysplastic pelvis by X-ray (67%).

    Additional characteristics useful in evaluation of older children and adults include mental retardation (99%); mouth usually open (65%); dental abnormalities (65%); blepharitis (undetermined frequency); rhagades (56%); furrowed tongue (50%); short broad neck (45%); and strabismus (14–23%).

**Complications:** Those associated with the various clinical features of the condition.

**Associated Findings:** Respiratory infections, epilepsy (10%), duodenal obstruction (8%), and leukemia.

**Etiology:** Presence of an additional chromosome number 21 or part of its long arm, including band q22.1 in all or some of the body cells. In most cases, 21 trisomy is due to a free trisomy (95%), resulting from non-disjunction during meiosis in one of the parents, which correlates with advanced maternal age. Banding techniques make individual differences visible, and these heteromorphisms have been used to identify the supernumerary chromosome as paternal or maternal. Non-disjunction in a maternal first meiotic division is the most common (60%) finding. Paternal non-disjunctions have been observed in about 20% of the cases. The percentage of second division errors in maternal oogenesis is much lower than the percentage of first division errors. In paternal gametogenesis, the first and second division errors are nearly equal.

    Mosaicism is observed in two percent of 21 trisomies. Two cell lines are usually found; one with a free trisomy and one with a normal karyotype. Mosaicism is considered a postzygotic event, occuring after fertilization. Great phenotypic variability is observed in these individuals; ranging from near-normal to the classic 21 trisomy phenotype.

    About five percent of cases are due to a translocation. These can occur *de novo* or be transmitted by one of the parents. Translocations are usually of the centric fusion or Robertsonian type, involving most frequently a chromosome 14 (14/21 translocation) or a 21 or 22 (21/21 or 22/21 translocation).

**Different types of translocations in Chromosome 21, trisomy 21**

| Type | Distribution | |
|---|---|---|
| 1. t(21q Dq) | 54 per 100 (55% de novo) | |
| | t(21q/14q) | 58.5 % |
| | t(21q/13q) | 22 % |
| | t(21q/15q) | 19.5% |
| 2. t(21q Gq) | 41 per 100 (95% de novo) | |
| | t(21q21q) | 84 % |
| | t(21q22q) | 16 % |
| 3. Others (tandem translocations) | 5 per 100 (22% de novo) | |

**Pathogenesis:** Unknown.

**POS No.:** 3100

**CDC No.:** 758.0

**Sex Ratio:** Slight male preponderance.

**Occurrence:** About 1:770 live births in Caucasian, American Negro and Japanese populations. Strongly maternal-age-dependent, with 1:2500 births in mothers age 20 or less, and 1:55 in mothers age 45 or more. Risk of occurrence rises rapidly after maternal age 35.

Prevelance: 1:1000 in 1st year of life; 1:1400 by school age; 1:2200 in 10–14 year group; 1:3300 to 1:2000 in the general population.

**Risk of Recurrence for Patient's Sib:** Most authors consider that for young mothers the risk is 1–2% in free trisomies, while for older mothers the risk is inherent to maternal age.

**Risk of Recurrence for Patient's Child:** 1:2 (50%)

**Age of Detectability:** An increasing number of 21 trisomy fetuses are being diagnosed in the second and third trimester of pregnancy by the finding of fetal abnormalities on routine echographic examination; e.g. hydrops fetalis, cystic hygroma colli, duodenal obstruction, prune belly anomaly and cardiac defects. The association of nuchal edema and macroglossia is especially suggestive of the diagnosis. The echographic diagnosis of one of these types of malformations should lead to a second or third trimester amniocenthesis and fetal chromosome analysis.

**Gene Mapping and Linkage:** See *Gene Map*.

**Prevention:** None known. Genetic counseling indicated. An extensive recent literature discusses the possible benefits of systematic amniocentesis in pregnancies with low alpha-fetoprotein maternal serum values at the beginning of the second trimester of pregnancy, where risk has been estimated at 1:300. Lowered alpha-fetoprotein serum levels are not, however, diagnostic nor are they specific to trisomy 21.

**Treatment:** As may be indicated.

**Prognosis:** Shortened life expectancy: about one-third die during 1st year; one-half by age 3 or 4; remainder's life expectancy is reduced. Congenital heart disease, a major cause of early death, may be correctable by surgery. Mental retardation at moderate or severe level is almost universal, even in cases with mosaicism. Rarely, higher intelligence levels are seen and, in a rare mosaic, intelligence may reach the normal level.

**Detection of Carrier:** When a translocation is detected in the parents, the risk of recurrence depends on the type of translocation and on the sex of the carrier parent. For a t(21q21q) in the parents, all gametes are abnormal and produce only monosomic or trisomic zygotes. When the translocation occurs between a 21 and a D or a 22, the risk is different according to the sex of the parent carrier. If the mother is the carrier, the risk is about 16%, while if the father is the carrier the risk is lower than five percent.

**Support Groups:**
New York; National Down Syndrome Society
Chicago; National Down Syndrome Congress
MD; Cumberland; Down Syndrome Association
MD; Oxon Hill; Down Syndrome Letters c/o George Johnson

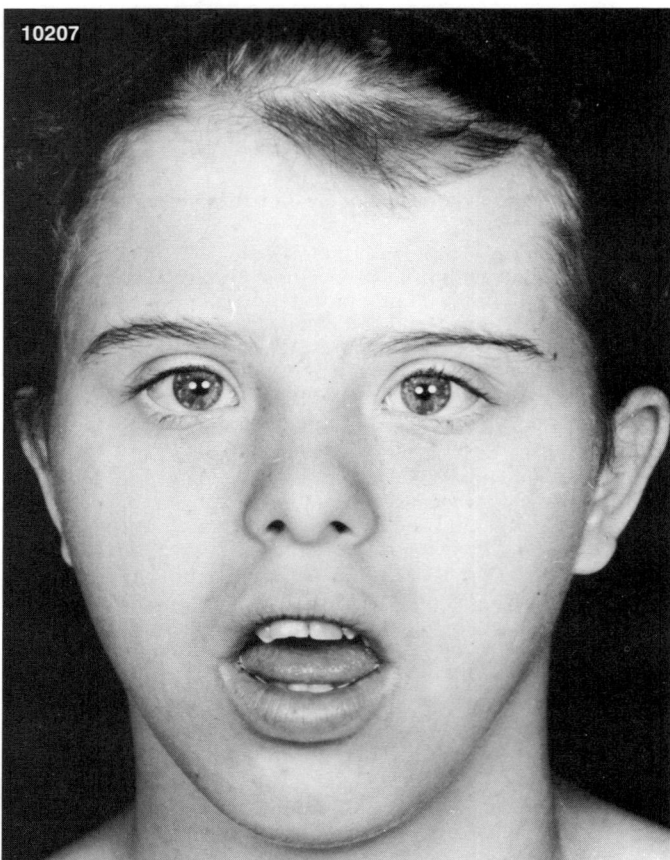

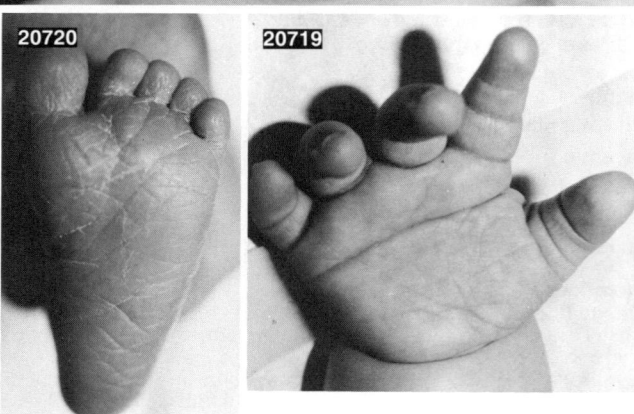

**0171**-10207: Down syndrome in a young adult. **20719:** Simian crease. **20720:** Increased space between the 1st and 2nd toes.

MD; Silver Spring; Parents of Down Syndrome Children
NY; Bellmore; Association for Children with Down Syndrome
TX; Houston; Parents of Children with Down Syndrome
WA; Milton; Caring, Inc.
ENGLAND: Birmingham; National Center for Down Syndrome

**References:**
Penrose LS, Smith GF: Down's anomaly. London: J. & A. Churchill, 1966.
Hamerton JL: Robertsonian translocations in man: evidence for prezygotic selection. Cytogenetics 1968; 7:260.

Mikkelsen M: Down anomaly: new research aspects of an old and well known syndrome. In: Medical genetics: past, present and future. New York: Alan R. Liss, 1985:293–307

Wald NJ, et al.: Maternal serum screening for Down's syndrome in early pregnancy. Br Med J 1988; 297:883–887.

FR030                                                          **Jean-Pierre Fryns**

## CHROMOSOME 22, MONOSOMY 22                                 0172

**Includes:** Chromosome 22, monosomy-G syndrome type II

**Excludes:** N/A

**Major Diagnostic Criteria:** Demonstration of complete or partial monosomy 22, plus several of the more common clinical features.

**Clinical Findings:** Low birthweight, growth and developmental retardation, microcephaly, seizures, hypotonia, ptosis, hypertelorism, epicanthus, flat nasal bridge, bifid uvula, large low-set ears, cutaneous syndactyly of toes, increased acetabular or iliac angles, cardiac anomalies.

**Complications:** Mental retardation.

**Associated Findings:** **Immunodeficiency, thymic agenesis.**

**Etiology:** Deletion of all or part of the long arm of chromosome 22.

**Pathogenesis:** Unknown.

**CDC No.:** 758.990

**Sex Ratio:** Undetermined, but both sexes affected.

**Occurrence:** Undetermined, although partial deletions are rare and full deletions are seldom if ever reported.

**Risk of Recurrence for Patient's Sib:** Increased if partial monosomy due to parental translocation.

**Risk of Recurrence for Patient's Child:** One case of parental transmission of partial monosomy reported.

**Age of Detectability:** At birth or by karyotype analysis of fetal cells.

**Gene Mapping and Linkage:** See *Gene Map.*

**Prevention:** None known. Genetic counseling indicated.

**Treatment:** Unknown.

**Prognosis:** Early death reported in some cases. Mental retardation varies from mild to severe.

**Detection of Carrier:** Balanced translocation or mosaic detectable by karyotype analysis.

**References:**
Warren R, et al.: Identification by fluorescent microscopy of the abnormal chromosomes associated with the G-deletion syndromes. Am J Hum Genet 1973; 25:77–81.

Kelley RI, et al.: The association of DiGeorge anomalad with partial monosomy of chromosome 22. J Pediatr 1982; 101:197–200.

B0021                                                      **Digamber S. Borgankar**

## CHROMOSOME 22, MONOSOMY 22Q                               2537

**Includes:**
Chromosome 22, monosomy 22q12-qter
Chromosome 22, monosomy 22q11
DiGeorge sequence with chromosome 22q11 deletion

**Excludes:** **Chromosome 22, ring 22 (2477)**

**Major Diagnostic Criteria:** Mental and physical retardation associated with epicanthal folds, deep set eyes, full eyebrows, and upper eyelids.

**Clinical Findings:** Skeletal and limb deformities include kyphosis or lordosis and short fingers. In addition to the DiGeorge sequence (see **Immunodeficiency, thymic agenesis,** defects in development of the thymus, parathyroids and great vessels as a result of a disturbed development of the third and fourth pharyngeal

pouches, and an association with partial monosomy of the proximal part of the long arm of chromosome 22 (22q11).

**Complications:** Unknown.

**Associated Findings:** Neurologic symptoms (hypotonia, ataxia, and epilepsy) were reported. In some patients, a broad bulbous nose, long eyelashes, and long philtrum were noteable findings.

**Etiology:** In the majority of patients the 22q deletion is the unbalanced product of parental autosomal reciprocal translocation involving 22q and another autosome or X-chromosome. In one report, a familial pericentric inversion of chromosome 22 with a recombinant subject presenting a pure partial 22q monosomy syndrome (22q12→qter) was described.

**Pathogenesis:** Unknown.

**CDC No.:** 758.990

**Sex Ratio:** M1:F1

**Occurrence:** About 20 cases have been documented.

**Risk of Recurrence for Patient's Sib:** Not increased if parental chromosomes are normal. Increased risk (possibly 5–10%) if an autosomal reciprocal translocation involving 22q and another autosome, or a pericentric inversion in chromosome 22, is present in one of the parents.

**Risk of Recurrence for Patient's Child:** Mental retardation in surviving patients makes reproduction unlikely.

**Age of Detectability:** At birth or in early childhood. Prenatal diagnosis by CVS or amniocentesis is possible.

**Gene Mapping and Linkage:** See *Gene Map.*

**Prevention:** None known. Genetic counseling indicated.

**Treatment:** Symptomatic.

**Prognosis:** Long-term survival is dependent on the severity of internal malformations, including the possible cardiac defects in the DiGeorge Sequence. More than one-half of the patients do not survive the first months of life.

**Detection of Carrier:** By cytogenetic examination.

**References:**
de la Chapelle A, et al: A Deletion in Chromosome 22 can cause DiGeorge Syndrome. Hum Genet 1981; 57:253–256.

Migliorini AM, et al: Fetal phenotype in a case of partial trisomy 21 and partial monosomy 22 detected prenatally. J Med Genet 1981; 18:383–398.

Watt JL, et al: A familial pericentric inversion of chromosome 22 with a recombinant subject illustrating a "pure" partial monosomy syndrome. J Med Genet 1985; 22:283–287.

Cannizzaro LA, Emanuel BS: In situ hybridization and translocation breakpoint mapping: DiGeorge syndrome with partial monosomy of chromosome 22. Cytogenet Cell Genet 1985; 39:179–183.

Schwanitz G, Zerres K: Partial Monosomy 22 as result of an X/22 translocation in a Newborn with DiGeorge syndrome. Ann Génét 1987; 30:2:80–84.

Kaplan JC, et al: Human Chromosome 22. J Med Genet 1987; 24:65–78.

FR030                                                          **Jean-Pierre Fryns**
CH043                                                    **Krysztyna Chrzanowska**

**Chromosome 22, monosomy 22q11**
  *See CHROMOSOME 22, MONOSOMY 22q*
**Chromosome 22, monosomy 22q12-qter**
  *See CHROMOSOME 22, MONOSOMY 22q*
**Chromosome 22, monosomy-G syndrome type II**
  *See CHROMOSOME 22, MONOSOMY 22*
**Chromosome 22, partial trisomy 22**
  *See CAT EYE SYNDROME*

## CHROMOSOME 22, RING 22     2477

**Includes:** Ring 22

**Excludes:** Chromosome 22, other anomalies

**Major Diagnostic Criteria:** As with other autosomal ring chromosomes, no specific clinical syndrome is associated with ring chromosome 22. Mental retardation, muscular hypotonia and motor incoordination are the only constant features. Cytogenetic analysis confirms the diagnosis.

**Clinical Findings:** Craniofacial dysmorphism may include **Microcephaly** (60%), almond-shaped eyes, epicanthus, hypertelorism, palpebral ptosis (30%), low-set eyebrows, bulbous nose, high-arched palate, and large ears in normal position. Growth and physical development are normal in the majority of patients.

**Complications:** Unknown.

**Associated Findings:** **Syndactyly** of fingers and toes. Internal malformations are rare, i.e., polycystic kidneys, stenosis of the ureteropelvic junction, heart defects, and microphthalmia.

**Etiology:** Familial transmission of r(22) was documented in four reports. In all other patients the ring chromosome formation occurred *de novo*. The variability in the phenotype of r(22) patients is explained by the differences in breakpoint in the ring chromosome formation and the secondary mitotic variability of the ring chromosome.

**Pathogenesis:** Unknown.

**CDC No.:** 758.990

**Sex Ratio:** M12:F28 (observed).

**Occurrence:** More than 40 cases have been reported.

**Risk of Recurrence for Patient's Sib:** Not increased if parental chromosomes are normal. The presence of a r(22), even in a mosaic state, should be carefully excluded in the parents.

**Risk of Recurrence for Patient's Child:** Familial transmission of the r(22) has been documented with variable phenotypic effects in different generations. Mental retardation in the majority of patients makes reproduction unlikely.

**Age of Detectability:** At birth, or by prenatal diagnosis by CVS or amniocenthesis.

**Gene Mapping and Linkage:** See *Gene Map*.

**Prevention:** None known. Genetic counseling indicated.

**Treatment:** Symptomatic.

**Prognosis:** The long term life prognosis is good. As in other chromosomal syndromes, prognosis is dependent of the presence of associated internal anomalies.

**Detection of Carrier:** Chromosome studies.

**References:**
Fryns JP, Van den Berghe H: Ring chromosome 22 in a mentally retarded child and mosaic 45,XX,-15,-22,+t(15;22) (p11;q11)/46,XXr(22)/46,XX karyotype in the mother. Hum Genet 1979; 47: 213–216.
Crusi A, Engel E: Diagnostic prénatal de trois cas de chromosome G en anneau: un 21 et deux 22, dont un de novo. Ann Génét 1986; 29:253–260.

FR030        **Jean-Pierre Fryns**

## CHROMOSOME 22, SUPERNUMERARY DER 22, T(11:22)     2043

**Includes:** Chromosome 47 XX or XY,+der(22)t(11;22)(q23;q11) or (q25;q13)

**Excludes:**
    **Cat eye syndrome** (0544)
    **Chromosome 11, partial trisomy 11q** (0161)
    **Chromosome 22, trisomy mosaicism** (2478)

**Major Diagnostic Criteria:** Mental deficiency, malformed ears with preauricular pits or tags, high-arched or cleft palate, micrognathia, congenital heart defect, and demonstration of the cytogenetic abnormality.

**Clinical Findings:** The following table is based on 85 chromosomally proven cases. Their mean birth weight was 2730 g (n=40). Moderate to severe mental deficiency was reported in all cases.

### Clinical Findings in 85 Cases

| | |
|---|---|
| Malformed ears with preauricular pits or tags | 50% |
| Highly arched or cleft palate | 50% |
| Micrognathia | 50% |
| Congenital heart disease | 50% |
| Undescended testes | 50% |
| Small penis | 50% |
| Hypotonia | 33% |
| Microcephaly | 25% |
| Craniofacial asymmetry | 25% |
| Large, beaked nose | 25% |
| Dislocated hips | 25% |
| Long philtrum | 10% |
| Absent or hypoplastic kidney | 10% |
| Imperforate anus | 10% |
| Abnormal placement of anus | 10% |
| Extra ribs | 10% |

**Complications:** Cardiac failure.

**Associated Findings:** Diaphragmatic hernia, **Hernia, inguinal**, excess nuchal skin, **Uvula, cleft**, and clubfoot.

**Etiology:** Duplication of the distal long arm of chromosome 11 (region 11q23 or 11q25→11qter) and the short arm and proximal long arm of chromosome 22 (region 22pter→22q11 or q13) due to supernumerary der(22) t(11;22). Proband receives the supernumerary der(22) as a result of 3:1 meiotic segregation in a translocation carrier parent. In the 85 families reported, the unbalanced chromosome was derived from the mother in 82 and from the father in three.

**Pathogenesis:** Unknown.

**POS No.:** 3628

**CDC No.:** 758.990

**Sex Ratio:** M7:F5

**Occurrence:** Undetermined but presumed rare. However, 11/22 translocation is thought to be one of the most common reciprocal translocations in man. At least 110 unrelated families reported from Europe and the United States with three instances known where the balanced 11/22 translocation occurs "de novo" in a carrier parent.

**Risk of Recurrence for Patient's Sib:** Depends on the sex of the translocation carrier parent. If the mother has the balanced 11/22 translocation, recurrence risk if 2–6%. If the father is the translocation carrier, recurrence risk is 2–4%.

**Risk of Recurrence for Patient's Child:** Unknown.

**Age of Detectability:** Prenatally by chromosome analysis utilizing chorionic villus sampling or amniocentesis, or at birth.

**Gene Mapping and Linkage:** See *Gene Map*.

**Prevention:** None known. Genetic counseling indicated.

**Treatment:** Symptomatic for congenital defects; special education.

**Prognosis:** One-quarter die within the first year of life. Of 80 known patients in follow-up, 62 were living at the last contact. The oldest known survivor is 20 years of age.

**Detection of Carrier:** Chromosome analysis.

**References:**
Fraccaro M, et al: The 11q;22q translocation: a European collaborative analysis of 43 cases. Hum Genet 1980; 56:21–51.
Zackai EH, Emanuel BS: Site-specific reciprocal translocation, t(11; 22)(q23;q11), in several unrelated families with 3:1 meiotic disjunction. Am J Med Genet 1980: 7:507–521.
Schinzel A, et al: Incomplete trisomy 22. Familial 11/22 translocation with 3:1 meiotic disjunction. Delineation of a common clinical picture and report of nine new cases from six families. Hum Genet 1981; 56:249–262. †
Iselius L, et al: The 11q;22q translocation: a collaborative study of 20 new cases and analysis of 110 families. Hum Genet 1983; 64:343–355. *
Lin AE, et al: Congenital heart disease in supernumerary der(22) t(11;22) syndrome. Clin Genet 1986; 29:61–67.

D0025                                **Alan E. Donnenfeld**
ZA000                                **Elaine H. Zackai**
EM000                                **Beverly S. Emanuel**

---

## CHROMOSOME 22, TRISOMY MOSAICISM           2478

**Includes:** N/A

**Excludes:**
    **Cat eye syndrome** (0544)
    Chromosome 22, incomplete or rearranged supernumerary
    **Turner syndrome** (0977)

**Major Diagnostic Criteria:** Demonstration of trisomy 22 (most likely in fibroblasts), hemidystrophy and webbed neck, plus other signs often associated with **Turner syndrome**. Non-mosaic trisomy 22 may show a somewhat different clinical spectrum.

**Clinical Findings:** Hemidystrophy, often linked with unilateral hearing loss; a shortened limb, particularly a leg; hypoplastic digits; abnormal palmar flexion creases; dysplasia or agenesis of nails; and linear skin pigmentations. Eyelid ptosis, webbed neck, low posterior hairline, malformations of great vessels (particularly of the aortic arch); and cubitus valgus and multiple pigmented skin nevi similar to those seen in **Turner syndrome**. IQ's cluster in the 60–70 range. Sexual infantilism, streak gonads, and unilateral ovarian and fallopian tube agenesis have been noted (and may be linked with renal defects). While the phenotype is still being defined, the diagnosis currently hinges on the demonstration of trisomy 22, which is least likely to be found in lymphocytes.

Two infants with non-mosaic trisomy 22 showed strikingly similar facies. A 1,560 gm. term neonate with **Eye, hypertelorism**, downward slanting palpebral fissures, epicanthic folds, **Cleft palate**, broad flat nose, malformed ears and preauricular pits, no pterygium nor short neck, wide spaced nipples, bilateral cryptorchidism, hypoplastic genitalia, distal tapering of fingers, hypoplastic nails and six arch patterns on the fingertips died shortly before his third birthday after a history of recurrent respiratory infections and feeding difficulties.

**Complications:** Cardiovascular malformations, renal malformations, shortened leg, or unilateral hearing loss.

**Associated Findings:** Mental subnormality; sexual infantilism.

**Etiology:** Presence of an extra complete chromosome 22.

**Pathogenesis:** Clinical signs suggest pathogenic mechanisms similar to those resulting in **Turner syndrome**.

**POS No.:** 3703

**CDC No.:** 758.520

**Sex Ratio:** M<1:F1. More prevalent in females.

**Occurrence:** Trisomy 22 conceptuses are miscarried during the early stages of pregnany. Complete trisomy 22 might rarely servive up to term, but is not compatible with life over a long period. Among spontaneous abortions, trisomy 22 represents the second most common trisomy and is found in approximately 10%

of specimens. In contrast (in a series of nearly 53,000 amniocenteses), non-mosaic trisomy 22 was not found among 1,200 chromosomal defects detected, whereas trisomy 22 mosaicism was found in three instances. Although rare, the tendency for trisomic cells to be prevalent in fibroblasts rather than lymphocytes is likely to have resulted in under ascertainment.

**Risk of Recurrence for Patient's Sib:** Unknown.

**Risk of Recurrence for Patient's Child:** Unknown.

**Age of Detectability:** At birth, or by prenatal diagnosis.

**Gene Mapping and Linkage:** See *Gene Map*.

**Prevention:** None known. Genetic counseling indicated.

**Treatment:** Treatment of cardiovascular malformations, hearing loss, asymmetry of limbs (particularly the legs), treatment of delayed puberty, and special schooling as needed.

**Prognosis:** Presumably normal life span, if treatment of threatening congenital malformations is effective.

**Detection of Carrier:** By cytogenetic analysis and clinical examination.

**Special Considerations:** Patients, particularly neonates with hemidystrophy or unilateral congenital malformations, should undergo cytogenetic analysis of fibroblasts. If, in addition, there are clinical signs suggestive of **Turner syndrome**, trisomy 22 mosaicism should be suspected. In three instances, trisomy 22 was found only in fibroblasts. and in one instance it was found in 10% of lymphocytes, (whereas 2% of lymphocytes were missing a chromosome 22). In another instance, trisomy 22 was found in a large proportion of amniocytes, but after delivery, it was found in only one of 27 lymphocytes studied.

**References:**
Shokeir MHK: Complete trisomy 22. Clin Genet 1978; 14:139–146.
Schinzel A: Incomplete trisomy 22: mosaic-trisomy 22 and the problem of full trisomy 22. Hum Genet 1981; 56:269–273.
Wertelecki W, et al.: Trisomy 22 mosaicism syndrome and Ullrich-Turner stigmata. Am J Med Genet 1986; 23:739–749. * †
Voiculescu I, et al.: Trisomy 22 in a newborn with multiple malformations. Hum Genet 1987; 76:298–301.

WE029                                   **W. Wertelecki**

**Chromosome 45,X syndrome**
    *See TURNER SYNDROME*
**Chromosome 47,XX or XY,+der(22)t(11;22)(q23;q11) or (q25;q13)**
    *See CHROMOSOME 22, SUPERNUMERARY DER 22, T(11:22)*
**Chromosome 47,XXX karyotype**
    *See CHROMOSOME X, TRIPLO-X*
**Chromosome 48,XXXX females**
    *See CHROMOSOME X, POLY-X*
**Chromosome 49,XXXXX females**
    *See CHROMOSOME X, POLY-X*
**Chromosome E1-trisomy syndrome**
    *See CHROMOSOME 18, TRISOMY 18*

---

## CHROMOSOME INSTABILITY, NIJMEGEN TYPE           2551

**Includes:**
    Cancer (lymphoreticular)-immunodeficiency-microcephaly
    Chromosome 7, rearrangements
    Chromosome 14, rearrangements
    Immunodeficiency-microcephaly-malignancy
    Microcephaly-immunodeficiency-lymphoreticular
        malignancy
    Nijmegen chromosome breakage syndrome
    Seemanova syndrome
    Weemaes chromosome breakage syndrome

**Excludes:**
    **Ataxia-telangiectasia** (0094)
    **Bloom syndrome** (0112)
    **Dubowitz syndrome** (0299)
    **Microcephaly, autosomal recessive with normal intelligence**
        (2838)

**Major Diagnostic Criteria:** Growth retardation and **Microcephaly**, both of prenatal onset, and a history of recurrent infection. Ataxia and telangiectasia are always absent.

The laboratory features are equally important for diagnosis. The serum alpha-fetoprotein (AFP) level is consistently normal. Chromosome studies reveal an increased proportion of cells with diverse chromosome rearrangements involving, particularly, chromosomes 7 and 14.

**Clinical Findings:** This syndrome, named after the city of Nijmegen in The Netherlands, is distinct from **Ataxia-telangiectasia** (AT). Like AT, the Nijmegen syndrome is characterized by immunodeficiency, rearrangements of chromosomes 7 and 14, increased radiosensitivity of chromosomes and cells, and radioresistance of DNA replication. Unlike AT, the Nijmegen syndrome involves growth retardation, **Microcephaly**, and bird-like facies. The serum AFP is always elevated in AT, but never in Nijmegen syndrome.

**Microcephaly** in the Nijmegen syndrome is mild to moderate in degree, and intelligence can be normal. Growth retardation is commonplace. The face appears narrow and bird-like, with relative prominence of the nose. The ears may look low and the chin recessed. Additional malformations may be present, such as congenital hip dislocation, fifth finger clinodactyly, and renal anomalies. Mild mental retardation is debatable; it may or may not be part of this syndrome.

The laboratory findings are remarkable. There is humoral and cellular immunodeficiency. IgG, IgA, IgD, and IgE levels may be decreased or absent. The T lymphocytes can be reduced in number with decreased response to phytohemagglutinin (PHA) and lymphocyte mitogens other than PHA. Chromosome rearrangements are elevated in lymphocytes and fibroblasts, with inversions and translocations nonrandomly involving chromosomes 7 and 14, with break points in chromosome bands 7p13, 7q34, 14q11.2, and 14q32. Chromosome damage and cell death are abnormally pronounced after X-irradiation in the $G_2$ phase of the cell cycle. However, X-irradiation inhibits DNA synthesis less in the Nijmegen syndrome than under normal circumstances.

**Complications:** Infections from immunodeficiency include oral candida, otitis media, pneumonia, gastroenteritis, urinary tract infections, and osteomyelitis. Recurrent otitis media without prompt, effective treatment can, in turn, produce conductive hearing loss.

**Associated Findings:** Right choanal atresia and cleft lip-palate, each in a single patient.

**Etiology:** Possibly autosomal recessive inheritance.

**Pathogenesis:** Undetermined. Some patients show slightly increased chromosomal instability in lymphocyte cultures.

**MIM No.:** *25126

**POS No.:** 4374

**CDC No.:** 758.990

**Sex Ratio:** M1:F1

**Occurrence:** Over a dozen cases have been documented; most of them from the Netherlands or Czechoslovakia.

**Risk of Recurrence for Patient's Sib:**
See Part I, *Mendelian Inheritance.*

**Risk of Recurrence for Patient's Child:**
See Part I, *Mendelian Inheritance.* No patient is known to have reproduced.

**Age of Detectability:** At birth and thereafter the syndrome can be suspected clinically and confirmed by the demonstration of elevated rearrangements of chromosomes 7 and 14, decreased response to PHA, and normal serum AFP level. Prenatal diagnosis is theoretically feasible by chorionic villus sampling, amniocentesis, or fetal blood sampling.

**Gene Mapping and Linkage:** Unknown. The chromosome break points in 14q11.2, 7q34, and 7p13 probably involve the $\alpha$-, $\beta$- and lambda-chain gene loci for the T-cell receptor (TCR) and the break point in 14q32, the immunoglobulin heavy-chain gene locus.

**Prevention:** None known. Genetic counseling indicated.

**Treatment:** Supportive measures against infection, such as immunoglobulin substitution and antibiotic therapy.

**Prognosis:** Some patients have died during infancy and early childhood of pneumonia, lymphoid leukemia, or lymphosarcoma. Otherwise, impact on life span is unknown.

**Detection of Carrier:** Unknown.

**Special Considerations:** This condition is among the more recent well-delineated chromosome instability disorders, joining **Ataxia-telangiectasia, Bloom syndrome, Pancytopenia syndrome, Fanconi type,** and **Xeroderma pigmentosum** as autosomal recessive phenotypes. The only autosomal dominant chromosome instability disorder known is the dysplastic nexus (familial atypical multiple male melanoma syndrome) syndrome (see **Cancer, malignant melanoma, familial**).

Given that the immunologic, cytogenetic, and radiobiologic features are very similar to those in AT, the gene for the Nijmegen syndrome may be allelic or otherwise related to that for AT. As in AT, there is probably genetic heterogeneity in the Nijmegen syndrome, with multiple forms of the disease.

The Nijmegen syndrome, like AT, predisposes to lymphoid leukemia and lymphoma. The far more frequent heterozygous carrier may pose a public health problem by also predisposing to malignancy.

The Nijmegen syndrome also resembles the **Dubowitz syndrome**, which is characterized by microcephaly, growth retardation, odd facies, and, in some cases, immunodeficiency. The Nijmegen and Dubowitz syndromes may be related diseases or even synonymous.

**References:**

Hustinz TWJ, et al.: Karyotype instability with multiple 7/14 and 7/7 rearrangements. Hum Genet 1979; 49:199–208.

Weemaes CMR, et al.: A new chromosomal instability disorder: the Nijmegen breakage syndrome. Acta Paediatr Scand 1981; 70:557–564.

Taalman RDFM, et al.: Hypersensitivity to ionizing radiation, in a new chromosomal breakage disorder, the Nijmegen breakage disorder. Mutat Res 1983; 112:23–32.

Seemanová E, et al.: Familial microcephaly with normal intelligence, immunodeficiency and risk for lymphoreticular malignancies: a new autosomal recessive disorder. Am J Med Genet 1985; 20:639–548.

Conley ME, et al.: A chromosome breakage syndrome with profound immunodeficiency. Blood 1986; 67:1251–1256

Hecht F, et al.: T-cell cancer breakpoints at genes for T-cell receptor on chromosomes 7 and 14. Cancer Genet Cytogenet 1986; 20:181–183.

Teebi AS, et al.: Autosomal recessive nonsyndromal microcephaly with normal intelligence. Am J Med Genet 1987; 26:355–359.

Weemaes CMR, et al.: Variants of ataxia ateleangiectasia or new chromosome breakage syndrome? In: Vossen J, Griscelli C, eds: Progress in immunodeficiency research and therapy. Kerkrade, The Netherlands: Int Group Immunodeficiencies, 1987:313–318.

Wegner R-D, et al.: A new chromosomal instability disorder confirmed by complementation studies. Clin Genet 1988; 33:20–32.

Taalman RDFM, et al.: further delineation of the Nijmegen breakage syndrome. Am J Med Genet 1989; 32:425–431.

SA020                          Avery A. Sandberg
HE008                          Barbara K. Hecht
HE007                              Frederick Hecht
PA043                         Eberhard Passarge

---

## CHROMOSOME MOSAICISM, 45,X/46,XY TYPE   0173

**Includes:**
Gonadal dysgenesis, asymmetric
Gonadal dysgenesis, mixed
Gonosomal intersexuality
Mosaic gonadal dysgenesis

**Excludes:**
**Androgen insensitivity syndrome, incomplete** (0050)
**Gonadal dysgenesis, XY type** (0437)
**Hermaphroditism, true** (0971)
**Steroid 5 alpha-reductase deficiency** (3062)

**Steroid** all other deficiencies
All other forms of male pseudohermaphroditism

**Major Diagnostic Criteria:** A mosaic 45,X/46,XY chromosome complement: The diagnosis is likely if an individual has a unilateral streak gonad and a contralateral testis, or bilateral dysgenetic testes and müllerian derivatives. If lymphocyte cultures of an individual with ambiguous external genitalia, a unilateral streak gonad, a contralateral testis, and a uterus are 46,XY, it is reasonable to assume the presence of 45,X/46,XY mosaicism. Normal testicular differentiation need not be present, but recognizable seminiferous tubules should be. By contrast, if oocytes are present, a diagnosis of true hermaphroditism is appropriate.

**Clinical Findings:** In individuals with a 45,X cell line and at least one cell line containing a Y chromosome, the phenotype ranges from almost normal males with cryptorchidism or penile hypospadias to females indistinguishable from those with the 45,X Turner syndrome.

45,X/46,XY individuals may be grouped into one of three clinical categories, namely those with 1) unambiguous female external genitalia, 2) ambiguous external genitalia (sex of rearing in doubt), or 3) almost normal male external genitalia. The spectrum of phenotypes is continuous, however, because no sharp demarcation between categories is possible. Somatic features of the Turner syndrome may be present in any 45,X/46,XY individual. The anomalies present cover the same spectrum as in 45,X individuals, but usually fewer anomalies are detected. It is important to exclude cardiac, vertebral, renal and auditory abnormalities.

1) *Unambiguous female external genitalia.* About 5% of patients with gonadal dysgenesis and unambiguous external genitalia have 45,X cells and cells containing a Y chromosome. These 45,X/46,XY individuals have well-differentiated female external genitalia, vagina, and müllerian derivatives. At puberty they fail to undergo normal secondary sex development. Gonadoblastomas and dysgerminomas may develop from the dysgenetic gonads.

2) *Ambiguous external genitalia.* Most 45,X/46,XY individuals have ambiguous external genitalia, specifically phallic enlargement, posterior labioscrotal fusion and a urogenital orifice leading superiorly to the urethra and inferiorly to a vagina. An important diagnostic feature is that müllerian derivatives (cervix, uterine corpus and fallopian tubes) are usually present; these are absent in most genetic forms of male pseudohermaphroditism. Occasionally the uterus is rudimentary or a fallopian tube fails to develop on the side on which a testis is present; however, a fallopian tube is usually present on the side containing the streak gonad. Most 45,X/46,XY individuals with ambiguous external genitalia have gonads consisting of a unilateral streak gonad and a contralateral dysgenetic testis (mixed or asymmetric gonadal dysgenesis). The streak gonads are usually similar in appearance to those of 45,X individuals, although sometimes relatively more mesonephric remnants or hilar cells are present. The testicular tissue is rarely normal in amount or in histologic appearance. However, a few seminiferous tubules can usually be identified. The likelihood that a gonad of such a patient will undergo neoplastic transformation is about 15–20%. Breast development in a 45,X/46,XY individual with ambiguous external genitalia suggests the presence of a gonadoblastoma or dysgerminoma, tumors that may produce hormones.

3) *Almost normal male external genitalia.* Some 45,X/46,XY patients may have almost normal male external genitalia, the only abnormalities being hypospadias or unilateral cryptorchidism. Compared with other 45,X/46,XY individuals, testicular development is relatively more normal, wolffian derivatives more normal, and müllerian derivatives less likely to be present. Pubertal virilization may occur, and fertility seems possible.

**Complications:** Neoplastic transformation of the streak gonad or dysgenetic testis. Secondary sex development is usually not normal; infertility.

**Associated Findings:** Somatic features of **Turner syndrome** may be present.

**Etiology:** Usually believed to arise by mitotic nondisjunction. However, structural abnormalities of the Y chromosome are often present. These abnormalities (eg dicentric chromosomes) suggest that the mosaicism may sometimes be initiated through formation of a structurally abnormal Y chromosome, with the 45,X line arising only secondarily. The line containing the structurally abnormal line may or may not persist.

**Pathogenesis:** The various associated phenotypes may reflect different tissue distributions of the 45,X and 46,XY cell lines. A streak gonad would thus presumably reflect the presence of 45,X cells, whereas a testis might more likely reflect 46,XY cells. However, this logical assumption has not been proven.

**MIM No.:** 15825

**CDC No.:** 758.800

**Sex Ratio:** N/A

**Occurrence:** Rare, but a definite consideration in the evaluation of genital ambiguity.

**Risk of Recurrence for Patient's Sib:** Probably negligible.

**Risk of Recurrence for Patient's Child:** Patients are usually infertile.

**Age of Detectability:** At birth if ambiguous external genitalia are present; otherwise at puberty because of lack of normal secondary sex development.

**Gene Mapping and Linkage:** See *Gene Map.*

**Prevention:** None known. Genetic counseling indicated.

**Treatment:** External genital reconstruction may be necessary, particularly if a child has genital ambiguity. Streak gonads and dysgenetic testes should be removed because of the danger of neoplastic transformation. This procedure should be undertaken without delay once the diagnosis is made. In 45,X/46,XY individuals with almost normal male external genitalia, scrotal testes should probably be retained. However, such individuals may or may not have an increased risk for neoplastic transformation and, hence, should be followed carefully. Hormone administration may be necessary. Individuals reared as females require estrogens; individuals reared as males may require androgens.

**Prognosis:** Presumably normal life span, provided life-threatening anomalies do not coexist or a malignant neoplasm does not develop. Infertility.

**Detection of Carrier:** Unknown.

**Special Considerations:** Familial recurrences are rare; however, in at least one family 45,X/47,XYY mosaicism was detected in two and perhaps three sibs whose parents were consanguineous.

This mosaicism has been detected in amniotic fluid fibroblasts obtained by amniocentesis. Fetuses usually show no phenotypic abnormalities at birth, and sex seems far more likely to be male than female (16 of 17 cases in one series).

**References:**
Pfeiffer RA, et al.: Die nosologische Sellung, des XO/XY- Mosaizimus. Arch Gynaekol 1968; 206:369–410.
German J: Abnormalities of human sex chromosomes. V. A unifying concept in relation to the gonadal dysgeneses. Clin Genet 1970; 1:15.
Hsu LYF, et al.: Familial chromosomal mosaicism, genetic aspects. Ann Hum Genet 1970; 33:343–349.
Simpson JL, Photopulos G: The relationship of neoplasia to disorders of abnormal sexual differentiation. In: Bergsma D, et al. eds: BD:OAS. New York: Alan R Liss, Inc for The National Foundation-March of Dimes, 1976:15–50.
Simpson JL: Disorders of sexual differentiation: etiology and clinical delineation. New York: Academic Press Inc, 1976.
Hsu LYF, Perlis TE: United States survey on chromosome mosaicism and pseudomosaicism in prenatal diagnosis. Prenatal Diagnosis 1984; 4:97–130.

SI018                                                   **Joe Leigh Simpson**

## CHROMOSOME TETRAPLOIDY 2238

**Includes:**
Chromosome, tetraploid/diploid mosaicism
Contraceptives, oral, and chromosome tetraploidy
Polyploid phenotype

**Excludes:**
Chromosome 13, trisomy 13 (0168)
Chromosome 18, trisomy 18 (0160)
Chromosome triploidy (0169)

**Major Diagnostic Criteria:** Low birth weight, multiple defects including **Microcephaly**, unusual facies, early death and demonstration of a tetraploid (4N) chromosome complement.

**Clinical Findings:** Near term gestation, slightly low birth weight, diminished viability, microcephaly, prominent narrow forehead, beaked nose, microphthalmia/anophthalmia, short palpebral fissures, **Eye, hypertelorism**, low-set ears with dysplastic cartilage, micrognathia, positional or structural limb defects, arachnodactyly, genital ambiguity, cryptorchidism, hypotonia, congenital heart disease, hypoplasia/aplasia of the olfactory tract, hypoplasia/aplasia of the optic tract, microgyria, rudimentary pituitary gland, **Anencephaly**, and meningomyelocele.

**Complications:** Perinatal death. Early death with longest reported survival three months. Some mosaic tetraploids have survived longer.

**Associated Findings:** None known.

**Etiology:** Presence of four complete chromosome sets instead of the normal two. It has been postulated that the ratio between different chromatin portions and/or the balance between chromosomes may influence phenotypic expression more than absolute chromosome numbers.

Based on duplication of the sex chromosome complement, i.e., XXXY or XXXX, and duplication of parental polymorphisms, the most common mechanism for tetraploidy is thought to be normal chromosome duplication followed by an error in cytoplasmic cleavage. Other mechanisms may include trispermy, fertilization of a haploid ovum by a diploid and haploid spermatozoa, and fertilization of a diploid ovum by two haploid spermatozoa, or by a single diploid spermatozoon.

**Pathogenesis:** Unknown.

**POS No.:** 3115

**CDC No.:** 758.585

**Sex Ratio:** Undetermined. Of five reported cases, four have been male (92, XXYY).

**Occurrence:** Five cases of tetraploidy and five cases of mosaic tetraploidy have been reported.

**Risk of Recurrence for Patient's Sib:** Undetermined but presumed very small.

**Risk of Recurrence for Patient's Child:** Affected individuals are not expected to survive to reproduce.

**Age of Detectability:** At birth, or prenatally.

**Gene Mapping and Linkage:** See *Gene Map.*

**Prevention:** None known. Genetic counseling indicated.

**Treatment:** Unknown.

**Prognosis:** Unknown.

**Detection of Carrier:** Cytogenetic studies help to determine the timing of the chromosome aberration and rule out low grade parental mosaicism (diploid/tetraploid) as the basis of the chromosomal anomaly.

**Special Considerations:** Polyploidy has been considered a cultural artifact in many prenatal studies. However, with an increased recognition of live born infants with tetraploidy or tetraploidy mosaicism, interpretation of such prenatal chromosome findings seems more tenuous. Fetoscopy for prenatal blood sampling may be warranted to confirm or exclude these questionable diagnoses.

An increased incidence of polyploidy has been noted when oral contraceptives were stopped within six months prior to conception. In two of the five reported cases of tetraploidy, oral contraceptives were being taken at the time of conception; in one case, these medications were stopped only six months prior to conception. Certainly, further research is needed before any definite correlation can be made.

**References:**
Golbus MS, et al.: Tetraploidy in a liveborn infant. J Med Genet 1976; 13:329–332. *
Kajii T, et al.: Origin of triploidy and tetraploidy in man: 11 cases with chromosome markers. Cytogenet Cell Genet 1977; 18:109–125.
Pitt D, et al.: Tetraploidy in a liveborn infant with spina bifida and other anomalies. J Med Genet 1981; 18:309–311.
Sheppard DM, et al.: Tetraploid conceptus with three prenatal contributions. Hum Genet 1982; 62:371–374.
Scarbrough PR, et al.: Tetraploidy: a report of three live-born infants. Am J Med Genet 1984; 19:29–37.
Wilson GW, et al.: MCA/MR syndrome in a female infant with tetraploidy mosaicism: review of the human polyploid phenotype. Am J Med Genet 1988; 30:953–961.

SC004                                      **Paula R. Scarbrough**

**Chromosome triploid/diploid mosaicism**
*See CHROMOSOME TRIPLOIDY*

## CHROMOSOME TRIPLOIDY 0169

**Includes:** Chromosome triploid/diploid mosaicism

**Excludes:**
Chromosome 13, trisomy 13 (0168)
Chromosome 18, trisomy 18 (0160)
Chromosome tetraploidy (2238)

**Major Diagnostic Criteria:** Multiple congenital anomalies (MCA) syndrome with severe intrauterine growth retardation (mean birthweight 1800 gr), fetal edema and contrastingly large placenta. Relatively large skull with incomplete ossification of the calvarium; small facies with microretrognathia and/or cleft lip/cleft palate.

**Clinical Findings:** Central nervous system (CNS) malformations are invariably present and include hydrocephaly, holoprosencephaly, cortical and cerebellar hypoplasia. Syndactyly of fingers and toes, simian creases, short halluces (frog-like position of hands and feet) and rocker-bottom deformity. Renal dysplasia with cortical cysts and urinary tract malformations leads to oli-

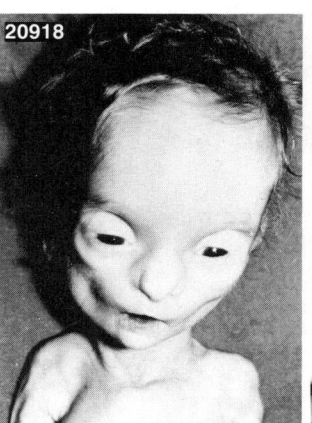
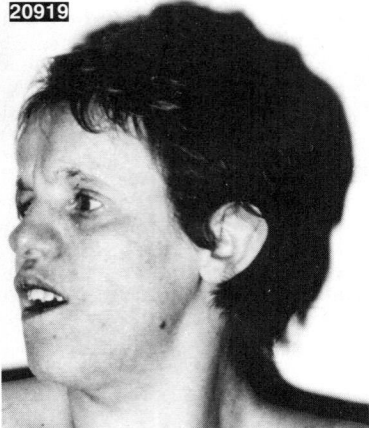

**0169A-20918:** Chromosome triploidy syndrome; infant with full triploidy. **20919:** Facial appearance in a mosaic/normal triploid adult severely retarded female.

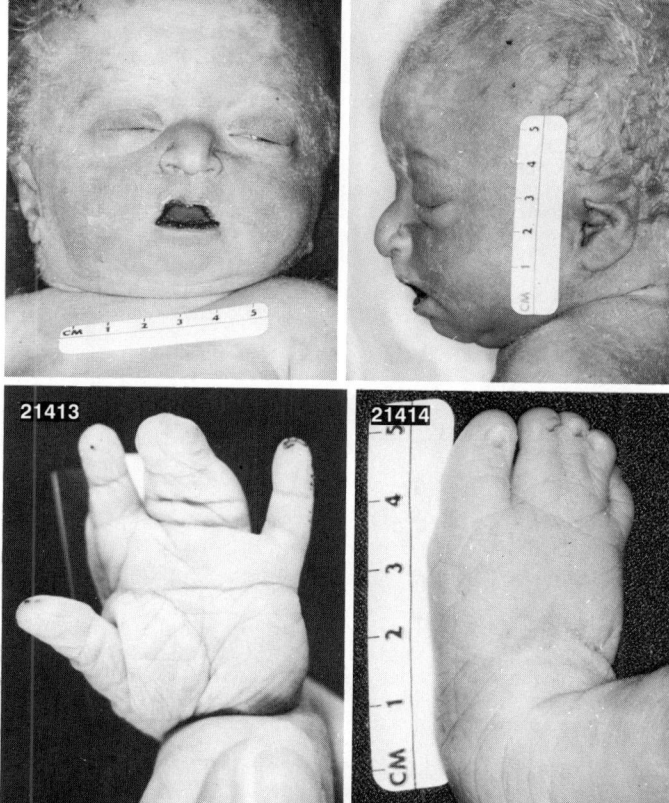

**0169B**-21411–12: Newborn with triploidy (69,XXY); note excessive lanugo, epicanthal folds, microphthalmia, beaked nose, small mouth, receding jaw, and low-set, malformed ears. 21413: Complete syndactyly of the third and fourth fingers and simian line. 21414: Syndactyly of second, third and fourth toes.

goamnios, meningocoele, omphalocoele and/or other abdominal wall defects.

Ocular anomalies are variable i.e. anopthalmia, microphthalmia, buphthalmia, colobomata and cataracts. A great number of other, mainly internal malformations were reported: abnormal lung lobulation, cardiac defects (septal defects, hypoplasia of pulmonary artery), thyroid and thymic hypoplasia, hernia diaphragmatica, pancreatic dysplasia (see also **Chromosome 13, trisomy 13**, and **Chromosome 18, trisomy 18**), and intestinal malrotation. Ovarian hypoplasia in females, hypospadias and testicular germinal hypoplasia in males. Enlarged and/or hydatidiform placenta. Partial hydatidiform mole is found in 80% of triploids (versus 1 in 1000 normal pregnancies) and was found to be associated with a double paternal contribution. The longer gestation in triploidy is a consequence of the presence of these pseudo-molar changes in the placenta. Hypersegmentation of neutrophilic nuclei; similar to that found in trisomy 13.

**Complications:** Unknown.

**Associated Findings:** None known.

**Etiology:** Triploid (3n) chromosome complement i.e. presence of three complete sets of chromosomes instead of the normal 2n.

**Pathogenesis:** The triploidy may arise in different ways: dispermy, digyny and diandry. Dispermy (fertilization of a haploid egg by two haploid sperms) is found in 60% of triploidies. The remaining 40% result from digyny (fertilization of a diploid egg due to maternal non disjunction by a haploid sperm) and diandry (fertilization of a haploid egg by a diploid sperm due to paternal nondisjunction). Hypo- or hypertriploidy is found in less than 10% of triploidies. There is consistent evidence that the occurrence of triploidy is increased in pregnancies which occur soon after oral contraceptives are stopped and after preconceptional abdominal irradiation.

**POS No.:** 3114

**CDC No.:** 758.586

**Sex Ratio:** M1.5:F1 (based on a review of 225 cases).

**Occurrence:** One percent of all human conceptuses are triploid. Triploidy is found in 15% of all chromosomally abnormal fetuses (late first trimester abortions and second or third trimester stillbirths). The incidence of liveborn triploids is 1:10.000 newborns.

**Risk of Recurrence for Patient's Sib:** Negligible.

**Risk of Recurrence for Patient's Child:** Lethal condition in full triploidy; severe mental retardation in diploid/triploid mosaic individuals. Affected individuals are unlikely to reproduce.

**Age of Detectability:** At birth by the presence of a typical MCA syndrome associated with severe intrauterine growth retardation. The echographic finding of severe intrauterine growth retardation, fetal edema, oligoamnios and a large placenta in the second or third trimester of pregnancy is a strong indication for amniocentesis and fetal karyotyping.

**Gene Mapping and Linkage:** See *Gene Map*.

**Prevention:** None known. Genetic counseling indicated.

**Treatment:** Unknown.

**Prognosis:** Death in the neonatal period. Survival after the neonatal period is exceptional. Some diploid/triploid individuals were reported to survive for several decades.

**Detection of Carrier:** Unknown.

**References:**
Uchida JA, et al: Triploidy and chromosomes. Am J Obstet Gynecol 1985; 151:65–69. *
Pettenati MJ, et al: Diploid-triploid mosaicism: report of necropsy findings. Am J Med Genet 1986; 24:23–38.
Sherard J, et al: Long survival in a 69,XXY triploid male. Am J Med Genet 1986; 25:307–312.

FR030
KL007

**Jean-Pierre Fryns**
**Alice Kleczkowska**

**Chromosome trisomy 17-18 syndrome**
*See CHROMOSOME 18, TRISOMY 18*
**Chromosome X monosomy X**
*See TURNER SYNDROME*

---

**CHROMOSOME X, POLY-X**            **3007**

**Includes:**
    Aneuploidy, chromosomal
    Chromosome 48,XXXX females
    Chromosome 49,XXXXX females

**Excludes:** N/A

**Major Diagnostic Criteria:** Chromosomal abnormality with more than three X chromosomes. Female patients may have nonspecific skeletal and other dysmorphic features.

**Clinical Findings:** Facial features sometimes resemble those seen in **Chromosome 21, trisomy 21**. Mild shortness of stature, delayed skeletal maturation, short neck, **Microcephaly**, flat nasal bridge, radioulnar synostosis, prognathism, low-set ears, mild-to-moderate mental retardation.

**Complications:** Depends on the skeletal and other dysmorphic features, as well as the degree of mental retardation if present.

**Associated Findings:** Eye defects, ear defects, webbed neck, joint defects, and dental anomalies.

**Etiology:** Nondisjunction in successive meiotic divisions of a parent.

**Pathogenesis:** Presumably related to the chromosomal aneuploidy.

**POS No.:** 3105, 3106

**CDC No.:** 758.990

**Sex Ratio:** M0:F1 (affects only females).

**Occurrence:** About 1,000 karyotyped individuals with these anomalies have been reported.

**Risk of Recurrence for Patient's Sib:** Probably 0.5 to 1% for any chromosomal aneuploidy.

**Risk of Recurrence for Patient's Child:** No affected individuals are known to have reproduced.

**Age of Detectability:** Usually during childhood, on the basis of congenital anomalies.

**Gene Mapping and Linkage:** See *Gene Map*.

**Prevention:** None known. Genetic counseling indicated.

**Treatment:** As indicated by the somatic features.

**Prognosis:** Variable.

**Detection of Carrier:** Possibly through karyotyping.

**References:**
Carr DH, et al.: An XXXX sex chromosome complex in two mentally defective females. Canad Med Asso J 1961; 84:131–137.
Archidiacono N, et al.: X pentasomy: a case review. Hum Genet 1979; 52:69–77.
Borgaonkar DS: Chromosomal variation in man: a catalog of chromosomal variants and anomalies, ed 5. New York: Alan R. Liss, 1989.

B0021                                    **Digamber S. Borgaonkar**

---

## CHROMOSOME X, TRIPLO-X                                    3006

**Includes:**
    Aneuploidy, chromosomal
    Chromosome 47,XXX karyotype

**Excludes:** N/A

**Major Diagnostic Criteria:** Females with three X-chromosomes.

**Clinical Findings:** Variable phenotype ranging from mostly normal to mildly dysmorphic (with or without fertility problems) to severely retarded individuals; **Eye, hypertelorism**; widely spaced nipples; skeletal anomalies, brachycephaly or **Microcephaly**; and moderate-to-severe mental retardation.

**Complications:** Depending on the severity of problems at presentation.

**Associated Findings:** Frequent fertility problems and mental subnormality has been reported. Bilateral renal agenesis and Mullerian anomalies were reported by Hogge et al (1989).

**Etiology:** Nondisjunction in parental meiotic divisions; however, no parental age relationship has been found.

**Pathogenesis:** Presumably related to the chromosomal aneuploidy.

**CDC No.:** 758.990

**Sex Ratio:** M0:F1 (affects only females).

**Occurrence:** Incidence is 1–2:3,000. One-to-two thousand karyotyped cases have been reported.

**Risk of Recurrence for Patient's Sib:** For any subsequent chromosomal aneuploidy, usually 0.5 to 1%.

**Risk of Recurrence for Patient's Child:** Unknown. Some patients have had chromosomally abnormal offspring.

**Age of Detectability:** On blood karyotyping at any age, or by prenatal diagnosis.

**Gene Mapping and Linkage:** See *Gene Map*.

**Prevention:** None known. Genetic counseling indicated.

**Treatment:** None required unless indicated because of somatic and psychologic problems.

**Prognosis:** Usually excellent.

**Detection of Carrier:** Possibly through karyotyping.

**References:**
Barr ML, et al.: The triple-X female: an appraisal based on a study of 12 cases and a review of the literature. Can Med Assoc J 1969; 101:247–258.
Zizka J, et al.: XXYY son of a triplo-X mother. Humangenetik 1975; 26:159–160.
Borgaonkar DS: Chromosomal variation in man: a catalog of chromosomal variants and anomalies, ed 5. New York, Alan R. Liss, 1989.
Hogge WA, et al.: Bilateral renal agenesis and Mullerian anomalies in a 47,XXX fetus. Am J Med Genet 1989; 33:242–243.

B0021                                    **Digamber S. Borgaonkar**

**Chromosome Xq duplication-mental retardation, X-linked**
    *See X-LINKED MENTAL RETARDATION-Xq DUPLICATION*
**Chromosome XXY**
    *See KLINEFELTER SYNDROME*

---

## CHROMOSOME XYY                                    2552

**Includes:**
    Chromosome XYY Males
    Chromosome XYY, 47,XYY Males

**Excludes:** Chromosome Y polysomy (others)

**Major Diagnostic Criteria:** Male phenotype with 47,XYY karyotype.

**Clinical Findings:** Although the first report of an XYY male was made in 1961, medical and lay interest in this chromosomal abnormality was only aroused with the 1965 report of an increased prevalence of the XYY constitution among tall and mentally retarded incarcerated males. Since that time multiple single case studies and retrospective surveys have contributed additional, although possibly biased, information about the XYY phenotype. Prospective developmental studies of 59 47,XYY males identified as newborns are in progress in several centers, and early data from these studies are now available.

Most affected individuals are phenotypically normal males. However, a variety of abnormal clinical features have been reported. Most of these anomalies are minor, and as yet no anomalies have consistently been seen in XYY males identified by random newborn screening. The most frequently reported physical feature is excessive height. At birth, growth parameters are unremarkable, but height above the 50th percentile is usually attained by early childhood. Nodulocystic acne, large deciduous and permanent teeth, and subtle neurologic abnormalities such as intention tremor and incoordination are probably associated with the XYY condition. Neurologic studies comparing XYY men to normal controls have demonstrated both significantly lower nerve conduction velocities and lower alpha-wave frequency on EEG. An increased PR interval on EKG has also been demonstrated. Dermatoglyphic studies have shown a significantly lower mean total ridge count. Varied genital abnormalities such as cryptorchidism, hypospadias, and small testes have been reported, and abnormal testicular histology, including decreased spermatogenesis, spermatogenic arrest, and Sertoli-cell-only configuration, has been found. However, in most XYY men gonadal development and testicular size are normal, and many XYY males have fathered children. Results of endocrine investigations are inconclusive and often contradictory. No consistent abnormality of androgens, pituitary gonadotropins, or growth hormone have been revealed in studies to date.

Data compiled from multicenter prospective studies of XYY infants identified from newborn surveys show cognitive development (performance and verbal IQ) to be within normal limits and not significantly different from sibs or controls. Despite this fact, educational difficulties occur in approximately 50% of these individuals. Language development is most often affected, and decreased speed in information processing has been noted. Moderate impairment in sensorimotor integration skills is also present. In contrast, data from psychologic testing of 12 Danish XYY men identified by examination of the top 15% of the height distribution of all males born during a specified period of time in Copenhagen showed full scale IQs significantly lower (P<0.001) than those of controls matched for age, height, and social class.

The relationship of the XYY karyotype to psychologic disturbance and criminality is the subject of multiple investigations. In prospective studies of children, the overall incidence of behavior problems is not significantly different than that of controls or 47,XXY individuals. The prevalence of XYY males is increased in Western mental-penal institutions perhaps as much as 20 times above the newborn prevalence rate. The causes of increased antisocial behavior in adult XYY males are uncertain, and whether a tendency to personality disorders exists has not been satisfactorily determined. Early reports characterized the XYY male as overly aggressive. However, the initial impression that these men were more likely to exhibit aggressive behavior against other people has not been substantiated. In general, crimes committed are not dissimilar to those committed by XY men, the most common crimes being theft, arson, and burglary. Other behavioral features frequently attributed to the XYY male include impulsivity, immaturity, and increased anxiety. Schizoid-type personality traits have been noted in several studies. None of these behavioral tendencies has been consistently noted in the neonatally ascertained groups, but, at present, these children have not reached adulthood.

**Complications:** Increased risk for difficulties with language development, questionable increased risk for behavioral disability, questionable increased risk for infertility.

**Associated Findings:** Various bone and joint abnormalities reported as single incidences, including **Radial-ulnar synostosis** in three black XYY males, varicose veins, and **Hernia, inguinal.**

**Etiology:** The origin of the extra Y chromosome is always paternal and results from nondisjunction in the second meiotic division. Mitotic nondisjunction after fertilization results in mosaicism. There are no clearly defined factors predisposing to XYY. No parental age effect has been shown. Familial predisposition to nondisjunction has been postulated, and, in fact, the first reported male with XYY was studied because he had a trisomy 21 daughter. There are also several single case reports of XYY and autosomal trisomy in the same patient.

**Pathogenesis:** The additive gene dosage effect of Y-linked genes is uncertain, although there is evidence that characteristics such as height and tooth size are influenced by an additional Y chromosome.

Although no one physical, neuropsychologic, or social factor has consistently been associated with the increased frequency of XYY males in mental-penal institutions, many of these individuals report a disordered or disrupted childhood environment. Investigators have postulated a decreased ability of XYY males to adapt to stress, with a nonsupportive environment predisposing to socially unacceptable behavior.

**CDC No.:** 758.990

**Sex Ratio:** M1:F0

**Occurrence:** Neonatal chromosome surveys show an incidence of approximately 1:1,000 in caucasian and Japanese populations. The incidence in blacks is lower, although not well established. Prevalence in mental-penal institutions may be as high as 20:1,000.

**Risk of Recurrence for Patient's Sib:** Risk for nondisjunction in subsequent pregnancies may be as high as 1%.

**Risk of Recurrence for Patient's Child:** Risk for aneuploidy seems low, with sons of XYY males usually having a normal chromosome constitution.

**Age of Detectability:** Prenatally by chromosomal analysis of amniotic fluid cells or chorionic villi. Fluorescent staining is often used to confirm the presence of an extra Y chromosome.

**Gene Mapping and Linkage:** Unknown.

**Prevention:** None known. Genetic counseling indicated.

**Treatment:** "Anticipatory guidance" offering early intervention for learning disabilities and psychologic abnormalities.

**Prognosis:** Life span is presumably normal.

**Detection of Carrier:** Unknown.

**Special Considerations:** Whether or not an XYY syndrome exists is controversial. Certainly the only consistent physical feature has been tall stature. Much publicity has been given to characteristics such as subnormal mentality and aggressive criminal behavior that were present in some of the early reported cases. At present, reports from prospective studies of XYY males identified as newborns show mental ability not significantly different from controls, but learning disabilities and, in some study groups, behavioral problems are increased. Studies on XYY males identified in a random population survey show a slight but statistically significant decrease in IQ and an increased frequency of criminal behavior. Thus, the genetic counseling of parents of an XYY fetus presents a dilemma. Most geneticists advocate full disclosure of the diagnosis and current data on growth and development of these individuals. At present, parents can be advised that their XYY sons are more likely to be tall and have decreased athletic abilities, and they are at increased risk for learning and possibly behavioral difficulties. Long-term prognosis attained from prospectively studied XYY newborns is still incomplete, since the oldest of these boys is now in late adolescence. A supportive family environment with anticipation and early intervention of learning or behavioral difficulties is advocated.

**References:**

Robinson A, et al., eds: Sex chromosome aneuploidy: prospective studies on children. BD:OAS XV(1). New York: March of Dimes Birth Defects Foundation, 1979:1–281.

Stewart DA, ed: Children with sex chromosome aneuploidy: follow-up studies. BD:OAS XVIII(4). New York: March of Dimes Birth Defects Foundation, 1982:1–251.

Theilgaard A: A psychological study of the personalities of XYY- and XXY- men. Acta Psych Scand [suppl 315] 1984; 69:1–133.

Sandberg AA, ed: The XYY syndrome. In: The Y chromosome, part B: clinical aspects of Y chromosome abnormalities. New York: Alan R. Liss, 1985:247–373. *

Ratcliffe SG, Paul N, eds: Prospective studies on children with sex chromosomal aneuploidy. BD:OAS XXII(3). New York: March of Dimes Birth Defects Foundation, 1986:1–328. *

M0039
WE005

**Cynthia A. Moore**
**David D. Weaver**

**Chromosome XYY Males**
*See CHROMOSOME XYY*
**Chromosome XYY, 47,XYY Males**
*See CHROMOSOME XYY*
**Chromosome, abnormal centromere and chromatid apposition**
*See ROBERTS SYNDROME*
**Chromosome, Marker X**
*See X-LINKED MENTAL RETARDATION, FRAGILE X SYNDROME*
**Chromosome, nucleolar organizer region, familial unbalanced**
*See CHROMOSOME, NUCLEOLAR ORGANIZER REGION, TRANSLOCATION*

## CHROMOSOME, NUCLEOLAR ORGANIZER REGION, TRANSLOCATION 2538

**Includes:**

Chromosome, nucleolar organizer region, familial unbalanced
Chromosome, translocation or insertion of NOR

**Excludes:**

Long arm of an acrocentric chromosome onto another chromosome.

**Major Diagnostic Criteria:** Translocations involving the nucleolar organizer region (NOR) occur in clinically normal individuals. Diagnosis is confirmed by silver staining of the chromosomes.

In a human karyotype, a maximum of ten secondary constrictions can be observed, one each on the short arms of the acrocentric chromosomes 13, 14, 15, 21, and 22. Each of these short arms has a short proximal chromatic segment (normal staining), the satellite, and achromatic secondary constriction, the

NORMAL Q-BANDED AND NOR CHROMOSOME #2

NORMAL Q-BANDED AND NOR CHROMOSOME #13

TRANSLOCATED NOR CHROMOSOME #2

DELETED NOR CHROMOSOME #13

**2538-20664:** Normal, translocated and deleted NOR regions.

stalk. The achromatic stalks contain active ribosomal DNA and represent the sites for the 18S + 28S ribosomal cistron. Using silver staining, the stalks stain deeply and are referred to as *AgNORs*. The size of the AgNOR is proportional to the stalk length: Chromosomes with very short stalks stain less frequently and carry the least amount of silver deposits. The NORs show a considerable range of polymorphic variants with respect to size, shape, and number, which can vary from individual to individual.

Singh et al (1986) reported a translocation of the short arm of a chromosome 13, including the NOR, onto the long arm of chromosome 2: 46,XY,-2,der(2),t(2;13)(q37;p11)pat. The unbalanced NOR was found to be present in six of 11 members of three generations. Previously, there have been reports of reciprocal translocations involving NORs and chromosomes 3, 5, and 9 (Hausmann et al, 1977; Dev et al, 1979), Cosper et al (1985) reported an insertion of a NOR and a centromere into chromosome 11 at band 11q21.

Stetten et al (1986) reported a unique finding of the satellited X chromosome in a woman with **Turner syndrome** and mosaic karyotype. Schmid et al (1984) and Bajnoczky et al (1985) have reported NOR on the long arm of the Y chromosome. All of the family members carrying satellited Y chromosomes were healthy; the abnormal phenotype of the propositus was interpreted as coincidence (Bajnoczky et al, 1985). Watt et al (1984) reported an inserted NOR on chromosome 12 in members of three generations with no physical anomaly.

**Clinical Findings:** Carriers of unbalanced nonreciprocal translocations of NOR on a chromosome have not been reported to have any appreciable clinical abnormalities. In a case with an unbalanced reciprocal translocation where other autosomes have a deletion, the clinical features would be those seen in a monosomy of that chromosome. NORs do not have mendelian genes that produce clinical abnormalities.

**Complications:** Carriers may be at risk for spontaneous abortions or miscarriages; otherwise, clinically normal carrier offspring will be born.

**Associated Findings:** None known.

**Etiology:** Unknown.

**Pathogenesis:** Unknown.

**CDC No.:** 758.990

**Sex Ratio:** M1:F1

**Occurrence:** Undetermined but presumed rare. Usually familial, but new translocations may occur.

**Risk of Recurrence for Patient's Sib:** If parent is a carrier, 1:2 or 50% for each sib to be a carrier; otherwise, not increased.

**Risk of Recurrence for Patient's Child:** 1:2 (50%).

**Age of Detectability:** At birth, or prenatally by chromosomal analysis.

**Gene Mapping and Linkage:** rDNA or 18S + 28S rDNA on the short arm of acrocentric chromosomes.

**Prevention:** None known. Genetic counseling indicated.

**Treatment:** Unknown.

**Prognosis:** Normal life span and intelligence.

**Detection of Carrier:** Chromosomal analysis with silver staining technique.

**References:**
Hausmann I, et al.: Reciprocal or non-reciprocal human chromosome translocations? The identification of reciprocal translocations by silver staining. Hum Genet 1977; 38:1–5.
Dev VG, et al.: Partial translocation of NOR and its activity in a balanced carrier and in her cri-du-chat fetus. Hum Genet 1979; 51:277–280.
Bardhan S, et al.: Possible association between radiation exposure and chromosome changes. Lancet 1981; II:362–363.
Schmid M, et al.: Satellited Y chromosomes: structure, origin, and clinical significance. Hum Genet 1984; 67:72–85.
Watt JL, et al.: A familial insertion involving an active nucleolar organiser within chromosome 12. J Med Genet 1984; 21:379–384.
Bajnoczky K, et al.: Coincidence of paternal 13pYq translocation and maternal increased 13p NOR activity in a child with arthrogryposis and other malformations. Acta Paediatr Hung 1985; 26:151–156.
Cosper P, et al.: Familial insertion of nucleolar organizer regions and centromere material into the long arm of 11. Am J Hum Genet 1985; 37:A89.
Singh DN, et al.: Familial unbalanced nucleolar organizer region (NOR) translocated chromosome 2. Berlin: Proc Seventh Int Cong Hum Genet 1986:68.
Stetten G, et al.: Translocation of the nucleolus organizer region to the human X chromosome. Am J Hum Genet 1986; 39:245–252.

SI025                                              **Dharmdeo N. Singh**

**Chromosome, ovulation induction trisomy**
*See OVULATION INDUCTION TRISOMY*
**Chromosome, tetraploid/diploid mosaicism**
*See CHROMOSOME TETRAPLOIDY*
**Chromosome, translocation or insertion of NOR**
*See CHROMOSOME, NUCLEOLAR ORGANIZER REGION, TRANSLOCATION*
**Chromosomes, balanced double translocations**
*See CHROMOSOMES, COMPLEX REARRANGEMENTS*
**Chromosomes, complex double translocations**
*See CHROMOSOMES, COMPLEX REARRANGEMENTS*

## CHROMOSOMES, COMPLEX REARRANGEMENTS          2535

**Includes:**
    Chromosomes, balanced double translocations
    Chromosomes, complex double translocations
    Chromosomes, complex translocations
    Chromosomes, multiple breaks and rearrangements
    Chromosomes, multiple reciprocal translocations

**Excludes:**
    Chromosome rearrangements, acquired complex
    Chromosome rearrangements in leukemias and cancer
    Chromosome rearrangements with less than three
        chromosome breaks

**Major Diagnostic Criteria:** The diagnosis should be considered whenever congenital anomalies and/or mental retardation of unknown etiology are encountered. Family history of first trimester

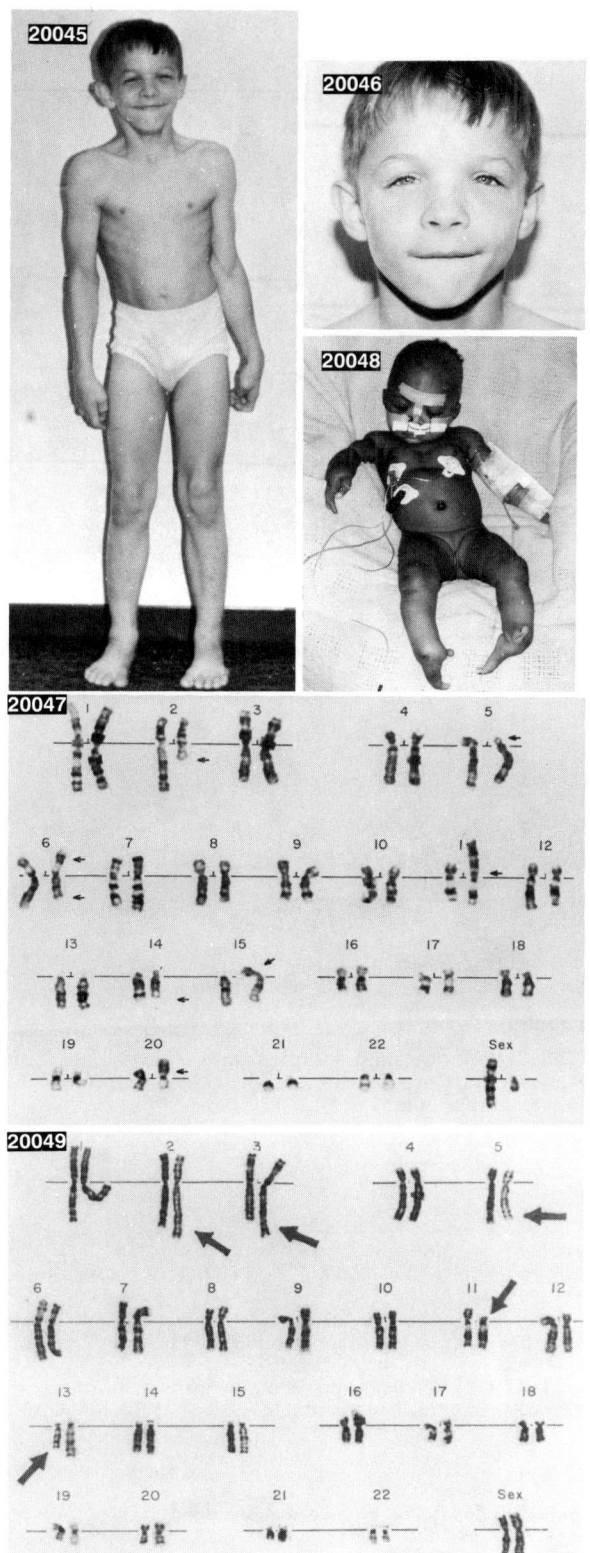

miscarriages and/or previous children with congenital anomalies of unknown etiology may represent a clue to the diagnosis in the familial cases. Otherwise, there are no characteristic phenotypic features; the latter vary with the different break points and derivative chromosomes. Karyotyping of two different tissues is necessary as well as karyotypes of the parents and determination of the break points by at least two banding techniques.

**Clinical Findings:** None is characteristic. In the reported patients, mental retardation was a frequent feature. Decreased growth rate leading to short stature and **Microcephaly** was also common. Seizures, aniridia, cataracts, cleft lip and/or cleft palate, hearing loss, congenital heart defects, scoliosis, intestinal malrotation, limb abnormalities, contractures, **Syndactyly**, hypospadias and minor anomalies have been reported.

**Complications:** Feeding problems and failure to thrive.

**Associated Findings:** Difficult to determine because of the different chromosomes involved.

**Etiology:** Unknown.

**Pathogenesis:** Possibly transient chromosome instability in the gamete (or zygote).

**CDC No.:** 758.990

**Sex Ratio:** M1:F1

**Occurrence:** Some 50 cases have been reported, including several prenatal reports.

**Risk of Recurrence for Patient's Sib:** Presumed to be increased in the familial subgroup.

**Risk of Recurrence for Patient's Child:** Increased in the familial subgroup. About 10% risk for an abnormal liveborn and 48% risk for an early miscarriage. In the *de novo* subgroup, there has been no known reproduction by an affected individual.

**Age of Detectability:** At birth, depending upon the severity of the clinical manifestations, or prenatally by cytogenetic studies. Restriction fragment length polymorphisms and DNA probes should be of use for more accurate determination of the break points and the resultant chromosome rearrangements.

**Gene Mapping and Linkage:** See *Gene Map.*

**Prevention:** None known. Genetic counseling indicated.

**Treatment:** Palliative for specific clinical features. Intensive infant stimulation for existing developmental delay.

**Prognosis:** Depends on the severity of the clinical features.

**Detection of Carrier:** By cytogenetic studies.

**Special Considerations:** While the phenomenon of congenital complex chromosome rearrangements is rare in man, it appears that both the clinical and cytogenetic diagnosis are rather difficult. Patients are often misdiagnosed, leading to inaccurate genetic counseling in regard to phenotype, prognosis and recurrence risk.

**References:**

Buchanan PD, et al.: A complex translocation involving chromosomes 3, 11, and 14 with an interstitial deletion, del (14) (q13q22) in a child with congenital glaucoma and cleft lip and palate. BD:OAS XIV(6C). New York: March of Dimes Birth Defects Foundation, 1978:317–322.

Pai GS, et al.: Complex chromosome rearrangements. Clin Genet 1980; 18:436–444.

Kleczkowska A, et al.: Complex chromosomal rearrangements (CCR) and their genetic consequences. J Hum Genet 1982; 30:199–214.

Kim HJ, et al.: Prenatal diagnosis of a de novo complex chromosomal rearrangement involving four chromosomes. Prenat Diagn 1986; 6:211–216.

Kousseff BG, et al.: Complex chromosome rearrangements and congenital anomalies. Am J Med Genet 1987; 26:771–782. *

Gorski JL, et al.: Reproductive risks for carriers of complex chromosome rearrangements: analysis of 25 families. Am J Med Genet 1988; 29:247–261.

K0018                                                      **Boris G. Kousseff**

**Chromosomes, complex translocations**
*See CHROMOSOMES, COMPLEX REARRANGEMENTS*

**2535**-20045: A boy with a complex chromosomal rearrangement; note fronto-pelvic tilt. 20046: Note facial features including downward slanting palpebral fissures and telecanthus. 20047: G-banded karyotype of patient in 20045. Arrows indicate break points. 20048: Infant with complex chromosomal rearrangements. Note the cleft lip, telecanthus and ectrodactyly. 20049: G-banded karyotype of infant in 20048. Arrows indicate break points.

**Chromosomes, multiple breaks and rearrangements**
*See CHROMOSOMES, COMPLEX REARRANGEMENTS*
**Chromosomes, multiple reciprocal translocations**
*See CHROMOSOMES, COMPLEX REARRANGEMENTS*
**Chronic osteopathy with hyperphosphatasia**
*See OSTEOECTASIA*
**CHRPE in adenomatous polyposis (Intestinal polyposis, type III)**
*See RETINA, CONGENITAL HYPERTROPHY OF RETINAL PIGMENT EPITHELIUM*
**CHRPE, isolated**
*See RETINA, CONGENITAL HYPERTROPHY OF RETINAL PIGMENT EPITHELIUM*
**Chwechweechwe**
*See ANEMIA, SICKLE CELL*
**Chylomicron retention disease**
*See LIPID TRANSPORT DEFECT OF INTESTINE*
**Cigarette smoking, fetal effects of**
*See FETAL EFFECTS OF MATERNAL CIGARETTE SMOKING*

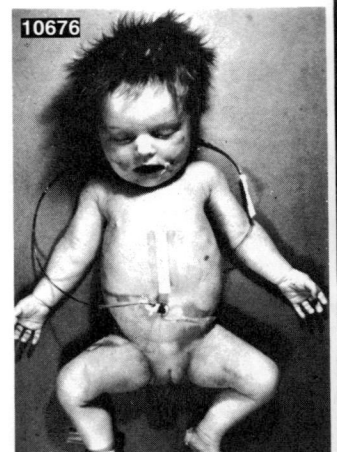
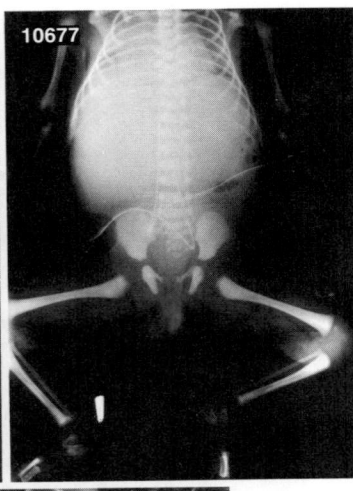
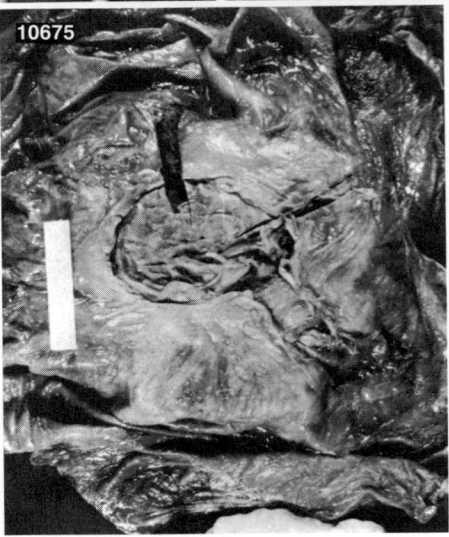

## CIRCUMVALLATE PLACENTA SYNDROME        0187

**Includes:**
    CNS depression-hemorrhage-skeletal syndrome
    Placenta, circumvallate

**Excludes:**  N/A

**Major Diagnostic Criteria:**  Polyhydramnios, CNS depression, neonatal hemorrhage, skeletal abnormalities.

**Clinical Findings:**  Neonatal death occurred in three sibs due to respiratory insufficiency. All three pregnancies were complicated by polyhydramnios, and each infant showed cutaneous and intracranial hemorrhage, marked CNS depression, and skeletal abnormalities, including thin ribs and overtubulation of long bones. Other findings include brachycephaly, frontal bossing, flat nasal bridge, hyperextensible joints, and hyperelastic skin. No specific coagulation defect was found, and electron microscopy did not reveal a morphologic defect of capillaries. There was no disease in the mother to explain polyhydramnios. The placenta of only one of the three cases was examined, and it was reported to be circumvallate with characteristic fibrin deposition.

**Complications:**  Neonatal hemorrhage, aspiration pneumonia, respiratory distress, cardiac arrest, neonatal death.

**Associated Findings:**  None known.

**Etiology:**  Possibly autosomal recessive inheritance.

**Pathogenesis:**  A maternofetal incompatibility, leading to fibrin deposition and formation of a circumvallate placenta, or repeated marginal placental hemorrhages, leading to circumvallate placenta, are possibilities.

**MIM No.:**  21555

**Sex Ratio:**  Presumably M1:F1

**Occurrence:**  Familial cases documented in at least three kinships.

**Risk of Recurrence for Patient's Sib:**
    See Part I, *Mendelian Inheritance.* Possibly 100% if maternofetal incompatibility exists.

**Risk of Recurrence for Patient's Child:**
    See Part I, *Mendelian Inheritance.*

**Age of Detectability:**  At birth.

**Gene Mapping and Linkage:**  Unknown.

**Prevention:**  None known. Genetic counseling indicated.

**Treatment:**  Careful surveillance of such mothers for polyhydramnios and circumvallate placenta and their infants for CNS depression, skeletal anomalies, and neonatal hemorrhage. Treatment of anoxia and hemorrhage. Supportive measures to prevent further CNS depression and hemorrhage.

**Prognosis:**  Poor. At least three cases died in the neonatal period.

**Detection of Carrier:**  Unknown.

**0187**-10676: Physical appearance immediately after death. 10677: X-ray shows mild shortness and overtubulation of long bones, with thin gracile ribs and bell-shaped thorax. 10675: Circumvallate placenta.

**References:**
Morgan J: Circumvallate placenta. J Obstet Gynaecol Br Commwlth 1955; 62:899–900.
Naftolin F, et al.: The syndrome of chronic abruptio placentae, hydrorrhea and circumvallate placenta. Am J Obstet Gynecol 1973; 116:347.
Deacon JSR, et al.: Polyhydramnios and neonatal hemorrhage in three sisters. A circumvallate placenta syndrome? In: BD:OAS 1974; X(7):41–49.

GI005                                    **Enid F. Gilbert-Barnes**

**Cirrhosis with deposition of abnormal glycogen, familial**
*See GLYCOGENOSIS, TYPE IV*
**Cirrhosis, congenital pigmentary**
*See HEMOCHROMATOSIS, IDIOPATHIC*
**Cirrhosis, juvenile (some)**
*See ALPHA(1)-ANTITRYPSIN DEFICIENCY*
**Cirsoid aneurysm of external ear**
*See EAR, ARTERIOVENOUS FISTULA*
**Cistinuria**
*See CYSTINURIA*

## CITRULLINEMIA                                    0174

**Includes:**
Argininosuccinate synthetase deficiency
Citrullinuria

**Excludes:**
**Aciduria, argininosuccinic** (0087)
**Pyruvate carboxylase deficiency with lactic acidemia** (0850)

**Major Diagnostic Criteria:** Elevation of plasma, urinary, and cerebrospinal fluid citrulline levels.

**Clinical Findings:** Most patients appear normal in the newborn period, but after feedings are begun, poor sucking, vomiting, and lethargy are noted. Muscle tone may be increased or decreased, and there may be grunting or rapid respirations. Some patients also have hepatomegaly with increased SGOT. Seizures follow, and eventually the baby lapses into deep coma, with progressive apnea requiring assisted ventilation; eventually death follows.

Less common are patients who present after the neonatal period with progressive feeding problems, vomiting, ataxia, and seizures. Some patients also have hepatomegaly with increased liver enzymes.

If the patient with either the neonatal or later-onset form survives the initial insult, recurrent crises occur, usually precipitated by intercurrent infection or by excessive protein intake. Each form is potentially life-threatening.

During any acute episode, the plasma ammonia level is several times normal, with values over 1,000 mg/dl common (normal for neonates, less than 100). Secondary increases in glutamine, alanine, and often lysine are seen. Serum arginine is low, and the BUN may be low or normal. Plasma citrulline levels are markedly elevated, often 40 times normal, while urinary excretion may reach several grams per day. CSF citrulline is also increased, but to a lesser extent than in blood.

**Complications:** Most surviving patients have a significant degree of mental retardation. Recurrent bouts of hyperammonemia are usual.

**Associated Findings:** None known.

**Etiology:** Autosomal recessive inheritance. Deficiency of argininosuccinate synthetase (ASS) enzyme, which mediates the ATP and magnesium-dependent reversible reaction between L-citrulline and L-aspartate to form argininosuccinate, AMP, and inorganic pyrophosphate. The enzyme is normally detectable in liver and fibroblast tissues.

**Pathogenesis:** Deficiency of ASS enzyme causes ammonia toxicity, which in turn results in the clinical findings described.

**MIM No.:** *21570

**Sex Ratio:** M1:F1

**Occurrence:** Undetermined but presumably rare. Established literature. A late-onset form has been frequently reported in Japanese populations (Walser, 1983).

**Risk of Recurrence for Patient's Sib:**
See Part I, *Mendelian Inheritance.*

**Risk of Recurrence for Patient's Child:**
See Part I, *Mendelian Inheritance.*

**Age of Detectability:** Elevated plasma citrulline levels after protein containing feeding begun. Detection is possible prenatally. In the late onset form, clinical findings do not appear until childhood or as late as age 48 in one case.
*Prenatal diagnosis:* Enzymatic analysis of cultured amniotic fluid cells will detect the defect. Some increase in citrulline content has also been found in amniotic fluid. A recent study reports rapid detection of citrullinemia in a 9-week fetus by testing incorporation of $^{14}$C-citrulline in villus tissue.

**Gene Mapping and Linkage:** ASS (argininosuccinate synthetase) has been mapped to 9q34-qter.

**Prevention:** None known. Genetic counseling indicated.

**Treatment:** *Acute:* Hemodialysis or peritoneal dialysis to help clear ammonia; high-caloric fluid to help minimize tissue catabolism. Arginine stimulates step 1 of the urea cycle, encouraging protein synthesis and nitrogen elimination via pyrimidines. Nitrogen excretion is enhanced by sodium benzoate (conjugates with glycine, excreted as hippuric acid) and sodium phenylacetate (conjugates with glutamine, excreted as phenylacetylglutamine).
*Chronic:* Dietary protein restriction with high-caloric intake. Supplementary arginine as needed; sodium benzoate and sodium phenylacetate may also be helpful.

**Prognosis:** Most patients who live beyond the neonatal period are mentally retarded. There is a good correlation between the duration of the neonatal hyperammonemia and the severity of both mental retardation and brain CT abnormalities (increase in ventricular and sulcus size, and in areas of low density). In one series, eight surviving patients aged 41 ± 7 months had IQs that measured 41 ± 8 (mean ± SEM).

**Detection of Carrier:** Intermediate levels of ASS enzyme have been found in the fibroblasts of parents of affected children.

**Special Considerations:** Fasting blood ammonia levels may be normal. If a urea cycle defect is suspected and the fasting level is normal, a protein load of 1.5 g of protein per kilogram is given, by nasogastric tube if necessary. The ammonia determination, made about 2 hours afterward, will reveal a severalfold increase.

**References:**
Coude FX, et al.: Secondary citrullinemia with hyperammonemia in four neonatal cases of pyruvate carboxylase deficiency. Pediatrics 1981; 68:914 (only).
Brusilow SW, et al.: Neonatal hyperammonemic coma. Adv Pediatr 1982; 29:69–103. *
Fleisher LD, et al.: Citrullinemia: prenatal diagnosis of an affected fetus. Am J Hum Genet 1983; 35:85–90.
Walser M: Urea cycle disorders and other hereditary hyperammonemic syndromes. In Stanbury, JB, et al., eds: The metabolic basis of inherited disease, 5th ed. New York: McGraw-Hill, 1983:402–438.
Brusilow SW, et al.: Treatment of episodic hyperammonemia in children with inborn errors of urea synthesis. N Engl J Med 1984; 310:1630–1634.
Kleijer WJ, et al.: First-trimester (chorion biopsy) diagnosis of citrullinemia and methylmalonicaciduria. Lancet 1984; II:1340 (only).
Msall M, et al.: Neurologic outcome in children with inborn errors of urea synthesis. N Engl J Med 1984; 310:1500–1505. *

AMO04                                          **Mary G. Ampola**

**Citrullinuria**
See *CITRULLINEMIA*
**Clark-Baraitser X-linked mental retardation**
See *X-LINKED MENTAL RETARDATION, CLARK-BARAITSER TYPE*
**Classic hemophilia**
See *HEMOPHILIA A*
**Classic migraine**
See *MIGRAINE*
**Clear cell carcinoma of the kidney**
See *CANCER, RENAL CELL CARCINOMA*
**Clear cell sarcoma of the kidney (CCSK)**
See *CANCER, WILMS TUMOR*
**Cleft chin**
See *FACE, CHIN FISSURE*
**Cleft ear lobe**
See *EAR LOBE, CLEFT*
**Cleft larynx**
See *LARYNGO-TRACHEO-ESOPHAGEAL CLEFT*

## CLEFT LIP                                        0178

**Includes:**
Cheilopalatoschisis
Cheiloschisis
Cleft palate-cleft lip (isolated)
Harelip
Intrauterine healed clefts
Lip, cleft
Lip, indentations of upper

**Excludes:**
**Cleft palate** (0180)

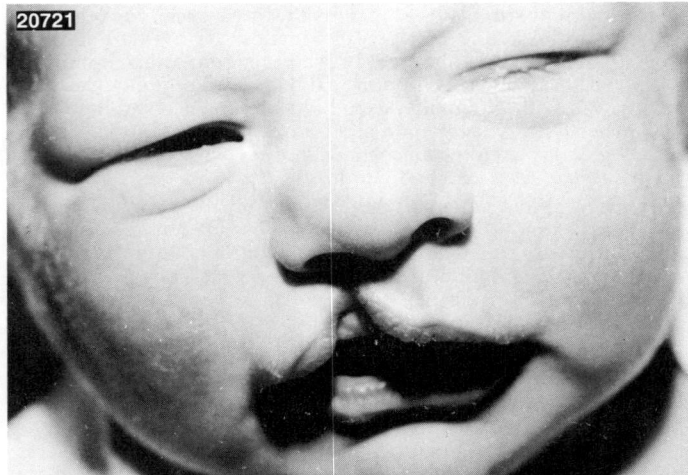

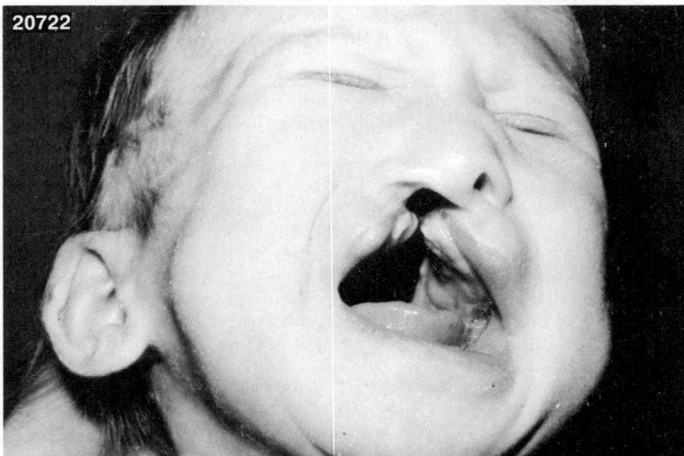

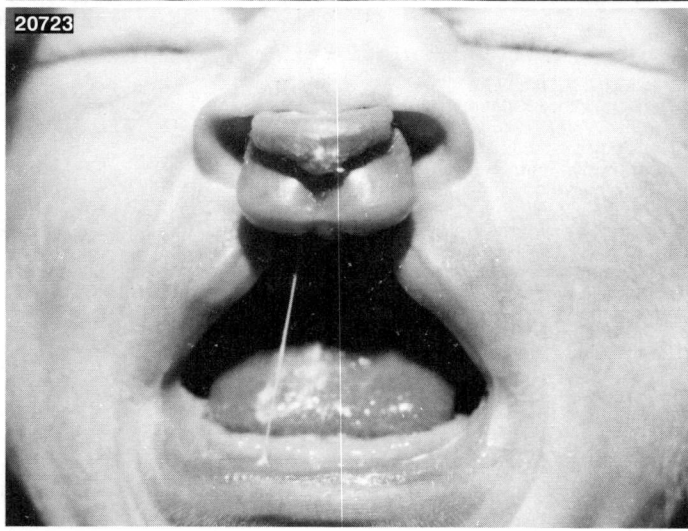

**0178**-20721: Unilateral cleft lip. 20722: Unilateral cleft lip and palate. 20723: Bilateral cleft lip and palate.

**Lip, median cleft of upper** (0595)
**Maxilla, median alveolar cleft** (0631)
**Major Diagnostic Criteria:** Cleft lip with or without cleft palate.

**Clinical Findings:** Findings include incomplete or complete clefts of the upper lip, which may be unilateral or bilateral and may extend posteriorly to include the maxillary alveolar process and hard and soft palates. In some cases, the ala of the nose may be deficient on the cleft side.

**Complications:** In the presence of a cleft of the palate, the following complications can occur: difficulty in sucking; inadequate intake of formula, resulting from excessive swallowing of air and leading to a false sense of fullness; serous otitis media and conductive hearing loss; aspiration; and hypernasal speech. In cases of cleft lip without cleft palate, no complications are known to occur.

**Associated Findings:** Congenital heart disease is known to be associated with unilateral cleft lip and palate (5%) and bilateral cleft lip and palate (12%). Deformity of the lower limbs is seen in 11% of patients with cleft lip and palate. Asymmetry of the ears is seen in 21% of cases.

**Etiology:** There are a large number of syndromes in which cleft lip and palate (CLP) may be one of the features. For most of these, the cause is unidentified. A few are associated with recognizable chromosomal aberrations, and about one-third are caused by major mutant genes. Each of these syndromes is rare, and together they may account for perhaps 5% of all cases, most of the rest being multifactorially determined.

It has been hypothesized that CLP is polygenic with a threshold effect such that the number of genes needed to exceed the developmental threshold and produce cleft is greater in females than in males and such that affected females have a greater risk for having affected children (with boys being at greatest risk), than do affected males for having affected offspring. Concordance for cleft lip in monozygotic twins (33%) is greater than for isolated cleft palate, suggesting that the genetic contribution to causation is larger and more significant than the environmental contribution. In spite of many attempts to demonstrate environmental factors associated with CLP, no association has been convincingly demonstrated between CLP and such things as season, geographic location (except for racial groups), social class, maternal age or parity, or paternal age. A number of prenatal factors have been tentatively implicated, such as pernicious vomiting during pregnancy, drugs (antiepileptic drugs are currently under suspicion), maternal bleeding, toxemia of pregnancy, and toxoplasma; but none is firmly supported. Recently, diazepam intake during pregnancy has been shown not to increase the risk of oral clefts in the fetus.

**Pathogenesis:** Parents of children with CLP tend to have less prominent maxillae, an increased bizygomatic diameter and more rectangular or trapezoid-shaped faces than controls. There is embryologic evidence that a small portion of the primary palate forms initially by an epithelial invagination process, and the major portion is formed by the coalescence of facial processes through epithelial fusion and mesenchymal consolidation. Studies on the embryogenesis of clefts of the primary palate in man and experimental animals have indicated that clefts result from a failure of the epithelial fusion-mesenchymal consolidation process. The process may fail at different stages as follows: failure of the embryonic facial processes to come into contact; failure of epithelial fusion despite contact of the processes; failure of mesenchymal consolidation; and rupture of the primary palate subsequent to fusion.

Certain underlying developmental alterations are of significance in some cases of CLP. These alterations are reduced facial mesenchyme; increased facial width; and distortion or malposition of the facial processes. Evidence supporting this is indirect and has been gathered from epidemiologic and other studies.

**MIM No.:** 21590

**CDC No.:** 749.1, 749.2

**Sex Ratio:** Depends on ethnic background and severity of the defect. The more severe the cleft, the greater the male preponderance.

## Sex Ratio by Family Background and Severity

| Caucasian | CL – CP | M62:F38 |
|---|---|---|
| | CL + CP | M66:F34 |
| Japanese | CL – CP | M45:F55 |
| | CL + CP | M66:F34 |
| American black | CL – CP | M39:F61 |
| | CL + CP | M48:F52 |

**Occurrence:** Caucasian, 1:1,000 births; Orientals, 1:700 births; Africans, 1:2,500 births.

**Risk of Recurrence for Patient's Sib:** Five percent for female proband and 3.9% for male proband.

**Risk of Recurrence for Patient's Child:** Four percent. If one parent and a child are affected, the risk of having another affected child is about 15%.

**Age of Detectability:** Prenatally by medical imaging forward projection of maxilla. At birth by physical examination.

**Gene Mapping and Linkage:** Unknown.

**Prevention:** None known. Genetic counseling indicated.

**Treatment:** When a cleft palate coexists with the cleft lip, there may be respiratory and feeding difficulties. For the former, the infant should be kept prone (face down) until he or she seems to be able to tolerate lying on the back. Feeding difficulties may be managed by feeding the infant in an upright position using a modified nipple.

The cleft lip and associated cleft palate can be closed at the usual age for such repairs. A lip adhesion is usually performed first, followed by definitive lip repairs at a later age. The palate is often closed at a separate surgery. Secondary surgery to correct residual nasal defects, abnormalities of the vermillion border and scar reduction is usually necessary. Mandibular orthognathic surgery may be necessary.

Presurgical orthopedics is recommended for cases with complete unilateral and bilateral cleft lip and palate. Repositioning of the floating premaxilla should be attempted before lip surgery is attempted. The insertion of ventilation tubes to drain middle ear fluid and to restore normal hearing may be necessary.

Speech therapy following surgical closure of the cleft palate is indicated if a residual speech problem is diagnosed after surgery. Orthodontics may be needed.

**Prognosis:** Good to excellent results depend on the availability of tissue and the degree of deficiency.

**Detection of Carrier:** Unknown.

**Support Groups:**
MA; Quincy; Prescription Parents, Inc.
CANADA: Ontario; Toronto; Canadian Cleft Lip and Palate Family Association

**References:**
Fraser FC: The genetics of cleft lip and cleft palate. Am J Hum Genet 1970; 22:336.
Fraser FC, Pashayan HM: Relation of face shape to susceptibility to congenital cleft lip: a preliminary report. J Med Genet 1970; 7:112.
Ross RB, Johnston MC: Cleft lip and palate. Baltimore: Williams & Wilkins, 1972.
Pashayan HM, McNab M: Simplified method of feeding infants born with cleft palate with or without cleft lip. Am J Dis Child 1979; 133:145.
Geis N, et al.: The prevalence of congenital heart disease among the population of a metropolitan cleft lip and palate clinic. Cleft Palate J 1981; 18:19.
Crawford FC, Sofaer JA: Cleft lip with or without cleft palate: identification of sporadic cases with a high degree of genetic predisposition. J Med Genet 1987; 24:163–169.

J0027
**Ronald J. Jorgenson**
*Hermine M. Pashayan*

**Cleft lip-polydactyly**
*See ORO-FACIO-DIGITAL SYNDROME, THURSTON TYPE*

**Cleft lip-tetramelia-deformed ears-ectodermal dysplasia**
*See ODONTO-TRICHOMELIC SYNDROME*
**Cleft lip/palate with split hand or split foot**
*See ECTRODACTYLY-ECTODERMAL DYSPLASIA-CLEFTING SYNDROME*
**Cleft lip/palate-abnormal thumbs-microcephaly**
*See ORO-CRANIO-DIGITAL SYNDROME*
**Cleft lip/palate-acrofacial dysostosis-triphalangeal thumb**
*See ACROFACIAL DYSOSTOSIS-CLEFT LIP/PALATE-TRIPHALANGEAL THUMB*
**Cleft lip/palate-craniocynostosis-malformed extremities**
*See HERRMANN-PALLISTER-OPITZ SYNDROME*

## CLEFT LIP/PALATE-ECTODERMAL DYSPLASIA-SYNDACTYLY 0179

**Includes:**
Ectodermal dysplasia-cleft lip/palate-syndactyly
Rosselli-Gulienetti syndrome
Syndactyly-cleft lip/palate-ectodermal dysplasia

**Excludes:**
Acrocephalosyndactyly type III (0229)
Cleft lip/palate-filiform fusion of eyelids (0176)
Ectrodactyly-ectodermal dysplasia-clefting syndrome (0337)
Ectodermal dysplasia-ectrodactyly-macular dystrophy (2793)
Ectodermal dysplasia, Hay-Wells type (2590)
Ectrodactyly-ectodermal dysplasia-clefting syndrome (0337)
Pili torti-cleft lip/palate-syndactyly (3126)
Pterygium syndrome, popliteal (0818)

**Major Diagnostic Criteria:** Congenital adhesions, such as synblepharon, fused labia, symmetric (kissing) skin ulcers, and syndactyly; cleft palate with or without cleft lip; scarring alopecia; dysplastic nails; mental retardation.

**Clinical Findings:** Mental retardation; alopecia, scarring type; deformed nails; cleft palate; genital hypoplasia; cleft lip; photophobia; adhesions between eyelids; syndactyly, toes and fingers; hypoplasia of enamel, missing teeth; hypohidrosis; renal anomalies; and abnormal EEG have all been reported.

**Complications:** Chronic scalp infection; congenital symmetric ulceration of skin in gluteal cleft or other areas of skin apposition; blepharitis.

**Associated Findings:** Persistent low-grade inflammation of scalp results in a chronic scarring process and gradual loss of hair from central area of scalp. Growth of nails is slow and irregular.

**Etiology:** Possibly autosomal recessive inheritance.

**Pathogenesis:** Undetermined. The physical defects are present at birth, and developmental retardation is usually obvious within the first few weeks of life. Sweat glands, hair follicles, and sebaceous glands are present. In the affected area of scalp the hair follicles and sebaceous glands are rare to absent, rete ridges are poorly developed, and the epidermis is thin.

**MIM No.:** 22500

**POS No.:** 3141

**Sex Ratio:** Presumably M1:F1

**Occurrence:** Up to nine affected individuals from three families have been documented.

**Risk of Recurrence for Patient's Sib:**
See Part I, *Mendelian Inheritance.*

**Risk of Recurrence for Patient's Child:**
See Part I, *Mendelian Inheritance.*

**Age of Detectability:** At birth.

**Gene Mapping and Linkage:** Unknown.

**Prevention:** None known. Genetic counseling indicated.

**Treatment:** Surgical correction of cleft palate and lip is indicated in view of overall prognosis. Appropriate hygienic measures to reduce risk of secondary infection of scalp and eyelids. Care in institution may be indicated in view of severe mental retardation.

**Prognosis:** Life span may be normal or only slightly reduced if infancy is survived.

**Detection of Carrier:** Unknown.

**Support Groups:**
MA; Quincy; Prescription Parents, Inc.
CANADA: Ontario; Toronto; Canadian Cleft Lip and Palate Family Association

*We are grateful to H. Brock Armstrong for his contribution to a previous version of this article.*

**References:**
Rosselli D, Gulienetti R: Ectodermal dysplasia. Br J Plast Surg 1961; 14:190–204.
Bowen P, Armstrong HB: Ectodermal dysplasia, mental retardation, cleft lip/palate and other anomalies in three sibs. Clin Genet 1976; 9:35–42. *
Ogur G, Yuksel M: Association of syndactyly, ectodermal dysplasia, and cleft lip and palate: report of two sibs from Turkey. J Med Genet 1988; 25:37–40.

B0030                                                    **Peter A. Bowen**

## CLEFT LIP/PALATE-FILIFORM FUSION OF EYELIDS          0176

**Includes:**
Ankyloblepharon filiforme adnatum-cleft palate
Eyelid fusion-cleft lip/palate

**Excludes:**
**Cleft lip/palate-lip pits or mounds** (0177)
**Ectodermal dysplasia, Hay-Wells type** (2590)
**Pterygium syndrome, popliteal** (0818)

**Major Diagnostic Criteria:** Cleft lip or cleft palate with filiform fusion of the eyelids.

**Clinical Findings:** Multiple connective tissue bands, 0.3–5.0 mm in width, extend from the white line of one lid to that of the other lid, posterior to the cilia and anterior to the meibomian orifices. No associated anomalies are found in the globes.

Filiform fusion of the eyelids may be an isolated phenomenon or may be seen with cleft lip or cleft palate. In other cases, pits of the lower lip have been found. Filiform adhesions may be single, multiple, unilateral, or bilateral. They may also be seen in **Pterygium syndrome, popliteal**.

**Complications:** Those usually associated with the clefts, since the lid adhesions are corrected by simply severing the attachments.

**Associated Findings:** A few patients have had patent ductus arteriosus.

**Etiology:** Possibly autosomal dominant inheritance with extremely variable expression. Most cases are isolated. Most reported cases have been from India and Germany. Affected identical twins have been reported.

**Pathogenesis:** Undetermined, but apparently not related to the simple persistence of normal union of the lids. Failure of fusion of primary and secondary palates.

**MIM No.:** 10625

**POS No.:** 3139

**Sex Ratio:** M1:F1

**Occurrence:** Rare. Thirty cases of isolated ankyloblepharon; fewer than ten cases of familial association of binary combination of ankyloblepharon with clefting.

**Risk of Recurrence for Patient's Sib:**
See Part I, *Mendelian Inheritance.*

**Risk of Recurrence for Patient's Child:**
See Part I, *Mendelian Inheritance.*

**Age of Detectability:** At birth by physical examination.

**Gene Mapping and Linkage:** Unknown.

**Prevention:** None known. Genetic counseling indicated.

**Treatment:** Surgical repair of clefts. Snip filiform adhesions of lids at birth. Speech therapy and orthodontic treatment.

**Prognosis:** Excellent. Does not appear to diminish lifespan.

**Detection of Carrier:** Unknown.

**Support Groups:**
MA; Quincy; Prescription Parents, Inc.
CANADA: Ontario; Toronto; Canadian Cleft Lip and Palate Family Association

**References:**
Lemtis H, Neubauer H: Ankyloblepharon filiforme et membraniforme adnatum. Klin Monatsbl Augenheilkd 1959; 135:510–516.
Long JC, Blandford SE: Ankyloblepharon filiforme adnatum with cleft lip and palate. Am J Ophthalmol 1962; 53:126.
Sood NN, et al.: Ankyloblepharon filiforme adnatum with cleft lip and palate. J Pediatr Ophthalmol 1968; 5:30.
Ehlers N, Jensen IK: Ankyloblepharon filiforme congenitum associated with hare-lip and cleft palate. Acta Ophthalmol 1970; 48:465–467.
Akkermans CH, Stern LM: Ankyloblepharon filiforme adnatum. Br J Ophthalmol 1979; 63:129–131.

G0038                                                    **Robert J. Gorlin**

**Cleft lip/palate-frontonasal dysplasia-postaxial polysyndactyly**
*See ACRO-FRONTO-FACIO-NASAL DYSOSTOSIS*

## CLEFT LIP/PALATE-LIP PITS OR MOUNDS               0177

**Includes:**
Cleft lip/palate-mucous cysts of lower lip
Lip pits or mounds and cleft lip or palate
van der Woude syndrome

**Excludes:**
**Cleft lip** (0178)
**Pterygium syndrome, popliteal** (0818)

**Major Diagnostic Criteria:** For an isolated case, pits of the lower lip associated with cleft lip or palate. Pits in the proband and cleft lip or palate in pedigree, or cleft lip or palate in the proband; pits in pedigree are sufficient for diagnosis.

**Clinical Findings:** Most frequently found are two paramedian fistulas or pits on the lower lip, sometimes secreting small amounts of viscous saliva. Some are mere depressions, while others are channels 10–15 mm deep. Rarely, only one pit is present, which may be either centrally located or lateral to the midline of the lower lip. Pits are frequently associated with cleft of the lip, or cleft palate, or cleft lip and palate. There is significant association between the types of clefts in parents and their

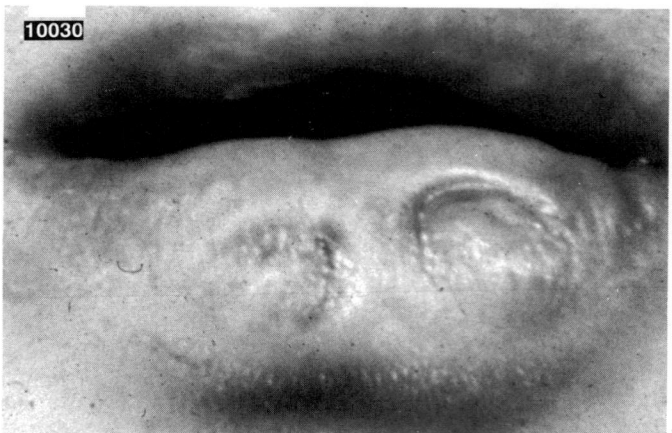

0177-10030: Lip pits.

children. Conical elevations, instead of sinuses, are observed. These are mainly associated with cleft palate (40%).

**Complications:** Feeding, respiratory, speech, and middle ear fluid infection or retention of fluid are associated with oral clefts in untreated patients.

**Associated Findings:** Frequently associated with missing or peg-shaped lateral upper incisors if cleft lip is present. Missing premolars and bilateral clubfeet have been described.

**Etiology:** Autosomal dominant inheritance with 80% penetrance. Shprintzen et al. (1980) observed 100% penetrance. Expressivity is variable: pits (69.6%) and clefts (36%) in affected persons.

**Pathogenesis:** Small invaginations appear on the embryonal mandibular process in normal embryos 7.5–12.5 mm long. A mutant gene prevents the normal obliteration of these "lateral sulci," which results in labial pits. The same mutant gene prevents closure of primary or secondary palate.

**MIM No.:** *11930

**POS No.:** 3140

**Sex Ratio:** M1:F1 (Caucasians).

**Occurrence:** 1:100,000 to 1:80,000 (Caucasians: Czechoslovakia and United States; estimation based on hospital records). Finland: 2.3% of cleft palate patients and 2.5% of patients with cleft lip (and palate).

**Risk of Recurrence for Patient's Sib:**
See Part I, *Mendelian Inheritance*. Ten percent if sporadic.

**Risk of Recurrence for Patient's Child:**
See Part I, *Mendelian Inheritance*.

**Age of Detectability:** At birth.

**Gene Mapping and Linkage:** VWS (Van der Woude syndrome) has been mapped to 1q32-q41.

**Prevention:** None known. Genetic counseling indicated.

**Treatment:** Plastic surgery for lip pits and clefts. Speech therapy, orthodontic treatment, and attention to hearing problems are essential.

**Prognosis:** Satisfactory results are achieved with plastic surgery and make possible normal social intercourse. Average life span is unaffected.

**Detection of Carrier:** Microforms: some cases of paramedian conical elevations of lower lip, cleft uvula, missing or malformed upper lateral incisors, canines, or premolars in members of pedigree with incidence of lip pits.

**Special Considerations:** As the risk for clefts is considerably higher in this syndrome, genetic counseling is markedly different from genetic advice given in "common" cleft lip or palate. The risk is for pits alone, cleft lip or palate alone, or combinations of the defects.

**Support Groups:**
MA; Quincy; Prescription Parents, Inc.
CANADA: Ontario; Toronto; Canadian Cleft Lip and Palate Family Association

**References:**
van der Woude A: Fistula labii inferioris congenita and its association with cleft lip and palate. Am J Hum Genet 1954; 6:244–256.
Červenka J, et al.: The syndrome of pits of the lower lip and cleft lip and/or palate: genetic considerations. Am J Hum Genet 1967; 19:416–432. *
Schneider EL: Lip pits and congenital absence of second premolars: varied expression of the lip pits syndrome. J Med Genet 1973; 10:346–349.
Janku P, et al.: The van der Woude syndrome in a large kindred: variability, penetrance, genetic risks. Am J Med Genet 1980; 5:117–123.
Shprintzen RJ, et al.: The penetrance and variable expression of the van der Woude syndrome: implications for genetic counseling. Cleft Palate J 1980; 17:52–57. *
Ranta R, Rintala AE: Correlations between microforms of the van der Woude syndrome and cleft palate. Cleft Palate J 1983; 20:158–162. †
Schinzel A, Klausler M: The van der Woude syndrome. J Med Genet 1986; 23:291–294. *

CE003 **Jaroslav Červenka**

**Cleft lip/palate-mucous cysts of lower lip**
*See CLEFT LIP/PALATE-LIP PITS OR MOUNDS*

## CLEFT LIP/PALATE-OLIGODONTIA-SYNDACTYLY-HAIR DEFECTS 2898

**Includes:**
Hair defects-cleft lip/palate-oligodontia-syndactyly
Oligodontia-cleft lip/palate-syndactyly-hair defects
Syndactyly-cleft lip/palate-oligodontia-hair defects

**Excludes:**
Cleft lip/palate-ectodermal dysplasia-syndactyly (0179)
Ectrodactyly-ectodermal dysplasia-clefting syndrome (0337)
Oculo-dento-osseous dysplasia (0737)
Oro-facio-digital syndrome I (0770)
Pili torti-cleft lip/palate-syndactyly (3126)

**Major Diagnostic Criteria:** **Cleft lip** and/or **Cleft palate**, dental anomalies, trichodysplasia, and **Syndactyly**.

**Clinical Findings:** Bilateral cleft lip/palate, absence of deciduous teeth, hypodontia of permanent teeth, small and abnormally shaped teeth, diastema, prominent eyes, congenital lagophthalmia, prominent and everted lower lip, hypoplasia of premaxilla, large nose with wide nasal root, coarse scalp hair with three hair whorls, wide eyebrows, long eyelashes, synophrys, pili torti, and bilateral **Syndactyly** of the first two fingers.

**Complications:** Difficulty in nursing, swallowing, respiration, and phonation.

**Associated Findings:** None known.

**Etiology:** Presumably autosomal dominant or X-linked dominant inheritance with variable expression.

**Pathogenesis:** Unknown.

**Sex Ratio:** Presumably M1:F1.

**Occurrence:** Two Chilean patients reported. One 4 10/12-year-old girl belonging to a sibship of four from nonconsanguineous parents has been described. Her father was normal, but the mother presented mildly coarse scalp hair, slight hypertelorism, somewhat large nose and wide nasal root, thin upper lip, small teeth, and diastema between the upper abnormally shaped central incisors.

**Risk of Recurrence for Patient's Sib:**
See Part I, *Mendelian Inheritance*.

**Risk of Recurrence for Patient's Child:**
See Part I, *Mendelian Inheritance*.

**Age of Detectability:** At birth, by physical examination.

**Gene Mapping and Linkage:** Unknown.

**Prevention:** None known. Genetic counseling indicated.

**Treatment:** Surgical repair of cleft lip/palate; speech therapy.

**Prognosis:** Normal life span.

**Detection of Carrier:** Unknown.

**Special Considerations:** This condition belongs to the trichoodontic subgroup of ectodermal dysplasias as classified by Freire-Maia (1971, 1977).

A similar condition but with probable autosomal recessive inheritance, **Pili torti-cleft lip/palate-syndactyly**, was described in 1987.

**Support Groups:**
MA; Quincy; Prescription Parents, Inc.
CANADA: Ontario; Toronto; Canadian Cleft Lip and Palate Family Association

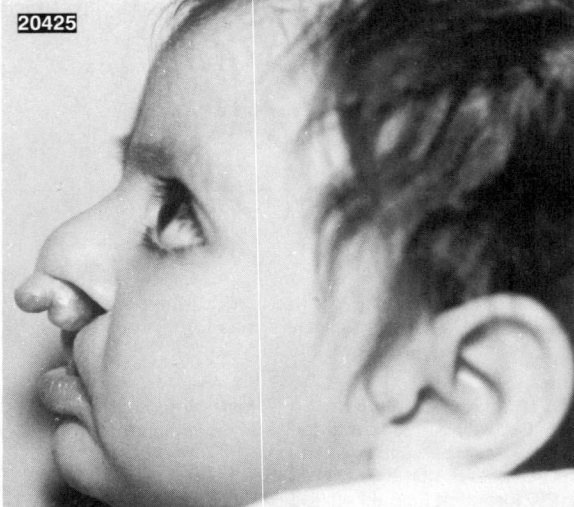

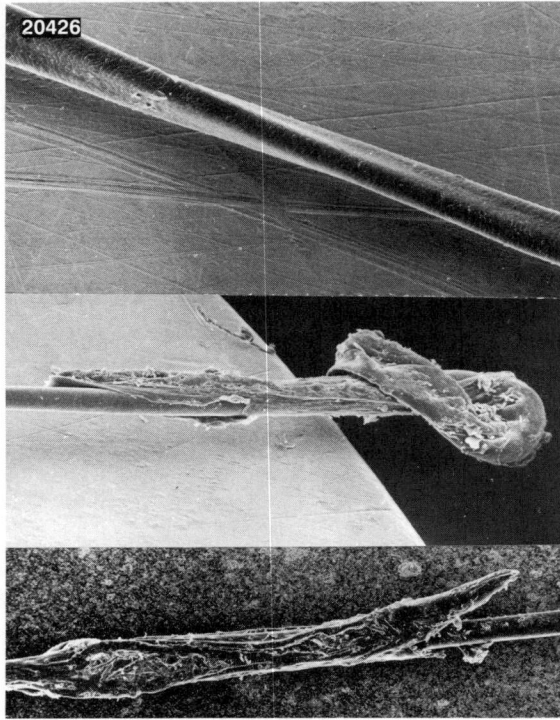

**2898**-20425: Affected girl at nine months; note bilateral cleft lip, prominent eye, wide eyebrow, long eyelashes, somewhat large ear, and prominent and everted lower lip. 20426: Scanning electron microscopic appearance of hair shafts showing twisting on the long axis (pili torti), dystrophic bulb, and longitudinal splitting.

**References:**
Freire-Maia N: Ectodermal dysplasias. Hum Hered 1971; 21:309–312.
Freire-Maia N: Ectodermal dysplasias revisited. Acta Genet Med Gemellol 1977; 26:121–131.
Martinez RB, et al.: Cleft lip/palate-oligodontia-syndactyly-hair alterations, a new syndrome: review of the conditions combining ectodermal dysplasia and cleft lip/palate. Am J Med Genet 1987; 27:23–31.

**Marta Pinheiro**

Cleft lip/palate-popliteal pterygium-digital and genital anomalies
    *See PTERYGIUM SYNDROME, POPLITEAL*
Cleft lip/palate-syndactyly-pili torti
    *See PILI TORTI-CLEFT LIP/PALATE-SYNDACTYLY*
Cleft of soft and hard palates (isolated)
    *See CLEFT PALATE*

---

## CLEFT PALATE                    0180

**Includes:**
    Cleft of soft and hard palates (isolated)
    Palate, cleft, submucous with a bifid uvula

**Excludes:**
    **Abruzzo-Erickson syndrome** (2365)
    **Cleft lip** (0178)
    **Uvula, cleft** (0184)
    **Velo-cardio-facial syndrome** (2129)
    Other syndromes, sequences, or associations with cleft palate

**Major Diagnostic Criteria:**  Cleft of the soft palate, cleft of the soft and hard palates, or submucous cleft palate.

**Clinical Findings:**  Findings include cleft of soft palate and hard palate, which may extend to the incisive canal. A submucous cleft of the palate is considered the mildest clinical form of expression and is always associated with a bifid uvula. The submucous cleft is manifested by the presence of a thin median raphe covered by mucosa in the area of the soft palate. There is failure of fusion of the underlying muscles. A notch is palpable at the junction of the hard and soft palates, replacing the posterior palatal spine. The vomer may lie unattached or be attached to either of the palatal processes.

**Complications:**  Difficulty in sucking (100% of cases that involve the soft and hard palates); inadequate intake of formula, resulting from excessive swallowing of air and leading to a false sense of fullness; serous otitis media and conductive hearing loss. Life-threatening aspiration can be a problem if the infant regurgitates while lying on his back. Hypernasal speech may result if repair of the palate does not provide adequate velopharyngeal closure.

**Associated Findings:**  Congenital heart disease occurs in 4.3% of the individuals.

**Etiology:**  Cleft palate is one of a number of relatively common defects that are clearly familial but cannot be made to fit all the expectations for Mendelian inheritance. Allelic restriction and multifactorial models have been proposed for all forms of orofacial clefting.
    Twin studies have shown a rather low concordance rate in MZ co-twins (23.5% vs. 10% in DZ co-twins) suggesting that the

---

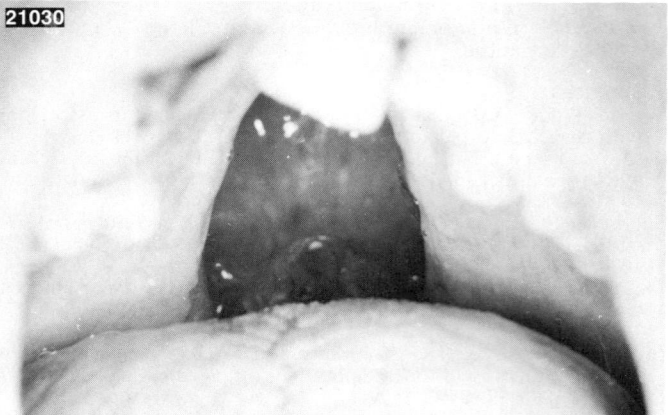

0180-21030:  Cleft palate.

environmental contribution to causation is larger than the genetic contribution.

**Pathogenesis:** At the time of primary palate formation, ridge-like palatal shelves extend from the medial aspects of the maxillary processes. The direction of growth of these shelves is downward and towards the midline, with the tongue between the shelves. A considerable amount of controversy exists regarding the mechanism by which the tongue is withdrawn and regarding the force that moves the shelves into their horizontal position. Upon completion of shelf elevation and opposition in the midline, fusion begins between the opposing epithelial surfaces and is followed by a breakdown of the epithelial seam and the consolidation of the secondary palate by mesenchymal penetration. The breakdown of the epithelial seam entails the death of a large number of cells in the presence of a large number of hydrolytic enzymes for the breakdown of cellular debris. Shelf elevation and fusion in the future hard palate region begin earlier in the male than in the female embryo. There is, however, little or no difference in the timing of closure in the soft palate region.

Precise timing is required for the palatal shelves to alter their direction of growth and to make contact and fuse. Animal studies have shown that experimental interference with a number of developmental processes will produce cleft palate. Failure of the shelves to make contact is the most common mechanism for cleft formation. The failure of shelf contact may result from a number of developmental disturbances that include insufficient growth of the palatal shelves or lack of shelf elevation. Narrow palatal shelves, especially if associated with wide facial structures, could result in contact failure.

Elevation of the palatal shelves is preceded by a number of developmental changes, and a delay in this process will frequently lead to a cleft of the palate. It is felt that the single most important event is active or passive withdrawal of the tongue from between the shelves. This withdrawal of the tongue is preceded by extension of the head. Other factors (mostly noted in animal studies) that may play a role are reduced shelf force and loss of amniotic fluid. This fluid loss leads to the collapse of the embryonic membrane onto the embryo, which can occur secondary to amniotic sac puncture or through the use of drugs such as cortisone. It is believed that these may affect fusion capability.

Submucous cleft palate is considered by some to be a less severe expression of the clefting process and is known to occur frequently in relatives of cleft palate individuals. The defect is thought to be due to an inadequate consolidation of mesenchyme across the midline.

**MIM No.:** 11954, 11957

**CDC No.:** 749.0

**Sex Ratio:** M1:F1.2 for soft palate only; M1:F2.3 for soft and hard palates.

**Occurrence:** 45:100,000 births, with little if any racial variation.

**Risk of Recurrence for Patient's Sib:** About 6% for sibs of male proband; About 3% for sibs of female proband; About 13% after two affected sibs.

**Risk of Recurrence for Patient's Child:** About 6.0%.

**Age of Detectability:** At birth by examination of the intraoral cavity.

**Gene Mapping and Linkage:** Unknown. Several investigators have obtained data indicating that a gene involved in susceptibility to cortisone-induced cleft palate in the A/J mouse strain is linked to the H-2 region or major histocompatibility complex. The differences among inbred strains of mice in susceptibility to cortisone-induced cleft palate have been attributed to genetically determined differences in fetal facial mesenchymal glucocorticoid receptor levels. Similar studies in man have not shown this type of correlation.

**Prevention:** None known. Genetic counseling indicated. Use of drugs such as cortisome and dilantin during the first 10 weeks of pregnancy may increase the risk of having a child cleft palate.

**Treatment:** It is important to provide a simple and effective feeding method to avoid the very common feeding problems associated with ineffective sucking of the infant in the immediate postnatal and presurgical period. Use a single hole nipple that has been crosscut. Feed the infant in the sitting position to reduce nasal regurgitation. Burp the infant after the intake of 1/2 ounce of formula in order to get rid of the ingested air and avoid the sense of fullness and colic. When placed in the crib, the infant should be kept in the prone position to avoid aspiration of formula.

The cleft palate can be closed at the usual age for such repairs. Secondary surgery may be needed for normal speech.

The insertion of pressure-equalization tubes to drain middle ear fluid and to restore normal hearing may be necessary. Speech therapy following surgical closure of the cleft palate is indicated if a residual speech problem is diagnosed after surgery. Orthodontic treatment may be necessary.

**Prognosis:** Excellent except in cases in which the palatal shelves are very deficient.

**Detection of Carrier:** Unknown.

**Support Groups:**
MA; Quincy; Prescription Parents, Inc.
CANADA: Ontario; Toronto; Canadian Cleft Lip and Palate Family Association

**References:**
Ross RB, Johnston MC: Cleft lip and palate. Baltimore: Williams and Wilkins, 1972.
Goldman AS, et al.: Human fetal palatal corticoid receptors and teratogens for cleft palate. Nature 1978; 272:464.
Pashayan HM, McNab M: Simplified method of feeding infants born with cleft palate with or without cleft lip. Am J Dis Child 1979; 33:145.
Jenkins M, Stady C: Dominant inheritance of cleft of the soft palate. Hum Genet 1980; 53:341.
Geiss N, et al.: The prevalence of congenital heart disease among the population of a metropolitan cleft lip and palate clinic. Cleft Palate J 1981; 18:19.
Shields ED, et al.: Cleft palate: a genetic and epidemiologic investigation. Clin Genet 1981; 20:13–24.
Meininger MG, Christ JE: Real-time ultrasonography for the prenatal diagnosis of facial clefts. BD:OAS XVIII(1). New York: March of Dimes Birth Defects Foundation, 1982:161–167.
Pashayan HM: What else to look for in a child born with a cleft of the lip and/or palate. Cleft Palate J 1983; 20:54–82.

J0027

**Ronald J. Jorgenson**
*Hermine M. Pashayan*

**Cleft palate, occult submucous**
*See PALATOPHARYNGEAL INCOMPETENCE*
**Cleft palate, X-linked**
*See ABRUZZO-ERICKSON SYNDROME*
**Cleft palate-cleft lip (isolated)**
*See CLEFT LIP*

## CLEFT PALATE-DYSMORPHIC FACIES-DIGITAL DEFECTS, MARTSOLF TYPE  2579

**Includes:**
Polydactyly-Robin anomaly-skeletal dysplasia
Skeletal dysplasia-Robin anomaly-polydactyly

**Excludes:**
Cleft palate-micrognathia-glossoptosis (0182)
Pierre-Robin anomaly syndromes, other
Oto-palato-digital syndrome, II (2258)

**Major Diagnostic Criteria:** The dysmorphic facies exhibits a square forehead, "pixie-like" ears, telecanthus, small mouth, **Cleft palate**, and marked micrognathia. There is rhizomelic brachymelia, short index fingers bilaterally, postaxial hexadactyly of the feet, joint laxity, and skeletal anomalies.

**Clinical Findings:** Rhizomelic brachymelia is present at birth, as are the cleft palate, small mouth, micrognathia, short neck, redundant skin folds, and the bilaterally short index fingers. At birth the head circumference is within the average range, with the length less than the third percentile. As growth progresses, all of

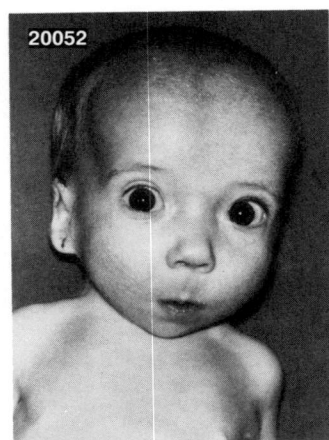

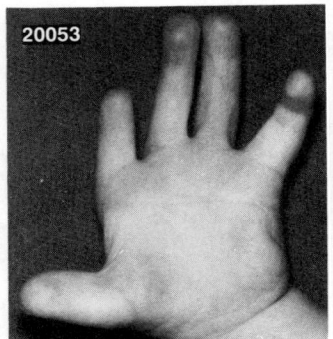

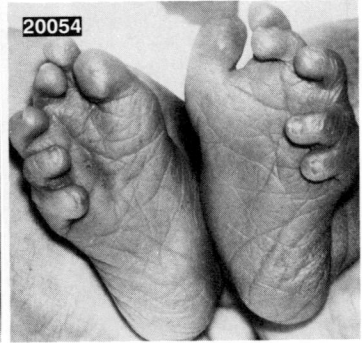

**2579A**-20052: Note square forehead, abnormal ears, hypertelorism, small mouth, micrognathia, short and webbed neck and the appearance of widely spaced nipples. 20053: Single palmar crease, broad varus thumb, short index finger and short middle phalanx of the third and fifth fingers. 20054: Broad halluces with valgus deformity, postaxial hexadactyly, normal nails.

the physical parameters, including head circumference, become less than the third percentile.

The prominent square forehead becomes more evident after the newborn period. The anterior fontanelle, which is still patent by 18 months of age, is at about the midpoint of the skull rather than more anteriorally placed. Hair texture is fine. The ears, which are normally positioned, are "pixie-like", with wide flat helices and very narrow canals. Telecanthus is present. Palpebral fissure length is within the normal range. Relative hypertelorism is present.

Chest circumference is compatible with other growth parameters, but the internipple distance falls within the low-normal range, although maintaining the expected internipple distance/chest circumference rate of 25%. A wide split $S_2$ with a II/VI systolic ejection murmur is heard on cardiac auscultation, which is compatible with an **Atrial septal defect**. EKG shows increased QRS voltage in $V_2$ and $V_3$.

All of the limbs are short, with the greatest involvement in the proximal segments. Malformations of the hands and feet are symmetric. The thumbs are broad with a varus deflection. There is hypoplasia of the third and fifth middle phalanges and absence of the middle phalanges of the index fingers. The halluces are broad with a valgus deflection. There is bilateral postaxial hexadactyly of the feet. All nails are normal. There is generalized joint laxity and redundant skin over the extremities.

X-ray studies show some frontal flatness of the skull. There is reversal of the normal cervical lordosis with questionable upper cervical vertebral abnormalities. Several lumbar vertebrae have coronal clefts. The lumbar vertebral bodies appear rounded. The

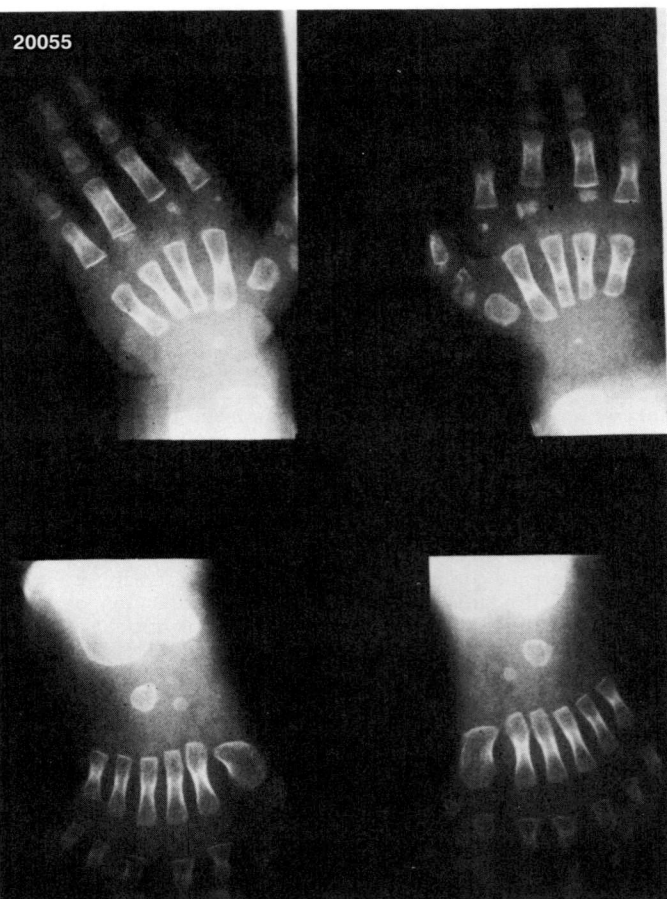

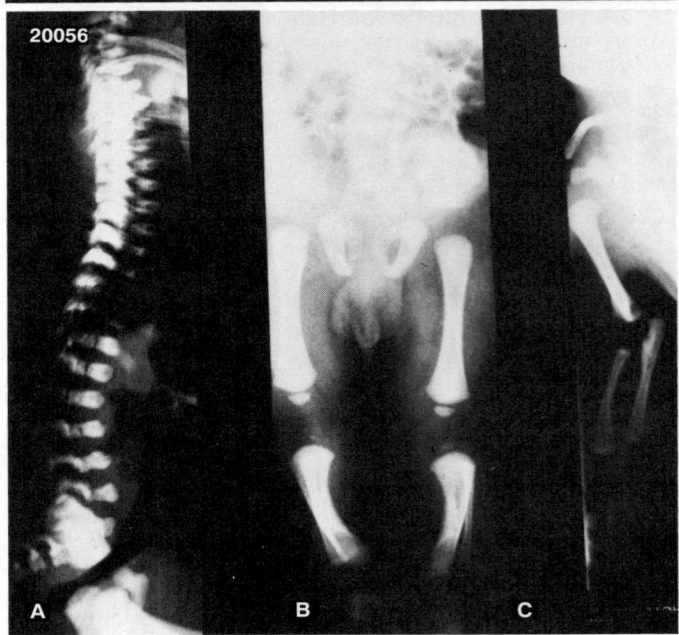

**2579B**-20055: Upper: abnormal first metacarpals, abnormal epiphyses of proximal phalanges, extra ossification center in thumbs, absent middle phalanges of index fingers, and hypoplasia of right third middle phalanx. Lower: bilateral abnormal first ray and hexadactyly. 20056: A. Spine showing reversal of normal curvature, increased sacral angle and minor bony anomalies. B. Abnormal flattened acetabula, short tubular bones, tibial bowing. C. Short tubular bones in the arm.

lumbosacral angle is increased. The acetabular roof is flattened with squaring of the ilium bilaterally. The pelvic outlet is narrow. The radii and ulnae are short. The first metacarpal bilaterally is short and broad. Each thumb has an extra ossicle lying medial to the interphalangeal joint. The middle phalanx of each index finger is missing. The right middle phalanx is hypoplastic. Some of the proximal phalangeal epiphyses are present at birth and appear malformed as they develop. The tibial shortness and bowing is most evident at birth. Each foot has a sixth digital ray on the fibular side. The first metatarsals are broad and slightly short. There is an extra ossicle lying medial to the first right metatarsophalangeal joint. The proximal phalanx of the left hallux is either displaced medially or unossified with an extra ossicle present.

Audiometry reveals normal hearing. Chromosome studies are normal. Metabolic screens reveal no abnormalities. Developmental assessment at 14 months showed a 7–8 month delay.

**Complications:** The long term complications are unknown, but orthopedic and dental complications may occur.

**Associated Findings:** None known.

**Etiology:** Unknown.

**Pathogenesis:** Unknown.

**POS No.:** 3923

**Sex Ratio:** Unknown.

**Occurrence:** One case was reported from central Canada.

**Risk of Recurrence for Patient's Sib:** Unknown.

**Risk of Recurrence for Patient's Child:** Unknown.

**Age of Detectability:** At birth.

**Gene Mapping and Linkage:** Unknown.

**Prevention:** None known. Genetic counseling indicated.

**Treatment:** Surgical closure of palate. Orthopedic and dental observation to detect any complication secondary to skeletal abnormalities and dental problems secondary to small mandible. Developmental assessments to determine progress.

**Prognosis:** Unknown.

**Detection of Carrier:** Unknown.

**Support Groups:**
MA; Quincy; Prescription Parents, Inc.
CANADA: Ontario; Toronto; Canadian Cleft Lip and Palate Family Association

**References:**
Martsolf JT, et al.: Skeletal dysplasia, Robin anomalad, and polydactyly. Syndrome Ident 1977; 5:14–18.

MA043      **John T. Martsolf**

**Cleft palate-exomphalos syndrome (CPEX)**
*See CLEFT PALATE-OMPHALOCELE*
**Cleft palate-growth failure-ectodermal dysplasia**
*See DONLAN SYNDROME*
**Cleft palate-growth/mental retardation-microcephaly-unusual facies**
*See WEAVER-WILLIAMS SYNDROME*
**Cleft palate-hand malformation**
*See DIGITO-PALATAL SYNDROME, STEVENSON TYPE*
**Cleft palate-joint contractures-Dandy-Walker malformation**
*See AASE-SMITH SYNDROME*

## CLEFT PALATE-MICROGNATHIA-GLOSSOPTOSIS    0182

**Includes:**
Glossoptosis-micrognathia-cleft palate
Micrognathia-glossoptosis-cleft palate
Pierre Robin syndrome
Pierre Robin-heart malformation-clubfoot, congenital
Robin anomaly, isolated
Robin sequence

**Excludes:**
**Arthro-ophthalmopathy, hereditary, progressive, Stickler type** (0090)
**Cleft palate** (0180)
**Cleft palate-micrognathia-glossoptosis** (0182)
**Mandibulofacial dysostosis** (0627)
**Oculo-auriculo-vertebral anomaly** (0735)

**Major Diagnostic Criteria:** Micrognathia and glossoptosis with a U-shaped cleft of the palate.

**Clinical Findings:** Micrognathia associated with glossoptosis and in 80% of cases with a U-shaped cleft of the palate, leading to feeding and respiratory problems in the neonatal period. X-ray of the mandible shows the ramus height and the mandibular body to

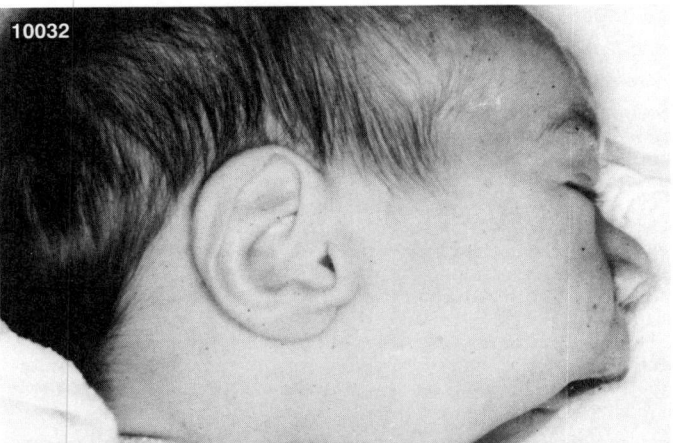

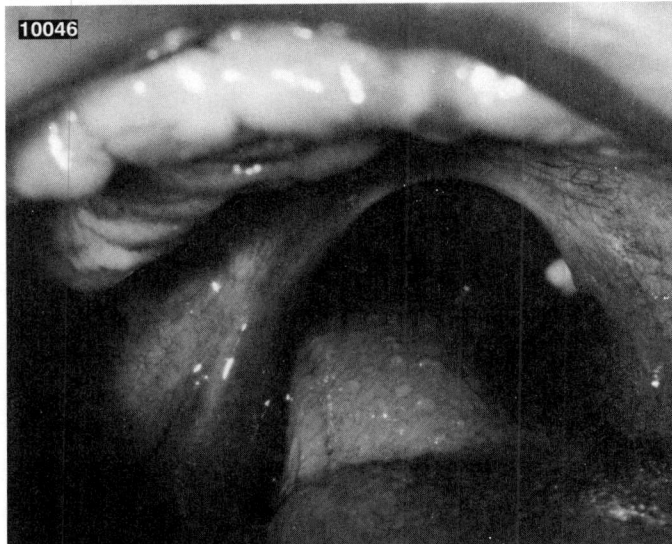

**0182-10032:** Severe microretrognathia. **10046:** U-shaped cleft palate.

be significantly smaller than normal with an obtuse mandibular angle.

**Complications:**  Moderate-to-severe degree of respiratory and feeding problems is directly correlated with the degree of micrognathia and glossoptosis.

Brain damage secondary to hypoxia and upper airway obstruction. Cor pulmonale secondary to airway obstruction.

**Associated Findings:**  Congenital heart disease is associated in about 14% of cases.

**Etiology:**  Possibly autosomal recessive inheritance, although an apparent X-linked variant involving heart malformation and clubfoot has been reported (Gorlin et al, 1970).

**Pathogenesis:**  Hypoplasia of the mandible, allowing the tongue to be posteriorly located and thereby impairing the closure of the posterior palatal shelves, which must grow over the tongue to meet in the midline.

**MIM No.:**  26180, 31190

**POS No.:**  3371

**CDC No.:**  524.080

**Sex Ratio:**  Presumably M1:F1, except for X-linked form.

**Occurrence:**  Over 75 cases have been documented.

**Risk of Recurrence for Patient's Sib:**  Undetermined, but rare.

**Risk of Recurrence for Patient's Child:**  Undetermined, but rare.

**Age of Detectability:**  At birth by clinical examination.

**Gene Mapping and Linkage:**  Unknown.

**Prevention:**  None known. Genetic counseling indicated.

**Treatment:**  Management in the newborn period involves treating respiratory and feeding difficulties. For the former, the infant should be kept prone (face down) at all times. Respiration should be monitored and an oral airway kept nearby. Intubation may be necessary if the above measures are unsuccessful. Tongue-lip adhesion (Beverly Douglas procedure) and tracheostomy should be used only if necessary to maintain an adequate airway. Feeding difficulties may be managed by feeding the infant in an upright position using a modified nipple. Gavage feeding may be unnecessary.

The cleft palate can be closed at the usual age for such repairs. Secondary surgery may be needed for normal speech. The mandible exhibits tremendous "catch-up" growth during the first two to four years, making orthognathic mandibular surgery necessary.

**Prognosis:**  Good if airway and feeding problems are handled aggressively from the start. Mental retardation and CNS damage may occur secondary to anoxia and upper airway obstruction in the newborn period.

**Detection of Carrier:**  Unknown.

**Support Groups:**
MA; Quincy; Prescription Parents, Inc.
CANADA: Ontario; Toronto; Canadian Cleft Lip and Palate Family Association

**References:**
Gorlin RJ, et al.: Robin's syndrome: A probable X-linked recessive subvariety exhibiting persistence of left superior vena cava and atrial septal defect. Am J Dis Child 1970; 119:176–178.
Hanson JW, Smith DW: U-shaped palatal defect in the Robin anomaly: developmental and clinical relevance. J Pediatr 1975; 87:30.
Lewis MB, Pashayan HM: Management of infants with Robin anomaly. Clin Pediatr 1980; 19:519.
Geis N, et al.: The prevalence of congenital heart disease among the population of a metropolitan cleft lip & palate clinic. Cleft Palate J 1981; 18:19.
Heaf DP, et al.: Nasopharyngeal airways in Pierre Robin syndrome. J Pediatr 1982; 100:698.
Sheffield LJ, et al.: A genetic follow-up study of 64 patients with the Pierre Robin complex. Am J Med Genet 1987; 28:25–37.

J0027                                          **Ronald J. Jorgenson**
                                               *Hermine M. Pashayan*

**Cleft palate-multiple anomalies, Abruzzo-Erickson type**
*See ABRUZZO-ERICKSON SYNDROME*

## CLEFT PALATE-OMPHALOCELE                              2809

**Includes:**
Cleft palate-exomphalos syndrome (CPEX)
Exomphalos-cleft palate
Omphalocele-cleft palate

**Excludes:**  Chromosome 13, trisomy 13 (0168)

**Major Diagnostic Criteria:**  The combination of **Cleft palate** and exomphalos with or without other congenital abnormalities.

**Clinical Findings:**  Three sisters with **Cleft palate** and **Omphalocele** died at ages two, four, and twelve months. Birth weights were below 3,000 g. The parents were normal and nonconsanguineous.

**Complications:**  Three sibs died of pneumonia in the first few weeks of life.

**Associated Findings:**  Bicornuate uterus in one patient and **Hydrocephaly** in another.

**Etiology:**  Possibly autosomal recessive inheritance.

**Pathogenesis:**  Unknown.

**MIM No.:**  25832

**POS No.:**  3835

**Sex Ratio:**  M0:F3 (observed).

**Occurrence:**  One family with three affected sisters has been documented.

**Risk of Recurrence for Patient's Sib:**
See Part I, *Mendelian Inheritance.*

**Risk of Recurrence for Patient's Child:**
See Part I, *Mendelian Inheritance.* Affected individuals are not expected to survive to reproduce.

**Age of Detectability:**  *In utero* by prenatal ultrasound and alpha-fetoprotein levels, or at birth by physical examination.

**Gene Mapping and Linkage:**  Unknown.

**Prevention:**  None known. Genetic counseling indicated.

**Treatment:**  Symptomatic. Surgical repair of omphalocele and cleft palate.

**Prognosis:**  All three infants died in the first year of life.

**Detection of Carrier:**  Unknown.

**Support Groups:**
MA; Quincy; Prescription Parents, Inc.
CANADA: Ontario; Toronto; Canadian Cleft Lip and Palate Family Association

**References:**
Czeizel A: New lethal omphalocele-cleft palate syndrome? Hum Genet 1983; 64:99 only.

CZ001                                          **Andrew Czeizel**
J0027                                          **Ronald J. Jorgenson**

## CLEFT PALATE-PERSISTENCE OF BUCCOPHARYNGEAL MEMBRANE              0181

**Includes:**
Atresia of nasopharynx, congenital
Intraoral bands-cleft uvula
Syngnathism, congenital

**Excludes:**
Hypoglossia-hypodactylia (0451)
Larynx, atresia (0571)

**Major Diagnostic Criteria:**  Intraoral bands associated with a cleft uvula or cleft palate.

**Clinical Findings:**  A partial or complete closure of the oral cavity and, in some cases, the nasopharynx is associated with different degrees of a cleft palate.

*Type I:* Intraoral bands or septum are located in the area anterior to the foramen caecum of the tongue.

*Type II:* Intraoral bands connect the sublingual plica with the oropharynx, leaving the tongue behind the bands or medial to the bands.

*Type III:* Intraoral septum and absence of the tongue.

**Complications:** Dysphagia, suffocation.

**Associated Findings:** Extra digits, heart anomalies, adrenal neuroblastoma, and absence of thyroid.

**Etiology:** Unknown.

**Pathogenesis:** Partial or total persistence of the buccopharyngeal membrane separating the ectodermal and endodermal portions of the primitive oral cavity in embryos 2–3 mm long. The tongue develops normally, and the palatine shelves fuse after the disappearance of the buccopharyngeal membrane.

**Sex Ratio:** Presumably M1:F1

**Occurrence:** Undetermined but rare.

**Risk of Recurrence for Patient's Sib:** Unknown.

**Risk of Recurrence for Patient's Child:** Unknown.

**Age of Detectability:** At birth by physical examination of the oral cavity and pharynx.

**Gene Mapping and Linkage:** Unknown.

**Prevention:** None known. Genetic counseling indicated.

**Treatment:** Surgical. Speech therapy if speech problems occur following palatal closure.

**Prognosis:** In severe cases, poor.

**Detection of Carrier:** Unknown.

**Support Groups:**
MA; Quincy; Prescription Parents, Inc.
CANADA: Ontario; Toronto; Canadian Cleft Lip and Palate Family Association

**References:**
Kouyoumdjian AO, McDonald JJ: Association of congenital adrenal neuroblastoma with multiple anomalies including an unusual oropharyngeal cavity (imperforate buccopharyngeal membrane?). Cancer 1951; 4:784.
Hayward JR, Avery JK: Variation in cleft palate. J Oral Surg 1957; 15:320.
Hub M, Jirásek JE: Persistence of the central part of the membrane buccopharyngicae. Cas Lek Cesk 1960; 99:1297.
Gorlin RJ, et al.: Syndromes of the head and neck, 2nd ed. New York: McGraw-Hill, 1976.
Flannery DB: Syndrome of imperforate oropharynx with costovertebral and auricular anomalies. Am J Med Genet 1989; 32:189–191.

JI001                                                            **Jan E. Jirásek**

---

## CLEFT PALATE-STAPES FIXATION-OLIGODONTIA          0183

**Includes:** Stapes fixation-oligodontia-cleft palate

**Excludes:** Symphalangism (dominant)-stapes fixation

**Major Diagnostic Criteria:** Cleft palate; stapes fixation; oligodontia; and carpal, tarsal, metatarsal anomalies.

**Clinical Findings:** A family has been reported in which two of four sibs have this syndrome. The parents were second cousins. Both female sibs had cleft soft palate, which had been repaired at about age 10 years and both exhibited mild primary telecanthus. Neither girl had more than three to four deciduous teeth, and neither had permanent dentition. The two male sibs were normal.

Hearing loss was noted prior to puberty, and audiometric testing demonstrated a bilateral conductive hearing loss. Exploratory surgery revealed bilateral fixation of the stapes footplate in both girls. The hearing loss in each patient was satisfactorily corrected by stapedectomy. X-ray examination of the hands and feet showed the following: the third toe was the longest on both feet; there was shortening of the first metatarsal, which was fused with the navicular bone. The second and third cuneiforms, the

talus and navicular, and the talus and calcaneus were fused. The talus was malformed, and there was underdevelopment of the joint surface of the tibia. In the hands there was underdevelopment of the navicular bones bilaterally.

**Complications:** Progressive hearing loss.

**Associated Findings:** Unknown.

**Etiology:** Possibly autosomal recessive inheritance.

**Pathogenesis:** Unknown.

**MIM No.:** 21630

**POS No.:** 3145

**Sex Ratio:** M0:F2 (observed)

**Occurrence:** Single reported family of Swedish extraction with two affected sisters.

**Risk of Recurrence for Patient's Sib:**
See Part I, *Mendelian Inheritance.*

**Risk of Recurrence for Patient's Child:**
See Part I, *Mendelian Inheritance.*

**Age of Detectability:** Childhood.

**Gene Mapping and Linkage:** Unknown.

**Prevention:** None known. Genetic counseling indicated.

**Treatment:** Stapedectomy or hearing aid for deafness; dentures for oligodontia; surgery for cleft palate.

**Prognosis:** Good for normal life span.

**Detection of Carrier:** Unknown.

**Support Groups:**
MA; Quincy; Prescription Parents, Inc.
CANADA: Ontario; Toronto; Canadian Cleft Lip and Palate Family Association

**References:**
Gorlin RJ, et al.: Cleft palate, stapes fixation and oligodontia: a new autosomal recessively inherited syndrome. In: BD:OAS VII(7). New York: March of Dimes Birth Defects Foundation, 1971:87–88. * †

K0023                                                    **Frederick K. Kozak**
                                                        *Cor W.R.J. Cremers*

---

**Cleft, facial cleft syndrome, Malpuech type**
*See FACIAL CLEFTING SYNDROME, GYPSY TYPE*
**Cleft, maxillary median alveolar**
*See MAXILLA, MEDIAN ALVEOLAR CLEFT*
**Clefting (facial)-hypertelorism-microtia-conductive deafness**
*See HYPERTELORISM-MICROTIA-FACIAL CLEFT-CONDUCTIVE DEAFNESS*
**Clefting syndrome-craniosynostosis-mental retardation**
*See CRANIOSYNOSTOSIS-MENTAL RETARDATION-CLEFTING SYNDROME*

---

## CLEFTING-ECTROPION-CONICAL TEETH          2759

**Includes:**
Eyelids, lower ectropion-clefting-conical teeth
Teeth, conical-clefting-ectropion

**Excludes:**
Acrofacial dysostosis (0017)
Acrofacial dysostosis, Nager type (2167)
Acrofacial dysostosis, postaxial type (2126)
Ectodermal dysplasia, Rapp-Hodgkin type (3056)
Ectodactyly-ectodermal dysplasia-clefting syndrome (0337)
Hypodontia-nail dysgenesis (0511)
Mandibulofacial dysostosis (0627)
Teeth, lobodontia (0607)

**Major Diagnostic Criteria:** The cardinal features of this disorder are **Cleft lip** with or without **Cleft palate**, ectropion of the lower eyelids, and conical teeth (see **Teeth, lobodontia**) subject to premature carious decay. A key negative finding is the absence of limb anomalies.

**Clinical Findings:** The clinical signs are often evident in the newborn period. These signs consist of a combination of oral clefting, ectropion, and ectodermal dysplasia. Bilateral or unilateral **Cleft lip** with or without **Cleft palate**, is present in 24% of individuals. The outer canthal region is not flush with the globe, but separated from it by a flap of conjunctiva, producing ectropion (40%). There is often associated lateral displacement of the lacrimal puncta, with an increased inner canthal distance. The teeth are conical shaped (48%) and subject to premature carious decay. The timing of tooth eruption appears to be normal. In infancy and childhood, the hair is sparse and fine with similarly sparse eyebrows and eyelashes. In the older child and adult, the hair is often curly and may be wiry.

Clinical variability is common within the family described. In one-fourth of the family members, only one of the three cardinal features was present.

**Complications:** The marked tendency to dental caries has required premature extraction of the teeth in many family members. Oral clefting causes an increased frequency of otitis media and conductive hearing loss.

**Associated Findings:** None known.

**Etiology:** Autosomal dominant inheritance with marked variability of expression is likely. The presence of two simultaneous monogenic conditions; one with cleft lip with or without cleft palate and the other affecting structures of ectodermal origin, cannot be ruled out. Multifactorial influences cannot be excluded.

**Pathogenesis:** Unknown.

**MIM No.:** 11958

**POS No.:** 3667

**Sex Ratio:** M1:F1

**Occurrence:** One Dutch Mennonite kindred has been reported in the literature, and a second kindred from Kentucky has been described.

**Risk of Recurrence for Patient's Sib:**
See Part I, *Mendelian Inheritance.*

**Risk of Recurrence for Patient's Child:**
See Part I, *Mendelian Inheritance.*

**Age of Detectability:** Usually clinically evident in the newborn period; however, 15% of affected individuals will only have a dental anomaly, in which case the clinical signs will not be obvious until later in infancy.

**Gene Mapping and Linkage:** Unknown.

**Prevention:** None known. Genetic counseling indicated.

**Treatment:** Surgical repair of facial clefts. Surgery may be required for ectropion. Scrupulous dental hygiene is necessary to avoid or delay carious decay.

**Prognosis:** Normal life span and intelligence.

**Detection of Carrier:** Careful clinical examination of all first-degree relatives will help indicate those who are minimally affected.

**Special Considerations:** The facial features of this syndrome are strikingly similar to those of **Acrofacial dysostosis, postaxial type**; however, limb reduction defects have not been noted in any affected individuals. Hypodontia has previously been reported in Dutch Mennonites, and hypodontia with facial clefting has been described.

H. Zellweger, in personal communications to R. Gorlin et al (1976), reported seeing a mother and son with clefting, ectropion, and limb reduction defects. At least four additional sporadic cases have been observed.

**References:**
Gorlin RJ, et al.: Syndromes of the head and neck. New York: McGraw-Hill, 1976.
Allanson JE, McGillivray BC: Familial clefting syndrome with ectropion and dental anomaly without limb anomalies. Clin Genet 1985; 27:426–429.
Falace PB, Hall BD: Congenital euryblepharon with ectropion and dental anomaly: an autosomal dominant clefting disorder with

marked variability of expression. Proceedings of the Greenwood Genetic Centre 1989; 8:208 only.

AL010

**Judith E. Allanson**

---

## CLEFTS, LOWER MEDIAN LIP, MANDIBLE AND TONGUE      0636

**Includes:**
    Mandibular cleft, median
    Median clefts of lower lip, mandible and tongue
    Tongue, median cleft

**Excludes:**
    **Oro-facio-digital syndrome** (0770)
    **Tongue, cleft** (0952)

**Major Diagnostic Criteria:** Median clefting of the lower lip that may involve the mandible, tongue, and neck.

**Clinical Findings:** Clefting is variable in degree, minimally involving the lower lip. In many cases, there is complete cleavage of the mandible, tongue, and structures of the midneck down to the hyoid bone. Clefting of the lower lip and mandible sometimes occurs without tongue involvement.

**Complications:** Unknown.

**Associated Findings:** Ankyloglossia, cleft upper lip, dysplastic ears, iris coloboma, cervical tags, hypodontia, congenital heart defects, and malformations of the sternum and extremities. Cleft of the lower lip and mandible may be part of a more complex association that includes acrocephaly, choanal atresia, cleft palate, malar hypoplasia, and bilateral colobomas of the lower lids.

**Etiology:** Unknown.

**Pathogenesis:** Mesodermal penetration into the mandibular process, leading to persistence of the central groove which, together with two lateral grooves, is present in 5-6 mm embryos.

**CDC No.:** 749.190, 750.140

**Sex Ratio:** Presumably M1:F1

**Occurrence:** 1:600 cases of orofacial clefting.

**Risk of Recurrence for Patient's Sib:** Undetermined but presumed low.

**Risk of Recurrence for Patient's Child:** Undetermined but presumed low.

**Age of Detectability:** At birth, by physical examination.

**Gene Mapping and Linkage:** Unknown.

**Prevention:** None known.

**Treatment:** Surgical correction of defect.

**Prognosis:** Undetermined. May be associated with increased neonatal morbidity.

**Detection of Carrier:** Unknown.

**References:**
Monroe CW: Midline cleft of the lower lip, mandible and tongue with flexion contracture of the neck. Plast Reconstr Surg 1966; 38:312–316.
Fujino H, et al.: Median cleft of lower lip, mandible, and tongue with midline cervical cord. Cleft Palate J 1970; 7:679–684.
Salinas CF, et al.: Colobomas of lower lids, malar hypoplasia, antimongoloid slant and clefting. Syndrome Identification 1976; 4:5–7.

SA012
J0027

**Carlos F. Salinas**
**Ronald J. Jorgenson**

**Cleidocranial dysostosis**
*See CLEIDOCRANIAL DYSPLASIA*

## CLEIDOCRANIAL DYSPLASIA                    0185

**Includes:**
   Cleidocranial dysostosis
   Dysplasia, cleidocranial
   Dysplasia, osteodental
   Marie-Sainton disease

**Excludes:**
   **Craniofacial dysostosis** (0225)
   **Pyknodysostosis** (0846)

**Major Diagnostic Criteria:** Brachycephaly and bossing of the cranium with evidence of delayed closure of the fontanels and sutures. Aplasia of all or a part of one or both clavicles and abnormal shoulder movements. Dental anomalies, including maleruption or supernumerary dentition.

**Clinical Findings:** Proportionate mild-to-moderate short stature with narrow, drooping shoulders. The skull is brachycephalic; there is bossing of the frontal, parietal, and occipital areas; and there is failure or delayed closure of the fontanels and sutures. Wormian bones may be present. The accessory sinuses and mastoids may be late or hypoplastic in development. Oral features include a high-arched palate with or without cleft; nonunion of the mandibular symphysis; delayed eruption or failure of eruption of the deciduous, permanent, and supernumerary teeth. Mentality is usually normal. Partial or complete aplasia of the clavicles unilaterally or bilaterally with associated muscle defects allows a remarkable range of shoulder movements. Many individuals can approximate the shoulders in front of their chest. The hands may show a number of anomalies: asymmetric length of fingers with long second metacarpals, tapering distal phalanges, and accessory proximal metacarpal epiphyses. Other skeletal deformities include delayed ossification of the pubic bone, coxa vara or valga, genu valgum, scoliosis, cervical ribs, vertebral malformations, and small scapulae. A host of other minor anomalies have been reported.

**Complications:** Cyst formation around unerupted, often inverted or displaced teeth may of itself cause problems and lead to gross destruction and pathologic fracture. Pregnancy usually requires cesarean section because of pelvic dysplasia.

**Associated Findings:** Syringomyelia.

**0185-10928:** Note ability to closely approximate shoulders. 10932: Wormian bones. 10930: Clavicular defect. 10931: Dental X-ray shows supernumerary, impacted teeth.

**Etiology:** Autosomal dominant inheritance with wide variability of expression but high penetrance. About one-third of the cases appear to represent new mutations.

**Pathogenesis:** Unknown.

**MIM No.:** *11960

**POS No.:** 3146

**CDC No.:** 755.555

**Sex Ratio:** M1:F1

**Occurrence:** Over 500 cases have appeared in the medical literature.

**Risk of Recurrence for Patient's Sib:**
   See Part I, *Mendelian Inheritance.*

**Risk of Recurrence for Patient's Child:**
   See Part I, *Mendelian Inheritance.*

**Age of Detectability:** At birth by physical and X-ray examinations.

**Gene Mapping and Linkage:** Unknown.

**Prevention:** None known. Genetic counseling indicated.

**Treatment:** Protective head gear while fontanels remain open. Appropriate dental management and surgical closure of cleft palate when indicated.

**Prognosis:** Normal life span.

**Detection of Carrier:** Unknown.

**Special Considerations:** Because of the wide variability in clinical expression, it may be necessary to obtain selected X-rays to detect affected cases in which expressivity is low. **Pyknodysostosis** shows wide skull sutures and delayed closure of the fontanels as in cleidocranial dysplasia, but is differentiated by the presence of acro-osteolysis, by generalized skeletal sclerosis with a tendency to fractures, and by an autosomal recessive mode of inheritance. Crouzon disease is distinguished by craniosynostosis, a parrot-beaked nose, normal clavicles, and symphysis pubis.

*The Center is grateful to Charles I. Scott, Jr., who prepared the original version of this article.*

**References:**
Forland M: Cleidocranial dysostosis; a review of the syndrome and report of a sporadic case with hereditary transmission. Am J Med 1962; 33:792.
Kalliala E, Taskinen PJ: Cleidocranial dysostosis; report of six typical cases and one atypical case. Oral Surg 1962; 15:808–822.
Dore DD, et al.: Cleidocranial dysostosis and syringomyelia: review of the literature and a case report. Clin Orthop Related Res 1987; 214:229–234.

MY001                                          **Terry L. Myers**

**Cleidocranial dysplasia-micrognathia, Yunis-Varon type**
   See *YUNIS-VARON SYNDROME*
**Cleidocranial dysplasia-micrognathia-no thumb-distal aphalangia**
   See *YUNIS-VARON SYNDROME*
**Cleidocranial dysplasia-parietal foramina**
   See *PARIETAL FORAMINA-CLAVICULAR HYPOPLASIA*
**Click-murmur syndrome**
   See *MITRAL VALVE PROLAPSE*
**Clioquinol induced subacute myelo-optico neuropathy**
   See *NEUROPATHY, MYELO-OPTICO, SUBACUTE TYPE*
**Cloacal dysgenesis with female virilization**
   See *URORECTAL SEPTUM MALFORMATION SEQUENCE*
**Cloacal exstrophy**
   See *EXSTROPHY OF CLOACA SEQUENCE*
**Cloacal membrane, persistence of**
   See *URORECTAL SEPTUM MALFORMATION SEQUENCE*
**Clomaphene ovulation induction and conjoined twins**
   See *TWINS, CONJOINED, TERATOGENICITY*
**Clomid△, ovulation induction trisomy**
   See *OVULATION INDUCTION TRISOMY*
**Clomiphene. ovulation induction trisomy**
   See *OVULATION INDUCTION TRISOMY*
**Clorurorrea**
   See *DIARRHEA, CONGENITAL CHLORIDE*

**Clotting factor V**
See *FACTOR V DEFICIENCY*
**Clotting factor XII**
See *FACTOR XII DEFICIENCY*
**Clouston ectodermal dysplasia**
See *ECTODERMAL DYSPLASIA, HIDROTIC*
**Cloverleaf skull syndrome**
See *CRANIOSYNOSTOSIS, KLEEBLATTSCHADEL TYPE*
**Cloverleaf tongue**
See *TONGUE, FOLDING OR ROLLING*
**Club hand (radial)**
See *HAND, RADIAL CLUB HAND*

## CNS ARTERIOVENOUS MALFORMATION 0186

**Includes:**
>  Arteriovenous malformations: spinal, cortical, and
>  cerebellar
>  Central nervous system arteriovenous malformation
>  Cystic arteriovenous malformations
>  Vein of Galen aneurysm

**Excludes:**
>  Hemangioblastoma
>  Intracranial aneurysm of childhood
>  **Sturge-Weber syndrome** (0915)
>  **Von Hippel-Lindau syndrome** (0995)

**Major Diagnostic Criteria:** A demonstration of the abnormal CNS vasculature by angiogram determines the diagnosis.

**Clinical Findings:** *Intracranial arteriovenous malformation (AVM)*: intracranial hemorrhage (40%); seizures (30%); hemiparesis or other neurologic defect (33%); headache (14%); and bruit (22%).

*Intraspinal AVM*: subarachnoid hemorrhage with back pain and sudden onset of paraplegia. Bruit may be heard over spine.

*Vein of Galen aneurysm*: heart failure in newborn; hydrocephalus in infancy.

**Complications:** A neurologic deficit may occur from bleeding of the AVM or from anoxia of adjacent brain tissue. Repeated bleeding may lead to communicating hydrocephalus.

**Associated Findings:** Of those affected, 5–10% have a subarachnoid hemorrhage.

**Etiology:** Unknown.

**Pathogenesis:** A direct artery-to-vein connection occurs without an intervening capillary bed. Blood shunted through the malformation leads to anoxia of the adjacent brain and produces an epileptogenic cortex.

**CDC No.:** 747.800

**Sex Ratio:** Presumably M1:F1

**Occurrence:** Unknown.

**Risk of Recurrence for Patient's Sib:** Unknown.

**Risk of Recurrence for Patient's Child:** Unknown.

**Age of Detectability:** Twenty percent of the affected individuals become symptomatic in first decade.

**Gene Mapping and Linkage:** Unknown.

**Prevention:** None known. Genetic counseling indicated.

**Treatment:** Surgical excision is possible; anticonvulsants may control seizures. Management of a child with AVM depends on the surgical accessibility of the lesion and the symptom complex produced.

**Prognosis:** There is a 15% risk of death once symptoms occur. Vein of Galen aneurysm is usually fatal for newborns.

**Detection of Carrier:** Unknown.

*The author is grateful to the late Kenneth Shulman for his contribution to an earlier version of this article.*

**References:**
Perret G, Nishioka H: Report on the cooperative study of intracranial aneurysms and subarachnoid hemorrhage. Section IV. Arteriovenous malformation. An analysis of 545 cases of craniocerebral arteriovenous malformations and fistulae reported to the cooperative study. J Neurosurg 1966; 25:467.
Matson DD: Neurosurgery of infancy and childhood, 2nd ed. Springfield: Charles C. Thomas, 1969.
Boynton RC, Morgan BC.: Cerebral arteriovenous fistula with possible hereditary telangiectasia. Am J Dis Child 1973; 125:99.
Bartal AD, et al.: Excision of the vein of Galen complicated by congestive heart failure. Neurochirurgia (Stuttg) 1974; 17:16.
Laing JW, Smith RR: Intracranial arteriovenous malformation in sisters: a case report. J Miss State Med Assoc 1974; 15:203–206.
Barre RG, et al.: Familial vascular malformation or chance occurrence? Neurology 1978; 28:98–100.
Snead OC III, et al.: Familial arteriovenous malformation. Ann Neurol 1979; 5:585–587.
Mori K, et al.: Clinical analysis of arteriovenous malformations in children. Childs Brain 1980; 6:13.
Aberfeld DC, Rao KR: Familial arteriovenous malformation of the brain. Neurology 1981; 31:184–186.

SH007                                       **Kenneth Shapiro**

**CNS depression-hemorrhage-skeletal syndrome**
See *CIRCUMVALLATE PLACENTA SYNDROME*

## CNS NEOPLASMS 0188

**Includes:**
>  Astrocytoma including optic nerve glioma
>  Central nervous system neoplasms
>  Ependymoma
>  Germinomas
>  Hamartoma of CNS
>  Medulloblastoma
>  Neoplasms of CNS
>  Papilloma of choroid plexus
>  Pinealomas, ectopic

**Excludes:**
>  **Cancer, glioma, familial** (2839)
>  **Neurofibromatosis** (0712)
>  Tumors rising in greatest preponderance after the age of
>  puberty

**Major Diagnostic Criteria:** In all tumors except optic gliomas and in some tumors involving the pineal gland, tumor biopsy or biopsy during tumor removal for microscopic identification is essential. Diagnosis of optic glioma can be made when there is an enlarged optic foramen and with a typical computer tomographic (CT) scan or air study.

**Clinical Findings:** As the most frequent solid tumors occurring in childhood, brain tumors constitute an important segment of pediatric oncology. Neurologic manifestations may be mild and easily overlooked or misinterpreted, particularly in the very young, because of the remarkable plasticity of the immature nervous system and the expandability of the infant skull. The majority of tumors produce increased intracranial pressure, usually the consequence of obstructive hydrocephalus. Specific neurologic deficits correspond to tumor location. The posterior fossa is the site of two-thirds of childhood tumors, and each of the four common tumors in this location produces a characteristic syndrome. Supratentorial tumors occupy the cerebral hemisphere, the suprasellar area, and the pineal gland. The tumor presentation during the first year of life is ordinarily as megalocephaly due to obstructive hydrocephalus. Finding of papilledema and an enlarging head should make one suspect a tumor rather than congenital hydrocephalus. After age 1 year, signs of increased intracranial pressure, nausea, vomiting, and lethargy predominate; the gradual development of neurologic signs is consistent with the tumor's location. Papilledema provides unequivocal evidence of increased intracranial pressure. Decreased visual acuity as a consequence of long-standing papilledema may be noticed by an observant parent or when vision fails in school. Abducens palsy, either unilateral or bilateral, may not lead to the complaint of diplopia. An uncorrectable refractive error in a child indicates a tumor of the optic nerve, chiasm, or tract. Generalized convulsions are relatively infrequent because of localization of the tumor in the posterior fossa.

*Focal neurologic abnormalities:* Posterior fossa tumors predominate.

*Cerebellar astrocytomas:* These are the most frequent posterior fossa tumors, preferentially involving the cerebellar hemispheres. About 50% of these tumors have an associated cyst within which a neoplastic mass may be confined to a relatively small nodule. A minority involve the vermis. Cerebellar hemisphere dysfunction is represented by ipsilateral hypotonia, incoordination and intention tremor, and nystagmus. With unilateral herniation of the ipsilateral cerebellar tonsil, a stiff neck and head tilt ensue.

*Medulloblastoma:* This has a decided predilection for males, occupying the cerebellar vermis and producing a syndrome of truncal ataxia. Because of the rapid growth of the tumor and the early obstruction of the fourth ventricle, there is an early increase in intracranial pressure.

*Brainstem gliomas:* These are present without increased intracranial pressure. Histologically, these tumors are low-grade astrocytomas, diffusely involving fiber tracts of the medulla and pons. The hallmark of brainstem glioma is cranial nerve involvement, at first unilateral, but soon thereafter bilateral. Most frequently the seventh and the sixth nerves are involved, followed by ninth and tenth, with fifth and eighth last. There is associated cerebellar dysmetria and, on the basis of corticospinal tract involvement, hemiparesis.

*Ependymomas:* Ependymomas originate within the fourth ventricle, obstructing it and producing increased intracranial pressure. By compressing the floor of the fourth ventricle in the region of the area postrema these tumors can produce intractable vomiting.

*Tumors of the cerebral hemisphere:* Several glial tumors arise in the cerebral hemispheres: astrocytomas, ependymomas, and subependymal giant cell astrocytomas. Seizures, frequently focal motor, are an early finding, with gradual hemiparesis and hemianopsia.

*Suprasellar tumors:* By either compressing or invading structures lying above and within the sella turcica, suprasellar tumors involve the optic chiasm, hypothalamus, third ventricle, and pituitary gland. Tumors frequently found include craniopharyngioma, astrocytomas arising from the optic chiasm and optic nerve, and germinomas (ectopic pinealomas). Impairment of hypothalamic function may cause a variety of clinical abnormalities. One unusual condition is the diencephalic syndrome with growth failure, cachexia, and dwarfism. Diabetes insipidus, visual failure, and hypopituitarism are characteristic of germinomas. The most frequent tumor, craniopharyngioma, ordinarily manifests as visual loss and headaches.

*Pinealomas:* These represent a clinically distinct syndrome of paresis of upward gaze, the so-called Parinaud syndrome. The masses in the region of the pineal gland may include astrocytoma, true pineal tumors or germinomas, and mixed teratomas.

*Papillomas:* Papillomas of choroid plexus arise in the plexus of the lateral ventricles (L > R) and produce increased intracranial pressure and hydrocephalus due to oversecretion of CSF and recurrent bleeding, which cause obstruction of the absorbing mechanisms. Surgical removal and cure are possible.

The diagnosis and management of CNS neoplasms have been revolutionized by the development of the CT scan. Done without risk or discomfort, this procedure permits imaging of the brain, with tumor density clearly distinguishable from brain.

In addition, plain skull X-rays and EEG may be useful. As a preoperative assessment, an angiogram that shows the blood supply of the tumor and adjacent blood vessels is useful. Pneumoencephalography, radionucleotide scanning, and ventriculography have been largely replaced by the CT scan.

**Complications:** Progressive neurologic deficit, progressive increase in intracranial pressure, visual loss, hypopituitary growth failure.

**Associated Findings: Neurofibromatosis** is frequently present in children with gliomas of the optic nerve and cerebral gliomas. Tuberous sclerosis is associated with subependymal giant cell astrocytomas.

**Etiology:** Undetermined. Embryonic cell rests lead to hamartomas. Persistence of granular layer may lead to medulloblastoma. Pathogenesis of tumor type is unknown. Papilloma of choroid plexus may be recessive.

**Pathogenesis:** Undetermined. Papilloma of the choroid plexus can lead to hydrocephalus; this is caused by overproduction of CSF.

**MIM No.:** 26050

**CDC No.:** 191.000

**Sex Ratio:** M>1:F1

**Occurrence:** Approximately 1–2.8:100,000; dependent on age, sex, and race. Second most common type of neoplasm of childhood.

**Risk of Recurrence for Patient's Sib:** Unknown.

**Risk of Recurrence for Patient's Child:** Unknown.

**Age of Detectability:** Neoplasms have been detected in premature newborns.

**Gene Mapping and Linkage:** Unknown.

**Prevention:** None known. Genetic counseling indicated.

**Treatment:** Possibilities include surgical removal for craniopharyngiomas, supratentorial gliomas, cerebellar astrocytomas, and medulloblastomas; radiotherapy for pineal tumors, germinomas, supratentorial gliomas, and postoperative medulloblastomas; chemotherapy.

**Prognosis:** Best in isolated gliomas, particularly those that are cystic, of the cerebellum, or are optic nerve tumors; an 80–90% cure rate can be effected. Worst in medulloblastoma, which tends to spread throughout the subarachnoid space. With radical surgical removal and total CNS radiation, 5-year survival may be obtained in 30% of patients.

**Detection of Carrier:** Unknown.

*The author is grateful to the late Kenneth Shulman for his contribution to an earlier version of this article.*

**References:**
Golden GS, et al.: Malignant glioma of the brain-stem. J Neurol Neurosurg Psychiatry 1972; 35:732.
DeGirolami U, Schmidek H: Clinocopathological study of 53 tumors of the pineal region. J Neurosurg 1973; 39:455.
Hoffman HJ, et al.: Management of craniopharyngioma in children. J Neurosurg 1977; 47:218–227.
Gold EB, Gordis L: Patterns of incidence of brain tumors in children. Ann Neurol 1979; 5:565–568.
Shapiro K, et al.: Craniopharyngiomas in childhood. J Neurosurg 1979; 50:617–623.
McLaurin RL, ed: Pediatric neurosurgery, surgery of the developing nervous system. New York: Grune & Stratton, 1982.
Kun LE, Mulhern RK: Neuropsychologic function in children with brain tumors: II. Serial studies of intellect and time after treatment. Am J Clin Oncol (CCT) 1983; 6:651–656.
Shapiro K, Katz M: The recurrent cerebellar astrocytoma. Childs Brain 1983; 10:168–176.

SH007

**Kenneth Shapiro**

**COACH syndrome**
*See OCULO-ENCEPHALO-HEPATO-RENAL SYNDROME*

---

**COAGULATION DEFECT, FAMILIAL MULTIPLE FACTORS**                                                    **2674**

**Includes:**
Factors II, VII, IX, and X deficiency
Factors V and VIII deficiency
Factors VII and VIII deficiency
Factors VII and X deficiency
Factors VIII and IX deficiency
Factors VIII, IX, and XI deficiency
Factors IX and XI deficiency
Protein C inhibitor deficiency

**Excludes:**
  Acquired coagulation factor inhibitors
  Acquired multiple coagulation factor defects

**Major Diagnostic Criteria:** Mild-to-moderate congenital hemorrhagic disorder; various abnormalities in *in vitro* testing, depending on the defect.

**Clinical Findings:** Ecchymoses, epistaxis, bleeding after trauma and surgery. May have hemarthroses and menorrhagia, but these manifestations are unusual. Diagnosis is suspected by finding an abnormal partial thromboplastin time and sometimes an abnormal prothrombin time. Diagnosis is established by functional assay of the coagulation factors.

**Complications:** Secondary to bleeding.

**Associated Findings:** **Carotid body tumor** with Factors VII and X deficiency.

**Etiology:** Usually autosomal recessive or possibly autosomal dominant inheritance:

### Inheritance of Coagulation Defect, Familial Multiple Factors

Factors II, VII, IX, X deficiency - possibly autosomal recessive.
Factors V and VIII deficiency - autosomal dominant.
Factors VII and VIII deficiency - autosomal dominant, or autosomal recessive plus recessive sex linked.
Factors VII and X deficiency - autosomal recessive.
Factors VIII and IX deficiency - autosomal dominant, or recessive sex linked.
Factors VIII, IX and XI deficiency - autosomal dominant.
Factors IX and XI deficiency - autosomal recessive.

**Pathogenesis:** Reduced coagulant activity of two or more coagulation factors, which can affect the intrinsic and extrinsic coagulation pathways.

**MIM No.:** 13443, 13451, 13452, 13454, *22730, 22731

**Sex Ratio:** Presumably M1:F1, except for X-linked sub-types.

**Occurrence:** Only a few families at most have been documented with any given combination. Combined Factors V and VIII deficiency is the most common and has been reported in about 30 families.

**Risk of Recurrence for Patient's Sib:**
  See Part I, *Mendelian Inheritance.*

**Risk of Recurrence for Patient's Child:**
  See Part I, *Mendelian Inheritance.*

**Age of Detectability:** At birth.

**Gene Mapping and Linkage:** F2L (coagulation factor II (prothrombin)-like) has been tentatively mapped to Xpter-q25.

**Prevention:** None known. Genetic counseling indicated.

**Treatment:** Through administration of the indicated blood components.

**Prognosis:** Normal life span.

**Detection of Carrier:** Factor assays of plasma.

**References:**
Kroll AJ, et al.: Hereditary deficiencies of clotting factors VII and X associated with carotid-body tumors. New Engl J Med 1964; 270:6–13.
McMillan CW, Roberts HR: Congenital combined deficiency of coagulation factors II, VII, IX and X. New Engl J Med 1966; 274:1313–1315.
Girolami A, et al.: Combined congenital deficiency of factor V and factor VIII: report of a further case with some considerations on the hereditary transmission of this disorder. Acta Haematol (Basel) 1976; 55:234–243.
Soff GA, Levin J: Familial multiple coagulation factor deficiencies. Semin Thromb Hemostas 1981; 7:112–148.
Rahim Adam KA, et al.: Combined factor V and factor VIII deficiency with normal protein C and protein C inhibitor: a family study. Scand J Haemat 1985; 34:401–405.
Vehar GA, et al.: Factor VIII and factor V: biochemistry and patho-
physiology. In: Scriver CR, et al, eds: The metabolic basis of inherited disease, 6th ed. New York: McGraw-Hill, 1989:2155–2170.

C0068

James J. Corrigan

**Coarctation of the aortic isthmus**
  *See AORTA, COARCTATION, INFANTILE TYPE*
**Coarctation, postductal**
  *See AORTA, COARCTATION*
**Coarctation, preductal**
  *See AORTA, COARCTATION*
**Coats disease**
  *See RETINA, COATS DISEASE*
**Cobalamin E disease (cb1E)**
  *See METHYLCOBALAMIN DEFICIENCY*
**Cobalamin F disease**
  *See VITAMIN B(12) LYSOSOMAL TRANSPORT DEFECT*
**Cobalamin G disease (cb1G)**
  *See METHYLCOBALAMIN DEFICIENCY*
**Cobalamin malabsorption**
  *See VITAMIN B(12) MALABSORPTION*
**Cobalamin, defect in lysosomal release of**
  *See VITAMIN B(12) LYSOSOMAL TRANSPORT DEFECT*
**Cocaine, fetal effects of**
  *See FETAL EFFECTS FROM MATERNAL COCAINE ABUSE*
**Cochlear deafness-myopia-oligophrenia**
  *See DEAFNESS-MYOPIA*
**Cochlear hearing loss**
  *See DEAFNESS*

## COCKAYNE SYNDROME 0189

**Includes:**
  Cockayne syndrome type I
  Cockayne syndrome type A

**Excludes:**
  **Cockayne syndrome, type II** (2787)
  **Progeria** (0825)
  **Werner syndrome** (0998)
  **Xeroderma pigmentosum** (1005)

**Major Diagnostic Criteria:** Cachectic dwarfism associated with a small head and senile appearance. There is progressive mental retardation, as well as neurological and retinal degeneration. The pronounced photosensitivity of the patients can also be observed

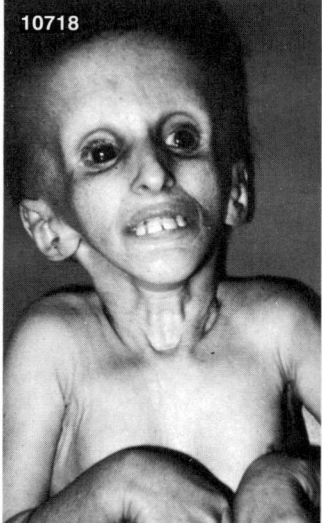
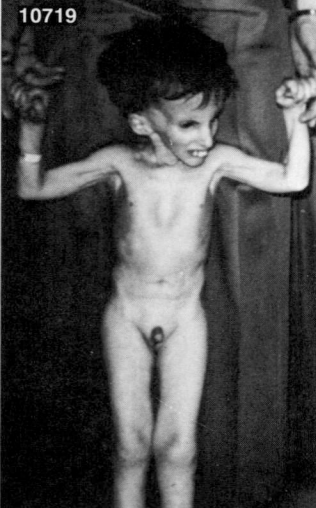

**0189-10718:** Pinched facies, sunken eyes, thin nose and sparse hair. **10719:** Short stature, decreased subcutaneous fat, and relatively long limbs in this 21-year-old male.

at the cellular level as hypersensitivity of cultured cells to the effects of ultraviolet light.

**Clinical Findings:** The onset of symptoms occurs in late infancy after six to twelve months of apparently normal development. The rate of growth and physical and mental development is then drastically and progressively reduced, resulting in severe dwarfism and mental retardation. Cachexia is marked by a loss of subcutaneous fat. The loss of adipose tissue from the face together with microcephaly, prognathism, malformed ears, beaked nose and sunken eyes gives rise to a characteristic wizened senile-like appearance.

Ocular lesions commonly include speckled pigmentation of the fundus, cataract, retinal atrophy and progressive retinal pigmentary degeneration. Other neurological abnormalities are also progressive. These include mental retardation, cerebellar movement disturbances, spasticity and sensorineural deafness. The progressive dementia, apraxic gait and progressive urinary incontinence have been attributed to normal pressure hydrocephalus.

Neuropathological investigations have revealed cerebellar atrophy, thickening of the leptomeninges and patchy demyelination. Radiological findings show intracranial calcifications, thickening of the calvarium, dental caries, and diverse skeletal abnormalities including steepening of the iliac angle in a small pelvis, slender clavicles and ribs and osteoporosis.

The severe sensitivity of the skin to sunlight seen in nearly all patients, results in a scaly rash, scarring, pigmentation and atrophy of exposed areas. Fibroblasts cultured from patients' skin are hypersensitive to the lethal effects of ultraviolet light. This is associated with a failure of RNA and DNA synthesis to recover to normal rates following UV irradiation. The defect in RNA synthesis, which probably results from an as yet unidentified defect in a DNA repair enzyme, provides a simple and rapid diagnostic test for Cockayne syndrome, which can also be used prenatally in affected families.

**Complications:** Unknown.

**Associated Findings:** Ultraviolet photosensitivity.

**Etiology:** Autosomal recessive inheritance with 100% penetrance.

**Pathogenesis:** Undetermined. Appears to be in an enzyme involved in the repair of cellular DNA following damage by ultraviolet light or chemical mutagens. This defect is an obvious cause of photosensitivity but the relationship to other symptoms of the disorder is as yet obscure. Other theories include a suggestion that the condition is a leukodystrophy, or a defect in DNA ligase.

**MIM No.:** *21640

**POS No.:** 3149

**CDC No.:** 759.820

**Sex Ratio:** M1:F1

**Occurrence:** Over 60 cases have been reported; in Europe, USA and Japan.

**Risk of Recurrence for Patient's Sib:**
See Part I, *Mendelian Inheritance.*

**Risk of Recurrence for Patient's Child:**
See Part I, *Mendelian Inheritance.*

**Age of Detectability:** Clinical symptoms usually become apparent within the first year, distinguishing this condition from **Cockayne syndrome, type II** in which the sysmptons can de detected by physical examination at birth. Cellular tests can be carried out prenatally in affected families.

**Gene Mapping and Linkage:** Unknown.

**Prevention:** None known. Genetic counseling indicated.

**Treatment:** Unknown. It has been suggested that relief of the normal pressure hydrocephalus might ameliorate some of the symptoms.

**Prognosis:** Progressive degeneration, with death usually in childhood, and in most cases before the age of 20.

**Detection of Carrier:** Unknown.

**Special Considerations:** The biochemical abnormality in the cellular response to ultraviolet light has enabled three genetically distinct complementation groups to be identified. A clinically atypical case has been described with no symptoms until the age of 5. At age 25 this patient had no ocular lesions, normal mental status and had had a successful pregnancy.

**Support Groups:** NY; North Valley Stream; Share and Care

**References:**
Cockayne EA: Dwarfism with retinal atrophy and deafness. Arch Dis Child 1936; 11:1–8.
Guzzetta F: Cockayne-Neill-Dingwall syndrome. In: Vinken PJ, Bruyn GW, eds: Handbook of clinical neurology. vol. 13. Amsterdam: North-Holland, 1972:431–440. *
Brumback RA, et al.: Normal pressure hydrocephalus. recognition and relationship to neurological abnormalities in Cockayne's syndrome. Arch Neurol 1978; 35:337–345.
Houston CS, et al.: Identical male twins and brother with Cockayne syndrome. Am J Med Genet 1982; 13:211–223. †
Lehmann AR, et al.: Prenatal diagnosis of Cockayne's syndrome. Lancet 1985; I:486–488.

LE049                                    **Alan R. Lehmann**

**Cockayne syndrome type A**
  *See COCKAYNE SYNDROME*
**Cockayne syndrome type I**
  *See COCKAYNE SYNDROME*
**Cockayne syndrome, early onset type**
  *See COCKAYNE SYNDROME, TYPE II*
**Cockayne syndrome, type B**
  *See COCKAYNE SYNDROME, TYPE II*

---

**COCKAYNE SYNDROME, TYPE II**                **2787**

**Includes:**
  Cockayne syndrome, early onset type
  Cockayne syndrome, type B

**Excludes:**
  **Cerebro-oculo-facio-skeletal syndrome** (0140)
  **Cockayne syndrome** (0189)
  **Seckel syndrome** (0881)

**Major Diagnostic Criteria:** Cockayne syndrome II is distinguished from Cockayne syndrome I by a prenatal onset of findings.

**Clinical Findings:** Affected children have prenatal onset of growth failure, with birth weights between 1,540 and 2,550 g at or near term. Congenital **Microcephaly** and cryptorchidism are also present. Other findings that develop during the first year include cataracts, sunken eyes, sparse hair, kyphosis, flexion contractures of joints, and deafness. All affected children have been severely retarded and exhibited failure to thrive. X-rays have demonstrated only acetabular anomalies, minimal flaring of ends of the long bones, and normal bone ages. Autopsies in two children demonstrated multiple brain abnormalities (diffuse dysmyelination, cerebral calcifications, and atrophic cerebellum) in both, and accessory left renal artery and absent testes in one.

**Complications:** Aspiration pneumonia as a result of poor feeding ability or gastroesophageal reflux.

**Associated Findings:** None known.

**Etiology:** Presumably autosomal recessive inheritance.

**Pathogenesis:** It is likely that the basic defect is related to cellular sensitivity to UV light, with failure of recovery of DNA and RNA synthesis occurring in UV-exposed cells. Although at least two complementation groups of cells in Cockayne syndrome have been demonstrated, it is unknown whether they correspond to classic Cockayne syndrome and to Cockayne syndrome type II.

**MIM No.:** 21641

**POS No.:** 3149

**CDC No.:** 759.820

**Sex Ratio:** M3:F1 (observed).

**Occurrence:** Four cases with prenatal onset of findings have been reported.

**Risk of Recurrence for Patient's Sib:**
See Part I, *Mendelian Inheritance.*

**Risk of Recurrence for Patient's Child:**
See Part I, *Mendelian Inheritance.*

**Age of Detectability:** At birth, by physical examination.

**Gene Mapping and Linkage:** Unknown.

**Prevention:** None known. Genetic counseling indicated.

**Treatment:** Supportive.

**Prognosis:** Mental retardation is severe; death occurred by age 3 1/2 years in one case and by age eight months in a second case.

**Detection of Carrier:** Unknown.

**Special Considerations:** Houston et al. (1982) reported sibs with what they called *early-onset Cockayne syndrome* in that one affected boy had **Microcephaly**, cataracts, and mental retardation at age one year. Birth weight and length were unknown. However, the two sibs had normal birth weights with slowness of growth and development occurring in infancy. Therefore, it is difficult to determine whether these cases should also be considered to be examples of Cockayne syndome type II. It has also been suggested that **Cerebro-oculo-facio-skeletal syndrome** be consisdered within this classification, although no studies on UV radiation effects on fibroblasts have been reported.

**Support Groups:** NY; North Valley Stream; Share and Care

**References:**
Lowry RB, et al.: Cataracts, microcephaly, kyphosis, and limited joint movement in two siblings: a new syndrome: J Pediatr 1971; 79:282–284. †
Houston CS, et al.: Identical male twins and brother with Cockayne syndrome. Am J Med Genet 1982; 13:211–223.
Lehmann AR: Three complementation groups in Cockayne syndrome. Mutat Res 1982; 106:347–356.
Moyer DB, et al.: Cockayne syndrome with early onset of manifestations. Am J Med Genet 1982; 13:225–230. *
Patton MA, et al.: Early onset Cockayne's syndrome: case reports with neuropathological and fibroblast studies. J Med Genet 1989; 26:154–159.

T0007 **Helga V. Toriello**

## COFFIN-LOWRY SYNDROME 0190

**Includes:** Short stature-head/face anomalies-kyphoscoliosis-retardation

**Excludes:** **Coffin-Siris syndrome** (2025)

**Major Diagnostic Criteria:** All males and up to two-thirds of females may show severe mental retardation, short stature, and a face with a prominent forehead, full outer eyebrows, hypertelorism, down-slanting palpebral fissures, a short nose, and a thick lower lip. Kyphoscoliosis will become obvious with increasing age. All males and all females have characteristic short, puffy, tapering, hyperextensible fingers.

**Clinical Findings:** Birth weight is probably normal. Development is slow from the start. Few males achieve useful speech, and mental retardation is usually severe. Mental retardation in females can also be severe, but it may be mild or absent. The personality is pleasant. Mental activity does not seem to deteriorate with age.

The characteristic appearance of the face may be recognized in early childhood. The forehead is square and the eyebrows are prominent, especially in their outer parts. The eyes are more or less down-slanting and set wide apart. The nose is short and bulbous, with a thick nasal septum. The lips are full, especially the lower, which is often everted over a small jaw. The mouth and ears are large. The facial features may become coarser with increasing age.

All the fingers are wide proximally and taper distally. There is true brachydactyly. The fingers are puffy with an excess of soft

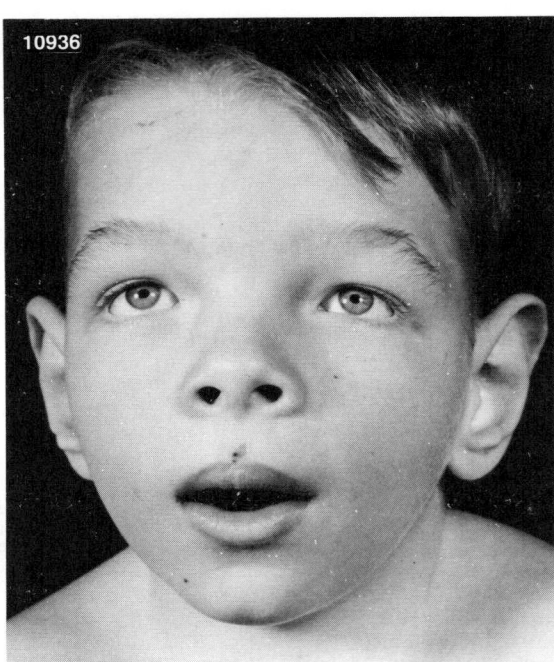

0190-10936: Note hypertelorism, prominent supraorbital ridges, broad nasal bridge, anteverted nostrils, open-mouth facies with pouty lower lip, protuberant ears.

tissue. This, and the hyperextensible joints, give a most characteristic feel, which has been likened to a bunch of sausages.

Short stature is the rule, with height just below the third centile: This may be accentuated in and beyond adolescence by scoliosis, kyphosis, or a mixture of the two. Puberty occurs normally.

The syndrome is X-linked, so the pattern of inheritance may be that of affected individuals in the family connected only through females. Some manifestations (e.g., short stature, scoliosis, mental retardation) may be more marked in males than in females.

X-ray findings include thickened facial bones with hyperostosis frontalis interna, narrowed intervertebral spaces, anterior defects in the vertebral bodies, kyphoscoliosis, and tufting of the distal phalanges, giving a drumstick appearance.

**Complications:** The most severe complications relate to kyphoscoliosis which may compromise breathing.

**Associated Findings:** Dental malocclusion with small, abnormal teeth is common. **Pectus carinatum** with or without **Pectus excavatum** may be seen. Some patients show a generalized connective tissue laxity (beyond that in the fingers) with hyperextensible large joints, flat feet, a clumsy gait, and hernias. Two patients have been reported with mitral insufficiency. Occasional findings are seizures and deafness.

**Etiology:** X-linked semidominant inheritance, with many isolated or sporadic cases.

**Pathogenesis:** The coarsening of the facies and increasing spinal deformity with increasing age have suggested an underlying storage disorder. None has been demonstrated so far, and there has been no evidence from skin biopsy material to support a generalized connective tissue dysplasia.

**MIM No.:** *30360

**POS No.:** 3150

**Sex Ratio:** M1:F1

**Occurrence:** Undetermined, but probably more common than the 40 or so published cases would indicate.

**Risk of Recurrence for Patient's Sib:**
See Part I, *Mendelian Inheritance.* Risks to sibs of an apparent sporadic case are not known. It is safest, at present, to assume the risks are the same as in familial cases.

**Risk of Recurrence for Patient's Child:**
See Part I, *Mendelian Inheritance.* No male is known to have reproduced, and would be unlikely to do so because of the severity of the mental retardation.

**Age of Detectability:** May be recognized at birth, but more likely to be detected in early childhood.

**Gene Mapping and Linkage:** CLS (Coffin-Lowry syndrome) has been mapped to Xp22.2-p22.1.

**Prevention:** None known. Genetic counseling indicated.

**Treatment:** Orthopedic measures may be useful to prevent or correct kyphoscoliosis.

**Prognosis:** Undetermined. The oldest reported patient is a woman who died at age 49 years of cardiac failure complicating mitral insufficiency. Males may survive into the third and fourth decades despite severe spinal deformity.

**Detection of Carrier:** Clinical examination may show minimal or subtle signs in the face and hands of carrier females.

**References:**

Coffin GS, et al.: Mental retardation with osteocartilaginous anomalies. Am J Dis Child 1966; 112:205–213.
Lowry B, et al.: A new dominant gene mental retardation syndrome. Am J Dis Child 1971; 121:496–500.
Procopis PG, Turner B: Mental retardation, abnormal fingers and skeletal anomalies: Coffin's syndrome. Am J Dis Child 1972; 124: 258–261.
Temtamy SA, et al.: The Coffin-Lowry syndrome: an inherited facio-digital mental retardation syndrome. J Pediatr 1975; 86:724–731. * †
Hunter AGW, et al.: The Coffin-Lowry syndrome. Experience from four centres. Clin Genet 1982; 21:321–335. * †
Partington MW, et al.: A family with the Coffin Lowry syndrome revisited: localization of CLS to Xp21-pter. Am J Med Genet 1988; 30:509–521.

PA026

M.W. Partington

## COFFIN-SIRIS SYNDROME                    2025

**Includes:** Fifth digit syndrome

**Excludes:**
**Chromosome 9, trisomy 9** (2452)
**Coffin-Lowry syndrome** (0190)
**De Lange syndrome** (0242)
**Ectodermal dysplasia**
**Ectrodactyly-ectodermal dysplasia-clefting syndrome** (0337)
**Gingival fibromatosis-digital anomalies** (0409)
**Nail-patella syndrome** (0704)
**Synostosis** (1522)
Teratogenesis secondary to antiepileptic drugs or alcohol

**Major Diagnostic Criteria:** Mental retardation, 100%; hypoplastic or absent fifth fingernails and phalanges, 100%; hypoplasia of other nails, 100%; feeding problems in infancy, 100%; joint laxity and/or hypotonia, 100%; retarded bone age, 80%; craniofacial anomalies, 100%.

**Clinical Findings:** Birth weight may be low. Poor feeding is prominent from birth. Developmental delay in all and postnatal growth deficiency in most become apparent during the first two years of life. A typical constellation of craniofacial anomalies includes microcephaly, eyebrow/eyelash hypertrichosis, a low nasal bridge, prominent lips, wide mouth or nose or both, sparse scalp hair, and a short philtrum. The facial features are individually variable but, taken together, are quite distinctive. The thick lips and scalp hypotrichosis appear to be either more or less prominent, respectively, with time.

**Complications:** Unknown.

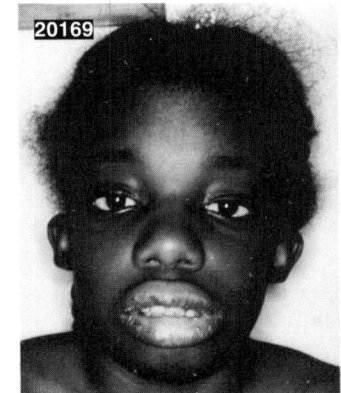
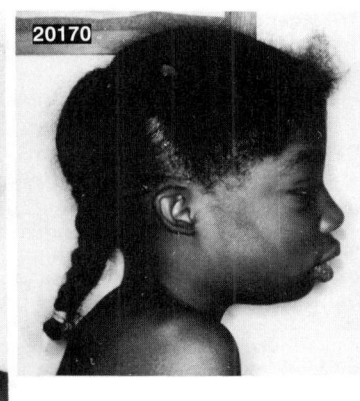
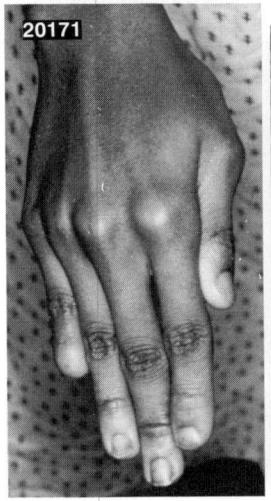
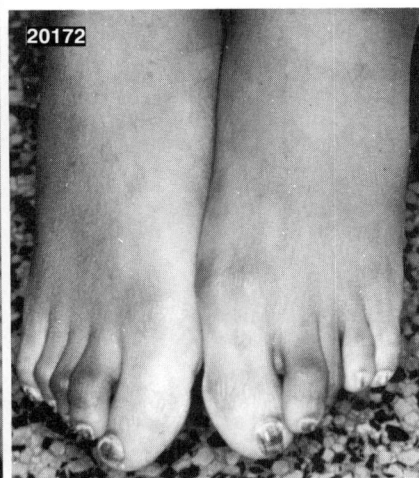

**2025-20169:** Coffin-Siris syndrome; note characteristic wide mouth with thick lips. **20170:** Lateral view of the face. **20171:** Short fifth finger with hypoplastic fingernail. **20172:** Dysplastic toenails.

**Associated Findings:** Dandy-Walker malformation or absent corpus callosum ( 8/22); congenital heart disease, (8/22); perforating ulcer disease, (2/22); urinary tract malformation, (4/22). A complex anemia, pericardial effusion of unknown etiology, and **Mitral valve prolapse** have been noted in one adolescent patient.

**Etiology:** Unknown. Familial cases have been reported.

**Pathogenesis:** Unknown.

**MIM No.:** 13590

**POS No.:** 3151

**Sex Ratio:** M1:F2

**Occurrence:** About two dozen cases have been reported in the literature.

**Risk of Recurrence for Patient's Sib:** Unknown.

**Risk of Recurrence for Patient's Child:** Unknown. There are no reported instances of an affected individual reproducing.

**Age of Detectability:** The diagnosis may be suspected at birth from the findings in the hands. Confirmatory facts of poor feeding and growth and developmental delay will require a variable number of months. Prenatal diagnosis may be possible.

**Gene Mapping and Linkage:** Unknown.

**Prevention:** None known. Genetic counseling indicated.

**Treatment:** There is no treatment known for the basic condition. Treatment for associated abnormalities is specific for the abnormality.

**Prognosis:** Dependent upon the presence and severity of associated abnormalities.

**Detection of Carrier:** Unknown.

**Special Considerations:** The **Mitral valve prolapse** discovered in one patient may be of significance. Evidence found in **Marfan syndrome, Ehlers-Danlos syndrome, Pseudoxanthoma elasticum, Von Willebrand disease**, and idiopathic scoliosis suggest that mitral valve prolapse is a manifestation of a generalized connective tissue defect. The association of joint laxity, limb-reduction defects, and nail hypoplasias may point to a generalized mesenchymal abnormality as the cause of the Coffin-Siris syndrome. In this regard it might be wondered if the cerebrovascular accident in the first patient of Coffin and Siris (1970) was a complication of mitral valve prolapse. A careful evaluation of every patient with the Coffin-Siris syndrome for the presence of mitral valve prolapse is indicated.

**References:**

Coffin GS, Siris E: Mental retardation with absent fifth fingernail and terminal phalanx. Am J Dis Child 1970; 119:433–439.
Camarasa F, et al.: Picture of the month. Am J Dis Child 1978; 132:1213–1214. †
Carey JC, Hall BD: The Coffin-Siris syndrome. Am J Dis Child 1978; 132:667–671.
Tunnessen WW, et al.: The Coffin-Siris syndrome. Am J Dis Child 1978; 132:393–395.
Schnizel A: The Coffin-Siris syndrome. Acta Paediatr Scand 1979; 68:449–452.
Lucaya J, et al: The Coffin-Siris syndrome: a report of four cases and a review of the literature. Padiatr Radiol 1981; 11:35–38.
Haspeslagh M, et al.: The Coffin-Siris syndrome: report of a family and further delineation. Clin Genet 1984; 26:374–378.
DeBassio WA, et al.: Coffin-Siris syndrome: neuropathologic findings. Arch Neurol 1985; 42:350–353.
Richieri-Costa A, et al.: Coffin-Siris syndrome in a Brazilian child with consanguineous parents. Rev Brasil Genet 1986; IX:169–177.

LA002                                          **Michael E. Labhard**

**Cogan ocular motor apraxia, congenital**
  *See OCULAR MOTOR APRAXIA, COGAN CONGENITAL TYPE*
**Cogan's microcystic dystrophy**
  *See CORNEAL DYSTROPHY, RECURRENT EROSIVE*

## COHEN SYNDROME                                    2023

**Includes:**
  Hypotonia-obesity-prominent incisors
  Incisors (prominent)-obesity-hypotonia
  Obesity-hypotonia-prominent incisors
  Pepper syndrome

**Excludes:**
  **Laurence-Moon syndrome** (0578)
  **Prader-Willi syndrome** (0823)
  **Retinopathy-microcephaly-mental retardation** (2846)

**Major Diagnostic Criteria:** At least five of the following: obesity, short stature, mental retardation, hypotonia, maxillary hypoplasia, short philtrum, micrognathia, narrow hands and feet, narrow and high-arched palate.

**Clinical Findings:** Micrognathia (100%), obesity (90%), hypotonia (90%), short philtrum (90%), narrow and high-arched palate (90%), narrow hands and feet (90%), short stature (82%), mental retardation (82%), maxillary hypoplasia (82%), joint hypermobility (73%), high nasal bridge (65%), **Microcephaly** (65%), prominent upper central incisors (considered to be a cardinal feature of Cohen syndrome but was present in only 62% of the patients), delayed puberty (56%), down-slanting palpebral fissures (55%), cubitus valgus (55%), genua valgum (48%), lordosis (45%), pes planus (42%), strabismus (42%), protruding and dysplastic ears

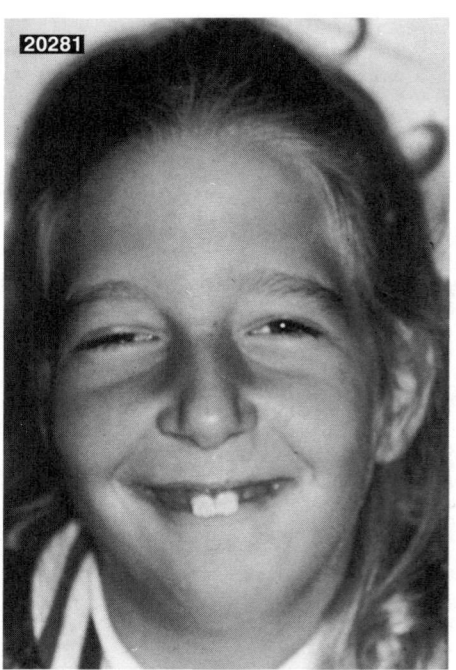

**2023A**-20281: Note prominent incisors, high nasal bridge, downward slanting palpebral fissures and maxillary hypoplasia.

(42%), myopia (33%), kyphosis (29%), heart anomalies (29%), leukopenia (19%), hand syndactyly (19%), hypoplasia of the thenar and hypothenar eminences (19%), simian creases (16%), short metacarpals and metatarsals (16%), and hypoplastic penis and testes (16%).

Malformations and findings less often reported include neonatal feeding difficulties, reduced fetal activity, delayed bone age, seizures, epicanthal folds, prominent root of the nose, low hair-

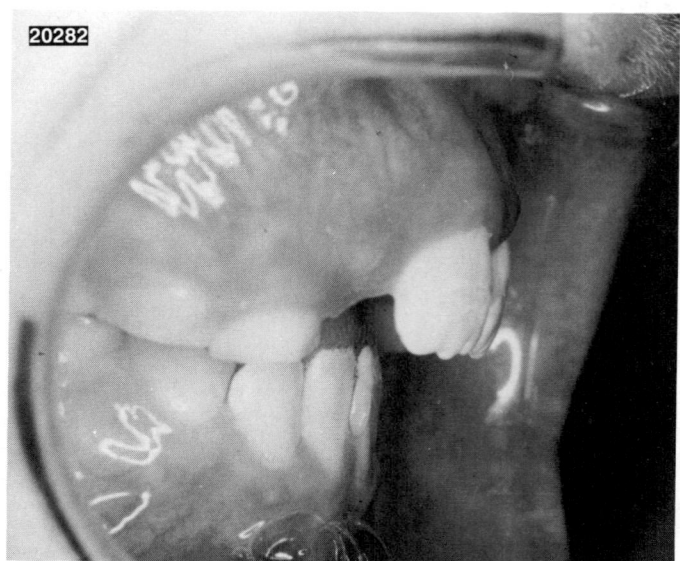

**2023B**-20282: Intraoral view of anterior teeth showing large overjet, minimal overbite, and class II relationship.

line, small tongue, enamel hypoplasia, submucous cleft, gingival hyperplasia, mottled retina, iris coloboma, chorioretinal dystrophy with bull's-eye-like maculae and pigmentary deposits, optic atrophy, microcornia, poor visual acuity, prominent choroidal vessels, hip dislocation, cryptorchidism, high-pitched voice, spina bifida oculta, and pectus excavatum.

**Complications:** Those patients with optic atrophy and chorioretinal dystrophy are at risk of becoming blind. Decreased visual acuity presents a problem for school performance and limits the patient's mobility. The oral findings produce crowding of the teeth and the characteristic facial appearance of Cohen syndrome.

**Associated Findings:** Poor school performance, walking difficulties due to genua valgum and pes planus, nystagmus, hearing deficiencies, hypertelorism, auricular tags, alternating exotropia, basal skull kyphosis, **Arthritis, rheumatoid**, and pseudoepiphyses in metacarpals 2 and 5. Recently, periureteric obstruction and epilepsy were reported.

**Etiology:** Possibly autosomal recessive inheritance, although sporadic cases have been reported, and the question of genetic heterogeneity has been raised on several occasions. In seven different instances, consanguinity was reported in the parents of affected children. There are also at least two families in which the Cohen syndrome appears to be inherited in an autosomal dominant fashion.

With the exception of one patient reported by Fuhrmann-Rieger et al. (1984), who had a chromosomal duplication (or insertion) on 15q11–13, no chromosomal abnormality has been reported in patients with Cohen syndrome.

**Pathogenesis:** Unknown.

**MIM No.:** *21655

**POS No.:** 3152

**Sex Ratio:** M1:F1

**Occurrence:** About 40 affected patients have been reported, out of whom at least 13 have been isolated cases. Sack and Friedman (1986) have suggested that the disorder may have a relatively high frequency in the Ashkenazi Jews, since five of the patients come from four such Jewish families.

**Risk of Recurrence for Patient's Sib:**
See Part I, *Mendelian Inheritance.*

**Risk of Recurrence for Patient's Child:**
See Part I, *Mendelian Inheritance.* Keeping in mind that two apparently autosomal dominant families exist, the risk could be between close to zero and 1:2.

**Age of Detectability:** The disorder should be recognizable at birth; it becomes more accentuated as the child grows older.

**Gene Mapping and Linkage:** Unknown.

**Prevention:** None known. Genetic counseling indicated.

**Treatment:** Orthopedic surgery if the joint malformations are severe; orthodontic treatment for the teeth anomalies (the upper incisors are not larger than normal; they are positioned forward on the maxilla); special education classes if necessary.

**Prognosis:** Slight-to-severe mental retardation has been observed in 90% of patients. Life span does not seem to be affected.

**Detection of Carrier:** Since at least two families exist with patients affected in more than one generation, a careful clinical examination of all relatives of an affected patient should be done to identify anyone who may be minimally affected.

**Special Considerations:** Since delayed puberty has been claimed to be a finding in Cohen syndrome, several investigators have evaluated their patients biochemically. Except for patient 2 of Carey and Hall (1978), who had isolated gonadotropins deficiency, no abnormalities have been found.

**References:**
Cohen MM Jr, et al.: A new syndrome with hypotonia, obesity, mental deficiency, and facial, oral, ocular and limb anomalies. J Pediatr 1973; 83:280–284.
Carey JC, Hall BD: Confirmation of the Cohen syndrome. J Pediatr 1978; 93:239–244.
Balestrazzi P, et al.: The Cohen syndrome: clinical and endocrinological studies of two new cases. J Med Genet 1980; 17:430–432.
Fuhrmann-Rieger A, et al.: Duplication of insertion in 15q11–13 associated with mental retardation, short stature and obesity: Prader-Willi or Cohen syndrome? Clin Genet 1984; 25:347–352.
North C, et al.: The clinical features of the Cohen syndrome: further case reports. J Med Genet 1985; 22:131–134.
Wilson S, et al.: Cohen syndrome: case report. Pediatr Dentistry 1985; 7:326–328.
Sack J, Friedman E: The Cohen syndrome in Israel. Isr J Med Sci 1986; 22:766–770.
Young ID, Moore JR: Intrafamilial variation in Cohen syndrome. J Med Genet 1987; 24:488–492.

ES000                                                    **Victor Escobar**

**Coital headache**
*See MIGRAINE*
**Cola-colored babies**
*See FETAL EFFECTS OF POLYCHLORINATED BIPHENYL (PCB)*

---

# COLD HYPERSENSITIVITY                                        2140

**Includes:**
   Cold-induced systemic reactions
   Cold urticaria, familial
   Idiopathic urticaria a-frigore (iUF)
   Urticaria syndromes, acquired

**Excludes:** Cold air-induced airway hyperreactivity in asthmatic children

**Major Diagnostic Criteria:** Urticaria, angioedema, and occasionally symptoms of hypotension after cold exposure. As much as 70% of cold-induced systemic reactions are the result of aquatic activities. Patients with cold hypersensitivity can show a coalescent wheal in response to local cold stimulation, such as an ice cube, within 3 minutes or less. In one study, 68% of individuals with a positive history showed a positive test, whereas 32% of the patients had a negative test or took longer than three minutes. In the absence of a positive test, history is sufficient to recommend prophylaxis or avoidance of cold exposure.

**Clinical Findings:** Development of an urticarial rash in areas exposed to cold or localized angioedema after exposure to cold. Less commonly, patients develop local urticaria or angioedema followed by hypotension after cold exposure. Studies have suggested that the mean age of onset of the disease is approximately 25.1 years, with a range of one to 74 years. The mean duration of symptomatology is approximately 6.3 to 9 years, the range being from 3 weeks to 37 years. Although symptoms of cold hypersensitivity disappear in most patients, a small percentage have recurrence several years later. Multiple studies have not revealed a specific causative factor and have not suggested that it is a precursor for any other specific disease complex. One individual has been described with cold hypersensitivity and C4 deficiency, elevated IgM, and proven deficiency of two half-null C4 haplotypes.

**Complications:** The hypotension can be significant and can create loss of consciousness. The urticaria can be quite uncomfortable, and the localized angioedema can be painful.

**Associated Findings:** A small percentage of patients will have heat urticaria concurrently with cold urticaria.

**Etiology:** There have been families described with classic autosomal dominant inheritance, but the majority of cases have been nonfamilial.

**Pathogenesis:** It has been proposed that C1-esterase inhibitor activity is low, but total C1-esterase inhibitor concentration is normal. Blocking histamine release diminishes the urticarial response to cold in patients with cold urticaria, therefore, it has been proposed that a portion of the etiology of cold-induced urticaria is through excessive histamine release.

**MIM No.:** *12010

**Sex Ratio:** M1:F1

**Occurrence:** The familial type is undetermined but presumed rare.

**Risk of Recurrence for Patient's Sib:**
See Part I, *Mendelian Inheritance*. Most cases are nonfamilial.

**Risk of Recurrence for Patient's Child:**
See Part I, *Mendelian Inheritance*. Most cases are nonfamilial.

**Age of Detectability:** The majority of patients have onset after age 20 years. There is no test for cold urticaria prior to clinical symptomatology.

**Gene Mapping and Linkage:** Unknown.

**Prevention:** Prophylactic use of cyproheptadine or doxepin have been effective in decreasing or suppressing the urticarial response to cold.

**Treatment:** Treatment prior to cold exposure with cyproheptadine or doxepin.

**Prognosis:** Cold hypersensitivity can be a chronic problem, but the majority of patients show decreased symptoms after six to nine years; some patients have had symptoms for as long as 37 years.

**Detection of Carrier:** Unknown.

**Special Considerations:** Several attempts have been made by different authors to categorize cold urticaria and to distinguish between acquired, familial, and those cases rarely associated with other conditions. At this time, no classification has been completely satisfactory in determining diagnostic criteria that can separate the different patterns. Therefore, the major consideration is to take an extended family pedigree and to determine if there are any other associated illnesses that may be the underlying basis for cold urticaria.

**References:**
Vlagopoulas T, et al.: Familial cold urticaria. Ann Allergy 1975; 34:366–369.
Wanderer AA, et al.: Primary acquired cold urticaria: double-blind comparative study of treatment with cyproheptadine, chlorpheniramine, and placebo. Arch Dermatol 1977; 113:1375–1377.
Bentley-Phillips CB, et al.: Cold urticaria: inhibition of cold-induced histamine release by doxantrazole. J Invest Dermatol 1978; 71:266–268.
Nilsson T, Back O: On the role of the C1-esterase inhibitor in cold urticaria. Acta Dermatol Venerol 1984; 64:197–202.
Neittaanmaki H: Cold urticaria: clinical findings in 220 patients. J Am Acad Dermatol 1985; 13:636–644.
Stafford CT, Jamieson DM: Cold urticaria associated with C4 deficiency and elevated IgM. Ann Allergy 1986; 56:313–316.
Wanderer AA, et al.: Clinical characteristics of cold-induced systemic reactions in acquired cold urticaria syndromes: recommendations for prevention of this complication and a proposal for a diagnostic classification of cold urticaria. J Allergy Clin Immunol 1986; 78:417–423.

BU007                                         **Bruce A. Buehler**

**Cold urticaria, familial**
*See COLD HYPERSENSITIVITY*
**Cold-induced systemic reactions**
*See COLD HYPERSENSITIVITY*
**Collagenase, excessive activity**
*See EPIDERMOLYSIS BULLOSUM, TYPE III*

---

### COLLAGENOMA, MULTIPLE CUTANEOUS, FAMILIAL     3166

**Includes:**
Cardiomyopathy-hypogonadism-collagenoma syndrome
Connective tissue nevus
Cutaneous collagenoma-cardiomyopathy-hypogonadism, familial

**Excludes:**
**Cardiomyopathy-genital defects** (2246)
Collagenoma, eruptive
Collagenoma, isolated (single)
**Hypergonadotropic hypogonadism with cardiomyopathy** (3195)
**Osteopoikilosis** (0781)

**Major Diagnostic Criteria:** Multiple cutaneous collagenomas.

**Clinical Findings:** Cutaneous nodules first appear over the back, chest and upper arms and often become more numerous after sexual maturation. Nodules vary in size from a few millimeters to several centimeters, and in number from a few to 100 or more. The nodules remain throughout life and progressively increase in number with advancing age. Number and size of nodules may increase during pregnancy.

Cardiovascular complications may first appear in early adulthood with hypertension and progress to heart enlargement with eventual cardiomyopathy by age 30 years. Atrial fibrillation may develop early and persist.

Hypogonadism has only been reported in males and is characterized by small testes and azoospermia. Penis is normal. Mild gynecomastia may occur. Females have shown normal fertility.

**Complications:** Congestive heart failure, infertility, systemic vasculitis, and **Diabetes mellitus**.

**Associated Findings:** Rarely, sensorineural hearing loss and atrophy of the iris.

**Etiology:** Presumably autosomal dominant inheritance.

**Pathogenesis:** A possible systemic autoimmune collagenosis is suspected.

**MIM No.:** 11525

**Sex Ratio:** Presumably M1:F1.

**Occurrence:** Four families, three caucasian and one black, have been reported in the literature, with two generations affected, and one unpublished additional family studied by Uitto (personal communication).

**Risk of Recurrence for Patient's Sib:**
See Part I, *Mendelian Inheritance*.

**Risk of Recurrence for Patient's Child:**
See Part I, *Mendelian Inheritance*.

**Age of Detectability:** Collagenomas usually appear between 14–19 years of age. Cardiomyopathy occurs later and may not be detected until adulthood and midlife. Hypogonadism should be apparent in the immediate post-pubertal period.

**Gene Mapping and Linkage:** Unknown.

**Prevention:** None known. Genetic counseling indicated.

**Treatment:** Specific treatment is directed to complications of cardiomyopathy and associated congestive heart failure and cardiac arrhythmias. Collagenomas are asymptomatic and no treatment is required. Cosmetic surgery is not appropriate and may lead to scarring.

**Prognosis:** Life span is normal in individuals with collagenomas and normal cardiovascular function. In those individuals with progressive cardiomyopathy and hypertension, death has occurred as early as age 40 years.

**Detection of Carrier:** Unknown.

**Special Considerations:** Expression in the families reported has varied greatly. In one family, cardiovascular complications dominated and only males appeared to have cardiomyopathy. Diabetes mellitus, arthritis, erythema multiforme, and urticaria in affected family members suggest an autoimmune component to the disease.

**References:**
Henderson RR, et al: Familial cutaneous collagenoma: report of cases. Arch Derm 1968; 98:23–27.
Hegedus SI, Schorr WF: Familial cutaneous collagenoma. Cutis 1972; 10:283–288.
Uitto J, et al: Familial cutaneous collagenoma: genetic studies on a family. Brit J Derm 1979; 101:185–195.
Sacks NH, et al: Familial cariomyopathy, hypogonadism, and collagenoma. Ann Intern Med 1980; 93:813–817.

LA007                                         **Roger L. Ladda**

**Collagenous plaques of the hands**
*See ACROKERATOELASTOIDOSIS*

Collodion baby
   *See ICHTHYOSIS*
Collodion baby (some)
   *See ICHTHYOSIS, CONGENITAL ERYTHRODERMIC*
   *also ICHTHYOSIS, LAMELLAR DOMINANT*
Collodion fetus (some)
   *See ICHTHYOSIS, LAMELLAR RECESSIVE*
Colloid bodies, familial
   *See OCULAR DRUSEN*
Coloboma of iris, choroid and retina
   *See EYE, MICROPHTHALMIA/COLOBOMA*
Coloboma, congenital
   *See EYELID, COLOBOMA*
Coloboma-nasopalpebral lipoma syndrome
   *See NASOPALPEBRAL LIPOMA-COLOBOMA SYNDROME*
Coloboma-obesity-polydactyly-hypogenitalism
   *See BIEMOND II SYNDROME*
Colobomatous microphthalmia, isolated
   *See EYE, MICROPHTHALMIA/COLOBOMA*
Colon (familial polyposis)-CNS tumors
   *See TURCOT SYNDROME*
Colon absence
   *See COLON, ATRESIA OR STENOSIS*
Colon agenesis
   *See COLON, ATRESIA OR STENOSIS*

## COLON, AGANGLIONOSIS                                    0192

**Includes:**
   Aganglionic megacolon
   Anal aganglionosis
   Hirschsprung disease
   Megacolon, aganglionic
   Rectal aganglionosis

**Excludes:**
   Functional megacolon
   Pseudo-Hirschsprung disease
   Psychogenic megacolon

**Major Diagnostic Criteria:** The diagnosis of aganglionic megacolon is based on a combination of physical and X-ray findings cited below and on the absence of submucosal and myenteric ganglion cells by full thickness rectal muscle biopsy or biopsy of the narrowed distal colon. (Deficiency of ganglion cells is observed in

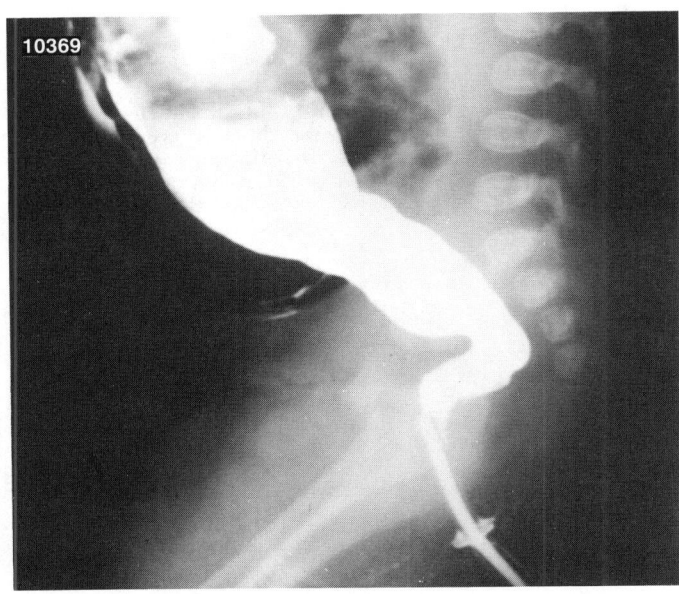

**0192-10369:** Recto-sigmoid transition in Hirschsprung disease.

the transitional segment, and proliferation or normal distribution of ganglion cells is observed in the colon proximal to the transitional zone.) A rectal suction biopsy may be done as a screening test; if ganglion cells are present in the superficial submucous plexus then a full thickness biopsy need not be done. In infants over age 6 months, rectal motility studies are employed in some centers to eliminate the diagnosis or to determine the need for biopsy.

**Clinical Findings:** Constipation occurs in all patients (100%), varying in severity from 1) inadequate or delayed passage of meconium to evidence of complete intestinal obstruction in the neonate to 2) chronic constipation in the absence of fecal soiling in the infant and child. Days or weeks may lapse before spontaneous defecation occurs. Obstipation accompanies constipation in 28% of patients with abdominal distension (85%) and vomiting (45%), nonbilious or bilious, depending on the degree of obstruction.
   *Physical examination:* Rectum is "snug" and empty by digital examination. A fecal mass may be palpated on bimanual examination or at the end of the examining finger. Explosive evacuation of fecal fluid and air on withdrawal of the finger is suggestive of rectal or rectosigmoid aganglionosis.
   *X-ray findings:* Intestinal distention is evident on three positional abdominal films. Absence of the normal rectal gas pattern on lateral films of the pelvis suggests colonic aganglionosis. The classic barium enema appearance of colonic aganglionosis demonstrates a narrowed distal aganglionic segment with a proximal dilated (ganglionic) segment. Barium enema is diagnostic in 81.5 of patients, suggestive in 14.6%, and nondiagnostic in 4.9%. Plain abdominal films obtained 24 hours following barium enema demonstrate retained barium. This examination suggests aganglionosis in the neonate who does not yet have dilation of the proximal (ganglionic) colon.

**Complications:** Enterocolitis (infants 35%; overall 14%) characterized by marked dilation of the colon with retention of air and liquid feces. Diarrhea may or may not be present. Infants are lethargic, febrile, and dehydrated. Perforation is rare.
   Physical underdevelopment or signs of malnutrition (18%). Characteristic features are muscular wasting of the limbs and hypoproteinemia. In severe cases infants may have dependent edema or anasarca.
   Obstructive uropathy (11%). Ureterovesical obstruction is a pressure phenomenon usually associated with a feces-filled rectosigmoid.
   Melena (5%) related to stercoral trauma.

**Associated Findings:** Imperforate anus (3%). (Aganglionosis associated with imperforate anus is probably secondary to vascular impairment of the colon following the pull-through procedure with a secondary resorption of ganglion cells.) Reported in six to ten percent of individuals with **Chromosome 21, trisomy 21.**

**Etiology:** Possibly autosomal recessive inheritance. Hyperthermia in early gestation has also been suggested as a factor (Lipson, 1988).

**Pathogenesis:** Congenital absence of the intramural myenteric parasympathetic nerve ganglia and sympathetic nerve plexus in a segment of colon that extends proximally from the anus for a varying distance. Aganglionosis is limited to the rectosigmoid in 70% of patients and is distal to the splenic flexure in 84%. Total colonic aganglionosis and small intestinal aganglionosis occur in 1–10% of various series.
   The aganglionic colon is unable to transmit the coordinated peristaltic waves from the proximal colon, producing variable degrees of physiologic intestinal obstruction. Hyperperistaltic activity results in increasing hypertrophy and dilation of the normal colon and possible enterocolitis if the obstruction is unrelieved.

**MIM No.:** 24920

**CDC No.:** 751.3

**Sex Ratio:** M2–3:F1

**Occurrence:** 1:8,000 live births. Caucasian, 90%; Black, less than 10%.

**Risk of Recurrence for Patient's Sib:** Familial frequency, 6%.

**Risk of Recurrence for Patient's Child:** Familial frequency, 6%.

**Age of Detectability:** At birth.

**Gene Mapping and Linkage:** Unknown.

**Prevention:** None known. Genetic counseling indicated.

**Treatment:** Definitive treatment is surgical. Diverting enterostomy in the proximal ganglionic zone is advised for the neonate or infant to allow complete decompression of the obstructed intestine. Patients with enterocolitis must be decompressed by a saline colonic irrigation prior to operation. Following restoration of normal colonic function, definitive surgical reconstruction is performed by 1) resection of aganglionic colon and abdominoperineal pull-through (Swenson) procedure; or 2) modification of the Swenson operation to avoid the tedious pelvic dissection, risk of parasympathetic nerve injury, and direct colonic anastomosis (Duhamel and Soave procedures).

**Prognosis:** Mortality during infancy is 20%. Mortality is secondary to a combination of findings: 1) late diagnosis with nutritional fluid and electrolyte complications, 2) enterocolitis during infancy, and 3) surgical complications. Normal life expectancy follows successful surgical reconstruction.

**Detection of Carrier:** Unknown.

**References:**

Kamijo K, et al.: Congenital megacolon: a comparison of spastic and hypertrophied segments with respect to cholinesterase activities and sensitivities to acetylcholine, DFP, and barium ion. Gastroenterology 1953; 24:173.

Bodian M, Carter CO: A family study of Hirschsprung's disease. Ann Hum Genet 1963; 26:261–277.

Passarge E: The genetics of Hirschsprung's disease. Evidence for heterogenous etiology and a study of sixty-three families. N Engl J Med 1967; 276:138–143.

Passarge E: Genetic heterogeneity and recurrence risk of congenital intestinal aganglionosis. In: Bergsma D, McKusick VA, eds: BD: OAS 1972; 63–67. Baltimore: Williams & Wilkins.

Kleinhaus S, et al.: Hirschsprung's disease: a survey of the members of the surgical section of The American Academy of Pediatrics. J Pediatr Surg 1979; 14:588–597. *

Lipson A, Harvey J: Three-generation transmission of Hirschsprung's disease. Clin Genet 1987; 32:175–178.

Lipson A: Hirschsprung's disease in the offspring of mothers exposed to hyperthermia during pregnancy. Am J Med Genet 1988; 29:117–124.

T0009 **Robert J. Touloukian**

**Colon, aganglionosis-pigmentary anomaly**
*See ALBINISM, WAARDENBURG TYPE-HIRSCHSPRUNG AGANGLIONOSIS*

## COLON, ATRESIA OR STENOSIS     0193

**Includes:**
Colon absence
Colon agenesis
Rectal atresia or stenosis

**Excludes:**
Colonic atresia or stenosis-aganglionosis and gastroschisis
**Exstrophy of cloaca sequence** (3193)
**Intestinal atresia or stenosis** (0531)
**Intestinal atresia, multiple** (2933)
Intestinal atresia-imperforate anus

**Major Diagnostic Criteria:** Low intestinal obstruction with X-ray confirmation of obstruction of colon.

**Clinical Findings:** Findings include signs of low intestinal obstruction with abdominal distention and obstipation. Vomiting of bile is a later finding. Stenosis with constipation as the paramount symptom may become clinically apparent later in infancy. X-rays show mechanical intestinal obstruction, whereas the barium enema demonstrates an unused colon ("microcolon") distal to the site of atresia. Complete or partial occlusion of the lumen of the colon occurs by 1) internal diaphragm (29%); 2) separation of the proximal and distal blind ends of the colon by a cord-like remnant of the bowel - the mesentery may not be intact (18%); 3) complete separation of the proximal and distal ends with defect in the mesentery (53%). Stenosis is relatively uncommon. Proximal and distal colon atresia are of equal frequency. Distal colonic atresia may be associated with severe malformation of the lower abdominal wall, pubis, anus, and rectum, with exstrophy of the bladder and cecovesical fistula ("exstrophy of the cloaca"). Duplication of the appendix, a portion of the colon, and terminal ileum also occurs with exstrophy of the cloaca.

**Complications:** Perforation of 1) antenatal intestine, with meconium peritonitis but no demonstrable intestinal perforation at the time of birth (10%); 2) proximal dilated colon segment at birth either with or without volvulus and infarction (10%); 3) distal colon segment coincident with barium enema examination (10%).

**Associated Findings:** Exstrophy of cloaca sequence, Gastroschisis.

**Etiology:** Possibly X-linked or autosomal dominant inheritance with reduced penetrance. Atresia is secondary to ischemia of the colon during the second or third trimester of pregnancy following mesenteric vascular injury or occlusion.

**Pathogenesis:** Vascular injury to the inferior mesenteric artery results in segmental atresia with normal rectum and perineum. Exstrophy of the cloaca results from a combination of an embryologic defect in hindgut development during the first trimester and a vascular accident with resorption of colon. Rectal atresia has been produced in experimental animals (rabbits) by mesenteric vascular occlusion.

**MIM No.:** 30365

**Sex Ratio:** M1:F1

**Occurrence:** 10.5% of atresia involve the colon. Incidence: 1:1,500 to 1:20,000 live births.

**Risk of Recurrence for Patient's Sib:**
See Part I, *Mendelian Inheritance*. Usually not increased.

**Risk of Recurrence for Patient's Child:**
See Part I, *Mendelian Inheritance*. Usually not increased.

**Age of Detectability:** Symptoms and signs of intestinal obstruction secondary to atresia are recognized at birth or during the initial week of life. Stenosis may be first detected in childhood or even adulthood.

**Gene Mapping and Linkage:** Unknown.

**Prevention:** None known. Genetic counseling indicated.

**Treatment:** Surgical correction of the intestinal defect with restoration of continuity; temporary enterostomy precedes abdominoperineal pull-through procedure. The surgeon must resect dilated bulbous obstructed proximal colon in attempts to preserve the ileocecal valve and avoid water and electrolyte losses and nutritional complications.

**Prognosis:** Normal life span except when late intestinal complications of primary or secondary operations occur.

**Detection of Carrier:** Unknown.

**Support Groups:** OH; Solon; National Support Group for Exstrophy

**References:**

Benson CD, et al.: Congenital atresia and stenosis of the colon. J Pediatr Surg 1968; 3:253–257.

Erskine JM: Colonic stenosis in the newborn: the possible thromboembolic etiology of intestinal stenosis and atresia. J Pediatr Surg 1970; 5:321–333.

Boles ET, et al.: Atresia of the colon. J Pediatr Surg 1976; 11:69–75. *

Benawra R, et al.: Familial occurrence of congenital colonic atresia. J Pediatr 1981; 99:435–436.

T0009 **Robert J. Touloukian**

## COLON, DUPLICATION    0194

**Includes:**

    Colonic "cyst"
    Rectal duplication

**Excludes:** Colon diverticulum

**Major Diagnostic Criteria:** Palpable abdominal mass due to duplication of colon, or rectum, or caudal twinning.

**Clinical Findings:** Variable, manifesting in the newborn period in infancy, or in childhood. Findings include the following characteristics: palpable abdominal or rectal mass with or without abdominal distention (40%); intestinal obstruction with vomiting of bile and abdominal distention (20%); rectal bleeding (10%); duplication of the external genitalia and anal orifice associated with tubular duplication of the colon, terminal ileal duplication, double bladder, and urethra (about 30%).

**Complications:** Presacral rectal duplication causes pressure symptoms, rectal prolapse, or bleeding. Tubular duplications of the colon fill with feces, become dilated, and compress the normal colon and urinary tract structures.

**Associated Findings:** Tubular duplications of the entire colon and rectum represent abortive twinning and are accompanied by duplication of the external genitalia, anus, bladder, and urethra (about 90%).

**Etiology:** Spherical and tubular duplications of the colon are not well explained by either the "solid core" or "diverticulum" theory of an embryologic defect in hindgut development. Complete duplication of the colon and rectum with doubling of the genitalia, bladder and urethra represents a caudal twinning with duplication of the hindgut and genital and lower urinary tracts.

**Pathogenesis:** Duplications of the colon arise from the mesenteric surface of the normal colon and have 1) colonic mucosal (90%) or heterotopic mucosal lining, usually gastric (about 10%); 2) smooth muscle coat shared with a segment of the parent colon; 3) a common mesentery; 4) an internal communication with the parent colonic lumen (80)% and a blind duplication (20%).

**Sex Ratio:** M1:F2

**Occurrence:** Thirty percent of all duplications in the alimentary tract arise from the colon. More than 50 cases of double colon, anus, bladder, urethra, and external genitalia have been reported.

**Risk of Recurrence for Patient's Sib:** Unknown.

**Risk of Recurrence for Patient's Child:** Unknown.

**Age of Detectability:** Caudal twinning of colon duplication is recognized at birth. Other forms of colon duplication are diagnosed either at birth or in childhood.

**Gene Mapping and Linkage:** Unknown.

**Prevention:** None known. Genetic counseling indicated.

**Treatment:** Surgical correction, by 1) total excision of the duplications, 2) partial excision of the duplication and stripping of the mucosa, or 3) a reentry procedure to relieve signs of intestinal obstruction and to provide adequate internal drainage of the duplication.

**Prognosis:** Normal life span except when late intestinal complications of primary or secondary operations occur.

**Detection of Carrier:** Unknown.

**Special Considerations:** Emphasis is placed on avoiding major resection of normal colon with long tubular duplications, since adequate internal drainage is obtained by partial resection and reentry procedure. Patients with complete tubular duplications of the colon should also be investigated for associated urinary tract duplications or anomalies. "Solid core" theory: growth of the hindgut accelerates during the sixth or seventh week of gestation with proliferation of epithelial cells and occlusion of the lumen. Vacuolation and coalescence of these cells fail to occur normally, leaving a cyst or tube, which eventually becomes a duplication. "Diverticulum" theory: a bud of intestinal epithelium penetrates the subepithelial connective tissue in the 4–23-mm embryo, form-

ing a secondary lumen, eventually lined by colonic epithelium and a smooth muscle layer.

**References:**

Ravitch MM: Hindgut duplication - doubling of colon and genital urinary tract. Ann Surg 1953; 137:588–601. *
Soper RT: Tubular duplication of the colon and distal ileum: case report and discussion. Surgery 1968; 63:998–1004.
McPherson AG, et al.: Duplication of the colon. Br J Surg 1969; 56:138–142.
Grosfeld JL, et al.: Enteric duplications in infancy and childhood: an 18-year review. Ann Surg 1970; 172:83–90.

T0009                            **Robert J. Touloukian**

**Colon, familial polyposis**
    *See INTESTINAL POLYPOSIS, TYPE I*
**Colonic "cyst"**
    *See COLON, DUPLICATION*

## COLOR BLINDNESS, BLUE MONOCONE-MONOCHROMATIC    0195

**Includes:**

    Achromatopsia, X-chromosomal linked incomplete
    Blue monocone-monochromatic, color blindness
    Cone monochromatism

**Excludes:** Color blindness, total (0198)

**Major Diagnostic Criteria:** Congenital absence of red and green cone function (by psychophysical and/or electrophysiological methods) occurs with normal rod function without evidence of progressive disease. An X-linked inheritance pattern suggests diagnosis. Luminosity, foveal dark adaptation and acuity data indicate the presence of blue-sensitive cones with a maximum sensitivity at about 440 nm.

**Clinical Findings:** Blue monochromats have a severe color defect but can distinguish blue and blue-green colors from yellow-green, yellow and orange-red colors. In addition, there is congenital reduced distance visual acuity (20/80 - 20/100), better near vision (Jaeger 1–4 point), with or without nystagmus, light aversion and myopia. The ophthalmoscopic appearance is normal or occasionally shows minimal pigment clumping in the macular area. At low luminance levels, these individuals function as complete achromats (198); at high luminance levels they function as blue-cone monochromats.

**Complications:** Affected individuals with X-linked achromatopsia have a serious visual handicap in school. In adult life, failure to qualify for a drivers license may limit activity. Prospective employers may need reassurance that this condition is nonprogressive.

**Associated Findings:** None known.

**Etiology:** X-linked recessive inheritance. The defect is probable a combination of **Color blindness, red-green protan series** and **Color blindness, red-green deutan series** defects.

**Pathogenesis:** Alterations in the red and green visual pigment cluster. It is assumed that blue-cone monochromats have the normal allotment of normal blue cones (and normal rods) and have few or no green and red pigment-bearing cones.

**MIM No.:** 30370

**Sex Ratio:** M1:F0 (Affected males are hemizygous; no homozygous females reported.)

**Occurrence:** Incidence 2–3:100,000 male live births.

**Risk of Recurrence for Patient's Sib:**
    See Part I, *Mendelian Inheritance.*

**Risk of Recurrence for Patient's Child:**
    See Part I, *Mendelian Inheritance.*

**Age of Detectability:** The presence of congenital nystagmus and photophobia with normal fundus appearance in infancy arouses suspicion of the diagnosis, particularly if the family history is positive; it is otherwise detected when reduced visual acuity is noted at 2–3 years. If the family history is negative, differentiation from **Color blindness, total** may require color vision examination at the age of 8 or older.

**Gene Mapping and Linkage:** CBBM (color blindness, blue monochromatic) has been mapped to Xq28.

**Prevention:** None known. Genetic counseling indicated.

**Treatment:** Although primary treatment is unavailable, special education which uses materials for the visually handicapped may help affected individuals.

**Prognosis:** Nonprogressive.

**Detection of Carrier:** Female heterozygotes, by the Lyon hypothesis, should display varying degrees of color or brightness anomalies. Approximately half of the carrier females have demonstrated mildly abnormal anomaloscope results. Carriers may also show dark adaptation or ERG abnormality, especially for a red light flash or for flicker stimuli.

**References:**

Alpern M, et al.: Pi-1 cone monochromatism. Arch Ophthalmol 1965; 74:334–337.
Spivey BE: The X-linked recessive inheritance of atypical monochromatism. Arch Ophthalmol 1965; 74:327–333.
Pokorny J, et al.: Congenital and acquired color vision defects. New York: Grune and Stratton, 1979. *
Smith VC, et al.: X-linked incomplete achromatopsia with more than one class of function cones. Invest Ophthalmol & Vis Sci 1983; 24:451–457.
Lewis RA, et al.: Mapping X-linked ophthalmic disease III. Arch Ophthalmol 1987; 105:1055–1059.
Nathans J, et al.: Molecular genetics of human blue cone monochromacy. Science 1989; 245:831–838. *

P0001
SM002

**Joel Pokorny**
**Vivianne C. Smith**

## COLOR BLINDNESS, RED-GREEN DEUTAN SERIES      0196

**Includes:**
  Color defect, deutan series
  Deuteranopia
  Red-green deutan series color blindness

**Excludes:  Color blindness, red-green protan series** (0197)

**Major Diagnostic Criteria:** 90–95% of all deutan individuals will fail a validated plate screening test for red-green defect. Clinical diagnosis of the precise defect is accomplished by an anomaloscope which measures the Rayleigh equation for a 1° or 2° field. The Rayleigh equation is a colorimetric equation in which a 589 nm light is matched in visual appearance to a mixture of two other lights: 545 nm and 670 nm. The instrument is designed so that the normal observer sets an equal proportion of 545 nm and 670 nm light to match the 589 nm. The deuteranomalous trichromat sets a narrow match with a high proportion, (about 0.75 - 0.80) of 545 nm light. The extreme deuteranomalous accepts a wide range of mixture including normal and deuteranomalous proportions. The deuteranope has a full range match: he can match 545 nm to the 589 nm light or 670 nm to the 589 nm light. Brightness settings of the 589 nm light indicate normal values for deutans. A classic laboratory diagnostic criterion for the dichromatic defect, deuteranopia, is the existence of a spectral neutral point: a spectral wavelength (c. 500 nm) which the deuteranope cannot distinguish from a neutral white. Deuteranomalous trichromats do not have such neutral points although blue-green lights (wavelengths c. 500 nm) do appear almost neutral in color.

**Clinical Findings:** Individuals with a deutan color defect have normal visual acuity but show color confusions for the shades of purple, grey and bluish blue-green. Such individuals show difficulty in discriminating between shades of green, yellow, orange and red. Spectral brightness sensitivity is normal. The severity of chromatic discrimination loss varies between the different alleles: in simple deuteranomaly there is relatively good discrimination but in deuteranopia discrimination is usually poor. Inter-familial variation is greater than intra-familial variation. The ability to discriminate colors improves dramatically as the field of view is increased. The chromatic discrimination loss is evidenced by failure on clinical plate screening tests as well as by clinical color discrimination tests.

**Complications:** There are no serious complications. However, affected individuals are prohibited from certain occupations in transport and in the Armed Forces for which color signal recognition is required. Additionally, affected individuals may find themselves handicapped in certain occupations which involve skill at color recognition or discrimination.

**Associated Findings:** None known.

**Etiology:** X-linked recessive inheritance. The allele for normal trichromacy is dominant to the deuteranomalous allele which, in turn, is dominant to that for the extreme deuteranomaly, which is dominant to the allele for deuteranopia. Males inheriting one defective gene express the defect (hemizygote). Females inheriting one defective gene are usually normal (See Detection of Carrier). Females inheriting two defective genes express the least severe defect. Deutans have the normal "red" and "blue" cone pigments but have an abnormal "green" cone pigment. Current research suggests that the severity of the defect, ranging from simple deuteranomaly to deuteranopia, reflects the amount of abnormal photopigment or the number of photoreceptors containing abnormal photopigment.

**Pathogenesis:** Unknown.

**MIM No.:** *30380

**Sex Ratio:** M16:F>1

**Occurrence:** Deuteranomalous trichromats: 1:20 male and 1:300 female live births.
  Deuteranopia: 1:70 male and 1:10,000 female live births. The incidence is less common among the Japanese (3.9%) and even much lower (1%) among Fiji Islanders and Eskimos.
  Prevalence 6500:100,000 of the U.S. male population.

**Risk of Recurrence for Patient's Sib:**
  See Part I, *Mendelian Inheritance.*

**Risk of Recurrence for Patient's Child:**
  See Part I, *Mendelian Inheritance.*

**Age of Detectability:** School age on routine screening or when family member or teacher notes color vision weakness.

**Gene Mapping and Linkage:** GCP (green cone pigment (color blindness, deutan)) has been mapped to Xq28.

**Prevention:** None known. Genetic counseling indicated.

**Treatment:** A controversial treatment is the prescription of the X-chrom lens. The X-chrom lens is a colored filter (deep red) which absorbs green light. The filter is made up as a contact lens for one (non-dominant) eye. The other eye may be fitted with a neutral grey lens. Use of the X-chrom lens may allow the affected individual to pass plate screening tests. The manufacturer claims that affected individuals experience a new perceptual world which they enjoy. It must be emphasized, however, that color discrimination is not improved by wearing the X-chrom lens nor is the color defect cured by wearing this lens. The X-chrom lens should not be worn for night driving. On the other hand, some affected individuals might find that a colored filter held before one eye and used in serial comparison may be helpful in distinguishing color samples (eg, for histology or geology).

**Prognosis:** Nonprogressive.

**Detection of Carrier:** Minimal color discrimination abnormalities have been detected in heterozygous females with one normal allele. In red-green flicker photometry, such heterozygotes require significantly more green than the normal subject for minimum flicker.
  The marked variablility and infrequent incidence of color defect in carrier females (normal heterozygotes) is explained by some authorities on the basis of the Lyon hypothesis.

**References:**

Porter IH, et al.: Linkage between glucose-6-phosphate dehydroge-nase and colour-blindness. Nature 1962; 193:506 (only).

Waardenburg PJ: Colour sense and dyschromatopsia. In: Waarden-burg PJ, et al., eds: Genetics and ophthalmology, vol II. Assesn, Netherlands: Royal Van Gorcum, 1963: 1425–1566.

Pokorny J, et al.: Congenital and acquired color vision defects. New York: Grune & Stratton, 1979. *

Pokorny J, Smith VC: New observations concerning red-green color defect. J Color Res & Appl 1982; 7:159–164.

Nathans J, et al.: Molecular genetics of human color vision: The genes encoding blue, green and red pigments. Science 1986; 232:193–202. *

Nathans J, et al.: Molecular genetics of inherited variations in human color vision. Science 1986; 232:203–232.

P0001                             **Joel Pokorny**
SM002                        **Vivianne C. Smith**

## COLOR BLINDNESS, RED-GREEN PROTAN SERIES    **0197**

**Includes:**

Protanopia
Red-green protan series color blindness

**Excludes:**  **Color blindness, red-green deutan series** (0196)

**Major Diagnostic Criteria:**  Most (90–95%) of all protan individu-als will fail a validated plate screening test for red-green defect. Clinical diagnosis of the precise defect is accomplished by using a device called an anomaloscope which measures the Rayleigh equation for a 1° or 2° field. The Rayleigh equation is a colorimetric equation in which a 589 nm light is matched in visual appearance to a mixture of two other lights: 545 nm and 670 nm. The instrument is designed so that the normal observer sets an equal proportion of 545 nm and 670 nm light to match the 589 nm. The protanomalous trichromat sets a narrow match with a high proportion (about 0.75 - 0.80) of 670 nm light. The extreme protanomalous accepts a wide range of mixture including normal and protanomalous proportions. The protanope has a full range match: he can match 545 nm to the 589 nm light or 670 nm to the 589 nm light. Brightness settings of the 589 nm light indicate reduced sensitivity at 670 nm.

A classic laboratory diagnostic criterion for the dichromatic defect, protanopia is the existence of a spectral neutral point; a spectral wavelength (c. 495 nm) which the protanope cannot distinguish from a neutral white. Protanomalous trichromats do not have such neutral points although blue-green lights (wave-lengths c. 495 nm) do appear almost neutral in color.

**Clinical Findings:**  Individuals with a protan color defect have normal visual acuity but show color confusions of shades of red, grey and bluish blue-green. Such individuals show difficulty in discriminating between shades of green, yellow and orange. Spectral brightness sensitivity is abnormal: protans have reduced sensitivity to long wavelength (red) lights. From simple prota-nomaly with relatively good discrimination to protanopia, where discrimination is usually poor, the severity of chromatic discrim-ination loss varies between the different alleles. Inter-familial variation is greater than intra-familial variation. The ability to discriminate colors improves dramatically as the field of view is increased. The chromatic discrimination loss is evidenced by failure on clinical plate screening tests as well as by clinical color discrimination tests.

**Complications:**  There are no serious complications. However, affected individuals are prohibited from certain occupations in transport and in the Armed Forces for which color signal recog-nition is required. Additionally, affected individuals may find themselves handicapped in certain occupations which involve skill at color recognition or discrimination.

**Associated Findings:**  None known.

**Etiology:**  X-linked recessive inheritance. The allele for normal trichromacy is dominant to the protanomalous allele, which, in turn, is dominant to that for the extreme protanomaly, which is dominant to the allele for protanopia. Males inheriting one defective gene express the defect (hemizygote). Females inherit-ing one defective gene are usually normal (see Detection of Carrier). Females inheriting two defective genes express the least severe defect.

Protans have the normal "green" and "blue" cone pigments but have an abnormal "red" cone pigment. Current research suggests that the severity of defect, ranging from simple protanomaly to protanopia, reflects the amount of abnormal photopigment or number of photoreceptors containing abnormal photopigment.

**Pathogenesis:**  Unknown.

**MIM No.:**  *30390

**Sex Ratio:**  M16:F>1

**Occurrence:**  Protanomalous trichromats 1:100 male and 3:10,000 female live births.

Protanopia: 1:100 male and 1:10,000 female live births. The incidence is less common among the Japanese (3.9%) and even much lower (1%) among Fiji Islanders and Eskimos.

Prevalence 200:100,000 of the male U.S. population.

**Risk of Recurrence for Patient's Sib:**
See Part I, *Mendelian Inheritance.*

**Risk of Recurrence for Patient's Child:**
See Part I, *Mendelian Inheritance.*

**Age of Detectability:**  School age on routine screening or when family member or teacher notes color vision weakness.

**Gene Mapping and Linkage:**  RCP (red cone pigment (color blind-ness, protan)) has been mapped to Xq28.

**Prevention:**  None known. Genetic counseling indicated.

**Treatment:**  A controversial treatment is the prescription of the X-chrom lens. The X-chrom lens is a colored filter (deep red) which absorbs green light. The filter is made up as a contact lens for one (non-dominant) eye. The other eye may be fitted with a neutral grey lens. Use of the X-chrom lens may allow the affected individual to pass plate screening tests. The manufacturer claims that affected individuals experience a new perceptual world which they enjoy. It must be emphasized, however, that color discrim-ination is not improved by wearing the X-chrom lens; nor is the color defect cured by wearing this lens. The X-chrom lens should not be worn for night driving. On the other hand, some affected individuals might find that a colored filter held before one eye and used in serial comparison may be helpful in distinguishing color samples (eg, for histology or geology).

**Prognosis:**  Nonprogressive.

**Detection of Carrier:**  Minimal color discrimination abnormalities have been detected in heterozygous females with one normal allele. In red-green flicker photometry, such heterozygotes require significantly more red than the normal subject for minimum flicker (the Schmidt sign).

**Special Considerations:**  The marked variability and infrequent incidence of color defect in carrier females (normal heterozygotes) is explained by some authorities on the basis of the Lyon hypoth-esis.

**References:**

Waardenburg PJ: Colour sense and dyschromatopsia. In: Waarden PJ, et al.: Genetics and ophthalmology. vol II. Assen, Netherlands: Royal Van Gorcum, 1963: 1425–1566.

Pokorny J, et al.: Congenital and acquired color vision defects. New York: Grune & Stratton, 1979. *

Pokorny J, Smith VC.: New observations concerning red-green color defect. J Color Res & Appl 1982; 7:159–164.

Nathans J, et al.: Molecular genetics of human color vision: The genes encoding blue, green and red pigments. Science 1986; 232:193–202. *

Nathans J, et al.: Molecular genetics of inherited variations in human color vision. Science 1986; 232:203–232.

P0001                             **Joel Pokorny**
SM002                        **Vivianne C. Smith**

## COLOR BLINDNESS, TOTAL 0198

**Includes:**
Achromatism
Achromatopsia, incomplete
Achromatopsia-amblyopia
Day blindness
Rod monochromatism

**Excludes:**
**Color blindness, blue monocone-monochromatic** (0195)
**Color blindness** (other)

**Major Diagnostic Criteria:** Congenital absence of cone function (by psychophysical and/or electroretinographic methods) with normal rod function without evidence of progressive retinal disease in one or more siblings suggests diagnosis of achromatopsia.

**Clinical Findings:** Complete achromats are unable to distinguish surfaces solely on the basis of their color, eg, a complete achromat cannot distinguish a blue from a red when matched for scotopic brightness, even when large color areas are used. Incomplete achromats show residual weak color perception that is optimal for large color surfaces and strong, highly saturated colors. In addition, complete and incomplete achromats have a serious reduction of visual acuity (20/80 - 20/200), photophobia (painless light aversion) and nystagmus. In general, the ophthalmoscopic appearance of the retina is normal or presents minute pigment clumping in or about the macular area, as well as a loss of the foveal reflex. Pallor of the optic disc occurs in 20% of the affected individuals. Peripheral visual fields may be normal or slightly constricted, especially to colored targets. Central visual fields may present, on occasion, a small central scotoma.

**Complications:** Affected individuals, with occasional exceptions, have a serious visual handicap in school. In adult life, failure to qualify for a driving license may limit activity. Prospective employers may need reassurance that this condition is nonprogressive.

**Associated Findings:** None known.

**Etiology:** Autosomal recessive inheritance. There may be two or three different autosomal recessive genes for complete and incomplete achromatopsia since there are at least two functionally distinguishable forms of autosomal recessive incomplete achromatopsia. Complete achromatopsia presents an enigma in that studies suggest that there are two types or photoreceptors in such eyes: one type functions at high levels of illumination and has some characteristics of normal cones but maintains the action spectrum of rods; the other type functions at low levels of illumination (normal rods).

**Pathogenesis:** Undetermined. There seems to be a deficiency in the number, morphology, and variety of the cones in the retina of affected individuals.

**MIM No.:** *21690

**Sex Ratio:** M1:F1

**Occurrence:** Europe 0.00025 to 0.00055; Japan 0.0041 to 0.0069; relatively higher where high incidence of consanguinity exists.

**Risk of Recurrence for Patient's Sib:**
See Part I, *Mendelian Inheritance.*

**Risk of Recurrence for Patient's Child:**
See Part I, *Mendelian Inheritance.*

**Age of Detectability:** In infancy the presence of congenital nystagmus and photophobia with a normal fundus arouses suspicion of the diagnosis, particularly if other siblings are affected; otherwise, the condition is detected when reduced visual acuity is noted between 2–3 years. Differentiation of complete and incomplete subtypes requires a color vision examination after the age of eight.

**Gene Mapping and Linkage:** Unknown.

**Prevention:** None known. Genetic counseling indicated.

**Treatment:** Undetermined. Affected individuals may be helped by special education or materials for the visually handicapped.

**Prognosis:** Nonprogressive.

**Detection of Carrier:** No defects have been reported in carriers.

**References:**
Sloan LL: The photopic retinal receptors of the typical achromat. Am J Ophthalmol 1958; 46:81–86.
Alpern M, et al.: The enigma of total typical monochromacy. Am J Ophthalmol 1960; 50:996–1011.
Waardenburg PJ: Achromatopsia congenita. In: Waardenburg PJ, et al., eds: Genetics and ophthalmology. vol II. Assen, Netherlands: Royal van Gorcum, 1963:1695–1718. *
Pokorny J, et al.: Classification of complete and incomplete autosomal recessive achromatopsia. Grafe's Arch Clin Exp Ophthalmol 1982; 219:121–130. *

P0001                               **Joel Pokorny**
SM002                     **Vivianne C. Smith**

## COLOR BLINDNESS, YELLOW-BLUE TRITAN 0199

**Includes:**
Blue colorblindness
Tritan defect, incomplete
Tritanomaly
Tritanopia
Yellow-blue color defect

**Excludes:**
**Color blindness** (other)
**Optic atrophy, Kjer type** (3069)

**Major Diagnostic Criteria:** There are no validated plate tests for rapid detection of tritan defect. Colorimetry, increment thresholds, family history and ophthalmoscopic evaluation are used to provide a diagnosis.

1. By colorimetry, using the Moreland equation (480 nm +580 nm = 500 nm + 430 nm): the affected individual can match 480 nm to 430 nm or to 500 nm with a 1° field of view. Alternately, this match of 480 nm to a mixture of 430 nm plus 500 nm is grossly abnormal.

2. By increment threshold, using the TNO tritan test: the affected individual does not perceive a small violet color field superimposed on a bright yellow background field.

3. Normal visual acuity has no sign of macular or optic disc disorder.

4. Family history is consistent with autosomal dominant inheritance.

**Clinical Findings:** Affected individuals have normal visual acuity but show color confusion of violet and orange-pink shades. They are unable to discriminate between shades of blue and blue-green. There is great intra- and inter-familial variability in color weakness among different tritan individuals. The majority of tritans show marked color discrimination losses for small color surfaces, but may have almost normal discrimination for large color surfaces. Affected individuals show color weakness on clinical color discrimination tests.

**Complications:** Unknown.

**Associated Findings:** None known.

**Etiology:** Autosomal dominant inheritance. Prior suggestions of the existence of a subtype of tritan defect, "tritanomaly," with X-linked recessive inheritance, have not been substantiated.

**Pathogenesis:** Unknown.

**MIM No.:** *19090, 30400

**Sex Ratio:** M1:F1.

**Occurrence:** Incidence 1–5:10,000 Caucasian live births. The population frequency of tritan defect is still in dispute. New population screening series using TNO tritan test are needed.

**Risk of Recurrence for Patient's Sib:**
See Part I, *Mendelian Inheritance.*

**Risk of Recurrence for Patient's Child:**
See Part I, *Mendelian Inheritance.*

**Age of Detectability:** Affected individuals are rarely aware of their color vision abnormality until it is brought to their attention by other family members.

**Gene Mapping and Linkage:** BCP (blue cone pigment) has been provisionally mapped to 7q22-qter.

**Prevention:** None known. Genetic counseling indicated.

**Treatment:** Unknown.

**Prognosis:** A congenital and stationary aberration of color perception is most common.

**Detection of Carrier:** Unknown.

**References:**

Wright WD: Characteristics of tritanopia. J Opt Soc Am 1952; 42:509–521.

Waardenburg PJ: Colour sense and dyschromatopsia. In: Waardenburg PJ, et al., eds: Genetics and ophthalmology. vol II. Assen, Netherlands: Royal Van Gorcum, 1963: 1425–1566.

Pokorny J, et al., eds.: Congenital and acquired color vision defects. New York: Grune & Stratton, 1979. *

Pokorny J, et al.: Color matching in autosomal dominant tritan defect. J Opt Soc Am 1981; 71:1327–1334.

Miyake Y, et al.: Differential diagnosis of congenital tritanopia and dominantly inherited juvenile optic atrophy. Arch Ophthalmol 1985; 103:1496–1501.

Went LN, Pronk N: The genetics of tritan disturbances. Hum Genet 1985; 69:255–262.

P0001
SM002

**Joel Pokorny**
**Vivianne C. Smith**

**Color defect, deutan series**
*See COLOR BLINDNESS, RED-GREEN DEUTAN SERIES*
**Colorectal cancer**
*See CANCER, COLORECTAL*

## COLPOCEPHALY 2012

**Includes:** Vesiculocephaly

**Excludes:**
Hydrocephaly (0481)
Lissencephaly syndrome (0603)

**Major Diagnostic Criteria:** Mental retardation, microcephaly, seizures and a characteristic CT scan or pneumoencephalogram.

**Clinical Findings:** Microcephaly and mental retardation are constant features. A variety of motor abnormalities may be present. Spasticity is frequent, though some infants may initially be hypotonic. Seizures are common and may be difficult to control. Pneumoencephalogram or CT scan of the brain shows frontal horns of a relatively normal size and markedly dilated occipital horns.

**Complications:** Unknown.

**Associated Findings:** None known.

**Etiology:** Unknown. Possibly an intrauterine insult which occurs between the second and sixth month of pregnancy. The timing of the insult is probably more important than its cause.

**Pathogenesis:** The lateral ventricles, starting about the second month of gestation, develop as cavities of the telencephalon after the closure of the neural sulcus and the formation of the neural tube. This cavity then undergoes changes in shape and size to approximate the adult configuration. Growth of the ventricular wall is an important factor in reducing the ventricular size. Fibers of the corpus callosum, the forceps and the tapetum, the internal parieto-occipital fissure and the calcarine fissure, all contribute in reducing and shaping the occipital horns. By the sixth month of gestation this sequence of events is largely completed. Interruption of development during this sequence of events results in the persistence of the fetal configuration of the occipital horns. The resultant malformation is termed colpocephaly.

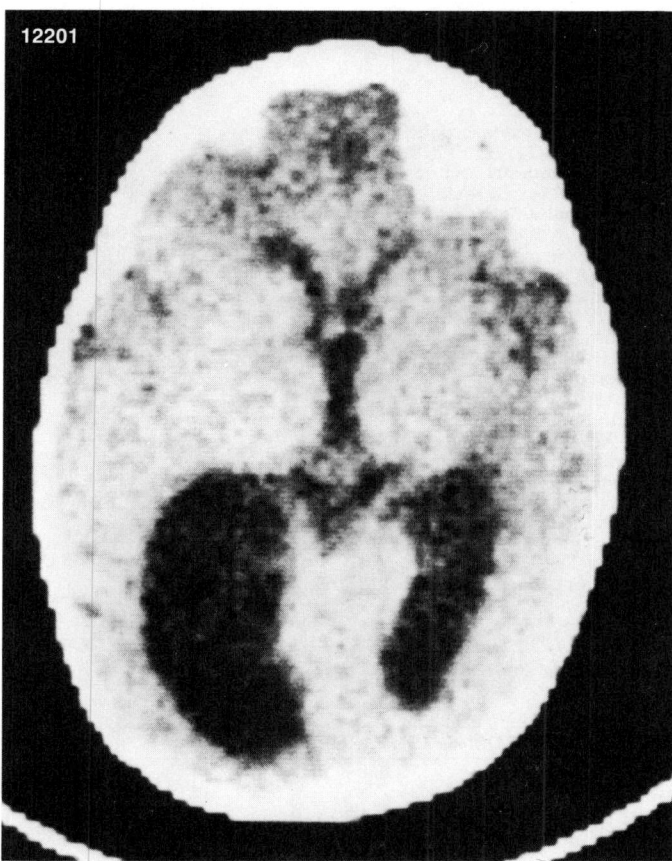

2012-12201: CT scan of colpocephaly.

**Sex Ratio:** Presumably M1:F1.

**Occurrence:** Unknown. One Center identified at least eight cases within two years. The condition is not yet coded separately in diagnostic reports, and therefore may be underestimated.

**Risk of Recurrence for Patient's Sib:** Unknown.

**Risk of Recurrence for Patient's Child:** Unknown.

**Age of Detectability:** Anytime after birth, by CT scan or pneumoencephalogram.

**Gene Mapping and Linkage:** Unknown.

**Prevention:** None known. Genetic counseling indicated.

**Treatment:** No definitive treatment. Special education, prevention of contractures, and anti-convulsant medications may be indicated.

**Prognosis:** Depends upon severity. Many patients will need life-long custodial care.

**Detection of Carrier:** Unknown.

**Special Considerations:** Colpocephaly should be regarded as a morphologic entity without a single etiology. The condition probably represents the end result of a variety of insults and disease processes that act on the developing brain at a critical time so as to interrupt maturation.

**References:**

Benda CE: Microcephaly. Am J Psychol 1940; 97:1135–1146.

Yakovlev PI, Wadsworth RC: Schizencephalies: a study of the congenital clefts in the cerebral mantle. 1. clefts without fused lips. J Neuropathol Exp Neurol 1946; 5:116–130.

Rebollo MA: A contribution to the study of the development of lateral ventricles. Acta Neurol Latino Am 1956; 2:99–106.

Garg BP: Colpocephaly: an error of morphogenesis? Arch Neurol 1982; 39:243–246. *

GA018

**Bhuwan P. Garg**

**Combined carboxylase deficiency, late-onset**
    See BIOTINIDASE DEFICIENCY
**Combined duodenal and gastric ulcer**
    See PEPTIC ULCER DISEASES, NON-SYNDROMIC
**Combined immunodeficiency with immunoglobulins**
    See IMMUNODEFICIENCY, NEZELOF TYPE
**Combined mesoectodermal dysplasia**
    See DERMAL HYPOPLASIA, FOCAL
**Commissural lip pits (isolated trait)**
    See LIP, PITS OR MOUNDS
**Common atrium**
    See ATRIAL SEPTAL DEFECTS
**Common migraine**
    See MIGRAINE
**Communicating hydrocele**
    See HERNIA, INGUINAL
**Communication interauriculaire**
    See ATRIAL SEPTAL DEFECTS
**Compelling helio-ophthalmic outburst syndrome**
    See ACHOO SYNDROME
**Complement C1 esterase inhibitor deficiency**
    See ANGIOEDEMA, HEREDITARY
**Complement C1 esterase inhibitor dysfunction**
    See ANGIOEDEMA, HEREDITARY
**Complement C5 dysfunction**
    See IMMUNODEFICIENCY, PLASMA-ASSOCIATED DEFECT OF
        PHAGOCYTOSIS

---

**COMPLEMENT COMPONENT 1, DEFICIENCY OF**        3210

**Includes:**
    Immunodeficiency, total C1q deficiency
    Immunodeficiency, functional C1q deficiency
    Immunodeficiency, C1r/C1s deficiency

**Excludes:**
    Acquired C1 deficiency
    C1 deficiency associated with other conditions
    **Lupus erythematosus, systemic** (2515)

**Major Diagnostic Criteria:** C1, the first complement component of the classical pathway, is composed of three subunits: C1q, C1r, and C1s. C1 deficiencies can be due to deficiencies of C1q or of both C1r and C1s; deficiency of either C1r or C1s alone apparently does not occur. The basic criteria are low or absent $CH_{50}$ levels that are normalized by the addition of normal C1 or the deficient C1 subunit(s). Levels of the deficient C1 subunit(s) are generally low or absent by immunologic assay, although there are exceptions.

**Clinical Findings:** Two forms of C1q deficiency exist. One form is total C1q deficiency, where the amount of C1q, as measured by immunoassay, is decreased. The other form is functional C1q deficiency. Here, an altered form of C1q is produced. The altered C1q shares partial antigenic identity with normal C1q, but has a reduced molecular weight and does not form a functional C1 molecule with the C1r and C1s subunits. Functional C1q deficiency is expressed as a co-dominant allele. However, heterozygotes have normal $CH_{50}$ levels and are clinically normal; **Lupus erythematosus, systemic**-like (SLE-like) syndromes are seen only in homozygotes for the abnormal protein.

C1q deficiency is also seen in patients with certain immunodeficiencies and blood dyscrasias. The etiology of this condition has been hypothesized to be increased C1q catabolism and increased extravascular C1q pools. In immunodeficiency states, this C1q deficiency can be corrected by administration of exogenous gammaglobulin or by bone marrow transplantation.

Findings may vary widely between patients, ranging from a nearly normal clinical picture to a serious condition with abundant findings. C2, C4, and C1 esterase inactivator levels are generally higher than normal. The alternate complement pathway is normal. Leukopenia and thrombocytopenia have been reported. In C1q deficiency, proteinuria, albuminuria, or microscopic hematuria may be present.

**Complications:** Either type of deficiency may result in an SLE-like syndrome. This syndrome may include: vasculitis, alopecia, arthralgias and arthritis, recurrent fever, and mesangioproliferative glomerulonephritis. Renal biopsies have revealed IgG, IgM, C3, C5, and fibrin deposition. ANA titers, rheumatoid factor, anti-Sm antibodies, and circulating immune complexes may be positive, while LE cells are generally negative. Other complications reported in C1q deficiency include: vesicular and poikilodermatiod skin lesions on the face and extremities; skin photosensitivity; mucocutaneous ulceration; stomatitis; positive antibodies versus native DNA, smooth muscle, and $HB_sAG$. **Raynaud disease** has also been reported in C1r/C1s deficiency. Another common complication of either type of deficiency is recurrent bacterial and fungal infections. These infections may include life-threatening meningitis and sepsis.

**Associated Findings:** **Rothmund-Thomson syndrome** has been reported in conjunction with C1q deficiency.

**Etiology:** Total C1q deficiency may or may not be a hereditary trait; no pattern of inheritance is seen in many cases. Functional C1q deficiency appears to be inherited and expressed as a co-dominant allel. C1r/C1s deficiency shows autosomal recessive inheritance. Heterozygotes show mildly depressed C1r and C1s, with approximately one-half normal C1 hemolytic activity.

**Pathogenesis:** It has been hypothesized that the SLE-like syndrome commonly occuring with these deficiencies may result from an inability to neutralize certain infectious agents and immune complexes.

**MIM No.:** *12055, *12057, *12058, *21695

**Sex Ratio:** Presumably M1:F1.

**Occurrence:** Undetermined. A recent summary list 13 reported cases of C1q deficiency and nine reported cases of C1r/C1s deficiency.

**Risk of Recurrence for Patient's Sib:**
    See Part I, *Mendelian Inheritance.*

**Risk of Recurrence for Patient's Child:**
    See Part I, *Mendelian Inheritance.*

**Age of Detectability:** Clinical features are generally evident within the first decade of life.

**Gene Mapping and Linkage:** C1QA (complement component 1, q subcomponent, alpha polypeptide) has been provisionally mapped to 1p.
    C1QB (complement component 1, q subcomponent, beta polypeptide) has been provisionally mapped to 1p.
    C1S (complement component 1, s subcomponent) has been mapped to 12p13.
    C1R (complement component 1, r subcomponent) has been mapped to 12p13.

**Prevention:** None known. Genetic counseling indicated.

**Treatment:** Plasmaphoresis or oral or parenteral corticosteroids may lead to an improvement in condition during the period of treatment, but clinical features generally return upon cessation of therapy. In one patient with C1r/C1s deficiency, a renal transplant was performed. Following the transplant, this patients C1s, total C1, and $CH_{50}$ were either normal or elevated; post-transplant C1r values were not reported.

**Prognosis:** Highly variable due to the range of expression of clinical findings. Prognosis may range from very good in patients showing few or no findings to poor in patients with severe recurrent infections and SLE-like symptoms.

**Detection of Carrier:** Examination of relatives $CH_{50}$, C1 hemolytic activity, and levels of C1 subunits may reveal carriers in certain cases.

**References:**
Day NK, Good RA: Deficiencies of the complement system in man. BD:OAS XI. New York: March of Dimes Birth Defects Foundation, 1975:306–311.

Guenther LC: Inherited disorders of complement. J Am Acad Derm 1983; 9:815–839.

Nusinow SR, et al: The hereditary and acquired deficiencies of complement. Med Clin North Am 1985; 69:487–504.

Loos M, Heinz HP: Component deficiencies 1: the first component: C1q,C1r, C1s. Prog Allergy 1986; 39:212–31. *

Rother K: Summary of reported deficiencies. Prog Allergy 1986; 39:202–211.

HA081
SC039

**Michael T. Halpern**
**Stanley A. Schwartz**

## COMPLEMENT COMPONENT 2, DEFICIENCY OF      2201

**Includes:**

Autoimmune disease, deficiency of C2
C2 deficiency

**Excludes:**

**Angioedema, hereditary** (0054)
C2 deficiency, acquired
**Lupus erythematosis, systemic** (2515)

**Major Diagnostic Criteria:** Functional and immunochemical determinations of all nine complement (C) components indicate that, with the exception of C2 (which may be undetectable or dramatically reduced in the heterozygote), all C components are within normal limits. In some instances, inherited C2 deficiency may be associated with low levels of Factor B of the alternative pathway.

**Clinical Findings:** Inherited C2 deficiency has been found to occur in conjunction with a wide variety of diseases, such as renal disease, recurrent infections, skin rashes, **Cancer, Hodgkin disease, familial**, fatal dermatomyositis, and anaphylactoid purpura.

**Complications:** Increased frequency of infections.

**Associated Findings:** About half have autoimmune disease, most commonly **Lupus erythematosis, systemic**, Henoch-Schonlein purpura, or polymyositis.

**Etiology:** Autosomal recessive inheritance.

**Pathogenesis:** A failure of synthesis, rather than synthesis of inactive analog. According to Cole et al (1985), a "specific and selective pretranslational regulatory defect in C2 gene expression."

**MIM No.:** *21700

**Sex Ratio:** M1:F4

**Occurrence:** The most frequent complement deficiency state. The frequency of the C2 deficiency gene in the general population is 1.2%, and the frequency of homozygous C2 deficiency has been calculated to be between 1:10,000 and 1:30,000

**Risk of Recurrence for Patient's Sib:**
See Part I, *Mendelian Inheritance.*

**Risk of Recurrence for Patient's Child:**
See Part I, *Mendelian Inheritance.*

**Age of Detectability:** May be detected at any age, but usually upon recognition of associated conditions(s).

**Gene Mapping and Linkage:** C2 (complement component 2) has been mapped to 6p21.3.

**Prevention:** None known. Genetic counseling indicated.

**Treatment:** Will depend on the type of disease associated with the deficiency.

**Prognosis:** Varies with the associated conditions.

**Detection of Carrier:** Examination of first degree relatives for C2 levels.

**References:**
Day NK, et al.: Inherited deficiencies of the complement system. In: Good RA, Day SB, eds: Biological amplification systems in immunology. London: Plenum Medical, 1977:229.

Jersild C, et al.: Complement and the major histocompatibility systems. In: Good RA, Day SB, eds: Biological amplification systems in immunology. London: Plenum Medical, 1977:229.

Ross SC, Densen P: Complement deficiency states and infection: epidemiology, pathogenesis and consequences of neisserial and other infections in an immune deficiency. Medicine 1984; 63:243.

Cole FS, et al.: The molecular basis for genetic deficiency of the second component of human complement. New Engl J Med 1985; 313:11–16.

Efthimiou J, et al.: Heterozygous C2 deficiency associated with angioedema, myasthenia gravis, and systemic lupus erythematosus. Ann Rheum Dis 1986; 45:428–430.

Callen JP, et al.: Subacute cutaneous lupus erythematosus in multiple members of a family with C2 deficiency. Arch Dermat 1987; 123:66–70.

DA028

**Noorbibi K. Day**

## COMPLEMENT COMPONENT 3, DEFICIENCY OF      2219

**Includes:**

Immunodeficiency, complement component 3
C3b inactivator deficiency (Factor I)
CR3 deficiency
Essential hypercatobolism of C3
Factor I ("Eye")

**Excludes:**

Properdin deficiency
Complement component deficiencies, other
C3 NEF

**Major Diagnostic Criteria:** Severe chronic or recurrent pyogenic infections, usually with gram positive organisms, are the most frequently observed problems. The patients most closely resemble clinically those with hypogammaglobulinemia Autoimmune diseases and immune complex mediated diseases (vasculitis, glomerulonephritis) are also seen. Neutrophilia may be found. Defects in opsonization, phagocytosis, chemotaxis, platelet aggregation, bactericidal activity and macrophage-monocyte migration may be observed upon laboratory testing. Almost complete absence of total hemolytic complement activity (CH50) is the laboratory hallmark of the deficiency state. Specific absence of C3, factor D. C3b inactivator, and/or complement receptors 1, 2, and 3 (CR1, CR2, CR3) may be detected depending on the specific component deficiency in an individual patient.

**Clinical Findings:** The frequency of C3 deficiency states is unknown but presumed to be uncommon. The clinical signs and symptoms of patients with deficiencies related to C3 may occur at any age from the newborn period to the second decade of life. The pyogenic manifestations usually occur within the first year of life while the autoimmune and immune complex manifestations occur later, occasionally into the second decade. The clinical problems are related to the immunological defects resulting from the absence of the various biologic products of C3 and its activation. In addition to the functional defects mentioned before, amplification of the general inflammatory response may be impaired. The various specific defects resulting from the failure of C3 activation

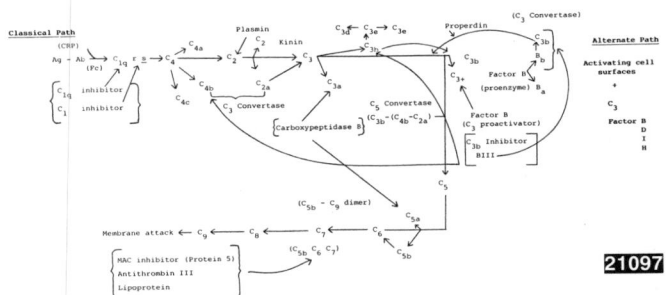

**2219-21097:** Classical and alternate pathways of the complement system.

may include the absence of C3b, C3b inactivator (Factor I), C3e, C3a, C3d, and Bd.

Patients who present clinically are homozygous for C3 deficiency. The presentation primarily includes pneumonia, septicemia and meningitis. In addition, the patients frequently demonstrate skin infections (impetigo), chronic otitis, sinusitis and mastoiditis. There may be an absence of leucocytosis. Other syndromes and diseases described include various types of maculopapular rashes, urticaria, arthralgias, vasculitis, autoimmune diseases such as **Lupus erythematosis, systemic**, other rheumatoid syndromes and autoimmune hemolytic anemia. Membranoproliferative and other forms of glomerulonephritis also occur. The bacterial agents associated with the infectious aspects of the deficiency are usually of the encapsulated variety, Streptococcus pneumonia and Neisseria meningitidis being amont the most common organisms. Other organisms frequently noted are *Hemophilus* influenza, *Klebsiella*, *Proteus*, *Pseudomonas*, *Staphlococcus* aureus, and B Hemolytic streptococci.

The laboratory findings are related to 1.) the specific infection. 2.) the immunologic defect and 3.) the severely decreased or absent total hemolytic complement activity along with the absence of C3 activity and the specific component. In the presence of a CR1 or CR3 deficiency the hemolytic complement ($CH_{50}$) activity as well as C3 components are usually normal.

**Complications:** Those associated with chronic or recurrent infection, and may include CNS damage secondary to meningitis, or chronic lung disease as a consequence of recurrent pneumonia.

**Associated Findings: Lupus erythematosis, systemic** has been associated with CR1 deficiency, delayed umbilical cord separation with CR3 deficiency, and partial lipodystrophy with Factor I (C3b inactivator) deficiency. The association with autoimmune disease, including autoimmune hemolytic anemia, has been previously mentioned.

**Etiology:** Presumably autosomal dominant inheritance. Some investigators have suggested autosomal recessive inheritance.

**Pathogenesis:** The pathogenesis of the C3 deficiency states is a result of C3's central role in the complement system which mediates certain host defense mechanisms and the inflammatory response. The complement system consists of two interacting pathways, the classical, initiated primarily by antigen and antibody and the alternate, initiated by endotoxin and/or activating cell surfaces including bacteria.

C3, which is synthesized in the liver, is the central protein in both pathways. Both paths result in the cleavage of C3 and subsequent late component activation with engagement of the lytic action of these terminal components.

Host defense mechanisms which are dependent on, or modified by, complement activation include opsonization, phagocytosis, chemotaxis, immune adherance, processing and clearance of immune complexes, direct lysis of cells and targets such as envelope viruses and both gram positive and negative bacteria, amplification of the general inflammatory response and the recognition of eukaryotic cells as foreign by the host. In addition, there may be as yet unrecognized immunoregulatory functions of complement proteins, their alleles or their activation fragments.

The activation products of C3 serve important biologic functions. C3a (anaphylatoxin) increases smooth muscle contraction, increases vascular permeability, aggregates platelets, and degranulates mast cells and basophilis. C3b and IC3b opsonize particles, solubilize immune complexes, facilitate phagocytosis, release lysosomal enzymes (C3b) and stimulate B cell lymphokine production. C3e releases neutrophils from the bone marrow and Bd inhibits migration of monocytes and macrophages. Cellular receptors for C3 fragments designated CR1, CR2, and CR3 exist on erythrocytes, neutrophils, macrophages, monocytes, some T and B cells and glomerular podocytes. They are important in providing ligand binding sites for complement proteins and help in processing circulating immune complexes, facilitate phagocytosis, immune adherance and neutrophil-cidal properties, as well as aid in self recognition.

**MIM No.:** *12070, *21703

**Sex Ratio:** M1:F1

**Occurrence:** Undetermined. Established literature.

**Risk of Recurrence for Patient's Sib:**
See Part I, *Mendelian Inheritance*.

**Risk of Recurrence for Patient's Child:**
See Part I, *Mendelian Inheritance*.

**Age of Detectability:** At birth.

**Gene Mapping and Linkage:** C3 (complement component 3) has been mapped to 19p13.3-p13.2.
IF (complement component I) has been mapped to 4q24-q25.

**Prevention:** None known. Genetic counseling indicated.

**Treatment:** Symptomatic care of the disease process and/or infection. Plasma infusions will restore the various component levels temporarily and may aid in the acute treatment of infectious states. Vaccinations with *hemophilus* influenza B and pneumococcal vaccines are recommended.

**Prognosis:** Variable, depends on the nature, frequency, and severity of the type of infections.

**Detection of Carrier:** Carriers will often have decreased $CH_{50}$ and C3 levels.

**References:**
Alper CA, et al: Increased susceptability to infection associated with abnormalities of complement mediated function and of the third component of complement (C3). New Eng J Med 1970; 282:349–354.
Guenther LC: Inherited disorders of complement. J Amer Acad Derm 1983; 9:815–839. *
Arnauot MA, Colten HR: Complement C3 receptors: structure and function. Mol Immuno 1984; 21:1191–1199.
Feldbush TL, et al: Role of complement in the immune response. Fed Proc 1984; 43:2548–2552.
McLean R, Winkelstein J: Genetically determined variation in the complement system: relationship to disease. J Ped 1984; 105:179–188.
Fries LF, et al: Inherited deficiencies of complement and complement related proteins. Immuno and Immunopath 1986; 40:37–49. *

KA044                                              **Donald B. Kaufman**

---

## COMPLEMENT COMPONENT 4, DEFICIENCY OF          2220

**Includes:** Autoimmune disease, deficiency of C4

**Excludes:**
> **Angioedema, hereditary** (0054)
> C4 deficiency, acquired
> **Lupus erythematosis, systemic** (2515)

**Major Diagnostic Criteria:** Functional and immunochemical determinations of all nine complement (C) components indicate that, with the exception of C4 (which may be undetectable or dramatically reduced in the heterozygote), all C components are within normal limits.

**Clinical Findings:** C4 plays an important, indirect role in host defense functions mediated by the classic pathway such as immune adherence, chemotactic factor generation, immune complex solubilization, and bactericidal activity. C4 appears to be independent of activation of the classic pathway to neutralize viruses.

**Complications:** Over 60% of the patients studied with inherited C4 deficiency have **Lupus erythematosis, systemic**, and 85% have some autoimmune disease. Deficiency of C4 is also associated with infections. Meningitis, bacteremia, and infections with herpes virus have also been reported.

**Associated Findings:** Reduced C1 if immune complexes are present.

**Etiology:** Autosomal recessive inheritance, although in some families C4 deficiency has been described as inherited as an autosomal dominant.

**Pathogenesis:** Unknown.

**MIM No.:** *12079, *12081, *12082, *12083

**Sex Ratio:** Presumably M1:F1.

**Occurrence:** About a dozen cases have been documented.

**Risk of Recurrence for Patient's Sib:**
See Part I, *Mendelian Inheritance.*

**Risk of Recurrence for Patient's Child:**
See Part I, *Mendelian Inheritance.*

**Age of Detectability:** By one month of age.

**Gene Mapping and Linkage:** C4A (complement component 4A) has been mapped to 6p21.3.

C4B (complement component 4B) has been mapped to 6p21.3.

C4BP (complement component 4 binding protein) has been mapped to 1q32.

HLA studies of families of C4-deficient individuals indicate that C4 loci on chromosome 6 is linked closely to the loci of C2 and Factor B on the major histocompatibility complex. Genetic polymorphism of C4 is not controlled by codominant alleles at a single locus, but is controlled by two different loci linked to HLA. It has been shown that two different genetic loci are responsible for C4 electrophoretic variants. One locus has the alleles S and S° recessive to S, and the other has alleles F and f° with f° recessive to F. The C4s locus and the C4f locus are closely linked to HLA-B. Furthermore, individuals who have the C4f pattern are also Chido blood group negative (Ch [a- ]), and individuals who have the C4s pattern are always Rodgers negative (Rg [a-]). The studies demonstrated that the Chido (Cha) and Rodgers (Rga) erythrocyte antigens are in fact distinct antigenic components of C4. At least 13 alleles have been described for C4F and 22 for the slowly moving, migrating, basic products.

**Prevention:** None known. Genetic counseling indicated.

**Treatment:** Type of treatment will depend on the disease that occurs in conjunction with the C4 deficiency.

**Prognosis:** Varies with associated conditions and complications.

**Detection of Carrier:** Immunochemical determination.

**References:**

Day NK, et al.: Inherited deficiencies of the complement system. In: Good RA, Day SB, eds: Biological amplification systems in immunology. London: Plenum Medical, 1977:229.

Jersild C, et al.: Complement and the major histocompatibility systems. In: Good RA, Day SB, eds: Biological amplification systems in immunology. London: Plenum Medical, 1977:229.

Ross SC, Densen P: Complement deficiency states and infection: epidemiology, pathogenesis and consequences of neisserial and other infections in an immune deficiency. Medicine 1984; 63(5):243.

DA028                                            **Noorbibi K. Day**

**Complement component C1, regulatory components, deficiency of**
*See ANGIOEDEMA, HEREDITARY*

---

## COMPLEMENT COMPONENT, ALTERNATIVE PATHWAYS, DEFICIENCIES OF                1525

**Includes:**
    Deficiencies of C3
    Deficiencies of C5
    Deficiencies of C6
    Deficiencies of C7
    Deficiencies of C8
    Deficiencies of C9
    Deficiencies of P
    Deficiencies of B
    Deficiencies of D
    Deficiencies of H
    Deficiencies of I

**Excludes:**
    Deficiencies of C1q
    Deficiencies of C1r
    Deficiencies of C1s
    Deficiencies of C4
    Deficiencies of C2

*Nomenclature and Classification:*
Proteins of the classical pathway and the late-acting components are designated by numbers e.g. C2, C3, whereas proteins of the alternative pathway (AP) are generally designated by letters, e.g. P (Properdin), B (Factor B). Whereas the classical pathway of complement is activated mainly by antigen-antibody complexes, the alternative pathway is activated, in the absence of antibody, usually by carbohydrate containing substances, e.g. bacterial endotoxin. Complement component C3 is cleaved in the alternative pathway by Factor B and Factor D and the complement cascade is activated to form the membrane attack complex, C5-C9, resulting in cell lysis.

*Associated Diseases:* Whereas deficiencies of the early components are associated with autoimmune disorders, deficiencies of the late acting components and AP proteins are often associated with life threatening bacterial infections. Complete deficiencies of all late acting components and control proteins have been documented.

*C3 Deficiency (C3D):* Approximately ten patients have been reported with C3D. Both hemolytic and immunochemical C3 levels in serum are undetectable. Opsonization, chemotactic factor generation and bactericidal complement activity are usually defective.

*Clinical Findings:* Recurrent pyogenic infections, glomerulonephritis.

*Genetics:* Autosomal recessive inheritance. C3 locus mapped to chromosome 19 and is polymorphic. Two major alleles F and S defined with as many as 20 other rare allotypes. C3F may be associated with **Arthritis, rheumatoid** and arteriosclerosis.

*C5 Deficiency (C5D)* A deficiency described in ten individuals from four families (one Asian, three Black). Individuals lack hemolytic and immunochemical C5 in serum chemotactic factor generation and bactericidal activity is usually defective.

*Clinical Findings:* Recurrent disseminated *Neisserial* infections, glomerulonephritis, **Lupus erythematosis, systemic**.

*Genetics:* Autosomal recessive inheritance. Chromosomal assignment not determined. Non HLA-linked. Limited polymorphism in Melanesians only.

*Deficiency (C6D):* Approximately 20 individuals reported with this disorder. Mainly occurs in North American Blacks. C6 individuals identified by lack of hemolytic and immunochemical C6 in serum. Opsonization and chemotactic generating activity normal. Defective bactericidal activity.

*Clinical Findings:* High frequency of systemic *Neisseria* infections. **Lupus erythematosis, systemic** may occur.

*Genetics:* Autosomal recessive inheritance. Non HLA-linked. Linked to C7. High degree of polymorphism. Two high frequency structural alleles.

*C7 Deficiency (C7D):* Approximately 20 individuals reported with this disorder. C7D individuals identified by lack of serum C7 protein. Defective complement bactericidal activity always present. Complement dependent opsonization and chemotactic factor generation usually not impaired.

*Clinical Findings:* Variety of clinical disorders associated with C7D. Usually recurrent disseminated *Neisseria* infections.

*Genetics:* Autosomal recessive inheritance. Locus non HLA-linked. Linked to C6. Limited polymorphism. No association of a particular allotype with disease.

*C8 Deficiency:* Disorder has been reported in ten individuals. Two types of C8D: 1.) No functional activity and C8 protein in serum. 2.) C8 protein detectable in serum with no functional activity due to lack of the beta subunit. Bactericidal activity of serum undetectable. Opsonization and chemotactic activity normal.

*Clinical Findings:* Disseminated *Neisseria* infections most common; may be associated with **Lupus erythematosis, systemic** and **Xeroderma pigmentosum**.

*Genetics:* Autosomal recessive inheritance. Non HLA-linked polymorphic protein. No disease association observed with a particular allotype.

*C9 Deficiency (C9D):* This disorder is rare in Caucasians, but more common in Japanese (estimated frequency of 0.036 percent). Total complement hemolytic activity essentially normal.

*Clinical Findings:* None identified. Adverse transfusion reactions may occur if C9D individual is transfused with normal plasma.

*Genetics:* Autosomal recessive inheritance. Non HLA-linked.

*Properdin Deficiency (PD):* Occurrence in one family with serum P levels of less than two percent of normal.

*Clinical Findings:* Meningococcal infections.

*Genetics:* Possibly X-linked recessive inheritance.

*H Deficiency (HD):* Reported in one Asian family. Immunochemical analysis revealed less than 5% of normal levels of H (BIH).

*Clinical Findings:* Glomerulonephritis.

*Genetics:* Autosomal recessive inheritance. Non HLA-linked.

*I Deficiency (ID):* Reported in two patients. Absence of immunochemical I in serum. C3 levels usually low.

*Clinical Findings:* Recurrent pyogenic infections.

*Genetics:* Autosomal recessive inheritance. Non HLA linked.

*B Deficiency (BD):* Total deficiency not described. Inheritance of a deficient allele suggested in families from studies of inheritance of B allotypes.

*Genetics:* Autosomal recessive inheritance. HLA-linked on chromosome 6. Polymorphic protein with two common allotypes F and S and two rarer F1 and S1 detected. No association of disease with particular allotype.

**References:**
O'Neill GJ: Complement component polymorphism. In: Whaley K, ed: Methods in complement for clinical immunologists. Edinburgh: Churchill Livingston, 1985:266.

Rynes R, Pickering RJ: Inherited complement component deficiencies in man. In: Whaley K, ed: Methods in complement for clinical immunologists. Edinburgh: Churchill Livingston, 1985:292.

Frank MM: Complement in the pathophysiology of human disease. New Engl J Med 1987; 316:1525.

ON001                                           **Geoffrey O'Neill**

**Complex glycerol kinase deficiency syndrome**
*See GLYCEROL KINASE DEFICIENCY*
**Complex IV deficiency of the mitochondrial respiratory chain**
*See MYOPATHY-METABOLIC, MITOCHONDRIAL CYTOCHROME C OXIDASE DEFICIENCY*
**Compression syndrome of peripheral nerves, hereditary**
*See NEUROPATHY, HEREDITARY WITH PRESSURE PALSIES*
**Concrescence of roots of teeth**
*See TEETH, ROOT CONCRESCENCE*
**Conductive hearing loss**
*See DEAFNESS*
**Condylomata acuminata, congenital**
*See PAPILLOMA VIRUS, CONGENITAL INFECTION*
**Cone dystrophy, X-linked with tapetal-like sheen**
*See RETINA, CONE DYSTROPHY, X-LINKED*
**Cone monochromatism**
*See COLOR BLINDNESS, BLUE MONOCONE-MONOCHROMATIC*
**Cone-rod degeneration, progressive**
*See RETINA, COMBINED CONE-ROD DEGENERATION*
**Cone-rod dystrophy (degeneration)**
*See RETINA, COMBINED CONE-ROD DEGENERATION*
**Congenital AIDS-related syndrome (CARS)**
*See FETAL ACQUIRED IMMUNE DEFICIENCY SYNDROME (AIDS) INFECTION*
**Congenital anterior staphyloma**
*See EYE, ANTERIOR SEGMENT DYSGENESIS*
**Congenital central hypoventilation syndrome (CCHS)**
*See HYPOVENTILATION, CONGENITAL CENTRAL ALVEOLAR TYPE*
**Congenital dermal melanocytosis (CDM)**
*See SKIN, CUTANEOUS MELANOSIS: MONGOLIAN SPOT*
**Congenital hypertrophy of the retinal pigment epithelium (CHRPE)**
*See RETINA, CONGENITAL HYPERTROPHY OF RETINAL PIGMENT EPITHELIUM*
**Congestive cardiomyopathy, familial**
*See CARDIOMYOPATHY, FAMILIAL DILATED*
**Conical cornea**
*See EYE, KERATOCONUS*
**Conjoined twins**
*See TWINS, CONJOINED*
**Conjunctival dermoid**
*See OCULAR DERMOIDS*
**Conjunctivitis, familial pseudomembranous**
*See EYE, LIGNEOUS CONJUNCTIVITIS*

**Connective tissue disorder, Marden-Walker type**
*See MARDEN-WALKER SYNDROME*
**Connective tissue disorder-joint stiffening-short stature**
*See WINCHESTER SYNDROME*
**Connective tissue nevus**
*See COLLAGENOMA, MULTIPLE CUTANEOUS, FAMILIAL*
**Conradi-Hunermann disease**
*See CHONDRODYSPLASIA PUNCTATA, MILD SYMMETRIC TYPE*
**Constitutional giant granulations of leukocytes, hereditary**
*See CHEDIAK-HIGASHI SYNDROME*
**Constitutional granular gigantism**
*See CHEDIAK-HIGASHI SYNDROME*
**Constricting bands, congenital**
*See AMNIOTIC BANDS SYNDROME*
**Continuous muscle fiber activity, hereditary**
*See ISAACS-MERTENS SYNDROME*
**Contraceptives, oral, and chromosome tetraploidy**
*See CHROMOSOME TETRAPLOIDY*
**Contractural arachnodactyly (some cases)**
*See MARFAN SYNDROME*
**Contractural arachnodactyly, congenital**
*See ARACHNODACTYLY, CONTRACTURAL BEALS TYPE*

---

**CONTRACTURE, DUPUYTREN**                    **0301**

**Includes:**
> Dupuytren disease
> Fibromatosis, palmar
> Palmar fibromatosis

**Excludes:**   Camptodactyly (2255)

**Major Diagnostic Criteria:** A nodule in the palmar fascia or an interphalangeal band producing a flexion deformity of the proximal interphalangeal joint.

**Clinical Findings:** Subcutaneous palmar nodules and flexion contractures of the fingers at the proximal interphalangeal (PIP) and metacarpophalangeal joints. Web space contractures draw pairs of digits together. Skin pits are attached to palmar bands. Knuckle pads and the Peyronie fibrous contracture of the penis are sometimes associated. Hand contractures are bilateral in 90% of cases.

**Complications:** Varying loss of function in affected hands.

**Associated Findings:** Knuckle pads are seen in 25% of cases, plantar involvement in 20%, and penile lesions in 3%.

**Etiology:** In some families, autosomal dominant inheritance with variable penetrance. The nodules, contractures and unaffected aponeurosis contain increased amounts of type III collagen. Also, increased incidence in patients with alcoholic liver disease, treated seizures, and diabetic disorders.

**Pathogenesis:** Fibrofatty tissue anterior to the palmar aponeurosis is replaced by centrifugal fibrosis which results in fixation of

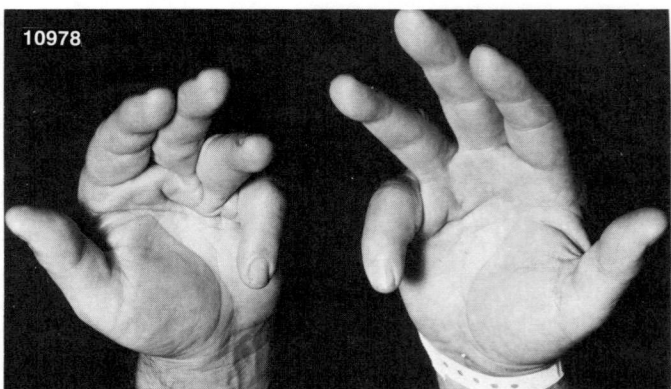

0301-10978: Dupuytren contracture.

skin, aponeurosis,and joint contracture, but not tendons in synovial sheaths. Contracture of newly produced mature collagen, possibly by a specialized cell (the myofibroblast), results in thickening of nodules and bands and progressively flexed digits at the metacarpophalangeal and PIP joints with hyperextension of the distal interphalangeal joint in advanced stages.

**MIM No.:** *12690

**Sex Ratio:** Under age 40, M4:F1; over age 40, M2:F1

**Occurrence:** Almost exclusively in people of European descent; increasing in frequency from four percent under age 20 years to 20% over age 60 years of age. Over 4,000 cases reported in the literature.

**Risk of Recurrence for Patient's Sib:**
See Part I, *Mendelian Inheritance.*

**Risk of Recurrence for Patient's Child:**
See Part I, *Mendelian Inheritance.*

**Age of Detectability:** Uncommon under age 20; onset in the sixth decade in about 50% of cases.

**Gene Mapping and Linkage:** Unknown.

**Prevention:** None known. Genetic counseling indicated.

**Treatment:** Surgical excision of fibrotic tissue is indicated. About one-third of patients with a strong family history, plantar lesions, knuckle pads, or a penile contracture (peyronie disease) have a severe form of the disease and higher incidence of recurrence after surgical excision.

**Prognosis:** Normal for life span and intelligence, variable disability in affected hands. Progressive contracture at a variable rate.

**Detection of Carrier:** Unknown.

**References:**

Hueston JT: Dupuytren's contracture. Baltimore: William & Wilkins, 1963.
Mikkelsen AO: Dupuytren's disease - initial symptoms, age of onset and spontaneous course. Hand 1977; 9:11–15.
Chice HF, McFarlane RM: Pathogenesis of Dupuytren's contracture. J Hand Surg 1987; 3:1–8.
McGrouther DA: Microanatomy of Dupuytren's contracture. Hand 1982; 14:215–222. †
Noble J, et al.: Diabetes mellitus in etiology of Dupuytren's disease. J Bone Joint Surg 1984; 66B:322–325.
Hurst LC, et al.: Pathology of Dupuytren's contracture: effect of prostaglandins on myofibroblast. J Hand Surg 1986; V.11A:18–22.

OS001                                                    **A. Lee Osterman**

**Contractures, congenital arthrogrypotic type**
*See ARTHROGRYPOSES*

## CONTRACTURES, CONGENITAL LETHAL FINNISH TYPE                                        2275

**Includes:**
Contractures, multiple, Finnish type
Lethal congenital contracture syndrome

**Excludes:**
**Hydrops fetalis, non-immune** (2198)
**Pena-Shokeir syndrome** (2080)
**Pterygium syndrome, multiple lethal** (2274)
**Pterygium syndrome, popliteal, lethal** (3233)

**Major Diagnostic Criteria:** Fetal hydrops, intrauterine death, joint contractures, micrognathia, pulmonary hypoplasia, and muscular atrophy.

**Clinical Findings:** The condition is prenatally lethal. The mean gestational age for 12 cases ending before term is 29 weeks. During gestation there is fetal edema at least from 16 weeks onward. In addition, some ascites, pleural fluid, and placental edema are present, but often massive subcutaneous edema is the most marked finding. The fetal edema is replaced by polyhydramnios later in gestation. Fetal movements are scanty.

Clinical findings include intrauterine growth retardation, un-

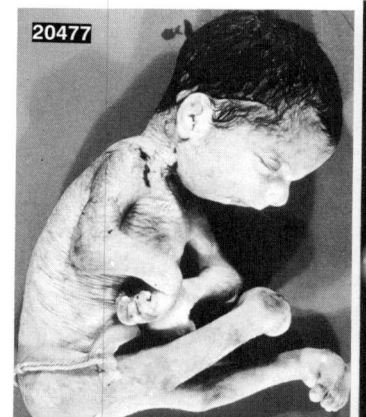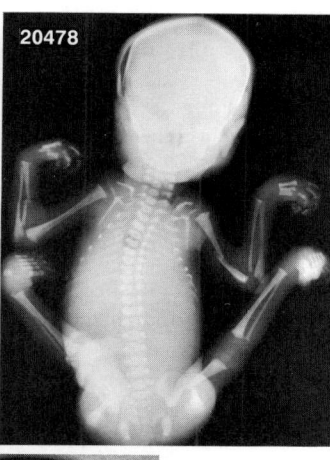
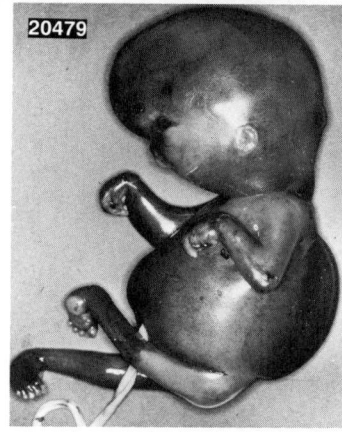

**2275-20477:** 28-week fetus with severe micrognathia and multiple contractures. **20478:** X-ray of 28-week fetus showing "breech hips," general thinning of the bones and fractures. **20479:** 18-week fetus with severe hydrops.

usual facies with **Eye, hypertelorism,** apparently low-set auricles, and severe micrognathia. The limbs are of normal size and proportion, with severe deformities because of multiple congenital contractures. The pattern of these contractures is fairly constant, with severe flexion contractures of the elbows, wrists, hips, and knees in marked hyperextension. Occasional pterygia are observed, most often in elbows and neck.

Constant autopsy findings have been severe pulmonary hypoplasia and hypoplastic heart. In all studied cases, there has been degeneration and loss of spinal motor neurons and gliosis. The muscles have been atrophic and replaced by fat and fibrous tissue consistent with neurogenic atrophy.

X-rays confirm hydrops, contractures, and muscular atrophy. There is also bilateral dislocation of the hips. The contours of long bones are normal but sometimes markedly thin.

In about half of fetuses the ribs have been extremely thin, appearing string-like. Fractures of long bones have been seen in three fetuses.

**Complications:** Unknown.

**Associated Findings:** Calcifications in the kidneys, high vertebrae, and dislocation of a vertebra.

**Etiology:** Autosomal recessive inheritance.

**Pathogenesis:** Neuronal loss and gliosis in spinal cord and brainstem is the primary event, which causes fetal inactivity, congenital contractures and hydrops, and muscular atrophy.

**MIM No.:** 25331

**POS No.:**  3658

**Sex Ratio:**  M1:F1

**Occurrence:**  Twenty-three cases in 13 families have been observed in Finland.

**Risk of Recurrence for Patient's Sib:**
See Part I, *Mendelian Inheritance.*

**Risk of Recurrence for Patient's Child:**
See Part I, *Mendelian Inheritance.*

**Age of Detectability:**  Prenatal diagnosis is possible by ultrasound from the 16–18th week of gestation on the basis of marked hydrops and diminished fetal movements.

**Gene Mapping and Linkage:**  Unknown.

**Prevention:**  None known. Genetic counseling indicated.

**Treatment:**  Unknown.

**Prognosis:**  Prenatally lethal.

**Detection of Carrier:**  Unknown.

**Special Considerations:**  Some observers consider this condition to be a variant of **Pena-Shokeir syndrome**.

**References:**
Herva R, et al.: A lethal autosomal recessive syndrome of multiple congenital contractures. Am J Med Genet 1985; 20:431–439.
Kirkinen P, et al.: Early prenatal diagnosis of a lethal syndrome of multiple contractures. Prenatal Diag 1987; 7:189–196.
Herva R, et al.: A syndrome of multiple congenital contractures: neuropathological analysis on five fetal cases. Am J Med Genet 1988; 29:67–76.

HE036                                              **Riitta Herva**

## CONTRACTURES, HERRMANN-OPITZ ARTHROGRYPOSIS TYPE                          0470

**Includes:**
Herrmann-Opitz arthrogryposis syndrome
VSR syndrome

**Excludes:**
**Arthrogryposes** (all others)
**Chondrodysplasia punctata, X-linked dominant type** (2730)
**Kniest dysplasia** (0557)
**Kuskokwin syndrome** (0560)
**Metatropic dysplasia** (0656)
Mietens syndrome

**Major Diagnostic Criteria:**  Appropriate skeletal findings in multiple areas (craniofacial, skeleton, limbs, vertebrae) and congenital joint contractures.

**Clinical Findings:**  The syndrome represents a generalized bone dysplasia manifested by congenital joint contractures. The three reported affected persons showed: shortness of stature, mesomelic shortness of upper limbs, rhizomelic shortness of lower limbs, craniofacial dysostosis (with trigonocephaly, prominent zygomatic bones, broad maxillary and mandibular bones and cleft palate), costovertebral anomalies (inluding scoliosis, sagittal cleft of vertebral bodies, and broad ribs), and flexion contractures at the elbow, wrist, finger, and ankle joints. Intelligence was normal.

**Complications:**  Limitation of movements including intrauterine activity; cutaneous dimples and dislocations at contracted joints; abnormal flexion creases; respiratory infections due to decreased mobility of chest.

**Associated Findings:**  Postterm delivery; inguinal hernia.

**Etiology:**  Persumably autosomal dominant inheritance.

**Pathogenesis:**  Many of the clinical manifestations can be related to a primary skeletal abnormality (of unknown type) of a generalized nature.

**POS No.:**  3252

**Sex Ratio:**  Presumably M1:F1

**Occurrence:**  One family reported with three cases.

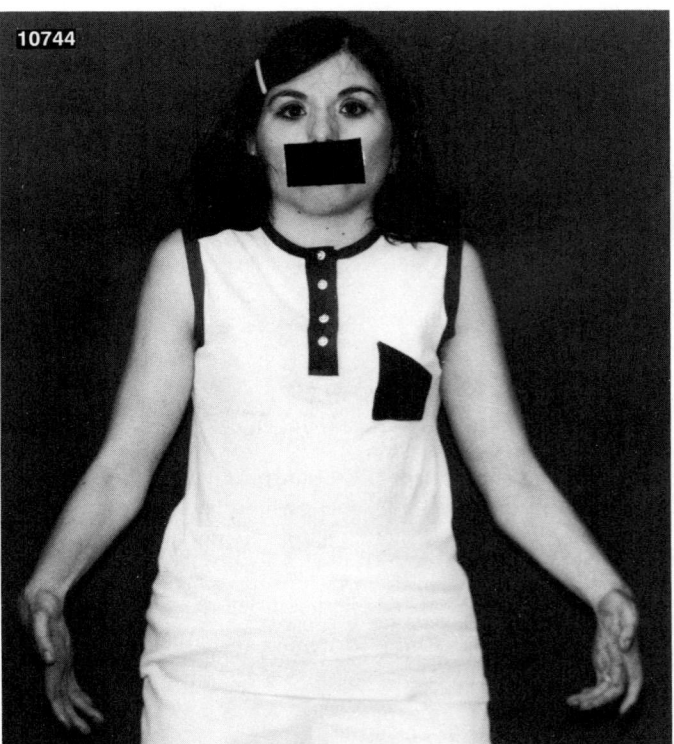

**0470**-10744:  Note broad zygomatic arch and nasal bones, short forearms, contractures of the shoulders, elbows, and finger joints with secondary muscular atrophy.

**Risk of Recurrence for Patient's Sib:**
See Part I, *Mendelian Inheritance.*

**Risk of Recurrence for Patient's Child:**
See Part I, *Mendelian Inheritance.*

**Age of Detectability:**  At birth. Prenatal diagnosis is perhaps possible, but has not been attempted.

**Gene Mapping and Linkage:**  Unknown.

**Prevention:**  None known. Genetic counseling indicated.

**Treatment:**  Intensive orthopedic treatment including multiple surgical procedures to correct contractures; cleft palate repair. Supportive care for neonatal feeding and respiratory infections.

**Prognosis:**  Good. Adequate recovery of joint mobility is possible.

**Detection of Carrier:**  Mildly affected individuals might be identified by X-ray, facial dysmorphism, and careful examination of dermatoglyphics.

**Special Considerations:**  Important to distinguish from many other forms of arthrogryposis, because recurrence risk is high.

**References:**
Herrmann J, Opitz JM: The VSR syndrome. BD:OAS;X(9). New York: March of Dimes Birth Defects Foundation, 1974:277. * †

WI044                                              **David R. Witt**

**Contractures, multiple with arachnodactyly**
*See ARACHNODACTYLY, CONTRACTURAL BEALS TYPE*
**Contractures, multiple, Finnish type**
*See CONTRACTURES, CONGENITAL LETHAL FINNISH TYPE*
**Contractures-hyperkeratosis**
*See RESTRICTIVE DERMATOPATHY*

**Contractures-mental retardation, X-linked-muscle atrophy-apraxia**
*See X-LINKED MENTAL RETARDATION-MUSCLE ATROPHY-
CONTRACTURES-APRAXIA*

## CONTRACTURES-MUSCLE ATROPHY-OCULOMOTOR APRAXIA      2832

**Includes:**

Apraxia, oculomotor-contractures-muscle atrophy
Muscle atrophy-contractures-oculomotor apraxia
Oculomotor apraxia-contractures-muscle atrophy
Wieacker syndrome
Wieacker-Wolff syndrome

**Excludes:**

**Arthrogryposes** (0088)
**Diplegia, congenital facial** (0376)
**Ocular motor apraxia, Cogan congenital type** (0191)
Mental retardation with muscle atrophy
**Muscular dystrophy**
**Myopathies** (1500)
**Myotonic dystrophy** (0702)
**Neuropathy, hereditary motor and sensory**
**Spinal muscular atrophy** (0895)

**Major Diagnostic Criteria:** Congenital contractures of the feet with pes calcaneovalgus and heel gait are apparent clinically. Progressive neural muscle atrophy, beginning in the lower limbs, can be confirmed by muscle and nerve biopsies. Other striking symptoms are ptosis, oculomotor apraxia, dysarthria, and a progressive mental deterioration. Only males are affected.

**Clinical Findings:** At birth, affected males show multiple contractures of the feet, resulting in a pes calcaneovalgus with heel gaits. Further development is characterized by motor and speech retardation. In affected adults, the speech is stuttering and unintelligible because of severe dysarthria. Eye symptoms include bilateral ptosis and sluggish reactions of the pupils to light and convergence. Vertical and horizontal eye movements are defective, resembling **Ocular motor apraxia, Cogan congenital type**.

During childhood, neurologic examination reveals a progressive weakness of the upper and lower limbs with a pronounced muscle atrophy, leading to severe progressive deformities of the hands and feet in later years. Muscle biopsy excludes a muscle dystrophy, and nerve biopsy should confirm the neural origin of muscle atrophy. Mental retardation is progressive, but seems to be influencable by educational support.

**Complications:** Severe and progressive contractures of the foot and hand joints, kyphoscoliosis.

**Associated Findings:** Paresis of the nervus facialis with lagophthalmus, strabismus, and hyperopia.

**Etiology:** X-linked recessive inheritance.

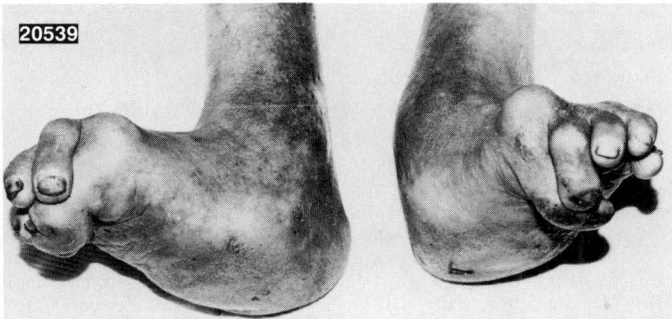

**2832-20539:** Contractures-muscle atrophy-oculomotor apraxia, Wieacker type; note severe, congenital contractures of the feet.

**Pathogenesis:** Unknown. Most of the symptoms can be explained by a progressive neuropathy due to motor neuron disorders, also involving cranial nerves. Onset is prenatal.

**MIM No.:** *31458

**Sex Ratio:** M1:F0

**Occurrence:** One family with seven affected males in three generations has been documented.

**Risk of Recurrence for Patient's Sib:**
See Part I, *Mendelian Inheritance.*

**Risk of Recurrence for Patient's Child:**
See Part I, *Mendelian Inheritance.*

**Age of Detectability:** All affected individuals were evident at birth on the basis of their congenital contractures.

**Gene Mapping and Linkage:** Linkage analysis with restriction fragment length polymorphisms (RFLPs) revealed close linkage with the DNA sequence DXYS1, localized at Xq13-Xq21.1

**Prevention:** None known. Genetic counseling indicated.

**Treatment:** Physical therapy to prevent progressive contractures, surgical corrections of contractures, early support to minimize mental handicap, and speech therapy.

**Prognosis:** Normal life span. Physical handicaps and mental retardation require special education.

**Detection of Carrier:** All affected individuals are related through females who do not show even minor symptoms of the syndrome. There is a possibility of detection by restriction fragment analysis if linkage can be confirmed.

**References:**

Wieacker P, et al.: A new X-linked syndrome with muscle atrophy, congenital contractures, and oculomotor apraxia. Am J Med Genet 1985; 20:597–606.
Turner G, et al.: Second international workshop on the fragile X and on X-linked mental retardation. (Conference Report) Am J Med Genet 1986; 23:11–67.
Wieacker P, et al.: Close linkage of the Wieacker-Wolff syndrome to the DNA segment DXYS1 in proximal Xq. Am J Med Genet 1987; 28:245–253.

WI058            **Peter Wieacker**
WO019           **Gerhard Wolff**

**Contralateral subclavian steal syndrome**
*See AORTA, ISOLATION OF SUBCLAVIAN ARTERY FROM AORTA*
**Conus, congenital**
*See OPTIC DISK, TILTED*

## CONVULSIONS, BENIGN FAMILIAL NEONATAL      3216

**Includes:**

Convulsions, fifth day fits
Fifth day fits
Epilepsy, benign neonatal
Seizures, benign familial neonatal-infantile
Seizures, dominant benign neonatal

**Excludes:**

Convulsions, neonatal, related to anoxic causes
Convulsions, neonatal, related to infection
Convulsions, neonatal, related to metabolic causes
Convulsions, neonatal, related to toxins
Convulsions, neonatal, related to vascular causes
**Neuropathy, heritable isoniazide type (INH)** (2044)
**Seizures, vitamin B(6) dependency** (0991)

**Major Diagnostic Criteria:** Seizures in an otherwise healthy and neurologically normal infant, with onset commonly by two to eight days of age. Electroencephalograms are usually normal interictally, and other evaluations including lumbar puncture, neuroimaging studies, and metabolic parameters are unremarkable. Family history is strongly positive for early-onset seizure activity in other individuals who are neurodevelopmentally normal.

**Clinical Findings:** Bjerre and Corelius (1968) published the first English language description of a family in which 14 members in five generations had frequent seizures during the first weeks of life, but then had a favorable neurodevelopmental outcome. Subsequent reports of at least 17 other families have appeared. In these families, the onset of seizure activity usually occurs on day two or three of life, although delayed onset of up to 15 days has been reported. Rare cases have not developed seizure activity until up to one to four months of age.

The seizures are commonly multifocal clonic or tonic-clonic, and are often multiple, with up to 40 or more episodes per day. Pyridoxine is ineffective, and often an incomplete response to anticonvulsants is seen. Prenatal and perinatal histories reveal no specific risk factors for seizures, and extensive evaluations to search for other etiologies are negative. Between seizures, the infants appear normal and feed well. Interictal electroencephalograms are commonly normal, although there have been instances of focal epileptiform discharges reported. Duration of the seizure activity is variable, with spells sometimes ceasing within a few days of onset, and commonly no seizures are seen after 6–8 months of age. Exceptionally, persistent seizures for up to 14 months have been reported.

Long-term outcome is excellent. In 137 individuals from 18 different families, only four are reported to have subnormal intelligence (2.9%) although details are not given. Subsequent nonfebrile seizures developed in fourteen of 137 (10.2%), an incidence which is significantly greater than the risk for epilepsy in the population as a whole (0.5–1.0%). Deaths were reported in one infant, a twin, during what was described as a cyanotic episode by Pettit and Fenichel (1980), and in two infants in Bierre and Corelius's family, although the latter two deaths were in the early 20th century, with the causes of death noted as obscure and possibly secondary to other factors.

**Complications:** Although the risk for mental retardation is approximately that of the general population, the risk for subsequent epilepsy is clearly increased.

**Associated Findings:** None known.

**Etiology:** Autosomal dominant inheritance with high penetrance and variable expressivity.

**Pathogenesis:** Unknown.

**MIM No.:** *12120

**Sex Ratio:** M1:F1

**Occurrence:** At least 116 cases from 18 kindreds have been reported, although incidence in the population overall has not been established. Cases have been reported both in Caucasian and Oriental families.

**Risk of Recurrence for Patient's Sib:**
See Part I, *Mendelian Inheritance*. There appears to be no difference in severity between maternal and paternal transmission, as has been suggested for other forms of epilepsy.

**Risk of Recurrence for Patient's Child:**
See Part I, *Mendelian Inheritance*.

**Age of Detectability:** Clinically manifest in infancy.

**Gene Mapping and Linkage:** EBN (epilepsy, benign neonatal) has been provisionally mapped to 20q.

**Prevention:** None known. Genetic counseling indicated.

**Treatment:** Evaluation must be undertaken to exclude other treatable and potentially lethal etiologies for seizures, such as meningitis and metabolic abnormalities, even in at-risk infants. Anticonvulsant therapy should be used to decrease or stop seizure occurrence during the neonatal period, but in most instances long-term treatment with anticonvulsants past a few weeks or months will not be required.

**Prognosis:** Usually excellent, although the risk for subsequent epilepsy is increased at 10.2%.

**Detection of Carrier:** Unknown.

**Special Considerations:** The benign outcome of neonatal seizures in these families stands in sharp contrast to the often pessimistic prognosis for many infants with neonatal seizures in

whom mortality is approximately 15%, and morbidity in the form of neurologic sequelae is 35%. A favorable prognosis is also reported in the poorly described entity of *fifth day fits*; seizures occurring between the third and seventh days of life in otherwise healthy infants, and which in one report have been linked to low cerebrospinal fluid zinc levels.

**References:**
Bjerre I, Corelius E: Benign familial neonatal convulsions. Acta Paediat Scand 1968; 57:557–561. *
Carton D: Benign familial neonatal convulsions. Neuropaediatric 1978; 9:167–171.
Quattlebaum TG: Benign familial convulsions in the neonatal period and early infancy. J Pediatr 1979; 95:257–259.
Pettit RE, Fenichel GM: Benign familial neonatal seizures. Arch Neurol 1980; 37:47–48.
Tibbles JAR: Dominant benign neonatal seizures. Dev Med Child Neurol 1980; 22:664–667.
Zonana J, et al.: Familial neonatal and infantile seizures: An autosomal dominant disorder. Am J Med Genet 1983; 16:595–599. *
Cunniff C, et al.: Autosomal dominant benign neonatal seizures. Am J Med Genet 1988; 30:963–966.
Leppert M, et al.: Benign familial neonatal convulsions linked to genetic markers on chromosome 20. Nature 1989; 337:647–648.

GR034
KA008

**May L. Griebel**
**Raymond S. Kandt**

**Convulsions, fifth day fits**
See CONVULSIONS, BENIGN FAMILIAL NEONATAL
**Convulsive disorder, familial, of prenatal or early onset**
See EPILEPSY, FAMILIAL
**Cooley anemia**
See THALASSEMIA
**Cooper-Jabs syndrome**
See AURAL ATRESIA-DYSMORPHIC FACIES-SKELETAL DEFECTS
**Copper retention**
See HEPATOLENTICULAR DEGENERATION
**Copper toxicosis, inherited**
See HEPATOLENTICULAR DEGENERATION
**Copper transport disease**
See MENKES SYNDROME
**Coproporphyrinogen oxidase deficiency**
See PORPHYRIA, COPROPORPHYRIA
**Coprostanic acidemia**
See ACIDEMIA, TRIHYDROXYCOPROSTANIC
**Cor triatriatum**
See HEART, COR TRIATRIATUM
**Cor triatriatum sinistrum**
See HEART, COR TRIATRIATUM
**Cor triloculare biatriatum**
See VENTRICLE, SEPTUM DEXTROPOSITION AND DOUBLE INLET LEFT VENTRICLE
**Coralliform cataract**
See CATARACT, AUTOSOMAL DOMINANT CONGENITAL
**Cori disease**
See GLYCOGENOSIS, TYPE III
**Cornea guttata**
See CORNEAL DYSTROPHY, ENDOTHELIAL

---

**CORNEA PLANA**              **0205**

**Includes:** Sclerocornea

**Excludes:** Inflammatory keratopathies

**Major Diagnostic Criteria:** Nonprogressive, noninflammatory flattened cornea.

**Clinical Findings:** Corneal curvature is less than normal. The stroma usually demonstrates diffuse opacification, frequently more marked posteriorly and centrally, although opacities range from minimal peripheral opacification to total opacification of the cornea resembling the appearance of sclera. There is scleralization of the limbus and absence of a defined corneoscleral interface so that the diameter of the cornea appears subnormal. The flattened cornea results in a shallow anterior chamber. The lid may appear ptotic (Streiff sign). The iris pattern may be absent or abnormal. Other extensive abnormalities of the eye may coexist causing certain authors to classify cornea plana with anterior chamber cleavage syndromes (including **Rieger syndrome**).

**Complications:**  Reduced visual acuity due to stromal opacification, abnormal refractive error, angle closure, glaucoma.

**Associated Findings:**  Posterior embryotoxon, iris coloboma and stromal abnormalities, abnormally shaped pupils, congenital cataract, retinal coloboma, glaucoma, strabismus, and bony and tooth abnormalities. Changes consistent with sclerocornea have been described in **Fetal alcohol syndrome**.

**Etiology:**  Usually autosomal dominant inheritance; less commonly autosomal recessive inheritance. Single case reports exist of association with 17p,10q translocation and **Chromosome 18, trisomy 18.**

**Pathogenesis:**  Failure of normal "cleavage" of the anterior chamber structures during embryonic life. Abnormalities in Descemet membrane anterior portion suggest abnormality occurs before the fifth month of gestation.

**MIM No.:**  *12140, *21730

**Sex Ratio:**  M1:F1

**Occurrence:**  Less than 75 cases reported; the majority in Finland.

**Risk of Recurrence for Patient's Sib:**
See Part I, *Mendelian Inheritance.*

**Risk of Recurrence for Patient's Child:**
See Part I, *Mendelian Inheritance.*

**Age of Detectability:**  During Childhood.

**Gene Mapping and Linkage:**  Unknown.

**Prevention:**  None known. Genetic counseling indicated.

**Treatment:**  Surgery for cataract, glaucoma and corneal opacification, as indicated.

**Prognosis:**  Poor for vision.

**Detection of Carrier:**  By slit lamp examination.

**References:**
Goldstein JE, Cogan DG: Sclerocornea and associated congenital anomalies. Arch Ophthalmol 1962; 67:761–768.
Duke-Elder S: System of ophthalmology, vol. 3, pt. 2. congenital deformities. London: Henry Kimpton, 1964.
Bloch W: Different types of sclerocornea, their hereditary modes and concomitant congenital malformations. J Genet Hum 1965; 14:133–172.
Henkind P, et al.: Mesodermal dysgenesis of the anterior segment: Rieger's anomaly. Arch Ophthalmol 1965; 73:810–817.
Reese AB, Ellsworth RM: The anterior chamber cleavage syndrome. Arch Ophthalmol 1966; 75:307–318.
Howard RD, Abrahams IW: Sclerocornea. Am J Ophthalmol 1971; 71:1254–1260.
Eriksson AW, et al.: Congenital cornea plana in Finland. Clin Genet 1973; 4:301–310.
Waring GO, Rodriques MM: Ultrastructure and successful keratoplasty of sclerocornea in Mieten's syndrome. Amer J Ophthalmol 1980; 90:469–475.

G0006                                              **Morton F. Goldberg**
SU001                                                    **Joel Sugar**

## CORNEA, CENTRAL CLOUDY DYSTROPHY OF FRANCOIS                                              3184

**Includes:**  Central cloudy corneal dystrophy of Francois

**Excludes:**
Cornea farinata
**Corneal dystrophy, macular type** (0212)
**Dermo-chondro-corneal dystrophy, Francois type** (0282)
Dystrophia corneae filiformis profunda
Posterior crocodile shagreen
Posterior polymorphous dystrophy

**Major Diagnostic Criteria:**  Bilateral dystrophy of the cornea with symmetrical central distribution of hazy stromal opacification.

**Clinical Findings:**  The diagnosis has been made in patients between the ages of eight and 70 years. Due to the subtle nature of the corneal changes as well as the fact that generally no decrease in visual acuity occurs, it is not clear if corneal changes can be found at an earlier age. The opacifications which are polygonal or rounded in shape with indistinct borders are primarily central and most often seen in the most posterior one-third of the stroma although one can observe them to extend anterior to Bowman's layer. Relatively clear stroma is seen between the opacities. No vascularization or corneal inflammation occurs and corneal thickness is normal. The corneal epithelium and endothelium as well as their respective basement membranes are spared.

**Complications:**  Unknown.

**Associated Findings:**  One case of combined central cloudy stromal dystrophy and fleck dystrophy of the cornea has been described (Collier, 1964). A case of pseudoxanthoma elasticum and central cloudy dystrophy of François has also been reported (Collier, 1965). In one study, only affected members of a family were found to have mild intraocular pressure elevations and the oldest affected member of the family had frank primary open angle glaucoma with visual field loss (Bramse, 1976).

**Etiology:**  Possibly autosomal dominant inheritance, but most reported cases have been sporadic.

**Pathogenesis:**  Unknown.

**Sex Ratio:**  M1:F1

**Occurrence:**  Undetermined but presumed rare. Often an incidental finding.

**Risk of Recurrence for Patient's Sib:**
See Part I, *Mendelian Inheritance.*

**Risk of Recurrence for Patient's Child:**
See Part I, *Mendelian Inheritance.*

**Age of Detectability:**  All cases have been diagnosed at between 8–70 years of age. Due to the subtle nature of the disease, it is not clear whether it is present at a younger age.

**Gene Mapping and Linkage:**  Unknown.

**Prevention:**  None known. Genetic counseling indicated.

**Treatment:**  None necessary, except for periodic assessment of visual acuity.

**Prognosis:**  Good.

**Detection of Carrier:**  Carriers will show the corneal changes.

**References:**
Collier M: Dystrophie mouchetee du parenchyme corneen avec dystrophie nuageuse centrale. Bull Soc Ophtal 1964; 608–611.
Collier M: Dystrophie nuageuse centrale et dystrophie ponctiforme predescemetique dans une meme famille. Bull Soc Ophtal 1965; 575–579.
François J: Heredofamilial corneal dystrophies. Trans Ophthalm Soc UK 1966; 86:400–410.
Strachan IM: Cloudy central corneal dystrophy of François. Br J Ophthalmol 1969; 53:192–194.
Bramsen TX, et al: Central cloudy dystrophy of François. Acta Ophthalmol 1976; 54:221–224.
Waring G, et al: Corneal dystrophies. Surv Ophthalmol 1982; 23:71–117.

PA051                                              **Stephen E. Pascucci**
LE052                                                **Michael A. Lemp**

**Cornea, conical**
See *EYE, KERATOCONUS*
**Cornea, enlarged**
See *CORNEA, MEGALOCORNEA*
**Cornea, juvenile epithelial degeneration of**
See *CORNEAL DYSTROPHY, JUVENILE EPITHELIAL, MEESMANN TYPE*

## CORNEA, MEGALOCORNEA 0637

**Includes:**
Anterior megalophthalmos
Cornea, enlarged
Keratomegalia
Megalocornea

**Excludes:**
Buphthalmos
**Glaucoma, congenital** (0414)
Keratoglobus

**Major Diagnostic Criteria:** Corneal diameter over 13 mm with normal intraocular pressure; no evidence of primary glaucoma. Corneal endothelial cell density is normal while in congenital glaucoma it is reduced.

**Clinical Findings:** Symmetric, bilateral, nonprogressive increase in the corneal diameter ( > 13 mm). The cornea is transparent, and occasionally has increased curvature resulting in astigmatism. The anterior chamber is deep, and there may be mesodermal abnormalities in the chamber angle and atrophy of the iris stroma. Attenuation of the dilator muscle of the pupil, which is relatively common, results in meiosis. Cataract frequently occurs, and may cause reduction in visual acuity. Lens subluxation has also been reported.

**Complications:** Glaucoma, cataract.

**Associated Findings:** An associated mosaic dystrophy of the cornea (possibly of different types) has been reported in three separate pedigrees. Megalocornea also occurs in **Marfan syndrome.** Two pedigrees have been described, both with mental retardation associated with megalocornea.

**Etiology:** Usually X-linked recessive inheritance, but may also be by autosomal recessive or autosomal dominant inheritance.

**Pathogenesis:** Unknown.

**MIM No.:** *30930

**CDC No.:** 743.220

**Sex Ratio:** M1:F< 1

**Occurrence:** Undetermined but presumed rare.

**Risk of Recurrence for Patient's Sib:**
See Part I, *Mendelian Inheritance.*

**Risk of Recurrence for Patient's Child:**
See Part I, *Mendelian Inheritance.*

**Age of Detectability:** At birth.

**Gene Mapping and Linkage:** MGC1 (megalocornea 1 (X-linked)) has been provisionally mapped to Xq12-q26.

**Prevention:** None known. Genetic counseling indicated.

**Treatment:** Correction of refractive error; therapy for the secondary glaucoma and cataract when indicated.

**Prognosis:** Good.

**Detection of Carrier:** Unknown.

**References:**
Riddell WJB: Uncomplicated hereditary megalocornea. Ann Eugen 1941; 11:102–107.
Young AI: Megalocornea and mosaic dystrophy in identical twins. Am J Ophthalmol 1968; 66:734–735.
Neuhäuser G, et al.: Syndrome of mental retardation, hypotonic cerebral palsy and megalocorneae, recessively inherited. Z Kinderheilkd 1975; 120:1–18.
Skuta GL, et al.: Corneal endothelial cell measurements in megalocornea. Arch Ophthalmol 1983; 101:51–53.

**Morton F. Goldberg**
**Joel Sugar**

G0006
SU001

## CORNEAL ANESTHESIA-RETINAL DEFECTS-UNUSUAL FACIES-HEART DEFECT 2836

**Includes:**
Corneal hypesthesia-retinal anomalies-deafness-unusual facies
Ductus arteriosus, patent-eye anomalies-unusual facies-deafness
Retinal anomalies-corneal hypesthesia-deafness-unusual facies

**Excludes:**
Choroidal atrophy, isolated central areolar
Cornea, neurotrophic ulceration because of trigeminal defect
Corneal hypesthesia, secondary or isolated

**Major Diagnostic Criteria:** At least some of the cardinal defects are present at birth or shortly thereafter. **Ductus arteriosus, patent,** corneal hypesthesia, **Eye, hypertelorism,** unusual facies, and sensorineural hearing loss were present early in the two reported sibs. Some degree of mental retardation was common to all three patients, as were retinal changes.

**Clinical Findings:** Clinical signs may be present at birth. **Ductus arteriosus, patent** may (1/2) require intervention, and corneal hypesthesia can eventuate in ulceration. Upslanting palpebral fissures, frontal bossing, depressed nasal root and bridge, anteverted nares, and midfacial hypoplasia were present in the two reported sibs, while **Eye, hypertelorism** was the feature common to all three known patients. Deafness is of the sensorineural type. The retinal defects are apparently not progressive, and include absence of the choriocapillaris and retinal pigment epithelium in a focal, peripapillary distribution. Mild mental retardation is common. Craniofacial pattern profiles show hypertelorism, large interorbital width/head width index, increased facial width, growth retardation of the cranial base, marked maxillary retrusion, and very small mandibular angle.

**Complications:** Corneal ulceration. Speech impairment may result from the hearing loss, and the **Ductus arteriosus, patent** may require treatment.

**Associated Findings:** None known.

**Etiology:** Probably autosomal dominant inheritance. Variable expressivity is indicated by the milder form of the condition noted in the mother in the reported family.

**Pathogenesis:** Unknown.

**MIM No.:** 12243

**Sex Ratio:** Presumably M1:F1.

**Occurrence:** Documented in a brother and sister, and in their mother.

**Risk of Recurrence for Patient's Sib:**
See Part I, *Mendelian Inheritance.*

**Risk of Recurrence for Patient's Child:**
See Part I, *Mendelian Inheritance.*

**Age of Detectability:** At birth.

**Gene Mapping and Linkage:** Unknown.

**Prevention:** None known. Genetic counseling indicated.

**Treatment:** Preventive measures, including tarsorrhaphy if necessary, to prevent corneal ulceration. Special education. Hearing aids. Treatment of **Ductus arteriosus, patent** as necessary.

**Prognosis:** Apparently consistent with a normal life span.

**Detection of Carrier:** By clinical examination.

**References:**
Ramos-Arroyo MA, et al.: Congenital corneal anesthesia with retinal abnormalities, deafness, unusual facies, persistent ductus arterio-

sus, and mental retardation: a new syndrome? Am J Med Genet 1987; 26:345–354.

H0003                                      **M.E. Hodes**
RA023                        **Maria A. Ramos-Arroyo**
CL020                    **G. Gregory Clark**
SA042                   **Sudha S. Saksena**

**Corneal clouding-cutis laxa-mental retardation**
*See CUTIS LAXA-GROWTH DEFECT, DE BARSY TYPE*
**Corneal dystrophy, band-shaped**
*See EYE, KERATOPATHY, BAND-SHAPED*
**Corneal dystrophy, congenital hereditary stationary**
*See CORNEAL DYSTROPHY, ENDOTHELIAL, CONGENITAL HEREDITARY*
**Corneal dystrophy, crystalline**
*See CORNEAL DYSTROPHY, SCHNYDER CRYSTALLINE*

## CORNEAL DYSTROPHY, ENDOTHELIAL    0208

**Includes:**
    Cornea guttata
    Endothelial corneal dystrophy
    Fuchs endothelial dystrophy

**Excludes:**
    **Corneal dystrophy, endothelial, congenital hereditary** (0207)
    **Corneal dystrophy, polymorphous posterior** (0213)

**Major Diagnostic Criteria:** Many tiny excrescences on Descemet membrane, progressive with age.

**Clinical Findings:** This disorder biomicroscopically resembles adult senile Fuchs endothelial dystrophy in that there are numerous tiny (0.04–0.08 mm) tightly packed distributed excrescences on Descemet membrane, which give an appearance of endothelial dimples. They may first appear during adolescence. Vision is rarely affected.

**Complications:** Reduced visual acuity infrequently occurs.

**Associated Findings:** Anterior polar cataract.

**Etiology:** Probably autosomal dominant inheritance. High penetrance, variable expressivity, and age dependency with increased severity for females has been reported.

**Pathogenesis:** May be related to abnormal calcium metabolism.

**MIM No.:** *13680

**Sex Ratio:** M1:F1

**Occurrence:** Undetermined but considered common.

**Risk of Recurrence for Patient's Sib:**
    See Part I, *Mendelian Inheritance.*

**Risk of Recurrence for Patient's Child:**
    See Part I, *Mendelian Inheritance.*

**Age of Detectability:** Adolescence. Histopathologic changes probably begin earlier.

**Gene Mapping and Linkage:** Unknown.

**Prevention:** None known. Genetic counseling indicated.

**Treatment:** None usually indicated. Penetrating keratoplasty in those developing corneal edema.

**Prognosis:** Normal for life and intelligence. Usually good for vision.

**Detection of Carrier:** Slit lamp examination.

**Special Considerations:** Considerable debate still exists in the classification and nomenclature of corneal dystrophy. Naming and classification codes are therefore not always consistent.

**References:**
Maumenee AE: An introduction to corneal dystrophies. In: Bergsma D, ed: Part VIII. Eye, BD:OAS, VII,3. Baltimore: Williams and Wilkins Co. for The National Foundation-March of Dimes, 1971:3.
Krachmer JH, et al.: Corneal endothelial dystrophy: a study of 64 families. Arch Ophthalmol 1978; 96:2036–2039.
Krachmer JH, et al.: Inheritance of endothelial dystrophy of the cornea. Ophthalmologica 1980; 181:301–313.
Krachmer JH, et al.: Inheritance of endothelial dystrophy of the cornea. Ophthalmologica 1980; 181:301–313.
Rosenblum P, et al.: Hereditary Fuchs' dystrophy. Am J Ophthalmol 1980; 90:455–462.
Bourne WM, et al.: The ultrastructure of Descemet's membrane III: Fuchs' dystrophy. Arch Ophthalmol 1982; 100:1952–1955.

G0006                     **Morton F. Goldberg**
SU001                      **Joel Sugar**

## CORNEAL DYSTROPHY, ENDOTHELIAL, CONGENITAL HEREDITARY    0207

**Includes:**
    Corneal dystrophy, congenital hereditary stationary
    Maumenee congenital corneal edema
    Maumenee corneal dystrophy

**Excludes:**
    **Corneal dystrophy, endothelial** (0208)
    **Corneal dystrophy, polymorphous posterior** (0213)
    **Corneal dystrophy, stromal, congenital hereditary** (3198)

**Major Diagnostic Criteria:** Corneal stromal edema in the absence of elevated intraocular pressure or excrescences on Descemet membrane.

**Clinical Findings:** In the progressive form diffuse clouding and thickening of the corneal stroma are present at birth and progress minimally. Epithelial irregularity occurs but large bullae and corneal vascularization are usually not seen. Excrescences are not seen in Descemet membrane. In the dominant form corneal changes are not evident at birth but develop over the first one to two years of life heralded by tearing and photophobia.

**Complications:** Reduced visual acuity, nystagmus (infrequent).

**Associated Findings:** Unknown.

**Etiology:** Autosomal dominant or autosomal recessive inheritance. The dominant form may in fact be a variant of **Corneal dystrophy, polymorphous posterior**.

**Pathogenesis:** Decreased-to-absent endothelial cells.

**MIM No.:** *12170, *21770

**Sex Ratio:** M1:F1

**Occurrence:** About 75 cases reported, with as many as 39 cases in a single family. At least one Black family reported.

**Risk of Recurrence for Patient's Sib:**
    See Part I, *Mendelian Inheritance.*

**Risk of Recurrence for Patient's Child:**
    See Part I, *Mendelian Inheritance.*

**Age of Detectability:** At birth.

**Gene Mapping and Linkage:** Unknown.

**Prevention:** None known. Genetic counseling indicated.

**Treatment:** Penetrating keratoplasty if visual acuity impaired.

**Prognosis:** Normal for life and intelligence. Fair for vision depending on degree of involvement.

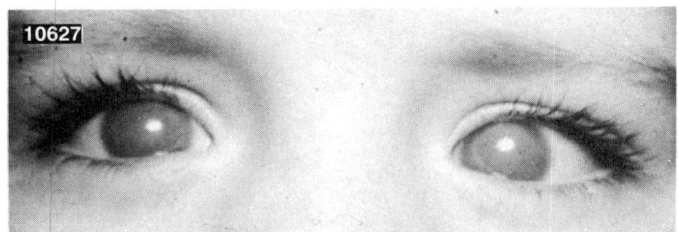

**0207**-10627: Congenital diffuse corneal clouding from corneal dystrophy.

**Detection of Carrier:**  Slit lamp examination.

**References:**
Maumenee AE: Congenital hereditary corneal dystrophy. Am J Ophthalmol 1960; 50:1114–1124.
Pearce WG, et al.: Congenital endothelial corneal dystrophy: clinical, pathological and genetic study. Br J Ophthalmol 1969; 53:577–591.
Judisch GF, Maumenee IH: Clinical differentiation of recessive congenital hereditary endothelial dystropy and dominant hereditary endothelial dystrophy. Am J Ophthalmol 1978; 85:606–612.
Kirkness CM, et al.: Congenital hereditary corneal oedema of Maumenee: its clinical features, mamagement, and pathology. Brit J Ophthalmol 1987; 71:130–144.

SU001                                          **Joel Sugar**
G0006                                   **Morton F. Goldberg**

**Corneal dystrophy, epithelial basement membrane**
  *See CORNEAL DYSTROPHY, RECURRENT EROSIVE*
**Corneal dystrophy, epithelial-skin and skeletal changes**
  *See CORNEO-DERMATO-OSSEOUS SYNDROME*
**Corneal dystrophy, gelatinous drop-like**
  *See AMYLOIDOSIS, CORNEAL*

---

## CORNEAL DYSTROPHY, GRANULAR        0209

**Includes:**
  Granular corneal dystrophy
  Groenouw type I corneal dystrophy

**Excludes:**
  **Corneal dystrophy, lattice type** (0211)
  **Corneal dystrophy, macular type** (0212)
  **Corneal dystrophy, Reis-Bucklers type** (0215)

**Major Diagnostic Criteria:**  Slit-lamp appearance of discrete, white opacities in anterior, axial, corneal stroma.

**Clinical Findings:**  Juvenile onset of multiple, bilateral, progressive, central, anterior, stromal opacities, which are usually grey or white and sharply defined. They may take the form of small disks, doughnuts, clubs, nodules, dots, etc. The peripheral cornea remains uninvolved. Recurrent painful epithelial erosions with secondary opacification and vascularization may occur, but are unusual. Decreased visual acuity often occurs between the 3rd to the 5th decades of life.

**Complications:**  Decreased corneal transparency.

**Associated Findings:**  None known.

**Etiology:**  Autosomal dominant inheritance.

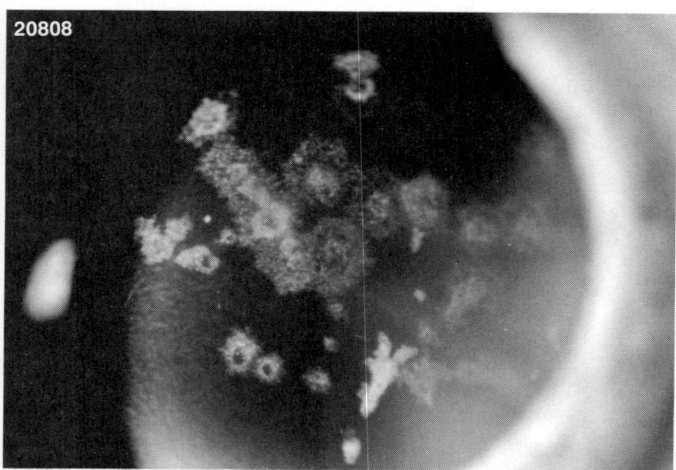

0209-20808:  Corneal dystrophy, granular.

**Pathogenesis:**  Hyaline degeneration of the corneal stroma. Microfibrillar protein is present in the granules and corneal phospholipid content is elevated.

**MIM No.:**  *12190

**Sex Ratio:**  M1:F1

**Occurrence:**  Undetermined but presumed rare.

**Risk of Recurrence for Patient's Sib:**
  See Part I, *Mendelian Inheritance.*

**Risk of Recurrence for Patient's Child:**
  See Part I, *Mendelian Inheritance.*

**Age of Detectability:**  Onset in juvenile period, but as late as age 20.

**Gene Mapping and Linkage:**  Unknown.

**Prevention:**  None known. Genetic counseling indicated.

**Treatment:**  Lamellar, or occasionally penetrating, keratoplasty, depending on depth of stromal opacities.

**Prognosis:**  Good for successful keratoplasty, though recurrences have been reported.

**Detection of Carrier:**  Unknown.

**References:**
Sornson ET: Granular dystrophy of the cornea: an electron microscopic study. Am J Ophthalmol 1965; 59:1001–1007.
Teng CC: Granular dystrophy of the cornea: a histochemical and electron microscopic study. Am J Ophthalmol 1967; 63:772–791.
Francois J: Heredofamilial corneal dystrophies. In: Symposium on surgical and medical management of congenital anomalies of the eye. St. Louis: CV Mosby Co., 1968.
Maumenee AE: An introduction to corneal dystrophies. In: Bergsma D, ed: Part VIII. Eye. BD:OAS, VII, 3. Baltimore: Williams and Wilkins Co. for The National Foundation-March of Dimes, 1971:3–12.
Herman SJ, Hughes WF: Recurrence of hereditary corneal dystrophy following keratoplasty. Am J Ophthalmol 1973; 75:689–694.
Brownstein S, et al.: Granular dystrophy of the cornea. Am J Ophthalmol 1974; 77:701–710.
Rodrigues MM, et al: Microfibrillar protein and phospholipid in granular corneal dystrophy. Arch Ophthalmol 1983; 101:802–810.

G0006                                   **Morton F. Goldberg**
SU001                                          **Joel Sugar**

**Corneal dystrophy, hereditary deep**
  *See CORNEAL DYSTROPHY, POLYMORPHOUS POSTERIOR*

---

## CORNEAL DYSTROPHY, JUVENILE EPITHELIAL, MEESMANN TYPE      0210

**Includes:**
  Cornea, juvenile epithelial degeneration of
  Juvenile epithelial corneal dystrophy
  Meesmann corneal dystrophy

**Excludes:**
  **Corneal dystrophy, recurrent erosive** (0214)
  Whorl-like corneal dystrophy

**Major Diagnostic Criteria:**  The appearance of homogeneous fine clear vesicles in the corneal epithelium.

**Clinical Findings:**  Fine punctate opacities, seen only with magnification, appear in the corneal epithelium bilaterally during the first few years of life. They frequently remain asymptomatic, but may cause an irritative sensation and may stain with topically applied fluorescein solution. Vision may be slightly reduced, due to corneal astigmatism or mild scarring. The opacities are diffusely located in the central area of the corneal epithelium and, in reflected light, resemble tiny vesicles or droplets. In advanced cases, the droplets may assume a vortex or whorl pattern.

**Complications:**  Corneal scarring with reduced visual acuity.

**Associated Findings:**  None known.

**Etiology:**  Autosomal dominant inheritance.

**Pathogenesis:** Primary abnormality of epithelial cell ground substance.

**MIM No.:** *12210

**Sex Ratio:** M1:F1

**Occurrence:** Several kindreds documented, including one kindred dating back to 1620, which accounted for 120 cases in Schleswig-Holstein.

**Risk of Recurrence for Patient's Sib:**
See Part I, *Mendelian Inheritance.*

**Risk of Recurrence for Patient's Child:**
See Part I, *Mendelian Inheritance.*

**Age of Detectability:** First few years of life.

**Gene Mapping and Linkage:** Unknown.

**Prevention:** None known. Genetic counseling indicated.

**Treatment:** Lamellar or penetrating keratoplasty in advanced cases.

**Prognosis:** Vision is sometimes significantly affected in adult, advanced cases. Prognosis for keratoplasty is guarded.

**Detection of Carrier:** Unknown.

**References:**
Snyder WB: Hereditary epithelial corneal dystrophy. Am J Ophthalmol 1963; 55:56–61.
Kuwabara T, Ciccarelli EC: Meesmann's corneal dystrophy: a pathological study. Arch Ophthalmol 1964; 71:676–682.
Alkemade PP, van Balen AT: Hereditary epithelial dystrophy of the cornea: Meesmann type. Br J Ophthalmol 1966; 50:603–605.
Maumenee AE: An introduction to corneal dystrophies. In: Bergsma D, ed: Part VIII. Eye. BD:OAS VII, 3. Baltimore: Williams and Wilkins Co. for The National Foundation-March of Dimes, 1971:3–12.
Fine BS, et al.: Meesman's epithelial dystrophy of the cornea. Am J Ophthalmol 1977; 83:633–642.

G0006
SU001

**Morton F. Goldberg**
**Joel Sugar**

## CORNEAL DYSTROPHY, LATTICE TYPE      0211

**Includes:**
    Amyloidosis, corneal, lattice
    Biber-Haab-Dimmer degeneration
    Lattice corneal dystrophy

**Excludes:**
    **Amyloidosis, corneal** (2147)
    **Amyloidosis, Finnish type** (2145)
    **Corneal dystrophy, granular** (0209)
    **Corneal dystrophy, macular type** (0212)
    Interstitial keratitis
    Prominent corneal nerves

**Major Diagnostic Criteria:** Slit-lamp appearance of opaque and translucent stromal lines.

**Clinical Findings:** Progressive, bilateral opacifications of the corneal stroma, having the form of fine lines or dots, particularly occupying the midperiphery and the anterior portions of the stroma. The process begins at about age 5, causing significant loss of vision by age 40 to 60. Corneal sensitivity is diminished, and recurrent painful erosions are common.

**Complications:** Reduced visual acuity due to decreased corneal transparency.

**Associated Findings:** None known.

**Etiology:** Autosomal dominant inheritance.

**Pathogenesis:** Possibly amyloid degeneration in the cornea of the stroma or corneal nerves. Cystine crystals have been reported to precede the amyloid deposition, but this has not been validated. Identity of the amyloid proteins is uncertain with AP present but AA demonstrated but not confirmed.

**MIM No.:** *12220

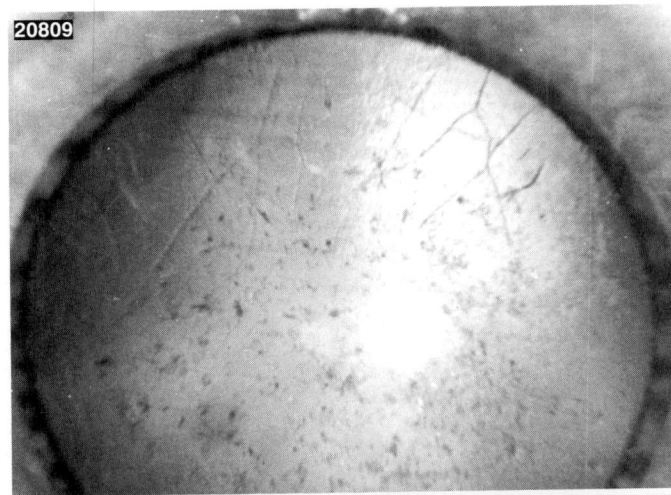

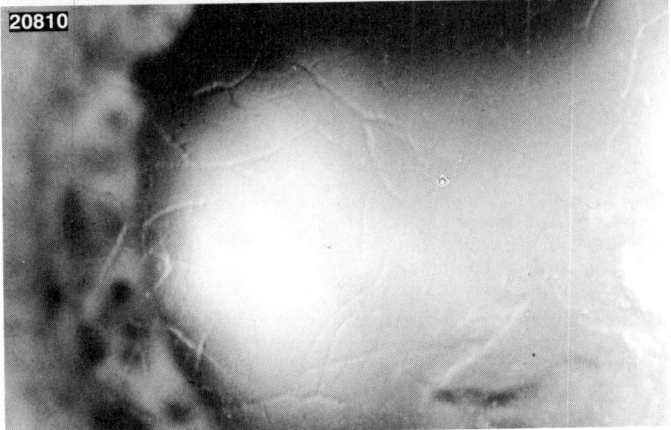

0211-20809–10: Corneal dystrophy, lattice.

**Sex Ratio:** M1:F1

**Occurrence:** Undetermined but probably rare. Established literature.

**Risk of Recurrence for Patient's Sib:**
See Part I, *Mendelian Inheritance.*

**Risk of Recurrence for Patient's Child:**
See Part I, *Mendelian Inheritance.*

**Age of Detectability:** Onset at about age five.

**Gene Mapping and Linkage:** Unknown.

**Prevention:** None known. Genetic counseling indicated.

**Treatment:** Keratoplasty, lamellar or penetrating, depending on depth and severity of stromal opacities; soft contact lenses. Recurrences have been noted in corneal grafts.

**Prognosis:** Good for successful keratoplasty.

**Detection of Carrier:** Unknown.

**Special Considerations:** Three types of lattice corneal dystrophy occur. Those with neuropathic amyloidosis are later in onset, corneal opacities are fewer and more peripheral. Those without systemic disease are earlier in onset, corneal opacities are more numerous and central. Unilateral corneal involvement in family members of individuals with bilateral involvement as well as unilateral sporadic cases have been reported. Hida et al (1987) reported a third variant.

**References:**

Klintworth GK: Lattice corneal dystrophy: an inherited variety of amyloidosis restricted to the cornea. Am J Pathol 1967; 50:371–379.

Smith ME, Zimmerman LE: Amyloid in corneal dystrophies: differentiation of lattice from granular and macular dystrophies. Arch Ophthalmol 1968; 79:407–412.

Meretoja J: Comparative histopathological and clinical findings in eyes with lattice corneal dystrophy of two different types. Ophthalmologica 1972; 165:15–37.

Herman SJ, Hughes WF: Recurrence of hereditary corneal dystrophy following keratoplasty. Am J Ophthalmol 1973; 75:689–694.

Rabb MF, et al.: Unilateral lattice dystrophy of the cornea. Trans Am Acad Ophthalmol Otolaryngol 1974; 78:440–444.

Rodrigues MM, et al.: Lack of evidence for AA reactivity in amyloid deposits of lattice corneal dystrophy and corneal amyloid degeneration. Invest Ophthalmol Vis Sci 1984; 25:6 (suppl).

Hida T, et al.: Clinical features of a newly recognized type of lattice corneal dystrophy. Am J Ophthalmol 1987; 104:241–248.

G0006
SU001

**Morton F. Goldberg**
**Joel Sugar**

## CORNEAL DYSTROPHY, MACULAR TYPE                    0212

**Includes:**

Fehr corneal dystrophy
Groenouw type II corneal dystrophy
Macular corneal dystrophy
Spotted corneal dystrophy

**Excludes:**

**Corneal dystrophy, granular** (0209)
**Corneal dystrophy, lattice type** (0211)
**Mucopolysaccharidosis** (all forms)

**Major Diagnostic Criteria:** Clouding of cornea with slit-lamp evidence that the irregular clouding involves all layers of the corneal stroma with extension from limbus to limbus. The anterior limiting membrane of the cornea is normal, but Descemet's membrane and the corneal endothelium are involved.

**Clinical Findings:** Variably dense, progressive, bilateral clouding of the corneal stroma begins between the ages of 5 and 9, and extends diffusely from the Bowman to Descemet membrane and from limbus to limbus. There are ill-defined stromal accentuations of the cloudiness called macules. Sensitivity of the cornea may be reduced, and recurrent epithelial erosions can cause photophobia and painful episodes. The corneal stroma is thinner than normal. Visual acuity is significantly reduced by the 4th decade of life.

**Complications:** Decreased visual acuity due to corneal opacities.

**Associated Findings:** None known.

**Etiology:** Autosomal recessive inheritance.

**Pathogenesis:** Remains ill defined. There is an accumulation of a keratan sulfate or keratan sulfate related molecule. At least some cases seem to be due to defective keratan sulfate proteoglycan.

**MIM No.:** *21780

**Sex Ratio:** M1:F1

**Occurrence:** Frequency varies with community, ranging from 1:500 to rare.

**Risk of Recurrence for Patient's Sib:**
See Part I, *Mendelian Inheritance.*

**Risk of Recurrence for Patient's Child:**
See Part I, *Mendelian Inheritance.*

**Age of Detectability:** Usually 9th to 20th year, but occasionally infancy or after 60 years of age.

**Gene Mapping and Linkage:** Unknown.

**Prevention:** None known. Genetic counseling indicated.

**Treatment:** Penetrating keratoplasty.

**Prognosis:** Progressive. Good for successful keratoplasty. Disease may recur in grafts.

**Detection of Carrier:** Unknown.

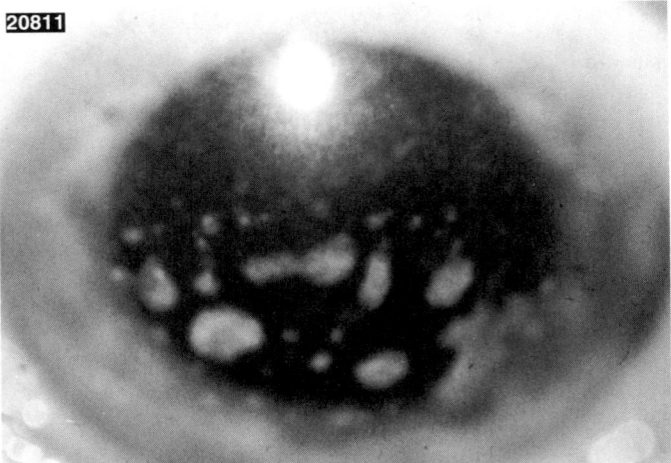

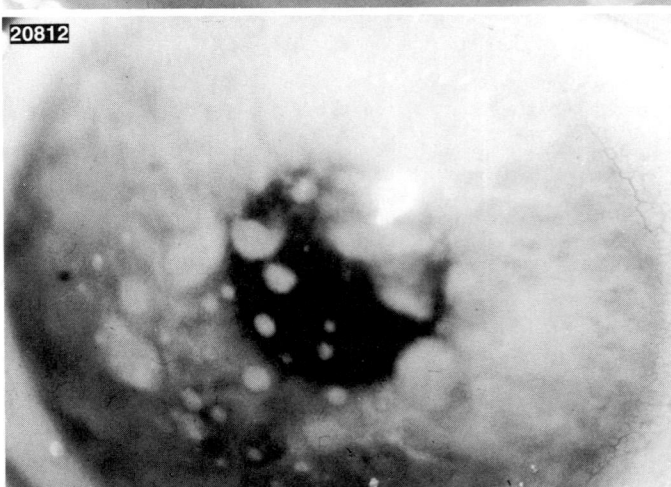

**0212**-20811–12:   Corneal dystrophy, macular.

**Support Groups:**   New York; Association for Macular Diseases

**References:**

Duke-Elder S: System of ophthalmology, vol. 8, part 2. Diseases of the outer eye. London: Henry Kimpton, 1965.

Goldberg MF, et al.: Corneal dystrophies associated with abnormalities of mucopolysaccharide metabolism. Arch Ophthalmol 1965; 74:516–520.

Morgan G: Macular dystrophy of the cornea. Br J Ophthalmol 1966; 50:57.

Teng CC: Macular dystrophy of the cornea: a histochemical and electron microscopic study. Am J Ophthalmol 1966; 62:436.

Hassell JR, et al.: Macular corneal dystrophy: failure to synthesize a mature keratan sulfate proteoglycan. Proc Natl Acad Sci USA 1980; 77:3705–3707.

Klintworth GK: Current concept of macular corneal dystrophy. BD: OAS; 18. New York: March of Dimes Birth Defects Foundation, 1982:463.

Maumenee AE: An introduction to corneal dystrophies. In: Bergsma D, ed: Part VIII. Eye. BD:OAS; 18. New York: March of Dimes Birth Defects Foundation, 1982:463.

Morgan G: Macular dystrophy of the cornea. Br J Ophthalmol 1966; 50:57.

Teng CC: Macular dystrophy of the cornea: a histochemical and electron microscopic study. Am J Ophthalmol 1966; 62:436.

Yang CJ, et al.: Immunohistochemical evidence of heterogeneity in macular corneal dystrophy. Am J Ophthalmol 1988; 106:65–71.

Thonar EJ, et al.: Absence of normal keratan sulfate in the blood of patients with macular corneal dystrophy. Am J Ophthalmol 1986; 102:561–569.

G0006                    **Morton F. Goldberg**
SU001                            **Joel Sugar**
KL008              **Gordon K. Klintworth**

## CORNEAL DYSTROPHY, POLYMORPHOUS POSTERIOR     0213

**Includes:**
    Corneal dystrophy, hereditary deep
    Polymorphous posterior corneal dystrophy
    Schlichting syndrome

**Excludes:**
    **Corneal dystrophy, endothelial, congenital hereditary** (0207)
    **Corneal dystrophy, endothelial** (0208)

**Major Diagnostic Criteria:** Small, bilateral, congenital "vesicles" in the posterior limiting membranes of the cornea may be confirmed by slit lamp exam.

**Clinical Findings:** Small, bilateral, congenital, nonprogressive "vesicular" lesions in the region of the corneal endothelium and Descemet membrane. These lesions appear clinically to be endothelial depressions or vesicles as in endothelial corneal dystrophy, but these histologically involve the Descemet membrane and the deep stroma, are fewer and larger (about 0.2 mm average with largest diameter about 0.75 mm) and also more irregular in size. There are usually no other symptoms.

**Complications:** Usually none; rarely, diffuse corneal edema.

**Associated Findings:** Broad iridocorneal adhesions and glaucoma have been reported.

**Etiology:** Autosomal dominant inheritance. Sporadic cases occur.

**Pathogenesis:** Undetermined. May be related to abnormal calcium metabolism.

**MIM No.:** *12200

**Sex Ratio:** M1:F1. One large kindred showed a greater number of females.

**Occurrence:** A dozen or so kindreds documented, with as many as 39 cases in one family.

**Risk of Recurrence for Patient's Sib:**
    See Part I, *Mendelian Inheritance.*

**Risk of Recurrence for Patient's Child:**
    See Part I, *Mendelian Inheritance.*

**Age of Detectability:** Has been detected in pre-school children.

**Gene Mapping and Linkage:** Unknown.

**Prevention:** None known. Genetic counseling indicated.

**Treatment:** Usually none required; rarely, penetrating keratoplasty.

**Prognosis:** Normal for life and intelligence. Vision may be variably reduced (not affected in most cases, but at least one individual was legally blind).

**Detection of Carrier:** Slit lamp examination.

**References:**
Morgan G, Patterson A: Pathology of posterior polymorphous degeneration of the cornea. Br J Ophthalmol 1967; 51:433–437.
Rubenstein RA, Silverman JJ: Hereditary deep dystrophy of the cornea associated with glaucoma and ruptures in Descemet's membrane. Arch Ophthalmol 1968; 79:123–126.
Strachan IM, Maclean H: Posterior polymorphous dystrophy of the cornea. Br J Ophthalmol 1968; 52:270–272.
Hogan MJ, Bietti G: Hereditary deep dystrophy of the cornea (polymorphous). Trans Am Ophthalmol Soc 1969; 67:234–264.
Cibis GW, et al.: The clinical spectrum of posterior polymorphous dystrophy. Arch Ophthalmol 1977; 95:1529–1537.
Chan CC, et al.: Similarities between posterior polymorphous and congenital hereditary endothelial dystrophies. Cornea 1982; 1:155–172.
Rodrigues MM, et al.: Posterior polymorphous corneal dystrophy:

recent developments. BD:OAS 18(6). White Plains: The National Foundation- March of Dimes, 1982:479–491.

G0006                     **Morton F. Goldberg**
SU001                           **Joel Sugar**

## CORNEAL DYSTROPHY, RECURRENT EROSIVE     0214

**Includes:**
    Cogan microcystic dystrophy
    Corneal dystrophy, epithelial basement membrane
    Erosive corneal dystrophy, hereditary recurrent
    Map-dot-fingerprint corneal dystrophy
    Mycrocystic dystrophy
    Recurrent erosive corneal dystrophy

**Excludes:**
    **Corneal dystrophy, endothelial** (0208)
    Epithelial erosions secondary to corneal trauma
    Primary stromal corneal dystrophies with secondary erosions

**Major Diagnostic Criteria:** Recurrent, painful corneal erosions begin in childhood. The small (1–2 mm) epithelial erosions are found without stromal dystrophies or antecedent corneal trauma.

**Clinical Findings:** Vision and corneal sensation are rarely impaired, but a foreign body sensation, epithelial filaments, small patches of epithelial edema, and fluorescein staining may all occur. Pain may occur just upon awakening, at the time of lid opening. Small epithelial cysts, fingerprint lines in the corneal epithelium, and grey map-like thickenings of epithelial basement membrane occur.

**Complications:** Corneal infection.

**Associated Findings:** None known.

**Etiology:** Autosomal dominant inheritance.

**Pathogenesis:** Unknown.

**MIM No.:** *12182, *12240

**Sex Ratio:** M1:F1

**Occurrence:** About a dozen kinships have been documented.

**Risk of Recurrence for Patient's Sib:**
    See Part I, *Mendelian Inheritance.*

**Risk of Recurrence for Patient's Child:**
    See Part I, *Mendelian Inheritance.*

**Age of Detectability:** Four to six years of age.

**Gene Mapping and Linkage:** Unknown.

**Prevention:** None known. Genetic counseling indicated.

**Treatment:** An emollient at night to prevent adhesion of the lid to the cornea, nocturnal use of a hypertonic ointment to prevent epithelial edema, topical antibiotics and cycloplegics and firm bandaging when indicated.

**Prognosis:** Very good in most cases.

**Detection of Carrier:** Unknown.

**References:**
Duke-Elder S: System of ophthalmology, vol. 8, part 2. Diseases of the outer eye. London: Henry Kimpton, 1965.
Valle O: Hereditary recurring corneal erosions: a familial study with special reference to Fuchs' dystrophy. Acta Ophthalmol (Kbh.) 1967; 45:829–836.
Bron AJ, Tripathi R: Cystic disorders of the corneal epithelium. Br J Ophthalmol 1973; 57:361–375.
Cogan DG, et al.: Microcyctic dystrophy of the cornea: a partial explanation for its pathogenesis. Arch Ophthal. 1974; 92:470–474.
Laibson PR, Krachmer JH: Familial occurrence of dot (microcystic), map, fingerprint dystrophy of the cornea. Invest Ophthalmol 1975; 14:397–399.

G0006                     **Morton F. Goldberg**
SU001                           **Joel Sugar**

## CORNEAL DYSTROPHY, REIS-BUCKLERS TYPE 0215

**Includes:**
Annular corneal dystrophy
Reis-Bucklers corneal dystrophy
Ring-like corneal dystrophy

**Excludes:**
Corneal dystrophy, granular (0209)
Corneal dystrophy, recurrent erosive (0214)
Neuroparalytic keratitis

**Major Diagnostic Criteria:** Recurrent painful corneal desquamation begins in childhood. Ring-like or annular opacities develop in the region of Bowman membrane.

**Clinical Findings:** The juvenile onset of painful, recurring, bilateral desquamations of the cornea followed by annular opacifications of Bowman membrane. Corneal sensitivity and visual acuity are reduced. There may be a remission in early adult life, followed by a later relapse.

**Complications:** Reduced visual acuity due to corneal opacities.

**Associated Findings:** Strabismus.

**Etiology:** Autosomal dominant inheritance.

**Pathogenesis:** Basement membrane and hemidesmosomes are absent over areas of destruction of the Bowman layer. Corneal erosions and early recurrences in grafts suggest a primary epithelial abnormality.

**MIM No.:** *12150

**Sex Ratio:** M1:F1

**Occurrence:** Undetermined but presumed rare.

**Risk of Recurrence for Patient's Sib:**
See Part I, *Mendelian Inheritance.*

**Risk of Recurrence for Patient's Child:**
See Part I, *Mendelian Inheritance.*

**Age of Detectability:** About five years of age.

**Gene Mapping and Linkage:** Unknown.

**Prevention:** None known. Genetic counseling indicated.

**Treatment:** Lamellar keratoplasty or superficial keratectomy.

**Prognosis:** Good following keratoplasty, but reoccurs. Peeling of the subepithelial fibastic material is more effective. Relapsing corneal erosions have been reported between ages 8–20, and again in a more severe form at about age 40–50.

**Detection of Carrier:** By clinical examination.

**References:**
Paufique L, Bonnet M: La dystrophie cornéenne hérédo-familiale de Reis-Bücklers. Ann Oculist (Paris) 1966; 199:14–37.
Griffith DG, Fine BS: Light and electron microscopic observations in a superficial corneal dystrophy: probable early Reis-Bücklers' type. Am J Ophthalmol 1967; 63:1659–1666.
Maumenee AE: An introduction to corneal dystrophies. In: Bergsma D, ed: Part VIII. Eye. BD:OAS; VII (3). Baltimore: Williams and Wilkins Co. for The National Foundation-March of Dimes, 1971:3–12.
Bron AJ, Tripathi RC: Corneal disorders. In: Goldberg MF, ed: Genetic and metabolic eye disease. Boston: Little, Brown, and Co., 1974.
Perry HD, et al.: Reis-Bücklers dystrophy: a study of eight cases. Arch Ophthalmol 1979; 97:664–670.

G0006
SU001

**Morton F. Goldberg**
**Joel Sugar**

## CORNEAL DYSTROPHY, SCHNYDER CRYSTALLINE 0216

**Includes:**
Central crystalline corneal dystrophy
Corneal dystrophy, crystalline
Crystalline corneal dystrophy
Schnyder crystalline corneal dystrophy

**Excludes:**
Bietti marginal crystalline dystrophy
Cornea urica
Cystinosis (0238)
Dysproteinemias

**Major Diagnostic Criteria:** The appearance of needle-shaped crystals in the subepithelial area of the corneal stroma in a circular pattern.

**Clinical Findings:** In infancy, slowly progressive (or stationary), bilateral, needle-shaped crystals collect in the subepithelial region of the cornea. These crystals are distributed centrally or paracentrally in a circular or disk-shaped pattern and may be white or variegated, dull or scintillating. There is minimal irritation or loss of vision. Xanthelasmata, arcus juvenilis or senilis, and Vogt limbal girdles may coexist. Occasionally, hypercholesterolemia may be found. At least 2 different pedigrees have been reported with associated dystrophies of long bones. Genu valgum is a prominent finding in these cases.

**Complications:** Infrequently, decreased visual acuity occurs if the opacities overlie the visual axis.

**Associated Findings:** Joint abnormalities.

**Etiology:** Autosomal dominant inheritance.

**Pathogenesis:** Undetermined. Possibly related to abnormal lipid metabolism. Crystals are cholesterol.

**MIM No.:** *12180

**Sex Ratio:** M1:F1

**Occurrence:** About 50 cases reported; 21 cases in one family.

**Risk of Recurrence for Patient's Sib:**
See Part I, *Mendelian Inheritance.*

**Risk of Recurrence for Patient's Child:**
See Part I, *Mendelian Inheritance.*

**Age of Detectability:** In infancy.

**Gene Mapping and Linkage:** Unknown.

**Prevention:** None known. Genetic counseling indicated.

**Treatment:** Corneal grafting and surgery of the knees, when indicated.

**Prognosis:** Usually good for vision; keratoplasty usually successful if required.

**Detection of Carrier:** By slit lamp examination.

**References:**
Fry WE, Pickett WE: Crystalline dystrophy of cornea. Trans Am Ophthalmol Soc 1950; 48:220–227.
Malbran JL, et al.: Hereditary crystalline degeneration of cornea. Ophthalmologica 1953; 126:369–378.
Luxenberg M: Hereditary crystalline dystrophy of the cornea. Am J Ophthalmol 1967; 63:507–511.
Delleman JW, Winkelman JE: Degeneratio cornea cristallinea hereditaria: a clinical, genetic, and histologic study. Ophthalmologica 1968; 155:409–426.
Goldberg MF: A review of selected inherited corneal dystrophies associated with systemic diseases. In: Bergsma D, ed: Part VIII. Eye. BD:OAS VII (3). Baltimore: Williams and Wilkins Co. for The National Foundation- March of Dimes, 1971:13–25.
Kaden R, Feurle G: Schnydersche Hornhautdystrophie and Hyperipidamie: Albrecht v. Graefes. Arch Clin Exp Ophthalmol 1976; 198:129–138.

G0006
SU001

**Morton F. Goldberg**
**Joel Sugar**

## CORNEAL DYSTROPHY, STROMAL, CONGENITAL HEREDITARY 3198

**Includes:** Stromal dystrophy of the cornea, congenital hereditary

**Excludes:**
Anterior segment mesenchymal dysgenesis
**Corneal dystrophy, endothelial** (0208)
**Corneal dystrophy, endothelial, congenital hereditary** (0207)
Cloudy cornea at birth, other causes

**Major Diagnostic Criteria:** Bilateral congenital feathery opacification of the corneal stroma, with normal appearing epithelium, Bowman membrane, corneal thickness, Descemet membrane, and corneal endothelium.

**Clinical Findings:** Corneal clouding is noted at birth and is more marked centrally. Patients develop nystagmus, and estimates of vision in reported cases range from 20/100 to 20/500. Some patients have esotropia and others have high myopia. On slit-lamp biomicroscopy, the cornea is found to be of normal thickness; the corneal epithelium, Descemet membrane, and endothelium appear normal; corneal opacities have a feathery but confluent appearance and are more prominent in the anterior stroma. On light microscopy, the pathologic changes are limited to the stroma where collagen lamellae are separated from each other in a fine reticular manner resulting in a widespread fibrillary appearance. On electron microscopy, collagen filaments measure only 150 Angstroms in diameter (normal 190–340 Angstroms) and are present in one of two patterns of lamellar groupings: tightly packed, or loosely and haphazardously arranged. The anterior portion of Descemet membrane does not show the normal banding pattern.

**Complications:** Poor visual acuity with amblyopia, nystagmus and strabismus.

**Associated Findings:** None known.

**Etiology:** Autosomal dominant inheritance.

**Pathogenesis:** Because of the confinement of pathologic changes to the corneal stroma, and the abnormalities in collagen fibril size and arrangement, it is believed that congenital hereditary stromal dystrophy is a disorder of stromal fibrillogenesis.
An early embryonic short-lived disturbance of the corneal endothelium may lead to an abnormal anterior portion of Descemet membrane; since normal stromal fibrillogenesis is dependent on a normal endothelium, the same transient endothelial dysfunction may account for the stationary stromal opacification.

**Sex Ratio:** M1:F1

**Occurrence:** Two families have been reliably studied clinically and histopathologically. One Europian family has been extensively studied and reported several times, lastly by Witschel and co-workers (1978) who also described another patient from an American family. Other families have been reported but the clinical and pathologic findings in affected members have not been adequately documented.

**Risk of Recurrence for Patient's Sib:**
See Part I, *Mendelian Inheritance.*

**Risk of Recurrence for Patient's Child:**
See Part I, *Mendelian Inheritance.*

**Age of Detectability:** At birth.

**Gene Mapping and Linkage:** Unknown.

**Prevention:** None known. Genetic counseling indicated.

**Treatment:** Penetrating keratoplasty should be performed as early as possible to prevent the development of amblyopia. Reported cases have been operated on after age five or six years, but by that time had developed amblyopia, nystagmus, and strabismus. Vision could only be modestly improved even though grafts remained clear for several years and up to 16 years in one case. Opacities in the remaining host corneal rim have remained stable over time.

**Prognosis:** Poor for vision if penetrating keratoplasty is delayed. No experience is available with penetrating keratoplasty and adequate amblyopia treatment early in infancy.

**Detection of Carrier:** Unknown.

**Special Considerations:** This condition must be differentiated from **Corneal dystrophy, endothelial, congenital hereditary** which is a progressive corneal disease with endothelial dysfunction, increased corneal thickness, and secondary Bowman membrane and epithelial changes; and stromal collagen fibrils are of normal or larger diameter.

**References:**
Witschel H, et al: Congenital hereditary stromal dystrophy of the cornea. Arch Ophthalmol 1978; 96:1043–1051.

TR009     **Elias I. Traboulsi**
FI033     **Ben S. Fine**

**Corneal dystrophy-dermo-chondro of Francois**
*See DERMO-CHONDRO-CORNEAL DYSTROPHY, FRANCOIS TYPE*
**Corneal dystrophy-gum hypertrophy**
*See GINGIVAL FIBROMATOSIS-CORNEAL DYSTROPHY*
**Corneal dystrophy-hyperkeratosis-short stature-brachydactyly**
*See CORNEO-DERMATO-OSSEOUS SYNDROME*
**Corneal dystrophy-poor eruption of teeth-gingival fibromatosis**
*See GINGIVAL FIBROMATOSIS-CORNEAL DYSTROPHY*

## CORNEAL DYSTROPHY-SENSORINEURAL DEAFNESS 0206

**Includes:**
Deafness, sensorineural-corneal dystrophy
Perceptive deafness-corneal dystrophy

**Excludes:**
Avascular syphilitic intrastitial keratosis
**Corneal dystrophy, endothelial, congenital hereditary** (0207)
Corneal dystrophy-abnormal calcium metabolism-hearing loss
Corneal dystrophy-hearing loss-mental retardation-obesity
**Glaucoma, congenital** (0414)
**Mucopolysaccharidosis I-H** (0674)

**Major Diagnostic Criteria:** Corneal dystrophy and sensorineural hearing loss.

**Clinical Findings:** The only family known consists of two sisters and their half-brother. The parents in both unions (the father was the same) were first cousins. Diffuse bluish-white opacities of the cornea and decreased vision from birth were seen in all three children. The corneal epithelium surface appeared to be rough in one and bedewed in two. All three stroma were diffusely edematous and thickened. The cornea was not vascularized. Audiometry showed bilateral progressive sensorineural hearing loss, especially for the high tones (2/3) beginning in late childhood.

**Complications:** Unknown.

**Associated Findings:** Intraocular pressure was elevated in one of three children. Recurrent bilateral otitis media (1/3). Intelligence was normal.

**Etiology:** Probably autosomal recessive inheritance.

**Pathogenesis:** An increased diameter of collagen fibrils in the stroma, a thinned Descemet membrane, and ultrastructural anomalies suggestive of defective endothelium were inferred from other cases, as was a degeneration of the stria vascularis and a loss of ganglion cells in the organ of Corti.

**MIM No.:** 21740

**POS No.:** 3153

**Sex Ratio:** M1:F2

**Occurrence:** One reported family with three affected individuals.

**Risk of Recurrence for Patient's Sib:**
See Part I, *Mendelian Inheritance.*

**Risk of Recurrence for Patient's Child:**
See Part I, *Mendelian Inheritance.*

**Age of Detectability:** Early adolescence.

**Gene Mapping and Linkage:** Unknown.

**Prevention:** None known. Genetic counseling indicated.

**Treatment:** Treatment of glaucoma and perhaps corneal transplants; glycerin instillation to improve vision. Hearing aids, speech and language therapy, and special schooling to mitigate the effects of deafness. Avoidance of prolonged periods of excessive noise and ototoxic drugs is very important.

**Prognosis:** Vision will deteriorate more rapidly than hearing.

**Detection of Carrier:** Unknown.

**References:**
Harboyan G, et al.: Congenital corneal dystrophy, progressive sensorineural deafness in a family. Arch Ophthalmol 1971; 85:27–32.

DA026                        **Sandra L.H. Davenport**
*Cor W.R.J. Cremers*

**Corneal dystrophy-spinocerebellar degeneration**
*See SPINOCEREBELLAR DEGENERATION-CORNEAL DYSTROPHY*
**Corneal hypesthesia-retinal anomalies-deafness-unusual facies**
*See CORNEAL ANESTHESIA-RETINAL DEFECTS-UNUSUAL FACIES-HEART DEFECT*
**Corneal leukoma-acromegaloid phenotype-cutis verticis**
*See ACROMEGALOID PHENOTYPE-CUTIS VERTICIS GYRATA-CORNEAL LEUKOMA*
**Corneal opacities-dyslipoproteinemia**
*See LECITHIN-CHOLESTEROL ACYL TRANSFERASE DEFICIENCY*
**Corneal opacities-gingival fibromatosis**
*See GINGIVAL FIBROMATOSIS-CORNEAL DYSTROPHY*
**Corneal-cerebellar syndrome**
*See SPINOCEREBELLAR DEGENERATION-CORNEAL DYSTROPHY*
**Cornelia de Lange Syndrome**
*See DE LANGE SYNDROME*

---

**CORNEO-DERMATO-OSSEOUS SYNDROME**      **2760**

**Includes:**
Brachydactyly-corneal dystrophy-hyperkeratosis-short stature
Corneal dystrophy, epithelial-skin and skeletal changes
Corneal dystrophy-hyperkeratosis-short stature-brachydactyly
Ectodermal dysplasia, corneo-dermato-osseous type
Hyperkeratosis-corneal dystrophy-short stature-brachydactyly

**Excludes:**
Corneal dystrophy, endothelial
Hyperkeratosis palmoplantaris
Lecithin-cholesterol acyl transferase deficiency (0580)
Tyrosinemia II, Oregon type (2009)

**Major Diagnostic Criteria:** Skin biopsy specimens show hyperkeratosis and acanthosis. Corneal biopsy specimens demonstrate mild dysplastic epithelial changes. X-rays show shortening of almost all hand bones, cortical thickening, and bulbous radial heads.

**Clinical Findings:** A unique nodular corneal dystrophy is present in adulthood, although the earliest age of onset is not certain. Affected persons complain of photophobia, reduced night vision, and varying visual acuity decreases. During the first month of life a skin disorder becomes apparent, with thickened, erythematous, scaly lesions on palms, soles, elbows, knees, and knuckles. There is scaling and occasional crusting of the scalp. Nails show distal onycholysis. There is mild shortness of stature: women average 155 cm, men 163 cm. There is **Brachydactyly** and single palmar creases. The proximal interphalangeal joints show soft tissue swelling. Teeth tend to be soft and subject to decay, with enamel dysplasia (although this is variable). Affected persons seem to be born 1–2 months premature.

**Complications:** Prematurity seems to be the rule. Visual problems are also to be expected. Loss of teeth and other dental problems occur frequently.

**Associated Findings:** A generalized erythroderma, carpal tunnel syndrome, and glomerulonephritis have each occurred in single affected family members. Their relationship to the syndrome is uncertain.

**Etiology:** Probably autosomal dominant inheritance. Three instances of male-to-male transmission have been reported.

**Pathogenesis:** Appears to belong to the broad group of ectodermal dysplasias.

**MIM No.:** 12244

**POS No.:** 4114

**Sex Ratio:** M1:F1

**Occurrence:** One kindred with seven affected persons over three generations has been reported.

**Risk of Recurrence for Patient's Sib:**
See Part I, *Mendelian Inheritance.*

**Risk of Recurrence for Patient's Child:**
See Part I, *Mendelian Inheritance.*

**Age of Detectability:** Skin changes which appear in the first month, combined with prematurity, can suggest the condition.

**Gene Mapping and Linkage:** Unknown.

**Prevention:** None known. Genetic counseling indicated.

**Treatment:** Symptomatic.

**Prognosis:** Normal life span with limited functional impairment aside from visual difficulties. In one patient in whom a corneal transplantation was performed, there was a tendency for recurrence as the donor epithelium was replaced.

**Detection of Carrier:** Unknown.

**References:**
Stern JK, et al.: Corneal changes, hyperkeratosis, short stature, brachydactyly, and premature birth: a new autosomal dominant syndrome. Am J Med Genet 1984; 18:67–77.

LU001                              **Mark Lubinsky**

**Cornification, disorder of (one form)**
*See ICHTHYOSIFORM ERYTHROKERATODERMA, ATYPICAL WITH DEAFNESS*
**Cornification, disorder of, bullous type (DOC 3)**
*See ICHTHYOSIFORM HYPERKERATOSIS, BULLOUS CONGENITAL*
**Cornification, disorder of, congenital erythrodermic type (DOC 5)**
*See ICHTHYOSIS, CONGENITAL ERYTHRODERMIC*
**Cornification, disorder of, harlequin type (DOC 6)**
*See ICHTHYOSIS, HARLEQUIN FETUS*
**Cornification, disorder of, lamellar dominant (DOC 6)**
*See ICHTHYOSIS, LAMELLAR DOMINANT*
**Cornification, disorder of, Netherton type (DOC 9)**
*See ICHTHYOSIS, LINEARIS CIRCUMFLEXA*
**Cornification, disorder of, neutral lipid storage type (DOC 12)**
*See STORAGE DISEASE, NEUTRAL LIPID TYPE*
**Cornification, disorders of, lamellar recessive (DOC 4)**
*See ICHTHYOSIS, LAMELLAR RECESSIVE*
**Coronal dentin dysplasia**
*See TEETH, DENTIN DYSPLASIA, CORONAL*
**Coronary arterial calcinosis**
*See ARTERY, CORONARY CALCINOSIS*
**Coronary arteries, anomalous origin from pulmonary artery**
*See ARTERY, CORONARY, ANOMALOUS ORIGIN FROM PULMONARY ARTERY*
**Coronary arteries, congenital medial sclerosis of**
*See ARTERY, CORONARY CALCINOSIS*
**Coronary arteriovenous fistula**
*See ARTERY, CORONARY, ARTERIOVENOUS FISTULA*
**Coronary artery sclerosis**
*See ARTERY, CORONARY CALCINOSIS*
**Coronary artery, single left or right**
*See ARTERY, SINGLE CORONARY*
**Coronary artery-cameral shunt**
*See ARTERY, CORONARY, ARTERIOVENOUS FISTULA*
**Coronary calcification of infancy**
*See ARTERY, CORONARY CALCINOSIS*
**Coronary disease, and hyperapobetalipoproteinemia**
*See HYPERAPOBETALIPOPROTEINEMIA*

**Coronary sclerosis, juvenile or infantile**
*See ARTERY, CORONARY CALCINOSIS*

---

## CORPUS CALLOSUM AGENESIS 0220

**Includes:**
  Agenesis of corpus callosum
  Agenesis of corpus callosum, partial

**Excludes:**
  **Aicardi syndrome** (2320)
  **Corpus callosum agenesis-sensorimotor neuropathy, familial**
    (3032)
  Forebrain defects

**Major Diagnostic Criteria:** X-ray studies showing a large dorsal displaced third ventricle separating the lateral ventricles so that they assume a "bat-wing" appearance. CAT scan shows separation of lateral ventricles.

**Clinical Findings:** Diagnosed in childhood in the investigation of mental retardation or macrocephaly. Most show severe, but nonprogressive retardation, not incompatible with life. Abnormalities of cerebrospinal fluid circulation are present in a large number of subjects with hydrocephaly. Rarely associated is cleft palate or lip. If corpus callosum is partially developed, this will occur anterior with the defects posterior. The septum pellucidum is absent; the fornix is abnormal with a well-developed longitudinal bundle. Some affected individuals are apparently symptom-free; their diagnosis is as an incidental finding. Defective integrative performance for visual and fine motor tasks may be apparent with careful testing of patients who are otherwise symptom-free.

**Complications:** Hydrocephaly is usually of the communicating variety.

**Associated Findings:** A small brain is a common associated defect in mentally retarded patients. The interhemispheric defect may be filled by a lipoma or cyst derived from the third ventricle or arachnoid membranes. Hippocampal commissure is absent; anterior commissure is present. A wide variety of non-CNS abnormalities have been reported.

**Etiology:** Mendelian inheritance or chromosomal defects seldom play a part in humans, except in two reports documenting X-linked familial occurrence. In the mouse, absence of the corpus callosum and presence of a longitudinal callosal bundle may be autosomal recessive.

**Pathogenesis:** The corpus callosum does not develop until the 12th week, when the first fibers appear anteriorly near the lamina terminalis. Crossing of fibers is complete by 22 weeks. A vascular cause has been suggested, but, if this were acting, more widespread defects of the hemispheres would be anticipated. An interference with this process would account for the pathology.

**MIM No.:** *30410

**POS No.:** 3154

**Sex Ratio:** Unknown.

**Occurrence:** Unknown.

**Risk of Recurrence for Patient's Sib:** Unknown.

**Risk of Recurrence for Patient's Child:** Unknown.

**Age of Detectability:** Variable: first year, 82%; second year, 6.5%. Nearly 90% in first 2 years of life

**Gene Mapping and Linkage:** Unknown.

**Prevention:** None known. Genetic counseling indicated.

**Treatment:** Treatment of **Hydrocephaly** and seizures if they occur.

**Prognosis:** Most patients do not die because of the absence of the corpus callosum. Mental retardation is nonprogressive.

**Detection of Carrier:** Unknown.

**Special Considerations:** Secondary loss of the corpus callosum occurs in extreme degrees of hydrocephaly and may also be found in cases of spina bifida with multiple coincidental malformations of brain and viscera.

**References:**
Menkes JH, et al.: Hereditary partial agenesis of corpus callosum. Arch Neurol 1964; 11:198–208.
Loeser JD, Alvord EC Jr: Clinicopathological correlations in agenesis of the corpus callosum. Neurology 1968; 18:745.
Probst FP: Congenital defects of the corpus callosum. Morphology and encephalographic appearances. Acta Radiol [Diagn] [Suppl] (Stockh) 1973; 1–152.
Parrish ML, et al.: Agenesis of the corpus callosum: a study of the frequency of associated oral formations. Ann Neurol 1979; 6:349–354.
Lynn RB, et al.: Agenesis of the corpus callosum. Arch Neurol 1980; 37:444–445.
Kaplan P: X-linked recessive inheritance of agenesis of the corpus callosum. J Med Genet 1983; 20:122–124.

SH007                                          **Kenneth Shapiro**

---

## CORPUS CALLOSUM AGENESIS-SENSORIMOTOR NEUROPATHY, FAMILIAL 3032

**Includes:**
  Agenesis of the corpus callosum-anterior horn cell disease
  Andermann syndrome
  Charlevoix disease (one type)
  Neuronopathy, sensorimotor-agenesis of the corpus callosum
  Sensorimotor neuronopathy-agenesis of the corpus callosum

**Excludes:**
  Agenesis of the corpus callosum-macrocephaly
  **Corpus callosum agenesis** (0220)
  Neuropathy, peripheral (other)

**Major Diagnostic Criteria:** Complete agenesis of the corpus callosum, mental retardation, slowly progressive peripheral neuropathy, and specific dysmorphic features.

**Clinical Findings:** In areas of high incidence, such as the Charlevoix-Lac-St.-Jean region of Québec, or in sibs of an affected child, the diagnosis may be suspected and established at 4–6 months of age. The infants are hypotonic, particularly in the lower extremities, areflexic, and have a characteristic square face. They may learn to walk with aid or braces by ages 4–8 years, then become weaker and are confined to a wheelchair by ages 10–13 years. There is striking footdrop. Severe contractures of the feet and hands. The thumbs are digitalized, perhaps because of subluxation. Areflexia, hypotonia, weakness, and wasting are present in 100% of patients. Cerebellar dysfunction is present in 37% of patients, nystagmus in 29%, sensory abnormalities in 18% (this is probably an underestimate related to mental retardation), strabismus in 24%, seizures in 22%, and asymmetric ptosis in 42%.

Dysmorphic features are progressive and include long, triangular, asymmetric face; hypoplastic maxilla; large angle of the mandible; low hairline; long distance from the lip to the chin; short neck; brachycephaly (see **Craniosynostosis**); high-arched palate; and **Eye, hypertelorism**.

Moderate mental retardation is present, with IQs of 45–60 in the majority, but with exceptional patients in the borderline or low-normal range. In the teens and 20s, episodes of hallucinatory psychosis and a tendency to speak less have been noted in some patients, but there is no evidence for progressive mental deterioration.

Patients usually die in the third or fourth decade from cardiopulmonary complications due to extreme scoliosis.

Pneumoencephalography and CT scans show complete agenesis of the corpus callosum, although in some undoubtedly affected probands or sibs this structure may be present. Electrodiagnostic tests show denervation with absent sensory potentials and some slowing of motor conduction velocity. CSF protein is mildly elevated (65–80 mg%).

Pathologic studies show many greatly enlarged axons with few neurofilaments and neurotubules and disproportionately thin myelin sheaths. These enlarged axons are present in anterior and posterior nerve roots and in the sciatic nerve. Axons of anterior horn cells within the spinal cord are normal; and examination of the brain shows only agenesis of the corpus callosum, with absence of the septum pellucidum.

**Complications:** A severe, progressive scoliosis leads to pain and cardiorespiratory complications. Urinary incontinence may develop in the third decade.

**Associated Findings:** None known.

**Etiology:** Autosomal recessive inheritance. Two hundred thirty-seven cases from the Charlevoix-Lax-St.-Jean area of Québec have been traced to a common ancestral couple who married in Québec City in the 17th century, demonstrating a founder effect.

**Pathogenesis:** The syndrome combines a major malformation of the CNS that is generally present with a unique peripheral neuropathy. The pathologic changes result from swelling and subsequent collapse of axons. A number of additional minor malformations are found. No chromosomal abnormalities have been demonstrated.

**MIM No.:** *21800

**POS No.:** 3911

**Sex Ratio:** M1:F1

**Occurrence:** In the Charlevoix-Saguenay-Lac-St.-Jean area of Québec, the prevalence of the disease is 68:100,000 (based on 237 reported cases in a population of 350,000). The incidence at birth is 44:100,000, with a gene frequency of 1:50, or two percent, in this population. The carrier frequency in the population at risk is 4%.

In addition to the French-Canadian patients described above, affected sibs born to consanguineous Algerian parents, an Italian patient presented by Battistella et al (1986), and American sibs examined by Najdu (1982) have been reported.

**Risk of Recurrence for Patient's Sib:**
See Part I, *Mendelian Inheritance.*

**Risk of Recurrence for Patient's Child:**
See Part I, *Mendelian Inheritance.* Because of their severe disability and retardation, the patients do not reproduce, and there is no record of any pregnancy involving an affected male or female.

**Age of Detectability:** Prenatal diagnosis based on ultrasound diagnosis of agenesis of the corpus callosum has been suggested, but has never been demonstrated, since all pregnancies in which it was carried out resulted in a normal child. Postnatal diagnosis varies with the index of suspicion, but can be made during infancy.

**Gene Mapping and Linkage:** Unknown.

**Prevention:** None known. Genetic counseling indicated.

**Treatment:** Orthopedic measures include bracing or the use of crutches and treatment of scoliosis by Harrington rods. Antiepileptic and antipsychotic agents may be required as appropriate.

**Prognosis:** Most patients die in the third or fourth decade, usually from cardiorespiratory complications of scoliosis. It is not entirely clear whether mental deterioration occurs. The absence of CNS abnormalities other than the callosal agenesis in one autopsied case does not suggest a progressive cerebral deterioration.

**Detection of Carrier:** Unknown.

**Special Considerations:** This syndrome is due to an unusual association of a fixed congenital anomaly with a progressive peripheral neuropathy that has very unusual and quite specific pathologic changes. The neuropathy, dysmorphic features, and mental retardation may occur in some patients whose corpus callosum is present.

**References:**

Andermann F, et al.: Familial agenesis of the corpus callosum with anterior horn cell disease: a syndrome of mental retardation, areflexia, and paraparesis. Trans Am Neurol Assoc 1972; 97:242–244.

Andermann E, et al.: Three familial midline malformation syndromes of the central nervous system: agenesis of the corpus callosum and anterior horn cell disease; agenesis of the cerebellar vermis; and atrophy of the cerebellar vermis. BD:OAS XI(2). New York: March of Dimes Birth Defects Foundation, 1975:269–293. †

Andermann E: Agenesis of the corpus callosum. In: Myrianthopoulos NC, ed: Handbook of clinical neurology, vol 42: Neurogenetic directory, part 1. Amsterdam: North Holland, 1981:6–9.

Andermann E: Sensorimotor neuronopathy with agenesis of the corpus callosum. In: Myrianthopoulos NC, ed: Handbook of clinical neurology, vol 42: Neurogenetic directory, part 1. Amsterdam: North Holland 1981:100–103. * †

Giroud M, Langevin P: Agenesie du corps calleux et atteinte de la corne anterieure de la moelle: une affection rare. Pediatrie 1982; 37:113–117.

Nagy JR: Familial agenesis of the corpus callosum with sensorimotor neuronopathy: genetic and epidemiological studies. M.Sc. thesis, Montreal: McGill University, 1982. *

Larbrisseau A, et al.: The Andermann syndrome: agenesis of the corpus callosum associated with mental retardation and progressive sensorimotor neuronopathy. Can J Neurol Sci 1984; 11:257–261. *

Battistella PA, et al: La sindrome di Andermann: primo caso Italiano. Chieti, Italy: Proc XIIth Nat Cong Neuropediatr 1986:161.

AN016                                                        **Eva Andermann**
AN018                                               **Frederick Andermann**

**Corpus callosum, agenesis of-chorioretinal abnormality**
See *AICARDI SYNDROME*

**Corrected transposition of great vessels/arteries**
See *VENTRICLES, INVERTED WITH TRANSPOSITION OF GREAT ARTERIES*

**Cortical cataract**
See *CATARACT, AUTOSOMAL DOMINANT CONGENITAL*

---

## CORTICAL HYPEROSTOSIS, INFANTILE                    0221

**Includes:** Caffey disease

**Excludes:**
Cherubism (0539)
Secondary hyperostoses, e.g., hypervitaminosis A

**Major Diagnostic Criteria:** Young infants show irritability and painful soft tissue swelling over affected bone, with elevated temperature. Subperiosteal new bone formation is found on X-ray of affected region. The mandible, clavicle, and ulna are most frequently affected. Only diaphyses are involved; metaphyses are normal.

**Clinical Findings:** Soft tissue swelling generally occurs under age 5 months and may even be prenatal. Hyperirritability accompanies the swelling of soft tissues, especially overlying the mandible. The swelling is tender but not warm or discolored. Onset is generally sudden in original sites and in recurrences; symptoms may resolve in one site while appearing in another. A mild-to-moderate temperature elevation is generally present. Spontaneous resolution occurs within weeks or months. White blood cell response is variable and not diagnostic. Hemoglobin is usually slightly low; erythrocyte sedimentation rate is elevated, and alkaline phosphatase is frequently elevated. Occasionally, thrombocytosis and elevated IgA and IgM occur alone or in combination. Initially, the soft tissue swelling is all that is visible by X-ray. The cortical hyperostoses may be present at the clinical onset, indicating prior disease. Progressive, variable, external cortical thickening is found in the affected bones. One bone may show severe alteration while an adjacent one is unaffected. In the mandible, massive thickening resembles the structureless appearance of fibrous dysplasia, but serial subperiosteal layers of new bone may be identified in appropriate projections. In the scapulae, the changes may simulate neoplasia. Cranial changes include focal resorption of the outer table of bone, resembling neuroblastoma as well as external hyperostoses. Affected orbital bones may produce proptosis. All bones have been affected except phalanges, round bones, and vertebrae. The mandible (80%), clavicle (50%), and ulna are the most commonly affected bones.

**Complications:** In exceptional cases, radioulnar synostosis with radial head dislocation; leg length discrepancy; bony bridging of adjacent affected ribs; proptosis; exophthalmos (rare); ipsilateral diaphragmatic paralysis or Erb paralysis associated with scapular involvement. Bowing of affected bones may occur after recovery. Pleural reactions occur when ribs are involved.

**Associated Findings:** None known.

**Etiology:** Autosomal dominant inheritance with incomplete penetrance and varying expression. Craniomandibular osteopathy in the canine is suggested as an animal model by Thornburg (1979). A viral agent has been suspected because of inflammatory changes on biopsy, apparent early immunity, and failure of response to anti-infectious agents. Milk allergy is postulated but unproved; collagen disease is also suggested.

The disease is sometimes familial, generally sporadic. An infectious cause is possible, although careful studies have failed to identify bacterial or viral infection. Endogenous prostaglandin disturbance is possible. X-ray findings may sometimes resemble those of a neoplasm from which this condition needs to be distinguished.

Several typical cases, except for lack of mandibular involvement, have occurred in infants receiving long-term prostaglandin E (PGE) therapy. Improvement has been observed in five cases of clinical Caffey disease after indomethacin treatment; PGE levels were high initially and were normal at end of therapy.

**Pathogenesis:** Undetermined. Early inflammatory reaction of periosteum with polymorphonuclear infiltration. Periosteal fibrous layers lose definition and merge with adjacent soft tissue, while inflammatory reaction extends into it and contiguous muscles. Some focal resorption of cortical bone was observed histologically but not on X-ray except in calvarium in rare cases. Subsequent production of subperiosteal new bone. Obliterating intimal proliferation in small arteries of affected bone and fascia has been described.

**MIM No.:** *11400

**POS No.:** 3430

**CDC No.:** 756.530

**Sex Ratio:** M1:F1

**Occurrence:** An early report indicates 3:1,000 patients under age 6 months in hospitals and clinics; a more recent review lists a high of 48:100,000 admissions to hospitals. A series of cases may be observed over a period of several months, and then years may pass before another case heralds the onset of another series. Eleven cases have been reported in two generations of one family.

**Risk of Recurrence for Patient's Sib:**
See Part I, *Mendelian Inheritance.*

**Risk of Recurrence for Patient's Child:**
See Part I, *Mendelian Inheritance.*

**Age of Detectability:** Onset almost invariably before age 5 months. Usually detected within the first 6 months, with recovery by the end of the first year.

**Gene Mapping and Linkage:** Unknown.

**Prevention:** None known. Genetic counseling indicated.

**Treatment:** Symptomatic treatment for fever and irritability. In progressive or severe cases, steroids produce remission within 3 days; relapses after cessation of treatment for 10 days are not uncommon. Steroids may be contraindicated in patients with elevated platelet counts. Anti-inflammatory agents (e.g., aspirin, indomethacin) may be useful if prostaglandin excess is involved.

**Prognosis:** Good. Recovery is usually complete, life span is normal, and intelligence is unimpaired. Rare chronic cases and cases with late onset have been described. Extremely rare deaths have occurred, but the relationship of the death to the primary disease is uncertain.

**Detection of Carrier:** Unknown.

**References:**
Caffey J: Infantile cortical hyperostosis: a review of the clinical and radiographic features. Proc R Soc Med 1957; 50:347.
Finsterbusch A, Rang M: Infantile cortical hyperostosis. Follow-up of 29 cases. Acta Paediatr Scand 1975; 216:727.
Thornburg LP: Animal model of human disease. Infantile cortical hyperostosis (Caffey-Silverman syndrome). Am J Path 1979; 95:575.
Saul RA, et al.: Caffey's disease revisited. Further evidence for autosomal dominant inheritance with incomplete penetrance. Am J Dis Child 1982; 136:56.
MacLachlan AK, et al.: Familial infantile cortical hyperostosis in a large Canadian family. Canad Med Assoc J 1984; 130:1172–1174.
Silverman FN: Pediatric X-ray. In: Caffey J, ed: Diagnosis, ed 8. Chicago: Year Book Medical Publishers, 1984. *

BE008
**Peter Beighton**
*Frederic N. Silverman*

**Cortical hyperostosis-syndactyly**
See SCLEROSTEOSIS
**Cortical thickening-skeletal bowing-bone fragility-ichthyosis**
See SKELETAL BOWING-CORTICAL THICKENING-BONE FRAGILITY-ICTHYOSIS
**Corticosteroid-binding globulin abnormalities**
See STEROID, BINDING GLOBULIN ABNORMALITIES
**Corticosteroid-binding globulin, decreased**
See STEROID, BINDING GLOBULIN ABNORMALITIES
**Corticosteroid-binding globulin, increased**
See STEROID, BINDING GLOBULIN ABNORMALITIES
**Corticosterone methyl oxidase type I deficiency**
See STEROID 18-HYDROXYLASE DEFICIENCY
**Corticosterone methyl oxidase type II deficiency**
See STEROID 18-HYDROXYSTEROID DEHYDROGENASE DEFICIENCY
**Cortisol resistance, familial**
See GLUCOCORTICOID RESISTANCE
**Cortisol resistance, primary**
See GLUCOCORTICOID RESISTANCE
**Costovertebral dysplasia**
See SPONDYLOTHORACIC DYSPLASIA
**Costovertebral dysplasia-hydrocephalus-Sprengel anomaly**
See HYDROCEPHALUS-COSTOVERTEBRAL DYSPLASIA-SPRENGEL ANOMALY
**Costovertebral segmentation anomalies**
See SPONDYLOCOSTAL DYSPLASIA
**Costovertebral segmentation defect-mesomelia**
See ROBINOW SYNDROME
**Cough syrup induced goiter**
See GOITER, GOITROGEN INDUCED
**Coumadin embryopathy**
See FETAL WARFARIN SYNDROME
**Counterwing teeth**
See TEETH, MESIOPALATAL TORSION OF CENTRAL INCISORS
**COVESDEM syndrome**
See ROBINOW SYNDROME
**Cowden disease**
See GINGIVAL MULTIPLE HAMARTOMA SYNDROME
**Coxa vara (hip, congenital)**
See HIP, CONGENITAL COXA VARA
**Coxa vara, idiopathic**
See HIP, CONGENITAL COXA VARA
**Coxa vara, infantile**
See HIP, CONGENITAL COXA VARA
**CR3 deficiency**
See COMPLEMENT COMPONENT 3, DEFICIENCY OF

## CRANDALL SYNDROME 3257

**Includes:**
Alopecia-deafness-hypogonadism
Deafness-alopecia-hypogonadism
Hypogonadism-deafness-alopecia

**Excludes:**
**Deafness-pili torti, Bjornstad type** (2015)
**Ectodermal dysplasia**
**Sohval-Soffer syndrome** (3258)

**Major Diagnostic Criteria:** The combination of alopecia, neurosensory deafness, and hypogonadism.

**Clinical Findings:** Alopecia consisting of absent body hair and eyebrows; eyelashes were short, curled and sparse, and head hair was sparse with pili torti. Neuro-sensory deafness, which was diagnosed in early childhood and was progressive. Short stature.

Two of three affected sibs also had hypogonadism, highly pitched voice, and increased carrying angle. Testicular biopsy demonstrated depletion of interstitial cells; laboratory studies suggested that gonadotropin insufficiency was the cause of hypogonadism. Growth hormone release was also diminished.

**Complications:** Unknown.

**Associated Findings:** None known.

**Etiology:** Probably autosomal recessive inheritance, although X-linked recessive inheritance has not been ruled out.

**Pathogenesis:** Unknown.

**MIM No.:** 26200

**Sex Ratio:** M3:F0 observed.

**Occurrence:** One sibship of three affected males has been reported.

**Risk of Recurrence for Patient's Sib:**
See Part I, *Mendelian Inheritance.*

**Risk of Recurrence for Patient's Child:**
See Part I, *Mendelian Inheritance.*

**Age of Detectability:** If family history is positive, within the first year of life by the presence of alopecia. Otherwise at puberty when the hypogonadism becomes evident.

**Gene Mapping and Linkage:** Unknown.

**Prevention:** None known. Genetic counseling indicated.

**Treatment:** Unknown.

**Prognosis:** Life span is probably unaffected. Mental development is near normal, with IQ's between 87–97 in the three affected boys.

**Detection of Carrier:** Unknown.

**Special Considerations:** Although these individuals were reported by Reed et al (1967) as having **Deafness-pili torti, Bjornstad type,** they were prepubertal at the time and the hypogonadism had not yet become evident.

**References:**
Reed WB, et al.: Hereditary syndrome with auditory and dermatologic manifestations. Arch Derm 1967; 95:456 only.
Crandall B, et al.: A familial syndrome of deafness, alopecia, and hypogonadism. J Pediatr 1973; 82:461–465.

T0007                                   **Helga V. Toriello**

**Cranial meningoceles**
*See MENINGOCELE*
**Cranial meningoencephaloceles**
*See ENCEPHALOCELE*
**Cranial sclerosis-osteopathia striata-macrocephaly**
*See OSTEOPATHIA STRIATA-CRANIAL SCLEROSIS-
MEGALENCEPHALY*

---

## CRANIO-CARPO-TARSAL DYSPLASIA, WHISTLING FACE TYPE                                   0223

**Includes:**
Carpo-tarsal and cranial dystrophy
Freeman-Sheldon syndrome
Whistling face syndrome
Windmill vane hand syndrome

**Excludes:** N/A

**Major Diagnostic Criteria:** Flat, immobile facies with sunken eyes, bulging cheeks, and pursed lips. Ulnar deviation of hands and finger contractures.

**Clinical Findings:** Hypotonia in infancy with flat face, deep-set eyes, full cheeks, and protuding lips as in whistling. Hypertelorism, convergent strabismus, a mild degree of blepharophimosis, and antimongoloid obliquity of the palpebral tissues are the major ocular findings. The small nose has notched alae at the proximal attachment (coloboma alae). The philtrum is long. The central parts of the cheek bulge excessively, resembling that seen

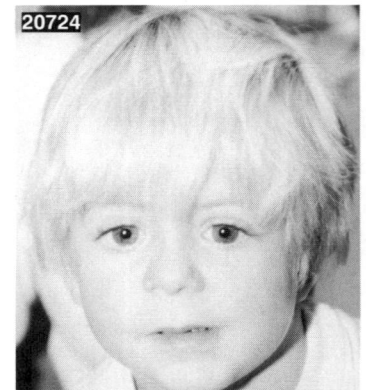
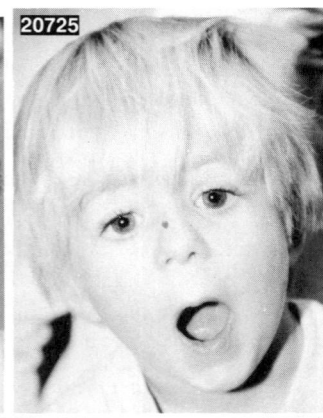
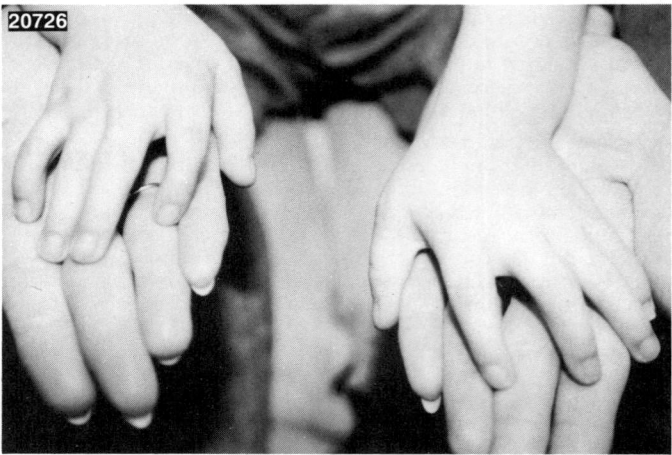

**0223-20724:** Cranio-carpo-tarsal dysplasia, whistling face type; note small nose, long philtrum, and H-shaped groove on the chin. **20725:** Subject is trying to open mouth and smile. **20726:** Ulnar deviation of the fingers.

---

when whistling, due to muscle atrophy. Oral findings are microstomia and high-arched palate. There is a fibrous band or elevation that is demarcated by two paramedian grooves, forming an H- or V-shaped, scar-like structure extending from the middle of the lower lip to the chin. Thickening of the skin and subcutaneous tissues over the flexor surface of hands, flexion contractures of the fingers, especially the metacarpophalangeal joint of the thumbs. Talipes equinovarus and a short neck are also found.

**Complications:** Walking difficulties. Growth retardation. Feeding problems due to severe microstomia.

**Associated Findings:** Ocular abnormalities.

**Etiology:** Autosomal dominant inheritance. Some families show autosomal recessive inheritance.

**Pathogenesis:** Undetermined. Possibly a myopathic arthrygryposis.

**MIM No.:** *19370, 27772

**POS No.:** 3156

**CDC No.:** 759.800

**Sex Ratio:** M1:F1

**Occurrence:** Over 65 cases reported.

**Risk of Recurrence for Patient's Sib:**
See Part I, *Mendelian Inheritance.*

**Risk of Recurrence for Patient's Child:**
See Part I, *Mendelian Inheritance.*

**Age of Detectability:** Neonatal period.

**Gene Mapping and Linkage:** Unknown.

**Prevention:** None known. Genetic counseling indicated.

**Treatment:** Orthopedic correction of talipes equinovarus. Surgical correction of severe microstomia may be necessary. Ulna deviation does *not* require correction, as it improves as the patient grows older.

**Prognosis:** After surgery, walking improves. General health is not impaired.

**Detection of Carrier:** Unknown.

**Support Groups:** UT; Bountiful; Freeman-Sheldon Parent Support Group

**References:**

Freeman EA, Sheldon JH: Cranio-carpotarsal dystrophy: undescribed congenital malformation. Arch Dis Child 1938; 13:277–283.

Červenka J, et al.: Craniocarpotarsal dysplasia or whistling face syndrome. Arch Otolaryngol 1970; 91:183–187.

Sauk JJ Jr, et al.: Electromyography of oral-facial musculature in craniocarpotarsal dysplasia (Freeman-Sheldon syndrome). Clin Genet 1974; 6:132–137.

Wettstein A, et al.: A family with whistling-face syndrome. Hum Genet 1980; 55:177–189.

Kouseff BG, et al.: Autosomal recessive type of whistling face syndrome in twins. Pediatrics 1982; 69:328–331.

O'Keefe M, et al.: Ocular abnormalities in the Freeman-Sheldon syndrome. Am J Ophthal 1986; 102:346–348.

Sánchez JM, Kaminker CP: New evidence for genetic heterogeneity of the Freeman-Sheldon syndrome. Am J Med Genet 1986; 25:507–512.

Wang T-R, Lin S-J: Further evidence for genetic heterogeneity of whistling face or Freeman-Sheldon syndrome in a Chinese family. Am J Med Genet 1987; 28:471–475.

SE007                                    **Heddie O. Sedano**

## CRANIO-DIAPHYSEAL DYSPLASIA                    **0224**

**Includes:**
Diaphyseal and cranial dysplasia
Dysplasia, cranio-diaphyseal

**Excludes:**
**Craniometaphyseal dysplasia** (0228)
**Diaphyseal dysplasia** (0290)
**Frontometaphyseal dysplasia** (0394)
**Pyle disease** (0847)
**Sclerosteosis** (0880)

**Major Diagnostic Criteria:** Severe hyperostosis and sclerosis of the skull bones, including the mandible. Diaphyseal widening and sclerosis of the tubular bones, ribs, and clavicles.

**Clinical Findings:** Severe craniofacial dysmorphism (leontiasis ossea) caused by thickening of the cranial bones; small stature. On X-ray, cranial hyperostosis and sclerosis with diaphyseal distention of the tubular bones.

**Complications:** Nasal obstruction, symptoms of cranial nerve compression leading to failure of vision, deafness, facial paralysis, mental retardation, seizures.

**Associated Findings:** None known.

**Etiology:** Autosomal recessive inheritance.

**Pathogenesis:** On cross-section, the bone is dense and the spongiosa is reduced in amount. Increased amounts of dense, lamellated bone are found, but the intrinsic structure of the compact bone is normal.

**MIM No.:** *21830

**POS No.:** 3157

**Sex Ratio:** M1:F1

**Occurrence:** Fewer than ten cases have been reported.

**Risk of Recurrence for Patient's Sib:**
See Part I, *Mendelian Inheritance.*

**Risk of Recurrence for Patient's Child:**
See Part I, *Mendelian Inheritance.*

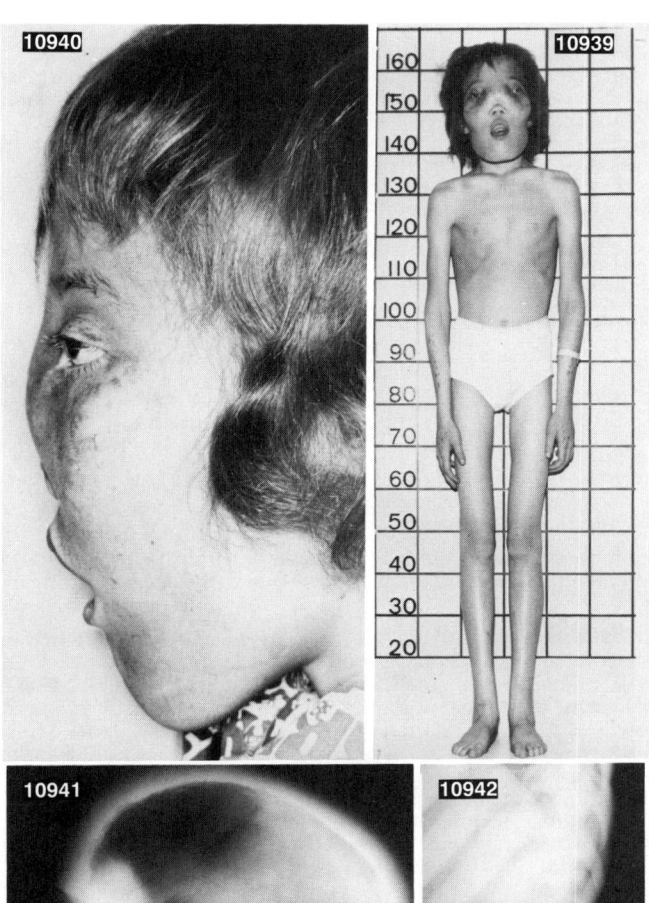

0224-10940–39: Enlarged head and facial features in tall, thin 12-year-old male; subcutaneous tissues are reduced and muscles are hypoplastic. 10941: Lateral skull X-ray shows enormously thickened cranial bones. 10942: Lateral view of the lumbar spine shows hypermineralized vertebral bodies.

**Age of Detectability:** Early infancy by X-rays of the skull and long bones.

**Gene Mapping and Linkage:** Unknown.

**Prevention:** None known. Genetic counseling indicated.

**Treatment:** Unknown.

**Prognosis:** The disease is progressive, leading to early death in the second or third decades of life.

**Detection of Carrier:** Unknown.

**References:**
Halliday J: Rare case of bone dystrophy. Br J Surg 1949; 37:52–63.
Joseph R, et al.: Dysplasie craniodiaphysaire progressive. Ses relations avec la dysplasie diaphysaire progressive de Camurati-Engelmann. Ann Radiol (Paris) 1958; 1:477–490.
Macpherson R: Craniodiaphyseal dysplasia, a disease or group of diseases? J Assoc Anad Radiol 1974; 25:22–23.
Tucker AS, et al.: Craniodiaphyseal dysplasia: evolution over a five-year period. Skeletal Radiol 1976; 1:47–53.

SP007                                                    **Jürgen W. Spranger**

---

## CRANIO-DIGITAL SYNDROME-MENTAL RETARDATION, SCOTT TYPE                                          2831

**Includes:**
  Scott craniodigital syndrome-mental retardation
  X-linked mental retardation, Scott type

**Excludes:**
  **Acrocephalopolysyndactyly**
  **Acrocephalosyndactyly**

**Major Diagnostic Criteria:** The combination of mental and growth retardation, distinctive facies, and **Syndactyly** of fingers and toes.

**Clinical Findings:** All known cases have had facial anomalies consisting of brachycephaly; prominent eyebrows; dark eyelashes; small, pointed nose; small mandible; hirsutism; mild soft tissue syndactyly affecting fingers 2, 3, and 4 and toes 2 and 3; and growth and mental retardation. Each child also had varus deformity of the foot and spina bifida occulta of L-5/S-1. The facial features and syndactyly are present at birth, whereas the growth retardation, primarily affecting height, occurs by age one year. X-ray findings include brachycephaly without craniosynostosis, **Eye, hypertelorism,** and wormian bones of the skull. Dermatoglyphics are also unusual in that the palmar axial triradius is distally placed and is associated with a large hypothenar pattern.

**Complications:** Unknown.

**Associated Findings:** None known.

**Etiology:** Presumably X-linked recessive inheritance, although autosomal recessive inheritance cannot be ruled out.

**Pathogenesis:** Unknown.

**MIM No.:** 31286

**Sex Ratio:** M3:F0 (observed).

**Occurrence:** Reported in three brothers in North America.

**Risk of Recurrence for Patient's Sib:**
  See Part I, *Mendelian Inheritance.*

**Risk of Recurrence for Patient's Child:**
  See Part I, *Mendelian Inheritance.*

**Age of Detectability:** At birth, by physical examination

**Gene Mapping and Linkage:** Unknown.

**Prevention:** None known. Genetic counseling indicated.

**Treatment:** Unknown.

**Prognosis:** IQs of the three affected boys ranged from 35 to 50. Life span does not appear to be affected.

**Detection of Carrier:** In the reported family, the mother and maternal grandmother had syndactyly of toes 2 and 3 and very mild syndactyly of fingers 2 and 3. Since this trait is common in the general population, it may be segregating as a separate autosomal dominant trait, or indicate carrier status.

**References:**
Scott CR, et al.: A new craniodigital syndrome with mental retardation. J Pediatr 1971; 78:658–663.

T0007                                                    **Helga V. Toriello**

---

## CRANIO-ECTODERMAL DYSPLASIA                                          2127

**Includes:**
  Cranio-ectodermal syndrome
  Levin syndrome
  Sensenbrenner-Dorst-Owens syndrome
  Skeletal dysplasia-sparse hair-dental anomalies
  Teeth (anomalies)-skeletal dysplasia-sparse hair

**Excludes:**
  **Chondroectodermal dysplasia** (0156)
  **Coffin-Siris syndrome** (2025)
  **Dermo-odontodysplasia** (2763)
  **Ectodermal dysplasia, hidrotic** (0334)
  **Growth retardation-alopecia-pseudoanodontia-optic atrophy** (2293)
  **Hypodontia-nail dysgenesis** (0511)
  **Incontinentia pigmenti** (0526)
  **Oculo-dento-osseous dysplasia** (0737)
  **Odonto-onychodysplasia-alopecia** (2890)
  **Odonto-trichomelic syndrome** (2887)
  **Rothmund-Thomson syndrome** (2037)
  **Schinzel-Giedion syndrome** (2123)
  **Tricho-dento-osseous syndrome** (0965)
  **Tricho-odonto-onychial dysplasia** (2889)
  **Tricho-rhino-phalangeal syndrome, type I** (0966)

**Major Diagnostic Criteria:** A characteristic pattern of clinical features including dolichocephaly, sparse slow-growing hair, dental anomalies, rhizomelic shortening of the limbs, and brachydactyly, in association with characteristic X-ray findings.

**Clinical Findings:** Mild growth deficiency of prenatal or postnatal onset is usually present. The head is dolichocephalic with frontal bossing; craniosynostosis of the sagittal suture often occurs. The scalp hair is sparse, thin, and slow-growing. Epicanthal folds, ocular hypotelorism, anteverted nares, full cheeks, and everted lower lip produce a characteristic facial appearance. Hyperopia, myopia, or nystagmus may occur. Oral anomalies include hypodontia, microdontia, taurondontia, dental fusion, and enamel dysplasia. The thorax is typically short with **Pectus excavatum.** There is rhizomelic shortening of the extremities, especially in the arms, and joint laxity. Brachydactyly is characteristic, and clinodactyly, cutaneous syndactyly, and altered palmar crease patterns may be seen. Intellectual development appears to be normal.

Typical X-ray features include mild generalized osteoporosis and shortening of the limbs, with short, wide hands and feet. The phalanges, especially the distal ones, are short. Long bones exhibit thin cortex, slightly widened metaphyses, and flattened epiphyseal ossification centers. The capital femoral epiphyses ossify later than expected. Vertebral bodies exhibit an infantile appearance in childhood with convex upper and lower borders. Premature fusion of the sutures of the body of sternum may occur.

**Complications:** Unknown.

**Associated Findings:** Congenital heart disease and multiple lingual frenula have been reported. The brain of one child who died was found to have widened sulci and narrowed frontal lobe gyri.

**Etiology:** Autosomal recessive inheritance.

**Pathogenesis:** Unknown.

**MIM No.:** *21833

**POS No.:** 3170

**Sex Ratio:** M1:F1

**Occurrence:** About a half-dozen cases have been reported.

**Risk of Recurrence for Patient's Sib:**
  See Part I, *Mendelian Inheritance.*

**Risk of Recurrence for Patient's Child:**
  See Part I, *Mendelian Inheritance.*

**Age of Detectability:** In infancy.

**Gene Mapping and Linkage:** Unknown.

**Prevention:** None known. Genetic counseling indicated.

**Treatment:** Craniosynostosis may require surgical treatment. Dental, ocular, and orthopedic abnormalities should be appropriately managed.

**Prognosis:** Of the first six children reported, three died by age seven years from heart failure (1) or recurrent pneumonia.

**Detection of Carrier:** Unknown.

**References:**

Sensenbrenner JA, et al.: New syndrome of skeletal, dental, and hair anomalies. BD:OAS XI(2). New York: March of Dimes Birth Defects Foundation, 1975:372–379.
Levin LS, et al.: A heritable syndrome of craniosynostosis, short thin hair, dental abnormalities, and short limbs: cranioectodermal dysplasia. J Pediatr 1977; 90:55–61. *
Gellis SS, Feingold M: Cranioectodermal dysplasia. Am J Dis Child 1979; 133:1275–1276. †
Freire-Mahia N, Pinheiro M: Ectodermal dysplasias: a clinical and genetic study. New York: Alan R. Liss, 1984:67–108.

FR017                       **J.M. Freidman**

**Cranio-ectodermal syndrome**
*See CRANIO-ECTODERMAL DYSPLASIA*
**Cranio-facio-cardio-skeletal syndrome**
*See DERMO-FACIO-CARDIO-SKELETAL SYNDROME*

## CRANIO-FRONTO-NASAL DYSPLASIA      2185

**Includes:**
Craniofrontal dysplasia
Frontonasal dysplasia with coronal craniosynostosis
Moreno syndrome

**Excludes:**
**Face, median cleft face syndrome** (0635)
**Fronto-facio-nasal dysplasia** (2979)
**Oro-facio-digital syndrome I** (0770)
**Polysyndactyly-dysmorphic craniofacies, Greig type** (2925)

**Major Diagnostic Criteria:** Eye, **hypertelorism**, broad nasal root, absent nasal tip, synostosis of coronal suture, wide mouth, **Syndactyly**, broad first digits, split nails, clavicle malformation, sternum malformation, and axial skeletal malformation. In the familial case, hypertelorism may be the minimal manifestation of the gene.

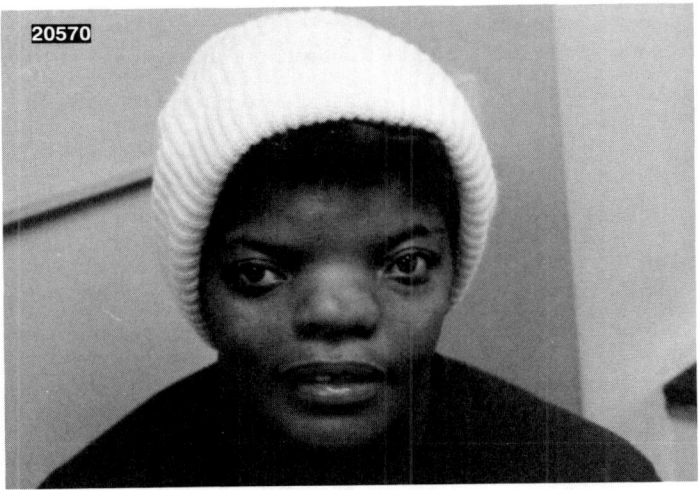

**2185-20570:** Cranio-fronto-nasal dysplasia; note the ocular hypertelorism, broad nose with grooved nasal tip, tall and broad forehead, and midface hypoplasia.

**Clinical Findings:** Cranio-fronto-nasal dysplasia (CFND) is a highly variable disorder. The characteristic craniofacial anomalies include true ocular hypertelorism, broad nose with bifid tip or grooved nasal tip, a tall, broad forehead, with frontal prominence and midface hypoplasia.

Mild facial manifestations may include only hypertelorism, broad nasal root, poorly defined nasal tip, and wide mouth. Moderate forms usually include a groove or a broad expanse of skin separating the nose into two eminences. Severe forms include median cleft of lip and palate. The craniosynostosis and other findings may vary in severity also. The broadening of the first digits and split nails may be related and represented in severe form by preaxial polydactyly. Thin concave nails with median longitudinal groove represent a mild manifestation and may occur on digits other than the first. The syndactyly is usually minor webbing and may be accompanied by clinodactyly. The clavicles are long, producing the appearance of a narrow thoracic outlet and resulting in mild webbing of the neck and sloping of shoulders. Pectus excavatum or pectus carinatum may be present. Other skeletal malformations include shallow vertebral bodies, asymmetric sacrum, asymmetric pubic bones, and small iliac bones. Scoliosis and lordosis may be present.

Generally, females have been described as being more severely affected than have males, but severely affected males have been reported, as have mildly affected females.

**Complications:** Facial deformity, ocular dysfunction secondary to extreme hypertelorism, and potentially secondary to the craniosynostosis. Digital anomalies seldom present more than a cosmetic problem.

**Associated Findings:** There appears to be an increased incidence of fetal wastage among the offspring of affected individuals. Occasionally, associated anomalies include ear malformations, cleft lip, and development delay.

**Etiology:** Probably autosomal dominant inheritance with widely variable expression (Kwee and Lindhout, 1988).

**Pathogenesis:** The CFND mutation may be analogous to semilethal mutations of the mouse T-locus.

The facial malformation appears to be due to either broadening of the median facial structures (derivatives of embryonic facial segment) or shortening of the lateral facial structures (branchial arch derivatives). The increased clavicle length is due to persistence of two ossification centers.

**MIM No.:** 12292, 30411

**Sex Ratio:** M1:F1.94

**Occurrence:** Undetermined. Established literature.

**Risk of Recurrence for Patient's Sib:** If a parent is affected, empirically estimated to be 70%. If parents are normal, there is low risk of recurrence.

**Risk of Recurrence for Patient's Child:** Empirically estimated to be 70%.

**Age of Detectability:** At birth, in most cases; prenatal detection by ultrasound may be possible.

**Gene Mapping and Linkage:** Unknown.

**Prevention:** None known. Genetic counseling indicated.

**Treatment:** Craniectomy is indicated for the coronal synostosis. The facial deformity is amenable to cosmetic surgery.

**Prognosis:** Aside from fetal loss, life span appears to be normal. Growth is usually normal. Mental retardation appears to be an infrequent problem. The facies is so striking that it may present a psychological problem.

**Detection of Carrier:** By clinical examination.

**References:**

Hunter AGW, Rudd NL: Craniosynostosis II. Teratology 1977; 15:301–310.
Cohen MM: Craniofrontonasal Dysplasia. BD:OAS XV(5B) New York: March of Dimes Birth Defects Foundation, 1979:85–89. *
Slover R, Sujansky E: Frontonasal dysplasia with coronal synostosis in three sibs. BD:OAS XV(5B). New York: March of Dimes Birth Defects Foundation, 1979:75–83.

Rollnick B, et al.: A pedigree: possible evidence for the metabolic interference hypothesis. Am J Hum Genet 1981; 33:823–826.

Kwee ML, Lindhout D: Frontonasal dysplasia, coronal craniosynostosis, pre- and postaxial polydactyly and split nails: a new autosomal dominant mutant with reduced penetrance and variable expression? Clin Genet 1983; 24:200–205.

Reynolds JF, et al.: Craniofrontonasal dysplasia: a new family. Proc Greenwood Genet Center 1983; 2:115.

Reich EW, et al.: Craniofrontal dysplasia: clinical delineations. (Abstract) Am J Hum Genet 1985; 37:A72.

Sax CM, Flannery DB: Craniofrontonasal dysplasia: clinical and genetic analysis. Clin Genet 1986; 29:508–515. * †

Morris CA, et al.: Delineation of the male phenotype in craniofrontonasal syndrome. Am J Med Genet 1987; 27:623–631.

Kwee ML, Lindhout D: Inheritance of cranio-fronto-nasal syndrome. (Letter) Am J Med Genet 1988; 30:841–842.

FL001
SA044
TH017
UR001

David B. Flannery
Christina M. Sax
T.F. Thurmon
S.A. Ursin

**Cranio-oculo-dental syndrome**
See ACROCEPHALOSYNDACTYLY TYPE III
**Cranio-oro-digital syndrome**
See ORO-CRANIO-DIGITAL SYNDROME
also OTO-PALATO-DIGITAL SYNDROME, II
**Cranioacrofacial syndrome**
See VENTRICULAR SEPTAL DEFECT

## CRANIODIAPHYSEAL DYSPLASIA, LENZ-MAJEWSKI TYPE 2508

**Includes:**
Bone density (increased)-syndactyly
Dwarfism, hyperostotic, Lenz-Majewski type
Lenz-Majewski hyperostotic dwarfism

**Excludes:**
Camurati-Engelmann syndrome
**Cortical hyperostosis, infantile** (0221)
**Cranio-diaphyseal dysplasia** (0224)
**Fibrous dysplasia, polyostotic** (0391)
**Progeria** (0825)

**Major Diagnostic Criteria:** Characteristic pattern of progressive hyperostosis, characteristic facies, cutis laxa, hypoplastic middle phalanges, and interdigital webbing.

**Clinical Findings:** Short stature, failure to thrive, emaciation, loose atrophic skin with prominent veins, delayed closure of fontanels, broad angular forehead, hypertelorism, prominent mandible, dental enamel dysplasia, short hands, proximal symphalangism and interdigital webbing, cryptorchidism, mental retardation, and delayed skeletal maturation.

**Complications:** Nasal obstruction.

**Associated Findings:** **Hypospadias, Hernia, inguinal**, and hyperextendable joints.

**Etiology:** Possibly autosomal dominant inheritance. Advanced paternal age has been noted. Most cases are sporadic, and no parental consanguinity has been reported.

**Pathogenesis:** Undetermined. Possibly a connective tissue disorder.

**MIM No.:** 15105

**POS No.:** 3045

**CDC No.:** 756.480

**Sex Ratio:** Presumably M1:F1

**Occurrence:** About a half-dozen cases have been documented.

**Risk of Recurrence for Patient's Sib:** Unknown.

**Risk of Recurrence for Patient's Child:** No patient known to have reached reproductive age.

**Age of Detectability:** At birth, or possibly prenatally by ultrasonography.

**Gene Mapping and Linkage:** Unknown.

**Prevention:** None known. Genetic counseling indicated.

**Treatment:** Unknown.

**Prognosis:** Death may occur in infancy or childhood. Survival to adolescence is known in one case.

**Detection of Carrier:** Unknown.

**References:**

Braham RL: Multiple congenital anomalies with diaphyseal dysplasia (Camurati-Engelmann's syndrome). Oral Surg 1969; 27:20–26.

Kaye CI, et al.: Cutis laxa, skeletal anomalies, and ambiguous genitalia. Am J Dis Child 1974; 127:115–117.

Lenz WD, Majewski F: A generalized disorder of the connective tissues with progeria, choanal atresia, symphalangism, hypoplasia of dentine and craniodiaphyseal hypostosis. BD:OAS X(12). New York: March of Dimes Birth Defects Foundation, 1974:133–136.

MacPherson RI: Craniodiaphyseal dysplasia: a disease or group of diseases? J Canad Assoc Radiol 1974; 25:22–23.

Robinow M, et al.: The Lenz-Majewski hyperostotic dwarfism. J Pediatr 1977; 91:417–421. †

Gorlin RJ, Whitley CB: Lenz-Majewski syndrome. Radiology 1983; 149:129–131. †

Hood OJ et al.: Cutis laxa with craniofacial, limb, genital and brain defects. J Clin Dysmorphol 1984; 2:23–26.

R0004
T0007

Meinhard Robinow
Helga V. Toriello

**Craniofacial anomalies-polysyndactyly**
See POLYSYNDACTYLY-DYSMORPHIC CRANIOFACIES, GREIG TYPE

## CRANIOFACIAL DYSOSTOSIS 0225

**Includes:**
Crouzon syndrome
Facial and cranial dysostosis
Pseudo-Crouzon disease

**Excludes:**
**Acrocephalosyndactyly type I** (0014)
**Acrocephalosyndactyly type III** (0229)
**Acrocephalosyndactyly type V** (2284)
**Gorlin-Chaudhry-Moss syndrome** (0440)
Isolated craniostenosis and craniostenosis syndromes

**Major Diagnostic Criteria:** Brachycephalic cranial deformity resulting from premature craniosynostosis, especially of the coronal and sagittal sutures, as well as cranial base abnormalities; exophthalmos with shallow orbits; maxillary hypoplasia with relative mandibular prognathism.

**Clinical Findings:** *Skull:* 1) Craniosynostosis especially of the coronal, sagittal, and occasionally lambdoidal sutures with palpable ridging and digital impressions; 2) widening of the hypophyseal fossa and small paranasal sinuses may be observed in some cases; 3) brachycephaly; 4) bifid uvula or cleft palate; and 5) bilateral atresia of the auditory meatus.
*Facies:* 1) ocular hypertelorism; 2) exophthalmos with shallow orbits; 3) divergent strabismus, nystagmus, and optic nerve damage; 4) psitticorhina (beak nose) with deviated septum; 5) maxillary hypoplasia with relative mandibular prognathism; 6) short upper lip; 7) class III malocclusion with V-shaped maxillary dental arch and maxillary anterior crowding.
*Other Findings:* 1) mental retardation; 2) bilateral anterior subluxation of the head of the radius

**Complications:** Increased intracranial pressure and optic atrophy. Nasopharyngeal obstruction may lead to respiratory compromise in infants.

**Associated Findings:** A variety of other low-frequency anomalies may be observed including **Craniosynostosis, Kleeblattschadel type**.

**Etiology:** Autosomal dominant inheritance with complete penetrance and variable expressivity. Up to 50% of reported cases arise

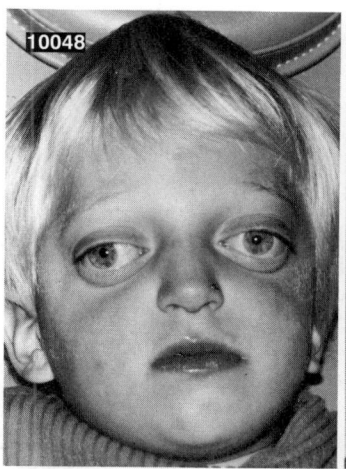
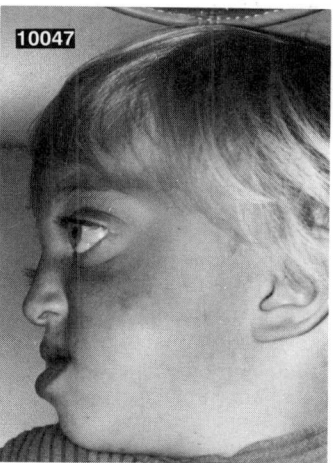
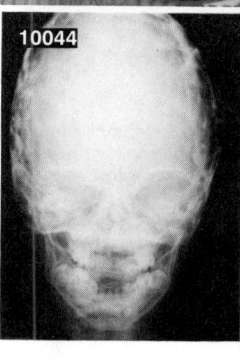
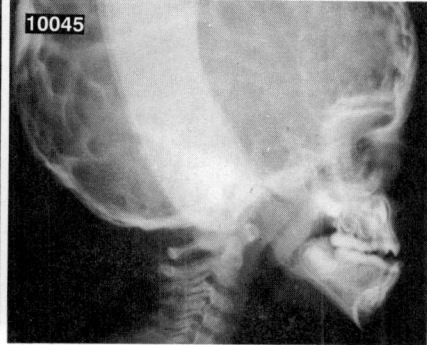

**0225-10047—48:** Note ocular proptosis and mid-face hypoplasia. **10044:** Skull X-ray shows high vertex; increased digital markings; premature suture synostosis; ocular hypertelorism; and large, shallow orbits. **10045:** Digital impressions in the skull.

as fresh mutations. These sporadic cases have been associated with increased paternal age.

**Pathogenesis:** Premature synostosis of the coronal, sagittal, and sometimes lambdoidal sutures together with sphenobasilar synchondrosis. Order and rate of progression determine degree of deformity and disability produced. Premature synostosis commences during the first year of life and is usually complete by 2–3 years in most instances.

**MIM No.:** *12350

**CDC No.:** 756.040

**Sex Ratio:** M1:F1

**Occurrence:** Undetermined but uncommon.

**Risk of Recurrence for Patient's Sib:**
See Part I, *Mendelian Inheritance.*

**Risk of Recurrence for Patient's Child:**
See Part I, *Mendelian Inheritance.*

**Age of Detectability:** At birth or during the first year of life, by physical and X-ray examination.

**Gene Mapping and Linkage:** Unknown.

**Prevention:** None known. Genetic counseling indicated.

**Treatment:** Surgical intervention mandatory in cases with rapid progression (increased intracranial pressure, progressive mental retardation, optic nerve involvement). Cosmetic surgery in selected cases.

**Prognosis:** Normal for life span.

**Detection of Carrier:** Since expressivity is variable, some individuals may have only minimal involvement. X-rays of the skull should detect premature synostosis in minimally affected family members by age 10 years.

**Special Considerations:** Although the skull is brachycephalic, cranial deformity is variable, depending on the order and rate of progression of sutural involvement. Other forms of craniostenosis and craniostenosis syndromes, both genetic and nongenetic, are known to occur. The use of the term "pseudo-Crouzon syndrome" to describe isolated cases of craniostenosis without the other features of craniofacial dysostosis should be avoided.

**References:**
Bertelson TI: The premature synostosis of the cranial sutures. Acta Ophthalmol [Suppl](Copenh) 1958; 51.
Vulliamy DG, Normandale PA: Craniofacial dysostosis in a Dorset family. Arch Dis Child 1966; 41:375–382.
Cohen MM Jr: An etiologic and nosologic overview of craniosynostosis syndromes. In: Bergsma D, ed: Malformation syndromes. BD: OAS 1975; XI(2):137. Amsterdam: Excerpta Medica, for The National Foundation-March of Dimes.
Kreiborg S, ed: Crouzon syndrome. Scand J Plast Reconstruc Surg [Suppl] 1981; 18:1–198.
Peterson-Falzone SJ, et al.: Nasopharyngeal dysmorphology in the syndromes of Apert and Crouzon. Cleft Palate J 1981; 18:237–249.
Rosen HM, Whitaker LA: Cranial base dynamics in craniofacial dysostosis. J Maxillofac Surg 1984; 12:56–61.

0B003                                                          **Jane O'Brien**

## CRANIOFACIAL DYSOSTOSIS-DIAPHYSEAL HYPERPLASIA                                                 **0226**

**Includes:** Stanescu osteosclerosis

**Excludes:**
**Cranio-diaphyseal dysplasia** (0224)
**Pyknodysostosis** (0846)
**Tubular stenosis** (0976)

**Major Diagnostic Criteria:** Thick cortices of long bones, small skull with thin cranium, and short stature. This condition appears to be distinct because of normal phalanges. An interesting feature is the depressed sutures.

**Clinical Findings:** Craniofacial dysostosis with small, brachycephalic, sometimes asymmetric skull; thin cranial bones with lack of pneumatization; depressions over frontoparietal and occipitoparietal sutures; narrow maxilla with obtuse angle; small mandible; shallow orbits with prominent eyes; and rather prominent bulbous nose. Mild-to-moderate short stature with disproportionately rhizomelic shortening of limbs and dense long bones with thick cortices. Hands are short without cone epiphyses or osteolysis of phalanges. Teeth are small and crowded with enamel hypoplasia. Some affected individuals have flat roof of palate, sacralization of S-1, kyphoscoliosis, pectus excavatum, exostoses, and fractures. Intelligence has been normal.

**Complications:** Short stature, increased thickening of cortices with age, mitral ilium, and growth retardation.

**Associated Findings:** Dermatoglyphic findings may include single flexion crease.

**Etiology:** Presumably autosomal dominant inheritance.

**Pathogenesis:** Affected individuals may be short at birth. Stature remains below normal. Cortical thickness increases with age and may not be present in infancy. Histology unknown.

**MIM No.:** 12290

**POS No.:** 3159

**CDC No.:** 756.040

**Sex Ratio:** M1:F1

**Occurrence:** Rare; about 15 cases reported.

**Risk of Recurrence for Patient's Sib:**
See Part I, *Mendelian Inheritance.*

**Risk of Recurrence for Patient's Child:**
See Part I, *Mendelian Inheritance.*

**Age of Detectability:** Probably at birth; definitely during early childhood.

**Gene Mapping and Linkage:** Unknown.

**Prevention:** None known. Genetic counseling indicated.

**Treatment:** Unknown.

**Prognosis:** Apparently normal life span with normal intelligence.

**Detection of Carrier:** Unknown.

**References:**
Hall JG: Craniofacial dysostosis - either Stanesco dysostosis or a new entity. In: Bergsma D, ed: Skeletal dysplasias. BD:OAS X(12). Amsterdam: Excerpta Medica, for The National Foundation - March of Dimes, 1974:521.
Maximilian C, et al.: Syndrome de dysostose cranio-facial avec hyperplasie diaphysaire. J Genet Hum 1981; 29:129–139.
Dipierri JE, Guzman JD: A second family with autosomal dominant osteosclerosis - type Stanescu. Am J Med Genet 1984; 18:13–18. *

HA014                                                **Judith G. Hall**

## CRANIOFACIAL DYSSYNOSTOSIS                         0227

**Includes:** Craniosynostosis-craniofacial dysostosis-other anomalies

**Excludes:**
 **Craniotelencephalic dysplasia** (2791)
 Craniosynostosis syndromes with craniofacial dysostoses, other

**Major Diagnostic Criteria:** Premature synostosis of lambdoid sutures and of posterior part of sagittal suture causing deformity of the skull with prominent forehead and small, flat or bulging occiput. Dysostosis of basal structures of the skull causing (secondary) anomalies of the face.

**Clinical Findings:** A dolichocephalic or brachyturricephalic configuration of the skull is present from birth, with protuberant forehead and small, flat or bulging occiput. The deformity becomes more pronounced during infancy. Osseous ridges are palpable over the lambdoid sutures and the posterior part of the sagittal suture, suggesting premature closure. The coronal suture may close prematurely, contributing to asymmetry of skull and face. Microcephaly is less often seen than macrocephaly; an abnormal hair pattern may be present. The facial appearance is characterized by hypoplastic supraorbital ridges, antimongoloid slanting of palpebral fissures, anteverted nostrils, short maxilla, micrognathia, and posteriorly rotated, sometimes dysplastic auricles. The palate usually is high and narrowly arched. Ocular signs include strabismus, nystagmus and optic atrophy. Shortness of stature was seen in all patients except one. Motor development is delayed; mental retardation is seen in most affected children. Seizures may occur; EEG recordings are abnormal. X-ray findings include brachycephaly, frontal bossing, synostosis of lambdoid sutures and posterior part of sagittal suture, posteriorly located anterior fontanel, short base of skull, steep slope of the base of anterior fossa, small posterior fossa. Cerebral malformation (agenesis of the corpus callosum) and hydrocephalus have been reported.

**Complications:** Increased intracranial pressure from craniosynostosis or hydrocephalus soon after birth; mental retardation; seizures; cerebral palsy.

**Associated Findings:** Congenital heart defect; other anomalies.

**Etiology:** Presumably autosomal recessive inheritance.

**Pathogenesis:** The condition probably reflects an etiologically heterogeneous but pathogenetically similar group of disorders. It is not possible to decide at present if the syndrome represents a dysostosis of cranial and facial structures or a dysmorphic syndrome with mental retardation. The mental retardation observed in the patients reported may represent ascertainment bias.

**MIM No.:** 21835
**POS No.:** 3160
**Sex Ratio:** Presumably M1:F1
**Occurrence:** Less than a dozen cases reported. About half of Spanish ancestry.
**Risk of Recurrence for Patient's Sib:**
See Part I, *Mendelian Inheritance.*
**Risk of Recurrence for Patient's Child:**
See Part I, *Mendelian Inheritance.*
**Age of Detectability:** Infancy; craniosynostosis may be detected with prenatal ultrasonography.
**Gene Mapping and Linkage:** Unknown.
**Prevention:** None known. Genetic counseling indicated.
**Treatment:** Craniosynostectomy at an early age; shunting procedures for progressive hydrocephalus; anticonvulsants, physiotherapy, special education.
**Prognosis:** Development may be normal following surgical intervention. Hydrocephalus sometimes arrests spontaneously. Associated anomalies impact the outcome.
**Detection of Carrier:** Unknown.

**References:**
Neuhäuser G, et al.: Studies of malformation syndromes of man XXXIX: a craniosynostosis-craniofacial dysostosis syndrome with mental retardation and other malformations: "craniofacial dyssynostosis." Eur J Pediatr 1976; 123:15–28. *
Cohen MM Jr: Craniosynostosis and syndromes with craniosynostosis: incidence, genetics, penetrance, variability, and new syndrome updating. In: BD:OAS 1979; XV:13–63.

NE012                                               **Gerhard Neuhäuser**

## CRANIOFACIAL-DEAFNESS-HAND SYNDROME               2761

**Includes:** Hand and craniofacial anomalies-sensorineural deafness

**Excludes:**
 **Cranio-carpo-tarsal dysplasia, whistling face type** (0223)
 **Oro-facio-digital syndrome**
 **Waardenburg syndromes** (0997)

**Major Diagnostic Criteria:** **Eye, hypertelorism**, sensorineural hearing loss, absence or hypoplasia of nasal bone confirmed by X-ray, and ulnar deviation of hands with variable digital flexion contractures.

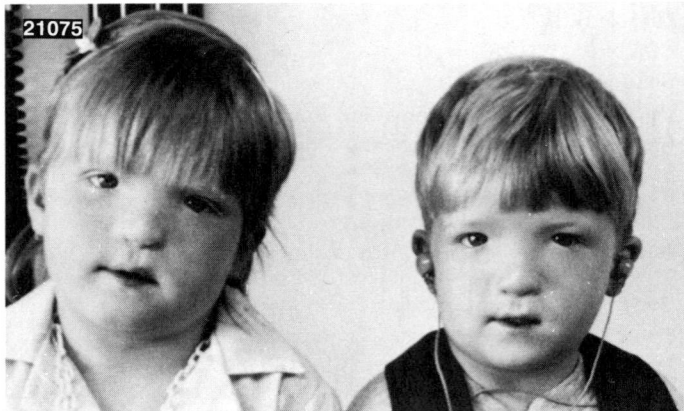

**2761-21075:** Sibs with the Craniofacial-Deafness-Hand syndrome.

**Clinical Findings:** The major clinical findings are present at birth and consist of a very distinct facial appearance. The head circumference is normal, but patients have significant hypertelorism, downslanting palpebral fissures, a small nose with slit-like nares, and a small "pursed" mouth. The facial profile is flat, and patients have a high forehead. There may be ulnar deviation of the hands. The remainder of the physical examination is entirely normal.

Early testing will reveal a profound sensorineural hearing loss. Because of a small upper airway secondary to small nares, absent nasal bone, and small oral passages, the patients may develop chronic upper airway obstruction, which could result in cor pulmonale. Adenoidectomy has greatly improved the airway obstruction. Early diagnosis of deafness is important for proper communication training, which should start as early as possible. All affected persons have had normal intelligence.

**Complications:** Chronic upper airway obstructions, communication problems if deafness is diagnosed too late, and minimal dexterity limitation because of ulnar deviation of hands and flexion contractures.

**Associated Findings:** None known.

**Etiology:** Autosomal dominant inheritance.

**Pathogenesis:** Unknown.

**MIM No.:** 12288

**POS No.:** 3601

**Sex Ratio:** Presumably M1:F1 (M1:F2 observed).

**Occurrence:** A mother and daughter have been reported in the literature, and an affected son was subsequently born to the same mother.

**Risk of Recurrence for Patient's Sib:**
See Part I, *Mendelian Inheritance.*

**Risk of Recurrence for Patient's Child:**
See Part I, *Mendelian Inheritance.*

**Age of Detectability:** At birth.

**Gene Mapping and Linkage:** Unknown.

**Prevention:** None known. Genetic counseling indicated.

**Treatment:** Hearing aids and auditory training. Monitoring of blood gases during infancy and evaluation for adenoidectomy if chronic upper airway obstruction. Possible of physical therapy for ulnar deviation and flexion contractures.

**Prognosis:** Normal life span, with sensorineural hearing loss the most significant functional impairment.

**Detection of Carrier:** Unknown.

**References:**
Sommer A, et al.: Previously undescribed syndrome of craniofacial, hand anomalies and sensorineural deafness. Am J Med Genet 1983; 15:71–77.

S0010                                    **Anne Marie Sommer**

**Craniofacial-genital-dental syndrome (CFGD)**
*See BRANCHIO-SKELETO-GENITAL SYNDROME*
**Craniofrontal dysplasia**
*See CRANIO-FRONTO-NASAL DYSPLASIA*
**Craniomandibular dermatodysostosis**
*See MANDIBULOACRAL DYSPLASIA*

---

## CRANIOMETAPHYSEAL DYSPLASIA          0228

**Includes:**
Dysplasia, craniometaphyseal
Schwartz-Lelek syndrome (one form)

**Excludes:**
**Cranio-diaphyseal dysplasia** (0224)
**Diaphyseal dysplasia** (0290)
**Frontometaphyseal dysplasia** (0394)
**Metaphyseal dysplasia-maxillary hypoplasia-brachydactyly** (2768)
**Pyle disease** (0847)
**Sclerosteosis** (0880)

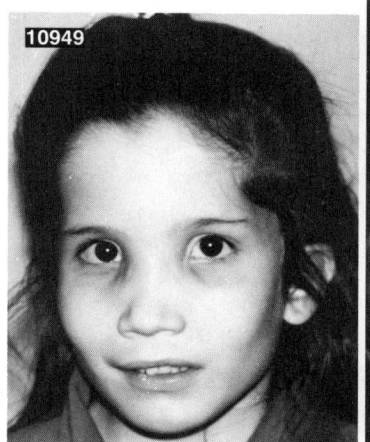 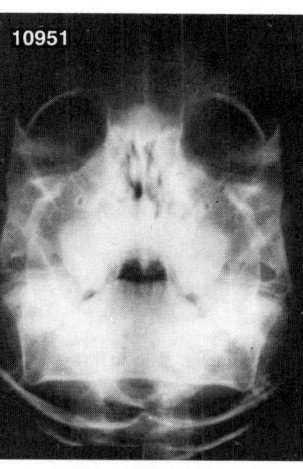

**0228**-10949: Frontonasal swelling and ocular hypertelorism. 10951: Osteosclerotic changes in the skull.

---

**Major Diagnostic Criteria:** Hyperostosis or sclerosis of the cranial bones, especially the frontal and occipital parts of the cranial vault; club-shaped metaphyseal flare of the tubular bones. Metaphyseal undermodeling is minimal in the first year of life. Varying degrees of diaphyseal sclerosis are present at this period.

**Clinical Findings:** Facial dysmorphism with frontonasal swelling, hypertelorism, mandibular enlargement. X-rays show cranial hyperostosis and metaphyseal undermodeling.

Craniometaphyseal dysplasia, dominant, must not be confused with **Pyle disease** in which the skull is only minimally affected.

Craniometaphyseal dysplasia, recessive, must not be confused with **Cranio-diaphyseal dysplasia** in which the skull shows even more sclerosis and in which there is no metaphyseal modeling defect.

**Complications:** Nasal obstruction; symptoms of cranial nerve compression such as conductive hearing loss, optic atrophy, facial paralysis; sensorineural hearing loss.

**Associated Findings:** None known.

**Etiology:** Genetic heterogeneity is present. Cases with autosomal dominant inheritance are clinically and on X-ray less severely affected than cases in which autosomal recessive transmission must be assumed.

**Pathogenesis:** Undetermined. Probably failure to resorb newly formed bone.

**MIM No.:** *12300, *21840

**POS No.:** 3162

**Sex Ratio:** M1:F1

**Occurrence:** More than 50 caes have been reported.

**Risk of Recurrence for Patient's Sib:**
See Part I, *Mendelian Inheritance.*

**Risk of Recurrence for Patient's Child:**
See Part I, *Mendelian Inheritance.*

**Age of Detectability:** Early infancy by X-ray of skull and long bones.

**Gene Mapping and Linkage:** Unknown.

**Prevention:** None known. Genetic counseling indicated.

**Treatment:** Operative removal of hyperostotic tissue for cosmetic purposes, hearing aids, and supportive treatment.

**Prognosis:** Normal life expectancy, but incapacitating progressive hyperostosis of the skull bones and ensuing cranial nerve compression. Normal adult body height. Regression of cranial hyperostosis has also been observed in adolescence and early adulthood.

**Detection of Carrier:** Unknown.

**Special Considerations:** Gorlin et al (1969) has suggested that a patient described by Schwartz (1960) as having craniometaphyseal dysplasia actually had a unique condition which became described as *Schwartz-Lelek syndrome*.

**References:**
Schwartz E: Craniometarphyseal dysplasia. Am J Roentgen 1960; 84:461–466.
Spranger J, et al.: Die kraniometaphysäre Dysplasie (Pyle). Z Kinderheilkd 1965; 93:64–79.
Holt JF: The evolution of craniometaphyseal dysplasia. Ann Radiol (Paris) 1966; 9:209–214.
Gorlin RJ, et al.: Genetic craniotubular bone dysplasias and hyperostoses: a critical analysis. BD:OAS V(4). New York: March of Dimes Birth Defects Foundation, 1969:79–95.
Beighton P, et al.: Craniometaphyseal dysplasia: variability of expression within a large family. Clin Genet 1979; 15:252–258.
Penchaszadeh VB, et al.: Autosomal recessive craniometaphyseal dysplasia. Am J Med Genet 1980; 4:43–55.
Shea J, et al.: Craniometaphyseal dysplasia: the first successful surgical treatment for associated hearing loss. Laryngoscope 1981; 91: 1369–1374.
Carnevale A, et al.: Autosomal dominant craniometaphyseal dysplasia. Clin Genet 1983; 23:17–22.

SP007                                   **Jürgen W. Spranger**

**Craniopagus**
  *See TWINS, CONJOINED*
**Craniorachischisis**
  *See ANENCEPHALY*
**Cranioskeletal dysplasia**
  *See HAJDU-CHENEY SYNDROME*

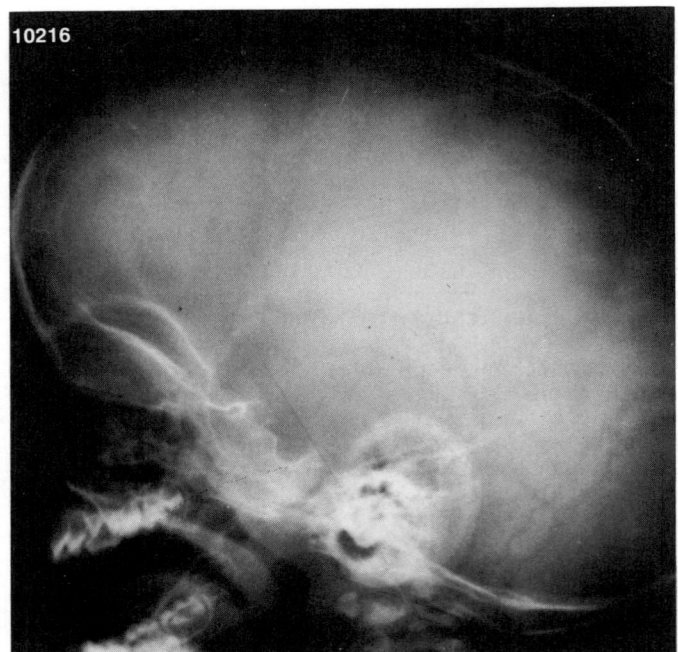

10216

**0230**-10216: Craniosynostosis involving saggital suture.

# CRANIOSYNOSTOSIS                                   0230

**Includes:**
  Brachycephaly
  Lambdoid suture closure, premature
  Oxycephally
  Plagiocephaly
  Scaphocephaly
  Turricephaly

**Excludes:**
  **Acrocephalosyndactyly type I** (0014)
  **Acrocephalosyndactyly type III** (0229)
  **Acrocephalosyndactyly type V** (2284)
  **Craniofacial dysostosis** (0225)

**Major Diagnostic Criteria:** Abnormally shaped head with premature closure of suture(s) by X-ray examination.

**Clinical Findings:** This is a disorder of the shape or form rather than the size of the cranial vault. The skull cannot enlarge at right angles to the prematurely closed suture. Rather, it expands parallel to such a closed suture with compensatory growth at the site of patent sutures; sagittal suture closure produces scaphocephaly, a long narrow head. Plagiocephaly is a unilateral coronal closure. Turricephaly represents a closure of both the coronal and sagittal sutures, with bony growth at the fontanel producing a pointed skull. All premature closures are present at birth but are accentuated by cranial growth during the first months of life. A closed suture tends to be ridged and palpable.

**Complications:** Mental subnormality, rare in sagittal closure, is more frequent in untreated bilateral coronal or multiple suture closure. Papilledema and secondary optic atrophy may also complicate the latter.

**Associated Findings:** Cleft palate, spina bifida.

**Etiology:** Both autosomal recessive and autosomal dominant inheritance have been reported.

**Pathogenesis:** The fusion of a cranial suture, possibly because of increased tension on the underlying dura matter, may be the result of a deformity of the skull base. Presumably this defect involves mesenchyme separating growing bony plates.

**MIM No.:** *12310, *21850

**CDC No.:** 756.000

**Sex Ratio:** M1:F<1; sagittal closure more common in males.

**Occurrence:** Hundreds of cases have been documented. Recessive cases reported among the Amish of Ohio.

**Risk of Recurrence for Patient's Sib:**
  See Part I, *Mendelian Inheritance*.

**Risk of Recurrence for Patient's Child:**
  See Part I, *Mendelian Inheritance*.

**Age of Detectability:** Newborn to first year of life. Prenatal medical imaging shows fused sutures, and ultrasonography shows unusual oval-shaped head with biparietal diameter more than 3 SD below mean.

**Gene Mapping and Linkage:** CRS (craniosynostosis) has been mapped to 7p21.

**Prevention:** None known. Genetic counseling indicated.

**Treatment:** Surgical repair is indicated in all multiple suture closures to prevent increased pressure and mental retardation. In sagittal synostosis, surgery may be indicated up to age 1 year for cosmetic effect.

**Prognosis:** Good with appropriate therapy; 75% of children have satisfactory results.

**Detection of Carrier:** Unknown.

**Special Considerations:** The tendency to group all varieties of synostosis together has recently become a controversial feature in the literature, especially when surgical indications are involved. The most prevalent form, sagittal synostosis, does not have a high risk of increased pressure or mental retardation. However, in those centers where pediatric neurosurgery is performed, surgical repair of the sagittal closure may be indicated solely for cosmetic reasons.

**References:**
Moss ML: The pathogenesis of premature cranial synostosis in man. Acta Anat (Basel) 1959; 37:351.
Freeman JM, Borkowf SB: Craniostenosis: review of literature and report of 34 cases. Pediatrics 1962; 30:57.
Anderson FM, Geiger L: Craniosynostosis: a survey of 204 cases. J Neurosurg 1965; 22:229–240.
Shillito J Jr, Matson DD: Craniosynostosis; a review of 519 surgical patients. Pediatrics 1969; 42:829–853.
Armendares S: On the inheritance of craniostenosis. Study of thirteen families. J Genet Hum 1970; 18:121–134.
Kosnik EJ, et al.: Familial inheritance of coronal craniosynostosis. Dev Med Child Neurol 1975; 17:630–633.
Hunter AGW, Rudd NL: Craniosynostosis: sagittal synostosis; its genetics and associated clinical findings in 214 patients who lacked involvement of the coronal suture(s). Teratology 1976; 14:185–193.
Cohen MM: Genetic perspectives on craniosynostosis and syndromes with craniosynostosis. J Neurosurg 1977; 47:886–898.

SH007                                                    **Kenneth Shapiro**

## CRANIOSYNOSTOSIS, KLEEBLATTSCHADEL TYPE        0555

**Includes:**
   Cloverleaf skull syndrome
   Kleeblattschadel craniosynostosis

**Excludes:**
   **Craniosynostosis** (other)
   **Thanatophoric dysplasia** (0940)

**Major Diagnostic Criteria:** Intrauterine craniosynostosis with a trilobar skull configuration.

**Clinical Findings:** Facial malformations include high forehead, severe proptosis or exophthalmos, beaked nose, midfacial hypoplasia, and downward displacement of ears. These abnormalities can be seen as 1) an isolated finding; 2) associated with other minor localized malformations (vertebral anomaly, elbow or knee ankylosis, hand and foot syndactyly); 3) associated with **Thanatophoric dysplasia**; or 4) in families with inherited craniosynostosis (**Craniofacial dysostosis, Acrocephalosyndactyly type I, Acrocephalopolysyndactyly,** and **Acrocephalosyndactyly type V**).

**Complications:** Most severely affected individuals are stillborn or die in infancy. Eyes are severely exophthalmic, and corneas are

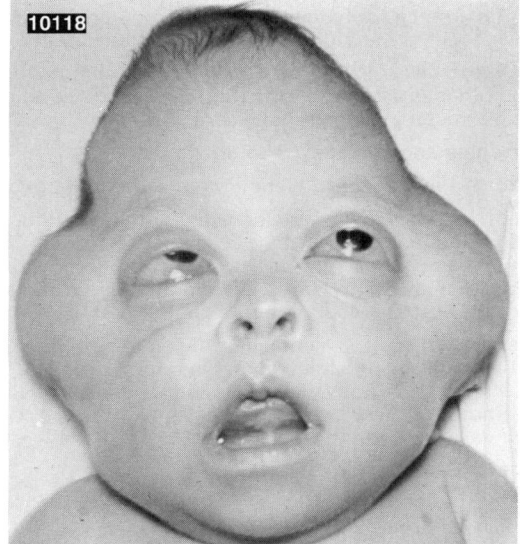

**0555-10118:** Note clover-leaf skull deformity and secondary facial changes.

exposed to trauma. If patients survive untreated, increased intracranial pressure leads to CNS complications and severe mental retardation.

**Associated Findings:** Thanatophoric dysplasia, Craniofacial dysostosis, Acrocephalosyndactyly type I, Acrocephalopolysyndactyly, and Acrocephalosyndactyly type V.

**Etiology:** This anomaly occurs in a heterogeneous group including as many as seven clinically overlapping conditions. If isolated or associated with minor anomalies, it appears to be sporadic with unknown etiology.

**Pathogenesis:** Abnormal shape of cranial base because of abnormal endochondral ossification and premature fusion of sutures. Subsequent brain growth results in bulging in areas of least resistance.

**MIM No.:** 14880, 27367

**POS No.:** 3271

**CDC No.:** 756.030

**Sex Ratio:** M1:F1

**Occurrence:** About 100 cases have been reported.

**Risk of Recurrence for Patient's Sib:** Not increased if isolated defect.

**Risk of Recurrence for Patient's Child:** Not increased if isolated defect.

**Age of Detectability:** At birth or prenatally. Prenatal diagnosis has been reported in both isolated cases and cases associated with **Thanatophoric dysplasia**, using ultrasound with a careful search for cranial bone anomaly, **Hydrocephaly**, and other bony abnormalities.

**Gene Mapping and Linkage:** Unknown.

**Prevention:** None known. Genetic counseling indicated.

**Treatment:** Neurosurgery for craniosynostosis in mild cases; total calvariectomy may be necessary to correct skull deformity. Careful ophthalmic management from birth to avoid trauma to eyes.

**Prognosis:** Poor in severe cases.

**Detection of Carrier:** Unknown.

**Special Considerations:** Kleeblattschadel anomaly appears to be a morphologic feature seen in numerous disorders. The skull is quite variable in shape, size, and evolution, depending on which sutures are affected and at what stage in development they fuse.

**References:**
McCorquodale M, et al.: Kleeblattschadel anomaly and partial trisomy for chromosome 13(47,XY,+der(13), t(3,13)(q24; q14) Clin Genet 1980; 17:409–414.
Turner PT, et al.: Generous craniectomy for kleeblattschadel anomaly. Neurosurgery 1980; 65:555–558.
Rogers GL, et al.: The management of the kleeblattschadel syndrome. Ann Ophthalmol 1981; 13:1173–1175.
Kremens B, et al.: Thanatophoric dysplasia with cloverleaf skull: case report and review of the literature. Eur J Pediatr 1982; 139:298–303.
Sano J, et al.: Cloverleaf skull syndrome: review of the literature. Acta Pathol Jpn 1982; 32:887–900.
Chervenak FA, et al.: Antenatal sonographic findings of thanatophoric dysplasia with cloverleaf skull. Am J Obstet Gynecol 1983; 984–985.
Horton WA, et al.: Discordance for the kleeblattschadel anomaly in monozygotic twins with thanatophoric dysplasia. Am J Med Genet 1983; 15:97–101.

HA014                                                    **Judith G. Hall**

## CRANIOSYNOSTOSIS-ARACHNODACTYLY-HERNIA    2915

**Includes:**

Arachnodactyly-craniosynostosis-hernia
Hernia-craniosynostosis-arachnodactyly
Shprintzen-Goldberg syndrome

**Excludes:**

**Acrocephalosyndactyly**
**Craniofacial dysostosis** (0225)
**Craniosynostosis** as a component of other conditions
**Marfan syndrome** (0630)

**Major Diagnostic Criteria: Craniosynostosis** of multiple cranial sutures; mandibular hypoplasia; maxillary hypoplasia; multiple

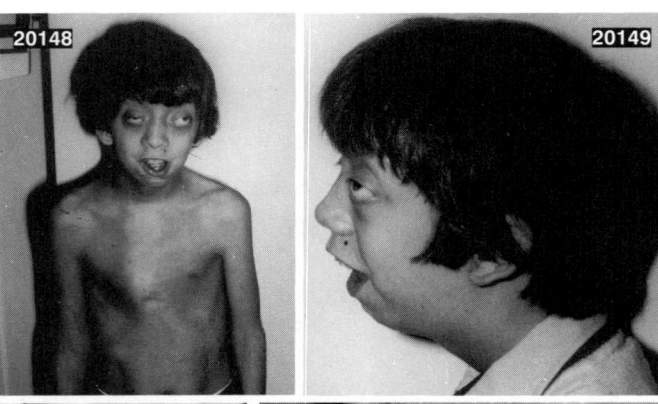

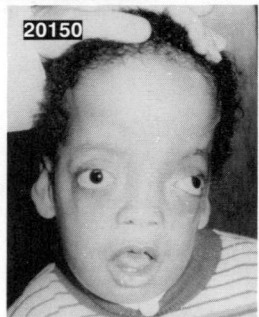
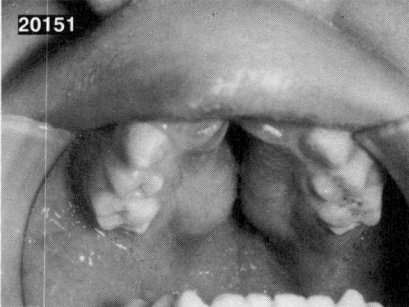

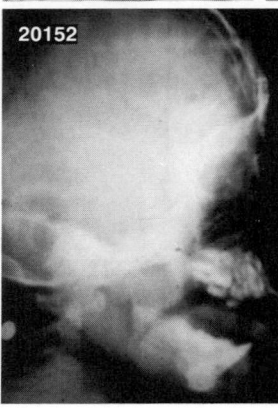
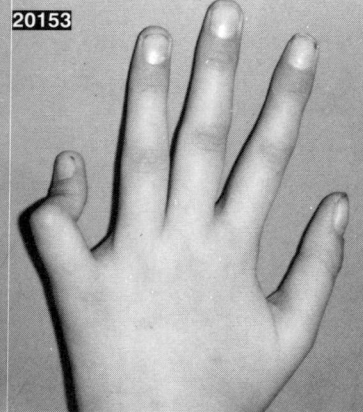

**2915-20148–50:** Note asymmetric facies and exophthalmos from cranial synostosis. **20148:** Pectus carinatum and wide diastasis recti. **20151:** Severe soft tissue hypertrophy of the palatal shelves forms a "pseudocleft." **20152:** Lateral skull X-ray shows hypoplastic maxilla and mandible with marked concavity of the body of the mandible. **20153:** Arachnodactyly and camptodactyly.

abdominal hernias; arachnodactyly; **Eye, hypertelorism**; exophthalmos; mental retardation; soft, low-set, posteriorly rotated ears; **Mitral valve prolapse**, joint contractures; **Foot, talipes equinovarus (TEV)**, **Pectus excavatum** or **Pectus carinatum**.

**Clinical Findings:** Craniosynostosis with an abnormally shaped cranium is present at birth. Obstructive apnea may also be present and is caused by an extremely small pharyngeal airway secondary to severe basicranial kyphosis. Both the maxilla and the mandible are hypoplastic, with the mandible showing a marked concavity of the body. Exophthalmos is accompanied by strabismus. The hard palatal shelves show severe soft tissue hypertrophy ("pseudocleft"). Infantile hypotonia has been a constant feature, as has developmental delay and mental retardation, which is usually severe in spite of surgical correction of the craniosynostosis. Speech and language impairment are particularly severe. Multiple large abdominal **Hernia** are the rule, including inguinal, umbilical, and diastasis recti. Arachnodactyly is also present from birth and may be accompanied by multiple digital contractures, which may improve with age. **Mitral valve prolapse** is common. Many joints may be abnormal, probably secondary to connective tissue abnormalities.

**Complications:** Severe obstructive apnea could lead to sudden death if untreated. The severe abnormalities of the maxilla and mandible combined with the severe hypotonia may result in deglutition problems. Because of the severely kyphotic cranial base, optic atrophy and increased intracranial pressure may occur in spite of early craniectomy. Delayed motor milestones are secondary to both cognitive impairment and joint limitation.

**Associated Findings:** Conductive hearing loss, drooling.

**Etiology:** Unknown.

**Pathogenesis:** The findings associated with this syndrome suggest some type of connective tissue abnormality, which might account for most or all of the anomalies. However, biochemical testing of tissue samples from two patients has not yielded any specific abnormalities.

**POS No.:** 3669

**Sex Ratio:** Unknown. All reported patients to date have been male.

**Occurrence:** Presumably rare, but it is also possible that many affected infants do not survive the neonatal period and are undiagnosed.

**Risk of Recurrence for Patient's Sib:** Undetermined but presumed low.

**Risk of Recurrence for Patient's Child:** Undetermined but probably low. Affected individuals are not likely to reproduce.

**Age of Detectability:** At birth. Severe cranial abnormalities, hernias, and other structural abnormalities may be detectable on fetal ultrasound imaging or fetoscopy. Otherwise.

**Gene Mapping and Linkage:** Unknown.

**Prevention:** None known. Genetic counseling indicated.

**Treatment:** Craniectomies are indicated to relieve craniosynostosis, and abdominal hernias may be treated surgically. Tracheostomy may be necessary for obstructive apnea. Joint contractures may improve with age and physical therapy. Speech and language therapy is indicated if cognitive functioning permits.

**Prognosis:** No adult patients have been reported; all known patients are children or adolescents. Therefore, complete information on life span is unavailable. Cognitive status of all known patients indicates a very poor prognosis for normal intellectual functioning.

**Detection of Carrier:** Unknown.

**References:**

Sugarman G, Vogel MW: Craniofacial and musculoskeletal abnormalities: a questionable connective tissue disease. Synd Ident 1981; 7:16–17.

Shprintzen RJ, Goldberg RG: A recurrent pattern syndrome of craniosynostosis associated with arachnodactyly and abdominal hernias. J Craniofac Genet Dev Biol 1982; 2:65–74.

Cohen MM Jr: Craniosynostosis. New York: Raven, 1986.

SH040                               **Robert J. Shprintzen**
G0008                               **Rosalie B. Goldberg**

**Craniosynostosis-bifid hallux syndrome**
*See CRANIOSYNOSTOSIS-FOOT DEFECTS, JACKSON-WEISS TYPE*
**Craniosynostosis-craniofacial dysostosis-other anomalies**
*See CRANIOFACIAL DYSSYNOSTOSIS*

## CRANIOSYNOSTOSIS-FIBULAR APLASIA, LOWRY TYPE        2184

**Includes:**

Fibular aplasia-craniosynostosis, Lowry type
Lowry syndrome

**Excludes:**
  **Craniosynostosis-radial aplasia syndrome** (0231)
  **Hermann-Pallister-Opitz syndrome** (2177)

**Major Diagnostic Criteria:** The combination of craniosynostosis and fibular aplasia.

**Clinical Findings:** Two cases have been reported. Findings in one or both include craniosynostosis, sagittal and/or coronal (2); large posterior fontanelle (1); prominent eyes (2); strabismus (1); highly arched or cleft palate (2); low-set ears (1); short, webbed neck (1); short sternum (1); cryptorchidism (2); chordee of penis (1); pilonidal dimple (1); transverse palmar creases (2); absent fibulae (2); and equinovarus (2).

**Complications:** The younger of the two affected children died soon after birth of respiratory distress. It is not known if neonatal complications are more frequent.

**Associated Findings:** None known.

**Etiology:** The occurrence in two sibs born of consanguineous parents suggests autosomal recessive inheritance.

**Pathogenesis:** Unknown.

**MIM No.:** 21855

**POS No.:** 3171

**Sex Ratio:** M2:F0 (observed in the two known cases).

**Occurrence:** Reported in two brothers of consanguineous parents.

**Risk of Recurrence for Patient's Sib:**
See Part I, *Mendelian Inheritance.*

**Risk of Recurrence for Patient's Child:**
See Part I, *Mendelian Inheritance.*

**Age of Detectability:** At birth; prenatal diagnosis using ultrasound may also be possible.

**Gene Mapping and Linkage:** Unknown.

**Prevention:** None known. Genetic counseling indicated.

**Treatment:** Craniectomy for correction of the craniosynostosis may be indicated.

**Prognosis:** The one surviving child was mentally normal at five years of age.

**Detection of Carrier:** Unknown.

**References:**
Lowry RB: Congenital absence of the fibula and craniosynostosis in sibs. J Med Genet 1972; 9:227–229.

T0007                               **Helga V. Toriello**

## CRANIOSYNOSTOSIS-FOOT DEFECTS, JACKSON-WEISS TYPE        2511

**Includes:**

Acrocephalosyndactyly, Robinow-Sorauf type
Craniosynostosis-bifid hallux syndrome
Craniosynostosis-midface hypoplasia-foot abnormalities
Jackson-Weiss craniosynostosis
Robinow-Sorauf syndrome

**Excludes:**
  **Acrocephalopolysyndactyly** (0013)
  **Acrocephalosyndactyly**
  **Craniofacial dysostosis** (0225)

**Major Diagnostic Criteria:** Craniosynostosis, abnormalities of facial bones in association with varus deformities of the great toes, and tarsal fusion. Although the literature suggests that no thumb anomalies occur, in the family reported by Escobar and Bixler (1977a,b) big thumbs with varus deformities were observed.

**Clinical Findings:** An unusual spectrum of craniofacial and foot anomalies has been described in this syndrome. However, with the exception of the clinical and X-ray appearance of the feet, no consistent manifestations have been observed. In some families, the craniofacial anomalies suggest Crouzon disease (see **Craniofacial dysostosis**) associated with foot anomalies, while in others, different types of **Acrocephalosyndactyly** can be observed.

The most commonly reported malformations include acrocephaly, **Craniosynostosis**, maxillary hypoplasia, deep-flattened nasal bridge, flat occiput, parrot-beaked nose, **Hydrocephaly**, deviation of nasal septum, anomalies of the external ear, hypertelorism, downward slanting of the palpebral fissures, ptosis of eyelids, strabismus, **Cleft palate**, and high-arched palate. Other less commonly observed anomalies include limitation of joint movement, genu valgum, **Syndactyly** (both "webbing" and "mitten" types), bone fusion abnormalities, absent phalanges, **Brachydactyly**, clinodactyly, **Camptodactyly**, big toes (possible duplication), hallux valgus, and broad and short first metatarsals. Dermatoglyphic alterations have been reported, and a low IQ has been present in a few patients.

Cephalometric analysis shows that both the maxilla and the mandible are small, both in ramus height and in body length. Also prominent are a marked upward slant of the lesser wings of the sphenoid, a depressed sella turcica, and small posterior and anterior cranial fossae. Posterior facial height is normal. X-ray analysis of the hands shows a generalized brachydactyly. The metacarpophalangeal pattern profile analysis (MCPP) is unique; it is highly correlated (r = .93) with the mean pattern generated from X-rays of **Acrocephalosyndactyly type V** patients.

**Complications:** Severe headaches, visual disturbances, and raised intracranial pressure secondary to **Craniosynostosis**. Mental retardation of variable degrees has been reported. Ambulatory difficulties may be present due to the feet abnormalities. The palatal clefting may require special feeding considerations.

**Associated Findings:** The outlook for normal central nervous system function is variable, but most patients are of average or above average intelligence.

**Etiology:** Four separate reports have fully described three families affected with what appears to be a separate acrocephalosyndactyly syndrome. The initial report by Cross and Opitz (1969) suggested autosomal recessive inheritance, but further study of the family by Jackson et al (1976) demonstrated autosomal dominant mode of transmission with variable expression and incomplete penetrance. This has since been confirmed by Robinow and Sorauf (1975) and by Escobar and Bixler (1977a,b).

**Pathogenesis:** Unknown.

**MIM No.:** 12315, *21850, 18075

**POS No.:** 3512

**CDC No.:** 756.057

**Sex Ratio:** M1:F1

**Occurrence:** Three families have been fully described and several others have been reported.

**Risk of Recurrence for Patient's Sib:**
See Part I, *Mendelian Inheritance.*

**Risk of Recurrence for Patient's Child:**
See Part I, *Mendelian Inheritance.*

**Age of Detectability:** At birth, with affected individuals showing craniosynostosis with or without foot deformities.

**Gene Mapping and Linkage:** Unknown.

**Prevention:** None known. Genetic counseling indicated.

**Treatment:** Surgery for the craniosynostosis, cleft palate, and foot and hand deformities. Speech therapy may be necessary.

**Prognosis:** After surgery and with proper follow up, life span seems to be normal. No mental retardation has been present in adult patients who did not undergo craniofacial surgery during childhood.

**Detection of Carrier:** Clinical examination. Cephalometric and metacarpophalangeal analyses seem to be useful in identifying "normal" heterozygote carriers.

**References:**

Cross HE, Opitz JM: Craniosynostosis in the Amish. J Pediatr 1969; 75:1037–1044.

Robinow M, Sorauf R: Acrocephalopolysyndactyly, type Noack, in a large kindred. BD:OAS XI(5). New York: March of Dimes Birth Defects Foundation, 1975:99–106.

Jackson CE, et al.: Craniosynostosis, midface hypoplasia, and foot abnormalities: an autosomal dominant phenotype in a large Amish kindred. J Pediatr 1976; 88:963–968.

Escobar V, Bixler D: Are the acrocephalosyndactyly syndromes variable expressions of a single gene defect? BD:OAS XIII(3C). New York: March of Dimes Birth Defects Foundation, 1977a:139–154.

Escobar V, Bixler D: On the classification of the acrocephalosyndactyly syndromes. Clin Genet 1977b; 12:169–178.

ES000                                          **Victor Escobar**

---

**Craniosynostosis-hypertrichosis-facial and other anomalies**
*See GORLIN-CHAUDHRY-MOSS SYNDROME*
**Craniosynostosis-malformed extremities-cleft lip/palate**
*See HERRMANN-PALLISTER-OPITZ SYNDROME*

---

## CRANIOSYNOSTOSIS-MENTAL RETARDATION-CLEFTING SYNDROME                 2790

**Includes:** Clefting syndrome-craniosynostosis-mental retardation

**Excludes:** Craniosynostosis (other syndromes)

**Major Diagnostic Criteria:** Craniosynostosis, mental retardation, **Cleft lip**, **Cleft palate**, and choroidal coloboma.

**Clinical Findings:** Cleft lip and palate and choroidal colobomas would be suggestive in a child with developmental delay and oxycephaly. The head circumference is likely to be small, with some flattening of the occiput. The other facial features are those found in other craniosynostoses and include a broad forehead, mild hypertelorism, beak-shaped nose, and protuberant ears. It would be necessary to look for renal pathology, especially a cystic dysplasia. Mild mesomelic shortening of the forearms and legs and a dry skin are possible added features. Mental retardation is moderate to severe.

**Complications:** Mental retardation and renal dysfunction.

**Associated Findings:** None known.

**Etiology:** Possibly autosomal recessive inheritance.

**Pathogenesis:** Unknown.

**MIM No.:** 21865

**Sex Ratio:** M1:F1 (observed).

**Occurrence:** An affected brother and sister have been documented in the literature.

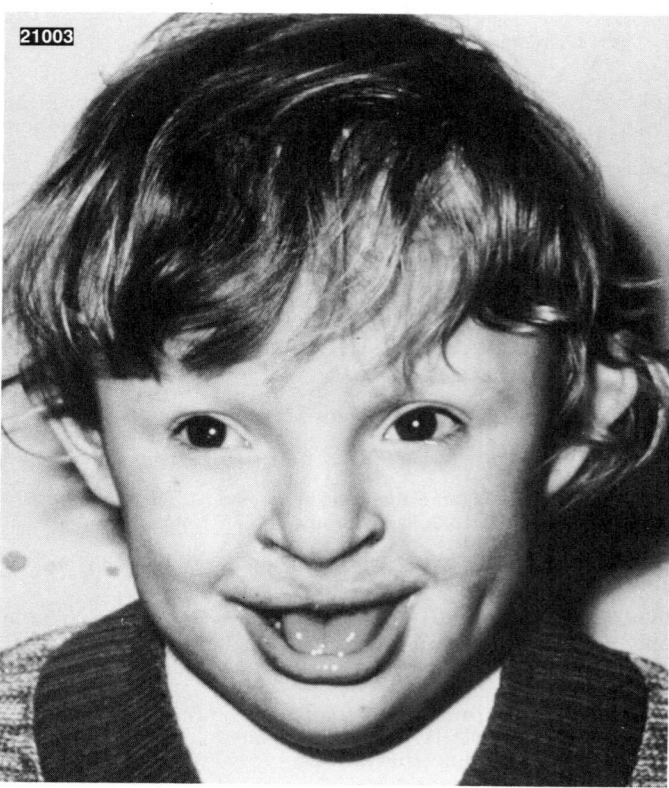

2790-21003: Note the broad forehead, mild hypotelorism, repaired cleft lip and palate, and anteverted ears.

**Risk of Recurrence for Patient's Sib:**
See Part I, *Mendelian Inheritance.*

**Risk of Recurrence for Patient's Child:**
See Part I, *Mendelian Inheritance.*

**Age of Detectability:** Prenatal diagnosis is possible through detection of the cleft lip and palate. It is difficult to make a diagnosis at birth, however, because the sutures, which close prematurely, might only close during the first few years of life and not at birth.

**Gene Mapping and Linkage:** Unknown.

**Prevention:** None known. Genetic counseling indicated.

**Treatment:** Unknown.

**Prognosis:** Mental retardation, renal failure.

**Detection of Carrier:** Unknown.

**References:**

Baraitser M, et al.: A new craniosynostosis-mental retardation syndrome diagnosed by fetoscopy. Clin Genet 1982; 22:12–15.

BA058                                        **Michael Baraitser**

**Craniosynostosis-midface hypoplasia-foot abnormalities**
*See CRANIOSYNOSTOSIS-FOOT DEFECTS, JACKSON-WEISS TYPE*

## CRANIOSYNOSTOSIS-RADIAL APLASIA SYNDROME     0231

**Includes:**
> Baller-Gerold syndrome
> Radial aplasia-craniosynostosis

**Excludes:**
> **Acrocephalosyndactyly**
> **Pancytopenia syndrome, Fanconi type** (2029)
> **Thrombocytopenia-absent radius** (0941)

**Major Diagnostic Criteria:** Craniosynostosis of one or more sutures and radial aplasia (probably bilateral).

**Clinical Findings:** Craniosynostosis present in all cases, but different sutures involved in different cases. Turribrachycephaly with steep forehead, high nasal bridge, and prominent mandible have been described. Epicanthal folds, ocular hypotelorism, and small dysplastic ears have been present. Radial aplasia or hypoplasia is present bilaterally in all cases. The thumb is hypoplastic, or absent. Metacarpal and carpal bones are fused, hypoplastic, or absent. Ulna is short and curved with radial deviation of the hand. Vertebral anomalies, rib anomalies, genitourinary anomalies, prenatal hearing loss, imperforate anus with or without fistula, delayed development, and scaling skin have been described. Intelligence is normal. One child had sudden unexplained death, and at autopsy polymicrogyria of the brain and subaortic valvular hypertrophy were present.

**Complications:** Craniosynostosis can lead to brain compression, but in this condition it is not clear whether the anomaly of the calvaria is primary or secondary to a deficit in brain growth. Delayed fine motor development in hands may occur because of arm and hand anomalies.

**Associated Findings:** None known.

**Etiology:** Presumably autosomal recessive inheritance. Consanguinity was present in two families, and male and female sibs were affected in another family.

**Pathogenesis:** Unknown.

**MIM No.:** *21860

**POS No.:** 3165

**Sex Ratio:** Presumably M1:F1

**Occurrence:** Some eight cases have been documented.

**Risk of Recurrence for Patient's Sib:**
> See Part I, *Mendelian Inheritance.*

**Risk of Recurrence for Patient's Child:**
> See Part I, *Mendelian Inheritance.*

**Age of Detectability:** Prenatally by ultrasound.

**Gene Mapping and Linkage:** Unknown.

**Prevention:** None known. Genetic counseling indicated.

**Treatment:** Prenatal diagnosis may be possible at 16–20 weeks (looking for radius). Surgical correction of synostosis if signs of increased cranial pressures or for cosmetic indications. Urologic evaluation to rule out obstructive anomaly. Spine X-ray to rule out vertebral anomaly that could lead to scoliosis. Corrective orthopedic surgery, physical and occupational therapy.

**Prognosis:** Would appear to be good if CNS is normal.

**Detection of Carrier:** Unknown.

**References:**
Greitzer LJ, et al.: Craniosynostosis-radial aplasia syndrome. J Pediatr 1974; 84:723–724.
Cohen MM: An etiologic and nosologic overview of craniosynostosis syndromes. In: Bergsma D, ed: Malformation syndromes. BD:OAS; XI(2):137. Amsterdam: Excerpta Medica, for The National Foundation-March of Dimes, 1975.
Anyane-Yeboa K, et al.: Baller-Gerold syndrome craniosynostosis-radial aplasia syndrome. Clin Genet 1980; 17:161–166. *
Pelias MZ, et al.: A sixth report (eighth case) of craniosynostosis-radial aplasia syndrome. Am J Med Genet 1981; 10:133–139. *

HA014            **Judith G. Hall**

## CRANIOTELENCEPHALIC DYSPLASIA     2791

**Includes:**
> Brain anomalies-frontal bone protuberance
> Forehead, bony protuberance-brain anomalies

**Excludes:**
> **Craniofacial dyssynostosis** (0227)
> **Holoprosencephaly** (0473)
> **Septo-optic dysplasia** (2018)
> **Walker-Warburg syndrome** (2869)

**Major Diagnostic Criteria:** The combination of frontal bone protuberance and brain anomalies.

**Clinical Findings:** Anomalies are limited to the craniofacial region. All affected children have had craniosynostosis, with a bony protuberance on the forehead. In 2/4 cases, a frontal encephalocele was also present. Microphthalmia (2/4), preauricular skin tags (1/4), and hypotelorism (1/4), likely secondary to the skull defect, have also been reported. CT examinations in two infants revealed **Hydrocephaly** (2/2), agenesis of the corpus callosum (1/2), hypoplastic cerebellum (1/2), and optic nerve hypoplasia with or without orbital hypoplasia (2/2). Autopsy in one child demonstrated lissencephaly with micropolygyria, absent olfactory nerves, hypoplastic optic nerves, absent corpus callosum, partial fusion of frontal lobes, aqueductal stenosis, neuronal heteropia in the cerebellum, and absent medullary pyramids.

**Complications:** Unknown.

**Associated Findings:** None known.

**Etiology:** Possibly autosomal recessive inheritance.

**Pathogenesis:** The craniosynostosis is thought to be secondary to abnormal brain growth; therefore, the primary defect is likely related to cerebral dysgenesis.

**MIM No.:** 21867

**POS No.:** 3639

**Sex Ratio:** M1:F3 (observed).

**Occurrence:** Four cases have been reported in detail (two affected sisters and two sporadic cases) from France, Canada, and the United States.

**Risk of Recurrence for Patient's Sib:**
> See Part I, *Mendelian Inheritance.*

**Risk of Recurrence for Patient's Child:**
> See Part I, *Mendelian Inheritance.*

**Age of Detectability:** At birth, although prenatal diagnosis by ultrasound is probably possible.

**Gene Mapping and Linkage:** Unknown.

**Prevention:** None known. Genetic counseling indicated.

**Treatment:** Surgical correction of craniosynostosis and corrective alignment of the frontal bone may be indicated.

**Prognosis:** All patients have been severely retarded, with the oldest reported child at 36 months being at an 18-month developmental level. Two affected children died by age nine months.

**Detection of Carrier:** Unknown.

**Special Considerations:** It has been suggested that craniotelencephalic dysplasia is the same condition as **Craniofacial dyssynostosis**, albeit a more severe presentation of the same basic defect. Additional reports of sibs will be necessary to confirm this hypothesis.

There are also many similarities to the **Walker-Warburg syndrome**, with the presence of craniosynostosis in craniotelencephalic dysplasia differentiating the two conditions. However, if the craniosynostosis is secondary to abnormal brain development, then the difference between the two conditions may simply be variability rather than heterogeneity.

**References:**
Daum S, et al.: Dysplasie telencephalique avec excroissance de l'os frontal. Sem Hop Paris 1958; 34:1893–1896.
Jabbour JT, Taybi H: Craniotelencephalic dysplasia. Am J Dis Child 1964; 108:627–632.

Hughes HE, et al.: Craniotelencephalic dysplasia in sisters: further delineation of a possible syndrome. Am J Med Genet 1983; 14:557–565. * †

T0007                                                               **Helga V. Toriello**

**Cranium bifidum**
  *See ENCEPHALOCELE*
**Crease, single palmar**
  *See SKIN CREASE, SINGLE PALMAR*
**CREST syndrome**
  *See SCLERODERMA, FAMILIAL PROGRESSIVE*
**Cretinism induced by extrinsic goitrogens**
  *See CRETINISM, ENDEMIC, AND RELATED DISORDERS*
**Cretinism, agoitrous**
  *See THYROID, DYSGENESIS*
**Cretinism, athyreotic**
  *See THYROID, DYSGENESIS*

---

## CRETINISM, ENDEMIC, AND RELATED DISORDERS            3167

**Includes:**
  Cretinism induced by extrinsic goitrogens
  Deafness, from extrinsically caused iodine disorder
  Fetal hypothyroidism of extrinsic origin
  Goiter, from extrinsically caused fetal iodine disorder
  Iodine deficiency, extrinsic, and fetal injury
  Mental retardation, from extrinsically caused iodine disorder
  Myxedematous endemic cretinism
  Nervous system endemic cretinism
  Spastic diplegia, from extrinsically caused iodine disorder

**Excludes:**
  Cretinism, sporadic nongoitrous
  Dwarfism and brain defects from other causes
  Embryonic errors of thyroid development
  Inborn errors of thyroid function
  Iodine, failure to concentrate
  Thyroglobulin metabolism, defects in
  **Thyroid, dysgenesis** (0946)
  **Thyroid, hormone resistance** (0257)
  **Thyroid, iodotyrosine deiodinase deficiency** (0543)
  **Thyroid, peroxidase defect** (0947)
  **Thyrotropin unresponsiveness** (0948)

**Major Diagnostic Criteria:**  Mental retardation, dwarfism, and/or congenital hypothyroidism, in areas with iodine deficiency or exposure to goitrogens.

**Clinical Findings:**  Endemic cretinism is perhaps the earliest recognized environmentally induced teratogenicity. Two syndromes exist. The first, sometimes identified as *nervous system endemic cretinism*, is characterized by mental deficiency and/or deaf mutism, sometimes with neuromuscular disorders, diplegia and squint, but without hypothyroidism. The second, sometimes identified as *myxedematous endemic cretinism*, has thyroid hypoplasia leading to persisting hypothyroidism beginning *in utero* and continuing from birth, with mental deficiency, abnormal skeletal maturation, and dwarfing, resembling that seen in sporadic cretinism. Both types have been seen in endemic goiter areas, and although either syndrome may be characteristic in a particular area, both may occur in the same area. Endemic cretinism represents only the extreme stage of a broader spectrum of developmental abnormalities, most significantly, mental retardation. T4 levels are usually low.

**Complications:**  Rarely, neonatal goiters are large enough to cause tracheal obstruction.

**Associated Findings:**  Abortions and stillbirths are increased in iodine deficiency pregnancies.

**Etiology:**  Fetal thyroid deficiency, either due to maternal dietary iodide deficiency and/or exposures to substance interfering with thyroid metabolism, *including even excessive iodine*. Drug goitigens include iodine-containing cough mixtures, amiodarone (antiarrhythmic), and lithium (used in the treatment of mood disorders).

**Pathogenesis:**  The observation that endemic cretinism may be more refractory to treatment than congenital hypothyroidism from intrinsic thyroid defects suggests that maternal thyroid (or iodine) deficiency contributes to irreversable fetal injury beyond that caused by intrinsic fetal thyroid deficiency.

**Sex Ratio:**  M1:F1

**Occurrence:**  A quarter of the world's population subsists on an iodine deficient diet. These are in inland areas not served by markets providing iodized salt, where iodine is not present in the soil. The largest problem is in Asia where 400,000,000 people are at risk, but the problem is also extensive in Latin America (especially mountainous areas), central Africa, Papau New Guinea, and other areas. In iodine deficiency areas, the combined incidence of the two cretinism syndromes may total 1–6%. Cretinism rapidly disappeared in iodine deficient areas of the United States and Europe with the marketing of iodized salt.

**Risk of Recurrence for Patient's Sib:**  Related to exposure.

**Risk of Recurrence for Patient's Child:**  Related to exposure. Endemic cretins are often the offspring of goitrous, and less often hypothyroid, mothers.

**Age of Detectability:**  At birth, but the condition is often undetected until several months of age.

**Gene Mapping and Linkage:**  N/A

**Prevention:**  Both forms can be prevented by iodine supplementation, usually provided in table salt, and or avoidance of goitrogenic environmental exposures. Pre-pregnancy injection of iodized oil before pregnancy will prevent iodine deficiency cretinism, but injections in the first trimester of pregnancy will not. An iodized oil injection can correct iodine deficiency for 3–5 years. Periodic oral administration of iodized oil has a comparable effect, and is increasingly used instead of injections. Population studies of urinary iodine levels and goiter frequency are the usual methods of detecting areas at risk for endemic cretinism and related disorders.

**Treatment:**  Administration of thyroid hormone for hypothyroidism, but iodine administration during pregnancy may not be fully successful. Many cretins, especially of the neurologic form, are euthyroid. In endemic cretinism areas, thyroid is started too late to have full effect.

**Prognosis:**  Thyroid hormone will correct hypothyroidism, but mental and developmental retardation persist. Prognosis is worse in the myxedematous form.

**Detection of Carrier:**  Mothers are usually iodine deficient and often goitrous.

**Special Considerations:**  An International Council for Control of Iodine Deficiency Disorders coordinates Agency interests in this problem.

**References:**
Warkony J: Iodine deficiency. Teratology 1985; 31:309–311.
Hetzel BS: Progress in the prevention and control of iodine-deficiency disorders. Lancet 1987; II:266.
Hetzel AI, Dunn JT, Stanbury JB, eds: Major health issues: the prevention and control of iodine deficiency disorders. Amsterdam: Elsevier, 1987. *

R0018                                                               **Franz W. Rosa**

**Cretinism, sporadic nongoitrous**
  *See THYROID, DYSGENESIS*

## CREUTZFELDT-JAKOB DISEASE 3244

**Includes:**

Heidenhain variant
Spastic pseudosclerosis
Subacute spongiform encephalopathy

**Excludes:**

**Alzheimer disease**
**Gerstmann-Straussler syndrome** (3245)
Kuru
Multi-infarct dementia
**Pick disease of the brain** (3243)

**Major Diagnostic Criteria:** Rapidly progressive dementia with onset in middle-age and associated with myoclonus, heightened startle reaction, and a variety of pyramidal and extrapyramidal features. Although CNS involvement is diffuse, focal neurologic signs and symptoms may be present depending on sites of maximal cerebral involvement. Brain computerized tomography (CT) or magnetic resonance imaging (MRI) may show cerebral atrophy or ventricular enlargement. The electroencephalogram (EEG) is distinctive, showing periodic sharp wave complexes and is frequently the most helpful diagnostic test in supporting the clinical impression. Diagnosis is confirmed by postmortem examination or rarely from biopsy of the brain which shows spongiform degeneration. The disease has been shown to be prion associated, and horizontal transmission has been demonstrated.

**Clinical Findings:** The onset of clinical symptoms is usually in the sixth or seventh decade. Although there may be variations in the clinical symptomatology, three clearly identifiable phases are recognized. The initial or prodromal phase usually lasts several weeks to months and is characterized by the insidious onset of vague physical and behavioral symptoms. Apprehension, fatigue, apathy, depression, dizziness, forgetfulness, insomnia, and complaints of generalized weakness are common. A functional disorder is often entertained. The prodromal symptoms are followed by a second phase of rapidly accumulating neurological deficits that include the subacutedevelopment of a cortical dementia in conjunction with characteristic pyramidal and extrapyramidal signs. Multiple cognitive impairments are seen, frequently with prominent aphasia. Myoclonus, exaggerated tendon reflexes, and a heightened startle reaction are characteristic. A wide variety of additional symptoms can be seen, including focal motor and sensory findings. This phase usually lasts 1–4 months.

Several clinical variants have been described, primarily reflecting predominant differential clinical features of this second phase of the illness. Preferential involvement of occipital cortices with prominent visual symptoms or cortical blindness is referred to as the *Heidenhain* variant; an ataxic form of the disease presents with primarily cerebellar involvement. Although the frequency with which lower motor neuron findings occur is controversial, most investigators do recognize a clinical variant with prominent amyotrophy and fasciculations. This usually occurs late in the disease and is more likely to be seen in disease of longer than average duration. The clinical differences are usually obscured when the third and terminal phase supervenes which is characterized by mutism, unresponsiveness, increased myoclonus, seizures, autonomic disturbances and usually decerebrate rigidity. The patient may survive in coma for several months; death is usually from infectious causes, most frequently pneumonia.

Jakob et al (1950) and his predecessors described the first reported family, the Backer kindred. Multiple well documented and pathologically confirmed pedigrees having apparently autosomal transmission have since been described. About 15% of all cases are familial. Although the clinical findings are generally similar in the familial and sporadic forms, onset of disease is usually earlier in familial cases and the course is more protracted. There tends to be a somewhat lower frequency of myoclonus, although it is still prominent at 79%.

Routine laboratory studies of the blood, serum, and urine are normal. CSF is generally normal (80%), although an increased protein or slight lymphocytosis can be seen. CSF immunoreactivity with prion-associated proteins has been demonstrated and is being investigated as a potential diagnostic tool. Neuroimaging studies (brain CT or MRI) may be normal or show mild diffuse atrophy; the usefulness of positron emission tomography (PET) is undetermined.

The most helpful diagnostic test is the EEG which demonstrates characteristic periodic sharp wave complexes (PSWC). These are frequently triphasic waves, having an amplitude of 50–200 uV, and a characteristic frequently of 1–2 per second. Levy et al have comprehensively reviewed the literature regarding EEG findings. They report that PSWC often appeared in the EEG before myoclonus is evident, and occurred within 12 weeks of onset of illness in 88% patients. In the approximately 10% of patients who had an unusually long course, PSWC appeared in only 55%. The earlier the onset of PSWC, the shorter the disease duration. There is no clear association of the PSWC with myoclonic jerks. Levy et al maintain that the absence of PSWC in the EEG after 12 weeks duration is a point strongly against the diagnosis of CJD, unless it is a rare subtype of long duration. In addition to PSWC, generalized slowing of the background is seen.

Neuropathological examination confirms the clinical diagnosis and is quite distinctive. Three findings are characteristic: (1) prominent neuronal degeneration and cell loss, (2) astrocytic proliferation and gliosis, and (3) varying degrees of spongiform change in the grey matter resulting from cytoplasmic vacuolization in glia. Although not invariably found, the spongiform changes are considered the most salient characteristic. No vascular or inflammatory changes are seen. Prion associated proteins and immunoreactivity have been demonstrated in neuropathological specimens.

**Complications:** Rapidly progressive dementia leads to loss of employment and disruption of familial and interpersonal relationships. Visual impairment and blindness is not uncommon due to involvement of occipital cortices.

**Associated Findings:** Vertigo, diplopia, cortical blindness, vertical gaze palsy, lower motor neuron findings, sleep disturbances (hyper and hyposomnia), diaphoresis, loss of abdominal cutaneous reflexes, and subjective sensory complaints can be seen. There is an apparent association with increased previous surgical procedures, trauma, and other major medical illnesses. Associations with HLA specificities DRw53 and DQw3 have been reported. Familial **Retinitis pigmentosa** has been reported in at least one pedigree.

**Etiology:** Although most cases appear sporadic, approximately 15% of all cases are familial in a pattern consistent with autosomal dominant inheritance.

**Pathogenesis:** Previously considered a disease transmitted by an "unconventional slow virus", CJD is now considered a prion associated disease. Horizontal transmission to nonhuman primates by cerebral inoculation has been demonstrated by many investigators. Iatrogenic human-to-human transmission via corneal transplants, human growth hormone injections, and from implantation of contaminated stereotactic electrodes has been documented. At least two conjugal cases have been reported, but this appears to be exceedingly rare. The mechanism for familial expression of the disease is unknown but both pathogenesis and transmission are thought to be related to the prion protein gene on chromosome 20. Whether there is a susceptibility locus or perhaps a "mutant" gene that is sufficient for development of the disease is unknonw.

**MIM No.:** *12340

**Sex Ratio:** M1:F1

**Occurrence:** This condition has been estimated to affect 1: 1,000,000 persons per year. World wide distribution is seen, although increased frequencies have been reported in Libyan born Israelis, and in Chile.

**Risk of Recurrence for Patient's Sib:**

See Part I, *Mendelian Inheritance*. In well documented pedigrees, percentages of siblings affected have been reported to vary between 27–80%.

**Risk of Recurrence for Patient's Child:**
See Part I, *Mendelian Inheritance*. This risk has not been adequately studied.

**Age of Detectability:** Onset is usually in the sixth or seventh decade, although patients as young as 20 have been reported. Earlier onset has been seen in association with iatrogenic infection. Familial cases have a significantly earlier age of onset than sporadic cases, and tend to have a more protracted course (average age of death is 51 in familial vs. 58 in sporadic cases). Anticipation phenomena alone cannot explain this earlier onset given, the short duration of the disease.

**Gene Mapping and Linkage:** Unknown. Owen et al (1989) reported an apparently rare Msp1 polymorphism in the prion protein (PrP) gene on chromosome 20 that appears to track with an autosomal dominant dementing illness with onset in middle age in a family with a neuropathologically confirmed history.

**Prevention:** None known. Genetic counseling indicated.

**Treatment:** None currently available to treat the primary disease. Supportive medical care, educational and supportive assistance to the families, and symptomatic treatment of complications as needed.

**Prognosis:** The disease is rapidly progressive and invariably fatal, with a mean duration of illness of eight months. Ninety percent of patients die within a year of symptom onset. The familial form appears to take a slightly longer course than sporadic cases, with mean duration of illness being 11 months.

**Detection of Carrier:** Unknown. Careful investigation of pedigrees may disclose persons at risk.

**Special Considerations:** Pruisner and others have investigated the role of prions in the development of a variety of diseases. Prions are transmissible pathogens that cause degenerative diseases in humans and animals (e.g. scrapie, transmissible mink encephalopathy, Kuru, **Gerstmann-Straussler syndrome**). Pathological features include neuronal vacuolation (spongiform changes), astrocytic proliferation and gliosis, and deposition of amyloid plaques. Westaway et al (1989) discuss the unique attributes of prion diseases which include infectious, sporadic and genetic manifestations, as well as progression to death, all in the absence of a detectable immune response. Prions are composed largely of a protein encoded by a cellular host gene, which distinguishes them from viruses. The human and mouse prion protein (PrP) genes have been shown to be located on chromosomes 20 and 2, respectively, which are homologous. The PrP gene of mice is linked to a gene controlling scrapie incubation times. The PrP gene of long incubation period mice encodes a variant prion protein. An amino acid substitution has recently been genetically linked to the development of **Gerstmann-Straussler syndrome**. Although prion diseases resemble viral illnesses in some respects, there is compelling evidence that they are genetically controlled diseases.

**References:**
Jakob H, et al.: Hereditary form of Creutzfeldt-Jakob disease (Backer family). Arch Psychiat 1950; 184:653–674.
May WW, et al.: Creutzfeldt-Jakob disease II: clinical, pathologic and genetic study of a family. Arch Neurol Psychiat 1968; 19:137–149.
Masters CL, et al.: Creutzfeldt-Jakob disease: patterns of worldwide occurrence and the significance of familial and sporadic clustering. Ann Neurol 1979; 5:177–188.
Masters CL, et al.: The familial occurrence of Creutzfeldt-Jakob disease and Alzheimer's disease. Brain 1981; 104:535–558.
Owen F, et al.: Insertion in prion protein gene in familial Creutzfeldt-Jakob disease. Lancet 1989; 51–52.
Westaway D, et al.: Unraveling prion diseases through molecular genetics. Trends Neurosci 1989; 12:331–337.

EA005                                                          **Nancy Lorraine Earl**

**Cri du chat syndrome**
See CHROMOSOME 5, MONOSOMY 5p
**Crigler-Najjar syndrome, type I**
See UDP-GLUCURONOSYLTRANSFERASE, SEVERE DEFICIENCY
TYPE I

**Crigler-Najjar syndrome, type II**
See HYPERBILIRUBINEMIA, UNCONJUGATED
**Criswick-Schepens syndrome**
See RETINA, VITREORETINOPATHY, FAMILIAL EXUDATIVE
**Crohn disease**
See INFLAMMATORY BOWEL DISEASE
**Crome syndrome**
See CATARACT-RENAL TUBULAR NECROSIS-ENCEPHALOPATHY, CROME TYPE
**Cronkhite-Canada syndrome**
See POLYPOSIS-ALOPECIA-PIGMENTATION-NAIL DEFECTS
**Cross syndrome**
See GINGIVAL FIBROMATOSIS-DEPIGMENTATION-MICROPHTHALMIA
**Croup, congenital**
See LARYNGOMALACIA
**Crouzon syndrome**
See CRANIOFACIAL DYSOSTOSIS

## CRYOGLOBULINEMIA                                              3138

**Includes:**
Essential cryoglobulinemia, familial
Meltzer-Franklin syndrome
Mixed cryoglobulinemia, familial

**Excludes:**
Cryoglobulinemia associated with chronic infections
Cryoglobulinemia associated with collagen-vascular disorders
Cryoglobulinemia associated with lymphoproliferative diseases

**Major Diagnostic Criteria:** The clinical syndrome of mixed cryoglobulinemia consists of recurrent palpable purpura (100% of patients), polyarthralgias (73%), and renal disease (55%). In general, the cryoglobulins have rheumatoid factor activity and contain IgM and polyclonal IgG.

**Clinical Findings:** *Skin:* purpuras, leg ulcers, cold urticaria, papules, hemorrhagic bullae, arthralgias, **Raynaud disease**, gangrene. *Kidney:* proteinuria, nephrotic syndrome, renal failure, hypertension, glomerulonephritis. *Neurologic:* polyneuropathy, demyelination, footdrop. *Liver:* hepatomegaly, chronic active hepatitis, lymphadenopathy, splenomegaly. Gastrointestinal, cardiac, pulmonary, and other organs may also be involved.

**Complications:** Chronic renal failure, hypertension, infections, systemic vasculitis

**Associated Findings:** None known.

**Etiology:** Autosomal dominant inheritance of cryoglobulinemia in three families (association with deficiency of C4 in one family) but presumably autosomal recessive inheritance in four sisters of one family. Sibs or parents may be asymptomatic.

**Pathogenesis:** Organ damage is related to the cryoglobulins, but the etiology of the cryoglobulinemia has by definition not been found in patients with (essential) mixed cryoglobulinemia.

**MIM No.:** *12355

**Sex Ratio:** M3:F7 (observed) in mixed cryoglobulinemia. M13: F11 (observed) in three families with dominant inheritance. M0:F4 (observed) in one family with presumed recessive inheritance.

**Occurrence:** About 30 inherited cases reported in the literature.

**Risk of Recurrence for Patient's Sib:**
See Part I, *Mendelian Inheritance*.

**Risk of Recurrence for Patient's Child:**
See Part I, *Mendelian Inheritance*.

**Age of Detectability:** Average age of onset is 50 (range 20–79) years.

**Gene Mapping and Linkage:** Unknown.

**Prevention:** None known. Genetic counseling indicated.

**Treatment:** The clinical disorder may be treated with immunosuppressive agents and plasmapheresis. End-stage renal disease is treated by chronic hemodialysis or continuous peritoneal dialysis and renal transplantation.

**Prognosis:** Good, although they may have many episodes of illness.

**Detection of Carrier:** By plasma cryoglobulins.

**Special Considerations:** Familial (mixed essential) cryoglobulinemia excludes by definition patients with a known cause of cryoglobulinemia.

**References:**
Sitomer G, et al.: Cryoglobulinemia: an inherited molecular disease? Am J Med 1963; 34:565–571.
Dammacco F, et al.: Cryoglobulinemia in four sisters. Acta Haematol 1978; 59:215–222.
Gorevic PD, et al.: Mixed cryoglobulinemia: clinical aspects and long-term follow-up of 40 patients. Am J Med 1980; 69:287–308.
Nightingale SD, et al.: Inheritance of mixed cryoglobulinemia. Am J Hum Genet 1981; 33:735–744.
Berliner S, et al.: Familial cryoglobulinemia and C4 deficiency. Scand J Rheumatol 1984; 13:151–154.

KA042                                               **Bernard S. Kaplan**

**Cryptophthalmos syndrome, Fraser type**
*See FRASER SYNDROME*
**Cryptophthalmos-other malformations**
*See FRASER SYNDROME*
**Cryptophthalmos-syndactyly**
*See FRASER SYNDROME*
**Cryptophthalmus**
*See EYE, CRYPTOPHTHALMOS WITH OTHER MALFORMATIONS*
**Cryptothyroidism**
*See THYROID, DYSGENESIS*
**Cryptotia**
*See EAR, CRYPTOTIA*
**Crystalline aculeiform or frosted cataract**
*See CATARACT, AUTOSOMAL DOMINANT CONGENITAL*
**Crystalline corneal dystrophy**
*See CORNEAL DYSTROPHY, SCHNYDER CRYSTALLINE*
**Cup ear**
*See EAR, CUPPED*
**Cupramin^, fetal effects of**
*See FETAL D-PENICILLAMINE SYNDROME*
**Curly hair-ankyloblepharon-nail dysplasia syndrome (CHANDS)**
*See CHANDS*
**Currarime triad**
*See TERATOMA, SACROCOCCYGEAL TERATOMA*
**Curry-Hall syndrome**
*See ACROFACIAL DYSOSTOSIS*
**Curth-Macklin syndrome**
*See ICHTHYOSIS HYSTRIX, CURTH-MACKLIN TYPE*
**Cushing disease-atrial myxoma-pigmentation**
*See NEVI-ATRIAL MYXOMA-MYXOID NEUROFIBROMAS-EPHELIDES*
**Cushing symphalangism**
*See SYMPHALANGISM*
**Cushing syndrome, familial**
*See NEVI-ATRIAL MYXOMA-MYXOID NEUROFIBROMAS-EPHELIDES*
**Cutaneous albinism**
*See ALBINOIDISM*
**Cutaneous albinism without deafness**
*See ALBINISM, CUTANEOUS*
**Cutaneous albinism-deafness**
*See ALBINISM, CUTANEOUS-DEAFNESS*
**Cutaneous amyloidosis, familial, dominant type**
*See AMYLOIDOSIS, FAMILIAL LICHEN*
**Cutaneous collagenoma-cardiomyopathy-hypogonadism, familial**
*See COLLAGENOMA, MULTIPLE CUTANEOUS, FAMILIAL*
**Cutaneous elastolysis, generalized congenital**
*See CUTIS LAXA*
**Cutaneous hypomelanosis**
*See ALBINOIDISM*
**Cutaneous hypopigmentation**
*See ALBINOIDISM*
**Cutaneous malignant melanoma, hereditary**
*See CANCER, MALIGNANT MELANOMA, FAMILIAL*
**Cutaneous melanosis (diffuse)**
*See SKIN, CUTANEOUS MELANOSIS, DIFFUSE*
**Cutaneous melanosis: mongolian spot**
*See SKIN, CUTANEOUS MELANOSIS: MONGOLIAN SPOT*
**Cutaneous porphyria**
*See PORPHYRIA CUTANEA TARDA*

**Cutaneous sebaceous neoplasms-keracanthomas-GI and other cancers**
*See CANCER, SEBACEOUS GLAND TUMOR-MULITPLE VISCERAL CARCINOMA*
**Cutaneous T-cell lymphomas**
*See LEUKEMIA/LYMPHOMA, T-CELL*
**Cutaneous, cartilaginous, and corneal lesions**
*See DERMO-CHONDRO-CORNEAL DYSTROPHY, FRANCOIS TYPE*

---

## CUTIS LAXA                                               0233

**Includes:**
> Alpha(1)-antitrypsin deficiency and connective tissue defect
> Chalastoderma
> Cutaneous elastolysis, generalized congenital
> Dermatochalasia
> Dermatomegaly
> Penicillamine, fetal effects of

**Excludes:**
> Acquired or secondary cutaneous elastolysis
> Circumscribed cutaneous elastolysis
> **Ehlers-Danlos syndrome** (0338)

**Major Diagnostic Criteria:** Generalized cutaneous laxity with typical changes in the elastin in skin biopsy specimens.

**Clinical Findings:** This systemic disease has a reduction of elastin fibers with laxity of the skin, which hangs in loose folds in all areas, producing a "hound-dog facies." Deepening of the voice is characteristic. Dermal changes are usually apparent at birth or develop during infancy. The dermal changes may remain static or may progress. Cardiac and pulmonary involvement is not uncommon.

**Complications:** Cardiac failure caused by gross pulmonary emphysema or structural cardiac abnormalities, liability to chest infections, diverticulae of the gut and bladder, blepharochalasis, ectropion, external hernia, rectal and vaginal prolapse, and lax vocal cords are encountered in this condition.

**Associated Findings:** A nasal abnormality consisting of a short columella and a hooked nose is frequently present. Widespread dental caries and developmental retardation have been noted in at least one kinship (Patton et al, 1987).

**Etiology:** It is probable that there are two or more separate genetic forms of the condition - a "benign" autosomal dominant inheritance with variable penetrance and a "malignant" autosomal recessive inheritance. These have not yet been completely delineated.

Cutis laxa has been the source of great semantic confusion, as this name has also been applied to the **Ehlers-Danlos syndrome** and to various localized or secondary forms of lax skin. It is likely that the incidence of visceral involvement is quite different in various forms of cutis laxa.

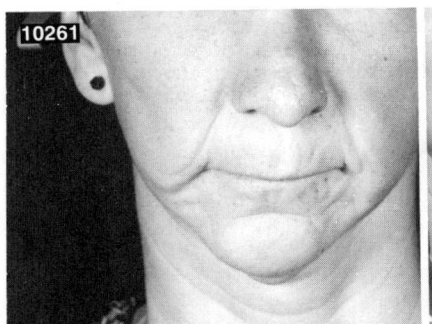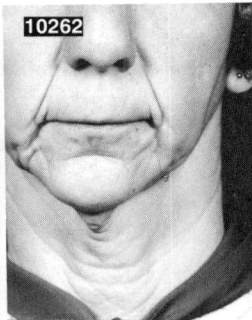

**0233A-10261:** Premature wrinkling and skin laxity in a 16-year-old female. **10262:** More profound laxity in an adult.

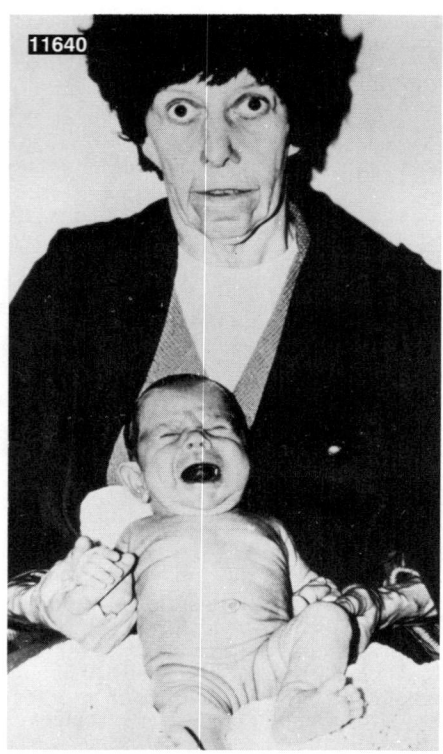

**0233B-11640:** Mother and infant daughter with cutis laxa.

---

There are scattered reports of infants with lax skin, associated with articular and skeletal abnormalities. These probably represent further separate genetic entities, which are excessively rare and poorly understood.

There are several reports of children with a cutis laxa phenocopy who were born to mothers who received D-penicillamine during pregnancy. Subsequent studies have revealed that penicillamine can inhibit cross-linkage of elastin in vitro. Cutis laxa with pulmonary emphysema has also been reported in alpha$_1$-antitrypsin deficiency caused by homozygous P1 null.

An X-linked inherited form of cutis laxa with decreased lysyl oxidase activity has been reported but should be considered a form of **Ehlers-Danlos syndrome** (type IX).

**Pathogenesis:** The dermal and visceral changes are due to the abnormality of elastin. It is not known whether this is the basic defect or merely a reflection of an underlying biochemical lesion. Diminution in absolute numbers of elastic fibers in the skin and viscera occurs. These fibers are fragmented, granular, and have increased thickness and electron density with marked granularity. In the X-linked form, dermal elastin is histologically normal, whereas collagen fibrils have an abnormal architecture. Activity of lysyl oxidase in skin biopsy specimens was shown to be decreased in two affected cousins.

**MIM No.:** *12370, *21910

**POS No.:** 3180

**CDC No.:** 757.370

**Sex Ratio:** M1:F1

**Occurrence:** Over 50 cases reported in the world literature.

**Risk of Recurrence for Patient's Sib:**
See Part I, *Mendelian Inheritance.*

**Risk of Recurrence for Patient's Child:**
See Part I, *Mendelian Inheritance.*

**Age of Detectability:** Usually at birth or in infancy. A few cases of late onset have been reported.

**Gene Mapping and Linkage:** Unknown.

**Prevention:** None known. Genetic counseling indicated.

**Treatment:** Plastic surgery may be required to correct the dermal changes. The initial results are usually good, but repeated operations may be required.

**Prognosis:** Normal intelligence. Probably normal life span if there is no cardiac or pulmonary involvement. Death may occur in childhood if these complications are severe or progressive.

**Detection of Carrier:** Unknown.

**References:**
Goltz RW, et al.: Cutis laxa - a manifestation of generalized elastolysis. Arch Dermatol 1965; 92:373–376.
Marshall J, et al.: Post-inflammatory elastolysis and cutis laxa: a report on a new variety of this phenomenon and a discussion of some syndromes characterized by elastolysis. S Afr Med J 1966; 40:1016–1019.
Beighton P: The dominant and recessive forms of cutis laxa. J Med Genet 1972; 9:216–220. * †
Schanderyl W, et al.: Alpha-1-antitrypsin deficiency of the Pi 00 type and connective tissue defect. Inserm 1975; 40:97–108.
Solomon L, et al.: Neonatal abnormalities associated with D- penicillamine treatment during pregnancy. N Engl J Med 1977; 296:54–55.
Weir EK, et al.: Cardiovascular abnormalities in cutis laxa. Eur J Cardiol 1977; 5:255–261.
Agha A, et al.: Two forms of cutis laxa presenting in the newborn period. Acta Paediatr Scand 1978; 67:775–780.
Philip AGS: Cutis laxa with intrauterine growth retardation and hip dislocation in a male. J Pediatr 1978; 93:150–151.
Byers PH, et al.: X-linked cutis laxa. Defective cross-link formation in collagen due to decreased lysyl oxidase activity. N Engl J Med 1980; 2:61–65.
Marchase P, et al.: A familial cutis laxa syndrome with ultrastructural abnormalities of collagen and elastin. J Invest Dermatol 1980; 75:399–402.
Fitzsimmons JS, et al.: Variable clinical presentation of cutis laxa. Clin Genet 1985; 28:284–295.
Patton MA, et al.: Congenital cutis laxa with retardation of growth and development. J Med Genet 1987; 24:556–561.
Beighton P, et al.: International nosology of heritable disorders of connective tissue, Berlin, 1986. Am J Med Genet 1988; 29:581–594.

BE008                                      **Peter Beighton**

---

**Cutis Laxa with maternal D-penicillamine exposure**
*See FETAL D-PENICILLAMINE SYNDROME*
**Cutis laxa, X-linked**
*See OCCIPITAL HORN SYNDROME*
**Cutis laxa-bone dystrophy**
*See CUTIS LAXA-DELAYED DEVELOPMENT-LIGAMENTOUS LAXITY*

---

## CUTIS LAXA-DELAYED DEVELOPMENT-LIGAMENTOUS LAXITY                                     2977

**Includes:**
> Cutis laxa-bone dystrophy
> Cutis laxa-growth deficiency syndrome
> Cutis laxa-intrauterine growth retardation
> Delayed development-cutis laxa
> Delayed development-cutis laxa-ligamentous laxity
> Intrauterine growth retardation-cutis laxa-hip dislocation
> Joint hypermobility-cutis laxa-retarded development
> Joint laxity-retarded development-cutis laxa
> Ligamentous laxity-cutis laxa-delayed development

**Excludes:**
> **Cutis laxa** (other)
> **Ehlers-Danlos syndrome** (0338)
> **Osteodysplastica gerodermia, Bamatter type** (2099)

**Major Diagnostic Criteria:** Cutis laxa with impairment of postnatal growth, variable mental retardation, and ligamentous laxity.

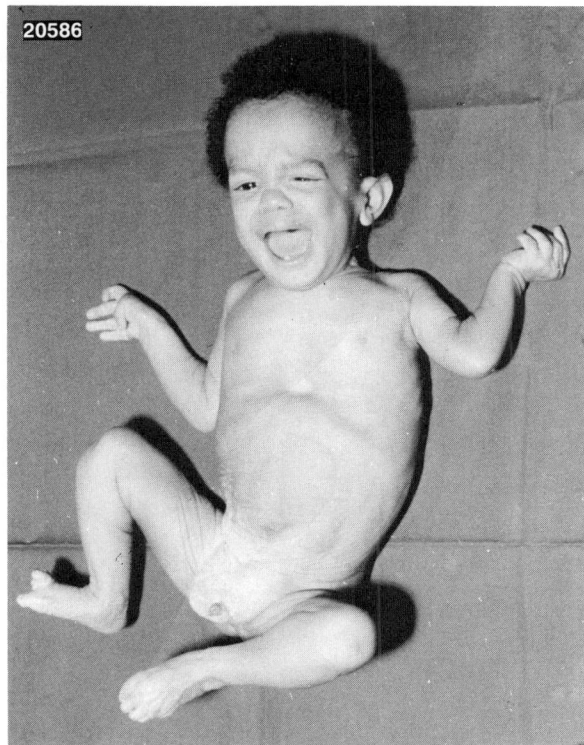

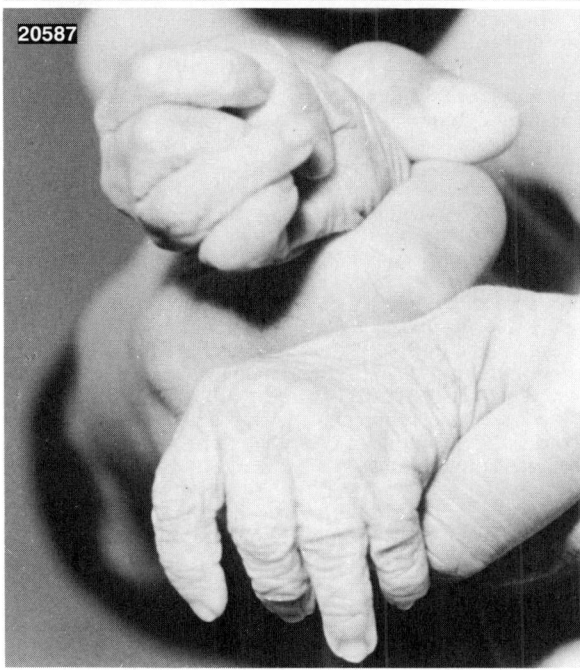

**2977-20586:** Redundant skin, inguinal hernias, and thumb clasping in this 11-month-old male. **20587:** Hands show marked cutis laxa and clasped thumbs.

**Clinical Findings:** Cutis laxa is normally apparent in the neonatal period, and delayed physical and intellectual development are early features. Ligamentous laxity, hypotonia, and dislocation of hips are commonly present. Facial dysmorphism with sagging jowls, epicanthic folds, upturned nares, eversion of lower lids, and abnormal ear folds should be apparent early.

**Complications:** **Hernia, hiatal** or **Hernia, inguinal** may occur.

**Associated Findings:** Some patients show craniofacial dysmorphic features including a widely patent anterior fontanelle; broad, depressed nasal bridge; true or apparent **Eye, hypertelorism**; large, low-set ears; and a high-arched palate.

Wide anterior fontanelle, proximally placed thumbs, clasped thumbs, cardiac murmur, speech disturbance, talipes, edema of hands and feet, osteoporosis, kyphoscoliosis, pes planus, and genu valgum have been reported in a few patients.

Joint dislocation, particularly congenital dislocation of the hip; urinary tract disorders; cutaneous telangiectatic vessels, blue sclerae, palmar simian creases, and thumb anomalies.

**Etiology:** Autosomal recessive inheritance.

**Pathogenesis:** Cutis laxa is associated with fragmentation of elastin fibers. No definite evidence of abnormalities of copper or lysyl oxidase.

**MIM No.:** *21920

**POS No.:** 3181

**Sex Ratio:** M1:F2 observed. Possibly lethal in males. One report includes two brother-sister sib pairs.

**Occurrence:** A few dozen cases have been documented in the literature. Reportedly frequent in Saudi Arabia.

**Risk of Recurrence for Patient's Sib:**
See Part I, *Mendelian Inheritance.*

**Risk of Recurrence for Patient's Child:**
See Part I, *Mendelian Inheritance.*

**Age of Detectability:** Clinical examination at birth or in early life should confirm cutis laxa and other features.

**Gene Mapping and Linkage:** Unknown.

**Prevention:** None known. Genetic counseling indicated.

**Treatment:** Surgical correction of hernias and joint dislocations. Special education.

**Prognosis:** Mental retardation is variable, and there is insufficient information on growth later in life. Cutis laxa is unlikely to affect life span, but some reduction can be expected if the mental retardation is severe.

**Detection of Carrier:** Unknown.

**References:**
Debné R, et al.: Cutis Laxa-avec dystrophies osseuses. Bull Soc Med Hop Paris 1937; 53:1038.
Philip AGS: Cutis laxa with intrauterine growth retardation and hip dislocation in a male. J Pediatr 1978; 93:150–151.
Karrar ZA, et al.: Cutis laxa, intrauterine growth retardation and bilateral dislocation of the hips: a report of five cases. In: Papadatos CJ, Bartsocas CS, eds: Skeletal dysplasias. New York: Alan R. Liss, 1982:215–221.
Sakati NO, Nyhan WL: Congenital cutis laxa and osteoporosis. Am J Dis Child 1983; 137:452–454.
Sakati NO, et al.: Syndrome of cutis laxa, ligamentous laxity, and delayed development. Pediatrics 1983; 72:850–856. *
Fitzsimmons JS, et al.: Variable clinical presentation of cutis laxa. Clin Genet 1985; 28:284–295.
Allanson J, et al.: Congenital cutis laxa with retardation of growth and motor development: a recessive disorder of connective tissue with male lethality. Clin Genet 1986; 29:133–136.
Patton MA, et al.: Congenital cutis laxa with retardation of growth and development. J Med Genet 1987; 24:556–561.
Goldblatt J, et al.: Cutis laxa, retarded development and joint hypermobility syndrome. Dysmorphol Clin Genet 1988; 1:142–144. *

FI022
G0056

**J.S. Fitzsimmons**
**Jack Goldblatt**

## CUTIS LAXA-GROWTH DEFECT, DE BARSY TYPE 2138

**Includes:**
> Corneal clouding-cutis laxa-mental retardation
> Cutis laxa-growth deficiency syndrome
> De Barsy-Moens-Dierckx syndrome
> De Barsy syndrome
> Progeroid syndrome of De Barsy

**Excludes:**
> **Cutis laxa-delayed development-ligamentous laxity** (2977)
> **Ehlers-Danlos syndrome** (0338)
> **Progeria** (0825)

**Major Diagnostic Criteria:** The combination of cutis laxa, cloudy cornea, athetoid movements, progeroid aspect, and short stature should suggest the diagnosis.

**Clinical Findings:** In 15 affected individuals, findings have been large dysplastic ears (14/14); cutis laxa (14/14); atrophy of the skin (14/14); muscular hypotonia (14/14); frontal bossing (13/13); progeroid facies (12/14); intrauterine growth retardation (10/14); postnatal short stature (11/13); hyperflexibility of small joints (11/11); brisk deep tendon reflexes (10/11); athetoid movements (10/11); translucent vein pattern (11/14); mental retardation (10/12); corneal clouding (9/14); thin lips (9/9); sparse hair (7/8); degeneration of the elastic and collagenous fibers (7/8); cataract (5/14); joint dislocations (3/7); and large fontanelles (5/7).

**Complications:** Unknown.

**Associated Findings:** Older children become clearly microcephalic (see **Microcephaly**). The following findings have been reported in two affected individuals each: dilatations of ventricles, seizures, arthrochalasis, punctate calcification. Findings in only one affected individual each include **Hernia, inguinal**, microcorneae, congenital heart defect, underdeveloped genitalia, and vesicoureteric reflux with enlarged ureters.

**Etiology:** Autosomal recessive inheritance.

**Pathogenesis:** Skin biopsies demonstrated a paucity of dermal elastin fibers, elastic fibers were frayed and reduced in number and density. In one patient the collagen fibril network was normal; with normal amino acid content and a normal electrophoretic pattern of collagen constituents in cultured skin fibroblasts. The chemotactic migration of cultured fibroblasts was diminished. Immunologic investigations revealed in this patient an impaired granulocyte function. However, that does not explain all of the findings (e.g. mental retardation, short stature).

**MIM No.:** *21915

**POS No.:** 3181

**Sex Ratio:** M9:F6 (observed)

**Occurrence:** About 20 cases reported. Wide geographic distribution.

**Risk of Recurrence for Patient's Sib:**
See Part I, *Mendelian Inheritance.*

**Risk of Recurrence for Patient's Child:**
See Part I, *Mendelian Inheritance.*

**Age of Detectability:** At birth, by physical examination.

**Gene Mapping and Linkage:** Unknown.

**Prevention:** None known. Genetic counseling indicated.

**Treatment:** Symptomatic.

**Prognosis:** Intellectual development has ranged from normal to severely retarded. The effect of this condition on life span is unknown; the oldest reported patient was 23 years of age at last follow-up.

**Detection of Carrier:** Unknown.

**References:**
De Barsy AM, et al.: Dwarfism, oligophrenia and degeneration of the elastic tissue in skin and cornea: a new syndrome? Helv Paediatr Acta 1968; 23:305–313.
Hoefnagel D, et al.: Congenital athetosis, mental deficiency, dwarf-ism, and laxity of skin and ligaments. Helv Paediatr Acta 1971; 26:397–402.
Bartsocas CS, et al.: De Barsy syndrome. In: Papadatos CJ, Bartsocas CS, eds: Skeletal dysplasia. New York: Alan R. Liss, 1982:157–160.
Saul R: Unknown case (R.F.W.). Proc Greenwood Genet Center 1983; 2:70–71.
Kunze J, et al.: De Barsy syndrome: an autosomal recessive, progeroid syndrome. Eur J Pediatr 1985; 144:348–354. * †
Pontz BF, et al.: Biochemical, morphological and immunological findings in a patient with a cutis laxa-associated inborn disorder (De Barsy syndrome). Eur J Pediatr 1986; 145:428–434.

KU008                                    **Jürgen Kunze**
T0007                               **Helga V. Toriello**

**Cutis laxa-growth deficiency syndrome**
*See CUTIS LAXA-DELAYED DEVELOPMENT-LIGAMENTOUS LAXITY also CUTIS LAXA-GROWTH DEFECT, DE BARSY TYPE*
**Cutis laxa-intrauterine growth retardation**
*See CUTIS LAXA-DELAYED DEVELOPMENT-LIGAMENTOUS LAXITY*

## CUTIS MARMORATA 2296

**Includes:**
> Cutis marmorata telangiectatica congenita (CMTC)
> Livedo reticularis
> Marble skin
> Marbling effect of newborn skin
> Van Lohuizen syndrome

**Excludes:**
> **Rothmund-Thomson syndrome** (2037)
> **Skin** (other cutaneous color disorders)

**Major Diagnostic Criteria:** A cutaneous blue or purple mottling or marbling pattern, most pronounced when the infant has been chilled or exposed to low environmental temperature.

**Clinical Findings:** When the newborn infant is exposed to low environmental temperature, but sometimes even in a neutral thermal range, a marbling pattern appears over most of the body surface. This is an evanescent, lacy, red or blue reticulated pattern resembling a net or a branching configuration. The marbling usually disappears when the infant is rewarmed. It is most frequent in preterm infants, but may be observed also in full term infants. The condition uncommon after several months of age, although it is sometimes discernible even in older children.

*Cutis marmorata telangiectatica congenita* (CMTC), or *Van Lohuizen syndrome*, which appears to be a distinct entity (South & Jacobs, 1978; Greist & Probst, 1980; and Powell & Daniel, 1984), is a persistent type of cutis marmorata characterized by generalized or segmental reticular telangiectasias and phlebectasias, sometimes associated with ulceration with crust. Unlike the common cutis marmorata, the mottling of CMTC is more striking and independent of environmental temperature. The condition can have a poor prognosis, owing to the frequent occurrence of thrombosis, atrophy/hypertrophy, bleeding, infection, and gangrene.

Histologic examination shows skin atrophy and dilated capillaries and veins, as well as phlebectasia and perivascular mononuclear cell infiltration in the dermis and hypodermis.

Most cases have been sporadic, although some familial patterns have been noted. Differential diagnosis should take into account the possible effects of maternal antinuclear antibody transported across the placenta to the fetus, specifically neonatal lupus (see **Lupus erythematosis, systemic**).

**Complications:** Usually, this is an intermittent and isolated phenomenon. When permanent, it may be a sign of hypothermia, sepsis, or hypothyroidism.

**Associated Findings:** In a more persistent form, cutis marmorata can be a feature of other syndromes including **Limb and scalp defects, Adams-Oliver type, Thyroid, dysgenesis, De Lange syndrome, Chromosome 18, trisomy 18**, and occasionally in **Chromosome 21, trisomy 21** and **Angio-osteohypertrophy syndrome**.

One-half of the published cases of *Cutis marmorata telangiectatica congenita* have been associated with other congenital anomalies including mental retardation, CNS abnormalities, spina bifida, glaucoma and corneal clouding, **Eye, hypertelorism, Cleft lip, Cleft palate**, dystrophic teeth, high-arched palate, micrognathia, **Ductus arteriosus, patent**, neonatal ascites, and other skeletal and skin anomalies.

**Etiology:** Unknown. An accentuated physiologic vasomotor reaction of the skin in some infants.

**Pathogenesis:** The mottling configuration is due to dilatation of the capillaries and venules in the darker areas.

**MIM No.:** 21925

**POS No.:** 3832

**CDC No.:** 757.390

**Sex Ratio:** Presumably M1:F1.

**Occurrence:** Undetermined but presumed rare, particularly in full term infants.

**Risk of Recurrence for Patient's Sib:** Unknown.

**Risk of Recurrence for Patient's Child:** Unknown.

**Age of Detectability:** At birth.

**Gene Mapping and Linkage:** Unknown.

**Prevention:** None known. Genetic counseling indicated.

**Treatment:** Unknown.

**Prognosis:** Excellent. The condition usually disappears after a few months of age.

**Detection of Carrier:** Unknown.

**References:**

Solomon LM, Esterly NB: Neonatal dermatology. Philadelphia: W.B. Saunders, 1973:45.

South DA, Jacobs AH: Cutis marmorata telangiectatica congenita. J Pediatr 1978; 93:944–949.

Vaughan VC, et al.: Textbook of pediatrics, 11th ed. Philadelphia: W.B. Saunders, 1979:1860.

Greist C, Probst E: Cutis marmorata telangiectatica congenita or neonatal lupus. Arch Dermatol 1980; 116:1102–1103.

Kurczynski TW: Hereditary cutis marmorata telangiectatica congenita. Pediatrics 1982; 70:52–53.

Powell ST, Daniel WP, Sr.: Cutis marmorata telangiectatica congenita: report of nine cases and a review of the literature. Cutis 1984; 34:305–312. *

ME034
RE025

**Paul Merlob**
**Salomon H. Reisner**

**Cutis marmorata telangiectatica congenita (CMTC)**
*See CUTIS MARMORATA*
**Cutis verticis gyrata-neurologic deficiency**
*See CUTIS VERTICIS GYRATA*
**Cutis verticis gyrata-thyroid aplasia-neurologic deficiency**
*See CUTIS VERTICIS GYRATA*
**Cutis verticis-gyratacorneal leukoma-acromegaloid phenotype**
*See ACROMEGALOID PHENOTYPE-CUTIS VERTICIS GYRATA-CORNEAL LEUKOMA*

| **CUTIS VERTICUS GYRATA** | **2295** |
|---|---|

**Includes:**
  Cutis verticis gyrata-neurologic deficiency
  Cutis verticis gyrata-thyroid aplasia-neurologic deficiency

**Excludes:**
  **Acromegaloid phenotype-cutis verticis gyrata-corneal leukoma** (0018)
  Cutis verticis gyrata as a sign of other diseases
  Cutis verticis gyrata secondary to physical irritation
  Cutis verticis gyrata secondary to tumors of the scalp
  **Pachydermoperiostosis** (0788)

**Major Diagnostic Criteria:** The cardinal finding is a folding and furrowing of the scalp. In some cases, it extends onto the forehead and the nape of the neck. Most cases have additional findings that permit classification into one of the major subtypes.

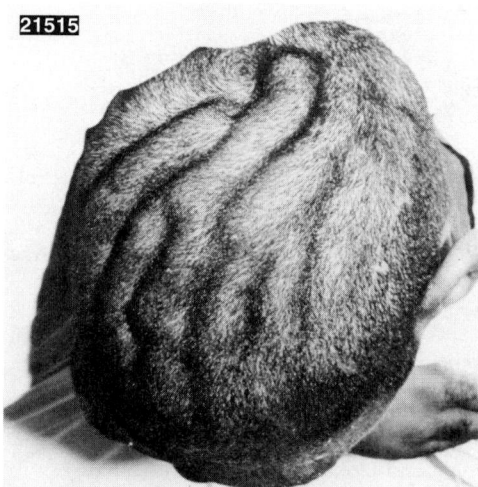

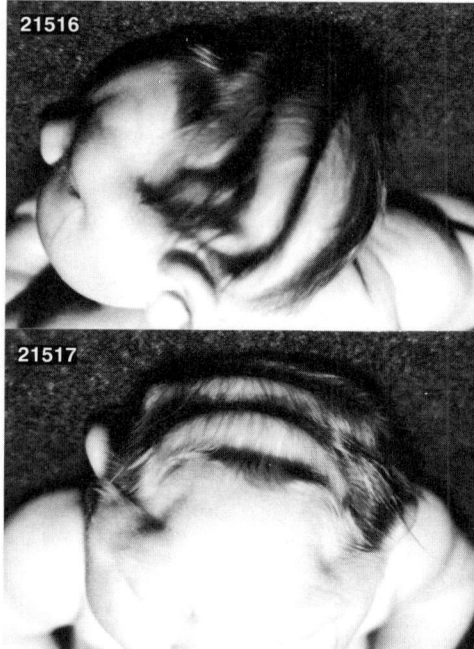

**2295-21515:** Top view of scalp shows folds and furrows running in an antero-posterior direction. **21516–17:** Scalp of an infant with fetal brain disruption syndrome showing scalp folds running in a coronal direction.

**Clinical Findings:** Cutis verticis gyrata may be present at birth in cases with neurologic deficiency, but is not noticed until puberty in most cases. The skin is generally thickened. Other congenital problems in these cases include mental retardation, spasticity, strabismus, nystagmus, epilepsy, **Microcephaly**, thyroid aplasia, and short stature.

The few cases of "pure" cutis verticis gyrata in the literature are not described in sufficient detail to determine if additional findings were really absent or simply not noticed.

**Complications:** Cutis verticis gyrata is a cosmetic defect and a hygienic problem.

**Associated Findings:** None known.

**Etiology:** Autosomal recessive inheritance, but there is a marked excess of males with thyroid aplasia, which suggests that X-linked inheritance may be responsible for those cases.

**Pathogenesis:** Unknown.

**MIM No.:** 21930, 30420

**POS No.:** 3662

**Sex Ratio:** M1:F1 except for some families with neurologic deficit and thyroid aplasia, in which nearly all affected individuals are male.

**Occurrence:** Over 50 cases have been reported by Akesson from Sweden. Reports from other sources have been rare.

**Risk of Recurrence for Patient's Sib:**
See Part I, *Mendelian Inheritance.*

**Risk of Recurrence for Patient's Child:**
See Part I, *Mendelian Inheritance.*

**Age of Detectability:** At birth, although many cases are not diagnosed until puberty.

**Gene Mapping and Linkage:** Unknown.

**Prevention:** None known. Genetic counseling indicated.

**Treatment:** Surgical reduction of the affected scalp skin is of value for hygiene and cosmesis.

**Prognosis:** Cutis verticis gyrata with neurologic deficiency is a chronic handicapping condition in most cases.

**Detection of Carrier:** Clinical examination may indicate some carriers.

**References:**
Rosenthal JW, Kloepfer HW: An acromegaloid, cutis verticis gyrata, corneal leukoma syndrome: a new medical entity. Arch Ophthalmol 1962; 68:36–40.
Akesson HO: Cutis verticis gyrata and mental deficiency in Sweden: epidemiologic and clinical aspects. Acta Med Scand 1964; 175:115–127.
Akesson HO: Cutis verticis gyrata and mental deficiency in Sweden: genetic aspects. Acta Med Scand 1965; 177:459–464.
Akesson HO: Cutis verticis gyrata, thyroaplasia and mental deficiency. Acta Genet Med Gemellol 1965; 14:200–204.

TH017
UR001

T.F. Thurmon<br>S.A. Ursin

**Cycad nut, effects of**
*See AMYOTROPHIC LATERAL SCLEROSIS, GUAM TYPE*
**Cycas circinalis (cycad nut), effects of**
*See AMYOTROPHIC LATERAL SCLEROSIS, GUAM TYPE*
**Cyclic AMP-dependent kinase**
*See GLYCOGENOSES*
**Cyclic neutropenia**
*See NEUTROPENIA, CYCLIC*

## CYCLOPIA 0234

**Includes:**
Cebocephaly
Ethmocephaly
Synopthalmia

**Excludes:**
**Aprosopia** (2487)
Cephalopagus twins with fused eyes
**Holoprosencephaly** (0473)

**Major Diagnostic Criteria:** Variable fusion of the optic vesicles.

**Clinical Findings:** Cyclopia results from maldevelopment of the embryonic forebrain. There are variable degrees of malformation of the brain, particularly failure of division of the telencephalon. Any degree of fusion of the optic vesicles, eyelids and lacrimal structures may occur. The nose is usually either absent or replaced by a proboscis-like structure above the eye.

**Complications:** Agenesis of corpus callosum, olfactory tracts, nasal bones, turbinates, vomer or premaxilla; cleft lip and palate.

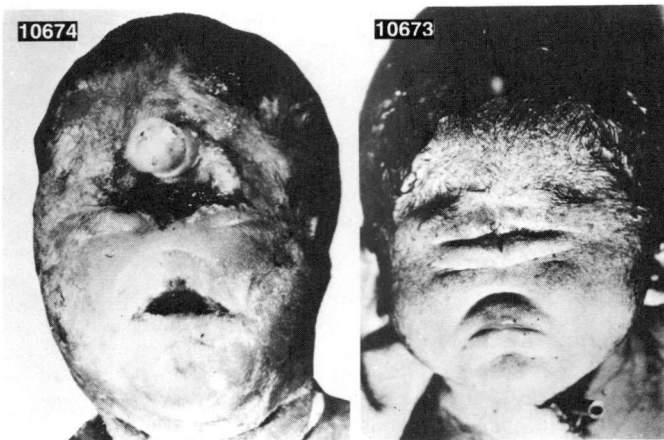

0234-10674: Cyclopia with proboscis. 10673: Cyclopia without proboscis.

**Associated Findings:** Polydactyly, sirenomelia, **Hernia, umbilical,** and spina bifida.

**Etiology:** Etiologically heterogeneous with evidence for autosomal recessive and chromosomal (18p-,+13) etiologies. Maternal diseases have been implicated, including cytomegalovirus (CMV) infection, and numerous noxious stimuli during early embryonic development have caused cyclopia in experimental animals.

**Pathogenesis:** Disturbance in the activity of the prosencephalic organizing center of the embryo resulting in failure of development of the anterior end of the neural tube and of the frontonasal process.

**MIM No.:** *23610

**Sex Ratio:** M1:F<1

**Occurrence:** Estimated 1:40,000.

**Risk of Recurrence for Patient's Sib:** Rare, but an increased incidence of spontaneous abortions occurs in families producing cyclopia.

**Risk of Recurrence for Patient's Child:** Affected individuals are not expected to survive to reproduce.

**Age of Detectability:** Prenatally or at birth.

**Gene Mapping and Linkage:** Unknown.

**Prevention:** None known. Genetic counseling indicated.

**Treatment:** Unknown.

**Prognosis:** Most affected individuals die at birth or within a few hours, although one reported patient survived 10 years.

**Detection of Carrier:** Unknown.

**Special Considerations:** Transitional malformations between synophthalmos and arrhinencephalia are sometimes broadly classified under the term **Holoprosencephaly**.

**References:**
Sedano HO, Gorlin RJ: The oral manifestations of cyclopia. Oral Surg 1963; 18:823.
Cohen MM Jr, Gorlin RJ: Genetic considerations in a sibship of cyclopia and clefts. BD:OAS9; V(2). White Plains: March of Dimes - Birth Defects Foundation, 1969:113.
Gardner DG, Lim H: The oral manifestations of cyclopia. Oral Surg 1971; 32:910–917.
Latham RA: Mechanism of maxillary growth in the human cyclops. J Dent Res 1971; 50:929–933.
Holme LB, Driscoll S, Atkins L: Genetic heterogeneity of cebocephaly. J Med Genet 1974; 11:35–40.
Burck U, et al.: Holoprosencephaly in monozygotic twins. Am J Med Genet 1981; 9:13–17.

Byrne PJ, et al.: Cyclopia and congenital cytomegalovirus infection. Am J Med Genet 1987; 28:61–65.

J0027                                                    Ronald J. Jorgenson

**Cylindromas of the scalp**
  *See SCALP, CYLINDROMAS*
**Cylindromatosis**
  *See SCALP, CYLINDROMAS*
**Cyst (adrenal)-ectodermal dysplasia**
  *See ECTODERMAL DYSPLASIA-ADRENAL CYST*
**Cyst of septum pellucidum**
  *See BRAIN, MIDLINE CAVES*
**Cyst of the spinal cord associated with posterior mediastinal cyst**
  *See SPINAL CORD, NEURENTERIC CYST*
**Cyst, developmental**
  *See ORAL DERMOIDS*
**Cyst, dysontogenetic**
  *See ORAL DERMOIDS*
**Cyst, epidermoid**
  *See ORAL DERMOIDS*
**Cyst, teratoid**
  *See ORAL DERMOIDS*
**Cystathionine beta-synthase deficiency**
  *See HOMOCYSTINURIA*
**Cystathioninemia**
  *See CYSTATHIONINURIA*

## CYSTATHIONINURIA                                    0236

**Includes:**
  Cystathioninemia
  Gamma-cystathionase deficiency

**Excludes:**
  Cystathioninuria associated with B(12) deficiency
  Cystathioninuria associated with other amino acid
    anomalies
  Cystathioninuria-defects of homocystine methylation

**Major Diagnostic Criteria:**  Concentrations of cystathionine persistently elevated in blood and urine. Cystathioninuria associated with other amino acid abnormalities should be exluded by metabolic studies.

**Clinical Findings:**  No consistent presentation has been described. Signs and symptoms range from nephrogenic diabetes insipidus and acromegaly to severe mental retardation, heart disease, thrombocytopenia, renal lithiasis, and convulsions. There have been individual reports of clubfoot, anomalous ears, and hyperactivity. The majority of individuals have no symptoms, suggesting that the metabolic defect may not cause clinical illness.

Cystathioninuria in the range of 160 to 1,400 mg per day depending on size of patient and methionine intake. Plasma concentrations range from about 10 to 100 $\mu$mole per liter. Normally, cystathionine is undetectable in the urine and plasma.

**Complications:**  Renal lithiasis has been reported in at least two individuals.

**Associated Findings:**  A variety of serious conditions such as thrombocytopenia and heart disease have been reported, although these cannot at present be related to the biochemical defect. Possibly all findings are coincidental; a causal relationship between signs and cystathionine excess has not been demonstrated.

**Etiology:**  Autosomal recessive inheritance. Deficiency of gamma-cystathionase with cystathionine levels increased above control values in blood and urine. There is no apparent deficiency of cysteine, one of the products of the cystathionase reaction.

**Pathogenesis:**  A defect in liver gamma-cystathionase, the enzyme that catalyzes the formation of cysteine and alpha-ketobutyrate from cystathionine. The excessive cystathionine levels can be reduced to normal or near normal in most patients with large doses of vitamin $B_6$, the cofactor of this enzyme. This indicates that the pyridoxal binding site is altered in these patients. Other patients are unresponsive.

**MIM No.:**  *21950

**Sex Ratio:**  M1:F1

**Occurrence:**  A prevalence of 1:333,000 to 1:70,000 has been determined from screening studies. About 4–5 dozen patients have been reported.

**Risk of Recurrence for Patient's Sib:**
  See Part I, *Mendelian Inheritance.*

**Risk of Recurrence for Patient's Child:**
  See Part I, *Mendelian Inheritance.*

**Age of Detectability:**  During the newborn period.

**Gene Mapping and Linkage:**  CTH (cystathionase) has been provisionally mapped to 16.

**Prevention:**  None known. Genetic counseling indicated.

**Treatment:**  Blood and urine cystathionine concentration can be decreased to near zero by high doses of vitamin $B_6$ (pyridoxine hydrochloride), e.g. 5 to 10 mg/kg in divided doses orally, per day. The significance of this, or desirability, is unknown.

**Prognosis:**  Unknown.

**Detection of Carrier:**  Some heterozygotes have elevated cystathionine excretion. L-methionine loading of 100 mg/kg may evoke cystathioninuria in carriers. Abnormal activity of cystathionase has been demonstrated in lymphoblastoid cells of a parent.

**Special Considerations:**  Problem areas include: the mechanism of $B_6$ effect, and whether or not the biochemical defect is related to the various disorders described or is coincidental. Patients continue to be reported and discussed who present with some medical problem, while others have no apparent clinical problem - occasionally in the same family. Since this also occurs in other aminoacidurias, the wise approach is to consider this an open question.

In most patients reported, administration of high doses of vitamin $B_6$ has resulted in marked decrease in the aminoaciduria. In vivo and in vitro studies led to the proposal that this could be accounted for by a defective structure of the protein apoenzyme; this causes the improper binding of the coenzyme, pyridoxal phosphate. This suggestion remains to be confirmed.

**References:**
Frimpter GW, et al.: Cystathioninuria: management. AM J Dis Child 1967; 113:115.
Tada K, et al.: Cystathioninuria not associated with vitamin $B_6$ dependency: a probably new type of cystathioninuria. Tohoku J Exp Med 1968; 95:235–242.
Frimpter GW: Recurrent urinary tract calculi possibly due to inherited cystathioninuria. Aerospace Med 1973; 44:1300–1301.
Pascal TA, et al.: Vitamin $B_6$-responsive and unresponsive cystathioninuria: two variant forms. Science 1975; 190:1209–1211.
Pascal TA, et al.: Cystathionase deficiency: evidence for genetic heterogeneity in primary cystathioninuria. Pediatr Res 1978; 12:125–133.
Mudd SH, Levy HL: Disorders of transsulfuration. In: Stanbury JB, et al., eds: The metabolic basis of hereditary disease, ed 5. New York: McGraw-Hill, 1983:522–559.
Schaumburg H, et al.: Sensory neuropathy from pyridoxine abuse. A new megavitamin syndrome. New Engl J Med 1983; 309:445–448.
Nyhan WL: Cystathioninuria. In: Abnormalities in Amino Acid Metabolism in Clinical Medicine. Norwalk: Appleton-Century-Crofts, 1984:235–240.

LE032                                                    Harvey L. Levy
VI006                                                 Jaclyn M. Vidgoff

**Cystathioninuria due to MTHFR deficiency**
  *See HOMOCYSTINURIA, N(5,10) METHYLENE
    TETRAHYDROFOLATE DEFICIENCY TYPE*
**Cystatin C**
  *See AMYLOIDOSIS, ICELANDIC TYPE*
**Cystic adenomatoid dysplasia of the lung**
  *See LUNG, CONGENITAL LOBAR ADENOMATOSIS*
**Cystic adenomatoid malformation of the lung**
  *See LUNG, CONGENITAL LOBAR ADENOMATOSIS*
**Cystic arteriovenous malformations**
  *See CNS ARTERIOVENOUS MALFORMATION*
**Cystic artery anomalies**
  *See GALLBLADDER, ANOMALIES*

**Cystic dilation of common duct, congenital**
  See BILE DUCT CHOLEDOCHAL CYST
**Cystic dilation of renal collecting tubules**
  See KIDNEY, MEDULLARY SPONGE KIDNEY
**Cystic disease of renal pyramids**
  See KIDNEY, MEDULLARY SPONGE KIDNEY
**Cystic disease of the renal medulla**
  See KIDNEY, NEPHRONOPHTHISIS-MEDULLARY CYSTIC DESEASE
**Cystic duct agenesis**
  See GALLBLADDER, AGENESIS
**Cystic dysplasia**
  See KIDNEY, RENAL DYSPLASIA, POTTER TYPE II

## CYSTIC FIBROSIS 0237

**Includes:**
  Cystic fibrosis of pancreas
  Fibrocystic disease of pancreas
  Mucoviscidosis
  Pancreatic fibrosis

**Excludes:** Gluten sensitive enteropathy (0423)

**Major Diagnostic Criteria:** Clinical findings may include some combination of malabsorption, failure to thrive, or recurrent respiratory infections. Diagnosis is confirmed by quantitative analysis of sweat electrolyte levels with sodium and chloride each exceeding 60 mEq/L.

Short of direct DNA analysis of the known mutation, the quantitative pilocarpine iontophoresis (Gibson-Cooke) technique for sweat stimulation and salt concentration measurement is the only acceptable clinical test. It is diagnostic in 98% of patients, especially when combined with characteristic pulmonary disease or pancreatic deficiencies. False positive sweat tests have been reported to be associated with several other disorders, such as hypothyroidism and fucosidosis. Absence of trypsin and increased viscosity has been found in digestive fluid in 85% of children. Low serum vitamin A and E levels may also be useful.

**Clinical Findings:** This generalized disorder affects the sweat glands and the exocrine glands of the body with production of abnormal secretions resulting in excessively high sweat electrolytes, pancreatic insufficiency, chronic pulmonary disease, and cirrhosis of the liver. Greater than 95% of patients have sweat sodium and chloride levels greater than twice normal (60 mEq/L), which may lead to salt loss and heat prostration.

Most patients (80%) are "pancreas insufficient" with pancreatic enzyme deficiencies (trypsin, lipase, and amylase) in the GI tract preventing proper digestion and absorption of fats, fat-soluble vitamins, and proteins causing malnutrition, failure to thrive, anemia, and hypoproteinemia with edema. Some patients do have residual pancreatic function.

Ninety-nine percent of patients who survive infancy go on to develop chronic pulmonary disease which may include hyperinflation, persistent cough, recurrent bronchitis, bronchiolitis, bronchiectasis, pneumonia, atelectasis, pneumothorax, and fibrosis. About 25% have chronic sinusitis and nasal polyps develop in 10%. Adult males show azoospermia secondary to vas deferens aplasia or hypoplasia.

**Complications:** Chronic pulmonary disease. Secondary infection (especially due to Pseudomonas aeroginosa) and organ dysfunction may occur following inspissation and blockage of any collecting system in the body, such as the liver or testicle.

**Associated Findings:** Intestinal obstruction due to meconium ileus occurs at birth in 5–10%. Perforation of the bowel and meconium peritonitis may be associated with ileal stenosis or atresia or meconium plug syndrome. Cirrhosis of the liver secondary to biliary obstruction occurs in 1–5%. Portal hypertension and esophageal varices may occur. Repeated episodes of rectal prolapse may occur in 5–10%.

**Etiology:** Autosomal recessive inheritance. The gene frequency in the general Caucasian population in the United States is estimated to be 1:50 with a carrier frequency of 1:20 to 1:25. About 70% of mutations involve the deletion of three base pairs with resultant loss of a phenylalanine at residue 508. Other less common mutations may be associated with residual pancreatic exocrine function.

**Pathogenesis:** The primary defect appears to be defective chloride transport in the apical membrane of several epithelia. There is evidence that the modulation of a chloride channel is abnormal. The CF protein has properties which are consistent with membrane association and is believed to be involved in adenosine triphosphate (ATP) binding.

**MIM No.:** *21970

**POS No.:** 3792

**CDC No.:** 277.000, 277.010

**Sex Ratio:** M1:F1

**Occurrence:** About 1:2000 among United States whites; rarer in blacks and Asians; most common in Northern Europeans.

**Risk of Recurrence for Patient's Sib:**
  See Part I, *Mendelian Inheritance.*

**Risk of Recurrence for Patient's Child:**
  See Part I, *Mendelian Inheritance.* Affected males are usually infertile. Pregnancies have occurred to some affected females. Such females have a 1:20 chance of having a carrier mate (unless he has a family history of cystic fibrosis) and thus a 1:40 chance of having an affected child.

**Age of Detectability:** Usually at several months of age by sweat electrolyte determination or at birth by direct DNA analysis. Collection of sufficient sweat may be difficult prior to one month of age. Prenatal diagnosis using direct mutation analysis and restriction fragment length polymorphisms (RFLP) analysis of DNA in CVS or in amniotic fluid is possible with 98–99% accuracy or nearly 100% accuracy by mutation analysis, in pregnancies at 25% risk. Prenatal diagnosis for couples at less than 1:4 risk is also possible using direct mutation analysis in association with DNA linkage disequilibrium studies and/or measurement of microvillar intestinal enzymes in amniotic fluid.

**Gene Mapping and Linkage:** CF (cystic fibrosis) has been mapped to 7q31-q32.
  The linkage map is as follows:
  Cen------met--XV2C--KM19--CF--D7S8(J3.11)-------tel.

**Prevention:** None known. Genetic counseling indicated.

**Treatment:** Pancreatic enzyme replacement, supplemental oral salt, pulmonary postural drainage, and antibiotic therapy.

**Prognosis:** Average life expectancy is about 20 years, with males generally surviving longer than females. However, this depends on the severity of the disorder in each case.

**Detection of Carrier:** Relatives of affected individuals can be tested for the likelihood of carrier status using DNA polymorphisms. Carrier detection in the general population may become available in the future.

**Support Groups:**
  MD; Bethesda; Cystic Fibrosis (CF) Foundation
  OH; Cleveland; International Cystic Fibrosis (Mucoviscidosis) Association
  CANADA: Ontario; Toronto; Canadian Cystic Fibrosis Foundation
  ENGLAND: Kent; Bromley; Cystic Fibrosis Research Trust

**References:**
Stern RC, et al.: Course of cystic fibrosis in 95 patients. J Pediatr 1976; 89:406–411.
Wood RE, et al.: Cystic fibrosis. Am Rev Respir Dis 1976; 113:833–878.
Taussig L, ed: Cystic fibrosis. New York: Thieme-Stratton, 1984. *
Beaudet AL, et al.: Linkage disequilibrium, cystic fibrosis, and genetic counseling. Am J Hum Genet 1989; 44:319–326.
Boat TF, et al.: Cystic fibrosis. In: Scriver CR, et al, eds: The metabolic basis of inherited disease, 6th ed. New York: McGraw-Hill, 1989: 2649–2681. *
Kerem B, et al.: Identification of the cystic fibrosis gene: genetic analysis. Science 1989; 245:1073–1080.
Li, M, et al.: Regulation of chloride channels by protein kinase C in normal and cystic fibrosis airway epithelia. Science 1989; 244:1353–1356.

Riordan JR, et al.: Identification of the cystic fibrosis gene: Cloning and characterization of complementary DNA. Science 1989; 245:1066–1073.

Rommens JM, et al.: Identification of the cystic fibrosis gene: Chromosome walking and jumping. Science 1989; 245:1059–1065.

Lemna WK, et al: Mutation analysis for heterozygote detection and the prenatal diagnosis of cystic fibrosis. New Engl J Med 1990; 322:291–296.

GR011  **Frank Greenberg**
FE014  **Gerald Feldman**

**Cystic fibrosis of pancreas**
  *See CYSTIC FIBROSIS*
**Cystic hamartoma of liver**
  *See LIVER, HAMARTOMA*
**Cystic hydrocalicosis, congenital**
  *See KIDNEY, RENAL DYSPLASIA, POTTER TYPE II*

---

## CYSTIC HYGROMA                                    3284

**Includes:**
> Cystic hygroma, post-natal
> Cystic lymphnagioma
> Hygroma axillare
> Hygroma colli cysticum
> Lymphangioma, cavernous
> Lymphangioma, cystic
> Lymphangioma, multifocal
> Ranula congenita

**Excludes:**
> **Encephalocele** (0343)
> **Hemangiomas of the head and neck** (2514)
> **Lipomas, familial symmetric** (0600)
> **Neck, branchial cleft, cysts or sinuses** (0117)
> **Neck, cystic hygroma, fetal type** (2252)
> **Thyroglossal duct remnant** (0945)

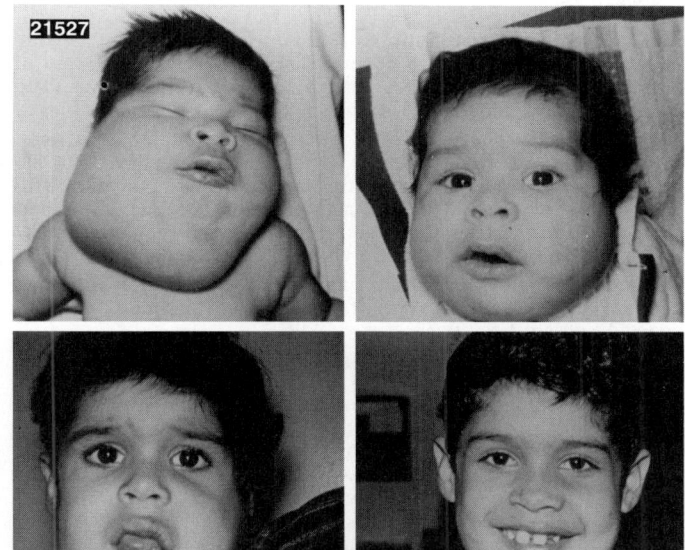

**3284-21527:** Child born with a giant cystic hygroma of the face and neck. Note the extent of the lesion at birth and the greatly improved appearance after four surgeries and orthodontic treatment. Appearance at the bottom right at 7 years of age is almost normal.

**Major Diagnostic Criteria:** A cystic mass of the neck which is diffuse and non-tender. The mass may be large or small and may extend to the face or mediastinum. Other primary locations may be in the axillae or groin.

**Clinical Findings:** This benign mass is often congenital and is most frequently found in the neck. If large it can extend to the face, mouth and chest. This lesion was first described by Redenbacker in 1828 who named it *ranula congenita*. The term cystic hygroma was first used to descibe this lesion in 1843 and it was in 1872 that Koester first suggested that these lesions were lymphatic in origin. While today it is recognized that cystic lymphangioma is a more accurate name for this lesion, the term cystic hygroma is firmly entrenched in the literature.

Cystic hygromas are most frequently found at birth in the neck. When small or medium in size they are generally asymtomatic unless they grow to a large size. Large masses can be life threatening and are difficult to remove. Few resolve spontaneously. Surgical removal is the treatment of choice; often multiple surgeries are required. Recurrence of the lesion may occur. If airway obstruction is present, a tracheostomy will be needed. Growth is unpredictable and the lesions may spread into neighboring tissues.

On physical examination, the lesion is soft and irregular and usually can be palpated in the posterior triangle of the neck. It is easily transilluminated. Fluid obtained from the lesion is usually clear or straw-colored, although bloody or blood tinged fluid may be found, either from sponatneous hemorrhage or close association with capillaries and/or cavernous venous spaces.

The axilla, shoulder, sacrum or retroperitoneum are rarely involved.

**Complications:** Hemorrhage, infection, airway obstruction and dysphagia. Nerve palsies occur rarely. Large masses involving the mouth and face cause abnormal mandibular development which may require orthodontic correction and possibly corrective jaw surgery.

**Associated Findings:** None known.

**Etiology:** These lesions occur early in developement, at about 40 days gestation, and result from the failure of the embryonic lymphatics to connect with the venous system. The lesions become canalized, continue to grow, and may infiltrate surrounding tissues producing pressure and sometimes necrosis, and forming cystic structures in the process.

**Pathogenesis:** Unknown. The developing lesions may be unilocular or multilocular with a thin transparent wall. Hemorrhage or infection may produce a thickened wall. The wall is lined with flat endothelial cell with varying amounts of fibrous stroma and areas of thrombus. The usual fluid content is clear or straw colored but may be brown or purulent if hemorrhage or infection has occurred. In the most severe cases the proliferating endothelial lined sacs infiltrate surrounding tissues causing anatomical distortion and difficulty in removal.

**CDC No.:** 239.200, 744.900

**Sex Ratio:** M1:F1

**Occurrence:** Constitute 5.6% of all benign tumors of infancy and childhood.

**Risk of Recurrence for Patient's Sib:** Unknown. Presumably low.

**Risk of Recurrence for Patient's Child:** Unknown. Presumably low.

**Age of Detectability:** By ultrasound examination at 16 weeks gestation. Most are apprarent at birth or within the first year of life. Rarely will these lesions become apparent in later childhood or adulthood.

**Gene Mapping and Linkage:** Unknown.

**Prevention:** None known. Genetic counseling indicated.

**Treatment:** Surgical removal is the treatment of choice if the mass is large or symtomptomatic. Large lesions may require multiple surgeries.

**Prognosis:** Good for life span and intellect. Overall prognosis depends on the size, location and growth of the lesion. Small and medium size lesions are genrally asymptomatic; large lesions may require intervention and are often difficult to manage. These may recur despite multiple surgeries. If airway obstruction results, the condition can be life threatening.

**Detection of Carrier:**  Unknown.

**References:**
Goetsch E: Hygroma colli cysticum and hygroma axillare. Arch Surg 1938; 36:394–479.
Marshall D, Rabuzzi DD: Cystic lymphangioma with enlarged tongue: a case report. Am J Orthod 1977; 71:685–688.
Farman AG, et al.: Mandibulo-facial aspects of the cervical cystic lymphangioma (cystic hygroma). Br J Oral Surg 1978–79; 16:125–134.
Emery PJ, et al.: Cystic hygroma of the head and neck: a review of 37 cases. J Laryngol Otol 1984; 98:613–619.
Som PM, et al.: Cystic hygroma and facial nerve paralysis: a rare association. J Computer assisted Tomography 1984; 8:110–113.
Seashore JH, et al.: Management of giant cystic hyromas in infants. Am J Surg 1985; 149:459–465.

BU032                                           **Mary Louise Buyse**

**Cystic hygroma of mesentery**
*See MESENTERIC CYSTS*
**Cystic hygroma of the neck (posterior)**
*See NECK, CYSTIC HYGROMA, FETAL TYPE*
**Cystic hygroma, post-natal**
*See CYSTIC HYGROMA*
**Cystic kidney disease-cataract-blindness**
*See KIDNEY, POLYCYSTIC DISEASE-CATARACT-BLINDNESS*
**Cystic kidney, type I**
*See KIDNEY, POLYCYSTIC DISEASE, RECESSIVE*
**Cystic lymphangiomas of orbit**
*See ORBITAL AND PERIORBITAL LYMPHANGIOMA*
**Cystic lymphnagioma**
*See CYSTIC HYGROMA*
**Cystic polyps**
*See INTESTINAL POLYPOSIS, JUVENILE TYPE*
**Cystic teratoma**
*See ORAL DERMOIDS*
**Cystine storage disease**
*See CYSTINOSIS*
**Cystine-lysine-arginine-ornithinuria**
*See CYSTINURIA*

## CYSTINOSIS                                        0238

**Includes:**
   Adult non-nephropatic cystinosis
   Benign cystinosis
   Cystine storage disease
   Early onset or infantile cystinosis
   Intermediate (late-onset) cystinosis
   Juvenile or adolescent cystinosis
   Nephropathic cystinosis
   Late-onset cystinosis

**Excludes:**
   **Cystinuria** (0239)
   **Renal tubular syndrome, Fanconi type** (0864)

**Major Diagnostic Criteria:**  The initial symptoms of renal tubular dysfunction usually occur at 8–12 months of age but in late-onset cystinosis, these symptoms might not occur until a later age (e.g., 4–26 years of age). In either case, slowly progressive glomerular damage occurs. The diagnosis of cystinosis is made by demonstrating cystine crystals in conjunctivae, bone marrow, lymph nodes or rectal mucosa. The precise biochemical diagnosis is made by finding an 80–100-fold increase in the free (non-protein) cystine content of peripheral leukocytes or cultured skin fibroblasts.

**Clinical Findings:**  The most characteristic presentation occurs at 8 to 12 months of age, with symptoms related to impaired tubular reabsorption of water, phosphate, sodium, potassium, bicarbonate, glucose, and amino acids. The defect in water reabsorption usually accounts for the presenting symptoms of the disease, which are polyuria, polydipsia, and recurrent unexplained fever. The renal loss of phosphate is associated with hypophosphatemic

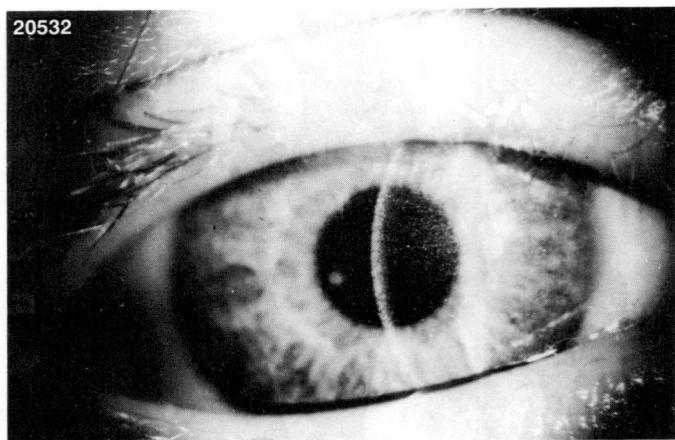

20532

0238-20532:   Cystinosis; note refractile bodies seen on slit lamp examination of the eye.

rickets, resistant to the usual antirachitic doses of vitamin D. The loss of bicarbonate and potassium results in chronic acidosis and hypokalemia. Affected children have severe growth retardation. Although it was originally thought that children with cystinosis all had a very fair complexion, many affected dark-skinned persons have now been identified.

These children develop progressive glomerular damage, which if untreated progresses to end-stage renal disease with uremia within the 1st decade of life. In other families (late-onset cystinosis), attenuated clinical expression permits survival into the 2nd or 3rd decade. In still other families, the kidney is spared and the disorder is benign.

In all three types of cystinosis, cystine crystal deposition can be demonstrated in conjunctivae, bone marrow, lymph nodes, and leukocytes. A characteristic retinopathy is observed in patients with nephropathic cystinosis but does not occur in benign cystinosis. The intracellular cystine content of free (nonprotein) cystine is approximately 100 times normal. This can be demonstrated in either peripheral leukocytes or cultured skin fibroblasts. The excess cystine is stored in lysosomes.

**Complications:**  These children have impairment of both renal tubular and glomerular function. They also have rickets, acidosis, hypokalemia, growth retardation, and often hypothyroidism. Individuals who have lived past ten years of age have had increased photophobia and decreasing visual acuity. Neurological involvement and diabetes mellitus have also been noted.

**Associated Findings:**  Several patients have been found to have cerebral atrophy with dilation of the ventricles and subarachnoid space when studies by CT scan or MRI.

**Etiology:**  Autosomal recessive inheritance. It is known that most cells from these patients contain 100 times the normal content of free-cystine and that the cystine is compartmentalized within lysosomes. It is also known that the major source of the cystine which accumulates within the lysosomes is from protein which has been degraded within the lysosomes. It is assumed that the cystine deposition leads to the renal tubular and glomerular damage and to the other complications of this disease.

**Pathogenesis:**  The exact pathogenesis of this disease is presumed to be related to the accumulation of cystine. The cystine storage occurs by 20 weeks' gestation, but cystine crystals do not develop until after birth. The retina begins to show signs of degeneration by 20 weeks' gestation.

The exact metabolic error which leads to cystine accumulation is a defect in the lysosomal efflux of cystine from the lysosome to the cytosol.

**MIM No.:**  *21975, *21980, *21990

**POS No.:** 3780

**Sex Ratio:** M1:F1

**Occurrence:** In a recent study in France, the incidence was estimated as 0.039:1,000 live births in Brittany and 0.003:1,000 live births in the rest of France. In West Germany, the minimal incidence has been reported as 0.006:1,000 live births. Such data is not available from other countries.

**Risk of Recurrence for Patient's Sib:**
See Part I, *Mendelian Inheritance.*

**Risk of Recurrence for Patient's Child:**
See Part I, *Mendelian Inheritance.*

**Age of Detectability:** It is possible to diagnose cystinosis in utero by estimating the free-cystine content of chorionic villi or cultured amniotic fluid cells. The diagnosis can be made at birth by measuring the placenta or leukocyte cystine content. Cystine crystals cannot be demonstrated until 2–4 months of age.

**Gene Mapping and Linkage:** Unknown.

**Prevention:** None known. Genetic counseling indicated.

**Treatment:** Systematic correction of the renal tubular losses is accomplished by fluid, potassium, and alkali replacement, and moderate doses of vitamin D (usually 5,000–10,000 units or its equivalent per day). Renal transplantation is routinely done in cystinotic children at the time of end-stage failure. Two patients have survived 20 years post-transplantation. Cysteamine is effective in improving growth and delaying the progression of renal glomerular damage in these patients.

**Prognosis:** In the past, children with nephropathic cystinosis usually died before 10 years of age, unless renal transplantation was performed. Patients with late-onset cystinosis survive for variable lengths of time. Patients with benign cystinosis appear to have a normal life expectancy. The prognosis of children who have had renal transplantation appears to be be better than that of children who have received renal transplants secondary to other causes of renal failure.

**Detection of Carrier:** Heterozygotes can be detected by a four to five fold increase in the intracellular content of free cystine in their polymorphonuclear leukocytes.

**Support Groups:** CA; Oakland; Cystinosis Foundation, Inc.

**References:**
Gahl WA, et al.: Cystine transport is defective in isolated leukocyte lysosomes from patients with cystinosis. Science 1982; 217:1263–1265.
Gahl WA, et al.: The course of nephropathic cystinosis after age 10 years. J Pediatr 1986; 109:605–608.
Schneider JA, Schulman JD: Cystinosis and the Fanconi syndrome. In Andreoli TE, et al, eds: Physiology of membrane disorders, ed 2. New York: Plenum Medical Book Co., 1986:985–997.
Gahl WA, et al.: Cysteamine therapy for children with nephropathic cystinosis. New Engl J Med 1987; 316:971–977.
Kaiser-Kupfer MI, et al.: Removal of corneal crystals by topical cysteamine in nephropathic cystinosis. New Engl J Med 1987; 316:775–779.
Smith ML, et al.: Prenatal diagnosis of cystinosis utilizing chorionic villus sampling. Prenatal diagnosis 1987; 7:23–26.
Smolin LA, et al.: An improved method for heterozygote detection of cystinosis, using polymorphonuclear leukocytes. Am J Hum Genet 1987; 41:266–275.
Pellett OL, et al.: Lack of complementation in somatic cell hybrids between fibroblasts from patients with different forms of cystinosis. PNAS 1988; 85:3531–3534.
Smolin LA, et al.: A comparison of the effectiveness of cysteamine and phosphocysteamine in elevating plasma cysteamine concentration and decreasing leukocyte free cystine in nephropatic cystinosis. Pediatr Res 1988; 23:616–620.
Trauner DA, et al.: Neurologic and cognitive deficits in children with cystinosis. J Pediatr 1988; 112:912–914.

**Jerry A. Schneider**

---

**CYSTINURIA**                                                    **0239**

**Includes:**
Cistinuria
Cystine-lysine-arginine-ornithinuria
Cystinuria and dibasic aminoaciduria

**Excludes:**
**Cystinosis** (0238)
Protein intolerance-defective transport dibasic amino acids
**Homocystinuria** (0474)
**Hyperdibasic aminoaciduria** (0491)
**Hypercystinuria** (0490)

**Major Diagnostic Criteria:** Urinary cyanide-nitroprusside test yields magenta red color. Non-specific cystine-lysine-arginine-ornithinuria by paper chromatography, paper electrophoresis or column chromatography; normal or decreased plasma concentrations of cystine and dibasic amino acids; exaggerated renal clearance of cystine and dibasic amino acids are necessary for diagnosis.

**Clinical Findings:** Formation of radio-opaque cystine calculi in renal pelvis, ureter or bladder; cystine crystalluria, dependent on urinary volume; renal or ureteral colic, hematuria, dysuria, and urinary tract infections secondary to cystine stone formation.

**Complications:** Renal insufficiency and uremia secondary to infection, obstruction and surgical intervention.

**Associated Findings:** Possibly short stature and/or increased incidence of mental retardation or psychiatric disturbance; hyperuricemia.

**Etiology:** Autosomal recessive inheritance with heterogeneity. There are at least three variants (Types I, II, III) due to allelic mutations. Cystinuria also occurs in dogs.

**Pathogenesis:** The mutation affects "carrier protein" (or "reactive site" probably on brush border side) of proximal renal tubule and small intestinal mucosa which mediates the shared transport of cystine, lysine, arginine and ornithine. Defective renal tubular reabsorption of cystine produces excessive urinary excretion, crystalluria and lithiasis due to limited solubility of cystine in urine (maximum solubility about 300 mg/liter). Cystine excretion is directly influenced by sodium intake. Shortened stature may be a consequence of impaired lysine nutrition.

**MIM No.:** *22010

**Sex Ratio:** M1:F1

**Occurrence:** 1:10,000 live births

**Risk of Recurrence for Patient's Sib:**
See Part I, *Mendelian Inheritance.*

**Risk of Recurrence for Patient's Child:**
See Part I, *Mendelian Inheritance.* Estimated 1:100.

**Age of Detectability:** Probably at birth. Diagnosis of phenotype (homozygous or heterozygous) is difficult before six months of age because the immaturity of renal reabsorption in infancy exaggerates the phenotype in heterozygotes.

**Gene Mapping and Linkage:** Unknown.

**Prevention:** None known. Genetic counseling indicated.

**Treatment:** High fluid intake; alkalinization of the urine to increase cystine solubility; oral administration of D-penicillamine (1–2 gm/24 hr in divided doses); surgical removal of renal, ureteral or vesical calculi. Management of renal insufficiency includes base replacement, low-protein diet, dialysis. Low sodium diet (150 mmol/day) in refractory cases.

**Prognosis:** Life span shortened by more than 10 years in affected males and by less than 10 years in affected females; death due to renal failure.

**Detection of Carrier:** Type I heterozygotes detectable only by studies of intestinal absorption or transport of cystine and dibasic amino acids. These account for about 2/3 of all carriers. Type II and Type III heterozygotes excrete increased amounts of cystine and dibasic amino acids in urine.

**Special Considerations:** There is no evidence that the several different genotypes responsible for cystinuria lead to clinically different syndromes. Clinical phenotype in genetic compounds for these allelic mutations is indistinguishable from that for homozygotes. Rare cystine calculi may be formed by Type II or Type III heterozygotes, suggesting that such individuals should also be encouraged to maintain a high urinary output. Since patients with cystinuria may form mixed stones and even noncystine stones, all patients with renal tract calculi should have a nitroprusside test to exclude this disorder. D-penicillamine is effective in prevention and dissolution of stones but also produces a variety of deleterious effects including serum sickness, leukopenia, thrombocytopenia, and a reversible nephrotic syndrome.

**References:**

Thier SO, Segal S. Cystinuria. In Stanbury JB, et al, eds.: The metabolic basis of inherited disease, 5th ed. New York: McGraw-Hill, 1983:1774–1791.

Smith A, Wilcken B: Homozygous cystinuria in New South Wales. Med J Aust 1984; 141:500

Giugliani R, et al.: Heterozygous cystinuria and urinary lithiasis. Am J Med Genet 1985; 22:703–715.

Scriver CR, et al.: Modifier manifestations of cystinuria gene. J Pediatr 1985; 106:411–416.

Jaeger P, et al.: Anticystinuric effects of glutamine and dietary sodium restriction. New Engl J Med 1986; 315:1120–1123.

Segal S, Thier SO: Cystinurias. In: Scriver CR, et al, eds: The metabolic basis of inherited disease, 6th ed. New York: McGraw-Hill, 1989: 2479–2498.

G0052
SC050

**Paul Goodyer**
**Charles R. Scriver**
*Leon E. Rosenberg*

**Cystinuria and dibasic aminoaciduria**
  *See CYSTINURIA*
**Cystinuria without dibasic aminoaciduria**
  *See HYPERCYSTINURIA*
**Cystinuria, some forms of atypical**
  *See ARGININEMIA*
**Cysts (multiple)**
  *See FETAL MULTIPLE CYSTS ANOMALY*
**Cysts of the nasopharynx, congenital**
  *See NASOPHARYNGEAL CYSTS*
**Cysts of the renal medulla, congenital**
  *See KIDNEY, NEPHRONOPHTHISIS-MEDULLARY CYSTIC DESEASE*
**Cysts, glottic**
  *See LARYNX, CYSTS*
**Cysts, inclusion of the oral mucosa of the newborn**
  *See MUCOSA, ORAL INCLUSION CYSTS OF THE NEWBORN*
**Cysts, saccular**
  *See LARYNX, CYSTS*
**Cysts, solitary liver**
  *See LIVER, CYST, SOLITARY*
**Cysts, true, benign**
  *See SPLEEN, CYSTS*
**Cytochrome C oxidase deficiency**
  *See MYOPATHY-METABOLIC, MITOCHONDRIAL CYTOCHROME C OXIDASE DEFICIENCY*
**Cytochrome P450, subfamily I (aromatic compound-inducible)**
  *See CANCER, LUNG, FAMILIAL*
**Cytochrome-b-negative granulomatous disease**
  *See GRANULOMATOUS DISEASE, CHRONIC X-LINKED*
**Cytochrome-b-positive autosomal granulomatous disease**
  *See GRANULOMATOUS DISEASE, CHRONIC X-LINKED*
**Cytomegalic adrenocortical hypoplasia**
  *See ADRENAL HYPOPLASIA, CONGENITAL*
**Cytomegalic inclusion disease, congenital**
  *See FETAL CYTOMEGALOVIRUS SYNDROME*
**Cytomegalovirus (CMV) infection**
  *See FETAL CYTOMEGALOVIRUS SYNDROME*
**Cytomegalovirus infection, fetal effects of**
  *See FETAL BRAIN DISRUPTION SEQUENCE*
**Cytomegalovirus, fetal effects of**
  *See FETAL CYTOMEGALOVIRUS SYNDROME*
**Cytosol factor, deficiency of**
  *See GRANULOMATOUS DISEASE, CHRONIC X-LINKED*
**Cytosolic tyrosine transaminase deficiency**
  *See TYROSINEMIA II, OREGON TYPE*

# ❖ D ❖

D Trisomy syndrome
  See CHROMOSOME 13, TRISOMY 13
D-glucose-6-phosphate ketol isomerase (E.C.5.3.1.9), deficiency of
  See ANEMIA, GLUCOSE PHOSPHATE ISOMERASE DEFICIENCY
D-penicillamine, fetal effects of
  See FETAL D-PENICILLAMINE SYNDROME
Dacryostenosis, congenital
  See NASOLACRIMAL DUCT OBSTRUCTION
Dalmatian hypouricemia
  See RENAL HYPOURICEMIA
Damane^, fetal effects
  See FETAL BENZODIAZEPINE EFFECTS
Danazol, maternal exposure and fetal virilization
  See FETAL EFFECTS FROM MATERNAL EXTRINSIC ANDROGENS
Danbolt syndrome
  See ACRODERMATITIS ENTEROPATHICA
Danbolt-Closs syndrome
  See ACRODERMATITIS ENTEROPATHICA
Dandy-Walker cyst-spondylocostal dysostosis-visceral defects
  See SPONDYLOCOSTAL DYSOSTOSIS-VISCERAL DEFECTS-
    DANDY WALKER CYST
Dandy-Walker malformation-joint contractures-cleft palate
  See AASE-SMITH SYNDROME
Dandy-Walker syndrome
  See HYDROCEPHALY
Danish type amyloidosis
  See AMYLOIDOSIS, DANISH CARDIAC TYPE
Danocrine^, maternal exposure and fetal virilization
  See FETAL EFFECTS FROM MATERNAL EXTRINSIC ANDROGENS
Dappled metaphysis syndrome
  See SPONDYLOEPIMETAPHYSEAL DYSPLASIA, STRUDWICK TYPE

## DARIER DISEASE                                    2865

**Includes:**
  Darier-White disease
  Keratosis follicularis
  Skin, Darier disease

**Excludes:**
  Acrokeratosis verruciformis (3256)
  Focal acantholytic dermatosis (Grover disease)
  Nevus, epidermal nevus syndrome (0593)
  Pemphigus, benign familial (3255)
  Skin, keratosis follicularis spinulosa decalvans (2867)

**Major Diagnostic Criteria:** Multiple keratotic papules and plaques occurring in a seborrheic distribution with characteristic histopathology of suprabasilar acantholysis with individually dyskeratotic cells.

**Clinical Findings:** The onset is typically between ages eight and 15 years, but may range from very early childhood through adulthood. The onset is often insidious, and the disorder is slowly progressive, with development of more lesions and involvement of new areas. In some patients the onset is fulminant due to a precipitating factor, most commonly intense sunlight exposure.

The eruption is characterized by hyperkeratotic papules and plaques. The primary lesion is a small, often inflamed papule surmounted by a gray-brown crust. In extensive disease, papules are numerous and coalesce to form vegetating plaques. Although the eruption may occur anywhere on the body, commonly it falls in a seborrheic distribution, i.e., scalp, ears, retroauricular areas, face, neck, upper chest, and back. Involvement of the flexures, especially the axillae, inframammary region, and groin is also common. In these occluded areas the disease is more plaque-like, with erythematous erosions or moist vegetating lesions. Involvement of the extremities is often accentuated on sun-exposed sites. Some patients develop extensive, confluent areas of warty hyperkeratoses. Flat-topped, wart-like papules may be present on the dorsum of the hands and tiny, seed-like, hyperkeratotic papules on the palms.

Although the scalp is commonly involved, the hair itself is unaffected. Nail involvement is one of the cardinal features and includes 1) longitudinal white streaks, 2) subungual hyperkeratoses, 3) thickening of the nail plate, 4) thinning of the nail plate with distal splintering, and 5) subungual splinter hemorrhages.

The oral mucosa is also involved, with a characteristic, cobblestone texture, particularly on the alveolar ridges, palate, tongue, and buccal mucosa. Similar, asymptomatic mucosal involvement has been observed in the hypopharynx, larynx, and rectum.

The epidermal histopathology is characterized by the combination of acantholysis and abnormal cornification. Focal suprabasilar acantholysis leads to the development of clefts or lucanae, the base of which form villous projections lined by a single layer of cells. Acantholytic cells within the lacunae show signs of premature abnormal keratinization. "Corps ronds," demonstrating a darkly staining central nucleus surrounded by clear cytoplasm, are prominent in the upper epidermis. "Grains," i.e., small, densely staining, anucleate cells, predominate in the parakeratotic stratum corneum overlying the clefts. Similar histopathologic changes are present in other clinical disorders, such as epidermal nevi, warty dyskeratomas, benign familial pemphigus (Hailey-Hailey disease), and focal acantholytic dermatosis (Grover disease). Therefore, the diagnosis of Darier disease cannot be made by histopathology alone, but must be considered in the context of the entire clinical presentation.

**Complications:** Acute sunburn may precipitate this condition. Severe superinfection of lesions may occur, particularly with herpes simplex virus (Kaposi varicelliform eruption). Salivary duct obstruction is reported.

**Associated Findings:** Several studies have demonstrated some impairment of T-cell function. Other possible noncutaneous manifestations are neuropsychiatric disorders and bone cysts. In one study, 5 of 51 patients were reported to be mentally subnormal, and another 8 of 51 had a psychiatric illness, while another kindred with 12 affected family members had four members with psychotic illnesses and three with mental deficiency. while bone cysts have been reported, a prospective survey of 31 patients failed to detect any bone cysts. Renal and testicular agenesis has also been reported.

**Etiology:** Autosomal dominant inheritance with full penetrance but expression 1) may be limited to nails or oral mucosa, 2) may be delayed until adulthood, and 3) may undergo extended periods of remission.

**Pathogenesis:** Unknown. Sunlight is an important provocative factor; the action spectrum responsible is predominantly in the UV-B range. Although several studies have described abnormalities of T-cell function, both the cause of the deficit and its relationship to the pathogenesis of the epidermal abnormality is unclear. Other theories postulate an abnormality in vitamin A metabolism or abnormal proteolytic activity.

**MIM No.:** *12420

**CDC No.:** 757.900

**Sex Ratio:** M1:F1

**Occurrence:** The disease has been reported to occur in a wide variety of ethnic groups, with an estimated prevalence rate in Denmark of 1:100,000.

**Risk of Recurrence for Patient's Sib:**
See Part I, *Mendelian Inheritance*.

**Risk of Recurrence for Patient's Child:**
See Part I, *Mendelian Inheritance*.

**Age of Detectability:** Usually during childhood but may be delayed into adulthood. Expression may be limited to nails or oral mucosa, and severity may wax and wane.

**Gene Mapping and Linkage:** Unknown.

**Prevention:** None known. Genetic counseling indicated. Diligent use of sunscreens and protective clothing will help to avoid sun-induced disease.

**Treatment:** Mild eruptions may respond to topical therapies, including retinoic acid (Retin-A) and glucocorticoids. Oral synthetic retinoids (e.g., etretinate or isotretinoin) may be indicated for severe flares. Doses should be adjusted to the lowest effective amount (e.g., etretinate, 0.3 mg/kg) and treatment continued only for as long as necessary to avoid long-term toxicity. Due to its teratogenicity and long half-life, etretinate is contraindicated in women of childbearing potential (see **Fetal retinoid syndrome**).

**Prognosis:** The disorder tends to become more widespread with age. Intelligence may be subnormal in some patients.

**Detection of Carrier:** Family members must be carefully examined, with special attention to nails and oral mucosa to detect mildly affected individuals.

**References:**
Svendsen IB, Albrechtsen B: The prevalence of dyskeratosis follicularis (Darier's disease) in Denmark: an investigation of the heredity in 22 families. Acta Dermato-Venerol 1959; 39:256–269.

Getzler NA, Flint A: Keratosis follicularis: a study of one family. Arch Dermatol 1966; 93:545–549.

Zaias N, Ackerman AB: The nail in Darier-White disease. Arch Dermatol 1973; 107:193–199. †

Prindeville DE, Stern D: Oral manifestations of Darier's disease. J Oral Surg 1976; 34:1001.

Beck AL Jr, et al.: Darier's disease: a kindred with a large number of cases. Br J Dermatol 1977; 97:335–339.

Jegasothy BV, Humeniuk JM: Darier's disease: a partially immunodeficient state. J Invest Dermatol 1981; 76:129–132.

Starink TM, Woerdeman MJ: Unilateral systematized keratosis follicularis: a variant of Darier's disease or an epidermal nevus (acantholytic dyskeratotic epidermal nevus)? Br J Dermatol 1981; 105:207–214.

Crisp AJ, et al: The prevalence of bone cysts in Darier's disease: a survey of 31 cases. Clin Exp Dermatol 1984; 9:78–83.

Matsuoka LY, et al.: Renal and testicular agenesis in a patient with Darier's disease. Am J Med 1985; 78:873–877.

WI013                                      **Mary L. Williams**

**Darier-White disease**
*See DARIER DISEASE*
**Dark dot disease**
*See SKIN CREASES, RETICULATE PIGMENTED FLEXURES, DOWLING-DEGOS TYPE*
**Darwin tubercle**
*See EAR, DARWIN TUBERCLE*

**Davidson disease**
*See MICROVILLUS INCLUSION DISEASE*
**Davies disease**
*See VENTRICLE, ENDOMYOCARDIAL FIBROSIS OF RIGHT*
*also VENTRICLE, ENDOMYOCARDIAL FIBROSIS OF LEFT*
**Day blindness**
*See COLOR BLINDNESS, TOTAL*
**De Barsy syndrome**
*See CUTIS LAXA-GROWTH DEFECT, DE BARSY TYPE*
**De Barsy-Moens-Dierckx syndrome**
*See CUTIS LAXA-GROWTH DEFECT, DE BARSY TYPE*
**de la Chapelle skeletal dysplasia**
*See SKELETAL DYSPLASIA, DE LA CHAPELLE TYPE*

---

## DE LANGE SYNDROME                              0242

**Includes:**
  Brachmann-de Lange syndrome
  Cornelia de Lange Syndrome
  Typus degenerativus Amstelodamensis

**Excludes:** Chromosome 3, trisomy 3q2 (2430)

**Major Diagnostic Criteria:** Physical and mental retardation, hirsutism and synophrys, microcephaly, long or protruding philtrum, anteverted nostrils, small or grossly malformed hands, and webbing of 2nd and 3rd toes.

**Clinical Findings:** Mild to severe mental retardation. Spasticity may be present in the severely retarded children. Growth retardation with low birthweight even at term. Generalized hirsutism, synophyrys, long eyelashes. Microcephaly, usually brachycephaly. Anteverted nostrils, prominent philtrum, thin lips turned down at angles of mouth. Limitation of extension of elbows. Single transverse palmar crease, proximally placed thumbs, clinodactyly of 5th finger. Severely malformed upper limbs, ranging from small hands to oligodactyly of phocomelia, and webbing of 2nd and 3rd toes. Neonatal feeding or respiratory problems are often noted. Recurrent respiratory infection, a short neck, low-pitched cry, undescended testes, delayed eruption and wide spacing of teeth are common. Cardiac defects are also common, but hypospadias, cleft palate, recurrent convulsions, herniae and other malformations are less common.

**Complications:** Neonatal feeding or respiratory difficulties.

**Associated Findings:** None known.

**Etiology:** Unknown in the great majority of cases. Autosomal dominant and recessive inheritance has been suggested. Chromosomal abnormalities have been reported in 16 of about 150 patients, but no specific chromosome is involved in all.

**Pathogenesis:** Unknown.

**MIM No.:** 12247

**POS No.:** 3183

**CDC No.:** 759.820

**Sex Ratio:** M1:F1

**Occurrence:** Estimated 1:>10,000 live births.

**Risk of Recurrence for Patient's Sib:**
See Part I, *Mendelian Inheritance*. Empiric risk of about two percent.

**Risk of Recurrence for Patient's Child:**
See Part I, *Mendelian Inheritance*. Only recently have there been reports of children born to affected individuals (Leavitt et al, 1985).

**Age of Detectability:** At birth.

**Gene Mapping and Linkage:** Unknown.

**Prevention:** None known. Genetic counseling indicated.

**Treatment:** Symptomatic, e.g. anticonvulsants for those with seizures, tranquilizers for behavioral disorders.

**Prognosis:** Diminished life expectancy; few known patients are adults; increased susceptibility to infections.

**Detection of Carrier:** Unknown. Rarely, recognized by demonstrating a balanced translocation in either parent.

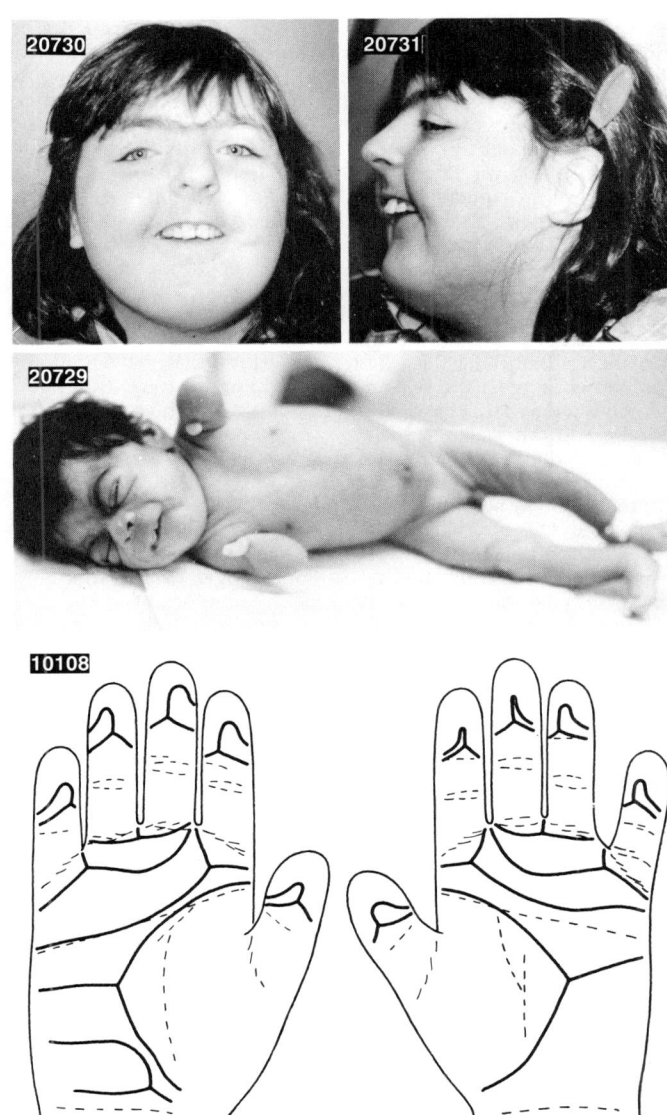

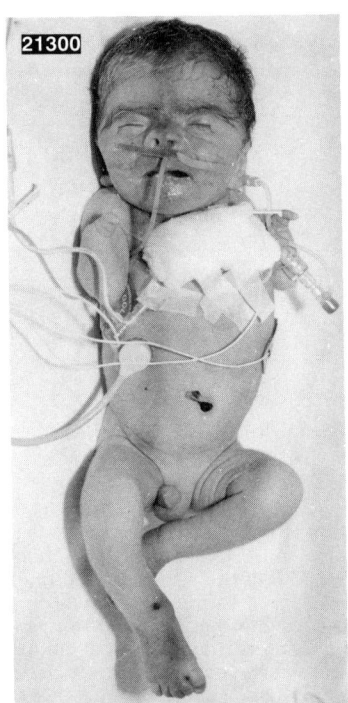

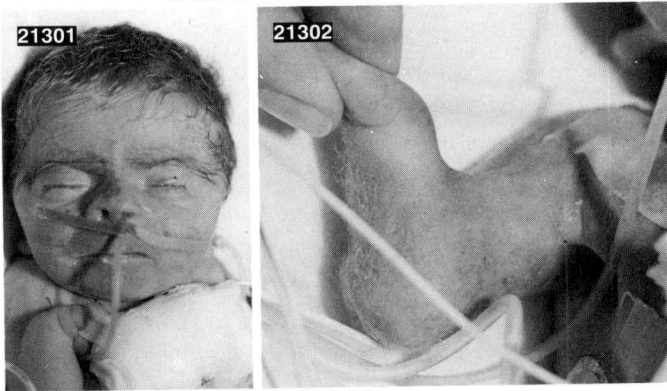

**0242A**-20730–31: De Lange syndrome; note this 12-year-old with synophrys, anteverted nares, thin upper lip and microcephaly. 20729: This affected infant has hirsutism, synophrys, broad philtrum, and micromelia. 10108: Dermatoglyphics in De Lange syndrome.

**0242B**-21300: Male infant with similar findings to the original subject first described by Dr. Brachmann in 1916. Note typical facial features including synophrys, thin and downcurved lips, and limb defects. 21301: Close-up of the facial features of the infant shown in 21300. Also note monodactyly from ulna ray defect. 21302: Close-up of the right arm of the infant shown in 21300. Note the severe shortening, ulnar pterygium, and monodactyly caused by the severe ulnar ray defect.

**Special Considerations:** While this syndrome was long known by the name Cornelia de Lange who published the first account in 1933, Dr. W. Brachmann first described the condition in 1916 (Opitz, 1985).

**Support Groups:**
AK; Sitka; Reaching Out
CT; Collinsville; Cornelia de Lange Syndrome (CdLS) Foundation

**References:**
Pashayan H, et al.: Variability of the de Lange syndrome. J Pediatr 1969; 75:853–858.
Berg JM, et al.: The de Lange syndrome. Oxford: Pergamon Press, 1970.

Beck B, Mikkelson M: Chromosomes in the Cornelia de Lange syndrome. Hum Genet 1981; 59:271–276.
Preus M, Rex AP: Definition and diagnosis of the Brachmann - de Lange syndrome. Am J Med Genet 1983; 16:301–312.
Hawley PP, et al.: Sixty-four patients with Brachmann-de Lange syndrome. Am J. Med Genet 1985; 20:453–459.
Leavitt A, et al.: Cornelia de Lange syndrome in a mother and daughter. Clin Genet 1985; 157–161.
Opitz JM: The Brachmann-de Lange syndrome. Am J Med Genet 1985; 22:89–102.
Fryns JP, et al.: The Brachmann-de Lange syndrome in two siblings of normal parents. Clin Genet 1987; 31:413–415.
Naguib KK, et al.: Brachmann-de Lange syndrome in sibs. J Med Genet 1987; 24:627–631.

SI001                                **Margaret W. Siber**

**De Morsier syndrome**
*See SEPTO-OPTIC DYSPLASIA*
**de Toni-Fanconi-Debre syndrome (some cases)**
*See MYOPATHY-METABOLIC, MITOCHONDRIAL CYTOCHROME C*
*OXIDASE DEFICIENCY*
**De Vaal disease**
*See IMMUNODEFICIENCY, SEVERE COMBINED*
**Deaf**
*See DEAFNESS*

---

## DEAFNESS                                   1512

**Includes:**

    Cochlear hearing loss
    Conductive hearing loss
    Deaf
    Hard of hearing
    Perceptive hearing loss
    Retrocochlear hearing loss.
    Sensorineural hearing loss

Deafness includes any degree of hearing loss since any degree implies loss of some important function in the ear or its neural connections. About 10% of the adult population, and about 5% of school-age children, have hearing impairment in one or both ears. It is generally accepted that genetic hearing loss of some type is present in between 1:600 and 1:2,000 of all children. The clinician should be aware, however, that hearing-impaired people may use the term quite differently. *Deaf* people are those whose hearing, even with the best amplification, is not good enough to understand speech. *Hard of hearing* describes the rest of the hearing-impaired population. This distinction is useful in determining the appropriate mode of communication and education, but not medically in determining etiology.

The approach to an etiologic diagnosis is to determine whether the hearing loss is syndromic or nonsyndromic, genetic or nongenetic. Otolaryngologists are trained to search for nongenetic hearing loss, and most textbooks of otolaryngology contain extensive information about ototoxic drugs, trauma, and other nongenetic causal mechanisms.

The diagnostician must sort out where the problem is, when it started, how quickly it progressed, and what it is associated with. The site of lesion can be inferred from audiologic testing. A *conductive loss* implies a problem in the outer or middle ear, which "conduct" the sound waves to the cochlea for interpretation and transmission to the brain. A *sensorineural or perceptive loss* is at the level of the cochlea (where the sensory cells are located) or its neural connections in the cochlear nerve, brainstem, or auditory cortex. A sensorineural impairment may therefore be further divided into a *cochlear* or *retrocochlear* (ie. central) loss.

Age at onset and progression of hearing loss are important for determining which syndrome may be involved, but obtaining precise information may require considerable research. A common etiology listed on school medical history forms is "high fever" during infancy or early childhood. This is a most unlikely etiology unless it is associated with meningitis, mumps, or other known causes of ototoxicity, including drugs used for milder infections. When a child is first tested audiometrically, the level of hearing may be underestimated using behavioral techniques, since the child learns to respond to sound over time. Brainstem audiometry is very useful in early infancy, but this is a neurophysiologic test that detects transmission of certain kinds of sounds to the brainstem. It implies nothing about whether the cortex can detect and interpret the signals.

Congenital impairments are usually thought to be stable, but that may not always be the case. Viable rubella (see **Fetal rubella syndrome**) and syphilis organisms (see **Fetal syphilis syndrome**), which further damage hearing, have been demonstrated in the cochlea postnatally. Among genetic causes, progressive loss may be due to a single gene with unknown pathogenetic influence, as in the dominant progressive hearing loss of later life to accumulation of a chemical substance, such as mucopolysaccharide (see **Mucopolysaccharidosis**), which is a major component of the tecto-

rial membrane in the cochlea; to bony overgrowth impinging on nerves, as in craniometaphyseal dysplasia; or to tumors, as in **Neurofibromatosis**. Sudden hearing losses are usually due to nongenetic casues such as trauma, vascular accidents, or infections, such as mumps. However, the so-called idiopathic losses may also be genetic but occur prior to the onset of other diagnostic symptoms. An individual with type III **Usher syndrome** (onset of hearing loss postnatally) described several episodes of sudden loss years apart, the first prior to the recognition of **Retinitis pigmentosa** symptoms.

The otologist and audiologist should help to identify as accurately as possible the site of lesion. The audiologist can help review previous testing and give suggestions about validity and needed studies to complete the auditory profile. Vestibular testing can aid in identifying the extent of labyrinthine involvement and sometimes suggest the reason for an apparent ataxia. Computed or polytomography can give information about the shape of the middle and inner ears, which may be important in deciding, for instance, whether a baby's hearing loss is secondary to anoxia, ototoxicity, or a problem prior to the second trimester. Other studies such as serology for syphilis or an EKG to identify the prolonged QT interval of **Cardio-auditory syndrome**, should be done only if the history, pedigree, and physical examination warrant them. A thorough dysmorphologic examination and review of past medical history are equally important.

Associated features of particular importance when hearing impairment is involved are vision and mental capacity. Because all hearing-impaired people rely heavily on vision, a thorough initial ophthalmologic examination and periodic subsequent examinations are important. Most screening school, pediatric, and even ophthalmologic examinations do not test for diminution in night or peripheral vision, which are associated with **Retinitis pigmentosa**, so parents and older affected individuals should be alerted to watch for these. Mental capability is especially difficult to assess in hearing-impaired individuals, since verbal language learning is primarily auditory. Therefore, in evaluating a developmental or intellectual assessment, the physician should find out how much experience the tester has had with hearing-impaired people and give more credence to performance than verbal scores.

Hearing tests of parents and other family members are essential. A case in point was a child with **Craniofacial dysostosis** inherited from her mildly affected father. Her mother and some relatives, however, turned out to have unsuspected hearing losses almost identical to hers. The proband had inherited a dominant disorder from each parent, and the hearing loss was not attributable to **Craniofacial dysostosis**.

Clues to pathogenesis of losses at various locations as well as to expected associated findings may be provided by the embryologic origin of the involved structures. The ear is derived from all three primitive layers: ectoderm-skin of pinna, canal, and outer layer of the eardrum (from the branchial arches), and inner ear or membranous labyrinth (from the otic placode); mesoderm-cartilage of pinna, middle layer of the eardrum, and any bones such as the middle ear ossicles and the bony labyrinth, which surrounds the fragile membranes of the inner ear (may be influenced by neural crest); and endoderm-lining of the middle ear cavity, which is continuous with that of the nose and mouth through the eustachian tube.

In branchial arch syndromes, therefore, the entire outer and middle ear structures may be affected, but not the inner ear unless some other problem is present. Such is the case in **Mandibulofacial dysostosis** in which the inner ear should be normal, and early fitting of a bone conduction hearing aid can allow the child to attain normal oral language development. The footplate of the stapes, however, fits snugly into the annular ligament, which is induced by the membranous labyrinth, so stapes fixation may occur when dysplasia of the inner ear is present as is sometimes the case in **Deafness with perilymphatic gusher**. Since the inner ear structures are from ectoderm, one might expect neural elements to be affected in other parts of the body as well as the ear. In **Waardenburg syndromes**, for instance, **Colon, aganglionosis** has been noted secondarily to missing colonic ganglion cells derived from neural crest.

Congenital malformations of the ear occur once in every 3,800 live births, and such changes are unilateral in over 90% of cases (Lapayowker, 1974). In a French study of 714 children, minor malformations of the external ear were observed in 9.3%; the three categories of these were protruding, severed, or pendulous ears. Anomalies of the lobe occurred in 4.4% of the series and included an absent, attached, or grooved lobe (Fontaine, 1982). Earlobe creasing develops with age, while both the shape of the earlobe and the onset of creasing are dependent on race (Overfield & Call, 1983).

Most outer and middle ear structures are formed by the fourth month of gestation, though cochlear structures are still undergoing major development through the fifth month. Therefore, any teratogens or genes acting in the first trimester could disrupt formation of any ear part, whereas those in the second trimester would primarily cause inner ear damage. Those children affected in the second trimester usually have normal conductive hearing, but a variable high-frequency sensorineural loss.

As with all other diagnostic challenges for geneticists, single gene, chromosomal anomalies, and environmental factors must be considered. Except for the hearing loss associated with **Cleft palate**, no multifactorial model has been proposed for any particular hearing impairment, though certainly a combination of genetic and environmental factors can occur. One example of this is ototoxicity that causes profound deafness in a person already hard of hearing due to a genetic syndrome (Davenport et al, 1979). Noise-induced hearing loss and chronic recurrent otitis media also involve a genetic predisposition.

The work-up of hearing impairment, therefore, requires no set battery of tests. Rather, the clinician should work with the otolaryngology team to find out as much as possible about hearing loss in the proband and relatives and to relate this information to the clinical findings in an effort to match the resulting profile to potential diagnoses.

**References:**
Lapayowker MS: Congenital anomalies of the middle ear. Radiol Clin North Am 1974; 12:463–471.
Konigsmark BW, Gorlin RJ: Genetic and metabolic deafness. Philadelphia: W.B. Saunders, 1976.
Davenport SLH, et al.: Dominant hearing loss, white hair, contractures, hyperkeratotic papillomata, and depressed chemotaxia. BD: OAS XV(5B). New York: March of Dimes Birth Defects Foundation 1979:227–237.
Fontaine G: Les anomalies morphologiques du pavillon de l'oreille chez l'enfant (a propos d'une nouvelle observation). LARC Med 1982; 2:772–774.
Overfield T, Call EB: Earlobe type, race, and age: effects on earlobe creasing. J Am Geriatr Soc 1983; 31:479–481.
Regenbogen LS, Coscas GJ: Oculo-auditory syndromes. New York: Masson, 1985.

DA026                                    **Sandra L.H. Davenport**

**Deafness (bilateral conductive)-absent incus-stapes**
See EAR LOBE, HYPERTROPHIC THICKENED
**Deafness (conduction)-multiple synostoses**
See SYMPHALANGISM
**Deafness (conductive)-hypertelorism-microtia-facial clefting**
See HYPERTELORISM-MICROTIA-FACIAL CLEFT-CONDUCTIVE DEAFNESS
**Deafness (conductive)-malformed external ear**
See EAR, LOW-SET
**Deafness (conductive)-thickened ear lobes**
See EAR LOBE, HYPERTROPHIC THICKENED
**Deafness (nerve)-nephrosis-hypoparathyroidism**
See NEPHROSIS-NERVE DEAFNESS-HYPOPARATHYROIDISM, BARAKAT TYPE
**Deafness (neural)-atypical atopic dermatitis**
See DEAFNESS-ATOPIC DERMATITIS
**Deafness (sensorineural) with X-linked ocular albinism**
See ALBINISM, OCULAR-LATE-ONSET-SENSORINEURAL DEAFNESS, X-LINKED

## DEAFNESS (SENSORINEURAL), MIDFREQUENCY          0267

**Includes:**
Deafness, mid-tone neural
Midfrequency nerve loss, hereditary
Midfrequency sensorineural deafness
"U"-shaped hearing loss

**Excludes:**
Deafness (sensorineural), progressive high-tone (0269)
Muscle wasting of hands-sensorineural deafness (0450)

**Major Diagnostic Criteria:** Sensorineural hearing loss in the midfrequencies. There is usually good discrimination considering the audiogram, with no tone decay. No other hereditary defects are found.

**Clinical Findings:** Midfrequency sensorineural hearing loss is demonstrated by audiometry in members of a family. Several of the affected families show members with hereditary hearing loss, but not all audiometric patterns are "U"-shaped. Some are high-tone, others low-tone, and some flat. The hearing loss reported has been nonprogressive in some families and progressive in others. Other than the hearing impairment, the medical history, physical examination, neurologic and otolaryngologic examinations are normal. Vestibular testing, including caloric examination, is normal. In most of the affected people the hearing loss progressed slowly over the years, paralleling that of presbycusis.

**Complications:** Mild paranoia, possibly associated with hearing loss, has been reported.

**Associated Findings:** None known.

**Etiology:** Probably autosomal dominant inheritance.

**Pathogenesis:** In most cases a mild-to-moderate hearing loss in early school life is noted. Frequently the hereditary hearing impairment is known in other members of the family. The tone decay tests are usually negative, tending to eliminate an eighth nerve lesion. Speech discrimination is remarkably good for the amount of hearing lost in the critical frequencies. In the families with the nonprogressive loss this can be explained by a learning process.

**MIM No.:** *12470

**Sex Ratio:** M1:F1 (In 5 families, 36 males: 28 females observed)

**Occurrence:** Documented in at least five kindreds.

**Risk of Recurrence for Patient's Sib:**
See Part I, Mendelian Inheritance.

**Risk of Recurrence for Patient's Child:**
See Part I, Mendelian Inheritance.

**Age of Detectability:** In infancy if computerized brain wave response is used; 4–6 years of age if audiometry is employed.

**Gene Mapping and Linkage:** Unknown.

**Prevention:** None known. Genetic counseling indicated.

**Treatment:** Hearing aids occasionally needed for socially adequate hearing.

**Prognosis:** Normal life span, with minimal handicap.

**Detection of Carrier:** Unknown.

**Special Considerations:** In several families some members showed a "U"-shaped deafness, while others showed a high-tone or flat deafness. In some families all showed a "U"-shaped loss. Some families have progressive hearing loss, in others nonprogressive. The kindreds have not been large enough to determine whether one, two, or more types of genetic problems are involved.

**References:**
Martensson B: Dominant hereditary nerve deafness. Acta Otolaryngol (Stockh) 1960; 52:270–274.
Williams F, Roblee LA: Hereditary nerve deafness. Arch Otolaryngol 1962; 75:69–77.
Konigsmark BW, et al.: Dominant midfrequency hearing loss. Ann Otol Rhinol Laryngol 1970; 79:42.

Bieber FR, Nance WE: Hereditary hearing loss. In: Jackson LG, Schimke RN, (eds): Clinical genetics. New York: John Wiley, 1979.

BI004

**Frederick R. Bieber**

## DEAFNESS (SENSORINEURAL), PROGRESSIVE HIGH-TONE        0269

**Includes:**
    Albrecht syndrome
    Hearing loss, hereditary progressive high-tone neural

**Excludes:** Deafness (sensorineural), midfrequency (0267)

**Major Diagnostic Criteria:** Progressive high-tone loss of hearing develops in children of families with an affected parent.

**Clinical Findings:** During childhood a high-tone hearing loss develops. Recruitment is not demonstrable. Other than slight evidence of tone decay in the high tones, there is no evidence of nerve involvement by this method. As the children with the trait become older the hearing impairment spreads, suggesting that the gene has the ability to change the rate of presbycusis.

**Complications:** Unknown.

**Associated Findings:** In one large kindred a parallel finding of nasal septal deviation was reported.

**Etiology:** Autosomal dominant inheritance with complete penetrance.

**Pathogenesis:** No recruitment and minimal tone decay suggests degeneration of the spiral ganglia cells rather than dissolution of the hair cells in the organ of Corti.

**MIM No.:** *12480

**Sex Ratio:** M1:F1

**Occurrence:** Undetermined. Established literature. Several large kindreds documented.

**Risk of Recurrence for Patient's Sib:**
    See Part I, *Mendelian Inheritance.*

**Risk of Recurrence for Patient's Child:**
    See Part I, *Mendelian Inheritance.*

**Age of Detectability:** As soon as patient is able to take a pure-tone audiometric examination, namely, age 3–6 years, depending on intelligence.

**Gene Mapping and Linkage:** Unknown.

**Prevention:** None known. Genetic counseling indicated.

**Treatment:** Undetermined. Possibly lip-reading or hearing aid in middle age.

**Prognosis:** Life span not affected. No patients developed total deafness, and all could function with a hearing aid or lip-reading.

**Detection of Carrier:** Unknown.

**References:**
Crowe SJ, et al.: Observations on the pathology of high-tone deafness. Bull Johns Hopkins Hosp 1934; 54:315–380.
Dolowitz DA, Stephens FE: Hereditary nerve deafness. Ann Otol Rhinol Laryngol 1961; 70:851.
Glorig A, Davis H: Age, noise, and hearing loss. Trans Am Otol Soc 1961; 49:262–280.
Huizing EH, et al.: Studies on progressive hereditary perceptive deafness in a family of 335 members. I. Genetical and general audiological results. Acta Otolaryng 1966; 61:35–41.
Huizing EH, et al.: Studies on progressive hereditary perceptive deafness in a family of 335 members. II. Characteristic patterns of hearing deterioration. Acta Otolaryng 1966; 61:161–167.
Paparella MM, et al.: Familial progressive sensorineural deafness. Arch Otolaryng 1969; 90:44–51.
Nance WE, McConnell FE: Status and progress of research in hereditary deafness. Adv Hum Genet 1974; 4:173–250.
Bieber FR, Nance WE: Hereditary hearing loss. In: Jackson LG, Schimke RN, eds: Clinical genetics. New York: John Wiley, 1979.

BI004

**Frederick R. Bieber**

## DEAFNESS (SENSORINEURAL), RECESSIVE EARLY-ONSET        0270

**Includes:** Neural deafness, recessive early-onset

**Excludes:**
    **Deafness (sensorineural), recessive profound** (0271)
    **Deafness** (other)

**Major Diagnostic Criteria:** Severe hearing loss with evidence either by history or by audiogram that some hearing was present during early childhood. Evidence of recessive transmission.

**Clinical Findings:** During the first several years of life there is some hearing, evidenced by the child learning to speak a few words. Hearing deteriorates, and by 5 or 6 years of age there is severe hearing loss. Audiometric testing when the child is 5 years old generally shows a 60–100 db symmetric sensorineural hearing loss. Hearing loss is so severe that no other audiometric tests can be done.

    Caloric vestibular tests show a normal response. Physical and neurologic examinations show no abnormalities except for the hearing loss. Laboratory tests, including temporal bone tomograms, are normal.

**Complications:** Unknown.

**Associated Findings:** None known.

**Etiology:** Autosomal recessive inheritance.

**Pathogenesis:** Hearing loss is probably due to degeneration, possibly of the hair cells in the organ of Corti as suggested by the following indirect evidence: neurologic examination shows no abnormalities; the vestibular system is also normal; and the inner ear is normal by tomogram.

**MIM No.:** 22160

**Sex Ratio:** M1:F1

**Occurrence:** Not described in general U.S. population. In Mennonite population of Lancaster, PA, risk is 1:500 live births. Genetic heterogeneity is likely.

**Risk of Recurrence for Patient's Sib:**
    See Part I, *Mendelian Inheritance.*

**Risk of Recurrence for Patient's Child:**
    See Part I, *Mendelian Inheritance.*

**Age of Detectability:** One or two years of age.

**Gene Mapping and Linkage:** Unknown.

**Prevention:** None known. Genetic counseling indicated.

**Treatment:** The disease should be diagnosed as early as possible, and hearing aids used during the period when the child is acquiring speech.

**Prognosis:** Average life span and intelligence.

**Detection of Carrier:** Unknown.

**References:**
Barr B, Wedenberg E: Prognosis of perceptive hearing loss in children with respect to genesis and use of hearing aid. Acta Otolaryngol (Stockh) 1964; 59:462–474.
Mengel MC, et al.: Recessive early-onset neural deafness. Acta Otolaryngol (Stockh) 1967; 64:313–326.

BI004

**Frederick R. Bieber**

## DEAFNESS (SENSORINEURAL), RECESSIVE PROFOUND      0271

**Includes:**
> Deafness, congenital I
> Deafness, congenital II
> Deafness, severe isolated congenital

**Excludes:**
> Acquired deafness
> **Deafness** (other)
> Deafness occurring with other somatic anomalies or defects

**Major Diagnostic Criteria:** Sensorineural deafness, severe-to-profound. Nonprogressive deafness present at birth or during early months of life. The diagnosis cannot be considered conclusive unless hearing loss is determined in a sibling.

**Clinical Findings:** Deafness is sensorineural and essentially symmetric bilaterally, is present at birth or shortly thereafter, and is nonprogressive after it becomes manifest. Audiometry shows severe hearing loss, ranging from no response to 80 db average in the speech frequencies. Because of the profundity of the loss, affected persons were in the past placed in manual (signing or finger spelling) programs and were not trained to speak intelligibly. From this situation arose the term "deaf-mutism", which is a misnomer; none of these people are inherently "mute" except insofar as they have not had oral speech training. It is probable that as many as 45% of this group have no responses to standard audiometry, and the remainder chiefly respond only to the low frequencies: 250, 500, and 1,000 Hz. Occasionally there is residual hearing throughout the audiometric range, but it is severely reduced to levels > 80 db.

Normal vestibular function is usually considered characteristic of this deafness, but some evidence suggests that 35% of this group have no response to rotation tests. Polytomography thus far has not been successful in identifying the pathology of this deafness.

**Complications:** Defective speech and language development results unless early training is instituted. Emotional problems can occur if the hearing loss is not recognized early and the child is not treated appropriately.

**Associated Findings:** None known.

**Etiology:** Autosomal recessive inheritance with variable penetrance; several genes are probably involved, and these are capable of variable expression in either the homozygote or heterozygote. No interaction need occur when two different recessive genes are involved.

**Pathogenesis:** No specific histopathology has been identified for this type of deafness, but recessive deafness has been related to the cochleosaccular membranous labyrinth degeneration described by Scheibe. Ormerod suggests that the pathology may resemble that of albino animals with recessive deafness, in which there is attempted maturity of the ear structures, with subsequent degeneration of the scala media. In some, this occurs soon after birth.

**MIM No.:** *22070, *22080

**Sex Ratio:** M1:F1

**Occurrence:** Phenotype frequency 1:5,000 to 1:330. Comprises 23% of all deafness and up to 68% of all congenital deafness (Morton, 1960).

**Risk of Recurrence for Patient's Sib:** See Table 1 in Fraser (1976).

**Risk of Recurrence for Patient's Child:**
See Part I, *Mendelian Inheritance*.

**Age of Detectability:** When deafness occurs at birth or in the first months of life, it should be identifiable by hearing tests.

**Gene Mapping and Linkage:** HOAC (hypoacusis 2 (autosomal recessive)) is ULG4.

**Prevention:** None known. Genetic counseling indicated.

**Treatment:** Speech and language dysfunction may be ameliorated by early training in language through auditory or manual learning techniques and oral speech training.

**Prognosis:** Normal for life span; probability is that hearing loss will be stable during life unless other exogenous effects act upon it. The prognosis for speech and language development is fairly good provided that intensive auditory or manual training techniques are instituted before age two years.

**Detection of Carrier:** Reportedly, it may be possible by Bekesy audiometric tests, which reveal erratic dips in the audiometric configuration.

**References:**
Morton NE: The mutational load due to detrimental genes in man. Am J Hum Genet 1960; 12:348–364.
Anderson H, Wedenberg E: Audiometric identification of normal hearing carriers of genes for deafness. Acta Otolaryngol (Stockh) 1968; 65:535.
Taylor IG, et al.: A study of the causes of hearing loss in a population of deaf children with special reference to genetic factors. J Laryngol Otol 1975; 89:899–904.
Fraser GR: The causes of profound deafness in childhood. Baltimore: Johns Hopkins University Press, 1976.
Northern JL, Downs MP: Hearing in children, 2nd ed. Baltimore: Williams & Wilkins, 1978.
Bieber FR, Nance WE: Hereditary hearing loss. In: Jackson LG, Schimke RN, eds: Clinical genetics: a sourcebook for physicians. New York: John Wiley, 1979.
Kabarity A, et al.: Autosomal recessive 'uncomplicated' profound deafness in an Arabic family with high consanguinity. Hum Genet 1981; 57:444–446.

BI004      **Frederick R. Bieber**

## DEAFNESS (SENSORINEURAL)-DYSTONIA      0266

**Includes:**
> Dystonia, atypical torsion
> Dystonia-neural deafness, familial

**Excludes:**
> **Deafness-hyperuricemia-ataxia** (0508)
> Dystonia, progressive with diurnal variation
> Dystonia, X-linked, described in Panay, Philippines
> **Hepatolenticular degeneration** (0469)
> Myoclonus-cerebellar ataxia-deafness, familial
> **Torsion dystonia** (0957)

**Major Diagnostic Criteria:** Based on the one known pedigree, there is progressive sensorineural hearing loss recognized first in early childhood, followed by dysarthria and deterioration of handwriting. Severe progressive dystonia resulting in loss of function and death in the second or third decade. Mental retardation may be a part of this syndrome.

**Clinical Findings:** The eight-year-old male proband had deafness, severe dysarthria, striking deterioration of handwriting, occasional bizarre posturing of the head and neck, and hyperactive behavior. The pregnancy, perinatal period, as well as early growth and development, were reportedly normal. Audiometric testing at 2 years confirmed a sensorineural hearing loss. At 7 years his parents noticed increasing distortion of his handwriting as well as dystonic movements of his left hand and neck. By 9 years he could not walk, was confined to a wheelchair with severe retrocollis in the upright position and was unable to articulate. Although he had a brief period of clinical improvement with L-dopa therapy, he continued to deteriorate and died at 11 years of age.

Although the parents of the proband are clinically normal, the proband's maternal uncle reportedly had hearing loss from age 6, subsequent progressive dystonic posturing, and died in his 20s. The proband's healthy 26-year-old sister had a 6-year-old son who had severe bilateral sensorineural hearing loss, lack of normal language development and severe psychomotor retardation.

**Complications:** Severe articulation defect, delay in receptive language when the auditory channel is used. Hyperactive, manipulative behavior, occasional attempts at self-mutilation. Feeding difficulties which may result in aspiration and respiratory failure. Deterioration of the intellectual function. Total functional loss and confinement to a wheelchair and ultimately bedridden.

**Associated Findings:** Emotional lability.

**Etiology:** Probably X-linked recessive inheritance in this single family.

**Pathogenesis:** Histopathologic examination of the proband's brain revealed neuronal loss and gliosis in both caudate nuclei, putamen and globus pallidus. Examination of the temporal bone revealed severe degeneration of the sensory epithelium and supporting cells in the basal turn of the cochlea, and absence of the organ of Corti.

At the present there is evidence that noradrenergic brain mechanisms may be involved in dystonia and, in contrast to a generally accepted notion, idiopathic dystonia may not be a primary disorder of the basal ganglia. It has been suggested that the increased concentration of norepinephrine in the red nucleus is the result of compensatory overactivity of the midbrain noradrenergic system in response to the primary neuronal loss in the locus ceruleus.

**MIM No.:** 30505

**Sex Ratio:** M3:F0

**Occurrence:** Rare; three members of one reported family with this combination of findings.

**Risk of Recurrence for Patient's Sib:**
See Part I, *Mendelian Inheritance.*

**Risk of Recurrence for Patient's Child:**
See Part I, *Mendelian Inheritance.*

**Age of Detectability:** Onset of hearing loss is evident by late infancy or early childhood.

**Gene Mapping and Linkage:** Unknown.

**Prevention:** None known. Genetic counseling indicated.

**Treatment:** Attempts of treatment with L-dopa, haloperidol, and GABA have brought a relative remission of symptoms for a brief period of time. Physical therapy to prevent contractures and to alleviate the pulmonary insufficiency in the final stage of the disease.

**Prognosis:** Progressive deterioration with total function loss and death before the second decade.

**Detection of Carrier:** Unknown.

**Support Groups:**
CA; Beverly Hills; Dystonia Medical Research Foundation
NY; Melville; Dystonia Foundation
CANADA: BC; Vancouver; Dystonia Medical Research Foundation

**References:**
Lee LV, et al: Torsion dystonia in Panay, Philippines. Adv Neurol 1976; 14:137–151.
Scribanu N, Kennedy C: Familial syndrome with dystonia, neural deafness, and possible intellectual impairment: clinical course and pathological findings. Adv Neurol 1976; 14:235–243. *
Hornykiewicz O, et al.: Brain neuro-transmitters in dystonia musculorum deformans. New Engl J Med 1986; 315:347–353.
Eldridge R: Letter. New Engl J Med 1987; 316:279.
Jankovic J, Svendsen CN: Letter. New Engl J Med 1987; 316:278–279.

SC052                                          **Nina Scribanu**

**Deafness (sensorineural)-imperforate anus-hypoplastic thumbs**
*See ANUS-HAND-EAR SYNDROME*
**Deafness (sensorineural)-renal tubular acidosis**
*See RENAL TUBULAR ACIDOSIS*
**Deafness (sensorineural)-retinitis pigmentosa**
*See USHER SYNDROME*

## DEAFNESS WITH PERILYMPHATIC GUSHER    3116

**Includes:**
Deafness-stapes fixation
Nance deafness
Perilymphatic gusher during stapes surgery
Stapes ankylosis and perilymphatic gusher-deafness
Stapes fixation-deafness
X-linked mixed deafness syndrome

**Excludes:**
**Deafness** (other)
Perilymphatic gusher from other causes
Perilymphatic gushers in other syndromes

**Major Diagnostic Criteria:** Perilymphatic gusher with or without stapes fixation, progressive mixed deafness with vestibular hypofunction, and dilated labyrinth with or without dilated internal auditory canal in a pattern of X-linked inheritance.

**Clinical Findings:** Perilymph is cochlear fluid that closely resembles and is probably derived from cerebrospinal fluid. The cochlea and vestibule are abnormally dilated and somewhat misshapen, either causing or resulting from an overabundance of perilymph. The increase in perilymphatic fluid results from increased flow through an abnormally patent cochlear aqueduct or increased leakage around the nerve sheaths, which enter the cochlea through an abnormally dilated internal auditory canal. The increased perilymphatic pressure pushes out on the stapes, which may wedge itself against an overhanging lip, causing fixation at high pressures. Other cases indicate congenital ankylosis of the stapes. At operation to mobilize the stapes, a small puncture or even just moving the stapes can yield a gush of fluid, which is hard to stop, hence the name *perilymphatic gusher*. Other causes of perilymphatic gusher are discussed by Glasscock (1973).

The hearing loss usually has the typical trough or "cookie-bite" configuration seen in stapes fixation from other causes, such as otosclerosis, except that the loss is not just conductive. The sensorineural component appears to be cochlear in origin and is progressive with or without surgery.

**Complications:** Surgical mobilization of the stapes usually results in a gusher, with sudden decompression of the cochlea. Most operated patients have lost further hearing after surgery though a progressive sensorineural loss is present regardless of surgery. Therefore, the benefits of surgery should be very carefully weighed.

**Associated Findings:** Olson and Lehman (1968) reported abnormal electroencephalograms and psychiatric disturbances in two maternal half-brothers.

**Etiology:** X-linked inheritance.

**Pathogenesis:** Possibly inherited size and shape of the internal auditory canal and cochlear aqueduct, which in turn leads to increased perilymphatic pressure. Whether the sensorineural hearing loss is also due to increased pressure or to some other pathogenetic mechanism is not known.

**MIM No.:** *30440

**Sex Ratio:** M1:F0

**Occurrence:** Four kindreds have been reported, two in the eastern United States, one in The Netherlands, and one in South Africa.

**Risk of Recurrence for Patient's Sib:**
See Part I, *Mendelian Inheritance.*

**Risk of Recurrence for Patient's Child:**
See Part I, *Mendelian Inheritance.*

**Age of Detectability:** At birth if family history is known. Otherwise, the diagnosis should be suspected in a male of any age who has mixed hearing loss and especially in young males with clinical evidence of stapes fixation but no definite sensorineural loss.

**Gene Mapping and Linkage:** DFN3 (deafness, conductive, with fixed stapes) has been mapped to Xq13-q21.2.

**Prevention:** None known. Genetic counseling indicated.

**Treatment:** Surgery has been aimed at ablating the cochlear aqueduct if that is the major source of fluid as reported by Brown Farrior and Endicott (1971). In Glasscock's hands, surgically decreasing the diameter of the internal auditory canal resulting in stemming the flow of fluid into the cochlea but no improvement in hearing. Because sudden decompression of the cochlea can result in further damage to the hearing, the benefits and risks of surgery should be carefully considered in any male with a preoperative diagnosis of stapes fixation.

Schooling and vocational planning should be aimed at appropriate education for progressive hearing loss, emphasizing auditory training in the early years to solidify rules of oral language grammar and usage, as well as speech training. However, in later years, written language and sign language may be the most important means of communication.

**Prognosis:** Hearing loss is progressive.

**Detection of Carrier:** Cremers and Juygen (1983) demonstrated a similar but milder hearing loss in four of nine obligate heterozygote females. No other carrier detection is known.

**References:**
Olson NR, Lehman RH: Cerebrospinal fluid otorrhea and the congenitally fixed stapes. Laryngoscope 1968; 78:352–359.
Brown Farrior J, Endicott JN: Congenital mixed deafness: cerebrospinal fluid otorrhea. Ablation of the aqueduct of the cochlea. Laryngoscope 1971; 81:684–699.
Glasscock ME: The stapes gusher. Arch Otolaryngol 1973; 98:82–91.
Thorpe P, et al.: X-linked deafness in a South African kindred. S Afr Med J 1974; 48:587–590.
Jensen J, et al.: Inner ear malformations with otoliquorrhea: tomographic findings in three cases with a mixed hearing impairment. Arch Otorhinolaryngol 1977; 214:271–282.
Cremers CWRJ, Huygen PLM: Clinical features of female heterozygotes in the X-linked mixed deafness syndrome (with perilymphatic gusher during stapes surgery). Int J Pediatr Otorhinolaryngol 1983; 6:179–185.
Cremers CWRJ, et al.: X-linked progressive mixed deafness with perilymphatic gusher during stapes surgery. Arch Otolaryngol 1985; 111:249–254.

DA026      **Sandra L.H. Davenport**

**Deafness with preauricular pits or sinuses**
*See DEAFNESS-EAR PITS*
**Deafness, congenital I**
*See DEAFNESS (SENSORINEURAL), RECESSIVE PROFOUND*
**Deafness, congenital II**
*See DEAFNESS (SENSORINEURAL), RECESSIVE PROFOUND*

## DEAFNESS, DOMINANT LOW-FREQUENCY    0256

**Includes:**
Hearing loss, familial, progressive, low-frequency
Konigsmark syndrome

**Excludes:**
Deafness (sensorineural), progressive high-tone (0269)
Deafness (sensorineural), midfrequency (0267)

**Major Diagnostic Criteria:** A progressive neural hearing loss detected by audiometric testing involving low frequencies in the latter half of the first or the second decade of life in a family with evidence for autosomal dominant inheritance of low-frequency hearing loss.

**Clinical Findings:** Hearing loss usually noted by second to fourth decades; detected as a slowly progressive hearing loss. Audiometric testing identifies affected persons. The hearing loss may be congenital, since the youngest patient tested was 7 years old and had a 25-db low-frequency hearing loss.

Younger affected persons show hearing loss involving frequencies up to about 2,000 Hz. With increasing age the higher frequencies also deteriorate, until finally in old age there is a severe hearing loss involving all frequencies. However, there is moderate individual variation: some affected persons in their

middle decades show a severe hearing loss, and some older affected persons have only a moderate loss.

The tone decay test generally is negative, suggesting that there is no eighth nerve involvement. However, the small increment sensitivity index generally is positive in affected persons, suggesting a cochlear locale for the hearing loss.

Physical, neurologic, and laboratory examinations are normal, as is vestibular testing.

**Complications:** Unknown.

**Associated Findings:** None known.

**Etiology:** Autosomal dominant inheritance.

**Pathogenesis:** Unknown.

**MIM No.:** *12490

**Sex Ratio:** M1:F1

**Occurrence:** Several kindreds have been reported. This hearing loss may be fairly common but is found only when looked for.

**Risk of Recurrence for Patient's Sib:**
See Part I, *Mendelian Inheritance.*

**Risk of Recurrence for Patient's Child:**
See Part I, *Mendelian Inheritance.*

**Age of Detectability:** After age 5 years, when audiometric testing can be done.

**Gene Mapping and Linkage:** Unknown.

**Prevention:** None known. Genetic counseling indicated.

**Treatment:** A hearing aid is indicated when the hearing loss becomes a problem.

**Prognosis:** Normal for life span and intelligence.

**Detection of Carrier:** Unknown.

**References:**
Iinuma T, et al.: Sensorineural hearing loss for low tones. Arch Otolaryngol 1967; 86:110–116.
Vanderbilt University Hereditary Deafness Study Group: Dominantly inherited low-frequency hearing loss. Arch Otolaryngol 1968; 88:242–250.
Konigsmark BW, et al.: Dominant low-frequency hearing loss. Laryngoscope 1971; 81:759–771.
Leon, PE, et al.: Low frequency hereditary deafness in man with childhood onset. Am J Med Genet 1981; 33:209–214.
Parving A: Inherited low-frequency hearing loss. Scand Audiol 1984; 13:47–56.

BI004      **Frederick R. Bieber**

**Deafness, fetal aminoglycoside ototoxicity**
*See FETAL AMINOGLYCOSIDE OTOTOXICITY*
**Deafness, from extrinsically caused iodine disorder**
*See CRETINISM, ENDEMIC, AND RELATED DISORDERS*
**Deafness, knuckle pads and leukonychia**
*See KNUCKLE PADS-LEUKONYCHIA-DEAFNESS*
**Deafness, mid-tone neural**
*See DEAFNESS (SENSORINEURAL), MIDFREQUENCY*

## DEAFNESS, PFAENDLER TYPE    0243

**Includes:**
Deafness, semilethal (misnomer)
Deafness-mental retardation-possible sterility

**Excludes:**
Deafness-hypogonadism (2322)
Deafness (other)

**Major Diagnostic Criteria:** Congenital severe sensorineural deafness with a preponderance of males. Mental deficiency was present in 40%. Possible sterility was present.

**Clinical Findings:** A systematic study of all individuals with recessive deafness in Werdenberg, Switzerland, was undertaken using records at the Institute for the Deaf and church and state archives. Five large pedigrees of 8 to 12 generations were established, but with statistical analysis concentration was on the period 1876 to 1950. A total of 172 individuals with hearing impairment were identified, of which 89% were profoundly deaf and 11% had a moderately severe sensorineural loss with a small conductive component with or without differences between the two ears. A sample of 37 individuals were personally examined. Some cases of conductive hearing loss in nonaffected family members were ascribed to otitis media, raising the question of otitis media contributing to the conductive loss since most were children during the preantibiotic era.

Consanguinity was established in 9 of 89 (10.1%) of sibships. In 30% one parent was definitely or probably not a member of the kindred. Of the 844 sibs of affected persons, 17% of the brothers compared with 9% of the sisters died before the age of 7 years. This was significantly different from the relative mortalities for Switzerland as a whole during the same period. Since only 9.5% of sibs were affected and since the mortality among males was higher than expected, a semilethal gene was postulated rather than two different genes.

**Complications:** Slight mental deficiency was present in 40% of affected and in some unaffected persons. "Hypogenitalism was almost always present"; however, no further mention of this complication was made by Pfaendler and Schnyder (1960). In subsequent writing, (Pfaendler, 1963) stated that no visible signs of hypogonadism were present, but the patients seldom married or had children. While the authors emphasized variable expression of the gene, citing the two types (degrees) of hearing loss and variable mental ability, they did not investigate the presumed sterility.

**Associated Findings:** Strabismus was present in 5/37 examined cases, and one case each ptosis and heterochromia were found.

**Etiology:** Possibly autosomal recessive inheritance.

**Pathogenesis:** Unknown.

**MIM No.:** 22100

**Sex Ratio:** M1.34:F1

**Occurrence:** 1–10:1,000 in examined populations, but apparently confined to eastern Switzerland.

**Risk of Recurrence for Patient's Sib:**
See Part I, *Mendelian Inheritance.*

**Risk of Recurrence for Patient's Child:**
See Part I, *Mendelian Inheritance.*

**Age of Detectability:** Infancy.

**Gene Mapping and Linkage:** Unknown.

**Prevention:** None known. Genetic counseling indicated.

**Treatment:** Auditory training, hearing aids if useful, and deaf education must begin early. While there was a definite difference observed among affected persons regarding mental ability, one must presume equal access to appropriate education since they were all from extended families in a confined area. However, lack of auditory training and deaf education could influence the impression of mental retardation without specific testing.

**Prognosis:** Life span is normal, and deafness is apparently nonprogressive.

**Detection of Carrier:** Unknown.

**Special Considerations:** The cause of the presumed sterility is not known. Some affected people apparently did have children, but it is not known if the offspring were affected. Lack of appropriate genetic counseling may have influenced the choice not to marry.

Pfaendler's original work postulated that a less-than-expected proportion of affected siblings was attributable to a semilethal effect of the gene. Recent researchers have suggested that the finding could be more easily explained by inadvertent inclusion of sporadic nongenetic or non-recessive cases (Fraser, 1976, pp 64).

**References:**
Pfaendler U: Une forme semiletale de la surdimutite recessive dans differentes populations de la Suisse orientale. Bull Acad Suisse Sci Med 1960; 16:255–217.
Pfaendler U, Schnyder E: La surdi-mutite recessive dans le Werdenberg (canton de Saint-Gall, Suisse). J Génét Hum 1960; 9:158–214. *
Pfaendler U: Le deficit de sourds-muets dans les fratries atteintes. Arch Klaus-Stift Vererb-Forsch 1963; 38:96.
Fraser GR: The causes of profound deafness in childhood. Baltimore: Johns Hopkins University Press, 1976.

DA026                                    **Sandra L.H. Davenport**

**Deafness, semilethal (misnomer)**
*See DEAFNESS, PFAENDLER TYPE*
**Deafness, sensorineural, congenital, unilateral**
*See DEAFNESS, UNILATERAL INNER EAR*
**Deafness, sensorineural-corneal dystrophy**
*See CORNEAL DYSTROPHY-SENSORINEURAL DEAFNESS*
**Deafness, sensorineural-hand muscle wasting**
*See MUSCLE WASTING OF HANDS-SENSORINEURAL DEAFNESS*
**Deafness, sensorineural-renal tubular acidosis**
*See RENAL TUBULAR ACIDOSIS-SENSORINEURAL DEAFNESS*
**Deafness, severe isolated congenital**
*See DEAFNESS (SENSORINEURAL), RECESSIVE PROFOUND*

**DEAFNESS, STREPTOMYCIN-SENSITIVITY**          **0272**

**Includes:**
Dihydrostreptomycin-sensitive deafness
Streptomycin-sensitivity deafness

**Excludes:** Fetal aminoglycoside ototoxicity (2992)

**Major Diagnostic Criteria:** Sensorineural hearing loss after streptomycin injections in an individual with normal renal function.

**Clinical Findings:** Early onset of tinnitus and moderately severe-to-profound hearing loss, usually following small doses of streptomycin sulfate (4–30 gm). Audiometry shows sensorineural hearing loss of 50–100 db. Caloric testing shows either normal responses or directional preponderance. Sibs and parents who did not receive streptomycin have normal audiograms.

**Complications:** Vestibular dysfunction.

**Associated Findings:** None known.

**Etiology:** Hearing loss was once presumed to be due to an abnormal sensitivity to streptomycin or dihydrostreptomycin, familial in nature, with the exact mode of transmission uncertain. The extrinsic causative factor was presumed to be the chemical streptomycin sulfate. The reported ototoxic dosage range was given as 12–325 gm. However, this wide range may include at the lower end of the spectrum persons who previously had other ototoxic drugs causing subclinical hair cell loss in the inner ear, or initial loss of hair cells subserving high frequencies beyond the reach of conventional audiometry (i.e. beyond 8000 cps), followed by further hair cell loss due to streptomycin, sufficient to cause clinically detectable hearing loss. On the other hand, some of the patients showing hearing loss in the lower dosage ranges may actually be those who demonstrate streptomycin sensitivity.

Research failed to support a familial or genetic differential sensitivity to these drugs, and attention focused more upon the general toxic nature of the aminoglycoside class of drugs **Fetal aminoglycoside ototoxicity**). Recently Higashi (1989), however, has suggested that a high susceptibility of cochlea to streptomycin is transmitted primarily through females by extranuclear inheritance.

**Pathogenesis:** Unknown. See **Fetal aminoglycoside ototoxicity**.

**MIM No.:** 18515

**Sex Ratio:** Presumably M1:F1.

**Occurrence:** A half-dozen or so reports have been published over the past 25 years.

**Risk of Recurrence for Patient's Sib:** Unknown.

**Risk of Recurrence for Patient's Child:** Unknown.

**Age of Detectability:** Presumably dependent upon exposure.

**Gene Mapping and Linkage:** Unknown.

**Prevention:** Avoidance of streptomycin whenever other drugs are effective and in patients with a possible family history of streptomycin sensitivity.

**Treatment:** Hearing conservation, i.e. avoidance of further exposure to ototoxic drugs, avoidance of acoustic trauma and noise exposure and prompt treatment of ear infections. A hearing aid, lip-reading and speech training may be helpful.

**Prognosis:** Hearing loss is permanent. There is no effect on life expectancy.

**Detection of Carrier:** Unknown.

**References:**
Prabziác M, et al.: Familial sensitivity to streptomycin. J Laryngol Otol 1964; 78:1037–1043.
Viljoen DL, et al.: Familial aggregation of streptomycin ototoxicity: autosomal dominant inheritance? J Med Genet 1983; 20:357–360.
Higashi K: Unique inheritance of streptomycin-induced deafness. Clin Genet 1989; 35:433–436. *

BE028                                    **LaVonne Bergstrom**

## DEAFNESS, TUNE                                    0273

**Includes:**
Dysmelodia
Tune deafness

**Excludes:** N/A

**Major Diagnostic Criteria:** Inability to recognize or reproduce (by singing or playing an instrument that is dependent on accurate pitch production) a tune or any series of pitches presented in sequence. These individuals have normal speaking voices, normal hearing, and are usually free of neurologic deficits.

**Clinical Findings:** The affected individual is able to sing only in a monotone and apparently cannot be taught to sing in tune, although usually able to reproduce the rhythm of the song. Apparently these individuals can be taught to play the piano or other instruments, for which ability to distinguish correct pitch is not essential to producing an accurate rendition of the music. Audiometric tests are normal, and such individuals often can distinguish differences in pure tone frequencies in isolation, but may be unable to make such discriminations when pitches are presented in groups, as in chords, or in sequence. In fact, cases have been recorded of individuals who had superior pitch discrimination but apparently could not learn the simplest tune. The speaking voice of tune-deaf individuals shows all the pitch and modulation characteristics of normal persons. No laryngeal motor abnormalities have been suspected or detected. Appreciation and enjoyment of music may be present, and such individuals may be quite sensitive to the beauties of other forms of art. Often, however, tune-deaf persons do not enjoy music.

**Complications:** Unknown.

**Associated Findings:** None known.

**Etiology:** Probably autosomal dominant inheritance. One or more dominant or recessive genes has been proposed. However, the influence of environment has not been disproved. The possibility of fetal or neonatal insult producing a specific learning disability has not been considered but cannot be ruled out.

**Pathogenesis:** Undetermined. It has been suggested that tune deafness is analogous to dyslexia or that there is some deficit in the feedback mechanism that prevents the individual from imitating a tone or series of tones. There is no information to suggest that neurologic or other learning deficits are more common in the tune deaf than in the general population.

**MIM No.:** *19120

**Sex Ratio:** Undetermined. Possibly M1:F1, although one study of school children showed 7% of boys and only 1% of girls to be "monotones." However, this could be culturally determined.

**Occurrence:** 1:20 of the adult population.

**Risk of Recurrence for Patient's Sib:**
See Part I, *Mendelian Inheritance.*

**Risk of Recurrence for Patient's Child:**
See Part I, *Mendelian Inheritance.*

**Age of Detectability:** In early childhood or by school years.

**Gene Mapping and Linkage:** Unknown.

**Prevention:** None known. Genetic counseling indicated.

**Treatment:** There is some evidence that intensive coaching of children aged 3–5 years can significantly improve pitch discrimination.

**Prognosis:** Some tune deaf individuals may outgrow or overcome their deficiency by about age 12 years. The reason for this is unknown.

**Detection of Carrier:** Unknown.

**References:**
Kalmus H: Inherited sense defects. Sci Am (May) 1952; 186:64–69.
Shuter R: Hereditary and environmental factors in musical ability. Eugen Rev 1966; 48:149.
Cuddy LL: Practice effects in the absolute judgment of pitch. J Acoust Soc Am 1968; 43:1069–1076. *
Kalmus H, Fry DB: On tune deafness (dysmelodia): frequency, development, genetics and musical background. Ann Hum Genet 1980; 43:369–382. *

BE028                                    **LaVonne Bergstrom**

## DEAFNESS, UNILATERAL INNER EAR                      0274

**Includes:** Deafness, sensorineural, congenital, unilateral

**Excludes:**
Acquired sensorineural hearing loss
**Deafness** (other)
Syndromes that include unilateral sensorineural hearing loss

**Major Diagnostic Criteria:** Unilateral, moderate-to-severe, congenital sensorineural hearing loss in a family with unilateral or bilateral hearing loss and no other abnormalities.

**Clinical Findings:** Smith (1939) reported a family of four generations in which nine individuals were "stone deaf" in one ear and two were "deaf-mutes" with bilateral losses. Those two were a woman, who went deaf after a measles infection, and her grandson, who had no known cause of deafness and whose father had "perfect hearing." The same woman had a daughter and granddaughter with unilateral deafness. Though no audiometric results were reported, a total loss would have to be sensorineural rather than conductive. Vestibular responses were normal by caloric testing.

Everberg (1960) documented several families with hearing impairment in which at least one person had a unilateral loss. One of the families (family XIII) had 12 bilateral losses, one unilateral only, and one with no hearing on one side but a high frequency loss on the other. Family XIII may not be the same as that reported by Smith.

**Complications:** Unknown.

**Associated Findings:** None known.

**Etiology:** Possibly autosomal dominant inheritance with variable expression.

**Pathogenesis:** Unknown.

**MIM No.:** 12500

**Sex Ratio:** M1:F1

**Occurrence:** Seventeen cases in two kinships documented.

**Risk of Recurrence for Patient's Sib:**
See Part I, *Mendelian Inheritance.*

**Risk of Recurrence for Patient's Child:**
See Part I, *Mendelian Inheritance.*

**Age of Detectability:** Bilateral hearing loss should be detectable in infancy. Unilateral loss may escape detection for many years, since the normal ear allows for normal speech and language development. It should be looked for in first degree relatives of individuals with known unilateral or bilateral hearing losses.

**Gene Mapping and Linkage:** Unknown.

**Prevention:** None known. Genetic counseling indicated.

**Treatment:** For unilateral loss, preferential seating in classrooms so that the normal ear is closest to the speaker(s). For bilateral hearing loss, hearing aide plus auditory training and deaf education.

**Prognosis:** Normal for life span and intelligence.

**Detection of Carrier:** Unknown.

**References:**
Smith AB: Unilateral hereditary deafness. Lancet 1939; II:1172–1173.
Everberg G: Further studies on hereditary unilateral deafness. Acta Otolaryngol (Stockh) 1960; 51:615.

DA026                                     **Sandra L.H. Davenport**

**Deafness-albinism-block locks**
*See ALBINISM-BLACK LOCKS-DEAFNESS*
**Deafness-alopecia-hypogonadism**
*See CRANDALL SYNDROME*

## DEAFNESS-ATOPIC DERMATITIS                    0245

**Includes:**
   Atopic dermatitis and (sensorineural) hearing loss
   Deafness (neural)-atypical atopic dermatitis
   Dermatitis (atopic)-deafness
   Hearing loss (sensorineural)-hereditary atopic dermatitis

**Excludes: Deafness** (other)

**Major Diagnostic Criteria:** Congenital, moderate, nonprogressive, sensorineural hearing loss with atopic dermatitis.

**Clinical Findings:** Two distinct types (A and B) may exist based on severity and shape of the audiogram, onset and distribution of atopic dermatitis, and pattern of inheritance. Konigsmark et al. (1968) described a sibship with congenital, nonprogressive, mild-to-moderate, slightly sloping sensorineural hearing loss and atypical atopic dermatitis, which began in late childhood and involved the forearms, elbows, antecubital fosse, and waist.
   One kindred each was described by Frentz et al. (1976) and Larsen et al. (1978) with congenital, moderate sensorineural hearing loss having a "basin-shaped" audiogram and typical atopic dermatitis beginning in infancy. The audiograms from the two families were almost superimposable and involved a 10–15 db conductive component at all frequencies. The atopic dermatitis involved hands, wrists, forearms, ankles, and legs. IgE levels were high.

**Complications:** Unknown.

**Associated Findings:** None known.

**Etiology:** Type A appears to be autosomal recessive inherited; and type B, by autosomal dominant inheritance.

**Pathogenesis:** Unknown.

**MIM No.:** 22170

**Sex Ratio:** M1:F1

**Occurrence:** Rare. Type A: 3 of 4 sibs affected. Type B: In the Frentz et al. (1976) kindred, two brothers had hearing loss and atopic dermatitis, four other members of the maternal family had atopic dermatitis, and both boys plus six paternal family members had keratoderma palmoplantaris. In the Larsen et al. (1978) kindred, three had combined hearing loss and atopic dermatitis (a father and two sons), one had hearing loss alone, and seven had atopic dermatitis alone.

**Risk of Recurrence for Patient's Sib:**
   See Part I, *Mendelian Inheritance.*

**Risk of Recurrence for Patient's Child:**
   See Part I, *Mendelian Inheritance.* Type A, each child would be a

carrier but not affected by the gene; type B, 1:2 (50%) will be affected with hearing loss, atopic dermatitis, or both.

**Age of Detectability:** Type A atopic dermatitis appears at about age 10 years; and type B appears in infancy. Hearing loss in either should be detectable in infancy but may not be suspected until speech delay is present.

**Gene Mapping and Linkage:** Unknown.

**Prevention:** None known. Genetic counseling indicated.

**Treatment:** Local therapy for the atopic dermatitis; hearing aide plus auditory training for the hearing loss.

**Prognosis:** Normal for life span and intelligence.

**Detection of Carrier:** Unknown.

**References:**
Konigsmark BW, et al.: Familial neural hearing loss and atopic dermatitis. JAMA 1968; 204:953–957.
Frentz G, et al.: Congenital perceptive hearing loss and atopic dermatitis. Acta Otolaryngol (Stockh) 1976; 82:242–245.
Larsen FS, et al.: Atopic dermatitis and congenital deafness. Br J Dermatol 1978; 99:325–328.

DA026                                     **Sandra L.H. Davenport**

**Deafness-cataract-muscular atrophy-skeletal defects**
*See OTO-OCULO-MUSCULO-SKELETAL SYNDROME*
**Deafness-Charcot-Marie-Tooth disease**
*See CHARCOT MARIE TOOTH DISEASE-DEAFNESS*
**Deafness-cutaneous albinism**
*See ALBINISM, CUTANEOUS-DEAFNESS*

## DEAFNESS-DIABETES                          0246

**Includes:** Diabetes mellitus-deafness

**Excludes:**
   **Diabetes (insipidus/mellitus)-optic atrophy-deafness** (0550)
   Deafness as a result of infection in the ear of a diabetic

**Major Diagnostic Criteria:** A progressive, often subclinical hearing loss involving predominantly the high frequencies in a diabetic subject.

**Clinical Findings:** Studies during the past 20 years have given conflicting evidence as to the existence of a connection between diabetes mellitus and hearing impairment. This association is certainly one to be expected, based on current knowledge of neurological and vascular complications of diabetes. Many investigators have found some evidence for a slowly progressive, bilateral, sensorineural hearing impairment that affects predominantly the higher frequencies. The decrease in auditory function is similar to that found in presbycusis, except that the hearing loss in diabetes is premature. More recent studies of deafness and diabetes have tended to discredit this association. For the most part, these have been carefully controlled studies of both insulin- and non-insulin-dependent diabetics of wide age ranges. Hearing assessments were performed using pure tone averages, speech audiometry, impedence audiometry, threshold tone decay, and brainstem evoked response audiometry. In general, no differences in hearing thresholds were found between diabetic subjects and normal controls, and there were no significant abnormalities of hearing related to the presence of neurological or vascular complications of diabetes or duration and control of the disease. However, some investigators point to the possibility of widespread subclinical tone decay abnormalities at frequencies above 2,000 Hz, although firm evidence for this has not been established.

**Complications:** Same as those of diabetes generally.

**Associated Findings:** None known.

**Etiology:** Most investigators conclude that the onset of hearing impairment is secondary to the pathologic effects of diabetes itself rather than being a genetically determined defect that is linked or associated with a diabetogenic gene.

**Pathogenesis:** Both sensory neuropathy and vascular degeneration alone or in combination have been proposed as the cause of hearing impairment in diabetes. More recent histopathologic investigations conclude that the hearing deficits in diabetes are primarily microvascular, which may be an important factor in causing neuronal degeneration. Specific pathologic changes found include periodic acid-Schiff-positive thickenings of the capillary walls of the striae vascularis and the modiolus, thickened walls and a narrow lumen in the internal auditory artery, atrophy of the spinal ganglion in the basal and middle turns of the cochlea, and demyelination and beading of the eighth nerve sheath.

**Sex Ratio:** M1:F1

**Occurrence:** Figures vary between 0 and 95% of the diabetic population; 0–1:25,000 in Western countries.

**Risk of Recurrence for Patient's Sib:** Unknown.

**Risk of Recurrence for Patient's Child:** Unknown.

**Age of Detectability:** About 30 years of age or later.

**Gene Mapping and Linkage:** Type I (insulin-dependent) diabetes has strong associations with specific HLA haplotypes. No differences in hearing impairment have been noted between types I and II (non-insulin-dependent) diabetes.

**Prevention:** None known. Genetic counseling indicated.

**Treatment:** Hearing aid and control of diabetes mellitus.

**Prognosis:** Hearing loss will increase with age but does not lead to complete deafness and, in fact, may often be subclinical.

**Detection of Carrier:** Detection of the diabetic condition plus possible hearing loss.

**Special Considerations:** A detailed assessment of hearing impairment in diabetes is necessary, since previous studies have used widely varying testing procedures and statistical analyses. In recent years diabetes has been shown to be a heterogenous group of disorders distinguished by insulin dependence, severity of complications, the presence of genetic markers, and immunologic characteristics such as autoimmunity. These factors need to be accounted for in any study of the effects of diabetes. Because of the similarities between hearing loss in diabetes and that of presbycusis and progressive hereditary nerve deafness, a genetic etiology of deafness in diabetes must also be investigated.

**References:**
Makishima K, Tanaka K: Pathological changes of the inner ear and central auditory pathway in diabetics. Ann Otol Rhinol Laryngol 1971; 80:218–228. †
Axelsson A, et al.: Hearing in diabetics. Acta Otolaryngol (Stockh) 1978; [Suppl] 356:1–10. *
Taylor IG, Irwin J: Some audiological aspects of diabetes mellitus. J Otolaryngol 1978; 92:99–113.
Gibbin KP, Davis CG: A hearing survey in diabetes mellitus. Clin Otolaryngol 1981; 6:345–350.
Sieger A, et al.: Auditory function in children with diabetes mellitus. Ann Otol Rhinol Laryngol 1983; 92:237–241.
Khardori R, et al.: Brainstem auditory and visual evoked potentials in Type 1 (insulin-dependent) diabetic patients. Diabetol 1986; 29:362–365.

SH046                                          **Kathleen Shaver**

**Deafness-diabetes-optic atrophy**
*See DIABETES (INSIPIDUS/MELLITUS)-OPTIC ATROPHY-DEAFNESS*

## DEAFNESS-DIABETES-PHOTOMYOCLONUS-NEPHROPATHY 0255

**Includes:**
>    Diabetes-deafness-photomyoclonus-nephropathy
>    Nephropathy-diabetes-deafness-photomyoclonus
>    Photomyoclonus-deafness-diabetes-nephropathy

**Excludes:**
>    Amaurosis
>    Jakob-Creutzfeld syndrome
>    **Nephritis-deafness (sensorineural), hereditary type** (0708)

**Major Diagnostic Criteria:** Photomyoclonus, deafness, cerebral dysfunction, diabetes mellitus, and nephropathy.

**Clinical Findings:** Thirteen affected patients in five generations of one family have been described. Four suffered from the complete syndrome; the others had only a part of the syndrome. Photomyoclonic seizures began about age 20 years, followed by progressive sensorineural deafness at about age 30–35 years, and progressive dementia, cerebellar symptoms, hemiparesis, and aphasic and agnosic deficits in the fourth decade. At this time, diabetes mellitus and low-grade glomerulo- and pyelonephritis were also diagnosed. Terminally bizarre myoclonus and bulbar signs were seen. No audiometric findings were described.

**Complications:** Extreme emaciation, progressive unresponsiveness.

**Associated Findings:** One patient died from bronchopneumonia.

**Etiology:** Presumably autosomal dominant inheritance.

**Pathogenesis:** In the brain, particularly in the cerebral and cerebellar cortices, generalized neural loss was revealed. Furthermore, the accumulation of abnormal lipids in the brain, most striking in dentate and inferior olivary nuclei, and in the kidney suggests marked lipidosis.

**MIM No.:** 17250

**Sex Ratio:** M4:F9 (All four patients with complete syndrome were female).

**Occurrence:** Single reported kindred with multiple affected individuals in several generations.

**Risk of Recurrence for Patient's Sib:**
See Part I, *Mendelian Inheritance.*

**Risk of Recurrence for Patient's Child:**
See Part I, *Mendelian Inheritance.*

**Age of Detectability:** About the third to fourth decades of life.

**Gene Mapping and Linkage:** Unknown.

**Prevention:** None known. Genetic counseling indicated.

**Treatment:** Supportive therapy, anticonvulsant medication, tube feeding.

**Prognosis:** Poor.

**Detection of Carrier:** Unknown.

**References:**
Herrmann C Jr, et al.: Hereditary photomyoclonus associated with diabetes mellitus, deafness, nephropathy and cerebral dysfunction. Neurology 1964; 14:212–221.

SH046                                          **Kathleen Shaver**
                                               *Cor W.R.J. Cremers*

**Deafness-digito-naso syndrome, Keipert type**
*See NASO-DIGITO-ACOUSTIC SYNDROME, KEIPERT TYPE*

## DEAFNESS-DIVERTICULITIS-NEUROPATHY 0265

**Includes:**
> Diverticulitis-deafness-neuropathy
> Groll-Hirschowitz syndrome
> Neuropathy-deafness-diverticulitis

**Excludes:**
> Deafness (progressive sensorineural)-sensory radicular
> neuropathy
> Diverticulitis of small intestine-steatorrhea-macrocytic
> anemia

**Major Diagnostic Criteria:** Sensorineural deafness in childhood, absent gastric motility, small bowel diverticulitis, and progressive sensory neuropathy.

**Clinical Findings:** A kindred has been reported in which three of six sibs showed the symptoms of this syndrome. The ages of onset of the progressive bilateral sensorineural deafness were 8, 3, and 9 years, respectively. At ages 10, 5, and 18 years, respectively, the deafness became total. Histologic examination of the temporal bones in the first case showed a type of cochleosaccular degeneration like that seen in the Scheibe-type malformation. A history of hearing loss was present on the paternal side in three generations, but was mild and had a much later onset (40 years or more). Vestibular function was normal in all three sibs. Abdominal cramps, vomiting, steatorrhea, and hypoalbuminemic edema were present. There was progressive loss of gastric antral motility and multiple diverticula of the ileum and lower jejunum. Inflammation in the diverticula resulted in extensive small bowel ulceration at the mesenteric border diagnosed at autopsy in the first patient (age 18 years), at laparotomy in the second, and is probably present in the third girl. Progressive peripheral neurophathy was seen in all three sibs.

Tendon reflexes at knees and ankles were hypoactive or absent. Two sibs had decreased or absent corneal reflexes. Two sibs suffered damage to the fingertips or feet with loss of sensation. Bilateral pes cavus was noted in the father and in two of the affected sibs. Autonomic dysfunction was manifest by lack of gastric motility and tachycardia. Demyeclination of fibers of the tenth cranial nerve were noted in the autopsy of sib 1. Spinal fluid protein was elevated in sibs 2 and 3 (85 mg/dl and 61 mg/dl, respectively). Sensory and motor nerve conduction velocities were diminished in sibs 2 and 3 and in the father. Sural nerve biopsy in sib 2 showed demyelination. Two sibs developed acanthosis nigricans, which responded to topical retinoic acid. A pair of sisters with a similar clinical history was recently described by Potasman et al (1985).

**Complications:** Steatorrhea and low serum proteins with hypoalbuminemic edema. Possible damage to joints or extremities due to unperceived injury.

**Associated Findings:** None known.

**Etiology:** Postulated to be autosomal recessive inheritance, with parental consanguinity noted in one family. The findings of pes cavus delayed nerve conduction velocity and mild deafness in the father suggest the possibility of autosomal dominant transmission of these features. It is possible that the gastrointestinal disorder in this sibship is due to a separate genetic entity. The neurologic signs in one sib clearly preceded the malabsorption, precluding a major role of malnutrition in the etiology of the neuropathy.

**Pathogenesis:** Unknown.

**MIM No.:** 22140

**Sex Ratio:** M0:F5 (observed)

**Occurrence:** Two reported families with three affected sibs in one and two in the other.

**Risk of Recurrence for Patient's Sib:**
> See Part I, *Mendelian Inheritance.*

**Risk of Recurrence for Patient's Child:**
> See Part I, *Mendelian Inheritance.*

**Age of Detectability:** Childhood or adolescence.

**Gene Mapping and Linkage:** Unknown.

**Prevention:** None known. Genetic counseling indicated.

**Treatment:** Oral antibiotic therapy, medium-chain triglyceride diet with methacholine chloride. Improvement of the acanthosis nigricans with topically applied vitamin A acid.

**Prognosis:** Poor because of the progressive nature of this disorder. Four of five reported affected individuals have died of complications of the disease.

**Detection of Carrier:** Unknown.

**References:**
Groll A, Hirschowitz BI: Steatorrhea and familial deafness in two siblings. Clin Res 1966; 14:47.

Groll A, Hirschowitz BI: Steatorrhea and absent gastric antral motility in three female siblings with familial deafness. Ann Intern Med 1968; 68:1147.

Hirschowitz BI, et al.: Hereditary nerve deafness in three sisters with absent gastric motility, small bowel diverticulitis and ulceration, and progressive sensory neuropathy. In: Bergsma D, ed: G.I. tract including liver and pancreas. BD:OAS; VIII(2):. Baltimore: Williams & Wilkins, 1972:27–41.

Montes LF, et al.: Acanthosis nigricans and hypovitaminosis A. Response of topical vitamin A acid. J Cutan Pathol 1974; 1:88.

Potasman I, et al.: The Groll-Hirschowitz syndrome. Clin Genet 1985; 28:76–79.

K0015
**Bruce Korf**
*Cor W.R.J. Cremers*

## DEAFNESS-EAR DEFECTS-FACIAL PALSY 2762

**Includes:**
> Ear defects-deafness-facial palsy
> Facial palsy-ear defects-deafness

**Excludes:**
> Ear, microtia-atresia (0664)
> External ear malformation-deafness syndromes (other)
> Hypertelorism-microtia-facial cleft-conductive deafness (0506)

**Major Diagnostic Criteria:** Conductive deafness due to stapedial abnormalities, microtia, and facial palsy.

**Clinical Findings:** Bilateral conductive deafness with stapedial abnormalities, facial paralysis and variable malformations of the external ears. Profound deafness is present at birth, and the anatomic nature of the middle ear defect is revealed at operation. The external ear malformations comprise variable but significant microtia. Facial palsy, which is congenital, is variable and may be unilateral or bilateral. General health is good, and there are no additional concomitants.

**Complications:** Unknown.

**Associated Findings:** None known.

**Etiology:** Presumably autosomal dominant inheritance.

**Pathogenesis:** Unknown.

**POS No.:** 4430

**Sex Ratio:** Presumably M1:F1.

**Occurrence:** A mother and her three offspring (two daughters and a son) have been reported. The family, who reside in Cape Town, South Africa, are of Indian heritage.

**Risk of Recurrence for Patient's Sib:**
> See Part I, *Mendelian Inheritance.*

**Risk of Recurrence for Patient's Child:**
> See Part I, *Mendelian Inheritance.*

**Age of Detectability:** At birth by recognition of external ear abnormalities.

**Gene Mapping and Linkage:** Unknown.

**Prevention:** None known. Genetic counseling indicated.

**Treatment:** Otologic operation on the middle ear structures is of questionable value in the improvement of hearing. Special educational facilities are necessary because of the profound degree of deafness.

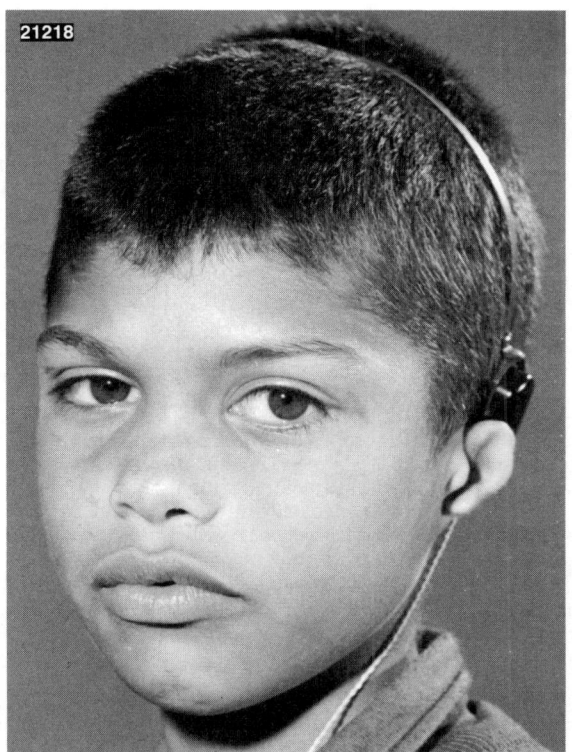

**2762-21218:** Note this boy with conductive deafness, malformation of the external ear, and bilateral facial palsy.

**Prognosis:** Unknown.

**Detection of Carrier:** Unknown.

**References:**
Sellars S, Beighton P: Autosomal dominant inheritance of conductive deafness due to stapedial anomalies, external ear malformations and congenital facial palsy. Clin Genet 1983; 23:376–379.

BE008                                                    **Peter Beighton**

## DEAFNESS-EAR PITS                                                   0247

**Includes:**
> Deafness with preauricular pits or sinuses
> Ear malformations-lateral/branchial cervical fistulas-deafness
> Ear pits and external ear malformations with deafness
> Preauricular appendages and deafness

**Excludes:**
> **Branchio-oto-renal dysplasia** (2224)
> **Ear, pits** (0329)
> **Mandibulofacial dysostosis** (0627)
> **Oculo-auriculo-vertebral anomaly** (0735)

**Major Diagnostic Criteria:** Preauricular pits with a conductive, sensorineural, or mixed hearing loss that has been present since birth.

**Clinical Findings:** The patient may have a normal pinna, a lop-ear deformity, or the ear may be low-set. A small pit or sinus is present just in front of the anterior extremity of the helix just superior to the takeoff of the crus helicis. This pit frequently becomes infected, but even in the absence of infection a small amount of fluid may discharge from or can be expressed from the pit. Occasionally, the pit communicates with the middle ear, and this can be demonstrated by injecting radiopaque dye and showing the dye in the middle ear by mastoid films or petrous pyramid polytomography. Often the sinus communicates with the external auditory canal. Ear pits may be multiple. They are usually bilateral. Facial palsy occurs rarely. Some patients have typical branchial cleft cysts and sinuses or fistulas in the neck. Preauricular appendages, which may be fleshy or also contain cartilage, are quite common.

Two types of congenital hearing loss may be seen in this entity and may indeed represent two separate clinical syndromes. In some pedigrees, sensorineural hearing loss is noted, in others conductive or mixed hearing loss is seen. In other pedigrees, however, all types of hearing loss occur. In the cases in which sensorineural hearing loss occurs, other etiologies, such as acoustic trauma and ototoxic drugs, were ruled out. The sensorineural hearing loss may be profound. Exploratory tympanotomy has been done in a few patients with conductive hearing loss and malformed ossicles; specifically, absence of the lenticular process of the incus was found. In these instances the air-bone gap on the audiogram will be about 40–60 db, and impedance testing will confirm ossicular discontinuity or fixation, since ossicular fixation is also theoretically possible in these instances. The findings will be distinctly different from those found in middle ear effusions. The pathologic findings at autopsy include abnormal facial nerve position; hypoplastic semicircular canals and cochlea; and decreased spiral ganglion cell and cochlear neuron population. Apparently in some pedigrees certain family members show other branchial cleft cysts or sinuses without the ear manifestations.

**Complications:** Infection of the preauricular sinus. With profound sensorineural or severe mixed hearing losses, failure to develop speech and language occurs unless the condition is recognized and early therapy is instituted. Psychologic disturbance may occur because of the cosmetic deformity, especially if it is severe.

**Associated Findings:** Hemifacial microsomia, micrognathia, microtia occasionally, lateral soft palate fistulas, mandibulofacial dysostosis, narrow external canals, cystathioninuria with brain abnormalities and pituitary disorders. Colobomata of upper eyelids, epibulbar dermoids, hemivertebrae of the cervical spine, and spina bifida (Goldenhar syndrome, see **Occulo-auriculo-vertebral anomaly**) occur very rarely. Frequency of preauricular pits and appendages approaches 100%. Renal anomalies are frequent.

**Etiology:** On occasions, by autosomal dominant inheritance with almost 100% expressivity of branchial fistulas and preauricular pits. The penetrance of hearing loss is reduced, but the degree of its reduction is unknown. Sporadic cases occur, and it is possible that some of these are either autosomal recessive or multifactorial.

**Pathogenesis:** Unknown.

**MIM No.:** *12510

**CDC No.:** 744.090

**Sex Ratio:** M1:F<1

**Occurrence:** Undetermined, but established literature.

**Risk of Recurrence for Patient's Sib:**
> See Part I, *Mendelian Inheritance.*

**Risk of Recurrence for Patient's Child:**
> See Part I, *Mendelian Inheritance.*

**Age of Detectability:** At birth, although an associated conductive or mild sensorineural hearing loss may escape detection for some time.

**Gene Mapping and Linkage:** Unknown.

**Prevention:** None known. Genetic counseling indicated.

**Treatment:** If the preauricular pits become infected, warm compresses and antibiotics are needed. Repeated infections are an indication for surgical excision. Before excising the tract it is important to be sure that it does not communicate with the middle ear or ear canal. Failure to do so will leave a deep potential cyst or sinus tract that will become infected, enlarge, and conceivably cause cholesteatoma formation with all of its attendant complications. In addition, the fistulous tract may run close to the facial nerve. In excising the tract great care must be taken not to injure the nerve. If there is conductive hearing loss, petrous pyramid polytomography may delineate the middle ear anomaly. Surgical repair of the ossicular abnormality is often possible and may be performed on one side at about age 4–5 years. Repair of the other middle ear may be deferred until adult life if serviceable hearing is obtained on one side. If this is not possible, or if the patient has a sensorineural loss, hearing aids and rehabilitative measures are indicated. Cervical branchial cleft remnants should also be excised, with medical treatment being used as a temporary expedient only in those instances in which infection occurs. Concomitant defects when present may require treatment.

**Prognosis:** Good for normal life. Fair for restoration to serviceable hearing in instances in which there is a potentially repairable middle ear defect. In mild-to-moderate sensorineural hearing losses, there is a good prognosis for adequate function in school and occupation with hearing aids and aural rehabilitation. In severe, mixed, or profound sensorineural hearing losses, patients may be limited in speech and oral language but may function well with the use of sign language and lip-reading.

**Detection of Carrier:** Unknown.

**Special Considerations:** As with any external ear malformation, a hearing loss must be considered to be present until proven otherwise. Preauricular ear pits are part of several syndromes, including the **Branchio-oto-renal dysplasia** and **Chromosome 4** syndromes. If the patient should have a tympanic perforation, such a communication might be demonstrated by injecting methylene blue or another harmless colored substance into the sinus opening and watching for its appearance in the middle ear. A bitter substance, such as a local or topical anesthetic, could be instilled through a tiny catheter into the sinus, and, if the patient tastes it, this might suggest that the substance traversed the middle ear and the eustachian tubes into the pharynx.

**References:**

McLaurin JW, et al.: Hereditary branchial anomalies and associated hearing impairment. Laryngoscope 1966; 76:1277–1288.
Rowley PT: Familial hearing loss associated with branchial fistulas. Pediatrics 1969; 44:978–985.
Fitch N, et al.: The temporal bone in the preauricular pit, cervical fistula, hearing loss syndrome. Ann Otol Rhinol Laryngol 1976; 85:268–275. *
Smith PG, et al.: Clinical aspects of the branchio-oto-renal syndrome. Otolaryngol Head Neck Surg 1984; 92:468–475. *

BE028                                     **LaVonne Bergstrom**

**Deafness-functional heart disease**
*See CARDIO-AUDITORY SYNDROME*
**Deafness-gingival fibromatosis**
*See GINGIVAL FIBROMATOSIS-DEAFNESS, JONES TYPES*

---

## DEAFNESS-GOITER                              0249

**Includes:**
 Goiter-sensorineural deafness
 Pendred syndrome
 Thyroid hormone organification defect IIB
 Thyroid hormonogenesis, genetic defect in

**Excludes:**
 Associations of deafness with endemic goiter (endemic cretinism)
 Defective iodotyrosine coupling
 Defective organification
 **Thyroid, iodide transport defect** (0542)
 **Thyroid, iodotyrosine deiodinase deficiency** (0543)
 Thyroidal and peripheral iodotyrosine deiodinase deficiency

**Major Diagnostic Criteria:** Perceptive deafness and goiter, with proven discharge of radioiodide with perchlorate or thiocyanate.

**Clinical Findings:** The sensorineural deafness is congenital, or at least of very early onset, and is probably not progressive. It is perceptive and of profound degree; almost invariably the two

sides are affected symmetrically. There is variable preservation of hearing in the low tones, which occasionally permits appreciation of speech and normal education. However, special education is almost always necessary. Vestibular function is often impaired to a variable extent.

The block in thyroxine synthesis is at the stage of incorporation of iodide into organic form in the thyroglobulin molecule and is detected by demonstrating a discharge of radioiodide from the thyroid gland by perchlorate or thiocyanate. This block is incomplete and of very variable degree, and, because of this, the thyroid disorder of Pendred syndrome may take many forms. Thus lifelong euthyroidism is the rule, although hypothyroidism may occur in infancy or following surgical removal of the thyroid. Because of the difficulty in hormone synthesis, hyperplasia of the thyroid gland is usual, though to a much lesser degree in males than females. Surgery is often unsatisfactory since regrowth of the remnant is common, and some affected persons have had four or more operations.

In common with other types of goiter associated with defects in thyroxine synthesis, the histologic picture is extremely pleomorphic and has given rise to suspicions of malignant change, though these are probably unjustified; at any rate, no well documented cases of fatally evolving metastasis have been reported.

**Complications:** Mental and physical retardation may occur in rare cases when pronounced hypothyroidism occurs in infancy. Death in infancy may very occasionally be due to respiratory obstruction caused by thyroid enlargement.

**Associated Findings:** None known.

**Etiology:** Autosomal recessive inheritance.

**Pathogenesis:** Undetermined. It has been suggested that the defect in organification occurs because the major components (thyroid peroxidase, iodide, thyroglobulin, and hydrogen peroxide) necessary for iodination fail to come together at the proper site at the cell-colloid interface.

**MIM No.:** *27460

**POS No.:** 4093

**Sex Ratio:** M1:F>1

**Occurrence:** Incidence 0.07:1,000 live births in Great Britain. Occurs in other white populations and also in many other ethnic groups, including Japanese, blacks, and populations from India, with unknown frequency.

**Risk of Recurrence for Patient's Sib:**
 See Part I, *Mendelian Inheritance.*

**Risk of Recurrence for Patient's Child:**
 See Part I, *Mendelian Inheritance.* Several marriages between persons affected with Pendred syndrome have been reported. In such cases the risk is 1:1 (100%). In the vast majority of other cases the risk is extremely small, being confined to those who marry heterozygotes, in which case 1:2 (50%) of the children will be affected.

**Age of Detectability:** Deafness in early infancy (though often not detected until later). The condition could probably be detected at birth if the perchlorate discharge test were applied.

**Gene Mapping and Linkage:** Unknown.

**Prevention:** None known. Genetic counseling indicated.

**Treatment:** In cases in which there is pronounced thyroid hyperplasia, prophylactic therapy with exogenous thyroid hormone preparations is effective in obviating the need for surgery and the risk of involved complications.

Surgery may be necessary for troublesome goiter. There is no therapy for the deafness; only supportive educational measures and the provision of appropriate electronic hearing aids can be offered.

**Prognosis:** Virtually normal life span. There is some risk in the newborn period of suffocation from extremely pronounced thyroid hyperplasia and later in life from surgery of the thyroid gland. In rare cases the complications of gross hypothyroidism may threaten life. There is probably no or minimal risk of malignant neoplasia of the thyroid gland.

**Detection of Carrier:** Unknown.

**References:**

Fraser GR, et al.: The syndrome of sporadic goitre and congenital deafness. Q J Med 1960; 29:279–295.

Fraser GR: Association of congenital deafness with goiter (Pendred's syndrome); a study of 207 families. Ann Hum Genet 1965; 28:201–249.

Niepomniszcze H, et al.: Biochemical studies on the iodine organification defect of Pendred's syndrome. Acta Endocrinol (Copenh) 1978; 89:70–79.

*G.R. Fraser*

---

## DEAFNESS-HYPERPROLINURIA-ICHTHYOSIS      0258

**Includes:**

    Ichthyosis-deafness-renal disease
    Renal disease-deafness-ichthyosis

**Excludes:**

    **Hyperprolinemia** (0502)
    Hyperprolinemia-microscopic hematuria
    Ichthyosis-strabismus-sensorineural deafness
    **Nephritis-deafness (sensorineural), hereditary type** (0708)
    Renal anomalies-hearing loss

**Major Diagnostic Criteria:** Hearing loss and ichthyosis with either renal disease or hyperprolinuria or a relative with those conditions.

**Clinical Findings:** Various combinations of renal disease, hearing loss, ichthyosis, and hyperprolinuria were found in 23 of 78 examined members of a kindred. Two of three children, born of a consanguineous union of affected parents, showed all elements of the syndrome except hearing loss. In no family members were all symptoms present. Thirteen of 67 tested family members had a sensorineural hearing loss, 8 had a nephropathy, 6 had ichthyosis and 4 had a proline defect. Two of the family members had 3 traits, 5 had 2 traits, 15 had only 1 trait.

The hearing loss is mainly in the frequencies above 4000 cycles/second and is slowly progressive. The degree of hearing loss was > 50 db in persons over 50 years of age and > 30 db in younger people.

Advanced renal disease with chronic renal failure was present in the proband and his younger sister. Six other persons had renal calculi. Histopathologic examination of kidney specimens obtained from the proband showed glomerular and periglomerular sclerosis. The interstitial tissue was infiltrated largely by lymphocytes. The small arteries and arterioles showed variable degrees of medial hypertrophy and subendothelial sclerosis. Electron microscopy showed a thickening of the mesangial basement membrane. Plasma proline levels were elevated in three persons, and prolinuria was noted in two family members.

**Complications:** Uremia.

**Associated Findings:** None known.

**Etiology:** Possibly autosomal dominant inheritance with variable expressivity.

**Pathogenesis:** Unknown.

**POS No.:** 3198

**Sex Ratio:** M13:F10

**Occurrence:** Twenty-three individuals identified in one kindred.

**Risk of Recurrence for Patient's Sib:**
    See Part I, *Mendelian Inheritance.*

**Risk of Recurrence for Patient's Child:**
    See Part I, *Mendelian Inheritance.*

**Age of Detectability:** Childhood and adolescence.

**Gene Mapping and Linkage:** Unknown.

**Prevention:** None known. Genetic counseling indicated.

**Treatment:** Treatment of renal calculi and uremia. A hearing aid, speech and language therapy, and special schooling may be of help.

**Prognosis:** In absence of uremia, no decrease of life span.

**Detection of Carrier:** Close examination of the apparently unaffected individual may reveal minimal expression.

**Special Considerations:** Some researchers consider this condition to be a variation of **Nephritis-deafness (sensorineural), hereditary type** or **Hyperprolinemia.**

**References:**

Goyer RA, et al.: Hereditary renal disease with neurosensory hearing loss, prolinuria and ichthyosis. Am J Med Sci 1968; 256:166–179.

KE018

**Janice Key**
*Cor W.R.J. Cremers*

**Deafness-hyperuricemia-ataxia**
*See PHOSPHORIBOSYL PYROPHOSPHATE (PRPP) SYNTHETASE ABNORMALITY*

---

## DEAFNESS-HYPOGONADISM      2322

**Includes:** Hypogonadism-deafness

**Excludes:**

    **Alstrom syndrome** (0041)
    **Deafness with perilymphatic gusher** (3116)
    **Kallmann syndrome** (2301)
    **Noonan syndrome** (0720)

**Major Diagnostic Criteria:** Congenital severe mixed (sensorineural and conductive) hearing loss with primary hypogonadism in a male.

**Clinical Findings:** Myhre et al (1982) reported a single kindred with five affected males having congenital severe mixed hearing loss, primary hypogonadism, thickened calvarium without other bony abnormalities, normal intelligence (except a single mildly retarded boy) and antisocial behavior with poor academic performance. A single male in another family was included because of similar clinical findings.

Audiogram showed air conduction in the profound range at the limit of the audiometer, and bone conduction was in the severe range with a "basin-shaped" curve. One boy underwent middle ear exploration, and fixation of the stapedial footplate was noted. On manipulation of the stapes, a profuse flow of CSF (possibly perilymph) was noted, and the surgery was terminated. Tomograms showed narrowing of the internal auditory canal, possibly accounting for the sensorineural component of the hearing loss.

**Complications:** Marked retardation in development of secondary sex characteristics and genital development was reported. Primary hypogonadism was manifested by low levels of plasma testosterone in adult subjects; a plasma testosterone response to HCG stimulation in two teenagers was less than what would occur in prepubertal males having one gonad; and an abnormal testicular biopsy specimen with aberrant spermatogenesis was found in one male. Infertility was reported in the single married male.

**Associated Findings:** Calvarial thickening in frontal, parietal, and upper occipital bones, with narrowing of the internal auditory canals. Marked antisocial and immature behavior may result in criminal offenses.

**Etiology:** X-linked recessive inheritance.

**Pathogenesis:** Unknown.

**MIM No.:** 30435

**POS No.:** 4115

**Sex Ratio:** M1:F0

**Occurrence:** One kindred with five affected males has been reported.

**Risk of Recurrence for Patient's Sib:**
    See Part I, *Mendelian Inheritance.*

**Risk of Recurrence for Patient's Child:**
    See Part I, *Mendelian Inheritance.* Affected individuals may not be able to reproduce.

**Age of Detectability:** Hearing loss should be detectable in infancy. Hypogonadism may not be noted until age of expected puberty.

**Gene Mapping and Linkage:** Unknown.

**Prevention:** None known. Genetic counseling indicated.

**Treatment:** Hearing aide plus auditory training and deaf education for the hearing loss. Gonadotropin therapy to accelerate sexual maturation. Psychosocial counseling and support.

**Prognosis:** Normal for life span and, usually, for intelligence. Academic performance may be poor, and severe psychosocial problems may be present.

**Detection of Carrier:** Unknown.

**References:**
Myhre SA et al.: Congenital deafness and hypogonadism: a new X-linked recessive disorder. Clin Genet 1982; 22:299–307.

DA026                                    **Sandra L.H. Davenport**

## DEAFNESS-KERATOPACHYDERMIA-DIGITAL CONSTRICTIONS                                    0259

**Includes:**
Digital constrictions-keratopachydermia-deafness
Keratopachydermia-digital constrictions-deafness
Mutilating keratoderma
Vohwinkel syndrome

**Excludes:**
Ainhum
**Deafness (sensorineural), progressive high-tone** (0269)
Keratosis palmaris et plantaris with ainhum
Pseudoainhum

**Major Diagnostic Criteria:** Palmoplantar keratoderma, congenital deafness, and distal digital constrictions.

**Clinical Findings:** Onset in infancy or early childhood of a diffuse palmoplantar keratoderma with honeycombed small depressions, starfish-shaped keratoses of the dorsa of hands and feet, and linear keratoses of elbows and knees. Digital band-like constrictions of the distal interphalangeal creases develop after age 4–5 years. Patients show congenital cochlear type of sensorineural high-frequency hearing loss that is not progressive. Loudness discomfort level is normal, and tone decay is absent. One patient is reported with deaf-mutism. X-rays may show constriction of phalangeal bone(s), trophic bony atrophy, and verrucous nodules of soft tissue.

**Complications:** Amputation of distal digit(s) because of gangrene or chronic sepsis.

**Associated Findings:** Diffuse nonscarring alopecia, **Hair, alopecia areata**, ridged dystrophic nails, syndactylia, transient plantar blisters, and hyperhidrosis.

**Etiology:** Autosomal dominant inheritance.

**Pathogenesis:** Unknown.

**MIM No.:** *12450

**POS No.:** 3199

**Sex Ratio:** Theoretical, M1:F1; observed, female preponderance (M1:F7 in one series).

**Occurrence:** Undetermined. Established literature.

**Risk of Recurrence for Patient's Sib:**
See Part I, *Mendelian Inheritance.*

**Risk of Recurrence for Patient's Child:**
See Part I, *Mendelian Inheritance.*

**Age of Detectability:** Deafness in infancy or early childhood. Keratoderma in infancy or early childhood. Digital constrictions as early as age 4–5 years to as late as adolescense or early adulthood.

**Gene Mapping and Linkage:** Unknown.

**Prevention:** None known. Genetic counseling indicated.

**Treatment:** Soaks of 10–40% urea solution followed by abrasive filing of hyperkeratosis; 40% salicylic acid plaster with débridement of hyperkeratoses. Excision of keratoses with full thickness skin grafting. Surgical amputation of gangrenous or septic digit(s). Specially fitted shoes, avoidance of trauma.

**Prognosis:** Normal for life span and intelligence.

**Detection of Carrier:** Unknown.

**References:**
Gibbs RC, Frank SB: Keratoma hereditaria mutilans (Vohwinkel). Differentiating features of conditions with constriction of digits. Arch Dermatol 1966; 94:619–625.
McGibbon DH, Watson RT: Vohwinkel's syndrome and deafness. J Laryngol Otol 1977; 91:853–857.
Lemont H, Schachter R: Vohwinkel's disease case report. J Am Podiatry Assoc 1978; 68:598–600.
Janaki VR, et al.: Keratoderma hereditaria mutilans of Vohwinkel. Indian Pediatr 1979; 16:287–289.
Aksu F, Mietens C: Keratopachydermie mit Schnuerfurchen in Fingern und Innenohrschwerhoerigkeit. Paediat Prox 1980; 23:303–310. †
Reddy BSN, Gupta SK: Mutilating keratoderma of Vohwinkel. Int J Dermatol 1983; 22:530–533.
Cole RD, et al.: Vohwinkel's keratoma hereditarium multilans. Int J Dermatol 1984; 23:131–134.

FE011                                    **Judith Ferry**
                                    *William C. Gentry, Jr.*

## DEAFNESS-MALFORMED EARS-MENTAL RETARDATION                                    2345

**Includes:**
Ears (malformed)-deafness-mental retardation
Mental retardation-ears (malformed)-deafness

**Excludes:**
**Deafness-ear pits** (0247)
**Deafness-malformed, low-set ears** (0254)
Ears, low-set, as part of other syndromes
**Ear, microtia-atresia** (0664)
**Hypertelorism-microtia-facial cleft-conductive deafness** (0506)

**Major Diagnostic Criteria:** Malformed, low-set ears; progressive sensorineural conductive hearing loss; and mental retardation in the absence of other abnormalities.

**Clinical Findings:** Variable degrees of malformed pinnae, hypoplastic auditory canal, congenital or early-onset conductive-sensorineural progressive deafness (in a range of 30–80 dB), although normal hearing is present in mildly affected patients. Moderate mental retardation is observed in the majority of patients. Polytomographic studies may show hypopneumatization, fused ossicles, plate of the stapes abnormally thick in both sides, and increased density of the cochlea and of the otic capsule.

This is a sensorineural conductive deafness with pinna anomalies. It can be easily distinguished from other types of deafness by its progressive course and typical X-ray findings. Mental retardation seems to be a consistent feature, unlike other types of deafness with auricular defects.

**Complications:** Progressive deafness.

**Associated Findings:** None known.

**Etiology:** Autosomal recessive inheritance.

**Pathogenesis:** Unknown.

**MIM No.:** *22130

**Sex Ratio:** M1:F1

**Occurrence:** Nine cases have been reported from three kinships.

**Risk of Recurrence for Patient's Sib:**
See Part I, *Mendelian Inheritance.*

**Risk of Recurrence for Patient's Child:**
See Part I, *Mendelian Inheritance.*

**Age of Detectability:** Pinna malformations at birth; deafness in childhood or early adulthood.

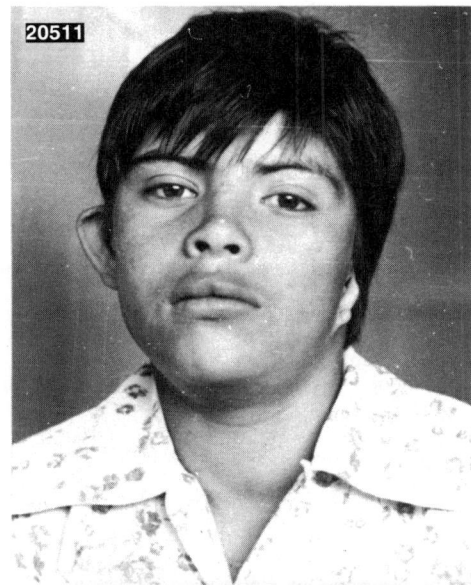

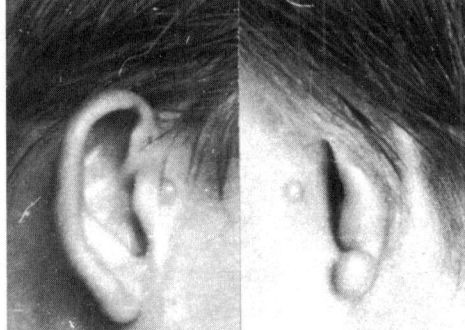

**2345-20511:**  Note variable degrees of malformed pinnae in the same subject.

**Gene Mapping and Linkage:**  Unknown.

**Prevention:**  None known. Genetic counseling indicated.

**Treatment:**  Plastic surgery of the dysplastic external ear could be of benefit in some cases. Hearing aids also can be useful. Special education may be helpful.

**Prognosis:**  Normal life span.

**Detection of Carrier:**  Unknown.

**References:**
Mengel MC, et al.: Conductive hearing loss and low-set ears as a possible recessive syndrome. J Med Genet 1969; 6:14–21.
Cantú JM, et al.: Autosomal recessive sensori-neural conductive deafness, mental retardation, and pinna anomalies. Hum Genet 1978; 40:231–234. *

CR023
CA011

**Diana García-Cruz**
**José María Cantú**

## DEAFNESS-MALFORMED, LOW-SET EARS                    **0254**

**Includes:**  Ears, malformed and low-set-deafness

**Excludes:**  Low-set ears in other syndromes with structural abnormalities

**Major Diagnostic Criteria:**  Malformed external ears and a conductive hearing loss in the absence of other major structural abnormalities are necessary to make the diagnosis.

**Clinical Findings:**  Malformed external ears are found in all cases, with the degree of deformity varying from mild cup-shaped deformity to marked flop-eared deformity. Fifty percent of the affected also have low-set ears. All those affected have a mild-to-moderate hearing loss. This is always a conductive loss and is usually worse in the more affected external ear. Mental retardation is present in 50% of the affected. Cryptorchism is found in 100% of the males.

**Complications:**  Deafness.

**Associated Findings:**  None known.

**Etiology:**  Autosomal recessive inheritance.

**Pathogenesis:**  Unknown developmental factors causing structural changes in middle ear bones and external pinna. Pathogenesis of mental retardation also unknown.

**MIM No.:**  *22130

**POS No.:**  3449

**Sex Ratio:**  M1:F1

**Occurrence:**  Rare. Nine cases from three kinships, including two from a Mennonite isolate and one case in which parents were third cousins, have been documented.

**Risk of Recurrence for Patient's Sib:**
See Part I, *Mendelian Inheritance.*

**Risk of Recurrence for Patient's Child:**
See Part I, *Mendelian Inheritance.*

**Age of Detectability:**  External ear deformity at birth; deafness in infancy.

**Gene Mapping and Linkage:**  Unknown.

**Prevention:**  None known. Genetic counseling indicated.

**Treatment:**  Some affected individuals may benefit from ear surgery. Special education for those mildly retarded may be of help. Hearing aids are often useful adjuncts to such special education.

**Prognosis:**  Normal for life span.

**Detection of Carrier:**  Unknown.

**References:**
Konigsmark BW: Hereditary deafness in man (second of three parts). N Engl J Med 1969; 281:713.
Mengel MC, et al.: Conductive hearing loss and malformed low-set ears, as a possible recessive syndrome. J Med Genet 1969; 6:14–21.
Cantu JM, et al.: Autosomal recessive sensorineural-conductive deafness and pinna anomalies. Hum Genet 1978; 40:231–234.

ME018                                        **Marvin C. Mengel**

**Deafness-mental retardation-possible sterility**
*See DEAFNESS, PFAENDLER TYPE*
**Deafness-metaphyseal dysostosis**
*See METAPHYSEAL DYSOSTOSIS-DEAFNESS*
**Deafness-mitral regurgitation-skeletal malformations**
*See MITRAL REGURGITATION-DEAFNESS-SKELETAL DEFECTS*

## DEAFNESS-MYOPIA 0251

**Includes:**
Cochlear deafness-myopia-oligophrenia
Eldridge syndrome
Myopia-cochlear deafness-intellectual impairment
Oligophrenia-cochlear deafness-myopia
Myopia-hearing loss

**Excludes:**
**Alstrom syndrome** (0041)
**Deafness-myopia-cataract-saddle nose, Marshall type** (0261)
**Diabetes (insipidus/mellitus)-optic atrophy-deafness** (0550)
Hearing loss-polyneuropathy-optic atrophy
Myopia-hearing loss-peripheral neuropathy-skeletal
 abnormalities
**Nephritis-deafness (sensorineural), hereditary type** (0708)
Retinal changes-deafness-muscular wasting-mental
 retardation

**Major Diagnostic Criteria:** Cochlear deafness (30–100 dB), myopia, intellectual impairment.

**Clinical Findings:** The natural history of the hearing impairment has not been fully documented, but it is probably present at birth and progresses little thereafter. The hearing loss is cochlear in origin. The vestibular function is normal. The eye changes are those of severe myopia diagnosed at age 4–6 years. EEG and CSF findings provide no consistent evidence of local or diffuse disease of the brain. Nonverbal IQ scores are in the range of 71 to 82. Difficulties in the proper evaluation of mental status in the presence of marked sensory deprivation must be recognized.

**Complications:** Unknown.

**Associated Findings:** None known.

**Etiology:** Autosomal recessive inheritance.

**Pathogenesis:** Probably an enzyme deficiency.

**MIM No.:** 22120

**Sex Ratio:** M1:F1

**Occurrence:** Undetermined. Higher in some isolated populations, such as Amish communities, because of consanguinity.

**Risk of Recurrence for Patient's Sib:**
See Part I, *Mendelian Inheritance.*

**Risk of Recurrence for Patient's Child:**
See Part I, *Mendelian Inheritance.*

**Age of Detectability:** Probably in newborn period if hearing loss is congenital and brainstem auditory evoked responses are used. Myopia may also be detectable in infancy or early childhood.

**Gene Mapping and Linkage:** Unknown.

**Prevention:** None known. Genetic counseling indicated.

**Treatment:** With early detection of hearing loss, corrective lenses, hearing aids, and appropriate education for the hearing impaired, improvement in functional prognosis might be possible.

**Prognosis:** Normal for life span. Independent living might not be possible.

**Detection of Carrier:** Unknown.

**Special Considerations:** The question of intellectual and/or psychiatric impairment must be regarded with caution in any child with both hearing and vision loss. It appears, however, that glasses provided satisfactory correction in the affected children. Therefore, educational efforts should be aimed at deaf education, careful assessment of intellectual abilities, and behavioral management.

**References:**
Eldridge R, et al.: Cochlear deafness, myopia, and intellectual impairment in an Amish family. Arch Otolaryngol 1968; 88:49–54. * †

DA026                                    **Sandra L.H. Davenport**

## DEAFNESS-MYOPIA-CATARACT-SADDLE NOSE, MARSHALL TYPE 0261

**Includes:**
Cataract-deafness-myopia-saddle nose
Marshall syndrome
Myopia-cataract-saddle nose-hypertelorism-short stature-
 deafness
Saddle nose-deafness-myopia-cataract

**Excludes:**
**Arthro-ophthalmopathy, hereditary, progressive, Stickler type** (0090)
**Facio-oculo-acoustic-renal syndrome (FOAR syndrome)** (0732)
**Fetal syphilis syndrome** (0385)
**Oto-oculo-musculo-skeletal syndrome** (0785)
**Retina, hyaloideoretinal degeneration of Wagner** (0479)

**Major Diagnostic Criteria:** Saddle nose, hypertelorism, high myopia, cataract, and sensorineural hearing loss. The extent of variability is not yet clear.

**Clinical Findings:** All patients have a severely depressed nasal bridge with anteverted nostrils. Wide-set eyes, myopia, congenital and juvenile cataracts, and a moderate-to-severe sensorineural hearing loss are frequent features of this syndrome. Esotropia, hypertropia, high-arched or cleft palate, and retinal detachment have also been noted. The upper incisors protrude in a number of cases. X-ray examinations revealed absent or small nasal bones. The facial appearance is thought to be due to faulty devlopment of the ethmoid bone, which also causes a short anterior cranial fossa. The saddle-nose deformity, which resembles syphillitic saddle nose and often leads to initial referral, becomes less obvious as the patient matures. As infants, the children may "snort" as they breathe, but by age 1–2 years this upper-airway sound disappears. The degree of myopia is usually > -10 D. In some cases there was a sudden maturation of cataract with glaucoma, necessitating surgery. The moderate-to-severe sensorineural hearing loss is progressive in some cases. By X-ray examination, the internal auditory canals were somewhat narrowed. In one case polytomography of the inner ears was normal. In another case vestibular function was normal as assessed by caloric stimulation with ice water.

**Complications:** Retinal detachment.

**Associated Findings:** None known.

**Etiology:** Autosomal dominant inheritance with variable expression.

**Pathogenesis:** Unknown.

**MIM No.:** *15478

**POS No.:** 3200

**Sex Ratio:** M1:F1

**Occurrence:** Six pedigrees with at least 21 affected members have been reported.

**Risk of Recurrence for Patient's Sib:**
See Part I, *Mendelian Inheritance.*

**Risk of Recurrence for Patient's Child:**
See Part I, *Mendelian Inheritance.*

**Age of Detectability:** Early childhood.

**Gene Mapping and Linkage:** Unknown.

**Prevention:** None known. Genetic counseling indicated.

**Treatment:** Surgical treatment of cataract. A hearing aid can be useful in some cases. Special education because of the hearing loss may be necessary. Plastic surgery may be of benefit for the saddle nose deformity.

**Prognosis:** Probably good for normal life span.

**Detection of Carrier:** Unknown.

**Special Considerations:** The nosologic relationship between this condition, **Arthro-ophthalmopathy, hereditary, progressive, Stickler type**, and **Retina, hyaloideoretinal degeneration of Wagner** have been the subject of considerable debate. For a systematic discussion of this issue, see Aymé & Preus, 1984.

**References:**

Marshall D: Ectodermal dysplasia. Report of a kindred with ocular abnormalities and hearing defect. Am J Ophthalmol 1958; 45:143–156. †

Keith CG, et al.: Abnormal facies, myopia, and short stature. Arch Dis Child 1972; 47:787–793. †

Zellweger H, et al.: The Marshall syndrome: report of a new family. J Pediatr 1974; 84:868–871.

O'Donnell JJ, et al.: Generalized osseous abnormalities in the Marshall syndrome. In: Bergsma D, ed: Cytogenetics, environment and malformation syndromes. BD:OAS 1976; XII(5):299. New York: Alan R. Liss, for The National Foundation - March of Dimes, 1976; 299–314. * †

Logan DC: Marshall syndrome: a case report. Missouri Speech-Language and Hearing Assoc 1980; 13:3–4.

Aymé S, Preus M: The Marshall and Stickler syndromes: objective rejection of lumping. J Med Genet 1984; 21:34–38. *

DA026

**Sandra L.H. Davenport**
*Cor W.R.J. Cremers*

**Deafness-nephritis**
*See NEPHRITIS-DEAFNESS (SENSORINEURAL) HEREDITARY TYPE*

---

## DEAFNESS-NEPHRITIS-MACROTHROMBOPATHIA    3046

**Includes:**
Epstein syndrome
Macrothrombopathia-deafness-nephritis
Nephritis-deafness-macrothrombopathia

**Excludes:**
**Immunodeficiency, Wiskott-Aldrich type** (0523)
**Leukocyte, May-Hegglin anomaly** (2681)
**Nephritis-deafness (sensorineural), hereditary type** (0708)

**Major Diagnostic Criteria:** The combination of thrombocytopenia, nephritis, and hearing loss.

**Clinical Findings:** A bleeding disorder is the presenting feature, with age of onset ranging from four months to ten years. This is characterized by epistaxis, with consistently low platelet counts. The platelets are large in most cases, although they were of normal size in one report (Eckstein et al, 1975). Deafness is also present in all reported individuals, ranging from moderate (30–40 dB) to severe sensorineural loss. Age of diagnosis ranged from two to 22 years. Nephritis, on the other hand, did not affect all individuals, having been reported in 12/17 patients. Age of onset of the nephritis ranged from four to 25 years. Renal biopsies revealed mixed glomerulonephritis and interstitial nephritis. In some individuals, the condition remained stable, whereas in others it was progressive and led to death in the third decade.

**Complications:** Cerebral hemorrhage, anemia, and hypertension are common complications.

**Associated Findings:** One patient had cystic medial necrosis and an aortic valve anomaly; two others had eczema.

**Etiology:** Autosomal dominant inheritance with variable expression and possible incomplete penetrance.

**Pathogenesis:** Unknown.

**MIM No.:** *15365

**POS No.:** 3864

**Sex Ratio:** Presumably M1:F1.

**Occurrence:** Three families and two sporadic cases have been described, for a total of 17 reported patients.

**Risk of Recurrence for Patient's Sib:**
See Part I, *Mendelian Inheritance.*

**Risk of Recurrence for Patient's Child:**
See Part I, *Mendelian Inheritance.*

**Age of Detectability:** By age ten years.

**Gene Mapping and Linkage:** Unknown.

**Prevention:** None known. Genetic counseling indicated.

**Treatment:** Hearing aid for hearing loss as indicated; renal transplant may be indicated in cases of severe renal failure. Cortisone and splenectomy had little effect.

**Prognosis:** Variable in that some individuals died of bleeding or renal complications in their 20s; others had a stable course, and yet others showed improvement. The oldest reported patient was alive at age 63 years.

**Detection of Carrier:** Unknown.

**Special Considerations:** This may actually represent a group of disorders in that platelet morphology differed between the reports of Epstein et al (1972), Bernheim et al (1976), and Parsa et al (1976), who found giant platelets, and the report of Eckstein et al (1975), who found normal-sized platelets.

**References:**

Epstein CJ, et al.: Hereditary macrothrombocytopathia, nephritis, and deafness. Am J Med 1972; 52:299–310.

Eckstein JD, et al.: Hereditary thrombocytopenia, deafness, and renal disease. Ann Intern Med 1975; 82:639–645.

Bernheim J, et al.: Thrombocytopenia, macrothrombopathia, nephritis and deafness. Am J Med 1976; 61:145–150.

Parsa KP, et al.: Hereditary nephritis, deafness, and abnormal thrombopoiesis. Am J Med 1976; 60:665–672.

Hansen MS, et al.: Megathrombocytopenia associated with glomerulonephritis, deafness, and aortic cystic medianecrosis. Scand J Haematol 1978; 21:197–205.

T0007

**Helga V. Toriello**

**Deafness-nephrosis-urinary tract and digital defects**
*See NEPHROSIS-DEAFNESS-URINARY TRACT AND DIGITAL DEFECTS*
**Deafness-ocular and facial anomalies-proteinuria**
*See FACIO-OCULO-ACOUSTIC-RENAL SYNDROME (FOAR SYNDROME)*
**Deafness-onycho-osteo dystrophy**
*See DEAFNESS-TRIPHALANGEAL THUMBS-ONYCHODYSTROPHY*

---

## DEAFNESS-ONYCHO-OSTEO-DYSTROPHY-RETARDATION-SEIZURES (DOORS)    0262

**Includes:**
DOOR(S) syndrome
Nails (abnormal)-deafness-retardation-seizures-dermatoglyphics
Thumbs-onychodystrophy-distal osteodystrophy-seizure-retardation

**Excludes:**
**Acidemia, 2-oxoglutaric** (2565)
**Deafness-onychodystrophy** (0252)
**Deafness-triphalangeal thumbs-onychodystrophy** (2151)
**Digito-reno-cerebral syndrome** (2792)
**Onychodystrophy-coniform teeth-sensorineural hearing loss** (2034)

**Major Diagnostic Criteria:** Triphalangy of thumbs and/or great toes, hypoplasia of the distal phalanges of other fingers and toes, hypoplastic, rudimentary or absent nails, congenital sensorineural deafness, mental retardation, seizure disorder, and digital arch patterns.

**Clinical Findings:** The constellation of findings include: (1) Long thumbs with two skin creases, abnormal in appearance, opposable, with a small extra distal phalanx in about 70% of cases. (2) Great toes are generally long and have large distal phalanx; in some cases an extra phalanx (triphalangy) may also be present. (3) Hypoplastic or absent distal phalanges of other fingers and toes. (4) Hypoplastic, rudimentary, or absent finger- and toe-nails. (5) Congenital, bilateral sensorineural deafness. (6) Seizure disorder beginning in the first year of life, usually of grand-mal type. (7) Profound to mild mental retardation, with IQ range from 10 to 70. (8) Arch patterns on all fingers and toes.

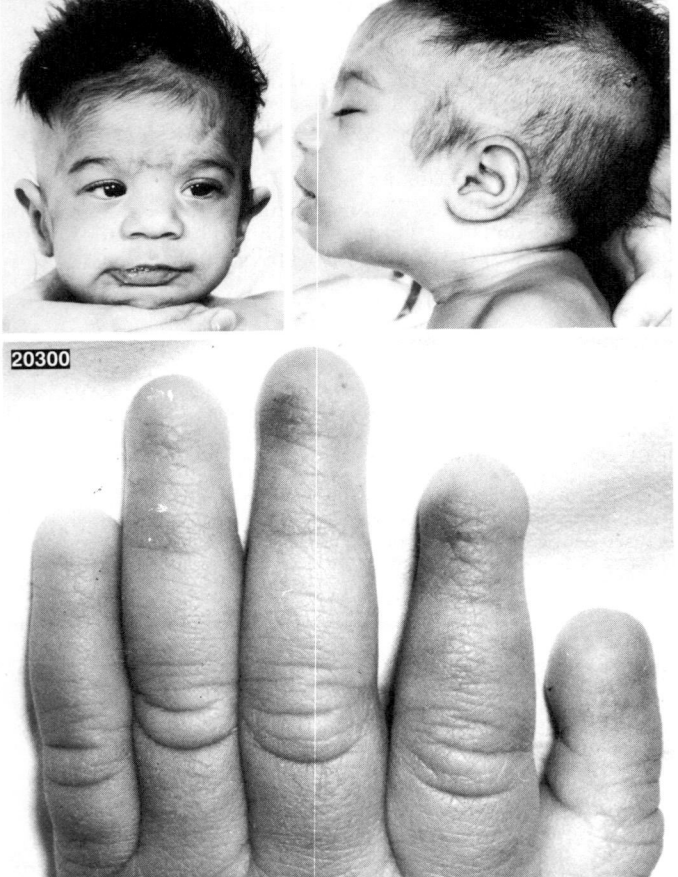

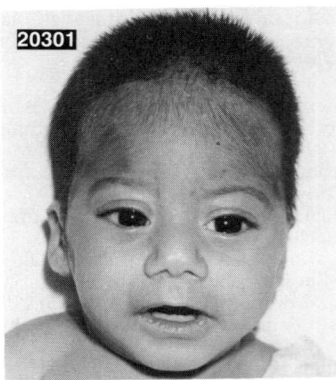

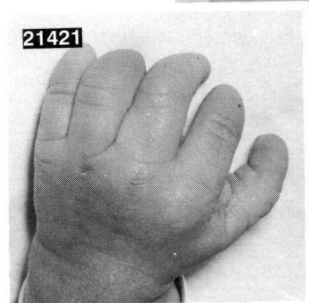
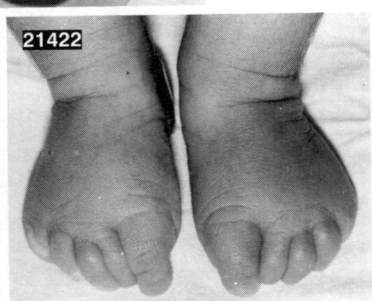

**0262A-20298–99:** Deafness-onychodystrophy-digital anomalies; note characteristic facies with broad nasal alae, a "square" nasal tip, a long upper lip, and a thin, vermilion border. **20300:** Note absent nails and reduction of the terminal phalanges.

**0262B-20301:** Characteristic facies include broad nasal alae, a square nasal tip, and a long upper lip with a thin vermilion border. **21421–22:** Absent nails, reduced terminal phalanges and a proximally placed thumb.

Patients are born at term with normal birth weight and do not present any problems of neonatal adaptation. Developmental milestones, other than of speech, are generally achieved at normal times. Physical growth and head size are within normal percentiles. Phalangeal abnormalities are clinically distinct and need to be confirmed by radiological studies. Parental consanguinity has been reported in 50% of families. Unaffected first degree relatives do not show any signs.

**Complications:** Profound deafness leads to mutism. Seizures if not properly controlled may lead to further deterioration of intellectual function. Severe hypotonia, leading to facial and cranial asymmetry and lumbar lordosis; status epilepticus; recurrent respiratory infections.

**Associated Findings:** Downward slanted eyes, ptosis of upper eyelids, ocular hypertelorism, low-set ears, large nostrils, highly arched palate, hypoplastic dentition, micrognathia, craniosynostosis, abnormal CAT scan of brain.

A raised level of organic acid 2-oxoglutarate was found in the plasma and urine of three patients; and an increased frequency of chromatid and chromosome breaks was reported in cultured lymphocytes of two patients and their mother.

**Etiology:** Autosomal recessive inheritance.

**Pathogenesis:** Unknown.

**MIM No.:** *22050

**POS No.:** 3733

**Sex Ratio:** M1:F1

**Occurrence:** Rare. Eight cases reported; Five of Latin ancestry (2 from Puerto Rico, 1 from Venezuela, 1 from Cuba, 1 from Spain).

**Risk of Recurrence for Patient's Sib:**
See Part I, *Mendelian Inheritance.*

**Risk of Recurrence for Patient's Child:**
See Part I, *Mendelian Inheritance.*

**Age of Detectability:** Long abnormal thumbs, dystrophic nails, and distinctive dermatoglyphic features could be noted soon after birth leading to suspicion of the condition. Seizures begin during the first year inviting medical attention to the infant. Hearing problems can be detected in the first three months. A mother who had one child with the condition, recognized the condition in her next newborn by the appearance of the thumbs and nails.

**Gene Mapping and Linkage:** Unknown.

**Prevention:** None known. Genetic counseling indicated.

**Treatment:** Management of seizures, habitation treatment for deafness, and supportive educational measures.

**Prognosis:** Profound to mild impairment of intelligence. Early death can occur due to respiratory infection or status epilepticus, but many patients have reached teenage years.

**Detection of Carrier:** Unknown.

**Special Considerations:** The designation "DOOR(S)" has been applied to a wide range of conditions and syndromes. **Deafness-onychodystrophy,** reported by Feinmesser and Zelig (1961), is characterized by dystrophic nails and sensorineural deafness but no osteodystrophy, triphalangeal thumbs, mental retardation or other associated abnormalities. **Deafness-triphalangeal thumbs-onychodystrophy,** described by Goodman et al (1969) and (Moghadam

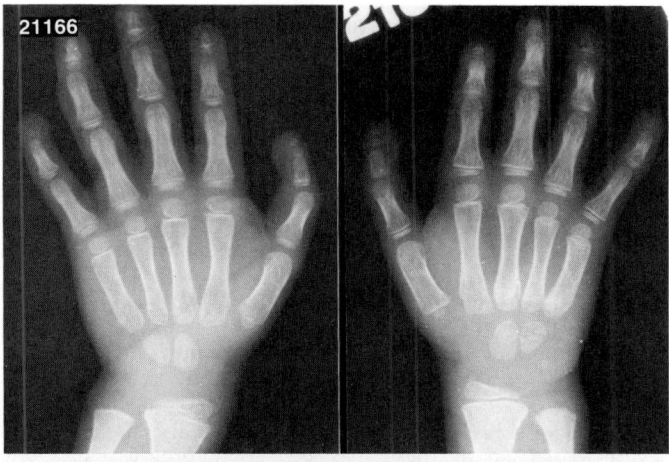

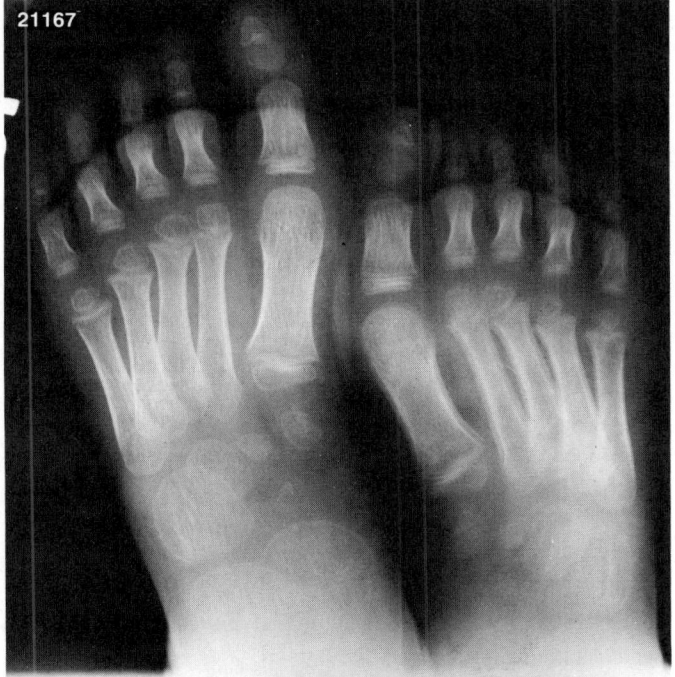

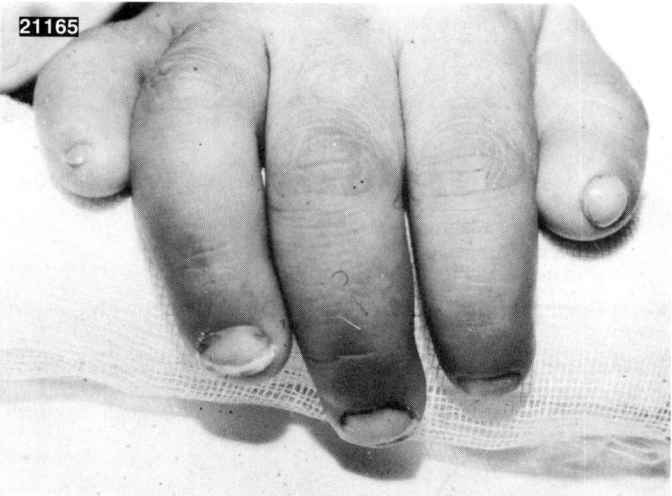

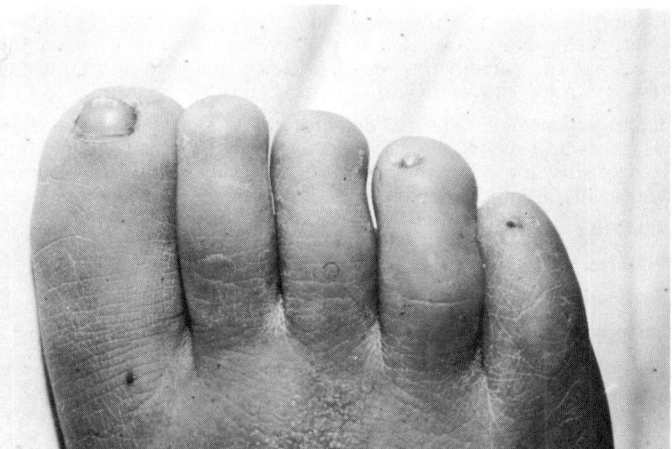

**0262D**-21165: Abnormal thumbs and hypoplastic nails (top); long great toes and hypoplastic nails (bottom).

**0262C**-21166: Triphalangy of the thumbs and hypoplasia of the distal phalanges of the other digits. 21167: Triphalangy of the great toes and absence of the terminal phalanges of the other toes.

and Statten, 1972) includes triphalangeal thumbs and underdeveloped tufts of the terminal phalanges besides onychodystrophy and sensorineural deafness. No additional abnormalities were to be found. **Digito-reno-cerebral syndrome**, described by Eronen et al. (1985), as an autosomal recessive condition with considerable similarity to the DOOR syndrome. Additional features were cystic dysplasia of the kidneys with rudimentary nephrons and cartilagenous tissue, unilateral renal agenesis, enlarged adrenals and thymus, and dilated cerebral ventricles.

The acronym "DOOR(S)", however, applies only the condition described in this article, and other related syndromes should be delineated, and differential diagnosis made, on the basis of clinical manifestations and modes of inheritance.

**References:**

Feinmesser M, Zelig S: Congenital deafness associated with onychodystrophy. Arch Otolaryngol 1961; 74:507–508.

Goodman RH, et al.: Hereditary congenital deafness with onychodystrophy. Arch Otolaryngol 1969; 90:474–477.

Qazi AH, Smithwick EM: Triphalangy of thumbs and great toes. Am J Dis Child 1970; 120:255–257.

Walbaum R, et al.: Surdite familiale avec osteo-onycho-dysplasie. J Genet Hum 1970; 18:101–108.

Moghadam H, Statten P: Hereditary sensorineural hearing loss with onychodystrophy. Canad Med Ass J 1972; 107:310–312.

Cantwell RJ: Congenital sensory neural deafness associated with onycho-osteodystrophy and mental retardation (DOOR syndrome). Hum Genet 1975; 26:261–265.

Qazi QH, Nangia BS: Abnormal distal phalanges and nails, deafness, mental retardation, seizure disorder: a new familial syndrome. J Pediatr 1984; 104:391–394. *

Patton MA, et al.: DOOR syndrome (deafness, onycho-osteodystrophy, and mental retardation): elevated plasma and urinary 2-oxoglutarate in three unrelated patients. Am J Med Genet 1987; 26:207–215.

QA000
WI057

**Qutub H. Qazi
Robin M. Winter**

## DEAFNESS-ONYCHODYSTROPHY     0252

**Includes:**
Nail dystrophy and sensorineural deafness
Onychodystrophy-deafness

**Excludes:**
**Deafness-onycho-osteo-dystrophy-retardation-seizures (DOOR)** (0262)
**Nails, anonychia, hereditary** (0066)
**Nails, pachyonychia congenita** (0789)
**Nail-patella syndrome** (0704)

**Major Diagnostic Criteria:** Sensorineural deafness with nail dystrophy.

**Clinical Findings:** Characterized by profound deafness, bilateral, of sensorineural type; normal or hypoactive labyrinth; and the nails of all fingers and toes show dystrophic changes from birth. Strabismus may be found.

**Complications:** Unknown.

**Associated Findings:** None known.

**Etiology:** Autosomal recessive inheritance, pleiotropic. The parents of the one involved family were both first cousins on the maternal and second cousins on the paternal side in a family of Jews from Egypt (coefficient of consanguinity F = 0.078).

**Pathogenesis:** Ectodermal defect involving ears and nails. Both deafness and dystrophic changes of the nails were found in two female sibs, the other members of the family being free of these anomalies. Strabismus was found in both sibs and mother.

**MIM No.:** *22050

**POS No.:** 3581

**Sex Ratio:** M1:F1

**Occurrence:** Presumably rare.

**Risk of Recurrence for Patient's Sib:**
See Part I, *Mendelian Inheritance*.

**Risk of Recurrence for Patient's Child:**
See Part I, *Mendelian Inheritance*.

**Age of Detectability:** At birth, although hearing loss may escape immediate notice.

**Gene Mapping and Linkage:** Unknown.

**Prevention:** None known. Genetic counseling indicated.

**Treatment:** Habilitation treatment for deafness.

**Prognosis:** Probably normal life span.

**Detection of Carrier:** Unknown.

**Special Considerations:** For a discussion of the delineation of this and related conditions, see **Deafness-onycho-osteo-dystrophy-retardation-seizures (DOORS)**.

**References:**
Cockayne EA: Inherited abnormalities of skin and its appendages. London: Oxford University Press, 1933:265.
Roberts JAF: An introduction to medical genetics, ed 2. London: Oxford University Press, 1959:140.
Feinmesser M, Zelig S: Congenital deafness associated with onychodystrophy. Arch Otolaryngol 1961; 74:507–508. * †
Goodman RM, et al.: Hereditary congenital deafness with onychodystrophy. Arch Otolaryngol 1969; 90:474–477.
Sanchez O, et al.: The deafness, onycho-osteo-dystrophy, mental retardation syndrome: two new cases. Hum Genet 1981; 58:228–230.

SH046           **Kathleen Shaver**
*Moshe Feinmesser*

**Deafness-onychodystrophy, dominant form**
*See ONYCHODYSTROPHY-CONIFORM TEETH-SENSORINEURAL HEARING LOSS*

## DEAFNESS-OPTIC NERVE ATROPHY, PROGRESSIVE     0253

**Includes:** Optic atrophy-deafness, progressive

**Excludes:**
**Deafness-polyneuropathy-optic atrophy** (0268)
**Diabetes (insipidus/mellitus)-optic atrophy-deafness** (0550)
**Optic atrophy, Leber type** (0579)
**Optico-cochleo-dentate degeneration** (0759)
Sylvester disease
Other syndromes including hearing loss and retinitis pigmentosa

**Major Diagnostic Criteria:** Congenital severe to profound sensorineural hearing loss in association with slowly progressive optic nerve atrophy and the absence of other anomalies or symptoms.

**Clinical Findings:** Profound bilateral sensorineural hearing loss of 60 to over 90 db, most marked in the midfrequencies, may be present from early childhood. Older individuals reported more severe losses, so deafness may be slowly progressive. Optic atrophy may be present in the first decade, but most individuals do not report vision loss until adulthood (ages 24–64 years). Vision loss is slowly progressive. Funduscopy showed paleness of the optic disk, with distinct margins, normal macular reflex, and normal retinal periphery. Neurologic examination is normal, except for deafness and optic nerve atrophy. Polytomography of the optic foramina, the chiasmatic region, and the temporal bone is normal.

**Complications:** Unknown.

**Associated Findings:** Deutan color defect.

**Etiology:** Autosomal dominant inheritance. Male to male transmission has been described.

**Pathogenesis:** Unknown.

**MIM No.:** 12525

**POS No.:** 3196

**Sex Ratio:** M1:F1

**Occurrence:** Undetermined. Seven kindreds have been independently described.

**Risk of Recurrence for Patient's Sib:**
See Part I, *Mendelian Inheritance*.

**Risk of Recurrence for Patient's Child:**
See Part I, *Mendelian Inheritance*.

**Age of Detectability:** Possible in the first or second decade of life.

**Gene Mapping and Linkage:** Unknown.

**Prevention:** None known. Genetic counseling indicated.

**Treatment:** Because of the severity of the sensorineural hearing loss, special education and hearing aids are necessary. Appropriate vocational planning for adulthood is essential.

**Prognosis:** Probably good for normal life span. Vision decreases progressively to blindness. Hearing loss usually is congenital and may be progressive.

**Detection of Carrier:** Unknown.

**References:**
Gernet HH: Hereditare Opticusatrophie in Kombination mit Taubheit. Ber Dtsch Ophthal Ges 1963; 65:545–547.
Michal S, et al.: Atrophy optique hérédo-familiale dominante associée à la surdi-mutité. Ann Oculiste (Paris) 1968; 201:431–435.
Kollarits CR, et al.: The autosomal dominant syndrome of progressive optic atrophy and congenital deafness. Am J Ophthalmol 1974; 87:789–792.
Konigsmark BW, et al.: Dominant congenital deafness and progressive optic nerve atrophy: occurrence in four generations of a family. Arch Ophthalmol 1974; 91:99–103. †
Deutman AF, Baarsma GS: Optic atrophy and deafmutism, dominantly inherited. Docum Ophthal Proc Series 1978; 17:145–154.
Grehn F, et al.: Dominant optic atrophy with sensorineural hearing loss. Ophthal Paediat Genet (Amsterdam) 1982; 1:77–88. †

Mets MB, Mhoon E: Probable autosomal dominant optic atrophy with hearing loss. Ophthal Paediat Genet (Amsterdam) 1985; 1/2:85–89. *

DA026                                    **Sandra L.H. Davenport**
                                          *Cor W.R.J. Cremers*

**Deafness-peripheral pulmonary stenoses-brachytelephalangy**
*See KEUTEL SYNDROME*

---

## DEAFNESS-PILI TORTI, BJORNSTAD TYPE                    2015

**Includes:**
    Bjornstad syndrome
    Pili torti-sensorineural hearing loss

**Excludes:**
    **Alopecia**
    **Deafness** (other)
    **Hypogonadism-partial alopecia** (2797)

**Major Diagnostic Criteria:** Suggested by the combination of pili torti with or without alopecia and bilateral sensorineural hearing loss.

**Clinical Findings:** To date, pili torti, with or without alopecia of scalp and body hair, has been a constant. Eyelashes and eyebrows are unaffected. The hair is twisted when examined microscopically. Sensorineural deafness, when present, has been bilateral and is usually, but not always, congenital.

**Complications:** Delayed speech development.

**Associated Findings:** Crandall et al. (1973) reported three male sibs with hypogonadism as an associated finding to the pili torti and deafness. The boys had originally been reported as having Bjornstad pili torti deafness. The male sibs in the report of Cremers et al. (1979) (their family No. 3) may also have had this

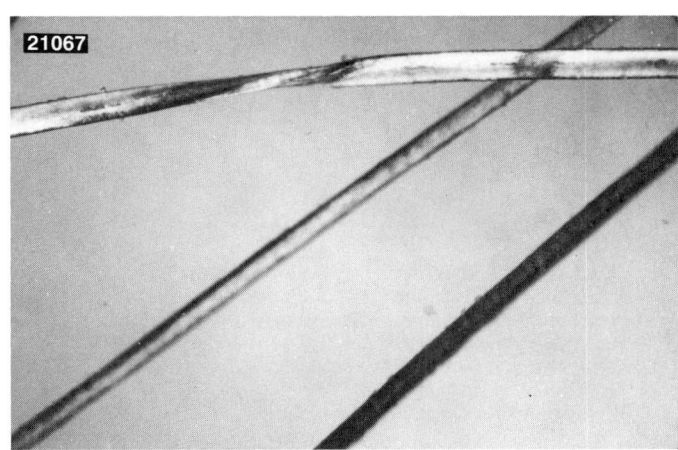

**2015B-21067:** The shaft of the superior hair is microscopically twisted around its own axis.

---

condition. This is likely an autosomal recessive trait, distinct from that reported by Bjornstad.

**Etiology:** Autosomal dominant inheritance in one form. The entity may be heterogeneous. In Bjornstad's (1965) report, only three of five affected individuals had positive family history; an aunt in one case and one sib each in two others. Reed et al. (1967) reported an affected mother and son. Cremers et al. (1979) reported two families, each with four generations of affected individuals. However, only two of 14 were deaf; 11 of 14 were female. The pedigrees were not complete enough to determine whether X-linked dominant inheritance was a possibility.

**Pathogenesis:** Unknown. Other than twisting, no other hair abnormality has been described.

**MIM No.:** 26200

**POS No.:** 3038

**Sex Ratio:** M1:F4

**Occurrence:** About 25 cases in less than a half-dozen families have been reported.

**Risk of Recurrence for Patient's Sib:** Unknown. May be as high as 50%, depending upon etiology.

**Risk of Recurrence for Patient's Child:** Unknown. May be as high as 50%, depending upon etiology.

**Age of Detectability:** Usually by the second year of life.

**Gene Mapping and Linkage:** Unknown.

**Prevention:** None known. Genetic counseling indicated.

**Treatment:** Unknown.

**Prognosis:** Life span and intellect are apparently not impaired.

**Detection of Carrier:** Deafness is not always present. Carriers with normal hearing can be detected by examination of the hair for the characteristic twisting.

**References:**
Bjornstad RT: Pili torti and sensory-neural loss of hearing. Proceedings of the Seventh Meeting of the Northern Dermatological Society. Copenhagen: Northern Dermatological Society, 1965:1–10.
Reed WB, et al.: Hereditary syndromes with auditory and dermatological manifestations. Arch Dermatol 1967; 95:456–461.
Robinson GC, Johnston MM: Pili torti and sensory neural hearing loss. J Pediatr 1967; 70:621–623.
Crandall BF, et al.: A familial syndrome of deafness, alopecia, and hypogonadism. J Pediatr 1973; 82:461–465. *
Cremers CWRJ, Geerts SJ: Sensorineuronal hearing loss and pili torti. Ann Otol Rhinol Laryngol 1979; 88:100–104. *

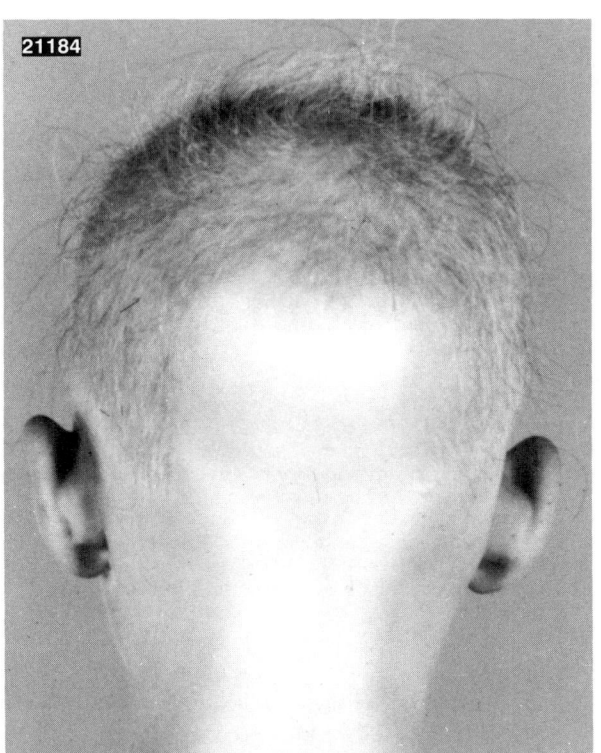

**2015A-21184:** 11-year-old boy with sensorineural deafness and pili torti.

T0007                                          **Helga V. Toriello**

## DEAFNESS-POLYNEUROPATHY-OPTIC ATROPHY     0268

**Includes:**
> Charcot-Marie-Tooth disease with optico-acoustic degeneration
> Optic atrophy-nerve deafness-distal neurogenic amyotrophy
> Polyneuropathy-deafness-optic atrophy
> Rosenberg-Chutorian syndrome

**Excludes:**
> **Deafness-optic nerve atrophy, progressive** (0253)
> **Diabetes (insipidus/mellitus)-optic atrophy-deafness** (0550)
> **Neuropathy, hereditary motor and sensory, type I** (2104)
> **Neuropathy, hereditary motor and sensory, type II** (2105)
> **Optic atrophy, infantile heredofamilial** (0755)
> **Optic atrophy, Leber type** (0579)
> **Phytanic acid storage disease** (0810)

**Major Diagnostic Criteria:** Sensorineural deafness, polyneuropathy, and optic atrophy.

**Clinical Findings:** Five patients in two families have been described with this symptom complex: in one family, two brothers and their nephew (son of sister); in another family, a brother and sister. Three patients presented in infancy with hearing loss, and two cases manifested at age 8 years with hand deformity (ulnar deviation, muscle weakness, and wasting). Bilateral optic atrophy, especially temporal sided, resulting in loss of visual acuity beginning with nyctalopia, was seen in four of five; bilateral sensorineural hearing loss was seen in all five; dysarthria or rhinolalia in four of five. Gait was deteriorated (broad-based, ataxic) in four of five. Distal amyotrophy of the upper limbs was seen in four of five and of the lower limbs in three of five. Distal sensory impairment was reported in three of five; peripheral nerve conduction velocity was lowered in three of five. Muscle biopsy showed features of neurogenic atrophy in two of five; this was also revealed by electromyogram in two of five. Demyelination was seen in sural nerve biopsy in two of five. Bone deformity, including tarsal bone, chest, and spine (scoliosis), occurred in three of five. All patients had normal intelligence.

**Complications:** The impaired speech may be secondary to deafness. Bone deformities may be due to muscle atrophy.

**Associated Findings:** Communication handicaps occur, which influence school performance.

**Etiology:** Autosomal recessive inheritance is likely in the sib pair described by Iwashita et al. (1970). Inheritance may be X-linked recessive in the family reported by Rosenberg and Chutorian (1967). Genetic heterogeneity probably exists.

**Pathogenesis:** The loss of visual acuity and the hearing loss are caused by optic and acoustic nerve degeneration. The optic atrophy is believed to be due to retrobulbar neuritis. The amyotrophy may be due to motor neuron disease.

**MIM No.:** 25865, 31107

**POS No.:** 3196

**Sex Ratio:** M4:F1 (observed)

**Occurrence:** At least five patients from two families have been described.

**Risk of Recurrence for Patient's Sib:**
> See Part I, *Mendelian Inheritance.*

**Risk of Recurrence for Patient's Child:**
> See Part I, *Mendelian Inheritance.*

**Age of Detectability:** In early infancy if auditory brainstem testing and acoustic reflex testing are done.

**Gene Mapping and Linkage:** Unknown.

**Prevention:** None known. Genetic counseling indicated.

**Treatment:** A hearing aid may be of help. Special instruction will be needed. Support by cane, braces, and special shoes.

**Prognosis:** Poor for vision and hearing because of the progressive nature of the syndrome.

**Detection of Carrier:** Unknown.

**Special Considerations:** The two described families are similar but not identical. It is difficult to be sure about the exact nosologic classification of this condition. These two families differ in the following areas: *1) Age of onset and severity of deafness.* The Rosenberg and Chutorian cases have onset in early childhood and progress to profound deafness by age 5 years. Iwashita's cases have onset around puberty and result in a moderate loss. *2) Nerve conduction velocities.* The velocities are abnormal for Iwashita's cases, but normal for the family reported by Rosenberg and Chutorian.

**References:**
Rosenberg RN, Chutorian A: Familial optico-acoustic nerve degeneration and polyneuropathy. Neurology 1967; 17:827–832.
Iwashita H, et al.: Optic atrophy, neural deafness and distal neurogenic amyotrophy. Arch Neurol 1970; 22:357–364.
Konigsmark BW, Gorlin RJ: Optic atrophy, polyneuropathy and sensorineural deafness. In: Genetic and metabolic deafness. Philadelphia: W.B. Saunders, 1976:108–110.
Pauli RM: Sensorineural deafness and peripheral neuropathy. (letter) Clin Genet 1984; 26:383–384.

MI029        **Joyce Mitchell**
*Cor W.R.J. Cremers*

**Deafness-short stature-vitiligo-muscle wasting-achalasia**
> *See DEAFNESS-VITILIGO-MUSCLE WASTING*
**Deafness-stapes fixation**
> *See DEAFNESS WITH PERILYMPHATIC GUSHER*
**Deafness-symphalangism, Herrmann type**
> *See SYMPHALANGISM*

## DEAFNESS-TRIPHALANGEAL THUMBS-ONYCHODYSTROPHY     2151

**Includes:**
> Deafness-onycho-osteo dystrophy
> Onychodystrophy-digital malformation-deafness
> Onycho-osteo dystrophy-deafness
> Triphalangeal thumbs-onychodystrophy and digital malformations

**Excludes:**
> **Deafness-onychodystrophy** (0252)
> **Deafness-onycho-osteo-dystrophy-retardation-seizures (DOORS)** (0262)
> **Onychodystrophy-coniform teeth-sensorineural hearing loss** (2034)
> Ectodermal dysplasia-sensorineural deafness-other anomalies

**Major Diagnostic Criteria:** Sensorineural deafness, dystrophic nails of fingers and toes, abnormally long thumbs with an extra distal phalanx (triphalangeal), and pointed distal phalanges with underdeveloped tufts.

**Clinical Findings:** Absent, rudimentary, or hypoplastic fingernails and toe-nails are noticeable at birth. Thumbs are abnormally long and shaped like fingers. X-rays of the hands show triphalangeal thumbs with an extra small distal phalanx. The distal phalanx of the little finger may be missing. The distal phalanges of the other fingers show underdevelopment of the tufts, giving the phalanges pointed-end appearance. X-rays of the feet may show either absent or underdeveloped distal phalanges. Deafness is recognized a few months after birth; it is bilateral and sensorineural. Individual variability in the expression of deafness and skeletal defects have been observed. No abnormalities of physical growth or mentation have been reported. Teeth and hair are normal. Digital abnormalities are clinically distinct but need to be confirmed by X-ray studies. Tomograms of the petrous pyramids show normal structures of the middle and inner ears. Dermatoglyphics were not reported.

**Complications:** Profound deafness leading to mutism.

**Associated Findings:** None known.

**Etiology:** In two families reported thus far, mother and son pairs were affected; in one, the mother was more mildly affected than her son. Although an autosomal dominant inheritance has been proposed, X-linked dominant inheritance cannot be ruled out until further observations become available.

**Pathogenesis:** An ectodermal defect could explain the coexistence of auditory and nail abnormalities.

**MIM No.:** *22050

**Sex Ratio:** Presumably M1:F1

**Occurrence:** Undetermined but presumed rare.

**Risk of Recurrence for Patient's Sib:**
See Part I, *Mendelian Inheritance.*

**Risk of Recurrence for Patient's Child:**
See Part I, *Mendelian Inheritance.*

**Age of Detectability:** Long, abnormal thumbs and dystrophic nails could be noted soon after birth, leading to suspicion of the condition. X-ray evidence could also be obtained. Hearing problem can be detected before six months of age.

**Gene Mapping and Linkage:** Unknown.

**Prevention:** None known. Genetic counseling indicated.

**Treatment:** Habitation treatment for deafness and supportive educational measures.

**Prognosis:** Normal for life span, intelligence, and fertility. Early recognition of the condition by skeletal and nail abnormalities may lead to earlier intervention in speech training.

**Detection of Carrier:** Clinical examination of first degree relatives.

**Special Considerations:** This condition is frequently confused with **Deafness-onycho-osteo-dystrophy-retardation-seizures (DOORS)**.

**References:**
Goodman RH, et al.: Hereditary congenital deafness with onychodystrophy. Arch Otolaryngol 1969; 90:474–477. * †
Moghadam H, Statten P: Hereditary sensorineural hearing loss with onychodystrophy. Canad Med Assoc J 1972; 107:310–312.

QA000                                            **Qutub H. Qazi**

**Deafness-urticaria-amyloidosis**
*See URTICARIA-DEAFNESS-AMYLOIDOSIS*

---

**DEAFNESS-VITILIGO-MUSCLE WASTING                 0275**

**Includes:**
Deafness-short stature-vitiligo-muscle wasting-achalasia
Muscle wasting-deafness-vitiligo
Rozycki syndrome
Vitiligo-deafness-muscle wasting

**Excludes:**
**Esophagus, achalasia** (0363)
**Oto-oculo-musculo-skeletal syndrome** (0785)

**Major Diagnostic Criteria:** Deafness, vitiligo, muscle wasting, achalasia.

**Clinical Findings:** Two children, a boy and a girl, in a family with a consanguineous marriage and sporadic deafness in another part of the family, have been described with the features of this syndrome. The initial manifestation was early childhood deafness. In both sibs there was sensorineural hearing loss > 100 db. The achalasia was the cause of frequent vomiting and difficulty in swallowing. Depigmented areas of vitiligo were present on their necks and torsos. Marked muscle wasting was noted in the hands, feet, and legs. Short stature was present only in the boy. Morphologic studies of a biopsy of the boy's anterior tibialis muscle revealed typical groups of small fibers indicative of a neuropathic process. Electromyographic studies performed on both patients were indicative of a neuropathic process with additional evidence of myopathy. Changes in EEG, globulin levels, thymol turbidity test, and cephalin-cholesterol flocculation were found. The dermatoglyphics revealed a rare radial loop on R2 of the boy and on R4 of the girl.

**Complications:** Failure to thrive and recurrent pneumonia due to achalasia.

**Associated Findings:** None known.

**Etiology:** Probably autosomal recessive inheritance.

**Pathogenesis:** Unknown.

**MIM No.:** *22135

**POS No.:** 3855

**Sex Ratio:** M1:F1 (observed)

**Occurrence:** One reported family with two affected sibs. McKusick (1973) has reported on related conditions.

**Risk of Recurrence for Patient's Sib:**
See Part I, *Mendelian Inheritance.*

**Risk of Recurrence for Patient's Child:**
See Part I, *Mendelian Inheritance.*

**Age of Detectability:** Early childhood.

**Gene Mapping and Linkage:** Unknown.

**Prevention:** None known. Genetic counseling indicated.

**Treatment:** Esophageal dilation by dilatator or surgical intervention to relieve esophageal obstruction. A hearing aid and special education at a school for the deaf.

**Prognosis:** Unknown.

**Detection of Carrier:** Unknown.

**References:**
Rozycki DL, et al.: Autosomal recessive deafness, associated with short stature, vitiligo, muscle wasting and achalasia. Arch Otolaryngol 1971; 93:194–197.
McKusick VA: Congenital deafness and Hirschsprung's disease. (letter). New Engl J Med 1973; 288:691 (only).

SH046                                          **Kathleen Shaver**
                                             *Cor W.R.J. Cremers*

**Debrancher deficiency**
*See GLYCOGENOSIS, TYPE III*
**Deciduous skin, idiopathic**
*See SKIN PEELING SYNDROME*
**Deficiencies of B**
*See COMPLEMENT COMPONENT, ALTERNATIVE PATHWAYS, DEFICIENCIES OF*
**Deficiencies of C3**
*See COMPLEMENT COMPONENT, ALTERNATIVE PATHWAYS, DEFICIENCIES OF*
**Deficiencies of C5**
*See COMPLEMENT COMPONENT, ALTERNATIVE PATHWAYS, DEFICIENCIES OF*
**Deficiencies of C6**
*See COMPLEMENT COMPONENT, ALTERNATIVE PATHWAYS, DEFICIENCIES OF*
**Deficiencies of C7**
*See COMPLEMENT COMPONENT, ALTERNATIVE PATHWAYS, DEFICIENCIES OF*
**Deficiencies of C8**
*See COMPLEMENT COMPONENT, ALTERNATIVE PATHWAYS, DEFICIENCIES OF*
**Deficiencies of C9**
*See COMPLEMENT COMPONENT, ALTERNATIVE PATHWAYS, DEFICIENCIES OF*
**Deficiencies of D**
*See COMPLEMENT COMPONENT, ALTERNATIVE PATHWAYS, DEFICIENCIES OF*
**Deficiencies of H**
*See COMPLEMENT COMPONENT, ALTERNATIVE PATHWAYS, DEFICIENCIES OF*
**Deficiencies of I**
*See COMPLEMENT COMPONENT, ALTERNATIVE PATHWAYS, DEFICIENCIES OF*
**Deficiencies of P**
*See COMPLEMENT COMPONENT, ALTERNATIVE PATHWAYS, DEFICIENCIES OF*
**Deficiency of ATP:AMP phosphotransferase (E.C.2.7.4.3)**
*See ANEMIA, ADENYLATE KINASE DEFICIENCY*

**Deficiency of radial rays and radius and phocomelia**
*See RADIAL DEFECTS*
**Dehydrogenase deficiency, glucose-6-phosphate**
*See GLUCOSE-6-PHOSPHATE DEHYDROGENASE DEFICIENCY*
**Deiodinase deficiency**
*See THYROID, IODOTYROSINE DEIODINASE DEFICIENCY*

## DEJERINE-SOTTAS DISEASE                    2054

**Includes:**
   Hereditary motor sensory neuropathy (HMSN), type III
   Hypertrophic interstitial neuropathy of Dejerine-Sottas
   Neuropathy, motor sensory, hereditary
   Onion bulb neuropathy
   Progressive hypertrophic interstitial neuritis of childhood

**Excludes:**
   **Cerebro-hepato-renal syndrome** (0139)
   **Leukodystrophy, globoid cell type** (0415)
   **Metachromatic leukodystrophies** (0651)
   **Myopathies** (1500)
   **Neuropathy, hereditary motor and sensory, type I** (2104)
   **Phytanic acid storage disease** (0810)
   **Polymyositis, infantile**
   **Spinal muscular atrophy** (0895)

**Major Diagnostic Criteria:** Childhood onset of subnormal to much-delayed motor development with gradually progressive hypotonia, distal weakness, areflexia, stocking-glove sensory loss, palpable enlargement of peripheral nerves, and atrophy affecting the lower extremities before the upper extremities. Cranial nerve involvement is variable and never the predominant feature. Laboratory findings include elevated cerebrospinal fluid (CSF) protein, markedly slowed nerve conduction velocities, and onion bulb formation detected by nerve biopsy.

**Clinical Findings:** The onset of the disease in classic cases is prior to age 30 years and, as described by Dyck et al. (1984), usually begins in infancy. Cases of adult onset reported in the literature prior to studies with nerve conduction velocities of both probands and their families may have been improperly diagnosed HMSN type I. Typically, walking is delayed up to age 48 months or more, and affected children are often never able to run, jump, or skip. Gradually, hand function becomes impaired, with weakness and atrophy in the upper and lower extremities. Muscle cramping may occur, and fasciculations are seen in up to one-third of the patients. Early in the course the atrophy may be asymmetric, with delays of three to four years noted between onset of symptoms in one upper extremity versus the other. Although all three of Dejerine's patients had facial nerve involvement, cranial nerve deficit is never a prominent feature. In infancy bulbar involvement may predispose to aspiration pneumonia, but generally swallowing and rectovesical sphincter control are well preserved. Cranial nerve deficits overall are reported in 15% of patients. Additionally, pupillary abnormalities, including miosis, sluggish constriction to light, and Argyll-Robertson pupils, are found in greater than 25% of patients. Deep tendon reflexes are either markedly decreased or absent, and plantar responses are flexor unless there is a myelopathy secondary to spinal cord compression from hypertrophic nerve roots or from gross spinal deformity. Abdominal and cremasteric reflexes are likewise sluggish or absent.

Sensory loss is usual but is rarely the presenting complaint. Commonly, the distal extremities are most affected, with vibratory, joint position, and touch-pressure sensations primarily involved. The Romberg sign is usually positive. Although Dyck et al. (1984) noted no loss of pain or temperature discrimination, other authors have found these sensations to be mildly impaired. Extremity pains described variously as shooting, sharp to dull, and aching are reported in 25% of patients.

Ataxia and intention tremor have been reported in 15–20% of patients, although it may be difficult to decide whether they are due to weakness or to impaired cerebellar function. Scanning speech, nystagmus, and impaired check and rebound responses have been seen. When found in association with ataxia and tremor, these features suggest cerebellar dysfunction. Some peripheral nerves are enlarged such that they are readily palpable or visible, especially the great auricular, sural, median, and ulnar nerves. However, nerves may not be palpable in affected younger children or in obese individuals.

Blood and CSF laboratory tests are normal except for elevated CSF protein. Nerve conduction velocities are markedly slowed. Auditory evoked potentials were abnormal in two cases. Nerve biopsy material reveals extensive hypomyelination, demyelination, and remyelination of peripheral nerves with onion bulb formation composed of cytoplasmic processes of interdigitating Schwann cells, which are separated by longitudinally oriented collagen fibers. The nerve appears gelatinous on cross section with interstitial metachromasia. Demyelination is periaxial, discontinuous, and segmental, with abnormal variability in the ratio of axis cylinder diameter to total fiber diameter and in the frequency distribution of myelinated fibers. Once thought to be pathognomonic for Dejerine-Sottas disease, onion bulbs are now known to be associated with any disease process involving repetitive segmental demyelination and remyelination, and they have been produced experimentally by such maneuvers as administration of lead salts and repeated application of tourniquets to nerves.

**Complications:** Skeletal deformities are common, with greater than 30% having foot deformities, most commonly pes cavus, and greater than 20% having kyphoscoliosis, sometimes quite severe. Clubfeet or clawing of the hands or feet has also been described. The most severely affected patients become wheelchair bound, and fine finger manipulations such as turning a key or holding eating and writing utensils may become impossible. Spinal cord compression caused by enlarged nerve roots has been demonstrated by myelography in seven patients.

**Associated Findings:** Early bilateral cataracts were reported in three Hindu sisters.

**Etiology:** Autosomal recessive inheritance. Kinships previously reported as autosomal dominant probably represent **Neuropathy, hereditary motor and sensory, type I**.

**Pathogenesis:** Because Dejerine-Sottas disease is inherited and because it has a similar pathology as is seen in **Phytanic acid storage disease**, it has been assumed that the pathogenesis is a metabolic abnormality, perhaps of the Schwann cells, resulting in defective myelin synthesis. Analysis of sural nerve and liver revealed a possible systemic disorder of cerebroside sulfate metabolism. In addition, an abnormality of axonal flow of dopamine-$\beta$-hydroxylase in sural nerve has been demonstrated, suggesting that axis cylinders may be primarily involved in the disease process. It currently is not known if the demyelination is secondary to neuronal atrophy or whether it represents concomitant Schwann cell metabolic aberration.

**MIM No.:** *14590

**Sex Ratio:** M1:F1

**Occurrence:** Because of varying diagnostic criteria and the tendency in the past by some authors to classify any patient with nerve hypertrophy or onion bulbs as having Dejerine-Sottas disease, its true incidence is unclear. Preliminary studies suggest a prevalence of about 8:1,000,000.

**Risk of Recurrence for Patient's Sib:**
   See Part I, *Mendelian Inheritance.*

**Risk of Recurrence for Patient's Child:**
   See Part I, *Mendelian Inheritance.*

**Age of Detectability:** During childhood.

**Gene Mapping and Linkage:** Unknown.

**Prevention:** None known. Genetic counseling indicated.

**Treatment:** Treatment is symptomatic, including optimal nutrition, prompt treatment of infections, physical therapy, and appropriate use of orthotic devices. Patients should be counseled to avoid postures that promote pressure neuropathy. Quinine sulfate may provide relief of nocturnal cramping. Spinal examinations to detect scoliosis need to be performed regularly. For the patient with evidence of a radiculopathy or myelopathy, laminectomy with decompression of hypertrophic nerve roots may be indicated.

**Prognosis:** The clinical course is usually one of slow progression, with resultant gait abnormalities or confinement to a wheelchair in the third or later decades. Predicted degree of disability may best be estimated by extrapolating from the course of each individual patient and affected relatives, if any. With attentive chronic care, life span may be only minimally altered. More severely affected individuals are eventually both wheelchair bound and limited in upper extremity function. The most severely affected patient described by Dejerine and Sottas lived for 31 years after becoming symptomatic. Intelligence remains normal.

**Detection of Carrier:** Careful physical examination, electromyography with nerve conduction velocities, and nerve biopsy can help detect individuals, including sibs, who are only mildly affected.

**References:**
Austin JH: Observations on the syndrome of hypertrophic neuritis (the hypertrophic interstitial radiculo-neuropathies). Medicine 1956; 35:187–237. *
O'Brien MD: Hypertrophic neuropathy: a report of Dejerine-Sottas disease in two sibs. Guy's Hosp Rep 1968; 117:79–87.
Pleasure DE, Towfighi J: Onion bulb neuropathies. Arch Neurol 1972; 26:289–301.
Carlin L, et al.: Hypertrophic neuropathy with spinal cord compression. Surg Neurol 1982; 18:237–240.
Dyck PJ, et al., eds: Peripheral neuropathy. Philadelphia: W.B. Saunders, 1984. *

GR034
KA008

**May L. Griebel**
**Raymond S. Kandt**

**Del Castillo syndrome**
*See GERM CELL APLASIA*
**Delayed development-cutis laxa**
*See CUTIS LAXA-DELAYED DEVELOPMENT-LIGAMENTOUS LAXITY*
**Delayed development-cutis laxa-ligamentous laxity**
*See CUTIS LAXA-DELAYED DEVELOPMENT-LIGAMENTOUS LAXITY*
**Delleman-Oorthuys syndrome**
*See OCULO-CEREBRO-CUTANEOUS SYNDROME*
**Delta phalanx**
*See THUMB, TRIPHALANGEAL*
**Delta-1-Pyrroline-5-carboxylate dehydrogenase deficiency**
*See HYPERPROLINEMIA*

## DELTA-AMINOLEVULINIC ACID DEHYDRASE DEFICIENCY     3091

**Includes:**
    Lead poisoning, susceptibility to
    Porphobilinogen synthase partial deficiency
    Porphyria, acute hepatic

**Excludes:**
    Delta-aminolevulinate dehydrase deficiency of lead poisoning
    **Porphyria, acute intermittent** (0820)
    Porphyria of homozygous porphobilinogen synthase deficiency
    **Tyrosinemia**

**Major Diagnostic Criteria:** Diagnosis is established by finding diminished erythrocyte levels of delta-aminolevulinate dehydrase; the normal mean is about 2.5 $\mu$mole of porphobilinogen formed per milliliter of erthrocytes per hour. The test must be interpreted cautiously because of a reported fourfold variation in control values.

**Clinical Findings:** The heterozygous state is not accompanied by pathologic symptoms; the oldest reported individual was 68 years old. The homozygous state is a recessive form of **Porphyria, acute intermittent** and is a clinically separate entity.

**Complications:** The condition is benign, but there is increased sensitivity to lead poisoning.

**Associated Findings:** One of ten reported biochemically affected individuals had iron deficiency anemia. Her enzyme activity was

the highest of the ten, presumably because of less heme feedback inhibition. The other nine individuals were healthy.

**Etiology:** Autosomal dominant inheritance.

**Pathogenesis:** There is no pathologic presentation. There are normal levels of both precursors and products of the enzyme.

**MIM No.:** *12527

**Sex Ratio:** M1:F1

**Occurrence:** One family with ten affected individuals in three generations has been reported. Because of the benign character of this partial enzyme deficiency, its discovery is serendipitous, and the occurrence is undoubtedly underestimated.

**Risk of Recurrence for Patient's Sib:**
See Part I, *Mendelian Inheritance.*

**Risk of Recurrence for Patient's Child:**
See Part I, *Mendelian Inheritance.*

**Age of Detectability:** This partial deficiency can be detected during the first year of life, assuming there are adequately age-matched controls.

**Gene Mapping and Linkage:** ALAD (aminolevulinate, delta-, dehydratase) has been mapped to 9q34.
The diminished enzyme activity may involve a regulatory and not structural gene.

**Prevention:** None known. Genetic counseling indicated. Avoiding lead exposure prevents environmental exacerbations.

**Treatment:** No treatment is necessary in the absence of lead exposure.

**Prognosis:** Excellent.

**Detection of Carrier:** The benign condition described here is the carrier state.

**Special Considerations:** Moderate lead exposure may result in severe poisoning, because lead inhibits delta-aminolevulinic dehydrase activity. Lead replaces the zinc cofactor, which stabilizes the sulfhydryl groups under aerobic conditions. The enzyme is also inhibited by a substrate analog, succinyl acetone, a metabolite accumulating in patients with tyrosinemia.
The homozygous deficiency has been reported in two families with **Porphyria, acute intermittent**.

**References:**
Bird TD, et al.: Inherited deficiency of delta-aminolevulinic acid dehydratase. Am J Hum Genet 1979; 31:662–668.
Doss M, et al.: New type of hepatic porphyria with porphobilinogen synthase defect and intermittent acute clinical manifestation. Klin Wochenschr 1979; 57:1123–1127.
Doss M, et al.: Acute hepatic porphyria syndrome with porphobilinogen synthase defect. Int J Biochem 1980; 12:823–826.
Doss M, Müller WA: Acute lead poisoning in inherited porphobilinogen synthase (delta-aminolevulinic acid dehydrase) deficiency. Blut 1982; 45:131–139.
Eiberg H, et al.: Delta-aminolevulinatedehydratase: synteny with ABO-AK1-ORM (and assignment to chromosome 9). Clin Genet 1983; 23:150–154.
Beaumont C, et al.: Assignment of the human gene for delta-aminolevulinate dehydrase to chromosome 9 by somatic cell hybridization and specific enzyme immunoassay. Ann Hum Genet 1984; 48(Pt 2):153–159.
Wang A-L, et al.; Delta-aminolevulinate dehydratase: induced expression and regional assignment of the human gene to chromosome 9q13-qter. Hum Genet 1985; 70:6–10.

VI006

**Jaclyn M. Vidgoff**

**Delta-storage pool disease**
*See ALBINISM, OCULOCUTANEOUS, HERMANSKY-PUDLAK TYPE*
**Dementia (progressive)-lipomembranous polycystic osteodysplasia**
*See OSTEODYSPLASIA, LIPOMEMBRANOUS POLYCYSTIC-DEMENTIA*
**Dementia-lobar atrophy and neuronal cytoplasmic inclusions**
*See PICK DISEASE OF THE BRAIN*
**DeMorsier dysplasia olfactogenitalis**
*See KALLMANN SYNDROME*

**Demyelinating disease**
  See MULTIPLE SCLEROSIS, FAMILIAL
**Dens invaginatus**
  See TEETH, DENS INVAGINATUS
**Dens telescopes**
  See TEETH, DENS INVAGINATUS
**Dental and bone defects**
  See SINGLETON-MERTEN SYNDROME
**Dental ankylosis**
  See TEETH, MOLAR REINCLUSION
**Dental defects-trichodermodysplasia**
  See TRICHO-DERMODYSPLASIA-DENTAL DEFECTS
**Dental eruption, arrested**
  See TEETH, ANKYLODONTIA, MULTIPLE HERITABLE TYPE
**Dental lamina cyst**
  See MUCOSA, ORAL INCLUSION CYSTS OF THE NEWBORN
**Dental-cataract-oto-brachydactyly defects**
  See CATARACTS-OTO-DENTAL DEFECTS
**Dentatorubral-pallidoluysian atrophy**
  See DENTATORUBROPALLIDOLUYSIAN DEGENERATION,
  HEREDITARY

## DENTATORUBROPALLIDOLUYSIAN DEGENERATION, HEREDITARY      3283

**Includes:**
  Dentatorubral-pallidoluysian atrophy
  Epilepsy, familial myoclonus-choreoathetosis
  Naito-Oyanagi disease

**Excludes:**
  Dentatorubropallidoluysian degeneration (atrophy),
    sporadic
  Dyssynergia cerebellaris myoclonica (dentatorubral atrophy)
  **Huntington disease** (0478)
  **Machado-Joseph disease** (2996)
  **Mucolipidosis I** (0671)
  **Myoclonic epilepsy-ragged red fibers** (3225)
  **Neuronal ceroid-lipofuscinoses (NCL)** (0713)
  Olivopontocerebellar atrophy
  Progressive pallidal atrophy
  **Seizures, progressive myoclonic, Lafora type** (2601)
  **Seizures, progressive myoclonic, Unverricht-Lundborg type**
    (2602)

**Major Diagnostic Criteria:** Myoclonus epilepsy with dementia (myoclonus-epilepsy syndrome), sometimes associated with choreoathetosis and/or cerebellar ataxia. Combined degeneration of the dentatorubral and pallidoluysian systems.

**Clinical Findings:** Onset is often with an ataxic gait and slurred speech in the typical adult patient. Younger patients, however, tend to have seizures and early dementia as the beginning symptoms.
  Major signs include dementia, dysarthria, and gait and limb ataxia, present in most patients. These are followed, in order of frequency, by mild to moderate pyramidal signs, myoclonus and opsoclonus, convulsions, and choreoathetosis.
  EEG has been abnormal, with spike-wave complexes, in all patients tested with onset under age 20 years. EEG tends to be normal in patients with later onset. CT scan may show atrophy of the brain stem and cerebellum with ventricular dilatation and occasional focal or diffuse lesions of the white matter.
  Expression is highly variable and depends on the age of onset. Younger patients tend to present the myoclonus-epilepsy syndrome. Patients with onset in late adult life show cerebellar ataxia and choreoathetosis, often without myoclonus and/or epilepsy.

**Complications:** Younger patients may die in status epilepticus. Bronchopneumonia is a complication of dysphagia and the cause of death in some patients.

**Associated Findings:** Nystagmus. Abnormal eye movements (slow horizontal saccades and saccadic pursuit, horizontal nystagmus on lateral gaze, limitation of vertical gaze, and impaired convergence) have been reported.

**Etiology:** Autosomal dominant inheritance with incomplete penetrance. A few asymptomatic (obligate) carriers have been reported.

**Pathogenesis:** Unknown.

**MIM No.:** *12537

**Sex Ratio:** Presumably M1:F1.

**Occurrence:** More than 25 Japanese kindreds have been documented, including 28 autopsied cases, have been reported.

**Risk of Recurrence for Patient's Sib:**
  See Part I, *Mendelian Inheritance.*

**Risk of Recurrence for Patient's Child:**
  See Part I, *Mendelian Inheritance.*

**Age of Detectability:** Onset ranges from three to 69 years of age, with a mean of 30.3 years.

**Gene Mapping and Linkage:** Unknown.

**Prevention:** None known. Genetic counseling indicated.

**Treatment:** No treatment has been able to affect progression or prognosis.

**Prognosis:** Variable but usually poor. Age at time of death has ranged from 20–77 years of age, with a mean of 41.4 years.

**Detection of Carrier:** Unknown.

**References:**
Titeca J, Van Bogaert L: Heredo-degenerative hemiballismus: a contribution to the question of primary atrophy of the Corpus Luysii. Brain 1946; 69:251–263.
Kobayashi H, et al.: An autopsy case of the characteristic degeneration of the dentate nucleus with choreic movement and psychic symptoms. Clin Neurol (Tokyo) 1975; 15:724–730.
Oyanagi S, et al.: A neuropathological study of 8 autopsy cases of degenerative type of myoclonus epilepsy, with special reference to latent combination of degeneration of the pallido-luysian system. Adv Neurol Sci 1976; 20:410–424.
Tanaka Y, et al.: Combined degeneration of the globus pallidus and the cerebellar nuclei and their efferent systems in two siblings of one family. Brain Nerve (Tokyo) 1977; 29:95–104.
Iizuka R, et al.: A clinico-pathological observation on spino-cerebellar degeneration. Adv Neurol Sci 1978; 22:1267–1280.
Takahata N, et al.: Familial chorea and myoclonus epilepsy. Neurology 1978; 28:913–919.
Goto I, et al.: Dentatorubropallidoluysian degeneration. Neurology 1982; 32:1395–1399.
Naito H, Oyanagi S: Familial myoclonus epilepsy and choreoathetosis: hereditary dentatorubral-pallidoluysian atrophy. Neurology 1982; 32:798–807. * †
Iwabuchi K, et al.: Two familial cases of DRPLA with pseudo-Huntington's chorea. Clin Neurol (Tokyo) 1985; 25:1052–1060.
Nakano T, et al.: An autopsy case of DRPLA clinically diagnosed as Huntington's chorea. Brain Nerve (Tokyo) 1985; 37:767–774.
Akashi T, et al.: Dentatorubro-pallidoluysian atrophy: a cliniconeuro-pathological study. Clin Psychiat (Japan) 1987; 16:1163–1172.

SE020                    **Jorge Sequeiros**
YU004                   **Tatsuhiko Yuasa**

**Dentes incluses**
  See TEETH, IMPACTED
**Dentin dysplasia type III**
  See TEETH, ODONTOBLASTIC DYSPLASIA, FOCAL
**Dentin dysplasia, coronal**
  See TEETH, DENTIN DYSPLASIA, CORONAL
**Dentin dysplasia, radicular**
  See TEETH, DENTIN DYSPLASIA, RADICULAR
**Dentin dysplasia, type I**
  See TEETH, DENTIN DYSPLASIA, RADICULAR
**Dentin dysplasia, type II**
  See TEETH, DENTIN DYSPLASIA, CORONAL
**Dentin dysplasia-sclerotic bone/skeletal anomalies**
  See DENTINO-OSSEOUS DYSPLASIA

## DENTINO-OSSEOUS DYSPLASIA 0280

**Includes:** Dentin dysplasia-sclerotic bone/skeletal anomalies
**Excludes:**
**Branchio-skeleto-genital syndrome** (0118)
Calcinosis
**Ehlers-Danlos syndrome** (0338)
Fibrous dysplasia of dentin
**Osteogenesis imperfecta** (0777)
**Teeth, dentin dysplasia, coronal** (0277)
**Teeth, dentin dysplasia, radicular** (0278)
**Teeth, dentinogenesis imperfecta** (0279)

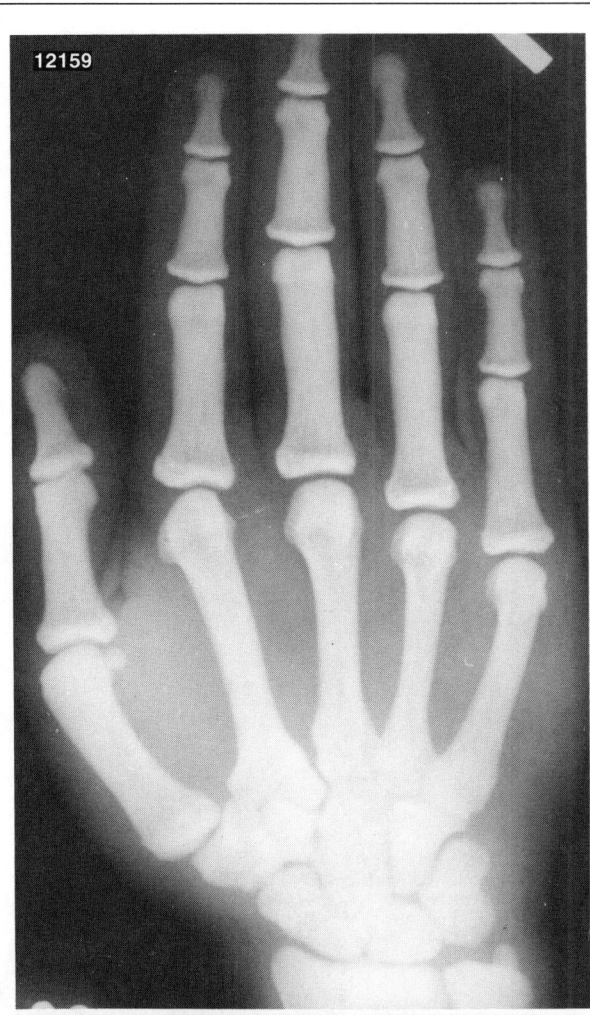

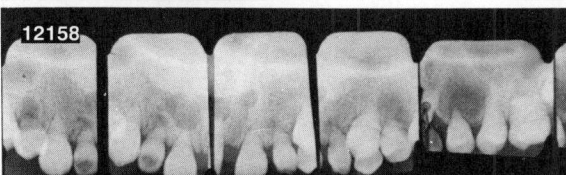

**0280-12159:** Hand X-ray of 13-year-old female shows carpal bones with dense mineralization; the metacarpal bones have thickened cortical bones with narrowing of the medullary space; the epiphyseal spaces are closed in the metacarpals prematurely. **12158:** Dental changes are characteristic of dentin dysplasia, radicular type.

**Teeth, odontodysplasia** (0739)

**Major Diagnostic Criteria:** Teeth with short roots, normal-colored crowns, obliteration of pulp chambers, and thickened, dense cortices of long bones.

**Clinical Findings:** Both dentitions are affected with dentin dysplasia, radicular type, in which the teeth are of normal color and by X-ray show short abnormal roots, lack pulp chambers or have small demilune-shaped pulp chambers and numerous periapical radiolucencies. These latter lesions are areas of granulation tissue. In addition, all affected patients have dense, thickened cortical layers of bone, affecting primarily the long bones; fine trabecular pattern of medullary bone; calcified epiphyseal disks; abnormalities of carpal bones, with large sesamoid bones in the hand; exostoses of hand and wrist bones; and medial displacement of thumbs.

**Complications:** Spontaneous exfoliation of teeth.

**Associated Findings:** None known.

**Etiology:** Autosomal dominant inheritance.

**Pathogenesis:** Histologically, the teeth are identical with those seen in radicular dentin dysplasia, with pulpal foci of tubular dentin-type denticles surrounded by normal dentin of the radicular sheath. Each denticle is capped by a vascular channel. Epithelial root sheath fragments and invades dental papilla, where mesenchymal cells are stimulated to transform into functional odontoblasts and to lay down foci of dentin that subsequently become incorporated into the dentin of the developing roots.

**MIM No.:** *12544

**POS No.:** 3989

**Sex Ratio:** M1:F1

**Occurrence:** Rare; one large kindred reported.

**Risk of Recurrence for Patient's Sib:**
See Part I, *Mendelian Inheritance.*

**Risk of Recurrence for Patient's Child:**
See Part I, *Mendelian Inheritance.*

**Age of Detectability:** By X-ray examination, at time of eruption of teeth at age 9–18 months.

**Gene Mapping and Linkage:** Unknown.

**Prevention:** None known. Genetic counseling indicated.

**Treatment:** Prosthetic replacement of teeth.

**Prognosis:** Does not appear to decrease life span. Risk for early loss of teeth.

**Detection of Carrier:** Unknown.

**References:**
Morris ME, Augsburger RH: Dentine dysplasia with sclerotic bone and skeletal anomalies inherited as an autosomal dominant trait. a new syndrome. Oral Surg 1977; 43:267–283. * †

M0019
WI043

**Merle E. Morris
Carl J. Witkop, Jr.**

**Dentinogenesis imperfecta, Brandywine type**
*See TEETH, DENTINOGENESIS IMPERFECTA*
**Dentinogenesis imperfecta, Mayflower type**
*See TEETH, DENTINOGENESIS IMPERFECTA*
**Dentinogenesis imperfecta, Shields type II, III**
*See TEETH, DENTINOGENESIS IMPERFECTA*

## DENTO-FACIO-SKELETAL DEFECTS, ACKERMAN TYPE    2093

**Includes:**
Ackerman syndrome
Glaucoma, juvenile-unusual upper lip and dental roots
Molar roots, pyramidal-juvenile glaucoma-unusual upper lip

**Excludes:**
Glaucoma, juvenile
**Knuckle pads-leukonychia-deafness** (0558)

**Major Diagnostic Criteria:** A combination of juvenile glaucoma, decreased body hair, minor facial anomalies (entropion, flat philtrum) and hand anomalies (syndactyly, clinodactyly, fingernail changes) are suggestive of the diagnosis. Although the authors described taurodontism in all affected individuals, this may have been a separate trait in this family.

**Clinical Findings:** In possibly five affected individuals, the following findings were observed: entropion of lower lids (1); glaucoma, juvenile type (2); thickening and widening of the philtrum (1); taurodontism (5); knuckle pads (1); syndactyly, 3rd and 4th fingers and/or 2nd and 3rd toes (2); clinodactyly (1); decreased body hair (3); sensorineural hearing loss (1); and possibly ridging (horizontal) of the fingernails (1).

**Complications:** Unknown.

**Associated Findings:** None known.

**Etiology:** Unknown. Although the taurodontism occurred in an autosomal dominant pattern, only male sibs were reportedly affected with the other anomalies.

**Pathogenesis:** Unknown. Both mesodermal and ectodermal structures are involved.

**MIM No.:** 20097

**Sex Ratio:** M5:F0 (observed).

**Occurrence:** Reported in one family.

**Risk of Recurrence for Patient's Sib:** Unknown.

**Risk of Recurrence for Patient's Child:** Unknown.

**Age of Detectability:** At birth, by physical examination.

**Gene Mapping and Linkage:** Unknown.

**Prevention:** None known. Genetic counseling indicated.

**Treatment:** If indicated, treatment for glaucoma and hearing loss.

**Prognosis:** Life span and intellect appear unimpaired.

**Detection of Carrier:** Unknown.

**Special Considerations:** In the report of the family, both maternal and paternal relatives were affected with taurodontism in an autosomal dominant pattern, whereas only the male siblings had other anomalies. It is therefore unknown whether taurodontism is part of the phenotype autosomal dominant taurodontism and the anomalies present in the boys are separate traits segregating in the family. It may also be possible that the boys are homozygotes for the autosomal dominant taurodontism gene.

**References:**
Ackerman JL, et al.: Taurodont, pyramidal and fused molar roots associated with other anomalies in a kindred. Am J Phys Anthropol 1973; 38:681–694.

T0007                                    **Helga V. Toriello**

**Dento-oculo-osseous dysplasia**
*See OCULO-DENTO-OSSEOUS DYSPLASIA*
**Dentocranioocular syndrome**
*See ACROCEPHALOSYNDACTYLY TYPE III*
**Denys-Drash syndrome**
*See WILMS TUMOR-PSEUDOHERMAPHRODITISM-
GLOMERULOPATHY, DENYS-DRASH TYPE*
**Depakene, fetal effects from**
*See FETAL VALPROATE SYNDROME*
**Depigmentation-gingival fibromatosis-microphthalmia**
*See GINGIVAL FIBROMATOSIS-DEPIGMENTATION-
MICROPHTHALMIA*

**Depressive disorders**
*See MOOD AND THOUGHT DISORDERS*
**Depressor anguli oris muscle, hypoplasia of**
*See CARDIOFACIAL SYNDROME-ASSYMETRIC FACIES*

## DERMAL HYPOPLASIA, FOCAL    0281

**Includes:**
Combined mesoectodermal dysplasia
Ectodermal and mesodermal dysplasia, congenital
Ectodermal and mesodermal dysplasia with osseous involvement
Focal dermal dysplasia syndrome
Focal dermato-phalangeal dysplasia
Goltz-Gorlin syndrome
Goltz syndrome

**Excludes:**
**Incontinentia pigmenti** (0526)
**Nevus, epidermal nevus syndrome** (0593)
**Rothmund-Thomson syndrome** (2037)

**Major Diagnostic Criteria:** Dermal hypoplasia with protrusion of fat; areas of underdevelopment and thinning of the skin, forming reticular, vermiform, cribriform, or sometimes linear streaks.

**Clinical Findings:** Widespread foci of dermal hypoplasia with herniation of fat and red streaking of the skin (100%). Frequent papillomas of the lips, gums, anus, and vulvae; sparsity of hair;

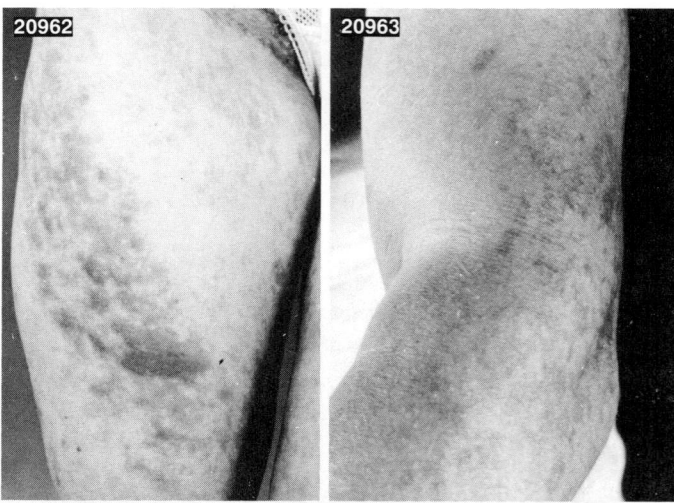

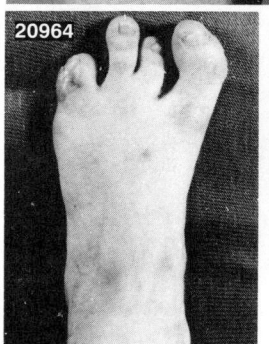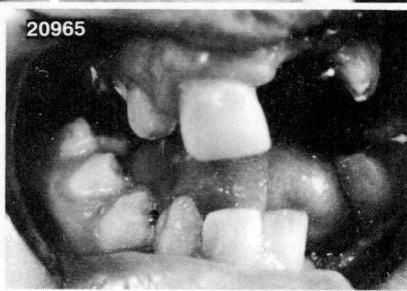

**0281-20962:** Focal dermal hypoplasia showing herniation of fat and skin discoloration. **20963:** Pigmented atrophic lesions on the forearm. **20964:** Irregular size of the toes; this also occurs in the fingers. **20965:** Dental abnormalities and cleft palate.

small stature; asymmetry of face, trunk, and limbs; mental retardation; and a variety of cutaneous, skeletal, ocular, oral, dental, or soft tissue defects as follows.

*Cutaneous abnormalities:* Area of underdevelopment and thinning of the skin; reticular, vermiform, cribriform, frequently linear, localized herniations of subcutaneous fat through the attenuated dermis; total absence of the skin from various sites at birth; linear or reticular areas of hyper- or hypopigmentation of the skin; telangiectasia; and papillomas of the lips, gums, base of tongue, circumoral area, anus, vulvar, inguinal, axillary, and periumbilical skin. There is an initial inflammatory or desquamative phase, with blistering and crusting, urtication, or intense reddening of the skin on stroking. Lichenoid, follicular, hyperkeratotic papules; keratotic lesions on palms and soles; radial folds around the mouth follow. Disorders of sweating (hypo- or hyperhidrosis), especially of palms and soles, occur. Scalp hair is sparse and brittle, and hair may be totally lacking from small areas of the scalp or pubis. Localized poliosis may be present. Fingers and toenails are absent or poorly developed, dystrophic, spooned, grooved, or hypopigmented.

*Skeletal defects:* Small stature; microcrania; rounded skull; pointed chin; thinness and deviation of nasal septum; prognathism; spinal anomalies; kyphosis; scoliosis; fusion and sacralization of vertebrae; spina bifida occulta; anomalies of vertebrae; rudimentary tail; asymmetric development of face, trunk, or limbs; absence of part of limb; deformity of bones; anomalies of hands and feet; hypoplasia or absence of digits; polydactyly; claw hand; split hand; syndactyly; fusion of phalanges; camptodactyly; clinodactyly; valgus deformity; generalized osteoporosis. Characteristic X-ray; and findings include linear striations of long bones ("osteopathia striata") and widening of the symphysis pubis.

*Ocular anomalies:* Anophthalmia; aniridia; wide spacing of eyes; strabismus; nystagmus; heterochromia; blue sclerae; irregularity of pupils; colobomas of iris, choroid, retina, and optic nerve; subluxation of lens; microphthalmia; patchy hypo- or hyperpigmentation of retina; optic atrophy; clouding of cornea or vitreous; ectropion; ptosis; and blockage of tear ducts with epiphora.

*Oral and dental anomalies:* Prognathism, underdevelopment of mandible; overbite; microdontia; dysplasia of teeth; agenesis of teeth; extra incisor; irregular spacing and malocclusion; enamel defects with caries; notching of upper and lower incisors; harelip; high-arched palate; defect in alveolar ridge; median cleft of tongue; double lingual frenulum; hemihypoplasia of tongue; absence of labial sulcus; and hypertrophy of gums. *Soft tissue defects:* Asymmetry of face; notching or underdevelopment of alae nasi; protrusion and asymmetry of ears; hypoplasia of helix; auricular appendage; combined neurosensory and conductive hearing loss; branchial cleft; mental retardation; thenar and hypothenar hypoplasia; diastasis recti; omphalocele; defect in abdominal musculature; hernia; inguinal, umbilical, and rectal prolapse; asymmetry of breast, with lateral displacement of areola; cardiac anomaly (aortic stenosis?) (atrial septal defect with pulmonary hypertension); abnormalities of kidney and ureter; and papilloma of stomach wall.

While some affected individuals have been mentally retarded, others have been notably intelligent. They may be severely handicapped by skeletal deformities and show marked cosmetic deformity because of the cutaneous, ocular, and skeletal anomalies.

**Complications:** Dependent on associated defects.

**Associated Findings:** Mental retardation, epileptiform seizures.

**Etiology:** Presumably X-linked dominant inheritance with lethality in males. Mosaicism is offered as an explanation for linear lesions in the skin and long bones.

**Pathogenesis:** The preponderance of affected girls and the possibility of increased miscarriages in mothers suggest that the syndrome in its fullest expression is lethal in males. The chromosomes of the peripheral blood have been normal in seven reported cases. The hand anomalies suggest that the abnormal development in this condition occurs before the eighth week of gestation, because the digits normally have elongated and separated by that time.

**MIM No.:** *30560

**POS No.:** 3204

**Sex Ratio:** M11:F150 (observed)

**Occurrence:** More than 160 reported cases.

**Risk of Recurrence for Patient's Sib:**
See Part I, *Mendelian Inheritance*. Reports of up to five cases in one sibship; frequent maternal history of abortions, miscarriages, and stillbirths. Father/daughter transmission has been reported.

**Risk of Recurrence for Patient's Child:**
See Part I, *Mendelian Inheritance*.

**Age of Detectability:** At birth.

**Gene Mapping and Linkage:** DHOF (dermal hypoplasia, focal) has been provisionally mapped to X.

**Prevention:** None known. Genetic counseling indicated.

**Treatment:** Ocular, dental, and orthopedic procedures may be indicated.

**Prognosis:** Only risk to life may be from soft tissue defects, especially cardiac and renal. These are uncommon features of this syndrome.

**Detection of Carrier:** Unknown.

**References:**
Goltz RW, et al.: Focal dermal hypoplasia syndrome: a review of the literature and report of two cases. Arch Dermatol 1970; 101:1–11. *
Feinberg A, Menter MA: Focal dermal hypoplasia (Goltz syndrome) in a male: a case report. S Afr Med J 1976; 50:554–555.
Happle R, Lenz W: Striation of bones in focal dermal hypoplasia: manifestation of mosaicism? Br J Dermatol 1977; 96:133–138.
Kunze J, et al.: Diaphragmatic hernia in a female newborn with focal dermal hypoplasia and marked asymmetric malformations (Goltz-Gorlin syndrome). Eur J Pediatr 1979; 64:24–29.
Uitto AU, et al.: Focal dermal hypoplasia: abnormal characteristics of skin fibroblasts in culture. J Invest Dermatol 1980; 75:170–175.
Burgdorf AU, et al.: Focal dermal hypoplasia in a father and daughter. J Am Acad Dermatol 1981; 4:273–277.

G0021                                                   **Robert Goltz**

**Dermal melanocytosis**
    *See NEVUS OF OTA*
**Dermatitis (atopic)-deafness**
    *See DEAFNESS-ATOPIC DERMATITIS*
**Dermatitis, congenital erosive and vesicular**
    *See ALOPECIA-SKIN ATROPHY-ANONYCHIA-TONGUE DEFECT*

---

## DERMATO-OSTEOLYSIS, KIRGHIZIAN TYPE     3044

**Includes:**
    Kirghizian dermato-osteolysis
    Kozlova-Altschuler-Kravchenko syndrome

**Excludes:**
    **Fibromatosis, juvenile hyaline** (0411)
    **Hajdu-Cheney syndrome** (2022)
    **Myositis ossificans progressiva** (0700)

**Major Diagnostic Criteria:** The combination of skin ulceration, oligodontia, visual impairment or blindness, and skeletal changes with eventual healing of the skin ulcers should assist in distinguishing this condition from other, similar disorders.

**Clinical Findings:** Onset of the condition is during infancy, with the appearance of skin or mucosal ulcerations. By age one year, the disorder resembles a chronic inflammatory disease, with episodic fever, arthralgia, and keratitis. Deeper skin ulcerations may also occur around joints, with subsequent effects on the bone. The disorder is self-limiting, however, in that viscera are spared and the condition improves within ten years, with subsequent healing of the skin defects. Oligodontia and keratitis are also features of the condition.

**Complications:** Skeletal anomalies such as osteolytic changes, swelling of metaphyses, modeling defects of diaphyses, with resultant limb asymmetry and scoliosis, are likely secondary to the invasive skin ulcers. Dystrophic nails are likely the result of nail bed ulceration. Visual impairment or blindness secondary to keratitis also occurs.

**Associated Findings:** None known.

**Etiology:** Presumably autosomal recessive inheritance.

**Pathogenesis:** Possibly a self-limiting mesoectodermal dysplasia.

**MIM No.:** 22181

**POS No.:** 3604

**Sex Ratio:** M1:F1

**Occurrence:** Five affected sibs have been documented.

**Risk of Recurrence for Patient's Sib:**
See Part I, *Mendelian Inheritance.*

**Risk of Recurrence for Patient's Child:**
See Part I, *Mendelian Inheritance.*

**Age of Detectability:** Symptoms should become apparent by age one year.

**Gene Mapping and Linkage:** Unknown.

**Prevention:** None known. Genetic counseling indicated.

**Treatment:** Antibiotics and anti-inflammatory drugs only provided transient symptomatic improvement; they had no effect on the overall course of the disease.

**Prognosis:** Other than residual scarring, the prognosis for this condition is good. Intellectual development and reproduction are not impaired, life span appears to be normal.

**Detection of Carrier:** Unknown.

**References:**
Kozlova SI, et al.: Self-limited autosomal recessive syndrome of skin ulceration, arthroosteolysis with pseudoacromegaly, keratitis, and oligodontia in a Kirghizian family. Am J Med Genet 1983; 15:205–210.

T0007                                                    **Helga V. Toriello**

## DERMATOARTHRITIS, FAMILIAL HISTIOCYTIC        **2158**

**Includes:**
Histiocytic dermatoarthritis, familial
Zayid-Farraj syndrome

**Excludes:**
**Dermo-chondro-corneal dystrophy, Francois type** (0282)
Giant cell reticulohistiocytoma
Lipoid dermatoarthritis
Multicentric reticulohistiocytosis
**Xanthomatosis, cerebrotendinous** (2395)

**Major Diagnostic Criteria:** A combination of a papulonodular cutaneous eruption, a progressively deforming and destructive polyarthritis, and extra-corneal ocular lesions, with familial occurrence.

**Clinical Findings:** Based on the six reported cases, clinical features may manifest any time in the first two decades of life. The cutaneous lesions are generally the first to appear, usually around ages 4–5 years, and consist of multiple soft-to-firm, smooth, nonulcerating, coalescing tender nodules, violaceous-to-brown in color, and ranging in size from 5 to 30 mm. They are distributed mainly on the face, ears, and dorsa of hands and feet, and occur in all cases (100%).

A symmetric, progressive, and deforming arthritis usually follows. This affects especially the small joints of the hands. On X-ray, there is marked periarticular bony resorption. Arthritis occurs in all cases (100%).

The ocular lesions include bilateral glaucoma, uveitis, and cataracts. Response to standard management is minimal. Blindness may result. Frequency of the ocular lesions is high (75%).

Variability in the clinical expression of the trait occurs with a wide-ranging degree of severity. For example, a single kindred may show severe deforming arthritis with numerous cutaneous nodules, while another kindred may have very mild symptoms that are only apparent on direct enquiry. The variable degree of expression could also manifest in relation to the cutaneous and ocular lesions. Careful examination of all family members is essential.

The natural history of this disorder proceeds from an active phase, when constitutional symptoms of fever and malaise are encountered, to a period of decreasing activity resulting, after several years, in a quiescent phase.

The condition is not associated with hypercholesterolemia or any disorder in lipid metabolism.

**Complications:** Cutaneous disfigurement and lichenification of skin; deformity and mutilation of joints, especially those of the hands; poor vision and possible blindness.

**Associated Findings:** Hoarseness of voice and possible deafness (25%).

**Etiology:** Autosomal dominant inheritance with variable expression.

**Pathogenesis:** Unknown.

**MIM No.:** *14273

**Sex Ratio:** M1:F1

**Occurrence:** Four cases in one family from Jordan, and two cases from Italy, have been reported.

**Risk of Recurrence for Patient's Sib:**
See Part I, *Mendelian Inheritance.*

**Risk of Recurrence for Patient's Child:**
See Part I, *Mendelian Inheritance.*

**Age of Detectability:** Usually clinically evident by ages 10–15 years; however, it is usually present by ages 4–5 years.

**Gene Mapping and Linkage:** Unknown.

**Prevention:** None known. Genetic counseling indicated.

**Treatment:** Physical therapy to minimize deformity. Symptomatic and surgical management of cutaneous, joint, and ocular lesions, including pain and fever. No curative therapy is known.

**Prognosis:** Normal life span. Physical handicaps resulting from joint deformity (75–100%) and loss of vision may occur. Intelligence is normal.

**Detection of Carrier:** Clinical examination of first degree relatives.

**Special Considerations:** The association of cutaneous nodules and a deforming, destructive arthritis, as two of the major diagnostic features in familial histiocytic dermatoarthritis (FHD), brings into consideration the differential diagnosis of multicentric reticulohistiocytosis (MR). Despite this resemblance, a number of

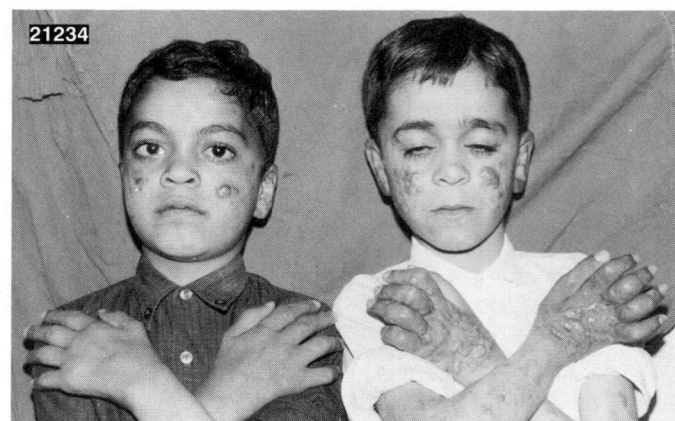

**2158A-21234:** Note multiple nodules on the face, ears, hand and forearms.

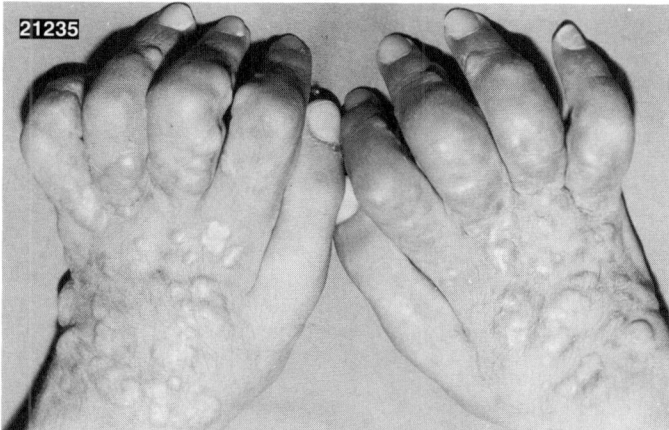

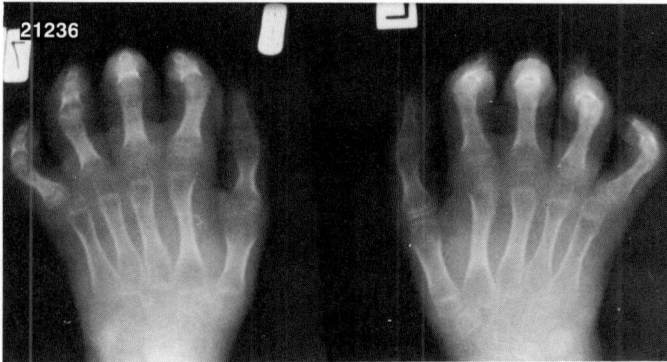

**2158B-21235:** Coalescing cutaneous nodules of the hands. 21236: X-ray of the hands shows bony deformities and subarticular bony resorption.

significant clinical and pathologic features separate the two conditions. Unlike FHD, in MR the condition occurs in adults, has a female predominance, and shows no ocular lesions and no hereditary mode of transmission. Furthermore, the histopathologic features are distinct. In FHD, the cutaneous lesions show a histiocytic granulomatous-type reactive process, while the histologic hallmark of MR is the multinucleated giant cell with a distinctive PAS-positive eosinophilic ground-glass cytoplasm.

**References:**
Zayid I, Farraj S: Familial histiocytic dermatoarthritis: a new syndrome. Am J Med 1973; 54:793–800. * †
Ringel E, Moschella S: Primary histiocytic dermatoses. Arch Dermatol 1985; 121:1531–1541.
Valente M, et al.: Familial histiocytic dermatoarthritis: histologic and ultrastructural findings in two cases. Am J Dermatopath 1987; 9:491–496.

ZA003                                       **Ismail Zayid**

**Dermatochalasia**
*See CUTIS LAXA*
**Dermatoglyphics absent-nail and simian crease anomalies**
*See ECTODERMAL DYSPLASIA, BASAN TYPE*
**Dermatolipoma**
*See EYE, DERMOLIPOMA*
**Dermatomegaly**
*See CUTIS LAXA*
**Dermatoosteopoikilosis**
*See OSTEOPOIKILOSIS*
**Dermatorrhexis cutis hyperelastica**
*See EHLERS-DANLOS SYNDROME*

# DERMO-CHONDRO-CORNEAL DYSTROPHY, FRANCOIS TYPE                    0282

**Includes:**
  Chondro-dermo-corneal dystrophy of Francois
  Corneal dystrophy-dermo-chondro of Francois
  Cutaneous, cartilaginous, and corneal lesions
  Francois dermochondrocorneal dysplasia

**Excludes:**
  **Mucopolysaccharidosis**
  **Wolman disease** (1003)
  Xanthomatoses

**Major Diagnostic Criteria:** Corneal opacities, deformities of hands and feet, and xanthoma-like nodules of skin.

**Clinical Findings:** Abnormal ossification of the cartilage of the hands and feet occurs, leading to marked deformities. Dermal nodules, resembling xanthomata, appear over the dorsal surface of the fingers, posterior surface of the elbows, and on the pinnae. The corneal lesion is characterized by a central epithelial collection of white, irregular opacities, causing moderately reduced visual acuity. The stroma, endothelium, and periphery of the cornea remain uninvolved.

**Complications:** Reduced visual acuity.

**Associated Findings:** Abnormal EEG, seizures. Involvement of the gingival and palatal membranes reported (Caputo et al, 1988)

**Etiology:** Autosomal recessive inheritance. Nonfamilial cases reported.

**Pathogenesis:** Unknown.

**MIM No.:** *22180

**POS No.:** 3205

**Sex Ratio:** Presumably M1:F1

**Occurrence:** François reported two sibs (brother and sister) affected with this syndrome in 1949. Jensen, who thought an unusual patient represented this disorder, similarly used the name "dermo-chondro-corneal dystrophy." However, the disorder he described is thought to be different in that the corneal lesions resembled pterygia and not epithelial opacities, the skin nodules resembled those of the Urbach-Wiethe syndrome (lipoid proteinosis) and not xanthomata, and the bony changes were mild. Remky and Engelbrecht (1967) have described the disorder in both of unlike-sex twins, and have identified a hypercholesterolemic early stage, involvement of the entire skeleton except the vertebrae and skull, and abnormal EEG with seizures.

**Risk of Recurrence for Patient's Sib:**
  See Part I, *Mendelian Inheritance.*

**Risk of Recurrence for Patient's Child:**
  See Part I, *Mendelian Inheritance.*

**Age of Detectability:** Unknown.

**Gene Mapping and Linkage:** Unknown.

**Prevention:** None known. Genetic counseling indicated.

**Treatment:** Unknown.

**Prognosis:** Unknown.

**Detection of Carrier:** Unknown.

**References:**
François J: Dystrophie dermo-chondro-cornéenne familiale. Ann Oculiste (Paris) 1949; 182:409–442.
Jensen VJ: Dermo-chondro-corneal dystrophy: report of a case. Acta Ophthalmol (Copenh) 1958; 36:71–78.
François J: Heredity in ophthalmology. St. Louis: C.V. Mosby, 1961.
Remky H, Engelbrecht G: Dystrophia dermo-chondro-cornealis (François). Klin Mbl Augenheilk 1967; 151:319–331.
Caputo R, et al.: Dermochondrocorneal dystrophy (François syndrome). Arch Dermatol 1988; 124:424–428.

SU001                                       **Joel Sugar**
G0006                                  **Morton F. Goldberg**

## DERMO-FACIO-CARDIO-SKELETAL SYNDROME 2337

**Includes:**
 Cantu syndrome
 Cardio-dermo-facio-skeletal syndrome
 Cranio-facio-cardio-skeletal syndrome
 Facio-dermo-cardio-skeletal syndrome
 Skeletal-dermo-facio-cardio syndrome

**Excludes:** Noonan syndrome (0720)

**Major Diagnostic Criteria:** Short stature, macrocranium, peculiar facies, cardiac anomalies, cutis laxa with characteristic wrinkled palms and soles, and skeletal defects.

**Clinical Findings:** The affected patients have delayed psychomotor development (IQ: 60–68) and a typical appearance mainly characterized by short stature; macrodolichocephaly with prominent forehead; scanty, thin, hypopigmented hair; coarse facies; hypertelorism; exophthalmos; flat nasal bridge; short nose with anteverted nostrils, long philtrum; low-set ears; short neck; short, wide thorax; cardiac murmur; prominent abdomen, cutis laxa; ecchymoses on the legs; wrinkled palms and soles; and joint hyperelasticity.
 X-ray findings include macrodolichocephaly; prominent frontal bone; diminished pneumatization of the mastoid and sphenoid cells; hypertelorism; malar bone hypoplasia; mild cardiomegaly; slender ribs, broader in the middle portion; small vertebral bodies; hypoplastic pelvis; subperiostic cystic lesions more evident in phalanges; slender bones with thin cortices; and delayed bone age.
 The peculiar facies, due to skull-face disproportion and prominent forehead, is caused by the macrodolichocephaly, which seems to be a constitutional feature of this syndrome. The cardiologic defects are nonspecific and include pulmonary stenosis and auricular communication.

**Complications:** Multiple ecchymoses due to fragile skin vessels.

**Associated Findings:** Astigmatism, hypermetropia, and amblyopia.

**Etiology:** In the four patients described, paternal age was advanced, suggesting autosomal dominant inheritance.

**Pathogenesis:** Unknown.

**MIM No.:** 11462

**Sex Ratio:** M0:F4 (observed).

**Occurrence:** Four sporadic cases have been reported.

**Risk of Recurrence for Patient's Sib:**
 See Part I, *Mendelian Inheritance.*

**Risk of Recurrence for Patient's Child:**
 See Part I, *Mendelian Inheritance.*

**Age of Detectability:** In early childhood.

**Gene Mapping and Linkage:** Unknown.

**Prevention:** None known. Genetic counseling indicated.

**Treatment:** Symptomatic.

**Prognosis:** Good. The cardiac defect is not severe enough to cause excessive problems, and the mild mental impairment permits nearly normal behavior.

**Detection of Carrier:** Unknown.

**References:**
Cantú JM, et al.: Individualization of a syndrome with mental deficiency, macrocranium, peculiar facies and cardiac and skeletal anomalies. Clin Genet 1982; 22:172–179. *

C0064
CA011

José Sánchez-Corona
José María Cantú

**Dermo-gu-cervico syndrome**
*See CERVICO-DERMO-GU SYNDROME, GOEMINNE TYPE*

## DERMO-ODONTODYSPLASIA 2763

**Includes:** Ectodermal dysplasia, dermo-odontodysplasia

**Excludes:** Ectodermal dysplasia (other)

**Major Diagnostic Criteria:** Dry and thin skin, dental alterations, onychodysplasia.

**Clinical Findings:** Hypodontia, microdontia, persistence of deciduous teeth, dysplastic and brittle finger- and toenails, dry and slow-growing scalp hair, circumscribed area of alopecia at the top of the head, sparse axillary and pubic hair, thin moustache, dry and thin skin, transpalmar creases, palpebral ptosis, prognathic mandible, fissures and scaling at plantar regions.

**Complications:** Feeding problems due to malocclusion and diastemas between present teeth; embarrassment and shyness due to dental alterations.

**Associated Findings:** None known.

**Etiology:** Presumably autosomal dominant inheritance with variable expression. Since all the affected are the offspring of an affected parent and, in the segregation sibships, the ratio of affected to normal is 6:6 among the women and 4:5 among the men (total ratio of 10:11), the hypothesis of an autosomal dominant gene is the most plausible. The expressivity of the gene in most of the heterozygotes may be termed mild; it is more severely expressed in the propositus.

**Pathogenesis:** Defective formation of several derivatives of the embryonic ectoderm and absence of malformations suggest that this condition must be classified as a pure ectodermal dysplasia.

**MIM No.:** 12564

**Sex Ratio:** M1:F1

**Occurrence:** A Caucasian Brazilian family was verified to have 11 affected persons (seven women and four men) in four generations.

**Risk of Recurrence for Patient's Sib:**
 See Part I, *Mendelian Inheritance.*

**Risk of Recurrence for Patient's Child:**
 See Part I, *Mendelian Inheritance.*

**Age of Detectability:** During childhood, by physical examination.

**Gene Mapping and Linkage:** Unknown.

**Prevention:** None known. Genetic counseling indicated.

**Treatment:** Prosthetic replacement and orthodontic treatment; skin emollients.

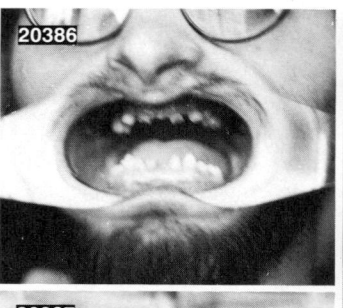
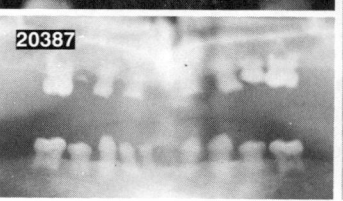
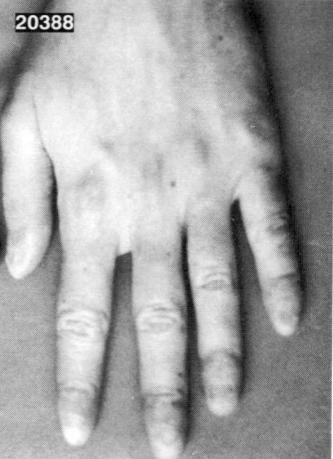

**2763-20386:** Dermo-odontodysplasia: note hypodontia, microdontia and persistent deciduous teeth. **20387:** X-ray of dental defects. **20388:** Dystrophic fingernails.

**Prognosis:** Normal for life span.

**Detection of Carrier:** Unknown.

**References:**
Pinheiro M, Freire-Maia N: Uma displasia ectodérmica pura devida a gene autossômico dominante. Ciênc Cult (suppl) 1982; 34:764.

Pinheiro M, Freire-Maia N: Dermoodontodysplasia: an eleven-member, four generation pedigree with an apparently hitherto undescribed pure ectodermal dysplasia. Clin Genet 1983; 24:58–68.

Freire-Maia N, Pinheiro M: Ectodermal dysplasias: a clinical and genetic study. New York: Alan R. Liss, 1984.

PI008                                              **Marta Pinheiro**

**Dermodistortive urticaria**
   See *URTICARIA, DERMO-DISTORTIVE TYPE*
**Dermoid cyst**
   See *TERATOMAS*
**Dermoid cyst of stomach**
   See *STOMACH, TERATOMA*
**Dermoid cyst of the salivary gland**
   See *SALIVARY GLAND, DERMOID CYST*
**Dermoid cyst or teratoma of head or neck**
   See *NECK/HEAD, DERMOID CYST OR TERATOMA*
**Dermoid cysts of nose of both skin and dural origin**
   See *NOSE/NASAL SEPTUM DEFECTS*
**Dermoid cysts, orbital and periorbital**
   See *ORBITAL AND PERIORBITAL DERMOID CYSTS*
**Dermoid of the cornea**
   See *OCULAR DERMOIDS*
**Dermoids of the head and neck**
   See *NECK/HEAD, DERMOID CYST OR TERATOMA*
**Dermoids, oral**
   See *ORAL DERMOIDS*
**Dermolipoma**
   See *EYE, DERMOLIPOMA*
**DES, fetal effects**
   See *FETAL DIETHYLSTILBESTROL (DES) EFFECTS*
**DeSanctis-Cacchione syndrome**
   See *XERODERMA PIGMENTOSUM-MENTAL RETARDATION*
**Desbuquois syndrome**
   See *LARSEN SYNDROME*
**Desiccacytosis, hereditary**
   See *ANEMIA, HEMOLYTIC, RED CELL MEMBRANE DEFECTS*
**Desmin defect**
   See *MYOPATHY OR CARDIOMYOPATHY DUE TO DESMIN DEFECT*
**Desquamation of the newborn**
   See *ICHTHYOSIS, LAMELLAR RECESSIVE*
**Deuteranopia**
   See *COLOR BLINDNESS, RED-GREEN DEUTAN SERIES*
**Developmental coxa vara**
   See *HIP, CONGENITAL COXA VARA*
**Developmental dyslexia**
   See *DYSLEXIA*
**Deviation on coup de vent**
   See *HAND, ULNAR DRIFT*
**DeVries hyperglycinuria**
   See *IMINOGLYCINURIA*

## DEXTROCARDIA-BRONCHIECTASIS-SINUSITIS SYNDROME                                    0285

**Includes:**
Bronchiectasis-dextrocardia-sinusitis syndrome
Bronchiectasis, sinusitis, and dextrocardia
Immotile cilia syndrome
Kartagener syndrome
Sinusitis-dextrocardia-bronchiectasis syndrome

**Excludes:**
Isolated dextrocardia
**Situs inversus viscerum** (0888)

**Major Diagnostic Criteria:** Clinical diagnosis can be considered definite in the isolated patient with no affected relatives if he or she has had thick nasal secretions since infancy, pansinusitis, and partial or complete situs inversus. Homozygotes can also be identified from the morphology of cilia or sperm examined by electron microscopy. A significant decrease in the number of inner

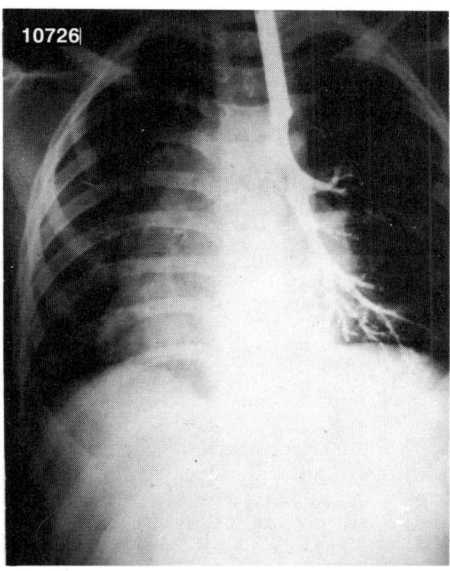

0285-10726:   Bronchiectasis and dextrocardia.

and outer dynein arms is a consistent finding. The ultrastructure of cilia can be used to identify homozygous individuals with bronchiectasis and sinusitus.

**Clinical Findings:** Affected persons may have all or any combination of these physical features: partial or complete situs inversus, thick nasal secretions from infancy through adulthood, pansinusitis from childhood, chronic serous otitis media and bronchiectasis. Some features are the progressive complications involving the respiratory epithelium that develop at different ages in each patient. Often the situs inversus is unrecognized for many years. Cardiac anomalies may be present, especially if the situs inversus is incomplete. Affected adult males may be sterile due to immotile spermatozoa.

**Complications:** Anosmia, a mild conductive hearing loss, nasal polyps, pneumonia, and bronchiectasis; infertility due to immotile sperm.

**Associated Findings:** **Asplenia syndrome** and cardiac anomalies.

**Etiology:** Autosomal recessive inheritance.

**Pathogenesis:** The primary defect in the respiratory epithelium appears to be abnormalities of the number, orientation, and structure of the microtubules in the cilia. The abnormal motility of the cilia leads to blockage of the paranasal sinuses, the eustachian tube, and the lobes of the lung, and these areas become infected. The occurrence of situs inversus does not appear to be related to the abnormality of the cilia.

**MIM No.:** *24440

**POS No.:** 3763

**CDC No.:** 746.800

**Sex Ratio:** M1:F1

**Occurrence:** Several hundred cases have been documented.

**Risk of Recurrence for Patient's Sib:**
See Part I, *Mendelian Inheritance.*

**Risk of Recurrence for Patient's Child:**
See Part I, *Mendelian Inheritance.*

**Age of Detectability:** Most patients have thick mucoid rhinorrhea and recurrent respiratory infections in the first year of life. A newborn displays respiratory distress and atelectasis of left middle lobe. The abnormality of the cilia can be determined upon examination of cross-sections of cilia by electron microscopy. Biopsy of the nasal epithelium removes these cilia.

**Gene Mapping and Linkage:** Unknown.

**Prevention:** None known. Genetic counseling indicated.

**Treatment:** Otitis media, acute sinusitis, and pneumonia should be carefully looked for and vigorously treated. Early treatment of respiratory complications may prevent bronchiectasis. A transient low level of serum IgG, if identified, should be treated. Patients with bronchiectasis benefit from the removal of the affected lobes or segments.

Long-term treatment of chronic serous otitis, including continuous drainage and ventilation, and use of hearing aid may be warranted.

**Prognosis:** For life: good, unless the patient has either a severe cardiac anomaly or extensive bronchiectasis. Although the actual life span is not known, most patients reach adulthood. For function: pulmonary function tests show that although the severity is variable, ventilatory obstruction occurs in all patients. Mildly affected individuals can without difficulty engage in vigorous physical activity. Although patients complain most about the constant rhinorrhea and chronic cough, they are often unaware of their anosmia and mild hearing loss. Infertility may be a problem because of immotile sperm. Infertility appears to be more common among affected males than among affected females.

**Detection of Carrier:** Obligatory heterozygotes do not show a decrease in the number of dynein arms in cross-sections of cilia examined by electron microscopy.

**Special Considerations:** This syndrome includes both developmental structural abnormalities and thick mucoid secretions throughout the entire respiratory epithelium. These seemingly unrelated problems are the pleiotropic effects of a single mutant gene. Family studies have shown a wide phenotypic variability within a sibship. For example, the index patient displays many features of this syndrome, while his brother has only thick nasal secretions and sinusitis; his sister has only situs inversus. Yet, all three sibs are considered examples of Kartagener syndrome. Bronchiectasis, sinusitis, and azoospermia also occur in Young syndrome, but the affected individuals do not have situs inversus or abnormalities of cilia ultrastructure.

**References:**

Holmes LB, et al.: A reappraisal of Kartagener's syndrome. Am J Med Sci 1968; 255:13–28. †

Hartline JV, Zelkowitz PS: Kartagener's syndrome in childhood. Am J Dis Child 1971; 121:349.

Afzelius BA: A human syndrome caused by immotile cilia. Science 1976; 193:317–319. *

Schneeberger EE, et al.: Heterogeneity of ciliary morphology in the immotile-cilia syndrome in man. J Ultrastruct Res 1980; 73:34–43.

Moreno A, Murphy EA: Inheritance of Kartagener syndrome. Am J Med Genet 1981; 8:305–313.

Walter RJ, et al.: Cell motility and microtubules in cultured fibroblasts from patients with Kartagener syndrome. Cell Motil 1983; 3:185–197.

Eavey RD, et al.: Kartagener's syndrome: a blinded, controlled study of cilia ultrastructure. Arch Otolaryngol Head Neck Surg 1986; 112:646–650. * †

Sturgess JM, Thompson MW: Genetic aspects of immotile cillia syndrome. Am J Med Genet 1986; 25:149–160.

H0019                                             **Lewis B. Holmes**

**Dextroposition of ventricular septum-double inlet left ventricle**
*See VENTRICLE, SEPTUM DEXTROPOSITION AND DOUBLE INLET LEFT VENTRICLE*
**Di- and trihexosyl ceramide lipidosis**
*See FABRY DISEASE*

## DIABETES (INSIPIDUS/MELLITUS)-OPTIC ATROPHY-DEAFNESS                                             0550

**Includes:**
Deafness-diabetes-optic atrophy
Diabetes insipidus-diabetes mellitus-optic atrophy-deafness (DIDMOAD)
Diabetes mellitus-otpic atrophy
Juvenile diabetes mellitus-optic atrophy-deafness
Optic atrophy-juvenile diabetes-deafness
Recessive optic atrophy-hearing loss-juvenile diabetes
Wolfram syndrome

**Excludes:**
Alstrom syndrome (0041)
Ataxia, Friedreich type (2714)
Bardet-Biedl syndrome (2363)
Cockayne syndrome (0189)
Diabetes insipidis, neurohypophyseal type (2611)
Diabetes mellitus, insulin dependent type (0549)
Laurence-Moon syndrome (0578)
Optic atrophy or deafness by themselves or with other syndromes
Phytanic acid oxidase deficiency, infantile type (2278)
Phytanic acid storage disease (0810)

**Major Diagnostic Criteria:** Diabetes mellitus, optic atrophy, mild-to-moderate high-frequency hearing impairment, and diabetes insipidus. The presence of at least two clinical findings is suggestive of this diagnosis.

**Clinical Findings:** In the majority of cases, diabetes mellitus first appears before age 10 years. Initially the diabetes may be controlled by diet, but it usually progresses to require insulin therapy. Decreased visual acuity due to optic atrophy usually occurs between six and 20 years of age and is progressive. Neurohypophyseal diabetes insipidus occurs in 1/3 of patients, usually appearing before the second decade of life, and responds to vasopressin administration. The optic atrophy is characterized by white disks and occasionally by periperal retinal pigmentation. Mild-to-moderate high-frequency sensorineural hearing impairment is usually diagnosed between 10 and 20 years of age and is often not suspected until audiograms are performed.

**Complications:** Complete blindness due to optic atrophy occurs in most patients. Vestibular abnormalities and ataxia are often seen. Vascular complications of diabetes mellitus may appear as may ketoacidosis, dehydration, megacystis, megaureter, hydronephrosis, renal failure, delayed growth and pubertal development.

**Associated Findings:** Problems with coordination and ataxia, cerebellar dysfunction, vertigo, anosmia, retinal pigmentation, abnormal pupillary reaction to photic stimulation, nystagmous, color blindness, EEG changes, dysautonomia, esophageal dysphagia, dilation and secondary muscular atrophy of the bladder and colon, sclerosis of bladder and bladderneck, aminoaciduria and hyperalaninuria have been reported.

**Etiology:** Autosomal recessive inheritance, pleiotropic. Several families with multiple sibs and normal parents, some of whom were consanguineous, have been reported.

**Pathogenesis:** Undetermined. Several studies have supported the neuropathologic nature of the disorder, including degeneration of the optic nerve, supraoptic and paraventricular nuclei, and the eighth nerve. Other pathologic studies have supported cellular degeneration without inflammation. Recent evidence of endocrine organ autoimmunity in some patients has led others to believe that this syndrome may result from an autoimmune process. The diabetes mellitus does not appear to be HLA linked.

**MIM No.:** *22230

**POS No.:** 3516

**Sex Ratio:** M1:F1

**Occurrence:** Since this entity was first recognized as a hereditary syndrome by Wolfram and Wagener in 1938, well over 150 cases have been reported. It has been estimated that this syndrome occurs in about 1:150 juvenile-onset diabetics.

**Risk of Recurrence for Patient's Sib:**
See Part I, *Mendelian Inheritance.*

**Risk of Recurrence for Patient's Child:**
See Part I, *Mendelian Inheritance.*

**Age of Detectability:** Variable. The first symptoms of diabetes mellitus develop between three and 10 years of age, and optic atrophy and sensorineural hearing impairment may not occur until much later.

**Gene Mapping and Linkage:** Unknown.

**Prevention:** None known. Genetic counseling indicated.

**Treatment:** Insulin therapy is usually required for management of diabetes mellitus. Vasopressin administration corrects the polyuria of diabetes insipidus if the diabetes mellitus is in resonable control. Surgical reconstruction or decompression maybe necessary to correct urinary tract abnormalities. Audiological augmentation may assist deafness.

**Prognosis:** Some patients die at an early age during a diabetic coma. Others may have a shortened life span due to the complications of diabetes. Intelligence is normal.

**Detection of Carrier:** Of the parents tested, some have demonstrated the obvious presence of diabetes mellitus (Gunn T, 1976) and others have not (Najjar S.S. et al 1985). Fundoscopic examinations as well as audiological and water deprivation testing of parents have been normal (Najjar S.S. et al 1985). Given this information, detection of a carrier by clinical criteria seems unlikely.

**Special Considerations:** Although insulin treatment improves patient's condition, there are numerous reports of patients withdrawing from insulin therapy up to several months without serious clinical sequalae. This implies that the secretion of insulin may be variable in these patients. If severe urinary tract dilation exists, the findings of coexisting secondary nephrogenic diabetes insipidus cannot be excluded.

**References:**
Wolfram DJ, Wagener HP: Diabetes mellitus and simple optic atrophy among siblings: report of four cases. Mayo Clin Proc 1938; 13:715–718.

Cremers CWRJ, et al.: Juvenile diabetes mellitus, optic atrophy, hearing loss, diabetes insipidus, atonia of the urinary tract and bladder, and other abnormalities (Wolfram syndrome): a review of 88 cases from the literature with personal observations on 3 new patients. Acta Paediatr Scand (suppl) 1977; 264:3–16.

Stanley CA, et al.: Wolfram syndrome not HLA linked. New Engl J Med 1979; 301:1398–1399.

Deschamps I, et al.: HLA-DR₂ and DIDMOAD syndrome. Lancet 1983; II:109.

Kahardori R, et al.: Diabetes mellitus and optic atrophy in two siblings: a report on a new association and a review of the literature. Diabetes Care 1983; 6:67–70.

Monson JP, Boucher BJ: HLA-type and islet cell antibody status in family with (diabetes insipidus and mellitus, optic atrophy, and deafness) DIDMOAD syndrome. Lancet 1983; I:1286–1287.

Najjar SS, et al.: Association of diabetes insipidus, diabetes mellitus, optic atrophy, and deafness: the Wolfram or DIDMOAD syndrome. Arch Dis Child 1985; 60:823–828.

Fishman L, Ehrlich RM: Wolfram syndrome: report of four new cases and a review of the literature. Diabetes Care 1986; 9:405–408. *

NA014
PH003
SH046

Jennifer L. Najjar
John A. Phillips, III
Kathleen Shaver

## DIABETES INSIPIDIS, NEUROHYPOPHYSEAL TYPE   2611

**Includes:**
Diabetes insipidus, acquired central
Diabetes insipidus, primary central
Diabetes insipidus, cranial type
Diabetes insipidus, idiopathic

**Excludes:**
**Diabetes (insipidus/mellitus)-optic atrophy-deafness** (0550)
**Diabetes insipidus, vasopressin resistant types I and II** (0287)
Psychogenic polydipsia and polyuria

**Major Diagnostic Criteria:** Hypotonic urine <300 mOsm/liter; when serum is hypertonic (>295 mOsm/liter) in the absence of renal tubular abnormalities and psychogenic polydipsia and polyuria. Serum vasopressin levels are generally <2 μg/liter when serum is >295 mOsm/liter. Patients respond to administered vasopressin.

**Clinical Findings:** Polydipsia and polyuria associated with urine < serum osmolality. One may encounter growth retardation in children due to inadequate caloric intake, and mental retardation secondary to dehydration and electrolyte abnormalities (hypernatremia).

**Complications:** Unknown.

**Associated Findings:** Megalocystis, megaureter, hydronephrosis, hypernatremic and dehydration. Central diabetes insipidus is seen in **Diabetes (insipidus/mellitus)-optic atrophy-deafness** in association with other findings, including, diabetes mellitus, optic atrophy, and blindness.

**Etiology:** Autosomal dominant and X-linked recessive inheritance. Idiopathic when no organic or familial case is identified.

**Pathogenesis:** Various insults involving the hypothalamic-pituitary axis (i.e. intracranial tumor, hysticocytosis, meningitis) can cause acquired neurohypophyseal diabetes insipidus (DI). In the few cases studied at autopsy, familial neurohypophyseal DI (autosomal dominant type) appears to be associated with degeneration of the supraoptic and paraventricular nuclei, areas responsible for vasopressin and oxytocin secretion.

**MIM No.:** *12570, *30490

**Sex Ratio:** Autosomal dominant type, M1:F1; X-linked recessive type, M1:F<1.

**Occurrence:** Undetermined but presumed rare. Established literature.

**Risk of Recurrence for Patient's Sib:**
See Part I, *Mendelian Inheritance.*

**Risk of Recurrence for Patient's Child:**
See Part I, *Mendelian Inheritance.*

**Age of Detectability:** Neonatal period through the first or second decade of life due to variable expression.

**Gene Mapping and Linkage:** ARVP (arginine vasopressin) has been provisionally mapped to 20.
OT (prepro-oxytocin-neurophysin I) has been provisionally mapped to 20.
MNS (MNS blood group) has been DISCONTINUED.
A linkage of autosomal dominant neurohypophyseal DI to DNA polymorphisms detected by the vasopressin gene, which maps to chromosome 20, is suggested by the observation of a lod score of 2.7 at theta = 0 (unpublished data in press). Linkage between autosomal dominant DI and the MN blood group and with **Huntington disease** is suggested by observation of a lod score of 1.17 at theta = 0 (Pedersen, 1985).

**Prevention:** None known. Genetic counseling indicated.

**Treatment:** Vasopressin subcutaneously, intramuscularly, or intranasally should be given to older patients. In children younger than age two years, treatment with thiazide diuretics is preferred. Thiazide therapy must be accompanied by a low-salt, potassium-supplemented diet. A thiazide diuretic is the preferred treatment in infants with DI, because it permits some hypotonic urine flow and thereby enables adequate caloric intake in the form of breastmilk or formula. Patients who demonstrate partial neuro-hypophyseal DI may respond to chlorpropramide, which acts as a secretagogue for vasopressin.

**Prognosis:** Good, given careful attention to the prevention of fluid and electrolyte disturbances.

**Detection of Carrier:** Unknown.

**References:**
Forssman H: Two different mutations of the X chromosome causing diabetes insipidus. Am J Hum Genet 1955; 7:21–27.
Crigler JF: Commentary on the use of pitressin in infants with neurogenic diabetes insipidus. J Pediatr 1976; 88:295–296.
Kaplowitz PB: Radioimmunoassay of vasopressin in familial central diabetes insipidus. J Pediatr 1982; 100:76–81.
Robertson GL: Thirst and vasopressin function in normal and disordered states of water balance. J Lab Clin Med 1983; 101:351–371.
Najjar SS: Association of diabetes insipidus, diabetes mellitus, optic atrophy and deafness: Wolfam or DIDMOAD syndrome. Arch Dis Child 1985; 60:823–828.
Pedersen EB: Familial cranial diabetes: a report of five families: genetic, diagnostic and therapeutic aspects. Quart J Med 1985; 57:883–896.

NA014                                    **Jennifer L. Najjar**
PH003                                **John A. Phillips, III**

**Diabetes insipidus, acquired central**
*See DIABETES INSIPIDIS, NEUROHYPOPHYSEAL TYPE*
**Diabetes insipidus, congenital nephrogenic, types I, II**
*See DIABETES INSIPIDIS, VASOPRESSIN RESISTANT TYPES I AND II*
**Diabetes insipidus, cranial type**
*See DIABETES INSIPIDIS, NEUROHYPOPHYSEAL TYPE*
**Diabetes insipidus, idiopathic**
*See DIABETES INSIPIDIS, NEUROHYPOPHYSEAL TYPE*
**Diabetes insipidus, primary central**
*See DIABETES INSIPIDIS, NEUROHYPOPHYSEAL TYPE*
**Diabetes insipidus, renal type**
*See DIABETES INSIPIDUS, VASOPRESSIN RESISTANT TYPES I AND II*

---

## DIABETES INSIPIDUS, VASOPRESSIN RESISTANT TYPES I AND II           0287

**Includes:**
Diabetes insipidus, congenital nephrogenic, types I, II
Diabetes insipidus, renal type
Nephrogenic diabetes insipidus
Vasopressin-resistant

**Excludes:**
Acquired polyuria due to renal disease
Neurohypophyseal diabetes insipidus (idiopathic and familial)
Psychogenic polydipsia and polyuria

**Major Diagnostic Criteria:** In both nephrogenic diabetes insipidus (DI) types I and II, serum vasopressin levels are normal to elevated (6 pg/ml) in spite of dilute urine (<300 mOsm/liter) and there is no response to administered vasopressin. Urinary tract obstruction, renal tubular diseases (i.e., sickle cell disease, amyloidosis), toxic conditions (i.e., hypercalcemia, hypokalemia, hyperglycemia, lithium, demeclocycline exposure), and psychogenic polydipsia must be excluded.

**Clinical Findings:** Polyuria and polydipsia, with urine < serum osmolality. Urine osmolality is commonly ≤ 100 mOsm/liter. Growth retardation can occur in children due to inadequate caloric intake. Mental retardation secondary to dehydration and electrolyte abnormalities (hypernatremia) is often seen.

**Complications:** Unknown.

**Associated Findings:** Megalocystis, megaureter, hydronephrosis, hypernatremic dehydration.

**Etiology:** Nephrogenic DI type I (common), X-linked recessive inheritance;
Nephrogenic DI type II (rare), autosomal dominant inheritance.

**Pathogenesis:** There is a lack of response to endogenous and exogenous vasopressin, resulting in an inability to concentrate urine.

**MIM No.:** *30480, *12580

**Sex Ratio:** Type I, M1:F<1; type II, M1:F1

**Occurrence:** Unknown. Established literature.

**Risk of Recurrence for Patient's Sib:**
See Part I, *Mendelian Inheritance.*

**Risk of Recurrence for Patient's Child:**
See Part I, *Mendelian Inheritance.*

**Age of Detectability:** Usually neonatal or early infancy.

**Gene Mapping and Linkage:** DIR (diabetes insipidus, renal) has been mapped to Xq28.

**Prevention:** None known. Genetic counseling indicated.

**Treatment:** Vasopressin administration is ineffective. Optimal therapy consists of adequate fluid replacement, treatment with thiazide diuretics, low-salt diet, and supplemental potassium. Infants of an affected parent should be monitored closely as neonates to detect appearance of the disease prior to severe dehydration.

**Prognosis:** Good, given careful attention to the prevention of fluid and electrolyte disturbances.

**Detection of Carrier:** Female carriers of the X-linked variety (type I) may demonstrate a partial impairment of urinary concentration during water deprivation or after vasopressin administration.

**Special Considerations:** Although X-linked recessive is the usual mode of inheritance of nephrogenic DI type I, several instances of male-to-male transmission implicate more than one genetic defect. In type I disease, there is impairment of renal tubule cAMP production. This could occur secondary to absence of the renal receptor for vasopressin. In type II disease, urinary cAMP response to vasopressin is preserved, implicating an abnormality distal to cAMP production. Diagnosis of both types I and II is difficult in neonates because the concentration of urine is normally impaired at that age. Differentiation of vasopressin resistance from psychogenic polydipsia can be accomplished by measurement of vasopressin levels or infusion of hypertonic saline. Incorrect diagnosis of vasopressin resistance can occur when other toxic or metabolic conditions are present, causing polyuria.

**References:**
Robinson MG, Kaplan SA: Inheritance of vasopressin-resistant (nephrogenic) diabetes insipidus. Am J Dis Child 1960; 99:164–174.
Bodl HH, Crawford JD: Nephrogenic diabetes insipidus in North America: the Hopewell hypothesis. N Engl J Med 1969; 280:750–754.
Rosenberg LE: Hereditary diseases with membrane defects. In: Dowben RM, ed: Biological membranes. Boston: Little Brown, 1969:255.
Ten Bensel RW, Petus ER: Progressive hydronephrosis, hydroureter, and dilatation of the bladder in siblings with congenital nephrogenic diabetes insipidus. J Pediatr 1970; 77:439–443.
Bell NH, et al.: Demonstration of a defect in the formation of adenosine 3-prime, 5-prime-mono-phosphate in vasopressin-resistant diabetes insipidus. Pediatr Res 1974; 8:223–230.
Ohzeki T, et al.: Familial cases of congenital nephrogenic diabetes insipidus type II: remarkable increment of urinary adenosine 3', 5'-monophosphate in response to antidiuretic hormone. J Pediat 1984; 104:593–595.
Kobrinsky NL, et al.: Absent factor VIII response to synthetic vaso-pressin analogue (DDAVP) in nephrogenic diabetes insipidus. Lancet 1985; I:1293–1294.
Kambouris M, et al.: Localization of the gene for X-linked nephrogenic diabetes insipidus to Xq 28. Am J Med Genet 1988; 29:239–246.

NA014                                  **Jennifer L. Najjar**
PH003                                **John A. Phillips, III**

**Diabetes insipidus-diabetes mellitus-optic atrophy-deafness (DIDMO**
*See DIABETES (INSIPIDUS/MELLITUS)-OPTIC ATROPHY-DEAFNESS*
**Diabetes mellitus and spondyloepiphyseal dysplasia**
*See EPIPHYSEAL DYSPLASIA, MULTIPLE-DIABETES MELLITUS*
**Diabetes mellitus, adult onset**
*See DIABETES MELLITUS, NON-INSULIN DEPENDENT TYPE*

## DIABETES MELLITUS, INSULIN DEPENDENT TYPE     0549

**Includes:**
   Diabetes mellitus, juvenile type
   Diabetes mellitus, ketosis-prone type
   Diabetes mellitus, type I
   Insulin-dependent diabetes mellitus (IDDM)

**Excludes:**
   **Diabetes (insipidus/mellitus)-optic atrophy-deafness** (0550)
   **Diabetes mellitus, non-insulin dependent type** (2327)
   **Diabetes mellitus** (other)
   **Diabetes mellitus, maturity onset of the young (MODY)** (2326)
   Diabetes mellitus secondary to pancreatectomy
   Diabetes mellitus secondary to pituitary/adrenocortical anomalies
   **Renal glycosuria** (0861)

**Major Diagnostic Criteria:** A decreased glucose tolerance and no increase in plasma immunoreactive insulin are essential for the diagnosis of diabetes mellitus. In association with the classic symptoms of polyuria and polydipsia and in the absence of obvious endocrinopathy or stress from recent illness, trauma, or surgery, an abnormal increase in blood sugar plus glycosuria can usually be considered diagnostic. Antibodies to pancreatic islet β cells is commonly present at the time of diagnosis. Glycosolated hemoglobin is usually elevated at the onset of the clinical illness.

**Clinical Findings:** Insulin-dependent diabetes mellitus (IDDM) is now considered likely to be an autoimmune disease highly associated with the HLA DR3 and DR4 alleles. The onset, in comparison with NIDDM, is clinically relatively abrupt, marked by hyperglycemia, glucosuria, weight loss or failure to gain weight in the past weeks or months, a tendency to develop ketoacidosis if untreated and an absolute requirement for insulin to correct the metabolic abnormalities. The natural history probably begins with a predisposition to autoimmune disease associated with specific HLA DR3 or DR4 alleles; months or years later a triggering event such as a viral illness, leads to the development of an autoimmune state directed at the β cell with the presence of β cell antibodies. After a further period of months or years the onset of clinical symptoms appears when approximately 90% of the β cells have been destroyed; ketoacidosis will follow if insulin therapy is not instituted. Following the onset of insulin therapy at 0.75 to 1.0 units of insulin/kg body weight/day, a period of partial remission generally occurs after 2–6 weeks. The remission period, which may last several months to several years, is characterized by a reduced insulin requirement (usually less than 0.5 units of insulin/kg/day).

   Thereafter, with progression of the autoimmune process, the destruction of β cells becomes complete, β cell antibodies disappear and insulin requirements average 1.0 u/kg/day. In the period when the autoimmune process is underway, but prior to the onset of clinical symptoms, glucose tolerance may be normal except under the stress of trauma, illness, surgery or the administration of adrenocortical hormones. If IDDM is diagnosed in the latter part of this period, insulin requirements are generally less than 0.5 u/kg/day and the partial remission period is rarely observed. If the diagnosis and therapy begins after clinical symptoms have occurred and glucose tolerance is clearly abnormal, the partial remission period is more likely to occur. During the period of partial remission, episodes of hypoglycemia and ketoacidosis are less common than in the ensuing years of the individual's life. Variation in insulin requirements occur in association with emotional disorders, illness, periods of increased physical activity and during adolescence.

   Symptoms occur with the following frequency ranges: polyuria (75–80%); polydipsia (70–80%); weight loss or failure to gain weight (50–60%); lassitude and malaise (40–50%); polyphagia (40–50%); nocturia (35–40%); abdominal pain (10–15%); hyperventilation (5–10%).

   Laboratory findings include: abnormal glucose tolerance (100%); glycosuria ultimately (100%); initial glycosuria (60–80%); ketosis with ketonuria, initially (20–25%); metabolic acidosis (15–20%); hypoglycemia (< 5%).

**Complications:** Ketoacidosis, coma, cerebral edema and hypoglycemia.

**Associated Findings:** Vascular changes in many organs, most notably in the eyes and kidneys. The onset of these changes occurs with clinical significance 5–15 years after adolescence, and without regard to the duration of the disease in the preadolescent. Other autoimmune conditions are more frequent than in the general population. Autoimmune thyroiditis is the most common, and autoimmune Addison disease is also seen. Antibodies to gastric parietal cells, antinuclear antibody (ANA) and rheumatoid factor have also been found with greater frequency than in the general population.

**Etiology:** Probably multifactorial; presence of genetic plus environmental factors seems highly probable. An association with certain HLA antigens has been noted, especially HLA DR3 and DR4. There is increasing evidence that some form of autoimmunity has an etiologic role. Occurs in dogs and mice.

**Pathogenesis:** A relative or absolute insulin deficiency alters glucose metabolism and some degree of cellular unresponsiveness to insulin also exists. Thus abnormalities of insulin receptors and of the glucose transport system may be involved. Genetic defects in the insulin receptor mechanism include receptor mRNA expression, conversion of the receptor precursor protein, blocking of insertion of the receptor into the cell membrane, reduction in insulin binding, and abnormalities in the tyrosine kinase which is an intracellular portion of the receptor complex.

   Glucose transporter (GT) proteins represent a group of enzymes found in various tissues. One of these GT's found in skeletal muscle, cardiac muscle and adipose tissue of the diabetic rat is particularly responsive to insulin. Reduced muscle glucose transporter mRNA and its related protein may be related to the cellular unresponsiveness to insulin in individuals with diabetes. Further work indicates that the liver type GT is found in the pancreatic β cells and is located predominantly in the microvilli facing adjoining endocrine cells.

**MIM No.:** 22210

**Sex Ratio:** M1:F1 in children; M1:F2 in older patients.

**Occurrence:** There is strong evidence for an increasing prevalence in persons less than 15 years of age: from an estimated prevalence of 1:2,500 children under 15 years of age in the 1930's, the prevalence reached about 1:1,000 in the 1960's and is now about 1:600. The prevalence of diabetes of all types is about 1:60. Type 1 diabetes (IDDM) constitutes about 5% of all diabetes mellitus.

   In the past two decades, the incidence of Type I diabetes in children less than five years of age appears to be increasing more rapidly than the overall increase in Type I diabetes.

**Risk of Recurrence for Patient's Sib:** If one child in a family has Type 1 diabetes, the risks for the other children are proportional to the degree of sharing of HLA haplotypes. With no sharing, the risk is 1%, with one shared haplotype the risk is about 5% and with two shared haplotypes the risk is 10–20%.

**Risk of Recurrence for Patient's Child:** Unknown. Appears to be related to the HLA haplotype of the child in relation to that of the parent with diabetes.

**Age of Detectability:** Although rarely seen in the first year of life in the past, there appears to be an increasing frequency of clinical disease in infancy.

**Gene Mapping and Linkage:** Unknown.

**Prevention:** None known. Genetic counseling indicated.

**Treatment:** Insulin required as a secondary prevention. Dietary restrictions, varying from concern for excessive simple carbohydrate to carefully prescribed diets, are considered useful in management. The extent of restriction depends on the philosophic view of the physician. Support in behavioral and social areas is of greatest consequence in the successful management of children with diabetes mellitus. More emphasis is required in these areas than in any other aspect of the illness.

   Immunosuppressive therapy (especially with cyclosporine A) at the onset of clinical symptoms has been demonstrated to reduce or abolish the requirement for exogenous insulin as long as the immunosuppressive agent is administered. This therapeutic approach is currently considered an experimental one in the United States.

**Prognosis:** If untreated, death in approximately six months. With appropriate treatment and dialysis or transplantation for renal failure, the long term mortality is uncertain.

**Detection of Carrier:** Unknown.

**Support Groups:**
New York; American Diabetes Association
New York; Juvenile Diabetes Foundation (JDF) International
CANADA: Ontario; Toronto; Canadian Diabetes Association
ENGLAND: London; International Diabetes Federation

**References:**
Bottazzo GF, et al.: In situ characterization of autoimmune phenomena and expression of HLA molecules in the pancreas in Diabetic Insulitis. New Engl J Med 1985; 313:353–359.
Eisenbarth GS: Type I Diabetes Mellitus: a chronic autoimmune disease. New Engl J Med 1986; 314:1360–1368. *
Chantelau EA, et al.: Intensive insulin therapy justifies simplication of the diabetes diet: a prospective study in insulin dependent diabetic patients. Am J Clin Nutr 1987; 45:958–962.
Kohrman AF, et al.: Diabetes Mellitus, in Rudolph AM, ed; Pediatrics, 18th ed. East Norwalk, CT: Appleton & Lang, 1987. *
Krolewski AS, et al.: Epidemiologic approach to the etiology of Type I Diabetes Mellitus and its complications. New Engl J Med 1987; 317:1390–1398. *
Rotter JI, Rimoin DL: The Genetics of diabetes. Hospital Practice 1987; 22:79–88. *
Bougneres JC, et al.: Factors associated with early remission of Type I Diabetes in children treated with Cyclosporine. New Engl J Med 1988; 318:663–670.
Brownlee M, et al.: Advanced glycosylation end products in tissue and the biochemical basis of Diabetic complications. New Engl J Med 1988; 318:1315–1321.
Diabetes Control and Complications Trial Research Group: Are continuing studies of metabolic control and microvascular complications in insulin-dependent diabetes mellitus justified? New Engl J Med 1988; 318:246–249.
Herold KC, Rubenstein AH: Immunosuppression for insulin-dependent diabetes. New Engl J Med 1988; 318:701–703.
Krolewski AS, et al.: Predisposition to hypertension and susceptibility to renal disease in Insulin-dependent Diabetes Mellitus. New Engl J Med 1988; 318:140–145.
Baum JD, et al.: National survey of childhood-onset diabetes, 1988. British Diabetic Association, Poster Session, September 7, 1989.
Kahn CR, Goldstein BJ: Molecular defects in insulin action. Science 1989; 245:13–14 *
Orci L, et al.: Localization of the Pancreatic Beta Cell Glucose Transporter to Specific Plasma Membrane Domains. Science 1989; 245: 295–297.
Becerra JE, et al.: Diabetes mellitus during pregnancy and the risks for specific birth defects. Pediatrics 1990; 85:1–9.

WE010                                    **William B. Weil, Jr.**

**Diabetes mellitus, juvenile type**
*See DIABETES MELLITUS, INSULIN DEPENDENT TYPE*
**Diabetes mellitus, ketosis-prone type**
*See DIABETES MELLITUS, INSULIN DEPENDENT TYPE*

---

## DIABETES MELLITUS, MATURITY ONSET OF THE YOUNG (MODY)                                    2326

**Includes:**
Juvenile diabetes mellitus, mild
Mason type diabetes
Maturity-onset diabetes of the young (MODY)
Maturity-onset type hyperglycemia of the young (MOHY)
Non-insulin-dependent diabetes of the young (NIDDY)

**Excludes:**
**Diabetes mellitus, insulin dependent type** (0549)
Non-insulin-dependent diabetes with age of onset over age 24 years

**Major Diagnostic Criteria:** Diagnosis of diabetes is made using National Diabetes Data Group criteria (Tattersall, 1974). MODY patients must also meet the following criteria (Barbosa, 1978): (1) age of onset for at least one family member ≤ 25 years; (2) correction of fasting hyperglycemia for at least two years without insulin; and (3) non-ketotic diabetes.

**Clinical Findings:** MODY diabetics have a form of diabetes milder than that found in **Diabetes mellitus, insulin dependent type** and often milder than that of individuals with non-MODY type non-insulin-dependent diabetes. Patients may be entirely asymptomatic at time of diagnosis. Most are not obese, though some cases may be moderately overweight. The MODY type of diabetes, by definition, is non-ketotic under basal non-stressed conditions, but, as with any form of diabetes, may become complicated by ketoacidosis in the face of severe stresses, such as infection.

**Complications:** Development of diabetic complications varies greatly among individuals. Genetic factors may play a role, since certain families appear more prone to complications than others. Some MODY cases show no sign of neuropathy, macrovascular, or microvascular complications; even after many years with diabetes. After 15 years with diabetes, about one-third show evidence of macrovascular complications (cardiovascular disease, circulatory problems) and about 20% show microvascular complications (retinopathy, nephropathy). Perhaps as much as 20% of MODY diabetics will eventually require insulin to control their hyperglycemia.

**Associated Findings:** None known.

**Etiology:** Autosomal dominant inheritance in many families. However, sporadic cases and cases in families that do not show clear evidence for autosomal dominant inheritance have been reported. These cases, along with pathophysiologic differences between families, have led several researchers to suggest etiologic heterogeneity for MODY.

**Pathogenesis:** Pathogenesis appears to be heterogeneous, but probably runs true within families. Some MODY cases show decreased and/or delayed insulin response to a glucose challenge. These appear to be the cases at highest risk to progress to insulin-requiring diabetes. Other MODY cases show normal or elevated insulin release in response to glucose. In children with hyperinsulinism, the response may return to normal following the pubertal growth spurt. In some MODY cases, a small change in weight (less than 10 pounds) can exacerbate glucose intolerance, and many MODY diabetics are of normal weight. Some individuals/families with abnormal insulins may have a type of diabetes which initially presents as a MODY type diabetes.

**MIM No.:** *12585

**Sex Ratio:** M1:F1

**Occurrence:** Undetermined, but thought to be rare compared with both **Diabetes mellitus, insulin dependent type** and **Diabetes mellitus, non-insulin dependent type**. The condition appears to be unusually frequent among blacks. Since mild cases may be undetected in the population, exact incidence rates will be difficult to obtain.

**Risk of Recurrence for Patient's Sib:**
See Part I, *Mendelian Inheritance.*

**Risk of Recurrence for Patient's Child:**
See Part I, *Mendelian Inheritance.*

**Age of Detectability:** Early childhood to 25 years of age.

**Gene Mapping and Linkage:** Unknown.

**Prevention:** None known. Genetic counseling indicated. In some individuals with abnormal glucose tolerance, maintenance of ideal body weight may be useful in slowing or preventing progression to frank diabetes.

**Treatment:** Since hyperglycemia is mild, at least initially, initial treatment is usually with a modified diabetic diet and/or oral hypoglycemic agents. Some individuals progress to requiring insulin treatment for control of hyperglycemia.

**Prognosis:** May be variable. The initial families studied had a mild form of MODY, with mild or no complications. The prognosis is good for MODY diabetics in such families. Other families appear to have a greater risk for diabetic complications, although the exact nature of this risk is currently unknown. The prevalence of diabetic complications, overall, is probably less than in NIDDM cases generally. Perhaps as many as 20% will ultimately require insulin to control their diabetes.

**Detection of Carrier:**  Unknown.

**Special Considerations:**  While initially thought to be a single, etiologically homogeneous entity, MODY diabetes now appears to be more heterogeneous than first expected. Clearly, MODY is not inherited as a simple autosomal dominant in all MODY pedigrees. Additionally, in some MODY families the primary defect appears to be associated with normo- or hyperinsulinism, while in others, decreased insulin response is common. The combined evidence suggests that there probably are several genetic or pathologic pathways that ultimately result in MODY diabetes.

The mildness of MODY diabetes, at least initially, makes the study of this disorder difficult. MODY diabetics may not be diagnosed until many years after the onset of diabetes, and then may be classified as **Diabetes mellitus, non-insulin dependent type** unless other family members were clearly identified at an earlier age. In addition, undoubtedly some affected members of a MODY family do not manifest their predisposition until after 25 years of age, and this must be true for sporadic cases as well.

**Support Groups:**

New York; American Diabetes Association
New York; Juvenile Diabetes Foundation (JDF) International
CANADA: Ontario; Toronto; Canadian Diabetes Association
ENGLAND: London; International Diabetes Federation

**References:**
Tattersall RB: Mild familial diabetes with dominant inheritance. Quart J Med 1974; 43::339–357.
Barbosa J, et al.: Plasma glucose, insulin, glucagon, and growth hormone in kindreds with maturity-onset type of hyperglycemia in young people. Ann Intern Med 1978; 88:595–601. *
Fajans SS, et al.: Clinical and etiological heterogeneity of idiopathic diabetes mellitus. Schweiz Med Wschr 1979; 109:1774–1785.
Serjeantson SE, Zimmer P: Analysis of linkage relationships in maturity-onset diabetes of young people and independent segregation of C6 and HLA. Hum Genet 1982; 62:214–216.
Tattersall RB: The present status of maturity-onset type of diabetes mellitus. In: Kobbering J, Tattersall RB, eds: Genetics of diabetes mellitus. New York: Academic Press, 1982:261–270.
Owerbach D, et al.: DNA insertion sequences near the insulin gene are not associated with maturity-onset diabetes of young people. Diabetologia 1983; 25:18–20.
Winter WE, et al.: Maturity-onset diabetes of youth in black Americans. New Engl J Med 1987; 316:285–291.

VA019
R0036

**Constance M. Vadheim**
**Jerome I. Rotter**

## DIABETES MELLITUS, MUTANT INSULIN TYPES          2328

**Includes:**

Human insulin Chicago
Human insulin Los Angeles
Human insulin Wakayama
Hyperproinsulinemia
Insulins, structurally abnormal

**Excludes:**

Diabetes mellitus, insulin dependent type (0549)
Diabetes mellitus, maturity onset of the young (MODY) (2326)
Diabetes mellitus, non-insulin dependent type (2327)

**Major Diagnostic Criteria:**  Hyperinsulinemia with normal or elevated plasma glucose levels but a normal glucose response to exogenous insulin. Hyperproinsulinemia commonly, but not always, occurs as well. Definitive diagnosis is made by the demonstration of an abnormally migrating insulin using reversed-phase high performance liquid chromatography (RP-HPLC).

**Clinical Findings:**  Can vary from overt non-insulin-dependent diabetes (NIDDM) to reactive hypoglycemia to complete absence of symptoms. Most probands studied so far have been recognized because of NIDDM with hyperinsulinemia and/or hyperproinsulinemia. Family members have subsequently been identified who are also hyperinsulinemic but have no clinical evidence of abnormal glucose regulation. All individuals have a normal glucose response to exogenous insulin and have no evidence of insulin resistance. In addition, there is a reduced C-peptide/insulin ratio.

**Complications:**  Impaired glucose tolerance; non-ketotic, non-insulin-dependent diabetes.

**Associated Findings:**  None known.

**Etiology:**  Autosomal dominant inheritance has been documented in several families.

**Pathogenesis:**  The mutant insulins thus far described are the result of point mutations within the insulin gene. Some (insulin Chicago, insulin Los Angeles) are the result of mutations in the B-chain coding region of the insulin gene. The hyperinsulinemia appears to result from decreased degradation, as the point mutations alter the insulin-receptor-binding portion of the molecule directly, or indirectly, through conformational changes, thus decreasing insulin degradation. Insulin Wakayama, the result of a point mutation in the insulin A-chain, also reduces binding to the insulin receptor and results in accumulation of the mutant insulin in plasma. Because of the mutation, there is also markedly reduced biological activity. It may require some degree of superimposed insulin resistance for hyperglycemia and/or diabetes to subsequently develop. Other mutant insulins result from mutations occurring at the dibasic amino acid site connecting the C-peptide and the insulin A-chain coding regions. The latter mutations result in the inability to cleave the C-peptide from the insulin A-chain and are subsequently associated with hyperproinsulinemia.

**Sex Ratio:**  M1:F1

**Occurrence:**  Only a handful of people with mutant insulins have thus far been identified. It appears that less than one-half of one percent of diabetes mellitus, non-insulin dependent type, can be attributed to mutant insulins. It is possible that mutant insulins are more common in certain ethnic groups, as demonstrated by the high proportion of cases reported from Japan.

**Risk of Recurrence for Patient's Sib:**

See Part I, *Mendelian Inheritance.* 50%, if parent affected, for hyperinsulinemia or hyperproinsulinemia. Unknown risk for overt diabetes or glucose intolerance.

**Risk of Recurrence for Patient's Child:**

See Part I, *Mendelian Inheritance.* 50% for hyperinsulinemia or hyperproinsulinemia. Unknown risk for overt diabetes or glucose intolerance.

**Age of Detectability:**  At birth.

**Gene Mapping and Linkage:**  Mutations occur within the insulin gene, which is located on the distal short arm of chromosome 11 and is linked to the beta globin locus.

**Prevention:**  None known. Genetic counseling indicated.

**Treatment:**  Exogenous insulin therapy and/or diet therapy in those individuals with overt diabetes or impaired glucose tolerance.

**Prognosis:**  Good, particularly with recent advances in diabetes therapy.

**Detection of Carrier:**  Reversed-phase, high-performance liquid chromatography (RP-HPLC) is probably the most definitive way to identify carrier individuals. However, within a family in which a mutant insulin has already been demonstrated, significant hyperinsulinemia alone can probably be used for carrier detection. In addition, in those individuals or families where the mutation has altered a known DNA restriction endonuclease site, carrier detection can be done at the DNA level. This can also be done using the polymerase chain reaction, specific oligonucleotide probes, and dot blot hybridization.

**Support Groups:**

New York; American Diabetes Association
New York; Juvenile Diabetes Foundation (JDF) International
CANADA: Ontario; Toronto; Canadian Diabetes Association
ENGLAND: London; International Diabetes Federation

**References:**

Gabbay KH, et al.: Familial hyperproinsulinemia: partial characterization of circulating proinsulin-like material. Proc Natl Acad Sci USA 1979; 76:2881–2885.
Haneda M, et al.: Familial hyperinsulinemia due to a structurally abnormal insulin: definition of an emerging new clinical syndrome. New Engl J Med 1984; 310:1288–1294.
Tager HS: Lilly Lecture 1983, Abnormal products of the human insulin gene. Diabetes 1984; 33:693–699.
Seino S, et al.: Identification of insulin variants in patients with hyperinsulinemia by reversed-phase, high-performance liquid chromatography. Diabetes 1985; 34:1–7.
Nanjo K, et al.: Mutant insulin syndrome: identification of two families with [Leu$^{A3}$] insulin and determination of its biological activity. Transaction of the Association of American Physicians 1986; 99:132–142.
Sanz N, et al.: Prevalence of insulin gene mutation in non-insulin dependent diabetes mellitus. New Engl J Med 1986; 314:1322 only.
Awata T, et al.: Identification of nucleotide substitution in gene encoding [Leu$^{A3}$] insulin in third Japanese family. Diabetes 1988; 37:1068–1070.
Miyano M, et al.: Use if in vitro DNA amplification to screen family members for an insulin gene mutation. Diabetes 1988; 37:362–366.
Vinik A, Bell G: Mutant insulin syndromes. Hormone and Metabolic Res 1988; 20:1–10.

RA017
R0036

Leslie J. Raffel
Jerome I. Rotter

## DIABETES MELLITUS, NON-INSULIN DEPENDENT TYPE   2327

**Includes:**

Diabetes mellitus, adult onset
Diabetes mellitus, type II
Non-insulin dependent diabetes mellitus (NIDDM)

**Excludes:**

**Diabetes mellitus, insulin dependent type** (0549)
**Diabetes mellitus, maturity onset of the young (MODY)** (2326)
**Diabetes mellitus, mutant insulin types** (2328)

**Major Diagnostic Criteria:**   Diagnosis is based on: 1) presence of symptoms such as polydipsia, polyuria, ketonuria, rapid weight loss, along with hyperglycemia; or 2) elevated fasting glucose on at least two occasions with a venous plasma glucose ≥140 mg/dl or a venous whole blood glucose ≥120 mg/dl; or 3) abnormal oral glucose tolerance testing with the two-hour sample and at least one other sample having a venous plasma glucose ≥200 mg/dl or a venous whole blood glucose ≥180 mg/dl.

**Clinical Findings:**   The patient often has a history of polydipsia, polyuria, unexplained weight loss, and fatigue. However, studies indicate that twice as many individuals will be detected if the entire adult population is screened. Often the patients are obese.

**Complications:**   Microvascular complications, including diabetic retinopathy and nephropathy are common. If untreated, these may result in blindness and end-stage kidney failure in some patients. Neuropathy, producing sensory loss in the lower extremities, is also common. The combination of microvascular changes and neuropathy can combine to produce chronic ulceration of the lower extremities. This may result in gangrene requiring amputation. Atherosclerosis occurs at an earlier age than usual, and can result in stroke and myocardial infarction.

**Associated Findings:**   None known.

**Etiology:**   Family studies and twin studies have clearly demonstrated that genetic factors play a significant role in disease. The specific mode(s) of inheritance is not known. NIDDM probably includes a heterogeneous group of disorders, all of which produce abnormalities of glucose intolerance. Some individuals with

NIDDM have elevated insulin levels, others have normal insulin levels, and still others have diminished insulin levels. Most patients have evidence of insulin resistance.

Environmental factors are also important in NIDDM, as evidenced by significant increases in incidences when primitive populations (e.g., the Micronesian population) change from a traditional rural environment and diet to a more urban, Westernized life-style. Obesity is also an environmental risk factor. In Western societies, however, the common environment, including diet and life-style, seems to be "diabetogenic" enough that genetic factors play the primary role in determining disease occurrence.

**Pathogenesis:**   Insulin resistance appears to be an important factor in many patients. Additionally, alterations in insulin secretion may be implicated.

**Sex Ratio:**   Probably M1:F1, after correction for differences in age and obesity between males and females.

**Occurrence:**   Lifetime prevalence estimales of 5% or more for diabetes and an additional 5–10% for impaired glucose tolerance in the United States and Europe. Much higher in certain populations (e.g., Micronesia, American Indian), with rates increasing with age (up to 60% of adults in the latter populations)

**Risk of Recurrence for Patient's Sib:**   10–15% for NIDDM; 25–30% for impaired glucose tolerance.

**Risk of Recurrence for Patient's Child:**   10–15% for NIDDM; 25–30% for impaired glucose tolerance.

**Age of Detectability:**   Most commonly during the fourth to sixth decade of life. Earlier presentation may also occur.

**Gene Mapping and Linkage:**   Restriction fragment length polymorphisms at several different loci have been reported to be associated with NIDDM, including the insulin receptor gene (chromosome 19p), the apolipoprotein B gene (chromosome 2p; see **Abetalipoproteinemia**), the **Apolipoprotein A-I and C-III deficiency states** gene cluster (chromosome 11q), and the HepG21/erythrocyte glucose transporter gene (chromosome 1p). Results have varied depending upon the ethnic or racial groups studied, and are preliminary.

**Prevention:**   None known. Genetic counseling indicated.

**Treatment:**   Treatment varies in different individuals. Some patients can be well controlled by weight loss and diet therapy alone. For others, the combination of diet and oral hypoglycemic agents is effective, and still other patients require exogenous insulin therapy.

Various specialized treatments are necessary for the complications of NIDDM. These include laser surgery for retinal microaneurysms, and dialysis for renal failure, among others.

**Prognosis:**   Good, for most patients. Depends to a large, but still not fully defined, extent on the degree of compliance with medical management. Morbidity is commonly related to the complications of NIDDM.

**Detection of Carrier:**   Oral glucose tolerance tests after the age of 30 to 40 should be performed periodically on the first-degree relatives of a NIDDM patient. These tests may detect some individuals with impaired glucose tolerance before the overt development of diabetes and, thus, early clinical intervention may be provided.

**Support Groups:**

New York; American Diabetes Association
New York; Juvenile Diabetes Foundation (JDF) International
CANADA: Ontario; Toronto; Canadian Diabetes Association
ENGLAND: London; International Diabetes Federation

**References:**

Fajans SS, et al.: Clinical and etiologic heterogeneity of idiopathic diabetes mellitus. Diabetes 1978; 27:1112–1125.
National Diabetes Data Group International Workgroup: Classification of diabetes mellitus and other categories of glucose intolerance. Diabetes 1979; 28:1039–1057. *
Zimmet P, et al.: Diabetes and environmental interactions. In: Melish JS, Anno J, Baba S, eds.: Genetic environmental interactions in diabetes mellitus. Amsterdam: Excerpta Medica, 1982:9–17.
Rotter JI, et al.: Genetics of diabetes mellitus. In: Ellenberg M, Rifkin

H, eds.: Diabetes mellitus, theory and practice, 3rd edition. New York: Medical Examination Publishing Co, 1983:481–503. *

Rotter JI, et al.: Genetics, diabetes mellitus heterogeneity and coronary heart disease. In: Rao DC, et al., eds: Genetic epidemiology of coronary heart disease. New York: Alan R. Liss, 1984:445–478. *

Haffner SM, et al.: Hyperinsulinemia in a population at high risk for non-insulin-dependent diabetes mellitus. New Engl J Med 1986; 315:220–224.

Haffner SM, et al.: Increased insulin concentrations in nondiabetic offspring of diabetic patients. New Engl J Med 1988; 319:1297–1301.

Li SR, et al.: Association of genetic variant glucose transporter with non-insulin-dependent diabetes mellitus. Lancet 1988; II:368–370.

McClain DA, et al.: Restriction fragment length polymorphism in insulin receptor gene and insulin resistance in NIDDM. Diabetes 1988; 37:1071–1075.

Kahn CR, Goldstein BJ: Molecular defects in insulin action. Science 1989; 245:13–14 *

Xiang K-S, et al.: Insulin-receptor and apolipoprotein genes contribute to development of NIDDM in Chinese Americans. Diabetes 1989; 38:17–23.

Becerra JE, et al.: Diabetes mellitus during pregnancy and the risks for specific birth defects. Pediatrics 1990; 85:1–9.

Bogardus C, Lillioja S: Where all the glucose doesn't go in non-insulin-dependent diabetes mellitus. New Engl J Med 1990; 322:262–263.

Shulman GI, et al.: Quantitation of muscle glycogen synthesis in normal subjects and subjects with non-insulin-dependent diabetes by 13C nuclear magnetic resonance spectroscopy. New Engl J Med 1990; 322:223–228.

RA017
R0036

**Leslie J. Raffel**
**Jerome I. Rotter**

**Diabetes mellitus, type I**
*See DIABETES MELLITUS, INSULIN DEPENDENT TYPE*
**Diabetes mellitus, type II**
*See DIABETES MELLITUS, NON-INSULIN DEPENDENT TYPE*
**Diabetes mellitus-deafness**
*See DEAFNESS-DIABETES*
**Diabetes mellitus-otpic atrophy**
*See DIABETES (INSIPIDUS/MELLITUS)-OPTIC ATROPHY-DEAFNESS*
**Diabetes, fetal effects from maternal**
*See FETAL EFFECTS FROM MATERNAL DIABETES*
**Diabetes, lipoatrophic-acrorenal field defect-ectodermal dysplasia**
*See AREDYLD SYNDROME*
**Diabetes-deafness-photomyoclonus-nephropathy**
*See DEAFNESS-DIABETES-PHOTOMYOCLONUS-NEPHROPATHY*
**Diabetes-hypogonadism-alopecia-deafness-retardation-EKG anomalies**
*See HYPOGONADISM-DIABETES-ALOPECIA-DEAFNESS-RETARDATION-EKG ANOMALIES*
**Diabetes-Rieger anomaly-lipodystrophy-short stature**
*See LIPODYSTROPHY-RIEGER ANOMALY-SHORT STATURE-DIABETES*
**Diacyclothrombopathia IIb-IIIa**
*See THROMBASTHENIA, GLANZMANN-NAEGELI TYPE*
**Dialysis-associated amyloidosis**
*See AMYLOIDOSIS, HEMODIALYSIS-RELATED*
**Diamond-Blackfan syndrome**
*See ANEMIA, HYPOPLASTIC CONGENITAL*
**Diaphorase deficiency**
*See METHEMOGLOBINEMIA, NADH-DEPENDENT DIAPHORASE DEFICIENCY*
**Diaphragm abnormally high**
*See DIAPHRAGM, EVENTRATION*
**Diaphragm of esophagus, congenital**
*See ESOPHAGUS, STENOSIS*
**Diaphragm, congenital relaxation of**
*See DIAPHRAGM, EVENTRATION*

## DIAPHRAGM, EVENTRATION        0288

**Includes:**
> Diaphragm abnormally high
> Diaphragm, congenital relaxation of
> Pleura and peritoneum, muscle deficiency between
> Zwerchfell eventration

**Excludes:**
> Absence of one leaf of diaphragm
> **Diaphragmatic hernia** (0289)
> Traumatic rupture of diaphragm

**Major Diagnostic Criteria:** Diaphragm (abnormally high but intact) arching smoothly from its normal costal attachments

**Clinical Findings:** If diaphragm is only slightly elevated, there may be no symptoms. If diaphragm is markedly elevated, there is limited expansion of the lung and atelectasis on the ipsilateral side. In small infants there may be a dangerous shift of the mediastinum to the contralateral side with further impairment of respiratory function by compression of the lung on the opposite side. Tachypnea is the first symptom which may progress to severe "respiratory fatigue" and death. Congenital absence of muscle in the diaphragm is the least common cause of eventration but usually produces very severe symptoms that are incompatible with life early in the newborn period. Partial eventration is seen in 65%, majority on the right side. Left side is usually complete. There is an occasionally bilateral involvement with poor prognosis.

The acquired form of eventration resulting from obstetric delivery may be either temporary or permanent depending on whether the phrenic nerve is merely stretched or irreversibly damaged or avulsed. Symptoms may develop a few days after birth but usually in the neonatal period. If the infant tolerates the restricted expansion of the lungs, a period of observation may be indicated, hoping for spontaneous improvement. If the symptoms persist with progressive fatigue of the infant or if the infant requires extra oxygen or has feeding difficulties due to shortness of breath, a surgical repair should not be delayed.

Acquired eventration, secondary to perinatal trauma, will often recover normal function and position within one year with conservative management. Acquired eventration occur equally on either side. Older children often present with chronic complaints and/or recurrent pneumonias. The eventration described in older individuals is often felt to be associated with age, malnutrition and tight abdominal clothing.

An anteroposterior X-ray of the chest shows an elevation of the involved leaf of the diaphragm with a normal position of the opposite leaf. Fluoroscopy shows paradoxical motion of the involved leaf of the diaphragm. On inspiration the involved leaf rises while the uninvolved leaf is depressed and during expiration the reverse occurs. Paradoxical motion also can be demonstrated by an X-ray taken in full inspiration and compared to one taken in full expiration. Penumoperitonograph with nitrous oxide or carbon dioxide may allow separation of abdominal masses from eventration. Ultrasonography is a rapid technique for diagnosis.

**Complications:** Ipsilateral atelectasis, mediastinal shift, tachypnea.

**Associated Findings:** None known.

**Etiology:** Unknown.

**Pathogenesis:** Most likely failure of development of adequate muscular tissue in septum transversum with presence of pleura and peritoneum.

**CDC No.:** 756.620

**Sex Ratio:** Presumably M1:F1

**Occurrence:** Unknown.

**Risk of Recurrence for Patient's Sib:** Unknown.

**Risk of Recurrence for Patient's Child:** Unknown.

**Age of Detectability:** At birth.

**Gene Mapping and Linkage:** Unknown.

**Prevention:** None known. Genetic counseling indicated.

**Treatment:** Under controlled, intubation anesthesia a thoracotomy is performed on the affected side. A central ellipse of the abnormal diaphragm is resected and the defect closed by overlapping the remaining 2 layers using nonabsorbable sutures. The repaired diaphragm after plication should be at the level of a normal diaphragm. A thoracotomy tube is placed on low suction for removal of any serum and protection against the possibility of an unrecognized postoperative pneumothorax. There is little evidence to support repair of an asymptomatic eventration.

**Prognosis:** Excellent if surgical plication is performed when needed before the infant has deteriorated from chronic oxygen insufficiency, prolonged atelectasis and associated pneumonia. Follow-up many years later show the plicated diaphragm remains at a normal level and is relatively fixed, showing little motion with deep inspiration and expiration.

**Detection of Carrier:** Unknown.

**References:**

Baffles, T. G.: Eventration of the diaphragm. In Mustard, W.T. et al eds: Pediatric Surgery. Chicago: Yearbook Medical Publishers, 1969; 350.
Bishop, H. C. and Koop, C. E.: Acquired eventration of the diaphragm in infancy. Pediatrics 1958; 22:1088.
Jewett, T. C., Jr. and Thomson, N. B., Jr.: Iatrogenic eventration of the diaphragm in infancy. J Thorac Cardiovasc Surg 1964; 48:861.
Wayne ER et al. Eventration of the diaphragm. J Ped Surg 1974; 9:643–651.
Othersen HB, Lorenzo RL: Diaphragmatic paralysis and eventration: newer approaches to diagnosis and operative correction. J Pediatric Surgery 1977; 12:309–315. *

BR021                                            **Diane Broome**

**Diaphragmatic defects-distal digital hypoplasia**
  *See FRYNS SYNDROME*
**Diaphragmatic esophageal hiatus hernia**
  *See HERNIA, HIATAL*

## DIAPHRAGMATIC HERNIA                              0289

**Includes:**
Anterolateral diaphragmatic hernia
Bochdalek hernia
Foramen of Morgagni hernia
Hemidiaphragm, congenital absence of
Hernia, diaphragmatic, congenital
Parasternal hernia
Posterolateral diaphragmatic hernia
Retrosternal diaphragmatic hernia
Subcostosternal hernia

**Excludes:**
Congenital short esophagus
**Diaphragm, eventration** (0288)
**Esophagus, chalasia** (0366)
Esophageal stricture
**Hernia, hiatal** (0471)
Lax cardia
Parahiatal hernia
Phrenic nerve palsy
Traumatic hernia of diaphragm

**Major Diagnostic Criteria:** *Posterolateral hernia:* demonstration on X-ray of abdominal viscera in chest with surgical confirmation of posterolateral diaphragmatic defect.
*Retrosternal hernia:* demonstration on X-ray of abdominal viscera displaced into lower anterior mediastinum.

**Clinical Findings:** *Posterolateral diaphragmatic hernia:* Severely affected infants have dyspnea and cyanosis from birth. Symptoms progress as swallowed air distends the hollow viscera, misplaced in the chest, causing further cardiopulmonary compression. Early onset of symptoms and high mortality correlate with the degree of associated pulmonary hypoplasia. Infants with compressed but fully developed lungs have more respiratory reserve and develop symptoms usually after the first 24 hours of life, when initial feedings and swallowed air increase the mass lesion in the chest. Defects in the left leaf of the diaphragm predominate 7:1. Less than one-half of the posterolateral hernias are contained by a hernia sac. Physical findings frequently include a scaphoid abdomen, cardiac dextroposition, decreased breath sounds, dullness to chest percussion on the affected side, and, occasionally, bowel sounds in the thorax. On X-ray, loops of air-filled bowel and solid viscera may be seen in the chest, whereas congenital lobar emphysema is distinguished by an even distribution of air in the affected lobe, the diaphragm remains visible in cystic adenomatoid malformation of the lungs, and pulmonary compression from increased intraluminal bowel air is associated with a distended rather than scaphoid abdomen. Contrast studies are diagnostic if the infant's condition permits. Acidosis, arterial hypoxia, and hypercarbia are usual laboratory findings in symptomatic infants.
*Retrosternal diaphragmatic hernia:* Affected infants may present with dyspnea in the first hours of life, but more often symptoms are recognized much later in infancy or childhood. These anterior hernias are probably limited in size by the adjacent pericardium and by the usual presence of a containing hernia sac. Right-sided hernias predominate, and they are seldom large enough to produce serious symptoms from mass compression in the chest. Symptoms may relate to moderate pulmonary compression or to partial bowel obstruction. Pulmonary hypoplasia is not commonly associated. Diagnosis is often first suspected from routine chest X-rays.

**Complications:** *Posterolateral hernia:* Preoperative: pneumothorax on ipsilateral or, more commonly, contralateral side of hernia; pneumomediastinum; hypoxia; acidosis; death. Bowel obstruction or volvulus and infarction can occur with late onset of symptoms. Postoperative: inability to be adequately ventilated due to pulmonary hypoplasia and persistent fetal circulation, apparently in proportion to the delay in closure of the pleuroperitoneal canals and consequent duration and extent of compression interference with fetal lung development. Also pneumothorax on either side, bowel obstruction, and inferior vena cava compression.
*Retrosternal hernia:* Preoperative: bowel obstruction, recurrent lung infections. Postoperative: bowel obstruction, recurrence of hernia, hemorrhage, infection (all frequent).

**Associated Findings:** *Posterolateral hernia:* occurs about twice as frequently in isolation as in association with other congenital anomalies, principally neural tube defects, but also cardiovascular, genitourinary, and gastrointestinal malformations. Other lethal anomalies are present in 16% of cases; karyotypic abnormality reported in 4% of cases.
*Retrosternal hernia:* associated malformation of cardiovascular, genitourinary, and CNS systems are common.

**Etiology:** Probably multifactorial inheritance.

**Pathogenesis:** *Posterolateral hernia:* thought to develop in the 8th to 12th week of fetal life. The formation of the diaphragm, the return of the gut from the yolk stalk, and the differentiation of the lung buds all take place during this period. An imbalance in timing is thought to result in thoracic migration of the gut with incomplete closure of the diaphragm and compression of the undeveloped lung buds.

**MIM No.:** 14234

**CDC No.:** 756.610

**Sex Ratio:** Posterolateral hernia, M2:F1; retrosternal hernia, undetermined.

**Occurrence:** Posterolateral hernia, 16–21:100,000 births; retrosternal hernia, probably less than 1:1,000,000 live births.

**Risk of Recurrence for Patient's Sib:** Reported 0.9–2% for posterolateral form; not increased for retrosternal. Neural tube defects in 1.8% of sibs in posterolateral form.

**Risk of Recurrence for Patient's Child:** Unknown.

**Age of Detectability:** Prenatal detection by ultrasonography in the third trimester reported in up to 97% of cases; at birth with chest X-ray.

**Gene Mapping and Linkage:** Unknown.

**Prevention:** None known. Genetic counseling indicated.

**Treatment:** Surgical repair: transthoracic or transabdominal reduction of displaced viscera into abdomen with repair of defect in diaphragm. Prosthetic enlargement of abdomen with later staged reconstruction may be required for some complicated posterolateral defects associated with pulmonary hypoplasia. Treatment of persistent fetal circulation/pulmonary hypoplasia complex. There have been reports of successful extracorporal membrane oxygenation.

**Prognosis:** Probably normal life span without disability if repair is uncomplicated, pulmonary development is normal, and other anomalies do not coexist. Effect of associated pulmonary hypoplasia on life span is unknown.

**Detection of Carrier:** Unknown.

**Special Considerations:** Postoperative survival is 11% when found with polyhydramnios and only 55% even when not so associated, being limited by other major anomalies, chiefly pulmonary hypoplasia and persistent fetal circulation. Premature delivery has not been found helpful due to the addition of pulmonary parenchymal immaturity. Successful repair of experimentally induced lesions in animals raises the hope of congenital diaphragmatic defects being the first application of complex fetal surgery.

**References:**
Wolff G: Familial congenital diaphragmatic defect: review and conclusions. Hum Genet 1980; 54:1–5.
Norio R, et al.: Familial congenital diaphragmatic defects: aspects of etiology, prenatal diagnosis and treatment. Am J Med Genet 1984; 17:471–483.
Adzick NS, et al.: Diaphragmatic hernia in the fetus: prenatal diagnosis and outcome in 94 cases. J Pediatr Surg 1985; 20:357–361.
Czeizel A, Koracs M: A familial study of congenital diaphragmatic defects. Am J Med Genet 1985; 21:105–115.

GA025                                    **Arthur R. Garrett**

**Diaphyseal aclasis**
*See EXOSTOSES, MULTIPLE CARTILAGINOUS*
**Diaphyseal and cranial dysplasia**
*See CRANIO-DIAPHYSEAL DYSPLASIA*

## DIAPHYSEAL DYSPLASIA                               0290

**Includes:**
    Camurati-Engelmann syndrome
    Engelmann disease
    Osteopathia hyperostotica scleroticans multiplex infantilis
    Progressive diaphyseal dysplasia
    Ribbing disease
    Schwartz-Lelek syndrome (one form)

**Excludes:**
    **Cortical hyperostosis, infantile** (0221)
    Diaphyseal sclerosis, hereditary multiple
    **Endosteal hyperostosis** (0497)
    **Fetal retinoid syndrome** (2261)
    **Melorheostosis** (0641)

**Major Diagnostic Criteria:** X-ray changes consisting of marked symmetric thickening of the cortices of the leg bones with consequent narrowing of the medullary canals are the predominant feature.

**Clinical Findings:** The manifestations are variable. Some patients are severely handicapped, while others are virtually asymptomatic. Characteristically, the disorder presents in midchildhood with muscular pain, weakness, wasting, and a wide-based, waddling gait. Occasionally, varus or valgus deformities of the knees are present, together with scoliosis or increased lumbar lordosis. Puberty may be delayed. Intelligence is normal.

X-ray features include involvement of the tubular bones of the lower limbs principally, but the upper limbs may also be affected. The axial skeleton and extremities are usually spared. The diaphyseal cortices are thickened by periosteal and endosteal prolifera-

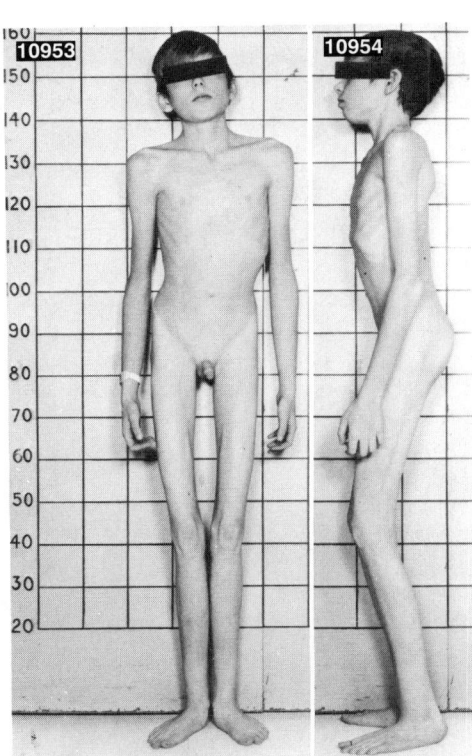

**0290A**-10953–54: Thin body habitus, dorsal scoliosis, flexion deformities at the elbows, knees and hips.

tion, but the metaphyses and epiphyses are unaffected. Infrequently, the skull is involved, with calvarial widening and basal sclerosis.

**Complications:** Crippling leg pain may incapacitate the individual. Fracture of a long bone is a rare complication. Cranial nerve compression and raised intracranial pressure are occasional complications.

**Associated Findings:** None known.

**Etiology:** Autosomal dominant inheritance. Most reports are of sporadic cases, which are presumably new mutations.

**Pathogenesis:** There appears to be decreased or absent osteoclastic activity and corticosteroids appear to stimulate osteoclasis and decrease lamellar bone deposition.

**MIM No.:** *13130

**POS No.:** 3206

**CDC No.:** 756.550

**Sex Ratio:** M1:F1

**Occurrence:** More than 100 cases have been reported.

**Risk of Recurrence for Patient's Sib:**
    See Part I, *Mendelian Inheritance.*

**Risk of Recurrence for Patient's Child:**
    See Part I, *Mendelian Inheritance.*

**Age of Detectability:** The youngest reported patient was recognized at age 4 months.

**Gene Mapping and Linkage:** Unknown.

**Prevention:** None known. Genetic counseling indicated.

**Treatment:** A good response to steroid therapy has been reported in 12 affected persons (Naveh et al., 1985) and in other isolated instances.

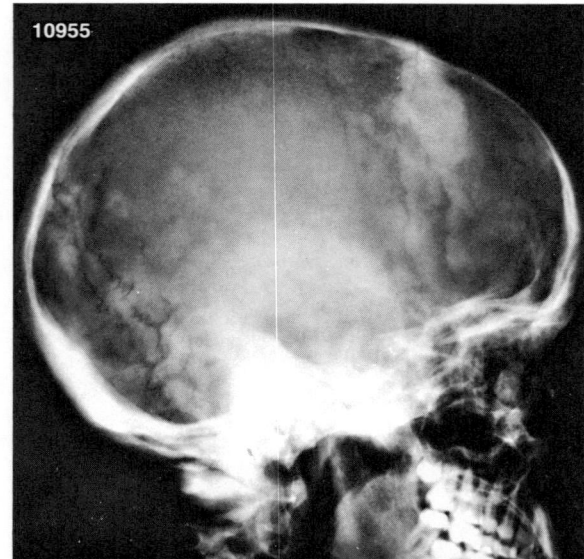

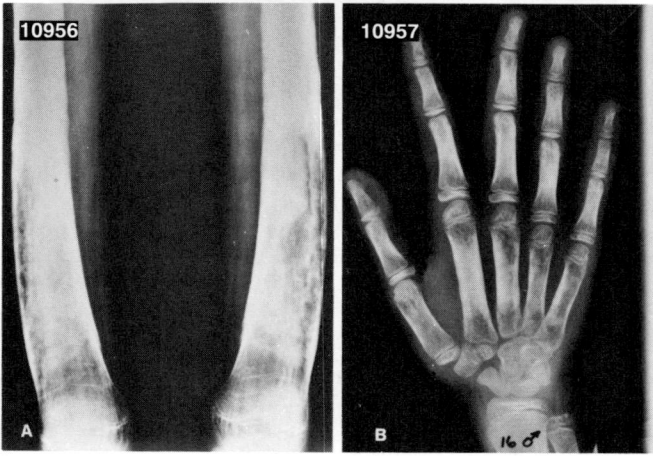

**0290B-10955:** Focal sclerosis with more marked thickening in the base than the vault. **10956:** Swollen diaphyses, particularly in the distal portions; irregular cortical thickening; sclerosis. **10957:** Wide, poorly modeled metacarpals and phalanges; irregular sclerotic shafts.

**Prognosis:** Life span does not appear to be shortened, though there may be a crippling disability. There is some evidence that progression of the bone lesions ends with the cessation of growth.

**Detection of Carrier:** Unknown.

**Special Considerations:** Gorlin et al have suggested that a patient reported by Lelek in 1961 as an example of Camurati-Engelmann disease actually had a distinct condition which they termed *Schwartz-Lelek syndrome* (see **Craniometaphyseal dysplasia**).

**References:**

Clawson DK, Loop JW: Progressive diaphyseal dysplasia (Engelmann's disease). J Bone Joint Surg 1964; 46:143–147.

Allen DT, et al.: Corticosteroids in the treatment of Engelmann's disease: progressive diaphyseal dysplasia. Pediatrics 1970; 46:523–531.

Sparkes RS, Graham CB: Camurati-Engelmann disease: genetics and clinical manifestations with a review of the literature. J Med Genet 1972; 9:73–85.

Minford AMB, et al.: Engelmann's disease and the effect of corticosteroids: a case report. J Bone Joint Surg 1981; 63B:597–600.

Naveh Y, et al.: Progressive diaphyseal dysplasia: genetics and clinical and radiologic manifestations. Pediatrics 1984; 74:399–405. * †

Naveh Y, et al.: Progressive diaphyseal dysplasia: evaluation of corticosteroid therapy. Pediatrics 1985; 75:321–323.

VI005                                  **Denis L. Viljöen**

**Diarrhea with hypoplastic villus atrophy**
*See MICROVILLUS INCLUSION DISEASE*

## DIARRHEA, CONGENITAL CHLORIDE        0148

**Includes:**
    Alkalosis with diarrhea
    Chloride diarrhea, congenital
    Clorurorrea

**Excludes:**
    Infectious gastroenteridides
    Mucous colitis

**Major Diagnostic Criteria:** Fecal chloride concentration is above 60 mEq/l in the newborn and above 100 mEq/l later. Stools are solid, and Cl- concentrations < 60 mEq/l occur only in chronic dehydration. Serum and urinary Cl- concentrations are very low.

**Clinical Findings:** The pregnancy is uniformly complicated by hydramnios, and the child is often premature. Watery diarrhea begins from the first day of life. Meconium usually cannot be found. Abdomen is often distended. Volvulus has been a complication in a few patients during the newborn period.

**Complications:** Excessive neonatal loss of weight, with dehydration and jaundice. Hyponatremia and hypochloridemia develop rapidly and, later, hypokalemia and metabolic alkalosis.

**Associated Findings:** None known.

**Etiology:** Autosomal recessive inheritance of a defect in the Cl-/HCO$_3$- exchange mechanism in the distal ileum and the colon.

**Pathogenesis:** Impairment or net Cl- reabsorption in ileum and colon is apparently responsible for osmotic diarrhea, with high Cl- concentration and low net fecal HCO$_3$- excretion associated with metabolic alkalosis.

**MIM No.:** *21470

**Sex Ratio:** M1:F1

**Occurrence:** 1:30,000 live births in Finland; rarer elsewhere. Over 30 probands outside Finland, and a similar number in Finland.

**Risk of Recurrence for Patient's Sib:**
    See Part I, *Mendelian Inheritance.*

**Risk of Recurrence for Patient's Child:**
    See Part I, *Mendelian Inheritance.*

**Age of Detectability:** At birth or neonatally.

**Gene Mapping and Linkage:** Unknown.

**Prevention:** None known. Genetic counseling indicated.

**Treatment:** The newborn should receive extra free water (150 ml/day), together with 10 mEq of Cl-/kg (approximately 2 mEq as KCl, the rest as NaCl). Later, adjustment of the daily intake of salt solution (both NaCl and KCl; Na:K = 5:1 - 1:1) will ensure that serum potassium and acid-base balance are normal and Cl- is excreted into the urine. Early treatment is life-saving. Inhibitors of prostaglandin synthesis are beneficial against **Bartter syndrome**-like complications.

**Prognosis:** Patients have died from superimposed infection during the first few years of life; growth failure and retarded mental development have been noted as well. Aggressive treatment should be given from birth, compatible with normal development.

**Detection of Carrier:** Unknown.

**Special Considerations:** This diagnosis must be considered in any patient with neonatal diarrhea; it demonstrates that chloride transport in intestine is genetically controlled and chemically mediated. No associated defect in renal handling of chloride indicates that the renal tubular reabsorptive mechanism for chloride is distinct from that in the intestine.

**References:**
Darrow DC: Congenital alkalosis with diarrhea. J Pediatr 1945; 26:519–532.
Gamble JL, et al.: Congenital alkalosis with diarrhea. J Pediatr 1945; 26:509–518.
Norio R, et al.: Congenital chloride diarrhea, an autosomal recessive disease. Genetic study of 14 Finnish and 12 other families. Clin Genet 1971; 2:182–192.
Holmberg C, et al.: Colonic electrolyte transport in health and in congenital chloride diarrhea. J Clin Invest 1975; 56:302–310.
Minford AMB, Barr DGD: Prostaglandin synthesis inhibitor in an infant with congenital chloride diarrhea. Arch Dis Child 1980; 55:70–72.
Booth IW, et al.: Defective jejunal brush-border Na+/H+ exchange: a cause of congenital secretory diarrhoea. Lancet 1985; I:1066–1069.

SC050
SI016                                          **Charles R. Scriver**
                                               **Olli G. Simell**

**Diastema, dental medial**
*See TEETH, DIASTEMA, MEDIAN INCISAL*
**Diastema-radial hypoplasia-triphalangeal thumbs-hypospadias**
*See RADIAL HYPOPLASIA-TRIPHALANGEAL THUMBS-HYPOSPADIAS-DIASTEMA*

## DIASTEMATOMYELIA                              0292

**Includes:**
Diplomyelia with bony spur
Split notocord syndrome

**Excludes:** Spinal cord, neurenteric cyst (0894)

**Major Diagnostic Criteria:** Clinical and X-ray findings that lead to myelography show a double column of contrast material surrounding the divided spinal cord with a central dark radiolucent zone of varying extent between the two halves.

**Clinical Findings:** Most frequent initial symptoms are gait disturbance with weakness and atrophy of one or both lower limbs. Bladder dysfunction may ensue. Pain in the back or the legs is infrequent. Examination of the lower back will show a skin abnormality: a patch of hair, a cutaneous dimple, hemangioma, or a subcutaneous fat pad (66% of cases). When X-rays show spina bifida, scoliosis, or kyphoscoliosis with widening of the interpediculate distances in the region of the spinal cord anomaly, the diagnosis is confirmed. Hemivertebrae or fused vertebrae may also be seen. The finding of a bony spur is not to be expected in every case, because the spur may be fibrous or cartilaginous.

**Complications:** Progressive neurologic deficit with bladder dysfunction and upper urinary tract pathology.

**Associated Findings:** Spina bifida distal to the diastematomyelia present in >50%. Scoliosis in nearly all patients (4.9% of scoliosis patients have diastematomyelia). An increased risk of neural tube defects has been reported in families of children with diastematomyelia or spinal dysraphism.

**Etiology:** Autosomal dominant inheritance has been suggested from reports of affected sisters in two kinships.

**Pathogenesis:** May result from hydromyelia in the embryo and lead to disruption of the roof plate and separation of cord lateral masses. Alternately, it may represent an accessory neurenteric canal. During the closure of the neural tube from the primitive neuroectoderm in the third to fourth week of gestation, aberrant mesodermal cells protrude into the neural tissue on its ventral surface instead of becoming arranged around its periphery. Ninety-five percent of the cases reported are below the T6 level. The spinal cord may be duplicated, but usually it has a single dorsal and ventral cell mass with lateral roots and no medial roots. Each hemicord is covered with pia, arachnoid, and dura. A frequently associated pathologic finding is an enlarged central canal (hydromyelia) cephalad to the diastematomyelia.

**MIM No.:** 22250

**CDC No.:** 742.520
**Sex Ratio:** M1:F2.4
**Occurrence:** Presumed rare. Several kinships have been reported.
**Risk of Recurrence for Patient's Sib:**
See Part I, *Mendelian Inheritance.*
**Risk of Recurrence for Patient's Child:**
See Part I, *Mendelian Inheritance.*
**Age of Detectability:** Usually 1–15 years, although occasionally an affected individual is an adult.
**Gene Mapping and Linkage:** Unknown.
**Prevention:** None known. Genetic counseling indicated.
**Treatment:** Surgical removal of the bony spur is indicated at any age if the lesion is symptomatic, and it should be removed in all children when spinal column growth is anticipated which may cause later symptoms. Tethering of the spinal cord below the spur is present in approximately 10% of affected persons and may require a separate operation.
**Prognosis:** Surgical results are satisfactory in preventing further neurologic loss, with the possibility of improving the presurgical status.
**Detection of Carrier:** Unknown.

**References:**
Bremer JL: Dorsal intestinal fistula; accessory neurenteric canal; diastematomyelia. Arch Pathol 1952; 54:132.
Cohen J, Sledge CB: Diastematomyelia. An embryological interpretation with report of a case. Am J Dis Child 1960; 100:257.
Hendrick EB: On diastematomyelia. In: Progress in neurosurgery. Basel: Karger, 1971:277–288.
Winter RB, et al.: Diastematomyelia and congenital spine deformities. J Bone Joint Surg 1974; 56A:27.
Carter CO, et al.: Spinal dysraphism: genetic relation to neural tube malformations. J Med Genet 1976; 13:343–350.
Kennedy PR: New data on diastematomyelia. J Neurosurg 1979; 51:355–361.

SH007                                          **Kenneth Shapiro**

**Diastrophic dwarfism**
*See DIASTROPHIC DYSPLASIA*

## DIASTROPHIC DYSPLASIA                         0293

**Includes:**
Diastrophic dwarfism
Diastrophic variant

**Excludes:**
Achondroplasia (0010)
Arthrogryposes (0088)

**Major Diagnostic Criteria:** Short-limbed dwarfism with clubfeet and one of the other characteristic abnormalities of diastrophic dysplasia.

**Clinical Findings:** *Clinical features:* Short-limbed dwarfism present at birth, with more rhizomelia than mesomelia. The name *diastrophic,* meaning *twisted* in Greek, was given by Lamy and Maroteaux because of the characteristic progressive scoliosis, combined with clubfeet and deformities of the joints. Scoliosis is not present at birth, but manifests by childhood. The scoliosis is progressive and frequently severe. It is not caused by malformation of vertebrae. Nearly all of these infants have clubfeet, which may be recalcitrant to treatment. Other joint abnormalities include limitation of mobility with or without a tendency to subluxation and dislocations of joints. Hip and knee dislocation frequently develop upon weight bearing. Frequently, the children walk on tiptoe because of the joint deformities. Degenerative joint disease frequently results. Typical hand deformities include brachydactyly and symphalangism of the proximal interphalangeal joint of fingers 2 through 5. The thumbs, by contrast, are proximally placed and subluxed in abduction, producing the characteristic

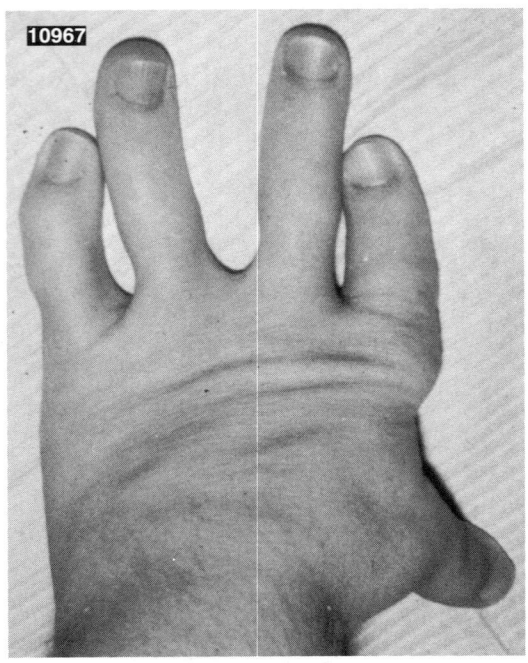

0293A-10967: Short fingers; proximal thumb (hitchhiker thumb).

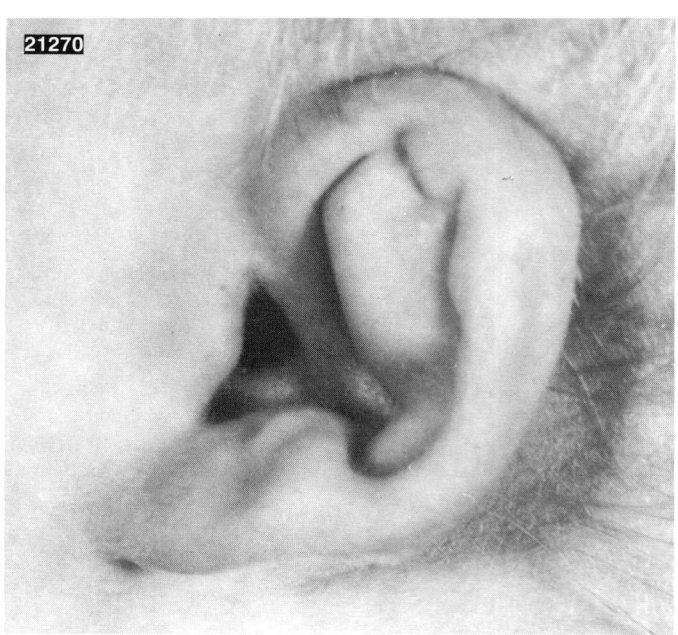

0293C-21270: Cystic swelling of the auricle.

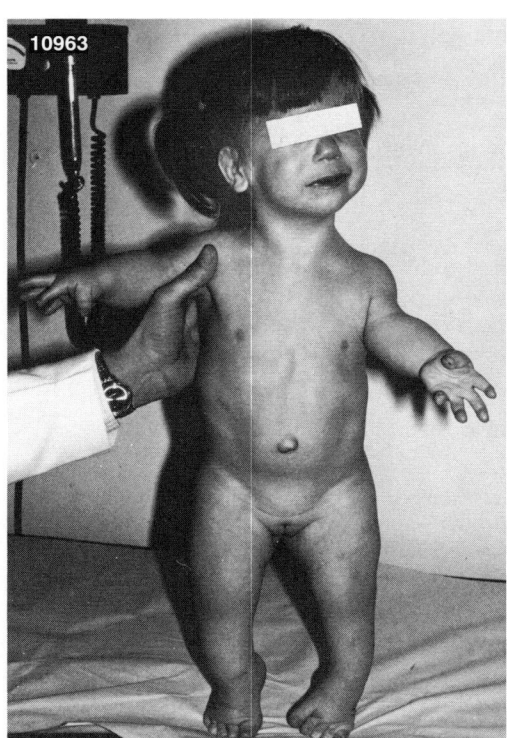

0293B-10963: Note short limbs, clubfeet, tiptoe stance, and hitchhiker thumbs.

"hitch-hiker" thumbs. Kyphosis may be a problem, and there is a tendency to subluxation of the cervical spine. Malformation of the external ear is common. Swelling of the ear usually develops in the first few weeks of life. There is an inflammatory reaction, and the tissue may feel cystic and fluctuant. The swelling resolves after 3–4 weeks, typically leaving the pinnae thickened, deformed, and hard, with calcifications in the cartilage. The ear canals may be narrowed, but hearing is usually normal. Cleft palate is present in one-third of these individuals. Some have micrognathia and are diagnosed as having Pierre Robin sequence. Lower frequency abnormalities include facial hemangiomata, anterior chamber eye malformation, craniosynostosis, a rasping cry, intracranial calcification, laryngeal or tracheal stenosis, and congenital heart disease. Intelligence is normal.

 *X-ray features:* Shortened tubular bones with metaphyseal flaring and undermodeling. Epiphyseal ossification is delayed, especially in the proximal femur. Paradoxically, the carpals may show accelerated maturation, and carpal centers may be irregular in shape. Epiphyses may be stippled in the neonate. Most epiphyses become broad in later life. The first metacarpal is short, frequently oval or delta shaped. The pelvis shows none of the signs of achondroplasia, although the acetabulae are frequently wide and irregular, and the sacrosciatic notches may be absent. The spine may show narrowing of the interpedicular distances caudally. Calcification of costal cartilages may occur.

**Complications:** The orthopedic deformities may interfere with walking and predispose the individual to degenerative arthritis. Cervical spine instability may lead to spinal cord injury. Clubfoot is notoriously difficult to treat and may require multiple procedures.

**Associated Findings:** Respiratory distress and feeding difficulties may be associated with the cleft palate.

**Etiology:** Autosomal recessive inheritance.

**Pathogenesis:** Histology of growth plate reveals irregular distribution of chondrocytes in the reserve zone and abnormal fibrous and cystic areas in the matrix.

**MIM No.:** *22260
**POS No.:** 3185
**CDC No.:** 756.445

**Sex Ratio:**  M1:F1

**Occurrence:**  Undetermined, but one of the more common skeletal dysplasias.

**Risk of Recurrence for Patient's Sib:**
See Part I, *Mendelian Inheritance.*

**Risk of Recurrence for Patient's Child:**
See Part I, *Mendelian Inheritance.*

**Age of Detectability:**  At birth. Prenatal diagnosis is possible.

**Gene Mapping and Linkage:**  Unknown.

**Prevention:**  None known. Genetic counseling indicated.

**Treatment:**  Orthopedic surgery, plastic and oral surgery, physical therapy. Intra-auricular injection of steroids may decrease the amount of ear deformity.

**Prognosis:**  Usually normal life span and intellectual development. There is wide variability of expression of the disorder. Neonatally lethal instances have been reported. Final adult height: females 105–123 cm, males 88–128 cm.

**Detection of Carrier:**  Unknown.

**Special Considerations:**  There is wide variablity in expression of diastrophic dysplasia. In the past it had been proposed that there was a distinct milder form of diastrophic dysplasia. There is no reason to consider "diastrophic variant" to be anything more than a milder expression of the same genetic entity.

**References:**

Lamy M, Maroteaux P: Le nanisme diastrophique. Presse Med 1960; 68:1977–1980.

Walker BA, et al.: Diastrophic dwarfism. Medicine 1972; 51:41–60. *

Horton WA, et al.: The phenotypic variability of diastrophic dysplasia. J Pediatr 1978; 93:609–613.

Lachman R, et al.: Diastrophic dysplasia: the death of a variant. Radiology 1981; 140:79–86.

Butler MG, et al.: Metacarpophalangeal pattern profile analysis in diastrophic dysplasia. Am J Med Genet 1987; 28:685–689.

Gollop TR, Eigier A: Prenatal ultrasound diagnosis of diastrophic dysplasia at 16 weeks. Am J Med Genet 1987; 27:321–324.

FL001                                                **David B. Flannery**

**Diastrophic variant**
*See DIASTROPHIC DYSPLASIA*
**Diazepam, fetal effects**
*See FETAL BENZODIAZEPINE EFFECTS*
**Diazoxide, fetal effects**
*See FETAL EFFECTS FROM MATERNAL VASODILATOR*
**Dibasic amino aciduria II**
*See HYPERDIBASIC AMINOACIDURIA*
**Dibucaine resistant variant E1a**
*See CHOLINESTERASE, ATYPICAL*
**Dicarboxylic aciduria due to LCAD**
*See ACYL-CoA DEHYDROGENASE DEFICIENCY, LONG CHAIN TYPE*
**Dicephalus**
*See TWINS, CONJOINED*
**Dienestrol, fetal effects**
*See FETAL DIETHYLSTILBESTROL (DES) EFFECTS*
**Diethylstilbestrol, fetal effects**
*See FETAL DIETHYLSTILBESTROL (DES) EFFECTS*
**Differentiated carcinoma of the papillary type**
*See CANCER, THYROID, FAMILIAL PAPILLARY CARCINOMA OF*
**Diffuse segmental bronchomalacia**
*See BRONCHOMALACIA*
**Diffuse T-cell lymphoma**
*See LEUKEMIA/LYMPHOMA, T-CELL*
**Diffuse undifferentiated lymphoma**
*See LYMPHOMA, BURKITT TYPE*
**DiGeorge anomaly**
*See IMMUNODEFICIENCY, THYMIC AGENESIS*
**DiGeorge sequence with chromosome 22q11 deletion**
*See CHROMOSOME 22, MONOSOMY 22q*
**DiGeorge syndrome**
*See IMMUNODEFICIENCY, THYMIC AGENESIS*
**Digit, hyperphalangy of index finger**
*See DIGITO-PALATAL SYNDROME, STEVENSON TYPE*
**Digital anomalies-gingival fibromatosis-hepatosplenomegaly**
*See GINGIVAL FIBROMATOSIS-DIGITAL ANOMALIES*

**Digital constrictions-keratopachydermia-deafness**
*See DEAFNESS-KERATOPACHYDERMIA-DIGITAL CONSTRICTIONS*
**Digital defects-albinism-microcephaly**
*See ALBINISM-MICROCEPHALY-DIGITAL DEFECTS*
**Digital defects-nephrosis-deafness urinary tract defects**
*See NEPHROSIS-DEAFNESS-URINARY TRACT AND DIGITAL DEFECTS*

## DIGITAL DEFECTS-NODULAR ERYTHEMA-EMACIATION, NAKAJO TYPE      2807

**Includes:**

Emaciation-erythema (nodular)-digital defects, Nakajo type
Erythema (nodular)-digital defects-emaciation, Nakajo type
Nakajo nodular erythema with digital changes
Nakajo syndrome
Nodular erythema-digital changes
Osteoperiostosis, secondary hypertrophic with pernio

**Excludes:**  Cockayne syndrome (0189)

**Major Diagnostic Criteria:**  The combination of nodular erythema with progressive emaciation, typical facial appearance, and large hands.

**Clinical Findings:**  The initial finding is the development of nodular erythema, which predominantly affects the face, ears, and extremities. These lesions are pink to dark red and elevated; brown pigmentation usually remains after the disappearance of the erythema. Although birth weight and early growth are normal, growth eventually slows, and weight and height often fall below the tenth percentile. The atrophy of facial muscles leads to the characteristic facial appearance of large eyes, nose, lips, and ears. The hands also appear large, with long fingers that have thickened interphalangeal joints. Cardiomegaly and hypertrophy of phalangeal periosteum are occasionally found (10–20%). Laboratory findings include anemia, elevated erythrocyte sedimentation rate, and serum gamma globulin.

**Complications:**  Unknown.

**Associated Findings:**  None known.

**Etiology:**  Possibly autosomal recessive inheritance.

**Pathogenesis:**  Unknown.

**MIM No.:**  25604

**Sex Ratio:**  M8:F4 (observed in 12 affected cases).

**Occurrence:**  A dozen cases have been reported since the 1930s, all from Japan.

**Risk of Recurrence for Patient's Sib:**
See Part I, *Mendelian Inheritance.*

**Risk of Recurrence for Patient's Child:**
See Part I, *Mendelian Inheritance.*

**Age of Detectability:**  The erythema appears between the ages of two months and five years. The progressive emaciation and slow-down in growth occur soon after.

**Gene Mapping and Linkage:**  Unknown.

**Prevention:**  None known. Genetic counseling indicated.

**Treatment:**  Treatment with prednisolone and vitamin E appeared to be beneficial in some cases.

**Prognosis:**  Although 2/12 individuals were mentally retarded, most have normal or above-normal intelligence. The oldest patient died at age 42 years of unknown causes.

**Detection of Carrier:**  Unknown.

**References:**

Kitano Y, et al.: A syndrome with nodular erythema, elongated and thickened fingers, and emaciation. Arch Dermatol 1985; 121:1053–1056.

T0007                                            **Helga V. Toriello**

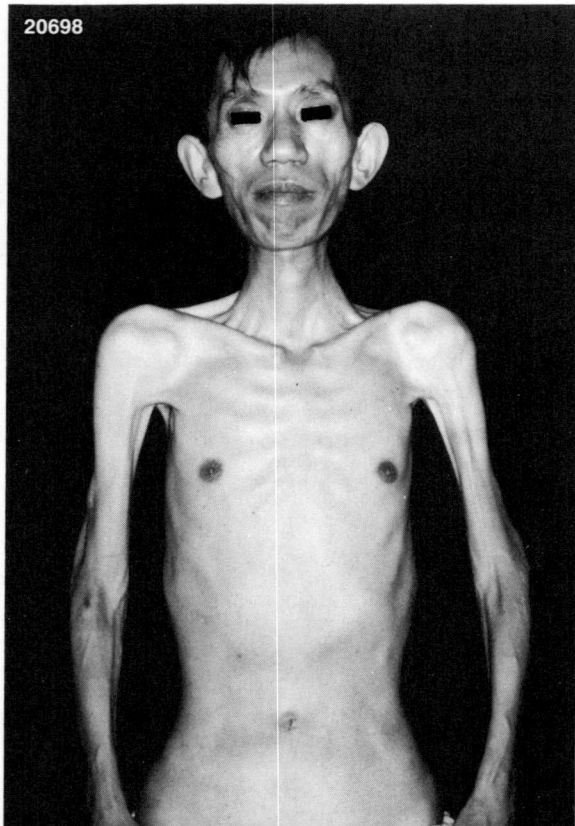

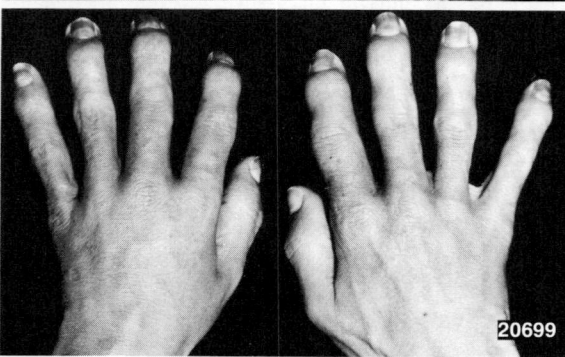

**2807-20698:** Digital defects-nodular erythema-emaciation, Nakajo type; loss of adipose tissue and muscle atrophy. **20699:** Hand deformities.

---

## DIGITAL FIBROMA, RECURRING IN INFANTS & CHILDREN                    2402

**Includes:**
Digital fibromatosis, infantile
Digital fibrous tumors of childhood, recurring
Fibroma, digital, recurring in infants and children
Finger, recurring fibroma
Toe, recurring fibroma

**Excludes:** Digital tumors and fibromatosis (other)

**Major Diagnostic Criteria:** A congenital or acquired benign tumor of a finger or toe, excluding thumb and great toe, whether recurrent or not, in the pediatric age group. The tumors are hard

and covered with epidermis. Biopsy or excision and light microscopic examination establish the diagnosis.

**Clinical Findings:** Tumors have a distinctive light microscopic appearance, consisting of benign spindle cells with prominent intracytoplasmic eosinophilic inclusion bodies.

**Complications:** Troublesome local recurrences are a feature, and sometimes amputation is necessary for their control. Metastases have not been recorded.

**Associated Findings:** None known.

**Etiology:** Unknown.

**Pathogenesis:** The true histogenesis of these benign spindle cell tumors has been demonstrated by electron microscopy. The ultrastructural features of the inclusion-bearing tumor cells are those of myofibroblasts. The ultrastructural morphology and topography of the inclusions suggests that they are derived from contractile microfibrils, possibly caused by an enzyme defect within neoplastic cells, leading to deranged assembly of filamentous proteins. The age incidence of these tumors ranges from birth to 15 years, with the majority occurring under age two years. One atypical case has been reported on the arm of a 44-year-old male.

**Sex Ratio:** M5:F7 (observed).

**Occurrence:** Seven cases were found in one large pediatric unit over a 35 year period. Over 70 cases are described in the English literature.

**Risk of Recurrence for Patient's Sib:** Presumably low.

**Risk of Recurrence for Patient's Child:** Unknown.

**Age of Detectability:** At birth, although diagnosis has been made as late as age 44.

**Gene Mapping and Linkage:** Unknown.

**Prevention:** None known. Genetic counseling indicated.

**Treatment:** Local surgical removal to amputation for recurrences.

**Prognosis:** Normal life span; local recurrences in 45% of cases and spontaneous remission in 3% of cases.

**Detection of Carrier:** Unknown.

**References:**
Reye RDK: Recurring digital fibrous tumours of childhood. Arch Pathol 1965; 80:228–231.
Rosenberg HS, et al.: The fibromatoses of infancy and childhood. In: Rosenberg HS, Bolande RP, eds: Perspectives in paediatric pathology, vol 4. Chicago: Year Book Medical Publishers, 1978:269–348.
Mortimer G, Gibson AAM: Recurring digital fibroma. J Clin Pathol 1982; 35:849–854. * †

M0036                                                    **Gabriel Mortimer**

**Digital fibromatosis, infantile**
  *See DIGITAL FIBROMA, RECURRING IN INFANTS & CHILDREN*
**Digital fibrous tumors of childhood, recurring**
  *See DIGITAL FIBROMA, RECURRING IN INFANTS & CHILDREN*
**Digital-facio-oro syndrome**
  *See ORO-FACIO-DIGITAL SYNDROME, WHELAN TYPE*
**Digital-oro-cranio syndrome**
  *See ORO-CRANIO-DIGITAL SYNDROME*
**Digital-oro-facio syndrome**
  *See ORO-FACIO-DIGITAL SYNDROME, BARAITSER-BURN TYPE*
**Digital-oro-facio syndrome III**
  *See ORO-FACIO-DIGITAL SYNDROME, SUGARMAN TYPE*
**Digital-oro-palatal syndrome**
  *See ORO-PALATAL-DIGITAL SYNDROME, VARADI TYPE*
**Digital-oto-palato syndrome**
  *See OTO-PALATO-DIGITAL SYNDROME, II*
**Digito-facio-genital syndrome**
  *See AARSKOG SYNDROME*
**Digito-naso-acoustic syndrome, Keipert type**
  *See NASO-DIGITO-ACOUSTIC SYNDROME, KEIPERT TYPE*
**Digito-oto-palatal syndrome**
  *See OTO-PALATO-DIGITAL SYNDROME, I*

## DIGITO-PALATAL SYNDROME, STEVENSON TYPE 2194

**Includes:**

Catel-Manzke syndrome
Cleft palate-hand malformation
Digit, hyperphalangy of index finger
Hand malformation-palatal syndrome
Hyperphalangy (symmetric)
Robin sequence with hyperphalangy
Stevenson syndrome

**Excludes:**

**Brachydactyly** (0114)
**Cleft palate-micrognathia-glossoptosis** (0182)
Osteochondrodystrophy-hyperphalangy

**Major Diagnostic Criteria:** The combination of micrognathia, **Cleft palate**, and a specific hand malformation, in which an accessory bone is located between the proximal phalanges of fingers 2 and 3, is required for the diagnosis.

**Clinical Findings:** This condition is readily recognized at birth because of the unique hand malformation. The accessory phalangeal ossification center causes the index finger to deviate to the radial side at the metacarpophalangeal joint and to the ulnar side at the first interphalangeal joint. The associated abnormalities include micrognathia (80%), cleft palate (80%), cardiac defects (40%), clubfeet (30%), and vertebral anomalies (30%). The calvarium appears globular; the eyes are prominent with or without epicanthus, the pinnae may be cupped, misshapen, or low-set, the neck is short; and the chest may be misshapen. Abnormal palmar creases and clinodactyly of the fifth fingers are often present. Barring asphyxia or other neonatal complications, development is normal. Several patients have had short stature.

**Complications:** The presence of cleft palate and micrognathia increases the risk for asphyxial episodes, aspiration, otitis with hearing loss, and nutritional deprivation.

**Associated Findings:** Poor growth may result from feeding difficulty, developmental impairments from asphyxial episodes, and hearing loss from ear infections.

**Etiology:** Possibly X-linked recessive inheritance, although female cases have been reported.

**Pathogenesis:** Unknown.

**MIM No.:** 30238

**Sex Ratio:** M13:F2 (observed).

**Occurrence:** Over a dozen cases have been documented.

**Risk of Recurrence for Patient's Sib:**

See Part I, *Mendelian Inheritance.*

**Risk of Recurrence for Patient's Child:**

See Part I, *Mendelian Inheritance.*

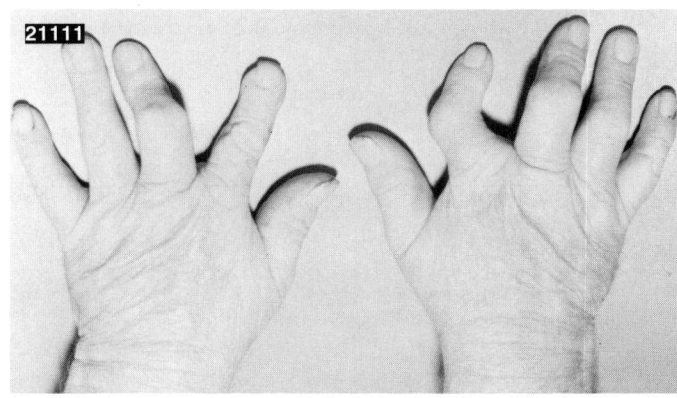

**2194B-21111:** Appearance of hands in an adult with digito-palatal syndrome showing characteristic digital malformation on the right. Other digits have contractures as well.

**Age of Detectability:** At birth.

**Gene Mapping and Linkage:** Unknown.

**Prevention:** None known. Genetic counseling indicated.

**Treatment:** Prompt attention must be given to airway maintenance and nutritional support during infancy. Surgical correction of cleft palate, cardiac defect, and the digital malformation.

**Prognosis:** Mortality is increased during infancy because of asphyxia from glossoptosis. The outlook for normal mental function in survivors is good.

**Detection of Carrier:** Unknown.

**References:**

Stevenson RE, et al.: A digitopalatal syndrome with associated anomalies of the heart, face and skeleton. J Med Genet 1980; 17:238–242.
Sundaram V, et al.: Hyperphalangy and clinodactyly of the index finger with Pierre Robin anomaly: Catel-Manzke syndrome; a case report and review of the literature. Clin Genet 1982; 21:407–410.
Brude E: Pierre Robin sequence and hyperphalangy-a genetic entity (Catel-Manzke syndrome). Eur J Pediatr 1984; 142:222–223.
Dignan P St J, et al.: Pierre Robin anomaly with an accessory

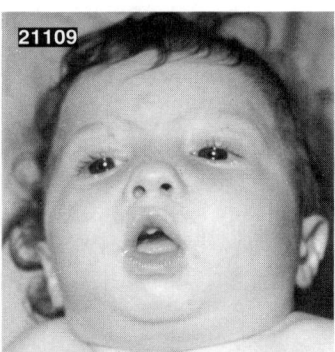
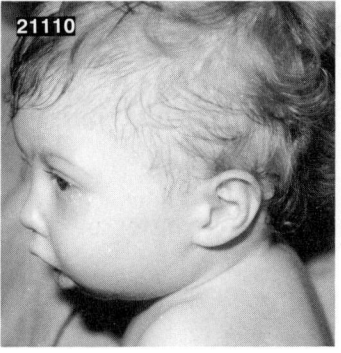

**2194A-21109–10:** 16-month-old male child with micrognathia and rounded facies.

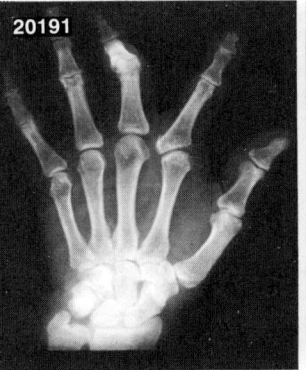
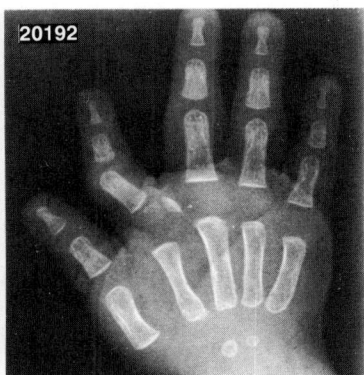

**2194C-20191:** Hand X-ray of a 57-year-old male with digito-palatal syndrome; note angulation of the digits and malformation of the first phalanx of the index finger. **20192:** Hand X-ray of a 2-month-old infant male showing accessory bone at base of the second digit and hypoplasia of the second metacarpal and phalanges.

metacarpal of the index fingers: the Catel-Manzke syndrome. Clin Genet 1986; 29:168–173.

Thompson EM, et al.: A male infant with the Catel-Manzke syndrome and dislocatable knees. J Med Genet 1986; 23:271–273.

ST021                                          **Roger E. Stevenson**

## DIGITO-RENO-CEREBRAL SYNDROME                    2792

**Includes:**
  Brachydactyly due to absence of distal phalanges
  Cerebral-digito-reno syndrome
  Eronen-Somer-Holmberg syndrome
  Reno-digito-cerebral syndrome

**Excludes:**
  **Acrodysostosis** (0016)
  **Brachydactyly**
  **Radial-renal-ocular syndrome** (2643)
  **Coffin-Siris syndrome** (2025)
  **Fetal hydantoin syndrome** (0382)
  Onychodystrophy, all forms

**Major Diagnostic Criteria:**  Congenital absence of distal phalanges and nails of all fingers and toes. Renal cystic dysplasia. Cerebral malformation associated with profound mental retardation.

**Clinical Findings:**  Prenatal history is uneventful; however, one female patient was small for gestational age. The affected infants have complete absence of nails and absence of distal phalanges of fingers (digits 2 to 5), of all toes, and of middle phalanges of toe 5. Associated anomalies consist of dysmorphic facies with coarse facial features; short, wide nose with full tip and wide base; bushy hair; and low-set, cup-shaped ears. Oral findings include high-arched palate and hypertrophic gums.

  CNS manifestations consist of marked muscular hypotonia, **Microcephaly**, blindness, convulsions, and profound mental retardation. Ultrasound and brain scan show a dilated ventricle. EEG reveals multiple spiked foci, and ophthalmologic examination shows optic nerve atrophy. Brain stem evoked potentials are absent.

  Urogenital abnormalities include dysplasia of kidneys, marked phimosis, and dysplastic uterus. Renal biopsy reveals cystic dysplasia with rudimentary nephrons and cartilaginous tissue.

  Other findings observed are sacral dimple, **Ductus arteriosus, patent**, and foramen ovale.

  Biochemical examinations and chromosomes are normal. X-rays of the hands and feet reveal absence of distal phalanges.

**Complications:**  Profound mental retardation without meaningful movements, and prolonged epileptic seizures in spite of antiepileptic medication. Recurrent respiratory infections. Early death.

**Associated Findings:**  Hip dislocation, enlarged thymus, adrenal glands of unusual shape.

**Etiology:**  Possibly autosomal recessive inheritance.

**Pathogenesis:**  Unknown.

**MIM No.:**  22276

**POS No.:**  3446

**Sex Ratio:**  Presumably M1:F1; M1:F2 observed.

**Occurrence:**  One family (two females and a male cousin of healthy, multiply consanguineous parents) has been documented.

**Risk of Recurrence for Patient's Sib:**
  See Part I, *Mendelian Inheritance.*

**Risk of Recurrence for Patient's Child:**
  See Part I, *Mendelian Inheritance.* Affected individuals are not expected to reproduce.

**Age of Detectability:**  At birth.

**Gene Mapping and Linkage:**  Unknown.

**Prevention:**  None known. Genetic counseling indicated.

**Treatment:**  Anticonvulsants for seizures. Physiotherapy. Symptomatic therapy for respiratory tract infections.

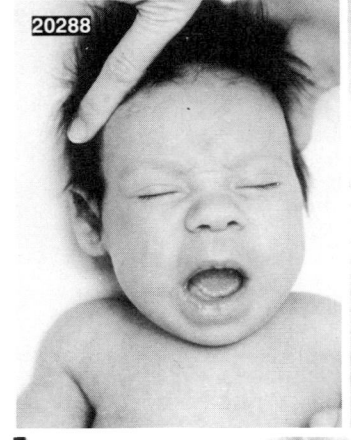
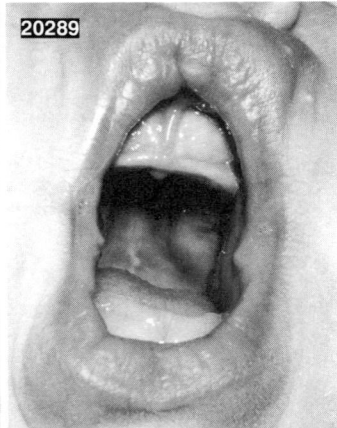
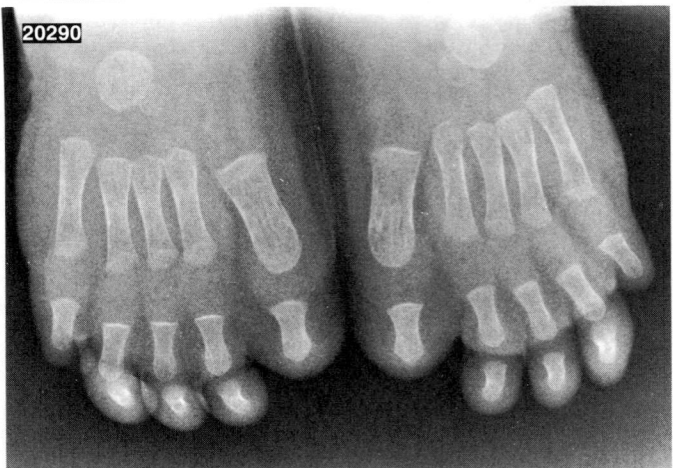
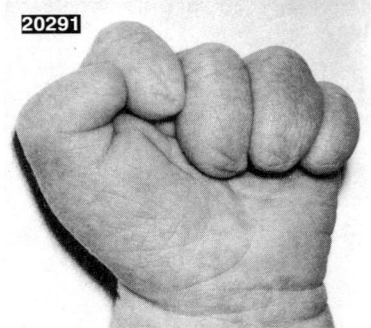
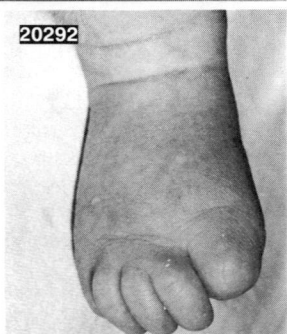

**2792-20288:**  Digito-reno-cerebral syndrome: note short, wide nose; bushy hair; cup-shaped ear; and hypertrophic gums. **20289:**  Marked hypertrophy of the gums and high-arched palate. **20290:**  Foot X-ray; note absent distal phalanges. **20291–92:**  Note absence of all nails and distal phalanges of the fingers and the toes.

**Prognosis:**  Of the three reported patients, one died neonatally, one died at age two years in an epileptic seizure, and one was still alive at age five years.

**Detection of Carrier:**  Unknown.

**References:**
Eronen M, et al.: A digito-reno-cerebral syndrome. Am J Med Genet 1985; 22:281–285.

ER004                                          **Marianne P. Eronen**

**Digito-talar dysmorphism**
*See HAND, ULNAR DRIFT*

## DIGITO-TALAR DYSMORPHISM      2267

**Includes:** Arthrogryposis, digito-talar dysmorphism

**Excludes:**
**Arthrogryposes** (0088)
**Cranio-carpo-tarsal dysplasia, whistling face type** (0223)
**Hand, ulnar drift** (2410)
**Thumb, clasped** (0175)

**Major Diagnostic Criteria:** Ulnar deviation of fingers, clasped thumbs, vertical tali, and short stature.

**Clinical Findings:** Bilateral contraction deformities of variable severity of the hands and feet are present at birth. Hands typically have significant ulnar deviation of the digits, with some degree of rotation at the phalangeal joints. The thumbs are adducted and webbed. The skin of the palms and digits appears tight and smooth but not fixed to the underlying tissues. Feet have vertical tali, and contractures of the soft tissues may produce further deformities.

Short stature is common, and other skeletal anomalies may include tortuous clavicles, **Pectus excavatum**, and scoliosis.

No chromosome abnormalities are present, and the affected individuals are not mentally retarded. Facial muscles appear normal.

**Complications:** Untreated individuals may have significant physical disabilities.

**Associated Findings:** None known.

**Etiology:** Autosomal dominant inheritance with complete penetrance.

**Pathogenesis:** Unknown.

**MIM No.:** *12605

**POS No.:** 3419

**CDC No.:** 755.510

**Sex Ratio:** M1:F1

**Occurrence:** Two or three kindreds have been documented.

**Risk of Recurrence for Patient's Sib:**
See Part I, *Mendelian Inheritance*.

**Risk of Recurrence for Patient's Child:**
See Part I, *Mendelian Inheritance*.

**Age of Detectability:** At birth.

**Gene Mapping and Linkage:** Unknown.

**Prevention:** None known. Genetic counseling indicated.

**Treatment:** Surgical correction of defects, combined with appropriate physical therapy, will markedly reduce the disability.

**Prognosis:** Life span and intelligence not decreased.

**Detection of Carrier:** Unknown.

**References:**
Sallis JG, Beighton P: Dominantly inherited digito-talar dysmorphism. J Bone Joint Surg 1972; 54B:509–515.
Stevenson RE, et al.: Dominantly inherited ulnar drift. BD:OAS XI(5). New York: March of Dimes Birth Defects Foundation, 1975:75–77.
Dhaliwal AS, Myers TL: Digitotalar dysmorphism. Orthopaedic Rev 1985; 14:90–94.

MY000          **Terry L. Myers**

**Digitofacial-mental retardation syndrome**
*See RUBINSTEIN-TAYBI BROAD THUMB-HALLUX SYNDROME*
**Digits, congenital contractures of the**
*See HAND, ULNAR DRIFT*
**Digits, short**
*See BRACHYDACTYLY*
**Dihydrobiopterin synthetase deficiency**
*See BIOPTERIN SYNTHESIS DEFICIENCY*

## DIHYDROPTERIDINE REDUCTASE DEFICIENCY      2001

**Includes:**
Hyperphenylalaninemia due to abnormal biopterin metabolism
Phenylketonuria II
PKU, atypical
Quinoid dihydropteridine reductase deficiency

**Excludes:**
**Biopterin synthesis deficiency** (2002)
Hyperphenylalaninemia, transient
Hyperphenylalaninemias, other
**Phenylketonuria** (0808)

**Major Diagnostic Criteria:** Progressive cerebral deterioration occurs despite excellent dietary control of phenylalanine concentrations in the blood. The diagnosis is readily confirmed by the prompt fall in the elevated serum concentration of phenylalanine following the administration of synthetic tetrahydrobiopterin, readily distinguishing the patient from those with classic phenylketonuria (PKU).

**Clinical Findings:** Hyperphenylalaninemia is detected in neonatal screening. Generally, affected infants are thought to have PKU except in programs in which all patients tentatively diagnosed as having PKU are screened for a defect in biopterin metabolism. In spite of the careful dietary treatment usually successful in PKU, these patients degenerate. This progressive course usually leads to the diagnosis. Marked hypotonia, spasticity and dystonic posturing are common features as well as seizures, myoclonus and EEG abnormalities. Drooling is commonly encountered. The retardation of psychomotor development is usually profound.

Tetrahydrobiopterin is an obligatory cofactor for phenylalanine hydroxylase. In the course of the hydroxylase reaction the cofactor is converted to a quininoid dihydrobiopterin. Its regeneration to the tetrahydro-form is catalyzed by dihydropteridine reductase.

**2267-21217:** The affected family with various abnormalities of the hands and feet.

The enzyme defect may be demonstrated by an assay of the enzyme activity in biopsied liver or cultured fibroblasts.

Tetrahydrobiopterin is also the cofactor for the hydroxylation of tryptophan and tyrosine, essential for the synthesis of serotonin, norepinephrine and dopamine. Levels of 5-hydroxyindoleacetic acid, vanillyl mandelic acid, and homovanillic acid in cerebrospinal fluid and urine are low.

**Complications:** Severe mental retardation; seizures.

**Associated Findings:** None known.

**Etiology:** Autosomal recessive inheritance.

**Pathogenesis:** Deficiency of the activity of dihydropteridine reductase interferes with the conversion of phenylalanine to tyrosine and thus a metabolic milieu identical to that of the patient with classic PKU. In addition defective hydroxylation of tryptophan and tyrosine interferes with the synthesis of neurotransmitters essential for nervous system function.

**MIM No.:** *26163

**Sex Ratio:** M1:F1

**Occurrence:** Undetermined but presumed rare. About two dozen cases have been documented.

**Risk of Recurrence for Patient's Sib:**
See Part I, *Mendelian Inheritance.*

**Risk of Recurrence for Patient's Child:**
See Part I, *Mendelian Inheritance.*

**Age of Detectability:** As in classic PKU, usually within 48 hours if protein intake is normal; by six days, virtually all cases should be detectable. Prenatal diagnosis is possible (Dahl, et al, 1988).

**Gene Mapping and Linkage:** QDPR (quinoid dihydropteridine reductase) has been mapped to 4p15.3.

**Prevention:** None known. Genetic counseling indicated.

**Treatment:** Synthetic tetrahydropbiopterin or a low phenylalanine diet should prevent the consequences of hyperphenynlalaninemia. It is recommended that in either case the patient be given 5-hydroxytryptophan and dihydroxyphenylalanine, along with a peripheral decarboxylase inhibitor such as carbidopa.

**Prognosis:** Usually grave. In those patients detected before the onset of symptoms, treatment should be effective.

**Detection of Carrier:** Unknown.

**References:**
Bartholome K, Byrd DJ: L-dopa and 5-hydroxytryptophan therapy in phenylketonuria with normal phenylalanine hydroxylase activity. Lancet 1975; II:1042–1043.
Kaufman S, et al.: Phenylketonuria due to a deficiency of dihydropteridine reductase. New Engl J Med 1975; 293:785–790. *
Smith I, et al.: New variant of phenylketonuria with progressive neurological illness unresponsive to phenylalanine restriction. Lancet 1975; I:1108–1111.
Brewster TG, et al.: Dihydropteridine reductase deficiency associated with severe neurologic disease and mild hyperphenylalaninemia. Pediatrics 1979; 63:94–99.
Butter I-J, et al.: Neurotransmitter defects and treatment of disorders of hyperphenylalaninemia. J Pediatr 1981; 98:729–733.
Lockyer J, et al.: Structure and expression of human dihydropteridine reductase. Proc Nat Acad Sci 1987; 84:3329–3333.
Nyhan WL: Hyperphenylalaninemia and defective metabolism of tetrahydrobiopterin. In: Nyhan WL, ed: Diagnostic recognition of genetic disease. Philadelphia: Lea & Febiger, 1987:107–112. *
Dahl H.-H, et al.: The use of restriction fragment length polymorphisms in prenatal diagnosis of dihydropteridine reductase deficiency. J Med Genet 1988; 25:25–28.

NY000                                                    **William L. Nyhan**

**Dihydrostreptomycin, fetal effects**
*See FETAL AMINOGLYCOSIDE OTOTOXICITY*
**Dihydrostreptomycin-sensitive deafness**
*See DEAFNESS, STREPTOMYCIN-SENSITIVITY*
**Dihydrotestosterone receptor deficiency**
*See ANDROGEN INSENSITIVITY SYNDROME, INCOMPLETE*
*also ANDROGEN INSENSITIVITY SYNDROME, COMPLETE*

**Dilacerated teeth**
*See TEETH, DILACERATED*
**Dilantin^, fetal effects of**
*See FETAL HYDANTOIN SYNDROME*
**Dilated composite odontome**
*See TEETH, DENS INVAGINATUS*
**Dilution, pigmentary**
*See ALBINOIDISM*

---

## DIPHALLIA                                                      2910

**Includes:**
Diphallus
Penis, double ("reduplicated")
Primary diphallia
Secondary diphallia

**Excludes:**
Double clitoris
Double "monster" diphallia
Penile skin tag
Pseudo-diphallia (lipoma or other tumors simulating penis)
Psychogenic diphallia (penis tatoo on single penis)
Quadruple penis
Triple penis

**Major Diagnostic Criteria:** A complete or partial duplication of the penis without primary diphallia (PD) or with secondary diphallia (SD) duplication of other wolffian duct structures. In primary diphallia, the penes may be complete, well formed, independent structures or may be incompletely fused and parts may be absent. In secondary diphallia, the penes lie in a superior and inferior ("over and under") configuration and may be complete or partial duplications of the normal penis as well as other structures.

**Clinical Findings:** Primary diphallia (68%) is twice as common as secondary diphallia (32%). PD is associated with malformations characterized by failure of fusion or agenesis of structures (e.g., **Bladder exstrophy**, omphalocele, diastasis pubis, sacral agenesis, imperforate anus, bifid or cleft scrotum). Anomalies of the pelvic bones are often present (e.g., pubic diastasis, sacral agenesis, hemisacrum, spina bifida with or without **Meningomyelocele**). SD is associated with additional duplications of normally single organs (e.g.,urinary bladder, colon, supernumerary kidneys). Scrotal anomalies (bifid, cleft) often accompany both PD and SD.

**Complications:** Renal failure due to nonfunctioning kidneys, noncommunicating urinary tract drainage, and recurrent genitourinary infections are common. Reproductive insufficiency relating to inadequate or anomalous erectile tissues is usually present.

**Associated Findings:** Only 36% of cases have normal or adequate urinary and reproductive function.

**Etiology:** Unknown.

**Pathogenesis:** PD represents a primary failure of the bilateral penile primordia to fuse and form the genital tubercle during the fourth week. This is accompanied by the incomplete formation of other structures. SD can be considered as the result of normal penile anlagen fusion and normal genital tubercle formation but with the subsequent fission of the genital tubercle.

**CDC No.:** 752.860

**Sex Ratio:** M1:F0

**Occurrence:** 1:19,000,000 births, estimated; 1:30,000 necropsies.

**Risk of Recurrence for Patient's Sib:** Undetermined but presumed low.

**Risk of Recurrence for Patient's Child:** Unknown.

**Age of Detectability:** During the newborn period, or prenatally by fetal ultrasonography.

**Gene Mapping and Linkage:** Unknown.

**Prevention:** None known. Genetic counseling indicated.

**Treatment:** Surgical repair of the urinary tract is usually required at birth (64%), followed by excision of the most vestigial penis and

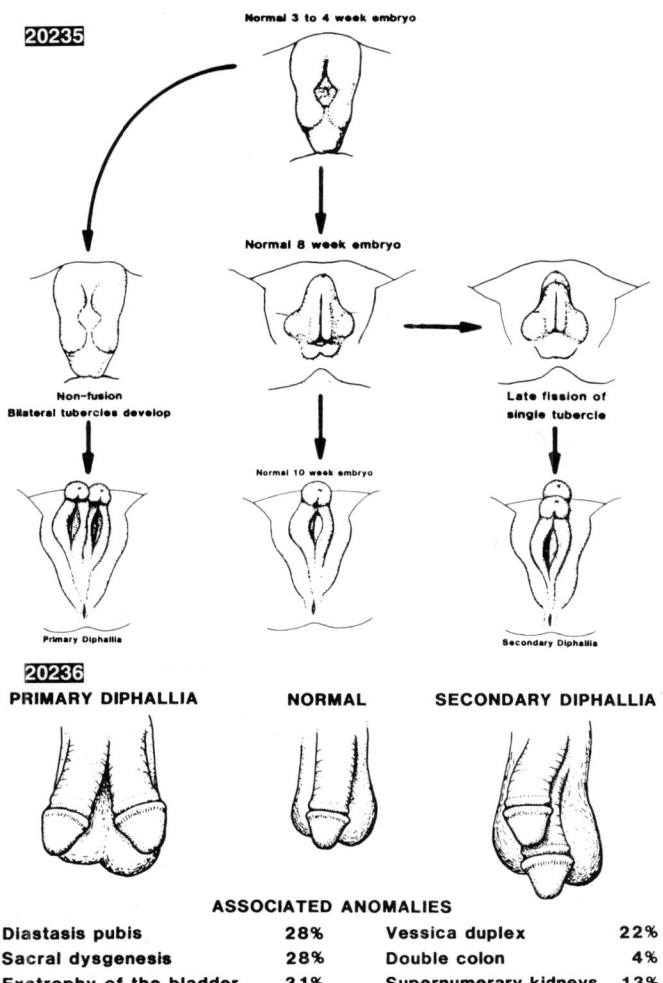

20235

Normal 3 to 4 week embryo

Normal 8 week embryo

Non-fusion
Bilateral tubercles develop

Late fission of
single tubercle

Normal 10 week embryo

Primary Diphallia

Secondary Diphallia

20236

| PRIMARY DIPHALLIA | NORMAL | SECONDARY DIPHALLIA |

**ASSOCIATED ANOMALIES**

| | | | |
|---|---|---|---|
| Diastasis pubis | 28% | Vessica duplex | 22% |
| Sacral dysgenesis | 28% | Double colon | 4% |
| Exstrophy of the bladder | 31% | Supernumerary kidneys | 13% |
| Imperforate Anus | 39% | Bifid or double ureters | 4% |
| Renal agenesis/dysgenesis | 16% | | |
| Urethral stenosis | 8% | | |
| Abdominal wall defects | 18% | | |
| Intestinal atresias | | | |
| Vesico-rectal fistuli | | | |

**2910-20235:** Embryological basis for classification of diphallia into primary and secondary types. Primary diphallia results in failure of fusion of the genital anlagen such that two side by side tubercles develop. In secondary diphallia a single tubercle is formed but subsequently undergoes fission in such a manner that "over and under" penes develop. **20236:** Primary and secondary diphallia: the penes in PD develop "side by side" while in SD the penes are in "over and under" positions. The associated anomalies are described in PD (left column) and in SD (right column).

plastic repair of the remaining penis. Care must be taken to assure urethral patency and proper urinary tract drainage.

**Prognosis:** Favorable if a functional renal system is present and the remaining phallus is of satisfactory size and is accompanied by an adequate quantity of properly developed erectile tissue. A normal penis is present in 34% of cases. In 46% of cases, only the corpora spongiosum is present.

**Detection of Carrier:** Unknown.

**Special Considerations:** X-ray examination of both the genitourinary and the skeletal systems is important. In PD, pelvic girdle anomalies are frequent, including anomalies of the sacrum and distal neural tube.

**References:**
Blanco S: Diphallus (double penis). J Urol 1954; 53:786–790.
Cohen SJ: Diphallus with duplication of the colon and bladder. Proc R Soc Med 1968; 61:305 only.
Johnson CF, et al.: Duplication of penis. Urology 1974; 4:722–725.
Hollowell JG, et al.: Embryologic considerations of diphallus and associated anomalies. J Urol 1977; 117:728–732.
McLeod NA, et al.: Clinical and embryological considerations of diphallia. Teratology 1980; 21:55A.

BL002                                    **Will Blackburn**

**Diphallus**
  *See DIPHALLIA*
**Diphosphoglycerate mutase (2,3) deficiency of erythrocyte**
  *See ERYTHROCYTE, DIPHOSPHOGLYCERATE MUTASE (2,3) DEFICIENCY*
**Diphtheria toxin sensitivity (DTS)**
  *See DIPHTHERIA, SUSCEPTIBILITY TO*

## DIPHTHERIA, SUSCEPTIBILITY TO          3079

**Includes:** Diphtheria toxin sensitivity (DTS)

**Excludes:** Susceptibility or resistance to other bacterial exotoxins

**Major Diagnostic Criteria:** The presence of a pseudomembrane in the posterior oropharynx is a distinctive clinical feature of diphtheria which, however, can occur with several other infections. Other clinical signs include discomfort at the site of primary infection with progression to a shock-like state due to toxic complications. Definitive diagnosis depends upon demonstration and culture of the etiologic agent, *Corynebacterium diphtheriae*. The Schick test, which consists of intradermal inoculation of very dilute exotoxin, was previously used to distinguish susceptibility or immunity to diphtheria. This test is no longer used.

**Clinical Findings:** Disease manifestations tend to be related to the site of primary infection and production of an exudative pseudomembrane. Thus infection can be restricted to the nasal mucosa, pharynx, or larynx with extension to contiguous sites. Symptoms are usually local with low grade fever. Toxic effects can eventually result in peripheral vascular collapse.

**Complications:** Myocarditis and peripheral neuritis can occur as a consequence of diphtheria.

**Associated Findings:** Cutaneous diphtheria has been described in the tropics.

**Etiology:** The causative agent is *Corynebacterium diphtheriae*, a nonmotile, gram positive, nonsporulating, club-shaped rod. Three strains, mitis, gravis and intermedius, have been identified on the basis of culture morphology. Pathogenicity is due to the production of an exotoxin protein whose synthesis is dependent upon the presence of a lysogenic bacteriophage containing the gene. Spread of disease is principally dependent upon microdeplet transmission.

**Pathogenesis:** Infection generally occurs via mucous membranes, primarily involving the upper respiratory tract. Growth of the organism at the local site combined with an inflammatory response by the host result in the development of a characteristic pseudomembrane. However the effects of exotoxin can be manifested at distal sites including the heart and peripheral nerves. Death usually results from respiratory embarassment or alternatively due to cardiac or nervous system complications.

**MIM No.:** *12615

**Sex Ratio:** M1:F1

**Occurrence:** Showing a predilection for temperate regions, diphtheria cases are rare in the United States.

**Risk of Recurrence for Patient's Sib:** While the risk of transmission of an infectious disease is relatively increased within a family, unimmunized siblings are no more or less susceptible to infection than the index case.

**Risk of Recurrence for Patient's Child:** Unknown.

**Age of Detectability:** Diphtheria can occur at any age.

**Gene Mapping and Linkage:** DTS (diphtheria toxin sensitivity) has been mapped to 5q23.

**Prevention:** Immunization confers protection from disease.

**Treatment:** The definitive treatment for diphtheria is administration of horse serum antitoxin. Coadministration of antibiotics has not been shown to be efficacious.

**Prognosis:** Early diagnosis and administration of antitoxin can reduce the morbidity and mortality of disease.

**Detection of Carrier:** The carrier state for the organisms can persist for a long time or may even be permanent. Susceptibility to diphtheria toxin appears to be a property of all humans.

**References:**
Creagan RP, et al.: Genetic analysis of the cell surface: association of human chromosome 5 with sensitivity to diphtheria toxin in mouse-human somatic cell hybrids. Proc Natl Acad Sci 1975; 72:2237–2241.

George DL, Francke U: Regional mapping of human genes for hexosaminidase B and diphtheria toxin sensitivity on chromosome 5 using mouse X human hybrid cells. 1977; 3:629–638.

Chang T-M, Neville DM Jr: Demonstration of diphtheria toxin receptors on surface membranes from both toxin-sensitive and toxin-resistant species. 1978; 253:6866–6871.

Gupta RS, Siminovitch L: Isolation and characterization of mutants of human diploid fibroblasts resistant to diphtheria toxin. 1978; 75:3337–3340.

M0046
SC039

**Arnold S. Monto**
**Stanley A. Schwartz**

## DIPLEGIA, CONGENITAL FACIAL                    0376

**Includes:**
Facial diplegia, congenital
Facial diplegia (6th and 7th cranial nerves)
Moebius syndrome
Nuclear hypoplasia congenital (6th and 7th cranial nerves)
Oromandibular-limb hypogenesis syndrome

**Excludes:**
**Charlie M syndrome** (2170)
Facial palsy, traumatic bilateral
**Hypoglossia-hypodactylia** (0451)
**Palsy, congenital facial** (0377)
**Muscular dystrophy**
**Muscular dystrophy, facio-scapulo-humeral** (2049)
**Myasthenic syndrome, familial infantile type** (2913)
**Myopathies**
**Myotonic dystrophy** (0702)

**Major Diagnostic Criteria:** A nonprogressive, congenital syndrome characterized by facial diplegia, usually bilateral.

**Clinical Findings:** The outstanding finding is the simultaneous, usually bilateral, palsy of the face and the horizontal gaze mechanisms. When the palsy is incomplete, the lower face and platysma tend to be spared. The weakness may cause difficulty in feeding in the neonatal period. There may be drooling of saliva, lodging of food in the cheeks, and indistinct speech at a later age. The facies is mask-like, and the mouth constantly held open. Approximately 75% of the patients have paralysis of cranial nerve VI and consequent weakness of the lateral rectus muscle, usually bilateral and complete. External ophthalmoplegia, which is rarely complete, has been reported in 25% of cases and the medial rectus muscle may underact secondarily.

Hypoplasia of the tongue, weakness of the palate, and masseters are noted occasionally.

There are no diagnostic laboratory tests; however, electromyography and nerve conduction studies are helpful in ruling out anterior horn cell disease, myotonic dystrophy, and other generalized neuromuscular disorders that are also associated with masked, expressionless facies. Computed tomography may reveal enlarged basal cisterns; MRI scans may also show hypoplasia of VI and VII N nuclei.

**Complications:** An infant may have difficulty in feeding secondary to weakness of the facial muscles. Corneal exposure may result from incomplete closure of the lids. Bulbar paralysis may result in aspiration of secretions, producing bronchopneumonia.

**Associated Findings:** Limb defects ranging from **Syndactyly** to brachydactyly and talipes equinovarus. Congenital absence of the pectoralis muscles with or without absence of the breast or with ipsilateral hand deformity (**Poland syndrome**) may be present. Ear lobe deformities and deafness may occur. Mental retardation may be an occasional concomitant.

**Etiology:** Most cases are sporadic, although autosomal dominant inheritance is possible. Affected sibs have occured in two families; recessive inheritance with consanguinity was possible in one of these families. When the syndrome includes skeletal malformations, the empiric recurrence risk for offspring is in the region of 2%. One family with three affected generations had a reciprocal translocation between chromosome 1 and 13. Only affected members had abnormal karyotypes. Positive maternal gestational history for intake of drugs, trauma, and illness in the first trimester has been reported.

**Pathogenesis:** Undetermined. Nuclear hypoplasia accounting for the cranial nerve paralysis has been documented in a few well-studied cases. Electromyographic studies tend to verify a supranuclear or nuclear cause for the palsies noted on examination. There have been some reports of hypoplasia of the VI and VII cranial nerve nuclei and of the facial nerve, and abnormalities of the facial and extraocular muscles, suggesting a possible neural or neuroectodermal cases, especially in view of the associated pectoralis muscle and limb deformaties. A vascular etiology has also been proposed (see **Poland syndrome**).

**MIM No.:** 15790

**CDC No.:** 352.600

**Sex Ratio:** M1:F1

**Occurrence:** Over 100 cases have been documented; 46 in one kindred alone.

**Risk of Recurrence for Patient's Sib:**
See Part I, *Mendelian Inheritance.*

**Risk of Recurrence for Patient's Child:**
See Part I, *Mendelian Inheritance.*

**Age of Detectability:** At birth by physical examination.

**Gene Mapping and Linkage:** Unknown.

**Prevention:** None known. Genetic counseling indicated.

**Treatment:** A special diet may be helpful to prevent aspiration. Occasionally tube feeding may be necessary in the neonatal period to overcome poor suck and to maintain nutrition.

Early recognition and treatment of associated malformations or complications such as lagophthalmos and corneal exposure may be helpful. As most children display abnormalities of speech due to the facial paralysis, speech therapy at an early age may be beneficial.

**Prognosis:** Good if complications can be avoided. Compatible with a normal life span.

**Detection of Carrier:** Unknown.

**Special Considerations:** Hypoglossia-hypodactylia, Hanhart syndrome, Glossopalatine ankylosis syndrome, **Charlie M syndrome**, and Moebius syndrome are grouped together under the category of *Oromandibular-limb hypogenesis syndrome*. These are clearly overlapping conditions of unknown etiology. While we recognize that these may be variants of an environmentally (or other) induced spectrum of anomalies, the *Encyclopedia* has placed Hanhart syndrome and Glossopalatine ankylosis under the title **Hypoglossia-hypodactylia** and has separate articles on Moebius syndrome (**Diplegia, congenital facial**) and **Charlie M syndrome**.

## References:

Henderson JL: Congenital facial diplegia syndrome: clinical features, pathology and aetiology; review of 61 cases. Brain 1939; 62:381–403.

Baraitser M: Genetics of Moebius syndrome. J Med Genet 1977; 14:415–417.

Ziter FA, et al.: Three generation pedigree of a Moebius syndrome variant with chromosome translocations. Arch Neurol 1977; 34:437–442.

Meyerson MD, Foushee DR: Speech, language and hearing in Moebius syndrome: a study of 22 patients. Dev Med Child Neurol 1978; 20:357–365.

Baraitser M: Heterogeneity and pleiotropism in the Moebius syndrome (letter). Clin Genet 1982; 21:290 only.

Stabile M, et al.: Abnormal B.A.E.P. in a family with Moebius syndrome: evidence for supranuclear lesion. Clin Genet 1984; 25:459–463.

Traboulsi EI, Maumenee IH: Extraocular muscle aplasia in Moebius syndrome. J Pediatr Ophthalmol Strabismus 1986; 23:120–122.

HA053
L0010

**Robert H.A. Haslam**
**R. Brian Lowry**

**Diplomyelia with bony spur**
 *See DIASTEMATOMYELIA*
**Diprosopus**
 *See TWINS, CONJOINED*
**Dipygus**
 *See TWINS, CONJOINED*
**Disaccharide intolerance I**
 *See SUCRASE-ISOMALTASE DEFICIENCY*
**Disaccharide intolerance II**
 *See LACTASE DEFICIENCY, CONGENITAL*
**Disaccharide intolerance III**
 *See LACTASE DEFICIENCY, PRIMARY*
**Discogenic scoliosis**
 *See SPINE, SCOLIOSIS, IDIOPATHIC*
**Discoid cataract**
 *See CATARACT, COPPOCK*
**Disequilibrium syndrome**
 *See DYSEQUILIBRIUM SYNDROME*
**Dislocation of the nasal septum**
 *See NOSE, DISLOCATED NASAL SEPTUM*
**Disseminated dermatofibrosis-osteopoikilosis**
 *See OSTEOPOIKILOSIS*
**Disseminated lipogranulomatosis**
 *See LIPOGRANULOMATOSIS*
**Disseminated sclerosis**
 *See MULTIPLE SCLEROSIS, FAMILIAL*
**Disseminated superficial actinic porokeratosis (DSAP)**
 *See SKIN, POROKERATOSIS*
**Distal arthrogryposis**
 *See ARTHROGRYPOSIS, DISTAL TYPES*
**Distal arthrogryposis, type IIA**
 *See CAMPTODACTYLY-CLEFT PALATE-CLUB FOOT, GORDON TYPE*
**Distal muscular dystrophy**
 *See MUSCULAR DYSTROPHY, DISTAL*
**Distal renal tubular acidosis**
 *See RENAL TUBULAR ACIDOSIS*

## DISTICHIASIS 0296

**Includes:**
 Eyelash, distichiasis
 Eyelashes, two rows of
**Excludes:**
 Distichiasis-heart defect-peripheral vascular disease/anomalies (2311)
 Distichiasis-lymphedema
 Entropion
 Tetrastichiasis
 Trichiasis
 Tristichiasis

**Major Diagnostic Criteria:** The presence of a second (accessory) row of eyelashes occupying the posterior lid margin, in the position of the meibomian gland openings accompanied by the absence of tarsal secretion even following lid massage.

**Clinical Findings:** The accessory eyelashes are most often present on all four eyelids but may be present merely on one, two, or three of them. They vary widely in number and tend to be shorter and more delicate than normal eyelashes. Although some patients are asymptomatic, most complain of constant irritation or a gritty or foreign-body sensation in the eye.

**Complications:** Continued irritation results in conjunctivitis with photophobia, blepharospasm, hyperlacrimia, chronic mucopurulent discharge, and rhinorrhea or keratitis with corneal erosion, ulceration, abscess formation, staining, pigmentation, vascularization, dulling, clouding, scarring, or opacification.

**Associated Findings:** Ectropion, entropion, ptosis, short palpebral fissure, epicanthus, absent or deficient tarsi with vertically short eyelids, thickened lid margins, visual abnormalities, blindness, microphthalmus, and a variety of minor dysmorphic and skeletal abnormalities.

**Etiology:** Autosomal dominant inheritance with a high degree of penetrance.

**Pathogenesis:** Both normal and atrophic meibomian glands with aberrant lashes are demonstrated on histopathologic examination of excised tissue. In some locations, the aberrant lashes are present in glands whose excretory ducts open into the upper one-half of the hair follicle in a manner similar to sebaceous glands but have the histologic structure of meibomian glands. However, in other locations, the glands are not fully developed and may appear rudimentary. Often well-developed Moll glands are observed at the posterior row of the pseudocilia, and an increased number of Krause glands may be observed in the conjunctivae.

**MIM No.:** *12630

**CDC No.:** 743.630

**Sex Ratio:** M1:F1

**Occurrence:** Rare. No reliable incidence or prevalence rates have been published. One large clinic in Vienna, with an annual attendance of more than 20,000 is reported to have seen 4 cases between 1886 and 1906.

**Risk of Recurrence for Patient's Sib:**
 See Part I, *Mendelian Inheritance.*

**Risk of Recurrence for Patient's Child:**
 See Part I, *Mendelian Inheritance.*

**Age of Detectability:** Should be detectable at birth but is usually difficult to recognize.

**Gene Mapping and Linkage:** Unknown.

**Prevention:** None known. Genetic counseling indicated.

**Treatment:** Distichiasis: none necessary unless disabling symptoms and/or complications occur. If only a few accessory lashes are present, simple epilation or electrolysis may suffice, however, surgical resection and plastic repair or cryotherapy are usually required. Ocular defect: correction of remedial problems. Skeletal and dysmorphic features: none.

**Prognosis:** Good with appropriate treatment. Intellect and life span are unaffected.

**Detection of Carrier:** Unknown.

**Special Considerations:** This condition should not be confused with trichiasis, which is an anterior row of eyelashes pointing inward. Although entropion (i.e., inwardly turning lid margin) may also cause the anterior lashes to point inward, its occurrence together with true distichiasis has also been reported.

## References:

Khunt H: Ueber distichiasis (congenita) vera. Z Aughen 1899; 2:46–57.
Pico G: Congenital ectropion and distichiasis: etiologic and hereditary factors: a report of cases and review of the literature. Trans Am Ophthalmol Soc 1957; 55:663–700. * †
Fox SA: Distichiasis. Am J Ophthalmol 1962; 53:14–18.
Deutsch AR: Distichiasis and epicanthus: a study of one family. Am J Ophthalmol 1971; 3:168–173.
Shammas HF, et al.: Atypical serum cholinesterase in a family with congenital distichiasis. J Med Genet 1976; 13:514–515.

G0046

**Stanley Goldstein**

## DISTICHIASIS-HEART DEFECT-PERIPHERAL VASCULAR DISEASE/ANOMALIES 2311

**Includes:**
Heart and vascular defects-distichiasis
Vascular anomalies-congenital heart defects-distichiasis

**Excludes:**
**Distichiasis** (0296)
**Distichiasis-lymphedema syndrome** (2039)
Tetrastichiasis
Tristichiasis

**Major Diagnostic Criteria:** The presence of distichiasis with evidence of accompanying congenital heart disease and altered peripheral circulation.

**Clinical Findings:** The prominent clinical features encountered in the single family with five cases reported thus far include distichiasis (100%); congenital heart defect (60%); lower limb edema (60%); inflammation of the legs (40%); prolonged venous filling time (80%); symptoms suggestive of venous disease (60%); accompanied by varicose veins (40%); prolonged reactive hyperemia time (60%); symptoms suggestive of arterial vasospastic disease (20%); photophobia (80%); vertebral anomalies (80%).

**Complications:** The accessory lashes may cause constant irritation to the eyes resulting in inflammation of the lids with erythema, photophobia, hyperlacrimia, blepharospasm, chronic mucopurulent discharge, rhinorrhea and corneal erosion, ulceration, clouding or scarring. Of greater consequence is the four fold increase in incidence of inflammatory episodes in the lower extremities (40%) as compared to that reported for **Distichiasis-lymphedema syndrome**. Varicose veins and varicose ulcerations may result from chronic venous disturbance but no complications have, as yet, been encountered from the arterial vasospastic disease. The vertebral anomalies can produce kyphosis which may be progressive.

**Associated Findings:** Microphthalmia and blindness (20%), astigmatism (60%), strabismus (40%), high-arched palate (60%), supernumerary teeth (20%), delayed dentition (20%), broad neck (40%), micrognathia (40%), clinodactyly (20%), short stature (20%), synphoresis (20%), abnormal dermatoglyphics (20%) and orthostatic proteinuria (40%).

**Etiology:** Presumably autosomal dominant inheritance with a high degree of penetrance.

**Pathogenesis:** Basic mechanism is unknown. Distichiasis appears to be identical to that of the isolated form. The edema is probably secondary to both chronic venous disease and lymphatic hypoplasia, although the role of the lymphatics has not been investigated in this entity.

**MIM No.:** 12632

**POS No.:** 3652

**Sex Ratio:** M2:F3

**Occurrence:** Reported in one family; a mother and four children.

**Risk of Recurrence for Patient's Sib:**
See Part I, *Mendelian Inheritance*.

**Risk of Recurrence for Patient's Child:**
See Part I, *Mendelian Inheritance*.

**Age of Detectability:** The distichiasis should be detectable at birth but is usually difficult to recognize. The congenital heart disease should be recognizable at birth or within the first 3–4 months of life. The peripheral vascular anomalies may not become apparent until the mid-teens or early adult life. Many of the ocular, dysmorphic and skeletal features are identifiable during childhood. The vertebral anomalies, however, are easily overlooked, unless searched for, and are frequently mistaken for juvenile epiphysitis.

**Gene Mapping and Linkage:** Unknown.

**Prevention:** None known. Genetic counseling indicated.

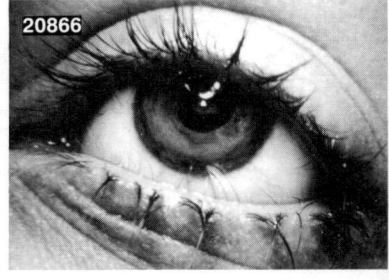
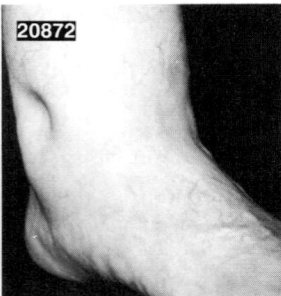
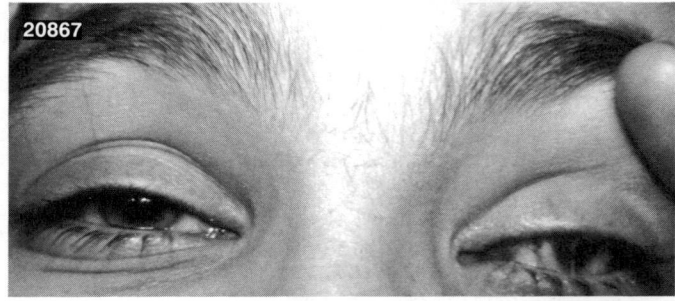
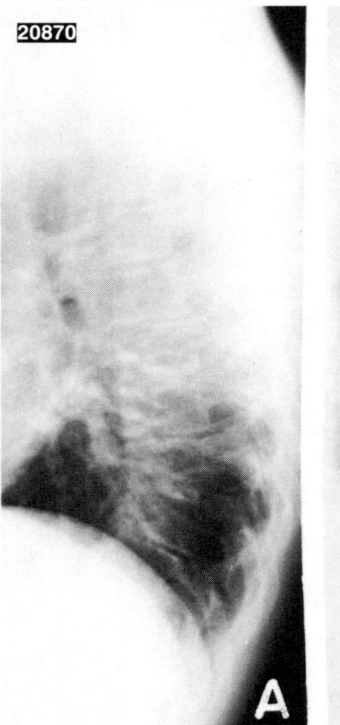
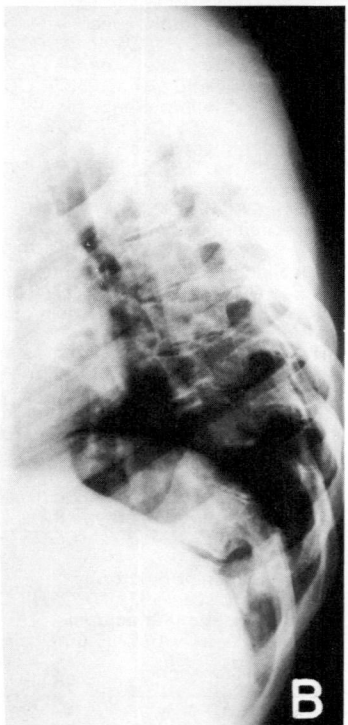

**2311-20866:** Distichiasis-heart defect-peripheral vascular disease; note accessory row of eyelashes along the posterior lid margins (distichiasis) curving inward toward the globe. **20867:** Microphthalmia OS. **20870:** Vertebral X-rays obtained at 15 (A) and 21 (B) years of age demonstrating anterior scalloping and fusion of T9, 10, 11, and an "H" shaped T8, calcifications in disc spaces T9–10 and T10–11, and progressive scoliosis. **20872:** Marked pitting edema and venous distension.

**Treatment:** Distichiasis requires no treatment unless disabling symptoms and/or complications occur. Simple epilation or electrolysis may suffice if only a few accessory lashes are present. However, surgical resection and plastic repair or cryotherapy are usually required.

Congenital heart disease is treated with standard diagnostic, medical and surgical intervention. Peripheral vascular anomalies may require Jobst stockings for edema and medical management of inflammatory episodes. Surgical intervention is usually not indicated. Possibly, long term aspirin and dipyridamole therapy for prophylaxis against the development of inflammatory episodes. Other treatments are as indicated by clinical problems.

**Prognosis:** Good with appropriate treatment. Intelligence and life span are unaffected.

**Detection of Carrier:** Unknown.

**Support Groups:** Dallas; American Heart Association

**References:**
Goldstein S, et al.: Distichiasis, congenital heart defects, and mixed peripheral vascular anomalies. Am J Med Genet 1985; 20:283–294. * †

G0046                                                    **Stanley Goldstein**
QA000                                                    **Qutub H. Qazi**

## DISTICHIASIS-LYMPHEDEMA SYNDROME          2039

**Includes:**
Eyelash, distichiasis-lymphedema syndrome
Lymphedema-distichiasis
Spinal achnoid cysts-distichiasis-lymphedeme, hereditary

**Excludes:**
**Distichiasis** (0296)
**Distichiasis-heart defect-peripheral vascular disease/anomalies** (2311)
**Lymphedema I** (0614)

**Major Diagnostic Criteria:** The combination of distichiasis, lymphedema of the lower limbs, pterygium colli, lower lid ectropion, extradural spinal cyst, and vertebral anomalies should suggest the diagnosis. With a positive family history, only one or two of the above features need be present.

**Clinical Findings:** Distichiasis (100%); vertebral anomalies [of those X-rayed] (100%); lymphedema of the lower extremities (80%); neck webbing (40%); extradural spinal cyst, certain or possible (35%); and ectropion (30%).

Dale (1987) demonstrated that the lymphedema associated with distichiasis is the uncommon "bilateral hyperplasia" form. Lymphography shows abundant and dilated lymphatics in both legs, and a thoracic duct is either absent or, if present, is obstructed or deformed.

Abnormal vertebral findings have included increased interpedicular distance, incomplete neural arch formation, increased density of the vertebral bodies, and kyphosis. Lymphangiograms have demonstrated hypoplastic lymph channels.

**Complications:** Photophobia and corneal irritation secondary to distichiasis, numbness and tingling of the lower extremities, and scoliosis.

**Associated Findings:** Present in only one patient each were astigmatism, **Heart, truncus arteriosus**, **Hernia, inguinal**, and cryptorchidism.

**Etiology:** Autosomal dominant inheritance. Males tend to be more severely affected than females.

**Pathogenesis:** The spinal cysts are thought to result from herniation of the arachnoid through dural diverticulae.

**MIM No.:** *15340

**POS No.:** 3744

**Sex Ratio:** M1:F1

**Occurrence:** About 20 cases have been documented.

**Risk of Recurrence for Patient's Sib:**
See Part I, *Mendelian Inheritance.*

**Risk of Recurrence for Patient's Child:**
See Part I, *Mendelian Inheritance.*

**Age of Detectability:** Diagnosis of this condition may be difficult at birth, unless distichiasis or ectropion are present, and there is a positive family history of this condition. The edema does not appear until later childhood/early teens in most cases (5–20 years in the reported cases), nor does the extradural spinal cyst generally become symptomatic until this period.

**Gene Mapping and Linkage:** Unknown.

**Prevention:** None known. Genetic counseling indicated.

**Treatment:** Surgical treatment of the spinal cysts if symptoms occur, epilation of irritating eyelashes, and use of elastic stockings to control edema.

**Prognosis:** Life span and intellect are apparently unaffected.

**Detection of Carrier:** Unknown.

**References:**
Falls HF, Kertesz ED: A new syndrome combining pterygium colli with developmental anomalies of the eyelids and lymphatics of the lower extremities. Trans Ophth Soc 1964; 62:248–275.
Chynn KY: Congenital spinal extradural cyst in two siblings. Am J Roentgenol Radium Ther Nucl Med 1967; 101:204–215.
Robinow M, et al: Distichiasis-lymphedema. Am J Dis Child 1970; 119:343–347. *
Schwartz JF, et al: Hereditary spinal arachnoid cysts, distichiasis, and lymphedema. Ann Neurol 1980; 7:340–343. *
Dale RF: Primary lymphedema when found with distichiasis is of the type defined as bilateral hyperplasia by lymphography. J Med Genet 1987; 24:170–171.

T0007                                                    **Helga V. Toriello**

**Distomolar**
*See TEETH, SUPERNUMERARY*
**Diverticular aneurysm of the left ventricle**
*See VENTRICLE, DIVERTICULUM*
**Diverticulitis-deafness-neuropathy**
*See DEAFNESS-DIVERTICULITIS-NEUROPATHY*
**Diverticulosis of the left ventricle**
*See VENTRICLE, DIVERTICULUM*
**Diverticulum of larynx**
*See LARYNGOCELE*
**Diverticulum of left ventricle**
*See VENTRICLE, DIVERTICULUM*
**Diverticulum of right ventricle**
*See VENTRICLE, DIVERTICULUM*
**'Doggennose'**
*See NOSE, BIFID*
**Dominant dystrophic epidermolysis bullosa (DDEB)**
*See EPIDERMOLYSIS BULLOSUM, TYPE III*

## DONLAN SYNDROME          2369

**Includes:**
Cleft palate-growth failure-ectodermal dysplasia
Ectodermal dysplasia-growth failure-pancreatic insufficiency
Growth failure-ectodermal dysplasia-pancreatic insufficiency
Pancreatic insufficiency-growth failure-ectodermal dysplasia

**Excludes:**
**Cystic fibrosis** (0237)
**Ectodermal dysplasia, Christ-Siemens-Touraine type** (0333)
**Ectrodactyly-ectodermal dysplasia-clefting syndrome** (0337)

**Major Diagnostic Criteria:** The combination of pancreatic insufficiency, soft palate cleft, micrognathia, and eczema should suggest the diagnosis.

**Clinical Findings:** Posterior cleft palate, micrognathia, growth failure, eczema, and dental hypoplasia. In addition, one child had surgery for an annular pancreas. Laboratory studies revealed stool trypsin deficiency in both. Growth hormone, sweat chloride, and chromosome studies were normal.

**Complications:** Unknown.

**Associated Findings:** None known.

**Etiology:** The occurrence in brother and sister with negative family history suggests autosomal recessive inheritance.

**Pathogenesis:** Unknown.

**Sex Ratio:** M1:F1 (observed).

**Occurrence:** Two cases have been reported.

**Risk of Recurrence for Patient's Sib:**
See Part I, *Mendelian Inheritance.*

**Risk of Recurrence for Patient's Child:**
See Part I, *Mendelian Inheritance.*

**Age of Detectability:** At birth.

**Gene Mapping and Linkage:** Unknown.

**Prevention:** None known. Genetic counseling indicated.

**Treatment:** Viokase improved both growth and eczema.

**Prognosis:** Unknown.

**Detection of Carrier:** Unknown.

**References:**
Donlan MA: Growth failure, cleft palate, ectodermal dysplasia, and apparent pancreatic insufficiency: new syndrome. BD:OAS XIII(3B). New York: March of Dimes Birth Defects Foundation, 1977:230–231.

T0007                                                    **Helga V. Toriello**

**Donohue syndrome**
  *See LEPRECHAUNISM*
**DOOR(S) syndrome**
  *See DEAFNESS-ONYCHO-OSTEO-DYSTROPHY-RETARDATION-SEIZURES (DOORS)*

---

## DOPAMINE BETA-HYDROXYLASE DEFICIENCY, CONGENITAL                                            2883

**Includes:** Autonomic noradrenergic and adrenomedullary failure (some)

**Excludes:**
  Autonomic failure, progressive (PAF)
  Baroreceptor failure
  Dopamine beta-hydroxylase, plasma decreased (some)
  **Dysautonomia I, Riley-Day type** (0307)
  **Ehlers-Danlos syndrome** (0338)
  Hypotension, orthostatic idiopathic (IOH)
  Neuralgia, glossopharyngeal or vagal
  **Menkes syndrome** (0643)
  Parkinsonism
  Shy-Drager syndrome
  Strionigral or cerebellar degenerations (other)

**Major Diagnostic Criteria:** Severe orthostatic hypotension in the first two decades of life is the main presenting symptom. Baroreflex testing shows absence of the phase IV pressure overshoot in the Valsalva maneuver, establishing the diagnosis of autonomic failure. Despite the autonomic failure, baroreflex regulation of the heart rate is not impaired. Pressure responses to cold and isometric exercise are absent. In contrast to other forms of chronic autonomic failure, there is a normal sweating pattern, which shows that sympathetic cholinergic function is intact. Further pharmacologic testing reveals that sympathetic innervation of the pupils is also disturbed, but that parasympathetic innervation of the pupils, heart, and gastric parietal cells is intact. The combined data can be explained by isolated noradrenergic sympathetic dysfunction as a cause for autonomic failure. Evidence for dopamine beta-hydroxylase deficiency is obtained from measurements of plasma catecholamines; norepinephrine and epinephrine are not detectable, and dopamine is grossly elevated. The venous-arterial ratio of dopamine is grossly elevated (1.3–1.5) as evidence of peripheral production of this catecholamine. Since epinephrine is absent, the patient also has adrenomedullary failure. Spontaneous episodes of hypoglycemic coma and supersensitivity to exogenous insulin suggest diminished insulin antagonism, which may be due to adrenomedullary failure. Adrenocortical function (cortisol and aldosterone) is intact. Plasma dopamine beta-hydroxylase (DBH) activity is not detectable, but this cannot be used as a key diagnostic criterion, since variations in plasma dopamine beta-hydroxylase in a randomly selected population are genetically determined. Very low amounts are found in 3–4% of the population, and this trait in healthy individuals is inherited as an autosomal recessive.

**Clinical Findings:** Immediately after birth the baby may be cyanotic and hypotonic. Episodes of vomiting may lead to dehydration, with hypothermia and hypoglycemic coma in the first year of life. Mild ptosis of the eyelids and skeletal muscle hypotonia are present and probably also reflect loss of noradrenergic innervation. Furthermore, the two described patients have a nasal voice, a high-arched palate, and hyperflexible joints. Facial muscle weakness is apparent clinically. Deep tendon reflexes are sluggish. No other sensory or motor abnormalities are present. Pupils react normally to light and accommodation. Smell, taste, and tear production are also normal. Mental and physical development, including sexual maturation, are normal. The hands show **Brachydactyly**. In the second decade of life episodes of blurred vision, dizziness, faintness, and occasionally syncope are reported. Routine clinical and laboratory investigations are all normal. The electrocardiogram shows normal sinus rhythm, but T waves in precordial leads may be flat or negative, probably also reflecting noradrenergic denervation of the heart, since this abnormality disappears after administration of a beta$_1$-adrenoceptor agonist. Routine cytogenetic analysis does not show any abnormality.

**Complications:** The consequences of spontaneous hypoglycemic coma in the first year of life and traumatic lesions resulting from syncope caused by orthostatic hypotension.

**Associated Findings:** **Eyelid, ptosis, congenital,** hyperflexible joints, sluggish deep tendon reflexes, **Brachydactyly,** facial muscle weakness.

**Etiology:** Autosomal recessive inheritance or possibly sporadic.

**Pathogenesis:** Dopamine beta-hydroxylase deficiency. Norepinephrine and epinephrine are not detectable in plasma, urine, and cerebrospinal fluid, whereas dopamine, the precursor of norepinephrine, is grossly elevated in these fluids. L-dopa, the precursor of dopamine, is also increased in plasma and cerebrospinal fluid. Furthermore, metabolites of norepinephrine and epinephrine in urine (normetanephrine, metanephrine, 3-methoxy-4-hydroxyphenylethylene glycol, and free vanilmandelic acid) are also not detectable, whereas metabolites of dopamine (homovanillic acid and 3-methoxy-tyramine) are elevated. 3-Methoxy-4-hydroxyphenylethylene glycol in cerebrospinal fluid is also absent, and homovanillic acid is elevated. Dopamine beta-hydroxylase cannot be demonstrated functionally (in plasma) or immunologically (in skin biopsy material). Copper, the cofactor for dopamine beta-hydroxylase, is not deficient; plasma copper and ceruloplasmin are normal, and urinary copper excretion is not increased. A number of ways to manipulate the plasma level of norepinephrine in normal individuals (hypoglycemia, standing, head-up or -down tilting, or administration of tyramine, yohimbine, or clonidine), resulted in changes in dopamine instead of the expected increments or decrements in norepinephrine. This shows that central, preganglionic and postganglionic sympathetic neurotransmission is intact but that dopamine, rather than norepinephrine, is the neurotransmitter in this syndrome.

**MIM No.:** *22336, 14650

**Sex Ratio:** M1:F1

**Occurrence:** Two cases have been decribed, although there is an extensive literature on plasma DBH-related disorders.

**Risk of Recurrence for Patient's Sib:**
See Part I, *Mendelian Inheritance.*

**Risk of Recurrence for Patient's Child:**
See Part I, *Mendelian Inheritance.*

**Age of Detectability:** At birth, or through prenatal diagnosis.

**Gene Mapping and Linkage:** DBH (dopamine beta-hydroxylase (dopamine beta-monooxygenase)) has been mapped to 9q34.

**Prevention:** None known. Genetic counseling indicated.

**Treatment:** Treatment of orthostatic hypotention. Postural therapy, sodium chloride, fluorocortisone, pindolol, clonidine, and metoclopramide have been used with varying success. The orthostatic hypotension can be cured with the unphysiological aminoacid L-threo-3,4-dihydroxyphenylserine (L-threo-DOPS). DOPS can be converted into norepinephrine by dopa-decarboxylase (aromatic L-aminoacid decarboxylase), the enzyme which normally converts L-dopa into dopamine and which is not deficient in this syndrome.

**Prognosis:** Life span and intelligence are not affected. Physical handicaps (orthostatic hypotension) pose limitations on a normal life-style in the first half of the day.

**Detection of Carrier:** Unknown.

**References:**

Robertson D, et al.: Isolated failure of autonomic noradrenergic neurotransmission: evidence for impaired beta-hydroxylation of dopamine. New Engl J Med 1986; 314:1494–1497.

Man in 't Veld AJ, et al.: Congenital dopamine beta-hydroxylase deficiency; a novel orthostatic syndrome. Lancet 1987; I:183–187.

Man in 't Veld AJ, et al.: Congenital dopamine beta-hydroxylase deficiency. Lancet 1987; I:693.

Man in 't Veld AJ, et al.: effect of an unnatural noradrenaline precursor on sympathetic control of orthostatic hypotension in dopamine beta-hydroxylase deficiency. Lancet 1987; II:1172–1175.

Man in 't Veld AJ, et al.: Patients with dopamine beta-hydroxylase deficiency: a lesson in catecholamine physiology. Am J Hypertension 1988; 1:231–238.

MA076                                    **Arie J. Man in 't Veld**

**Dorsal cyst or sac**
   *See BRAIN, MIDLINE CAVES*
**Double chambered right ventricle**
   *See VENTRICLE, DOUBLE CHAMBERED RIGHT*
**Double inlet left ventricle with ventricular inversion**
   *See VENTRICLE, SEPTUM DEXTROPOSITION AND DOUBLE INLET LEFT VENTRICLE*
**Double inlet left ventricle without ventricular inversion**
   *See VENTRICLE, SEPTUM DEXTROPOSITION AND DOUBLE INLET LEFT VENTRICLE*
**Double outlet l. ventricle-atresia of r. ventricular infundibulum**
   *See VENTRICLE, DOUBLE OUTLET LEFT*
**Double outlet left ventricle-pulmonary stenosis**
   *See VENTRICLE, DOUBLE OUTLET LEFT*
**Double outlet left ventricle-ventricular septal defect**
   *See VENTRICLE, DOUBLE OUTLET LEFT*
**'Double uterus' (misnomer)**
   *See MULLERIAN FUSION, INCOMPLETE*
**Dowling-Degos disease (DDD)**
   *See SKIN CREASES, RETICULATE PIGMENTED FLEXURES, DOWLING-DEGOS TYPE*
**Down syndrome**
   *See CHROMOSOME 21, TRISOMY 21*
**Doyne discoid cataract**
   *See CATARACT, COPPOCK*
**Doyne honeycombed retinal degeneration**
   *See OCULAR DRUSEN*
**DR syndrome**
   *See RADIAL-RENAL-OCULAR SYNDROME*
**Drash syndrome**
   *See WILMS TUMOR-PSEUDOHERMAPHRODITISM-GLOMERULOPATHY,DENYS-DRASH TYPE*
**Drepanocytic anemia**
   *See ANEMIA, SICKLE CELL*
**Drug-induced insulin resistance**
   *See SKIN, ACANTHOSIS NIGRICANS*
**Drusen ocular**
   *See OCULAR DRUSEN*
**Drusen of Bruch membrane**
   *See OCULAR DRUSEN*
**Duane anomaly-radial ray abnormalities-deafness**
   *See EYE, DUANE RETRACTION SYNDROME*
**Duane retraction syndrome**
   *See EYE, DUANE RETRACTION SYNDROME*
**Duane syndrome-radial defects**
   *See RADIAL-RENAL-OCULAR SYNDROME*
**Dubin-Johnson syndrome**
   *See HYPERBILIRUBINEMIA, CONJUGATED*

## DUBOWITZ SYNDROME                                    0299

**Includes:** Growth retardation-microcephaly-characteristic facies

**Excludes:**
   **Dubowitz syndrome** (0299)
   **Fetal alcohol syndrome** (0379)
   Nanocephaly
   **Seckel syndrome** (0881)

**Major Diagnostic Criteria:** Low birth weight, postnatal growth retardation, microcephaly and characteristic facial features which include high forehead, broad nasal bridge, telecanthus, ptosis, blepharophimosis and micrognathia.

**Clinical Findings:** All reported patients have had low birth weight, postnatal growth retardation, and microcephaly. Mental retardation of a mild degree is frequently encountered. The characteristic dysmorphic facial features include: sparse hair, high sloping forehead, flat supraorbital ridges, broad nasal bridge in line with the forehead, telecanthus, ptosis, blepharophimosis with short palpebral fissures, epicanthal folds and micrognathia. The voice is usually high-pitched and hoarse. The lateral portions of the eyebrows may be hypoplastic. Eczema, poor dietary intake, vomiting and chronic diarrhea may occur during the 1st year. Internal abnormalities have not been detected. Hypospadias or cryptorchidism may be encountered in affected males.

**Complications:** Shy personality.

**Associated Findings:** Prolapse of rectum due to chronic diarrhea, arterial anomalies, aplastic anemia, infection of eczema, failure to thrive, poor school performance.

**Etiology:** Autosomal recessive inheritance.

**Pathogenesis:** Unknown.

**MIM No.:** *22337

**POS No.:** 3187

**Sex Ratio:** M1:F1

**Occurrence:** About 40 cases reported in the literature. Occurs in Caucasions and Orientals.

**Risk of Recurrence for Patient's Sib:**
   See Part I, *Mendelian Inheritance.* Affected monozygotic twins and siblings have been reported.

**Risk of Recurrence for Patient's Child:**
   See Part I, *Mendelian Inheritance.*

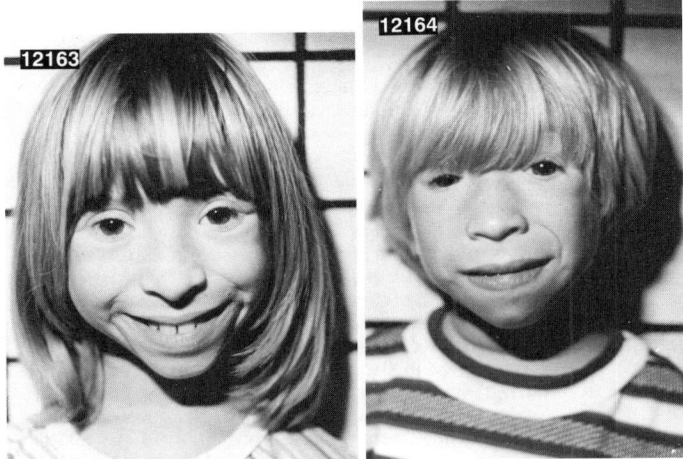

**0299**-12163: Dysmorphic features include wide nasal bridge, telecanthus, prominent nose and micrognathia. 12164: Affected brother has ptosis, blepharophimosis, telecanthus, broad nasal bridge and micrognathia.

**Age of Detectability:** Neonatal period.

**Gene Mapping and Linkage:** Unknown.

**Prevention:** None known. Genetic counseling indicated.

**Treatment:** Surgery for ptosis or ocular abnormality; special education.

**Prognosis:** Probably normal life span.

**Detection of Carrier:** Unknown.

**References:**
Dubowitz V: Familial low birth weight dwarfism with an unusual facies and a skin eruption. J Med Genet 1965; 2:12–17. †
Grosse R, et al.: The Dubowitz syndrome. Z Kinderheilkd 1971; 110:175–187.
Opitz JM, et al.: Studies of malformation syndromes in man XXIV B: the Dubowitz syndrome. Further observations. Z Kinderheilkd 1973; 116:1–12.
Parrish J, Wilroy RS: The Dubowitz syndrome: the psychological status of ten cases at follow-up. Am J Med Genet 1980; 6:3–8.
Moller KT, Gorlin RJ: The Dubowitz syndrome: a retrospective. J Craniofa Genet Develop Biol Suppl 1985; 1:283–286.
Kuster W, Majewski F: The Dubowitz syndrome. Europ J Pediat 1986; 144:574–578.
Winter RM: Dubowitz syndrome. J Med Genet 1986; 23:11–13.

WI021                                      **R.S. Wilroy, Jr.**

**Duchenne muscular dystrophy**
*See MUSCULAR DYSTROPHY, CHILDHOOD PSEUDOHYPERTROPHIC*
**Duchenne muscular dystrophy (atypical cases)**
*See MYOPATHY, MALIGNANT HYPERTHERMIA*
**Duchenne-like autosomal recessive muscular dystrophy**
*See MUSCULAR DYSTROPHY, AUTOSOMAL RECESSIVE PSEUDOHYPERTROPHIC*
**Duct, thyroglossal remnant**
*See THYROGLOSSAL DUCT REMNANT*
**Ductal cyst**
*See EPIGLOTTIS, VALLECULAR CYST*
**Ductal cyst of the salivary gland**
*See SALIVARY GLAND, DUCTAL CYST*

## DUCTUS ARTERIOSUS, PATENT                    0800

**Includes:**
 Patent ductus arteriosus
 Persistent ductus arteriosus

**Excludes:**
 **Aortico-pulmonary septal defect** (0083)
 **Fetal effects of nonsteroidal anti-inflammatory drugs (NSAIDS)** (3281)
 **Heart, truncus arteriosus** (0972)

**Major Diagnostic Criteria:** The presence of classic clinical and laboratory findings with the characteristic continuous murmur. Selective aortogram, if necessary, is the procedure of choice to confirm the diagnosis.

**Clinical Findings:** Patent ductus arteriosus (PDA), in its pathologic manifestation, represents the postnatal patency of a normal fetal vessel between the left pulmonary artery and the aorta. In fetal life, most of the blood from the right ventricle bypasses the nonaerated lungs through this channel. Functional closure of the ductus usually occurs within hours or days after birth. The hemodynamic changes and clinical manifestations of its persistence depend on the magnitude of the pulmonary blood flow. The amount of left-to-right shunt is related to the size of the ductal lumen and the resistance in the pulmonary vascular bed. Infants and small children with a large ductus and low pulmonary vascular resistance have the highest pulmonary blood flow and pressures. The large pulmonary venous return results in relative mitral valve stenosis and increases in left ventricular end diastolic pressure and volume. The degree of right ventricular overloading depends on the magnitude of pulmonary artery pressure. The aortic diastolic runoff lesion characteristically results in widening of the systemic arterial pulse pressure. These patients are usually symptomatic early in life with the clinical findings of a large extracardiac left-to-right shunt. Tachypnea, frequent respiratory infections, growth retardation and congestive heart failure (sometimes resulting in pulmonary edema) are common findings. Bounding peripheral pulses or pulses of normal amplitude in the presence of congestive heart failure are highly suggestive of this lesion. Infants with PDA have variable murmurs, depending on the systolic and diastolic pressure differences between the aorta and pulmonary artery. The majority lack the diastolic component of the continuous murmur typically heard in older children or the diastolic component is short. A diastolic mitral flow murmur of the apex is usually present. Small premature babies, particularly those with respiratory disease, may have a "silent" ductus.

After one year of age, the great majority of cases are asymptomatic with normal growth and development. The left-to-right shunt is of small-to-moderate size and the pulmonary artery pressure is usually normal. The typical and diagnostic continuous machinery-like murmur is present in more than 90% of the cases. This murmur is maximal in the second and third left intercostal space and left subclavian area. It is often associated with a systolic thrill also present over the suprasternal notch area. The characteristic ductus murmur has a crescendo-decrescendo configuration peaking around the second sound and often obscures it. The second sound is normally split and the pulmonic component may be slightly accentuated.

The X-ray findings are dependent on the hemodynamic situation. Infants with left-to-right shunts usually have cardiomegaly, increased vascular markings and left atrial enlargement. The ascending aorta may appear enlarged and the pulmonary trunk prominent. Sometimes the ductus itself is visible as a short, convex density just below the aortic knob. In older children, the X-rays are often normal or show mild cardiomegaly with only slight increase of the pulmonary arterial markings. The ductus (or ductus infundibulum) is often apparent as a discrete density distal to the aortic knob or as an extra density between the aortic knob and pulmonary trunk. This may be apparent in patients with otherwise normal roentgenographic findings. The EKG in infancy commonly shows biventricular hypertrophy and left atrial enlargement. In contrast, older children's EKGs are normal or show left ventricular hypertrophy of the volume overload type.

Echocardiac findings of a PDA result from the increased pulmonary blood flow. The left atrium enlarges as a function of increased pulmonary venous return. The left ventricle is dilated and hyperkinetic. Two dimensional echocardiograph can visualize the patent ductus and rule out associated cardiac lesions. Doppler examination can demonstrate turbulent flow in the pulmonary artery. Color doppler can clearly show a continuous jet entering at the origin of the left pulmonary artery.

Cardiac catheterization is sometimes necessary to confirm the presence of the extracardiac left-to-right shunt and associated cardiac lesions. Direct passage of the catheter through the ductus is often possible.

**Complications:** Death from congestive heart failure and pneumonia; development of high pulmonary vascular resistance resulting in the reversal of the shunt (Eisenmenger physiology); aneurysm of the ductus arteriosus; subacute bacterial endocarditis later in life.

**Associated Findings:** Approximately 15% have an additional cardiac lesion. The most common are **Ventricular septal defect**, **Aorta, coarctation**. A high incidence of extracardiac congenital anomalies are present as part of **Fetal rubella syndrome**.

**Etiology:** Presumably multifactorial inheritance. Since the ductus arteriosus represents the distal left sixth aortic arch, a normal vessel during fetal life, the question of etiology is concerned not with its existence but with the possible causes of its patency. Rubella, prematurity and hypoxia are the main known factors. Rubella infection in the first trimester of pregnancy leads to congenital defects in 70–80%. About one-half of these include heart malformations, of which patent ductus or pulmonary artery coarctations are by far the most common. The importance of arterial oxygen tension after birth for the closure of the ductus seems to be established from the clinical and experimental experience. Perinatal respiratory distress or a reduced oxygen tension at high altitude leads to a higher frequency of the malformation. There is also some evidence for genetic factors in its presence (families with several cases of PDA have been reported).

**Pathogenesis:** Unknown.

**MIM No.:** 16910

**CDC No.:** 747.000

**Sex Ratio:** M1:F2 (M1:F1 in rubella-related PDA)

**Occurrence:** Approximately 1:830 live births.

**Risk of Recurrence for Patient's Sib:** Empiric risk about 3%.

**Risk of Recurrence for Patient's Child:** If mother is affected, empiric risk is about 4%. If father is affected, empiric risk is about 2%.

**Age of Detectability:** From birth, by heart murmur, echocardiography/Doppler, or aortogram.

**Gene Mapping and Linkage:** Unknown.

**Prevention:** Vaccine for rubella; prevention of prematurity and neonatal hypoxemia. Genetic counseling is indicated.

**Treatment:** Surgical division or ligation of the ductus. Indomethacin, an inhibitor of prostaglandin synthesis, has been successfully used for the pharmacological closure of PDA in premature newborns. Transcatheter occlusion of the PDA has been accomplished.

**Prognosis:** Generally good. After successful surgical repair, normal life expectancy. Surgical mortality less than 1%, higher in infancy (in particular when associated with other cardiac lesions). In undetected cases, increasing mortality in the fourth decade of life and onwards due to the development of pulmonary vascular changes or subacute bacterial endocarditis.

**Detection of Carrier:** Unknown.

**Special Considerations:** PDA in a premature infant is likely to close spontaneously, even if heart failure has occurred. In symptomatic full-term infants, spontaneous closure seldom occurs.

**References:**
Cassels DE: The ductus arteriosus. Springfield, IL: C.C. Thomas, 1973.
Friedman WF, et al.: Pharmacologic closure of patent ductus arteriosus in the premature infant. New Engl J Med 1976; 295:526–529.
Heymann MA, Rudolph AM: The ductus arteriosus. Report of the 75th Ross conference of pediatric research. Columbus, OH: Ross Laboratories, 1978. *
Allen HD, et al.: Use of echocardiography in newborns with patent ductus arteriosus: a review. Ped Cardiol 1982; 3:65–70.
Nora JJ, Nora AH: Maternal transmission of congenital heart disease. Am J Cardiol 1987; 59:459–463. *

VI001                                    **Benjamin E. Victorica**

**Ductus arteriosus, patent-eye anomalies-unusual facies-deafness**
  *See CORNEAL ANESTHESIA-RETINAL DEFECTS-UNUSUAL FACIES-HEART DEFECT*
**Ductus arteriosus, prenatal closure with NSAID exposure**
  *See FETAL EFFECTS OF NONSTEROIDAL ANTI-INFLAMMATORY DRUGS (NSAIDS)*
**Duffy blood group positive**
  *See MALARIA, VIVAX, SUSCEPTIBILITY TO*
**Duncan disease**
  *See IMMUNODEFICIENCY, X-LINKED LYMPHOPROLIFERATIVE DISEASE*
**Dunnigan syndrome**
  *See LIPODYSTROPHY, FAMILIAL LIMB AND TRUNK*
**Duodenal atresia**
  *See DUODENUM, ATRESIA OR STENOSIS*
**Duodenal atresia of the first segment, hereditary**
  *See PYLORODUODENAL ATRESIA, HEREDITARY*
**Duodenal stenosis**
  *See DUODENUM, ATRESIA OR STENOSIS*
**Duodenal ulcer (DU)**
  *See PEPTIC ULCER DISEASES, NON-SYNDROMIC*
**Duodenal ulcer-leukonychia-gallstones**
  *See ULCER-LEUKONYCHIA-GALLSTONES*
**Duodenal ulcer-tremor syndrome**
  *See TREMOR-DUODENAL ULCER SYNDROME*

## DUODENUM, ATRESIA OR STENOSIS          0300

**Includes:**
  Duodenal atresia
  Duodenal stenosis

**Excludes:**
  Duodenal bands and rotational abnormalities
  Gastric atresia or stenosis
  **Intestinal atresia or stenosis** (0531)
  **Pancreas, annular** (0062)
  **Stomach, pyloric atresia** (0910)

**Major Diagnostic Criteria:** Upper abdominal or gastric distension occurs during the first 24–36 hours of life, usually associated with bile-stained emesis. A characteristic "double-bubble" appearance of abdominal X-rays, with little or no air elsewhere in the abdomen, is frequently noted. In partial obstruction, a contrast study of the stomach and duodenum may be required for diagnosis.

**Clinical Findings:** In more than 80% of affected patients, the atresia or stenosis occurs distal to the opening of the ampulla of Vater into the duodenum. Annular pancreas and rotational abnormalities are frequently associated with duodenal atresia and stenosis occurring in 20–30% of the cases. Half of the patients are premature or small-for-date infants. The types of atresias are classified as follows:
*Type I:* Atresia with an intact membrane producing marked discrepancy in size between the proximal and distal segments.
*Type II:* The two blind ends of the duodenum are connected by a short fibrous cord.
*Type III:* There is no connecting fibrous cord between the blind ends.
  Stenosis can be caused either by an intraluminal membrane with a perforation, or by a "wind-sock" anomaly with a membrane which may be stretched to the point of the distal obstruction but that actually occurs proximally and so might be missed at the time of surgery.
  Bile stained emesis is the first symptom, occuring in over 80% of patients. Distension in the upper abdomen is evident. Meconium is passed in one-half of patients prior to operation. Jaundice with elevation of the unconjugated bilirubin occurs in most patients, especially if there is delay in diagnosis. Polyhydramnios occurs in half of the patients, and this diagnosis can be made prenatally by ultrasound.

**Complications:** Emesis, aspiration, pneumonia, sepsis, and electrolyte depletion.

**Associated Findings:** Approximately one-third of all cases have **Chromosome 21, trisomy 21.** Malrotation of the intestinal tract and **Pancreas, annular** occur in 20–30% of patients. Congenital heart disease occurs in 20%. **Tracheoesophageal fistula,** distal jejunal and ileal atresias and stenosis, and renal malformations are less common.

**Etiology:** Possibly autosomal recessive inheritance in some instances. One such kindred reported.

**Pathogenesis:** The condition may be due to a persistence of a "solid cord" state of a small segment of duodenum during embryologic development in the first trimester. However, some theories implicate vascular injury and compression of the duodenum by surrounding organs such as annular pancreas or rotational abnormalities.

**MIM No.:** 22340

**Sex Ratio:** M1:F1

**Occurrence:** Incidence 1:10,000 live births.

**Risk of Recurrence for Patient's Sib:** Same as for general population unless inherited form.

**Risk of Recurrence for Patient's Child:** Same as for general population unless inherited form.

**Age of Detectability:** Most of the patients will be diagnosed in the first days of life. In the cases of duodenal stenosis, 25% can be diagnosed in the first few days of life; another 25% in the first

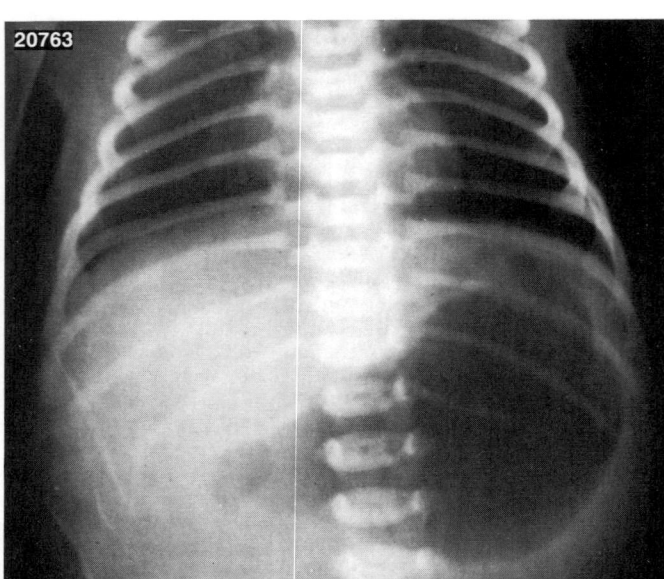
20763

**0300-20763:** Duodenum, atresia or stenosis; note the double bubble sign on this X-ray.

month, and an additional 25% in the remainder of the first year. The remainder would be detectable throughout the subsequent years of life.

**Gene Mapping and Linkage:** Unknown.

**Prevention:** None known. Genetic counseling indicated.

**Treatment:** Duodenal duodenostomy for atresias and stenosis with excision of the wind-sock deformity when present. Nasogastric decompression and/or gastrostomy with routine postoperative care, including parenteral alimentation, is necessary.

**Prognosis:** Death occurs from malnutrition or aspiration if obstruction is not relieved. Death is usually attributed to associated anomalies or respiratory complications. Most of the patients with duodenal atresias, diaphragms, or stenosis survive with good postoperative care.

**Detection of Carrier:** Unknown.

**References:**
Schnaufer L: Duodenal atresia, stenosis and annular pancreas. In Welch K, et al.: Pediatric surgery, ed 4. Philadelphia: W.B. Saunders, 1986.

BE049                                                    **Arthur S. Besser**

**Dupen△, fetal effects**
  *See FETAL D-PENICILLAMINE SYNDROME*
**Duplicate labiale**
  *See LIP, DOUBLE*
**Duplication of colon, external genitalia and lower urinary tract**
  *See INTESTINAL DUPLICATION*
**Dupuytren contracture, congenital**
  *See CAMPTODACTYLY*
**Dupuytren's disease**
  *See CONTRACTURE, DUPUYTREN*

**Includes:**
  Chondrodysplasias
  Osteodysplasias
  Skeletal dysplasia
  Stature, short

Skeletal growth is a complex process that is influence by numerous genetic and environmental factors from early embryonic life through the end of puberty. Dwarfism is caused by prolonged or permanent disturbances in this process, resulting in dramatic short stature. The term is not applied to normal variations in growth patterns that result in mild short stature, i.e. familial short stature and constitutional delay of growth. Dwarfism can be classified in many different ways; however, separation into proportionate and disproportionate dwarfism based on whether the body proportions are normal or not is most useful clinically.

Proportionate dwarfism that is evident at or before birth is a feature of many multiple congenital anomaly/malformation syndromes and almost all syndromes resulting from chromosomal aberrations and from exposure to teratogens. In most instances the growth deficiency probably reflects a generalized disturbance of cellular metabolism that adversely affects the morphogenesis and growth of multiple tissues and organ systems, including the skeleton. The diagnosis of such infants is usually based on the particular pattern of anomalies that the infant exhibits, the prenatal history, and results of chromosomal analysis. Prognosis and recurrence risks depend on the particular syndrome. There is generally no treatment that can restore growth to normal.

Growth deficiency of the proportionate type may also accompany multisystem syndromes of postnatal onset such as **Progeria** or **Cockayne syndrome**. As above, the deficiency reflects a generalized cellular abnormality. Typically, however, proportionate dwarfism of postnatal onset suggests deficient stimulation of an otherwise normally growing skeleton. Defects in the hypothalamic-growth hormone-somatomedin axis, such as isolated growth hormone deficiency, or panhypopituitarism, produce this clinical picture. Developmental defects of midline cranial structures, such as **Septo-optic dysplasia** or **Cleft lip** and **Cleft palate**, may be associated with hypothalamic dysfunction with growth hormone deficiency. Many inborn errors of metabolism are associated with substantial proportionate short stature due to the secondary effects of the metabolic abnormality on the hormonal axis or on the growing skeleton itself. Evaluation of children in this category should thus be aimed at identifying an endocrine and metabolic cause for the growth deficiency. In many cases, growth can be restored toward normal if the abnormality can be corrected, e.g. growth hormone replacement for growth hormone deficiency.

Disproportionate dwarfism is characterized by limb-to-trunk disproportion, resulting in either short limb or short trunk dwarfism. These disorders comprise a very large group of mostly inherited conditions called *skeletal dysplasias*. The abnormalities reside in the growing skeleton. The disorders can be subdivided into *osteodysplasias* and *chondrodysplasias*. The former result from defects that are expressed in bone cells, such as type I collagen abnormalities expressed by osteoblasts in **Osteogenesis imperfecta** or the osteoclast dysfunction that occurs in **Osteopetrosis**. The chondrodysplasias are disorders of endochondral ossification, and abnormalities of the growth plate have been described in many instances.

Many of the skeletal dysplasias present at or before birth, of which a large number are lethal, e.g. **Osteogenesis imperfecta** type II and **Thanatophoric dysplasia**. In contrast, growth deficiency may not be evident before age two years or even later in, for example, **Pseudoachondroplastic dysplasia**. The manifestations are limited to the skeleton in some conditions, but other connective tissues such as ligaments, eyes, skin, and so forth may be involved in other conditions. Thus, although disproportionate dwarfism is common to many of these disorders, the clinical presentations of the specific conditions are unique.

The diagnosis is commonly based on the clinical, genetic, and

X-ray findings; however, special studies, such as collagen analysis or growth plate assessment, are becoming increasingly important. Management should be tailored to the individual disorder; however there are currently no methods to normalize bone growth in any of the skeletal dysplasias. Prenatal diagnosis using ultrasonography to examine the fetal skeleton growth is available.

**Support Groups:**
CA; San Bruno; Little People of America, Inc. (LPA)
MD; Bethesda; Human Growth Foundation (HGF)
MD; Silver Spring; Parents of Dwarfed Children

**References:**
Rimoin DL, Horton WA: Short stature, parts I and II. J Pediatr 1978; 92:523–528, 697–704.
Smith DW: Recognizable patterns of human malformation. Philadelphia: W.B. Saunders, 1982.
Horton WA: Disproportionate short stature. In: Kelley V, ed: Practice of pediatrics. New York: Harper and Row, 1983:1–15.
Schaff-Blass E, et al.: Advances in diagnosis and treatment of short stature, with special reference to the role of growth hormone. J Pediatr 1984; 104:801–813.
Byers PH: Disorders of collagen biosynthesis and structure. In: Scriver CR, et al, eds: The metabolic basis of inherited disease, 6th ed. New York: McGraw-Hill, 1989:2805–2842.
Phillips JA, III: Inherited defects in growth hormone synthesis and action. In: Scriver CR, et al, eds: The metabolic basis of inherited disease, 6th ed. New York: McGraw-Hill, 1989:1965–1984.

H0033                                                    **William A. Horton**

## DWARFISM (SHORT LIMBED)-PETERS ANOMALY OF THE EYE                          2812

**Includes:**
Eye (Peters anomaly) associated with short-limbed dwarfism
Ophthalmo-mandibulo-melic dwarfism
Peters anomaly-short limbed dwarfism
Peters plus
Pillay syndrome

**Excludes:**
**Eye, anterior segment dysgenesis** (0439)
**Fetal alcohol syndrome** (0379)
**Ophthalmo-mandibulo-melic dwarfism** (3259)
**Walker-Warburg syndrome** (2869)

**Major Diagnostic Criteria:**  Short-limbed dwarfism, Peters anomaly, round facies, thin upper lip, and variable psychomotor delay.

**Clinical Findings:**  *Rhizomelic dwarfism:* round face with thin upper lip, hypoplastic columella, micrognathia, narrow palpebral fissures. *Corneal clouding secondary to Peters anomaly:* glaucoma, lens opacity, narrow external auditory canals, motor and intellectual delay. *Genitourinary abnormalities:* increased frequency of pyelonephritis in one patient, cryptorchidism in one patient.

**Complications:**  Visual loss from corneal and lens opacities and glaucoma. Hearing loss, perhaps secondary to multiple episodes of otitis media.

**Associated Findings:**  Persistent hyaloid system of the eye.

**Etiology:**  Usually autosomal recessive inheritance.

**Pathogenesis:**  Unknown.

**MIM No.:**  26154, *16490

**POS No.:**  4483

**Sex Ratio:**  Presumably M1:F1.

**Occurrence:**  Four boys and two girls, including three patients of van Schooneveld et al (1984), have been reported.

**Risk of Recurrence for Patient's Sib:**
See Part I, *Mendelian Inheritance.*

**Risk of Recurrence for Patient's Child:**
See Part I, *Mendelian Inheritance.*

**Age of Detectability:**  At birth.

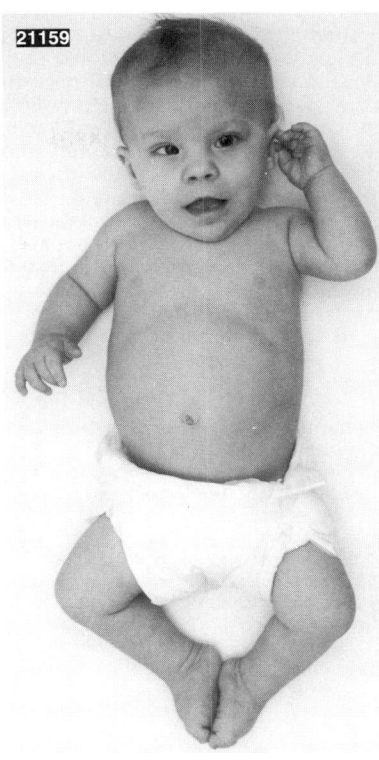

**2812A**-21159:  Affected infant at age one year; note thin upper lip, hypoplastic columella, round face and short limbs.

**Gene Mapping and Linkage:**  Unknown.

**Prevention:**  None known. Genetic counseling indicated.

**Treatment:**  Management of ocular conditions to promote normal visual development. Management of recurrent otitis media and pyelonephritis. Special education as needed.

**Prognosis:**  Guarded for vision.

**Detection of Carrier:**  Unknown.

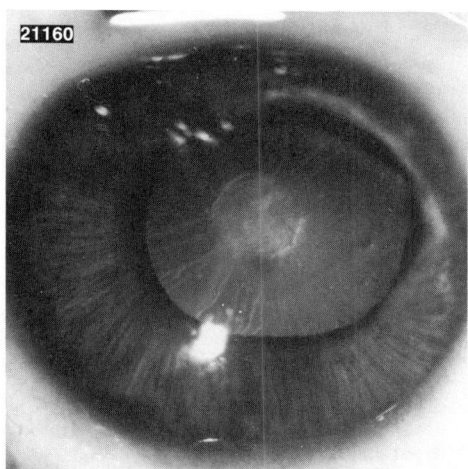

**2812B**-21160:  Round central corneal opacity due to lens adherence and many fine iris processes extending to the opacity.

**Special Considerations:** The *Peters plus* patients reported by van Schooneveld et al (1984) also had short stature and Peters anomaly. Dr. Schooneveld kindly provided further information and photographs of her patients (personal communication, July 18, 1986). Her patient No. 9, and possibly patient No. 6, as well as an additional patient (22.367) whom she has seen since the publications, could be diagnosed as having the disorder presented above. A different facial appearance (possibly due to age), including cleft lip with or without palate and abnormal ears, excludes the other *Peters plus* patients from the present diagnosis at this time.

*Ophthalmo-mandibulo-melic dwarfism*, or *Pillay syndrome* (Pillay, 1964), documented in three members of one family, also consists of corneal opacity and limb shortening. If this proves to be a related condition, then this syndrome may show a high degree of variability.

**References:**

Pillay VK: Ophthalmo-mandibulo-melic dysplasia: an hereditary syndrome. J Bone Joint Surg 1964; 46A:858–862.
Krause U, et al.: A case of Peters' syndrome with spontaneous corneal perforation. J Pediatr Ophthalmol 1969; 6:145–149.
van Schooneveld MJ, et al.: Peters'-plus: a new syndrome. Ophthalmic Pediatr Genet 1984; 4:141–146.
Kivlin JD, et al.: Peters' anomaly as a consequence of genetic and nongenetic syndromes. Arch Ophthalmol 1986; 104:61–64. *
Ponder SW, et al.: Cornelia de Lang syndrome with Peters anomaly and fat malabsorption. Dysmorphol Clin Genet 1988; 2:2–5.
Thompson EM, Winter RM: A child with sclerocornea, short limbs, short stature and distinct facial appearance. Am J Med Genet 1988; 30:719–724.

KI021
FI006
Jane D. Kivlin
Robert M. Fineman

**Dwarfism, acromesomelic, Campailla-Martinelli type**
*See ACROMESOMELIC DYSPLASIA, CAMPAILLA-MARTINELLI TYPE*
**Dwarfism, campomelic**
*See CAMPOMELIC DYSPLASIA*
**Dwarfism, deformity with mesomelic**
*See DYSCHONDROSTEOSIS*
**Dwarfism, dysplasia spondyloepiphysaria tarda**
*See SPONDYLOEPIPHYSEAL DYSPLASIA, LATE*

## DWARFISM, DYSSEGMENTAL, ROLLAND-DESBUQUOIS TYPE   2690

**Includes:**
Anisospondylic camptomicromelic dwarfism
Dyssegmental dwarfism
Dyssegmental dysplasia, mild type
Rolland-Desbuquois syndrome

**Excludes:**
**Dwarfism, dyssegmental, Silverman-Handmaker type** (2935)
**Kniest dysplasia** (0557)
**Oto-spondylo-megaepiphyseal dysplasia** (2304)
Spondylocostal dysostosis

**Major Diagnostic Criteria:** Micromelic skeletal dysplasia with less pronounced dwarfism than in **Dwarfism, dyssegmental, Silverman-Handmaker type** and survival into early infancy. Disproportionate short stature, unusual facial appearance, short neck, narrow thorax, short and bent extremities, and decreased joint mobility. **Cleft palate** is common. The diagnosis is established primarily by X-ray on the basis of anisospondyly of the vertebral bodies.

**Clinical Findings:** In common with **Dwarfism, dyssegmental, Silverman-Handmaker type**, the anomaly is immediately obvious at birth, although the clinical picture is less severe, the dwarfism and the micromelia both being less marked. Body length at birth varies between 35 and 50 cm, and weight varies between 2,100 and 4,500 g. Five minutes after delivery, most of the patients record Apgar scores of between 8 and 10.

The children usually have flat facies with micrognathia, and the neck is short. Narrowing of the chest is less pronounced than in the severe form of dyssegmental dysplasia. The limbs are uni-

formly shortened and most of the joints have reduced mobility. Nonskeletal malformations are, however, only rarely observed.

X-ray features show a greater degree of variability, with some of the dysplastic changes being less marked. The vertebral column represents the major diagnostic feature. The vertebral bodies show moderate anisospondyly, with coronal clefting of the lower thoracic and lumbar vertebrae. Apart from slight hypoplasia, the iliac bones are largely normal. The long bones are less noticeably shortened, but they also show mild midshaft angulation together with metaphyseal flaring and cupping. In individual cases the clavicles may appear long. Shortening of the ribs varies from case to case, resulting in differences in the narrowing of the chest. Scapular changes, however, have not been reported. Chondro-osseous morphology is characterized by prominent patches of broad collagen fibers. There may be foamy Kniest-like changes observed in resting cartilage, but the growth plate and calcification process appear normal.

**Complications:** Narrowing of the thorax leads to respiratory problems such as tachypnea or frequent pulmonary infections. Death due to cardiac failure arising from the underlying respiratory failure.

**Associated Findings:** **Cleft palate**, hirsutism, encephalocele (1/11), or a hernia may also be present.

**Etiology:** Presumably autosomal recessive inheritance.

**Pathogenesis:** The cause of the defects seen in the spine is assumed to be a disturbance in segmentation. Despite the fact that histologic data are often lacking, the dwarfism indicates that an additional enchondral growth disorder, albeit less marked, is also involved.

**MIM No.:** 22440
**POS No.:** 4282
**Sex Ratio:** M1:F3

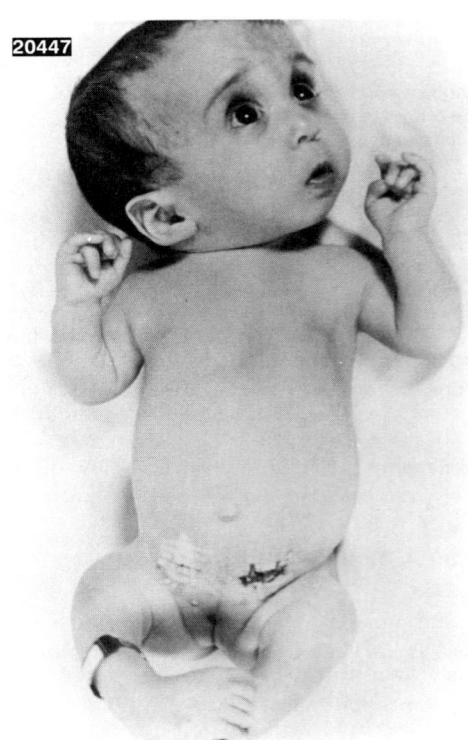

**2690-20447:** Dyssegmental dysplasia, Rolland-Desbuquois type; note unusual facies, short neck, short and bent limbs, and narrow thorax.

**Occurrence:** About a dozen cases have been reported in the literature. With respect to ethnic origin, West Europeans predominate. Two cases have also been described among Navajo Indians.

**Risk of Recurrence for Patient's Sib:**
See Part I, *Mendelian Inheritance.*

**Risk of Recurrence for Patient's Child:**
See Part I, *Mendelian Inheritance.* Affected individuals are not expected to survive to reproduce.

**Age of Detectability:** At birth.

**Gene Mapping and Linkage:** Unknown.

**Prevention:** None known. Genetic counseling indicated.

**Treatment:** No effective treatment is known. Respiratory infections should be treated accordingly. If such associated findings as cleft palate or hernia are present, surgery may be required.

**Prognosis:** Thus far, all of the patients reported have died at the latest in early childhood.

**Detection of Carrier:** Unknown.

**Special Considerations:** The variable clinical picture and the variations in the course of the disease clearly indicate a heterogeneity of dyssegmental dysplasia. Because of the different prognoses, however, an differentiation should be made between this condition, **Kniest dysplasia**, **Oto-spondylo-megaepiphyseal dysplasia**. Differentiation from spondylocostal dysostosis, can be made on the basis of the additional rib lesions involved.

**References:**
Rolland JC, et al.: Nanisme chondrodystrophique et division palatine chez un nouveau-né. Ann Pediatr 1972; 19:139–143.
Gorlin RJ, Langer LO, Jr: Dyssegmental dwarfism: lethal anisospondylic camptomicromelic dwarfism. BD:OAS XIV(6B). New York: March of Dimes Birth Defects Foundation, 1978:193–197.
Bueno M, et al.: Dysplasie dyssegmentaire: a propos de 2 cas familiaux d'evolution letale. Arch Fr Pediatr 1984; 41:269–271.
Fasanelli S: Dyssegmental dysplasia. Skeletal Radiol 1985; 14:173–177.
Aleck KA, et al.: Dyssegmental dysplasia: clinical, radiographic, and morphologic evidence of heterogeneity. Am J Med Genet 1987; 27:295–312.

ST054
AL006

**Hartmut R. Stoess**
**Kirk Aleck**

---

## DWARFISM, DYSSEGMENTAL, SILVERMAN-HANDMAKER TYPE — 2935

**Includes:**
Anisospondylic camptomicromelic dwarfism, lethal
Dyssegmental dysplasia, Silverman type
Silverman-Handmaker dwarfism

**Excludes:**
**Dwarfism, dyssegmental, Rolland-Desbuquois type** (2690)
**Kniest dysplasia** (0557)
**Thanatophoric dysplasia** (0940)

**Major Diagnostic Criteria:** Congenital lethal chondrodysplasia with disproportionate short stature; unusual facial appearance; short neck; narrow thorax; short, bent extremities; and decreased joint mobility. **Cleft palate** (5/16) and **Encephalocele** (4/16) are seen in some patients.

X-ray evaluation shows severe segmentation defects of the vertebral spine (anisospondyly), visible on both anteroposterior and lateral views of the spine. In addition, shortening and bending of the long bones, unusual appearing ilia, abnormal scapulae, and occipital skull defects are seen.

**Clinical Findings:** Dyssegmental dysplasia, evident at birth, is characterized by severe disproportionate dwarfism with marked micromelia and bowed limbs. The feet are in the talipes position. The length at birth varies between 20 and 39 cm, and birth weight varies between 800 and 2,700 g. In addition, the face is flat with micrognathia and microphthalmia, and the nose is flattened. The neck is very short and the thorax severely narrowed, with resulting hypoplasia of the lungs. Mobility of the joints is reduced.

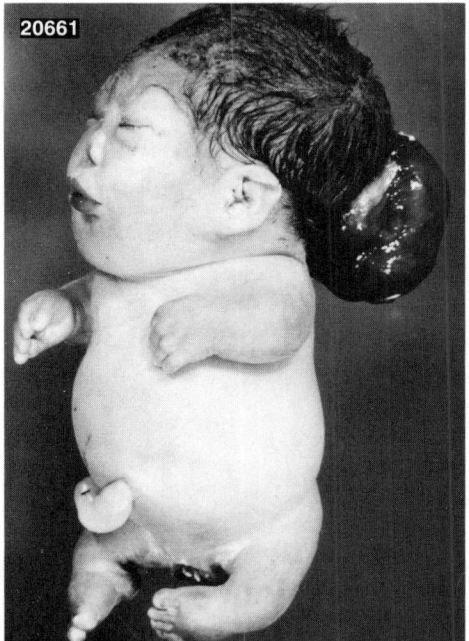

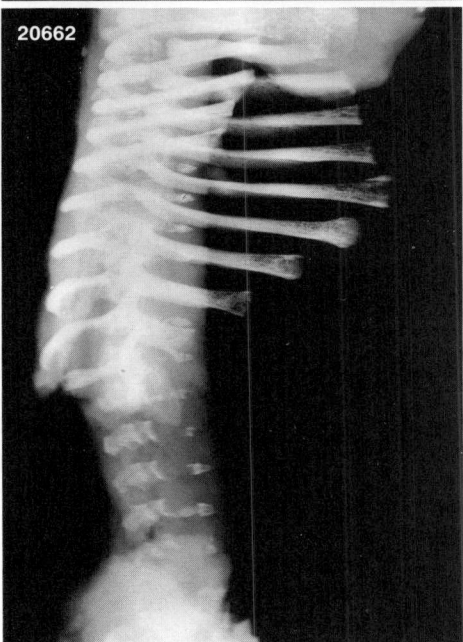

**2935A-20661:** Dwarfism, dyssegmental dysplasia, Silvermann-Handmaker type; note this 33-week-old stillborn girl with small chest, short limbs and encephalocele. **20662:** Note anisospondyly of the spine on lateral view.

---

A lumbosacral kyphosis is often observed. The predominant features on X-ray are the changes affecting the vertebral column, which is shortened in overall length and reveals, in addition to pronounced segmentation defects of the vertebral bodies (anisospondyly), vertebral arch anomalies. The iliac bones are small and rounded, with irregular borders. The greatly shortened long bones reveal irregularly structured epiphyses with unsharply delimited mineralization zones and widened metaphyses. In the middle of the shaft there is a camptomelic-like angulation of

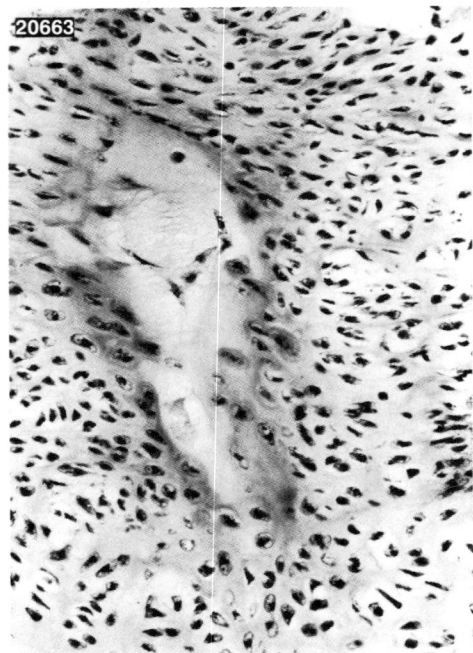

**2935B**-20663: Note highly cellular resting cartilage with foci of mucoid transformation (PAS × 200).

varying degree. The radius and fibula are noticeably shortened compared with the ulna and tibia. The short tubular bones are thickened and widened and show epiphyseal and metaphyseal defects. The scapulae are small and have irregular borders. There is a disproportion between the hypoplastic joint surface and the

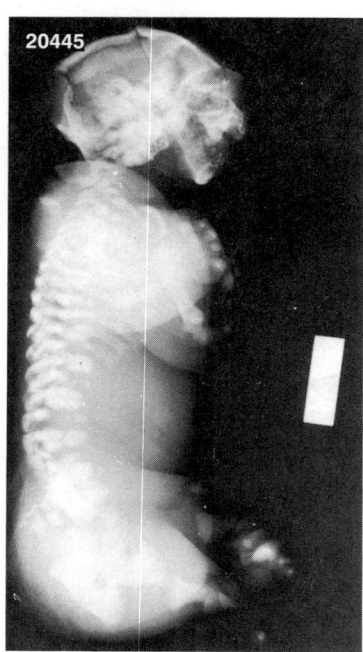

**2935C**-20445: X-ray shows severe segmentation defects of the spine.

humerus. In about one-third of the cases such additional anomalies as encephalocele, cleft palate, urologic defects, and hirsutism are present. Histomorphologically the cartilage is highly cellular. The resting cartilage reveals mucoid degeneration with circumscribed reduction of chondrocytes and focal, highly fibrous canaliculi. Typical differentiation with formation of a proliferation zone and columnization does not occur. Enchondral ossification is completely disordered.

**Complications:** All affected individuals have died within the first 48 hours of life, death being due to respiratory failure, resulting from the too narrow thorax with its short, almost perpendicular ribs.

**Associated Findings:** Further supplementary diagnostic features that vary in frequency are **Cleft palate**, occipital ossification defects or occipital meningoencephaloceles with displacement of brain tissue, hernias, hydronephrosis, hydroureter, cardiac lesions, hirsutism, talipes, or hydramnion.

**Etiology:** Probably autosomal recessive inheritance.

**Pathogenesis:** Pathomorphologically, in addition to segmentation defects of the spine, there is enchondral growth disturbance with combined structural and probably also functional-biochemical defects of cartilage and bone tissue. Histomorphologic findings and the sparse biochemical data point to a generalized disturbance of connective tissue metabolism.

**MIM No.:** 22441

**POS No.:** 4281

**Sex Ratio:** M1:F1

**Occurrence:** Seventeen cases have been reported in the literature. Hispanics are heavily represented. Only a few cases have been reported from Central Europe.

**Risk of Recurrence for Patient's Sib:**
See Part I, *Mendelian Inheritance.*

**Risk of Recurrence for Patient's Child:**
See Part I, *Mendelian Inheritance.* Affected individuals are not expected to survive to reproduce.

**Age of Detectability:** At birth. With a relevant family history and selective examination with ultrasound, intrauterine diagnosis may be possible.

**Gene Mapping and Linkage:** Unknown.

**Prevention:** None known. Genetic counseling indicated.

**Treatment:** Unknown.

**Prognosis:** Patients are not viable. They are either stillborn, die during delivery, or within 48 hours of birth.

**Detection of Carrier:** Unknown.

**References:**
Silvermann FN: Forms of dysostotic dwarfism of uncertain classification. Ann Radiol 1969; 995–1005.
Handmaker SD, et al.: Dyssegmental dwarfism: a new syndrome of lethal dwarfism. BD:OAS XIII(3D). New York: March of Dimes Birth Defects Foundation, 1977:79–90.
Fasanelli S, et al.: Dyssegmental dysplasia. Skeletal Radiol 1985; 14:173–177.
Stoess HR: Dyssegmentale Dysplasie: Fallbeschreibung und Literaturübersicht. Pathologe 1985; 6:88–95.
Kim HJ, et al.: Prenatal diagnosis of dyssegmental dwarfism. Prenatal Diag 1986; 143–150.
Aleck KA, et al.: Dyssegmental dysplasias: clinical, radiographic, and morphologic evidence of heterogeneity. Am J Med Genet 1987; 27:295–312.

ST054
AL006

**Hartmut R. Stoess**
**Kirk Aleck**

**Dwarfism, hyperostotic, Lenz-Majewski type**
*See CRANIODIAPHYSEAL DYSPLASIA, LENZ-MAJEWSKI TYPE*

## DWARFISM, LARON                    0302

**Includes:**
    Growth hormone receptor deficiency, suspected
    Human growth hormone, dwarfism with high plasma
        immunoreactive
    Laron pituitary dwarfism
    Pituitary dwarfism II

**Excludes:**
    **Dwarfism, osteodysplastic primordial, Majewski-Ranke type**
        (2582)
    **Dwarfism, osteodysplastic primordial, Majewski-Winter type**
        (2581)
    **Dwarfism, panhypopituitary** (0303)
    **Growth hormone deficiency, isolated** (0447)
    Panhypopituitarism
    Proportionate short stature, other causes of
    **Seckel syndrome** (0881)

**Major Diagnostic Criteria:**    Proportionate dwarfism with elevated basal plasma human growth hormone (hGH); low plasma somatomedin activity; and absent response to exogenous hGH administration.

**Clinical Findings:**    Proportionate short stature with growth retardation commencing in early infancy. Normal birthweight and slightly decreased birth length. With growth retardation there are accompanying delays in bone maturation and dental eruption; sexual maturation also is delayed but eventually complete. There may be early delays in motor development. Intelligence is usually normal, though average IQ may be reduced.

Physically, patients resemble each other closely. Craniofacial disproportion due to maxillary and mandibular hypoplasia results in large-appearing head, saddle nose, and "sign of the sunset"

eyes. Hair growth may be slow and the hair sparse; the teeth may be discolored and brittle. Hands and feet are relatively small, as apparently are the male genitalia. The truncal obesity and high-pitched voice characteristic of pituitary dwarfs are present. Physically patients cannot be differentiated from those with isolated hGH deficiency, but they are significantly shorter on the average.

Metabolically, affected individuals they are characterized by an elevation of basal immunoreactive hGH levels. However, as in normal individuals, hGH levels are variable and multiple blood samples may have to be analyzed to document elevation. Plasma hGH concentrations rise further in response to provocative stimuli, but fail to be suppressed normally with hyperglycemia. Serum somatomedin levels are low and there is no response to exogenous hGH. Also, there is no sustained response in linear growth with administration of exogenous hGH. Other metabolic parameters show little or no response to hGH administration though variability has been noted. Abnormal glucose metabolism is present, with hypersensitivity to insulin, insulinopenia and spontaneous hypoglycemia during infancy and childhood.

**Complications:**    Spontaneous hypoglycemia of infancy and childhood.

**Associated Findings:**    None known.

**Etiology:**    Autosomal recessive inheritance.

**Pathogenesis:**    There may be two forms: one with deficient or defective growth hormone receptors, and one with a defect in the structural gene for somatomedin C. Daughaday and Trivedi (1987) found that the serum growth hormone binding protein is absent in Laron dwarfism, suggesting a close relationship between the cellular receptor and the serum binding protein.

**MIM No.:**    *26250

**POS No.:**    3207

**Sex Ratio:**    M1:F1

**Occurrence:**    Originally described in oriental Jews, but affected individuals in other ethnic groups have been described. At least several dozen cases have been documented.

**Risk of Recurrence for Patient's Sib:**
    See Part I, *Mendelian Inheritance.*

**Risk of Recurrence for Patient's Child:**
    See Part I, *Mendelian Inheritance.*

**Age of Detectability:**    Clinically in early infancy with appearance of growth retardation or hypoglycemia. May be detectable at birth by hGH measurement. However, hGH levels are elvated normally during the first 2–4 weeks of life.

**Gene Mapping and Linkage:**    Unknown.

**Prevention:**    None known. Genetic counseling indicated.

**Treatment:**    No effective treatment available for short stature.

**Prognosis:**    Good for general health; marked dwarfism a certainty.

**Detection of Carrier:**    Unknown.

**References:**
Rabinowitz D, Merimee TJ: Isolated human growth hormone deficiency and related disorders. Isr J Med Sci 1973 9:1601.
Laron Z, et al.: Syndrome of familial dwarfism and high plasma immunoreactive growth hormone. Isr J Med Sci 1974; 10:1247–1254.
Golde DW, et al.: Peripheral unresponsiveness to human growth hormone in Laron dwarfism. New Engl J Med 1980; 303:1156–1159.
Daughaday WH, Trivedi B: Absence of serum growth hormone binding protein in patients with growth hormone receptor deficiency (Laron dwarfism). Proc Nat Acad Sci 1987; 84:4636–4640.
Geffner ME, et al.: Tissues of the Laron dwarf are sensitive to insulin-like growth factor I but not to growth hormone. J Clin Endocr Metab 1987; 64:1042–1046.

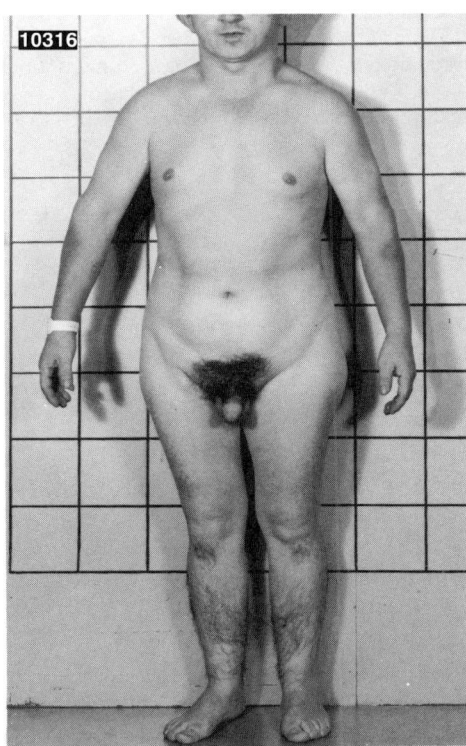

**0302-10316:**    Proportionate short stature with high basal levels of hGH, low sulfation factor activity, and peripheral insensitivity to hGH.

B0025

**Zvi Borochowitz**
*David L. Rimoin*

## DWARFISM, LETHAL, SHORT-LIMBED PLATYSPONDYLIC TYPE     2766

**Includes:** Vertebral body hypoplasia-lethal short-limbed dwarfism

**Excludes:**
    **Achondrogenesis**
    **Thanatophoric dysplasia**

**Major Diagnostic Criteria:** Severe neonatal short-limbed skeletal dysplasia with "wafer-thin" vertebral bodies and tubular long bones.

**Clinical Findings:** Horton et al (1979) described a distinct form of lethal short-limbed dwarfism previously classified under the rubric of "variant thanatophoric dysplasia." The phenotype resembles thanatophoric dysplasia. The head is large, the chest small, and the abdomen protuberant. Extreme shortening of the limbs causes truncal length to appear normal, although truncal length is actually decreased for gestational age. All patients have died of pulmonary hypoplasia during the newborn period. Initially two subtypes, the Torrance and San Diego types, were described based on histologic parameters, but the limited number of cases makes the existence of subtypes uncertain.

On X-ray these infants show decreased ossification of the basicranium, uniformly thin vertebral bodies, which appear "wafer-like" or discoid on lateral projection, short thin ribs, and tubular long bones with enlarged and cupped metaphyses. The proximal tibiae are not hypoplastic, and the fibulae are not widened, as in **Thanatophoric dysplasia**.

**Complications:** Pulmonary hypoplasia is lethal during the neonatal period.

**Associated Findings:** None known.

**Etiology:** Presumably an inherited condition of undetermined etiology.

**Pathogenesis:** An error in endochondral ossification. Histologically, resting cartilage from epiphyseal or apophyseal sites shows enlarged chondrocytes with an abundant clear cytoplasm, giving a "ballooned" appearance to the cells. The growth plate changes included poor column formation in some sections to relatively normal column formation with excessive retention of cartilage anlage in the metaphyseal bone.

**Sex Ratio:** Presumably M1:F1

**Occurrence:** Undetermined but presumed rare.

**Risk of Recurrence for Patient's Sib:**
    See Part I, *Mendelian Inheritance.*

**Risk of Recurrence for Patient's Child:**
    See Part I, *Mendelian Inheritance.*

**Age of Detectability:** Prenatally, probably during the second trimester.

**Gene Mapping and Linkage:** Unknown.

**Prevention:** None known. Genetic counseling indicated.

**Treatment:** Unknown.

**Prognosis:** All cases have been lethal in the neonatal period.

**Detection of Carrier:** Unknown.

**References:**
Horton WA, et al.: Further heterogeneity within lethal neonatal short-limbed dwarfism: the platyspondylic types. J Pediatr 1979; 94:736–742.

H0025
H0033
                                **O.J. Hood**
                      **William A. Horton**

**Dwarfism, mesomelic Robinow type**
    *See ROBINOW SYNDROME*
**Dwarfism, metatropic, type II**
    *See KNIEST DYSPLASIA*

## DWARFISM, MICROCEPHALIC PRIMORDIAL WITH CATARACTS     2584

**Includes:** Osteodysplastic primordial dwarfism, type IV

**Excludes:**
    **Dwarfism, osteodysplastic primordial, Majewski-Ranke type (2582)**
    **Dwarfism, osteodysplastic primordial, Majewski-Winter type (2581)**
    **Seckel syndrome (0881)**

**Major Diagnostic Criteria:** The combination of intrauterine growth retardation, **Microcephaly**, and cataracts.

**Clinical Findings:** Growth failure of prenatal onset, **Microcephaly**, downslanting palpebral fissures, enamel hypoplasia, short hands and feet, and clinodactyly. Frequent respiratory infections were common during infancy, and decreased levels of IgG was were demonstrated in both of the known cases. Cataracts developed before the age of four years. X-ray findings included marked delay of ossification (bone age at four years was interpreted as being consistent with age five months) and brachymesophalangy. Mental retardation was present in the two reported patients.

**Complications:** The susceptibility to respiratory infections is likely secondary to a mild immune deficiency.

**Associated Findings:** None known.

**Etiology:** The presence of the condition in sibs suggests autosomal recessive inheritance.

**Pathogenesis:** Unknown. Histologic exam of bone and cartilage demonstrated hypertrophic chondrocytes and fibrous-appearing matrix.

**POS No.:** 4187

**Sex Ratio:** M0:F2 (observed).

**Occurrence:** Two cases have been reported.

**Risk of Recurrence for Patient's Sib:**
    See Part I, *Mendelian Inheritance.*

**Risk of Recurrence for Patient's Child:**
    See Part I, *Mendelian Inheritance.*

**Age of Detectability:** At birth, although prenatal ultrasound may detect intrauterine growth failure.

**Gene Mapping and Linkage:** Unknown.

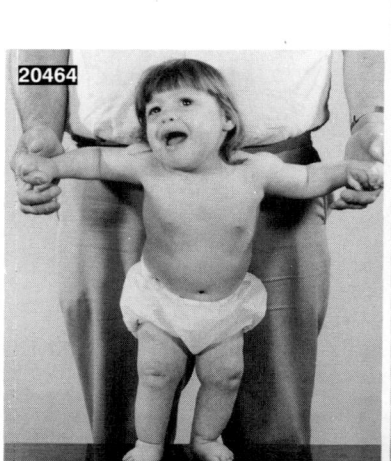
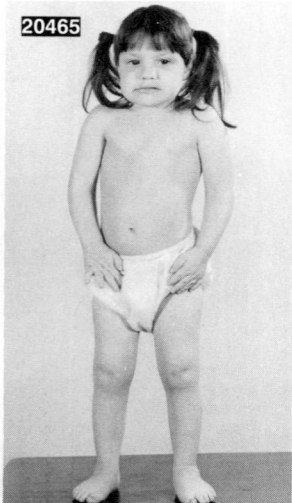

**2584-20464–65:** Two sisters; note microcephaly, downslanted palpebral fissures, proportionate short stature and small hands and feet.

**Prevention:**  None known. Genetic counseling indicated.

**Treatment:**  Supportive.

**Prognosis:**  Mental retardation is moderate to severe, life span is unknown, although one child died of pneumonia at age 5 1/2 years.

**Detection of Carrier:**  Unknown.

**References:**
Toriello HV, et al.: An apparently new syndrome of microcephalic primordial dwarfism and cataracts. Am J Med Genet 1986; 25:1–8. †

T0007                                      **Helga V. Toriello**

**Dwarfism, microcephalic-taurodontism-short rooted teeth**
*See TAURODONTISM-SHORT ROOTED TEETH-MICROCEPHALIC DWARFISM*

## DWARFISM, MULIBREY TYPE              2081

**Includes:**
> Dwarfism-pericarditis
> Mulibrey nanism
> Pericardial constriction-growth failure

**Excludes:**  Silver syndrome (0887)

**Major Diagnostic Criteria:**  Short stature (>2 SD for bone age and sex), and two of the following four features: symptoms of pericardial constriction, yellow pigment in ocular fundi, fibrous dysplasia of the long bones, and J-shaped sella turcica.

**Clinical Findings:**  Thirty cases with this condition have been described. The average birth weight is 2.58 kg and birth length is 45.6 cm, both less than the tenth percentile. The other major findings, found in 50–100% of affected individuals, are short stature (97%); hypotonia (70%); triangular face with prominent forehead (100%); hypoplasia of choriocapillaris or yellow pigment in fundi (90%); small tongue (62%); highly pitched voice (90%); prominent veins on the head and neck (83%); elevated venous pressure (77%); liver enlargement (100%); cutaneous capillary hemangiomata, particularly on the limbs (60%); delayed onset of puberty in females (100%); proven pericardial constriction (33%); and fibrous dysplasia of the tibia (27%).

Dental findings have included dental crowding and hypodontia of the second bicuspid. Other X-ray findings have included missing or small frontal, maxillary, and/or sphenoidal sinuses; long, shallow sella turcica; horizontal nuchal plane; frontal bossing; vertical nasal bone; and delayed bone age (although two affected individuals were considered to have advanced bone ages). Abnormal EKGs and large cerebral ventricles and cisterna are also common.

**Complications:**  Fractures and pseudarthrosis secondary to tibial fibrous dysplasia, limited physical capacity, increased susceptibility to respiratory infections, ascites, edema or pulmonary congestion, and cardiac failure secondary to the pericardial constriction.

**Associated Findings:**  One affected individual each had facial asymmetry with deafness on the affected side, and **Cancer, Wilms tumor.**

**Etiology:**  Autosomal recessive inheritance.

**Pathogenesis:**  The tissues involved are predominantly of mesodermal origin; there is characteristic replacement with collagenous connective tissue and scar formation. However, biochemical, physiologic, or histologic studies have not demonstrated the primary defect.

**MIM No.:**  *25325

**POS No.:**  3328

**Sex Ratio:**  M1:F1

**Occurrence:**  More than 30 cases have been reported; most of Finnish ethnic origin.

**Risk of Recurrence for Patient's Sib:**
See Part I, *Mendelian Inheritance.*

**Risk of Recurrence for Patient's Child:**
See Part I, *Mendelian Inheritance.*

**Age of Detectability:**  At birth, by physical exam.

**Gene Mapping and Linkage:**  Unknown.

**Prevention:**  None known. Genetic counseling indicated.

**Treatment:**  Pericardiectomy to relieve the pericardial constriction, treatment with diuretics to prevent and/or alleviate ascites and hepatic congestion.

**Prognosis:**  Intelligence is usually not impaired. Onset of cardiac symptoms is variable, and can range from birth to late teens. The oldest patient was 24 years of age at the time of the report.

**Detection of Carrier:**  Unknown.

**References:**
Perheentupa J, et al: Mulibrey nanism: review of 23 cases of a new autosomal recessive syndrome. BD:OAS XI(2). New York: March of Dimes Birth Defects Foundation, 1975:3–17. * †
Cumming GR, et al: Constrictive pericarditis with dwarfism in two siblings (mulibrey nanism). J Pediatr 1976; 88:569–572. *
Voorhess M, et al: Growth failure with pericardial constriction. Am J Dis Child 1976; 130:1146–1148.
Myllarniemi S, et al: Craniofacial and dental study of mulibrey nanism. Cleft Palate J 1978;369–377.
Simila S, et al: A case of mulibrey nanism with associated Wilms' tumor. Clin Genet 1980; 17:29–30.

T0007                                      **Helga V. Toriello**

## DWARFISM, OCULO-PALATO-CEREBRAL TYPE      2808

**Includes:**
> Oculo-palatal-cerebral dwarfism
> Persistent hypertrophic primary vitreous in OPC dwarfism

**Excludes:**
> Arthro-ophthalmopathy, hereditary, progressive, Stickler type (0090)
> Norrie disease (0721)
> Retina, hyaloideoretinal degeneration of Wagner (0479)

**Major Diagnostic Criteria:**  Persistent hypertrophic primary vitreous with or without secondary ocular changes, **Microcephaly** with mental retardation, spastic quadriplegia, midline **Cleft palate**, connective tissue abnormality, and disproportionate short stature.

**Clinical Findings:**  There is considerable variability in clinical presentation. The ocular findings are present at birth and range from unilateral persistent hypertrophic primary vitreous without secondary changes to bilateral involvement with secondary glaucoma, cataracts, leukoma adherans, and eventual bulbar atrophy. Central nervous system involvement ranges from borderline intelligence to severe mental retardation and from increased muscle tone of the lower extremities, to quadriplegia. A variable degree of **Microcephaly** was observed and brain atrophy was documented in one patient. The neurologic examination is abnormal at birth.

A midline cleft of the soft palate was present in all patients. All patients had soft skin and the veins were visible. Joint hypermobility was present, and one patient had moderate kyphoscoliosis. The two known males were cryptorchid. The known female patient went through normal puberty.

Stature was 2.5 to 4.0 SD below the mean. The limbs were relatively short, but there were no signs of skeletal dysplasia. The hands and feet were small.

**Complications:**  Ocular changes may progress to bulbar atrophy. Contractures may develop. Kyphoscoliosis and otitis media secondary to **Cleft palate** may be factors in lower respiratory infections.

**Associated Findings:**  The three affected sibs had severe steroid-dependent asthma. No other cases of atopy are known in the family. Neonatal hypotonia, large pointed ears, deafness, and **Hernia, umbilical,** have also been noted.

**Etiology:**  Probably autosomal recessive inheritance. The parents are first cousins once removed, the patients are of both sexes, and

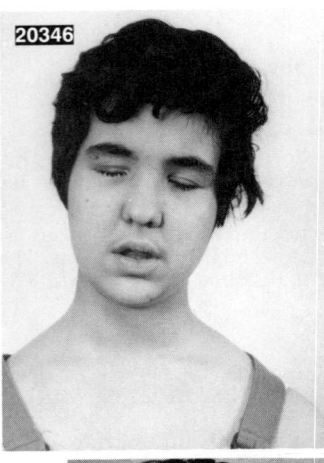
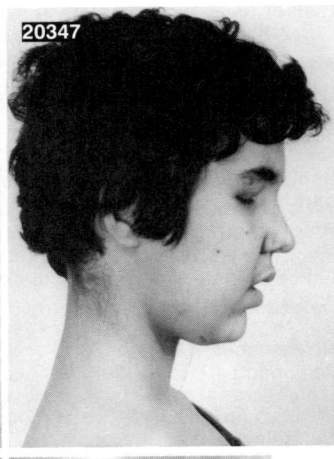
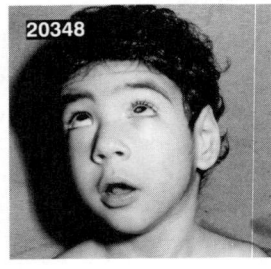
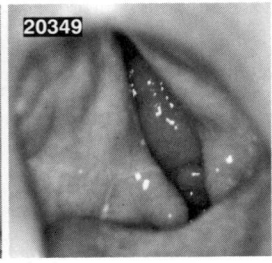

**2808-20346–47:** Dwarfism, oculo-palatal-cerebral type; slender neck and sloping shoulders on frontal and lateral views. **20348:** Retrolental opacity and pointed ear. **20349:** Midline cleft palate.

the parents are normal. Nevertheless, in view of the clinical variability and the milder manifestations in the female patient, X-linked transmission remains a possibility.

**Pathogenesis:** A neuro-mesodermal dysgenesis has been postulated.

**MIM No.:** 25791

**POS No.:** 3993

**Sex Ratio:** M2:F1 (observed).

**Occurrence:** One family of Moroccan Jewish origin was reported with three affected sibs.

**Risk of Recurrence for Patient's Sib:**
See Part I, *Mendelian Inheritance.*

**Risk of Recurrence for Patient's Child:**
See Part I, *Mendelian Inheritance.*

**Age of Detectability:** At birth. All patients had low birth weight, cleft palate, and ocular and neurologic manifestations.

**Gene Mapping and Linkage:** Unknown.

**Prevention:** None known. Genetic counseling indicated.

**Treatment:** Early surgical intervention may prevent blindness. Repair of **Cleft palate**. Physical therapy and surgery to prevent contractures. Removal of intra-abdominal testicles.

**Prognosis:** Related to severity of CNS involvement and extent of kyphoscoliosis. Milder cases should have normal life span.

**Detection of Carrier:** Unknown.

**Special Considerations:** In view of the considerable variability in the clinical manifestations, cases may exist without the typical ocular or neurologic manifestations. Cases of familial **Microcephaly** and **Cleft palate** with and without short stature are well documented, and some may be further examples of this syndrome in whom the expression is incomplete.

The association of severe asthma with this syndrome may be coincidental, but if the view that asthma is autosomal recessive is accepted then the association may be significant.

**References:**
Frydman M, et al.: Oculo-palato-cerebral dwarfism: a new syndrome. Clin Genet 1985; 27:414–419.

FR034                                                        **Moshe Frydman**

**Dwarfism, omodysplasia**
*See OMODYSPLASIA*

---

## DWARFISM, OSTEODYSPLASTIC PRIMORDIAL, MAJEWSKI-RANKE TYPE                                  **2582**

**Includes:**
Bird-headed dwarfism, osteodysplastic, type III
Microcephalic primordial dwarfism, type II
Osteodysplastic primordial dwarfism, type II

**Excludes:**
**Dwarfism, microcephalic primordial with cataracts** (2584)
**Dwarfism, osteodysplastic primordial, Majewski-Winter type** (2581)
**Seckel syndrome** (0881)

**Major Diagnostic Criteria:** The combination of intrauterine growth retardation, **Microcephaly**, prominent nose, micrognathia, and characteristic skeletal changes on X-ray.

**Clinical Findings:** Intrauterine growth retardation (average birth weight is less than 2,000 g), relative **Microcephaly** (OFC disproportionate to height), beaked nose, relatively large eyes, micrognathia, dysplastic ears, clinodactyly, and cryptorchidism.

Postnatal growth retardation and mental retardation occurred in all cases. The limbs are described as short during the first years of life, but later appear more proportionate. X-ray findings include epiphyseolysis, pseudepiphysis, triangular epiphyses, metaphyseal flaring, retarded ossification, and a high, narrow pelvis. These osteodysplastic changes improve with age, so skeletal survey during the first year of life may be necessary to confirm the diagnosis.

**Complications:** Unknown.

**Associated Findings:** Occasional findings include upwardslanting or downslanting palpebral fissures, blepharophimosis, enamel hypoplasia, hip dysplasia, and dislocated radial head.

**Etiology:** Unknown. Verloes (1987) reported sibs whose parents were first cousins.

**Pathogenesis:** Unknown.

**MIM No.:** 21072

**POS No.:** 3345

**Sex Ratio:** M1:F4 (observed).

**Occurrence:** Eight cases have been reported, all from Europe.

**Risk of Recurrence for Patient's Sib:** Unknown.

**Risk of Recurrence for Patient's Child:** Unknown.

**Age of Detectability:** At birth, although prenatal ultrasound may detect severe growth retardation.

**Gene Mapping and Linkage:** Unknown.

**Prevention:** None known. Genetic counseling indicated.

**Treatment:** Supportive.

**Prognosis:** Mental retardation is mild to moderate, life span is unknown since all affected cases have been children, although none had any additional health problems.

**Detection of Carrier:** Unknown.

**References:**
Majewski F, et al.: Studies of microcephalic primordial dwarfism: the osteodysplastic type II or primordial dwarfism. Am J Med Genet 1982; 12:23–35. †
Verloes A, et al.: Microcephalic osteodysplastic dwarfism (type II-like) in siblings. Clin Genet 1987; 32:88–94. †
Willems PJ, et al.: A new case of the osteodysplastic primordial dwarfism type II. Am J Med Genet 1987; 26:819–824.

T0007                                      **Helga V. Toriello**

## DWARFISM, OSTEODYSPLASTIC PRIMORDIAL, MAJEWSKI-WINTER TYPE                    2581

**Includes:**
 Bird-headed dwarfism, osteodysplastic, type I
 Bird-headed dwarfism, osteodysplastic, type III
 Brachymelic primordial dwarfism
 Osteodysplastic primordial dwarfism, types I and III

**Excludes:**
 **Alopecia-skeletal anomalies-short stature-mental retardation** (2782)
 **Dwarfism, microcephalic primordial with cataracts** (2584)
 **Dwarfism, osteodysplastic primordial, Majewski-Ranke type** (2582)
 **Seckel syndrome** (0881)

**Major Diagnostic Criteria:** The combination of intrauterine growth retardation, **Microcephaly**, alopecia, characteristic facial appearance, and X-ray changes of the spine, pelvis, and long bones.

**Clinical Findings:** Marked intrauterine growth retardation; **Microcephaly** with premature suture closure; low, receding forehead; prominent occiput at birth; alopecia; hyperkeratotic skin; large eyes; prominent nose; thick lips, micrognathia; low-set ears, short

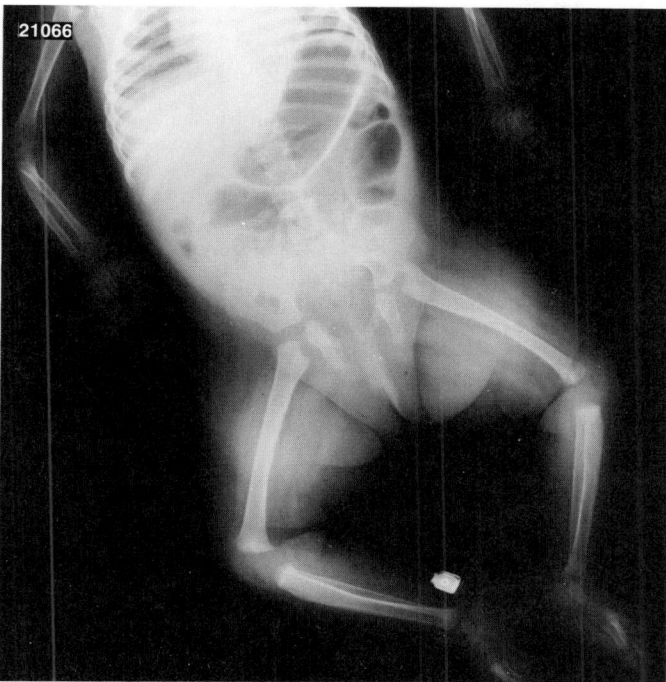

**2581-21066:** Postmortem X-ray at one year showing changes of both types I and III including platyspondyly, small pelvis with horizontal acetabular roofs, enlarged proximal femoral metaphyses, left dislocated hip and poor modeling of long bones.

neck; and large hands and feet with short fingers and clinodactyly of the fifth fingers. X-ray abnormalities include elongated clavicles, platyspondyly, cleft cervical vertebrae, dysplastic pelvis with hypoplastic iliac wings and horizontal acetabular roof, enlarged proximal femoral metaphyses with medial spurs, dislocated elbows and hips, short long bones, and bowed humeri/femora. Some of these changes may be age related; originally Majewski et al (1982) distinguished between types I and III; however, Winter et al (1985) reported a case with X-ray findings of both types, suggesting that they are the same condition. Internal anomalies in autopsied cases have included partial **Corpus callosum agenesis**, small testes, and absent or small ovaries.

**Complications:** Susceptibility to infection.

**Associated Findings:** None known.

**Etiology:** All reported cases have been sporadic.

**Pathogenesis:** Unknown.

**MIM No.:** 21073

**POS No.:** 3387

**Sex Ratio:** M1:F1

**Occurrence:** Four cases have been reported.

**Risk of Recurrence for Patient's Sib:**
 See Part I, *Mendelian Inheritance.*

**Risk of Recurrence for Patient's Child:**
 See Part I, *Mendelian Inheritance.*

**Age of Detectability:** At birth, although prenatal ultrasound may detect growth delay and skeletal changes.

**Gene Mapping and Linkage:** Unknown.

**Prevention:** None known. Genetic counseling indicated.

**Treatment:** Supportive.

**Prognosis:** Mental retardation and early death appear to be the rule; 3/4 died within their first year of age, the fourth case was two months at the time of the report.

**Detection of Carrier:** Unknown.

**References:**
Bass HN, et al.: Case report 33. Syndrome Ident 1975; 3:12–14.
Majewski F, Spranger J: Uber einen neuen Typ des primordiaten Minderwuchses: der brachymele primordiale Minderwuchs. Monatssch Kinderheilkd 1976; 124:499–503.
Majewski F, et al.: Studies of microcephalic primordial dwarfism: an intrauterine dwarf with platyspondyly and anomalies of pelvis and clavicles-osteodysplastic primordial dwarfism type III. Am J Med Genet 1982; 12:37–42.
Winter RM, et al.: Osteodysplastic primordial dwarfism: report of a further patient with manifestations similar to those seen in patients with types I and III. Am J Med Genet 1985; 21:569–574. * †

T0007                                      **Helga V. Toriello**

## DWARFISM, PANHYPOPITUITARY                    0303

**Includes:**
 Asexual ateleotic dwarfism
 Ateliotic dwarfism
 Hanhart dwarfism
 Panhypopituitarism, X-linked
 Pituitary dwarfism III
 Pituitary dwarfism IV

**Excludes:**
 Dwarfism due to biologically inactive hGH
 **Dwarfism, pituitary with abnormal sella turcica** (0304)
 **Dwarfism** (other)
 **Growth hormone deficiency, isolated** (0447)
 Pituitary, congenital absence of

**Major Diagnostic Criteria:** Proportionate dwarfism becoming evident at about age six months and characterized by consistently decreased human growth hormone (hGH) response to recognized stimuli such as clonidine, L-dopa, arginine, or insulin-induced

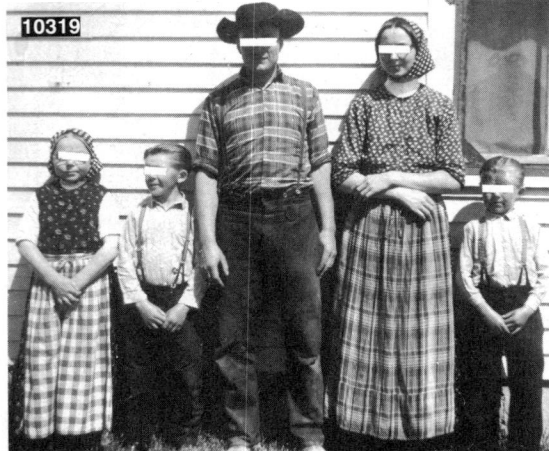

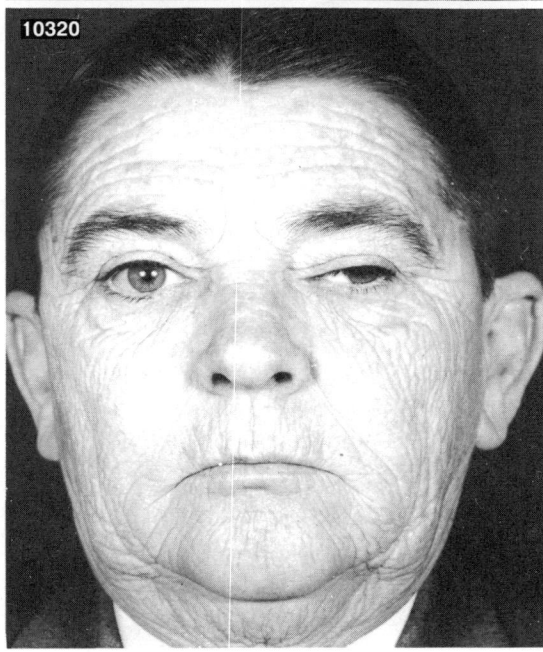

**0303**-10319: Familial panhypopituitarism in a Hutterite sibship. Left to right: affected female age 31, affected male age 27, normal brother age 25, normal sister, age 24 and affected male age 20. 10320: Marked wrinkling of the face and congenital ptosis in a 53-year-old male.

hypoglycemia together with evidence of at least one other tropic hormone deficiency: gonadotropins, adrenocorticotropic hormone (ACTH) or thyroid-stimulating hormone (TSH).

**Clinical Findings:** A deficiency of human growth hormone (hGH) and at least one other pituitary hormone including gonadotropins followed in order of frequency by adrenocorticotropic hormone (ACTH) and thyroid stimulating hormone (TSH) occur in panhypopituitary dwarfism. However, the particular pattern may vary among families and even among affected members of the same family. The clinical findings depend on which pituitary hormone deficiencies are present. The hGH deficiency results in dwarfism; excess subcutaneous adipose tissue, a high-pitched peculiar voice, soft wrinkled skin, and childlike facies. The growth retardation is not usually evident prior to six months of age, and is proportionate although adults retain childlike proportions, ie

relatively long trunk and short legs. The deficiency is associated with a marked delay in skeletal bone age. Metabolically, the lack of hGH leads to glucose intolerance, decreased lipolysis, a relative insulinopenia, and diminished serum somatomedin levels. Gonadotropin deficiency results in complete lack of secondary sexual characteristics. Females demonstrate primary amenorrhea; and males, small testes and phallus. When present, ACTH deficiency may contribute to severe hypoglycemic attacks in infancy and childhood. TSH deficiency usually does not result in severe hypothyroidism but may occasionally produce definite signs, including slow reflexes, hypometabolism, and epiphyseal dysplasia.

Since patients with isolated growth hormone deficiency usually have delayed puberty, it may be difficult to differentiate panhypopituitary from isolated growth hormone deficient patients in late adolescence. Treatment with growth hormone often stimulates spontaneous puberty in isolated growth hormone deficient patients and may help in this distinction.

**Complications:** Related to particular hormone deficiencies present. In addition, psychological problems arise as a result of small stature.

**Associated Findings:** None known.

**Etiology:** Most cases occur sporadically, and the majority are probably not genetic. However, both autosomal recessive and X-linked recessive inheritance have been described; and all three forms are clinically and metabolically indistinguishable.

**Pathogenesis:** In most cases a hypothalamic defect is likely, since, in these cases, the pituitary responds to synthetic hypothalamic-releasing factors. In the remainder, a structural, degenerative, or secretory defect of the pituitary is postulated.

**MIM No.:** *26260, *31200

**POS No.:** 3101

**Sex Ratio:** M1:F1 in sporadic and autosomal recessive forms. Only males affected in X-linked recessive form.

**Occurrence:** About ten thousand cases in the United States.

**Risk of Recurrence for Patient's Sib:**
See Part I, *Mendelian Inheritance*. In a sporadic nongenetic case, and the risk of recurrence is negligible.

**Risk of Recurrence for Patient's Child:**
See Part I, *Mendelian Inheritance*. Fertility is rare due to gonadotropin deficiency.

**Age of Detectability:** Growth retardation is usually not apparent before 6 months of age, but if suspected, hGH and other hormone deficiencies can be identified at birth.

**Gene Mapping and Linkage:** PHP (panhypopituitarism) has been provisionally mapped to X.

**Prevention:** None known. Genetic counseling indicated.

**Treatment:** Replacement with hGH and other secondarily deficient hormones, i.e. thyroxine, cortisone, estrogens, testosterone. In some cases it may be possible to induce fertility by appropriate gonadotropin therapy.

**Prognosis:** Depends on adequacy of treatment. Relatively normal stature and correction of hormonal deficiency states may result from early diagnosis and appropriate treatment.

**Detection of Carrier:** Unknown.

**References:**
Rosenfield RL, et al.: Idiopathic anterior hypopituitarism in one of monozygotic twins. J Pediatr 1967; 70:115–117.
Rimoin DL, Schimke RN: Genetic disorders of the endocrine glands. St. Louis: CV Mosby, 1971:11–65.
Rimoin DL: Hereditary forms of growth hormone deficiency and resistance. In: Bergsma D, ed: Growth problems and clinical advances. BD:OAS, vol. XII, no 6. New York: Alan R. Liss, Inc. for The National Foundation-March of Dimes, 1976:15–29.
McArthur RG, et al.: The natural history of familial hypopituitarism. Am J Med Genet 1985; 22:553–566.

H0033
H0025
**William A. Horton**
**O.J. Hood**

**Dwarfism, pituitary**
*See GROWTH HORMONE DEFICIENCY, ISOLATED*

## DWARFISM, PITUITARY WITH ABNORMAL SELLA TURCICA                                                    0304

**Includes:**
Pituitary dwarfism-sella turcica defect
Sella turcica defect-pituitary dwarfism

**Excludes:**
**Dwarfism, Laron** (0302)
**Dwarfism, panhypopituitary** (0303)
**Growth hormone deficiency, isolated** (0447)
Pituitary, congenital absence of the

**Major Diagnostic Criteria:**  Characteristically abnormal sella turcica on X-ray associated with evidence of pituitary insufficiency.

**Clinical Findings:**  Two sets of sibs have been reported with severe growth failure, spontaneous hypoglycemia, and laboratory evidence of human growth hormone (hGH), adrenocorticotropic hormone (ACTH) and thyroid-stimulating hormone (TSH) deficiencies. Skull X-rays show a small sella turcica. Hypoglycemia can be severe during infancy and may result in mental retardation if the child survives. Gonadotropin deficiency may also be part of this syndrome.

**Complications:**  Related to hormone deficiencies.

**Associated Findings:**  None known.

**Etiology:**  Probable autosomal recessive inheritance.

**Pathogenesis:**  Presumably a defect in the hypothalamic-pituitary axis.

**MIM No.:**  26270

**Sex Ratio:**  Presumably M1:F1

**Occurrence:**  Rare. About three families reported.

**Risk of Recurrence for Patient's Sib:**
See Part I, *Mendelian Inheritance.*

**Risk of Recurrence for Patient's Child:**
See Part I, *Mendelian Inheritance.*

**Age of Detectability:**  At birth, if suspected, but growth failure is not usually apparent before six months of age.

**Gene Mapping and Linkage:**  Unknown.

**Prevention:**  None known. Genetic counseling indicated.

**Treatment:**  Replacement of hGH and secondarily deficient hormones, i.e. thyroxine, cortisone, and estrogen or androgen when needed.

**Prognosis:**  Unknown.

**Detection of Carrier:**  Unknown.

**Special Considerations:**  Lateral X-rays of the skull are recommended in all questionable cases of pituitary dwarfism.

**References:**
Ferrier PE, Stone EF: Familial pituitary dwarfism associated with an abnormal sella turcica. Pediatrics 1969; 43:858–865.
Rimoin DL, Schimke RN: Genetic disorders of the endocrine glands. St. Louis: CV Mosby, 1971:11–65.
Sipponen P, et al.: Familial syndrome with panhypopituitarism, hypoplasia of the hypophysis and a poorly developed sella turcica. Arch Dis Child 1978; 53:664–667.

H0033
H0025

**William A. Horton**
**O.J. Hood**

**Dwarfism, Seckel type**
*See SECKEL SYNDROME*

## DWARFISM, SHORT-RIB, BEEMER TYPE                              2818

**Includes:**
Short-rib syndrome, Beemer type
Skeletal dysplasia, short rib dwarfism, Beemer type

**Excludes:**
**Asphyxiating thoracic dysplasia** (0091)
**Short rib-polydactyly syndrome, type I** (0884)
**Short rib-polydactyly syndrome, type II** (0883)

**Major Diagnostic Criteria:**  Short ribs and short limbs are apparent clinically in the absence of **Polydactyly**. There are no kidney abnormalities, and genital abnormalities may be present (1/4). X-ray metaphyses are normal and there are no disproportionate, short tibiae.

**Clinical Findings:**  Clinical signs are manifest at birth. Affected children are stillborn or die very short after birth. They are hydropic and have a short stature (38.5–40 cm), short ribs, and short limbs with lung hypoplasia. Most of them have a median **Cleft lip** and **Cleft palate**; cleft lip alone is possible also. A complicated heart malformation may be present. **Omphalocele** is present; no kidney abnormalities are found. Abnormalities of the external genitalia may also be present.

On X-ray the ribs are very short, as are the tubular bones. Disproportionate, short tibiae are absent. Pelvic bones are normal. There is platyspondyly. Metaphyses are normal, and there is no premature ossification of the epiphyses.

On autopsy the epiphyseal growth zone shows disorganization of the proliferative and hypertrophic cartillage. The formation of trabecular bone is grossly abnormal with broad bony spicules. There are no intracytoplasmic inclusions in the chondrocytes.

**Complications:**  All have been stillborn or have died immediately after birth due to lung hypoplasia.

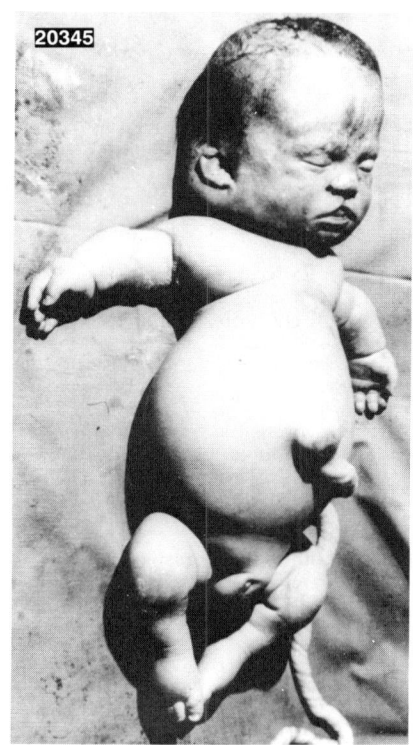

2818-20345:  Note short ribs with protuberant abdomen, median cleft lip and the absence of polydactyly.

**Associated Findings:** Intestinal malrotation (2/4); polymicrogyria and internal **Hydrocephaly** (1/4); and arrhinencephaly, epiglottis and larynx hypoplastic (one case).

**Etiology:** Probably autosomal recessive inheritance.

**Pathogenesis:** Unknown.

**MIM No.:** 26986

**POS No.:** 3586

**Sex Ratio:** M2:F2 (observed).

**Occurrence:** Four cases have been documented in the literature: two sib cases, one single case from The Netherlands (unrelated), and one case from the United States. Two unpublished sibling cases have also been seen in the Netherlands.

**Risk of Recurrence for Patient's Sib:**
See Part I, *Mendelian Inheritance.*

**Risk of Recurrence for Patient's Child:**
See Part I, *Mendelian Inheritance.* Affected individuals are not expected to survive to reproduce.

**Age of Detectability:** During pregnancy by ultrasound at about the 18th to 20th week. Clinically evident immediately after birth.

**Gene Mapping and Linkage:** Unknown.

**Prevention:** None known. Genetic counseling indicated.

**Treatment:** Unknown.

**Prognosis:** Affected individuals have been stillborn or have died immediately after birth.

**Detection of Carrier:** Unknown.

**Special Considerations:** Heterogeneity may exist. There are reports of children with very similar clinical findings but with **Polydactyly**. Patients have also been described who have almost identical clinical findings without polydactyly but with renal abnormalities. There are clear-cut clinical and X-ray differences between **Short rib-polydactyly syndrome** and asphyxiating thoracic dystrophy.

**References:**
Wladimiroff JW, et al.: Early diagnosis of skeletal dysplasia by real-time ultrasound. Lancet 1981; I:661–662.
Beemer FA, et al.: A new short rib syndrome: report of two cases. Am J Med Genet 1983; 14:115–123. *
Passarge E: Letter to the editor: familial occurrence of a short rib syndrome with hydrops fetalis but without polydactyly. Am J Med Genet 1983; 14:403–405.
Yang SS, et al.: Three conditions in neonatal asphyxiating thoracic dysplasia (Jeune) and short rib polydactyly syndrome spectrum: a clinicopathologic study. Am J Med Genet 1987; (Suppl 3:191–209)

BE006                                        **Frits A. Beemer**

**Dwarfism, short-trunk with retarded ossification**
*See SPONDYLOEPIPHYSEAL DYSPLASIA CONGENITA*
**Dwarfism, Silver-Russell type**
*See SILVER SYNDROME*
**Dwarfism, six-fingered**
*See CHONDROECTODERMAL DYSPLASIA*
**Dwarfism, Thanatophoric**
*See THANATOPHORIC DYSPLASIA*
**Dwarfism-congenital medullary stenosis**
*See TUBULAR STENOSIS*
**Dwarfism-cortical thickening of tubular bones**
*See TUBULAR STENOSIS*

## DWARFISM-DYSMORPHIC FACIES-RETARDATION, PITT TYPE                                          2814

**Includes:**
> Face, unusual-mental retardation-intrauterine growth retardation
> Growth retardation, intrauterine-mental retardation-unusual facies
> Mental retardation-unusual facies-intrauterine growth retardation
> Pitt syndrome
> Pitt-Rogers-Danks syndrome

**Excludes:** Dwarfism, intrauterine, other

**Major Diagnostic Criteria:** Intrauterine and postnatal growth retardation; moderate-to-severe mental retardation; characteristic facies with prominent eyes, telecanthus, beaked nose, short and featureless philtrum, flat maxilla, and large mouth.

**Clinical Findings:** Affected children were small at birth (<10th percentile for weight and length), and grew slowly (height <third percentile). The head was proportionately small, and there was moderate-to-severe developmental delay without neurologic regression. Four of the five reported patients developed seizures, and their behavior was described as hyperactive, with two displaying head nodding.

The facies were striking, with prominent eyes, telecanthus, upward (3/5) or downward (2/5) slanting palpebral fissures, large or beaked nose, flat maxilla, and short and featureless philtrum with a large mouth (long intercommisural distance). Hypoplastic

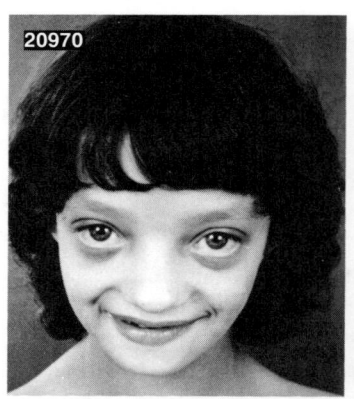
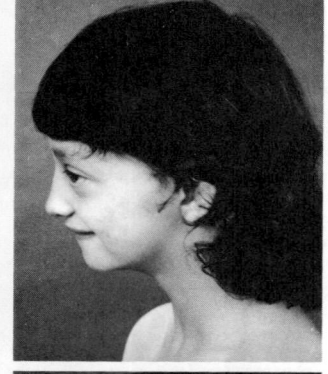
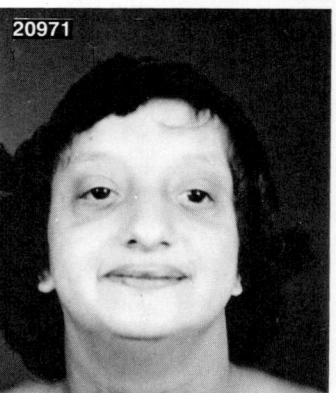
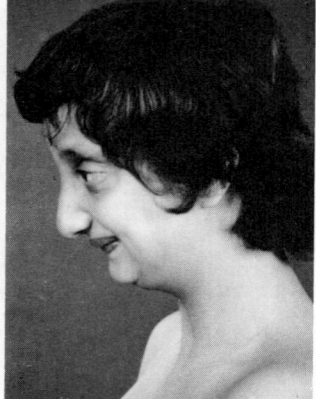

**2814-20970:** Microcephaly, prominent eyes, telecanthus, beaked nose, short, featureless philtrum, macrostomia and thick lower lip. **20971:** Affected sister of girl in 20970 with similar facies, microcephaly, growth and mental retardation.

female genitalia (3/5), radioulnar synostosis (2/5), and unusual dermatoglyphics were other reported features.

**Complications:** Unknown.

**Associated Findings:** None known.

**Etiology:** Presumably autosomal recessive inheritance.

**Pathogenesis:** Unknown.

**MIM No.:** 26235

**POS No.:** 3646

**Sex Ratio:** M1:F4 (observed).

**Occurrence:** Five cases, including two female sibs, have been reported.

**Risk of Recurrence for Patient's Sib:**
See Part I, *Mendelian Inheritance.*

**Risk of Recurrence for Patient's Child:**
See Part I, *Mendelian Inheritance.*

**Age of Detectability:** Small size at birth; characteristic facies could be diagnosed in the newborn.

**Gene Mapping and Linkage:** Unknown.

**Prevention:** None known. Genetic counseling indicated.

**Treatment:** As for any child with intellectual disability and hyperactive behavior.

**Prognosis:** Moderate-to-severe mental retardation. Life span does not appear to be affected.

**Detection of Carrier:** Unknown.

**References:**
Pitt DB, et al.: Mental retardation, unusual face, and intrauterine growth retardation: a new recessive syndrome? Am J Med Genet 1984; 19:307–313.
Donnai D: A further patient with the Pitt-Rogers-Danks syndrome of mental retardation, unusual face, and intrauterine growth retardation. Am J Med Genet 1986; 24:29–32.
Oorthuys JWE, Bleeker-Wagemakers EM: A girl with Pitt-Rogers-Danks syndrome. Am J Med Genet 1989; 32:140–141.

BA062                                                    **Agnes Bankier**

**Dwarfism-pericarditis**
*See DWARFISM, MULIBREY TYPE*
**Dwarfism-polydactyly-dysplastic nails**
*See CHONDROECTODERMAL DYSPLASIA*

---

## DWARFISM-STIFF JOINTS                                    2033

**Includes:**
Eye anomalies-dwarfism-stiff joints
Joints, stiff-dwarfism-eye defects
Moore-Federman syndrome

**Excludes:**
**Achondroplasia** (0010)
**Dyschondrosteosis** (0308)
**Hypochondroplasia** (0510)
**Leri pleonosteosis syndrome** (2102)
**Mucopolysaccharidosis IV** (0678)

**Major Diagnostic Criteria:** Short stature, joint stiffness, and ocular findings distinguish this syndrome from other skeletal dysplasias.

**Clinical Findings:** All affected individuals have been from the same family, and had short stature by the age of five years, with onset soon after birth in one case. Growth pattern and sexual maturation were normal, however, with a pubertal growth spurt occurring appropriately.

Joint stiffness affecting both flexion and extension also commonly occurred by six years of age, with involved joints including interphalangeal, elbow, knee, and wrist joints. No structural bony defects were noted on X-ray, however. Other common features include hyperopia, asthma occurring by age seven years, hoarse voice, hepatomegaly of unknown cause, and taut skin. When

measurements were done, the span was less than the height, and the crown-pubis measurement was greater than one-half the height, indicating that the shortness of stature was attributable to short legs.

Ocular findings in addition to the hyperopia included cataracts and glaucoma in one-half of the cases.

**Complications:** Retinal detachment occurred in a few cases.

**Associated Findings:** None known.

**Etiology:** Autosomal dominant inheritance with variable expressivity.

**Pathogenesis:** Unknown.

**MIM No.:** *12720

**POS No.:** 3318

**Sex Ratio:** M2:F4 (observed).

**Occurrence:** Reported in six members of one family in North America.

**Risk of Recurrence for Patient's Sib:**
See Part I, *Mendelian Inheritance.*

**Risk of Recurrence for Patient's Child:**
See Part I, *Mendelian Inheritance.*

**Age of Detectability:** By five to six years of age.

**Gene Mapping and Linkage:** Unknown.

**Prevention:** None known. Genetic counseling indicated.

**Treatment:** Treatment of ocular complications and asthma is indicated.

**Prognosis:** Life span is apparently unaffected; intellectual development is normal.

**Detection of Carrier:** Unknown.

**Special Considerations:** This condition is similar to **Leri pleonosteosis syndrome** which is also an autosomal dominant condition; however, asthma, hepatomegaly, and ocular findings have not been described in that condition. Interestingly, in the Leri pleonosteosis, the thumbs are described as broad and dorsiflexed, whereas in the Moore-Federman syndrome, the great toes are broad and dorsiflexed, indicating that although they may distinct conditions, they may share a pathogenetic pathway.

**References:**
Moore WT, Federman DD: Familial dwarfism and "stiff joints". Arch Intern Med 1965; 115:398–404. * †

T0007                                               **Helga V. Toriello**

---

## DYGGVE-MELCHIOR-CLAUSEN SYNDROME              0306

**Includes:** Smith-McCort dwarfism

**Excludes:**
**Mucopolysaccharidosis IV** (0678)
**Mucopolysaccharidosis** (other)
spondyloepiphyseal dysplasias, other

**Major Diagnostic Criteria:** Truncal dwarfism with characteristic skeletal abnormalities on X-ray, particularly of the vertebral bodies, pelvic and hand bones.

**Clinical Findings:** Short trunk type of dwarfism, protruding sternum, barrel chest, accentuated spinal curves, restricted joint mobility, waddling gait. Mental retardation in most cases, frequently associated with microcephaly.

X-rays show characteristic skeletal changes with flat, anteriorly pointed vertebral bodies. In younger patients, the superior and inferior end-plates of the vertebral bodies are notched. Short and broad ilia with defective ossification of their basilar portions and irregularly ossified (lace-like) crests; laterally displaced capital femoral epiphyses; irregular carpal bones, shortened metacarpal bones and phalanges with accessory ossification centers in various metacarpals and phalanges become apparent between the ages of one and 13 years. Odontoid hypoplasia occurs.

The Dyggve-Melchior-Clausen syndrome was originally thought

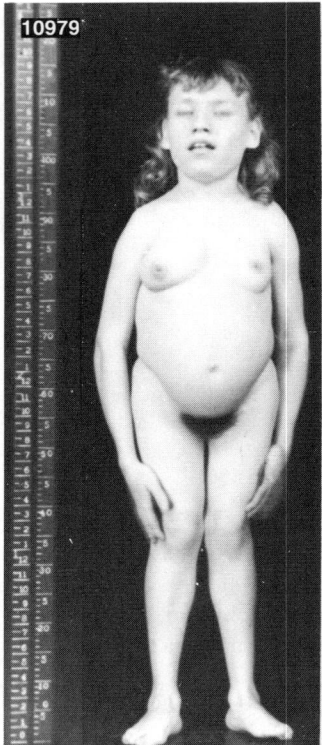
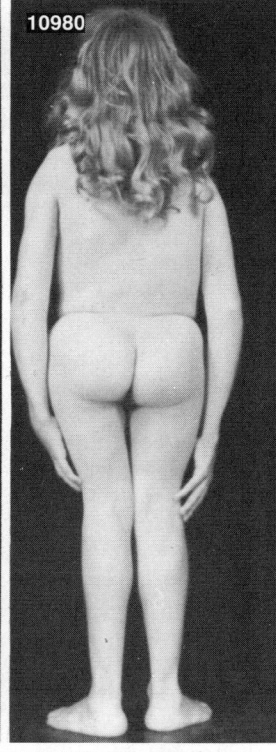

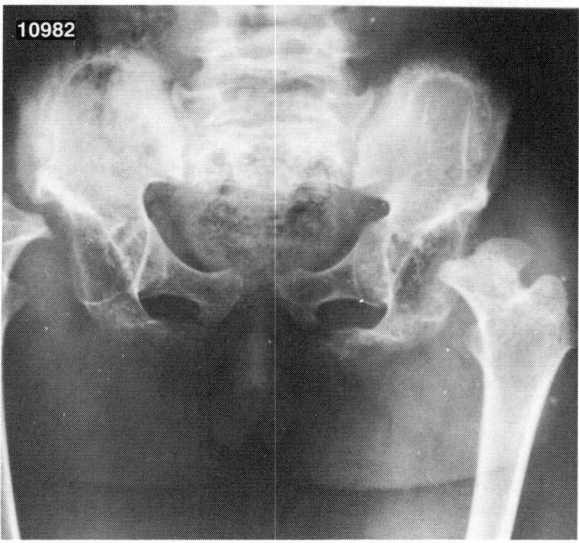

**0306**-10979–80: Short trunk, lumbar lordosis, marked hip dislocation, relatively long limbs. 10982: Hips are dislocated with poorly developed femoral heads, necks and acetabula; increased transverse diameter of pelvic inlet relative to vertical height; lacey appearance of the iliac crests.

to be a **Mucopolysaccharidosis**. Normal urinary excretion of acid mucopolysaccharides and failure to demonstrate mucopolysaccharide storage by microscopic and biochemical means make this improbable. Most patients are mentally retarded. Spranger et al (1976) have, however, delineated a similar entity, which they designate Smith-McCort dwarfism, which differs only in that affected individuals are not mentally retarded.

**Complications:** Usual sequelae of marked intellectual impairment.

**Associated Findings:** None known.

**Etiology:** Autosomal recessive inheritance.

**Pathogenesis:** Abnormalities in the growth plate, include randomly oriented bundles of loosely woven parallel fibers of type II collagen and cytoplasmic inclusions in chondrocytes, disrupt normal endochondral ossification. Studies suggest a deficiency of a specific sulfatase and/or a protease involved in proteoglycan degradation.

**MIM No.:** *22380

**POS No.:** 3188

**Sex Ratio:** M1:F1

**Occurrence:** Undetermined. Reported in Greenland, Norway, and Lebanon.

**Risk of Recurrence for Patient's Sib:**
See Part I, *Mendelian Inheritance.*

**Risk of Recurrence for Patient's Child:**
See Part I, *Mendelian Inheritance.*

**Age of Detectability:** In infancy.

**Gene Mapping and Linkage:** Unknown.

**Prevention:** None known. Genetic counseling indicated.

**Treatment:** Spinal fusion when atlanto-axial instability is present, and appropriate orthopedic care.

**Prognosis:** The life expectancy is unknown. The oldest patients with mental retardation are in their 20s; several patients without mental retardation are in their 40s.

**Detection of Carrier:** Unknown.

**References:**
Spranger J, et al.: . Radiology 1975; 114:415–422.
Spranger J, et al.: Heterogeneity of Dyggve-Melchior-Clausen dwarfism. Hum Genet 1976; 33:279–287.
Toledo SPA, et al.: Dyggve-Melchior-Clause syndrome: genetic studies and report of affected sibs. Am J Hum Genet 1979; 4:255–261.
Bonatede RP, Beighton P: The Dyggve-Melchior-Clausen syndrome in adult siblings. Clin Genet 1978; 14:24–30.
Hall-Craggs MA, Chapman M: Case Report 431: Radiological Studies. Skeletal Radiology 1978; 16:422–424. †
Horton WA, Scott CI: Dyggve-Melchior-Clausen syndrome. J Bone Joint Surg 1982; 64A:408–415.
Beck M, et al.: Dyggve-Melchior-Clausen syndrome: normal degradation of proteodermatan sulfate, proteokeratan sulfate and heparan sulfate. Clin Chim Acta 1984; 141:7–15.

HE006
H0033

Jacqueline T. Hecht
William A. Horton

**Dysalbuminemic hyperthyroxinemia**
*See ANALBUMINEMIA*

## DYSAUTONOMIA I, RILEY-DAY TYPE      0307

**Includes:**
Dysautonomia, familial
Hereditary sensory and autonomic neuropathy III (HSAN III)
Riley-Day syndrome

**Excludes:**
**Biemond I syndrome** (3034)
**Immunodeficiency, common variable type** (0521)
Pain, congenital indifference to

**Major Diagnostic Criteria:** The disease can be suspected on the basis of family history and the appearance of swallowing deficits, aspiration pneumonia, unusual postures and limb movements, and altered states of consciousness in the newborn. In addition, indifference to pain may be detected.

There is no single diagnostic test. There is an abnormal response to intradermal histamine in which there is a thin red

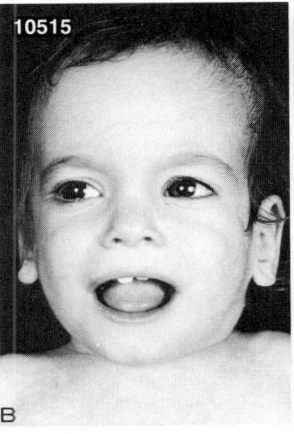
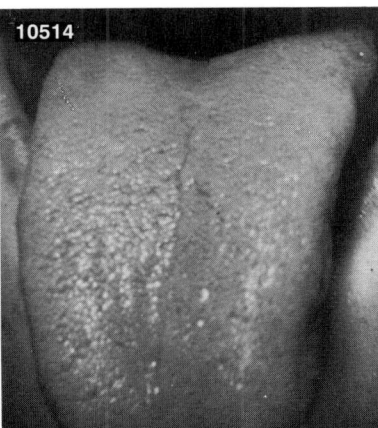

**0307-10515:** 3½-year-old with dysautonomia; note skin blotching and wet hair from excess sweating. **10514:** Absent fungiform papillae.

border but no surrounding flare as there is in the normal newborn. Simply scratching the skin does not result in the usual flared response. There are also pharmacologic abnormalities, particularly a hypersensitivity to both cholinergic and adrenergic agents. Fetal diagnosis by amniotic fluid bile content is being explored.

**Clinical Findings:** The process presents as a complex. There are no symptoms or signs that are by themselves pathognomonic of the disease. The constant features include an absence of overflow tears (alacrima), usually an absence of the fungiform papillae of the tongue, vasomotor instability, hypoactive or absent deep tendon reflexes, and relative indifference to pain. In younger children feeding difficulties are very frequent. In addition physical retardation, episodic vomiting, marked emotional instability, scoliosis and disturbances of GI motility are frequent. The most common neurologic feature is the insensitivity to pain. Older patients have a progressive sensory loss. Mental retardation is very uncommon.

The incidence of these features is as follows: absence of fungiform papillae (100%); absence of overflow tears (100%); vasomotor disturbance [blotching] (98%); abnormal sweating (97%); episodic fever (92%); incoordination and unsteadiness (90%); scoliosis (90%); swallowing difficulty in infancy (85%); physical retardation (78%); elevated blood urea nitrogen (BUN) (76%); episodic vomiting (67%); breath-holding attacks (66%); marked emotional instability (65%); bowel disturbance (49%).

"Atypical" cases, in which one or more major features are lacking, are being described with increasing frequency.

**Complications:** The complications may come from the insensitivity to pain, scoliosis, or from the GI disturbance, particularly the swallowing deficit. Repeated aspirations and episodes of pneumonia are a common complication. Failure of somatic growth is an integral part of the process; whether it is secondary or primary is not clear. Corneal abrasions and keratitis are frequent.

**Associated Findings:** None known.

**Etiology:** Autosomal recessive inheritance.

**Pathogenesis:** Undetermined. There are features that suggest that the central and peripheral autonomic nervous system are involved in a defect in neurotransmission. Whether some biochemical abnormality of neuronal maturation or maintenance is at fault has not been clearly established. There is a possible depletion of substance-P in the substantia gelatinosa. Whether there is a genetic defect involving β-nerve growth factor is unclear.

**MIM No.:** *22390

**POS No.:** 3189

**CDC No.:** 742.810

**Sex Ratio:** M1:F1

**Occurrence:** Occurs primarily in Ashkenazi Jewish families in Israel where the incidence has been calculated at 1:3,703.

**Risk of Recurrence for Patient's Sib:**
See Part I, *Mendelian Inheritance.*

**Risk of Recurrence for Patient's Child:**
See Part I, *Mendelian Inheritance.*

**Age of Detectability:** In the neonatal period, but often the definitive diagnosis is not made until later in life.

**Gene Mapping and Linkage:** Unknown.

**Prevention:** None known. Genetic counseling indicated.

**Treatment:** There is no known treatment for the disease. Complications may be treated, as exemplified by the use of antibiotics for repeated episodes of pneumonia. Progressive scoliosis must be monitored and treated vigorously. When anesthetics are used during surgery, particular care must be taken to avoid vasomotor dysfunction.

**Prognosis:** The prognosis varies but many cases die in childhood or early adult life from the complications of defects in swallowing and secondary pneumonia. Fundoplication and gastrostomy are often required.

**Detection of Carrier:** Unknown.

**Support Groups:** New York; The Dysautonomia Foundation, Inc.

**References:**
Riley CM: Familial dysautonomia. Adv Pediatr 1957; 9:157.
Brunt PW, McKusick VA: Familial dysautonomia: a report of genetic and clinical studies, with a review of the literature. Medicine 1970; 49:343–374.
Pearson J, Pytel BA: Quantitative studies of sympathetic ganglia and spinal cord intermedio-lateral gray columns in familial dysautonomia. J Neurol Sci 1978; 39:47.
Pearson J, et al.: Tyrosine hydroxylase immunoreactivity in familial dysautonomia. Science 1979; 206:71.
Schwartz JP, Breakefield XO: Altered nerve growth factor in fibroblasts from patients with familial dysautonomia. Proc Natl Acad Sci (USA) 1980; 77:1154–1158.
Axelrod FB, et al.: Progressive sensory loss in familial dysautonomia. Pediatrics 1981; 67:517–522.
Pearson J, et al.: Renal disease in familial dysautonomia. Kidney Int 1980; 17:102–112.
Axelrod FB, et al.: Neonatal recognition of familial dysautonomia. J Pediat 1987; 110:946–948.

GI010                                                **Herbert Gilmore**

**Dysautonomia, familial**
*See DYSAUTONOMIA I, RILEY-DAY TYPE*
**Dysautonomia, type II, familial**
*See NEUROPATHY, CONGENITAL SENSORY WITH ANHIDROSIS*
**Dyscephaly with congenital cataract and hypotrichosis**
*See OCULO-MANDIBULO-FACIAL SYNDROME*
**Dyschondroplasia**
*See ENCHONDROMATOSIS*
**Dyschondroplasia-hemangiomatosis (some cases)**
*See ENCHONDROMATOSIS AND HEMANGIOMAS*

---

**DYSCHONDROSTEOSIS**                                    **0308**

**Includes:**
Dwarfism, deformity with mesomelic
Leri-Weill disease
Madelung deformity
Mesomelic dwarfism-Madelung deformity

**Excludes:**
Madelung deformity due to trauma or infection
**Mesomelic dysplasia** (all others)
**Turner syndrome** (0977)

**Major Diagnostic Criteria:** The wrist deformity often referred to as Madelung deformity in a person with mesomelic short stature. In a family in which one or more individuals have the condition, a relative with Madelung deformity and normal stature would be considered affected.

**Clinical Findings:** Mild disproportionate short stature is accompanied by mesomelia of both limbs. Usual adult height varies between 137 and 152 cm. A marked modeling deformity of the wrists produces bowing of the forearm and wrists with lateral and dorsal bowing of the radius, most marked distally. Motion is limited at the elbow and wrist. The radius is short and thickened. A V-shaped deformity of the wrist appears on X-ray with slanting at the distal radial contour and dorsal dislocation of the ulna. There is wedging of the carpal bones between the deformed radius and protruding ulna, resulting in a triangular configuration with the lunate at the apex. Inconstant features include humeral neck deformities, exostoses of the proximal medial tibia, shortening and thickening of the metacarpals and phalanges, coxa valga, cubitus valgus, lateral subluxation of the patella, osteoarthritis of large joints, and lumbar spine stenosis.

**Complications:** Limitation of elbow and wrist motion, occasional osteoarthrosis.

**Associated Findings:** None known.

**Etiology:** Autosomal dominant inheritance; more severe in females. Male-to-male transmission has been observed.

**Pathogenesis:** Unknown.

**MIM No.:** *12730

**POS No.:** 3190

**Sex Ratio:** An apparent excess of females may be attributable to bias of ascertainment.

**Occurrence:** Undetermined. Most common form of mesomelic dwarfism.

**Risk of Recurrence for Patient's Sib:**
See Part I, *Mendelian Inheritance.*

**Risk of Recurrence for Patient's Child:**
See Part I, *Mendelian Inheritance.*

**Age of Detectability:** Mid-to-late childhood because of short stature or wrist deformity.

**Gene Mapping and Linkage:** Unknown.

**Prevention:** None known. Genetic counseling indicated.

**Treatment:** Orthopedic surgery for wrist if Madelung deformity is severe.

**Prognosis:** Normal life span.

**Detection of Carrier:** Unknown.

**Special Considerations:** There is some controversy as to whether there is a distinct, heritable, isolated form of Madelung deformity in the absence of a generalized bone dysplasia. A more severe form of mesomelic dwarfism, similar to **Mesomelic dysplasia, Langer type** may occur in an individual who is homozygous for the dyschondrosteosis gene.

**References:**

Langer LO: Dyschondrosteosis: a hereditable bone dysplasia with characteristic roentgenographic features. Am J Roentgenol Radium Ther Nucl Med 1965; 95:178–188.

Felman AH, et al.: Dyschondrosteose. Mesomelic dwarfism of Leri and Weill. Am J Dis Child 1970; 20:329–331.

Espiritu C, et al.: Mesomelic dwarfism as the homozygous expression of dyschondrosteosis. Am J Dis Child 1975; 29:375–377.

Kaitila II, et al.: Mesomelic skeletal dysplasias. Clin Orthop 1976; 114:94.

Hecht F, Hecht BK: Linkage of skeletal dysplasia gene to t(2;8)(q32–3) chromosome translocation breakpoint (letter). Am J Med Genet 1984; 18:779–780.

Jackson LG: Dyschondrosteosis: clinical study of a sixth generation family (abstract). Proc Greenwood Genet Center 1985; 4:147–148. *

B0025

*Zvi Borochowitz*
*Ralph S. Lachman*
*David L. Rimoin*

**Dyschondrosteosis, as heterozygote state**
See MESOMELIC DYSPLASIA, LANGER TYPE
**Dyschromatosis universalis hereditaria**
See DYSKERATOSIS CONGENITA
**Dyscoria**
See PUPIL, DYSCORIA
**Dysencephalia splanchnocystica**
See MECKEL SYNDROME

---

## DYSEQUILIBRIUM SYNDROME 2421

**Includes:**
> Cerebellar atrophy
> Cerebellar disorder (nonprogressive)-mental retardation
> Cerebellar hypoplasia
> Disequilibrium syndrome

**Excludes:**
> **Acidemia, gamma-hydroxybutyric** (2113)
> **Angelman syndrome** (2086)
> **Cerebellar ataxia**
> **Cerebral palsy** (2931)
> **Marinesco-Sjogren syndrome** (2031)

**Major Diagnostic Criteria:** Early onset of hypotonia, imbalance, mental retardation, and cerebellar hypoplasia.

**Clinical Findings:** Initially hypotonic with delayed motor development. Independent walking delayed until ages six to 15 years. Gait broadly based and unsteady with frequent uncompensated falls. Severe expressive language delay and dysarthria. Increased muscle stretch reflexes and positive Babinski responses may develop later. Nystagmus is not characteristic. Balance (equilibrium) is the main cerebellar function affected, although intention tremor and athetosis were present in four Hutterite sibs described

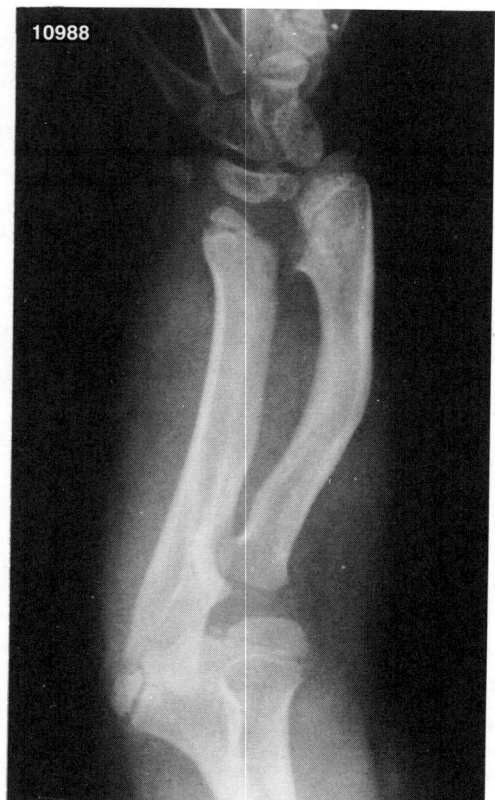

0308-10988: Note uneven fusion of distal epiphyses of radius and ulna.

by Pallister and Opitz (1985). Two of their patients also had borderline small heads, whereas the remainder have had a normal head circumference. Mental retardation (mild to moderate) was present in 15/15 Hutterite and 11/13 Swedish patients. Height is below average. Some but not all affected individuals studied by X-ray have had hypoplasia of the cerebellar hemispheres and vermis. One of two Hutterite sisters who were studied in depth also had dilation of the third and lateral ventricles on a CT scan of her head. Both sisters had generalized grade II dysrhythmia on their electroencephalograms and normal electromyographic (EMG) studies. The EMG was normal in 7/9 Swedish cases. Pneumoencephalography in the Swedish cases showed hypoplastic vermis, helping to differentiate this condition from congenital ataxia.

**Complications:** Cataracts were present in 3/13 Swedish cases and epilepsy in 2/13 compared with 1/15 for either in the Hutterites.

**Associated Findings:** Strabismus was noted in 11/15 Hutterite and 6/13 Swedish cases.

**Etiology:** Autosomal recessive inheritance. Both the Swedish and Hutterite cases belong to inbred goups in which multiply affected sibships with and without parental consanguinity have been observed. The clinical and X-ray findings are nonspecific, and it is likely that nongenetic cases (phenocopies) occur. The empiric risk for recurrence in a sib of a sporadic patient in an outbred population has not been determined.

**Pathogenesis:** Reduced numbers of granule neurons in the cerebellar cortex with or without demonstrable hypoplasia of the vermis and hemispheres could explain the hypotonia and dysequilibrium. However, these findings are nonspecific (Sarnat and Alcala, 1980), as may also be the finding of low levels of serum dopamine-β-hydroxylase by Gustavson, et al.(1977). No evidence for adverse pre- or perinatal factors was found in a controlled study by Rasmussen et al. (1985). Dysequilibrium syndrome appears to be a distinct pathological entity from **Acidemia, gamma-hydroxybutyric**, although they share the same clinical features. Gibson et al (1985) demonstrated normal organic acid excretion and normal lymphocyte succinic semialdehyde dehydrogenase activities in three patients.

**MIM No.:** *22405

**POS No.:** 3714

**Sex Ratio:** Presumably M1:F1. There have been six males and 11 females among documented cases in the Hutterites, compared with ten males and three females in the Swedish study.

**Occurrence:** Seventeen cases have been documented in Hutterites and thirteen among Swedes.

**Risk of Recurrence for Patient's Sib:**
See Part I, *Mendelian Inheritance.*

**Risk of Recurrence for Patient's Child:**
See Part I, *Mendelian Inheritance.*

**Age of Detectability:** Hypotonia and delayed motor development are usually noted during the first year of life.

**Gene Mapping and Linkage:** Unknown.

**Prevention:** None known. Genetic counseling indicated.

**Treatment:** Supports held by hands are necessary for a variable period before independent walking is mastered. Speech therapy may be helpful in those who are only mildly retarded. Ocular problems (strabismus, cataracts) should be treated if they interfere with vision. Anticonvulsant medication for control of seizures when indicated.

**Prognosis:** Life span may be normal or only slightly reduced. The disorder is nonprogressive, and most affected individuals eventually learn to walk without support.

**Detection of Carrier:** Clinical examination of first degree relatives.

**References:**
Hagberg B, et al.: The dysequilibrium syndrome in cerebral palsy: clinical aspects and treatment. Acta Paediatr Scand 1972; 61[Suppl 226]:1–63.

Gustavson K-H, et al.: Low serum dopamine-(beta)-hydroxylase activity in the dysequilibrium syndrome. Clin Genet 1977; 11:270–272.
Sarnat HB, Alcala H: Human cerebellar hypoplasia. Arch Neurol 1980; 37:300–305.
Schurig V, et al.: Nonprogressive cerebellar disorder with mental retardation and autosomal recessive inheritance in Hutterites. Am J Med Genet 1981; 9:43–53.
Gibson KM, et al.: Clinical correlation of Dysequilibrium syndrome and 4-hydroxybutyric aciduria. J Inherit Metab Dis 1985; 8:58 only.
Pallister PD, Opitz JM: Disequilibrium syndrome in Montana Hutterites. Am J Med Genet 1985; 22:567–569.
Rasmussen F, et al.: The dysequilibrium syndrome: a study of the etiology and pathogenesis. Clin Genet 1985; 27:191–195.

B0030                                              **Peter A. Bowen**

**Dyserythropoietic anemia, HEMPAS type**
*See ANEMIA, DYSERYTHROPOIETIC, TYPE II*
**Dyserythropoietic anemia, type I**
*See ANEMIA, DYSERYTHROPOIETIC, TYPE I*
**Dyserythropoietic anemia, type II (HEMPAS)**
*See ANEMIA, HEMOLYTIC, RED CELL MEMBRANE DEFECTS*
**Dyserythropoietic anemia, type III**
*See ANEMIA, DYSERYTHROPOIETIC, TYPE III*
**Dysfibrinogenemia, congenital**
*See FIBRINOGENS, ABNORMAL CONGENITAL*
**Dysfluency**
*See STUTTERING*
**Dysgammaglobulinemia antibody deficiency syndrome**
*See IMMUNODEFICIENCY, X-LINKED WITH HYPER IgM*
**Dysgammaglobulinemia type IV**
*See IMMUNOGLOBULIN A DEFICIENCY*
**Dysgammaglobulinemia, type I**
*See IMMUNODEFICIENCY, X-LINKED WITH HYPER IgM*
**Dysgammaglobulinemia-deficient 7S and elevated 19S gammaglobulins**
*See IMMUNODEFICIENCY, X-LINKED WITH HYPER IgM*
**Dysgenesis mesostromal**
*See EYE, ANTERIOR SEGMENT DYSGENESIS*
**Dysgenesis neuroepithelialis retinae**
*See RETINA, AMAUROSIS CONGENITA, LEBER TYPE*
**Dysgenesis of inner ear**
*See EAR, INNER DYSPLASIAS*

## DYSKERATOSIS CONGENITA                              2024

**Includes:**
Dyschromatosis universalis hereditaria
Dyskeratosis congenita, autosomal recessive type
Dyskeratosis congenita, Scoggins type
Zinsser-Cole-Engman syndrome

**Excludes:**
**Mucosa (oral/eye), intraepithelial dyskeratosis, benign** (0538)
**Pancytopenia syndrome, Fanconi type** (2029)

**Major Diagnostic Criteria:** The classic triad consists of a reticular pattern of hyper- and hypopigmentation of the skin, progressive nail dystrophy and mucosal leukoplakia. Pancytopenia due to bone marrow failure may be a common and important component of the syndrome.

**Clinical Findings:** The usual onset of symptoms is in early childhood, virtually all cases expressing the full phenotype by puberty. Nail dystrophy has been reported at birth. The frequencies of the most common findings are: cutaneous pigmentary anomaly (100%), atrophic changes over dorsum of the hands and palms leading to loss of dermatoglyphics (93%), hyperkeratosis of the palms and soles (74%), hyperhidrosis (74%), nail dystrophy (98%), mucosal leukoplakia, mostly of the tongue and buccal surface (87%). Atresia of the lacrimal puncta with chronic epiphora occur in about 80% of the patients. Alopecia, sparse eyebrows and eyelashes, extensive dental caries with early loss of teeth, dysphagia, hyposthenic build, microcephaly with reduced intelligence, acrocyanosis, small testes and penis occur in 40%-50% of the cases. Bone marrow failure leading to pancytopenia may be seen in nearly half of all patients, and thrombocytopenia has been the presenting symptom in a few.

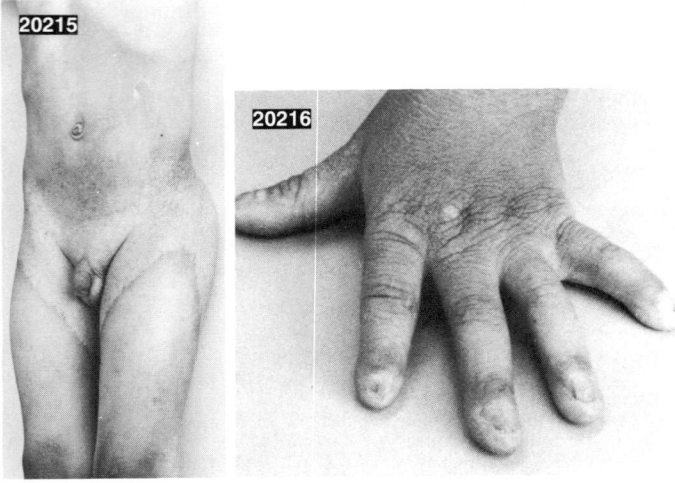

**2024-20215:** Bathing trunk distribution of reticulated hyperpigmentation in a 4-year-old Black male with dyskeratosis congenita. **20216:** Nail dystrophy.

**Complications:** Increased incidence (16%) of solid neoplasms, mainly carcinomas, which often arose in the areas of leukoplakia. One case of Hodgkin's disease and no leukemias have been reported. At least two patients have had multiple primaries. Immune dysfunction leading to opportunistic infections and gastrointestinal bleeding have been the causes of death in several patients.

**Associated Findings:** Abnormal sella turcica, intracranial calcification, abnormal EEG, corneal ulceration, bilateral cataracts, enlarged thyroid gland, sharp or pinched facial appearance with beaked nose, esophageal stenosis and webs, aseptic necrosis of the femoral heads, excessive bony trabeculation with fracture on minimal trauma, urethral stenosis, horseshoe kidneys have been seen in occasional patients.

**Etiology:** X-linked recessive inheritance is most common on the basis of preponderance of affected males with typical pedigree patterns. However, etiologic heterogeneity is evident from reports of affected male and female sib-pairs born of consanguineous unions, and of male-to-male transmission in at least two families. A significant proportion of reported cases have occurred sporadically.

**Pathogenesis:** Undetermined. Reports of excessive spontaneous chromosome breakage and of increased spontaneous sister chromatid exchanges have been inconsistent. An impaired ability to remove photoadducts induced by ultraviolet light following trimethyl psoralen treatment, and the increased sensitivity to ionizing radiation-induced $G_2$ chromatid breakage point towards a DNA repair defect as a possible pathogenic mechanism. A bone marrow stem cell defect has been proposed as an explanation for the pancytopenia.

**MIM No.:** *30500, 12755, 22423.

**POS No.:** 3191

**Sex Ratio:** M10:F1

**Occurrence:** Over 120 cases are known worldwide. The disease has been seen in all major racial and ethnic groups.

**Risk of Recurrence for Patient's Sib:**
See Part I, *Mendelian Inheritance.*

**Risk of Recurrence for Patient's Child:**
See Part I, *Mendelian Inheritance.*

**Age of Detectability:** Usually in early childhood, although nail dysplasia is occasionally present at birth.

**Gene Mapping and Linkage:** DKC (dyskeratosis congenita) has been mapped to Xq27-q28.

**Prevention:** None known. Genetic counseling indicated.

**Treatment:** Symptomatic. Bone marrow transplantation has been done in four patients with fatal outcome in each.

**Prognosis:** Life expectancy is generally shortened. Several patients died of opportunistic infections and gastrointestinal bleeding, primarily in the second decade, and of malignancies; mostly in the third and fourth decades.

**Detection of Carrier:** Unknown.

**References:**
Sirinavin C, Trowbridge AA: Dyskeratosis congenita: clinical features and genetic aspects: report of a family and review of the literature. J Med Genet 1975; 12:339–354.
Carter DM, et al.: Psoralen-DNA cross-linking photoadducts in dyskeratosis congenita: delay in excision and promotion of sister chromatid exchange. J Invest Dermatol 1979; 73:97–101.
Connor JM, Teague RH: Dyskeratosis congenita: report of a large kindred. Br J Dermatol 1981; 105:321–325.
Friedland M, et al.: Dyskeratosis congenita with hypoplastic anemia: a stem cell defect. Am J Hematol 1985; 20:85–87.
Juneja HS, et al.: Abnormality of platelet size and T-lymphocyte proleferation in an autosomal recessive form of dyskeratosis congenita. Eur J Haematol 1987; 39:306–310.
DeBauche DM, et al.: Hypersensitivity to X-irradiation-induced G2 chromatid damage in dyskeratosis congenita. Am J Hum Genet 1988; 43:22A.
Pai GS, et al.: Etiologic heterogeneity in dyskeratosis congenita. Am J Med Genet 1989; 32:63–66.

CA040
PA006

Nancy J. Carpenter
G. Shashidhar Pai

**Dyskeratosis congenita, autosomal recessive type**
See DYSKERATOSIS CONGENITA
**Dyskeratosis congenita, Scoggins type**
See DYSKERATOSIS CONGENITA
**Dyskeratosis, intraepithelial**
See MUCOSA (ORAL/EYE), INTRAEPITHELIAL DYSKERATOSIS, BENIGN

**DYSLEXIA**     **3005**

**Includes:**
Developmental dyslexia
Reading disorder, developmental
Reading disorder, specific
Word blindness, congenital

**Excludes:** Mental retardation

**Major Diagnostic Criteria:** Impairment in the development of reading or spelling skills that is not due to general intellectual retardation or to inadequate schooling. Functionally this is defined as a significant discrepancy between cognitive potential (as measured by intelligence tests) and academic achievement (as measured by tests of reading skill).

**Clinical Findings:** Clinical findings that would permit early (preacademic) identification have not been found. Abnormality in the planum temporale has been reported in several postmortem specimens, but neuroimaging and neurophysiologic studies have not consistently supported anatomic deviations.

Nonspecific neurobehavioral signs of developmental dysfunction-hyperactivity, immaturity, gross and fine motor delays (clumsiness), and evidence of central processing dysfunction (e.g., deviant language development or visual-perceptual dysfunction)-may be present before academics are attempted. However, specific clinical signs are not evident until the child begins to learn to read. Early diagnosis may be delayed by the inability of the child to meet diagnostic criteria for "significant" discrepancy or by the presence of confounding circumstances.

Children with dyslexia have marked impairment in the development of reading skills and poor academic performance in tasks requiring reading skills. Reading is slow, with reduced comprehension, and is characterized by omissions, substitutions, and word distortions. The constellation of clinical manifestations varies, although similar patterns of dysfunction have been described in families. Attempts at defining subtypes remain to be validated, although there appear to be at least four subtypes: visual perception, linguistic processing, articulatory/graphomotor, and mixed. Although males are more commonly affected than females, sex does not relate to severity.

Long-term follow-up studies suggest that most children ultimately attain literacy, but persistent deficits in reading, spelling, and the written language may be noted. These deficits may be of little functional import or may cause significant handicap. Outcomes are only partially determined by the primary impairment. Frequently the associated factors, e.g., self-esteem, hyperactivity, social interaction, and family function, are of greater significance.

**Complications:** School achievement may be so impaired that school failure results. Mental health disturbances, such as feelings of inadequacy, insecurity, and withdrawal, are not infrequent. More severe disorders of conduct or mood are seen less commonly. Alcoholism, depression, and other dysfunctions may be noted in adolescence and adulthood. It is not clear whether the adverse outcomes are related to the primary dysfunction or to secondary problems arising from poor self-esteem.

**Associated Findings:** Minimal brain dysfunction, attention deficit disorder (with or without hyperactivity), developmental language disorder, developmental arithmetic disorder.

**Etiology:** Studies suggest substantial familial clustering. Studies of twins have found a 90% concordance for monozygotic and 32% concordance for dizygotic twins. However, it is likely that the imprecision of the diagnostic criteria and the lack of definition of the pathophysiology obscure a number of dyslexia syndromes. As a result, several different modes of inheritance have been proposed.

**Pathogenesis:** Unknown. Multiple mechanisms likely. Acquired forms exist.

**MIM No.:** *12770

**Sex Ratio:** M3–4:F1, although questions have been raised about the completeness of verification of female cases.

**Occurrence:** The estimated prevalence among school children is 10 to 15%. Reading retardation may be increased in children of lower socioeconomic status who attend inner city schools.

**Risk of Recurrence for Patient's Sib:** Unknown.

**Risk of Recurrence for Patient's Child:** Unknown.

**Age of Detectability:** Early school age (5–8 years).

**Gene Mapping and Linkage:** A possible linkage between reading disability and chromosome 15 was reported. However, repeating the analysis with chromosome 15-specific DNA probes failed to confirm the preliminary findings.

**Prevention:** None known. Genetic counseling indicated.

**Treatment:** No treatment has been shown to be effective in all cases. The complex and pervasive nature of dyslexia usually requires a comprehensive, coordinated, multimodal approach that addresses educational, parental, and child factors. Educational remediation is most commonly used, although proof of efficacy is lacking. Alteration of the environment to circumvent the impairment is thought to have a positive effect on mental health. Treatment must also address the associated behavioral and emotional dysfunctions.

**Prognosis:** Generally good for function. Mental health outcomes variable.

**Detection of Carrier:** Unknown.

**Special Considerations:** Further advances in understanding the familial nature of dyslexia will require a better definition of the condition. Defining dyslexia is complicated by a lack of universal agreement to an operational definition. This may be attributed to several reasons: 1) persistence in trying to define a single dyslexia syndrome; 2) using a heterogeneous outcome to define the syndrome rather than the disordered function; 3) the varied amount and quality of school experiences in children of differing ages; 4) the inability to determine the effect of confounding factors such as socioeconomic status, cultural biases, and concurrent behavioral disturbance; and 5) substantial disagreement over the measures used to define the syndrome(s).

Reading is a complex neurologic function. Disordered reading is likely to result from a variety of dysfunctions. Clinical heterogeneity is noted in presentation, ranging from word blindness to inefficient, but functional, reading. The "gifted" dyslexic child may have high scores on intellectual testing but only average reading scores. Whether the child with a reading inefficiency has the same dysfunction as the child who manifests obvious reading disability is unknown.

Similar variation is noted in neuropsychologic function and in studies of the type of errors made by dyslexics. Attempts to define dyslexia with a single neuropsychologic profile have been unsuccessful. All dyslexics do not make the same type of reading errors. Studies of dyslexia subtypes have been limited because of referral populations, restrictive selection criteria, cross-sectional designs, incomplete evaluations, and varied population characteristics, such as age.

**References:**
Benton A, Pearl D, eds: Dyslexia: an appraisal of current knowledge. New York: Oxford University, 1978.
Omenn GS, Weber BA: Dyslexia: search for phenotypic and genetic heterogeneity. Am J Med Genet 1978; 1:333–342.
Lewitter FI, et al.: Genetic models of reading disability. Behav Genet 1980; 10:9–30.
Haslam RHA, et al.: Cerebral asymmetry in developmental dyslexia. Arch Neurol 1981; 38:679–682.
DeFries, JC, et al.: Evidence for a genetic aetiology in reading disability of twins. Nature 1987; 329:537–539.

SH051
M0045

**Bruce K. Shapiro**
**Peggy S. Monahan**

**Dysmelia**
  *See LIMB REDUCTION DEFECTS*
**Dysmelodia**
  *See DEAFNESS, TUNE*
**Dysmorphic facies-ataxia-trichodysplasia**
  *See ATAXIA-DYSMORPHIC FACIES-TRICHODYSPLASIA*
**Dysmyelinogenic leukodystrophy**
  *See ALEXANDER DISEASE*

## DYSOSTEOSCLEROSIS                                    0310

**Includes:**
  Albers-Schonberg
  Osteosclerosis-platyspondyly
  Platyspondyly-osteosclerosis

**Excludes:**
  **Osteopetrosis** (all forms)
  **Pyknodysostosis** (0846)

**Major Diagnostic Criteria:** Dense osteopetrotic bones with platyspondyly and phalangeal tuft resorption. This disorder may be confused with the more typical forms of osteopetrosis, but can be distinguished by the presence of platyspondyly, superior and inferior irregularity of vertebral ossification, clinical findings of a high incidence of developmental defects of the teeth, and the absence of hematologic complications.

**Clinical Findings:** Short stature with increased bone fragility. Delayed eruption of primary teeth, hypodontia, and early loss of teeth with poorly calcified chalky enamel. Sclerosis of the base of the skull may lead to optic atrophy, other cranial nerve involvement, and upper motor neuron lesions. X-ray evaluation reveals generalized increased density of the cartilaginous bones, including the base of the skull. Platyspondyly and sclerosis of the vertebrae are characteristic features. The metaphyses of long bones are expanded with exaggerated linear growth lines, and there is phalangeal tuft resorption. Recurrent infections of the mandible may occur.

**Complications:** Optic atrophy and other cranial nerve involvement; increased predisposition to bone fractures as in osteopetrosis.

**Associated Findings:** Progressive mental deterioration and upper motor neuron disease may occur.

**Etiology:** Autosomal recessive inheritance. One pedigree reported with apparent X-linked recessive inheritance.

**Pathogenesis:** There is a lack of resorption of calcified cartilage at the growth plate, which is surrounded only by thin rims of bone. Bone from the orbital roof has been shown to be of a woven nature. The primary defect appears to involve the replacement of calcified cartilage by mature bone.

**MIM No.:** *22430

**POS No.:** 3728

**Sex Ratio:** Presumably M1:F1

**Occurrence:** Unknown.

**Risk of Recurrence for Patient's Sib:**
See Part I, *Mendelian Inheritance.*

**Risk of Recurrence for Patient's Child:**
See Part I, *Mendelian Inheritance.*

**Age of Detectability:** Early childhood, when X-rays are performed for fractures or cranial nerve involvement.

**Gene Mapping and Linkage:** Unknown.

**Prevention:** None known. Genetic counseling indicated.

**Treatment:** Routine treatment of fractures; repair and capping of teeth; unroofing of the optic canal may be necessary to retard visual loss.

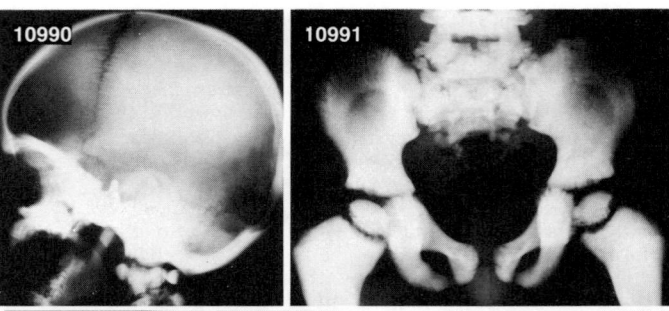

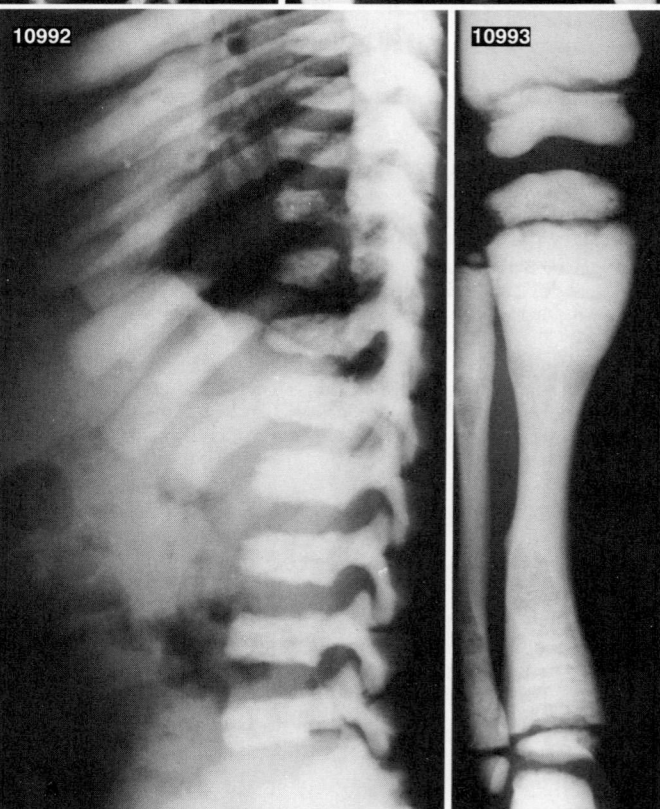

**0310B-10990:** Lateral view of the skull shows sclerosis is most prominent in the basilar portion. **10991:** Irregularities of iliac crests and acetabular roofs; increased striations extend from these areas. **10992:** Marked sclerosis and platyspondyly; ribs lack normal modeling of distal ends. **10993:** Long bones have abnormally molded metaphyses with relatively milder epiphyseal changes; diaphyses show narrowing of the marrow cavity.

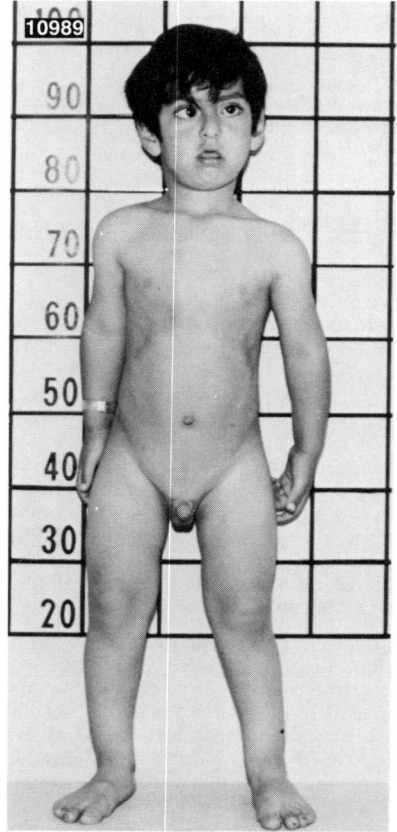

**0310A-10989:** Note disproportionately short limbs and slight bowing of the long bones.

**Prognosis:** No adults have yet been reported.

**Detection of Carrier:** Unknown.

**References:**

Roy C, et al.: Un nouveau syndrome osseux avec anomalies cutanées et troubles neurologiques. Arch Fr Pediatr 1968; 25:893–905.

Spranger J, et al.: Die Dysosteosklerose: eine Sonderform der generalisierten Osteosklerose. Fortschr Rontgenstr 1968; 109:504–512.

Leisti J, et al.: Dysosteosclerosis. BD:OAS; XI(6). New York: March of Dimes Birth Defects Foundation, 1975;349.

Pascual-Castroviego, et al.: X-linked dysosteosclerosis. Eur J Pediat 1977; 126:127–138.

Houston CS, et al.: Dysosteosclerosis. Am J Roentgen 1978; 130:988–991.

B0025                                    **Zvi Borochowitz**
                                          *Ralph S. Lachman*
                                          *David L. Rimoin*

**Dysostosis enchondralis metaepiphysaria, Catel-Hempel type**
  *See CHONDRODYSTROPHIC MYOTONIA, SCHWARTZ-JAMPEL TYPE*
**Dysostosis mandibulofacial**
  *See MANDIBULOFACIAL DYSOSTOSIS*
**Dysostosis, acrofacial**
  *See ACROFACIAL DYSOSTOSIS*

## DYSOSTOSIS, CHEIROLUMBAR                    2692

**Includes:**
  Cheirolumbar dysostosis
  Wackenheim syndrome

**Excludes:**
  **Acrodysostosis** (0016)
  Brachydactyly-hypertension
  **Parathyroid hormone resistance** (0830)
  Pippow syndrome
  Pseudopseudohypoparathyroidism

**Major Diagnostic Criteria:**  The association of a narrowed lumbar canal and shortness of one or several phalanges, with or without one or more metacarpals. May be unilateral or bilateral.

**Clinical Findings:**  May be well tolerated in minor forms. More severe forms provoke subjective and objective symptoms of radicular pain, sciatica, neurogenic claudication, and even cauda equina paralysis. No significant laboratory findings or alterations of dermatoglyphics or karyotype have been noted.

**Complications:**  Arthrosis in digital and lumbar articulations. Paralysis in the field of the cauda equina.

**Associated Findings:**  In the extremities, the shortening may also involve the feet (phalanges and metatarsals). The anomaly is then an acrolumbar dysostosis. In the spinal canal, the narrowing may also involve the cervical segment and, more rarely, the thoracic segment. The anomaly is then a cheirocervicolumbar or cheirothoracolumbar dysostosis.

**Etiology:**  Autosomal dominant inheritance of the severe form. In a given family with the severe form, 50% are normal. The other 50% have brachycheiry or lumbar stenosis or both (in two families described).

**Pathogenesis:**  Unknown.

**Sex Ratio:**  Presumably M1:F1.

**Occurrence:**  Well-tolerated minor forms are probably frequent. Two kinships with a severe familial form have been documented.

**Risk of Recurrence for Patient's Sib:**
  See Part I, *Mendelian Inheritance.*

**Risk of Recurrence for Patient's Child:**
  See Part I, *Mendelian Inheritance.*

**Age of Detectability:**  After 10 years of age.

**Gene Mapping and Linkage:**  Unknown.

**Prevention:**  None known. Genetic counseling indicated.

**Treatment:**  Laminectomy to enlarge the spinal canal is indicated only in cases with neurologic deficiency or severe neurogenic claudication.

**Prognosis:**  Life span not affected. The neurologic prognosis depends on the severity of the lumbar canal narrowing and the response to surgical treatment.

**Detection of Carrier:**  Clinical and X-ray examinations of hands and lumbar spines.

**Special Considerations:**  Cheirolumbar dysostosis is determined by hypoplasia of phalanges, metacarpals, and posterior arches. There is no specific malformation of the bones. In both locations

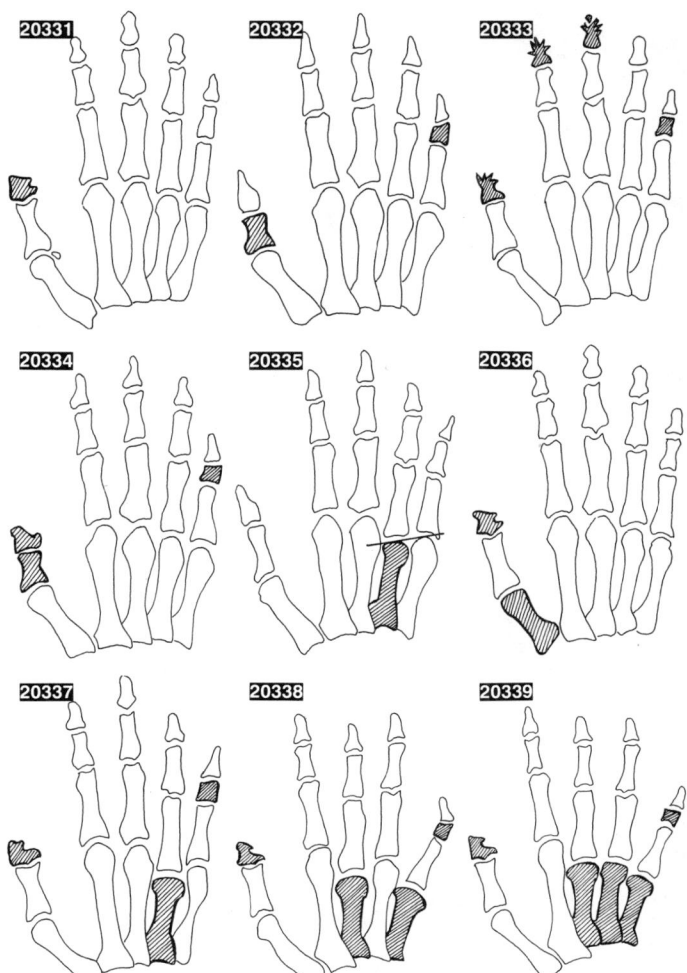

**2692A-**20331–39: Nonexhaustive varieties of brachyphalangia and brachymetacarpia occurring in patients with cheirolumbar dysostosis.

(hands and vertebrae), the anomaly consists of shortness and broadness of the bones. There are numerous methods for measuring the lengths of the phalanges and metacarpals, and the diameters of the lumbar canal.

**References:**
Wackenheim A: Une dysostose cheirolumbaire (brachymétacarpophalangie et dysostose sténosante de l'arc vertébral postérieur). J Radiol 1978; 59:563–566.
Wackenheim A: Disostosis chiro-lombare. Radiol Med (Torino) 1979; 65:1–21.
Wackenheim A, ed: Cheirolumbar dysostosis. Heidelberg: Springer-Verlag, 1980.
Wackenheim A: Cheirolumbar dysostosis: developmental brachycheiry and narrowness of the lumbar canal. In: Wackenheim A, Babin E, eds: The narrow lumbar canal. Heidelberg: Springer-Verlag, 1980:147–155.
Kretzschmar R: Zur Rontgenologie der cheirolumbalen Dysostose. Radiologie 1989; 29:447–450.
Wackenheim A: Disostosi cheirolombare: eredita Mendaliana in una famiglia. Rivista di Neuroradiologia 1989; 2:11–20.

WA050                                    **A. Wackenheim**

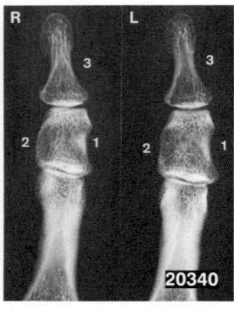
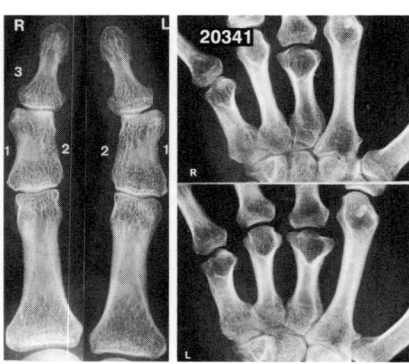
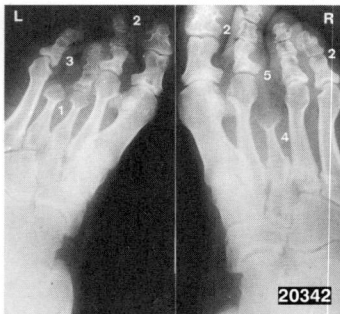
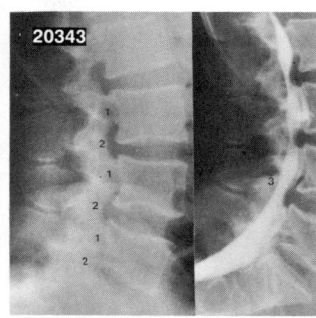

**2692B-20340:** Brachymesophalangia in two patients with cheirolumbar dysostosis. 1: Concave cubital aspect of the middle phalanx on both sides. 2: Convex radial aspect of the middle phalanx on both sides. 3: Radially bent distal phalanx. **20341:** Bilateral brachymetacarpia. **20342:** Brachymetatarsia in a patient with cheirolumbar dysostosis. 1: Brachymetatarsia of the third and fourth rays. 2: Very marked diffuse brachyphalangia. 3: Surgically amputated phalanges of the fourth ray. 4: Brachymetatarsia of the third ray. 5: Surgically amputated phalanges of the third ray. **20343:** Constitutional stenosis of the lumbar canal in a patient with cheirolumbar dysostosis. 1: Short pedicles. 2: Narrow intervertebral foramina. 3: Narrow dural sac.

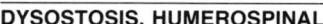

## DYSOSTOSIS, HUMEROSPINAL               2698

**Includes:**

    Humerospinal dysostosis
    Skeletal dysplasia, humerospinal dysostosis

**Excludes:**

    **Atelosteogenesis** (2521)
    **Chondrodysplasia punctata, mild symmetric type** (0153)
    **Chondrodysplasia punctata, rhizomelic type** (0154)
    **Chondrodysplasia punctata, X-linked dominant type** (2730)
    **Dwarfism, dyssegmental, Rolland-Desbuquois type** (2690)
    **Dwarfism, dyssegmental, Silverman-Handmaker type** (2935)
    **Fibrochondrogenesis** (2694)
    **Kniest dysplasia** (0557)
    **Kniest-like dysplasia** (2799)
    **Metatropic dysplasia** (0656)
    Malsegmentations of the spine-coronal cleft vertebrae (other)

**Major Diagnostic Criteria:** Bifid distal humeral metaphyses, subluxation in the elbow joints, coronal cleft vertebrae, and congenital heart disease.

**Clinical Findings:** At birth: congenital heart disease, talipes equinovarus, dislocated knees, elbow deformities, short humeri, narrow thorax, lumbar hyperlordosis, hypertelorism, and limitation of joint movements.

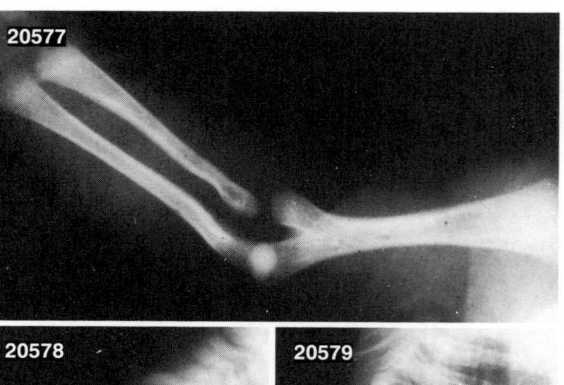
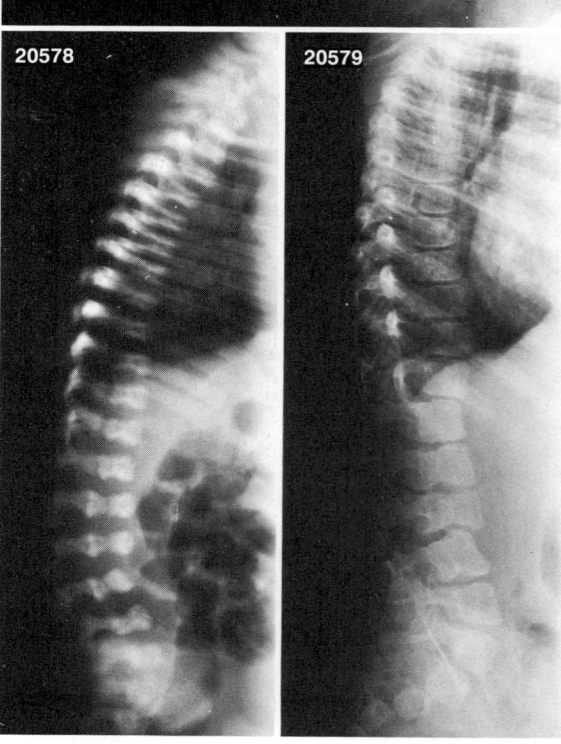

**2698-20577:** Dysostosis, humerospinal; note bifid distal end of the humerus in a six-week-old infant. **20578:** Mid-coronal clefts of the vertebral bodies in this two-week-old infant. **20579:** Dysplastic lumbar vertebral bodies in a 13-month-old infant.

**Complications:** Shortening of stature, spine malalignments, limitation of joint movements, and those of congenital heart disease. Death, possible early in life, because of congenital heart disease.

**Associated Findings:** None known.

**Etiology:** Unknown.

**Pathogenesis:** Unknown.

**POS No.:** 4077

**Sex Ratio:** Presumably M1:F1.

**Occurrence:** Undetermined but presumed rare.

**Risk of Recurrence for Patient's Sib:** Unknown.

**Risk of Recurrence for Patient's Child:** Unknown.

**Age of Detectability:** At birth, by X-ray.

**Gene Mapping and Linkage:** Unknown.

**Prevention:** None known. Genetic counseling indicated.

**Treatment:** Orthopedic and rehabilitative treatment to prevent or correct limb and spine deformities.

**Prognosis:** Probably normal for life span in patients who are free of severe cardiac malformation.

**Detection of Carrier:** Unknown.

**References:**

Kozlowski KS, et al.: Humero-spinal dysostosis with congenital heart disease. Am J Dis Child 1974; 127:407–410.

Cortina H, et al.: Humero-spinal dysostosis. Pediatr Radiol 1979; 8:188–190.

K0021 **K.S. Kozlowski**

**Dysostosis, peripheral**
*See ACROMESOMELIC DYSPLASIA, MAROTEAUX-MARTINELLI-CAMPAILLA TYPE*

**Dysostosis, peripheral-nasal hypoplasia-mental retardation (PNM)**
*See ACRODYSOSTOSIS*

## DYSPLASIA EPIPHYSEALIS HEMIMELICA　0311

**Includes:**

Carpal osteochondroma
Epiphyseal osteochondroma, benign
Hemimelic skeletal dysplasias
Osteochondroma, intra-articular of the astragalus
Osteochondroma of the distal femoral epiphysis
Tarsomegaly
Trevor disease

**Excludes:**

**Enchondromatosis** (0345)
**Epiphyseal dysplasia, multiple** (0358)
**Exostoses, multiple cartilaginous** (0685)
**Metachondromatosis** (0650)

**Major Diagnostic Criteria:** Hemimelic involvement of one or more epiphyses, tarsal or carpal centers.

**Clinical Findings:** A developmental disorder of childhood in which there is asymmetric cartilaginous overgrowth of one or more epiphysis or of a tarsal or carpal bone. It is usually limited to the medial or lateral half of a single limb, although the entire epiphysis may at times be involved. The usual presentation is with unilateral swelling about the inner or outer aspects of the ankles or knees, pain, deformity, or limitation of motion. The medial side is affected twice as often as the lateral side. Multiple lesions did occur in two of three cases, but involvement of the upper limbs is rare.

Observed frequencies are talus, 61.5%; distal femoral epiphysis, 45.5%; proximal tibial epiphysis, 26.5%; tarsal navicular, 24.5%; medial cuneiform, 17.5%; distal fibular epiphysis, 17.5%; and femoral capital epiphysis, 8.8%. The deformities and size of lesions increase with the growth of epiphyses. The earliest X-ray changes are premature appearance of the osseous centers on the affected side. Thereafter, an irregular radio-opacity develops on one side of the epiphysis. The lesions appear as irregular, lobulated osseous masses protruding from one side of the epiphysis. The final appearance may be similar to an exostosis. There are no characteristic laboratory changes and no known systemic associations.

**Complications:** Deformity of the affected bone due to unequal involvement of the epiphyses. The most common deformities are genu valgum or varum and valgus or equinus deformity of the ankle. Pain and limitation of motion may occur at the involved joint. Pain may result from an osteochondral fracture. Occasionally, inequality of limb size, both shortening and lengthening, may occur.

**Associated Findings:** None known.

**Etiology:** Undetermined. There is no familial aggregation. The disorder is thought to be an embryopathy of limb bud formation occurring at about the fifth week of fetal development.

**Pathogenesis:** Thought to result from an ectopic focus of proliferating cartilage on the epiphyseal side of the growth plate, with subsequent enchondral ossification. Both by gross inspection and microscopically the lesions are indistinguishable from osteocartilaginous exostosis. There are no reports of malignant degeneration.

**MIM No.:** 12780

**POS No.:** 3742

**Sex Ratio:** M3:F1

**Occurrence:** Unknown.

**Risk of Recurrence for Patient's Sib:** Not thought to be increased.

**Risk of Recurrence for Patient's Child:** Not thought to be increased.

**Age of Detectability:** May be detected from birth to adult life, with the most frequent ages of detection being 2 and 14 years, by X-ray.

**Gene Mapping and Linkage:** Unknown.

**Prevention:** None known. Genetic counseling indicated.

**Treatment:** This is a localized deformity in an otherwise normal child and requires early orthopedic correction to avoid deformities of the affected limb. The involved epiphysis should be excised in patients having pain, deformity, unequal limb length, or limitation of motion.

**Prognosis:** Normal for life span and intelligence. Function is also good after early orthopedic correction.

**Detection of Carrier:** Unknown.

**Special Considerations:** Secondary metaphyseal abnormalities such as bone spurs, or streaking and bowing of the metaphysis as in enchondromatosis may develop. Active growth of lesions may occur in adult life. The lesions in this condition are distinguished from those in multiple exostoses only by their epiphyseal location and lack of diaphyseal migration.

**References:**

Trevor, D.: Tarso-epiphysial aclasis: a congenital error of epiphyseal development. J Bone Joint Surg 1950; 32B:204–213.

Kettelkamp DB, et al.: Dysplasia epiphysealis hemimelica: a report of fifteen cases and review of the literature. J Bone Joint Surg 1966; 48A:746–766.

Theodorou S, Lanitis G: Dysplasia epiphysialis hemimelica (epiphyseal osteochondromata). Report of two cases and review of the literature. Helv Paediatr Acta 1968; 23:195–204.

Carlson DH, Wilkenson RH: Variability of unilateral epiphyseal dysplasia. Radiology 1979; 133:369.

Widemann HR, et al.: Dysplasia epiphysealis hemimelica. Eur J Pediatr 1981; 136:311–316.

Connor JM, et al.: Dysplasia epiphysialis hemimelica. J Bone Joint Surg 1983; 65B:350–354.

LA006 **Ralph S. Lachman**

**Dysplasia epiphysealis punctata**
*See CHONDRODYSPLASIA PUNCTATA, X-LINKED DOMINANT TYPE*

**Dysplasia epiphysialis multiplex**
*See EPIPHYSEAL DYSPLASIA, MULTIPLE*

**Dysplasia olfactogenitalis of DeMorsier**
*See KALLMANN SYNDROME*

**Dysplasia spondyloepiphysaria tarda**
*See SPONDYLOEPIPHYSEAL DYSPLASIA, LATE*

**Dysplasia, arterio-hepatic**
*See ARTERIO-HEPATIC DYSPLASIA*

**Dysplasia, cleidocranial**
*See CLEIDOCRANIAL DYSPLASIA*

**Dysplasia, congenital thymic type**
*See IMMUNODEFICIENCY, X-LINKED SEVERE COMBINED*

**Dysplasia, cranio-diaphyseal**
*See CRANIO-DIAPHYSEAL DYSPLASIA*

**Dysplasia, craniometaphyseal**
*See CRANIOMETAPHYSEAL DYSPLASIA*

**Dysplasia, osteodental**
*See CLEIDOCRANIAL DYSPLASIA*

**Dysplasia-gigantism syndrome, X-linked**
*See SIMPSON-GOLABI-BEHMEL SYNDROME*

**Dysplastic nevus syndrome**
*See CANCER, MALIGNANT MELANOMA, FAMILIAL*

**Dysplastic spondylolisthesis and spondylolysis**
*See SPINE, SPONDYLOLISTHESIS AND SPONDYLOLYSIS*
**Dysprothrombinemia**
*See HYPOPROTHROMBINEMIA*
**Dyssegmental dwarfism**
*See DWARFISM, DYSSEGMENTAL, ROLLAND-DESBUQUOIS TYPE*
**Dyssegmental dysplasia, mild type**
*See DWARFISM, DYSSEGMENTAL, ROLLAND-DESBUQUOIS TYPE*
**Dyssegmental dysplasia, Silverman type**
*See DWARFISM, DYSSEGMENTAL, SILVERMAN-HANDMAKER TYPE*
**Dyssynergia cerebellaris myoclonica (some cases)**
*See SEIZURES, PROGRESSIVE MYOCLONIC, UNVERRICHT-
LUNDBORG TYPE*
**Dystonia musculorum deformans**
*See TORSION DYSTONIA*
**Dystonia, atypical torsion**
*See DEAFNESS (SENSORINEURAL)-DYSTONIA*
**Dystonia-neural deafness, familial**
*See DEAFNESS (SENSORINEURAL)-DYSTONIA*
**Dystopia canthorum**
*See HYPERTELORISM-HYPOSPADIAS SYNDROME*
**Dystopic lipidosis, hereditary**
*See FABRY DISEASE*
**Dystrophia myotonica**
*See MYOTONIC DYSTROPHY*

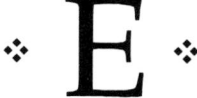

Eagle-Barrett syndrome
*See PRUNE-BELLY SYNDROME*
Ear abnormalities-short stature-elbow/hip dislocation
*See AURICULO-OSTEODYSPLASIA*
Ear anomalies-contractures-dysplasia of bone with kyphoscoliosis
*See ARACHNODACTYLY, CONTRACTURAL BEALS TYPE*
Ear bump
*See EAR, EXCHONDROSIS*
Ear defects-deafness-facial palsy
*See DEAFNESS-EAR DEFECTS-FACIAL PALSY*
Ear lobe sinuses
*See EAR LOBE, PIT*

## EAR LOBE, ATTACHED — 0323

**Includes:** Earlobe attachment: attached vs unattached

**Excludes:** **Ear, lobe, absent** (0320)

**Major Diagnostic Criteria:** Attachment of ear lobe to head.

**Clinical Findings:** Lower part of ear attached directly onto head with no free-hanging lobes. There may be considerable variation in the shape of the lower part of ear.

**Complications:** Unknown.

**Associated Findings:** None known.

**Etiology:** Possibly autosomal dominant inheritance, although probably polygenic.

**Pathogenesis:** Unknown.

**MIM No.:** 12890

**Sex Ratio:** M1:F1

**Occurrence:** About 1:7 in Germany.

**Risk of Recurrence for Patient's Sib:**
See Part I, *Mendelian Inheritance.*

**Risk of Recurrence for Patient's Child:**
See Part I, *Mendelian Inheritance.*

**Age of Detectability:** At birth.

**Gene Mapping and Linkage:** Unknown.

**Prevention:** None known. Genetic counseling indicated.

**Treatment:** None indicated.

**Prognosis:** Normal for life span, intelligence, and function.

**Detection of Carrier:** Unknown.

**References:**
Powell EF, Whitney DD: Ear lobe inheritance: an unusual 3-generation photographic pedigree-chart. J Hered 1937; 28:185–186.
Dutta P, Granguly P: Further observations on ear lobe attachment. Acta Genet Statist Med 1965; 15:77–86.
Lai LYC, Walsh RJ: Observations on ear lobe types. Acta Genet Statist Med 1966; 16:250–257.
Mohanraju C, Mukherjee DP: Ear lobe attachment in an Andhra village and other parts of India. Hum Hered 1973; 23:288–297.

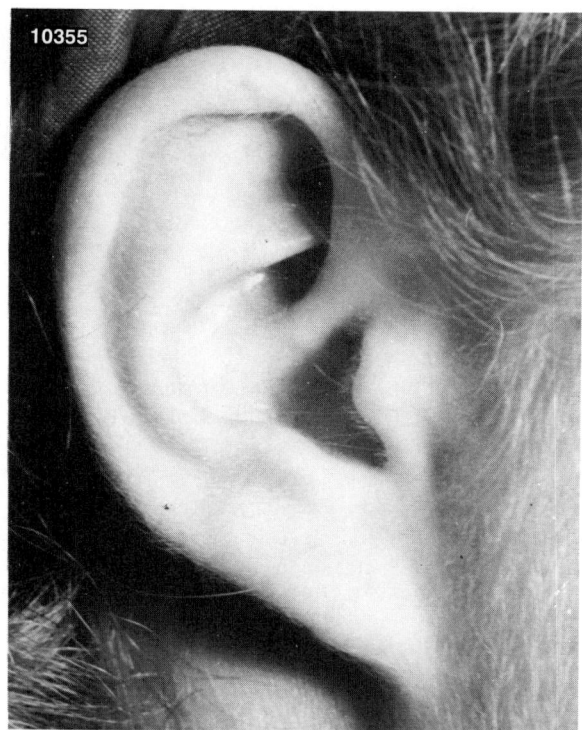
10355

0323-10355: Attached earlobe.

Winchester AM: Genetics: a survey of the principles of heredity, ed 3. Boston: Houghton Mifflin, 1977.

WI034

**A.M. Winchester**

## EAR LOBE, CLEFT — 0321

**Includes:** Cleft ear lobe

**Excludes:**
Atresia (alone)
**Deafness-ear pits** (0247)
**Ear, Darwin tubercle** (0241)
Ear flare
Ear lobe crease
**Ear lobe, pit** (0322)
**Ear, microtia-atresia** (0664)

**Major Diagnostic Criteria:** Longitudinal cleft of lobule.

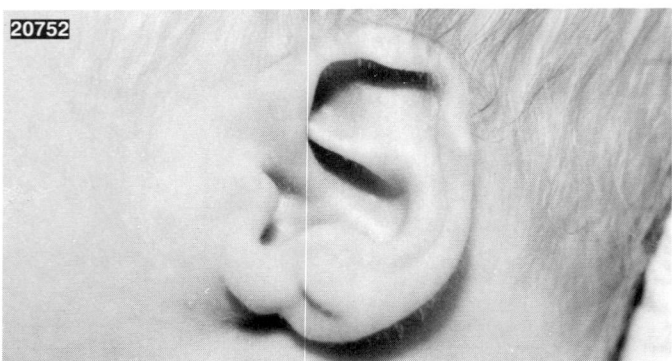

0321-20752: Ear lobe, cleft.

**Clinical Findings:** Coloboma lobuli. The ear lobe is cleft longitudinally. The cleft may be partial, but usually extends to, but not through, the incisura intertragica. The deformity may be unilateral or bilateral.

**Complications:** Unknown.

**Associated Findings:** None known.

**Etiology:** Unknown.

**Pathogenesis:** Unknown.

**Sex Ratio:** Presumably M1:F1

**Occurrence:** Unknown.

**Risk of Recurrence for Patient's Sib:** Unknown.

**Risk of Recurrence for Patient's Child:** Unknown.

**Age of Detectability:** At birth.

**Gene Mapping and Linkage:** Unknown.

**Prevention:** None known. Genetic counseling indicated.

**Treatment:** Plastic surgical repair may be indicated.

**Prognosis:** Good for life span, intelligence, and function if isolated defect of outer ear; otherwise, dependent on concomitant defects.

**Detection of Carrier:** Unknown.

**References:**
Converse JM, ed: Reconstructive plastic surgery. Vol. 3. Philadelphia: W.B. Saunders, 1964.
Rubin A, ed: Handbook of congenital malformations. Philadelphia: W.B. Saunders, 1967.

BE028                                                    **LaVonne Bergstrom**

## EAR LOBE, HYPERTROPHIC THICKENED                    0324

**Includes:**
   Deafness (bilateral conductive)-absent incus-stapes
   Deafness (conductive)-thickened ear lobes
   Earlobes (thick)-deafness from incudostapedial
      abnormalities
   Hypertrophic ear lobes
**Excludes:**
   Atresia (alone)
   **Deafness-ear pits** (0247)
   **Ear, Darwin tubercle** (0241)
   Ear flare
   **Ear lobe, pit** (0322)
   **Ear, microtia-atresia** (0664)
**Major Diagnostic Criteria:** Disproportionately large, thick ear lobes.

**Clinical Findings:** The ear lobe is disproportionately large for the overall size of the ear, is thickened, and feels fibrotic in the center of the lobule. Affected persons have an associated congenital conductive hearing loss. The eardrum is normal. At tympanotomy a malformed incus that does not articulate with the stapes is found. Histologic examination of the incus shows a nest of connective tissue fibers at its distal end.

**Complications:** Hearing loss and possible secondary speech disorder.

**Associated Findings:** Malformed incus that does not articulate with the stapes.

**Etiology:** Autosomal dominant inheritance.

**Pathogenesis:** Exploration of the middle ear has shown curvature of the long crus of the incus and absence of the head of the stapes with a fibrous band connecting the two bones.

**MIM No.:** *12898

**Sex Ratio:** M1:F1

**Occurrence:** Unknown. Documented in two kindreds.

**Risk of Recurrence for Patient's Sib:**
   See Part I, *Mendelian Inheritance.*

**Risk of Recurrence for Patient's Child:**
   See Part I, *Mendelian Inheritance.*

**Age of Detectability:** At birth, although conductive hearing loss might not be suspected for several years.

**Gene Mapping and Linkage:** Unknown.

**Prevention:** None known. Genetic counseling indicated.

**Treatment:** If this is an isolated defect, no treatment is usually needed. If conductive hearing loss is present, computed tomography should be done to assess the anatomic configuration of the middle ear, and, if it seems favorable, exploratory tympanotomy and surgical correction should be performed, if feasible. If not feasible, if unsuccessful, or if the patient has a sensorineural hearing loss, hearing aids should be fitted, and aural rehabilitation should be undertaken.

**Prognosis:** Good for life span, intelligence and function if isolated defect of outer ear; otherwise, dependent on concomitant defects.

**Detection of Carrier:** Unknown.

**Special Considerations:** External ear anomalies should also prompt the physician to look for anomalies of other systems and to follow the infant for possible mental retardation. Careful genetic and clinical studies of the family should be carried out if accompanying defects are found.

**References:**
Escher F, Hirt H: Dominant hereditary conductive deafness through lack of incus-stapes junction. Acta Otolaryngol (Stockh) 1968; 65:25–32.
Konigsmark BW: Hereditary deafness with external-ear abnormalities: a review. Johns Hopkins Med J 1970; 127:228.
Wilmot TJ: Hereditary conductive deafness due to incus-stapes abnormalities and associated with pinna deformity. J Laryngol 1970; 84:469–479.
Prasad U, Chin YH: Bilateral congenital absence of incus. J Laryngol Otol 1980; 94:773.

BE028                                                    **LaVonne Bergstrom**

## EAR LOBE, PIT                                                    0322

**Includes:**
Ear lobe sinuses
Earring holes, natural

**Excludes:** N/A

**Major Diagnostic Criteria:** Pit in ear lobe.

**Clinical Findings:** Pit about 1 mm deep in ear lobes at about the point where they would normally be pierced for earrings. The holes do not completely penetrate the lobe.

**Complications:** Unknown.

**Associated Findings:** None known.

**Etiology:** Autosomal dominant inheritance with variable expressivity and incomplete penetrance. In about one-half of the cases the pit is in only one lobe, and in a few cases the gene is carried without showing pits in either lobe.

**Pathogenesis:** Unknown.

**MIM No.:** 12900

**Sex Ratio:** M1:F1

**Occurrence:** Rare. Natural "earring" holes have been reported in one kinship.

**Risk of Recurrence for Patient's Sib:**
See Part I, *Mendelian Inheritance.*

**Risk of Recurrence for Patient's Child:**
See Part I, *Mendelian Inheritance.*

**Age of Detectability:** At birth.

**Gene Mapping and Linkage:** Unknown.

**Prevention:** None known. Genetic counseling indicated.

**Treatment:** None indicated.

**Prognosis:** Normal for life span, intelligence, and function.

**Detection of Carrier:** Unknown.

**References:**
Edmonds HW, Keeler CE: Natural "ear-ring" holes; inherited sinuses of ear lobe. J Hered 1940; 31:507–510.
Winchester AM: Genetics: a survey of the principles of heredity, ed 3. Boston: Houghton Mifflin, 1977:450.

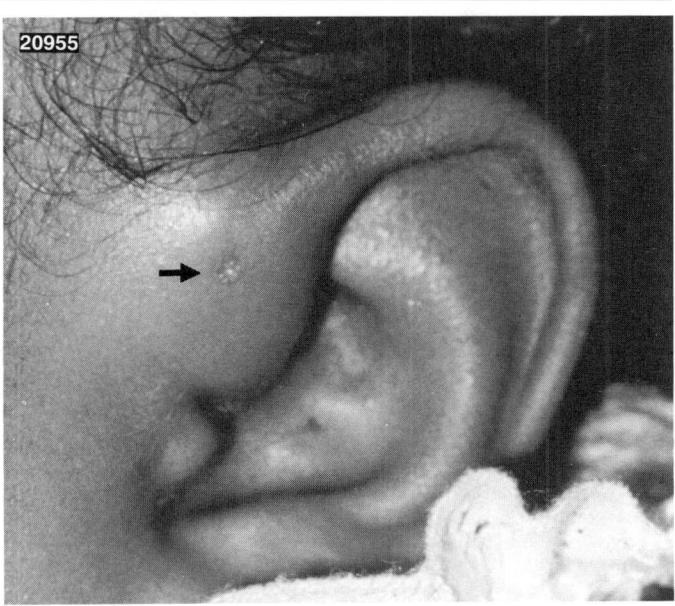

0322-20955:   Pre-auricular pit.

Ramirez M-L, Cantu JM: Two distinct autosomal dominant traits in the pinna. BD:OAS; 18(3B). New York: March of Dimes Birth Defects Foundation, 1982:243–246.

WI034                                                    **A.M. Winchester**

**Ear lobe-syndactyly-polydactyly syndrome**
*See SYNDACTYLY-POLYDACTYLY-EAR LOBE SYNDROME*
**Ear malformations-cervical fistulas/nodules-mixed hearing loss**
*See BRANCHIO-OTO-RENAL DYSPLASIA*
**Ear malformations-lateral/branchial cervical fistulas-deafness**
*See DEAFNESS-EAR PITS*
**Ear pit-deafness syndrome**
*See BRANCHIO-OTO-RENAL DYSPLASIA*
**Ear pits and external ear malformations with deafness**
*See DEAFNESS-EAR PITS*
**Ear wax types**
*See EAR, CERUMEN VARIATIONS*
**Ear without helix**
*See EAR, LOP*

## EAR, ABSENT TRAGUS                                              0312

**Includes:** Tragus, of ear, absent

**Excludes:**
Atresia (alone)
**Deafness-ear pits** (0247)
**Ear, Darwin tubercle** (0241)
Ear flare
**Ear lobe, pit** (0322)
**Ear, microtia-atresia** (0664)

**Major Diagnostic Criteria:** Absent tragus of ear.

**Clinical Findings:** Usually seen only in conditions in which the mandible is also absent or markedly hypoplastic.

**Complications:** Unknown.

**Associated Findings:** Agnathia or severe micrognathia. Sporadic cases of hearing loss have been reported.

**Etiology:** Unknown.

**Pathogenesis:** Unknown.

**Sex Ratio:** Presumed M1:F1

**Occurrence:** Presumed rare.

**Risk of Recurrence for Patient's Sib:** Unknown.

**Risk of Recurrence for Patient's Child:** Unknown.

**Age of Detectability:** At birth.

**Gene Mapping and Linkage:** Unknown.

**Prevention:** None known. Genetic counseling indicated.

**Treatment:** If isolated defect, no treatment is needed.

**Prognosis:** Good for life span, intelligence and function if isolated defect of outer ear, otherwise dependent upon concomitant defects.

**Detection of Carrier:** Unknown.

**Special Considerations:** Anomalies of the external ear should suggest the possibility of an anomaly of the middle ear as well. Hearing should be assessed as soon as possible and appropriate therapy instituted. The anatomy of the middle and inner ear should be determined by computed tomography of the temporal bones if there is an associated hearing loss.

**References:**
Converse JM, ed: Reconstructive plastic surgery. vol. 3. Philadelphia: W.B. Saunders, 1964.

BE028                                                    **LaVonne Bergstrom**

## EAR, ANEURYSM OF INTERNAL CAROTID ARTERY    0530

**Includes:**
Aneurysm of middle ear
Carotid artery aneurysm
Internal carotid artery aneurysm of middle ear
Middle ear aneurysm of internal carotid artery

**Excludes:**
Aneurysm of the lateral dural sinus
Arteriovenous aneurysm of internal carotid artery
**Ear; Chemodectoma of middle ear** (0145)
Posttraumatic carotid artery aneurysm in middle ear

**Major Diagnostic Criteria:** Aneurysm of the middle ear demonstrated by carotid angiography.

**Clinical Findings:** The patient may present with spontaneous bleeding from the ear or profuse bleeding after mild trauma. There may be a history of, or symptoms suggesting, acute suppurative ear disease or chronic adhesive otitis. Profuse, pulsatile, bright red bleeding follows attempted myringotomy. The patient may complain of pulsatile tinnitus, deafness, vertigo, or facial nerve weakness. CNS symptoms, headache, vomiting, convulsions, and cranial nerve palsies may be seen with extensive aneurysms. The patient may have had previous middle ear exploration or mastoidectomy associated with severe bleeding from the middle ear during surgery. In some cases there may be associated bleeding from the nose.

Physical examination may show a red bulge and visible pulsation behind the tympanic membrane. Pneumatic otoscopy under operating microscope magnification may show blanching with pressure. Often a bruit can be heard over the skull or over the carotid artery system in the neck. Facial paresis or palsy may be present as well as nystagmus. Caloric examination may demonstrate asymmetric response or absent response to stimuli on the involved side. Conductive, sensorineural, or mixed hearing loss is often present, and complete hearing loss may occur.

Clinical examination usually does not reveal the true nature of the problem which, however, becomes evident on carotid angiography. Angiography is diagnostic and delineates the extent of the aneurysm and rules out multiple aneurysms, since their incidence in all intracranial aneurysm patients is 13–25%. Computerized tomography of the petrous bone with contrast enhancement may also be helpful. Magnetic resonance imaging is now the diagnostic study of choice, since there is no radiation given and the soft tissue delineation is good.

**Complications:** Anemia, shock, hypoxemia, and death from hemorrhage; facial or vestibular paresis or palsy; hearing loss; bone erosion; CNS symptoms, e.g. seizures, coma, and cranial nerve palsies.

**Associated Findings:** Strabismus was reported in only one case. In another, a large anomalous trigeminal or auditory artery and a rudimentary vertebral artery were found in association with absence of the opposite carotid artery system.

**Etiology:** Unknown.

**Pathogenesis:** This is a type of the berry aneurysm seen elsewhere intracranially, possibly caused by a developmental deficiency in the medial layer of arteries, or weaknesses in the wall where embryonic capillary plexuses opened. However, there is considerable disagreement about both of these concepts.

**Sex Ratio:** Presumably M1:F1

**Occurrence:** Ten cases have been documented.

**Risk of Recurrence for Patient's Sib:** Unknown.

**Risk of Recurrence for Patient's Child:** Unknown.

**Age of Detectability:** Variable. Detected when aural bleeding occurs, but it would be possible to suspect the diagnosis in a patient who has a feeling of stuffiness in the ear, pulsatile tinnitus, hearing loss, vertigo, or facial weakness. The presence of a pulsatile middle ear mass in a child is especially suspicious.

**Gene Mapping and Linkage:** Unknown.

**Prevention:** None known. Genetic counseling indicated.

**Treatment:** Ligation of the homolateral common carotid artery may be effective. However, surgical exposure of the middle ear via a tympanotomy, mastoidectomy, or temporal bone resection with control of the carotid artery in the neck may be necessary. Resection or clipping of the aneurysm can then be accomplished. Cryoprobe therapy is not effective. Ligation of the internal carotid artery may be necessary; in about 25% of patients various motor, sensory and speech deficits, or even death may ensue.

Tight packing of the external auditory canal or mastoid cavity (if there is one) with hemostatic gauze or sponge material or ordinary dry strip packing, digital compression of the carotid artery in the neck, blood transfusions and other supportive measures may be needed for management of acute hemorrhage prior to definitive diagnosis and therapy.

**Prognosis:** Death may result from exsanguinating hemorrhage. This occurred in two of eight reported cases, as compared with a mortality rate of 44–55% in other intracranial aneurysms. Complete hearing loss may occur secondary to bone erosion from the aneurysm, from tight emergency aural packing, or from necessary definitive surgery. Facial paresis or palsy, vestibular loss, and CNS damage also occur but less frequently.

The likelihood of rebleeding is high in patients in whom only emergency tamponade is performed, but rebleeding has not been reported after definitive surgery.

**Detection of Carrier:** Unknown.

**Special Considerations:** Patients with profuse aural bleeding should be controlled by emergency and supportive measures and then given definitive diagnostic measures and definitive therapy promptly, as the probability of rebleeding is high.

**References:**
Ehni G, Barrett JH: Hemorrhage from the ear due to an aneurysm of the internal carotid artery. New Engl J Med 1960; 262:1323.
Grinker RR, Sahs AL: Neurology. 6th ed. Springfield: Charles C Thomas, 1966.
Allen GW: Angiography in otolaryngology. Laryngoscope 1967; 77:1909.
Conley J, Hildyard V: Aneurysm of the internal carotid artery presenting in the middle ear. Arch Otolaryngol 1969; 90:35. *
Stallings JO, McCabe BF: Congenital middle ear aneurysm of internal carotid. Arch Otolaryngol 1969; 90:39. *
Sinnreich AI, et al.: Arterial malformations of the middle ear. Otolaryngology Head and Neck Surg 1984; 92:194–206.

BE028                                         **LaVonne Bergstrom**

## EAR, ARTERIOVENOUS FISTULA    0313

**Includes:**
Aneurysm serpentina of external ear
Angioma cavernosum of external ear
Arteriovenous aneurysm of external ear
Cirsoid aneurysm of external ear
Venous aneurysm of external ear, pulsating

**Excludes:**
Chondroma of ear
Dermoid of ear
Fibroma of external ear
Hemangioma of ear
Lymphangioma of ear
**Nevus flammeus** (0715)

**Major Diagnostic Criteria:** The history of an enlarged, pinkish-to-bluish, distorted, pulsatile auricle manifesting itself at birth or within the first two decades of life plus physical findings of the above signs (perhaps with overlying bruit). Retrograde arteriography may be helpful, but is not essential to the diagnosis. Unlike acquired arteriovenous fistulae occurring in other body regions, there is no related cardiac hypertrophy or failure. This is probably due to the smaller caliber of the arteriovenous communications of the external ear.

**Clinical Findings:** Enlargement and distortion of the auricle or a part thereof. This has a pinkish-to-bluish discoloration, is often pulsatile, may have a bruit, and usually involves adjacent portions of cheek, scalp, or neck. In 3 of 8 cases, necrosis and hemorrhage occurred from the affected auricle. Ipsilateral increase in facial bone growth has occasionally been observed, usually with the more extensive arteriovenous fistulae. Retrograde arteriography demonstrates increased vascularity of the involved auricle.

**Complications:** Perichondritis of auricle; necrosis (ulceration of auricle) in 3 of 8 cases; hemorrhage from auricle in 3 of 8 cases.

**Associated Findings:** None known.

**Etiology:** Unknown.

**Pathogenesis:** Normally there are rich anastomoses between the internal carotid and external carotid arteries along the walls of the external auditory meatus. This vascular network along with venous channels differentiates from an embryonal plexus of fine tubules. Most of these channels become obliterated. Congenital arteriovenous fistulae result from failure of obliteration of these embryonal connections. The progressive enlargement of this lesion is apparently due to the ability of arteriovenous fistulae to stimulate the formation of collateral circulation.

**Sex Ratio:** M3:F5 (observed)

**Occurrence:** Eight cases have been documented.

**Risk of Recurrence for Patient's Sib:** Unknown.

**Risk of Recurrence for Patient's Child:** Unknown.

**Age of Detectability:** From birth through the second decade by means of physical examination.

**Gene Mapping and Linkage:** Unknown.

**Prevention:** None known. Genetic counseling indicated.

**Treatment:** The only successful treatment is complete excision of the involved auricle with plastic or prosthetic reconstruction of the auricle. Attempts at ligation of feeding vessels have been unsuccessful in that some channels are invariably overlooked. It is possible that embolization of the vessels, using new techniques, might be successful.

**Prognosis:** With adequate excision of the lesion, a normal life span can be anticipated. In the untreated patient, death from auricular hemorrhage is possible.

**Detection of Carrier:** Unknown.

**References:**
Dingman RO, Grabb WC: Congenital arteriovenous fistulae of the external ear. Plast Reconstr Surg 1965; 35:620.

BE028                                          **LaVonne Bergstrom**

## EAR, AUDITORY CANAL ATRESIA                        **0097**

**Includes:** Auditory canal, atresia of

**Excludes:**
Ear, microtia-atresia (0664)
Postsurgical stenosis of external auditory canal
Posttraumatic stenosis of external auditory canal

**Major Diagnostic Criteria:** Atresia of external auditory canal.

**Clinical Findings:** The appearance of the pinna is not diagnostic. The patient may have a normal pinna or one that is somewhat low-set, large, small, or with a minor variation such as a prominent anthelix or folded-over helix. The canal may be completely atretic, without a visible meatus, or may appear patent, only to funnel down to complete atresia at about the osseous-cartilaginous junction of the ear canal. Membranous occlusion has also been reported. Limited information is available regarding polytomography or other X-ray findings in the ears. X-rays demonstrate the bony atresia but have been otherwise normal except for one report in which the middle ear in the unilateral case was smaller than that on the normal side. Vestibular testing by rotation has been done in a few cases and was reported to be normal. At surgical exploration one or more of the following middle ear anomalies have been noted: fixation of the malleus to the tympanic plate, stapes footplate fixation, fusion of the malleus and incus, abnormal course of the facial nerve, hypoplasia of the middle ear space, retrodisplacement of the ossicles in reference to the bony posterior canal wall, and absence of the annulus tympanicus. Most patients with external auditory canal atresia are otherwise normal.

**Complications:** Maximum conductive hearing loss with significant speech and language handicap if bilateral.

**Associated Findings:** Somatic malformations, mild hypertelorism, epicanthal folds, flattened midface, submucous cleft palate, micrognathia, mild syndactyly of some of the toes and fingers, clubfoot, congenital dislocation of the hip, cardiac anomalies, hydronephrosis, hypospadias, mental retardation, microcephaly, frontal bossing, ptosis, chromosome 18q-, absent IgA. (All the foregoing are inconstant.) If an eardrum is present deep to the atresia plate, cholesteatoma development is a theoretical possibility. Some reported cases have had chromosome 18q- or 16r. The association of auditory canal atresia with the *Oculo-auriculo-vertebral anomaly* is frequent.

**Etiology:** Autosomal dominant inheritance.

**Pathogenesis:** Undetermined. There may be failure of recanalization of the primitive auditory canal, or recanalization may be partial.

**MIM No.:** *10876

**Sex Ratio:** M1:F1

**Occurrence:** Unknown. Two families documented.

**Risk of Recurrence for Patient's Sib:**
See Part I, *Mendelian Inheritance.*

**Risk of Recurrence for Patient's Child:**
See Part I, *Mendelian Inheritance.*

**Age of Detectability:** Potentially at birth, but if a careful newborn physical examination is not performed, it may be missed since the meatus and cartilaginous canal may appear normal. In these instances the defect may not be known until the hearing loss is discovered.

**Gene Mapping and Linkage:** Unknown.

**Prevention:** None known. Genetic counseling indicated.

**Treatment:** If the atresia is bilateral the infant should be fitted with a hearing aid. At about age 4 or 5 years corrective surgery to create a canal and correct middle ear malformations should be done on one side unless high-resolution computerized tomography of the petrous pyramid shows that there is a coincidental inner ear malformation or that the middle ear malformation is so severe that it precludes successful surgery. If the atresia is unilateral, surgery should be deferred until adult life when the individual can decide whether or not he wishes to undergo surgery, fully understanding the risks involved.

**Prognosis:** Generally good for life unless the patient has serious concomitant defects. Fair for obtaining serviceable hearing after surgery. Possible complications of surgery include failure to have improvement in hearing, otitis media and perforation of the tympanic membrane graft, injury to the inner ear with loss of hearing, injury to the facial nerve resulting in facial palsy or paralysis, persistent perilymph leak from the oval window if a fixed stapes and abnormally patent cochlear aqueduct coexist, and recurrent meningitis if a perilymph fistula persists.

**Detection of Carrier:** Unknown.

**References:**
Crabtree JA: Tympanoplastic techniques in congenital atresia. Arch Otolaryngol 1968; 88:63–70.
Hoenk BE, et al.: Cholesteatoma auris behind a bony atresia plate. Arch Otolaryngol 1969; 89:470–477.

Stewart JM, et al.: Absent IgA and deletions of chromosome 18. J Med Genet 1970; 7:11–19.

Bergstrom L, et al.: External auditory atresia and the deleted chromosome. Laryngoscope 1974; 84:1905–1917. *

Robinow M, Jahrsdoerfer RA: Autosomal dominant atresia of the auditory canal and conductive deafness. Am J Med Genet 1979; 4:89–94. *

BE028                                              **LaVonne Bergstrom**

## EAR, CERUMEN VARIATIONS                              0141

**Includes:**

    Bran ear wax
    Cat ear wax
    Cerumen variation
    Ear wax types
    Honey ear wax
    Oily ear wax
    Rice ear wax

**Excludes:** N/A

**Major Diagnostic Criteria:** Cerumen in the external ear canal is classified as either sticky and honey-colored (wet type) or dry and gray (dry type). Stickiness is the most important differentiating criterion. Wet cerumen has also been called "honey ear wax," "oily ear wax," or "cat ear wax," whereas the dry type is also known as "rice-bran ear wax."

**Clinical Findings:** Human cerumen is readily classifiable as wet or dry by direct otologic examination. Occasionally an intermediate type is encountered. Cerumen is the product of the secretions of ceruminous and sebaceous glands, with the variation due to the ceruminous components. The secretory cells of people with wet cerumen show more cytoplasmic lipid droplets and pigment granules and more have striated cuticular borders than do the cells of individuals with dry cerumen. Wet cerumen has three times more lipid and one-third as much protein as the dry type. Dry cerumen has a greater proportion of lysozyme and IgG than does the wet type; however, the latter finding may be related to the increased protein content of dry cerumen.

**Complications:** Loss of hearing acuity if either type accumulates and occludes the external auditory canal. Coughing may be associated with movement of dry, hard cerumen within the ear canal.

**Associated Findings:** Cerumen type is thought to reflect differences in apocrine gland function, with wet type indicative of increased secretion. This has been related to axillary odor in 77.3% of those with wet cerumen. Wet cerumen has been rare in Japan, and the odor traditionally has been considered to be pathologic in that population. Increased risk of arteriosclerosis in individuals with wet cerumen has been suggested. Petrakis (1971) reported an association between wet cerumen and increased incidence of breast cancer. A direct relationship was not supported in studies by Ing et al. (1973), but further investigations by Petrakis have indicated that wet cerumen is related to increased secretory activity of the breast, which may then be related to exposure of breast tissue to carcinogens.

**Etiology:** Single gene, two allele system with dry cerumen expressed as a recessive inherited trait. The allele for wet cerumen is usually a complete dominant, but heterozygotes with an intermediate phenotype have been described.

**Pathogenesis:** Unknown.

**MIM No.:** *11780

**Sex Ratio:** M1:F1

**Occurrence:** The proportion of wet:dry phenotypes shows considerable variation among different ethnic groups. The following are representative composite findings for gene and phenotype frequencies for dry cerumen. In most studies, phenotype was classified as either wet or dry, so only figures for dry are given.

### Frequencies in 1,000 Live Births in Different Ethnic Groups

| Ethnic Group | Dry Type | Dry Allele |
| --- | --- | --- |
| North Chinese | 958 | 0.96 |
| Koreans | 924 | 0.96 |
| Japanese | 837 | 0.92 |
| American Indians | 513 | 0.82 |
| American Whites | 44 | 0.21 |
| American Blacks | 20 | 0.07 |
| Germans | 31 | 0.18 |

**Risk of Recurrence for Patient's Sib:** Depends upon the genotype of the parents.

**Risk of Recurrence for Patient's Child:** Depends upon the genotype of the parents.

**Age of Detectability:** Within the first year of life.

**Gene Mapping and Linkage:** Unknown.

**Prevention:** None known. Genetic counseling indicated.

**Treatment:** Either type of cerumen may become impacted and require removal. Removal of excess cerumen is best done with instruments under direct observation (using an operating microscope). The most useful instruments are wire loops, dull curettes, and Hartmann forceps. Irrigation and suctioning are also used.

**Prognosis:** Cerumen type does not appear to affect life span, intelligence, or function.

**Detection of Carrier:** In most cases, heterozygotes are phenotypically indistinguishable from homozygotes for the wet allele. An intermediate phenotype was found in 0.5% of Japanese and 5.3% of Germans. These are presumably heterozygotes. Otherwise, heterozygosity may be inferred from family studies.

**Special Considerations:** The straightforward inheritance pattern and ease of typing have made this a useful polymorphism for linkage analysis. Because of the variation in frequency of the 2 types in different populations, cerumen type has also been used as an anthropologic marker. A biologic basis for the polymorphism has not been determined, but Omoto (1974) has suggested that dry cerumen developed in the Mongolian population and had a selective advantage in the extremely cold climate. Frequencies in other populations would then represent a combination of migration and genetic drift.

**References:**

Kataura A, Kataura K: The comparison of free and bound amino acids between dry and wet types of cerumen. Tohoku J Exp Med 1967; 91:215–225.

Kataura A, Kataura K: The comparison of lipids between dry and wet types of cerumen. Tohoku J Exp Med 1967; 91:237.

Petrakis NL, et al.: Cerumen in American Indians: genetic implications of sticky and dry types. Science 1967; 158:1192–1193.

Hyslop NE Jr: Ear wax and host defense (editorial). New Engl J Med 1971; 284:1099–1100.

Petrakis NL: Cerumen genetics and human breast cancer. Science 1971; 173:347–349.

Ing R, et al.: Evidence against association between wet cerumen and breast cancer. Lancet 1973; I:41.

Omoto K: Polymorphic traits in peoples of eastern Asia and the Pacific. In: Ramot B, et al. (eds): Genetic diseases and polymorphisms in man. New York: Academic Press, 1974:69–89.

Petrakis NL, et al.: Epidemiology of breast fluid secretion: associations with breast cancer risk factors and cerumen type. J Natl Cancer Inst 1981; 67:277–284.

SM008                                              **Shelley D. Smith**

## EAR, CHEMODECTOMA OF MIDDLE EAR      **0145**

**Includes:**

Glomus jugulare tumors
Glomus tympanicum tumors
Glomus vagale tumors
Paragangliomas of the middle ear and temporal bone

**Excludes:**

**Carotid body tumor** (0127)
**Hemangiomas**

**Major Diagnostic Criteria:** A middle ear mass is seen in most patients. Histologic confirmation is characterized by the presence of chief cells or epithelioid cells in a vascular stroma. Chromaffin staining or fluorescent microscopy will detect the presence of catecholamines. Preoperative tissue sampling is to be avoided because of associated biopsy hemorrhage. Presumptive diagnosis is based upon clinical observations and history along with audiometric and neuroradiographic imaging including: CT scanning, MR imaging and angiography.

**Clinical Findings:** Most (98%) of associated symptoms are aural. Included among these are: hearing loss (63%), pulsatile or non-pulsatile tinnitus (56%), bleeding (35%), infection associated pain (35%), unsteadiness or vertigo (22%). Cranial nerve involvement is noted in 3% of patients with VII nerve palsy present in 33% of these cases. 18% of cranial palsies result from intracranial extension. Metastases are observed in 1%, and recurrence is rare once primary lesion is removed.

Clinical findings include an abnormal otoscopic exam in 97%. A bleeding mass, aural polyp, or a middle ear vascular blushing mass may be seen. Blanching of the mass may be noted with pneumatic otoscopy (Brown's sign). Dysfunction of cranial nerves IX, X, XI may be variably observed due to involvement of the jugular foramen. Encroachment along the irregular skull base may disrupt other cranial nerves (V, VIII and XII in particular).

Conventional X-rays and tomograms are of limited use but both would demonstrate bone erosion. Contrast enhanced CT scanning is optimal for demonstrating the extent of tumor invasion, particularly intracranial extension. MRI, while demonstrating soft tissue tumor mass, does not demonstrate the bony destruction. Arteriography will demonstrate feeding vessels as well as contralateral cerebral crossfilling. Venography plays no role in evaluation today.

Glomus tumors are most commonly found in Caucasian females on the left side. Glomus tumors have been associated with the MEN syndromes, especially medullary thyroid carcinomas (see **Endocrine neoplasia, multiple type II**).

**Complications:** Cranial nerve palsies; chronic otitis media.

**Associated Findings:** Catecholamine secretion is noted in less than 5% of patients and may result in hypertension, tachycardia, and anxiety.

**Etiology:** Unknown.

**Pathogenesis:** Unknown.

**MIM No.:** *16800

**Sex Ratio:** Females predominate by up to M1:F5

**Occurrence:** Undetermined but presumed rare.

**Risk of Recurrence for Patient's Sib:** Familial tendency noted but unknown inheritance pattern.

**Risk of Recurrence for Patient's Child:** Unknown.

**Age of Detectability:** Usually not until early adult life.

**Gene Mapping and Linkage:** Unknown.

**Prevention:** None known. Genetic counseling indicated.

**Treatment:** Surgical extirpation for both intracranial and extracranial tumor mass is the principal treatment. Preoperative embolism may decrease the vascular supply. Radiation therapy should be considered adjunctive only and individually tailored.

**Prognosis:** Unknown.

**Detection of Carrier:** Unknown.

**References:**

Spector GJ: Glomus jugulare tumors: Self-instruction package on Continuing Medical Education. Amer Acad Otolaryngol Head Neck Surg 1978, Rochester, Minnesota.

Fisch U: Infratemporal fossa approach for glomus tumors of the temporal bone. Ann Otol Rhinol Laryngol 1982; 91:474–479.

Montague ED: Therapy of glomus tumors of the ear and base of skull (radiation procedures); Glasscock ME III, Kveton JF: Therapy of glomus tumors of the ear and base of skull (surgical procedures). In: Thawley SE et al., eds: Comprehensive management of head and neck tumors. Philadelphia: W.B. Saunders, 1986:219–246.

Pensak ML, et al.: Perioperative evaluation and care of patients with lesions involving the skull base. Otolaryngol Head Neck Surg 1986; 94:497–503.

Smith PG, et al.: Clinical evaluation of glomus tumors of the ear and the base of skull. In: Thawley SE, et al., eds: Comprehensive management of head and neck tumors. Philadelphia: W.B. Saunders, 1986:207–218.

PE021                                     **Myles L. Pensak**

## EAR, CHOLESTEATOMA OF TEMPORAL BONE      **0150**

**Includes:**

Cholesteatoma, congenital
Cholesteatoma, primary
Cholesteatoma, true
Cholesteatoma of temporal bone
Petrous pyramid cholesteatoma
Temporal bone cholesteatoma

**Excludes:** Acquired cholesteatoma

**Major Diagnostic Criteria:** Otoscopic examination reveals a whitish mass, either circumscribed or filling the middle ear, behind an intact tympanic membrane. A gradually progressive facial nerve palsy in the absence of chronic ear infection may suggest the condition.

**Clinical Findings:** Features vary according to site of lesion.

*Middle ear or mastoid cholesteatoma* is usually seen in children. Most have a conductive hearing loss but occasionally hearing is normal. In 80% of cases the otoscopic examination reveals a whitish mass, either circumscribed or totally filling the middle ear space, behind an intact tympanic membrane. The age of the patient at the time of diagnosis is usually between 3 and 14 years.

*Primary cholesteatoma* originating in the petrous pyramid is detected in about 90% of cases because of a facial palsy of gradual onset and progression. There is usually a homolateral profound sensorineural deafness, and a loss of caloric response. The patient's age at the time of recognition of the cholesteatoma is usually between 35 and 55.

Multidirectional tomography and/or high-resolution computed tomography of the temporal bone are the studies of choice in defining the exact location of the lesion and the extent of bone erosion.

**Complications:** Conductive hearing loss occurs in about three-fourths of cases of primary cholesteatoma of the middle ear and mastoid; a slowly progressive facial palsy and a profound sensorineural hearing loss develops in about 90% of petrous pyramid cholesteatoma patients.

**Associated Findings:** None known.

**Etiology:** Unknown.

**Pathogenesis:** The consensus of clinical researchers is that the cholesteatoma can be attributed to the presence of an embryonic epidermal rest within the middle ear, attic, mastoid, or petrous pyramid. However, Aimi, (1983) may have explained the presence of the epidermal rest by his tympanic isthmus theory. Once this stratified squamous epithelium starts to grow, it sloughs off in layers as a normal growth process. This results in a gradually enlarging enclosed mass of desquamated keratinized epithelium. Whether necrosis of contiguous bony structures results from the pressure of an expansile mass or from a chemical and enzymatic lysis is undetermined.

**Sex Ratio:** M1:F1

**Occurrence:** Unknown.

**Risk of Recurrence for Patient's Sib:** Unknown.

**Risk of Recurrence for Patient's Child:** Unknown.

**Age of Detectability:** Cholesteatoma of middle ear and mastoid, 3–14 years; of petrous pyramid, 35–55 years.

**Gene Mapping and Linkage:** Unknown.

**Prevention:** None known.

**Treatment:** Complete surgical excision followed by periodic postoperative recheck for early detection of any residual or recurrent cholesteatoma which will require secondary excision.

**Prognosis:** Normal life span for treated cases. Unknown for untreated cases.

**Detection of Carrier:** Unknown.

**Special Considerations:** Multidirectional tomography or high-resolution computer tomography provide accurate information regarding ossicular destruction and are helpful in differentiating primary cholesteatoma from the acquired form.

**References:**
Cawthorne T, Griffith A: Primary cholesteatomata of the temporal bone. Arch Otolaryngol 1961; 73:252.
Derlacki EL, Clemis JD: Congenital cholesteatoma of the middle ear and mastoid. Ann Otol Rhinol Laryngol 1965; 74:706. *
Derlacki EL, et al.: Congenital cholesteatoma of the middle ear and mastoid: a second report presenting seven additional cases. Laryngoscope 1968; 78:1050.
Derlacki EL: Congenital cholesteatoma of the middle ear and mastoid: a third report. Arch Otolaryngol 1973; 97:177.
Derlacki EL: Congenital cholesteatoma of the middle ear and mastoid: a fourth report. In: Shambaugh GE Jr, Shea JJ, eds: The Shambaugh fifth international workshop on middle ear micro-surgery and fluctuant hearing loss. Huntsville: Strode, 1977.
Derlacki EL: Congenital cholesteatoma update. In: Shambaugh GE Jr, Shea JJ, eds: Proceedings of the sixth Shambaugh international workshop on otomicroscopy and third Shea fluctuant hearing loss symposium. Huntsville: Strode, 1981.
Aimi K: Role of the tympanic ring in the pathogenesis of congenital cholesteatoma. Laryngoscope 1983; 93:1140. *
McDonald TJ, Cody DTR, Ryan RE Jr: Congenital cholesteatoma of the ear. Ann Otol Rhinol Laryngol 1984; 93:637.

DE022                                          **Eugene L. Derlacki**

## EAR, CRYPTOTIA                                              0232

**Includes:** Cryptotia

**Excludes:**
    **Deafness-ear pits** (0247)
    **Ear, Darwin tubercle** (0241)
    Ear flare
    **Ear lobe, pit** (0322)
    **Ear, microtia-atresia** (0664)

**Major Diagnostic Criteria:** The upper margin of the pinna is buried under the scalp.

**Clinical Findings:** The superior portion of the auricle is covered with scalp. Usually the cartilaginous framework and remainder of the ear are intact and said to be fairly normal. The anomaly may be unilateral or bilateral. Audiometry reported to be normal in one case (Kantu et al, 1972).

**Complications:** Unknown.

**Associated Findings:** None known.

**Etiology:** Bilateral symmetry and familial incidence suggest a genetic etiology.

**Pathogenesis:** Unknown.

**CDC No.:** 744.280

**Sex Ratio:** M13:F1 (observed)

**Occurrence:** At least 21 cases have been documented in the literature (Kantu et al, 1972).

**Risk of Recurrence for Patient's Sib:** Unknown.

**Risk of Recurrence for Patient's Child:** Unknown.

**Age of Detectability:** At birth.

**Gene Mapping and Linkage:** Unknown.

**Prevention:** None known. Genetic counseling indicated.

**Treatment:** Plastic surgical repair may be indicated.

**Prognosis:** Good for life span, intelligence, and function if isolated defect of outer ear; otherwise dependent upon concomitant defects.

**Detection of Carrier:** Unknown.

**Special Considerations:** Anomalies of the external ear should suggest the possibility of an anomaly of the middle ear as well. Hearing should be assessed as soon as possible and appropriate therapy instituted. The anatomy of the middle and inner ear should be determined by computed tomography. Facial nerve location must considered during surgical repair.

**References:**
Converse JM, ed. Reconstructive plastic surgery. Philadelphia: W.B. Saunders Co., Vol. 3, 1964:1006.
Rubin A: Handbook of congenital malformations. Philadelphia: W.B. Saunders Co., 1967:227–247. Kantu K, et al.: Cryptotia. Laryngoscope 1972; 82:161–165.

BE028                                          **LaVonne Bergstrom**

## EAR, CUPPED                                                 0314

**Includes:** Cup ear

**Excludes:**
    Atresia (alone)
    **Deafness-ear pits** (0247)
    Ear flare
    **Ear lobe, pit** (0322)
    **Ear, microtia-atresia** (0664)

**Major Diagnostic Criteria:** Pinna folded forward over the external auditory meatus.

**Clinical Findings:** The pinna is cupped forward over the external auditory meatus in varying degrees. The helix is short, and extends downward rather than upward. The surface of the ear which normally faces the side of the head is posterolateral or lateral. The ear lobe is also at right angles to the head. The ear appears small, but is actually of normal size. The condition is nearly always bilateral. Hearing is usually normal. Congenital hearing loss may occur in conjunction with cleft lip; may be conductive, sensorineural or mixed. Polytomograms in one patient showed ossicular malformations; bilateral vestibular and cochlear dysplasias. Cup ear has also been seen in the congenital rubella syndrome with first arch anomalies, conductive or profound sensorineural hearing loss, and Mondini cochlear dysplasia in one case.

**Complications:** No medical complications, but pyscho-social complications have been reported.

**Associated Findings:** Pierre Robin micrognathia and conductive hearing loss occurs in **Lacrimo-auriculo-dento-digital syndrome;** some patients showing mild or severe conductive or sensorineural hearing loss. Tympanometry suggests ossicular fixation in patients having a conductive component.

**Etiology:** Autosomal dominant inheritance with regular penetrance and variable expressivity. May be sporadic.

**Pathogenesis:** Undetermined. Possible arrest at a fetal stage of development. Congenital rubella was reported in three cases.

**MIM No.:** *12860

**Sex Ratio:** M1:F1

**Occurrence:** At least 25 cases reported in the literature.

**Risk of Recurrence for Patient's Sib:**
See Part I, *Mendelian Inheritance.*

**Risk of Recurrence for Patient's Child:**
See Part I, *Mendelian Inheritance.*

**Age of Detectability:** At birth.

**Gene Mapping and Linkage:** Unknown.

**Prevention:** None known. Genetic counseling indicated.

**Treatment:** Plastic surgical repair may be indicated. If pinna can be unfolded during the first three weeks of life, with use of dental compound and surgitaping for three weeks, many cupped pinnae may be at least partially restored esthetically.

**Prognosis:** Good for life span, intelligence and function if it is an isolated defect of the outer ear; otherwise, dependent upon concomitant defects.

**Detection of Carrier:** Unknown.

**References:**
Potter EL: A hereditary ear malformation transmitted through five generations. J Hered 1937; 28:255–258.
Erich JB, Abu-Jamra FN: Congenital cup-shaped deformity of the ears transmitted through four generations. Mayo Clinic Proc 1965; 40: 597–602.
Peterson DM, Schimke RN: Hereditary cup-shaped ears and the Pierre Robin syndrome. J Med Genet 1968; 5:52–55.
Rogers BO: Microtic, lop, cup and protruding ears: four directly inheritable deformities. Plast Reconstr Surg 1968; 41:208–231.
Hollister DW, et al.: The lacrimo-aurieulo-dento-digital syndrome. J Pediatr 1973; 83:438.
Bergstrom L: Anomalies of the ear. In: English GM, ed: Otolaryngology. New York: Harper and Row, 1979:6–7,12–13.

BE028                                          **LaVonne Bergstrom**

## EAR, DARWIN TUBERCLE                                      0241

**Includes:** Darwin tubercle

**Excludes:**
Darwin pointed pinnae (outward pointed projections of ears)
Small enlargement of the ear rim at the Darwin ear point

**Major Diagnostic Criteria:** Tubercle on posterosuperior helix.

**Clinical Findings:** A variable-sized tubercle on the posterosuperior helix, presenting as a projection from the inner rim of the ear at about its midpoint. The cartilage is thickened at this point to form a tubercle that can be distinctly seen.

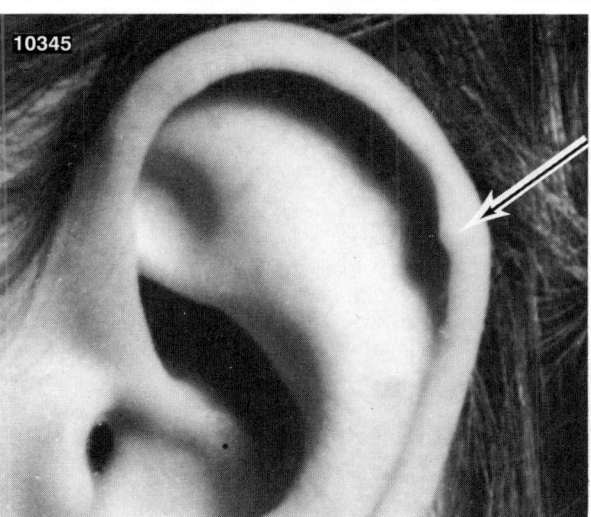

**0241**-10345: Darwin tubercle.

**Complications:** Unknown.

**Associated Findings:** None known.

**Etiology:** Autosomal dominant inheritance with variable expressivity. Expression varies from a small tubercle to larger infolded point with a series of intermediate forms. Some have the tubercle in only one ear. A few carry the gene without expressing the trait in either ear.

**Pathogenesis:** Unknown.

**MIM No.:** 12440

**CDC No.:** 744.280

**Sex Ratio:** M55:F45. Possibly sex plays some role in the degree of expressivity of the gene.

**Occurrence:** Finland, about 50%; Germany, about 20%; and England, about 55%.

**Risk of Recurrence for Patient's Sib:**
See Part I, *Mendelian Inheritance.*

**Risk of Recurrence for Patient's Child:**
See Part I, *Mendelian Inheritance.*

**Age of Detectability:** At birth.

**Gene Mapping and Linkage:** Unknown.

**Prevention:** None known. Genetic counseling indicated.

**Treatment:** Unknown.

**Prognosis:** Normal for life span, intelligence, and function.

**Detection of Carrier:** Physical examination.

**References:**
Winchester AM: Genetics: a survey of the principles of heredity, ed 4. Boston: Houghton Mifflin, 1977. * †

WI034                                          **A.M. Winchester**

**Ear, dysgenesis of**
*See EAR, MICROTIA-ATRESIA*

## EAR, ECTOPIC PINNA                                      0316

**Includes:** Pinna, ectopic placement of pinna

**Excludes:**
Atresia (alone)
**Deafness-ear pits** (0247)
**Ear, Darwin tubercle** (0241)
Ear flare
**Ear lobe, pit** (0322)
**Ear, microtia-atresia** (0664)

**Major Diagnostic Criteria:** Normally contoured pinna found in a displaced position without relationship to the external auditory canal, eardrum, and middle ear, which are in normal position; or normally contoured pinna with associated canal, drum, and middle ear all displaced from their usual position.

**Clinical Findings:** Ectopic placement of the pinna on the head without displacement of the external auditory canal and with normal eardrum and middle ear has been reported in perhaps two cases in the literature. In one case, there was no evidence of auricular structures or auricular appendages at the normal site, and the opposite pinna was completely normal in form and location. The ectopic ear was also normal in contour, except that it seemed attached anteriorly to the forehead and temple by a thick pedicle of tissue. The ear was above its normal position. In other instances, the ear canal and middle ear have been displaced with the pinna.

**Complications:** Malformation of the middle ear and eustachian tube.

**Associated Findings:** None known.

**Etiology:** Unknown.

**Pathogenesis:** Undetermined. Possible intrauterine trauma that led to transplantation of pinna precursor to another area of skull;

or amniotic fibrous adhesions that pulled developing pinna into abnormal position.

**CDC No.:** 744.230

**Sex Ratio:** Presumably M1:F1

**Occurrence:** Unknown.

**Risk of Recurrence for Patient's Sib:** Unknown.

**Risk of Recurrence for Patient's Child:** Unknown.

**Age of Detectability:** At birth.

**Gene Mapping and Linkage:** Unknown.

**Prevention:** None known. Genetic counseling indicated.

**Treatment:** Plastic surgical repair may be indicated. If conductive hearing loss is present, computed tomography of the temporal bone should be done to assess the anatomic configuration of the middle ear, and if this seems favorable, exploratory tympanotomy and surgical correction should be performed. If not feasible, or if unsuccessful, or if the patient has a sensorineural hearing loss, hearing aids should be fitted and aural rehabilitation undertaken. Reconstructive surgery of the middle ear should be performed at about age 5 years in patients with bilateral ectopic pinna, but not until adolescence in patients with unilateral ectopy.

**Prognosis:** Good for life span, intelligence, and function if isolated defect of outer ear; otherwise, dependent on concomitant defects.

**Detection of Carrier:** Unknown.

**References:**
Smith CR, et al.: Congenital gross displacement of the pinna. Arch Otolaryngol 1967; 86:49.

BE028                                                    **LaVonne Bergstrom**

**Ear, enlarged scapha and lobule**
*See EAR, MACROTIA*

## EAR, EUSTACHIAN TUBE DEFECTS                          0370

**Includes:**
   Eustachian tube atresia
   Eustachian tube cysts
   Eustachian tube diverticuli
   Eustachian tube tumors

**Excludes:**
   Carcinoma and other acquired tumors of the nasopharynx
   Functional defects secondary to cleft palate

**Major Diagnostic Criteria:** An abnormality of the eustachian tube; either histological, pathological or embryological, which alters its normal function and usually results in intractable serous or chronic otitis media. Subsequent hearing loss is of a conductive nature.

**Clinical Findings:** Congenital defects of the eustachian tube usually present as persistent serous otitis media or chronic otitis media resistant to antibiotic therapy. Perforation of the tympanic membrane or cholesteatoma may result. Hearing loss is of a conductive nature. A cyst or tumor may be seen in the protympanum or nasopharynx.

**Complications:** Hearing loss secondary to persistent otitis media or perforation of the tympanic membrane. Cholesteatoma may also occur.

**Associated Findings:** None known.

**Etiology:** Unknown.

**Pathogenesis:** Unknown.

**CDC No.:** 744.250

**Sex Ratio:** Presumably M1:F1

**Occurrence:** Undetermined. Presumed rare.

**Risk of Recurrence for Patient's Sib:** Unknown.

**Risk of Recurrence for Patient's Child:** Unknown.

**Age of Detectability:** Usually in childhood, but actual etiology may not be discovered until much later.

**Gene Mapping and Linkage:** Unknown.

**Prevention:** None known. Genetic counseling indicated.

**Treatment:** Surgical removal of hamartoma or dermoid cyst. Ventilation of middle ear with tympanotomy tube to prevent otitis media with effusion, chronic otitis and possible subsequent retraction cholesteatoma.

**Prognosis:** Good, unless due to a neoplasm. An operative risk may be permanent hearing loss.

**Detection of Carrier:** Unknown.

**Special Considerations:** Defects of the eustachian tube vary and include diverticuli, dermoid cysts, hamartomas, and the hypothesized hypercompliant auditory tube ("floppy tube"). Eustachian tubes can be fused, shortened, rudimentary, abnormally narrow, or completely absent. A defect in branchial arch I, II, or III, or pharyngeal pouch I may occur. There is a paucity of histopathologic material on defects of the eustachian tube. Numerous temporal bones have been examined histologically by Schuknecht and no eustachian tube abnormalities have been found in cases of: chondrodysplasia, meatal atresia, cretinism, **Craniofacial dysostosis, Mucopolysaccharidosis I, Osteogenesis imperfecta,** phocomelia, **Fetal rubella syndrome, Bone, Paget disease, Otosclerosis,** renal rickets, osteomalacia, or temporal bone fractures. Abnormalities of the eustachian tube have been observed in: otocephaly, **Cyclopia,** anencephaly, **Klippel-Feil anomaly,** and congenital atresia of the ear.

**References:**
Altman F: Malformations of the eustachian tube, the middle ear, and its appendages. Arch Otolaryngol 1951; 54:241–246.
Altman F: The ear in severe malformations of the head. Arch Otolaryngol 1957; 66(6):7–25.
Eichel BS, Hallberg OE: Hamartoma of the middle ear and eustachian tube. Laryngoscope 1966; 76:1810–1815.
Proctor B: Embryology and anatomy of the eustachian tube. Arch Otolaryngol 1967; 86:51–62.
Schuknecht HF, Kerr AG: Pathology of the eustachian tube. Arch Otolaryngol 1967; 86:45–50.
Rood SR, Doyle WJ: An extreme morphologic variation of the auditory tube cartilage: a case report. Cleft Palate J 1981; 18:293–298.
Arcand P, Abela A: Dermoid cyst of the eustachian tube. J Otol 1985; 14:187–191.

K0023                                                 **Frederick K. Kozak**

## EAR, EXCHONDROSIS                                      0317

**Includes:**
   Ear bump
   Exchondrosis of pinna

**Excludes:**
   Atresia (alone)
   **Deafness-ear pits** (0247)
   **Ear, Darwin tubercle** (0241)
   Ear flare
   **Ear lobe, pit** (0322)
   **Ear, microtia-atresia** (0664)

**Major Diagnostic Criteria:** Bump at lower end of posterior surface of ear next to scalp.

**Clinical Findings:** A cartilaginous bump occurs on the posteromedial surface of the pinna close to its scalp attachment ("posterior ear bump").

**Complications:** Unknown.

**Associated Findings:** None known.

**Etiology:** Autosomal dominant inheritance.

**Pathogenesis:** Unknown.

**MIM No.:** *13350

**CDC No.:** 744.230

**Sex Ratio:** M1:F1

**Occurrence:** Unknown. Reported in one family.

**Risk of Recurrence for Patient's Sib:**
See Part I, *Mendelian Inheritance.*

**Risk of Recurrence for Patient's Child:**
See Part I, *Mendelian Inheritance.*

**Age of Detectability:** At birth.

**Gene Mapping and Linkage:** Unknown.

**Prevention:** None known. Genetic counseling indicated.

**Treatment:** Plastic surgical repair may be indicated.

**Prognosis:** Good for life span, intelligence, and function if isolated defect of outer ear; otherwise, dependent on concomitant defects.

**Detection of Carrier:** Unknown.

**Special Considerations:** Anomalies of the external ear should suggest the possibility of an anomaly of the middle ear as well, but this external observation itself is not evidence of other anomalies.

**References:**
Gates RR: Human Genetics. Vol. 1. New York: Macmillan, 1947:249.

BE028                                              **LaVonne Bergstrom**

## EAR, EXOSTOSES                                   0318

**Includes:**
> Aural exostoses
> Exostoses of external auditory canal
> Hyperostoses of auditory canal
> Ivory exostoses of ear canal
> Osteomata, multiple compact

**Excludes:** Osteomata of external auditory canal

**Major Diagnostic Criteria:** Clinical findings include small, multiple, bilateral, symmetric, sessile bony masses in the external auditory canals next to the sulcus tympanicus. These occur in a child or infant who is too young for exposure to the classic exogenous factors thought to be of importance in the etiology of noncongenital exostoses.

**Clinical Findings:** Exostoses are usually asymptomatic; rarely do they become large enough to obstruct or nearly obstruct the external auditory canal so that cerumen and desquamated canal debris become impacted medial to the exostosis. This may cause a conductive hearing loss or external otitis. In coincidental or secondary suppurative otitis media and tympanic membrane rupture, large exostoses may cause obstruction to drainage and may interfere with evaluation and treatment. During otoscopic examination, rounded, sessile, hard, bony nodules protruding from the bony external auditory canal wall near the sulcus tympanicus are observed: These are usually multiple and bilateral. Often the exostoses are on opposing walls of the canal, most commonly the posterior and anterior, at the approximate locations of the tympanomastoid and tympanosquamous sutures. The floor of the canal is said to be seldom involved. The skin covering them is usually normal, unless self-induced trauma or infection has occurred. Occasionally exostoses of the external auditory canal may be associated with multiple exostoses in other locations, e.g., the orbit or mandible.

Hyperostoses are similar but more diffuse, annular, or segmented bony thickenings of the external canal. Hyperostosis of other bones of the skull and face may be associated. There is considerable confusion in distinguishing between exostoses and osteomata of the external auditory canal. Osteomata tend to be unilateral, often pedunculated, and usually occur at the junction of the bony and cartilaginous canals. Osteomata are generally single, but multiple compact osteomata have been described. Osteomata are believed to be rarer than exostoses, but are more likely to be associated with complications such as infection and hearing loss. As in exostoses and hyperostoses, familial syndromes are known in which osteomata of the external ear canal

occur. Mastoid X-rays and computerized tomography are useful adjuncts to physical examination when surgery is necessary for the following reasons: to determine the extent of involvement, to delineate the course of the facial nerve, and to see if concomitant middle or inner ear anomalies or pathology, such as cholesteatoma, are present.

It may be useful to search for generalized bone disease in certain cases. However, no abnormalities of calcium or phosphorus metabolism have been described in aural exostoses per se. The pathology of the bony tissue in exostoses is felt to be distinct from that of osteomata. Osteomata usually show a thin shell of compact bone over a trabecular, fibrous center, whereas exostoses and hyperostoses are felt to comprise a circumscribed hypertrophy of the periosteal bone.

**Complications:** May include, in order of frequency, cerumen impaction, otitis externa, conductive hearing loss, otitis media, cholesteatoma, and ossicular disruption. All of these complications are rare. Perforation of the tympanic membrane or damage to the facial nerve may occur as a complication of surgery for exostoses.

**Associated Findings:** Rarely; exostoses or hyperostoses of other bones.

**Etiology:** Undetermined. Possibly multifactorial inheritance.

**Pathogenesis:** Unknown.

**MIM No.:** 12830

**CDC No.:** 744.230

**Sex Ratio:** M3:F1 (observed)

**Occurrence:** Although frequently found in prehistoric Indian skulls, no ethnic predominance is known in living racial groups. The older literature indicates that this condition comprises about 1:270 to 1:200 cases of aural disease.

**Risk of Recurrence for Patient's Sib:**
See Part I, *Mendelian Inheritance.*

**Risk of Recurrence for Patient's Child:**
See Part I, *Mendelian Inheritance.*

**Age of Detectability:** Not found until symptomatic, or by otoscopy during a routine otolaryngologic examination.

**Gene Mapping and Linkage:** Unknown.

**Prevention:** None known. Genetic counseling indicated.

**Treatment:** Small exostoses and hyperostoses are best treated with periodic observation and careful aural hygiene (avoidance of self-cleaning or trauma to the ear canal). Keeping water out of the ear is especially important, since many otologists feel that water, particularly swimming in cold salt water, may cause or aggravate aural exostoses. Large, obstructing exostoses should be removed using an endaural approach, reflecting a tympanomeatal skin flap over the exostoses and removing them with a high-speed drill and dental burs, followed by the usual postoperative packing and care. Occasionally, a postauricular approach may be preferable. For those extremely rare cases in which middle ear complications occur, tympanoplasty and ossicular reconstruction are used. If a cholesteatoma should occur, mastoidectomy of a type dictated by the extent of the pathology will be needed.

**Prognosis:** Ear function is usually normal unless obstruction or infection supervene, in which instances conductive hearing loss, tympanic membrane rupture, otitis media, cholesteatoma and ossicular disruption or destruction may occur. Although it is extremely unlikely that this disease would go undetected until cholesteatoma formation, should this occur, it is possible that CNS complications of cholesteatoma, such as brain abscess or meningitis, could result and endanger the patient's life.

**Detection of Carrier:** Unknown.

**References:**
Hrdlicka A: Ear exostoses. Smithsonian Miscellaneous Collections. 1935; 93:1–100.
Mawson SR: Diseases of the ear. Baltimore: Williams & Wilkins, 1963.
Canciullo R, Bozzi A: Osteomi ed esostosi del condotto uditivo esterno. Otorinolaringol Ital 1967; 36:294.

Shambaugh GE Jr: Surgery of the ear, ed 2. Philadelphia: W.B. Saunders, 1967.
Ballenger JJ: Diseases of the nose, throat and ear. Philadelphia: Lea & Febiger, 1969.
DiBartolomeo JR: Exostoses of the external auditory canal. Ann Otol Rhinol Laryngol 1969; 88(suppl):61.

BE028                                                                LaVonne Bergstrom

**Ear, external, congenital sinuses of**
*See EAR, PITS*
**Ear, floppy helix of**
*See EAR, LOP*

## EAR, HAIRY                                                      0319

**Includes:**
    Hairy ears
    Hairy pinnae
    Hypertrichosis pinnae auris
**Excludes:** Hairy tragus and meatus acusticus externus in males alone

**Major Diagnostic Criteria:** Hairy ears.

**Clinical Findings:** Up to 1-inch-long, coarse hairs growing closely together on the helix of the ears. In the population in India the common site is in the sulcus at the side of the ears, while in the Israeli population and in Malta, hair frequently occurs at the top of the ear.

**Complications:** Unknown.

**Associated Findings:** In India, 68.9% association with hairy tragus and with higher frequency of baldness. Frequency of hairy tragus alone, 34.6%. Strong association with age in all populations.

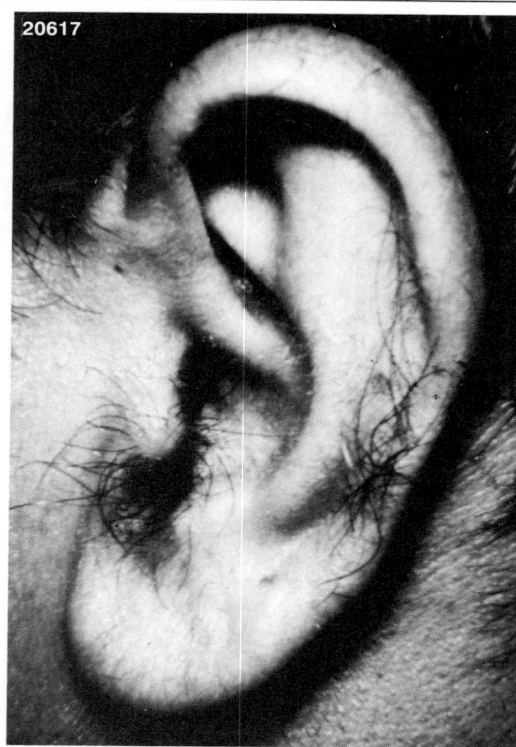

**0319-20617:** Ear, hairy.

**Etiology:** It has been proposed but not sufficiently documented that this trait is Y-linked, i.e., the responsible gene is situated on the Y chromosome. A high proportion of brothers, fathers, and paternal grandfathers of probands are affected at age of expression of the trait. Male relatives from the maternal side are affected only exceptionally, mainly coincidentally, because of the high frequency of the trait in some populations in India.

Recently the two-gene hypothesis was suggested which involves two nonallelic genes, one of which is situated on the nonhomologous part and the other on homologous part of the Y chromosome (the homologous part of the X chromosome sharing also a corresponding allele). Penetrance is almost complete in older men (above age 60 years). Based on our present knowledge of the genetic content of the Y chromosome, the hairy ear trait probably exhibits sex-modified autosomal inheritance.

**Pathogenesis:** Unknown.

**MIM No.:** 13950

**Sex Ratio:** M1:F0

**Occurrence:** The overall mean prevalence in the Indian population is 16.8% (excluding Asian groups of India and the people of the sub-Himalayan region). The higher prevalence was observed in All-Brahmins and All-Kayasthas: 23% to 27%. In West Bengal 60% of males between ages 70 and 79 years were affected. In Israel the prevalence in males was only 1.1% to 25.8%, depending on the age at examination.

**Risk of Recurrence for Patient's Sib:** Almost all male sibs are affected at an older age.

**Risk of Recurrence for Patient's Child:** Almost all sons of male patients are affected.

**Age of Detectability:** Around 20 years of age and later.

**Gene Mapping and Linkage:** Unknown.

**Prevention:** None known. Genetic counseling indicated.

**Treatment:** Cosmetic.

**Prognosis:** Normal for life span, intelligence, and function.

**Detection of Carrier:** Unknown.

**References:**
Dronamraju KR: Hypertrichosis of the pinna of the human ear, Y-linked pedigrees. J Genet 1960; 57:23.
Stern C, et al.: New data on the problem of Y-linkage of hairy pinnae. Am J Hum Genet 1964; 16:455–471.
Chakravartti MR: Hairy pinnae in Indian populations. Acta Genet (Basel) 1968; 18:511–518.
Rao DC: Two-gene hypothesis for hairy pinnae of the ear. Acta Genet Med Gemellol (Roma) 1969; 19:448–453.
Rao, DC: A contribution to the genetics of hypertrichosis of the ear rims. Hum Hered 1970; 20:486–492.
Rao DC: Hypertrichosis of the ear rims: two remakes on the two-gene hypothesis. Acta Genet Med Gemellol (Roma) 1972; 21:216–220. *

CE003                                                            Jaroslav Červenka

## EAR, INNER DYSPLASIAS                                          0315

**Includes:**
    Abiotrophies of inner ear
    Bing-Siebenmann dysplasia
    Dysgenesis of inner ear
    Heredodegenerations of inner ear
    Hypoplasia of inner ear
    Mondini-Alexander malformation of inner ear
    Scheibe cochleosaccular degeneration of inner ear

**Excludes:** Ear, labyrinth aplasia (0562)

**Major Diagnostic Criteria:** Severe-to-profound unilateral or bilateral congenital hearing loss with varying degrees of bony dysplasia of the inner ear detectable by high resolution computerized tomography of the petrous pyramid. Some types of membranous dysplasia may be inferred from the audiometric pattern or abnormal vestibular testing.

**Clinical Findings:** Although there is considerable anatomic variation in the inner ear dysplasias, the clinical picture is usually that of moderately severe-to-profound hearing loss. There is considerable evidence from animal studies that one type of dysplasia, the cochleosaccular degeneration of Scheibe, may occur in the early neonatal period. By light microscopy, the ears appear normal at birth. Improved techniques for testing hearing in newborn and young infants suggest that a similar phenomenon may occur in some cases of human deafness in which no known exogenous causes of hearing loss can be found. The infant usually babbles and vocalizes normally until about age 6–9 months, when his production of vocalization diminishes and changes in pitch. An alert parent may suspect the hearing loss early because of failure to respond to loud, nonvibratory sounds; but often the hearing loss is not suspected or detected until speech and language fail to develop.

Attempts have been made to correlate pathology with audiometric patterns; these have been most successful in cases in which cochleosaccular degeneration occurs. In this entity, atrophy of the stria vascularis, degeneration of the organ of Corti, and rolling up of the tectorial membrane are constant features and are most marked in the basal turn of the cochlea, where higher frequencies are represented. In the apical turn, where low frequencies are localized, these structures appear less distorted or may even appear normal. The Reissner membrane may be collapsed, or the endolymphatic compartment may be dilated. The audiogram often shows residual hearing only in the low frequencies. However, in the Mondini-Alexander malformation, audiometric patterns have been quite variable, from profound hearing loss to normal hearing. In this classic malformation, the bony cochlea is shorter than the normal 2 1/2 - 2 3/4 turns, and may be only 1 or 1 1/2 turns long. Varying degrees of membranous inner ear malformations are seen. There may be dilatation of the saccule, endolymphatic duct, and sac. The bony vestibular labyrinth may show anomalies of the semicircular canals. Varying degrees of hypodevelopment of the acoustic and vestibular ganglia and fibers are seen. The otic capsule may be poorly developed; stapes footplate fixation, other middle ear anomalies, or external auditory atresia may be associated.

Petrous pyramid polytomography has shown that at least 11 of 15 possible combinations of inner ear anomalies occur. Therefore, the classic categories need augmentation or revision. These 11 combined anomalies of the inner ear structures, in order of frequency of occurrence (and preceded by an asterisk if they might affect hearing) are: (1) semicircular canal(s); (2) * cochlea, vestibule and semicircular canal(s); (3) vestibule and semicircular canals; (4) * cochlea, internal meatus, vestibule and semicircular canal(s); (5) * cochlea alone; (6) internal meatus only; (7) * cochlea and vestibule; (8) * cochlea and semicircular canal(s); (9) * cochlea and internal meatus; (10) * cochlea, internal meatus and semicircular canals; and (11) * internal meatus and semicircular canals.

Diminished vestibular function (caloric tests) is seen in some of these patients but is rarely symptomatic, since it is present from birth or early life. A membranous cochlear dysplasia associated with nonprogressive high-tone or basin-shaped loss and good speech discrimination was postulated.

In the Bing-Siebenmann dysplasia, the bony cochlea and vestibular portions of the inner ear are well formed, but the membranous components of both the inner ear and systems are malformed. X-rays of the inner ear are normal. The organ of Corti consists of a small mound of undifferentiated cells; some remains of the tectorial membrane are present. Reissner membrane is usually collapsed but may be ballooned out so that the cochlear duct is dilated. Aplasia of the membranous vestibular labyrinth may be seen. It has been shown that the Scheibe and Mondini malformations may be unilateral, and presumably the other malformations may also be unilateral. In these instances, the patient would have normal speech and language development, and the unilateral hearing loss might not be discovered until school age or later.

Asymmetry of malformation is common, and the patient may have, for example, a Scheibe malformation of one ear and a Mondini malformation of the other. In these instances, the degree

or pattern of hearing loss and the X-ray findings may well be different on the two sides.

**Complications:** Unknown.

**Associated Findings:** Scheibe malformation may be found in **Waardenburg syndromes**, **Cardio-auditory syndrome**, **Chromosome 13, trisomy 13**, **Usher syndrome**, **Phytanic acid storage disease**, sensory radicular neuropathy, osteitis deformans of Paget, and **Fetal rubella syndrome**. Mondini-Alexander malformation may be found in **Deafness-goiter**, **Klippel-Feil anomaly**, **Cervico-oculo-acoustic syndrome**, **Chromosome 18, trisomy 18**, and **Charge association**. Bing-Siebenmann malformation may be found with mental retardation or **Retinitis pigmentosa**. Many of these inner ear dysplasias are isolated defects.

**Etiology:** Unknown, unless associated with a specific genetic syndrome. Varied when part of a syndrome, e.g. Scheibe malformation is usually autosomal recessive.

**Pathogenesis:** Unknown in humans. Inner ear studies in one 7-week-old embryo aborted because of maternal rubella suggest that Scheibe malformation could occur in utero. Animal studies of Scheibe malformation show progressive degeneration of a normal-appearing cochlea and saccule. Pathogenesis of other inner ear dysplasias is unknown; it is postulated to be an arrest of embryologic development in some instances. However, in other cases the pathology is bizarre and does not correspond to any known normal phase of inner ear development.

**CDC No.:** 744.030

**Sex Ratio:** Presumably M1:F1 unless related to a condition with a different known sex ratio.

**Occurrence:** Accounts for 3–4% of profound congenital deafness.

**Risk of Recurrence for Patient's Sib:** As per associated condition(s).

**Risk of Recurrence for Patient's Child:** As per associated condition(s).

**Age of Detectability:** Bony dysplasias may be diagnosed by petrous pyramid polytomography shortly after birth or as soon as the hearing loss is discovered. Membranous dysplasias cannot be detected except at autopsy, although, if associated with a known genetic disease, they may be inferred as soon as the physical findings of the syndrome are manifest.

**Gene Mapping and Linkage:** Unknown.

**Prevention:** None known. Genetic counseling indicated.

**Treatment:** Hearing aids; auditory and other special training for the hearing impaired. Hearing conservation, treatment, or training as appropriate for associated defects.

**Prognosis:** A life prognosis depends on the other associated defects. The ability of the hearing-impaired patient to function in society is directly related to prompt diagnosis and prompt and vigorous habilitation and training. Most of these individuals have usable residual hearing.

**Detection of Carrier:** Unknown.

**References:**

Ormerod FC: The pathology of congenital deafness. J Laryngol 1960; 74:919.

Schuknecht HF: Pathology of sensorineural deafness of genetic origin. In: McConnell F, Ward P, eds: Deafness in childhood. Nashville: Vanderbilt University Press, 1967:69.

Valvassori GE, et al.: Inner ear anomalies: clinical and histopathological considerations. Ann Otol Rhinol Laryngol 1969; 78:929.

Lindsay JR: Inner ear pathology in congenital deafness. Otolaryngol Clin North Am 1971; 4:249.

Paparella MM: Mondini's deafness: a review of histopathology. Ann Otol Rhinol Laryngol 1980; 89:(suppl) 67.

Schuknecht HF: Mondini's dysplasia: a clinical and pathological study. Ann Otol Rhinol Laryngol 1980; 89 (suppl.): 65.

BE028                                    **LaVonne Bergstrom**

## EAR, LABYRINTH APLASIA                                                     0562

**Includes:**
  Agenesis of inner ear
  Inner ear, aplasia
  Michel malformation of inner ear

**Excludes:**
  Ear dysplasias, inner
  Inner ear, obliteration by bone after suppurative
    labyrinthitis

**Major Diagnostic Criteria:**  Total absence of hearing and vestibular response, either unilateral or bilateral, and X-rays that show absence of inner ear structure and internal auditory meatus.

**Clinical Findings:**  Labyrinthine aplasia is a developmental anomaly that occurs as a result of dysplasia of the petrous bone. The degree of hearing loss may not be suspected until the child or infant fails to respond to sound after an adequate trial with powerful hearing aids. The pinna, external canal, and tympanic membrane are nearly always normal, and facial nerve function is usually intact. Vestibular symptoms are usually absent, but caloric examination shows no peripheral vestibular response. If the deformity is unilateral and involves only the inner ear, the hearing loss may go undetected for a number of years, since the child uses his normal ear to acquire speech and language. The total hearing loss may be found only after school screening audiometry shows a hearing loss which is confirmed by further testing. Aplasia of the inner ear may be suggested by absence of bony inner ear cavities and the internal auditory meatus on standard mastoid X-ray. It is confirmed by computerized tomography of the petrous bone, which generally shows a normal middle ear and external canal. At autopsy, the petrous bone may show aplasia or hypoplasia. Aplasia is rare. At times there may be spaces in the bony labyrinth that do not, however, in any way resemble inner ear structures. In Michel's original case, the stapes and stapedius tendon were also absent.

**Complications:**  Inability to acquire speech and language through the auditory route, even with amplification, if the defect is bilateral.

**Associated Findings:**  Absence of stapes and stapedius tendon. Mental retardation is said by Ormerod to occur "often." However, some of the developmental delay may have been secondary to total hearing deficit.

**Etiology:**  Unknown, except in those cases of maternal ingestion of thalidomide during pregnancy.

**Pathogenesis:**  Unknown.

**CDC No.:**  744.030

**Sex Ratio:**  Presumably M1:F1

**Occurrence:**  Thought to occur in about 1% of the 1:1,000–2,000 congenitally deaf children who have severe to profound sensorineural hearing loss (Ormerod, 1960).

**Risk of Recurrence for Patient's Sib:**  Unknown.

**Risk of Recurrence for Patient's Child:**  Undetermined for idiopathic cases. No recurrence is expected in the offspring of Thalidomide cases.

**Age of Detectability:**  In infancy, by computerized tomography of petrous bone. Magnetic resonance imaging to rule out absence of auditory nerve.

**Gene Mapping and Linkage:**  Unknown.

**Prevention:**  None known. Genetic counseling indicated.

**Treatment:**  Unilateral: hearing conservation to prevent injury to the normal ear. Bilateral: prompt institution of non-auditory methods for language acquisition. Electrode placement in cochlear nuclei, if there is no auditory nerve, may prove helpful.

**Prognosis:**  Normal for life span. With age and related changes in the central vestibular system or with acquired visual problems, e.g., cataracts of old age, some symptomatic vestibular problems, possibly disabling, might occur if the defect is bilateral.

**Detection of Carrier:**  Unknown.

**Special Considerations:**  The patient may show no response to sound at all if the malformation is bilateral. Behavioral audiometry, play conditioning, reflex responses, evoked response audiometry, and psychogalvanometric skin response audiometry all fail to elicit valid hearing responses. Tactile responses to low frequencies presented by bone conduction may be falsely interpreted as true hearing responses. Apparent lack of response to amplified sound is an indication for computed tomography. Absence of the inner ear will then indicate that training should be redirected into manual and visual methods as early as possible so that acquisition of language and its dependent skills, reading and writing, may be optimum. In the few instances in which the mother ingested thalidomide during early pregnancy, the external ear, internal auditory canal, and facial nerve all may be abnormal or absent. In thalidomide ears, there may be absence of the internal auditory canal, inner ear, facial nerve, and VIII cranial nerves.

**References:**
Ormerod FC: The pathology of congenital deafness. J Laryngol 1960; 74:919–950.
Schuknecht HF: Pathology of sensorineural deafness of genetic origin. In: McConnell F, Wards PH, eds: Deafness in childhood. Nashville: Vanderbilt University Press, 1967:69–90. *
Valvassori EE, et al.: Inner ear anomalies: clinical and histopathological considerations. Ann Otol Rhinol Laryngol 1969; 78:929–938 *.

BE028                                                    **LaVonne Bergstrom**

## EAR, LOBE, ABSENT                                                         0320

**Includes:**  Lobe, ear, absent

**Excludes:**
  Atresia (alone)
  **Deafness-ear pits (0247)**
  **Ear, Darwin tubercle (0241)**
  Ear flare
  **Ear lobe, pit (0322)**
  **Ear lobe, attached (0323)**
  **Ear, microtia-atresia (0664)**

**Major Diagnostic Criteria:**  Hypoplastic or absent ear lobe.

**Clinical Findings:**  The ear lobe is either absent or hypoplastic.

**Complications:**  Unknown.

**Associated Findings:**  Often noted in conjunction with syndromes, e.g., **Seckel syndrome.**

**Etiology:**  Unknown.

**Pathogenesis:**  Unknown.

**CDC No.:**  744.230

**Sex Ratio:**  Presumably M1:F1

**Occurrence:**  Undetermined. Said to be more frequent in Blacks and Filipinos.

**Risk of Recurrence for Patient's Sib:**  Unknown.

**Risk of Recurrence for Patient's Child:**  Unknown.

**Age of Detectability:**  At birth.

**Gene Mapping and Linkage:**  Unknown.

**Prevention:**  None known. Genetic counseling indicated.

**Treatment:**  If this is an isolated defect, no treatment is needed.

**Prognosis:**  Good for lifespan, intelligence, and function if isolated defect of outer ear; otherwise, dependent on concomitant defects.

**Detection of Carrier:**  Unknown.

**Special Considerations:**  Anomalies of the external ear should suggest the possibility of an anomaly of the middle ear as well. Hearing should be assessed as soon as possible, and appropriate therapy should be instituted.

**References:**
Smith DW: Recognizable patterns of human malformation: genetic, embryologic and clinical aspects (Major Problems in Clinical Pediatrics). Philadelphia: W.B. Saunders, 1970.

BE028                            **LaVonne Bergstrom**

## EAR, LONG, NARROW, POSTERIORLY ROTATED     0325

**Includes:** Ear, posteriorly rotated

**Excludes:**
Atresia (alone)
**Deafness-ear pits** (0247)
**Ear, Darwin tubercle** (0241)
Ear flare
**Ear lobe, pit** (0322)
**Ear, microtia-atresia** (0664)

**Major Diagnostic Criteria:** Posterior rotation of ear around axis of external auditory meatus.

**Clinical Findings:** The ear's configuration is normal except that the ear is somewhat elongated. It may be slightly low-set or at the normal height but rotated from the perpendicular more than 10% backward around an axis that goes through both external auditory meati. This may be associated with syndromes such as the broad thumb-hallux syndrome and is suggested in osteogenesis imperfecta. In the latter case, it may be caused by the bulging of the squama of the temporal bone.

**Complications:** Unknown.

**Associated Findings:** See **Rubinstein-Taybi broad thumb-hallux syndrome** and **Osteogenesis imperfecta.**

**Etiology:** Unknown.

**Pathogenesis:** Unknown.

**CDC No.:** 744.246

**Sex Ratio:** Presumably M1:F1

**Occurrence:** Unknown.

**Risk of Recurrence for Patient's Sib:** Unknown.

**Risk of Recurrence for Patient's Child:** Unknown.

**Age of Detectability:** At birth.

**Gene Mapping and Linkage:** Unknown.

**Prevention:** None known. Genetic counseling indicated.

**Treatment:** If this is an isolated defect, no treatment is usually needed.

**Prognosis:** Good for life span, intelligence and function if isolated defect of outer ear, otherwise dependent upon concomitant defects.

**Detection of Carrier:** Unknown.

**Special Considerations:** Anomalies of the external ear should suggest the possibility of an anomaly of the middle ear as well. Hearing should be assessed as soon as possible, and appropriate therapy should be instituted. The anatomy of the middle and inner ear should be determined by computed tomography. External ear anomalies should also prompt the physician to look for anomalies of other systems and to follow the infant for possible mental retardation. Careful genetic and clinical studies of the family should be carried out if accompanying defects are found.

**References:**
Converse JM, ed: Reconstructive plastic surgery. Vol. 3. Philadelphia: W.B. Saunders, 1964.

BE028                            **LaVonne Bergstrom**

## EAR, LOP                             0326

**Includes:**
"Bat ear"
Ear, floppy helix of
Ear without helix

**Excludes:**
Atresia (alone)
**Deafness-ear pits** (0247)
**Ear, Darwin tubercle** (0241)
Ear flare
**Ear lobe, pit** (0322)
**Ear, microtia-atresia** (0664)

**Major Diagnostic Criteria:** Floppy helix; poor development of scapha and anthelix.

**Clinical Findings:** The concha appears large, while the anthelix and scapha are poorly developed so that the ear protrudes, giving a floppy appearance to the helix or the appearance that there is no anthelix at all. In some instances, the helix droops to a degree sufficient to cover the concha. The condition may be unilateral, but is usually bilateral and fairly symmetric.

**Complications:** No medical complications; psychosocial complications have been reported.

**Associated Findings:** Reduplicated darwin tubercle, absence of the lobule, microtia, macrotia, curling or displacement of the ear, facial asymmetry, **Chromosome 21, trisomy 21**, occasionally conductive or sensorineural hearing loss, micrognathia, imperforate anus, or triphalangeal thumbs.

**Etiology:** Autosomal dominant inheritance in some cases, in others possible arrest at a fetal stage of development. Reason for increased clinical occurrence in males is unknown.

**Pathogenesis:** Rogers (1968) has suggested that the lop ear resembles a fetal stage of pinna development, suggesting arrest of development at that stage.

**MIM No.:** 12880

**CDC No.:** 744.230

**Sex Ratio:** M3:F1

**Occurrence:** In the only known study, 21:108,744 pediatric hospital admissions.

**Risk of Recurrence for Patient's Sib:**
See Part I, *Mendelian Inheritance.*

**Risk of Recurrence for Patient's Child:**
See Part I, *Mendelian Inheritance.*

**Age of Detectability:** At birth.

**Gene Mapping and Linkage:** Unknown.

**Prevention:** None known. Genetic counseling indicated.

**Treatment:** Plastic surgical repair may be indicated. During first 3 weeks of life, with dental compound and Steritape lop ear often can be corrected, by taping the ear to the side of the head. If conductive hearing loss is present, computerized tomography of the middle and inner ears should be done to assess the anatomic configuration of the middle ear, and, if it seems favorable, exploratory tympanotomy and surgical correction should be performed, if feasible. If not feasible, if unsuccessful, or if the patient has a sensorineural hearing loss, hearing aids should be fitted, should be and aural rehabilitation should be undertaken.

**Prognosis:** Good for life span, intelligence, and function if isolated defect of outer ear; otherwise, dependent on concomitant defects.

**Detection of Carrier:** Unknown.

**Special Considerations:** External ear anomalies should also prompt the physician to look for anomalies of other systems and to follow the infant for possible mental retardation. Careful genetic and clinical studies of the family should be carried out if accompanying defects are found.

**References:**
MacCollum DW: The lop ear. JAMA 1938; 110:1427–1430.
Converse JM, ed: Reconstructive plastic surgery. Vol. 3. Philadelphia: W.B. Saunders, 1964.
Rogers BO: Microtic, lop, cup and protruding ears: four directly inheritable deformities. Plast Reconstr Surg 1968; 41:208.
Konigsmark BW: Hereditary deafness with external-ear abnormalities: a review. Johns Hopkins Med J 1970; 127:228.

BE028                                          **LaVonne Bergstrom**

## EAR, LOW-SET                                          0327

**Includes:**
> Low-set ear
> Deafness (conductive)-malformed external ear

**Excludes:**
> Atresia (alone)
> **Deafness-ear pits** (0247)
> **Ear, Darwin tubercle** (0241)
> Ear flare
> **Ear lobe, pit** (0322)
> **Ear, microtia-atresia** (0664)

**Major Diagnostic Criteria:**   An ear that is set below an arbitrary line drawn between the lateral canthus of the eye and the occipital protuberance is considered low-set. Associated backward rotation of pinna.

**Clinical Findings:**   By definition, an ear is low-set when the helix meets the cranium below a line drawn between the outer canthus of the eye and the occipital protuberance. When the head is level, the external auditory meatus is normally at about the level of the ala nasi. Low-set ears may be normal in configuration and merely set below the landmarks outlined; they have some tendency toward backward rotation around an axis passing through both external auditory meati. However, usually low-set ears are also somewhat small and have associated minor malformations. The condition is usually bilaterally symmetric.

**Complications:**   Unknown.

**Associated Findings:**   Seen in many individuals with various syndromes as well as in normal individuals. Often the ears are somewhat small and deformed in varying degrees. In some instances conductive hearing loss is associated. Mental retardation and hypogonadism have been reported in inherited cases.

**Etiology:**   Probably multifactorial.

**Pathogenesis:**   Unknown.

**MIM No.:**   *22130

**CDC No.:**   744.245

**Sex Ratio:**   Presumably M1:F1

**Occurrence:**   Undetermined. Nine inherited cases have been reported in three isolated kinships. Also observed, in varying degrees, in association with various syndromes and in the general population.

**Risk of Recurrence for Patient's Sib:**
> See Part I, *Mendelian Inheritance*.

**Risk of Recurrence for Patient's Child:**
> See Part I, *Mendelian Inheritance*.

**Age of Detectability:**   At birth.

**Gene Mapping and Linkage:**   Unknown.

**Prevention:**   None known. Genetic counseling indicated.

**Treatment:**   If this is an isolated defect, no treatment is usually needed. If conductive hearing loss is present, petrous pyramid computerized tomography should be done to assess the anatomic configuration of the middle ear, and, if it seems favorable,

exploratory tympanotomy and surgical correction should be performed, if feasible. If not feasible, if unsuccessful, or if the patient has a sensorineural hearing loss, hearing aids should be fitted, and aural rehabilitation should be undertaken.

**Prognosis:**   Good for life span, intelligence, and function if the defect is isolated to the outer ear; otherwise, dependent on concomitant defects.

**Detection of Carrier:**   Unknown.

**Special Considerations:**   Anomalies of the external ear should suggest the possibility of an anomaly of the middle ear as well. Hearing should be assessed as soon as possible, and appropriate therapy should be instituted. The anatomy of the middle and inner ear should be determined by computed tomography. External ear anomalies should also prompt the physician to look for anomalies of other systems and to follow the infant for possible mental retardation. Careful genetic and clinical studies of the family should be carried out if accompanying defects are found.

**References:**
Converse JM, ed: Reconstructive plastic surgery. Vol. 3. Philadelphia: W.B. Saunders, 1964.
Mengel MC, et al.: Conductive hearing loss and malformed low-set ears, as a possible recessive syndrome. J Med Genet 1969; 6:14–21.
Konigsmark BW: Hereditary deafness with external-ear abnormalities: a review. Johns Hopkins Med J 1970; 27:228.
Cantu JM, et al.: Autosomal recessive sensorineural-conductive deafness and pinna anomalies. Hum Genet 1978; 40:231–234.

BE028                                          **LaVonne Bergstrom**

## EAR, MACROTIA                                          0619

**Includes:**
> Ear, enlarged scapha and lobule
> Macrotia

**Excludes:**
> **Deafness-ear pits** (0247)
> **Ear, Darwin tubercle** (0241)
> Ear flare
> **Ear lobe, pit** (0322)
> **Ear, microtia-atresia** (0664)

**Major Diagnostic Criteria:**   Very much enlarged pinna, particularly in area of the scapha.

**Clinical Findings:**   The patient has a very large, but generally well-shaped auricle without other malformations of the ear. The ear is, however, somewhat disproportionate in that the most exaggerated portion is the scapha. The other parts of the ear are also somewhat larger than normal, especially the lobule. Occasionally the ear may protrude somewhat. A variant of this may be seen in Marfan syndrome in which the cartilage is somewhat floppy in addition to the ear being large. The condition is usually bilateral and symmetric.

**Complications:**   Embarrassment or psychologic disturbance due to the excessive size of the ears.

**Associated Findings:**   **Marfan syndrome**, ectopia lentis, defects of the media of arteries, and other complex malformation syndromes.

**Etiology:**   Autosomal dominant inheritance in some cases.

**Pathogenesis:**   Unknown.

**MIM No.:**   *12860

**CDC No.:**   744.200

**Sex Ratio:**   Presumably M1:F1

**Occurrence:**   Unknown.

**Risk of Recurrence for Patient's Sib:**
> See Part I, *Mendelian Inheritance*.

**Risk of Recurrence for Patient's Child:**
> See Part I, *Mendelian Inheritance*.

**Age of Detectability:**   At birth.

**Gene Mapping and Linkage:** Unknown.

**Prevention:** None known. Genetic counseling indicated.

**Treatment:** Plastic surgical repair may be indicated.

**Prognosis:** Good for life span, intelligence, and function if an isolated defect of outer ear; otherwise dependent on concomitant defects.

**Detection of Carrier:** Unknown.

**Special Considerations:** Anomalies of the external ear should suggest the possibility of an anomaly of the middle ear as well. Hearing should be assessed as soon as possible, and appropriate therapy should be instituted. The anatomy of the middle and inner ear should be determined by computerized tomography of the temporal bone if there is hearing loss.

**References:**

Rogers BO: Microtic, lop, cup and protruding ears: four directly inheritable deformities. Plast Reconst Surg 1968; 41:208–231.

Ver Meulen VR: Macrotia - the over-sized ear: a method for reduction. Laryngoscope 1970; 80:1053–1063. *

BE028

**LaVonne Bergstrom**

---

## EAR, MICROTIA-ATRESIA                                    0664

**Includes:**

Anotia

Ear, dysgenesis of

Microtia-atresia

Microtia-meatal atresia-conductive deafness

Ossicles, malformed and conductive hearing loss

Pinna, hypogenesis of, with associated atresia of external ear

Thalidomide external ear malformation

**Excludes:**

**Alopecia-anosmia-deafness-hypogonadism, Johnson type** (2765)

Atresia of the external auditory canal, isolated

**Branchio-oto-renal dysplasia (2224)**

**Deafness-ear defects-facial palsy (2762)**

**Ear, cryptotia (0232)**

Pinna malformation, isolated

Post-traumatic or postsurgical auricular deformity

Stenosis of the external auditory canal

Auricular malformations, other

**Major Diagnostic Criteria:** Deformed or absent pinna with an atretic ear canal and, with most forms, conductive hearing loss.

**Clinical Findings:** The right ear is more frequently involved than the left; 1/6 of the patients have bilateral deformity. In a few instances microtia with or without atresia may be seen on one side and atresia alone on the contralateral side. The pinna may be only slightly smaller than normal and have the general configuration of a normal ear. In most instances, the auricle appears crumpled and grossly deformed; with only a few fleshy and cartilaginous rem-

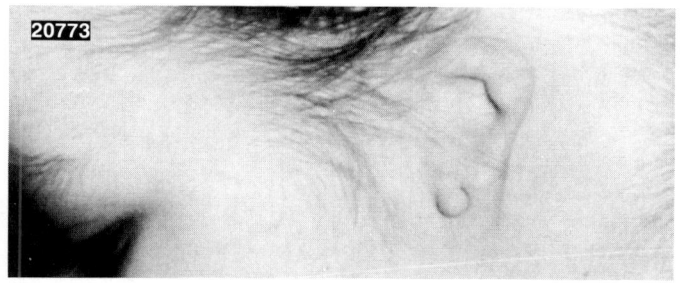

**0664A-20773:** Microtia.

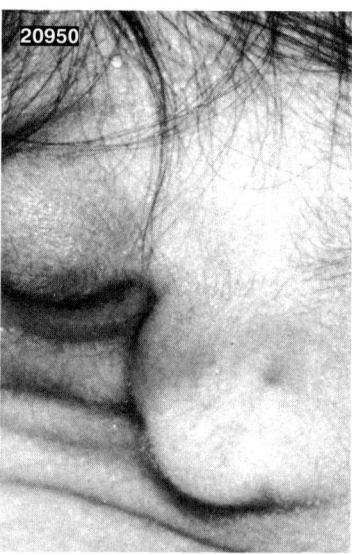

**0664B-20950:** Microtia.

---

nants, resembling the embryologic hillocks that eventually form the pinna. Occasionally, the external ear is entirely absent (anotia). The external auditory canal may be absent, narrowed throughout its length, or show a funnel-like narrowing to complete atresia a few millimeters medial to the concha. Occasionally, a tiny opening can be found anterior, inferior, or, in some instances, posterosuperior to the normal canal position. Often such openings end blindly, but in rare instances, they communicate with a tympanic membrane. Evidently, some of these deformed misplaced canals contain ceruminous glands, since cerumen can be found in the lumen. However, others are more correctly termed preauricular pits. Various parts of the ear may be deformed. In some instances the helix is deficient; in others the lobule is deformed. The tragus may show varying degrees of malformation. Preauricular appendages may be associated. In the rare instances in which anotia occurs, there may be no palpable space between the mastoid tip and the condyloid process of the mandible due to growth of the temporomandibular joint posteriorly. In these instances, severe middle ear anomalies, hypoplasia, or aplasia of the middle ear may be associated, making reconstruction of the hearing mechanism difficult or impossible. The mastoid process may be poorly developed. Occasionally thick soft tissue is found at surgery where the drumhead should be; but more commonly, a bony atresia plate of varying thickness is present. In extremely rare cases, a true tympanic membrane lies just medial to the atretic area, which may be associated with a cholesteatoma and widespread bone destruction. A conductive hearing loss with an air-bone gap of 40–60 db is nearly always present, even when the auditory canal is patent. This is due to associated ossicular or middle ear malformation. In some instances a sensorineural hearing loss is also present, caused by a concomitant inner ear anomaly. Vestibular evaluation by rotational testing has been reported to be normal. X-ray study using high resolution computerized tomography of middle and inner ear is essential in planning surgical therapy and in offering a prognosis. If X-rays reveal a severely deformed or aplastic middle ear or significant inner ear malformations, surgery may not be beneficial. The X-rays may also outline an abnormal course of the facial nerve in the temporal bone, a commonly associated anomaly.

At operation, a narrow or nonexistent space for an external auditory canal may be found. The middle ear cleft and mastoid may be normal in size or hypoplastic. The malleus and incus are often deformed, fused, or fixed to the bony atresia plate. The incus may be absent. Abnormal bony prominences are often present in the middle ear. The stapes may be deformed or the footplate fixed. There may be discontinuity at the incudostapedial junction. The round window may be absent.

**Complications:** Conductive hearing loss due to atresia or to associated middle ear anomalies. Frequency approaches 100%. Malposition, anomaly, or hypoplasia of the facial nerve with or without partial or complete facial palsy. Otitis media and mastoiditis may be found at surgery.

**Associated Findings:** Hypoplasia of the ipsilateral mandible and face due to malformation of the entire first branchial arch complex; narrowing of the osseous portion of the eustachian tube, absence of the torus tubarius (very rare), abnormal widening of the eustachian tube. Inner ear anomalies are found in 12–50%. Absence or hypoplasia of parotid gland. Absence of homolateral tonsil. Preauricular pits and appendages, branchial cysts, hypoplasia, and displacement of the tensor tympani muscle and tendon, absence of the lesser petrosal nerve, cleft palate, teratoid tumors of the tonsil; various craniofacial, skeletal, spinal, and visceral anomalies. See also **Oculo-auriculo-vertebral anomaly**.

**Etiology:** Non-syndromic microtia shows autosomal dominant inheritance in a minority of families. Occasionally it occurs in sibs with normal parents. Most cases are not isolated. Chromosome 18q- and also 18 trisomy have been found in some patients. Thalidomide has caused microtia and anotia with cranial nerve palsies and aplasia of the inner ear. Rubella and other intrauterine infections have been implicated. Absence or malfunction of an inductive "organizer" has been postulated. Condition has been seen in pigs, cattle, goats, sheep, horses, rabbits, and mice.

**Pathogenesis:** Disturbances of development of the first branchial groove and of the hillocks of the pinna, nearly all of which are also formed from first and second branchial arch structures. The core of the mesoderm which forms in the primitive canal area may fail to recanalize and form an atresia plate. Since the first branchial arch develops abnormally, other structures derived from it (the malleus, incus, tensor tympani, and mandible) may also be deformed. The second branchial arch may also be involved, resulting in stapes and facial nerve anomalies. The pathogenesis of associated visceral or skeletal anomalies is probably related to exogenous factors that affect the growth of other organ systems that are developing during the same embryonic period.

**MIM No.:** *25180

**CDC No.:** 744.010

**Sex Ratio:** M>1:F1. Some investigators believe that the apparent increased incidence in males is due only to the fact that females cover the deformity with their hair.

**Occurrence:** 1:10,000 to 1:20,000 births (Melnick and Myriantho-poulos, 1979). Said to be relatively frequent in Navajo Indians: 1:1,200 live births (Jaffe, 1969).

**Risk of Recurrence for Patient's Sib:**
See Part I, *Mendelian Inheritance*.

**Risk of Recurrence for Patient's Child:**
See Part I, *Mendelian Inheritance*.

**Age of Detectability:** At birth. In cases in which the canal is patent, a middle ear anomaly is almost invariably present with maximum conductive hearing loss. In these cases the hearing loss may be overlooked for a long time, but it should be suspected and can be diagnosed at birth.

**Gene Mapping and Linkage:** Unknown.

**Prevention:** None known. Genetic counseling indicated.

**Treatment:** Pinna, canal, and middle ear reconstruction. If the defect is bilateral, hearing aids should be fitted until the hearing mechanism is reconstructed. If surgical restoration of hearing is not possible or fails, fitting of hearing aids, preferential seating in school, and speech therapy are advisable. In bilateral cases, surgical reconstruction can be performed on one side at about age

five years, but in unilateral cases surgery should be delayed until adolescence.

**Prognosis:** Good for life unless serious associated defects exist. Restoration of serviceable hearing occurs in 50–67%. Facial nerve injury or external ear canal stenosis occurs as a complication of surgery in some patients. In a few patients, inner ear damage resulting in total hearing loss occurs.

**Detection of Carrier:** Unknown.

**Special Considerations:** The child with microtia-atresia deserves careful evaluation of the anatomy of the external canal, middle, and inner ear. Hearing should be thoroughly tested, even if there is no atresia. Bilateral computerized axial tomography should be done, since middle or inner ear anomalies may occur in the contralateral or ipsilateral ear. The patient should also have a careful general evaluation to rule out significant occult defects.

**References:**
Converse JM, ed: Reconstructive plastic surgery, vol 3. Philadelphia: W.B. Saunders Co., 1964:1084–1106.
d'Avignon M, Barr B: Ear abnormalities and cranial nerve palsies in thalidomide children. Arch Otolaryngol 1964; 80:136–140.
Crabtree JA: Tympanoplastic techniques in congenital atresia. Arch Otolaryngol 1968; 88:63–70.
Naunton RF, Valvassori GE: Inner ear anomalies: their association with atresia. Laryngoscope 1968; 78:1041–1049.
Hoenk, BE, et al.: Cholesteatoma auris behind a bony atresia plate. Arch Otolaryngol 1969; 89:470–477.
Jaffe BF: The incidence of ear diseases in the Navajo Indians. Laryngoscope 1969; 79:2126–2134.
Melnick M, Myrianthopoulos N, eds: External ear malformations: epidemiology, genetics and natural history. BD:OAS XV(9): New York: Alan R. Liss, 1979:1–140. *
Strisciuglio P, et al.: Microtia with meatal atresia and conductive deafness: mild and severe manifestations in the same sibship. J Med Genet 1986; 23:459–460.

BE028                                                    **LaVonne Bergstrom**

---

**Ear, middle-genitourinary anomalies**
*See RENAL-GENITAL-MIDDLE EAR ANOMALIES*

---

## EAR, MOZART TYPE                                                0328

**Includes:** Mozart ear

**Excludes:**
Atresia (alone)
**Deafness-ear pits** (0247)
Ear flare
**Ear lobe, pit** (0322)
**Ear, Darwin tubercle** (0241)
**Ear, microtia-atresia** (0664)

**Major Diagnostic Criteria:** Bulging superior margin of pinna caused by fusion of crura of the anthelix and the crus helicis.

**Clinical Findings:** This condition is said to have been present in the composer Mozart and in his father and son. The two crura of the anthelix and the crus of the helix are fused, giving a bulging appearance to the cartilaginous framework of the anterosuperior portion of the pinna. The anthelix is also somewhat larger than usual. (None of the usually published portraits of Mozart demonstrate this malformation, although one family portrait suggests it.)

**Complications:** Unknown.

**Associated Findings:** None known.

**Etiology:** Possible autosomal dominant inheritance.

**Pathogenesis:** Unknown.

**MIM No.:** 12840, 12850

**CDC No.:** 744.230

**Sex Ratio:** Presumably M1:F1

**Occurrence:** Undetermined. One United Kingdom study disclosed two cases among 2,227 patients attending hospital ear and medical clinics.

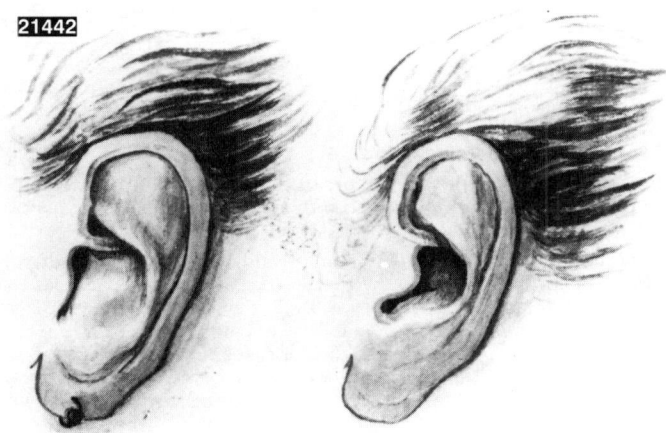

**0328-21442:** Mozart's ear is shown in detail on the left contrasted with a normal ear on the right. It is believed that this drawing of the Mozart ear deformity is from Mozart's son, who inherited the ear defect from his father.

**Risk of Recurrence for Patient's Sib:**
See Part I, *Mendelian Inheritance.*

**Risk of Recurrence for Patient's Child:**
See Part I, *Mendelian Inheritance.*

**Age of Detectability:** At birth.

**Gene Mapping and Linkage:** Unknown.

**Prevention:** None known. Genetic counseling indicated.

**Treatment:** If this is an isolated defect, no treatment is usually needed.

**Prognosis:** Good for life span, intelligence, and function if isolated defect of outer ear; otherwise, dependent on concomitant defects.

**Detection of Carrier:** Unknown.

**Special Considerations:** While there are no good illustrations of the actual ear of Wolfgang Amadeus Mozart, Sr. (he is thought to have concealed the condition), his son Wolfgang Jr. was said to have inherited the condition, and the pictures used today are actually those of the younger Mozart. Anomalies of the external ear should suggest the possibility of an anomaly of the middle ear as well. A range of other ear fold and flare variations have been reported of which the Mozart ear may be one expression.

A recent theory holds that Mozart died of a congenital renal anomaly. Some observers hold that the characteristic ear may in fact be part of that larger birth defect. A comprehensive review of this condition, and associated historical debates, can be found in Davies (1987). Arthur Everett Rappoport, M.D., professor emeritus of pathology at Northeastern Ohio Universities and now of Vero Beach, FL, has also made a major study of the topic and has spoken extensively on the "Amadeus murder mystery myth."

**References:**
Gates RR: Human genetics, vol. 1. New York: Macmillan, 1946.
Davies PJ: Mozart's left ear, nephropathy and death. Med J Aust 1987; 147:581–586.

BE028                                             **LaVonne Bergstrom**

**Ear, nose, digital anomalies-gingival fibromatosis**
*See GINGIVAL FIBROMATOSIS-DIGITAL ANOMALIES*

## EAR, OSSICLE AND MIDDLE EAR MALFORMATIONS          0773

**Includes:**
    Middle ear malformations with hearing loss
    Nerve malformations of middle ear
    Ossicle malformations
    Vascular malformations of middle ear

**Excludes:**
    Ear, anomalies of the external or internal
    Ear malformations associated with other branchial
      derivatives
    Middle ear malformations associated with other syndromes

**Major Diagnostic Criteria:** The malformations may be asymptomatic and present as an incidental finding during ear surgery for unrelated disease. However, middle ear malformations may be associated with nonprogressive conductive, and rarely with mixed conductive and sensorineural, hearing loss since birth.

**Clinical Findings:** Malformations of the middle ear are of major importance to both the patient and the otologist. When these malformations are associated with hearing loss since birth they may lead to an impaired speech development, and many of the affected children may be labeled mentally retarded, causing a serious social problem. Awareness of these malformations and the normal variations of the middle ear structures is extremely important during ear surgery to provide the necessary treatment and to avoid further destruction.

*Middle ear malformations with hearing loss::* There is usually a nonprogressive conductive hearing loss since birth or since the earliest recollection of childhood. One should suspect a middle ear malformation if another malformation is present or if there is a family history of a pharyngeal arch anomaly. Audiometrically, congenital conductive deafness tends to produce a more severe conductive loss, around 70 dB, than that in the usual acquired cases of deafness. The air conduction curve tends to be flat through the speech frequencies, while the bone conduction is on a top line with the Carhart notch, not present on the graph. A wide variation in the contour of the tympanogram curve is demonstrated by impedence audiometry, which may indicate ossicular discontinuity in the lateral components of the ossicular chain.

*Middle ear malformation without hearing loss:* usually discovered incidentally during ear surgery for unrelated diseases.

In addition to audiometric tests, examination of the tympanic membrane may reveal some of the middle ear malformations. These malformations can be evaluated preoperatively by high-resolution thin section axial CT scans and by multidirectional tomography.

**Complications:** Due to hearing impairment, delayed or slow mental development may occur. The severity is proportional to the hearing impairment. Recurrent meningitis may complicate subarachnoid-tympanic fistulae that may accompany stapes footplate defects.

**Associated Findings:** Defects of other derivatives of the same pharyngeal arches (I and II).

**Etiology:** Unknown except for rare, isolated cases of congenital rubella or syphilis, although these are more likely to be associated with other systemic manifestations.

**Pathogenesis:** Middle ear malformations are related to faulty developmental processes during embryonic life. The middle ear structures develop from the first and second pharyngeal arches and the intervening first pharyngeal pouch. The middle ear begins to form in the third embryonic week, and the tympanic cavity is almost completely formed by 13 weeks. The ossicles are fully formed in the cartilage and begin to ossify in the 16th week; they reach adult form in the 35th week. The head of the malleus and the body and short process of the incus arise from the first pharyngeal arch. The long process of the incus and the stapes, with the exception of the inner portion of the footplate, arise from the second arch. The anterior process of the malleus arises from ossification; the medial part of the stapes footplate is derived from a portion of the otic capsule.

*Ossicular malformations:* The malleus is the most commonly malformed ossicle. It is often fused to the incus. It also may be fixed by bone to the walls of the epitympanum. In addition to bony fixation to the malleus, the incus may also be fused to the head of the stapes or fixed to the medial wall of the epitympanum with its long process is almost always deformed. Anomalies of the stapes include footplate fixation, bony fusion of the head to the promontory, absence of the head and the crura, columella-type malformation, small form, and total absence. Some cases of deformed footplate may be associated with subarachnoid-tympanic fistulae in which cases recurrent meningitis may be a complication. Absence of the oval window is uncommon and is usually associated with absence of the stapes footplate, absent stapedius tendon, absent pyramidal prominence, deformed or absent incus and malleus, facial nerve anomalies, and/or absent chorda tympani. Absence of the oval window is associated with conductive or mixed conductive and sensorineural hearing loss.

*Soft tissue malformations:* Congenital absence of the stapedial muscle and tendon is found in eight of 1,000 operations on the middle ear; it may be associated with absence of the pyramidal prominence. A congenital defect in the posterior and inferior bony walls of the middle ear may lead to herniation of the jugular bulb into the tympanic cavity just below the oval window. This occurs in approximately one ear per 400. The stapedial artery may rarely persist as a moderately large vessel crossing the anterior stapes footplate. This occurs in approximately one ear per 1,000. Congenital dehiscence of the bony facial canal in the region of the oval window is present in 31% of normal temporal bones. An anomalous course of the facial nerve is most often an inferior displacement below the oval window across the promontory. An aberrant course of the facial nerve is present in 24% of ears with middle ear malformations.

**CDC No.:** 744.020

**Sex Ratio:** M1:F1

**Occurrence:** Defects sufficient to interfere with hearing function, about 1:40,000 live births. A surgically significant malformation sufficient to distort surgical landmarks, probably 1:100 births. Prevalence, one in 1:50,000 to 1:33,000.

**Risk of Recurrence for Patient's Sib:** Not increased except in rare cases of ossicular malformations that have an autosomal dominant inheritance.

**Risk of Recurrence for Patient's Child:** Not increased except in rare cases of ossicular malformations that have an autosomal dominant inheritance.

**Age of Detectability:** Early childhood in cases of significant hearing loss.

**Gene Mapping and Linkage:** Unknown.

**Prevention:** None known. Genetic counseling indicated.

**Treatment:** Otologic surgery or amplification; speech and language training.

**Prognosis:** Normal for life span. There is no progression of the structural malformation or the hearing loss after birth.

**Detection of Carrier:** Unknown.

**References:**
Hough JV: Congenital malformations of the middle ear. Arch Otolaryngol 1963; 78:335–343.
Sando I, Wood RP: Congenital middle ear anomalies. Otolaryngol Clin North Am 1971; 4:291–318.
Edwards WG: Congenital conditions of the middle-ear cleft. In: Ballantyne J, Groves J, eds: Diseases of the ear, nose and throat, Vol 2, ed 4. 1979:129–157.
Jahrsdoerfer RA: Congenital malformation of the ear. Ann Otol Rhinol Laryngol 1980; 89:348–352.
Jahrsdoerfer RA: The facial nerve in congenital middle ear malformations. Laryngoscope 1981; 91:1217–1225.

FA014                                    **Anwar I. Farhood**

---

**Includes:**
Ear, external, congenital sinuses of
Preauricular fistulae

**Excludes:**   Deafness-ear pits (0247)

**Major Diagnostic Criteria:** A preauricular or anterior helicine pit or sinus in an individual in whom there is a positive family history for the trait.

**Clinical Findings:** A usually shallow pit, which may be funnel-like or cystic, is located in the descending limb of the helix of the ear or just anterior to it. Occasionally, the pit may extend 1 or 2 cm as a sinus tract and rarely may communicate with the middle ear. The trait is unilateral in about 75% of cases and bilateral in about 25% of cases, with right and left sides being involved about equally in unilateral cases. The tracts are lined with squamous or columnar epithelium. If the lining is squamous, the usual skin appendages may be present. The pits often discharge a milky substance and are prone to become infected. Occasionally, a chronic infection may appear granulomatous.

**Complications:** Infection in the sinus.

**Associated Findings:** Branchial fistulas, cleft palate, spina bifida, imperforate anus, renal defects. It is possible that the association of all but branchial fistulas with ear pits is coincidental.

**Etiology:** Autosomal dominant inheritance with incomplete penetrance. One of identical twins may have the trait and the other may not.

**Pathogenesis:** Undetermined. It has been theorized that preauricular pits represent abortive accessory ear canals or that they represent areas of failure of fusion of the primitive ear hillocks. However, there is considerable disagreement about this. Both of these theories are somewhat attractive in view of the fact that ear pits are often seen in patients with microtia.

**MIM No.:** *12870

**Sex Ratio:** M1:F2 (observed)

**Occurrence:** Incidence 1:50 live births in African tribes, 1:500 live births in Europeans. Prevalence 0.9% among British draftees, 0.2% among white races, 5.2% among American blacks, 4.0% among African blacks, 1:1,000 in India. "Very prevalent" among the Chinese (exact figures not cited).

**Risk of Recurrence for Patient's Sib:**
See Part I, *Mendelian Inheritance.*

**Risk of Recurrence for Patient's Child:**
See Part I, *Mendelian Inheritance.*

**Age of Detectability:** At birth.

**Gene Mapping and Linkage:** Unknown.

**Prevention:** None known. Genetic counseling indicated.

**Treatment:** Medical treatment if pits become infected; incision and drainage if an abscess forms; excision of the tract if infection is recurrent or chronic.

**Prognosis:** Normal for life span, intelligence, and function.

**Detection of Carrier:** Unknown.

**References:**
Quelprud T: Ear pit and its inheritance: fistula auris congenita, described in 1864, still a genetical and embryological puzzle. J Hered 1940; 31:379–384.
Stiles KA: Inheritance of pitted ear. J Hered 1945; 36:53–61.
Ewing MR: Congenital sinuses of external ear. J Laryngol 1946; 61:18–23.
Martins AG: Lateral cervical and preauricular sinuses: their transmission as dominant characters. Br Med J 1961; 1:255–256.
Simpkiss MJ, Lowe A: Congenital abnormalities in the African newborn. Arch Dis Child 1961; 36:404–406.
Bhalla V, et al.: Familial transmission of preauricular fistula in a seven generation Indian pedigree. Hum Genet 1979; 48:339–341.

BE028                                    **LaVonne Bergstrom**

Ear, posteriorly rotated
*See EAR, LONG, NARROW, POSTERIORLY ROTATED*

## EAR, PROMINENT ANTHELIX 0330

**Includes:**
Anthelix, prominent
Wildermuth ear

**Excludes:**
Atresia (alone)
**Deafness-ear pits** (0247)
**Ear, Darwin tubercle** (0241)
Ear flare
**Ear lobe, pit** (0322)
**Ear, microtia-atresia** (0664)

**Major Diagnostic Criteria:** Prominent anthelix.

**Clinical Findings:** Prominence of the anthelix with a very poorly formed helix is seen.

**Complications:** Unknown.

**Associated Findings:** This condition may be seen in a number of syndromes, some of which have multiple anomalies. A sensorineural or conductive hearing loss may be present in some instances and is probably due to associated middle ear anomalies.

**Etiology:** Unknown.

**Pathogenesis:** Unknown.

**CDC No.:** 744.230

**Sex Ratio:** Presumably M1:F1

**Occurrence:** Unknown.

**Risk of Recurrence for Patient's Sib:** Unknown.

**Risk of Recurrence for Patient's Child:** Unknown.

**Age of Detectability:** At birth.

**Gene Mapping and Linkage:** Unknown.

**Prevention:** None known. Genetic counseling indicated.

**Treatment:** If this is an isolated defect, no treatment is usually needed. If a conductive hearing loss is present, computed tomography should be done to assess the anatomic configuration of the middle ear, and, if it seems favorable, exploratory tympanotomy and surgical correction should be performed, if feasible. If not feasible, if unsuccessful, or if the patient has a sensorineural hearing loss, hearing aids should be fitted, and aural rehabilitation should be undertaken.

**Prognosis:** Good for life span, intelligence, and function if the defect is confined to the outer ear; otherwise, it is dependent upon concomitant defects.

**Detection of Carrier:** Unknown.

**Special Considerations:** Anomalies of the external ear should suggest the possibility of an anomaly of the middle ear as well.

**References:**
Rubin A, ed: Handbook of congenital malformations. Philadelphia: W.B. Saunders, 1967.
Konigsmark BW: Hereditary deafness with external-ear abnormalities: a review. Johns Hopkins Med J 1970; 127:228.

BE028 **LaVonne Bergstrom**

## EAR, SMALL WITH FOLDED-DOWN HELIX 0331

**Includes:** Ear, with folded-down helix (incompletely developed)
**Excludes:**
Atresia (alone)
**Deafness-ear pits** (0247)
**Ear, Darwin tubercle** (0241)
Ear flare
**Ear lobe, pit** (0322)
**Ear, microtia-atresia** (0664)

**Major Diagnostic Criteria:** Small ear with poorly developed helix folded down close to pinna.

**Clinical Findings:** The ear is small, and the helix is folded down close to the pinna in a plane parallel to the top of the head. The helix is poorly developed. Congenital absence of the incus-stapes articulation and deformity of the incus and stapes may be present, causing conductive hearing loss. A similar malformation is part of a number of syndromes.

**Complications:** Unknown.

**Associated Findings:** Absence of incus-stapes articulation and deformities of incus and stapes. Also seen in **Chromosome 21, trisomy 21**.

**Etiology:** Possibly autosomal dominant inheritance.

**Pathogenesis:** Unknown.

**MIM No.:** 12850

**CDC No.:** 744.280

**Sex Ratio:** Presumably M1:F1

**Occurrence:** Unknown. Unusual varieties of folding of the helix and other parts of the ear have been described in the literature.

**Risk of Recurrence for Patient's Sib:**
See Part I, *Mendelian Inheritance*.

**Risk of Recurrence for Patient's Child:**
See Part I, *Mendelian Inheritance*.

**Age of Detectability:** At birth.

**Gene Mapping and Linkage:** Unknown.

**Prevention:** None known. Genetic counseling indicated.

**Treatment:** Plastic surgical repair may be indicated. Within the first three weeks of life, the pinna may be molded on dental compound and surgitaped to the head for 3 weeks.

**Prognosis:** Good for life span, intelligence, and function if isolated defect of outer ear; otherwise, dependent on concomitant defects.

**Detection of Carrier:** Unknown.

**Special Considerations:** Anomalies of the external ear should suggest the possibility of an anomaly of the middle ear as well. Hearing should be assessed as soon as possible, and appropriate therapy should be instituted. The anatomy of the middle and inner ear should be determined by computed tomography. External ear anomalies should also prompt the physician to look for anomalies of other systems. Careful genetic and clinical studies of the family should be carried out if accompanying defects are found.

**References:**
Converse JM, ed: Reconstructive plastic surgery. Vol. 3. Philadelphia: W.B. Saunders, 1964.
Rogers BO: Microtic, lop, cup and protruding ears: four directly inheritable deformities. Plast Reconstr Surg 1968; 41:208.
Ahuja YR, Gupta M: Inheritance of an unusual ear type in man. Acta Genet Med Gemellol 1970; 19:454–456.
Konigsmark BW: Hereditary deafness with external-ear abnormalities: a review. Johns Hopkins Med J 1970; 127:228.
Schruddle J, Petrovici V: Beidaeitige symmetrische Ohrmuschelbildung mit dominanten Erbganz. HNO 1979; 27:38–40.

BE028 **LaVonne Bergstrom**

Ear, with folded-down helix (incompletely developed)
*See EAR, SMALL WITH FOLDED-DOWN HELIX*

**Earlobe attachment: attached vs unattached**
See EAR LOBE, ATTACHED
**Earlobes (thick)-deafness from incudostapedial abnormalities**
See EAR LOBE, HYPERTROPHIC THICKENED
**Early onset or infantile cystinosis**
See CYSTINOSIS
**Earring holes, natural**
See EAR LOBE, PIT
**Ears (low-set)-reduced mouth and jaws**
See AGNATHIA-MICROSTOMIA-SYNOTIA
**Ears (malformed)-deafness-mental retardation**
See DEAFNESS-MALFORMED EARS-MENTAL RETARDATION
**Ears, malformed and low-set-deafness**
See DEAFNESS-MALFORMED, LOW-SET EARS
**Eaton-McKusick syndrome**
See MESOMELIC DYSPLASIA, WERNER TYPE
**Ebstein anomaly of tricuspid valve**
See TRICUSPID VALVE, EBSTEIN ANOMALY
**Ebstein anomaly with maternal lithium exposure**
See FETAL LITHIUM EFFECTS
**Ecchymotic type Ehlers-Danlos syndrome**
See EHLERS-DANLOS SYNDROME
**Ectodermal and mesodermal dysplasia with osseous involvement**
See DERMAL HYPOPLASIA, FOCAL
**Ectodermal and mesodermal dysplasia, congenital**
See DERMAL HYPOPLASIA, FOCAL
**Ectodermal dysplasia, 'acquired'**
See FETAL EFFECTS OF POLYCHLORINATED BIPHENYL (PCB)
**Ectodermal dysplasia, anhidrotic**
See ECTODERMAL DYSPLASIA, CHRIST-SIEMENS-TOURAINE TYPE
**Ectodermal dysplasia, anhidrotic, autosomal recessive**
See ECTODERMAL DYSPLASIA, PASSARGE TYPE
**Ectodermal dysplasia, anhidrotic-palate and lip anomalies**
See ECTODERMAL DYSPLASIA, RAPP-HODGKIN TYPE

---

## ECTODERMAL DYSPLASIA, BASAN TYPE     0102

**Includes:**
> Basan syndrome
> Dermatoglyphics absent-nail and simian crease anomalies
> Ectodermal dysplasia-hypotrichosis
> Hypohidrosis-defective teeth-unusual dermatoglyphics
> Jorgenson syndrome

**Excludes:**
> **Dyskeratosis congenita** (2024)
> **Ectodermal dysplasia, Christ-Siemens-Touraine type** (0333)
> **Ectodermal dysplasia, hidrotic** (0334)

---

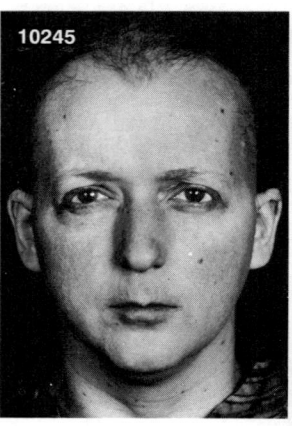 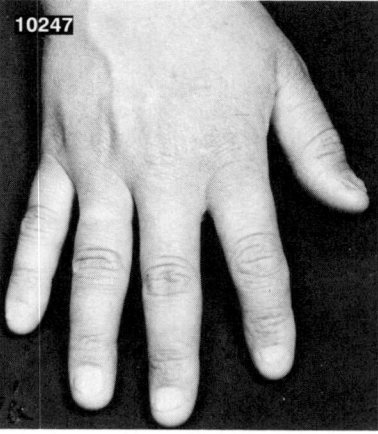

**0102**-10245: Characteristic facies includes narrow nose, long philtrum, thin vermilion border of the upper lip, sparse lashes, brows, and scalp hair. **10247:** Thick nails with longitudinal ridges and thick skin over the dorsal interphalangeal joints.

**Major Diagnostic Criteria:** Hypohidrosis, hypotrichosis, very fine dermal ridges over the hands and feet, single palmar flexion creases, and dysplastic nails.

**Clinical Findings:** Dry skin over the entire body, very fine dermal ridges over the hands and feet, single palmar flexion creases, short fingernails and toenails with thick longitudinal ridges, hypotrichosis, hypohidrosis, and dryness of mucous membranes. Body hair, eyebrows, and eyelashes are sparse from birth. Scalp hair in members of one family was normally thick at birth, but was coarse and grew slowly; it was shed rapidly toward the end of the second decade of life. Affected individuals sweat evenly over their entire bodies, although the amount of sweat is less than normal in quantity. The conjunctivae are dry, and conjunctivitis is frequent.

Facial features of affected members of one family were strikingly similar, characterized by thin alae nasi, long philtrums, and thin upper lips. Teeth of these individuals were lost early in life because of uncontrollable decay. The enamel appeared to be normal in thickness and density, but reportedly developed brown spots that eventually coalesced and decayed over the labial and buccal surfaces.

**Complications:** Nausea and flushing due to hypohidrosis; inability to tolerate heat; decreased libido.

**Associated Findings:** None known.

**Etiology:** Autosomal dominant inheritance.

**Pathogenesis:** Defective formation of several derivatives of the embryonic ectoderm suggest that this disorder may be properly classified as an ectodermal dysplasia. The onset of the dysplasia is probably later than that of several others of this set of disorders since it is the late-forming structures only that are affected. The late age of hair loss is unexplained, but the associated dental decay may be secondary to sparse oral secretions.

**MIM No.:** *12920

**POS No.:** 3822

**CDC No.:** 757.340

**Sex Ratio:** M1:F1

**Occurrence:** Rare; at least three kinships reported.

**Risk of Recurrence for Patient's Sib:**
See Part I, *Mendelian Inheritance.*

**Risk of Recurrence for Patient's Child:**
See Part I, *Mendelian Inheritance.*

**Age of Detectability:** At birth.

**Gene Mapping and Linkage:** Unknown.

**Prevention:** None known. Genetic counseling indicated.

**Treatment:** Avoidance of heat; lacrimal duct expansion may aid tearing; salves, creams, and artificial tears to keep conjunctivae moist.

Wigs are necessary in early adult life; early aggressive dental care is needed to reduce the spread of caries.

**Prognosis:** Good. The sweating dysfunction is not severe enough to cause excessive problems. Vision is the most severely compromised function.

**Detection of Carrier:** Unknown.

**Support Groups:** IL; Mascoutah; National Foundation for Ectodermal Dysplasias (NFED)

**References:**
Basan M: Ektodermale dysplasie: fehlendes papillarmuster, nagel-veranderungen und vierfingerfurche. Arch Clin Exp Dermatol 1965; 222:546–557.
Jorgenson RJ: Ectodermal dysplasia with hypotrichosis, hypohidrosis, defective teeth and unusual dermatoglyphics (Basan syndrome?). In: BD:OAS 1974; X(4):323–325. New York: Alan R. Liss. * †
Reed T, Schreiner RL: Absence of dermal ridge patterns: genetic heterogeneity. Am J Med Genet 1983; 16:81–88.

J0027          **Ronald J. Jorgenson**

**Ectodermal dysplasia, Berlin type**
See BERLIN SYNDROME

# ECTODERMAL DYSPLASIA, CHRIST-SIEMENS-TOURAINE TYPE

**0333**

**Includes:**

Christ-Siemens-Touraine syndrome
Ectodermal dysplasia, anhidrotic
Ectodermal dysplasia, hypohidrotic
Ectodermal polydysplasia
Hypohidrosis-hypodontia-hypotrichosis
"Toothless man of Sind"
"Whitaker Negroes"

**Excludes: Ectodermal dysplasia** (other)

**Major Diagnostic Criteria:** Hypohidrosis, hypodontia, hypotrichosis, charactistic facial appearance.

**Clinical Findings:** There is a life-long inability to sweat in response to heat, although some stress-related sweat function may be seen. The scalp hair, brows, lashes, axillary hair and pubic hair are sparse. Facial (beard) hair is present. Hair that is present may be excessively light in color. Periorbital skin is wrinkled and may be more deeply pigmented than surrounding skin. Teeth may be absent or only a few conical ones, representing the canines and incisors, may be present. Persistence of primary dentition and delayed eruption have been reported. There is frontal bossing, a depressed nasal bridge and loss of vertical height of the lower third of the face. This latter feature is secondary to hypodontia. Other features may include hyperconvex nails, foul-smelling nasal discharge, growth problems, and other skin changes.

**Complications:** Desquamation of skin in neonatal period, repeated episodes of high fever especially due to heat intolerance, constipation, dry corneas, otitis media, repeated upper respiratory infections (pneumonia, bronchitis), susceptibility to infections, and difficulties with eating are common problems. Hypogammaglobulinemia and propensity to allergies and atopic dermatitis have also been reported.

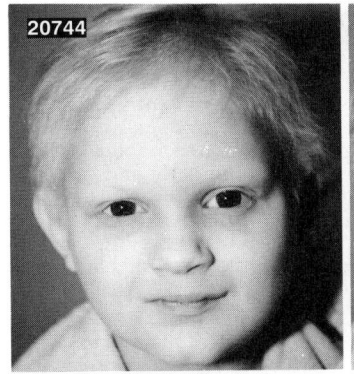
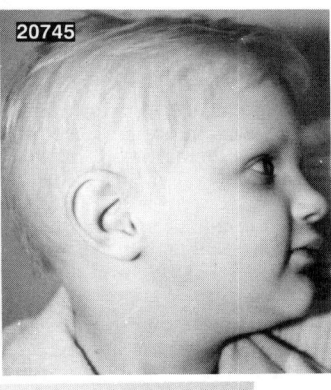
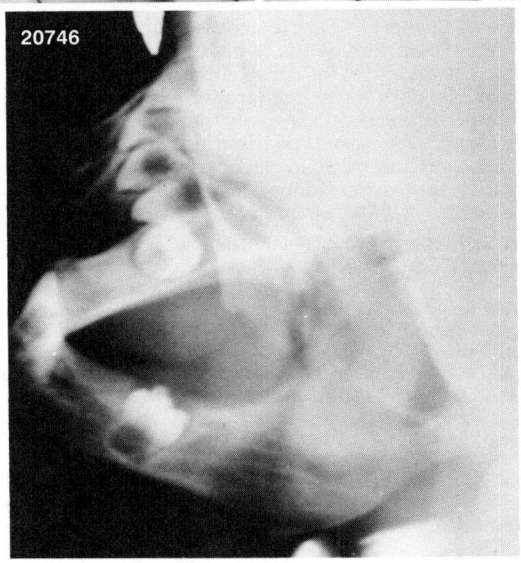

**0333B-**20744–45: Ectodermal dysplasia, Christ-Siemans-Touraine type; note sparse hair and dry periorbital skin. 20746: X-ray of the mandible shows absent teeth.

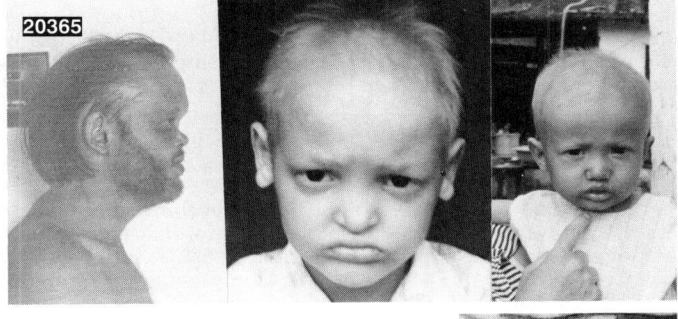
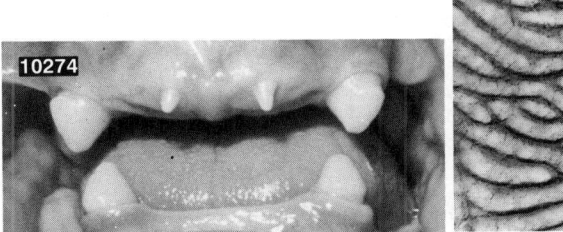

**0333A-**20365: Frontal and lateral views of affected males at different ages; note hypotrichosis, frontal bossing, protruding lips, saddle nose, abnormal auricles and apparently normal beard. 10274: Missing and conical teeth. 20366: Absence of sweat pores at the fingertip of an affected male.

**Associated Findings:** Glaucoma, vaginal atresia and learning disability have been reported. This latter feature may be secondary to brain damage suffered during prolonged episodes of high fever.

**Etiology:** Both autosomal recessive and X-linked recessive inheritance have been reported.

**Pathogenesis:** Defects in more than one ectodermal structure suggests that there is a primary defect in the ectoderm or the mesoderm underlying the defective structures.

**MIM No.:** *22490, *30510

**POS No.:** 3208

**CDC No.:** 757.340

**Sex Ratio:** Presumably M1:F1, because even in the X-linked form females show mild manifestations.

**Occurrence:** 1–7:10,000.

**Risk of Recurrence for Patient's Sib:**
See Part I, *Mendelian Inheritance.*

**Risk of Recurrence for Patient's Child:**
See Part I, *Mendelian Inheritance.*

**Age of Detectability:** Neonatal period by dry, sloughing skin or unexplained fever. Most cases are detected in early childhood because of heat intolerance or dental defects.

**Gene Mapping and Linkage:** EDA (ectodermal dysplasia, anhidrotic (hypohydrotic)) has been mapped to Xq12-q13.1.

**Prevention:** None known. Genetic counseling indicated.

**Treatment:** Most treatment is restorative or preventive in nature. Missing teeth are replaced with dentures or bridges, with dental implants being used in the past few years. Impacted nasal secretions and ear wax must be removed regularly and carefully. Some ointments seem to improve the dry skin. Artificial tears and wigs are useful in some cases. Because of the dyshidrosis, a cool environment must be maintained. Air conditioning, sponge baths, cool cloths, and large amounts of dietary fluids are necessary in warm weather.

**Prognosis:** Good for function, intelligence, and life span. However, cases of brain damage as a consequence of high fever, and of sudden infant death syndrome (SIDS), have been reported.

**Detection of Carrier:** None for autosomal recessive type. About 70% of female carriers of the X-linked recessive type may have mild manifestations of at least some of the diagnostic signs. Heterozygotes also have been reported to show a pattern of lyonization that corresponds, over the back for example, to lines of Blaschko. Sweat pore distribution and function, size and number of teeth and microscopic appearance of hair have all been investigated for carrier identification, but none is universally applicable.

**Support Groups:** IL; Mascoutah; National Foundation for Ectodermal Dysplasias (NFED)

**References:**

Weech AA: Hereditary ectodermal dysplasia (congenital ectodermal defect). Am J Dis Child 1929; 37:766–790. *

Gorlin RJ, et al.: Hypohidrotic ectodermal dysplasia in females. Z Kinderheilk 1970; 108:1–11. *

Verbov J: Hypohidrotic (or anhidrotic) ectodermal dysplasia - an appraisal of diagnostic methods. Br J Derm 1970; 83:341–348.

Bartlett RC, et al.: Autosomal recessive hypohidrotic ectodermal dysplasia. dental manifestations. Oral Surg 1972; 33:736–742.

Airenne P: X-linked hypohidrotic ectodermal dysplasia in Finland. Proc Finn Dent Soc 1981; 77(Suppl I)1–106.

Hotzes J, et al.: Anhidrotic ectodermal dysplasia: therapeutic attempts. Dermatologica 1982; 164:54–61.

Happle R, Frosch PJ: Manifestation of the lines of Blaschko in women heterozygous for X-linked hypohidrotic ectodermal dysplasia. Clin Genet 1985; 27:468–471.

Soderholm A-L, Kaitila I: Expression of X-linked hypohidrotic ectodermal dysplasia in six males and in their mothers. Clin Genet 1985; 28:136–144.

Clarke A: Hypohidrotic ectodermal dysplasia. J Med Genet 1987; 24:659–663.

Executive and Scientific Advisory Boards of the National Foundation for Ectodermal Dysplasias: Scaling skin in the neonate: a clue to the early diagnosis of X-linked hypohidrotic ectodermal dysplasia (Christ-Siemens-Touraine syndrome). J Pediatr 1989; 114:600–602.

J0027                      **Ronald J. Jorgenson**

## ECTODERMAL DYSPLASIA, CONGENITAL FACIAL, SETLEIS TYPE     2095

**Includes:**
Bitemporal aplasia cutis congenita
"Forceps marks" scarring and unusual facies, temporal
Temporal "forceps marks" scarring and unusual facies
Facial ectodermal dysplasia
Setleis syndrome

**Excludes:**
Ectodermal dysplasia, hidrotic (0334)
Ehlers-Danlos syndrome (0338)

**Major Diagnostic Criteria:** Bitemporal skin depressions resembling forceps marks, associated with a "leonine" facial expression.

**Clinical Findings:** Craniofacial abnormalities that have occurred in all eleven reported patients include bitemporal skin depressions consistent with aplasia cutis congenita; periorbital puffiness which

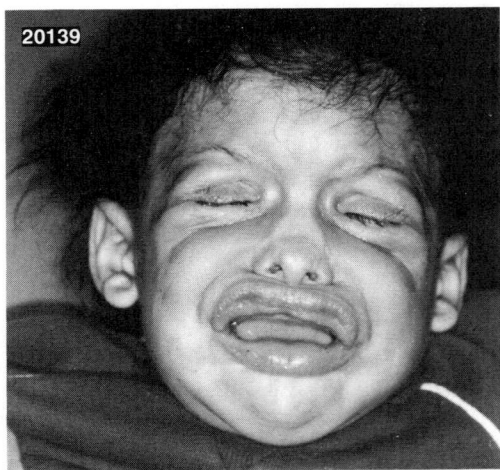

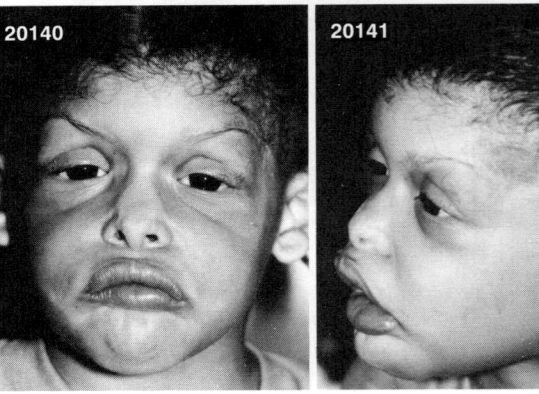

2095-20139: Characteristic facies of Setleis syndrome at age 15 months. Note redundant facial soft tissue; periorbital puffiness; thin, flaring eyebrows; flattened nasal bridge with bulbous tip; and prominent vermilion border of the lip. 20140: Subject shown in 20139 at 31 months of age. 20141: Lateral view of facies at 31 months of age, showing bitemporal depressions resembling forceps marks.

is responsible for an aged appearance; eyebrows that angle sharply upward and outward, but which are deficient laterally; abnormalities of the eyelashes, including distichiasis of the upper lids and astichiasis of the lower lids; abnormalities of the nose, including a flat nasal bridge, a bulbous tip, and a nasal septum extending below the alae nasae; and increased mobility of the skin and connective tissue of the upper lip, associated with severely redundant facial soft tissue.

The bitemporal depressions are quite striking in affected newborns, and have prompted parents of at least three of the patients to maintain that forceps were used during delivery, even though the obstetric record did not support this. Further, the facial stigmata are so characteristic that photographs of one patient might very well be substituted for another.

**Complications:** Blepharitis has occurred in four of eight affected individuals, secondary to irritation caused by the eyelash abnormalities.

**Associated Findings:** Craniofacial features noted in some of the patients have included strabismus (1/11); downward obliquity of the palperbal fissures; small, malformed ears; and abnormalities of the hair, including alopecia, thin scalp hair, and low frontal hair line. Extracranial abnormalities have included hypo- or hyperpigmentation (cafe-au-lait spots, vitiliginous areas, etc), abnormal palmar creases, abnormal nipples, and imperforate anus. Mental retardation was present in one chilld. Otherwise, growth and development has been normal.

**Etiology:** Autosomal recessive inheritance.

**Pathogenesis:** This condition is primarily an ectodermal defect. skin biopsy of the temporal area in one individual has shown thinned epidermis, and absent dermal structures, such as the pilo-sebaceous apparatus, sweat glands, and hair follicles. This picture is consistent with aplasia cutis congenita.

**MIM No.:** *22726

**POS No.:** 3407

**CDC No.:** 757.346

**Sex Ratio:** M4:F7 (observed).

**Occurrence:** The families of eight reported patients are from Puerto Rico, with seven of the eight coming from the towns of San Sebastion and Aguadilla. The remaining three were of other ethnic backgrounds.

**Risk of Recurrence for Patient's Sib:**
See Part I, *Mendelian Inheritance*.

**Risk of Recurrence for Patient's Child:**
See Part I, *Mendelian Inheritance*.

**Age of Detectability:** In the neonatal period, by physical examination.

**Gene Mapping and Linkage:** Unknown.

**Prevention:** None known. Genetic counseling indicated.

**Treatment:** Symptomatic treatment of blepharitis; epilation of aberrant eyelashes may be helpful. The facial features tend to become more normal with age. Because of this, plastic surgery for correction of the craniofacial abnormalities should be postponed as long as possible.

**Prognosis:** Life span and intellect are usually unimpaired.

**Detection of Carrier:** Unknown.

**Support Groups:** IL; Mascoutah; National Foundation for Ectodermal Dysplasias (NFED)

**References:**
Setleis H, et al: Congenital ectodermal dysplasia of the face. Pediatr 1963; 32:540–547. †
Rudolph RI, et al.: Bitemporal aplasia cutis congenita: occurrence with other cutaneous abnormalities. Arch Dermatol 1974; 110:615–618.
Rudolph RI, et al.: Emendation to "Bitemporal aplasia cutis congenita". Arch Dermatol 1974; 110:636 only.
Marion RW, et al: Autosomal recessive inheritance in the Setleis bitemporal "forceps marks" syndrome. Am J Dis Child 1987; 141: 895–897.
Clark RD, et al.: Expanded phenotype and ethnicity in Setleis syndrome. Am J Med Genet 1989; 34:354–357. *

T0007
MA032

**Helga V. Toriello**
**Robert W. Marion**

**Ectodermal dysplasia, corneo-dermato-osseous type**
*See CORNEO-DERMATO-OSSEOUS SYNDROME*
**Ectodermal dysplasia, dermo-odontodysplasia**
*See DERMO-ODONTODYSPLASIA*
**Ectodermal dysplasia, euhidrotic-refractive errors**
*See TRICHODENTAL DYSPLASIA WITH REFRACTIVE ERRORS*

## ECTODERMAL DYSPLASIA, HAY-WELLS TYPE 2590

**Includes:**
Ankyloblepharon-ectodermal defects-cleft lip and palate (AEC)
Hay-Wells syndrome

**Excludes:**
**Chands** (3039)
**Cleft lip/palate-ectodermal dysplasia-syndactyly** (0179)
**Cleft lip/palate-filiform fusion of eyelids** (0176)
**Ectrodactyly-ectodermal dysplasia-clefting syndrome** (0337)
**Ectodermal dysplasia, Rapp-Hodgkin type** (3056)

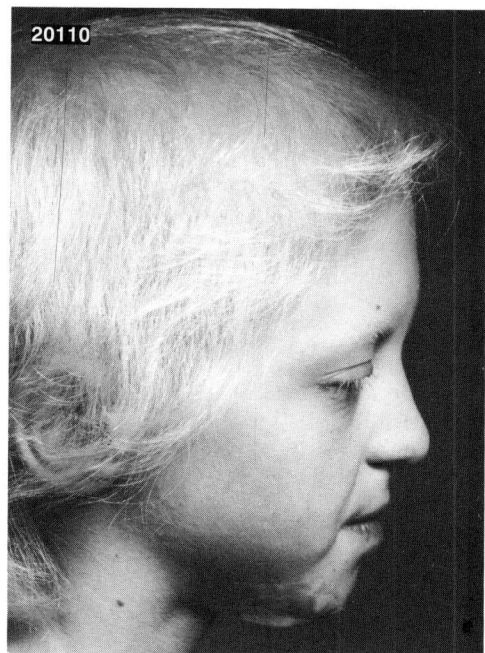

**2590-20110:** Lateral view of face showing maxillary hypoplasia and pale blond, wiry, coarse scalp hair.

**Eyelid, ankyloblepharon** (0060)
**Pterygium syndrome, popliteal** (0818)

**Major Diagnostic Criteria:** Ankyloblepharon filiform adnatum, scalp erythema or erosions at birth with predisposition to infections, sparse coarse hair or alopecia, hypodontia, dystrophic nails, mild hypohidrosis, maxillary hypoplasia, and cleft lip/palate or velopharyngeal incompetence are the most constant features. Palmoplantar keratoderma is often present in adults.

**Clinical Findings:** The condition is evident at birth. Of the 12 patients described in the literature, all have had sparse hair that is described as coarse, wiry, and brittle. Several patients had progressive shedding of hair, so that all four adults had almost total alopecia, while two of seven children had patchy alopecia.

All 12 patients have had abnormalities of nails, which varied from complete absence of nails in one patient, to a combination of absent and dystrophic nails in two patients, to only dystrophic nails in the remaining nine patients. All patients have had hypodontia; teeth were small and pointed with decreased enamel. Some patients had partial congenital anodontia, while others lost their teeth because of severe caries.

Eleven of the twelve patients had **Cleft palate**, while one had only velopharyngeal incompetence. **Cleft lip** occurred in four of the 12 patients.

**Eyelid, ankyloblepharon** was present in 11 of the 12 patients; in the remaining patient, no information from early childhood was available. These bands can be surgically divided with ease, and there is one report of spontaneous separation. Residua of the bands may appear as small papules along the borders of the eyelids. In seven of 12 patients, one or more lacrimal puncta were absent or hypoplastic, and six of 12 patients complained of blepharitis and/or photophobia.

Dry skin was described in eight of 12 patients, but only three noticed decreased sweating. This was never severe enough to result in hyperthermia or exercise intolerance. Of six patients who had skin biopsies, four had a patchy decrease in the number of sweat glands. Four of five adults had sparse body hair, but sparse lashes and brows were noted at all ages. Plantar and palmar keratoderma were present in four of five adults but in none of the children.

For nine patients who had complete medical information available from childhood, six had significant scalp infections, especially in infancy.

Five of six adults and older children were noted to have maxillary hypoplasia with a relatively prominent chin; four also had a broad nasal bridge. Distinctive facial features were not noted in infancy except for one infant who had a broad nasal bridge.

Two patients had unilateral cupped ears; one had bilateral cupped ears plus bilateral congenital stenosis of the ear canals. One patient with normally formed ears developed a web in one canal. Mild conductive hearing loss was present only in patients with ear canal obstruction. One patient had partial neural hearing loss, but his unaffected mother also had partial deafness. Intellect has been normal in all patients.

**Complications:** Ear infections related to cleft palate. Conductive hearing loss due to ear canal stenosis or webs. Blepharitis, dental caries, and scalp infections are medical complications. Cleft lip, sparse hair or alopecia, and dystrophic nails may be of cosmetic concern.

**Associated Findings:** Only two patients had partial syndactyly of toes 2 and 3, and one of these patients also had **Syndactyly** of toes 3 and 4 (unilateral) and fingers 3 and 4 (bilateral). One patient had a supernumerary nipple, and another had ectopic breast tissue in the axilla. Only one patient had skin hyperpigmentation of the upper extremities. One patient had choanal atresia and one other patient had a granuloma of the vocal cord. One male had **Hypospadias**.

**Etiology:** Possibly autosomal dominant inheritance with variable expression. Four of the 12 reported cases were sporadic. No instance of incomplete penetrance is known.

**Pathogenesis:** Unknown.

**MIM No.:** 10626

**POS No.:** 3524

**CDC No.:** 757.346

**Sex Ratio:** M1:F1

**Occurrence:** Twelve cases have been described in the literature. Families were from Great Britain, the United States, and Canada (French-Canadian).

**Risk of Recurrence for Patient's Sib:**
See Part I, *Mendelian Inheritance.*

**Risk of Recurrence for Patient's Child:**
See Part I, *Mendelian Inheritance.*

**Age of Detectability:** In infancy.

**Gene Mapping and Linkage:** Unknown.

**Prevention:** None known. Genetic counseling indicated.

**Treatment:** Surgical correction of ankyloblepharon, cleft lip/palate, ear canal stenosis, or webs; good dental hygiene; antibiotics for scalp infections.

**Prognosis:** Normal life span.

**Detection of Carrier:** Clinical examination.

**Support Groups:** IL; Mascoutah; National Foundation for Ectodermal Dysplasias (NFED)

**References:**

Bowen P, Armstrong HB: Ectodermal dysplasia, mental retardation, cleft lip/palate and other anomalies in 3 sibs. Clin Genet 1976; 9:35–42.

Hay RJ, Wells RS: The syndrome of ankyloblepharon, ectodermal defects and cleft lip and palate: an autosomal dominant condition. Br J Dermatol 1976; 94:227–289. *

Rosenman Y, et al.: Ankyloblepharon filiforme adnatum: congenital eyelid- band syndromes. Am J Dis Child 1980; 134:751–753.

Freire-Maia N, Pinheiro M: Ectodermal dysplasias: a clinical and genetic study. New York: Alan R. Liss, 1984.

Spiegel J, Colton A: AEC syndrome: ankyloblepharon, ectodermal defects, and cleft lip and palate. J Am Acad Dermatol 1985; 12:810–815.

Greene SL, et al.: Variable expression in ankyloblepharon-ectodermal defects-cleft lip and palate syndrome. Am J Med Genet 1987; 27:207–212. *

Shwayder TA, et al.: Hay-Wells syndrome. Proceed Greenwood Genet Center 1987; 6:98 only.

MI002                                **Virginia V. Michels**

## ECTODERMAL DYSPLASIA, HIDROTIC      0334

**Includes:**

Clouston ectodermal dysplasia
Fischer-Jacobsen-Clouston syndrome
Hair and nails, hereditary dystrophy
Jacobsen syndrome
Ungual ectodermal dysplasia

**Excludes:**

**Dyskeratosis congenita** (2024)
**Ectodermal dysplasia** (other)
Hidrotic ectodermal dysplasia-deafness

**Major Diagnostic Criteria:** Variable sparsity of head and body hair and dystrophy of nails.

**Clinical Findings:** Sparse, thin, fragile hair with reduced tensile strength on the head, eyebrows and body. Dystrophic, thick nails with subungual infections (sometimes hypoplastic or missing). Thick rough skin on palms and soles with brownish pigmentation. Normal sweat glands and teeth. Thickening of skull bones, tufting of terminal phalanges. Electron microscope shows disorganization of the hair fibrils with loss of cuticular cortex. Variable expressivity, especially of the hair defect.

**Complications:** Unknown.

**Associated Findings:** Possibly dental anomalies.

**Etiology:** Autosomal dominant inheritance with complete penetrance.

**Pathogenesis:** Structural defect of keratin resulting from a change in molecular structure involving loss of high molecular weight components of the matrix protein.

**MIM No.:** *12950

**POS No.:** 3209

**CDC No.:** 757.340

**Sex Ratio:** M1:F1

**Occurrence:** Rare. Most common in areas settled by French families carrying the gene, e.g. near Montreal and New Orleans.

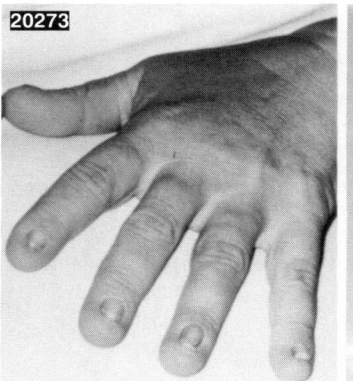 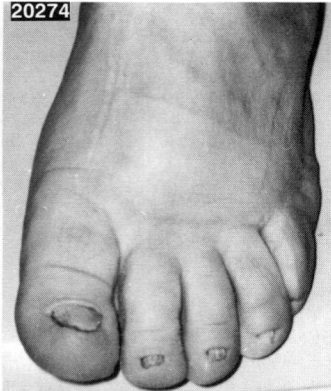

**0334A-20273:** Small and dystrophic fingernails with convex ends. **20274:** Small, dystrophic toenails with longitudinal striations.

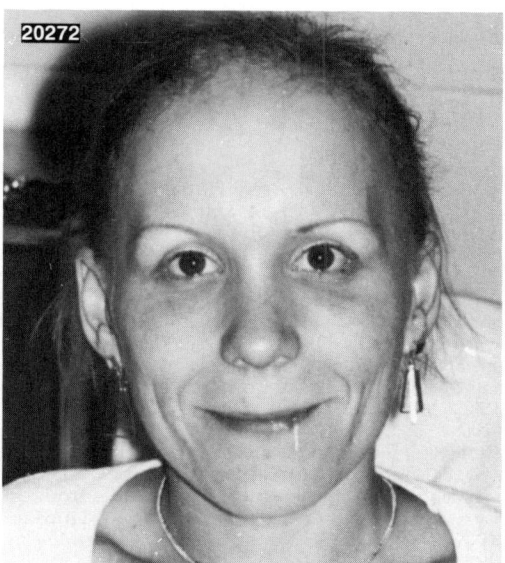

**0334B**-20272: Note sparse hair, scanty eyelashes and brows.

**Risk of Recurrence for Patient's Sib:**
See Part I, *Mendelian Inheritance.*

**Risk of Recurrence for Patient's Child:**
See Part I, *Mendelian Inheritance.*

**Age of Detectability:** In neonatal period.

**Gene Mapping and Linkage:** Unknown.

**Prevention:** None known. Genetic counseling indicated.

**Treatment:** Undetermined. Wigs and gloves may be cosmetically and psychologically helpful.

**Prognosis:** Normal life span.

**Detection of Carrier:** Unknown.

**Special Considerations:** Some researchers have suggested that there is evidence of reproductive overcompensation.

**Support Groups:** IL; Mascoutah; National Foundation for Ectodermal Dysplasias (NFED)

**References:**
Clouston HR: A hereditary ectodermal dystrophy. Can Med Assoc J 1929; 21:18–31.
Williams M, Fraser FC: Hidrotic ectodermal dysplasia-Clouston's family revisited. Can Med Assoc J 1967; 96:36–38.
Gold RJM, Kachra Z: The molecular defect in hydrotic ectodermal dysplasia. In: Brown AC, ed: The first human hair symposium. New York: Medcom Press, 1974:260–276.
Rajagopalan KV, Tay CH: Hidrotic ectodermal dysplasia: study of a large Chinese pedigree. Arch Derm 1977; 113:481–484.
Escobar V, et al.: Clouston syndrome: an ultrastructural study. Clin Genet 1983; 24:140–146.

FR009                                                    **F. Clarke Fraser**

Ectodermal dysplasia, hypohidrotic
    *See ECTODERMAL DYSPLASIA, CHRIST-SIEMENS-TOURAINE TYPE*
Ectodermal dysplasia, hypohidrotic, autosomal recessive
    *See ECTODERMAL DYSPLASIA, PASSARGE TYPE*

---

**ECTODERMAL DYSPLASIA, NAEGELI TYPE**          **0703**

**Includes:**
   Chromatophore nevus of Naegeli
   Franceschetti-Jadassohn syndrome
   Incontinentia pigmenti of Naegeli
   Melanophoric nevus
   Naegeli-Franceschetti-Jadassohn syndrome
   Naegeli syndrome
   Palmoplantar hyperkeratosis-reticular pigmentation
   Reticular pigmented dermatosis
   Skin, Naegeli syndrome

**Excludes:**
   **Berlin syndrome** (0105)
   **Dyskeratosis congenita** (2024)
   **Incontinentia pigmenti** (0526)

**Major Diagnostic Criteria:** Cutaneous hyperpigmentation, plantar and palmar hyperkeratosis, dental alteration, and discomfort provoked by heat.

**Clinical Findings:** Affected individuals have cutaneous hyperpigmentation in reticular, "sheeting", and/or macular patterns. Onychodystrophy is present, and dental anomalies consisting of yellow spotting of the enamel, supernumerary teeth, and abnormal shape have been described. Palms and soles are hyperkeratotic, and dermal ridges are hypoplastic. Hyperlucent tympanic membranes and sparse hair have been described. Functional hypohidrosis is common.
   Although this condition closely resembles **Dyskeratosis congenita** and **Incontinentia pigmenti**, and may share a common pathogenesis, the mode of inheritance and age of onset should assist in differential diagnosis.

**Complications:** Heat intolerance caused by diminished sweat gland function.

**Associated Findings:** Reported in one affected patient each; abnormal EEG, osteoporosis, cataract, short stature, underdeveloped secondary sexual characteristics, and blistering of the heels in infancy.

**Etiology:** Autosomal dominant inheritance.

**Pathogenesis:** This is an ectodermal defect. Skin biopsies have shown hyperpigmentation of the epidermis and secondary pigmentary incontinence. Numerous melanin granules may be present in the upper dermis. Eccrine glands are present, suggesting that the hypohidrosis is functional.

**MIM No.:** *16100

**POS No.:** 4118

**CDC No.:** 757.900

**Sex Ratio:** M1:F1

**Occurrence:** Two kindreds have been documented.

**Risk of Recurrence for Patient's Sib:**
   See Part I, *Mendelian Inheritance.*

**Risk of Recurrence for Patient's Child:**
   See Part I, *Mendelian Inheritance.*

**Age of Detectability:** By the end of the second year, although possibly at birth if blistering on the heels occurs.

**Gene Mapping and Linkage:** Unknown.

**Prevention:** None known. Genetic counseling indicated.

**Treatment:** Unknown.

**Prognosis:** Average life span. Reproductive fitness seems unimpaired. Pigmentation decreases, sweating ability increases, and the hyperkeratosis and nail changes improve with age, usually after the second decade.

**Detection of Carrier:** Unknown.

**References:**
Naegeli O: Familiärer chromatophorennäevus. Schwei Med Wochenschr 1927; 57:48 only.
Franceschetti A, Jadassohn W: A propos de ''l'incontinentia pigmenti'', délimitation de deux syndromes différents figurant sous le même terme. Dermatologica 1954; 108:1–28.
Curth HO, Warburton D: The genetics of incontinentia pigmenti. Arch Dermatol 1965; 92:229–235.
Sparrow GP, et al.: Hyperpigmentation and hypohidrosis (the Naegeli-Franceschetti-Jadassohn syndrome): report of a family and review of the literature. Clin Exp Dermatol 1976; 1:127–141.

T0007                           **Helga V. Toriello**

**Ectodermal dysplasia, odonto-onychodermal dysplasia type**
*See ODONTO-ONYCHODERMAL DYSPLASIA*
**Ectodermal dysplasia, odonto-onychodysplasia-alopecia type**
*See ODONTO-ONYCHODYSPLASIA-ALOPECIA*

## ECTODERMAL DYSPLASIA, PASSARGE TYPE     3120

**Includes:**
Ectodermal dysplasia, hypohidrotic, autosomal recessive
Ectodermal dysplasia, anhidrotic, autosomal recessive

**Excludes:**
Ectodermal dysplasia, Christ-Siemens-Touraine type (0333)
Ectodermal dysplasia (other)

**Major Diagnostic Criteria:** Trichodysplasia, hypodontia, hypohidrosis, and characteristic face.

**Clinical Findings:** Sparse, brittle, lightly pigmented, and lanugo-like scalp hair; absent or scanty eyebrows, lashes and body hair; hypodontia, anodontia, conical teeth; hypohidrosis (with severe heat intolerance); thin, smooth, dry and hypoplastic skin (with dermatoglyphic changes, rudimentary nipples, and slight pigmented areolae); characteristic facies with saddle nose, frontal bossing, prominent auricles, and wrinkling especially about the eyes and mouth; the skin around the orbits may also be darker. Hypoplasia of lacrimal ducts; decreased function of lacrimal glands. Dystrophic nails, and tapered fingers have also been noted.

**Complications:** Hyperthermia due to reduced number of sweat glands; respiratory infections due to atrophy of the mucous glands of the respiratory tract; hoarseness or laryngitis-like speech; photophobia; chronic rhinitis.

**Associated Findings:** Sensorineural hearing loss and orbital hypertelorism have been reported.

**Etiology:** Autosomal recessive inheritance.

**Pathogenesis:** Unknown.

**MIM No.:** *22490

**Sex Ratio:** Presumably M1:F1.

**Occurrence:** At least 40 cases have been described. Females outnumber males, but this is probably due to a diagnostic bias: when sporadic affected males are seen, they are diagnosed as having the X-linked form.

**Risk of Recurrence for Patient's Sib:**
See Part I, *Mendelian Inheritance.*

**Risk of Recurrence for Patient's Child:**
See Part I, *Mendelian Inheritance.*

**Age of Detectability:** During the neonatal period, mainly by unexplained fever. Most cases are diagnosed during childhood.

**Gene Mapping and Linkage:** Unknown.

**Prevention:** None known. Genetic counseling indicated.

**Treatment:** Prosthetic replacement and orthodontic treatment; wigs are cosmetically and psychologically helpful. Limited exercise in heat. Use of false tears for dryness of eyes.

**Prognosis:** After early life, during which hyperthermic crisis may be severe, prognosis is good.

**Detection of Carrier:** Some heterozygotes present subclinical manifestations of the condition (e.g., low sweat pore count).

**Support Groups:** IL; Mascoutah; National Foundation for Ectodermal Dysplasias (NFED)

**References:**
Passarge E, et al: Anhidrotic ectodermal dysplasia as autosomal recessive trait in an inbred kindred. Humangenetik 1966; 3:181–185.
Gorlin RJ, et al: Hypohidrotic ectodermal dysplasia in females: a critical analysis and argument for genetic heterogeneity. Z Kinderheilkd 1970; 108:1–11.
Bartlett RC, et al: Autosomal recessive hypohidrotic ectodermal dysplasia: dental manifestations. Oral Surg 1972; 33:736–742.
Kratzsch R: Ektodermale Dysplasie vom anhidrotischen Typ bei zwei Schwestern. Klin Pädiatr 1972; 184:328–332.
Passarge E, Fries E: Autosomal recessive hypohidrotic ectodermal dysplasia with subclinical manifestation in the heterozygote. BD: OAS XII(3C). New York: March of Dimes Birth Defects Foundation, 1977:95–100.
Kleinebrecht J, et al: Sweat pore counts in ectodermal dysplasias. Hum Genet 1981; 54:437–439.
Anton-Lamprecht I, et al.: Autosomal recessive anhidrotic ectodermal dysplasia: report of a case and discrimination of diagnostic features. BD:OAS XXIV (2). New York: March of Dimes Birth Defects Foundation, 1988:183–195.

PI008                           **Marta Pinheiro**
FR033                     **Newton Freire-Maia**

**Ectodermal dysplasia, pilo-dento-ungular type**
*See PILO-DENTO-UNGULAR DYSPLASIA WITH MICROCEPHALY*

## ECTODERMAL DYSPLASIA, RAPP-HODGKIN TYPE     3056

**Includes:**
Ectodermal dysplasia, anhidrotic-palate and lip anomalies
Hair, wiry, uncombable, straw-like-palate/lip anomalies
Rapp-Hodgkin ectodermal dysplasia

**Excludes:**
Ectrodactyly-ectodermal dysplasia-clefting syndrome (0337)
Ectodermal dysplasia, Christ-Siemens-Touraine type (0333)
Ectodermal dysplasia, Hay-Wells type (2590)
Ectodermal dysplasia, Passarge type (3120)

**Major Diagnostic Criteria:** Hypohidrotic ectodermal dysplasia with anomalies of palate and lip and wiry, uncombable, straw-like hair. SEM of hair shows pili canaliculi, irregular twists, and diminished height between cuticula margins. Polarizing light studies show alternating dark and light bands.

**Clinical Findings:** Various clefts of the lip, palate, or uvula; dysplastic nails, very sparse hair, and hypospadias are present at birth.
Hair will grow very slowly and apparently abundantly due to wiry and uncombable characteristics. At a closer examination the hair is sparse, coarse to touch, and generally dull in appearance with a straw-like color. Mothers will usually cut children's hair or nails only once or twice a year. Children have speech problems and otitis media due to cleft palate or submucous cleft. They also may have a breathy voice associated with the absence of normal mucosal covering of the vocal folds. Hypodontia and microdontia of primary and permanent teeth are observed; small mouth and hypoplastic alae nasi have been reported. The sweating activity is limited, although some patients perspire abundantly by the scalp. Premature baldness in males and females has been observed.

**Complications:** Hyperthermia due to limited sweating. Recurrent otitis media or chronic otitis media probably associated with the **Cleft palate** defect. Purulent conjunctivitis, epiphora due to aplasia of the lacrimal canaliculi, and scalp may have ulcer-like lesions.

**Associated Findings:** Atretic ear canal, hearing deficits, dental caries, epiphora, and flattening of epidermal ridges.

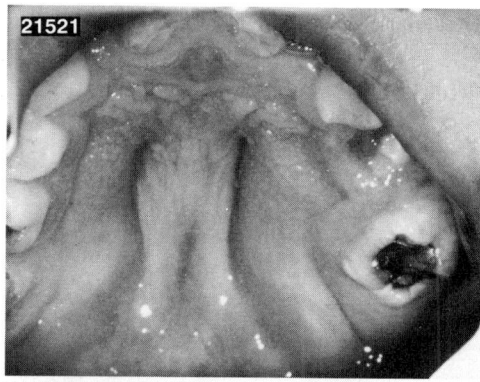

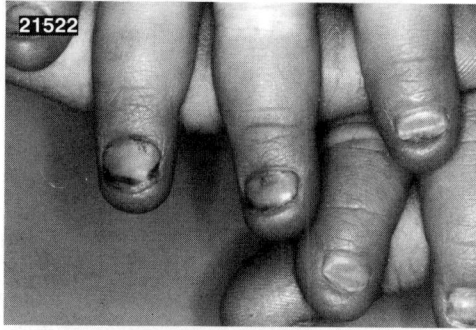

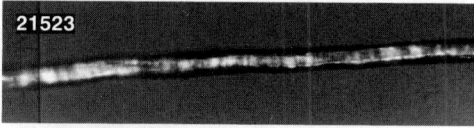

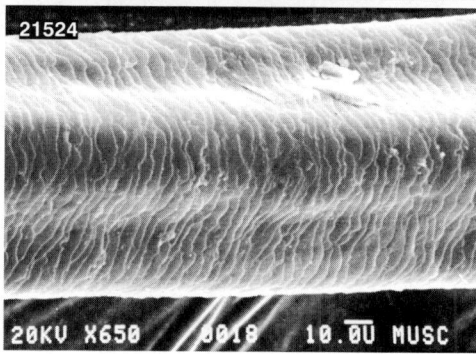

**3056**-21521: Midline submucous cleft palate. 21522: Dysplastic nails. 21523: Note bands of birefringency and nonbirefringency in the hair. 21524: Scanning electron micrograph of hair shows "pili canaliculi" and cuticular abnormalities.

**Etiology:** Autosomal dominant inheritance with variable expression. Recently male-to-male transmission was demonstrated in three generations.

**Pathogenesis:** Unknown.

**MIM No.:** *12940

**POS No.:** 3137

**Sex Ratio:** M1:F1

**Occurrence:** A few dozen cases have been documented.

**Risk of Recurrence for Patient's Sib:**
See Part I, *Mendelian Inheritance.*

**Risk of Recurrence for Patient's Child:**
See Part I, *Mendelian Inheritance.*

**Age of Detectability:** Possibly at birth. However, the condition is most obvious in late infancy, with hair changes, hypodontia, and hypohidrosis.

**Gene Mapping and Linkage:** Unknown.

**Prevention:** None known. Genetic counseling indicated.

**Treatment:** Cleft lip/palate repair; speech therapy; dental treatment, prevention of caries, cosmetic dentistry for misshapen teeth and dentures. Hair is more manageable with oil-based ointments.

**Prognosis:** Normal life span and intelligence.

**Detection of Carrier:** Unknown.

**Special Considerations:** Rapp-Hodgkin syndrome shows a great degree of variability, and the majority of patients consult cleft lip/palate teams for evaluation and treatment. The anomalies associated with the cleft have been, to some extent, overlooked. If a case is suspected, it is advisable to use SEM and polarizing microscopy hair studies to confirm the diagnosis. Hair studies are relatively simple, and hair changes are constant findings. The observations on the absence of normal mucosal coverings of the vocal folds suggest that antihistamines should be avoided, because they may further dry the mucosal covering.

**Support Groups:** IL; Mascoutah; National Foundation for Ectodermal Dysplasias (NFED)

**References:**
Rapp RS, Hodgkin WE: Anhidrotic ectodermal dysplasia: autosomal dominant inheritance with palate and lip anomalies. J Med Genet 1968; 5:269–272. * †
Wannarachue N, et al.: Ectodermal dysplasia and multiple defects (Rapp-Hodgkin type). J Pediatr 1972; 81:1217–1218.
Stasiowska B, et al.: Rapp-Hodgkin ectodermal dysplasia syndrome. Arch Dis Child 1981; 56:793–795. * †
Silengo MC, et al.: Distinctive hair changes (pili torti) in Rapp-Hodgkin ectodermal dysplasia syndrome. Clin Genet 1982; 21:297–300. * †
Meyerson MD: The effect of syndrome diagnosis on speech remediation. BD:OAS XXI(2). New York: March of Dimes Birth Defects Foundation, 1985:47–68.
Schroeder HW, Jr., Sybert VP: Rapp-Hodgkin ectodermal dysplasia. J Pediatr 1987; 110:72–75.
Salinas CF, Montes GM: Rapp-Hodgkin syndrome: observations on ten cases and characteristic hair changes (pili canaliculi). In: BD: OAS XXIV(2). New York: March of Dimes Birth Defects Foundation, 1988:149–168.

SA012
J0027

**Carlos F. Salinas
Ronald J. Jorgenson**

**Ectodermal dysplasia, tetramelic**
*See ODONTO-TRICHOMELIC SYNDROME*
**Ectodermal dysplasia, tricho-dermodysplasia-dental defects**
*See TRICHO-DERMODYSPLASIA-DENTAL DEFECTS*
**Ectodermal dysplasia, tricho-odonto-onychial type**
*See TRICHO-ODONTO-ONYCHIAL DYSPLASIA*
**Ectodermal dysplasia, tricho-onychodysplasia-xeroderma type**
*See TRICHO-ONYCHODYSPLASIA-XERODERMA*
**Ectodermal dysplasia-acrorenal field defect-lipoatrophic diabetes**
*See AREDYLD SYNDROME*

---

**ECTODERMAL DYSPLASIA-ADRENAL CYST**     **2833**

**Includes:**
Adrenal cyst-ectodermal dysplasia
Cyst (adrenal)-ectodermal dysplasia
Odonto-onychohypohidrotic dysplasia with midline scalp defect

**Excludes:**
**Ectodermal dysplasia** (others)
**Odonto-onychodermal dysplasia** (2618)
**Onycho-trichodysplasia-neutropenia** (2331)
**Tricho-odonto-onychial dysplasia** (2889)

**Major Diagnostic Criteria:** Aplasia cutis verticis, hypohidrosis, nipple/breast hypoplasia, onychodysplasia, and delayed dental eruption with minor tooth anomalies. The association of adrenal cyst in the propositus might represent evidence of fetal avascular dysplasia.

**Clinical Findings:** The boy presented with acute fever, gross hematuria, and left flank pain. Initially urinary tract infection was suspected, but investigation showed the presence of a 3 x 4-cm adrenal cyst. Subsequent surgical pathologic examination showed the cyst to be of adrenal cortex origin.

The boy and his mother shared all the major diagnostic criteria mentioned above. They both had similar aplasia cutis verticis, onychodysplasia, and hypohidrosis as documented by pilocarpine iontophoresis sweat volume collection. The boy had delayed dental eruption with minor tooth anomalies, and the mother had had all her teeth capped, making evaluation of her dentition impossible. The boy had nipple hypoplasia of a significant cosmetic degree. The mother had both nipple and breast hypoplasia and was unable to nurse either of her two children successfully. While the mother had no evidence of adrenal cyst, she did have a history of left renal abscess and hypertension of undetermined cause. There was also evidence of ectodermal dysplasia in two maternal uncles by history of hypohidrosis and dentition problems.

**Complications:** Those due to adrenal and peritoneal cysts. The mother was unable to lactate. The son had psychologic problems because of hypoplastic nipples, and his condition required plastic surgery.

**Associated Findings:** None known.

**Etiology:** Possibly autosomal dominant inheritance.

**Pathogenesis:** Unknown. Possibly fetal avascular dysplasia involving ectodermal and mesodermal anlage.

**MIM No.:** 12955

**CDC No.:** 757.346

**Sex Ratio:** Presumably M1:F1.

**Occurrence:** A mother and son have been documented in the literature.

**Risk of Recurrence for Patient's Sib:**
See Part I, *Mendelian Inheritance.*

**Risk of Recurrence for Patient's Child:**
See Part I, *Mendelian Inheritance.*

**Age of Detectability:** At birth, by clinical examination. Ultrasound examination could show the presence of adrenal or renal malformation if suspected. Subtle fetal avascular dysplasia might be missed, leaving the subject susceptible to future renal or adrenal problems.

**Gene Mapping and Linkage:** Unknown.

**Prevention:** None known. Genetic counseling indicated.

**Treatment:** Prosthetic and orthodontic treatment. Surgical removal of cysts. Plastic surgery for nipple/breast hypoplasia.

**Prognosis:** Life span and intellectual development are presumably unaffected.

**Detection of Carrier:** By careful physical examination, followed by ultrasound examination of adrenal/renal organs if indicated.

**Special Considerations:** It is unknown whether adrenal and peritoneal cysts, renal abscesses, and hypertension are components of the condition or are coincidental findings (cf. Freire-Maia and Pinheiro, 1984:58–59). Although the hypothesis of an autosomal dominant gene, as suggested by Tuffli and Laxova (1983), is more plausible, the hypothesis of an X-linked gene cannot be discarded.

**Support Groups:** IL; Mascoutah; National Foundation for Ectodermal Dysplasias (NFED)

**References:**
Tuffli GA, Laxova R: New, autosomal dominant form of ectodermal dysplasia. Am J Med Genet 1983; 14:381–384.

Freire-Maia N, Pinheiro M: Ectodermal dysplasias: a clinical and genetic study. New York: Alan R. Liss, 1984.

TU015  **Gorden A. Tuffli**
PI008  **Marta Pinheiro**
FR033  **Newton Freire-Maia**

**Ectodermal dysplasia-cleft lip/palate-syndactyly**
*See CLEFT LIP/PALATE-ECTODERMAL DYSPLASIA-SYNDACTYLY*
**Ectodermal dysplasia-ectrodactyly-clefting syndrome**
*See ECTRODACTYLY-ECTODERMAL DYSPLASIA-CLEFTING SYNDROME*

## ECTODERMAL DYSPLASIA-ECTRODACTYLY-MACULAR DYSTROPHY     2793

**Includes:**
EEM syndrome
Ohdo-Hirayama-Terawaki syndrome

**Excludes:**
Bardet-Biedl syndrome (2363)
Dermal hypoplasia, focal (0281)
Ectrodactyly-ectodermal dysplasia-clefting syndrome (0337)
Growth retardation-alopecia-pseudoanodontia-optic atrophy (2293)
Laurence-Moon syndrome (0578)
Oculo-dento-osseous dysplasia (0737)
Oculo-mandibulo-facial syndrome (0738)

**Major Diagnostic Criteria:** The combination of ectodermal dysplasia in the form of scant hair and small or missing teeth, ectrodactyly (terminal transverse limb defects), and macular dystrophy.

**Clinical Findings:** All affected individuals have had sparse and short scalp, eyebrow, and eyelash hair. Teeth are often described as being small and widely spaced, and partial anodontia can occur. The limb defect usually affects the hands and includes variable degrees of terminal transverse defects and **Syndactyly.** The feet are less often and less severely affected; the only defect is usually syndactyly. However, one case had missing distal phalanges of two toes, whereas another had a bifid distal phalanx of the great toe. The macular dystrophy was characterized by pigmentary changes. Growth and intellect are usually normal.

**Complications:** Unknown.

**Associated Findings:** None known.

**Etiology:** Autosomal recessive inheritance.

**Pathogenesis:** Unknown.

**MIM No.:** *22528

**POS No.:** 3580

**Sex Ratio:** M1:F1

**Occurrence:** Fewer than a dozen cases have been documented; most from Japan and Denmark.

**Risk of Recurrence for Patient's Sib:**
See Part I, *Mendelian Inheritance.*

**Risk of Recurrence for Patient's Child:**
See Part I, *Mendelian Inheritance.*

**Age of Detectability:** At birth by the presence of the limb defect. Prenatal diagnosis by ultrasound is possible.

**Gene Mapping and Linkage:** Unknown.

**Prevention:** None known. Genetic counseling indicated.

**Treatment:** Supportive.

**Prognosis:** Intellectual development is normal in most cases (although one child had an IQ of 81); life span seems unaffected.

**Detection of Carrier:** Unknown.

**Special Considerations:** Kuster et al (1987) described a single patient with short stature, alopecia developing at age 20 years, macular degeneration, multiple dental caries, and small hands and feet. The authors believed this to be a distinct condition.

**Support Groups:** IL; Mascoutah; National Foundation for Ectodermal Dysplasias (NFED)

**References:**
Albrectsen B, Svendsen IB: Hypotrichosis, syndactyly, and retinal degeneration in two siblings. Acta Derm Venereol (Stockh) 1956; 1:96–101.
Hayakawa M, et al.: A case of central and pericentral retinopathy pigmentosa with abnormalities of hair, hands and teeth. Ganka 1979; 21:433–438.
Ohdo S, et al.: Association of ectodermal dysplasia, ectrodactyly, and macular dystrophy: the EEM syndrome. J Med Genet 1983; 20:52–57. *
Kuster W, et al.: Alopecia, macular degeneration, and growth retardation: a new syndrome? Am J Med Genet 1987; 28:477–481.

T0007                                    **Helga V. Toriello**

**Ectodermal dysplasia-exocrine pancreatic insufficiency**
 *See JOHANSON-BLIZZARD SYNDROME*
**Ectodermal dysplasia-growth failure-pancreatic insufficiency**
 *See DONLAN SYNDROME*
**Ectodermal dysplasia-hearing loss (sensorineural)-digital defects**
 *See ONYCHODYSTROPHY-CONIFORM TEETH-SENSORINEURAL HEARING LOSS*
**Ectodermal dysplasia-hypotrichosis**
 *See ECTODERMAL DYSPLASIA, BASAN TYPE*
**Ectodermal dysplasia-skeletal anomalies-growth/mental retardation**
 *See ALOPECIA-SKELETAL ANOMALIES-SHORT STATURE-MENTAL RETARDATION*

## ECTODERMAL DYSPLASIAS                     1503

Ectodermal dysplasias form a complex nosologic group of conditions which involve one or more of the "classic" structures of hair, teeth, nails, and sweat glands, with or without malformations and other ectodermal defects.

Ectodermal dysplasia definition and classification systems have been proposed, but they have been complicated by a lack of consensus on such a basic element as pathogenesis. The number of conditions which may be considered ectodermal dysplasias is, however, large, and appears to be growing.

**Support Groups:** IL; Mascoutah; The National Foundation for Ectodermal Dysplasias

**References:**
Freire-Maia N, Pinheiro M: Ectodermal dysplasias: a clinical and genetic study. New York, Alan R. Liss, 1984.
Freire-Maia N, Pinheiro M: Ectodermal dysplasias: a review of the conditions described after 1984 with an overall analysis of all the conditions belonging to this nosologic group. Rev Brasil Genet 1987; 10:403–414.

FR033                                  **Newton Freire-Maia**
PI008                                     **Marta Pinheiro**

**Ectodermal polydysplasia**
 *See ECTODERMAL DYSPLASIA, CHRIST-SIEMENS-TOURAINE TYPE*
**Ectopia cordis**
 *See HEART, CORDIS ECTOPIA*
**Ectopia lentis, congenital**
 *See LENS, ECTOPIC*
**Ectopic anus**
 *See ANORECTAL MALFORMATIONS*

## ECTRODACTYLY                                  0336

**Includes:**
  Fingers, absence of
  Split-hand deformity
  Lobster claw deformity
  Monodactyly
  "Ostrich-footed" tribe
  Tetramelic monodactyly

**Excludes:**
  **Hypoglossia-hypodactylia** (0451)
  **Brachydactyly** (0114)
  **Amniotic bands syndrome** (0874)
  **Ectrodactyly-ectodermal dysplasia-clefting syndrome** (0337)
  **Lacrimo-auriculo-dento-digital syndrome** (2180)

**Major Diagnostic Criteria:** Absence of one or more (central) digits.

**Clinical Findings:** Ectrodactyly refers to a heterogeneous group of hand and foot malformations. The clinical findings range from partial to complete absence of a finger to the cleft hand or foot deformity (absence of the third digit with clefting into the proximal portion of the hand or foot and syndactyly of the remaining digits on each side of the cleft) to monodactyly (absence of all but the fifth digit). Simple absence of a finger usually represents a sporadic event, occurs unilaterally and without foot involvement. The cleft hand/foot and monodactyly malformations appear to reflect different degrees of severity of a common developmental defect and are distinct from the isolated absent finger. This type of anomaly usually occurs bilaterally, foot involvement is frequent

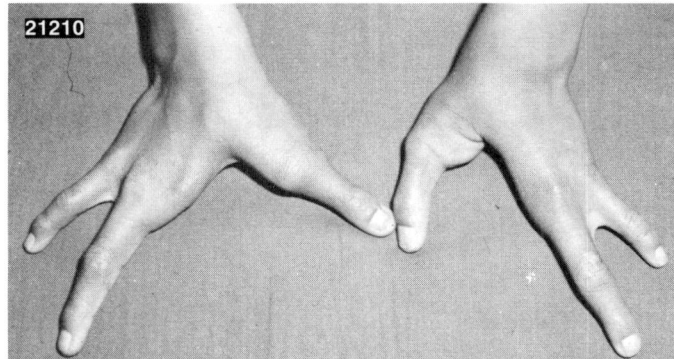

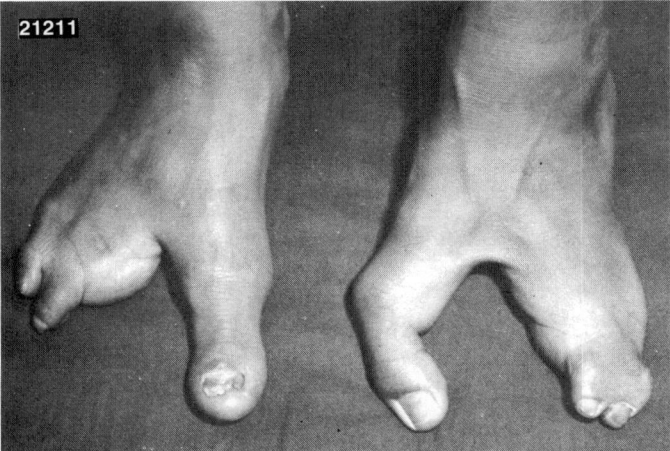

**0336A**-21210: Ectrodactyly of the hands. 21211: Ectrodactyly of the feet.

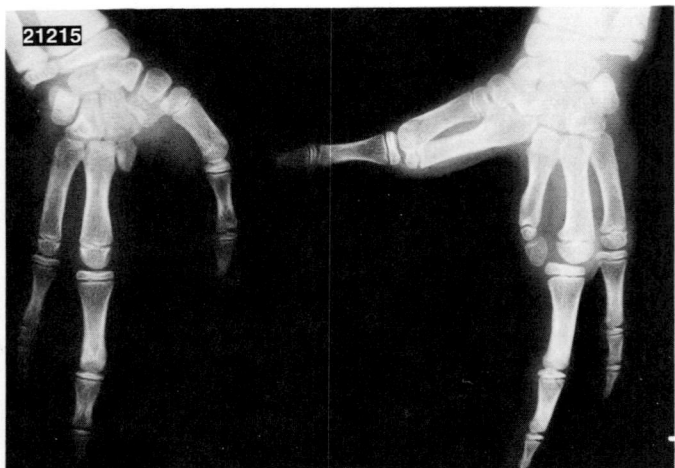

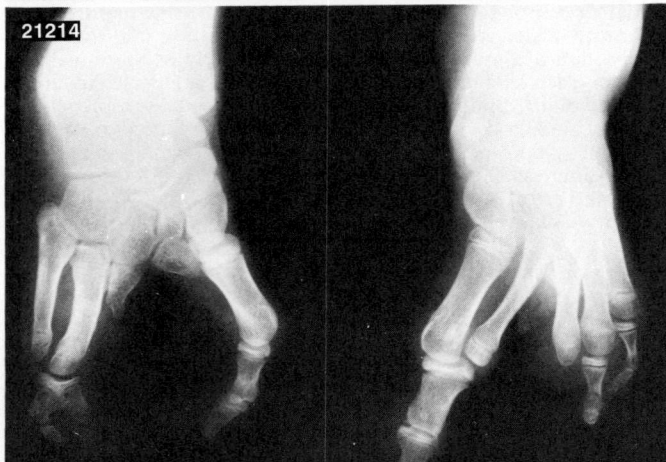

0336B-21215: X-ray of ectrodactyly of the hands.   21214: X-ray of ectrodactyly of the feet.

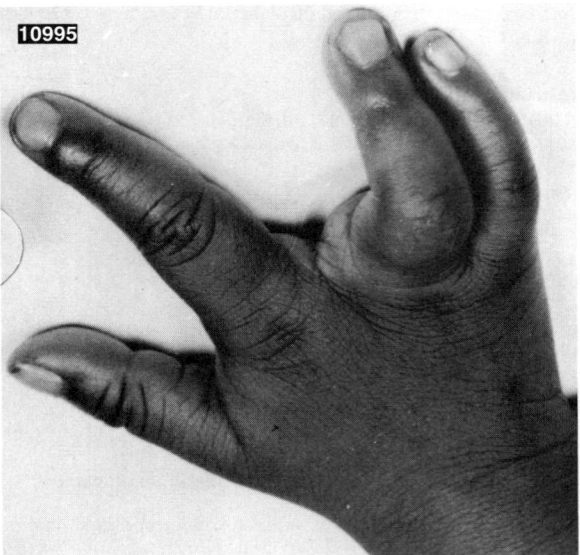

0336C-10995:  Ectrodactyly.

and may occur alone, and a positive family history is obtained in about one-half of the cases. Several genetically distinct traits probably manifest this anomaly.

**Complications:**  Diminished function related to severity of defect.

**Associated Findings:**  Absence of long bones of the upper and lower limbs has been reported (Hoyme et al, 1987)

**Etiology:**  The sole absence of a digit usually occurs sporadically. Cleft hand/foot and monodactyly deformities often by autosomal dominant inheritance with considerable variability in expression. Pedigrees consistent with autosomal recessive inheritance (only sibs affected and consanguinity present) have been reported; however, these cases are very rare. Clefting or monodactyly, bilaterality and foot involvement suggest a dominant trait.

**Pathogenesis:**  Presumably suppression of the central and, in more severe cases, also radial rays in the developing limbs.

**MIM No.:**  *18360, 22530, 27341

**POS No.:**  3210

**CDC No.:**  755.250, 755.350

**Sex Ratio:**  M1:F1

**Occurrence:**  About 70 pedigrees reported prior to 1965. In Denmark, estimated 1:90,000.

**Risk of Recurrence for Patient's Sib:**
  See Part I, *Mendelian Inheritance.*

**Risk of Recurrence for Patient's Child:**
  See Part I, *Mendelian Inheritance.*

**Age of Detectability:**  At birth. Syndactyly and lobster claw deformity detected prenatally by ultrasonography and fetoscopy.

**Gene Mapping and Linkage:**  Unknown.

**Prevention:**  None known. Genetic counseling indicated.

**Treatment:**  Reconstructive surgery when applicable.

**Prognosis:**  Intelligence and life span are normal. Function is dependent on severity of deformity.

**Detection of Carrier:**  Unknown.

**Special Considerations:**  In the sporadic case, it is important to distinguish ectrodactyly from atypical split-hand deformity which is suggested by unilateral hand involvement, lack of foot abnormalities and the presence of hypoplastic digits on the axial portion of the hand. All reported cases of the latter deformity have been sporadic.

**References:**
Maisels DD. Lobster claw deformities of the hand. Hand. 1970; 2:79–82.
David TS. The differential diagnosis of the cleft hand and cleft foot malformations. Hand. 1974; 6:58–61.
Temtamy SA, McKusick VA. The genetics of hand malformations. New York: Alan R. Liss, 1978.
Bujdoso G, Lenz W: Monodactylous splithand-splitfoot: a malformation occurring in three distinct genetic types. Europ J Pediat 1980; 133:207–215.
Henrion R, et al. Prenatal diagnosis of ectrodactyly. Lancet. 1980; 2:319 (only).
Viljoen D, Beighton P: The split-hand and split-foot anomaly in a Central African Negro population. Am J Med Genet 1984; 19:545–552.
Mufti MH, Wood SK: Ectrodactyly in sisters and half sisters. J Med Genet 1987; 24:220–224.
Hoyme HE, et al.: Autosomal dominant ectrodactyly and absence of long bones of upper or lower limbs: further clinical delineation. J Pediat 1987; 111:538–543.

H0033                                               **William A. Horton**
H0025                                               **O.J. Hood**

## ECTRODACTYLY-ANONYCHIA 0065

**Includes:** Anonychia-ectrodactyly

**Excludes:**
Anonychia-absence and blistering of skin and mucous membranes
**Ectrodactyly-ectodermal dysplasia-clefting syndrome** (0337)
**Nail-patella syndrome** (0704)
**Nails, anonychia, hereditary** (0066)

**Major Diagnostic Criteria:** Characteristic nail and digital abnormalities.

**Clinical Findings:** Nail anomalies; usually complete absence of nail and nail bed with index and middle fingers commonly affected. Thumbnail often present only on the proximal, lateral corners of the nail fold; radial half of the ring fingernail usually absent; little fingernail usually normal; toe anonychia parallels the anonychia in corresponding fingers. The nail anomaly is usually present from birth, nonprogressive and symmetric digitally.

Digital anomalies occur in about one-third of the affected individuals. They are nearly always asymmetric and are often restricted to one hand or one foot. The digital anomalies are bizarre, including absence of one or more digits, absence of corresponding metacarpal bones, syndactyly, or polydactyly.

**Complications:** Unknown.

**Associated Findings:** None known.

**Etiology:** Possibly autosomal dominant inheritance (nonallelism of this syndrome and nail-patella genes).

**Pathogenesis:** Unknown.

**MIM No.:** 10690

**POS No.:** 4357

**Sex Ratio:** M1:F1

**Occurrence:** Undetermined but apparently rare.

**Risk of Recurrence for Patient's Sib:**
See Part I, *Mendelian Inheritance.*

**Risk of Recurrence for Patient's Child:**
See Part I, *Mendelian Inheritance.*

**Age of Detectability:** At birth.

**Gene Mapping and Linkage:** Unknown.

**Prevention:** None known. Genetic counseling indicated.

**Treatment:** Occupational and physical therapy (appliances and the like) as needed.

**Prognosis:** Does not appear to affect normal life span.

**Detection of Carrier:** Unknown.

**References:**
Lees DH, et al.: Anonychia with ectrodactyly: clinical and linkage data. Ann Hum Genet 1957; 22:69–79.
Rahbari H, et al.: Anonychia with ectrodactyly Arch Derm 1975; 111(11):1482–1483.
Yesudian P, et al.: Anonychia with ectrodactyly: a south Indian pedigree study. Int J Dermatol 1977; 16(7):599–604.

MI038                                    **Giuseppe Micali**

**Ectrodactyly-brachydactyly-triphalangeal thumb**
*See THUMB, TRIPHALANGEAL-BRACHYECTRODACTYLY*
**Ectrodactyly-cleft palate (ECP) syndrome**
*See ECTRODACTYLY-ECTODERMAL DYSPLASIA-CLEFTING SYNDROME*

## ECTRODACTYLY-ECTODERMAL DYSPLASIA-CLEFTING SYNDROME 0337

**Includes:**
Cleft lip/palate with split hand or split foot
Ectrodactyly-cleft palate (ECP) syndrome
Ectodermal dysplasia-ectrodactyly-clefting syndrome
EEC syndrome
Rudiger syndrome

**Excludes:**
**Cleft lip/palate-ectodermal dysplasia-syndactyly** (0179)
**Cleft lip/palate-oligodontia-syndactyly-hair defects** (2898)
**Ectodermal dysplasia-ectrodactyly-macular dystrophy** (2793)
**Ectodermal dysplasia, Rapp-Hodgkin type** (3056)
**Limb and scalp defects, Adams-Oliver type** (0459)
**Odonto-trichomelic syndrome** (2887)
**Pili torti-cleft lip/palate-syndactyly** (3126)
**Roberts syndrome** (0875)

**Major Diagnostic Criteria:** Ectrodactyly, lacrimal gland or duct atresia, and ectodermal dysplasia are features of the syndrome, with cleft lip and palate being slightly less consistent.

**Clinical Findings:** The EEC syndrome shows a wide range of variation. Ectrodactyly, while not an obligatory feature, is common. The third digit is most commonly absent or dysplastic. When present, it is often fused to adjacent digits. The first digit is usually unaffected. The feet and hands are involved, although affectation is not always bilaterally symmetric. In the absence of ectrodactyly, there may be syndactyly or onychodystrophy. Aplasia of the lacrimal gland and stenosis of the nasolacrimal duct are common, while absent orifices of the Meibomian glands, hypertelorism, and epicanthus may be seen. Superficial features of ectodermal dysplasia include fine, sparse scalp hair that is blonde and grays early. Intraoral features include hypodontia, microdontia, and enamel dysplasia. The lip and palate are frequently cleft, and various renal anomalies may exist, including hydronephrosis, hydroureters, pyelonephritis, renal agenesis, and renal duplication.

**Complications:** The lacrimal defects lead to abnormal tearing with concomitant susceptibility to ocular infections, conjunctivitis, and scarring of the conjunctiva, which may lead to decreased vision. Photophobia may also be present. A reported susceptibility to caries may be caused by decreased salivation. The skin is often dry and atopic eczema may be present, although sweat function does not seem to be compromised.

**Associated Findings:** Brown macules over the trunk and limbs and palmoplantar hyperkeratosis may be seen. Some affected persons have had psychomotor retardation, microencephaly, or

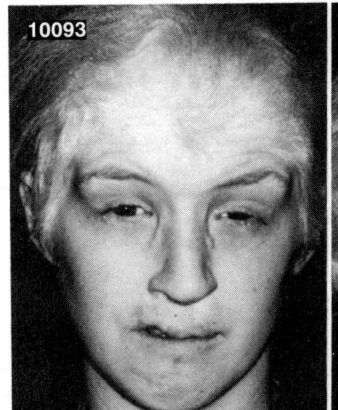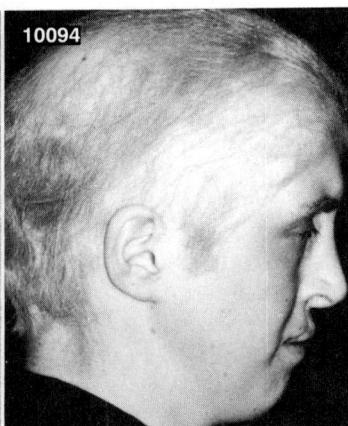

**0337A**-10093–94:  Scanty hair and malar hypoplasia.

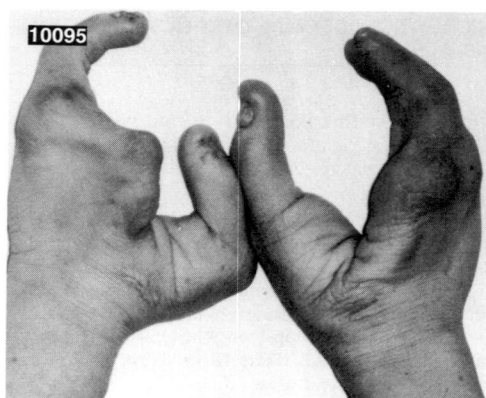

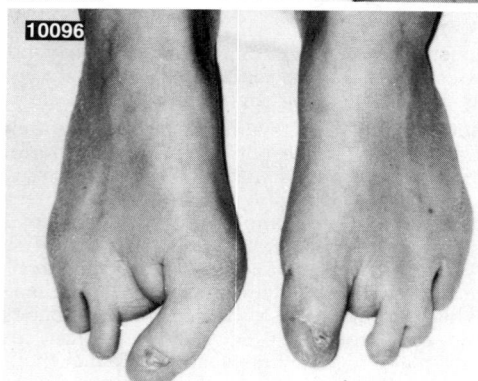

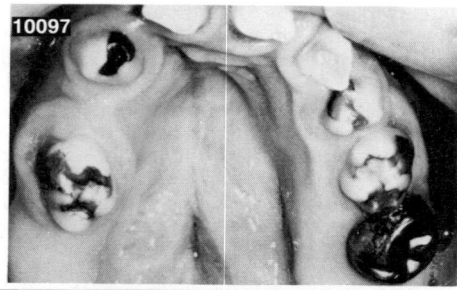

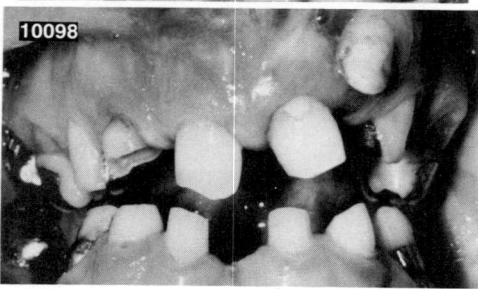

**0337B-10095:** Lobster-claw configuration of the hands. **10096:** Ectrodactyly of the feet. **10097–98:** Oligodontia and enamel hypoplasia.

hearing loss. Urinary tract and genital anomalies have also been reported.

**Etiology:** Autosomal dominant inheritance with incomplete penetrance and variability in expression. Autosomal recessive inheritance has been suggested in some families.

**Pathogenesis:** Defects of the hair and teeth point toward a primary defect in ectoderm. The ectrodactyly and clefting suggest a defect in mesodermal migration. Digit aplasia may result from deficient migration of limb mesoderm, while syndactyly may result from a shift of mesoderm from one digit to another. Growth hormone deficiency has also been suggested.

**MIM No.:** *12990, 12983

**POS No.:** 3211

**Sex Ratio:** M1:F1

**Occurrence:** Presumably rare, but established literature.

**Risk of Recurrence for Patient's Sib:**
See Part I, *Mendelian Inheritance.*

**Risk of Recurrence for Patient's Child:**
See Part I, *Mendelian Inheritance.*

**Age of Detectability:** At birth, although prenatal detection is possible.

**Gene Mapping and Linkage:** Unknown.

**Prevention:** None known. Genetic counseling indicated.

**Treatment:** All the listed structural defects are amenable to surgical correction, although success in correcting the ectrodactyly will depend on its extent. Nasolacrimal duct drainage can be improved by placement of tubes. Orthodontic treatment and speech therapy may be needed following surgery to correct the clefting.

**Prognosis:** Normal growth, development, and life span. Manual dexterity is limited by the extent of ectrodactyly.

**Detection of Carrier:** When the gene is clinically nonpenetrant, carriers may be able to be detected by X-ray examination of the hands or feet or through minimal manifestations of cleft lip and palate (velopharyngeal insufficiency, submucous cleft palate).

**Special Considerations:** Opitz et al (1980) reported briefly on a large kindred without cleft lip or ectodermal features. It is not clear how this condition, sometimes called the ECP syndrome, relates to the present condition often called EEC syndrome. The terminology is further confused by the fact that **Ectodermal dysplasia-ectrodactyly-macular dystrophy** is also known as the EEM syndrome.

**References:**
Rudiger RA, et al.: Association of ectrodactyly, ectodermal dysplasia, and cleft lip-palate. Am J Dis Child 1970; 120:160–163.
Bixler D, et al.: The ectrodactyly-ectodermal dysplasia-clefting (EEC) syndrome. Clin Genet 1971; 33:43–51.
Preus M, Fraser FC: The lobster claw defect with ectodermal defects, cleft lip/palate, tear duct anomaly and renal anomalies. Clin Genet 1973; 4:369–375.
Rosenmann R, et al.: Ectrodactyly, ectodermal dysplasia and cleft palate (EEC syndrome): report of a family and review of the literature. Clin Genet 1976; 9:347–353.
Schmidt R, Nitowsky HM: Split hand and foot deformity and the syndrome of ectrodactyly, ectodermal dysplasia, and clefting (EEC). Hum Genet 1977; 39:15–25. †
Opitz JM, et al.: The ECP syndrome, another autosomal dominant cause of monodactylous ectrodactyly. Europ J Pediat 1980; 133:217–220.
Kuster W, et al.: EEC syndrome without ectrodactyly? Report of 8 cases. Clin Genet 1985; 28:130–135. †
Knudtzon J, Aarskog D: Growth hormone deficiency associated with the ectrodactyly-ectodermal dysplasia-clefting syndrome and isolated septum pellucidum. Pediatrics 1987; 79:410–412.
Rollnick BR, Hoo JJ: Genitourinary anomalies are a component manifestation in the ectodermal dysplasia, ectrodactyly, cleft lip/palate (EEC) syndrome. Am J Med Genet 1988; 29:131–136.

J0027                                                    **Ronald J. Jorgenson**

## ECTRODACTYLY-POLYDACTYLY 2794

**Includes:** Polydactyly-ectrodactyly

**Excludes:**
**Acro-renal-mandibular syndrome** (2778)
**Polydactyly**
**Tibial hypoplasia/aplasia-ectrodactyly** (2388)

**Major Diagnostic Criteria:** The coexistence of defects of both ulnar and middle rays of the hand.

**Clinical Findings:** In the reported affected sibship, two sibs had postaxial **Polydactyly** of the hand, bilateral in one, and unilateral in the other; one sib had absence of all digits on one hand; and the fourth sib had absence of distal phalanges of toes 2 and 3 and partial **Syndactyly** of fingers 3 and 4 unilaterally.

**Complications:** Unknown.

**Associated Findings:** None known.

**Etiology:** Possibly autosomal recessive inheritance.

**Pathogenesis:** A defect of the distal mesoderm of the limb bud was postulated.

**MIM No.:** 22529

**POS No.:** 4153

**CDC No.:** 755.250, 755.0

**Sex Ratio:** M1:F1

**Occurrence:** One sibship in Belgium has been documented.

**Risk of Recurrence for Patient's Sib:**
See Part I, *Mendelian Inheritance.*

**Risk of Recurrence for Patient's Child:**
See Part I, *Mendelian Inheritance.*

**Age of Detectability:** At birth by physical examination. Prenatal diagnosis using ultrasound or fetoscopy may also be possible.

**Gene Mapping and Linkage:** Unknown.

**Prevention:** None known. Genetic counseling indicated.

**Treatment:** Surgical intervention may be indicated.

**Prognosis:** The limb defect is the only anomaly. Growth, intellect, and life span are normal.

**Detection of Carrier:** Unknown.

**References:**
van Regemorter N, et al.: Familial ectrodactyly and polydactyly: variable expressivity of one single gene - embryological considerations. Clin Genet 1982; 22:206–210.

T0007                                   **Helga V. Toriello**

**Ectrodactyly-tibial hemimelia**
*See TIBIAL HYPOPLASIA/APLASIA-ECTRODACTYLY*
**Ectromelia, unilateral-psoriasis-CNS anomalies**
*See LIMB REDUCTION-ICHTHYOSIS*
**Ectropion**
*See EYELID, ECTROPION, CONGENITAL*
**Eczema, atopic**
*See SKIN, ATOPY, FAMILIAL*
**Eczema-thrombocytopenia-diarrhea-infection syndrome**
*See IMMUNODEFICIENCY, WISKOTT-ALDRICH TYPE*
**Edema (vs. Lymphedema)**
*See LYMPHEDEMA I*
**Edentate hypertrichosis**
*See HAIR, HYPERTRICHOSIS, LANUGINOSA*

## EDINBURGH MALFORMATION SYNDROME 3041

**Includes:** Typus Edinburgensis

**Excludes:** **De Lange syndrome** (0242)

**Major Diagnostic Criteria:** The combination of abnormal facial appearance, apparent **Hydrocephaly**, retardation, and failure to thrive.

**Clinical Findings:** Normal birth weight, length, and head circumference. However, facial features are unusual and include frontal bossing, apparent microophthalmia, small nose with anteverted nares, long philtrum, thin and downturned lips, and apparently low-set ears. Additional features include long and silky hair, long hands and feet, and, in one child, flexion contractures and ulnar deviation of the fingers. Hyperbilirubinemia (2/5), poor feeding (2/5), nasal obstruction (5/5), and increased muscle tone (1/5) can also occur. Death occurred by age one year in all cases. Autopsy demonstrated **Hydrocephaly** in one case and micropolygyria in another.

**Complications:** Bronchopneumonia occurred in four cases.

**Associated Findings:** None known.

**Etiology:** In the reported family, four sibs had either affected children or affected grandchildren. Therefore, although autosomal dominant inheritance with reduced penetrance is possible, a subtle chromosome rearrangement could be responsible.

**Pathogenesis:** Unknown.

**MIM No.:** 12985

**POS No.:** 3948

**Sex Ratio:** M1:F4 (observed).

**Occurrence:** Five patients from one family from Edinburgh have been reported.

**Risk of Recurrence for Patient's Sib:**
See Part I, *Mendelian Inheritance.*

**Risk of Recurrence for Patient's Child:**
See Part I, *Mendelian Inheritance.*

**Age of Detectability:** At birth by physical examination.

**Gene Mapping and Linkage:** Unknown.

**Prevention:** None known. Genetic counseling indicated.

**Treatment:** Supportive as indicated.

**Prognosis:** All affected children died before age one year.

**Detection of Carrier:** Unknown.

**References:**
Habel A: "Typus Edinburgensis?" Pediatrics 1974; 53:425–430.

T0007                                   **Helga V. Toriello**

**Edwards syndrome**
*See CHROMOSOME 18, TRISOMY 18*
**EEC syndrome**
*See ECTRODACTYLY-ECTODERMAL DYSPLASIA-CLEFTING SYNDROME*
**EEG (unusual)-alopecia-epilepsy-mental retardation**
*See ALOPECIA-EPILEPSY-OLIGOPHRENIA, MOYNAHAN TYPE*
**EEM syndrome**
*See ECTODERMAL DYSPLASIA-ECTRODACTYLY-MACULAR DYSTROPHY*
**Effie pygmy growth deficiency**
*See GROWTH DEFICIENCY, AFRICAN PYGMY TYPE*
**Ehlers-Danlos features with progeroid facies**
*See PROGEROID SYNDROME WITH EHLERS-DANLOS FEATURES*
**Ehlers-Danlos gravis**
*See EHLERS-DANLOS SYNDROME*

## EHLERS-DANLOS SYNDROME                    0338

**Includes:**
    Arterial type Ehlers-Danlos syndrome
    Arthrochalasis multiplex congenita
    Dermatorrhexis cutis hyperelastica
    Ecchymotic type Ehlers-Danlos syndrome
    Ehlers-Danlos gravis
    Hydroxylysine deficient collagen disease
    Joint laxity, Ehlers-Danlos syndrome
    Lysyl oxidase deficiency
    Ocular-scoliotic type Ehlers-Danlos syndrome
    Periodontosis type Ehlers-Danlos syndrome
    Platelet/fibronectin abnormality-Ehlers-Danlos syndrome
    Procollagen peptidase deficiency
    Procollagen protease deficiency
    Proteodermatan sulfate, defective biosynthesis of
    Proto-collagen lysyl hydroxylase deficiency
    Sack type Ehlers-Danlos syndrome

**Excludes:**
    **Articular hypermobility, familial** (3220)
    Congenital ligamentous laxity
    **Cutis laxa** (0233)
    **Cutis laxa-growth defect, De Barsy type** (2138)
    **Larsen syndrome** (0570)
    **Nephrosis-hydrocephalus-thin skin-blue sclera-growth defect**
      (2187)
    **Occipital horn syndrome** (3219)
    **Progeroid syndrome with Ehlers-Danlos features** (3012)

**Major Diagnostic Criteria:** Some degree of "loose" or fragile connective tissues, especially affecting the joints and skin. Biochemical documentation of specific enzyme deficiency in these disorders when known.

**Clinical Findings:** This is a heterogeneous group of connective tissue disorders which share hyperextensibility of joints and, often, skin. Nine distinct entities can be recognized on clinical, genetic, and biochemical grounds.

*ED-I, Gravis type,* is characterized by generalized and severe joint hypermobility. Musculoskeletal deformities, eg pes planus, may occur. Skin hyperextensibility and easy bruising are severe. Increased fragility leads to skin splitting and subsequent "cigarette paper"-like scarring particularly over the forehead, elbows, knees, and shins. Varicose veins occur commonly, as do molluscoid pseudotumors and subcutaneous spheroids. Generalized tissue friability may result in difficulty with wound healing following trauma or surgery as well as premature rupture of fetal membranes.

*ED-II, Mitis type,* resembles but is milder than ED-I. Joint laxity is often confined to the hands and feet; cutaneous involvement is minimal. There is a slight tendency toward bruising but little scar formation. Varicose veins are uncommon, and tissue friability is rarely a problem.

*ED-III, Benign hypermobile type,* shows severe hypermobility of all joints usually without musculoskeletal deformities. Skin changes are minimal.

*ED-IV, Arterial, ecchymotic, or Sack type,* is potentially lethal due to the tendency toward spontaneous rupture of large and intermediate sized arteries and perforation of the bowel. The skin is very thin and easily bruised, with prominent underlying veins, but stretchability is increased only slightly. See also **Nephrosis-hydrocephalus-thin skin-blue sclera-growth defect**.

*ED-V, X-linked type,* manifests only moderate joint hypermobility in contrast to marked hyperextensibility of the skin. Cutaneous bruisability and fragility are moderately increased.

*ED-VI, Ocular-scoliotic type,* is characterized by severe scoliosis and ocular fragility in addition to moderate joint and skin involvement. Rupture of the sclera and cornea or retinal detachment often result from minor trauma.

*ED-VII, Arthrochalasis multiplex congenita,* exhibits short stature and extreme generalized joint hypermobility. Subluxations of hips, knees, elbows and feet are common. Infants with this disorder are floppy. There is moderate skin stretchability and

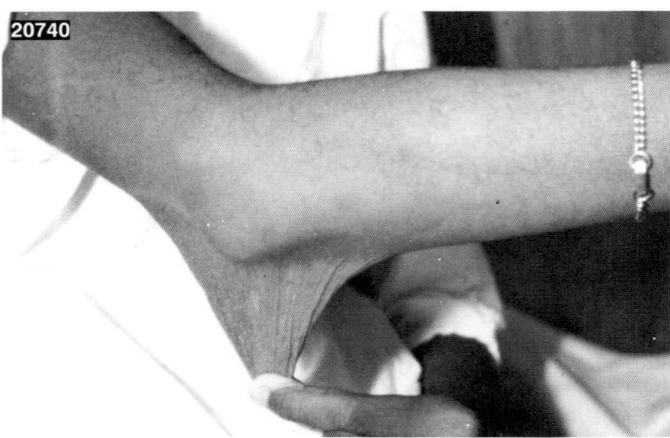

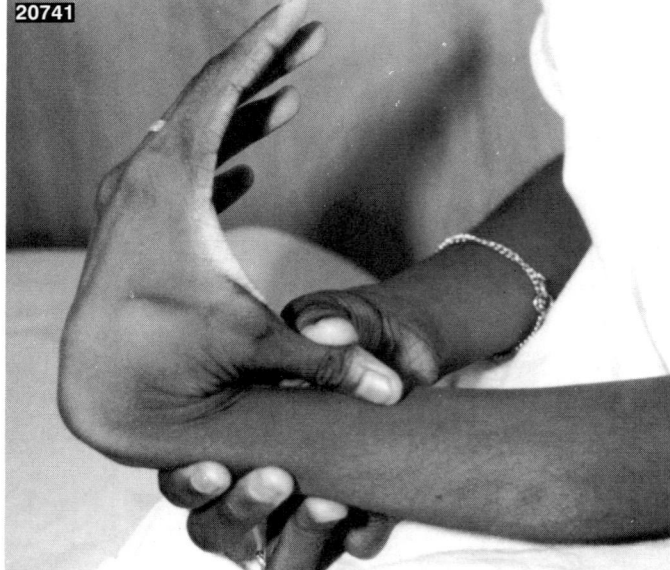

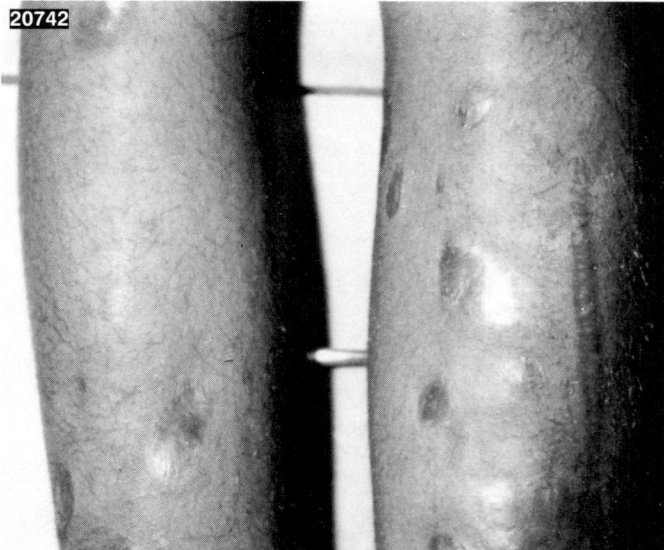

**0338A**-20740: Ehlers-Danlos syndrome; note hyperextensible skin. 20741: Hyperextensible joints. 20742: Cigarette paper-like scars.

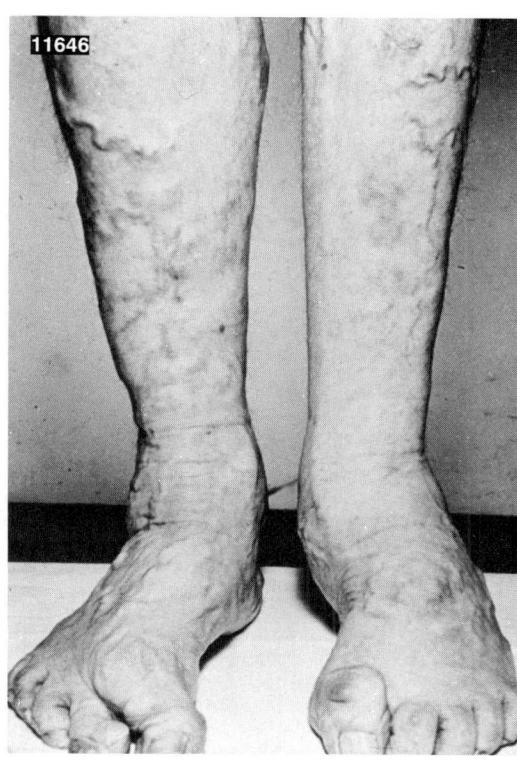

**0338B-11646:** Varicose veins and bruising on legs and feet in Ehlers-Danlos syndrome.

bruisability. Abnormal facies including hypertelorism, epicanthal folds and scooped out midfacies may be part of this disorder.

*ED-VIII, Periodontitis type,* shows mild skin and joint hyperextensibility, bruising, and moderate skin friability. The major feature is severe and generalized periodontitis leading to extensive resorption of alveolar bone and premature loss of teeth.

*ED-IX, now vacant.* See **Occipital horn syndrome.**

*ED-X, Fibronectin abnormality,* shows mild skin changes and defective collagen-induced platelet aggregation.

*ED-XI, now vacant.* See **Articular hypermobility, familial.**

**Complications:** Variable with age.

**Associated Findings:** Variable with type.

**Etiology:** ED-I, II, III, VIII: autosomal dominant inheritance. In one case with demonstrated defective synthesis of Type III collagen, there was a partial defect in both parents.

ED-IV, VII: Evidence for autosomal dominant inheritance in some, autosomal recessive inheritance in others.

ED-V: X-linked recessive inheritance.

ED-VI: autosomal recessive inheritance.

**Pathogenesis:** The friability and hyperextensibility result from defective connective tissue, most likely a collagen abnormality. Specific defects in collagen synthesis have been identified in ED VI, VII and possibly in ED-IV and X.

ED-VI-deficiency of lysyl hydroxylase

ED-VII-deficiency of procollagen (Type I) alpha 2 structural defect, possible procollagen N-peptidase deficiency.

ED-IV-possible synthesis of abnormal or reduced type III collagen.

ED-X-possible abnormal fibronectin.

**MIM No.:** *13000, 13001, 13002, *13005, 13006, *13008, 13009, *14790, 22531, 22532, *22535, 22536, *22540, 22541, *30415, *30520

**POS No.:** 3212

**CDC No.:** 756.85040

**Sex Ratio:** M1:F1 except the X-1inked forms in which only males are affected.

**Occurrence:** 1:150,000 in the United Kingdom. Undetermined elsewhere; extensive literature.

**Risk of Recurrence for Patient's Sib:**
See Part I, *Mendelian Inheritance.*

**Risk of Recurrence for Patient's Child:**
See Part I, *Mendelian Inheritance.*

**Age of Detectability:** Early childhood.

**Gene Mapping and Linkage:** LOX (lysyl oxidase; ?cutis laxa-X; ?Ehlers-Danlos V) has been provisionally mapped to X.

**Prevention:** None known. Genetic counseling indicated.

**Treatment:** Avoid trauma. Wear protective padding over bony prominences. Meticulous surgical, dental and obstetric care. Repair of superficial lacerations with tape rather than suture. Angiography may be hazardous, particularly in ED-IV.

**Prognosis:** Life span is reduced in ED-IV but probably normal in other types. Intelligence is normal.

**Detection of Carrier:** Unknown.

**Special Considerations:** The Ehlers-Danlos syndrome is among the heritable disorders of connective tissue covered by the International Nosology developed in Berlin in 1986 (Beighton et al, 1988).

**Support Groups:** MI; Southgate; Ehlers Danlos National Foundation

**References:**
Beighton P: The Ehlers-Danlos syndrome. London: William Heinemann, 1970.
Arneson MA, et al.: A new form of Ehlers-Danlos syndrome: fibronectin corrects defective platelet function. JAMA 1980; 244:144–147.
Horton WA, et al.: Familial joint instability syndrome. Am J Med Genet 1980; 6:221–228.
Steinmann B, et al.: Evidence for a structural mutation of procollagen type I in a patient with the Ehlers-Danlos syndrome type VII. J Biol Chem 1980; 255:8887–8893.
Byers PH, et al.: Molecular mechanisms of connective tissue abnormalities in the Ehlers-Danlos syndrome. Coll Res 1981; 5:475–489.
Hollister DW: Clinical features of Ehlers-Danlos syndrome types VIII and IX. AAOS symposium on heritable disorders of connective tissue. St Louis: CV Mosby, 1982:102–113.
Beighton P, Curtis D: X-linked Ehlers-Danlos syndrome type V: the next generation. Clin Genet 1985; 27:471–478.
Stolle CA, et al.: Synthesis of an altered type II procollagen in a patient with type IV Ehlers-Danlos syndrome. J Biol Chem 1985; 260:1937–1944.
De Paepe A, et al.: Ehlers-Danlos syndrome type I: a clinical and ultrastructural study of a family with reduced amounts of collagen type III. Brit J Derm 1987; 117:89–97.
Beighton P, et al.: International nosology of heritable disorders of connective tissue, Berlin, 1986. Am J Med Genet 1988; 29:581–594.

H0033                         **William A. Horton**
H0025                             **O.J. Hood**

**Ehlers-Danlos syndrome IX (obsolete)**
*See OCCIPITAL HORN SYNDROME*
**Ehlers-Danlos syndrome XI (obsolete)**
*See ARTICULAR HYPERMOBILITY, FAMILIAL*
**Ehlers-Danlos, type IV (possible form)**
*See NEPHROSIS-HYDROCEPHALUS-THIN SKIN-BLUE SCLERA-GROWTH DEFECT*
**Eisenberg supravalvar aortic stenosis**
*See AORTIC STENOSIS, SUPRAVALVAR*
**Eisenmenger complex**
*See VENTRICULAR SEPTAL DEFECT*
**EKG, prolonged QT interval-deafness-sudden death**
*See CARDIO-AUDITORY SYNDROME*
**Elastodosis marginalis**
*See ACROKERATOELASTOIDOSIS*
**Elastoma intrapapillarea perforans verruciforme**
*See SKIN, ELASTOSIS PERFORANS SERPIGINOSA*

**Elastosis dystrophica**
  See *PSEUDOXANTHOMA ELASTICUM*
**Elastosis perforans serpiginosa**
  See *SKIN, ELASTOSIS PERFORANS SERPIGINOSA*
**Elbow/hip dislocation-ear abnormalities-short stature**
  See *AURICULO-OSTEODYSPLASIA*
**Eldridge syndrome**
  See *DEAFNESS-MYOPIA*
**Electron transfer flavoprotein (ETF) deficiency**
  See *ACIDEMIA, GLUTARIC ACIDEMIA II*
**Electron transfer flavoprotein (ETF), partial deficiencies of**
  See *ACIDEMIA, ETHYLMALONIC-ADIPIC*
**Electron transfer flavoprotein, alpha subunit, deficiency of**
  See *ACIDEMIA, GLUTARIC ACIDEMIA II*
**Elejalde acrocephalopolydactylous dysplasia**
  See *ACROCEPHALOPOLYDACTYLOUS DYSPLASIA*
**'Elephant man' (possible diagnosis)**
  See *PROTEUS SYNDROME*
**Elfin faces-hypercalcemia**
  See *WILLIAMS SYNDROME*

---

## ELLIPTOCYTOSIS                                              2665

**Includes:**

  Elliptocytosis, hereditary
  Hemolytic elliptocytosis
  Malaysian-Melanesian elliptocytosis
  Melanesian ovalocytosis
  Ovalocytosis, hereditary
  Ovalocytoses, Malaysian-Melanesian type
  Pyropoikilocytosis

**Excludes:**

  Autoimmune hemolytic anemia
  Elliptocytosis associated with aplastic anemia
  Elliptocytosis associated with defective erythropoiesis
  Elliptocytosis associated with defective metaplasia
  Elliptocytosis associated with defective myeloid
  **Spherocytosis** (0892)

**Major Diagnostic Criteria:** Patients will have some degree of hemolysis with a variety of abnormally shaped erythrocytes. These are quite variable among the syndromes, but always include some ovalocytic erythrocytes, frequently include more exaggerated elliptocytes, and may include some fragmented poikilocytes. Splenomegaly is sometimes present. Positive family histories are obtained from most families. Diagnosis is based on the peripheral blood morphology. The patients have anemias of varying severity, ranging from fully compensated with a minimally elevated reticulocyte count to moderately severe anemia with a high reticulocyte count and reduced serum haptoglobin. Hereditary elliptocytosis must be distinguished from elliptocytosis associated with acquired or congenitally defective erythropoiesis. The latter anemias are of greater clinical severity and lack the compensatory reticulocytosis.

**Clinical Findings:** Elliptocytosis is clearly a group of disorders and is therefore quite heterogeneous. Although the majority of patients are afflicted with a mild, chronic anemia that may first be noticed during childhood, adolescence, or adulthood, a minority of patients are afflicted with a more severe anemia that is first detected during early childhood or even infancy. Certain infants with a moderately severe anemia with poikilocytic erythrocytes will develop into a more indolent and typical form of elliptocytosis as they mature.

The clinical findings are generally related to the anemia, and while most patients are compensated to normal or near-normal hemoglobin levels, some will have evidence of ongoing hemolysis, elevated reticulocyte count, reduced serum haptoglobin level, or elevated unconjugated bilirubin. Only rare patients suffer sufficient anemia to require regular transfusions.

Only those patients with clinically significant anemia require surgical splenectomy. The operation does not alter the underlying erythrocyte abnormality, but permits the abnormal erythrocytes to circulate longer, thereby increasing the peripheral blood counts. Most patients require no therapy. Many patients are aware of other relatives with a history of anemia and splenectomy, and it is

likely that most cases represent autosomal dominant traits. Individuals with moderately severe anemia and poikilocytic erythrocytes and have no known affected relatives may be homozygotes for a recessive disorder.

The Melanesian form of elliptocytosis affects the native peoples of Malaya and Australia and is distinctly different from the other forms of elliptocytosis. Melanesian elliptocytosis should not be considered a disease, since the affected individuals are not anemic and their erythrocytes are unusually rigid and resistant to penetration by malaria merozoites.

**Complications:** All patients are susceptible to the transient parvovirus-induced aplastic anemia and can have a significant fall in hematocrit during the 7–10-day period of erythroid aplasia. Patients are at increased risk for forming pigmented gallstones, leg ulcers, and postsplenectomy sepsis.

**Associated Findings:** None known.

**Etiology:** Usually (95%) autosomal dominant inheritance, resulting in a defect in the erythrocyte membrane skeleton. Pyropoikilocytosis is probably an autosomal recessive condition.

**Pathogenesis:** Much recent research has pinpointed several molecular defects as the causes of the different forms of elliptocytosis. Nearly all cases of pyropoikilocytosis and approximately 50% of elliptocytosis affecting Blacks is associated with inheritance of abnormalities in the N-terminal domain of alpha-spectrin, with a resulting decrease in the affinity of dimer:dimer associations. Abnormalities in another membrane-skeleton component, protein 4.1, have been identified in several Caucasian families. The common feature of the different defects leads to a reduced ability of the affected erythrocytes to regain the normal biconcave shape after deformation in the circulation. The molecular explanation for Melanesian elliptocytosis has not been identified.

**MIM No.:** 13045, *13050, *13060, *16690, 26614

**CDC No.:** 282.100

**Sex Ratio:** M1:F1

**Occurrence:** Elliptocytosis has been reported in virtually all ethnic groups. The disease is most common among Blacks, individuals of Mediterranean ancestry, and Melanesians in Australia, Malaysia, and the Pacific islands. The overall prevalence is 1:2,000 among Blacks in the United States. Pyropoikilocytosis is rare and has been identified primarily among Blacks.

**Risk of Recurrence for Patient's Sib:**
  See Part I, *Mendelian Inheritance.*

**Risk of Recurrence for Patient's Child:**
  See Part I, *Mendelian Inheritance.*

**Age of Detectability:** Usually clinically evident during childhood, although severe cases can be identified during infancy and very mild cases may escape notice until adulthood.

**Gene Mapping and Linkage:** EL1 (elliptocytosis 1 (Rh-linked); band 4.1 protein) has been mapped to 1pter-p34.

Some forms of elliptocytosis and most forms of pyropoikilocytosis are linked to the alpha-spectrin gene on chromosome 1. Other forms of ovalocytosis and elliptocytosis are linked to protein 4.1. The gene for protein 4.1 resides on the short arm of chromosome 1 near the locus for the Rh antigen gene. The close proximity of the 4.1 and Rh genes is probably the explanation for the apparent linkage between certain forms of elliptocytosis and the Rh blood type.

**Prevention:** None known. Genetic counseling indicated.

**Treatment:** Surgical splenectomy is warranted in the minority of cases in which clinically significant anemia is evident. In severe cases, splenectomy can be done in early childhood.

**Prognosis:** Normal life span with normal quality is expected in 99% of cases.

**Detection of Carrier:** Detection of carriers of recessive forms of the disease is currently done on an experimental basis by analysis of proteolytic digests of spectrin (Marchesi et al, 1987).

**Special Considerations:** The disorder is heterogeneous with regard to inheritance and clinical severity.

## References:

Dacie JV: The hemolytic anemias: congenital and acquired, ed 2. New York: Grune & Stratton, 1960.*

Lecomte MC, et al.: Hereditary pyropoikilocytosis and elliptocytosis in a Caucasian family: transmission of the same molecular defect in spectrin through three generations with different clinical expression. Hum Genet 1987; 77:329–334.

Marchesi SL, et al.: Mutant forms of spectrin alpha subunits in hereditary elliptocytosis. J Clin Invest 1987; 80:191–198.

McGuire M, et al.: Distinct variants of erythrocyte protein 4.1 inherited in linkage with elliptocytosis and the Rh type in the white families. Blood 1988; 72:287–293.

Lux SE, Becker PS: Disorders of the red cell membrane skeleton: hereditary spherocytosis and hereditary elliptocytosis. In: Scriver CR, et al, eds: The metabolic basis of inherited disease, 6th ed. New York: McGraw-Hill, 1989:2367–2408.

AG000                                                    **Peter Agre**

**Elliptocytosis with transverse siltlike changes**
   *See ANEMIA, HEMOLYTIC, RED CELL MEMBRANE DEFECTS*
**Elliptocytosis, hereditary**
   *See ANEMIA, HEMOLYTIC, RED CELL MEMBRANE DEFECTS*
   *also ELLIPTOCYTOSIS*
**Ellis-van Creveld syndrome**
   *See CHONDROECTODERMAL DYSPLASIA*
**Elsahy syndrome**
   *See BRANCHIO-SKELETO-GENITAL SYNDROME*
**Elsahy-Waters syndrome**
   *See BRANCHIO-SKELETO-GENITAL SYNDROME*
**Emaciation-erythema (nodular)-digital defects, Nakajo type**
   *See DIGITAL DEFECTS-NODULAR ERYTHEMA-EMACIATION, NAKAJO TYPE*
**Embryoma of head or neck**
   *See NECK/HEAD, DERMOID CYST OR TERATOMA*
**Embryopathy**
   *See FETAL EFFECTS OF POLYCHLORINATED BIPHENYL (PCB)*
**Emery-Dreifuss muscular dystrophy, autosomal dominant type**
   *See HAUPTMANN-THANHAUSER SYNDROME*

---

## EMERY-DREIFUSS SYNDROME                            2491

**Includes:**
   Humeroperoneal neuromuscular disease
   Muscular dystrophy, tardive with contractures

**Excludes:**
   **Hauptmann-Thanhauser syndrome** (3246)
   **Muscular dystrophy, adult pseudohypertrophic** (0687)
   **Muscular dystrophy, childhood pseudohypertrophic** (0689)
   **Muscular dystrophy, limb-girdle** (0691)
   Neuromuscular disorders, other
   Rigid spine syndrome

**Major Diagnostic Criteria:**   Onset of slowly progressive humeroperoneal muscle weakness in the first decade. Contractures, predominantly of elbows, with limitation of neck flexion. Absence of pseudohypertrophy. Cardiomyopathy, causing conduction deficits that lead to arrhythmias and atrial arrest.

**Clinical Findings:**   There is onset of mild upper extremity proximal muscle weakness in the first decade, with contractures involving the neck, elbows, and ankles as an early and prominent feature. These may not be significant enough to bring the child to medical attention. In the upper limbs there is usually marked wasting and weakness of the humeral muscles with the shoulders less severely affected. In the lower extremities, distal musculature may be affected before proximal musculature. Most cases have had peroneal wasting and weakness. Muscle hypertrophy does not occur. Though the usual pattern of weakness is humeroperoneal in distribution, humeropelvic, scapuloperoneal, and facioscapulohumeral distributions have been described. The course is slowly progressive with ambulation into the 4th, 5th, and 6th decades. Cardiomyopathy causing arrhythmias and atrial paralysis can be recognized and treated with a permanent ventricular demand pacemaker to prevent sudden death. Some authors feel that atrial conduction defects may also affect female carriers.

Diagnostic laboratory findings include mildly elevated creatine kinase (CK) and a myopathic pattern on electromyogram (EMG). The muscle biopsy demonstrates primary myopathic features. In cross section the contour of muscle fibers is rounded instead of polygonal. The diameters of fibers vary within each fasciculus. Large muscle fibers are abundant, and type 1 fibers predominate. There are centrally-placed nuclei, abundant lipid bodies, and occasional splitting of large fibers. Many type 1 fibers display a moth-eaten appearance. The endomysial connective tissue is increased. Ultrastructural studies confirm the primary myopathic changes.

**Complications:**   There is slowly progressive muscular weakness and stiffness, but atrial conduction abnormalities leading to heart block and permanent atrial paralysis are the most serious problems.

**Associated Findings:**   Color blindness.

**Etiology:**   Usually X-linked recessive inheritance, with the responsible gene linked to color-blindness and DNA markers in the Xq27-qter region. This condition appears to be allelic to the X-linked forms of scapuloperoneal and humeroperoneal muscular dystrophies (Thomas et al, 1972; Waters et al, 1975) in that they also map to Xq28 (Thomas et al, 1986; Yates et al, 1986; Romeo et al, 1988).

**Pathogenesis:**   Progressive, slow muscle fiber degeneration (myopathy), although occasionally neurogenic changes have been reported.

**MIM No.:**   *31030, 31285

**POS No.:**   4385

**Sex Ratio:**   M1:F0

**Occurrence:**   More than 21 families have been reported in the literature.

**Risk of Recurrence for Patient's Sib:**
   See Part I, *Mendelian Inheritance.*

**Risk of Recurrence for Patient's Child:**
   See Part I, *Mendelian Inheritance.*

**Age of Detectability:**   In the first decade of life. DNA diagnosis is now possible, based on genetic linkage analysis with DNA markers mapped on the distal part of the long arm of the X chromosome.

**Gene Mapping and Linkage:**   EMD (Emery-Dreifuss muscular dystrophy) has been mapped to Xq27.3-q28.

**Prevention:**   None known. Genetic counseling indicated.

**Treatment:**   Physical therapy to prevent contractures. Orthoses may be helpful depending on disability. Shortening of the Achilles tendon may require surgery. Cardiac involvement should be monitored from an early age. A pacemaker is recommended in all patients who have ventricular rates less than 50 beats per minute.

**Prognosis:**   Dependent primarily on the severity of cardiac disease. The cardiac conduction defect is usually manifested clinically by sinus bradycardia and prolongation of the PR interval on EKG. Most affected individuals survive into the middle ages with varying degrees of incapacity and no apparent intellectual deficits.

**Detection of Carrier:**   Based on genetic linkage analysis. Creatine kinase may be slightly elevated in carrier females, and this information may be used in conjunction with linked DNA markers for carrier detection.

**Special Considerations:**   Except for the possibility of more variability in age of onset and degree of severity, the autosomal dominant form of this condition (see **Hauptmann-Thanhauser syndrome**) appears clinically identical to this condition.

Differential diagnosis includes a second type of X-linked progressive humeroperoneal weakness in which early contractures are not a feature, and mental retardation is present (Bergia et al, 1986).

Emery-Dreifuss syndrome differs from **Hauptmann-Thanhauser syndrome** in that it is usually X-linked and myopathic, while the latter condition is usually autosomal dominant and neurogenic. **Hauptmann-Thanhauser syndrome** usually has a later onset, and cardiac conduction defects are not a constant feature. These distinctions are not always clear-cut, and because of the variability within individual families, Emery (1989) has suggested that the term Emery-Dreifuss *syndrome* be confined to the combination of early contractures, humeroperoneal muscle weakness, and cardiomyopathy. Cases would then be classified as either myopathic or neurogenic in origin, and as inherited in either an X-linked recessive or autosomal dominant fashion.

**Support Groups:** New York; Muscular Dystrophy Association (MDA)

**References:**

Emery AE, Dreifuss TF: Unusual type of benign X-linked muscular dystrophy. J Neurol Neurosurg Psychiatry 1966; 29:338–342.

Thomas PK, et al.: X-linked scapuloperoneal syndrome. J Neurol Neurosurg Psychiat 1972; 35:208–215.

Waters DP, et al.: Cardiac features of an unusual X-linked humeroperoneal neuromuscular disease. New Engl J Med 1975; 293:1017–1022.

Rowland LP, et al.: Emery-Dreifuss muscular dystrophy. Ann Neurol 1979; 5:111–117.

Dickey RP, et al.: Emery-Dreifuss muscular dystrophy. J Pediatr 1984; 104:555–559.

Miller RG, et al.: Emery-Dreifuss muscular dystrophy with autosomal dominant transmission. Neurology 1985; 35:1230–1233.

Bergia B, et al.: Familial lethal cardiomyopathy with mental retardation and scapuloperoneal muscular dystrophy. J Neurosurg Psychiatry 1986; 49:1423–1426.

Graham JM Jr, et al.: Autosomal dominant limb-girdle muscular dystrophy with a progressive cardiomyopathy: report of a large family and delineation of natural history. Am J Med Genet 1986; 25:720–721.

Johnston AW, McKay E: X-linked muscular dystrophy with contractures. J Med Genet 1986; 23:591–595.

Merlin L, et al.: Emery-Dreifuss muscular dystrophy: report of five cases in a family and review of the literature. Muscle Nerve 1986; 9:481–485.

Thomas NST, et al.: Localization of the gene for Emery-Dreifuss muscular dystrophy to the distal long arm of the X chromosome. J Med Genet 1986; 23:596–598.

Yates JRW, et al.: Emery-Dreifuss muscular dystrophy: localization to Xq 27.3 qter confirmed by linkage to the factor VIII gene. J Med Genet 1986; 587–590.

Emery AEH: X-linked muscular dystrophy with early contractures and cardiomyopathy (Emery-Dreifuss type). Clin Genet 1987; 32:360–367.

Romeo G, et al.: Mapping of the Emery-Dreifuss gene through reconstruction of crossover points in two Italian pedigrees. Hum Genet 1988; 80:59–62.

Emery AE: Emery-Dreifuss syndrome. J Med Genet 1989; 26:637–641.

GR000
RA015
N0007
I0000

John M. Graham, Jr.
Eileen Rawnsley
Richard Nordgren
Victor V. Ionasescu

**Emery-Nelson syndrome**
   See ACROFACIAL DEFECTS, EMERY-NELSON TYPE
**EMG syndrome**
   See BECKWITH-WIEDEMANN SYNDROME
**Emphysema, congenital lobar**
   See LUNG, EMPHYSEMA CONGENITAL LOBAR
**Emphysema, familial**
   See ALPHA(1)-ANTITRYPSIN DEFICIENCY
**Emphysema, localized congenital**
   See LUNG, EMPHYSEMA CONGENITAL LOBAR
**EN-arthropathy-BHL syndrome**
   See SARCOIDOSIS
**Enalapril, fetal effects**
   See FETAL ANGIOTENSIN CONVERTING ENZYME (ACE)
      INHIBITION RENAL FAILURE
**Enamel and dentin defects from tetracycline**
   See TEETH, DEFECTS FROM TETRACYCLINE
**Enamel and dentin staining from erythropoietic porphyria**
   See PORPHYRIA, ERYTHROPOIETIC
**Enamel aplasia, chronologic**
   See TEETH, ENAMEL HYPOPLASIA
**Enamel hypocalcification-onycholysis-hypohidrosis**
   See AMELO-ONYCHO-HYPOHIDROTIC SYNDROME

**Enamel hypoplasia, hereditary**
   See TEETH, AMELOGENESIS IMPERFECTA
**Enamel hypoplasia-taurodontism-tight hair-cortical sclerosteosis**
   See TRICHO-DENTO-OSSEOUS SYNDROME
**Enamel shelf teeth**
   See TEETH, ENAMEL AND DENTIN DEFECTS FROM
      ERYTHROBLASTOSIS FETALIS
**Enamel, hypoplastic-hypocalcified with taurodontism**
   See TEETH, AMELOGENESIS IMPERFECTA
**Enamel, hypoplastic-hypomaturation**
   See TEETH, AMELOGENESIS IMPERFECTA
**Enamel, hypoplastic-hypomaturation-taurodontism**
   See TEETH, AMELOGENESIS IMPERFECTA
**Encephalitis, Venezuelan equine**
   See FETAL VENEZUELAN EQUINE ENCEPHALITIS INFECTION
**Encephalo-cranio-cutaneous lipomatosis**
   See PROTEUS SYNDROME

## ENCEPHALOCELE      0343

**Includes:**
   Cranial meningoencephaloceles
   Cranium bifidum

**Excludes:**
   **Hydrocephaly** (0481)
   **Meckel syndrome** (0634)
   **Meningocele** (0642)
   **Orbital ephaloceles** (0762)
   **Schisis association** (2249)

**Major Diagnostic Criteria:** A midline mass with underlying bony defect of skull is present.

**Clinical Findings:** An encephalocele usually presents as a mass in the midline of the parietal or occipital skull, that is usually skin covered. Frontal encephaloceles are present in the midline (nasion), in the medial wall of the orbit, or as a cystic mass in the nasopharynx. All are present at birth. The infant's neurologic testing is abnormal in those instances of large encephaloceles containing major amounts of brain. The defect in the skull is confirmed by X-ray.

**Complications:** If the encephalocele is not skin-covered, meningitis may occur. Improper manipulation of nasal encephaloceles may also lead to meningitis.

**Associated Findings:** Posterior encephaloceles are associated with abnormalities of the cerebrospinal fluid (CSF) pathways, leading to **Hydrocephaly** in greater than 50% of the cases. Two instances of associated myelomeningocele, one lipoma of the cauda equina, and one **Klippel-Feil anomaly** are recorded. Many occipital encephaloceles exist as part of **Meckel syndrome**, with associated polycystic kidneys and microcephaly. Other midline

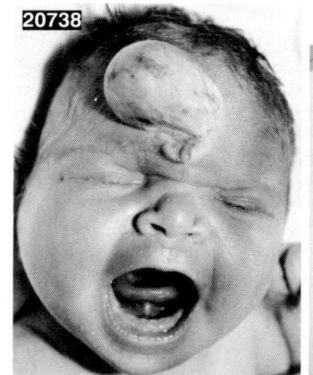
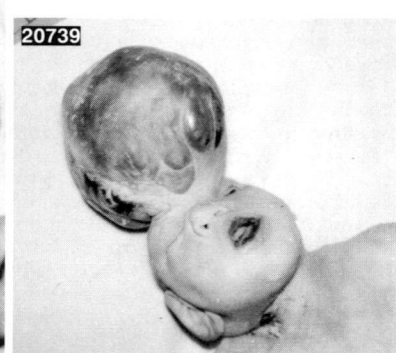

**0343-20738:** Encephalocele; this newborn has a small anterior encephalocele. **20739:** Large encephalocele.

closure defects including cleft lip and palate and **Corpus callosum agenesis** are occasionally found.

**Etiology:** Unknown.

**Pathogenesis:** The basis of the cerebral defect is a failure of closure of the midline with brain protrusion or overgrowth. Many large lesions contain primarily the cranial meninges and CSF with little brain, suggesting a primary mesodermal failure.

**POS No.:** 3720

**CDC No.:** 742.0

**Sex Ratio:** M1:F1

**Occurrence:** Variable but estimated at 1:2000 live births. Highest in Ireland. Unusually high incidence of frontal encephaloceles in Thailand.

**Risk of Recurrence for Patient's Sib:** CNS anomaly in subsequent sibs; 6%. May vary with ethnic group and geographic region.

**Risk of Recurrence for Patient's Child:** Unknown.

**Age of Detectability:** Prenatally, by elevated alpha-fetoprotein in amniotic fluid; lucent shadow associated with fetal head on amniography; bulge or gap near the parietal bone on ultrasonography.

**Gene Mapping and Linkage:** Unknown.

**Prevention:** None known. Genetic counseling indicated.

**Treatment:** Surgical closure as soon after birth as possible, but as an emergency if the encephalocele is open and draining CSF.

**Prognosis:** Related to presence and amount of brain within the sac. Approximately 20% of children will be mentally subnormal or neurologically handicapped. With occipital lesions, successful treatment of the hydrocephaly affects prognosis.

**Detection of Carrier:** Unknown.

**References:**

Blumenfeld R, Skolnick EM: Intranasal encephaloceles. Arch Otolaryngol 1965; 82:527.
Lorber J: The prognosis of occipital encephalocele. Dev Med Child Neurol (suppl) 1967; 13:75.
Dedo HH, Sooy FA: Endaural encephalocele and cerebrospinal fluid otorrhea. Ann Otol Rhinol Laryngol 1970; 79:168.
Dedo HH, Sooy FA: Endaural brain hernia (encephalocele): diagnosis and treatment. Laryngoscope 1970; 80:1090.
Mealey J Jr, et al.: The prognosis of encephaloceles. J Neurosurg 1970; 32:209.
Miskin M, et al.: Prenatal ultrasonic diagnosis of occipital encephalocele. Am J Obstet Gynecol 1978; 130:585.
Rahman NU: Nasal encephalocele. J Neurol Sci 1979; 42:73–85.

SH007                                      **Kenneth Shapiro**

**Encephalocele, orbital**
  *See ORBITAL CEPHALOCELES*
**Encephalochoristoma nasofrontalis**
  *See NOSE, GLIOMA*
**Encephalofacial angiomatosis**
  *See STURGE-WEBER SYNDROME*
**Encephalopathy**
  *See MYOPATHY, MITOCHONDRIAL-ENCEPHALOPATHY-LACTIC ACIDOSIS-STROKE*

## ENCEPHALOPATHY, NECROTIZING                    0344

**Includes:**
  Encephalopathy, subacute necrotizing
  Leigh disease
  Infantile necrotizing encephalomyelopathy
  Subacute necrotizing encephalomyelopathy (SNE)

**Excludes:**
  **Acidemia, ethylmalonic-adipic** (2377)
  **Acidemia, glutaric acidemia I** (0421)
  **Acidemia, glutaric acidemia II, neonatal onset** (2289)
  **Acidemia, methylmalonic** (0658)

**Acidemia, propionic** (0826)
**Biotinidase deficiency** (2591)
**Brain, spongy degeneration** (0115)
**Fructose-1,6-diphosphatase deficiency** (0396)
**Glycogenosis, type Ia** (0425)
**Hepatolenticular degeneration** (0469)
**Joubert syndrome** (2908)
Lactic acidosis, congenital (other)
**Leukodystrophy, globoid cell type** (0415)
**Metachromatic leukodystrophies** (0651)
Mitochondriopathies (other)
**Multiple sclerosis, familial** (2598)
**Myopathy-metabolic, mitochondrial cytochrome C oxidase deficiency** (2707)
**Neuroaxonal dystrophy, infantile** (2701)
**Neuronal ceroid-lipofuscinoses (NCL)** (0713)
**Spinocerebellar degeneration-corneal dystrophy** (2619)
Striatal necrosis, infantile
Wernicke encephalopathy

**Major Diagnostic Criteria:** Definitive diagnosis still requires autopsy. Clinical features vary with the course of the disease and the age of onset. The following features are highly suggestive of SNE and represent the most common clinical picture: insidious onset of weight loss, weakness, hypotonia, and variable degrees of psychomotor retardation in a child under 2 years of age. These features are associated with symptoms and signs suggestive of brainstem lesions (nystagmus, abnormal eye movements, sluggish pupils, and respiratory alterations). The presence of lactic acidosis (with hyperpyruvatemia, hyperalaninemia, and hyperalaninuria), inexorable and step-wise progression, and the exacerbation of symptoms when the child is catabolically stressed also represent components of the common clinical picture. The additional presence of lucencies in the basal ganglia and/or brain stem by cranial CT scan, or similarly placed lesions on magnetic resonance imaging, makes the diagnosis highly likely. However, other clinical pictures of SNE include: an acute onset associated with seizures, older age of onset often associated with movement disorders (clumsiness, tremor, falling, inability to walk, ataxia), adult onset, or chronic disease punctuated by spontaneous remissions of any of the previous symptoms. The remissions, however, are usually brief and incomplete. When the clinical picture is that of a progressive disorder characterized by peripheral neuropathy, hypotonia, and possibly loss of deep tendon reflexes, SNE can easily be confused with metachromatic leukodystrophy, neuroaxonal dystrophy, or globoid cell leukodystrophy (especially if extensor spasms occur).

**Clinical Findings:** Based on a review by Pincus (1972), key findings are:
  *Age at onset* of symptoms [N=86]: Less than 12 months (60%); Less than 24 months (91%); Greater than 24 months (9%).
  *Rhythm of onset* [N=86]: Insidious (71%); Subacute (14%); Acute (15%).
  *Course length* [N=83]: Less than 12 months (52%); Less than 24 months (66%); Greater than 24 months (33%).
  *Course rhythm* [N=83]: Chronic unremitting (55%); Chronic remitting (28%); Subacute unremitting (14%); Acute unremitting (2%).
  *Signs and symptoms* [N=86]: Respiratory problems [Hyperventilation, sobbing, apnea, dyspnea, tachypnea, respiratory failure, deep sighs, Cheyne-Stokes, ataxic respirations] (78%); Cranial nerve deficits [Abnormal eye movements, sluggish pupils, bulbar palsies, etc.] (66%); Hypotonia (59%); Movement disorder [Cerebellar or extrapyramidal] (40%); Blindness (36%); Babinski sign(s) (35%); Seizures (31%); Absent tendon reflexes (24%); Spasticity (15%); Microcephaly (6%); Low-grade fever (?%).
  *Laboratory findings*: The findings most suggestive of SNE are a blood and CSF lactic acidosis, and lesions of the basal ganglia (especially the putamina), thalamus, or brainstem as identified by cranial CT scans or magnetic resonance imaging. The lactic acidosis is often intermittent, therefore a normal lactic acid does not exclude SNE. CSF is more likely to be acidotic than blood. Likewise, pyruvatemia, hyperalaninuria, low serum bicarbonate, and respiratory alkalosis provide supplementary evidence in favor

of SNE, but are not diagnostically helpful when normal. Enzyme activity, as measured in cultured skin fibroblasts, may be deficient for one of the following enzymes or enzyme systems: the pyruvate dehydrogenase complex (PDHC), cytochrome c oxidase, NADH coenzyme Q reductase, or pyruvate carboxylase. On at least one occasion, cytochrome c oxidase was normal in fibroblasts, but abnormal in other tissues (DiMauro et al, 1987). A specific enzyme deficiency cannot be determined in all cases. A minority of the cases have generalized aminoaciduria, elevated cerebrospinal-fluid protein, and mild lymphocytic CSF reaction. Several cases have had evidence of peripheral nerve dysfunction, and one controversial case had "ragged red" muscle fibers. A deficiency of brain thiamine triphosphate was seen in 5/5 cases studied. Urine adenosine triphosphate-thiamine pyrophosphate (ATP-TPP) phosphoryl transferase inhibitor, i.e., the "urine inhibitor," was initially present in all autopsy-proven cases. A negative result was thought to exclude the diagnosis of SNE. However, further studies revealed at least 20% false-negative rate. The test for the urine inhibitor may also be falsely negative if the specimen is not tested within two weeks of collection or if the patient has been treated with a thiamine derivative. There is a 6.4% false-positive rate. In general, the urine inhibitor test is *not useful* for the diagnosis of individual cases. Analysis of urine organic acids helps to exclude many disorders similar to SNE. Abnormalities of brainstem conduction on brainstem auditory evoked responses and prolonged latency on visual evoked responses are present in many cases.

**Complications:** Progressive and usually fatal.

**Associated Findings:** Hypertrophic cardiomyopathy (7 of 12 cases studied specifically, and 8 other possible cases from the literature).

**Etiology:** Probably autosomal recessive inheritance. Parental consanguinity is frequent. SNE has not been reported in 2 successive generations. A single report describes two male half siblings, suggesting X-linked inheritance or autosomal recessive inheritance with both fathers being carriers.

**Pathogenesis:** A biochemical defect of oxidative metabolism is probable, but a single specific biochemical marker has not been discovered. Hyperalaninuria in the presence of elevated plasma alanine, pyruvate, and lactate has suggested an abnormality in the pyruvate dehydrogenase complex (of which the pyruvate decarboxylase subunit is thiamine pyrophosphate dependent). In some cases, it is not clear whether these biochemical changes are due to a primary or secondary disturbance in the catabolism of pyruvate (eg hyperventilation by itself may cause elevation of blood lactate and pyruvate). Lipoamide dehydrogenase deficiency, another component of the pyruvate dehydrogenase complex, has also been associated with SNE. Absence of pyruvate carboxylase has been reported in several instances of SNE and could cause lactic acidosis, hyperpyruvatemia and hyperalaninemia; however, the reliability of the pyruvate carboxylase determination has been criticized and other patients with SNE have had normal pyruvate carboxylase.

ATP-TTP phosphoryl transferase catalyzes the formation of thiamine triphosphate (TTP). An inhibitor of ATP-TPP phosphoryl transferase has been demonstrated in the urine of patients with SNE, and absence of brain TTP has been documented in several cases of SNE. The pathology of SNE shows a close resemblance to the CNS lesions of Wernicke encephalopathy, a disorder related to thiamine deficiency. It is not yet clear how a disorder of thiamine metabolism could account for SNE but there is evidence to support a coenzyme-independent role of thiamine in nervous tissue.

A deficiency of the mitochondrial enzyme cytochrome c oxidase was demonstrated in the muscle of a case with SNE. Subsequently DiMauro et al (1987) demonstrated cytochrome c oxidase deficiency in brain and several other tissues from five children with Leigh disease. This deficiency, through its effect on the cerebral energy state, could account for many of the findings in SNE.

The possibility of several distinct subtypes of SNE resulting in a similar pathological picture is another explanation for the abnormalities of pyruvate dehydrogenase complex, pyruvate carboxyl-ase, cytochrome c oxidase, and ATP-TPP phosphoryl transferase. Although several patients with SNE have had deficient enzymes of oxidative metabolism, other patients have had seemingly identical deficiencies, but have not had SNE. The relationship of SNE to a hyperendorphin state (single case report) remains speculative.

**MIM No.:** *25600

**Sex Ratio:** M1.8:F1.0

**Occurrence:** More than 130 cases have been described and it has been suggested that as many as 100 more have been diagnosed at postmortem examination and have not been reported.

**Risk of Recurrence for Patient's Sib:**
See Part I, *Mendelian Inheritance.*

**Risk of Recurrence for Patient's Child:**
See Part I, *Mendelian Inheritance.*

**Age of Detectability:** Most cases have onset under two years of age.

**Gene Mapping and Linkage:** Unknown.

**Prevention:** When an enzyme deficiency (e.g. cytochrome c oxidase deficiency) is detected in an affected child, prenatal testing may be possible during subsequent pregnancies. Therefore, it is reasonable to store cultured skin fibroblasts from an affected child in the event that additional specific enzyme deficiencies causing SNE are discovered. Genetic counseling is indicated.

**Treatment:** Initial enthusiasm for various therapies has been tempered by recognition of the considerable variability in the natural history of SNE. No effective form of treatment is available. Therapies that have met with anecdotal success include biotin 10 mg daily (cofactor for pyruvate carboxylase), lipoic acid 25–50 mg/kg/day (cofactor for lipoamide dehydrogenase), thiamine 50–100 mg daily, ketogenic diet, sodium bicarbonate or citrate from 2–20 or more mEg/kg/day, acetazolamide 10–20 mg/kg/day, and aspartate 80 mg/kg/day. Due to its neurotoxicity, dichloroacetate is not suitable for chronic treatment of lactic acidosis. Seizures may be treated with antiepileptic agents and the ketogenic diet. Respiratory support may be given although remissions are extremely rare once respiratory failure has occurred.

**Prognosis:** Usually fatal, although the course may be variable.

**Detection of Carrier:** Unknown.

**Special Considerations:** Pathology of the lesions in the central nervous system has been similar to Wernicke encephalopathy. Symmetrical, necrotic lesions with loosening of the neuropil, capillary proliferation, and relative preservation of the neurons most commonly occur in the pontine tegmentum but also in the medulla and midbrain. The next most common sites of involvement are the spinal cord, followed closely by the basal ganglia and the visual system. Dendrites and myelin are generally more damaged than axons or neuronal cell bodies. In contrast to Wernicke encephalopathy, the mamillary bodies are rarely involved in SNE while the substantia nigra is commonly involved in SNE (more than half the cases of SNE in Montpetit's Series, 1971).

In Wernicke encephalopathy, the mamillary bodies are almost always affected, while the substantia nigra is almost never affected.

**References:**
Montpetit VJA, et al.: Subacute necrotizing encephalomyelopathy: a review and a study of two families. Brain 1971; 94:1–30.
Pincus JH: Subacute necrotizing encephalomyelopathy (Leigh's disease): a consideration of clinical features and etiology. Develop Med Child Neurol 1972; 14:87–101. *
Gray F, et al.: Adult form of Leigh's disease: a clinicopathological case with CT scan examination. J Neurosurg Psychiatry 1984; 47: 1211–1215.
Evans OB: Lactic acidosis in childhood (Parts I and II). Pediat Neurol 1985; 1:325–328, and 2:5–12.
Koch TK: Magnetic resonance imaging (MRI) in subacute necrotizing encephalomyelopathy (Leigh's disease). Ann Neurol 1986; 19:605–607. †
DiMauro S, et al.: Cytochrome c oxidase deficiency in Leigh syndrome. Ann Neurol 1987; 22:498–506. *

Hinman LM, et al.: Deficiency of pyruvate dehydrogenase complex (PDHC) in Leigh's disease fibroblasts: an abnormality in lipoamide dehydrogenase affecting PDHC activation. Neurology 1989; 39:70–75.

KA008
DS000

**Raymond S. Kandt**
**Bernard D'Souza**

**Encephalopathy, subacute necrotizing**
*See ENCEPHALOPATHY, NECROTIZING*
**Encephalopathy, subacute spongiform, Gerstmann-Straussler type**
*See GERSTMANN-STRAUSSLER SYNDROME*
**Encephalopathy-cataract-renal tubular necrosis**
*See CATARACT-RENAL TUBULAR NECROSIS-ENCEPHALOPATHY, CROME TYPE*
**Encephalotrigeminal angiomatosis**
*See STURGE-WEBER SYNDROME*
**Enchondral dysostosis**
*See EPIPHYSEAL DYSPLASIA, MULTIPLE RIBBING TYPE*

## ENCHONDROMATOSIS 0345

**Includes:**

Dyschondroplasia
Internal chondromatosis
Multiple enchondromatosis
Ollier syndrome
Osteochondromatosis

**Excludes:**

**Dysplasia epiphysealis hemimelica** (0311)
**Enchondromatosis and hemangiomas** (0346)
**Exostoses, multiple cartilaginous** (0685)
**Metachondromatosis** (0650)
Osteochondromata
**Spondylometaphyseal dysplasia with enchondromatous changes** (2595)

**Major Diagnostic Criteria:** A wide variety of bone abnormalities may occur. The diagnosis is confirmed by X-ray evidence of typical enchondromata.

**Clinical Findings:** Both expansion of the enchondromas and their interference with endochondral ossification produce a wide variety of skeletal deformities that affect primarily the tubular bones. Frequent deformities include phalangeal enlargement, asymmetric limb shortening, bowing of long bones, and ulnar deviation of the wrist. Involvement is asymmetric and usually bilateral. Severity ranges from minimal involvement of one limb to marked and generalized deformities. Tumor growth is sporadic

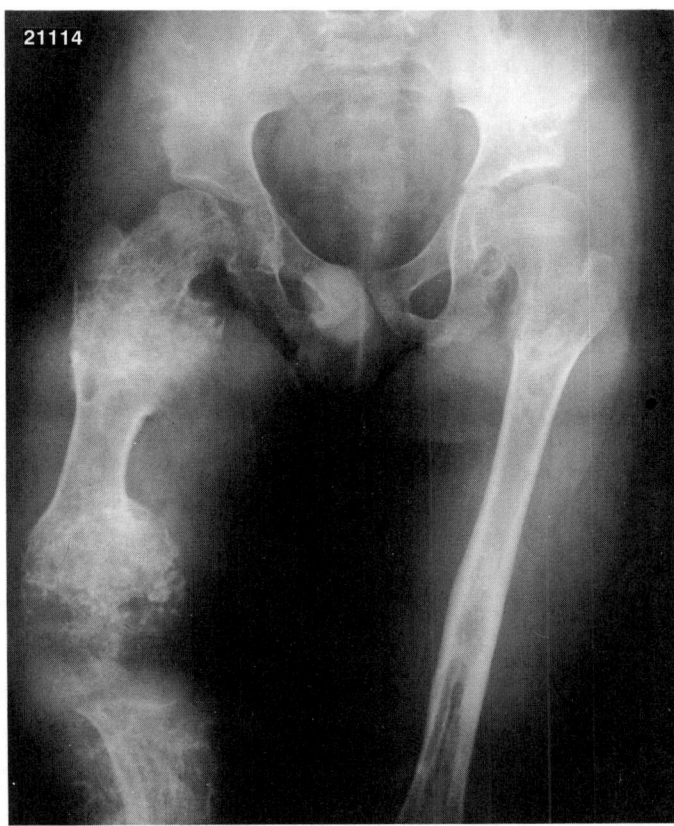

**0345B-**21114: Severe changes of enchondromatosis in the hip of this 5-year-old child.

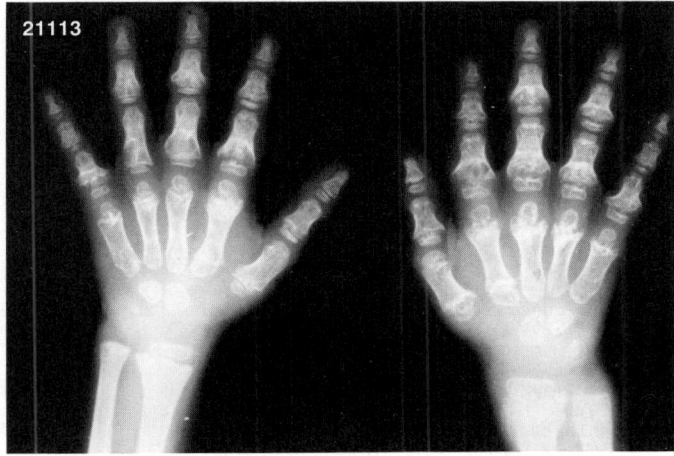

**0345A-**21113: X-ray of the hands of a 5-year-old shows changes of enchondromatosis.

through adolescence after which lesions tend to stabilize and may partially regress as cartilage is replaced by mature bone. During adulthood sarcomatous degeneration can occur, but is uncommon.

Lesions seen on X-ray films vary from minute foci of incompletely calcified cartilage extending linearly from the growth plate into the metaphysis to large tumorous masses of cartilage producing massive metaphyseal enlargement. Irregular calcifications are found within the tumor. Cortical thinning and disruption often occur in overlying bone and may be associated with abnormal metaphyseal modeling. Radiolucent defects may extend into the shaft of the bone.

**Complications:** Fracture through lesion; chondrosarcoma.

**Associated Findings:** Generalized irregular vertebral lesions or platyspondyly. ovarian juvenile granulosa cell tumor and precocious pseudopuberty.

**Etiology:** All cases appear to be sporadic.

**Pathogenesis:** Enchondromas extending from the growth plate into the metaphysis continue to proliferate, causing distortion of the metaphysis and interference with normal endochondral ossification.

**MIM No.:** 16600

**POS No.:** 3121

**CDC No.:** 756.410

**Sex Ratio:** M1:F1

**Occurrence:** Unknown.

**Risk of Recurrence for Patient's Sib:** Unknown.

**Risk of Recurrence for Patient's Child:** Unknown.

**Age of Detectability:** At birth or during early childhood.

**Gene Mapping and Linkage:** Unknown.

**Prevention:** None known. Genetic counseling indicated.

**Treatment:** Orthopedic management of deformities; X-ray examination for malignant degeneration if clinically indicated (pain or rapid enlargement in an adult).

**Prognosis:** Good.

**Detection of Carrier:** Unknown.

**Special Considerations:** Care should be taken to exclude the presence of hemangiomas, which distinguishes this from **Enchondromatosis and hemangiomas**. The distinction is important, since the present condition has a good prognosis while the latter implies more severe deformities and an increased risk of malignancy (30–40%).

**References:**

Langenskiäld A: The stages of development of the cartilaginous foci in dyschondroplasia (Ollier's disease). Acta Orthop Scand 1967; 38: 174.

Manizer F, et al.: The variable manifestations of multiple enchondromatosis. Pediatr Radiol 1971; 99:377–388. *

Kaufman HJ: Enchondromatosis. Semin Roentgenol 1973; 8:176–177.

Feldman F: Cartilaginous lesions of bones and soft tissues. CRC Crit Rev Clin Radiol Nucl Med 1974; 4:477–551.

Spranger J, et al.: Two peculiar types of enchondromatosis. Pediatr Radiol 1978; 7:215.

Shapiro F: Ollier's disease. An assessment of angular deformity, shortening and pathological fracture in 21 patients. J Bone Joint Surg 1982; 64A:95.

Horton WA: Abnormalities of bone structure. In: Emery AEH, Rimoin DR, eds: Principles and practices of medical genetics. Edinburgh: Churchill Livingstone, 1983:752–764. *

LA006
H0033
H0025

**Ralph S. Lachman**
**William A. Horton**
**O.J. Hood**

## ENCHONDROMATOSIS AND HEMANGIOMAS                    0346

**Includes:**

Dyschondroplasia-hemangiomatosis (some cases)
Hemangiomas-enchondromatosis
Maffucci syndrome

**Excludes:**

**Angio-osteohypertrophy syndrome** (0055)
**Dysplasia epiphysealis hemimelica** (0311)
**Enchondromatosis** (0345)
**Exostoses, multiple cartilaginous** (0685)
**Nevus, blue rubber bleb nevus syndrome** (0113)
**Metachondromatosis** (0650)

**Major Diagnostic Criteria:** Coexisting hemangiomas and enchondromas verified by X-ray or microscopic examination.

**Clinical Findings:** The cardinal feature of this syndrome is the coexistence of hemangiomas and enchondromas. Superficial or cavernous hemangiomas are usually detected at or shortly after birth. They are usually located on the limbs (97%); however, lingual, umbilical, and GI hemangiomas are also reported. The size of the lesions is not stationary, and they range from a few millimeters to massive clusters, deforming an entire limb. Multiple enchondromas appear in early childhood, and may be clinically heralded by the development of asymmetry of the limbs or face or by irregular expansion of the small bones of the hands or feet. X-ray examination typically discloses multiple enchondromas occurring as discrete lesions or in irregular clusters. With time, massive distortion of a long bone by the enchondromas may occur. Though asymmetry of the enchondral bones of the base of the skull may occur, these lesions do not appear to produce the massive distortion seen at other sites. There is, for the most part, no correlation between the sites of hemangiomas and enchondromas. Either may be unilateral or bilateral in distribution.

Other clinical findings include enchondromas (100%) bilateral,

62%, and unilateral, 38%; hemangiomas (100%) bilateral, 56%, and unilateral, 44%; sarcomatous degeneration, 30%; phlebectasia, 25%; phleboliths, 43%.

**Complications:** Physical handicap because of limb deformities; malocclusion if face and jaw are involved; pathologic fractures; GI bleeding. Malignant degeneration of hemangiomas or enchondromas to angiosarcoma or osteosarcoma may occur.

**Associated Findings:** Vitiligo; GI hemangiomas; other malignant tumors, 7%; benign tumors 7%; lymphangiomas.

**Etiology:** Possibly autosomal dominant inheritance.

**Pathogenesis:** Two major pathogenetic mechanisms have been proposed. First, both the hemangiomas and enchondromas may result from mesodermal dysplasia of the anlagen of vessels and bones in the affected areas. Second, enchondromas may result from failure of resorption of part of the cartilage growth plate of the epiphysis. This failure may be induced by an abnormality of the blood supply to the bone or by the presence of vascular anomalies, i.e., hemangiomas within the bone. Careful examination has, on occasion, revealed the coexistence of osseous hemangioma and enchondroma at the same site.

**MIM No.:** 16600

**POS No.:** 3759

**CDC No.:** 756.420

**Sex Ratio:** M1:F1

**Occurrence:** Approximately 100 cases reported.

**Risk of Recurrence for Patient's Sib:** Unknown

**Risk of Recurrence for Patient's Child:** Unknown.

**Age of Detectability:** At birth or shortly after.

**Gene Mapping and Linkage:** Unknown.

**Prevention:** None known. Genetic counseling indicated.

**Treatment:** Orthopedic and surgical intervention to minimize deformities. Surveillance for GI lesion and sarcomatous change. Psychosocial support can be helpful.

**Prognosis:** Patients may have nearly normal life span with normal intelligence. Progression of deformities tends to cease by adolescence, although sarcomas may develop later on, and the occurrence of enchondromas may be exacerbated by fractures.

**Detection of Carrier:** Unknown.

**Special Considerations:** The accurate recognition of this condition is crucial in view of the increased incidence of malignancy in this disorder.

The term "enchondromatosis" is preferable to the less specific "dyschondroplasia." It should be noted that early reports use the terms interchangeably.

**References:**

Carleton A, et al.: Maffucci's syndrome. Q J Med 1942; 11:203.

Anderson IF: Maffucci's syndrome: report of a case with review of the literature. S Afr Med J 1965; 39:1066–1070.

Lewis RJ: Maffucci's syndrome: functional and neoplastic significance. J Bone Joint Surg [Am] 1973; 7:1465–1469.

Sun T-C, et al.: Chondrosarcoma in Maffucci's syndrome. J Bone Joint Surg 1985; 67A:1214–1219.

T0006

MY001

**Kathleen Toomey**
*David W. Hollister*
**Terry L. Myers**

**End-organ unresponsiveness to 1,25 dihydroxycholecalciferol**
*See RESISTANCE TO 1,25 DIHYDROXY VITAMIN D*
**End-organ unresponsiveness to vitamin D**
*See RESISTANCE TO 1,25 DIHYDROXY VITAMIN D*
**Endemic Burkitt lymphoma**
*See LYMPHOMA, BURKITT TYPE*
**Endocardial cushion defects**
*See HEART, ENDOCARDIAL CUSHION DEFECTS*
**Endocardial fibroelastosis (EFE) of left ventricle**
*See VENTRICLE, ENDOCARDIAL FIBROELASTOSIS OF LEFT VENTRICLE*

**Endocardial fibroelastosis (EFE) of right ventricle**
*See VENTRICLE, ENDOCARDIAL FIBROELASTOSIS OF RIGHT VENTRICLE*
**Endocrine adenomatosis, multiple, type I**
*See ENDOCRINE NEOPLASIA, MULTIPLE TYPE I*
**Endocrine adenomatosis, multiple, type II**
*See ENDOCRINE NEOPLASIA, MULTIPLE TYPE II*
**Endocrine adenomatosis, multiple, type IIb**
*See ENDOCRINE NEOPLASIA, MULTIPLE TYPE III*
**Endocrine disorders-epilepsy-mental deficiency**
*See BORJESON-FORSSMAN-LEHMANN SYNDROME*

---

## ENDOCRINE NEOPLASIA, MULTIPLE TYPE I                0350

**Includes:**

Endocrine adenomatosis, multiple, type I
Forbes-Albright syndrome (some cases)
Hyperparathyroidism, hereditary (some cases)
Wermer syndrome
Zollinger-Ellison syndrome (some cases)

**Excludes:**

Endocrine neoplasia, multiple type II (0351)
Endocrine neoplasia, multiple type III (0352)

**Major Diagnostic Criteria:** Hyperactivity of more than one endocrine gland, i.e. thyroid, parathyroid, pituitary, adrenal, pancreas, and the like, in a member of a family in which various tumors of endocrine glands have been found, strongly suggests the diagnosis.

**Clinical Findings:** The age of diagnosis ranges from the second to the seventh decades of life, rarely in childhood. The presenting symptoms depend upon which endocrine organ is initially involved and whether or not hormonal hypersecretion is clinically significant. More than one endocrine gland may be affected simultaneously; alternatively, years may elapse between clinical symptoms caused by a single gland dysfunction and symptoms caused by other glands. Affected glands include pituitary, parathyroid, and pancreas. Adrenal cortex and thyroid follicular cell involvement is probably either secondary or coincidental. Bronchial and intestinal carcinoids also have been described.

Pituitary adenomas may give rise to symptoms of acromegaly or the Cushing syndrome if hyperfunctioning. Amenorrhea or galactorrhea or both may be seen (Forbes-Albright syndrome). Headache and visual disturbances secondary to an expanding intrasellar mass are not uncommon.

Parathyroid adenomas are usually multiple; diffuse hyperplasia of all glands may be seen. The parathyroid is the most commonly affected gland in the syndrome (> 80%). Symptoms may be typical of hyperparathyroidism, or the elevated blood calcium and parathyroid hormone levels may be discovered only by laboratory screening. Parathyroid carcinoma is rare.

Pancreatic adenomas or adenocarcinomas arise from the islet cells, and symptoms depend on which cell type is involved; i.e., insulinomas, glucagonomas, or gastrinomas. There may be diffuse islet cell hyperplasia or multiple tumor nodules, frequently malignant. Intractable or recurrent peptic ulceration, or both, may result from excess gastrin secretion (Zollinger-Ellison syndrome).

Adrenal cortical hyperplasia or adenomas are not as common, but may be associated with hypercorticism, hyperaldosteronism, or with symptoms related to excessive sex steroids. It is questionable whether the adrenal is primarily involved or becomes secondarily hypertrophied as a consequence of excess pituitary ACTH secretion or ectopic ACTH secretion from pancreatic tumors or others.

Thyroid involvement is less common, and the lesions are not consistent, i.e., adenomas, thyroiditis, and colloid goiter all have been described.

**Complications:** Include all those classically associated with hormonal hypersecretion. Ectopic peptide hormone production may be a feature. Carcinoid tumors arising from the bronchi, thymus, or upper small intestine may be responsible for excessive secretion of serotonin and the carcinoid syndrome. Pancreatic cholera or the watery diarrhea syndrome has been seen.

**Associated Findings:** Epithelial thymomas, schwannomas, and multiple benign lipomas have been described.

**Etiology:** Autosomal dominant inheritance with virtually complete penetrance, if the entire age range and variable expressivity are taken into account.

**Pathogenesis:** Possibly a two-step model involving an abnormality of a plasma-membrane receptor in the affected endocrine glands. The somatic mutation may involve depression of a primitive gene coding for a protein that promotes the growth of the endocrine glands. This "primitive gene" may be an oncogene.

**MIM No.:** *13110

**Sex Ratio:** M1:F1

**Occurrence:** Undetermined. Established literature.

**Risk of Recurrence for Patient's Sib:**
See Part I, *Mendelian Inheritance.* Extensive hormone assays may be necessary to exclude diagnosis, even in asymptomatic first-degree relatives.

**Risk of Recurrence for Patient's Child:**
See Part I, *Mendelian Inheritance.*

**Age of Detectability:** Between 10 and 60 years of age. Screening of at-risk relatives with hormone assays (perhaps with discretionary use of provocative or suppressive tests), serum calcium levels, and visual-field examinations at yearly intervals is advised.

**Gene Mapping and Linkage:** MEN1 (multiple endocrine neoplasia I) has been mapped to 11q12-q13.

**Prevention:** None known. Genetic counseling indicated.

**Treatment:** Pituitary lesions may be treated surgically or with appropriate radiotherapy. If hyperparathyroidism or hyperadrenalcorticism develops, all parathyroid or adrenal tissue should be removed; the recurrence risk is high. The Zollinger-Ellison syndrome has responded to total gastrectomy, and, rarely, metastatic lesions have disappeared. In view of the fact that the tumors are often not resectable and/or widespread metastatic disease is present, $H_2$-blockers such as cimetidine or substituted benzimidazole derivatives are commonly used for symptomatic relief. Other pancreatic lesions should be treated by surgical excision. Thyroid lesions are usually not malignant and may be managed conservatively. Other miscellaneous tumors (carcinoids, thymomas) should be removed. Lipomas are benign and require no therapy.

After surgical removal of a gland, hormone replacement therapy is indicated. If the parathyroid glands are totally removed, vitamin D and calcium will be necessary. Autotransplantation of a single parathyroid into an accessible site has occasionally been useful to avoid life-long supplementation. Nonresectable or metastatic lesions may respond to chemotherapy. Prostaglandin inhibitors may be helpful in control of pancreatic cholera.

**Prognosis:** Good for nonmalignant facet of disease, if symptoms detected early. Poor for pancreatic malignancy, although long-term survivors of Zollinger-Ellison syndrome have been described.

**Detection of Carrier:** Periodic serum calcium, phosphorus, prolactin, and pancreatic polypeptide screening for at-risk individuals.

**References:**

Prosser PR, et al.: Prolactin-secreting pituitary adenomas in multiple endocrine adenomatosis, type I. Ann Intern Med 1979; 91:41–44.

Betts JB, et al.: Hyperparathyroidism: a prerequisite for Zollinger-Ellison syndrome in multiple endocrine adenomatosis type 1 - report of a further family and a review of the literature. Q J Med 1980; 49:69–76.

Stacpoole PW, et al.: A familial glucagonoma syndrome: genetic, clinical and biochemical features. Am J Med 1981; 70:1017–1026.

Lamers CB, et al.: Omeprazole in Zollinger-Ellison syndrome. N Engl J Med 1984; 310:758–761.

Schimke RN: Genetic aspects of multiple endocrine neoplasia. Annu Rev Med 1984; 35:25–31.

Schimke RN: Multiple endocrine neoplasia: search for an oncogenic trigger (Editorial). New Engl J Med 1986; 314:1315–1316.

Wolfe MM, Jensen RT: Zollinger-Ellison syndrome: current concepts in diagnosis and management. New Engl J Med 1987; 317:1200–1209.

SC016

R. Neil Schimke

## ENDOCRINE NEOPLASIA, MULTIPLE TYPE II 0351

**Includes:**

Medullary thyroid carcinoma and pheochromocytoma
  syndrome
Medullary thyroid carcinoma syndrome (most cases)
MEN II syndrome
MEN IIa syndrome
Endocrine adenomatosis, multiple, type II
Pheochromocytoma and amyloid-producing medullary
  thyroid carcinoma
PTC syndrome
Sipple syndrome

**Excludes:**

Endocrine neoplasia, multiple type I (0350)
Endocrine neoplasia, multiple type III (0352)
Pheochromocytoma, familial
Pheochromocytoma occurring with other syndromes

**Major Diagnostic Criteria:**  The presence of pheochromocytoma, medullary thyroid carcinoma, or both, in any member of a family in which others have shown similar lesions suggests the diagnosis. An elevated plasma calcitonin level alone is *not* sufficient for diagnosis, since this hormone may be ectopically secreted by lung tumors, pancreatic tumors, and even a sporadic pheochromocytoma.

**Clinical Findings:**  Age of diagnosis is variable but may range from childhood to seventh decade. Patients may present with symptoms related to catecholamine excess, including headache, palpitations, diaphoresis, flushing, and either labile or sustained hypertension secondary to pheochromocytoma. The pheochromocytoma, however, may be asymptomatic. Pheochromocytomas are bilateral and occasionally, extraadrenal. Malignant degeneration is rare.

Medullary thyroid carcinoma is invariably multifocal, but the nodules may or may not be palpable and may or may not be detectable by radioactive scanning. Measurements of plasma calcitonin, with or without stimulation, may be the only means of diagnosis of the asymptomatic patient. The tumor may elaborate ectopic hormones, including ACTH. The carcinoid syndrome, as well as the watery diarrhea syndrome, have been seen with these tumors.

Parathyroid hyperplasia or adenomatosis is frequently seen; but is rarely symptomatic.

**Complications:**  Include those associated with catecholamine-induced hypertension, e.g., cardiac disease, renal damage, strokes, and symptoms associated with parathyroid hormone excess. Ectopic hormone production by the medullary carcinoma may lead to a variety of problems, depending upon the peptide secreted.

**Associated Findings:**  Gliomas, glioblastomas, and meningiomas have been reported. Other tumors and nonmalignant lesions are probably no more common than in the general population.

**Etiology:**  Autosomal dominant inheritance, with high penetrance and variable expressivity.

**Pathogenesis:**  A heritable defect in neural crest differentiation has been suggested, but the presence of rather consistent parathyroid hyperplasia suggests a more complex etiology. The various tumors are clonal in origin.

**MIM No.:**  *17140

**Sex Ratio:**  M1:F1

**Occurrence:**  Undetermined. Extensive literature.

**Risk of Recurrence for Patient's Sib:**

See Part I, *Mendelian Inheritance.* An apparently sporadic case

should not be considered a new mutation until extensive family testing has been undertaken.

**Risk of Recurrence for Patient's Child:**

See Part I, *Mendelian Inheritance.*

**Age of Detectability:**  Between early childhood and 60 years.

**Gene Mapping and Linkage:**  MEN2A (multiple endocrine neoplasia IIA) has been mapped to 10p11.2-q11.2.

**Prevention:**  None known. Genetic counseling indicated. Catecholamine assays may reveal pheochromocytoma before hypertension adversely affects the cardiovascular system. Elevated baseline plasma calcitonin levels suggest the presence of thyroid tumors. Provocative stimulation of calcitonin secretion with calcium, pentagastrin, or both is useful in detecting early stages of thyroid disease, i.e., c-cell hyperplasia. Serum calcium and parathyroid hormone levels may be useful in preventing long-term complications of hyperparathyroidism.

**Treatment:**  Surgical excision of both adrenals if tumors are present, since lesions are usually bilateral. Surgical removal of entire thyroid, with or without local neck dissection for medullary thyroid tumor. Plasma calcitonin levels may be useful in determining adequacy of resection and aid in detection of metastases. Radiation therapy may be useful with metastatic disease. To avoid reoperation all parathyroids should be removed if hyperparathyroidism develops.

$\alpha$- and $\beta$-adrenergic receptor blocking agents may be used if pheochromocytoma is unresectable for any reason. Nonresectable thyroid tumors producing ACTH may require adrenalectomy. The watery diarrhea syndrome may respond to prostaglandin synthesis inhibitors. After surgery, appropriate hormone and vitamin replacement is necessary.

**Prognosis:**  Good for pheochromocytoma. Good for medullary thyroid tumor if resected before metastatic disease evident; poor otherwise, although long-lived exceptions have been seen.

**Detection of Carrier:**  Age-related probability tables have been constructed for the thyroid tumor.

**References:**

Wells SA, Jr, et al.: Provocative agents and the diagnosis of medullary carcinoma of the thyroid gland. Ann Surg 1978; 188:139–141.
Gagel RF, et al.: Age-related probability of development of hereditary medullary thyroid carcinoma. J Pediatr 1982; 101:941–946.
Rogier P, et al.: Medullary thyroid carcinomas: prognostic factors and treatment. Int J Radiat Oncol Biol Phys 1983; 9:161.
Schimke RN: Genetic aspects of multiple endocrine neoplasia. Annu Rev Med 1984; 35:25–31.
Castiglione C, et al.: Assignment of multiple endocrine neoplasia type 2A to chromosome 10 by linkage. Nature 1987; 328:528–530.
Gagel RF, et al.: The clinical outcome of prospective screening for multiple endocrine neoplasia type 2a: an 18-year experience. New Engl J Med 1988; 318:478–484.

SC016

R. Neil Schimke

## ENDOCRINE NEOPLASIA, MULTIPLE TYPE III 0352

**Includes:**

Endocrine adenomatosis, multiple, type IIb
Ganglioneuromatosis of the alimentary tract
MEN IIb syndrome
Neuromata, mucosal-endocrine tumors
Mucosal neuroma syndrome
Pheochromocytoma-medullary thyroid carcinoma-multiple
  neuroma

**Excludes:**

Endocrine neoplasia, multiple type I (0350)
Endocrine neoplasia, multiple type II (0351)
Mucosal neuromas (other)
Neurofibromatosis (0712)
Pheochromocytoma (other)

**Major Diagnostic Criteria:**  Not known with certainty, since sufficiently detailed family studies have not been reported; i.e.,

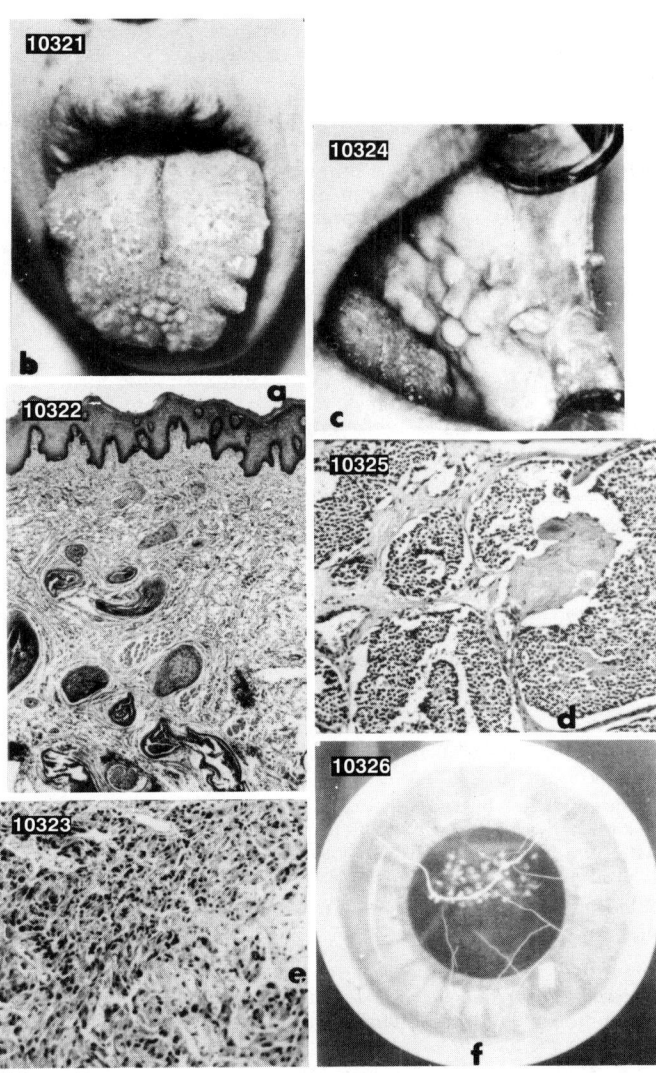

**0352**-10321: Nodules of lips and tongue. 10324: Nodules of buccal mucosa. 10322: Photomicrograph of mucosal neuroma. 10325: Medullary carcinoma of thyroid with amyloid production. 10323: Pheochromocytoma. 10326: Thickened corneal nerves.

whether or not all affected individuals invariably have the typical physiognomy. When present, the facies is virtually pathognomonic of underlying malignancy, with prominent blubbery lips and pseudoprognathism. Neuromas of conjunctivae, nasal, labial, and buccal mucosa, and the tongue are frequently present. Muscular hypotonia and a Marfan-like habitus are common. Feeding difficulties may be seen in early childhood.

**Clinical Findings:** The physiognomy is frequently striking and diagnostic. Affected patients may have some or all of the following: neuromas of conjunctiva, nasal, labial, and buccal mucosa, the tongue and other parts of the GI tract including colon, with or without megacolon; esthenic habitus; muscular hypotonia; café-au-lait spots or diffuse freckling; large blubbery lips and pseudoprognathism; kyphosis, lordosis, pes cavus, genu valgum, and generalized joint laxity; and absent flare response to intradermal histamine.

Medullary thyroid carcinoma is a constant feature, with all the attendant symptoms (see **Endocrine neoplasia, multiple type II**).

Prophylactic surgery is warranted simply on the basis of the facies.

Pheochromocytoma is frequently bilateral and may be asymptomatic.

Intestinal symptoms are related to colonic ganglioneuromas (megacolon) or are secondary to excessive prostaglandin or VIP (vasoactive intestinal polypeptide) secreted by the thyroid tumor which may cause diarrhea.

Parathyroid hyperplasia probably never occurs.

**Complications:** These are similar to those of **Endocrine neoplasia, multiple type II**. Joint laxity may give rise to orthopedic problems. Fluid and electrolyte disturbances result from altered bowel motility. A laryngeal tumor may cause vocal problems. It is conceivable that additional tumors derived from the neural crest will be reported. Ectopic hormone production may be less common, but in view of the small number of cases reported, this may be fortuitous.

**Associated Findings:** None known.

**Etiology:** Autosomal dominant inheritance. Penetrance unknown but probably high. Variable expressivity possible.

**Pathogenesis:** A defect in the differentiation of certain neural crest derivatives.

**MIM No.:** *16230

**POS No.:** 3319

**Sex Ratio:** M1:F1

**Occurrence:** Undetermined; probably not as common as types I and II.

**Risk of Recurrence for Patient's Sib:**
See Part I, *Mendelian Inheritance*. A sporadic case may be a new mutant, but caution must be exercised since penetrance has not been defined.

**Risk of Recurrence for Patient's Child:**
See Part I, *Mendelian Inheritance*.

**Age of Detectability:** As early as infancy and as late as 40 years; detection at birth may be possible. Examination of at-risk relatives for neuromas, and hormone assays should be done.

**Gene Mapping and Linkage:** MEN2B (multiple endocrine neoplasia IIB) has been provisionally mapped to 10pter-q11.2.

**Prevention:** None known. Genetic counseling indicated.

**Treatment:** Symptomatic; surgical removal of malignant tumors. X-ray therapy may be useful with metastatic thyroid cancer.

**Prognosis:** Dependent on tumor type and stage when detected. The thyroid tumor behaves in a much more malignant fashion than in **Endocrine neoplasia, multiple type II**, although there have been reports of an indolent course in some individuals.

**Detection of Carrier:** Carrier probably always shows typical facies. Calcium-pentagastrin stimulated calcitonin useful for thyroid tumor. Urine catecholamines for hypertensive at-risk relatives.

**References:**
Khairi MR, et al.: Mucosal neuromas, pheochromocytoma and medullary thyroid carcinoma: multiple endocrine neoplasia, type 3. Medicine (Baltimore) 1975; 54:89–112.
Carney JA, et al.: The parathyroid glands in multiple endocrine neoplasia type 2b. Am J Pathol 1980; 99:387–398.
Jones BA, et al.: Early diagnosis and thyroidectomy in multiple endocrine neoplasia, type 2b. J Pediatr 1983; 102:219–223.
Kullberg BJ, Nieuwenhuijzen Kruseman AC: Multipe endocrine neoplasia type 2b with a good prognosis. Arch Intern Med 1987; 147:1125–1127.

SC016                                           **R. Neil Schimke**

**Endocrine overactivity-spotty pigmentation-myxomas**
*See NEVI-ATRIAL MYXOMA-MYXOID NEUROFIBROMAS-EPHELIDES*
**Endomyocardial fibrosis (EMF) of left ventricle**
*See VENTRICLE, ENDOMYOCARDIAL FIBROSIS OF LEFT*
**Endomyocardial fibrosis (EMF) of right ventricle**
*See VENTRICLE, ENDOMYOCARDIAL FIBROSIS OF RIGHT*

**Endophytum type retinoblastoma**
  *See RETINOBLASTOMA*
**Endosteal hyperostosis**
  *See HYPEROSTOSIS, WORTH TYPE*

## ENDOSTEAL HYPEROSTOSIS                    0497

**Includes:**
  Hyperostosis corticalis generalisata
  Hyperphosphatasemia tarda
  Sclerosteosis
  Van Buchem disease

**Excludes:**
  **Hyperostosis, Worth type** (2691)
  **Osteopetrosis, malignant recessive** (0780)
  **Pachydermoperiostosis** (0788)
  **Sclerosteosis** (0880)

**Major Diagnostic Criteria:**   A widened chin can be observed in the adolescent or adult, but the diagnosis is made by X-ray study of the skull and long bones. The regular thickening of the diaphyseal cortex without increased diameter is characteristic, as well as the prominence of the mandible and thickening of the skull roof and base.

**Clinical Findings:**   Thickening and widening of the chin can be observed in the adolescent and becomes very striking in the adult. A thickened clavicle also may be palpable in adolescents but the hands and feet have normal dimensions. X-ray examination reveals symmetric thickening of the diaphyseal cortex of the long bones without increased diameter. The base and roof of the skull are thick but all sinuses are pneumatized. The prominence and thickening of the mandible are typical. The spinal processes of the vertebrae are sclerotic as are vertebral bodies, but to a lesser degree. In affected children hyperostosis is present in the skull and diaphyseal cortex but the mandibular changes are not yet characteristic. The serum alkaline phosphatase is often elevated.

**Complications:**   The osteosclerosis of the base of the skull often causes compression of cranial nerves. Paralysis of the facial nerve and sensorineural deafness are frequent. Spontaneous fractures and anemia do not occur.

**Associated Findings:**   None known.

**Etiology:**   Autosomal recessive inheritance. Another form of hyperostosis corticalis generalisata, first described by Worth and Wollin (1966), seems to be inherited as an autosomal dominant trait. In this form, the deformity of the mandible is mild and a torus palatinus is often present. X-rays show a smilar but milder involvement of the skull and long bones and sclerosis of the pelvis and vertebrae. The serum alkaline phosphatase concentration is normal (Maroteaux, et al, 1971).
  Kenny and Linarelli (1966) and Caffey (1967) have described another dominant syndrome: congenital stenosis of medullary spaces in tubular bone. In this syndrome, the marrow cavity is filiform and the growth of the long bones is reduced.
  The recessive type described is very similar to the sclerosteosis frequent in South Africa (many of the Afrikaners had their origin in Holland where Van Buchem's patients were studied, 1962). The main distinguishing feature is the syndactyly of the second and third finger, absent in hyperostosis corticalis generalisata (Beighton, 1979).

**Pathogenesis:**   In two of Van Buchem's patients, the plasma calcitonin was markedly elevated, but it was normal in two other patients. No conclusion is possible relative in the action of calcitonin in the pathogenesis of hyperostosis corticalis.

**MIM No.:**   *23910

**POS No.:**   3256

**Sex Ratio:**   M1:F1

**Occurrence:**   About 30 affected persons reported in the literature. The majority lived in Holland with possible origins on the island of Urk in the Zuider Zee.

**Risk of Recurrence for Patient's Sib:**
  See Part I, *Mendelian Inheritance.*

**Risk of Recurrence for Patient's Child:**
  See Part I, *Mendelian Inheritance.*

**Age of Detectability:**   The condition may be recognized in childhood, but most often it is detected in the adult.

**Gene Mapping and Linkage:**   Unknown.

**Prevention:**   None known. Genetic counseling indicated.

**Treatment:**   Surgical decompression may be attempted for cranial nerve involvement. Supportive therapy may also be recommended.

**Prognosis:**   Life expectancy is apparently normal.

**Detection of Carrier:**   Unknown.

**References:**

Van Buchem FS, et al.: Hyperostosis corticalis generalisata: report of seven cases. Am J Med 1962; 33:387–397.
Kenny FM, Linarelli L: Dwarfism and cortical thickening of tubular bones: transient hypocalcemia in a mother and son. Am J Dis Child 1966; 111:201–207.
Caffey JP: Congenital stenosis of medullary spaces in tubular bones and calvaria in two proportionate dwarfs, mother and son, coupled with transitory hypocalcemic tetany. Am J Roentgen 1967; 100:1–14.
Maroteaux P, et al.: L'hyperostose corticale généralisée à transmission dominante (type Worth). Arch Fr Pediatr 1971; 28:685–698. *
Van Buchem ESP, et al: Hyperostosis corticalis generalisata familiaris (van Buchem disease). New York: Elsevier, 1976.

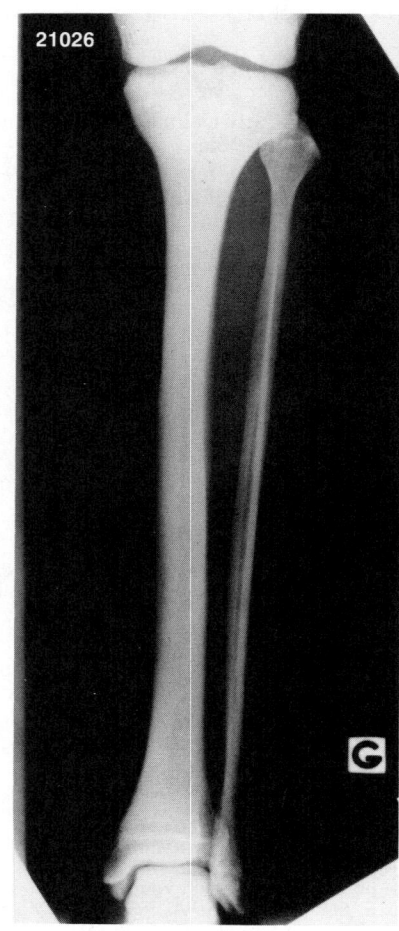

**0497-21026:**   Endosteal hyperostosis.

Gorlin RJ, Glass L: Autosomal dominant osteosclerosis. Radiology 1977; 125:547–548.
Beighton P, et al.: The syndromic status of sclerosteosis and van Buchem disease. Clin Genet 1986; 25:175–181.

MA034                                                    **Pierre Maroteaux**

**Endostosis cranii**
    See HYPEROSTOSIS FRONTALIS INTERNA
**Endothelial corneal dystrophy**
    See CORNEAL DYSTROPHY, ENDOTHELIAL
**Endothelioma capitis of Kaposi**
    See SCALP, CYLINDROMAS
**Engelmann disease**
    See DIAPHYSEAL DYSPLASIA
**Enteric cysts**
    See INTESTINAL DUPLICATION
**Enterogenous cysts**
    See INTESTINAL DUPLICATION
**Enterokinase deficiency, primary**
    See INTESTINAL ENTEROKINASE DEFICIENCY
**Enteropathy, familial**
    See MICROVILLUS INCLUSION DISEASE
**Enteropathy, gluten-induced**
    See GLUTEN-SENSITIVE ENTEROPATHY
**Enteropeptidase deficiency**
    See INTESTINAL ENTEROKINASE DEFICIENCY
**Enteroumbilical fistula**
    See OMPHALOMESENTERIC DUCT ANOMALIES
**Entropion of lid, congenital**
    See EYELID, ENTROPION

## EOSINOPHILIA, FAMILIAL                                2666

**Includes:** N/A

**Excludes:**
    Eosinophilia secondary to other illness or injury
    Eosinophilic gastroenteritis
    Eosinophilic leukemia
    Hypereosinophilic syndrome
    Loffler syndrome
    Pulmonary eosinophilia

**Major Diagnostic Criteria:** According to Naiman et al (1964), three criteria must be met for diagnosis: 1) significant eosinophilia must be present with an indirect eosinophil count of >400/mm³ (determined by multiplying the total leukocyte count by the percentage of eosinophils in the differential count) or a direct eosinophil count of >440/mm³; 2) more than one generation in the family must be affected; and 3) other recognized causes of eosinophilia must be excluded.

**Clinical Findings:** Familial eosinophilia is asymptomatic. Patients do not suffer from an increased incidence of infections, congenital anomalies, or other illnesses. The major finding is that of an increased number of eosinophils in the peripheral blood (usually >400/mm³). Eosinophil morphology and total leukocyte count are normal. Bone marrow examination may reveal an increased number of eosinophil precursors. Wide fluctuations in the blood eosinophil count may occur in response to infection or even spontaneously. No adverse effects from these fluctuations have been reported.

**Complications:** Unknown.

**Associated Findings:** In two of the 17 families reviewed by Naiman et al (1964) mild ovalocytosis in erythrocytes was noted in family members affected with eosinophilia.

**Etiology:** Autosomal dominant inheritance.

**Pathogenesis:** Appears to be a benign condition. caused by disordered regulation of eosinophil production in the bone marrow.

**MIM No.:** *13140

**Sex Ratio:** M1:F1

**Occurrence:** Naiman et al (1964) reviewed reports up to 1964 and found 17 families containing 119 affected members (out of a total

of 167 members) who satisfied the diagnostic criteria defined above. At least one case has been reported since that review.

**Risk of Recurrence for Patient's Sib:**
    See Part I, *Mendelian Inheritance.*

**Risk of Recurrence for Patient's Child:**
    See Part I, *Mendelian Inheritance.*

**Age of Detectability:** In early infancy.

**Gene Mapping and Linkage:** Unknown.

**Prevention:** None known. Genetic counseling indicated.

**Treatment:** None required.

**Prognosis:** Normal life span.

**Detection of Carrier:** Due to the autosomal dominant mode of inheritance, the carrier state is associated with significant eosinophilia.

**Special Considerations:** It is important that all other possible underlying causes of eosinophilia be excluded before making the diagnosis. The diagnostic criterion that more than one generation be affected helps to exclude many of these other causes, although unrecognized familial endemics of parasitic disease must still be ruled out. The absence of major organ dysfunction serves to distinguish familial eosinophilia from the idiopathic hypereosinophilic syndrome.

**References:**
Naiman JL, et al.: Hereditary eosinophilia: report of a family and review of the literature. Am J Hum Genet 1964; 16:195–203. *
Zeni G, et al.: In tema di ipereosinofilia constituzionale familiare idiopatica. Acta Med Patav 1964; 24:589–602.
Beeson PB, Bass DA: The eosinophil. Philadelphia: W.B. Saunders, 1977.

CU012                                                    **John T. Curnutte**

**Ependymoma**
    See CNS NEOPLASMS
**Epi-laryngeal cyst**
    See EPIGLOTTIS, VALLECULAR CYST
**Epiblepharon, inferior**
    See EYELID, EPIBLEPHARON
**Epiblepharon, superior**
    See EYELID, EPIBLEPHARON
**Epibulbar dermoid**
    See OCULAR DERMOIDS
**Epicanthus inversus**
    See BLEPHAROPTOSIS-BLEPHAROPHIMOSIS-EPICANTHUS
        INVERSUS-TELECANTHUS
**Epidermal dysplasia, type I, late fetal**
    See APLASIA CUTIS CONGENITA-GASTROINTESTINAL ATRESIA
**Epidermal nevus syndrome**
    See NEVUS, EPIDERMAL NEVUS SYNDROME
**Epidermoid cysts**
    See SPLEEN, CYSTS
**Epidermolysis bullosa atrophicans II (EBA)**
    See EPIDERMOLYSIS BULLOSUM, TYPE II
**Epidermolysis bullosa atrophicans, atresia type**
    See EPIDERMOLYSIS BULLOSUM, TYPE II
**Epidermolysis bullosa atrophicans, generalisata gravis subtype**
    See EPIDERMOLYSIS BULLOSUM, TYPE II
**Epidermolysis bullosa atrophicans, generalisata mitis type**
    See EPIDERMOLYSIS BULLOSUM, TYPE II
**Epidermolysis bullosa atrophicans, inversa type**
    See EPIDERMOLYSIS BULLOSUM, TYPE II
**Epidermolysis bullosa atrophicans, letalis with pyloric subtype**
    See EPIDERMOLYSIS BULLOSUM, TYPE II
**Epidermolysis bullosa atrophicans, localisata type**
    See EPIDERMOLYSIS BULLOSUM, TYPE II
**Epidermolysis bullosa atrophicans, muscular atrophy type**
    See EPIDERMOLYSIS BULLOSUM, TYPE II
**Epidermolysis bullosa dystrophica III (EBD)**
    See EPIDERMOLYSIS BULLOSUM, TYPE III
**Epidermolysis bullosa dystrophica neurotrophica**
    See EPIDERMOLYSIS BULLOSUM, TYPE III
**Epidermolysis bullosa dystrophica, Bart subtype**
    See EPIDERMOLYSIS BULLOSUM, TYPE III
**Epidermolysis bullosa dystrophica, Cockayne-Touraine subtype**
    See EPIDERMOLYSIS BULLOSUM, TYPE III

**Epidermolysis bullosa dystrophica, Fine subtype**
*See EPIDERMOLYSIS BULLOSUM, TYPE III*
**Epidermolysis bullosa dystrophica, Hallopeau Siemens subtype**
*See EPIDERMOLYSIS BULLOSUM, TYPE III*
**Epidermolysis bullosa dystrophica, inversa subtype**
*See EPIDERMOLYSIS BULLOSUM, TYPE III*
**Epidermolysis bullosa dystrophica, Pasini subtype**
*See EPIDERMOLYSIS BULLOSUM, TYPE III*
**Epidermolysis bullosa dystrophica, pretibial subtype**
*See EPIDERMOLYSIS BULLOSUM, TYPE III*
**Epidermolysis bullosa dystrophica, progressiva subtype**
*See EPIDERMOLYSIS BULLOSUM, TYPE III*
**Epidermolysis bullosa dystrophica, Winship subtype**
*See EPIDERMOLYSIS BULLOSUM, TYPE III*
**Epidermolysis bullosa junctionalis, disentis type**
*See EPIDERMOLYSIS BULLOSUM, TYPE II*
**Epidermolysis bullosa letalis**
*See EPIDERMOLYSIS BULLOSUM, TYPE II*
**Epidermolysis bullosa letalis-pyloric atresia**
*See EPIDERMOLYSIS BULLOSUM, TYPE II*
**Epidermolysis bullosa Mendes da Costa**
*See EPIDERMOLYSIS BULLOSUM, TYPE I*
**Epidermolysis bullosa of hands and feet**
*See EPIDERMOLYSIS BULLOSUM, TYPE I*
**Epidermolysis bullosa simplex Cockayne/Toursine**
*See EPIDERMOLYSIS BULLOSUM, TYPE I*
**Epidermolysis bullosa simplex herpetiformis, Dowling-Meara**
*See EPIDERMOLYSIS BULLOSUM, TYPE I*
**Epidermolysis bullosa simplex Koebner type**
*See EPIDERMOLYSIS BULLOSUM, TYPE I*
**Epidermolysis bullosa simplex Niemi**
*See EPIDERMOLYSIS BULLOSUM, TYPE I*
**Epidermolysis bullosa simplex Ogna type (EBSI)**
*See EPIDERMOLYSIS BULLOSUM, TYPE I*
**Epidermolysis bullosa simplex Weber-Cockayne**
*See EPIDERMOLYSIS BULLOSUM, TYPE I*
**Epidermolysis bullosa simplex with GGT deficiency**
*See EPIDERMOLYSIS BULLOSUM, TYPE I*
**Epidermolysis bullosa simplex, lethal type**
*See EPIDERMOLYSIS BULLOSUM, TYPE I*
**Epidermolysis bullosa, recessive dystrophic**
*See EPIDERMOLYSIS BULLOSUM, TYPE III*
**Epidermolysis bullosa-deafness**
*See EPIDERMOLYSIS BULLOSUM, TYPE III*
**Epidermolysis bullosa-localized skin absence-nail deformity**
*See EPIDERMOLYSIS BULLOSUM, TYPE III*

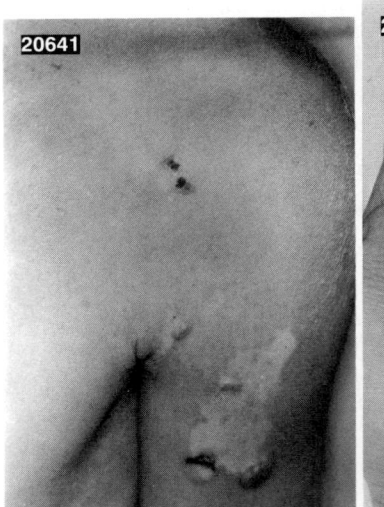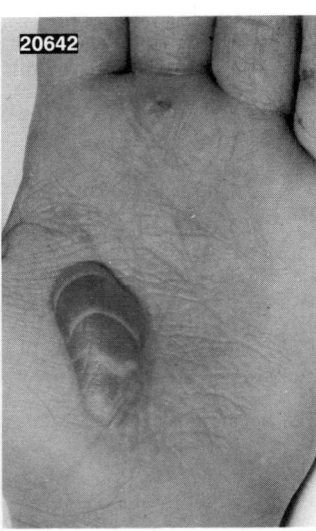

**2560**-20641: Typical grouping of lesions in epidermolysis bullosa simplex herpetiformis, Dowling Meara subtype. 20642: Intraepidermal bullous epidermolysis bullosa simplex subtype.

## EPIDERMOLYSIS BULLOSUM, TYPE I    2560

**Includes:**
Epidermolysis bullosa of hands and feet
Epidermolysis bullosa Mendes da Costa
Epidermolysis bullosa simplex Cockayne/Toursine
Epidermolysis bullosa simplex herpetiformis, Dowling-Meara
Epidermolysis bullosa simplex Koebner type
Epidermolysis bullosa simplex, lethal type
Epidermolysis bullosa simplex Niemi
Epidermolysis bullosa simplex Ogna type (EBSI)
Epidermolysis bullosa simplex Weber-Cockayne
Epidermolysis bullosa simplex with GGT deficiency
Hyperpigmentation-punctate palmoplantar keratoses-blistering

**Excludes:**
Epidermolysis bullosa, junctional
**Epidermolysis bullosum** (other)
**Poikiloderma, hereditary acrokeratotic, Kindler-Weary type** (3038)

**Major Diagnostic Criteria:** Recurrent traumatically induced blistering of the skin, usually with onset at birth or during infancy. Healing of lesions without atrophy or scarring. Electron microscopic confirmation of intraepidermal bullae.

**Clinical Findings:** Blistering usually begins during the first week of life or once the child becomes ambulant. Blisters may be generalized or localized to the extremities depending on the subtype. The lesions are induced by minor trauma. Healing occurs without scarring or atrophy. The mucous membranes, mainly the oral mucosa, may be involved in infancy, but these lesions rarely persist. Nail involvement is very rare.

There are nine subtypes of epidermolysis bullosa (EBS), with minor specific differentiating factors, which may be clinical, biochemical, or histologic.

*EBS Koebner*: generalized intraepidermal bullae.
*EBS Weber-Cockayne*: Lesions localized to hands and feet, worse in summer. Later onset, once child is ambulant.
*EBS with GGT deficiency*: Galactosylglucosyltransferase deficiency. Histologically, dissolution of tonofilaments.
*EBS Ogna*: Bruising associated with blisters.
*EBS with mottled pigmentation*: Lesions mainly on extremities. Speckled hyperpigmentation. Blisters caused by cytolysis in hyperpigmented basal cells.
*EBS herpetiformis Dowling-Meara*: Generalized distribution. Herpetiformis grouping of lesions. Lesions clear with fever.
*EBS Niemi*: Clinically the same as EBS Koebner. Histologically cytolysis of basal cells with clumping of tonofibrils.
*EBS Mendes da Costa*: Associated **Microcephaly**. X-linked recessive inheritance.
*EBS lethal type*: Death from unknown causes in infancy. Autosomal recessive inheritance.

All types of EBS are characterized histologically by intraepidermal blistering, i.e., a clearance phase within the subnuclear layer of the basal layer of the epidermis. Subtle variations may be seen in the different subtypes.

The natural history of EBS is continual blistering, with a tendency to slight improvement during adulthood. Life span is unaltered except in the newly recognized lethal form in which death occurs within the first year of life. Lesions are often worse during the summer. There is uniformity in the clinical features of sibs, and the subtype of EBS breeds true within a family.

**Complications:** Impetiginization of blisters.

**Associated Findings:** Focal hyperkeratotic pitting of fingertips may be seen within EBS with mottled pigmentation. **Microcephaly** with EBS Mendes da Costa.

**Etiology:** Autosomal dominant inheritance except for EBS Mendes da Costa, which is by X-linked recessive inheritance, and EBS lethal type, which is by autosomal recession inheritance. Clearance of basal layer of epidermis with trauma to form bullae.

**Pathogenesis:** Unknown.

**MIM No.:** *13180, 13188, *13190, *13195, 13196

**CDC No.:** 757.330

**Sex Ratio:** M1:F1, except for X-linked form.

**Occurrence:** Over a dozen, often large, kindreds have been documented, although the Dystrophic Epidermolysis Research Association (DEBRA) estimates that 50,000 Americans, mostly children, have the condition.

**Risk of Recurrence for Patient's Sib:**
See Part I, *Mendelian Inheritance.*

**Risk of Recurrence for Patient's Child:**
See Part I, *Mendelian Inheritance.*

**Age of Detectability:** Onset is at birth or during infancy. Possible prenatal diagnosis by fetal skin sampling via fetoscopy; 97% accuracy by glutamic pyruvic transaminase (GPT) typing of fetal blood in EBS Ogna.

**Gene Mapping and Linkage:** EBDCT (epidermolysis bullosa dystrophica (Cockayne-Touraine)) is unassigned.
EBS1 (epidermolysis bullosa simplex (Ogna)) has been provisionally mapped to 8.

**Prevention:** None known. Genetic counseling indicated.

**Treatment:** Symptomatic treatment with topical emollients, vitamin preparations, corticosteroids, and antiseptics.

**Prognosis:** Normal life span in all subtypes, except for the newly described lethal type in which death occurs during infancy.

**Detection of Carrier:** Unknown.

**Special Considerations:** EBS is a heterogeneous condition; however, the nine subtypes are consistent within a family. Most of the EBS subtypes are autosomal dominant, and these demonstrate complete penetration with invariable expression. See also **Poikiloderma, hereditary acrokeratotic, Kindler-Weary type**, which is sometimes classified as a variant of EBS with mottled pigmentation.

In an attempt to determine the actual incidence and prevalence of Epidermolysis Bullosa, the United States National Institutes of Heath has established a National Patient Registry and four Clinical Centers. For more information, contact D. Martin Carter, M.D., Ph.D., Laboratory of Investigative Dermatology, National EB Registry, HOS W202, the Rockefeller University, 1230 York Avenue, New York, NY 10021.

**Support Groups:** NY; Brooklyn; Dystrophic Epidermolysis Bullosa Research Asso. of America (DEBRA)

**References:**

Olaisen B, Gedde-Dahl T Jr: GPT-EBS(1) linkage group: general linkage relations. Hum Hered 1974; 24:178–185.
Eady RA, Tidman MJ: Diagnosing epidermolysis bullosa. Br J Dermatol 1983; 108:621–626.
Gedde-Dahl TJ, Anton Lamprech I: Epidermolysis bullosa. In: Emery A, Rimoin D, eds: Principles and practices of medical genetics. Edinburgh: Churchill Livingstone, 1983:672–687.
Fine JD: Epidermolysis bullosa: clinical aspects, pathology and recent advances in research. Int J Dermatol 1986; 25:143–157.
Beighton P, et al.: International nosology of heritable disorders of connective tissue, Berlin, 1986. Am J Med Genet 1988; 29:581–594.

WI055 **Ingrid M. Winship**

## EPIDERMOLYSIS BULLOSUM, TYPE II     2561

**Includes:**
Epidermolysis bullosa atrophicans, atresia type
Epidermolysis bullosa atrophicans, generalisata gravis subtype
Epidermolysis bullosa atrophicans, generalisata mitis type
Epidermolysis bullosa atrophicans, inversa type
Epidermolysis bullosa atrophicans, letalis with pyloric subtype
Epidermolysis bullosa atrophicans, localisata type
Epidermolysis bullosa atrophicans, muscular atrophy type
Epidermolysis bullosa atrophicans II (EBA)
Epidermolysis bullosa junctionalis, disentis type

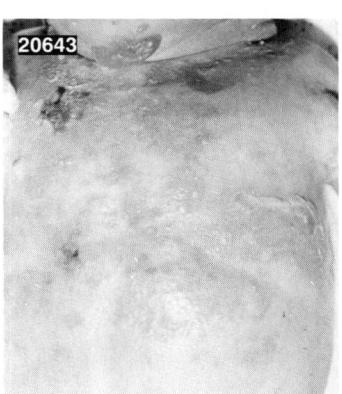
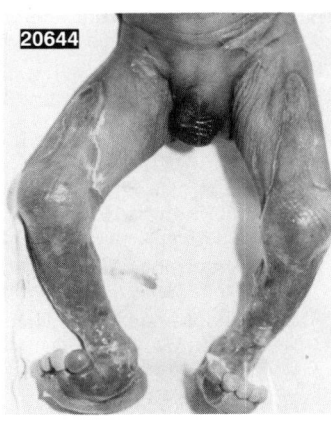

**2561-20643:** Multiple bullae in the epidermolysis bullosa atrophicans generalista mitis subtype. **20644:** Note denuded areas of skin where junctional bullae have deroofed in an infant with epidermolysis bullosa atrophicans generalista gravis subtype.

Epidermolysis bullosa letalis
Epidermolysis bullosa letalis-pyloric atresia
Generalized atrophic benign epidermolysis bullosa, Herlitz type
Herlitz-Pearson junctional epidermolysis bullosa
Junctional epidermolysis bullosa
Ureterovesical stenosis

**Excludes:** Epidermolysis bullosum (other)

**Major Diagnostic Criteria:** Traumatically induced blistering of the skin, onset at birth. Atrophy of the skin without scarring. Electron microscopic confirmation of a cleavage plane within the dermoepidermal junction.

**Clinical Findings:** The bullae of epidermolysis bullosa atrophicans (EBA) begins *in utero,* and the skin lesions present at or soon after birth. As blisters become deroofed, denuded areas remain. The distribution of skin lesions is generalized, except in EBA generalisata gravis, when hands and feet may be spared. In EBA inversa the groin, genitals, axillae, and shins are affected, while in EBA localisata the shins and soles only are affected. Nail involvement may be in the form of dystrophy or clubbing. Hypoplastic dental enamel and severe caries are associated.

Various clinical concomitants have been associated with the different subtypes. Pyloric atresia is accepted as a syndromic component of one type of lethal EBA. EBA generalisata mitis, generalised atrophic benign EB (GABEB), and EB junctionalis discutis are all associated with alopecia. Shagrun nevocytic nevi are seen in GABEB, while nevoid and palmar hyperkeratoses are a component of the discutis subtype.

All types of EBA have junctional blistering, i.e., a cleavage plane between the basal lamina and the plasma membrane of the basal cells, identifiable by electron microscopy. In addition, the hemidesmosomes are hypoplastic and lack the subbasal dense plate.

The natural history differs greatly among the several types. EBA generalisata gravis and EBA letalis with pyloric atresia are rapidly fatal in infancy. Conversely, life span is good in the other types, although quality of life is poor.

There is uniformity in the clinical features of sibs, and the type of EBA breeds true within a family.

**Complications:** 1) Early death in the two lethal types, usually as a result of septicemia, dehydration, or respiratory failure; 2) severe dental caries; 3) local skin infection; 4) esophageal strictures as a result of mucosal blistering.

**Associated Findings:** None known.

**Etiology:** Autosomal recessive inheritance. Cleavage of dermoepidermal junction with trauma (or spontaneously) to form bullae. Although EBA is a heterogeneous group of conditions, the various types are consistent within a family.

**Pathogenesis:** Unknown.

**MIM No.:** 22665, *22670, 22673

**CDC No.:** 757.330

**Sex Ratio:** M1:F1

**Occurrence:** Undetermined; established literature. The Dystrophic Epidermolysis Research Association (DEBRA) estimates that 50,000 Americans, mostly children, have epidermolysis.

**Risk of Recurrence for Patient's Sib:**
See Part I, *Mendelian Inheritance.*

**Risk of Recurrence for Patient's Child:**
See Part I, *Mendelian Inheritance.*

**Age of Detectability:** At birth, or prenatal diagnosis by fetal skin sampling.

**Gene Mapping and Linkage:** Unknown.

**Prevention:** None known. Genetic counseling indicated.

**Treatment:** Topical treatment with emollients, vitamin preparations, and corticosteroids. Systemic corticosteroids of limited value. Phenytoin is not recommended.

**Prognosis:** Early death in the two lethal forms.

**Detection of Carrier:** Unknown.

**Special Considerations:** In an attempt to determine the actual incidence and prevalence of Epidermolysis Bullosa, the United States National Institutes of Heath has established a National Patient Registry and four Clinical Centers. For more information, contact D. Martin Carter, M.D., Ph.D., Laboratory of Investigative Dermatology, National EB Registry, HOS W202, the Rockefeller University, 1230 York Avenue, New York, NY 10021.

**Support Groups:** NY; Brooklyn; Dystrophic Epidermolysis Bullosa Research Asso. of America (DEBRA)

**References:**
Pearson RW, et al.: Epidermolysis bullosa hereditaria letalis: clinical and histological manifestations and course of the disease. Arch Dermatol 1974; 109:349–355.
Bull MJ, et al.: Epidermolysis bullosa - pyloric atresia: an autosomal recessive syndrome. Am J Dis Child 1983; 137:449–451.
Eady RA, Tidman MJ: Diagnosing epidermolysis bullosa. Br J Dermatol 1983; 105:621–626.
Löfberg L, et al.: Prenatal exclusion of Herlitz syndrome by electron microscopy of foetal skin biopsies obtained at fetoscopy. Acta Dermatol Venereol (Stockh) 1983; 63:185–189.
Egan N, et al.: Junctional epidermolysis bullosa and pyloric atresia in two siblings. Arch Derm 1985; 121:1186–1188.
Beight P, et al.: International nosology of heritable disorders of connective tissue, Berlin, 1986. Am J Med Genet 1988; 29:581–594.

WI055                                           **Ingrid M Winship**

---

## EPIDERMOLYSIS BULLOSUM, TYPE III        2562

**Includes:**
Albopapuloid dominant dystrophic epidermolysis bullosa
Bart syndrome
Collagenase, excessive activity
Dominant dystrophic epidermolysis bullosa (DDEB)
Epidermolysis bullosa-deafness
Epidermolysis bullosa dystrophica, Bart subtype
Epidermolysis bullosa dystrophica, Cockayne-Touraine subtype
Epidermolysis bullosa dystrophica, Fine subtype
Epidermolysis bullosa dystrophica, Hallopeau Siemens subtype
Epidermolysis bullosa dystrophica, inversa subtype
Epidermolysis bullosa dystrophica neurotrophica
Epidermolysis bullosa dystrophica, Pasini subtype
Epidermolysis bullosa dystrophica, pretibial subtype
Epidermolysis bullosa dystrophica, progressiva subtype

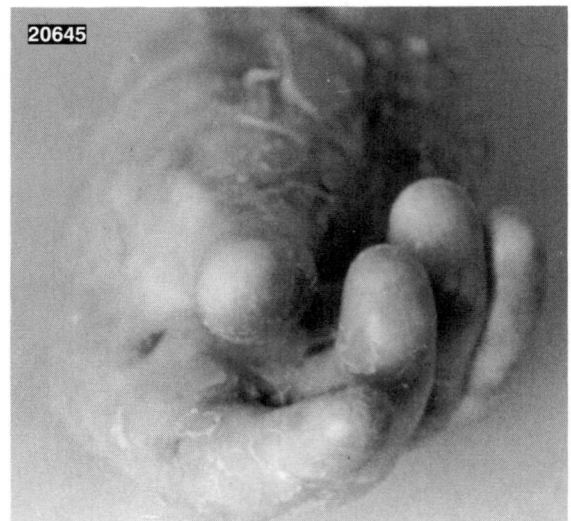

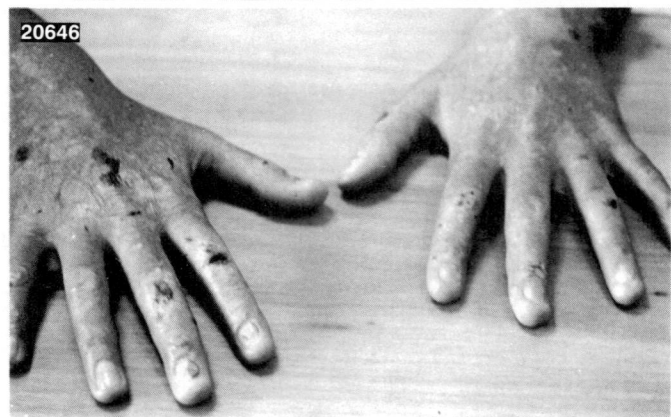

**2562-20645:** Mitten deformity of a hand in a young man with epidermolysis bullosa dystrophica Hallopeau Siemons (mutilans).
**20646:** Blisters, scars, and nail dystrophy in a man with the Cockayne-Touraine subtype.

Epidermolysis bullosa dystrophica, Winship subtype
Epidermolysis bullosa dystrophica III (EBD)
Epidermolysis bullosa-localized skin absence-nail deformity
Epidermolysis bullosa, recessive dystrophic
Recessive dystrophic epidermolysis bullosa (RDEB)
Scarring epidermolysis bullosa

**Excludes:** Epidermolysis bullosum (other)

**Major Diagnostic Criteria:** Blistering of skin, usually from birth or soon after. Slow healing of blisters with residual scaring. Milia and atrophy distinguishes these epidermolysis bullosa dystrophica (EBD) types.

**Clinical Findings:** Onset of blistering is at birth or soon thereafter. EBD pretibial and EBD progressiva differ in that presentation is in late childhood or adolescence.

In EBD, bullous skin lesions arise either as a result of trauma or spontaneously. The common feature in all types is that healing of the skin is slow and results in dystrophic scars, milia, and areas of atrophy.

The distribution of lesions varies in the different types. The table below outlines the distribution of the lesions, the clinical concomitants in each type, and the pattern of inheritance.

| Type | Inheritance | Distribution | Clinical concomitant |
|---|---|---|---|
| EBD Cockayne-Touraine | AD | Dorsum of extremities | Malignant change in scars |
| EBD Pasini | AD | Limbs | Albopapuloid patches on trunk in adolescence |
| EBD pretibial | AD | Pretibial | Occasional albopapuloid lesions |
| EBD Bart | AD | Generalized | Congenital absence of skin; skin ulceration |
| EBD inversa | AR | Intertriginous | Anal and esophageal distribution strictures; sideropenic anemia |
| EBD progressiva | AR | Distal extremities | Progressive deafness |
| EBD Hallopeau-Siemens | AR | Distal extremities | Esophageal strictures |
| EBD local | AR | Distal extremities | Esophageal strictures |
| EBD general | AR | Generalized | Esophageal strictures |
| EBD mutilans | AR | Generalized | Syndactyly, contractures, strictures |
| EBD Fine | AR | Proximal arms and legs | Centripetal progression of symmetric bullae |
| EBD Winship | AR | Generalized | Alopecia, short stature, contractures |

In addition to the skin lesions, the nails are dystrophic in all types of EBD. Nails that have been repeatedly shed due to sublingual blisters may not regenerate. Tooth involvement in EBD Hallopeau-Siemens and EBD Winship types is in the form of hypoplastic enamel. The mucous membranes are frequently affected in all types.

There are two major groups of scarring EBD: those inherited as an autosomal dominant trait and those that are autosomal recessive. In general, the phenotype of the autosomal recessive types is more severe. While life span is not reduced, the quality of life is markedly impaired in all the dystrophic types, especially in EBD Hallopeau-Siemens (mutilans).

The cleavage plane in EBD, as seen by electron microscopy, is below the basal lamina, which forms the root of the blister. Dermal collagen is the blister floor. Various reports of nonspecific alterations in dermal collagen have been made. Anchoring fibrils are reduced in number and are structurally abnormal in all types of EBD in both blistered and nontraumatized skin.

Although there is considerable heterogeneity in EBD, the type breeds true within a kindred.

**Complications:** 1) Esophageal strictures occur as a result of mucous membrane involvement, notably in EBD Hallopeau-Siemens. 2) Corneal ulceration may occur. 3) Urethral strictures have been reported rarely. 4) Squamous carcinomas may occur in the dystrophic scars of EBD Cockayne-Touraine. 5) Severe dental caries occurs in those types with hypoplastic enamel.

**Associated Findings:** None known.

**Etiology:** *Autosomal dominant inheritance:* EBD Cockayne-Touraine, EBD Pasini, EBD pretibial, EBD Bart.

*Autosomal Recessive inheritance:* EBD inversa, EBD progressiva, EBD Hallopeau-Siemens, EBD Fine, EBD Winship.

Cleavage below the basal lamina results in subepidermal bullae.

**Pathogenesis:** Type VII collagen defect and consequent defective anchoring fibrils are postulated to be etiologic factors in both autosomal dominant and autosomal recessive types. An increase

in collagenase activity is thought to be a causal factor in autosomal recessive EBD Hallopeau-Siemens. Deranged glycosaminoglycan metabolism in EBD Pasini.

**MIM No.:** *13170, *13175, 13185, *13200, *22645, *22650, *22660

**CDC No.:** 757.330

**Sex Ratio:** EBD, M1:F1; EBD Hallopeau-Siemens, M3:F1.

**Occurrence:** Undetermined but presumed rare, although the Dystrophic Epidermolysis Research Association (DEBRA) estimates that 50,000 Americans, mostly children, have epidermolysis.

**Risk of Recurrence for Patient's Sib:**
See Part I, *Mendelian Inheritance.*

**Risk of Recurrence for Patient's Child:**
See Part I, *Mendelian Inheritance.*

**Age of Detectability:** At birth, or by prenatal diagnosis by fetal skin sampling via fetoscopy in EBD Hallopeau-Siemens.

**Gene Mapping and Linkage:** EBR3 (epidermolysis bullosa progressiva) is ULG4.

CLG (collagenase, epidermolysis bullosa, dystrophic, (autosomal recessive)) has been mapped to 11q21-q22.

**Prevention:** None known. Genetic counseling indicated.

**Treatment:** *Topical:* emollients, antibiotics, vitamin creams, and corticosteroids.

*Systemic:* vitamin E (corticosteroids are not recommended).

Diphenylhydantoin, which decreases collagenase activity, is of limited value in EBD Hallopeau-Siemens. Retinoids have limited success in recessive dystrophic epidermolysis bullosa.

**Prognosis:** Life span is not reduced.

**Detection of Carrier:** Unknown.

**Special Considerations:** EBD, or all the scarring forms of EB, have been considered as a group rather than splitting them into their distinct entities. It is important in terms of genetic counseling to divide these into the broader categories of autosomal dominant or autosomal recessive inheritance. Within each subgroup, penetrance is complete and expression is variable.

Bart syndrome, or EBD Bart, has been included as a type of EBD, although unpublished histologic data suggest that this may be a simplex type.

In an attempt to determine the actual incidence and prevalence of Epidermolysis Bullosa, the United States National Institutes of Heath has established a National Patient Registry and four Clinical Centers. For more information, contact D. Martin Carter, M.D., Ph.D., Laboratory of Investigative Dermatology, National EB Registry, HOS W202, the Rockefeller University, 1230 York Avenue, New York, NY 10021.

**Support Groups:** NY; Brooklyn; Dystrophic Epidermolysis Bullosa Research Asso. of America (DEBRA)

**References:**
Bauer EA, et al.: The role of human skin collagenase in epidermolysis bullosa. J Invest Dermatol 1977; 68:119–124.
Gedde-Dahl TJ, Anton-Lamprecht I: Epidermolysis bullosa. In: Emory A, Rimoin D, eds: Principals and practices of medical genetics. Edinburgh: Churchill Livingstone, 1983.
Fine JD: Epidermolysis bullosa: clinical aspects, pathology and recent advances in research. Int J Dermatol 1986; 25:143–157.
Destro M, et al.: Recessive dystrophic emidermolysis bullosa. Arch Ophthal 1987; 105:1248–1252.
Beighton P, et al.: International nosology of heritable disorders of connective tissue, Berlin, 1986. Am J Med Genet 1988; 29:581–594.

WI055                                     **Ingrid M Winship**

**Epidermolytic hyperkeratosis**
*See KERATOSIS PALMARIS ET PLANTARIS OF UNNA-THOST
also ICHTHYOSIFORM HYPERKERATOSIS, BULLOUS CONGENITAL*
**Epiglottic cyst**
*See EPIGLOTTIS, VALLECULAR CYST*

## EPIGLOTTIS, VALLECULAR CYST                                   2588

**Includes:**
> Ductal cyst
> Epiglottic cyst
> Epi-laryngeal cyst
> Laryngeal retention cyst
> Vallecular cyst

**Excludes:**
> Cystadenoma
> Epiglottitis
> **Esophagus, duplication** (0368)
> Hemangioma
> **Laryngocele** (0575)
> **Laryngomalacia** (0576)
> Lingual thyroid
> **Lung, bronchogenic cyst** (2702)
> Lymphang. .ma
> **Macroglossia** (0618)
> Saccular cyst
> **Thyroglossal duct remnant** (0945)
> Tongue, base of, tumor-dermoid or teratoma

**Major Diagnostic Criteria:** A vallecular cyst can usually be seen in the upper airway by direct visualization. Diagnosis is confirmed by endoscopy and aspiration.

**Clinical Findings:** Although benign, vallecular cysts in the neonate can fill the entire airway and be life threatening. Neonates often have inspiratory stridor and some degree of respiratory distress. Suprasternal, intercostal or substernal retractions may be present. The cry may be normal, muffled, hoarse, shrill, weak, or even inaudible, depending on the amount of obstruction. Airway distress is often made worse by supine positioning, by agitation, or with feeding. Patients will have poor weight gain secondary to the dysphagia. Aspiration is common. Cyanosis may be present and may be worsened by agitation or feeding.

The vallecular cyst arises from the lingual surface of the epiglottis, vallecula, or base of tongue. A careful detailed history usually suggests location of the lesion in the upper airway. The cyst is easily visualized at the base of the tongue. X-ray examination of the soft tissues of the neck in the anteroposterior and lateral planes usually shows a mass in the pre-epiglottic area.

Endoscopy, however, is needed to confirm the diagnosis. Direct laryngoscopy will show a pale, yellowish-white, smooth-surfaced cyst filling the vallecula. Aspiration may help to confirm its cystic nature.

The size of the cysts varies from 2–3 mm up to several cm, and there may be several located adjacent to one another. They can be globular, bilobed, or trilobed. Serous, turbid or serosanguinous fluid or mucus fills the cyst. Most commonly, cysts are lined with stratified squamous epithelium. Cuboidal, columnar, and ciliated columnar epithelia have also been reported.

Other indirect diagnostic studies include barium swallow, fluoroscopy, computerized tomographic (CT) scan, MRI, and thyroid scan.

**Complications:** Complete airway obstruction requiring emergent tracheotomy. Pneumonia may occur secondary to aspiration. Poor weight gain may be secondary to dysphagia. Secondary infection of the cyst may cause epiglottitis or an epiglottic abscess.

**Associated Findings:** None known.

**Etiology:** Unknown.

**Pathogenesis:** There are several theories. Vallecular cysts may form secondary to ductal obstruction with secondary cyst formation. The cysts are lined with mucous glands and expand in response to glandular secretions. Vallecular cysts may also be due to angiomatous or lymphatic malformations. Others believe that the growth is not a laryngeal malformation, but rather represents a secondary disturbance in the development of the larynx which may be of teratomatous or branchiogenic origin.

**Sex Ratio:** M1:F1

**Occurrence:** Undetermined but presumed rare, although this is the most common cyst of the larynx.

**Risk of Recurrence for Patient's Sib:** Presumably not increased.

**Risk of Recurrence for Patient's Child:** Presumably not increased.

**Age of Detectability:** Vallecular cysts are more common in adults, but symptoms in the neonate are often more clinically apparent. Symptoms can be present at birth.

**Gene Mapping and Linkage:** Unknown.

**Prevention:** None known. Genetic counseling indicated.

**Treatment:** Aspiration of the cyst may help to confirm the diagnosis, but aspiration alone is associated with a high incidence of recurrence. Puncture of the cyst to allow decompression has been advocated, but has a high risk of pulmonary aspiration and should not be done until the airway is secured.

Definitive treatment requires marsupialization of the cyst with either laryngeal microinstruments or by carbon dioxide laser. Removal at the base with a tonsillar snare may also be done.

**Prognosis:** Recurrence is rare if adequate marsupialization is done. Development of the child should be normal, unless there has been prolonged anoxia.

**Detection of Carrier:** Unknown.

**References:**
Keenleyside HB, Greenway RE: Management of pre-epiglottic cysts. Can Med Assoc J 1968; 99:645–649.
DeSanto LW, et al.: Cysts of the larynx: classification. Laryngoscope 1970; 80:145–176.
Canty TG, Hendren WH: Upper airway obstruction from foregut cysts of the hypopharynx. J Pediatr Surg 1975; 10:807–812.
Richardson MA, Cotton RT: Anatomic abnormalities of the pediatric airway. Pediatr Clin North Am 1984; 31:821–834.
Henderson LT, et al.: Airway-obstructing epiglottic cyst. Ann Otol Rhinol Laryngol 1985; 94:473–476.
Myer CM: Vallecular cyst in a newborn. Ear Nose and Throat J 1988; 67:122–124.

MY003                     **Charles M. Myer III**
SH050                      **Sally Shott**

**Epignathus**
> *See TERATOMAS*
> *also NECK/HEAD, DERMOID CYST OR TERATOMA*

**Epilepsy evoked by factors like eating and somatosensory stimuli**
> *See EPILEPSY, REFLEX*

**Epilepsy of childhood with occipital spike-waves, benign partial**
> *See EPILEPSY, BENIGN OCCIPITAL*

**Epilepsy of childhood with Rolandic spikes**
> *See EPILEPSY, BENIGN CHILDHOOD WITH CENTROTEMPORAL EEG FOCUS (BEC)*

**Epilepsy of childhood, benign partial**
> *See EPILEPSY, BENIGN CHILDHOOD WITH CENTROTEMPORAL EEG FOCUS (BEC)*

## EPILEPSY, BENIGN CHILDHOOD WITH CENTROTEMPORAL EEG FOCUS (BEC)          3217

**Includes:**
> Epilepsy of childhood, benign partial
> Epilepsy of childhood with Rolandic spikes
> Rolandic epilepsy
> Sylvian seizures

**Excludes:**
> Epilepsy, Jacksonian
> Seizures, centrecephalic
> Seizures, complex partial
> Seizures, temporal lobe

**Major Diagnostic Criteria:** Predominantly partial or secondarily generalized seizures affecting mainly the facial, oropharyngeal and upper extremity musculature with onset between ages two and 13 years, primarily between ages five to 9 years. Affected children are developmentally and intellectually normal. Seizures are without neuropsychological sequelae and are not related to progressive cerebral disease of any type. Interictal electroencephalograms (EEG's) are characterized by centrotemporal (Rolandic) spike or sharp-wave discharges. With or without treatment the seizure activity generally ceases within 2–3 years of its onset or during puberty, and 95% of patients are seizure-free after the age of 15 years.

**Clinical Findings:** The predominant types of seizures associated with benign epilepsy of childhood with centrotemporal EEG foci (BEC) are partial seizures or secondarily generalized tonic-clonic seizures in 68 to 74% of cases with the remainder reported as generalized tonic-clonic from the onset. From 55–75% of the episodes occur, however, either during sleep or during transitions from sleep to wakefulness, and therefore partial onset in an even larger number of cases may be missed. In 58% of seizures, full consciousness is maintained although speech arrest based on motor interference with speech (anarthria) is seen in 39%. Not uncommonly (31%), the seizure awakens the child who later can describe hearing and seeing his family without being able to communicate with them. Hemifacial signs including jerking of facial muscles or deviation of the mouth occur in 48%. Oropharyngeal signs such as salivation, guttural sounds, mouth movements, unusual buccal-oral sensations, contraction of the jaw, difficulty moving the tongue, inability to swallow, and feelings of suffocation are seen in 53%. Involvement of an upper extremity is reported in 21% whereas only 8% report clonic movements of a lower extremity. Notably rare or absent are complex automatisms as seen with complex partial seizures, visceral auras, psychic or perceptual symptoms, or amnesia and postictal confusion except in those cases of generalized tonic-clonic convulsions. The character of the seizures seems to vary somewhat with age with younger children having less localized spells and older children having strictly localized and very brief seizures, usually isolated to the face or oropharyngeal region.

Interictal EEG phenomena are an essential part of the diagnosis of BEC. Characteristically, clusters of stereotyped bi- or triphasic sharp waves or slow spike discharges of variable amplitudes of up to 300 microvolts or greater occur in the midtemporal region with spread to the central or Rolandic area. Frequency of the epileptiform discharges is increased during drowsiness and sleep. They are unilateral or bilateral and, when bilateral, occur either synchronously or independently. Laterality may also shift on serial EEG's. Maximum voltage often is found over the upper bank of the Sylvian fissure. In all cases, the background is well preserved. Rare patients have, as well, generalized bilaterally synchronous spike-wave discharges, most commonly during activation procedures.

Commonly BEC responds well to anticonvulsant medication with 65% of seizures quickly controlled by therapy. In 21%, seizures persist up to one year, eventually being controlled by increased medication, while in 14% seizures may last for greater than one year or recur after one or several years. Only 8%, however, have 20 seizures or more. With or without treatment, most patients have no further seizures after age 15 years. EEG abnormalities usually normalize although this normalization may lag behind cessation of seizure activity. Rare patients have been reported with recurrence or persistence of seizure activity into adulthood, primarily generalized tonic-clonic, and often with a precipitant such as ethanol. There is a single report of a patient who suffered recurrent partial seizures as an adult in association with typical Rolandic discharges on EEG.

Family history is commonly positive for children with BEC with studies ranging from 13 to 68% of probands having immediate family or relatives with seizures. In one study of 19 children with BEC, 13 (68%) had relatives with seizures in childhood although only 4 of the 38 parents at risk had had seizures. Of 34 siblings, 32 had EEG's, and 11 of 32 (34%) had Rolandic discharges. Five of the 11 siblings with Rolandic discharges had seizures, but six of the 11 did not have seizures despite having had an abnormal EEG. Rolandic discharges have rarely been reported in parents who have never had seizures.

**Complications:** Prolonged seizures lasing greater than 30 minutes or a postictal Todd's paralysis are rarely seen.

**Associated Findings:** None known.

**Etiology:** Autosomal dominant inheritance with variable, age-dependent penetrance.

**Pathogenesis:** Unknown.

**Sex Ratio:** M1:F1

**Occurrence:** BEC is now thought to be the most common type of partial motor epilepsy in childhood with an incidence reported in Sweden of 21:100,000 in children less than 15 years of age. Of all epilepsy reported in childhood, BEC accounts for from 15.7 to 23.9%.

**Risk of Recurrence for Patient's Sib:**
See Part I, *Mendelian Inheritance.*

**Risk of Recurrence for Patient's Child:**
See Part I, *Mendelian Inheritance.*

**Age of Detectability:** Commonly manifest during early school years (ages 5–9 years). Cases with onset prior to age two years or greater than 13 years of age are extremely rare.

**Gene Mapping and Linkage:** Unknown.

**Prevention:** None known. Genetic counseling indicated.

**Treatment:** Most authors recommend treatment following the occurrence of the second seizure in an affected child. However, there is a theoretical debate about the efficacy of treatment since outcome appears to be excellent with or without treatment or with or without complete seizure control once treatment is initiated. Certainly the simultaneous use of several anticonvulsants with the attendant risk of increased side effects in an effort totally to control a child with more recalcitrant BEC may not be warranted.

**Prognosis:** Excellent, with almost all patients seizure-free after age 15 years with normal intelligence and neurologic function.

**Detection of Carrier:** Unknown. Rare parents with Rolandic discharges as adults are described, but since the occurrence of Rolandic discharges is age-dependent, EEG's of parents will commonly be normal.

**Special Considerations:** The genetic significance of the unusual simultaneous occurrence on EEG of Rolandic discharges concomitantly with 3/sec spike-and-wave discharges as seen in absence epilepsy is unknown. The EEG findings themselves suggest an inherited predisposition toward two different types of seizures, one focal and one generalized.

**References:**
Lombroso CT: Sylvian seizures and midtemporal spike foci in children. Arch Neurol 1967; 17:52–59.
Loiseau P, Beaussart P: The seizures of benign childhood epilepsy with Rolandic paroxysmal discharges. Epilepsia 1973; 14:381–389. *
Heijbel J, et al.: Benign epilepsy of children with centrotemporal EEG foci: a study of incidence rate in outpatient care. Epilepsia 1975; 16:657–664.
Heijbel J, et al.: Benign epilepsy of childhood with centrotemporal EEG foci: a genetic study. Epilepsia 1975; 16:285–293. *
Beaussart M, Faou R: Evolution of epilepsy with Rolandic paroxysmal foci: a study of 324 cases. Epilepsia 1978; 19:337–342.
Cavazzuti GB: Epidemiology of different types of epilepsy in school age children of Modena, Italy. Epilepsia 1980; 21:57–62.

GR034
KA008

**May L. Griebel**
**Raymond S. Kandt**

**Epilepsy, benign neonatal**
*See CONVULSIONS, BENIGN FAMILIAL NEONATAL*

## EPILEPSY, BENIGN OCCIPITAL　　　　　3218

**Includes:**
Epilepsy of childhood with occipital spike-waves, benign partial
Epilepsy-occipital spike-wave complexes suppressed by eye-opening
Scoto-epilepsy

**Excludes:**
Basilar artery migraine
**Epilepsy, benign childhood with centrotemporal EEG focus (BEC) (3217)**

**Major Diagnostic Criteria:** As defined by Gastaut (1982) benign occipital epilepsy (BOE) of childhood is diagnosed by a combination of clinical features and electroencephalographic (EEG) findings. Clinically, onset is in early childhood with remission usually before age 19 years. Ictal symptoms include a variety of visual complaints followed by seizures which are predominantly hemiclonic. The post-ictal period may be marked by severe headache. The interictal EEG is characterized by high amplitude spike-wave discharges occurring when visual fixation is prevented or when eyes are closed.

**Clinical Findings:** Age of onset of BOE ranges from 23 months to nine years with a peak occurrence from 4–8 years and a mean age of onset of six years. Gastaut reported visual symptomatology as the initial event in most seizures of this type with amaurosis occurring in 65% of cases, phosphenes in 58%, figurative hallucinations in 23%, and illusions in 12%. Other investigators have reported a lower incidence of visual symptoms, including Beaumanoir's 44%, but the difficulty of accurate assessment of visual symptoms in small children is well recognized. The seizures can remain simple partial in nature or can be followed by hemiclonic motor events in 44%, complex partial seizures in 19%, and generalized tonic-clonic seizures in 8%. Of Gastaut's original cases, 36% complained of headache sometimes associated with nausea and vomiting following the seizures; others have reported migrainous symptoms preceding the spells. Exclusive night-time occurrence of seizures in BOE has been noted in from 33% to 66% of cases. Institution of treatment successfully suppressed seizure activity in only 53% of Gastaut's cases. However, the course is usually benign with 92% of patients achieving full remission of their seizures before the age of 19 years.

Although Gastaut reported normal neuropsychiatric status in almost all of his patients, other authors have described learning difficulties or mental handicaps in from 30% to 62% of patients. Beaumanoir also noted a variety of visual handicaps including strabismus with amblyopia, severe myopia with congenital nystagmus, and unilateral macular degeneration in 50% of her cases. Only five of Beaumanoir's 18 cases had normal ophthalmological and psychometric examinations.

The interictal EEG in patients with BOE contains paroxysms of high amplitude, 200–300 $\mu$V spike-wave discharges at 2–3 cps occurring virtually continuously only when the eyes are closed or when visual fixation is prevented. Eye opening in an illuminated room either totally or greatly suppresses the discharges. Maintaining central vision in the dark by focusing on a red spot of light inhibits the abnormalities. The spike-wave discharges occur either in the occipital or occipital-posterior temporal regions and are unilateral or bilateral, synchronous or asynchronous, symmetrical or asymmetrical. Photic stimulation does not enhance the occurrence of the discharges and in some cases has decreased their frequency. Unlike in benign epilepsy of childhood with centrotemporal focus, sleep does not increase the frequency of discharges in BOE.

Gastaut reported a positive family history for epilepsy in 47% and for migraine headaches in 19% of his cases. Other authors have found the incidence of epilepsy in family members to vary from 6% to 35%. A large family study revealed EEG abnormalities in 57% of family members including the typical occipital spike-wave pattern in 26%. The latter was more evident in younger members, supporting the idea that BOE has age-dependent expression.

**Complications:** Unknown.

**Associated Findings:** Visual deficits, learning disabilities, and mental handicaps have been reported in up to 50% of cases.

**Etiology:** Autosomal dominant inheritance with age-dependent expression and variable penetrance.

**Pathogenesis:** Unknown.

**MIM No.:** 13209

**Sex Ratio:** M1:F1

**Occurrence:** More than 70 cases have been reported, but incidence is unknown.

**Risk of Recurrence for Patient's Sib:**
See Part I, *Mendelian Inheritance.*

**Risk of Recurrence for Patient's Child:**
See Part I, *Mendelian Inheritance.*

**Age of Detectability:** Usually manifest no later than nine years of age.

**Gene Mapping and Linkage:** Unknown.

**Prevention:** None known. Genetic counseling indicated.

**Treatment:** Just over one-half of cases respond readily to anticonvulsant medications. Even if seizures are incompletely controlled, however, generally seizure frequency is fairly low, and the seizures spontaneously resolve in late adolescence. Careful ophthalmologic examination and neuropsychologic testing to optimize academic curricula are indicated in selected patients.

**Prognosis:** Excellent for remission of seizures, but visual or learning deficits may limit outcome.

**Detection of Carrier:** Unknown. Given age dependency for expression of the trait, EEG's are unlikely to be abnormal past adolescence.

**Special Considerations:** The clinical and EEG features of BOE may overlap with basilar artery migraine, which is often associated with visual loss, or may resemble the occasional occurrence of a migrainous event followed by a seizure. Camfield et al (1978) attributed the EEG findings and clinical seizures in their patients to ischemia resulting from severe migraine and stated that the seizures required the migrainous aura to become manifest. The relationship between migraine and epilepsy in general and specifically the relationship between the syndrome as described by Camfield and BOE as described by Gastaut is uncertain.

**References:**
Camfield PR, et al.: Basilar migraine, seizures, and severe epileptiform EEG abnormalities. Neurology 1978; 28:584–588.
Panayiotopoulos CP: Inhibitory effect on central vision of occipital lobe seizures. Neurology 1981; 31:1331–1333.
Gastaut H: A new type of epilepsy: benign partial epilepsy of childhood with occipital spike-waves. Clinical Electroencephalography 1982; 13:13–22. *
Beaumanior A: Infantile epilepsy with occipital focus and good prognosis. Eur Neurol 1983; 22:43–52.
Newton R, Aicardi J: Clinical findings in children with occipital spike-wave complexes suppressed by eye-opening. Neurology 1983; 33: 1526–1529.
Kuzniecky R, Rosenblatt B: Benign occipital epilepsy: a family study. Epilepsia 1987; 28:346–350. *

GR034
KA008

**May L. Griebel
Raymond S. Kandt**

**Epilepsy, centralopathic**
*See SEIZURES, CENTRALOPATHIC*
**Epilepsy, centrencephalic**
*See SEIZURES, CENTRALOPATHIC*

## EPILEPSY, FAMILIAL                                    1504

**Includes:**

Convulsive disorder, familial, of prenatal or early onset
Epilepsy-yellow teeth
Epilepsy, photogenic-spastic diplegia-mental retardation
Epilepsy-Telangiectasia

**Excludes:**

Convulsions, benign familial neonatal (3216)
Epilepsy, benign childhood with centrotemporal EEG focus
   (BEC) (3217)
Epilepsy, benign occipital (3218)
Epilepsy, reflex (3239)
Seizures, centralopathic (0135)
Seizures, febrile (2568)
Seizures, in females, Juberg-Hellman type (2479)
Seizures, myoclonic, juvenile Janz type (2567)
Seizures, progressive myoclonic, Lafora type (2601)
Seizures, progressive myoclonic, Unverricht-Lundborg type
   (2602)
Seizures, vitamin B(6) dependency (0991)
Seizures-ichthyosis-mental retardation (0741)

**Major Diagnostic Criteria:** Epilepsy refers to the occurrence of two or more seizures that are not due to a proximate cause. For example, two seizures due to two episodes of acute head trauma are not epileptic seizures, whereas repetitive seizures occurring after the acute effects of the head trauma have resolved are posttraumatic epileptic seizures. Seizures represent paroxysmal and disordered electric discharges of central nervous system gray matter. They are classified according to their mode of onset: local (partial seizures) or generalized from onset (generalized seizures). The three most common types of partial seizures are *simple partial*, *complex partial*, and *complex partial seizures with secondary generalization*. The most common generalized seizures are tonic-clonic seizures and absence seizures.

By contrast, epileptic syndromes are those in which various seizure types may occur as part of the syndrome (e.g., the concurrence of myoclonic seizures, generalized tonic-clonic seizures, and occasionally absence seizures in **Seizures, myoclonic, juvenile Janz type**). Although the disorders listed in the *Excludes* section represent varieties of familial epilepsy, their individualities warrant specific articles as referenced above. In addition to these well-recognized syndromes, there are a number of uncommon epileptic syndromes, the distinguishing characteristics of which are evident from their names, several of which are listed above and cross-referenced below.

The paroxysmal alterations of consciousness or abnormal movements of seizures can be mimicked by several nonepileptic conditions, the most common of which is breathholding spells, occurring in 4–5% of young children. Other entities that are confused with seizures include cardiac arrhythmias, sleep-related events (e.g. night terrors), migrainous disorders, movement disorders (e.g. **Tourette syndrome**), psychological disorders, daydreaming, and gastrointestinal disorders.

**MIM No.:** 21720, 22675, 22680, 22685

**References:**

Lombroso CT, Lerman P: Breath holding spells. Pediatrics 1967;
   39:563–581.
Commission on Classification and Terminology of the International
   League Against Epilepsy. Proposal for revised clinical and electro-
   encephalographic classification of epileptic seizures. Epilepsia 1981;
   22:489–501.
Commission on Classification and Terminology of the International
   League Against Epilepsy. Proposal for classification of epilepsies
   and epileptic syndromes. Epilepsia 1985; 26:268–278.
Rothner AD: "Not everything that shakes is epilepsy": The differential
   diagnosis of paroxysmal nonepileptiform disorders. Cleveland
   Clinic J Med 1989; 56:S206–S213.

KA008                                            **Raymond S. Kandt**

**Epilepsy, familial myoclonus-choreoathetosis**
   *See DENTATORUBROPALLIDOLUYSIAN DEGENERATION,
   HEREDITARY*
**Epilepsy, juvenile myoclonic, Janz type**
   *See SEIZURES, MYOCLONIC, JUVENILE JANZ TYPE*
**Epilepsy, myoclonic-ragged red fibers**
   *See MYOCLONIC EPILEPSY-RAGGED RED FIBERS*
**Epilepsy, myoclonus, Lafora type**
   *See SEIZURES, PROGRESSIVE MYOCLONIC, LAFORA TYPE*
**Epilepsy, photogenic-spastic diplegia-mental retardation**
   *See EPILEPSY, FAMILIAL*

## EPILEPSY, REFLEX                                       3239

**Includes:**

Epilepsy evoked by factors like eating and somatosensory
   stimuli
Language-induced epilepsy
Musicogenic epilepsy
Photogenic epilepsy
Reading epilepsy
Stimulus-evoked epilepsy

**Excludes:**

Photoconvulsive response on EEG without clinical seizures
Primary generalized epilepsy with photosensitivity

**Major Diagnostic Criteria:** A common feature in all types of reflex epilepsy, which may be evoked by any of a variety of stimuli, is that seizures develop in a stereotyped fashion following the presentation or occurrence of a very specific stimulation. Although persons with epilepsy who have spontaneous seizures may also have seizures precipitated by certain influences such as fatigue, hyperventilation, or flashing lights; spontaneous seizures per se do not occur in pure reflex epilepsy. Affected individuals have no evidence otherwise of neurologic dysfunction, and resting electroencephalograms (EEG's) are normal.

**Clinical Findings:** Vary dependent upon the type of stimulus needed to evoke seizures. Age at presentation ranges from infancy in seizures induced by eating or hot baths to adolescence and early adulthood in reading and photic-induced seizures; the two most common types of reflex epilepsies. The onset of reading-induced seizures is generally in the second and third decades. Photosensitivity is rarely seen under the age of six years, and the onset of photic-induced epilepsy is commonly between the ages of eight and nineteen years.

Attacks in reading epilepsy occur when subjects are reading either aloud or silently. The duration of stimulation required to elicit a seizure varies both for individual subjects and between subjects; in the Forster (1977) series, it ranged from 1–40 minutes. Stimulus material, according to Forster, needs to be meaningful and unfamiliar. Attacks begin with an interruption of reading, myoclonic jerks of the jaw and tongue, and vocalization if the subject has been reading aloud. This simple partial (focal) motor seizure may be followed by a brief period of loss of consciousness; generalized tonic-clonic seizures may also occur. During simple partial seizures, affected subjects are often unable to speak but are alert and can execute nonverbal commands. Jaw and tongue myoclonus are accompanied by abnormal EEG discharges.

The triggering phenomenon for photic-induced seizures is flickering light from a variety of sources, such as sunlight filtering through leaves on a tree or reflected off of water or snow. Oscilloscopes, televisions, and video games all have been implicated as precipitants. Most commonly, the resultant seizures are generalized tonic-clonic in nature. The EEG usually demonstrates a photoconvulsive response when photic stimulation is presented.

Myriad other stimuli have been reported to induce seizures in individual cases, including church bells or certain frequencies, nursery rhymes, somatosensory stimuli, card games, thinking, mathematical computation, and eating.

**Complications:** Educational and career opportunities may be severely limited in specific instances such as in reading epilepsy. Eating-induced epilepsy may lead to severe malnutrition.

**Associated Findings:** None known.

**Etiology:** Autosomal dominant inheritance with variable, age-dependent penetrance. Greater expressivity in females has been suggested in photic-induced epilepsy.

**Pathogenesis:** Unknown.

**MIM No.:** 13210, 13230

**Sex Ratio:** M1:F1 for reading epilepsy. M1:F1.5 for photic-induced epilepsy.

**Occurrence:** Over a dozen families have been reported in the literature.

**Risk of Recurrence for Patient's Sib:**
See Part I, *Mendelian Inheritance.*

**Risk of Recurrence for Patient's Child:**
See Part I, *Mendelian Inheritance.*

**Age of Detectability:** Commonly manifest during second and third decades for both photic-induced and reading epilepsies.

**Gene Mapping and Linkage:** Unknown.

**Prevention:** None known. Genetic counseling indicated.

**Treatment:** Treatment measures undertaken often involve manipulation of the environment or avoidance of the known precipitant, and must be specific for the type of reflex epilepsy present. For example, use of polarized sunglasses out of doors may be sufficient to prevent seizures evoked by flickering sunlight. If the precipitant is difficult to avoid, a trial of anticonvulsant medication may be attempted although efficacy has been reported to be limited in reflex epilepsies. For example, in reading epilepsy, anticonvulsants may prevent secondarily generalized tonic-clonic seizures without decreasing the initial simple partial seizures. Forster has described the use of detailed conditioning techniques involving stimulus and threshold alterations.

**Prognosis:** Generally excellent. In individual patients, however, educational and career options may be severely limited by their specific seizure stimuli.

**Detection of Carrier:** Unknown.

**Support Groups:** MD; Landover; Epilepsy Foundation of America

**References:**
Davidson S, Watson CW: Hereditary light sensitive epilepsy. Neurology 1956; 6:233–261.

Daly RF, Forster FM: Inheritance of reading epilepsy. Neurology 1975; 25:1051–1054.

Forster FM: Reflex epilepsy, behavioral therapy and conditional reflexes. Springfield, IL, Charles C. Thomas, 1977. *

Newmark ME, Penry JK: Photosensitivity and epilepsy: a review. New York: Raven Press, 1979.

GR034
KA008

**May L. Griebel**
**Raymond S. Kandt**

**Epilepsy-alopecia-pyorrhea-mental retardation**
*See ALOPECIA-SEIZURES-MENTAL RETARDATION, SHOKEIR TYPE*
**Epilepsy-amelogenesis**
*See AMELO-CEREBRO-HYPOHIDROTIC SYNDROME*
**Epilepsy-gingival fibromatosis-cherubism**
*See GINGIVAL FIBROMATOSIS-CHERUBISM-SEIZURES, RAMON TYPE*
**Epilepsy-occipital spike-wave complexes suppressed by eye-opening**
*See EPILEPSY, BENIGN OCCIPITAL*
**Epilepsy-Telangiectasia**
*See EPILEPSY, FAMILIAL*
**Epilepsy-yellow teeth**
*See EPILEPSY, FAMILIAL*
*also AMELO-CEREBRO-HYPOHIDROTIC SYNDROME*
**Epiloia**
*See TUBEROUS SCLEROSIS*
**Epimerase deficiency, galactose (GALE)**
*See GALACTOSE EPIMERASE DEFICIENCY*
**Epiphyseal changes and high myopia**
*See ARTHRO-OPHTHALMOPATHY, HEREDITARY, PROGRESSIVE, STICKLER TYPE*
**Epiphyseal damage with constitutional symptoms**
*See INFLAMMATORY DISEASE, NEONATAL BATES-LORBER TYPE*

**Epiphyseal dysplasia multiplex**
*See EPIPHYSEAL DYSPLASIA, MULTIPLE, RECESSIVE TARDA TYPE*

## EPIPHYSEAL DYSPLASIA, MULTIPLE     0358

**Includes:**
Dysplasia epiphysialis multiplex
Fairbank disease
Polyosteochondrite (Turpin and Coste)

**Excludes:**
Arthro-ophthalmopathy, hereditary, progressive, Stickler type (0090)
Chondrodysplasia punctata, mild symmetric type (0153)
Chondrodysplasia punctata, X-linked dominant type (2730)
Pseudoachondroplastic dysplasia (0828)
Spondyloepiphyseal dysplasia congenita (0897)
Spondyloepiphyseal dysplasia, late (0898)

**Major Diagnostic Criteria:** Clinical signs include short hands and feet, waddling gait, and joint limitations. The diagnosis can be made by demonstrating the small, irregular epiphyses of the long bones and hands.

**Clinical Findings:** Multiple epiphyseal dysplasia with waddling gait or articular limitations manifests itself between the second and fifth years of life. However, the diagnosis of this condition is often late, motivated by discomfort secondary to osteoarthritic changes. Clinically, the limbs appear relatively short, but the stature is not much decreased (close to 150 cm in the adult). The shortness of the hand and foot is the most striking. The mobility of the hip joint and sometimes of the shoulder or other articulations is restricted.

On X-ray examination the epiphyses of the long bones and the carpal and tarsal bones are small, irregular, and sometimes fragmented. These changes become progressively more marked with time. The metaphyses of the long bones are normal in this type, but the metacarpals and phalanges are slightly short and their metaphyseal limits are irregular. The vertebral bodies are usually normal, but sometimes show minimal irregularities of the plates.

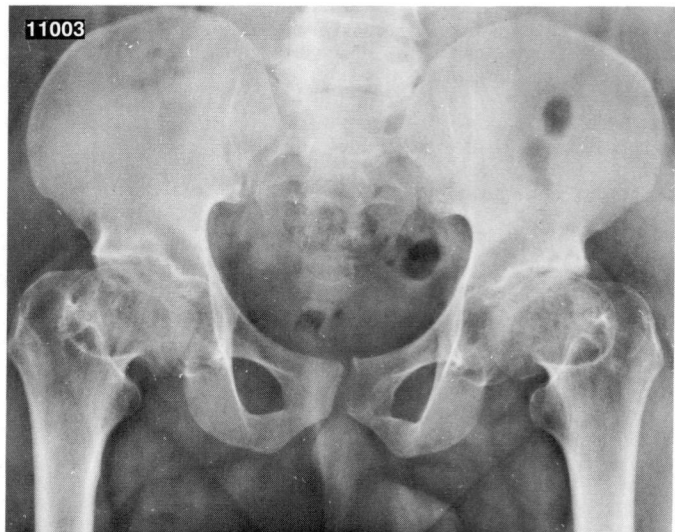

**0358-11003:** Note affected hips and secondary degenerative joint disease.

**Complications:** Osteoarthritic changes appear with advancing age, and these are almost constant in the adult, especially in the hip.

**Associated Findings:** Chondrodysplastic rheumatism is sometimes observed in the adult.

**Etiology:** Autosomal dominant inheritance.

**Pathogenesis:** The appearance of the chondrocytes is similar to that in pseudoachondroplasia, but the alterations are less marked. The swelling of the endoplasmic reticulum, with a sketch of a periodic structure, is visible and suggests an accumulation of an abnormal protein. However, unlike pseudoachondroplasia, the proteoglycans of the cartilage seem normal by electrophoretic analysis.

**MIM No.:** *13240

**POS No.:** 3214

**CDC No.:** 756.570

**Sex Ratio:** M1:F1

**Occurrence:** Undetermined. Established literature.

**Risk of Recurrence for Patient's Sib:**
See Part I, *Mendelian Inheritance.*

**Risk of Recurrence for Patient's Child:**
See Part I, *Mendelian Inheritance.*

**Age of Detectability:** In childhood by articular limitation or gait disorder.

**Gene Mapping and Linkage:** Unknown.

**Prevention:** None known. Genetic counseling indicated.

**Treatment:** Orthopedic surgery of the hip may be indicated (osteotomy of the pelvis or the collum femoris) or sometimes osteotomy of the leg (correction of genu varum or valgum).

**Prognosis:** Normal life span.

**Detection of Carrier:** X-ray films of the hips and knees allow the detection of the inapparent forms.

**Special Considerations:** The described type conforms to Fairbank's description (1947), but the heterogeneity of the multiple epiphyseal dysplasia is not fully delineated (Spranger, 1976). For example, an autosomal recessive form is probable, and some difference by X-ray from the dominant form (flat femoral head, no metaphyseal irregularities of the metacarpals and phalanges) exists. In this form, the chondrocytes contain inclusions probably of lysosomal origin with granular or filamentous material.

**References:**
Fairbank HAT: Dysplasia epiphysialis multiplex. Br J Surg 1947; 34:225–232.
Maroteaux P, et al.: Essai de classification des dysplasies spondylo-épiphysaires. Simep édit Lyon, 1968. *
Kahn MF, et al.: Le rhumatisme chondrodysplasique. Semin Hop Paris 1970; 46:1938–1953.
Murphy MC, et al.: Multiple epiphyseal dysplasia. Report of a pedigree. J Bone Joint Surg 1973; 55A:814–820.
Maroteaux P, et al.: Dysplasie poly-épiphysaire probablement récessive autosomique. Apport de l'étude ultrastructurale dans l'isolement de cette forme autonome. Nouv Presse Med 1975; 4:2169–2172.
Spranger J: The epiphyseal dysplasias. Clin Orthop 1976; 114:46–60. *

MA034                                             **Pierre Maroteaux**

## EPIPHYSEAL DYSPLASIA, MULTIPLE RIBBING TYPE      2699

**Includes:**
> Enchondral dysostosis
> Microepiphyseal dysplasia
> Multiple epiphyseal dysplasia, flat epiphyses type
> Multiple epiphyseal dysplasia, mild

**Excludes:**
> **Arthro-ophthalmopathy**
> **Epiphyseal dysplasia, multiple** (0358)
> **Pseudoachondroplastic dysplasia** (0828)
> **Spondyloepiphyseal dysplasia congenita** (0897)
> **Spondyloepiphyseal dysplasia, late** (0898)

**Major Diagnostic Criteria:** Flattened, small capital femoral epiphyses with variable involvement of other epiphyses accompanied by mild short stature.

**Clinical Findings:** The Ribbing type of multiple epiphyseal dysplasia (MED) may manifest in childhood as mild short stature or an abnormal waddling gait resulting from dysplasia of the hip. Other patients are not recognized until adulthood, when they present with early osteoarthritis of the hip and are recognized to be short as well. The short stature and disproportion (short limbed) may be of only mild degree, with height at the lower end of the normal curve. The hands and feet show a greater degree of involvement than do the long bones. Clinically there is no involvement of the spine.

On X-ray, a generalized mild epiphyseal dysplasia is seen. The hips are the most severely involved joint, followed by the joints of the hands and feet. The epiphyses are small and flattened, but do not exhibit the highly irregular surfaces seen in the more severe **Epiphyseal dysplasia, multiple**. Very mild spinal involvement consisting of Schmorl nodes or end-plate irregularity without loss of vertebral body height may be recognized.

**Complications:** Osteoarthritic changes of the hip appear in the second decade and worsen with time. Osteochondritis of the hip has been seen in some children. The degree of short stature is mild.

**Associated Findings:** None known.

**Etiology:** Autosomal dominant inheritance.

**Pathogenesis:** Presumably a defect in endochondral ossification, but there are no specific morphologic abnormalities of the growth plate. No biochemical defects have been identified.

**MIM No.:** *13240

**CDC No.:** 756.570

**Sex Ratio:** M1:F1

**Occurrence:** Established literature, but inexact delineation makes occurrence count difficult. Presumably rare.

**Risk of Recurrence for Patient's Sib:**
See Part I, *Mendelian Inheritance.*

**Risk of Recurrence for Patient's Child:**
See Part I, *Mendelian Inheritance.*

**Age of Detectability:** During childhood.

**Gene Mapping and Linkage:** Unknown.

**Prevention:** None known. Genetic counseling indicated.

**Treatment:** Orthopedic surgery.

**Prognosis:** Normal life span.

**Detection of Carrier:** Unknown.

**References:**
Spranger J: The epiphyseal dysplasias. Clin Orthop 1976; 114:46–60.
Maroteaux P: Multiple epiphyseal dysplasias. In: Maroteaux P, ed: Bone diseases of children. Philadelphia: J.B. Lippincott, 1979:69–74.
Rimoin DL, Lachman RS: The Chondrodystrophies. In: Rimoin DL, Emery AEH, eds: Principles and practice of medical genetics. New York: Churchill Livingstone, 1983:721–722.

H0025                                      **O.J. Hood**
H0033                                **William A. Horton**

## EPIPHYSEAL DYSPLASIA, MULTIPLE, RECESSIVE TARDA TYPE · 2017

**Includes:**
Epiphyseal dysplasia multiplex
Juberg-Holt type recessive multiple epiphyseal dysplasia tarda

**Excludes:**
**Diastrophic dysplasia** (0293)
**Epiphyseal dysplasia, multiple** (0358)
**Epiphyseal dysplasia, multiple ribbing type** (2699)
**Mucopolysaccharidosis IV** (0678)
**Pseudoachondroplastic dysplasia** (0828)
**Spondyloepiphyseal dysplasia, late** (0898)

**Major Diagnostic Criteria:** Defective epiphyseal development of the long bones but not of the vertebrae, short stature; micromelia, stubby hands, joint discomfort, limitation of joint motion.

**Clinical Findings:** Micromelia might be the initial sign of the disorder, especially in a child known to be at risk. Difficulty in walking and later in running will probably be the first evidence in a sporadic case. Short stature and stubby hands will become apparent. Patients describe joint discomfort, most notably in the knees and hips. The gait may be characterized by short steps, waddling, and lordosis of the lumbosacral spine. Limited range of joint motion may be present.

All epiphyses of the tubular bones may be flattened and irregular to some degree, with the most prominent changes being evident in the metacarpals, metatarsals, phalanges, proximal femora, and distal radii. The same bones may be strikingly short and broad. In contrast, the diaphyses and metaphyses of the long tubular bones may be normal. The carpals and tarsals may be slightly irregular. A cleft or double-layered patella occurs. The spine shows only minimal abnormalities, with all vertebral bodies being slightly decreased in vertical height.

**Complications:** Difficulty in walking and running, degenerative arthritis.

**Associated Findings:** Short fingers, ulnar deviation of digits 2 and 3, abnormal position of thumb with flexion at the metacarpophalangeal articulation, extension at the interphalangeal articulation, and cubitus varus.

Pfeiffer et al (1973) reported three sons of third-cousin parents with epiphyseal dysplasia of femoral heads, myopia, and deafness.

**Etiology:** Autosomal recessive inheritance.

**Pathogenesis:** Unknown.

**MIM No.:** *22690, 22695

**CDC No.:** 756.570

**Sex Ratio:** M1:F1

**Occurrence:** Undetermined. Reported from Great Britain, Germany, Czechoslovakia, Norway, and the United States (Michigan and Indiana).

**Risk of Recurrence for Patient's Sib:**
See Part I, *Mendelian Inheritance.*

**Risk of Recurrence for Patient's Child:**
See Part I, *Mendelian Inheritance.*

**Age of Detectability:** Within the first two years of life, by difficulty in ambulation.

**Gene Mapping and Linkage:** Unknown.

**Prevention:** None known. Genetic counseling indicated.

**Treatment:** Orthopedic surgery.

**Prognosis:** Probably normal for life span.

**Detection of Carrier:** Unknown.

**References:**
Hunt DD, et al.: Multiple epiphyseal dysplasia in two siblings. J Bone Joint Surg 1967; 49A:1611–1627.
Juberg RC, Holt JF: Inheritance of multiple epiphyseal dysplasia, tarda. Am J Hum Genet 1968; 20:549–563. * †
Gamboa I, Lisker R: Multiple epiphyseal dysplasia tarda: a family with autosomal recessive inheritance. Clin Genet 1974; 6:15–19.
Weaver DD, et al.: Juberg-Holt type recessive multiple epiphyseal dysplasia tarda in an Amish family. (Abstract) Am J Hum Genet 1978; 30:71A.

JU000                                          **Richard C. Juberg**

## EPIPHYSEAL DYSPLASIA, MULTIPLE-DIABETES MELLITUS · 3048

**Includes:**
Diabetes mellitus and spondyloepiphyseal dysplasia
IDDM-MED syndrome
MED-IDDM syndrome
Wolcott-Rallison syndrome

**Excludes:**
**Dyggve-Melchior-Clausen syndrome** (0306)
**Mucopolysaccharidosis IV** (0678)
**Spondyloepiphyseal dysplasia congenita** (0897)
**Spondyloepiphyseal dysplasia, late** (0898)

**Major Diagnostic Criteria:** Infancy-onset diabetes mellitus with multiple epiphyseal dysplasia distinguishes this condition from other epiphyseal dysplasias.

**Clinical Findings:** All affected children have had diabetes mellitus diagnosed in early infancy. Short stature and walking difficulties are noted after age one year, with X-rays demonstrating delayed epiphyseal ossification. In later years, the children have a short-trunk dwarfism with normal face, short and broad chest, increased lumbar lordosis, genu valga, and occasional calcaneovalgus positioning of the feet. One child had seizures, one had **Microcephaly** and mental retardation, and three had apparently normal mental development. Renal failure occurred in three patients. Ectodermal changes, including tooth discoloration (2/7), skin hyperpigmentation (2/7), and dry, scaly skin (3/7), were also noted.

**Complications:** Joint pain, ketoacidosis (uncommon).

**Associated Findings:** Neutropenia was present in one patient.

**Etiology:** Autosomal recessive inheritance.

**Pathogenesis:** Unknown. Thought to affect both chondrocytes and endocrine function.

**MIM No.:** *22698

**POS No.:** 3917

**Sex Ratio:** M1:F1

**Occurrence:** Three sibships have been described.

**Risk of Recurrence for Patient's Sib:**
See Part I, *Mendelian Inheritance.*

**Risk of Recurrence for Patient's Child:**
See Part I, *Mendelian Inheritance.*

**Age of Detectability:** Within the first few weeks of life by the presence of diabetes mellitus.

**Gene Mapping and Linkage:** Unknown.

**Prevention:** None known. Genetic counseling indicated.

**Treatment:** Treatment of the diabetes as indicated; orthopedic intervention may also be required.

**Prognosis:** Variable in that death occurred at ages six weeks (from infection), 2.4 years (from renal insufficiency), and 11 years (from renal failure) in 3/7 patients. Intellectual impairment can occur, but is not invariable. The oldest reported patient was aged 15 years.

**Detection of Carrier:** Unknown.

**References:**
Wolcott CD, Rallison ML: Infancy-onset diabetes mellitus and multiple epiphyseal dysplasia. J Pediatr 1972; 80:292–297.
Groumy P, et al.: Syndrome de transmission récessive autosomique associant un diabéte congénital et des désordres de la croissance des épiphyses. Arch Fr Pediatr 1980; 37:323.

Stoss H, et al.: Wolcott-Rallison syndrome: diabetes mellitus and spondyloepiphyseal dysplasia. Eur J Pediatr 1982; 138:120–129.

T0007 **Helga V. Toriello**

**Epiphyseal osteochondritides**
*See JOINTS, OSTEOCHONDRITIS DISSECANS*
**Epiphyseal osteochondroma, benign**
*See DYSPLASIA EPIPHYSEALIS HEMIMELICA*
**Episkopi blindness**
*See NORRIE DISEASE*

---

## EPISPADIAS                                         2008

**Includes:** Penis, epispadias

**Excludes:**
Bladder, agenesis of
**Bladder exstrophy** (3015)
**Exstrophy of cloaca sequence** (3193)
Exstrophy, duplicated
Pseudoextrophy
Vesico-intestinal fissure

**Major Diagnostic Criteria:** By physical examination. In a child without **Bladder exstrophy**, the presence of an urethral meatus at a dorsal location proximal to the tip of the phallus is the most important diagnostic feature. Intravenous pyelography (IVP), cystourography, and renal scanning are important to establish the extent of involvement.

**Clinical Findings:** Epispadias is a rare congenital anomaly in which the urethral meatus is displaced more proximally on the dorsal surface of the phallus. The urethera is delineated by the pink, smooth epithelium covering the anterior surface of a stubby penis that ends in a cleft glans. Embryologically, it represents a mild degree of a spectrum of anomalies of the extrophy complex. In all cases typical pelvic skeletal abnormality is evident; pubic bones are separated from each other. There is usually no orthopedic disability. The degree of musculoskeletal derangement coincides with the degree of urinary defect.

Epispadias can usually be classified by the location of the meatus into balanic or glandular, penile and penopubic forms. The only recognized female form is the subsymphyseal epispadias which corresponds to the male penopubic form. *Balanic epispadias* is the rarest and mildest form, in which the defect extends anteriorly from the meatus to the corona of the glans penis. The glans penis is split dorsally and flattened in a spade-shaped formation. The penis is short and stubby, and may show upward curvature (dorsal chordee). The foreskin may be confined to the ventral aspect. The patients are usually continent.

In *penile epispadias*, the urethral meatus terminates along the shaft of the penis. The distal urethera remains as an open epithelial-lined groove. The penis is short, flattened and curved anteriorly due to dorsal chordee. These patients are generally continent.

*Penopubic epispadias*, the most common form, has an opening along the entire length of the penis; extending through the sphincter of the bladder neck. The patient is often incontinent with constant dribbling, unless he is in the supine position. The anterior bladder wall may prolapse through the urinary opening; the bladder itself is dystrophic and reflux is common.

In *female suprasymphyseal epispadias*, the urethra is short; failure of the labia to fuse anteriorly results in a bifid clitoris. There are varying degrees of incontinence; its severity is determined by the patient's bladder capacity. Duplication of the vagina or uterus is rarely seen, but the possibility of a vaginal septum should be excluded by endoscopy.

**Complications:** Urinary incontinence, usually seen in penopubic epispadias in males and suprasymphyseal epispadias in females, occurs in 60% of the cases.

Infertility: although the penis is capable of a normal erection, since it is tethered close to the abdominal wall, intercourse may be difficult. Males usually do not father children; females may become pregnant.

Vesicoureteral reflux is seen in 75% of the cases.

**Associated Findings:** Duplication of the vagina, absent or septate vagina, and bicornuate uterus are rare in female patients with epispadias.

Vaginal hernias may be associated with epispadias.

**Etiology:** Unknown.

**Pathogenesis:** This developmental abnormality occurs between the 12–16 mm stage in embryogenesis. It has been suggested by Muecke (1964) that the persistence of the cloacal membrane would form a membranous center in the infraumbilical abdominal wall and divert mesodermal flow to either side as well as caudally (wedge effect). This membranous wall eventually becomes dehiscent; the structures lying directly behind it will be turned inside out and lie on the surface of the lower anterior abdominal wall. If this dehiscence occurs after the urorectal septum has partitioned the cloaca, classical exstrophy will result. If the persistence of the cloacal membrane is partial, an inferior epispadias results.

**CDC No.:** 752.610

**Sex Ratio:** M5:F1

**Occurrence:** Incidence 1:100,000 live births.

**Risk of Recurrence for Patient's Sib:** As in the general population; one sibship involving two siblings has been reported.

**Risk of Recurrence for Patient's Child:** Most males with this condition do not reproduce. At least 33 children have been born to 26 mothers who had epispadias; none had the deformity.

**Age of Detectability:** At birth.

**Gene Mapping and Linkage:** Unknown.

**Prevention:** None known. Genetic counseling indicated.

**Treatment:** Treatment is surgical. Surgery is aimed at the reconstruction of the existing urethera and bladder neck as well as straightening and lengthening the penis, cosmetic and functional considerations, and restoration of continence. Surgery is performed in two stages; the first stage consists of elimination of chordee; penile lengthening; approximation of pubic bones with bilateral ilial osteotomies; advancement of urethral meatus to the base of penile dorsum. The second stage consists of reconstruction of a neourethera. This procedure is recommended only in patients with continence. Incontinent patients may require a urinary deversion procedure. These patients use their urethra to channel seminal fluid only. Reconstructive surgery for the urethra is not indicated since neourethra is prone to stricture. If significant vesicoureteric reflux persists, ureteric reimplantation may be needed.

**Prognosis:** Due to a gradual increase in vesicourethral muscular development and power there is usually slow improvement at puberty. Maturity usually contributes to continence, but the correction of severe incontinence remains a problem. A well-developed bladder with good capacity and musculature is a prerequisite for satisfactory continence.

**Detection of Carrier:** Unknown.

**Special Considerations:** There is a close relationship among all forms of the exstrophy-epispadias complex. Embryologically they share a similar background: the persistence of the cloacal membrane. The timing and the degree of persistence of the cloacal membrane will determine the severity of the spectrum of anomalies which reflect varying degrees of severity, ie exstrophy, to a lesser degree of anomaly, ie epispadias.

**Bladder exstrophy** is the most frequent malformation within this spectrum. The milder form of the malformation, balanic epispadias, is much less common.

**References:**
Duckett JW Jr: Epispadias. Urol Clin North Am 1978; 5:107–126.
Woodhouse CR, Kellet MJ: Anatomy of the penis and its deformities in exstrophy and epispadias. J Urol 1984; 132:1122–1124.
Diamond DA, Jeffs RD: Cloacal exstrophy: a 22 year experience. J Urol 1985; 133:779–782.
Kramer SA, et al.: Long-term follow-up of cosmetic appearance and genital function in male epispadias: review of 70 patients. J Urol 1986; 135:543–547.

Muecke EC: Exstrophy, epispadias and other anomalies of the bladder. In: Walsh PC, et al., eds: Campbell's urology, 5th ed. Philadelphia: W.B. Saunders, 1986:1856–1880.

BI012
SA008
**Nesrin Bingol**
**Inge Sagel**

**Epispadias-exstrophy complex (one component)**
*See BLADDER EXSTROPHY*
**Epithelial cysts**
*See SPLEEN, CYSTS*
**Epithelial dystrophy, central areolar pigment**
*See EYE, MACULAR DYSTROPHY, NORTH CAROLINA TYPE*
**Epithelial thymomas, pseudorosette type**
*See CANCER, THYMOMA*
**Epithelioma adenoides cysticum (EAC)**
*See EPITHELIOMAS, HEREDITARY MULTIPLE CYSTIC*

## EPITHELIOMA, MULTIPLE SELF-HEALING SQUAMOUS 0359

**Includes:**

Ferguson-Smith epithelioma
Self-healing squamous cell epithelioma, multiple familial

**Excludes:** Keratoacanthoma

**Major Diagnostic Criteria:** Common findings include more than one tumor with the histologic appearance of squamous epithelioma, a history of self-healing tumors in patient and family members, and characteristic scars.

**Clinical Findings:** Multiple cutaneous tumors, histologically indistinguishable from well-differentiated squamous epithelioma are important features. They principally affect the circumoral region, the nose and ears, and, less frequently, the scalp, hands, forearms, and legs. Each tumor starts in normal skin as a small papule, which enlarges, ulcerates, and eventually heals. It leaves deep, pitted scars with irregular, overhanging crenellated borders. Individual tumors last for several months; additional tumors appear in even greater numbers. Tumors infiltrate the dermis and have been seen in local lymphatics.

**Complications:** Severe trauma resulting from excessive radiotherapy or surgery.

**Associated Findings:** None known.

**Etiology:** Autosomal dominant inheritance.

**Pathogenesis:** Undetermined. Tumors are thought to arise in pilosebaceous follicles.

**MIM No.:** *13280

**Sex Ratio:** M1:F1

**Occurrence:** Eleven families have been reported from Scotland and a similar number from North America and elsewhere. Thought to have arisen as a unique mutation in Central Scotland before 1745. Most families have Scottish ancestry.

**Risk of Recurrence for Patient's Sib:**
See Part I, *Mendelian Inheritance.*

**Risk of Recurrence for Patient's Child:**
See Part I, *Mendelian Inheritance.*

**Age of Detectability:** After puberty; 90% of affected men and women have their first lesion by 41 and 34 years of age, respectively.

**Gene Mapping and Linkage:** Unknown.

**Prevention:** None known. Genetic counseling indicated.

**Treatment:** Individual tumors should be excised as soon as they become apparent. Larger tumors may be excised or curetted after freezing with liquid nitrogen. Radiotherapy is contraindicated.

**Prognosis:** Normal for life span, intelligence, and function. Tumors have never metastasized.

**Detection of Carrier:** Unknown.

**References:**

Currie AR, Smith JF: Multiple primary spontaneous-healing squamous-cell carcinomata of the skin. J Pathol Bacteriol 1952; 64:827–839.
Ferguson-Smith MA, et al.: Multiple self-healing squamous epithelioma. BD:OAS; VII(8). New York: March of Dimes Birth Defects Foundation, 1971:157–163.
Schmatzler L: Epithéliomatose familiale de Ferguson-Smith. A propos de 2 cas familiaux. Ann Derm Vener 1977; 104:206.
Haydey RP, et al.: Treatment of keratoacanthomas with oral 13-cis-retinoic acid. N Engl J Med 1980; 303:560–562.
Jackson IT, et al.: Self-healing squamous epithelioma: a family affair. Brit J Plastic Surg 1983; 36:22–28.

FE007
**Malcolm A. Ferguson-Smith**

## EPITHELIOMAS, HEREDITARY MULTIPLE CYSTIC 2392

**Includes:**

Ancell-Spiegler-Brooke cylindromas
Brooke-Fordyce trichoepithelioma
Brooke tumor
Epithelioma adenoides cysticum (EAC)
Spiegler-Brooke tumors
Trichoepitheliomas, multiple
Turban tumors

**Excludes:**

**Gingival multiple hamartoma syndrome** (0412)
**Nevoid basal cell carcinoma syndrome** (0101)
Trichoepithelioma, solitary
**Tuberous sclerosis** (0975)

**Major Diagnostic Criteria:** Typical skin lesions in a characteristic facial distribution.

**Clinical Findings:** Lesions consisting of translucent papules and nodules mainly located on the face, but, occasionally, also found on the scalp, neck, and upper trunk. With these lesions gradually increase in number and size. Such lesions are skin-colored or slightly pink, and their diameter is between two and 30 mm. Facial lesions usually involve the nasolabial folds, nose, forehead, upperlip, and sometimes the external ears. The lesions grow slowly and only rarely ulcerate or invade deeply. A few telangiectatic vessels may be present on the surface of the larger lesions, but the lesions are generally asymptomatic. Histologically the lesions are usually well circumscribed. Horn cysts are the most characteristic feature, and they consist of a fully keratinized center surrounded by basophilic cells that appear similar to the cells of basal cell epithelioma. The keratinization in the horn cysts is abrupt and complete. Besides the horn cysts, the second major component is the presence of islands of basophilic cells with the appearance of basalioma cells, arranged usually in a lace-like or adenoid network but occasionally also as solid aggregates exhibiting peripheral palisading.

**Complications:** In some patients the lesions result in disfigurement, causing significant cosmetic problems.

**Associated Findings:** Renal and pulmonary cysts, infiltrating lobular breast carcinoma, and carcinoma of the cervix have been concurrently described in affected patients. Nail dystrophy has been reported in one case. In an affected family, one member developed basal cell carcinoma.

**Etiology:** Autosomal dominant inheritance with high penetrance in females and reduced penetrance in males.

**Pathogenesis:** Unknown. One group of subjects from a family with affected members in four generations, presenting also with the Mediterranean form of G6PD deficiency, was studied. It was found that females heterozygous for G6PD deficiency had both G6PD-deficient cells and G6PD normal cells in the same tumor, indicating a multicellular origin.

**MIM No.:** *13270, 31310

**Sex Ratio:** M<1:F1. Because of reduced male penetrance and expressivity, the disorder is more commonly seen in females.

**Occurrence:** Undetermined but presumed rare. Related conditions have been reported in Finland and Greenland.

**Risk of Recurrence for Patient's Sib:**
See Part I, *Mendelian Inheritance.*

**Risk of Recurrence for Patient's Child:**
See Part I, *Mendelian Inheritance.*

**Age of Detectability:** Usually during the second decade of life.

**Gene Mapping and Linkage:** Unknown.

**Prevention:** None known. Genetic counseling indicated.

**Treatment:** Both dermabrasion and carbon dioxide ($CO_2$) laser vaporization have proven to be effective in the treatment of the lesions.

**Prognosis:** The disorder runs a benign course, with no shortening of life span. The degeneration of the skin lesions into basal cell carcinoma is still in debate.

**Detection of Carrier:** Unknown.

**Special Considerations:** The association of this condition with *Ancell-Spiegler-Brooke cylindromas* (*turban tumors*) has been reported frequently. This association is strengthened by instances of both conditions in the same patient, and of trichoepitheliomas in one and cylindromas in another member of the same family. The two are probably phenotypic manifestations of the same entity.

**References:**
Brooke HG: Epithelioma adenoides cysticum. Br J Dermatol 1892; 4:269–286.
Fordyce JA: Multiple benign cystic epithelioma of the skin. J Cutan Genitourinary Dis 1892; 10:459–473.
Gartler SM, et al.: Glucose-6-phosphate dehydrogenase mosaicism as a tracer in the study of hereditary multiple trichoepithelioma. Am J Hum Genet 1966; 18:282–287.
Ziprkowski L, Schewach-Millet M: Multiple trichoepithelioma in a mother and two children. Dermatologica 1966; 132:248–256.
Welch JP, et al.: Ancell-Spiegler cylindromas (turban tumours) and Brooke-Fordyce trichoepitheliomas: evidence for a single genetic entity. J Med Genet 1968; 5:29–35.
Rasmussen JA: A syndrome of trichoepitheliomas, milias, and cylindromas. Arch Dermatol 1975; 111:610–614.
Anderson DE, Howell JB: Epithelioma adenoides cysticum: genetic update. Br J Dermatol 1976; 95:225–232.
Sandbank M, Bashan D: Multiple trichoepithelioma and breast carcinoma. Arch Dermatol 1978; 114:1230.
Wheeland R, et al.: Carbon dioxide ($CO_2$) laser vaporization for the treatment of multiple trichoepithelioma. J Dermatol Surg Oncol 1984; 10:470–475.
Merrick Y, et al.: Familial clustering of salivary gland carcinoma in Greenland. Cancer 1986; 57:2097–2102.
Autio-Harmainen H, et al.: Familial occurrence of malignant lymphoepithelial lesions of the parotid gland in a Finnish family with dominantly inherited trichoepithelioma. Cancer 1988; 61:161–166.

MI038                                                  **Giuseppe Micali**

**Epstein pearls**
*See MUCOSA, ORAL INCLUSION CYSTS OF THE NEWBORN*
**Epstein syndrome**
*See DEAFNESS-NEPHRITIS-MACROTHROMBOPATHIA*
**Epstein-Barr virus-induced lymphoproliferative disease in males**
*See IMMUNODEFICIENCY, X-LINKED LYMPHOPROLIFERATIVE DISEASE*
**Epulis, congenital**
*See TEETH, EPULIS, CONGENITAL*
**Erb muscular dystrophy**
*See MUSCULAR DYSTROPHY, LIMB-GIRDLE*
**Ermine phenotype**
*See ALBINISM-BLACK LOCKS-DEAFNESS*
**Eronen-Somer-Holmberg syndrome**
*See DIGITO-RENO-CEREBRAL SYNDROME*
**Erosive corneal dystrophy, hereditary recurrent**
*See CORNEAL DYSTROPHY, RECURRENT EROSIVE*
**Eruption failure of the permanent dentition**
*See TEETH, ANKYLODONTIA, MULTIPLE HERITABLE TYPE*
**Erythema (nodular)-digital defects-emaciation, Nakajo type**
*See DIGITAL DEFECTS-NODULAR ERYTHEMA-EMACIATION, NAKAJO TYPE*

**Erythema chronicum migrans**
*See FETAL EFFECTS FROM LYME DISEASE*
**Erythema infectiosum**
*See FETAL PARVOVIRUS INFECTION*
**Erythema migrans**
*See FETAL EFFECTS FROM LYME DISEASE*
**Erythema nuchae**
*See NEVUS FLAMMEUS*
**Erythema palmare hereditarium**
*See SKIN, PALMO-PLANTAR ERYTHEMA*
**Erythema palmo-plantar**
*See SKIN, PALMO-PLANTAR ERYTHEMA*
**Erythematokeratotic phacomatosis**
*See SKIN, ERYTHROKERATODERMIA, PROGRESSIVA SYMMETRICA*
**Erythroblastic endopolyploidy-multinucleated normoblasts**
*See ANEMIA, DYSERYTHROPOIETIC, TYPE II*

## ERYTHROBLASTOSIS FETALIS                           3063

**Includes:**

Alloimmune hemolytic disease of the newborn
Anemia, hemolytic
Blood group, Rhesus system (Rh)
Hemolytic disease resulting from Rh incompatibility
Isoimmune hemolytic disease of the newborn
Rh incompatibility

**Excludes:**
**Anemia** (other hemolytic)
**Hyperbilirubinemia, unconjugated** (0487)

**Major Diagnostic Criteria:** Hemolytic disease is present at birth, accompanied by mild-to-severe anemia, reticulocytosis, erythroblastemia, and **Hyperbilirubinemia, unconjugated.** The direct antiglobulin (Coombs) test is characteristically positive, indicating the presence of immunoglobulin bound to the surface of the erythrocytes.

**Clinical Findings:** The severity of clinical manifestations is extremely variable, with the level of maternal antibody and the antibody specificity being the major determinants. The mildest forms are characterized by an inapparent hemolytic process without anemia. The most severe forms may produce generalized edema, heart failure, and a rapidly fatal course. Although jaundice is almost invariably a prominent clinical feature, this finding is usually absent at birth because of the rapid clearance of bilirubin from the fetal circulation by the placenta. Visible jaundice is usually present within the first 24 hours of life in patients with significant hemolytic disease.

Findings at birth are primarily attributable to the degree of anemia. The most severely affected infants present the picture of **Hydrops fetalis** with marked pallor, edema, and swelling of the chest and abdomen caused by effusion of fluid. The placentas of these infants are often large, pale, and edematous. Manifestations of severe anemia at birth most frequently accompany hemolytic disease resulting from Rh (D) incompatibility.

Infants with alloimmune hemolysis caused by ABO incompatibility most often develop jaundice during the first 24 hours of life, but without clinical evidence of anemia. Affected infants commonly exhibit splenic and hepatic enlargement. If severe anemia is present, hepatosplenomegaly may in part be caused by congestive changes of heart failure. The presence of spherocytes is a characteristic finding in infants with ABO alloimmune hemolytic disease, but this finding is not observed in Rh-associated disease.

**Complications:** Heart failure, which may occur *in utero* in the most severe forms of the disease, occurs as a result of severe anemia. More severely affected infants may also develop petechiae and purpura accompanied by hemorrhagic complications. These infants often have low platelet counts and, in some instances, hypofibrinogenemia and changes in other coagulation factors, suggesting the presence of disseminated intravascular coagulation. High levels of unconjugated bilirubin in these infants pose the serious risk of causing neurologic damage as a result of entry of the bilirubin into the brainstem and basal ganglia of the brain, producing encephalopathic changes.

**Associated Findings:** None known.

**Etiology:** Autosomal dominant inheritance.

**Pathogenesis:** Transplacental passage of maternal antibody with specificity for one or more red cell surface antigens present on the infant's erythrocytes. Maternal antibody formation may be stimulated by a mismatched blood transfusion or by sensitization due to fetal erythrocytes that enter the maternal circulation. Antibody-coated erythrocytes in the fetus and infant undergo rapid destruction in the spleen and other reticuloendothelial organs because of immaturity of the bilirubin-conjugating mechanism in newborn infants. This hemolytic process may result in high levels of unconjugated bilirubin.

**MIM No.:** *11170

**Sex Ratio:** M1:F1

**Occurrence:** The most severe forms of the disease have been observed in infants of Rh-negative women with sensitization to the D factor. This is explained by the early expression of the D group on fetal erythrocytes and by its high level of immunogenicity. Significant racial differences have been demonstrated in the incidence of the D factor, with approximately 85% of the European population, 93% of the Black population, and more than 99% of the Chinese having this factor. This distribution correlates well with the incidence of Rh alloimmune hemolytic disease, which is approximately three times more frequent in white individuals than in Blacks, and is rare among Chinese.

**Risk of Recurrence for Patient's Sib:**
See Part I, *Mendelian Inheritance*. In the case of D factor-associated alloimmune disease, the severity of disease in subsequent pregnancies is usually equal or greater for Rh-positive infants. A relationship of this kind does not occur, however, in hemolytic disease resulting from ABO incompatibility.

**Risk of Recurrence for Patient's Child:**
See Part I, *Mendelian Inheritance*.

**Age of Detectability:** When a severely affected fetus is anticipated, prenatal studies can reliably demonstrate the presence of hemolysis, anemia, and hyperbilirubinemia in the fetus.

**Gene Mapping and Linkage:** RH (Rhesus blood group) has been mapped to 1p36.2-p34.

**Prevention:** The widespread practice of administering antifactor D (Rhogam) to Rh-negative women following the delivery or abortion or an Rh-positive infant or fetus has virtually abolished Rh-related alloimmune hemolytic disease.

**Treatment:** For the known seriously affected fetus *in utero*, fetal salvage can be improved by intrauterine transfusion of erythrocytes that are transfusion-compatible with the mother's serum. Plasmapheresis to diminish levels of circulating antibody has also been shown to be beneficial in highly sensitized mothers. Management of infants detected at birth is directed toward ameliorating the anemia and preventing complications of unconjugated hyperbilirubinemia. For the mildly affected infant, bilirubin levels can usually be maintained within acceptable levels by the use of phototherapy. When this measure is inadequate, exchange transfusions using red cells that are transfusion-compatible with the maternal serum will allow larger amounts of bilirubin to be removed while also correcting anemia and removing antibody-coated red cells, which can be a further source of unconjugated bilirubin in the infant.

**Prognosis:** The outlook for survival is guarded for severely affected fetuses requiring intrauterine transfusion. Infants with severe anemia accompanied by heart failure and other elements of the hydrops fetalis syndrome also often have a poor outcome. For other affected infants, phototherapy combined with exchange transfusions virtually always make it possible to maintain the serum bilirubin within acceptable levels, and these infants usually have no demonstrable long-term sequelae of the disease.

**Detection of Carrier:** Rh-negative women, who are at greatest risk of having affected infants, are routinely tested as part of their prenatal assessment.

**References:**

Naiman J: Current management of hemolytic disease of the newborn infant. J Pediatr 1972; 80:1049–1059.

Bock J: Intrauterine transfusion in severe hemolytic disease. Acta Obstet Gynecol Scand [Suppl] 1976; 53(suppl):1–40.

Herman M, Kjellman J: Rh-prophylaxis with immunoglobulin anti-D administered during pregnancy and after delivery. Acta Obstet Gynecol Scand 1976; 49(Suppl)1–11.

Bowman J: The management of Rh-isoimmunization. Obstet Gynecol 1978; 52:1–16.

Harman C, et al.: Severe Rh disease: poor outcome is not inevitable. Am J Obstet Gynecol 1983; 145:823–829.

H0024

**George R. Honig**

## Erythroblastosis fetalis and staining of enamel and dentin
*See TEETH, ENAMEL AND DENTIN DEFECTS FROM ERYTHROBLASTOSIS FETALIS*

## ERYTHROCYTE ALDOLASE-A DEFICIENCY      2662

**Includes:** Aldolase-A deficiency, erythrocyte

**Excludes:** N/A

**Major Diagnostic Criteria:** Based on the demonstration of severely defective erythrocyte aldolase in terms of catalytic activity, abnormal kinetics, or thermostability.

**Clinical Findings:** Of the few known cases, one had chronic, nonspherocytic hemolytic anemia in a setting of a galaxy of malformations. It is not clear if any of the latter symptoms were related other than fortuitously to aldolase deficiency. A second unrelated patient exhibited the hemolytic syndrome without other manifestations.

**Complications:** All individuals with chronic hemolysis have an increased risk of developing cholelithiasis, and may have worsening of anemia during infection or stress such as surgery.

**Associated Findings:** None known.

**Etiology:** Probably autosomal recessive inheritance, although some believe the condition to be dominant. A structural gene mutation was postulated in one of the few known cases. In one case, parents were related as first cousins.

**Pathogenesis:** The mature erythrocyte depends on the conversion of glucose to lactate to maintain ATP and meet energy needs. Molecular lesions of glycolysis, when severe, impair the necessary flow of glycolytic intermediates.

**MIM No.:** *10385

**Sex Ratio:** Presumably M1:F1

**Occurrence:** Three cases have been reported from two families.

**Risk of Recurrence for Patient's Sib:**
See Part I, *Mendelian Inheritance*.

**Risk of Recurrence for Patient's Child:**
See Part I, *Mendelian Inheritance*.

**Age of Detectability:** At birth.

**Gene Mapping and Linkage:** ALDOA (aldolase A, fructose-bisphosphate) has been provisionally mapped to 16q22-q24.

**Prevention:** None known. Genetic counseling indicated.

**Treatment:** Supplements of folate are indicated. Presumably splenectomy can be considered if anemia is severe and transfusions are required. Its potential benefit is unsubstantiated and, by analogy with other glycolytic erythroenzymopathies, could result in partial benefit, but with ongoing vigorous hemolysis.

**Prognosis:** Unknown.

**Detection of Carrier:** Investigation of aldolase catalytic activity, kinetics, and thermostability.

**References:**

Penhoet E, et al.: Multiple forms of fructose diphosphate aldolase in mammalian tissues. Proc Nat Acad Sci 1966; 56:1275–1282.

Beutler E, et al.: Red cell aldolase deficiency and hemolytic anemia: a new syndrome. Trans Assoc Am Physicians 1973; 86:154–166.

Lowry RB, Hanson JW: Aldolase A deficiency with syndrome of growth and developmental retardation, midfacial hypoplasia, hepatomegaly, and consanguineous parents. BD:OAS XIII(3B). New York: March of Dimes Birth Defects Foundation, 1977:222–228.

Miwa S, et al.: Two cases of red cell aldolase deficiency associated with hereditary hemolytic anemia in a Japanese family. Am J Hematol 1981; 11:425–437.

Hurst JA, et al.: A syndrome of mental retardation, short stature, hemolytic anemia, delayed puberty, and abnormal facial appearance: similaritiesto a report of aldolase A deficiency. Am J Med Genet 1987; 28:965–970.

Kishi H, et al.: Human aldolase A deficiency associated with hemolytic anemia: thermolabile aldolase due to a single base mutation. Proc Nat Acad Sci 1987; 84:8623–8627.

VA024                                   **William N. Valentine**

**Erythrocyte hexokinase deficiency hemolytic anemia**
*See ANEMIA, HEMOLYTIC, ERYTHROCYTE HEXOKINASE DEFICIENCY*
**Erythrocyte membrane defects**
*See ANEMIA, HEMOLYTIC, RED CELL MEMBRANE DEFECTS*
**Erythrocyte phosphoglycerate kinase deficiency**
*See ANEMIA, HEMOLYTIC, ERYTHROCYTE PHOSPHOGLYCERATE KINASE DEFICIENCY*

## ERYTHROCYTE TRIOSEPHOSPHATE ISOMERASE DEFICIENCY                                2686

**Includes:**
Anemia, hemolytic, due to triose isomerase deficiency
Triose phosphate isomerase deficiency
Triosephosphate isomerase deficiency

**Excludes:** Anemia, hemolytic (others)

**Major Diagnostic Criteria:** Severely deficient patients have chronic nonspherocytic hemolytic anemia, severe neurologic deficits chiefly motor in type, and sometimes other evidence of multisystem disease. Triosephosphate isomerase activity is severely diminished in erythrocytes, leukocytes, plasma, spinal fluid, and all other tissues in which the isomerase has been assayed.

**Clinical Findings:** Chronic nonspherocytic hemolytic anemia is present from birth. Severe neurologic dysfunction appears most often around age six months but sometimes not until age two years. This includes diffuse weakness, hypotonia, and absent limb reflexes and may progress to unintelligible speech and fixed deformities of the hands and legs. When tested, intellect has been preserved, sensory impairment absent, and brain scans and EEG normal. Pyramidal tract signs, dystonia, and dyskinesia point to brainstem and basal ganglion involvement, but the cerebal cortex appears unaffected. Sudden death, presumably due to cardiac arrythmias, and clinically increased susceptibility to infection have also been reported.

**Complications:** Neurologic dysfunction, sudden death, increased infections.

**Associated Findings:** None known.

**Etiology:** Autosomal recessive inheritance of defective alleles encoding triosephosphate isomerase results in severe tissue deficiency of the enzyme in all body tissues studied. A structural gene abnormality is believed to be involved, and in two unrelated patients a single amino acid substitution, Glu-104→Asp-104, has been documented, giving rise to an unstable enzyme.

**Pathogenesis:** Precise effects of the generalized enzyme deficiency are undetermined. In terms of hemolytic anemia, severe enzyme deficiency obviously disrupts glycolysis, and, in addition, dihydroxyacetone phosphate accumulates to a marked degree in red cells. In two unrelated patients, a GC→GG transversion in the codon for amino acid 104 resulted in a thermolabile enzyme.

**MIM No.:** *19045

**Sex Ratio:** M1:F1

**Occurrence:** About 25 patients have been reported in the literature.

**Risk of Recurrence for Patient's Sib:**
See Part I, *Mendelian Inheritance.*

**Risk of Recurrence for Patient's Child:**
See Part I, *Mendelian Inheritance.*

**Age of Detectability:** Hemolytic anemia is present at birth. Detectability depends on obtaining specific enzyme assay of erythrocytes.

**Gene Mapping and Linkage:** TPI1 (triosephosphate isomerase 1) has been mapped to 12p13.

**Prevention:** None known. Genetic counseling indicated.

**Treatment:** None available other than folate administration, as in other hemolytic syndromes, and attention to preventable sequelae of the severe neurologic deficits such as fixed contractures.

**Prognosis:** One patient has lived to young adulthood. Death usually occurs in childhood.

**Detection of Carrier:** Demonstration of partial (usually about one-half normal) enzyme activity in heterozygote erythrocytes.

**References:**
Schneider AS, et al.: Hereditary hemolytic anemia with triosephosphate isomerase deficiency. New Engl J Med 1965; 272:229–235.

Valentine WN, et al.: Hereditary hemolytic anemia with triosephosphate isomerase deficiency: studies in kindreds with coexistent sickle cell trait and erythrocyte glucose-6-phosphate dehydrogenase deficiency. Am J Med 1966; 41:27–41.

Neel JV, et al.: Rate of spontaneous mutation at human loci encoding protein structure. Proc Natl Acad Sci USA 1980; 77:6037–6041.

Clay SA, et al.: Triose phosphate isomerase deficiency. Am J Dis Child 1982; 136:800–802.

Valentine WN, Paglia DE: Erythrocyte enzymopathies, hemolytic anemia, and multisystem disease: an annotated review. Blood 1984; 64:583–591.

Poll-The BT, et al.: Neurological findings in triosephosphate isomerase deficiency. Ann Neurol 1985; 17:439–443.

Daar IO, et al.: Human triose-phosphate isomerase deficiency: a single amino acid substition results in a thermolabile enzyme. Proc Nat Acad Sci 1986; 83:7903–7907.

Bellingham AJ, et al.: Prenatal diagnosis of a red-cell enzymopathy: triose phosphate isomerase deficiency. Lancet 1989; II:419–421.

VA024                                  **William N. Valentine**

## ERYTHROCYTE, DIPHOSPHOGLYCERATE MUTASE (2,3) DEFICIENCY                        2664

**Includes:**
Bisphosphoglycerate mutase, (E.C.2.7.5.4) deficiency
Blood, diphosphoglycerate mutase (2,3) deficiency
Diphosphoglycerate mutase (2,3) deficiency of erythrocyte

**Excludes:** N/A

**Major Diagnostic Criteria:** Absent or near absent 2,3-diphosphoglycerate (2,3-DPG) and near-absent assayable activity of 2,3-DPG mutase and phosphatase activity in the erythrocyte must be documented. Both of the latter activities reside in the same protein.

**Clinical Findings:** Patients are asymptomatic but have mild erythrocytosis by laboratory parameters.

**Complications:** Unknown.

**Associated Findings:** Mild increases in erythrocyte counts and hemoglobin concentration.

**Etiology:** Autosomal recessive inheritance.

**Pathogenesis:** The mild erythrocytosis is secondary to a near lack of 2,3-DPG, which results in increased affinity of hemoglobin for oxygen and hence somewhat less $O_2$ delivery to tissues at a given partial pressure. Erythropoietin production and some expansion of the erythron is the result.

**MIM No.:** *22280

**Sex Ratio:** Presumably M1:F1

**Occurrence:** While a possible deficiency has been indirectly inferred in several individuals and sibships, only one kindred is unequivocably documented and thoroughly studied.

**Risk of Recurrence for Patient's Sib:**
See Part I, *Mendelian Inheritance.*

**Risk of Recurrence for Patient's Child:**
See Part I, *Mendelian Inheritance.*

**Age of Detectability:** At any age by special laboratory assays.

**Gene Mapping and Linkage:** BPGM (2,3-bisphosphoglycerate mutase) has been mapped to 7q31-q34.

**Prevention:** None known. Genetic counseling indicated.

**Treatment:** None indicated.

**Prognosis:** No ill effects have been documented.

**Detection of Carrier:** Assay of 2,3-DPG mutase and phosphatase showed partial deficiencies.

**References:**
Benesch R, Benesch RE: Intracellular organic phosphates as regulators of oxygen release by haemoglobin. Nature 1969; 221:618–622.
Rosa R, et al.: Diphosphoglycerate mutase and 2,3-diphosphoglycerate phosphatase activities of red cells: comparative electrophoretic study. Biochem Biophys Res Commun 1973; 51:536–542.
Rosa R, et al.: The first case of a complete deficiency of diphosphoglycerate mutase in human erythrocytes. J Clin Invest 1978; 62:907–915.

VA024                                                    **William N. Valentine**

---

## ERYTHROCYTE, LACTATE TRANSPORTER DEFECT          2945

**Includes:**
Lactate transporter defect, myopathy due to
Lactate transporter deficiency
Lactate transporter myopathy, metabolic
Myopathy (metabolic), lactate transporter defect

**Excludes:**
Lactic acidemia
Lactic acidosis

**Major Diagnostic Criteria:** 1) Defective erythrocyte lactate efflux or influx (less than 40% normal). 2) In addition, delayed blood lactate declines after an appropriately conducted ischemic forearm exercise test (less than 4% decline/minute). Item one establishes the red cell defect; item two argues indirectly for the same defect in skeletal muscle.

**Clinical Findings:** Patients may have muscle pain and easy fatigue on heavy exercise, and may exhibit a mildly to moderately elevated serum creatine kinase level. Neurologic examination, muscle biopsy material, and electromyography are likely to be normal.

**Complications:** Affected patients may have an increased risk of exercise and anesthetic-induced rhabdomyolysis.

**Associated Findings:** None known.

**Etiology:** Possibly autosomal recessive inheritance.

**Pathogenesis:** During heavy exercise, exceeding the aerobic capacity, lactic acid builds up rapidly intramuscularly, and the acidosis comprises both the contraction-relaxation apparatus and the regenerative metabolism. In the absence of the lactate transporter, the efflux is limited by diffusion and other carriers to perhaps 10–15% the normal rate so that fatigue and cramping occur earlier and last longer.

**MIM No.:** 24534

**Sex Ratio:** Presumably M1:F1.

**Occurrence:** Undetermined.

**Risk of Recurrence for Patient's Sib:** Unknown.

**Risk of Recurrence for Patient's Child:** Unknown.

**Age of Detectability:** Should be detectable at any age by red cell assay; normal values in infants and children have not been established.

**Gene Mapping and Linkage:** Unknown.

**Prevention:** Episodes should be preventable by avoidance of extreme exercise.

**Treatment:** Avoidance of extreme exercise may be sufficient.

**Prognosis:** Probably no compromise of ordinary daily functioning, physical activity, or life span.

**Detection of Carrier:** Undetermined. At this point it is still possible that the deficient patients thus far identified are heterozygotes, carrier cases, or that a more complete defect may yet be found.

**Special Considerations:** Although at this point the defect is only directly demonstrable in the red cell, the entity may be considered a metabolic myopathy because only exercising muscle produces a rapid rise of lactic acid to extreme levels (30 mM). Occurrence of extracellular acidosis (in contrast to intramuscular acidosis) would depend on the genetic relation between the red cell and the hepatic lactate transporter. If the latter is coded by a different gene, then lactate uptake and conversion to glucose in the liver will be unimpaired, and lactic acidosis will not occur, even on extreme exercise.

**References:**
Fishbein WN: Lactate transporter defect: a new disease of muscle. Science 1986; 234:1254–1256.
Fishbein WN, et al.: Clinical assay of the human erythrocyte lactate transporter: principles, procedure, and validation. Biochem Med 1988; 39:338–350.
Fishbein WN, et al.: Clinical assay of the human erythrocyte lactate transporter: analysis and display of normal human data. Biochem Med 1988; 39:351–359.
Fishbein WN, et al.: Erythrocyte lactate transporter deficiency: a common metabolic myopathy. Can J Sports Sci 1988; 13:12P.
Fishbein WN: Metabolic myopathy due to lactate transporter defect. Neurology 1989; 39(Suppl 1):258 only.

FI028                                                    **William Fishbein**

**Erythrodontia**
  *See PORPHYRIA, ERYTHROPOIETIC*
**Erythrogenesis imperfecta**
  *See ANEMIA, HYPOPLASTIC CONGENITAL*
**Erythrohepatic protoporphyria**
  *See PORPHYRIA, PROTOPORPHYRIA*
**Erythroid hypoplastic anemia, congenital**
  *See ANEMIA, HYPOPLASTIC CONGENITAL*
**Erythroid multinuclearity, familial**
  *See ANEMIA, DYSERYTHROPOIETIC, TYPE III*
**Erythrokeratoderma figurata, congenital familial, in plaques**
  *See SKIN, ERYTHROKERATODERMIA, VARIABLE*
**Erythrokeratodermia figurata, congenital familial, in plaques**
  *See SKIN, ERYTHROKERATODERMIA, PROGRESSIVA SYMMETRICA*
**Erythrokeratodermia variabilis Mendes da Costa**
  *See SKIN, ERYTHROKERATODERMIA, VARIABLE*
**Erythrokeratodermia-ataxia**
  *See GIROUX-BARBEAU SYNDROME*
**Erythrokeratolysis hiemalis**
  *See SKIN, ERYTHROKERATOLYSIS HIEMALIS*
**Erythrophagocytic lymphohistiocytosis, familial**
  *See LYMPHOHISTIOCYTOSIS, FAMILIAL ERYTHROPHAGOCYTIC*
**Erythropoietic porphyria, congenital**
  *See PORPHYRIA, ERYTHROPOIETIC*
**Erythropoietic protoporphyria (EPP)**
  *See PORPHYRIA, PROTOPORPHYRIA*
**Erythroreticulosis, hereditary benign**
  *See ANEMIA, DYSERYTHROPOIETIC, TYPE III*
**Escobar syndrome**
  *See PTERYGIUM SYNDROME, MULTIPLE*
**Eskatlith^ induced goiter**
  *See GOITER, GOITROGEN INDUCED*
**Eskatlith^, fetal effects**
  *See FETAL LITHIUM EFFECTS*
  *also TRICUSPID VALVE, EBSTEIN ANOMALY*

Esophageal atresia-tracheoesophageal fistula
*See TRACHEOESOPHAGEAL FISTULA*
Esophageal chalasia
*See ESOPHAGUS, CHALASIA*
Esophageal cyst
*See ESOPHAGUS, DUPLICATION*
Esophageal diverticulum
*See ESOPHAGUS, DIVERTICULUM*
Esophageal duplication
*See ESOPHAGUS, DUPLICATION*
Esophageal duplication (mediastinal cyst of foregut origin)
*See INTESTINAL DUPLICATION*
Esophageal hiatus hernia
*See HERNIA, HIATAL*
Esophageal lobe
*See LUNG, ABERRANT LOBE*
Esophageal stenosis
*See ESOPHAGUS, STENOSIS*
Esophageal stricture, congenital
*See ESOPHAGUS, STENOSIS*
Esophageal web or veil
*See ESOPHAGUS, STENOSIS*
Esophagotrachea, persistent
*See LARYNGO-TRACHEO-ESOPHAGEAL CLEFT*

## ESOPHAGUS, ACHALASIA                              0363

**Includes:**
Achalasia, esophageal
Cardiospasm
Megaesophagus

**Excludes:**
Esophagitis
Stricture of esophagus secondary to reflux

**Major Diagnostic Criteria:** A large, poorly emptying esophagus without evidence of distal esophagitis or stricture by X-ray and endoscopic examination is diagnostic of achalasia. This is an unusual diagnosis to be made in the young child, but if one follows the rule of investigating persistent respiratory, deglutition, or regurgitation complaints by barium swallow examination, it will not be overlooked. The classic esophageal manometric findings are elevation of the lower esophageal sphincter pressure, failure of the lower esophageal sphincter to relax with swallowing, and the lack of peristalsis in the body of the esophagus.

**Clinical Findings:** Persistent vomiting and recurrent aspiration pneumonia are the most frequent problems in infants and young children. Dysphagia and recurrent vomiting are the most frequent symptoms in older children. Failure to thrive or weight loss, heart-burn, choking, odynophagia, and nighttime cough are other frequent presentations.

**Complications:** Repeated aspiration pneumonitis, dysphagia, or regurgitation with evidence of poor nutrition are common presenting complications.

**Associated Findings:** Familial glucocorticoid deficiency and familial recessive deafness have been reported. Rarely, the very large, almost constantly filled esophagus may produce symptoms of pressure on the airway.

**Etiology:** Possibly autosomal recessive inheritance.

**Pathogenesis:** This lesion begins with cardiospasm and leads eventually to secondary changes in the esophagus. Many investigators have proposed abnormalities in the myenteric plexuses and the distal esophagus. A study by Cassella et al. (1964) demonstrated, by electron microscopy, that the only persistent change in this condition was a Wallerian type of degeneration of the vagus nerve. Protracted distal obstruction causes marked muscular hypertrophy of the esophagus. Inherent peristaltic defects that may be present are not helped in any way by this hypertrophy. Long periods of time may be required for resolution of this hypertrophic muscle following relief of the obstruction at the junction.

**MIM No.:**  *20040

**CDC No.:**  750.480

**Sex Ratio:** M1:F1, except in familial cases in which report M2:F1.

**Occurrence:** Undetermined. About ten kinships reported with familial patterns.

**Risk of Recurrence for Patient's Sib:**
See Part I, *Mendelian Inheritance.*

**Risk of Recurrence for Patient's Child:**
See Part I, *Mendelian Inheritance.* There is one reported case of possible vertical transmission.

**Age of Detectability:** During infancy or childhood.

**Gene Mapping and Linkage:** Unknown.

**Prevention:** None known. Genetic counseling indicated.

**Treatment:** Treatment options include pneumatic dilation, esophageal myotomy, or esophageal myotomy with an anti-reflux procedure. Controversy exists as to whether pneumatic dilation or esophageal myotomy should be the initial treatment for achalasia. Because of the significant occurrence of gastroesophageal reflux following myotomy, some investigators favor an anti-reflux procedure at the time of myotomy.

**Prognosis:** Vantrappen and Hellemans (1980) compared the "late" results of forceful dilation and operative treatment of achalasia. Approximately 75% of the patients in either treatment group had "good" or "excellent" results. Recurrence of symptomatic achalasia can occur many years after either procedure. Poor results, generally defined as persistence or worsening of symptoms, occur in 5 to 10% of patients. Esophageal carcinoma develops in one to 7% of patients.

**Detection of Carrier:** Unknown.

**References:**
Cassella RR, et al.: Achalasia of the esophagus: pathologic and etiologic considerations. Am Surg 1964; 160:474–487.
Csendes A, et al.: A prospective randomized study comparing forceful dilatation and esophagomyotomy in patients with achalasia of the esophagus. Gastroenterology 1980; 80:789–795.
Vantrappen G, Hellemans J: Treatment of achalasia and related motor disorders. Gastroenterology 1980; 79:144–154.
Bosher LP, Shaw A: Achalasia in siblings. Am J Dis Child 1981; 135:709–710.
Berquist WE, et al.: Achalasia: diagnosis, management, and clinical course in 16 children. Pediatrics 1983; 71:798–805.
Nakayama DK, et al.: Pneumatic dilatation and operative treatment of achalasia in children. J Pediatr Surg 1987; 22:619–622.

R0055                                    **Charles C. Roberts**
AS000                                    **Keith W. Ashcraft**

## ESOPHAGUS, ATRESIA                               0364

**Includes:** Atresia, esophageal

**Excludes:**
**Esophagus, atresia and tracheoesophageal fistula** (0365)
**Esophagus, stenosis** (0369)
**Tracheoesophageal fistula** (0960)

**Major Diagnostic Criteria:** Excessive salivation, regurgitation, and obstruction in the esophagus as tested by catheter and X-ray in the immediate newborn period.

**Clinical Findings:** This defect is first detectable in the immediate neonatal period. The presence of prematurity and polyhydramnios should suggest to the physician that an appropriately sized catheter be passed and X-rays taken to rule out the presence of esophageal atresia in the immediate postnatal period.

"Excessive salivation" is noted shortly after birth and is only apparently excessive because the child cannot swallow his secretions. Regurgitation with feedings is characteristic. If the lesion remains untreated, dehydration or starvation follows.

Children suspected of having this lesion should have a stiff 10 or 12 French catheter passed via the nose or mouth into the esophagus. An obstruction 9 to 13 cm from the nares or upper alveolar ridge confirms the presence of atresia. A tube being passed further than this does not exclude atresia since the tube may coil in an

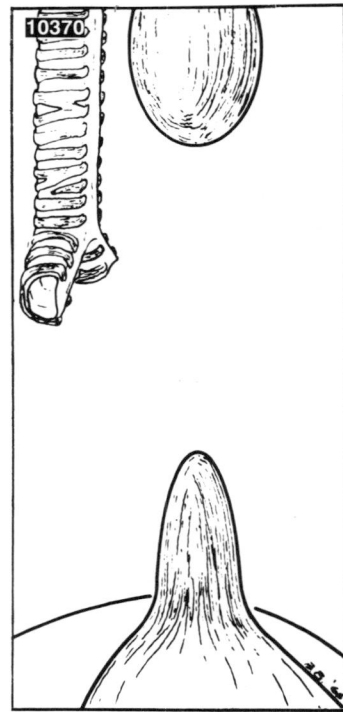

**0364**-10370: Esophageal atresia.

atretic proximal esophagus. A portable upright chest X-ray with the tube in place should be taken in every infant in whom there is any question of esophageal atresia. This will 1) demonstrate the relative length of the upper pouch, 2) confirm the absence of a distal tracheoesophageal fistula, 3) document the status of the lungs, 4) demonstrate abnormalities in cardiac configuration, and 5) show skeletal abnormalities such as hemivertebra. The injection of 1 cc of dilute barium into the upper esophagus can be helpful in instances where the diagnosis is not clear from the passage of a radio-opaque catheter. If barium enters the trachea it confirms the presence of a tracheoesophageal fistula. It is helpful to put 1/2 cc of Dionosil into the upper esophagus for clearer identification of the pouch and perhaps demonstration of a fistula from the proximal esophagus to the trachea.

**Complications:** If untreated, the lesion is invariably fatal through either dehydration or starvation.

**Associated Findings:** Numerous severe congenital anomalies are associated with approximately half of the patients born with esophageal atresia. In order of frequency, these include congenital heart disease; GI anomalies; GU anomalies; imperforate anus; skeletal deformities, including many arm and hand abnormalities; cleft defects of the face; CNS lesions such as meningoceles or **Hydrocephaly** and **Chromosome 21, trisomy 21.** One-third are premature.

**Etiology:** The esophagus develops abnormally in the 4th embryonic week. Because of the frequency of associated anomalies that are also explainable on the basis of an unknown embryologic insult at approximately the same time, it is felt that this is a random, generalized insult to embryogenesis.

**Pathogenesis:** Atresia of the esophagus occurs at the end of the first month of gestational life. The inability to swallow prevents the fetus from participating in the normal turnover of amniotic fluid and may result in polyhydramnios and through this mechanism lead to premature birth. After birth, saliva cannot be swallowed and will be regurgitated through the mouth and nose.

Feedings likewise will be taken usually with voracity, only to be returned a few moments later.

**CDC No.:** 750.300

**Sex Ratio:** M1:F1

**Occurrence:** 1:32,000 live births.

**Risk of Recurrence for Patient's Sib:** Presumably not increased.

**Risk of Recurrence for Patient's Child:** Presumably not increased.

**Age of Detectability:** At birth by passage of nasogastric tube with chest X-ray. Third-trimester alpha-fetoprotein elevated in amniotic fluid. Amniography in third trimester shows hydramnios and a lack of intestinal contrast. Fetography at this time shows lack of swallowing of opacified amniotic fluid.

**Gene Mapping and Linkage:** Unknown.

**Prevention:** None known. Genetic counseling indicated.

**Treatment:** Initial treatment consists of establishing of a feeding gastrostomy and determining the length, if possible, of the upper and lower esophageal segments. Bougienage to lengthen both upper and lower segments may be carried out to stretch the two ends so that they can be primarily connected. If this is not elected it is perfectly reasonable to bring the upper esophageal segment out as a cervical esophagostomy and do a later interposition of colon or gastric tube to replace the atretic esophageal segment. This should probably be delayed until at least age 1 year. Perhaps as many as 50% of patients are amenable to bougienage and primary anastomosis.

**Prognosis:** Once surgically corrected, this lesion should not interfere with the normal life span, but complications of the interposed segment or of anastomotic stricture due to associated gastroesophageal reflux may require repetitive dilatations or other operative procedures.

**Detection of Carrier:** Unknown.

**References:**

Seppala M: Increased alpha-fetoprotein amniotic fluid associated with a congenital esophageal atresia of the fetus. Obstet Gynecol 1973; 42:613.

Mahour GH, et al.: Elongation of the upper pouch and delayed anatomic reconstruction in esophageal atresia. J Ped Surg 1974; 9:373.

Hendren WH, Hale JR: Electromagnetic bougienage to lengthen esophageal segments in congenital esophageal atresia. N Engl J Med 1975; 293:428.

Holder TM: Esophageal atresia and tracheoesophageal fistula. In: Ashcraft KA, Holder TM, eds.: Pediatric Esophageal Surgery. Orlando, FL: Grune and Stratton, 1986:29.

R0055　　　　　　　　　　　　　　　　　　　　　**Charles C. Roberts**
AS000　　　　　　　　　　　　　　　　　　　　**Keith W. Ashcraft**

## ESOPHAGUS, ATRESIA AND TRACHEOESOPHAGEAL FISTULA　　　　　　　　　　　　　　　　　　0365

**Includes:**

　Atresia of esophagus with or without tracheoesophageal atresia

　Tracheoesophageal fistula with or without esophageal atresia

**Excludes:**

　Esophageal strictures, congenital or acquired

　Stenosis and tracheoesophageal fistula due to trauma

**Major Diagnostic Criteria:** The diagnosis should be considered when the baby chokes on feedings. Failure to pass a No. 8 or 10 French catheter into the stomach followed by a plain X-ray of the chest demonstrating a coiled catheter at the upper pouch of the atretic esophagus establishes the diagnosis. It is rare that a contrast study needed to confirm the diagnosis of esophageal atresia. Meticulous care under fluoroscopic control with the slow injection through a tube in the upper esophageal pouch with 0.5

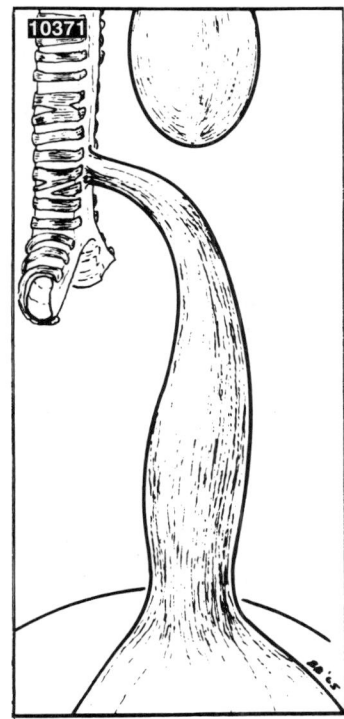

**0365**-10371: Esophageal atresia with distal tracheoesophageal fistula.

---

to 1 cc of barium is carried out. Immediate aspiration of the barium then follows.

An EKG and echocardiogram is necessary, since a high percentage of infants with esophageal atresia have serious life-threatening cardiac anomalies. Some may be asymptomatic and must be ruled out before repair of the atresia is undertaken.

**Clinical Findings:** Excessive salivation and choking, coughing, and regurgitation when feeding. Abdominal distention due to increased air passing through the fistula into the stomach. Clinical manifestations of pneumonitis due to reflux of gastric secretions through the fistula into the lungs or atelectasis due to aspiration of saliva and mucus into the tracheobronchial tree may occur. Further pulmonary difficulties follow because of an elevated diaphragm secondary to gastric dilation and pulmonary pathology. Infants with esophageal atresia and absent tracheoesophageal fistula will have a gasless, flat abdomen.

**Complications:** Aspiration, pneumonitis, sepsis, dehydration, electrolyte imbalance.

**Associated Findings:** Severe cardiac anomalies occur in about 40% of the cases; with other gastrointestinal malformations occur in 20%, imperforate anus in 4–5%, and **Vater association** in 4–5%. Severe skeletal, renal, and neurologic anomalies occur in decreasing frequency.

**Etiology:** Possibly autosomal recessive inheritance. Developmental problems in the fetus may also be a factor.

**Pathogenesis:** The anomaly occurs between the third and sixth weeks of fetal life. Obstruction due to vascular anomalies by compression of the esophagus, or failure of closure of the laryngotracheal groove are thought to be the cause.

**MIM No.:** 18996

**CDC No.:** 750.310

**Sex Ratio:** M1:F1

**Occurrence:** 1:3,000–5,000 live births. Occurrence of the various types of esophageal atresia with or without a fistula: distal fistula, 85–87%; upper fistula, 1–3%; double fistula, 1%; esophageal atresia without a fistula, 8%.

**Risk of Recurrence for Patient's Sib:** If parents are normal with one affected child, 1% risk for next child to be affected. If more than one child has the condition, risk for subsequent siblings increases to 20%.

**Risk of Recurrence for Patient's Child:** If one parent is affected, there is a 3.6% risk for the child.

**Age of Detectability:** Newborn period.

**Gene Mapping and Linkage:** Unknown.

**Prevention:** None known. Genetic counseling indicated.

**Treatment:** 1. Preoperative management includes an environment with temperature control for the infant, semi-Fowler position, sump catheter with constant suction of the upper pouch, intravenous therapy, and antibiotics. Identification of severe cyanotic congenital cardiac disease with possible cardiac shunt surgery before the esophageal repair may be necessary.

2. Immediate operative repair for any infant with a birth weight of over 2.5 kg without significant pneumonia or other major congenital anomalies. A right thoracotomy and an extrapleural dissection is performed, with suture ligation and division of the fistula with an end-to-end anastomosis of the two ends of the esophagus. Esophageal myotomies have been performed to increase the length of the esophagus when the distance is too great for a safe anastomosis.

3. Delayed primary repair is used in an infant with a birth weight of 4 to 5 1/2 lb who is well or in infants with a higher birth weight with pneumonia or congenital anomaly. Preoperative management is continued until the birth weight increases or the pneumonia or congenital anomaly is stabilized. A preoperative gastrostomy tube placed under a local anesthesia may be performed. The gastrostomy tube is not used for feeding. The tube is used to prevent reflux of gastric secretions into the lung. The infant may be fed using parenteral hyperalimentation or passing a tube through the gastrostomy into the duodenum.

4. Staged repair in an infant with a birth weight under 4 lb or a higher birth weight with severe pneumonia or severe congenital anomaly. Preoperative treatment is continued. A gastrostomy with or without division and ligation of a large fistula may be performed. If the fistula is large enough to cause severe gastric dilation and reflux into the lungs, this treatment would be appropriate. When the infant gains weight and the condition improves, a primary anastomosis is performed.

5. Treatment of the other congenital anomalies may be necessary in the newborn period, such as a colostomy for an imperforate anus.

6. Follow-up care of an esophageal repair includes esophagram 3 to 6 months after leaving the hospital and later if suggestion of gastroesophageal reflux, esophageal stricture, or any feeding difficulties occur.

**Prognosis:** Excellent. Complications of esophageal stricture or leak demands further care. The mortality in esophageal atresia surgery is related to the serious cardiac anomalies or when the esophageal repair is performed in a low-birth-weight infant or in an infant with pneumonia or serious congenital anomalies.

**Detection of Carrier:** Examination of relatives for evidence of this trait.

**References:**

David TJ, O'Callaghan SE: Esophageal atreasia in the southwest of England. J Med Genet; 1975; 12:1–11.

Van Staey M, et al.: Familial congenital esophageal atresia: personal case report and review of the literature. Hum Genet 1984; 66:260–266.

Evans JA, et al.: Tracheal agenesis and associated malformations. A comparison with a tracheoesophageal fistula and the VACTERL association. Am J Med Genet 1985; 21:21–34.

Randolph, AJ: Esophageal atresia and stenosis. In Welsh K, et al.: Pediatric surgery, ed 4. Chicago: Yearbook Medical, 1986:682–694.

BE049                                                    **Arthur S. Besser**

## ESOPHAGUS, CHALASIA                                     0366

**Includes:**
  Esophageal chalasia
  Gastroesophageal reflux without hiatus hernia
  Reflux, esophageal

**Excludes:**  Gastroesophageal reflux associated with hiatus hernia

**Major Diagnostic Criteria:**  Gastroesophageal reflux has been defined as the frequent passage of stomach contents into the esophagus. Gastroesophageal reflux can be demonstrated by barium contrast studies and by a gastric scintiscan. Barium studies can also exclude other mechanical causes for spitting up or vomiting, such as pyloric stenosis. Demonstration of acid reflux into the esophagus after an acid load (Tuttle test) is a more accurate measure of reflux than radiography. Extended esophageal pH monitoring is widely used and offers the advantages of prolonged observation. Upper endoscopy and esophageal biopsy are used to identify esophagitis occurring secondary to acid reflux.

**Clinical Findings:**  The "spitty baby" is a very common pediatric problem. The vast majority of infants outgrow their problem without complications. Spitting up or vomiting after a feeding is the most frequent symptom. The vomiting can sometimes be projectile. It is aggravated by lying recumbent, bouncing, or crying with a full stomach. Vomiting may also occur several hours after a feeding. Choking, coughing, or wheezing can occur either secondary to laryngospasm or from aspiration. Esophagitis from acid reflux can lead to irritability, occult bleeding and anemia, hematemesis, and esophageal stricture. Poor growth or failure to thrive can occur with massive esophageal reflux. If the infant is not vomiting large amounts of the daily feedings, other causes for poor growth need to be considered, even if gastroesophageal reflux is demonstrated. Gastroesophageal reflux has also been implicated as a possible cause of apnea and crib death.

**Complications:**  Complications are unusual. They can occur without overt vomiting or spitting up. The most frequent complications are choking, aspiration, and esophagitis. Apnea has also been demonstrated to occur with episodes of gastroesophageal reflux.

**Associated Findings:**  The most common associated condition is pylorospasm. Gastroesophageal reflux has also been associated with pyloric stenosis, slow gastric emptying, Sandifer syndrome (head tilt), and finger clubbing with protein-losing enteropathy.

**Etiology:**  Multifactorial. It is best viewed as the result of an incompetence of the lower esophageal sphincter mechanism.

**Pathogenesis:**  Werlin et al (1980) demonstrated that gastroesophageal reflux can occur with a low basal sphincter pressure, with inappropriate relaxation of the lower esophageal sphincter, or with an increase in abdominal pressure. In addition, the angle at which the esophagus enters the stomach, the ligamentous attachments to the diaphragm, and the H configuration of the collapsed distal esophagus may all play a role in preventing gastroesophageal reflux. How rapidly refluxed contents are cleared by the esophagus also play a role in the symptomatology.

**CDC No.:**  750.480

**Sex Ratio:**  M1:F1

**Occurrence:**  Undetermined but presumably common.

**Risk of Recurrence for Patient's Sib:**  Unknown.

**Risk of Recurrence for Patient's Child:**  Unknown.

**Age of Detectability:**  Newborn period.

**Gene Mapping and Linkage:**  Unknown.

**Prevention:**  None known. Genetic counseling indicated.

**Treatment:**  Primary treatment of gastroesophageal reflux consists of simple medical maneuvers. If these are unsuccessful and

the symptoms of gastroesophageal reflux are significant, pharmacologic agents can be tried. There is a greater experience with bethanechol in the treatment of pediatric gastroesophageal reflux, but metoclopramide has also been used. The effectiveness of these agents has not been clearly established, however. In the unusual situation where medical therapy is unsuccessful and the complications do not allow the patient to "outgrow" the reflux, an operative fundoplication can be performed. The success rate with the fundoplication is approximately 95%.

**Prognosis:**  The vast majority of infants and children will outgrow their gastroesophageal reflux as the lower esophageal sphincter mechanism "matures." The small minority of patients with persistent reflux may require fundoplication to prevent a late complication of esophageal stricture, estimated to occur in 5% of patients. The prognosis after surgical correction is excellent.

**Detection of Carrier:**  Unknown.

**References:**
Neuhauser EBD, Berenberg W: Cardioesophageal relaxation as a cause of vomiting in infants. Radiology 1947; 48:480.
Boix-Ochoa J, Canals J: Maturation of the lower esophagus. J Pediatr Surg 1976; 11:749.
Werlin SL, Dodds WS, Hogan WJ, Arndorfer RC: Mechanisms of gastroesophageal reflux in children. J Pediatr, 1980; 97:244.
Herbst JJ: Gastroesophageal reflux. J Pediatr 1981; 98:859.

R0055                                                **Charles C. Roberts**
AS000                                                 **Keith W. Ashcraft**

## ESOPHAGUS, DIVERTICULUM                                 0367

**Includes:**
  Esophageal diverticulum
  Pharyngoesophageal diverticulum
  True esophageal diverticulum

**Excludes:**
  Esophageal diverticula, pulsion or tension
  **Esophagus, duplication** (0368)
  Traumatic esophageal pseudodiverticulum

**Major Diagnostic Criteria:**  Dysphagia, regurgitation, and barium contrast study of the esophagus showing the diverticulum. Esophagoscopy can also document a diverticulum.

**Clinical Findings:**  Esophageal diverticula usually produce symptoms, at a very early age, of either esophageal obstruction or aspiration or obstruction of airway. Regurgitated food may be old and is unchanged by gastric acid. There may be a mass lesion visible in the neck if the diverticulum is high, or by chest X-ray if it is low. The obstructive symptoms at the thoracic inlet may be severe and are notably intermittent. Since the lesion makes aspiration easy, pneumonitis may be the prominent presenting feature. Barium swallow will often show contrast material in a pouch or external pressure on the esophagus if the pouch should be filled with food.

**Complications:**  Aspiration is the most common complication. Complete airway obstruction may occur. Starvation, a late complication, may result from neglect.

**Associated Findings:**  Gastroesophageal reflux may be present.

**Etiology:**  Undetermined. May be associated with the embryonic vacuolization of the esophageal wall.

**Pathogenesis:**  A true diverticulum is generally located in the upper one-third of the esophagus and contains mucosa, submucosa, and muscular coats, thus differentiating it from an acquired pulsion diverticulum. Obstruction secondary to a filled diverticulum produces the symptoms that call attention to the malformation. The diverticulum presumably enlarges through a process of stretching from entrapped secretions or fluid over a period of months or years.

**CDC No.:**  750.420

**Sex Ratio:**  Presumably M1:F1

**Occurrence:**  Undetermined but presumed rare.

**Risk of Recurrence for Patient's Sib:** Unknown.

**Risk of Recurrence for Patient's Child:** Unknown.

**Age of Detectability:** Infancy and early childhood.

**Gene Mapping and Linkage:** Unknown.

**Prevention:** None known. Genetic counseling indicated.

**Treatment:** Surgical excision is the only treatment of any benefit.

**Prognosis:** The prognosis is excellent, once surgical treatment has been carried out. While esophageal diverticula are extremely rare lesions, they may be fatal as a result of airway obstruction.

**Detection of Carrier:** Unknown.

**References:**
Ravitch MM: Diverticulum of the esophagus. In: Ravitch, et al., eds: Pediatric surgery. Chicago: Year Book Medical Publishers, 1979.
Othersen HB Jr: Esophageal lesions. In: Holder TM, Ashcraft KW, eds: Pediatric surgery. Philadelphia: W.B. Saunders, 1980.

R0055              **Charles C. Roberts**
AS000            **Keith W. Ashcraft**
H0013            **Thomas M. Holder**

## ESOPHAGUS, DUPLICATION         0368

**Includes:**
> Esophageal cyst
> Esophageal duplication
> Neurenteric cyst

**Excludes:**
> **Esophagus, diverticulum** (0367)
> **Lung, bronchogenic cyst** (2702)

**Major Diagnostic Criteria:** Wheezing is the most common symptom of esophageal duplication, presumably by producing pressure upon the airway. Dysphagia is the next most common complaint, although the duplication has to be massive before this will occur. Most duplications are discovered incidentally upon chest X-ray, when a mass is found in the mediastinum. Barium contrast study of the esophagus will show a smooth indentation of the esophageal lumen by the enlarged duplication. These may be located anywhere from the thoracic inlet to the diaphragm.

**Clinical Findings:** Respiratory distress, as a result of either partial obstruction of the esophagus or actual pressure upon the trachea, is the most frequent presenting complaint. Dysphagia is the next most common symptom. Occasionally, ulceration resulting in bleeding will be the presenting feature. A number of these lesions are incidental findings on chest X-rays, and on very careful questioning absolutely no symptoms can be elicited referable to the lesion. A duplication is generally found in the older child or adult and will appear on X-ray as a posterior, usually well-rounded, mediastinal mass. A smooth filling defect in the esophagus on barium study suggests extrinsic pressure.

**Complications:** Persistent wheezing is the most common complication. Anemia may be present because of ulceration of the mucosa overlying the duplication. Failure to thrive because of dysphagia may be noted.

**Associated Findings:** Abnormalities of the vertebral bodies can be found in association with neurenteric cyst. The second most common association is an additional duplication of the small intestine.

**Etiology:** Unknown.

**Pathogenesis:** It is suspected that vacuoles develop in the thickened endoderm of the primitive foregut and persist as a cystic duplication. Proof for this theory is lacking, but support is gained from the fact that a common muscular wall is shared by the true esophagus and by the duplicated segment. These lesions grow with the child, and most are separate, although rarely there may be a small communication with the esophageal lumen. They frequently fill with a thin fluid and gradually enlarge. The lining may occasionally contain respiratory epithelium. Most are

squamous lined, and all are located within the muscle of the esophageal wall.

**CDC No.:** 750.430

**Sex Ratio:** M1:F1

**Occurrence:** Unknown.

**Risk of Recurrence for Patient's Sib:** Unknown.

**Risk of Recurrence for Patient's Child:** Unknown.

**Age of Detectability:** In infancy.

**Gene Mapping and Linkage:** Unknown.

**Prevention:** None known. Genetic counseling indicated.

**Treatment:** Surgical excision is usually possible without much difficulty. Occasionally the lumen of the esophagus will be entered, and a temporary feeding gastrostomy may be indicated.

**Prognosis:** Excellent. Respiratory wheezing and dysphagia usually disappear very promptly.

**Detection of Carrier:** Unknown.

**References:**
Wrenn EL Jr: Alimentary tract duplications. In: Holder TM, Ashcraft KW, eds: Pediatric surgery. Philadelphia: W.B. Saunders, 1980:36.

R0055            **Charles C. Roberts**
AS000           **Keith W. Ashcraft**

## ESOPHAGUS, STENOSIS         0369

**Includes:**
> Diaphragm of esophagus, congenital
> Esophageal stenosis
> Esophageal stricture, congenital
> Esophageal web or veil

**Excludes:**
> Esophageal lesions, acquired
> Lower esophageal lesions such as Schatzke ring
> Strictures secondary to reflux esophagitis
> Upper esophageal web of Plummer-Vinson syndrome

**Major Diagnostic Criteria:** In order to establish the diagnosis, X-rays of an upper or middle stenotic esophageal lesion are necessary. Gastroesophageal reflux should not be present on X-ray or by pH measurement in the esophagus, or the lesion will probably be attributable to reflux esophagitis.

**Clinical Findings:** Neonatal dysphagia, coughing, and choking with feedings are manifestations of congenital esophageal stenosis.

**Complications:** Failure to thrive is the most common complication of this lesion. Aspiration may occur, and pneumonia may be the most common symptom. Rarely the child may reach the state at which solid food lodges in the narrowed area of the esophagus, which otherwise had gone unnoticed.

**Associated Findings:** None known.

**Etiology:** Probably the result of a developmental malformation of the esophagus. Since gastroesophageal reflux is so common in children there is a tendency to attribute any esophageal stenosis to this etiology. It is unlikely that gastroesophageal reflux would produce esophagitis and stricture in the newborn, since this usually occurs in the somewhat older child.

**Pathogenesis:** It has been postulated that most of these lesions occur at the point where the esophagus gives origin to the tracheobronchial tree, i.e., the bifurcation of the trachea. Esophageal stenosis is unusual, but the documented cases show a firm, fibrous ring or web of mucosa varying only in length. The obstruction results in dilation proximal to the stenosis with subsequent hypertrophy of the muscle.

**CDC No.:** 750.340

**Sex Ratio:** M1:F1

**Occurrence:** Unknown.

**Risk of Recurrence for Patient's Sib:** Unknown.

**Risk of Recurrence for Patient's Child:** Unknown.

**Age of Detectability:** Usually in the neonatal period.

**Gene Mapping and Linkage:** Unknown.

**Prevention:** None known. Genetic counseling indicated.

**Treatment:** Repeated dilatation may be effective, but local resection of the esophageal lesion with end-to-end anastomosis may be needed.

**Prognosis:** The prognosis is excellent once the condition is corrected.

**Detection of Carrier:** Unknown.

**References:**

Gross RE: Surgery of infancy and childhood. Philadelphia: W.B. Saunders, 1953.
Ashcraft KW, Holder TM: Lesions of the esophagus and stomach in infants and children. In: Practice of surgery. Hagerstown, Maryland: Harper & and Row, 1976.

AS000                                                    **Keith W. Ashcraft**

**Essential carpotarsal osteolysis**
*See OSTEOLYSIS, ESSENTIAL*
**Essential cryoglobulinemia, familial**
*See CRYOGLOBULINEMIA*
**Essential familial hyperlipemia**
*See HYPERCHYLOMICRONEMIA*
**Essential fructosuria**
*See FRUCTOSURIA*
**Essential hypercatobolism of C3**
*See COMPLEMENT COMPONENT 3, DEFICIENCY OF*
**Essential osteolysis-nephropathy**
*See OSTEOLYSIS, CARPAL-TARSAL AND CHRONIC PROGRESSIVE GLOMERULOPATHY*
**Estren-Dameshek variant of Fanconi anemia**
*See ANEMIA, HYPOPLASTIC CONGENITAL*
*also PANCYTOPENIA SYNDROME, FANCONI TYPE*
**ETF dehydrogenase, partial deficiencies of**
*See ACIDEMIA, ETHYLMALONIC-ADIPIC*
**ETF:ubiquinone oxidoreductase (ETF:QO) deficiency**
*See ACIDEMIA, GLUTARIC ACIDEMIA II*
**ETF:ubiquinone oxidoreductase, partial deficiencies of**
*See ACIDEMIA, ETHYLMALONIC-ADIPIC*
**Ethmocephaly**
*See CYCLOPIA*
*also HOLOPROSENCEPHALY*
**Ethylmalonic aciduria due to SCAD**
*See ACYL-CoA DEHYDROGENASE DEFICIENCY, SHORT CHAIN TYPE*
**Ethylmalonic-adipic aciduria**
*See ACIDEMIA, ETHYLMALONIC-ADIPIC*
**Etretinate, fetal effects of**
*See FETAL RETINOID SYNDROME*
**Eulenburg disease**
*See PARAMYOTONIA CONGENITA*
**Eunuchoidism, familial hypogonadotrophic**
*See HYPOGONADOTROPIC HYPOGONADISM*
**Euryopia**
*See EYE, HYPERTELORISM*
**Eustachian tube atresia**
*See EAR, EUSTACHIAN TUBE DEFECTS*
**Eustachian tube cysts**
*See EAR, EUSTACHIAN TUBE DEFECTS*
**Eustachian tube diverticuli**
*See EAR, EUSTACHIAN TUBE DEFECTS*
**Eustachian tube tumors**
*See EAR, EUSTACHIAN TUBE DEFECTS*
**Eversion of sacculus**
*See LARYNX, VENTRICLE PROLAPSE*
**Eversion of ventricle**
*See LARYNX, VENTRICLE PROLAPSE*
**Ewing sarcoma of bone**
*See CANCER, EWING SARCOMA*
**Exchondrosis of pinna**
*See EAR, EXCHONDROSIS*
**Exencephaly**
*See ANENCEPHALY*
**Exertional headache, benign**
*See MIGRAINE*

**Exomphalos-cleft palate**
*See CLEFT PALATE-OMPHALOCELE*
**Exomphalos-macroglossia-gigantism syndrome**
*See BECKWITH-WIEDEMANN SYNDROME*
**Exophytum type retinoblastoma**
*See RETINOBLASTOMA*
**Exostoses of external auditory canal**
*See EAR, EXOSTOSES*

---

## EXOSTOSES, MULTIPLE CARTILAGINOUS          0685

**Includes:**

Diaphyseal aclasis
Multiple cartilaginous exostoses
Multiple exostoses

**Excludes:**

**Dysplasia epiphysealis hemimelica** (0311)
**Enchondromatosis** (0345)
**Metachondromatosis** (0650)

**Major Diagnostic Criteria:** Cartilage-capped exostoses at site of actively growing bone.

**Clinical Findings:** Characterized by numerous cartilage-capped exostoses clustered around areas of actively growing bone. The most common sites of involvement are the juxtaepiphyseal areas of the tubular bones, ribs, pelvis, and scapula, while the vertebral bodies, the patella, and the skull are usually unaffected. Seventy-five percent of patients have recognizable bony deformities. Most commonly, these are forearm deformities (50%), bowed radius with shortened ulna (43%), valgus ankles (45%), short stature (41%), conical ulna (25%), genu valgum (21%), radiohumeral dislocation (8%), scoliosis (4%), pelvic deformities (4%), and thoracic deformities (3%). The short stature is mild and due to shortness of the lower limbs. The arm span is also decreased. Bony deformities occur in bones affected with exostoses and are thought to be due to a "squandering" of linear growth for lateral growth. Growth of the exostoses keeps pace with active skeletal growth by enchondral growth and ceases with calcification of the cartilage cap. On X-ray, an isolated exostosis jutting from the diaphyseal shaft or a characteristic club-shaped appearance may be observed. Bone scan may helpful in detecting malignant degeneration.

**Complications:** Vertebral exostoses may cause spinal cord compression; pelvic exostoses may cause urinary obstruction or fetal

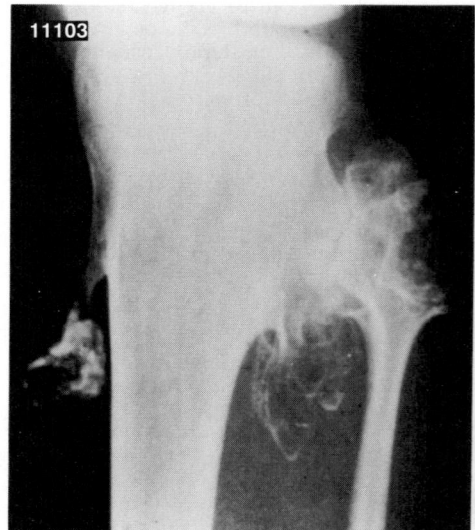
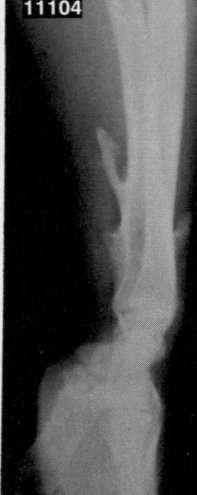

0685-11103–04:  Bony exostoses.

malposition; exostoses may be fractured and require removal; peripheral nerves and tendons may be compressed. Malignant degeneration may occur in about 10% of cases. Subcutaneous bursa may develop over the exostosis.

**Associated Findings:** Osteoma cutis, **Myositis ossificans progressiva, Turner syndrome, Chondroectodermal dysplasia, Parathormone resistance, Tricho-rhino-phalangeal syndrome, type II.**

**Etiology:** Autosomal dominant inheritance with complete penetrance. About 40% of cases are sporadic. The pattern of involvement with exostoses is usually not transmitted; offspring may not show the same distribution of the exostoses as their affected parent. Homozygosity results in increased number of lesions and rapid evolution.

**Pathogenesis:** On X-ray the lesions are initially recognized as an asymmetric or beaked overgrowth of the cortex immediately adjacent to the epiphyseal plate. Thereafter, this projection may be followed by normal bone growth, leaving an isolated exostosis jutting from the diaphyseal shaft, or an asymmetric increase in width may occur producing the characteristic club-shaped appearance. The exostosis, grossly and microscopically, is identical with the adjacent bone, with an outer cortex, inner marrow, and covering cartilage cap. Growth proceeds by enchondral ossification. The exostosis migrates with the diaphysis.

**MIM No.:** *13370

**POS No.:** 3184

**CDC No.:** 756.470

**Sex Ratio:** Presumably M1:F1, although earlier literature reported a male preponderance.

**Occurrence:** Krooth et al (1961) reported an incidence of 1:1,000 on Guam. Prevalence reported as 1:90,000 patient visits per year in a general hospital; 1:7,000 patient visits per year in an orthopedic hospital. No ethnic predisposition has been reported.

**Risk of Recurrence for Patient's Sib:**
See Part I, *Mendelian Inheritance.*

**Risk of Recurrence for Patient's Child:**
See Part I, *Mendelian Inheritance.*

**Age of Detectability:** At birth; 80% detected within the first decade of life.

**Gene Mapping and Linkage:** Unknown.

**Prevention:** None known. Genetic counseling indicated.

**Treatment:** Resection of exostoses, which interfere with movement, are painful, fractured, and compress nerves or tendons, or for cosmesis. Chondrosarcomas are resistant to radiotherapy and should be treated by surgical excision.

**Prognosis:** Normal life expectancy unless chondrosarcomas develop. Malignant degeneration has been reported to occur after trauma. Chondrosarcomas increase in size slowly and metastasize late.

**Detection of Carrier:** Unknown.

**References:**
Jaffe HL: Hereditary multiple exostoses. Arch Pathol 1943; 36:335.
Krooth RS, et al.: Diaphyseal aclasis (multiple exostoses) on Guam. Am J Hum Genet 1961; 13:340–347.
Solomon L: Hereditary multiple exostoses. Am J Hum Genet 1964; 16:351–363.
Lanzenskiold A: The development of multiple cartilaginous exostoses. Acta Orthop Scandinav 1967; 38:259.
Giedion A, et al.: The widened spectrum of multiple cartilaginous exostoses (MCE). Pediat Radiol 1975; 3:93.
Shapiro F, et al.: Hereditary multiple exostoses: anthropometric, roentgenographic and clinical aspects. J Bone Joint Dis 1979; 61A: 815.
Voutsinas S, Wynne-Davies R: The infrequency of malignant disease in diaphyseal aclasis and neurofibromatosis. J Med Genet 1983; 20:345–349.

LA006                                               **Ralph S. Lachman**

## EXOSTOSES-ANETODERMIA-BRACHYDACTYLY TYPE E                                    2764

**Includes:**
Anetodermia-exostoses-brachydactyly type E
Brachydactyly type E-Anetodermia-exostoses

**Excludes:**
**Exostoses, multiple cartilaginous** (0685)
**Macular coloboma-brachydactyly** (0621)
**Tricho-rhino-phalangeal syndrome, type II** (0967)

**Major Diagnostic Criteria:** The combination of anetodermia, multiple exostoses, and type E **Brachydactyly.**

**Clinical Findings:** Of ten affected family members, only two had all three findings of anetodermia (macular atrophy), multiple exostoses, and **Brachydactyly.** One or multiple exostoses were present in seven of ten individuals; these occurred between ages five and 33 years. Anetodermia were present in six individuals, and developed around ages 6–7 years. Histologically the epidermis was atrophic, whereas the dermis showed infiltration by mastocytes. Brachydactyly type E occurred in two individuals.

**Complications:** Unknown.

**Associated Findings:** None known.

**Etiology:** Autosomal dominant inheritance is suggested by the presence of the condition in three generations of one family.

**Pathogenesis:** Mollica et al. (1984) suggested that the main effect was on tissues of mesodermal origin.

**MIM No.:** 13369, 25045

**POS No.:** 3202

**CDC No.:** 756.470

**Sex Ratio:** Presumably M1:F1.

**Occurrence:** Reported in three generations of one family from Sicily.

**Risk of Recurrence for Patient's Sib:**
See Part I, *Mendelian Inheritance.*

**Risk of Recurrence for Patient's Child:**
See Part I, *Mendelian Inheritance.*

**Age of Detectability:** At birth by the presence of brachydactyly; otherwise, ages 5–33 years.

**Gene Mapping and Linkage:** Unknown.

**Prevention:** None known. Genetic counseling indicated.

**Treatment:** Supportive.

**Prognosis:** Life span and intellectual development appear to be unaffected.

**Detection of Carrier:** Unknown.

**Special Considerations:** Anetoderma was also seen in two Egyptian sisters with metaphyseal dysplasia and optic atrophy (Temtamy SA, et al, 1974).

**References:**
Temtamy SA, et al.: Metaphyseal dysplasia, anetoderma and optic atrophy: an autosomal recessive syndrome. In: Bergsma D, ed: Skeletal dysplasias. Amsterdam: Excerpta Medica, 1974:61–71.
Mollica F, et al.: New syndrome: exostoses, anetodermia, brachydactyly. Am J Med Genet 1984; 19:665–667.

T0007                                               **Helga V. Toriello**

**Expanded rubella syndrome**
*See FETAL RUBELLA SYNDROME*
**Exstrophia splanchnica**
*See EXSTROPHY OF CLOACA SEQUENCE*

## EXSTROPHY OF CLOACA SEQUENCE                    3193

**Includes:**
    Cloacal exstrophy
    Exstrophia splanchnica
    Omphalocele-exstrophy-imperforate anus-spina bifida
        (OEIS)

**Excludes:**
    **Bladder exstrophy** (3015)
    **Colon, atresia or stenosis** (0193)
    **Epispadias** (2008)

**Major Diagnostic Criteria:** Exstrophy of the bladder with intestinal epithelium between the hemibladders, phallic separation with epispadias, separation of the pubic arch anteriorly, and rudimentary hindgut with imperforate anus.

**Clinical Findings:** Exstrophy of the cloaca represents the most severe manifestation of the epispadias-exstrophy spectrum of ventral body wall defects (See **Epispadias** and **Bladder exstrophy**). The anomaly resembles classical bladder exstrophy on initial inspection, but the defect is more extensive and much more complex. Laterally are hemibladders with the posterior mucosal wall of the bladders exposed. Intervening is a strip of intestinal mucosa. The distal ileum, often prolapsed, opens to the surface at the cephalad margin of this strip and a blind segment of colon opens at the caudal margin. One or more vermiform appendices may open on the intestinal epithelium. The anorectal region is absent (See **Colon, atresia or stenosis**). In both male and female patients, the phallus is bifid and the pubic rami are widely separated. The ureteral orifices are located low on the lateral bladder mucosa. In the female, the uterus is frequently bicornuate and the vagina is duplex ending blindly or as orifices on the bladder mucosa. Some 90% of patients have an associated

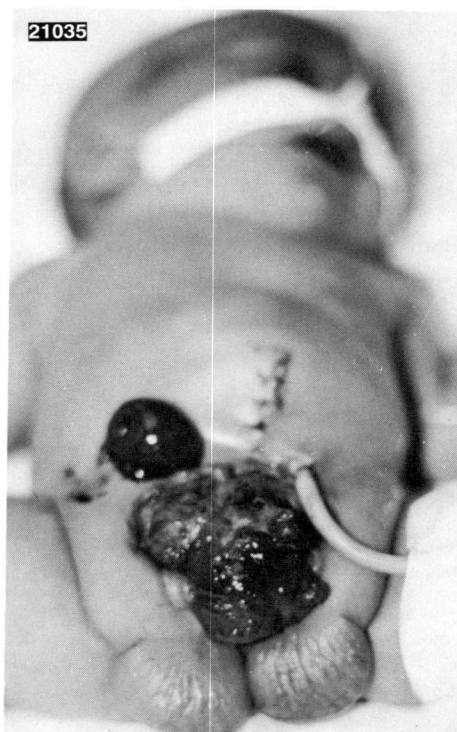

**3193-21035:** Exstrophy of the cloaca. An omphalocele has been repaired and a colostomy placed. Note the exposed bladder mucosa and bifid penis and scrotum.

**Omphalocele,** while spinal dysraphism with or without **Meningomyelocele** is present in 40%. Other commonly associated abnormalities include upper urinary tract anomalies, single umbilical artery, and lower limb defects.

**Complications:** Fluid loss, electrolyte imbalance, and infection (especially in the presence of an omphalocele) are immediate and life-threatening complications. Additional complications include short gut syndrome, fecal and or urinary incontinence, chronic urinary tract infection, vesicoureteral reflux, hydronephrosis, neurologic impairment secondary to neural tube defects, musculoskeletal abnormalities secondary to vertebral defects, and difficulties with social adjustment. There is an increased potential for malignant changes in the exstrophic bladder mucosa.

**Associated Findings:** Congenital hip dislocation, cryptorchidism, **Colon, duplication,** congenital heart defects.

**Etiology:** Unknown. All cases have been sporadic.

**Pathogenesis:** The embryology of exstrophy of the cloaca has not been clearly determined. There are several embryologic failures that must be explained: failure of separation of the gastrointestinal and genitourinary tracts, failure of closure of the anterior body wall, and failure of formation of the distal midgut and distal colon.

Normally, at approximately the seventh week of gestation, the urorectal septum divides the cloaca into an anterior urogenital sinus and a posterior anorectal canal by migrating caudally to fuse with the cloacal membrane. The divided cloacal membrane ruptures forming the urethral and anal orifices. The infraumbilical abdominal wall is postulated to form by mesodermal ingrowth between the ectodermal and endodermal layers of the cloacal membrane.

In exstrophy of the cloaca, a disturbance of the normal process probably occurs during the fifth week of gestation before descent of the urorectal septum and before fusion of the genital tubercles has taken place. Various proposed etiologies include abnormal or arrested mesodermal ingrowth leading to an unstable cloacal membrane which ruptures prematurely and abnormal growth and persistence of the cloacal membrane producing a wedge effect which inhibits the medial migration of mesoderm to form the infraumbilical wall. Thomalla and coworkers have produced cloacal exstrophy by $CO_2$ laser injury to the tail bud region of the chick embryo. They postulated that exstrophy of the cloaca is produced by the untimely rupture of the cloacal membrane, perhaps secondary to an ischemic insult.

Although herniation of hindgut between the hemibladders and foregut and or midgut into an omphalocele can be explained as the result of intra-abdominal pressure, other bowel abnormalities are more difficult to explain. Rectal or hindgut atresia may be secondary to vascular insufficiency since frequently the inferior mesenteric artery is absent. Abnormal mechanical stress on the vasculature from anterior herniation of abdominal contents may be a factor. Malformations of the midgut, namely absence of the ileum and proximal colon, have not been satisfactorily explained. The intestinal portion interposed between the hemibladders is usually cecum which leads to tethering of the ileocecal loop and again possible vascular compromise. Zarabi and Rupani (1986) proposed a dual origin of the midgut from both yolk sac and allantois with the allantois contributing the distal limb of the midgut. Accordingly, abnormalities of the allantois may lead to failure of ascent and alignment with the yolk sac. The allantois then persists as an underdeveloped limb of midgut which can impede the caudal migration of the urorectal septum. There is pathologic evidence to support this hypothesis in at least one case.

**Sex Ratio:** Previously assumed to be M1:F1, several large series have now reported a male preponderance of M2:F1.

**Occurrence:** The incidence is 1:200,000 to 1:250,000 live births.

**Risk of Recurrence for Patient's Sib:** Presumably not increased.

**Risk of Recurrence for Patient's Child:** Unknown. There are no reports of reproduction.

**Age of Detectability:** The diagnosis in a fetus should be suspected whenever there is an elevated maternal serum or amniotic fluid alpha-fetoprotein and presence of an acetylcholinesterase isozyme in the amniotic fluid in addition to absence of an identifiable bladder with or without presence of an omphalocele by ultrasonography.

**Gene Mapping and Linkage:** Unknown.

**Prevention:** None known. Genetic counseling indicated.

**Treatment:** Treatment goals include preservation of renal function, management of shortened bowel, control of urinary and fecal incontinence, reconstruction of the abdominal wall and genitalia, and management of neurologic and or musculoskeletal abnormalities. Gender assignment should be made early, and needs to be based on the size and status of the phallus.

Surgical reconstruction is performed in stages with immediate attention given to closure of an omphalocele or neural tube defect. The first stage also includes separation of the gastrointestinal tract from the bladder with creation of an ileostomy or colostomy. Bladder closure may be performed initially or as a delayed procedure in conjunction with bilateral iliac osteotomies; early closure in the first 2–3 days of life is preferred. Further stages include bladder neck reconstruction, antireflux procedures such as ureteral reimplant, and finally, genital reconstruction.

**Prognosis:** The mortality rate has decreased from 100% to less than 50% in the years following the first successful surgical correction in 1960. Urinary continence of 3–4 hours duration has been achieved in some patients and with newly-developed surgical methods, there is hope for fecal continence. There is an increased risk for deterioration of the upper urinary tract due to chronic infection and vesicoureteral reflux and a small but definitely increased risk for malignant change in the exstrophic bladder.

**Detection of Carrier:** Unknown.

**Special Considerations:** The major goal of management is survival with achievement of acceptable social interaction. With the continually improving surgical techniques now in use, the potential for functional and productive lives is high. However, management of this problem is difficult and is best approached by a multispecialty team with continued support and encouragement for the parents as well as the patient. Initial gender assignment should be given careful consideration since more than 80% of genetic males with this condition have phalluses that cannot be made functionally adequate. Most XY males should be given a female gender assignment, appropriate reconstruction of the genitalia, and bilateral orchiectomy.

**References:**
Flanigan RC, et al: Cloacal exstrophy. Urology 1984; 23:227–233. *
Diamond DA, Jeffs RD: Cloacal exstrophy: a 22-year experience. J Urol 1985; 133:779–782. *
Thomalla JV, et al: Induction of cloacal exstrophy in the chick embryo using the $CO_2$ laser. J Urol 1985; 134:991–995.
Zarabi CM, Rupani M: A hypothesis on the allantoic origin of the distal midgut. Anat Rec 1986; 215:65–70.
Jeffs RD: Exstrophy, epispadias, and cloacal and urogenital sinus abnormalities. Pediatr Clin North Am 1987; 34:1233–1257.

M0039
WE005

**Cynthia A. Moore
David D. Weaver**

**Exstrophy of the bladder**
  See BLADDER EXSTROPHY
**Extensor pollicis brevis or longus**
  See THUMB, CLASPED
**Extensor pollicis longus, congenital absence of**
  See THUMB, CLASPED
**External ophthalmoplegia congenita**
  See OPHTHALMOPLEGIA, FAMILIAL STATIC
**External ophthalmoplegia-myopia**
  See OPHTHALMOPLEGIA EXTERNA-MYOPIA
**Extraadenoidal cysts**
  See NASOPHARYNGEAL CYSTS
**Extracardiac shunt to proximal pulmonary artery**
  See AORTA, ISOLATION OF SUBCLAVIAN ARTERY FROM AORTA
**Extrahepatic biliary atresia-discontinuity of bile duct**
  See BILIARY ATRESIA

**Extraocular muscles, congenital fibrosis**
  See EYE, FIBROSIS OF THE EXTRAOCULAR MUSCLES, GENERALIZED
**Extraocular muscular dystrophy, progressive**
  See OPHTHALMOPLEGIA, PROGRESSIVE EXTERNAL
**Extremities (malformed)-craniocynostosis-cleft lip/palate**
  See HERRMANN-PALLISTER-OPITZ SYNDROME
**Exudative detachment of retina, central**
  See RETINA, MACULAR DEGENERATION, VITELLIRUPTIVE
**Exudative vitreoretinopathy**
  See RETINA, VITREORETINOPATHY, FAMILIAL EXUDATIVE
**Eye (Peters anomaly) associated with short-limbed dwarfism**
  See DWARFISM (SHORT LIMBED)-PETERS ANOMALY OF THE EYE
**Eye anomalies-dwarfism-stiff joints**
  See DWARFISM-STIFF JOINTS
**Eye defects-diffuse renal mesangial sclerosis**
  See RENAL MESANGIAL SCLEROSIS-EYE DEFECTS
**Eye movement disorder**
  See BROWN SYNDROME
  also EYE, DUANE RETRACTION SYNDROME
**Eye, absent**
  See EYE, ANOPHTHALMIA
**Eye, Aland disease**
  See FORSIUS-ERIKSSON SYNDROME
**Eye, anisocoria**
  See PUPIL, ANISOCORIA

## EYE, ANISOMETROPIA                                         0059

**Includes:**
  Anisometropia
  Berg syndrome
  Hyperopia (bilateral) with marked difference between eyes
  Hyperopia, unilateral
  Myopia (bilateral) with marked difference between eyes
  Myopia, unilateral

**Excludes:**
  Lens, aphakia (0084)
  Cornea plana (0205)
  Eye, keratoconus (0552)
  Glaucoma, congenital (0414)
  Microphthalmos, unilateral
  Tumors distorting shape of eyeball
  Unilateral refractive error secondary to disease

**Major Diagnostic Criteria:** Usually a difference of 1.50 diopters by spherical equivalent will be symptomatic. However, large unilateral astigmatic errors can induce amblyopia despite little or no difference in the spherical equivalents of the two eyes.

**Clinical Findings:** A child with anisometropia may be amblyopic; this form of amblyopia is most often detected with preschool vision screening. The degree of amblyopia is proportional to the difference between the two eyes. Older patients may complain of visual fatigue.

**Complications:** Amblyopia; strabismus, due to suppression of the eye by the CNS; Aniseikonia (the difference in size of retinal images), and resultant loss of fine depth perception; Visual fatigue (asthenopia).

**Associated Findings:** Myelinated nerve fibers in highly myopic eyes, which is associated with a worse prognosis for vision. Small hyperemic disc in a highly hyperopic eye, but function is usually normal.

**Etiology:** The difference in refractive error is largely due to a difference in the axial length of the eye rather than differences in the lens power or corneal curvature. The cause of a difference in growth of the two eyes without other pathology is unknown. Examples of apparent autosomal dominant and autosomal recessive inheritance have been reported.

**Pathogenesis:** Structural weakness of the sclera in resisting intraocular pressure may be a cause.

**Sex Ratio:** M1:F1

**Occurrence:** Undetermined but apparently uncommon.

**Risk of Recurrence for Patient's Sib:**
See Part I, *Mendelian Inheritance*.

**Risk of Recurrence for Patient's Child:**
See Part I, *Mendelian Inheritance*.

**Age of Detectability:** Many cases are probably congenital. Differential growth could occur in infancy; the eye grows most rapidly in the first 18 months of life.

**Gene Mapping and Linkage:** Unknown.

**Prevention:** None known. Genetic counseling indicated.

**Treatment:** Correcting the refractive error, if done early enough, can prevent amblyopia. If amblyopia and/or strabismus have developed, earlier treatment is more successful. Scleral reinforcement for high myopia is controversial.

**Prognosis:** Less favorable for vision with a more severe refractive error, and presence of strabismus. Myelinated nerve fibers are associated with least favorable prognosis.

**Detection of Carrier:** By eye examination.

**Special Considerations:** Many pathologic conditions and syndromes can cause anisometropia. The complications listed above compound the visual loss caused by these conditions.

**References:**
Francois J: Refraction errors. In: Heredity in ophthalmology. St. Louis: CV Mosby, 1961. *
Waardenburg PJ, et al.: Genetics in ophthalmology. Oxford: Blackwell Scientific Publications, 1961.
Kivlin J, Flynn JT: Therapy of anisometropic amblyopia. J Pediatr Ophthalmol 1981; 19:47–56.
Ellis GS, et al.: Myelinated nerve fibers, axial myopia, and refractory amblyopia. J Pediat Ophthalmol Strabism 1987; 24:111–119.

KI021                                    **Jane D. Kivlin**

## EYE, ANOPHTHALMIA               0067

**Includes:**
    Anophthalmia, clinical
    Anophthalmos, true or primary
    Eye, absent

**Excludes:**
    Anophthalmia, degenerative or consecutive
    **Anophthalmia-limb anomalies** (3172)
    **Anophthalmia-limb defects, Waardenburg type** (2784)
    **Eye, microphthalmia/coloboma** (0661)
    Secondary anophthalmia
    Surgical anophthalmia

**Major Diagnostic Criteria:** Anophthalmia, strictly speaking, means the total absence of eye tissue. This is rare. It occurs if there is complete failure of formation of the primary optic vesicle, in which case it is called a true or primary anophthalmia. It is usually bilateral. Only upon histologic examination of the entire orbital contents can the absence of all ocular tissue be ascertained. Anophthalmia is observed clinically and is confirmed by microscopic examination.

**Clinical Findings:** The ocular adnexa are usually present, structurally intact, but smaller than normal. Tears are produced upon crying from functionally normal lacrimal glands. The orbit is shallow and lined with conjunctiva. The ophthalmic artery is the only structure ordinarily observed to course through the underdeveloped optic foramen.

**Complications:** Complete loss of vision in the affected eye.

**Associated Findings:** Chromosomal aberrations (e.g., **Chromosome 13, trisomy 13**), developmental disturbances including absence of the optic nerves and chiasm, rudimentary optic tracts, gliotic lateral goniculus, thinned calcarine cortex, absent lacrimal puncta, ankyloblepharon, microphthalmia of opposite eye, malformations of the brain, face, and limbs (for a discussion of "crooked fingers" see **Anophthalmia-limb defects, Waardenburg type**), posterior orbital encephalocele, and congenital cyst of the orbit; also seen in the Villaret and Weyers-Thier oculovertebral

syndromes, and in **Klinefelter syndrome**, and other complex malformation syndromes.

**Etiology:** Autosomal recessive inheritance, usually in association with consanguinity. In conjunction with other defects it can be transmitted as an autosomal dominant, X-linked recessive, or is found sporadically with a chromosomal aberration. It has also been found in association with drugs, vitamin A deficiency, and congenital infections, such as cytomegalovirus, within the third trimester of gestation.

**Pathogenesis:** Ectodermal elements of the eye are missing; minute traces of mesodermal elements may be present. Lack of differentiation of the optic plate following the development of the rudimentary forebrain, which results in failure of formation of the optic vesicle. One theory postulates pressure upon the head of the embryo by thickened amnion with suppression of growth of the optic vesicles.

**MIM No.:** *20690

**CDC No.:** 743.000

**Sex Ratio:** M1:F1

**Occurrence:** Several pedigrees reported.

**Risk of Recurrence for Patient's Sib:**
See Part I, *Mendelian Inheritance*.

**Risk of Recurrence for Patient's Child:**
See Part I, *Mendelian Inheritance*.

**Age of Detectability:** At birth.

**Gene Mapping and Linkage:** Unknown.

**Prevention:** None known. Genetic counseling indicated.

**Treatment:** Cosmetic improvement can rarely be achieved through progressive dilatation of the orbit by successive implants of increasingly larger size during the period of rapid growth for proper development and for maintenance of a prosthesis. Surgical reconstruction of the socket as necessary.

**Prognosis:** Good when defect is isolated; dependent upon the severity of the coexistent findings when part of other syndromes.

**Detection of Carrier:** Unknown.

**References:**
Joseph R: A pedigress of anophthalmos. Brit J Ophthal 1957; 41:541–543.
Roy FH: Cosmetic treatment of bilateral anophthalmos. Am J Ophthalmol 1969; 67:580.
Fargueta JS, et al.: Posterior orbital encephalocele with anophthalmos and other brain malformations. J Neurosurg 1973; 38:215.
Welter DA, et al.: Klinefelter's syndrome with anophthalmos. Am J Ophthalmol 1974; 77:895.
McCarthy RW, et al.: Anophthalmia and cytomegalovirus. Am J Ophthalmol 1980; 90:558.
Brunquell PJ, et al.: Sex-linked hereditary bilateral anophthalmos. Arch Ophthalmol 1984; 102:108.

RA004                                  **Elsa K. Rahn**

## EYE, ANTERIOR SEGMENT DYSGENESIS      0439

**Includes:**
    Anterior chamber cleavage syndrome
    Congenital anterior staphyloma
    Dysgenesis mesostromal
    Goniodysgenesis
    Hypodontia-mesoectodermal dysgenesis of iris and cornea
    Iridocorneal mesodermal dysgenesis
    Iridogoniodysgenesis
    Mesoectodermal dysgenesis of anterior segment
    Mesoectodermal dysgenesis of iris and cornea
    Peters anomaly
    Peters plus
    Posterior embryotoxon
    Posterior marginal dysplasia of cornea

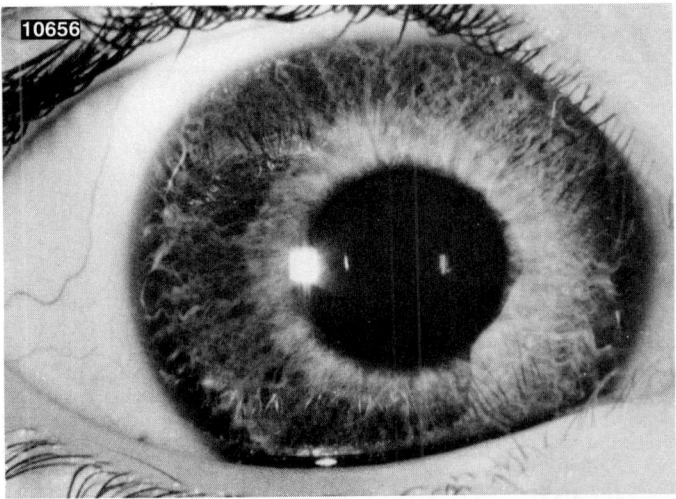

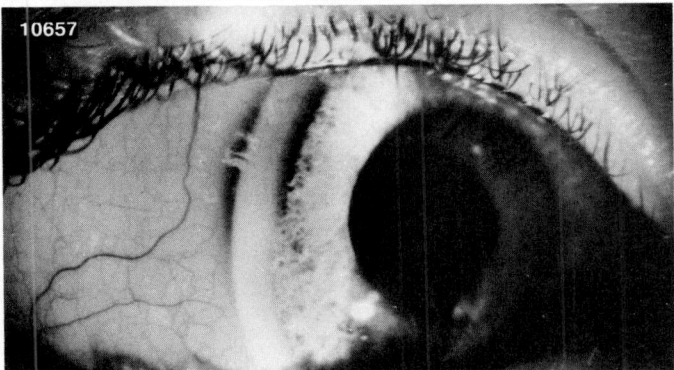

**0439-10656—57:** Slit-lamp examination of the cornea shows hypoplasia of the anterior stromal leaf of the cornea, trabecular iris adhesions, anterior displacement and thickening of Schwalbe ring.

**Excludes:**
   **Aortc stenosis-corneal clouding-growth and mental retardation** (2819)
   **Dwarfism (short limbed)-Peters anomaly of the eye** (2812)
   Essential iris atrophy
   **Glaucoma, congenital** (0414)
   **Ophthalmo-mandibulo-melic dwarfism** (3259)
   Polycoria
   **Rieger syndrome** (2139)

**Major Diagnostic Criteria:** The congenital presence of some degree of mesodermal dysplasia of the anterior ocular segment. The least severe form is merely the presence of posterior embryotoxon.

**Clinical Findings:** This congenital defect represents a mesodermal dysplasia of the anterior ocular segment. It may present as any one of several forms depending upon the severity of the dysplasia; hence the confusion of the appropriate term to apply. Goniodysgenesis is suggested as the most useful term.

*Posterior embryotoxon* is the mildest form in which there is an unusual prominence and forward displacement of the Schwalbe line, which stands out like an encircling glass rod inside the limbus. This can easily be seen by external inspection or slit-lamp examination and it is estimated to be present to some degree in 15% of individuals. When dense bands of iris tissue extend and attach to this posterior embryotoxon, it is referred to as the Axenfeld anomaly.

*Peters anomaly* is the term most frequently used when the mesodermal dysgenesis of the anterior ocular segment includes a central corneal stromal opacity with a defect in the posterior stroma and the Descemet membrane.

*Congenital anterior staphyloma* is a severe degree of the entity in which there is disorganization of the anterior chamber with a staphylomatous opaque cornea. These eyes usually have severe glaucoma and eventually become atrophic.

**Complications:** Glaucoma, cataracts, subluxated or dislocated lenses, opacification of cornea, phthisis bulbi.

**Associated Findings:** Dental anomalies, short stature, abdominal wall, skeletal and cardiovascular malformations. Myopathies and mental retardation may also occur. Some families have consistent associations of eye defects with specific malformations.

*Peters plus* consists of Peters' anomaly, short stature, brachymorphy, mental retardation, abnormal ears, and cheilo(gnatho)palatoschisis (Van Schooneveld et al, 1984). Autosomal recessive inheritance is presumed. Cases described by Kivlin et al (1986) and Thompson and Winter (1988) (see **Dwarfism (short limbed)-Peters anomaly of the eye**) are thought to be a different disorder by these authors.

**Etiology:** Autosomal dominant inheritance in many cases, often with extreme variability in expression. One member of a family may have a severe form whereas only minimal signs will be present in another family member. Some cases are associated with chromosomal aberrations, and Peters plus appears to be transmitted through autosomal recessive inheritance.

**Pathogenesis:** Presumed to be a developmental aberration of the mesodermal and possibly ectodermal germ layers of the anterior ocular segment.

**MIM No.:** *10725

**CDC No.:** 743.480

**Sex Ratio:** M1:F1

**Occurrence:** Undetermined but presumed rare.

**Risk of Recurrence for Patient's Sib:**
   See Part I, *Mendelian Inheritance.*

**Risk of Recurrence for Patient's Child:**
   See Part I, *Mendelian Inheritance.*

**Age of Detectability:** At birth.

**Gene Mapping and Linkage:** ASMD (anterior segment mesenchymal dysgenesis) has been provisionally mapped to 4q.

**Prevention:** None known. Genetic counseling indicated.

**Treatment:** Control of glaucoma, cataract extraction, corneal transplant, enucleation to relieve pain or cosmesis.

**Prognosis:** Normal for life span and intelligence; poor for vision only in severe cases, especially in Peters anomaly.

**Detection of Carrier:** Unknown.

**References:**
Alkemade PPH: Dysgenesis mesodermalis of the iris and cornea. Springfield: Charles C Thomas, 1969:95.
Waring GO, et al.: Anterior chamber cleavage syndrome: a stepladder classification. Surv Ophthalmol 1975; 20:3–27. *
Van Schooneveld MJ, et al.: Peters' Plus: a new syndrome. Ophthalm Paediatr Genet 1984; 3:141–146.
Kivlin JD, et al.: Peters' anomaly as a consequence of genetic and nongenetic syndromes. Arch Ophthalmol 1986; 104:61–54.

HA041

**David J. Harris**
*Morton E. Smith*

## EYE, CARUNCLE ABERRATIONS 0130

**Includes:**
Caruncle aberrations
Caruncle, absence of
Caruncle, hypoplasia of
Caruncle, hyperplasia of
Caruncle, notch or cleavage of
Caruncle, supernumerary

**Excludes:**
Caruncle, melanosis of
Cysts, orbital and periorbital dermoid

**Major Diagnostic Criteria:** Anatomic variation from normal caruncle.

**Clinical Findings:** The caruncle is the round mass of opaque pink tissue at the inner canthus that contains sebaceous, sweat, and lacrimal glands, as well as small hairs. Anomalies are congenital, but may not be detected for years.

**Complications:** Hairs on abnormal caruncular tissue occasionally irritate the eye. Absence or hypoplasia usually occurs in association with other congenital anomalies, such as ptosis and epicanthus, **Waardenburg syndromes**, **Anophthalmia-limb anomalies**, coloboma of the lid, or abnormal extraocular muscles. Cleavage of the caruncle has occurred in association with **Mandibulofacial dysostosis**.

**Associated Findings:** Anomalies of the adjacent semilunar fold of the conjunctiva, but not with anomalies of the lacrimal system.

**Etiology:** Unknown.

**Pathogenesis:** The caruncle develops as an outgrowth from the posterior surface of the lower lid and is first visible in an embryo of 57mm crown-rump length.

**Sex Ratio:** Presumably M1:F1

**Occurrence:** Undetermined but apparently rare.

**Risk of Recurrence for Patient's Sib:** Unknown.

**Risk of Recurrence for Patient's Child:** Unknown.

**Age of Detectability:** At birth, although frequently unnoticed initially.

**Gene Mapping and Linkage:** Unknown.

**Prevention:** None known. Genetic counseling indicated.

**Treatment:** Surgical repair.

**Prognosis:** Nonprogressive.

**Detection of Carrier:** Unknown.

**Special Considerations:** The caruncle and plica semilunaris correspond to the nictitating membrane found in many animals.

**References:**
Waardenburg PJ, et al.: Genetics in ophthalmology. Oxford: Blackwell Scientific Publications, 1961.*
Mansour K, van Bijsterveld OP: Supernumerary caruncle: report of a case. Ann Ophthalmol 1984; 16:677–678.

KI021 **Jane D. Kivlin**

**Eye, cataracts**
*See CATARACTS*

## EYE, CRYPTOPHTHALMOS WITH OTHER MALFORMATIONS 0003

**Includes:**
Ablepharon
Cryptophthalmos
Eyelid, absent

**Excludes:**
**Eyelid, ankyloblepharon** (0060)
**Cryptophthalmos syndrome, Fraser type** (2271)

**Major Diagnostic Criteria:** Absence or complete fusion of eyelid.

**Clinical Findings:** In the most severe form bilateral absence of eyelids occurs without recognizable differentiation of the lids and its associated lashes and brows. The skin of the forehead and face are fused with an occasionally visible horizontal line within the area of the absent eyelids. In its less severe form ablepharon may be unilateral, or incomplete, in which case only the upper or lower lid is lacking.

**Complications:** Unknown.

**Associated Findings:** Lid colobomas in unilateral involvement, absent lacrimal glands, ocular deformities such as anophthalmos, microphthalmos and anterior segment abnormalities, dermoids, cleft lip and palate, umbilical hernia, ear and nose aberrations, laryngeal atresia, syndactyly, urogenital malformations, ventral hernias, meningoencephalocele, basal encephalocele, tricuspid atresia, ventricular and atrial septal defects, transposition of great vessels, right aortic arch and aberrant right subclavian artery have been reported.

**Etiology:** Autosomal recessive inheritance. Sporadic cases have been reported.

**Pathogenesis:** Possibly agenesis from a primary failure in induction, or secondary to abnormal intrauterine factors such as increased amniotic pressure causing localized obstruction, or response to infectious or other teratogenic substances.

**MIM No.:** *21900

**POS No.:** 3179

**CDC No.:** 743.630

**Sex Ratio:** M1:F1

**Occurrence:** About 100 cases reported.

**Risk of Recurrence for Patient's Sib:**
See Part I, *Mendelian Inheritance.*

**Risk of Recurrence for Patient's Child:**
See Part I, *Mendelian Inheritance.*

**Age of Detectability:** At birth.

**Gene Mapping and Linkage:** Unknown.

**Prevention:** None known. Genetic counseling indicated.

**Treatment:** If laryngeal atresia is present, immediate tracheotomy for relief of airway obstruction. Surgical restoration of existing anatomy of eyelids in partial cases, protection against exposure and further destruction of remaining eye structures, cosmetic and functional repair of other malformations are indicated.

**Prognosis:** Poor for vision on affected side. Life expectancy related to severity of associated anomalies.

**Detection of Carrier:** Unknown.

**References:**
Gorlin RJ, Cervenka J: Syndromes of facial clefting. Scand J Plast Reconstr Surg 1974; 8:13.
Goldhammer Y, Smith JL: Cryptophthalmos syndrome with basal encephalocele. Am J Ophthalmol 1975; 80:146.
Thomas, IT, et al.: Isolated and syndromic cryptophthalmos. Am J Med Genet 1986; 25:85–98. *

RA004 **Elsa K. Rahn**

## EYE, DERMOLIPOMA             0284

**Includes:**
    Dermatolipoma
    Dermolipoma
    Lipodermoid

**Excludes:**
    **Lipomas, familial symmetric** (0600)
    **Ocular dermoids** (0591)
    **Orbital and periorbital dermoid cysts** (0761)

**Major Diagnostic Criteria:** Clinical diagnosis based on presence of subconjunctival tumor on superotemporal aspect of globe. Histopathologic features are consistent with a choristoma comprised predominantly of fat and a variable amount of squamous epithelium and dermal appendages.

**Clinical Findings:** Dermolipoma is a subconjunctival tumor, yellowish-pink in color, with a smooth surface located on the superotemporal aspect of the globe. Besides the visible anterior component, they have a posterior component which interdigitates with the levator palpebrae and recti muscles. Most dermolipomas are detected soon after birth as unilateral or bilateral masses. Presence of dermal appendages, particularly attached hairs, are characteristic. As a rule, the unsightly appearance of the tumor is the only symptom.

**Complications:** On occasion enlargement of the tumor or presence of attached hairs may cause irritation of the external eye.

**Associated Findings:** **Oculo-auriculo-vertebral anomaly**.

**Etiology:** Sporadic.

**Pathogenesis:** Ectopic overgrowth of tissues usually found at the interface of ectoderm and mesoderm.

**Sex Ratio:** M1:F1

**Occurrence:** Comprise less then 1% of orbital tumors.

**Risk of Recurrence for Patient's Sib:** Unknown.

**Risk of Recurrence for Patient's Child:** Unknown.

**Age of Detectability:** Soon after birth.

**Gene Mapping and Linkage:** Unknown.

**Prevention:** None known. Genetic counseling indicated.

**Treatment:** No treatment is necessary in most cases. Surgical excision is recommended when the tumor creates a significant cosmetic blemish or it incites irritation of the external eye.

**Prognosis:** No visual impairment. Normal life expectancy.

**Detection of Carrier:** Unknown.

**Special Considerations:** Should be distinguished from ectopic lacrymal gland which is usually unilateral and has a lobulated appearance and prolapsed orbital fat which is an acquired defect without attached dermal appendages.

**References:**
Duke-Elder S: System of ophthalmology, vol. 3, Congenital deformities. London: Henry Kimpton, 1964:823.
Crawford JC: Conjunctival tumors. In: Duane TD, ed: Clinical ophthalmology, vol. 4. Hagerstown, MD: Harper & Row, 1986. *

WE035                          **Avery H. Weiss**

## EYE, DUANE RETRACTION SYNDROME      3180

**Includes:**
    Duane anomaly-radial ray abnormalities-deafness
    Duane retraction syndrome
    Eye movement disorder
    Ocular retraction syndrome
    Okihiro syndrome
    Paralysis of sixth nerve, congenital
    Retraction syndrome
    Stilling-Turk-Duane syndrome
    Strabismus, Duane type
    Wildervack syndrome

**Excludes:**
    Acquired Duane retraction syndrome
    Acquired sixth nerve paralysis
    **Radial-renal-ocular syndrome** (2643)

**Major Diagnostic Criteria:** A congenital eye movement disorder. Depending on the type of the syndrome, there is marked limitation or absence of abduction, variable limitation of adduction, or both, and palpebral fissure narrowing and globe retraction on attempted adduction. Other congenital malformations are present in 30–50% of patients with this syndrome.

**Clinical Findings:** This is primarily a disorder of horizontal eye movements. It is unilateral in 80–85% of cases. This condition is more common in females than in males, and the left eye is more frequently affected. A head turning is present in some patients.

Huber distinguished three types of Duane retraction syndrome based on electromyographic recordings. *Duane type I* (the most common) consists of limited or absent abduction with relatively normal adduction; *Duane type II* consists of limited or absent adduction with normal abduction; and *Duane type III* consists of limited or absent abduction and adduction. Palpebral fissure narrowing and globe retraction on attempted adduction is common in all types. Vertical eye movements, most frequently in the upward direction, are more often noted in types II and III. Most patients with Duane syndrome are orthophoric in primary position of gaze. When strabismus is present, it is usually convergent in type I and divergent in type II.

**Complications:** Strabismus; abnormal head position with a face turn; amblyopia. Amblyopia is rare, and is usually seen when there is an associated anisometropia.

**Associated Findings:** Approximately 30–50% of the patients with Duane syndrome have one or more associated congenital defects, primarily involving ocular, skeletal, auricular, and neural structures.

Epibulbar dermoids (usually as part of **Oculo-auriculo-vertebral anomaly**), nystagmus, ptosis, anisocoria, microphthalmia, and optic nerve hypoplasia are among the most common associated ocular defects. Skeletal defects include fusion of vertebrae (See **Klippel-Feil anomaly**), cleft vertebrae, spina bifida, scoliosis, congenital absence of ribs, other rib malformations, hypoplasia of the bony orbit, **Cleft palate**, facial anomalies with asymmetry and hemimicrosomia, hypoplasia of one or more extremities, hypoplasia of the thumb, **Polydactyly**, and **Radial-ulnar synostosis**. The combination of *Duane syndrome-radial ray abnormalities-deafness* has become known as *Okihiro syndrome* (Hayes et al 1985). The association of radial anomalies (usually hypoplasia or absence of the thumb), urologic anomalies (vesicoureteral reflux, bladder diverticulum, renal ectopia and other renal abnormalities), and Duane syndrome constitute the **Radial-renal-ocular syndrome**. Congenital ear and hearing abnormalities include sensorineural deafness, preauricular skin tags, malformed pinna, hypoplastic external ear canal, and anomalous ossicles. The triad of Duane syndrome, **Klippel-Feil anomaly**, and congenital sensorineural deafness forms the *Wildervack syndrome*.

Associated central nervous system disorders consist of convulsive disorders, generalized hypotonia, congenital facial palsy, and other neurologic disorders of both cerebral and cerebellar structures. Genitourinary anomalies include renal agenesis, bifid ureter, cryptorchidism, atrophic testicles, and bladder exstrophy. In addition, congenital pyloric stenosis, and cardiopulmonary anomalies have been reported in some patients with Duane syndrome.

No large series studied with CT scan or nuclear magnetic resonance of the brain has been reported.

**Etiology:** The large majority of cases are apparently sporadic, with only 5–10% familial incidence. When Duane syndrome is associated with **Klippel-Feil anomaly** and deafness, it is by autosomal dominant inheritance with variable expressivity.

**Pathogenesis:** It appears that Duane retraction syndrome and associated congenital anomalies are the result of a teratogenic event during the second month of gestation. The development of the ocular motor nerves occurs between the 4th and 8th week of gestation and coincides with the differentiation of the other structures most commonly affected in Duane syndrome. Relatively recent autopsy studies have shown a brainstem abnormality. In a case of bilateral Duane type III, there was bilateral absence of the abducens nuclei and nerves and the lateral rectus muscles were partially innervated by branches from the inferior division of the oculomotor nerves. In another case of unilateral Duane type I, the abducens nucleus on the affected side contained no cell bodies of motorneurons, but in its rostral portion there were many small cell bodies believed to represent internuclear neurons. In this last case, the abducens nerve on the affected side was absent and the lateral rectus was innervated by branches from the inferior division of the oculomotor nerve. These findings are consistent with the results of electromyographic studies and explain both the limitation of abduction and the globe retraction caused by co-contraction of medial and lateral recti on attempted adduction.

**MIM No.:** *12680

**Sex Ratio:** M2:F3

**Occurrence:** Duane's original report (1905) described 54 cases, and other accounts have since appeared in the literature.

**Risk of Recurrence for Patient's Sib:**
See Part I, *Mendelian Inheritance.* In sporadic cases (majority) the risk for the patient's sibs is no greater than in the general population.

**Risk of Recurrence for Patient's Child:**
See Part I, *Mendelian Inheritance.* In sporadic cases (majority) the risk for the patient's children is no greater than in the general population.

**Age of Detectability:** During infancy. Some cases escape detection until adolescence.

**Gene Mapping and Linkage:** Unknown.

**Prevention:** None known. Genetic counseling indicated.

**Treatment:** In the majority of cases, no surgery is necessary unless the patient has strabismus in primary position of gaze, or marked head turns.

**Prognosis:** Vision is virtually always normal unless there is associated anisometropia.

**Detection of Carrier:** Unknown.

**References:**
Duane A: Congenital deficiency of abduction associated with impairment of adduction, retraction movements, contractions of the palpebral fissure and oblique movements of the eye. Arch Ophthalmol 1905; 34:133–159.
Pfaffenbach DD, et al: Congenital anomalies in Duane's retraction syndrome. Arch Ophthalmol 1972; 88:635–639. *
Huber A: Electrophysiology of the retraction syndromes. Br J Ophthalmol 1974; 58:293–300.
Hotchkiss MG, et al: Bilateral Duane's retraction syndrome. Arch Ophthalmol 1980; 98:870–874.
Miller NR, et al: Unilateral Duane's retraction syndrome (type 1). Arch Ophthalmol 1982; 100:1468–1472.
Hayes A, et al: The Okihiro syndrome of Duane anomaly, radial ray abnormalities, and deafness. Am J Med Genet 1985; 22:273–280.
Miller NR: Duane syndrome. In: Walsh and Hoyt's Clinical Neuro-Ophthalmology, vol 2, 4th ed. Baltimore: Williams and Wilkins, 1985:691–698. *
MacDermot K, Winter RM: Radial ray defect and Duane anomaly: report of a family with autosomal dominant transmission. Am J Med Genet 1987; 27:313–319.

CH042                                              **Georgia A. Chrousos**

**Eye, fetal fibrovascular sheath of lens, persistent**
*See EYE, VITREOUS, PERSISTENT HYPERPLASTIC PRIMARY*

## EYE, FIBROSIS OF THE EXTRAOCULAR MUSCLES, GENERALIZED 3185

**Includes:**
 Abiotrophic ophthalmoplegia externa
 Blepharoptosis-absent eye movements
 Extraocular muscles, congenital fibrosis
 Fibrosis of the extraocular muscles, congenital
 Generalized fibrosis syndrome
 Ophthalmoplegia, congenital
 Ocular fibrosis syndrome, congenital
 Ptosis-inferior rectus fibrosis, congenital hereditary
 Rectus muscle, congenital fibrosis of the inferior

**Excludes:**
 **Brown syndrome** (3179)
 Double elevator palsy
 **Eye, Duane retraction syndrome** (3180)
 Myasthenia gravis
 **Ophthalmoplegia, progressive external** (0752)
 Orbital periostitis
 Strabismus fixus
 Thyroid ophthalmopathy of Grave

**Major Diagnostic Criteria:** Fibrosis of the extraocular muscles and blepharoptosis are present at birth. Ocular misalignment is present, usually downgaze with exotropia. Ocular rotations are absent or severely restricted. Forced ductions are positive (abnormal). Familial occurrence is frequent.

**Clinical Findings:** The presentation of this disorder will vary depending on the severity of fibrosis, the number of extraocular muscles involved, and the presence or absence of bilaterality. Usually, fibrosis occurs in and prevents function of all extraocular muscles and ptosis is present. The eyes are usually in a down turned, diverged position, and rotations are absent. Less severe and less frequent variations are congenital fibrosis of the inferior rectus muscle or the inferior rectus and levator palpebri muscles. All forms rarely may present unilaterally. The forced duction test is always abnormal. The extraocular muscles may have anomalous insertions. Fibrosis may involve other orbital structures, especially connective tissue, and may lead to secondary enophthalmos.

**Complications:** Amblyopia, anomalous head positioning with secondary cervical spine degeneration and cervical muscle contractures.

**Associated Findings:** Usually not associated with other ocular or systemic abnormalities. Rare cases of associated ocular and systemic anomalies have been summarized by Kalpakian et al (1986), including one patient with **Prader-Willi syndrome**.

**Etiology:** Autosomal dominant inheritance with variability in expression. Numerous reports of isolated occurrence exist, as well as rare cases of possible recessive and X-linked recessive inheritance.

**Pathogenesis:** Extraocular muscle biopsies reveal replacement of normal contractile muscle tissue by fibrous tissue either partially or completely. Histopathology, including electron microscopy, of five cases is presented in Harley et al (1978).

**MIM No.:** *13570

**Sex Ratio:** M1:F1

**Occurrence:** Undetermined but presumed rare. A few dozen cases have been documented.

**Risk of Recurrence for Patient's Sib:**
See Part I, *Mendelian Inheritance.*

**Risk of Recurrence for Patient's Child:**
See Part I, *Mendelian Inheritance.*

**Age of Detectability:** At birth.

**Gene Mapping and Linkage:** Unknown.

**Prevention:** None known. Genetic counseling indicated.

**Treatment:** Surgery is indicated in the presence of an anomalous head posture. Extraocular muscle surgery will correct the hypotropia and a frontalis sling will elevate the lids and expose the pupils. Care should be taken to protect the corneas post-operatively.

**Prognosis:** Good. The condition is stable.

**Detection of Carrier:** Ptosis evaluation for strabismus and ptosis.

**References:**
Harley RD, et al: Congenital fibrosis of the extraocular muscles. J Pediatr Ophthalmol Strabismus 1978; 15:346–358.
Kalpakian B, et al: Congenital ocular fibrosis syndrome associated with the Prader-Willi syndrome. J Pediatr Ophthalmol Strabismus 1986; 23:170–173.

HU016
JA016

**Lee R. Hunter**
**Mohammad S. Jaafar**

## EYE, GOLDMANN-FAVRE DISEASE       3137

**Includes:**
> Favre hyaloideoretinal degeneration
> Favre microfibrillar vitreoretinal degeneration
> Goldmann-Favre disease
> Hyaloideotapetoretinal degeneration
> Retinoschisis-early hemeralopia

**Excludes:**
> **Arthro-ophthalmopathy, hereditary, progressive, Stickler type (0090)**
> **Retina, hyaloideoretinal degeneration of Wagner (0479)**
> **Retinitis pigmentosa (0869)**
> **Retinoschisis (0871)**

**Major Diagnostic Criteria:** Early onset of nightblindness, bilateral symmetrical pigmentary retinopathy, peripheral and foveal retinoschisis, vitreous degeneration, and opacified/sheathed peripheral retinal vessels. The electroretinogram is nonrecordable or markedly abnormal.

**Clinical Findings:** Patients of either gender present typically during the first two decades of life with nightblindness associated with a bilateral, often subtle, pigmentary retinopathy. Retinoschisis of the periphery and broad zones of lattice-like degeneration leading to retinal hole formation may be evident. Associated ocular findings include vitreous syneresis with an optically empty, "liquefied" vitreous cavity, and occasional vitreous bands and epiretinal membranes. Patients may develop cataracts at an early age. Rhegmatogenous retinal detchment is an occasional sequela. Foveal retinoschisis and angiographically demonstrable cystoid macular edema has been reported in some patients. Peripheral retinal vessels appear opaque or sclerotic but typically demonstrate leakage on fluorescein angiography. The electroretinogram is either non-recordable or markedly abnormal even early in life. Visual acuity may remain relatively stable during the first two decades but usually shows progressive deterioration latter. Histopathologic findings in a full-thickness eye-wall biopsy showed degeneration of the sensory retina with relatively normal retinal pigment epithelium and choriocapillaris; a thick epiretinal membrane was present in an area of retinoschisis.

**Complications:** Cataracts, macular edema, rhegmatogenous retinal detachment.

**Associated Findings:** None known.

**Etiology:** Autosomal recessive inheritance.

**Pathogenesis:** Degeneration of the vitreous and neurosensory retina.

**MIM No.:** *26810

**Sex Ratio:** M1:F1

**Occurrence:** Fewer than two dozen cases have been reported.

**Risk of Recurrence for Patient's Sib:**
> See Part I, *Mendelian Inheritance.*

**Risk of Recurrence for Patient's Child:**
> See Part I, *Mendelian Inheritance.*

**Age of Detectability:** Clinical presentation during first two decades of life. Could be detected earlier in younger sibs of known affected patients.

**Gene Mapping and Linkage:** Unknown.

**Prevention:** None known. Genetic counseling indicated.

**Treatment:** Prophylactic treatment of asymptomatic retinal breaks to prevent retinal detachment.

**Prognosis:** Normal for life span and intelligence. Poor for vision.

**Detection of Carrier:** Unknown.

**References:**
Goldmann H: Biomicroscopie du corps vitré et du fond de l'oeil. Bull Mem Soc Fr Ophtalmol 1957; 70:265.
Favre M: A propos de deux cas de degénérescence hyaloideorétinienne. Ophthalmologica 1958; 135:604–609.
François J, et al.: Dégénérescence hyaloideo-tapéto-rétinienne de Goldmann-Favre. Ophthalmologica 1974; 168:81–96.
Fishman GA, et al.: Diagnostic features of the Favre-Goldmann syndrome. Br J Ophthalmol 1976; 60:345–353. *
Peyman GA, et al.: Histopathology of Goldmann-Favre syndrome obtained by full-thickness eye-wall biopsy. Ann Ophthalmol 1977; 9:479–484.

F0013
TR009

**David J. Forster**
**Elias I. Traboulsi**

## EYE, HYPERTELORISM       0504

**Includes:**
> Euryopia
> Greig syndrome
> Hypertelorism of eyes
> Ocular hypertelorism

**Excludes:**
> **Hypertelorism-hypospadias syndrome (0505)**
> **Hypertelorism-microtia-facial cleft-conductive deafness (0506)**
> Pseudohypertelorism (e.g. secondary to epicanthus or telecanthus)

**Major Diagnostic Criteria:** Increased interpupillary or interorbital distance, as determined by X-ray of the facial and orbital bones, for the patient's age, sex and race. Telecanthus often accompanies hypertelorism, but one should not be misled by the clinical impression of hypertelorism frequently produced by telecanthus in the presence of normal ocular separation.

**Clinical Findings:** Increased interorbital distance with increased interpupillary distance can be found as a primary defect or secondary to other developmental malformations of the cranium and face. Typically, the nasal bridge is broad and often depressed and the forehead prominent. Exotropia frequently occurs, making measurement of the interpupillary distance difficult. (It can be accomplished, however, by alternate fixation on a common point.) Usually mentality is not affected. The condition is usually bilaterally symmetric.

**Complications:** Occasionally, narrowing of the optic canals produces optic atrophy. Frequently the wide-set orbits lead to exotropia.

0504-10636: Ocular hypertelorism.

**Associated Findings:** Abnormal dentition, acrocyanosis, arched palate, enlarged terminal phalanges, rudimentary clavicles, syndactyly and undescended testes.

**Etiology:** Most primary hypertelorism occurs sporadically, although families with apparent autosomal dominant or recessive inheritance have been described. Secondary hypertelorism has been described as a part of many birth defects and complex malformation syndromes.

**Pathogenesis:** Undetermined. Disproportionate growth, embryonic fixation and secondary effects of other malformations are implicated in some cases.

**MIM No.:** *14540

**CDC No.:** 756.085

**Sex Ratio:** Presumably M1:F1.

**Occurrence:** Undetermined, in part because objective criteria are poorly established. In one family, the condition was traced through five generations.

**Risk of Recurrence for Patient's Sib:**
See Part I, *Mendelian Inheritance.*

**Risk of Recurrence for Patient's Child:**
See Part I, *Mendelian Inheritance.*

**Age of Detectability:** Variable. Usually in infancy or early childhood.

**Gene Mapping and Linkage:** Unknown.

**Prevention:** None known. Genetic counseling indicated.

**Treatment:** Extraocular muscle surgery to reduce strabismus; plastic surgery to decrease associated surface malformations.

**Prognosis:** Primary hypertelorism is usually associated with a normal life span. The prognosis in secondary hypertelorism is dictated by the primary cause.

**Detection of Carrier:** Unknown.

**References:**
Bojlen K, Brems T: Hypertelorism (Greig). Acta Path Microbiol Scand 1938; 15:217–258.
Jöhr, P: Valeurs moyennes et limites normales en fonction de l'âge, le quelques mésures de la tête et de la region orbitaire. J Génét Hum 1953; 2:247–256.
Duke-Elder S: System of Ophthalmology. vol. 3, part 2. Congenital defects, St. Louis: CV Mosby, 1963:1053–1057.
Christian, JC, et al.: Familial telecanthus with associated congenital anomalies. BD:OAS;V(2). New York: The National Foundation-March of Dimes, 1969:82–83.

DE034
BE026

**Monte A. Del Monte**
**Donald R. Bergsma**

## EYE, IRIDOPLEGIA, FAMILIAL　　2287

**Includes:**
Mydriasis, congenital
Pupils, fixed, dilated

**Excludes:**
Iris trauma
Mydriasis, pharmacologic
Myotonic pupil in Charcot-Marie-Tooth disease
Peninsula pupil
Pupil, fixed dilated, familial cranial nerve III mydriasis

**Major Diagnostic Criteria:** Fixed, dilated pupils, which are essentially unchanged following instillation of constricting or dilating drops, combined with an absence of significant neurologic impairments, history of ocular trauma, or use of mydriatics.

**Clinical Findings:** The presence of mid-dilated pupils at birth, with no evidence of iris transillumination. Funduscopic examination, evaluation by slit-lamp, and intraocular pressure are normal. Ocular motility is intact. Instillation of mydriatic and miotic drops do not produce an appreciable change in pupillary size. Affected individuals develop photophobia and may have a poor ability to

accommodate, although vision remains intact. There is no evidence of significant neurologic impairments or ocular trauma.

**Complications:** Photophobia; decreased accommodative abilities.

**Associated Findings:** Bilateral subdural effusions that resolved over a three-month period, muscular hypotonia, motor delays, and a ventricular septal defect were identified in one patient in infancy. Mild hypotonia and fine motor problems persisted in early childhood. These findings were suspected to be unrelated to the pupillary defect. Intellectual abilities were normal in all known cases.

**Etiology:** Autosomal or X-linked dominant inheritance.

**Pathogenesis:** Localized, structural abnormality of the intraocular musculature of the iris.

**MIM No.:** 15942

**Sex Ratio:** M1:F2

**Occurrence:** Undetermined but presumed rare.

**Risk of Recurrence for Patient's Sib:**
See Part I, *Mendelian Inheritance.*

**Risk of Recurrence for Patient's Child:**
See Part I, *Mendelian Inheritance.*

**Age of Detectability:** At birth.

**Gene Mapping and Linkage:** Unknown.

**Prevention:** None known. Genetic counseling indicated.

**Treatment:** Use of glasses for accommodative loss and photophobia.

**Prognosis:** Good visual status.

**Detection of Carrier:** Unknown.

**References:**
Keltner JL, et al.: Myotonic pupils in Charcot-Marie-Tooth disease: successful relief of symptoms with 0.025% pilocarpine. Arch Ophthalmol 1975; 93:1141–1148.
Caccamise WD, Townes PL: Bilateral congenital mydriasis. Am J Ophthalmol 1976; 81:515–517.
Bosanquet RC, Johnson GJ: Peninsula pupil: anomaly unique to Newfoundland and Labrador? Arch Ophthalmol 1981; 99:1824–1826.
Hersh JH, et al.: Familial iridoplegia. J Pediatr Ophthalmol and Strabismus 1987; 24:49–50.

HE024
D0023

**Joseph H. Hersh**
**Craig Douglas**

## EYE, KERATOCONUS　　0552

**Includes:**
Conical cornea
Cornea, conical
Keratoconus

**Excludes:** Lenticonus (0585)

**Major Diagnostic Criteria:** Asymmetric myopic astigmatism with any of the physical signs cited below or with a positive family history for full-blown keratoconus or conical cornea.

**Clinical Findings:** Noninflammatory, progressive ectasia of the central cornea results in myopic astigmatism, conical projection of the corneal apex, a surrounding ring of iron-containing pigment (Fleischer ring), protrusion of the lower lid by the conical cornea on downward gaze (Munson sign), vertical stretch marks in the posterior stroma, and ruptures in the Descemet and Bowman membranes. Abnormal reflexes are seen with the keratoscope, retinoscope, ophthalmoscope, or ophthalmometer (keratometer). Occasionally, acute ectasia, caused by sudden rupture of Descemet membrane and the endothelium, occurs allowing aqueous to penetrate and cause total opacification of the stroma. The corneal thinning is usually bilateral but asymmetric, and begins at about puberty. There are variable stages of remission and exacerbation.

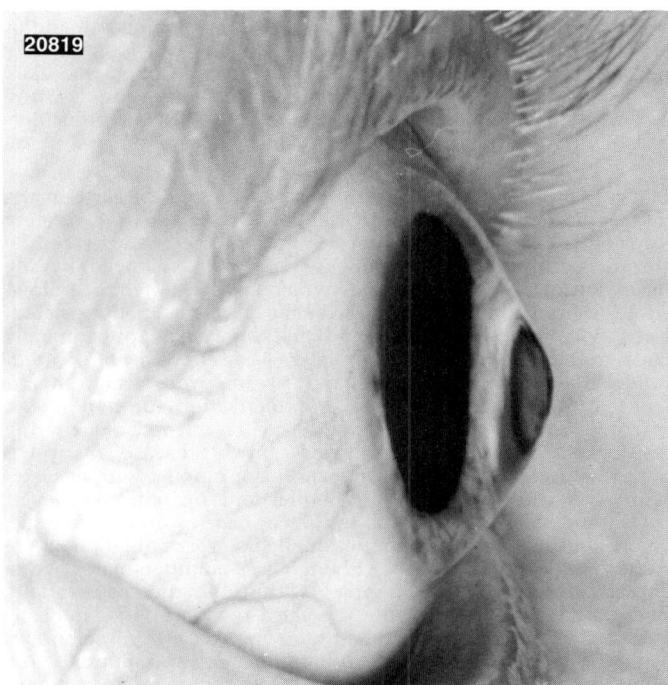

0552-20819:   Cornea, keratoconus.

**Complications:**   Acute ectasia, reduced visual acuity.

**Associated Findings:   Marfan syndrome, Chromosome 21, trisomy 21,** pigmentary retinopathy, **Retina, amaurosis congenita, Leber type,** atopic dermatitis, vernal conjunctivitis, **Ehlers-Danlos syndrome** types I and IV, and other disorders.

**Etiology:**   Autosomal recessive, autosomal dominant, and X-linked recessive inheritance has been reported. Eye rubbing has also been cited as a cause.

**Pathogenesis:**   Possibly related to degenerative processes in the basement membrane of the corneal basal epithelium or in Bowman membrane. Possibly to abnormalities in the stromal collagen itself. Various abnormalities of protein synthesis by stromal keratocytes have been suggested but not consistently identified suggesting that keratoconus has different possible etiologies in different patients.

**MIM No.:**   24450

**Sex Ratio:**   M4:F6

**Occurrence:**   Undetermined. High incidence of acute ectasia in **Chromosome 21, trisomy 21,** and in **Retina, amaurosis congenita, Leber type.**

**Risk of Recurrence for Patient's Sib:**
See Part I, *Mendelian Inheritance.*

**Risk of Recurrence for Patient's Child:**
See Part I, *Mendelian Inheritance.*

**Age of Detectability:**   Variable. At birth in inherited types.

**Gene Mapping and Linkage:**   Unknown.

**Prevention:**   None known. Genetic counseling indicated.

**Treatment:**   Pressure patch for acute ectasia, contact lens for early cases with irregular astigmatism, keratoplasty in advanced cases.

**Prognosis:**   Variable; good following keratoplasty.

**Detection of Carrier:**   Refraction reveals asymmetric myopic astigmatism in affected family members.

**References:**
Duke-Elder S: System of ophthalmology, vol. 8, part 2. Diseases of the outer eye. London: Henry Kimpton, 1965.
Karel I: Keratoconus in congenital diffuse tapetoretinal degeneration. Ophthalmologica (Basel) 1968; 155:8–15.
Goldberg MF: A review of selected inherited corneal dystrophies associated with systemic diseases. BD:OAS;VII(3). Baltimore: Williams and Wilkins, for The National Foundation-March of Dimes, 1971:13–25.
Kim JO, Hassard DTR: On the enzymology of the cornea. Can J Ophthalmol 1973; 8:151–156.
Krachmer JH, et al.: Keratoconus and related noninflammatory corneal thinning disorders. Ophthalmol 1984; 28:293–322.
Rehany U, Shoshan S: In vitro incorporation of proline into keratoconic human corneas. Invest Ophthalmol Vis Sci 1984; 25:1254–1257.
Yue BYJT, et al.: Heterogeneity in keratoconus: possible biochemical basis. Proc Soc Exp Biol Med 1984; 175:336–341.

G0006                                                    **Morton F. Goldberg**
SU001                                                          **Joel Sugar**

---

**EYE, KERATOPATHY, BAND-SHAPED**                              **0553**

**Includes:**
    Band keratitis
    Band-shaped keratopathy
    Corneal dystrophy, band-shaped
    Keratopathy, band-shaped

**Excludes:**
    **Eye, anterior segment dysgenesis** (0439)
    Vogt limbal girdle

**Major Diagnostic Criteria:**   White band in Bowman membrane occupying the interpalpebral space and having characteristic small, dark clear spaces or lacunae.

**Clinical Findings:**   Slow, progressive development of a white band in Bowman membrane, beginning near the limbus in the interpalpebral space and extending centrally. Rarely, the band begins centrally and extends horizontally to the peripheral cornea. There is usually a clear space between the ends of the band and the limbus. Small, dark, pathognomonic clear spaces or lacunae are present. Corneal sensation is usually intact. Irritative episodes do not occur unless calcified plaques erode the overlying epithelium. If the band occupies the visual axis, acuity can be diminished.

**Complications:**   Epithelial erosions, decreased visual acuity.

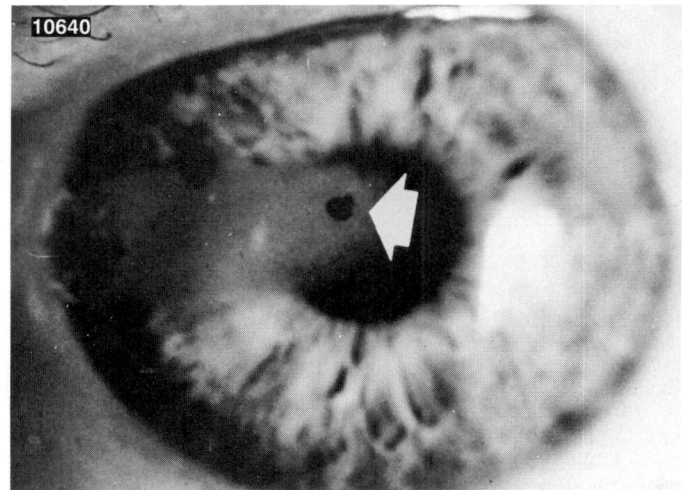

0553-10640:   Note clear fenestration in white haze (arrow).

**Associated Findings:** Band keratopathy may develop secondary to a variety of conditions, including: ocular disease e.g. juvenile iridocyclitis and rheumatoid arthritis (Still disease), **Norrie disease**, uveitis in adults, syphilitic interstitial keratitis, longstanding glaucoma; chronic corneal trauma, e.g. exogenous irritants; hypercalcemia, regardless of its etiology; hypophosphatasia; or **Gout** (rare). Also "familial" cases of primary band keratopathy (juvenile or senile).

**Etiology:** Possibly autosomal recessive inheritance. Heterogeneity exists. X-linked recessive band keratopathy, as reported by Duke-Elder and Leigh, is in reality **Norrie disease** with secondary corneal calcification.

**Pathogenesis:** Possibly supersaturation of the interpalpebral cornea with calcium salts, due to evaporation of water in this location, or loss of carbon dioxide to the atmosphere in the interpalpebral location with consequent elevation of the pH and precipitation of calcium salts, or deposition of calcium salts in the interpalpebral area by the massaging action of the lids.

**MIM No.:** *21750

**Sex Ratio:** M1:Fl

**Occurrence:** Undetermined. At least three hereditary kinships have been documented.

**Risk of Recurrence for Patient's Sib:**
See Part I, *Mendelian Inheritance.*

**Risk of Recurrence for Patient's Child:**
See Part I, *Mendelian Inheritance.*

**Age of Detectability:** Two forms exist. One with onset of corneal changes in infancy, the other with no changes until old age.

**Gene Mapping and Linkage:** Unknown.

**Prevention:** Prevention of congenital syphilis, corneal trauma or hypercalcemia. Genetic counseling if inherited.

**Treatment:** Treatment of primary ocular disease and of hypercalcemia, chelation of corneal calcium with topically applied EDTA which is successful in removing corneal calcium.

**Prognosis:** Depends upon underlying systemic or local disease.

**Detection of Carrier:** Unknown.

**References:**
Wagener HP: The ocular manifestations of hypercalcemia. Am J Med Sci 1956; 231:218.
Lessel S, Norton EW: Band keratopathy and conjunctival calcification in hypophosphatasia. Arch Ophthalmol 1964; 71:497–499.
Duke-Elder S, Leigh AG: System of ophthalomology. vol. 8, part 2. Diseases of the outer eye. London: Henry Kimpton, 1965.
Fishman RS, Sunderman FW: Band keratopathy in gout. Arch Ophthalmol 1966; 75:367–369.
Warburg M: Norrie's disease: a congenital progressive oculo-acoustico-cerebral degeneration. Acta Ophthalmol (suppl.) (Kbh.) 1966; 89:1–147.
Goldberg MF: A review of selected inherited corneal dystrophies associated with systemic diseases. BD:OAS;VII(3). Baltimore: Williams and Wilkins, for The National Foundation-March of Dimes, 1971:13–25.

G0006
SU001

**Morton F. Goldberg**
**Joel Sugar**

## EYE, LIGNEOUS CONJUNCTIVITIS                    3186

**Includes:**
Conjunctivitis, familial pseudomembranous
Ligneous conjunctivitis
Membranous conjunctivitis

**Excludes:**
**Amyloidosis**
Lipoid proteinosis
Pyogenic granuloma

**Major Diagnostic Criteria:** Chronic, often bilateral, conjunctivitis accompanied by induration of the eyelids and the formation of pseudomembranes or membranes on the tarsal, palpebral, and/or bulbar surfaces. The normal conjunctival mucosa is eventually replaced by thickened, tough, nodular masses of "wood-like" consistency. There may be secondary corneal ulceration, scarring or perforation. Similar recurrent lesions may involve other mucous membranes lining the vagina, cervix, larynx, gingiva, vocal cords, trachea, and nose.

**Clinical Findings:** Clinical signs generally manifest early in the first decade of life, although cases have been reported ranging from birth to 85 years. The earlier findings are characterized by chronic epiphora with conjunctival injection followed by the formation of pseudomembranes which appear as white, yellow-white, or red firm masses that can be sessile or pedunculated, often with an overlying mucoid discharge. An approximately equal number of bilateral and unilateral cases have been reported.

Secondary corneal changes may lead to severe visual impairment due to corneal thinning, vascularization, ulceration and scarring. Corneal perforation may occur requiring a penetrating keratoplasty. During the acute phase of the disease, many patients present with systemic signs and symptoms of upper respiratory tract infection, urinary tract infection, tonsillitis, and fever.

Histologically, the ligneous lesions appear as an eosinophilic, amorphous material containing small foci of granulation tissue and hyperplastic epithelium with interspersed inflammatory cells. Foreign bodies may be trapped within the mucoid exudate. Immunohistologic studies have revealed the amorphous deposits to be comprised of serum components including fibrin, albumin, activated T-cells, plasma cells, B-lymphocytes, and immunoglobulins. Vascular endothelial cells within the ligneous membranes showed marked degenerative changes and a thick, multilaminated basement membrane. These changes may allow the formation of ligneous membranes secondary to vascular leakage.

In the chronic phase of the disease, mucous membranes lining other parts of the body may become involved. Development of the upper respiratory tract may lead to stridor and asphyxia. In general, the disease takes a chronic course, lasting many years with frequent recurrences. Spontaneous resolution has occurred in a few reported cases, but recurrence is common even following attempts at therapy.

**Complications:** Visual impairment secondary to corneal vascularization, ulceration, scarring, and/or perforation. Attemps to peel off the membranous lesions may result in bleeding. Multiple polypoid membranous lesions of the larynx, vocal cords, trachea, and nose may lead to airway compromise. Cervical and vaginal lesions may also be symptomatic.

**Associated Findings:** Similar membranous lesions of other mucosal surfaces.

**Etiology:** Possibly autosomal recessive inheritance. Autosomal dominant inheritance with mild expressivity was suggested in one reported family.

**Pathogenesis:** Theories include streptococcal infection, a hypersensitivity reaction, a disturbance in glycosaminoglycan and collagen metabolism, and a primary vasculopathy with formation of excess basement membrane material and secondary vascular leakage.

**MIM No.:** 21709

**Sex Ratio:** M1:F1

**Occurrence:** About 75 cases have been documented, many from Turkey.

**Risk of Recurrence for Patient's Sib:**
See Part I, *Mendelian Inheritance.*

**Risk of Recurrence for Patient's Child:**
See Part I, *Mendelian Inheritance.*

**Age of Detectability:** Frequently detectable during infancy, but the onset has been reported in adults as well as in the elderly.

**Gene Mapping and Linkage:** Unknown.

**Prevention:** None known. Genetic counseling indicated.

**Treatment:** Early reports of the presence of mucopolysaccharides in the lesions led to treatment with hyaluronidase, but the efficacy of this treatment has not been confirmed. Frequent irrigation of the conjunctival sac and application of topical vasoconstrictors and topical disodium cromoglycate have been reported to be helpful. Surgical removal of the pseudomembranes and membranes are generally followed by recurrences but may establish a histopathologic diagnosis. Surgical approaches have included placing a pursestring suture around the base of the membrane as well as scleral and mucous membrane grafting. The use of systemic immunosuppressive chemotherapy with azothiaprine has been promising in rare cases. Selected patients have benefited from excisional biopsy and topical cyclosporine.

**Prognosis:** Good for life span, although membranous involvement of larynx and upper respiratory tract may cause airway embarrassment. Visual prognosis varies considerably, and depends upon secondary corneal involvement.

**Detection of Carrier:** Unknown.

**References:**

Bouisson M: Ophthalmie sur-aigue avec formation de pseudomembranes a la surface de la conjonctive. Ann Oculist (Paris) 1847; 17:100–104.

Borel MG: Un nouveau syndrome palpebral. Bull Soc Ophthalmol Fr 1933; 46:168–180.

Bateman JB, et al: Ligneous conjunctivitis; an autosomal recessive disorder. J Pediatr Ophthalmol Strabismus 1986; 23:137–140.

Hidayat AA, Riddle PJ: Ligneous conjunctivitis: a clinical pathologic study of seventeen cases. Ophthalmology 1987; 94:949–959.

Holland EJ, et al.: Immunohistologic findings and results of treatment with cyclosporine in ligneous conjunctivitis. Am J Ophthalmol 1989; 107:160–166.

PE023          **Jay S. Pepose**

## EYE, MACULAR DYSTROPHY, NORTH CAROLINA TYPE    3282

**Includes:**

Epithelial dystrophy, central areolar pigment
Lefler-Wadsworth-Sidbury syndrome
North Carolina macular dystrophy (NCMD)
Pigment epithelial and choroidal degeneration, dominant central

**Excludes:**

Eye, fundus dystrophy, Sorsby type
**Retina, fundus flavimaculatus** (0400)
**Retina, macular degeneration, vitelliruptive** (0622)

**Major Diagnostic Criteria:** Marked opthalmoscopic variability is present, ranging from only a few small (<50μ), flat specks in the fovea; to yellow specks; to large (1–2 disc diameters), single, well-circumscribed white colobomatous lesions in the macular area. The peripheral retina is variably abnormal with scattered whitish-yellowish flecks which appear similar to peripheral **Ocular drusen.**

**Clinical Findings:** Based on a single pedigree of over 1,400 individuals in eight generations, most of whom reside in the mountains of North Carolina, affected individuals may be completely asymptomatic or may have a central scotoma causing vision to decrease to the 20/200 level. Median visual acuity is 20/50. Visual acuity and ophthalmoscopic findings are generally stable, and have been unchanged in a number of patients over 20 years. Subretinal neovascularization does not occur. Nystagmus and cataracts are absent. Electrophysiologic (electroretinography and electrooculography) and color vision testing yield normal results in most patients.

**Complications:** Poor vision in patients with moderate to severe retinal involvement.

**Associated Findings:** Aminoaciduria has been reported in some affected individuals.

**Etiology:** Autosomal dominant inheritance. It has been suggested, based on a number of double first cousin marriages, that the aminoaciduria may be a separate autosomal recessive condition.

**Pathogenesis:** Unknown.

**MIM No.:** *13655

**Sex Ratio:** Presumably M1:F1, although Frank et al (1974) did report gender difference in a related population.

**Occurrence:** Documented in one large kindred, although the central areolar pigment epithelial dystrophy described by Hermsen & Judisch (1984) in Iowa is part of this same kindred, and the central pigment epithelial and choroidal degeneration reported by Leveille et al (1982) may also be related.

**Risk of Recurrence for Patient's Sib:**

See Part I, *Mendelian Inheritance.*

**Risk of Recurrence for Patient's Child:**

See Part I, *Mendelian Inheritance.*

**Age of Detectability:** The youngest patient observed with this dystrophy was three months old, although the condition may be detectable at birth or early infancy.

**Gene Mapping and Linkage:** Unknown.

**Prevention:** None known. Genetic counseling indicated.

**Treatment:** Low vision aids for severely affected individuals.

**Prognosis:** Fair for vision; not a progressive condition. Vision is often much better than expected from the ophthalmoscopic appearance of the lesions.

**Detection of Carrier:** By clinical examination.

**References:**

Sorsby A, Crick RP: Central areolar choroidal sclerosis. Br J Ophthalmol 1953; 37:129–139.

Lefler WH, et al.: Hereditary macular degeneration and aminoaciduria. Am J Ophthalmol 1971; 71:224–230.

Frank HR, et al.: A new dominant progressive foveal dystrophy. Am J Ophthalmol 1974; 78:903–916.

Leveille AS, et al.: Autosomal domiant central pigment epithelial and choroidal degeneration. Ophthalmology 1982; 89:1407–1413.

Hermsen VM, Judisch GF: Central areolar pigment dystrophy. Ophthalmologica 1984; 189:69–72.

Small KW: North Carolina macular dystrophy, revisited. Ophthalmology 1989; 96:1747–1754. * †

SM022          **Kent W. Small**

## EYE, MELANOSIS OCULI, CONGENITAL    0640

**Includes:**

Melanosis oculi, congenital
Ocular melanocytosis, congenital

**Excludes:**

**Cancer, malignant melanoma, familial** (2318)
Melanosis oculi, acquired
Nevus
**Nevus of Ota** (0716)
**Optic disk, melanocytoma** (0639)
Precancerous melanosis

**Major Diagnostic Criteria:** Congenital hyperpigmentation of episclera, sclera and uveal tract.

**Clinical Findings:** Diffuse or localized areas of blue or slate grey pigmentation of episclera and sclera present at birth in one eye. More frequent in dark races (blacks and orientals). Involvement of ipsilateral uveal tissues causes heterochromia of the iris and fundus (subtle finding in brown-eyed individuals). Same pigmentation may be present in the conjunctiva (sometimes extending onto the superficial cornea) or within the optic nerve. Association of congenital ocular melanosis with pigmentation within the periorbital dermis is known as oculodermal melanocytosis (**Nevus of Ota**).

**Complications:** May rarely be associated with ipsilateral glaucoma.

**Associated Findings:** Probably higher incidence of uveal melanoma (conjunctival or orbital less common) in eyes with congenital melanosis oculi particularly when it occurs in whites. Tumors

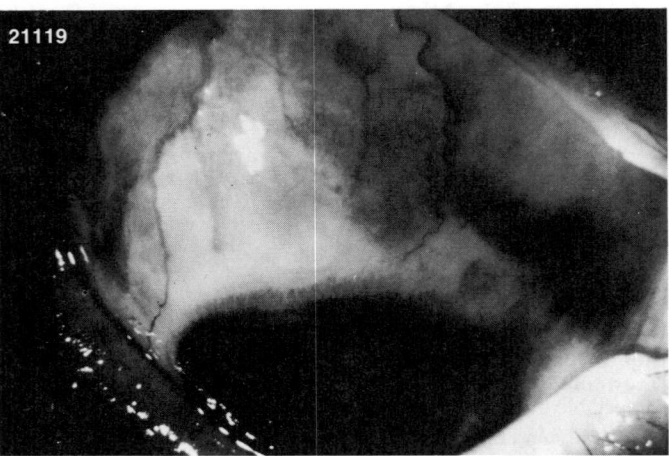

21119

**0640-21119:** Slit lamp photograph of external eye shows patchy hyperpigmentation of the episclera and sclera.

may be multifocal. Primary meningeal melanomas more frequent than in normal population.

**Etiology:** Unknown.

**Pathogenesis:** Unknown.

**Sex Ratio:** M1:F1

**Occurrence:** 38:1,000. Occurs more commonly in dark-complexioned individuals, e.g. blacks and Orientals.

**Risk of Recurrence for Patient's Sib:** Unknown.

**Risk of Recurrence for Patient's Child:** Unknown.

**Age of Detectability:** Present at birth, but episcleral pigmentation may be subtle or not appreciated until adolescence.

**Gene Mapping and Linkage:** Unknown.

**Prevention:** None known. Genetic counseling indicated.

**Treatment:** Unknown.

**Prognosis:** Good, no visual impairment unless melanoma develops. Patients with ocular melanocytosis should be examined periodically for suspected melanoma.

**Detection of Carrier:** Unknown.

**Special Considerations:** Hyperpigmentation in ocular structures derived from mesenchyme (sclera, uvea), but not those derived from neuroectoderm (pigment epithelium). Giant macromelanosomes have been demonstrated within cytoplasm of iris melanocytes which implies defect in melanogenesis similar to X-linked albinism or neurofibromatosis.

**References:**
Sang DN, et al.: Nevus of Ota with contralateral cerebral melanoma. Arch Ophthalmol 1977; 95:1820–1824.
Pomerantz GA, et al.: Multifocal choroidal melanoma in ocular melanocytosis. Arch Ophthalmol 1981; 99:857–863.
Gonder JR, et al.: Ocular melanocytosis. a prospective study to determine the incidence of ocular melanocytosis. Ophthalmology 1982; 89:950–952.
Gonder JR, et al.: Uveal malignant melanoma associated with ocular and oculodermal melanocytosis. Ophthalmology 1982; 89:953–960.
Hamilton RF, et al.: Posterior corneal pigmentation in melanosis oculi. Arch Ophthalmol 1983; 101:1909–1911.
Rennie IG, Blechan SS: Melanosis oculi: an ultrastructural study of an affected iris. Arch Ophthalmol 1983; 101:1912–1916.
Velasquez N, Jones IS: Ocular and oculodermal melanocytosis associated with uveal melanoma. Ophthalmology 1983; 90:1472–1476.
Folberg R, et al.: Benign conjunctival melanocytic lesions: clinicopathologic features. Ophthalmology 1989; 96:436–461.

WE035

**Avery H. Weiss**

**EYE, MICROPHTHALMIA/COLOBOMA** **0661**

**Includes:**
Choroid, coloboma
Coloboma of iris, choroid and retina
Colobomatous microphthalmia, isolated
Iris, coloboma
Microphthalmia, colobomatous isolated
Retina, coloboma
Uveal coloboma

**Excludes:**
Amniotic bands syndrome (0874)
Anemia, hypoplastic congenital (0051)
Arachnodactyly, contractural Beals type (0085)
Charge association (2124)
Dermal hypoplasia, focal (0281)
Eye, cryptophthalmos (0003)
Eye, vitreous, persistent hyperplastic primary (0994)
Gingival fibromatosis-depigmentation-microphthalmia (0413)
Humero-radial synostosis (0477)
Lenz microphthalmia syndrome (3171)
Meckel syndrome (0634)
Microphthalmia with cataracts and developmental delay

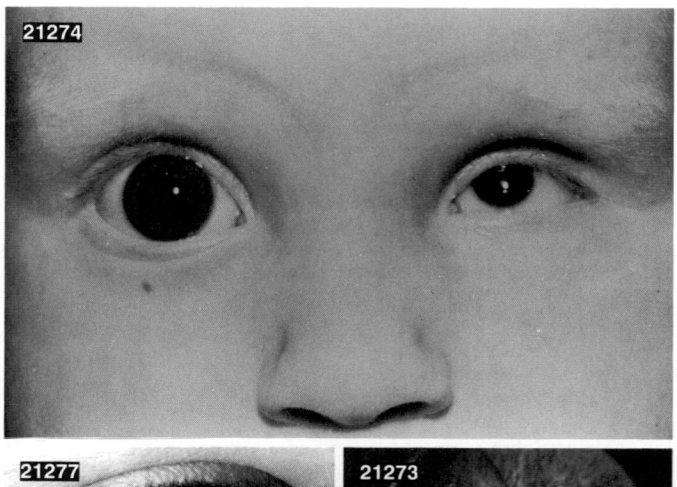
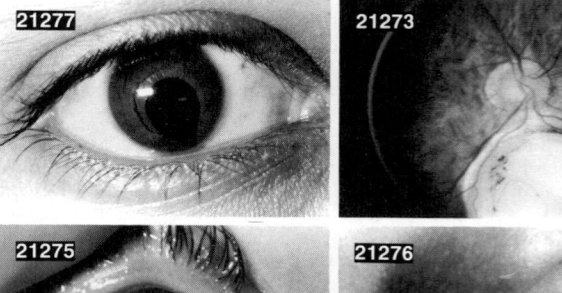
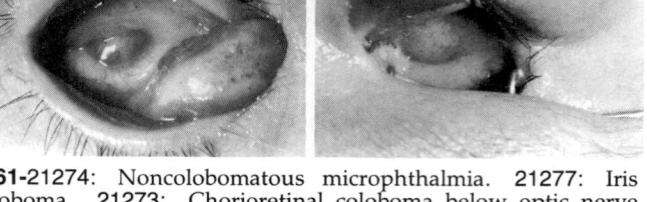

**0661-21274:** Noncolobomatous microphthalmia. **21277:** Iris coloboma. **21273:** Chorioretinal coloboma below optic nerve head. **21275:** Microphthalmia with cyst. **21276:** Clinical anophthalmia; no ocular structures identified by ultrasound or CAT scan.

Microphthalmia and congenital falciform retinal folds
Microphthalmia and developmental delay
Microphthalmia and multisystem disorders malformations
**Mucopolysaccharidosis II** (0676)
Nanophthalmia
**Nevoid basal cell carcinoma syndrome** (0101)
**Nevus, epidermal nevus syndrome** (0593)
**Oculo-mandibulo-facial syndrome** (0738)
**Renal tubular syndrome, Fanconi type** (0864)
**Rubinstein-Taybi broad thumb-hallux syndrome** (0119)
Saraux syndrome
**Walker-Warburg syndrome** (2869)
X-linked microcephaly, microphthalmia, and other ocular
abnormalities

**Major Diagnostic Criteria:** Microphthalmia: smaller than normal axial length (less than 20 mm) of eye by A-scan ultrasonography (normals vary with age).

Colobomatous microphthalmia: smaller than normal axial length of eye by ultrasound associated with coloboma of iris and/or choroid and/or optic nerve.

**Clinical Findings:** The term microphthalmia is derived from the Greek origins *micro* meaning small and *ophthalmos* eye and refers to a congenital malformation in which the volume of the eye is reduced; the spectrum ranges from mild reduction in the anteroposterior axis to histologically-documented anophthalmia following serial sectioning of the orbit. Nanophthalmia is used to describe a microphthalmic eye with normal intraocular structures and is a distinct genetic malformation. The diagnosis of microphthalmia can often be suspected by inspection; microcornea or high hyperopia may be useful clues for the clinician. However, as microcornea may occur without microphthalmia and, conversely, microphthalmia may occur in association with a normal-sized cornea, a clinical diagnosis may be inaccurate. In addition, many microphthalmic eyes are highly myopic. Ultrasonography, with precise measurement of the anteroposterior axis, now permits, and in fact is essential for, a biometric diagnosis in-vivo. The specific criterion for microphthalmia depends on the normal values of the laboratory performing the test; however, as most normal adult eyes range from 21.50 to 27.00 mm, an axial length of less than 20 mm should be considered abnormal. Extreme microphthalmia may be difficult to distinguish from true anophthalmia even with the use of computed tomography. The term clinical anophthalmia is therefore used to indicate clinical absence of the globes. Severe microphthalmia can be distinguished from anophthalmia by serial sectioning of the orbit to determine the presence or absence of rudimentary ocular structures. These malformations may be unilateral or bilateral; asymmetry is common.

The general categories of microphthalmia are colobomatous and noncolobomatous. Although uveal (iris, choroid, and/or optic nerve) colobomata may occur in the absence of microphthalmia, the two conditions frequently are associated and, presumably, are etiologically and embryologically related.

Microphthalmia, with or without colobomata, can be a manifestation of many different disorders, including genetic, environmental, or those of unknown cause. In addition to a complete ophthalmological examination, all affected individuals should have a carefully obtained history, including a genetic pedigree, and a careful physical examination. In selected cases, a karyotype may be obtained.

Autosomal dominant colobomatous microphthalmia, without associated systemic malformations, has been well established. Variable expressivity has been observed; from small iris or choroidal coloboma to clinical anophthalmia or microphthalmia with cyst, and incomplete penetrance has been documented. The parents of children with isolated colobomatous microphthalmia should be carefully examined for small, visually insignificant colobomata. In a family with an autosomal dominant inheritance pattern, it has been estimated that any individual with a normal ocular exam has an 8.6% chance of having an affected child. Pedigrees supporting autosomal recessive inheritance of microphthalmia are few and lack careful documentation of the ocular status of the parents. The best evidence for this pattern is based on

a large study of the Japanese population with microphthalmia by Fujiki et al (1982); segregation analysis indicated a recessive form of inheritance in 12%. However, there was no differentiation between the colobomatous and noncolobomatous forms and associated malformations were not discussed. Although environmental influences would seem plausible in sporadic cases of colobomatous microphthalmia, few have been established as embryopathic agents. Thalidomide may cause this ocular malformation as well as phocomelia. Intrauterine vitamin A deficiency in humans has also been implicated; this observation has been supported by the finding of colobomatous microphthalmia in the offspring of rats deprived of vitamin A during pregnancy.

Although usually associated with other ocular malformations, noncolobomatous microphthalmia may occur as an autosomal dominant disorder. A three-generation family with noncolobomatous microphthalmia has been observed; penetrance was incomplete and expressivity was variable from unilateral microphthalmia to clinical bilateral anophthalmia. Isolated autosomal dominant microphthalmia more commonly occurs with associated ocular malformations such as congenital cataracts or myopia and corectopia. Isolated microphthalmia has been reported with microcornea and with normal-sized corneas. High hyperopia is an important clinical clue to both diagnoses. Patients with microcornea, in the absence of other malformations, are prone to develop uveal effusions and/or angle-closure glaucoma from progressive narrowing of the anterior chamber; consistent follow-up is necessary for early detection. Patients with normal-sized corneas probably have a different syndrome; they have a crowded posterior pole with horizontal folding of the retina and diminution of the capillary-free zone. Microphthalmia with congenital retinal detachment also may be inherited as an autosomal recessive disorder. Congenital cataracts associated with microphthalmia likewise may be inherited in this pattern. X-linked noncolobomatous microphthalmia with cataracts has been described; the relationship of this disease to **Lenz microphthalmia syndrome** is uncertain.

**Complications:** Secondary glaucoma, retinal detachment (uncommon).

**Associated Findings:** A variety of associated ocular and systemic abnormalities may be observed.

**Etiology:** Autosomal recessive, dominant, or X-linked recessive inheritance. Intrauterine insults and chromosomal rearrangements may be associated, but multisystem abnormalities are usually evident. It has been estimated that 15–30% of patients with microphthalmia coloboma have **Charge association**.

Viral embryopathies such as cytomegalovirus, Epstein-Barr virus, varicella, and herpes virus may be associated with microphthalmia. Although less well documented, maternal fever during pregnancy and prenatal irradiation also have been implicated. In animal models, ocular teratogens causing microphthalmia have included folic acid deficiencies (rat), irradiation (rat), exposure to nickel carbonyl (rat), and elevated incubation temperatures (chick).

In addition to the numerous syndromes associated with colobomatous or noncolobomatous microphthalmia, sporadic cases with no demonstrable etiology are common. The study by Fujiki and colleagues of 1,313 cases of patients with microphthalmia and their families indicated, by segregation analysis, that approximately 15% were autosomal recessive and 22% were autosomal dominant; the remainder were of unknown etiology and considered sporadic. Using a test for polygenic inheritance, the authors found that microphthalmia was between multifactorial and simple recessive inheritance.

Multiple chromosomal aberrations, including triploidy, trisomies, duplications, and deletions, may be associated with colobomatous microphthalmia. Although some disorders, such as trisomy 13 (Patau syndrome) or the 4q-(Wolf-Hirschhorn) syndrome, have specific clinical features which may alert the physician to the diagnosis, many of these chromosomal syndromes are nonspecific. The physician, whether an ophthalmologist or a pediatrician, should consider the possibility of a chromosomal disorder in individuals who have developmental delay, colobomatous microphthalmia, and one other dysmorphic feature. Although most chromosomal abnormalities associated with microphthalmia exhibit colobomata, the 10q+ and the ring-B syndromes have been reported with noncolobomatous forms. Warburg and Friedrich (1987) reviewed the chromosomal abnormalities associated with ocular coloboma microphthalmia, and their article provides an extensive bibliography on the subject.

**Pathogenesis:** Colobomata result from incomplete closure of the fetal fissure, a process that is normally completed by the sixth week of gestation; the resulting "typical" coloboma is located inferonasally. The embryological processes that determine the size of the eye are poorly understood. Cystic eye and anophthalmia are extreme forms of this dysembryogenesis.

**MIM No.:** *12020, 21682, 30970

**CDC No.:** 743.100, 743.430

**Sex Ratio:** M1:F1

**Occurrence:** Microphthalmia appears to be a relatively common ocular malformation in all races; the high incidence which would be unusual for a disorder caused by a single gene suggests multiple etiologies. Because of the difficulty in collecting accurate data, few studies have documented the incidence in the general population or the prevalence in the blind. In a prospective study of more than 50,000 pregnancies in the United States, the incidence of anophthalmia/microphthalmia was found to be 0.22 per thousand births and that of coloboma to be 0.26 per thousand. Prevalence among blind adults has been calculated at 0.6% and 1.9%. Among children it accounts for a greater proportion of blindness with 3.2% to 11.2% of cases (Table 1). The differences in prevalence may reflect the race or population studied; the highest prevalence (11.2%) was found in the 1980 survey of the causes of blindness among Japanese schoolchildren:

#### TABLE 1
#### Prevalence of Microphthalmia and Coloboma in the Legally Blind

| STUDY: | McDonald (1965) | National Society to Prevent Blindness (1980) | Fraser and Friedmann (1967) | Fujiki and colleagues (1982) |
|---|---|---|---|---|
| | all ages | all ages | <5 years | <22 years | school children |
| microph-thalmia | 0.012 | | | | |
| coloboma | 0.007 | | | | |
| combined | 0.019 | 0.006 | 0.062 | 0.032 | 0.112 |

#### Risk of Recurrence for Patient's Sib:
See Part I, *Mendelian Inheritance*. Genetic counseling for patients with microphthalmia or their parents is difficult. A careful history, including prenatal influences, and a family pedigree are essential to determine if environmental agents or hereditary factors were causative. Specifically, the family should be asked if there have been any cases of anophthalmia, microphthalmia, or blindness, and if there is any consanguinity. A chromosomal analysis should be performed on patients who have colobomatous microphthalmia, developmental delay, and at least one other dysmorphic feature. If no specific syndrome can be identified, the recurrence risk for the parents of an affected child is approximately 2%; if one parent is affected, the risk increases to 14%.

#### Risk of Recurrence for Patient's Child:
See Part I, *Mendelian Inheritance*.

#### Age of Detectability: At birth.

#### Gene Mapping and Linkage: Unknown.

#### Prevention: None known. Genetic counseling indicated. Avoidance of medications and exposure to teratogens during pregnancy is recommended.

#### Treatment: Correction of refractive errors. Cataract extractions if associated. Corneal transplantation in selected cases.

**Prognosis:** Visual impairment in microphthalmia varies from little or none to complete loss as in anophthalmia and best correlates with the degree of microphthalmia and the associated abnormalities; cataracts, optic nerve hypoplasia, and/or colobomata of the macula or optic nerve may cause appreciable visual impairment.

**Detection of Carrier:** Examination of parents of children with isolated colobomatous microphthalmia may reveal small, visually non-significant, uveal colobomas.

**References:**
MacDonald AE: Causes of blindness in Canada: an analysis of 24,605 cases registered with the Canadian National Institute for the Blind. Can Med Assoc J 1965; 92:264–278.
Fraser GR, Friedman AI: The causes of blindness in childhood. Baltimore: Johns Hopkins, 1967.
Lamba PA, Sood NN: Congenital microphthalmos and colobomata in maternal vitamin A deficiency. J Pediatr Ophthalmol 1968;5:115–117.
National Society to Prevent Blindness: Vision problems in the U.S. New York: National Society to Prevent Blindness, 1980.
Pagon RA: Ocular coloboma. Surv Ophthalmol 1981;25:223–236.
Warburg M: Diagnostic precision in microphthalmia and coloboma of heterogeneous origin. Ophthalm Paediatr Genet 1981;1:37–42.
Fujiki K, et al: Genetic analysis of microphthalmos. Ophthalmol Paed Genet 1982;1:139–149.
Spitznas M, et al: Hereditary posterior microphthalmos with papillomacular fold and high hyperopia. Arch Ophthalmol 1983;101:413–417.
Warburg M: Ocular coloboma and multiple congenital anomalies. The CHARGE association. Ophthalm Paediatr Genet 1983;3:189–199.
Feldman ST, et al: Corneal transplantations in microphthalmia eyes. Am J Ophthalmol 1987;104:164–167.
Warburg M, Freidrich U: Coloboma and microphthalmos in chromosomal aberrations. Ophthalm Paediatr Genet 1987;8:105–118.

BA042                                          **J. Bronwyn Bateman**

---

### EYE, ORBITAL TERATOMA, CONGENITAL          3159

#### Includes:
Fetus in fetu
Orbital teratoma
Orbitopagus parasiticus
Teratoid cyst of the orbit, congenital

#### Excludes:
Eye, congenital cystic
**Eye, microphthalmia/coloboma** (0661)
**Orbital and periorbital dermoid cysts** (0761)
Orbital extension of an intracranial teratoma
Microphthalmos with cyst

**Major Diagnostic Criteria:** Severe proptosis and orbital enlargement at birth with a normally developed eye. The orbital tumor does not generally communicate with the intracranial cavity. The tumor is composed of elements from all three germinal layers.

**Clinical Findings:** Orbital teratomas are unilateral (only one bilateral case reported), large orbital tumors present at birth in a healthy child. They represent <1% of all orbital tumors in children. The eye, which is pushed typically forward and upward, is normally developed, but may become blind because of either optic nerve compression or complications from anterior segment exposure. The mass is tense, fluctuant, and transilluminates easily. The lids are stretched and the conjunctiva is chemotic. Computed tomography and orbital echography shows multiple cystic cavities, solid regions, and occasional tumor calcification. Histopathologically, any tissue derived from all three germinal layers may be found. Two cases of complete fetus implanted in the orbit (fetus *in fetu* or *orbitopagus parasiticus*) have been reported.

**Complications:** Blindness may result from optic nerve compression by the tumor. However, several cases with preservation of the eye, and some remaining vision have been reported following tumor resection. The extreme proptosis may lead to corneal

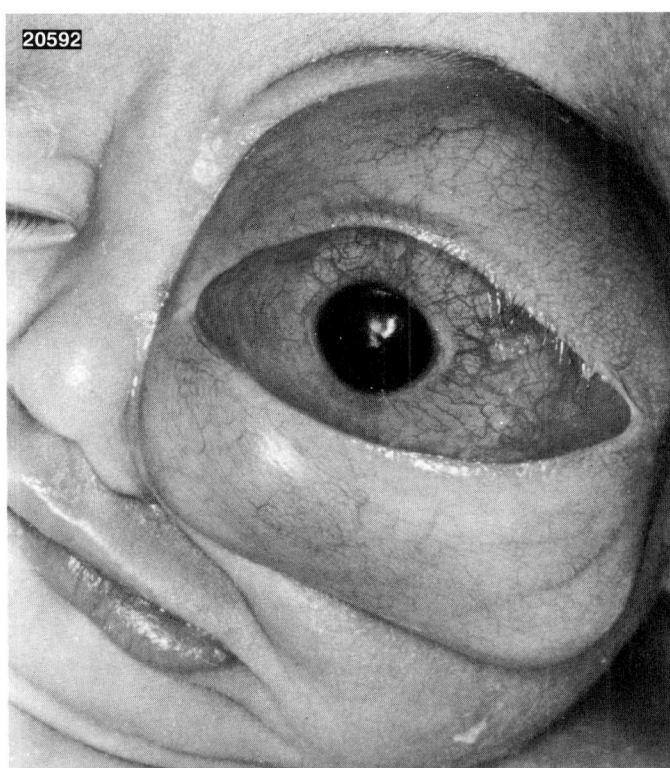

**3159-20592:** Newborn infant with large congenital orbital teratoma. Globe is severely proptosed with corneal exposure and widely expanded palpebral aperture.

exposure, ulceration, and secondary infection. All except one reported case of congenital orbital teratomas were benign.

**Associated Findings:** None known.

**Etiology:** Unknown.

**Pathogenesis:** Ovarian teratomas are thought to be parthenogenic tumors that arise from a single germ cell following meiotic division. A similar mechanism may account for the development of orbital teratomas.

**Sex Ratio:** M1:F2

**Occurrence:** About 50 cases have been reported in the literature.

**Risk of Recurrence for Patient's Sib:** Presumably not increased.

**Risk of Recurrence for Patient's Child:** Presumably not increased.

**Age of Detectability:** At birth. Intrauterine demonstration by ultrasound is feasible in principle.

**Gene Mapping and Linkage:** Unknown.

**Prevention:** None known. Genetic counseling indicated.

**Treatment:** Because tumors are benign, tumor resection with attempted preservation of the eye should be performed as early as feasible. Awaiting surgery, medical management of ocular proptosis to prevent complications of corneal exposure and to minimize optic nerve stretching and compression.

**Prognosis:** Ambulatory vision may be achieved if optic nerve damage has not occurred.

**Detection of Carrier:** Unknown.

**References:**
Hoyt WF, Joe S: Congenital teratoid cyst of the orbit: a case report and review of the literature. Arch Ophthalmol 1962; 68:196–201.

Linder D, et al: Parthenogenic origin of benign ovarian teratomas. New Engl J Med 1975; 292:63.
Mamalis N, et al: Congenital orbital teratoma: a review and report of two cases. Surv Ophthalmol 1985; 30:41–46. *
Itani K, et al: Conservative surgery in orbital teratoma. Orbit 1986; 5:61–65.

TR009                                                    **Elias I. Traboulsi**

## EYE, PUPILLARY MEMBRANE PERSISTENCE          0845

**Includes:**
> Anterior tunica vasculosa lentis persistence
> Pupillary membrane persistence

**Excludes:**
> Cataract, anterior capsular
> **Eye, anterior segment dysgenesis** (0439)
> **Rieger syndrome** (2139)

**Major Diagnostic Criteria:** Strands or sheets of iris, with one or both ends attached to the iris collarette, and usually crossing a portion of the pupil. Most clearly seen with the slit lamp following dilatation.

**Clinical Findings:** A variety of tissue remnants in the pupillary space are found in 95% of newborns, and less frequently in older age groups. These are usually asymptomatic fine strands attached to the iris collarette (lesser circle). Occasionally, hyperplasia of the iris stroma or imperforate pupil membrane results, but most iris attachments have no functional significance.

Less often strands attach to the anterior lens capsule, at which point there may be a white plaque dense enough to require surgery. Isolated pigment splotches on the lens capsule also occur. Rarely, central anterior synechiae to the posterior cornea are the end result. When white opacities of the cornea are associated, the picture is not unlike mesodermal dysgenesis of the anterior segment.

**Complications:** Amblyopia, if the membrane is dense enough to preclude foveal fixation.

**Associated Findings:** Corneal and lenticular opacities.

**Etiology:** A defect in embryogenesis of undetermined cause, for which a few pedigrees have been reported. Autosomal dominance was noted in one kindred, which had members with irregular tissue in the pupillary space in four generations.

**Pathogenesis:** Failure of the normal process of atrophy of the pupillary arcades and associated mesodermal tissue.

**MIM No.:** 17890

**Sex Ratio:** M1:F1

**Occurrence:** Several dozen cases documented in the literature.

**Risk of Recurrence for Patient's Sib:**
> See Part I, *Mendelian Inheritance.*

**Risk of Recurrence for Patient's Child:**
> See Part I, *Mendelian Inheritance.*

**Age of Detectability:** At birth.

**Gene Mapping and Linkage:** Unknown.

**Prevention:** None known. Genetic counseling indicated.

**Treatment:** Usually none is required; if strands at anterior lens capsule are dense, surgery may be needed. Removal and visual rehabilitation are necessary in infancy if amblyopia occurs.

**Prognosis:** Life span normal; excellent ocular prognosis.

**Detection of Carrier:** Unknown.

**References:**
Cassady JR, Light A: Familial persistent pupillary membranes. Arch Ophthalmol 1957; 58:438–448. *
Duke-Elder S: System of ophthalmology. vol. 3, part 2. Congenital deformities. London: Henry Kimpton, 1964:775–782.
Reynolds JD, et al.: Hyperplastic persistent pupillary membrane: surgical management. J Ped Ophthal Strabismus 1983; 20:149–152.

CR012                                                    **Harold E. Cross**

**Eye, superior oblique tendon sheath syndrome of Brown**
*See BROWN SYNDROME*
**Eye, superior orbital click syndrome**
*See BROWN SYNDROME*

## EYE, VITREOUS, PERSISTENT HYPERPLASTIC PRIMARY       0994

**Includes:**
Eye, fetal fibrovascular sheath of lens, persistent
Hyaloid artery, persistence of
Vitreous, persistent hyperplastic primary (PHPV)

**Excludes:**
**Retinal dysplasia** (0866)
**Retinoblastoma** (0870)
**Retinopathy of prematurity** (0872)

**Major Diagnostic Criteria:** White reflex (leukocoria) and a retrolental fibrovascular mass in a microphthalmic eye. Less severe forms of the disease occur with variable degrees of fibrovascular proliferation.

**Clinical Findings:** When severe, this entity is detected immediately after birth on the basis of the white pupil (leukocoria). This condition occurs in full-term infants, is unilateral and there is always some degree of microphthalmos. The anterior chamber is shallow and the blood vessels on the iris are prominent. A dehiscence in the posterior lens capsule may be present or a complete cataract may exist. Characteristically, there is a retrolental fibrovascular mass into which the ciliary processes are pulled. The hyaloid artery is sometimes observable. Computed tomography (CT) scan and ultrasound may be helpful in making the diagnosis and differentiating PHPV from **Retinoblastoma**.

**Complications:** Vitreous hemorrhage, retinal detachment, secondary glaucoma, cataract, phthisis bulbi.

**Associated Findings:** Patients with PHPV have normal systemic findings. One exception is a case reported by Traboulsi et al (1986) in a patient with **Oculo-dento-osseous dysplasia**.

**Etiology:** Unknown.

**Pathogenesis:** Persistence of the entire hyaloid system, with hyperplasia of its associated tissue. Dysplastic retina is often seen within the retina on histopathologic examination.

**CDC No.:** 743.580

**Sex Ratio:** Presumably M1:F1.

**Occurrence:** Undetermined but presumed rare.

**Risk of Recurrence for Patient's Sib:** Unknown.

**Risk of Recurrence for Patient's Child:** Unknown.

**Age of Detectability:** At birth, or in the first year of life in mild variants.

**Gene Mapping and Linkage:** Unknown.

**Prevention:** None known. Genetic counseling indicated.

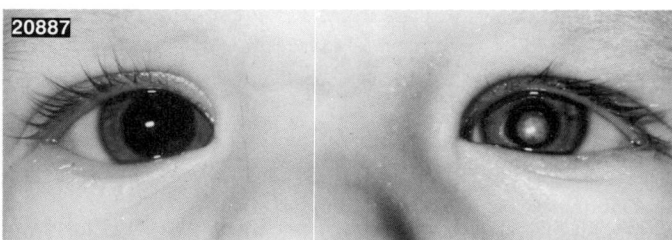

**0994-20887:** Persistence and hyperplasia of the primary vitreous (PHPV) OD; the left eye is microphthalmic with cataract.

**Treatment:** Removal of the cataractous lens and severing of the stalk to remove traction on the ciliary body rarely improves vision, but may prevent eventual phthisis, and is the treatment of choice.

**Prognosis:** Normal for life span and intelligence; poor for vision in the affected eye.

**Detection of Carrier:** Unknown.

**References:**
Duke-Elder S: System of ophthalmology. In: Congenital deformities, vol. III, pt. 2. St. Louis: C.V. Mosby, 1964:770–775.
Gass JD: Surgical excision of persistent hyperplastic primary vitreous. Arch Ophthalmol 1970; 83:163–168.
Nankin SJ, Scott WE: Persistent hyperplastic primary vitreous: rotoextraction and other surgical experience. Arch Ophthal 1977; 95:240–243.
Goldberg MF, Mafee M: Computed tomography for diagnosis of persistent hyperplastic primary vitreous (PHPV). Ophthalmology 1983; 30:442–451.
Stark WJ, et al.: Persistent hyperplastic primary vitreous: surgical treatment. Ophthalmology 1983; 30:452–457.
Traboulsi EI, et al.:Persistent hyperplastic primary vitreous and recessive oculo-dento-osseous dysplasia. Am J Med Genet 1986; 24:95–100.

ME032

**Marilyn B. Mets**
*Morton E. Smith*

**Eye-muscle-brain syndrome**
*See MUSCLE-EYE-BRAIN SYNDROME*
**Eyebrow-cheek-ichthyosis syndrome**
*See ICHTHYOSIS-CHEEK-EYEBROW SYNDROME*
**Eyelash, distichiasis**
*See DISTICHIASIS*
**Eyelash, distichiasis-lymphedema syndrome**
*See DISTICHIASIS-LYMPHEDEMA SYNDROME*
**Eyelashes (long)-mental retardation**
*See TRICHOMEGALY-RETARDATION-DWARFISM-RETINAL PIGMENTARY DEGENERATION*
**Eyelashes, congenital underdevelopment of**
*See EYELID, MADAROSIS*
**Eyelashes, two rows of**
*See DISTICHIASIS*
**Eyelid fusion**
*See EYELID, ANKYLOBLEPHARON*
**Eyelid fusion-cleft lip/palate**
*See CLEFT LIP/PALATE-FILIFORM FUSION OF EYELIDS*
**Eyelid tumor**
*See OCULAR DERMOIDS*
**Eyelid, absent**
*See EYE, CRYPTOPHTHALMOS WITH OTHER MALFORMATIONS*

## EYELID, ANKYLOBLEPHARON       0060

**Includes:**
Ankyloblepharon filiforme adnatum
Ankyloblepharon, external
Ankyloblepharon, internal
Eyelid fusion

**Excludes:** Cleft lip/palate-filiform fusion of eyelids (0176)

**Major Diagnostic Criteria:** Partial adhesion of the ciliary edges of the eyelids.

**Clinical Findings:** The lid margins are variably fused. Internal ankyloblepharon is characterized by failure of separation of the lid borders medially thereby shortening the interpalpebral fissure. In external ankyloblepharon the lid fusion is at the lateral canthus. Ankyloblepharon filiforme adnatum consists of one or more stretchable bands of tissue which connect the upper and lower edges of the lids at the grey line restricting the opening of the interpalpebral fissure. These strands are composed of fibrovascular connective tissue surrounded by epithelium without inflammatory changes. Sebaceous glands and hair follicles may also be found within them.

**Complications:** Unknown.

**Associated Findings:** Cleft palate, harelip, anophthalmia, microphthalmia, ptosis, microcephaly, patent ductus arteriosus, lower lip fistulae, interventricular septal defect, syndactyly, and ear anomalies.

**Etiology:** Autosomal dominant inheritance has been noted in some families. Autosomal recessive transmission is suggested in Khanna's (1957) report of ankyloblepharon filiforme adnatum, although most cases appear sporadic.

**Pathogenesis:** Believed to arise from aberration of mesodermal or ectodermal origin during lid fusion. Theories of intrauterine inflammation or trauma from fingernails have been refuted.

**MIM No.:** 12357

**CDC No.:** 743.635

**Sex Ratio:** M1:Fl

**Occurrence:** Undetermined.

**Risk of Recurrence for Patient's Sib:**
See Part I, *Mendelian Inheritance.*

**Risk of Recurrence for Patient's Child:**
See Part I, *Mendelian Inheritance.*

**Age of Detectability:** At birth.

**Gene Mapping and Linkage:** Unknown.

**Prevention:** None known. Genetic counseling indicated.

**Treatment:** The shortened interpalpebral fissure can be lengthened by plastic surgery of the fused canthal areas. This is seldom necessary, unless extreme, since the cosmetic appearance tends to improve with age. The adhesions in ankyloblepharon filiforme adnatum may be broken with a muscle hook if thin and narrow. Broader and thicker bands are excised.

**Prognosis:** No deterrent to health or function.

**Detection of Carrier:** Unknown.

**References:**
Khanna VD: Ankyloblepharon filiforme adnatum. Am J Ophthal 1957; 43:774.
Allerman CH, Stern LM: Ankyloblepharon filiforme adnatum. Brit J Ophthal 1979; 63:129–131.
Rosenman Y, et al.: Ankyloblepharon filiforme adnatum: congenital eyelid-band syndromes. Am J Dis Child 1980; 134:751–753.

RA004                                          **Elsa K. Rahn**

**Eyelid, blepharophimosis tetrad**
*See BLEPHAROPTOSIS-BLEPHAROPHIMOSIS-EPICANTHUS INVERSUS-TELECANTHUS*

---

## EYELID, COLOBOMA                           2941

**Includes:** Coloboma, congenital

**Excludes:**
Ablepharon
Microblepharon

**Major Diagnostic Criteria:** Full thickness deletion defects of the eyelid.

**Clinical Findings:** Colobomas typically manifest in a triangular configuration, although they may occasionally assume a quadrilateral, W, or irregular shape. Partial thickness colobomas may occur in the lower eyelid. Such partial thickness defects may retain orbicularis oculi muscle, tarsal elements, cilia, or glandular structures. Such retained tissues are usually malformed and malpositioned. The coloboma edge is rounded and covered with conjunctiva. Defect size may range from a small indentation at the eyelid margin to absence of almost the entire eyelid, suggesting ablepharon.

Colobomas are most frequently encountered at the medial aspect of the upper eyelid or at the lateral aspect of the lower eyelid. Typically unilateral, colobomas may also be bilateral and on occasion have involved all four eyelids. Symmetric defects are not uncommon, and multiple colobomas may occur on one eyelid.

**Complications:** Complications relate to corneal exposure from the coloboma defect. The larger the defect, the greater is the risk of maintained corneal dessication. Upper eyelid colobomas are more prone to exposure, while lower eyelid colobomas frequently cause trichiasis. Exposure becomes significant when more than one-third of either eyelid is missing.

**Associated Findings:** Eyelid colobomas have been associated with a myriad of ocular, periorbital, and facial defects. Associations have included microphthalmos, corneal opacification (from exposure), corectopia, coloboma of the iris or choroid, anterior polar **Cataract**, lens subluxation, epibulbar dermoid, caruncle malformation, symblepharon, nasolacrimal obstruction, eyebrow malformation, orbital dermoids, **Mandibulofacial dysostosis**, **Oculo-auriculo-vertebral anomaly**, **Cleft lip**, and **Cleft palate**.

**Etiology:** Although rarely hereditary, occasionally an autosomal dominant pedigree is observed.

**Pathogenesis:** Congenital eyelid colobomas result from delayed or incomplete union of mesodermal sheets of the frontonasal and maxillary processes.

**CDC No.:** 743.636

**Sex Ratio:** M1:F1

**Occurrence:** Undetermined but presumed rare.

**Risk of Recurrence for Patient's Sib:**
See Part I, *Mendelian Inheritance.* Mendelian only in those occasional cases with hereditary predisposition.

**Risk of Recurrence for Patient's Child:**
See Part I, *Mendelian Inheritance.* Mendelian only in those occasional cases with hereditary predisposition.

**Age of Detectability:** At birth.

**Gene Mapping and Linkage:** Unknown.

**Prevention:** None known. Genetic counseling indicated.

**Treatment:** Since most colobomas are small, ophthalmic plastic surgical correction can proceed electively during the first four years of life if Bell phenomenon is intact. During this interval, medical management is essential to avoid exposure. In mild cases, lubricating ointment and drops given frequently may prove sufficient. In more severe cases a moisture chamber or bandage soft contact lens may also be required. Surgery is urgent if significant corneal exposure ensues despite conservative measures.

**Prognosis:** No impairments unless part of a malformation syndrome.

**Detection of Carrier:** Unknown.

**Special Considerations:** The clinically apparent size of a coloboma may be misleading. The disrupted orbicularis oculi muscle causes the surrounding normal eyelid elements to retract horizontally away from the defect. This artifactually expands the coloboma. The true extent of the defect may be determined by simply approximating the defect's edges.

**References:**
Kidwell E, Tenzel R: Repair of congenital colobomas of the lids. Arch Ophthalmol 1979; 97:1931.
Patipa M, et al.: Surgical management of congenital eyelid coloboma. Ophthalmic Surg 1982; 13:212.
Kohn R: Congenital anomalies of the eyelids, socket, and orbit. In: Hornblass A, ed: Ophthalmic and orbital plastic and reconstructive surgery, Vol I. Baltimore: Williams & Wilkins, 1988.
Kohn R: Textbook of ophthalmic plastic and reconstructive surgery. Philadelphia: Lea & Febiger, 1988.

K0025                                          **Roger Kohn**

## EYELID, ECTROPION, CONGENITAL 0371

**Includes:** Ectropion

**Excludes:** Congenital tarsal kink

**Major Diagnostic Criteria:** Congenital ectropion denotes eversion of either eyelid present from birth.

**Clinical Findings:** The eyelid margins are everted to varying degrees, exposing the palpebral conjunctiva. Congenital ectropion is more common in the lower than the upper eyelid, because the tarsal plates of the latter are stronger and because the effects of gravity predispose to eversion of the lower eyelid. Primary congenital ectropion of the lower eyelid is an extraordinarily rare condition with occasional familial associations. Congenital ectropion is more commonly seen as a disorder secondary to other conditions as noted under Associated Findings.

Congenital ectropion of the upper eyelid presents as a total eversion. This is postulated to arise from birth trauma interfering with venous drainage. The resultant chemosis everts the eyelid and triggers orbicularis oculi muscle spasm. Orbicularis oculi muscle hypotonia has also been suggested as an etiology.

**Complications:** Ectropion of the lower eyelid may result in pooling of tears and epiphora. If associated with lagophthalmos (incomplete eyelid closure), exposure keratitis and corneal ulceration may result.

**Associated Findings:** Most cases of congenital ectropion are secondary to such conditions as microphthalmos, buphthalmos, euryblepharon, tumors of the eyelid, or as part of **Blepharoptosis-blepharophimosis-epicanthus inversus-telecanthus**. Rare cases of congenital ectropion may also result from excessive horizontal eyelid length.

A syndrome of **Clefting-ectropion-conical teeth** has also been reported in two families and four sporadic cases.

**Etiology:** Most cases appear sporadic. A few kindreds with this syndrome are compatible with autosomal dominant inheritance.

**Pathogenesis:** Lower eyelid, vertical cutaneous insufficiency or excessive horizontal eyelid length; upper eyelid, total eversion of the upper eyelid compromising venous return, which results in chemosis and orbicularis oculi spasm or hypotonia.

**CDC No.:** 743.610

**Sex Ratio:** Presumably M1:F1

**Occurrence:** Undetermined but presumably rare.

**Risk of Recurrence for Patient's Sib:**
See Part I, *Mendelian Inheritance*. Mendelian only for the exceedingly rare hereditary cases, otherwise unknown.

**Risk of Recurrence for Patient's Child:**
See Part I, *Mendelian Inheritance*. Mendelian only for the exceedingly rare hereditary cases, otherwise unknown.

**Age of Detectability:** At birth.

**Gene Mapping and Linkage:** Unknown.

**Prevention:** None known. Genetic counseling indicated.

**Treatment:** Ophthalmic plastic surgical correction. The specific procedure is based on the specific etiology of the ectropion. Additional conservative measures to prevent exposure keratitis is also essential.

**Prognosis:** Good following surgical correction.

**Detection of Carrier:** Unknown.

**Special Considerations:** Ectropion may gradually evolve during the first several years of life as sequelae of anterior lamellar shrinkage from such dermatologic disorders as **Ichthyosis**, **Darier disease**, spinulosa decalvans, erythroderm ichthyosiforme congenitum, **Xeroderma pigmentosum**, and lamellar exfoliation of the newborn.

**References:**
Mortada A: Lamella exfoliation of the newborn and ectropion of the eyelids. Ophthalmologica 1966; 152:68.
Gupta K, Kumar K: Euryblepharon with ectropion. Am J Ophthalmol 1968; 66:554.
Johnson C, McGowan B: Persistent congenital ectropion of all four eyelids with megaloblepharon. Am J Ophthalmol 1969; 67:252.
Stern E, et al.: Conservative management of congenital eversion of the eyelids. Am J Ophthalmol 1973; 75:319.
Rodrigue D: Congenital ectropion. Can J Ophthalmol 1976; 11:355.
Kohn R: Congenital anomalies of the eyelids, socket, and orbit. In: Hornblas A, ed: Ophthalmic and orbital plastic and reconstructive surgery, Vol I. Baltimore: Williams & Wilkins, 1988.
Kohn R: Textbook of ophthalmic plastic and reconstructive surgery. Philadelphia: Lea & Febiger, 1988.

K0025        **Roger Kohn**

## EYELID, ENTROPION 0372

**Includes:** Entropion of lid, congenital

**Excludes:**
Entropion of iris
**Eyelid, epiblepharon** (0355)
Secondary entropion

**Major Diagnostic Criteria:** Inversion of eyelid.

**Clinical Findings:** The tarsus of the eyelid is inverted or turned inward toward the globe with resultant rubbing of the lashes against the cornea. It usually affects the lower lid and is more often bilateral than unilateral. It may be found as an isolated phenomenon or in association with other anomalies, especially epicanthus and epiblepharon. The latter has been postulated to cause, in some instances, entropion. In the presence of anomalies of the globe, such as microphthalmia or anophthalmia, both upper and lower lids may be secondarily inverted.

**Complications:** Keratitis and traumatic pannus are seen from trauma of the lashes rubbing against the cornea.

**Associated Findings:** Epicanthus, epiblepharon, downward obliquity of the palpebral fissures, anophthalmia, microphthalmia, polytrichia, bone defects of skull and clubfeet.

**Etiology:** Autosomal dominant inheritance has been reported.

**Pathogenesis:** Defective development of the tarsal plate, hypertrophy of the tarsus, hypertrophy of the palpebral portion of the orbicularis muscle, and attachments of the orbicularis and inferior rectus muscles into the skin of the lid have all been implicated as possible factors in the pathogenesis of entropion. In combination with epiblepharon, the excess fold of skin may cause backward pressure on the ciliary margin with inward turning of the lid. Lack of support to the lid margins in the presence of small or absent globes may result in the inward turning from a mechanical defect.

**CDC No.:** 743.620

**Sex Ratio:** M1:F1

**Occurrence:** Undetermined but presumed rare.

**Risk of Recurrence for Patient's Sib:**
See Part I, *Mendelian Inheritance*.

**Risk of Recurrence for Patient's Child:**
See Part I, *Mendelian Inheritance*.

**Age of Detectability:** At birth.

**Gene Mapping and Linkage:** Unknown.

**Prevention:** None known. Genetic counseling indicated.

**Treatment:** Surgical repair is usually necessary in entropion. The type of procedure is dependent upon the area and extent of involvement and associated complications.

**Prognosis:** Good.

**Detection of Carrier:** Unknown.

**References:**
Bacskulin J, Bacskulin E: Beitrag zur klinik und therapie des kongenitalen entropiums. Ophthalmologica 1966; 151:555.
Hiles DA, Wilder LW: Congenital entropion of the upper lids. J Pediatr Ophthalmol 1969; 6:157.

RA004        **Elsa K. Rahn**

## EYELID, EPIBLEPHARON                                    0355

**Includes:**
>    Epiblepharon, inferior
>    Epiblepharon, superior

**Excludes:**
>    Blepharochalasis
>    **Eyelid, entropion** (0372)

**Major Diagnostic Criteria:** A horizontal fold of skin on eyelid which is often exaggerated in downward gaze.

**Clinical Findings:** Both inferior and superior epiblepharon occur. It is a horizontal fold of skin in the tarsal region of the lid. Accessory lid structures are usually normal. The excess skin overhangs the lower portion of the upper lid or overlaps the upper portion of the lower lid. It is most evident near the medial canthi. The overriding of skin may extend to the lid border causing an inturning of the lashes. This is often exaggerated in downward gaze. Symptoms are more likely to arise if the condition persists. Infants with epiblepharon characteristically have chubby cheeks, prominent eyes and a narrow interpupillary distance. Epiblepharon is usually bilateral but asymmetric. Inferior epiblepharon tends to disappear with facial growth.

**Complications:** Increased lacrimation, photophobia, bulbar conjunctival infection and keratitis.

**Associated Findings:** Paresis of the inferior oblique muscle, eyelid entropion, hypertrophy of the tarsus, and epicanthus.

**Etiology:** For superior epiblepharon, autosomal dominant inheritance has been demonstrated. Inferior epiblepharon has a familial tendency, and is probably also an autosomal dominant.

**Pathogenesis:** It has been suggested that epiblepharon results from incomplete development of the fascial planes, absence of the tarsus, hypertrophy of the marginal portion of the orbicularis, and from anomalous strands of insertions of the vertical recti muscles into the skin of the lids. Superior epiblepharon, in addition to the preceding, has been felt to result from a Z-shaped kink in the orbicularis fibers or insertion of the levator tendon too close to the lid margin.

**MIM No.:** 13145, 13146

**CDC No.:** 743.630

**Sex Ratio:** Presumably M1:F1

**Occurrence:** Undetermined. Superior epiblepharon is considered relatively rare, whereas inferior epiblepharon is more common; 10% of Chinese students in one study.

**Risk of Recurrence for Patient's Sib:**
>    See Part I, *Mendelian Inheritance.*

**Risk of Recurrence for Patient's Child:**
>    See Part I, *Mendelian Inheritance.*

**Age of Detectability:** At birth for inferior epiblepharon.

**Gene Mapping and Linkage:** Unknown.

**Prevention:** None known. Genetic counseling indicated.

**Treatment:** The overlapping portion of skin may be excised in epiblepharon for either cosmetic purposes or, if repeated keratitis occurs, from inturned lashes. The application of collodion, adhesive, or cellophane tapes from the lower lid to the cheek may be of some help to pull the skin fold away from the lid as a temporizing measure. Inferior epiblepharon usually corrects itself spontaneously within the 1st year of life with growth and development of the facial and orbital bone. Its persistence is rare. Irritation of the cornea, if it occurs, is usually temporary and may be lessened by the application of a protective ointment. Superior epiblepharon more often requires surgical correction than inferior epiblepharon.

**Prognosis:** Excellent for both types.

**Detection of Carrier:** Unknown.

**References:**
Swan KC: Syndrome of congenital epiblepharon and inferior oblique insufficiency. Am J Ophthalmol 1955; 39:130.

Levitt JM: Epiblepharon and congenital entropion. Am J Ophthalmol 1957; 44:112.
Karlin BD: Congenital entropion, epiblepharon, and antimongoloid obliquity of the palpebral fissure. Am J Ophthalmol 1960; 50:487.
Duke-Elder S: System of ophthalmology, vol. 3, part 2. Congenital deformities. London: Henry Kimpton, 1964:857.
Hu D-N: Ophthalmic genetics in China. Ophthal Paediat Genet 1983; 2:39–45.

RA004                                          **Elsa K. Rahn**

## EYELID, MADAROSIS                                    0623

**Includes:**
>    Eyelashes, congenital underdevelopment of
>    Madarosis

**Excludes:**
>    **Ectodermal dysplasia**
>    Hyperkeratosis follicularis spinulosa decalvans
>    Hypotrichosis, generalized
>    Hypomelia-hypotrichosis-facial hemangioma
>    **Oculo-mandibulo-facial syndrome** (0738)

**Major Diagnostic Criteria:** Hypoplasia (severe diminution or absence) of lashes. Lack of primary cause, such as trauma, inflammation, mycotic infection, neurotic epilation, or systemic disease such as forms of alopecia, idiopathic hypoparathyroidism, xeroderma pigmentosa, or mandibulofacial dysostosis.

**Clinical Findings:** In congenital underdevelopment of the lashes, the cilia are replaced by fine hairs, and there can be absence of the intermarginal area of the lid. The nails and sweat glands are usually normal.

**Complications:** Ocular pain if associated with distichiasis (eyelashes growing in abnormal locations on lid margin and rubbing against cornea).

**Associated Findings:** Distichiasis.

**Etiology:** The two families described have displayed dominant inheritance. The family described by Traquair (1912) also had distichiasis.

**Pathogenesis:** Unknown.

**Sex Ratio:** Presumably M1:F1.

**Occurrence:** Undetermined but presumed rare.

**Risk of Recurrence for Patient's Sib:**
>    See Part I, *Mendelian Inheritance.*

**Risk of Recurrence for Patient's Child:**
>    See Part I, *Mendelian Inheritance.*

**Age of Detectability:** At birth.

**Gene Mapping and Linkage:** Unknown.

**Prevention:** None known. Genetic counseling indicated.

**Treatment:** None to replace lashes. Cryotherapy to ablate irritating distichiasis.

**Prognosis:** Normal life span.

**Detection of Carrier:** Unknown.

**Special Considerations:** Has been reported in cattle and dogs. Many forms of hypotrichosis spare the eyelashes.

**References:**
Traquair HM: A case congenital deficiency of cilia and intermarginal area of both lower lids with distichiasis. Ophthalmic Rev 1912; 31:138–140.
Urrets-Zavalia A Jr, Jimenez ES: Hereditary ciliary and superciliary hypotrichosis of a dominant character. Br J Ophthalmol 1958; 42:694–696.*

KI021                                          **Jane D. Kivlin**

## EYELID, PTOSIS, CONGENITAL 0834

**Includes:**
> Blepharoptosis, congenital
> Myogenic stiff ptosis
> Neurogenic flaccid ptosis
> Palsy, double elevator
> Ptosis, congenital
> Ptosis-epicanthus
> Ptosis-superior rectus weakness

**Excludes:**
> **Blepharoptosis-blepharophimosis-epicanthus inversus-telecanthus** (2103)
> **Horner syndrome** (0475)
> **Jaw-winking syndrome** (0548)
> **Ophthalmoplegia, progressive external** (0752)
> **Ophthalmoplegia, total with ptosis and miosis** (0753)
> Pseudoptosis
> Ptosis, periodic with cyclic oculomotor spasm
> Ptosis secondary to myasthenia gravis or myotonic dystrophy
> Third nerve paralysis

**Major Diagnostic Criteria:** No sharp cutoff exists for diagnosing mild bilateral cases. Unilateral cases can be detected by comparison with the fellow lid. Diagnosis is most obvious on upward gaze. Differentiation between myogenic and neurogenic ptosis is best made by electromyographic examination. The phenylephrine 10% test is also helpful in establishing the diagnosis.

**Clinical Findings:** Simple ptosis is characterized by drooping of and inability to raise the upper eyelid associated in one-third of cases with weakness of upward movement of the eye. Approximately 80% are unilateral. This type of simple ptosis accounts for approximately 80% of all congenital ptosis. It is stationary throughout life and unaccompanied by visual defects unless the lid covers the pupil causing amblyopia, or weakness of the recti muscles causes strabismus. The degree of ptosis varies among cases and may be noticeable only on upward gaze. Elevation of the eyebrow and backward head tilt are frequent compensatory maneuvers. The skin of the lid is smooth without the normal tarsal fold. Presence of a lid crease suggests levator aponeurosis dehiscence, a traumatic non-hereditary form of the condition.

**Complications:** Postural anomalies, with changes in neck musculature and the cervical spine, due to hyperextension of the head (particularly in bilateral cases). Amblyopia (particularly in unilateral cases, or with associated strabismus).

**Associated Findings:** Occasional association with micrognathia, hereditary edema of the limbs, general mental and physical degeneration, arachnodactyly, **Turner syndrome, Chromosome 18, monosomy 18q,** and a wide variety of congenital neurologic and cranial malformations have been described.

**Etiology:** Autosomal dominant inheritance with approximately 60–70% penetrance.

**Pathogenesis:** Most cases are due to abnormal peripheral differentiation of the levator muscle (which embryologically develops from the superior rectus). Other cases, particularly those with ophthalmoplegia (other than paresis of the superior rectus), are due to agenesis or aplasia of the appropriate midbrain nuclei. Fibrosis of the atrophic muscle usually occurs.

**MIM No.:** *17830

**CDC No.:** 743.600

**Sex Ratio:** M1:F1

**Occurrence:** Common in several large kindreds, including the Metcalfs of Lafayette, Tennessee, and a possibly related Georgia mountain family.

**Risk of Recurrence for Patient's Sib:** If parent is affected 1:3 for each offspring to be affected, 1:2 for inheriting the gene; otherwise not increased.

**Risk of Recurrence for Patient's Child:** 1:3 for each offspring to be affected, 1:2 for inheriting the gene.

**Age of Detectability:** Most cases are diagnosable at birth.

**Gene Mapping and Linkage:** There is probable linkage to the genes for the MN blood group system.

**Prevention:** None known. Genetic counseling indicated.

**Treatment:** Many surgical procedures have been described, with the facia lata or nupramyd sling being used most frequently. Results are good on simple ptosis, but often poor when accompanied by defective eye motility. Early treatment is necessary to prevent amblyopia or postural changes where these are a consideration. Crutch spectacles.

**Prognosis:** Normal life span. Condition is nonprogressive.

**Detection of Carrier:** Clinical examination of first degree relatives.

**References:**
Berke RN: Congenital ptosis: a classification of 200 cases. Arch Ophthalmol 1949; 41:188–197.
Rank BK, Thomson JA: The genetic approach to hereditary congenital ptosis. Aust New Zeal J Surg 1959; 28:274–279.
Duke-Elder, S: System of ophthalmology (normal and abnormal development). vol. 3, part 2. Congenital deformities. St. Louis: C.V. Mosby, 1963:887–888.
Beard C: Ptosis. St. Louis: C.V. Mosby, 1969:40–50,81–107.
Smith B, et al.: Surgical treatment of blepharoptosis. Am J Ophthalmol 1969; 68:92–106.
Spacth EB: An analysis of the causes, types, and factors important to the correction of congenital blepharoptosis. Am J Ophthalmol 1971; 71:696–717.
Anderson RL, Gordy DD: Aponeurotic defects in congenital ptosis. Trans Am Acad Ophthalmol Otolaryngol 1979; 86:1493–1500.
Crawford JS: Congenital ptosis: examination and treatment. In: Transaction of the New Orleans Acad Ophthalmol. New York: Raven Press, 1986:173–191.
McCord CD, Jr.: The evaluation and treatment of the patient with congenital ptosis. Clin Plast Surg 1988; 15:169–184.

DE034
BE026

**Monte A. Del Monte**
**Donald R. Bergsma**

## EYELID, PUNCTA AND CANALICULI, SUPERNUMERARY 0844

**Includes:** Supernumerary puncta and canaliculi

**Excludes:**
> **Lacrimal canaliculus atresia** (0563)
> **Lacrimal sac fistula** (0565)
> **Nasolacrimal duct obstruction** (0705)

**Major Diagnostic Criteria:** Supernumerary puncta and canaliculi.

**Clinical Findings:** Extra puncta and canaliculi in close anatomic proximity to the normal punctum and canaliculus. More than one extra punctum and canaliculus may be present. These supernumerary structures may communicate with the normal lacrimal drainage system or may end blindly. Some cases of double puncta may represent a side opening from a single canaliculus.

**Complications:** Epiphora from obstruction of the nasolacrimal system is more common in these cases. Most patients, though, are asymptomatic.

**Associated Findings:** Abnormalities of the orbital bones, **Eyelid, coloboma,** and **Blepharoptosis-blepharophimosis-epicanthus inversus-telecanthus.**

**Etiology:** Undetermined. In one kindred, autosomal dominant inheritance was demonstrated through three generations.

**Pathogenesis:** Irregular outbudding of the superior end of the ectodermal core, thereby engulfing this tissue into mesoderm.

**Sex Ratio:** Presumably M1:F1.

**Occurrence:** Undetermined but presumed rare.

**Risk of Recurrence for Patient's Sib:** Unknown.

**Risk of Recurrence for Patient's Child:** Unknown.

**Age of Detectability:** At birth.

**Gene Mapping and Linkage:** Unknown.

**Prevention:** None known. Genetic counseling indicated.

**Treatment:** Generally, no treatment is required because patients are asymptomatic.

**Prognosis:** Good.

**Detection of Carrier:** Unknown.

**References:**
Chignell A: Double punctum and canaliculus. Am J Ophthalmol 1968; 65:736.
Kohn R: Textbook of ophthalmic plastic and reconstructive surgery. Philadelphia: Lea & Febiger, 1988.

K0025                                              **Roger Kohn**

**Eyelid, winking upon movement of jaw**
   *See JAW-WINKING SYNDROME*
**Eyelids, lower ectropion-clefting-conical teeth**
   *See CLEFTING-ECTROPION-CONICAL TEETH*
**Eyes, interpupillary distance**
   *See TELECANTHUS, HEREDITARY*

# F

**F syndrome**
*See ACROPECTOROVERTEBRAL DYSPLASIA*

## FABRY DISEASE                                            0373

**Includes:**

> Alpha-galactosidase A deficiency
> Angiokeratoma, diffuse
> Ceramide trihexosidase deficiency
> Di- and trihexosyl ceramide lipidosis
> Dystopic lipidosis, hereditary
> Fabry-Anderson disease
> Glycolipid lipidosis
> Ruiter-Pompen-Wyers syndrome

**Excludes:**

> **Alpha-N-acetylgalactosaminidase deficiency** (3254)
> Angiokeratoma Mibelli
> Erythromelalgia
> Rheumatic fever
> **Telangiectasia, osler hemorrhagic** (2021)

**Major Diagnostic Criteria:** Hemizygotes can be diagnosed by a history of acroparesthesia and the presence of the characteristic skin lesions (angiokeratoma) and corneal opacities. Birefringent lipid can be observed histologically in biopsied tissues, bone marrow macrophages, or urinary sediment. Heterozygotes are usually asymptomatic or may manifest attenuated symptoms; about 80% of obligate heterozygotes have the characteristic cor-neal lesions. Clinically diagnosed hemizygotes and heterozygotes should be confirmed biochemically by the demonstration of deficient alpha-galactosidase A activity in plasma, isolated leukocytes, tears, or cultured fibroblasts or by increased levels of trihexosyl ceramide in urinary sediment, plasma, or cultured fibroblasts.

**Clinical Findings:** Clinical onset of the disease in hemizygous males usually occurs during childhood or adolescence. Typically, onset is characterized by periodic, excruciating acroparesthesias, which may become more frequent and severe with age. These painful episodes may last from several hours to days and usually are associated with a low-grade fever and an elevation of the erythrocyte sedimentation rate. Affected individuals describe these pains as burning, tingling sensations that begin in the fingers and toes and then radiate proximally. The acroparesthesias usually are triggered by fever, fatigue, or changes in environmental temperature or humidity. During the second and third decades of life, these painful episodes often become less frequent and usually are exacerbated by febrile episodes. They frequently have led to the misdiagnosis of rheumatic fever or erythromelalgia. In addition, affected individuals may experience a chronic discomfort in their extremities, which usually occurs in the late afternoon or evening.

The cutaneous vascular lesions, angiokeratomas, usually appear during childhood and progressively increase in number and size with age. Characteristically, they are most dense between the umbilicus and knees and do not blanch with pressure. Variants without angiokeratomas also have been reported. Hypohidrosis presumably results from involvement of the sweat glands. Ocular manifestations include aneurysmal dilation and tortuosity of conjunctival and retinal vessels as well as characteristic corneal and lenticular opacities. The corneal lesions, which must be observed by slit-lamp microscopy, are characterized by whorled streaks emanating from a central vortex. A phenocopy of the Fabry keratopathy occurs in patients receiving long-term chloroquine or amiodarone therapy. The lenticular opacity involves the anterior capsule and occurs in a propeller-like distribution.

With increasing age, the major symptoms result from involvement of the renal-cardiovascular system. In childhood, casts, red cells, and lipid inclusions with characteristic, birefringent "Maltese crosses" appear in the urinary sediment. Proteinuria, isosthenuria, and gradual deterioration of renal function and development of azotemia occur in the second to fourth decades. Cardiovascular findings may include hypertension, left ventricular hypertrophy, myocardial ischemia or infarction, and cerebral vascular disease. Common electrocardiographic abnormalities include left ventricular hypertrophy, ST segment changes, T-wave inversion, and a short PR interval. Mitral valve involvement is common.

Nausea, vomiting, diarrhea, and abdominal or flank pain are common gastrointestinal symptoms. Other less frequent symptoms include lymphedema of the legs and dyspnea, neurologic defects secondary to small-vessel ischemia, and infarction in cortical and brainstem areas. Personality changes may occur late in the disease course. Musculoskeletal system findings include a

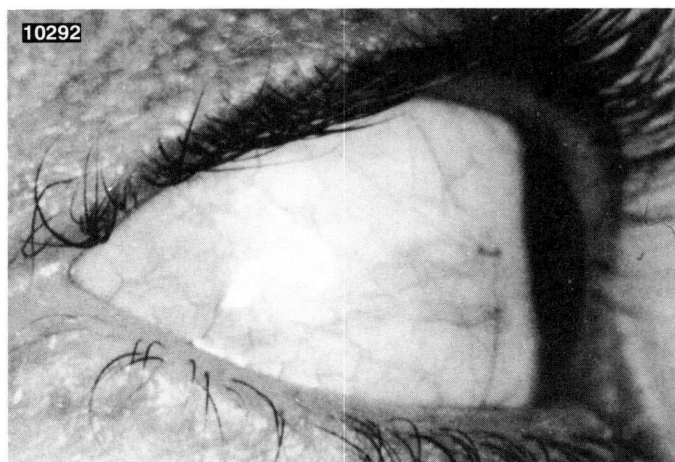

10292

**0373-10292:** Microaneurysms and telangiectasias of bulbar conjunctiva.

permanent deformity of the distal interphalangeal joint of the fingers, osteoporosis of dorsal vertebrae, and avascular necrosis of the head of femur or talus. Affected males have a mild hypochromic microcytic anemia, presumably due to decreased red cell survival. Many hemizygotes appear to have growth retardation or delayed puberty. Affected individuals may complain of fatigue and weakness and may be incapacitated for prolonged periods of time. Death most often results from uremia or vascular disease of the heart or brain during the fourth decade of life.

Heterozygous females may be totally asymptomatic or may manifest many of the same symptoms as the hemizygous males in attenuated form. Isolated single angiokeratoma with or without corneal opacities are present in the majority of these carriers of the Fabry gene. Most heterozygotes experience a normal life span. With advanced age, heterozygotes may become symptomatic, and death may result from renal or cardiac insufficiency secondary to glycosphingolipid accumulation. Rare heterozygous females as severely affected as hemizygous males have been described.

**Complications:** Renal insufficiency leading to uremia. Cardiovascular and cerebrovascular complications may include seizures, intranuclear ophthalmoplegia, and central retinal artery occlusion.

**Associated Findings:** Subacute bacterial endocarditis, chronic bronchitis. A high incidence of mitral valve prolapse has been reported in hemizygotes and heterozygotes.

**Etiology:** X-linked recessive inheritance with complete penetrance and variable clinical expressivity in hemizygous males. Expressivity in heterozygous females ranges from typically asymptomatic individuals to rare females with severe manifestations of the disease.

**Pathogenesis:** Fabry disease is characterized by the systemic accumulation of the glycosphingolipid globotriaosylceramide (trihexosylceramide); the primary site of deposition is in the endothelium of blood vessels. A related glycosphingolipid, galabiosylceramide (digalactosyl ceramide), is deposited to a lesser extent in certain tissues, including the heart and kidney. In addition, patients who are blood group B antigen positive accumulate the blood group B-1 glycolipid and experience a more rapid disease progression.

The primary metabolic defect is the defective activity of the lysosomal hydrolase alpha-galactosidase A, which normally catabolizes these three glycosphingolipids. Although globotriaosylceramide is synthesized in all non-neural cells (and in certain cell types in the nervous system), the major sites of synthesis are in hepatocytes and bone marrow. Globotriaosylceramide synthesized in the liver is secreted in association with the low-density lipoproteins (LDL). The plasma globotriaosylceramide level in affected males is four- to ten-fold that in normal individuals. Presumably, the accumulated plasma globotriaosylceramide gains access to vascular endothelial cells by the LDL receptor-mediated uptake pathway. The progressive glycosphingolipid deposition in the vascular endothelium results in ischemia and infarction, the major causes of pathology in this disease.

**MIM No.:** *30150

**POS No.:** 3023

**Sex Ratio:** M1:F+0

**Occurrence:** For hemizygotes, the estimated incidence is about 1:40,000. Of the over 300 cases reported, most have occurred in Caucasians of Western European extraction; however, Oriental, Black, Egyptian, and Latin American patients have been described. The disease has not been reported in American Indians.

**Risk of Recurrence for Patient's Sib:**
See Part I, *Mendelian Inheritance.*

**Risk of Recurrence for Patient's Child:**
See Part I, *Mendelian Inheritance.*

**Age of Detectability:** Antenatal and postnatal diagnosis of hemizygotes can be accomplished by determining the alpha-galactosidase A activity in plasma, leukocytes, or tears. The level of alpha-galactosidase A can be determined in chorionic villi obtained in the first trimester of pregnancy or in amniocytes cultured from amniotic fluid obtained in the second trimester.

**Gene Mapping and Linkage:** GLA (galactosidase, alpha) has been mapped to Xq21.3-q22.

**Prevention:** None known. Genetic counseling indicated.

**Treatment:** Painful Fabry crises may be relieved and prevented by low maintenance doses of diphenylhydantoin or carbamazepine. Treatment of renal, cardiovascular, pulmonary, neurologic, and musculoskeletal problems remains symptomatic at present. Kidney transplantation can be undertaken in appropriate individuals. Enzyme replacement therapy may be feasible in the future.

**Prognosis:** Average reported life span of affected males prior to hemodialysis or renal transplantation was 40 years. Asymptomatic heterozygotes usually have a normal life span; however, symptomatic heterozygotes have been reported to expire in the fourth and fifth decades of life.

**Detection of Carrier:** Heterozygotes for Fabry disease can be biochemically identified by 1) increased levels of globotriaosylceramide in urinary sediment or cultured fibroblasts; 2) intermediate levels of alpha-galactosidase A activity in plasma, lymphocytes, tears, isolated hair roots, or cultured fibroblasts; 3) demonstration of normal and mutant cell lines following single cell cloning of fibroblasts; 4) clinical examination for isolated angiokeratoma; and 5) slit-lamp examination for the characteristic corneal dystrophy.

**Special Considerations:** Hemizygotic variants without the classic skin lesions have been reported. Interfamilial variation in the clinical manifestations suggests multiple mutant alleles at the X-linked locus for this disorder. Survival of uremic patients can be prolonged by hemodialysis or renal transplantation. Enzyme therapy is experimental at present and is limited by the availability of the purified human enzyme; further experience will determine its therapeutic effectiveness.

**References:**
Lockman L, et al.: Relief of the painful crises of Fabry's disease by diphenylhydantoin. Neurology 1973; 23:871–875.
Johnson DL, et al.: Fabry disease: diagnosis of hemizygotes and heterozygotes by alpha-galactosidase A activity in tears. Clin Chim Acta 1975; 63:81–90.
Desnick RJ, et al.: Enzyme therapy in Fabry disease: differential in vivo plasma clearance and metabolic effectiveness of plasma and splenic alpha-galactosidase A isozymes. Proc Natl Acad Sci USA 1979; 76:5326–5330.
Desnick RJ, Sweeley CC: Fabry's disease. Defective alpha-galactosidase A. In: Stanbury JB et al., eds: The metabolic basis of inherited disease, 5th ed. New York: McGraw-Hill, 1982:906–944.
Bishop DF, et al.: Human α-galactosidase A: nucleotide sequence of a cDNA clone encoding the mature enzyme. Proc Natl Acad Sci USA 1986; 83:4859–4863.
Friedlaender MM, et al.: Renal biopsy in Fabry's disease eight years after successful renal transplantation.

DE024                                        **Robert J. Desnick**

**Fabry-Anderson disease**
*See FABRY DISEASE*
**Face (dysmorphic)-skeletal defects-torsion dystonia**
*See BLEPHARO-NASO-FACIAL SYNDROME*
**Face, absence of facial structures**
*See APROSOPIA*
**Face, acromegaloid appearance**
*See ACROMEGALOID FACIAL APPEARANCE SYNDROME*

---

**FACE, CHIN FISSURE**                                     **0146**

**Includes:**
Chin cleft
Chin dimple
Chin groove or furrow
Chin fissure
Cleft chin
Fissure of chin, Y-shaped
Fovea mentalis
Incisura mentalis types I, II, III, IV
Sulcus mentalis

**Excludes:**

Cleft tongue, syndromes related to
**Cranio-carpo-tarsal dysplasia, whistling face type** (0223)
Median clefts of lower lip, mandible, and tongue
Mental fold

**Major Diagnostic Criteria:** Permanent depression of the soft tissue part of the chin.

**Clinical Findings:** Chin fissures are single visible depressions of the soft tissue part of the chin. Four different types of chin fissures can be distinguished clinically and genetically. The most common type is a perpendicular furrow in the midline of the chin (incisura mentalis) ranging from a superficial depression in the area of the gnathion to a more pronounced furrow. Less commonly a steep fissure (sulcus mentalis) or a round dimple with a center of varying depth (fovea mentalis) is observed. Very rarely, a Y-shaped fissure in the middle of the chin is found. Bony defects of the underlying mental tubercle may or may not be associated with fissures in the soft tissues and may even be present without a furrow of the overlying skin. Fissures of the chin may not be present at birth but arise later during childhood or early adulthood. They may disappear later in life or after trauma.

**Complications:** Unknown.

**Associated Findings:** In one family reported by Güenther (1939), 4 of 6 individuals had preauricular fistulas in addition to a Y-shaped fissure of the chin.

**Etiology:** Autosomal dominant inheritance with high degree of penetrance and variable expressivity for all types.

**Pathogenesis:** Fissures of the chin may occur by partial fusion of the mental muscles with the overlying skin. Local absence of subcutaneous fat and muscular tissue in the area of the gnathion may cause an adhesion of the dermis to the periosteum by means of collagen bundles or even a ligament. These developmental variations leading to chin furrows may be determined around the end of the first trimester.

**MIM No.:** *11900

**Sex Ratio:** About M2:F1

**Occurrence:** About 14 to 21% in males and 9 to 15% in females in German populations. The first type (incisura mentalis) was 8.4% in males and 4.2% in females. The second type (sulcus mentalis) was present in 0.73% and 0.04%; fovea mentalis was found in 0.27% and 0.16%; and the Y-shaped fissure in 0.15% and 0.08% of males and females, respectively.

**Risk of Recurrence for Patient's Sib:**
See Part I, *Mendelian Inheritance.*

**Risk of Recurrence for Patient's Child:**
See Part I, *Mendelian Inheritance.*

**Age of Detectability:** Fissures are sometimes present at birth, but they more commonly become visible in childhood or early adulthood.

**Gene Mapping and Linkage:** Unknown.

**Prevention:** None known. Genetic counseling indicated.

**Treatment:** Plastic surgery for cosmetic reasons.

**Prognosis:** Furrows may disappear with age or after trauma. No effect on longevity or function.

**Detection of Carrier:** Unknown.

**Special Considerations:** Chin fissures, especially the first type (sulcus mentalis), are a common finding in the general population and should be considered as normal variations of chin form. The steep furrow (sulcus mentalis) resembling a cleft of the soft tissue part of the chin may only represent a more pronounced expression of the common furrow. Güenther (1939) reported 4 out of 6 individuals of one family as having, in addition to a Y-shaped fissure, preauricular fistulas, suggesting a specific syndrome. However, this association was probably caused by two different traits. Preauricular fistulas are also known to be transmitted in an autosomal dominant pattern.

*The author wishes to thank Gordon G. Keyes for his contribution to an earlier version of this article.*

**References:**

Günther H: Anomalien und Anomaliekomplexe in der Gegend des ersten Schlundbogens. Z Menschl Vererb Konstitutions 1939; 23:43–52.

Lebow MR, Sawin PB: Inheritance of human facial features: a pedigree study involving length of face, prominent ears and chin cleft. J Hered 1941; 32:127–132.

Pfannenstiel D: Zur morphologie und genetik der mund-und kinnregion. Arch Julius Klaus-Stift Vererb-Forsch 1952; 27:1.

J0027

**Ronald J. Jorgenson**

**Face, coarse with full lips-deafness-mental retardation**
*See FOUNTAIN SYNDROME*
**Face, diffuse symmetric lipomatosis of**
*See NECK/FACE, LIPOMATOSIS*
**Face, dysmorphic-pterygia-short stature-mental retardation**
*See PTERYGIA-DYSMORPHIC FACIES-SHORT STATURE-MENTAL RETARDATION*
**Face, dysmorphic-skeletal defects-aural atresia**
*See AURAL ATRESIA-DYSMORPHIC FACIES-SKELETAL DEFECTS*
**Face, interpupillary distance**
*See TELECANTHUS, HEREDITARY*

---

## FACE, MEDIAN CLEFT FACE SYNDROME          0635

**Includes:**

Fronto-nasal dysplasia
Median cleft face syndrome

**Excludes:**

**Eye, cryptophthalmos** (0003)
**Hypertelorism-hypospadias syndrome** (0505)
**Nose, glioma** (0726)

**Major Diagnostic Criteria:** Ocular hypertelorism, broad nasal root, and variable degree of median nasal groove.

**Clinical Findings:** Patients consistently manifest true ocular hypertelorism. Anterior cranium bifidum occultum may be present, and the anterior hairline may assume a widow's peak configuration, which is a V-shaped extension of the hair onto the center of the forehead. The severity of median clefting varies from absence of the nasal tip to separation of the nose into two parts. Less common physical features include brachycephaly, micro-

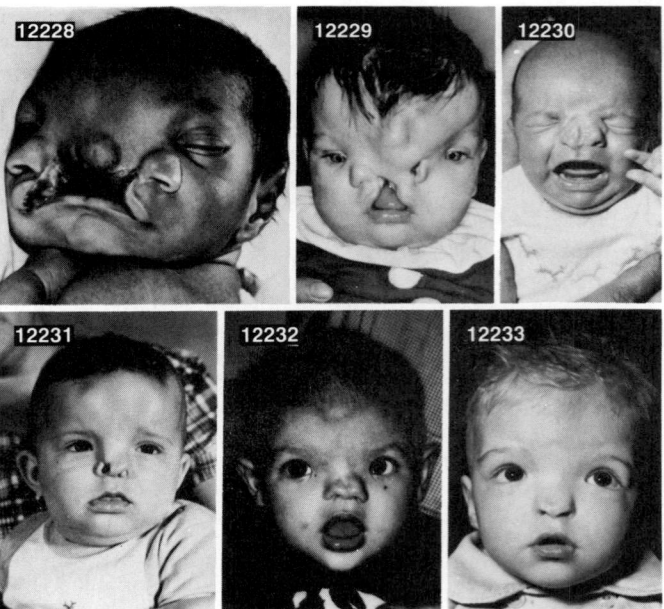

**0635**-12228–33:   Variability in the medial facial cleft syndrome.

phthalmia, epibulbar dermoids, colobomas of the upper eyelid, congenital cataracts, preauricular skin tags, hypoplastic frontal sinuses, clinodactyly, camptodactyly, and cryptorchidism. Approximately 20% of those affected are mentally retarded, usually to a mild degree.

**Complications:** Feeding problems if cleft lip and/or palate is present. Central nervous system problems if associated with encephalocele or meningocele. Psychological problems may develop if facial reconstruction is delayed.

**Associated Findings:** Encephalocele associated with cranium bifidum frontalis, agenesis of the corpus callosum, meningocele or meningoencephalocele.

**Etiology:** Virtually all cases are sporadic.

**Pathogenesis:** This syndrome involves the central portion of the face and can be viewed as persistence of the paired medial fronto-nasal processes rather than normal fusion.

**POS No.:** 3288

**Sex Ratio:** M1:F1

**Occurrence:** Unknown.

**Risk of Recurrence for Patient's Sib:** Probably not increased.

**Risk of Recurrence for Patient's Child:** Probably not increased.

**Age of Detectability:** At birth.

**Gene Mapping and Linkage:** Unknown.

**Prevention:** None known.

**Treatment:** Surgery for repair of cleft lip and palate, hypertelorism, and nose. Psychiatric help may be indicated.

**Prognosis:** Normal life span.

**Detection of Carrier:** Unknown.

**References:**
Sedano H, et al.: Frontonasal dysplasia. J Pediatr 1970; 76:906.
DeMyer W: Median facial malformations and their implications for brain malformations. BD:OAS XI(7). New York: Alan R. Liss Inc. for The National Foundation-March of Dimes, 1975:155.

WI021                                              **R.S. Wilroy, Jr.**

**Face, midface retraction-X-ray and renal anomalies-hypertrichosis**
  *See SCHINZEL-GIEDION SYNDROME*
**Face, unusual-mental retardation-intrauterine growth retardation**
  *See DWARFISM-DYSMORPHIC FACIES-RETARDATION, PITT TYPE*
**Face-limb syndrome (one form)**
  *See CHARLIE M SYNDROME*
**Faces (flat) with hand and foot deformity**
  *See ACROFACIAL DEFECTS, EMERY-NELSON TYPE*

---

## FACES SYNDROME                                          2242

**Includes:** Facial dysmorphology-anorexia-cachexia-eye and skin lesions

**Excludes:** Lentigines syndrome, multiple (0586)

**Major Diagnostic Criteria:** A combination of unusual facies, anorexia, cachexia, eye and skin defects, and musculoskeletal defects.

**Clinical Findings:** A combination of the following features should be present for a clinical diagnosis of this syndrome. *Facial features*: anteverted nares; bifid tip of nose; nasal speech; and short palate. *Eyes*: ptosis of eyelids; **Retinitis pigmentosa**; xanthalesma. *Musculoskeletal*: bilateral **Syndactyly** of hands and feet; severe generalized muscle wasting; atrophy of temporal and interossei muscles; **Pectus excavatum** and asymmetry of chest; genu varum; pes planus. *Skin*: multiple lentigines; café-au-lait spots. *Other*: thyroid anomalies.

The acronym "FACES" syndrome stands for Facial dysmorphia, Anorexia, Cachexia, Eye and Skin anomalies. An outstanding feature of this syndrome is the severe cachexia and anorexia which may appear during the teens or before. Failure to demonstrate a distorted attitude toward food, an absence of previous overweight, as well as the lack of other physical, psychological and

laboratory abnormalities makes the diagnosis of anorexia nervosa doubtful.

**Complications:** Thyroid anomalies in two of the three reported patients consisted of papillary carcinoma of the thyroid in one and diffuse enlargement in the other. No serum lipid abnormalities were associated with the ocular xanthomata noted in two of the patients.

**Associated Findings:** None known.

**Etiology:** Possibly autosomal dominant inheritance, although X-linked dominant inheritance cannot be ruled out.

**Pathogenesis:** Unknown.

**POS No.:** 3622

**Sex Ratio:** M0:F3 (observed in the reported mother and her two daughters).

**Occurrence:** Reported in one Jewish Yemenite family with an affected mother and two daughters.

**Risk of Recurrence for Patient's Sib:**
  See Part I, *Mendelian Inheritance.*

**Risk of Recurrence for Patient's Child:**
  See Part I, *Mendelian Inheritance.*

**Age of Detectability:** Presumably late in childhood.

**Gene Mapping and Linkage:** Unknown.

**Prevention:** None known. Genetic counseling indicated.

**Treatment:** Treatment of thyroid anomalies.

**Prognosis:** Unknown.

**Detection of Carrier:** Unknown.

**References:**
Friedman E, Goodman RM: The "FACES" syndrome: a new syndrome with unique facies, anorexia, cachexia, and eye and skin lesions. J Craniofac Genet Dev Biol 1984; 4:227–231.

G0026                                              **Richard M. Goodman**

**Facial and cranial dysostosis**
  *See CRANIOFACIAL DYSOSTOSIS*
**Facial and ocular anomalies-proteinuria-deafness**
  *See FACIO-OCULO-ACOUSTIC-RENAL SYNDROME (FOAR SYNDROME)*

---

## FACIAL CLEFT, LATERAL                                    0374

**Includes:**
  Facial cleft, transverse
  Macrostomia

**Excludes:** Facial cleft, oblique (0375)

**Major Diagnostic Criteria:** Lateral facial cleft extending from either corner of the mouth.

**Clinical Findings:** The facial cleft extends laterally from the corner of the mouth, with the usual lateral limit being the anterior edge masseter muscle. Both unilateral (92%) and bilateral (8%) clefts occur. They are commonly associated with hypoplasia of ipsilateral soft palate and tongue. Preauricular tags (16/16) are almost always associated. Other associated defects include absence of ipsilateral parotid duct opening (70%), ear deformities (56%), masseter involvement (56%), hypoplastic zygoma (25%), and hypoplastic maxilla (6%).

**Complications:** Temporo-zygomatic clefts, psychological effect of the cosmetic deformity.

**Associated Findings:** Sometimes present in **Acrocephalosyndactyly type I**, **Craniofacial dysostosis**, and Weyer-Thier syndromes; associated occasionally with lateral canthal dystropia, polydactyly, syndactyly, absence of fingers, hypoplasia of temporal bone and muscle, cleft lip and palate, dorsal sinus of nose, grooves above ears, amniotic bands, nasal dermoids, congenital heart anomalies, and mental retardation.

Lateral clefts are the major sign in 16% (16/102) of first and second branchial arch syndrome, and a frequent component in more complex expressions of this syndrome. Lateral clefts are present in **Oculo-auriculo-vertebral anomaly** (40%) and often present in **Mandibulofacial dysostosis.**

**Etiology:** Unknown.

**Pathogenesis:** Persistent separation of embryonic maxillary and mandibular processes.

**Sex Ratio:** M2:F9 (11 cases of lateral cleft); M63:F39 (102 cases of more complicated temporo-zygomatic clefts.)

**Occurrence:** Incidence 18:100,000 live births (Michigan area); 1:100–300 of all facial clefts. Prevalence 0.76:100,000 population in Brazil's Rio area.

**Risk of Recurrence for Patient's Sib:** Unknown.

**Risk of Recurrence for Patient's Child:** Unknown.

**Age of Detectability:** At birth by visual examination.

**Gene Mapping and Linkage:** Unknown.

**Prevention:** None known. Genetic counseling indicated.

**Treatment:** Operative closure of cleft. Repair and therapy as needed for associated anomalies.

**Prognosis:** Normal life span.

**Detection of Carrier:** Unknown.

**References:**
Blackfield HM, Wilde NJ: Lateral facial clefts. Plast Reconstr Surg 1950; 6:68.
Grabb WC: The first and second branchial arch syndrome. Plast Reconstr Surg 1965; 36:485.
Pitanguy I, Franco T: Nonoperated facial fissures in adults. Plast Reconstr Surg 1967; 39:569.
Mansfield OT, Herbert DC: Unilateral transverse facial cleft: a method of surgical closure. Br J Plast Surg 1972; 25:29.
Converse JM, et al.: On hemi-facial microsomia: the first and second branchial arch syndrome. Plast Reconstr Surg 1973; 51:268.
Tessier P: Anatomical classification of facial, cranio-facial and latero-facial clefts. J Maxillo Fac Surg 1976; 4:69.

MI016                                    **Stephen H. Miller**

## FACIAL CLEFT, OBLIQUE                        0375

**Includes:**
  Maloschisis
  Naso-maxillary cleft
  Naso-ocular cleft
  Oro-ocular cleft

**Excludes:**
  **Cleft lip** (0178)
  **Cleft palate** (0180)
  **Face, median cleft face syndrome** (0635)
  **Facial cleft, lateral** (0374)

**Major Diagnostic Criteria:** Facial cleft extending from or near the oral cavity to the eye.

**Clinical Findings:** Oblique facial clefts are variable in pattern and extent. They may be unilateral or bilateral. In some cases the nostril may be involved. When the cleft involves the orbital margin, the eyelid usually fails to develop, leaving the eye globe exposed.

**Complications:** Cleft lip, cleft palate, or lateral facial cleft.

**Associated Findings:** **Hydrocephaly, Encephalocele,** structural abnormalities of the eye, **Arthrogryposes,** talipes, adactyly, genitourinary anomalies.

**Etiology:** Undetermined. Possibly a result of amniotic band.

**Pathogenesis:** Failure of penetration of ectomesenchyme between the lateral nasal and maxillary processes with failure of obliteration of the nasolacrimal groove. Some cases may result from early rupture of the amnion.

**Sex Ratio:** M1:F1

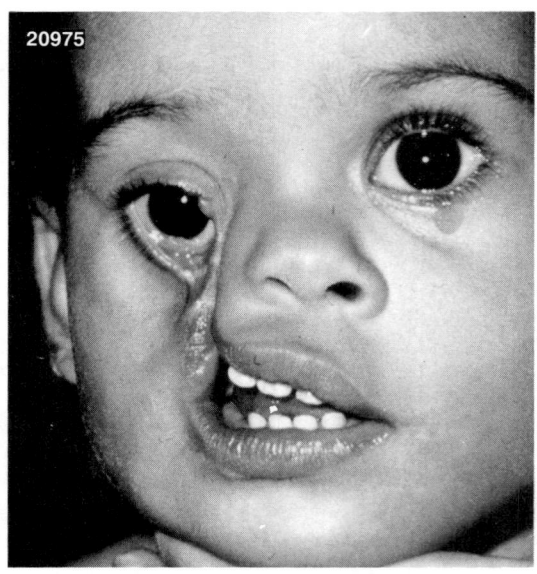

0375A-20975:  Unilateral oblique facial cleft.

**Occurrence:** 1:1300 cases of orofacial clefting.

**Risk of Recurrence for Patient's Sib:** Unknown. Presumably low.

**Risk of Recurrence for Patient's Child:** Unknown. Presumably low.

**Age of Detectability:** At birth by clinical evaluation.

**Gene Mapping and Linkage:** Unknown.

**Prevention:** None known. Genetic counseling indicated.

**Treatment:** Surgical correction.

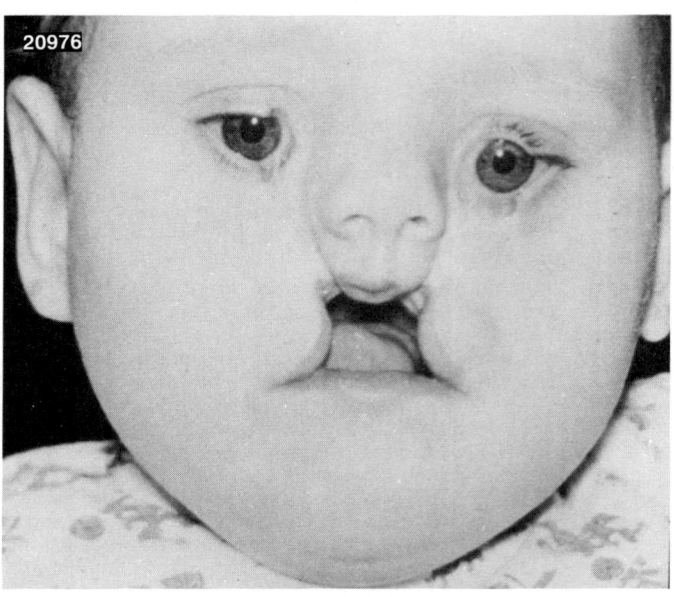

0375B-20976:  Bilateral oblique facial cleft.

**Prognosis:** Depends on the severity and the nature of the associated anomalies.

**Detection of Carrier:** Unknown.

**Special Considerations:** Alar clefts or colobomas may represent incomplete forms of the condition.

**References:**
Pitanguy I, Franco T: Plast Reconstr Surg 1967; 39:569–577. †
Boo-Chai K: The oblique facial cleft: a report of 2 cases and a review of 41 cases. Br J Plast Surg 1970; 23:352–359. *
Dey DL: Oblique facial clefts. Plast Reconstr Surg 1973; 52:258–263.

J0027      **Ronald J. Jorgenson**

**Facial cleft, transverse**
*See FACIAL CLEFT, LATERAL*

## FACIAL CLEFTING SYNDROME, GYPSY TYPE    2767

**Includes:**
Cleft, facial cleft syndrome, Malpuech type
Malpuech facial clefting syndrome

**Excludes:**
**Aarskog syndrome** (0001)
**Cleft lip** (0178)
**Face, median cleft face syndrome** (0635)
**Hypertelorism-hypospadias syndrome** (0505)

**Major Diagnostic Criteria:** Hypertelorism, **Cleft lip/Cleft palate**, urogenital anomalies, and growth and mental retardation.

**Clinical Findings:** Birth weights of the four described individuals ranged between 2.6 and 2.9 kg, and pregnancies were near or at term. All had growth retardation, with stature by early childhood of 3–5 SD below normal. All children had **Eye, hypertelorism**, unilateral or bilateral clefting of lip/palate, and urogenital anomalies. In three of the four, the kidneys were affected, with hypoplasia, malrotation, and ectopia. Vesicoureteral reflux (2/4), testis ectopia (2/3 males), micropenis with hypospadias (1/3 males), and vesical diverticulosis (1/4) were also described. All children were mentally retarded, with IQs between 45 and 60.

**Complications:** Unknown.

**Associated Findings:** None known.

**Etiology:** Possibly autosomal recessive inheritance.

**Pathogenesis:** Unknown.

**MIM No.:** 15435

**POS No.:** 3682

**Sex Ratio:** M3:F1 (observed).

**Occurrence:** Reported in four members of one family of inbred Gypsies in France.

**Risk of Recurrence for Patient's Sib:**
See Part I, *Mendelian Inheritance.*

**Risk of Recurrence for Patient's Child:**
See Part I, *Mendelian Inheritance.*

**Age of Detectability:** At birth, although potentially prenatal by ultrasound if severe oligohydramnios secondary to renal anomalies is present.

**Gene Mapping and Linkage:** Unknown.

**Prevention:** None known. Genetic counseling indicated.

**Treatment:** Treatment of potential complications of renal anomalies is indicated.

**Prognosis:** Growth and mental retardation are severe. Although the oldest living child was aged 10 years at the time of the report, there were seven older relatives who were not examined, and three sibs who were stillborn.

**Detection of Carrier:** Unknown.

**Support Groups:**
MA; Quincy; Prescription Parents, Inc.

CANADA: Ontario; Toronto; Canadian Cleft Lip and Palate Family Association

**References:**
Malpuech G, et al.: A previously undescribed autosomal recessive multiple congenital anomalies/mental retardation (MCA/MR) syndrome with growth failure, lip/palate cleft(s), and urogenital anomalies. Am J Med Genet 1983; 16:475–480. *

T0007      **Helga V. Toriello**

**Facial defects-brachydactyly-growth defect**
*See GROWTH DEFICIENCY-FACIAL DEFECTS-BRACHYDACTYLY*
**Facial diplegia (6th and 7th cranial nerves)**
*See DIPLEGIA, CONGENITAL FACIAL*
**Facial diplegia, congenital**
*See DIPLEGIA, CONGENITAL FACIAL*

## FACIAL DYSMORPHIA-JOINT HYPEREXTENSIBILITY SYNDROME    2172

**Includes:** Joint hyperextensibility-facial dysmorphia syndrome

**Excludes:** Dysmorphic facies (other)

**Major Diagnostic Criteria:** Unusual facies, joint hyperextensibility, fifth finger clinodactyly, short stature, and mental retardation.

**Clinical Findings:** Birth weight is low, and the baby feeds poorly and has choking spells. The facial findings are present at birth and become more well defined with age: prominent forehead, hypertelorism, epicanthus, ptosis, small nose, downturned angles of the mouth, and prominent chin. The ears are large and low-set. There is clinodactyly of the fifth fingers. Growth is poor and development is slow, leading to short stature and mental retardation. Hypotonia is present, and the joints are hyperextensible.

**Complications:** Unknown.

**Associated Findings:** None known.

**Etiology:** Presumably autosomal recessive inheritance.

**Pathogenesis:** Unknown.

**POS No.:** 4239

**Sex Ratio:** M2:F0 (observed).

**Occurrence:** One family with two affected brothers has been reported.

**Risk of Recurrence for Patient's Sib:**
See Part I, *Mendelian Inheritance.*

**Risk of Recurrence for Patient's Child:**
See Part I, *Mendelian Inheritance.*

**Age of Detectability:** At birth.

**Gene Mapping and Linkage:** Unknown.

**Prevention:** None known. Genetic counseling indicated.

**Treatment:** Unknown.

**Prognosis:** Unknown.

**Detection of Carrier:** Unknown.

**References:**
Morillo-Cucci G, et al.: Two male sibs with a previously unrecognized syndrome: facial dysmorphia, hyperextensibility of joints, clinodactyly, growth retardation and mental retardation. BD:OAS XI(2). New York: March of Dimes Birth Defects Foundation, 1975:380–383.

TH017      **T.F. Thurmon**
UR001      **S.A. Ursin**

**Facial dysmorphology-anorexia-cachexia-eye and skin lesions**
*See FACES SYNDROME*
**Facial ectodermal dysplasia**
*See ECTODERMAL DYSPLASIA, CONGENITAL FACIAL, SETLEIS TYPE*
**Facial hemiatrophy, progressive**
*See HEMIFACIAL ATROPHY, PROGRESSIVE*
**Facial palsy, congenital partial**
*See PALSY, CONGENITAL FACIAL*

**Facial palsy, congenital unilateral or bilateral**
  See *PALSY, CONGENITAL FACIAL*
**Facial palsy, congenital with exposure to retinoids**
  See *FETAL RETINOID SYNDROME*
**Facial palsy, familial recurrent peripheral**
  See *PALSY, LATE-ONSET FACIAL, FAMILIAL*
**Facial palsy, late-onset**
  See *PALSY, LATE-ONSET FACIAL, FAMILIAL*
**Facial palsy, partial-urinary abnormalities**
  See *UROFACIAL SYNDROME*
**Facial palsy-ear defects-deafness**
  See *DEAFNESS-EAR DEFECTS-FACIAL PALSY*
**Facial paralysis, familial congenital peripheral**
  See *PALSY, CONGENITAL FACIAL*
**Facial paresis, partial, unilateral**
  See *CARDIOFACIAL SYNDROME-ASSYMETRIC FACIES*
**Facial-oculo syndrome**
  See *OCULO-FACIAL SYNDROME, BENCZE TYPE*
**Facial-oculo-cerebro syndrome**
  See *OCULO-CEREBRO-FACIAL SYNDROME, KAUFMAN TYPE*
**Facial-oculo-mandibulo syndrome**
  See *OCULO-MANDIBULO-FACIAL SYNDROME*
**Facio-audio-osymphalangism**
  See *SYMPHALANGISM*
**Facio-auriculo-vertebral spectrum**
  See *OCULO-AURICULO-VERTEBRAL ANOMALY*
**Facio-cardio-cutaneous syndrome**
  See *CARDIO-FACIAL-CUTANEOUS SYNDROME*

---

### FACIO-CARDIOMELIC DYSPLASIA, LETHAL    3190

**Includes:** Cardiomelic-facio dysplasia, lethal
**Excludes:**
  **Aase-Smith syndrome** (3029)
  **Acrofacial dysostosis, Nager type** (2167)
  **Aortic valve atresia** (0079)
  **Chromosome 18, trisomy 18** (0160)
  **Cleft palate-micrognathia-glossoptosis** (0182)
  **Heart-hand syndrome** (0455)
  **Mandibulofacial dysostosis** (0627)
  **Pancytopenia syndrome, Fanconi type** (2029)
  Pierre Robin sequence
  **Thrombocytopenia-absent radius** (0941)

**Major Diagnostic Criteria:** Pregnancy complicated by polyhydramnios, congenital mesoacromelic dwarfism, facial dysmorphy, severe cardiac defects, limb and digital anomalies. Survival has averaged nine days.

**Clinical Findings:** Low birthweight and short height; peculiar facies due to epicanthal folds, microretrognathia, microstomia, microglossia, and glossoptosis; dysplastic auricles with enlarged auricular lobule, short webbed neck; cardiac defects including (postmortem data): enlarged right atrium, dilated right ventricle, small left atrium, hypertrophic and hypoplastic ventricle; hypoplastic ascending aorta, with atretic valve; pulmonary artery originated from the right ventricle, widely open interventricular septum and atretic mitral valve, persistence of the left superior vena cava (in one patient); truncus arteriosus communis, **Ductus arteriosus, patent**, patent foramen ovale, and high interventricular communication (in other patient). Upper and lower mesomelic hypoplasia, wide and short hands radially deviated, digital anomalies (thumb hypoplasia, brachymetacarpalia, brachymesophalangy and clinodactyly, wide gap between 1st and 2nd toes), talipes, with hypoplastic heels.
  Two out of the three reported patients died at the fourth day of life, the other died at 20 days of age.
  X-ray findings include mandibular hypoplasia, radial and ulnar hypoplasia, brachymetacarpalia, brachymetatarsalia, fibular, tibial, and calcaneous hypoplasia, and delayed bone age.

**Complications:** Those derived from the cardiac defect, leading to failure and death.

**Associated Findings:** Hepatosplenomegaly.

**Etiology:** Possibly autosomal recessive inheritance. Since only males were found to be affected, sex limited influence cannot be ruled out.

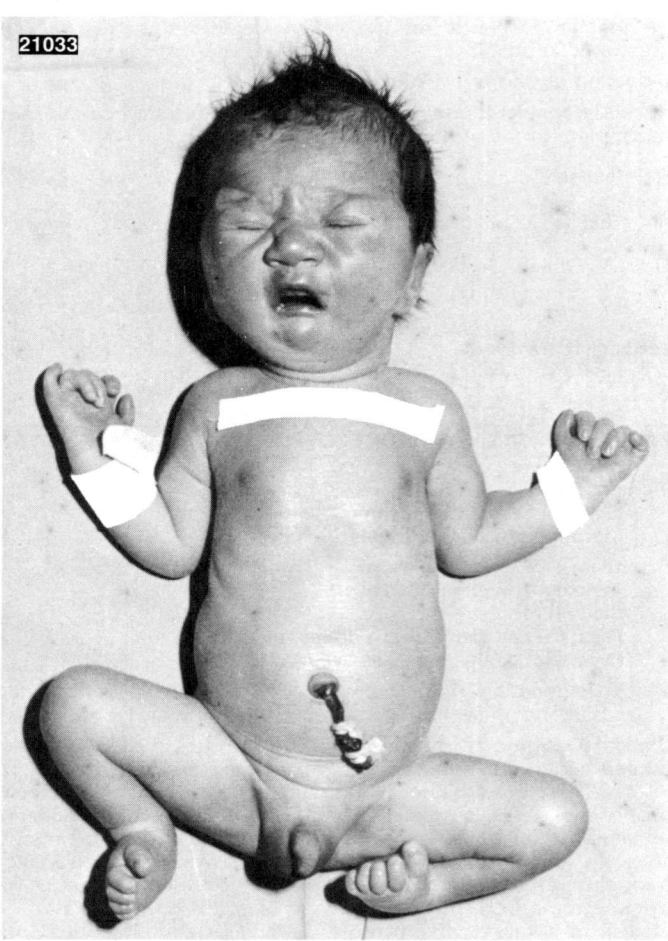

3190-21033: Facio-cardiomelic dysplasia, lethal; note microstomia, severe microretrognathia, hypoplastic thumbs, radial deviation of the hands and bilateral talipes.

---

**Pathogenesis:** Unknown.
**MIM No.:** 22727
**POS No.:** 3228
**Sex Ratio:** M3:F0 observed.
**Occurrence:** Three brothers have been reported in the literature.
**Risk of Recurrence for Patient's Sib:**
  See Part I, *Mendelian Inheritance.*
**Risk of Recurrence for Patient's Child:**
  See Part I, *Mendelian Inheritance.*
**Age of Detectability:** At birth.
**Gene Mapping and Linkage:** Unknown.
**Prevention:** None known. Genetic counseling indicated.
**Treatment:** Surgery if indicated. Supportive.
**Prognosis:** Lethal, with survival an average of nine days.
**Detection of Carrier:** Unknown.

**References:**
Cantu JM, et al: Lethal faciocardiomelic dysplasia: a new autosomal recessive disorder. BD:OAS XI(5). New York: March of Dimes Birth Defects Foundation, 1975:91–98.

CR023
CA011

**Diana García-Cruz**
**José María Cantú**

**Facio-dental-skeletal anomalies-joint contractures-hyperostosis**
*See FRONTOMETAPHYSEAL DYSPLASIA*
**Facio-dermo-cardio-skeletal syndrome**
*See DERMO-FACIO-CARDIO-SKELETAL SYNDROME*
**Facio-digital-oro syndrome**
*See ORO-FACIO-DIGITAL SYNDROME, BARAITSER-BURN TYPE*
**Facio-digito-genital dysplasia**
*See AARSKOG SYNDROME*
**Facio-fronto-nasal dysplasia**
*See FRONTO-FACIO-NASAL DYSPLASIA*
**Facio-genito-popliteal syndrome**
*See PTERYGIUM SYNDROME, POPLITEAL*

## FACIO-NEURO-SKELETAL SYNDROME                    2339

**Includes:**
  Fragoso-Cantu syndrome
  Neuro-facio-skeletal syndrome
  Marfanoid mental retardation syndrome
  Skeletal-neuro-facio syndrome

**Excludes:**
  **Homocystinuria** (0474)
  **Marfan syndrome** (0630)
  Marfanoid phenotype, all other syndromes with
  **X-linked mental retardation, Marfanoid habitus type** (2921)

**Major Diagnostic Criteria:** Psychomotor retardation, typical flat and coarse facies, and Marfanoid phenotype: tall stature, long and slim limbs, arm span larger than height, "arachnodactyloid" hands and feet, little subcutaneous fat, and muscle hypotonia.

**Clinical Findings:** Psychomotor retardation (IQ: 30–50); cortical and subcortical atrophy; flat, coarse facies; dolichocephaly; low posterior hairline; synophrys; hypertelorism and peculiar palpebral fissures; broad nose with bifid columella; malar hypoplasia; marked philtrum; characteristic small mouth; high palate; broad chin; large ears with attached lobes; telangiectasia; back hirsutism; pectus excavatum; muscle hypoplasia; mild hypotonia; dolichostenomelia; "arachnodactyloid" hands (long but not slender); hypotrophic thenar and hypothenar eminences; and long flat feet. Despite the Marfanoid phenotype neither cardiac nor ocular manifestation of the **Marfan syndrome** are present.
  CT scan of the brain may reveal cortical and subcortical atrophy. X-rays show osteopenia, asynchronous osseous maturation, retarded bone age in childhood (by 2–3 years); other findings include a thinning of the metacarpals, metatarsals, phalanges, long bones, and ribs; a persistent thymus; cardiomegaly; partial fusion of L-2, L-3, and L-4; hemivertebra at L-3; rachischisis L-2, L-4, L-5, and S-1; and retrospondylolisthesis.

**Complications:** Unknown.

**Associated Findings:** Psychomotor retardation; generalized muscular weakness during childhood.

**Etiology:** Presumably autosomal recessive inheritance. Parental consanguinity has not been definitely established in the parents of any of the affected patients.

**Pathogenesis:** Unknown.

**MIM No.:** 24877

**POS No.:** 3698

**Sex Ratio:** M5:F2 (observed).

**Occurrence:** Seven cases (including two sporadic males), from three families, have been documented.

**Risk of Recurrence for Patient's Sib:**
  See Part I, *Mendelian Inheritance.*

**Risk of Recurrence for Patient's Child:**
  See Part I, *Mendelian Inheritance.*

**Age of Detectability:** At birth, by physical examination.

**Gene Mapping and Linkage:** Unknown.

**Prevention:** None known. Genetic counseling indicated.

**Treatment:** Physical therapy and special education may be useful.

**Prognosis:** Good for life span but poor for intellectual performance. Affected children and young adults are usually not fully incapacitated. Nevertheless, affected children may have mild-to-severe hypotonia and severe difficulty with walking.

**Detection of Carrier:** Unknown.

**References:**
Fragoso R, Cantú JM: A new psychomotor retardation syndrome with peculiar facies and Marfanoid habitus. Clin Genet 1984; 25:187–190. *

FR031                                           **Rubén Fragoso**
CA011                                         **José María Cantú**

## FACIO-OCULO-ACOUSTIC-RENAL SYNDROME (FOAR SYNDROME)                    0732

**Includes:**
  Deafness-ocular and facial anomalies-proteinuria
  Facial and ocular anomalies-proteinuria-deafness
  FOAR syndrome
  Ocular and facial anomalies-proteinuria-deafness
  Proteinuria-ocular and facial anomalies-deafness
  Renal-facio-oculo-acoustic syndrome

**Excludes:**
  **Charge association** (2124)
  **Deafness-myopia-cataract-saddle nose, Marshall type** (0261)
  **Oro-facio-digital syndrome, Mohr type** (0771)
  Renal disease, congenital-deafness-myopia
  **Waardenburg syndromes** (0997)

**Major Diagnostic Criteria:** Myopia, coloboma, hypertelorism, severe congenital sensorineural hearing loss, and proteinuria.

**Clinical Findings:** Three patients, two of whom were sister and brother, have been described. The most prominent eye symptoms were myopia, cataract, coloboma, and total retinal detachment causing blindness. Furthermore, posterior staphyloma, small corneas, hypoplasia of iris stroma, choroidal atrophy, coloboma of iris and lens, rubeosis iridis, heterochromia, congenital pupillary membrane, underdeveloped filtration angle, and laterally displaced inferior canaliculi were reported. Telecanthus, hypertelorism, a flat bridge of the nose, highly arched palate, and brownish teeth were noted in both patients. Proteinuria was found in both; bilateral ureteral reflux and dilatation were found in one. Severe sensorineural hearing loss was diagnosed in both.

**Complications:** Low psychomotor development was noted in one patient. No speech was present.

**Associated Findings:** Epiphyseal dysplasia of the femoral heads has been noted.

**Etiology:** Possibly autosomal recessive inheritance.

**Pathogenesis:** Unknown.

**MIM No.:** 22729

**POS No.:** 3338

**Sex Ratio:** M1:F1

**Occurrence:** Undetermined but presumably rare.

**Risk of Recurrence for Patient's Sib:**
  See Part I, *Mendelian Inheritance.*

**Risk of Recurrence for Patient's Child:**
  See Part I, *Mendelian Inheritance.*

**Age of Detectability:** In early infancy.

**Gene Mapping and Linkage:** Unknown.

**Prevention:** None known. Genetic counseling indicated.

**Treatment:** Unknown.

**Prognosis:** The severe eye anomalies will eventually lead to blindness.

**Detection of Carrier:** Unknown.

**References:**
Murdoch JL, Mengel MC: An unusual eye-ear syndrome with renal abnormality. BD:OAS VII(4). Baltimore: Williams & Wilkins for The National Foundation-March of Dimes, 1971:136 only.
Holmes LB, Schepens CL: Syndrome of ocular and facial anomalies, telecanthus and deafness. J Pediatr 1972; 81:552–555.
Ozer FL: A possible "new" syndrome with eye and renal abnormalities. BD:OAS X(4). Baltimore: Williams & Wilkins for The National Foundation-March of Dimes, 1974:168 only.
Fraser GR: The causes of profound deafness in childhood: a study of 3535 individuals with severe auditory handicaps present at birth or of childhood onset. Baltimore: Johns Hopkins University, 1976.

MI029            **Joyce Mitchell**
*Cor W.R.J. Cremers*

**Facio-oro-digital syndrome**
*See ORO-FACIO-DIGITAL SYNDROME, WHELAN TYPE*
**Facio-oro-digital syndrome III**
*See ORO-FACIO-DIGITAL SYNDROME, SUGARMAN TYPE*
**Facio-palato-osseous syndrome**
*See OTO-PALATO-DIGITAL SYNDROME, II*
**Facio-scapulo-humeral dystrophy**
*See MUSCULAR DYSTROPHY, FACIO-SCAPULO-HUMERAL*
**Facio-scapulo-humeral dystrophy, infantile**
*See MUSCULAR DYSTROPHY, FACIO-SCAPULO-HUMERAL*
**Facioauriculoradial dysplasia**
*See LIMB-OTO-CARDIAC SYNDROME*
**Faciogenital dysplasia**
*See AARSKOG SYNDROME*
**Factor I ("Eye")**
*See COMPLEMENT COMPONENT 3, DEFICIENCY OF*
**Factor II deficiency**
*See HYPOPROTHROMBINEMIA*

## FACTOR V DEFICIENCY     2668

**Includes:**
Clotting factor V
Labile factor deficiency
Owren parahemophilia
Parahemophilia
Proaccelerin deficiency

**Excludes:**
Acquired factor V deficiency
**Coagulation defect, familial multiple factors** (2674)
Factor V inhibitors

**Major Diagnostic Criteria:** Mild-to-moderate congenital hemorrhagic disorder due to a deficiency of coagulation Factor V; prolonged prothrombin time and partial thromboplastin time; reduced level of Factor V on specific assay.

**Clinical Findings:** A rare, mild-to-moderate hemorrhagic disorder affecting both sexes. Only homozygous patients have a bleeding diathesis. Ecchymosis, epistaxis, menorrhagia, gastrointestinal bleeding, and hemorrhages following trauma and surgery are frequent manifestations. Cerebral hemorrhage is very rare.

**Complications:** Central nervous system hemorrhage; death due to uncontrolled bleeding; antibodies against Factor V as a consequence of treatment.

**Associated Findings:** A prolonged bleeding time has been reported in a few patients.
Bilateral duplication of genitourinary collecting system, duplication of the left renal vein pelvis and ureter, **Ductus arteriosus, patent, Atrial septal defects, Ventricular septal defect, Syndactyly,** short stature, and **Epidermolysis bullosum.**

**Etiology:** Autosomal recessive inheritance.

**Pathogenesis:** Factor V participates in the prothrombin converting complex, which is composed of phospholipids, Factor Xa, Factor V, and calcium ions.

**MIM No.:** *22740
**Sex Ratio:** M1:F1

**Occurrence:** About 75 cases have been reported in the world literature.

**Risk of Recurrence for Patient's Sib:**
See Part I, *Mendelian Inheritance.*

**Risk of Recurrence for Patient's Child:**
See Part I, *Mendelian Inheritance.*

**Age of Detectability:** At birth.

**Gene Mapping and Linkage:** F5 (coagulation factor V) has been mapped to 1q21-q25.

**Prevention:** None known. Genetic counseling indicated.

**Treatment:** Factor V replacement using fresh or fresh-frozen plasma.

**Prognosis:** Normal life span.

**Detection of Carrier:** Factor V assay.

**References:**
Owren PA: Parahaemophilia, haemorrhagic diathesis due to absence of a previously unknown clotting factor. Lancet 1947; I:446–448.
Seeler RA: Parahemophilia. Factor V deficiency. Med Clin North Am 1972; 56:119–125.
Mammen EF: Congenital coagulation disorders. Semin Thromb Hemostas 1983; 19:17–18.
Jenny RJ, et al.: Complete cDNA and derived amino acid sequence of human factor V. Proc Nat Acad Sci 1987; 84:4846–4850.

C0068        **James J. Corrigan**

## FACTOR VII DEFICIENCY     2669

**Includes:**
Factor VII variants
Hypoproconvertinemia
Serum prothrombin conversion accelerator deficiency
Stable Factor deficiency

**Excludes:**
Acquired factor VII deficiency
Combined deficiencies
Factor VII inhibitors

**Major Diagnostic Criteria:** Moderate-to- evere congenital hemorrhagic disorder; prolonged prothrombin time; normal partial thromboplastin time; reduced plasma level of coagulation Factor VII activity. Variants have Factor VII protein present but reduced activity.

**Clinical Findings:** Homozygous patients have bleeding manifestations from birth. Affects both sexes. These include bleeding from the umbilical cord, epistaxis, ecchymosis, melena, hematemesis, hemarthrosis (males), menorrhagia, and bleeding following trauma and surgery. Central nervous system hemorrhage has been reported in 19% of patients. Factor VII activity is usually less than 10 units/dl. Heterozygotes are generally asymptomatic.

There is a poor relationship between severity of bleeding manifestations and level of Factor VII activity. Other tests of hemostatic function, including the bleeding time, are generally normal.

**Complications:** Neurologic complications secondary to central nervous system bleeding; chronic joint disease due to hemarthrosis; death; antibodies against Factor VII as a consequence of treatment.

**Associated Findings:** The condition has been reported in patients with various anomalies of chromosome 13.

**Etiology:** Autosomal recessive inheritance. Deficiency of coagulation Factor VII activity and protein or Factor VII activity with the protein present, using immunologic methods (Factor VII variants).

**Pathogenesis:** When activated by tissue factor, Factor VII initiates the extrinsic coagulation pathway to activate Factor X. Factor VII can also be activated by thrombin, Factor Xa, and Factor XIIa.

**MIM No.:** *22750

**Sex Ratio:** M1:F1

**Occurrence:** About 75 patients have been reported in the world literature.

**Risk of Recurrence for Patient's Sib:**
See Part I, *Mendelian Inheritance.*

**Risk of Recurrence for Patient's Child:**
See Part I, *Mendelian Inheritance.*

**Age of Detectability:** At birth.

**Gene Mapping and Linkage:** F7 (coagulation factor VII) has been mapped to 13q34.

**Prevention:** None known. Genetic counseling indicated.

**Treatment:** Fresh or fresh-frozen plasma; prothrombin complex concentrates.

**Prognosis:** Normal life span.

**Detection of Carrier:** Factor VII coagulant activity levels between 40 and 60 units/dl.

**References:**
Marder VJ, Shulman NR: Clinical aspects of congenital Factor VII deficiency. Am J Med 1964; 37:182–194.
Ragni MV, et al.: Factor VII deficiency. Am J Hematol 1981; 10:79–88.
Mammen EF: Congenital coagulation disorders. Semin Thromb Hemostas 1983; 9:19–21.
Fukushima Y, et al.: Activity and antigen of coagulation factors VII and X in five patients with abnormal chromosome 13. Jpn J Hum Genet 1987; 32:91–96.

C0068                                              **James J. Corrigan**

**Factor VII variants**
*See FACTOR VII DEFICIENCY*
**Factor VIII deficiency**
*See HEMOPHILIA A*
**Factor IX defeciency-sideroblastic anemia**
*See ANEMIA, SIDEROBLASTIC*
**Factor IX deficiency**
*See HEMOPHILIA B*

## FACTOR X DEFICIENCY                              2670

**Includes:**
   Factor X variants
   Stuart-Prower Factor deficiency

**Excludes:**
   Acquired factor X deficiency
   Factor X inhibitors

**Major Diagnostic Criteria:** Prolonged prothrombin time and partial thromboplastin time; low plasma level of Factor X; variants have Factor X protein detected but reduced coagulant activity.

**Clinical Findings:** Homozygous patients have bleeding from the umbilical cord, ecchymosis, epistaxis, menorrhagia, hematuria, and, rarely, hemarthrosis. Bleeding also occurs with trauma and surgery. Central nervous system involvement is very rare. Both sexes are affected. Homozygous patients usually have less than 2 units/dl of Factor X activity; heterozygotes have levels between 40 and 68 units/dl. Heterozygotes are usually asymptomatic.

**Complications:** Death secondary to bleeding; antibodies against Factor X as a consequence of treatment.

**Associated Findings:** None known.

**Etiology:** Autosomal recessive inheritance. Deficiency of coagulation Factor X activity. Factor X protein may be detected in the variants, but the protein exhibits no coagulant activity.

**Pathogenesis:** Factor X is activated by Factor VIIa and by the complex composed of Factor IXa, Factor VIIIa, and phospholipids, and becomes a component of the prothrombin converting complex, which converts prothrombin to thrombin.

**MIM No.:** *22760

**Sex Ratio:** M1:F1

**Occurrence:** Fewer than 50 cases have been reported in the world literature.

**Risk of Recurrence for Patient's Sib:**
See Part I, *Mendelian Inheritance.*

**Risk of Recurrence for Patient's Child:**
See Part I, *Mendelian Inheritance.*

**Age of Detectability:** At birth.

**Gene Mapping and Linkage:** F10 (coagulation factor X) has been mapped to 13q34.

**Prevention:** None known. Genetic counseling indicated.

**Treatment:** Fresh or fresh frozen plasma; prothrombin complex concentrates.

**Prognosis:** Normal life span expected.

**Detection of Carrier:** Factor X coagulant activity between 40 and 68 units/dl.

**References:**
Mori K, et al.: Congenital Factor X deficiency in Japan. Tohoku J Exp Med 1981; 133:1–19.
Mammen EF: Congenital coagulation disorders. Semin Thromb Hemostas 1983; 9:31–33.
Girolami A, et al.: Factor X Padua: a 'new' congenital factor X abnormality with a defect only in extrinsic system. Acta Haemat 1985; 73:31–36.
Sumer T, et al.: Severe congenital factor X deficiency with intracranial haemorrhage. Europ J Pediat 1986; 145:119–120.

C0068                                              **James J. Corrigan**

**Factor X variants**
*See FACTOR X DEFICIENCY*

## FACTOR XI DEFICIENCY                             2671

**Includes:**
   Hemophilia C
   Plasma thromboplastin antecedent (PTA) deficiency
   PTA deficiency

**Excludes:**
   Acquired factor XI deficiency
   Factor XI inhibitors

**Major Diagnostic Criteria:** Mild congenital hemorrhagic disease due to reduced plasma coagulant activity of Factor XI; prolonged partial thromboplastin time, normal prothrombin time, and normal bleeding time.

**Clinical Findings:** Both sexes are affected. Bleeding usually only follows surgery or severe trauma and is rarely spontaneous. Epistaxis, menorrhagia, and excessive bleeding after childbirth have been described. The severity of the bleeding may not be closely correlated with the degree of the deficiency as measured by Factor XI assay. A large percentage of patients are of Jewish descent (especially Ashkenazi Jews). Only homozygous patients have a hemorrhagic diathesis.

**Complications:** Antibodies against Factor XI as a consequence of treatment. Death due to bleeding is very rare.

**Associated Findings:** None known.

**Etiology:** Autosomal recessive inheritance. Deficiency of plasma coagulation Factor XI.

**Pathogenesis:** Factor XI is required in the intrinsic coagulation pathway. It is activated to Factor XIa by Factor XIIa. Factor XIa will then activate Factor IX.

**MIM No.:** *26490

**Sex Ratio:** M1:F1

**Occurrence:** Incidence is estimated at 1:10,000,000. Almost all affected individuals have been of Jewish extraction. Rosenthal (1964) reported on 72 cases from 46 Jewish families.

**Risk of Recurrence for Patient's Sib:**
See Part I, *Mendelian Inheritance.*

**Risk of Recurrence for Patient's Child:**
See Part I, *Mendelian Inheritance.*

**Age of Detectability:** At birth for severe deficiency (<1 unit/dl); ages 9–12 months for moderate-to-mild (1/20 unit/dl) deficiency.

**Gene Mapping and Linkage:** F11 (coagulation factor XI) has been provisionally mapped to 4q35.

**Prevention:** None known. Genetic counseling indicated.

**Treatment:** Fresh or fresh-frozen plasma.

**Prognosis:** Normal life span.

**Detection of Carrier:** Heterozygotes' Factor XI coagulant activity is between 30 and 65 units/dl.

**Special Considerations:** The level of Factor XI activity is low in normal newborns. Adult levels are not achieved until about age nine months. Thus, moderate and mild deficiencies may not be diagnosed until after the newborn period.

**References:**
Rosenthal RL: Haemorrhage in PTA (factor XI) deficiency. (Abstract) Proc 10th Inter Cong Hematol., Stockholm, 1964.
Zacharski LR, French EE: Factor XI (PTA) deficiency in an English-American kindred. Thromb Haemost 1978; 39:215–222.
Mammen EF: Congenital coagulation disorders. Semin Thromb Hemostas 1983; 9:34–35.
Saito H: Contact factors in health and disease. Semin Thromb Hemostas 1987; 13:36–49.

C0068                                      **James J. Corrigan**

## FACTOR XII DEFICIENCY                                      2672

**Includes:**
Clotting factor XII
Hageman factor deficiency

**Excludes:**
Acquired factor XII deficiency
Factor XII inhibitors

**Major Diagnostic Criteria:** Congenital coagulation factor deficiency not associated with a hemorrhagic disease; prolonged partial thromboplastin time, normal prothrombin time, and normal bleeding time; reduced plasma level of Factor XII.

**Clinical Findings:** The disorder is usually discovered by coincidence through prolonged partial thromboplastin times. A few patients have had thromboembolic episodes. Affects both sexes. Homozygotes have Factor XII levels of less than 1 unit/dl. Reduced fibrinolytic activity of plasma.

**Complications:** Possible thromboembolic disease.

**Associated Findings:** None known.

**Etiology:** Autosomal recessive inheritance.

**Pathogenesis:** Factor XII is activated to XIIa, which initiates the intrinsic coagulation pathway. Factor XIIa activates Factor XI.

**MIM No.:** *23400

**Sex Ratio:** M1:F1

**Occurrence:** About 170 cases have been reported.

**Risk of Recurrence for Patient's Sib:**
See Part I, *Mendelian Inheritance.*

**Risk of Recurrence for Patient's Child:**
See Part I, *Mendelian Inheritance.*

**Age of Detectability:** At birth.

**Gene Mapping and Linkage:** F12 (coagulation factor XII (Hageman)) has been mapped to 5q33-qter.

**Prevention:** None known. Genetic counseling indicated.

**Treatment:** Unknown.

**Prognosis:** Normal life span.

**Detection of Carrier:** Factor XII levels are between 15 and 80 units/dl.

**References:**
Ratnoff OD, Saito H: Surface mediated reactions. Curr Top Hematol 1972; 2:1–57.
Mammen EF: Congenital coagulation disorders. Semin Thromb Hemostas 1983; 9:36–41.
Bernardi F, et al.: Factor XII gene alteration in Hageman trait detected by TaqI restriction enzyme. Blood 1987; 69:1421–1424.

C0068                                      **James J. Corrigan**

## FACTOR XIII (FIBRIN STABILIZING FACTOR)              2673

**Includes:**
Factor XIII deficiency
Fibrin stabilizing factor, A subunit
Fibrinase deficiency
Fibrinogen and factor XIII
Fibrinoligase deficiency
Plasma transglutaminase

**Excludes:**
Acquired factor XIII deficiency
Factor XIII inhibitors

**Major Diagnostic Criteria:** Congenital hemorrhagic disorder characterized by poor wound healing and late wound bleeding; poor fibrin clot stability in vitro. Specific *in vitro* testing is required. Clot stability in 5 M urea solution or weak acids can be used for a qualitative the assessment. All other tests of hemostasis are normal.

**Clinical Findings:** Only homozygous patients have a bleeding diathesis, and then only if the Factor XIII level in the plasma is less than 1 unit/dl. Umbilical cord bleeding is a characteristic early sign. Other bleeding manifestations include ecchymoses, hematomas, hemarthroses, and delayed bleeding following trauma and surgery. Intracranial bleeding has occurred in 25% of patients, usually following minor injury. Abnormal wound healing has been described in about 25% of all cases.

**Complications:** Death from bleeding; neurologic deficits due to intracranial bleeding; poor wound healing; and acquired inhibitors (antibodies) to Factor XIII following treatment.

**Associated Findings:** Male fertility may be affected.

**Etiology:** Usually autosomal recessive inheritance.

**Pathogenesis:** Factor XIII is responsible for the stabilization of fibrin monomers following their spontaneous polymerization. Factor XIII is converted to XIIIa by thrombin and catalyzes a transamidation reaction between the fibrin chains.

**MIM No.:** *13457

**Sex Ratio:** M1:F1

**Occurrence:** About 100 cases have been documented.

**Risk of Recurrence for Patient's Sib:**
See Part I, *Mendelian Inheritance.*

**Risk of Recurrence for Patient's Child:**
See Part I, *Mendelian Inheritance.*

**Age of Detectability:** At birth.

**Gene Mapping and Linkage:** F13A1 (coagulation factor XIII, A1 polypeptide) has been mapped to 6p25-p24.

**Prevention:** None known. Genetic counseling indicated.

**Treatment:** Fresh or fresh-frozen plasma; cryoprecipitates.

**Prognosis:** Normal life span.

**Detection of Carrier:** By Factor XIII level.

**References:**
Kitchens CS, Newcomb TF: Factor XIII. Medicine 1979; 58:413–429.
Mammen EF: Congenital coagulation disorders. Semin Thromb Hemostas 1983; 9:10–12.
Berliner S, et al.: Hereditary factor XIII deficiency: report of four families and definition of the carrier state. Brit J Haemat 1984; 56:495–505.

Frydman M, et al.: Male fertility in factor XIII deficiency. Fertil Steril 1986; 45:729–731.

Lorand L, et al.: Autoimmune antibody (IgG Kansas) against fibrin stabilizing factor (factor XIII) system. Proc Nat Acad Sci 1988; 85:232–236.

Chung D, Ichinose A: Hereditary disorders related to fibrinogen and factor XIII. In: Scriver CR, et al, eds: The metabolic basis of inherited disease, 6th ed. New York: McGraw-Hill, 1989:2135–2154.

C0068                                                           **James J. Corrigan**

**Factor XIII deficiency**
    *See FACTOR XIII (FIBRIN STABILIZING FACTOR)*
**Factors II, VII, IX, and X deficiency**
    *See COAGULATION DEFECT, FAMILIAL MULTIPLE FACTORS*
**Factors V and VIII deficiency**
    *See COAGULATION DEFECT, FAMILIAL MULTIPLE FACTORS*
**Factors VII and VIII deficiency**
    *See COAGULATION DEFECT, FAMILIAL MULTIPLE FACTORS*
**Factors VII and X deficiency**
    *See COAGULATION DEFECT, FAMILIAL MULTIPLE FACTORS*
**Factors VIII and IX deficiency**
    *See COAGULATION DEFECT, FAMILIAL MULTIPLE FACTORS*
**Factors VIII, IX, and XI deficiency**
    *See COAGULATION DEFECT, FAMILIAL MULTIPLE FACTORS*
**Factors IX and XI deficiency**
    *See COAGULATION DEFECT, FAMILIAL MULTIPLE FACTORS*
**Fairbank disease**
    *See EPIPHYSEAL DYSPLASIA, MULTIPLE*
**Falciform detachment, congenital**
    *See RETINAL FOLD*
**Falciform retinal fold**
    *See RETINAL DYSPLASIA*
**Familial Amyloidotic Polyneuropathy (FAP)**
    *See AMYLOIDOSES*
**Familial articular hypermobility, dislocating type**
    *See ARTICULAR HYPERMOBILITY, FAMILIAL*
**Familial articular hypermobility, uncomplicated type**
    *See ARTICULAR HYPERMOBILITY, FAMILIAL*
**Familial atypical mole-malignant melanoma (FAMMM)**
    *See CANCER, MALIGNANT MELANOMA, FAMILIAL*
**Familial cavernous malformations of the CNS and retina (FCMCR)**
    *See RETINA, CAVERNOUS HEMANGIOMA*
**Familial chronic mucocutaneous candidiasis (FCMC)**
    *See CANDIDIASIS, FAMILIAL CHRONIC MUCOCUTANEOUS*
**Familial congenital bowing with short bones**
    *See KYPHOMELIC DYSPLASIA*
**Familial dysbetalipoproteinemia**
    *See HYPERLIPOPROTEINEMIA, BROAD BETA TYPE*
**Familial fat-induced hyperlipemia**
    *See HYPERCHYLOMICRONEMIA*
**Familial hemophagocytic lymphohistiocytosis**
    *See LYMPHOHISTIOCYTOSIS, FAMILIAL ERYTHROPHAGOCYTIC*
**Familial hyperchylomicronemia**
    *See HYPERCHYLOMICRONEMIA*
**FAMMM syndrome of Lynch**
    *See CANCER, MALIGNANT MELANOMA, FAMILIAL*
**Fanconi anemia, I**
    *See PANCYTOPENIA SYNDROME, FANCONI TYPE*
**Fanconi nephronophthisis**
    *See KIDNEY, NEPHRONOPHTHISIS-MEDULLARY CYSTIC DESEASE*
**Fanconi pancytopenia, type I**
    *See PANCYTOPENIA SYNDROME, FANCONI TYPE*
**Fanconi renotubular syndrome I, childhood and infantile forms**
    *See RENAL TUBULAR SYNDROME, FANCONI TYPE*
**Fanconi renotubular syndrome II, adult form**
    *See RENAL TUBULAR SYNDROME, FANCONI TYPE*
**Fanconi syndrome-intestinal malabsorption-galactose intolerance**
    *See RENAL TUBULAR SYNDROME, FANCONI TYPE*
**Fanconi-like radioulnar hypoplasia-hypoplastic anemia**
    *See WT SYNDROME*
**Fanconi-like syndrome**
    *See RENAL TUBULAR SYNDROME, FANCONI TYPE*
**Farabee brachydactyly**
    *See BRACHYDACTYLY*
**Farber disease**
    *See LIPOGRANULOMATOSIS*
**Fascial dystrophy**
    *See STIFF SKIN SYNDROME*
**Fatal intrahepatic cholestasis**
    *See JAUNDICE, INTRAHEPATIC CHOLESTATIC, BYLER TYPE*

**Fatty acid oxidation disorders**
    *See VISCERA, FATTY METAMORPHOSIS*
**Fatty alcohol:NAD+ oxidoreductase (FAO), deficiency of**
    *See SJOGREN-LARSSON SYNDROME*
**Favism**
    *See GLUCOSE-6-PHOSPHATE DEHYDROGENASE DEFICIENCY*
**Favre hyaloideoretinal degeneration**
    *See EYE, GOLDMANN-FAVRE DISEASE*
**Favre microfibrillar vitreoretinal degeneration**
    *See EYE, GOLDMANN-FAVRE DISEASE*
**Fazio-Londe disease**
    *See PALSY, PROGRESSIVE BULBAR OF CHILDHOOD*
**Febrile convulsions, simple and complex (complicated)**
    *See SEIZURES, FEBRILE*
**Fechtner syndrome**
    *See NEPHRITIS-DEAFNESS (SENSORINEURAL), HEREDITARY TYPE*
**Feet, congenital 'rocker-bottomed'**
    *See FOOT, VERTICAL TALUS*
**Feet, ulceration and loss of sensation**
    *See ACRO-OSTEOLYSIS, NEUROGENIC*
**Fehr corneal dystrophy**
    *See CORNEAL DYSTROPHY, MACULAR TYPE*
**Female pseudo-Turner syndrome**
    *See NOONAN SYNDROME*
**Female pseudohermaphritism from maternal extrinsic androgens**
    *See FETAL EFFECTS FROM MATERNAL EXTRINSIC ANDROGENS*
**Female pseudohermaphroditism**
    *See STEROID 21-HYDROXYLASE DEFICIENCY*
**Female Turner syndrome with normal XX karyotype**
    *See NOONAN SYNDROME*
**Feminizing male pseudohermpahroditism (Jones)**
    *See ANDROGEN INSENSITIVITY SYNDROME, INCOMPLETE*
**Feminizing testes syndrome, complete**
    *See ANDROGEN INSENSITIVITY SYNDROME, COMPLETE*
**Femoral bowing-fibula aplasia/hypoplasia-poly-, syn-, oligodactyly**
    *See SKELETAL DYSPLASIA, FUHRMANN TYPE*
**Femoral duplication**
    *See MESOMELIC DYSPLASIA, WERNER TYPE*
**Femoral dysgenesis, bilateral**
    *See FEMORAL HYPOPLASIA-UNUSUAL FACIES SYNDROME*
**Femoral dysgenesis, bilateral-Robin anomaly**
    *See FEMORAL HYPOPLASIA-UNUSUAL FACIES SYNDROME*

---

**FEMORAL HYPOPLASIA-UNUSUAL FACIES SYNDROME**                           **2027**

**Includes:**

    Femoral dysgenesis, bilateral
    Femoral dysgenesis, bilateral-Robin anomalie
    Femoral-facial syndrome

**Excludes:**

    Bone dysplasias with short femurs, other
    **Chondrodysplasia punctata, rhizomelic type** (0154)
    **Fibula, congenital absence of** (2229)
    **Kyphomelic dysplasia** (2754)
    **Roberts syndrome** (0875)

**Major Diagnostic Criteria:**    Bilateral femoral hypoplasia associated with characteristic facial features, including a short nose with a broad tip and hypoplastic alae nasi, a long philtrum, a thin upper lip, upward-slanting palpebral fissures, and micrognathia; small stature due to short lower limbs.

**Clinical Findings:**    Normal intelligence; cleft palate; abnormally shaped or small ears; upper extremity anomalies including Sprengel deformity, limited shoulder and elbow motion; radiohumeral and radioulnar synostosis; pes equinovarus deformity; poly-, oligo-, or syndactyly involving toes; rib, vertebral, and sacral anomalies.

**Complications:**    Mostly orthopedic complications, due to abnormalities of the extremities. Others include feeding problems resulting from cleft palate and urinary complications, such as recurrent urinary infections and urinary incontinence.

**Associated Findings:**    Congenital heart disease, astigmatism, esotropia, short third, fourth, and fifth metatarsals, cryptorchidism, inguinal hernia, hypoplastic external genitalia, polycystic or absent kidneys.

**Etiology:** Unknown. Some cases have been attributed to fetal constraint or maternal diabetes. Most cases have been sporadic.

**Pathogenesis:** Unknown. Oligohydramnios resulting in severe intrauterine compression may explain the clinical picture in some cases. Teratogenic effects of insulin (as has been shown in chickens) or unstable maternal glucose homeostasis may be considered in this regard for those patients born to diabetic mothers.

**MIM No.:** 13478

**POS No.:** 3232

**CDC No.:** 755.380

**Sex Ratio:** M:2:F:3

**Occurrence:** Undetermined but presumed rare.

**Risk of Recurrence for Patient's Sib:** Unknown.

**Risk of Recurrence for Patient's Child:** May be increased.

**Age of Detectability:** At birth, by clinical and X-ray examination; prenatally by ultrasound.

**Gene Mapping and Linkage:** Unknown.

**Prevention:** None known. Genetic counseling indicated.

**Treatment:** Mainly orthopedic; otherwise treatment depends on clinical findings outside the skeletal system such as cleft palate, congenital heart disease, genitourinary malformations.

**Prognosis:** Life span appears to be normal in most cases in the absence of serious complications.

**Detection of Carrier:** Unknown.

**Special Considerations:** Some investigators question the existence of this syndrome as a separate entity. There is also disagreement with regard to existence of patients who have femoral abnormality without characteristic facial features.

**References:**
Daentl DL, et al.: Femoral hypoplasia - unusual facies syndrome. J Pediatr 1975; 86:107–111
Hurst D, Johnson DF: Femoral hypoplasia - unusual facies syndrome. Am J Med Genet 1980; 5:255–258
Lampert RP: Dominant inheritance of femoral hypoplasia - unusual facies syndrome. Clin Genet 1980; 17:255–258.
Lord J, Beighton P: The femoral hypoplasia - unusual facies syndrome: a genetic entity? Clin Genet 1982; 20:267–275.
Johnson JP, et al.: Femoral hypoplasia unusual facies syndrome in infants of diabetic mothers. J Pediatr 1983; 102:866–872
Burn J, et al.: The femoral hypoplasia - unusual facies syndrome. J Med Genet 1984; 21:331–340.

SA033                                                       **Burhan Say**

**Femoral-facial syndrome**
See *FEMORAL HYPOPLASIA-UNUSUAL FACIES SYNDROME*
**Femur-fibula-ulna (FFU) syndrome**
See *FIBULA, CONGENITAL ABSENCE OF*
**Ferguson-Smith epithelioma**
See *EPITHELIOMA, MULTIPLE SELF-HEALING SQUAMOUS*
**Ferrell-Okihiro-Halal syndrome**
See *RADIAL-RENAL-OCULAR SYNDROME*
**Ferrochelatase deficiency**
See *PORPHYRIA, PROTOPORPHYRIA*
**Fertile eunuch syndrome**
See *GONADOTROPIN DEFICIENCIES*
also *HYPOGONADOTROPIC HYPOGONADISM*

## FETAL ACQUIRED IMMUNE DEFICIENCY SYNDROME (AIDS) INFECTION                                      2497

**Includes:**
AIDS, perinatal
Congenital AIDS-related syndrome (CARS)
Human immunodeficiency virus (HIV), congenital infection
Human T lymphotrophic virus (HTLV) III, congenital infection
Lymphadenopathy associated virus (LAV) congenital infection

**Excludes:**
AIDS, pediatric, of non-maternal origin
Immune deficiencies, congenital, from other causes
Immunosuppressive exposures
Malnutrition, primary severe
Lymphoreticular malignancy
Transient passive HIV seropositivity in infancy

**Major Diagnostic Criteria:** Exposure in the perinatal period to an infected mother and, in addition: 1) identification of the virus in blood or tissues, or 2) presence of HIV antibody in an infant or child who has abnormal immunologic test results indicating both humoral and cellular immunodeficiency (increased immunoglobulin levels, depressed T4 (T-helper) absolute cell count, absolute lymphopenia, decreased T4/T8 ratio, and who have one or more specific clinical symptoms (infectious, oncologic, neurologic) associated with HIV, or 3) clinical symptoms meeting the Centers for Disease Control (CDC) criteria for pediatric AIDS.

**Clinical Findings:** In many cases of pediatric AIDS with perinatal transmission, the mother has not had AIDS manifestations and the infant is often the first symptomatic person in the family to be recognized. Although almost all infants born of mothers with HIV infection have a positive transient positive serology from passive maternal transfer of anti HIV IgG antibodies, most will lose this by one year of age, indicating that infection has not been transmitted. Prospective data is limited, and it is not yet possible to fully describe the course of infection. Of those who have been reported with the manifestation, the average age of onset is about six months. As in adults, the average duration of infection before manifestations become apparent is not fully established.

In addition to the disease characteristic in adults (Pneumocystis carinii pneumonia, and other opportunistic protozoal, viral and fungal infections. Kaposi's sarcoma and other tumors are uncommon in pediatric AIDS), HIV infected children are frequently noted to have lymphoid interstitial pneumonitis (LIP), recurrent severe bacterial infection, herpes simplex, toxoplasmosis, and cryptosporidiosis which may have onset in the first few months of life. Wasting and anemia are characteristic. Some clinical features are similar to those of children with severe combined immunodeficiency; these include oral and esophageal candidiasis, chronic diarrhea, and eczematoid rashes. In addition, HIV-infected infants may have lymphoadenopathy, hepatosplenomegaly, progressive neurologic degenerative diseases, cardiomyopathy and renal disease. Immune test findings are similar to those in HIV-infected adults, and may include decreased T-helper cell numbers, decreased T-helper to T-suppressor cell ratios, hypergammaglobulinemia (more pronounced in children), lymphopenia (less common), and/or thrombocytopenia. Even when gamma globulin levels are elevated, specific antibody responses are frequently defective. In about 10% of cases, HIV serology is negative.

**Complications:** The most obvious complications are those resulting from immune deficiency. Infections, both opportunistic and non-opportunistic, chronic diarrhea, pulmonary disorders, lymphadenopathy, and hepato-splenomegaly are among the consequences of the immunologic dysfunction. Developmental delay, neurologic disorders, and B-cell lymphomas are also seen in HIV-infected children.

**Associated Findings:** Thrombocytopenia and a reticulonodular lung pattern on chest X-ray. Neuroradiologically, calcification of the basal ganglia, progressive cerebral atrophy, and enlargement of the ventricular system has been reported.

In addition, a specific dysmorphism has been reported (Marion et al.,1986) with features which include: 1) growth failure, with height and weight less than fifth percentile, which is intrauterine in origin in 25%; 2) **Microcephaly**, with head circumference less than fifth percentile; 3) prominent, boxlike forehead; 4) flattened nasal bridge which, in profile appears "scooped out"; 5) prominent eyes; 6) mild upward or downward obliquity of the eyes; 7) blue tinged sclerae; 8) ocular hypertelorism; 9) short nose with flattening of the columella; 10) prominent philtrum; and 11) prominent or normally formed vermilion border of the upper lip. Findings have been noted prior to the onset of symptoms of immune deficiency, and have been seen in newborns, in whom successful prediction of HIV seropositivity has been accomplished. The significance of these observations has been a topic of debate (Qazi et al, 1988; Blanche et al, 1989), and the observed features must be distinguised from possible drug or alcohol abuse exposure dysmorphia, as well as the racial characteristics of high risk groups.

**Etiology:** Transmission of HIV infection from an infected mother. About 75% of mothers are intravenous drug users, and most of the others are infected sexually. Distinguishing parturitional infection from prenatal infection is difficult, although it may eventually become important in defining potential neonatal preventive measures. Although many newborn are infected without breast feeding, the observation of the importance of breast feeding in HTLV 1 leukemia infections, and the documentation of breast feeding HIV infection in several cases where the mother appeared not to have contracted AIDS until after pregnancy, render credence to possible risk with breast feeding.

**Pathogenesis:** HIV can infect T-helper lymphocytes, some neurologic cells, and macrophages. It is unclear whether B lymphocytes can be infected or function defectively solely because of a deficiency of T-helper lymphocytes. The T4 receptor on the infected cells appears to be the site of virus entry; HIV replicates more rapidly in activated T-helper cells. The virus' effects on the immune system are complex and contribute to a wide array of secondary infections, hematologic disorders, and malignancies. Its effects on the neurologic system can range from subclinical dysfunction to rapidly progressive neurologic degeneration.

**Sex Ratio:** Presumably M1:F1.

**Occurrence:** The first pediatric AIDS case was reported in 1982. By December 19, 1988, 1,298 United States pediatric AIDS cases had been reported to CDC; about 78% acquired perinatally. Several follow-up samples have determined that AIDS reporting is better than 90% complete. Most of the reports were from New York, New Jersey and Florida, but the trend is for these to become more widespread. Prospective data are still limited for quantitating the course of perinatal HIV exposures. Publication of prospectively followed-up offspring of seropositive mothers in 12 locations involve about 300 births, with most followed up for less than a year. Practically all infants born of seropositive mothers are seropositive at birth. Prospective data suggests that about one-half have lost their positive antibody status by age one year. However, life table analysis was insufficient to clarify whether the proportion is distorted by including infants that have not reached a year of age. Retrospective case data are more extensive. The mean age of diagnosis is 9.3 months. From the limited prospective data it appears that about 10% of offspring of seropositive mothers have AIDS prior to age nine months. A projection of the retrospective mean to the preliminary prospective data would indicate that approximately 20% will develop AIDS. Data on population frequencies of perinatal HIV *infection* are unavailable. A survey of 1,000,000 newborns nationwide is underway. A report of completed data from 18 states and territories for 1988 (George et al, 1989) found seroprevalences ranging from 0.03 to 0.66%. To identify actual fetal infection, other tests are needed that are at this time not widely available (hybridization for messenger RNA, polymerase chain reaction identifiers for the viral genome).

**Risk of Recurrence for Patient's Sib:** In three small studies of offspring subsequent to perinatal AIDS cases, about one-half developed AIDS. Discordance in twins for transplacental HIV acquisition has been reported.

**Risk of Recurrence for Patient's Child:** The duration of HIV infection surveillance is insufficient to determine whether a significant number of individuals congenitally infected will survive to the reproductive period (as frequently happens with HTLV 1 infections).

**Age of Detectability:** Although infection can be detected at birth (Rogers et al, 1989), the diagnosis is often difficult, especially in seropositive children without clear symptoms, until after passive antibodies disappear (these may last as long as 15 months). As antigen tests and culture techniques become more widely available, the earlier recognition of infection will become more feasible.

**Gene Mapping and Linkage:** N/A

**Prevention:** Avoiding contaminated needles and drug administration materials, and avoiding sexual exposure to HIV-infected sex partners. Identifying infections in high risk women, with avoidance of pregnancies, where this is an acceptable choice.

**Treatment:** Many treatments for the complicating infections and other manifestations are available, but none curative of the primary infection. Specific therapies may modify or alleviate specific secondary infections. Maintenance therapy with intravenous gamma globulin has been reported to modify secondary disease symptoms. Steroids are used as therapy for LIP. Azidothymidine (AZT) is the first agent approved for specific treatment by the Food and Drug Administration, but the duration of experience is limited. Trials in the pediatric age group are underway. AZT treatment of pediatric AIDS appears to be particularly effective, especially against the prevalent neurological findings, but not curative. AZT trials are being initiated in pregnant women. Other treatments are under exploration.

**Prognosis:** Once congenital AIDS is established, diminishing health until death is inexorable, although treatment may alleviate specific infections. Recurrence of infections is the rule. Death often occurs in a few months, although some cases have survived for several years. In general the earlier the onset, the more fulminating the course. *Pneumocystis caranii* pneumonia in infants is the main contributor to early mortality. In cases where this is avoided, survival is longer.

**Detection of Carrier:** HIV infection can be determined by isolation of the virus in blood or body tissues, antigen detection in blood or body tissues, presence of HIV antibody as indicated by repeated reactive screening test (e.g., enzyme immunoassay), plus a positive confirmatory test (e.g., Western blot, immunoflourescence assay).

**Special Considerations:** Pediatric AIDS cases do not require isolation, as the risk of transmission is very low. The usual precautions should be observed, however, in wearing gloves and avoiding finger pricks when exposed to possibly infected blood.

All health care personnel are encouraged to report AIDS cases to their public health departments. Report AZT pregnancy exposures to the manufacturer, Burrough's Wellcome; a registry of these exposures is being followed to assess effects.

**Support Groups:** Los Angeles; World Hemophilia AIDS Center

*The authors wish to thank Janine M. Jason, Chief of Epidemiology Studies Section, Division of Host Factors, Centers for Disease Control, and Susan Mankoff of the CDC's AIDS Program, for their assistance in the preparation of this article. Nothing in this article, however, represents an official statement of the United States Government or of any employee or branch thereof.*

**References:**

Marion RW, et al.: Human T-cell lymphotropic virus type III (HTLV-III) embryopathy: a new dysmorphic syndrome associated with intrauterine HTLV-III infection. Am J Dis Child 1986; 140:638–640. †

Barbour SD: Acquired immunodeficiency syndrome of childhood. Pediatric Clinics of North America 1987; 2:247–268. *

Borkowsky W, et al.: Human-immunodeficiency-virus infections in infants negative for anti-HIV by enzyme-linked immunoassay. Lancet 1987; I:1168–1170.

Centers for Disease Control: Classification system for human immunodeficency virus infection in children under 13 years of age. Morbidity and Mortality Weekly Report 1987; 36:225–235.

Minkoff H, et al.: Pregnancies resulting in infants with acquired immunodeficiency syndrome or AIDS-related complex: follow-up of mothers, children and subsequently born siblings. Obstet Gynecol 1987; 69:288–291.

Mok JQ, et al.: Infants born to mothers seropositive for human immunodeficiency virus: preliminary findings from a multicentre European study. Lancet 1987; I:1164–1167.

Rogers MF, et al.: Acquired immunodeficiency syndrome in children: report of the Centers for Disease Control National Surveillance, 1982 to 1985. Pediatrics 1987; 79:1008–1014.

United States Department of Health and Human Services: Report of the Surgeon General's Workshop on Children with HIV Infection and Their Families, April 6–9, 1987. DHHS Publication No. HRS D-MC 87-1.

Qazi QH, et al.: Lack of evidence for craniofacial dysmorphism in perinatal human immunodeficiency virus infection. J Pediatr 1988; 112:7–11. †

American Academy of Pediatrics Task Force on Pediatric AIDS: Perinatal human immunodeficiency virus infection. Pediatrics 1988; 82:841–944.

George R, et al.: National survey of HIV seroprevalence in women delivering live children in the United States. Fifth International Congress on AIDS, Montreal, June 7, 1989 (Abstract WAO 12).

Blanche S, et al.: A prospective study of infants born to women seropositive for human immunodeficiency virus type 1. New Engl J Med 1989; 320:1643–1648.

Rogers MF, et al.: Use of the polymerase chain reaction for early detection of the proviral sequences of human immunodeficiency virus in infants born to seropositive mothers. New Engl J Med 1989; 320:1649–1654.

Ryder RW, et al.: Perinatal transmission of the human immunodeficiency virus type 1 to infants of seropositive women in Zaire. New Engl J Med 1989; 320:1637–1642.

Update: acquired immunodeficiency syndrome - United States 1989. MMWR 1990; 39:81–86.

| R0018 | **Franz W. Rosa** |
| MA032 | **Robert W. Marion** |
| WI056 | **Andrew A. Wiznia** |
| QA000 | **Qutub Qazi** |

**Fetal akinesia deformation sequence, Pena-Shokeir I phenotype**
*See PENA-SHOKEIR SYNDROME*

---

## FETAL ALCOHOL SYNDROME           0379

**Includes:** Alcohol, fetal effects of

**Excludes:** Fetal effects (other)

**Major Diagnostic Criteria:** Prenatal and postnatal growth deficiency, microcephaly, irritability, moderate mental deficiency, short palpebral fissures, midface hypoplasia and major organ system malformations in a child exposed in utero to alcohol.

**Clinical Findings:** Babies exposed in utero to alcohol are often light for dates and may be preterm as well. Head circumference, weight, and length are all reduced relative to the duration of the pregnancy. There is no postnatal catch up of the prenatal growth deficiency. Furthermore, postnatal weight and height may diverge from the lower centiles. Bone age is not usually delayed.

Neurodevelopmental disorders are very variable. Irritability in the neonatal period and moderate mental retardation with hyperactivity, distractibility, short attention span, and speech delay are the most characteristic.

The facial dysmorphism includes a narrow forehead, short palpebral fissures, epicanthus, ptosis, midface hypoplasia, short nose, long and smooth philtrum, thin upper lip, and hypoplastic mandibula.

Structural malformations affect a minority of alcohol damaged babies. Any organ may be affected, but the most common malformations are microphthalmia, cleft palate, cardiac septal defects, fused cervical vertebrae, hemangiomas, and malformed ears.

Any subcombination of anomalies can occur, depending on alcohol exposure dose and timing during pregnancy and on individual differences in embryofetal and maternal vulnerability to the effects of alcohol. Developmental delay and CNS dysfunctions are the most sensitive indicators of gestational alcohol intake. The behavioral, intellectual and motor impairments can occur in the absence of the craniofacial malformations but appear to be closely related to the body growth deficit. Major organ malformations have been observed only in offspring of severe chronic alcoholic mothers.

**Complications:** Unknown.

**Associated Findings:** Microphthalmia, strabismus, **Pectus excavatum**, ungual hypoplasia, hirsutism at birth, diaphragmatic defects, altered palmar crease patterns and inability to extend metacarpal-phalangeal joints are possible. Few cases of major limb

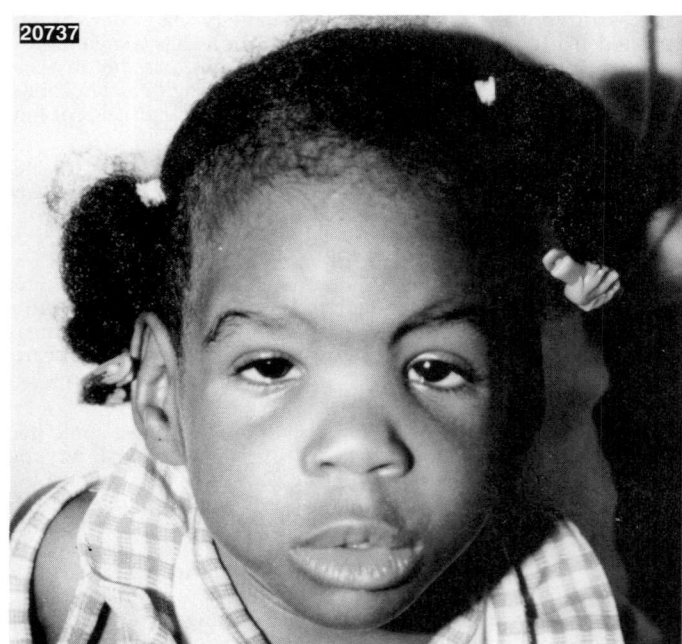

0379-20737: Fetal alcohol syndrome; note short palpebral fissures, flat nasal bridge, long philtrum and thin vermilion border of the upper lip.

---

malformations have been reported. An increased incidence of life-threatening bacterial infections, and a propensity to minor infections are observed. A possible association of in utero alcohol exposure with embryonic carcinomas has been suggested.

**Etiology:** Alcohol and its major metabolite, acetaldehyde, readily cross the placenta. Both can be directly teratogenic. Because the enzymes necessary for drug biotransformation are absent in the embryo, it is exposed to both compounds long after they have been cleared from the maternal system. There are other indirect ways in which alcohol can impair embryofetal development, such as malnutrition, hypothermia, dehydration, placental dysfunction, impaired hormone synthesis, and end-organ responsiveness.

**Pathogenesis:** It is likely that alcohol-related developmental abnormalities, including those observed in the brain, can be explained in terms of cellular growth restriction during critical periods of rapid growth. Alcohol would be a rather weak, nonspecific teratogen that can affect most cell types. It has been demonstrated experimentally on the rat that decreased development of the neural plate and its derivatives account for the craniofacial malformations. In nonhuman primate infants, ethanol-related behavioral teratogenesis occurs without accompanying physical anomalies, and early gestational exposure appears to be more damaging to cognitive function. The amount of alcohol per day or per week necessary to cause detectable damage has not been clearly established. In nonhuman primate infants, measurable teratogenic effects from weekly exposures occur only at intoxicating doses of ethanol.

**POS No.:** 3218

**CDC No.:** 760.710

**Sex Ratio:** M1:F1

**Occurrence:** Occurs in approximately one percent of newborns in Western countries. This figure fluctuates depending on local habits in alcohol consumption. Among heavy drinkers, probably one-third give birth to affected children.

**Risk of Recurrence for Patient's Sib:** Depends on the maternal alcohol consumption during the pregnancy.

**Risk of Recurrence for Patient's Child:** Depends on the maternal alcohol consumption during the pregnancy.

**Age of Detectability:** Detectability in utero can be expected through growth retardation, microcephaly and major organ malformations, which could be detected prenatally by ultrasound. Maternal serum $\gamma$-glutamyltransferase level is also a good predictor of the outcome. Severely affected cases can be easily diagnosed at birth. The mildest cases will be suspected later in development.

**Gene Mapping and Linkage:** Unknown.

**Prevention:** Alcohol related mental retardation is now considered to be the most frequent preventable cause of mental retardation. Since the discontinuing of drinking after pregnancy is discovered may be too late to prevent embryonic injury, women who have the potential to become pregnant should avoid drinking. Stopping alcohol abuse after the first trimester cannot modify the risk of malformations, but is likely to reduce the occurrence of central nervous system dysfunction. Ethanol ingested through breast milk has a slight but detrimental effect on motor development (but not mental development) and should be avoided.

**Treatment:** Surgical correction of major defects.

**Prognosis:** Life span probably reduced. No correction of the growth deficiency or mental retardation to be expected.

**Detection of Carrier:** Unknown.

**Support Groups:** MD; Rockville; National Clearinghouse for Alcohol Information

**References:**
Lemoine P, et al.: Les enfants de parents alcoliques: anomalies observées. Ouest Med 1968; 21:476–482.
Streissguth AP: Fetal alcohol syndrome: an epidemiologic perspective. Am J Epid 1978; 107:467–478. *
Iosub S, et al.: Fetal alcohol syndrome revisited. Pediatrics 1981; 68:475–479.
Kennedy LA: The pathogenesis of brain abnormalities in the fetal alcohol syndrome: an integrating hypothesis. Teratology 1984; 29: 363–368.
Larsson G, et al.: Prospective study of children exposed to variable amounts of alcohol in utero. Arch Dis Child 1985; 60:316–321.
Mulvihill JJ: Fetal alcohol syndrome. In: Sever JL, Brent RL, eds: Teratogen update: environmentally induced birth defect risks. New York: Alan R. Liss, 1986:13–18. *
Halmesmäki E, et al.: Patterns of alcohol consumption during pregnancy. Obstet Gynecol 1987; 69:594–597.
Clarren SK, et al.: Physical anomalies and developmental delays in nonhuman primate infants exposed to weekly doses of ethanol during gestation. Teratology 1988; 37:561–569.
Graham JM, et al.: Independent dysmorphology evaluations at birth and four years of age for children exposed to varying amounts of alcohol in utero. Pediatrics 1988; 81:772–778.
Little RE, et al.: Maternal alcohol use during breast-feeding and infant mental and motor development at one year. New Engl J Med 1989; 321:425–430.
Zajac CS, et al.: Changes in red nucleus neuronal development following maternal alcohol exposure. Teratology 1989; 40:567–570.

AYO10                                                **Ségolène Ayme**

## FETAL AMINOGLYCOSIDE OTOTOXICITY          **2992**

**Includes:**
Amikacin, fetal effects
Amikin^, fetal effects
Aminoglycoside, fetal effects
Deafness, fetal aminoglycoside ototoxicity
Dihydrostreptomycin, fetal effects
Garamycin^, fetal effect
Genticin^, fetal effects
Gentamycin, fetal effects
Kanamycin, fetal effects
Kantrex^, fetal effects
Klebcil^, fetal effects
Netilmycin, fetal effects
Netromycin^, fetal effects
Streptomycin, fetal effects
Tobramycin, fetal effects
Tobrex^, fetal effects

**Excludes:** Deafness, streptomycin-sensitivity (0272)

**Major Diagnostic Criteria:** Sensorineural hearing deficiency and vestibular disturbance in offspring with maternal systemic exposure to streptomycin, kanamycin, gentamycin, tobramycin, amikacin, netilmicin, or other aminoglycosides.

**Clinical Findings:** Approximately 40 cases of congenital hearing loss with or without vestibular disturbances after maternal exposures to antituberculous use of streptomycin or dihydrostreptomycin, and ten cases after maternal exposure to kanamycin, have been reported. Knowledge that direct administration of these and other aminoglycosides causes ototoxicity indicates a potential hazard with all aminoglycosides. Although there is some inconsistency in the reports, the ototoxicity is characteristically bilateral and permanent. The ototoxicity may be delayed or progressive for several months after discontinuing administration. See also **Deafness, streptomycin-sensitivity**.

**Complications:** As with other forms of congenital deafness, delayed recognition may lead to learning impairments.

**Associated Findings:** None known.

**Etiology:** Maternal systemic exposure to aminoglycosides. High doses injected for a long period of time carry the highest risk. Maternal renal impairment increases risks. Aminoglycosides given orally for gut sterilization are poorly absorbed. Extensive topical use on open dermatologic lesions can produce systemic exposures. Early exposure in pregnancy appears to be more injurious, although adverse effects have also been reported with late exposure. Genetic susceptibility may be a factor (see **Deafness, streptomycin-sensitivity**).

**Pathogenesis:** Injury to the organ of Corti and eighth nerve toxicity. Aminoglycosides may be retained in the inner ear endolyph, explaining delayed injury.

**Sex Ratio:** Presumably M1:F1.

**Occurrence:** Various studies have estimated the risk to be from 5–15% of streptomycin exposures, although both the numerators (type of injury included) and the denominators are variable. Injury is more frequent with higher doses for longer durations, and streptomycin is now used much less than formerly. Use of newer types of aminoglycosides is infrequent but increasing. All carry a warning not to employ during pregnancy, which should reduce exposures.

**Risk of Recurrence for Patient's Sib:** Unknown.

**Risk of Recurrence for Patient's Child:** Unknown.

**Age of Detectability:** For early detection, sensitive hearing tests should be employed in those exposed.

**Gene Mapping and Linkage:** Unknown.

**Prevention:** Avoidance of aminoglycosides during pregnancy unless the potential benefits outweigh the risks.

**Treatment:** Hearing augmentation and training as for other types of sensorineural deafness.

**Prognosis:** Hearing impairment is generally irreversible.

**Detection of Carrier:** Unknown.

**References:**
Warkany J: Antituberculosis drugs. Teratology 1979; 20:133–138.
Schardein JL: Chemically induced birth defects. New York: Marcel Dekker, 1985:370–371.

R0018
GR039

Franz W. Rosa
Theresa Reed Greene

## FETAL AMINOPTERIN SYNDROME     0380

**Includes:**
> Aminopterin, fetal effects of
> Four-amino-pteroyl-glutamic acid, fetal effects of
> Methotrexate, fetal effects of

**Excludes:** Pseudoaminopterin syndrome (2628)

**Major Diagnostic Criteria:** Congenital malformations in the off-spring whose mother had aminopterin or similar drug during pregnancy.

**Clinical Findings:** Aminopterin taken by a woman in the first trimester of pregnancy can cause depression of fetal hematopoiesis, necrosis of the liver or adrenals or fetal death. In an older embryo, the drug may induce congenital malformations such as hydrocephaly, meningoencephalocele, cleft lip, and cleft palate. If the fetus lives to near term, anencephaly, partial craniostenosis, particularly cranial dysplasia (lack of ossification of the cranial bones), have been observed. Facial anomalies, posterior cleft palate, clubhands and clubfeet also occur. In case of survival the disease picture can improve and ossification of the skull bones progresses slowly. Shortening of the forearms and coxa vara deformity of the hips may persist. There may be mental retardation.

A methyl derivative of amniopterin; methotrexate, used as an abortifacient or in the treatment of psoriasis during early pregnancy can result in anomalies of the skull, hypertelorism and finger defects similar to malformations produced by aminopterin.

**Complications:** Unknown.

**Associated Findings:** None known.

**Etiology:** Aminopterin ingestion during pregnancy. Dose range in reported cases varied from 6 to 12 mg over a 2–5 day period. A methyl derivative of amniopterin methotrexate, used as an abortifacient or in the treatment for psoriasis during early pregnancy can result in anomalies of the skull, hypertelorism and finger defects similar to malformations produced by aminopterin.

**Pathogenesis:** Thought to be related to folic acid deficiency.

**POS No.:** 3219

**Sex Ratio:** M1:F1

**Occurrence:** Undetermined.

**Risk of Recurrence for Patient's Sib:** Related to subsequent exposure.

**Risk of Recurrence for Patient's Child:** Related to maternal exposure.

**Age of Detectability:** At birth or early infancy; third trimester X-rays show delayed ossification of calvarium and hydramnios.

**Gene Mapping and Linkage:** Unknown.

**Prevention:** Avoidance of aminopterin during pregnancy.

**Treatment:** Unknown.

**Prognosis:** Varies with kind and severity of defects present.

**Detection of Carrier:** Unknown.

**References:**
Meltzer HJ: Congenital anomalies due to attempted abortion with 4-amino-pteroylglutamic acid. JAMA 1956; 161:1253.
Milunsky A, et al.: Methotrexate-induced congenital malformations. J Pediatr 1968; 72:790.
Shaw EB, Steinbach HL: Aminopterin-induced fetal malformation:

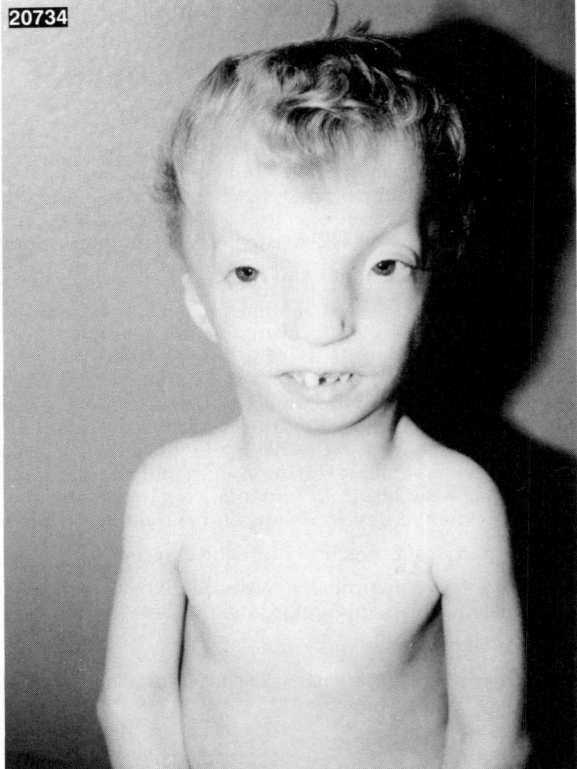

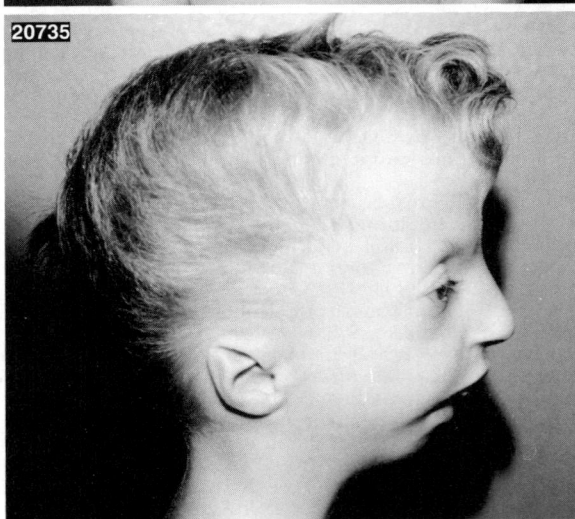

0380-20734–35: Fetal aminopterin syndrome; note 5-year-old with hypertelorism, shallow orbits, low supraorbital ridges, up-swept scalp hair, low-set pointed ears, wide glabella and pegged teeth. Micrognathia is evident on the lateral view.

survival of infant after attempted abortion. Am J Dis Child 1968; 115:477.
Baker H: Some hazards of methotrexate treatment of psoriasis. Trans St Johns Hosp Dermatol Soc 1970; 56:111.
Netzloff ML, et al.: Maternal aminopterin ingestion. Am J Dis Child 1973; 125:459.
Howard MJ, Rudd NL: The natural history of aminopterin-induced embryopathy, in Bergsma D, Lowry RB (eds): BD:OAS; XIII(3C). Natural History of Specific Birth Defects. New York, Alan R. Liss Inc for The National Foundation-March of Dimes, 1977:85.

Warkany J: Aminopterin and methotrexate folic acid deficiency. Teratology 1978; 17:353.

Shaw EB, Rees EL: Fetal damages due to maternal aminopterin ingestion: Follow-up at 17 1/2 years of age. Am J Dis Child 1980; 134:1172.

WA027                                                    Josef Warkany

## FETAL ANGIOTENSIN CONVERTING ENZYME (ACE) INHIBITION RENAL FAILURE                                 2962

**Includes:**

Captopril, fetal effects
Capoten^, fetal effects
Enalapril, fetal effects
Hypertension, maternal treatment, fetal ACE inhibitors
Lisinopril, possible fetal effects
Primivil^, possible fetal effects
Vasotec^, fetal effects
Zestril^, possible fetal effects

**Excludes:**

**Fetal effects** (other)
Fetal effects of maternal indomethacin exposure
Neonatal anuria from other causes
Oligohydramnios from other causes

**Major Diagnostic Criteria:** Perinatal oliguria or anuria with maternal angiotension enzyme (ACE) inhibitor treatment of maternal hypertension.

**Clinical Findings:** Angiotensin-converting enzyme (ACE) inhibition agents are employed to treat hypertension. Hypertensive disease of pregnancy and its treatment is often complicated by fetal anoxia, intrauterine growth retardation, neonatal respiratory distress, and increased perinatal mortality (see **Fetal developmental retardation with maternal hypertension**). However, neonatal anuria has seldom been reported unless an ACE inhibitor has been included in the maternal regimen. As of September 1989, 20 cases of perinatal renal failure associated with concurrent maternal exposure to ACE inhibitors have been reported. Oligohydramnios is an intrauterine signal of this renal failure. In neonates, the hypotension associated with the anuria may be refractory to treatment until the ACE inhibition subsides. In surviving cases, usually supported by peritoneal dialysis, hypotension and oliguria subside during the first week. Seven of the 20 cases died perinatally. Autopsies did not show renal pathology. Five of the cases were with captopril (Capoten^), and 15 with enalapril (Vasotec^). No cases have yet been reported with the more recently introduced ACE inhibitor lisinopril (Primivil^).

**Complications:** Perinatal death, intrauterine growth retardation, respiratory distress.

**Associated Findings:** Two cases had **Ductus arteriosus, patent.** Neonatal characteristics from oligohydramnios, including inadequate lung expansion and limb contractures, may be seen.

**Etiology:** ACE inhibitors are new antihypertensive agents, employed to manage the hypertensive effects of angiotension.

**Pathogenesis:** In animal studies, ACE inhibition caused fetal hypotension. Hypotension/reduced renal perfusion may lead to renal failure. During pregnancy the placenta can remove the renal wastes. Oliguric oligohydramnios may cause positional contractures in the fetus, and interference with pulmonary development. Postnatally renal failure occurs unless measures are taken to maintain the infants renal balance until ACE levels return. Nephrogenesis appears normal, and the renal failure appears to be functional and transient.

**Sex Ratio:** Presumably M1:F1.

**Occurrence:** Pregnancy ACE inhibitor exposures up to delivery have been projected to be 3,200 in the United States in 1988. Adverse outcomes have not been determined. Most case reports have been from outside the United States.

**Risk of Recurrence for Patient's Sib:** Presumably related to maternal ACE inhibitor exposure.

**Risk of Recurrence for Patient's Child:** Presumably related to maternal ACE inhibitor exposure.

**Age of Detectability:** Oligohydramnios may be detected prenatally. Other cases are detected by hypotension and anuria from birth.

**Gene Mapping and Linkage:** N/A

**Prevention:** Data are insufficient for risk benefit guidelines. Until further data are available, existing animal data and the cases reported suggest that ACE inhibitor use should be discontinued during pregnancy if possible.

**Treatment:** Peritoneal dialysis of the newborn until diuresis occurs reflecting the return of ACE function. Pregnant women on ACE inhibitors should deliver their babies where intensive neonatal care is available.

**Prognosis:** In surviving infants the blood pressure usually normalizes and renal output returns in a few days, but renal dysfunction has persisted for several weeks in some cases. Follow-up is insufficient to determine the extent of permanent renal dysfunction. Intrauterine growth retardation, oligohydramnios positional contractures, and respiratory hypoplasia may be sequelae.

**Detection of Carrier:** N/A

**Special Considerations:** Any pregnancy ACE inhibitor exposures should be reported to the Food and Drug Administration, HFD 733, by telephone at (301) 443 2306; or by mail to HFD 733, Rockville MD 20857.

*This article reflects the views of the author and is not an official statement of the Food and Drug Administration or any Governmental organization.*

**References:**

Guignard JP, et al: Persistent anuria in a neonate: side effect of captopril. Int J Pediatr Nephrol 1981; 2:133 only.

Broughton Pipkin F, et al: The effect of captopril (SQ 14,225) upon mother and fetus in the chronically cannulated ewe and in the pregnant rabbit. J Physiol 1982; 232:415–432.

Miller JA, et al.: Management of severe hypertension in pregnancy by a combined drug regime including captopril: case report. New Zealand Med J 1983; 96:796 only.

Boutroy M, et al: Captopril administration in pregnancy impairs fetal angiotensin converting enzyme activity and neonatal adaptation. Lancet 1984; II:935–936.

Rothberg A, Lorenz R: Can captopril cause fetal and neonatal renal failure? Pediatric pharmacology 1984; 4:189–192.

Schubiger G, et al.: Enalapril for pregnancy-induced hypertension: acute renal failure in a neonate. Annals Int Med 1988; 108:15–16.

Broughton-Pipkin F, et al.: ACE inhibitors in pregnancy. Lancet 1989; II:96–97.

Mehta N, Modi N, et al.: ACE inhibitors in pregnancy. (Letters) Lancet 1989; II:96–97.

Rosa FW, et al.: Neonatal anuria with maternal angiotensin-converting enzyme inhibition. Obstet Gynecol 1989; 74:371–374. *

Scott AA, Purohit DM: Neonatal renal failure: a complication of maternal antihypertensive therapy. Am J Obstet Gynecol 1989; 160:1223–1224.

R0018                                                    Franz W. Rosa

**Fetal ascites-macrosomia-Wilms tumor**
*See OVERGROWTH-RENAL HAMARTOMA, PERLMAN TYPE*

## FETAL BARBITURATE EFFECTS                               2930

**Includes:**

Antiepileptic drugs (some), fetal effects
Barbiturate effects, fetal

**Excludes:**

Dysmorphia caused by concurrent drug exposures
Epilepsy, parental, dysmorphia due to
**Fetal alcohol syndrome** (0379)

**Major Diagnostic Criteria:** Possible dysmorphia or cardiovascular defects caused by first trimester barbiturate exposure.

**Clinical Findings:** Some authorities have stated that a dysmorphic syndrome, resembling or identical to **Fetal hydantoin syn-**

drome, is seen with maternal barbiturate use. Others believe barbiturates are the antiepileptic agent least likely to have teratogenic risks. In the Collaborative Perinatal Project, an association of aortic stenosis with two high dose rapidly metabolized barbiturates (secobarbital and amobarbital) was observed (Rosa, 1986). However, this could have resulted from concurrent exposures, or by chance due to the multiplicity of possible associations examined. This and other association of dysmorphia, cardiovascular defects, and **Cleft lip** with barbiturates has not been confirmed.

Several clinical studies suggest antiepileptic teratogenesis is higher with combinations (usually including phenobarbital) than with monotherapy. However, the risk of spina bifida with valproate exposure appears to be reduced by concomitant phenobarbital exposure. Hemorrhagic disease of the newborn due to vitamin K deficiency has been observed with maternal barbiturate exposure and exposure to other antiepileptics. As with benzodiazapines and other neurofunctional agents, neonatal depression and withdrawal symptoms are seen, but long-term sequelae of maternal barbiturate exposure are difficult to assess. Barbiturate animal teratogenesis has been reported, but at dosages greatly exceeding those used clinically. There are also distinct variations between animal species and strains.

**Complications:**  Unknown.

**Associated Findings:**  None known.

**Etiology:**  Presumably maternal exposure to barbiturates.

**Pathogenesis:**  There are many theories for varying teratogenicity of these agents. Rapidity of metabolism to potentially teratogenic intermediate metabolites and observed lowering of folic acid levels may be important. Increased teratogenicity of hydantoin with concurrent barbiturate exposure might be due to accelerated production of teratogenic metabolites. Reduced teratogenicity of valproate with concurrent phenobarbital use may be due to phenobarbital accelerating the catabolism of valproate.

**Sex Ratio:**  Presumably M1:F1.

**Occurrence:**  Phenobarbital teratogenicity, if it exists, is not as prominent as that from the hydantoins and the methadiones. Secobarbital and amobarbital exposures are infrequent, and an association found with **Aorta, coarctation** has not been confirmed in other data. Although in the general population benzodiazepines are now favored over barbiturates for tranquilization, because of their wider margin of safety and lower sedative effect (see **Fetal benzodiazepine effects**), barbiturate exposure is still widespread. Barbiturate abuse is confounded by association with maternal alcohol and other substance abuse. Therefore, sufficient data should find a crude association of barbiturates with **Fetal alcohol syndrome**, although the association could be indirect unless proved otherwise by multivariate analysis.

**Risk of Recurrence for Patient's Sib:**  Unknown.

**Risk of Recurrence for Patient's Child:**  Unknown.

**Age of Detectability:**  Possibly by infancy or early childhood.

**Gene Mapping and Linkage:**  Unknown. Genetically determined factors such as slow epoxide metabolization may increase susceptibility.

**Prevention:**  Barbiturate use in pregnancy should be limited to essential indications, mainly antiepileptic use. Combinations should be avoided when possible. Amobarbital and secobarbital use in early pregnancy should be avoided. Associations do not appear to be strong enough to justify therapeutic abortion for accidental exposures. It remains to be shown whether supplementation with folic acid can improve antiepileptic risk benefits. Vitamin K should always be administered to the newborn.

**Treatment:**  Unknown.

**Prognosis:**  Undetermined. Possibly similar to that of **Fetal hydantoin syndrome**.

**Detection of Carrier:**  Unknown.

**References:**
Bethenod M, Frederic A: Les enfants des antiepileptics. Pediatrie 1973; 30:227–248.

Hanson JW, Smith DW: The fetal hydantoin syndrome. J Pediatr 1975; 87:285–900.
Siep M: Growth retardation, dysmorphic facies and minor malformations following massive exposure to phenobarbitone in utero. Acta Paediatr Scand 1976; 65:617–621.
Heinonen OP, et al.: Birth defects and drugs in pregnancy. Littleton, MA: PSG Publishing, 1977.
Lindhout D, et al.: Hazards of fetal exposure to drug combinations. In: Janz D, et al., eds: Epilepsy, pregnancy and the child. New York: Raven, 1982:275–281.
Robert E, Rosa FW: Valproate and birth defects. (Letter) Lancet 1983; II:937 only.
Rosa FW: Human barbiturate teratology. (Abstract) Teratology 1986; 33:27A only.
Finell RH, et al.: Strain differences in phenobarbital-induced teratogenesis in mice. Teratology 1987; 177–186.

R0018                                          **Franz W. Rosa**
FR030                                     **Jean-Pierre Fryns**

---

**FETAL BENZODIAZEPINE EFFECTS**                     **2929**

**Includes:**
  Alprazolam, fetal effects
  Ativan^, fetal effects
  Benzodiazepine, fetal effects
  Chlordiazepoxide, fetal effects
  Dalmane^, fetal effects
  Diazepam, fetal effects
  Flurazepam, fetal effects
  Halcion^, fetal effects
  Hypotonia "floppy baby" syndrome (some)
  Librium^, fetal effects
  Lorazepam, fetal effects
  Oxazepam, fetal effects of
  Restoril^, fetal effects
  Serax^, fetal effects
  Temazepam, fetal effects
  Tranquilizer, fetal effects (some)
  Tranxene^, fetal effects
  Triazolam, fetal effects
  Valium^, fetal effects
  Xanax^, fetal effects

**Excludes:**  **Fetal effects** (other concurrent exposures)

**Major Diagnostic Criteria:**  Possible characteristic dysmorphology with high-level maternal benzodiazepine exposure.

**Clinical Findings:**  Hypotonia ("floppy baby" syndrome) and "withdrawal" agitation, which are often surprisingly persistent, are well recognized with prolonged maternal benzodiazepine exposure persisting up to term. Even with severe neonatal depression, neurologic follow-up has usually been normal. However, reported follow-up beyond the neonatal period is exceptional. Despite numerous studies going back more than twenty years, a consensus does not exist on whether lasting fetal injury results from maternal benzodiazepine exposure.

A 1987 report from Sweden raised the question once again. Seven infants were described with high-level diazepam and oxazepam exposure throughout pregnancy (all mothers denying concurrent alcohol exposure). All infants had at least six of the following: telecanthus, epicanthal folds, slanted eyes, uptilted nose, dysplastic auricles, high-arched palate, wide-spaced nipples, and webbed neck. Pronounced myopathy and expressionless face were also said to be characteristic. Growth and developmental retardation, choreiform and athetoid symptoms, and encephalopathy are described. Other features in the seven infants were submucous **Cleft palate** in two, convulsions in two, neonatal abstinence syndrome in two, Dandy-Walker syndrome and **Lissencephaly syndrome** in one infant who died in the fourth week of life, **Hydrocephaly** in another infant who also died in the fourth week of life, **Microcephaly** in one surviving infants, and reduced head size in two others. The five surviving infants have had limited follow-up. The findings were distinct enough for the authors to feel they were able to identify the exposure from this appearance. However, denominators are unclear for establishing the proportion of children with these findings who have actually had the exposure, or the proportion of exposed infants who have these findings.

An exposure denominator is particularly difficult to establish because of varying dosages, concurrent exposures, and unreliable maternal recall. Because benzodiazepine abuse is strongly associated with alcohol, epidmiologic data should provide an indirect association of benzodiazepine with fetal alchohol syndrome. We are unaware of any current epidemiologic data base adequate to distinguish whether this association would be due to the benzodiazepine or to confounding factors, especially alcohol abuse. Only careful clinical studies can examine this question, and maternal benzodiazepine abuse should be confirmed through serologic levels.

The dysmorphic endpoint is also difficult, because it involves multiple findings rather than a single, distinct, easily enumerated outcome. These features also are seen in spontaneous case reports and in exposure studies, but observations are inadequate to clarify benzodiazepine causation.

Follow-up of 511 maternal exposures did not find a diminution of IQ (Hartz, 1975). However, these studies dilute high-dose exposures with large numbers of low-dose exposures and use an index that would not identify cranial nerve or other types of neurologic injury. Czeizel (1987) reported normal outcomes even with high-dose exposures, but long-term follow-up may be limited.

**Cleft lip,** with or without **Cleft palate** also was a suspected association with diazepam exposure, based on animal studies and early epidemiology in Atlanta and Finland, but this was not supported by later, more extensive data from Boston, the National Institutes of Health/Kaiser Permanente, and FDA exposure cohort data from Michigan. Unfortunately, a dysmorphic syndrome is unlikely to be recognizable in these databases, which analyze sharply defined endpoints. In a Yale case control study a statistically significant 3.7-fold association of central nervous system anomalies with first-trimester tranquilizer exposures (mainly diazepam) was found.

In laboratory studies, in addition to the cleft findings, chlordiazepoxide or diazepam induced a variety of malformations in hamsters. Rats and primates were unreactive except for postnatal behavioral effects in the former.

**Complications:** Respiratory difficulties, hypothermia, and hyperbilirubinemia have been found as neonatal effects of maternal benzodiazepine exposures prior to delivery.

**Associated Findings:** None known.

**Etiology:** Presumably benzodiazepine exposures.

**Pathogenesis:** Because of immature metabolic and excretory capacities, blood levels of benzodiazepines may persist for 7–10 days after birth.

The central concern in the described lasting dysmorphy appears to be central nervous system pathology. The basal ganglia, cranial nerve nuclei, cerebellum, and cortex appear to be involved.

Some laboratory studies point to a GABA as well as a benzodiazepine receptor involvement.

**Sex Ratio:** Presumably M1:F1.

**Occurrence:** Benzodiazepines are the most widely used tranquilizers during pregnancy, and are employed as anticonvulsants (usually in combinations). High doses are likely to be associated with abuse.

**Risk of Recurrence for Patient's Sib:** Unknown.

**Risk of Recurrence for Patient's Child:** Unknown.

**Age of Detectability:** By the neonatal period.

**Gene Mapping and Linkage:** Unknown. Genetic factors in benzodiazepine metabolism could play a role in the reported findings.

**Prevention:** Because benzodiazepine tranquilization is seldom essential, and teratogenic findings are uncertain, the benefits of any use during pregnancy should be balanced against possible risks. However, with therapeutic or accidental short-term expo-

sures, the attributable risk for long-term adverse outcomes appears to be limited.

**Treatment:** Neonatal respiratory depression may require intubation and respiratory assistance. Feeding assistance may be required.

**Prognosis:** Unknown.

**Detection of Carrier:** Unknown.

**References:**

Rosenberg L, et al.: Lack of relation of oral clefts to diazepam use during pregnancy. New Engl J Med 1983; 309:1282–1285.

Grimm VE: A review of diazepam and other benzodiazepines in pregnancy. In: Yanai J, ed: Neurobehavioral teratology. New York: Elsevier Science, 1984:153–162. *

Strong PH, Mills JL: Oral clefts and diazepam during pregnancy. New Engl J Med 1984; 311:919–920.

Weber LWD: Benzodiazepines in pregnancy: academic debate or teratogenic risk? Int J Biol Res Preg 1985; 6:151–157.

Czeizel A, Lendway A: In-utero exposure to benzodiazepines. Lancet 1987; I:627–628.

Laegreid L, et al.: Abnormalities in children exposed to benzodiazepines in utero. Lancet 1987; I:108–109. * †

Laegreid L, et al.: Teratogenic effects of benzodiazepine use during pregnancy. J Pediatr 1989; 114:126–131.

R0018                                             **Franz W. Rosa**

---

## FETAL BRAIN DISRUPTION SEQUENCE                    **2254**

**Includes:**

>   Brain (fetal) disruption sequence
>   Cytomegalovirus infection, fetal effects of
>   Monozygotic co-twin, fetal effects of vascular obstruction

**Excludes:**  Cutis verticus gyrata (2295)

**Major Diagnostic Criteria:**  Congenital **Microcephaly** with overlapping cranial sutures, prominent occipital bone, rugation of the scalp, and X-ray or autopsy evidence of partial brain destruction.

**Clinical Findings:**  The clinical features of this disruption sequence vary greatly in severity and include mild to profound microcephaly, overlapping of cranial bones, rugation of the scalp and an occiput overriding the calvaria in a keel-like fashion. Usually neurological deficiencies are present including hypertonia, hyperreflexia, lethargy, lack of visual pursuit, a high-pitched cry and, if the child survives, developmental delay. Computed tomography of the head, or autopsy, will show partial brain destruction of varying degree with fluid replacement, or significant brain atrophy. The scalp hair pattern is normal.

**Complications:**  Usually secondary to the neurological problems, e.g., feeding difficulty, aspiration, pneumonia, apnea, and bradycardia; or from other defects produced by the same mechanism that caused the brain destruction in the first place.

---

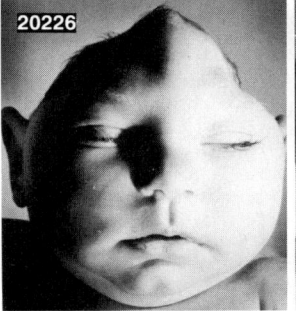 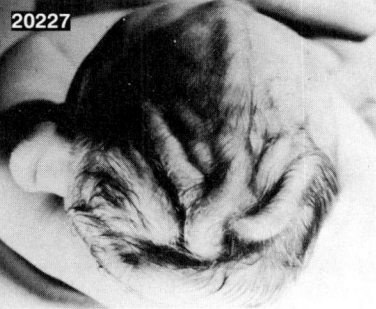

**2254-20226:**  Profound microcephaly and overriding sutures. **20227:**  Marked rugations of the scalp.

**Associated Findings:** None known.

**Etiology:** Any environmental agent or disruptive mechanism which will lead to brain necrosis, including prenatal cytomegalovirus infection and vascular obstruction secondary to intrauterine demise of a monozygotic co-twin.

**Pathogenesis:** Presumably fetal brain growth is normal for the first 12 weeks or so. Subsequently, but prior to birth, there is partial destruction of the brain which leads to microcephaly, diminished intracranial pressure, and collapse of the fetal skull. The collapse of the skull produces the characteristic cranial phenotype. The exact neurologic impairment will depend on the location and extent of the brain lesion(s).

**Sex Ratio:** Presumably M1:F1.

**Occurrence:** Undetermined but presumed rare.

**Risk of Recurrence for Patient's Sib:** Related to underlying etiology, but probably less than 1%.

**Risk of Recurrence for Patient's Child:** Probably not increased.

**Age of Detectability:** At birth.

**Gene Mapping and Linkage:** Unknown.

**Prevention:** Avoid teratogens during pregnancy, have prepregnancy immunizations, and receive appropriate prenatal care during pregnancy.

**Treatment:** Appropriate treatment of secondary problems arising as a result of the neurologic deficiency.

**Prognosis:** Depends on the extent and location of the brain disruption. If severe, it may lead to death during infancy.

**Detection of Carrier:** Unknown.

**Special Considerations:** This disorder is a form of **Hydranencephaly**, but it differs by collapse of the skull. The cause of the mechanism producing the reduced intracranial pressure leading to the skull collapse is not known.

**References:**
Russell LJ, et al.: In utero brain destruction resulting in collapse of the fetal skull, microcephaly, scalp rugae and neurologic impairment: the fetal brain disruption sequence. Am J Med Genet 1984; 17:509–521. * †

WE005                                           **David D. Weaver**

## FETAL CARBAMAZEPINE EXPOSURE          **2991**

**Includes:**
   Carbamazepine exposure, fetal effects
   Tegretal^, fetal exposure

**Excludes:**
   Epilepsy, maternal, fetal effects
   Epilepsy, maternal, fetal effects of concurrent treatment
   **Fetal effects** (other)

**Major Diagnostic Criteria:** Possible association of maternal carbamazepine exposure with reduced head size, spina bifida or **Encephalocele**.

**Clinical Findings:** Distinguishing the effects of specific antiepileptic agents from the effects of the maternal condition, and from concomitant exposures, is difficult. The relative safety of various antiepileptic regimens remains to be clarified, although it is generally accepted that maternal epilepsy should be treated as necessary.

In 1981 Hiilesmaa reported from Finland that 20 infants born with maternal carbamazepine exposure had an average head circumference of 338 mm, and for 26 born with maternal carbamazepine combinations with phenobarbital or primidone 342 mm, compared to 348 mm in 143 controls and 349 mm in 55 with phenytoin monotherapy. The reduction in head size with carbamazepine monotherapy was statistically significant (p <.01, and in combinations p <.05). The head size deficiency was still apparent at 18 months age. This finding received support in 1987 from a monotherapy cohort study from Sweden, France and Italy.

Carbamazepine was found to be associated with significantly reduced head size as well as weight for gestational age (the latter was not found in the Finnish study) compared to phenytoin, phenobarbital and valproic acid. This was after adjustment for country of birth and maternal age. The total number of monotherapy exposures was 250 for phenobarbital, 153 for phenytoin, 70 for carbamazepine, and 62 for valproic acid (55% of the births had head measurements).

Association of spina bifida with maternal carbamazepine exposure has also been suggested. This association is not as clear as the association of valproic acid with spina bifida (see **Meningomyelocele**). In eight of 20 published and unpublished maternal antiepileptic cohort studies, spina bifida cases have been reported with maternal carbamazepine exposure. In the 1,457 maternal carbamazepine exposures without confounding valproate exposure in all 20 studies, 11 instances of spina bifida have been observed (1:132 exposures; about ten times the expected number in the populations in which these studies were performed). Five of the spina bifidas were with 582 carbamazepine monotherapies, and six with carbimazepine combined with phenobarbital and/or phenytoin. Outside these cohorts four encephalocele isolated case reports have been received by FDA with maternal carbamazepine exposure. Two of these were with valproic acid combinations. Only one encephalocele has been reported with maternal valproate exposure not in combination with carbamazepine.

Jones et al (1989) reported a specific pattern of minor craniofacial defects, fingernail hypoplasia, and developmental delay among eight children born of 54 women who reported carbamazepine exposure early in their pregnancy.

**Complications:** Unknown.

**Associated Findings:** None known.

**Etiology:** Fetal exposure to carbamazepine.

**Pathogenesis:** Unknown. Folic acid inhibition has been reported with carbamazepine as well as with other antiepileptic exposures.

**Sex Ratio:** Presumably M1:F1.

**Occurrence:** Eleven of 1,457 exposures, unconfounded by concurrent valproic acid.

**Risk of Recurrence for Patient's Sib:** Unknown.

**Risk of Recurrence for Patient's Child:** Unknown.

**Age of Detectability:** Spina bifida may be detectable prenatally.

**Gene Mapping and Linkage:** Genetic factors may be important in the metabolism of antiepileptics as well as susceptibility to spina bifida and other antiepileptic effects.

**Prevention:** The limited available data suggest that intensive antenatal surveillance of maternal carbamazepine exposures is warrented.

**Treatment:** Unknown.

**Prognosis:** Unknown.

**Detection of Carrier:** Unknown.

**Special Considerations:** The FDA Division of Epidemiology and Surveillance encourages additional studies and reports of maternal carbamazepine exposures.

**References:**
Hiilesmaa V, et al.: Fetal head growth retardation associated with maternal antiepileptic drugs. Lancet 1981; I:1392–1393.
Lindhout D, Meinardi H: Spina bifida and in-utero exposure to valproate. Lancet 1984; II:396 only.
Lindhout D, et al.: Teratogenicity of anticonvulsant drug combinations with special emphasis on epoxidation (of carbamazepine). Epilepsia 1984; 25:77–83.
Bertollini R, et al.: Anticonvulsant drugs in monotherapy: effects on the fetus. Eur J Epidemiol 1987; 3:164–171.
Kaneko S, et al.: Teratogenicity of antiepileptic drugs: analysis of possible risk factors. Epilepsia 1988; 29:459–467.
Bod M: Teratogenic evaluation of anticonvulsants in a population-based Hungarian material. Teratology 1989; 40:277 only.
Jones KL, et al.: Pattern of malformations in the children of women treated with carbamazepine during pregnancy. New Engl J Med 1989; 320:1661–1666. †

Jones KL, et al.: Teratogenic effects of carbamazepine. (Letters) New Engl J Med 1989; 321:1480–1481.

R0018
LI030

**Franz W. Rosa**
**D. Lindhout**

**Fetal carbon monoxide syndrome**
*See FETAL EFFECTS FROM MATERNAL CARBON MONOXIDE EXPOSURE*

## FETAL CYTOMEGALOVIRUS SYNDROME                    0381

**Includes:**
  Cytomegalic inclusion disease, congenital
  Cytomegalovirus (CMV) infection
  Cytomegalovirus, fetal effects of
  Salivary gland virus infection

**Excludes:**  Transplacental infections (other)

**Major Diagnostic Criteria:**  Intrauterine growth retardation associated with hepatosplenomegaly, purpura, jaundice, erythroblastemia, and thrombocytopenia in the neonatal period. Intracranial calcification and microcephaly with or without generalized systemic disease may also be present. Infection beyond the neonatal period is associated with an infectious mononucleosis-like syndrome, isolated hepatomegaly, or severe pulmonary infection.

**Clinical Findings:**  Cytomegalovirus, when transmitted in utero to the conceptus, may be associated with a spectrum of infection ranging from asymptomatic viruria to severe systemic disease that involves the brain, lungs, liver, spleen, and bone marrow.

Manifestations with frequencies of over 50% include hepatosplenomegaly (90%), thrombocytopenia or petechia (70%), jaundice (60%), and hemolytic anemia (55%). Manifestations with frequencies of less than 50% include microcephaly (40%), intrauterine growth retardation (35%), cerebral calcifications (25%), metaphysitis (25%), and pneumonia (25%).

**Complications:**  When cytomegalovirus infection is mild, there may be no permanent sequelae. Approximately 3% of all newborn infants excrete cytomegalovirus, but only 5% of these infants

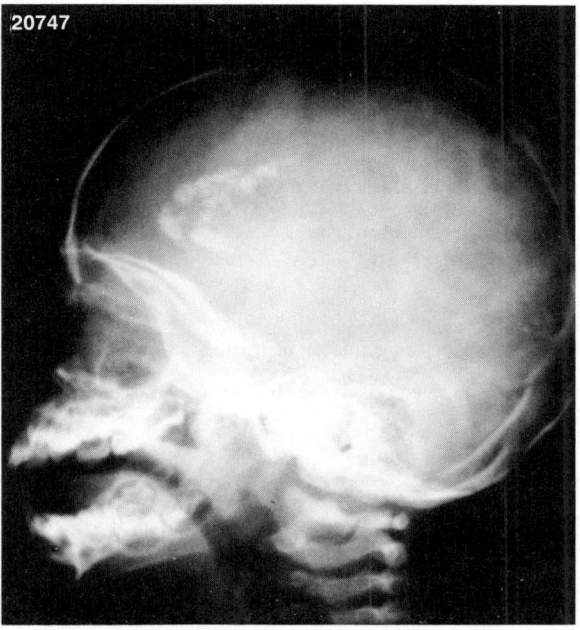

**0381-20747:**  Fetal cytomegalovirus syndrome; note X-ray showing intraventricular calcifications.

show clinical symptoms in the newborn period. If the disease is clinically detectable at birth, approximately 80% of infants have sequelae related to the CNS. These include varying degrees of mental retardation, spasticity, hyperactivity, and convulsive seizures. Microcephaly may be present at birth but may not become apparent until age 18 months.

Hepatosplenomegaly is the most common manifestation at birth and may persist up to 4 years. Despite extensive involvement of the liver at the time of infection, chronic liver problems are rare. The major histologic findings in liver biopsy specimens with clinical and chemical evidence of liver dysfunction include varying degrees of portal fibrosis, hepatitis with giant cells, and cholangitis. As many as 15% of asymptomatic newborn infants who excrete CMV in their urine show signs of deafness later in life.

**Associated Findings:**  Microgyria, porencephaly, hypoplasia of the cerebellar hemisphere, absence of olfactory bulbs and tracts, hearing loss with inner ear involvement, **Pulmonary valve, stenosis**, **Mitral valve stenosis**, **Atrial septal defects**, chorioretinitis, **Hydrocephaly**, congenital ascites, and seizures have all been observed.

**Etiology:**  Transplacental transmission of human-specific cytomegalovirus. Organism can be cultured in vitro only in human fibroblast cells. Fine structure of a particle from culture material reveals a capsomere-like herpes simplex virus. The nucleoprotein is DNA. Cytomegaloviruses are species-specific and infect man, monkeys, and rodents.

**Pathogenesis:**  Symptomatic infection usually takes place in utero in the first half of pregnancy by transplacental transmission. Primary CMV infection in the mother poses a 30–40% risk of infant infection. Cytomegalovirus multiplies within cells and destroys them. Cytomegalovirus can cause a disseminated necrotizing, calcifying encephalitis. Infection may be acquired in the early postnatal period via transfusion of whole fresh blood or transcervically causing postnatal pneumonia and deafness.

**POS No.:**  3220

**CDC No.:**  771.210

**Sex Ratio:**  M1:F1

**Occurrence:**  1:3,500 live births.

**Risk of Recurrence for Patient's Sib:**  Secondary intrauterine infection is rare but is documented, both from maternal endogenous reactivation and reinfection.

**Risk of Recurrence for Patient's Child:**  Unknown.

**Age of Detectability:**  Although a variety of tests are available to aid in the diagnosis of congenital cytomegalovirus infection, isolation of the organism remains the most reliable method. For technical reasons, many laboratories rely on less specific tests. Characteristic inclusion cells are only seen in 30% of cases, and other types of cells may be easily confused with true cytomegalic cells. It should be remembered that although serum macroglobulins are usually elevated, infants with infection may have normal IgM levels. Enzyme-linked immunosorbent assay (ELISA) was positive in 73% of pregnant women with documented primary cytomegalovirus infections. The ELISA assay was positive in 69% of babies proven by culture to be congenitally infected as opposed to 5.7% of unaffected control newborn infants. At present, positive antibody tests are helpful, but false negatives do occur. In general, the strongest evidence of fetal cytomegalovirus syndrome is the presence of documented rising titers during the first half of pregnancy in the mother, clinical features consistent with cytomegalovirus infection in the infant, and positive CMV studies in the infant.

**Gene Mapping and Linkage:**  Unknown.

**Prevention:**  Avoid exposure to cytomegalovirus during pregnancy.

**Treatment:**  Unknown.

**Prognosis:**  Many infants with severe infection die during the newborn period as a result of cerebral involvement. Others may die with superimposed infections. Infants with severe infection in the newborn period have had seizures, are spastic, and are sometimes mentally retarded. Infants with mild disease at birth may develop within normal limits but are at risk for hearing loss.

**Detection of Carrier:**  Primary cytomegalovirus infection in the mother, who may be asymptomatic. There are documented endogenous recurrences causing affected sibs, suggesting reactivation of a previous infection in the mother. The presence of CMV antibodies does not guarantee that recurrence will not occur.

**Special Considerations:**  There are no clinical manefestations that can completely differentiate this in utero infection from many others. Cerebral calcifications may be periventricular but may also be flat, disseminated calcifications, as occurs in toxoplasmosis. Chorioretinitis occurs much less frequently than with toxoplasmosis; it is usually peripheral but may also be macular. Microcephaly without evidence of systemic involvement may be caused by cytomegalovirus.

**References:**

Huang ES, et al.: Molecular epidemiology of cytomegalovirus infections in women and their infants. New Engl J Med 1980; 303:958–962.
Stagno S, et al.: Congenital cytomegalovirus infection. The relative importance of primary and recurrent maternal infection. New Engl J Med 1982; 306:945–949.
Kumar ML, et al.: Postnatally acquired cytomegalovirus infections in infants of CMV-excreting mothers. J Pediatr 1984; 104:669–673.
Pass RF, et al.: Increased rate of cytomegalovirus infection among parents of children attending day-care centers. New Engl J Med 1986; 314:1414–1418.
Stagno S, et al.: Primary cytomegalovirus infection in pregnancy. Incidence, transmission to fetus, and clinical outcome. J Am Med Asso 1986; 256:1904–1908.
Boldogh I, et al.: Activation of proto-oncogenes: an immediate early event in human cytomegalovirus infection. Science 1990; 247:561–564.

BU007                                            **Bruce A. Buehler**
SH032                                       **Henry R. Shinefield**

## FETAL D-PENICILLAMINE SYNDROME                    2260

**Includes:**

> Chalastoderma with exposure to D-penicillamine
> Cupramin^, fetal effects of
> Cutis laxa with maternal D-penicillamine exposure
> D-penicillamine, fetal effects of
> Dupen^, fetal effects
> Immunodeficiency, thymic agenesis from exposure to D-penicillamine
> Penicillamine, fetal effects

**Excludes:**

> **Arthrogryposes** (0088)
> **Ehlers-Danlos syndrome** (0338)
> **Immunodeficiency, thymic agenesis** (0943)

**Major Diagnostic Criteria:**  In utero exposure to D-penicillamine in an infant with cutaneous hyperextensibility, joint hyperflexibility or contractures.

**Clinical Findings:**  D-penicillamine is an agent used for treating **Hepatolenticular degeneration**, heavy metal poisoning, **Cystinuria**, **Arthritis, rheumatoid**, and other collagen diseases. Six pregnancies with maternal D-penicillamine exposures have resulted in infants with generalized cutaneous hyperextensibility, and an "Ehlers-Danlos" like appearance. At least three of the **Cutis laxa** patients also had low-set ears and micrognathia. One of these had **Immunodeficiency, thymic agenesis** with interrupted aortic arch, hypoplastic left ventricle, and absent parathyroids. One of the infants with cutis laxa had joint hyperflexibility; another had joint contractures. Three additional infants without cutis laxa had brain injury, two had **Hydrocephaly**, and two had joint contractures, probably secondary to intrauterine paralysis. Brain injury and contractures have been described in experimental animal studies.

**Complications:**  Two cutis laxa cases died following abdominal surgery in infancy for undisclosed reasons. The case with

**Immunodeficiency, thymic agenesis** died from the cardio-vascular anomaly. Four of the cutis laxa patients had **Hernia, inguinal**. One of the cases with hydrocephalus, also had intraventricular hemorrhage and died at 18 hours of age. Another case with brain injury died from "crib death" at age four months.

**Associated Findings:**  None known.

**Etiology:**  All of the cases had maternal penicillamine exposure continued throughout pregnancy. The effects may be dose-related. The influence of disturbed heavy metal metabolism from the treatment or from the maternal condition being treated (**Hepatolenticular degeneration**) must be considered.

**Pathogenesis:**  Penicillamine interferes with condensation of both collagen and elastin crosslinks by compressing free lysine-derived aldehydes. Cutis laxa improved in two of the patients after birth. This suggests that exposure to penicillamine is needed to maintain the cutis laxa. Penicillamine acts in **Hepatolenticular degeneration** by chelation of excess free copper, and it also chelates other heavy metals, such as zinc, which may be necessary for normal fetal development. In laboratory studies, rats have been protected against the teratogenicity of copper administration by penicillamine chelation and/or copper replacement. This is not practical when penicillamine is used in the human treatment of **Hepatolenticular degeneration**, and may not be practical with other treatment procedures in humans.

**Sex Ratio:**  Presumably M1:F1.

**Occurrence:**  All ten known adverse outcomes are described above. At least 44 normal outcomes have been observed with penicillamine exposure throughout pregnancy. No abnormalities were observed with 38 additional maternal exposures discontinued in the first trimester.

**Risk of Recurrence for Patient's Sib:**  None without penicillamine exposure.

**Risk of Recurrence for Patient's Child:**  None without penicillamine exposure.

**Age of Detectability:**  All cases have been detected at birth.

**Gene Mapping and Linkage:**  N/A

**Prevention:**  Penicillamine should not be used for treating conditions other than **Hepatolenticular degeneration** when there is risk of pregnancy. However, because **Hepatolenticular degeneration** is a grave threat to the mother as well as the fetus, for which few alternative therapies are available, and because most outcomes have been favorable with treatment, penicillamine therapy may be continued in as low a dose as possible (1 gm or less daily).

Maternal exposures to penicillamine should be reported to the Food and Drug Administration's Division of Drug and Biological Product Experience, Rockville, Maryland.

**Treatment:**  Surgery for **Hernia, inguinal** and **Hydrocephaly**.

**Prognosis:**  Five of the ten cases were fatal in the perinatal period or infancy. Cutis laxa resolved in two infants by four months of age. The remaining infant with hydrocephaly improved after ventricular catheterization.

**Detection of Carrier:**  Unknown.

**References:**

Mjolnerod OK, et al.: Congenital connective tissue defect probably due to D-penicillamine treatment during pregnancy. Lancet 1977; 1:673–675.
Solomon L, et al.: Neonatal abnormalities associated with D-penicillamine during pregnancy. New Engl J Med 1977; 296:54–55.
Walshe JM: Pregnancy in Wilson's disease. Q J Med 1977; 46:73–83.
Harpey JP, et al.: Cutis laxis and low serum zinc after antenatal exposure to penicillamine. Lancet 1983; 2:858.
Keen CL, et al.: Teratogenic effects of D-penicillamine in rats: relation to copper deficiency. Drug-Nutrient Interactions 1983; 2:17–34.
Gal P, Ravenel SD: Congenital contractures and hydrocephalus associated with penicillamine, delalutin therapy and maternal surgery during gestation. J Clin Dysmorph 1984; 2:9–11.
Rosa FW: Teratogen update: Penicillamine. Teratogen 1986; 33:127–131. *

R0018                                            **Franz W. Rosa**

## FETAL DEVELOPMENTAL RETARDATION WITH MATERNAL HYPERTENSION                    2961

**Includes:**

Hypertension, maternal, and fetal developmental retardation

Intrauterine growth retardation, and maternal hypertension

Placental hypoperfusion fetal developmental retardation

Preeclampsia, and fetal developmental retardation

**Excludes:**

**Fetal angiotensin converting enzyme (ACE) inhibition renal failure** (2962)

Fetal developmental retardation from other causes

**Major Diagnostic Criteria:**   Intrauterine growth retardation with maternal blood pressure over 130/80 or a rise of 30 mm systolic or 15 mg diastolic during pregnancy, or other evidence of utero-placental arteral hypoperfusion. Related placental hypoperfusion can occur without hypertension.

**Clinical Findings:**   Maternal hypertension occurs in about seven percent of pregnancies. About three quarters of hypertensive pregnancies develop during the last trimester (preeclampsia) and a quarter are continuations of hypertension antedating pregnancy. Preeclampsia tends to be more frequent with the first pregnancy. Preexisting hypertension increases stepwise with succeding pregnancies. Pregnancy hypertension is the most common factor identified with adverse pregnancy outcome, associated with about a third of perinatal mortality and a third of low birth weight. Low birth weight is from premature delivery and/or low-weights for dates. The latter is associated with long term developmental retardation, directly proportional to the weight deficiency for dates. Head size tends to be reduced. This developmental retardation is similar to that with other extra-circulatory or respiratory causes of intrauterine growth retardation.

**Complications:**   Stillbirth is frequent in severe cases. Other neonatal complications largely relate to premature induction of delivery to manage the condition.

**Associated Findings: Ductus arteriosus, patent,** neutropenia, thrombocytopenia, and gastrointestinal hypomobility.

**Etiology:**   Hypertension with onset predating pregnancy is most often essential hypertension, renovascular or nephritic in origin. The causes of preeclampsia and essential hypertension are unknown. Dietary, obesity, low socio-economic status, familial and racial factors exist. Blacks are more susceptible to essential hypertension and preeclampsia. Some adverse fetal effects are attributed to antihypertensive medications, but controlled studies indicate that outcomes tend to be better with selected antihypertensives than without mediation.

**Pathogenesis:**   Imbalance of maternal homeostasis; reduced maternal plasma volume; decreased placental perfusion; uteroplacental arterial vasoconstriction, probably thromboxane related; failure of normal parturitional refractoriness to angiotensin, adrenergics, and perhaps other vasospastic influences; placental fibrin thrombi; infarctions and reduced placental size are associated. Inadequate fetal oxygen supply causes intrauterine respiratory distress and meconium aspiration. Intrauterine growth retardation includes retardation of brain development at a critical period, which is only partially reversible after birth. Uteroplacental vasoconstriction and placental fibrinization are caused by thromboxane A2 and inhibited by prostacyclin.

**Sex Ratio:**   Presumably M1:F1.

**Occurrence:**   About 70% of pregnancy hypertension develops during pregnancy and is otherwise known as toxemia, preeclampsia, or eclampsia. Thirty percent of maternal hypertension exists before pregnancy, usually as essential hypertension. In developed countries hypertensive disease of pregnancy is a leading cause of intrauterine growth retardation and its developmental sequelae. An additional proportion of pregnancies are likely to have similar placental perfusion problems without maternal hypertension.

**Risk of Recurrence for Patient's Sib:**   Unknown. Although there is an increased risk for recurrence of placental hypoperfusion intrauterine growth retardation, subsequent pregnancies are at less risk for preeclampsia than are first pregnancies.

**Risk of Recurrence for Patient's Child:**   Women from placental hypoperfusion fetal growth retardation pregnancies, with or without hypertension, are at increased risk of having these conditions in their own pregnancies.

**Age of Detectability:**   At birth or prenatally.

**Gene Mapping and Linkage:**   Unknown.

**Prevention:**   Early detection and management of increased blood pressure is one of the most important components of prenatal care. Avoidance of obesity prior to pregnancy is desirable. Dietary management of hypertension during pregnancy has not been effective. Adequate rest is desirable. Cesarean section when the infant has reached 1,500 g may be considered safer for the infant and the mother than continuing pregnancy in refractory maternal hypertension cases. The benefits of early induction of delivery to the mother and the infant must be balanced against the risks to the infant of early induction. Preliminary studies of low dose aspirin (60 mg/day, after the first trimester) show promise in preventing preeclampsia and related placental hypoperfusion fetal developmental retardation, and trials are currently expanding.

**Treatment:**   Antihypertensive therapy with methyldopa, beta-adrenergic blockers, and hydralazine has been demonstrated to decrease fetal injury from hypertension, even though signs of antihypertensive effects on the fetus are sometimes reported and the effects of the maternal and placental problems may not be completely alleviated. Use of thiazide diuretics has been controversial, and most studies do not show they are beneficial. Treatment with newer antihypertensive mechanisms, including calcium channel blockers and angiotensin conversion enzyme inhibitors, has not been fully evaluated. Perinatal renal failure has been observed with the latter (see **Fetal developmental retardation with maternal hypertension**). Beta-adrenergic blockers cause fetal bradacardia.

**Prognosis:**   Intrauterine growth retardation includes retardation of brain development at a critical period, which is only partially reversible after birth.

**Detection of Carrier:**   N/A

**Special Considerations:**   The importance of hypertensive complications of pregnancy must be kept in mind when evaluating the risk of antihypertensive agents. Large-scale, well-controlled clinical trials are highly desirable for antihypertensive agents and other means of managing this problem.

**References:**

Grant NF, et al.: A study of angiotensin II pressor response throughout primigravid pregnancy. J Clin Invest 1973; 52:2682–2689.

Lin C, et al.: Fetal outcome in hypertensive disorders of pregnancy. Am J Obstet Gynecol 1980; 142:225–260. *

Brazy JE, et al.: Neonatal manifestations of severe maternal hypertension occurring before the 36th week of pregnancy. J Pediatr 1982; 100:265–271.

Ferris TF: How should hypertension during pregnancy be managed? Med Clin North Am 1984; 68:491–503.

Rubin PC: Treatment of hypertension in pregnancy. Clin Obstet Gynecol 1986; 13:307–317.

Wallenberg HCS, et al.: Low-dose aspirin prevents pregnancy-induced hypertension and pre-eclampsia in angiotensis-sensitive primigravidae. Lancet 1986; I:1–3.

Lees KR, Rubin PC: Prescribing in pregnancy: treatment of cardiovascular diseases. Br Med J 1987; 294:359–360.

Benigni A, et al.: Effects of low-dose aspirin on fetal and maternal generation of thromboxane by platelets in women at risk for pregnancy-induced hypertension. New Engl J Med 1989; 321:357–362.

Schiff E, et al.: The use of aspirin to prevent pregnancy-induced hypertension and lower the ratio of thromboxane A prostacylin in relative high risk pregnancies. New Engl J Med 1989; 321:351–356.

R0018                                                          **Franz W. Rosa**

## FETAL DIETHYLSTILBESTROL (DES) EFFECTS     **2297**

**Includes:**
> Adenocarcinoma of the vagina, fetal DES effects
> DES, fetal effects
> Diethylstilbestrol, fetal effects
> Dienestrol, fetal effects
> Hexestrol, fetal effects
> Nonsteroidal synthetic estrogens, fetal effects
> Reproductive tract injuries in DES daughters
> Stilbestrol^, fetal effects

**Excludes:** Fetal effects of steroid estrogens or progesterones

**Major Diagnostic Criteria:** Structual and functional reproductive abnormalities, generally detected after the first decade of life, following maternal use of diethylstilbestrol (Stilbestrol^ or "DES") during pregnancy. DES was introduced in the 1940 to prevent fetal wastage, and its use was discontinued in the 1970s following documentation of its teratogenic effects. Two other non-steroidal estrogens, dienestrol and hexestrol, may have similar effects.

**Clinical Findings:** The most common abnormalities found in DES-exposed daughters are nonmalignant changes in the lower genital tract. Among patients studied, one-third to one-half showed vaginal epithelial changes (adenosis) and/or cervical eversion or ectropion. This means that the normal vaginal squamous epithelium has been replaced by müllerian-derived columnar or mucosal epithelium. Vaginal adenosis rarely occurs in women who have not had fetal DES exposure, and it is more likely to occur in those women who were exposed either early in gestation or to a high dose of DES. These vaginal epithelial changes are benign and resolve spontaneously over time secondary to squamous metaplasia.

Cervical abnormalities (collars, ridges, hoods, and protuberances) have been found in one-fourth to one-half of DES-exposed daughters. Structural abnormalities of the uterus and fallopian tubes have also been documented on hysterosalpingogram, including a "T-shaped" uterus. Kaufman et al. (1984) reported uterine cavity defects, intrauterine defects, or both in up to one-half of the women studied. These upper tract structural abnormalities occurred more often among the women who also had adenosis in the lower tract.

The rarest, yet most serious, sequelae occurring in DES-exposed daughters is clear cell adenocarcinoma of the vagina or cervix. Case-control studies in the early 1970s linked this rare and potentially fatal tumor to fetal DES exposure and heralded the concern about DES teratogenicity. Fortunately, this tumor appears to occur in less than 1:1,500 DES-exposed daughters.

A number of functional reproductive abnormalities have also been reported among DES-exposed daughters. These women have an approximately three- to four-fold increase in risk for having any "adverse pregnancy outcome," consisting primarily of premature delivery, ectopic pregnancy, or spontaneous abortion. Those women with structural uterine abnormalities documented on hysterosalpingogram have an even greater likelihood of having one of these abnormal pregnancy outcomes. Despite this, Barnes et al. (1980) found that 82% of DES-exposed daughters have gone on to have a term liveborn infant. Other functional abnormalities, such as infertility or menstrual irregularities, have been reported in some studies but not confirmed by others.

Less information is available on long-term sequelae in DES-exposed sons. Gill et al. (1976) reported that penile and testicular abnormalities, such as meatal stenosis, hypospadias, hypotrophic testes, and cryptorchidism have been found more commonly among DES-exposed sons compared with unexposed controls. A higher frequency of sperm abnormalities has also been found, including lower sperm count and motility, altered motility, and altered morphology. These findings are based on a relatively small number of men and cannot be considered generalizable or conclusive at the present time.

**Complications:** Among females, reproductive outcomes appear altered following fetal DES exposure. It remains unclear whether this is soley attributable to underlying structural abnormalities of the reproductive tract.

**Associated Findings:** Fetal DES exposure does not increase the risk for structural malformations outside of the reproductive tract.

**Etiology:** Fetal DES exposure, especially first trimester exposure, is considered responsible for the structural changes and very likely the functional changes described above. Although clear cell adenocarcinoma can occur in the absence of in utero DES exposure, this exposure is present in 63% of reported cases.

Precancerous vaginal adenosis occured in 73% of women exposed before the 9th week of gestation but in only 7% exposed after the 17th week. Total dose of DES received by cancer patients varied from 1.5 mg to 225 mg, but risk appears unrelated to dose.

**Pathogenesis:** Vaginal epithelial changes may occur on the basis of DES interfering with the normal migration of vaginal squamous cells up toward the cervix. Consequently, the original müllerian-derived columnar epithelium persists. A pathogenetic mechanism for the other abnormalities is not known.

**Sex Ratio:** Although equal numbers of male and female fetuses were exposed to DES in utero, most studies have focused on DES-exposed daughters. The greater number and variety of abnormalities found in the DES daughters may be attributed either to limited information on DES-exposed sons, or to selective teratogenic effect of DES on female fetuses.

**Occurrence:** DES was prescribed in two to three million pregnancies between the late 1940's and 1971, before its use was banned. Since all exposed individuals have not been studied or followed systematically since birth, the frequency of all DES effects is not known. Among the sample of DES daughters who have undergone examination, vaginal epithelial changes were found in approximately one-third to one-half, while clear cell adenocarcinoma of the vagina occurred in less than 1:1,500. Reproductive tract injuries in DES daughters leading to adverse pregnancy outcomes is more frequent.

**Risk of Recurrence for Patient's Sib:** Some investigators suggest that the increased risk for an unfavorable pregnancy outcome among DES-exposed daughters can be attributed to a genetic predisposition toward fetal wastage rather than the teratogenic effect of DES. In other words, a mother receiving DES during pregnancy was treated because she had a history of reproductive failures, and she might pass this tendency on to all her offspring. However, when comparing reproductive outcomes among DES-exposed and -unexposed sibs, the exposed sibs still had a higher frequency of adverse pregnancy outcomes, suggesting that DES rather than "genetics" was the contributing risk factor.

**Risk of Recurrence for Patient's Child:** See above.

**Age of Detectability:** Vaginal epithelial changes among DES-exposed daughters are presumably present at birth, but are generally not noted until the time of the first internal pelvic examination. Most cases of clear cell adenocarcinoma have been diagnosed by the time the affected DES-exposed daughter reached age 22 years, but the earliest case ever detected was at age seven years. Functional changes are not apparent until after puberty.

**Gene Mapping and Linkage:** N/A

**Prevention:** Avoidance of DES during pregnancy.

**Treatment:** Adenosis is benign and does not require therapy. Other sequelae, such as adenocarcinoma, are treated according to appropriate medical or surgical indications. DES-exposed daughters who achieve a pregnancy should be monitored closely, given the increased risk for an unfavorable pregnancy outcome.

**Prognosis:** Life span is unaffected except in those rare individuals who develop adenocarcinoma of the vagina. The quality of life is unaltered outside of the increased risk for unfavorable pregnancy outcomes.

**Detection of Carrier:** N/A

**Support Groups:**   NY; New Hyde Park; DES Action National

**References:**
Gill WB, et al.: Structural and functional abnormalities in the sex organs of male offspring of mothers treated with diethylstilbestrol (DES). J Reprod Med 1976; 16:147–153.
Barnes AB, et al.: Fertility and outcome of pregnancy in women exposed in utero to diethylstilbestrol. New Engl J Med 1980; 302:609–613.
Herbst AL: Diethylstilbestrol and other sex hormones during pregnancy. Obstet Gynecol 1981; 58:35S–40S.
Stillman RJ: In utero exposure to diethylstilbestrol: adverse effects on the reproductive tract and reproductive performance in male and female offspring. Am J Obstet Gynecol 1982; 142:905–921.
Kaufman RH, et al.: Upper genital tract abnormalities and pregnancy outcome on diethylstilbestrol-exposed progeny. Am J Obstet Gynecol 1984; 148:973–984.
McFarlane MJ, et al.: Diethylstilbestrol and clear cell vaginal carcinoma. Am J Med 1986; 81:855–863.

P0021                                                      **Barbara Pober**

---

## FETAL EFFECT FROM HEPATITIS B INFECTION          3008

**Includes:**

    Hepatitis B infection, perinatal transmission
    Perinatal transmission of hepatitis B infection

**Excludes:**   Hepatic diseases with negative HB antigenicity, other childhood

**Major Diagnostic Criteria:**   Persisting hepatitis B (HB) antigenicity in infants of mothers who are actively infected with HB virus. Most affected infants, like their mothers, remain asymptomatic carriers, but many develop hepatitis, cirrhosis, and hepatic cancer in childhood or later life.

**Clinical Findings:**   HB infection is indigenous in extensive areas of Africa and Asia due to parturitional or fetal transmission. Only about five percent of infants developing the infection are antigen positive at birth. However, this does not rule out prenatal infection, since the infection may be focal in hepatocytes and modified by antibody levels from the mother. Some cases infected with HB lose their positive viral status. Many who remain infected do not have clinical manifestations but become asymptomatic carriers. The most serious outcomes are chronic hepatitis, cirrhosis, and hepatic cancer.

**Complications:**   Individuals who remain infected may become asymptomatic carriers.

**Associated Findings:**   None known.

**Etiology:**   Infection by parturitional contamination or postnatal infection is more frequent than transplacental transmission. In one study transplacental infection was found in two of 30 abortuses of infected mothers. Prenatal infection is also assumed when an infected infant is born from a mother who has had acute hepatitis in early pregnancy but has become antigen negative before delivery. Positive cord blood may be due to parturitional contamination and does not reliably indicate fetal infection, since infant systemic blood may be negative. Postnatal conversion may not rule out prenatal transmission. Why perinatal HB is indigenous in some populations but rare in others is unclear. Concurrent factors in the etiology of hepatic cancer, such as diet and aflatoxin exposure, are suspected.

**Pathogenesis:**   HB DNA enters into somatic cell DNA sequences to cause progressive hepatic disease or to remain in a carrier state.

**Sex Ratio:**   Presumably M1:F1.

**Occurrence:**   An estimated 200,000,000 persons worldwide are actively infected with HB, mostly in areas of high indigenicity where perinatal transmission accounts for a high proportion. Approximately 1,000,000 persons are actively infected in the United States. The risk of perinatal transmission from HB surface antigen-positive mothers is from 20–50%, depending on maternal ethnic background and life-style. If the mother is HB e antigen positive at the time of delivery, there is a 90% risk that the infant

will be chronically infected. In a New Orleans study, active maternal infection was found in 0.6% of Caucasians and Blacks, but in 8.8% of Orientals (presumably many from Viet Nam). Although rare in Western countries, on a worldwide basis childhood hepatic cancer from HB is second only to lung cancer as an environmentally caused cancer. The familial transmission from generation to generation may resemble that of HTLV 1 leukemia. In the United States, maternal infection is often a result of sharing drug abuse needles (as is the case with AIDS).

**Risk of Recurrence for Patient's Sib:**   High for infection. The risks of hepatic disease are the same in all affected sibs.

**Risk of Recurrence for Patient's Child:**   Probably high for infection.

**Age of Detectability:**   Determination whether infection was prenatal cannot be made with precision. In infants developing the infection, HB antigen is demonstrable at birth in about five percent. In the remainder with perinatal infection, positive antigenicity develops in the first few months of life.

**Gene Mapping and Linkage:**   HVBS4 (hepatitis B virus integration site 4) has been provisionally mapped to 2.
HVBS8 (hepatitis B virus integration site 8) has been provisionally mapped to 17p12-p11.2.

**Prevention:**   Passive and active neonatal HB immunization has extensive potential for preventing perinatal infection and interrupting vertical transmission. After immunization of neonates of mothers with active infection, the proportion developing antigenicity is reduced from about 75 to 5%. Although the failure rate may be related to prenatal infection, the distinction between prenatal and postnatal infection is not a practical determinant in whether to provide neonatal immunization.

Primary prevention is through avoiding infections in fertile women. Sharing of drug abuse needles must be avoided.

**Treatment:**   Unknown.

**Prognosis:**   Loss of positive infant antigenicity is infrequent. Most remain asymptomatic carriers. Childhood HB hepatitis has a poor prognosis, with cirrhosis and cancer progressing to death.

**Detection of Carrier:**   Infectivity is most strongly indicated by actual detection of HB DNA virus (HBV DNA). HB e antigen appears to be a better indicator of the infectious state than does HB surface antigen. Although maternal HBV DNA assay may predict the efficacy of HB immunization, neonatal immunization appears warranted when any of these indicators are detected in the mother.

**References:**
Papaevangelou G, et al.: Transplacental transmission of hepatitis B by symptom free chronic carrier mothers. Lancet 1974; II:746–748.
World Health Organization: Prevention of liver cancer. WHO Tech Rep Ser 1983;691. *
Lee S-D, et al.: Prevention of maternal-infant hepatitis B virus transmission by immunization: the role of serum hepatitis B virus DNA. Hepatology 1986; 6:369–373.
London WT, O'Connell AT: Transplacental transmission of hepatitis B virus. Lancet 1986; I:1037–1038.
Chen D-S, et al.: A mass vaccination program in Taiwan against hepatitis B virus infection in infants of hepatitis B surface antigen-carrier mothers. J Am Med Asso 1987; 257:2597–2603.
Stevens CE, et al.: Yeast-recombinant hepatitis B vaccine: efficacy with hepatitis B immune globulin in prevention of perinatal hepatitis B virus transmission. J Am Med Asso 1987; 257:2612–2616. *
Summers PE, et al.: The pregnant hepatitis B carrier: evidence favoring comprehensive antepartum screening. Obstet Gynecol 1987; 69:701–704.
Immunization Practices Committee: Prevention of perinatal transmission of hepatitis B virus: prenatal screening of all pregnant women for hepatitis B surface antigen. MMWR 1988; 37:341–346.
Schalm SW, et al.: Prevention of hepatitis B infection in newborns through mass screening and delayed vaccination of all infants of mothers with hepatitis B surface antigen. Pediatrics 1989; 83:1041–1048.

WR003                                                      **Janet Wright**
R0018                                                    **Franz W. Rosa**

## FETAL EFFECTS FROM ANGEL DUST (PHENCYCLIDINE OR PCP)    2986

**Includes:**

Angel dust, fetal effects
PCP, fetal effects
Phencyclidine, fetal effects

**Excludes:**  Heroin/methadone prenatal exposure

**Major Diagnostic Criteria:**  A prenatal history of exposure to phencyclidine (PCP) or angel dust; positive urine toxicology screens in mother at time of delivery or in infant (usually within three days of delivery); irritability; tremors; darting eye movements; hypersensitivity to light and sounds during the neonatal period; smooth gross motor planning and movements are absent, and there especially is noted continued fine motor incoordination demonstrated by unsteady awkward movements of arms and hands in an attempt to obtain objects during the early childhood years.

**Clinical Findings:**  Infants exposed prenatally to PCP demonstrate increased periods of irritability, jitteriness, darting eye movements, and periodic episodes of indistinct staring. Seizures, diarrhea, and vomiting are not usually observed. Height, weight, and head circumference are not abnormal.

During the first year of life these infants have erratic sleep/wake cycles, hypertonia, and may have sporadic episodes of intense screaming with associated total extension of trunk and extremities. Tremors gradually subside and are replaced by unsteady movements of the body with hands held in a semiextended posture when approaching objects. Impairments of the sensory and proprioceptive systems seem apparent. Sucking and swallowing is usually not a problem. During the second year, the infant has continued difficulties in executing coordinated gross and fine motor movements, often bumping into walls and doors. The sleep/wake cycle improves; the irritability and screaming episodes lessen. Activity levels are high, and the infants often demonstrate poor interpersonal skills in spite of residing in consistent nurturing environments. The caretakers describe them as very independent.

By age 24 months, the majority of affected infants form words that are very indistinct. This improves over time; however, articulation and fine motor coordination remain abnormal even by age 60 months. Cognitive and language skills generally fall below average, into the mildly retarded range. Play skills are unusual in that some of these children demonstrate a lack of creative or pretend play and persist in a motor act in spite of failing, i.e., stacking blocks.

In spite of their grossly normal acquisition of motor milestones, affected infants appear to have continual problems with motor planning and articulation. Their overall intellectual and social development is also delayed.

**Complications:**  Increased activity levels and global developmental delays are present when affected individuals enter elementry school.

**Associated Findings:**  There is one reported case in which an infant exposed prenatally to PCP had dysmorphic feature consisting of wide-set eyes and triangular-shaped face with prominent forehead and a small chin. Unexplained wheezing (asthma-type episodes) has been reported.

**Etiology:**  Fetal exposure to phencyclidine or PCP.

**Pathogenesis:**  Impairment to CNS functioning appears to be global. May be related to interference of neurotransmitter systems.

**POS No.:**  3509

**Sex Ratio:**  M1:F1

**Occurrence:**  Undetermined. PCP is a commonly used drug in urban areas.

**Risk of Recurrence for Patient's Sib:**  Unknown.

**Risk of Recurrence for Patient's Child:**  Unknown.

**Age of Detectability:**  During the newborn period.

**Gene Mapping and Linkage:**  N/A

**Prevention:**  Abstinence from PCP use.

**Treatment:**  Medications to calm the irritable infant must be judiciously chosen. PCP acts as a CNS stimulant and depressant. Thus phenobarbitol, a CNS depressant, is contraindicated. Advise using no medications to calm infants. However, environmental interventions to calm infant are helpful: swaddling, pacifiers, and holding. During early childhood, enriched, structured, consistent settings are imperative.

**Prognosis:**  Children exposed to PCP are usually healthy and would be expected to have a normal life span. Intelligence is frequently impaired, usually within the low normal to mildly retarded range.

**Detection of Carrier:**  N/A

**References:**

Balster RL, Chait LD: The behavioral pharmacology of phencyclidine. Clin Toxicol 1976; 9:513.

Golden NL, et al.: Angel dust: possible effects on the fetus. Pediatrics 1980; 65:18–20.

Strauss AA, et al.: Neonatal manifestations of maternal phencyclidine (PCP) abuse. Pediatrics 1981; 68:550–552.

Chasnoff IJ, et al.: Phencyclidine: effects on the fetus and neonate. Dev Pharmacol Ther 1983; 6:404–408.

Howard J, et al.: The long-term effects on neurodevelopment in infants exposed prenatally to PCP. In: Clouet DH, ed: Phencyclidine: an update. National Institute on Drug Abuse Research Monograph No. 64, 1986:237–251.

H0055                                                    **Judith Howard**

## FETAL EFFECTS FROM LYME DISEASE    3212

**Includes:**

Bannwarth syndrome
Borrelia burgdorferi infection
Erythema chronicum migrans
Erythema migrans
Fetal effects of maternal Lyme disease
Lyme borreliosis
Lyme disease
Spirochete, fetal effects of maternal Lyme disease
Tick-borne meningopolyneuritis.

**Excludes:**

Congenital infections, other
**Palsy, late-onset facial, familial** (0378)

**Major Diagnostic Criteria:**  The clinical syndrome associated with congenital Lyme disease is not well defined. The diagnosis is confirmed by 1) *Borrelia burgdorferi*-specific IgM in cord blood or patient's sera immediately after delivery, 2) direct culture of *B. burgdorferi* from the placenta or the newborn, or 3) histological identification of *B. burgdorferi* in infant tissues using specific immunofluorescent techniques.

**Clinical Findings:**  Lyme disease is transmitted through the bite of the Ixodid tick. Maternal infection is manifested by the characteristic erythema chronicum migrans rash and associated flu-like symptoms 3 to 30 days after a tick bite. Erythema chronicum migrans (ECM) does not necessarily occur at the site of the tick bite. Satellite lesions may accompany ECM, which must be differentiated from local inflammation that occurs immediately after the tick bite. Some patients (10–30%) have no history of tick bite or ECM. In these patients, early Lyme disease is characterized by flu-like symptoms, including low-grade fever, chronic fatigue, headache, regional lymphadenopathy, myalgias, and arthralgias.

Although Lyme is often a mild, self-limited illness, approximately 80% of untreated patients will develop articular symptoms (migrating large-joint polyarthralgias) weeks to months after onset of the ECM. Symptoms may progress to include neurological involvement in 18% of patients (palsy, polyradiculoneuritis, peripheral paresthesias, and aseptic meningitis with lymphocytic pleocytosis) or cardiac involvement in 10% of patients (conduction defects, carditis). Months to years after the tick bite, approximately 60% of untreated patients will develop objective arthritic signs which may progress onto an established monoarticular arthritis resembling rheumatoid arthritis. Joints commonly affected include knees, shoulders, temporomandibular joints, ankles, hips, and elbows.

Pregnant women from endemic areas who have recent onset of an erythematous rash and arthritic symptoms should be evaluated for Lyme disease. The diagnosis of Lyme disease should not be based on serology alone. Current serological tests are not sensitive in early Lyme disease, and in highly endemic areas 5–10% of the population will be asymptomatically seropositive. In addition, it is also estimated that some five percent or more of patients with chronic Lyme disease may still test negative (Dattwyler et al, 1988). Therefore, diagnosis should rely primarily on compatible clinical history and examination.

**Complications:**  Two neonatal deaths have been reported, one infant having aortic coarctation, endocardial fibroelastosis, and persistent left vena cava draining into the coronary sinus. A second infant died of respiratory depression several days postpartum without major structural anomalies. Individual case reports of cortical blindness, syndactyly, intrauterine fetal death, prematurity and newborn rash have been reported.

**Associated Findings:**  None known.

**Etiology:**  Transplacental infection with *B. burgdorferi*.

**Pathogenesis:**  Unknown.

**Sex Ratio:**  Presumably M1:F1.

**Occurrence:**  Lyme disease is the most common tick-borne illness in the United States. In 1988, 4,572 cases of Lyme disease were reported to state health departments in the United States. The incidence of Lyme disease is dependent on the local prevalence of the tick vector. The Pacific coastal regions, upper Midwest, New England and Mid-Atlantic states, and parts of Europe are endemic for this disease. In heavily endemic areas (central Wisconsin, southern New York, eastern Massachusetts, northern New Jersey, and southern Connecticut), the annual incidence of Lyme disease can approach 1%. As many as 10% of individuals in these areas have serological evidence of past exposure to the spirochete. The risk of transplacental infection in a woman with active Lyme disease is currently unknown.

**Risk of Recurrence for Patient's Sib:**  Undetermined but presumed to be negligible if parent is successfully treated.

**Risk of Recurrence for Patient's Child:**  Unknown.

**Age of Detectability:**  Immediately postpartum using serological and pathological identification.

**Gene Mapping and Linkage:**  N/A

**Prevention:**  Pregnant mothers in endemic areas should be counseled to avoid tick bites through the use of insect repellents, long-legged pants, and daily personal inspection. Early tick removal probably decreases risk of infection. Pregnant women should be aware of the early symptoms of Lyme disease to allow prompt diagnosis and treatment. Antibiotic prophylaxis is untested and not recommended. No known direct person-to-person or animal-to-person transmission has been documented. Occurrence of Lyme disease in household members or in household pets, however, should alert the physician to the potential for exposure in the mother.

**Treatment:**  Successful therapy requires prolonged use of antibiotics with good tissue penetration. In pregnant women with early Lyme disease, penicillin 500 mg p.o. q.i.d. for three weeks is the current treatment of choice. In established or severe Lyme disease, intravenous antibiotic treatment (ceftriaxone, 2 g daily for 2 weeks, or penicillin G, 20 megaunits daily for 10 to 14 days) may be required. In newborns with suspected infection, effective antibiotic therapy has not been established. Adjusted dosage with intravenous ceftriaxone or penicillin is suggested at this time.

**Prognosis:**  Unknown.

**Detection of Carrier:**  N/A

**Special Considerations:**  The risk of adverse pregnancy outcome in mothers infected with *B. burgdorferi* is not known, and this syndrome is not recognized by all authorities. One retrospective study found that 5 of 19 infected mothers had adverse outcomes occurring during infection at all trimesters of pregnancy. No specific clinical syndrome was delineated. Two postpartum deaths associated with maternal infection have been reported. Unlike congenital syphilis, no inflammatory changes were noted at autopsy, and spirochetes were rarely found in histological specimens. In one case, the mother was inadequately treated with oral penicillin. In a small, prospective study of births from endemic and nonendemic areas, no increased rate of malformations or adverse outcomes was found in endemic patients.

Until additional studies clarify this issue, physicians should be aware of the possibility of congenital infection. Physicians should be alert for Lyme disease occurring during pregnancy, and pregnant women with suspected illness should be treated early. At this time, oral antibiotics (with the exception of the tetracyclines) can be used in uncomplicated Lyme disease, but patients should be followed closely for treatment failure. Physicians must balance the unknown risk of Lyme disease to the fetus with the known risk of adverse drug reactions to antibiotics.

Current serologic tests for diagnosing Lyme disease include a specific, whole-cell enzyme-linked immunoassay (ELISA), and a specific immunofluorescent assay (IFA). These tests are highly specific, but have low sensitivity. False-positives may be caused by infections with other spirochete pathogens, including *Treponema pallidum*. Unlike syphilis serology, Lyme disease serology can remain elevated after successful treatment. In endemic areas, high seropositivity rates can be expected in asymptomatic pregnant women who are presumably not at risk. Asymptomatic seropositivity may reflect past exposure and does not necessarily warrant treatment.

**Support Groups:**
CT; Farmington; Connecticut Pregnancy Exposure Information Service
CT; Tolland (P.O. Box 462); Lyme-Borreliosis Association

**References:**
Centers for Disease Control: Update: Lyme disease and cases occurring during pregnancy, United States. MMWR, 1985; 34:376–378.
Schlesinger PA, et al.: Maternal-fetal transmission of the Lyme disease spirochete, *Borrelia burgdorferi*. Ann Intern Med 1985; 103:67–68.
Malawista SE, Steere AC: Lyme disease: infectious in origin, rheumatic in expression. Adv Intern Med 1986; 31:147–166.
Markowitz LE, et al.: Lyme disease during pregnancy. J Am Med Asso 1986; 255:3394–3396.
Anonymous: Treatment of Lyme disease. Med Lett 1988; 30:65–66.
Dattwyler RJ, et al.: Seronegative Lyme disease: dissociation of specific T- and B-lymphocyte responses to *Borrelia burgdorferi*. New Engl J Med 1988; 319:1441–1446.
Weber K, et al. *Borrelia burgdorferi* in a newborn despite oral penicillin for Lyme Borreliosis during pregnancy. Pediatr Infect Dis J 1988; 7:286–289.
Lyme disease - United States, 1987 and 1988. MMWR 1989; 38:668–672.
Markby DP: Lyme disease facial palsy: differentiation from Bell's palsy. Br Med J 1989; 299:605–606.
Steere AC: Lyme disease. New Engl J Med 1989; 321:586–596.

M0049                                    **Patrick S. Moore**

---

**FETAL EFFECTS FROM MATERNAL CARBON MONOXIDE EXPOSURE**                    **2510**

**Includes:**
 Carbon monoxide, fetal effects of
 Fetal carbon monoxide syndrome

**Excludes:**
 **Microcephaly** (0659)
 Tetraplegia

**Major Diagnostic Criteria:**  CNS and/or musculoskeletal anomalies in the infant of a woman exposed to carbon monoxide (CO) in pregnancy.

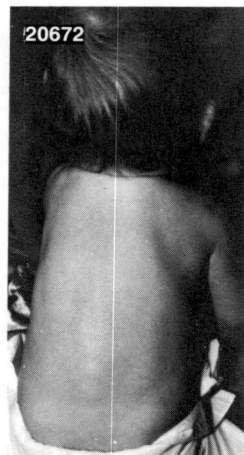

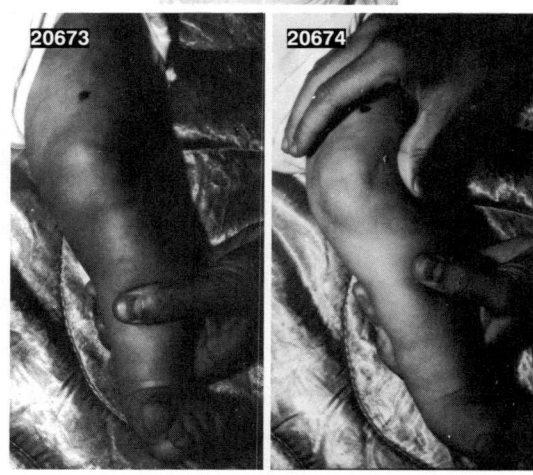

**2510-20672:** Fetal carbon monoxide syndrome; note anteriorly rotated shoulders with reduced muscle mass. **20673-74:** Note loose ligaments in the knee at 8 months of age; the lower limb deviates laterally approximately 20 degrees.

---

**Clinical Findings:** The literature yields five cases of first CO trimester intoxication with coma and subsequent survival of the fetus. Musculoskeletal abnormalities, as well as encephalopathy, are associated with exposure at this time in development. Most of the cases are not well documented, and although all followed maternal first-trimester coma, the reports are not sufficient to exclude other possible effects such as maternal medication. Three of the reports are from Europe during the period of **Fetal thalidomide syndrome**, and a 1957 case with severe limb deformities appears compatible with that diagnosis. Another case may be compatible with FFU syndrome (see **Fibula, congenital absence of**), another with **Osteogenesis imperfecta**, and a fourth case with **Chromosome 21, trisomy 21**.

1) *The case of Zourbas, 1947*: maternal coma for nine hours from stove gas, at the end of the third month of gestation, resulted in an infant with micrognathia and glossoptosis, and encephalopathy characterized by difficulty swallowing, and inability to suck, necessitating spoon feeding; at eight months, just prior to death from aspiration pneumonia, the infant was in a vegetative state, markedly hypertonic save for markedly hypotonic neck musculature. No autopsy was performed.

2) *The case of Lombard, 1956*: maternal coma for 1 1/2 hours from "butane" gas at two months, delivery at seven months of an infant with "mongolism" who died at three days of age. Autopsy revealed sclerosis of the pancreas.

3) *The case of Gere and Szekeres, 1955, reported by Ingalls*: "severe CO poisoning", maternal effect unspecified, at 5–7 weeks, seen at age 10 years: normal intellect, with severe anomalies of the extremities; the right arm was normal, the left was hemimelic, with a short cone-shaped humerus and no digital remnants; the left femur was absent, the right femur short and deformed with immobile flexion contractures at the hip and knee; the tibias were bowed, and fibulae and lateral toes were absent.

4) *The case of Bette, 1957*: maternal coma for two hours at nine weeks gestation, resulting in an infant with equinovarus deformity, upper limb reduction deformities with contractures at the elbows and fingers, subluxed hips, but without signs of encephalopathy.

5) *The case of Corneli, 1955, described by Beaudoing*: maternal intoxication, extent not described, in the first month, resulting in an infant with bilateral foot deformation, hip dysplasia, and abnormal bone fragility.

There are two cases of first trimester exposure not causing coma:

*The case of Copel et al, 1982*: maternal exposure overnight in a room heated with a defective coal furnace, with malaise and headache, alerted because of the toxic condition of her children, at eight weeks pregnancy, carboxyhemoglobin (COHb) of 24.5% one hour after exposure; infant with normal developmental milestones at six months of age.

*Personal case - Z.H.*: mother worked in an automotive garage with no ventilation of exhaust fumes; during the first trimester (winter) it was heated with a homemade LP gas heater. She recalled in her third month a race car running "full out", filling the garage with fumes; she had to leave the garage frequently to avoid fumes, and had frequent headaches. At birth, the infant was hypotonic in all four extremities and neck, and had hypoactive deep tendon reflexes, and wasting of muscle groups, particularly the proximal of all extremities; he had adducted shoulders, flexion contractures of 30° in the elbows and knees, and 45° at the hips. Both feet had passively correctable calcaneovalgus deformities. Ligament laxity was noted, particularly the left knee. The contractures were mostly resolved by three months of age. He was not comfortable in the prone position, and spent infancy supine or on his side. At eight months of age he had micrognathia, thickened lateral palatine ridges, internally rotated shoulders with decrease scapular muscle mass, and an unstable right knee; the lower leg could be laterally deviated 20 degrees. The elbows were mildly unstable, with a lateral deviation of 5–10 degrees possible. At age 5 he is reportedly of normal intellect, and knock-kneed.

There are five cases of survival of the fetus after maternal CO intoxication in the second trimester: all cases resulted from maternal coma; one was premature; all infants had encephalopathy, with one neonatal death, and three of the remaining survivors in a vegetative state, the eldest reported at eight years as profoundly retarded; spastic extremities were noted in three, athetosis in one, microcephaly in one, and profound hypotonic neck musculature in one. Autopsy findings in the case of neonatal death revealed massive parenchymal destruction of the brain with symmetrical temporal microgyria; in the case of spastic athetosis, abnormalities included damage of the globus pallidus, striatum, red zone of the substantia nigra, and lateral nucleus of thalamus, with diffuse loss of neurons and polymicrogyria affecting frontal and anterior central regions of the cortex in the case with spastic athetosis.

Seven third trimester cases resulted in three neonatal deaths, profound mental retardation in three, ventriculomegaly in three, microcephaly in two, athetosis in two, convulsions in two, and normal intellect but with spastic athetoid cerebral palsy in an individual who died at age 81 years. The findings in six autopsies include marked injury to the basal ganglia in five cases, areas of cortical destruction in four; and extensive damage to the centrum semiovale in four.

**Complications:** Those associated with static encephalopathy and **Cerebral palsy**.

**Associated Findings:** None known.

**Etiology:** Evidence is compelling that the cause of CO toxicity is not merely hypoxia secondary to reduction of the oxygen carrying capacity of hemoglobin expressed as the percentage of Hb combined with CO. CO is a direct metabolic poison, through competitive inhibition with O2 of cytochrome oxidase in the mitochondria, the site of cellular respiration. Low levels of CO may exert toxic effects even in the absence of hypoxic effects.

**Pathogenesis:** CO is tasteless, odorless, colorless, non-irritating, and may not be associated with smoke; many deaths are reported yearly from the indoor use of sterno and charcoal fires, as well as defective furnace flues. The affinity of CO for adult hemoglobin (Hb) is on the average 240 times that of oxygen. Air containing 0.1% CO (1000 ppm) results in 50% COHb at equilibrium. CO first dissolves in plasma prior to combining with Hb, and it is the dissolved component which poisons cellular respiration. At high concentrations, lethal levels may be obtained in minutes. The victim may have no warning; there is no sense of dyspnea, since CO does not stimulate the respiratory center as CO2 does; to a person in a fire, an obviously emotionally charged environment, the first symptoms may be confusion, loss of consciousness or fatal dysrhythmia - hence the reason why people with opportunity do not escape fires - and why no one should ever enter a burning structure without a self-contained breathing apparatus.

Tissues with the highest metabolic rates are poisoned first: the basal ganglia, other CNS tissue, and the heart (the bundle of His has an extremely high metabolic rate - hence the major morbidity from dysrhythmias). Myoglobin is three times more avid for CO than hemoglobin.

In pregnancy, the mother may die of acute poisoning (within minutes) with the fetus expiring from anoxia with little detectable fetal COHb at necropsy; fetal hemoglobin is even more avid for CO than adult hemoglobin, but the equilibration time between maternal and fetal circulation is 3–5 hours. Chronic maternal exposure results in near-equivalent fetal COHb levels. Non-fatal poisonings may result in both toxic and anoxic effects.

In adults and children, the sequelae after severe poisoning are protean. After apparent recovery from exposure, death from demyelinization may occur, as well as basal ganglia syndromes, psychoses, hyperactivity, dysgraphia, vision impairment, agnosias, apraxias, seizures and personality change. Autopsy findings after acute intoxication typically include necrosis of the basal ganglia. Rhabdomyolysis is a rare sequela of CO poisoning in the adult (and may occur even in the absence of coma), as is myocarditis. Hyperglycemia is a common sequela, of limited duration, from presumed pancreatic toxicity; it is notable that one first trimester exposure resulted in an infant with pancreatic sclerosis.

A significant increase of COHb occurs after exposure to methylene chloride, a solvent found in furniture strippers and household aerosols.

**Sex Ratio:** M1:F1

**Occurrence:** The incidence of CO poisoning was estimated as 15.3:100,000 in France in 1979, with an estimated misdiagnosis of 30% of cases when first seen. A 1973 study estimated that 10,000 Americans required treatment for CO poisoning each year, exclusive of suicides, which would approximate an incidence of 5:100,000. The fire fatality rate was estimated at 12,000 for 1982; more than 70% of these deaths were caused by CO poisoning rather than burns, cyanide, or respiratory effects of smoke inhalation. There are little data available for estimating the actual rate of non-fatal CO exposure; morbidity may be significant. No data are available on the rate of exposure of pregnant women.

**Risk of Recurrence for Patient's Sib:** Negligible in the absence of additional CO exposure.

**Risk of Recurrence for Patient's Child:** Negligible in the absence of CO exposure.

**Age of Detectability:** Fetal ultrasonography may detect signs of severe effects such as cortical atrophy and intrauterine growth retardation, as well as more subtle effects, such as severe limitation of extension of the extremities. Abnormalities such as **Microcephaly** would become evident only with growth of the fetus, presumed normal at the time of the exposure.

**Gene Mapping and Linkage:** N/A

**Prevention:** The diagnosis, and hence definitive treatment, of acute CO poisoning depends on both public and physician awareness of its possibility. Anyone escaping from a burning structure should be presumed to have significant carbon monoxide poisoning, and be provided 100% oxygen if available, until appropriate diagnostic tests prove otherwise. Clinically, the first symptom of severe poisoning may be confusion or fatal cardiac dysrhythmia; because blood CO2 levels initially are normal, there is no dyspnea or hyperpnea; these effects explain why people with opportunity do not escape fires, and why many with significant poisoning may never receive treatment. The half-life of COHb is 5–6 hr. in room air, 1 1/2 hr. in 100% 02, and 23 minutes or less in hyperbaric oxygen at 2–2.5 atmospheres; the last is the treatment of choice for significant poisoning.

**Treatment:** Physical and orthopedic therapy as required.

**Prognosis:** Dependent on the extent of CNS damage.

**Detection of Carrier:** N/A

**Special Considerations:** The carboxyhemoglobin levels of inhaling cigarette smokers generally are in the range of 4–10%, the highest recorded at 20%. The concentration of CO in cigarette smoke is approximately the same as non-catalyzed automobile exhaust (20,000–60,000 ppm vs 30,000–80,000 ppm), and a smoke-filled room approximates that of a major traffic interchange (25–100 ppm vs 50–100 ppm). 24 hours exposure to 50 ppm of CO results in blood COHb of 8%. It is possible that the adverse affects associated with cigarette smoking in pregnancy are due to the effects of carbon monoxide rather than nicotine and other substances present in cigarette smoke. The average decrease in weight of the neonate of a smoking mother is 200 gm. (the average decrease of weight of infants born during the Dutch famine in the winter of 1944 was 240 gm.)

Animal models have demonstrated embryotoxic, but not teratogenic effects in the mouse and rat; in the rabbit, 9–18% COHb decreased weight and markedly increased stillbirths and neonatal deaths, with a significant number born without a limb. This teratogenic effect was not confirmed in subsequent rabbit experiments. In the guinea pig, Corneli (1955) reported paralysis of the posterior trunk and malformations of posterior paws.

**References:**
Corneli F: Contributo sperimentale all'azione teratogenica dell'ossido di carbonio en mammiferi. Ortop e Traumatol 1955; 23:261.
Longo LD: Carbon monoxide in the pregnant mother and fetus and its exchange across the placenta. Ann NY Acad Sci 1970; 174:313–341. *
Myers RAM, et al.: Carbon monoxide poisoning: the injury and its treatment. JACEP 1979; 479–484. *
Werler MM, et al.: Smoking and pregnancy. Teratol 1985; 32:473–481.

R0003                                                  **Richard M. Roberts**

## FETAL EFFECTS FROM MATERNAL COCAINE ABUSE          2603

**Includes:** Cocaine, fetal effects of

**Excludes:**
**Fetal alcohol syndrome** (0379)
Fetal effects of other stimulants, narcotics and alcohol

**Major Diagnostic Criteria:** Documentation of maternal abuse of cocaine during gestation; demonstration of byproducts of cocaine in the urine of the newborn infant who manifests clinical features of fetal cocaine exposure.

**Clinical Findings:** Clinical manifestations of fetal cocaine exposure depend on the gestational age of the fetus, the dose and the route of administration, and the chronicity of cocaine abuse. Human fetuses exposed to cocaine in the first trimester have been reported by several investigators to have major malformations. Four types of abnormalities have been identified; cranio-facial, central nervous system, cardiac, and genito-urinary system.

In 50 cases of cocaine abusing mothers, one stillborn with **Anencephaly**, one offspring with **Encephalocele**, one with parietal bone defect, and two infants with congenital heart disease were identified (Bingol et al 1987). Also, nine cases of genitourinary malformation with hydrops and **Prune-belly syndrome** have been reported (Chasnoff, 1985; Bingol, 1987). Exposure to cocaine during pregnancy may produce growth retardation resulting in small-for-gestational-age as well as premature infants.

Increased fetal wastage, such as spontaneous abortions and stillbirths associated with abruptio placentae, have been reported. Neonatally, infants may manifest seizures and signs of intracranial hemorrhage. Withdrawal symptoms from cocaine, e.g. tremulousness and hyperexcitability, are seen in some newborns; although more severe symptoms may be associated with maternal polydrug use or alcohol abuse. Long term effects on growth, fine motor or mental development, and behavior are unknown.

**Complications:** Unknown.

**Associated Findings:** None known.

**Etiology:** Single or multiple doses of cocaine abuse during pregnancy, in form of snuffing of cocaine hydrochloride, intravenous administration, or inhalation of free-base cocaine any time during gestation. Other possibilities include substances which are used for adulteration of cocaine, e.g., lidocaine, lactose, mannitol, baking soda, and the like.

**Pathogenesis:** Cocaine is known to cause an immediate but transient rise in blood pressure and vasoconstriction of placental vessels. These may contribute to abruptio placentae and to an interruption of the blood supply to the various fetal tissues, causing deformation or disruption of morphogenesis. Maternal or fetal cardiac arrhythmias caused by cocaine may also be responsible for hypoxia of the fetal tissues, as well as hydrops. Vasoconstriction at the uteroplacental complex coupled with the anorexic effect of cocaine might explain the growth retardation observed in experimental animals and in the offspring of cocaine-abusing mothers. Cocaine also causes seizures even after a single administration by lowering the seizure threshold and by adrenergic stimulation. Certain individuals who are genetically deficient in liver and plasma cholinesterases, which metabolize cocaine to its byproducts, may be especially sensitive to its effects.

**Sex Ratio:** M1:F1

**Occurrence:** In a sample group of 1,226 urban, young, low-income Black and Hispanics in Boston, Zuckerman (1989) reported 18% of pregnant women used cocaine on the basis of interview responses, urine assay, or both. Twenty-four percent of the women who used cocaine during their pregnancy as determined by urine assay denied any use. These women would have been misclassified if urine assay had not been performed.

**Risk of Recurrence for Patient's Sib:** Undetermined but presumed linked to maternal cocaine abuse.

**Risk of Recurrence for Patient's Child:** Undetermined but presumed linked to maternal cocaine abuse.

**Age of Detectability:** Prenatally by ultrasonography to detect fetal malformations, fetal ascites, and, in some cases, placental abruption. At birth by urine toxicology and physical examination.

**Gene Mapping and Linkage:** N/A

**Prevention:** Education and counseling of women of reproductive age; avoidance of cocaine in any form during pregnancy. Pregnant women who abuse cocaine should be informed of the serious consequences of the drug, and should be counseled.

**Treatment:** Abruptio placentae may require an emergency cesarean. Arrhythmias may be treated with antiarrhythmic drugs. Seizure disorder may require anticonvulsants. Surgical correction of major defects may be indicated.

**Prognosis:** Life span is reduced in some cases of fetal ascites and major malformations.

**Detection of Carrier:** Unknown.

**Special Considerations:** Animal experiments have shown that cocaine hydrochloride is teratogenic, when administered in nontoxic doses, to gravid CF-1 mice on days 7–12 of gestation. Eye defects occurred when administered during early gestation. Skeletal defects occurred when the drug was administered later in gestation (Mahalik, 1980). In rats, Fantel (1982) reported reduction

in maternal and fetal weight, increased resorption frequency, and fetal edema, but no teratogenicity at high doses. Swiss-Webster mice showed decreased fetal weight but no congenital malformations.

**References:**
Mahalik MP, et al.: Teratogenic potential of cocaine hydrochloride in CF-1 mice. J Pharm Sci 1980; 69:703–706.
Fantel AG, Macphail BJ: The teratogenicity of cocaine. Teratology 1982; 26:17–19.
Acker D, et al.: Abruptio placentae associated with cocaine use. Am J Obstet Gynecol 1983; 146:220–221.
Chasnoff J, et al.: Cocaine use in pregnancy. New Engl J Med 1985; 313:666–669.
Cregler LL, Mark H: Medical complications of cocaine abuse. New Engl J Med 1986; 315:1495–1500.
Bingol N, et al.: Teratogenicity of cocaine in humans. Pediatrics 1987; 110:93–96.
Chavez GF, et al.: Maternal cocaine use during early pregnancy as a risk factor for congenital urogenital anomalies. J Am Med Asso 1989; 262:795–798.
Graham K, et al.: Determination of gestational cocaine exposure by hair analysis. J Am Med Asso 1989; 262:3328–3330.
Hadeed AJ, Siegel SR: Maternal cocaine use during pregnancy: effect on the newborn infant. Pediatrics 1989; 84:205–210.
Shepard TH: Catalog of teratogenic agents, ed 6. Baltimore: Johns Hopkins University Press, 1989.
Zuckerman B, et al.: Effects of maternal marijuana and cocaine use on fetal growth. New Engl J Med 1989; 320:762–768.

BI012                                                   **Nesrin Bingol**
FU008                                               **Magdalena Fuchs**

## FETAL EFFECTS FROM MATERNAL DIABETES          2498

**Includes:**
  Diabetes, fetal effects from maternal
  Infant of diabetic mother (IDM)
  Infant of gestational diabetic mother (IGDM)
  Pedersen hypothesis

**Excludes:**
  **Caudal regression syndrome** (3211)
  Large for date infants without maternal or gestational diabetes

**Major Diagnostic Criteria:** Newborn infants of both insulin dependent and gestational diabetic mothers.

**Clinical Findings:** Often, infants of diabetic mothers (IDMs) and infants of gestational diabetic mothers (IGDMs) are large for dates with obese, plethoric, and cushingoid appearance and visceromegaly (enlarged heart, liver, spleen, kidneys, and umbilical cord). The head may appear disproportionately small because the brain size does not increase relative to body size or gestational age. Excessive body weight is a result of increased body fat; determinations of fat cell size, skin fold thickness and body composition indicate that an IDM can have up to twice as much fat as an infant of a non-diabetic mother. The excessive fat is laid down predominantly during the third trimester; IDMs delivered earlier are rarely macrosomic.

Although less pathognomonic, IDMs, but not IGDMs, are, on the other hand, often small for dates. This is especially likely in long-standing maternal diabetes with severe vascular problems, including hypertension.

Most IDMs (40–60%) and 80% of IGDMs have an uneventful neonatal period. The frequency of neonatal problems (metabolic, hematologic, anatomic) is much higher in IDMs than IGDMs.

Metabolic and hematologic problems of IDMs include hypoglycemia, hypocalcemia, hypomagnesemia, hyperbilirubinemia, polycythemia, and hyperuricemia. Anatomic problems include a high incidence of Respiratory Distress Syndrome, congenital malformations and vascular thrombosis. Also, transient anomalies such as small left colon, transient hypertrophic subaortic stenosis, and transient hematuria, may be encountered.

The prevalence of congenital malformations among insulin-dependent IDMs is two- to threefold higher compared with nondiabetics, and closely related to the severity of the mother's diabetes and the control of maternal diabetes. The frequency of malformations among offspring has been reported to be 4.4% in White classes B and C; 9.7% in class D; and 16.7% in class F; with an overall prevalence of 6.4% in all diabetic offspring compared with 2% in the general population. No statistically significant difference was observed between the frequency of anomalies among IGDMs and offspring of nondiabetics.

There is no pathognomonic congenital malformation syndrome for IDMs. The spectrum of congenital malformations in diabetic embryopathy is large, highly variable and includes:

*Central Nervous System*: neural tube defects, **Anencephaly, Microcephaly,** and **Hydrocephaly.**

*Cardiovascular*: **Heart, transposition of great vessels, Ventricular septal defect, Aorta, coarctation, Atrial septal defects,** single umbilical artery; and hypertrophic subaortic stenosis (transient).

*Renal*: hydronephrosis, renal agenesis, ureteral duplication, multicystic dysplasia.

*Gastrointestinal*: duodenal atresia, anorectal atresia, and small left colon (transient).

*Genital*: hypospadias, maldescended testis, hypoplastic genitalia, and ovarian cysts.

*Skeletal*: **Caudal regression syndrome,** ribs and vertebral anomalies.

*Facial*: **Cleft lip, Cleft palate.** *Ear*: aplasia, atresia, low-set ears, large ears, and hairy ears. *Eyes*: cataracts, iris coloboma, and optic nerve hypoplasia.

**Complications:** *Vascular thrombosis*: polycythemia and hyperviscosity in IDMs and IGDMs are the main contributing factor of vascular thrombosis. Renal vein thrombosis, cerebral, retinal, coronal, pulmonary, adrenal, mesenterial and peripheral (limbs) thrombosis may also appear.

*Birth injury*: the presence of an excessive-size fetus in a mother with a small-to-normal size pelvis may result in prolonged labor, dystocia, or birth injury; particularly when a vaginal delivery is attempted. Fractures (clavicle, ribs, humerus), nerve palsy (facial, brachial, phrenic) and hemorrhage (intracranial, etc.) may be encountered.

*Late complications*: diabetes. There is greater risk for the offspring of diabetic mother to develop diabetes mellitus later in life.

*Obesity*: IDMs who are large for gestational age at birth, at age seven years and also at age 14–17 years, are found to be obese, with a weight/height ratio exceeding 1.2. In contrast, IDMs appropriate for gestational age at birth did not show a comparable tendency to obesity.

*Neuropsychologic impairment*: Because of the lack of appropriate prospective studies, the effect of a diabetic pregnancy on an offspring's neuropsychologic outcome is still not definitively known. Retrospective studies revealed conflicting results, but suggest that rather than diabetes per se, unfavorable antepartum events, together with perinatal complications, are the principal determinants of poor long-term outcome for IDMs.

**Associated Findings:** Occipital encephalocele, holoprosencephaly, **Heart, tetralogy of Fallot,** hypoplastic left heart, single ventricle, anomalous pulmonary venous return, **Pulmonary valve, stenosis, Mitral valve atresia,** gastrointestinal malrotation, volvulus, omphalocele, gastroschisis, **Polydactyly, Syndactyly,** clinodactyly, choanal atresia, absence depressor anguli oris muscle, fused orbits, and situs inversus.

Increased incidence of spontaneous abortions, stillbirths and preterm deliveries,

**Etiology:** IDMs survive an unusual genetic and environmental intrauterine milieu. The pregnancy has a diabetogenic effect, which becomes apparent in the second trimester by increasing demands for insulin, and a gradually increasing risk of ketoacidosis throughout the remainder of the pregnancy. This is the result of placental production of hormones that antagonize the actions of insulin (HPL, estrogens, progesterone, cortisol). Both experimental and clinical studies suggest that malformations in IDMs arise from an early teratogenic insult in a genetically predisposed individual. On the other hand, diabetes mellitus has

several effects on pregnancy: excessive ponderal gain, hydramnios, preeclampsia, and ultrastructural placental changes. Altered maternal metabolism is believed to be the main cause of the different fetal and neonatal problems of IDMs.

**Pathogenesis:** No single, unifying pathogenic mechanism has been clearly defined to explain the diverse problems observed in IDMs. The most accepted hypothesis is the maternal hyperglycemia-fetal hyperinsulinism theory. Diabetic women, even those under close observation, experience higher blood glucose concentrations during periods of the diurnal cycle than do nondiabetic women. This episodic maternal hyperglycemia is the major predisposing factor to an altered fetal state, leading ultimately to the various clinical manifestations of the IDM. Intermittent maternal hyperglycemia results in fetal hyperglycemia because of the direct relationship between the maternal and fetal blood glucose concentrations. Fetal hyperglycemia stimulates release of insulin by fetal islet cells, giving rise to persistent hyperinsulinism in the fetus.

Prior to age seven weeks, the alterations in the fetal environment are thought to be teratogenic, and to contribute to the increased incidence of congenital malformations in IDMs.

Later in pregnancy, the altered milieu promotes aberrant fetal physiology, which may explain many of clinical signs of IDMs. Fetal hyperinsulinism has multiple effects on the fetus: it promotes glucose uptake in a variety of organs and tissues, including adipose tissue, leading to macrosomia, fetal hypoglycemia, increased risk for neonatal hypoglycemia, and it may have an inhibitory effect on the normal enzyme-inducing action of cortisol on the fetal pneumocytes production of surfactant. This may delay normal fetal lung maturation and increase the risk of RDS.

The *Pedersen hypothesis* (maternal hyperglycemia-fetal hyperinsulinism) has been extended by Freinkel et al (1984, 1985), who have examined the role of other nutrients that provide a substrate mixture for the fetus. There are many findings which support the heterogeneity of the diabetic state and suggest that control of both glucose and fetal growth is multifactorial. Freinkel et al conclude that mixed nutrients (e.g., amino acids, free fatty acids) other than glucose are important in fetal/neonatal metabolic control, as well as in "fuel-mediated" teratogenesis.

**POS No.:** 4499

**Sex Ratio:** M1:F1

**Occurrence:** Some 0.3% of pregnancies are IDM. A similar proportion are labeled IGDM, but this varies with the criteria used. Even milder degrees of maternal hyperglycemia which occur in as much as 20% of pregnancies appear to be related to increased perinatal mortality and morbidity; but like IGDM, not to teratologic factors. Congenital malformations are three times more frequent in IDM than in nondiabetic outcomes, and now represent more than 40% of IDM perinatal deaths (as deaths from other causes have been reduced by better management).

**Risk of Recurrence for Patient's Sib:** Dependent on optimal metabolic control of the mother prior to conception and during pregnancy.

**Risk of Recurrence for Patient's Child:** Not increased unless IDM or IGDM.

**Age of Detectability:** At birth or possibly through prenatal diagnosis.

**Gene Mapping and Linkage:** Unknown.

**Prevention:** Hyperglycemia and hyperketonemia may both singly, and in combination, be of teratological significance. The routine screening of all diabetic pregnancies with first trimester glycosylated hemoglobin, early second trimester alpha-fetoprotein determination, along with fetal ultrasonography for a general anatomic survey, are useful methods for prenatal diagnosis of congenital malformations. Clinical and laboratory data also suggest that excellent prepregnant glycemic control will provide the intrauterine milieu necessary for normal embryogenesis and, therefore, possible prevention of congenital malformations in IDMs.

Although it is still uncertain whether glycemic control will prevent congenital malformations, careful glycemic control in later pregnancy will improve perinatal mortality and morbidity. Even management of mild maternal hyperglycemia by diet has an important effect.

Selective caesarian section can prevent perinatal problems from associated preeclampsia, or dystocia with exceptionally large babies.

**Treatment:** Intensive metabolic control of diabetes prior to conception and throughout pregnancy is extremely important to minimize maternal and fetal morbidity and mortality. Conception can be attempted as soon as prepregnancy evaluation is complete and a very good glycemic control is achieved. Maintenance of a hemoglobin A1c value of 7% or below, and of a mean blood glucose level of 84 mg/dl/day during pregnancy should be considered very good overall control. Monitoring at one or two week intervals throughout the pregnancy should include evaluation of maternal ophthalmologic, renal, neurologic, and cardiovascular functions, together with prevention of preeclampsia, ketoacidosis, and urinary tract infections, and maintenance of fetal well-being. Ultrasonography is useful in following fetal development. The timing and route of delivery should be carefully established to prevent asphyxia and injuries at birth.

Regardless of their size and maturity, IDMs should be cared for in an intensive care nursery. Careful observation with determinations of baseline glucose, hematocrit, electrolytes, and bilirubin, and thereafter, serial blood sugar evaluations for 1,2,4,6 and 12 hours, are essential to prevent or promptly treat the metabolic and hematologic problems of IDMs. Special attention must be given to body temperature, airway patency, oxygenation, acid-base status, respiratory and cardiac functions, and early oral feeding.

Prompt and adequate therapy is necessary in the presence of hyaline membrane disease, congestive heart failure, renal vein thrombosis, small left colon, or other congenital malformations.

**Prognosis:** Prior to 1922 and the discovery of insulin, only one-half of infants delivered of a diabetic mother survived. Today, perinatal mortality for the IDMs treated by a team of experts is approaching that of the nondiabetic.

**Detection of Carrier:** N/A

**References:**
Cornblath M, Schwartz R: Infant of the diabetic mother. In: Quilligan EJ, Kretchmer N, eds: Fetal and maternal medicine. New York: John Wiley, 1980:609–635. †
Vohr B, et al.: Somatic growth of children of diabetic mothers with reference to birth size. J Pediatr 1980; 97:196–199.
Cowett RM, Schwartz R: The infant of the diabetic mother. Pediatr Clin North Am 1982; 29:1213–1231.
Mills JL: Malformations in infants of diabetic mothers. Teratology 1982; 25:385–394.
Freinkel N, et al.: The honeybee syndrome: implications of the teratogenicity of mannose in rat-embryo culture. New Engl J Med 1984; 310:223–230.
Freinkel N, et al.: Gestational diabetes mellitus: heterogeneity of maternal age, weight, insulin secretion, HLA antigens, and islet cell antibodies and the impact of maternal metabolism on pancreatic B-cell and somatic development in the offspring. Diabetes 1985; 34(suppl 2):1–7.
Molsted-Pedersen L, Pedersen JF: Congenital malformations in diabetic pregnancies: clinical viewpoints. Acta Paediatr Scand 1985; 320(Suppl):79–84.
Levin ME, et al.: Pregnancy and diabetes: team approach. Arch Intern Med 1986; 146:758–767. *
Reece EA, Hobbins JC: Diabetic embryopathy: pathogenesis, prenatal diagnosis and prevention. Obstet Gynecol Surv 1986; 41:325–335. *
Tallarigo L, et al.: Relation of glucose tolerance to complications of pregnancy in nondiabetic women. New Engl J Med 1986; 315:989–992 (see also editorial pages 1025–1026).
Mills JL, et al.: Lack of relation of increased malformation rates in infants of diabetic mothers to glycemic control during organogenesis. New Engl J Med 1988; 318:671–676.
Petersen MB, et al.: Early growth delay in diabetic pregnancy: relation to psychomotor development at age four. Brit Med J 1988; 296:598–600.

ME034
RE025

**Paul Merlob**
**Salomon H. Reisner**

## FETAL EFFECTS FROM MATERNAL EXTRINSIC ANDROGENS  2734

**Includes:**
Androgen, fetal effects
Androgenic substance, maternal exposure and fetal virilization
Danazol, maternal exposure and fetal virilization
Danocrine^, maternal exposure and fetal virilization
Female pseudohermaphritism from maternal extrinsic androgens
Progestins, maternal exposure and fetal virilization
Testosterones, maternal exposure and fetal virilization
Virilization of the female from maternal extrinsic androgens

**Excludes:**
**Fetal vasodilator-exposure hypertrichosis** (2927)
**Steroid 21-hydroxylase deficiency** (0908)
Virilization due to androgens of maternal or fetal origin

**Major Diagnostic Criteria:** Virilization of the female fetus characterized by cliteral enlargement and fused labia following maternal exposure to androgenic substances.

**Clinical Findings:** With maternal extrinsic exposure to androgenic substances continuing until after the development of androgen receptors around eight weeks of embryogenesis, virilization of the female fetus occurs. This is manifested by varying degrees of labial fusion, and cliteral enlargement. In marked cases, the newborn may have the superficial appearance of being male (female pseudohermaphritism). Other than genital dysplasia from **Fetal diethylstilbestrol (DES) effects**, this is the only well established congenital effect of extrinsic maternal sex hormonal exposure.

**Complications:** Unknown.

**Associated Findings:** None known.

**Etiology:** Maternal exposure to testosterones, testosterone derivative progestins, danazol or other androgenic substances, continuing beyond eight weeks of embryogenesis. Other chemicals

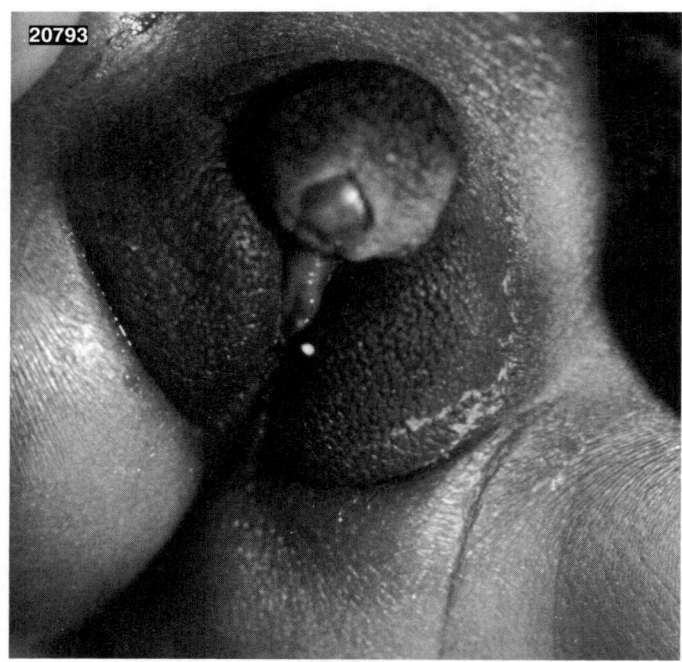

**2734-20793:** Fetal androgen effects: note large clitoris and masculinization effects in an infant exposed to progesterone in utero.

including some insecticides are androgenic, but fetal virilization from these exposures has not been confirmed.

**Pathogenesis:** The mechanism of extrinsic androgenic exposure effect on the female fetus is similar to the effect of excess androgens of adrenal or neoplastic origin in the female fetus or mother, or of fetal testosterone on the male fetus. Androgen receptors develop around eight weeks of embryogenesis.

**Sex Ratio:** Apparent only in females.

**Occurrence:** Over a hundred occurrences with testosterone derivative (19-nor) progestins have been reported. Only a few cases have been reported with 21 C progesterones (progesterone, hydroxyprogesterone, medroxyprogesterone). Twenty cases with maternal danazol exposure are known to the FDA. Only a small proportion of exposures and occurrences are likely to be reported.

**Risk of Recurrence for Patient's Sib:** Related to maternal exposure.

**Risk of Recurrence for Patient's Child:** Unknown.

**Age of Detectability:** During the newborn period.

**Gene Mapping and Linkage:** N/A

**Prevention:** Avoidance of extrinsic maternal androgenic exposures. Testing for pregnancy before beginning therapy with androgenic substances.

**Treatment:** Virilization of the female fetus is surgically correctable, usually with limited residual effects.

**Prognosis:** Long term development sequelae in the female have not been confirmed.

**Detection of Carrier:** N/A

**References:**

Grumbach M, et al: The effects of androgens on fetal sexual development. Fertil Steril 1960; 11:157–179.

Wilkens L: Masculinization of the female fetus due to orally given progestogins. J Am Med Asso 1960; 172:1028–1030.

Shardein J: Congenital abnormalities and hormones during pregnancy: a clinical review. Teratology 1980; 22:251–270.

Wilson GJ, Brent RL: Are female sex hormones teratogenic? Am J Obstet Gynecol 1981; 141:567–580.

Rosa FW: Virilization of the female fetus with maternal danazol exposure. Am J Obstet Gynecol 1984; 149:99 only.

R0018                                                Franz W. Rosa

---

## FETAL EFFECTS FROM MATERNAL HYPERTHERMIA     2385

**Includes:**
> Fetal effects of hyperpyrexia
> Heat, fetal effects from maternal hyperthermia
> Hyperthermia, fetal effects from maternal
> Maternal hyperthermia, fetal effects from

**Excludes:**
> **Anencephaly** (0052)
> **Encephalocele** (0343)
> **Meningomyelocele** (0693)

**Major Diagnostic Criteria:** Hyperthermic teratogenic effects are not expected to produce a single malformation syndrome, but would differ according to the stage of morphogenesis of the affected pregnancy; neural tube defects (NTD) in embryos exposed at the time of neural groove formation and closure (four to six weeks gestation as measured from the first day of the last menstrual period); as well as abnormalities of morphogenesis to 18 weeks gestation. Microphthalmia, midface hypoplasia, and mental retardation with abnormal neurologic examination are reported in retrospective and case report studies.

**Clinical Findings:** One hundred and sixty-eight cases from neural tube defects (NTD) clinics in the Pacific Northwest and Southeastern United States were examined retrospectively and revealed a hyperthermic episode at the time of neural groove closure in approximately 10% of cases; **Anencephaly, Encephalocele,** and **Meningomyelocele.** With regard to the 17 encephalocele

cases, in five cases the exposure was intermittent spiking fever to 39.4°C or higher and in one case exposure was to a hot tub for one hour. A similar percentage of exposures was noted in a Japanese study of human embryos in which recall bias was eliminated: febrile illness was reported in 16 of 113 embryos affected with exencephaly or myeloschisis; in eight of ten cases in which the timing of the febrile episode was known, it occurred during neural tube closure.

Eight retrospective cases of hyperthermia at six to eight weeks gestation (Smith et al, 1978) showed pre- and postnatal growth deficiency in four of eight cases and CNS abnormalities (mental retardation in 7/7, microencephaly in 3/8, hypotonia in 5/8, hypertonia in 2/8, infantile seizures in 4/7, and abnormal EEG in 3/8). Facial abnormalities included microphthalmia in 5/8, midface hypoplasia in 3/8, cleft palate in 3/8. In addition, clinodactyly was noted in 4/7 and micropenis in 2/4.

Five retrospective cases of hyperthermia at nine through 18 weeks gestation showed psychomotor retardation in 3/4, hypotonia in 4/4, neurogenic arthrogryposis in 3/5, and CNS malformations (cerebral dysgenesis, a possible anterior motor horn cell problem, and cortical atrophy) in 4/4. Frazer and Skelton (1978) reported a strikingly significant excess of cases of microphthalmia associated with fever in pregnancy versus no recorded fever.

**Complications:** Maternal hyperthermia from other than an infectious cause may progress to heat shock and death. Postulated effects in humans documented in animal models include premature labor, miscarriage, failure of implantation, and embryonic death.

**Associated Findings:** None known.

**Etiology:** Women experiencing elevated core body temperatures include: 1) those with hyperpyrexia from infectious processes (such as pyelonephritis, a common morbidity of pregnancy; the human febrile response maximum is 41.5°C); 2) those who expose themselves to high environmental temperatures beyond subjective discomfort (such as laundry workers or inexperienced or overzealous sauna and hot tub users or sunbathers); and 3) those whose prolonged physical activity generates high core body temperatures (such as marathon runners).

**Pathogenesis:** The effects of hyperthermia at the cellular level are not well understood. Three mechanisms may explain putative teratogenicity: 1) selective death of dividing cells; 2) redistribution of protein synthesis to heat shock proteins by embryonic or fetal cells with subsequent interference in differentiation; and 3) synergistic or additive effects with other potential teratogens, including ionizing radiation and drugs.

With regard to the first mechanism, *in vitro* mammalian cell death curves are logarithmic with straight slopes at 43°C or above. In the range of 41 to 43°C, the Arrhenius curves are not straight, indicating a different mechanism of cell death; heat inactivation energies in this range are compatible with those calculated for depurination of DNA and for inactivation of DNA repair enzymes. Hyperthermia below 43°C appears to interfere with the process of DNA replication (S phase) and mitosis. Mitotic and S-phase cells have been shown to be selectively killed *in vitro* and *in vivo* within the normal mammalian febrile response.

Edwards and Wanner (1977) describe a striking linear relationship between reduction in weight of the guinea pig brain with increasing hyperthermic exposure, and demonstrated selective death of mitotic and S-phase brain cells as the mechanism of the resultant microcephaly.

With regard to the second mechanism, any noxious stimulus to eukaryotic cells, including temperature elevation, induces so-called heat shock protein synthesis at the cost of usual cellular synthetic activity; the heat shock proteins are thought to stabilize the cell under stress, producing thermotolerance and resistance to other noxious conditions. This diversion of intracellular activity may play a role in abnormal morphogenesis.

The last mechanism accounts for the utility of hyperthermia as an antineoplastic modality; the antineoplastic effects of hyperthermia are synergistic with ionizing radiation and cytotoxic chemotherapeutic agents such as adriamycin. The degree of additive or synergistic effects of hyperthermia with ionizing radiation on various neoplasms is called the *thermal enhancement ratio*. Robins et al (1985) currently employ a radiant heat apparatus to routinely produce whole-body hyperthermia of 41.8°C with little morbidity in lightly anesthetized patients. The interaction of hyperthermia with known or suspected human teratogens is unknown but possible; one instance of **Fetal hydantoin syndrome** occurred with unusually severe manifestations in a woman with a first trimester hyperthermic exposure.

Individuals who have high fevers usually feel sick but do not feel hot, because the subjective sense of heat is dependent on the hypothetical hypophyseal "body thermostat" whose set point is thought to be elevated by the action of pyrogens. On the contrary, such individuals feel subjectively cold after the thermostat is "reset" higher, and shivering, one of the body's mechanisms for producing heat, will ensue until the fever is generated. Only if the hypothalamic center is quickly reset to normal will the sensation of heat be appreciated, as following a fever spike. Antipyretics are thought to act by inhibiting the pyrogen effect on the set point.

In contrast, healthy individuals with high body temperatures from environmental exposure or exercise may not feel sick but they do feel hot. The body commands behavioral means (the urge to get out of the sun, hot tub, sauna) as well as physiologic means (perspiration and dilation of the epidermal capillaries) to maintain homeothermy; the behavioral response may be consciously repressed with resultant increase in body temperature to toxic levels. Edwards and Wanner (1977) found the core body temperature of a marathon runner to be 41.9°C. Many marathon runners have died by forcing their bodies to generate more heat than their physiologic cooling mechanisms could cope with.

**POS No.:** 3532

**Sex Ratio:** Presumably M1:F1

**Occurrence:** The occurrence of febrile illness in pregnancy at specified levels (such as 40°C) is unknown. If 10% of human NTD are presumed to be associated with hyperthermia, then the incidence is estimated as one-tenth that of NTD (1:10,000 if the incidence of NTD is 1:1000).

**Risk of Recurrence for Patient's Sib:** Unknown.

**Risk of Recurrence for Patient's Child:** Unknown.

**Age of Detectability:** Maternal serum alpha-fetoprotein determination may be prudent in any pregnancy with presumed hyperthermic exposure at the time of neural tube formation. Diagnostic ultrasound examination may detect signs associated with hyperthermic insult as early as 13–14 weeks gestation (as measured from the first day of the last menstrual period). Microphthalmia would become evident only with growth of the fetus, since the eyes would be presumed normal at the time of the hyperthermic insult.

**Gene Mapping and Linkage:** N/A

**Prevention:** The toxic threshold in human pregnancy is unknown. In pregnancy, prudent management of fever may include measures to keep the core body temperature below the potentially toxic range-perhaps 40°C. Patient education with regard to physical causes of elevated core body temperature may follow a common sense plan: prolongation of exposure to hot environments or vigorous physical exercise beyond discomfort (the subjective sensation of feeling uncomfortably hot) may create potentially toxic core body temperatures. A woman may monitor any activity of concern by taking her temperature (rectal or vaginal, not oral) immediately after the activity; she should be aware that her response may alter with ingestion of drugs or alcohol.

**Treatment:** Appropriate management of malformations, developmental delay, and mental retardation.

**Prognosis:** Dependent on the severity of the malformation.

**Detection of Carrier:** N/A

**Special Considerations:** Hyperthermia within the normal febrile response has proven teratogenic in virtually every animal model studied: rats, mice, hamsters, rabbits, chicks, guinea pigs, sheep, swine, marmosets, and bonnet monkeys. The CNS appears most sensitive to insult. Time and temperature thresholds have been reported for several species. Abortifacient and embryolethal effects have also been documented in many species.

It has been argued that the fact that the incidence of NTD is lowest in those countries where presumed environmental hyperthermic episodes could occur most frequently (Finland in saunas and Japan in hot baths) stands a priori evidence that hyperthermia is not an important human teratogen. However, the contrary may be true. Because of presumed hyperthermic exposure, the genetic component responsible for the NTD may have been selected against more vigorously than in gene pools in which such environmental stress is not frequently present early in gestation. The frequency of a comparatively rare gene in a population may be altered from Hardy-Weinberg equilibrium in comparatively few generations only if an allele is selected against in its heterozygous state; lowering the threshold of expression of the heterozygous multigenic interacting alleles presumed to be associated with NTD might increase the rate at which they are eliminated from the gene pool in a given population, the fitness of affected heterozygotes being close to zero.

The assumption that individuals in cultures other than Japan and Finland have similar exposure in the same hot environment may be invalid. The Finnish use of the sauna is conservative. Saxen et al (1982) determined that the "vast majority" of pregnant Finns visit the sauna at least weekly, with an estimated average stay of 20 minutes (probably two 10-minute innings) at 70 to 90°C, with core body temperature elevations to 37.5–38.5°C. Results in the novice from a different culture are different. Sohar et al (1976) reported that of 60 inexperienced Israelis agreeing to have a sauna for as long as they could tolerate, 13 stayed for 20 minutes, and had rectal temperatures of >39.0°C, the highest being 40.2°C.

Abnormalities attributed to hyperthermia due to extended exposure to hot tub or sauna from retrospective studies characteristically show prolonged periods of exposure. One woman had a 35-minute sauna with a five-minute cooling period and fainted at the end of exposure; another related exposure in a tub was at 106°F (41.1°C) for nearly one hour.

The Collaborative Perinatal Project (Sever, 1982) revealed a statistically significant association of symptomatic urinary tract infection (UTI) in the second and third trimesters with stillbirth, intrauterine growth retardation, poor motor ability at age eight months, and a lower IQ at age seven years. The lack of associated findings with first trimester UTI was thought to be due to the paucity of women who joined the study in the first trimester. Clarren et al (1979) analyzed the data from women who recalled a fever of at least 38.9°C in the first trimester, and 165 women (selected on the average at midgestation) with positive histories did not have children with significantly increased rates of malformations compared with controls. The recall appears to be an underestimate: one episode of fever per 111 woman-years of women in the study. In McDonald's (1958) prospective study on congenital defects in 3,216 pregnancies, the only occupation significantly associated with increased birth defects was that of laundry workers: of 27 pregnancies, there was one case each of **Anencephaly**, **Hydrocephaly** (type unspecified, possibly cortical atrophy), congenital heart disease, and **Hypospadias**. There was also an excess of febrile episodes in women who had children with major defects (14% vs. 4.2%).

**References:**

McDonald AD: Maternal health and congenital defect: a prospective investigation. New Eng J Med 1958; 258:767–773.

Maron MB, et al.: Thermoregulatory responses during competitive marathon running. J Appl Physiol 1977; 42:909–914.

Sohar E, et al.: Effects of exposure to Finnish sauna. Israel J Med Sci 1976; 12:1275–1282.

Edwards MJ, Wanner RA: Extremes of temperature. In: Wilson JG, Fraser FC, eds: Handbook of teratology, Vol 1. New York: Plenum, 1977;421–444.

Miller P, et al.: Maternal hyperthermia as a possible cause of anencephaly. Lancet 1978; I:519–521.

Halperin LR, Wilroy RS: Maternal hyperthermia and neural tube defects. Lancet 1978; II:212–213.

Chance PF, Smith DW: Hyperthermia and meningomyelocele and anencephaly. Lancet 1978; I:769–770.

Fraser FC, Skelton J: Possible teratogenicity of maternal fever. Lancet 1978; II:634.

Smith DW, et al.: Hyperthermia as a possible teratogenic agent. J Pediat 1978; 92:878–883.

Clarren SK, et al.: Hyperthermia: a prospective evaluation of possible teratogenic agent in man. J Pediat 1979; 95:81–83.

Fisher NL, Smith DW: Occipital encephalocele and early gestational hyperthermia. Pediatrics 1981; 68:480–483.

Sever JL: Infections in pregnancy: highlights from the collaborative perinatal project. Teratology 1982; 25:227–237.

Saxen L, et al.: Sauna and congenital defects. Teratology 1982; 25:309–313.

Shiota K: Neural tube defects and maternal hyperthermia in early pregnancy. Am J Med Genet 1982; 12:281–288.

Robins HI, et al.: A nontoxic system for 41.8°C whole-body hyperthermia: results of a phase I study using a radiant heat device. Cancer Res 1985; 45:3937–3944.

Warkany J: Hyperthermia. Teratology 1986; 33:367–371.

Lipson A: Hirschsprung disease in the offspring of mothers exposed to hyperthermia during pregnancy. Am J Med Genet 1988; 29:117–124.

R0003                                        **Richard M. Roberts**

---

## FETAL EFFECTS FROM MATERNAL LEAD EXPOSURE    3194

**Includes:**

Intrauterine death due to transplacental lead exposure

Intrauterine developmental retardation from fetal lead exposure

Lead, fetal effects from maternal exposure

Lead, effects of postnatal exposure

**Excludes:** Developmental retardation from other causes

**Major Diagnostic Criteria:** Intrauterine developmental retardation following fetal lead exposure.

**Clinical Findings:** Except in major exposures, the findings are not diagnostic and are most often associated with inconspicuous exposures. Therefore the evidence of the extent of fetal lead toxicity must depend on careful epidemiologic studies giving attention to numerous confounding factors.

Lead has long been recognized to be poisonous, more often from accumulation during chronic exposure rather than acute exposures. Lead crosses the placenta. It has long been observed that occupational and other recognized high dose maternal lead exposure increases abortions and stillbirths. Mental retardation and stunting among surviving children has been observed. More recently it has been recognized that widespread ubiquitous lead exposure is a major environmental factor in even more ubiquitous handicapped neurologic development. Multivariate analysis has shown developmental handicap associated with cord blood levels of less than 25 micrograms/dl after stratifying for socioeconomic level and other confounding factors associated with lead exposure. It is difficult to distinguish between the role of prenatal and postnatal exposure, but both clearly can play a role.

**Complications:** Unknown.

**Associated Findings:** None known.

**Etiology:** The greatest source of lead is in the atmosphere from burning lead alkyl additives in automotive fuels. In 1975 it was reported that the atmospheric lead levels in some areas were rising by 5% annually. Since 1976 the Enviromental Protection Agency reports that atmospheric lead emissions have been dropping annually, falling from 169,000 tons in 1976 to 9,500 in 1986. Other sources are widespread, including lead contamination of food and water, plumbing, medicines, waterproofing, varnishes, lead dryers, chrome pigments, antifouling paints, insecticides, wood preservatives, smelting, and numerous occupational exposures.

**Pathogenesis:** Unknown.

**Sex Ratio:** Presumably M1:F1

**Occurrence:** As with other forms of intrauterine developmental retardation, reduction of intellectual capacity has been demonstrated in all IQ ranges so that the frequency is much more widespread than when defined by the mental retardation by population IQ disbribution. Lead may have been one of the most

important environmental reproductive toxicities in the United States during this century. In some urban areas of other countries, the risk is likely to be increasing.

**Risk of Recurrence for Patient's Sib:** Unknown.

**Risk of Recurrence for Patient's Child:** Unknown.

**Age of Detectability:** May be detected in individuals by high lead levels in the mother or the neonate. Usually detectable only through sophisticated epidemiologic studies of neonatal lead levels and childhood development.

**Gene Mapping and Linkage:** N/A

**Prevention:** Reduction of leaded gasoline use has been the most important factor in avoiding fetal exposure. Careful attention to other maternal exposures is important.

**Treatment:** Calcium disodium edetate chelation of lead in women high levels has been used on a small scale.

**Prognosis:** Unknown.

**Detection of Carrier:** Blood lead levels may detect mothers at risk.

**References:**

Angle CR, McIntyre MS: Lead poisoning during pregnancy: fetal tolerance of calcium disodium edetate. Am J Dis Child 1964; 108:436–439.

Scanlon JW: Dangers to the human fetus from certain heavy metals in the environment. Rev Environ Health 1975; 2:29–64.

Moore MR, et al.: A retrospective analysis of blood-lead in mentally retarded children. Lancet 1977; I:717–719.

Schardein JL: Chemically induced birth defects. New York: Marcel Dekker, 1985:619–622.

Bellinger O, et al.: Longitudinal analysis of prenatal and postnatal lead exposure and cognitive development. New Engl J Med 1987; 316: 1037–1043.

Dietrich KN, et al.: Low level fetal lead exposure effect on neuorbehavioral development in early infancy. Pediatrics 1987; 80:721–730.

McMichael AJ, et al.: Port Pirie cohort study: environmental exposure to lead and childrens abilities at the age of four years. New Engl J Med 1988; 319:468–475.

Agency for Toxic Substances and Disease Registry: The nature and extent of lead poisoning in children in the United States: a report to Congress. Chapter I B. Quantitative examination of lead exposure and toxicity in children and pregmant women and strategies for abatement. Pages I 1–41. United States Dept of Health and Human Services, Atlanta GA, 1988.

Jones RR: The continuing hazard of lead in drinking water. Lancet 1989; II:669–670.

Shukla R, et al.: Fetal and infant lead exposure: effects on growth in stature. Pediatrics 1989; 84:604–612.

Surveillance for occupational lead exposure: United States, 1987. MMWR 1989; 38:642–646.

Needleman HL, et al.: The long-term effects of exposure to low doses of lead in childhood: an 11-year follow-up report. New Engl J Med 1990; 322:83–88. *

R0018                                        **Franz W. Rosa**

---

## FETAL EFFECTS FROM MATERNAL PKU        2236

**Includes:**

Folling disease

Hyperphenylalaninemia, mild

Maternal hyperphenylalaninemia

Maternal phenylketonuria

Oligophrenia phenylpyruvica

Phenylalanine hydroxylase deficiency

Phenylketonuria

PKU

**Excludes:**

**Fetal rubella syndrome** (0384)

**Fetal syphilis syndrome** (0385)

**Fetal toxoplasmosis syndrome** (0387)

**Microcephaly** (0659)

**Major Diagnostic Criteria:** Maternal phenylketonuria has an adverse effect on the fetus and results in mental retardation and microcephaly in most offspring of affected women. An increased frequency of congenital heart disease and low birth weight among offspring has also been a feature of maternal phenylketonuria.

An increased concentration of blood phenylalanine in the mother is the critical diagnostic feature. Urine from the mother may also contain phenylketones, as determined by the ferric chloride and dihydrophenylhydrazine tests.

**Clinical Findings:** Microcephaly is usually evident at birth. Low birth weight and congenital heart disease may also be present. The heart disease may be severe and untreatable, or it may be less severe. Developmental delay is often identifiable by the end of the first year of life, and the child is usually considered to be mentally retarded sometime during middle childhood years. Other neurologic features include hyperactive behavior, increased muscle tone, and increased deep tendon reflexes.

The frequency of defects in the offspring seems to relate to the phenylalanine elevation in the mother. When the mothers have classic phenylketonuria [blood phenylalanine $\geq$ 1,200 $\mu$M ($\geq$ 20 mg/dl)], frequencies are: 1) mental retardation (92%); 2) microcephaly (73%); 3) congenital heart disease (10%); and 4) birth weight $\leq$ 2,500 gm (40%).

With high atypical phenylketonuria [blood phenylalanine 1,000–1,150 $\mu$M (16–19 mg/dl)] in the mother, these frequencies seem to be 1) mental retardation (75%); 2) microcephaly (68%); 3) congenital heart disease (11%); and 4) birth weight $\leq$ 2,500 gm (50%).

With lower degrees of atypical phenylketonuria or mild hyperphenylalaninemia [blood phenylalanine 200–800 $\mu$M (3–13 mg/dl)] in the mother, the frequencies of complications in these offspring may not be greater than expected in the general population.

**Complications:** Those due to the presence of congenital heart defects and those that are associated with mental retardation.

**Associated Findings:** None known.

**Etiology:** The biochemical abnormalities of phenylketonuria (e.g. increased blood phenylalanine level) which are transferred to the fetus.

**Pathogenesis:** Virtually nothing is known about the cause of fetal effects in maternal phenylketonuria other than their association with the maternal biochemical abnormalities. Offspring of monkeys in which an increased blood phenylalanine level was induced by feeding phenylalanine during pregnancy had behavioral and performance deficits at birth and during the early months of life. Neurochemical studies performed on the brain from an infant of a mother with phenylketonuria revealed lipid changes similar to those found in the brain in untreated phenylketonuria, suggesting a common pathogenesis.

**MIM No.:** *26160

**POS No.:** 3533

**Sex Ratio:** M1:F1

**Occurrence:** About 500 cases known throughout the world.

**Risk of Recurrence for Patient's Sib:** ~ 100%.

**Risk of Recurrence for Patient's Child:** Unknown.

**Age of Detectability:** At birth, or shortly thereafter. Risk for having offspring damaged by maternal PKU is detectable by diagnosing PKU in the woman before or during pregnancy.

**Gene Mapping and Linkage:** PAH (phenylalanine hydroxylase) has been mapped to 12q22-q24.2.

**Prevention:** Low phenylalanine diet with control of the maternal biochemical abnormalities during pregnancy, preferably begun prior to conception.

**Treatment:** Low phenylalanine diet with control of the maternal biochemical abnormalities during pregnancy, preferably begun prior to conception.

**Prognosis:** The few known results of optimally treated pregnancies are encouraging and suggest that biochemical control in the mother, if begun prior to conception and continued through the pregnancy, may prevent all of the adverse fetal effects.

**Detection of Carrier:** Measurement of plasma phenylalanine and tyrosine under the appropriate conditions and determination of the ratio of phenylalanine to tyrosine (P/T); P/T $\geq$ 1.2 usually indicates the carrier state, while P/T $\leq$ 1.0 usually indicates the homozygous normal state. DNA analysis with RFLP determination using the cloned phenylalanine hydroxylase gene may be informative in some families.

**Support Groups:**
CA; Los Altos; PKU Parents Group
ENGLAND: Kent; Bexley; National Society for Phenylketonuria

**References:**
Woo SLC: Prenatal diagnosis and carrier detection of classical phenylketonuria by gene analysis. Pediatrics 1984; 74:412–423.
Drogari E, et al.: Timing of strict diet in relation to fetal damage in maternal phenylketonuria. Lancet 1987; II:927–930.
Levy HL: Maternal phenylketonuria: review with emphasis on pathogenesis. Enzyme 1987; 38:312–320.
Rohr FJ, et al.: The New England Maternal PKU Project: prospective study of untreated and treated pregnancies and their outcomes. J Pediatr 1987; 110:391–398.
Waisbren SE, et al.: The New England maternal PKU Project: identification of at-risk women. Am J Pub Hlth 1988; 78:789–792.

LE032                                                           **Harvey L. Levy**

---

**FETAL EFFECTS FROM MATERNAL VASODILATOR       2927**

**Includes:**
Blood pressure, fetal effects of maternal hypertension medication
Diazoxide, fetal effects
High blood pressure, maternal, fetal effects of medication
Hyperstat^, fetal effects
Hypertension medication, fetal effects
Hypertrichosis, fetal effect from maternal vasodilator
Loniten^, fetal effects
Minoxidil, fetal effects
Proglycem^, fetal effects
Vasolidator, fetal effects

**Excludes:**
**Chromosome 3, trisomy 3q2** (2430)
**Fetal effects from maternal extrinsic androgens** (2734)
Hair, neonatal lanugal

**Major Diagnostic Criteria:** Neonatal hypertrichosis with maternal exposure to minoxidil or diazoxide.

**Clinical Findings:** Three cases of fetal hypertrichosis with maternal exposures to antihypertensive vasodilators have been reported. Two of these exposures were to minoxidil and one to diazoxide. One infant exposed to minoxidil and other antihypertensives had generalized hypertrichosis most pronounced in the sacral area, lower legs, and forearms. The infant also had an omphalocele, ventricular septal defect, depressed nasal bridge, low-set ears, micrognathia, clinodactyly of the little fingers, undescended testicles, and a circumferential mid-phallic constriction. The hypertrichosis subsided over a two-month period. The second case also exposed to minoxidil and other antihypertensives had hypertrichosis described as a general increase of bristly hair, longest in the sacral area. The infant was otherwise robust, and the female genitalia were normal. The hypertrichosis subsided over a period of 3 months, and at follow-up at age two years the infant was surviving and well. The third infant had maternal exposure to diazoxide in the last trimester of pregnancy. Hypertrichosis did not develop until the second week, and when most florid, involved the forehead, cheeks, sacrum, buttocks, and doral surfaces of the arms and legs. This infant also had a ring of alopecia around the scalp from birth, which became more obvious with the contrasting hypertrichosis. When the infant was last seen at age five months, the hypertrichosis was less but the alopecia remained. The infant was otherwise normal.

**Complications:** Unknown.

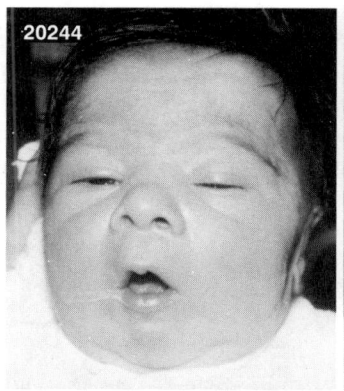
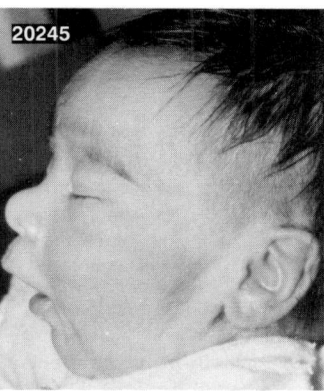
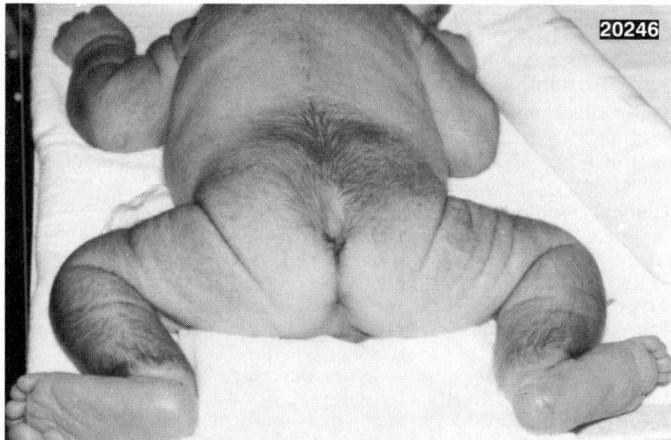

**2927-20244–46:** Hypertrichosis associated with in utero minoxidil exposure.

**Associated Findings:** Three other last-trimester diazoxide exposure outcomes were reported. These infants did not have hypertrichosis, but two of them also had areas of alopecia. They otherwise had normal development. At the time of this writing only one other birth with maternal exposure to minoxidil (along with other antihypertensive agents) is known; the newborn lacked hypertrichosis but died of transposition of the great vessels on the second day. It is speculative whether the other defects observed in this case and in one of the above cases of maternal exposures to minoxidil were due to the agent, to concurrent agents, to the maternal condition, or to another factor.

**Etiology:** Maternal exposure to antihypertensive vasodilators: minoxidil, and diazoxide (Hypertrichosis also occurs in persons directly receiving these agents).

**Pathogenesis:** Unknown. The hypertrichosis is not androgenic in distribution. Vasodilation of peripheral arterioles may contribute to the condition.

**Sex Ratio:** Presumably M1:F1.

**Occurrence:** Five cases have been reported. No cohort of pregnancy experience with these agents is available with which to assess the frequency distribution of adverse and normal outcomes. In isolated case reports, normal outcomes are seldom reported.

**Risk of Recurrence for Patient's Sib:** Unknown. Presumably related to exposure.

**Risk of Recurrence for Patient's Child:** Unknown. Presumably related to independent exposure.

**Age of Detectability:** During the first two weeks of life.

**Gene Mapping and Linkage:** N/A

**Prevention:** Data are insufficient to assess the risk benefits of employing minoxidil in women refractory to other antihypertensive agents. Diazoxide is now used infrequently because of its hyperglycemic effects.

**Treatment:** Unknown.

**Prognosis:** One of three patients died of associated anomalies. The hypertrichosis subsided without complications in the first few months of life in the other two infants.

**Detection of Carrier:** Unknown.

**Special Considerations:** All United States pregnancy exposures to minoxidil should be reported to the Food and Drug Administration at (301) 443–6410 for follow-up investigation.

**References:**
Miller RDG, Chouksey SK: Effects of fetal exposure to diazoxide in man. Arch Dis Child 1972; 47:537–543.
Kaler SG, et al.: Hypertrichosis and congenital anomalies associated with maternal use of minoxidil. Pediatrics 1987; 79:434–436. *
Rosa FW, et al.: Fetal minoxidil exposure. (Letter) Pediatrics 1987; 80:120 only.

KA041
R0018
ID000

**Stephen G. Kaler**
**Franz W. Rosa**
**Juhana Idanpaan-Heikkila**

## FETAL EFFECTS FROM METHIMAZOLE AND CARBIMAZOLE                    2926

**Includes:**
> Antithyroid fetal effects, scalp and urachal
> Carbimazole fetal effects, scalp and urachal
> Methimazole, fetal effects, scalp and urachal
> Scalp defects from fetal exposure
> Tapazole^, fetal effects
> Urachal defects from fetal exposure

**Excludes:** Cutis aplasia without antithyroid exposure

**Major Diagnostic Criteria:** Infant scalp and urachal defects caused by maternal treatment with antithyroid agents (methimazole or carbimazole).

**Clinical Findings:** In 1971, Milham and Elledge (1972) identified two exposures to methimazole among 11 mothers having offspring with scalp defect recorded on Washington State birth certificates. In one of the exposed pregnancies fraternal twins occurred, both having scalp defects. In 1975 Mujtaba and Burrow reported two infants with scalp defects born from one of four women treated with methimazole. The Centers for Disease Control Atlanta Metropolitan Area Birth Defect Monitoring System reported to Milham a case with methimazole exposure, The Netherlands Adverse Drug Reactions Office communicated a case, and another case was communicated of an infant born in Hong Kong (exposed to carbimazole, which metabolizes to methimazole). Two additional isolated methimazole scalp defect case reports have been received by the Food and Drug Administration.
The scalp defects are described as single or multiple, circumscribed, midline, vertex or parietal, and in one case exposing the meninges, probably by overlying the anterior fossa. Two of the cases also had urachal defects, in one described as a "patent urachus" and in the other as a "patent vitelline" duct. No affected infants have been observed in association with maternal use of propylthiouracil; a more common treatment for hyperthyroidism.
A Japanese cohort study (Momotani et al, 1984) of 243 methimazole or carbimazole pregnancy exposures found no scalp defects, and only two defect outcomes of any kind (a malformed earlobe and omphalocele). Although a cohort of this size is insufficient to rule out an elevated *relative* risk for a rare defect picked up in a case registry, it does show that the *absolute* risk of scalp or other

defects with these exposures is low. The omphalocele possibly could be of significance relative to the urachal defects reported elsewhere. In the Netherlands, no additional scalp defects could be found among 24 mothers receiving first trimester methimazole or carbimazole, nor could any additional antithyroid exposures be found among 13 scalp defects occurring among 49,091 births occurring between 1959 and 1986 (Van Dijke et al, 1987).

**Complications:** Unknown.

**Associated Findings:** Neonatal goiter is seen in the newborn of mothers with hyperthyroidism. When this is associated with transient neonatal hyperthyroidism, it is an effect of placental passage of long-acting thyroid stimulator immunoglobulin responsible for the maternal hyperthyroidism. Hypothyroid goiters, usually transient, also are seen in infants of mothers treated with antithyroid agents.

**Etiology:** Fetal exposure to the maternal antithyroid agents methimazole or carbimazole.

**Pathogenesis:** Unknown.

**Sex Ratio:** Presumably M1:F1.

**Occurrence:** The overall frequency of antithyroid use during pregnancy in the United States is about 1:5,000 pregnancies. Until recently methimazole was used in about one-third of treatments. Although 11 exposures with this rare defect strongly suggest an association, the absence of scalp defects among two cohorts totaling 267 exposures indicates that this is not a frequent outcome.

**Risk of Recurrence for Patient's Sib:** Unknown. Presumably related to further exposure.

**Risk of Recurrence for Patient's Child:** Unknown. Presumably related to independent exposure.

**Age of Detectability:** In infancy.

**Gene Mapping and Linkage:** N/A

**Prevention:** Propylthiouracil is preferred to methimazole for managing hyperthyroidism during pregnancy, because it appears to have less transplacental transmission (Marchant et al, 1977).

**Treatment:** Usually not required, since most defects heal spontaneously. Large defects may require surgical repair or grafting.

**Prognosis:** Good for life span and function.

**Detection of Carrier:** Unknown.

**Special Considerations:** This is the first example of initial detection of any type of teratogenicity by follow-up of an unusual frequency in a birth defect register (Washington State).

Birth defects with maternal antithyroid exposure should be reported to the Division and Epidemiology and Surveillance of the Food and Drug Administration, Rockville, MD 20851.

**References:**
Milham S, Elledge W: Maternal methimazole and congenital defects in children. Teratology 1972; 5:125.
Mujtaba Q, Burrow GN: Treatment of hyperthyroidism in pregnancy with propylthiouracil and methimazole. Obstet Gynecol 1975; 48: 282–286.
Marchant B, et al.: The placental transfer of propylthiouracil, methimazole and carbimazole. J Clin Endocrinol Metab 1977; 1187–1193.
Munro DS, et al.: The role of thyroid stimulating immunoglobulins of Grave's disease in neonatal thyrotoxicosis. Br J Obstet Gynaecol 1978; 18–83.
Ramsay I, et al.: Thyrotoxicosis in pregnancy: results of treatment by antithyroid drugs combined with T4. Clin Endocrinol 1983; 18:73–85.
Cooper DS: Antithyroid drugs. New Engl J Med 1984; 311:1353–1362.
Momotani N, et al.: Maternal hyperthyroidism and congenital malformation in offspring. Clin Endocrinol 1984; 20:695–700.
Burrow GN: The management of thyrotoxicosis in pregnancy. New Engl J Med 1985; 562–565.
Milham S: Scalp defects in infants of mothers treated for hyperthyroidism with methimazole or carbimazole during pregnancy. Teratology 1985; 32:321. *

Van Dijke CP, et al.: Methimazole, carbimazole, and congenital skin defects. Ann Int Med 1987; 106:60–61.

MI037
R0018
**Samuel Milham**
**Franz W. Rosa**

## FETAL EFFECTS FROM VARICELLA-ZOSTER          **2499**

**Includes:**
 Chickenpox, fetal effects
 Fetal varicella-zoster syndrome
 Varicella-zoster, fetal effects
 Varicella embryopathy

**Excludes:**
 **Amniotic bands syndrome** (0874)
 **Cataract**
 Chorioretinitis
 Fetal disruption syndromes of other viral etiology
 **Microcephaly** (0659)
 Microphthalmia

**Major Diagnostic Criteria:** Focal cutaneous ulceration or scarring with cicatrix formation, and disruption of underlying structures, in the fetus of a mother with gestational varicella-zoster virus infection.

**Clinical Findings:** The hallmark of fetal varicella-zoster syndrome is disruption and scarring of the skin and underlying structures. The scars may be thick and hypertrophic, resembling keloids, and adjacent skin may be indurated and erythematous. The cutaneous involvement may follow a dermatome distribution. Extremities may have severe reduction deformities and paralytic atrophy.

Thirty-one infants have been described following maternal varicella- zoster infection between eight and 20 weeks gestation. Death in the period from birth to 20 months occurred in 9/31; in infancy 7/17. Cicatrix formation 28/31; hypoplastic limbs 20/31; muscular atrophy 17/31; small for gestational age 11/31. CNS abnormalities (including cortical atrophy, ventriculomegaly, **Mi-**

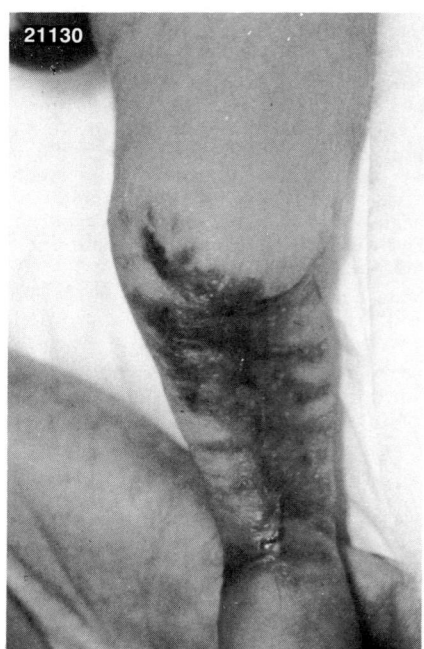

**2499A-21130:** Limb reduction, cicatrix formation in an infant exposed to varicella in utero.

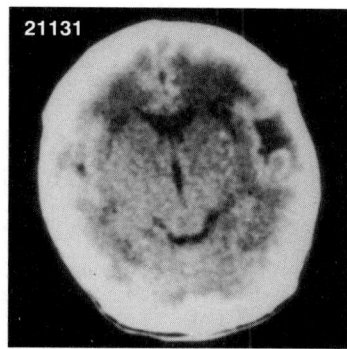

**2499B-21131:** CT scan of the head of the child shown in 21130 showing focal cortical atrophy.

crocephaly) 14/31; delayed development 7/24; microphthalmia (bilateral or unilateral) 9/31; cataracts and nystagmus 5/31; recurrent respiratory infection (8/24); healed chorioretinitis 10/31; and facial asymmetry 4/31. Occasional findings include adherence of pinna to scalp, rudimentary digits, unilateral facial nerve palsy, micrognathia, disfiguring microstomia, obliteration of the nose, scoliosis, small left colon, urinary and fecal incontinence, hypoplastic clavicle, scapula, and humerus; dysphagia, phrenic nerve palsy, lack of iris pigmentation (unilateral), absent swallow, and prominent ears.

Autopsy findings included necrotizing encephalitis; penumonitis; pancreatic and adrenal scarring; unilateral hydronephrosis; focal atresia of the sigmoid colon; widespread infiltrative calcified lesions in the liver, lung, spleen and diaphragm; absent kidneys; hypoplastic thymus; and retinal calcifications.

**Complications:** Fetal demise due to fatal maternal varicella-zoster pneumonia or encephalitis.

**Associated Findings:** Unilateral hearing deficit, **Cleft palate**, gastroesophageal reflux, undescended testis, pilonidal sinus, **Hernia, inguinal**, and incomplete duplication of the ureter.

**Etiology:** The varicella-zoster (V-Z) virus is a DNA virus of the family *herpesviridae*. After primary infection (chickenpox), the V-Z virus is thought to remain quiescent in the sensory nerve ganglia; reactivation may occur with waning humeral immunity, or with immunosuppression, in the form of shingles (zoster), or more severely, the rare zoster-varicellosus, in which the vesicles are not limited to sensory nerve dermatomes, but become widespread.

**Pathogenesis:** Infection with chickenpox is initiated through close contact with an individual with chickenpox or shingles; airborne inoculum is presumed an important route of infection as well as direct contact with vesicular fluid. The risk for developing the disease after exposure may be higher than 90% in susceptible individuals. The incubation period is usually two weeks, with a viremic phase prior to the familiar papulovesicular cutaneous eruption. Affected individuals are highly contagious from two days prior to eruption of vesicles until all vesicles are crusted, when virus is no longer detectable.

The clinical course is usually benign, but occasionally the lesions may become hemorrhagic and confluent with widespread visceral and CNS involvement. The severe musculoskeletal abnormalities of the congenital syndrome may be the result of both tissue necrosis and denervation. The latter has been demonstrated with nerve conduction and electromyography in one severely affected infant. Neonatal chickenpox may have a fulminant course with widespread necrotic lesions in the brain, liver, lung, kidney, heart, and eye. The severity of neonatal cases is thought to be linked to absence of protective maternal IgG antibody; near-term maternal infection more than five days prior to delivery was not associated with neonatal mortality in 27 of 27 reported cases in which the baby subsequently developed varicella. However, when the maternal symptoms began four days or less prior to delivery, seven of 23 affected infants died of fulminant infection.

One-quarter of maternal cases are thought to result in intrauterine infection. Seven of 33 infants had positive immunologic response in the Paryani and Arvin (1986) prospective study, and all were subsequent to second and third trimester maternal cases, indicating that fetal infection is a common occurrence and is usually benign. None of seven infants tested whose mother had first trimester infections, however, had positive immunologic tests, including the one infant severely affected with the syndrome (limb atrophy with cicatrices, bilateral chorioretinitis, cortical atrophy, and unilateral hydronephrosis); the fetal immune response to viral infection may not be competent in the first trimester. Current immonologic tests on infants with first trimester exposure are not useful for confirmation of viral infection. The immaturity of the immune system is also manifest by case reports of shingles in infants whose mothers had chickenpox in pregnancy, indicating premature senescence of immunity following the presumed primary infection *in utero*.

Shingles (zoster) is caused by reactivation of the varicella-zoster virus along sensory nerve dermatomes, thought to occur after humoral and cellular immune response wanes. Viremia has not been proven; a degree of dissemination of lesions was noted in one-third of 88 patients without cancer. There are three case reports in the literature of abnormalities in infants following maternal shingles; the defects were limited to the eye and CNS, and in two of these other viral etiology was not excluded. No cases of the full syndrome following maternal shingles have been noted, supportive of the theory that viremia is uncommon.

The risk to the fetus of maternal chickenpox infection appears to be different at various stages of pregnancy. Twenty-seven of 31 fetuses affected with the syndrome occurred after maternal disease at sixteen weeks gestation or less, and four between 17 to 20 weeks. The syndrome in its most severe form has been reported only in the first half of pregnancy. Only two case reports have documented abnormalities after 20 weeks gestation; after maternal varicella at 23 weeks, the infant was affected with dense nuclear cataracts; and after the mother had varicella at 28 weeks gestation, the infant was born with bleeding skin ulcers, and subsequently required tenotomy for progressive equinovarus deformity of the affected extremity. The ulcers resolved with scarring and cicatrix formation. Thus the examination of data with regard to the first one-half versus the second one-half of pregnancy may be more appropriate than the traditional first, second and third trimester comparisons, since the first half of the second trimester appears to be a period at risk for the full syndrome. This period of risk may be explained by the impaired transfer of maternal IgG across the placenta prior to 28 weeks.

**POS No.:** 3530

**Sex Ratio:** Theoretically M1:F1. M1:F4 observed.

**Occurrence:** Chickenpox is a disease primarily of children in temperate countries, and of young adults in the semitropics and tropics. Five to 10% of adults in the United States are thought to be susceptible to chickenpox; however, 16% of Puerto Rican women of childbearing age in New York City were seronegative, reported in 1976. In Germany (FDR), 5.2% of women 16–40 years were seronegative in a 1981 study. In Southampton, England, 7.8% of mothers (86 of 1,106) were seronegative at delivery, reported in 1986. In Israel, 19% of young adults were reported seronegative in 1978; in West Bengal, the mean age for chickenpox was 23.7 years, reported in 1976.

The incidence of chickenpox during pregnancy is 70:10,000 in the United States, estimated in a 1968 study. The incidence of chickenpox in the 15–19 year age group in the United States is 2.91:1,000, and in the 20+ year age group, 33:100,000 estimated in a 1986 study. The incidence of maternal varicella in the critical period of four days prior to delivery was 3:5,000 deliveries per year at Southampton, England, reported in 1986. The incidence of shingles in women age 15–45 years is estimated to be 2.16:1,000 in the United States and 3:1,000 in Great Britain. The incidence of fetal varicella syndrome following first trimester infection in two similar prospective studies was 1:38 term neonates, with evidence of fetal effects (microcephaly) in another. The incidence of the syndrome following maternal shingles in these studies was 0:22 first and second trimester cases.

**Risk of Recurrence for Patient's Sib:** Not increased in the absence of infection.

**Risk of Recurrence for Patient's Child:** Not increased in the absence of infection.

**Age of Detectability:** Diagnostic ultrasound examination may detect signs of fetal varicella syndrome as early as 14 weeks gestation (as measured from the first day of the last menstrual period). Serial examination of fetal morphology as well as growth is prudent; microphthalmia, for example, would become evident only with growth of the fetus, since the eyes would be presumed normal at the time of the infection.

Ultrasonic assessment of one severely affected infant suggested a meningomyelocele; at birth a transparent skin lesion extended from the iliac crest to the lumbosacral area, possibly the result of a severe bullous lesion of the skin visualized at the time of ultrasonic evaluation. Because the integrity of the skin is presumed breached in affected fetuses, it is possible that a rise in alpha fetoprotein in both amniotic fluid and maternal serum occurs. Because of the marked difficulty in growing the virus, its detection in amniotic fluid may be dependent on visualization of viral particles with EM; development of a specific recombinant DNA probe may facilitate confirmation of *in utero* infection.

**Gene Mapping and Linkage:** N/A

**Prevention:** Primary prevention is through the establishment of immunity to the virus prior to conception. The Oka vaccine is not available for general use in the United States at this time. A combined vaccine (measles, mumps, rubella, and chickenpox) has proven effective, and hopefully the single and combined vaccines will soon be licenced in the United States. Routine obstetric care in the future most likely will include varicella as well as rubella testing with appropriate immunization of women at risk.

*Passive immunization*: Varicella-zoster immune globulin (VZIG) may prevent infection in exposed individuals when given within 48–96 hours of exposure. Treatment of exposed non-immune pregnant women appears warranted on the basis of the significant risk of fatal maternal varicella-zoster pneumonia. Enders (1984) reported that VZIG given to seven pregnant seronegative women 24 to 72 hours after exposure prevented infection, while of five pregnant seronegative women who did not receive VZIG, four developed chickenpox. Administration to mothers at term and infants whose mothers develop varicella four days or less prior to delivery to two days after delivery appears warranted, as it may prevent a fulminant course. The 1986 Redbook (American Academy of Pediatrics) recommends one vial of 125u per 10 kg. weight (neonatal dose: 1 vial), to a maximum of 5 vials, given intramuscularly, and denotes as candidates for therapy the immunocompromised, normal non-immune individuals at least 15 years old, prematures at least 28 weeks gestation whose mother lacks immunity, and prematures less than 28 weeks or less than 1,000 gm regardless of maternal immunity, if significant exposure has occurred.

**Treatment:** Antiviral therapy has been employed during pregnancy when the health of the mother is seriously threatened (varicella pneumonia), and in the neonate at risk of fulminant infection.

**Prognosis:** Dependent on the extent and characterization of the morphologic disruptions. Limited scarring abnormalities should have excellent prognosis, whereas abnormalities of the brain will have a guarded prognosis. Most severely affected infants have not survived.

**Detection of Carrier:** N/A

**Special Considerations:** Confirmation of *in utero* infection in infants of mothers with second and third trimester infections has been accomplished with specific lymphocyte transformation in response to varicella-zoster virus antigen; or varicella IgM antibody in the neonate, or persistence of significant titers of varicella-zoster IgG antibody after age seven months with no history of clinical varicella.

Any pregnancy complicated by chickenpox may be regarded as high-risk. Maternal morbidity in the Paryani and Arvin prospec-

tive study of 43 women included four who developed pneumonia, (one required mechanical ventilation, and one died), four of 42 had premature labor during the acute phase of the infection, and two of these delivered prematurely. One of 11 women with varicella in the first trimester had an infant with severe fetal varicella syndrome, manifested by microcephaly, cortical atrophy, chorioretinitis, hydroureter and hydronephrosis of the left kidney, severe gastroesophageal reflux, right lower leg scarring and deformation, who died of recurrent aspiration pneumonia; another infant had microcephaly, but no other signs of the syndrome.

Enders'(1984) prospective study confirmed serologicaly 35 pregnant women with chickenpox in the first trimester; of these, four terminated the pregnancy and four miscarried, leaving 27 who delivered normal neonates (viral studies on the abortuses were negative). Ten womens had chickenpox at 4–7 months gestation, and all delivered normal infants. Seventeen women had zoster at 3–7 months gestation, and all had normal infants.

The 1951–1952 prospective British study (Manson et al, 1960) showed that of 76 first trimester cases confirmed by medical examination, three miscarried (no information on the fetus available), three were stillborn, and of liveborns, two died before the age of two, and another was mentally retarded. Maternal morbidity was not reported.

Another prospective cohort study (Siegel, 1973) of cases reported to the health department in 1957–1964 in New York City yielded 32 cases of first trimester chickenpox, five of whom miscarried (no information on the fetus available), and two neonates affected with abnormalities associated with the fetal V-Z syndrome: one with microcephaly, the other a congenital cataract; of 60 second trimester cases, there were four fetal deaths. Of these nine fetal deaths, three occurred within two weeks of maternal disease, two within 3–5 days, one was associated with maternal chickenpox encephalitis, and one with fatal maternal chickenpox pneumonia at 20 weeks. No deaths occurred in 52 third trimester cases; one infant was congenitally deaf, and another had unilateral renal agenesis and the remaining kidney was hypoplastic. About one-half of cases were Puerto Rican-American.

The Genetics Section of the Dept. of OB/GYN at the University of Wisconsin, Milwaukee Clinical Campus, has initiated a registry of prospectively ascertained maternal chickenpox cases. In the first year, it examined four first-trimester cases with diagnostic ultrasound prior to 20 weeks, with no abnormalities detected.

**References:**
Siegel M: Congenital malformations following chickenpox, measles, mumps, and hepatitis. J Am Med Asso 1973; 226:1521–1524.
Weller T: Varicella and herpes zoster. New Engl J Med 1983; 309:1362-1368; 1434–1440.
Enders G: Varicella-zoster virus infection in pregnancy. Prog Med Virol 1984; 29:166–96.
Hanshaw JB, et al.: Viral diseases of the fetus and newborn, 2 ed. Philadelphia: W.B. Saunders, 1985. * †
Paryani SG, Arvin AM: Intrauterine infection with varicella-zoster virus after maternal varicella. New Engl J Med 1986; 314:1542–1546. *

R0003                                                     **Richard M. Roberts**

**Fetal effects of hyperpyrexia**
*See FETAL EFFECTS FROM MATERNAL HYPERTHERMIA*

---

## FETAL EFFECTS OF MATERNAL CIGARETTE SMOKING    2960

**Includes:**
   Cigarette smoking, fetal effects of
   Intrauterine growth retardation (some)
   Smoking, cigarette, fetal effects

**Excludes:** Intrauterine growth retardation from other causes

**Major Diagnostic Criteria:** Low birth weight in children of mothers who smoke cigarettes.

**Clinical Findings:** The main finding is a low birth weight for the gestational age of the infant. There is an approximate 200 g deficit in birth weight among infants born to women who smoked 10–20

cigarettes per day throughout pregnancy. Affected infants are shorter and have smaller head circumferences. Maternal smoking is also associated with less frequent, yet more severe, pregnancy outcomes including early and late fetal deaths and abnormal placentation.

**Complications:** Unknown.

**Associated Findings:** Studies on the relationship between maternal smoking and birth defects are inconsistent; there is no strong evidence that smoking causes any specific type of structural defect. Respiratory disorders, behavioral problems, and decreased congnitive function are reported to be more frequent among children of women who smoked during pregnancy; however, these problems may result from exposures during childhood rather than gestation.

**Etiology:** The exact components of cigarette smoke that affect fetal growth are not known; nicotine, carbone monoxide, and thiocyanate have been implicated.

**Pathogenesis:** There is evidence suggesting that nicotine-mediated uteroplacental vessel constriction causes growth retardation through decreased perfusion of fetal tissues. It has also been proposed that fetal hypoxia resulting from maternal carbon monoxide ingestion plays a causal role.

**Sex Ratio:** Presumably M1:F1.

**Occurrence:** The rate of low birth weight, defined as <2,500 g, is approximately 14% among women who smoke in comparison to 8% among nonsmokers. Placental problems, including placenta previa, abruptio placentae, and intrapartum hemorrhage, occur among approximately 4% of smoking women.

**Risk of Recurrence for Patient's Sib:** Unknown.

**Risk of Recurrence for Patient's Child:** Unknown.

**Age of Detectability:** At birth. Prenatal diagnosis by ultrasound may be possible.

**Gene Mapping and Linkage:** N/A

**Prevention:** Abstention from smoking cigarettes during pregnancy. Women who stop smoking after the first trimester deliver infants with birth weights close to infants of nonsmoking women.

**Treatment:** Unknown.

**Prognosis:** There are no known specific problems among growth-retarded infants of smokers. Perinatal mortality increases with decreasing birth weight for infants of both smokers and nonsmokers.

**Detection of Carrier:** Unknown.

**Special Considerations:** There are many factors other than maternal smoking that affect the risk of intrauterine growth retardation, fetal death, and abnormal placentation. The association of maternal smoking and these adverse reproductive outcomes remain after other factors are statistically controlled.

**References:**
Butler N, et al.: Cigarette smoking in pregnancy: its influence on birth weight and perinatal mortality. Br Med J 1972; 2:127–130.
Meyer MB, et al.: Perinatal events associated with maternal smoking. Am J Epidemiol 1976; 103:464–476.
Harrison GG, et al.: Association of maternal smoking with body composition of the newborn. Am J Clin Nutr 1983; 38:757–762.
Werler MM, et al.: Smoking and pregnancy. Teratology 1985; 32:473–481.

WE039                                  **Martha M. Werler**

**Fetal effects of maternal Lyme disease**
*See FETAL EFFECTS FROM LYME DISEASE*

## FETAL EFFECTS OF NONSTEROIDAL ANTI-INFLAMMATORY DRUGS (NSAIDS)   3281

**Includes:**
> Ductus arteriosus, prenatal closure with NSAID exposure
> Ibuprofen, fetal effects
> Indocin^, fetal effects
> Indomethacin, fetal effects
> Mefenamic acid, fetal effects
> Motrin^, fetal effects
> Naprosyn^, fetal effects
> Naproxen, fetal effects
> Oligohydramnios, fetal, with NSAID exposure
> Oliguria, neonatal, with NSAID exposure
> Perinatal effects of nonsteroidal anti-inflammatory drugs (NSAIDS)
> Ponstel^, fetal effects
> Prostaglandin synthesis inhibition, fetal effects

**Excludes:**
> Fetal angiotensin converting enzyme (ACE) inhibition renal failure (2962)
> Fetal exposure to other types of anti-inflammatory agents

**Major Diagnostic Criteria:** Premature closure or partial closure of the ductus arteriosus with third trimester NSAID exposure. Oligohydramnious and neonatal oliguria with third trimester NSAID exposure.

**Clinical Findings:** NSAIDS are usually administered as analgesics and anti-inflammatory agents, but in pregnancy they have been specifically used as tocolytics (to avoid threatened premature delivery) and to treat polydydramnios. In the neonate, NSAIDS are used to close a persisting **Ductus arteriosus, patent.** Both the effect in suppressing the production of amniotic fluid, and of closing the ductus, can have adverse fetal effects. Maternal NSAID exposure can produce oligohydramnios (Hendricks et al, 1989; Bond et al, 1989), with its associated adverse effects on fetal lung development, and limb mobility (joint contractures).

Persisting after birth, transient neonatal anuria or oliguria can be associated with fluid retention, hyponatremia, hyperkalemia, cardiac arrhythmias, and cardiac failure (Mogilner et al, 1982; Alun-Jones & Williams, 1986; Heijden et al, 1988; Simeoni et al, 1989). Maternal NSAID administration can also cause constriction and sometimes closure of the fetal ductus arteriosus with associated pulmonary hypertension, and pulmonic and tricuspid regurgitation (Moise et al, 1988; Kirshon et al, 1989a, 1989b).

**Complications:** Those associated with oligohydramnious/renal failure amd ductus constriction.

**Associated Findings:** Where NSAIDS are used for threatened premature delivery in pregnancies compromised by other complications, the effect of those complications, most characteristically intrauterine growth retardation, may be associated.

**Etiology:** Maternal exposure to NSAIDS-acting prostaglandin synthesis inhibition.

**Pathogenesis:** Most NSAIDS exert their effects through suppression of prostaglandins; thromoxane and leukotriene synthesis from arachiodonic acid (Mortensen & Rennebohm, 1989). These metabolites have wide effects on inhibiting inflammatory reactions, associated pain, induction of labor, blood coagulation, maintenance of urinary function, maintenance of ductus patency, and many other effects. NSAIDS tend to block these effects, potentially causing both beneficial and adverse effects related to dose, indication, and timing of administration.

**Sex Ratio:** Presumably M1:F1.

**Occurrence:** Related to dose, duration, and indication of NSAID therapy. Denominator and numerator data is currently inadequate to quantify risks.

**Risk of Recurrence for Patient's Sib:** Unknown.

**Risk of Recurrence for Patient's Child:** N/A

**Age of Detectability:** Oliguria and ductus constriction can be detected prenatally.

**Gene Mapping and Linkage:** N/A

**Prevention:** Avoid unessential exposures. In cases of necessary exposure, follow amniotic fluid volume and fetal circulation closely and discontinue use if indicated.

**Treatment:** Careful management of neonatal renal failure, associated electrolyte imbalance, and cardiac complications.

**Prognosis:** Neonatal anuria is transient and resolves spontaneously if cardiac failure does not occur from fluid overload and electrolyte imbalance.

**Detection of Carrier:** N/A

**References:**

Mogilner BM, et al.: Hydrops fetalis caused by maternal indomethacin treatment. Acta Obstet Gynecol Scand 1982; 61:183–185.

Alun-Jones C, Williams J: Hyponatremia and fluid retention in a neonate associated with maternal naproxen overdosage. J Toxicol-Clin Toxicol 1986; 24:257 only.

Heijden AJ, et al.: Renal functional impairment in preterm neonates related to intrauterine indomethacin exposure. Pediatr Res 1988; 5:644–648.

Moise J, et al.: Indomethacin in the treatment of premature labor: effects on the fetal ductus arteriosus. New Engl J Med 1988; 319:327–331.

Bond A, et al.: Chronic indomethacin administration and oligohydramnios. Proceedings of the Society for Perinatal Obstetricians, February 1989, Abstract 352.

Hendricks SK, et al.: Association of prostaglandin synthesis inhibitors with antenatal development of olighydramnios in a high risk preterm labor population. Proceedings of the Society for Perinatal Obstetricians, February 1989, Abstract 353.

Kirshon B, et al.: Indomethacin therapy in the treatment of polyhydramnos. Proceedings of the Society for Perinatal Obstetricians, February 1989a, Abstract 13.

Kirshon B, et al.: Indomethacin effect on the fetal ductus arteriosus in polyhydramnios. Proceedings of the Society for Perinatal Obstetricians, February 1989b, Abstract 245.

Marales WJ, et al.: Efficacy and safety of indomethacin versus ritodrine in the management of preterm labor: a randomized study. Obstet Gynecol 1989; 74:567–572.

Mortensen ME, Rennebohm RM: Clinical pharmacology and use of nonsteroidal anti-inflammatory drugs. Pediatr Clinics of North Am 1989; 36:1113–1137.

Simeoni U, et al.: Neonatal renal dysfunction and intrauterine exposure to prostaglandin synthesis inhibitors. Eur J Pediatr 1989; 148:371–373.

R0018                                                    **Franz W. Rosa**

---

# FETAL EFFECTS OF POLYCHLORINATED BIPHENYL (PCB)                                           2733

**Includes:**

    Cola-colored babies
    Ectodermal dysplasia, "acquired"
    Embryopathy
    PCB fetopathy
    Polychlorinated biphenyl (PCB), fetal effects of
    Yucheng, congenital
    Yusho, congenital

**Excludes:** Fetal effects (other)

**Major Diagnostic Criteria:** Thus far, the syndrome has only been seen in two Asian outbreaks in which women consumed cooking oil contaminated by polychlorinated biphenyls (PCBs) that were in turn contaminated with polychlorinated dibenzofurans (PCDFs); thus criteria include a history of exposure to these chemicals at high doses. The illness is called *Yusho* in Japan, and *Yucheng* in Taiwan; both words mean "oil disease". The syndrome has not been seen among workers exposed to "clean" PCBs or in the general population. There have not been any known exposures to PCDFs alone.

**Clinical Findings:** The most common and most distinctive physical findings are diffuse hyperpigmentation, pigmentation and hypoplasia of the nails, and meibomian gland hypertrophy and hypersecretion. Low birth weight is common; natal teeth, neonatal acne, and hyperbilirubinemia also occur. The syndrome is best described as an acquired ectodermal dysplasia, since a variety of ectodermal structures (hair, nails, teeth, pigment cells) can be affected.

Continued exposure after birth occurs if the child is breast-fed, since the chemicals are fat soluble and appear in the fat of breast milk. The syndrome has appeared as long as five years after exposure to the mother has ceased, since she stores the chemicals in fat tissue and does not excrete them well except into the fetus or into breast milk.

Follow-up information is available on less than 150 children. Of 39 affected children in Taiwan, eight died in the neonatal or perinatal period.

**Complications:** PCBs are toxic to the thymus and also concentrate to some degree in lung tissue, and thus these children suffer increased frequency of infections, especially of the skin and lower respiratory tract.

**Associated Findings:** Mild-to-severe developmental delay, the mechanism of which is unclear, and an associated behavioral disorder that may be secondary to the developmental effects.

**Etiology:** There is a clear causal relationship between ingestion of thermally degraded PCBs (which contain PCDFs) by a woman during or previous to pregnancy and the syndrome in her offspring. The specific roles of the PCBs, PCDFs, or individual isomers and congeners of the agents are not known.

**Pathogenesis:** Individual features of the syndrome reflect the varied toxicities of the chemicals. Some portion of the toxicity is thought to reflect the interaction with the aryl hydrocarbon hydroxylase receptor, but the role of receptor interaction in human toxicity is unclear.

**Sex Ratio:** M1:F1

**Occurrence:** Over 150 cases have been reported in two Asian outbreaks. There is probably a direct relationship to the dose of chemicals ingested by the mother and, to a lesser degree, to the proximity in time of the pregnancy to the exposure. The condition has not been observed outside of the documented outbreaks. There is high risk among affected women.

**Risk of Recurrence for Patient's Sib:** Pregnancies subsequent to one affected by exposure are less likely to be affected, and breast-feeding probably lowers subsequent risk (although it should nevertheless be avoided).

**Risk of Recurrence for Patient's Child:** For males, probably none. For females, there is a theoretic risk from stored chemical acquired prenatally and from breast-feeding.

**Age of Detectability:** During the newborn period.

**Gene Mapping and Linkage:** N/A

**Prevention:** Avoidance of exposure to PCBs or PCDFs.

**Treatment:** No successful treatment for primary condition. Standard treatment for associated conditions.

**Prognosis:** The growth deficit in the less severely affected children has moderated during school age, but in some cases the developmental delay and the ectodermal changes persist. Very few of the Japanese children, who were born in 1968 and after, have been followed. One hundred seventeen (of perhaps 130 alive) of the Taiwanese children are in follow-up, but the oldest of them was born in 1978.

**Detection of Carrier:** N/A

**Special Considerations:** PCBs and PCDFs are potent inducers of mixed function oxidase enzymes, and thus drug treatment of these children, particularly with anticonvulsants, must be monitored carefully. Breast-feeding is generally discouraged.

**References:**

Rogan WJ: PCBs and cola-colored babies: Japan, 1968, and Taiwan, 1979. Teratology 1982; 26:259–262.

Hara I: Health status and PCBs in blood of workers exposed to PCBs and of their children. Environ. Health Perspect 1985; 59:85–90.

Hsu ST, et al.: Discovery and epidemiology of PCB poisoning in

Taiwan: a four-year followup. Environ. Health Perspect 1985; 59:5–10.

Miller RW: Congenital PCB poisoning: a reevaluation. Environ. Health Perspect 1985; 60:211–214.

Lan SJ, Yen YY: Study of the effects of PCBs poisoning on the growth of primary school children [in Chinese; English summary]. Kaohsiung J Med Sci 1986; 2:682–687.

Lan SJ, et al.: The effects of PCB poisoning; a study of a transplacental Yu-Cheng baby: report of a case [in Chinese; English summary]. Kaohsiung J Med Sci 1987; 3:64–68.

Lan SJ, et al.: A study on the birth weight of transplacental Yu-Cheng babies [in Chinese; English summary]. Kaohsiung J Med Sci 1987; 3:273–282.

Rogan WJ, et al.: Congenital poisoning by polychlorinated biphenyls and their contaminants in Taiwan. Science 1988; 241:334–336.

Rogan WJ: Yucheng. In: Kimbrough RD, Jensen AA, eds: Halogenated biphenyls, terphenyls, naphthalenes, dibenzodioxins and related products, ed 2. New York: Elsevier/North Holland, 1989:401–417.

R0050                                           **Walter J. Rogan**

**Fetal face syndrome**
  *See ROBINOW SYNDROME*
**Fetal herpes infection**
  *See FETAL HERPES SIMPLEX VIRUS INFECTION*

---

## FETAL HERPES SIMPLEX VIRUS INFECTION          **2988**

**Includes:**
  Fetal herpes infection
  Herpes simplex virus infection, congenital
  Intrauterine herpes simplex virus infection

**Excludes:**
  **Fetal cytomegalovirus syndrome** (0381)
  **Fetal effects from varicella-zoster** (2499)
  Herpes simplex virus infection, intrapartum

**Major Diagnostic Criteria:** Vesicular rash present at birth or appearing shortly thereafter, **Microcephaly**, chorioretinitis, and microphthalmia. The diagnosis is best established by isolating herpes simplex virus, usually from skin vesicles.

**Clinical Findings:** Congenital abnormalities of the skin, central nervous system, and eyes are the most prominent features. An almost universal finding is a vesicular rash that is apparent at birth in the majority of patients or that may initially manifest within the first 3–5 days of life. The vesicular lesions may be localized to one area or, more commonly, may have a generalized distribution. Recurrent vesicular eruptions may occur in survivors. Other dermatologic features include bullous formation and cutaneous scars involving the face, scalp, trunk, or extremities, either of which may occur in about 10–15% of affected newborns.

About 60% of patients have **Microcephaly**. Intracranial cortical or periventricular calcifications occur in about 15% of cases, and these may be present at birth or detected later in infancy. Manifestations of extensive brain damage such as cerebral and cerebellar necrosis, brain atrophy, and **Hydranencephaly** are common and can be detected by computed tomography during the first week of life or at autopsy.

The most common ocular abnormalities are chorioretinitis (40–50%) followed by microphthalmia (25%). Lesions encountered less frequently include cloudy corneas, cataracts, and retinal dysplasia.

Two thirds of these patients are born prematurely, most after 32–37 weeks gestation. Intrauterine growth retardation is also found in about one fourth of all newborns. Hepatosplenomegaly with elevation of hepatic enzyme concentrations may be present. X-rays of the long bones may reveal metaphyseal lucencies or other abnormalities.

The diagnosis is best established by isolating the virus from one or more body sites such as skin vesicles, cerebrospinal fluid, or brain biopsy specimens. Infection is usually caused by herpes simplex virus type 2; infection by the type 1 virus has been reported in only five patients to date. Serologic tests are of limited value in this condition. Detection of viral antigens in tissue specimens or autopsy material by immunohistochemical techniques may be helpful in some cases.

**Complications:** Neonatal seizures are common (30%). Disseminated infection may develop in some patients. Calcifications of the skin, lungs, adrenal glands, liver, or umbilical cord may be present. Other potential complications include bacterial sepsis and respiratory distress syndrome.

**Associated Findings:** Absence of scalp skin, short digitis, hip dislocation, **Ductus arteriosus, patent**, hypoplastic kidney, **Hernia, inguinal**, and Dandy-Walker malformation have been rarely noted.

**Etiology:** Intrauterine infection with type 2 herpes simplex virus or, occasionally, type 1.

**Pathogenesis:** Herpes simplex virus can potentially infect the developing fetus by either crossing the placental barrier or ascending from an infected birth canal into the uterus. Observations supporting a transplacental route of transmission include the association of primary herpes simplex virus infection with viremia, the presence of herpetic placental lesions such as vesicles, infarcts, or necrotizing villous inflammation in some patients, and the demonstration that transplacental transmission occurs when animals such as rabbits or hamsters are experimentally infected. Some patients were born to mothers whose membranes had spontaneously ruptured hours to days prior to delivery, thus suggesting that an ascending infection had occurred. Rarely, patients with disease manifestations at birth are born to mothers with recurrent genital herpes, a condition not known to be associated with viremia in normal hosts and whose membranes remain intact until the time of delivery, thereby suggesting that the virus may be capable of causing an ascending infection across intact membranes. The congenital abnormalities in this condition are a direct result of intrauterine infection or its postinfectious residuals.

**MIM No.:** 14242, *14245

**Sex Ratio:** M1:F1.5 observed.

**Occurrence:** About 70 infants with this condition have been reported, almost all from the United States. Its true frequency is probably higher, since some cases are likely to go unrecognized while others may develop a severe intrauterine infection that results in a spontaneous abortion. By using immunohistochemical techniques for the detection of herpes simplex virus antigen, some investigators have shown that a latent form of this infection is very common in apparently normal placental tissues and in organs of neonates dying from a variety of unexplained problems such as cystic brain, interstitial pneumonia, and intrauterine growth retardation, although no viral cytologic abnormalities or positive viral cultures were observed in these tissues. This suggests that fetal herpetic infection may be much more common than currently believed.

**Risk of Recurrence for Patient's Sib:** Unknown. No cases in sibs have been reported.

**Risk of Recurrence for Patient's Child:** Unknown.

**Age of Detectability:** Abnormalities are present at birth. Occasionally, vesicles may not appear until 3–5 days of age.

**Gene Mapping and Linkage:** HV1S (herpes simplex virus type 1 sensitivity) has been inconsistently mapped to 3 or 11p11-qter.

Based on limited data, it appears that region 11p11-qter carries genes for host factors required for productive herpes simplex virus type 1 infection.

**Prevention:** None known. Genetic counseling indicated.

**Treatment:** Intravenous acyclovir or vidarabine should be used, because disseminated infection may occur.

**Prognosis:** The mortality rate is about 40%. About 40 to 50% of survivors will have significant long-term residual abnormalities such as psychomotor retardation, seizures, spasticity, deafness, or blindness.

**Detection of Carrier:** Genital cultures for herpes simplex virus will identify women who are asymptomatic shedders of this virus.

**Special Considerations:** Counseling pregnant women about intrauterine herpes simplex virus infection is complicated by the fact that fetal infection may follow primary or recurrent disease and can occur at any time in gestation. Only about one-third of cases have a history suggestive of maternal herpes infection during pregnancy. Isolation of the virus from amniotic fluid obtained at amniocentesis does not necessarily imply fetal infection. An accurate estimate of the risk of congenital malformations following maternal herpes infection during pregnancy is not currently possible but appears to be very small. Women at highest risk are those with primary infection during the first trimester.

### References:

Zervoudakis IA, et al.: Herpes simplex in the amniotic fluid of an unaffected fetus. Obstet Gynecol 1980; 55:16S–17S.

Francke U, Francke B: Requirement of the human chromosome 11 long arm for replication of herpes simplex virus type 1 in nonpermissive Chinese hamster X human diploid fibroblast hybrids. Somatic Cell Mol Genet 1981; 7:171–191.

Christie JD, et al.: Hydranencephaly caused by congenital infection with herpes simplex virus. Pediatr Infect Dis 1986; 5:473–478.

Harris HH, et al.: Intrauterine herpes simplex infection resembling mechanobullous disease in a newborn infant. J Am Acad Dermatol 1986; 15:1148–1155. †

Robb JA, et al.: Intrauterine latent herpes simplex virus infection: latent neonatal infection. Hum Pathol 1986; 17:1210–1217.

Hutto C, et al.: Intrauterine herpes simplex virus infections. J Pediatr 1987; 110:97–101. * †

Baldwin S, Whitley RJ: Teratogen update: intrauterine herpes simplex virus infection. Teratology 1989; 39:1–10. *

FR039
SE021

**Bishara J. Freij**
**John L. Sever**

---

## FETAL HYDANTOIN SYNDROME 0382

**Includes:**

    Dilantin^, fetal effects of
    Hydantoin anticonvulsants, fetal effects of
    Mephenytoin, fetal effects of
    Mesantoin^, fetal effects of
    Phenytoin, fetal effects of

**Excludes:** Fetal damage from other anticonvulsants

**Major Diagnostic Criteria:** Diagnosis may be considered in any infant exposed prenatally to hydantoin anticonvulsants. Hypoplasia of nails and distal phalanges with growth deficiencies have been the most consistent findings. Developmental delay, cleft lip and palate, and midfacial hypoplasia are consistent with the diagnosis.

**Clinical Findings:** The most consistent clinical manifestations have been prenatal and postnatal growth deficiency with evidence of nail hypoplasia and sometimes hypoplasia of the distal phalanges of both hands and feet. The most consistent dysmorphic features have included a flat nasal bridge with mild epicanthic folds, mild hypertelorism, and strabismus. Less commonly the philtrum is underdeveloped; there is mild webbing of the neck, ptosis, and cleft lip and palate. There is an increased frequency of low-arched digital dermal ridge patterns and occasionally, finger-like thumbs. The exact incidences of developmental delays and mental retardation are difficult to ascertain, but rates approximate 30% of children with findings of hydantoin teratogenesis. The presence of microencephaly places the child at a higher risk of having developmental disabilities.

**Complications:** Failure to thrive in infancy. Mild-to-moderate mental retardation in approximately one-third of the affected individuals.

**Associated Findings:** Cardiac, genital-urinary tract, and central nervous system anomalies.

**Etiology:** Maternal exposure to hydantoin anticonvulsants.

**Pathogenesis:** Possible relationship to enzyme activity of epoxide hydrolase in the exposed fetus. Based on one case of heteropaternal twins, it appears that fetal metabolism of Dilantin is a significant contributing factor to the teratogenesis. Several investigators have suggested that epoxide hydrolase, an enzyme

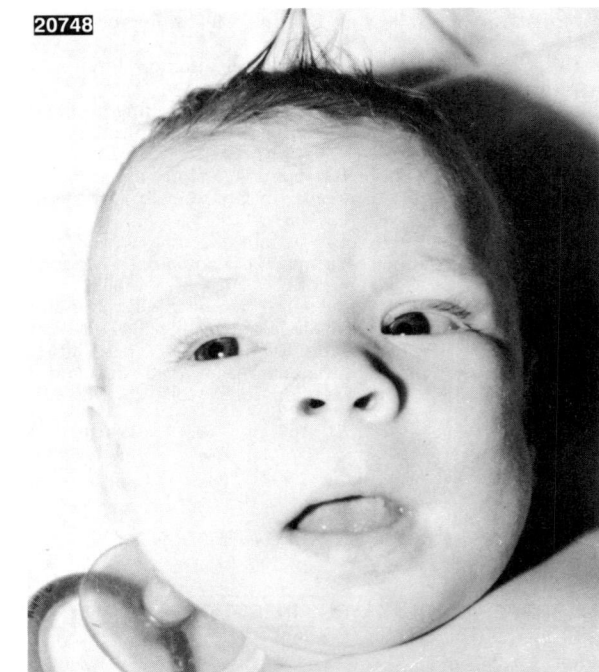

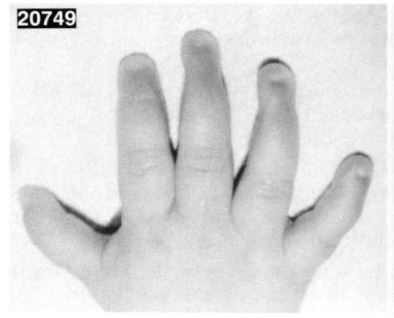 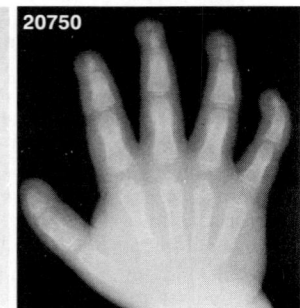

**0382-20748:** Fetal hydantoin syndrome; note epicanthal fold, short nose with broad depressed bridge and strabimus in this 3-month-old exposed to hydantoin in utero. **20749:** Distal hypoplasia of the nails and digits. **20750:** Narrow distal phalanges and hyperphalangism.

---

that converts the arene oxide form of hydantoin to a hydroxylated form, may be involved in the biochemical etiology. Individuals with clinical evidence of hydantoin teratogenesis have been demonstrated to have low leukocyte epoxide hydrolase and decreased fibroblast epoxide hydrolase activities. Unaffected sibs have shown higher epoxide hydrolase levels in comparison to their affected sibs.

**POS No.:** 3221

**CDC No.:** 760.750

**Sex Ratio:** M1:F1

**Occurrence:** The full pattern of abnormalities described for fetal hydantoin syndrome have been documented in approximately 7–10% of exposed infants. This figure includes growth retardation and distal digital hypoplasia as the most consistent features. Within the same family, there are documented cases of affected and unaffected sibs exposed to comparable maternal serum levels. This has led to the postulation that enzyme differences either fetal or fetal and maternal have determined which infant will show clinical symptoms of hydantoin teratogenesis.

**Risk of Recurrence for Patient's Sib:** Unknown.

**Risk of Recurrence for Patient's Child:** Minimal in the absence of maternal exposure to hydantoin anticonvulsants during pregnancy.

**Age of Detectability:** Possibly in utero based on growth retardation. Definitely at birth or during early infancy.

**Gene Mapping and Linkage:** Unknown.

**Prevention:** Avoidance of hydantoin anticonvulsants during pregnancy. Appropriate counseling of risks should be given prior to pregnancy, including information on the lack of confirmed safety with other antiepileptics with the possible exception of phenobarbital.

**Treatment:** Surgical correction of major defects may be necessary. Otherwise, educational intervention to maximize abilities.

**Prognosis:** Depends on severity of involvement.

**Detection of Carrier:** Levels of epoxide hydrolase have allowed experimental carrier testing.

**References:**

Hanson JW, Smith DW: The fetal hydantoin syndrome. J Pediatr 1975; 87:285.

Hanson JW, Buehler BA: Fetal hydantoin syndrome: current status. J Pediatr 1982; 101:816–818.

Phelan MC, et al.: Discordant expression of fetal hydantoin syndrome in heteropaternal dizygotic twins. N Engl J Med 1982; 307:99–101.

Finnell RH, Chernoff GF: Genetic background: the elusive component in the fetal hydantoin syndrome. Am J Med Genet 1984; 19:459–462.

Strickler SM, et al.: Genetic predisposition to phenytoin-induced birth defects. Lancet 1985; II:746–749.

BU007
HA028

Bruce A. Buehler
James W. Hanson

**Fetal hypothyroidism of extrinsic origin**
*See CRETINISM, ENDEMIC, AND RELATED DISORDERS*

## FETAL LITHIUM EFFECTS                                    2732

**Includes:**

Goiter with maternal lithium exposure, congenital
Ebstein anomaly with maternal lithium exposure
Eskatlith^, fetal effects
Lithium, fetal effects
Lithobid^, fetal effects
Lithone^, fetal effects

**Excludes:** Tricuspid valve, Ebstein anomaly (0332)

**Major Diagnostic Criteria:** Ebstein anomaly or congenital goiter with history of maternal lithium exposure.

**Clinical Findings:** Teratogenic findings in animals exposed to lithium led to concern for possible human teratogenicity since its use began in the 1960s for managing manic-depressive psychosis. Although use has increased steadily, only limited pregnancy exposure data exist to assess risks. In an early Scandinavian Health Service study of 40 women with lithium therapy, two had malformations (neither had heart defects). A hospital study in Denmark found no defects among 18 exposed infants. In a more recent Swedish cohort study by Kallen and Tandberg (1983), four heart defects (none of these were Ebstein anomaly) occurred among 59 maternal exposures. A Food and Drug Administration (FDA) analysis of Michigan Medicaid data, no defects were identified among 14 maternal exposures. In another small cohort study based on outcomes of 50 maternal lithium exposures prospectively reported to the California Teratogen Information Center, two defects occurred: meningomyelocele and a **Hernia, inguinal.** No heart defects have been reported.

An early retrospective study of 118 exposed infants by Schou (1976) did not confirm any distinct risk. Nine defects were reported of which six were cardiovascular and two were **Tricuspid**

valve, **Ebstein anomaly.** Since that time, eight more cases of Ebstein anomaly have been reported with maternal lithium exposure. No Ebstein anomaly case has occurred in the cohort data limited to the studies described above. Although four heart defects were excessive in the first small cohort, there have been no heart defects in the additional small cohorts.

Case control studies have little power to detect lithium teratogenicity because of the infrequency of exposure in women who complete pregnancies. Limited data available to the FDA indicate that use is currently about 1:4,000 completed pregnancies. In United States epidemiologic data available to the FDA, no lithium exposures were identified among 2,500 cardiovascular defects.

The rarity of Ebstein anomaly (about 1:20,000 births) and nine reports with lithium exposure suggest an association. Even with a 50-fold relative risk, the attributable risk would be only 1:400 exposures. Other heart defects may also be associated, but the case exposure data suggest that the risk may be on the low side of the wide confidence limits provided by the limited cohort data.

Congenital goiters have been reported with two maternal lithium exposures (lithium is a known goitrogen).

**Complications:** Transient neonatal hypotonicity and cyanosis have been observed when lithium is continued until the time of delivery.

**Associated Findings:** A study of the births with maternal lithium exposure found 29% of births were premature, but large for the duration of gestation.

**Etiology:** Maternal exposure to lithium.

**Pathogenesis:** Unknown.

**Sex Ratio:** Undetermined but presumably M1:F1.

**Occurrence:** Ninety percent of births with maternal lithium exposure are likely to be normal. The frequency of Ebstein anomaly is likely to be less than 1%.

**Risk of Recurrence for Patient's Sib:** N/A

**Risk of Recurrence for Patient's Child:** N/A

**Age of Detectability:** Ebstein anomaly may be detectable by prenatal echocardiography.

**Gene Mapping and Linkage:** N/A

**Prevention:** Lithium should probably be used during pregnancy only in women who have had recent or recurrent mania and in those cases kept at a dosage less than 1 g daily, monitoring serologic levels if possible. Use should be suspended temporarily with signs of approaching labor to avoid toxic levels in the newborn.

**Treatment:** Unknown.

**Prognosis:** Depends on the severity of the cardiac lesion. In reported cases, these tend to be severe. In a follow-up of 67 babies born without defects who reached age five years, Schou (1976) found no increase in physical or mental problems.

**Detection of Carrier:** Unknown.

**Special Considerations:** Lithium pregnancy exposures should be reported prospectively to Motherisk, 555 University Avenue, Toronto, CANADA, M56 1X8, or by telephone to (416) 597–1500.

**References:**

Schou MA, et al.: Occurrence of goiter during lithium treatment. Br Med J 1968; 3:710–713.

Schou MA, et al.: Lithium in pregnancy: hazards to women given lithium during pregnancy and delivery. Br Med J 1973; 2:137–138.

Schou MA: What happened to lithium babies? A follow up study of children born without malformations. Acta Psychiatr Scand 1976; 54:193–197.

Weinstein M: Lithium treatment of women during pregnancy and in the post delivery period. In: Johnson FN, ed: Handbook of lithium therapy. Baltimore: University Park, 1980:421–429.

Allen LD, et al.: Prenatal echocardiography screening for Ebstein's anomaly in mothers on lithium therapy. Lancet 1982; II:857–856.

Kallen BA, Tandberg A: Lithium and pregnancy: a cohort study of manic depressive women. Acta Psychiatr Scand 1983; 68:1984–1989. *

Yoder MD, et al.: Infants of mothers treated with lithium during

pregnancy have an increased incidence of prematurity, macrosomia, and perinatal mortality. Pediatr Res (program issue) 1984.
Warkany J: Lithium. Teratology 1988; 38:293–297.
Cunniff CM, et al.: Pregnancy outcome in women treated with lithium. Teratology 1989; 39:447–448.

R0018                                                    Franz W. Rosa

## FETAL METHYLMERCURY EFFECTS                          2495

**Includes:**
  Methylmercury, organic, fetal effects of
  Minamata disease
  Organomercurials (phenyl and alkylmercury), fetal effects
  Hunter-Russell syndrome
**Excludes:**
  **Cerebral palsy** (2931)
  **Microcephaly** (0659)

**Major Diagnostic Criteria:** Grossly abnormal neurologic signs in the first weeks or months of life. The final diagnosis requires determining the type and level of mercury in biologic samples of urine, hair, and blood.

**Clinical Findings:** Based on data from two large epidemics in Japan and Iraq, methylmercury profoundly affects the developing fetal brain as well as the central nervous system. The signs and symptoms in 22 cases of prenatal methylmercury intoxication in Japan were mental disturbance, ataxia, gait impairment, and speech disturbances. Chewing and swallowing disturbances were also seen in all affected patients.

Other findings included increased tendon reflexes (82%), pathologic reflexes (54%), involuntary movement (73%), increased salivation (77%), and forced laughing (27%).

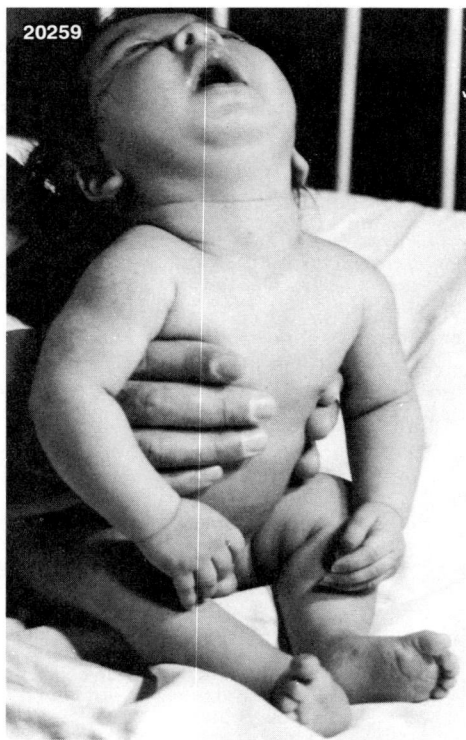

**2495-20259:** Note head lag, hypotonia and early signs of cerebral palsy in this 4-month-old infant with fetal methylmercury exposure.

In two separate studies in Iraq, blindness was found in five of 15 prenatally exposed infants and **Microcephaly** was detected in eight of 32 children who were examined over a five-year period after the poisoning.

Experimental studies on animal models have shown embryotoxic and teratogenic effects that were due to prenatal methylmercury poisoning. The predominant malformations and abnormal neurologic findings in prenatally exposed animal and human fetuses to methylmercury were **Cleft palate**, micrognathia, **Microcephaly**, and **Cerebral palsy**.

While there is overwhelming evidence in experimental animals and in man that short-chain alkylmercury compounds can pass through the placenta and are teratogenic to the fetus, there are no data implicating inorganic mercury in embrotoxicity. Moreover, Magos et al (1985) concluded that in rats, equimolar doses of ethylmercury compounds slowly decompose to inorganic mercury. In addition, the histochemical visualization of inorganic mercury showed no silver-mercury deposits in the granular layer, where the cerebellar damage was largely localized. Thus, inorganic mercury or dealkylation cannot be responsible for granular layer damage in alkylmercury intoxication.

**Complications:** By far the most common and severe complications of fetal methylmercury poisoning are those related to the central and peripheral nervous system. Although clinical improvement is possible, the damage to the nervous system is permanent. Marked improvement of ataxia, weakness, and visual and sensory changes were noticed in a follow-up study of 49 children poisoned with methylmercury in the 1971–1972 Iraqi epidemic.

**Associated Findings:** None known.

**Etiology:** Prenatal exposure to methylmercury.

**Pathogenesis:** Both Japanese and Iraqi autopsy examination revealed a reduction of brain size and major permanent disruption of the cerebral and cerebellar cytoarchitecture consisting of multiple nests of heterotopic neurons. These changes disrupt the normal synaptic circuitry in the brain, which may explain some of the behavioral or electrophysiologic defects reported in the victims.

**POS No.:** 4315

**Sex Ratio:** M1:F1

**Occurrence:** Related to prenatal exposure to methylmercury. Prevalence has been highest when heavy exposure to methylmercury occurred through ingestion of poisoned fish or inadvertent misuse of grain treated with the poison as a fungicide.

Since the 1971–1972 Iraqi epidemic of methylmercury poisoning, most countries have banned the use of the substance as a fungicide. Recent isolated cases have been due to accidental or suicidal ingestion.

**Risk of Recurrence for Patient's Sib:** Not increased in the absence of exposure.

**Risk of Recurrence for Patient's Child:** Not increased in the absence of exposure.

**Age of Detectability:** In the first weeks or months of life.

**Gene Mapping and Linkage:** N/A

**Prevention:** Avoid prenatal exposure to methylmercury.

**Treatment:** Partial removal of methylmercury from tissues may be achieved by administering drugs such as dimercaprol, penicillamine polythiol resin, selenium, and vitamin E. In addition, extracorporeal hemodialysis and/or exchange transfusion may be effective in removing methylmercury from the body.

**Prognosis:** Permanent nervous system damage.

**Detection of Carrier:** N/A

**Special Considerations:** Ethylmercury-treated grain was also reported to cause similar effects in ten offspring in Russia. Fetal mercury concerns are not limited to methyl and ethyl mercury, although these forms are particularly toxic. Other forms of mercury have caused fetal injury in all species tested, and are known to cause insidious neurotoxicity in humans. Human cases of pregnancy wastage and developmental retardation with maternal exposure to organic mercury compounds have been reported worldwide. As with lead, the fetus is particularly susceptible, but may not manifest injury until later in childhood. Exposure is through dental amalgamation; fish high in the food chain; mercury compound medicinals, spermicides, cosmetics, and soaps (use now curtailed in the United States); and occupational exposures from mercury catalysts and wastes in the pulp and paper factory, chlorine and caustic soda manufacturing, thermometer manufacturing, paint, ceramics, herbicides, fungicides, and electrical apparatus industries. Environmental exposure to toxic mercury appears to be increasing because of fossil fuel use, industrial wastes, and conversion to more toxic forms by methogenic bacteria in water.

Hunter & Russell (1954) report several detailed cases of focal cerebral and cerebellar atrophy due to adult industrial exposure to methylmercury compounds.

**References:**

Hunter D, et al.: Poisoning by methylmercury compounds. Quart J Med 1940; 130:193–213.
Hunter D, Russell DS: Focal and cerebellar atrophy in a human subject due to organic mercury compounds. J Neurol Neurosurg Psychiat 1954; 17:235–241.
Harada Y: Study group on Minamata disease. In: Katsuma M, ed: Minamata disease. Kumamoto: Japan University, 1968:92–121.
Amin-Zaki L, et al.: Perinatal methylmercury poisoning in Iraq. Am J Dis Child 1976; 130:1070–1076.
Amin-Zaki L, et al.: Methylmercury poisoning in Iraqi children: clinical observations over two years. Br Med J 1978; 1:613–616.
Amin-Zaki L, et al.: Prenatal methylmercury poisoning, clinical observation over five years. Am J Dis Child 1979; 133:172–177.
Elhassani SB: The many faces of methylmercury poisoning. J Toxicol Clin Toxicol 1983; 19:875–906. *
Magos L, et al.: The comparative toxicology of ethyl and methylmercury. Arch Toxical 1985; 57:260–267.
Melkonian R, Baker D: Risks of industrial mercury exposure in pregnancy. Obstet and Gynecol Rev 1989; 43:637–641.
Schardein JL, Keller K: Potential human developmental toxicants and the role of animal testing in their identification and characterization: mercury. CRC Critical Reviews in Toxicology 1989; 19:284–286.

EL013                                                    **Sami B. Elhassani**

---

## FETAL MONOZYGOUS MULTIPLE PREGNANCY DYSPLACENTATION EFFECTS                    2958

**Includes:**
Infarction defects in surviving monozygous twins
Intrauterine growth retardation (one type)
Intrauterine mortality in monozygous multiple pregnancies
Transfusion, twin-to-twin
Twin-to-twin transfusion

**Excludes:**
Intrauterine fetal defects from other causes
Intrauterine fetal developmental retardation from other causes
Intrauterine mortality from other causes

**Major Diagnostic Criteria:** Disparate weight for dates and developmental retardation sequelae in monozygous multiple births. Intrauterine mortality in one of monozygous twins with infarction-caused defects in the survivor.

**Clinical Findings:** Fetal developmental retardation in the lower weight member of twins born with disparate birth weights relates to discrepant placentation in monozygous twins. In addition, the developmentally retarded twin can be the consequence of blood loss through placental anastomoses. The smaller twin is born with findings and sequelae similar to other types of extrinsic intrauterine growth retardation. This donor member in twin-to-twin placental transfusion may be anemic. The recipient twin may be hyperemic. The degree of developmental retardation is proportional to the weight discrepancy at birth. Where IQ has been employed as a measurement, there are about two points deficit per 100 gms birth weight deficit compared to the "identical" twin.

Monozygotic twins have higher intrauterine mortality than dizygotic twins. Surviving members of monozygotic pairs have been observed to have defects apparently due to infarction, producing hydranencepaly or porencephaly, intestinal atreasia, renal cortical necrosis, **Kidney, horseshoe**, terminal limb defects, coronary thrombosis, cutis aplasia, and hemifacial microsomia (see **Oculo-auriculo-vertebral anomaly**).

**Complications:** In surviving monozygous pairs, a sudden twin-to-twin transfusion may take place at delivery, with acute congestive heart failure in the recipient. The donor may be in acute hemorrhagic shock. With sudden massive twin-to-twin transfusion, the recipient is at greater risk than the donor.

**Associated Findings:** Monozygotic twins have higher rates of several types of defects than dizygotic twins. Acardia is a defect unique to monozygous twinning.

**Etiology:** Unknown. Several instances of familial monozygotic twinning have been reported, and Derom et al (1987) suggested autosomal dominant inheritance for a subset of these cases.

**Pathogenesis:** Monozygous multiple births tend to be associated with disparate placentation. Monochorionic placental anastomoses allow one to transfuse the other. If one twin dies, transfusion of thromboplastin to the survivor may lead to infarction causing hyrdranencephaly or porencephaly, and other vascular obstruction-related defects.

**MIM No.:** 27641

**Sex Ratio:** M5.7:F1 (17 of 20 like-sexed twins with hydranencephaly/porencephaly were male).

**Occurrence:** Monozygous twinning is found in about 1:200 deliveries. Varying degrees of disparate birth weight related to placentation problems are found in a high proportion of monozygous twins, although milder degrees do not have easily measurable developmental sequelae. Although monozygous twins more frequently have defects than do singletons, denominators are limited to a few hundred monozygous twins in each of various studies, so the numbers for comparing specific defects are small. Dyzygous multiple births do not appear to have higher malformation rates than singletons except for those related to prematurity: **Hernia, inguinal, Ductus arteriosus, patent**, and undescended testicles. Often one twin (more likely monozygotic) "disappears" in early pregnancy. In a review of 188 monozygous twins, seven were associated with a recognized deceased twin. Two of the seven were reported to have a major brain problem.

**Risk of Recurrence for Patient's Sib:** The risk of recurrence of monozygotic twinning is about two-fold (or about 1%).

**Risk of Recurrence for Patient's Child:** Unknown.

**Age of Detectability:** Variable.

**Gene Mapping and Linkage:** Unknown.

**Prevention:** None known. Genetic counseling indicated.

**Treatment:** Unknown.

**Prognosis:** Follow-up studies of monozygous twins with markedly disparate birth weights show that the developmental retardation in the lower birth weight infant persists. Because of identical genetic endowment and similar postnatal environments, this finding has provided insights into the probable sequelae of other types of intrauterine growth retardation which cannot be studied with such perfect controls. Cases with hydranencephaly or porencephaly usually die in infancy.

**Detection of Carrier:** Unknown.

**Special Considerations:** For a possibly related disorder, see the pathogenesis of **Leukemia, acute lymphocytic, familial**.

**Support Groups:**
MD; Rockville; National Organization of Mothers of Twin Clubs
RI; Providence; The Twins Foundation

**References:**

Benirschke K: The pathology of the human placenta. New York: Springer-Verlag, 1974:187–236.
Myrianthopoulos NC: Congenital malformations in twins: epidemio-

logic survey. BD:OAS XI(8). New York: March of Dimes Birth Defects Foundation, 1975.

Melnick M: Brain damage in survivor after death of monozygotic co-twin. Lancet 1977; II:1287.

Hoyme HE, et al.: Vascular etiology of disruptive structural defects in monozygous twins. Pediatrics 1981; 67:288. *

Jung JH, et al.: Congenital hydranencephaly/porencephaly due to vascular disruption in monozygous twins. Pediatrics 1984; 73:467–9.

Derom C, et al.: Increased monozygotic twinning rate after ovulation induction. Lancet 1987; I:1236–1238.

R0018                                                          **Franz W. Rosa**

## FETAL MULTIPLE CYSTS ANOMALY                    2509

**Includes:**

    Cysts (multiple)
    Multiple cysts anomaly, abnormal karyotype other than 45,X
    Postmortem dermatolysis, multiple cysts

**Excludes:**

    Fetal hydrops
    Hygroma colli cysticum
    **Mesenteric cysts** (0645)
    **Michelin tire baby syndrome** (2642)
    Nuchal cysts syndrome with 45,X karyotype
    **Turner syndrome** (0977)

**Major Diagnostic Criteria:** Multiple cysts filled with fluid are seen in the affected fetus. Generalized subdermic edema and collection of fluid in the same space are common observations. Fetuses appear to have a skeletal dysplasia characterized by mildly shortened long bones and abnormally placed (downward) ribs, which are flatter than normal and produce a bell-shaped chest. Most fetuses have large effusions involving all the cavities of the body, most noticeably the peritoneal space. The cysts and the subdermic collection of fluid deform the fetal body, making it appear like the "Michelin man" with pronounced creases. The anomaly is probably due to a severe alteration of the fluid management by the fetal cardiovascular system and in many ways resembles anasarca in adults and the fetal hydrops seen in isoimmune fetal disease (although this does not show the formation of cysts). The skin is very thick due to the subdermic edema. The fetus usually dies before the 24th week of gestation, and it appears that the most likely cause is heart failure. The anomaly is very homogenous in its manifestations. Most affected fetuses look very much alike, but the disease is very heterogenous in the associated abnormalities, and probably in its etiology.

**Clinical Findings:** This anomaly is usually found by sonography without any maternal signs. The anomaly has a wide variation, which is already noted in the literature. The fetus has generalized edema, commonly associated with pleural, pericardial, and peritoneal effusions. As a consequence of the accumulation of fluid in the subdermic tissues, the fetus develops cystic cavities filled with fluid, producing a very typical appearance. The edema is more marked above the waist, with severe deformation of the head and neck. Most of these fetuses die during the second trimester, although a few of them live until the middle of the third. The amount of amniotic fluid remains normal in most cases. A few cases may be associated with polyhydramnios. The fetuses have a bell-shaped chest, which is smaller than normal. The lungs are hypoplastic and incompletely lobulated. The heart rhythm is normal, but it becomes bradycardic and dysrhythmic as the condition progresses and the accumulation of fluid becomes more noticeable. Probably the anomaly is more common than is recognized by sonography and by direct examination, because many of the affected will become unrecognizable due to postmortem changes.

**Complications:** Fetal death. Maternal eclampsia was present in one case.

**Associated Findings:** The anomaly could be divided in four groups regarding the presence of associated factors: 1) chromosomal abnormalities, i.e., **Chromosome 13, trisomy 13** and **Chromo-**

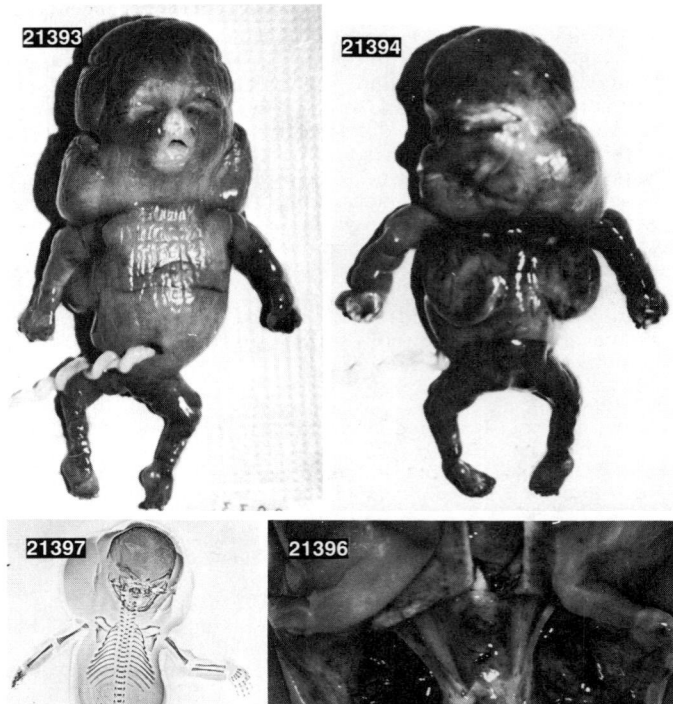

**2509**-21393–94: Fetuses with the recessive type of multiple cysts; note the generalized edema; the nuchal, cephalic and thoracic cysts. **21394**: Note the separation and clear differentiation between the nuchal and thoracic cysts. **21397**: Xeroradiograph of a fetus with the recessive type of multiple cysts; note the large nuchal cyst, generalized edema, the bell-shaped rib cage, the abnormal shape of the scapulae, the mildly shortened tubular bones and the flat, sharp metaphyses. **21396**: Internal aspect of the nuchal cysts; the cavities are formed by dissection of the subcutaneous planes creating a space between the subdermis and the muscular planes without the formation of vesicular sacs.

**some 21, trisomy 21**; 2) a group of multiple congenital malformation syndromes, i.e., **Pterygium syndrome, multiple** and **Roberts syndrome**; 3) consequences of postmortem dermatolysis; and 4) hydrops fetalis, which has recently been reported possibly to be associated with maternal and fetal infection by parvovirus B19, and produces generalized edema with pericardial, pleural, and peritoneal effusions. Two of the reported fetuses also had an aplastic crisis diagnosed by fetal blood sampling.

**Etiology:** Presumably heterogeneous. Probably a nonspecific anomaly when it occurs associated with other chromosomal abnormalities and with multiple congenital malformations. It is possible for several etiologic factors to produce a similar anomaly that may include an autosomal recessive gene, lytic changes following fetal death, infection by parvovirus B19. Although it has been proposed that some of the cases are due to an autosomal recessive gene, no definitive proof exists of the gene. The infectious etiology of fetal hydrops appears to be well established, but unfortunately descriptions of the fetuses are not clear enough to indicate how similar they are to those thought to have the recessive gene.

The postmortem dermatolysis and the formation of cysts is well documented in fetuses who did not have cysts or hydrops before death, but developed soon after dying. The cysts and fluid accumulation in these cases is not as dramatic as is seen in the supposedly recessive cases. Some of the known cases have been associated with other chromosomal abnormalities and inherited syndromes; this probably constitutes an indication that the hydrops and the cysts are the consequences of a common process that can occur in abnormal fetuses, perhaps in response to the abnormality affecting them.

**Pathogenesis:** If the three etiologic factors previously mentioned are correct, they could produce multiple cysts anomaly and hydrops fetalis by three different or by one common pathogenetic mechanism. In the case of the proposed autosomal recessive anomaly, probably a profound abnormality occurs in the fluid control by the cardiovascular system that allows for the accumulation of fluid from very early in gestation in the subcutaneous space, creating cystic cavities, generalized edema, and effusions, which probably are due to the terminal heart failure caused by the severe imbalance of fluid management seen in these fetuses.

In the cases of the fetuses infected by parvovirus and with fetal hydrops, evidence indicates that the virus not only colonizes all tissues but produces severe tissue alterations, including aplastic anemia and pronounced erythroblastic reaction, hepatitis, and eosinophilic changes in the hematopoietic cell nuclei. This virus is known to be present in asymptomatic blood donors and to induce aplastic crises in patients with sickle cell anemia and hereditary spherocytosis. The affected mother may have arthralgia with or without a rash, and the virus could produce erythema infectiosum, which was recognized in Scotland in the mothers of affected fetuses.

It has been shown that after the viral infection, the maternal serum alpha-fetoprotein was higher than normal. This may be an indication of the infection.

The possibility that the virus is a secondary or associated factor cannot be determined at this time. In this case an immunologically impaired fetus, if infected by the virus, will develop the anomaly, whereas an immunologically intact fetus will survive with minimal sequelae.

When it occurs as a postmortem change, it is due to dermatolysis of the subcutaneous tissue with the subsequent accumulation of fluid.

**Sex Ratio:** Presumably M1:F1

**Occurrence:** Common as a group, but prevalence is undetermined. In the case of the anomaly associated with parvovirus, seasonal occurrence is possible. The formation of postmortem cysts appears to be a common phenomenon after fetal death and is more noticeable on the posterior aspect of the neck, where it becomes evident soon after heart activity ceases. The exact pathogenetic mechanism is not known; it may involve a deposit of lymph due to an abnormal pattern of circulation after death.

**Risk of Recurrence for Patient's Sib:**

See Part I, *Mendelian Inheritance*. In the case of the infectious type, risk will depend on the recurrence of the condition in the population and the ability of the mother to mount an adequate defense. When associated with other chromosomal abnormalities and genetic syndromes, the risk of recurrence depends on the pattern of inheritance and etiology of the condition.

**Risk of Recurrence for Patient's Child:** Affected individuals are not expected to survive to reproduce.

**Age of Detectability:** The earliest detected case was at 11 weeks gestation. Ultrasonographic examination of the fetus has been the most reliable method of detection.

**Gene Mapping and Linkage:** Unknown.

**Prevention:** None known. Genetic counseling indicated.

**Treatment:** Unknown.

**Prognosis:** All known cases have died before completion of gestation.

**Detection of Carrier:** Unknown.

**Special Considerations:** While reported over the past 15 years, diagnosis of the anomaly is difficult to make. Those who probably have the recessive type appear to be phenotypically more similar to those who have other chromosomal abnormalities than to those

who have parvovirus infection, who look more like the fetuses with immune and nonimmune hydrops. The demonstration that the fetus is not infected by the virus and the presence of well-delineated large cysts involving the base of the neck and upper aspect of the back, and at times cysts on the extremities, speak of the recessive type. The presence of hydrops with prominent cysts and the demonstration of the virus, by viral cultures or by DNA analysis, favor the virus as the most likely etiology.

Special care should be taken when examining these fetuses not to assume that all of them have the 45,X karyotype; rather they may be associated with other factors, which should be clearly considered before a final diagnosis is made.

**References:**
van der Putte SCJ: Lymphatic malformation in human fetuses. Virchows Arch [Pathol Anat] 1977; 376:233–246.
Bieber FR, et al.: Prenatal detection of a familial nuchal bleb simulating encephalocele. BD:OAS XV(5A). New York: March of Dimes Birth Defects Foundation, 1979:51–61.
Chervenak FA, et al.: Cystic hygroma. New Engl J Med 1983; 309:822–825.
Elejalde BR, et al.: Nuchal cysts syndromes: etiology, pathogenesis and prenatal diagnosis. Am J Med Genet 1985; 21:417–432.

EL014                            **Maria Mercedes de Elejalde**
EL002                                 **B. Rafael Elejalde**

**Fetal paramethadione syndrome**
*See FETAL TRIMETHADIONE SYNDROME*

---

## FETAL PARVOVIRUS INFECTION        2980

**Includes:**
> Fifth disease
> Erythema infectiosum
> Parvovirus (B19)-induced fetal aplastic anemia-hydrops fetalis

**Excludes:**
> Erythroblastosis fetalis-hydrops (immunologic hydrops fetalis)
> **Fetal rubella syndrome** (0384)
> **Hydrops fetalis, non-immune** (2198)
> Hydrops fetalis-cytomegalovirus infection

**Major Diagnostic Criteria:** The fetal hydrops due to intrauterine parvovirus infection is associated with a severe anemia. Amphophilic and eosinophilic intranuclear inclusions are present in red cell progenitors, and excess iron is present in the liver. The diagnosis is confirmed by the presence of IgM-specific antibody to human parvovirus (B19) in the fetal serum and by identifying parvovirus DNA in the fetal tissues using a radiolabeled or biotin labelled DNA probe.

**Clinical Findings:** Human specific parvovirus causes erythema infectiosum. Infections in adults may be subclinical and atypical. Transplacental infection can occur at any time during pregnancy. Of 26 deaths due to B19 hydrops fetalis, 17 were at 10–20 weeks, seven at 20–30 weeks, and two were over 30 weeks.

Fetal infection results in abortion, stillbirth, or neonatal death if hydrops fetalis develops. Hydrops fetalis is the most frequent abnormality and is associated with a severe fetal anemia, which has been shown by cord blood sampling to be aplastic in type. There is also a nonimmunologic hemolytic anemia with excess iron in the fetal liver and occasional liver damage. Raised levels of alpha-fetoprotein in the maternal serum have been reported in five of six cases developing hydrops fetalis. Histologic examination shows amphophilic and eosinophilic inclusions in red cell progenitors (probably late normoblasts). Electron microscopy shows the amphophilic inclusions to contain viral particles. Pronormoblasts, myeloblasts, and myelocytes are increased and are detected in many organs. Excessive iron deposition is present in the liver. The diagnosis is confirmed by the presence of IgM-specific antibody to human parvovirus in the fetal serum. Dot hybridization and radio/biotin labeled human parvovirus DNA probes will reveal viral DNA in fetal tissues, even if they have been preserved in formaldehyde solution and embedded in paraffin wax.

Childhood cases are characterized by fever for several days, which drops concurrently with eruption of a generalized rash, most prominent on the face. More than one-third of pregnant women are susceptible to the infection. As with rubella, susceptible pregnant women are likely to be infected from exposure to childhood cases in epidemics.

**Complications:** All recorded cases of fetal hydrops due to parvovirus have been fatal unless treated by transfusion.

**Associated Findings:** Polyhydramnios, hepatosplenomegaly, liver disease including neonatal hepatitis (one case). A single case with transplacental infection at six weeks gestation has shown myocarditis, myositis, and ocular malformations similar to those in **Fetal rubella syndrome**. A large study had previously failed to reveal an increased incidence of antibodies to human parvovirus in malformed infants.

**Etiology:** Caused by human-specific parvovirus, which is a single-strand DNA virus, the virus particle being 22 nm in size.

**Pathogenesis:** The virus crosses the placenta during maternal viremia, which occurs even in asymptomatic maternal infection. It has a special affinity for rapidly dividing cells, particularly the red cell precursors. The late normoblasts appear to be those most severely infected. As the virus inhibits host cell multiplication, it produces maturation arrest, causing a reticulocytopenia and aplastic anemia. Parvoviruses destroy the host cell, and it is this cytolysis of normoblasts that results in increased iron in the liver. The severe anemia produces fetal cardiac failure (i.e., hydrops fetalis). The fetus is susceptible to B19-induced anemia because it has both a short red cell lifespan and hyperplastic erythropoiesis. It increases its red cell mass 34-fold between the third and sixth months; the same period during which hydrops is most common.

The virus also damages hepatocytes and probably other rapidly reduplicating tissues. It has been detected within myocardial cells. Culture of the virus is difficult, but it will replicate in bone marrow cultures rich in erythroid progenitors. It requires cellular factors present only in the S-phase of mitosis.

**Sex Ratio:** M1:F1

**Occurrence:** Depends on the prevalence of parvovirus infection in the community. During an epidemic, a small series indicated that 30% of fatal hydrops fetalis cases of previously unknown etiology were due to parvovirus infection in utero.

At least 26 fatal hydrops cases have been reported, 16 in the United Kingdom and Europe, ten in the United States. The number of infected live-born infants is undetermined.

The risk to the fetus in maternal infection is variable. Two large studies have indicated that it is low (10%). Smaller series studying maternal parvovirus infection in pregnancy suggest that 20–30% of these mothers suffered abortion or intrauterine death. The remaining mothers delivered apparently normal infants. None of these infants had IgM-specific antibodies to parvovirus at birth, so it is possible that transplacental infection had not occurred in these pregnancies. However, follow-up indicated that 50% (4/7) were persistent secretors of IgG-specific antibody even at age 15 months. If persistent IgG-specific antibody indicates in utero infection then transplacental infection rates may be as high as 60%, with a lethal outcome in one-half of these.

**Risk of Recurrence for Patient's Sib:** None (the mother is henceforth immune).

**Risk of Recurrence for Patient's Child:** Related to parvovirus exposure.

**Age of Detectability:** At birth, or antenatally by scan.

**Gene Mapping and Linkage:** N/A

**Prevention:** No vaccine is currently available to prevent maternal infection.

**Treatment:** Possibly exchange transfusion in utero to correct anemia.

**Prognosis:** All cases of untreated parvovirus-induced hydrops fetalis have resulted in death. The proportion of infected fetuses to survive is undetermined. Long-term follow-up is required to exclude late teratogenic effects in fetuses born to infected mothers. This is especially important in those infants with persistently raised specific IgG levels at age 12 months, as these infants were probably infected in utero.

**Detection of Carrier:** Parvovirus infection in pregnant women.

**Special Considerations:** Only 50–75% of pregnant women are immune to B19. Any pregnant women in contact with B19, or who develop a rash known not to be rubella, should have her specific antibodies to B19 (IgM and IgG) measured (at the Centers for Disease Control in the United States, or PHLS, London, in the United Kingdom). This will establish her immune status and exclude or confirm recent B19 infection. If this diagnostic test is unavailable, ultrasound examination of the fetus should be carried out to exclude hydrops fetalis. Raised alphafetoprotein levels have been reported in hydropic cases and could also be monitored.

All aborted, stillborn, or hydropic infants born during an epidemic of erythema infectiosum should be assessed for fetal parvovirus infection. This is necessary to assess the actual risk this virus poses to human pregnancy.

**References:**

Mortimer PP, et al.: Human parvovirus and the fetus. Lancet 1985; II:1012 only. *
Anand A, et al.: Human parvovirus infection in pregnancy and hydrops fetalis. New Engl J Med 1987; 316:183–187. * †
Gray ES, et al.: Human parvovirus and fetal anaemia. Lancet 1987; I:1144 only.
Weiland HT, et al.: Parvovirus B19 associated with fetal abnormality. Lancet 1987; I:682–683. †
Rodis JF, et al.: Human parvovirus infection in pregnancy. Obstet Gynecol 1988; 72:733–738.
Schwarz TF, et al.: Human parvovirus B19 in pregnancy. Lancet 1988; 2:566–567.
Centers for Disease Control: Risk associated with human parvovirus B19 infection. MMWR 1989; 38:81–88. (reprinted in J Am Med Asso 1989; 261:1406- 1408, 1555–1563) *
Metzman R, et al.: Hepatic disease associated with intrauterine parvovirus infection in a newborn premature infant. J Pediatr Gastroenterol Nutr 1989; 9:112–114.

GR037                                                    **Elizabeth Gray**

---

## FETAL PRIMIDONE EMBRYOPATHY                              2982

**Includes:**
Mysoline, fetal effects of
Phenytoin-type embryopathy
Primidone, fetal effects of

**Excludes:** Fetal hydantoin syndrome (0382)

**Major Diagnostic Criteria:** Craniofacial dysmorphology similar to that found in **Fetal hydantoin syndrome**, cleft lip and/or cleft palate, and cardio-aortic defects.

**Clinical Findings:** Experience is limited for primidone, since it is less commonly used than phenytoin, phenobarbital, and carbamazepine, and is usually used in combination with other antiepilepics. Primidone is structurally related and partially metabolized to phenobarbital.

Forty-three unpublished or published reports of major births defect outcomes with maternal primidone exposure (mostly without exposure denominators) are available to the United States Food and Drug Administration. Any conclusions based upon this data must be regarded as suggestive only, since they a based upon anecdotal reports and not upon the results of systematic research. Nevertheless, of these report, fifteen are with monotherapy. Defects reported include phenytoin type dysmorphia (four cases with monotherapy, as well as additional cases with combination therapy), **Cleft lip** and **Cleft palate** (eight cases, all combination), **Cleft palate** (two monotherapy), **Aorta, coarctation** (three mono, one combination), dextrocardia (two mono), miscellaneous or unspecified heart defects (five combinations), gastroschisis, **Microcephaly** (two combinations), **Anencephaly** (one mono), **Oculo-auriculo-vertebral anomaly** (one mono), and neonatal hemorrhages (two mono). Two cases of spina bifida have been reported among 344 cohort exposures, but one of these was confounded by concurrent valproic acid and carbamazepine, either of which appear to be independently associated with spina bifida.

**Complications:** As with other diole and triole exposures, hemorrhagic disease of the newborn has been observed.

**Associated Findings:** None known.

**Etiology:** Primidone exposure, either as monotherapy or in combinations, possibly with genetic susceptibility.

**Pathogenesis:** Undetermined. As with phenytoin and barbiturates, the teratogen is possibly an epoxide metabolite, in genetically slow epoxide metabolizers. Folic acid interference is another possible factor. Probably dose related. Possibly related to increased epoxide production from concurrent exposure enzyme induction of the agent and its primary metabolites. Depression of vitamin K dependent clotting factors is suspected to cause hemorrhagic risks.

**Sex Ratio:** M1:F1

**Occurrence:** Most defect reports lack exposure denominators from which frequency of occurrence can be obtained. Nine exposure cohorts totaling 344 exposures include mostly combinations so that it is not possible to separate the teratogenicity of primidone from concurrent exposures. The most careful cohort study, by Rating et al (1982), showed an increased frequency of minor dysmorphic features and microcephaly, especially among combinations, but also observed with monotherapy.

**Risk of Recurrence for Patient's Sib:** Presumably increased with primidone exposure.

**Risk of Recurrence for Patient's Child:** Unknown.

**Age of Detectability:** Cranial dysmorphy and some other defects can be detected prenatally. Functional neurologic defects may not be recognized at birth.

**Gene Mapping and Linkage:** Unknown.

**Prevention:** Monotherapy may be safer than combinations if adequate to control seizures. Evidence is inadequate to show other antiepileptic exposures are safer than primidone. Vitamin K should be administered parturitionally to decrease hemorrhagic risks.

**Treatment:** Surgical repairs where feasable.

**Prognosis:** Usually good. Mental retardation is unusual.

**Detection of Carrier:** Tests for slow epoxide metabolizers are available.

**References:**
Rudd NL, Freedom RM: A possible primidone embryopathy. J Pediatr 1979; 94:835–837.
Majewski R, et al.: The teratogenicity of hydantoins and barbiturates in humans, with considerations on the etiology of malformations and cerebral disturbances in the children of epileptic parents. Int J Biol Res Pregnancy 1981; 2:37–45.
Myhre SA, Williams R: Teratogenic effects associated with maternal primidone therapy. J Pediatr 1981; 99:160–163.
Rating D, et al.: Teratogenic and pharmcacokinetic studies of primidone during pregnancy and in the offspring of epileptic women. Acta Paediatr Scand 1982; 71:301–315.
Kraus CM, et al.: Four siblings with similar malformations after exposure to phenytoin and primidone. J Pediatr 1984; 105:750–755.
Cohen A, Mudel G: The fetal primidone syndrome. Harefuah 1988; 114:171–173.

**Franz W. Rosa**

## FETAL RADIATION SYNDROME                                   0383

**Includes:**
  Radiation, fetal effects of
  Radiation embryopathy
  Radiation teratogenesis
  Radon gas, fetal effects of

**Excludes:** Radiation prior to conception, fetal effects of

**Major Diagnostic Criteria:** Radiation embryopathy consists of severe mental retardation, usually with small head circumference. There are no pathognomonic features. The relationship to ionizing radiation exposure is revealed only through epidemiologic study which shows that the rate for the effect exceeds normal expectations.

**Clinical Findings:** Inability to perform simple calculations, to make simple conversation, or to care for oneself. The radiation dose received should be determined as accurately as possible. The data from study of Japanese survivors exposed prenatally to the automic bomb show the effect primarily when exposure occurred at 8–15 weeks of gestational age. There appears to be a threshold at 20–40 rads, possibly above 50 rads. Such exposures are far above those from diagnostic radiology. MRI reveals jumbled islands of ectopic cerebral cortex. Supporting observations concerning exposure level may be provided through biodosimetry; e.g., dicentric chromosomes or increased somatic cell mutation in blood cells. Small head size is seen ten times more often than severe mental retardation, at doses as low as 10–19 rad.

**Complications:** Leukemia may also be induced at the same level of exposure. If a child is seen with leukemia and severe mental retardation or small head size, inquiry should be made about exposure to ionizing radiation at 8–15 weeks of gestational age.

**Associated Findings:** Changes in the posterior capsule of the ocular lens; i.e., a polychromatic sheen seen on slit-lamp examination.

**Etiology:** Exposure to sufficient doses of ionizing radiation from radiotherapy, or accidental exposure, as from nuclear reactors, or from nuclear weapons.

**Pathogenesis:** Severe mental retardation is due to disturbance in the development and function of neurons which normally migrate from near the ventricles to the cerebral cortex at 8–15 weeks of gestational age. Small head circumference without mental retardation may occur as an effect of lesser doses, or early in gestation, from destruction of glial cells.

**Sex Ratio:** M1:F1

**Occurrence:** Severe mental retardation among Japanese atomic-bomb survivors exposed at 8–15 weeks of gestational age occurred as follows:

### Severe Mental Retardation by Radiation Exposure

| Absorbed dose (rad) | Number exposed | Number affected |
| --- | --- | --- |
| 100+ | 9 | 6 |
| 50–99 | 13 | 4 |
| 10–49 | 50 | 4 |
| 1–9 | 69 | 3 |
| Controls | 257 | 2 |

This disorder has been observed only after therapeutic or heavy accidental radiation exposure.

In several studies, the relative risk of leukemia after intrauterine exposure late in gestation was 1.5.

**Risk of Recurrence for Patient's Sib:** Related to maternal exposure to radiation during each pregnancy.

**Risk of Recurrence for Patient's Child:** Related to maternal exposure to radiation during pregnancy.

**Age of Detectability:** Small head size is detectable at birth, and mental retardation is recognizable during the first year of life.

**Gene Mapping and Linkage:** N/A

**Prevention:** Avoidance of radiation exposures during early pregnancy. Therapeutic abortion should *not* be recommended following diagnostic abdominal radiation, since the increased risk, if any, to the fetus is extremely small.

**Treatment:** Persons with radiation-induced anomalies should avoid additional radiation exposures, which may be incompletely additive with regard to leukemogenesis among other late effects.

**Prognosis:** Retardation of intelligence may be minimal to severe.

**Detection of Carrier:** N/A

**Special Considerations:** There has recently been renewed public concern regarding the possible fetal effects of natural radon gas within homes and public buildings. Inhalation of radon can induce lung cancer in adults. Because inhaled radon particles do not penetrate beyond the pregnant woman's lungs, there would be no effect on the fetus.

**Support Groups:** CA; Berkeley; National Association of Radiation Survivors (NARS)

**References:**
Brent RL. Radiation teratogenesis. Teratol 1980; 21:281–298.
Monson RR, MacMahon B: Prenatal X-ray exposure and cancer in children. Prog Cancer Res Ther 1984; 26:97–105.
Otake M, Schull WJ: In utero exposure to A-bomb radiation and mental retardation: a reassessment. Br J Radiol 1984;57:409–414.
Miller RW: Effects of prenatal exposure to ionizing radiation. in Koval TM (ed): Some Issues Important In Developing Basic Radiation Protection Recommendations. Bethesda, Maryland, National Council on Radiation Protection and Measurements. March 1, 1985:62–74.
A report of a Task Group of Committee I of the International Commission on Radiological Protection: Developmental effects of irradiation of the brain of the embryo and fetus. ICRP Public 1986; 49:1–43. *
Miller RW, Boice JD Jr: Radiogenic cancer after prenatal or childhood exposure. in Upton AC, et al (eds): Radiation Carcinogenesis. New York, Elsevier North-Holland, 1986:379–386. *
Miller RW: Prenatal effects of exposure to ionizing radiation. J Washington Academy of Science 1988; 78:94–100.
Yoshimoto Y, et al.: Risk of cancer among children exposed in utero to A-bomb radiations, 1950–84. Lancet 1988; II:665–669.
Committee on the Biological Effects of Ionizing Radiations: Health effects of exposure to low loevels of ionizing radiation. BEIR V. Washington, D.C.: National Academy Press, 1990:352–362. *

MI035                                          **Robert W. Miller**

## FETAL RETINOID SYNDROME                                    2261

**Includes:**
    Accutane^, fetal effects of
    Etretinate, fetal effects of
    Facial palsy, congenital with exposure to retinoids
    Hypervitaminosis A, fetal effects from
    Isotretinoin, fetal effects of
    Microtia from exposure to retinoids
    Retinoic acid syndrome
    Retinoic fetal effects, experimental in animals
    Tegison^, fetal effects of
    Thymic agenesis from maternal exposure to retinoids
    Vitamin A megadose, retinol or retinaldehyde fetal effects
      of

**Excludes:** N/A

**Major Diagnostic Criteria:** Maternal exposure to isotretinoin, (Accutane^, 13-cis retinoic acid), etretinate (Tegison^), and pos-

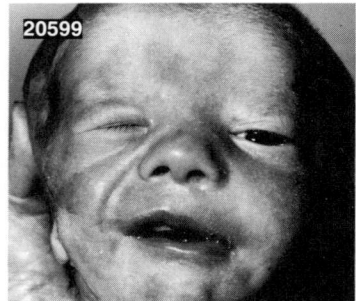 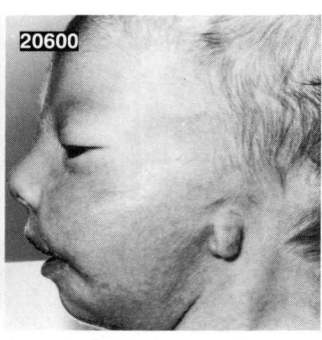

**2261-20599–20600:** Fetal retinoid syndrome in an infant exposed to 80 mg daily through 6 weeks of pregnancy; note left facial paralysis, ear tags, hypoplastic orbital ridges, sloping forehead, micrognathia and short nose. The external auditory canal is absent. In addition, this child had cleft palate, dysplastic pulmonary and aortic valves, enlarged scrotal sac, left simian crease, and decreased muscle mass in the limbs.

sibly to teratogenic dosage of vitamin A or other vitamin A congeners during pregnancy.

Characteristic findings in affected infants include low-set, small or absent external ears and canals; enlarged cerebral ventricles, **Microcephaly** or **Hydrocephaly**, facial palsy, thymic hypoplasia, and cardio-aortic defects.

**Clinical Findings:** From 1983 through 1988, 86 pregnancy outcomes with one or more of the characteristic findings have been reported with maternal isotretinoin exposures during pregnancy. Bilateral small or absent, low-set ears and canals is the most unique finding, since this is rare (although it has been seen in **Fetal thalidomide syndrome**). Most infants with microtia had unusual facies, with micrognathia, broad nose, and **Eye, hypertelorism**, as well as downward slanting, small palpebral fissures. **Cleft palate** has also been observed.

Central nervous pathology usually consists of dilated cerebral ventricles, usually with **Microcephaly** sometimes developing into moderate **Hydrocephaly**. This was described as lissencephaly in one case and as **Hydranencephaly** in another. Many of the patients have also had a posterior fossa cyst. Facial nerve palsy has also been reported. Several infants had oculomotor paralysis. Thymic aplasia accompanying all three major features has been reported in one infant. Microphthalmia was reported in two patients. At least one isotretinoin outcome was holoprosencephaly. Forty-one spontaneous abortions temporally related to maternal isotretinion exposure have been reported. Usually tissue was insufficient for morphologic examination. Absence of the ears was described in one induced abortion.

Three outcomes of pregnancies with hypervitaminosis A exposure have also been reported with microtia and abnormal facies. One of these was described as having **Oculo-auriculo-vertebral anomaly** with bilateral low, hypoplastic ears, atresia of the canals, right facial hemiatrophy, facial palsy, downward slanting palpebral fissures, micrognathia and bilateral epibulbar dermoids. Another of the infants with microtia had **Cleft palate** and **Cleft lip**. None of these three infants had heart or brain pathology. Cases with heart defects and **Cleft palate**, **Microcephaly**, holoprosencephaly, and **Sirenomelia sequence** have also been reported.

Topical retinoic acid (tretinoin, Retin-A^), has been presumed to be nonteratogenic because of the small dose absorbed (less than 0.5 mg daily) and because this has no measurable impact on serum levels. Because of the frequency of topical tretinoin exposure, many defects will occur by chance, and the small proportion reported are likely to be biased towards those resembling the isotretinoin experience. Three holoprosencephaly cases have been spontaneously reported to the FDA with maternal topical tretinoin exposure. Case control exposure studies are being explored to see if this is possibly a rare but actual increased risk.

Eleven infants born following maternal exposure to another retinoic acid derivative, etretinate (Tegison^ (Roche)), marketed for treating psoriasis), had craniofacial, nervous system and skeletal defects. Microtia was reported in one of these cases. Three of the neurologic defects were **Meningomyelocele**.

Parallel findings were produced experimentally in primates with retinoic acid, and in small animals by retinol (vitamin A), retinoic acid, isotretinoin, and etretinate.

**Complications:**  Sudden unexplained death has been reported in two infants with maternal isotretinoin exposure.

**Associated Findings:**  Cortical blindness has been present in several of the cases with micro/hydrocephaly. Auditory nerve injury was mentioned in only one case, and in others with microtia, auditory nerve function was apparently present, or not evaluated.

**Etiology:**  Vitamin A and its congeners have long been known to be teratogens in small animals. Retinoic acid 7.5 to 40 mg/kg day tested in 21 monkeys with term outcomes, produced cranio/facial defects in 19 of 21 exposed, microtia in 12, nervous system pathology in four, and defects of the extremities in seven. A cardio-aortic defect was described in one monkey, thymic agenesis in another. Isotretinoin (an isomer of retinoic acid) and etretinate (an aromatic retinoid) are prescribed systemically in humans, both with teratogenic warnings. The warning was strengthened with the information on human teratogenicity as quickly as this was observed in inadvertent maternal exposures. Isotretinoin has been associated with malformations in dosages of as little as 20 mg/day or more continued beyond the second week of embryogenesis. Retinoic acid, and to a lesser extent isotretinoin, are natural metabolites of vitamin A. Maternal exposures to high dosages of vitamin A are under little surveillance. The few adverse outcomes reported are too few to evaluate the relative role of retinol or its metabolites. Adverse outcomes with vitamin A involved exposures of 40,000 to 150,000 units per day for several months or more.

Creech Kraft et al (1989) reported that retinoic acid levels in an embryo were found to be several hundred times those in the sera following a maternal exposure to 50 mg isotretinoin daily discontinued three days before an induced abortion. Comparison determinations of retinoid levels in abortuses relative to maternal levels would be important in those 1) not exposed to therapeutic retinoids, 2) with maternal megadosages of vitamin A, 3) etretinate, and 4) spontaneous abortions incidental to topical tretinoin use.

**Pathogenesis:**  Undetermined. Vitamin A and derivatives are anoxidents and regulators of cellular development. Embryotoxic exposure may inhibit development of ectodermal and underlying mesodermal derivatives of the upper end of the neural crest.

**POS No.:**  3624

**Sex Ratio:**  M1:F1

**Occurrence:**  Among first trimester isotretinoin exposures continuing to term, about 23% will manifest this syndrome. The teratogenic proportion of those continuing the exposure beyond the missed menstrual period is higher than in those discontinuing the exposure prior to the missed menstrual period. Reported cases are assumed to represent only a fraction of actual occurrences.

**Risk of Recurrence for Patient's Sib:**  Presumably none in the absence of first trimester exposure.

**Risk of Recurrence for Patient's Child:**  Presumably none in the absence of first trimester exposure.

**Age of Detectability:**  Dilated cerebral ventricles may be detectable by prenatal sonograph. Less characteristic cases may escape detection at birth.

**Gene Mapping and Linkage:**  N/A

**Prevention:**  Isotretinoin and etretinate should be used with great caution, if at all, in fertile females. Every precaution should be taken to avoid pregnancy while taking isotretinoin, and to avoid taking isotretinoin while pregnant. Unlike isotretinoin, which has a half life of less than a day, etretinate and retinol have half lives of several months, and are stored and cumulative. Although their teratogenicity is less defined, pregnancy should be avoided within a year of exposure to etretinate. Although exposures to vitamin A beyond the recommended 5,000 units daily should be avoided, teratogenic observations have been insufficient to define risks with higher exposures.

**Treatment:**  Unknown.

**Prognosis:**  One-third of the outcomes involving birth defects have been fatal in the perinatal period. Survivors have had severe neurologic impairment and blindness. Less severe forms exist, but have not been sufficiently identified to determine their frequency and prognosis unless in follow-up of an identified exposure.

**Detection of Carrier:**  N/A

**Special Considerations:**  Although normal infants have been reported following maternal isotretinoin exposure, some were not exposed beyond the second week of embryogenesis, or were exposed to less than 0.5 mg/kg day. Difficulties defining the onset of pregnancy makes timing imprecise. Hypervitaminosis A exposure is difficult to define, and has not been under pharmaceutical surveillance. Milder degrees of central nervous system injury and isolated cardiac finding are indistinctive markers to associate with exposures, because of their frequency, even without exposure, and the unlikelihood of careful retrospective investigation when they do occur.

Any exposures to isotretinoin or etretinate, or to dosage of vitamin A exceeding 25,000 units daily should be prospectively reported to the Division of Epidemiology and Surveillance of the Food and Drug Administration, Rockville, MD, for evaluation and follow-up. Unusual birth defects occurring with topical retinoic acid exposure should also be reported. First trimester maternal retinol and retinoic acid level exposures should also be reported, along with periconceptional exposures to megadose vitamin A, isotretinoin, and etretinate. Consideration should be given to obtaining and reporting immediate fetal retinoid levels in any abortions with retinoid exposures.

**References:**

Shenefelt RE: Morphogenesis of malformations in hamsters caused by retinoic acid: relation to dose and stage of treatment. Teratology 1972; 5:103–118.

Fantel AG, et al.: Teratogenic effects of retinoic acid in pigtail monkeys. l. general features. Teratology 1977; 15:65–72.

Rosa FW: Teratogenicity of isotretinoin. Lancet 1983; 2:513 only.

Fernoff PM, Lammer EJ: Craniofacial features of isotretinoin embryopathy. J Pediatr 1984; 105:595–597.

Lammer EJ, et al.: Retinoic acid embriopathology. New Engl J Med 1985; 313:837–841.

Rosa FW, et al.: Teratogen update: Vitamin A consequences. Teratology 1986; 33:355–364.

Teratology Society: Recommendations for vitamin A use during pregnancy. Teratology 1987; 35:269–275.

Lammer EJ, et al.: Unusually high risk for adverse outcomes for pregnancy following fetal isotretinoin exposure. Am J Hum Genet 1988; 43(suppl):A58 only.

Abbott BD, et al.: Etiology of retinoic acid-induced cleft palate varies with the embryonic stage. Teratology 1989; 40:533–553.

Boyd AS: An overview of the retinoids. Am J Med 1989; 86:568–574.

Creech Kraft J, et al.: Human embryro retinoid concentrations after maternal intake of isotretinoin. New Engl J Med 1989; 321:262.

R0018                                                    **Franz W. Rosa**

---

**FETAL RUBELLA SYNDROME**                               **0384**

**Includes:**
    Rubella malformation syndrome
    Expanded rubella syndrome
    Gregg syndrome

**Excludes:**
    Cataract and sensorineural hearing loss, other causes
    **Fetal parvovirus infection** (2980)
    **Microcephaly** (0659)

**Major Diagnostic Criteria:**  Congenital rubella should be suspected in any neonate with intrauterine growth retardation,

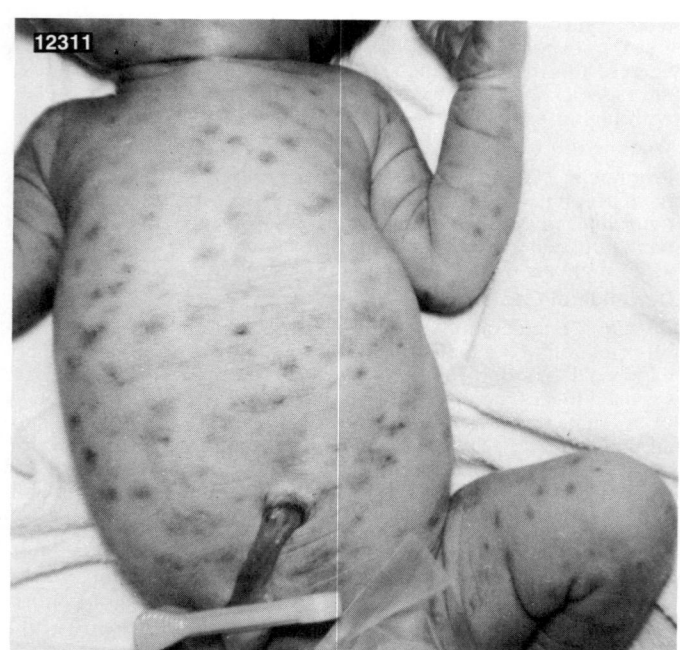
12311

0384-12311: Newborn with fetal rubella syndrome. Skin lesions are purple.

hepatosplenomegaly, purpura, or jaundice. Infants or children with microcephaly, cataract, retinopathy, sensorineural hearing loss, congenital heart disease and/or mental retardation should also be suspect. A history of rubella during pregnancy is helpful. The presence of retinopathy is most helpful in patients with unexplained congenital deafness. The diagnosis may be confirmed by isolation of rubella virus from a pharyngeal swab, cerebrospinal fluid, cataractous lens or other tissue. The presence in the serum of a newborn infant of specific rubella IgM antibody or persistence of any rubella antibody after 8–12 months of age (in the absence of postnatal rubella or rubella vaccination) is also diagnostic. The rubella hemagglutination inhibition (HI) and enzyme linked immunoassay (ELISA) antibody tests are widely available, convenient, and economical. The ELISA test appears to be more sensitive.

Children with congenital rubella may appear clinically normal at birth and during early infancy. All infants whose mothers are suspected of having had rubella during pregnancy should be studied for laboratory and clinical signs. Any positive finding warrants regular evaluation during infancy and early childhood with special emphasis on detection of ocular, audiologic and neurologic defects. Cardiac lesions are less likely to be overlooked. As the child grows older, diabetes mellitus is common.

**Clinical Findings:** Fetal infection with rubella virus may cause spontaneous abortion, stillbirth or a variety of birth defects occurring singly or in combination. Transient neonatal manifestations include low birthweight, hepatosplenomegaly, purpura, bulging unusually large anterior fontanel and metopic suture, corneal clouding, and jaundice. Laboratory studies during this period may also reveal thrombocytopenia, hemolytic or hypoplastic anemia, hepatitis, radiographic lesions in the metaphyseal portions of the long bones, pleocytosis and elevated protein levels in the cerebrospinal fluid, elevated serum IgM (and less frequently IgA) and persistence of rubella virus in many organs. Pneumonia, meningitis, encephalitis, and rarely an intermittent rash may develop during infancy.

Permanent manifestations include sensorineural deafness which may be bilateral or unilateral, mild to profound; congenital heart disease, almost always patent ductus arteriosus with or without pulmonary artery or valvular stenosis, septal defect or aortic arch abnormalities; cataract, unilateral or bilateral, with or without microphthalmia; retinopathy; glaucoma; and high myopia. Encephalitis may lead to varying degrees of psychomotor retardation with intellectual or motor impairment, including typical spastic cerebral palsy. Endocrine disorders, especially insulin-dependent diabetes mellitus and hypo- or hyperthyroidism may occur during childhood and adolescence. Progressive rubella panencephalitis is a rare manifestation occurring in late adolescence or early adulthood.

**Complications:** Rubella induced lesions appear to have the same risk of complications as do the same lesions from other causes.

**Associated Findings:** Hernia, inguinal, increased incidence of abnormal dermatoglyphic patterns, skin dimpling and pigmented macular skin lesions.

**Etiology:** Rubella virus is a moderate-sized, pleomorphic, ether-sensitive RNA-containing virus classified as a togavirus although its clinical and laboratory behavior is more like the paramyovirus group.

The infant with congenital rubella may shed virus in pharyngeal secretions, urine, stool and tears for months after birth; hence he must be considered contagious to all susceptible persons with whom he may have direct contact. Virus shedding is uncommon (< 10%) after one year of age and has not been reported after two years of age.

**Pathogenesis:** In postnatal rubella infection, viremia occurs for as long as one week before onset of the rash. Viremia also occurs in subclinical rubella. When a pregnant woman develops rubella before the 17th gestational week, placental infection following maternal viremia may lead to fetal viremia and disseminated fetal infection involving virtually every organ. Rubella virus infection of human fetal tissue inhibits mitosis, and elicits an inflammatory response in certain organs. Anomalies result from varying degrees of undergrowth or hypoplasia, inflammatory responses and their sequelae. Cataract, glaucoma, sensorineural hearing loss and neurologic impairment may progress after birth as a consequence of the continued virus infection. Rubella specific circulating immune complexes may play a pathogenic role in the endocrine and neurologic manifestations.

**POS No.:** 3222

**CDC No.:** 771.090

**Sex Ratio:** M1:F1

**Occurrence:** Depends on prevalence of rubella in the community; may exceed 1:100 live births during epidemic years or less than 1:10,000 live births during immediate postepidemic years or in communities where rubella vaccine has been widely distributed.

When laboratory-confirmed maternal rubella occurs before the 11th gestational week, 90% of the infants will be affected. From the 11th through 16th week, 35% of infants will be affected. For greater detail see Ueda et al (1979).

**Risk of Recurrence for Patient's Sib:** None. Rubella impacts only one pregnancy, leaving the mother immune and subsequent pregnancies protected.

**Risk of Recurrence for Patient's Child:** Probably none.

**Age of Detectability:** At birth or infancy if rubella virus is isolated from an infected child. Antibody studies on cord blood may be diagnostic. Hearing loss may be detected early by alert parents, nurse or pediatrician. However, in some cases clinical stigmata alone may not be detectable for months or rarely, several years. Amniocentesis has not been useful for distinguishing between an infected and uninfected fetus.

**Gene Mapping and Linkage:** Unknown.

**Prevention:** Rubella vaccination of all children.

**Treatment:** Some of the neonatal manifestations of congenital rubella are self-limited and resolve spontaneously, eg thrombocytopenic purpura, hepatitis, bone lesions, and hemolytic anemia. Therapy for specific defects requires the services of a variety of specialists. Ideally, a multidisciplinary team should provide the coordinated care necessary for the multihandicapped child. No variation from established procedures is required, ie early congestive heart failure is justification for cardiac catheterization, angiocardiography and surgical correction of a **Ductus arteriosus, patent** during infancy. Surgery for bilateral cataracts in the first weeks of life as indicated. Congenital glaucoma requires immediate surgery. Amplification and auditory training are indicated as soon as significant hearing loss is determined. Specialists in rehabilitation medicine, and education of the handicapped, should be an integral part of the treatment team.

Sensory deprivation from auditory or ocular defects compounds any intellectual deficit associated with the sequelae of congenital rubella encephalitis. Early efforts at habilitation and education should include intensive family counseling and activities designed to stimulate the intact senses.

Labeling of a child with congenital rubella as "suitable for custodial care" should be avoided. Because of the chronic virus infection and the sensory deficits, some infants exhibit a degree of psychomotor retardation which does not accurately reflect their potential for learning. A trial in a multidisciplinary diagnostic teaching program, geared to multihandicapped preschool children, may provide helpful information on a child's ability to learn. Severe behavioral disturbances appearing during adolescence are a particularly difficult management problem.

**Prognosis:** Varies critically with the timing of the maternal infection. For multihandicapped infants, especially those with neonatal thrombocytopenic purpura, the mortality rate is high. A death rate of 35% was observed during the first year of life in one group of 58 infants with purpura. The overall mortality for infants with manifestations of congenital rubella detected during the first year of life is 10–20%. For those who survive infancy, most may anticipate normal life span. The exceptions are those severely retarded nonambulatory children who require institutional care. When provided early with intensive treatment and special education, many multihandicapped children may make reasonable socio-economic adjustments. The usual causes of death during early infancy are congestive heart failure, sepsis and general debility. Children with rubella-associated diabetes mellitus are not clinically different from others with early onset insulin-dependent diabetes.

**Detection of Carrier:** N/A

*The author wishes to thank Saul Krugman for his contributions to an earlier version of this article.*

**References:**
Cooper LZ: Congenital rubella in the U.S. in Krugman S, Gershon A (eds): Progress in Clinical and Biological Research, vol 3: Infections of the fetus and newborn. New York, A. Russ, Inc, 1975:1.
Cederquist LL, et al: Prenatal diagnosis of congenital rubella. Br Med J 1977; 1:615.
Ueda K, et al.: Congenital rubella syndrome: correlation of gestation age at time of maternal rubella with type of defect. J Pediatr 1979; 94:763–765.
Miller E, et al. Consequences of confirmed maternal rubella at successive stages of pregnancy. Lancet 1982; II:781.
Rubella vaccination during pregnancy: United States 1971–1988. Morbid Mort Wkly Rpt 1989; 38:289–293.

C0039                                                    **Louis Z. Cooper**

---

**FETAL SYPHILIS SYNDROME**                              **0385**

**Includes:**
Angeborene lues
Luetic disease
Syphilis, prenatal

**Excludes:** N/A

**Major Diagnostic Criteria:** All body systems may be involved in the infected neonate. The major clinical signs are maculopapular bullous eruptions, condylomata lata, hemorrhagic rhinitis, hepatosplenomegaly, osteochondritis, meningoencephalitis, pneumonia, nephritis, and nephrosis. No overt evidence of infection

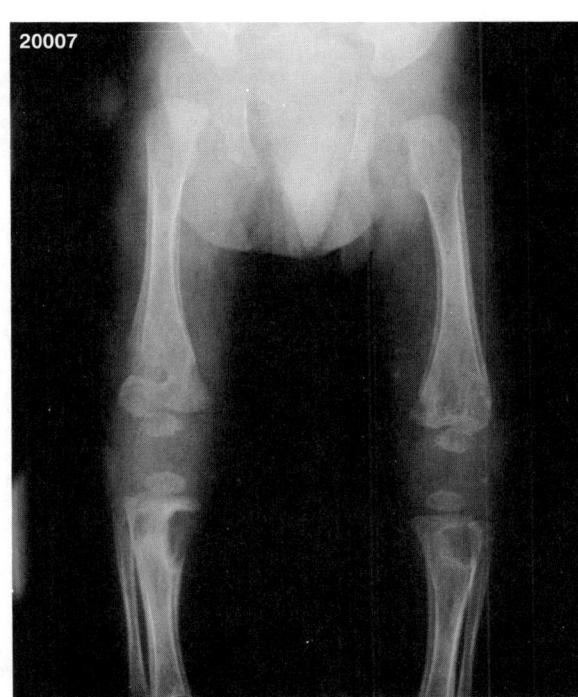

**0385-20007:** Periostitis and metaphyseal changes are evident in the long bones of an infant with fetal syphilis.

may be present at birth, but signs will usually appear within the first 3 months of life. The most rapid means of diagnosis remains dark-ground (microscopic) examination of moist skin lesions. Careful serologic testing and X-ray are the standard confirmatory investigations.

**Clinical Findings:** Twenty-five percent of untreated cases are stillborn. In the neonate, all organ systems may be variably involved. Early manifestations of congenital syphilis resemble those of secondary syphilis in the adult and are characterized by the following:

*Skin lesions:* Maculopapular, bullous, vesicular, eczematous or, annular cutaneous lesions are common and are localized to the circumoral or anogenital regions, palms, and soles. Desquamation is usual. Flat condylomata lata can occur in the perianal region. Mucous patches and fissures may be found on the lips and in the anal cleft, and involvement of the nasal mucosa results in purulent or hemorrhagic rhinitis (snuffles). If untreated, 90% of syphilitic infants will eventually have some skin manifestation.

*Osseous lesions:* Ninety percent of affected infants have bony lesions, which may only be radiographically demonstrable. Osteochondritis is commonly found in the long bones and occasionally involves the small bones of the hand (dactylitis). Diffuse periostitis of the long bones may develop. Extensive erosions of the upper medial tibial metaphyses produce a ragged or "rat-bite" X-ray appearance (Wimberger sign), and fracture through such areas may lead to the so-called "pseudoparalysis of Parrot."

*Miscellaneous early manifestations:* Meningeal inflammation occurs in 40% of individuals, resulting in raised spinal fluid protein levels and a pleocytosis. hemolytic anemia, hepatosplenomegaly, and jaundice are common features, whereas renal lesions are rare and manifest as nephritis or nephrotic syndrome. Pneumonia or signs of interstitial pneumonitis may occur.

*Late manifestations:* Manifestations that appear only after infancy are due to neonatal infection or untreated congenital syphilis. Some lesions are thought to be due to hypersensitivity reactions. Interstitial keratitis has its onset between ages 3 and 20 years. An intense inflammatory vascular infiltration associated with iritis can result in scarring and subsequent blindness. The late sequelae of early lesions are characteristic: saddle nose (rhinitis); "snail track" scars (snuffles); rhagades (perioral lesions); Clutton joints, saber shin, Hutchinson teeth, mulberry molars (osseous lesions); mental retardation, vestibular dysfunction, and sensorineural deafness (CNS involvement); aortic valvulitis (gummatous lesions).

**Complications:** Unknown.

**Associated Findings:** None known.

**Etiology:** Infection of a human fetus by *Treponema pallidum* at any stage of gestation. The previous belief that *T. pallidum* only infected the fetus after 20 weeks of gestation has been discarded following evidence of infection in 9-week abortuses. Immunocompetence in the fetus is only established after 20 weeks of gestation, and the clinical manifestations are secondary to this inflammatory response.

**Pathogenesis:** Infection may result in abortion, stillbirth, or delivery of a symptomatic baby or of a neonate who appears normal but develops signs in the early months of life. The lesions result from precisely timed insults to developing tissue by *Treponema* organisms (or an "allergic" manifestation thereof), resulting in the protean clinical manifestations.

**POS No.:** 3223

**CDC No.:** 090.000

**Sex Ratio:** M1:F1

**Occurrence:** After eight years of decline in the United States, the Center for Disease Control reports an increase for the period 1985–1987 from 108 to 268 cases. A shift away from the use of penicillin to other agents for the treatment of gonorrhea may be a factor in this increase.

**Risk of Recurrence for Patient's Sib:** Dependent on effective treatment of infected mother and the possibility of reinfection.

**Risk of Recurrence for Patient's Child:** Dependent upon maternal infection.

**Age of Detectability:** At birth or during early infancy.

**Gene Mapping and Linkage:** Unknown.

**Prevention:** Prompt treatment and reporting of all cases of early or latent syphilis, particularly during the antenatal period.

**Treatment:** *T. pallidum* retains a high sensitivity to penicillin, which is the drug of choice. For the infant or neonate, procaine penicillin 50,000 units/kg/day intramuscularly for 10 days is curative for all manifestations including the meningoencephalitic form. The use of benzathine penicillin is not advised, because the drug does not cross the blood-brain barrier effectively. A single dose of 4.8 million units of long-acting bicillin is recommended for affected adults. Erythromycin can be substituted in penicillin-sensitive individuals.

**Prognosis:** Dependent on the degree of tissue involvement and promptness of effective therapy.

**Detection of Carrier:** A positive Venereal Disease Research Laboratory (VDRL) titer will identify an asymptomatic carrier.

**Special Considerations:** Many serologic tests for *T. pallidum* are available. The interpretation of the results is confusing and complicated by the presence of both nontreponemal and treponemal antibodies, both of which can be transferred to the fetus in infected and noninfected pregnancies. In the presence of a positive maternal VDRL test (specificity = 99.4%), it is recommended that the total immunoglobulin M (IgM) fraction of cord blood be evaluated. Should the level exceed 0.20 g/liter, treponemal-specific IgM levels can be determined to exclude nontreponemal fetal infections. Raised treponemal-specific IgM antibodies together with positive X-ray evidence will confirm the diagnosis in the majority (90–95%) of cases. Following treatment, rising or static VDRL titers are the best indication of persistent infection and the need to continue therapy.

**References:**
Rudolph AH, Duncan WC: Syphilis: diagnosis and treatment. Clin Obstet Gynaecol 1975; 18:163–181. * †
Centers for Disease Control: CDC recommended treatment schedules. Morbid Mortal Weekly Rep 1976; 25:101.
Breasett M: The laboratory diagnosis of congenital syphilis: a review. Am J Technol 1979; 45:645–647.
Jones JE: Diagnostic evaluation of syphilis during pregnancy. Obstet Gynecol 1979; 54:611–614.
Center for Disease Control: Congenital syphilis in the United States 1983–1985. MMWR 1986; 35:625–628.

VI005        **Denis L. Viljöen**

## FETAL THALIDOMIDE SYNDROME    0386

**Includes:** Thalidomide, fetal effects

**Excludes:** **Thrombocytopenia-absent radius** (0941)

**Major Diagnostic Criteria:** Maternal ingestion of at least 100 mg of thalidomide at the critical stage of embryonic development (34–55 days after last menstrual period) and birth of an infant with reduction deformities of the limbs.

**Clinical Findings:** The development of almost any organ may be affected; however, the most obvious finding is reduction deformity of the limbs, ranging from hypoplasia of one or more digits to total absence of all limbs. The association of limb reduction, nasal hemangioma, anal atresia, duodenal stenosis, coloboma, and other defects sometimes included in the description of the thalidomide syndrome.

**Complications:** Deafness, blindness, and congenital defects of the heart, kidneys, GI tract, reproductive and other organs may occur. Severely involved fetuses were often stillborn or died perinatally.

**Associated Findings:** None known.

**Etiology:** Maternal ingestion of thalidomide at the sensitive period of embryonic development (4–6 weeks).

**Pathogenesis:** Unknown.

**POS No.:** 3224

**Sex Ratio:** M1:F1

**Occurrence:** Highest where thalidomide was most used. An iatrogenic epidemic occurred in 1958–1963.

**Risk of Recurrence for Patient's Sib:** Related to maternal exposure to thalidomide.

**Risk of Recurrence for Patient's Child:** Related to maternal exposure to thalidomide.

**Age of Detectability:** At birth for limb reduction deformities and immediately thereafter for anal atresia and duodenal stenosis. Other malformations, including those of hips and spine, may not be immediately diagnosed. Genital malformations may be detectable only at adolescence.

**Gene Mapping and Linkage:** Unknown.

**Prevention:** Avoidance of thalidomide in women of child-bearing age. Thalidomide is currently available only for restricted use for treatment of leprosy.

**Treatment:** Appropriate surgical or medical treatment of cardiac, renal and gastro-intestinal tract defects. Prostheses, mobility and self-help devices as indicated by the severity and distribution of limb deformities.

**Prognosis:** For those surviving early infancy, life span is considered normal if only limbs are involved. Heart, kidney, and other organ defects may affect life expectancy.

**Detection of Carrier:** Unknown.

**Special Considerations:** Thalidomide ($\alpha$-phthalimidoglutarimide) (Thalidomide, Contergan, Softenon, Distaval, Neurosedyn, Kevadon, Talimol, Isomia, and some sixty other proprietary names) was synthesized in 1954 in the laboratories of Chemie Grünenthal Stolberg, Federal Republic of Germany. The drug was first marketed widely from 1957, both on prescription and over the counter, as a sedative and hypnotic depending on dosage. In 1960–1961 reports of peripheral neuritis as a side effect in adults were published. Late in 1961 Wiedemann, (Sept. 16th), McBride,

(Dec. 16th) and Lenz, (Dec. 29th) directed attention to the increased incidence of reduction deformities of the limbs of newborn children. The last two authors attributed the increase to maternal ingestion of thalidomide in early pregnancy. The drug was withdrawn from the market in most countries by early 1962, although total withdrawal was delayed, particularly in Japan. Thereafter the incidence of limb deformities returned to the pre-thalidomide level. Probably a total of 8,000 to 10,000 neonates were affected.

*New Clinical Uses for Thalidomide*: Thalidomide is now used for the treatment of the Lepra Reaction (erythema nodosum leprosum) throughout the world. The compound has no effect on *B. leprae*. Thalidomide has also become the drug of choice for many cutaneous diseases, including discoid lupus erythematosis, actinea prurigo, and Weber Christian syndrome. In fact, the use of thalidomide has expanded greatly (Koch, 1985, provides 502 references).

Despite the awareness of Thalidomide teratogenicity, in a few instances the drug has been given to pregnant women. Great care must taken in the use of medications which may contain thalidomide, and pregnant women should be warned against the sharing of medications.

**References:**

Lenz W. Kindliche Missbildungen nach Medikament-einnahme während der Gravidität? Dtsch Med Wochenschr. 1961; 86:2555–2556.

McBride WG. Thalidomide and congenital abnormalities. Lancet. 1961; 2:1358.

Wiedemann HR. Hinweis auf eine derzeitige Häufung hypo-und aplastischer Fehlbildungen der Gliedmassen. Med Welt. 1961: 37: 1863–1866.

Sheskin J: Thalidomide in the treatment of Lepra reactions. Clin Pharmacol Therapeutice 1965; 6:303–306.

Swinyard CA, ed. Limb development and deformity: problems of evaluation and rehabilitation. Springfield: Charles C Thomas Co., 1969.

Koch HP: Thalidomide and Congeners as anti-inflammatory agents. Progress in Medical Chemistry 1985; 22:166–242.

SW004                                    **Chester A. Swinyard**

---

## FETAL TOXOPLASMOSIS SYNDROME          0387

**Includes:**

    Angeborene Toxoplasmose
    Chorioretinitis, toxoplasmic
    Toxoplasmosis, infantile

**Excludes:**

    **Erythroblastosis fetalis** (3063)
    **Fetal cytomegalovirus syndrome** (0381)
    **Fetal rubella syndrome** (0384)
    **Microcephaly with chorioretinopathy** (2333)

**Major Diagnostic Criteria:** Congenital toxoplasmosis has been classically described in terms of a triad of clinical signs: chorioretinitis, hydrocephaly or microcephaly, and intracranial calcifications. However, it is now recognized that there is a wide range of signs and symptoms from the neonate with severe disease to the asymptomically infected infant. Diagnosis can be confirmed by isolation of *Toxoplasma* (T) *gondii* from body fluids or tissues from a fetus or newborn, or by demonstration of toxoplasma IgM antibodies in cord or neonatal serum. In the absence of these data, the serologic titers of toxoplasma antibodies may be followed. These titers are compared with the mother's titer obtained at or soon after delivery. An uninfected infant's titer will decrease 50% each month after birth while an infected infant's titer will be maintained, rise, or transiently fall until the infant begins to produce antibodies.

**Clinical Findings:** Prospective studies have shown that most infants born with congenital toxoplasmosis are asymptomatic. However, the disease manifestations vary from stillbirths (8%) and severely affected newborns (10%) to the infected newborn without clinically apparent disease (75%). Prematurity is common, occurring in 25% of cases. The severity of toxoplasmosis in

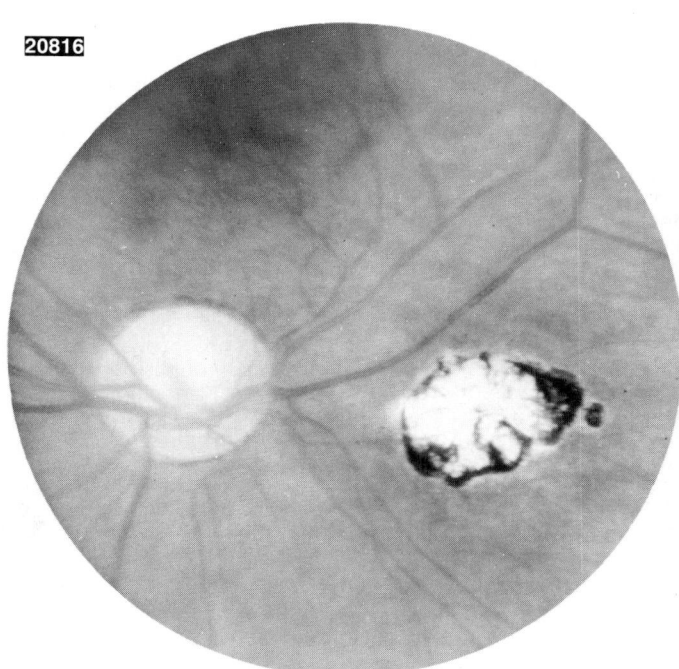

**0387-20816:**   Fetal toxoplasmosis syndrome; note chorioretinitis.

newborns appears to be related to the trimester during which the acute maternal infection occured. Infections acquired early in pregnancy seem to result in more severe fetal damage than those acquired during the third trimester. The latter infants are often asymptomatic at birth. Fortunately, the parasite is less likely to be transmitted to the fetus if the mother's acute infection is acquired during the first or second trimester than if it is acquired during the third trimester of pregnancy.

In the severely affected infant, central nervous system abnormalities such as microcephaly or hydrocephaly, chorioretinitis, periventricular calcifications, microphthalmia, seizures, and psychomotor retardation are common. Other manifestations seen in infants with active disease include jaundice, hepatosplenomegaly, maculopapular rash, purpura, fever, carditis, and pneumonitis. Mildly affected infants usually show ocular involvement in the form of chorioretinitis with absence of other signs and symptoms. Subsequent complications include recurrent chorioretinitis, psychomotor retardation, and seizures. Periventricular calcifications may be demonstrable. Infants with asymptomatic or subclinical infection are at risk for subsequently developing chorioretinitis and neurological deficits.

The diagnosis of acute toxoplasmosis infection may be established by several methods. In stillborns the diagnosis is supported by high toxoplasma antibodies in the mother and visualization or isolation of the organism from fetal tissue obtained at autopsy. In the severely affected infant cerebrospinal fluid shows xanthochromia, mononuclear pleocytosis, high protein content, and occasionally, eosinophilia. Leukocytosis or leukopenia may be present. Anemia, thrombocytopenia, and eosinophilia are other peripheral blood manifestations. High titers of toxoplasma antibodies in both the mother and infant are not diagnostic since all infants from mothers with antibody have maternal IgG toxoplasma antibodies whether infected or not. In the United States approximately 30% of obstetrical patients have toxoplasma antibodies and 3–4% of these women have high titers. Transferred antibody titers may be greatly elevated without infection in the infant. Since IgM antibodies are not transferred transplacentally, elevated IgM antibodies in the infant confirm the diagnosis. However, there is a percentage of false-negative results when using fluorescent tests for IgM antibodies (IgM-IFA) due to competition for antigenic sites when high titers of IgG antibodies are present. False-positive IgM-IFA test results have been obtained in sera containing rheumatoid factor. An IgM enzyme-linked immunosorbent assay (IgM-ELISA) has been shown to be both highly sensitive and specific for the diagnosis of congenital toxoplasmosis. Other widely used serologic tests include the Sabin-Feldman dye test, the complement fixation test, the indirect hemagglutination test, and the agglutination test. *T. gondii* may be isolated from blood, cerebrospinal fluid, bone marrow, tissues, and the placenta. The parasite can be isolated from both mildly and severely affected infants. Mildly affected infants, as well as those with subclinical infection, show both elevated total IgM levels and elevated IgM antibody levels specific for toxoplasma.

**Complications:** Neurologic manifestations are the major complications in survivors of the clinically apparent disease. Mental retardation is present in over 80%, seizures, spasticity, and palsy occur in over 70%, severely impaired eyesight occurs in about 60%, hydrocephaly or microcephaly is present in about 40%, and deafness is found in about 15%. Mildly affected infants with only ocular manifestations may progress to central nervous system involvement and recurrent chorioretinitis. Infants with subclinical infections also frequently develop later neurological and ocular symptoms (See Prognosis).

**Associated Findings:** None known.

**Etiology:** Transplacental transmission of *T. gondii* to the fetus occurs in approximately 40% of women who develop the infection during pregnancy.

**Pathogenesis:** There are three forms of the parasite, *T. gondii*: the tachyzoite, the tissue cyst, and the oocyst. The tachyzoite, an obligate intracellular form, is present in the acute stage of infection. It will invade all types of mammalian cells. The tissue cyst develops in host cells from tachyzoites and varies in size from those with only a few organisms to those containing several thousand. These cysts commonly are found in muscle and central nervous system tissue. The oocyst develops in the intestine of members of the cat family and is excreted in their feces.

Congenital infection occurs when there is transplacental spread of tachyzoites from mother to fetus. The tachyzoites proliferate in fetal cells resulting in cell death and areas of necrosis. Cysts may then develop within muscle, brain, retina, and other tissues and may exist within the host tissue for weeks to years. Factors which lead to cyst formation are uncertain. Extrinsic factors such as development of immunity or intrinsic changes in the organism itself may play a role. Chorioretinitis, whether primary or recurrent infection, follows rupture of cysts within the retina and results in an inflammatory response, resumption of tachyzoite multiplication, and progressive tissue necrosis. In the brain, active infection persists the longest. Hydrocephalus is the result of aqueductal obstruction. Periventricular necrosis follows dissemination of *T. gondii* in the ventricular system. As the necrosis progresses there is ventriculomegaly and marked elevation of protein in the ventricular fluid. Rupture of tissue cysts appears to be of minimal consequence in other tissues in the immunologically competent host.

**POS No.:** 3225

**CDC No.:** 771.210

**Sex Ratio:** M1:F1

**Occurrence:** Estimated at about 1:1000 deliveries in the United States, but varies in differing climates and among different ethnic groups.

**Risk of Recurrence for Patient's Sib:** No risk except to a twin, in the absence of further maternal infection.

**Risk of Recurrence for Patient's Child:** Dependent upon maternal exposure.

**Age of Detectability:** Recently prenatal diagnosis of congenital toxoplasmosis has been reported by a combination of fetal blood sampling at 20–24 weeks gestation for IgM specific antibodies, detection of parasitemia by inoculation of fetal blood and amniotic fluid into mice, and repeated ultrasound examination for fetal ventriculomegaly.

**Gene Mapping and Linkage:** Unknown.

**Prevention:** Measures for prevention of toxoplasma infection in pregnant women should be directed toward the two infectious forms of *T. gondii*, tissue cysts and oocysts. The tissue cyst can be rendered noninfective by cooking meat to 140° F (60° C) for at least 10 minutes. Freezing of meat is a less reliable method of killing the cyst. Hands and other surfaces which have come in contact with raw meat should be washed thoroughly. Contact with mucous membranes while handling meat should be avoided. Infection by the oocyst can be avoided by several measures. Pregnant women should avoid handling cat feces. Litter pans should be emptied daily and rinsed with nearly boiling water. Toxoplasma oocysts from soil or sand can be avoided by wearing disposable gloves and by strict hand washing after exposure. These oocysts become infective one to three days after excretion and remain viable in moist and shaded soil for as long as one year.

No vaccine is presently available. Treatment during pregnancy with pyrimethamine, sulfadiazine, and folinic acid has been employed in an attempt to decrease the incidence and severity of congenital toxoplasma infection. This therapy, however, is not utilized in the first trimester because of the possible teratogenicity of pyrimethamine. Abortion is an option especially if the infection was acquired early in pregnancy.

**Treatment:** All infants diagnosed with congenital toxoplasmosis, including subclinical infections, should be treated with pyrimethamine, sulfadiazine, and folinic acid. The therapy is principally effective against the actively multiplying tachyzoites; the tissue cysts are not affected. Bone marrow suppression, the main complication of the pyrimethamine-sulfadiazine combination, is avoided by folinic acid. Spiramycin, an antibiotic currently not available in the United States, has reportedly been effective in France.

**Prognosis:** A mortality rate of 12% regardless of clinical grouping was reported in one study. Marked ocular and central nervous system abnormalities including psychomotor retardation occur in greater than 80% of those with severe disease (See Clinical Findings). Infants with only chorioretinitis at diagnosis may later manifest symptoms of central nervous system involvement and recurrent chorioretinitis. Furthermore, in one study of 13 infants with subclinical infection (followed for a mean of over 8 years) 11 developed chorioretinitis including 3 with unilateral blindness, and 5 showed major (2) or minor (3) neurological sequelae.

**Detection of Carrier:** Unknown.

**Special Considerations:** Comparison of antibody titers in mother and infant can provide valuable diagnostic support in clinically suspected congenital toxoplasmosis. In the older child the likelihood that the infection was acquired after birth is greater. However, acquisition of T. gondii infection is slow in children in the United States, and the percentage of those with toxoplasma antibodies is usually less than the given age (e.g., less 10% in 10 year olds, etc.). The incidence of seropositivity varies substantially with place of residence especially outside the United States.

Toxoplasmosis can be transmitted from mother to fetus during either clinical or subclinical infection of the mother. Only 10–20% of women who become infected have clinical symptoms, most commonly fever and lymphadenopathy. In the clinically suspected disease, the time of acquisition is estimated to be 2 weeks prior to the onset of symptoms. In subclinical infections the time of acquisition is seldom known unless detected by seroconversion or substantial rise in antibody titers.

The advice of experts in interpreting serologic results is recommended, especially if clinical evidence is absent or not entirely characteristic.

**References:**

Wilson CB, et al.: Development of adverse sequelae in children born with subclinical congenital toxoplasma infection. Pediatrics 1980; 66:767–774.

Remington JS, Desmonts G: Toxoplasmosis. In: Remington JS, Klein JO, eds: Infectious diseases of the fetus and newborn infant. Philadelphia: W.B. Saunders, 1983:143–263. *

Desmonts G, et al.: Prenatal diagnosis of congenital toxoplasmosis. Lancet 1985; 1:500–504.

Frenkel JK: Toxoplasmosis. Pediatr Clin North Am 1985; 32:917–932.

Daffos F, et al.: Prenatal management of 746 pregnancies at risk for congenital toxoplasmosis. New Engl J Med 1988; 318:271–275.

M0039
WE005

Cynthia A. Moore
David D. Weaver

## FETAL TRIMETHADIONE SYNDROME                    0388

**Includes:**

Fetal paramethadione syndrome
Paradione^, fetal effects of
Paramethadione, fetal effects of
Tridione^, fetal effects of
Trimethadione, fetal effects of
Troxidone embryopathy

**Excludes:** Teratogenic effects of other anticonvulsant drugs

**Major Diagnostic Criteria:** The signs most commonly seen in the syndrome are upward-slanting eyebrows and marked, incomplete outfolding (otherwise described as overfolding) of the superior helix in posteriorly angulated ears. Most common effects include cardiac anomalies, pre- and postnatal growth deficiency, mental retardation, and cleft lip and/or palate.

**Clinical Findings:** Few cases have been reported since Feldman et al (1977) summarized findings in 40 fetuses exposed in pregnancy:

*CNS*: Mental retardation/developmental delay (10/18); speech abnormalities (7/18); anencephaly or meningomyelocele (3/43), and microcephaly (2/43).

*Craniofacial*: Malformed ears (20/43); cleft lip and/or palate (13/43); high arched palate (8/43); upward slanting eyebrows (7/18); broad nasal bridge (10/18); teeth irregularity (6/18).

*Growth*: Intrauterine growth retardation (12/24); short stature (8/18).

*Other*: Congenital heart defects (21/43); tracheoesophageal anomalies (5/43); renal anomalies (6/43); hypospadias (5/26); inguinal or umbilical hernia (8/43); gastrointestinal defects (6/43).

**Complications:** Stillbirth, neonatal death.

**Associated Findings:** Imperforate anus, facial hemangioma, branchial cleft, **Polydactyly**, oligodactyly, scoliosis, single flexion

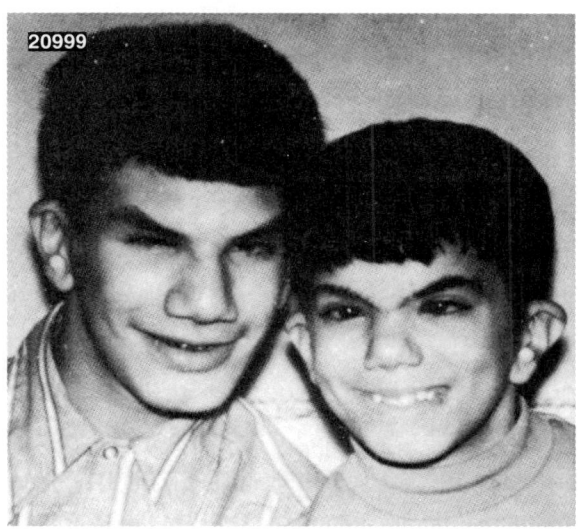

**0388-20999:** Fetal trimethadione syndrome; note broad nasal bridges, epicanthal folds and V-shaped eyebrows.

crease of fifth finger, webbed neck, micrognathia, **Eye, microphthalmia/coloboma**, single palmar crease, conductive hearing loss.

**Etiology:** Maternal ingestion of trimethadione or paramethadione during pregnancy.

**Pathogenesis:** In children and adults, therapy may cause exfoliative dermatitis, severe erythema multiforme, blood dyscrasias, hepatitis, ANA antibodies, nephritis, nephrosis, lymphadenopathy, and a myasthenia gravis-like syndrome. Patients must be monitored with monthly liver functions, blood count, and urinalysis.

**POS No.:** 3980

**Sex Ratio:** Presumably M1:F1

**Occurrence:** Presumed rare; since these anticonvulsants are now less used.

**Risk of Recurrence for Patient's Sib:** Related to further maternal exposure.

**Risk of Recurrence for Patient's Child:** Unknown, but likely to be negligible in the absence of maternal exposure.

**Age of Detectability:** The diagnosis may be confirmed, but not excluded, upon ultrasonographic demonstration of major malformations associated with the syndrome prior to 20 weeks gestation.

**Gene Mapping and Linkage:** Unknown.

**Prevention:** Para- and trimethadione should be used only when less toxic drugs (such as ethosuximide) have been ineffective in controlling absence seizures. In women of reproductive age, they should be used only after teratogenicity has been explained, as well as the option of termination of any pregnancy occurring during therapy. Should a woman desire pregnancy, she should be given the option of a period of suboptimal control with less toxic drugs, particularly for the period of organogenesis. She should also be informed that malformations and reduced intellect may be the likely result in any pregnancy exposed to these oxazolidines in the first trimester.

**Treatment:** Appropriate management of malformations, developmental delay and mental retardation.

**Prognosis:** Dependent on the type of malformations: severe cardiac anomalies may be incompatible with life. Survivors may be mentally retarded or of normal intelligence (highest IQ measured: 90).

**Detection of Carrier:** Unknown.

**Special Considerations:** In the eight families reported by German et al (1970) 32 pregnancies with first trimester exposure to para- or trimethadione (usually in conjunction with other antiepileptics) occurred: (7/32) pregnancies miscarried; one was a small-for-dates stillborn; and of 24 liveborns, 19 had major anomalies, with five neonatal deaths. After discontinuance of para- or trimethadione, (5/ 5) pregnancies resulted in normal infants in three of the families. One mother who had three severely affected infants (all died of effects) and two first trimester miscarriages while taking paramethadione in conjunction with other antiepileptics had a normal child after paramethadione was replaced by ethosuximide (Zarontin).

**References:**

German J, et al.: Trimethadione and human teratogenesis. Teratology 1970; 3:349–362.

Zackai EH, et al.: The fetal trimethadione syndrome. J Pediatr 1975; 87:280–284. * †

Feldman GL, et al.: The fetal trimethadione syndrome. Am J Dis Child 1977; 131:1389–1392. *

R0003

**Richard M. Roberts**

## FETAL VALPROATE SYNDROME      2496

**Includes:**
> Depakene^, fetal effects from
> Valproic acid, fetal damage from

**Excludes:** Fetal damage from other anticonvulsants

**Major Diagnostic Criteria:** The diagnosis may be considered in any infant exposed in utero to valproic acid (VPA) and who manifests spina bifida or a consistent craniofacial phenotype which may in turn be associated with other minor and major abnormalities.

**Clinical Findings:** Spina bifida is the most conspicuous consequence of embryonic VPA exposure. Other major manifestations that characterize children exposed in utero to VPA (Depakene^) are facial changes consisting of epicanthal folds that continued inferiorly and laterally to form a crease or groove under the orbit; flat nasal bridge; small upturned nose; long upper lip with a relatively shallow philtrum; a thin upper vermilion border; microstomia; and downturned angles of the mouth. In addition to the craniofacial changes, other anomalies have been found several times in exposed children: aplasia of first ribs, diastasis recti, hernias, dislocated hip, cardiac defects (**Heart, tetralogy of Fallot, Ventricular septal defect, Ductus arteriosus, patent**), hypoplastic or hyperconvex nails, hypospadias, arachnodactyly, overlapping fingers and toes, and neural tube defects. Developmental delay has been noted in several patients, but few data on long-term psychomotor development are available. Birth weight is normal. Adverse effects seem to be dose related. Infants with major malformations have the highest number of minor anomalies.

**Complications:** Distress during labor and low Apgar score.

**Associated Findings:** Dysplasia of sternum, trigonencephaly, **Thumb, triphalangeal**, inverted nipples, urinary tract malformations, bundle branch block, and alveolar cleft.

**Etiology:** Prenatal exposure to VPA during the first trimester of pregnancy. VPA crosses the human placenta and may gain the opportunity to exert a teratogenic effect.

**Pathogenesis:** VPA teratogenicity has been demonstrated experimentally in rabbits, rats, and mice. Induced anomalies include renal agenesis, **Cleft palate**, encephalocele, vertebral defects, rib fusion, and ablepharia. These effects are dose related, but were observed with doses several times higher than those given in clinical practice. It has been postulated that problems related to VPA intake may be mediated through alteration of trace metal status.

**POS No.:** 3650

**Sex Ratio:** M1:F1

**Occurrence:** Spina bifida is observed in 1–5% of maternal exposures; major anomalies including spina bifida in 5–10%; and some facial changes in nearly half of the exposed children. Some published VPA spina bifida cases have had family histories of spina bifida.

Some 175 neural tube defects with maternal VPA exposure have been reported internationally, in births from 1974 through 1988. The extent of underreporting is unknown. All but seven (three anencephalies, four encephaloceles) were spina bifida.

**Risk of Recurrence for Patient's Sib:** Not increased in the absence of exposure.

**Risk of Recurrence for Patient's Child:** Not increased in the absence of exposure.

**Age of Detectability:** At birth, or prenatally by ultrasound for major organ malformations.

**Gene Mapping and Linkage:** Unknown.

**Prevention:** Even given that VPA is a potential teratogen, good control of seizures in pregnancy is highly desirable. Therefore, decisions on therapy must rest on clinical judgment. Women receiving VPA therapy must be informed of the risk, and have their VPA serum concentrations monitored. A high serum concentration may thus be avoided.

**Treatment:** Surgical correction of major defects.

**Prognosis:** Depends on associated major defects.

**Detection of Carrier:** Unknown.

**Special Considerations:** Total VPA serum concentration seems to decrease during pregnancy although dosage remains the same. During the first trimester, VPA serum concentrations are consistently above the so-called therapeutic range (50 to 80 $\mu$g) with a daily dose of 1,500 mg. Considerable fluctuations of serum concentrations between doses are observed, with high peak concentrations of free VPA that probably increase the embryotoxic potential of VPA.

**References:**
Robert E, Guibaud P: Maternal valproic acid and congenital neural tube defects. Lancet 1982; II:937 only. *

DiLiberti JH, et al.: The fetal valproate syndrome. Am J Med Genet 1984; 19:473–481. * †

Jäger-Roman E, et al.: Fetal growth, major malformations, and minor anomalies in infants born to women receiving valproic acid. J Pediatr 1986; 108:997–1004. †

Lindhout D, Schmidt D: In-utero exposure to valproate and neural tube defects. Lancet 1986; I:1392–1393.

Lammer EJ, et al.: Teratogen update: valproic acid. Teratology 1987; 35:465–473.

Winter RM, et al.: Fetal valproate syndrome: is there a recognizable phenotype? J Med Genet 1987; 24:692–695. †

Ardinger HH, et al.: Verification of the fetal valproate syndrome phenotype. Am J Med Genet 1988; 29:171–185. †

AY010                          **Ségolène Aymé**

**Fetal varicella-zoster syndrome**
*See FETAL EFFECTS FROM VARICELLA-ZOSTER*

## FETAL VENEZUELAN EQUINE ENCEPHALITIS INFECTION      2731

**Includes:**
> Encephalitis, Venezuelan equine
> Infection, Venezuelan equine encephalitis
> Venezuelan equine encephalitis (VEE)

**Excludes:** Hydroanencephalia caused by thrombosis

**Major Diagnostic Criteria:** Venezuelan equine encephalitis (VEE) occurred as an epidemic during a season of very heavy rains in 1962, followed by an increase in insect (mosquito) vectors. The epidemic was signaled first by the appearance of many dead horses and monkeys. The epidemic swept over large areas of Venezuela, attacking many kinds of animals. Both human children and adults were affected, with high mortality in children. In adults, VEE was often a benign disease, with slight, nonspecific symptoms for a week or so, but in more severe cases the condition produced neurologic symptoms such as somnolence, loss of consciousness, or abnormal reflexes.

The diagnosis is established by laboratory tests, such as finding and identifying the virus in pharyngeal swabs or in blood, or by finding neutralizing antibodies. In the mild cases, the diagnosis is epidemiologically based on the presence of the patient in the area affected by an epidemic of VEE. The severity of maternal disease was not related to the occurrence of fetal cerebral necrosis.

**Clinical Findings:** In spite of severe loss of parts of the cerebral tissue or extensive cerebral necrosis, affected newborns lived from 15 minutes to seven days, with a clinical picture of dyspnea, anoxia, convulsions, and septicemia. The cerebral necrosis was an unexpected finding during autopsy. The severity of the clinical symptoms seemed to be related to the interval between maternal disease and birth. In cases of two-week to four-month intervals between maternal disease and birth, birth weights were 2,500 to 3,050 g, and the principal symptoms were dyspnea and anoxia. One child, born five months after the maternal encephalitis, had no active movements and complete arreflexia; the infant lived four hours with respiratory support. After a five-month interval, one case was stillborn, with severe associated malformations.

Previous to birth, the condition was not suspected by the mothers or by the examining doctors. In only one instance, after a pregnancy of eight months with maternal encephalitis in the third month, did the mother note the lack of fetal growth. The mother never noted movements, and the fetus was stillborn, with a weight of 1,400 g.

**Complications:** It was surprising that the four infants who had nearly total necrosis of both hemispheres lived from two to seven days. They had been diagnosed as only having dyspnea and anoxia, and the causes of death had been attributed to broncopneumonia or pulmonary atelectasia. In another case of stillbirth five months after the maternal encephalitis, there was a total lack of nervous tissue, the medulla measuring only 2 mm in diameter, and there was no nervous tissue in the retina, which was formed by only two sheets of pigmented epithelium. In general, the brain tissue in infants born soon (two weeks) after the encephalitis attack had fresh necrosis. After 1–5 weeks, the infants showed absorption of necrotic tissue and even a fibrous organization around islets of necrotic nervous tissue. After five months of life there were only thin membranes surrounding cystic spaces, appearing similar to **Hydranencephaly.**

**Associated Findings:** There were no other anomalies except in the one stillborn with **Microcephaly**, microphthalmia, fixed contractions of several joints, and coxofemoral luxation. The weights of the other affected fetuses were between 2,500 and 3,550 g.

**Etiology:** The relation between the acute attack of maternal encephalomyelitis and the cerebral necrosis is apparent. Diagnosis of maternal disease was made on clinical grounds, and the diagnosis of the epidemic was established by laboratory tests.

**Pathogenesis:** The virus is believed to pass the placental barrier. Presumably this was associated with an increase of virulence that developed specifically during the 1962 epidemic, when the virus frequently changed from one host to another. This produced disease in animals who were not affected by encephalitis. The great multiplication of the insect vectors seems to have been responsible for this effect. In 1962, transmission occurred directly from humans to humans, without the intervention of an insect vector (mosquito). London et al (1977) subsequently induced cerebral malformations in rhesus monkey fetuses by inoculating the virus directly into the brain tissue.

**Sex Ratio:** Presumably M1:F1.

**Occurrence:** Seven cases have been reported, all in 1962, of which six were found on routine autopsy. Since these cases were found in offsprings of mothers from an area of a VEE epidemic, new cases are expected only in areas of such an epidemic. Spontaneous abortions are increased when mothers contract VEE in the first trimester.

**Risk of Recurrence for Patient's Sib:** Minimal in the absence of further maternal exposure.

**Risk of Recurrence for Patient's Child:** Minimal in the absence of maternal exposure.

**Age of Detectability:** The fetal effects are detected during infancy.

**Gene Mapping and Linkage:** N/A

**Prevention:** Pregnant women should avoid areas of known epidemics of encephalomyelitis, especially of the Venezuelan type.

**Treatment:** Unknown.

**Prognosis:** Affected newborns died within seven days.

**Detection of Carrier:** Unknown.

**References:**
Wenger F: Necrosis cerebral masiva del feto en casos de encefalitis Equina Venezolana. Invest Clin 1967; 21:15–31. *
London WT, et al.: Congenital cerebral and ocular malformations, induced in rhesus monkeys by Venezuelan equine encephalitis virus. Teratology 1977; 16:285–295.
Moreland AF, et al.: Effects of influenza, mumps and Western equine encephalitis viruses on fetal rhesus monkeys (*Macaca mulatta*). Teratology 1979; 20:53–64.
Moreland AF, et al.: Fetal mortality and malformations associated with

experimental infections of Western equine encephalomyelitis vaccine virus in rhesus monkeys (*Macaca mulatta*). Teratology 1979; 20:65–74.
Wenger F, et al.: Venezuelan equine encephalitis: its relation to severe cerebral malformations. In: Sever JL, Brent RL, eds: Teratogen update: environmentally induced birth defect risks. New York: Alan R Liss, 1986:107–111. * †

WE037                                          **Franz Wenger**

## FETAL WARFARIN SYNDROME            0389

**Includes:**
    Anticoagulant, oral, embryopathy
    Coumadin embryopathy
    Vitamin K-antagonist embryopathy
    Warfarin, fetal effects of

**Excludes:**
    **Chondrodysplasia punctata, mild symmetric type** (0153)
    **Chondrodysplasia punctata, rhizomelic type** (0154)

**Major Diagnostic Criteria:** Documented history of maternal ingestion of vitamin K-antagonist anticoagulant in therapeutic doses during the first trimester of pregnancy in association with one or more common malformations, i.e. hypoplastic nose, stippled epiphyses, or eye abnormality. Second or third trimester ingestion of vitamin K antagonists may be associated with either CNS and/or eye anomalies.

**Clinical Findings:** Summary of 24 cases with first trimester exposure:

1) The only consistent feature is nasal hypoplasia and depression of the bridge of the nose, resulting in a flattened, upturned

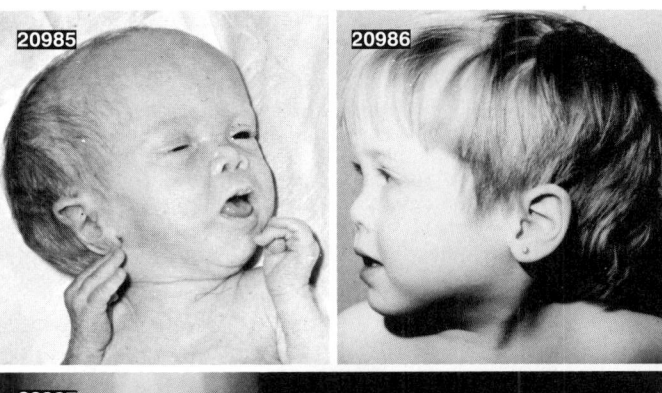

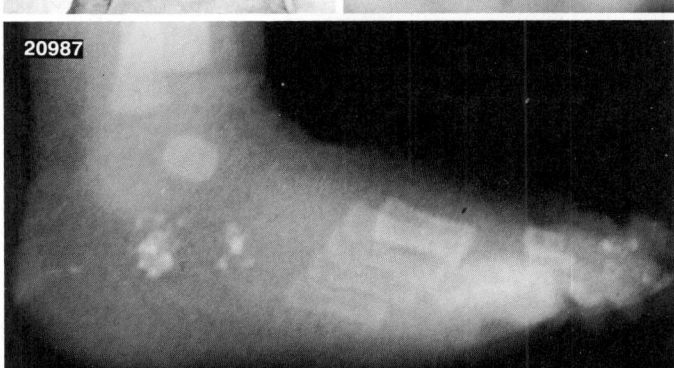

**0389A-20985–86:** Fetal Warfarin syndrome at birth and at age 3 years. Facial changes include midface and nasal hypoplasia. **20987:** X-ray of the foot at birth showing stippling of the calcaneus. Stippling was also present at the proximal femoral head and in the paraspinous region.

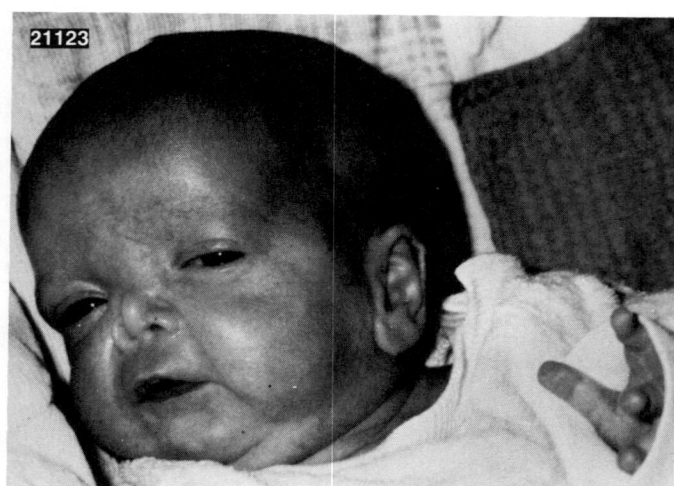

**0389B-21123:** This is a child with Warfarin embryopathy. Note the hypoplastic nose and small distal phalanges.

appearance. A deep groove between the alae nasi and the tip of the nose is often present, probably secondary to undergrown cartilage. The nares and air passages are usually small, resulting in neonatal respiratory distress secondary to upper airway obstruction in about one-half of the patients. True choanal stenosis was documented in only four subjects.

2) Stippling in uncalcified epiphyseal regions, and in certain cartilages and soft tissues was present in all but two patients when looked for at an appropriate age (stippling may not be evident after the first year of life). The stippling, which is seen on X-ray, occurs primarily in the axial skeleton, at the proximal femurs, and in the calcanei.

3) Four of 24 (17%) subjects had significant eye abnormalities (i.e. blindness, optic atrophy and microphthalmia). However, all four were exposed to coumarin derivatives in all three trimesters.

4) In 12 of 24 (50%) subjects, variable degrees of hypoplasia of the extremities were reported, ranging from severe rhizomelic dwarfing to dystrophic nails and shortened fingers.

Infants exposed to vitamin K antagonists in the second and third trimesters seem to have an increased risk of CNS structural anomalies. In addition, an increased number of stillborns and abortions occur in women taking vitamin K antagonists in the second and third trimesters. If taken until delivery, excessive bleeding in both mother and child may occur.

Other Findings: scoliosis (4/24) - 17%; significant development retardation (5/16) - 31%; blindness (3/24) - 12%; deafness (3/24) - 12%; CHD (2/24) - 8%; and seizures (1/24) - 4%. Overall, one half (12/24) apparently had no severe disability. All patients with developmental retardation, blindness and deafness were exposed in all three trimesters. Dandy-Walker cyst and agenesis of the corpus calosum may be associated with late first trimester exposure.

**Complications:** Infants may have bleeding problems at birth if mother is still on anticoagulants.

**Associated Findings:** Small nasal passages enlarge with age. Scoliosis may develop if the vertebrae were involved with stippling.

**Etiology:** A critical period of embryologic exposure is associated with embryopathic manifestations. All 24 patients in whom Warfarin embryopathy was demonstrable were exposed between the sixth and ninth week of gestation; there is no other common time of exposure. Exposure in the second and third trimesters appear to be associated with a different set of problems.

**Pathogenesis:** Initially, it was proposed that the abnormalities were due to fetal microhemorrhage and subsequent calcification of

the hemorrhagic regions. This is unlikely because the critical time period is 6–9 weeks of gestation when clotting factors affected by Vitamin K antagonists are not yet demonstrable in the embryo. A mechanism involving a vitamin K dependent protein seems likely. During the second and third trimester, vitamin K dependent clotting factors are present. In the second and third trimester bleeding in the fetus from vitamin K antagonists having crossed the placenta and resulting in anticoagulation of the fetus could result in intracranial hemorrhage in utero and subsequent CNS anomalies.

**POS No.:** 3227

**Sex Ratio:** M1:F1

**Occurrence:** Not all women taking oral anticoagulants during the critical period have affected infants. The best available estimate based on published data is that if coumadin derivatives are used during pregnancy, one-sixth of the pregnancies will result in an abnormal liveborn infant, one-sixth will result in spontaneous abortions or stillbirths, and, two-thirds will have normal outcome; however the risk of an abnormal birth with first trimester exposure may be as low as 5% and with second trimester, even lower.

**Risk of Recurrence for Patient's Sib:** Related to maternal exposure.

**Risk of Recurrence for Patient's Child:** Related to maternal exposure.

**Age of Detectability:** At birth (stippling may be gone by one year of age so X-rays should be taken at birth). Prenatal diagnosis with ultrasound looking for short limbs, small nose, stippling or structural CNS.

**Gene Mapping and Linkage:** Unknown.

**Prevention:** None known. Genetic counseling indicated.

**Treatment:** The use of heparin during gestation does not result in a significantly better outcome of pregnancy. However the above anomalies would be avoided with preconceptual counseling. Scoliosis prevention.

**Prognosis:** Varies with severity of defects. Of significantly affected liveborn infants, those with hemorrhage or CNS abnormalities generally do poorly, whereas one-half of those with embryopathy have done very well.

**Detection of Carrier:** Unknown.

**References:**
Hall HG, et al.: Maternal and fetal sequelae of anticoagulation during pregnancy. Am J Med 1980; 68:122–140. *
Stevenson RE, et al.: Hazards of oral anticoagulants during pregnancy. JAMA 1980; 243:1549–1551.
Harrod JJE, et al.: Warfarin embryopathy in siblings. Obstet Gynecol 1981; 57:673–676.
Kort HI, et al.: An appraisal of warfarin therapy during pregnancy. S Afr Med J 1981; 60:578.
Chong MKB, et al.: Follow-up study of children whose mothers were treated with warfarin during pregnancy, Br J Obstet Gynaecol 1984; 91:1070–1073.
Iturbe-Alessio I, et al.: Risk of anticoagulant therapy in pregant women with artificial heart valves. New Engl J Med 1986; 315:1390–1393.

HA014                                         **Judith G. Hall**

**Fetus in fetu**
*See EYE, ORBITAL TERATOMA, CONGENITAL*

## FEVER, FAMILIAL MEDITERRANEAN (FMF)      2161

**Includes:**
Hyperimmunoglobulinaemia D and periodic fever
Mediterranean fever, familial (FMF)
Paroxysmal polyserositis, familial
Periodic disease
Periodic fever
Periodic peritonitis
Polyserositis, benign paroxysmal
Polyserositis, recurrent

**Excludes:** Periodic or cyclic disorders, other

**Major Diagnostic Criteria:** Hyperimmunoglobulinemia D and periodic fever
Recurrent episodes of fever, peritonitis, or pleuritis.

**Clinical Findings:** In most instances, symptoms appear at about 5–10 years of age. Acute attacks commonly last 1–2 days, but they may be prolonged as much as 10 days. Frequency of attacks varies, although in most cases they take place about every 2–4 weeks. Attacks appear to be more frequent in the winter, and practically none occur during pregnancy. Spontaneous remissions of long duration may occur. Fever and abdominal pain are almost always present. During acute episodes, the fever may be as high as 40°C. Abdominal pain may start as a localized phenomenon, but it soon spreads to other parts of the abdomen, resulting in one or more needless laparotomies. Many patients also have chest pain. However, acute pleuritic pain may occur without associated abdominal discomfort.

**Complications:** Drug addiction, psychologic problems such as depression, gallbladder disease; rarely **Amyloidosis**, except in the Middle East or Mediterranean population (amyloidosis is found in about 25% of the patients with FMF in Israel).

**Associated Findings:** Joint pain (involving one or more joints), rarely with findings suggesting acute arthritis; painful, erythematous skin lesions, commonly over the lower extremities, disappearing in 1–2 days; pericarditis, hematuria, mild splenomegaly, and hepatomegaly.

**Etiology:** Autosomal recessive inheritance. The condition is not restricted to, but predominantly occurs in, Sephardic Jews (less common in Ashkenazi Jews), Armenians, Arabs, Turks (i.e., Middle East and Mediterranean populations).

**Pathogenesis:** Undetermined. Matzner and Brzezinski (1984) studied levels of chemotactic activity in peritoneal fluid obtained from normal women and patients with FMF, finding less than 10% activity for C5a inhibitor in the FMF patients. It may be that uninhibited accumulation of neutrophils due to deficiency of this inhibitor results in localized inflammation.
Baraket et al (1984) developed a provocative test using metaraminol on the basis of their hypothesis that FMF may be the result of an inborn error of catecholamine matabolism. In a controlled, double-blind study, they used a 10 mg dose of metaraminol infusion on 21 patients with FMF to stimulate endogenous cathecolamine release. All patients with FMF responded with a typical disease-like attack (somewhat milder in nature) within 48 hours. No such reaction was observed among 21 control subjects.
The six cases of *Hyperimmunoglobulinaemia D and periodic fever* reported by van der Meer et al (1984) had high serum IgD levels, while such levels are rare among FMF patients, suggesting that these may be different conditions.

**MIM No.:** *24910

**Sex Ratio:** M6:F4

**Occurrence:** Uncommon except in Middle East and Mediterranean populations. One study reported on over 1,000 cases in a follow-up study. Extensive literature.

**Risk of Recurrence for Patient's Sib:**
See Part I, *Mendelian Inheritance.*

**Risk of Recurrence for Patient's Child:**
See Part I, *Mendelian Inheritance.*

**Age of Detectability:** In Childhood or adolescence.

**Gene Mapping and Linkage:** Unknown.

**Prevention:** None known. Genetic counseling indicated.

**Treatment:** Colchicine administration by mouth reduces the number of acute attacks. Due to the side effects of this drug in some patients, such as azospermia, colchicine can be recommended only for patients with severe FMF. If started early, colchicine may also be used to abort acute attacks. Kidney transplants are recommended for patients with amyloidosis.

**Prognosis:** Very good, except for patients who develop amyloidosis.

**Detection of Carrier:** Unknown.

**References:**
Sohar E, et al.: Familial Mediterranean fever. Am J Med 1967; 43:227–253.
Dinarello CA, et al.: Colchicine therapy for familial Mediterranean fever: a double-blind-trial. New Engl J Med 1974; 291:934–937.
Meyerhoff J: Familial Mediterranean fever: report of a large family, review of the literature, and discussion of the frequency of amyloidosis. Medicine (Baltimore) 1980; 59:66–77. *
Baraket MH, et al.: Metaraminol provocative test: a specific test for Familial Mediterranean Fever. Lancet 1984; I:656–657.
Matzner Y, Brzezinski, A: C5a-inhibitor deficiency in peritoneal fluids from patients with familial Mediterranean fever. New Engl J Med 1984; 311:287–290. *
van der Meer JWM, et al: Hyperimmunoglobulinemia D and periodic fever: a new syndrome. Lancet 1984; I:1087–1090.
Barakat MH, et al.: Familial Mediterranean fever in Arabs: a study of 175 patients and a review of the literature. Q J Med 1986; 60:837–847.
Zemer D, et al.: Colchicine in the prevention and treatment of the amyloidosis in familial Mediterranean fever. New Engl J Med 1986; 314:1001–1005.
Schwabe AD, Nishizawa A: Recurrent polyserositis (familial Mediterranean fever) in a Japanese. Jap J Med 1987; 26:370–372.
Shohat M, et al.: Hypothesis: familial Mediterranean Fever: a genetic disorder of the Lipocortin family? Am J Med Genet 1989; 34:163–167.

SA033      **Burhan Say**

## FG SYNDROME, OPITZ-KAVEGGIA TYPE      0754

**Includes:** Opitz-Kaveggia FG syndrome

**Excludes:**
**Acropectorovertebral dysplasia** (0022)
**Anus-hand-ear syndrome** (0072)

**Major Diagnostic Criteria:** A male with characteristic facies, mental retardation, hypotonia, macrocephaly, camptodactyly, and severe constipation.

**Clinical Findings:** Normal intrauterine growth, and an occipitofrontal circumfrence that ranges from the 50th percentile to >98th percentile at birth and postnatally, and may lead to the false impression of hydrocephaly; postnatal growth failure, with adult heights of 145–160 cm; congenital hypotonia of variable degree, with squints and ptosis; hypotonic mouth-breathing facies with highly arched palate, micrognathia, inverted V shape of upper lip, protruding tongue with drooling, and malocclusion; sloping shoulders with winged scapulae, mild-to-moderate pectus excavatum, and repeated attacks of pneumonia; lumbar hyperlordosis, distended abdomen with marked constipation; at times cryptorchidism; hyperextensible joints, clubfeet, simian creases, crowding of toes, and deep creases of soles; at times, with a history of hypoactive fetal movements; a characteristic facial appearance with a high broad forehead, hypertelorism with prominent nose, upsweep of frontal hair, relatively large mouth with thick lips; mild posterior rotation of small auricles, with minor anomalies of auricular differentiation; minor anomalies of limbs with broad thumbs and big toes, minimal cutaneous syndactyly of 3rd and 4th fingers, at times mild joint contractures; imperforate anus (usually membranous) or other anal anomalies such as anal stenosis occur. Severe constipation is found in all patients.

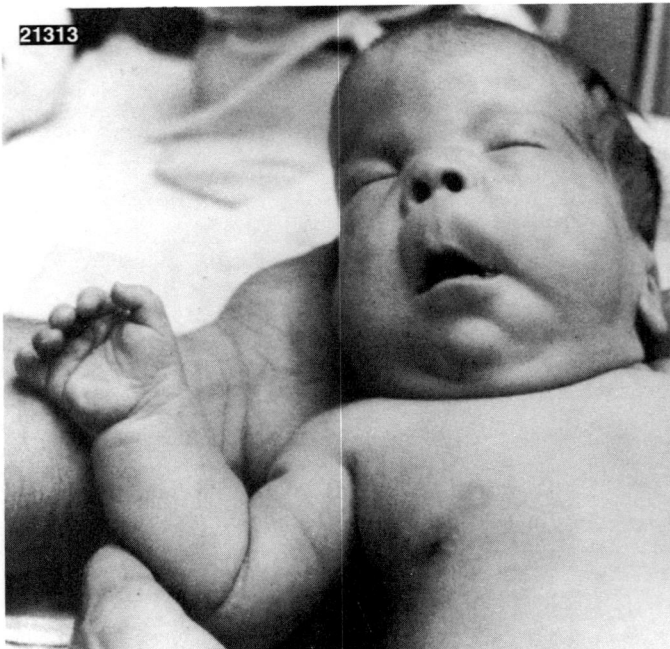

**0754-21313:** Premature male with characteristic facies; note high forehead, prominent nose, low-set ears, long philtrum and inverted v-shaped upper lip.

Affected individuals have IQs around 50; agenesis of corpus callosum was seen in one patient and suspected in another. One patient had seizures. All survivors have shown a hyperactive, mischievous, easy-going and affable personality. Pyloric stenosis has been seen in two patients; hypoplastic left heart, **Ventricular septal defect**, generalized dilation of the urinary tract, and severe craniosynostosis were each seen in one patient.

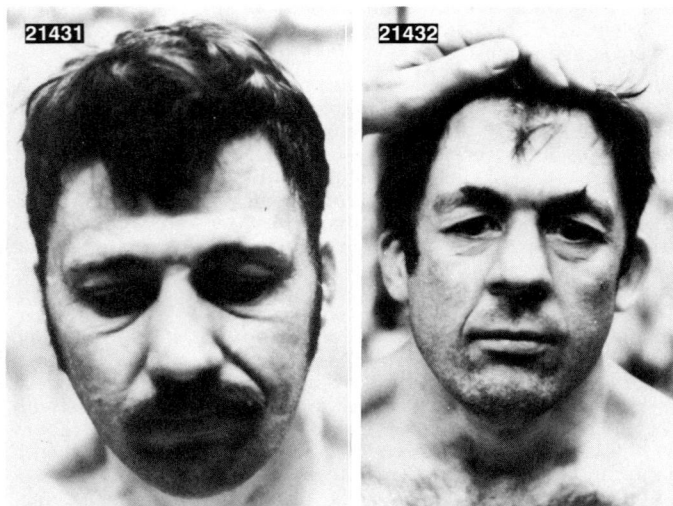

**0754B-21431–32:** Two affected brothers with the characteristic facies including a high forehead, hypertelorism, prominent nose, and large mouth with thick lips.

**Complications:** Pneumonia and constipation due to hypotonia.

**Associated Findings:** Frequently a breech presentation. Sensorineural deafness, inperforated anus, and pigmentary dysplasia have been reported.

**Etiology:** X-linked recessive inheritance.

**Pathogenesis:** Undetermined. A true multiple congenital anomaly/mental retardation (MCA/MR) syndrome. Histological studies of the skin of a patient who had a pigmentary dysplasia showed a reduction of collagen fibers, and relative increase of the elastic fibers. This may explain hyperelastic skin and hyperextensible joint, and may contribute to hypotonia. Many findings involve midline structures, and may reflect developmental effects on the midline.

**MIM No.:** *30545

**POS No.:** 3566

**Sex Ratio:** M1:F0

**Occurrence:** More than 25 cases have been documented in the literature.

**Risk of Recurrence for Patient's Sib:**
See Part I, *Mendelian Inheritance.*

**Risk of Recurrence for Patient's Child:**
See Part I, *Mendelian Inheritance.* Ability to reproduce is doubtful.

**Age of Detectability:** At birth.

**Gene Mapping and Linkage:** Unknown.

**Prevention:** None known. Genetic counseling indicated.

**Treatment:** Surgical treatment of anal defects; treatment of congestive heart disease (CHD) if present, seizures, constipation and pneumonia.

**Prognosis:** Four of 15 reported cases died neonatally (one of CHD and one of amniotic aspiration and hyaline membrane disease), one affected individual died at 4 1/2 months of age of an unstated cause, and two others at about two years of age of pneumonia. The remainder have been mentally retarded.

**Detection of Carrier:** Unknown.

**Special Considerations:** One affected individual had unusual histologic brain abnormalities: dense, subependymal infiltrates of glial cells, granulocytes, lymphocytes and histiocytes; especially in a perivascular distribution. Diagnosis may be difficult in isolated sporadic cases.

**References:**

Opitz JM, Kaveggia EG: Studies of malformation syndromes of man XXXIII: the FG syndrome: an X-linked recessive syndrome of multiple congenital anomalies and mental retardation. Z Kinderheilk 1974; 117:1–18.

Keller MA, et al.: A new syndrome of mental deficiency with craniofacial, limb and anal abnormalities. J Pediatr 1976; 88:589–591.

Riccardi VM, et al.: Studies of malformation syndromes of man. XXXIII B: The FG syndrome: further characterization, report of a third family, and of a sporadic case. Am J Med Genet 1977; 1:47–58.

Opitz JM, et al.: Studies of malformation syndromes of humans. XXXIIIC: The FG syndrome. Am J Med Genet 1982; 12:147–154.

Neri G, et al.: Sensorineural deafness in the FG syndrome: report on four new cases. Am J Med Genet 1984; 19:369–377.

Richieri-Costa A: FG syndrome in a Brazilian child with additional previously unreported signs. Am J Med Genet (suppl) 1986; 2:247.

Thompson EM, Baraitser M: FG syndrome. J Med Genet 1987; 24:139–143.

LU001                                                    **Mark Lubinsky**

**Fiber-type disproportion myopathy**
*See MYOPATHY, DISPROPORTIONATE FIBER TYPE I*
**Fibrin stabilizing factor, A subunit**
*See FACTOR XIII (FIBRIN STABILIZING FACTOR)*
**Fibrinase deficiency**
*See FACTOR XIII (FIBRIN STABILIZING FACTOR)*
**Fibrinogen and factor XIII**
*See FACTOR XIII (FIBRIN STABILIZING FACTOR)*

## FIBRINOGENS, ABNORMAL CONGENITAL        0004

**Includes:** Dysfibrinogenemia, congenital

**Excludes:**
  Acquired dysfibrinogenemia
  Afibrinogenemia, congenital
  Fibrin degradation products
  Fibrinogen degradation
  Hypofibrinogenemia

**Major Diagnostic Criteria:** Over one-half of the families with dysfibrinogenemia do not have any symptoms. These families are identified by abnormal laboratory tests. Approximately 33% experience hemorrhagic symptoms, and 13% experience bleeding and thrombosis or just thrombosis. The diagnosis can be confirmed by a long thrombin time not related to the presence of heparin or fibrinogen degradation products. The Reptilase test is also prolonged. The fibrinogen concentration as measured by functional assays is almost invariably reduced by 50% compared with the concentration determined by physical/chemical or immunologic techniques.

**Clinical Findings:** The symptoms associated with dysfibrinogenemia have been quite varied. Bleeding, thrombosis, wound dehiscence, and recurrent abortions are the major findings in these patients. The majority have been asymptomatic. In patients who have thrombosis associated with their dysfibrinogenemia, both venous and arterial thromboses have been reported.

**Complications:** Individuals who have dysfibrinogenemia with a clinical bleeding tendency usually receive plasma products, primarily cryoprecipitate, for bleeding episodes. These products have the potential of transmitting hepatitis or HIV infections.

**Associated Findings:** Infusion induced hepatitis.

**Etiology:** Autosomal dominant inheritance. In two families (dysfibrinogenemia Metz and dysfibrinogenemia Detroit) the propositi are homozygous for the abnormal fibrinogen.

**Pathogenesis:** The molecular abnormality that accounts for the abnormal function of these fibrinogens is either a single amino acid substitution or a partial deletion of one of the fibrinogen chains. The most common amino acid substitution occurs within the first 19 amino acids of the amino terminus of the A-alpha chain. To date, over 150 different abnormal fibrinogens have been reported.

**MIM No.:** *13482, *13483, *13485

**Sex Ratio:** M1:F1

**Occurrence:** All of the known variants of fibrinogen are of uncommon or rare occurrence.

**Risk of Recurrence for Patient's Sib:**
  See Part I, *Mendelian Inheritance.*

**Risk of Recurrence for Patient's Child:**
  See Part I, *Mendelian Inheritance.*

**Age of Detectability:** The vast majority of affected individuals are detected during routine coagulation screening tests. Those individuals who are symptomatic usually have symptoms in early childhood, although in several instances the abnormal fibrinogen was not detected until bleeding during adolescence or adulthood.

**Gene Mapping and Linkage:** FGA (fibrinogen, A alpha polypeptide) has been mapped to 4q28.
  FGB (fibrinogen, B beta polypeptide) has been mapped to 4q28.
  FGG (fibrinogen, gamma polypeptide) has been mapped to 4q28.
  Dysfibrinogenemia has been associated with hemophilia A.

**Prevention:** None known. Genetic counseling indicated.

**Treatment:** Administration of human cryoprecipitate rich in human fibrinogen is the treatment of choice. Therapy is only necessary for active bleeding or as prophalyxis for bleeding in patients who have invasive procedures or surgery and have a previous bleeding history. Patients with thrombotic disease are treated with antithrombotic therapy. Those individuals who have more than one thrombotic episode may need to have antithrom-

botic therapy for the rest of their lives. A functional fibrinogen concentration of greater than 100 mg/dl is usually sufficient to prevent hemorrhage during major surgical procedures. It is imperative that the fibrinogen be maintained at approximately 100 mg/dl during the postoperative period.

**Prognosis:** Most patients are not substantially handicapped by this defect.

**Detection of Carrier:** Asymptomatic family members of individuals with dysfibrinogenemia can be easily identified by performing a thrombin time and a functional assay and a physical, chemical or immunologic assay of plasma fibrinogen.

**Special Considerations:** Several cases of the abnormal fibrinogens (dysfibrinogenemia) are hypodysfibrinogenemias. These must be differentiated from congenital hypofibrinogenemia. The best technique is the use of the different fibrinogen assays that show discrepant values between the functional and the physical, chemical or immunologic methods in dysfibrinogenemia but have comparable values in the congenital hypodysfibrinogenemia.

**References:**
Gralnick HR: Congenital disorders of fibrinogen. In: Hematology, vol 14, ed 3. 1986:1399–1410.
McDonagh J, Carrell N: Disorders of fibrinogen structure and function. In: Coleman R et al., eds: Hemostasis and Thrombosis, ed 2. Philadelphia: JB Lippincott, 1987:301–317.

GR033                               **Harvey R. Gralnick**

**Fibrinoid leukodystrophy**
  *See ALEXANDER DISEASE*
**Fibrinoligase deficiency**
  *See FACTOR XIII (FIBRIN STABILIZING FACTOR)*
**Fibroblast interferon deficiency**
  *See INTERFERON DEFICIENCY*

## FIBROCHONDROGENESIS        2694

**Includes:** Skeletal dysplasia, fibrochondrogenesis

**Excludes:**
  **Achondrogenesis, Langer-Saldino type** (0008)
  **Kniest-like dysplasia** (2799)
  **Skeletal dysplasia, Schneckenbecken type** (2632)
  **Skeletal dysplasia** (other)
  **Thanatophoric dysplasia** (0940)

**Major Diagnostic Criteria:** Lethal neonatal dwarfism with characteristic clinical, radiologic, and histopathologic features.

**Clinical Findings:** A rare lethal neonatal dwarfism. Most published cases have been stillborns or died shortly after birth. On clinical grounds, these cases cannot be distinguished from the other known lethal short-limb dysplasias. The skull is brachycephalic but proportionate, with flat face, **Cleft palate**, and narrow chest. On X-ray the skull is collapsed with enlarged scalp; there is diffuse platyspondly, the cervical vertebrae are undermineralized, with superior-inferior clefting defects in the cervical and lumbar regions. The ribs are short and cupped. The pelvic bones are hypoplastic, with medial acetabular spike. The long bones are short, with a dumbbell-like shape and metaphyseal flare in both the proximal and the distal ends. The fibulae are disproportionately short.

**Complications:** Intrauterine or neonatal death.

**Associated Findings:** None known.

**Etiology:** Autosomal recessive inheritance. Two cases occured in an uncle-niece marriage.

**Pathogenesis:** Pathologic examination of cartilage has demonstrated abnormal growth plate. The resting chondrocytes are large and round with fibroblastic appearance. Dense fibrous matrix swirled around groups of chondrocytes. Ultrastructurally, a paucity of rough endoplasmic reticulum was noted.

**MIM No.:** *22852

**POS No.:** 3642

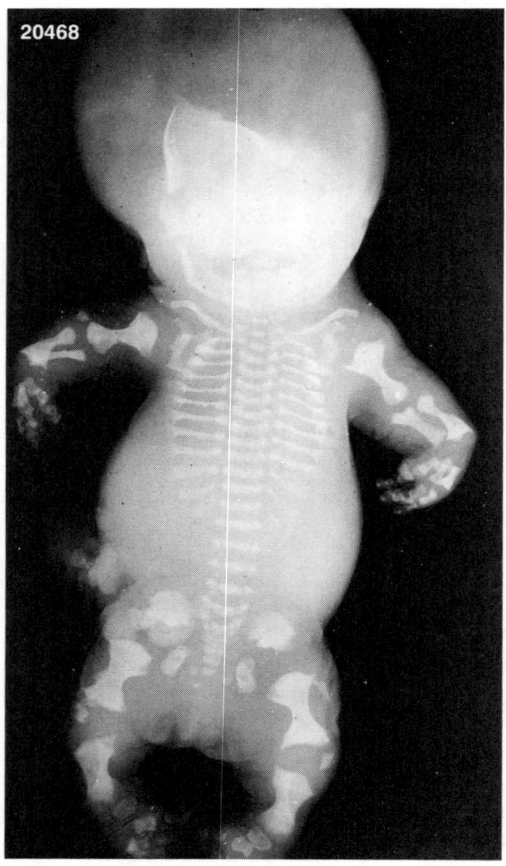

**2694A-20468:** Fibrochondrogenesis; X-ray of stillborn; note short dumbbell-like long bones with extra articular ossifications. The ribs are short and cupped. Vertebral bodies are flattened. Ilia are hypoplastic with medial and lateral spikes.

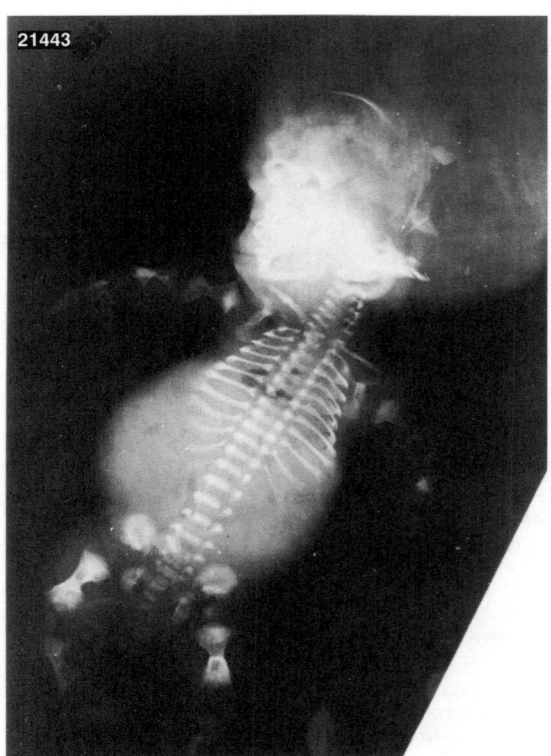

**2694B-21443:** X-ray of stillborn at 37 weeks gestation; note short ribs, hypoplastic pelvis with ovoid ilia and flat spiky acetabula. Diffuse platyspondyly is present. The long bones have a dumbbell-like configuration.

---

chondrodysplasia with distinctive cartilage histopathology. Am J Med Genet 1984; 19:265–275.

B0025 **Zvi Borochowitz**

**Sex Ratio:** M1:F4 (observed in the five patients reported to date).

**Occurrence:** Some five cases have been reported, with single case reports from regions including Japan and Italy.

**Risk of Recurrence for Patient's Sib:**
See Part I, *Mendelian Inheritance.*

**Risk of Recurrence for Patient's Child:**
See Part I, *Mendelian Inheritance.* Affected individuals are not expected to survive to reproduce.

**Age of Detectability:** At birth. Prenatal diagnosis through mid-trimester (14–16 weeks gestation) ultrasound is potentially available.

**Gene Mapping and Linkage:** Unknown.

**Prevention:** None known. Genetic counseling indicated.

**Treatment:** Unknown.

**Prognosis:** Fatal in the neonatal period.

**Detection of Carrier:** Unknown.

**References:**
Lazzaroni-Fossati F, et al.: La Fibrochondrogenèse. Arch Fr Pediatr 1978; 35:1096–1104.
Eteson JD, et al.: Fibrochondrogenesis: radiologic and histologic studies. Am J Med Genet 1984; 19:277–290.
Whitley BC, et al.: Fibrochondrogenesis: lethal, autosomal recessive

Fibrocystic disease of pancreas
 *See CYSTIC FIBROSIS*
Fibrodysplasia of arteries
 *See ARTERY, RENAL FIBROMUSCULAR DYSPLASIA*
Fibrodysplasia ossificans progressiva
 *See MYOSITIS OSSIFICANS PROGRESSIVA*
Fibroma, digital, recurring in infants and children
 *See DIGITAL FIBROMA, RECURRING IN INFANTS & CHILDREN*
Fibromatosis, gingival
 *See GINGIVAL FIBROMATOSIS*
Fibromatosis, gingival-progressive deafness
 *See GINGIVAL FIBROMATOSIS-DEAFNESS, JONES TYPES*

---

**FIBROMATOSIS, JUVENILE HYALINE**     **0411**

**Includes:**
 Gingival fibromatosis-multiple hyaline fibromas
 Hyaline fibromas-gingival fibromatosis
 Hyalinosis, systemic (Ishikawa-Hori)
 Mesenchymal dysplasie of Puretic
 Murray syndrome
 Murray-Puretic syndrome
 Murray-Puretic-Drescher syndrome
 Puretic syndrome

**Excludes:**
 **Enchondromatosis** (0345)
 **Enchondromatosis and hemangiomas** (0346)
 **Gingival fibromatosis** (0407)

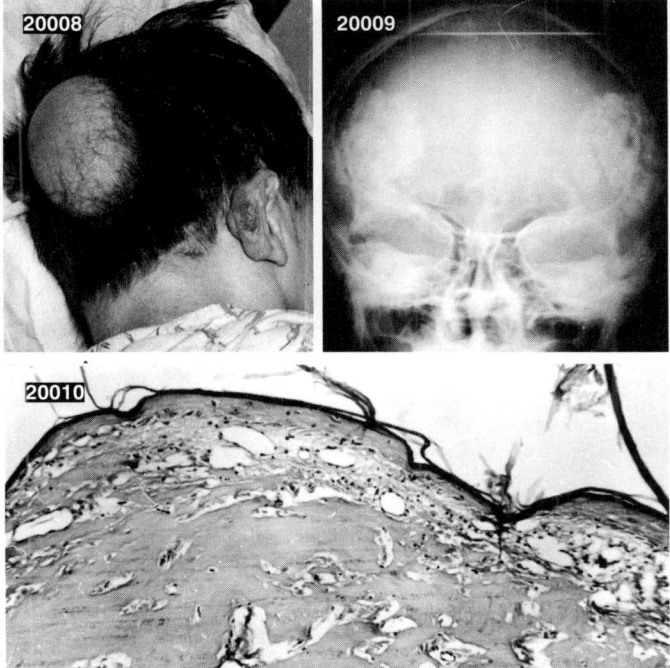

**0411-20008:** 19-year-old male with posterior scalp tumor and translucent nodules on the posterior pinna.  **20009:** Skull X-ray shows the calcification of the tumors in the parieto-occipital region.  **20010:** Tumor histology shows homogeneous eosinophilic masses and "chondroid" cells in the dermis.

Gingival fibromatosis, symmetric
**Gingival fibromatosis-corneal dystrophy** (0408)
**Gingival fibromatosis-deafness, Jones types** (2315)
**Gingival fibromatosis-depigmentation-microphthalmia** (0413)
**Gingival fibromatosis-digital anomalies** (0409)
**Gingival fibromatosis-hypertrichosis** (0410)
**Gingival multiple hamartoma syndrome** (0412)
**Mucolipidosis II** (0672)
**Mucopolysaccharidosis**
**Neurofibromatosis** (0712)
**Scalp, cylindromas** (0235)
**Skin, lipoid proteinosis** (0599)
**Tuberous sclerosis** (0975)
**Winchester syndrome** (1000)

**Major Diagnostic Criteria:**  From early infancy multiple cutaneous and subcutaneous nodules, nodes and tumors, some of which ulcerate and/or calcify, coarse face, gingival hypertrophy, progressive flexural contractures of large joints, cystic defects, muscle atrophy, delayed bone maturation and sexual development, stunted growth, normal mental development. The diagnosis can be suspected from typical clinical signs and from characteristic histological and histochemical findings of the skin and gingival lesions.

**Clinical Findings:**  Gingival enlargement may be present at birth or develops during the first 2 years of life. All of the gingivae have a hard, firm, slowly enlarging lesion. In early childhood, sub- and periungual growths appear and slowly enlarge. Multiple firm, painless, elastic or hard nodules adherent to the overlying skin

develop by coalescence and growth of white miliary nodules. These slowly enlarge and may reach orange-sized pendulous tumors. They also appear on the tip of the nose, on chin and perianal areas. Gelatinous or hemorrhagic blisters may appear suddenly, later transforming into hard translucent nodules. Lichenoid, sclerodermiform and dysseborrhoic lesions are found. Tumors usually appear first on the head, face, shoulders and digits. Those involving the trunk, back, thighs, and legs usually develop later in childhood. The scalp tumors resemble turban tumors. There have been no café-au-lait spots, hypertrichosis, epilepsy, neurofibromata, hemangiomas, osteochondromata, dermoids, juvenile aponeurotic fibromata, keloids or oligophrenia in the cases reported. X-rays may show destructive long bone and joint lesions. Laboratory tests are normal.

In one patient multiple polypoid lesions of the nasal cavity arose from the septum and produced nasal deformity. There was close histological similarity between the associated gingival and cutaneous tissues and the nasal masses examined.

**Complications:**  Malocclusion, interference with speech, nasal deformity and obstruction, local irritation depending on site of tumor involvement. Recurrent bacterial infections of the skin, middle ear, eyes and nose.

**Associated Findings:**  Painful flexion contractures of limbs are often noted. Pseudoarthrosis; kyphoscoliosis; coarse face, bulbous nose deformity.

**Etiology:**  Autosomal recessive inheritance with variable expression and penetrance. Both mild and severe forms of the syndrome can be seen.

**Pathogenesis:**  Slowly enlarging gingivae result from deposits of PAS-positive amorphous substance in the lamina propria without inflammatory infiltrates. The tumors are composed of a hyaline homogenous amorphous, acidophilic, PAS-positive, ground substance in which are embedded abundant blood vessels and ovoid-to-spindle-shaped "chondroid" cells forming minute streaks. Fine silver staining fibers are between cells. The sections have the appearance of pseudocartilage but only minute amounts of hyaluronic acid are found on electrophoresis of tumor extracts. True cartilage, elastic, or nervous tissue has not been observed in tumors.

At the ultrastructural level, thin collagenous fibers are noted within the hyaline areas along with ruthenium red-positive material in the form of granules, filaments and cross-banded aggregates of chondroitin sulfate-proteoglycan and/or glycoprotein. Entangled tubular structure within the fibroblast cytoplasm have been noted in addition to dilated rough endoplasmic reticulum forming so-called fibril-filled balls. Fibrils range from 6 - 10nm in diameter indicating the presence of both actin and intermediate type filaments, but an absence of 15nm thick myelin filaments. In an overall context there appears to be less collagen per unit volume in skin tissue when examined biochemically.

**MIM No.:**  *22860, *26570

**Sex Ratio:**  M1:F1

**Occurrence:**  About forty cases reported; 26 cases from 19 families are published in detail. Parental consanguinity was presented in six families. There is no difference in the prevalence in various ethnic groups and geographic locations. There are reports of patients originated from United States, various parts of Europe (middle and south), Japan, North Eastern Africa, Arabia and India.

**Risk of Recurrence for Patient's Sib:**
See Part I, *Mendelian Inheritance.*

**Risk of Recurrence for Patient's Child:**
See Part I, *Mendelian Inheritance.*

**Age of Detectability:**  Usually clinically evident in early infancy, fully developed syndrome in early childhood.

**Gene Mapping and Linkage:**  Unknown.

**Prevention:**  None known. Genetic counseling indicated.

**Treatment:**  Extraction of teeth and gingivectomy may be necessary. Surgical removal of tumors has met with variable success; several have recurred at surgical site. Tenotomy of contractured joints help temporarily. Steroid given systemically or locally can have some satisfactory effect as well as physical therapy on joints lesions and motility. Prosthetic replacement of teeth may also be recommended.

**Prognosis:** At least one case has survived to sixth decade of life. The contractures of joints cause deformity and usually complete stiffness. Surgical excision of tumors has met with only partial success as tumors tend to recur.

**Detection of Carrier:** Unknown.

**Special Considerations:** The original cases were described by Murray in 1871 and were thought by later investigators to be examples of **Neurofibromatosis**. Neurofibromatosis can affect gingivae but the neurofibromata are usually localized and do not involve all of the gums as is seen in this disease. Ungual fibromata may occur in both conditions. **Tuberous sclerosis** may have nodular tumors of the face and nose in addition to a generalized pebbly appearing lesion of the gums. The nodules in tuberous sclerosis usually do not reach the size seen in this disease and the histologic picture is different. **Enchondromatosis** and **Enchondromatosis and hemangiomas** can be differentiated from this disease by the occurrence in the former diseases of hemangiomas and true cartilage and osseous containing tumors.

**References:**

Murray J: On three peculiar cases of molluscum fibrosum in children family (neurofibromatosis). Med Chir Trans 1873; 38:235–253.
Puretić S, et al.: A unique form of mesenchymal dysplasia. Br J Dermatol 1962; 74:8–19. *
Woyke S, et al.: Ultrastructure of a fibromatosis hyalinica multiplex juvenilis. Cancer 1970; 26:1157.
Witkop CJ, Jr: Heterogeneity in gingival fibromatosis. BD:OAS;VII(7). Baltimore, Williams and Wilkins, 1971:210.
Kitano Y: Juvenile hyalin fibromatosis. Arch Dermatol 1976; 112:86–88.
Remberger K, et al.: Fibromatosis hyalinica multiplex (Juvenile hyaline fibrmatosis). Cancer, 1985; 56:614–624.
Fayad MN, et al.: Juvenile hyaline fibromatosis: two new patients and a review of the literature. Am J Med Genet 1987; 26:123–131.

WI043
PU005
PU006

**Carl J. Witkop, Jr.**
**Zvonimir Puretić**
**Višnja Milavec-Puretić**

**Fibromatosis, palmar**
  See CONTRACTURE, DUPUYTREN
**Fibromuscular atresia of antrum**
  See STOMACH, PYLORIC ATRESIA
**Fibromuscular dysplasia of arteries**
  See ARTERY, RENAL FIBROMUSCULAR DYSPLASIA
**Fibromuscular dysplasia with medial fibroplasia**
  See ARTERY, RENAL FIBROMUSCULAR DYSPLASIA
**Fibromuscular hyperplasia**
  See ARTERY, RENAL FIBROMUSCULAR DYSPLASIA
**Fibromuscular subaortic stenosis**
  See HEART, SUBAORTIC STENOSIS, FIBROUS
**Fibroplasia retrolental**
  See RETINOPATHY OF PREMATURITY
**Fibroplastic renal artery disease**
  See ARTERY, RENAL FIBROMUSCULAR DYSPLASIA
**Fibrosarcoma**
  See CANCER, SOFT TISSUE SARCOMA
**Fibrosis of the extraocular muscles, congenital**
  See EYE, FIBROSIS OF THE EXTRAOCULAR MUSCLES, GENERALIZED

## FIBROUS DYSPLASIA, MONOSTOTIC 0390

**Includes:** Jaffe-Lichtenstein disease

**Excludes:**
  Aneurysmal bone cyst
  **Fibrous dysplasia, polyostotic** (0391)
  Ossifying fibroma
  Unicameral bone cyst

**Major Diagnostic Criteria:** A solitary pseudocystic lesion of bone usually develops during childhood or adolescence. This disorder is suspected on X-ray findings, but the diagnosis can only be made by biopsy and histologic confirmation.

**Clinical Findings:** This disease is characterized by a solitary pseudocystic lesion of bone which usually develops during childhood or adolescence. The individual lesion is identical to that found in polyostotic fibrous dysplasia, but it is isolated to one area and is not associated with extraskeletal manifestations. The lesions are most common in the craniofacial bones, ribs, vertebrae, and long bones. Craniofacial lesions can produce deformities secondary to the presence of a mass, or difficulty in chewing because of maxillary enlargement. Lesions in the ribs are usually discovered incidentally on routine chest X-rays. Involvement of the vertebrae may produce low back pain. Those lesions affecting the long bones usually present as a mass. The earliest radiographic changes are loss of density in the site where bone is being replaced by fibrous tissue. Later the whole shaft may exhibit a ground-glass appearance with expansion of the medullary cavity and internal atrophy of the cortical walls. Diagnosis can only be made on microscopic confirmation of the typical lesion consisting of whorls of fibrous tissue with interspersed islands of bony trabeculae and calcified cartilage.

The term "Jaffe-Lichtenstein syndrome" should be restricted to those cases of fibrous dysplasia that are monostotic. The polyostotic form of the disease (see **Fibrous Dysplasia, polyostotic**) is often associated with endocrine and skin manifestations and probably represents a completely distinct entity. This disorder may appear identical on X-ray to unicameral bone cysts, aneurysmal bone cysts and ossifying fibromas. The diagnosis can only be confirmed on histologic examination of biopsied tissue.

**Complications:** Unknown.

**Associated Findings:** None known.

**Etiology:** Unknown.

**Pathogenesis:** According to one theory drawn from histological findings, fibrous dysplasia is due to dysfunction of bone-forming mesenchyme with formation of abnormal osteoblasts. The mesenchymal cells seem to differentiate into bone-forming cells as in early stages of membranous ossification during bone development. But, unlike membranous ossification, in fibrous dysplasia the normal process of bone remodeling is impaired, probably due to a lack of osteoblastic differentiation.

**Sex Ratio:** M1:F1

**Occurrence:** Unknown.

**Risk of Recurrence for Patient's Sib:** All observed cases have been sporadic.

**Risk of Recurrence for Patient's Child:** Unknown.

**Age of Detectability:** Can be detected in early childhood by skeletal X-rays.

**Gene Mapping and Linkage:** Unknown.

**Prevention:** None known. Genetic counseling indicated.

**Treatment:** Orthopedic procedures such as curettage of the lesion and packing with bone chips.

**Prognosis:** Normal for life span. Lesions may progressively increase in size. Regrowth has often occurred following curettage, which has apparently been incomplete.

**Detection of Carrier:** Unknown.

**References:**
Jaffe HL, Lichtenstein L: Non-osteogenic fibroma of bone. Am J Pathol 1942; 18:205.
Harris WH, et al.: The natural history of fibrous dysplasia. J Bone Joint Surg [Am] 1962; 44:207.
Henry A: Monostotic fibrous dysplasia. J Bone Joint Surg 1969; 300:51B.
Gil-Carcedo LM, Gonzalez M: Monostotic fibrous dysplasia of the ethmoid. J Laryngol Otology 1986; 100:429–434.
Greco MA, Steiner GC: Ultrastructure of fibrous dysplasia of bone. Ultrastructural Path 1986; 10:55–66.

B0025
BE050

Zvi Borochowitz
Michael Beck
David L. Rimoin
David W. Hollister

## FIBROUS DYSPLASIA, POLYOSTOTIC                    0391

**Includes:**
Albright syndrome
McCune-Albright syndrome
Polyostotic fibrous dysplasia-skin pigmentation-sexual precocity

**Excludes:**
**Fibrous dysplasia, monostotic** (0390)
**Hyperparathyroidism, familial** (0499)
**Neurofibromatosis** (0712)

**Major Diagnostic Criteria:** The classic triad of this syndrome consists of polyostotic fibrous dysplasia, skin pigmentation, and sexual precocity. The diagnosis can be made based on the classic X-ray appearance of polyostotic fibrous dysplasia, with or without the associated skin or endocrine anomalies. Neither the skin lesions nor sexual precocity are required to make a diagnosis.

**Clinical Findings:** The skeletal disorder can occur alone or with the cutaneous or endocrine components. The bone disorder consists of patchy areas of rarefaction with a pseudocystic appearance. The lesions may be disseminated throughout the skeleton, and are frequently found in the lower limbs. They occur less frequently in the upper limbs and rarely in the skull. The skull may have a sclerotic overgrowth of bone at the base, which may be so dense that the sella cannot be visualized. Deforming overgrowth of the skull, jaw, or facial bones may occur. The skeletal lesions result in frequent fractures, deformity, and leg length discrepancy. In one series, 70% of the patients presented with a limp, leg fracture, or limb pain; 60% had leg length discrepancy; 85% experienced at least one fracture; and 40% experienced three or more fractures. Serum alkaline phosphatase levels are elevated in about one-third of the patients. The lesions are progressive, usually by extension or by the appearance of new lesions. The frequency of fractures does not change with age or the onset of puberty. Fracture healing is not delayed. The skeletal lesions consist of poorly differentiated fibrous tissue with fibrous bone trabeculae interspersed, and sometimes multiple islands of cartilage are found. Sarcomatous degeneration in an area of fibrous dysplasia has been described twice.

The skin lesions (large café-au-lait spots) are flat, brown, irregular patches (macules). They are frequently congenital, unilateral, segmental, and may overlie areas of bone involvement.

Precocious puberty occurs primarily in females, but several affected males are known. Approximately 50% of females with polyostotic fibrous dysplasia have sexual precocity. It usually presents as precocious menarche as early as 3 months of age. In contrast to other types of sexual precocity, the vaginal bleeding is usually scanty and irregular and precedes breast development and sexual hair growth by as much as 7 years. The ovaries contain follicles in various stages of development, sometimes with large follicular cysts. There is no evidence of ovulation or corpus luteum formation. Urinary gonadotropins are usually low to absent, but high peaks of urinary luteinizing hormone are detectable. Urinary estrogen, 17-hydroxycorticoid and 17-ketosteroid concentrations are elevated in some. Ovulation and regular periods occur at the regular time of puberty, and fertility is not impaired. Generally, affected males do not have sexual abnormalities, but precocious puberty is described in a few, one of whom had active spermatogenesis. Advanced skeletal maturation and accelerated growth in childhood may occur in patients with sexual precocity. Adult height, however, is usually normal or somewhat decreased. Diffuse or nodular thyroid enlargement is frequent, and mild hyperthyroidism is also common; parathyroid hyperplasia is described in several patients. A variety of other endocrine pathology has been described: gonadal and adrenal steroids are elevated in the plasma, growth hormone levels are elevated; and diabetes mellitus can occur.

Skeletal X-rays show hypo- or hypersclerotic cysts, which may be scattered throughout the skeleton. They are not bilaterally symmetric and may have a segmental distribution. They have a ground-glass appearance due to a myriad of thin, calcified trabeculae. The overlying cortex has variable thickness, and the periosteal surface is smooth. Other disorders, such as unicameral bone cysts, aneurysmal bone cysts, and non-ossified fibroma may have a similar appearance on X-ray. However, involvement of the entire bone, from epiphyseal plate to epiphyseal plate, and the increased density of the base of the skull is not found in these other disorders. Bending or bowing of the affected bones occurs as well as the classic deformity of the "shepherd's crook" malformation of the femoral neck.

**Complications:** The skeletal lesions may result in multiple fractures, leg length discrepancy, bowing of the limbs, a waddling gait, and persistent pain. The sclerotic lesions of the base of the skull may result in obliteration of the nasal sinuses, facial asymmetry, and rarely may impinge on the optic nerves, resulting in optic atrophy. Sarcomatous degeneration of the bony lesions has been described in two patients. The multiple fractures may result in disability, and multiple rib fractures may predispose to pneumonia.

**Associated Findings:** Gigantism has been reported.

**Etiology:** Autosomal dominant inheritance has been suggested in some reports.

**Pathogenesis:** It has been observed that the skin lesions follow the lines of Blaschko: a typical fountain-like, V-shaped pattern on the back, and a characteristic S-shape on the lateral and anterior aspects of the trunk. Because this cutaneous pattern visualizes the outgrowth of two different cell populations during early embryogenesis, it has been postulated that the condition is composed of two different cell lines. This would explain the asymmetric and disseminated distribution of the bone lesions, including the striking asymmetry of the face, and would account for why both central and peripheral endocrine dysfunctions are seen in different patients. The occurrence of incomplete forms of the syndrome may be attributed to a minor proportion of mutant cells within the mosaic. The occurrence of monozygotic twins is also consistent with this theory. Because most cases are sporadic, the disease is presumed to be caused by a dominant lethal gene. Cells with this gene can only survive by being mixed with normal cells. The mosaic may arise either from an early somatic mutation or from a gametic half chromatid mutation.

**MIM No.:** 17480

**POS No.:** 3373

**CDC No.:** 756.510

**Sex Ratio:** Presumably M1:F1

**Occurrence:** About fifty cases documented.

**Risk of Recurrence for Patient's Sib:** Most cases to date appear sporadic, including discordant identical twins.

**Risk of Recurrence for Patient's Child:** Unknown.

**Age of Detectability:** The disease may be detected at birth by the pigmented skin lesions; in infancy or childhood by sexual precocity; or in childhood or adolescence by the deformities, fractures, or leg length discrepancy resulting from the fibrous dysplasia of bone.

**Gene Mapping and Linkage:** Unknown.

**Prevention:** None known. Genetic counseling indicated.

**Treatment:** Orthopedic surgical correction for progressive deformity, nonunion of fractures, femoral shaft fractures in adults, or persistent pain. Medroxyprogesterone may be used for sexual precocity.

**Prognosis:** Normal life span. When the fibrous dysplasia is extensive early in life, the progression of the disorder is marked, and the prognosis is poor.

**Detection of Carrier:** Unknown.

**Special Considerations:** The association of polyostotic fibrous dysplasia, sexual precocity, and skin pigmentation is known as the McCune-Albright syndrome. However, the polyostotic fibrous dysplasia is the only invariable feature of this disorder and may occur alone or with one or both of the associated anomalies. Polyostotic fibrous dysplasia with or without the associated skin and endocrine manifestations should be considered as a unified syndrome.

**References:**

Alvarez-Arratia MC, et al.: A probable monogenic form of polyostotic fibrous dysplasia. Clin Genet 1983; 24:132–139.

D'Armiento M, et al.: McCune-Albright syndrome: evidence for autonomous multiendocrine hyperfunction. J Pediatr 1983; 102:584–586.

Comite F, et al.: Cyclical ovarian function resistant to treatment with an analogue of luteinizing hormone releasing hormone in McCune-Albright syndrome. New Engl J Med 1984; 311:1032–1036.

Happle R: The McCune-Albright syndrome: a lethal gene surviving by mosaicism. Clin Genet 1986; 29:321–324. *

Lee PA, et al.: McCune-Albright syndrome: long-term follow-up. JAMA 1986; 256:2980–2984. *

B0025
BE050

Zvi Borochowitz
Michael Beck
David L. Rimoin
David W. Hollister

**Fibrous subaortic stenosis**
*See HEART, SUBAORTIC STENOSIS, FIBROUS*
**Fibula aplasia/hypoplasia-femoral bowing-poly-, syn-, oligodactyly**
*See SKELETAL DYSPLASIA, FUHRMANN TYPE*
**Fibula dysplasia-anonychia-abnormal ears**
*See OTO-ONYCHO-PERONEAL SYNDROME*

## FIBULA, CONGENITAL ABSENCE OF 2229

**Includes:**
  Femur-fibula-ulna (FFU) syndrome
  Fibula, congenital deficiency of
  Proximal femoral focal deficiency

**Excludes:**
  **Acheiropody** (2486)
  **Achondrogenesis, Parenti-Fraccaro type** (0009)
  **Amniotic bands syndrome** (0874)
  **Atelosteogenesis** (2521)
  **Campomelic dysplasia** (0122)
  **Fetal thalidomide syndrome** (0386)
  Fibular dysplasia-brachydactyly
  **Mesomelic dysplasia** (all)
  Pseudothalidomide syndrome
  **Roberts syndrome** (0875)
  **Skeletal dysplasia, Fuhrmann type** (2696)
  Ulna and fibula, hypoplasia of

**Major Diagnostic Criteria:** Unilateral or bilateral short lower extremity frequently associated with anterior bowing of the lower leg, with skin dimpling and anomalies of the foot.

**Clinical Findings:** Fibula abnormality varies from a partial absence, with relatively normal-appearing limb, to absent fibula, with marked shortening of the femur, curved tibia, and serious foot anomalies. Generally three types have been recognized. *Type I* includes cases with unilateral or partial absence of the fibula, with mild or no bowing of the tibia (10% of the cases). The leg may

or may not be shortened. In *type II*, patients have unilateral absence of the fibula, anterior bowing of the tibia with dimpling, foot deformity with absent rays, and marked shortening of the leg. This form is observed in about 35% of cases. In *type III*, the remaining 55% of the patients have unilateral or bilateral absence of the fibula, with the same leg and foot deformities already described and other multiple skeletal defects, such as tarsal and metatarsal anomalies and upper extremity defects. Short femur of varying degrees appears to be a frequent finding in type II and III patients, as are talipes equinovarus or equinovalgus deformities and a tight band extending from the calcaneous to the upper portions of the tibia.

**Complications:** Orthopedic, including physical limitations caused by limb defects. Potential psychological problems have not yet been evaluated.

**Associated Findings:** Peromelia, **Syndactyly**, congenital dislocation of the head of radius, spina bifida, **Craniosynostosis**, cardiac anomalies, and renal anomalies have been observed in a few patients.

**Etiology:** Usually occurs as a sporadic event, although familial incidence has been reported in a small percentage of cases. Teratogens and mechanical factors have not been ruled out.

**Pathogenesis:** Embryologic studies indicate a developmental insult to the embryo at about the fifth or sixth week of intrauterine life. Similar anomalies have been successfully produced in experimental animals by various chemical substances, such as busulfan, if administered during a specific period of intrauterine development. Tibial bowing and foot deformities are probably the result of abnormal attachments of the fibular muscles, resulting in abnormal stresses on the developing tibia and the foot, respectively.

**MIM No.:** 22820

**Sex Ratio:** M2:F1

**Occurrence:** Fibula probably is the most frequently hypoplastic or absent long bone. Several hundred cases are on record.

**Risk of Recurrence for Patient's Sib:** Probably negligible.

**Risk of Recurrence for Patient's Child:** Unknown.

**Age of Detectability:** At birth; in mild cases diagnosis may be missed. Prenatal diagnosis is possible by ultrasound.

**Gene Mapping and Linkage:** Unknown.

**Prevention:** None known. Genetic counseling indicated.

**Treatment:** Orthopedic treatment directed to developing limbs suitable for weight bearing. Conservative measures for milder cases include casts and braces. Other patients may require early excision of tight band, plastic surgery, osteotomy of the tibia, or amputation.

**Prognosis:** Rehabilitation varies depending on the severity of the limb deficiency. Prognosis is good with regard to mental development and life span.

**Detection of Carrier:** Unknown.

**Special Considerations:** Partial or total congenital absence of the fibula is not an isolated entity. Patients commonly have other malformations and/or deformations of the affected limb. Fibular deficiency has also been observed as a component of several hereditary, well-defined syndromes, as well as sporadic and rather vague clinical entities.

**References:**

Thompson TC, et al.: Congenital absence of the fibula. J Bone Joint Surg 1957; 39A:1229–1236.

Kuhne D, et al.: Defekt von Femur und Fibula mit Amelia. Peromelia oder ulnaren Strahldefekten der Arme. Hum Genet 1967; 3:244–263. †

Warkany J: Congenital malformations: notes and comments. Chicago: Year Book Medical Publishers 1971:1002–1003.

Pappas AM, et al.: Congenital defects of the fibula. Orthop Clin North Am 1972; 3:187–199.

Fitch N: Congenital absence of fibula. J Pediatr 1975; 87:839. *

Coventry MG, et al.: Congenital absence of the fibula. J Bone Joint Surg 1981; 34-A:941–955. *

SA033                                                    **Burhan Say**

**Fibula, congenital deficiency of**
    See FIBULA, CONGENITAL ABSENCE OF
**Fibular and ulnar absence with severe limb deficiency**
    See LIMB DEFECT WITH ABSENT ULNA/FIBULA
**Fibular aplasia-craniosynostosis, Lowry type**
    See CRANIOSYNOSTOSIS-FIBULAR APLASIA, LOWRY TYPE
**Fickler-Winkler olivopontocerebellar atrophy**
    See OLIVOPONTOCEREBELLAR ATROPHY, RECESSIVE FICKLER-
    WINKLER TYPE
**Fifth day fits**
    See CONVULSIONS, BENIGN FAMILIAL NEONATAL
**Fifth digit syndrome**
    See COFFIN-SIRIS SYNDROME
**Fifth disease**
    See FETAL PARVOVIRUS INFECTION
**Fifth phacomatosis**
    See NEVOID BASAL CELL CARCINOMA SYNDROME
**Filippi syndrome**
    See SYNDACTYLY-MICROCEPHALY-MENTAL RETARDATION,
    FILIPPI TYPE
**Finger flexor tendons, short**
    See CAMPTODACTYLY-TRISMUS SYNDROME
**Finger, cold, hereditary**
    See RAYNAUD DISEASE
**Finger, recurring fibroma**
    See DIGITAL FIBROMA, RECURRING IN INFANTS & CHILDREN

---

**FINGERPRINTS, ABSENT**                                    **0393**

**Includes:** Hands, absent fingerprints

**Excludes:**
    **Dermal hypoplasia, focal** (0281)
    **Ectodermal dysplasia, Basan type** (0102)
    Keratosis palmaris and plantaris

**Major Diagnostic Criteria:** Complete absence of finger-, palm-, and toeprint dermatoglyphics from birth.

**Clinical Findings:** Complete absence of dermatoglyphics (finger-, palm-, and toeprints) from birth. Of 16 affected members in four generations, all had congenital milia, which lasted for about 6 months, and absent ridge formation. Bilateral webbing of the toes and bilateral flexion contractures of the fingers or the toes were present in all members either alone or in combination. Sweating of the affected areas was virtually absent. No other evidence of an ectodermal defect was present. Intelligence and other physical findings, including teeth and fingernails and patterns of illness, were not remarkable.

**Complications:** Painful fissures and discomfort of the palms and soles during hot or cold weather.

**Associated Findings:** None known.

**Etiology:** Autosomal dominant inheritance.

**Pathogenesis:** Highly speculative. Possibly an intrauterine epidermolytic process. This would be severe enough to lead to massive sloughing and would involve only the volar surfaces. If this process occurred, the new skin would lack ridges and the contractures would be induced by the fetal reparative activities.

**MIM No.:** *13600, *12554

**Sex Ratio:** M1:F1

**Occurrence:** Rare; but several kindreds have been documented.

**Risk of Recurrence for Patient's Sib:**
    See Part I, Mendelian Inheritance.

**Risk of Recurrence for Patient's Child:**
    See Part I, Mendelian Inheritance.

**Age of Detectability:** At birth.

**Gene Mapping and Linkage:** Unknown.

**Prevention:** None known. Genetic counseling indicated.

**Treatment:** Unknown.

**Prognosis:** Normal life span.

**Detection of Carrier:** Unknown.

**Special Considerations:** In the kindred reported by Reed and Schreiner (1983), nine of 22 members among five generations are known to be affected. They presented with many similarities, as well as many striking differences, compared with Baird's kindred (1964). The similarities include absence of dermal ridges, lack of sweating or sweat pores on the volar surfaces, and single transverse palmar creases. The differences included the presence at birth of several vesiculobullous lesions on the fingers and soles, abnormal nails with horizontal and vertical grooves, vertical splits, and distal attachment to the hyponychium. In cold weather the fingernails tend to pull away from the skin. Milia-like lesions were present at birth, but in contrast to Baird's patients, the lesions regressed within one week compared with 6 months. This seems to represent a different condition.

Clinical heterogeneity suggests that absent finger prints, patternless dermal ridges, and possibly **Ectodermal dysplasia, Basan type** may form a single nosologic group.

**References:**
Baird HW: Absence of fingerprints in four generations. Lancet 1968; II:1250 only.
David TJ: Congenital malformations of human dermatoglyphs. Arch Dis Child 1973; 48:191–198.
Schaumann B, Alter M: Dermatoglyphics in medical disorders. New York: Springer-Verlag, 1976:89–102.
Reed T, Schreiner RL: Absence of dermal ridge patterns: genetic heterogeneity. Am J Med Genet 1983; 16:81–88.

MI038                                                **Giuseppe Micali**

**Fingers, 'crooked fingers syndrome'**
    See ANOPHTHALMIA-LIMB ANOMALIES
**Fingers, absence of**
    See ECTRODACTYLY
**Fingers, congenital contracture of**
    See CAMPTODACTYLY
**Fingers, flexed**
    See CAMPTODACTYLY
**Fingers, hammer**
    See CAMPTODACTYLY
**Fingers, recurrent locking-growth defect**
    See HAND, LOCKING DIGITS-GROWTH DEFECT
**Finkel late-adult spinal muscular atrophy**
    See SPINAL MUSCULAR ATROPHY
**Finnish amyloidosis with lattice corneal dystrophy**
    See AMYLOIDOSIS, FINNISH TYPE
**Finnish nephrosis**
    See NEPHROSIS, CONGENITAL
**First and second branchial arch syndrome**
    See OCULO-AURICULO-VERTEBRAL ANOMALY
**Fischer-Jacobsen-Clouston syndrome**
    See ECTODERMAL DYSPLASIA, HIDROTIC
**Fish eye disease (obsolete; pejorative)**
    See LECITHIN-CHOLESTEROL ACYL TRANSFERASE DEFICIENCY
**Fish odor syndrome**
    See TRIMETHYLAMINURIA
**Fissure of chin, Y-shaped**
    See FACE, CHIN FISSURE
**Fissured tongue**
    See TONGUE, FISSURED
**Fistula of palate**
    See PALATE, FISTULA
**Fitzsimmons syndrome**
    See HYPERKERATOSIS PALMOPLANTARIS-SPASTIC PARAPLEGIA-
    RETARDATION
**Fitzsimmons-McLachlan-Gilbert syndrome**
    See HYPERKERATOSIS PALMOPLANTARIS-SPASTIC PARAPLEGIA-
    RETARDATION
**Five-Oxoprolinuria**
    See ACIDEMIA, PYROGLUTAMIC
    also ANEMIA, HEMOLYTIC, GLUTATHIONE SYNTHETASE
    DEFICIENCY
**Fleck retina disease (one form)**
    See RETINA, FUNDUS ALBIPUNCTATUS
**Fleck retina of Kandori**
    See RETINA, FLECKED KANDORI TYPE

**'Floating beta' disease**
 *See HYPERLIPOPROTEINEMIA, BROAD BETA TYPE*
**Floppy infant**
 *See MYOPATHIES*
**Floppy mitral valve**
 *See MITRAL VALVE PROLAPSE*
**'Floppy' infant (one type)**
 *See GLYCOGENOSIS, TYPE IIa*
**Floriform cataract**
 *See CATARACT, AUTOSOMAL DOMINANT CONGENITAL*
**Flowing hyperostosis**
 *See MELORHEOSTOSIS*
**Flurazepam, fetal effects**
 *See FETAL BENZODIAZEPINE EFFECTS*
**Flying fetus syndrome**
 *See UMBILICAL CORD, SHORT UMBILICAL CORD SYNDROME*
**Flynn-Aird syndrome**
 *See NEUROECTODERMAL SYNDROME, FLYNN-AIRD TYPE*
**FOAR syndrome**
 *See FACIO-OCULO-ACOUSTIC-RENAL SYNDROME (FOAR SYNDROME)*
**Focal dermal dysplasia syndrome**
 *See DERMAL HYPOPLASIA, FOCAL*
**Focal dermato-phalangeal dysplasia**
 *See DERMAL HYPOPLASIA, FOCAL*

## FOLATE MALABSORPTION                                2166

**Includes:**
 Folic acid, transport defect
 Transport defect involving folate malabsorption
**Excludes:**
 **Anemia, pernicious congenital** (2656)
 Cellular uptake disorders of folate
 Dihydrofolate reductase deficiency
 Glutamate formiminotransferase deficiency
 **Methylcobalamin deficiency** (2605)
 Methylmalonic aciduria with homocystinuria (cblC and cblD diseases)
 **Transcobalamin II deficiency** (2624)
 **Vitamin B(12) malabsorption** (0992)

**Major Diagnostic Criteria:** Low serum and cerebrospinal fluid folate levels. Increased urinary excretion of formiminoglutamic acid. Abnormal absorption of oral folates; no abnormality in the absorption of fat, glucose, or vitamin A. The megaloblastic anemia is unresponsive to physiologic doses of folate(s) by mouth but responsive to physiologic doses of parenteral folate(s).

**Clinical Findings:** Onset of megaloblastic anemia in the first few months of life.

**Complications:** Mild-to-severe mental retardation.

**Associated Findings:** Seizures reported in one-half of the cases. Other neurologic findings include cerebral calcifications, ataxia, athetosis, and peripheral neuropathy. Anorexia, stomatitis, glossitis, and vulvovaginitis have also been reported.

**Etiology:** Autosomal recessive inheritance. Evidence of parental consanguinity was found in three families.

One proband had four sibs (three females, one male) who died in infancy or childhood (Corbeel et al, 1982); another (Poncz et al, 1981) had one older sib who died at age three months.

**Pathogenesis:** The phenotype offers evidence for a specific folate carrier both in the intestine and at the level of the blood-brain barrier. Oxidized and reduced folates apparently use this transport system, since none were effectively absorbed by the patients. It is probable that a different mechanism determines uptake of folate(s) into blood cells, since a hematologic response occurs even in the presence of relatively low serum folate levels.

**MIM No.:** *22905

**Sex Ratio:** M1:F6 (observed).

**Occurrence:** Seven confirmed cases have been reported, two in one family.

**Risk of Recurrence for Patient's Sib:**
 See Part I, *Mendelian Inheritance.*

**Risk of Recurrence for Patient's Child:**
 See Part I, *Mendelian Inheritance.*

**Age of Detectability:** Within the first few months of life.

**Gene Mapping and Linkage:** Unknown.

**Prevention:** None known. Genetic counseling indicated.

**Treatment:** In at least four cases there was a clear hematologic response to pharmacologic doses of folic acid by mouth. Parenteral administration of folic acid seems to be effective in elevating serum folate levels and improving anemia, but has not been an effective means of elevating folate levels in the cerebrospinal fluid. Parenteral folinic acid (5-formyl-THF) may be more effective in raising CSF levels and might prevent mental retardation (Poncz et al., 1981).

**Prognosis:** Early childhood deaths in sibs in two families. In other probands, the natural history is unclear. The disorder is compatible with survival into adulthood (one case).

**Detection of Carrier:** Not clearly delineated. In some obligate carriers, the oral folate absorption response is blunted.

**Special Considerations:** Clinical heterogeneity of this disorder is likely associated with heterogeneity at the molecular level. In some patients, seizures were made worse by folate treatment, whereas in others, they were ameliorated. The one affected male had a partial deficiency in both humoral and cellular immunity.

**References:**
Poncz M, et al.: Therapy of congenital folate malabsorption. J Pediatr 1981; 98:76.
Corbeel L, et al.: Congenital folate malabsorption with mental retardation and cerebral calcifications. Pediatr Res 1982; 16:693 (abstr).
Corbeel L, et al.: Congenital folate malabsorption. Eur J Pediatr 1985; 143:284.
Urbach J, et al.: Congenital isolated folic malabsorption. Arch Dis Child 1987; 62:78.

BU039                                              **Janet A. Buchanan**
R0052                                           **David S. Rosenblatt**

**Folic acid, transport defect**
 *See FOLATE MALABSORPTION*
**Follicle-stimulating hormone (FSH), isolated deficiency of**
 *See GONADOTROPIN DEFICIENCIES*
**Follicular large cell lymphoma**
 *See LYMPHOMA, NON-HODGKIN*
**Follicular lymphoma**
 *See LYMPHOMA, NON-HODGKIN*
 *also LEUKEMIA/LYMPHOMA, B-CELL*
**Follicular mixed small cleaved and large cell lymphoma**
 *See LYMPHOMA, NON-HODGKIN*
**Follicular small cleaved lymphoma**
 *See LYMPHOMA, NON-HODGKIN*
**Follicular variant of papillary carcinoma**
 *See CANCER, THYROID, FAMILIAL PAPILLARY CARCINOMA OF*
**Folling disease**
 *See FETAL EFFECTS FROM MATERNAL PKU*
**Following disease**
 *See PHENYLKETONURIA*
**Fong disease**
 *See NAIL-PATELLA SYNDROME*
**Foot (split)-mandibular hypoplasia-renal anomalies**
 *See ACRO-RENAL-MANDIBULAR SYNDROME*
**Foot and hand deformity with flat facies**
 *See ACROFACIAL DEFECTS, EMERY-NELSON TYPE*
**Foot, claw-absent tendon jerks**
 *See NEUROPATHY, HEREDITARY MOTOR AND SENSORY, TYPE I*

## FOOT, CONGENITAL CLUBFOOT     1517

**Includes:**
> Metatarsus adductus
> Metatarsus varus
> Talipes calcaneovalgus

**Excludes:** Foot, talipes equinovarus (TEV) (2164)

**Clinical Findings:** *Congenital clubfoot* is a term used to describe a variety of abnormalities. *Metatarsus varus* or *adductus* denotes the forefoot to be adducted and often supinated while the heel and ankle remain in normal position. *Talipes calcaneovalgus* defines a dorsiflexed and everted foot. The bones are usually in a normal alignment relative to each other. *Talipes equinovarus* (see **Foot, talipes equinovarus (TEV)**) describes a complex anomaly including forefoot adduction and supination, heel varus, and ankle equinus. The muscles of the posterior and medial aspects of the leg are relatively shortened, and the fibrous capsules of affected joints are often thickened in their lateral aspects.

The newborn infant can usually be "bundled" into the uterine position. Such positioning will generally quiet the baby and has been called the *position of comfort*. Ascertainment of this position will often demonstrate how the fetal feet were wrapped around other body parts and molded into the deformed position.

**Complications:** If not fully corrected, abnormalities in gait.

**Associated Findings:** Clubfoot has a heterogeneous origin. When of deformational cause, other deformities may be found, especially dislocated hip and torticollis. Clubfoot, especially **Foot, talipes equinovarus (TEV)**, is typically found as a primary malformation in a large group of malformation syndromes, including **Femoral hypoplasia-unusual facies syndrome; Larsen syndrome; Pena-Shokeir syndrome; Chromosome triploidy; Cerebro-hepato-renal syndrome**, and many chromosomal deletion syndromes (including **Chromosome 4, monosomy 4p; Chromosome 9, partial monosomy 9p; Chromosome 13, monosomy 13q;** and **Chromosome 18, monosomy 18q**), and is occasionally seen in other syndromes, including **Aarskog syndrome; Bloom syndrome; Dubowitz syndrome; Chondroectodermal dysplasia; Homocystinuria; Mucopolysaccharidosis II; Mietens-Weber syndrome; Noonan syndrome; Seckel syndrome;** and **Weaver syndrome**. Clubfoot occurs as a secondary malformation in numerous neuromuscular disorders, including **Sacrococcygeal dysgenesis syndrome; Meningomyelocele,** and **Arthrogryposes**. Finally, clubfoot may be the result of bony dysplasia and may be found in conditions such as **Diastrophic dysplasia**.

**Etiology:** The heterogeneous origins of clubfoot have been discussed since the time of Hippocrates. Abundant evidence for intrinsic and extrinsic causes have been advanced. When clubfoot is isolated, a recurrence risk of 3–5% has been empirically observed. Specific pedigrees have demonstrated direct transmission of clubfoot from parents to children, whereas recessive transmission is proposed in other families. Concordance in monozygotic twinning is approximately 30% (as opposed to 3% in dizygotic twinning), which argues a mixed etiology of genetic and nongenetic factors. When clubfoot is part of a broader pattern of malformation or dysplasia, then the etiology becomes related to the process of anomaly in that condition.

**Pathogenesis:** Constraint-induced anomalies of the foot more often include metatarsus adductus or talipes calcaneovalgus than talipes equinovarus. The anomaly is usually supple, and the infant's "position of comfort" often helps to confirm the clinical suspicion of the deformational origin.

The foot of the 26–30-mm fetus is maintained in an equinovarus position because of a growth discrepancy between the fibula and tibia at that time. Several authors have suggested that the primary malformational form of clubfoot stems from an arrest in relative growth from this fetal period. A general condition leading to muscular imbalance about the ankle from either a neuropathic or myopathic cause produces clubfoot. Intrinsic anomalies of specific bones such as the talis or general bony dysplasias can also underlie equinovarus.

**MIM No.:** *11990

**Sex Ratio:** M2:F1

**Occurrence:** Given the heterogeneity in etiology and the numerous conditions subsumed in the definition of "clubfoot," it is not surprising that the occurrence varies by area of ascertainment and by clinical rigor in diagnosis. Incidence reports vary from lows of 6:10,000 in Germany, Switzerland, and Asia to highs of 6.8:100 in native Hawaiians. The North American and European average incidence has been estimated by Warkany (1971) as 18:10,000.

**Risk of Recurrence for Patient's Sib:**
See Part I, *Mendelian Inheritance*. Varying and depending on overall situation from 50% to essentially zero.

**Risk of Recurrence for Patient's Child:**
See Part I, *Mendelian Inheritance*. Varying and depending on overall situation from 50% to essentially zero.

**Age of Detectability:** During the neonatal period.

**Gene Mapping and Linkage:** Unknown.

**Prevention:** None known for isolated clubfoot. Genetic counseling may be indicated when clubfoot is associated with other malformations.

**Treatment:** Sequential casting of the foot back to neutral position will generally resolve cases of metatarsus adductus, talipes calcaneovalgus, and some cases of talipes equinovarus. Surgery may be required in persistent cases or when bony anomalies of the foot are present. When neuromuscular imbalance produces the clubfoot, surgical success may only be partial.

**Prognosis:** Dependent on the etiology and overall condition.

**Detection of Carrier:** In clubfoot due to chromosomal conditions, parental karyotyping may be appropriate. In most other situations carrier status cannot be determined except possibly when a parent has a clubfoot.

**References:**
Gardner ED: The development and growth of bones and joints. J Bone Joint Surg 1963; 45A:856–862.
Kite JH: The clubfoot. New York: Grune & Stratton, 1964. *
Tachdjiian MO: Diagnosis and treatment of congenital deformities of the musculoskeletal system in the newborn and infant. Pediatr Clin North Am 1967; 14:307–358.
Warkany J: The lower extremities. In: Warkany J, ed: Congenital malformations. Chicago: Yearbook Medical, 1971:1004–1009. †
Smith DW: Recognizable patterns of human deformation. Philadelphia: W.B. Saunders, 1981. *

CL006      **Sterling K. Clarren**

## FOOT, METATARSUS VARUS     2523

**Includes:**
> Metatarsus varus, type I
> Skewfoot

**Excludes:**
> **Foot, congenital clubfoot** (1517)
> **Foot, talipes equinovarus (TEV)** (2164)

**Major Diagnostic Criteria:** 1) Medial rotation and overlap of the cuneiform bones, with concomitant medial deviation of the metatarsals, particularly two through four, resulting in adduction of the anterior foot; 2) abnormal elevation of the longitudinal arch; 3) concavity of the medial border of the foot and convexity of the lateral border; 4) dorsal flexion and wide separation of the great toe from the second toe; 5) neutral position of the heel; and 6) a reflex rather than a straight angle at the intersection of two lines drawn from the midportions of the forefoot and the hindfoot, using the medial border as base.

**Clinical Findings:** Adduction and dorsal curvature of the forefoot, increased height of the longitudinal arch, medial concavity and lateral convexity of the borders, normal position of the heel, and possibly stiffness of the forefoot to attempted straightening should be evident. X-ray evidence of eversion at the tarsometatarsal level, bowing of the metatarsal bones, and delayed development of tarsal bones may be seen.

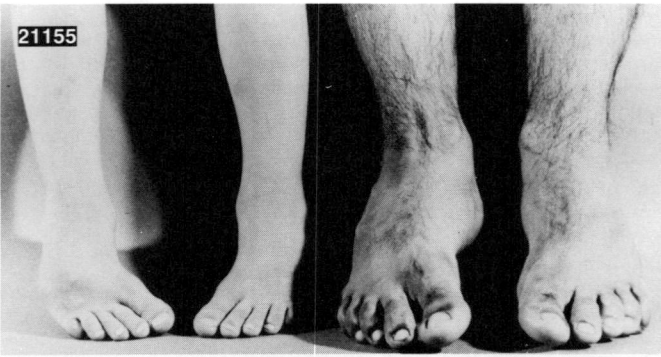

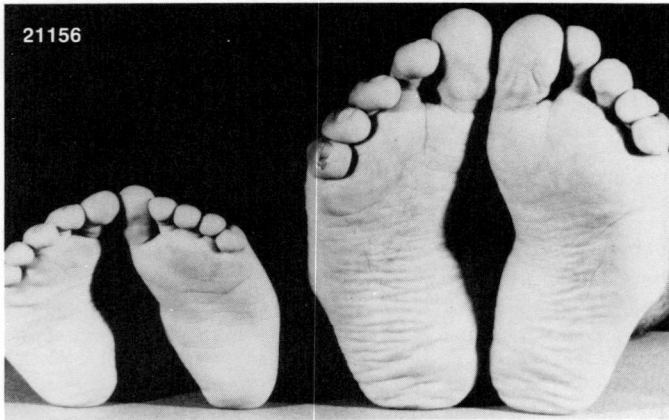

**2523**-21155: Propositus (left) and his father (right). Note medial angulation of the forefoot and dorsal flexion in both, and height of the longitudinal arch in the father. 21156: Propositus (left) and his father (right). Note concavity of the medial border and convexity of the lateral border.

**Complications:** Stiff-legged gait may result from associated knee and hip deformities. Toed-in gait and limited running ability depend on extent of defect.

**Associated Findings:** Esotropia (1/7), epicanthi (1/7), flat nasal bridge (1/7), clinodactyly of the fifth fingers (1/7), incomplete extension of first metacarpophalangeal joint (1/7), incomplete extension of elbow (1/7).

**Etiology:** Autosomal dominant inheritance with variable expression.

**Pathogenesis:** Unknown.

**MIM No.:** *15652

**CDC No.:** 754.520

**Sex Ratio:** M6:F2 (observed).

**Occurrence:** One kindred reported.

**Risk of Recurrence for Patient's Sib:**
See Part I, *Mendelian Inheritance.*

**Risk of Recurrence for Patient's Child:**
See Part I, *Mendelian Inheritance.*

**Age of Detectability:** Neonatally, by clinical findings.

**Gene Mapping and Linkage:** Unknown.

**Prevention:** None known. Genetic counseling indicated.

**Treatment:** Casting and orthopedic operative procedures.

**Prognosis:** Normal life span.

**Detection of Carrier:** By clinical and X-ray examination.

**References:**
Juberg RC, Touchstone WJ: Congenital metatarsus varus in four generations. Clin Genet 1974; 5:127–132. * †

JU000                                                        **Richard C. Juberg**

## FOOT, TALIPES EQUINOVARUS (TEV)                          2164

**Includes:**
    Talipes equinovarus, congenital idiopathic
    TEV
**Excludes:**
    **Amniotic bands syndrome** (0874)
    Disorders with generalized joint laxity
    Disorders with multiple joint involvement
    **Foot, congenital clubfoot** (1517)
    Leg malformations
    Metabolic disorders

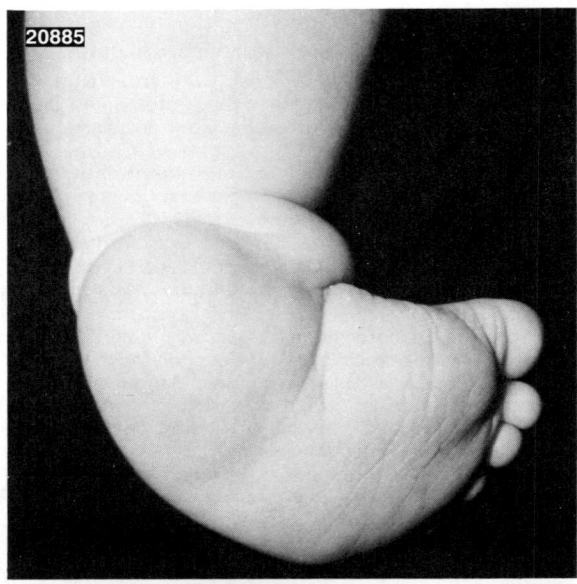

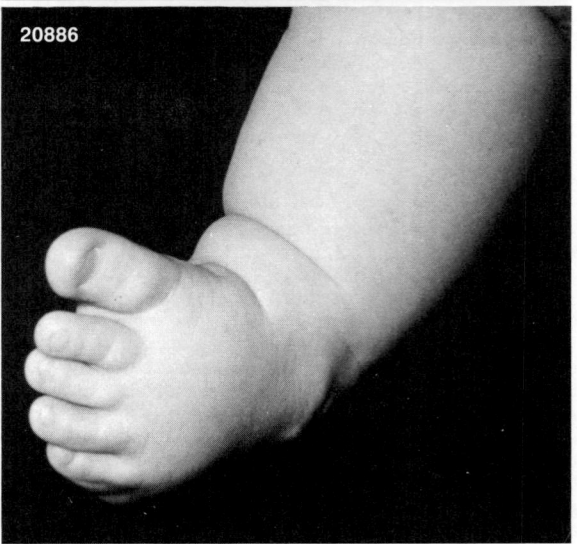

**2164**-20885: Note hindfoot equinus and varus with deep medial crease. 20886: Forefoot supination and adduction.

Metatarsus varus
Neuromuscular disease
Postural talipes equinovarus
Skeletal dysplasia
Talipes calcaneovalgus
Teratogen exposure, fetal effects of
TEV developing postnatally
TEV due to identifiable cause or part of a generalized
condition

**Major Diagnostic Criteria:** The forefoot is adducted, inverted, and supinated, the heel is inverted, and the ankle and subtalar joint are in the equinus position. The foot is rigid in that it cannot be passively brought to a neutral position.

**Clinical Findings:** The foot is malpositioned. Significant soft tissue contractures may be noted medially. Laterally, the skin may be thin and stretched, with decreased subcutaneous tissue. All the bones of the foot may be affected, but the talus and the bones of the foot adjacent to the talus are most severely involved. CT scan may be more sensitive than routine X-rays for defining the bony abnormalities. Circulation and sensation are usually normal.

About one-half of the cases of TEV are bilateral. In unilateral cases, right-sided defects are slightly more common. About one-fourth of the cases are considered to be severe; in these cases the foot is significantly smaller than normal, is quite rigid, often has a transverse crease medially, and usually requires surgery. In the remainder of cases, the more conventional clubfoot is more supple and often corrects with nonoperative treatment. Even with this milder deformity, however, the foot, the calf, and even the bones of the leg may be somewhat reduced in size.

There is some suggestion that familial cases are more likely to be bilateral and more likely to be difficult to treat and that bilateral cases are more likely to be more severe, independent of the family history.

**Complications:** Untreated, the deformity becomes progressively worse. Even with optimal treatment, there may be residual deformity, rigidity, and decreased size of the foot, calf, and leg. Orthoses may be required, gait abnormalities may persist, and the joint may be painful. In general, however, good-to-excellent functional results can be achieved.

**Associated Findings:** Increased joint laxity, inguinal hernias, and other minor abnormalities related to connective tissue have been noted with greater frequency in patients and first degree relatives. Careful examination of the hips to check for congenital dislocation should be performed. Cleft lip and palate and TEV may occur together with greater than expected frequency; one study found that 2% of patients with cleft lip and palate or cleft palate had clubfoot.

**Etiology:** Several lines of evidence suggest a genetic contribution to TEV and a multifactorial mode of inheritance. One study in twins found that MZ twins had a concordance rate of 32.5%, while DZ twins had a concordance rate of 2.9% (the same risk as singleton sibs); this tenfold increase in MZ twins is not consistent with other modes of inheritance. Consistent differences in incidence by race and sex have been found, and the recurrence risk is greater for sibs of the less frequently affected sex. The rate of decrease in risk to second and third degree relatives is also compatible with multifactorial inheritance.

The possible role of intrauterine molding (deformation) is controversial.

**Pathogenesis:** Considerable research has failed to demonstrate the primary abnormality leading to TEV. Intrauterine deformation, developmental arrest, regional growth disturbance in the area served by the tibial nerve, and abnormal tendon insertions have been advocated, as have primary defects in innervation of muscles, the muscles themselves, the bones (especially the talus), the joint, fascia, and the vascular supply. There is debate about whether TEV is increased among the firstborn or whether it is associated with breech presentation. One study found an increased rate of maternal hypertension and antepartum hemorrhage.

**MIM No.:** 11980

**CDC No.:** 754.500

**Sex Ratio:** M2:F1

**Occurrence:** The risk in the Caucasian population is about 1:1,000 (reported ranges between 0.64 and 1.24). One study in Hawaii found that people of Oriental descent had a lower risk (0.57:1,000) and that people of Polynesian descent had an increased risk (6.81:1,000). Increased rates have also been reported in Hungarian gypsies and in certain Mediterranean populations.

**Risk of Recurrence for Patient's Sib:** The overall risk is about 3%. If the propositus is male, the recurrence risk is 2%; if the propositus is female, the risk is 5%.

**Risk of Recurrence for Patient's Child:** Empiric data are sparse. Theoretically the same 3% risk for sibs should apply to other first degree relatives, including offspring. Three studies looked at the incidence of TEV in parents of affected children. Combining the data from these three populations shows that parents of affected males and females had TEV 2.6% and 3.3% of the time, respectively. However, in two of those studies the parents of female patients were affected less often than those of male patients. One paper looked at offspring of affected parents, but in a highly selected population. Subtracting the probands gave recurrence rates when fathers and mothers were affected of 5.3% and 16.7% respectively.

**Age of Detectability:** At birth. TEV may also be detected prenatally by ultrasound.

**Gene Mapping and Linkage:** Unknown.

**Prevention:** None known. Genetic counseling indicated.

**Treatment:** Orthopedic consultation should be sought in the immediate newborn period. Over a period of several weeks the foot is gently manipulated toward a more normal position; taping or casting is used to hold the foot progressively closer toward a neutral or slightly valgus position. Such conservative treatment is sufficient about half the time. If there is insufficient improvement after several months, surgery may be indicated. TEV has a tendency to recur, and careful monitoring, including splinting, may be necessary for several years.

**Prognosis:** Normal life span and intelligence. Function is usually good to excellent, but there may be residual deformity.

**Detection of Carrier:** Unknown. Thorough family history is important, as adults may initially be unaware of treatment they had received for foot deformities in infancy.

**Special Considerations:** There are several reports of TEV being diagnosed prenatally by ultrasound, but it is not known what percentage of cases can be diagnosed by this technique. Detection of clubfoot by ultrasound should lead to a careful search for other anomalies, and amniocentesis should be considered. It is not known whether the presence of clubfoot in the second trimester is more likely to be associated with multiple anomalies than clubfoot diagnosed at birth.

In general, the term *clubfoot* refers specifically to talipes equinovarus. However, some people also use this term to describe other foot deformities as well, including metatarsus varus and talipes calcaneovalgus. This difference in nosology should be kept in mind when reviewing the literature (see **Foot, congenital clubfoot**).

Postural TEV, in which an equinovarus foot can be brought into neutral position passively in the newborn period, has an incidence of about 0.5:1,000 and is more common in females (M.31:F1).

**References:**
Palmer RM, et al.: Studies of the inheritance of idiopathic talipes equinovarus. Orthop Clin North Am 1974; 5:99–108.
Lovell WW, et al.: The foot. In: Lovell WW, Winter RB, eds: Pediatric orthopaedics. Philadelphia: J.B. Lippincott, 1978.
Cowell HR, Wein BK: Genetic aspects of clubfoot. J Bone Joint Surg 1980; 62A:1381–1384.
Czeizel A, et al.: Confirmation of the multifactorial threshold model for congenital structural talipes equinovarus. J Med Genet 1981; 18:99–100.
Wynne-Davies R, et al.: Aetiology and interrelationship of some common skeletal deformities. J Med Genet 1982; 19:321–328.
Dietz FR: On the pathogenesis of clubfoot. Lancet 1985; I:388–390.

Dunn PM: Pathogenesis of clubfoot. Lancet 1985; I:635–636.
Hashimoto BE, et al.: Sonographic diagnosis of clubfoot in utero. J Ultrasound Med 1986; 5:81–83.

FL005
KA040

**Ellen A. Fleischnick**
**James R. Kasser**

## FOOT, VERTICAL TALUS                                 3142

**Includes:**   Feet, congenital "rocker-bottomed"

**Excludes:**
   **Arthrogryposes** (0088)
   Paralytic vertical talus
   Vertical talus associated with other congenital abnormalities

**Major Diagnostic Criteria:**   Isolated primary dislocation of the talonavicular joint, in which the navicular articulates with the dorsal aspect of the talus.

**Clinical Findings:**   To make a definite diagnosis, it is essential to demonstrate that the navicular is dislocated dorsally on the neck of the talus when the foot is maintained in extreme flexion. It is important to rule out other abnormalities that might lead to this abnormality, such as **Arthrogryposes**, neuromuscular abnormalities, and other congenital abnormalities. Bilateral as well as unilateral involvement may occur in the same family, with a wide range of severity.

**Complications:**   Posture abnormality.

**Associated Findings:**   Hip dislocation.

**Etiology:**   Autosomal dominant inheritance with variable expressivity. One-half of the reported cases have been sporadic.

**Pathogenesis:**   Possibly related to an embryologic fault during the first trimester of pregnancy.

**CDC No.:**   754.735, 755.616

**Sex Ratio:**   M1:F1

**Occurrence:**   About 100 cases have been reported since the condition was delineated in the 1960s. In one-half of the patients with primary vertical talus, there is a positive history of foot deformity in the first degree relatives.

**Risk of Recurrence for Patient's Sib:**
   See Part I, *Mendelian Inheritance.*

**Risk of Recurrence for Patient's Child:**
   See Part I, *Mendelian Inheritance.*

**Age of Detectability:**   At birth.

**Gene Mapping and Linkage:**   Unknown.

**Prevention:**   None known. Genetic counseling indicated.

**Treatment:**   Cast correction alone is not successful as the definitive treatment, and surgical treatment is indicated. A number of methods and technique of treatment have been described (Herndon & Heyman, 1963; Clark et al, 1977; Ogata et al, 1979). Reduction of the talonavicular dislocation combined with a complete posterior capsulotomy and heel cord lengthening has been shown to be a safe technique. Following this, a delayed lateral arthrodesis is indicated in those selected cases with persistent lateral subluxation of the calcaneus at the subtalar joint.

**Prognosis:**   Good following surgical correction.

**Detection of Carrier:**   By clinical examination of first degree relatives.

**References:**
Herndon CH, Heyman CH: Problems in the recognition and treatment of congenital conves pes valug. J Bone Joint Surg 1963; 45A:413.
Clark MW, et al.: Congenital vertical talus: treatment by open reduction and navicular excision. J Bone Joint Surg 1977; 59A:816.
Ogata K, et al.: Congenital vertical talus and its familial occurrence. Clin Orthop 1979; 139:129–132. †
Stern HJ, et al.: Autosomal dominant transmission of isolated congenital vertical talus. Am J Hum Genet 1987; 41:A86.

SH053                                             **Mordechai Shohat**

**Footless and handless families of Brazil**
   See *ACHEIROPODY*
**Foramen of Morgagni hernia**
   See *DIAPHRAGMATIC HERNIA*
**Forbes disease**
   See *GLYCOGENOSIS, TYPE III*
**Forbes-Albright syndrome (some cases)**
   See *ENDOCRINE NEOPLASIA, MULTIPLE TYPE I*
**Forceps marks scarring and unusual facies, temporal**
   See *ECTODERMAL DYSPLASIA, CONGENITAL FACIAL, SETLEIS TYPE*
**Forehead, bony protuberance-brain anomalies**
   See *CRANIOTELENCEPHALIC DYSPLASIA*
**Forelock (white) without deafness**
   See *ALBINISM, CUTANEOUS*

## FORSIUS-ERIKSSON SYNDROME                          3183

**Includes:**
   Aland Island disease
   Albinism, ocular, Forsius-Eriksson type
   Eye, Aland disease
   Forsius-Eriksson-Miyake syndrome
   Ocular albinism, Forsius-Eriksson type

**Excludes:**
   **Albinism, ocular** (0032)
   **Albinism, ocular, autosomal recessive type** (2010)
   **Albinoidism** (2359)
   **Nightblindness, congenital stationary, X-linked recessive** (0718)

**Major Diagnostic Criteria:**   *In males:* axial high myopia with astigmatism; foveal hypoplasia; impairment of central and night vision with nystagmus; and protanomalous color blindness. *In female heterozygotes:* minimal disturbance of color discrimination; electromyographically demonstrable nystagmus.

**Clinical Findings:**   In 1964, Forsius and Eriksson reported on a six-generation family from the Aland islands, Denmark, where seven blond males had decreased visual acuity, nightblindness nystagmus, high myopia, poor foveal reflexes, pale fundi, and protanomalous color vision defects. Some carrier females had mild nystagmus and decrease in visual acuity. For years this condition was thought to be a novel form of X-linked ocular albinism. None of the affected males or carrier females had macromelanosomes on skin biopsy (O'Donnell et al, 1980) and there was no pigment mottling in the fundus periphery of carrier females. Recent electrophysiologic studies (van Dorp et al, 1985) failed to show misrouting of the optic nerve fibers to the brain as seen in albinism. In addition, ERG recordings showed normal a-waves but reduced ("negative") b-waves, suggesting congenital stationary nightblindness.

**Complications:**   Poor visual acuity and color deficiency of the protanomalous variety.

**Associated Findings:**   None known.

**Etiology:**   X-linked inheritance.

**Pathogenesis:**   Unknown. Because of the normal a-wave and abnormal b-wave, a defect in (retinal) neural transmission is inferred.

**MIM No.:**   *30060

**Sex Ratio:**   M1:F0.

**Occurrence:**   Two families (Forsius and Eriksson, 1964; Warburg, 1964 (same family); Scialfa, 1967) with this condition have been reported in the literature. However, the condition appears to be X-linked congenital stationary nightblindness in a Scandinavian blond population.

**Risk of Recurrence for Patient's Sib:**
   See Part I, *Mendelian Inheritance.*

**Risk of Recurrence for Patient's Child:**
   See Part I, *Mendelian Inheritance.*

**Age of Detectability:**   Nystagmus and poor visual acuity are present early in life.

**Gene Mapping and Linkage:** AIED (Aland island eye disease (Forsius-Eriksson ocular albinism) has been provisionally mapped to Xp21.3-p21.2.

Recombination fraction of 0.12 with Xg blood group (Race and Sanger, 1968).

**Prevention:** None known. Genetic counseling indicated.

**Treatment:** Correction of error of refraction.

**Prognosis:** Poor but stable for vision.

**Detection of Carrier:** Nystagmus may be demonstrated electromyographically even if absent clinically. No peripheral retinal pigmentary changes as in X-linked Nettleship-Falls ocular albinism (see **Albinism, ocular**).

**Special Considerations:** It is most probable that the family described by Forsius and Eriksson has **Nightblindness, congenital stationary, X-linked recessive**. The color vision abnormalities may be coincidental. The absence of macromelanosomes in skin biopsies and the presumed normal optic pathways argue against this condition being a form of albinism. Rather, the X-linked congenital stationary nightblindness has occurred in a Scandinavian family with light complexion.

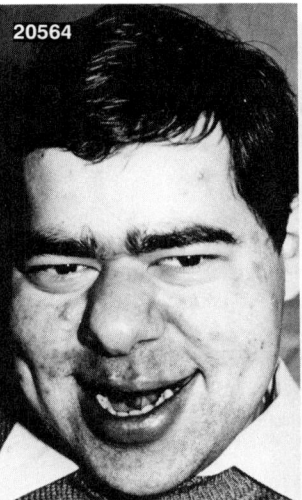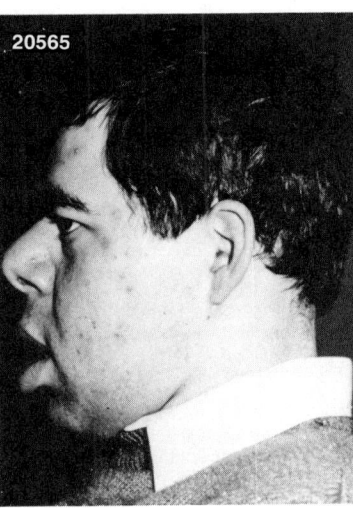

2580-20564–65: Fountain syndrome; note the characteristic coarse facies with swelling of the lips and cheeks.

**References:**

Forsius H, Eriksson AW: Ein neues augensyndrom mit X-chromosomaler transmission: eine Sippe mit fundusalbinismus, foveahypoplasie, nystagmus, myopie, astigmatismus und dyschromatopsie. Klin Mbl Augenheilk 1964; 144:447–457.

Warburg M: Ocular albinism and protanopia in the same family. Acta Ophthalmol 1964; 42:444–451.

Scialfa AC: Albinisme oculaire et dyschromatopsie. Arch Ophtalmol 1967; 27:483–494.

Elenius D, et al.: ERG in a case of X-chromosomal pigment deficiency of fundus in combination with myopia, dysanomatopsias, and defective dark adaptation. In: Proceedings of the 5th ISCERG symposium. New York: S. Karger AG, 1968:369–377.

Race RR, Sanger R: Blood groups in man. Philadelphia, FA Davis, 1968:549

O'Donnell FE, et al.: Forsius-Eriksson syndrome: its relation to the Nettleship-Falls X-linked ocular albinism. Clin Genet 1980; 17:403–408.

van Dorp DB, et al.: Aland eye disease: no albino misrouting. Clin Genet 1985; 28:526–531.

Miyake Y, et al.: Congenital stationary night blindness with negative electroretinogram: a new classification. Arch Ophthalmol 1986; 104:1013–1020.

Weleber RG, et al.: Aland Island disease (Forsius-Eriksson syndrome) associated with contiguous deletion syndrome at Xp21: similarity to incomplete congenital stationary night blindness. Arch Ophthalmol 1989; 107:1170–1179.

TR009                                    **Elias I. Traboulsi**

**Forsius-Eriksson-Miyake syndrome**
*See FORSIUS-ERIKSSON SYNDROME*

---

**FOUNTAIN SYNDROME**                            **2580**

**Includes:**
Deafness-coarse facies-mental retardation
Face, coarse with full lips-deafness-mental retardation
Mental retardation-deafness-coarse facies

**Excludes: Cheilitis granulomatosa, Melkersson-Rosenthal type (2083)**

**Major Diagnostic Criteria:** Mental retardation, sensorineural deafness, and plethoric swelling of the face with edematous infiltration of the subcutaneous tissue.

**Clinical Findings:** All patients have a variable degree of mental retardation, complete sensorineural deafness, and plethoric swelling of the face with edematous infiltration of the subcutaneous tissue, mostly of the lips and cheeks. Skeletal surveys showed marked thickness of the calvaria and confirmed the clinical impression of short, stubby hands, with broad and short phalanges and metacarpals with thickened cortices. Computerized tomography of the inner ear showed anatomic anomalies of the turns of the cochlea in two brothers.

**Complications:** Unknown.

**Associated Findings:** Short stature, hyperkyphosis, and infantile generalized seizures were documented in two or more patients.

**Etiology:** Possibly autosomal recessive inheritance.

**Pathogenesis:** Sensorineural deafness is anatomically related to a cochlear anomaly. Pathogenesis of the facial changes is largely unknown.

**POS No.:** 4162

**Sex Ratio:** M6:F1 (observed).

**Occurrence:** Seven cases (six sibs and one isolated patient) have been described in two reports.

**Risk of Recurrence for Patient's Sib:**
See Part I, *Mendelian Inheritance.*

**Risk of Recurrence for Patient's Child:**
See Part I, *Mendelian Inheritance.*

**Age of Detectability:** During the first years of life.

**Gene Mapping and Linkage:** Unknown.

**Prevention:** None known. Genetic counseling indicated.

**Treatment:** Antiepileptic treatment in the presence of early-onset generalized infantile seizures.

**Prognosis:** Life span is normal. Mental retardation, varying from mild to severe, has been present in all patients.

**Detection of Carrier:** Unknown.

**References:**

Fountain RB: Familial bone abnormalities, deaf mutism, mental retardation, and skin granulomas. Proc R Soc Med 1974; 67:878–879.

Fryns JP, et al.: Mental retardation, deafness, skeletal abnormalities, and coarse face with full lips: confirmation of the Fountain syndrome. Am J Med Genet 1987; 26:551–555. †

FR030                                    **Jean-Pierre Fryns**

**Four-amino-pteroyl-glutamic acid, fetal effects of**
*See FETAL AMINOPTERIN SYNDROME*
**Four-aminobutyric acid (GABA) aminotransferase deficiency**
*See GAMMA-AMINOBUTYRIC ACID (GABA) TRANSAMINASE DEFICIENCY*

**Four-finger line**
*See SKIN CREASE, SINGLE PALMAR*
**Four-hydroxy-L-proline oxidase deficiency**
*See HYDROXYPROLINEMIA*
**Four-hydroxyphenylpyruvate hydroxylase, deficiency of**
*See HAWKINSINURIA*
**Four-hydroxyphenylpyruvic acid oxidase deficiency**
*See TYROSINEMIA I*
**Fourth phacomatosis**
*See STURGE-WEBER SYNDROME*
**Fovea mentalis**
*See FACE, CHIN FISSURE*
**Fragile X chromosome**
*See X-LINKED MENTAL RETARDATION, FRAGILE X SYNDROME*
**Fragoso-Cantu syndrome**
*See FACIO-NEURO-SKELETAL SYNDROME*
**Franceschetti-Jadassohn syndrome**
*See ECTODERMAL DYSPLASIA, NAEGELI TYPE*
**Franceschetti-Klein syndrome**
*See MANDIBULOFACIAL DYSOSTOSIS*
**Francois dermochondrocorneal dysplasia**
*See DERMO-CHONDRO-CORNEAL DYSTROPHY, FRANCOIS TYPE*
**Francois dyscephalic syndrome**
*See OCULO-MANDIBULO-FACIAL SYNDROME*
*also INTESTINAL POLYPOSIS, TYPE III*

## FRASER SYNDROME                                      2271

**Includes:**

Cryptophthalmos-other malformations
Cryptophthalmos-syndactyly
Cryptophthalmos syndrome, Fraser type
Syndactyly-cryptophthalmos

**Excludes:**

Bowen syndrome of multiple malformations
**Eye, cryptophthalmos (0003)**

**Major Diagnostic Criteria:** Partial cutaneous **Syndactyly**; genital malformations, usually hypoplasias; renal malformations ranging from unilateral or bilateral dysplasia to unilateral or bilateral agenesis or hypoplasia; and **Eye, cryptophthalmos.** Cryptophthalmos is usually, but not always, present.

**Clinical Findings:** Recognized at birth by partial cutaneous **Syndactyly**; genital malformations, usually hypoplasias; renal malformations ranging from unilateral or bilateral dysplasia to unilateral or bilateral agenesis or hypoplasia; and **Eye, cryptophthalmos.** Cryptophthalmos is usually, but not always, present. Affected infants may be stillborn. Hair growth pattern may be abnormal.

**Complications:** Unilateral or bilateral blindness.

**Associated Findings:** Laryngeal stenosis, **Eye, hypertelorism**, lacrimal duct defect; aural malformations comprising outer ear atresia and/or middle ear defect; displacement of umbilicus.
Clitoral enlargement, bicornuate uterus, and vaginal and labial malformation in female. Hypospadias, cryptorchidism in male. Anal atresia, cerebral polymicrogyria, high palate/cleft palate, intestinal hypoplasia, and **Skin crease, single palmer**. Gonadoblastoma was reported in one patient.

**Etiology:** Autosomal recessive inheritance. The parents of affected children are sometimes, but not always, consanguineous. The condition has been described in monozygous twins.

**Pathogenesis:** Unknown.

**MIM No.:** *21900, 21120

**POS No.:** 3179

**Sex Ratio:** M1:F1

**Occurrence:** About 75 cases have been documented.

**Risk of Recurrence for Patient's Sib:**
See Part I, *Mendelian Inheritance.*

**Risk of Recurrence for Patient's Child:**
See Part I, *Mendelian Inheritance.*

**Age of Detectability:** At birth.

**Gene Mapping and Linkage:** Unknown.

**Prevention:** None known. Genetic counseling indicated.

**Treatment:** None, if renal agenesis is present. Surgical correction of cryptophthalmos is possible but has been of limited value if ocular malformation is also present. Genital, digital, and laryngeal malformations are surgically correctable.

**Prognosis:** Related to renal and respiratory conditions. Prognosis is excellent for survival if cryptophthalmos is the main abnormality. Severe bilateral renal dysplasia or agenesis implies no prospect for survival. Visual acuity is likely to be poor in many cases, even after surgical correction of lid malformation. Stillbirth and intrauterine fetal death have been recorded. There is no clear prognosis regarding mental retardation.

**Detection of Carrier:** Unknown.

**Special Considerations:** The designation *Fraser syndrome* is the preferred name for this condition in which multiple congenital malformations are found in the kidneys, the genitalia, the larynx, the ears and the digits (partial cutaneous syndactyly), and these are frequently but not invariably accompanied by cryptophthalmos and associated ocular abnormalities. The precise characterization of the syndrome is still evolving; many authors consider Fraser syndrome in cases of renal agenesis, hypoplasia, or dysplasia found in association with any of the above extra-renal malformations. It is generally recognized that cryptophthalmos is helpful but not essential for the diagnosis. The prognosis for recurrence in future pregnancies is considerably worse (1:4) than for isolated renal abnormalities, so that greater awareness of the syndrome is important for genetic counseling.
Fraser syndrome should also be contrasted with *Bowen syndrome of multiple malformations* (Bowen et al, 1964) which was reported in one or two families in the early 1960s.

**References:**

Fraser GR: Our genetical "load": a review of some aspects of genetic variation. Ann Hum Genet 1962; 25:387–415.
Bowen P, et al.: A familial syndrome of multiple congenital defects. Bull Johns Hopkins Hosp 1964; 114:402–414.
Lurie IW, Cherstvoy ED: Renal agenesis as a diagnostic feature of the cryptophthalmos - syndactyly syndrome. Clin Genet 1984; 25:528–533.
Mortimer G, et al.: Fraser syndrome presenting as monozygotic twins with bilateral renal agenesis. J Med Genet 1985; 22:76–78.
Koenig R, Spranger J: Cryptophthalmos-syndactyly syndrome without cryptophthalmos. Clin Genet 1986; 29:413–416.
Thomas IT, et al.: Isolated and syndromic cryptophthalmos. Am J Med Genet 1986; 25:85–98.
Gattuso J, et al.: The clinical spectrum of the Fraser syndrome: report of three new cases and review. J Med Genet 1987; 24:549–555. *
Boyd PA, et al.: Fraser syndrome: review of eleven cases with postmortem findings. Am J Med Genet 1988; 31:159–168.

M0036                                              **Gabriel Mortimer**

**Fraser-Ayme-Hall syndrome**
*See BRANCHIO-OTO-URETERAL SYNDROME*
**Freeman-Sheldon syndrome**
*See CRANIO-CARPO-TARSAL DYSPLASIA, WHISTLING FACE TYPE*
**Freiburg disease (head of second metatarsal)**
*See JOINTS, OSTEOCHONDRITIS DISSECANS*
**Freire-Maia syndrome**
*See ODONTO-TRICHOMELIC SYNDROME*
**Frey syndrome**
*See SWEATING, GUSTATORY*
**Friedreich ataxia (FA)**
*See ATAXIA, FRIEDREICH TYPE*
**Friedreich ataxia-Charcot-Marie-Tooth disease-deafness**
*See CHARCOT MARIE TOOTH DISEASE-DEAFNESS*
**Friedreich disease**
*See ATAXIA, FRIEDREICH TYPE*
**Friedreich disease, abortive type**
*See NEUROPATHY, HEREDITARY MOTOR AND SENSORY, TYPE I*
**Fromont anomaly**
*See POLYDACTYLY*
**Fronto-facio-nasal dysostosis**
*See FRONTO-FACIO-NASAL DYSPLASIA*

## FRONTO-FACIO-NASAL DYSPLASIA 2979

**Includes:**
Facio-fronto-nasal dysplasia
Fronto-facio-nasal dysostosis
Nasal-fronto-faciodysplasia

**Excludes:**
**Cranio-fronto-nasal dysplasia** (2185)
**Face, median cleft face syndrome** (0635)

**Major Diagnostic Criteria:** **Cleft lip** and **Cleft palate**; nasal hypoplasia and hypoplastic nasal wings; primary telecanthus; blepharophimosis, lagophthalmos, and S-shaped palpebral fissures; midface hypoplasia; and computed tomography of central nervous system showing cranium bifidum occultum or encephalocele.

**Clinical Findings:** Diagnosis can be established immediately after birth. Mental and neurologic development seems to be normal. The eye involvement seems to have great clinical variability. In some cases there is no eye involvement, but one patient showed cataract, microphthalmia, microcornea, and coloboma of iris.

Encephalocele and cranium bifidum occultum are closely related abnormalities, and this belief is supported by Cohen (1979), who pointed out that the pathogenesis encompasses frontal encephalocele, frontal lipoma, frontal teratoma, intrinsic nasal capsule abnormalities, early ossification of the lesser sphenoidal wings, craniosynostosis, and enlargement of the ethmoidal sinuses.

**Complications:** Feeding difficulties due to severe cleft palate.

**Associated Findings:** Brachycephaly, frontal lipoma, widow's peak, eyelid coloboma, limbic dermoid of eye, bifid nose, and absent eyelashes.

**Etiology:** Autosomal recessive inheritance. Parental consanguinity was present in all reported cases.

**Pathogenesis:** Unknown.

**MIM No.:** *22940

**POS No.:** 3511

**Sex Ratio:** M1:F2 (observed).

**Occurrence:** Three patients, all Brazilian, have been reported in the literature.

**Risk of Recurrence for Patient's Sib:**
See Part I, *Mendelian Inheritance.*

**Risk of Recurrence for Patient's Child:**
See Part I, *Mendelian Inheritance.*

**Age of Detectability:** Immediately after birth. Prenatal diagnosis is possible using ultrasound to detect facial clefts and encephalocele or cranium bifidum occultum.

**Gene Mapping and Linkage:** Unknown.

**Prevention:** None known. Genetic counseling indicated.

**Treatment:** Neurosurgery to correct encephalocele and cranium bifidum occultum and plastic surgery to correct clefts and eyelid defects.

**Prognosis:** There are no reasons to suspect that life span is shortened. The oldest patient has reached her teens.

**Detection of Carrier:** Unknown.

**References:**
Gollop TR: Fronto-facio-nasal dysostosis: a new autosomal recessive syndrome. Am J Med Genet 1981; 10:409–412.
Gollop TR, et al.: Fronto-facio-nasal dysplasia: evidence for autosomal recessive inheritance. Am J Med Genet 1984; 19:301–305.

G0044                                        **Thomaz R. Gollop**

**Fronto-nasal dysplasia**
*See FACE, MEDIAN CLEFT FACE SYNDROME*
**Frontodigital syndrome**
*See POLYSYNDACTYLY-DYSMORPHIC CRANIOFACIES, GREIG TYPE*

## FRONTOMETAPHYSEAL DYSPLASIA 0394

**Includes:** Facio-dental-skeletal anomalies-joint contractures-hyperostosis

**Excludes:**
**Craniometaphyseal dysplasia** (0228)
Craniotubular dysplasias (other)
**Osteodysplasty** (0775)
**Oto-palato-digital syndrome, I** (0786)
**Oto-palato-digital syndrome, II** (2258)
**Pyle disease** (0847)

**Major Diagnostic Criteria:** Peculiar facial appearance, dental abnormalities, multiple joint contractures, skeletal dysplasia with hyperostosis, abnormal pelvic appearance.

The similar clinical and X-ray findings suggest that osteodysplasty and frontometaphyseal dysplasia are the same condition. There are, however, subtle differences in the appearance of the vertebral bodies and hand bones of reported cases. Further observations are needed to show whether these differences are consistent or if they are variable manifestations of the same mutation.

**Clinical Findings:** Peculiar face with prominent supraorbital ridges; a small pointed chin; micrognathia/retrognathia; high-arched palate; malaligned, small teeth; unerupted or congenitally missing teeth. Relatively short trunk with a straight thoracic spine or thoracic lordosis, scoliosis; pectus excavatum or carinatum, winging of the scapulae; long extremities relative to trunk with long hands and feet, multiple joint contractures of the large and small joints, poorly developed musculature.

X-rays reveal diffuse hyperostosis of the calvaria and/or perisutural sclerosis, prominent supraorbital ridges, underdeveloped paranasal sinuses, especially the frontal sinuses, micrognathia with antegonial notching, and multiple dental abnormalities; abnormalities of the spine curvature: spina bifida occulta, and flattened vertebral bodies; irregular contours of the ribs; flared iliac wings and constricted mid-pelvis, coxa valga, wide femoral neck; metaphyseal flaring and bowed shafts of the long tubular bones; genu valgum/genu recurvatum; small carpal bones with pronounced underdevelopment of the proximal row; elongation

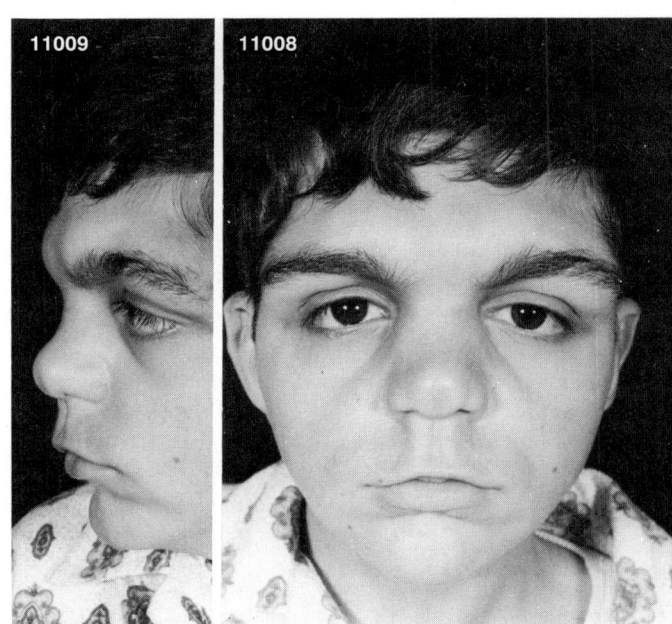

**0394**-11008–09:  Broad nasal bridge, thickened nares, prominent supraorbital ridge and small pointed chin.

and lack of metaphyseal modeling of the short tubular bones of the hands.

**Complications:** Progression of joint contractures, joint pain, muscular hypotrophy, hammer toe, progressive thickening of the cranial vault; combined sensorineural and conductive hearing loss; obstructive uropathy; and psychologic problems due to facial appearance.

**Associated Findings:** Impaired vision due to congenital esotropia and secondary amblyopia; hyperopia; bifid uvula, recurrent respiratory and middle ear infections; cardiac defects.

**Etiology:** Although autosomal dominant inheritance was initially reported, re-examination of previous case reports suggest X-linked inheritance with severe manifestation in males and extremely variable manifestation in females.

**Pathogenesis:** Unknown.

**MIM No.:** *30562

**POS No.:** 3236

**Sex Ratio:** M1:F<1.

**Occurrence:** About 20 cases have been documented.

**Risk of Recurrence for Patient's Sib:**
See Part I, *Mendelian Inheritance.*

**Risk of Recurrence for Patient's Child:**
See Part I, *Mendelian Inheritance.*

**Age of Detectability:** Early infancy with joint contractures. Skeletal changes, peculiar faces, and hearing loss detected in mid-childhood.

**Gene Mapping and Linkage:** Unknown.

**Prevention:** None known. Genetic counseling indicated.

**Treatment:** As appropriate for orthopedic, dental and hearing problems. Surgical removal of the frontal torus has been recommended for cosmetic reasons.

**Prognosis:** Psychomotor development and life span are normal in most patients. The complications listed above may interfere with the patient's physical and social performance.

**Detection of Carrier:** Skeletal X-rays may detect abnormal bone modeling or cranial hyperostosis in otherwise unaffected relatives.

**Special Considerations:** Superti-Ferga and Gimelli (1987), upon review of cases from the literature, have suggested that this condition may be same as **Oto-palato-digital syndrome.**

**References:**
Holt JF, et al.: Frontometaphyseal dysplasia. Radiol Clin North Am 1972; 10:225–243.
Medlar RC, Crawford AH: Frontometaphyseal dysplasia presenting as scoliosis: a report of a family with four cases. J Bone Joint Surg 1978; 60A:392–394.
Kanemura T, et al.: Frontometaphyseal dysplasia with congenital urinary tract malformations. Clin Genet 1979; 16:399–404.
Gorlin RJ, Winter RB: Frontometaphyseal dysplasia: evidence for X-linked inheritance. Am J Med Genet 1980; 5:81–84.
Jend-Rossman I, et al.: Frontometaphyseal dysplasia. J Oral Maxillofac Surg 1984; 42:743–748.
Superti-Furga A, Gimelli F: Frontometaphyseal dysplasia and the oto-palato-digital syndrome. Dysmorph Clin Genet 1987; 1:2–5.

J0010

Virginia P. Johnson<br>Jürgen W. Spranger

**Frontonasal dysplasia with coronal craniosynostosis**
 *See CRANIO-FRONTO-NASAL DYSPLASIA*
**Fructose intolerance, hereditary**
 *See FRUCTOSE-1-PHOSPHATE ALDOLASE DEFICIENCY*
**Fructose-1,6-bisphosphate aldolase B deficiency**
 *See FRUCTOSE-1-PHOSPHATE ALDOLASE DEFICIENCY*

## FRUCTOSE-1,6-DIPHOSPHATASE DEFICIENCY  0396

**Includes:** Hepatic fructose-1,6-diphosphatase deficiency

**Excludes:**
 **Fructose-1-phosphate aldolase deficiency** (0395)
 **Glycogen synthetase deficiency** (0424)
 **Glycogenosis, type Ia** (0425)
 **Glycogenosis, type III** (0426)
 **Pyruvate carboxylase deficiency with lactic acidemia** (0850)
 **Pyruvate dehydrogenase deficiency** (0851)

**Major Diagnostic Criteria:** Symptomatic hypoglycemia and lactic acidosis occur in the newborn. Hypoglycemia, lactic acidosis and ketosis occur after fasting and/or during febrile infections in an infant or a small child. Absence or severe deficiency of hepatic or jejunal fructose-1,6-diphosphatase is diagnostic. Enzyme assays on leukocytes or platelets were successfully done in some laboratories but not in others.

**Clinical Findings:** This inborn error of hepatic gluconeogenesis may present in the neonatal period with acute episodes of hyperventilation, apnea, convulsions, coma, lactic acidosis, hypoglycemia, ketosis, and hyperalaninemia, with a precipitous and often lethal course. In infancy or early childhood, such attacks occur in the fasting state and are often provoked by febrile infections. Peculiar EEG patterns during the acute episodes are reported. During the asymptomatic intervals, mild hepatomegaly (fatty infiltration, increased glycogen content) muscle hypotonia and hyperventilation may be noted. Psychomotor development is normal.

Blood glucose is low after fasting and may fall below 10–20 mg/dl. Lactate is usually elevated, and after fasting may be > 200 mg/dl. The lactate falls rapidly with correction of hypoglycemia. Alanine may be elevated, especially during acidosis. Glucagon fails to raise blood glucose after prolonged fasting but postprandially it raises blood glucose to normal. Adult onset was reported in a woman who presented with fatigue and emotional lability and had reactive and symptomatic hypoglycemia; her daughter had the same defect.

**Complications:** Unknown.

**Associated Findings:** None known.

**Etiology:** Autosomal recessive inheritance.

**Pathogenesis:** Blood glucose cannot be maintained after depletion of liver glycogen stores because of the defect in hepatic gluconeogenesis. Prolonged fasting is poorly tolerated. Mild intolerance to fructose, sorbitol and glycerol exists and is caused by the inhibition of hepatic glycogenolysis by certain phosphate esters.

**MIM No.:** *22970

**Sex Ratio:** M32F46 (observed)

**Occurrence:** Sixty-eight cases reported.

**Risk of Recurrence for Patient's Sib:**
See Part I, *Mendelian Inheritance.*

**Risk of Recurrence for Patient's Child:**
See Part I, *Mendelian Inheritance.*

**Age of Detectability:** Neonatal period.

**Gene Mapping and Linkage:** Unknown.

**Prevention:** None known. Genetic counseling indicated.

**Treatment:** Prompt correction of hypoglycemia and acidosis. *Caution: the infusion of sorbitol for suspected brain edema has been lethal in one child!* Treatment with folic acid has been suggested but remains to be proven beneficial in each patient. Avoid prolonged fasting, especially during febrile infections. Frequent meals, restriction of dietary fructose and sorbitol, reduction of fats are recommended. As weight reduction is difficult to achieve, caloric intake should be watched in order to prevent obesity.

**Prognosis:** Acute episodes are life-threatening. Growth, psychomotor and intellectual development seem unimpaired if acute episodes can be treated successfully.

**Detection of Carrier:** In the 3 parents examined, the activity of hepatic frutose-1,6-diphosphatase was reduced to approximately 1/2 of the normal or less. Possibly, heterozygotes can be identified by measuring fructose-1,6-diphosphatase in cultured or peripheral lymphocytes.

**Special Considerations:** This disorder may be difficult to distinguish initially from glycogen storage disease especially type I, but also type III. The blood lactate levels should distinguish it from type III, and the response to glucagon following an adequate carbohydrate intake should distinguish it from type I. Combined deficiency of fructose-1, 6-diphosphatase and glucose-6-phosphatase or glucose-6-phosphate dehydrogenase was reported.

**References:**
Baker L, Winegrad AI: Fasting hypoglycaemia and metabolic acidosis associated with deficiency of hepatic fructose-1,6-diphosphatase activity. Lancet 1970; II:13–16.
Ito M, et al.: Detection of heterozygotes for fructose-1,6-diphosphatase deficiency by measuring fructose-1,6 diphosphatase activity in their cultured peripheral lymphocytes. Clin Chim Acta 1984; 141:27–32.
Alexander D, et al.: Fructose-1,6-diphosphatase deficiency: diagnosis using leukocytes and detection of heterozygotes with radiochemical and spectrophotometric methods. J Inherit Metab Dis 1985; 8:174–177.
Gitzelmann R, et al.: Disorders of fructose metabolism. In: Scriver C, et al., eds: The metabolic basis of inherited disease. 6th ed. New York: McGraw-Hill, 1989. *

GI013                                             **Richard Gitzelmann**

## FRUCTOSE-1-PHOSPHATE ALDOLASE DEFICIENCY        **0395**

**Includes:**
Aldolase B deficiency
Fructose intolerance, hereditary
Fructose-1,6-bisphosphate aldolase B deficiency
Fructosemia

**Excludes:**
**Fructose-1,6-diphosphatase deficiency** (0396)
**Fructosuria** (0397)
Galactose and fructose intolerance

**Major Diagnostic Criteria:** Ingestion of fructose causes vomiting, jaundice, hypoglycemia, and seizures. An intravenous fructose tolerance test with 3 gm of fructose per m² in children and 0.25 gm of fructose per kg in adults leads to a sustained fall in blood glucose, hypoglycemic symptoms and hypophosphatemia. Blood glucose and inorganic serum phosphorus must be determined in 15-minute intervals up to 120 minutes. A fall in blood glucose of more than 40% from the initial value lasting for 1/2 hour or longer proves the diagnosis of fructose intolerance. This diagnosis is confirmed by the measurement of the ratio of the hepatic aldolase activities to fructose-1,6-diphosphate and fructose-1-phosphate, respectively, which is above 5.0 (normal ratio 1.4).

**Clinical Findings:** The major symptoms occur with continuous fructose exposure: failure to thrive, vomiting, hepatomegaly, jaundice, and seizures caused by hypoglycemia. The acute syndrome after fructose ingestion consists of nausea, vomiting, and all signs and symptoms of hypoglycemia and fructosuria. Hypoglucosemia develops rapidly after fructose intake and reaches its lowest values after 30–60 minutes. Children demonstrate symptoms faster than adults. At the same time, the level of serum inorganic phosphorus falls in a sustained manner. After massive doses of fructose, hyperbilirubinemia and a rise in serum levels of hepatic enzymes (e.g. sorbitol dehydrogenase and glutamate-pyruvate-transhydrogenase) may be seen. Transient aminoaciduria of the "hepatic type" may occur. The chronic syndrome is seen only during infancy. It is caused by prolonged intake of fructose, most often in the form of saccharose (table sugar or sucrose) and fruit juices.
Fructosuria is present after fructose intake. Later fibrosis and cirrhosis of the liver may develop together with ascites and

edema. If the condition is not recognized in due time, the babies may die in a cachectic state. Tubular acidosis has been described. The teeth are free from dental caries. All patients from the age of 6 months onward develop a strong aversion to all food stuffs that are sweet and contain fructose, and thus protect themselves from getting ill.

**Complications:** If fructose ingestion continues, cachexia, liver failure, and dehydration result.

**Associated Findings:** None known.

**Etiology:** Autosomal recessive inheritance of a deficiency of fructose-1-phosphate aldolase in liver, kidney, and mucosa of small bowel.

**Pathogenesis:** Since fructose-1-phosphate aldolase is needed only for the metabolism of fructose, patients with fructose intolerance are perfectly healthy as long as no fructose is ingested. Fructokinase is present in normal amounts, and fructose is phosphorylated primarily by the liver to fructose-1-phosphate, which accumulates intracellularly. Fructose-1-phosphate blocks glycogenolysis and gluconeogenesis leading, to hypoglucosemia. Fructose-1-phosphate impedes the action of phosphorylase and thus the formation of glucose-1-phosphate from glycogen. On the other hand, fructose-1-phosphate appears to inhibit the formation of fructose-1,6-diphosphate aldolase, which is also present in the liver. Hepatocellular damage is also believed to be caused by the accumulation of fructose-1-phosphate.

**MIM No.:**  *22960

**Sex Ratio:**  M1:F1

**Occurrence:**  Undetermined. Extensive literature.

**Risk of Recurrence for Patient's Sib:**
See Part I, *Mendelian Inheritance.*

**Risk of Recurrence for Patient's Child:**
See Part I, *Mendelian Inheritance.*

**Age of Detectability:** At birth, by fructose tolerance test or enzyme determination in liver biopsy.

**Gene Mapping and Linkage:** ALDOB (aldolase B, fructose bisphosphate) has been mapped to 9q21.3-q22.2.

**Prevention:** None known. Genetic counseling indicated.

**Treatment:** All fructose-containing foods must be completely avoided. Hypoglycemic attacks caused by the ingestion of fructose may be relieved instantaneously by the IV administration of glucose. There is no specific treatment for hepatocellular damage in fructose intolerance except complete avoidance of any fructose-containing substances.

**Prognosis:** The prognosis is very unfavorable when the condition is not recognized. The earlier fructose is started and continued, the faster the condition deteriorates. Babies with fructose intolerance who were persistently fed fructose died between 2 and 6 months of age. The cause of death is cachexia, liver failure and dehydration. Death due to hypoglycemia has not been described. No residual brain damage was found in any surviving child or adult with fructose intolerance.
Hepatocellular damage is usually reversible when the child is taken off fructose. Recovery is complete and life span is normal.

**Detection of Carrier:** The heterozygous carriers of fructose intolerance are not detectable clinically with the use of fructose tolerance tests. An intermediate ratio of hepatic fructose-1-phosphate to fructose-1,6-diphosphate aldolase activity between normal subjects and patients with fructose intolerance is to be expected, but has not yet been proven.

**Special Considerations:** Fructose intolerance is not the same as **Fructosuria**, another anomaly of fructose metabolism characterized by a lack of fructokinase. Another disorder of fructose metabolism distinct from fructose intolerance is fructose and galactose intolerance. Two sisters displayed severe hypoglycemic attacks after fructose and galactose ingestion, accompanied by hyperinsulinism, which is not present in fructose intolerance. Nausea and vomiting, typical for fructose intolerance, were absent in these two sibs, neither of whom developed a distaste toward sweet food stuffs.

**References:**

Odievre M, et al.: Hereditary fructose intolerance in childhood: diagnosis, management, and course in 55 patients. Am J Dis Child 1978; 132:605–608.
Mock DM, et al.: Chronic fructose intoxication after infancy in children with hereditary fructose intolerance. New Engl J Med 1983; 309:764–770.
Oberhaensli RD, et al.: Study of hereditary fructose intolerance by use of (31)P magnetic resonance spectroscopy. Lancet 1987; II:931–934.
Gitzelmann R, et al.: Disorders of fructose metabolism. In: Scriver C et al., eds: The metabolic basis of inherited disease, 6th ed. New York: McGraw-Hill, 1989; 399–424.

FR023                                                    **E. R. Froesch**

**Fructosemia**
*See FRUCTOSE-1-PHOSPHATE ALDOLASE DEFICIENCY*

---

## FRUCTOSURIA                                              0397

**Includes:**
    Essential fructosuria
    Hepatic fructokinase deficiency

**Excludes:** Fructose-1-phosphate aldolase deficiency (0395)

**Major Diagnostic Criteria:** The reducing sugar in the urine must be identified as fructose. Blood fructose levels after oral administration of fructose (1 gm/kg body weight) are markedly increased (above 25 mg/dl), and levels remain high four hours later. Following an oral fructose load, fructose appears rapidly in the urine. Glucose and galactose metabolism are normal.

**Clinical Findings:** Individuals are normal and asymptomatic except for the presence of a reducing sugar in the urine (positive Benedict, positive Fehling, positive Nylander qualitative tests, negative glucose-oxidase (Testape or Clinistix)) after meals containing either fructose or sucrose. It is important as a differential for diabetes mellitus.

**Complications:** Unknown.

**Associated Findings:** None known.

**Etiology:** Autosomal recessive inheritance of a deficiency of hepatic fructokinase.

**Pathogenesis:** Fructose is excreted in the urine because of elevated blood fructose levels due to lack of hepatic fructokinase which normally catalyzes the conversion of fructose to fructose-1-phosphate.

**MIM No.:** *22980

**Sex Ratio:** M1:F1

**Occurrence:** 1:130,000 of general population; 18:50 cases have occurred in Jews.

**Risk of Recurrence for Patient's Sib:**
See Part I, *Mendelian Inheritance.*

**Risk of Recurrence for Patient's Child:**
See Part I, *Mendelian Inheritance.*

**Age of Detectability:** Any age, dependent upon diet, if urine examined for reducing sugar (fructose).

**Gene Mapping and Linkage:** Unknown.

**Prevention:** None known. Genetic counseling indicated.

**Treatment:** None required.

**Prognosis:** Excellent; patients have a normal life expectancy.

**Detection of Carrier:** Unknown.

**Special Considerations:** Fructose is fermentable by yeast, yields a positive Seliwanoff reaction and is levorotatory. Its identity is confirmed by paper chromatographic techniques.

**References:**

Lasker M: Essential fructosuria. Hum Biol 1941; 13:51–63.
Laron Z: Essential benign fructosuria. Arch Dis Child 1961; 36:273–277.

Schapira F, et al.: La lésion enzymatique de la fructosuria bénigne. Enzym Biol Clin 1961–62; 1:170–175.
Gitzelmann R, et al.: Disorders of fructose metabolism. In: Scriver C et al., eds: The metabolic basis of inherited disease, 6th ed. New York: McGraw-Hill, 1989; 399–424.

K0004                                                    **Maurice D. Kogut**

---

## FRYNS SYNDROME                                           2265

**Includes:** Diaphragmatic defects-distal digital hypoplasia

**Excludes:**
    **Facio-cardiomelic dysplasia, lethal** (3190)
    Limb defects, isolated terminal transverse
    **Pena-Shokeir syndrome** (2080)
    **Roberts syndrome** (0875)

**Major Diagnostic Criteria:** Hydramnios, characteristic facies, narrow thorax, limb defects, and visceral defects.

**Clinical Findings:** Hydramnios in the second trimester of pregnancy with normal fetal growth; distinct craniofacial features with coarse face, broad flat nasal bridge, large nose with anteverted nostrils, short upper lip, macrostomia, **Cleft lip** and/or **Cleft palate**, microretrognathia, poorly shaped auricles with attached earlobes; narrow thorax, hypoplastic widely spaced nipples; distal limb hypoplasia with brachytelephalangy, hypoplastic to absent nails, and rudimentary development of terminal (and middle) phalanges most pronounced on rays IV-V.

Internal malformations include diaphragmatic defects (aplasia of posterolateral parts) with primary or secondary lung hypoplasia; G.I. anomalies (malrotations and non-fixation, duodenal or multiple atresias); Genito-urinary malformations with bicornuate uterus in the female.

**Complications:** Unknown.

**Associated Findings:** Cloudy corneae and microphthalmia, up-slanting of palpebral fissures, short neck with nuchal folds, transverse palmar creases, and club feet. Internal malformations include renal dysplasia and cortical cysts, cerebral malformations including Dandy-Walker cyst, and multiple cerebellar glioneural heterotopias.

**Etiology:** Autosomal recessive inheritance. Three pairs of sibs have been reported. Parents were first degree cousins in the case of one isolated patient.

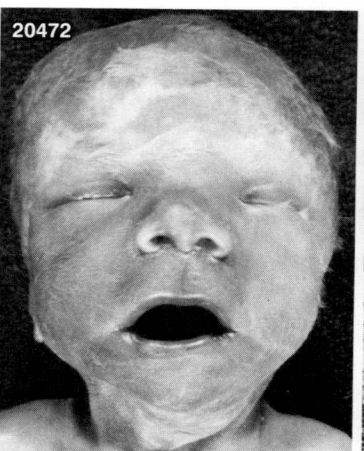
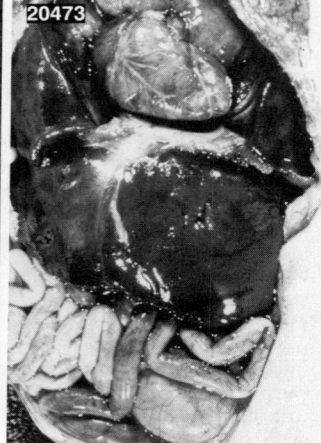

**2265-20472:** Broad, flat nasal bridge, large nose and macrostomia in a newborn. **20473:** Bilateral agenesis of the posterolateral diaphragm with herniation of abdominal organs into the thoracic cage.

**Pathogenesis:** Unknown. In most patients, the fibrous part of the diaphragm, originating from the septum transversum and the muscular portion of the diaphragm, were well developed. In contrast, the postero-lateral parts of the diaphragm, derived from the plicae pleuroperitoneales, were bilaterally absent. The formations of these plicae is induced by the outgrowth of both lungs. This suggests that lung hypoplasia with absence of lobulations might be the primary event, with secondary absence of formations and outgrowth of the plicae pleuroperitoneales.

**MIM No.:**  *22985

**POS No.:**  3608

**Sex Ratio:**  Presumably M1:F1.

**Occurrence:**  Estimated at 1:10,000 births. Three patients were detected in Leuven in a consecutive series of 900 perinatal autopsies.

**Risk of Recurrence for Patient's Sib:**
See Part I, *Mendelian Inheritance.*

**Risk of Recurrence for Patient's Child:**
See Part I, *Mendelian Inheritance.* Affected individuals are not expected to reproduce. Three survivors have been reported; all with severe mental retardation.

**Age of Detectability:**  Prenatal ultrasonographic diagnosis of associated diaphragmatic defects (present in 90% of patients) is feasible at about 15–18 weeks gestation. Fetoscopic diagnosis at 19–20 weeks by the presence of cleft lip/palate and distal digital hypoplasia. Elevated amniotic fluid AFP levels in the presence of renal anomalies.

**Gene Mapping and Linkage:**  Unknown.

**Prevention:**  None known. Genetic counseling indicated.

**Treatment:**  Postnatal correction of internal malformations is theoretically possible.

**Prognosis:**  Poor life prognosis in the presence of severe lung hypoplasia. This syndrome apparently represents a new entity among other syndrome with sublethal outcome.

**Detection of Carrier:**  Unknown.

**References:**
Fryns JP, et al.: A new lethal syndrome with cloudy corneae, diaphragmatic defects and distal limb deformities. Hum Genet 1979; 50:65–70. †
Lubinsky M, et al.: Fryns syndrome: a new variable multiple congenital anomaly (MCA) syndrome. Am J Med Genet 1983; 14:461–466. †
Meinecke P, et al.: Zwerchfelldefekte, kraniofaziale anomalien einschliesslich Lippen-Kiefer und/oder Gaumenspalte sowie Hypoplasien der Endphalangen ("Fryns-Syndrom") poster presentation. 4. Symposion Klinische Genetik in der Pädiatrie, Baden-Baden, 15. 17 Juli 1983. †
Fryns JP: Fryns syndrome: a variable MCA syndrome with diaphragmatic defects, coarse face, and distal limb hypoplasia. J Med Genet 1987; 24:271–274. * †
Samueloff A, et al.: Fryns syndrome: a predictable, lethal pattern of multiple congenital anomalies. Am J Obstet Gynec 1987; 156:86–88. †
Schwyzer U, et al.: Fryns syndrome in a girl born to consanguineous parents. Acta paediatr Scand 1987; 76:167–171. †
Moerman P, et al.: The syndrome of diaphragmatic hernia, abnormal face and distal limb anomalies (Fryns syndrome). Am J Med Genet 1988; 31:805–814. †
Bamforth JS, et al.: Congenital diaphragmatic hernia, course facies, and acral hypoplasia: Fryns syndrome. Am J Med Genet 1989; 32:93–99. †

FR030                                        **Jean-Pierre Fryns**

**Fuch coloboma**
*See OPTIC DISK, TILTED*
**Fuchs endothelial dystrophy**
*See CORNEAL DYSTROPHY, ENDOTHELIAL*

## FUCOSIDOSIS                                        0398

**Includes:**
  Alpha-L-fucosidase deficiency
  Mucopolysaccharidosis F

**Excludes:**
  **Aspartylglucosaminuria** (2042)
  **Fabry disease** (0373)
  **Galactosialidosis** (3110)
  **G(m2)-gangliosidosis with hexosaminidase A and B deficiency** (0433)
  **G(m2)-gangliosidosis with hexosaminidase A deficiency** (0434)
  **Mannosidosis** (2079)
  **Mucolipidosis**
  **Mucopolysaccharidosis**

**Major Diagnostic Criteria:**  Clinical findings are variable. Two main subtypes have been identified. Both show deterioration of the central nervous system. This syndrome is confirmed by a demonstration of absent α-L-fucosidase activity in leukocytes or cultured skin fibroblasts and increased urine or tissue levels of fucose-containing oligosaccharides and sphingolipids. Plasma should not be used for screening, since a small percentage of normal individuals have no detectable activity. Localized deficiencies limited to cultured fibroblasts have been encountered, while normal activity was preserved in leukocytes and plasma. The significance of these findings is unknown. Ultrastructural studies on biopsies from the skin or conjunctiva will settle the diagnosis in cases with questionably low enzyme activity.

**Clinical Findings:**  A great deal of clinical heterogeneity is apparent, but two main groups can be delineated. In type 1, corresponding to the original disease description, the children make fair progress in the first year of life but then have progressive cerebral degeneration, with weakness and hypotonia followed by

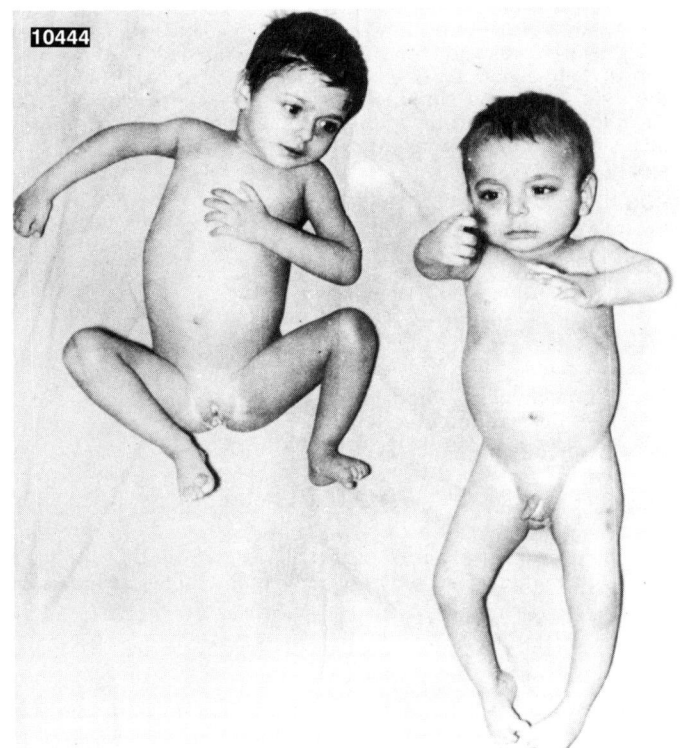

**0398-10444:**  Appearance of the first 2 patients identified as having fucosidosis.

spastic quadriplegia. They have thick skin, with abundant sweating and cardiomegaly. Seizures are not frequent. Of note is a markedly increased sodium and chloride level in sweat (3–9x N), and progressive impairment of gallbladder function. Spinal fluid is normal, and urinary mucopolysaccharides are not increased, but a number of fucose-containing oligosaccharides and glycopeptides have been detected. Faint corneal cloudiness may be present. There is a brachycephalic skull with frontal bulging, and lumbar kyphosis with hypoplasia and beaking of L-2 and L-3. Special features are an accumulation of fucose-containing oligosaccharides in urine, vacuolated lymphocytes, skin, liver and other tissues (intracellular), an increase of fucose-containing lipids in liver and brain, and an absence of α-L-fucosidase in tissue assays.

In type 2, the children present with delayed psychomotor development. Angiokeratomas, similar to those of Fabry disease, may appear around age 3 years. Coarse features and dwarfism may mimic a mucopolysaccharidosis. Neurologic symptoms include spasticity, contractures, peripheral neuropathy, and amyotrophy. There is no visceromegaly. Skeletal abnormalities are generally discrete, resembling those of **Mucopolysaccharidosis III**.

**Complications:** Chronic recurrent respiratory infection is a problem, as well as the easy dehydration and electrolyte depletion from sweat losses. In these children there is progressive weight loss, as well as signs of myocarditis. Decreased nerve conduction velocities of the median nerve suggest a carpal tunnel syndrome. Bull's eye retinopathy and **Megalencephaly** have also been reported.

**Associated Findings:** Thickened skin, muscle contractures.

**Etiology:** Autosomal recessive inheritance of a deficiency of α-L-fucosidase has been found in liver, lung, kidney, brain, skin fibroblasts, leukocytes and serum. Consanguinity reported in nine of the 30 families studied.

**Pathogenesis:** A gradual increase in the levels of fucose-containing oligosaccharides and glycolipids is noted in most tissues, including brain, apparently correlating with the above-mentioned deficiency of tissue fucosidase. More than 20 oligosaccharides and glycopeptides have been characterized in patients' urine. Changes are notable also in the mucous-secreting glands, skin, cornea, peripheral nerves and lymphocytes. The white matter of the brain shows demyelination and gliosis. Electron microscopic studies of the liver, skin, and conjunctiva cells have revealed cytoplasmic vacuoles surrounded by a single membrane containing granular inclusions and lamellar bodies.

**MIM No.:** *23000

**POS No.:** 3238

**Sex Ratio:** M1:F1

**Occurrence:** About fifty cases reported in the literature.

**Risk of Recurrence for Patient's Sib:**
See Part I, *Mendelian Inheritance.*

**Risk of Recurrence for Patient's Child:**
See Part I, *Mendelian Inheritance.*

**Age of Detectability:** Prenatal diagnosis is feasible. One affected fetus was mistaken for a heterozygote.

**Gene Mapping and Linkage:** FUCA1 (fucosidase, alpha-L-1, tissue) has been mapped to 1p35-p34.

**Prevention:** None known. Genetic counseling indicated.

**Treatment:** Attention to fluid requirements. Surgery for carpal tunnel syndrome or spinal cord compression (potential complications which are not yet reported). Use of antibiotics as indicated.

**Prognosis:** Death has occurred at around five years of age in type 1. Survival to adulthood can be expected in type 2 (a 33-year-old patient has been reported).

**Detection of Carrier:** Most heterozygotes have intermediate α-L-fucosidase activity in cultured skin fibroblasts or leukocytes. Overlap between heterozygous individuals and normals occasionally occurs. Until a statistically significant number of obligate heterozygotes has been studied, individuals with equivocal activities are best considered at risk.

**Special Considerations:** The six known α-L-fucosidase isozymes are barely detectable in both types of fucosidosis, which have both occurred in two different sibships of a large inbred family. Attempts to relate the clinical expression to the Lewis blood types have not been conclusive.

**References:**
Libert J, et al.: Fucosidosis: ultrastructural study of conjunctiva and skin and enzyme analysis of tears. Invest Ophthalmol 1976; 15:626–639.
Ikeda S, et al.: Adult fucosidosis: histochemical and ultrastructural studies of rectal mucosa biopsy. Neurology 1984; 34:451–456.
Blitzer MG, et al.: A thermolabile variant of alpha-L-fucosidase: chemical and laboratory findings. Am J Med Genet 1985; 20:535–539.
Johnson K, Dawson G: Molecular defect in processing alpha-fucosidase in fucosidosis. Biochem Biophys Res Commun 1985; 133:90–97.
Philippart M: Fucosidosis. In: Gomez MR, ed: Neurocutaneous diseases: a practical approach. Stoneham, MA: Butterworth, 1987:143–154. *
Williams PJ, et al.: Identification of a mutation in the structural α-L-fucosidase gene in Fucosidosis. Am J Hum Genet 1988; 43:756–763.

PH000                                    **Michel Philippart**

**Fuhrmann skeletal dysplasia**
*See SKELETAL DYSPLASIA, FUHRMANN TYPE*
**Fukuyama disease**
*See MUSCULAR DYSTROPHY, CONGENITAL WITH MENTAL RETARDATION*
**Fumarase deficiency**
*See ACIDURIA, FUMARIC*
**Fumaric acidemia**
*See ACIDURIA, FUMARIC*
**Fumarylacetoacetase deficiency**
*See TYROSINEMIA I*
**Fundus albipunctatus**
*See RETINA, FUNDUS ALBIPUNCTATUS*
**Fundus flavimaculatus with macular degeneration**
*See RETINA, FUNDUS FLAVIMACULATUS*
**Funnel chest**
*See PECTUS EXCAVATUM*

# ❖ G ❖

**G deletion syndrome**
*See CHROMOSOME 21, MONOSOMY 21*

## G SYNDROME                                                0401

**Includes:**
Hypertelorism-esophageal abnormality-hypospadias
Hypospadias-dysphagia syndrome
Opitz-Frias syndrome
Opitz G-syndrome
Opitz oculo-genito-laryngeal syndrome

**Excludes:**
**Aarskog syndrome** (0001)
**Hypertelorism-hypospadias syndrome** (0505)

**Major Diagnostic Criteria:** Characteristic appearance, unusual type of hypospadias, dysphagia and hoarse voice. Some heterozygotes may have no manifestations at all, one apparently affected male only had the characteristic facies; some heterozygotes only have stridor ("wheezers").

**Clinical Findings:** Findings range from congenital or neonatal lethality with multiple congenital anomalies, to a less severe form with functional swallowing problems which, if managed properly, may allow survival, to very mild forms with minimal or no functional impairment. These mild forms are usually ascertained on family studies. Most of the severely affected patients are males, although two lethally affected neonates were females, one in the original G family. The facial appearance is characteristic: hypertelorism with relatively flattened bridge of nose, prominence of parietal eminences and occiput with relatively dolichocephalic skull and large anterior fontanels, relatively narrow, slit-like palpebral fissures with slight mongoloid or antimongoloid slant, epicanthal folds with or without an accessory fold following the

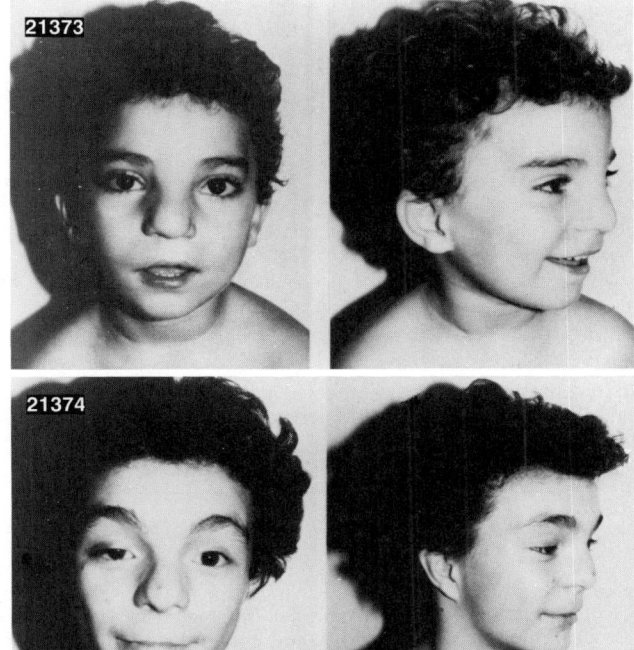

**0401B-21373:** Hypertelorism, downward slant of the palpebral fissures, prominent nasal root, short and large nose with hypoplastic alae and flattened tip, repaired cleft lip and palate, receding chin, anteflexed auricles and bitemporal constriction. **21374:** Hypertelorism, ptosis of the right eyelid, prominent nasal root, large and short nose, long upper lip with hypoplastic philtrum and thin upper vermilion border. Also note dry curly hair, an upsweep of the anterior hairline and thick eyebrows. These two boys shown in 21373 and 74 are not related.

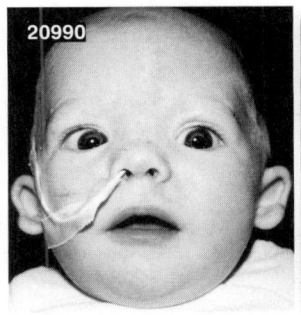
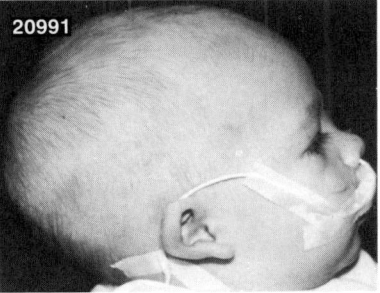

**0401A-20990:** G syndrome; note hypertelorism, anteverted nares, low-set ears and flat nasal bridge. **20991:** Lateral view demonstrates the dolichocephaly and prominent occiput.

upper lid partly to the outer canthus, strabismus, anteversion of nostrils, philtrum relatively flat and unapparent, with relatively severe micrognathia. Voice and cry are hoarse; usually no other external anomalies are evident except for hypospadias and occasional imperforate anus with rectourethral fistula. The hypospadias is unusual ranging in severity from mild coronal to perineoscrotal degrees, with chordee at times pulling tip of glans to anterior edge of anus. Labioscrotal folds may be incompletely fused but testes are usually descended; the two halves of the

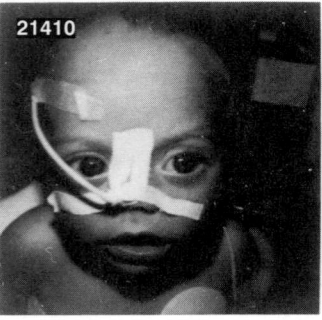
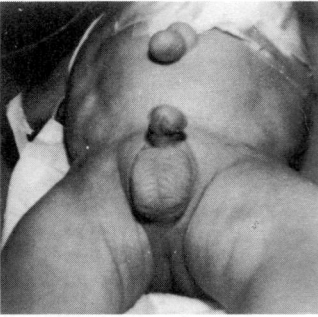
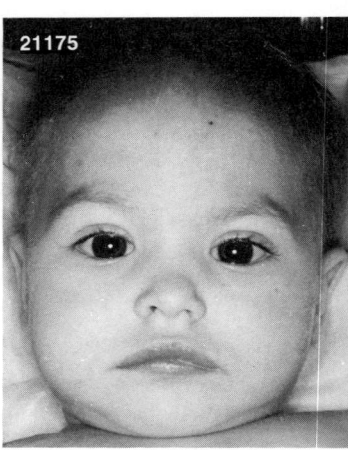
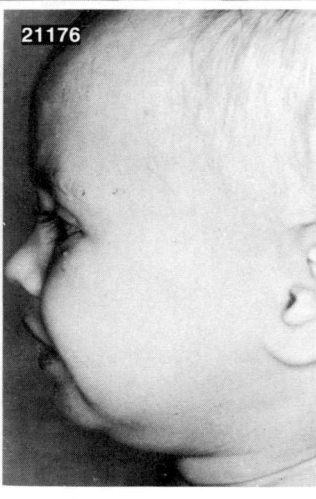

**0401C**-21410: This young affected male has hypertelorism, micrognathia, hypospadias and esophageal motor dysfunction. 21175–76: Characteristic facies include hypertelorism, anteverted nares, flat philtrum and micrognathia.

scrotum may be incompletely descended and cover the phallus. Cleft lip, palate, uvula or tongue has been seen in one-fourth of the cases, and a highly arched palate in about one third of cases. Bifid tip of tongue may also be present. The forehead may be prominent and a widow's peak may be observed. Rare anomalies are pectus carinatum, pectus excavatum, and cryptorchidism. About 10% of the cases present with deep sacral dimple, relatively long fingers and toes, clinodactyly and overlapping toes. Many patients have distal axial triradii and a low total ridge count on the fingers. Premonitory gestational signs may be fetal ascites and polyhydramnios detected by ultrasonography; mean birth weight is 3,200 gm.

The combination of characteristic facies and genital defects with hoarse or stridorous cry is diagnostic and should immediately lead the clinician to search for the potentially fatal esophageal functional defect which leads to repeated aspiration. In severe cases the infant sucks eagerly but chokes, coughs and becomes cyanotic, develops respiratory distress, increase in stridor, aspiration pneumonia, patchy atelectasis and emphysema, and in chronic cases bronchiectasis. Cinefluoroscopic studies should be done with a water soluble contrast medium; they usually show severely disordered esophageal motion with some or much of the bolus entering the trachea, and much gastroesophageal reflux which may be designated "hiatus hernia" and lead to surgical repair. In these severe cases the functional defects may have additional anatomic bases, ie laryngeal cleft with hypoplasia of epiglottis, vocal cords and larynx, high bifurcation of trachea, hypoplasia of one lung, duodenal stricture. The functional defect usually requires surgery (gastrostomy; in extreme cases ligation of the esophagus with cervical esophagostomy). Survivors mature in

their swallowing capacity in a few months to a year to the point where they can eat a normal diet, but continue to choke and aspirate if forced to drink fluids rapidly. They continue to have a relatively hoarse voice and stridor which leads to a false diagnosis of respiratory allergy and asthma.

Autopsy may show anomalous venous return to the heart, midline position of the heart with patency of foramen ovale and ductus arteriosus, nonlobed lungs, bifid renal pelvis with double ureter, Meckel diverticulum or absence of gallbladder.

**Complications:** Aspiration, pneumonia, death. Respiratory insufficiency may occur in cases of unilateral pulmonary hypoplasia.

**Associated Findings:** Mild mental retardation in about 50% of cases. Agenesis of the corpus callosum and umbilical hernia were reported in one case.

**Etiology:** Autosomal dominant inheritance.

**Pathogenesis:** Primarily operates on midline organs and structures, and less effectively on paramedian structures.

**MIM No.:** *14541

**POS No.:** 3239

**Sex Ratio:** Severe dysphagia-hypospadias complex is confined to males, although some females may have more or less severe pulmonary manifestations.

**Occurrence:** At least 30 cases documented.

**Risk of Recurrence for Patient's Sib:**
See Part I, *Mendelian Inheritance.*

**Risk of Recurrence for Patient's Child:**
See Part I, *Mendelian Inheritance.*

**Age of Detectability:** Any age, including neonatal, by physical examination.

**Gene Mapping and Linkage:** Unknown.

**Prevention:** None known. Genetic counseling indicated.

**Treatment:** Any child suspected at birth of having the G syndrome should be fed only water; fluoroesophagraphy should be performed with a contrast medium least harmful to the lungs. If a swallowing defect is demonstrated, a feeding jejunostomy should be established immediately. If the patient survives to 1 year of age the esophagus can probably be reanastomosed. Supportive pediatric care should supplement surgical management. Hypospadias repair is indicated if the patient survives past infancy.

**Prognosis:** In cases of severe dysphagia, death is usually due to aspiration and inanition. In successfully treated cases prognosis for life, growth and reproduction is presumably normal, although some individuals may be mildly mentally retarded.

**Detection of Carrier:** Most heterozygotes appear to be relatively healthy persons; some have lifelong stridor. Any suspected carrier (close relative of proband and presence of stridor) should have a chest film to rule out pulmonary anomalies.

**Special Considerations:** Because of the overlap in phenotypic features, some investigators have suggested that this condition and **Hypertelorism-hypospadias syndrome** may be variants of the same disorder. Sedano and Gorlin (1988) proposed a joint name of *Opitz oculo-genito-laryngeal syndrome.*

*The author wishes to thank John M. Opitz for his contributions to an earlier draft of this article.*

**References:**
Cordero JF, Holmes LB: Phenotypic overlap of the BBB and G syndromes. Am J Med Genet 1978; 2:145–152.
Cappa M, et al.: The Opitz syndrome: a new designation for the clinically indistinguishable BBB and G syndromes. Am J Med Genet 1987; 28:303–309.
Opitz JM: G syndrome: perspective in 1987 and bibliography. Am J Med Genet 1987; 28:275–285.
Williams CA, Frias JL: Apparent G syndrome presenting as neck and upper limb dystonia and severe gastroesophageal reflux. Am J Med Genet 1987; 28:297–302.

Sedano HO, Gorlin RJ: Opitz oculo-genital-laryngeal syndrome. (Letter) Am J Med Genet 1988; 30:847–849.

GI005                                          **Enid F. Gilbert-Barnes**

## G(M1)-GANGLIOSIDOSIS, TYPE 1                              **0431**

**Includes:**

Beta-galactosidase-1 deficiency
Cerebral G(M1)-gangliosidosis
Gangliosidosis, type 1 (generalized)
Neurovisceral lipidosis, familial
Pseudo-Hurler disease
Tay-Sachs with visceral involvement

**Excludes:**

**Fucosidosis** (0398)
**G(M1)-gangliosidosis, type 2** (0432)
**G(M1)-gangliosidosis, type 3** (3215)
**G(M2)-gangliosidosis with hexosaminidase A deficiency** (0434)
**Metachromatic leukodystrophies** (0651)
**Mucolipidosis**
**Mucopolysaccharidosis**
**Niemann-Pick disease** (0717)

**Major Diagnostic Criteria:** This diagnosis should be considered in a retarded infant with visceromegaly, skeletal changes similar to those found in **Mucopolysaccharidosis I-H**, and unusual facies. Further support would be given by the vacuolized lymphocytes and marrow cells, and renal biopsy if available. Urinary mucopolysaccharide levels are normal. Diagnosis rests with demonstration of the $G_{M1}$-ganglioside increase in brain and ganglioside and oligosaccharide increases in the viscera and in urine, plus the deficiency of $\beta$-galactosidase activity in brain, liver, cultured skin fibroblasts, or leukocytes.

**Clinical Findings:** Early and severe retardation of mental and motor development occurs in infancy with unusual facial appearance; flat nose, full forehead and the impression of wide-spaced eyes. Characteristic changes in the long bones by X-ray include first periosteal cloaking, then architectural modifications similar to those in Hurler disease, hypoplasia or beaking of the vertebral bodies. Enlargement of the liver and, less notably, the spleen, gingival hyperplasia, generalized edema, glomerular epithelial cytoplasmic vacuolization, foam cells in the marrow, and vacuolization of circulating lymphocytes are other findings. A cherry-red macula is seen in half of those affected. All have increased $G_{M1}$-ganglioside in brain and viscera, and deficient $\beta$-galactosidase in tissues and body fluids.

**Complications:** Growth and nutritional failure, progressive neurologic derangement, recurrent infection and seizures. Bronchopneumonia is a common complication and may be the immediate cause of death.

**Associated Findings:** Cataracts have been found in one patient.

**Etiology:** Autosomal recessive inheritance. The fundamental defect is felt to be a deficiency of lysosomal $\beta$-galactosidase in the brain and other organs.

**Pathogenesis:** $\beta$-galactosidase is known to be involved in the cleavage of galactose from ganglioside, galactose-containing mucopolysaccharides, and glycoproteins. Hence, a deficiency of this enzyme would constitute a reasonable basis for accumulation of these substrates in the tissue. It is probable that the neuronal gangliosidosis is responsible for the cumulative cerebral handicaps, the skeletal oligosaccharidosis is the setting for the bony deformities, and both elements contribute to the visceral histiocytosis with organomegaly.

**MIM No.:** *23050

**POS No.:** 3242

**CDC No.:** 330.100

**Sex Ratio:** M1:F1

**Occurrence:** More than 50 cases have been documented, but many others undoubtedly exist in unclassified categories in other studies. No increased frequency has been identified with any particular ethnic group, except for a suspicion of increased frequency on Malta.

**Risk of Recurrence for Patient's Sib:**
See Part I, *Mendelian Inheritance.*

**Risk of Recurrence for Patient's Child:** Affected individuals are not expected to survive to reproduce.

**Age of Detectability:** Prenatal diagnosis is possible; cultured amniotic fluid cells show absent $\beta$-galactosidase activity and also cytoplasmic vacuoles with phase-contrast microscopy. Biochemical diagnosis can be accomplished at birth, but clinical evidence is generally not present until early infancy.

**Gene Mapping and Linkage:** GLB1 (galactosidase, beta 1) has been mapped to 3pter-p21.

**Prevention:** None known. Genetic counseling indicated.

**Treatment:** The supportive treatment would be that for any of the debilitating, brain-handicapping sphingolipidosis disorders.

**Prognosis:** Most affected individuals do not survive beyond two years of age, although some have lived to age four.

**Detection of Carrier:** Identification of heterozygously involved individuals is possible by assay of $\beta$-galactosidase activity in leukocytes and cultured fibroblasts from skin biopsy.

**Special Considerations:** Critical progress has been made in the establishment of the phenotypic classification for unusual children formerly viewed as "atypically" involved in inborn error syndromes as discussed above and in the articles listed in the *Excludes* above. Definitive decisions dependent on careful analysis of tissue glycolipids and polysaccharides, plus enzyme assays. $\beta$-galactosidase abnormalities are common to several of these diseases, but thus far the deficiency has been most extreme in generalized gangliosidosis.

**References:**

Okada S, O'Brien JS: Generalized gangliosidosis: beta-galactosidase deficiency. Science 1968; 160:1002–1004.
Warner TGW, et al.: Diagnosis of $Gm_1$ gangliosidosis based on detection of urinary oligosaccharides with high performance liquid chromatography. Clin Chim Acta 1983; 127:313.
Giughiani R, et al.: GM(1) gangliosidosis: clinical and laboratory findings in eight families. Hum Genet 1985; 70:347–359.
Hoogeveen AT, et al.: GM1-gangliosidosis: defective recognition site on beta-galactosidase precursor. J Biol Chem 1986; 261:5702–5704.
O'Brien JS: Beta-galactosidase deficiency. In: Scriver CR, et al, eds: The metabolic basis of inherited disease, 6th ed. New York: McGraw-Hill, 1989:1797–1806.

0B001                                                  **John S. O'Brien**

## G(M1)-GANGLIOSIDOSIS, TYPE 2                              **0432**

**Includes:**

Gangliosidosis, generalized juvenile type
G(M1)-gangliosidosis, juvenile type
G(M1)-gangliosidosis of late onset without bony deformities
Lipidosis, late infantile systemic

**Excludes:**

**G(M1)-gangliosidosis, type 1** (0431)
**G(M1)-gangliosidosis, type 3** (3215)
Lipidosis, juvenile
Late infantile amaurotic idiocy (Jansky-Bielschowsky disease)
**Neuronal ceroid-lipofuscinoses (NCL)** (0713)
Sphingolipidoses (other)

**Major Diagnostic Criteria:** Clinical findings include spasticity and ataxia late in the first year of life, with progressive neurologic deterioration. Identification of marrow foam cells or neuronal lipidosis is helpful. Diagnosis depends on demonstration of increased $G_{M1}$-ganglioside in the brain and deficient $\beta$-galactosidase in tissues, leukocytes, or urine.

**Clinical Findings:** Affected children may have mental and motor retardation by 6–12 months of age, with progressive spasticity, ataxia, weakness, and then rigidity, seizures, and dementia. They die by 3 to 10 years of age (rarely later). The fundi are generally normal and the viscera are not enlarged. Foam cells are often found in the marrow, but the bones are normal or mildly dysplastic by X-ray, as is the face. Vacuolated cells in the liver, spleen, and glomeruli are notable in some of the patients, and lipidosis of the central and autonomic nervous system neurons is general. As in the generalized gangliosidosis syndrome, $G_{M1}$-ganglioside accumulates in the brain and oligosaccharides in the liver. β-galactosidase activity is deficient in the brain, liver, leukocytes, and cultured fibroblasts. Urinary oligosaccharides are elevated.

**Complications:** Seizures that may be difficult to manage and recurrent infections, particularly bronchopneumonia.

**Associated Findings:** None known.

**Etiology:** Autosomal recessive inheritance. The basic defect is β-galactosidase deficiency. Analysis of total enzyme, and its electrophoretic components, has not to date allowed any specific differentiation from the β-galactosidase deficiency of $G_{M1}$-gangliosidosis, type 1.

**Pathogenesis:** The enzyme deficiency presumably accounts for the neuronal handicap, which, in turn, lies behind the neurologic deterioration. The visceral changes are moderate but of the same basic origin.

**MIM No.:** 23060

**POS No.:** 3242

**CDC No.:** 330.100

**Sex Ratio:** M1:F1

**Occurrence:** More than 20 patients identified to date, with no special predilection in any particular ethnic group.

**Risk of Recurrence for Patient's Sib:**
See Part I, *Mendelian Inheritance.*

**Risk of Recurrence for Patient's Child:** Affected individuals are not expected to survive to reproduce.

**Age of Detectability:** The enzyme defect is identifiable in cultured fetal cells from amniocentesis or in the infant at any time after birth.

**Gene Mapping and Linkage:** Unknown.

**Prevention:** None known. Genetic counseling indicated.

**Treatment:** Supportive medical treatment as needed. Assistance to the family in the dilemma of a child with degenerative CNS disease.

**Prognosis:** Most patients die in early or middle childhood, but survival has been noted up to 20 years.

**Detection of Carrier:** Unknown. β-galactosidase assay of the circulating leukocytes has been abnormal in the parents of involved children.

**Special Considerations:** Children with this disease bear considerable resemblance to the clinical picture of so-called "late infantile amaurotic idiocy" (Jansky-Bielschowsky), although marrow foam cells are lacking and macular pigmentation is prominent in the latter condition. It is possible that some patients with $G_{M1}$-gangliosidosis, type 2, have been listed in earlier reports as examples of Jansky-Bielschowsky disease. The definitive examination obviously involves the enzyme assay.

**References:**

Derry DM, et al.: Late infantile systemic lipidosis (major monosialo-gangliosidosis delineation of two types). Neurology 1968; 18:340–347.

Suzuki K, et al.: Morphological, histochemical and biochemical studies on a case of systemic late infantile lipidosis (generalized gangliosidosis). J Neuropathol Exp Neurol 1968; 27:15.

O'Brien JS: Generalized gangliosidosis. BD:OAS;V(4). New York: The National Foundation-March of Dimes, 1969:190.

Wolfe LS, et al.: GM1-gangliosidosis without chondrodystrophy or visceromegaly. Neurology 1970; 20:23–43.

Booth CW, et al.: Intrauterine detection of Gm₁ gangliosidosis, type 2. Pediatrics 1973; 52:521.

Wenger DA, et al.: Adult GM1 gangliosidosis. Clin Genet 1980; 17:323–334.

Warner TGW, et al.: Diagnosis of G(M1)-gangliosidosis based on detection of urinary oligosaccharides with high performance liquid chromatography. Clin Chim Acta 1983; 127:313.

O'Brien JS: Beta-galactosidase deficiency. In: Scriver CR, et al, eds: The metabolic basis of inherited disease, 6th ed. New York: McGraw-Hill, 1989:1797–1806.

0B001

**John S. O'Brien**

## G(M1)-GANGLIOSIDOSIS, TYPE 3      3215

**Includes:** Gangliosidosis, generalized GM(1), adult type

**Excludes:**
**G(M1)-gangliosidosis, type 1** (0431)
**G(M1)-gangliosidosis, type 2** (0432)
**G(M2)-gangliosidosis with hexosaminidase A deficiency** (0434)

**Major Diagnostic Criteria:** Progressive cerebellar dysarthria and ataxia beginning in the juvenile period (teenage to 20+ years). Intellectual impairment is mild, but with time loss of intellectual function is evident. Seizures are uncommon, and vision remains unimpaired. Beta-galactosidase is deficient in all tissues.

**Clinical Findings:** Onset during the teenage to 20+ years period. Mental-motor retardation is present. Facial appearance is normal. Mild X-ray changes in long bones and vertebrae. Vacuolated lymphocytes and foam cells in the marrow are often present. Hepatomegaly, splenomegaly, cherry-red spot, **Retinitis pigmentosa**, startle response, **Microcephaly**, and macroglossia are *not* present. Neuronal lipidosis is evident, with mild visceral histiocytosis.

**Complications:** Unknown.

**Associated Findings:** None known.

**Etiology:** Autosomal recessive inheritance. Beta-galactosidase is deficient in all tissues.

**Pathogenesis:** Beta-galactosidase is known to be involved in the cleavage of galactose from ganglioside, galactose-containing mucopolysaccharides, and glycoproteins. Hence, a deficiency of this enzyme would constitute a reasonable basis for accumulation of these substrates in the tissues. It is probable that the neuronal gangliosidosis is responsible for the cumulative cerebral handicaps, the skeletal oligosaccharidosis is the setting for the bony deformities, and both elements contribute to the visceral histocytosis.

**MIM No.:** 23065

**Sex Ratio:** M1:F1

**Occurrence:** About 25 cases have been documented.

**Risk of Recurrence for Patient's Sib:**
See Part I, *Mendelian Inheritance.*

**Risk of Recurrence for Patient's Child:**
See Part I, *Mendelian Inheritance.*

**Age of Detectability:** In the teenage period and 20+ years. Biochemical diagnosis can be accomplished at birth, but clinical evidence is not present until adulthood.

**Gene Mapping and Linkage:** GLB1 (galactosidase, beta 1) has been mapped to 3p21-cen.

**Prevention:** None known. Genetic counseling indicated.

**Treatment:** The supportive treatment would be that for any of the debilitating, brain-handicapping sphingolipid disorders.

**Prognosis:** Decades of survival are possible after diagnosis.

**Detection of Carrier:** Identification of heterozygous individuals is possible by assay of beta-galactosidase activity in leukocytes and cultured fibroblasts from skin biopsy.

**References:**
Wenger DA, et al.: Adult GM1 gangliosidosis. Clin Genet 1980; 17:323–334.
Nakano T, et al.: Adult GM1-gangliosidosis-Clinical patterns and rectal biopsy. Neurology 1985; 35:815–880.
Ushiyama M, et al.: Type III (Chronic) GM1-gangliosidosis: histochemical and ultrastructural studies of rectal biopsy. J Neurol Sci 1985; 71:209–223.
Ikeda S, et al.: Ultrastructural findings of rectal and skin biopsies in adult GM1 gangliosidosis. Acta Pathol Jpn 1986; 36:1823–1831.

OB001                                                      **John S. O'Brien**

## GALACTOSIALIDOSIS                                              3110

**Includes:**
> Cherry-red spot-myoclonus with dementia
> G(M1)-gangliosidosis, type 4
> Goldberg syndrome
> Neuraminidase/beta-galactosidase expression
> Neuraminidase deficiency with beta-galactosidase deficiency
> Sialidosis type II, juvenile-onset form

**Excludes:**
> **G(M1)-gangliosidosis** (other)
> **Mucolipidosis**
> Sialidosis (other)

**Major Diagnostic Criteria:** Galactosialidosis is distinguished from primary, isolated deficiencies of either neuraminidase (sialidase) or beta-galactosidase by virtue of the fact that this disorder has a combined deficiency of both beta-galactosidase and neuraminidase in fibroblasts and leukocytes. Other lysosomal enzymes are normal. Affected patients have vacuoles in the hepatic parenchymal cells, bone marrow, and peripheral lymphocytes. Urinary sialyloligosaccharides are elevated without mucopolysacchariduria.

**Clinical Findings:** At least three clinical forms of this disease have been described. In the *early-infantile type*, the patients present at or soon after birth with severe edema, ascites, skeletal dysplasia, and ocular abnormalities. In the *late-infantile form*, the symptoms become apparent after age 6–12 months and consist of skeletal dysplasia, visceromegaly, macular cherry-red spots, and mental retardation. In the *juvenile/adult galactosialidosis form*, skeletal dysplasia, dysmorphic features, corneal clouding, cherry-red spots, and mental retardation become apparent sometime between childhood and adulthood. On clinical grounds it may be difficult to distinguish many galactosialidosis patients from sialidosis patients who also lack neuraminidase activity but have normal levels of beta-galactosidase activity.

**Complications:** Similar to other lysosomal disorders of glycoprotein and mucopolysaccharide metabolism. These may include mental retardation, nephrotic syndrome, growth disturbances, joint stiffness, and coarse features.

**Associated Findings:** Possibly recurrent respiratory infections and hearing loss.

**Etiology:** Autosomal recessive inheritance. The various forms of galactosialidosis are grouped together by virtue of the fact that all have a severe reduction in the intracellular levels of both neuraminidase and galactosidase. The combined deficiencies of these two lysosomal enzymes result from a lack of a "protective" glycoprotein required to stabilize the aggregation of the subunits of galactosidase and its complex with neuraminidase. Additionally, recent evidence indicates that the different clinical forms are the result of differences in either the amount or the degree of conversion of a 52-kd precursor to the final 32-kd glycoprotein. Thus, in the early infantile form there is a marked decrease in both the 52-kd precursor and the 32-kd product, whereas in the juvenile form there is relatively more of the 52-kd precursor but no 32-kd product.

**Pathogenesis:** Both neuroaminidase and galactosidase are lysosomal enzymes involved in the degradation of glycoproteins and sometimes gangliosides. There is a decreased ability of affected cells to degrade these natural substrates, which, in turn, results in the biochemical and clinical manifestations of the type usually associated with lysosomal storage diseases. Specifically, there is lysosomal storage of the undegraded substrates, clinical manifestations of abnormal storage, and a progressive, declining clinical course.

**MIM No.:**  *25654

**Sex Ratio:**  M1:F1

**Occurrence:** Undetermined but presumably rare. The juvenile form, which appears to be the most common, has been found mainly in patients of Japanese ancestry. Other forms do not appear to have a predilection in any particular ethnic group.

**Risk of Recurrence for Patient's Sib:**
See Part I, *Mendelian Inheritance.*

**Risk of Recurrence for Patient's Child:**
See Part I, *Mendelian Inheritance.*

**Age of Detectability:** The age of usual clinical diagnosis is dependent in part on the clinical form of the disease, i.e., the early-infantile patients showing gross abnormalities at or very shortly after birth whereas the juvenile/adult form can present over a wide age between infancy and adulthood. The enzyme alterations can be demonstrated at any age in all forms of the disease. Prenatal diagnosis has been carried out in at least the early-infantile form of the disease.

**Gene Mapping and Linkage:** GSL (galactosialidosis) has been provisionally mapped to 20.
Mueller et al. (1986) have presented evidence that the mutation in one patient with the early-infantile form of galactosialidosis was caused by a gene located on human chromosome 20. It is to be noted, however, that the 32-kd "protective protein," believed to be defective in at least some patients with this disorder, has been shown to be encoded on chromosome 22. The relationship of these findings is unclear at the present time.

**Prevention:** None known. Genetic counseling indicated.

**Treatment:** Unknown.

**Prognosis:** Dependent on the form of the disorder, i.e., early-infantile being the most severe, resulting in an early death, whereas the juvenile/adult form is characterized by a long period (sometimes 20 to 30 years) of normality before the appearance of clinical manifestations.

**Detection of Carrier:** As the beta-galactosidase and neuraminidase abnormalities in affected patients are secondary to a defect in a "protective protein," it may be difficult to identify carriers of this disorder. Obligate galactosialidosis heterozygotes have not been shown consistently to have reductions in either beta-galactosidase or neuraminidase levels.

**References:**
d'Azzo A, et al.: Molecular defect in combined beta-galactosidase and neuraminidase deficiency in man. Proc Natl Acad Sci USA 1982; 79:4535–4539.
Sakuraba H, et al.: Galactosidase-neuraminidase deficiency (galactosialidosis): clinical, pathological, and enzymatic studies in a postmortem case. Ann Neurol 1983; 13:497–503.
Loonen MCB, et al.: Combined sialidase (neuraminidase) and beta-galactosidase deficiency: clinical, morphological and enzymological observations in a patient. Clin Genet 1984; 26:139–149.
Verheijen FW, et al.: Human placental neuraminidase activation, stabilization and association with galactosidase and its "protective" protein. Eur J Biochem 1985; 149:315–321.
Mueller OT, et al.: Sialidosis and galactosialidosis: chromosomal assignment of two genes associated with neuraminidase-deficiency disorders. Proc Natl Acad Sci USA 1986; 83:1817–1821.
Palmeri S, et al.: Galactosialidosis: Molecular heterogeneity among distinct clinical phenotypes. Am J Hum Genet 1986; 38:137–148.
Takeda E, et al.: Involvement of thiol proteases in galactosialidosis. Clin Chim Acta 1986; 155:109–116.
Willemsen R, et al.: Immunoelectron microscopical localization of lysosomal β-galactosidase and its precursor forms in normal and mutant human fibroblasts. Eur J Cell Biol 1986; 40:9–15.
Nanba E, et al.: Galactosialidosis: a direct evidence that a 46-kilodalton

protein restores deficient enzyme activities in fibroblasts. Biochem Biophys Res Commun 1987; 144:138–142.

TH021                                                    George H. Thomas

### G(M1)-gangliosidosis of late onset without bony deformities
See G(M1)-GANGLIOSIDOSIS, TYPE 2
### G(M1)-gangliosidosis, juvenile type
See G(M1)-GANGLIOSIDOSIS, TYPE 2

---

## G(M2)-GANGLIOSIDOSIS WITH HEXOSAMINIDASE A AND B DEFICIENCY                                      0433

**Includes:**
G(M2)-gangliosidosis, variant zero
Sandhoff disease
Systemic G(M2)-gangliosidosis

**Excludes:**
G(M1)-gangliosidosis, type 1 (0431)
G(M1)-gangliosidosis, type 2 (0432)
G(M2)-gangliosidosis with hexosaminidase A deficiency (0434)
Neuronal ceroid-lipofuscinoses (NCL) (0713)

**Major Diagnostic Criteria:** Findings typical of Tay-Sachs disease (see **G(M2)-gangliosidosis with hexosaminidase A deficiency**) plus signs of systemic lipid storage such as foam cells within bone marrow. Both major forms of hexosaminidase, A and B, are deficient from serum and tissue.

**Clinical Findings:** By six months of age, psychomotor retardation; cherry-red macula, hypotonia, and exaggerated startle response are evident. The child fails to attain normal milestones, and by age 12–15 months develops seizures, blindness, loss of contact with the environment, and finally spastic tetraparesis. Occasionally, there is hepatosplenomegaly. Death results by age 2–3 years.

**Complications:** Relentlessly progressive and ultimately fatal disease with death from pneumonitis or septicemia.

**Associated Findings:** None known.

**Etiology:** Autosomal recessive inheritance.

**Pathogenesis:** Defective synthesis of the B chain of hexosaminidase, leading to deficiency of both hexosaminidase A, which is necessary for $G_{M2}$-ganglioside hydrolysis, and of hexosaminidase B which is needed for degradation of globoside. Nerve cells throughout the body progressively enlarge due to the accumulation of $G_{M2}$-ganglioside (Tay-Sachs ganglioside). Eventually, these cells and their axons undergo dissolution, and are replaced by glial tissue. Simultaniously, there is progressive accumulation of globoside within many of the visceral tissues. This neutral glycolipid is a normal component of many cell membranes including the erythrocyte, and in this disease accumulates in vascular endothelium and cells of the reticuloendothelial system. Both $G_{M2}$-ganglioside and globoside have an amino sugar (hexosamine) as the terminal sugar.

**MIM No.:** *26880

**POS No.:** 3244

**CDC No.:** 330.100

**Sex Ratio:** M1:F1

**Occurrence:** The gene frequency is thought to be about 1:500 in Jews and 1:278 in non-Jews, although no cases have been reported in Jewish children.

**Risk of Recurrence for Patient's Sib:**
See Part I, *Mendelian Inheritance*.

**Risk of Recurrence for Patient's Child:** Affected individuals are not expected to survive to reproduce.

**Age of Detectability:** Prenatally by amniocentesis or as early as clinically suspected.

**Gene Mapping and Linkage:** HEXB (hexosaminidase B (beta polypeptide)) has been mapped to 5q13.

**Prevention:** None known. Genetic counseling indicated.

**Treatment:** Unknown.

**Prognosis:** Progression to death.

**Detection of Carrier:** Enzyme determination of serum, white blood cells, or skin fibroblasts.

**Special Considerations:** Where the clinical presentation contains features of classic Tay-Sachs disease plus visceromegaly, this variant must be considered.

**References:**
Sandhoff K, et al.: Deficient hexosaminidase activity in an exceptional case of Tay-Sachs disease with additional storage of kidney globoside in visceral organs. Life Sciences 1968; 7:283–288.
O'Dowd BF, et al.: Molecular heterogeneity in the infantile and juvenile forms of Sandhoff disease (0-variant G(M2) gangliosidosis). J Biol Chem 1986; 261:12680–12685.
Bolhuis PA, et al.: Ganglioside storage, hexosaminidase lability, and urinary oligosaccharides in adult Sandhoff's disease. Neurology 1987; 37:75–81.
Cantor RM, et al.: Sandhoff disease heterozygote detection: a component of population screening for Tay-Sachs disease carriers. II: Sandhoff disease gene frequencies in American Jewish and non-Jewish populations. Am J Hum Genet 1987; 41:16–26.

K0010                                                  Edwin H. Kolodny

---

## G(M2)-GANGLIOSIDOSIS WITH HEXOSAMINIDASE A DEFICIENCY                                             0434

**Includes:**
G(M2)-gangliosidosis, type I
G(M2)-gangliosidosis, variant AB
G(M2)-gangliosidosis, variant B
Hexosaminidase A deficiency
Hexosaminidase activator deficiency
Tay-Sachs disease

**Excludes:**
Ceroidlipofuscinoses
Gaucher disease (0406)
G(M1)-gangliosidosis
G(M2)-gangliosidosis with hexosaminidase A and B deficiency (0433)
Leukodystrophy, adult onset progressive dominant type (2975)
Leukodystrophy, globoid cell type (0415)

**Major Diagnostic Criteria:** A physically normal appearance, psychomotor delay, increased startle response, and cherry red macula within the first year of life strongly suggests a neuronal storage disease. This disease is most common among Ashkenazi Jews. The diagnosis is confirmed by demonstrating a deficiency of hexosaminidase A in serum or tissues. The term Tay-Sachs disease is restricted to the infantile form of $G_{M2}$-gangliosidosis with hexosaminidase A deficiency.

**Clinical Findings:** The clinical picture is characterized by visual inattention and developmental retardation beginning within the first six months of life. Other early signs are hypotonia and poor head control. The child fails to turn over and sit, and becomes apathetic and unresponsive to exogenous stimuli. Only rarely may a child reach the stage of early crawling.

Blindness is noted toward the latter part of the first year, and a white halo is observed in the macula region of the eye, accentuating the normal red color of the fovea. There is often a dissociation between the child's responses to auditory stimuli, which may be exaggerated, and his response to visual stimuli. The exaggerated response to sound may initially look like a Moro reflex but can be an exaggerated jerk of the arms and legs to any sound stimulus.

Seizures are a later manifestation which may be quite refractory to any convulsant medication. EEG abnormalities appear toward the end of the 1st year of life and will develop into paroxysmal discharges which decrease as the child reaches a more advanced form of the disease.

As the disease progresses the child reaches a vegetative state, being quite hypertonic with exaggerated reflexes. The exaggerated response to sound diminishes and the child often develops megalencephaly. Death usually occurs by age two but a few children have lived to age three or four.

**Complications:** The disease is relentlessly progressive and ultimately fatal. Death is usually associated with aspiration pneumonia.

**Associated Findings:** None known.

**Etiology:** Autosomal recessive inheritance, with a high gene frequency in Ashkenazi Jews.

**Pathogenesis:** Failure of the degradation of $G_{M2}$-ganglioside. The enzymatic defect is the deficiency of hexosaminidase A, resulting from an absence of or defective synthesis of the $\alpha$-chain of this enzyme. $G_{M2}$-gangliosidosis is due to a failure of degradation of $G_{M2}$-ganglioside and a subsequent storage of this ganglioside in neurons throughout the body. The neuronal cell body is ballooned out by the accumulated ganglioside and other lipids complexed to it. These accumulations form membranous cytoplasmic bodies that are distinguished under the electron microscope by the appearance of multiple membrane-bound concentrically laminated structures. Eventually the neurons die and are replaced by gliosis. Some neurons, such as granular cells of the cerebellum, degenerate quite early in the course of the disease.

There is no appreciable accumulation of ganglioside in other organs. However, the metabolic defect is present in all tissues. The disease can be diagnosed in utero by demonstration of the enzymatic defect in amniotic cells as well as at birth from examination of serum or skin fibroblasts.

**MIM No.:** *27275, *27280

**POS No.:** 3244

**CDC No.:** 330.100

**Sex Ratio:** M1:F1

**Occurrence:** For Ashkenazi Jewish families, the theoretical incidence is 1:3,800 live births. The gene frequency in Ashkenazi families is 1:37. Occurrence is also fairly high among French-Canadians. The carrier rate for non-Jews is approximately 1:300, and is probably even lower for Sephardic Jews. Carrier screening programs and prenatal diagnosis have reduced the incidence of Tay-Sachs among Ashkenazi Jews. Prevalence is very low because of early death.

**Risk of Recurrence for Patient's Sib:**
See Part I, *Mendelian Inheritance.*

**Risk of Recurrence for Patient's Child:** Affected individuals are not expected to survive to reproduce.

**Age of Detectability:** By clinical examination at four to six months. Prenatal diagnosis is available.

**Gene Mapping and Linkage:** GM2A (GM2 ganglioside activator protein) has been provisionally mapped to 5.
HEXA (hexosaminidase A (alpha polypeptide)) has been mapped to 15q23-q24.

**Prevention:** None known. Genetic counseling indicated.

**Treatment:** There is no proven therapy at present.

**Prognosis:** The disease is progressive and death occurs by three to four years of age.

**Detection of Carrier:** The heterozygote can be detected by enzymatic assay of serum leukocytes or cultured skin fibroblasts. Carriers usually have 40–60% of the activity of control patients.

**Special Considerations:** Sandhoff referred to **G(M2)-gangliosidosis with hexosaminidase A and B deficiency** as variant 0 (since both hexosaminidase A and B are missing), and to classic Tay-Sachs as variant B (since hexosaminidase A is absent), but also identified a variant AB, in which both hexosaminidase A and B are increased. At least two variants of this rare condition, involving the ganglioside GM2 activator protein, have been documented (Li Y-T et al, 1983; Ohno and Suzuki, 1988).

**Support Groups:**
NY; Cedarhurst; National Tay-Sachs Parent Peer Group
MA; Newton; The National Tay-Sachs and Allied Diseases Association (NTSAD)

ENGLAND: Essex; Ilford; Tay-Sachs and Allied Diseases Association
SOUTH AFRICA: Lyndhurst; Tay-Sachs Association of South Africa

**References:**
O'Brien JS, et al.: Tay-Sachs disease. Detection of heterozygotes and homozygotes by serum hexosaminidase assay. New Engl J Med 1970; 283:15–20.
Kolodny EH: Tay-Sachs disease. In: Goodman RM, Motvlsky AG, eds: Genetic diseases among Ashkenazi Jews. New York: Raven Press, 1979:217.
Li Y-T, et al.: Differentiation of two variants of type-AB Gm-2-gangliosidosis using chromogenic substrates. Am J Hum Genet 1983; 35:520–522.
Myerowitz R, Hogikyan ND: Different mutations in Ashkenazi Jewish and non-Jewish French Canadians with Tay-Sachs disease. Science 1986; 232:1646–1648.
Bayleran J, et al.: Tay-Sachs disease with hexosaminidase A: characterization of the defective enzyme in two patients. Am J Hum Genet 1987; 41:532–548.
Myerowitz R, Costigan FC: The major defect in Ashkenazi Jews with Tay-Sachs disease is an insertion in the gene for the $\alpha$-chain of $\beta$-hexosaminidase. J Biol Chem 1988; 263:18587–18589.
Ohno K, Suzuki K: Mutation in G(M2)-gangliosidosis B₁ variant. J Neurochem 1988; 50:316–318.

K0010                                    **Edwin H. Kolodny**

**G(M2)-gangliosidosis, type I**
*See G(M2)-GANGLIOSIDOSIS WITH HEXOSAMINIDASE A DEFICIENCY*
**G(M2)-gangliosidosis, variant AB**
*See G(M2)-GANGLIOSIDOSIS WITH HEXOSAMINIDASE A DEFICIENCY*
**G(M2)-gangliosidosis, variant B**
*See G(M2)-GANGLIOSIDOSIS WITH HEXOSAMINIDASE A DEFICIENCY*
**G(M2)-gangliosidosis, variant zero**
*See G(M2)-GANGLIOSIDOSIS WITH HEXOSAMINIDASE A AND B DEFICIENCY*
**G6PD deficiency**
*See GLUCOSE-6-PHOSPHATE DEHYDROGENASE DEFICIENCY*
**GABA metabolic defect**
*See ACIDEMIA, GAMMA-HYDROXYBUTYRIC*
**GABA transaminase deficiency**
*See GAMMA-AMINOBUTYRIC ACID (GABA) TRANSAMINASE DEFICIENCY*

---

**GALACTOKINASE DEFICIENCY**                        **0402**

**Includes:**
Cataracts, due to galactokinase deficiency
Galactosemia II
GALK (Galactokinase deficiency)

**Excludes: Galactosemia (0403)**

**Major Diagnostic Criteria:** Cataracts occur in early infancy. Laboratory findings include hypergalactosemia, hypergalactosuria, and a normal blood spot test for galactose-l-phosphate uridyltransferase. Absence of erythrocyte galactokinase confirms the diagnosis.

**Clinical Findings:** Nuclear and/or zonular cataracts in early infancy, hypergalactosemia, and galactose-galactitol-glucose diabetes. Mental development is normal.

**Complications:** Nuclear and/or zonular cataracts. A peculiar type of polyneuropathy observed in an adult patient who refused treatment may represent a complication of untreated galactokinase deficiency of long standing.

**Associated Findings:** Pseudotumor cerebri and mental retardation have been reported, but a causal relationship to the biochemical defect remains to be established. An association of partial galactokinase deficiency and presenile cataracts has been reported, but in other studies the presumed higher prevalence of heterozygosity for galactokinase deficiency in patients with presenile cataracts was not found.

**Etiology:** Autosomal recessive inheritance. An allele coding for a variant (Philadelphia) galactokinase seems prevalent in American Blacks. Another variant has been reported in Italy. Transient galactokinase deficiency has been described in one infant.

**Pathogenesis:** Inability to metabolize galactose normally with resulting accumulation of galactitol in the intra- and extra-cellular fluids. Galactitol accumulation in the lens causes osmotic swelling, electrolyte imbalance, protein denaturation, and thus the formation of "sugar" cataract. Cultured fibroblasts and lymphoblasts have been found deficient in thymidine kinase activity.

**MIM No.:** *23020

**Sex Ratio:** Presumably M1:F1

**Occurrence:** Estimated 1:100,000 or less live births in Europe. Prevalence higher in countries of Southeastern Europe.

**Risk of Recurrence for Patient's Sib:**
See Part I, *Mendelian Inheritance.*

**Risk of Recurrence for Patient's Child:**
See Part I, *Mendelian Inheritance.*

**Age of Detectability:** Prenatal diagnosis is available. Newborns who are fed milk have hypergalactosemia, which can be discovered in the routine newborn screening program (microbiologic or enzymatic assay of galactose in dried blood spots), and galactosuria (testing for reducing substances in urine).

**Gene Mapping and Linkage:** GALK (galactokinase) has been mapped to 17q21-q22 or 17q23-q25.

**Prevention:** Early detection through mass screening of newborns for elevated blood galactose is possible, and immediate dietary treatment will prevent cataracts. Genetic counseling is indicated.

**Treatment:** Exclusion of milk, milk products, and all other sources of galactose and lactose from the diet. Cataracts cause severe visual handicap and those not responding to dietary treatment are removed surgically. Diet should be established prior to cataract operation as it may help in the prevention of recurring cataracts.

**Prognosis:** If treatment is begun early after birth and maintained for life, cataract formation is prevented. Early cataracts are reversible under galactose exclusion diet. Recurring cataracts may require discission. Life expectancy is normal, but may be impacted by the risks of amblyopia or blindness due to cataracts.

**Detection of Carrier:** Erythrocyte galactokinase approximately 50% of normal.

**References:**

Gitzelmann R: Hereditary galactokinase deficiency: a newly recognized cause of juvenile cataracts. Pediatr Res 1967; 1:14–23.

Gitzelmann R, Hansen RG: Galactose metabolism, hereditary defects and their clinical significance. In: Burman D, et al., eds: Inherited disorders of carbohydrate metabolism. Lancaster: MTP Press, 1980: 163–190.

Magnani M, et al.: A new variant of galactokinase. Hum Hered 1982; 32:329–334.

Magnani M, et al.: Red blood cell galactokinase activity and presenile cataracts. Enzyme 1983; 29:58–60.

Schoen RC, et al.: Thymidine-kinase activity of cultured cells from individuals with inherited galactokinase deficiency. Am J Hum Genet 1984; 36:815–822.

Soni T, et al.: Screening of a Philadelphia variant of galactokinase in racially unmixed black Africans. Am J Hum Genet 1988; 42:96–103.

Segal S: Disorders of galactose metabolism. In: Scriver C, et al., eds: The metabolic basis of inherited disease. New York: McGraw-Hill, 1989. *

GI013                                    **Richard Gitzelmann**

**Galactosamine-6-sulfatase deficiency**
*See MUCOPOLYSACCHARIDOSIS IV*

## GALACTOSE EPIMERASE DEFICIENCY                0357

**Includes:**
Epimerase deficiency, galactose (GALE)
UDP-galactose-epimerase deficiency
Uridine diphosphate galactose 4'-epimerase deficiency

**Excludes:**
**Galactokinase deficiency** (0402)
**Galactosemia** (0403)

**Major Diagnostic Criteria:** Absence or severe deficiency of epimerase from blood cells, a moderate increase of erythrocyte galactose-1-phosphate, and a normal blood spot test for galactose-1-phosphate uridyltransferase.

**Clinical Findings:** None in 12 individuals known to be affected by the mild form. In one infant with the severe form, jaundice, vomiting, failure to thrive, hepatomegaly, hypergalactosuria, and generalized hyperaminoaciduria were observed.

**Complications:** In the severe form, impairment of psychomotor development.

**Associated Findings:** None known.

**Etiology:** Autosomal recessive inheritance.

**Pathogenesis:** In the severe form, the patient is a galactose auxotroph, unable to synthesize galactose from glucose. Dietary galactose in excess of actual biosynthetic needs causes the accumulation of UDP-galactose and galactose-1-phosphate. The latter compound is a presumptive toxic metabolite in galactosemia. When the amount of ingested galactose does not meet biosynthetic needs, synthesis of galactosylated compounds such as galactoproteins and galactolipids is impaired.

**MIM No.:** *23035

**Sex Ratio:** M6:F7 (observed)

**Occurrence:** Undetermined. Cases reported from Switzerland, Japan, and Great Britain.

**Risk of Recurrence for Patient's Sib:**
See Part I, *Mendelian Inheritance.*

**Risk of Recurrence for Patient's Child:**
See Part I, *Mendelian Inheritance.*

**Age of Detectability:** Prenatal diagnosis is possible. Newborns who are fed milk have high levels of red blood cell galactose-1-phosphate; they may be discovered by screening tests for galactose or epimerase in blood spotted on filter paper.

**Gene Mapping and Linkage:** GALE (UDP-galactose-4-epimerase) has been mapped to 1p36-p35.

**Prevention:** None known. Genetic counseling indicated.

**Treatment:** Treatment is unnecessary in the majority of cases (mild form). Limitation of dietary galactose has been attempted in severe cases.

**Prognosis:** Normal life span in the majority of cases of the mild form. In the severe form, mental retardation appears to be inevitable.

**Detection of Carrier:** Erythrocyte epimerase activity is approximately 50% or less of normal.

**References:**

Gitzelmann R: Deficiency of uridine diphosphate galactose 4-epimerase in blood cells of an apparently healthy infant: preliminary communication. Helv Paediat Acta 1972; 27:125–130.

Mitchell B, et al.: Reversal of UDP-galactose 4-epimerase deficiency of human leukocytes in culture. Proc Natl Acad Sci USA 1975; 72:5026–5030.

Gitzelmann R, et al.: Uridine diphosphate galactose 4-epimerase deficiency. IV. report of eight cases in three families. Helv Paediatr Acta 1976; 31:441–452.

Gitzelmann R, Hansen RG: Galactose metabolism, hereditary defects and their clinical significance. In: Burman D, et al., eds: Inherited disorders of carbohydrate metabolism. Lancaster, U.K.: MTP Press, 1980:163–190.

Ichiba Y, et al.: Uridine diphosphate galactose 4-epimerase deficiency. Am J Dis Child 1980; 134:995.

Oyanagi K, et al.: Uridine diphosphate galactose 4-epimerase deficiency. Eur J Pediatr 1981; 135:303–304.

Gillett MG, et al.: Prenatal determination of uridine diphosphate galactose-4-epimerase activity. Prenatal Diag 1983; 3:57–59.

Henderson MJ, et al.: Further observations in a case of deficiency with a severe clinical presentation. J Inherit Metab Dis 1983; 6:17–20.

Sardharwalla IB, et al.: A patient with severe type of epimerase deficiency galactosemia. J Inherit Metab Dis 1988; 211 (suppl. 2):249–251.

GI013                                        **Richard Gitzelmann**

**Galactose-1-phosphate uridyl transferase deficiency**
*See GALACTOSEMIA*
**Galactose-glucose malabsorption**
*See GLUCOSE-GALACTOSE MALABSORPTION*

## GALACTOSEMIA                                        0403

**Includes:**
   Galactose-1-phosphate uridyl transferase deficiency
   Galactosemia-Duarte and Negro variants

**Excludes:** Galactokinase deficiency (0402)

**Major Diagnostic Criteria:** Demonstrated absence of galactose-1-phosphate uridyltransferase activity in red cells.

**Clinical Findings:** The infant affected with galactosemia usually appears normal at birth; the symptoms do not develop until milk feedings are given. Excluding patients diagnosed at birth, the findings in symptomatic patients revealed that most have hepatomegaly, jaundice, anorexia and weight loss. Cataracts, vomiting, abdominal distention, and lethargy are frequently reported. Less frequent are ascites, splenomegaly, and bulging anterior fontanel. Hemorrhagic phenomena and edema have been reported in a few instances.

One of the earliest signs is jaundice, which appears at 4–10 days of age and which may last for more than 6 weeks. Lethargy and hypotonia are frequent. Food may be refused; vomiting is common; diarrhea appears occasionally. The clinical course of some infants is fulminant; in these patients death may occur early from infection, inanition, or hepatic failure. The diagnosis of overwhelming sepsis is often suggested by clinical manifestations.

Galactosemia may vary in severity, but the symptoms in the majority of the cases reported have been severe. In a small number of milder cases, the diagnosis may be overlooked for weeks or months. Digestive difficulties, retarded physical and mental development, hepatic enlargement, cataracts, and perhaps intolerance to milk should suggest the possibility of galactosemia.

Mature cataracts are usually a late manifestation of the disease. Untreated children who survive beyond the first weeks usually manifest signs of mental retardation, which may be moderate or severe. Specific neurologic abnormalities are usually absent.

**Complications:** Overwhelming infection with Escherichia coli is the most common complication in infancy; if untreated, it often results in death. Additional complications include hypoglycemia, convulsions, gallstones, and gangrene of the limbs secondary to septicemia. A high incidence of hypergonadotropic hypogonadism has been reported in female galactosemia individuals.

**Associated Findings:** Late clinical manifestations can include ovarian failure, neurological abnormalities, and speech defects.

**Etiology:** Autosomal recessive inheritance. Presently available evidence suggests a structural change affecting the reactive site of the enzyme.

**Pathogenesis:** The absence of galactose-1-phosphate uridyltransferase causes galactose, galactose-1-phosphate, and galactitol to accumulate. It has been shown that galactose-1-phosphate may be inhibitory to certain enzyme systems. In galactokinase deficiency, galactose-1-phosphate does not accumulate, but galactitol does, and nuclear cataracts also occur. Therefore, it is assumed that the cataract of galactosemia results from galactitol accumulation and that galactose-1-phosphate is responsible for the other clinical manifestations. Bilirubin retention may be a result of injury to hepatic cells by metabolites of galactose. Mild hemolysis may be a contributing factor, but the anemia usually accompanying the disease is unexplained.

It has also been suggested that a decrease uridine diphosphate galactose (UDPGal) formation due to the absence of galactose-1-phosphate uridyltransferase is responsible for such late clinical manifestations as ovarian failure, neurological abnormalities, and speech defects.

**MIM No.:** *23040

**POS No.:** 3789

**Sex Ratio:** M1:F1

**Occurrence:** About 1:50,000–70,000 in the United Kingdom, United States, and Germany. Somewhat higher in Austria and Ireland, and considerably lower in Japan.

**Risk of Recurrence for Patient's Sib:**
   See Part I, *Mendelian Inheritance.*

**Risk of Recurrence for Patient's Child:**
   See Part I, *Mendelian Inheritance.*

**Age of Detectability:** Prenatally diagnosed by deficiency of galactose-1-phosphate uridyltransferase activity in cultured amniotic fluid cells. At birth by absence of enzyme in erythrocytes.

**Gene Mapping and Linkage:** GALT (galactose-1-phosphate uridylyltransferase) has been mapped to 9p13.

**Prevention:** None known. Genetic counseling indicated. Most states in the United States now screen newborns for galactosemia.

**Treatment:** Early exclusion of milk and milk products from the diet prevents appearance of the clinical manifestations of the disease. Later treatment eliminates most symptoms with the exception of matured cataracts and mental retardation. A number of milk substitutes, including casein hydrolysates and soybean products are, available. Fortunately, exogenous galactose is dispensable. Galactolipids and other essential galactose-containing compounds are provided endogenously from uridine diphoshoglucose via reversal of the epimerase system. Consequently, normal physical growth and maturation are possible. Appropriate therapy must be undertaken to control infection, to correct fluid and electrolyte imbalance, and to manage bleeding manifestations. The emotional aspects of long-term dietary therapy may require attention. Administration of uridine has also been proposed as an approach to the treatment of the late clinical manifestations.

**Prognosis:** With untreated galactosemia, the patient's mortality is high in the first few months of life. An untreated patient who survives often develops nuclear cataracts and mental retardation. Long-term follow-up indicates that individuals with galactosemia, even those diagnosed at birth, have significant complications that include neuropsycologic, neurologic, communication, and ovarian deficits.

**Detection of Carrier:** The heterozygote has about 50% of normal galactose-1-phosphate uridyltransferase activity in erythrocytes and is usually asymptomatic.

**Special Considerations:** Beutler (1965) reported a transferase deficiency (the Duarte variant) different from that commonly described. In the families studied, homozygotes had about one-half the normal erythrocyte enzyme activity; heterozygotes averaged about 75% of the normal amount. Homozygotes for this defect are asymptomatic. Pedigree analysis has suggested that the gene for the Duarte variant is an allele of the galactosemia gene. Other transferase variants have been described. Some are associated with clinical manifestations (Negro, Rennes, Indiana and Chicago). Others are not (Los Angeles, Berne).

**Support Groups:** NY; New City (#1 Ash Court); Parents of Galactosemia Children

**References:**
Woolf LI: Inherited metabolic disorders: galactosemia. In: Sobotka H, Steward CP, eds: Advances in clinical chemistry, vol. 5. New York: Academic Press, 1962.

Beutler E, et al.: A new genetic abnormality resulting in galactose-1-phosphate uridyltransferase deficiency. Lancet 1965; I:353–354.

Houghton S, Levy HL: Rennes-like variant of galactosemia: clinical and biochemical studies. J Pediatr 1975; 87:50–57.

Ng WG, et al.: Prenatal diagnosis of galactosemia. Clin Chim Acta 1977; 74:227.

Segal S: Disorders of galactose metabolism. In: Stanbury JB, et al., eds: The metabolic basis of inherited disease. 5th ed. New York: McGraw-Hill, l983:167.

Kaufman FR, et al.: Gonadal function in patients with galactosemia. J Inherit Metab Dis 1986; 9:140–146.

Ng WG, et al.: Deficit of uridine diphosphate galactose (UDPGal) in galactosemia (abstract). Am J Hum Genet 1987; 41(3) Suppl, A12.

Kaufman FR, et al.: Correlation of ovarian function with galactose-1-phosphate uridyl transferase levels in galactosemia. J Pediatr 1988; 112:754–756.

D0009
NG000

George N. Donnell
Won Gin Ng

**Galactosemia II**
*See GALACTOKINASE DEFICIENCY*
**Galactosemia-Duarte and Negro variants**
*See GALACTOSEMIA*

## GALACTOSIALIDOSIS      3110

**Includes:**
Cherry-red spot-myoclonus with dementia
G(M1)-gangliosidosis, type 4
Goldberg syndrome
Neuraminidase/beta-galactosidase expression
Neuraminidase deficiency with beta-galactosidase
    deficiency
Sialidosis type II, juvenile-onset form

**Excludes:**
**G(M1)-gangliosidosis** (other)
**Mucolipidosis**
Sialidosis (other)

**Major Diagnostic Criteria:** Galactosialidosis is distinguished from primary, isolated deficiencies of either neuraminidase (sialidase) or beta-galactosidase by virtue of the fact that this disorder has a combined deficiency of both beta-galactosidase and neuraminidase in fibroblasts and leukocytes. Other lysosomal enzymes are normal. Affected patients have vacuoles in the hepatic parenchyma cells, bone marrow, and peripheral lymphocytes. Urinary sialyloligosaccharides are elevated without mucopolysacchariduria.

**Clinical Findings:** At least three clinical forms of this disease have been described. In the *early-infantile type*, the patients present at or soon after birth with severe edema, ascites, skeletal dysplasia, and ocular abnormalities. In the *late-infantile form*, the symptoms become apparent after age 6–12 months and consist of skeletal dysplasia, visceromegaly, macular cherry-red spots, and mental retardation. In the *juvenile/adult galactosialidosis form*, skeletal dysplasia, dysmorphic features, corneal clouding, cherry-red spots, and mental retardation become apparent sometime between childhood and adulthood. On clinical grounds it may be difficult to distinguish many galactosialidosis patients from sialidosis patients who also lack neuraminidase activity but have normal levels of beta-galactosidase activity.

**Complications:** Similar to other lysosomal disorders of glycoprotein and mucopolysaccharide metabolism. These may include mental retardation, nephrotic syndrome, growth disturbances, joint stiffness, and coarse features.

**Associated Findings:** Possibly recurrent respiratory infections and hearing loss.

**Etiology:** Autosomal recessive inheritance. The various forms of galactosialidosis are grouped together by virtue of the fact that all have a severe reduction in the intracellular levels of both neuraminidase and galactosidase. The combined deficiencies of these two lysosomal enzymes result from a lack of a "protective" glycoprotein required to stabilize the aggregation of the subunits of galactosidase and its complex with neuraminidase. Addition-

ally, recent evidence indicates that the different clinical forms are the result of differences in either the amount or the degree of conversion of a 52-kd precursor to the final 32-kd glycoprotein. Thus, in the early infantile form there is a marked decrease in both the 52-kd precursor and the 32-kd product, whereas in the juvenile form there is relatively more of the 52-kd precursor but no 32-kd product.

**Pathogenesis:** Both neuroaminidase and galactosidase are lysosomal enzymes involved in the degradation of glycoproteins and sometimes gangliosides. There is a decreased ability of affected cells to degrade these natural substrates, which, in turn, results in the biochemical and clinical manifestations of the type usually associated with lysosomal storage diseases. Specifically, there is lysosomal storage of the undegraded substrates, clinical manifestations of abnormal storage, and a progressive, declining clinical course.

**MIM No.:** *25654

**Sex Ratio:** M1:F1

**Occurrence:** Undetermined but presumably rare. The juvenile form, which appears to be the most common, has been found mainly in patients of Japanese ancestry. Other forms do not appear to have a predilection in any particular ethnic group.

**Risk of Recurrence for Patient's Sib:**
See Part I, *Mendelian Inheritance.*

**Risk of Recurrence for Patient's Child:**
See Part I, *Mendelian Inheritance.*

**Age of Detectability:** The age of usual clinical diagnosis is dependent in part on the clinical form of the disease, i.e., the early-infantile patients showing gross abnormalities at or very shortly after birth whereas the juvenile/adult form can present over a wide age between infancy and adulthood. The enzyme alterations can be demonstrated at any age in all forms of the disease. Prenatal diagnosis has been carried out in at least the early-infantile form of the disease.

**Gene Mapping and Linkage:** GSL (galactosialidosis) has been provisionally mapped to 20.

Mueller et al. (1986) have presented evidence that the mutation in one patient with the early-infantile form of galactosialidosis was caused by a gene located on human chromosome 20. It is to be noted, however, that the 32-kd "protective protein," believed to be defective in at least some patients with this disorder, has been shown to be encoded on chromosome 22. The relationship of these findings is unclear at the present time.

**Prevention:** None known. Genetic counseling indicated.

**Treatment:** Unknown.

**Prognosis:** Dependent on the form of the disorder, i.e., early-infantile being the most severe, resulting in an early death, whereas the juvenile/adult form is characterized by a long period (sometimes 20 to 30 years) of normality before the appearance of clinical manifestations.

**Detection of Carrier:** As the beta-galactosidase and neuraminidase abnormalities in affected patients are secondary to a defect in a "protective protein," it may be difficult to identify carriers of this disorder. Obligate galactosialidosis heterozygotes have not been shown consistently to have reductions in either beta-galactosidase or neuraminidase levels.

**References:**

d'Azzo A, et al.: Molecular defect in combined beta-galactosidase and neuraminidase deficiency in man. Proc Natl Acad Sci USA 1982; 79:4535–4539.

Sakuraba H, et al.: Galactosidase-neuraminidase deficiency (galactosialidosis): clinical, pathological, and enzymatic studies in a post-mortem case. Ann Neurol 1983; 13:497–503.

Loonen MCB, et al.: Combined sialidase (neuraminidase) and beta-galactosidase deficiency: clinical, morphological and enzymological observations in a patient. Clin Genet 1984; 26:139–149.

Verheijen FW, et al.: Human placental neuraminidase activation, stabilization and association with galactosidase and its "protective" protein. Eur J Biochem 1985; 149:315–321.

Mueller OT, et al.: Sialidosis and galactosialidosis: chromosomal assignment of two genes associated with neuraminidase-deficiency disorders. Proc Natl Acad Sci USA 1986; 83:1817–1821.

Palmeri S, et al.: Galactosialidosis: Molecular heterogeneity among distinct clinical phenotypes. Am J Hum Genet 1986; 38:137–148.

Takeda E, et al.: Involvement of thiol proteases in galactosialidosis. Clin Chim Acta 1986; 155:109–116.

Willemsen R, et al.: Immunoelectron microscopical localization of lysosomal β-galactosidase and its precursor forms in normal and mutant human fibroblasts. Eur J Cell Biol 1986; 40:9–15.

Nanba E, et al.: Galactosialidosis: a direct evidence that a 46-kilodalton protein restores deficient enzyme activities in fibroblasts. Biochem Biophys Res Commun 1987; 144:138–142.

TH021                                              **George H. Thomas**

**Galactosylceramidase deficiency**
  *See LEUKODYSTROPHY, GLOBOID CELL TYPE*
**Galactosylceramide beta-galactosidase deficiency**
  *See LEUKODYSTROPHY, GLOBOID CELL TYPE*
**GALK (Galactokinase deficiency)**
  *See GALACTOKINASE DEFICIENCY*
**Gallbladder, absent**
  *See GALLBLADDER, AGENESIS*

## GALLBLADDER, AGENESIS                              2415

**Includes:**
  Cystic duct agenesis
  Gallbladder, absent

**Excludes:**
  **Biliary atresia** (0110)
  Cystic duct atresia
  **Gallbladder, anomalies** (0404)
  Gallbladder hypoplasia

**Major Diagnostic Criteria:**  Absence of gallbladder and cystic duct in the presence of normal or atretic hepatic and common bile ducts with (30%) or without (70%) additional anomalies. Condition may be suspected in nonvisualization of gallbladder during cholangiography in the absence of cystic duct disease or serious liver disease. Anomalous liver shape is commonly present.

**Clinical Findings:**  Most cases (70%) occur as an isolated anomaly without clinical signs or symptoms. In nine percent of children with gallbladder agenesis, the bile ducts are atretic. Additional serious anomalies are present in 21% of children with gallbladder agenesis but without bile duct atresia. In the latter group, the associated anomalies include **Ventricular septal defect** (13%), imperforate anus (13%), gut malrotation (12%), **Renal agenesis** (9%), **Syndactyly** (9%), **Kidney, horseshoe** (7%), duodenal atresia (6%), and, rarely, pancreatic agenesis.

**Complications:**  Unknown.

**Associated Findings:**  The anomaly is strongly associated with **Chromosome triploidy**, **Chromosome 13, trisomy 13**, and ring chromosome 13 (see **Chromosome 13, monosomy 13q3**).

**Etiology:**  Usually sporadic, but may be heritable and has been described in sibs. Viral disease has also been suggested.

**Pathogenesis:**  The cystic duct-gallbladder anlagen arises from the hepatic diverticulum from the foregut. Failure of the caudal wing of the hepatic diverticulum during the fourth week leads to both cystic duct and gallbladder agenesis.

**MIM No.:**  13704

**CDC No.:**  751.630

**Sex Ratio:**  Overall, M1:F2; gallbladder agenesis with bile duct atresia, M2:F1; gallbladder agenesis without associated bile duct atresia but with other anomalies, M1:F1

**Occurrence:**  As an isolated anomaly, 0.08% of the United States population.

**Risk of Recurrence for Patient's Sib:**
  See Part I, *Mendelian Inheritance.* Presumably low.

**Risk of Recurrence for Patient's Child:**
  See Part I, *Mendelian Inheritance.* Presumably low.

**Age of Detectability:**  In infancy.

**Gene Mapping and Linkage:**  Unknown.

**Prevention:**  None known. Genetic counseling indicated.

**Treatment:**  Unknown. Counseling of patient and parents to prevent unwarranted surgical exploration.

**Prognosis:**  Excellent when present as an isolated anomaly.

**Detection of Carrier:**  Unknown.

**References:**

Frey F, et al.: Agenesis of the gallbladder. Am J Surg 1967; 114:917–925.

Nadeau LA, et al.: Hereditary gallbladder agenesis: twelve cases in the same family. J Maine Med Assoc 1972; 63:1–4.

Lopez-Rasi A, Edmonds MC: Agenesis of the gallbladder. VA Med Monthly 1974; 101:849–853.

Ramenofsky ML, et al.: Agenesis of the gallbladder: a classification based on associated anomalies. Teratology 1982; 25:69A only.

Wilson JE, Deitrick JE: Agenesis of the gallbladder: case report and familial investigation. Surgery 1986; 99:106–108.

BL002                                              **Will Blackburn**

## GALLBLADDER, ANOMALIES                              0404

**Includes:**
  Cystic artery anomalies
  Gallbladder, bilobed
  Gallbladder, diverticulum of
  Gallbladder, duplication of
  Gallbladder, ectopic
  Gallbladder, floating

**Excludes:**
  **Bile duct choledochal cyst** (0149)
  Cholecystitis
  Cholelithiasis
  Cholesterolosis
  **Gallbladder, agenesis** (2415)
  Hydrops of gallbladder

**Major Diagnostic Criteria:**  Usually asymptomatic. Rarely a diagnosis of duplication is made by X-ray when two rows of stones are observed. "Floating" gallbladder causes sudden right-upper quadrant pain, nausea and vomiting if torsion occurs.

**Clinical Findings:**  *Duplication of gallbladder* (double gallbladder): The 2nd gallbladder may be alongside the normal organ or may reside in an unusual location, e.g. in the left lobe of the liver. The duplication is usually the same size as the normal organ. It commonly has a separate cystic duct empties independently into the common bile duct and, rarely, empties into a common "Y"-shaped cystic duct. There are no characteristic symptoms or signs to make it obvious. Diagnosis is usually made at operation or as an autopsy finding. Rarely, the diagnosis is made by X-ray; two rows of stones are seen on cholecystogram.

*Bilobed gallbladder* (bifid, partially divided gallbladder): This is a very rare defect in which two 2 cavities join into a single cystic duct. Two clinical types are noted; those with an internal septum dividing them and a truly paired fundic variety. These are usually asymptomatic.

*Diverticulum of gallbladder:* A diverticulum can be located anywhere along the free surface of the organ from neck to fundus. Rarely, stones may form in a narrow-necked diverticulum due to stasis.

*"Floating" gallbladder:* This anomaly refers to a gallbladder that hangs from a long mesentery, which attaches either to the entire organ, or more rarely, the neck and cystic duct only, letting the fundus hang free. Torsion may complicate the latter type with subsequent infarction (rare in childhood). These instances are characterized by right-upper quadrant pain, nausea, and vomiting.

*Anomalous location or ectopic gallbladder:* There are three specific types, each rarely observed: intrahepatic, left-sided, and retrodisplaced. The intrahepatic variety is of surgical significance because of the difficulty encountered during cholecystectomy for cholelithiasis and cholecystitis. The incidence of gallstone formation is considered to be quite high in cases of intrahepatic gallbladder.

*Anomalies of the cystic artery:* The cystic artery arises from the right hepatic artery in 75% of cases, the common hepatic artery in 15%, and the left hepatic artery in 10%. In 25% of cases a double cystic artery is observed.

**Complications:** Unknown.

**Associated Findings:** Ectopic tissue, particularly gastric mucosa and pancreas, may be found in duplicated or bilobed gallbladder.

**Etiology:** Unknown.

**Pathogenesis:** Unknown.

**CDC No.:** 751.640

**Sex Ratio:** Presumably M1:F1

**Occurrence:** Rare except for gallbladder agenesis, which occurs in 1:3300 live births, and duplication of gallbladder which occurs in 1:4000 live births.

**Risk of Recurrence for Patient's Sib:** Unknown.

**Risk of Recurrence for Patient's Child:** Unknown.

**Age of Detectability:** Unknown.

**Gene Mapping and Linkage:** Unknown.

**Prevention:** Unknown.

**Treatment:** Unknown.

**Prognosis:** Normal life span.

**Detection of Carrier:** Unknown.

**References:**

Gross RE: Congenital anomalies of the gallbladder: review of 148 cases with report of a double gallbladder. Arch Surg 1936; 32:131.
Flannery MG, Caster MP: Congenital abnormalities of the gallbladder. Surg Gynecol Obstet 1956; 103:439.

GR022  **Jay L. Grosfeld**
CL007  **H. William Clatworthy, Jr.**

**Gallbladder, bilobed**
  *See GALLBLADDER, ANOMALIES*
**Gallbladder, diverticulum of**
  *See GALLBLADDER, ANOMALIES*
**Gallbladder, duplication of**
  *See GALLBLADDER, ANOMALIES*
**Gallbladder, ectopic**
  *See GALLBLADDER, ANOMALIES*
**Gallbladder, floating**
  *See GALLBLADDER, ANOMALIES*
**Galloway syndrome**
  *See MICROCEPHALY-HIATUS HERNIA-NEPHROSIS, GALLOWAY TYPE*
**Gamma globulin (Gm) antigens**
  *See SERUM ALLOTYPES, HUMAN*
**Gamma-A-globulin, selective deficiency of**
  *See IMMUNOGLOBULIN A DEFICIENCY*

## GAMMA-AMINOBUTYRIC ACID (GABA) TRANSAMINASE DEFICIENCY  2984

**Includes:**

Acidemia, 4-aminobutyrate aminotransferase deficiency
Four-aminobutyric acid (GABA) aminotransferase deficiency
GABA transaminase deficiency
Gamma-aminobutyric acid aminotransferase deficiency
Gamma-aminobutyric acid transaminase deficiency

**Excludes:**

**Cerebral gigantism** (0137)
**Hyperbeta-alaninemia** (0486)
**Leukodystrophy, adult onset progressive dominant type** (2975)
**Leukodystrophy, globoid cell type** (0415)
**Pelizaeus-Merzbacher syndrome** (0803)

**Major Diagnostic Criteria:** Significantly elevated GABA and $\beta$-alanine concentrations in plasma and lumbar cerebrospinal fluid. Deficiency of 4-aminobutyric acid aminotransferase activity may be demonstrated in biopsied liver material, lymphocytes isolated from whole blood, or Epstein-Barr virus transformed cultured lymphoblasts.

**Clinical Findings:** Cardinal manifestations include severe psychomotor retardation, axial hypotonia, generalized hyperreflexia, convulsions, high-pitched cry, accelerated length-growth, and lethargy. Fasting plasma growth hormone levels are increased. Brain evoked responses may be suggestive of leukodystrophy, such as that seen in phenylketonuria. In one of two affected sibs in the index family, electroencephalography at age two weeks was normal, while at age seven months there was generalized low activity, predominant $\beta$ activity, and epileptic discharges. At age two years the EEG of this patient displayed generalized epileptic bursts. At the same time, CT scan of the brain showed enlarged ventricles, cisternae, and cortical sulci.

**Complications:** In the only family studied, one child died at age five days from an unknown cause, while two others died at approximately ages three years (patient A) and 1 year (patient B), the former with documented deficiency of 4-aminobutyric acid aminotransferase. Although definitive enzyme studies were absent, patient B was inferred to have the same enzyme deficiency due to a similar clinical course as his sib. One other sib was healthy. Thus, a high mortality rate may be associated with 4-aminobutyric acid aminotransferase deficiency. For the surviving patient, psychomotor retardation may be expected to be extreme. In patient A, psychomotor development was less than four weeks at the age of two years.

**Associated Findings:** Adiposity and intermittent hepatomegaly may be present. Autopsy of patient B revealed a well-developed panniculus adiposus, edema and congestion of the brain, large thymus, bilateral bronchopneumonia, and small necrotic regions in the liver. In the same patient, neuropathologic examination revealed poor or absent myelination in the white matter of the gyri. Even where well-myelinated, a spongy state of varying degree was present throughout the white matter.

**Etiology:** Autosomal recessive inheritance.

**Pathogenesis:** In mammalian tissues, the inhibitory neurotransmitter GABA is converted into succinic semialdehyde by 4-aminobutyric acid aminotransferase (E.C.2.6.1.19). GABA has been estimated to be present in nearly one third of human synapses. The inherited enzyme deficiency results in a significant accumulation of GABA and $\beta$-alanine in central nervous system tissues. A patient with an apparent defect in the degradation of $\beta$-alanine, who also had increased cerebrospinal fluid and plasma GABA levels, has been reported by Scriver et al. (1966 ). These data and the present cases suggest the existence of two different enzymes catalyzing the transamination of the structural homologues $\beta$-alanine and GABA and further suggest that $\beta$-alanine is an alternative substrate for 4-aminobutyric acid aminotransferase and GABA an alternative substrate for $\beta$-alanine aminotransferase. The clinical course of the patient described by Scriver et al (1966) was very similar to that displayed by patients A and B. Sjaastad et al (1976) presented a clinically normal adult with CSF homocarnosine levels about twice those of patient A. These findings indicate that the brain damage and encephalopathy in patients with 4-aminobutyric acid aminotransferase deficiency may well be a result of elevated GABA and possibly $\beta$-alanine concentrations in central nervous system tissue. The acceleration of length-growth may be a result of the growth hormone-releasing effect of GABA.

**MIM No.:** *13715

**Sex Ratio:** M1:F1

**Occurrence:** Two clinically affected sibs in a single family with one healthy child in four pregnancies. Definitive enzyme studies were performed in one case. Parental consanguinity cannot be completely ruled out, as both parents originate from the same small Flemish region.

**Risk of Recurrence for Patient's Sib:**
See Part I, *Mendelian Inheritance.*

**Risk of Recurrence for Patient's Child:**
See Part I, *Mendelian Inheritance.*

**Age of Detectability:** Birth to four days for patients A and B. The potential for prenatal diagnosis by means of chorionic villus sampling has been presented. The possibility of prenatal diagnosis by measurement of amniotic fluid levels of GABA and β-alanine may also exist.

**Gene Mapping and Linkage:** Unknown.

**Prevention:** None known. Genetic counseling indicated.

**Treatment:** Unknown.

**Prognosis:** Undetermined, although a high mortality rate appears likely. For the surviving patient, extreme psychomotor retardation seems probable.

**Detection of Carrier:** Levels of enzyme activities for 4-aminobutyric acid aminotransferase consistent with heterozygosity have been documented in extracts of lymphocytes and lymphoblasts obtained from the parents and healthy sib of patients A and B. Evidence of homozygosity for 4-aminobutyric acid aminotransferase deficiency was presented in the same tissues and biopsied liver material obtained from patient A.

**Special Considerations:** It may be worthwhile to request quantitative plasma amino acid analysis on patients presenting with psychomotor deficit, hypotonia, accelerated length-growth, and hyperreflexia. The detection of elevated levels of GABA and β-alanine would warrant the analysis of cerebrospinal fluid amino acid concentrations. The documentation of 4-aminobutyric acid aminotransferase activity in cells obtained from peripheral blood should simplify the assessment of other patients with this disease and preclude the necessity for liver biopsy.

**Support Groups:** KS; Kansas City; The Organic Acidemia Association

**References:**
Scriver CR, et al.: Hyper-β-alaninemia associated with β-aminoaciduria and γ-aminobutyricaciduria, somnolence and seizures. New Engl J Med 1966; 274:635–643.
Sjaastad O, et al.: Homocarnosinosis: a familial metabolic disorder associated with spastic paraplegia, progressive mental deficiency, and retinal pigmentation. Acta Neurol Scand 1976; 53:275–290.
Jaeken J, et al.: Gamma-aminobutyric acid-transaminase deficiency: a newly recognized inborn error of neurotransmitter metabolism. Neuropediatrics 1984; 15:165–169. *
Gibson KM, et al.: Demonstration of 4-aminobutyric acid aminotransferase deficiency in lymphocytes and lymphoblasts. J Inherit Metab Dis 1985; 8:204–208. *
Gibson KM, et al.: Inborn errors of GABA metabolism. Bioessays 1986; 4:24–27.
Sweetman FR, et al.: Activity of biotin dependent and GABA metabolizing enzymes in chorionic villus samples: potential for 1st trimester prenatal diagnosis. Prenatal Diagn 1986; 6:187–194.

GI019                                    **Kenneth M. Gibson**

**Gamma-aminobutyric acid aminotransferase deficiency**
*See GAMMA-AMINOBUTYRIC ACID (GABA) TRANSAMINASE DEFICIENCY*
**Gamma-aminobutyric acid transaminase deficiency**
*See GAMMA-AMINOBUTYRIC ACID (GABA) TRANSAMINASE DEFICIENCY*
**Gamma-cystathionase deficiency**
*See CYSTATHIONINURIA*
**Gamma-glutamyl cysteine synthetase deficiency**
*See ANEMIA, HEMOLYTIC, GAMMA-GLUTAMYL/CYSTEINE SYNTHETASE DEFICIENCY*
**Gamma-glutamyl transpeptidase deficiency**
*See GLUTATHIONURIA*
**Gamma-hydroxybutyric aciduria**
*See ACIDEMIA, GAMMA-HYDROXYBUTYRIC*
**Gamma-interferon deficiency**
*See INTERFERON DEFICIENCY*
**Gamma-trace, defect in metabolism of**
*See AMYLOIDOSIS, ICELANDIC TYPE*

**Ganglion nodosum tumor**
*See CAROTID BODY TUMOR*
**Ganglioneuromatosis of the alimentary tract**
*See ENDOCRINE NEOPLASIA, MULTIPLE TYPE III*
**Ganglioside neuraminidase deficiency**
*See MUCOLIPIDOSIS IV*
**Ganglioside sialidase deficiency**
*See MUCOLIPIDOSIS IV*
**Gangliosidosis, generalized GM, adult type**
*See G(M1)-GANCLIOSIDOSIS, TYPE 3*
**Gangliosidosis, generalized juvenile type**
*See G(M1)-GANGLIOSIDOSIS, TYPE 2*
**Gangliosidosis, type 1 (generalized)**
*See G(M1)-GANGLIOSIDOSIS, TYPE 1*
**GAPO syndrome**
*See GROWTH RETARDATION-ALOPECIA-PSEUDOANODONTIA-OPTIC ATROPHY*
**Garamycin^, fetal effect**
*See FETAL AMINOGLYCOSIDE OTOTOXICITY*
**Gardner syndrome**
*See INTESTINAL POLYPOSIS, TYPE III*
**Gardner-Silengo-Wachtel syndrome**
*See GENITO-PALAT0-CARDIAC SYNDROME*
**Gareis-Mason syndrome**
*See X-LINKED MENTAL RETARDATION-CLASPED THUMB*
**Gargoylism (obsolete/pejorative)**
*See MUCOPOLYSACCHARIDOSIS I-H*
**Gass syndrome**
*See RETINA, CAVERNOUS HEMANGIOMA*
**Gastric atresia**
*See STOMACH, PYLORIC ATRESIA*
**Gastric cancer**
*See CANCER, GASTRIC FAMILIAL*
**Gastric diverticulum, congenital**
*See STOMACH, DIVERTICULUM*
**Gastric emptying disorders, idiopathic**
*See INTESTINAL PSEUDO-OBSTRUCTION SYNDROMES*
**Gastric enterocystoma**
*See STOMACH, DUPLICATION*
**Gastric outlet obstruction, incomplete**
*See STOMACH, PYLORIC ATRESIA*
**Gastric teratoma**
*See STOMACH, TERATOMA*
**Gastric ulcer**
*See PEPTIC ULCER DISEASES, NON-SYNDROMIC*

---

**GASTROCUTANEOUS SYNDROME**                    **2981**

**Includes:**
Cafe-au-lait-ulcer, peptic/hiatal hernia-hypertelorism-myopia
Hernia, hiatal/ulcer, peptic-cafe-au-lait-hypertelorism-myopia
Hypertelorism-Ulcer, peptic/hiatal hernia-cafe-au-lait-myopia
Lentigines-peptic ulcer/hiatal hernia-hypertelorism-myopia
Ulcer, peptic/hiatal hernia-cafe-au-lait-hypertelorism-myopia

**Excludes:**
Intestinal polyposis, type II (2344)
Intestinal polyposis, type III (0536)
Skin pigmentation-gastrointestinal anomalies without peptic ulcer

**Major Diagnostic Criteria:** Peptic ulcer/**Hernia, hiatal**, multiple lentigines/cafe-au-lait spots, **Eye, hypertelorism**, myopia.

**Clinical Findings:** The familial occurrence of the gastrocutaneous syndrome was described in a large French-Canadian family. Of a total of 24 affected individuals (over 11 years) in the pedigree, 16 had had symptoms of peptic ulcer/hiatal hernia; five requiring operations. Symptoms had usually started in the second or third decade, rarely during adolescence. In all documented cases, the peptic ulcer was antral and the hiatal hernia was the sliding type.

Multiple lentigines with or without café-au-lait spots were present in all 16 ulcer patients and in four nonulcer patients. Lentigines were light brown and usually scattered over the back, shoulders, arms, and forearms and very rarely over the face; their histologic appearance is that of the lentigo simplex type of skin lesions. Usually one or two café-au-lait spots were located in the hip area, less frequently on the face, back, and thighs. Skin pigmentation in the index patient antedated the peptic ulcer for several years, whereas in others it paralleled their gastric symptomatology.

Apparent **Eye, hypertelorism** and myopia were present in 12 of the 16 ulcer patients and in two and four of the eight nonulcer patients, respectively. Adult-onset diabetes, congenital heart disease, and ischemic heart disease were present respectively in three, two, and five ulcer patients and were absent in the nonulcer individuals.

Dermatoglyphics in the index patient and her affected mother were unusual; they both had a high total ridge count and distal axial triradii. Similar changes were present in some other affected individuals.

**Complications:** Recurrent upper abdominal pain, hematemesis, melena.

**Associated Findings:** Round back, adenocarcinoma of the sigmoid, cancer of the "shoulder," hearing loss at age 50 years, breast cancer, superficial uterine adenomyomatosis, pelvic endometriosis, **Raynaud disease**, heterochromia, and clubfeet.

**Etiology:** Presumably autosomal dominant inheritance with high penetrance and variable expression.

**Pathogenesis:** Unknown. In at least the index patient and her affected mother, the peptic ulcer was associated with increased acid secretion; pentagastrin stimulation test showed a high maximal acid output in both.

**MIM No.:** 13727

**POS No.:** 3905

**Sex Ratio:** Presumably M1:F1.

**Occurrence:** Described in 24 members of one French-Canadian kindred.

**Risk of Recurrence for Patient's Sib:**
See Part I, *Mendelian Inheritance.*

**Risk of Recurrence for Patient's Child:**
See Part I, *Mendelian Inheritance.*

**Age of Detectability:** Usually in the second or third decade; rarely during adolescence.

**Gene Mapping and Linkage:** Unknown.

**Prevention:** None known. Genetic counseling indicated.

**Treatment:** Antacids, cimetidine, pyloroplasty-vagotomy, or gastrectomy depending on severity of the symptoms.

**Prognosis:** Probably less than normal life span in individuals with ischemic heart disease and diabetes.

**Detection of Carrier:** Unknown. The presence of multiple lentigines with or without café-au-lait spots in a young individual with a family history of the gastrocutaneous syndrome (before peptic ulcer symptoms) is suggestive.

**References:**
Rotter JI, Rimoin DL: The genetic syndromology of peptic ulcer. Am J Med Genet 1981; 10:315–321.
Halal F, et al.: Gastro-cutaneous syndrome: peptic ulcer/hiatal hernia, multiple lentigines/café-au-lait spots, hypertelorism, and myopia. Am J Med Genet 1982; 11:161–176. * †
Rotter JI, Rimoin DL: Additional comment on the ulcer multiple lentigines syndrome. (Letter) Am J Med Genet 1982; 11:251–252.
Halal F: Dermatoglyphics "in the gastrocutaneous syndrome." (Letter) Am J Med Genet 1983; 15:338–339.

HA074 **Fahed Halal**

**Gastroesophageal reflux without hiatus hernia**
*See ESOPHAGUS, CHALASIA*
**Gastrogen lactose intolerance**
*See LACTOSE INTOLERANCE*
**Gastrointestinal atresia-aplasia cutis congenita**
*See APLASIA CUTIS CONGENITA-GASTROINTESTINAL ATRESIA*
**Gastrointestinal atresia-aplasia cutis congenital**
*See SKIN, LOCALIZED ABSENCE OF*

**Gastrointestinal polyposis-ectodermal defects**
*See POLYPOSIS-ALOPECIA-PIGMENTATION-NAIL DEFECTS*

## GASTROSCHISIS 0405

**Includes:**
Abdominal wall defect
Aparoschisis

**Excludes:**
**Omphalocele** (0748)
Ruptured hernia
**Urachal anomalies** (2573)

**Major Diagnostic Criteria:** 1) A small abdominal wall defect. 2) A small abdominal cavity. 3) The umbilical cord is usually attached to the abdominal wall to the left of the defect. 4) The herniated organs usually consist of thickened small intestine. 5) Absence of a covering sac.

**Clinical Findings:** Infants with gastroschisis characteristically are of low birth weight, have a small abdominal cavity, a small abdominal wall defect without a remnant of a covering sac. The wall of the herniated small intestine is thick, edematous, matted and chronically inflamed. Uterine ultrasonography may identify the condition prenatally.

**Complications:** Dehydration, infection, hypothermia, metabolic acidoses, volvulus, and midgut infarction may occur in babies with gastroschisis. Complications related to associated anomalies are rare.

**Associated Findings:** None known.

**Etiology:** Two theories have been proposed to explain the etiology of gastroschisis: 1) Early intrauterine rupture of an omphalocele with complete resorption of the sac (Shaw, 1975); and 2) intrauterine vascular accident involving the omphalomesenteric artery (Hoyme et al, 1981).

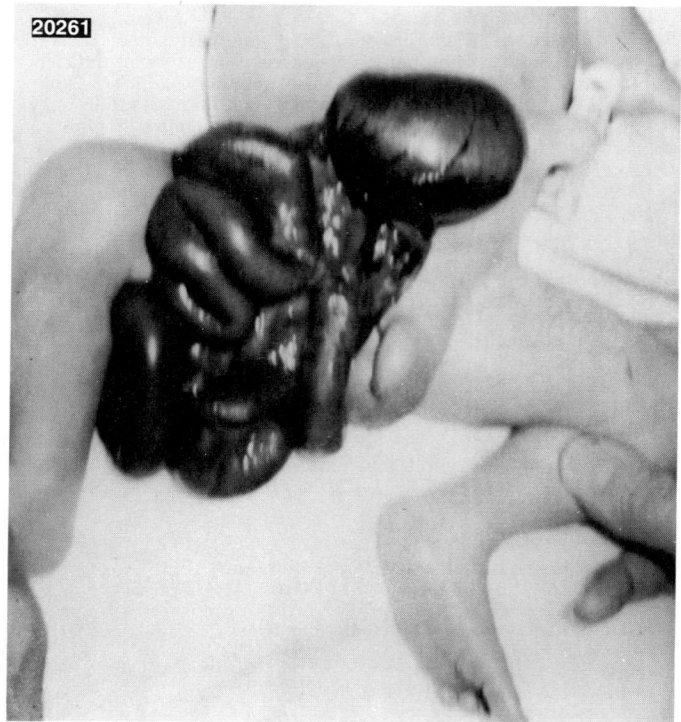

0405-20261: Gastroschisis; note the lesion is lateral to the umbilical cord.

**Pathogenesis:** Gastroschisis is associated with anatomic and histologic changes in the herniated intestine (Sherman and Asch, 1981). Such changes include shortening, edema, volvulus and midgut infarction. The shortening is related to the chronic intrauterine exposure of the bowel to the amniotic fluid, with subsequent serosal changes leading to fibrosis and contraction. Volvulus and midgut infarction may be related to nonfixation of the bowel and excess weight of the herniated intestine.

**CDC No.:** 756.710

**Sex Ratio:** M1:F1

**Occurrence:** 1:6,000 live births.

**Risk of Recurrence for Patient's Sib:** Minimal.

**Risk of Recurrence for Patient's Child:** Minimal.

**Age of Detectability:** At birth.

**Gene Mapping and Linkage:** Unknown.

**Prevention:** None known. Genetic counseling indicated.

**Treatment:** Surgical closure of the defect, either primarily or staged using silastic prosthesis.

**Prognosis:** Ninety-percent survival.

**Detection of Carrier:** Unknown.

**Special Considerations:** Over 90% of infants with gastroschisis can be expected to survive due to improved surgical technique and postoperative total parenteral nutrition.

**References:**
Shaw A: The myth of gastroschisis. J Pediatr Surg 1975; 10:235–244.
Seashore JH: Congenital abdominal wall defects. Clinics in Perinat 1978; 5:61–78.
Hoyme HE, et al.: The vascular pathogenesis of gastroschisis: intrauterine interruption of the omphalomesenteric artery. J Pediatr 1981; 98:228–231.
Sherman NJ, Asch MJ: Gastroschisis: current concept. J Calif Perinat Assoc 1981; 1:74–78.

SE006                                          **John H. Seashore**

## GAUCHER DISEASE                                          0406

**Includes:**
    Acid beta-glucosidase deficiency
    Cerebroside lipidosis
    Cerebrosidosis
    Gaucher disease, acute neuronopathic (type II)
    Gaucher disease, chronic neuronopathic (type III)
    Gaucher disease, infantile cerebral (type II)
    Gaucher disease, juvenile and adult cerebral (type III)
    Gaucher disease, noncerebral juvenile (type I)
    Glucocerebrosidase deficiency
    Glucocerebrosidosis
    Norrbottnian Gaucher disease

**Excludes:**
    **G(m1)-gangliosidosis, type 1** (0431)
    **G(M2)-gangliosidosis with hexosaminidase A deficiency** (0434)
    **Leukemia, chronic myeloid (CML)** (3092)
    **Niemann-Pick disease** (0717)
    Sea-blue histiocytosis
    Sphingolipidoses (other)

**Major Diagnostic Criteria:** The infantile patient presents with a characteristic appearance of neurologic abnormalities plus visceromegaly. In the chronic form, obscure splenomegaly or, in its absence, skeletal difficulties, suggests the diagnosis.

Gaucher cells (large histiocytic elements with a "wrinkled-appearing" cytoplasm) can usually be demonstrated on the initial marrow examination. Electron microscopy reveals characteristic tubular inclusions. Atypical Gaucher cells may occasionally present as Niemann-Pick cells or sea-blue histiocytes. In a few reports they have been identified sparsely in the marrow of obligatory heterozygotes. Rarely, cells of somewhat similar appearance may be found in the marrow of patients with chronic leukemia or hemolytic anemia.

Ultimately, it must be demonstrated that there is an increase in glucocerebrosides in the involved tissues or in the plasma, or a deficiency of β-glucosidase, glucocerebrosidase, or both in the tissue or the circulating white blood cells. Enzymic differentiation of neurologic and non-neurologic forms has recently been achieved in spleen, brain, and cultured fibroblasts. At least four different allelic mutations have been identified in the chronic form (type I). For optimal β-glucosidase activity, fibroblasts require taurocholate and leukocytes taurocholate and Triton X-100.

A lesser increase in glucocerebrosides and a partial deficiency of β-glucosidase have been observed in **Niemann-Pick disease**, especially in the juvenile form (Crocker group C) with normal sphingomyelinase activity.

**Clinical Findings:** In the so-called *acute* or *infantile* form of Gaucher disease (type II), the child presents a picture of "pseudobulbar palsy," with strabismus, difficulty in swallowing, laryngeal spasm, a common position of comfort with the head extended (resembling opisthotonos), and developmental retardation. Simultaneously, there is significant enlargement of the liver and spleen. There are episodes of troubled aspiration, with chronic bronchopneumonia and increasing debility. Most such infants die by 6 to 12 months of age; in a few (? "*subacute*" type) the neurologic handicaps may be milder in the early months, and survival may be possible until approximately 2 years of age.

Another group of patients who also have nervous system involvement have been labeled the *juvenile* type (type III). They show a gradually increasing dementia during middle-to-late childhood, often with behavioral changes, seizures, extrapyramidal and cerebellar signs, and difficulties because of pulmonary disease. Organomegaly is mild. Some aspects of this infrequent clinical picture remain obscure, and the diagnosis should be made with caution. This group seen more frequently in certain areas of Sweden. A rare variant presented without organomegaly and without glucosylceramide storage outside of the brain.

By far, the most common type of Gaucher disease is the *chronic* or *adult* form (type I), probably representing 90% of the total. In spite of the "adult" designation, the first symptoms may appear as early as one year of age. The presenting clinical features are abdominal enlargement (from the notable increase in spleen and liver size) and orthopedic difficulties. Symptoms in the bones and joints (pain, pathologic fractures, aseptic necrosis) result from the handicaps of a greatly expanded medullary cavity volume; X-rays show tubulation failure and areas of dissolution in the long bones and vertebrae. Yellow patches on the sclerae ("pingueculae") are seen in about 25% of the adults, and abnormal pigmentation of the face, neck, hands, or shins may occur. A variety of neurologic disorders was recently reported in adult patients.

**Complications:** In time, the marrow-suppressing effects of the continuing splenomegaly produce a lowering of all formed blood elements. When the thrombocytopenia reaches critical levels, various hemorrhagic symptoms appear, including easy bruising and epistaxis. Massive hepatomegaly may cause abdominal pain but does not appear to interfere with hepatic functions; portal hypertension is almost unknown. Splenic rupture is rarely reported. As mentioned, skeletal complications are common, with fractures of the femoral neck and the vertebral bodies most important, plus the secondary development of aseptic necrosis of the femoral head. In the infantile patient, pneumonia occurs, along with the effects of increasing cerebral handicap.

**Associated Findings:** Immunoglobulin abnormalities are rarely reported. Transient changes in Factor IX may contribute to bleeding problems. Elevated serum angiotensin-converting enzyme is common. A significant elevation of serum hexosaminidase B is detected in Gaucher type I homozygotes (but not heterozygotes) compared to Tay-Sachs heterozygotes.

**Etiology:** Autosomal recessive inheritance in each form of Gaucher disease. (In two families only, there is apparently dominant transmission of the chronic form.) There are no genetic interrelationships but in one family two siblings had the acute form and another the chronic form. In another family one child had the acute form and a second cousin the subacute form. Different molecular forms of β-glucocerebrosidase have been demonstrated in neurologic and non-neurologic phenotypes.

A reduction in the levels of β-glucosidase is found at many sites (e.g.,liver, spleen, white blood cells). In the chronic form, leukocytes contain substantial residual activity of glucocerebrosidase (20%) or β-glucosidase (up to 30%); fibroblasts have lower activity of glucocerebrosidase (15%) or β-glucosidase (10%). Severity of clinical symptoms is not always well correlated with the amount of enzyme deficit.

In patients with bone disease, there is also a consistent increase in acid phosphatase activity (isozyme 5, derived from osteoclasts), histochemically demonstrable in the cytoplasm of the Gaucher cells, with excretion producing an elevation in the serum level of tartrate-resistant acid phosphatase.

**Pathogenesis:** Glucocerebrosidase, which is firmly membrane-bound, is part of an enzyme system involving a membrane-bound factor C, a heat-stable glycoprotein factor P, and acidic phospholipids. The tissue deficiency of β-glucosidase, which seems to be the cerebroside-cleaving enzyme, correlates well with the cytoplasmic accumulation in histiocytes of glycolipid, which cannot be catabolized. There are two theories about the actual origin of the cellular cerebroside augmentation. The traditional view is that it arises from local in situ synthesis preeminently; it has been demonstrated that isolated normal spleen or liver slices are capable of normal cerebroside biosynthesis. Another hypothesis views the major source of stockpiled glycolipid as arising from the normal breakdown of white and red blood cells, the engulfed products of which are then blocked from further catabolism. The mechanism of the cerebral handicap in the infantile form is not well understood, but it is of interest to note that some neurons (e.g., in the thalamus) show mild distention with periodic acid-Schiff (PAS)-positive material. It has been speculated that psychosine (β-glucosylsphingosine), a minor accumulating metabolite, may be toxic to the neurons. The greatly increased amount of the special "Gaucher acid phosphatase" in the final stages of the disease probably reflects the severity of the bone involvement. A new variant has been identified with normal glucosylceramidase activity and a defect in the non-enzymic sphingolipid $A_{1a}$ activator protein.

**MIM No.:** *23080, 23090, 23100

**Sex Ratio:** M1:F1

**Occurrence:** Over 350 patients have been reported. About two-thirds of the patients with chronic Gaucher disease are of Ashkenazi Jewish ancestry, and, in this group, the carrier rates may be as high as 1:25. The observed incidence of clinically affected homozygotes is substantially less than expected from the carrier rate. It is not known if milder, atypical, or asymptomatic cases account for the difference.

**Risk of Recurrence for Patient's Sib:**
See Part I, *Mendelian Inheritance.*

**Risk of Recurrence for Patient's Child:**
See Part I, *Mendelian Inheritance.*

**Age of Detectability:** Prenatal diagnosis is possible in cell culture from amniotic fluid. For patients with infantile Gaucher disease, stiffness and irritability commonly begin by 2 to 3 months of age, organomegaly by 3 to 6 months, and respiratory distress by 3 months or soon after. In the chronic form, enlargement of the liver and spleen may be detected as early as one year of age.

**Gene Mapping and Linkage:** GBA (glucosidase, beta; acid) has been mapped to 1q21.

**Prevention:** None known. Genetic counseling indicated.

**Treatment:** Splenectomy provides useful permanent control of the hemorrhagic symptoms but should only be pursued when there are serious clinical issues in this area. Partial splenectomy may become a useful option in children if it can be validated with longer follow-up periods. Informed conservative orthopedic supervision can keep the skeletal complications to a minimum. Simple immobilization is required for the acute pain episodes.

Eventual "total hip replacement" operations may be necessary for management of the late effects in adult life.

Individuals and families need considerable general support and reassurance. Trials of enzyme replacement therapy and bone marrow transplantation are of only experimental relevance at this time.

**Prognosis:** There is only a 1- to 2-year survival in the infantile form. For the chronically involved patient, however, there should be no shortening of normal life expectancy.

**Detection of Carrier:** Heterozygote identification by β-glucosidase analysis on white blood cells or cultured fibroblasts is possible in about 90% of obligatory heterozygotes.

**Support Groups:** DC; Washington; National Gaucher Foundation (NGF)

**References:**
Lee RE, et al.: Gaucher's disease: clinical, morphologic, and pathogenetic considerations. Pathol Annu 1977; 12:309–339. * †
Chiao YB, et al.: Comparison of various β-glucosidase assays used to diagnose Gaucher's disease. Clin Chim Acta 1980; 105:41–50.
Daniels LB, et al.: Normal acid phosphatase and angiotensin converting enzyme activities in serum of a patient with Gaucher's disease. Clin Chem 1981; 27:1782–1783.
Desnick RJ, et al.: Gaucher disease: a century of delineation and research. New York: Alan R. Liss, 1982.
Nakagawa S, et al.: Changes of serum hexosaminidase for the presumptive diagnosis of type I Gaucher disease in Tay-Sachs carrier screening. Am J Med Genet 1983; 14:525–532.
Wenger DA, et al.: Biochemical studies in a patient with subacute neuropathic Gaucher disease without visceral glucosylceramide storage. Ped Res 1983; 17:344–348.
Choy FYM: Gaucher disease: comparative study of acid phosphatase and glucocerebrosidase in normal and type-1 Gaucher tissues. Am J Med Genet 1985; 21:519–528.
Lanir A, et al.: Gaucher disease: assessment with MR imaging. Radiology 1986; 161:239–244. †
Rubin M, et al.: Partial splenectomy in Gaucher's disease. J Ped Surg 1986; 21:125–128.
Fabbro D, et al.: Gaucher disease: genetic heterogeneity within and among the subtypes detected by immunoblotting. Am J Hum Genet 1987; 40:15–31.
Christomanou H, et al.: N-terminal amino-acid sequence of a sphingolipid activator protein missing in a new human Gaucher disease variant. Biol Chem Hoppe-Seyler 1987; 368:1193–1196.
Sorge J, et al.: Complete correction of the enzymatic defect of type I Gaucher disease fibroblast by retroviral-mediated gene transfer. Proc Nat Acad Sci 1987; 84:906–909.
Zimran A, et al.: Prediction of severity of Gaucher's disease by identification of mutations at DNA level. Lancet 1989; II:349–352.
Zlotogora J, et al.: Gaucher disease type I and pregnancy. Am J Med Genet 1989; 32:475–477.

PH000                                            **Michel Philippart**

**Gaucher disease, acute neuronopathic (type II)**
*See GAUCHER DISEASE*
**Gaucher disease, chronic neuronopathic (type III)**
*See GAUCHER DISEASE*
**Gaucher disease, infantile cerebral (type II)**
*See GAUCHER DISEASE*
**Gaucher disease, juvenile and adult cerebral (type III)**
*See GAUCHER DISEASE*
**Gaucher disease, noncerebral juvenile (type I)**
*See GAUCHER DISEASE*
**Gc plasma protein component**
*See PLASMA, GROUP-SPECIFIC COMPONENT*
**Gehrig's disease**
*See AMYOTROPHIC LATERAL SCLEROSIS*
*also AMYOTROPHIC LATERAL SCLEROSIS, FAMILIAL ADULT AND JUVENILE TYPES*
**Gelatinous drop-like corneal dystrophy**
*See AMYLOIDOSIS, CORNEAL*

## GELEOPHYSIC DWARFISM                    2020

**Includes:**
Acrofacial dysplasia
Mucopolysaccharidosis, "focal"

**Excludes:**
**Acromicric dysplasia** (2716)
**Tricho-rhino-phalangeal syndrome**
**Tricho-rhino-phalangeal syndrome, type II** (0967)

**Major Diagnostic Criteria:** The combination of short stature, pleasant facial appearance, bone dysplasia affecting the hands and feet, hepatomegaly, and cardiac involvement.

**Clinical Findings:** The average birth weight at term is 2.7 kg, and subsequent growth is slow, resulting in short stature in all reported patients. All patients have also had upward-slanting palpebral fissures, anteverted nares, long, flat philtrum, thin vermilion, short hands and feet, and cardiac anomalies, including **Atrial septal defects**, aortic valve insufficiency, **Pulmonary valve, stenosis, Mitral valve stenosis**, and ventricular hypertrophy. Other findings include facial hirsutism, apparent hypertelorism, slight micrognathia, delayed dentition, liver enlargement, and "tight" skin. Psychomotor retardation can occur, but is not a consistent feature.

X-ray findings have included short, plump, tubular bones, particularly in the hands and feet; capital femoral epiphyses which become small and irregular after age four years; and broad ribs.

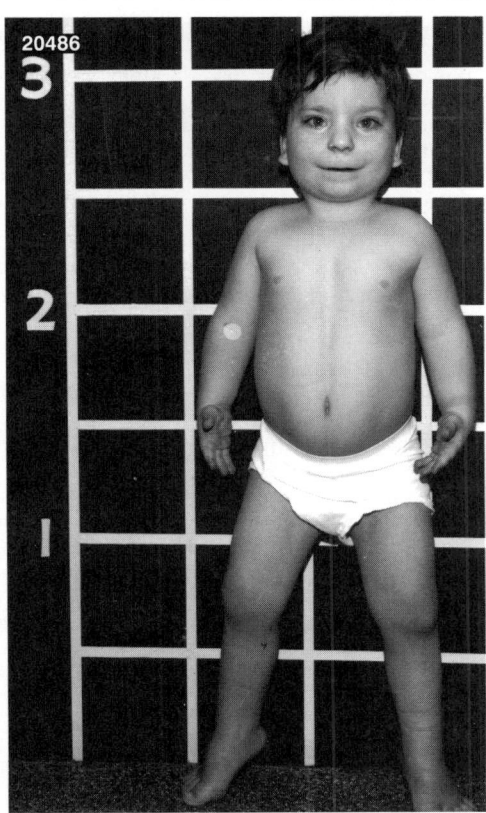

**2020A**-20486: Geleophysic dysplasia; patient at 4 years; note unusual facies, short hands and feet, and multiple joint contractures. The face has a happy appearance due to a prominent philtrum, short nose and upturned angles of the lips.

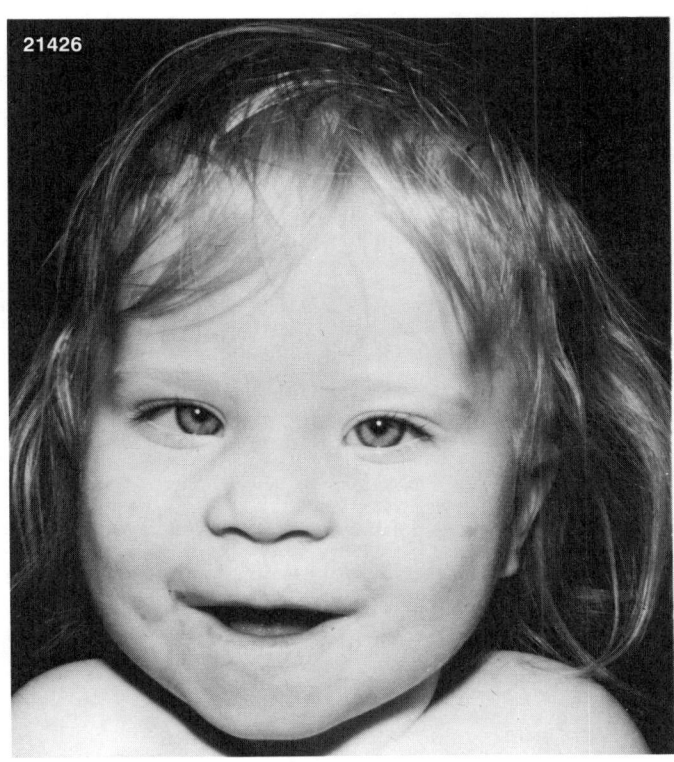

**2020B**-21426: Characteristic facies with short nose, a long upper lip, and upturned corners of the mouth.

**Complications:** Joint contractures, recurrent respiratory infections, delayed speech development (secondary to chronic otitis media) and cardiac failure are common.

**Associated Findings:** Findings each reported in only one patient include thick eyebrows, long eyelashes, low-set ears, tightly folded ears, increased anteroposterior diameter of the chest, **Hernia, umbilical**, diastasis recti, and seizures.

**Etiology:** Autosomal recessive inheritance.

**Pathogenesis:** This disorder is likely an aberration of glycoprotein metabolism, with lysosomal storage of probable glycoprotein occurring in fibroblasts of cardiac leaflets and hepatocytes, and possibly in other mesenchymal tissues.

**MIM No.:** *23105

**POS No.:** 3459

**Sex Ratio:** M1:F1

**Occurrence:** A dozen or so cases, including several sets of siblings, have been reported from widely different areas of the world.

**Risk of Recurrence for Patient's Sib:**
See Part I, *Mendelian Inheritance.*

**Risk of Recurrence for Patient's Child:**
See Part I, *Mendelian Inheritance.*

**Age of Detectability:** At birth, by noting small hands and feet.

**Gene Mapping and Linkage:** Unknown.

**Prevention:** None known. Genetic counseling indicated.

**Treatment:** Treatment of respiratory infections and cardiac disease as indicated.

**Prognosis:** Variable. Several patients are living and well in their second decade. The cause of death is usually cardiac failure, which has occurred between the ages of two and eight years. One patient was stillborn. The oldest reported living patient was 18 years of age at the time of the report.

**Detection of Carrier:** Unknown.

**Special Considerations:** Spranger et al (1984) discuss an earlier reported case of *acrofacial dysplasia, growth retardation, joint contractures, mitral valve incompetence, and focal hepatic storage of glycoprotein*. However, the facial appearance and X-ray changes were not typical of geleophysic dysplasia. This may represented a different, albeit closely related condition, although variable expression of the genetic defect causing geleophysic dysplasia could not be ruled out.

Spranger and his associates have also termed this condition a "*focal*" *mucopolysaccharidosis*, and coined the term "geleophysic" after noting the happy faces of the affected children (gelios meaning happy, and physis meaning nature).

**References:**
Spranger JW, et al.: Geleophysic dwarfism - a "focal" mucopolysaccharidosis? (letter) Lancet 1971; II:97–98.
Koiffman CP, et al.: Familial recurrence of geleophysic dysplasia. Am J Med Genet 1984; 19:483–486. †
Spranger JW, et al.: Acrofacial dysplasia resembling geleophysic dysplasia. Am J Med Genet 1984; 19:501–506.
Spranger JW, et al.: Geleophysic dysplasia. Am J Med Genet 1984; 19:487–499. †

T0007                                                    **Helga V. Toriello**

**Geminated teeth**
  *See TEETH, GEMINATED*
**Genee-Wiedemann syndrome**
  *See ACROFACIAL DYSOSTOSIS, POSTAXIAL TYPE*
**Generalized atrophic benign epidermolysis bullosa, Herlitz type**
  *See EPIDERMOLYSIS BULLOSUM, TYPE II*
**Generalized fibrosis syndrome**
  *See EYE, FIBROSIS OF THE EXTRAOCULAR MUSCLES, GENERALIZED*
**Generalized glycogenosis**
  *See GLYCOGENOSIS, TYPE IIa*
**Generalized lentigo**
  *See LENTIGINES SYNDROME, MULTIPLE*
**Genital ambiguity, pseudovaginal perineoscrotal hypospadias**
  *See STEROID 5 ALPHA-REDUCTASE DEFICIENCY*
**Genital anomaly-cardiomyopathy**
  *See CARDIOMYOPATHY-GENITAL DEFECTS*
**Genital-renal-middle ear anomalies**
  *See RENAL-GENITAL-MIDDLE EAR ANOMALIES*
**Genitalia, pigmentary changes-megalencephaly-intestinal polyposis**
  *See OVERGROWTH, RUVALCABA-MYHRE-SMITH TYPE*
**Genito-branchio-skeletal syndrome**
  *See BRANCHIO-SKELETO-GENITAL SYNDROME*
**Genito-facio-digital syndrome**
  *See AARSKOG SYNDROME*
**Genito-oculo-oligophrenic-dento-skeleto syndrome (GOODS)**
  *See BRANCHIO-SKELETO-GENITAL SYNDROME*

## GENITO-PALATO-CARDIAC SYNDROME                    2634

**Includes:** Gardner-Silengo-Wachtel syndrome

**Excludes:**
  **Campomelic dysplasia** (0122)
  **Smith-Lemli-Opitz syndrome** (0891)

**Major Diagnostic Criteria:** Male pseudohermaphroditism with micrognathia, **Cleft palate**, and conotruncal cardiac defect.

**Clinical Findings:** Male pseudohermaphroditism (12/13); **Cleft palate** (11/13); micrognathia (9/13); low-set ears (9/13); cardiac defect (7/13); conotruncal defect (4/7); **Ventricular septal defect** (3/7); prominent heels (4/13); **Microcephaly** (3/13); and neonatal death (8/10).

**Complications:** All but two cases were aborted or died in the neonatal period.

**Associated Findings:** Cleft alveolar ridge, **Cleft lip**, **Diaphragm, eventration**, **Hydrocephaly**, **Polydactyly**, and urinary tract defects.

**Etiology:** Unknown. Two affected sibs had duplication of the short arm of the X chromosome (46, dup(Xp)Y) which was inherited from the mother, suggesting a possible X-linked disorder.

**Pathogenesis:** Unknown.

**POS No.:** 4209

**Sex Ratio:** All cases have been 46,XY with all but two cases having female phenotype.

**Occurrence:** Over a dozen cases have been reported.

**Risk of Recurrence for Patient's Sib:** Unknown. Possibly 1:4 (25%).

**Risk of Recurrence for Patient's Child:** Unknown. Affected individuals are not expected to survive to reproduce.

**Age of Detectability:** Prenatally using amniocentesis and high resolution ultrasound to detect male pseudohermaphroditism and conotruncal cardiac defects.

**Gene Mapping and Linkage:** Unknown.

**Prevention:** None known. Genetic counseling indicated.

**Treatment:** Supportive.

**Prognosis:** Eight of 10 affected infants died in the newborn period.

**Detection of Carrier:** Undetermined, unless a chromosome abnormality is present.

**Special Considerations:** This disorder may be heterogeneous and may represent several different, but similar overlapping conditions. There is some overlap with **Smith-Lemli-Opitz syndrome** and with **Campomelic dysplasia**, both of which have male pseudohermaphroditism as common components. Camptomelic dysplasia can usually be distinguished by the presence of bowed femora and other skeletal defects.

Two patients in one family have had duplication of the short arm of the X chromosome suggesting the possibility of X-linkage. Thus far, nearly all cases have been genetic males with pseudohermaphroditism, which would be consistent with X-linkage. However, if pseudohermaphroditism is taken as a necessary finding, affected females may be missed.

**References:**
Wachtel SS: H-Y antigen and the biology of sex determination. New York: Grune and Stratton, 1983:224–225.
Greenberg F, et al.: The Gardner-Silengo-Wachtel or Genito-Palato-Cardiac syndrome: male pseudohermaphroditism with micrognathia, cleft palate, and conotruncal cardiac defect. Am J Med Genet 1987; 26:59–64.

GR011                                                    **Frank Greenberg**

**Genodermatose en cocarde of Degos**
  *See SKIN CREASES, RETICULATE PIGMENTED FLEXURES, DOWLING-DEGOS TYPE*
  *also SKIN, ERYTHROKERATOLYSIS HIEMALIS*
**Gentamycin, fetal effects**
  *See FETAL AMINOGLYCOSIDE OTOTOXICITY*
**Genticin^, fetal effects**
  *See FETAL AMINOGLYCOSIDE OTOTOXICITY*
**Gerbich-negative phenotype**
  *See ANEMIA, HEMOLYTIC, RED CELL MEMBRANE DEFECTS*
**Gerhardt syndrome**
  *See LARYNGEAL PARALYSIS*
  *also VOCAL CORD PARALYSIS*

## GERM CELL APLASIA 3163

**Includes:**

> Androgen insensitivity syndrome, incomplete (some)
> Del Castillo syndrome
> Sertoli-cell-only syndrome

**Excludes:**

> Five alpha-reductase deficiency
> **Gonadotropin deficiencies** (0438)
> **Gynecomastia due to increased aromatase activity, familial** (2308)
> **Hypogonadotropic hypogonadism** (2300)
> **Kallmann syndrome** (2301)
> **Klinefelter syndrome** (0556)
> **Leydig cell hypoplasia** (2298)
> Sex reversed males (46,XX)
> Testosterone biosynthesis, defects of

**Major Diagnostic Criteria:** 46,XY individuals with seminiferous tubules lacking in spermatogonia.

**Clinical Findings:** Traditionally considered phenotypically normal males who are sterile as result of seminiferous tubules lacking spermatogonia. Such testes are often smaller than normal. Tubular hyalinization and sclerosis are less common than in the Klinefelter syndrome. Leydig cell function is traditionally stated to be normal; thus, secondary sexual development is normal. Predictably, FSH is elevated, and LH is normal. However, varied expressivity is characteristic of this heterogenous syndrome. In fact, some individuals to whom the appellation has been applied show spermatozoa. Conversely, gynecomastia is not uncommon.

**Complications:** Infertility; lack of secondary sexual development in some cases.

**Associated Findings:** None known.

**Etiology:** Heterogeneous. In a few families, by X-linked recessive inheritance. Such individuals may or may not show **Androgen insensitivity syndrome, incomplete**. In other families, autosomal recessive genes produce germ cell aplasia in males and streak gonads in females. In yet other individuals the etiology is nongenetic (mumps, irradiation).

**Pathogenesis:** Although mutant gene(s) may deleteriously affect germ cell development, their mode(s) of action are unknown. Embryonic failure of germ call formation or persistence is presumed, but postnatal factors are also plausible. In some individuals the pathogenesis may involve androgen insensitivity. In nongenetic cases (mumps or irradiation) pathogenesis reflects the specific etiology; all presumably involve germ cell destruction.

**MIM No.:** 30570

**Sex Ratio:** M1:F0

**Occurrence:** Undetermined but presumably rare.

**Risk of Recurrence for Patient's Sib:** In general low, but dependent upon specific etiology.

**Risk of Recurrence for Patient's Child:** Unknown. This disorder is usually defined by sterility, making the question moot.

**Age of Detectability:** Usually at puberty because of lack of secondary sexual development.

**Gene Mapping and Linkage:** Unknown.

**Prevention:** None known. Genetic counseling indicated. Minimizing irradiation exposure may reduce forms due to that etiology. Mumps immunization.

**Treatment:** Normally virilized individuals showing azoospermia ordinarily need no treatment. However, hormonal replacement is obviously necessary if androgen deficiency exists in androgen sensitive individuals. Individuals with extreme oligospermia may be candidates for *in vitro* fertilization or other extracoital fertilization techniques that can take advantage of only a few viable sperm.

**Prognosis:** Life expectancy is presumably normal if somatic anomalies do not coexist. Affected individuals are raised as males, and develop a male sexual identity.

**Detection of Carrier:** Unknown.

**Special Considerations:** Germ cell aplasia is so heterogeneous that its existence as a distinct entity is in doubt. In addition, some authorities believe that many if not all cases merely represent **Androgen insensitivity (resistance), minimal**. Presumably, gynecomastia is an expression of androgen insensitivity in some individuals.

Of special note are five sibships, in each of which a female sib has shown germ cell failure (streak gonads) and a male sib has shown germ cell aplasia. In two (Smith et al, 1979; Granat et al, 1983), no somatic anomalies coexisted; the parents were consanguineous. In three other kindreds (Hamat et al, 1973; Al-Alwadi et al, 1985; Mikati et al, 1985) unique patterns of somatic anomalies coexisted, the coexistant somatic anomalies being variable. In aggregate, one can deduce that a number of genes are capable of producing germ cell failure in both males and females. These families suggest that germ cell aplasia should be considered more a histological condition than a distinct entity.

**References:**

Del Castillo EB, et al: Syndrome produced by absence of the germinal epithelium without impairment of the Sertoli or Leydig cells. J Clin Endocrinol 1947; 7:493–502.
Edwards JA, Bannerman RM: Familial gynecomastia. BD:OAS VII(6). New York: March of Dimes Birth Defects Foundation Birth Defects, 1971:193–195.
Hamat P, et al: Hypertension with adrenal genital, renal defects, and deafness. Arch Intern Med 1973; 131:563–569.
Smith A, et al: Three siblings with premature gonadal failure. Fertil Steril 1979; 32:528–530.
Granat M, et al: Familial gonadal germinative failure: endocrine and human leukocyte antigen studies. Fertil Steril 1983; 40:215–219.
Al-Alwadi SA, et al: Priminary hypergonadism and partial alopecia in three sibs with Mullerian hypoplasia in the affected females. Am J Med Genet 1985; 22:619–622.
Mikati MA, et al: Microcephaly, hypergonadotropic hypergonadism, short stature and minor anomalies: a new syndrome. Am J Med Genet 1985; 22:599–608.

SI018 **Joe Leigh Simpson**

**German amyloidosis**
*See AMYLOIDOSIS, ILLINOIS TYPE*
**German type amyloidosis**
*See AMYLOIDOSIS, FAMILIAL VISCERAL*
**Germinomas**
*See CNS NEOPLASMS*
**Geroderma osteodysplastica hereditaria (GOH)**
*See OSTEODYSPLASTICA GERODERMIA, BAMATTER TYPE*
**Gerodermia osteodysplastica**
*See OSTEODYSPLASTICA GERODERMIA, BAMATTER TYPE*

## GERSTMANN-STRAUSSLER SYNDROME 3245

**Includes:**

> Amyloidosis, cerebral, with spongiform encephalopathy
> Cerebellar ataxia-progressive dementia-amyloid deposits in CNS
> Encephalopathy, subacute spongiform, Gerstmann-Straussler type
> Gerstmann-Straussler-Scheinker disease
> Straussler disease
> Spinocerebellar ataxia with dementia and amyloid plaques
> Subacute spongiform encephalopathy

**Excludes:**

> **Alzheimer disease**
> **Creutzfeldt-Jakob disease** (3244)
> Kuru
> **Olivopontocerebellar atrophy**

**Major Diagnostic Criteria:** Gerstmann-Straussler Syndrome (GSS) is a rare, neurodegenerative familial disorder with onset in middle age and characterized clinically by cerebellar ataxia, progressive dementia, and absent lower extremity reflexes. Pathologically it is distinguished by extensive amyloid plaques with an unusual characteristic morphology and prion protein immuno-reactivity throughout the central nervous system.

**Clinical Findings:** Onset of clinical symptoms is usually in the fifth decade, with gait impairment or ataxia being the predominant symptom. Frequently, weakness and pain with dysesthesiae of the legs is also described. Gait difficulties gradually progress, with many patients becoming wheelchair dependent. Usually 1–2 years after the onset of gait disturbance, additional symptoms of dysarthria, scanning speech, difficulty swallowing, incoordination of all extremities, and general bradykinesia develop. Nystagmus may be seen. Deep tendon reflexes in the upper extremities are normal or hyperactive; they are absent in the lower extremities. Plantar responses are bilateral extensor. Although higher cognitive functions are initially not affected, memory impairment with a progressive dementia later supervenes, usually several years after the development of gait and cerebellar dysfunction. The course ranges from 2–10 years, from symptom onset to time of death.

Routine laboratory studies of the blood, serum, and urine are normal. Cerebrospinal fluid is usually normal, but increased protein has been reported. Neuroimaging studies (brain CT or MRI) may be normal or show mild diffuse atrophy; the usefulness of positron emission tomography (PET) is not known. EEG is generally normal. Clinical impression is supported by careful pedigree analysis of this strikingly familial disorder and confirmed by neuropathological examination of the brain. Macroscopic examination of the brain reveals only slight atrophy of the cerebrum and cerebellum; histopathological changes, however, are quite distinctive. These include plaques of several types throughout the nervous system, but most dramatic are massive multicentric amyloid and Kuru-type plaques found throughout grey and white matter, predominantly in the cerebellum. These show protease-resistant prion protein (PrP) and PrP-immunoreactivity. Systemic atrophy is seen with the spinocerebellar and corticospinal tracts and posterior columns of the spinal cord being affected. Neurofibrillary tangles are not seen. Spongiform changes occur in some cases, but are frequently mild and may be absent.

**Complications:** Seizures may be seen, but are rare.

**Associated Findings:** Congenital hip dysplasia has been described in one kindred; Parkinsonian symptoms as well as psychiatric symptoms of delusions and hallucinations have been reported.

**Etiology:** Autosomal dominant inheritance with age-dependent penetrance.

**Pathogenesis:** Although a familial disorder, GSS can also be horizontally transmitted to nonhuman primates by cerebral inoculation of brain homogenates from patients with the disease. It is now considered a prion-associated disease. The prion protein (PrP) gene on chromosome 20 is implicated in both the transmission and pathogenesis of GSS. It has recently been shown that PrP codon 102 is linked to the putative gene for GSS in two pedigrees and that substitution of leucine for proline at PrP codon 102 may lead to the development of GSS. Whether this represents a susceptibility locus, or perhaps a "mutant" gene sufficient for development of the disease is unknown.

**MIM No.:** 13744

**Sex Ratio:** M1:F1

**Occurrence:** Estimated at 1–10 per hundred million.

**Risk of Recurrence for Patient's Sib:**
See Part I, *Mendelian Inheritance.*

**Risk of Recurrence for Patient's Child:**
See Part I, *Mendelian Inheritance.*

**Age of Detectability:** Clinical onset of symptoms is between the third and sixth decades of life, generally during the fifth decade. Intra-family differences in symptom onset may be as great as 30 years.

**Gene Mapping and Linkage:** Linkage has recently been established with the PrP gene on the short arm of chromosome 20 in two unrelated pedigrees. Additionally, a mis-sense variant (sub-stitution of leucine for proline) at PrP codon 102 was found in both pedigrees.

**Prevention:** None known. Genetic counseling indicated.

**Treatment:** Unknown. Treatment is symptomatic, usually including ambulation aides. Supportive medical care, educational and supportive interventions for the family, and symptomatic treatment of complications are provided as needed.

**Prognosis:** The disease progresses over 1–10 years, from the onset of clinical symptoms to the time of death. Decreased life span is observed.

**Detection of Carrier:** Unknown. Careful pedigree analysis with neurological examination of relatives at risk may disclose early symptoms.

**Special Considerations:** Pruisner and others have investigated the role of prions in the development of a variety of diseases. Prions are transmissable pathogens that cause degenerative diseases in humans and animals (e.g. scrapie, transmissable mink encephalopathy, Kuru, CJD, GSS). Pathological features include neuronal vacuolation (spongiform changes), astrocytic proliferation and gliosis, and deposition of amyloid plaques. Westaway and colleagues' recent paper discusses the unique attributes of prion diseases which include infectious, sporadic and genetic manifestations, as well as progression to death, all in the absence of a detectable immune response. Prions are composed largely of a protein encoded by a cellular host gene, which distinguishes them from viruses. The human and mouse prion protein genes have been shown to be located on chromosomes 20 and 2, respectively, which are homologous. The PrP gene of mice is linked to a gene controlling scrapie incubation times. The PrP gene of long incubation period mice encodes a variant prion protein. An amino acid substitution has recently been genetically linked to the development of Gerstmann-Straussler syndrome. Additionally, a structural rearrangement of the PrP allele has been reported in a family with familial **Creutzfeldt-Jakob disease**. Although prion diseases resemble viral illnesses in some respects, there is compelling evidence that they are genetically controlled diseases.

**References:**

Gerstmann J, et al.: Ueber eine eigenartige hereditaer-familiaere Erkrankung des Zentralnervensystems. Z Gesamte Neurol Psych 1936; 154:736–762.

Masters CL, et al.: Creutzfeldt-Jakob disease virus isolations from the Gerstmann-Straussler syndrome with an analysis of the various forms of amyloid plaque deposition in the virus-induced spongiform encephalopathies. Brain 1981; 104:559–588.

Seitelberger F: Straussler's disease. Acta Neuropath 1981; 7:341–343.

Peiffer J: Gerstmann-Straussler's disease: atypical multiple sclerosis and carcinomas in a family of sheepbreeders. Acta Neuropath 1982; 56:87–92.

Hudson AJ, et al.: Gerstmann-Straussler-Scheinker disease with coincidental familial onset. Ann Neurol 1983; 14:670–678.

Kuzuhara S, et al.: Gerstmann-Straussler-Scheinker's disease. Ann Neurol 1983; 14:216–225.

Vinters HV, et al.: Gerstmann-Straussler-Scheinker disease: autopsy study of a familial case. Ann Neurol 1986; 20:540–543.

Collinge J, et al.: Diagnosis of Gerstmann-Straussler syndrome in familial dementia with prion protein gene analysis. Lancet 1989; II:15–17.

Hsiao K, et al.: Linkage of a prion protein missense variant to Gerstmann-Straussler syndrome. Nature 1989; 338:342–345.

Nochlin D, et al.: Familial dementia with PrP-positive amyloid plaques: a variant of Gerstmann-Straussler syndrome. Neurol 1989; 39:910–918.

Westaway D, et al.: Unraveling prion diseases through molecular genetics. Trends Neurosci 1989; 12:331–337.

EA005                                                        **Nancy Lorraine Earl**

**Gerstmann-Straussler-Scheinker disease**
*See GERSTMANN-STRAUSSLER SYNDROME*
**Gestant odontome**
*See TEETH, DENS INVAGINATUS*
**Gestational trophoblastic disease**
*See HYDATIDIFORM MOLE*

Gestational trophoblastic neoplasm
  See *HYDATIDIFORM MOLE*
Giaccai type acroosteolysis
  See *ACRO-OSTEOLYSIS, NEUROGENIC*
Giant cell chondrodysplasia
  See *ATELOSTEOGENESIS*
Giant pigmented hairy nevus (GPHN)
  See *NEVUS, CONGENITAL NEVOMELANOCYTIC*
Giedion-Langer syndrome
  See *TRICHO-RHINO-PHALANGEAL SYNDROME, TYPE II*
Giessen (AI) apolipoprolipoprotein variants
  See *HYPOALPHALIPOPROTEINEMIA*
Gigantism of cytoplasmic organelles, hereditary
  See *CHEDIAK-HIGASHI SYNDROME*
Gigantism of peroxidase granules, congenital
  See *CHEDIAK-HIGASHI SYNDROME*
Gigantism, cerebral
  See *CEREBRAL GIGANTISM*
Gigantism, hands and feet-nevi-hemihypertrophy-megalencephaly
  See *PROTEUS SYNDROME*
Gilbert syndrome
  See *HYPERBILIRUBINEMIA, UNCONJUGATED*
Gilbert-Dreyfus syndrome
  See *ANDROGEN INSENSITIVITY SYNDROME, INCOMPLETE*
Gilles de la Tourette syndrome
  See *TOURETTE SYNDROME*
Gillespie syndrome
  See *ANIRIDIA-CEREBELLAR ATAXIA-MENTAL DEFICIENCY*
Gingival cyst of the newborn
  See *MUCOSA, ORAL INCLUSION CYSTS OF THE NEWBORN*

---

## GINGIVAL FIBROMATOSIS 0407

**Includes:** Fibromatosis, gingival

**Excludes:**
  Dilantin and other causes of gingival enlargement
  **Fibromatosis, juvenile hyaline** (0411)
  Gingival dystrophy
  **Gingival fibromatosis-deafness, Jones types** (2315)
  **Gingival fibromatosis-digital anomalies** (0409)
  **Gingival fibromatosis-hypertrichosis** (0410)
  **Gingival fibromatosis-depigmentation-microphthalmia** (0413)
  Gingival fibromatosis, symmetric
  **Gingival multiple hamartoma syndrome** (0412)

**Major Diagnostic Criteria:** Hard, firm, noninflammatory enlargement of all of the gingivae. All of the gingivae usually involved at some stage in this disease. Early at the initiation of the enlargement, only a portion of the gingivae around erupting teeth may be involved or after surgical removal, recurrences may initially be localized. Local gingival fibromatosis has been observed in sibs and relatives in what appears to be a recessive form of the disease. Symmetric gingival fibromatosis usually involves only the molar area bilaterally, has its onset after 12 years of age, is generally less firm than gingival fibromatosis and is nonfamilial in most reported examples.

**Clinical Findings:** Generalized gingival enlargement involves all of the gingivae in both jaws. The gums are hard, firm and of normal color and have a normal or accentuated stippling resembling an orange peel. The gums may be smooth or partially lobulated around the necks of teeth. All teeth may be completely covered by the tissue, but more frequently the crowns are partly exposed. In untreated cases the gingivae may reach enormous size and protrude from mouth. The teeth may undergo root resorption within the gingiva.

Genetic heterogeneity exists. Dilantin^, lesions of the diencephalon, certain blood and endocrine disorders may have generalized gingival enlargement which follows the onset of these conditions. Has been reported in Caucasians and American Negroes.

**Complications:** Interference with tooth eruption and exfoliation. Difficulties in chewing, swallowing, speech and respiration. Drooling with secondary ulceration of extruded gingivae and lips. Gingival infection and dentigerous cysts develop around unerupted teeth.

**Associated Findings:** None. There is no statistically higher risk for oligophrenia or epilepsy in cases with only gingival fibromatosis. However, when accompanied by *hypertrichosis* the risk for these defects is considerable.

**Etiology:** Autosomal dominant inheritance. Approximately 80% of reported cases are familial and 20% reported as isolated cases or familial history not investigated.

**Pathogenesis:** Initiating event not fully understood but gingival enlargement is intimately associated with the presence of erupted teeth. As either the primary teeth, the secondary teeth or both begin to erupt there is a progressive enlargement of the gingivae. In most but not all cases, extraction of the teeth causes a regression and disappearance of the gingival lesion. Histologically, the tissue is composed of dense mature hyperplastic and hypertrophic collagen bundles in the lamina propria and submucosa. Evidence for inflammatory elements is absent or scanty foci of chronic inflammatory infiltrate are found between bundles of connective tissue or localized to secondarily traumatized or infected areas. The condition has been compared to a keloid as an overresponse of gingival connective tissue to the trauma of tooth eruption and erupted teeth.

**MIM No.:** 13530

**Sex Ratio:** M63:F73 (observed)

**Occurrence:** Thirty-six kindreds reported with about 136 affected members.

**Risk of Recurrence for Patient's Sib:**
  See Part I, *Mendelian Inheritance.*

**Risk of Recurrence for Patient's Child:**
  See Part I, *Mendelian Inheritance.*

**Age of Detectability:** At time of eruption of teeth. Approximately 50% begin at the eruption of primary teeth 6 months to 3 years and 50% at the time of eruption of the permanent teeth 5 to 12 years. Those that have their onset during eruption of the primary teeth also have involvement of the permanent dentition.

**Gene Mapping and Linkage:** Unknown.

**Prevention:** None known. Genetic counseling indicated.

**Treatment:** Conservative treatment should be tried first consisting of gingivectomy followed by good oral hygiene. Many cases tend to recur. These refractory cases can be treated by extraction of all teeth and gingivectomy. Prosthetic replacement of teeth may be necessary.

**Prognosis:** Good. Normal life span.

**Detection of Carrier:** Unknown.

**References:**
Rushton MA: Hereditary or idiopathic hyperplasia of the gums. Dent Practit 1957; 7:136–146.
Witkop CJ Jr: Heterogeneity in gingival fibromatosis. BD:OAS; VII(7). New York: March of Dimes Birth Defects Foundation, 1971:210–221. *
Jorgenson RJ, Cocker ME: Variation in the inheritance and expression of gingival fibromatosis. J Periodontol 1974; 45:472–477.

WI043                                        **Carl J. Witkop, Jr.**

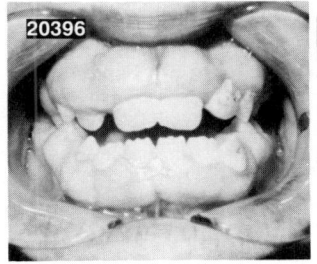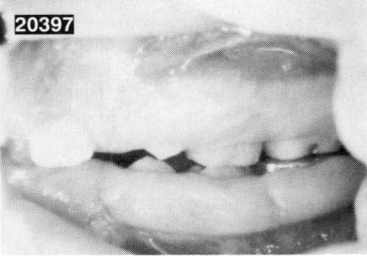

**0407-20396–97:** Gingival fibromatosis.

## GINGIVAL FIBROMATOSIS-CHERUBISM-SEIZURES, RAMON TYPE
**2610**

**Includes:**
> Cherubism-gingival fibromatosis-epilepsy-hypertrichosis
> Epilepsy-gingival fibromatosis-cherubism
> Ramon syndrome
> Ramon syndrome-juvenile Rheumatoid arthritis

**Excludes:**
> **Cherubism** (0539)

> **Fibromatosis, juvenile hyaline** (0411)
> **Gingival fibromatosis** (0407)
> **Gingival fibromatosis-corneal dystrophy** (0408)
> **Gingival fibromatosis-deafness, Jones types** (2315)
> **Gingival fibromatosis-depigmentation-microphthalmia** (0413)
> **Gingival fibromatosis-digital anomalies** (0409)
> **Gingival fibromatosis-hypertrichosis** (0410)
> **Gingival multiple hamartoma syndrome** (0412)

**Major Diagnostic Criteria:** The mildest form includes only gingival fibromatosis (with narrow palate and impacted teeth as secondary features) associated with mild mental deficiency. The full form includes gingival fibromatosis, mild mental deficiency, cherubism, partial epilepsy with secondary generalization, fibrous dysplasia of the mandible, retarded postnatal growth, moderate hypertrichosis, and juvenile **Arthritis, rheumatoid.** Electroencephalography is frequently abnormal; X-ray examination of the maxillary bones may reveal characteristic fibrous dysplasia, and rheumatic activity tests may be abnormal.

**Clinical Findings:** In most cases (5/6), clinical signs and symptoms manifest in the first year of life. The initial symptoms are variable. In some patients (3/6) the first signs of the syndrome are neuromotor retardation and delayed dental eruption due to gingival fibromatosis. In others (2/6) the first signs are convulsive seizures between 8–10 months of age. Only one patient has shown the first signs when of school age, i.e. gingival hypertrophy at age seven years and difficulty in learning. Excess gingival growth progresses slowly, leading to difficulty in closing the mouth, in addition to delayed dental eruption (which may occur as early as age four years), with many teeth remaining impacted. The fibrous dysplasia of the maxillae leads to enlargement of lower half of face, with a cherubic look (cherubism) occurring between ages three and six years. The convulsive seizures, which may start in the first year of life (2/6), but which may also appear as late as 30 months of age, are characterized as being of a partial type, with secondary generalization. Usually these are of benign evolution (4/5). In one of patient, however, the seizures could not be controlled with medication and evolved into myoclonic epilepsy.

All patients show difficulty in learning and mild mental retardation. Even though birth weight and height are normal, retarda-

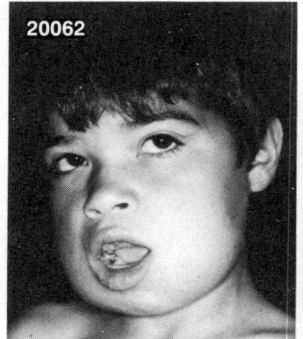
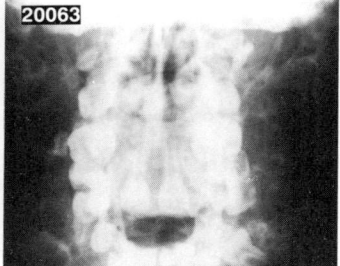

**2610-20062:** Note the cherubic facies, open mouth and gingival hypertrophy. **20063:** Note the "soap bubble" infiltration of a multilocular type with bone insufflation.

tion of physical growth may occur. In some patients (3/6) a clinical and laboratory picture of juvenile rheumatoid arthritis manifested during adolescence (between age 12 and 14 years). The clinical picture of the syndrome consists of 12 signs: mild mental retardation (6/6); gingival fibromatosis (5/6) with delayed dental eruption, impacted teeth, and narrow palate, occurring as secondary phenomena; partial epilepsy with secondary generalization (5/6), with the possibility of myoclonic epilepsy (1/6); cherubism (5/6), with characteristic maxillary fibrotic dysplasia (5/6); retarded postnatal growth (4/5); moderate hypertrichosis (3/6); and juvenile rheumatoid arthritis (3/6). In only one patient (belonging to the family reported by Ramon et al, 1967) was a wide fontanelle detected, persisting at age nine years.

Wide intrafamilial variability is possible, since in the family described by Ramon et al (1967) one of the patients showed only four of the 12 signs described (gingival hypertrophy, impacted teeth, delayed dentition and mental retardation), whereas his affected brother showed 11 of the 12 signs. On the other hand, despite the variable expressivity of the syndrome most patients (5/6) present with at least 9 of the 12 signs.

The EEG examination is characterized by disorganization and symmetrical or asymmetrical irregularity of background activity (4/4), by the presence of isolated spike-wave patterns in the R frontal region (1/4), or by the presence of diffuse bursts of slow spike-waves and slow polyspikewaves of 2–3 Hz, which are irregular but synchronous, asymmetrical and of sharp predominance in the left hemisphere (1/4).

X-rays of the face show the presence of a "soap bubble" infiltrating lesion of a multilocular type causing considerable bone distention with thinning of the cortical layer in both mandibular rami and in the maxillae (5/6).

A gingival biopsy specimen showed a similar aspect in all cases studied (3/6), with alterations of the epithelium and of the connective tissue. The epithelium was hyperplastic. The dermal papillae were long and thin and had a net-like appearance when cut transversally. Keratinization was of variable thickness. The lamina propria consisted of dense connective tissue that was rich in collagen, poor in blood vessels and showed a moderate number of fibroblasts. In the deeper zones of the lamina propria and in areas where the epithelial network was present, the collagen fibers were arranged in whorls or round clumps compressing the fibroblasts, which were of variable shapes. The blood vessels appeared like narrow slits with their lumens compressed by collagen.

Biopsy showed that the mandibular bony lesions were composed of soft tissue of variegated appearance. The striking feature of the connective tissue was the rearrangement of the collagen fibers in a characteristic halo around small blood vessels, very similar in appearance to the collagen arrangement found in the gingivae.

In the patients who developed juvenile rheumatoid arthritis, the test for C-reactive protein was positive and mucoprotein measurement showed elevated levels, whereas the result of the latex test was negative. These tests may be altered even in the absence of clinical and X-ray signs of rheumatoid arthritis.

**Complications:** Delayed dental eruption, gingival bleeding after small injuries, difficulty in closing the mouth because of the slow and continuous gingival growth, with gingivectomy becoming necessary at different times in life. The patients have difficulty in adapting to school and social activities, although they are well adapted to family routine. The patients with rheumatoid arthritis eventually become unable to walk and develop articular deformities. Even though in most patients the convulsive seizures are of benign evolution, it is possible that they may not be controlled even with the use of anticonvulsive drugs, with progression toward myoclonic and even grand mal epilepsy.

**Associated Findings:** Wide and persistent fontanelle was described in one patient.

**Etiology:** Autosomal recessive inheritance with variability in expression.

**Pathogenesis:** Unknown. The lesions detected in the connective tissue of the gingivae and of the maxillary bones are similar.

**MIM No.:** 26627

**POS No.:** 4211

**Sex Ratio:** M1:F1

**Occurrence:** Six cases from two families have been observed: one of Sephardic Jewish origin of Syrian parentage, and the other from a Brazilian rural zone and of Latin European origin.

**Risk of Recurrence for Patient's Sib:**
See Part I, *Mendelian Inheritance.*

**Risk of Recurrence for Patient's Child:**
See Part I, *Mendelian Inheritance.*

**Age of Detectability:** The first year of life for most patients (5/6). However, the syndrome may also manifest at school age.

**Gene Mapping and Linkage:** Unknown.

**Prevention:** None known. Genetic counseling indicated.

**Treatment:** Anticonvulsive drugs, gingivectomy, special education. Anti-inflammatory drugs for patients with arthritis.

**Prognosis:** Normal life span. Mental deficiency.

**Detection of Carrier:** Unknown. Heterozygotes do not show the signs and symptoms of the syndrome.

**References:**
Ramon Y, et al.: Gingival fibromatosis combined with cherubism. Oral Surg Oral Pathol 1967; 24:436–448.
Pina-Neto JM, et al.: Cherubism, gingival fibromatosis, epilepsy, and mental deficiency (Ramon syndrome) with juvenile rheumatoid arthritis. Am J Med Genet 1986; 25:433–441.

DE035                                    **João M. de Pina-Neto**

## GINGIVAL FIBROMATOSIS-CORNEAL DYSTROPHY        0408

**Includes:**
Corneal dystrophy-gum hypertrophy
Corneal dystrophy-poor eruption of teeth-gingival fibromatosis
Corneal opacities-gingival fibromatosis
Gingival fibromatosis-poor eruption of teeth-corneal dystrophy
Gingival hypertrophy-corneal dystrophy
Rutherfurd syndrome
Teeth, poor eruption-corneal dystrophy-gingival fibromatosis

**Excludes:**
Fibromatosis, juvenile hyaline (0411)
Gingival fibromatosis (0407)
Gingival fibromatosis, symmetric
Gingival fibromatosis-depigmentation-microphthalmia (0413)
Gingival fibromatosis-digital anomalies (0409)
Gingival fibromatosis-hypertrichosis (0410)
Gingival multiple hamartoma syndrome (0412)

**Major Diagnostic Criteria:** The presence of gingival fibromatosis and curtain-like corneal opacities affecting the upper half of the eye.

**Clinical Findings:** Generalized dense fibrotic enlarged gingivae cover the teeth which fail to erupt. Both primary and secondary teeth may be embedded within the fibrotic gums during the period of mixed dentition with root resorption of the primary teeth occurring within the gums. A few teeth of either dentition may erupt and be visible in the mouth and are frequently hypoplastic being peg- or cone-shaped. Curtain-like corneal opacities involve the superior portion of each cornea; the lower portion of the eye is usually spared. Complete visual loss due to vascularization of cornea occurs in the fifth decade.

**Complications:** Tooth fragments from incomplete exfoliation may remain within the gingivae. Dentigerous cysts and gingival infections. Loss of vision.

**Associated Findings:** Possibly oligophrenia. Two affected kindred members were also mentally retarded. Skull asymmetry and undescended testes noted in one infant.

**Etiology:** Autosomal dominant inheritance.

**Pathogenesis:** Undetermined. Dense fibrotic gingivae are present in infancy and primary teeth fail to erupt. The secondary dentition fails to appear but by X-rays full primary dentition undergoing root resorption may be present. Corneal opacities involving the upper portion of the eye vascularize with age.

**MIM No.:** *18090

**POS No.:** 4260

**Sex Ratio:** M1:F1

**Occurrence:** Reported by Rutherfurd in one English kindred with seven affected members. The same kindred was re-examined by Houston and Shotts (1966).

**Risk of Recurrence for Patient's Sib:**
See Part I, *Mendelian Inheritance.*

**Risk of Recurrence for Patient's Child:**
See Part I, *Mendelian Inheritance.*

**Age of Detectability:** Early infancy by clinically noting gingival fibromatosis and corneal opacities.

**Gene Mapping and Linkage:** Unknown.

**Prevention:** None known. Genetic counseling indicated.

**Treatment:** Gingivectomy, surgical removal of cysts.

**Prognosis:** Good except for visual defect. Probably does not affect longevity significantly. Patients have survived to sixth decade.

**Detection of Carrier:** Unknown.

**References:**
Rutherfurd ME: Three generations of inherited dental defect. Br Med J 1931; 2:9–11. †
Houston IB, Shotts N: Rutherfurd's syndrome; a familial oculodental disorder. Acta Paediatr Scand 1966; 55:233–238. †
Witkop CJ Jr: Heterogeneity in gingival fibromatosis. BD:OAS;VII(7). Baltimore: Williams & Wilkins, 1971:210–221.

WI043                                    **Carl J. Witkop, Jr.**

## GINGIVAL FIBROMATOSIS-DEAFNESS, JONES TYPES        2315

**Includes:**
Deafness-gingival fibromatosis
Fibromatosis, gingival-progressive deafness
Gingival fibromatosis-sensorineural hearing loss
Jones syndrome

**Excludes:**
Fibromatosis, juvenile hyaline (0411)
Gingival fibromatosis (0407)
Gingival fibromatosis-corneal dystrophy (0408)
Gingival fibromatosis-depigmentation-microphthalmia (0413)
Gingival fibromatosis-digital anomalies (0409)
Gingival fibromatosis-hypertrichosis (0410)
Phenytoin and other causes of gingival enlargement, effects of

**Major Diagnostic Criteria:** Gingival fibromatosis with progressive sensorineural hearing loss in an individual or family history of progressive sensorineural hearing loss.

**Clinical Findings:** Generalized gingival hyperplasia with possible delay in clinical eruption of the primary and secondary dentition. A sloping sensorineural hearing loss of 30–70 dB between 1,000–8,000 HZ may become symptomatic in the latter part of the second decade. A mild (20–40 dB), sloping hearing loss between 4,000–8,000 HZ was noted in the left ear of a 10-year-old girl. Her right ear had borderline acuity. Hearing loss was also noted in a 10-year-old male in another family, indicating that the hearing deficiency in this syndrome may be detectable in childhood. Of the 39 reported individuals, 15 had gingival fibromatosis only, while 24 had gingival fibromatosis and hearing loss.

**Complications:** Gingival hyperplasia may delay tooth eruption, render good oral hygiene difficult, and impair mastication.

**Associated Findings:** None known.

**Etiology:** Autosomal dominant inheritance.

**Pathogenesis:** Unknown.

**MIM No.:** *13555

**POS No.:** 3578

**Sex Ratio:** Approximately M2:F1.

**Occurrence:** Two families have been documented.

**Risk of Recurrence for Patient's Sib:**
See Part I, *Mendelian Inheritance.*

**Risk of Recurrence for Patient's Child:**
See Part I, *Mendelian Inheritance.*

**Age of Detectability:** As young as 10 years for the hearing loss, 1–3 years for evidence of delayed eruption of the primary dentition. The presence of gingival fibromatosis in a kindred should alert the clinician to a possible sensorineural hearing loss.

**Gene Mapping and Linkage:** Unknown.

**Prevention:** None known. Genetic counseling indicated.

**Treatment:** Gingivectomy to expose the crowns of the teeth. Lip reading or a hearing aid may be needed in middle age.

**Prognosis:** Normal life span and intelligence. Variable for auditory function.

**Detection of Carrier:** Unknown.

**Special Considerations:** Repeated gingivectomies may be necessary to insure exposure of the crowns of the teeth. Excessive pain or bleeding tendency are not usually encountered during surgery. The gingival overgrowth appears to be associated with the presence of the teeth and may not occur in their absence. Observed delayed tooth eruption suggests a change in the alveolar mucosa prior to tooth eruption.

**References:**

Jones G, et al.: Familial gingival fibromatosis associated with progressive deafness in five generations of a family. BD:OAS XIII(3B). New York: March of Dimes Birth Defects Foundation 1977:195–201.

Hartsfield JK Jr, et al.: Gingival fibromatosis with sensorineural hearing loss: an autosomal dominant trait. Am J Med Gen 1985; 22:623–627.

HA069
PA047

James K. Hartsfield, Jr.
Raj-Rajendra A. Patel

## GINGIVAL FIBROMATOSIS-DEPIGMENTATION-MICROPHTHALMIA     0413

**Includes:**
> Athetosis-gingival fibromatosis-depigmentation-microphthalmia
> Cross syndrome
> Depigmentation-gingival fibromatosis-microphthalmia
> Kramer syndrome
> Microphthalmia-gingival fibromatosis-depigmentation
> Oculocerebral syndrome with hypopigmentation
> Oligophrenia-gingival fibromatosis-depigmentation-microphthalmia

**Excludes:**
> **Fibromatosis, juvenile hyaline** (0411)
> **Gingival fibromatosis** (0407)
> Gingival fibromatosis, symmetric
> **Gingival fibromatosis-corneal dystrophy** (0408)
> **Gingival fibromatosis-deafness, Jones types** (2315)
> **Gingival fibromatosis-digital anomalies** (0409)
> **Gingival fibromatosis-hypertrichosis** (0410)
> **Gingival multiple hamartoma syndrome** (0412)

**Major Diagnostic Criteria:** Depigmentation, microphthalmia, oligophrenia, athetosis, and gingival fibromatosis. No information is available on the absence of one or more of these signs as possible variations in expressivity in this syndrome because all reported patients so far have shown the full clinical syndrome.

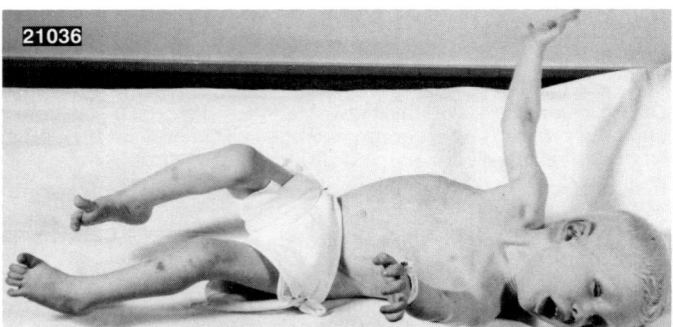

**0413A-**21036: Three-year-old male with gingival fibromatosis, depigmentation, and microphthalmia showing exaggerated Moro reflex and extended toes.

**Clinical Findings:** Gingival fibromatosis and a high-arched palate, constricted in the bicuspid region are found in conjunction with severe oligophrenia in children with athetosis, depigmentation and microphthalmia. Children have depigmentation at birth and small eyes, with coarse, jerky horizontal nystagmus. Diffuse, dense corneal opacities become heavily vascularized with spastic ectropion and injected palpebral conjunctivae. Head size is normal but dolichocephalic. By three months of age random athetoid movements, constant sucking sounds and weak high-pitched cry are noted and developmental parameters such as head holding, sitting and walking are not reached. Hyperextension of head and flexion contractures of limbs, shoulders and hips develop in late infancy. Exaggerated deep tendon reflexes and extensor plantar responses are present. Grasp and sucking reflexes are retained into childhood. No clonus is elicited. Children do not respond to sound or light. Depigmentation of all of the skin and hair is present and the hair shaft is thin. Hair bulbs have a decreased number of melanocytes with clumps of melanosomes within

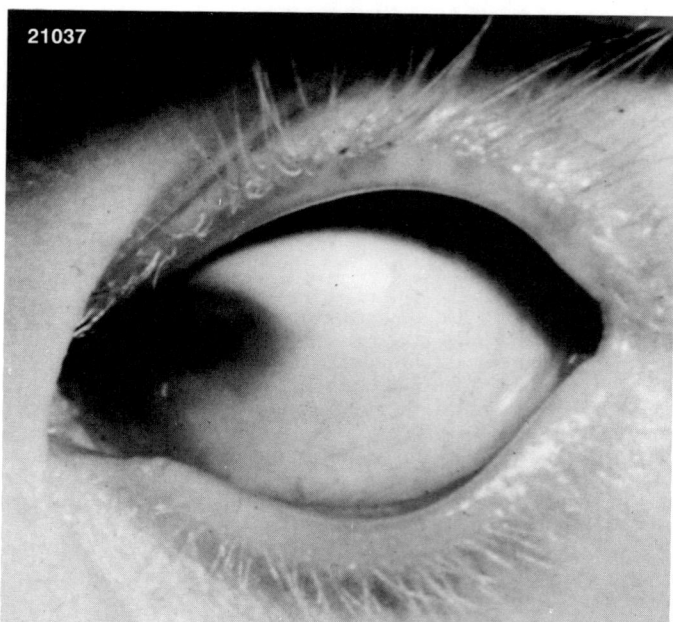

**0413B-**21037: Small globe, hypopigmented lashes and irregular scleralization of the cornea is evident.

melanocyte cytoplasm. The hair bulb tyrosine test is weakly positive showing tyrosinase is present. Melanocytes are seen arranged in a pinion gear fashion within the hair bulbs. Limited clinical and laboratory investigations have been done in this disease. The following tests were found normal: routine blood, urine, electroencephalogram, urine chromatography, fasting serum phenylalanine and tyrosine, cerebrospinal fluid glucose, protein, cells, lactic dehydrogenase and karyotype. One child had steep basilar angle compatible with compensated hydrocephaly on skull radiographs.

**Complications:**  Erythrodermia on even brief exposure to sunlight. Generalized sequelae of severe oligophrenia with institutionalization, growth and weight retardation, flexion contractures, underdeveloped secondary sex characteristics.

**Associated Findings:**  Cutaneous syndactyly 2nd-3rd toes, osseous thinning, hypochromic anemia, neutropenia, deafness.

**Etiology:**  Autosomal recessive inheritance.

**Pathogenesis:**  Unknown.

**MIM No.:**  *25780

**POS No.:**  3178

**Sex Ratio:**  Presumably M1:F1

**Occurrence:**  Three families reported.

**Risk of Recurrence for Patient's Sib:**
See Part I, *Mendelian Inheritance.*

**Risk of Recurrence for Patient's Child:**  Affected individuals are not expected to survive to reproduce.

**Age of Detectability:**  Neonatal period to early infancy by physical examination.

**Gene Mapping and Linkage:**  Unknown.

**Prevention:**  None known. Genetic counseling indicated.

**Treatment:**  Nursing care, protection from sunlight.

**Prognosis:**  Reduced life span. Three affected children died by age 10 years.

**Detection of Carrier:**  Unknown.

**References:**
Cross HE, et al.: A new oculocerebral syndrome with hypopigmentation. J Pediatr 1967; 70:398–406.
Passarge E, Fuchs-Mecke S: Oculocerebral syndrome with hypopigmentation. BD:OAS:I(2). Baltimore: Williams & Wilkins, 1971:466–467.
Witkop CJ Jr, et al.: Classification of albinism in man. BD:OAS;VII(8). Baltimore: Willaims & Wilkins, 1971:13.
Preus M, et al.: An oculocerebral hypopigmentation syndrome. J Génét Hum 1983; 31:323–328.

CRO12                                      **Harold E. Cross**
WI043                                      **Carl J. Witkop, Jr.**

---

## GINGIVAL FIBROMATOSIS-DIGITAL ANOMALIES          0409

**Includes:**
Digital anomalies-gingival fibromatosis-hepatosplenomegaly
Ear, nose, digital anomalies-gingival fibromatosis
Hepatosplenomegaly-gingival fibromatosis-digital anomalies
Laband syndrome
Nose, ear, digital anomalies-gingival fibromatosis
Phalangeal hypoplasia-gingival fibromatosis
Splenomegaly-gingival fibromatosis-digital anomalies
Zimmermann-Laband syndrome

**Excludes:**
**Deafness-onycho-osteo-dystrophy-retardation-seizures (DOORS)** (0262)
**Fibromatosis, juvenile hyaline** (0411)
**Gingival fibromatosis** (all others)
Gingival fibromatosis, symmetric
Gingival enlargement, other causes
**Gingival multiple hamartoma syndrome** (0412)

**Major Diagnostic Criteria:**  Gingival fibromatosis associated with soft bulky cartilage of the nose and ears, distal phalangeal dysplasia with nail absence or dysplasia, other skeletal anomalies and occasionally hepatosplenomegaly, mental retardation, and epilepsy.

**Clinical Findings:**  Development of gingival fibromatosis begins in childhood, usually with the eruption of primary teeth. Facial features include a narrow facies with hypertrophy of the soft tissue of the lips, tongue, nose and ears which progresses from mid-childhood through adolescence. Nail dysplasia or absence of nails is noted at birth. Characteristically, the thumbs and great toes are involved, although other nails and multiple distal phalangeal dysplasia has been described. The fingers demonstrate a "tree-frog-like" appearance. X-rays of the hands show shortened tubular bones, abnormally tapered and bulbous distal phalanges with enlargement of the bases of the terminal phalanges. Small and large joint hypermobility and arachnodactyly have been described in most reported cases.

**Complications:**  Massive overgrowth of gingiva has resulted in malocclusion, salivation with secondary lesions at commissures of lips, defects of mastication, speech and swallowing, exfoliation of teeth, secondary infections of gingivae, protrusion of lips with xerostomia. Hepatosplenomegaly has led to misdiagnosis of anemia and tumor. Joint dislocation may occur rarely. Splenomegaly may lead to hypersplenism.

**Associated Findings:**  One patient had giant oral melanotic nevus of palate and buccal mucosa. Rarely; seizures, pes cavus, and hypertrichosis.

**Etiology:**  Usually autosomal dominant inheritance. No affected parent in the cases of two carefully examined patients. Chromosomes found to be normal.

**Pathogenesis:**  Histological studies show increased amounts of mature collagenous connective tissue in submucosa and lamina propria of the gingiva and increased fibrous tissue in portal tracts.

**MIM No.:**  *13550

**Sex Ratio:**  M1:F1

**Occurrence:**  About 20 cases reported. Has been reported in persons of East Indian ancestry from India and West Indies most frequently, but it is also known in isolated cases in Caucasians. No cases among Mongoloids, Capoids, Australoids or Congoids reported.

**Risk of Recurrence for Patient's Sib:**
See Part I, *Mendelian Inheritance.*

**Risk of Recurrence for Patient's Child:**
See Part I, *Mendelian Inheritance.*

**Age of Detectability:**  Early infancy by clinical and X-ray examination of terminal phalanges and noting nose and ear defects. All signs of syndrome may not be present until eruption of teeth at 2–3 years of age.

**Gene Mapping and Linkage:**  Unknown.

**Prevention:**  None known. Genetic counseling indicated.

**Treatment:**  Good oral hygiene delays onset and reduces severity of gingival lesions. Excision of gingival tissue with pressure packs and good oral hygiene. May recur despite treatment.

**Prognosis:**  Not known if hepatosplenomegaly contributes to decreased longevity. Persons with trait have survived to sixth decade. There is a risk of mental retardation which was present in half the cases reported.

**Detection of Carrier:**  Unknown.

**References:**
Zimmermann: Uber anomalien des ektoderms. Vjschr Zahnheilk 1928; 44:419–434.
Läwen (Königsberg): Chirurgische demonstrationen. Demonstration von Bildern eines Falles von Elephantiasis gingivae (diffuse zahnfleischfibromatose, gingivitis hypertrophica, diffuse fibromatose entartung der gingiva) bei einem 15 jahrigen Jungen. Zentralbl Chir 1929; 56:626–629.
Laband PF, et al.: Hereditary gingival fibromatosis: report of an

affected family with associated splenomegaly and skeletal and soft tissue abnormalities. Oral Surg 1964; 17:339–351. †

Alvandar G: Elephantiasis gingivae. J All India Dent Assoc 1965; 37:349–353.

Witkop CJ Jr: Heterogeneity in gingival fibromatosis. BD:OAS;VII(7). New York: March of Dimes Birth Defects Foundation, 1971:210–221. †

Oikawa K, Cavaglia AMV: Laband syndrome: report of a case. J Oral Surg 1979; 37:120–122.

Chodirker BN, et al.: Zimmermann-Laband syndrome and profound mental retardation. Am J Med Genet 1986; 25:543–547.

WI043                                          **Carl J. Witkop, Jr.**
CH030                                          **Albert E. Chudley**

## GINGIVAL FIBROMATOSIS-HYPERTRICHOSIS    0410

**Includes:**

   Hair, excessive-gingival enlargement
   Hirsutism-gingival enlargement
   Hypertrichosis-gingival fibromatosis

**Excludes:**

   **Fibromatosis, juvenile hyaline** (0411)
   Gingival fibromatosis, symmetric
   **Gingival fibromatosis-corneal dystrophy** (0408)
   **Gingival fibromatosis-depigmentation-microphthalmia** (0413)
   **Gingival fibromatosis-digital anomalies** (0409)
   **Gingival multiple hamartoma syndrome** (0412)
   Other causes of gingival hyperplasia

**Major Diagnostic Criteria:**   Gingival enlargement with hirsutism.

**Clinical Findings:**   Hypertrichosis is noted first, usually within the first 2 years of life. The child develops excessive hair on head, face and body which tends to be black even in blond families. Enlargement of the gingiva is usually noted when teeth fail to appear on schedule. The patient has a slowly progressive firm fibrotic enlargement of gums which are covered with normal appearing mucosa, often showing normal "orange peel" stippling, which, in untreated cases may fill oral cavity and protrude from mouth. A few teeth may erupt only to be recovered by the expanding gingival tissue or the teeth may exfoliate prematurely. About one-half of children also have epileptic attacks or oligophrenia.

**Complications:**   Interference with chewing, respiration and speech. Failure of eruption or exfoliation of teeth. Periodontal

abscesses. Xerostomia and dribbling of saliva from mouth. Trauma to tongue and body secondary to epileptic seizures.

**Associated Findings:**   Patients with gingival fibromatosis and hypertrichosis have a high risk for epilepsy and oligophrenia in contrast to those patients with gingival fibromatosis without hirsutism. About one-half (22/52) reported cases have had either oligophrenia or epilepsy or both.

**Etiology:**   Usually autosomal dominant inheritance. Approximately one-fourth of the reported cases (12/52) have been sporadic with no family history.

All reported cases have been in Caucasians. There was one Filipino case. A recessive form may exist as several families have had sibs but not parents affected. It is in these nonfamilial cases where oligophrenia and epilepsy occur most frequently. It is not known if this is really a different entity from **Gingival multiple hamartoma syndrome** which it may resemble, especially before the age of onset of the breast lesions in a girl showing few of the signs associated with fibroadenoma syndrome. Family history and associated defects are important in distinguishing the two conditions.

**Pathogenesis:**   Undetermined. Gingival overgrowth with proliferation and hypertrophy of collagen fibers develops about the time of eruption of primary teeth. Anticonvulsive drugs have been reported to cause a phenocopy.

**MIM No.:**   13540

**POS No.:**   3323

**Sex Ratio:**   M1:F1

**Occurrence:**   Less than 60 cases reported.

**Risk of Recurrence for Patient's Sib:**
   See Part I, *Mendelian Inheritance.*

**Risk of Recurrence for Patient's Child:**
   See Part I, *Mendelian Inheritance.*

**Age of Detectability:**   Nearly all cases noted before two years of age. Most diagnosed before one year of age.

**Gene Mapping and Linkage:**   Unknown.

**Prevention:**   None known. Genetic counseling indicated.

**Treatment:**   Surgical excision with pressure dressings should be tried first. Many patients have recurrence. Extraction of teeth and gingivectomy usually prevent the recurrence of the gingival lesions except in very rare instances. Dilantin^ or other epileptic controlling therapy. Depilatory treatment for hirsutism. Full denture prosthesis, special education may be necessary if oligophrenia is present.

**Prognosis:**   Data on longevity not available. For gingival fibromatosis, excellent with adequate treatment; for epilepsy, fair with therapy; for oligophrenia, poor.

**Detection of Carrier:**   Unknown.

**References:**

Byars LT, Sarnat BG: Congenital macrogingivae (fibromatosis gingivae) and hypertrichosis. Am J Orthodont 1945; 31:48–51. *

Witkop CJ Jr: Heterogeneity in gingival fibromatosis. BD:OAS;VII(7). Baltimore: Williams and Wilkins, Dimes, 1971:210–221. †

Jorgenson RJ, Cocker ME: Variation in the inheritance and expression of gingival fibromatosis. J Periodontol 1974; 45:472–477.

Horning GM, et al.: Gingival fibromatosis with hypertrichosis: a case report. J Periodontol 1985; 56:344–347.

WI043                                          **Carl J. Witkop, Jr.**

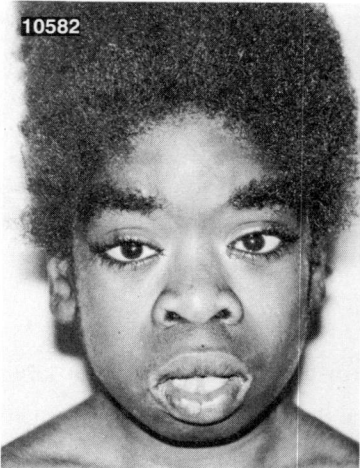
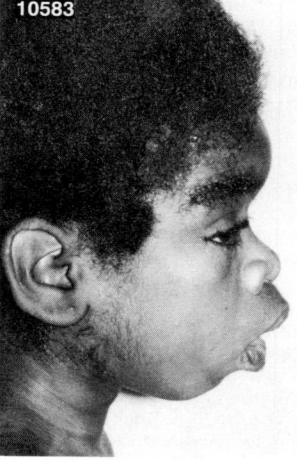

**0410**-10582–83:   Hypertrichosis and lip protrusion secondary to gingival fibromatosis.

**Gingival fibromatosis-hypertrichosis-fibroadenomas of breasts**
   *See GINGIVAL MULTIPLE HAMARTOMA SYNDROME*
**Gingival fibromatosis-multiple hyaline fibromas**
   *See FIBROMATOSIS, JUVENILE HYALINE*
**Gingival fibromatosis-poor eruption of teeth-corneal dystrophy**
   *See GINGIVAL FIBROMATOSIS-CORNEAL DYSTROPHY*
**Gingival fibromatosis-sensorineural hearing loss**
   *See GINGIVAL FIBROMATOSIS-DEAFNESS, JONES TYPES*
**Gingival granular cell tumor, congenital**
   *See TEETH, EPULIS, CONGENITAL*

**Gingival hyperkeratosis-hyperkeratosis palmoplantaris**
*See SKIN, HYPERKERATOSIS, FOCAL PALMOPLANTAR AND GINGIVAL*
**Gingival hypertrophy-corneal dystrophy**
*See GINGIVAL FIBROMATOSIS-CORNEAL DYSTROPHY*

## GINGIVAL MULTIPLE HAMARTOMA SYNDROME     0412

**Includes:**

Breast fibroadenomas-hypertrichosis-gingival fibromatosis
Cowden disease
Gingival fibromatosis-hypertrichosis-fibroadenomas of breasts
Hypertrichosis-gingival fibromatosis-fibroadenomas of breasts
Multiple hamartoma syndrome

**Excludes:**

**Fibromatosis, juvenile hyaline** (0411)
**Gingival fibromatosis** (0407)
Gingival fibromatosis, symmetric
**Gingival fibromatosis-corneal dystrophy** (0408)
**Gingival fibromatosis-deafness, Jones types** (2315)
**Gingival fibromatosis-depigmentation-microphthalmia** (0413)
**Gingival fibromatosis-digital anomalies** (0409)
**Gingival fibromatosis-hypertrichosis** (0410)
**Intestinal polyposis, type II** (2344)

**Major Diagnostic Criteria:** Multiple hamartomatous lesions especially consisting of mucosal and cutaneous papillomatosis and fibromatosis, fibrocystic breast disease in the female, and thyroid lesions.

**Clinical Findings:** Gingival fibromatosis appearing from birth to one year of age, hypertrichosis appearing from birth to five years of age and massive "virginal" bilateral enlargement of breasts after puberty. At birth the hair may be coarse and black, the affected child frequently being the only black-haired child in the sibship. Hypertrichosis involves trunk, face, arms and legs and may increase at menarche. Axillary and pubic hair have a normal female distribution. Breast enlargement seems to coincide with a "precipitating" event such as the first menarche, or breast development may be normal for a time with enlargement occurring later, in some at the time of first pregnancy. Initial growth is rapid, the breasts may double in size within a few months with a later slowing rate of enlargement so that 2 years have elapsed in some instances before the breasts reach a size sufficiently great to cause the patient to seek medical attention. In other examples, enlargement was so rapid that within an 8-month-span the breasts hung to a level of the pubes. The breast lesions are giant fibroadenomas which undergo early malignant degeneration. All affected women have fibrocystic breast disease which may become malignant. Precocious breast hypertrophy has been seen in only two females. Gynecomastia occurred in one male. There are usually no other indications of hypothalamic or gonadal dysfunction such as menstrual abnormalities, changes in features, voice, size of feet or hands, striae pigmentation, loss of libido or urinary symptoms. Gingival enlargement may be accompanied by hyperkeratosis or parakeratosis of the overlying epithelium or a generalized hyperkeratotic papillomatosis of lips, oral and pharyngeal mucosa. Mild mental retardation occurs in about 50%.

Patients have extensive facial trichilemmomas, and mucosal papillomatosis and fibromatosis. Verrucous lesions appear throughout the oral cavity, about all facial orifices, on the extensor surfaces of the limbs, and punctate keratoderma may be seen on palmar and plantar surfaces. Thyroid adenoma and goiter, thyroiditis, thyroid hypofunction and thyroid carcinoma occur more frequently in women. Gynecologic abnormalities include menstrual irregularity, miscarriage, stillbirth, uterine fibroid tumors and ovarian cyst. The GI tract may be involved with polyposis of the stomach, colon and rectum, submucosal neuroma, leiomyoma, diverticulae and perirectal abscess. Carcinoma of the colon developed in 1 patient. Other carcinomas include melanoma, squamous cell carcinoma and pleomorphic atypical malignancy of the lung. Skeletal abnormalities are diverse and include adenoid

facies, mandibular hypoplasia, high-arched palate, pectus excavatum, scoliosis and bone cysts.

**Complications:** Malignant degeneration of breast lesions, lordosis, rupture of breast cysts, difficulties in speech, mastication, swallowing and respiration, dentigerous cysts, retained tooth fragments within gingivae.

**Associated Findings:** In the thyroid: adenoma, goiter and carcinoma; in GU tract: uterine fibroids, ovarian cyst, carcinoma of the endometrium and ovaries, also miscarriage and stillbirth; in GI tract: benign and malignant GI tumors; in the skin: cutaneous neuromas, hemangiomas, lipomas, melanoma and squamous cell carcinoma. Carcinoma of the endometrium and ovaries. Pleomorphic atypical malignancy of the lung, pseudotumor cerebri and retinal glioma are also reported.

**Etiology:** Autosomal dominant inheritance.

**Pathogenesis:** Initial precipitating event is unknown. Children are born with coarse, black hair and are frequently the only black-haired children in the sibship. Gingival enlargement may be present at birth or noted by one year of age. Hirsutism may be congenital or develop as late as 4 to 5 years. Breast enlargement occurs after puberty at time of first menses or later and may occur at first pregnancy. Gingival lesions are composed of thick dense bundles of mature collagen bands in submucosa and lamina propria. The overlying epithelium is hyperkeratotic. Verrucous papillary growths arise about facial orifices, on the oral mucosa and on glabrous skin surfaces. Breast lesions have features of fibrocystic disease or giant fibroadenomas. Ductal carcinomas have been found in some cases. Thyroid tumors with histologic changes indistinguishable from carcinoma are reported. Chromosomal structure and numbers have been normal in 3 patients. An autosomal dominant mode of inheritance with variable expression was proposed for Cowden disease. Electron microscopic examinations of warty cutaneous lesions do not demonstrate viral particles.

**MIM No.:** *15835

**POS No.:** 3155

**Sex Ratio:** M11:F21 (observed)

**Occurrence:** Over 75 cases have been documented.

**Risk of Recurrence for Patient's Sib:**
See Part I, *Mendelian Inheritance.*

**Risk of Recurrence for Patient's Child:**
See Part I, *Mendelian Inheritance.*

**Age of Detectability:** For full syndrome, puberty to young adult. For gingival fibromatosis and hirsutism, birth to 4 years.

**Gene Mapping and Linkage:** MHAM (multiple hamartoma (Cowden syndrome)) is unassigned.

**Prevention:** None known. Genetic counseling indicated.

**Treatment:** Surgical removal of excess gingival tissue, although this often recurs. If lesion recurs, extraction of all teeth, then gingivectomy. Surgical removal of malignant tumors of breast, thyroid or GI tract if they arise. Full dentures, depilatories, plastic repair of breasts; special education for those with oligophrenia may be necessary. One percent 5-fluorouracil topically for skin lesions.

**Prognosis:** Good with early surgical removal of breast adenomas. Fair if malignant transformation has occurred.

**Detection of Carrier:** Unknown.

**Special Considerations:** It is not known if this condition is really a different entity from **Gingival fibromatosis-hypertrichosis**. Of 40 familial cases (M22:F18) with Gingival fibromatosis-hypertrichosis, none has been reported with breast lesions.

**References:**
Lloyd KM II, Dennis M: Cowden's disease: a possible new symptom complex with multiple system involvement. Ann Intern Med 1963; 58:136–142.
Witkop CJ Jr: Heterogeneity in gingival fibromatosis. BD:OAS;VII(7). Baltimore: William & Wilkins, 1971:210–221. †

Gentry WC Jr, et al.: The multiple hamartoma syndrome (Cowden's disease). Arch Dermatol 1974; 109:521–525. *

Nuss DD, et al.: Multiple hamartoma syndrome (Cowden's disease). Arch Dermatol 1978; 114:743–746.

Brownstein MH, et al.: The dermatopathology of Cowden's syndrome. Br J Dermatol 1979; 100:667–673.

Ruschak PJ, et al.: Cowden's disease associated with immunodeficiency. Arch Derm 1981; 117:573–575.

Elston DM, et al.: Multiple hamartoma syndrome (Cowden's disease) associated with non-Hodgkin's lymphoma. Arch Derm 1986; 122: 572–575.

Starink TM, et al.: The Cowden syndrome:a clinical and genetic study in 21 patients. Clin Genet 1986; 29:222–233.

WI043

**Carl J. Witkop, Jr.**
*William C. Gentry, Jr.*

## GIROUX-BARBEAU SYNDROME                2866

**Includes:**

> Ataxia-erythrokeratodermia
> Erythrokeratodermia-ataxia
> Ichthyosis-hepatosplenomegaly-cerebellar degeneration

**Excludes:**

> **Skin, erythrokeratodermia, progressiva symmetrica** (2863)
> **Skin, erythrokeratodermia, variable** (0361)
> **Skin, erythrokeratolysis hiemalis** (2862)
> **Skin, pityriasis rubra pilaris** (0811)
> **Skin, psoriasis vulgaris** (0833)

**Major Diagnostic Criteria:** Focal hyperkeratotic plaques are present during infancy and resolve by early adulthood. After age 40 years, progressive neurologic symptoms develop, including ataxia.

**Clinical Findings:** Giroux and Barbeau (1972) reported a large French-Canadian kindred that exhibited focal erythematous, hyperkeratotic plaques during infancy and childhood, followed by the development of a progressive neurologic syndrome in adulthood. Discrete configurations of erythema and scaling with a predilection for the external ears, extensor surfaces of elbows and knees, over wrists, ankles, and dorsum of hands and feet develop soon after birth. These improve in the summers and resolve by early adulthood. Palms and soles are always spared. After age 40 years, a progressive neurologic disorder of ataxia, nystagmus, dysarthria, and decreased tendon reflexes ensues. Some patients complain of muscle cramps. Cranial nerves are not affected. Before age 40 years, the only abnormal neurologic sign is hyporeflexia. Neurologic abnormalities were preceded by the skin eruption in all cases.

**Complications:** At an older age, progressive ataxia results in confinement to a wheelchair.

**Associated Findings:** None known.

**Etiology:** Autosomal dominant inheritance, fully penetrant.

**Pathogenesis:** Unknown.

**MIM No.:** *13319

**CDC No.:** 757.190

**Sex Ratio:** Presumably M1:F1; M14:F11, observed.

**Occurrence:** Giroux and Barbeau (1972) reported a single French-Canadian kindred with 25 affected patients spanning five generations.

**Risk of Recurrence for Patient's Sib:**
See Part I, *Mendelian Inheritance.*

**Risk of Recurrence for Patient's Child:**
See Part I, *Mendelian Inheritance.*

**Age of Detectability:** Skin manifestations are present soon after birth.

**Gene Mapping and Linkage:** Unknown.

**Prevention:** None known. Genetic counseling indicated.

**Treatment:** Unknown.

**Prognosis:** Skin manifestations usually resolve by the third decade. Neurologic manifestations are progressive and are ultimately disabling. Intelligence is unaffected.

**Detection of Carrier:** Careful skin examination for individuals less than age 20 years and history and neurologic examination after age 20 years. Skin lesions may resolve during the summer.

**Special Considerations:** A kindred with generalized scaling, hepatosplenomegaly, and late-onset cerebellar ataxia was reported by Dykes et al (1980); inheritance was consistent with either an X-linked or autosomal recessive trait. The skin eruption was nonerythrodermic, with flexural sparing and a prominent palmoplantar keratoderma. An increased number of desmosomes were seen in the granular and lower corneal cell layers. Both steroid sulfatase activity and serum phytanic acid levels were normal. The differences in clinical phenotype and inheritance indicate that this represents a distinct genetic entity.

**References:**

Giroux JM, Barbeau A: Erythrokeratodermia with ataxia. Arch Dermatol 1972; 106:183–188.

Dykes RJ, et al.: Syndrome of ichthyosis, hepatosplenomegaly, and cerebellar degeneration - steroid sulphatase activity. Br J Dermatol 1980; 102:353–354.

WI013

**Mary L. Williams**

**Gitlin syndrome**
*See IMMUNODEFICIENCY, SEVERE COMBINED*
**Glanzmann thrombasthenia**
*See THROMBASTHENIA, GLANZMANN-NAEGELI TYPE*
**Glaswolle-Haar and crystalline cataract**
*See HAIR, UNCOMBABLE-CRYSTALLINE CATARACT*

## GLAUCOMA, CONGENITAL                0414

**Includes:**

> Buphthalmos, congenital
> Glaucoma, infantile
> Glaucoma, primary
> "Ox eye" (buphthalmos)

**Excludes:**

> Angle closure glaucoma
> **Aniridia** (0057)
> **Dento-facio-skeletal defects, Ackerman type** (2093)
> **Eye, anterior segment dysgenesis** (0439)
> "Juvenile" glaucoma
> **Oculo-cerebro-renal syndrome** (0736)
> Primary open angle glaucoma
> Secondary glaucoma

**Major Diagnostic Criteria:** Elevated intraocular pressure or corneal enlargement, ruptures in Descemet membrane, and corneal edema.

**Clinical Findings:** This relatively rare form of glaucoma is diagnosed within the 1st year of life in 80% of cases. The early clinical signs include lacrimation, photophobia, irritability and pain, blepharospasm, corneal clouding (edema), corneal enlargement, horizontal ruptures in Descemet membrane, and cupping and atrophy of the optic disks. The globe eventually becomes enlarged. It is bilateral in 50–75% of cases and more common in males. Examination under anesthesia confirms the above findings plus increased intraocular pressure with poor outflow facilities.

**Complications:** Enlargement of globe with the development of axial myopia, visual loss, and anisometropic amblyopia.

**Associated Findings:** Congenital glaucoma is seen in association with a wide range of birth defects and complex malformation syndromes.

**Etiology:** Autosomal recessive inheritance in about thirty percent of all cases. Sporadic cases are more common.

**Pathogenesis:** May be due to failure of the normal cleavage process of the iris from the angle structures, with remaining underdeveloped mesodermal tissue blocking the outflow chan-

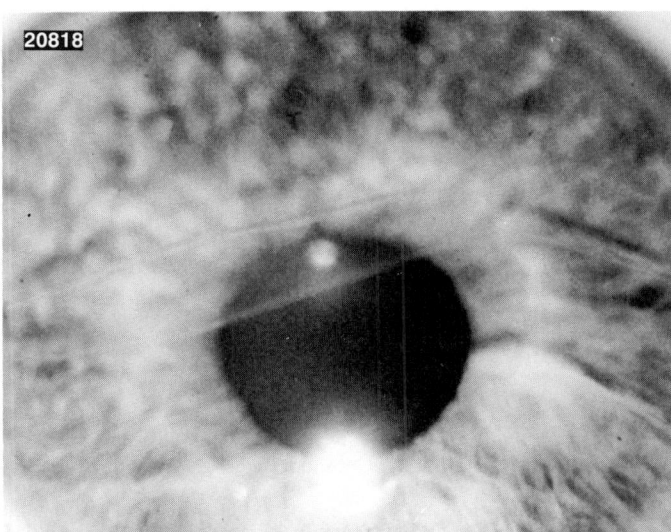

**0414-20818:** Glaucoma, congenital; cornea with Descemet ruptures.

nels, or to persistence of a thin "cellophane"-like membrane over the trabecular meshwork, or a combination of these.

**MIM No.:** *23130

**CDC No.:** 743.200

**Sex Ratio:** M3:F2

**Occurrence:** Incidence 1:10,000 births. Particularly prevalent in a Gypsy subpopulation of Slovakia.

**Risk of Recurrence for Patient's Sib:**
See Part I, *Mendelian Inheritance.* Unilaterally affected cases are more likely to be multifactorial.

**Risk of Recurrence for Patient's Child:**
See Part I, *Mendelian Inheritance.*

**Age of Detectability:** Sixty percent in the first six months of life. Eighty percent with the first year.

**Gene Mapping and Linkage:** Unknown.

**Prevention:** None known. Genetic counseling indicated.

**Treatment:** Medical treatment virtually ineffective. Surgery should be performed as early as possible and the procedure of choice is goniotomy. Other surgical procedures are often resorted to when repeated goniotomies fail.

**Prognosis:** If the pressure is elevated at birth, there is less chance of cure than if the symptoms appear after the 2nd month. Surgery can be successful in salvaging the eye in 80% of the latter cases. Vision may be poor, however, due to amblyopia and damaged optic nerve. Although spontaneous remissions have been reported, most infants go blind unless successful surgery is performed.

**Detection of Carrier:** Primary open angle glaucoma in adults is not related to congenital glaucoma, and parents of patients with congenital glaucoma do not show significant intraocular pressure elevation to topical corticosteroid challenge.

**References:**
Goldberg MF, ed: Genetic and metabolic eye disease. Boston: Little, Brown, 1974.
Ferak V, et al.: Population genetic aspects of primary congenital glaucoma. Hum Genet 1982; 61:198–200.
Demenais F: Further analysis of familial transmission of congenital glaucoma. Am J Hum Genet 1983; 35:1156–1160.
Kolker A, Hetherington J, eds: Becker and Shaffer's diagnosis and therapy of the glaucomas, 5th ed. St. Louis: C.M. Mosby, 1983.
Roy FH: Ocular differential diagnosis, 3rd ed. Philadelphia: Lea & Febiger, 1984.

BA041                                                    **Harold N Bass**

**Glaucoma, infantile**
*See GLAUCOMA, CONGENITAL*
**Glaucoma, juvenile-unusual upper lip and dental roots**
*See DENTO-FACIO-SKELETAL DEFECTS, ACKERMAN TYPE*
**Glaucoma, primary**
*See GLAUCOMA, CONGENITAL*
**GLI gene**
*See CANCER, GLIOMA, FAMILIAL*
**Glioblastoma multiforme, familial**
*See CANCER, GLIOMA, FAMILIAL*
**Glioma oncogene**
*See CANCER, GLIOMA, FAMILIAL*
**Glioma, nasal**
*See NOSE, GLIOMA*
**Glioma, of optic nerve**
*See ORBITAL NERVE GLIOMA*
**Glioma-polyposis**
*See TURCOT SYNDROME*
**Gliomas, familial aggregation**
*See CANCER, GLIOMA, FAMILIAL*
**Gliosis**
*See SYRINGOMYELIA*
**Globodontia-high frequency hearing loss**
*See OTO-DENTAL DYSPLASIA*
**Globoid cell leukodystrophy**
*See LEUKODYSTROPHY, GLOBOID CELL TYPE*
**Glomerular cysts**
*See KIDNEY, GLOMERULOCYSTIC*
**Glomerulocystic kidney**
*See KIDNEY, GLOMERULOCYSTIC*
**Glomerulocystic renal dysplasia**
*See KIDNEY, GLOMERULOCYSTIC*
**Glomus jugulare tumors**
*See CAROTID BODY TUMOR*
*also EAR, CHEMODECTOMA OF MIDDLE EAR*
**Glomus tumors, multiple**
*See SKIN TUMORS, MULTIPLE GLOMUS*
**Glomus tympanicum tumors**
*See EAR, CHEMODECTOMA OF MIDDLE EAR*
**Glomus vagale tumors**
*See EAR, CHEMODECTOMA OF MIDDLE EAR*
**Glossitis, benign migratory**
*See TONGUE, GEOGRAPHIC*

## GLOSSITIS, MEDIAN RHOMBOID                          0417

**Includes:**
    Candida albicans infection, chronic, median rhomboid glossitis
    Median rhomboid glossitis

**Excludes:**
    Central papillary atrophy
    Lingual tonsil
    **Thyroglossal duct remnant** (0945)
    **Tongue, geographic** (0954)

**Major Diagnostic Criteria:** A persistent ovoid or rhomboid, nodular, fissured, or smooth red mass or zone in the midline of the dorsum of the tongue, just anterior to the circumvallate papillae. It usually is somewhat elevated. Microscopic examination reveals nonkeratinized epithelium and a chronic inflammatory infiltrate.

**Clinical Findings:** An ovoid or rhomboid, fissured, or smooth red mass or zone in the midline of the dorsum of the tongue, just anterior to the V formed by the circumvallate papillae; usually somewhat elevated.

Microscopically, the epithelium generally is nonkeratinized and may be thin and flat or acanthotic with elongated rete ridges. A chronic inflammatory infiltrate of varying intensity is almost always present. Frequently there is degeneration of underlying muscle fibers and accumulation of dense collagen and hyaline material.

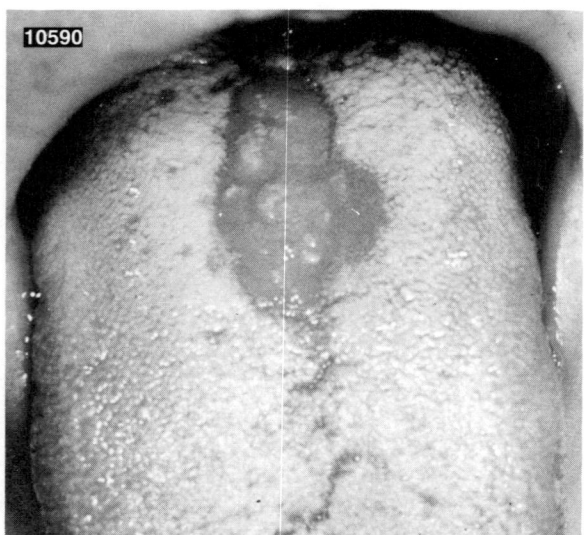
10590

**0417-10590:** Rhomboid glossitis.

**Complications:** Food and detritus accumulation in fissures may cause irritation.

**Associated Findings:** **Diabetes mellitus** has been suggested but not confirmed.

**Etiology:** Developmental defect of unknown etiology is the currently accepted theory. This is challenged by evidence suggesting many, if not most, cases arise through chronic *Candida albicans* infection. The two theories are not incompatible. The developmental defect theory offers an explanation for why only one particular zone of the dorsum of the tongue in a few individuals is the site of the persistent and characteristic lesions. Such a defect might render the site peculiarly susceptible to superficial infection by *Candida*.

If the developmental defect theory is correct, it should be detectable at birth or even in aborted fetuses older than eight weeks of gestation. However, the youngest age at which it has been seen is seven months.

**Pathogenesis:** Thought to be a failure of the lateral lingual tubercles to completely overgrow the tuberculum impar during the development of the tongue, resulting in a nonpapillated mucosa. However, most lesions biopsied in several investigations were found to harbor mycelia of *Candida albicans* in the superficial layers of the epithelium, suggesting an infectious pathogenesis.

**Sex Ratio:** M4:F1

**Occurrence:** 300:100,000 Caucasion births; 150:100,000 Blacks births.

**Risk of Recurrence for Patient's Sib:** Unknown.

**Risk of Recurrence for Patient's Child:** Unknown.

**Age of Detectability:** Not known to be recognized before seven months of age.

**Gene Mapping and Linkage:** Unknown.

**Prevention:** None known. Genetic counseling indicated.

**Treatment:** None indicated unless irritation causes discomfort. Then hygienic measures or topical fungicides may be of value. Only if the lesion is enlarging or causes persistent discomfort, or if the patient has an intractable fear that the lesion is cancerous, is excision recommended. If the tongue lesion responds to fungicidal therapy, endocrinopathy, especially diabetes mellitus, should be ruled out.

**Prognosis:** Excellent. Does not reduce longevity. Carcinoma arises rarely in this region of the tongue.

**Detection of Carrier:** Unknown.

**Special Considerations:** A similar but usually evanescent lesion occurs on the dorsum of the tongue, but more anteriorly and not always in the midline. Etiology of this focal glossitis and similar lesions of other oral mucosal sites includes heavy smoking and candidal infection. Temporary regression is the usual response to topical fungicides. Cessation of smoking usually leads to partial or complete regression of this type of lesion in the absence of other factors, such as endocrinopathy or inadequate denture hygiene.

**References:**
Martin HE, Howe ME: Glossitis rhombica mediana. Ann Surg 1938; 107:39–49.
Redman RS: Prevalence of geographic tongue, fissured tongue, median rhomboid glossitis, and hairy tongue among 3,611 Minnesota school children. Oral Surg 1970; 30:390–395.
Baughman RA: Median rhomboid glossitis: a developmental anomaly? Oral Surg 1971; 31:56–65.
Wright BA: Median rhomboid glossitis: not a misnomer. Oral Surg 1978; 46:806–814. *
van der Waal I, et al.: Median rhomboid glossitis caused by *candida*? Oral Surg 1979; 47:31–35.
Holmstrup P, Bessermann M: Clinical, therapeutic, and pathogenic aspects of chronic oral multifocal candidiasis. Oral Surg 1983; 56:388–395.

RE003                                                    **Robert S. Redman**

**Glossopalatine ankylosis syndrome**
*See HYPOGLOSSIA-HYPODACTYLIA*
**Glossoptosis-micrognathia-cleft palate**
*See CLEFT PALATE-MICROGNATHIA-GLOSSOPTOSIS*
**Glottic atresia**
*See LARYNX, ATRESIA*
**Glottic web**
*See LARYNX, WEB*
**Glucocerebrosidase deficiency**
*See GAUCHER DISEASE*
**Glucocerebrosidosis**
*See GAUCHER DISEASE*
**Glucocorticoid deficiency, familial isolated**
*See ADRENOCORTICAL UNRESPONSIVENESS TO ACTH, HEREDITARY*

## GLUCOCORTICOID RESISTANCE                              2952

**Includes:**
   Cortisol resistance, familial
   Cortisol resistance, primary
   Hypercortisolism (spontaneous) without Cushing syndrome
**Excludes:**
   Alcoholism
   Depression
   **Mood and thought disorders** (1532)
   **Nevi-atrial myxoma-myxoid neurofibromas-ephelides** (2572)
   Pseudo-Cushing state

**Major Diagnostic Criteria:** Biochemical evidence of increased secretion of cortisol (increased total and free plasma cortisol, increased 24-hour urinary excretion of 17-hydroxysteroids or free cortisol, and resistance to dexamethasone suppression) and no evidence of **Nevi-atrial myxoma-myxoid neurofibromas-ephelides** or other stigmata of hypercortisolism. Characteristically, the circadian rhythm of plasma cortisol is preserved as is the plasma cortisol response to insulin-induced hypoglycemia, indicating that the central regulation of secretion of ACTH and cortisol are qualitatively normal in these patients but at a higher set point.

**Clinical Findings:** The majority of reported patients with glucocorticoid resistance have been asymptomatic; all have been diagnosed as adults. The degree of cortisol hypersecretion varied from high (urinary free cortisol exceeding 1,500 $\mu$g/24 hours) to moderately elevated (250–1,000 $\mu$g/24 hours) and mildly elevated (90–250 $\mu$g/24 hours). All have had resistance to dexamethasone suppression, and normal or elevated plasma mineralocorticoid steroids (deoxycorticosterone, corticosterone) and androgens ($\Delta$)4-androstenedione, dehydroepiandrosterone, testosterone).

Two patients have been clearly symptomatic. An adult male with biochemical evidence of highly increased cortisol secretion had hypertension and hypokalemic alkalosis, with elevated levels of plasma deoxycorticosterone and corticosterone. A young adult female with biochemical evidence of moderate hypercortisolism developed facial hirsutism, male-type scalp baldness, and menstrual irregularities with elevated plasma concentrations of testosterone and androstenedione.

Clinical and biochemical variability is common even within families. In a single kindred there may be an individual with severe hypertension, electrolyte abnormalities, and profound hypercortisolism and individuals with mild or borderline elevations of cortisol, mineralocorticoid steroid, or androgen secretion and no evidence of hypermineralocorticoidism or hyperandrogenism.

**Complications:** Atherosclerotic arterial changes can develop from long-term untreated hypertension, resulting in cardiovascular, cerebrovascular, and possibly renal diseases.

Anovulation and infertility may result from chronic untreated hyperandrogenism in women with glucocorticoid resistance. In theory, polycystic ovarian disease can develop in these individuals as a result of the hyperandrogenism. Acne, hirsutism, and male-type baldness may also develop in such women.

**Associated Findings:** None known.

**Etiology:** Autosomal dominant inheritance.

**Pathogenesis:** Members of two families with glucocorticoid resistance had defects of their glucocorticoid receptors, explaining the partial glucocorticoid resistance observed. In the first family the glucocorticoid receptor had a low affinity for glucocorticoid hormones, suggesting decreased ability of the receptor to interact and form complexes with the hormone. In the second family a low concentration of glucocorticoid receptors was found. The severity of the syndrome has been correlated with the glucocorticoid receptor defect.

It appears that the glucocorticoid receptor abnormality observed may be generalized in all glucocorticoid target tissues, including the hypothalamic-pituitary unit. The decrease of glucocorticoid negative feedback at the hypothalamic-pituitary unit probably results in compensatory hypersecretion of corticortropin-releasing hormone (CRH) and ACTH and hyperstimulation of adrenocortical function. Hyperfunction of the adrenal zona fasciculata results in hypersecretion of both cortisol and several of its precursors that have mineralocorticoid activity (11-deoxycorticosterone, corticosterone, and so forth). The exposure of the kidney mineralocorticoid receptor to high levels of cortisol (which has some mineralocorticoid activity) and the mineralocorticoid cortisol precursors can explain the development of hypertension and hypokalemic alkalosis. Hyperstimulation of the adrenal zona reticularis, on the other hand, results in hypersecretion of adrenal androgens (δ4-androstenedione, δ5-dehydroepiandrosterone, and so forth). The exposure of the androgen receptor to high concentrations of adrenal androgens can explain the development of hirsutism, male pattern baldness, and menstrual irregularities.

**MIM No.:** *13804

**Sex Ratio:** M2:F1 (observed).

**Occurrence:** Unknown. Has been reported in families of Dutch or Japanese ancestry.

**Risk of Recurrence for Patient's Sib:**
See Part I, *Mendelian Inheritance*.

**Risk of Recurrence for Patient's Child:**
See Part I, *Mendelian Inheritance*.

**Age of Detectability:** Although the condition has only been reported in adults, it is believed that hypersecretion of cortisol characterizes all ages and should be detectable by the same approach as that applied in adults.

**Gene Mapping and Linkage:** GRL (glucocorticoid receptor) has been mapped to 5q31-q32.

**Prevention:** None known. Genetic counseling indicated.

**Treatment:** The symptomatic patients can be successfully treated with synthetic glucocorticoids that have negligible mineralocorticoid activity. Dexamethasone doses as high as three- to sixfold

above normal replacement (1.5–3 mg/day) have been used, successfully correcting the hypertension, hypokalemic alkalosis, and hyperandrogenism of symptomatic patients without causing any of the stigmata of Cushing syndrome (see **Nevi-atrial myxoma-myxoid neurofibromas-ephelides**).

**Prognosis:** Asymptomatic patients are expected to have a normal life span. Intelligence has been described as normal. No mood or behavior disturbances have been reported.

**Detection of Carrier:** Biochemical evidence of hypercorticolism by measuring 24 hour urinary free cortisol excretion and by measuring the plasma concentration of cortisol after a midnight oral dose of dexamethasone.

**Special Considerations:** Patients with glucocorticoid resistance and mild hypercortisolism (urinary free cortisol excretion less than 250/μg/24 hours) can be difficult to distinguish from patients with mild Cushing syndrome or pseudo-Cushing states such as depression or alcoholism. Careful history taking, including a psychiatric interview, and several biochemical tests will help with the differential diagnosis. Tests include evaluation of the cortisol circadian rhythm (maintained in glucocorticoid resistance and pseudo-Cushing states, lost in Cushing syndrome) and responsiveness to insulin-induced hypoglycemia (maintained in glucocorticoid resistance and pseudo-Cushing states, lost in Cushing syndrome). Exogenous bovine CRH could also in theory be employed in the differential diagnosis (maintained ACTH responses in cortisol resistance and pituitary Cushing's syndrome, blunted or abolished ACTH responses in depression and the ectopic ACTH syndrome). Recently, athletes have been shown to have mild hypercortisolism without evidence of Cushing syndrome and poor responsiveness of plasma ACTH to exogenous bovine CRH. History alone should differentiate these patients from those with glucocorticoid resistance.

**References:**
Vingerhoeds ACM, et al.: Spontaneous hypercortisolism without Cushing's syndrome. J Clin Endocrinol Metab 1976; 43:1128–1133.
Chrousos GP, et al.: Primary cortisol resistance in man: a glucocorticoid receptor-mediated disease. J Clin Invest 1982; 69:1261–1269.
Chrousos GP, et al.: Primary cortisol resistance: a family study. J Clin Endocrinol Metab 1983; 56:1243–1245.
Chrousos GP, et al.: Primary cortisol resistance: a family study and an animal model. J Steroid Biochem 1983; 19:567–576.
Chrousos GP, et al.: The clinical applications of corticotropin releasing factor. Ann Intern Med 1985; 102:344–358.
Iida S, et al.: Primary glucocorticoid resistance accompanied by a reduction in glucocorticoid receptors in two members of the same family. J Clin Endocrinol Metab 1985; 60: 967–972.
Lipsett MB, et al.: The defective glucocorticoid receptor in man and nonhuman primates. Recent Prog Horm Res 1985; 41:199–247.
Gold PW, et al.: Responses to corticotropin releasing hormone in the hypercortisolism of depression and Cushing's disease: pathophysiologic and diagnostic implications. New Engl J Med 1986; 314:1329–1335.
Lamberts SWJ, et al.: Familial cortisol resistance: differential diagnostic and therapeutic aspects. J Clin Endocrinol Metab 1986; 63:1328–1333.
Tomita M, et al.: Glucocorticoid receptors in Epstein Barr virus-transformed lymphocytes from patients with glucocorticoid resistance and a glucocorticoid resistant New World primate. J Clin Endocrinol Metab 1986; 62:1145–1154.
Luger A, et al.: Acute hypothalamic-pituitary-adrenal responses to the stress of treadmill exercise: physiologic adaptations to physical training. New Engl J Med 1987; 316:1309–1315.

CH040                                    **George P. Chrousos**

**Glucocorticoid-responsive hyperaldosteronism**
*See HYPERALDOSTERONISM, FAMILIAL GLUCOCORTICOID SUPPRESSIBLE*

## GLUCOGLYCINURIA　　　　　　　　　　　　　**0418**

**Includes:** Renal glucosuria-hyperglycinuria

**Excludes:**
　Acidemia, propionic (0826)
　Hyperglycinemia, nonketotic (0492)
　Renal glycosuria (0861)

**Major Diagnostic Criteria:** Glucosuria associated with reduced "venous" plasma threshold and normal $T_m$ (Reubi type B renal glucosuria).
　Renal hyperglycinuria, plasma concentration of glycine (Cgly) > 8.6 ml/min/1.73 m². No other evidence of renal tubular dysfunction.

**Clinical Findings:** Fourteen members in a Swiss pedigree of 45 members exhibited isolated glucosuria and hyperglycinuria. All but the 9 1/2-year-old male proband were healthy; the latter had a clinical condition compatible with cystic fibrosis. Investigations indicated that the glucosuria was the result of reduced tubular reabsorption; the plasma threshold for glucosuria was reduced (79 mg/dl), whereas the $T_m$ glucose was normal (386 mg/min/1.73 m²); a load:$T_m$ ratio of 4 was achieved. Hyperglycinuria was less well studied, but it was clearly documented when the plasma concentration of glycine was normal. No other disturbance of renal function was discovered. Intestinal transport was not investigated.

**Complications:** Unknown.

**Associated Findings:** None known.

**Etiology:** Probably autosomal dominant defect of renal tubule transport activity.

**Pathogenesis:** Deficiency of tubular absorptive mechanism(s) for both glucose and glycine.

**MIM No.:** 13807

**Sex Ratio:** M9:F5 (observed)

**Occurrence:** Reported in one Swiss kindred.

**Risk of Recurrence for Patient's Sib:**
　See Part I, *Mendelian Inheritance.*

**Risk of Recurrence for Patient's Child:**
　See Part I, *Mendelian Inheritance.*

**Age of Detectability:** Probably early infancy.

**Gene Mapping and Linkage:** Unknown.

**Prevention:** None known. Genetic counseling indicated.

**Treatment:** Unknown.

**Prognosis:** Normal life span; apparently harmless trait as described.

**Detection of Carrier:** Trait so far identified only in carriers.

**Special Considerations:** Reubi type B glucosuria describes reduced affinity (increased Km value) of transport system for glucose, assuming Michaelis kinetics for its uptake. This type of glucosuria is one predictable mode of expression for a mutant genotype affecting glucose transport. However, this type of glucosuria should not necessarily be associated with impaired glycine transport, since the two molecules do not share a common mode of transport. A selective defect in Na⁺ cotransport is a possibility.
　Glucoglycinuria has been described as being accompanied by a phosphate transport defect (Scriver et al., 1964); the transport defect was clearly of the "low-$T_m$" type.

**References:**
Reubi F: Physiopathologie et diagnostic diabète rénal. Rev Fr Etud Clin Biol 1956; 1:575–585.
Käser H, et al.: Glucoglycinuria: a new familial syndrome. J Pediatr 1962; 61:386–394.
Scriver CR, et al.: Hypophosphatemic rickets with renal hyperglycinuria, renal glucosuria, and glycylprolinuria: a syndrome with evidence for renal tubular secretion of phosphorus. Pediatrics 1964; 34:357–371.
Wyngaarden JB, Segal S: The hyperglycinurias. In: Stanbury JB, et al.,

eds: The metabolic basis of inherited disease, 2nd ed. New York: McGraw-Hill, 1966:341–352.

SC050　　　　　　　　　　　　　　　　　**Charles R. Scriver**

**Glucose-6-phosphate**
　*See GLYCOGENOSIS, TYPE Ia*

## GLUCOSE-6-PHOSPHATE DEHYDROGENASE
## DEFICIENCY　　　　　　　　　　　　　　**0420**

**Includes:**
　Dehydrogenase deficiency, glucose-6-phosphate
　Favism
　G6PD deficiency
　Hemolytic anemia, nonspherocytic, associated with G6PD deficiency
　Primaquine sensitive anemia

**Excludes:**
　Drug-induced hemolysis not associated with deficient G6PD
　Other causes of congenital nonspherocytic hemolytic anemia

**Major Diagnostic Criteria:** Hemolytic anemia, hemoglobinuria, and jaundice following ingestion or exposure to a hemolytic agent and demonstration of deficiency of erythrocyte glucose-6-phosphate dehydrogenase (G6PD).

**Clinical Findings:** Clinical findings are variable and depend on: 1) the molecular variant of G6PD present; 2) the presence of other, as yet undefined genetic abnormalities which may interact with G6PD deficiency (e.g. favism); 3) environmental factors, particularly the presence of oxidant drugs and chemicals. In general, the defect is characterized by episodic or chronic hemolytic anemia.
　*Episodic hemolysis* follows ingestion of an oxidant drug (e.g. primaquine), exposure to certain chemicals (e.g. naphthalene), or occurs during either viral or bacterial infections. Hemolysis begins two or three days after exposure to a hemolytic agent, with hemoglobinuria, jaundice, increasing anemia, and reticulocytosis. Occasionally, prostration, abdominal and back pain, and death occur. Heinz bodies may be found within the red cells during the early phases of hemolysis, but not later. Despite continued presence of the hemolytic agent, recovery may ensue, and a stage of compensated hemolysis be reached, characterized by normal hemoglobin levels but evidence of shortened erythrocyte survival.
　*Chronic unremitting hemolysis* present from birth (congenital nonspherocytic hemolytic anemia), with hyperbilirubinemia, anemia, reticulocytosis, and splenomegaly is encountered with the rare, severe variants of G6PD deficiency. Hemolysis in these patients may be exacerbated by exposure to hemolytic agents.
　Some, but not all, patients with the Mediterranean variant of G6PD undergo episodes of severe hemolysis following ingestion of fava beans or inhalation of fava bean pollen (Favism). Favism is also noted in South China, but not in the African (A-) G6PD variant.
　*Neonatal hyperbilirubinemia* occurs frequently in Oriental (China, Thailand) and Mediterranean (Greece, Italy, Israel) G6PD-deficient infants. Full-term American Blacks with G6PD deficiency are not unusually susceptible to hyperbilirubinemia, but premature infants are. In Greece, other undefined genetic or environmental factors may act in concert with G6PD deficiency to produce hyperbilirubinemia in as many as 43% of G6PD-deficient infants.

**Complications:** The expected sequelae of chronic jaundice or anemia may occur (e.g. gallstones, congestive heart failure). Intrauterine hemolysis leading to hydrops fetalis is exceedingly rare.

**Associated Findings:** Increased bacterial infections and abnormal glucose tolerance tests have been reported.

**Etiology:** X-linked recessive inheritance.

**Pathogenesis:** Deficiency of G6PD leads to diminished generation of NADPH, an essential reducing agent in the erythrocyte, and renders the cell incapable of converting GSSG to GSH. Devoid of its endogenous reducing power, the cell becomes susceptible to both exogenous (e.g. drugs) and endogenous (e.g. $H_2O_2$) oxidants. These oxidants may attack membrane, hemoglobin or enzyme S-H groups, may oxidize hemoglobin to methemoglobin, or may peroxidate membrane lipids. One consequence of the oxidative attack upon hemoglobin is the formation of intraerythrocytic Heinz bodies which represent aggregates of denatured hemoglobin. Removal of such inclusion bodies by the spleen may result in loss of cell membrane and partial cell fragmentation. The ultimate cause of hemolysis is not known, but it is thought to be the consequence of membrane injury either as a result of Heinz body formation or following a direct oxidative assault on structural components essential for membrane integrity.

**MIM No.:** *30590

**CDC No.:** 282.200

**Sex Ratio:** M1F<1. Severe phenotypic expression of deficiency almost always occurs in males or in homozygous females, who are numerically far less frequent than affected males. Heterozygous females demonstrate variable, intermediate levels of enzyme deficiency and are usually clinically normal.

**Occurrence:** For males: United States Blacks 10–14%; West Africa Blacks 5–20%; East Africa Blacks 2–27%; South Africa Blacks 0–5%; Italy 0–20%; Greece 0–32%; Saudi Arabia 5–65%; Iran 0–20%; Iraq 25%; Kurdistan 50%; Ashkenazic Jews 0.4%; Spain 0–1%; Great Britian 0%; China 0–5.5%; Japan 0%; Philippines 6.6%; India 0–19%; New Guinea 0–17%; Polynesia 0–0.2%.

**Risk of Recurrence for Patient's Sib:**
See Part I, *Mendelian Inheritance.*

**Risk of Recurrence for Patient's Child:**
See Part I, *Mendelian Inheritance.*

**Age of Detectability:** At birth by assay of erythrocyte G6PD.

**Gene Mapping and Linkage:** G6PD (glucose-6-phosphate dehydrogenase) has been mapped to Xq28.

**Prevention:** None known. Genetic counseling indicated.

**Treatment:** Avoidance of agents capable of inducing hemolysis. These include: Antimalarials-(primaquine, pamaquine, pentaquine); Sulfonamides-(sulfanilamide, sulfacetamide, sulfapyridine, sulfamethoxazole); Nitrofurans-(nitrofurantoin); Antipyretics and analgesics-(acetanilide); and others-(methylene blue, naphthalene, niridazole, trinitrotoluene, toluidine blue, phenylhydrazine, fava beans, and nalidixic acid).

Blood transfusions when necessary for acute hemolytic anemia. Cholecystectomy if gallstones occur. Splenectomy usually of little or no benefit in G6PD-deficient patients with chronic congenital nonspherocytic hemolytic anemia.

**Prognosis:** Most affected males will survive into adulthood and normal longevity is the rule except in the most severe cases. However, in one survey of American Blacks the incidence of G6PD deficiency was 12% in males overall but declined to 8% in those over 40 years of age, suggesting an unfavorable influence of G6PD deficiency on mortality. Heterozygous females appear to have a normal life expectancy.

**Detection of Carrier:** Heterozygous, carrier females are usually free of clinical manifestations of G6PD deficiency (but hemolysis may ensue in some following exposure to hemolytic agents) and identification therefore depends upon quantitative assay of the erythrocyte enzyme. In individual carriers, enzyme activity may range from the low levels found in G6PD-deficient males to levels indistinguishable from normal. Special tests are available to aid in identification of the latter group.

**Special Considerations:** More than 150 molecular variants of human G6PD have been described. Their differentiation has been on the basis of electrophoresis, pH maximal activity, substrate kinetics, and utilization of alternate substrates. Normally, Caucasians have the B+ isoenzyme, identified by its electrophoretic migration, as do approximately 70% of American Blacks. 18% of Blacks have the A+ isoenzyme which is structurally distinguished from the B+ by a single amino acid substitution of aspartic acid for asparagine. G6PD-deficient American Black males have a different A isoenzyme (A-), so named because its electrophoretic migration

is identical to the A+ isoenzyme. The activity of the A- enzyme may be normal in reticulocytes, but it declines rapidly as the cell ages. Thus the older erythrocytes are particularly liable to hemolysis. Caucasians with G6PD deficiency may have a B isoenzyme (B-) or one of the many other variants mentioned. Even reticulocytes from these patients are deficient in G6PD activity. Hemolysis upon exposure to an oxidant is, therefore, often more severe in this group.

Other tissues (WBC, lens, liver, skin, platelets) may demonstrate deficient G6PD activity but WBC G6PD is normal in G6PD-deficient Blacks. It has been suggested that there is a selective advantage of G6PD-deficiency in malarious areas (Roth et al, 1983).

**References:**
Yoshida A, et al.: Table of human glucose-6-phosphate dehydrogenase variants. Bull WHO 1971; 45:243–253.
Beutler E, Yoshida A: Human glucose-6-phosphate dehydrogenase variants: a supplementary tabulation. Ann Hum Genet 1973; 37:151–156.
Beutler E: Glucose-6-phosphate dehydrogenase deficiency. In: Wintrobe MM, ed: Red cell metabolism in hemolytic anemia. New York: Plenum Medical Book Co., 1978.
Luzzatto L, Testa U: Human erythrocyte glucose 6-phosphate dehydrogenase: structure and functions in normal and mutant subjects. In Piomelli S, Yachnin S, eds: Current topics in hematology, vol. 1. New York: Alan R. Liss, 1978:2–70.
Yoshida A, Beutler E: Human glucose-6-phosphate dehydrogenase variants: a supplementary tabulation. Am Hum Gen 1978; 41:347–355.
Piomelli S, Vora S: G6PD deficiency and related disorders of the pentose pathway. In: Nathan DG, Oski FA, eds: Hematology of infancy and childhood. 2nd ed, Philadelphia: W.B. Saunders, 1981: 608–642.
Roth EF Jr., et al.: Glucose-6-phosphate dehydrogenase deficiency inhibits in vitro growth of Plasmodium falciparum. Proc Nat Acad Sci 1983; 80:298–299.
Mallouh AA, Abu-Osba YK: Bacterial infections in children with glucose-6-phosphate dehydrogenase deficiency. J Pediat 1987; 111: 850–852.

ME019        **William C. Mentzer, Jr.**
*Louis K. Diamond*

**Glucose-6-phosphate dehydrogenase deficiency-sideroblastic anemia**
*See ANEMIA, SIDEROBLASTIC*
**Glucose-6-phosphate transport defect**
*See GLYCOGENOSIS, TYPE Ib*

---

## GLUCOSE-GALACTOSE MALABSORPTION       0419

**Includes:**
Galactose-glucose malabsorption
Intestinal monosaccharide intolerance

**Excludes:**
**Lactase deficiency, congenital** (0566)
**Lactase deficiency, primary** (0567)
**Lactose intolerance** (0569)
**Renal glycosuria** (0861)
**Sucrase-isomaltase deficiency** (0920)

**Major Diagnostic Criteria:** Specific intestinal monosaccharide intolerance for glucose and galactose, combined with osmotic diarrhea and flat oral glucose tolerance test. Intermittent glycosuria occurs with euglycemia. Confirmation can be done by demonstration of defect in uptake of glucose or galactose by jejunal mucosa in the absence of disaccharidase deficiency.

**Clinical Findings:** Severe diarrhea occurs in the neonatal period (nearly 100%). Intolerance to formula containing glucose or galactose in any form is common. The symptoms are ameliorated when fructose is used as a carbohydrate source (100%). Large amounts of glucose and galactose are found in feces (100%).

**Complications:** Severe dehydration and shock secondary to diarrhea; failure to thrive if undiagnosed and not treated with fructose-containing formula.

**Associated Findings:** Intermittent glycosuria.

**Etiology:** Autosomal recessive inheritance affecting specific glucose-galactose "carrier protein" in small intestine and kidney.

**Pathogenesis:** Intestinal transport defect leads to osmotic diarrhea and dehydration when glucose or galactose are ingested. Failure to thrive is produced by diarrheal episodes, inanition, and dehydration. A renal tubular defect is clinically insignificant. As patients mature and lactose-containing formulae become less part of the diet, diarrhea becomes less severe. Affected adults may have no symptoms from small amounts of malabsorbed monosaccharides because of the large surface area-to-volume ratio of the intestinal lumen.

**MIM No.:** *23160

**Sex Ratio:** M1:F1

**Occurrence:** About 20 cases cases reported in the literature.

**Risk of Recurrence for Patient's Sib:**
See Part I, *Mendelian Inheritance.*

**Risk of Recurrence for Patient's Child:**
See Part I, *Mendelian Inheritance.*

**Age of Detectability:** As soon after birth as oral lactose, glucose, or galactose is ingested.

**Gene Mapping and Linkage:** Unknown.

**Prevention:** Avoidance of malabsorbed monosaccharides or their precursor disaccharides in infancy and early childhood.

**Treatment:** Removal of glucose- or galactose-containing food from the diet. Oral or parenteral fluid replacement for dehydration.

**Prognosis:** Fatal if untreated. No shortening of life span if glucose and galactose are avoided. Symptoms seem to ameliorate with age.

**Detection of Carrier:** A reduced uptake of glucose by the jejunal mucosa was demonstrable in both parents of one affected child.

**Special Considerations:** The intestinal transport and absorption of glucose is completely defective, whereas renal tubular reabsorption of glucose is only modestly impaired, thus demonstrating that at least two systems mediate glucose reabsorption in the renal tubule in contrast to a single mechanism in the intestine (see **Glucoglycinuria** which affects only the kidney). Normal affinity but reduced capacity for intestinal glucose transport in jejunal mucosa of obligate heterozygotes implies that mutation affects the number of carrier molecules.

**References:**
Schneider AJ, et al.: Glucose-galactose malabsorption: report of a case with autoradiographic studies of a mucosal biopsy. New Engl J Med 1966; 274:305–312.
Meeuwisse GW, Dahlqvist A: Glucose-galactose malabsorption. A study with biopsy of the small intestinal mucosa. Acta Paediatr (Scand) 1968; 57:273–280.
Elsas LJ II, et al.: Renal and intestinal hexose transport in familial glucose-galactose malabsorption. J Clin Invest 1970; 49:576–585.
Stirling CE, et al.: Quantitative radioautography of sugar transport in intestinal biopsies from normal humans and a patient with glucose-galactose malabsorption. J Clin Invest 1972; 51:438.
Elsas LJ II, Lamb DW Jr: Familial glucose-galactose malabsorption: remission of glucose intolerance. J Pediatr 1973; 83:226–232.
Flier JS, et al.: Distribution of glucose transporter messenger RNA transcripts in tissue of rat and man. J Clin Invest 1987; 79:657–661.

EL009                                                                 **Louis J. Elsas, II**

**Glucosephosphate isomerase, deficiency of**
*See ANEMIA, GLUCOSE PHOSPHATE ISOMERASE DEFICIENCY*
**Glucosuria**
*See RENAL GLYCOSURIA*
**Glutamate-aspartate transport defect**
*See ACIDURIA, DICARBOXYLIC AMINOACIDURIA*

**Glutaric aciduria type I**
*See ACIDEMIA, GLUTARIC ACIDEMIA I*
**Glutaric aciduria type IIA, neonatal form**
*See ACIDEMIA, GLUTARIC ACIDEMIA II*
**Glutaric aciduria type IIB (mild and/or adult variants)**
*See ACIDEMIA, ETHYLMALONIC-ADIPIC*
**Glutaryl-CoA dehydrogenase deficiency**
*See ACIDEMIA, GLUTARIC ACIDEMIA I*
**Glutathionase deficiency**
*See GLUTATHIONURIA*
**Glutathione peroxidase deficiency, hemolytic anemia due to**
*See ANEMIA, HEMOLYTIC, GLUTATIONINE PEROXIDASE DEFICIENCY*
**Glutathione reductase deficiency, hemolytic anemia due to**
*See ANEMIA, HEMOLYTIC, GLUTATHIONE REDUCTASE DEFICIENCY*
**Glutathione synthetase deficiency**
*See ACIDEMIA, PYROGLUTAMIC*
**Glutathione synthetase deficiency, hemolytic anemia due to**
*See ANEMIA, HEMOLYTIC, GLUTATHIONE SYNTHETASE DEFICIENCY*

## GLUTATHIONURIA                                                    0422

**Includes:**
Gamma-glutamyl transpeptidase deficiency
Glutathionase deficiency

**Excludes:** N/A

**Major Diagnostic Criteria:** May include mental retardation, behavioral, and psychiatric problems. Laboratory studies show a marked increase in excretion of urinary glutathione, increased plasma glutathione concentrations, and normal concentration of erythrocyte glutathione. The urine may give a positive nitroprusside test. A severe reduction of the activity of gamma-glutamyl transpeptidase has been demonstrated in serum, urine, leukocytes, and cultured skin fibroblasts.

**Clinical Findings:** Three patients with this disorder have been described. One was an adult male with mild mental retardation and no other clinical abnormalities. Another was a 22-year-old female who spends most of her time in an institution for the retarded. This individual fed poorly as an infant. She walked and was toilet trained at a normal time, but speech was slow, and tantrums were prominent from age 3 to 5 years. Her IQ was in the low 60s on several testings. At age 12, behavioral problems became more severe, and an EEG showed mild, non-specific, diffuse dysrhythmia. Severe behavioral abnormalities continued, including self-inflicted injury, suicidal threats, and attacks on hospital staff and other patients. Physical examination was normal. A third patient was briefly described by O'Daley (1968). This patient was described as "a child suffering from a psychiatric disorder." Transpeptidase deficiency has been documented in this subject.

**Complications:** The few patients described have had some abnormality in mental function. Whether this is a consequence of the enzyme defect or a coincidental finding is undetermined.

**Associated Findings:** None known.

**Etiology:** Autosomal recessive inheritance of a generalized deficiency of gamma-glutamyl transpeptidase.

**Pathogenesis:** Unknown.

**MIM No.:** *23195

**Sex Ratio:** Presumably M1:F1

**Occurrence:** Three cases have been documented.

**Risk of Recurrence for Patient's Sib:**
See Part I, *Mendelian Inheritance.*

**Risk of Recurrence for Patient's Child:**
See Part I, *Mendelian Inheritance.*

**Age of Detectability:** Presumably at birth by enzyme assay of peripheral leukocytes or demonstration of glutathionuria. Since gamma-glutamyl transpeptidase activity is present in normal cultured amniotic fluid cells, antenatal diagnosis of this disorder might be possible.

**Gene Mapping and Linkage:** GGT1 (gamma-glutamyltransferase 1) has been mapped to 22q11.1-q11.2.

**Prevention:** None known. Genetic counseling indicated.

**Treatment:** Unknown.

**Prognosis:** The possibility that glutathionuria is usually a harmless disorder must be considered. However, the condition may cause or predispose to mental retardation and/or psychiatric problems.

**Detection of Carrier:** Both parents of one patient had moderate reductions in fibroblast transpeptidase activity. Other obligate heterozygotes have not been investigated.

**References:**
O'Daley S: An abnormal sulphydryl compound in urine. Irish J Med Sci 1968; 7:578–579.
Goodman SI, et al.: Serum gamma-glutamyl transpeptidase deficiency. Lancet 1971; I:243–235.
Schulman JD, et al.: Glutathionuria: inborn error of metabolism due to tissue deficiency of gamma-glutamyl transpeptidase. Biochem Biophys Res Commun 1975; 65:68–74.
Wright EC, et al.: Glutathionuria: gamma-glutamyl transpeptidase deficiency. J Inherit Metab Dis 1979; 2:3–7.

G0025                                 **Stephen I. Goodman**
PA032                                       **A.D. Patrick**
SC033                             **Joseph D. Schulman**

## GLUTEN-SENSITIVE ENTEROPATHY       0423

**Includes:**
Celiac disease
Celiac sprue
Enteropathy, gluten-induced
Idiopathic steatorrhea
Nontropical sprue
Sprue

**Excludes:** Intestinal malabsorption unrelated to gluten ingestion

**Major Diagnostic Criteria:** Flattened mucosa of the small bowel on a biopsy specimen. Remission of symptoms on a gluten-free diet. The small bowel may be challenged with gluten after the patient improves and a further biopsy specimen obtained; but this is a matter of judgment.

**Clinical Findings:** Diarrhea (90%); weight loss, usually progressive; growth retardation; abdominal distention; peripheral edema; anemia from iron deficiency or folic acid deficiency; steatorrhea; low serum carotene level (90%); delayed passage of barium through the small bowel; dilated jejunum; and a flattened small bowel mucosa on biopsy.

**Complications:** Osteomalacia and hypoprothrombinemia from malabsorption of vitamins D and K. Hypokalemia, hypocalcemia, and hypomagnesemia from fecal electrolyte losses. Bacterial overgrowth may occur in the upper GI tract.

**Associated Findings:** Dermatitis herpetiformis (about 70% of patients with dermatitis herpetiformis have flattening of the small bowel mucosa); vasculitis; GI lymphoma and adenocarcinoma; ulceration of the terminal ileum; other disorders that may have an autoimmune basis (e.g. autoimmune thyroid disease, insulin dependent diabetes.

**Etiology:** Gluten is toxic to the small bowel in genetically susceptible individuals. The toxic portion of gluten is thought to rest with the α-fraction of gliadin, the alcohol-soluble proteins of wheat endosperm. People of Irish or Northwestern European ancestry are a particularly susceptible group. Most likely there is more than one disease susceptibility locus. One locus appears to be linked to the HLA region on chromosome six, and the disease itself is associated with the HLA-B8, DR3, and DR7 alleles. A second hypothesized disease susceptibility gene may be related to a B-cell alloantigen or to a locus encoding the immunoglobulin heavy-chain constant regions (the Gm locus). The precise mode of

inheritance has not been proven. Genetic heterogeneity is suggested by HLA differences in young vs. older patients.

**Pathogenesis:** The damage to the small bowel mucosa becomes problematic during infancy soon after cereals are added to the diet or in young adulthood for unknown reasons. Direct exposure of the mucosal surface to gluten leads to the loss of villi and, hence, mucosal flattening. The proximal small bowel is more involved than the distal. How gliadin in gluten causes mucosal damage is not certain, but the immune response probably has the major role. Increased levels of circulating antigliadin antibodies, greater numbers of inflammatory cells in the small bowel lamina propria, and the association of gluten-sensitive enteropathy with autoimmune disorders support this hypothesis. A defect in the mucosal processing of gliadin (due to a missing enzyme, for example) with subsequent build-up of toxic intermediates is less likely a step in the development of mucosal flattening. Whatever the mechanism, the clinical manifestations are variable, ranging from none at all to severe malabsorption.

**MIM No.:** 21275

**Sex Ratio:** M1:F1.2–1.4 (M1:F2 in some registries).

**Occurrence:** 1:2,000 to 1:1,000 in much of Great Britain; 1:600 in West Ireland; 1:1,000 in Sweden and Norway.

**Risk of Recurrence for Patient's Sib:** Monozygotic twins, 70%; HLA-identical sibs, 30%; sibs overall, 10%.

**Risk of Recurrence for Patient's Child:** Perhaps 5–10%.

**Age of Detectability:** Small bowel biopsy has been performed in children under one year of age.

**Gene Mapping and Linkage:** One disease susceptibility locus appears to be linked to HLA on chromosome six. There is no definitive mapping of other disease loci.

**Prevention:** Gluten-free diet in relatives at risk, unless other information renders dietary restriction unnecessary.

**Treatment:** A gluten-free diet is the mainstay. Prednisone has been used in patients who do not respond to diet. Folic acid can be given to anemic patients, but this is usually unnecessary. Vitamin D supplementation in the presence of bone disease.

**Prognosis:** Usually normal life span. Children with severe malabsorption and growth retardation may remain short.

**Detection of Carrier:** Carrier detection in the usual sense (i.e., for single gene disorders) does not strictly apply to gluten-sensitive enteropathy, although HLA typing should identify asymptomatic family members carrying the presumed HLA-linked susceptibility gene. More important is the detection of asymptomatic relatives with abnormal small bowel mucosa, and this can be done reliably only with biopsy.

**Special Considerations:** Current genetic counseling for relatives at risk can perhaps be optimized by applying a two-locus model for the inheritance of the disease. Such a model, in which both disease susceptibility genes are recessively expressed, also fits the population prevalence data for the disease. The HLA-DR3 and DR7 associations are factored into the risk estimates by using Bayes' rule. Thus, sibs who share both HLA haplotypes with the patient or who have the HLA-DR3 marker in the unshared haplotypes have the highest risk for the disease (about 30%). Other combinations of HLA haplotypes in sibs of affected patients are associated with a lower risk, for example, less than 0.1% if no HLA haplotypes are shared, and HLA DR3 and DR7 markers are absent.

**Support Groups:**
WA; Seattle; The Gluten Intolerance Group of North America (GIG)
IA; Des Moines; Celiac-Sprue Association (CSA/USA)
NJ; Jersey City; American Celiac Society

**References:**
Falchuk ZM: Update on gluten-sensitive enteropathy. Am J Med 1979; 67:1085–1096. * †
Strober W: Genetic factors in gluten-sensitive enteropathy. In: JI Rotter, et al., eds: Genetics and heterogeneity of common gastrointestinal disorders. New York: Academic Press, 1980:243–259.

Kagnoff MF: Two genetic loci control the murine immune response to A-gliadin, a wheat protein that activates coeliac sprue. Nature 1982; 296:158–160.

Cacciari E, et al.: Short stature and celiac disease: a relationship to consider even in patients with no gastrointestinal tract symptoms. J Pediatr 1983; 103:708–711.

Lin HJ, et al.: Use of HLA marker associations and HLA haplotype linkage to estimate disease risks in families with gluten-sensitive enteropathy. Clin Genet 1985; 28:185–198.

Polanco I, et al.: Effect of gluten supplementation in healthy siblings of children with celiac disease. Gastroenterology 1987; 92:678–681.

Brocchi E, et al.: Endoscopic demonstration of loss of duodenal folds in the diagnosis of celiac disease. New Engl J Med 1988; 319:741–744.

Scott H, Brandtzaeg P: Gluten IgA antibodies and coeliac disease. Lancet 1989; I:382–383.

LI026
R0036

**Henry J. Lin**
**Jerome I. Rotter**

## Glycerokinase deficiency
*See GLYCEROL KINASE DEFICIENCY*

---

## GLYCEROL INTOLERANCE SYNDROME 2286

**Includes:** Hypoglycemia, glycerol-induced

**Excludes:**
**Fructose-1,6-diphosphatase deficiency** (0396)
**Glycerol kinase deficiency** (2310)

**Major Diagnostic Criteria:** Gastrointestinal and central nervous system (CNS) disturbances are precipitated by glycerol tolerance testing; these symptoms may or may not be associated with hypoglycemia. There is no demonstrable complete deficiency of glycerol kinase, fructose 1,6-diphosphatase, or other enzyme of carbohydrate metabolism, though partial deficiency of fructose 1,6-diphosphatase has been seen.

**Clinical Findings:** Infants with glycerol intolerance have had initial signs and symptoms of hypoglycemia between day one and 11 months of age. Episodes have followed either overnight fasting or fatty meals, or both. Hypoglycemia has occurred with oral glycerol tolerance testing and has been associated with symptoms of nausea, vomiting, diarrhea, euphoria, confusion, drowsiness, and unresponsiveness; hypophosphatemia, elevated serum uric acid, and ketonuria have also been observed. An intravenous (i.v.) glycerol tolerance test in one patient produced profound symptoms within four minutes, including rapid loss of consciousness and a seizure, followed by coma; glucose did not fall during this i.v. glycerol tolerance test, however. Similarly, a second oral glycerol tolerance test in the same patient resulted in CNS abnormalities without hypoglycemia. An oral challenge with a medium-chain triglyceride (Portagen) in this patient produced diarrhea and euphoria, without associated hypoglycemia. Another patient underwent glycerol tolerance testing on three different occasions: at 5 9/12 years, at 5 11/12 years after a six-week course of folic acid, and at 15 4/12 years; hypoglycemia was observed only after the initial tolerance test. Intellectual development was reportedly normal.

**Complications:** Significant CNS consequences could result from the profound symptomatic hypoglycemia reported in these patients.

**Associated Findings:** Patients were premature, with gestational ages ranging from 34 to 37 weeks and birth weights from 1,850 to 2,722 g.
One patient underwent liver biopsy, and histology showed a mosaic pattern of the hepatic parenchyma, with fibrous septae. Electron microscopy revealed lipid droplets in cytoplasm and nuclei, swollen mitochondria with matrix inclusions, and substantial glycogen stores.

**Etiology:** Unknown. Family history from one patient suggested hypoglycemia in two of four paternal uncles and was positive in another patient for a chronic convulsive disorder, and for mental retardation in a second cousin.

**Pathogenesis:** Several hypotheses have been proposed to explain the pathogenesis of glycerol kinase activity: 1) It was noted that glycerol caused a marked decrease in serum dopamine β-hydroxylase activity in one of these patients, and it was suggested that this reflected an influence of glycerol on nervous system activity. 2) Partial deficiencies of hepatic fructose 1,6-diphosphatase, glycerol 3-phosphate dehydrogenase, and glycerol 3-phosphate oxidase have been observed to be associated with elevated glycerol 3-phosphate and a possible increased sensitivity of the patient's fructose 1,6-diphosphatase to inhibition by glycerol 3-phosphate. It has been suggested that these factors may lead to a block in gluconeogenesis. 3) One may speculate that altered compartmentation of glycerol kinase in these patients could result in the metabolic abnormalities, especially in light of the clinical similarity between patients with glycerol intolerance and the juvenile form of glycerol kinase deficiency.

**Sex Ratio:** M2:F1

**Occurrence:** Three cases have been documented. All have been white with ethnicity recorded in only one: mother German-Jewish and father Russian-Jewish and Irish-Protestant.

**Risk of Recurrence for Patient's Sib:** Unknown.

**Risk of Recurrence for Patient's Child:** Unknown.

**Age of Detectability:** In the first year of life.

**Gene Mapping and Linkage:** Unknown.

**Prevention:** None known. Genetic counseling indicated.

**Treatment:** Frequent feedings and limitation of intake of fats, i.e., glycerol.
One patient was treated with folic acid (30 mg/day orally) and seemed to have an improvement in glycerol tolerance. The same patient appeared to outgrow glycerol intolerance by age 15, which has led to speculation that this may be a metabolic dysmaturity syndrome.
It has been suggested that treatment should include limitation of fructose intake, but both patients had normal fructose tolerance tests.

**Prognosis:** Probably good if treatment is followed. One patient was reported to outgrow the disorder by the teenage years.

**Detection of Carrier:** Unknown.

**References:**
Maclaren NK, et al.: Glycerol intolerance in a child with intermittent hypoglycemia. J Pediatr 1975; 86:43–49.
Wapnir RA, et al.: Glycerol-induced hypoglycemia: a syndrome associated with multiple liver enzyme deficiencies. Clinical and in vitro studies. Metabolism 1982; 31:1057–1064. *
Ginns EI, et al.: A juvenile form of glycerol kinase deficiency with episodic vomiting, acidemia, and stupor. J Pediatr 1984; 104:736–739.
Fort P, et al.: Long-term evolution of glycerol intolerance syndrome. J Pediatr 1985; 106:453–456.*
Wapnir RA, Stiel L: Regulation of gluconeogenesis by glycerol and its phosphorylated derivatives. Biochem Med 1985; 33:141–148.
McCabe ERB, Seltzer WK: Glycerol kinase deficiency: compartmental considerations regarding pathogenesis and clinical heterogeneity. In: Brauthar N, ed: Myocardial and sketal muscle bioenergetics. New York: Plenum Press 1986:481–493.
McCabe ERB: Disorders of glycerol metabolism. In: Scriver CR, et al, eds: The metabolic basis of inherited disease, 6th ed. New York: McGraw-Hill, 1989:945–963.

MC002

**Edward R.B. McCabe**

## GLYCEROL KINASE DEFICIENCY                    2310

**Includes:**
Adrenal hypoplasia-glycerol kinase deficiency
Complex glycerol kinase deficiency syndrome
Glycerokinase deficiency
Glyceroluria
Hyperglycerolemia
Liver glycerol kinase deficiency-hypertriglyceridemia
Liver glycerol kinase deficiency-pseudohypertriglyceridemia
Muscular dystrophy (Duchenne type)-glycerol kinase deficiency

**Excludes:**
**Adrenal hypoplasia, congenital** (0024)
**Adrenoleukodystrophy, X-linked** (2533)
Glycerol-induced hypoglycemia with normal glycerol kinase activity
**Glycerol intolerance syndrome** (2286)
Glyceroluria without hyperglycerolemia
Hypertriglyceridemia without hyperglycerolemia
**Muscular dystrophy, adult pseudohypertrophic** (0687)
**Muscular dystrophy, childhood pseudohypertrophic** (0689)

**Major Diagnostic Criteria:** The clinical findings vary with different clinical forms of this inborn error of metabolism. Therefore, the biochemical features are key to the diagnosis: hyperglycerolemia, glyceroluria, and demonstration of glycerol kinase deficiency in fibroblasts, leukocytes, lymphoblastoid cell line (LCL), liver, and/or kidney. Patients with associated myopathy have deletions involving the DMD locus (see **Muscular dystrophy, childhood pseudohypertrophic**) which are detectable with the dystropin cDNA and genomic probes in this region of Xp21.

**Clinical Findings:** Glycerol kinase deficiency has been subdivided into the infantile, juvenile, and adult (or benign) forms with the clinical characteristics consistent within individual pedigrees.

The *infantile form* is a contiguous gene syndrome which has been characterized by clinical evidence of adrenal cortical insufficiency, adrenal hypoplasia at autopsy, and developmental delay. Many patients have also had a dystrophic myopathy with elevated serum creatine kinase (CK) values. The myopathy is indistinguishable from the progressive Duchenne type seen in **Muscular dystrophy, childhood pseudohypertrophic**, or the milder Becker type seen in **Muscular dystrophy, adult pseudohypertrophic**.

The *juvenile form* has been reported in two boys who presented with episodes of vomiting, acidemia and stupor at four years of age. They showed no evidence of adrenal insufficiency and were developmentally normal. Clinically, these two boys resembled patients with **Glycerol intolerance syndrome**, though the latter have normal glycerol kinase activity.

The *adult form* (or benign form) has been diagnosed incidentally, with no consistent pattern of clinical abnormalities. These patients were discovered during investigation of their pseudohypertriglyceridemia when the clinical chemistry laboratory misinterpreted their hyperglycerolemia.

**Complications:** Adrenal or Addisonian crisis (see **Adrenoleukodystrophy, X-linked**) may occur in patients with the infantile form as a consequence of glucocorticoid and mineralocorticoid deficiency. These crises are life-threatening and are the presumed cause of death in patients not receiving replacement steroids.

**Associated Findings:** Patients with the infantile form may have the peculiar "pinched" facies with alternating strabismus, hypertelorism, and drooping mouth. X-ray evidence of decreased bone density may be seen and has been described as osteoporosis or osteopenia, and they may have pathologic fractures. Testes may be undescended or even absent. Fingers may be flexed and tapering, and skin may be thin and semitranslucent. **Ornithine transcarbamylase deficiency** was documented in one patient.

Abnormal electroencephalograms may be seen in patients with infantile or juvenile forms.

Individuals with the adult form have had a variety of associated problems, including diabetes mellitus, myocardial infarctions, osteoarthritis, laryngeal carcinoma in situ, and **Hypertriglyceri-**

demia, but others have had no reported medical problems. The associated abnormalities probably reflect a bias of ascertainment, representing those who have blood lipids examined and pseudohypertriglyceridemia recognized.

**Etiology:** Pedigrees with the infantile and adult forms were consistent with X-linked inheritance, and the two patients with the juvenile forms were both males.

**Pathogenesis:** The infantile or complex form is a microdeletion syndrome with the spectrum of clinical involvement dependent on the extent of the deletion in the Xp21 region. The glycerol kinase (GK), **Muscular dystrophy, childhood pseudohypertrophic** (DMD), and **Adrenal hypoplasia, congenital** (AHC or AHX) loci are clearly discrete. The juvenile and benign forms presumably represent isolated mutations of this locus, with the former perhaps representing a more significant mutation of the GK locus. However, it should be noted that concordance between the enzyme deficiency and clinical phenotype has not been possible in the two boys with the juvenile form, since these were the only affected individuals in their families, and these features could be coincidential.

**MIM No.:** *30703

**Sex Ratio:** Infantile forms, M>20:F1. Juvenile and adult forms, M≥10:F0.

**Occurrence:** At least 30 cases have been reported; more than 20 with the infantile form, two with the juvenile form, and eight or more with the adult form.

**Risk of Recurrence for Patient's Sib:**
See Part I, *Mendelian Inheritance.* Occasional heterozygous females show mild to more complete clinical expression as a consequence of lyonization.

**Risk of Recurrence for Patient's Child:**
See Part I, *Mendelian Inheritance.* Fertility has been demonstrated in the adult form.

**Age of Detectability:** In utero through adulthood. Adrenal hypoplasia and insufficiency are present in the fetus, and, therefore, the infantile form may be diagnosed in utero by low maternal estriols. Glycerol kinase activity is expressed in amniocytes, but no affected pregnancies have yet been monitored using this technique.

**Gene Mapping and Linkage:** GK (glycerol kinase deficiency) has been mapped to Xp21.3-p21.2.
The gene order in the Xpter region is Xpter ...AHC-GK-DMD...cen.

**Prevention:** None known. Genetic counseling indicated.

**Treatment:** Patients with the infantile form associated with congenital adrenal hypoplasia require mineralocorticoids and replacement therapy with glucocorticoids in order to prevent life-threatening adrenal crises. A diet low in fat, and therefore low in glycerol, may be useful in preventing episodes of vomiting, acidemia, and stupor in patients with the infantile form. A similar diet will lower blood glycerol in patients with the infantile form, but appears to have no beneficial clinical effect.

**Prognosis:** Patients with the infantile form have a good prognosis for survival if treated with steroid replacement. However, this does not appear to alter the other clinical findings. Patients with the juvenile form are abnormal only during episodes, which may be quite severe, but these episodes may decrease in frequency with a low-glycerol diet. The adult form seems to be clinically benign.

**Detection of Carrier:** If an X-chromosome deletion is present in the proband at the microscopic level or by DNA probes, these techniques may be useful for carrier detection. Enzymatic activity may be decreased in carrier women, but, as with most X-linked diseases, this is quite variable, and therefore, may not be used reliably to exclude the carrier status.

**Special Considerations:** The gene for glycerol kinase is an important linked marker for Duchenne muscular dystrophy (see **Muscular dystrophy, childhood pseudohypertrophic**, and this enzyme deficiency should be considered in those patients with Duchenne dystrophy and developmental delay. Adrenal function should be evaluated in all patients with glycerol kinase deficiency, since recognition and treatment may be life-saving.

The banded karyotype should be analyzed in all affected females to rule out X chromosome abnormalities.

### References:

Guggenheim MA, et al.: Glycerol kinase deficiency with neuromuscular, skeletal and adrenal abnormalities. Ann Neurol 1980; 7:441–449. *

Francke U, et al.: Congenital adrenal hypoplasia, myopathy and glycerol kinase deficiency: molecular evidence for deletions. Am J Hum Genet 1987; 40:212–227.

Kenwrick S, et al.: Molecular analysis of the Duchenne muscular dystrophy region using pulsed field gel electrophoresis. Cell 1987; 48:351–357.

Wise JE, et al.: Phenotypic features of patients with congenital adrenal hypoplasia and glycerol kinase deficiency. Am J Dis Child 1987; 141:744–747. *

Darras BT, Francke U: Myopathy in complex glycerol kinase deficiency patients is due to 3′ deletions of the dystrophin gene. Am J Hum Genet 1988; 43:126–130.

McCabe ERB et al.: Complementary cDNA probes for the Duchenne muscular dystrophy locus demonstrates a previously undetectable deletion in a patient with dystrophic myopathy, glycerol kinase deficiency, and congenital adrenal hypoplasia. J Clin Invest 1989; 83:95–99.

McCabe ERB: Disorders of glycerol metabolism. In: Scriver CR, et al, eds: The metabolic basis of inherited disease, 6th ed. New York: McGraw-Hill, 1989:945–956. *

MC002

**Edward R.B. McCabe**

**Glyceroluria**
*See GLYCEROL KINASE DEFICIENCY*
**Glycinemia, ketotic, I**
*See ACIDEMIA, PROPIONIC*
**Glycinuria with or without oxalate urolithiasis**
*See IMINOGLYCINURIA*
**Glycoaminoacid storage disease-angiokeratoma corporis diffusion**
*See ALPHA-N-ACETYLGALACTOSAMINIDASE DEFICIENCY*
**Glycogen deficiency syndrome with visceral fatty metamorphosis**
*See GLYCOGEN SYNTHETASE DEFICIENCY*
**Glycogen storage disease - zero**
*See GLYCOGEN SYNTHETASE DEFICIENCY*
**Glycogen storage disease, type I**
*See GLYCOGENOSIS, TYPE Ia*
**Glycogen storage disease, type Ib**
*See GLYCOGENOSIS, TYPE Ib*
**Glycogen storage disease, type Ic**
*See GLYCOGENOSIS, TYPE Ic*
**Glycogen storage disease, type IIa**
*See GLYCOGENOSIS, TYPE IIa*
**Glycogen storage disease, type IIb**
*See GLYCOGENOSIS, TYPE IIb*
**Glycogen storage disease, type IIb (McKusick)**
*See GLYCOGENOSIS, TYPE IIc*
**Glycogen storage disease, type IIc**
*See GLYCOGENOSIS, TYPE IIc*
**Glycogen storage disease, Type IId**
*See GLYCOGENOSIS, TYPE IId*
**Glycogen storage disease, type III**
*See GLYCOGENOSIS, TYPE III*
**Glycogen storage disease, type IV**
*See GLYCOGENOSIS, TYPE IV*
**Glycogen storage disease, type V**
*See GLYCOGENOSIS, TYPE V*
**Glycogen storage disease, type VI**
*See GLYCOGENOSIS, TYPE VI*
**Glycogen storage disease, type VII**
*See GLYCOGENOSIS, TYPE VII*
**Glycogen storage disease, type VIII**
*See GLYCOGENOSIS, TYPE VIII*
**Glycogen storage disease, type VIII (McKusick)**
*See GLYCOGEN STORAGE DISEASE, X-LINKED WITH NORMAL HEPATIC ENZYMES*
**Glycogen storage disease, type IXa**
*See GLYCOGENOSIS, TYPE IXa*
**Glycogen storage disease, type IXb**
*See GLYCOGENOSIS, TYPE IXb*

**Glycogen storage disease, type IXc**
*See GLYCOGENOSIS, TYPE IXc*

## GLYCOGEN STORAGE DISEASE, X-LINKED WITH NORMAL HEPATIC ENZYMES    2303

**Includes:**

Glycogen storage disease, type VIII (McKusick)
Hepatic glycogenosis with normal enzymes
Hepatic phosphorylase kinase deficiency
Phosphorylase kinase deficiency of liver

**Excludes:**

**Fructose-1,6-diphosphatase deficiency** (0396)
**Glycogenosis, type IIa** (0011)
**Glycogenosis, type III** (0426)
**Glycogenosis, type IXa** (0430)
**Glycogenosis, type IXb** (2878)

**Major Diagnostic Criteria:**   Hepatomegaly and increased hepatic glycogen content in males only during childhood; normal hepatic glycogenolytic enzymes.

**Clinical Findings:**   Affected males have hepatomegaly, delay in growth and sexual maturation, muscular weakness in childhood, and gouty arthritis. Hypoglycemia, acidosis, and hyperlipidemia are mild, if they occur at all. Weakness, growth retardation, and hepatomegaly spontaneously improve after puberty. However, puberty may be delayed until age 18 years.

**Complications:**   Unknown.

**Associated Findings:**   Brachycephaly, nerve deafness, and congenital cataracts were observed in a single patient.

**Etiology:**   X-linked inheritance.

**Pathogenesis:**   Probably due to defect in a hepatic and/or muscle enzyme involved in glycogen catabolism.

**MIM No.:**   *30600

**POS No.:**   3241

**CDC No.:**   271.000

**Sex Ratio:**   M1:F0

**Occurrence:**   About ten cases have been documented.

**Risk of Recurrence for Patient's Sib:**
See Part I, *Mendelian Inheritance.*

**Risk of Recurrence for Patient's Child:**
See Part I, *Mendelian Inheritance.*

**Age of Detectability:**   In infancy.

**Gene Mapping and Linkage:**   PHKA (phosphorylase kinase, alpha) has been provisionally mapped to Xq12-q13.
PHK (phosphorylase kinase deficiency, liver (glycogen storage disease type VIII)) has been mapped to X.

**Prevention:**   None known. Genetic counseling indicated.

**Treatment:**   Unknown.

**Prognosis:**   Good for survival; physical and social disability during childhood is variable.

**Detection of Carrier:**   Unknown.

**Special Considerations:**   This is not the only entity in which hepatic glycogenosis occurs without a definable enzymatic explanation. Sporadic occurrences of glycogen storage may not be distinguishable from this disease by current clinical or biochemical methods.

McKusick has placed this condition in his type VIII (see **Glycogenosis, type IXa**).

**Support Groups:**   IA; Durant; Association for Glycogen Storage Disease

### References:

Huijing F, Fernandes J: X-chromosome inheritance of liver glycogenosis with phosphorylase kinase deficiency. Am J Hum Genet 1969; 21:275–283.

Spencer-Peet J, et al.: Hepatic glycogen storage disease. Q J Med 1971; 157:95–114.

Keating JP, et al.: X-linked glycogen storage disease: a cause of hypotonia, hyperuricemia and growth retardation. Am J Dis Child 1985; 139:609–613.

KE023            **James P. Keating**

**Glycogen storage disease-deficient cardiac phosphorylase kinase**
*See GLYCOGENOSIS, TYPE IXc*

## GLYCOGEN SYNTHETASE DEFICIENCY      0424

**Includes:**

     Aglycogenosis
     Glycogen deficiency syndrome with visceral fatty
         metamorphosis
     Glycogen storage disease - zero
     Glycogenosis, type zero
     Hypoglycemia with deficiency of glycogen synthetase in
         liver
     UDPG-glycogen transferase

**Excludes:**

     **Fructose-1,6-diphosphatase deficiency** (0396)
     **Glycogenosis** (Other)
     Hyperinsulinism
     Nesideoblastosis

**Major Diagnostic Criteria:** Recurrent hypoglycemic convulsions occur during short periods of starvation. There is ketonuria with hypoglycemia and post-prandial glycosuria. Measurement of intermediary metabolites shows the characteristic diurnal profile with morning fasting hypoglycemia and hyperketonemia followed by post-prandial hyperglycemia and hyperlactatemia. There is glucose intolerance after oral glucose administration which is associated with hyperlactatemia. No increase in blood glucose occurs after glucagon administration when starved, although a small increase may be observed three hours after a meal. There is normal increase in blood glucose after oral galactose and oral alanine administration. Enzyme studies show very low levels of glycogen synthetase activity (uridine diphosphoglucose (UDPG) - glycogen transglucosylase activity). Glycogen content (around 0.5 to 0.6 gm/100 gm wet weight) below normal range. Both muscle glycogen content and glycogen synthetase activity are normal, as is red and white cell glucose synthetase activity. Hepatic glycogen synthetase cannot be activated by reaction with muscle glycogen synthetase or with control liver extract.

**Clinical Findings:** Birthweight may be less than the 10th percentile for gestation. Onset of lethargy, somnolence, unconsciousness, convulsions, sweating, poor feeding, poor weight gain during the neonatal period or, more characteristically, at the time of omission of night feeding in later infancy. Spontaneous resolution of symptoms may occur despite persistence of the biochemical defect. In these mildly affected individuals, growth and neurologic development may be normal. Hepatomegaly is not present. Clinical symptoms are often subtle in hypoglycemic infants.

**Complications:** Delayed motor development, mental retardation, and microcephaly occur in severely affected children. Short stature occurring in moderately affected children, is corrected with dietary treatment.

**Associated Findings:** None known.

**Etiology:** Autosomal recessive inheritance with complete penetrance and variable expressivity of glycogen synthetase deficiency.

**Pathogenesis:** Affected individuals have very low glycogen stores and are thus unable to release glucose from stored glycogen during starvation. The failure to manufacture glycogen prevents glucose from being trapped after feeding, which leads to hyperglycemia with overloading of glycolysis, resulting in hyperlactatemia. It is not clear why gluconeogenesis is unable to maintain normoglycemia during early starvation. Recurrent hypoglycemic convulsions can lead to permanent brain damage, although normal development has been reported in some patients.

**MIM No.:** *24060

**CDC No.:** 271.000

**Sex Ratio:** M1:F1

**Occurrence:** Less than a dozen cases have been documented.

**Risk of Recurrence for Patient's Sib:**
     See Part I, *Mendelian Inheritance.*

**Risk of Recurrence for Patient's Child:**
     See Part I, *Mendelian Inheritance.*

**Age of Detectability:** Newborn period by biochemical methods.

**Gene Mapping and Linkage:** Unknown.

**Prevention:** None known. Genetic counseling indicated.

**Treatment:** Administration of oral or intravenous glucose to correct hypoglycemic convulsions. Glucagon administration in hypoglycemia is contraindicated. Hypoglycemia and metabolic acidosis can be prevented by frequent administration of small meals (every fours hours; day and night) with normal or low carbohydrate content. A carbohydrate-rich diet will exacerbate hyperlactatemia and will lead to metabolic acidosis.

**Prognosis:** In severely affected children without treatment, there is poor neurologic prognosis. Treatment begun before irreversible brain damage leads to normal life expectancy and neurologic development.

**Detection of Carrier:** Unknown.

**Support Groups:** IA; Durant; Association for Glycogen Storage Disease

**References:**

Aynsley-Green A, et al. Hepatic glycogen synthetase deficiency. Arch Dis Child. 1977; 52:573–579.
Lewis GM, et al. Infantile hypoglycaemia due to inherited deficiency of glycogen synthetase in liver. Arch Dis Child. 1963; 38:40–48.
Aynsley-Green A, et al. The dietary treatment of hepatic glycogen synthetase deficiency. Helv Paediat Acta. 1977; 32:71–75.
Gitzelmann R, et al. Blood cell glycogen synthetase activities in hepatic glycogen synthetase deficiency. Clin Chim Acta. 1977; 79:219.
Aynsley-Green A, et al. Asymptomatic hepatic glycogen synthetase deficiency. Lancet I. 1978; 147–148.
Aynsley-Green A, et al. Hepatic glycogen synthetase deficiency. In: Randle PJ, Steiner DF, Whelan WJ, eds. Carbohydrate metabolism and its disorder. New York: Academic Press. 1981: 139.
Gitzelmann R, et al.: Hepatic glycogen synthetase deficiency not expressed in cultured skin fibroblasts. Clin Chim Acta. 1983; 130: 111–115.

SI003            **James B. Sidbury**
AY001            **A. Aynsley-Green**

## GLYCOGENOSES      1507

**Includes:**

     Cyclic AMP-dependent kinase
     Hemolytic disorders, glycogen metabolism related
     Lactate dehydrogenase, M isozyme
     Lactate transporter
     Phosphoglucomutase
     Phosphoglucose isomerase
     Phosphoglycerate kinase, M isozyme
     Phosphoglycerate mutase, M isozyme
     Phosphoglucose isomerase, Homberg type

Glycogenoses refers to the various inborn errors in the metabolism of glycogen. Historically, these have been known by the names of their discoverers, and more recently by a numbering system adopted and extended in this volume. One definition of these glycogen metabolism storage diseases, however, is a heritable disorder of glycogen metabolism which can be enzymatically defined. This definition excludes those conditions in which tissue glycogen accumulation is secondary, such as over-treatment of diabetes with insulin or administration of pharmacologic amounts of hydrocortisol or its analogues. This definition would also

**Table 1507-1**  Classification of Glycogenoses by Site and Enzyme Defect

| Type | Enzyme Defect | Encyclopedia Article or Reference |
|---|---|---|
| **Liver (L)** | | |
| I (L) | UDPG-glycogen transferase | 0424 **Glycogen synthetase deficiency** |
| IIa (L) | Glucose-6-phosphatase | 0425 **Glycogenosis, Type Ia** |
| IIb (L) | Glucose-6-phosphate translocase | 2168 **Glycogenosis, Type Ib** |
| IIc (L) | Phosphate-pyrophosphate translocase | 2871 **Glycogenosis, Type Ic** |
| III (L) | Amylo-1,6-glucosidase/oligo-1,4→1,4-glucantransferase[1] | 0426 **Glycogenosis, Type III** |
| IV (L) | Alpha-1,4 glucan-6-Alpha-glucosyltransferase | 0116 **Glycogenosis, Type IV** |
| V (L) | Hepatic phosphorylase | 0427 **Glycogenosis, Type VI** |
| VI (L) | Phosphorylase kinase[2] | 0430 **Glycogenosis, Type IXa** |
| **Generalized (L & M)** | | |
| I (M&L) | Amylo-1,6-glucosidase/oligo-1,4→1,4-glucan transferase | 0426 **Glycogenosis, Type III** |
| II (M&L) | Cyclic AMP-dependent kinase | See Hugo et al (1970) |
| III (M&L) | Phosphorylase kinase | 2878 **Glycogenosis, Type IXb** |
| IV (M&L) | Phsophoglucomutase | See Kobayashi et al (1986) |
| V (M&L) | Phosphoglucose isomerase | See Van Biervliet and Staal (1977) |
| VI (M&L) | Triose phosphate isomerase | 2686 **Erythrocyte triosephosphate isomerase deficiency** |
| **Muscle (M)** | | |
| Ia (M) | Lysosomal Alpha-1,4 glucosidase | 0011 **Glycogenosis, Type IIa** |
| Ib (M) | Late onset lysosomal Alpha-1,4 glucosidase | 2873 **Glycogenosis, Type IIb** |
| IIa (M) | Myophosphorylase kinase | 2878 **Glycogenosis, Type IXb** |
| IIb (M) | Myocardial myophosphorylase kinase | 2879 **Glycogenosis, Type IXc** |
| III (M) | Myophosphorylase | 2877 **Glycogenosis, Type V** |
| IV (M) | Phosphoglucose isomerase, Homberg type | See Bardosi et al (1985) |
| V (M) | Phosphoglucose isomerase inhibitor | 0429 **Glycogenosis, Type VIII** |
| VI (M) | Phosphofructokinase, M isozyme | 0428 **Glycogenosis, Type VII** |
| VII (M) | Phosphoglycerate kinase, M isozyme[2] | See Di Mauro, Dalakas & Miranda (1981) |
| VIII (M) | Phosphoglycerate mutase, M isozyme | See Di Mauro, Miranda et al (1981) |
| IXa (M) | Lactate dehydrogenase, M isozyme | See Kanno et al (1980) |
| IXb (M) | Lactate transporter | See Fishbein (1986) |

1 = Probably a promotor defect
2 = X-linked

exclude those instances or conditions which appear to be due to an enzyme defect but which can not yet be enzymatically defined. This would exclude the currently-accepted types IIc and IId glycogenosis.

Historically, deficiency of glucose-6-phophatase (see **Glycogenosis, type Ia**) was the first inborn error of metabolism to be enzymatically defined. Deficiency of the debrancher (see **Glycogenosis, type III**) and brancher (**Glycogenosis, type IV**) were the first inborn errors to be demonstrated to be associated with an abnormal product. The deficiency of lysosomal alpha glucosidase (see **Glycogenosis, type IIa**) was the first error of the lysosome to be defined. Finally, the deficiency of the muscle isozyme of phosphofructokinase (see **Glycogenosis, type VII**) was the first inborn error to be demonstrated to be the result of a deficiency of an isozyme.

Enzymatic definition of certain of the glycogenoses immediately clarified the normal metabolic pathway. For example, when **Glycogenosis, type V** was shown to be consequent to an absence of myophosphorylase, it was immediately evident that glycogen synthesis and breakdown did not result from reversing the direction of flow of phosphorylase. The fact that there was a glycogenosis due to a deficiency of phosphorylase which affected only muscle, and another glycogenosis with deficient phosphorylase which affected the liver and not the muscle, demonstrated separate and distinctive genetic control in liver and in muscle.

Since these early milestones in the biochemistry of human genetics, there has been steady progress both in the delineation and explanation of glycogenoses, but no true consensus on classification. At the present time, there are some 26 glycogenoses

identified by site(s) and enzyme defect. While the deficient enzyme is the ultimate descriptor of the cause of a particular glycogenosis, the name of the enzyme alone does not make a useful classification. Therefore, a type classification based upon both enzyme and clinical presentation has been proposed; an approach which may prove more useful to the clinician and clinical geneticist.

The proposed classification separates the glycogenoses into those which clinically affect the liver, the muscle, or both liver and muscle. Within this framework, the glycogenoses are ordered according to the proximity of the enzyme defect to glycogen. For example, the numbers given to lysosomal glucosidase is lowest, while lactic dehydrogenase is highest in the muscle group.

Some conditions reflect recent discoveries (phosphoglucose isomerase, Homberg type; lactate dehydrogenase, M isozyme; lactate transporter), and other (tricose phosphate isomerase; phosphoglucose isomerase; phosphoglycerate kinase, M isozyme) have been considered hemolytic disorders which have only recently been identified as glycogenoses.

**Support Groups:**  IA; Durant; Association for Glycogen Storage Disease

**References:**
Hugo G, et al: Loss of cyclic 3'5' - AMP dependent kinase and reduction of phosphorylase kinase in skeletal muscle. Biochem Biophys Res Comm 1970; 40:982–988.
Van Biervliet GM, Staal GEJ: Excessive hepatic glycogen storage in glucosephosphate isomerase deficiency. Acta Paediatr Scand 1977; 66:311–315.

Kanno T, et al: Hereditary deficiency of lactate dehydrogenase M-subunit. Clinica Chim Acta 1980; 108:267–276.

Di Mauro S, et al: Phosphoglycerate kinase deficiency: a new cause of recurrent myoglobinuria. Ann Neurology 1981; 10:90.

Di Mauro S, et al: Human muscle phosphoglycerate mutase deficiency: newly discovered matabolic myopathy. Science 1981; 212: 1277–1279.

Bardosi A, et al: Ultrastructural and histochemical abnormalities of skeletal muscle in a patient with a new variant (type Homburg) of glucosephosphate isomerase (GPI) deficiency. Clin Neuropathol 1985; 4:72–76.

Fishbein WN: Lactate transporter defect: a new disease of muscle. Science 1986; 234:1254–1256.

Kobayashi J, et al: A case of phosphoglucomutase deficiency with decreased muscle and serum carnitine. No To Hattatsu 1986; 18:310–315.

SI003                                             **James B. Sidbury**

**Glycogenosis, type zero**
*See GLYCOGEN SYNTHETASE DEFICIENCY*
**Glycogenosis, type I**
*See GLYCOGENOSIS, TYPE Ia*

## GLYCOGENOSIS, TYPE IA                          **0425**

**Includes:**
>    Glucose-6-phosphate
>    Glycogen storage disease, type I
>    Glycogenosis, type I
>    Hepatorenal glycogenosis
>    von Gierke disease

**Excludes:**
>    **Glycogenosis** (other)
>    Hepatomegaly of other etiologies
>    Hypoglycemia of other cause

**Major Diagnostic Criteria:** Fasting hypoglycemia; hypoglycemic seizures; large liver; poor rate of growth; no rise in blood glucose to glucagon, but an increase in blood lactate; high uric acid, cholesterol, and triglycerides; moderately elevated transaminases. Absent or low liver glucose-6-phosphatase.

**Clinical Findings:** In the neonatal period hypoglycemic seizures or hepatomegaly may be the cardinal findings. As feedings become less frequent or infections supervene, hypoglycemia and ketoacidosis will be seen. Delayed growth becomes apparent by age one year. Difficulty handling simple respiratory infections becomes a problem. Nose bleeds usually begin around age two years, often associated with URI. Motor development is usually somewhat delayed. As the child becomes older, hypoglycemia is seen primarily with infection and stress. Xanthomas develop in about 10% of patients. The physical examination reveals a short, cherub-faced individual with a protuberant abdomen. The liver, but not the spleen, is very large. Muscular tone is relatively poor. Chemical findings include low blood glucose and high blood lactate, urate, cholesterol, triglycerides, and transaminases. The bleeding time is prolonged and the platelets increased.

**Complications:** In the early years, death from rapidly evolving ketoacidosis precipitated by infection; later, short stature; after puberty, bleeding tendency, gout, and hepatomata.

**Associated Findings:** Uric acid renal stones usually after puberty. Renal failure from the late teens onward; hepatoblastoma.

**Etiology:** Autosomal recessive inheritance.

**Pathogenesis:** Absence of glucose-6-phosphatase in liver, kidney, and intestinal epithelium. Most findings result from secondary effect of chronic recurrent hypoglycemia.

**MIM No.:** *23220
**POS No.:** 3241
**CDC No.:** 271.000
**Sex Ratio:** M1:F1
**Occurrence:** Estimated to be 1:400,000 live births.

**Risk of Recurrence for Patient's Sib:**
See Part I, *Mendelian Inheritance.*

**Risk of Recurrence for Patient's Child:**
See Part I, *Mendelian Inheritance.*

**Age of Detectability:** At birth.

**Gene Mapping and Linkage:** Unknown.

**Prevention:** None known. Genetic counseling indicated.

**Treatment:** Frequent feedings containing glucose (glucose polymers, nasogastric drip supplying 6 mg glucose/min/kg body weight; corn starch, 1.75 g/kg q6h after pancreas produces sufficient amylase to split starch [8 months to 4.5 years]). Allopurinol for elevated serum uric acid. An alkalinizing agent (e.g., Polycitra) may be useful during periods of stress to prevent acidosis. Kidney transplant for renal failure.

**Prognosis:** Generally good. Malignant conversion of hepatomata is unusual. Frequency of renal failure from the late teens onward is not established.

**Detection of Carrier:** One report described the detection of a heterozygote by determining the glucose-6-phosphatase level through peroral intestinal biopsy.

**Support Groups:** IA; Durant; Association for Glycogen Storage Disease

**References:**
Greene HG, et al.: Continuous nocturnal intragastric feeding for management of type I glycogen storage disease. New Engl J Med 1976; 294:423–425.
Emmet M, Norins RG: Renal transplantation in type I glycogenosis: failure to improve glucose metabolism. JAMA 1978; 239:1642–1644.
Howell RR, et al.: Hepatic adenoma with type I glucogen storage disease. J Nucl Med 1978; 19:354–358.
Chen YT, et al.: Cornstarch therapy in type I glycogen storage disease. New Engl J Med 1984; 310:171–175.
Burchell A, et al.: Diagnosis of type Ia and type Ic glycogen storage disease in adults. Lancet 1987; I:1059–1062.
Ito E, et al.: Type Ia glycogen storage disease with hepatoblastoma in siblings. Cancer 1987; 59:1776–1780.

SI003                                             **James B. Sidbury**

## GLYCOGENOSIS, TYPE IB                          **2168**

**Includes:**
>    Glucose-6-phosphate transport defect
>    Glycogen storage disease, type Ib
>    Translocase 1 deficiency

**Excludes:**
>    **Glycogenosis, type Ia** (0425)
>    **Glycogenosis, type Ic** (2871)
>    **Glycogenoses** (1507)
>    Hepatomegaly of a variety of etiologies
>    Hypoglycemia of other etiologies

**Major Diagnostic Criteria:** The same as for **Glycogenosis, type Ia,** except that glucose-6-phosphatase is present in liver samples previously frozen or treated with detergents. In addition, these individuals have leukopenia, granulocytopenia, and a tendency toward local abcesses.

**Clinical Findings:** The same as for **Glycogenosis, type Ia,** with the addition of a tendency toward local abcesses, e.g., perianal, mouth, boils.

**Complications:** Rapidly developing ketoacidosis, bleeding tendency, short stature, and, in the postpubescent period, gout and hepatomata (adenoma). In addition, local infections can be a significant problem.

**Associated Findings:** Uric acid stones after puberty. Hypertension with hypertrophy of juxtaglomerular apparatus and glomerulonephritis in single cases.

**Etiology:** Autosomal recessive inheritance.

**Pathogenesis:** Deficient glucose-6-phosphate transport system (translocase 1) in the liver endoplasmic reticulum and granulocytes.

**MIM No.:** *23222

**POS No.:** 3241

**CDC No.:** 271.000

**Sex Ratio:** M1:F1

**Occurrence:** Estimated at 1:800,000 live births.

**Risk of Recurrence for Patient's Sib:**
See Part I, *Mendelian Inheritance*.

**Risk of Recurrence for Patient's Child:**
See Part I, *Mendelian Inheritance*.

**Age of Detectability:** After birth.

**Gene Mapping and Linkage:** Unknown.

**Prevention:** None known. Genetic counseling indicated.

**Treatment:** Frequent feedings containing glucose (glucose polymers, nasogastric drip supplying 6 mg glucose/min/kg body weight; corn starch, 1.75 g/kg q6hrs after pancreas produces sufficient amylase to split starch [eight months to 4.5 years of age]). Allopurinol for elevated serum uric acid. An alkalinizing agent (e.g., Polycitra) may be useful during periods of stress to prevent acidosis. Manage abcesses as for any other child. Renal failure is not known to be associated with this condition.

**Prognosis:** Generally good. Severity and frequency of infections is variable, and can affect prognosis.

**Detection of Carrier:** Unknown.

**Support Groups:** IA; Durant; Association for Glycogen Storage Disease

**References:**
Kuzuya T, et al.: An adult case of type Ib glycogen storage disease. New Engl J Med 1983; 308:566–569.
Ambruso DR, et al.: Infections and bleeding complications with glycogenosis type Ib. Am J Dis Child 1985; 139:691–697.
Koven NL, et al.: Impaired chemotaxis and neutrophil (polymorphonuclear leucocyte) function in glycogenosis Ib. Pediatr Res 1986; 20:438–442.
Ueno N, et al.: Impaired monocyte function in glycogen storage disease Ib. Eur J Pediatr 1986; 145:312–314.

SI003                                    **James B. Sidbury**

---

## GLYCOGENOSIS, TYPE IC                                    2871

**Includes:**
Glycogen storage disease, type Ic
Phosphate-pyrophosphate translocase
Translocase 2 deficiency

**Excludes:**
**Glycogenosis** (other)
Hepatosplenomegaly of a other etiologies
Hypoglycemia of other causes

**Major Diagnostic Criteria:** Clinical picture resembles a mild form of type Ia glycogenosis. Liver biopsy shows little glucose-6-phosphatase activity without freezing the tissue or using detergents. The inorganic pyrophosphatase pyrophosphate:glucose phosphotransferase and carboxyl phosphate:glucose phosphotransferase ratios are totally latent (i.e., no demonstrable activity without detergent).

**Clinical Findings:** In the neonatal period hypoglycemic seizures or hepatomegaly may be the cardinal findings. As feedings become less frequent or infections supervene, hypoglycemia and ketoacidosis will be seen. Delayed growth becomes apparent by age one year. Difficulty handling simple respiratory infections becomes a problem. Nose bleeds usually begin around age two years, often associated with URI. Motor development is usually somewhat delayed. As the child becomes older, hypoglycemia is seen primarily with infection and stress. Xanthomas develop in

about 10% of patients. The physical examination reveals a short, cherub-faced individual with a protuberant abdomen. The liver, but not the spleen, is very large. Muscular tone is relatively poor. Chemical findings include low blood glucose and high blood lactate, urate, cholesterol, triglycerides, and transaminases. Bleeding time is prolonged and the platelets increased. No evidence of leukocyte dysfunction has been documented.

**Complications:** Unknown.

**Associated Findings:** One patient had diabetes.

**Etiology:** Presumably autosomal recessive inheritance.

**Pathogenesis:** Absence of putative translocase specific for $P_i$, $PP_i$, and carboxyle P (Arion et al, 1980).

**MIM No.:** 23224

**POS No.:** 3241

**CDC No.:** 271.000

**Sex Ratio:** Presumably M1:F1.

**Occurrence:** Two cases, an eleven year old girl and a 52-year-old man, have been reported in the literature.

**Risk of Recurrence for Patient's Sib:**
See Part I, *Mendelian Inheritance*.

**Risk of Recurrence for Patient's Child:**
See Part I, *Mendelian Inheritance*.

**Age of Detectability:** Presumably shortly after birth.

**Gene Mapping and Linkage:** Unknown.

**Prevention:** None known. Genetic counseling indicated.

**Treatment:** See **Glycogenosis, type Ia**.

**Prognosis:** Unknown.

**Detection of Carrier:** Unknown.

**Support Groups:** IA; Durant; Association for Glycogen Storage Disease

**References:**
Arion WJ, et al.: Evidence for the participation of independent translocases for phosphate and glucase-6-phosphate in the microsomal glucose-6-phosphate system. J Biol Chem 1980; 255:10396–10406.
Nordle RC, et al.: Type Ic: a novel glycogenosis. J Biol Chem 1983; 258:9739–9744.
Nordlie RC, Sukalski KA: Multiple forms of type I glycogen storage disease: underlying mechanisms. Trends Biochem Sci 1986; 11:61–65.
Burchell A, et al.: Diagnosis of type Ia and type Ic glycogen storage diseases in adults. Lancet 1987; 11:1059–1062.

SI003                                    **James B. Sidbury**

---

## GLYCOGENOSIS, TYPE IIA                                    0011

**Includes:**
Acid maltase deficiency, infant onset
Alpha 1,4-glucosidase deficiency
Cardiac form of generalized glycogenosis
Cardiomegalia glycogenica diffusa
"Floppy" infant (one type)
Generalized glycogenosis
Glycogen storage disease, type IIa
Heart disease, glycogen
Lysosomal glucosidase deficiency
Myopathy-metabolic, acid maltase deficiency, infant onset
Pompe disease

**Excludes:**
**Glycogenosis** (other)
Heart diseases, other congenital
Idiopathic hypertrophy of the heart
**Ventricle, endocardial fibroelastosis of left ventricle** (0348)
**Ventricle, endocardial fibroelastosis of right ventricle** (0349)

**Major Diagnostic Criteria:** Absence of lysosomal α-1,4-glucosidase in all tissues except kidney. Massive accumulation of glycogen in lysosomes of affected tissues.

**Clinical Findings:** After one or two months of life, baby becomes progressively weak (floppy), loses reflexes, develops progressive cardiomegaly, and has an abnormal EKG with abnormally short conduction time. These infants usually die within the first two years of life.

Occasionally cardiomegaly is not a prominent feature and central nervous and neuromuscular involvement may lead to a picture like that of infantile **Spinal muscular atrophy** (Werdnig-Hoffmann disease). In this situation there may be profound muscular weakness and hypotonia.

EKG in the infantile (Pompe) form is considered characteristic with gigantic QRS complexes and a short PR interval. EMG is said to have pseudomyotonic bursts. Light microscopy of muscle shows a vacuolar myopathy with PAS positive material and the absence of acid phosphatase staining. Electron microscopy demonstrates membrane bound glycogen granules, presumably within lysosomes. The lack or absence of acid maltase can be confirmed in leukocytes as well.

**Complications:** Pneumonia frequently supervenes. It cannot be handled normally because of weakness of intercostal muscles and precipitates heart failure and death. Aspiration pneumonitis and macroglossia may be present.

**Associated Findings:** Cardiac arrhythmias often seen in the infantile form. Older patients show considerable heterogeneity; often with residual enzymatic activity at about the 10% level. The heart is usually not involved. Only striated and non-cardiac muscle is involved.

**Etiology:** Autosomal recessive inheritance.

**Pathogenesis:** Absence of lysosomal α-1,4-glucosidase activity. CRM protein and absence of the enzyme protein have been demonstrated in different patients. The absence of the enzyme in the lysosome results in a failure of breakdown of glycogen normally taken by the lysosomes.

**MIM No.:** *23230

**CDC No.:** 271.000

**Sex Ratio:** M1:F1

**Occurrence:** Estimated to be 1:400,000 live births.

**Risk of Recurrence for Patient's Sib:**
See Part I, *Mendelian Inheritance.*

**Risk of Recurrence for Patient's Child:** Affected individuals are not expected to survive to reproduce.

**Age of Detectability:** In utero, by fibroblasts and chorionic villi biopsy. Cultured cells are deficient in α-1,4-glucosidase activity; uncultivated cells show glycogen-filled lysosomes with electron microscopy.

**Gene Mapping and Linkage:** GAA (glucosidase, alpha, acid) has been mapped to 17q23.

**Prevention:** None known. Genetic counseling indicated.

**Treatment:** Supportive. Intravenous administration of placental lysosomal α-1,4-glucosidase and bone marrow transplant has not been effective.

**Prognosis:** Children with the infantile form almost always die within the first two years of life.

**Detection of Carrier:** Carrier detection can be done from leukocytes, skin fibroblasts, muscle, and urine. Enzyme levels intermediate between disease state and normal activity.

**References:**
Engel AG, et al.: The spectrum and diagnosis of acid maltase deficiency. Neurology 1973; 23:95–106.
Bexancron AM, et al.: Prenatal diagnosis of glycogenosis type II (Pompe's disease) using chorionic villi biopsy. Clin Genet 1985; 27:479–482.
Martiniuk F, et al.: Further regional localization of the genes for human acid alpha glucosidase (GAA), peptidase D (PEPD), and

alpha mannosidase B (MANB) by somatic cell hybridization. Hum Genet 1985; 69:109–111.
Renser AS, et al.: Defects in synthesis, phosphorylation, and maturation of acid alpha-glucosidase in glycogenosis type II. J Biol Chem 1985; 260:8336–8341.
Trend P, et al.: Acid maltase deficiency in adults. Brain 1985; 108:845–860.
Isaacs H, et al.: Acid maltase deficiency: a case study and review of the pathophysiological changes and proposed therapeutic measure. J Neurol Neurosurg Psych 1986; 49:1011–1018.
Reuser AJJ, et al.: Clinical diversity in glycogenosis type II. J Clin Invest 1987; 79:1689–1699.

SI003                                                    **James B. Sidbury**
HA015                                                    **Jerome S. Haller**

---

## GLYCOGENOSIS, TYPE IIB                                        2873

**Includes:**
    Acid maltase deficiency, adult onset
    Acid maltase deficiency, childhood onset
    Glycogen storage disease, type IIb
    Lysosomal alpha-1,4 glucosidase, late onset
    Myopathy-metabolic, acid maltase deficiency, late onset

**Excludes:**
    Muscle weaknesses of central origin
    **Myopathy**
    Neuropathies, peripheral (other)

**Major Diagnostic Criteria:** Myopathy with an onset in childhood or later, associated with a marked decrease (2–15%) in striated muscle lysosomal α-1,4-glucosidase.

**Clinical Findings:** The clinical picture ranges from a mild weakness, which may initially be noted when the child begins to walk, to an onset of myopathy, which may not be manifest until the third, fourth, or fifth decades. The myopathy is slowly progressive. Death is usually due to respiratory causes because of the progressive weakness of the intercostal muscles. One family reported with infantile and late-onset cases.

**Complications:** Hypostatic pneumonia.

**Associated Findings:** None known.

**Etiology:** Autosomal recessive inheritance.

**Pathogenesis:** Decreased muscle lysosomal α-1,4-glucosidase of striated muscle (2–15% of normal). The mechanism relating enzyme defect to observed symptoms is unclear.

**MIM No.:** *23230

**POS No.:** 3787

**CDC No.:** 271.000

**Sex Ratio:** M1:F1

**Occurrence:** Undetermined; extensive literature.

**Risk of Recurrence for Patient's Sib:**
See Part I, *Mendelian Inheritance.*

**Risk of Recurrence for Patient's Child:**
See Part I, *Mendelian Inheritance.*

**Age of Detectability:** At birth or prenatally, although the clinical onset has been reported as late as retirement age.

**Gene Mapping and Linkage:** GAA (glucosidase, alpha; acid) has been mapped to 17q23.

**Prevention:** None known. Genetic counseling indicated.

**Treatment:** Supportive. A high-protein, low-carbohydrate diet has been reported to be of benefit in two patients.

**Prognosis:** Course of disease is usually slow but progressive.

**Detection of Carrier:** By lymphocyte or muscle biopsy.

**Support Groups:** IA; Durant; Association for Glycogen Storage Disease

**References:**
Engel AG, et al.: The spectrum and diagnosis of acid maltase deficiency. Neurology 1973; 23:95–106.

Mehler M, DiMauro S: Residual acid maltase activity in late-onset acid maltase deficiency. Neurology 1977; 27:178–184.

Loonen MCB, et al.: A family with different clinical forms of acid maltase deficiency (glycogenosis type II): biochemical and genetic studies. Neurology 1981; 31:1209–1216.

Shauske S, DiMauro S: Late-onset acid maltase deficiency: biochemical studies of leucocytes. J Neurol Sci 1981; 50:57–62.

Slonim AE, et al.: Improvement in muscle function in acid maltase deficiency by high-protein therapy. Neurology 1983; 33:34–36.

Isaacs H, et al.: Acid maltase deficiency: a case study and review of the pathophysiological changes and proposed therapeutic measures. J Neurol Neurosurg Psychiatry 1986; 49:1011–1018.

SI003                                                    **James B. Sidbury**

## GLYCOGENOSIS, TYPE IIC                                          2874

**Includes:**
>  Cardiomyopathy due to lysosomal glycogen storage
>  Glycogen storage disease, type IIc
>  Glycogen storage disease, type IIb (McKusick)
>  Lysosomal glycogen storage disease without acid maltase deficiency
>  Myopathy (vacuolar) with glycogen

**Excludes:**
>  **Cardiomyopathy** (other)
>  **Glycogenosis, type IIa** (0011)
>  **Glycogenosis, type IIb** (2873)
>  **Glycogenosis, type IId** (2875)
>  **Myopathy** (other)

**Major Diagnostic Criteria:**  Weakness, fatigue, shortness of breath, cardiac enlargement, abnormal EKG, abnormal electromyography (EMG) with myotonic-like high-frequency discharges, elevated transaminases, and creatinine phosphokinase. Muscle biopsy shows vacuolar myopathy with glycogen.

**Clinical Findings:**  Onset of weakness can be from age two years onward. The cardiac symptoms; palpitation, shortness of breath; appear later, usually in the teens or after. EKG is abnormal, showing biventricular hypertrophy, **Arrhythmia, Wolff-Parkinson-White type**, and ST changes. X-rays show cardiomegaly. EMG has a myopathic pattern. Myopathy is slowly progressive.

**Complications:**  Heart failure, cardiac arrest.

**Associated Findings:**  Mental retardation was seen in one family. One infant had hydrops fetalis, nonimmunohemolytic.

**Etiology:**  Probably autosomal dominant inheritance. An X-linked form has also been suggested.

**Pathogenesis:**  Lysosomal storage of glycogen in the heart and striated muscle. It is unclear how lysosomal storage of glycogen interferes with myocardial function and conduction, or how it causes myopathy. Histologically, there was some muscle necrosis and fibrosis. All enzymes measured were normal. Maltase was increased.

**MIM No.:**  23233

**POS No.:**  3787

**Sex Ratio:**  Presumably M1:F1. The reported cases have been predominantly male, but females are affected and transmit the condition.

**Occurrence:**  Four cases from three families have been documented.

**Risk of Recurrence for Patient's Sib:**
> See Part I, *Mendelian Inheritance.*

**Risk of Recurrence for Patient's Child:**
> See Part I, *Mendelian Inheritance.*

**Age of Detectability:**  Shortly after birth.

**Gene Mapping and Linkage:**  Unknown.

**Prevention:**  None known. Genetic counseling indicated.

**Treatment:**  Symptomatic.

**Prognosis:**  Some patients have lived beyond the third decade.

**Detection of Carrier:**  Unknown.

**Special Considerations:**  It has been suggested that this condition is the same as Antopol disease (see **Glycogenosis, type IId**).

Since McKusick does not distinguish between early and late onset forms of **Glycogenosis, type II**, he has assigned the designation IIb to the condition described in this article.

**Support Groups:**  IA; Durant; Association for Glycogen Storage Disease

**References:**
Danon MJ, et al.: Lysosomal glycogen storage disease with normal acid maltase. Neurology 1981; 31:51–57.

Riggs JE, et al.: Lysosomal glycogen storage disease without acid maltase deficiency. Neurology 1983; 33:873–877.

Atkins J, et al.: Fatal infantile cardiac glycogenosis without acid maltase deficiency presenting as congenital hydrops. Eur J Pediatr 1984; 142:150 only.

Byrne E, et al.: Dominantly inherited cardioskeletal myopathy with lysosomal glycogen storage and normal acid maltase levels. Brain 1986; 109:523–536.

SI003                                                    **James B. Sidbury**

## GLYCOGENOSIS, TYPE IID                                          2875

**Includes:**
>  Antopol disease
>  Glycogen storage disease, Type IId
>  Lysosomal glycogen storage disease limited to the heart

**Excludes:**
>  Cardiomyopathies, other hypertrophic
>  **Glycogenosis, type IIa** (0011)
>  **Glycogenosis, type IIb** (2873)
>  **Glycogenosis, type IIc** (2874)
>  Heart disease, congenital

**Major Diagnostic Criteria:**  A child with cardiac hypertrophy, dyspnea, precordial pain, and arrhythmia.

**Clinical Findings:**  One patient failed to thrive poorly from birth and had intermittent paroxysmal tachycardia from age six months and heart failure at age 11 years; in another cardiomegaly was detected at age seven years. Two other boys were in their teens when they developed shortness of breath. A patient of Antopol et al (1940) had striated muscle involvement and hence may have been type IIc rather than IId.

**Complications:**  Heart failure.

**Associated Findings:**  **Arrhythmia, Wolff-Parkinson-White type**. Endocardial fibroelastosis was reported in one patient.

**Etiology:**  Possibly X-linked inheritance. All known patients have been male.

**Pathogenesis:**  Cardiomegaly, poor myocardial function, and accelerated conduction time seem to be consistently seen with lysosomal storage disease of the heart. The mechanism is unclear as is the cause of patches of myocardial fibrosis.

**MIM No.:**  23210

**POS No.:**  3787

**CDC No.:**  271.000

**Sex Ratio:**  M1:F0 (observed).

**Occurrence:**  Four cases from three families have been reported.

**Risk of Recurrence for Patient's Sib:**
> See Part I, *Mendelian Inheritance.*

**Risk of Recurrence for Patient's Child:**
> See Part I, *Mendelian Inheritance.*

**Age of Detectability:**  During infancy.

**Gene Mapping and Linkage:**  Unknown.

**Prevention:**  None known. Genetic counseling indicated.

**Treatment:**  Symptomatic.

**Prognosis:**  All known patients have died in their teens or earlier.

**Detection of Carrier:**  Unknown.

**Special Considerations:**  It has been suggested that this may be the same condition reported as **Glycogenosis, type IIc.**

**Support Groups:**  IA; Durant; Association for Glycogen Storage Disease

**References:**
Antopol W, et al.: Cardiac hypertrophy caused by glycogen storage disease in a 15-year-old boy. Am Heart J 1940; 20:546–556.
Mehrizi A, Oppenheimer EH: Heart failure associated with unusual deposition of glycogen in the myocardium. Bull Johns Hopkins Hosp 1960; 107:329–336.

SI003                                                  **James B. Sidbury**

---

## GLYCOGENOSIS, TYPE III                                          0426

**Includes:**
>   Amylo-1,6-glucosidase deficiency
>   Cori disease
>   Debrancher deficiency
>   Forbes disease
>   Glycogen storage disease, type III
>   Limit dextrinosis

**Excludes:**
>   **Glycogenosis** (other)
>   Hepatomegaly of other etiologies
>   Hypoglycemia of other etiologies
>   Myopathies of other etiologies

**Major Diagnostic Criteria:**  Hepatomegaly, which may be associated with hypoglycemia. The majority of cases are also associated with myopathy, mild in childhood, grossly symptomatic in the later years. The liver or liver and muscle have a deficiency of amylo-1,6-glucosidase and amylo-1,4 → 1,4-glucan-transferase.

**Clinical Findings:**  Rarely symptomatic in neonatal period. There is a wider spectrum of severity in type III than in type I. The course in the first 4–6 years of life may be clinically undistinguishable from type I except for the mild myopathy, which may be present in type III. There may be fasting hypoglycemia, failure to respond to glucagon in the fasting state but responding postprandially, no rise of lactate following glucagon, hyperlipemia, ketoacidosis with stress, poor handling of infections, epistaxis, bleeding tendency, and massive hepatomegaly. The short stature, cherubic face, and protuberant abdomen is similar to type I. Symptoms and findings can be minimal and easily overlooked. The hepatomegaly, short stature, bleeding tendency, and hypoglycemia subside at puberty. In adult life the myopathy becomes more prominant and progressive and may be associated with peripheral neuropathy. Ten percent of patients have only liver involvement.

**Complications:**  Bleeding with tooth extraction, and adenoid and tonsil removal, but almost never a problem during biopsies.

**Associated Findings:**  Occasionally clinical or symptomatic evidence of cardiac involvement. Secondary neuropathy may be seen in association with the myopathy, usually late in the progress of the disease.

**Etiology:**  Autosomal recessive inheritance. Absence or marked reduction of activity of amylo-1,6-glucosidase and amylo-1,4 → 1,4 glucan-transferase. Both activities are found on a single polypeptide. In the limited number of persons tested, the peptide appears to be absent. Liver-only involvement may be due to a mutation in the promoter unique to the liver.

**Pathogenesis:**  The diminution of the debrancher enzymes results in accumulation of glycogen that cannot be normally broken down, functionally deficient glycogen, and a residual abnormal glycogen, namely, short-chain glycogen or limit dextrin. The result is glucose deficiency during fasting until gluconeogenesis is adequate to supply total blood glucose needs.

**MIM No.:**  *23240

**POS No.:**  3241

**CDC No.:**  271.000

**Sex Ratio:**  M1:F1

**Occurrence:**  Highly variable. In general, probably less than glycogenosis Ia, i.e., 1:400,000 live births. In Israel, in 73% of cases of glycogen storage disease (estimated 1:5,420), all patients being non-Ashkenazim, mainly of North African extraction.

**Risk of Recurrence for Patient's Sib:**
See Part I, *Mendelian Inheritance.*

**Risk of Recurrence for Patient's Child:**
See Part I, *Mendelian Inheritance.*

**Age of Detectability:**  In utero.

**Gene Mapping and Linkage:**  Unknown.

**Prevention:**  None known. Genetic counseling indicated.

**Treatment:**  High-protein diet to utilize and stimulate gluconeogenesis; raw corn starch to maintain blood glucose.

**Prognosis:**  Unknown.

**Detection of Carrier:**  Unknown.

**Support Groups:**  IA; Durant; Association for Glycogen Storage Disease

**References:**
Levin S, et al.: Glycogen storage disease in Israel: a clinical, biochemical and genetic study. Israel J Med Sci 1967; 3:397–410.
Brown BI: Prenatal diagnosis of glycogen storage disease. Am J Hum Genet 1984; 36:1865.
Slonim AE, et al.: Myopathy and growth failure in debrancher enzymes deficiency: improvement with high-protein nocturnal enteral therapy. J Pediatr 1984; 105:906–911.
Moses SW, et al.: Neuromuscular involvement in glycogen storage disease type III. Acta Paediatr Scand 1985; 75:259–296.
Ding JH, et al.: Immunoblot analysis of glycogen debrancher enzyme in type III glycogen storage disease. Am J Hum Genet 1986; 39:47(Abst 013).
Borowitz SU, Green HL: Cornstarch therapy in a patient with Type III glycogen storage disease. J Pediatr Gastroenterol 1987; 6:631–634.
Chen Y-T, et al.: Glycogen debranching enzyme: purification, antibody characterization, and immunoblot analysis of type III glycogen storage disease. Am J Hum Genet 1987; 41:1002–1015.

SI003                                                  **James B. Sidbury**

---

## GLYCOGENOSIS, TYPE IV                                           0116

**Includes:**
>   Amylopectinosis
>   Andersen disease
>   Brancher deficiency
>   Cirrhosis with deposition of abnormal glycogen, familial
>   Glycogen storage disease, type IV
>   Myopathy-metabolic, brancher disease

**Excludes:**  All other forms of glycogen storage disease

**Major Diagnostic Criteria:**  Progressive liver failure with jaundice in infancy, hepatomegaly, ascites, moderate muscular weakness, and demonstration of abnormal glycogen accumulations and abnormal glycogen structure in liver and other tissues.

**Clinical Findings:**  Patients usually are discovered in infancy with cirrhosis of the liver and storage of abnormal glycogen. Occasionally muscular weakness and muscular contractures are present. Cirrhosis with associated hepatic failure is the most characteristic feature and is in conjunction with progressive accumulating ascites. Neuromuscular involvement is more common than is appreciated because patients suffer from severe liver disease. There is muscle weakness, loss of tendon stretch reflexes, and mental deterioration. An adult case of brancher deficiency mimicked limb girdle muscular dystrophy.

Laboratory features are those of progressive hepatic failure with cirrhosis, deepening icterus, and associated severe chronic illness. Liver biopsy will demonstrate accumulation of glycogen in the range of 2–4 gm%, with lesser amounts of glycogen in muscle and other tissues. The glycogen is abnormal in its structure, with a reduced number of 1,6 branch points. The glycogen resembles amylopectins of plant starch. The abnormal glycogen has been found in the CNS, the peripheral nervous system, and in muscle.

**Complications:** Hepatic failure, occasionally congestive heart failure or renal failure due to accumulation of glycogen or to an unusual foreign body reaction to an abnormal polysaccharide component. The adult cases have had a slowly progressive course of muscle weakness over many years.

**Associated Findings:** None known.

**Etiology:** Probably autosomal recessive inheritance. Defect of brancher enzyme in liver and other tissues. Brancher enzyme is also identified as amylo-(1,4 to 1,6) transglucosidase. The reduced branching makes glycogen much less soluble.

**Pathogenesis:** Accumulation of an abnormally structured polysaccharide quite similar to an amylopectin in liver, muscle, kidney, peripheral nerve, spinal cord, and brain. There is probably a foreign body reaction to the accumulation of this unusual polysaccharide component, which leads to significant hepatic fibrosis and advanced cirrhosis.

**MIM No.:** *23250

**CDC No.:** 271.000

**Sex Ratio:** Presumably M1:F1

**Occurrence:** Undetermined but presumed rare. About a half-dozen cases documented.

**Risk of Recurrence for Patient's Sib:**
See Part I, *Mendelian Inheritance.*

**Risk of Recurrence for Patient's Child:**
See Part I, *Mendelian Inheritance.*

**Age of Detectability:** Usually before one year of age when associated with progressive hepatic failure.

**Gene Mapping and Linkage:** Unknown.

**Prevention:** None known. Genetic counseling indicated.

**Treatment:** Unknown.

**Prognosis:** Death usually occurs from hepatic failure before the third year of life.

**Detection of Carrier:** Unknown.

**References:**
Andersen DH: Studies on glycogen disease with report of a case in which the glycogen was abnormal. In: Najjar VA, ed: Carbohydrate metabolism: a symposium on the clinical and biochemical aspects of carbohydrate utilization in health and disease. Baltimore: Johns Hopkins University Press, 1953:28.
Sidbury JB Jr., et al.: Type IV glycogenosis: report of a case proven by characterization of glycogen and studied at necropsy. Bull Johns Hopkins Hosp 1962; 111:157–181.
Howell RR, et al.: Type IV glycogen storage disease: branching enzyme deficiency in skin fibroblasts and possible heterozygote detection. J Pediatr 1971; 78:638–642.
Bannayan GA, et al.: Type IV glycogen storage disease: light microscopic and enzymatic study. Am J Clin Pathol 1976; 66:702–709.
McMaster KR, et al.: Nervous system involvement in type IV glycogenosis. Arch Pathol Lab Med 1979; 103:105.
Ferguson IT, et al.: WJK: An adult case of Andersen's disease - type IV glycogenosis: a clinical, histochemical, ultrastructural and biochemical study. J Neurol Sci 1983; 60:337–351. *

HA015                                                          **Jerome S. Haller**

## GLYCOGENOSIS, TYPE V 2877

**Includes:**
  Glycogen storage disease, type V
  McArdle disease
  Muscle glycogen phosphorylase deficiency
  Myophosphorylase deficiency

**Excludes:**
  **Glycogenosis, type VII** (0428)
  **Glycogenosis** (other)
  **Myopathy** (other)
  Psychoneurosis

**Major Diagnostic Criteria:** Deficient myophosphorylase in muscle.

**Clinical Findings:** Muscle pain and stiffness with vigorous exercise, which abates promptly if the exercise is stopped promptly. If the patient persists in exercise for a longer period, soreness and swelling of the muscle lasting 1–2 days will result, and gross myoglobinuria will be evident because of muscle breakdown. Affected individuals usually have elevated creatinine phosphokinase levels, even at rest; failure of the blood lactate to rise three to five-fold after one minute of anoxic forearm exercise is a useful screening test for the metabolic myopathies involving glycogen and glycolytic metabolism. The symptoms may become apparent in childhood, but more commonly in the teens and later. Muscle atrophy becomes slowly but progressively apparent.

**Complications:** Renal failure due to massive myoglobinuria. Syncope or seizures with prolonged vigorous exercise.

**Associated Findings:** The long duration of symptoms causes muscle atrophy.

**Etiology:** Autosomal recessive inheritance.

**Pathogenesis:** Absent or deficient activity of myophosphorylase. The muscle of some patients has cross reacting material protein; others have no phosphorylase protein or mRNA. Nuclear magnetic resonance (NMR) demonstrates a sharp fall in creatine phosphate and pH, with a rise in inorganic phosphate with anoxic exercise. Heterozygote showed a greater than normal acid production during aerobic exercise. Available glycogen is necessary for muscle oxidation metabolism; available glucose not as effective.

**MIM No.:** *23260

**POS No.:** 3241

**CDC No.:** 271.000

**Sex Ratio:** M1:F1

**Occurrence:** Over a dozen cases have been reported in an established literature.

**Risk of Recurrence for Patient's Sib:**
See Part I, *Mendelian Inheritance.*

**Risk of Recurrence for Patient's Child:**
See Part I, *Mendelian Inheritance.*

**Age of Detectability:** *In utero* (adult muscle isozyme has been found in a four-month-old fetus). More practically, by muscle biopsy after birth or by NMR at an age at which the child could cooperate in directed active exercise using a spectroscopic technique that permits quantitative and qualitative separation of phosphate forms of different energy levels *in situ.*

**Gene Mapping and Linkage:** PYGM (phosphorylase, glycogen (McArdle syndrome)) has been mapped to 11q12-q13.2.

**Prevention:** None known. Genetic counseling indicated.

**Treatment:** Physical rehabilitation counseling. A high-protein diet is reported to improve stamina.

**Prognosis:** Good for life span and function, but in later years the myopathy may become debilitating.

**Detection of Carrier:** By $P_i$ NMR.

References:

DiMauro S, et al.: McArdle disease: the mystery of reappearing phosphorylase activity in muscle culture: a fetal isozyme. Am Neurol 1978; 3:60–66.

Daegelen D, et al.: Absence of functional messenger RNA for glycogen phosphorylase in the muscle of two patients with McArdle's disease. Ann Hum Genet 1983; 47:107–115.

Lebo RV, et al.: High-resolution chromosome sorting and DNA spot-block analysis assign McArdle's syndrome to chromosome 11. Science 1984; 225:57–59.

Slonim AE, Goans PJ: Myopathy in McArdle's syndrome: improvement with a high protein diet. New Engl J Med 1985; 312:355–359.

Bogusky RT, et al.: McArdle's disease heterozygotes: metabolic adaptation assessed using [31]P-nuclear magnetic resonance. J Clin Invest 1986; 77:1881–1887.

Gautron S, et al.: Molecular mechanisims of McArdle's disease (muscle glycogen phosphorylase deficiency). J Clin Invest 1987; 79:275–281.

SI003                                          **James B. Sidbury**

---

## GLYCOGENOSIS, TYPE VI                                    0427

**Includes:**

> Glycogen storage disease, type VI
> Hepatic phosphorylase
> Hers disease
> Liver phosphorylase deficiency
> Phosphorylase deficiency glycogen-storage disease of liver

**Excludes:**

> **Glycogenosis** (other hepatic)
> Hepatomegaly of other etiologies

**Major Diagnostic Criteria:** Low leukocyte phosphorylase activity is helpful but a liver biopsy with assay of liver glycogen content and phosphorylase activity is definitive.

**Clinical Findings:** The clinical spectrum of these patients is relatively broad. They have very large livers, moderate to severe fasting hypoglycemia, hypotonia, growth retardation, cherubic facies, elevated cholesterol and triglycerides, variable urate elevation, normal blood lactate. There is a general tendency to improve with age; some decrease in abnormal distention occurs in adolescence.

**Complications:** Symptomatic fasting hypoglycemia.

**Associated Findings:** None known.

**Etiology:** Autosomal recessive inheritance.

**Pathogenesis:** Phosphorylase is the primary degradative enzyme of glycogen, hence reduced activity hampers the liver's ability to regulate blood glucose. Intermittent hypoglycemia results, and secondary increase in fatty acid mobilization and triglyceride formation can follow.

**MIM No.:** *23270

**POS No.:** 3241

**CDC No.:** 271.000

**Sex Ratio:** M1:F1

**Occurrence:** Undetermined. Less frequent than **Glycogenosis, type Ia.**

**Risk of Recurrence for Patient's Sib:**
See Part I, *Mendelian Inheritance.*

**Risk of Recurrence for Patient's Child:**
See Part I, *Mendelian Inheritance.*

**Age of Detectability:** Presumably at birth.

**Gene Mapping and Linkage:** PYGL (phosphorylase, glycogen; liver (Hers disease, glycogen storage disease type VI)) has been mapped to 14q11.2-q24.3.

**Prevention:** None known. Genetic counseling indicated.

**Treatment:** Frequent high carbohydrate feeding (3 gm/kg protein) in first four years if hypoglycemia is a problem. Cornstarch

---

therapy can be useful for management of h⌣ **Glycogenosis, type Ia).**

**Prognosis:** Undetermined. Adults have normal st⌣

**Detection of Carrier:** Detection by cDNA proble h⌣ attempted.

**Support Groups:** IA; Durant; Association for Glycogen Stor⌣ ease

References:

Williams HE, Field JB: Low leukocyte phosphorylase in hepat⌣ phosphorylax-deficiency glycogen storage disease. J Clin Invest 1961; 40:1841–1845.

Wallis PG, et al.: Hepatic phosphorylase defect: studies in peripheral blood. Am J Dis Child 1966; 111:278–282.

Hers HG, et al.: Glycogen storage disease: types II and VI glycogenoses. In Dickens F, et al, eds: Carbohydrate metabolism and its disorders. New York: Academic Press, 1968.

Newgard CB, et al.: Sequence analysis of the cDNA encoding human liver glycogen phosphorylase reveals tissue-specific codon usage. Proc Nat Acad Sci 1986; 83:8132–8136.

SI003                                          **James B. Sidbury**

---

## GLYCOGENOSIS, TYPE VII                                    0428

**Includes:**

> Anemia, hemolytic, phosphofructokinase deficiency
> Glycogen storage disease, type VII
> Hemolytic disease, PFK deficiency
> Hemolytic disease, phosphofructokinase deficiency
> Muscle phosphofructokinase deficiency
> Myopathy-hemolysis
> PFK, liver type
> Phosphofructokinase (PFK) deficiency
> Tarui disease

**Excludes:**

> **Muscular dystrophy**
> **Myopathy, central core disease type** (0134)
> **Myotonic dystrophy** (0702)

**Major Diagnostic Criteria:** The classical syndrome results in the association of myopathy and hemolysis. The diagnosis is established by the demonstration of reduced PFK activity in the erythrocytes. In cases where there is myopathy, PFK activity in muscle biopsy is absent. When hemolysis is present, this is demonstrated by an elevation of the reticulocyte count, but there is no anemia; instead mild polycythemia may be present. A few patients with an apparently similar defect have been described, in whom the defect was associated with hemolysis alone, myopathy alone, or even an asymptomatic state. A few cases have been reported with congenital progressive myopathy; however, the association with PFK deficiency is not completely established.

**Clinical Findings:** Myopathy and/or hemolysis. In a few asymptomatic individuals, however, the defect was detected fortuitously. This extreme variability can be easily explained by our current understanding of the molecular structure of PFK. This enzyme is a tetramer, that may contain either one or two subunits. In the muscle, PFK is a homogenous tetramer containing only the type M subunit; similarly, in the liver, PFK is also a homogenous tetramer, containing only the type L subunit. In the erythrocytes, the enzyme is a tetramer containing both the type M and the type L subunits. It has been shown that all five expected hybrid species $(L_4, L_3M_1, L_2M_2, L_1M_3$ and $M_4)$ are present in the erythrocyte.

Congenital absence of the M subunit results in myopathy and in hemolysis. Congenital absence of the L subunit is probably incompatible with life. However, some asymptomatic individuals have an unstable L subunit of the enzyme.; their erythrocytes lack the $L_4$ subunit, but all other hybrids are present.

Although a few patients have been reported with isolated myopathy, it appears likely that in these cases the hemolysis may have been missed, since this is characteristically not associated with anemia. Similarly, in one of the cases originally reported with isolated hemolysis, critical review demonstrated the absence of pathy. It appears therefore that there are two main types of [PFK] deficiency: one, due to total lack of the M subunit, results in classical syndrome of myopathy with hemolysis and erythrocytosis; another is due to an unstable L subunit, and is totally symptomatic. A third type has been recently described in a single family, that probably results from an unstable M subunit and is associated with late appearance of myopathy. The syndromes of isolated myopathy and of isolated hemolysis, when carefully studied, appear to be in reality classical cases, with both myopathy and hemolysis.

The *myopathy* of PFK deficiency is of the exertional type. In the ischemic exercise test both lactate and pyruvate fail to rise in the venous blood, as a consequence of the block in glycolysis. In the muscle a modest accumulation of glucose is observed (1.5 to 5%; normal <1.0%).

The *hemolysis* of PFK deficiency is very well compensated and it is characteristically associated with either normal or slightly increased red cell number. It has been shown that this modest polycythemia reflects the low level of 2–3 diphosphoglycerate, secondary to the partial block of glycolysis. This in turn results in hypoxia, since the oxygen dissociation curve is not shifted. The hypoxia stimulates further production of RBCs. Hence, paradoxically, in PFK deficiency there is an increased production of erythrocytes which, however, because of their defective glycolysis, are low in 2–3 DPG and thus not very effective in oxygen transport. The defect results in moderate hypoxia, but no anemia.

**Complications:** Unknown.

**Associated Findings:** None known.

**Etiology:** Autosomal recessive inheritance.

**Pathogenesis:** Myopathy results from inability of the muscle to glycolize in anaerobiosis. Hemolysis probably results from the reduced glycolytic rate.

**MIM No.:** *23280, *17186

**POS No.:** 3241

**CDC No.:** 271.000

**Sex Ratio:** M1:F1

**Occurrence:** The syndrome of myopathy and hemolysis is rare; less than 20 cases have been reported. The asymptomatic PFK defect, however, is probably rather frequent, since the few cases reported have been detected in very small surveys.

**Risk of Recurrence for Patient's Sib:**
See Part I, *Mendelian Inheritance.*

**Risk of Recurrence for Patient's Child:**
See Part I, *Mendelian Inheritance.*

**Age of Detectability:** Usually in adolescence, occasionally earlier.

**Gene Mapping and Linkage:** PFKM (phosphofructokinase, muscle type) has been provisionally mapped to 1cen-q32.
PFKL (phosphofructokinase, liver type) has been mapped to 21q22.3.

**Prevention:** None known. Genetic counseling indicated.

**Treatment:** Avoidance of vigorous or sudden burst of activity. Affected individuals can handle moderate, paced acitivity without symptoms. Vocational guidance toward sedentary employment is suggested. Lactate response and fatigue have not responded to fructose loading.

**Prognosis:** The syndrome of myopathy and hemolysis appears to remain stable with age and results only in minimal disability.

**Detection of Carrier:** Carriers can be detected by demonstration of reduced PFK activity in the erythrocytes (45–65% of normal) and, in the case of the classical syndrome, by the demonstration of reduced PFK activity in muscle biopsy as well (15–45% of normal).

**Support Groups:** IA; Durant; Association for Glycogen Storage Disease

**References:**
Tarnu S, et al: Phosphofructokinase deficiency in skeletal muscle: A new type of glycogenosis. Biophys Res Commun 1965; 19:517–523.
Vora S, et al: Isozymes of human phosphofructokinase: identification and subunit structural characterization of a new system. Proc Nat Acad Sci USA 1980; 77:62–66.
Vora S, et al: The molecular mechanism of the inherited phosphofructokinase deficiency associated with hemolysis and myopathy. Blood 1980; 55:629–635.
Vora S: Isozymes of phosphofructokinase. In: Current Topics in Biological and Medical Research. New York: Alan R Liss, 1982:119–167.
Vora S, et al: Heterogeneity of the molecular lesions in inherited phosphofructokinase deficiency. J Clin Invest 1983; 72:1995–2006.
Mineo I, et al.: Myogenic hyperuricemia: a common pathophysiologic feature of glycogenosis types III, V, and VI. New Engl J Med 1987; 317:75–80.
Vora S, et al: Characterization of the enzymatic defect in late onset muscle phosphofructokinase deficiency: new subtype of glycogen storage disease type VII. J Clin Invest 1987; 80:1479–1485.

PI010                                                    **Sergio Piomelli**

## GLYCOGENOSIS, TYPE VIII                                    0429

**Includes:**
Glycogen storage disease, type VIII
Phosphofructokinase, muscle type
Phosphoglucose isomerase inhibitor

**Excludes:**
**Glycogenosis** (other)
**Muscular dystrophy**
Myoglobinuria, idiopathic
**Myopathy** (others)
Neurogenic muscle disease

**Major Diagnostic Criteria:** Muscle pain, stiffness, and fatigue occur in adults after exercise. The lack of the expected rise in blood lactate during anoxic exercise is a useful screening test. Definitive diagnosis requires the demonstration of diminished lactate production by muscle homogenate with glucose-1-phosphate or glucose-6-phosphate substrate. Normal lactate production occurs when fructose-6-phosphate or fructose-1,6-diphosphate are added. The phosphohexoisomerase activity is normal.

**Clinical Findings:** Muscle pain, stiffness, and fatigability after exercise. Symptoms generally occur in the fourth decade. A few hours after moderately heavy exercise muscle pain and stiffness appear and remain during rest or at the end of the day. The symptoms are relieved by rest for several days. Myoglobinuria may occur after heavy exercise. The physical examination is normal and without muscle weakness or atrophy. The creatine phosphokinase is elevated. Blood lactate does not rise when the forearm is subjected to anoxic exercise, nor are there any associated muscle cramps. Lactate response is normal after an oral fructose load.

**Complications:** The condition appears to be progressive and interferes with the individual's ability to do physically active work.

**Associated Findings:** None known.

**Etiology:** Presumably autosomal recessive inheritance.

**Pathogenesis:** Presumably an inhibitor of phosphohexoisomerase is present in the muscle of these individuals.

**MIM No.:** *23280

**POS No.:** 3241

**CDC No.:** 271.000

**Sex Ratio:** Presumably M1:F1

**Occurrence:** Reported in two Japanese brothers.

**Risk of Recurrence for Patient's Sib:**
See Part I, *Mendelian Inheritance.*

**Risk of Recurrence for Patient's Child:**
See Part I, *Mendelian Inheritance.*

**Age of Detectability:** In the documented cases, at 35 years of age or older.

**Gene Mapping and Linkage:** PFKM (phosphofructokinase, muscle type) has been provisionally mapped to 1cen-q32.

**Prevention:** None known. Genetic counseling indicated.

**Treatment:** Avoidance of excessive physical activity. It is reported that fructose administered orally prevented the recurrence of symptoms.

**Prognosis:** Relatively rapidly debilitating after onset.

**Detection of Carrier:** Unknown.

**Special Considerations:** Victor McKusick has classified this condition as a form of **Glycogenosis, type VII**, and has applied the type VIII designation to a condition often classified as a variant of type IX (see **Glycogenosis, type IXa**). Glycogenosis, type VIII can be distinguished from **Glycogenosis, type VII** by the fact that type VIII does not involve hemolytic anemia and is responsive to fructose loading.

**Support Groups:** IA; Durant; Association for Glycogen Storage Disease

**References:**

Satoyoshi E, Kowa H: A new myopathy due to glycolytic abnormalities. Trans Am Neurol Assoc 1965; 90:46.

Satoyoshi E, Kowa H: A myopathy due to glycolytic abnormalities. Arch Neurol 1967; 17:248–256.

SI003                                    **James B. Sidbury**

---

## GLYCOGENOSIS, TYPE IXA                          0430

**Includes:**

Glycogen storage disease, type VIII (McKusick)
Glycogen storage disease, type IXa
Hepatic phosphorylase kinase deficiency
Liver phosphorylase kinase deficiency
Phosphorylase kinase deficiency of liver

**Excludes:**

**Glycogenosis** (other hepatic)
Hepatomegaly (other)

**Major Diagnostic Criteria:** Hepatomegaly, increased glycogen in the liver, deficient phosphophorylase kinase in the liver and leukocytes. No involvement of muscle.

**Clinical Findings:** A mild form of hepatic glycogenosis. Males are more prominently affected. They have a protuberant abdomen with significant hepatomegaly, retarded growth, and delayed puberty. Symptomatic hypoglycemia is unusual, lipids are moderately elevated, uric acid may be elevated, glucose response to glucagon is variable, and the transaminases are moderately elevated. The symptoms and findings return toward normal at puberty. Hemizygous females may have hepatomegaly and mild growth retardation until the age of 5 or 6 years, when all findings resolve. Clinical expressivity in female hemizygotes is not known.

**Complications:** Unknown.

**Associated Findings:** None known.

**Etiology:** X-linked inheritance, with limited expression in hemizygotes.

**Pathogenesis:** Deficiency in phosphorylase kinase activity in the liver. The liver and WBC enzyme in the affected patient has a Km 20-fold higher than controls; the Km is fourfold higher in hemizygotes.

**MIM No.:** *30600

**POS No.:** 3241

**CDC No.:** 271.000

**Sex Ratio:** M1:F<1. Expression in females, if any, is undetermined.

**Occurrence:** Probably less 1:400,000 live births.

**Risk of Recurrence for Patient's Sib:**
See Part I, *Mendelian Inheritance.*

**Risk of Recurrence for Patient's Child:**
See Part I, *Mendelian Inheritance.*

**Age of Detectability:** At birth.

**Gene Mapping and Linkage:** PHKA (phosphorylase kinase, alpha) has been provisionally mapped to Xq12-q13.

PHK (phosphorylase kinase deficiency, liver (glycogen storage disease type VIII)) has been mapped to X.

**Prevention:** None known. Genetic counseling indicated.

**Treatment:** Adjust carbohydrate and protein in diet for maximal growth.

**Prognosis:** Symptoms of affected males resolve at puberty; of hemizygotes, by ages 5 or 6 years.

**Detection of Carrier:** Measurement of the enzyme in leukocytes.

**Support Groups:** IA; Durant; Association for Glycogen Storage Disease

**References:**

Hug G, et al.: Deficient activity of dephosphophorylase kinase and accumulation of glycogen in the liver. J Clin Invest 1969; 48:704–705.

Huijing F: Glycogen-storage diseases type VIa: low phosphorylase kinase activity caused by a low enzyme-substrate affinity. Biochem Biophys Acta 1970; 206:199–201.

Schimke RN, et al.: Glycogen storage disease type IX: benign glycogenosis of liver and hepatic phosphorylase kinase deficiency. J Pediatr 1973; 83:1031–1034.

Chamberlain JS, et al.: Analysis of the phosphorylase B kinase deficiency locus in mice: linkage to the mdx and Duchenne muscular dystrophy genes. Abstract presented at the National Muscular Dystrophy Meeting 1986.

SI003                                    **James B. Sidbury**

---

## GLYCOGENOSIS, TYPE IXB                          2878

**Includes:**

Glycogen storage disease, type IXb
Myopathy, recessive phosphorylase kinase deficiency
Phosphorylase kinase deficiency, generalized

**Excludes:**

**Glycogenosis, type IXa** (0430)
**Glycogenosis** (other)
Hepatomegaly, other causes of
**Myopathy** (other)

**Major Diagnostic Criteria:** Deficient phosphorylase kinase in liver, muscle, leukocytes, and RBC.

**Clinical Findings:** A relatively mild disease characterized by hepatomegaly, cherubic facies, stunted growth, and weakness. No apparent cardiac involvement. Clinical chemistry is normal, except for elevated lipids and transaminases.

**Complications:** Unknown.

**Associated Findings:** None known.

**Etiology:** Autosomal recessive inheritance.

**Pathogenesis:** Deficient phosphorylase kinase activity depresses glycogen breakdown and thereby slows glycolysis.

**MIM No.:** *26175

**POS No.:** 3241

**CDC No.:** 271.000

**Sex Ratio:** M1:F1

**Occurrence:** Fewer than a dozen cases have been documented in the literature.

**Risk of Recurrence for Patient's Sib:**
See Part I, *Mendelian Inheritance.*

**Risk of Recurrence for Patient's Child:**
See Part I, *Mendelian Inheritance.*

**Age of Detectability:** At birth.

**Gene Mapping and Linkage:** Unknown.

**Prevention:** None known. Genetic counseling indicated.

**Treatment:** A relatively high carbohydrate diet, since one patient did poorly on a high protein diet.

**Prognosis:** Good.

**Detection of Carrier:** Unknown.

**Support Groups:** IA; Durant; Association for Glycogen Storage Disease

**References:**
Lederer B, et al.: The autosomal form of phosphorylase kinase deficiency in man: reduced activity of the muscle enzyme. Biochem Biophys Res Commun 1980; 92:169–174.
Lerner A, et al.: A new variant of glycogen storage disease: type IXc. Am J Dis Child 1982; 136:406–410.
Tuchman M, et al.: Clinical and laboratory observations in a child with hepatic phosphorylase kinase deficiency. Metabolism 1986; 35:627–633.

SI003                                              **James B. Sidbury**

## GLYCOGENOSIS, TYPE IXC                              2879

**Includes:**
Glycogen storage disease, type IXc
Glycogen storage disease-deficient cardiac phosphorylase kinase

**Excludes:**
**Carnitine deficiency, systemic** (2121)
**Glycogenosis, type IIa** (0011)
**Glycogenosis, type IXa** (0430)
Heart disease, congenital, nonmetabolic
Myocarditis
Myocardiopathy, familial hypertrophic
**Myopathy-metabolic, carnitine deficiency, primary and secondary** (0124)

**Major Diagnostic Criteria:** Enlarged heart, short PR interval, and deficient phosphorylase kinase in the heart only.

**Clinical Findings:** Very similar to **Glycogenosis, type IIa.** In the only reported case, there was enlarged heart; short PR interval, but no weakness or loss of reflexes; mildly elevated creatinine phosphokinase; and transaminases were not elevated.

**Complications:** Death from heart failure precipitated by upper respiratory infection.

**Associated Findings:** None known.

**Etiology:** Unknown.

**Pathogenesis:** Glycogen availability appears to be necessary for myocardial and normal conduction function.

**POS No.:** 3241

**CDC No.:** 271.000

**Sex Ratio:** M1:F0 (observed).

**Occurrence:** One case, a Japanese male infant, has been reported in the literature.

**Risk of Recurrence for Patient's Sib:** Unknown.

**Risk of Recurrence for Patient's Child:** Unknown.

**Age of Detectability:** Shortly after birth, by clinical examination.

**Gene Mapping and Linkage:** Unknown.

**Prevention:** None known. Genetic counseling indicated.

**Treatment:** Supportive.

**Prognosis:** The one known affected infant died at age five months.

**Detection of Carrier:** Unknown.

**Support Groups:** IA; Durant; Association for Glycogen Storage Disease

**References:**
Eishi Y, et al.: Glycogen storage disease confined to the heart with deficient activity of cardiac phosphorylase kinase: a new type of glycogen storage disease. Hum Pathol 1985; 2:193–197.

SI003                                              **James B. Sidbury**

**Glycolipid lipidosis**
See FABRY DISEASE
**Glycophorin deficiency**
See ANEMIA, HEMOLYTIC, RED CELL MEMBRANE DEFECTS
**Glycoprotein complex IIb-IIIa, deficiency of**
See THROMBASTHENIA, GLANZMANN-NAEGELI TYPE
**Glycoprotein neuraminidase, deficiency of**
See MUCOLIPIDOSIS I
**Glycoprotein p150,95 (CD11c/CD18) deficiency**
See GRANULOCYTE GLYCOPROTEIN CD11/CD18 DEFICIENCY
**Glycoprotein-glycosaminoglycan storage myopathy**
See MYOPATHY-METABOLIC, GLYCOPROTEIN-GLYCOSAMINOGLYCANS STORAGE TYPE
**Glycosuria, renal**
See RENAL GLYCOSURIA
**Goeminne syndrome**
See CERVICO-DERMO-GU SYNDROME, GOEMINNE TYPE
**Goiter with maternal lithium exposure, congenital**
See FETAL LITHIUM EFFECTS
**Goiter, congenital**
See THYROID, THYROGLOBULIN DEFECTS
**Goiter, familial**
See THYROID, PEROXIDASE DEFECT
**Goiter, familial (some forms)**
See THYROID, IODOTYROSINE DEIODINASE DEFICIENCY
also THYROID, IODIDE TRANSPORT DEFECT
**Goiter, from extrinsically caused fetal iodine disorder**
See CRETINISM, ENDEMIC, AND RELATED DISORDERS

## GOITER, GOITROGEN INDUCED                          0435

**Includes:**
Antithyroid drug goiter
Cough syrup induced goiter
Eskalith^ induced goiter
Goiter, neonatal, due to maternal goitrogenic agents
Iodide goiter
Lithium induced goiter
Lithobid^ induced goiter
Lithone^ induced goiter
Propylthiouracil (PTU) goiter

**Excludes:**
**Cretinism, endemic** (3167)
Endemic goiter
Enzymatic goiter, congenital
**Fetal effects from methimazole and carbimazole** (2926)
Goitrous cretinism
**Thyroid, dysgenesis** (0946)
Transient neonatal toxic goiter caused by maternal hyperthyroidism

**Major Diagnostic Criteria:** The presence of a goiter in a newborn infant with a history of maternal ingestion of antithyroid agents, or iodides, or iodide containing amniography dyes. Neonatal hypothyroid goiters caused by such antithyroid agents must be distinguished from transient hyperthyroid goiters caused by a maternal condition such as Graves disease.

**Clinical Findings:** Goiter (enlargement of thyroid); hypothyroidism may or may not accompany the goiter. Neonatal goiter has been observed by the use of iodinated antiseptics applied to the skin.

**Complications:** Mental retardation can result from the hypothyroidism, when present, but is seldom observed since severe hypothyroidism is uncommon. Occasionally large goiters may produce respiratory distress and asphyxia due to tracheal compression and, may interfere with delivery of the infant.

**Associated Findings:** None known.

**Etiology:** Maternal ingestion of antithyroid drugs (of which propylthiouracil is considered the drug of choice since it has the least transplacental transfer) or iodide in excess. Chronic intake of cough mixture containing potassium iodide is a frequent source of iodide excess to the fetus.

**Pathogenesis:** The fetal thyroid uptake of iodide transferred across the placenta starts at approximately the 12th week of gestation. Excess iodide in the fetal thyroid inhibits synthesis and release of thyroid hormone, thereby stimulating pituitary TSH followed by hypertrophy of the thyroid gland. Antithyroid drugs including PTU cross the placenta and can inhibit T4 synthesis, which causes excess TSH production and a resultant goiter.

**Sex Ratio:** M1:F1

**Occurrence:** With proper antithyroid treatment, significant neonatal goitrogenicity is infrequent.

**Risk of Recurrence for Patient's Sib:** Minimal in the absence of excess maternal iodides.

**Risk of Recurrence for Patient's Child:** Minimal in the absence of excess maternal iodides.

**Age of Detectability:** At birth or early neonatal period.

**Gene Mapping and Linkage:** N/A

**Prevention:** Definitive management of maternal hyperthyroidism before and during pregnancy, with reduction of antithyroid medications to the point where maternal T4 levels are at the upper end of normal. Iodides should be discontinued entirely. Mothers who are taking antithyroid drugs or iodides, which are secreted in milk, should not nurse their babies.

**Treatment:** Synthetic L-thyroxine should be given to the infant until goiter regresses, beginning at a dose of 25 micrograms.

**Prognosis:** Condition is not life-threatening unless the goiter mechanically interferes with respiration.

**Detection of Carrier:** N/A

**References:**
Chabriolle JP et al. Goiter and hyperthyroidism in the newborn after cutaneous absorption of iodine. Arch Dis Child. 1973; 53:495.
Refetoff S, et al.: Neonatal hyperthyroidism and goiter in one infant of each of two sets of twins due to maternal therapy with antithyroid drugs. J Pediat. 1974; 85:240.
Rauke M. Congenital goiter in a premature infant after ammiography. Monatssch Kinderheilk. 1977; 125:941.

SC016

R. Neil Schimke
*Robert M. Blizzard*

**Goiter, neonatal, due to maternal goitrogenic agents**
*See GOITER, GOITROGEN INDUCED*
**Goiter-double lip-blepharochalasis**
*See BLEPHAROCHALASIS-DOUBLE LIP-NONTOXIC GOITER*
**Goiter-sensorineural deafness**
*See DEAFNESS-GOITER*
**Goitrous hypothyroidism**
*See THYROID, THYROGLOBULIN DEFECTS*
**Golabi-Ito-Hall syndrome**
*See X-LINKED MENTAL RETARDATION, GOLABI-ITO-HALL TYPE*
**Golabi-Rosen syndrome**
*See SIMPSON-GOLABI-BEHMEL SYNDROME*
**Goldberg syndrome**
*See GALACTOSIALIDOSIS*
**Goldberg-Pashayan syndrome**
*See SYNDACTYLY-POLYDACTYLY-EAR LOBE SYNDROME*
**Goldenhar syndrome**
*See OCULO-AURICULO-VERTEBRAL ANOMALY*
**Goldenhar-Gorlin syndrome**
*See OCULO-AURICULO-VERTEBRAL ANOMALY*
**Goldmann-Favre disease**
*See EYE, GOLDMANN-FAVRE DISEASE*
**Gollop-Wolfgang syndrome**
*See TIBIAL HYPOPLASIA/APLASIA-ECTRODACTYLY*
**Goltz syndrome**
*See DERMAL HYPOPLASIA, FOCAL*
**Goltz-Gorlin syndrome**
*See DERMAL HYPOPLASIA, FOCAL*

**Gonadal agenesis**
*See AGONADIA*
**Gonadal differentiation (abnormal)-nephropathy-Wilms tumor**
*See WILMS TUMOR-PSEUDOHERMAPHRODITISM-GLOMERULOPATHY,DENYS-DRASH TYPE*
**Gonadal dysgenesis, asymmetric**
*See CHROMOSOME MOSAICISM, 45X/46,XY TYPE*
**Gonadal dysgenesis, mixed**
*See CHROMOSOME MOSAICISM, 45X/46,XY TYPE*

## GONADAL DYSGENESIS, XX TYPE  0436

**Includes:**
Ovarian dysgenesis, familial
XX form of pure gonadal dysgenesis
XX gonadal dysgenesis

**Excludes:**
Chromosome mosaicism, 45,X/46,xy type (0173)
Gonadal dysgenesis, XY type (0437)
Hypogonadotropic hypogonadism (2300)
Perrault syndrome (2350)
Turner syndrome (0977)

**Major Diagnostic Criteria:** Streak gonads in 46,XX individuals with female external genitalia and normal müllerian development. Fibrous streaks should either be demonstrated by laparoscopy or laparotomy or deduced on the basis of elevated gonadotropin levels (FSH > 40 miu/ml). A monosomic (45,X) cell line should be excluded.

**Clinical Findings:** Individuals with gonadal dysgenesis may have an apparently normal female (46,XX) chromosomal complement with female external genitalia. Their external genitalia and their streak gonads are indistinguishable from individuals who have gonadal dysgenesis and a 45,X chromosomal complement. The endocrine features and the lack of secondary sexual development are similar to other individuals with streak gonads. Estrogen levels are decreased; follicle-stimulating hormone (FSH) and luteinizing hormone (LH) levels are increased. Müllerian derivatives remain infantile yet well differentiated. Most individuals with XX gonadal dysgenesis are normal in stature. XX gonadal dysgenesis patients with features of the **Turner syndrome** phenotype probably have undetected **Chromosome mosaicism, 45x/46,XY type**.

The diagnosis is applied only to individuals whose gonads either consist of bilateral streak gonads or show endocrine evidence of ovarian failure (elevated FSH and LH levels). However, in several families one 46,XX sib had bilateral streak gonads, whereas another had primary amenorrhea and extreme ovarian hypoplasia with a few follicles. These observations suggest that a few oocytes may persist in some individuals who carry the abnormal allele, possibly explaining some familial aggregates of premature ovarian failure.

**Complications:** Hypogonadism; infertility.

**Associated Findings:** While sensorineural deafness was once considered an associated finding, its combination with ovarian dysgenesis is now recognized as **Perrault syndrome**.

**Etiology:** Autosomal recessive inheritance. At least 22 familial aggregates are known. In each aggregate, sibs were the only relatives affected, and in some families parents were consanguineous.

**Pathogenesis:** Undetermined. 45,X cells are unlikely to be present yet undetected in available tissues, although monosomy limited to germ cells cannot be excluded.

**MIM No.:** *23330

**POS No.:** 3809

**CDC No.:** 752.720

**Sex Ratio:** M0:F1

**Occurrence:** Rare, but the explanation for about 20% of individuals with primary amenorrhea.

**Risk of Recurrence for Patient's Sib:**
See Part I, *Mendelian Inheritance.* 1:4 (25%) for 46,XX sibs; 1:8 (12.5%) for all sibs.

**Risk of Recurrence for Patient's Child:**  All patients are infertile.

**Age of Detectability:**  At puberty because of primary amenorrhea.

**Gene Mapping and Linkage:**  Unknown.

**Prevention:**  None known. Genetic counseling indicated.

**Treatment:**  Treatment of hypogonadism by administration of estrogens. Assessment for auditory deficits. In the future, embryo transfer techniques might make it possible for the affected to carry a pregnancy. (The husband's sperm would "artificially" inseminate the donor female, and the resulting embryo would be flushed from the donor and transferred to the wife lacking ovaries.)

**Prognosis:**  Probably normal life span.

**Detection of Carrier:**  Unknown.

**Special Considerations:**  The frequent association of XX gonadal dysgenesis and neurosensory deafness suggests either genetic heterogeneity or, less likely, pleiotropy for the gene causing XX gonadal dysgenesis (see **Perrault syndrome**). In addition, in four other families, each apparently unique, 46,XX females with gonadal dysgenesis had a specific pattern of somatic abnormalities. None of these patterns have been associated with the Turner syndrome. In each family the anomalies were different, and in each an allele different from XX gonadal dysgenesis can be suspected (Simpson, 1978).

Most authors consider males, if affected, to show no gonadal findings. Moreover, in at least one family a brother of two affected sisters manifested azoospermia.

**References:**
Simpson JL, et al.: Gonadal dysgenesis in individuals with apparently normal chromosomal complements: tabulation of cases and compilation of genetic data. BD:OAS;VII(6). Baltimore: Williams & Wilkins, 1971:215–228.
Simpson JL: Disorders of sexual differentiation: etiology and clinical delineation. New York: Academic Press, 1976:293–296.
Simpson JL: Gonadal dysgenesis and sex chromosomal abnormalities: phenotypic-karyotypic correlations. In: Vallet HL, Porter IH, eds: Genetic mechanisms of sex determination. New York: Academic Press Inc, 1978:365–405.
Vesley DL, et al: Familial ovarian dysgenesis in 46,XX females. Am J Med Sci 1980; 280:157–166.
Aleem FA: Familial 46,XX gonadal dysgenesis. Fertil Steril 1981; 35:317–320.

SI018                                          **Joe Leigh Simpson**

**Gonadal dysgenesis, XX type, with deafness**
*See PERRAULT SYNDROME*
**Gonadal dysgenesis, XY female type**
*See GONADAL DYSGENESIS, XY TYPE*

## GONADAL DYSGENESIS, XY TYPE                          0437

**Includes:**
Gonadal dysgenesis, XY female type
Pure testicular dysgenesis
Swyer syndrome
Testis-determining factor, X-chromosomal
XY form of pure gonadal dysgenesis
XY gonadal dysgenesis

**Excludes:**
**Agonadia** (0029)
**Androgen insensitivity syndrome, complete** (0049)
**Campomelic dysplasia** (0122)
**Chromosome mosaicism, 45x/46,XY type** (0173)
**Gonadal dysgenesis, XX type** (0436)
**Leydig cell hypoplasia** (2298)
**Steroid 17 alpha-hydroxylase deficiency** (0903)
**Turner syndrome** (0977)

**Major Diagnostic Criteria:**  Streak gonads in a 46,XY individual with female external genitalia and normal müllerian derivatives. The diagnosis may be properly applied to 46,XY individuals who have normal female external genitalia or minimal clitoral hypertrophy and either gonadoblastomas or dysgerminomas.

**Clinical Findings:**  Individuals with a normal male (46,XY) chromosomal complement may show bilateral streak gonads, female external genitalia, and müllerian derivatives (uterus and fallopian tubes). No somatic abnormalities are present. The streak gonads in these individuals are usually histologically indistinguishable from the gonads of individuals with a 45,X complement. As a result of lack of gonadal development, these individuals do not menstruate and fail to develop breasts or pubic and axillary hair. Their external genitalia are female, yet sexually infantile. The uterus and fallopian tubes are likewise small yet well differentiated. Estrogen and testosterone levels are decreased; gonadotropin levels are increased (FSH > 40 miu/ml). In XY gonadal dysgenesis the streak gonads may undergo neoplastic transformation to dysgerminomas or gonadoblastomas. As many as 20–30% of XY gonadal dysgenesis patients have such a tumor, which may or may not be associated with virilization or feminization. Neoplasia is much more likely to develop if H-Y antigen is present.

**Complications:**  Effects of hypogonadism; infertility. Gonadal neoplasia is associated with 20–30% of individuals with XY gonadal dysgenesis. Feminization or masculinization may occur as a result of these tumors.

**Associated Findings:**  If features of the **Turner syndrome** phenotype are present, undetected **Chromosome mosaicism, 45,X/46,XY type** cells should be suspected. There is increased likelihood of developing parenchymal renal disorders, as evidenced by nephrotic syndrome nephritis in some patients. Campomelic dwarfism has occurred in some 46,XY individuals with female external genitalia and bilateral streak gonads, but this entity is presumably distinct.

**Etiology:**  In one form, X-linked recessive or male-limited autosomal dominant inheritance. Submicroscopic deletion of the portion of the Y short arm containing the Testis Determining Factor (TDF) seems to be responsible for many sporadic if not familial cases (Page et al, 1987). Wachtel (1980) suggests that the loss of the H-Y receptor is probably involved in an autosomal recessive form of XY gonadal dysgenesis.

**Pathogenesis:**  Extensive investigations indicate that 45,X cells are unlikely to be present; however, monosomy limited to germ cells cannot be excluded. H-Y antigen is present in some cases and absent in others, suggesting genetic heterogeneity irrespective of the role of H-Y antigen in sex determination. Lack of H-Y antigen could explain the phenotype on the basis of the indifferent gonad failing to differentiate into a fetal testis, leading to female internal and external genitalia. In H-Y positive cases, the same aberrant embryologic steps presumably occur; however, pathogenesis must involve another mechanism, possibly defective H-Y receptors.

**MIM No.:**  *30610, 23342

**POS No.:**  3809

**CDC No.:**  752.710

**Sex Ratio:**  M1:F0

**Occurrence:**  Close to 200 cases have been reported.

**Risk of Recurrence for Patient's Sib:**
See Part I, *Mendelian Inheritance.*

**Risk of Recurrence for Patient's Child:**  All patients are infertile.

**Age of Detectability:**  Usually at puberty because of primary amenorrhea. A few patients may be detected before puberty if screening is performed because other relatives are affected or if gonadoblastomas or dysgerminomas produce feminization, virilization, or pelvic pain.

**Gene Mapping and Linkage:**  TDF (testis determining factor) has been mapped to Yp11.3.

**Prevention:**  None known. Genetic counseling indicated.

**Treatment:** Treatment of lack of secondary sex development by administration of estrogen; removal of gonadal streaks to prevent neoplastic transformation. Following diagnosis, gonadal extirpation should be performed without delay. Neoplasia appears more likely in H-Y positive cases. The uterus should not be removed because embryo transfer techniques are now available. Renal status should be assessed. Dialysis or renal transplantation may be appropriate in some cases.

**Prognosis:** Probably normal life span, although gonadal streaks could undergo malignant transformation, and renal disease can be life-threatening. Infertility.

**Detection of Carrier:** Unknown.

**Special Considerations:** In at least three families one 46,XY sib had XY gonadal dysgenesis, whereas another sib had genital ambiguity, bilateral testes and müllerian derivatives (uterus and fallopian tubes). Possible explanations include 1) undetected 45,X cells in several family members (familial mosaicism), thus explaining the presence of a uterus (see **Chromosome mosaicism, 45,X/ 46,XY type**); 2) the gene controlling XY gonadal dysgenesis is capable of varied expressivity; or 3) a gene different from that producing XY gonadal dysgenesis is capable of varied expressivity.

XY gonadal dysgenesis associated with campomelic dwarfism is a different disorder, as is a related condition described by Brosnan et al (1980).

**References:**
Brosnan PG, et al.: A new familial syndrome of 46,XY gonadal dysgenesis with anomalies of ectodermal and mesodermal structures. J Pediatr 1980; 97:586–590.

Wachtel SS, et al.: H-Y antigen in 46,XY gonadal dysgenesis. Hum Genet 1980; 54:25–30.

Bricarelli FD, et al.: Sex-reversed XY females with campomelic dysplasia are HY negative. Hum Genet 1981; 57:15–22.

Simpson JL, et al.: XY gonadal dysgenesis: genetic heterogeneity based upon clinical observations, H-Y antigen status and segregation analysis. Hum Genet 1981; 58:91–97.

Simpson JL, et al.: Chronic renal disease, myotonic dystrophy, and gonadoblastoma in an individual with XY gonadal dysgenesis. J Med Genet 1982; 9:73.

Wachtel SS: H-Y antigen and the biology of sex determination. New York: Grune & Stratton, 1982

Mann JR, et al.: The X-linked recessive form of XY gonadal dysgenesis with a high incidence of gonadal germ cell tumors: clinical and genetic studies. J Med Genet 1983; 20:264–270.

Page DC, et al.: The sex-determining region of the human Y chromosome encodes a finger protein. Cell 1987; 51:1091–1104.

SI018                                    **Joe Leigh Simpson**

**Gonadal dysgenesis-cataracts-myopathy, familial congenital type**
   *See MYOPATHY-CATARACT-GONADAL DYSGENESIS*
**Gonadal mosaicism in pseudoachondroplasia**
   *See PSEUDOACHONDROPLASTIC DYSPLASIA*

## GONADOTROPIN DEFICIENCIES                    0438

**Includes:**
   **Dwarfism, panhypopituitary** (0303)
   Fertile eunuch syndrome
   Follicle-stimulating hormone (FSH), isolated deficiency of
   Luteinizing hormone (LH), deficiency of

**Excludes:**
   **Hypogonadotropic hypogonadism** (2300)
   **Kallmann syndrome** (2301)

**Major Diagnostic Criteria:** Deficiency of FSH or LH associated with otherwise normal pituitary function.

**Clinical Findings:** In isolated gonadotropin deficiency (IGD), the absence of pituitary gonadotropins results in failure of normal sexual maturation, infertility, and complete lack of secondary sexual characteristics in both sexes. In addition, however, there are at least two other variants of clinical interest.

A few patients with otherwise typical IGD have low LH levels but normal spermatogenesis and FSH levels. These patients have been termed fertile eunuchs and appear to have an isolated deficiency of LH. At least some may have a diminished FSH response to clomiphene citrate; this has been interpreted as a "reduced FSH reserve." Hence many authors feel that the fertile eunuch is only a clinical variant of the IGD syndrome. In addition, at least one female has been described with primary amenorrhea, poor sexual development, low FSH, but high LH. It is not clear if this represents a separate syndrome of isolated FSH deficiency or is a clinical variant of the IGD syndrome.

**Complications:** Unknown.

**Associated Findings:** None known.

**Etiology:** The vast majority of cases are sporadic, but autosomal recessive inheritance has been reported.

**Pathogenesis:** Most cases probably represent a hypothalamic defect in LRF release, but pituitary defects have also been postulated. The pathogenesis is likely heterogeneous.

**MIM No.:** 22907, 22830

**Sex Ratio:** M1:F1

**Occurrence:** Undetermined but presumed rare.

**Risk of Recurrence for Patient's Sib:** Generally very low, but may be as high as 25%.

**Risk of Recurrence for Patient's Child:** Negligible.

**Age of Detectability:** Usually during mid-adolescence when anticipated puberty fails to occur.

**Gene Mapping and Linkage:** Unknown.

**Prevention:** None known. Genetic counseling indicated.

**Treatment:** Replacement of secondarily deficient hormones, i.e. testosterone or estrogen, will result in development of secondary sexual characteristics. Treatment with a combination of human menopausal gonadotropins (HMG) and human chorionic gonadotropins (HCG) will also produce secondary sexual development and often fertility as well.

**Prognosis:** Appropriate treatment results in relatively normal life.

**Detection of Carrier:** Unknown.

**Special Considerations:** During adolescence it may be difficult to differentiate IGD from constitutional delay. Administration of LRF will often help to distinguish these two disorders since patients with constitutional delay usually show some rise in gonadotropins, whereas those with IGD usually do not. It is also possible that the prolactin response to thyrotropin-releasing hormone is abnormal in IGD, and may be helpful in differentiating this group from those with delayed puberty.

**References:**
Faiman C, et al.: 'The fertile eunuch' syndrome: demonstration of isolated luteinizing hormone deficiency by radio-immuno-assay technique. Mayo Clin Proc 1968; 43:661–667.

Bell J, et al.: Isolated deficiency of follicle-stimulating hormone: further studies. J Clin Endocrinol 1975; 40:790–794.

Rabinowitz D, Spitz IM: Isolated gonadotropin deficiency and related disorders. Isr J Med Sci 1975; 11:1011–1078.

Rabinowitz D, et al.: Isolated follicle-stimulating hormone deficiency revisited: ovulation and conception in presence of circulating antibody to follicle-stimulating hormone. N Engl J Med 1979; 300:126–128.

Spitz IM, et al.: The prolactin response to thyrotropin-releasing hormone differentiates isolated gonadotropin deficiency from delayed puberty. New Engl J Med 1983; 308:575–579.

Toledo SPA, et al.: Familial idiopathic gonadotropin deficiency: a hypothalamic form of hypogonadism. Am J Med Genet 1983; 15:405–416.

H0033                                    **William A. Horton**
H0025                                    **O.J. Hood**

**Gonadotropin deficiency, familial idiopathic (FIGD)**
   *See HYPOGONADOTROPIC HYPOGONADISM*
**Gonadotropin deficiency, isolated (one form)**
   *See HYPOGONADOTROPIC HYPOGONADISM*

**Gonadotropin unresponsiveness**
*See LEYDIG CELL HYPOPLASIA*
**Goniodysgenesis**
*See EYE, ANTERIOR SEGMENT DYSGENESIS*
**Goniodysgenesis-hypodontia**
*See RIEGER SYNDROME*
**Gonosomal intersexuality**
*See CHROMOSOME MOSAICISM, 45,X/46,XY TYPE*
**Good syndrome**
*See AGAMMAGLOBULINEMIA-THYMOMA SYNDROME*
**Goodman syndrome**
*See ACROCEPHALOPOLYSYNDACTYLY*
**Gordon syndrome**
*See CAMPTODACTYLY-CLEFT PALATE-CLUB FOOT, GORDON TYPE*
**Gorham osteolysis**
*See OSTEOLYSIS, CARPAL-TARSAL AND CHRONIC PROGRESSIVE GLOMERULOPATHY*
**Gorlin syndrome**
*See GORLIN-CHAUDHRY-MOSS SYNDROME*

## GORLIN-CHAUDHRY-MOSS SYNDROME          0440

**Includes:**
Craniosynostosis-hypertrichosis-facial and other anomalies
Gorlin syndrome

**Excludes:**
**Craniofacial dysostosis** (0225)
**Spherophakia-brachymorphia syndrome** (0893)

**Major Diagnostic Criteria:** Based on about six cases, the major findings include craniosynostosis, flat midface, hypertrichosis, hypodontia and small labia majora.

**Clinical Findings:** The original cases are sisters issuing from a nonconsanguineous marriage. Both had mild growth and mental retardation, midfacial flattening, painful ulceration of the skin near the metatarsal arch, hypertrichosis, umbilical hernia, mild microphthalmia, hypodontia, patent ductus arteriosus, and hypoplasia of the labia majora. Both sisters were brachycephalic due to premature closure of the coronal sutures. Additional, as yet unpublished isolated examples of the syndrome have been reported from Germany and the Netherlands.

**Complications:** Unknown.

**Associated Findings:** None known.

**Etiology:** Possibly autosomal recessive inheritance.

**Pathogenesis:** Unknown.

**MIM No.:** 23350

**POS No.:** 3173

**Sex Ratio:** Unknown.

**Occurrence:** Undetermined but presumed rare.

**Risk of Recurrence for Patient's Sib:**
See Part I, *Mendelian Inheritance.*

**Risk of Recurrence for Patient's Child:**
See Part I, *Mendelian Inheritance.*

**Age of Detectability:** At birth.

**Gene Mapping and Linkage:** Unknown.

**Prevention:** None known. Genetic counseling indicated.

**Treatment:** Unknown.

**Prognosis:** Undetermined. Mild intelligence deficit probable.

**Detection of Carrier:** Unknown.

**References:**
Gorlin RJ, et al.: Craniofacial dysostosis, patent ductus arteriosus, hypertrichosis, hypoplasia of labia majora, dental and eye anomalies-a new syndrome? J Pediatr 1960; 56:778–785.
Gorlin RJ: Gorlin-Chaudhry-Moss syndrome: an affirmation. Proc Greenwood Genet Center 1986; 5:138.
Ippel PF, Bijlsma JB: Confirmation of the Gorlin-Chaudhry-Moss

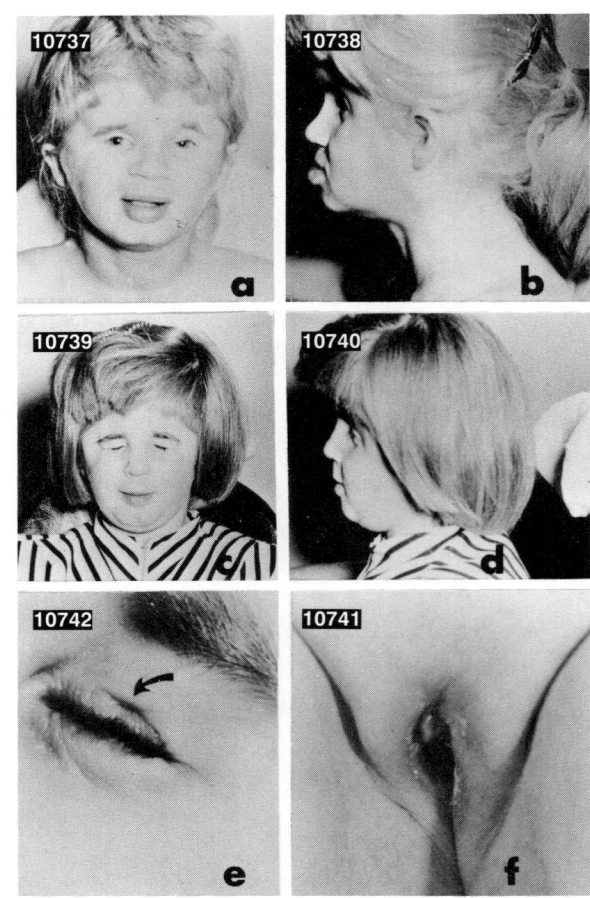

**0440**-10737–42: A,B) Pronounced maxillary hypoplasia and low-set frontal hairline. C,D) Milder maxillary hypoplasia, antimongoloid obliquity and hypotrichosis. E) Notched defect of upper eyelid. F) Hypoplastic labia majora with gaping fourchette.

syndrome. March of Dimes Clinical Genetics Conference, Philadelphia, June 8–11, 1986:30.

G0038                                          **Robert J. Gorlin**

**Gorlin-Psaume syndrome**
*See ORO-FACIO-DIGITAL SYNDROME I*
**Gorling-Goltz syndrome**
*See NEVOID BASAL CELL CARCINOMA SYNDROME*

## GOUT          0441

**Includes:**
Hyperuricemia, primary
Hyperuricemia, primary, familial
Hypoxanthine guanine phosphoribosyl transferase, deficiencies of

**Excludes:**
**Adenine phospho-ribosyl-transferase (APRT) deficiency** (3104)
Hyperuricemia, secondary

**Major Diagnostic Criteria:** The uric acid concentrations in plasma of persons with gout are over 6 mg/dl. However, a certain number of normal individuals have concentrations as high as 7 mg/dl. In the absence of impaired renal function, patients with gout seldom have concentrations higher than 8 to 12 mg/dl. These values reflect the concentrations of supersaturated solutions of sodium urate in plasma.

**Clinical Findings:** Primary gout refers to a heterogeneous group of conditions for which the diagnostic hallmark is hyperuricemia. With time, hyperuricemic individuals develop recurrent attacks of acute arthritis. Hematuria, crystalluria, urinary tract stones, and progressive nephropathy also occur regularly. Urate is deposited in tophi in soft tissues, especially around the joints and in cartilage. Chronic gout leads to deformities of the limbs and destruction of bone.

Some patients with gout have an increased rate of uric acid synthesis. This usually is true of patients who have clinical manifestations of hyperuricemia in childhood as well as of a certain proportion of adults with gout. A large number of adults appear to have hyperuricemia on the basis of diminished renal elimination of uric acid. Among those with increased rates of purine synthesis, some have been shown to have partial deficiencies of the enzyme hypoxanthine guanine phosphoribosyl transferase, which is completely deficient in **Lesch-Nyhan syndrome**. Initial distinction among these conditions can be made by quantitating the excretion of uric acid in the urine. Another subgroup of patients with overproduction of purine de novo has been shown to have an abnormality in the enzyme phosphoribosyl pyrophosphate (PRPS1) synthetase. This is an interesting disorder in that the patients have more activity than normal. An adult with overproduction gout generally excretes over 600 mg of uric acid per day.

**Complications:** Possible renal failure.

**Associated Findings:** Obesity, hypertensive cardiovascular disease, diabetes.

**Etiology:** Gout is clearly multifactorial and probably polygenic. Occasionally, this defect results from a single gene defect and the primary site of gene action is in the activity of the enzyme hypoxanthine guanine phosphoribosyl transferase or in that of PRPS1 synthetase. In either case there is increased synthesis of uric acid. There are individuals with increased rates of uric acid synthesis in whom the site of the defect has not been established. In others with gout it is apparent that the transport of urate in the renal tubule is abnormal. Genetic control of uric acid concentrations in normal individuals is almost certainly polygenic, and these influences are present in hyperuricemias as well. It seems likely that a number of the diseases we know as gout will ultimately be found to be determined by single gene defects. Some of these may be transmitted as autosomal dominants, and some as autosomal recessives. Hypoxanthine guanine phosphoribosyl transferase activity is determined by genes on the X chromosome; deficiency of this enzyme is transmitted as an X-linked recessive character. PRPS1 synthetase is also determined by a gene on the X-chromosome. This disorder is more likely to be expressed clinically in the female.

**Pathogenesis:** Most of the clinical manifestations of gout can be readily correlated with the occurrence of supersaturated solutions of urate in body fluids and consequent precipitation in tissues. The acute inflammatory reaction in the joint has been correlated with the physicochemical characteristics of the crystal encountered there, a needle-like crystal that is engulfed by leukocytes in the inflammatory process.

**MIM No.:** 13890, *30800, 31185

**Sex Ratio:** M95:F5 in large series. The hypoxanthine guanine phosphoribosyl transferase deficiency disease has not been seen in the female.

**Occurrence:** 1:500 to 1:330 in the United States and Europe. Higher among inhabitants of the Philippine and Marianas Islands. In the Maori of New Zealand, 1:12 males.

**Risk of Recurrence for Patient's Sib:**
See Part I, *Mendelian Inheritance*. Hyperuricemia has been found in 25–72% of relatives of gouty patients.

**Risk of Recurrence for Patient's Child:**
See Part I, *Mendelian Inheritance*. Hyperuricemia has been found in 25–72% of relatives of gouty patients.

**Age of Detectability:** The time of onset of hyperuricemia in individuals ultimately having clinical gout is quite variable. Clinical manifestations are rare before the menopause in the female.

**Gene Mapping and Linkage:** HPRT (hypoxanthine phosphoribosyltransferase) has been mapped to Xq26.

PRPS1 (phosphoribosyl pyrophosphate synthetase 1) has been mapped to Xq21-q27.

**Prevention:** None known. Genetic counseling indicated.

**Treatment:** Hyperuricemia can be controlled in many patients using uricosuric agents, such as probenecid, salicylates, or sulfinpyrazone. Allopurinol, the xanthine oxidase inhibitor, hydroxypyrazolo (3,4-D) pyrimidine is more uniformly effective even in patients otherwise difficult to control. It is the drug of choice in patients excreting large amounts of urate and may be the drug of choice in patients needing treatment for hyperuricemia. Control of hyperuricemia in this way will prevent nephropathy and stones, and prevent or resolve tophi. The number of attacks of acute arthritis in treated patients appears to be decreasing. Colchicine is the drug of choice in the treatment of acute gouty arthritis. Phenylbutazone, indomethacin, and adrenal steroids are also effective.

**Prognosis:** Progressive nephropathy may be lethal. Early prevention of nephropathy should lead to a normal life span.

**Detection of Carrier:** Unknown.

**References:**
Gutman AB, ed.: Proceedings of conference on gout and purine metabolism. Arthritis Rheum 1965; 8:614–621.
Kelley WN, et al.: A specific enzyme defect in gout associated with overproduction of uric acid. Proc Natl Acad Sci USA 1967; 57:1735–1739.
Becker MA, et al.: Variant human phosphoribosylpyrophosphate synthetase altered in regulatory and catalytic functions. J Clin Invest 1980; 65:109–120.
Seegmiller JE: Disorders of purine and pyrimidine metabolism. In: Emery, AEH, Rimoin DL, eds: Principles and practices of medical genetics. New York: Churchill Livingston, 1983:1286–1305.
Nyhan WL: Diagnostic recognition of genetic disease. Philadelphia: Lea & Febiger, 1987:8–19. *

NY000                                              **William L. Nyhan**

**Gowers form of dystrophy**
*See MUSCULAR DYSTROPHY, DISTAL*
**Gradient-type renal tubular acidosis**
*See RENAL TUBULAR ACIDOSIS*
**Grant syndrome**
*See SHORT STATURE-WORMIAN BONES-JOINT DISLOCATIONS*
**Granular cell epulis, congenital**
*See TEETH, EPULIS, CONGENITAL*
**Granular cell fibroblastoma, congenital**
*See TEETH, EPULIS, CONGENITAL*
**Granular cell myoblastoma, congenital**
*See TEETH, EPULIS, CONGENITAL*
**Granular cell tumor (WHO terminology)**
*See TEETH, EPULIS, CONGENITAL*
**Granular corneal dystrophy**
*See CORNEAL DYSTROPHY, GRANULAR*

## GRANULOCYTE GLYCOPROTEIN CD11/CD18 DEFICIENCY                    2970

**Includes:**
CD11/CD18 leukocyte glycoprotein deficiency syndrome
Glycoprotein p150,95 (CD11c/CD18) deficiency
Immunodeficiency, granulocyte glycoprotein deficiency
Infections, recurrent severe
Leukocyte adherence deficiency
LFA-1 (CD11a/CD18) deficiency
Mo1 (CD11b/CD18) deficiency

**Excludes:** Immunodeficiency (other)

**Major Diagnostic Criteria:** Decreased expression of one of the glycoproteins (CD11a, CD11b, CD11c, or CD18) on an individual's leukocyte membranes. Since all patients with this disorder have exhibited a deficiency of the CD11b glycoprotein (Mo1) on their monocytes and granulocytes, and anti-Mo1 monoclonal antibodies are commercially available (Coulter, Mo1; Ortho Diagnostics, OKM1; Becton-Dickinson, Leu 15), use of this monoclonal has become the standard means of establishing this diagnosis. There are certain normal individuals, however, who have unusually low quantities of this glycoprotein on their phagocyte plasma membranes at rest but who increase that quantity to normal levels upon exposure to degranulating stimuli. Such individuals' neutrophil function is normal. To avoid falsely diagnosing these patients as having the glycoprotein deficiency syndrome, the phagocytes should be treated with A23187 (1 $\mu$M concentration) prior to assaying for CD11b with the monoclonal probe. Severely affected individuals will have little or no antibody binding above background levels, while moderately affected individuals will have stimulated levels 5–10% of control.

**Clinical Findings:** Affected individuals present during infancy or early childhood with recurrent severe bacterial, viral, or fungal infections. Often they have had delayed umbilical cord separation. Peripheral neutrophil counts are usually elevated, with baseline WBCs in the range of 20,000–30,000 (80–90% PMNs), which rise to 50,000–120,000 with acute infections. Despite this leukocytosis there is very little pus formation at the sites of infection because of the phagocytes' inability to migrate properly. Most commonly, the infections involve the skin, mucous membranes, sinuses, and respiratory tract. Otitis media is very frequent.

**Complications:** Pneumonias and septicemia are quite common. The most frequent bacterial pathogens are *Staphylococcus aureus*, streptococci, *Escherichia coli*, *Proteus mirabilis*, and *Pseudomonas aeruginosa*. Less frequently, enteroviruses, *Aspergillis*, and *Candida* cause life-threatening infections. The severity and frequency of these infections correlates directly with the degree of deficiency of CD11/CD18 glycoproteins. In addition, these individuals often have impaired wound healing.

**Associated Findings:** None known.

**Etiology:** Autosomal recessive inheritance. All affected individuals are homozygotic. Heterozygotes are asymptomatic carriers.

**Pathogenesis:** Impairment of myeloid and lymphoid function due to the deficiency or complete absence of a family of three glycoprotein heterodimers normally present on the leukocyte plasma membrane. These three glycoproteins have unique $\alpha$ subunits and share a common $\beta$ subunit. Our current understanding is that the underlying defect is a failure to synthesize a normal $\beta$ subunit, which also results in improper posttranslational processing of the $\alpha$ subunit. As a result, neither is present on the cell membrane. LFA-1 (CD11a/CD18) is normally present on all leukocytes and is important for adhesion of the leukocyte to target cells (e.g., for cellular cytotoxicity), to endothelium, and to other leukocytes (e.g., to facilitate lymphocyte interactions). Mo1 (CD11b/CD18) is normally present on the surface of monocytes, neutrophils, and natural killer cells. Like LFA-1, it is an important mediator of cellular adhesion, facilitating margination, diapedesis, and chemotaxis. Mo1 is also the receptor for C3bi and thus is necessary for complement-mediated phagocytosis and superoxide generation. Glycoprotein p150,95 (CD11c/CD18) is normally present on the plasma membrane of monocytes and neutrophils and appears to facilitate adhesion of these cells to substrates.

The neutrophils and monocytes of affected individuals are unable to adhere properly to substrates and to other cells and thus have a markedly diminished capacity for migration, chemotaxis, and phagocytosis of particles. They are also unable to generate normal quantities of superoxide in response to certain particulate stimuli such as opsonized zymosan. As a result, inadequate numbers of phagocytes are able to get to the sites of infection, and those that do are unable to properly engulf and destroy the offending pathogens. In addition, antibody-directed cytotoxicity by T lymphocytes, killer cells, natural killer cells, and neutrophils is impaired. Some lymphocyte function such as delayed hypersensitivity responses are usually normal, but certain individuals

have been found to have diminished blastogenic activity in response to certain stimuli.

**MIM No.:** *11692, *12098, *15151, *15337, 16282

**Sex Ratio:** Presumably M1:F1.

**Occurrence:** Thirty-two cases have been reported in the literature.

**Risk of Recurrence for Patient's Sib:**
See Part I, *Mendelian Inheritance.*

**Risk of Recurrence for Patient's Child:**
See Part I, *Mendelian Inheritance.*

**Age of Detectability:** After 20 weeks gestation. Prenatal diagnosis has been reported in one case in which decreased expression of CD11/CD18 was detected on fetal PMNs obtained by amniocentesis.

**Gene Mapping and Linkage:** CD18 (lymphocyte function-associated antigen 1; macrophage antigen) has been mapped to 21q22.3.
CD11A (antigen CD11A (p180), lymphocyte function-associated antigen 1) has been mapped to 16p13.1
CD13 (antigen CD13 (p150)) has been provisionally mapped to 15q25-qter.
NM (neutrophil migration) has been provisionally mapped to 7q22-qter.
The gene for the $\beta$ subunit is located on chromosome 21.

**Prevention:** None known. Genetic counseling indicated.

**Treatment:** Infections should be treated promptly with broad-spectrum parenteral antibiotics. For serious infections, granulocyte transfusions should be given if available. These transfusions often result in rapid deferescence and a marked drop in the peripheral neutrophil count. Trimethoprim-sulfamethoxazole prophylaxis has been of variable efficacy. Allogeneic bone marrow transplantation has been curative in two patients and probably is the treatment of choice for severely affected individuals with histocompatible sibs.

**Prognosis:** Dependent on the degree of the deficiency. Moderately deficient individuals often live into adulthood, while many of the severely affected die in childhood.

**Detection of Carrier:** Analysis of the expression of CD11b/CD18 (Mo1) on the neutrophils or monocytes by flow cytometry. Carriers will have approximately 50% of the usual amount of the glycoprotein on their cell membranes following stimulation with a secretogogue such as FMLP or A23187.

**References:**
Bower TJ, et al.: Severe recurrent bacterial infections associated with defective adherence and chemotaxis in two patients with neutrophils deficient in a cell-associated glycoprotein. J Pediatr 1982; 101:932–940.
Anderson DC, et al.: Abnormalities of polymorphonuclear leukocyte function associated with a heritable deficiency of high molecular weight surface glycoproteins (GP138): common relationship to diminished cell adherence. J Clin Invest 1984; 74:536–551.
Arnaout MA, et al.: Deficiency of a leukocyte surface glycoprotein (LFA-1) in two patients with Mo1 deficiency. J Clin Invest 1984; 74:1291–1300.
Dana N, et al.: Deficiency of a surface membrane glycoprotein (Mo1) in man. J Clin Invest 1984; 73:153–159.
Koboyashi K, et al.: An abnormality of neutrophil adhesion: autosomal recessive inheritance associated with missing neutrophil glycoproteins. Pediatrics 1984; 73:606–610.
Anderson DC, et al.: The severe and moderate phenotypes of heritable Mac-1, LFA-1, deficiency: their quantitative definition and relation to leukocyte dysfunction and clinical features. J Infect Dis 1985; 152:668–689.

AX001
B0048

**Richard Axtell**
**Lawrence A. Boxer**

**Granulocytic leukemia, chronic**
*See LEUKEMIA, CHRONIC MYELOID (CML)*

## GRANULOMATOSIS-POLYSYNOVITIS, FAMILIAL SYSTEMIC 3141

**Includes:**

Granulomatous arthritis-iritis-rash, familial

Granulomatous arthritis, familial

Granulomatous arteritis-polyarthritis of juvenile onset, familial

Jabs syndrome

Synovitis-granulomatous-uveitis-cranial neoropathies, familial

**Excludes:** Sarcoidosis (2966)

**Major Diagnostic Criteria:** The articular feature is a symmetric, non-erosive polysynovitis, primarily affecting the hands, wrists, and ankles. Biopsy of the synovium reveals granulomatous inflammation. Patients are generally affected with iridocyclitis and may develop a granulomatous skin rash and/or cranial nerve palsy. Chest X-rays are normal.

**Clinical Findings:** Patients generally develop a boggy symmetric synovitis involving primarily the hands, wrists, and ankles. Other joints are affected less commonly. X-rays of the affected joints reveal no erosions or joint destruction, even in patients who have had the disease active for greater than 20 years. While mild limitation of range of motion has been described, physical disabilities are relatively minor. Chest X-rays are uniformly normal and reveal no evidence of classic sarcoidosis. Synovectomy or biopsy specimens of the synovium reveal granulomatous inflammation. Patients are anti-nuclear antibody negative, rheumatoid factor negative, and have a normal serum angiotensin converting enzyme level. An erythematous maculopapular rash may develop, which reveals granulomatous inflammation on biopsy. Cranial neuropathies may occur including sensorineural hearing loss or oculomotor paresis. A recurrent or chronic iridocyclitis is often seen.

**Complications:** Visual loss due to secondary complications of iridocyclitis, such as glaucoma and cataracts, may be seen.

**Associated Findings:** None known.

**Etiology:** Autosomal dominant inheritance with variability in expression. Sporadic cases have been reported.

**Pathogenesis:** Unknown. Granulomatous inflammation is present on biopsy.

**MIM No.:** *18658

**POS No.:** 4456

**Sex Ratio:** M1:F1

**Occurrence:** Five families and several sporadic cases have been reported.

**Risk of Recurrence for Patient's Sib:**

See Part I, *Mendelian Inheritance.*

**Risk of Recurrence for Patient's Child:**

See Part I, *Mendelian Inheritance.*

**Age of Detectability:** Usually clinically evident by 10–20 years of age.

**Gene Mapping and Linkage:** Unknown.

**Prevention:** None known. Genetic counseling indicated.

**Treatment:** Corticosteroids may be used to control the rash, uveitis, cranial neuropathy and vasculopathy.

**Prognosis:** Normal life expectancy. Minimal physical handicaps.

**Detection of Carrier:** Careful history and clinical examination including ophthalmologic examination and X-rays of the chest and symptomatic joints will help identify those relatives who are affected.

**Special Considerations:** Sporadic, non-familial cases have been described and are most often called childhood sarcoidosis. While it cannot be unequivocally demonstrated that these patients do not have sarcoidosis, the lack of pulmonary disease and normal ACE levels argue strongly against this.

An entity termed *familial granulomatous arteritis with polyarthritis of juvenile onset* (Rotenstein et al, 1982) has been described. This family had associated large vessel vasculitis, hypertension, and constitutional symptoms. It is not yet clear whether this represents the same or a different syndrome, but it is likely that they are within the same spectrum.

**References:**

North AF, et al: Sarcoid arthritis in children. Am J Med 1970; 48:449–455.

Rotenstein D, et al: Familial granulomatous arteritis with polyarthritis of juvenile onset. New Engl J Med 1982; 306:86–90.

Blau ED: Familial granulomatous arthritis, iritis, and rash. J Pediatr 1985; 107:689–693.

Jabs DA, et al: Familial granulomatous synovitis, uveitis, and cranial neuropathies. Am J Med 1985; 78:801–804.

Miller JJ: Early onset "sarcoidosis" and "familial granulomatous arthritis (arteritis)": the same disease. J Pediatr 1986; 109:387–388.

JA015                            **Douglas A. Jabs**
JA014                         **Ethylin Wang Jabs**

**Granulomatous arteritis-polyarthritis of juvenile onset**
*See ARTHRITIS-ARTERITIS SYNDROME*

**Granulomatous arteritis-polyarthritis of juvenile onset, familial**
*See GRANULOMATOSIS-POLYSYNOVITIS, FAMILIAL SYSTEMIC*

**Granulomatous arthritis, familial**
*See GRANULOMATOSIS-POLYSYNOVITIS, FAMILIAL SYSTEMIC*

**Granulomatous arthritis-iritis-rash, familial**
*See GRANULOMATOSIS-POLYSYNOVITIS, FAMILIAL SYSTEMIC*

**Granulomatous colitis**
*See INFLAMMATORY BOWEL DISEASE*

**Granulomatous disease, chronic autosomal recessive**
*See GRANULOMATOUS DISEASE, CHRONIC X-LINKED*

## GRANULOMATOUS DISEASE, CHRONIC X-LINKED 0443

**Includes:**

Cytochrome-b-negative granulomatous disease

Cytochrome-b-positive autosomal granulomatous disease

Cytosol factor, deficiency of

Granulomatous disease, chronic autosomal recessive

Xk-related chronic granulomatous disease

**Excludes:**

Immunodeficiency, hyper IgE type (2211)

Immunodeficiency, myeloperoxidase deficiency type (2214)

**Major Diagnostic Criteria:** Chronic granulomatous disease (CGD) is a congenital immunodeficiency syndrome characterized by susceptibility to infection by catalase-positive organisms. This susceptibility is due to the inability of the afflicted individual's phagocytes to undergo a respiratory burst and thereby generate the microbicidal oxidants necessary to kill phagocytized organisms. This results in chronic and recurrent infections with the development of granulomata composed of giant cells and lipid-filled histiocytes. Chemotaxis, phagocytosis, and degranulation are all normal in these individuals.

**Clinical Findings:** Age of presentation can be from one week to young adulthood, although 80% are diagnosed in the first year of life. The severity of the affliction can likewise be variable: some having frequent severe infections with death in early childhood; and some having relatively infrequent infections and surviving until middle age. The cause of this variability is not understood.

The infecting organisms are atypical for normal children and most commonly include *staphylococcus aureus*, enteric gram negative rods, *candida albicans*, and *aspergillus* species. These organisms can cause pyogenic infections and/or granulomas in any organ system but most frequently infect the lungs (often with abscess formation), the skin, the mucosa (recurrent stomatitis, candidal esophagitis, and so on) and the reticuloendothelial system (superative lymphadenitis, hepatic and splenic abcesses). Osteomyelitis, especially with *serratia marcescens*, is not uncommon. Less frequently involved are the meninges and urinary tract. Septicemia is infrequent, but is life-threatening when it does occur.

The total white blood count and absolute neutrophil count are normal or elevated but there is often an anemia of chronic inflammation present. Immunoglobulin and complement levels are normal or elevated.

**Complications:** Urinary tract disorders.

**Associated Findings:** None known.

**Etiology:** The appellation "chronic granulomatous disease" is applied to a collection of slightly different genetic disorders with a common phenotype: absence of a respiratory burst and a subsequent inability to kill catalase positive organisms.

Approximately 80% of cases are X-linked inherited in which the males are symptomatic and their mothers and carrier sisters are chimeras: as would be expected by the Lyon hypothesis. The carriers do not seem to have any increased susceptibility to disease despite the fact that one-half of their neutrophils are defective.

The remaining 20% of individuals with CGD appear to have inherited the disease in an autosomal recessive fashion.

**Pathogenesis:** The underlying neutrophil abnormality in CGD is an inability to undergo a respiratory burst, which is the mechanism by which microbicidal oxidants are produced. In normal phagocytes, the response to the ingestion of a pathogen is the activation of a membrane-bound flavoprotein oxidase which catalyzes the synthesis of superoxide by the following mechanism:

$$NADPH + 2O_2 \rightarrow 2O_2- + H^+ + NADP^+$$

This superoxide radical is then used to synthesize hydrogen peroxide, a reaction catalyzed by superoxide dismutase:

$$2O_2- + 2H^+ \rightarrow H_2O_2 + O_2$$

This hydrogen peroxide is then employed in the production of the halogen oxidants (usually hypochlorous acid) which appear to be the actual microbicidal chemicals. This reaction is catalyzed by the myeloperoxidase present in the specific granules:

$$H_2O_2 + HCl \rightarrow H^+ + OCl\cdot + H_2O$$

In the neutrophils of patients with CGD, there is a failure of the membrane-bound oxidase to catalyze the production of superoxide and as a result the necessary microbicidals are not endogenously generated. All microbes, however, produce small quantities of $H_2O_2$ and thus, once a microbe is ingested, this $H_2O_2$ can act as the substrate for the myeloperoxidase-catalyzed production of hypochlorous acid. Certain bacteria and fungi, however, contain catalase (an enzyme which reduces $H_2O_2$ to water and molecular oxygen) and these organisms secrete no $H_2O_2$. This is the reason why individuals with CGD do not have problems with catalase-negative organisms, but those with catalase: s. aureus, gram negative enterobacteria, candida and aspergillus species, cause chronic infections. The invading bacteria or fungi are opsonized and phagocytized but they are not killed and are released intact when the engulfing neutrophil dies. The macrophages of an afflicted individual likewise are unable to kill these organisms and this leads to the development of smouldering infections, abscesses, and the characteristic granulomata.

The exact nature of the defect in the initiating oxidase's function has been the object of considerable controversy. At present, it appears that in some individuals there is missing cytochrome, and that in others the protein is normal but the mechanism by which it is activated is defective.

**MIM No.:** *23370, *30640

**Sex Ratio:** M6:F1

**Occurrence:** Over 300 cases reported. Approximately 1:1,000,000

**Risk of Recurrence for Patient's Sib:**
See Part I, *Mendelian Inheritance*.

**Risk of Recurrence for Patient's Child:**
See Part I, *Mendelian Inheritance*.

**Age of Detectability:** Prenatally by the use of the NBT slide test on blood obtained from placental vessel puncture. Otherwise, can be detected clinically in the neonatal period.

**Gene Mapping and Linkage:** NCF1 (neutrophil cytosolic factor 1) has been provisionally mapped to 10.

CYBB (cytochrome b-245, beta polypeptide (chronic granulomatous disease)) has been mapped to Xp21.1.

**Prevention:** None known. Genetic counseling indicated.

**Treatment:** There is no way to rectify the biochemical defect present in the affected patient's neutrophils. Use of subcutaneous interferon gamma has resulted in partial correction of the phagocyte defect (Ezekowitz et al, 1988). The use of prophylactic antibiotics is believed to decrease the frequency of serious infections. Both trimethoprim-sulfamethoxazole (5 mg of TMP/kg/day divided BID) and penicillinase-resistant penicillins have been used and the former is felt to be superior. When either overt or occult (as evidenced by a fever without apparent source) infections occur, parenteral broad-spectrum antibiotics are indicated, covering for s. aureus and gram negative rods. Persistence of fever despite antibacterial therapy should prompt a search for sites of fungal infection and consideration of antifungal therapy. With life-threatening infections, granulocyte transfusions are a logical supportive maneuver, but their efficacy has not been definitively demonstrated. Surgical drainage of abscesses may be necessary, and surgical removal of granulomata may be necessary when they cause obstruction of organs such as the stomach, bowel, or ureters.

Bone marrow transplant offers the only possibility of cure for this affliction, and successful engraftment with the production of granulocytes capable of a respiratory burst has been reported.

**Prognosis:** Lifespan of affected individuals is variable and depends on the frequency and severity of the infections and the alacrity and appropriateness of therapy. Some die in infancy or early childhood and some are living to middle age.

**Detection of Carrier:** In those cases where the disorder is X-linked, carrier females will have two populations of neutrophils: one capable of a respiratory burst and superoxide production; and one that is incapable. In this situation, a nitroblue tetrazolium slide test will show that some of the cells are capable of oxidizing this yellow dye to purple and that some are not able to do so.

Those individuals who are heterozygous for the autosomal recessively inherited variety are not detectable by current methods.

**References:**

Gallin FI, et al.: Recent advances in chronic granulomatous disease. Ann Int Med 1983; 99:657–674.

Tauber AI, et al.: Chronic granulomatous disease: a syndrome of phagocyte oxidase deficiencies. Medicine 1983; 62:286–309.

Curnutte JT, et al.: Clinically significant phagocytic cell defects. In: Remington RS, et al., eds: current topics in infectious diseases. New York: McGraw-Hill, 1985:103–105.

Curnutte JT, et al.: Chronic granulomatous disease. In: Harris H, Hirschhorn K, eds: Advances in human genetics, vol 16. New York: plenum Publishers, 1987:229–297.

Ezekowitz RAB, et al.: Partial correction of the phagocyte defect in patients with X-linked chronic granulomatous disease by subcutaneous interferon gamma. New Engl J. Med 1988; 319:146–151.

Clark RA, et al.: Genetic variants of chronic granulomatous disease: prevalence of deficiencies of two cytosolic components of the NADPH oxidase system. New Engl J Med 1989; 321:647–652.

Forehand JR, et al.: Inherited disorders of phagocyte killing. In: Scriver CR, et al, eds: The metabolic basis of inherited disease, 6th ed. New York: McGraw-Hill, 1989:2779–2803.

AX001
B0048

**Richard Axtell**
**Laurence A. Boxer**

**Granulosis rubra nasi**
*See NOSE, GRANULOSIS RUBRA NASI*

**Graves disease**
*See THYROTOXICOSIS*

**Great veins, transposition of (complete)**
*See PULMONARY VENOUS CONNECTION, TOTAL ANOMALOUS*

**Great veins, transposition of (partial)**
*See PULMONARY VENOUS CONNECTION, PARTIAL ANOMALOUS*

**Great vessel transposition**
*See HEART, TRANSPOSITION OF GREAT VESSELS*

**Great vessels from right ventricle-posterior septal defect**
*See VENTRICLE, DOUBLE-OUTLET RIGHT WITH POSTERIOR SEPTAL DEFECT*

**Grebe chondrodysplasia**
*See GREBE SYNDROME*

## GREBE SYNDROME 0445

**Includes:**
    Achondrogenesis, type II (McKusick)
    Brazilian achondrogenesis
    Grebe chondrodysplasia
    Skeletal dysplasia, Grebe type

**Excludes:**
    **Achondrogenesis** (other)
    **Hypochondroplasia** (0510)

**Major Diagnostic Criteria:** Nonlethal short-limbed dwarfism. Limbs are short and deformed, often with valgus forearms, hands, and feet. The digits are extremely small, and polydactyly is common. X-rays show aplasia and hypoplasia of the limb bones.

**Clinical Findings:** Affected individuals are short (around 100 cm) and have marked hypomelia of upper and lower extremities. The limbs are progressively shortened from proximal to distal segments and tend to be obese. The hands are extremely short with stubby, toe-like fingers. Polydactyly (postaxial) has been described in about 60% of the reported cases. Shortening of the lower limbs is more severe than that of the upper limbs. The feet are short, broad, and in valgus position. Rudimentary toes may be present. Joint movements in the extremities are greatly reduced. All affected persons seem to be mentally normal.

Bones from the trunk and the head are apparently normal, but X-rays of the extremities show variable aplasia and hypoplasia of all bony elements. Bone abnormalities are bilateral, except in a few cases, in the phalanges and more severe distally. Bone structures seems to be unaffected, although the appearance of the epiphyseal centers of some bones is retarded.

**Complications:** Unknown.

**Associated Findings:** None known.

**Etiology:** Autosomal recessive inheritance.

**Pathogenesis:** Possibly a segmentation defect of the embryonic limb bud.

**MIM No.:** *20070

**POS No.:** 3755

**Sex Ratio:** M1:F1

**Occurrence:** Since the original report by Grebe (1952) in a German kindred, this condition has been documented in 47 cases from a highly inbred Brazilian population and in at least six individuals from a Miao Nationality Chinese consanguineous kindred. Only one affected individual has so far been identified in an English family in which a variable degree of brachydactyly was reported in a son and grandson.

A gene frequency of 2% in the Brazilian township was suggested. The prevalence of the affected individuals with the disorder at birth is probably 0.005:1000.

**Risk of Recurrence for Patient's Sib:**
    See Part I, *Mendelian Inheritance.*

**Risk of Recurrence for Patient's Child:**
    See Part I, *Mendelian Inheritance.* The risk of a skeletal abnormality in a heterozygote is probably less than 1:100.

**Age of Detectability:** At birth. Prenatal diagnosis may be possible by ultrasound.

**Gene Mapping and Linkage:** Unknown.

**Prevention:** None known. Genetic counseling indicated.

**Treatment:** Orthopedic care as indicated.

**Prognosis:** Quelce-Salgado (1968) reported that many of the affected Brazilians in his study were stillborn (11%) or died in infancy (38%). Survival to adulthood has been reported by other researchers.

**Detection of Carrier:** Unknown.

**Special Considerations:** Quelce-Salgado (1968) suggested that the mutant gene may have a slight effect on the heterozygotes. Curtis (1986) suggested brachydactyly as possible heterozygote expression in this disorder. Segregation of this disorder with

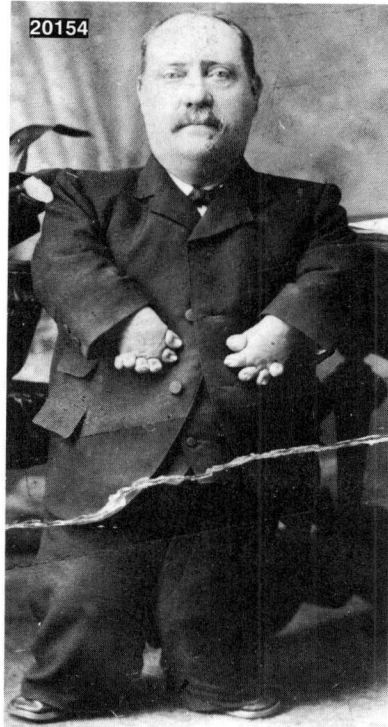

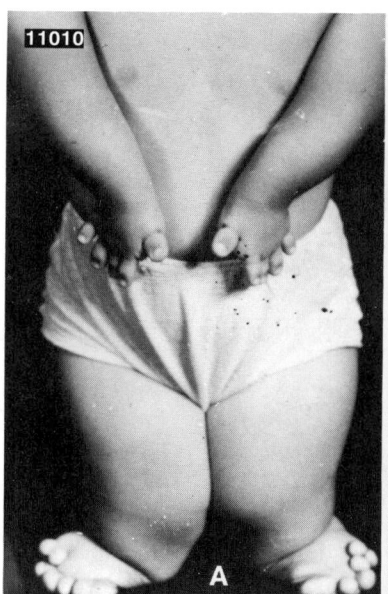
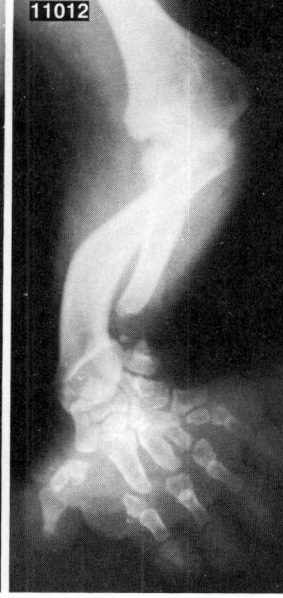

**0445-20154:** Grebe type of short-limbed disproportionate short stature; note stubby toe-like fingers and polydactyly. **11010:** Short limbs and postaxial polydactyly of the feet. **11012:** Markedly bowed and short radius, and hypoplastic ulna.

minor skeletal abnormalities in the heterozygotes may give an erroneous impression of an autosomal dominant trait with variable expression. Grebe syndrome is a distinct chondrodysplasia, not to be mistaken for a type of achondrogenesis affecting the limbs. Survival to adulthood is expected, and reproductive capability is probably not reduced.

**References:**
Grebe H: Die Achondrogenesis: ein einfach rezessives Erbmerkmal. Folia Hered Pathol 1952; 2:23–28.
Quelco-Salgado A: A rare genetic syndrome. Lancet 1968; I:1430 only.
Garcia-Castro JM, Perez-Comas A: Nonlethal achondrogenesis (Grebe-Quelce-Salgado type) in two Puerto Rican sibships. J Pediatr 1975; 87:948–952.
Romeo G, et al.: Grebe chondrodysplasia and similar forms of severe short-limbed dwarfism. BD:OAS;XII(3C). New York: March of Dimes Birth Defects Foundation, 1977:109–115.
Kumar D, et al.: Grebe chondrodysplasia and brachydactyly in a family. Clin Genet 1984; 25:68–72.
Curtis D: Heterozygote expression in Grebe chondrodysplasia. Clin Genet 1986; 29:455–456.
Teebi AS, et al.: Severe short-limb dwarfism resembling Grebe chondrodysplasia. Hum Genet 1986; 74:386–390.

KU009                                    **Dhavendra Kumar**

**Gregg syndrome**
  See *FETAL RUBELLA SYNDROME*
**Greig cephalopolysyndactyly syndrome**
  See *POLYSYNDACTYLY-DYSMORPHIC CRANIOFACIES, GREIG TYPE*
**Greig syndrome**
  See *EYE, HYPERTELORISM*
**Greither keratoderma**
  See *KERATOSIS PALMARIS ET PLANTARIS OF UNNA-THOST*
**Grey teeth**
  See *TEETH, DEFECTS FROM TETRACYCLINE*
**Griscelli syndrome**
  See *HYPOPIGMENTATION-IMMUNE DEFECT, GRISCELLI TYPE*
**Griseofulvin exposure and conjoined twins**
  See *TWINS, CONJOINED, TERATOGENICITY*
**Groenblad-Strandberg syndrome**
  See *PSEUDOXANTHOMA ELASTICUM*
**Groenouw type I corneal dystrophy**
  See *CORNEAL DYSTROPHY, GRANULAR*
**Groenouw type II corneal dystrophy**
  See *CORNEAL DYSTROPHY, MACULAR TYPE*
**Groll-Hirschowitz syndrome**
  See *DEAFNESS-DIVERTICULITIS-NEUROPATHY*
**Group-specific protein**
  See *PLASMA, GROUP-SPECIFIC COMPONENT*
**Growth defect-hydrocephalus-nephrosis-thin skin-blue sclera**
  See *NEPHROSIS-HYDROCEPHALUS-THIN SKIN-BLUE SCLERA-GROWTH DEFECT*
**Growth defect-locking digits**
  See *HAND, LOCKING DIGITS-GROWTH DEFECT*

---

## GROWTH DEFICIENCY, AFRICAN PYGMY TYPE          3100

**Includes:**
  Aka pygmy growth deficiency
  Effie pygmy growth deficiency
  Insulin-like growth factor deficiency
  Pigmy, African Baka of central Cameroon
  Short stature in the African pygmy
  Somatomedin C deficiency

**Excludes:**
  **Dwarfism, Laron** (0302)
  **Growth hormone deficiency, isolated** (0447)
  Growth retardation secondary to malnutrition
  **Leprechaunism** (0587)

**Major Diagnostic Criteria:** Growth hormone responses to provocative stimuli such as arginine infusion and insulin-induced hypoglycemia are normal in pygmies. Basal concentrations of insulin-like growth factors I and II (IGF1 and IGF2) may not be distinguishable from those of normal individuals in childhood. However, in adults, 70 to 80% of pygmies will have IGF1 concentrations in a hypopituitary range. IGF2 concentrations in serum are normal. Concentrations of IGF1 are significantly less than normal during adolescence, the period of accelerated growth in normal nonpygmy subjects.

**Clinical Findings:** The African pygmy may differ only slightly from others during childhood in terms of linear height and growth. In a large series comparing heights in 38 ethnic groups, pygmy children ranked only 18th, yet pygmy adults ranked last. The critical period that determines the final short stature of the pygmy appears to be puberty.

IGF1 is the principal agent responsible for pubertal growth acceleration. Adolescent pygmies do not have a normal increase of IGF1 concentration in serum during puberty, whereas normal adolescents of other groups have increases of IGF1 from two to two and a half times the adult level. Associated with this abnormality of IGF1 secretion, adolescent pygmies do not exhibit a growth spurt during puberty or exhibit only a blunted growth spurt.

**Complications:** Unknown.

**Associated Findings:** Since IGF1 is the principal factor mediating the anabolic effects of growth hormone (GH), several abnormalities can be expected: 1) Insulin secretion is reduced and 2) GH treatment, which does not increase IGF1 in the pygmy, will secondarily fail to increase insulin secretion, fail to alter urinary Ca and $PO_4$, and fail to cause normal nitrogen retention.

**Etiology:** Probably autosomal recessive inheritance. Sporadic cases have been reported.

**Pathogenesis:** Current work suggests a defective or absent gene that modulates IGF1 secretion, but no defect in the IGF1 gene itself. The ''modulator'' gene would be expressed at puberty. A gene modulating IGF2 secretion has been demonstrated in normal persons, but no data are yet available for the IGF1 gene and its postulated modulating genes.

Concentrations of a growth hormone binding protein, which is derived from the cellular receptor for GH, are described in pygmies. By this measurement pygmies have a deficiency of GH-receptor of 50% or greater. This probably accounts for low IGF I levels, i.e. reduced responsiveness to GH.

**MIM No.:** *14744, 26585

**Sex Ratio:** Presumably M1:F1.

**Occurrence:** Multiple pygmy tribes in Africa have been described, but most pygmies belong to one of two groups: the Aka or Effie. Two sporadic cases of dwarfism resembling the pygmy type have been described in the United States (Merimee and Rabinowitz, 1974).

**Risk of Recurrence for Patient's Sib:**
  See Part I, *Mendelian Inheritance*. One hundred percent in pygmy tribes, but no data are available on sporadic cases.

**Risk of Recurrence for Patient's Child:**
  See Part I, *Mendelian Inheritance*.

**Age of Detectability:** Impossible to detect in childhood in non-pygmies, since 35% of normal children have IGF1 serum levels significantly less than those of adults. A failure of IGF1 to increase appropriately during puberty despite normal sexual maturation is the major abnormality.

**Gene Mapping and Linkage:** IGF1 (insulin-like growth factor 1) has been mapped to 12q23.

**Prevention:** None known. Genetic counseling indicated. Not applicable in pygmy tribes in which short stature is the norm.

**Treatment:** Not applicable in pygmy tribes. In sporadic cases, high-dose GH treatment to augment IGF1 maximally would probably not succeed. If IGF1 becomes available, IGF1 injections should induce normal growth acceleration.

**Prognosis:** Factors other than stature appear to be unaffected.

**Detection of Carrier:** Apparent in pygmy tribes. Otherwise, undetermined.

**References:**
Merimee TJ, Rabinowitz D: Isolated human growth hormone deficiency and related disorders. New York: Intercontinental Medical Book Corporation, 1974:1–63.
Meredith HV: Research between 1960 and 1970 on the standing height

of young children in different parts of the world. Adv Child Dev Behav 1978; 12:1–59.

Merimee TJ, et al.: Insulin-like growth factors in pygmies: the role of puberty in determining final stature. New Engl J Med 1987; 316:906–911.

ME041 **Thomas J. Merimee**

## GROWTH DEFICIENCY-FACIAL DEFECTS-BRACHYDACTYLY      2175

**Includes:**
Brachydactyly-growth deficiency-dysmorphic faces
Facial defects-brachydactyly-growth defect

**Excludes:** Dysmorphic facies-brachydactyly (other)

**Major Diagnostic Criteria:** Growth deficiency, dysmorphic facies, and brachydactyly.

**Clinical Findings:** Birth weight is low and postnatal growth is poor, with height in the low normal range. Development is also in the low normal range. A peculiar face is noticed at birth: downward eye slant, epicanthus, ptosis, and hypertelorism. The ears are cup shaped and low-set. The hands are short, the middle phalanx being most shortened. There is ulnar deviation of the index finger and clinodactyly of the fourth and fifth fingers.

**Complications:** Unknown.

**Associated Findings:** None known.

**Etiology:** Presumed autosomal dominant inheritance.

**Pathogenesis:** Unknown.

**Sex Ratio:** Presumably M1:F1.

**Occurrence:** A mother and son have been reported.

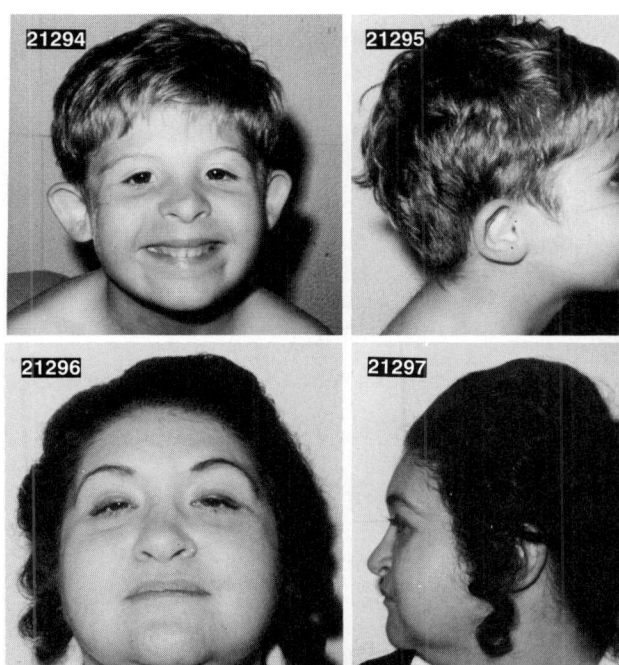

**2175A**-21294–97: Facial view of proband and his mother shows hypertelorism, downward slanting of the palpebral fissures, epicanthal folds, and cup-shaped ears.

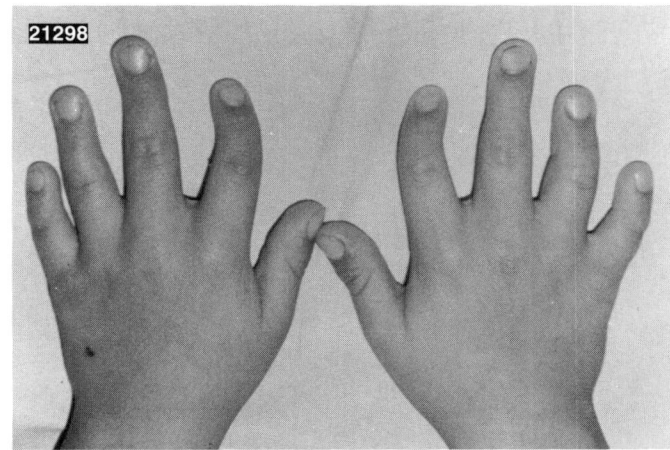

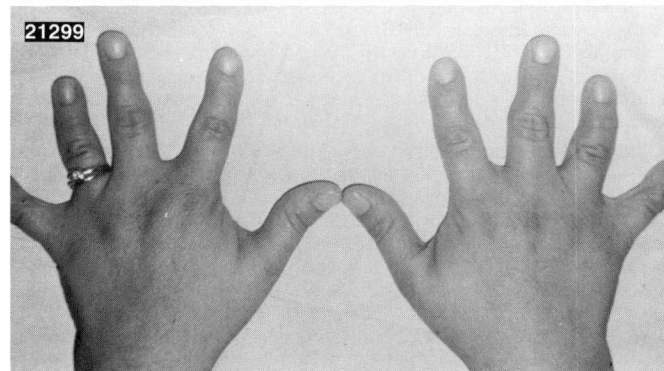

**2175B**-21298: Proband's hands show short hands with especially short middle phalanges, ulnar deviation of the index fingers and clinodactyly of the fourth and fifth fingers. 21299: Proband's mother's hands show short digits with the fourth digit being most affected.

**Risk of Recurrence for Patient's Sib:**
See Part I, *Mendelian Inheritance.*

**Risk of Recurrence for Patient's Child:**
See Part I, *Mendelian Inheritance.*

**Age of Detectability:** At birth.

**Gene Mapping and Linkage:** Unknown.

**Prevention:** None known. Genetic counseling indicated.

**Treatment:** Unknown.

**Prognosis:** Unknown.

**Detection of Carrier:** Unknown.

**References:**
Frias JL, et al.: Growth deficiency, facial dysmorphogenesis and brachydactyly: a new syndrome. BD:OAS XI(2). New York: March of Dimes Birth Defects Foundation, 1975:30–33.

TH017      **T.F. Thurmon**
UR001      **S.A. Ursin**

**Growth deficiency-facial erythema-chromosome instability**
*See BLOOM SYNDROME*
**Growth failure-ectodermal dysplasia-pancreatic insufficiency**
*See DONLAN SYNDROME*

## GROWTH HORMONE DEFICIENCY, ISOLATED 0447

**Includes:**
Dwarfism, pituitary
Illig-type growth hormone deficiency
Primordial dwarfism
Sexual ateleotic dwarfism

**Excludes:**
**Dwarfism, Laron** (0302)
**Dwarfism, panhypopituitary** (0303)
**Dwarfism, pituitary with abnormal sella turcica** (0304)
Dwarfism due to biologically inactive hGH
Pituitary, congenital absence of

**Major Diagnostic Criteria:** Proportionate dwarfism with evidence of human growth hormone (hGH) deficiency (poor response to recognized hGH stimuli, i.e. clonidine, L-dopa, arginine infusion, insulin-induced hypoglycemia) in the absence of other pituitary hormone deficiencies.

Since patients with isolated growth hormone deficiency (IGHD) usually have late puberty, it may be difficult to differentiate them from those with panhypopituitarism during late adolescence. Treatment with hGH often stimulates spontaneous puberty in IGHD patients and may be helpful in distinguishing these patients.

**Clinical Findings:** Isolated growth hormone deficiency (IGHD) refers to a heterogeneous group of disorders that differ clinically, biochemically and genetically. The most common IGHD type, IB, is characterized by proportionate dwarfism, excessive subcutaneous adipose tissue, particularly of the trunk, soft wrinkled skin, round doll-like facies and a peculiar high-pitched voice. Birth length and weight are normal, but hypoglycemic episodes may be a problem during infancy. Growth retardation begins at birth, but usually is not apparent before 6 months of age. Skeletal bone age is mildly retarded. Normal sexual development occurs but often is delayed until the late teens or early 20s. Fertility is normal. Metabolic abnormalities include glucose intolerance unassociated with ketosis or diabetic vascular complications, insulinopenia following glucose ingestion or arginine infusion, prolonged hypoglycemia following insulin infusion, and diminished lipolysis.

**0447-10332–33:** Phenotype of isolated deficiency of hGH, type 1. **10334:** Normal daughter of woman shown in **10333.**

hGH replacement results in correction of these abnormalities. In type IA, the clinical presentation is similar to IB, although some infants have been small at birth. These patients differ in that they develop high levels of hGH antibodies following therapy with hGH.

IGHD, type II, a rarer and less well-defined form, differs from IGHD, type I, in that patients lack the wrinkled skin and peculiar voice and tend to be somewhat more obese. Although they have glucose intolerance and decreased lipolysis, they demonstrate an increased rather than a decreased insulin response to glucose ingestion or arginine infusion and a relative resistance to insulin infusion. Furthermore, these metabolic abnormalities may not be corrected with hGH treatment. Hence, these patients show a relative resistance to the metabolic effects of both insulin and hGH. Probably IGHD, type II is a heterogeneous disorder, as patients have been described with different combinations of metabolic abnormalities.

**Complications:** Unknown.

**Associated Findings:** None known.

**Etiology:** *IGHD, type I*: Almost all families show autosomal recessive inheritance, but autosomal dominant inheritance may occur rarely in patients with this constellation of metabolic abnormalities.

*IGHD, type II*: Most cases are sporadic, but autosomal dominant inheritance has been recognized.

**Pathogenesis:** A variety of defects in the hypothalamic-pituitary axis has been postulated; all of them could ultimately lead to isolated growth hormone deficiency. Somatotropic cells have been identified in the pituitaries of several autopsied cases of IGHD, type I, suggesting a primary hypothalamic defect. In some families with IGHD, type IA, deletion of hGH genes has been found. A report by Laron et al (1985), however, suggests that the pathogenesis of anti-hGH is more complex.

**MIM No.:** *26240, *13925, *17310

**POS No.:** 3771

**Sex Ratio:** M1:F1

**Occurrence:** Over 100 cases documented.

**Risk of Recurrence for Patient's Sib:**
See Part I, *Mendelian Inheritance.*

**Risk of Recurrence for Patient's Child:**
See Part I, *Mendelian Inheritance.*

**Age of Detectability:** At birth, but usually not suspected before six months of age.

**Gene Mapping and Linkage:** GHI (growth hormone I) has been mapped to 17q22-q24.

**Prevention:** None known. Genetic counseling indicated.

**Treatment:** Replacement with hGH should be started as early as possible. Pregnant females with the disorder need cesarean section since children, whether affected or unaffected, will be of normal size at birth.

**Prognosis:** Good if detected early and patient responds to therapy.

**Detection of Carrier:** Unknown.

**References:**
Rimoin DL: Hereditary forms of growth hormone deficiency and resistance. BD:OAS;XII(6). New York: Alan R. Liss for the National Foundation-March of Dimes, 1976:15–29.
Donaldson MDC, et al.: Recessively inherited growth hormone deficiency in a family from Iraq. J Med Genet 1980; 17:288–290.
Phillips JA III, et al.: Molecular basis for familial isolated growth hormone deficiency. Proc Natl Acad Sci 1981; 78:6372–6375.
Van Gelderen HH, van der Hoog CE: Familial isolated growth hormone deficiency. Clin Genet 1981; 20:173–175.
Laron Z, et al.: Human growth hormone gene deletion without antibody formation or growth arresting during treatment. Isr J Med Sci 1985; 21:999–1006.

Tani N, et al.: A family case with autosomal dominant inherited pituitary dwarfism. Tohoko J Exp Med 1987; 152:319–324.

H0033                                  **William A. Horton**
H0025                                       **O.J. Hood**

**Growth hormone receptor deficiency, suspected**
*See DWARFISM, LARON*
**Growth retardation, intrauterine-mental retardation-unusual facies**
*See DWARFISM-DYSMORPHIC FACIES-RETARDATION, PITT TYPE*

---

## GROWTH RETARDATION-ALOPECIA-PSEUDOANODONTIA-OPTIC ATROPHY      2293

**Includes:**
    Alopecia-growth retardation-pseudoanodontia
    GAPO syndrome
    Teeth (pseudoanodontia)-growth retardation-alopecia

**Excludes:**
    Alopecia, isolated or in other combination
    Growth retardation, isolated or in other combination
    Optic atrophy, isolated or in other combination
    Pseudoanodontia, isolated or in other combination

**Major Diagnostic Criteria:** Growth retardation, alopecia, and pseudoanodontia. Optic atrophy is a less constant feature.

**Clinical Findings:** Scalp hair is present at birth, but after the first year of life, it is gradually lost over the next year or two and never regrows. Eyebrows and eyelashes as well as all body hair is lost or never develops. Breast development in females has been minimal.

There is frontal bossing, a high forehead, dilated scalp veins, mild midfacial hypoplasia, and delayed closure of the anterior fontanelle.

Birth weight is normal but birth length is somewhat reduced. Short stature becomes evident at the sixth month check-up. Body build is proportional. Bone age is significantly retarded; otherwise, skeletal alterations are unremarkable except for mild **Pectus excavatum**. **Hernia, umbilical** has been an essentially constant feature.

The jaws are crowded with both dentitions, neither of which erupts, hence pseudoanodontia.

**Complications:** Optic atrophy is variable in onset and has been noted on only about one-fourth of the patients reported. Nephrocalcinosis has been described in a few patients.

**Associated Findings:** Absent or occluded transverse sigmoid sinuses in a few cases.

**Etiology:** Autosomal recessive inheritance.

**Pathogenesis:** It has been suggested that this is a progeroid syndrome.

**MIM No.:** *23074

**POS No.:** 3640

**Sex Ratio:** M1:F1

**Occurrence:** Over a dozen patients have been reported. Although there are thought to be a larger number of Brazilian cases, other reports have originated from Denmark, Israel, Algeria, and the United States.

**Risk of Recurrence for Patient's Sib:**
    See Part I, *Mendelian Inheritance.*

**Risk of Recurrence for Patient's Child:**
    See Part I, *Mendelian Inheritance.*

**Age of Detectability:** Probably between one and two years of age, since scalp hair will have begun to be lost, and although present on X-ray examination no teeth will have erupted.

**Gene Mapping and Linkage:** Unknown.

**Prevention:** None known. Genetic counseling indicated.

**Treatment:** A wig may be worn, and dentures constructed. There is no evidence of an isolated growth hormone deficiency.

**Prognosis:** Normal life span. Optic atrophy variable in onset and severity.

**Detection of Carrier:** Unknown.

**References:**
Andersen TH, Pindborg JJ: Et tilfaelde af "pseudo-anodonti" i forbindelse med kraniedeformitet, dvaergvaekst og ektodermal displasi. Odont T 1947; 55:484–493.
Fuks A: Pseudoanodontia, cranial deformity, blindness, alopecia and dwarfism: a new syndrome. J Dent Child 1978; 45:155–157.
Tipton RE, Gorlin RJ: Growth retardation alopecia, pseudo-anodontia, and optic atrophy: the GAPO syndrome. Am J Med Genet 1984; 19:209–216.
Gagliardi ART: GAPO syndrome: report of three affected brothers. Am J Med Genet 1984; 19:217–224.
Manouvrier-Hanu S, et al.: The GAPO syndrome. Am J Med Genet 1987; 26:683–688.

G0038                                        **Robert J. Gorlin**

**Growth retardation-cortical blindness-postaxial polydactyly**
*See BLINDNESS (CORTICAL)-RETARDATION-POSTAXIAL POLYDACTYLY*
**Growth retardation-microcephaly-charcteristic facies**
*See DUBOWITZ SYNDROME*
**Growth retardation-Rieger anomaly**
*See SHORT SYNDROME*

---

## GROWTH-MENTAL DEFICIENCY, MYHRE TYPE      2176

**Includes:** Myhre syndrome

**Excludes:** Growth deficiency and mental deficiency (other)

**Major Diagnostic Criteria:** Short stature, muscle hypertrophy, and decreased joint mobility.

**Clinical Findings:** Findings noticed at birth include low birth weight, blepharophimosis, hypoplastic maxilla, prognathism, short philtrum, small mouth, heart malformation, and cryptorchidism. Growth is poor, leading to short stature. During childhood, hyperopia, mental retardation, sensorineural deafness, muscle hypertrophy, and decreased joint mobility are noticed. X-rays show thick calvarium, broad ribs, hypoplastic iliac wings, short tubular bones, platyspondyly, and large vertebrae with large pedicles.

**Complications:** Unknown.

**Associated Findings:** One affected boy had **Cleft palate, Hypospadias, Hernia, inguinal**, and hypertension.

**Etiology:** Presumably autosomal dominant inheritance, since both boys had fathers older than 35 years of age.

**Pathogenesis:** Unknown.

**MIM No.:** 13921

**POS No.:** 3631

**Sex Ratio:** Presumably M1:F1; M2:F0 observed.

**Occurrence:** Two reported cases have been reported, in unrelated males.

**Risk of Recurrence for Patient's Sib:**
    See Part I, *Mendelian Inheritance.*

**Risk of Recurrence for Patient's Child:**
    See Part I, *Mendelian Inheritance.*

**Age of Detectability:** In childhood.

**Gene Mapping and Linkage:** Unknown.

**Prevention:** None known. Genetic counseling indicated.

**Treatment:** Unknown.

**Prognosis:** Unknown.

**Detection of Carrier:** Unknown.

**References:**
Myhre SA, et al.: A new growth deficiency syndrome. Clin Genet 1981; 20:1–5.

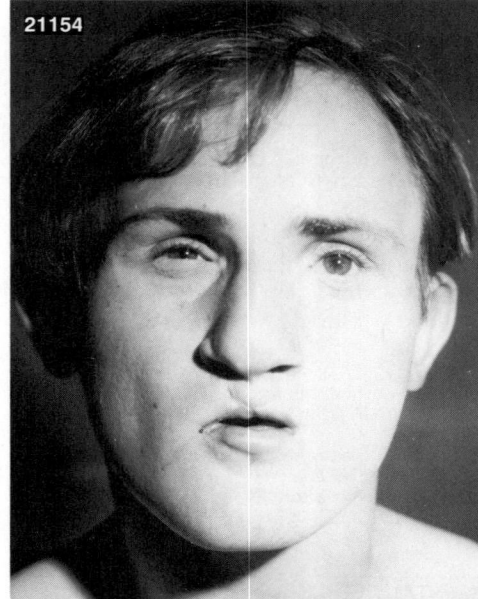

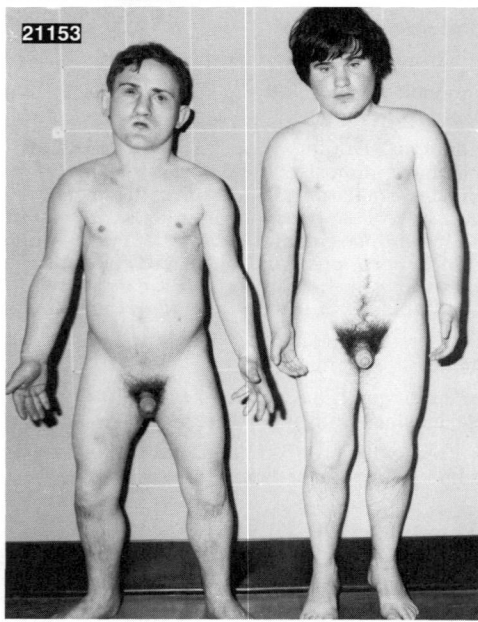

**2176**-21154: Blepharophimosis, small mid-face, prognathism, short philtrum, and small mouth. 21153: Short stature, unusual facies, muscle hypertrophy, and joint limitations.

Soljak MA, et al.: A new syndrome of short stature, joint limitation and muscle hypertrophy. Clin Genet 1983; 23:441–446.

TH017            **T.F. Thurmon**
UR001            **S.A. Ursin**

**Growth/mental retardation-microcephaly-unusual facies-cleft palate**
 See WEAVER-WILLIAMS SYNDROME
**Gruber syndrome**
 See MECKEL SYNDROME
**Gu-dermo-cervico syndrome**
 See CERVICO-DERMO-GU SYNDROME, GOEMINNE TYPE

**Guadalajara camptodactyly**
 See CAMPTODACTYLY SYNDROME, GUADALAJARA TYPE II
**Guadalajara camptodactyly, type I**
 See CAMPTODACTYLY SYNDROME, GUADALAJARA TYPE I
**Guam disease**
 See AMYOTROPHIC LATERAL SCLEROSIS, GUAM TYPE
**Guerin-Stern syndrome**
 See ARTHROGRYPOSES
**Guibaud-Vainsel syndrome**
 See OSTEOPETROSIS, MALIGNANT RECESSIVE
 also RENAL TUBULAR ACIDOSIS-OSTEOPETROSIS SYNDROME
**Gunther disease**
 See PORPHYRIA, ERYTHROPOIETIC
**GUSB deficiency**
 See MUCOPOLYSACCHARIDOSIS VII
**Gustatory sweating**
 See SWEATING, GUSTATORY

## GYNECOMASTIA DUE TO INCREASED AROMATASE ACTIVITY, FAMILIAL  2308

**Includes:**
 Aromatase
 Gynecomastia, early-onset

**Excludes:**
 **Androgen insensitivity (resistance), minimal** (2954)
 **Androgen insensitivity syndrome, incomplete** (0050)
 Gynecomastia-congenital virilizing adrenal hyperplasia
 Gynecomastia, pubertal transient
 Gynecomastia with or without hypogonadism, familial

**Major Diagnostic Criteria:** Slowly progressing gynecomastia occurring at an early age (between 8 and 11 years) concomitantly with pubertal changes, normal male habitus, and an elevated ratio of plasma estradiol-17$\beta$ to testosterone.

**Clinical Findings:** Gynecomastia accompanies male sexual differentiation between ages 8 and 11 years. Whereas the gynecomastia progresses steadily, the pubertal changes advance slowly. The body habitus is otherwise normal male, with normal pubic hair growth and normal testicular and penile size. Bone age is advanced. Thyroid and liver function tests, prolactin and gonadotropin levels, and Leydig cell functions are within normal limits.

**Complications:** Embarrassment due to breast enlargement.

**Associated Findings:** None known.

**Etiology:** Male-limited autosomal dominant inheritance; the phenotype is likely to escape clinical detection in the female.

**Pathogenesis:** Evidence has been provided for increased extraglandular aromatase activity in patients compared with that found in normal men. Aromatase is a cytochrome P450 enzyme which is present in many tissues such as skin, muscle, fat, and nerve; and catalyzes the aromatization of C19 androgens to C18 estrogens. It is induced by follicle-stimulating hormone. The postulated explanations for increased aromatase activity include 1) a mutant regulatory gene resulting in increased transcription of the P450-aromatase gene; 2) decreased catabolism of the enzyme; and 3) a persistence of fetal levels of both aromatase and sulfokinase enzyme activities. Interestingly, the increased estrogen formation in the Sebright Bantam chicken was shown to be due to an abnormal elevation in the level of peripheral aromatase activity.

**MIM No.:** *10791

**CDC No.:** 757.680

**Sex Ratio:** M1:F0 (observed).

**Occurrence:** About a dozen cases reported, including a Black kinship.

**Risk of Recurrence for Patient's Sib:**
 See Part I, *Mendelian Inheritance.*

**Risk of Recurrence for Patient's Child:**
 See Part I, *Mendelian Inheritance.*

**Age of Detectability:** About age 8–11 years, concurrent with male sexual differentiation.

**Gene Mapping and Linkage:** CYP19 (cytochrome P450, subfamily XIX (aromatization of androgens)) has been mapped to 15q21.

**Prevention:** None known. Genetic counseling indicated.

**Treatment:** Indications for surgery of gynecomastia include psychologic and cosmetic reasons. Supportive psychologic management may be needed.

**Prognosis:** Normal life span and intelligence.

**Detection of Carrier:** Unknown.

**Special Considerations:** An increased aromatase activity has been demonstrated in pubic skin fibroblasts from patients with isolated gynecomastia. It is postulated that the resulting elevation of estradiol concentration produces androgen-estrogen imbalance locally, leading to the appearance of gynecomastia.

**References:**

Hemsell DL, et al.: Massive extraglandular aromatization of plasma androstenedione resulting in feminization of a prepubertal boy. J Clin Invest 1977; 60:455–464.

Leshin M, et al.: Increased estrogen formation and aromatase activity in fibroblasts cultured from the skin of chickens with the Henny feathering trait. J Biol Chem 1981; 256:4341–4344.

Berkovitz GD, et al.: Familial gynecomastia with increased extraglandular aromatization of plasma carbon(19)-steroids. J Clin Invest 1985; 75:1763–1769. * †

Whitlock JP, Jr: The regulation of cytochrome P-450 gene expression. Ann Rev Pharm Toxicol 1986; 26:333–369.

Bulard J, et al.: Increased aromatase activity in pubic skin fibroblasts from patients with isolated gynecomastia. J Clin Endocrinol Metab 1987; 64:618–623.

Chen S, et al.: Human aromatase: cDNA cloning. Southern blot analysis and assignment of the gene to chromosome 15. DNA 1988; 7:27–38.

QA000                                                              **Qutub H. Qazi**

**Gynecomastia, early-onset**
*See GYNECOMASTIA DUE TO INCREASED AROMATASE ACTIVITY, FAMILIAL*

---

## GYRATE ATROPHY OF THE CHOROID AND RETINA          0449

**Includes:**
> Choroid, gyrate atrophy
> Hyperornithinemia with gyrate atrophy (HOGA)
> Ornithine-delta-aminotransferase deficiency
> Ornithine ketoacid aminotransferase deficiency
> Ornithinemia with gyrate atrophy of the choroid & retina
> Retina, gyrate atrophy

**Excludes:**
> **Choroideremia** (0925)
> **Hyperornithinemia-hyperammonemia-homocitrullinuria** (3169)
> **Retinitis pigmentosa** (0869)

**Major Diagnostic Criteria:** History of progressive loss of peripheral and night vision; characteristic funduscopic appearance; hyperornithinemia; and deficiency of ornithine-δ-aminotransferase in cultured skin fibroblasts.

**Clinical Findings:** Affected individuals usually are found to be myopic early in childhood and have reduced peripheral vision and problems with night vision early in the second decade of life. Continued reduction of the visual fields leads to tunnel vision and eventually to blindness in the fifth to sixth decade. Most patients develop posterior subcapsular cataracts in the second or third decade. Aside from these visual symptoms and a mild proximal muscle weakness demonstrable in less than 20% of patients, there are no other consistant symptoms.

Central visual acuity is relatively preserved until late in the course of the disease but may be impaired by cataracts. Psychophysical tests of retinal function confirm the irregularly progressive nature of this disorder. The electroretinogram usually is diminished in the first decade and completely extinguished by the second to third decade. The electrooculogram, dark adaptometry and tests of color vision also are progressively impaired.

Despite the lack of symptoms of muscle weakness, most patients have a myopathic electromyogram with short-duration, low amplitude motor unit action potentials in their proximal skeletal muscles. Electroencephalographic exam shows mild slowing in about 1/3 of patients.

Plasma ornithine concentrations are usually about ten-fold elevated (normal is $75 \pm 15 \mu M$) and there are modest but statistically significant reductions in plasma lysine, glutamate and glutamine. The remainder of the plasma amino acids are normal. Ornithine concentration in other body fluids including aqueous humor, cerebrospinal fluid, and urine also is increased about ten-fold. Plasma creatine and creatinine are often subnormal. In contrast to patients with the hyperornithinemia-hyperammonemia-homocitrullinemia, gyrate atrophy patients do not have elevated plasma ammonia concentrations nor do they excrete increased amounts of homocitrulline.

Clinical variability occurs with some patients retaining considerable visual function into the sixth - seventh decades while others have lost nearly all vision by the fourth decade. This variability plus the irregular rate of progression makes prediction of the course of the disease in any particular patient unreliable.

**Complications:** Mild proximal muscle weakness is present in less than 20% of patients. Many also have mild patchy alopecia.

**Associated Findings:** None known.

**Etiology:** Autosomal recessive inheritance. Heterozygotes are asymptomatic, have normal plasma amino acids, and about half normal OAT activity.

The primary biochemical abnormality is deficiency of ornithine-δ- aminotransferase (OAT) with affected individuals havaing <6% of normal OAT activity in cultured skin fibroblasts. In a few patients (<5% of total described), there is both *in vivo* and *in vitro* pyridoxine responsiveness. In these pyridoxine-responsive patients, plasma ornithine values decrease to less than 50% of initial values following institution of pharmacologic doses of pyridoxine-HCl. OAT activity in extracts of fibroblasts from pyridoxine-responsive patients increases to values as high as 30% of control when the concentration of pyridoxal phosphate in the assay is increased from 20 $\mu M$ to 1 mM.

**Pathogenesis:** The OAT-catalyzed reaction is a necessary step in ornithine and arginine catabolism and a block in this pathway accounts for ornithine accumulation. Ornithine is an inhibitor of glycine transaminidase, the enzyme which catalyzes the first step in creatine synthesis, and inhibition at this step probably accounts for the reduced levels of creatine and its precursor, guanidinoacetate. The pathophysiology of the ocular abnormalities is not known.

**MIM No.:** *25887

**Sex Ratio:** M1:F1

**Occurrence:** There are about 150 reported cases, approximately half of which are Finnish, while the remainder come from a wide variety of ethnic backgrounds.

**Risk of Recurrence for Patient's Sib:**
See Part I, *Mendelian Inheritance.*

**Risk of Recurrence for Patient's Child:**
See Part I, *Mendelian Inheritance.* In non-consanguineous matings; probably less than 1:200.

**Age of Detectability:** Deficiency of OAT is detectable in amniotic fluid cells or cultured skin fibroblasts at any age. The hyperornithinemia has been documented in children as early as one year of age, but may not be present in the first few weeks of life. Funduscopic abnormalities have been observed in children examined for the first time between one and two years of age.

**Gene Mapping and Linkage:** OAT (ornithine aminotransferase) has been mapped to 10q26.

**Prevention:** None known. Genetic counseling indicated.

**Treatment:** An initial trial of pharmacologic doses (500 mg/day in adults) of pyridoxine should be performed in all patients for four weeks. There should be no change in dietary protein during this time and a reduction of plasma ornithine by at least 50% indicates a positive result. The long-term consequences of pyridoxine therapy in responders has not been reported. For pyridoxine nonresponders (95% or more of all patients), restriction of dietary arginine (the major precursor of ornithine) reduces the ornithine accumulation and some patients have maintained near normal ornithine levels for several years on this diet. In some of these patients, the rate of chorioretinal degeneration has slowed or stopped, while others have had some progression of their funduscopic abnormalities. Thus, the efficacy of this experimental therapy is still unclear. Treatment with creatine has not prevented deterioration of visual function.

**Prognosis:** Normal lifespan and intelligence with progressive loss of visual function.

**Detection of Carrier:** Carriers have fibroblast OAT activity which averages about 50% of normal.

**Special Considerations:** The OAT gene has been cloned and several different mutant alleles have been discovered. This allelic heterogeneity probably accounts for some of the clinical variability. Diagnosis and carrier detection by direct DNA analysis will soon be possible but must be interpreted with care in view of the high level of allelic heterogeneity.

**References:**

Valle D, et al: Gyrate atrophy of the choroid and retina: amino acid metabolism and correction of hyperornithinemia with an arginine restricted diet. J Clin Invest 1980; 65:371–378.

Valle D, Simell O: The hyperornithinemias. In: Scriver CR, et al, eds: The metabolic basis of inherited disease, 6th ed. New York: McGraw-Hill, 1989:599–628.

Inana G, et al: Molecular cloning of human ornithine aminotransferase mRNA. Proc Natl Acad Sci (USA) 1986; 83:1203–1207.

Kaiser-Kupfer MI, Valle DL: Clinical biochemical and therapeutic aspects of gyrate atrophy. In: Osbourne N, Chader J, eds: Progress in Retinal Research. New York: Pergamon Press, 1987:179–206.

Vannas-Sulonen K, et al: Gyrate atrophy of the choroid and retina: the ocular disease progresses in juvenile patients despite normal or near normal plasma ornithine concentration. Ophthalmol 1987; 94:1428–1433.

Mitchell GA, et al.: An initiator codon mutation in ornithine-δ-aminotransferase causing gyrate atrophy. J Clin Invest 1988; 81:630–633.

Mitchell GA, et al.: Human ornithine-delta-aminotransferase: cDNA cloning and analysis of the structural gene. J Biol Chem 1988; 263:14228–14295.

Mitchell GA, et al.: At least two mutant alleles of ornithine-δ-aminotransferase cause gyrate atrophy of the choroid and retina in Finns. Proc Natl Acad Sci USA 1989; 86:197–201.

VA000
KA046

**David Valle**
**Muriel Kaiser-Kupfer**

# ❖ H ❖

**Haber syndrome (some)**
  *See SKIN CREASES, RETICULATE PIGMENTED FLEXURES,*
  *DOWLING-DEGOS TYPE*
**Haemamoeba vivax malaria**
  *See MALARIA, VIVAX, SUSCEPTIBILITY TO*
**Hageman factor deficiency**
  *See FACTOR XII DEFICIENCY*
**Hailey-Hailey disease**
  *See PEMPHIGUS, BENIGN FAMILIAL*
**Hair (absence)-microcephaly-developmental delay**
  *See ALOPECIA-MENTAL RETARDATION*
**Hair (black)-albinism-deafness**
  *See ALBINISM-BLACK LOCKS-DEAFNESS*
**Hair (silver)-psychomotor and developmental retardation**
  *See NEUROECTODERMAL MELANOLYSOSOMAL SYNDROME*
**Hair and nails, hereditary dystrophy**
  *See ECTODERMAL DYSPLASIA, HIDROTIC*
**Hair defect-photosensitivity-mental retardation**
  *See TRICHOTHIODYSTROPHY*
**Hair defects-cleft lip/palate-oligodontia-syndactyly**
  *See CLEFT LIP/PALATE-OLIGODONTIA-SYNDACTYLY-HAIR*
  *DEFECTS*
**Hair graying-premolar aplasia-hyperhidrosis**
  *See HYPERHIDROSIS-PREMATURE GREYING-PREMOLAR APLASIA*
**Hair(curly)-ankyloblepharon-nail dysplasia syndrome**
  *See CHANDS*
**Hair, 'bamboo'**
  *See ICHTHYOSIS, LINEARIS CIRCUMFLEXA*
**Hair, 'tiger tail'**
  *See TRICHOTHIODYSTROPHY*

## HAIR, ALOPECIA AREATA                    0038

**Includes:**
  Alopecia areata
  Alopecia totalis
  Alopecia universalis
  Ophiasis

**Excludes:**
  **Alopecia** (other forms)
  Scalp, congenital absence of

**Major Diagnostic Criteria:** Presence of circumscribed or extensive areas of complete nonscarring alopecia affecting the scalp, beard, or other hairy skin, including eyebrows or eyelashes.

**Clinical Findings:** Single or multiple, discrete or confluent plaques of asymptomatic, nonscarring alopecia are most commonly seen on the scalp, but hairy skin anywhere may be affected. Occasionally the condition may progress to generalized loss of hair. The majority of cases are mild, however, and normal regrowth usually occurs after a few months, although initial attempts at formation of hair produce fine nonpigmented hairs. Exclamation point hairs are usually seen in variable numbers at the margins of the bald areas. They are distinctive, short, and pigmented, tapering down to atrophic roots. Dystrophic changes in fingernails, usually pitting or longitudinal ridging of the nail plates, are commonly seen. Shedding of the nails rarely occurs

**Complications:** Cataracts rarely have been reported but may be a coincidental finding.

**Associated Findings:** Vitiligo, thyroid disorders and probably atopic dermatitis.

**Etiology:** Unknown.

**Pathogenesis:** Growth of hair is restrained in the growth period (anagen) of the hair cycle, which is characteristic. This can be seen in the shed hairs as tapering, depigmented hair roots. The number of telogen (resting) hairs is also increased, probably as a secondary phenomenon. Characteristic microscopic features are lymphocytic inflammatory infiltration of the connective tissue sheath enveloping affected hair bulbs and atrophic anagen hairs. Lymphocytic involvement, favorable response to corticosteroid therapy, and increased frequency of association with several conditions suggest that allergic, possibly autoimmune, mechanisms may be involved.

**MIM No.:** 10400

**CDC No.:** 757.400

**Sex Ratio:** M1:F1

**Occurrence:** An unpublished epidemiological study in Rochester, MN, disclosed an age specific incidence rate of 17:100,000 per year. Prevalence estimates in a Swedish population are 1:3300 to 1:1000. Estimates in the Rochester, MN, population over a 25-year period were 1%.

**Risk of Recurrence for Patient's Sib:** Studies show a familial incidence of approximately 10% for this disorder and of 20% for alopecia totalis.

**Risk of Recurrence for Patient's Child:** Unknown.

**Age of Detectability:** Anytime after birth but most commonly in the 3rd, 4th, or 5th decades. The average age at onset is 30 years, but 20% of patients are children. Detected by clinical evaluation, which may include gross and microscopic examination of the scalp and hairs.

**Gene Mapping and Linkage:** Unknown.

**Prevention:** None known. Genetic counseling indicated.

**Treatment:** Systemic corticosteroid therapy frequently will cause regrowth of hair but the effects are usually temporary. Intralesional injections of triamcinolone acetonide into affected scalp areas may result in regrowth of hair in stable, limited disease. A wig may aid psychosocial adjustment to the loss of hair.

Approximately 50% of the alopecia totalis patients treated with the topical dinitrochlorobenzene in acetone or ointment base to produce chronic contact dermatitis has permitted regrowth of scalp hair. This is not an easy treatment to carry out and should be done only by dermatologists experienced in this form of treatment. There have been questions raised concerning the long-term risks involved; to date, the author is unaware of any malignant tumors that have been related to this form of treatment. It should not be administered to pregnant women and suitable precautions should be taken by women of childbearing age to avoid conception during treatment.

Recently, reports have indicated that the application of a 1–5%

minoxidil solution has resulted in hair regrowth in individuals with male pattern baldness (See **Hair, baldness, common**). The effectiveness of this drug in the treatment of the present condition has not been confirmed.

**Prognosis:** Normal life span and general health. In mild disease regrowth of hair usually occurs spontaneously within a few months although recurrences are not uncommon. Progression to alopecia totalis is more common among children or when loss of hair is severe or widespread. Estimates of progression to alopecia totalis vary from 5–30% depending on the selection of cases and length of follow-up. Permanent regrowth of hair after the development of alopecia totalis is infrequent.

**Detection of Carrier:** Unknown.

**Special Considerations:** Estimates indicate that the probability of an affected patient having an affected relative is approximately 100 times greater than in the general population. In a few families, however, twins, sibs or consecutive members of 3 generations have been affected. A number of disorders have been related to the onset of alopecia areata, but they are either incidental or nonspecific precipitating factors. These include errors of refraction, foci of infection, psychic trauma and anxiety, physical trauma, or allergic reactions.

**References:**
Van Scott EJ: Morphologic changes in pilosebaceous units and anagen hairs in alopecia areata. J Invest Dermatol 1958; 31:35–43.
Muller SA, Winkelmann RK: Alopecia areata: an evaluation of 736 patients. Arch Dermatol 1963; 88:290–297. * †
Muller SA: Alopecia: syndromes of genetic significance. J Invest Dermatol 1973; 60:475–492. * †
Happle R, Sebulla K: Echternach-Happle E: dinitrochlorobenzene therapy for alopecia areata. Arch Dermatol 1978; 114:1629–1631.
Gilhar A, Krueger GG: Hair growth in scalp grafts from patients with alopecia areata and alopecia universalis grafted onto nude mice. Arch Dermatol 1987; 123:44–50.

MU007                                    **Sigfrid A. Muller**

## HAIR, ATRICHIA CONGENITA                           2346

**Includes:**
    Alopecia, congenital
    Hairlessness
    Hypotrichosis, congenital
**Excludes:**
    Atrichia with papular lesions
    **Hair, alopecia areata** (0038)
    **Hair, hypotrichosis** (3151)

**Major Diagnostic Criteria:** Congenital absence of hair in variable degrees with absence of hair follicles proved histopathologically.

**Clinical Findings:** There is a nonscarring alopecia characterized by an almost total absence of hair on the scalp. Commonly, however, there are scanty, thin, sparse, and hypopigmented hairs in the parietal regions. The eyebrows and eyelashes are also involved, and there is mild eyelid hyperpigmentation. The body hair is also scanty, and there is no development of axillary or pubic hair at pubescence. The microscopic analysis of scalp hair and eyebrows shows a very fine and thin constitution.

**Complications:** Unknown.

**Associated Findings:** None known.

**Etiology:** Both autosomal dominant and recessive inheritances have been described.

**Pathogenesis:** Unknown.

**MIM No.:** *24190

**CDC No.:** 757.400

**Sex Ratio:** M1:F1

**Occurrence:** About 20 kinships have been reported.

**Risk of Recurrence for Patient's Sib:**
    See Part I, *Mendelian Inheritance.*

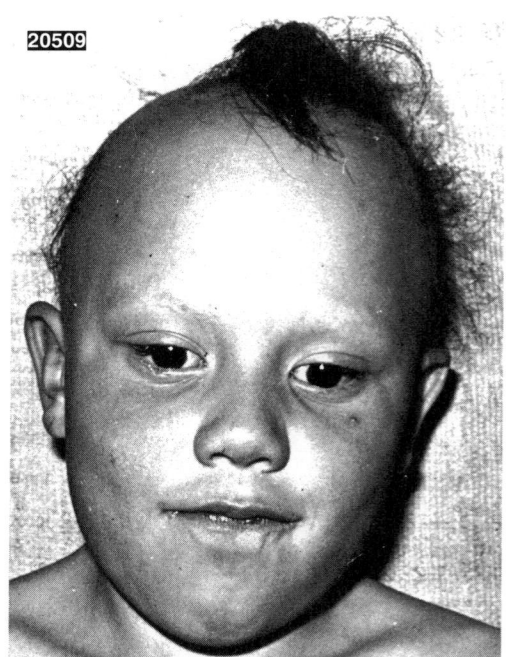

**2346-20509:** Hair, atrichia congenita; note thin, scanty and sparse hair, non-scarring alopecia with scanty eyebrows and eyelashes.

**Risk of Recurrence for Patient's Child:**
    See Part I, *Mendelian Inheritance.*

**Age of Detectability:** At birth.

**Gene Mapping and Linkage:** Unknown.

**Prevention:** None known. Genetic counseling indicated.

**Treatment:** Cosmetic use of wig or hairpieces.

**Prognosis:** Normal life span and health.

**Detection of Carrier:** Unknown.

**References:**
Cantú JM, et al.: Autosomal recessive inheritance of atrichia congenita. Clin Genet 1980; 17:209–212. *

C0064                                    **José Sánchez-Corona**
CA011                                      **José María Cantú**

## HAIR, BALDNESS, COMMON                              0099

**Includes:**
    Alopecia, chronic diffuse
    Alopecia, male or female pattern
    Androgen-genetic regional alopecia
    Androgenetic alopecia
    Hair, loss of
    Male pattern baldness
    Premature alopecia
    Seborrheic alopecia

**Excludes:** **Hair, alopecia areata** (0038)

**Major Diagnostic Criteria:** Chronic or progressive postpubertal loss of scalp hair.

**Clinical Findings:** An M-shaped frontal recession of the hair margin is usually followed by the development of a bald spot on the posterior crown in men. Enlargement and confluence of these bald areas may progress to a final stage at which only a peripheral fringe of scalp hair remains on the temporal and occipital portions of the scalp. Women with masculinizing syndromes or idiopathic hirsutism may have a similar loss of hair. However, common baldness in women is usually quite different clinically, in that alopecia is more diffuse and severe in the frontocentral scalp and only rarely, if ever, progresses to a smooth pate. Seborrhea and tenderness or discomfort of the scalp may be experienced.

**Complications:** Actinic keratosis and epitheliomas of scalp caused by sunlight.

**Associated Findings:** None known.

**Etiology:** Mode of transmission is not certain. It has been thought to be an autosomal dominant inherited trait in males and autosomal recessive in females who are bald only if homozygous. Some reports suggest autosomal dominant inheritance with incomplete penetrance and variable expressivity. Men are more commonly and severely affected than women. Androgens are necessary for phenotypic expression, as is aging.

**Pathogenesis:** It is likely that there is a single pathogenic entity in men and women. Usually the onset is gradual with increased loss of hair and thinning of the frontal and vertical scalp regions. The shed hairs are all telogen (resting) hairs and tend to be short and thinned because the anagen (growth) phase progressively shortens. An ascending obliterative fibrosis of the follicular connective tissue sheaths is seen histologically.

**MIM No.:** *10920

**CDC No.:** 757.480

**Sex Ratio:** Estimated at M1.5–2:F1.

**Occurrence:** Precise data are not available. Current estimates are that at least 50% of men and 25% of women of Caucasian ancestry will be affected. Blacks are less commonly affected, and American Indians and Orientals least of all.

**Risk of Recurrence for Patient's Sib:**
See Part I, *Mendelian Inheritance.*

**Risk of Recurrence for Patient's Child:**
See Part I, *Mendelian Inheritance.*

**Age of Detectability:** Average age at onset in Caucasian men is in the early 20s and in women a decade later. Detection is by clinical evaluation including gross and microscopic examination of the scalp and hairs.

**Gene Mapping and Linkage:** Unknown.

**Prevention:** None known. Genetic counseling indicated.

**Treatment:** Punch or strip autografts of the peripheral unaffected fringe of occipital and temporal scalp may be used to repopulate the bald areas with permanently growing hairs. Scalp reduction with excision of the bald occipital areas to decrease the numbers of punch autografts needed may be indicated. Approval by the Food and Drug Administration has been granted for the use of 2% minoxidil solution (Rogaine^, Upjohn Company) applied to the affected scalp of men. Approximately 40% of more than 1,800 men responded with cosmetically significant terminal hair regrowth during a 12-month study in 27 U.S. study centers. Younger, less severely involved men responded better. Anecdotal reports suggest it may also be useful in affected women. Loss of regrown hairs occurs a few weeks after the medication is stopped.

**Prognosis:** Normal life span, intelligence, and fertility. The end stages of the condition at which only a peripheral fringe of normal scalp hair outlines a bald pate will develop in at least 15% of Caucasian men. Degrees of baldness in women are rarely as severe as those that develop in men.

**Detection of Carrier:** Unknown.

**Special Considerations:** Delayed onset and variable expression make ascertainment difficult to determine. The distinction between normal growth of scalp hair and mild common baldness may be difficult to determine. Also, expression of the disorder will be more apparent in later decades but will merge with loss of hair thought to be unrelated and normal for aged persons.

**References:**
Hamilton JB: Patterned loss of hair in man: types and incidence. Ann NY Acad Sci 1951; 53:708–728. * †

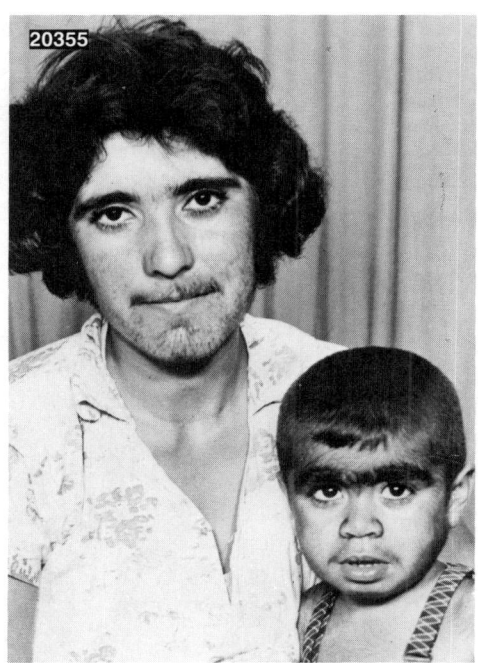

0507A-20355: Mother and son with hypertrichosis lanuginosa. The boy also has dental alterations.

Salamon T: Genetic factors in male pattern alopecia. In: Baccaredda-Boy A, et al., eds: Biopathology of pattern alopecia. New York: Karger, 1968:39–49.
Muller SA: Alopecia: syndromes of genetic significance. J Invest Derm 1973; 60:475–492. * †
Olson EA, et al: Safe response study of topical minoxidil in male-pattern baldness. J Amer Acad Dermatol 1986; 15:30–37.

MU007
**Sigfrid A. Muller**

**Hair, development in utero**
*See RESISTANCE TO 1,25 DIHYDROXY VITAMIN D*
**Hair, excessive-gingival enlargement**
*See GINGIVAL FIBROMATOSIS-HYPERTRICHOSIS*

## HAIR, HYPERTRICHOSIS, LANUGINOSA 0507

**Includes:**
> Edentate hypertrichosis
> Hypertrichosis lanuginosa, congenital
> Hypertrichosis universalis

**Excludes:**
> Acquired hypertrichosis or hirsutism
> **Gingival fibromatosis-hypertrichosis** (0410)
> **Hypertrichosis** (other)
> Localized hypertrichosis
> Senility or metabolic disorders (porphyria, mucopolysaccharidoses)

**Major Diagnostic Criteria:** Generalized hairiness in excess of the amount usually present in persons of the same sex, age, and race.

**Clinical Findings:** Excessive growth of hair on all parts of the body except the palms, soles, and mucous membranes. The teeth may be abnormal, but there are no systemic manifestations of the disorder. The undue hairiness is usually present at birth, and increases during infancy. It may partially resolve during later childhood.

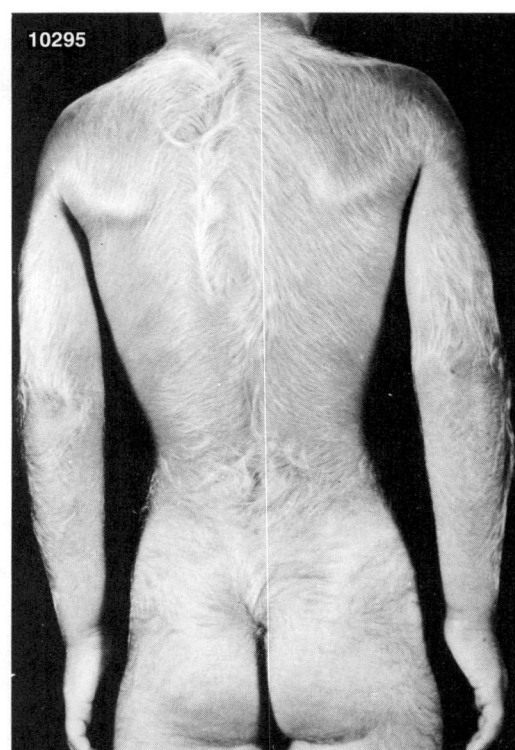

**0507B-10295:** Congenital hypertrichosis universalis.

Burma, his affected daughter Maphoon, and her son Moung Phoset.)

**References:**
Danforth CH: Studies on hair; with special reference to hypertrichosis. Arch Dermatol Syph (Chic.) 1925; 12:380–384.
Felgenhauer WR: Hypertrichosis lanuginosa universalis. J Genet Hum 1969; 17:1–44.
Beighton P: Congenital hypertrichosis lanuginosa. Arch Dermatol 1970; 101:669–672.
Freire-Maia N, et al.: Hypertrichosis lanuginosa in a mother and son. Clin Genet 1976; 10:303–306.

BE008                                                      **Peter Beighton**

---

**HAIR, HYPERTRICHOSIS, X-LINKED**                            **2314**

**Includes:**
   Hypertrichosis, congenital generalized
   Hypertrichosis, X-linked

**Excludes:**
   **Gingival fibromatosis-hypertrichosis (0410)**
   **Hair, hypertrichosis, lanuginosa (0507)**
   Hypertrichosis, acquired (usually endocrine or metabolic)
   Hypertrichosis, localized, sporadic or secondary
   Hypertrichosis, other forms of familial localized
   **Osteochondrodysplasia with hypertrichosis (2332)**

**Major Diagnostic Criteria:** Excessive generalized hairiness present at birth, becoming more dense at the first year of life and persisting through adulthood.

**Clinical Findings:** Excessive hair covering practically all the body, severely affecting the face, external ears, and trunk and more mildly affecting the lower limbs. No hair is found on the palms, soles, and mucous membranes. Females are less severely affected than males and have asymmetric hair distribution.

**Complications:** Psychosocial impact from the physical appearance.

**Associated Findings:** None known.

**Etiology:** Presumably X-linked dominant inheritance.

**Complications:** Psychosocial problems due to the unusual appearance of the patient.

**Associated Findings:** None known.

**Etiology:** Autosomal dominant inheritance. Expression is variable.

**Pathogenesis:** Undetermined. It is possible that the hair follicles are unduly responsive, or that a biosynthetic defect exists in one of the hormones that controls nonsexual hair growth.

**MIM No.:** *14570

**CDC No.:** 757.450

**Sex Ratio:** M1:F1

**Occurrence:** Less than 40 cases in the world literature. Reported in Britain, Europe, United States, Canary Isles, Burma, East Africa, and China.

**Risk of Recurrence for Patient's Sib:**
   See Part I, *Mendelian Inheritance.*

**Risk of Recurrence for Patient's Child:**
   See Part I, *Mendelian Inheritance.*

**Age of Detectability:** At birth.

**Gene Mapping and Linkage:** Unknown.

**Prevention:** None known. Genetic counseling indicated.

**Treatment:** Removal of unsightly hair by shaving or depilatory applications. Camouflage by bleaching or makeup.

**Prognosis:** Normal for life span, intelligence and function.

**Detection of Carrier:** Unknown.

**Special Considerations:** The undue hairiness poses serious cosmetic problems especially to women. Apart from variable abnormalities in the teeth, the condition is harmless. In the past, several affected individuals were well-known circus exhibitionists. (Jo-Jo, the Human Skye Terrier; Shwe-Maong, the dog-faced man of

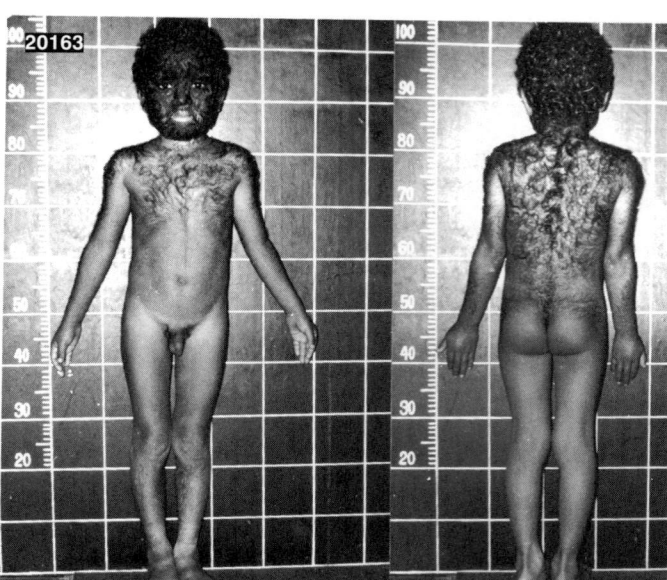

**2314-20163:** Note the pattern and distribution of hypertrichosis with excess hair on the face, trunk and genital region and mildly affected limbs.

**Pathogenesis:** Unknown.

**MIM No.:** 30715

**CDC No.:** 757.450

**Sex Ratio:** M1:F1.5 (observed).

**Occurrence:** Reported in 21 affected members of five generations of one family.

**Risk of Recurrence for Patient's Sib:**
See Part I, *Mendelian Inheritance.*

**Risk of Recurrence for Patient's Child:**
See Part I, *Mendelian Inheritance.*

**Age of Detectability:** At birth.

**Gene Mapping and Linkage:** Unknown.

**Prevention:** None known. Genetic counseling indicated.

**Treatment:** Removal of hair by depilatory applications, shaving, diathermy, or radiation; the use of bleaching or makeup.

**Prognosis:** Normal life span, no functional impairment, and normal intelligence.

**Detection of Carrier:** By observation of asymmetric hypertrichosis in females.

**Special Considerations:** In this severe and uncomplicated form of congenital generalized hypertrichosis, females show a "lionization" effect. Orthodox explanations for this spectacular, though very rare, entity include a simple, forward mutation of a gene with a very low mutation rate and the additive effect of at least two independent mutations. However, an alternative hypothesis of a back mutation awakening a very old "sleeping" gene is feasible, mainly because the excess of hair seems to be the consequence of a gene product surplus rather than a deficiency.

The term atavistic genes refers to those genes producing ancestral phenotypes and whose most probable origin is a retromutation that either switches on a gene already set off for at least one generation or reverts to normal an altered gene and, consequently, its product. Depending on the ancestor, atavistic genes are classified as intraspecies or interspecies. The latter would explain X-linked dominant hypertrichosis. Interspecies atavistic genes do not belong to the active DNA makeup of the species and, therefore, are independent of the functional genome. Other examples are supernumerary nipples, several forms of hypertrichosis, the ability to move the scalp and the ears, and the supracondylar foramen.

**References:**
Macías-Flores MA, et al.: A new form of hypertrichosis inherited as an X-linked dominant trait. Hum Genet 1984; 66:66–70. * †
Cantú JM, Ruiz D: On atavisms and atavistic genes. Ann Genet 1985; 28:133 only. *

CA011
CR019

**José-María Cantú
Diana García-Cruz**

## HAIR, HYPOTRICHOSIS                    3151

**Includes:**
Hypotrichosis, hereditary
Marie Unna type hypotrichosis
Trichodysplasia hereditary

**Excludes:**
**Hair, atrichia congenita** (2346)
Atrichia with papular lesions

**Major Diagnostic Criteria:** Short, sparse hair at birth; development during childhood of coarse, wiry hair; increasing sparseness of hair around time of puberty; absent eyelashes; sparse hair in axillary and pubic areas and in eyebrows in older children; no involvement of other ectodermal structures.

**Clinical Findings:** Scalp hair is sparse or absent at birth. During early childhood, terminal hairs slowly appear which are coarse, large, and irregularly twisted; the hairs are described by Stevanovic (1970) as resembling those of a horse's tail. From the time of puberty, hair becomes more sparse, especially on the vertex and to a greater extent in males. A high frontal and nuchal hairline is characteristic.

Extent of baldness is occasionally total in males and sometimes in females. Degree of alopecia is generally greater in males. Hair density does not exceed 10–60 hairs per cm².

Eyelashes are absent; eyebrows, axillary, and pubic hairs are very sparse. Beard hair in the male is generally sparse unpigmented vellus. Other ectodermal structures are normal. Somatic and sexual development are generally normal.

**Complications:** Unknown.

**Associated Findings:** Milia-like lesions were present in one kindred, described by Solomon et al (1971). These were shown to be follicles with keratin plugs.

**Etiology:** Autosomal dominant inheritance.

**Pathogenesis:** Light microscopic studies show deformity in root sheath of hair follicle and the cuticular layer of the hair. Not all hairs are involved, nor are they involved to same extent. On electron microscopy, intracellular cuticular defect was observed in osmiophilic band proximal to hair cortex. This band is normally rich in disulfide bonds. Question was raised as to whether a deficiency of disulfide bonds in the osmiophilic band leads to its fracture and focal separation within the cuticular cells. Other hypotheses have also been suggested.

**MIM No.:** *14655

**Sex Ratio:** M1:F1

**Occurrence:** A few dozen cases have been documented.

**Risk of Recurrence for Patient's Sib:**
See Part I, *Mendelian Inheritance.*

**Risk of Recurrence for Patient's Child:**
See Part I, *Mendelian Inheritance.*

**Age of Detectability:** At birth.

**Gene Mapping and Linkage:** Unknown.

**Prevention:** None known. Genetic counseling indicated.

**Treatment:** No reliable treatment has been reported.

**Prognosis:** Normal life span. Normal physical and sexual growth.

**Detection of Carrier:** Generally the diagnosis of affected individuals is made clinically. There have been no reports in the literature of skipped generations. Should the clinical diagnosis be in question, electron microscopy of hair shafts have been reported to show characteristic abnormalities, as described above.

**References:**
Unna M: Uber hypotrichosis congenita hereditaria. Derm Wschr 1925; 81:1167–1168.
Stevanovic DV: Hereditary hypotrichosis congenita Marie Unna type. Brit J Derm 1970; 83:331–337. †
Solomon LM, et al.: Hereditary trichodysplasia: Marie Unna's hypotrichosis. J Invest Derm 1971; 57:389–400. * †
Birnbaum PS, Baden HP: Heretable disorders of hair. Dermatol Clin 1987; 5:137–153.

FI031

**Cheryl Nagel Fialkoff**

**Hair, loss of**
*See HAIR, BALDNESS, COMMON*

## HAIR, MONILETHRIX                                              2906

**Includes:**  Monilethrix hair

**Excludes:**
**Aciduria, argininosuccinic** (0087)
**Ichthyosis, linearis circumflexa** (2858)
**Menkes syndrome** (0643)
Pili torti
Pseudomonilethrix
Trichorrhexis nodosa
**Trichothiodystrophy** (2559)

**Major Diagnostic Criteria:**  Appearance of the condition at birth or within first two years of life. Lanugo hair is normal, but regular hair is friable and beaded, characterized by elliptic nodes separated by constricted internodes lacking medulla.

**Clinical Findings:**  Short, friable hair may be present at birth. While the head is usually involved, the rest of the body may also be affected. The involvement may be patchy, involving the frontal area, vertex, or nape of the neck, or the entire scalp and other hairy areas may be affected. The hair is generally quite short and manifests as 5–10-mm long stubble which break off at the internodes. Follicular hyperkeratosis is common. The condition may improve at puberty or during pregnancy or it may remain unchanged throughout life. The nails and teeth are not involved.

**Complications:**  Psychologic difficulty, especially in women who are completely or partially bald.

**Associated Findings:**  None known.

**Etiology:**  Usually autosomal dominant inheritance with variable expression, although extensively affected kindreds have been reported with apparent recessive inheritance.

**Pathogenesis:**  Unknown.

**MIM No.:**  *15800, 25220

**CDC No.:**  757.410

**Sex Ratio:**  M1:F1

**Occurrence:**  Presumably rare, although it has been estimated that as many as twenty percent of families carry a recessive form of this condition.

**Risk of Recurrence for Patient's Sib:**
See Part I, *Mendelian Inheritance.*

**Risk of Recurrence for Patient's Child:**
See Part I, *Mendelian Inheritance.*

**Age of Detectability:**  May be detectable at birth.

**Gene Mapping and Linkage:**  Unknown.

**Prevention:**  None known. Genetic counseling indicated.

**Treatment:**  Emotional counseling as necessary. Retinoic acid and progesterone have been proposed as possible treatments.

**Prognosis:**  Apparently consistent with a normal life span.

**Detection of Carrier:**  By clinical examination.

**References:**
Baker H: An investigation of monilethrix. Br J Dermatol 1962; 74:24–30.
Moschella SL, et al.: Dermatology, ed 2. Philadelphia: W.B. Saunders, 1975:1199–1200. †
Schaap T, et al.: The genetic analysis of monilethrix in a large inbred kindred. Am J Med Genet 1982; 11:469–474. †
Fitzpatrick TB, et al.: Dermatology in general medicine, ed 3. New York: McGraw-Hill, 1987:629–630. * †

H0003                                              **M.E. Hodes**

**Hair, sparse, short, thin and brittle**
*See TRICHOTHIODYSTROPHY*
**Hair, wiry, uncombable, straw-like-palate/lip anomalies**
*See ECTODERMAL DYSPLASIA, RAPP-HODGKIN TYPE*
**Hair, uncombable**
*See HAIR, UNCOMBABLE-CRYSTALLINE CATARACT*

## HAIR, UNCOMBABLE-CRYSTALLINE CATARACT          2558

**Includes:**
Cataract, coralliform-uncombable hair (misnomer)
Cataract, crystalline-uncombable hair
Glaswolle-Haar and crystalline cataract
Hair, uncombable
Pili trianguli et canaliculi
Pili trianguli et canaliculi-crystalline cataract
Spun-glass hair and crystalline cataract
Uncombable hair and crystalline cataract

**Excludes:**
Hair abnormalities, isolated
Kinky hair-crystalline cataract
Pili torti-crystalline cataract
Woolly hair-crystalline cataract

**Major Diagnostic Criteria:**  Dry, blond, shiny hair that sticks out from the scalp in all directions and cannot be combed in combination with crystalline cataract. The diagnosis can be confirmed by scanning electron microscopy of the hair (pili trianguli et canaliculi) and by slit-lamp examination of the lens, respectively.

**Clinical Findings:**  The hair abnormality is noted in early infancy, from the first months of life on. It can be disappointing especially for the mother that the hairs cannot be managed, not even for a short time. The hairs can easily be torn without pain. The condition is limited to the scalp hair and ameliorates spontaneously when the child grows up. If one is not aware of the combination, cataract is not noticed until visual acuity has been diminished. In the only case described, the cataract, diagnosed at age four years, was progressive and had to be operated on when the girl was eight years old.
By slit-lamp examination, the cataracts show accumulations of crystal-like opacities, radiating out from the center of the nucleus towards the capsule. Photophobia can be an accompanying symptom.

**Complications:**  Visual handicap caused by progressive cataract.

**Associated Findings:**  None known.

**Etiology:**  Isolated uncombable hair probably has an autosomal dominant mode of inheritance, as is the case in crystalline cataract. It is unknown in the combination described.

**Pathogenesis:**  Unknown.

**MIM No.:**  *19148

**POS No.:**  4418

**Sex Ratio:**  Presumably M1:F1

**Occurrence:**  One girl with the combined condition, and about 50 cases of uncombable hair alone, have been reported.

**Risk of Recurrence for Patient's Sib:**  Unknown.

**Risk of Recurrence for Patient's Child:**  Unknown.

**Age of Detectability:**  Uncombable hair can be diagnosed as soon as lanugo hairs disappear (from age three months on). Careful ophthalmologic examination to prevent amblyopia by cataract is recommended.

**Gene Mapping and Linkage:**  Unknown.

**Prevention:**  None known. Genetic counseling indicated.

**Treatment:**  In contrast to uncombable hair that ameliorates with time, the cataract is progressive and must be operated on when vision is impaired.

**Prognosis:**  Normal life span, with good vision after cataract extraction and aphakic correction.

**Detection of Carrier:**  Careful ophthalmologic examination to detect the first symptoms of cataract will be helpful in early diagnosis. As long as the possibility of variable expression exists, it seems to be appropriate to investigate the hairs of the elder relatives with a crystalline cataract.

**Special Considerations:**  Since the first publication by Dupré (1973), about 50 cases of uncombable hair has been published. In none of them was a form of cataract mentioned. Crystalline

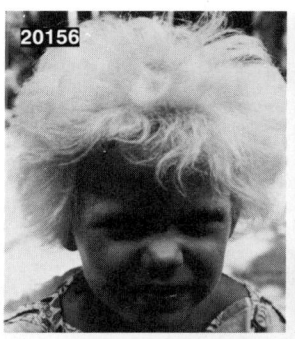
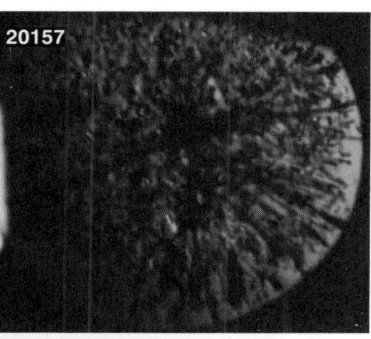
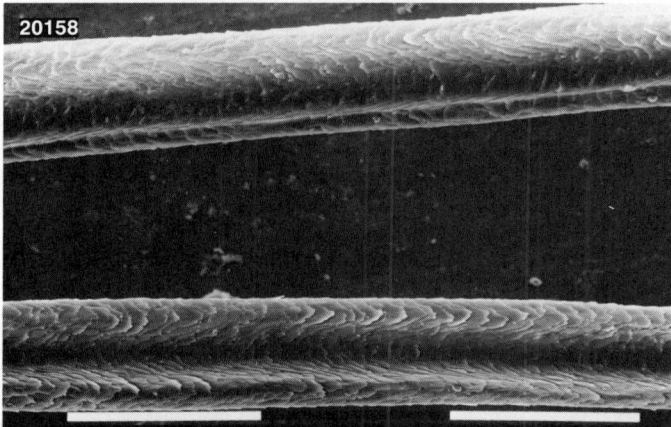
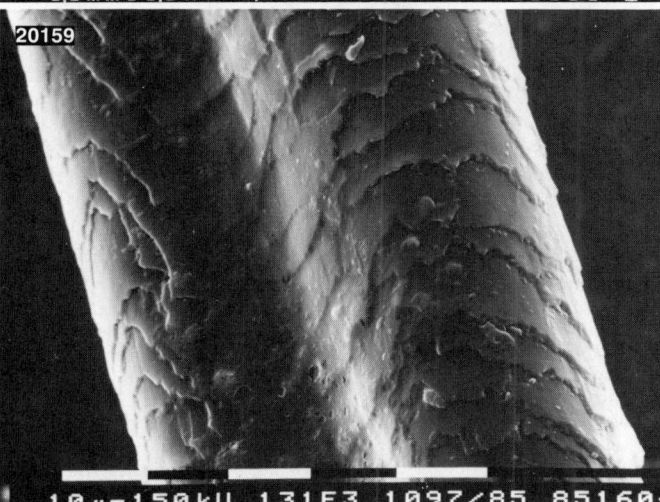

**2558**-20156: Note dry, blond, shiny, uncombable hair that sticks out in all directions from the scalp. 20157: Coralliform cataract. 20158–59: Scanning electron micrograph shows canal-like groove in uncombable hair (pili canaliculi).

cataract mostly occurs in elderly people and is not frequently described. Nevertheless, the possibility of coincidence in this combination exists.

### References:
François J: Congenital cataracts. Assen, The Netherlands: Royal Van Gorcum, 1963.
Dupré A, Bonafé JL: A new type of pilar dysplasia: the uncombable hair syndrome with pili trianguli et canaliculi. Acta Dermatol Res 1978; 261;217–218.
Shelley WB, Shelley ED: Uncombable hair syndrome: observations on response to biotin and occurrence in siblings with ectodermal dysplasia. J Am Acad Dermatol 1985; 13:97–102. †
Bleeker-Wagemakers EM, et al.: Uncombable hair syndrome and coralliform cataract. Berlin: Seventh Int Cong Hum Genet, 1986:240.
Herbert AA, et al.: Uncombable hair: evidence for dominant inheritance with complete penetrance based on scanning electron microscopy. Am J Med Genet 1987; 28:185–193.
Zegpi M, Roa I: The uncombable hair syndrome. Arch Path Lab Med 1987; 111:754–755.

BL021                              **E. M. Bleeker-Wagemakers**

**Hair-bone-nail-tooth dysplasia**
*See TRICHO-DENTO-OSSEOUS SYNDROME*
**Hair-brain syndrome**
*See TRICHOTHIODYSTROPHY*
**Hairlessness**
*See HAIR, ATRICHIA CONGENITA*
**Hairy cyst on head or neck**
*See NECK/HEAD, DERMOID CYST OR TERATOMA*
**Hairy ears**
*See EAR, HAIRY*
**Hairy melanocytic nevus, giant congenital**
*See NEVUS, CONGENITAL NEVOMELANOCYTIC*
**Hairy pinnae**
*See EAR, HAIRY*

---

**HAJDU-CHENEY SYNDROME**                          **2022**

**Includes:**
> Acro-osteolysis-osteoporosis-changes in skull and mandible
> Arthro-dento-osteodysplasia
> Cheney syndrome
> Cranioskeletal dysplasia
> Osteodysplasia with acro-osteolysis, hereditary

**Excludes:**
> **Acro-osteolysis, dominant type** (0021)
> **Acro-osteolysis, neurogenic** (3052)
> Acropathy, neurogenic ulcerative
> **Arthritis, rheumatoid** (2517)
> **De Lange syndrome** (0242)
> **Epidermolysis bullosum**
> Frostbite
> **Hyperparathyroidism, familial** (0499)
> Leprosy
> Mechanical injury, repetitive
> **Mucolipidosis**
> **Mucopolysaccharidosis**
> Osteodystrophy, renal
> **Osteolysis, carpal-tarsal and chronic progressive glomerulopathy** (0128)
> **Osteolysis, essential** (2596)
> Osteolysis, massive of Gorham
> Osteolysis, neurogenic
> **Osteolysis, recessive carpal-tarsal** (0129)
> Polyvinyl chloride polymer injury
> **Progeria** (0825)
> **Pyknodysostosis** (0846)
> **Scleroderma, familial progressive** (2154)
> **Skin, psoriasis vulgaris** (0833)
> Syphilis
> **Syringomyelia** (0924)
> Thermal injury
> **Winchester syndrome** (1000)

**Major Diagnostic Criteria:** Characteristic features include short stature, a dolichocephalic skull with distinctive facies, early loss of teeth, and progressive generalized skeletal dysplasia with prominent acro-osteolysis of the terminal phalanges. Since acro-osteolysis develops later in childhood and is the most distinctive feature, diagnosis has been delayed in most cases. No laboratory studies are available to confirm the diagnosis.

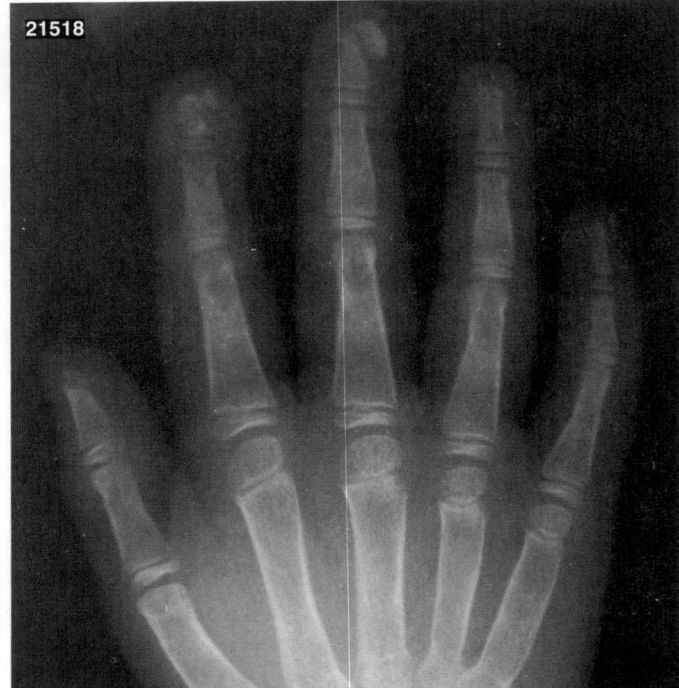

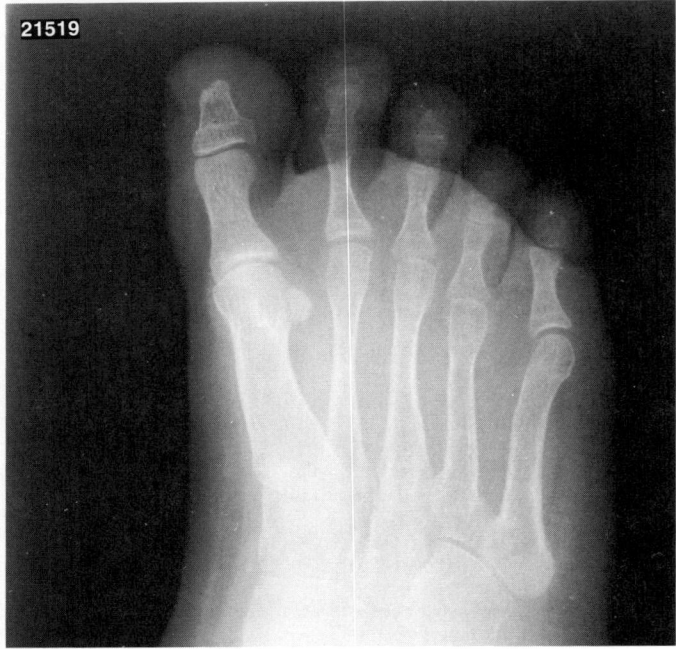

**2022-21518:** X-ray of the hand at age 10⅔ years shows destructive bony changes in the terminal phalanges (acro-osteolysis). 21519: Destructive bony changes in the terminal phalanges of the foot at 16¼ years.

**Clinical Findings:** The skeletal features at birth are not known. By early childhood, abnormalities of skull shape and long bone deformities are seen. There is a prominent occiput, localized posterior fossa thickening, persistent open sutures, and wormian bone formation. The frontal sinus is either absent or very small, and platybasia is seen in most adults. The skull is normal or slightly enlarged. Long bones demonstrate decreased tubulation often with unequal growth leading to bowing or deformity, such as valgus knees or dislocated radial heads. Fractures occur commonly in association with generalized osteoporosis, including vertebral compression. Joint laxity is common. Early loss of teeth commonly occurs. Adult height ranges from 140 to 170 cm.

A distinctive facial appearance is identifiable in childhood: short neck; small, recessed mandible; high-arched palate; dental maleruption and malocclusion; thick eyebrows with synophrys; long eyelashes; coarse hair; and low-set ears. Conductive hearing loss is common, most likely as a result of dysplastic changes of the ossicles. Feeding problems often occur secondary to micrognathia, with a tendency to frequent respiratory infections.

Two abnormal patterns of bone resorption occur, often together: One is a terminal resorption at the distal end of the terminal phalanx, and the other is the development of transverse lytic lesions across the midportion of the affected bone. X-ray periosteal changes are absent. These osteolytic patterns tend to be more severe in the hands than feet and usually start in the more distal bones with progression proximally. Metatarsal and metacarpal changes are uncommon. Pseudoclubbing is often seen as a result of telescoping of soft tissue around the shortened distal phalanx. All laboratory tests, including serum calcium, phosphorus, alkaline phosphatase, and serum proteins, are normal. Autoantibody tests and other indicators of acute or chronic inflammation, such as sedimentation rate and C-reactive protein, are normal. Since acro-osteolysis may also occur as an associated abnormality in connective tissue diseases, metabolic disorders, and vascular compromise, careful clinical assessment is needed. Most patients appear to have a normal life span; however, the original patient reported by Hajdu and Kauntze in 1948 died at age 49 years, 11 years after diagnosis, of progressive increased intracranial pressure secondary to basilar impression.

**Complications:** Short stature results from decreased growth in later life because of vertebral collapse. Generalized osteoporosis predisposes to fractures of the long bones, and dysplastic lesions may cause episodic skeletal pain. Altered skull skeletal growth with closed cranial sutures may lead to neurologic sequelae, such as decreased hearing, visual field defects, nystagmus, and sixth nerve palsy.

**Associated Findings:** *Syndactyly* may be seen rarely early in life, hernia is present in 5–15% of children, and one male developed **Thyrotoxicosis** at age 22 years.

**Etiology:** Possibly autosomal dominant inheritance, although most cases are sporadic.

**Pathogenesis:** Both generalized and striking osteolysis of the distal extremities suggest that there is an accelerated rate of bone removal. Bone matrix is normal, and no abnormalities of bone mineral metabolism have been demonstrated. Electron microscopy of bone and skin collagen is normal, and there is no evidence of mucopolysaccharidosis or endocrine imbalance. Bone biopsy specimens show marked fibrous and angiomatous changes, with some mast cells and many nerve fibers. Osteolysis apparently does not result from increased osteoclast activity, since these cells are essentially absent from most tissue sections. Using the tetracycline-labeling technique, one recent study showed very little new bone-forming activity in diseased areas (phalanges). Very recent histologic studies showed proliferation of mast cells in the hypervascular tissue surrounding bone islets which suggests that mast cells are elaborating local factors such as heparin or prostaglandin $D_2$, which promote osteolysis and reduce bone-forming capacity.

**MIM No.:** *10250

**POS No.:** 3013

**Sex Ratio:** M1:F1

**Occurrence:** About 30 cases have now been reported. Most are from either western or central Europe or the United States.

**Risk of Recurrence for Patient's Sib:**
See Part I, *Mendelian Inheritance.*

**Risk of Recurrence for Patient's Child:**
See Part I, *Mendelian Inheritance.*

**Age of Detectability:** Morphologic and skeletal features develop early and should suggest the diagnosis in childhood. X-ray changes of the skull, vertebral bodies, and long bones become more pronounced with growth, and the development of acro-osteolysis of the distal phalanges, usually after the first decade, is diagnostic.

**Gene Mapping and Linkage:** Unknown.

**Prevention:** None known. Genetic counseling indicated.

**Treatment:** Early vision and auditory assessment, and occupational and physical therapy programs, may forestall developmental delay and promote normal musculoskeletal function. Caloric supplementation early in life may ameliorate the effects of poor feeding and subsequent failure to thrive. Regular neurologic assessment is needed to detect complications as a result of osseous abnormalities.

**Prognosis:** A normal life span in most, although the first patient reported by Hajdu and Kauntze (1948) died 11 years after diagnosis as a result of basilar skull impression. Intelligence is unimpaired. Functional impairment may occur as a result of orthopedic and hand dysfunction or of neurologic complications.

**Detection of Carrier:** Careful clinical examination of all relatives may help to disclose variability in expression.

**Special Considerations:** Hajdu-Cheney syndrome may be more common than is generally thought. Heterogeneity of this syndrome seems to occur, and comprehensive study of all additional cases is essential to determine the prevalence of various features. Thus far, in spite of seemingly characteristic changes, few cases are diagnosed in childhood prior to the development of acro-osteolysis of the distal phalanges. This diagnosis should be considered in infants with unusual facies, joint laxity, and delayed growth and in later childhood with the development of generalized osteoporosis, multiple fractures, early loss of teeth, and acro-osteolysis.

**References:**

Hajdu R, Kauntze R: Cranioskeletal dysplasia. Br J Radiol 1948; 21:42–48.
Brown DM, et al.: The acro-osteolysis syndrome: morphologic and biochemical studies. J Pediatr 1976; 88:573–580.
Weleber RG, Beals RK: Hajdu-Cheney syndrome: report of 2 cases and review of literature. J Pediatr 1976; 88:243–249. *
Elias AN, et al.: Hereditary osteodysplasia with acro-osteolysis (the Hajdu-Cheney syndrome). Am J Med 1978; 65:627–636.
Udell J, et al.: Idiopathic familial acro-osteolysis: histomorphometric study of bone and literature review of the Hajdu-Cheney syndrome. Arthritis Rheum 1986; 29:1032–1038. * †

G0043 / **Donald P. Goldsmith**

**Halcion∧, fetal effects**
*See FETAL BENZODIAZEPINE EFFECTS*
**Hall-Pallister syndrome**
*See HYPOTHALAMIC HAMARTOBLASTOMA SYNDROME, CONGENITAL*
**Hallermann-Streiff syndrome**
*See OCULO-MANDIBULO-FACIAL SYNDROME*

---

**HALLERVORDEN-SPATZ DISEASE**      **2526**

**Includes:**
    Neuroaxonal dystrophy, late-infantile
    Stiff man syndrome (obsolete; pejorative)

**Excludes:**
    **Amyotrophic lateral sclerosis**
    **Ataxia, Friedreich type** (2714)
    Kernicterus
    **Neuroaxonal dystrophy, infantile** (2701)
    Parkinson disease, infantile
    **Torsion dystonia** (0957)

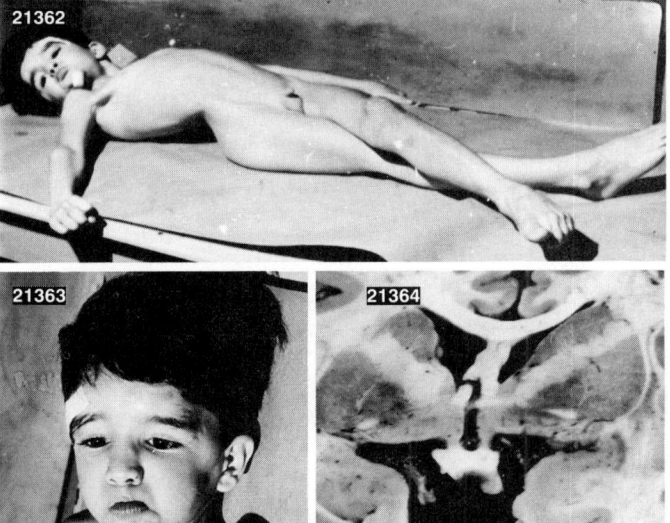

**2526A-21362:** Full body view of affected individual shows severe tonic extension of all the muscles. **21363:** Note the facial grimacing and multiple scars from self-inflicted trauma. **21364:** Coronal section of the brain at the level of the basal ganglia; note the pigmentation of the globus pallidus.

---

**Major Diagnostic Criteria:** Abnormal or absent speech (90%), motor abnormalities (88%), generalized spasticity (88%), rigidity (82%), dystonic feet (74%), mental retardation and deterioration (70%), deformed teeth (70%), hyperkinesis (64%), facial grimacing (44%), abnormal gait (walking on the tips of the toes) (38%), pyramidal signs (34%), dysphagia (26%), muscular atrophy (36%),

---

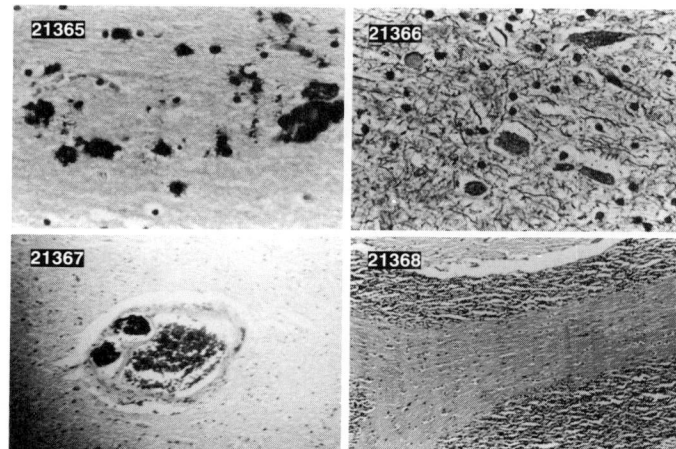

**2526B-21365:** Microscopic section of the globus pallidus illustrates the pigment granules which stain blue when stained for iron. **21366:** Microscopic view (500×) of the globus pallidus, stained according to the method of Bodian shows nerve fibers with partial demyelination, abnormal neurons and spheroids. **21367:** A small vessel from the central nervous system shows two of the accumulations of periodic acid Schiff (PAS) positive material in its wall. **21368:** Microscopic view of the cerebellum shows the reduced number of Purkinje cells.

Torsion dystonia (36%), optic atrophy (22%), nystagmus (16%), Retinitis pigmentosa (16%), behavioral changes (14%), seizures (12%), torticollis (10%), cerebellar signs (10%), skin pigmentation (8%), tremor (6%).

Individuals with these signs should not be considered affected by the syndrome until postmortem examination of the central nervous system is performed. The definitive diagnosis can be established only by demonstrating the histologic lesion in the CNS. Iron isotope scanning of the basal ganglia and MRI scanning are also important in confirming the diagnosis. This precaution is necessary because several conditions could produce similar neurologic symptomatology without having the same lesions.

The following are the histopathologic lesions considered typical of HSD (listed in descending order for the familial cases; the frequency in the sporadic ones is noted in parentheses: pigmentation of the globus pallidus (100%), formation of "spheroids" in the pallidus (90%), excessive pigmentation of the substantia nigra (86%), formation of "spheroids" in the substantia nigra (86%), abnormal Purkinje cells (52%), formation of "spheroids" in other areas, deposits of positive periodic acid-Schiff material in different areas of the brain (23%). The yellow "rusty" pigmentation of the globus pallidus and of the substantia nigra is the most characteristic sign of the condition and can be seen macroscopically during postmortem examinations of the brains of affected individuals.

Clinical Findings: The condition usually begins with dystonia, followed by dysphagia and difficulty speaking. The children become rigid and stiff within the first 2–3 years of the disease. Intellectual performance appears not to be impaired at first, but is limited by the inability of the affected individuals to communicate verbally. They remain bedridden for most of their lives and require special care and attention due to their severe functional limitations. One of the most noticeable manifestations of the condition is dysphagia, which makes it difficult for the affected to be fed by themselves or by others. These problems progress to be so severe that patients require feeding by tube or parenterally.

One of the most striking signs of the condition is facial grimacing, produced by extreme spasticity and contraction of the facial muscles, mainly of the masseters, the peri-buccal, and others in the mid-facial region.

The posture the patients take is characteristic, and is the reason for previously calling this condition "stiff man syndrome" and making it very difficult to care for them. Due to posture, they develop skin ulcers and at times aspirate, developing pneumonia, which is the most common cause of death.

The variation of manifestations within families is small, and usually an affected child looks very much like his or her affected brother or sister. The age of onset within families is very similar. There is a broader variation in the nonfamilial cases.

Complications: *Nutritional,* due to the eating difficulties; *traumatic* due to multiple falls resulting from lack of coordination, leading to fractures and superficial lesions of the skin, mostly in the face, knees, elbows, and ankles; *psychologic,* due to the isolation that these individuals suffer because of their inability to communicate verbally; and *functional,* due to the severe neurologic impairment, including seizures, difficulty in moving the patient, and positional ulcers.

Associated Findings: Reduced muscular mass is probably due to the lack of movements produced by spasticity and rigidity.

Etiology: Autosomal recessive inheritance.

Pathogenesis: Probably an inborn error of the metabolism that shows its effects on the basal ganglia by the "globoid degeneration" of the neurons and by the deposit of the macroscopically recognizable "rusty yellow" pigment in the same area, which is positive for periodic acid-Schiff reaction. This substance accumulates in the basal ganglia, in the arteries of almost all the organs, and in the reduced number of abnormal Purkinje cells.

The error may involve the dopamine-neuromelanin-lipofuscin metabolic pathway. This proposed pathogenetic mechanism is supported by 1) deposit of an iron-rich pigment in the globus pallidus; 2) partial depletion of neuromelanin in the neurons of the substantia nigra; 3) pigmentary abnormalities of the skin; and

4) alteration of the visual function described as Retinitis pigmentosa.

MIM No.: *23420

Sex Ratio: M1:F1

Occurrence: Sixty-four cases reported in the literature. Most of the families (81%) are of European origin.

Risk of Recurrence for Patient's Sib:
See Part I, *Mendelian Inheritance.*

Risk of Recurrence for Patient's Child:
See Part I, *Mendelian Inheritance.*

Age of Detectability: The mean age of onset is 8.3 years (SD 7.1 years). In several families signs of the condition were noticeable by the second year of life. Usually the first sign of the condition is the appearance of involuntary movements.

Gene Mapping and Linkage: Unknown. An allelic relationship with Neuroaxonal dystrophy, infantile (Seitelberger disease) has been proposed by Williamson et al (1982).

Prevention: None known. Genetic counseling indicated.

Treatment: At this time there is no adequate treatment for the condition. When affected individuals have seizures, antiepileptic medication is indicated. Treatment with L-dopa has not led to any improvement.

Prognosis: On average, patients live 11 years after the first sign of the condition is observed. The mean age of death is 19 years. This analysis is based on 54 cases; 41 familial and 13 sporadic. Of these, 28 were males and 26 were females.

All individuals are bedridden a few years after disease onset and remain completely dependent. In addition, they are more likely to develop respiratory tract infections and severe malnutrition due to the characteristics of the condition.

Detection of Carrier: Unknown.

Special Considerations: This condition should be considered in the differential diagnosis of all children who exhibit involuntary movements associated with dysphagia and difficulty speaking.

References:
Wigboldus JM, Bruyn GW: Hallervorden-Spatz disease. In: Vinken PJ, Bruyn GW, eds: Handbook of clinical neurology: diseases of the basal ganglia, Vol 6. Amsterdam: North Holland, 1968:604–631.
Hallervorden J, Spatz H: Eigenartige Erkrankung im extrapyramidalen System mit Besonderer Beteiligung des Globus pallidus und der Substantia nigra. Ein Beitrag zu den Beziehungen zwischen diesen beiden Zentren. Z Gesante Neurol Psychiatry 1976; 79:254–302.
Elejalde BR, et al.: Hallervorden-Spatz disease. Clin Genet 1979; 16:1–18.
Malmstrom-Groth AG, Kristensson K: Neuroaxonal dystrophy in childhood: report of two second cousins with Hallervorden-Spatz disease, and a case of Seitelberger's disease. Acta Paediat Scand 1982; 71:1045–1049.
Williamson K, et al.: Neuroaxonal dystrophy in young adults: a clinicopathological study of two unrelated cases. Ann Neurol 1982; 11:335–343.
Jankovic J, et al.: Late-onset Hallervorden-Spatz disease presenting as familial Parkinsonism. Neurology 1985; 35:227–234.
Schaffert DA, et al.: Magnetic resonance imaging in pathologically proven Hallervorden-Spatz disease. Neurology 1989; 39:440–442.

EL002
EL014
B. Rafael Elejalde
Maria Mercedes de Elejalde

Hallgren syndrome
*See USHER SYNDROME*
Hallux duplication-postaxial polydactyly-absent corpus callosum
*See ACROCALLOSAL SYNDROME, SCHINZEL TYPE*
Hallux-broad thumb syndrome
*See RUBINSTEIN-TAYBI BROAD THUMB-HALLUX SYNDROME*
Halo nevi
*See SKIN, VITILIGO*
Haltia-Santavuori disease (infantile NCL or INCL)
*See NEURONAL CEROID-LIPOFUSCINOSES (NCL)*
Hamartoma and nephroblastomatosis
*See OVERGROWTH-RENAL HAMARTOMA, PERLMAN TYPE*

**Hamartoma of CNS**
  *See CNS NEOPLASMS*
**Hamartoma of liver**
  *See LIVER, HAMARTOMA*
**Hamartoma, venous**
  *See NEVUS, BLUE RUBBER BLEB NEVUS SYNDROME*
**Hamartomatous polyps**
  *See INTESTINAL POLYPOSIS, JUVENILE TYPE*
**Hand and craniofacial anomalies-sensorineural deafness**
  *See CRANIOFACIAL-DEAFNESS-HAND SYNDROME*
**Hand and foot deformity with flat facies**
  *See ACROFACIAL DEFECTS, EMERY-NELSON TYPE*
**Hand malformation-palatal syndrome**
  *See DIGITO-PALATAL SYNDROME, STEVENSON TYPE*

## HAND, LOCKING DIGITS-GROWTH DEFECT     2638

**Includes:**
  Fingers, recurrent locking-growth defect
  Growth defect-locking digits
**Excludes:**
  Psudorheumatoid arthropathy
  **Synovitis, familial hypertrophic** (2155)
  Spondyloepiphyseal dysplasia tarda-progressive
    arthropathy
**Major Diagnostic Criteria:** Intrauterine growth retardation, proportionate short stature, and intermittant locking of the fingers.
**Clinical Findings:** Intrauterine growth retardation is evident at birth. Proportionate short stature is present continuously from birth. Problems with intermittent locking of fingers in flexion at the middle interphalangeal joint begin in early childhood. Initially the locking can be reduced by gentle traction. By age seven the locking becomes nonreduceable and remains for several days until spontaneous reduction occurs, usually during sleep. Metacarpal-phalangeal joints eventually become frozen. Thyroid studies are normal.
**Complications:** Locking of fingers becomes nonreducible. Metacarpal-phalangeal joints become frozen.
**Associated Findings:** The mother of the proband (who was also affected) had an **Atrial septal defect.**
**Etiology:** Presumably autosomal dominant inheritance.
**Pathogenesis:** Unknown.
**CDC No.:** 754.880
**Sex Ratio:** Presumably M1:F1 (both of the known cases have been female).

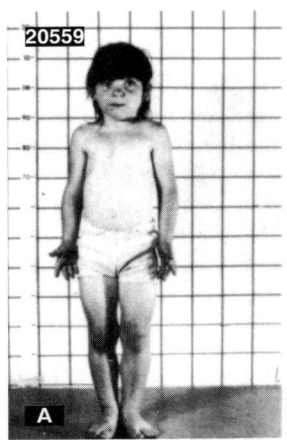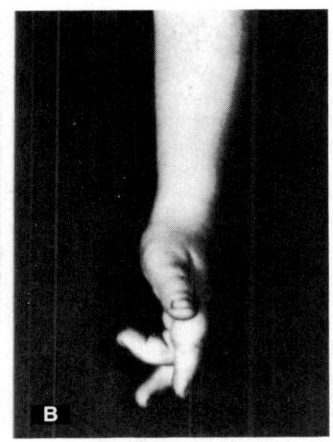

**2638**-20559: Hand, locking digits and growth defect: affected girl age 9 years (A) and left middle finger locked in flexion (B).

**Occurrence:** Two female members of one family have been reported.
**Risk of Recurrence for Patient's Sib:**
  See Part I, *Mendelian Inheritance.*
**Risk of Recurrence for Patient's Child:**
  See Part I, *Mendelian Inheritance.*
**Age of Detectability:** Clinically by 3–5 years of age.
**Gene Mapping and Linkage:** Unknown.
**Prevention:** None known. Genetic counseling indicated.
**Treatment:** Treatment with diazepam has had limited success in hastening reduction of locking of the fingers.
**Prognosis:** Intelligence is normal. Adult stature is approximately 130 cm. Life span is unknown.
**Detection of Carrier:** Unknown.

**References:**
Eng CEL, Strom CM: Familial proportionate short stature, intrauterine growth retardation, and recurrent locking of the fingers. Am J Med Genet 1987; 26:217–220. †

ST038             **Charles M. Strom**

## HAND, RADIAL CLUB HAND     2409

**Includes:**
  Aplasia and hypoplasia of the radius
  Club hand (radial)
  Phocomelia, deficiency of
  Preaxial upper limb deficiency
  Radial deficiency or defect
  Radial dysplasia
  Radial hemimelra
  Radial rays, deficiency of
  Radius, congenital absence of the
  Radius, deficiency of
**Excludes:** **Hand, ulnar drift** (2410)
**Major Diagnostic Criteria:** A short, often bowed forearm with radially deviated wrist.
**Clinical Findings:** A short forearm slightly bowed to radial side. A prominent knob distally represents the end of the ulna. The hand is radially deviated. The thumb, if present, is short or defective. Often, there are flexion contractures of the interphalangeal (IP) joints of the fingers, especially the index and long fingers. Wrist extensors are often absent or nonfunctioning. Hypoplasia or absence of carpal bones, especially scaphoid and trapezium may be noted. Ulna is often bowed; humeral shortening and abnormal elbow motion may be present.
   More often unilateral than bilateral; right side greater than left. In unilateral cases, the thumb on the opposite hand is often found to be hypoplastic or defective to some degree.
**Complications:** Grip strength is decreased due to absent or defective thumb as well as finger IP contractures. Pronation and supination are limited. Elbows often differ in extended position. Aesthetic disadvantages.
**Associated Findings:** **Cleft palate**, clubfoot, **Hydrocephaly**, hernia, kyphosis, sclerosis, hemivertebrae, rib deformity, aplasia or absent lung, and imperforated anus. High incidence of cardiac defects (see **Heart-hand syndrome**. Aplastic anemia (see **Pancytopenia syndrome, Fanconi type**) and platelet defects.
**Etiology:** Ninty percent of cases are sporadic. A portion of the remainder appear to be by autosomal dominant inheritance. Irradiation (see **Fetal radiation syndrome**), viral infections, and chemicals (see **Fetal thalidomide syndrome**) also appear to play a role. The dysplastic factor affects limbs in the first few weeks of fetal life.
**Pathogenesis:** There are four types of radial dysplasia: 1) short distal radius as the result of decreased growth rate of distal epiphysis; 2) hypoplastic radius resulting from defective growth in proximal and distal epiphysis; 3) partial absence of radius, usually

distal ulna; and 4) total absence of the radius. Lack of support for the radius results in radial deviation of the hand and carpus. The greater the carpal deviation, the less effective the forearm musculature. Tendon insertions, nerves, and blood supply may be abnormal.

**MIM No.:** 17910

**CDC No.:** 754.840

**Sex Ratio:** M1:F1

**Occurrence:** 1–3:100,000 live births.

**Risk of Recurrence for Patient's Sib:**
See Part I, *Mendelian Inheritance*. If sporadic, the risk is minimal.

**Risk of Recurrence for Patient's Child:**
See Part I, *Mendelian Inheritance*. If sporadic, the risk is minimal.

**Age of Detectability:** At birth.

**Gene Mapping and Linkage:** Unknown.

**Prevention:** None known. Genetic counseling indicated.

**Treatment:** Stretching casts or splints started soon after birth. Best results if surgery is performed in pre-school years. Surgery includes centralization of carpus over ulna, with soft tissue release and often tendon transfers. Ulnar osteotomy may be indicated if there is significant bowing.

**Prognosis:** If untreated, patients adapt to deformity but have limited function compared to treated patients. Radial drift of hand may recur after surgical treatment. Recentralization as well as ulnar osteotomy may be indicated. If unassociated with syndrome, normal intelligence and normal life span can be anticipated.

**Detection of Carrier:** Unknown.

**References:**
Reedy JJ, Bodner LM: Dominant inheritance of radial hemimelia. J Hered 1953; 44:254–256.
Kelikian, H: Congenital deformities of the hand and forearm. Philadelphia: W.B. Saunders, 1974:780–813.
Temtamy SA, McKusick VA: The genetics of hand malformation. New York: Alan R. Liss, 1978:44–48.
Bora FW, et al.: Radial club deformity. J Bone Joint Surg 1981; 63A:741–745. †
Green DP: Operative hand surgery: congenital hand deformities. New York: Churchill Livingstone, 1982:219–232.
Bora FW Jr: The pediatric upper extremity. Philadelphia: W.B. Saunders, 1986. †
Bayne LG, Klug MS: Long term review of the surgical treatment of radial deficiencies. J Hand Surgery 1987; 12A:169–179.

0S001
G0054

**A. Lee Osterman**
**W. Lea Gorsuch**

---

## HAND, ULNAR AND FIBULAR RAY DEFICIENCY, WEYERS TYPE    2292

**Includes:**
Hydronephrosis-oligodactyly
Oligodactyly-hydronephrosis
Weyers oligodactyly

**Excludes:**
Adactyly
Ectrodactyly (0336)
Ectrodactyly-ectodermal dysplasia-clefting syndrome (0337)
Hypoglossia-hypodactylia (0451)
Mesomelic dysplasia, Langer type (0646)
Micromesomelia
Mesomelic dysplasia, Nievergelt type (0647)
Skeletal dysplasia, boomerang dysplasia (2522)
Skeletal dysplasia, Fuhrmann type (2696)

**Major Diagnostic Criteria:** Oligodactyly involving both the fingers and the toes, deficiency of the ulnar and fibular rays characterized by severe hypoplasia or absence of these bones, and malformations of the kidneys and the spleen.

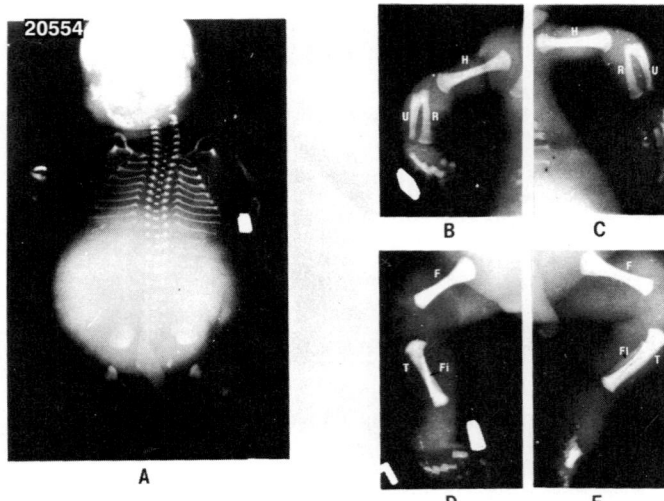

**2292A-20554:** X-ray of a stillborn infant affected by Weyers oligodactyly: A) whole body anterior posterior view; note the hypoplastic lateral vertebral processes, the thin clavicles and ribs, which are also more horizontal than normal. The scapulae are abnormally shaped. B, C) upper limbs; note the marked shortness of the bones, most noticeably the ulna. D,E) lower limbs, the bones are also very short, most markedly the fibulae.

---

**Clinical Findings:** The syndrome in its severe form is characterized by oligohydramnios, bilateral hydronephrosis, severe lung hypoplasia with bell-shaped chest, and intrauterine death. The condition is also compatible with postnatal life. The patients described by Blockey and Lawrie (1963) and by Lausecker (1954) survived at least to late childhood.

In addition to the major diagnostic criteria described by Weyers (1957), other associated malformations include antecubital pterygia, reduced sternal segments, cleft lip and palate, dental malformations, maxillary hypoplasia and a hypoplastic acromial end of the clavicle. In one case there were only two fingers on each hand, and in another there were two fingers on one hand and one on the other.

**Complications:** Depend upon the severity of disease and the time of its manifestations. Fetuses that are severely affected do not survive because severe renal damage impedes the formation of urine, producing all the complications of oligohydramnios for the fetus and for the management of the pregnancy. The most common of these complications are 1) severe pulmonary hypoplasia and, consequently, respiratory distress syndrome; 2) severe neonatal asphyxia incompatible with resuscitation at birth. Other complications arise from the malformations of the extremities and the functional limitation that results. Minor malformations of the urinary tract may be associated with infections and hydronephrosis after birth.

**Associated Findings:** Oligohydramnios, neonatal asphyxia.

**Etiology:** Probably autosomal recessive inheritance.

**Pathogenesis:** Impaired skeletal development of the fetus, which is most noticeable in the long bones but which also affects the spine, ribs, and membranous bones to a lesser degree. The same defect impairs the development of the kidney and the ureters, producing multicystic kidney disease and hydronephrosis. The most dramatic effect is severe interference with normal development of the ulna and the fibula, which are extremely short; shorter than the radius and the tibia. The selective impairment of the growth of these bones is peculiar and is probably related to the abnormal development of the fingers, which may be completely absent or severely hypoplastic.

2292B-20555: Ultrasonographic images of a fetus affected by Weyers oligodactyly. The picture marked 1 is the same as the one marked 2, but has the different structures labelled according to the following code: H, humerus; E, elbow; R, radius; U, ulna; W, wrist; M, metacarpal; F, finger; K, knee; T, tibia; A, ankle; F, fibula. A) shows the left arm, B) the right forearm, C) the left forearm; note the marked smallness of the ulna compared with the radius, which is also smaller than normal, D) the entire upper limb; note the shortness of the arm and forearm when compared with the hand. E,F) shows the right and the left legs; note the marked shortness of the fibula compared with the tibia, which is also shorter than normal.

The most likely explanation for the renal abnormalities is the obstruction of the ureters or of the collecting system in the early development of the fetus, resulting in a dysplastic kidney, multicystic kidneys, or hydronephrotic kidneys.

In his original report, Weyers (1957) described a strain of mice that showed manifestations similar to those of this syndrome.

**CDC No.:** 755.440, 755.510

**Sex Ratio:** M1:F1

**Occurrence:** Five cases have been reported. All malformations of the ulnar ray are rare, 1:100,000 in the Danish population, and only a fraction of those may have Weyers oligodactyly. It is likely that a very mild form of oligodactyly with mild shortening of the long bones, especially the ulna and the fibula, and minor renal abnormalities represent manifestations of the same condition that are not diagnosed.

**Risk of Recurrence for Patient's Sib:**
See Part I, *Mendelian Inheritance.*

**Risk of Recurrence for Patient's Child:**
See Part I, *Mendelian Inheritance.*

**Age of Detectability:** As early as the nineteenth week of gestation in utero by sonography. The fetal fingers can be counted at the twelfth week of gestation and the toes by the twentieth week. Hydronephrosis and multicystic kidneys can be seen as early as the sixteenth week of gestation. Other findings include generalized shortening of the long bones, below the third percentile. The shortening is most noticeable in the ulna and fibula, which are shorter than the radius and the tibia. The same fetus may have normal transverse growth of the skull and chest and an abnormally large abdomen because of severe hydronephrosis. The extremities are short and thick and their range of movement severely limited.

**Gene Mapping and Linkage:** Unknown.

**Prevention:** None known. Genetic counseling indicated.

**Treatment:** If the renal problems are due to obstruction and there is enough renal tissue to save, plastic reconstruction of the ureters may improve the prognosis. Kidney transplantation may also be indicated in rare instances.

**Prognosis:** In the presence of severe manifestation of the condition in utero, chances of survival are remote. The infant may die in utero or in the immediate neonatal period. For those free of severe renal malformations, the prognosis is good and compatible with a normal life span.

**Detection of Carrier:** Unknown.

**References:**

Lausecker H: Der angeborene defekt der Ulna. Virchows Arch Anat 1954; 325:211–226.
Weyers H: Das olygodactylie syndrom des menschen und seine parrallelmutation bei der hausmaus. Ann Pediatr 1957; 189:351–370.
Blockey NJ, Lawrie JH: An unusual symmetrical distal limb deformity in siblings. J Bone Joint Surg 1963; 45B:745–747.
Elejalde BR, et al.: Prenatal diagnosis of Weyers syndrome (deficient ulnar and fibular rays with bilateral hydronephrosis). Am J Med Genet 1985; 21:439–444.

EL014                      **Maria Mercedes de Elejalde**
EL002                          **B. Rafael Elejalde**

## HAND, ULNAR DRIFT           2410

**Includes:**

> Deviation on coup de vent
> Digito-talar dysmorphism
> Digits, congenital contractures of the
> Ulnar drift, congenital
> Wind blown hand
> Wind-mill vain hand

**Excludes:**

> **Arthritis, rheumatoid** (2517)
> **Arthrogryposes** (0088)
> **Arthrogryposis, amyoplasia type** (2281)
> **Contracture, Dupuytren** (0301)

**Major Diagnostic Criteria:** All fingers and sometimes the thumb are deviated toward ulnar border of hand. Not associated with bony deformity.

**Clinical Findings:** Ulnar drift of fingers, which increases as the child matures. Flexion contractures at metacarpal-phalangeal (MP) joints. There is often webbing of thumb to palm by a soft tissue bridge. Usually bilateral. May have decreased muscle mass and limited mobility of shoulders and forearm. Extensor tendons dislocated toward ulnar side at metacarpal heads. Ulnar dislocation of the extensor tendons at the metacarpal joints may be noted.

**Complications:** Most limiting disability due to thumb-in-palm deformity. There may also be limited pronation and supination of the forearm.

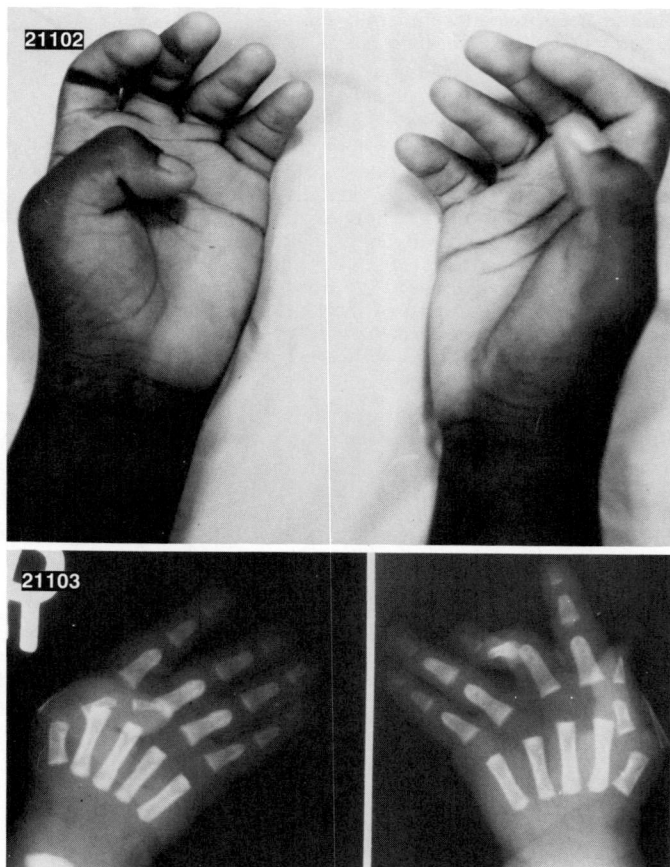

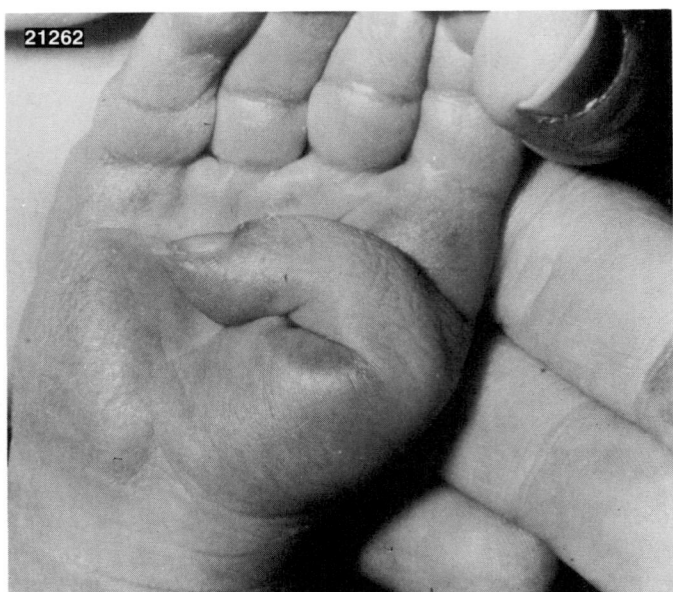

**2410B**-21262:  Ulnar deviation of the hand and pterygia.

**2410A**-21102:  Adult hand showing contractures and clasped thumb.  21103:  X-ray of neonate with ulnar drift of the digits, right thumb clasped into palm, and contracture of the left third digit.

**Associated Findings:**  Cranial facial malformation (see **Craniocarpo-tarsal dysplasia, whistling face type**). Foot deformities include vertical talus, clubfoot, rocker-bottom foot, and tightly constricted toes. There is frequently asymmetry of the chest and shoulders with scoliosis. Minor manifestations may present in the form of **Camptodactyly**, hammer toes.

**Etiology:**  Usually autosomal dominant inheritance with variable expressivity.

**Pathogenesis:**  Theories include 1) collagen deficiency which affects capsules of small joints of hands and feet; 2) abnormality of flexor, extensor mechanisms; and 3) Absence of the lateral portion of extensor tendon expansion.

**MIM No.:**  *12605

**CDC No.:**  754.880

**Sex Ratio:**  M1:F1

**Occurrence:**  Over 75 cases have been documented in the literature, including a large American black family (Stevenson, 1975).

**Risk of Recurrence for Patient's Sib:**
See Part I, *Mendelian Inheritance.*

**Risk of Recurrence for Patient's Child:**
See Part I, *Mendelian Inheritance.*

**Age of Detectability:**  At birth.

**Gene Mapping and Linkage:**  Unknown.

**Prevention:**  None known. Genetic counseling indicated.

**Treatment:**  Splinting initially within the first two years of life. Surgery is needed to release the thumb web contracture, and for flexor pollicis longus (FPL) lengthening, release of thumb intrinsics, MP flexion contracture and intrinsic release, and centralize extensor tendons. Over age four, metacarpal osteotomies are often needed.

**Prognosis:**  Normal life span and intelligence. Progressive hand deformity if untreated.

**Detection of Carrier:**  Unknown.

**References:**

Sallis JT, Beighton P: Dominantly inherited digitotalar dysmorphism. J Bone Joint Surg 1972; 54B:509–515.
Kelikian H: Congenital deformities of the hand and forearm. Philadelphia: W.B. Saunders, 1974:577–583.
Stevenson RE, et al.: Dominantly inherited ulnar drift. BD:OAS XI(5). New York: March of Dimes Birth Defects Foundation, 1975:75–77.
Powers RC, Ledbeller RH Jr: Congenital flexion and ulnar deviation of the metacarpophalangeal joints of the hand: a case report. Clin Orthop 1976; 116:173–175. *
Temtamy SA, McKusick VA: The genetics of hand malformation. New York: alan R. Liss, 1978:447–451.
Green DP: Operative hand surgery: congenital hand deformities. New York: Churchill Livingstone, 1982:346–351. *
Dhaliwal AS, Myers, TL: Digitotalar dysmorphism. Orthopaedic Rev 1985; 14:90–94.

OS001
G0054

**A. Lee Osterman**
**W. Lea Gorsuch**

---

**HAND-FOOT-GENITAL SYNDROME**     **2570**

**Includes:**  Hand-foot-uterus syndrome

**Excludes:**
   **Mullerian aplasia** (0682)
   **MURCS association** (2406)
   **Vaginal atresia** (0984)

**Major Diagnostic Criteria:**  An association of hand and foot abnormalities together with various genital abnormalities that include bifid uterus, septate vagina, double uterus and double cervix in the female, and hypospadias in the male. The most typical X-ray changes are the characteristic degree of shortening of

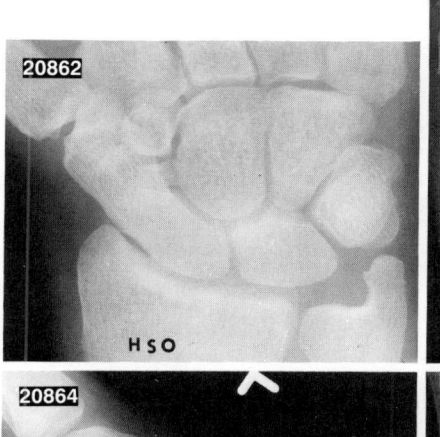
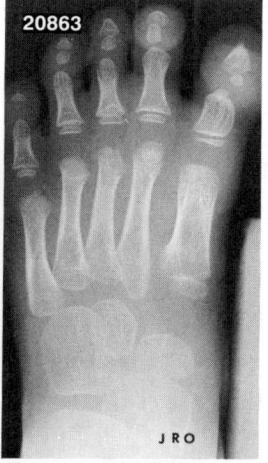
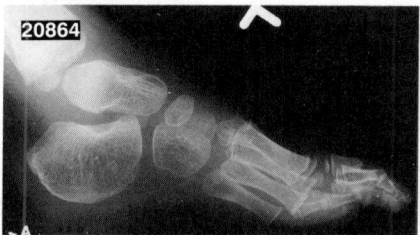
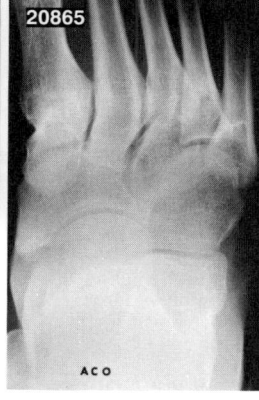

(20/26), fusion of cuneiforms to other tarsal bones (9/22), and delay in appearance of maturation of the medial intermediate cuneiform (12/12). The most characteristic findings are the carpal fusions, particularly trapezium scaphoid, and tarsal fusions involving the cuneiforms. Also, when a pattern profile is obtained, characteristic alterations in pattern are noted (Poznanski et al, 1975).

**Complications:** This is a relatively benign disorder with few complications. The major complications can occur because of the genital abnormalities. One child had a urinary infection associated with the abnormal insertion of the ureters.

**Associated Findings:** None known.

**Etiology:** Autosomal dominant inheritance, with some variability in expression seen in the first two families reported. The family reported by Giedion and Prader (1976) had three affected sibs with no definite abnormalities seen in the parents.

**Pathogenesis:** Unknown.

**MIM No.:** *14000

**POS No.:** 3237

**Sex Ratio:** M1:F1

**Occurrence:** Four kindreds have been reported.

**Risk of Recurrence for Patient's Sib:**
See Part I, *Mendelian Inheritance.*

**Risk of Recurrence for Patient's Child:**
See Part I, *Mendelian Inheritance.*

**Age of Detectability:** Usually during early childhood. One case may have been present in a neonate.

**Gene Mapping and Linkage:** Unknown.

**Prevention:** None known. Genetic counseling indicated.

**Treatment:** May require treatment for genitourinary abnormalities.

**Prognosis:** Normal life span and intelligence.

**Detection of Carrier:** Unknown.

**References:**
Poznanski AK, et al.: Radiographic findings in the hand-foot-uterus syndrome (HFUS). Radiology 1970; 95:129–134. * †
Stern AM, et al.: The hand-foot-uterus syndrome: a new hereditary disorder characterized by hand and foot dysplasia, dermatoglyphic abnormalities, and partial duplication of the female genital tract. J Pediatr 1970; 77:109–116. * †
Pinsky L: A community of human malformation syndromes involving the Mullerian ducts, distal extremities, urinary tract, and ears. Teratology 1973; 9:65–80.
Poznanski AK, et al.: A new family with the hand-foot-genital syndrome: a wider spectrum of the hand-foot-uterus syndrome. BD:OAS XI(4). New York: March of Dimes Birth Defects Foundation, 1975:127–135. †
Giedion A, Prader A: Hand-foot-uterus-(HFU) syndrome with hypospadias: the hand-foot-genital (HFG)-syndrome. Pediatr Radiol 1976; 4:96–102. * †
Elias S, et al.: The hand-foot-uterus syndrome: a rare autosomal dominant disorder. Fertil Steril 1978; 29:239–240.
Halal F: The hand-foot-genital syndrome: family report and update. Am J Med Genet 1988; 30:793–803. †

P0015                                        **Andrew K. Poznanski**

**Hand-foot-uterus syndrome**
  *See HAND-FOOT-GENITAL SYNDROME*
**Hand-heart syndrome**
  *See HEART-HAND SYNDROME*
**Handless and footless families of Brazil**
  *See ACHEIROPODY*
**Handmann disk anomaly**
  *See OPTIC DISC, MORNING GLORY ANOMALY*
**Hands, muscle wasting-sensorineural deafness**
  *See MUSCLE WASTING OF HANDS-SENSORINEURAL DEAFNESS*
**Hands, absent fingerprints**
  *See FINGERPRINTS, ABSENT*
**Hands, collagenous plaques of**
  *See ACROKERATOELASTOIDOSIS*

**2570-20862:** Hand-foot-uterus syndrome in an adult; the trapezium and scaphoid are fused. An os centrale is present. The ulnar styloid is very prominent. The appearance is typical of affected adults. **20863–64:** AP and lateral view of the foot of an affected 4-year-old boy; the calcaneus is very short and the medial and intermediate cuneiforms are not yet ossified. The distal phalanges of the toes are pointed, and the great toe lacks a tuft. There is a pseudoepiphysis in the proximal portion of the great toe, and the first metatarsal is short. **20865:** This affected adult shows fusion of the medial cuneiform to the first metatarsal and of the intermediate cuneiform to the second metatarsal.

---

the bones of the hand, which is seen on pattern profile analysis, and carpal, tarsal coalitions.

**Clinical Findings:** Relatively mild, and include a somewhat short thumb with a hypoplastic thenar eminence, a short fifth finger with clinodactyly, and small feet with occasional shortening of the great toe. A variety of uterine and genitourinary abnormalities are seen, including duplications of the genital tract. In one patient there was abnormal insertion of the ureter into the bladder without evidence of duplication. The hypospadias seen in males is usually glandular in type.

X-ray changes include a short first metacarpal (22/26), pointed distal phalanx of the thumb (13/26), pseudoepiphysis or notch of the first metacarpal (15/16), short middle phalanx of the fifth finger (24/26), clinodactyly of the fifth finger (22/26), pseudoepiphysis of the middle phalanx of the fifth finger (14/16), abnormally shaped scaphoid (14/20), trapezium scaphoid fusion (6/18), os centrale (4/18), relatively late trapezium and trapezoid (14/14), a short first metatarsal (15/26), a short and tuftless distal phalanx (20/26), pseudoepiphysis of the proximal phalanx (11/26), short and proximal phalanx (12/22), abnormal scaphoid (11/22), short calcaneus

**Hands, dystonic movements-mental retardation, X-linked**
*See X-LINKED MENTAL RETARDATION-DYSTONIC MOVEMENTS OF THE HANDS*
**Hanhart dwarfism**
*See DWARFISM, PANHYPOPITUITARY*
**Hanhart syndrome**
*See HYPOGLOSSIA-HYPODACTYLIA*
**Hapnes-Boman-Skeie syndrome**
*See ANGIOLIPOMATOSIS*
**Happy puppet syndrome (obsolete, pejorative)**
*See ANGELMAN SYNDROME*
**Hapsburg jaw**
*See MANDIBULAR PROGNATHISM*

## HAPTOGLOBIN 0452

**Includes:**

Hemoglobin-binding alpha globulins
Hemoglobin-binding beta globulins

**Excludes:** Heme-binding protein (hemopexin)

**Major Diagnostic Criteria:** Measurement of hemoglobin-binding capacity and electrophoretic determination of phenotype.

**Clinical Findings:** Haptoglobin (Hp) levels in plasma (expressed as the hemoglobin-binding capacity) normally vary over a wide range of about 30–180 dl although the level is fairly constant in any given healthy individual. Men have generally higher levels than women, and this may be due to a hormonal effect. Newborn infants usually have little or no demonstrable haptoglobin and adult levels are reached at about one year. In conditions associated with inflammatory reactions, neoplasia, or severe stress, the Hp level is usually increased, sometimes exceeding 1,000 dl. Conversely, in hemolytic states, Hp is either decreased or absent, unless the hemolysis is entirely extravascular. Hp is also decreased in severe liver disease, presumably because synthesis of Hp occurs in that organ. Measurements of Hp are of some value in following the course of liver disease and in determining the presence of increased intravascular hemolysis. However, hypohaptoglobinemia can occur in apparently normal subjects, including about 1% of White subjects, 10% of Black children, and about 4% of Black adults; therefore, decreased or absent Hp must be evaluated with caution.

The common electrophoretic phenotypes are Hp1S, Hp1F, Hp2, Hp2-1F, Hp2–1S, and Hp 1S-1F, representing homo- and heterozygosity for three codominant alleles, Hp$^{1F}$, Hp$^{1S}$, and Hp$^2$. Although there is considerable heterogeneity in the geographic distribution of these genes, there is no convincing evidence available for an association between Hp genetic type and disease.

**Complications:** Unknown.

**Associated Findings:** None known.

**Etiology:** Autosomal dominant inheritance of each allele.

**Pathogenesis:** Unknown.

**MIM No.:** *14010, 14020

**Sex Ratio:** M1:F1

**Occurrence:** Unknown.

**Risk of Recurrence for Patient's Sib:**
See Part I, *Mendelian Inheritance.*

**Risk of Recurrence for Patient's Child:**
See Part I, *Mendelian Inheritance.*

**Age of Detectability:** In infancy.

**Gene Mapping and Linkage:** HP (haptoglobin) has been mapped to 16q22.1.

**Prevention:** None known. Genetic counseling indicated.

**Treatment:** Unknown.

**Prognosis:** Normal life span.

**Detection of Carrier:** The haptoglobin phenotype is determined by performing electrophoresis in starch gel or acrylamide gel on serum to which hemoglobin has been added in excess of the binding capacity. The three common types have a characteristic appearance. About 10% of Blacks have a quantitatively altered Hp

2–1 type called Hp 2–1 (Mod), in which there is a shift in concentration of Hp 2–1 components toward the fastest moving bands. The inheritance of this phenotype is consistent with the existence of a third allele, Hp$^{2M}$. However, the possibility of a genetic event such as regulator gene mutation cannot be entirely ruled out.

**References:**
Giblett ER: Genetic markers in human blood. Oxford: Blackwell Scientific, 1969.
Kurosky A, et al.: Covalent structure of human haptoglobin: a serum protease homolog. Proc Natl Acad Sci 1980; 77:3388–3392.
Yang F, et al.: Identification and characterization of human haptoglobin cDNA. Proc Natl Acad Sci 1983; 80:5875–5879.
Maeda N, et al.: Duplication within the haptoglobin Hp2 gene. Nature 1984; 309:131–135.
McGill JR, et al.: Localization of the haptoglobin α and β genes (HPA and HPB) to human chromosome 16q22 by in situ hybridization. Cytogenet Cell Genet 1984; 38:155–157.
Maeda N, Smithies O: The evolution of multigene families: human haptoglobin genes. Annu Rev Genet 1986; 20:81–108.

B0037 **Barbara Bowman**

**HARD +/-E syndrome**
*See WALKER-WARBURG SYNDROME*
**Hard of hearing**
*See DEAFNESS*
**Hard syndrome**
*See WALKER-WARBURG SYNDROME*
**Harderoporphyria**
*See PORPHYRIA, COPROPORPHYRIA*
**Harelip**
*See CLEFT LIP*
**Harlequin fetus ichthyosis**
*See ICHTHYOSIS, HARLEQUIN FETUS*
**Harrington syndrome**
*See IMMUNODEFICIENCY, THYMIC AGENESIS*

## HARTNUP DISORDER 0453

**Includes:** Behavioral disturbance, reversible

**Excludes:** Pellagra

**Major Diagnostic Criteria:** Affected persons are usually asymptomatic, but may have mental or behavioral disturbances. A specific hyper-α-aminoaciduria, involving neutral and ring-structured amino acids occurs. Excluded are dicarboxylic and dibasic amino acids, the imino acids, and glycine. Excessive neutral amino acids are also found in the feces. For another form of the trait, the intestinal defect is absent (presumably because of a different allele). A third form (putative) has normal renal and mutant intestinal transport.

**Clinical Findings:** May be asymptomatic. Usually discovered by urine screening of healthy newborns or in patients with intermittent psychiatric disorder, or mild mental retardation. Photosensitivity of exposed areas of skin occurs after sufficient UV dosage. Intermittent clinical manifestation is characteristic. Conditioning factors, if they exist, have not been fully clarified, but marginal nutrition is suspected to be important in precipitating symptoms. Impaired nicotinic acid nutrition is implicated.

Plasma levels of tryptophan metabolites are slightly depressed. The same amino acids are affected by the intestinal and renal tubular transport defects.

**Complications:** Pellagra-like symptoms related to impaired endogenous synthesis of nicotinic acid, under marginal nutritional intake. Intermittent and reversible "psychosis" may occur.

**Associated Findings:** None known.

**Etiology:** Autosomal recessive inheritance. Unlike PKU, maternal Hartnup disorder has no ill effects on the fetus.

**Pathogenesis:** Deficiency of a group-specific membrane-transport system for certain aliphatic and ring-structured neutral α-amino acids. Transport of oligopeptides involving the same amino acids is normal.

Biochemical characteristics include specific hyper-α-aminoaciduria (it excludes the dibasic amino acids, the dicarboxylic amino acids, the imino acids, and glycine); and a high clearance (renal) mechanism for the aminoaciduria. Urine also contains excessive amounts of tryptophan derivatives, such as indoxyl sulfate, indole-3-acetic acid, and indolylacetyl glutamine, which are of intestinal origin, secondary to impaired intestinal absorption of tryptophan, and can be suppressed with neomycin.

**MIM No.:** *23450

**Sex Ratio:** M1:Fl (approximate).

**Occurrence:** About 1:14,500 live births (Massachusetts survey). Since many cases are asymptomatic, the "disease" prevalence is lower than the "trait" occurrence. The symptomatic trait occurs worldwide, but it is infrequently found in North America, where the high standard of nutrition may offset features that are likely to precipitate symptoms.

**Risk of Recurrence for Patient's Sib:**
See Part I, *Mendelian Inheritance.*

**Risk of Recurrence for Patient's Child:**
See Part I, *Mendelian Inheritance.*

**Age of Detectability:** At birth.

**Gene Mapping and Linkage:** Unknown.

**Prevention:** None known. Genetic counseling indicated.

**Treatment:** Good protein nutrition; nicotinic acid supplements to offset proposed deficiency in endogenous synthesis of coenzyme and prevent pellagra-like symptoms. Tryptophan methylester is absorbed and will repair CNS metabolite (5-HT, 5-H1AA) homeostasis.

**Prognosis:** Normal life span.

**Detection of Carrier:** No identifying characteristics under usual prevailing conditions. Renal $T_m$ should be lower than normal for amino acids, whose transport is affected by trait.

**References:**
Mahon BE, Levy HL: Maternal Hartnup disorder. Am J Med Genet 1986; 24:513–518.
Scriver CR, et al.: The Hartnup phenotype: Mendelian transport disorder, multifactorial disease. Am J Hum Genet 1987; 40:401–412. *
Levy HL: Hartnup disorder. In: Scriver CR, et al., eds: The metabolic basis of inherited disease, 6th ed. New York: McGraw-Hill, 1989; 2515–2528.

SC050                                          **Charles R. Scriver**

## HAUPTMANN-THANHAUSER SYNDROME          3246

**Includes:**
Emery-Dreifuss muscular dystrophy, autosomal dominant type
Muscular dystropy-muscular shortening
Muscular shortening and dystrophy
Rigid spine syndrome
Scapuloilioperoneal atrophy-cardiopathy
Spine, rigid spine syndrome

**Excludes:**
**Emery-Dreifuss syndrome** (2491)
**Muscular dystrophy** (other)

**Major Diagnostic Criteria:** Contractures and weakness of the neck muscles, long dorsal muscles and flexor muscles of the arms, with a pattern of autosomal dominant inheritance.

**Clinical Findings:** Hauptmann and Thanhauser (1941) studied a family of French-Canadian descent in which most of the members for three generations showed inability to flex the neck and back as well as extend their elbows. Neurological evaluation revealed shortness (contractures) of the neck muscles, long dorsal muscles, and flexor muscles of the arms. The proximal muscles of the arms and the gluteal muscles were underdeveloped and weak. Some members of this family manifested features of progressive muscular dystrophy with decrease or absence of deep tendon reflexes. However, most of the members of this family exhibited mainly shortening (contractures) and underdevelopment of neck and proximal muscles of the extremities, without any progressivity. The webbings, which was formed by the shortened upper trapezius, caused the neck to appear broader than usual. The cervical X-rays revealed that all the vertebrae were present. Routine urine and blood chemistry, done only in one patient, was normal. There was no heart involvement mentioned in any of the patients. However, other families with autosomal dominant muscular dystrophy and early contractures showed cardiomyopathy (Chakrabarti & Pearce, 1981; Fenichel et al, 1982; Miller et al, 1985). Becker (1986) distinguishes Hauptmann-Thannhauser dystrophy from **Emery-Dreifuss syndrome** on the basis of its autosomal dominant inheritance.

**Complications:** Unknown.

**Associated Findings:** None known.

**Etiology:** Autosomal dominant inheritance, with male to male transmission and high penetrance.

**Pathogenesis:** Unknown.

**MIM No.:** 15920, *18135

**Sex Ratio:** M1:F1

**Occurrence:** One French-Canadian kindred has been reported in the literature.

**Risk of Recurrence for Patient's Sib:**
See Part I, *Mendelian Inheritance.*

**Risk of Recurrence for Patient's Child:**
See Part I, *Mendelian Inheritance.*

**Age of Detectability:** During the first decade of life.

**Gene Mapping and Linkage:** Unknown.

**Prevention:** None known. Genetic counseling indicated.

**Treatment:** Unknown.

**Prognosis:** Good in most cases, with little or no progression of the disease.

**Detection of Carrier:** Unknown. Affected individuals are carriers of the disease.

**References:**
Hauptmann A, Thanhauser SJ: Muscular shortening and dystrophy: a heredofamilial disease. Arch Neurol Psychiat 1941; 46:654–664.
Chakrabarti A, Pearce JMS: Scapuloperoneal syndrome with cardiomyopathy: report of a family with autosomal dominant inheritance and unusual features. J Neurol Neurosurg Psychiat 1981; 44:1146–1152.
Fenichel GM, et al.: An autosomal domiant dystrophy with humeropelvic distribution and cardiomyopathy. Neurology 1982; 32:1399–1401.
Miller RG, et al.: Emery-Dreifuss muscular dystrophy with autosomal dominant transmission. Neurology 1985; 35:1230–1233.
Bailey RO, et al.: Benign muscular dystrophy with contractures: a new syndrome. Acta Neurol Scand 1986; 73:439–443.
Becker PE: Dominant autosomal muscular dystrophy with early contractures and cardiomyopathy (Hauptmann-Thannhauser). Hum Genet 1986; 74:184 only.
Emery AE: Emery-Dreifuss syndrome. J Med Genet 1989; 26:637–641.

I0000                                          **Victor V. Ionasescu**

## HAWKINSINURIA          2230

**Includes:**
Acidemia, Hawkinsinuria type
Four-hydroxyphenylpyruvate hydroxylase, deficiency of

**Excludes:** Tyrosinemia

**Major Diagnostic Criteria:** Clinical findings vary widely but include chronic acidosis, failure to thrive, or mental retardation. Laboratory studies are diagnostic; increased tyrosine products in the urine or plasma is a necessary finding. Increased excretion of 4-hydroxyphenyllactic acid, 4-hydroxyphenylpyruvic acid, and L-pyroglutamic acid are identified by gas chromatography. The

**21018**

① tyrotsine aminotransferase
② 4-OH-phenylpyruvate dioxygenase (EC 1.13.11.27)

**2230-21018:** Metabolic block in Hawkinsinuria.

---

specific compound designated "hawkinsin" with the structural identity of (2-L-cystein-S-yl-1,4-dihydroxycyclohex-5-en-1-yl)-acetic acid is recognizable in urine and plasma as a ninhydrin-reactive compound that is identifiable by amino acid chromatography, and by gas chromatography/mass spectroscopy.

**Clinical Findings:** Hawkinsinuria is a rare and unusual disorder of amino acid metabolism. The clinical picture can range from no detectable clinical symptoms to a spectrum of chronic acidosis, failure to thrive, probable mental retardation, and potential death. The degree of symptoms may be dependent upon the quantity of protein ingested during infancy. The greater the protein intake, the greater the degree of metabolic acidosis and clinical symptoms. Infants who have been breast-fed appear to have minimal symptoms. This has been postulated to be related to the lower protein concentration in breast milk compared with commercial infant formulas or cow's milk. It is likely that most patients with hawkinsinuria escape significant clinical symptoms during infancy. This theory is supported by preliminary information gained from sibs and other family members affected with the disorder who have no history of significant problems.

Hawkinsinuria is unusual as a disorder of metabolism because it is inherited as an autosomal dominant condition. Parents, sibs, and other family members of probands have been identified as having hawkinsinuria, a finding consistent with a single gene disorder.

**Complications:** Those related to symptoms during infancy: chronic metabolic acidosis, failure to thrive, poor head growth, and delayed development.

**Associated Findings:** Unusual body odor similar to a "swimming pool," and short stubby hair that grows poorly. Enlarged liver, anxiety, and irritability have been reported.

**Etiology:** Autosomal dominant inheritance.

**Pathogenesis:** The clinical symptoms are believed to result from a defect in the metabolism of a reactive intermediate that is formed during the reaction of 4-hydroxyphenylpyruvate dioxygenase (EC 1.13.11.27). The accumulation of the hawkinsin compound, or one of the other tyrosine intermediates, appears to be toxic and interferes with normal cellular growth. The accumulation of these compounds adds a significant quantity of anions to the plasma and results in metabolic acidosis. The degree of toxicity can be modulated by decreasing the tyrosine in the diet (by restricting phenylalanine and tyrosine intake and limiting protein ingestion) and decreasing the formation of the toxic intermediates.

**MIM No.:** *14035

**Sex Ratio:** M1:F1

**Occurrence:** Less than 1:100,000 in the general population. At least five kindreds have been documented.

**Risk of Recurrence for Patient's Sib:**
See Part I, *Mendelian Inheritance.*

**Risk of Recurrence for Patient's Child:**
See Part I, *Mendelian Inheritance.*

**Age of Detectability:** At birth.

**Gene Mapping and Linkage:** Unknown.

**Prevention:** None known. Genetic counseling indicated.

**Treatment:** Two forms of treatment have been suggested for symptomatic infants; restriction of tyrosine intake and ascorbic acid. Symptomatic infants have responded clinically to reduction of their phenylalanine and tyrosine intake to approximately 60 mg/kg/day and 50 mg/kg/day, respectively. This has resulted in correction of metabolic acidosis, decreased excretion of tyrosine products, improvement in clinical symptoms, and restoration of normal growth pattern. This dietary restriction can be accomplished by using a formula designated 3200 AB (Mead-Johnson) and by limiting other protein sources.

Ascorbic acid is of value because of its assistance in glutathione metabolism and its reported stabilizing effect on the enzyme 4-hydroxyphenylpyruvic acid oxidase. Once the children have reached 18 months to two years of age, they may not require specific dietary intervention and either subjectively adjust their own diet to a lower protein intake or are capable of taking increased quantities of protein without adverse effects.

**Prognosis:** For those individuals with hawkinsinuria who pass through the first 18 months of childhood, the prognosis is excellent. Adults identified with hawkinsinuria are functioning with intelligence and physical performance in the normal range.

**Detection of Carrier:** All reported individuals have been heterozygous for the condition. No persons homozygous for hawkinsinuria are known. Carriers of the gene can be detected by evaluation of the urine for the hawkinsin compound by applying techniques for amino acid analysis.

**References:**

Danks DM, et al.: A new form of prolonged transient tyrosinemia presenting with severe metabolic acidosis. Acta Pediatr Scand 1975; 64:209–214.

Niederwieser A, et al.: A new sulfur amino acid named hawkinsin, identified in a baby with transient tyrosinemia and her mother. Clin Chim Acta 1977; 76:345–356.

Niederwieser A, et al.: Excretion of cis- and trans-4-hydroxycyclohexylacetic acid in addition to hawkinsin in a family with a postulated defect of 4-hydroxyphenylpyruvate dioxygenase. Clin Chim Acta 1978; 90:195–200.

Wilcken B, et al.: Hawkinsinuria: a dominantly inherited defect of tyrosine metabolism with severe effects in infancy. New Engl J Med 1981; 305:865–869.

SC046                                              **C. Ronald Scott**

**Hay-Wells syndrome**
   *See ECTODERMAL DYSPLASIA, HAY-WELLS TYPE*
**Hayfever, atopic**
   *See SKIN, ATOPY, FAMILIAL*
**Head, rhomboid-shaped**
   *See PLAGIOCEPHALY*
**Headache, benign exertional**
   *See MIGRAINE*
**Headache, benign sexual**
   *See MIGRAINE*
**Headache, migraine**
   *See MIGRAINE*
**Hearing loss (sensorineural)-hereditary atopic dermatitis**
   *See DEAFNESS-ATOPIC DERMATITIS*

Hearing loss, familial, progressive, low-frequency
See DEAFNESS, DOMINANT LOW-FREQUENCY
Hearing loss, hereditary progressive high-tone neural
See DEAFNESS (SENSORINEURAL), PROGRESSIVE HIGH-TONE
Hearing loss-nephritis
See NEPHRITIS-DEAFNESS (SENSORINEURAL), HEREDITARY
TYPE
Heart and vascular defects-distichiasis
See DISTICHIASIS-HEART DEFECT-PERIPHERAL VASCULAR
DISEASE/ANOMALIES
Heart block with maternal systemic lupus erythematosis
See ARRHYTHMIA, FROM MATERNAL AUTOIMMUNE DISEASE,
CONGENITAL
Heart block with other maternal connective tissue diseases
See ARRHYTHMIA, FROM MATERNAL AUTOIMMUNE DISEASE,
CONGENITAL
Heart block, congenital complete
See ARRHYTHMIA, HEART BLOCK, CONGENITAL COMPLETE
Heart defects-blepharophimosis-mental retardation
See MENTAL RETARDATION-HEART DEFECTS-
BLEPHAROPHIMOSIS
Heart defects-hydrocephalus-dense bones
See HYDROCEPHALUS-HEART DEFECT-DENSE BONES, BEEMER
TYPE
Heart defects-polysyndactyly
See POLYSYNDACTYLY-CARDIAC MALFORMATIONS
Heart disease, glycogen
See GLYCOGENOSIS, TYPE IIa
Heart upper limb syndrome
See HEART-HAND SYNDROME
Heart, arcade formation of the leaflets and chordae
See MITRAL VALVE INSUFFICIENCY
Heart, complete d-transposition
See HEART, TRANSPOSITION OF GREAT VESSELS

---

## HEART, COR TRIATRIATUM        0204

**Includes:**
Cor triatriatum
Cor triatriatum sinistrum
Pulmonary vein, stenosis of the common

**Excludes:**
Cor triatriatum dextrum
Subtotal cor triatriatum

**Major Diagnostic Criteria:** Heart murmur or heart failure accompanied by elevation of pulmonary artery wedge pressure with demonstration of the abnormality by pulmonary arteriography.

**Clinical Findings:** *Anatomy:* Cor triatriatum is a rare cardiac anomaly wherein the left atrium is divided into 2 chambers, distal and proximal, by a fibromuscular septum. The more distal part of

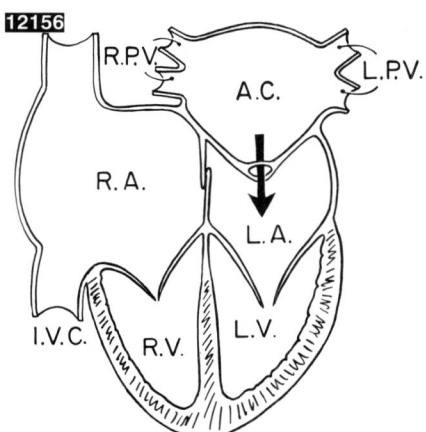

0204-12156: Drawing of cor triatriatum.

the left atrium receives the pulmonary veins and the more proximal part communicates with the mitral valve, left atrial appendage and the foramen ovale. There may be defects in the atrial septum allowing communication of either the proximal or, more rarely, the distal left atrial chamber with the right atrium. Right ventricular hypertrophy and dilatation are almost invariably found. A large number of variants of cor triatriatum have been described, including the association of cor triatriatum with total anomalous pulmonary venous connection and partial anomalous pulmonary venous connection. Cor triatriatum may be associated with other obstructive lesions on the left side of the heart. These include coarctation of the aorta, aortic stenosis, bicuspid aortic valve, parachute mitral valve, supravalvar stenosis of the left atrium and stenosis of the pulmonary veins.

*Physiology:* In those anatomic defects in which the blood from the distal atrial chamber enters into the right major atrial chamber directly or indirectly, hemodynamics are comparable to those in total anomalous pulmonary venous connection. When there are additional left-sided obstructive lesions the hemodynamic alterations are related to the combination of obstructive lesions. In the classic form of cor triatriatum the obstructive left atrial membrane causes elevated pressure in the accessory left atrial chamber which is transmitted to the pulmonary veins. This pressure is freely transmitted to the pulmonary capillary bed and results in pulmonary edema. Reflex pulmonary arteriolar constriction then reduces blood flow into the pulmonary capillary bed; it also results in pulmonary arterial hypertension, right ventricular hypertrophy and ultimately right ventricular failure.

Most individuals with classic cor triatriatum have onset of symptoms within the first years of life. However, a significant number of individuals are asymptomatic until the second or third decades of life. Symptoms include dyspnea, frequent respiratory infections and pneumonia. The signs of pulmonary hypertension, including a loud pulmonary component of the second heart sound, right ventricular heave and pulmonary ejection systolic click are invariably present. Right heart failure is often seen and reflected by hepatomegaly, distended neck veins and peripheral edema. Pulmonary rales are often present. A soft blowing systolic murmur is often heard along the left sternal border; less often a diastolic murmur is detected at the mitral area or a continuous murmur is heard. Rarely, a murmur is absent.

The EKG reflects systolic pressure overload of the right ventricle, tall R waves in the right precordial leads; tall peaked P waves are usual. Occasionally, the P wave is also broad and notched. The chest x-ray reflects a pulmonary venous obstruction. Fine diffuse reticular pulmonary markings fan out from the pulmonary hilus; Kerley B lines may be present. The main pulmonary artery and major branches are dilated. There are signs of right ventricular and right atrial enlargement.

Echocardiographic features are not pathognomonic because of the multiple anatomic expressions of cor triatriatum. An abnormal left atrial echo may be seen anterior and in proximity to the mitral valve. This echo moves briskly with atrial events. It is similar to the left atrial echo seen in TAPVC to coronary sinus and persistent LSVC connecting to coronary sinus. Cor triatriatum may produce mid-left atrial echo with slight motion. The left atrial echo may be thin and intermittent or absent.

At cardiac catheterization significant pulmonary hypertension and elevated pulmonary artery wedge pressure are routinely found. A shunt may be detected in the presence of a communication between the proximal and distal left atrial chambers and the right atrium.

The precise diagnosis is defined by selective pulmonary arteriography. Films must be programmed to accommodate the prolonged pulmonary transit time. As the pulmonary veins opacify, they drain into the accessory left atrial chamber; a significant delay is noted between the opacification of this chamber and that of the true left atrium and left ventricle. The obstructive membrane is best seen in the anterior-posterior view.

**Complications:** Death may occur from pulmonary edema and right heart failure; pulmonary congestive symptoms may be present as well as medial hypertrophy of the pulmonary arterioles. The latter is reversible after surgery.

**Associated Findings:** None known.

**Etiology:** Unknown.

**Pathogenesis:** Undetermined. One view suggests that the anomaly results from a faulty development of the atrial septum. The currently accepted theory is that the common pulmonary vein has failed to become incorporated into the left atrium in a normal fashion. However, the diversity of cor triatriatum variants favors multiple embryologic bases.

**CDC No.:** 746.820

**Sex Ratio:** M1:F1

**Occurrence:** 0.2% of congenital heart disease.

**Risk of Recurrence for Patient's Sib:** Unknown.

**Risk of Recurrence for Patient's Child:** Unknown.

**Age of Detectability:** From birth by selective angiography.

**Gene Mapping and Linkage:** Unknown.

**Prevention:** None known. Genetic counseling indicated.

**Treatment:** Resection of the obstructing left atrial membrane. The great anatomic variety that may be encountered in patients with cor triatriatum makes utilization of cardiopulmonary bypass and correction by direct vision desirable.

Symptomatic therapy for heart failure and pneumonia should be instituted. However, once heart failure occurs, the course is unaffected by medical management; surgical intervention should be performed as soon as possible.

**Prognosis:** Survival is related to the size of the orifice in the obstructing membrane: three months if the orifice is less than 3 mm, 16 years if the orifice is greater than 3 mm. Postoperative prognosis approaches normal.

**Detection of Carrier:** Unknown.

**Support Groups:** Dallas; American Heart Association

**References:**
Edwards JE: Malformation of the thoracic veins. In: Gould SE, ed: Pathology of the heart, 2nd ed. Springfield: Charles C Thomas, 1960:484.
Niwayama G: Cor triatriatum. Am Heart J 1960; 59:291.
Lucas RV Jr, Schmidt RE: Anomalous venous connection, pulmonary and systemic. In: Moss AJ, et al., eds: Heart disease in infants, children, and adolescents, 2nd ed. Baltimore: Williams & Wilkins Co., 1977:454–457. *

LU003

**Russell V. Lucas, Jr.**

---

**HEART, CORDIS ECTOPIA**　　　　　　　　**0335**

**Includes:**
Cervical, thoracic-thoracoabdominal ectopia cordis
Ectopia cordis
Heart, not in thorax

**Excludes:**
Cardiac malpositions within thorax
**Heart, pericardium agenesis** (0805)
**Pentalogy of Cantrell** (3121)
**Ventricle, diverticulum** (0988)

**Major Diagnostic Criteria:** Complete or partial thoracic ectopia cordis is apparent by physical examination. The thoracoabdominal type may be suspected if a pulse is apparent in an omphalocele, but ultrasonography or angiography may be necessary to demonstrate mild forms. In the rare isolated abdominal variety, the chest film will show an absence of the cardiac shadow, confirming the diagnosis.

**Clinical Findings:** While several forms of this entity exist, the common pathologic finding in all is partial or complete displacement of the heart from the thorax. This, in nearly all cases, is associated with a midline defect of the anterior body wall at some point.

Various classifications have been proposed based on the location of the displaced heart. There are 2 major clinical forms: the thoracic and thoracoabdominal types. The thoracic type is the most common and accounts for more than two-thirds of the reported cases. The usual anatomic arrangement consists of a completely cleft sternum, absence of the skin and parietal pericardium resulting in total extrusion of the heart with the apex displaced anteriorly and superiorly. Failure of union of the anterior thorax is usually associated with a similar defect in the anterior abdominal wall so that an omphalocele is present. An incomplete variant of the thoracic type exists and is sometimes referred to as the thoracocervical type. The sternum may be united in its inferior portion, but bifid superiorly with the heart being located in the upper thorax and neck. The skin is usually present, though the parietal pericardium may or may not be found. An abdominal defect is not usually present. This form is unusual and represents approximately 5% of the cases. The thoracoabdominal type is the second most common form, comprising 20–25% of the cases. Anatomically, the sternum is usually not fused in its inferior position and this is associated with an anterior defect of the diaphragm and abdominal wall resulting in herniation of the heart inferiorly.

When these defects comprise the thoracoabdominal type of ectopia cordis are accompanied by a deficiency of the diaphragmatic pericardium and a congenital intracardiac defect, the combination of these anomalies is known as the **Pentalogy of Cantrell**. Isolated abdominal and true cervical forms are exceedingly rare and are usually associated with other lethal malformations. The physical findings are striking and are usually indicative of the type of ectopia which is present. Diagnosis of the thoracoabdominal type may at times be difficult if there is only minimal herniation. Additional physical findings are largely dependent on the associated heart lesion. Eighty percent of the complete thoracic and thoracoabdominal forms will have intracardiac anomalies, ventricular septal defect being the most common.

If the diagnosis is not made from physical examination, a chest film may reveal inferior displacement of the heart in the thoracoabdominal type. With minimal herniation, the X-ray may be normal, though ventricular herniation may cause a slight dextrorotation due to the bilateral symmetry of the diaphragmatic defect. The EKG is of little aid in the diagnosis of ectopia cordis.

**Complications:** Cardiac embarrassment from compression or strangulation of cardiovascular structures, death from infection.

**Associated Findings:** Complex cyanotic congenital heart disease.

**Etiology:** Unknown.

**Pathogenesis:** Undetermined. The complete thoracic form is thought to be secondary to a failure of fusion of the right and left anterior body walls, resulting in a midline defect with cardiac extrusion and omphalocele. Thoracoabdominal ectopia is associated with a failure of development of the septum transversum allowing herniation of the heart through the diaphragm. The true cervical form of ectopia cordis apparently results from a failure of migration of the heart to the thorax from its original position near the mandibular arch.

**POS No.:** 3248

**CDC No.:** 746.880

**Sex Ratio:** M1:F1

**Occurrence:** Less than 200 cases of all forms reported to date.

**Risk of Recurrence for Patient's Sib:** Unknown.

**Risk of Recurrence for Patient's Child:** Unknown.

**Age of Detectability:** The severe forms may be detected prenatally by ultrasonography and by physical examination at birth. The mild thoracoabdominal forms may require ultrasonography or angiography.

**Gene Mapping and Linkage:** Unknown.

**Prevention:** None known. Genetic counseling indicated.

**Treatment:** General supportive care of the infant until surgical replacement of the heart into the thorax can be effected.

**Prognosis:** Depends upon the type of ectopia cordis and the associated malformations. Infants with the complete thoracic form die during the first days of life. Thoracoabdominal forms have been successfully repaired. The incomplete thoracic form is amenable to surgery and offers the best prognosis in that usually there is no associated cardiac malformation. With surgical correction and no associated lesion, a normal life span can be anticipated.

**Detection of Carrier:** Unknown.

**Support Groups:** Dallas; American Heart Association

**References:**
Kanagasuntheram R, Verzin JA: Ectopia cordis in man. Thorax 1962; 17:159–167. * †
Toyama WM: Combined congenital defects of the anterior abdominal wall, sternum, diaphragm, pericardium, and heart: a case report and review of the syndrome. Pediatrics 1972; 50:778–792.
Harrison M, et al.: Prenatal diagnosis and management of omphalocele and ectopia cordis. J Pediatr Surg 1982; 17:64–66.
Van Praagh R, et al.: Malpositions of the heart. In Adams FH, et al, eds: Heart disease in infants, children, and adolescents, 3rd ed. Baltimore: William & Wilkins, 1983:454–458.
Khoury MJ, et al.: Ectopia cordis, midline defects and chromosome abnormalities: an epidemiologic perspective. Am J Med Genet 1988; 30:811–817.

MI019      **Robert H. Miller**

## HEART, ENDOCARDIAL CUSHION DEFECTS    0347

**Includes:**
Atrioventricular canal, persistent common
Atrioventricularis communis
Endocardial cushion defects
Ostium primum atrial septal defect, persistent ostium primum
Ventricular septal defect, endocardial cushion defect type

**Excludes:**
Atrial septal defects, sinus venosus type
Fossa ovalis, defects at

**Major Diagnostic Criteria:** The presence of an atrial level left-to-right shunt (pulmonary ejection systolic murmur, diastolic tricuspid flow murmur, widely split and fixed components of the second sound at the base); an EKG which shows the combination of left axis deviation in the limb leads and mild-to-moderate right ventricular hypertrophy pattern in the precordial leads; and radiographic findings of an atrial level shunt are strongly suggestive of the diagnosis of the partial form of ECD (Endocardial Cushion Defect) with an atrial level communication. Left ventricular angiogram confirms the diagnosis. Clinical findings suggesting a ventricular level shunt (systolic thrill and loud harsh holosystolic murmur at the lower sternal border, mitral flow murmur) together with an EKG which shows left axis deviation and biventricular hypertrophy, and radiographic findings of a left-to-right shunt beyond the level of the atrioventricular valves suggest the diagnosis of partial form of ECD with interventricular communication. A left ventriculogram confirms the diagnosis. Symptoms in infancy or early childhood of recurrent pneumonitis, dyspnea, feeding difficulties, congestive heart failure, auscultatory findings of a loud, harsh precordial systolic murmur, diastolic flow murmurs (and sometimes also a widely split, fixed second sound at the base), EKG evidence of marked left axis deviation and biventricular enlargement together with radiographs showing moderate-to-marked cardiomegaly, hypervascularity of the lung fields and the absence of left atrial enlargement are strongly suggestive of the diagnosis of complete type of ECD. The left ventricular angiogram is usually diagnostic. In all types of ECD, an apical systolic murmur indicating mitral incompetence is usually, but not invariably, present.

**Clinical Findings:** ECD's comprise a group of pathogenetically related cardiac anomalies thought to be the result of abnormal development of the embryonic atrioventricular endocardial cushions. Pathologic and anatomic features characteristic of ECD and shared by all types to a varying degree are: the aortic cusp of the mitral valve is cleft and its origin is concave, rather than convex

towards the atrium as in the normal heart; the ventricular septum has a peculiar "scooped out" appearance; the left ventricular outflow tract is more narrow and elongated than normal; the superoinferior (anteroposterior) diameter of the ventricles is increased at the base. Usually a large, very characteristic interatrial communication, an interventricular communication, or both, is present. The clinical findings in individual cases are determined almost wholly by the type of defect present in the cardiac septum, eg whether there is an intracardiac shunt at the atrial or ventricular level or at both. The cleft mitral valve is usually (but not always) incompetent. The degree of incompetence has a significant, if not dominant, influence on the clinical course.

*ECD, partial type with interatrial communication:* the interatrial communication is usually quite large and located immediately above the level of the atrioventricular valves. While true atrial septal defects also may be present, the characteristic interatrial communication in ECD corresponds in position to the atrioventricular part of the cardiac septum which is absent in ECD. As compared to a normal heart, the medial portions of the two atrioventricular ostia are displaced apically. The atrial septum itself typically is normal and its lower free border, or upper rim of the interatrial communication, corresponds to the line of origin of the anterior mitral cusp of the normal heart. A portion of the ventricular septum of variable size, just below the atrioventricular ostia, is fibrous and contains short chordae tendineae which insert into the medial most portion of the cleft mitral valve.

In cases where the mitral valve is competent, the clinical picture closely resembles that seen in true atrial septal defects (ASD). There is evidence of a large left-to-right shunt at the atrial level with enlargement of the right atrium and the right ventricle and engorgement of the pulmonary arterial tree. Respiratory infections are common, and growth retardation, fatigability and dyspnea are seen more commonly and tend to occur at an earlier age than in cases with true ASD. As in ASD, an ejection type systolic murmur is audible at the left upper sternal border and the second sound at the base is distinctly split; with respiration this splitting varies little or none at all. A thrill, uncommon in ASD, is present much more often in ECD. Also present along the lower left sternal border is a lower frequency diastolic flow murmur, encompassing $S_3$ and $S_4$, which represents relative tricuspid stenosis. In somewhat more than half the cases, a high-pitched, blowing systolic murmur indicating the presence of mitral insufficiency, is present over the apex and transmitted to the axilla. With more severe degrees of valve incompetence, there may be an associated diastolic flow murmur of relative mitral stenosis.

The EKG with rare exceptions, shows a combination of left axis deviation of -40° to -130°, and a right bundle branch block pattern of right ventricular hypertrophy in the precordial leads. The PR interval is commonly prolonged. The vectorcardiogram characteristically shows a superiorly oriented, counterclockwise inscribed QRS loop in the frontal plane. In cases with significant mitral incompetence, evidence of combined ventricular hypertrophy is found.

On X-ray, the heart tends to be somewhat larger than in patients with ASD. The pulmonary trunk is enlarged and the vascularity is prominent and of a shunt type. Left atrial enlargement is absent except in those cases where the atrial communication is small and the mitral insufficiency is moderate to severe.

In contrast to the secundum type of ASD, the echocardiogram shows abnormal thickening of the right ventricular anterior wall and the interventricular septum. In addition, the right ventricular cavity is dilated, as in other types of ASD, and the septal motion may be flat to paradoxical. The mitral valve motion pattern may vary widely from normal to the typical motion pattern of ECD where the valve echocardiographically appears to traverse the septum during diastole.

Cardiac catheterization findings are similar to those found in ASD. An unusually low position of the cardiac catheter as it crosses from right atrium to left atrium may suggest the true nature of the defect. Significant elevation of right ventricular and pulmonary arterial pressures are more common than in ASD. Much more useful in the differentiation between ASD and ECD, however, is angiocardiography. In ASD the left ventricular angiogram is normal; in ECD the left ventriculogram in the frontal plane shows the elongated left ventricular outflow tract ("gooseneck") and the "scooped out" ventricular septum. The long, narrow left ventricular outflow tract is best appreciated during cardiac diastole, whereas during systole, the two halves of the cleft anterior mitral valve cusp bulge into the left atrium forming a notch indicating the position of the cleft. Mitral insufficiency, if present, is readily demonstrated.

*ECD, partial type with interventricular communication:* the clinical features of this anomaly closely resemble those seen in patients with defects of the basilar portion of the ventricular septum. Mitral incompetence is usually present. Electrocardiographically there is evidence of left ventricular volume overload as in other cases with ventricular septal defects, but the frontal plane axis is typically deviated leftward. In these cases with intact atrial septum, the anterior cusp of the mitral valve, while cleft, originates normally and the "gooseneck" may not be readily apparent on the left ventriculogram.

*ECD, partial type with interatrial and interventricular communications:* this type is uncommon and the clinical picture resembles that seen in cases where there is a combination of an atrial level and a ventricular level shunt. As in the other types, mitral incompetence is usually present.

*ECD, partial type with left ventricular to right atrial shunt:* this lesion is extremely uncommon. The clinical, EKG and radiographic findings are similar to those seen in cases with an atrial level shunt, a precordial systolic thrill is almost always present and radiographically the right atrium tends to be more distinctly enlarged. A left ventricular angiogram demonstrates the shunt, but cannot always differentiate it with certainty from cases with a ventricular septal defect and tricuspid valve insufficiency.

*ECD, partial type with isolated cleft of the mitral valve:* this anomaly is exceedingly rare and is only important when the mitral valve is incompetent. Such cases cannot be differentiated with certainty from other conditions with mitral insufficiency.

*ECD, complete type:* in this anomaly, the central portion of the cardiac septum is absent and there is a single atrioventricular ostium with free communication between the 4 cardiac chambers. The atrial component of the septal defect is similar to that seen in the partial form with interatrial communication, and the ventricular component of the defect is similar to that seen in the partial form with interventricular communication. In addition to the normal posterior cusp of the mitral valve and the anterior and posterolateral cusps of the tricuspid valve, there is a large anterior cusp which crosses the top of the ventricular septum and inserts on the left side on the anterior papillary muscle of the left ventricle and on the right side on the medial papillary muscle of the right ventricle. In some cases, the cusp is also attached to the top of the ventricular septum. In others, the large anterior cusp may combine with the normal right ventricular anterior tricuspid cusp, in which case the medial papillary muscle is absent. Opposite the large anterior cusp a somewhat smaller, posterior common cusp inserts; on the left side, onto the posterior left ventricular papillary muscle, and on the right side, usually onto the top of the ventricular septum and sometimes also to a number of small posterior right ventricular papillary muscles.

The common atrioventricular valve may be competent, particularly in very young infants. The complete type of ECD usually causes severe difficulties early in infancy, such as repeated respiratory infections, feeding difficulties, growth retardation, dyspnea and congestive heart failure. Most of the infants die within the first 2 years of life. Cyanosis is rare unless there is an associated obstruction of the right ventricular outflow tract, respiratory infection, heart failure or very high pulmonary vascular resistance. Cardiomegaly develops rapidly after birth. In general, the larger the ventricular component of the defect and the more pronounced the mitral insufficiency, the sicker the child. Extreme degrees of left axis deviation may be seen in the EKG, and marked right ventricular hypertrophy indicating high right ventricular pressures is common. In X-rays, the pulmonary vascularity indicates a large shunt, often with concomitant signs of failure and pneumonia. The heart is usually quite large. Few shunt lesions result in so much cardiomegaly. Signs of left atrial enlargement

are usually inapparent except in the presence of significant mitral valve incompetence.

The M-mode echocardiogram shows either very little or no interventricular septum. The diastolic atrioventricular valve motion is exaggerated and completely crosses the ventricular cavity; in systole the leaflets appear joined at the level of the aortic root. Many patients with the complete defect have pulmonary vascular obstructive disease; the echo of the pulmonary valve is accordingly abnormal, with loss of the "A" dip, flattening of the diastolic slope and a "W" pattern of systolic motion; the early closure occurs in the first one-third of the valve opening trace. In less severe forms of the defect, the valve motion pattern is less exaggerated and more septal representation is noted. Mitral echoes, ordinarily at the plane of the posterior aortic root, can be traced to the anterior border of the left ventricular outflow tract. Due to the unusual valve orientation, in most forms of the defect, the E-F slope is difficult to record and generally only the D-E slope is seen in diastole. 2-D echocardiography clearly demonstrates the anatomy of the various forms of the anomaly.

**Complications:** Congestive heart failure is unusual in infancy and early childhood in the partial form of ECD with an atrial level shunt. It is much more common in those cases where a ventricular level shunt is present, particularly in the complete type of ECD. In these forms, recurrent pneumonitis, growth retardation and dyspnea are also commonly seen. Bacterial endocarditis is uncommon. Increased pulmonary vascular resistance secondary to progressive pulmonary vascular changes tends to develop at a relatively early age, particularly in the complete type of ECD, and particularly also in patients with Down syndrome. Right ventricular hypertension is common. Such patients become progressively more cyanotic.

**Associated Findings:** None known.

**Etiology:** Multifactorial inheritance is presumed to occur in two-thirds of the cases; trisomy 21 is present in one-third of the cases. About 15% of the patients with chromosome 21 trisomy have some form of ECD, usually the complete type. ECD, usually the complete type, is also present in the majority of cases of **Asplenia syndrome** and, also to a lesser extent, in the polysplenia syndrome. There appears to be a strikingly higher offspring recurrence risk if the mother is affected (14:100), as opposed to the father being affected (1:100). This suggests further inheritance factors such as cytoplasmic and marked vulnerability to teratogens within the multifactorial mode.

**Pathogenesis:** Possibly due to partial or complete failure of fusion of the superior and inferior atrioventricular endocardial cushions. After fusion, the endocardial cushions normally bend to form an arc, the convexity of which is toward the atrial side. The atrial septum primum fuses with the high point of the arc, thus dividing it into two approximately equal parts. The right half contributes to the ventricular septum, the atrioventricular septum and the medial or septal cusp of the tricuspid valve. The left half of fused cushions plays an important role in the formation of the aortic or anterior cusp of the mitral valve. In ECD, the cushions fuse only in part or not at all, and the arc is usually not formed. The lower border of the atrial septum cannot reach the endocardial cushions; a large interatrial communication remains. In addition, the atrioventricular part of the cardiac septum is not formed. Failure of the left side of the endocardial cushions to fuse explains the cleft in the mitral valve cusp.

**CDC No.:** 745.6

**Sex Ratio:** M1:F1

**Occurrence:** Incidence approximately 1:2500 live births. Prevalence 1:25,000 of the infant and child population

**Risk of Recurrence for Patient's Sib:** Empiric risk: 3:100.

**Risk of Recurrence for Patient's Child:** If mother is affected, 14:100; if father is affected, 1:100.

**Age of Detectability:** In infancy.

**Gene Mapping and Linkage:** Unknown.

**Prevention:** None known. Genetic counseling indicated.

**Treatment:** Banding of the pulmonary trunk has been carried out in individuals with the complete type of ECD and with the partial form with interventricular communication; this is an effort to reduce pulmonary blood flow and prevent the development of peripheral vascular changes which result in increased resistance. Results of this procedure have been mediocre but, occasionally, fairly good results have been reported.

Children with the more severe forms of ECD usually need vigorous medical therapy for respiratory infections and congestive heart failure in early infancy. Corrective surgery should be carried out as early as possible, even in the more benign forms of the anomaly, particularly if the mitral valve is still competent. Once this valve has become insufficient, the surgical results tend to be mediocre.

**Prognosis:** The prognosis of the severe forms of the anomaly generally is poor: most of the infants die at an early age. The partial form with interatrial communication carries the best prognosis, particularly if the mitral valve is competent. When mitral insufficiency occurs, the prognosis is determined largely by the degree of such insufficiency. Pulmonary vascular changes resulting in high pulmonary vascular resistance tend to occur early in the severe forms of the anomaly.

**Detection of Carrier:** Unknown.

**Special Considerations:** Since the prognosis of ECD depends so much on the presence and severity of mitral incompetence, surgery should be carried out as early as is practically feasible, even when mild forms of the anomaly occur in children who are asymptomatic. In such cases it is advisable to simply close the intracardiac communication and not try to repair the cleft in the mitral valve. Such a repair may, in some, if not most cases, lead to impaired function of the anterior cusp. This repair may result in turbulence and consequent damage, thereby actually promoting the appearance of mitral insufficiency.

**Support Groups:** Dallas; American Heart Association

**References:**

Edwards JE, et al.: Persistent common atrioventricular canal. In: Edwards JE, ed: Congenital heart disease, correlation of pathologic anatomy and angiocardiography vol 1. Philadelphia: W.B. Saunders, 1965:208–224. *

Williams RG, Rudd M: Echocardiographic features of endocardial cushion defects. Circulation 1974; 49:418–422.

Goldberg SJ, et al.: Pediatric and adolescent echocardiography. Chicago: Year Book Medical Publishers, 1975:85–89.

Silverman NH, Snider AR: Two-dimensional echocardiography in congenital heart disease. Connecticut: Appleton-Century-Crofts, 1982.

Nora JJ, Nora AH: Maternal transmission of congenital heart disease. Am J Cardiol 1987; 59:459–463. *

N0003                                              **James J. Nora**

**Heart, narrowing of tricuspid orifice**
*See TRICUSPID VALVE, STENOSIS*
**Heart, noninverted transposition**
*See HEART, TRANSPOSITION OF GREAT VESSELS*
**Heart, not in thorax**
*See HEART, CORDIS ECTOPIA*

**Includes:**
Agenesis of pericardium
Left atrial herniation
Pericardial defects, congenital
Pericardium, congenital partial or complete absence of
Pericardium agenesis

**Excludes:** Heart, cordis ectopia (0335)

**Major Diagnostic Criteria:** Characteristic X-ray findings are suggestive; diagnostic pneumothorax is confirmatory if positive.

**Clinical Findings:** Although this entity was first described in 1559, more than one-half of the cases have appeared in the literature during the past two decades, suggesting that pericardial agenesis is not as rare as once believed. St. Pierre and Froment (1970) reviewed 153 cases from the literature up to 1970, and subdivided them as follows: total absence of pericardium (9%); left-sided defect (70%); partial (35%); total (35%); right-sided defect (4%); partial (4%); total (0%); diaphragmatic pericardial aplasia (17%).

Clinically, most patients are asymptomatic, but when symptoms occur, they are thought to be related to the specific defect. For example, in partial left-sided defects (foramen type) herniation of the left ventricle through the foramen can result in chest pain or even sudden death. Pressure on the coronary arteries from the rim of the foramen may produce angina. Some authors suggest that chest pain is related to mediastinal adhesions, torsion of the great vessels due to lack of stability of the heart, or the previously mentioned pressure on the coronary arteries.

In a review of the isolated partial left-sided type of defect, 16 of 27 cases were asymptomatic. Chest pain, occasionally associated with radiation to the left arm and dyspnea, was present in 8 cases. Other symptoms included occasional syncopal attacks, dyspnea without pain, and small hemoptyses.

Physical findings have also been vague and variable. Sometimes cardiac enlargement or hypermobility of the heart is present. Soft systolic murmurs are sometimes reported. EKG findings are present only in cases with associated heart malformations or malrotation of the heart.

The most useful diagnostic features are X-ray findings. Absence of the left side of the pericardium produces a very prominent aortic arch, pulmonary artery, and left atrial shadows. If herniation of the left atrium through a foramen has occurred, the radiograph may be interpreted as a dilatation of the pulmonary artery, atrial tumor or various hilar tumors, or lymph node enlargement. The X-ray frequently suggests cardiac enlargement. Complete defects produce morbid shifting of the heart without shifting of the trachea. A case of partial right-sided defect revealed radiolucent herniation of the lung into the pericardial cavity.

Fluoroscopy may reveal asynchronous pulsation of the left

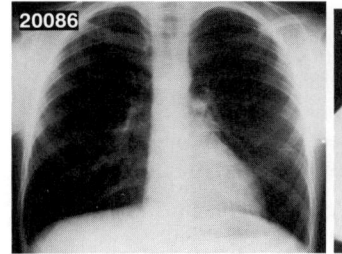
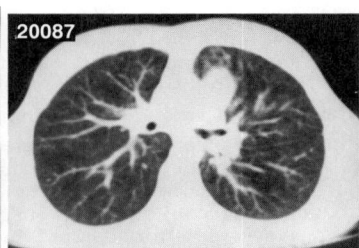

**0805-20086:** Chest X-ray of a 1-year-old boy showing rotation of the heart to the left with the right cardiac border overlying the spine. There is a slight bulge in the region of the pulmonary artery segment. **20087:** CT scan 2 cm caudal to the carina shows anterior extension of the pulmonary artery beyond the normal mediastinal border.

atrium with either partial or complete defects. A diagnostic pneumothorax may be useful in showing air entering the pericardial cavity. If positive, this procedure is diagnostic, but a negative result does not rule out a pericardial defect as it is sometimes difficult to introduce air through small pericardial defects or if pleuropericardial adhesions are present.

Cardiac catheterization and angiography may reveal a displaced left atrium if herniation has occurred and will rule out other cardiac abnormalities. In one case angiocardiography suggested an encysted pericardial effusion which on echocardiogram was disproved.

**Complications:** Sudden death has been associated with herniation and strangulation of the left ventricle. In the preantibiotic era, pleuropericarditis resulted from exposure of the unprotected heart to pulmonary infections.

**Associated Findings:** 30–40% have associated anomalies. Bronchogenic cyst is probably the most common, followed by associated cardiac defects including patent ductus arteriosus, bifid heart, **Heart, tetralogy of Fallot**, **Ventricular septal defect**, tricuspid incompetence, and bicuspid aortic valve. Cerebral anomalies have occurred in two patients. Congestive heart failure, when it occurs, is usually related to associated intracardiac defects.

**Etiology:** Unknown.

**Pathogenesis:** Undetermined, but generally thought to result from incomplete development of either the transverse septum or of the pleuropericardial folds, which in turn may be due to premature atrophy of the duct of Cuvier of the left side. This theory supports the left-sided defects, but fails to explain the infrequent right-sided defect.

**CDC No.:** 746.850

**Sex Ratio:** M3:F1

**Occurrence:** Over 200 cases have been reported.

**Risk of Recurrence for Patient's Sib:** No reported cases have occurred in more than one member of a family, or in twins.

**Risk of Recurrence for Patient's Child:** No reported cases have occurred in more than one member of a family, or in twins.

**Age of Detectability:** In infancy, by X-ray.

**Gene Mapping and Linkage:** Unknown.

**Prevention:** None known. Genetic counseling indicated.

**Treatment:** Many cases have not been treated. Partial defects, if small, may be closed primarily. In other cases adjacent tissues such as pleura have been used to close partial defects. In cases of left atrial herniation, some surgeons have done left atrial appendectomy. Some have favored the creation of a complete defect, if a partial defect exists, in hopes of preventing entrapment or incarceration of portions of the heart. The best treatment is probably restoration of normal anatomy if possible, thus preventing other complications of complete defects such as pleuropericarditis or adhesions of the heart, lung tissue and other adjacent tissues. Various surgical techniques have been discussed by Fosburg et al who favor anatomic closure.

**Prognosis:** The defects may be well tolerated and compatible with a normal life span. There is no effect on intellect and usually none on function. However, fatal complications such as herniation and strangulation of the left ventricle or left atrium and pleuropericarditis have been reported.

**Detection of Carrier:** Unknown.

**Special Considerations:** Reported cases continue to show the high incidence of complete left-sided defects (70%). The frequent lack of clinical symptoms and laboratory findings make the diagnosis difficult, but when suspected, a diagnostic pneumothorax may be performed and the size ascertained by cardiac catheterization. If symptoms are persistent or threatening, surgical exploration may be indicated.

**Support Groups:** Dallas; American Heart Association

**References:**

Saint Pierre A, Froment R: Absence totales et partielles du pericarde. Arch Mal Coeur 1970; 63:638–648. *

Mancada R, et al.: Diagnostic role of computed tomography in pericardial heart disease: congenital defects, thickening, neoplasms and effusions. Am Heart J 1982; 103:263–282. †

Gutierrez F, et al.: Diagnosis of congenital absence of left pericardium by MR imaging. J Comput Assist Tomogr 1985; 9:551–553.

Nasser WK: Congenital defects of the pericardium. In: Fowler NO, ed: The pericardium in health and disease. Mount Kisco, NY: Futura Publishing, 1985:51. *

Taysi K, et al.: Congenital absence of left pericardium in a family. Am J Med Genet 1985; 21:77–83.

N0004                   **Audrey H. Nora**
N0003                    **James J. Nora**

**Heart, shortened or defective valve tissue**
*See MITRAL VALVE INSUFFICIENCY*
**Heart, single transposition of great vessels**
*See HEART, TRANSPOSITION OF GREAT VESSELS*

## HEART, SUBAORTIC STENOSIS, FIBROUS      0916

**Includes:**

> Fibromuscular subaortic stenosis
> Fibrous subaortic stenosis
> Membranous subaortic stenosis
> Subaortic stenosis, discrete
> Subaortic stenosis, fibrous

**Excludes:** Heart, subaortic stenosis, muscular (0917)

**Major Diagnostic Criteria:** Identification, at left heart catheterization, of a pressure gradient between the left ventricular cavity and the aorta during systole, localized to the subaortic area of the left ventricular outflow tract.

Left ventricular angiocardiography identifies the discrete area of subvalvular stenosis.

**Clinical Findings:** The anatomic lesion consists of a membranous diaphragm or fibrous ring encircling the left ventricular outflow tract just beneath the base of the aortic valve. The clinical differentiation between stenosis of the aortic valve and fibrous subaortic stenosis is extremely difficult, and there are no clinical criteria that can be relied upon to distinguish the two forms of obstruction. Such differences in the clinical findings as do exist are of limited diagnostic help. Nevertheless, in the discrete form of subvalvular or fibrous subaortic stenosis, a systolic ejection sound is rarely heard, and the diastolic murmur of aortic regurgitation is more common than it is in valvular aortic stenosis. Also, valvular calcification is not observed on X-ray, even in adult patients with discrete subaortic stenosis. Dilation of the ascending aorta is common in patients with discrete subvalvular obstruction but is usually less prominent than in patients with valvular stenosis.

Echocardiography is most useful in the differentiation of valvular and subvalvular stenosis. The finding by single crystal methods of a fine, high-intensity echo in the left ventricular outflow tract may suggest the presence of a subaortic diaphragm. Multiple, thick echoes from a level near the annular attachment of the anterior mitral leaflet and below the sinuses of Valsalva have been observed with fibromuscular subaortic obstruction, as well as premature closure of the aortic valve associated with high frequency systolic vibrations. Cross-sectional echo studies reveal persistent, prominent echoes in the subaortic left ventricle in both systole and diastole. Echocardiography can also identify hypertrophic subaortic stenosis when it coexists with fixed subaortic stenosis, and distinguish between the two forms of obstruction.

Definitive differentiation between valvular and subvalvular obstruction is also accomplished by recording pressure tracings as a catheter is withdrawn across the outflow tract and valve or by localizing the site of obstruction with selective left ventricular angiocardiography. Even then the task may be difficult. Mild degrees of aortic valvular regurgitation are often observed in patients with fibrous subaortic stenosis; these are probably caused by thickening of the valve and impaired mobility of the cusps secondary to the trauma created by the high velocity jet passing through the subaortic diaphragm. Severe aortic regurgitation may result when these abnormal valve cusps are further deformed by the vegetations of bacterial endocarditis.

**Complications:** Aortic valve insufficiency, bacterial endocarditis, congestive heart failure, syncope, arrhythmias, and sudden death.

**Associated Findings:** Occasionally, valvular and subvalvular aortic stenosis coexist in the same patient, producing a tunnel-like narrowing of the left ventricular outflow tract.

**Etiology:** Presumably multifactorial inheritance.

**Pathogenesis:** Unknown.

**MIM No.:** 27195

**Sex Ratio:** M2:F1 (observed).

**Occurrence:** Undetermined. Probably <1:10,000 live births.

**Risk of Recurrence for Patient's Sib:** Unknown. Probably under 2%.

**Risk of Recurrence for Patient's Child:** Unknown. Probably under 2%.

**Age of Detectability:** From birth, by echocardiography and left heart catheterization and selective left ventricular angiocardiography.

**Gene Mapping and Linkage:** Unknown.

**Prevention:** None known. Genetic counseling indicated.

**Treatment:** Because of the likelihood of both progression of obstruction and aortic regurgitation, the presence of even mild-to-moderate subaortic stenosis warrants consideration of elective surgery. Surgical correction consists of excising the membrane or fibrous ridge. This may be expected to improve the hemodynamic state substantially and frequently may be totally corrective. In a small fraction of patients, secondary muscular hypertrophy of the outflow tract and a subaortic pressure gradient may persist following the operative relief of valvular or discrete subvalvular aortic stenosis. Ultimately, however, this form of outflow obstruction generally resolves as the secondary hypertrophy regresses.

**Prognosis:** The prognosis depends upon the severity of obstruction. Bacterial endocarditis or chronic trauma to the aortic valve leaflets may result in severe aortic regurgitation, which may become the predominant hemodynamic lesion. In these instances, the risk of surgical correction is increased, since the replacement of the aortic valve with a prosthesis may be necessary.

**Detection of Carrier:** Unknown.

**Support Groups:** Dallas; American Heart Association

**References:**
Braunwald E, et al.: Congenital aortic stenosis. I: clinical and hemodynamic findings in 100 patients. Circulation 1963; 27:426–462.
Edwards JE: Congenital malformations of the heart and great vessels. In: Gould SE, ed: Pathology of the heart and blood vessels, ed 3. Springfield, Illinois: Charles C Thomas, 1968:262–287.
Davis RH, et al.: Echocardiographic manifestations of discrete subaortic stenosis. Am J Cardiol: 1974; 33:277–280. *
Gale AW, et al.: Familial subaortic membranous stenosis. Aust New Zeal J Med 1974; 4:576–581.
DiSessa TG, et al.: Two dimensional echocardiographic evaluation of discrete subaortic stenosis from the apical long axis view. Am Heart J 1981; 6:774–782.
Friedman WF: Congenital aortic stenosis. In: Moss AJ, Adams FH, eds: Heart disease in infants, children and adolescents. Baltimore: Williams & Wilkins Co, 1983:171–188. *

FR019                                                       **William F. Friedman**

## HEART, SUBAORTIC STENOSIS, MUSCULAR    0917

**Includes:**
   Cardiomyopathy, hypertrophic obstructive
   Muscular subaortic stenosis
   Pseudoaortic stenosis
   Septal hypertrophy with obstruction, asymmetric
   Subaortic stenosis, idiopathic hypertrophic
   Subaortic stenosis, muscular
   Ventricle, functional obstruction of left
   Ventricular hypertrophy, hereditary

**Excludes:**
   Glycogenosis, type IIa (0011)
   Heart, subaortic stenosis, fibrous (0916)

**Major Diagnostic Criteria:** Midsystolic ejection murmur, cardiomegaly, left ventricular lift and a bifid carotid pulse. Common symptoms are fatigue, dyspnea, angina and syncope. Left ventricular hypertrophy is confirmed by X-ray and EKG. Left heart catheterization is needed to exclude cardiomyopathies other than from muscular subaortic stenosis and the discrete form of fibrous subaortic stenosis. A systolic intraventricular pressure gradient, either in the basal state or during provocation with isoproterenol, the Valsalva maneuver, or nitroglycerine can be demonstrated. Selective left ventricular angiography shows impingement in systole of the closed anterior leaflet of the mitral valve on the hypertrophied interventricular septum.

**Clinical Findings:** Marked hypertrophy of the left ventricle involving especially the ventricular septum and left ventricular outflow tract. The most important landmark in the understanding of muscular subaortic stenosis was the observations, both angiographically and echocardiographically, that abnormal systolic anterior movement of the mitral valve in proximity or contact with asymmetrically hypertrophied septum created the systolic pressure gradient. The principal determinants of the severity of obstruction are the force of LV contraction, the size of the cavity during systole and the transmural pressure which distends the outflow tract during systole. Since these factors are variable, the degree of obstruction may change from moment to moment.

The discovery of a heart murmur is usually the first clinical sign of muscular subaortic stenosis. The most common symptoms are easy fatigability, dyspnea, palpitations, angina, dizziness and syncope. Physical findings include cardiomegaly and a left ventricular lift, often with a double or triple apical impulse. Accentuation of the atrial contraction (A) wave may be noted in the jugular venous pulse. A prominent finding is a bifid carotid pulse with a rapid upstroke. Paradoxical splitting of the second heart sound and a fourth heart sound may be present. A midsystolic ejection type murmur is always present; occasionally, the regurgitant murmur of mitral incompetence is audible.

Abnormalities of the EKG include left ventricular hypertrophy with abnormally deep and broad Q waves related to gross septal hypertrophy and **Arrhythmia, Wolff-Parkinson-White type.** On X-ray, an enlarged, globular left ventricle is seen. Aortic dilatation is an uncommon finding. Evidence of right ventricular enlargement is seen in approximately half the patients.

On echocardiograph, the major abnormal finding is mitral valve systolic anterior motion apposing the mitral leaflet to the thickened septum and apparently producing the subaortic obstruction during ejection. Asymmetric septal hypertrophy, ie a septum which is greater than 1.3 times thicker than the posterior left ventricular wall, is routinely demonstrated echocardiographically. Asymmetric septal hypertrophy, without abnormal motion of the mitral valve, is present in patients with the asymptomatic or nonobstructive form of this cardiomyopathy. The disease complex appears to be inherited as an autosomal dominant trait. It should be cautioned that many normal newborns, infants of diabetic mothers, and patients with right ventricular outflow tract obstruction, sometimes have asymmetric septal hypertrophy.

At left heart catheterization, the obstruction can be localized to the left ventricular outflow tract by the demonstration of a pressure gradient between the left ventricular cavity and the subvalvar area. The zone of elevated pressure extends from the ventricular apex to the leaflets of the mitral valve. Variation of the magnitude of the systolic pressure gradient may occur in the course of a single hemodynamic study and distinguishes muscular subaortic stenosis from other forms of left ventricular obstruction. Analysis of the postextrasystolic pulse pressure response is a useful diagnostic test in these patients. In normal patients and in those with fixed forms of aortic stenosis the arterial pulse pressure in the cycle following a premature ventricular contraction is greater than normal. In patients with muscular subaortic stenosis, the postextrasystolic augmentation of the force of left ventricular contraction intensifies the obstruction and the arterial pulse pressure, following a premature ventricular contraction, does not exceed the pulse pressure of the control beat. A pressure gradient may be induced or intensified in these patients by isoproterenol infusion and the Valsalva maneuver. Angiographically, the site of obstruction can be seen as a radiolucent line in the frontal view representing contact of the leading edge of the anterior leaflet of the mitral valve with the hypertrophied muscular ventricular septum. In the left anterior oblique and lateral projections, the mitral leaflets do not swing posteriorly in a normal fashion but project into the outflow tract during mid and late systole.

**Complications:** Approximately 10% of patients with muscular subaortic stenosis have a systolic pressure gradient in excess of 10 mm Hg in the outflow tract of the right ventricle. In an occasional patient, the obstruction to right ventricular outflow is more severe than on the left. Progressive clinical deterioration with the onset of angina pectoris, syncope or symptoms of congestive heart failure may occur. Arrhythmias are the most common cause of sudden, unexpected death. Bacterial endocarditis is a rare complication.

**Associated Findings:** Infrequently, other congenital cardiovascular anomalies such as **Aorta, coarctation**, **Ventricular septal defect**, and **Ductus arteriosus, patent**.

**Etiology:** Probably autosomal dominant inheritance. It has been suggested that muscular subaortic stenosis represents only one part of the spectrum of an hypertrophic cardiomyopathy in which outflow tract obstruction may be severe, mild, or even absent. Asymmetric septal hypertrophy (ASH) is considered the characteristic anatomic abnormality that can be detected reliably and easily by either noninvasive or invasive diagnostic techniques. Conventionally, ASH is defined echocardiographically by a disproportionately thickened ventricular septum when compared to the postero-basal left ventricular free wall thickness. The disease spectrum includes many more patients with nonobstructive hypertrophy than those with ASH and left ventricular outflow tract obstruction (typical muscular subaortic stenosis). The spectrum of embraces three clinical subgroups of patients: 1) those who have no obstruction either at rest or after provocative maneuvers; 2) patients who develop obstruction after provocative maneuvers; and 3) patients who have obstruction to left ventricular outflow under resting conditions (classic muscular subaortic stenosis). It appears preferable that muscular subaortic stenosis not be considered as a clinical or physiologic entity, but rather as a form of cardiomyopathy characterized principally by asymmetric septal hypertrophy.

Family studies using echocardiography to detect disproportionate ventricular septal thickening have revealed that ASH is transmitted genetically as an autosomal dominant trait with a high degree of penetrance that occurs in an equal percentage in both sexes in preclinical and clinical forms. All clinical subtypes of the disorder may be observed in any one family.

**Pathogenesis:** Unknown.

**MIM No.:** *19260

**Sex Ratio:** M1:F1

**Occurrence:** Undetermined, but presumably <1:10,000 live births. Less than 1% of CHD. Probably somewhat more common than discrete forms of subaortic obstruction.

**Risk of Recurrence for Patient's Sib:**
See Part I, *Mendelian Inheritance*.

**Risk of Recurrence for Patient's Child:**
See Part I, *Mendelian Inheritance*.

**Age of Detectability:** From birth, by echocardiography and left heart catheterization and selective left ventricular angiocardiography.

**Gene Mapping and Linkage:** Unknown.

**Prevention:** None known. Genetic counseling indicated.

**Treatment:** Beta adrenergic and calcium channel blocking agents may temporarily alleviate symptoms in some patients. Digitalis is thought by some to be contraindicated. Left ventricular myotomy, with or without resection of a portion of the hypertrophied interventricular septum, may be expected to abolish or reduce the pressure gradient and may strikingly ameliorate symptoms in the great majority of patients who are severely disabled by their disease. However, the primary myocardial disease process is not amenable to surgical correction.

**Prognosis:** Variable. Patients who are asymptomatic tend to remain so, while those who are disabled at initial detection generally deteriorate or die. Familial cases may have a higher incidence of sudden death.

**Detection of Carrier:** Possibly by clinical examination of first degree relatives.

**Support Groups:** Dallas; American Heart Association

**References:**
Frank S, Braunwald E: Idiopathic hypertrophic subaortic stenosis: clincial analysis of 126 patients with emphasis on the natural history. Circulation 1968; 37:759–788. *
Abbasi AS, et al.: Echocardiographic diagnosis of idiopathic hypertrophic cardiomyopathy without outflow obstruction. Circulation 1972; 46:897–904.
Henry WL, et al.: Asymmetric septal hypertrophy (ASH): the unifying link in the IHSS disease spectrum: observations regarding its pathogenesis, pathophysiology and course. Circulation 1973; 47: 827–832.
Larter WL, et al.: The asymmetrically hypertrophied septum: further differentiation of its causes. Circulation 1976; 53:9–19.
Maron BJ: Cardiomyopathies. In: Moss' heart disease in infants, children and adolescents. Baltimore: Williams & Wilkins, 1983:757–780. *
Greaves SC, et al.: Inheritance of hypertropic cardiomyopathy: a cross-rectional and M mode echocardiographic study of 50 families. Brit Heart J 1987; 58:259–266.
Maron BJ, et al.: Hypertropic cardiomyopathy: interrelations of clinical manifestations, pathophysiology, and therapy. New Engl J Med 1987; 316:780–789.

FR019                                          **William F. Friedman**

## HEART, TETRALOGY OF FALLOT                              0938

**Includes:** Tetralogy of Fallot

**Excludes:**
Pulmonary atresia with intact ventricular septum
Ventricular septal defect-pulmonary valve stenosis-normal crista

**Major Diagnostic Criteria:** Cyanosis, systolic murmur, single second sound, normal heart size, right ventricular hypertrophy on EKG suggest tetralogy of Fallot. A right aortic arch in addition strengthens the diagnosis. Selective right ventricular angiocardiography is confirmatory, but echocardiography-Doppler studies are usually diagnostic.

**Clinical Findings:** The pathologic anatomy of this lesion consists of the combination of a large ventricular septal defect (VSD) and narrowing of the infundibulum. The right ventricular outflow tract stenosis may occur at the ostium of the infundibulum or may consist of a diminutive infundibulum throughout with a small annulus of the pulmonary valve. Valvar stenosis occurs in association with infundibular narrowing in 25% of patients.

Since the VSD is large, variations in the physiologic state depend upon the severity of the infundibular stenosis, which is the primary regulator of pulmonary blood flow. The course may be variable. The onset of cyanosis during the first month of life is associated with a severe course and progressive cyanosis. Most patients demonstrate cyanosis during the first 6 months; this usually becomes accentuated over 1–3 years. Clubbing of the fingers and toes may be present in cyanotic patients after 6 months of age. A loud systolic murmur over the upper left sternal border is characteristic; with severe tetralogy and marked diminution in pulmonary blood flow, the murmur may be short and of low intensity. The second sound is single and accentuated (due to aortic valve closure). Continuous murmurs may be present after infancy and indicate systemic-pulmonary collateral circulation or the presence of **Ductus arteriosus, patent**.

X-ray findings demonstrate a normal size heart and concavity in the area of the main pulmonary artery. A right aortic arch is present in 25% of patients. Left atrial enlargement is absent. With increasing degree of diminished pulmonary blood flow, pulmonary vascular markings are commensurately diminished. With marked increase in collateral blood flow, the lung fields present a reticular appearance.

EKG shows right ventricular hypertrophy and right axis deviation. Right atrial hypertrophy may be evident.

Echocardiographic findings parallel those of recognized anatomic derangement. The aorta is enlarged and aortic intercusp distance is increased. The anterior aortic wall is displaced anteriorly with respect to the ventricular septum and is not in continuity with it. This discontinuity represents aortic override in the area of the VSD. Right ventricular anterior wall is thickened and the right ventricular outflow tract is narrow. The pulmonary valve may be found in most patients and its presence rules out **Heart, truncus arteriosus** and **Pulmonary valve, atresia**. In other patients, the pulmonary valve is present but difficult to image. The right pulmonary artery is usually small, but may be of normal size. Doppler studies show a large right ventricular to pulmonary artery systolic gradient.

Cardiac catheterization with selective angiocardiography confirms and clarifies the anatomy of the infundibular stenosis, as well as the pulmonary artery size and branch stenoses. Oxygen saturation data indicate the pulmonary blood flow and degree of right-to-left shunt.

**Complications:** Episodes of paroxysmal hyperpnea, with death from severe episodes, brain abscess, bacterial endocarditis, and cerebral thrombosis.

**Associated Findings:** Rarely, **Chromosome 21, trisomy 21** or other complex malformation syndromes.

**Etiology:** Multifactorial inheritance.

**Pathogenesis:** Displacement of the conus septum anteriorly which produces infundibular stenosis. This results in inability to form the normal crista supraventricularis, and to close the interventricular septum.

**MIM No.:** 18750

**CDC No.:** 745.2

**Sex Ratio:** M3:F2

**Occurrence:** Estimated 1:1,000 in pediatric population. Ten percent of congenital heart disease.

**Risk of Recurrence for Patient's Sib:** About 2.5%.

**Risk of Recurrence for Patient's Child:** If mother is affected, empiric risk is 2.6%. If father is affected, empiric risk is 1.4%.

**Age of Detectability:** From birth, by selective angiocardiography.

**Gene Mapping and Linkage:** Unknown.

**Prevention:** None known. Genetic counseling indicated.

**Treatment:** Definitive surgery with infundibulectomy and closure of ventricular defect. Surgical palliation with anastomosis of subclavian-to-pulmonary artery (Blalock-Taussig operation) can be used to palliate. Treatment of paroxysmal hyperpnea episodes and prevention of dehydration.

**Prognosis:** Depends upon the severity of pulmonary stenosis and resultant degree of cyanosis. With surgical intervention, the prognosis is good. Infants who survive to undergo definitive surgical repair have good prognosis. Recent marked improvements in definitive and palliative operations have considerably

improved the success rate with severely cyanotic infants and some can undergo primary repair without palliative shunts.

**Detection of Carrier:** Unknown.

**Support Groups:** Dallas; American Heart Association

**References:**

Guntheroth WG: Tetralogy of Fallot. In: Adams FH, Emmanouilides GC eds: Heart disease in infants, children, and adolescents, 3rd ed. Baltimore: Williams & Wilkins, Co., 1983:215–227. *
Sanders SP: Echocardiography and related techniques in the diagnosis of congenital heart defects. Part III. Conotruncus and great arteries. Echocardiography: a review of cardiovascular ultrasound 1984; 1:443–493.
Der Kaloustian VM, et al.: Tetralogy of Fallot with pulmonary atresia in siblings. Am J Med Genet 1985; 21:119–122.
Hammon JW, et al.: Tetralogy of Fallot: selective operative management can minimize mortality. Ann Thor Surg 1985; 40:280–284.
Jones MC, Waldman JD: An autosomal dominant syndrome of characteristic facial appearance, preauricular pits, fifth finger clinodactyly, and tetralogy of Fallot. Am J Med Genet 1985; 22:135–141.
Graham TP Jr, et al.: Conotruncal abnormalities in the neonate. In: Long WA, ed: Fetal and Neonatal cardiology. Philadelphia: W.B. Saunders, 1989.

GR002                                   **Thomas P. Graham Jr.**

---

**HEART, TRANSPOSITION OF GREAT VESSELS          0962**

**Includes:**

Great vessel transposition
Heart, complete d-transposition
Heart, noninverted transposition
Heart, single transposition of great vessels
Heart, uncorrected transposition of great vessels
Transposition of great vessels
True transposition of great vessels

**Excludes:**

Atretic atrioventricular valve-transposition of great vessels
Ventricle, double inlet left
**Ventricle, double-outlet right with anterior septal defect** (0297)
**Ventricle, double-outlet right with posterior septal defect** (0298)
**Ventricles, inverted without transposition of great arteries** (0541)

**Major Diagnostic Criteria:** A newborn who shows: 1) cyanosis, 2) an EKG that is normal, or shows minimal signs of right ventricular hypertrophy, 3) a single second sound, 4) a normal or only questionably abnormal X-ray, and 5) no evidence of pulmonary disease, complete transposition is by far the most likely diagnosis. However, the confirmation of complete transposition, as well as associated anomalies, is by selective angiocardiography. Right and left ventriculography are recommended in most cases. The latter is especially important in ruling out obstructive malformations involving the subpulmonary and pulmonary valve areas. Diagnosis should never be based upon the location and course of the ascending aorta in the frontal view. At least 20% of the cases will show a great vessel relationship similar to that seen in cases of ventricular inversion.

**Clinical Findings:** In complete transposition, there are two functioning ventricles. The aorta, with the coronary arteries in turn arising from it, takes origin from the right ventricle, while the pulmonary trunk takes origin exclusively from the left ventricle. The anterior leaflet of the mitral valve is in continuity with pulmonary valvar tissue. Both AV valves are patent and have the corresponding structure of the right- and left-sided valves of the normal heart. If life is maintained after birth, some communication must exist between the systemic and pulmonary circulations. These potential communications are 1) patent foramen ovale or **Atrial septal defects**, 2) **Ventricular septal defect** (VSD), 3) **Ductus arteriosus, patent** (PDA), 4) any combination of the foregoing, 5) bronchial arteries. The communications may be large or small. In somewhat less than half the cases, the ventricular septum is intact. The anterior-posterior relationship between the aorta and pulmonary artery varies. Commonly, the pulmonary artery is situated posterior and to the left of the aorta or lies directly behind it. Uncommonly, the two great vessels lie side-to-side. The right coronary artery arises above the posterior aortic valve cusp and the left coronary artery arises above the left aortic cusp; the right or anterior cusp is the noncoronary one. Theoretically, many isolated lesions may be associated with complete transposition. Certain defects tend to occur with a higher degree of frequency than others. These are shunt lesions such as VSD or PDA. Less commonly, VSD and pulmonary stenosis occur. In the latter, there is a relatively high incidence of right aortic arch. Coarctation of the aorta, interruption of the aortic arch, hypoplasia of the right ventricle rarely occur with this condition.

The hemodynamic alterations vary according to the associated malformations. The pathologic arrangement of the two great vessels establishes the following two circulations: 1) the systemic venous blood enters the right atrium, proceeds to the right ventricle and passes out the aorta to the peripheral circulation where it returns to the systemic veins; 2) meanwhile, the pulmonary venous blood enters the left atrium, enters the left ventricle, then the pulmonary artery and back into the pulmonary veins. Thus, potentially there are two completely independent circulations. Since life depends on desaturated venous blood reaching the lungs and oxygenated blood reaching the peripheral arterial circulation, some means of communication between the two circulations must exist. The less the communication between the two circulations, the more systemic venous blood reaches the periphery without passing through the pulmonary capillary bed, and thus the more cyanotic the infant. When a large VSD or PDA is present, easy mixing between arterial and venous streams is possible. When pulmonary flow exceeds systemic flow because pulmonary vascular resistance is lower, a relatively large amount of highly oxygenated blood is available to mix with a relatively small amount of desaturated blood. Here, cyanosis may be minimal. However, in large communications, pulmonary resistance may eventually exceed systemic resistance, and the "Eisenmenger physiology" stage is reached. Pulmonary flow may also be diminished when pulmonary stenosis exists.

The typical history is that of a male infant (usually not a first-born child), who is noted to be cyanotic and tachypneic shortly after birth. Congestive heart failure follows, with hepatomegaly and increased tachypnea. The infant is often chubby, round-faced and has a higher than average birthweight. On auscultation, the first sound is followed by a short, soft systolic murmur and a loud single second sound. When a large VSD exists, the systolic murmur is of a loud regurgitant quality and both components of $S_2$ are noted. When pulmonary stenosis exists (usually with a VSD), the murmurs are again prominent. Congestive heart failure usually does not occur with the latter combination of defects.

The EKG usually indicates the size of the communication between the systemic and venous circulations. However, the EKG may be normal in the first two weeks of life. In patients with a small communication or shunt, the EKG usually reveals pure right ventricular hypertrophy. In patients with large communications, the EKG usually shows biventricular hypertrophy. Complete transposition is one form of transposition complex which shows Q waves in the left precordial leads. Left axis deviation may be present when the following lesions are associated: 1) coarctation or interruption of the aorta, 2) hypoplastic right ventricle, or 3) endocardial cushion defect.

The characteristic X-ray findings are prominent pulmonary vascularity of a shunt type together with a globular-shaped heart and a narrow mediastinum. The right heart in the posterior-anterior and left anterior oblique views is enlarged in nearly all cases. The left atrium is enlarged in the presence of increased flow. During the first one or two weeks of life, the heart and vasculature may appear normal or only slightly prominent. Other cyanotic or admixture lesions may mimic the X-ray findings in complete transposition. In cases with pulmonary stenosis and VSD, the vasculature appears normal or diminished. The cardiac silhouette often resembles **Heart, tetralogy of Fallot**.

The echocardiographic diagnosis of transposition of the great vessels rests on the identification of abnormal great vessel relationships, ie an anterior and rightward or midline aorta compared to a posterior pulmonary artery. Techniques for achieving this differentiation involve 1) using right and left transducer movements on single-crystal echocardiography to determine the rightward anterior great vessel, or 2) demonstrating simultaneous superimposition of 1 great vessel upon another, both in the same A-P plane, suggesting the lack of the normal spiral relationship. The latter finding has many false-positives in normal newborns. Several authors have utilized the longer pre-ejection period and shorter ejection time parameter measured in a systematic circuit in an attempt to use valve timing to separate aortas from pulmonary arteries. Nevertheless, the diagnosis of the transposed great vessel relationship regardless of situs is most reliably made using real-time cross-sectional echocardiography.

Cardiac catheterization will determine oxygen saturations in the four cardiac chambers and great arteries. The peripheral oxygen saturation is uniformly higher among patients with large communications versus those with small communications when pulmonary vascular resistance is less than systemic vascular resistance. Determination of pulmonary artery and left ventricular pressures is important in calculating the comparable systemic vascular resistance and pulmonary vascular resistance which determines ultimate operability. Oximetry data in the calculation of shunts is not reliable since the great artery and ventricular samples are strongly influenced by streaming and bidirectional shunting at one or more levels.

**Complications:** During the first year, death occurs from congestive heart failure and pneumonia in approximately 90% of the cases unless palliative surgery is performed. If the individual survives infancy, high pulmonary vascular resistance develops which eventually leads to "Eisenmenger physiology". In cases with severe pulmonary stenosis or atresia, clubbing and hypoxic spells occur as well as other symptoms.

**Associated Findings:** None known.

**Etiology:** Multifactorial inheritance.

**Pathogenesis:** Complete transposition is thought to be due to a single embryologic error; an error which takes place in the truncus arteriosus. In normal development there are two pairs of truncus swellings which actively partition the truncus: the major pair are termed dextrodorsal and sinistroventral conus swellings; the other pair (the intercalated valve swellings) form a pair of semilunar valve cusps of each great artery. It is postulated that complete (or d-) transposition is the result of the wrong truncus swellings becoming the major pair. The pulmonary and aortic intercalated valve swellings partition the truncus and respectively align themselves with the sinistroventral and dextrodorsal conus swellings. As a result, the aorta arises from the right ventricle anteriorly and the pulmonary artery from the left ventricle posteriorly. The conus septum develops normally; its derivatives, the crista supraventricularis, the medial portion of the tricuspid valve, and the medial papillary muscle are normal.

**CDC No.:** 745.1

**Sex Ratio:** Approximately M2:F1

**Occurrence:** Incidence estimated 1:2,000 live births. Prevalence < 1:2,000 in the pediatric population.

**Risk of Recurrence for Patient's Sib:** Estimated at 1.5%.

**Risk of Recurrence for Patient's Child:** Unknown. Reproductive fitness greatly diminished.

**Age of Detectability:** From birth, by selective angiocardiography.

**Gene Mapping and Linkage:** Unknown.

**Prevention:** None known. Genetic counseling indicated.

**Treatment:** *Palliative:* Creation of an atrial septal defect surgically (Blalock-Hanlon procedure) or medically by tearing the rim of the foramen ovale by the Rashkind procedure: a balloon-tipped catheter is passed via the femoral vein through the foramen ovale into the left atrium. Additional procedures are: surgical banding of the pulmonary artery among patients with excess blood flow to the lungs, or performing a shunt procedure, Blalock-Taussig or Waterston-Cooley, in patients with decreased pulmonary flow.

*Corrective*: The Mustard operation has been found to produce the best results and has superseded older techniques. At cardiopulmonary bypass, the atrial septum is removed and a pericardial graft is sutured into the atrium so that pulmonary venous blood is directed into the right ventricle and the systemic venous blood into the left ventricle.

Symptomatic therapy is recommended for congestive heart failure and pneumonia.

**Prognosis:** Death occurs in approximately 90% of affected individuals before six months of age, unless adequate intracardiac shunting is surgically provided. Those who survive infancy without operation are represented by the additional anomalies: pulmonary stenosis with VSD, or high pulmonary vascular resistance.

**Detection of Carrier:** Unknown.

**Support Groups:** Dallas; American Heart Association

**References:**

Elliot LP, et al.: Complete transposition of the great vessels. I. an anatomic study of sixty cases. Circulation 1963; 27:1105.

Mustard WT, et al.: The surgical management of transposition of the great vessels. J Thorac Cardiovasc Surg 1964; 48:953.

Gramiak R, et al.: Echocardiographic diagnosis of transposition of the great vessels. Radiology 1973; 106:187.

Sahn DJ, et al.: Multiple crystal cross-sectional echocardiography in the diagnosis of cyanotic congenital heart disease. Circulation 1974; 50:230.

Paul MH: Transposition of the great arteries. In: Adams FH, Emmanoulides GC, eds: Heart disease in infants, children, and adolescents, 3rd ed. Baltimore: Williams & Wilkins, 1983:296–333. *

EL004                                                    **Larry P. Elliott**

**Heart, tricuspid valve atresia**
  *See TRICUSPID VALVE, ATRESIA*
**Heart, tricuspid valve insufficiency**
  *See TRICUSPID VALVE, INSUFFICIENCY*

---

## HEART, TRUNCUS ARTERIOSUS                          0972

**Includes:** Truncus arteriosus (persistent) types I-III

**Excludes:**
  **Aortico-pulmonary septal defect** (0083)
  **Pulmonary artery, origin from ascending aorta** (0767)
  **Pulmonary valve, absent** (0836)

**Major Diagnostic Criteria:** Angiocardiography is the procedure of choice to confirm the diagnosis. Either selective ascending thoracic "aortography" or right ventriculography will delineate the anatomic abnormalities. Since in this malformation there is a certain degree of maldevelopment of the conus septum, the latter procedure will characteristically show absence of a well-developed right ventricular infundibulum.

**Clinical Findings:** The pathologic anatomy of this lesion is characterized by the presence of a large single arterial vessel at the base of the heart (without any remnant of either an atretic aorta or pulmonary trunk) from which the aortic arch, pulmonary and coronary arteries originate. The truncal valve is usually tricuspid but may be bicuspid or have four or more cusps. A large subvalvar ventricular septal defect is always present.

Three anatomic types have been described according to the site of origin of the arteries supplying the lungs. In the most common, type I, the pulmonary arteries arise from the left inferior aspect of the common arterial trunk by means of a short main stem. Less frequently, the pulmonary arteries arise close together from the dorsal wall (type II) or independently from either side of the truncus (type III). Cases previously defined as type IV are probably not true examples of truncus arteriosus. A right aortic arch is present in approximately 25% of the cases. Associated extracardiac anomalies are common.

The hemodynamic alterations and consequently the clinical manifestations will vary according to the magnitude of pulmonary blood flow. In the common types, with large unobstructed pulmonary arteries arising from the arterial trunk, pulmonary blood flow is greatly increased. This is the case in infants and small children with low resistance in the pulmonary vascular bed. They present with the physical findings of a large extracardiac left-to-right shunt. Cyanosis is only minimal or absent and the infants usually have congestive heart failure, frequent respiratory infections and growth retardation. A loud systolic murmur along the lower left sternal border is always present. It is characteristically preceded by a constant ejection click and ends before the second sound. The second sound is described as loud and single but "splitting" is not uncommon. A diastolic apical flow murmur is frequently present. Early diastolic murmurs of truncal valve insufficiency may also be present. Continuous, machinery-type murmurs are rare. With the development of a high pulmonary vascular resistance, the left-to-right shunt gradually diminishes, the patient becomes progressively more cyanotic and the apical diastolic flow murmur disappears.

The X-ray findings depend on which hemodynamic situation is present. In the usual case, with a large left-to-right shunt, cardiomegaly and prominent pulmonary vascularity are the rule. In the presence of a right aortic arch these findings are highly suggestive of persistent truncus arteriosus. If the pulmonary vascular resistance increases, the magnitude of the left-to-right shunt progressively diminishes. Consequently the cardiomegaly and pulmonary plethora decrease.

The EKG commonly shows normal mean QRS axis for age, atrial enlargement and biventricular hypertrophy. With high resistance in the pulmonary vascular bed, right axis deviation and right ventricular hypertrophy are usually present.

Abnormalities of the tetralogy/truncus group are characterized echocardiographically by the demonstration of preservation of mitral-aortic continuity with a lack of septal aortic continuity; that is, aortic override. M-mode echocardiographic differentiation between tetralogy and truncus requires the demonstration of a pulmonary valve. As this is often difficult to do in severe tetralogy, it is a hazardous differential diagnosis. Both lesions often have concomitant thickening of the right ventricular wall and enlargement of the right ventricular cavity. In many patients with truncus arteriosus, the degree of override is greater, and at times multiple abnormal truncal valve cusp echoes may be imaged to aid in the differential diagnosis. 2-D echocardiography allows visualization of the cono-truncal anatomy, and the pulmonary arteries originating from the truncus.

Cardiac catheterization will usually confirm the presence of high flow, high pressure, intra- and extracardiac, bidirectional shunt. Oximetry data are not reliable, since right ventricular, pulmonary artery, and aortic samples are strongly influenced by streaming. A left-to-right shunt at the ventricular level may go undetected, and aortic oxygen saturation may exceed pulmonary artery saturation.

**Complications:** Truncal valve insufficiency, death from congestive heart failure, and pneumonia, frequent development of high pulmonary vascular resistance leading eventually to the "Eisenmenger physiology." Subacute bacterial endocarditis later in life.

**Associated Findings:** A high incidence of extracardiac congenital anomalies has been reported (up to 50%). Most common are absence or hypoplasia of one kidney, absent gallbladder, hypoplastic lung, and cleft palate or bony abnormalities. **Immunodeficiency, thymic agenesis**.

**Etiology:** Probably multifactorial inheritance.

**Pathogenesis:** Most likely due to failure of division of the embryonic truncus arteriosus with consequent abnormal development of the truncoconal area, resulting in a single semilunar valve and a subvalvar ventricular septal defect. The difference between the described anatomic types may well result from the lack of development of the truncus septum alone (type I) or in association with nondevelopment of the aorticopulmonary septum (types II and III).

**CDC No.:** 745.000

**Sex Ratio:** M1:F1

**Occurrence:** Prevalence approaches 1:33,000. Approximately 1:200 cases of congenital heart defects

**Risk of Recurrence for Patient's Sib:** Predicted risk and empiric risk for truncus or developmentally related lesion 1:100.

**Risk of Recurrence for Patient's Child:** Unknown.

**Age of Detectability:** From birth, by 2-D echocardiography or selective angiocardiography.

**Gene Mapping and Linkage:** Unknown.

**Prevention:** None known. Genetic counseling indicated.

**Treatment:** Palliative banding of the pulmonary arteries to prevent the development of pulmonary vascular changes. Repair of the ventricular septal defect and construction of a pulmonary trunk with a valved external conduit or pulmonary homograft. Symptomatic therapy for congestive heart failure and pneumonia.

**Prognosis:** Depends upon the anatomic type, and in particular, the magnitude of the pulmonary blood flow. Prognosis is generally poor in infants with excessive blood flow to the lungs. Most of these children die within the first year. The few patients who survive infancy develop high pulmonary vascular resistance and have only a small increase in pulmonary blood flow. They have a better short-term prognosis, with a relatively normal life during childhood.

**Detection of Carrier:** Unknown.

**Support Groups:** Dallas; American Heart Association

**References:**
Raatikka M, et al.: Familial third and fourth pharyngeal pouch syndrome with truncus arteriosus. Pediatrics 1981; 67:173–175.
Rice MJ, et al.: Definitive diagnosis of truncus arteriosus by two-dimensional echocardiograph. Mayo Clin Proc 1982; 57:476–481. * †
DiDonato RM, et al.: Fifteen-year experience with surgical repair of truncus arteriosus. J Thorac Cardiovasc Surg 1985; 89:414–422.
Butto F, et al.: Persistent truncus arteriosus: Pathologic anatomy in 54 cases. Ped Cardiol 1986; 7:95–101. *

VI001                                    **Benjamin E. Victorica**

**Heart, uncorrected transposition of great vessels**
*See HEART, TRANSPOSITION OF GREAT VESSELS*

---

**HEART-HAND SYNDROME**                              **0455**

**Includes:**
    Atriodigital dysplasia
    Cardiac limb syndrome
    Cardiomelic syndrome
    Hand-heart syndrome
    Heart-upper limb syndrome
    Holt-Oram syndrome
    Upper limb cardiovascular syndrome

**Excludes:**
    Autosomal trisomies
    **Chondroectodermal dysplasia** (0156)
    **Heart-hand syndrome** (other)
    **Pancytopenia syndrome, Fanconi type** (2029)
    **Radial defects** (0853)
    **Thrombocytopenia-absent radius** (0941)
    **Vater association** (0987)

**Major Diagnostic Criteria:** Thumb anomaly (triphalangism, hypoplasia or absence) with congenital heart disease.

**Clinical Findings:** Congenital heart disease, usually secundum atrial septal defect (ASD), and skeletal anomalies of the upper limb, usually thumb hypoplasia, triphalangism or absence; upper limb phocomelia occasionally occurs. The 1st metacarpal has both a proximal and a distal epiphyseal ossification center and the carpal bones may be either absent or increased in number. The triphalangeal thumb is usually in the same plane as the fingers. The radius, ulna, and humerus may be abnormal; inability to supinate and pronate the hand is common. The scapulae and clavicles may also be anomalous and the pectoralis major absent;

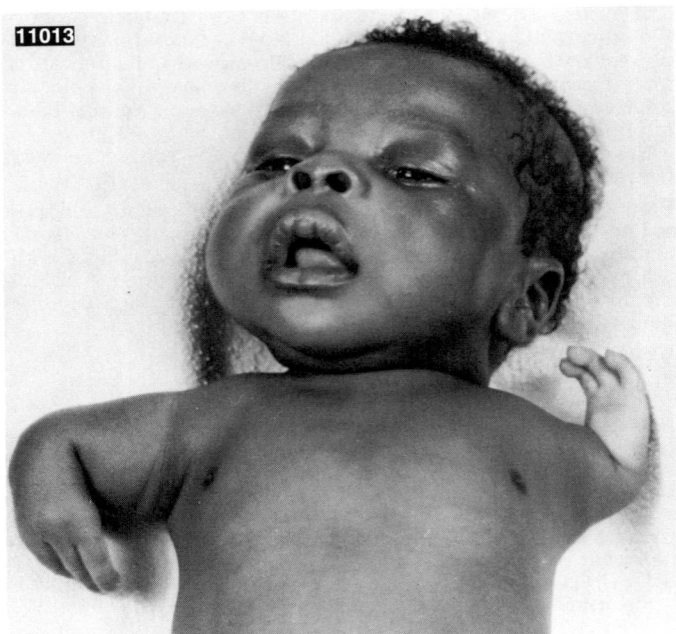

**0455A-11013:** Phocomelia of arms with three digits on each hand.

pectus excavatum has been reported. The lower limbs are not affected. Abnormalities of other systems have been reported infrequently. Mental retardation is not a characteristic of the syndrome.

The cardiac anomaly is ASD in over two-thirds of the cases; other congenital heart defects reported include the following: patent ductus arteriosus, coarctation of the aorta, ventricular septal defect (VSD), transposition of the great vessels, single coronary artery and prolapsed mitral valve. EKG may show a prolonged P-R interval; atrial arrythmias occur. Occasionally either the cardiac or upper limb anomalies occur alone. Families have been reported where VSD occurs consistently as the cardiac anomaly; this may indicate genetic heterogeneity in the heart-hand syndrome. A significant proportion of cases are sporadic. Careful studies of the heart and upper limb skeleton should be performed on family members prior to assuming a new mutation.

**Complications:** Functional limitations due to limb deformities.

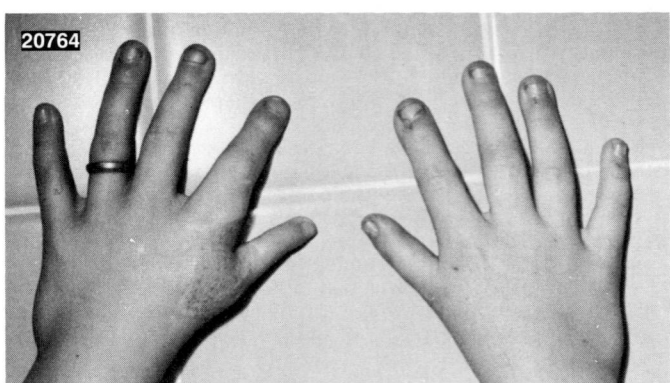

**0455B-20764:** Bilateral hypoplasia of the thumbs in this subject with an atrial septal defect.

**Associated Findings:** None known.

**Etiology:** Autosomal dominant inheritance with variable expression.

**Pathogenesis:** Undetermined. Similar skeletal and cardiac abnormalities are seen as a result of thalidomide embryopathy, the critical time being the 4th and 5th weeks of pregnancy. It is likely that in this syndrome the abnormal gene is active at this same stage in embryogenesis.

**MIM No.:** *14290

**POS No.:** 3247, 3990

**CDC No.:** 759.840

**Sex Ratio:** M1:F1

**Occurrence:** Uncommon, but cases have been reported from many different populations and in both Caucasians and Blacks.

**Risk of Recurrence for Patient's Sib:**
See Part I, *Mendelian Inheritance.*

**Risk of Recurrence for Patient's Child:**
See Part I, *Mendelian Inheritance.*

**Age of Detectability:** In infancy by clinical examination; prenatal detection is possible with ultrasonography.

**Gene Mapping and Linkage:** Unknown.

**Prevention:** None known. Genetic counseling indicated.

**Treatment:** Appropriate operative treatment for congenital heart disease and for skeletal anomalies.

**Prognosis:** Normal for intelligence. Life span and function depend upon cardiac and limb anomalies.

**Detection of Carrier:** Minimal expression may be detected by physical examination, EKG, and diagnostic imaging.

**Support Groups:** Dallas; American Heart Association

**References:**
Holt M, Oram S: Familial heart disease with skeletal malformations. Br Heart J 1960; 22:236–242.
Gall JC, Jr., et al.: Holt-Oram syndrome: clinical and genetic study of a large family. Am J Hum Genet 1966; 18:187–200.
Silver W, et al.: The Holt-Oram syndrome with previously undescribed associated anomalies. Am J Dis Child 1972; 124:911–914.
Smith AT, et al.: Holt-Oram syndrome. J Pediat 1979; 95:538–543.
Gladstone I, Sybert VP: Holt-Oram syndrome: penetrance of the gene and lack of maternal effect. Clin Genet 1982; 21:98–103. *
Van Regemorter N, et al.: Holt-Oram syndrome mistaken for thalidomide embryopathy: embryological considerations. Europ J Pediatr 1982; 138:77–80.
Zhang K-Z, et al.: Holt-Oram syndrome in China: a collective review of 18 cases. Am Heart J 1986; 111:572–577.

PA006                                              **G. Shashidhar Pai**

## HEART-HAND SYNDROME II                        3265

**Includes:** Tabatznik syndrome

**Excludes:** Heart-hand syndrome (other)

**Major Diagnostic Criteria:** The combination of upper limb anomalies and congenital cardiac arhythmias should suggest the diagnosis.

**Clinical Findings:** The upper limb malformations consist of sloping shoulders, hypoplastic deltoid muscles, short arms, and **Brachydactyly** D. On X-ray, bowing of the radius and ulna can be present, as well as absence of the ulnar styloid process. The cardiac arhythmias have been described as paroxsmal atrial fibrillation or tachycardia, and all individuals had abnormal EKG findings. Displacement of the heart to the right (2/4) and cardiomegaly (1/4) were also described.

**Complications:** Unknown.

**Associated Findings:** Scoliosis (see **Spine, scoliosis, idiopathic** may also be an associated feature. **Pectus excavatum** was present in one affected child.

**Etiology:** X-linked dominant inheritance is most likely.

**Pathogenesis:** Unknown.

**Sex Ratio:** M1:F1

**Occurrence:** One family has been documented.

**Risk of Recurrence for Patient's Sib:**
See Part I, *Mendelian Inheritance.*

**Risk of Recurrence for Patient's Child:**
See Part I, *Mendelian Inheritance.*

**Age of Detectability:** At birth, and potentially prenatally by ultrasound.

**Gene Mapping and Linkage:** Unknown.

**Prevention:** None known. Genetic counseling indicated.

**Treatment:** Supportive.

**Prognosis:** Life span appears to be unaffected.

**Detection of Carrier:** Unknown.

**References:**
Temtamy S, McKusick VA: The genetics of hand malformations. BD:OAS XIV(3). New York: March of Dimes Birth Defects Foundation, 1978:241–244.

T0007                                              **Helga V. Toriello**

## HEART-HAND SYNDROME III                        3266

**Includes:** Heart-hand syndrome, Spanish type

**Excludes:** Heart-hand syndrome (other)

**Major Diagnostic Criteria:** The combination of limb anomalies (most commonly **Brachydactyly**) with cardiac defects (sick sinus or intraventricular conduction defects) should suggest the diagnosis.

**Clinical Findings:** All affected individuals in the reported family had brachydactyly type C, characterized by hypoplasia of the middle phalanges (with occasional involvement of proximal phalanges or metacarpals as well) of digits 2–5 of hands and feet. Cardiac defects include sick sinus syndrome, incomplete bundle branch block, or anterior fascicular block. Individuals with the latter two cardiac conditions were asymptomatic.

**Complications:** The individual with sick sinus syndrome experienced syncope, palpitation, and dizziness.

**Associated Findings:** None known.

**Etiology:** Autosomal dominant inheritance.

**Pathogenesis:** Unknown.

**MIM No.:** *14045

**Sex Ratio:** M1:F1

**Occurrence:** One family from Spain has been reported.

**Risk of Recurrence for Patient's Sib:**
See Part I, *Mendelian Inheritance.*

**Risk of Recurrence for Patient's Child:**
See Part I, *Mendelian Inheritance.*

**Age of Detectability:** Potentially during infancy by the presence of brachydactyly; abnormal EKG findings would confirm the diagnosis.

**Gene Mapping and Linkage:** Unknown.

**Prevention:** None known. Genetic counseling indicated.

**Treatment:** Insertion of a cardiac pacemaker may be useful.

**Prognosis:** Mental development is normal; life span is unlikely to be affected.

**Detection of Carrier:** Unknown.

**References:**
De la Fuente SR, Prieto F: Heart-hand syndrome III: a new syndrome in three generations. Hum Genet 1980; 55:43–47.

T0007                                              **Helga V. Toriello**

## HEART-HAND SYNDROME IV                                    3272

**Includes:**

Cardiomelic dysplasia-mesoaxial hexadactyly
Mexican cardiomelic dysplasia
Mesoaxial hexadactyly-cardiac malformation
Postaxial polydactyly-dental-vertebral syndrome
Rogers syndrome

**Excludes:**

**Chondroectodermal dysplasia** (0156)
**Heart-hand syndrome** (others)
**Oculo-cerebro-facial syndrome, Kaufman type** (2179)

**Major Diagnostic Criteria:**  The combination of facial dysmorphism, cardiac defects, and **Polydactyly.**

**Clinical Findings:**  This condition has been reported in one pair of sibs (one male, one female). The propositus was 17 years old at the time of the report; his sister died at age six days and was determined to be affected retrospectively. The propositus was described as being small at birth, with bilateral polydactyly, dyspnea, and natal teeth observed. At age 13 years he had short stature (3rd centile), mental retardation, wide forehead, telecanthus, ocular torticollis, tented nares, lateral pits in the alae nasi, short philtrum, macrostomia, everted lower lip, dental diastemata and malocclusion, large pinnae, prominent antihelix, short neck, hypoplastic nipples, genital hypoplasia, mesoaxial hexadactyly, cutaneous **Syndactyly** (digits 2–3), thenar and hypothenar hypoplasia, right hallucal polysyndactyly, and flattened toenails. X-rays showed delayed bone age, osteopenia, cervical scoliosis, and thinning of the cortices. Cardiac evaluation revealed pulmonary stenosis, persistent ductus arteriosus, single atrium, and **Ventricular septal defect.** The deceased sister had low birthweight, hexadactyly, and cardiac anomalies.

**Complications:**  Unknown.

**Associated Findings:**  None known.

**Etiology:**  Autosomal recessive inheritance seems likely.

**Pathogenesis:**  Unknown.

**MIM No.:**  24967, 26354

**Sex Ratio:**  M1:F1

**Occurrence:**  One family from Mexico has been described.

**Risk of Recurrence for Patient's Sib:**
See Part I, *Mendelian Inheritance.*

**Risk of Recurrence for Patient's Child:**
See Part I, *Mendelian Inheritance.*

**Age of Detectability:**  At birth, although prenatal ultrasound may be useful if polydactyly can be demonstrated.

**Gene Mapping and Linkage:**  Unknown.

**Prevention:**  None known. Genetic counseling indicated.

**Treatment:**  Supportive.

**Prognosis:**  One child died in the neonatal period, the other was alive at 17 years of age. Mental retardation was moderate (IQ = 57).

**Detection of Carrier:**  Unknown.

**Special Considerations:**  A similar condition was reported by (Rogers et al. 1977), in that their patients also had short stature, prominent nose, malformed ears, short neck, broad appearing chest, polydactyly, and cardiac defects. Additional anomalies included fused teeth, webbed neck, vertebral anomalies, and renal defects. The polydactyly was postaxial in these patients, whereas the children described above had mesaxial polydactyly.

**References:**
Rogers JG, et al.: A postaxial polydactyly-dental-vertebral syndrome. J Pediatr 1977; 90:230–235.
Martinez R, et al.: A new probably autosomal recessive cardiomelic dysplasia with mesoaxial hexadactyly. J Med Genet 1981; 18:151–154.

T0007                                                    **Helga V. Toriello**

---

**Heart-hand syndrome, Spanish type**
*See HEART-HAND SYNDROME III*
**Heat, fetal effects from maternal hyperthermia**
*See FETAL EFFECTS FROM MATERNAL HYPERTHERMIA*
**Hecht syndrome**
*See CAMPTODACTYLY-TRISMUS SYNDROME*
**Heidenhain variant**
*See CREUTZFELDT-JAKOB DISEASE*
**Heine-Medin disease**
*See POLIO, SUSCEPTIBILITY TO*
**Heinz body anemia**
*See ANEMIA, HEINZ BODY*
**Helio-ophthalmic outburst syndrome**
*See ACHOO SYNDROME*
**Hemangiectatic hypertrophy**
*See ANGIO-OSTEOHYPERTROPHY SYNDROME*
**Hemangiolipomatosis**
*See ANGIOLIPOMATOSIS*
**Hemangioma of eyelids and orbit**
*See ORBITAL HEMANGIOMA*
**Hemangioma, salivary gland**
*See SALIVARY GLAND, HEMANGIOMA*
**Hemangioma, subglottic**
*See SUBGLOTTIC HEMANGIOMA*
**Hemangioma-thrombocytopenia**
*See HEMANGIOMAS OF THE HEAD AND NECK*

---

## HEMANGIOMA-THROMBOCYTOPENIA SYNDROME      0456

**Includes:**

Kasabach-Merritt syndrome
Thrombocytopenia-hemangioma syndrome
Vascular tumors-hemangioid cell derivation-spontaneous hemorrhage

**Excludes:**  Hemangioma with rapid growth, ulceration, without spontaneous hemorrhage

**Major Diagnostic Criteria:**  Hemangioma (small or large) with associated systemic hemorrhagic symptoms due to thrombocytopenia.

**Clinical Findings:**  Characterized by normal-appearing hemangioma suddenly increasing in size (in 100%), associated thrombocytopenia (100%), petechiae and ecchymoses (75%), marked decrease in hemoglobin and erythrocyte levels (75%), hypofibrinogenemia, and decreased prothrombin.

**Complications:**  In 21% of reported cases, death occurred from hemorrhage because of platelet sequestration within the capillary bed of the hemangioma.

**Associated Findings:**  Visceral hemangiomatosis, and high-output congestive heart failure.

**Etiology:**  Unknown.

**Pathogenesis:**  Consumption coagulopathy and microangiopathic hemolytic anemia; chronic localized coagulopathy or acute disseminated type of intravascular coagulopathy can take place; fibrinogen depletion occurs in some cases.

**MIM No.:**  14100

**Sex Ratio:**  M1:F1

**Occurrence:**  Reported in teaching hospital files as 1:500 reported hemangiomas.

**Risk of Recurrence for Patient's Sib:**  Unknown.

**Risk of Recurrence for Patient's Child:**  Unknown.

**Age of Detectability:**  Birth through 73 years; median age 5 weeks. Detected primarily through platelet counts.

**Gene Mapping and Linkage:**  Unknown.

**Prevention:**  None known. Genetic counseling indicated.

**Treatment:**  Systemic steroids, irradiation, surgical extirpation of tumor if feasible, and splenectomy may be used. Heparinization when fibrinogen is decreased; whole blood transfusions may also be needed. Preliminary reports indicate that treatment with argon laser may be beneficial.

**Prognosis:** Mortality rate is 21%, median age at death is five weeks, for treated cases only; statistics for untreated cases are unknown. The usual cause of death is hemorrhage. The size or the type of vascular tumor in no way determines the possible development of this syndrome.

**Detection of Carrier:** Unknown.

**References:**

Shim WK: Hemangiomas of infancy complicated by thrombocytopenia. Am J Surg 1968; 116:896–906.

Hagerman LJ, et al.: Giant hemangioma with consumption coagulopathy. J Pediatr 1975; 87:766–768.

Wind ES, Pillari G: Deep soft tissue hemangioma of infancy: Kasabach-Merritt syndrome. NY State J Med 1979; 79:373–374.

Stern JK, et al.: Benign neonatal hemangiomatosis. J Am Acad Dermatol 1981; 4:442–446.

Esterly NB: Kasabach-Merritt syndrome in infants. J Am Acad of Dermatol 1983; 8:504–513. * †

Larsen EC, et al.: Kasabach-Merritt syndrome: therapeutic considerations. Pediatrics 1987; 79:971–980.

WI022                                                    **Charles J. Wilson**

---

## HEMANGIOMAS OF THE HEAD AND NECK                   2514

**Includes:**

Arteriovenous hemangioma/malformation
Capillary hemangioma
Cavernous hemangioma
Hemangioma-thrombocytopenia
Hemangiomas, cavernous, of face and supraumbilical midline raphe
Kasabach-Merritt syndrome (some cases)
Neck/head, hemangiomas
Mixed hemangioma
Raphe, supraumbilical midline-cavernous facial hemangiomas
Strawberry nevus
Vascular malformations, familial

**Excludes:**

Angiofibroma, juvenile nasopharyngeal
**Cystic hygroma** (3284)
**Enchondromatosis and hemangiomas** (0346)
Hemangioendothelioma
**Hemangioma-thrombocytopenia syndrome** (0456)
Hemangiopericytoma
Lymphangioma
**Nevus flammeus** (0715)

**Major Diagnostic Criteria:** Mass lesion consisting of a benign nonreactive proliferation of capillaries or other blood vessel channels. The superficial lesion is reddish to bluish in color, from soft to firm in consistency, and blanches on compression, filling again with blood on relaxing compression. The deep lesion may be diagnosed by its distinctive features on angiography or by biopsy. Computed tomography is useful in determining the extent of deep involvement and the progressive change in the lesion.

**Clinical Findings:** The head and neck region is the site of 50% or more of all hemangiomas, and the lesions may be single or multiple. About 30–40% of the lesions are found at birth, but more typically they are noticed during the first month of life.

Lesions grow during the first year of life and then involute in approximately 90% of cases. Much variability exists in their clinical course from rapid spontaneous regression before age four years to slow regression and increased scarring beyond age two years, to rapid growth with ulceration, hemorrhage, airway obstruction, and functional and cosmetic disfigurement.

Cutaneous surfaces are most frequently involved, with the scalp being the most common site, followed by the neck and the face, respectively. Other sites include the mucosa in the upper aerodigestive tract (e.g., oral cavity, nasal septum, and larynx), parotid, orbit, and brain; greater than 50% of all salivary gland tumors before age 1 year are hemangiomas. Most cutaneous and mucosal

hemangiomas are not invasive, but those located in deep subcutaneous tissue, fascia, and muscle tend to be infiltrating.

Based on histopathologic features, these lesions may be further subclassified as capillary, cavernous, mixed, or arteriovenous hemangiomas. The capillary hemangioma is composed of capillaries lined by endothelial cells and surrounded by pericytes. The **Nevus flammeus**, or strawberry nevus are examples.

Cavernous hemangiomas consist of large, tortuous vascular spaces lined by endothelial cells. These lesions may be found in the skin or deep soft tissue. Those present at birth tend to involute, while the others tend to be permanent. The cavernous hemangioma is the second most common intramuscular hemangioma and is associated with a 9% recurrence rate. Mixed hemangiomas have the histopathologic features of both capillary and cavernous hemangiomas. They are associated with a 25% recurrence rate in the intramuscular location. These lesions do not involute and can involve bone.

Arteriovenous hemangiomas are referred to by some as *arteriovenous malformations* and are characterized by the finding of intimal thickening or by the demonstration of diverse arteriovenous connections in serial sections. Clinical features include a pulsatile mass and the physiologic findings of an arteriovenous shunt.

An alternative classification of pediatric vascular lesions is to divide these lesions into hemangiomas and vascular malformations based on clinical and cellular characteristics. Hemangiomas show rapid growth within endothelial proliferation and increased mass cells during the first few months of life but usually involute by one year of age. Vascular malformations grow with the child and show no endothelial proliferation, no increased numbers of mast cells, and no regression.

**Complications:** Cosmetic deformity commonly occurs; ulceration and hemorrhage are sometimes associated with the rapidly enlarging hemangioma and the nasal septal hemangioma. Functional deformity is less common but can result in stridor, upper airway obstruction, proptosis, and blindness. When extensive, hemangiomas can result in hemodynamic instability. Cerebellar and retinal hemangiomas associated with **Von Hippel-Lindau syndrome** may cause increased intracranial pressure and retinal detachment. Disseminated intravascular coagulopathy is a complication of **Hemangioma-thrombocytopenia syndrome.**

**Associated Findings:** Although rare, additional occult hemangiomas may occur, especially involving the larynx and the brain. Cutaneous hemangiomas occur in 40% of patients with a subglottic hemangioma and in 5–9% of patients with **Von Hippel-Lindau syndrome.** Multiple syndromes with their associated features, e.g., **Angio-osteohypertrophy syndrome, Von Hippel-Lindau syndrome, Beckwith-Wiedemann syndrome, Nevus, blue rubber bleb nevus syndrome,** and **Hemangioma-thrombocytopenia syndrome,** are related to head and neck hemangiomas.

**Etiology:** Often by autosomal dominant inheritance. Hemangiomas do occur in many syndromes, and may occur as isolated traits.

**Pathogenesis:** Aberrations of vasoformative mesoderm cause hemangiomas. Capillary hemangiomas are caused by arrest in the capillary network stage of embryogenesis; cavernous hemangiomas result from arrest in the early retiform stage. Arteriovenous hemangiomas result from arrest in the late retiform stage.

**MIM No.:** *14080, 14085

**Sex Ratio:** Overall, approximately M1:F2; in arteriovenous hemangiomas, M1:F1.

**Occurrence:** The overall incidence of hemangiomas is 62:1,000 in newborns. The incidence of strawberry mark is 20:1,000. At age one year, the prevalence is 120:1,000 children.

**Risk of Recurrence for Patient's Sib:** Generally indeterminate except in selected syndromes.

**Risk of Recurrence for Patient's Child:** Generally indeterminate except in selected syndromes.

**Age of Detectability:** Approximately 30–40% are detectable at birth, and up to 85% by the first year of life.

**Gene Mapping and Linkage:** Unknown.

**Prevention:** None known. Genetic counseling indicated.

**Treatment:** A period of observation is advisable if life-threatening complications are not imminent; 90% of congenital hemangiomas will involute after a short accelerated growth phase. Tracheotomy may be needed for airway support of an obstructive subglottic hemangioma. Up to 90% of the remaining capillary cavernous hemangiomas respond to a 2–3-week course of prednisone, 20–40 mg daily, with regression of the lesion within 2–3 weeks. Alternate-day therapy may be used to reduce steroid side effects and may be continued for 30–90 days. If the lesion enlarges on discontinuance of steroids, further courses may be given.

Radiation therapy was a widely accepted treatment for these lesions in the past, but has generally fallen into disfavor today. Sclerosing agents were also commonly used before, but now are controversial, although 95% ethanol is still advocated as an efficacious and relatively safe sclerosing agent. Embolization under angiographic control may be used as a primary treatment or as a preoperative adjunct in the arteriovenous hemangioma.

Surgery is reserved for persistent hemangioma involvement, especially after more conservative treatment has stabilized the lesion. Indications for surgery include airway obstruction; rapid growth; hemorrhage, ulceration, or impending cardiovascular decompensation; infection and tissue loss; and severe deformity. Laser therapy has shown promising results with some lesions. The tuned dye laser has shown good results with preservation of overlying skin.

**Prognosis:** Normal life span except in those with significant airway compromise or other life-threatening complications. Cosmetic deformity is often present, but may be lessened by treatment. Intelligence is normal.

**Detection of Carrier:** In selected syndromes, by clinical examination or procedures specific to the individual syndrome.

**Special Considerations:** Great degree of variability in the spectrum of this entity exists, with multiple classification systems proposed based on histopathologic, clinical, and prognostic features. The information presented here is based on the classification system of Edgerton (1976) and is widely accepted.

**References:**
Watson WL, McCarthy WD: Blood and lymph vessel tumors: a report of 1,056 cases. Surg Gynecol Obstet 1940; 71:569–588.
Edgerton MT: The treatment of hemangiomas: with special reference to the role of steroid therapy. Ann Surg 1976; 183:517–530.
Garfinkle TJ, Handler SD: Hemangiomas of the head and neck in children: a guide to management. J Otolaryngol 1980; 9:439–450. †
Pasyk KA, et al.: Familial vascular malformations: report of 25 members of one family. Clin Genet 1984; 26:221–227.
Persky MS: Congenital vascular lesions of the head and neck. Laryngoscope 1986; 96:1002–1015. *
Myer CM: Tumors of the head and neck in children. In: Thawley SE, et al.: Comprehensive management of head and neck tumors. Philadelphia: W.B. Saunders, 1987. *

ST049 **John A. Stith**

**Hemangiomas, cavernous, of face and supraumbilical midline raphe**
*See HEMANGIOMAS OF THE HEAD AND NECK*
**Hemangiomas-enchondromatosis**
*See ENCHONDROMATOSIS AND HEMANGIOMAS*
**Hemangiomata-cleft sternum**
*See STERNAL MALFORMATION-VASCULAR DYSPLASIA ASSOCIATION*
**Hemangiomatosis, generalized cavernous**
*See NEVUS, BLUE RUBBER BLEB NEVUS SYNDROME*
**Hemangiomatosis, multiple**
*See VON HIPPEL-LINDAU SYNDROME*
**Hematopoietic hypoplasia, generalized**
*See IMMUNODEFICIENCY, SEVERE COMBINED*
**Hematoporphyria congenita**
*See PORPHYRIA, ERYTHROPOIETIC*
**Heme synthase deficiency**
*See PORPHYRIA, PROTOPORPHYRIA*
**Hemeralopia**
*See NIGHTBLINDNESS, CONGENITAL STATIONARY, AUTOSOMAL DOMINANT*

**Hemeralopia-myopia, X-linked**
*See NIGHTBLINDNESS, CONGENITAL STATIONARY, X-LINKED RECESSIVE*
**Hemi 3 syndrome**
*See HEMIHYPERTROPHY*
**Hemicrania**
*See ANENCEPHALY*
**Hemidiaphragm, congenital absence of**
*See DIAPHRAGMATIC HERNIA*
**Hemidysplasia-ichthyosis, congenital**
*See LIMB REDUCTION-ICHTHYOSIS*

## HEMIFACIAL ATROPHY, PROGRESSIVE 2615

**Includes:**
> Parry-Romberg syndrome
> Facial hemiatrophy, progressive
> Romberg syndrome

**Excludes:**
> Lipodystrophy, cephalo-thoracic
> **Oculo-auriculo-vertebral anomaly** (0735)
> **Scleroderma, familial progressive** (2154)

**Major Diagnostic Criteria:** Unilateral impairment of facial growth, not present at birth.

**Clinical Findings:** Onset is usually in the first decade with the appearance of atrophy in the cheek, later spreading to involve the mandible and upper face. The process may involve skin, subcutaneous tissues, underlying musculature, and the facial skeleton. The left side is more commonly affected. Either increased skin pigmentation or vitiligo may be present and scalp involvement may cause blanching of hair or alopecia. Involvement of the upper face gives rise to "coup de sabre" appearance. Patches of skin pigmentation may also be present on the trunk and limbs. Skin biopsy during active phase of the process may show thickening of

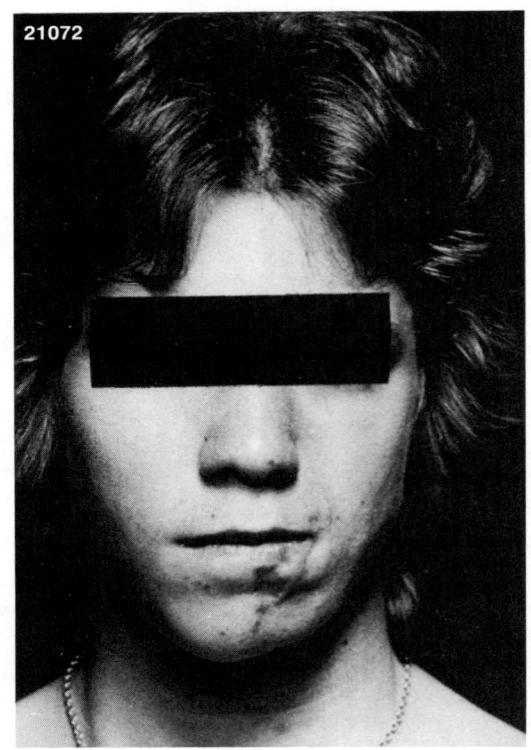

**2615-21072:** 16-year-old with mild hemifacial atrophy, mandibular hypoplasia and induration of the overlying skin.

collagen bundles and inflammatory cellular infiltrates; these non-specific changes resemble those of idiopathic scleroderma. There has been nosologic uncertainty since the beginning of the century regarding the relationship of progressive hemifacial atrophy to localized forms of scleroderma including morphea and linear scleroderma of childhood. Synovitis, **Raynaud disease**, renal involvement, and other aspects of progressive systemic sclerosis are not features of progressive hemifacial atrophy.

The condition slowly progresses, usually for a period of three to five years, and then tends toward inactivity with resultant growth abnormality being evident for the rest of the individual's life.

**Complications:** Delay in dental eruption, dental malocclusion, atrophy of half of tongue, enophthalmos, refractive error, and unilateral atrophy of facial musculature. Localized bony depressions in mandible, orbit, forehead and calvarium.

**Associated Findings:** Trigeminal neuralgia, **Horner syndrome**, heterochromia iridis, contralateral Jacksonian seizures, migraine-like headaches, and malocclusion.

**Etiology:** Most cases occur sporadically, but autosomal dominant inheritance has been suggested.

**Pathogenesis:** Cervical sympathectomy in rats gives rise to a comparable syndrome. Autoimmune phenomena reported in scleroderma have not been extensively studied but appear to be rare in progressive hemifacial atrophy.

**MIM No.:** 14130

**POS No.:** 3370

**Sex Ratio:** M2:F3

**Occurrence:** Undetermined but presumed rare.

**Risk of Recurrence for Patient's Sib:** Unknown.

**Risk of Recurrence for Patient's Child:** Unknown.

**Age of Detectability:** During the first decade of life or occasionally early in second decade.

**Gene Mapping and Linkage:** Unknown.

**Prevention:** None known. Genetic counseling indicated.

**Treatment:** Since this is a self-arresting disorder, no treatment should be initiated until the progress has stopped and the full extent of the deformity known. Then, plastic surgery and maxillofacial surgery can be performed as indicated. Subcutaneous silicone implantation or more extensive forms of plastic surgery have been used to augment areas of facial atrophy.

**Prognosis:** Good for life span and health, except in patients with extensive central nervous system involvement.

**Detection of Carrier:** Unknown.

**References:**
Wartenberg R: Progressive facial hemiatrophy. Arch Neurol Psychiatr 1945; 54:75–96.
Rogers BO: Progressive facial hemiatrophy (Romberg's disease): a review of 772 cases. In: Broadbent TR, ed: Transactions of the third international congress of plastic surgery. Amsterdam: Excepta Medica, 1964:681–689.
Rees TD: Facial atrophy. Clin Plast Surg 1976; 3:637–646.
Aracena T, et al.: Progressive hemiofacial atrophy (Parry-Romberg syndrome): report of two cases. Ann Ophthalmol 1979; 11:953–958.
Lewkonia RM, Lowry RB: Progressive hemifacial atrophy (Parry-Romberg syndrome): report with review of genetics and nosology. Am J Med Genet 1983; 14:385–390.

LE050
J0027
**Raymond M. Lewkonia**
**Ronald J. Jorgenson**

**Hemifacial hyperplasia with strabismus (HFH)**
*See OCULO-FACIAL SYNDROME, BENCZE TYPE*
**Hemifacial hypertrophy**
*See HEMIHYPERTROPHY*
**Hemifacial microsomia**
*See OCULO-AURICULO-VERTEBRAL ANOMALY*
**Hemigigantism**
*See HEMIHYPERTROPHY*

## HEMIHYPERTROPHY　　　　0458

**Includes:**
　Asymmetry, congenital
　Hemi 3 syndrome
　Hemifacial hypertrophy
　Hemigigantism
　Hemihypertrophy, isolated
　Hypertrophy, unilateral
　Overgrowth disorder, hemihypertrophy

**Excludes:**
　**Angio-osteohypertrophy syndrome** (0055)
　**Beckwith-Wiedemann syndrome** (0104)
　**Hemifacial atrophy, progressive** (2615)
　**Fibrous dysplasia, polyostotic** (0391)
　Macrodactylia fibromatosis
　**Neurofibromatosis** (0712)
　**Proteus syndrome** (2382)
　**Silver syndrome, X-linked** (2829)
　**Silver syndrome** (0887)
　Vascular anomalies, underlying

**Major Diagnostic Criteria:** Evidence of gross body asymmetry (total or partial) is easily perceptible by external examination and is due to enlargement of body side or segments. Mild forms of asymmetry are very common, often go unnoticed, and are normal variations.

**Clinical Findings:** Hemihypertrophy varies considerably in the severity and extent of involvement. External examination may show enlargement of an entire side (total hemihypertrophy) or specific regions of the body (partial or segmental), or occasionally different anatomic areas on both sides of the body (crossed). The hemihypertrophy may affect not only the visible portions of the body (skin, soft tissue, and musculoskeletal system), but also the internal organs. The enlarged side may show abnormal pigmentation and increased temperature of skin, dystrophic nails, hypertrichosis, precocious dentition with malocclusion, and larger pupils with iris heterochromia. There are no specific laboratory abnormalities and X-ray examination may show advanced bone

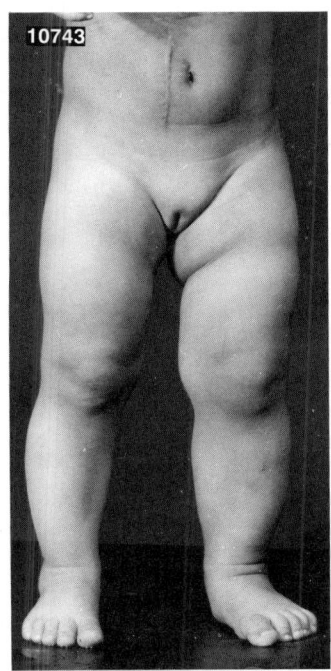

**0458**-10743:　Note enlargement of left lower limb.

age in the hypertrophied limbs and enlarged viscera (e.g. kidney on IVP). Approximately 20–30% of the reported cases of hemihypertrophy have hamartomatous lesions (e.g. pigmented nevi, hemangiomas) or various congenital defects, especially mental retardation and GU anomalies. There is an increased susceptibility to childhood neoplasms and premalignant lesions of the kidney, adrenal cortex and liver.

**Complications:** Leg-length discrepancy may lead to difficulty in walking.

**Associated Findings:** A predisposition to childhood cancers including **Cancer, Wilms tumor**, adrenocortical neoplasms, hepatoblastoma, and possibly other tumors. Medullary sponge kidney and other GU defects may impair renal function. Internal hamartomatous growths can cause liver failure, and hemangiomas may rupture. Adrenal hemorrhage has been reported in some cases.

**Etiology:** Undetermined. A few cases have been reported among sibs or successive generations on the maternal line. In addition, some cases have been reported with a variety of chromosomal abnormalities in blood leukocytes or skin fibroblasts (different forms of mosaicism and in one case a pair of elongated No. 16 chromosomes). Most cases studied have had no familial aggregation, chromosomal defect or unusual environmental exposures.

**Pathogenesis:** The nature of hemihypertrophy suggests origins in the very early stages of embryogenesis. The histopathology shows cellular hyperplasia rather than cellular hypertrophy, and skin biopsy has shown an increased growth rate of cultured keratinocytes and fibroblasts on the enlarged side. No metabolic or endocrine defect has been described.

**MIM No.:** 23500

**CDC No.:** 759.890

**Sex Ratio:** M1:F1

**Occurrence:** 1:14,300 births followed to age six, as reported from the registry of malformations in Birmingham, England. About 200 cases described in the literature.

**Risk of Recurrence for Patient's Sib:** No reliable data, but scattered case reports suggest a slightly increased risk.

**Risk of Recurrence for Patient's Child:** Possibly slightly increased risk among offspring of affected mothers.

**Age of Detectability:** Ordinarily, soon after birth, but severity of asymmetry may increase or diminish with advancing age.

**Gene Mapping and Linkage:** Unknown.

**Prevention:** None known. Genetic counseling indicated.

**Treatment:** Treatment is symptomatic and may involve corrective shoes, braces, and orthopedic procedures, such as epiphysiodesis, for leg-length asymmetry. Surgical procedures for correction of associated congenital and hamartomatous defects; careful follow-up with periodic clinical, X-ray, and sonographic examinations through childhood for early detection of abdominal neoplasia and surgical intervention in appropriate cases.

**Prognosis:** Average life span, though not affected by hemihypertrophy itself, may be diminished by associated disorders, such as neoplasia, renal anomalies, and hamartomas. Mental retardation occurs in some cases. Limb asymmetry may interfere to some extent with function, and renal anomalies may produce problems.

**Detection of Carrier:** Unknown.

**Special Considerations:** Diagnosis is made from clinical evidence of gross asymmetry between two sides of the body. The condition should be distinguished from 1) hemiatrophy, which shows unilaterally subnormal development, muscle weakness, or neurologic deficit; 2) hemihypertrophy secondary to hemangiomatous, lymphangiomatous, lipomatous, or osseous malformations; 3) hemihypertrophy or asymmetry associated with primary neurocutaneous disorders or multiple-defect syndromes in which body asymmetry is only one of several major anomalies. Hemihypertrophy shares with the neurocutaneous syndromes and the **Beckwith-Wiedemann syndrome** a susceptibility to hamartomatous growths and neoplasms, but the origins of hemihypertrophy are much less clearly genetic. One-third of the cases with childhood

neoplasms had tumors in a side that was externally unaffected by hemihypertrophy, suggesting that the oncogenic stimulus does not necessarily lateralize to the larger side. Components of this malformation - neoplasia syndrome may be spread over the family tree, as suggested by Meadows et al (1974), reporting a woman with congenital hemihypertrophy who had three children with **Cancer, Wilms tumor** and a fourth with a urinary tract defect.

Nudleman et al (1984) delineated a subtype termed Hemi 3 syndrome which appears to be a neural tube defect.

**References:**

Fraumeni JF Jr, et al.: Wilms' tumor and congenital hemihypertrophy: report of five new cases and review of literature. Pediatrics 1967; 40:886–899. * †
Meadows AT, et al.: Wilms' tumor in 3 children of a woman with congenital hemihypertrophy. New Engl J Med 1974; 291:23–25.
Pfister RC, et al.: Congenital asymmetry (hemihypertrophy) and abdominal disease. Radiology 1975; 116:686–683. †
Furukawa T, Shinohara T: Congenital hemihypertrophy: oncogenic potential of the hypertrophic side. Ann Neurol 1981; 10:199–201. †
Beals RK: Hemihypertrophy and hemihypotrophy. Clin Orthop 1982; 166:199–203.
Nudleman K, et al.: The hemi 3 syndrome: hemihypertrophy, hemihypaesthesia, hemiareflexia and scoliosis. Brain 1984; 107:533–546.
Viljoen D, et al.: Manifestations and natural history of idiopathic hemihypertrophy: a review of 11 cases. Clin Genet 1984; 26:81–87.

FR010                                              **Joseph F. Fraumeni, Jr.**

**Hemihypertrophy, isolated**
  *See HEMIHYPERTROPHY*
**Hemimelia**
  *See LIMB REDUCTION DEFECTS*
**Hemimelia-scalp skull defects**
  *See LIMB AND SCALP DEFECTS, ADAMS-OLIVER TYPE*
**Hemimelic skeletal dysplasias**
  *See DYSPLASIA EPIPHYSEALIS HEMIMELICA*
**Hemiplegia, infantile-porencephaly**
  *See BRAIN, PORENCEPHALY*
**Hemisacrum, familial type II**
  *See TERATOMA, PRESACRAL-SACRAL DYSGENESIS*
**Hemivertebrae, autosomal dominant multiple**
  *See SPONDYLOCOSTAL DYSPLASIA*
**Hemivertebrae, autosomal recessive multiple**
  *See SPONDYLOTHORACIC DYSPLASIA*

---

**HEMOCHROMATOSIS, IDIOPATHIC**                    **0460**

**Includes:**
  Bronze diabetes
  Cirrhosis, congenital pigmentary
  Iron overload disease
  Iron retention

**Excludes:**
  Hemochromatosis acquired from Bantu cirrhosis
  Hemochromatosis acquired from Kaschin Beck disease
  Hemochromatosis acquired from transfusions
  Hemochromatosis from high iron diet in alcoholic cirrhosis
  Hemochromatosis secondary to hyperplastic anemias

**Major Diagnostic Criteria:** Proof of large iron overload is requisite for the diagnosis. The desferrioxamine urinary iron excretion test is preferred. Either values over 6 mg/24 hrs in males, or over 4 mg in females, or values steadily increasing at 2–3 year intervals, and associated with normal erythrocyte output and survival, while on a normal diet, are required. Seroferritin also correlates with the iron stores: concentrations over 1,000 ng/ml are usually found (normal 15 to 250 ng/ml). Both tests should be obtained, as they are not necessarily liable to the same errors.

Familial involvement, though not prerequisite, is an important support for the diagnosis. HLA $A_3$ is found in 79% of the patients (N: 26) and $B_7$ in 53% (N: 20). In some geographical areas $B_{14}$ is found 25.5% as opposed to 3.4% in controls.

**Clinical Findings:** The early (1882) terms for the disease; bronze cirrhosis or bronze diabetes, point to the three major clinical features: hypertrophic cirrhosis, diabetes mellitus, and melano-dermia. After a silent asymptomatic progressive loading of about 15 gm of iron at a rate of 1–5 mg a day, the clinical disease generally becomes evident in the 4th decade (often later and with reduced frequency in females).

Clinical onset may begin with diabetes mellitus (50%) or one or several of the following: general weakness (45%); loss of libido (15%); pains in various locations mainly hepatalagia (30%); and a metallic gray hue or banal bronze tan (90%). Articular involvement as an opening symptom has also been underestimated.

Ultimately diabetes mellitus occurs in 60–80% of patients with hemochromatosis, and at least one-half of diabetics are or become insulin dependent. Endocrine deficiencies are in most instances dependent on pituitary insufficiency, mainly gonadotropic (Follicle-stimulating hormone (FSH) < 5 mouse units, low 17-ketosteroid urinary output), rarely adrenotropic or thyrotropic. Liver hypertrophic cirrhosis is regularly found, but portal hypertension is uncommon, as is liver cellular failure; functional hepatic tests remain within normal limits for a fairly long period. Cardiac involvement is frequently restricted to EKG findings: low voltage, flattening or inversion of T waves, and partial blocks. Articular pain with or without chondrocalcinosis on X-ray is relatively frequent. Iron and pyrophosphate may be found in the affected articulations.

Hemochromatosis is rarely noted before the age of 35 (90% occur after 35) but it may appear at any age. In early onset cases the rate of iron overloading is faster and the disease is more acute, but involves basically the same organ impairments and the same genetic transmission. The greatest difference is the outstanding severity of the cardiac involvement in children, for which there is no adequate explanation. This is frequently associated with congestive acute asystole. The hormonal involvement is also altered by the age at onset. Primary infantilism is associated with early onset, regressive infantilism with onset at puberty, and secondary gonadal atrophy in young men after a period of normal sexual life.

**Complications:** Nonspecific cellular insufficiencies ultimately result from the siderosclerosis of the various organs, including the usual complications of diabetes (when associated with hemochromatosis): ketonemic or hypoglycemic coma, thought to be due to variations in sensitivity to insulin may occur. The frequency of late degenerative sequelae is now considered comparable to that observed in late onset diabetes, since there is increased longevity of patients with hemochromatosis. Liver failure (edema, ascites, jaundice) and cirrhosis, with rare visceral hemorrhage due to portal hypertension. Cardiac damage, various types of dysrhythmias (ventricular extrasystoles, paroxysmal auricular or supraventricular tachycardia), acute bouts of pseudopericarditis with a prognosis much better than that for terminal congestive failure with biventricular dilatation and anasarca.

**Associated Findings:** Diabetes mellitus resulting from the co-existence in affected individuals of a familial predisposition to diabetes, and a low insulin output due to pancreatic siderosclerosis. Hepatoma or cholangioma is the major complication. It occurs with even higher frequency than in other types of cirrhosis (about 15%), independent of correct depletion therapy, generally after age 60.

**Etiology:** Autosomal recessive inheritance.

**Pathogenesis:** The one known constant consequence is progressive iron overloading eventually leading, usually after the age of 35, to organ damage presumably through siderosclerosis. It is unknown whether this is an inborn error of metabolism.

**MIM No.:** *23520

**Sex Ratio:** M1:F 0.1–0.2. This difference is attributable to iron loss in females (10–20 gm/lifetime).

**Occurrence:** Hundreds of cases documented worldwide. Tends to be infrequent in areas of prevailing iron deficiency and to concentrate where consanguinity is more common. Prevalence of heterozygous carriers in the general population ranges from two to eight percent in some areas of France (Normandy and Britany) and among the Mormons in the United States.

**Risk of Recurrence for Patient's Sib:**
See Part I, *Mendelian Inheritance.*

**Risk of Recurrence for Patient's Child:**
See Part I, *Mendelian Inheritance.*

**Age of Detectability:** Usually around the age of 40 when decompensation occurs, although the diagnosis has been made at as early as 29 months of age. In the sibship of an index case, theoretically the disease may be detected quite early through demonstration of an iron overload that steadily increases at yearly intervals and/or HLA identity.

**Gene Mapping and Linkage:** HFE (hemochromatosis) has been mapped to 6p21.3.

**Prevention:** None known. Genetic counseling indicated. Preventive venesection therapy, when started in the latent phase, prevents the organic injuries characteristic of the decompensation period.

**Treatment:** Removal of excess body iron through phlebotomies at weekly intervals progressively restores normal color to the skin, improves liver size and function, frequently improves cardiac condition, usually prevents enhancement of endocrine deficiencies, rarely reduces insulin requirements, and has generally little influence on articular involvement. Once returned to normal, a few venesections a year prevent resumption of iron overload. Desferrioxamine injections are a useful adjuvant and are the sole possible treatment when venesections are contraindicated. Continuous perfusion of large doses of desferrioxamine with a mini-pump system is beneficial when cardiac failure threatens the life of patients at the onset of the disease. Corticosteroids and alcoholic beverages should be avoided.

Supportive treatment for existing organ damage; oral hypoglycemic drugs and insulin in 70% of associated diabetes; testosterone for impotence; usual management of liver cirrhosis with rare indications for portocaval anastomosis. Hepatocarcinomas are a particular concern for older patients and should be diagnosed early since some evolve slowly and remain localized for long periods. Assay of plasmatic fetoprotein is indicated every three months; liver echotomograph every six months. A prospective vaccination against hepatitis B virus (HBV) is currently under investigation. The implication of HBV genome integration in patient's hepatocyte DNA found in about half of hepatitis carcinoma could be one of the factors involved in hepatocyte degenerescence.

**Prognosis:** Differs in early and late onset of the disease. The younger the patient is at clinical onset, the worse the prognosis. Overall, life expectancy after diagnosis, initially rather short, has been extended to about five years after the insulin era, and again needs to be reexamined now that sufficient time has elapsed since the introduction of venesection therapy. This is especially true when early diagnosis is achieved in the asymptomatic phase through family studies. Major causes of death may be summarized as: cardiac failure (30%), hepatic coma (15%), hematemeses (15%), hepatoma (15%), and diabetic coma (5%).

**Detection of Carrier:** Twenty-five percent of heterozygous carriers of the gene have slightly abnormal iron stores, rarely exceeding 2 gm, when on a normal diet. They may be detected by the finding of serum iron and unsaturated iron-binding capacity (UIBC) abnormalities. They may be differentiated from homozygotes by a normal (significantly less than 2 mg) urinary excretion of iron after desferrioxamine injection. Heterozygous carriers tend to stabilize with time.

**Special Considerations:** Ascertainment of a large enough iron overload using desferrioxamine and seroferritin is basic to the differentiation of patients with the disease (homozygotes) from healthy carriers of the mutant gene (heterozygotes). For this purpose neither histology nor plasma iron study is adequate. Histologic quantitation of iron is frequently misleading, particularly when the size of the liver is not taken into account. Impressive amounts of iron have been found on the smear coexistent with as little as 2–3 gm of iron excess. Serum iron and UIBC, similarly, have proved to be misleading. The maximum possible alterations are restricted by the actual quantity of circulating transferrin. These are reached at a level of iron overload well below the upper limit found in heterozygotes.

Use of histology and plasma findings as criteria for the diagnosis of the disease have contributed greatly to erroneous conclusions of dominant inheritance in idiopathic hemochromatosis.

A study of 72 patients with hemochromatosis designed to reexamine the influence of iron overload on the appearance of diabetes in this disease revealed no compulsory relationship between iron overload and diabetes.

**Support Groups:**

FL; West Palm Beach; Iron Overload Diseases Association, Inc. (IOD)
NY; Albany; The Hemochromatosis Research Foundation

**References:**

Saddi R, Feingold J: Idiopathic haemochromatosis and diabetes mellitus. Clin Genet 1974; 5:242–247.
Lipinski M, et al.: Idiopathic hemochromatosis: linkage with HLA. Tissue Antigens 1978; 11:471–474.
Ryder LP, et al., eds: HLA and disease registry (3rd report). Copenhagen: Munksgaard, 1979:26. *
Saddi R et al.: HLA(A3) (B7) linkage disequilibrium in hemochromatotic patients with or without insulin dependent diabetes. Tissue Antigens 1981; 17:473–479.
Bothwell TH, et al.: Hemochromatosis. In: Stanbury JB, et al., eds: The metabolic basis of inherited disease, 5th ed. New York: McGraw-Hill, 1983:1269–1298. *
Saddi R et al.: Hepatitis B vaccination and idiopathic hemochromatosis. Lancet 1985; II:1061–1062.
Siemons LJ, Mahler C: Hypogonadtropic hypogonadism in hemochromatosis: recovery of reproductive function after iron depletion. J Clin Endocr Metab 1987; 65:585–587.

SA006

**Raymond Saddi**
*Georges Schapira*

**Hemodialysis-related amyloidosis**
See AMYLOIDOSIS, HEMODIALYSIS-RELATED
**Hemoglobin H disease-mental retardation-multiple anomalies**
See MENTAL RETARDATION, HEMOGLOBIN H RELATED
**Hemoglobin Lepore syndromes**
See THALASSEMIA
**Hemoglobin variants, unstable with inclusion body formation**
See ANEMIA, HEINZ BODY
**Hemoglobin-binding alpha globulins**
See HAPTOGLOBIN
**Hemoglobin-binding beta globulins**
See HAPTOGLOBIN
**Hemolytic anemia due to glutathione peroxidase deficiency**
See ANEMIA, HEMOLYTIC, GLUTATHIONINE PEROXIDASE DEFICIENCY
**Hemolytic anemia due to glutathione reductase deficiency**
See ANEMIA, HEMOLYTIC, GLUTATHIONE REDUCTASE DEFICIENCY
**Hemolytic anemia due to glutathione synthetase deficiency**
See ANEMIA, HEMOLYTIC, GLUTATHIONE SYNTHETASE DEFICIENCY
**Hemolytic anemia, nonspherocytic, associated with G6PD deficiency**
See GLUCOSE-6-PHOSPHATE DEHYDROGENASE DEFICIENCY
**Hemolytic disease of newborn**
See TEETH, ENAMEL AND DENTIN DEFECTS FROM ERYTHROBLASTOSIS FETALIS
**Hemolytic disease resulting from Rh incompatibility**
See ERYTHROBLASTOSIS FETALIS
**Hemolytic disease, PFK deficiency**
See GLYCOGENOSIS, TYPE VII
**Hemolytic disease, phosphofructokinase deficiency**
See GLYCOGENOSIS, TYPE VII
**Hemolytic disorders, glycogen metabolism related**
See GLYCOGENOSES
**Hemolytic elliptocytosis**
See ELLIPTOCYTOSIS

## HEMOLYTIC-UREMIC SYNDROME 3148

**Includes:**

Hemolytic-uremic syndrome with recurrent episodes
Thrombotic microangiopathy, familial
Thrombotic thrombocytopenic purpura, familial

**Excludes:**

Hemolytic uremic syndrome, nonfamilial
Pneumoccoccus-associated hemolytic uremic syndrome
Shiga-associated hemolytic uremic syndrome
Verotoxin-associated hemolytic uremic syndrome

**Major Diagnostic Criteria:** Acute hemolytic anemia with fragmented erythrocytes, thrombocytopenia, and acute renal injury, in the absence of a typical prodrome. The hereditary forms of the syndrome are not differentiated until a second individual is affected in a kindred, with intrafamilial onset usually separated by more than one year. Renal biopsy findings show predominantly arteriolar involvement.

**Clinical Findings:** Presents with the features of the typical hemolytic uremic syndrome: acute hemolytic anemia, thrombocytopenia, and acute renal injury. The prodromal illness of bloody diarrhea with or without vomiting seen in typical, nonhereditary cases of hemolytic-uremic syndrome is usually absent. The onset may be insidious or acute, in a previously well patient. The anemia is Coombs negative, and the red blood cells are fragmented (microangiopathic hemolysis). Platelet counts are below 100,000/cmm and may be as low as 5,000/cmm. Urine output may be normal, decreased, or the patient may be anuric. Urine sediment contains red blood cells and red blood cell casts; proteinuria is invariably present. Seizures may occur, as may severe hypertension and cardiac failure. Within a single sibship, one sib may resemble hemolytic uremic syndrome, and the other thrombotic thrombocytopenic purpura. The ages of onset are remarkably similar for sibs within a sibship, but may range from a few months to the third decade of life from one family to another.

**Complications:** Chronic renal failure, central nervous system disease, severe hypertension, cardiac failure, and recurrent episodes reported in 12% of patients with the recessive inherited form. May recur after renal transplantation. Association with pregnancy in the autosomal dominant form of hemolytic uremic syndrome.

**Associated Findings:** None known.

**Etiology:** Autosomal recessive and autosomal dominant inheritance.

**Pathogenesis:** Defects in the metabolism of prostacyclin have been suggested. Defects in the function of complement occur in some kindreds. The most proximal defect seems to be in endothelial cells, especially in those of the renal arterioles and glomerular capillaries, but is is not known whether these are primary or secondary. It is believed that following endothelial injury, erythrocytes and platelets are damaged by fibrin strands in the microvessels of the kidneys. The damaged blood cells then release active compounds that may enhance the vessel injury, and they in turn may either accumulate in the microvessels or be removed from the circulation by the spleen. Endothelial cell swelling and intravascular thrombus formation result in reduction or cessation of blood flow with consequent tissue hypoxia and injury.

**MIM No.:** 23540, 27415

**Sex Ratio:** Presumably M1:F1. In the 38 recessive-form families known, there are 33 affected males and 46 affected females. In the nine dominant families reported there are 15 affected males and 20 affected females, with only males affected in some families and only females affected in others.

**Occurrence:** About 100 families are currently listed in the International Registry for the Hemolytic Uremic Syndrome. Hereditary forms account for fewer than five percent of all cases.

**Risk of Recurrence for Patient's Sib:**

See Part I, *Mendelian Inheritance.*

**Risk of Recurrence for Patient's Child:**
See Part I, *Mendelian Inheritance.* No affected individuals with the recessive form are known to have reproduced.

**Age of Detectability:** Patients can only be detected when they present with the syndrome; this may occur from a few months of age to adulthood. However, prostacyclin activity and complement function have been abnormal in affected patients and their family members.

**Gene Mapping and Linkage:** Unknown.

**Prevention:** None known. Genetic counseling indicated. There is a possible association with estrogen-containing oral contraceptives.

**Treatment:** Dialysis for acute renal failure. Judicious use of blood transfusions for anemia. Possible roles for infusion of fresh frozen plasma and plasmaphresis. Chronic hemodialysis or continuous peritoneal dialysis. Renal transplantation.

**Prognosis:** Of the 86 known patients with the recessive form, 30% were alive at last follow-up, and of these 12% were well, 6% were alive but in chronic renal failure, and 12% had recurrent episodes. Seventy percent were known to have died.

In the 34 reported cases of the dominant form, more than 90% were deceased and the remainder were either in chronic renal failure or had had a kidney transplant.

**Detection of Carrier:** Unknown.

**Special Considerations:** Affected individuals resemble patients with acquired hemolytic-uremic syndrome so closely that it is virtually impossible to assign a sporadic case to either of the inherited groups until a second sib or family member is afflicted. When sibs or family members with an acquired form of HUS become ill, each usually becomes sick within days or weeks of the other. This is in contrast to the hereditary forms in which the interval between the onset of illness may range from 1–14 years.

**References:**
Farr MJ, et al.: The haemolytic uraemic syndrome: a family study. Q J Med 1975; 44:161–188.
Kaplan BS, et al.: Hemolytic uremic syndrome in families. New Engl J Med 1975; 292:1090–1093.
Kaplan BS: Hemolytic uremic syndrome with recurrent episodes: an important subset. Clin Nephrol 1977; 8:495–498.
Remuzzi G, et al.: Familial deficiency of a plasma factor stimulating vascular prostacyclin activity. Thromb Res 1979; 16:517–525.
Carreras L, et al.: Familial hypocomplementemic hemolytic uremic syndrome with HLA-A3,B7 haplotype. J Am Med Asso 1981; 245:602–604.
Kaplan BS, Proesmans W: The hemolytic uremic syndrome of childhood and its variants. Semin Hematol 1987; 24:148–160.
Mattoo TK, et al.: Familial recurrent hemolytic-uremic syndrome. J Pediatr 1989; 114:814–816.

KA042                                     **Bernard S. Kaplan**
KA043                                     **Paige Kaplan**

**Hemolytic-uremic syndrome with recurrent episodes**
*See HEMOLYTIC-UREMIC SYNDROME*
**Hemophagocytic reticulosis**
*See IMMUNODEFICIENCY, RETICULOENDOTHELIOSIS WITH EOSINOPHILIA*

---

## HEMOPHILIA A                                     0461

**Includes:**
AHF deficiency
AHG deficiency
Classic hemophilia
Factor VIII deficiency
Hemophilia A-vascular abnormality

**Excludes:**
Coagulation factor deficiencies (other)
**Factor XI deficiency** (2671)
**Hemophilia B** (0462)
**Von Willebrand disease** (0996)

**Major Diagnostic Criteria:** Factor VIII coagulant assay with less than 20% of normal activity. The patients are categorized as severe with less than 1% of Factor VIII coagulant activity, moderate with 2–7%, and mild with 7–20%. Approximately one-half of known affected individuals are in the severe category.

**Clinical Findings:** In severely deficient patients, hemorrhage into joints, particularly knees, ankles, elbows, wrists, and hips, leads to progressive arthropathy in the absence of prompt Factor VIII infusion. The hemorrhages may occur into muscles leading to fibrosis and atrophy. In young children, oral hemorrhage following a cut tongue, lip, or frenulum is common. Hemorrhage into the central nervous system, in some instances following only trivial trauma, is a major cause of death. Patients frequently have bruises over the soft tissues and trunk. In mildly affected patients, hemorrhage may occur only in response to trauma or surgery.

**Complications:** Approximately 7–10% of the severely affected patients have such an abnormal coagulant molecule that the infusion of normal Factor VIII to achieve hemostasis results in the production of an IgG anti-Factor VIII antibody (inhibitor). The level of the inhibitor may be so great that no dose of Factor VIII is effective in achieving hemostasis.

Patients may develop non-A, non-B (NANB) hepatitis, and they may develop hepatitis B if not immunized. Approximately 90% of the patients have antibodies to hepatitis B. Delta hepatitis super-infection results in progressive liver disease and accounts for approximately 10–15% of the hemophiliac deaths on an annual basis.

The majority of the severely deficient patients who were treated with pooled, non-heat-treated Factor VIII concentrates between 1980 and 1984 have become infected with HIV. Approximately 2% of the severe hemophiliacs have developed AIDS.

**Associated Findings:** Egeberg (1965) reported a Norwegian family in which at least seven members had hemophilia A combined with a vascular abnormality with the features of **Von Willebrand disease**.

**Etiology:** X-linked recessive inheritance of decreased or absent Factor VIII coagulant activity due to an abnormal Factor VIII molecule. Approximately one-third of the cases are thought to be new mutations. The amino acid substitutions have not been identified. It is anticipated that the mild, moderate, and severe cases will have different genetic abnormalities.

**Pathogenesis:** The abnormal Factor VIII coagulant protein does not catalyze the conversion of Factor X to activated Factor X as quickly as the normal protein. Thus hemostasis is delayed with the consequent hemorrhage.

**MIM No.:** *30670, 30680

**CDC No.:** 286.000

**Sex Ratio:** M1:F0. Females have very rarely been described.

**Occurrence:** 1:10,000 live male births, without racial or ethnic variance. Prevalence is less than the birth frequency due to the relatively high death rate in patients prior to the advent of effective therapy around 1960.

**Risk of Recurrence for Patient's Sib:**
See Part I, *Mendelian Inheritance.*

**Risk of Recurrence for Patient's Child:**
See Part I, *Mendelian Inheritance.*

**Age of Detectability:** Factor VIII does not cross the placenta, and the absence of the coagulant activity can be diagnosed at birth. Prenatal diagnosis is possible.

**Gene Mapping and Linkage:** F8C (coagulation factor VIIIc, pro-coagulant component (hemophilia A)) has been mapped to Xq28.

**Prevention:** None known. Genetic counseling indicated.

**Treatment:** As soon as the diagnosis is made the patient should be immunized against hepatitis B.

The prompt infusion of intravenous Factor VIII at the earliest symptoms of bleeding will limit the extensiveness of the hemorrhage and subsequent joint destruction. Most severe patients receive self-administered home therapy and are infused with 20 U/kg at the first sign of bleeding. The half-life of Factor VIII is approximately 12 hours. For head or abdominal trauma, patients are infused prophylactically with 40 U/kg.

Factor VIII preparations are now routinely heated to destroy the HIV virus. Most treatment centers are using heat-treated concentrates, which can be rendered HIV-noninfectious, in preference to cryoprecipitate, which cannot be. Current heating techniques do not render the concentrates noninfectious for NANB hepatitis.

The patient who develop an inhibitor need to be treated at a specialized center. The current approaches to patients with inhibitors who are bleeding include infusions of materials that ''bypass'' Factor VIII, porcine Factor VIII, and various techniques of plasmaphoresis or Sepharose column absorption to remove the IgG inhibitor. The long-term elimination of the inhibitor can be achieved by inducing immune tolerance with daily Factor VIII infusions for 1 year or more.

Some patients with mild Factor VIII coagulation deficiency respond to desmopressin (DDAVP) infusions, with a two to four-fold release of Factor VIII coagulant from the vascular endothelium. Patients need to be individually tested for their response to desmopressin before it is used to treat a bleeding episode.

Liver transplantation for end-stage liver disease has resulted in the sustained cure of the Factor VIII deficiency in three affected individuals.

**Prognosis:** The prognosis for life with prompt therapy has been excellent in those patients who did not develop an inhibitor or liver disease. However, the current AIDS epidemic, with over 90% of the severely deficient patients having been infected with HIV, has introduced a large degree of uncertainty. Newly diagnosed patients who are treated exclusively with heat-treated materials will have a decreased risk of becoming HIV positive and should have a useful and unrestricted, active life.

**Detection of Carrier:** Female carriers are usually asymptomatic. Their Factor VIII activity is intermediate between the normal and the affected individual, but is quite variable and cannot serve as an adequate screening technique. Determination of the ratio of Factor VIII activity to the Factor VIII-associated antigen will identify approximately 80–90% of carriers. Restriction endonuclease polymorphisms can identify some carriers when the hemophilia gene is associated with a pattern of restriction endonuclease digestion fragments different than those of the nonaffected members of the family. Carrier detection has been done with both intragenic and extragenic mutations.

**Support Groups:**
Los Angeles; World Hemophilia AIDS Center
New York; The National Hemophilia Foundation (NHF)
New York; Hemophilia Research
CANADA: Ontario; Hamilton; Canadian Hemophilia Society
CANADA: Quebec; Montreal; World Federation of Hemophilia
ENGLAND: London; The Haemophilia Society
WEST GERMANY: Heidelberg; World Federation of Hemophilia Information Clearinghouse

**References:**
Egeberg O: An inherited hemorrhagic trait with characteristics resembling both mild hemophilia of type A and von Willebrands disease. Scand J Clin Lab Invest 1965; 17:25–32.
Hilgartner MW, ed: Hemophilia in the child and adult. Masson, 1982.
Bontempo FA, et al.: Liver transplantation in hemophilia A. Blood 1987; 69:1721.
Pecorara M, et al.: Hemophilia A: carrier detection and prenatal diagnosis by DNA analysis. Blood 1987; 70:531–535.
Sommer SS, Sobel JL: Application of DNA-based diagnosis to patient care: the example of hemophilia A. Mayo Clin Proc 1987; 62:387.

SE022                                    **Ruth Andrea Seeler**

**Hemophilia A-vascular abnormality**
*See HEMOPHILIA A*

---

## HEMOPHILIA B                                              0462

**Includes:**
Christmas disease
Factor IX deficiency
Plasma thromboplastin component deficiency

**Excludes:**
Coagulation factor deficiencies (other)
**Hemophilia A** (0461)
**Factor XI deficiency** (2671)
**Von Willebrand disease** (0996)

**Major Diagnostic Criteria:** Factor IX coagulant activity assay with less than 20% of normal activity. The severely deficient patients have less than 1% of normal activity, moderate 2–7%, and mildly affected 7–20%. Approximately 50% of the patients are in the mild category, 20–30% are moderate, and less than 20% of the Factor IX deficient patients are severe. The patients have normal bleeding times.

**Clinical Findings:** Similar to those seen in **Hemophilia A**, and depend on the individual's level of functional coagulation factor. Severely deficient patients may have spontaneous bleeding episodes into joints and muscles. Mildly affected patients frequently are not diagnosed until they sustain severe trauma or surgery.

**Complications:** Similar to those for **Hemophilia A**. Patients treated with multiple transfusions frequently have had hepatitis B as well as non-A, non-B (NANB) hepatitis. A smaller percentage of patients with hemophilia B are infected with the HIV virus. Factor IX-specific antibodies (inhibitors) may develop in patients with severe Factor IX deficiency.

**Associated Findings:** Chronic hepatitis resulting from NANB or hepatitis B with superimposed delta hepatitis. Chronic arthritides as a result of hemorrhage into joints and muscle atrophy or contractures due to muscle hemorrhages.

**Etiology:** X-linked inheritance.

**Pathogenesis:** The abnormal Factor IX protein does not function adequately in the coagulation cascade. In most cases Factor IX is detectable immunologically in normal levels, but functionally is deficient, indicating the presence of an abnormal Factor IX protein. Because of the different degrees of severity, a variety of genetic defects was anticipated and has recently been directly demonstrated.

It is recognized that the Factor IX-deficient patients who have developed inhibitors have deletion of part or all of the Factor IX gene.

**MIM No.:** *30690

**CDC No.:** 286.000

**Sex Ratio:** M1:F0

**Occurrence:** Approximately 1:50,000 live male births, possibly as high as 1:30,000 in the United Kingdom, without racial or ethnic variation. Prevalence is less because of the deaths that occurred prior to effective therapy in the early 1960s.

**Risk of Recurrence for Patient's Sib:**
See Part I, *Mendelian Inheritance.*

**Risk of Recurrence for Patient's Child:**
See Part I, *Mendelian Inheritance.*

**Age of Detectability:** Affected fetuses may be diagnosed prenatally using restrictive endonuclease polymorphisms. However, not all cases of Factor IX have polymorphism detectable by recombinant DNA technology. Affected severe patients may be diagnosed at birth by measuring the Factor IX coagulant level. For the mildly and moderately deficient patients, diagnosis at birth may not be possible because of the physiologically low levels of the vitamin K-dependent factors at birth. Assays should be run 24 hours after giving vitamin K.

**Gene Mapping and Linkage:** F9 (coagulation factor IX (Christmas disease)) has been mapped to Xq26.3-q27.1.

**Prevention:** None known. Genetic counseling indicated.

**Treatment:** Patients should be vaccinated against hepatitis B as soon as the diagnosis is made.

The prothrombin complex concentrates containing Factors II, VII, IX, and X are used to treat hemorrhages and prophylactically for surgical and dental procedures. The usual dose is 20–30 U/kg/day. Concentrates should be heat treated to prevent the transmission of HIV infection. Fresh-frozen plasma may be used, when concentrates are unavailable, for joint and soft tissue hemorrhage. The duration of therapy is dependent on extent of hemorrhage and location.

Factor IX-deficient patients do not respond to desmopressin.

Those patients who develop an inhibitor should be referred to hemophilia treatment centers experienced in the management of patients with inhibitors. Such patients may respond to the activated prothrombin complex concentrations such as Autoplex and FEIBA.

**Prognosis:** Prompt treatment of hemorrhage has resulted in marked diminution of chronic arthropathy and muscle atrophy. For those without chronic active hepatitis, HIV infection, or an inhibitor, a long and productive life can be expected.

**Detection of Carrier:** Female carriers are usually asymptomatic. Diagnosis by Factor IX level is usually not accurate. Several different polymorphisms have already been identified, and more are expected. When a restriction endonuclease polymorphism exists within a family, heterozygote detection is often possible.

**Support Groups:**
Los Angeles; World Hemophilia AIDS Center
New York; The National Hemophilia Foundation (NHF)
New York; Hemophilia Research
CANADA: Ontario; Hamilton; Canadian Hemophilia Society
CANADA: Quebec; Montreal; World Federation of Hemophilia
ENGLAND: London; The Haemophilia Society
WEST GERMANY: Heidelberg; World Federation of Hemophilia Information Clearinghouse

**References:**
Hilgartner MW, ed: Hemophilia in the child and adult. New York: Masson, 1982:1–303.
Poon M-C, et al.: Hemophilia B (christmas disease) variants and carrier detection analysis by DNA probes. J Clin Invest 1987; 79:1204–1209.
Thompson AR: Structure, function, and molecular defects of Factor IX. Blood 1986; 67:565.

SE022                                        **Ruth Andrea Seeler**

**Hemophilia C**
*See FACTOR XI DEFICIENCY*
**Hemorrhagic telangiectasia, hereditary**
*See TELANGIECTASIA, OSLER HEMORRHAGIC*
**HEMPAS**
*See ANEMIA, DYSERYTHROPOIETIC, TYPE II*
**Heparan sulfate sulfatase deficiency**
*See MUCOPOLYSACCHARIDOSIS III*
**Heparin cofactor deficiency**
*See ANTITHROMBIN III DEFICIENCY*
**Hepatic (liver) cysts**
*See LIVER, POLYCYSTIC AND MULTICYSTIC DISEASE, ADULT TYPE*
**Hepatic agenesis**
*See LIVER, AGENESIS*
**Hepatic arterial anomalies**
*See LIVER, ARTERIAL ANOMALIES*
**Hepatic carnitine palmitoyl transferase deficiency (some)**
*See MYOPATHY-METABOLIC, CARNITINE PALMITYL TRANSFERASE DEFICIENCY*
*also VISCERA, FATTY METAMORPHOSIS*
**Hepatic cholesteryl ester storage disease**
*See CHOLESTERYL ESTER STORAGE DISEASE*
**Hepatic cyst, nonparasitic**
*See LIVER, CYST, SOLITARY*
**Hepatic cyst, solitary**
*See LIVER, CYST, SOLITARY*
**Hepatic cyst, unilocular**
*See LIVER, CYST, SOLITARY*
**Hepatic ductular hypoplasia, syndromatic**
*See ARTERIO-HEPATIC DYSPLASIA*

**Hepatic dysfunction, constitutional**
*See HYPERBILIRUBINEMIA, UNCONJUGATED*
**Hepatic fibrosis, congenital**
*See KIDNEY, POLYCYSTIC DISEASE, RECESSIVE*

## HEPATIC FIBROSIS, CONGENITAL                    0605

**Includes:**
Kidney disease, autosomal recessive polycystic
Liver-kidney disease, infantile polycystic
Liver-kidney, polycystic disease, autosomal recessive type
Nephronophtisis-congenital hepatic

**Excludes:**
Banti syndrome
Caroli disease
Centrovenous occlusive disease
Cirrhosis
**Cystic fibrosis** (0237)
Extrahepatic portal vein thrombosis
**Liver, polycystic and multicystic disease, adult type** (3201)
Non-cirrhotic portal hypertension

**Major Diagnostic Criteria:** *Hepatic*: Evidence of portal hypertension, firm hepatomegaly, histology consistent with hepatic fibrosis.

*Renal*: Renal failure or insufficiency, nephromegaly, histology demonstrating collecting tubule ectasia.

**Clinical Findings:** *Hepatic*: The clinical features of congenital hepatic fibrosis vary from the total absence of symptoms with discovery during evaluation of renal disease or incidentally to severe portal hypertension. The most common presentation is with hepatomegaly. The liver is very firm, which can draw attention to relatively mild enlargement. The next most common presentation is with hematemesis, and next is splenomegaly. Impaired liver function is relatively uncommon. A few patients will demonstrate pruritus secondary to portosystemic shunting of bile salts and even fewer will exhibit portosystemic encephalopathy. Transaminase values are usually normal whereas alkaline phosphatase may be moderately increased.

Imaging techniques may be useful in establishing the diagnosis. Ultrasound with Doppler flow analysis will demonstrate splenomegaly with patent splenic and portal veins which often have reduced flow velocity. The liver is diffusely echogenic and may contain numerous cystic dilatations of the intrahepatic biliary tree. Some dilitations of the extrahepatic bile ducts and/or gall bladder may also be observed. Splenoportogram or superior mesenteric arteriogram may demonstrate abnormalities including duplication and "pruning" of small to mid-size branches of the portal vein or hepatic artery. Splenic pulp pressure and portal vein pressure are elevated. Wedged hepatic vein pressure may be normal because of the presinusoidal location of the flow resitance in these patients. Computerized tomography or percutaneous transhepatic cholangiogram may be useful in determining the nature and degree of ductal abnormalities.

Histologic confirmation of the diagnosis should be attempted. Finding characteristic changes is diagnostic, but biopsy may be negative because the lesion can be irregularly distributed through the hepatic mass. Broad bands of dense fibrosis extending between and separating lobules is pathognomonic for congenital hepatic fibrosis. Within the fibrous bands may be found numerous bile ducts which may be variably ectatic or cystic. Inflammation is minimal and when present is associated with ectatic bile ducts. Although fibrosis may completely encircle liver lobules, this lesion should be differentiated from cirrhosis by the normal architecture of the lobule. The fibrosis does not involve the central venule. The intrahepatic ducts are variably involved. Fusiform to saccular cystic dilation reminiscent of Caroli disease is often seen.

*Renal*: Virtually all patients with congenital hepatic fibrosis have polycystic kidney disease. The typical type of cystic renal lesion is identical to the autosomal recessive or "infantile" type of polycystic kidney disease and has been classified as *Potter type I* cystic kidney disease. In older children the appearance of the cystic renal lesions may be indistinguishable from medullary sponge kidney.

Cysts are located in cortical or medullary collecting tubules. Generally the cysts are small fusiform dilations; however, occasionally cysts may expand to large dimensions and resemble the autosomal dominant type of polycystic kidney disease.

The diagnosis of polycystic kidney lesion associated with congential hepatic fibrosis should be suspected when renal ultrasonography demonstrates increased echogenicity of the kidneys with loss of corticomedullary differentiation. The excretory urogram shows a delayed nephrogram with prolonged retention of contrast media in the ectatic collecting ducts. The diagnosis is confirmed by renal biopsy. Recent identification of a lectin, *Arachis hypogaea*, which is specific for distal nephron epithelia, has greatly enhanced the diagnostic capability of the renal biopsy.

Renal function may vary from marked reduction to normal levels of glomerular filtration rate. Deterioration of renal function in some patients may progress slowly over many years. In general, renal function is normal or minimally impaired when congenital hepatic fibrosis with cystic kidney disease is discovered in older children or adolescents. The urinalysis is often normal, but may contain blood or protein.

**Complications:** *Hepatic:* Complications of portal hypertension, including esophageal varices, hypersplenism, and gastrointestinal hemorrhage, are frequently observed. Cholangitis and hepatic abcess formation are uncommon. The disease tends to be progressive, and liver failure may be observed in young adults.
*Renal:* Oliguric or polyuric renal failure, hypertension, growth failure, metabolic bone disease, and anemia are frequent.

**Associated Findings:** Pancreatic cysts; splenic cysts; renal collecting system abnormalities including duplication, stenosis, and atresia; pulmonary hypoplasia and pulmonary arteriovenous malformations (Alvarez et al., 1981; Lieberman et al., 1971; Hartnett and Bennett, 1976).

An unusual family with congenital hepatic fibrosis, retinal hypoplasia, and nephronophthisis has been reported, and an unconfirmed example of congenital hepatic fibrosis and autosomal dominant kidney disease has also been described.

**Etiology:** Probably autosomal recessive inheritance.

**Pathogenesis:** Two principal theories place the primary defect in the formation of the ductular structures or the connective tissue. In one, obstruction of ducts (interlobular bile ducts or collecting tubules) during organogenesis results in a reactive proliferation of fibroblasts and formation of collagen. In the other, a primary defect in control of connective tissue formation is blamed. During early organogenesis when ductal budding, proliferation, and migration are underway, mesodermal elements, which must accompany the epithelial elements, undergo uncontrolled proliferation. The ductal changes are thought to be secondary to fibrosis and obstruction.

**MIM No.:** *26320

**CDC No.:** 751.610

**Sex Ratio:** M1:F1

**Occurrence:** Undetermined but presumably uncommon.

**Risk of Recurrence for Patient's Sib:**
See Part I, *Mendelian Inheritance.*

**Risk of Recurrence for Patient's Child:**
See Part I, *Mendelian Inheritance.*

**Age of Detectability:** Usually in the first decade, by clinical examination.

**Gene Mapping and Linkage:** Unknown.

**Prevention:** None known. Genetic counseling indicated.

**Treatment:** Conservative management of renal insufficiency and hypertension reduces early morbidity. Dialysis and renal transplantation may be required. Management of portal hypertension includes conservative measures to prevent gastrointestinal hemorrhage, such as abstaining from taking aspirin and ethanol, endoscopic sclerotherapy of varices, and surgical portal vein decompression. Liver transplantation may be required.

**Prognosis:** The initial outcome is dictated by the renal involvement. Severely affected individuals will exhibit renal failure in infancy. Later, gastrointestinal hemorrhage becomes more important. Few follow-up studies are available, but the disease is probably slowly progressive. Liver and sometimes renal transplantation may provide significant extension of life.

**Detection of Carrier:** Unknown.

**References:**
Kerr DNS, et al.: Congenital hepatic fibrosis. Q J Med 1961; 30:91–118.
Blyth H, Ockenden BG: Polycystic disease of kidneys and liver presenting in childhood. J Med Genet 1971; 8:257–284.
Lieberman E, et al.: Infantile polycystic disease of the kidneys and liver. Medicine 1971; 50:277–318.
Alvarez F, et al.: Congenital hepatic fibrosis in children. J Pediatr 1981; 99:370–375.
Witzleben CL, Sharp AR: "Nephronophthisis-congenital hepatic fibrosis": an additional hepatorenal disorder. Hum Pathol 1982; 13:728–733.
Cole BR, et al.: Polycystic kidney disease in the first year of life. J Pediatr 1987; 111:693–699.

WH007                                    **Peter F. Whitington**
ST055                                    **F. Bruder Stapleton**

**Hepatic fibrosis-polycystic kidneys-colobomata**
*See OCULO-ENCEPHALO-HEPATO-RENAL SYNDROME*
**Hepatic fructokinase deficiency**
*See FRUCTOSURIA*
**Hepatic fructose-1,6-diphosphatase deficiency**
*See FRUCTOSE-1,6-DIPHOSPHATASE DEFICIENCY*
**Hepatic glycogenosis with normal enzymes**
*See GLYCOGEN STORAGE DISEASE, X-LINKED WITH NORMAL HEPATIC ENZYMES*
**Hepatic hamartoma**
*See LIVER, HAMARTOMA*
**Hepatic hemangiomatosis**
*See LIVER, HEMANGIOMATOSIS*
**Hepatic infantile hemangioendothelioma**
*See LIVER, HEMANGIOMATOSIS*
**Hepatic lobes anomalous**
*See LIVER, ACCESSORY LOBE*
**Hepatic lobes, accessory**
*See LIVER, ACCESSORY LOBE*
**Hepatic phosphorylase**
*See GLYCOGENOSIS, TYPE VI*
**Hepatic phosphorylase kinase deficiency**
*See GLYCOGENOSIS, TYPE IXa*
*also GLYCOGEN STORAGE DISEASE, X-LINKED WITH NORMAL HEPATIC ENZYMES*
**Hepatic situs inversus**
*See LIVER, TRANSPOSITION*
**Hepatic storage disease**
*See HYPERBILIRUBINEMIA, CONJUGATED*
*also HYPERBILIRUBINEMIA, CONJUGATED, ROTOR TYPE*
**Hepatic venous anomalies**
*See LIVER, VENOUS ANOMALIES*
**Hepatitis B infection, perinatal transmission**
*See FETAL EFFECTS FROM HEPATITIS B INFECTION*
**Hepatitis, neonatal (some)**
*See ALPHA(1)-ANTITRYPSIN DEFICIENCY*
**Hepato-skeleto-cardiac syndrome**
*See ARTERIO-HEPATIC DYSPLASIA*
**Hepatoerythropoietic porphyria**
*See PORPHYRIA CUTANEA TARDA*

---

**HEPATOLENTICULAR DEGENERATION**                    **0469**

**Includes:**
Ceruloplasmin deficiency
Copper retention
Copper toxicosis, inherited
Hypoceruloplasminemia
Progressive lenticular degeneration
Wilson disease

**Excludes:**
**Cholestasis-lymphedema, Aagenaes type** (3118)
Arterioductular hypoplasia syndrome

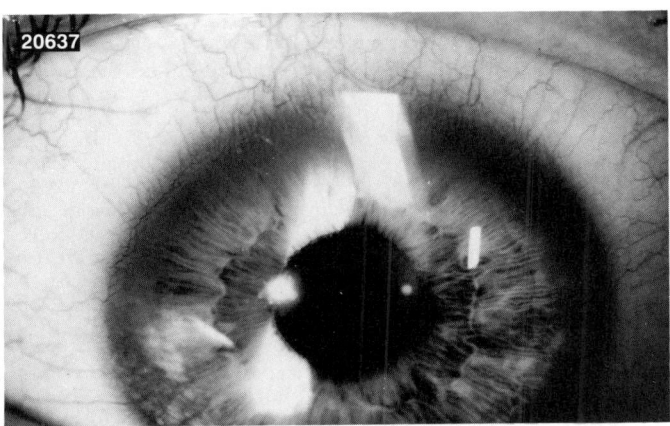

**0469-20637:** Hepatolenticular degeneration; Kayser-Fleischer ring. A brownish-red deposition of copper appears in Descemet's membrane in the deep layer at the periphery of the corneal stroma.

**Cerebro-hepato-renal syndrome** (0139)
Indian childhood cirrhosis
Primary biliary cirrhosis

**Major Diagnostic Criteria:** Serum ceruloplasmin is usually decreased (<20 mg%) but not in 100% of the cases. Liver copper levels exceed 300 $\mu$g/g dry weight; 5 mg of tissue is required for this chemical (not histologic) test. A definitive test is lack of incorporation of intravenously administered Cu[64] into ceruloplasmin during a 48-hour period. Cultured skin fibroblasts have also been found to accumulate copper.

With few exceptions, patients with neurologic presentation have copper deposition in the Descemet membrane of the cornea, forming the characteristic Kayser-Fleischer ring, which can be visualized by slit-lamp examination. Sunflower cataracts occur in 15–20% of the cases.

**Clinical Findings:** Patients appear to be healthy for at least 5 to 8 years. Those presenting with hepatic complications become symptomatic prior to puberty, sometimes by age 8 years, whereas neurologic presentation occurs later, with some presenting in the sixth decade. Hepatic dysfunction is characterized by "hepatitis" symptoms, elevated hepatic enzymes in the circulation, diminished synthesis of clotting factors, and hemolytic anemia. Neurologic symptoms are asymmetric and variable: dysarthria, drooling, ataxia, tremor, aberrant behavior, and movement disorders.

Wilson disease has been divided into at least three types: 1) an atypical, German-Mennonite form, in which obligate carriers have heterozygote levels of ceruloplasmin; 2) a late-onset, primarily neurological form, of Slavic origin; and 3) a juvenile-onset, primarily hepatic form, of Western European origin. In types two and three, heterozygotes have normal ceruloplasmin levels.

**Complications:** Thrombocytopenia and anemia may result from hypersplenism. Renal tubular and glomerular dysfunction occur frequently and may be the presenting symptom in some cases. Renal lithiasis can occur. Death may result from either hepatic or neurologic disease if the diagnosis and treatment are delayed.

**Associated Findings:** All signs and symptoms are secondary to copper accumulation and resulting toxic sequelae.

**Etiology:** Autosomal recessive inheritance.

**Pathogenesis:** Positive copper balance results from compromised biliary excretion of copper; there is a concomitant inability to incorporate copper into circulating ceruloplasmin. Excess copper is stored in the liver until the capacity of that organ is exceeded. Copper is then deposited in the basal ganglia (lenticula), cornea, renal tubules, and other organs. Intestinal absorption

(2 mg/day) is normal; biliary excretion (0.2–0.4 mg/day) is 10–20% of normal; urinary excretion (1 mg/day) is 25 times normal.

**MIM No.:** *27790

**POS No.:** 3251

**Sex Ratio:** M1:F1

**Occurrence:** 1–2:100,000 live births. Probably many undiagnosed and unrecognized cases exist.

**Risk of Recurrence for Patient's Sib:**
See Part I, *Mendelian Inheritance.*

**Risk of Recurrence for Patient's Child:**
See Part I, *Mendelian Inheritance.*

**Age of Detectability:** Biochemically, age six months; symptomatically, anywhere from ages 6–8 years to the sixth decade.

**Gene Mapping and Linkage:** WND (Wilson disease) has been mapped to 13q14.2-q21.

**Prevention:** None known. Genetic counseling indicated.

**Treatment:** D-penicillamine chelates copper (and other metal ions), allowing excretion in soluble form in the urine. Negative copper balance is difficult to maintain for more than one year, although the patients remain well, and this has suggested that penicillamine may form a detoxifying complex or induce the synthesis of metallothionein. This isomer is less likely to evoke untoward responses such as vitamin B6 deficiency and nephrotic syndrome than the D-L racemic mixture. There is a 3–6-month lag in clinical benefits following institution of chelation therapy. There are occasional reports of dramatic neurologic worsening immediately after therapy begins.

Adverse reactions to penicillamine are common, such as systemic lupus erythematosus (SLE) and nephritis, and triethylene tetramine (TETA) is therefore sometimes used as a substitute. See also **Fetal D-penicillamine syndrome.** Vitamin B6 deficiency can be treated with pyridoxine replacement. Acute arthritis is also a common complication of treatment, as are poor wound healing and skin lesions, some of which are only slowly reversible with cessation of therapy, if at all. Patients with reactions severe enough to preclude continuing therapy can be given triethylene tetramine; most symptoms will abate, except SLE.

During the interval of latency of response, adjunct therapies that might be helpful include albumin infusion to increase copper binding, peritoneal dialysis with albumin in the dialysate, exchange transfusions, and L-dopa to control the CNS symptoms.

Liver transplantation has been tried with reported success for severe hepatic failure.

Treatment with zinc supplements has received mixed reports of efficacy. Zinc is lost during penicillamine therapy, and administration of this metal ion creates a competitive environment, diminishing copper absorption by the intestine.

**Prognosis:** Asymptomatic individuals can remain healthy indefinitely with treatment. The prognosis for symptomatic individuals depends on the progression of the disease when diagnosis is made and treatment is instituted. Clinical symptoms can be reversed, but slurred speech is sometimes never completely cleared.

**Detection of Carrier:** Studies of ceruloplasmin uptake of Cu[64] can identify only 80–90% of heterozygotes. However, tests are advocated to identify presymptomatic homozygotes.

**Special Considerations:** Normal sheep and a mutant Bedlington terrier may serve as animal models of the human disease.

**Support Groups:**
NY; Bronx Foundation for the Study of Wilson's Disease
DC; Washington Wilson's Disease Association

**References:**
Scheinberg IH: A genetic defect in the transport of caeruloplasmin-copper from blood to bile as the possible pathogenesis of Wilson's disease. In: Blauer G, Sund H, eds: Transport by proteins. Berlin: Walter DeGruyter, 1978.
Chan WY, et al.: Genetic expression of Wilson's disease in cell culture: a diagnostic marker. Science 1980; 208:299–300.

Walshe JM: Treatment of Wilson's disease with trientine (triethylene tetramine) dihydrochloride. Lancet 1982; I:643–647.

Walshe JM: Wilson's disease: genetics and biochemistry: their relevance to therapy. J Inherited Metab Dis 1983; 6(suppl 1):51–58.

Van Caillie-Bertrand M, et al.: Wilson's disease: assessment of D-penicillamine treatment. Arch Dis Child 1985; 60:652–655.

Lingam S, et al.: Neurological abnormalities in Wilson's disease are reversible. Neuropediatrics 1987; 18:11–12.

Polson RJ, et al.: Reversal of severe neurological manifestations of Wilson's disease following orthotopic liver transplantation. Quart J Med 1987; 64:685–691.

Scheinberg IH, et al.: Penicillamine may detoxify copper in Wilson's disease. Lancet 1987; II:95 only.

Starosta-Rubinstein S, et al.: Clinical assessment of 31 patients with Wilson's disease. Arch Neurol 1987; 44:365–370.

VI006                                                    **Jaclyn M. Vidgoff**

**Hepatorenal glycogenosis**
  *See GLYCOGENOSIS, TYPE Ia*
**Hepatorenal tyrosinemia**
  *See TYROSINEMIA I*
**Hepatosplenomegaly-gingival fibromatosis-digital anomalies**
  *See GINGIVAL FIBROMATOSIS-DIGITAL ANOMALIES*
**Hereditary cerebral hemorrhage with amyloidosis (HCHWA)**
  *See AMYLOIDOSIS, ICELANDIC TYPE*
**Hereditary cutaneous malignant melanoma (HCMM)**
  *See CANCER, MALIGNANT MELANOMA, FAMILIAL*
**Hereditary motor sensory neuropathy (HMSN), type III**
  *See DEJERINE-SOTTAS DISEASE*
**Hereditary nonpolyposis colorectal cancer (HNPCC)**
  *See CANCER, SEBACEOUS GLAND TUMOR-MULITPLE VISCERAL CARCINOMA*
  *also CANCER, COLORECTAL*
**Hereditary sensory and autonomic neuropathy III (HSAN III)**
  *See DYSAUTONOMIA I, RILEY-DAY TYPE*
**Hereditary sensory and autonomic neuropathy IV (HSAN-IV)**
  *See NEUROPATHY, CONGENITAL SENSORY WITH ANHIDROSIS*
**Heredodegenerations of inner ear**
  *See EAR, INNER DYSPLASIAS*
**Heredopathia atactica polyneuritiformis**
  *See PHYTANIC ACID STORAGE DISEASE*
**Herlitz-Pearson junctional epidermolysis bullosa**
  *See EPIDERMOLYSIS BULLOSUM, TYPE II*
**Hermansky-Pudlak syndrome**
  *See ALBINISM, OCULOCUTANEOUS, HERMANSKY-PUDLAK TYPE*
**Hermaphroditism**
  *See HERMAPHRODITISM, TRUE*

---

## HERMAPHRODITISM, TRUE                                  0971

**Includes:**  Hermaphroditism

**Excludes:**
  **Chromosome mosaicism, 45,X/46,XY type** (0173)
  Pseudohermaphroditism, male and female, all forms

**Major Diagnostic Criteria:**  Histologically verified ovarian follicles and seminiferous tubules or spermatozoa. A 46,XX/46,XY or 46,XX/47,XXY complement does not alone warrant the diagnosis.

**Clinical Findings:**  True hermaphrodites have both ovarian and testicular tissue. Specifically: 1) There must be histologically verified ovarian follicles or proof of their prior existence (e.g., corpora albicantia); fibrous stroma will not suffice. 2) Testicular tubules or spermatozoa must be present; Leydig or hilar cells will not suffice. The diagnosis is applied irrespective of chromosome complement. Somatic anomalies are usually absent.

Most true hermaphrodites are 46,XX, but a few are 46,XY, 46,XX/46,XY, or 46,XX/47,XXY. Their external genitalia are usually ambiguous or predominantly male, with evidence of androgen insufficiency (e.g., hypospadias or bifid scrotum). About 70% are reared as males. A vagina and well-differentiated uterus are usually present. Fallopian tubes are less likely to be normal.

Gonadal tissue may be organized into separate ovary and testis, but more often combined into one or more ovotestes. Relative locations of ovarian and testicular tissue may be 1) bilateral, both ovarian and testicular tissue present on each side, usually in the form of ovotestes; 2) unilateral, both ovarian and testicular tissue

present only on one side, with gonadal tissue of the opposite type present on the contralateral side; or 3) alternate, ovarian tissue present on one side and testicular tissue present on the opposite side. The greater the proportion of testicular tissue in an ovotestis, the greater the likelihood of gonadal descent. In 80% of the ovotestes the testicular and ovarian components exist in end-to-end fashion. Thus, most testes can be detected externally because testicular tissue is softer and darker than ovarian tissue. In 20% of ovotestes the testicular tissue is limited to the hilar region. A vas deferens may be present near a testis or ovotestis, in which case no fallopian tube may be present on that side. Fallopian tubes adjacent to ovotestes often show occlusion of the fimbriated end. Spermatozoa are rarely present, but oocytes are often present. Leydig cell hyperplasia occurs in about one-third of cases, and seminiferous tubules may contain many Sertoli cells.

Endocrine features at puberty depend upon the extent of testicular or ovarian tissue present, but true hermaphrodites are more likely to feminize than to virilize. Most patients with a uterus menstruate. If the uterus is not connected to the urogenital sinus, hematometrocolpos may develop. In some true hermaphrodites with predominantly male external genitalia, menstruation has occurred in the form of cyclic hematuria. Squamous metaplasia of the endocervix is relatively common. The above description applies in general to true hermaphrodites; however, some data suggest that the phenotypes associated with different karyotypes may be dissimilar.

**Complications:**  Puberal virilization in individuals reared as females; puberal feminization in individuals reared as males. Neoplastic transformation of intraabdominal or inguinal testes has been reported.

**Associated Findings:**  None known.

**Etiology:**  True hermaphrodites are etiologically heterogeneous; 46,XX/46,XY or 46,XX/47,XXY true hermaphroditism presumably results from chimerism or mosaicism. The etiology of 46,XY true hermaphroditism is unknown, but phenotypic similarities with 46,XX/46,XY true hermaphrodites suggest that many apparent 46,XY true hermaphrodites may have undetected 46,XX cells. There is one report of X-chromatin-negative sibs with true hermaphroditism, but more extensive cytogenetic studies were not available.

The presence of testicular tissues in individuals lacking a Y (i.e., 46,XX true hermaphrodites) could be explained in at least four ways: 1) undetected mosaicism or chimerism, 46,XY cells thus being present but not detected; 2) translocation of Y-linked testicular determinants to an X chromosome; 3) translocation of Y-linked testicular determinants to an autosome; 4) mutant gene(s). Each may explain certain cases, but the most common etiology is undetermined.

The DNA sequence connoting the TDF on the Y short arm is not present in XX true hermaphrodites, even though it is present in XX males. This suggests that translocation of TDF is not responsible for XX true hermaphrodites. That another etiology exists would be consistent with coexistence of ovarian tissue, a phenomenon not observed in XX males. Perturbation of a mutant gene thus is raised as an etiologic possibility. 46,XX true hermaphroditism is usually not inherited and the prevalence of consangunity does not appear to be increased. However, in several families multiple sibs had 46,XX true hermaphroditism. The presence of both XX males and XX true hermaphrodites in more than one generation of another family has also occurred.

**Pathogenesis:**  The cellular pathogenesis depends upon the etiology of true hermaphroditism. 46,XX/46,XY true hermaphroditism presumably results from admixtures of 46,XX and 46,XY germ cells. Translocation of testicular determinants from the Y to an X or an autosome could explain the presence of testicular tissue in individuals who apparently lack a Y chromosome. As noted, however, such an explanation does not necessarily explain the presence of both ovarian and testicular tissue. Elaboration of diffusible compounds that affect surrounding undifferentiated gonadal tissue could potentially offer an explanation

**MIM No.:**  23560

**CDC No.:**  752.700

**Sex Ratio:** Unknown.

**Occurrence:** Over 400 cases have been documented.

**Risk of Recurrence for Patient's Sib:** Usually negligible. However, in the few families in which 46,XX true hermaphroditism appears to be inherited in autosomal recessive fashion, the recurrence risk is presumably 1:8 for all sibs, or 1:4 for 46,XX sibs.

**Risk of Recurrence for Patient's Child:** Affected individuals are infertile, except for four exceptions.

**Age of Detectability:** Usually at birth because of genital ambiguity, but some patients with relatively normal external genitalia may not be detected until puberty, at which time they fail to show normal secondary sexual development. Occasionally, 46,XX/46,XY true hermaphroditism is suspected by recognizing iridal heterochromia or by detecting two populations of erythrocytes during blood grouping analyses. If 46,XX/46,XY mosaicism is detected in utero, data are insufficient to state the likelihood that the fetus will be phenotypically abnormal, i.e., show true hermaphroditism.

**Gene Mapping and Linkage:** Unknown.

**Prevention:** None known. Genetic counseling indicated.

**Treatment:** Genital reconstruction. Extirpation of cryptorchid testes may be appropriate to prevent neoplastic transformation. Administration of hormones may be necessary.

**Prognosis:** Normal life span, provided neoplasia does not occur; infertility.

**Detection of Carrier:** Unknown.

**Special Considerations:** True hermaphroditism is usually not diagnosed before surgical exploration. Thus, female or male pseudohermaphroditism should initially be considered in an infant with genital ambiguity only after other diagnoses seem inappropriate. The diagnosis may be suspected on observation of chimerism, a gonad with tissue that shows two consistencies (a softer testicular portion and a firmer ovarian portion), squamous metaplasia of the endocervix, or a fallopian tube with fimbrial occlusion.

**References:**

Van Niekerk WA: True hermaphroditism. New York: Harper & Row, 1974.
Simpson JL: Disorders of sexual differentiation: etiology and clinical delineation. New York: Academic Press, 1976:237–252.
Simpson JL: True hermaphroditism, etiology and phenotypic considerations. BD:OAS XIV(6c). New York: Alan R. Liss, for The National Foundation-March of Dimes, 1978:9–35.
Tegenkamp TR, et al.: Pregnancy without benefit of reconstructive surgery in a bisexually active hermaphrodite. Am J Obstet Gynecol 1979; 135:427–428.
Van Niekerk WA, Retief AE: The gonads of human true hermaphrodites. Hum Genet 1981; 58:117–122.
Wachtel SS: H-Y antigen and the biology of sex determination. New York: Grune & Stratton, 1982:192–206.
Vergnaud G, et al.: A deletion map of the human Y based DNA hybridization. Am J Hum Genet 1986; 38:109–124.
Ramsey M, et al.: XX true hermaphroditism in Southern African blacks: an enigma of primary sexual differentiation. Am J Med Genet 1988; 43:4–13.

SI018                                                                    **Joe Leigh Simpson**

**Hernia uteri inguinale syndrome**
*See MULLERIAN DERIVATIVES IN MALES, PERSISTENT*
**Hernia, diaphragmatic, congenital**
*See DIAPHRAGMATIC HERNIA*

## HERNIA, HIATAL                                                        0471

**Includes:**
  Diaphragmatic esophageal hiatus hernia
  Esophageal hiatus hernia
  Hiatus hernia
  Paraesophageal hernia
  Short esophagus, most instances

**Excludes:**
  **Microcephaly-hiatus hernia-nephrosis, Galloway type** (2755)
  Short esophagus, congenital (rare)

**Major Diagnostic Criteria:** A hiatal hernia is the protrusion of the stomach through the esophageal hiatus of the diaphragm. Most commonly the esophagus and the stomach both prolapse. A much less common form is a paraesophageal hernia. In this condition, the lower esophagus maintains its normal position, and the proximal stomach herniates through the hiatus along side the esophagus. The diagnosis of a hiatal hernia can be made with a barium study, upper endoscopy, or esophageal manometry. The diagnosis by radiographic study requires demonstration of the stomach above the diaphragm. This is generally recognized by the presence of gastric folds, a mucosal notch, and a non-peristaltic pouch above the diaphragm. Diagnosis can be difficult. Hiatal hernia is confirmed endoscopically by noting gastric mucosa above the indentation of the diaphragm. Esophageal manometry can locate the lower esophageal sphincter pressure, and identify its relationship to the diaphragm by noting whether there are negative or positive deflections with inspiration. A negative deflection occurs with inspiration when the perfusion catheter is measuring pressures above the diaphragm, positive deflections occur below the diaphragm. Esophageal manometry also allows measurement of lower esophageal sphincter pressure.

**Clinical Findings:** The clinical significance of an hiatal hernia is related to its association with gastroesophageal reflux. Although, gastroesophageal reflux is more common in individuals with a hiatal hernia, the two terms are not synonymous. Gastroesophageal reflux can occur with or without an hiatal hernia. The clinical findings of a hiatal hernia are therefore, those of gastroesophageal reflux. The most common symptom is vomiting or "spitting up". Heartburn is a much less common symptom. The paraesophageal hernia can be associated with abdominal pain and vomiting. The risk of strangulation and infarction is significant and surgical correction needs to be considered in all cases of paraesophageal hernia.

**Complications:** Gastroesophageal reflux can lead to esophagitis, aspiration pneumonia, choking, and if there is a large amount of calories lost through vomiting, and failure to thrive. Occult blood loss, anemia, and an esophageal stricture are all unusual complications of an esophagus inflamed by acid reflux. A cause and effect relationship between gastroesophageal reflux and apnea and aborted sudden infant death syndrome has been suggested.

**Associated Findings:** Both pyloric stenosis and pylorospasm have been noted in association with gastroesophageal reflux. A peculiar head posturing, Sandifer syndrome, in association with gastroesophageal reflux is a recognized entity.

**Etiology:** Undetermined. Possibly autosomal dominant inheritance in instances of *short esophagus* which has been reported in several kindreds. Gastroesophageal reflux is presumably caused by a defective lower esophageal sphincter mechanism.

**Pathogenesis:** A structural defect exists at the esophageal hiatus. Because of the sling arrangement of the two arms of the right crus, their contraction with inspiration serves as a "pinchcock" mechanism to prevent reflux during the period of negative intrathoracic pressure. The angle of His has been suggested by some to be of significance in maintaining integrity of the gastroesophageal junction and prevention of reflux, although this mechanism certainly is controversial. The role of the phrenoesophageal ligament in keeping the gastroesophageal junction below the diaphragm is likewise a matter of controversy. It has been shown, however, that in the presence of herniation of the stomach into the chest, the phrenoesophageal ligament serves as a means of opening the gastroesophageal junction thereby producing easy reflux. This is, of course, related to the presence of the physiologic sphincter at the distal end of the esophagus and thus its placement into the chest favors reflux.

**MIM No.:** 14240

**CDC No.:** 750.600

**Sex Ratio:** M1:F1

**Occurrence:** Uncommon; associated with less than 20% of children who have significant gastroesophageal reflux.

**Risk of Recurrence for Patient's Sib:** Unknown.

**Risk of Recurrence for Patient's Child:** Unknown.

**Age of Detectability:** Anytime in childhood or infancy.

**Gene Mapping and Linkage:** Unknown.

**Prevention:** None known. Genetic counseling indicated.

**Treatment:** No treatment is necessaary unless there are symptoms of gastroesophageal reflux or esophagitis is demonstrated. Medical treatment of gastroesophageal reflux includes positional therapy, thickening of feedings, small more frequent feedings, or, if necessary, a trial of bethanechol or metoclopramide. The 30° prone position is the best position to minimize gastroesophageal reflux.

The effectiveness of bethanechol and metoclopramide is unclear. Surgical therapy is indicated only in those patients who have significant complications of gastroesophageal reflux and fail to respond to medical therapy. The usual operative therapy is a gastric fundoplication.

**Prognosis:** Approximately 80% of patients will respond to positional therapy and time. Surgical correction is successful in over 95% of the cases.

**Detection of Carrier:** Unknown.

**Special Considerations:** Some investigators have felt that hiatus hernia in childhood is not a congenital anomaly but is associated with a congenitally *short esophagus*. This, in all probability, is not the case. Barrett has demonstrated that a congenitally short esophagus does exist, but it is extremely rare, and most of the short esophagi associated with hiatus hernia are due to cicatricial shortening from reflux esophagitis. Muscle spasm from esophagitis also will accentuate any tendency toward shortening of the esophagus.

Perhaps the respiratory complications of gastroesophageal reflux associated with hiatus hernia are the most feared of complications. Sudden death may follow laryngospasm due to reflux, or chronic respiratory disorders may produce long-term disability. With the excellent outlook of fundoplication in the child and the low morbidity of surgical repair, more emphasis is being placed upon early correction and prevention of long-term or fatal complications.

**References:**
Carre IJ: The natural history of the partial thoracic stomach ("hiatus hernia"). Arch Dis Child 1959; 34:344–352.
Kinsbourne M: Hiatus hernia with contortions of the neck. Lancet 1964; I:1058–1061.
Darling DB: Hiatal hernia and gastroesophageal reflux in infancy and childhood: analysis of the radiologic findings. Am J Roentgenol Radium Ther Nucl Med 1975; 123:724–736.
Leape LL, et al.: Respiratory arrest in infants secondary to gastroesophageal reflux. Pediatr 1977; 60:924–928.
Herbst JJ, et al.: Gastroesophageal reflux in the "near miss" sudden infant death syndrome. J Pediatr 1978; 92:73–75.
McCauley RGK, et al.: Gastroesophageal reflux in infants and children: a useful classification and reliable physiologic technique for its demonstration. Am J Roentgenol 1978; 130:47–50.
Ashcraft KW, et al.: Treatment of gastroesophageal reflux in children by Thal fundoplication. J Thorac Cardiovasc Surg 1981; 82:706–712.
Silverman A, Roy CC: Pediatric Clinical Gastroenterology. C.V. Mosby Co., 1983.

R0055
AS000

**Charles C. Roberts**
**Keith W. Ashcraft**

Hernia, hiatal/ulcer, peptic-cafe-au-lait-hypertelorism-myopia
*See GASTROCUTANEOUS SYNDROME*

## HERNIA, INGUINAL 0529

**Includes:**
Communicating hydrocele
Hernia, inguinal direct or indirect
Hydrocele
Incarcerated hernia
Inguinal hernia
Sliding hernia
Strangulated hernia

**Excludes:**
Femoral hernia
Varicocele
Ventral hernia

**Major Diagnostic Criteria:** Presence or history of a mass in groin on straining or at rest. Persistent hydrocele in a child over 1 year of age. Palpation of inguinal ring is invalid in children for detection of hernia. An irreducible mass in the inguinal region is an incarcerated hernia until proven otherwise, although in the absence of symptoms, it may be a hydrocele of the spermatic cord (or of the canal of Nuck in females). Differential diagnosis must be made at operation.

**Clinical Findings:** Presence of a mass in the groin or scrotum in males and the groin in females. The mass may be intermittent and more evident on straining, crying, etc, or constant in the case of hydrocele with or without herniated viscera. An incarcerated hernia cannot be reduced and is painful and tender. In infants, incarcerated hernias may be asymptomatic until signs of intestinal obstruction or strangulation supervene. Persistent hydrocele in children over one year of age generally signifies the presence of a hernia. A hydrocele present in a toddler or infant at the end of the day, but absent in the morning, is a "communicating hydrocele" and also indicates a hernia.

**Complications:** Intestinal obstruction may result from incarceration. Strangulation or ischemic change in the bowel wall due to incarceration may result in intestinal perforation, shock, peritonitis, and death if not treated promptly. Testicular atrophy may result from obstruction of the testicular vessels by an incarcerated hernia. Ovarian atrophy may result from incarceration and ischemia of the ovary.

**Associated Findings:** Hernias are more frequent in premature infants; undescended testes.

**Etiology:** Persistence of the processus vaginalis

**Pathogenesis:** Most inguinal hernias in children are indirect. Less than 1% are direct. The indirect hernia is the result of a failure of obliteration of the processus vaginalis, a projection of the peritoneal cavity into the inguinal canal and scrotum. The processus vaginalis normally is obliterated, except around the testes where it becomes the tunica vaginalis. A hydrocele may form in the tunica vaginalis or in a more proximal part of the processus vaginalis that fails to obliterate (hydrocele of the cord). Failure of closure of the entire processus vaginalis may lead to a communicating hydrocele or a hernia, or both. Hydroceles are very common in the first months of life as the processus vaginalis is obliterating. If a hydrocele persists after one year of age, a hernia is present 95% of the time.

**CDC No.:** 550.000, 550.100, 550.900

**Sex Ratio:** M9:F1

**Occurrence:** Males: 20–30:1000 live births; Females: 3–4:1000 live births. 1:100 children under 12 years of age will have hernias, based upon data from a Newcastle, England Study.

**Risk of Recurrence for Patient's Sib:** Unknown.

**Risk of Recurrence for Patient's Child:** Unknown.

**Age of Detectability:** Any age from birth through infancy and childhood.

**Gene Mapping and Linkage:** Unknown.

**Prevention:** None known. Genetic counseling indicated.

**Treatment:** Treatment is surgical. Inguinal hernias should be repaired electively, preferably as an outpatient procedure. Operation consists of high ligation of the sac (processus vaginalis) at the level of the internal ring and excision of the sac distally. Suture of the deep muscle layers is rarely necessary. Hydroceles should be treated just as hernias with removal of the residual processus vaginalis down to and including part of the tunica vaginalis. When associated with undescended testes, orchidopexy should be carried out at the time of herniorrhaphy. A groin mass that cannot be reduced despite sedation and constant firm pressure toward the internal ring is an incarcerated hernia and requires immediate surgical repair.

**Prognosis:** Normal life expectancy with exceedingly rare recurrence.

**Detection of Carrier:** Unknown.

**Special Considerations:** Fifty percent of infants and children who have a symptomatic hernia on one side will have a patent processus vaginalis on the opposite side, but only a small percentage of these patients will ever develop a contralateral hernia. The question of exploring the opposite side at the time of herniorrhaphy is controversial. Many pediatric surgeons recommend exploration of the contralateral side in infants under two years of age because 1) there is some evidence that a contralateral hernia is more likely to develop if the first hernia appears in infancy rather than in childhood, 2) incarceration is more likely to be the first manifestation of an inguinal hernia in infants than in children, 3) physical examination for hernia is difficult and unreliable in infants, and 4) the risk of incarceration is 15 to 20 times higher in infants than it is in children. Routine bilateral exploration is recommended in girls of all ages because the incidence of clinical bilateral hernias is higher than in males, and there is no risk of damaging important structures during a negative exploration.

Direct inguinal hernia is very rare, occurring in 1% of cases or less. Repair is similar to adult or acquired direct hernia with so-called Cooper ligament repair.

The sliding hernia should be repaired with inversion of the sac by a purse string suture. Care in ligation of the sac in all females should be exercised to prevent injury to the fallopian tube in the neck of the sac.

One percent of girls who have inguinal hernias have the testicular feminization syndrome. This can be excluded by visualizing a normal tube and ovary through the opened sac.

**References:**
Potts WJ: Inguinal hernia in infants. Pediatrics 1948; 1:772.
Swenson O: Diagnosis and treatment of inguinal hernia. Pediatrics 1964; 34:412.
Harper RG, et al.: Inguinal hernia: a common problem of premature infants weighing less than 1000 grams at birth. Pediatrics 1975; 56:112.
Rowe MI, Lloyd DA: Inguinal hernia. In: Welch KJ, et al, eds: Pediatric surgery, 4th ed. Chicago: Year Book Medical Publishers, 1986:779–792.

SE006
                                                            **John H. Seashore**

**Hernia, inguinal direct or indirect**
*See HERNIA, INGUINAL*

---

## HERNIA, UMBILICAL 2575

**Includes:**
  Prominent umbilicus
  Supraumbilical (paraumbilical) hernia
  Umbilical hernia

**Excludes:**
  **Omphalocele** (0748)
  Umbilical granuloma
  Ventral hernia

**Major Diagnostic Criteria:** Visual and digital examinations of the umbilical stump establish the diagnosis of umbilical hernia. A protuberant and sharply rimmed mass covered by redundant but otherwise normal skin is diagnostic.

**Clinical Findings:** Usually there is a soft asymptomatic outpouching of the umbilicus, which protrudes and becomes tense when the infant cries and is usually reducible when the infant is relaxed. Umbilical hernias generally have a benign course and a high incidence of spontaneous closure in the early years of life. This natural history should be emphasized to the child's parents. Operative repair of childhood umbilical hernias needs to be done only for incarceration or if the hernia causes psychologic disturbance.

**Complications:** Despite the presence of bowel in the hernial sac, incarceration and strangulation are rare complications in the pediatric population. However, such complications are common in adults, especially in obese, multiparous women.

**Associated Findings:** None known.

**Etiology:** Embryologically, umbilical hernia is thought to result from interruption of the normal process of return, rotation, and fixation of the intestine to the posterior abdominal wall, thus leaving a part of the intestine in the umbilical coelom covered by amnion and chorion.

**Pathogenesis:** Skin and subcutaneous tissue covers the umbilical hernia sac protruding through separated rectal muscles.

**CDC No.:** 553.100

**Sex Ratio:** M1:F1

**Occurrence:** The incidence of umbilical hernia is increased several times in Black infants (31.8 percent of Black infants under six weeks of age, compared with 4.1 percent in White infants of the same age). Another predisposing factor is low birth-weight (84% in newborn infants weighing 1,000 to 15,000 grams compared with 21% in infants with a birth-weight over 2,500 grams). In addition, the condition often occurs in **Chromosome 13, trisomy 13, Chromo-**

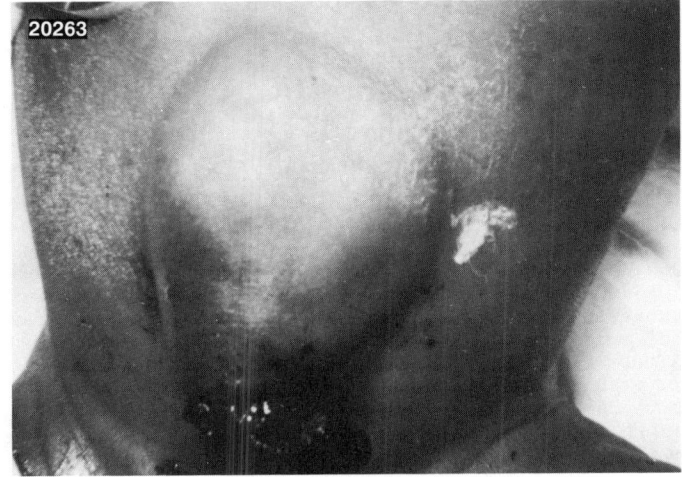

**2575-20263:** A large umbilical hernia.

some 18, trisomy 18, Williams syndrome, Mucopolysaccharidosis I-H, and athyrotic hypothyroidism sequence.

**Risk of Recurrence for Patient's Sib:** Depends on the recurrence of prematurity. If isolated, recurrence is unknown.

**Risk of Recurrence for Patient's Child:** Unknown.

**Age of Detectability:** At birth or in the first year of life.

**Gene Mapping and Linkage:** N/A

**Prevention:** None known. Genetic counseling indicated.

**Treatment:** Unknown.

**Prognosis:** Unknown.

**Detection of Carrier:** Unknown.

**References:**

Crump EP: Umbilical hernia: occurrence of the infantile type in Negro infants and children. J Pediatr 1952; 40:214–223.

Vohr BR, et al.: Umbilical hernia in the low-birth-weight infant (less than 1,500 gm). Pediatrics 1977; 90:807–808.

Elhassani SB: The umbilical cord: care, anomalies, and diseases. S Med J 1984; 77:730–736.

EL013                                           **Sami B. Elhassani**

**Hernia-craniosynostosis-arachnodactyly**
*See CRANIOSYNOSTOSIS-ARACHNODACTYLY-HERNIA*
**Herniation into the umbilical cord**
*See OMPHALOCELE*
**Herpes simplex virus infection, congenital**
*See FETAL HERPES SIMPLEX VIRUS INFECTION*
**Herrmann symphalangism-brachydactyly syndrome**
*See SYMPHALANGISM*
**Herrmann-Opitz arthrogryposis syndrome**
*See CONTRACTURES, HERRMANN-OPITZ ARTHROGRYPOSIS TYPE*
**Herrmann-Opitz syndrome**
*See HERRMANN-PALLISTER-OPITZ SYNDROME*

---

## HERRMANN-PALLISTER-OPITZ SYNDROME          2177

**Includes:**

Cleft lip/palate-craniosynostosis-malformed extremities
Craniosynostosis-malformed extremities-cleft lip/palate
Extremities (malformed)-craniosynostosis-cleft lip/palate
Herrmann-Opitz syndrome
Pallister-Herrmann-Opitz syndrome
Opitz-Pallister-Herrmann syndrome

**Excludes:**

**Craniosynostosis-fibular aplasia, Lowry type** (2184)
**Craniosynostosis-radial aplasia syndrome** (0231)
**Roberts syndrome** (0875)

**Major Diagnostic Criteria:** Mental retardation, craniosynostosis, cleft lip and palate, and both radial and fibular aplasia.

**Clinical Findings:** Two affected individuals have been reported. Findings present in both include craniosynostosis, mainly involving the coronal suture; hypertelorism; capillary hemangioma (midfacial in one, occipital in the other); protruding, dysplastic ears; cleft lip and palate; malocclusion; small scrotum and cryptorchidism; short ulnae; absent radii; valgus position of the hands; ankylosis of the knees; absent fibulae; and varus foot posture. Mental retardation was severe in one, mild in the other. In addition, one patient had depressed lower sternum, fused carpals, absent fourth and fifth fingers, duplicated distal phalanx of the third fingers, dysplastic femoral head and neck, dislocated hip, and hypoplastic third and fourth toes. A second affected individual had, in addition, simian creases, clinodactyly of the fifth finger, pterygia, and vertebral anomalies. An affected fetus has also been recently described; findings included coronal craniosynostosis, hypertelorism, beaked nose, micrognathia, small ears, short limbs with syndactyly and oligodactyly, pterygiae, imperforate urethra, and absent first ribs on X-ray.

**Complications:** Unknown.

**Associated Findings:** None known.

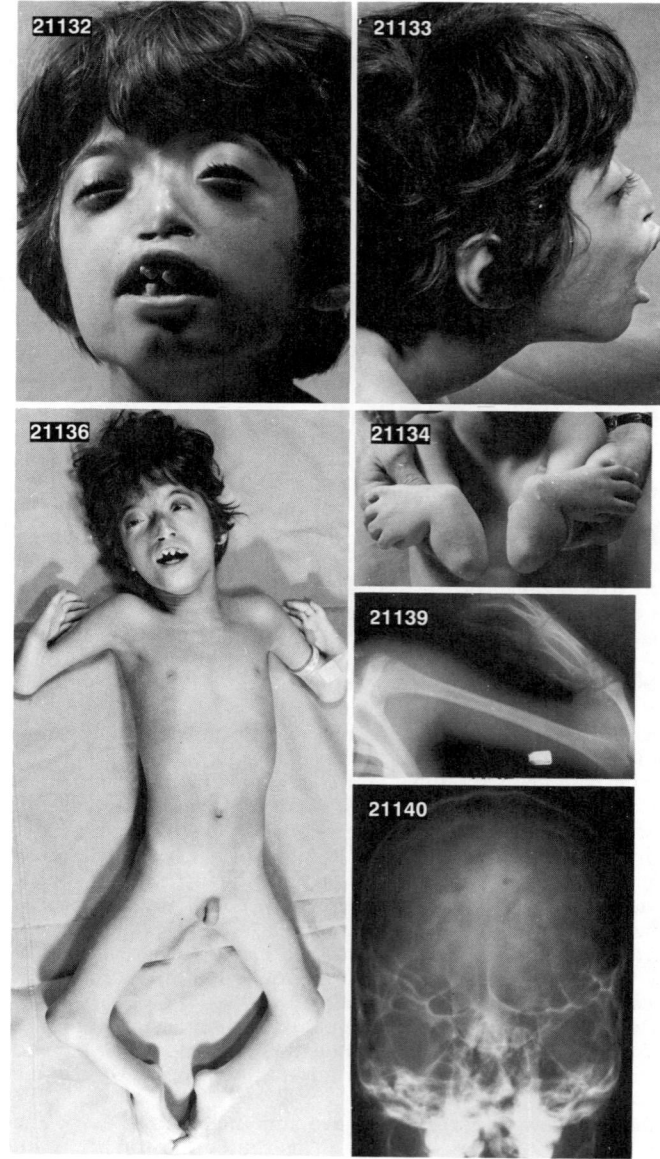

**2177-**21132–33: Facies show prominent eyes with shallow orbits, flattened and hypoplastic mid-face, repaired cleft lip and nasal deformity. 21136: Short stature, towering skull from craniosynostosis, aplasia of radii and fibulae with hypoplasia of ulnae and tibia. There are pterygia at the elbows and knees. 21134: Bilateral shortened forearms with radial clubbed hands. 21139: X-ray shows hypoplastic ulna and radial aplasia. 21140: Skull X-ray shows craniosynostosis, shallow orbits, and "beaten silver" appearance of the inner tables.

---

**Etiology:** Each patient was the only affected individual in his family; one had eight normal older sibs, one had three normal older sibs and one had two normal older sibs. In each case, the father was over the age of 35 (37, 39 and 42), suggesting that this condition may be an autosomal dominant inherited trait. Thus, each case would have been the result of a new mutation.

**Pathogenesis:** Unknown.

**POS No.:** 3175

**Sex Ratio:** M3:F0 (observed).

**Occurrence:** Three cases have been reported.

**Risk of Recurrence for Patient's Sib:**
See Part I, *Mendelian Inheritance.*

**Risk of Recurrence for Patient's Child:**
See Part I, *Mendelian Inheritance.*

**Age of Detectability:** At birth, although prenatal diagnosis using ultrasound may be possible.

**Gene Mapping and Linkage:** Unknown.

**Prevention:** None known. Genetic counseling indicated.

**Treatment:** Orthopedic management of the joint contractures; correction of the cleft lip and palate.

**Prognosis:** Two of the patients were nine and 11 years old at the time they were described, and were apparently healthy. Mental retardation was severe in one (IQ = 27), and the other had a borderline low IQ (IQ = 80). The third report was of a fetus that died in utero at 32 weeks.

**Detection of Carrier:** Unknown.

**References:**
Herrmann J, et al.: Craniosynostosis and craniosynostosis syndromes. Rocky Mt Med J 1969; 66:45–56.
Ladda RL, et al.: Craniosynostosis associated with limb reduction malformations and cleft/lip palate: a distinct syndrome. Pediatrics 1978; 61:12–15. * †
Anyane-Yeboa K, et al.: Herrmann-Opitz syndrome: report of an affected fetus. Am J Med Genet 1987; 27:467–470.

T0007                                                  **Helga V. Toriello**

**Hers disease**
*See GLYCOGENOSIS, TYPE VI*
**Heterotropic pigmented retinoblastoma**
*See JAW, NEUROECTODERMAL PIGMENTED TUMOR*
**Heterozygous protein C deficiency**
*See PROTEIN C DEFICIENCY*
**Hexestrol, fetal effects**
*See FETAL DIETHYLSTILBESTROL (DES) EFFECTS*
**Hexokinase deficiency hemolytic anemia**
*See ANEMIA, HEMOLYTIC, ERYTHROCYTE HEXOKINASE DEFICIENCY*
**Hexosaminidase A deficiency**
*See G(M2)-GANGLIOSIDOSIS WITH HEXOSAMINIDASE A DEFICIENCY*
**Hexosaminidase activator deficiency**
*See G(M2)-GANGLIOSIDOSIS WITH HEXOSAMINIDASE A DEFICIENCY*
**Hexosephosphate isomerase, deficiency of**
*See ANEMIA, GLUCOSE PHOSPHATE ISOMERASE DEFICIENCY*
**HHH syndrome**
*See HYPERORNITHINEMIA-HYPERAMMONEMIA-HOMOCITRULLINURIA*
**HHRH**
*See RICKETS, HEREDITARY HYPOPHOSPHATEMIC WITH HYPERCALCIURIA (HHRH)*
**Hiatus hernia**
*See HERNIA, HIATAL*
**Hiatus hernia-microcephaly-nephrosis, Galloway type**
*See MICROCEPHALY-HIATUS HERNIA-NEPHROSIS, GALLOWAY TYPE*
**HIE syndrome**
*See IMMUNODEFICIENCY, HYPER IgE TYPE*
**High blood pressure, maternal, fetal effects of medication**
*See FETAL EFFECTS FROM MATERNAL VASODILATOR*
**High phosphatidylcholine hemolytic anemia (HPCHA)**
*See ANEMIA, HEMOLYTIC, ERYTHROCYTE PHOSPHOLIPID DEFECT*
**High scapula**
*See SPRENGEL DEFORMITY*
**High sinus venosus with partial pulmonary venous connection**
*See ATRIAL SEPTAL DEFECTS*
**High sinus venosus without partial pulmonary venous connection**
*See ATRIAL SEPTAL DEFECTS*

## HIP, CONGENITAL COXA VARA                          2397

**Includes:**
Coxa vara (hip, congenital)
Coxa vara, idiopathic
Coxa vara, infantile
Developmental coxa vara

**Excludes:**
Coxa vara in other disorders
**Metaphyseal chondrodysplasia, type Schmid (0654)**

**Major Diagnostic Criteria:** A decrease in the neck-shaft angle of the femur for age as shown by X-ray studies (for adults, an angle less than 120°). Commonly the neck of the femur is short, and the greater trochanter is extended upward with malposition of the proximal femur. A complete X-ray study is necessary to diagnose this condition and distinguish it from similar conditions.

**Clinical Findings:** Coxa vara commonly becomes evident with the onset of walking when children show a painless limp or a waddling gait. Affected individuals are frequently short for their age. An excessive lordosis may also be noted. The Trendelenburg sign is positive, and abduction is limited. There may be mild flexion contractures of the hip as well. Older children and adolescents may experience pain and fatigue. Prior to walking, the major findings may be a deformity or asymmetry of the configuration of the hip and upper thigh when compared with the normal hip in patients with unilateral involvement.

**Complications:** Usually orthopedic in nature, such as pseudoarthrosis, especially if there is considerable delay in the treatment.

**Associated Findings:** Short stature, shortening of the affected limb.

**Etiology:** Autosomal dominant inheritance. Sporadic cases are also reported.

**Pathogenesis:** Most authorities feel that coxa vara is the result of a primary endochondral ossification defect of the subcapital epiphyseal plate that is probably due to unequal growth from the trochanteric apophysis and the capital epiphysis. Weight bearing may aggravate the varus deformity. The cause of the abnormal ossification itself is not clear. It may be the result of a primary defect within the cartilaginous anlage, or may be caused by an embryonic vascular disturbance.

**MIM No.:** *12275

**CDC No.:** 755.660

**Sex Ratio:** M1:F1

**Occurrence:** A Scandinavian study suggests 1:2,500 live births.

**Risk of Recurrence for Patient's Sib:**
See Part I, *Mendelian Inheritance.*

**Risk of Recurrence for Patient's Child:**
See Part I, *Mendelian Inheritance.*

**Age of Detectability:** Usually during infancy or early childhood.

**Gene Mapping and Linkage:** Unknown.

**Prevention:** None known. Genetic counseling indicated.

**Treatment:** In the majority of cases, surgical intervention is necessary. Conservative treatment may be considered in mild cases when varus deformity is not progressive and neck shaft angle approaches normal.

**Prognosis:** Depends on the severity of the deformity, age at diagnosis and first surgical intervention, and the success of operative correction. Recurrences after successful correction have been recorded.

**Detection of Carrier:** Unknown.

**Special Considerations:** A study involving 94 individuals with congenital coxa vara living in a Turkish village in Cyprus clearly demonstrated a dominant inheritance pattern for this entity, since the pathology could be traced back in both sexes for thirteen generations by history and four generations by X-ray. The severity of the condition varied in affected individuals. In addition to the hip pathology, the patients had bowing of the legs, short stature

(60%), hypoplastic bones (40%), protrusio acetabuli (22%), and nonspecific degenerative changes; usually in the hip and knee secondary to the coxa vara deformity.

**References:**
Martin H: Coxa vara congenita bei eineiigen Zwillingen. Arch Orthop Clin 1942; 42:230–240.
Almond HG: Familial infantile coxa vara. J Bone Joint Surg 1956; 38B:539–544.
Pylkkanen PV: Coxa vara infantum. Acta Orthop Scand 1960; 48(Suppl):1–120.
Say B, et al.: Hereditary congenital coxa vara with dominant inheritance? Hum Genet 1971; 11:266–268.
Say B, et al.: Dominant congenital coxa vara. J Bone Joint Surg 1974; 56B:78–85. †
Wynne-Davis R, et al.: Atlas of skeletal disorders, 1st ed. Edinburgh: Churchill Livingstone, 1985.

SA033                                              **Burhan Say**

---

## HIP, CONGENITAL DISLOCATED                              2163

**Includes:**
  Hip, congenital dislocated/relocatable
  Hip, congenital dislocations due to acetabular dysplasia
  Hip, congenital dislocations due to ligamentous laxity
  Hip, congenital dislocations due to uterine mechanical
    constraint
  Hip, congenital lax (subluxatable)

**Excludes:**
  Dislocated hip as part of a complex malformation syndrome
  Dislocated hip in joint and/or connective tissue disorders
  Dislocated hip associated with neuromuscular disease
  **Hip, dysplasia, Namaqualand type (2239)**

**Major Diagnostic Criteria:** In the newborn period, diagnosis of congenital dislocated hip (CDH) depends almost entirely on physical examination. X-rays are of limited value because of non-ossification of the femoral head and acetabulum. The role of CT scanning and ultrasound in the newborn period is presently being investigated. Ultrasound appears to be the most reliable imaging technique for diagnosing CDH in the newborn.

Beyond four months of age, diagnostic criteria include both physical signs and symptoms, and X-ray findings.

**Clinical Findings:** In the newborn, shortening of the leg and asymmetric thigh folds may be noted with unilateral CDH; limitation of abduction of the hip due to CDH is unusual. Two provocative tests, the Ortolani and Barlow maneuvers should be done routinely as part of the normal newborn examination. In the majority of cases of CDH, one or both of these tests will be

positive. They must be performed gently, however, to avoid damaging the hip.

In the Ortolani test, a dislocated hip is relocated. In this test, the hip is flexed 90° with approximately 60° of abduction. Gentle pressure is applied with the fingers over the greater trochanter, reducing the femur into the acetabulum with a palpable "clunk". If the Ortolani test is negative, the Barlow manuever is tried. The hip is flexed to 90° with neutral abduction; pressure is then applied over the medial thigh with the thumb. The test is positive if the examiner feels a "clunk" with the fingers over the greater trochanter; this indicates that the femoral head, located within the acetabulum at the start of the maneuver, can be dislocated. With practice, an examiner can differentiate the lax, subluxatable hip, which cannot be dislocated but does exhibit unusual instability. Palpable or audible clicks, without dislocation, are generally thought to be of no significance, but some authors believe that these hips need more careful follow-up to be sure they remain stable.

Screening of all newborns, including use of the provocative maneuvers described above, is mandatory. However, a normal newborn exam does not preclude development of CDH later. Thus evaluation for possible CDH should continue throughout infancy and early childhood. Particular care must be taken in following infants who have special risk factors, including an equivocal newborn examination, positive family history, history of in utero breech position (even if delivered by C-section), and presence of other congenital postural deformities such as torticollis or positional foot deformities; some physicians advocate routine X-rays at about six months of age in addition to clinical examinations in this selected sub-group. When CDH develops after the newborn period, the underlying etiology is still presumed to be the same as for congenital CDH.

The presenting signs of CDH beyond age four moneths include shortening of the leg (if unilateral), asymmetry of thigh folds (if unilateral), and limitation of abduction. Beyond 6 months of age, it is quite rare to find a positive Ortolani or Barlow test. X-rays are quite helpful, as both the superior and lateral migration of the proximal femur as well as failure of development of the acetabulum may be evident.

In older children, any of the following signs and symptoms should also suggest the possibility of CDH: easy fatigability, pain, limp, waddling gait, positive Trendelenburg sign (downward pelvic tilt when the standing patient bends the ipsilateral leg), hyperlordotic posture. Occasionally, children will have a clinically normal examination but suggestive symptoms and evidence of CDH on X-ray. If one hip is abnormal, the contralateral hip should be carefully examined.

**Complications:** Lax and dislocatable hips are of concern because of the risk of progression to frank dislocation. Dislocated hips, left untreated, lead to progressive deformity of the acetabulum and femoral head, possible formation of a false acetabulum, and progressive distortion of the joint capsule, ligaments, and surrounding muscles. Gait abnormalities and degenerative hip changes will occur if this condition is left untreated.

Treatment with excessive forced abduction of the hips may lead to avascular necrosis of the femoral head, with growth disturbance causing a deformity similar to that seen in **Epiphyseal dysplasia, multiple ribbing type**.

**Associated Findings:** Between 10 and 20% of patients with CDH have associated congenital anomalies, mostly other postural deformities of the musculoskeletal system such as foot deformities and, **Torticollis**.

**Etiology:** Multifactorial pattern of inheritance is most likely in the majority of patients. Contributing factors include acetabular dysplasia, ligamentous laxity, in utero mechanical forces, and female sex. Rarely, autosomal dominant inheritance has been noted in a large kindred.

**Pathogenesis:** Both genetic and environmental factors are important. Monozygotic twins have an increased concordance rate (30–50%) compared with dizygotic twins (3–5%), the latter being about the same risk as that of singleton siblings. A familial tendency toward acetabular dysplasia has been noted when

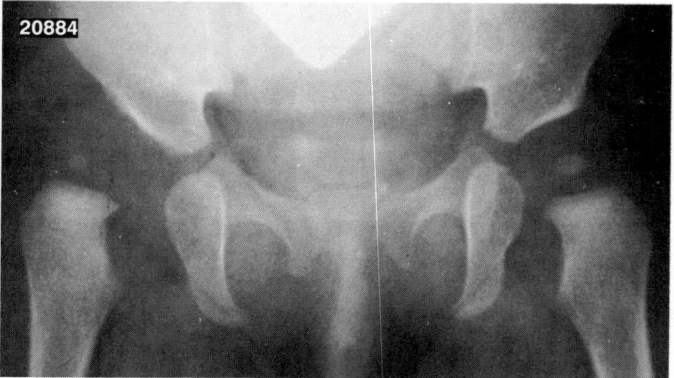

**2163-20884:** Hip, congenital dislocated; note right congenital dislocated hip with poorly formed acetabulum and lateral displacement of the femur.

X-rays of the parents have been examined. Increased rate of joint laxity has been found both in patients and in their relatives. The increased incidence of CDH in females may be at least partly due to hormonal influences on connective tissue, which would cause decreased joint laxity in males.

Other risk factors include being first-born and in utero breech position, reflecting mechanical factors acting on the hip joint. An increased incidence of CDH is found in some ethnic groups which swaddle their young, such as certain North American Indian tribes and Lapps. Since the incidence of "unstable" hips is almost ten times that of frankly dislocated hips at birth, the forced extension as in swaddling may cause dislocation of these initially unstable hips. There is a decreased incidence of CDH in some infants on their backs, with the child's hips in a flexed position; this position favors normal development of the initially unstable hips. Unilateral CDH more often affects the left hip, which may reflect in utero position.

**MIM No.:** 14270

**CDC No.:** 754.300

**Sex Ratio:** M1:F5 (approximately).

**Occurrence:** Dislocated hips occur with a frequency of about 1:1,000 in Caucasian North American and European populations. Unstable hips, including lax and dislocatable hips, have a frequency in newborns as high as 1 to 2% in some series. All require careful follow-up.

CDH is rare in African Blacks and the Chinese. The incidence in American Blacks may be about one-third of Whites. The incidence is higher in the Japanese and groups who swaddle their young.

**Risk of Recurrence for Patient's Sib:** Different studies report a range of recurrence risks, from 2% to 14%. A recurrence risk of about 5% is most often given. The risk is lower for brothers and higher for sisters. Whether siblings of a male proband are at increased risk is not clear.

**Risk of Recurrence for Patient's Child:** Published figures range from 3 to 12%, being lower for male offspring and higher for female offspring. The risk of an affected parent having a second affected child is between 10 and 36%.

**Age of Detectability:** At birth (most cases). Late cases still occur, even in patients having had a normal newborn examination.

**Gene Mapping and Linkage:** Unknown.

**Prevention:** None known. Genetic counseling indicated. Early diagnosis is mandatory to prevent later problems. Avoidance of forced hip extension in infancy may prevent some cases of late onset CDH.

**Treatment:** About half of all unstable hips detected in the immediate neonatal period become stable within the first week of life. Careful follow-up may be all that is necessary. Persistently lax, dislocatable, and dislocated hips are treated with one of a variety of devices designed to keep the femoral head reliably in the acetabulum. Dislocated/non-relocatable hips can be treated initially with gentle traction to relocate the joint and then a device to maintain position until the joint stabilizes. CDH not responding to the above measures, and late diagnosed CDH, particularly if the child is already walking, may require more aggressive therapy, including open reduction, and the results may be less satisfactory. Severe deformity of the hip joint may require eventual joint replacement in adult life.

**Prognosis:** Life span is not affected except as related to the risks of hospitalization and surgery, which should be minimal. CDH, which is diagnosed early, and which responds to therapy, may result in a virtually normal hip joint. Cases in which there is residual deformity, for whatever reason, can result in gait abnormalities, pain, and degenerative joint disease. Aseptic necrosis of the femoral head, the most serious risk of treatment, can also lead to joint deformity and sequalae.

**Detection of Carrier:** Unknown.

**Special Considerations:** There is little standardization of terminology in the literature, so that CDH may, in some articles, refer only to overtly dislocated hips, while in others it may refer to the entire spectrum of unstable and dislocated hips.

Routine screening of newborns began in the 1950's and 1960's. Thus information about the pathogenesis, incidence, recurrence risks, and the significance of unstable hips in the newborn is continuing to evolve.

**References:**
Wynne-Davies R: The epidemiology of congenital dislocation of the hip. Dev Med Child Neurol 1972; 14:515–517.
Wynne-Davies R: Heritable disorders in orthopedic practice. London: Blackwell Scientific Publications, 1973:193–196.
Horton WA: Common skeletal deformities. In: Emery AEH, Rimoin DL, eds: Principles and practice of medical genetics. New York: Churchill Livingstone, 1983:815–816.
Higuchi F: Genetic study on the congenital dislocation of the hip. Bull Tokyo Med Dent Univ 1984; 31:195–207.
Burke SW, et al.: Congenital dislocation of the hip in the American black. Clin Orthop 1985; 192:120–123.
Bernard AA, et al.: An improved screening system for the early detection of congenital dislocation of the hip. J Pediatr Orthop 1987; 7:277–282.

FL005
KA040

Ellen A. Fleischnick
James R. Kasser

**Hip, congenital dislocated/relocatable**
*See HIP, CONGENITAL DISLOCATED*

**Hip, congenital dislocations due to acetabular dysplasia**
*See HIP, CONGENITAL DISLOCATED*

**Hip, congenital dislocations due to ligamentous laxity**
*See HIP, CONGENITAL DISLOCATED*

**Hip, congenital dislocations due to utero mechanical constraint**
*See HIP, CONGENITAL DISLOCATED*

**Hip, congenital lax (subluxatable)**
*See HIP, CONGENITAL DISLOCATED*

---

## HIP, DYSPLASIA, NAMAQUALAND TYPE      2239

**Includes:** Namaqualand hip dysplasia

**Excludes:**
    **Epiphyseal dysplasia, multiple** (0358)
    **Hip, osteonecrosis, capital femoral epiphysis** (2288)
    Meyer arthropathy
    Mseleni joint disease
    **Spondyloepiphyseal dysplasia, late** (0898)

**Major Diagnostic Criteria:** Pain in the hip joint in late childhood and handicap in adulthood due to progressive fragmentation of the femoral capital epiphyses and degenerative arthropathy. The diagnosis is established on X-ray and through family studies.

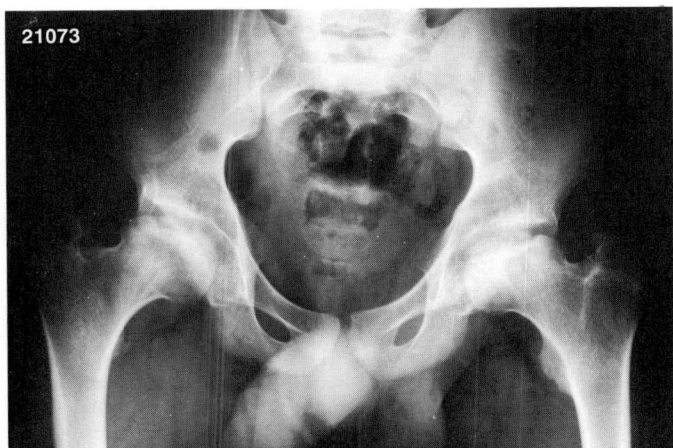

**2239-21073:** Dysplastic changes in the femoral heads.

**Clinical Findings:**   Pain and limitation of movement in the hip joints. X-rays show progressive flattening and fragmentation of the femoral capital epiphyses with subsequent secondary arthropathy. Variable, mild platyspondyly appears in 60% of affected persons.

**Complications:**   Degenerative arthropathy of the hip joints.

**Associated Findings:**   Spinal malalignment, usually mild, in 10% of affected persons. Exostoses on the lateral margins of the iliac bodies in 6%, and mild flattening of the femoral heads in 20%.

**Etiology:**   Autosomal dominant inheritance.

**Pathogenesis:**   Unknown.

**MIM No.:**   14267

**CDC No.:**   755.660

**Sex Ratio:**   M1:F1

**Occurrence:**   Forty-five affected persons have been documented from in five generations of a kindred of mixed ancestry in South Africa. The condition seems to be a "private syndrome" and the prevalence in the population of mixed ancestry in the Cape Province, South Africa is 1:60,000.

**Risk of Recurrence for Patient's Sib:**
See Part I, *Mendelian Inheritance.*

**Risk of Recurrence for Patient's Child:**
See Part I, *Mendelian Inheritance.*

**Age of Detectability:**   In late childhood, by X-ray studies.

**Gene Mapping and Linkage:**   Unknown.

**Prevention:**   None known. Genetic counseling indicated.

**Treatment:**   Orthopedic measures, including prosthetic hip joint replacement.

**Prognosis:**   Progressive handicap due to degenerative changes in hip joint. Life span and general health are unimpaired.

**Detection of Carrier:**   Unknown.

**References:**
Beighton P, et al.: Namaqualand hip dysplasia: an autosomal dominant entity. Am J Med Genet 1984; 19:161–169. *
Learmonth ID: Namaqualand hip dysplasia: orthopaedic implications. Clin Orthop 1987; 218:142–147.

BE008                                                          **Peter Beighton**

## HIP, OSTEONECROSIS, CAPITAL FEMORAL EPIPHYSIS    2288

**Includes:**
> Necrosis of the capital femoral epiphysis-primary coxa plana
> Legg-Calve-Perthes disease
> Osteochondritis deformans juvenilis
> Perthes disease
> Pseudocoxalgia

**Excludes:**
> Avascular or aseptic osteonecrosis of the femoral head, secondary
> Coxalgia
> **Hip, congenital coxa vara** (2397)
> Slipped capital femoral epiphysis
> Synovitis of the hip

**Major Diagnostic Criteria:**   The actual diagnosis is made by X-rays, but is usually considered on the basis of a typical but somewhat mild history of a limp, often accompanied by pain. When present, the pain is usually in the knee, hip, or leg. However, insofar as children often do not complain or localize pain, the only evidence may be a diminution in their usual level of physical activity.

The earliest X-ray evidence is a slightly smaller ossific nucleus or a widened cartilage space in the epiphysis. A medial joint space shown on X-ray to be increased by >2 mm over the normal size is considered diagnostic. Later, one may see a crescent-like submarginal strip of decreased density (Caffey sign), which is believed to be a subchondral fracture. During disease progression, broken

areas of radiodensity and radiolucency accompanied by some flattening and irregularity of the femoral head are noted. Often a sclerosed sequestrum of bone surrounded by more normal-appearing bone gives a characteristic "head within a head" appearance. Some degree of anterolateral subluxation of the femoral head frequently occurs, but may not be fully appreciated, especially during the early stages, unless multiple views, serial X-rays and/or arthrograms are obtained.

Acute synovitis of the hip may present with some of these early symptoms and X-ray signs, but arthrography and the lack of progression should clarify the diagnosis. Radionuclide scintography has produced conflicting results, showing both increased and decreased uptake. Bone densitometry may be emerging as an excellent diagnostic and monitoring tool.

**Clinical Findings:**   Despite the dramatic alterations shown on X-ray and even permanent deformities of the femoral head, neck, and acetabulum, there is a paucity of clinical symptoms. For most patients, the first symptom is a limp with or without pain. Only about 50% of patients experience any associated pain. Surprisingly, 15% localize the pain to the knee, but it can also be noted in the groin or inner thigh. Muscle spasm often causes decreased abduction and internal rotation of the hip, and a mild transient synovitis can be present in the early stages.

Only one leg is usually involved initially, but the disease is identified as bilateral in 7–15%. Onset on the opposite side frequently lags by an average interval of 12–18 months, with a range of two months to five years. This delay likely results in an underestimate of the number of cases that are ultimately bilateral.

Disease progression and recovery extends from 18 months to four years. Symptoms usually disappear quickly after treatment commences, and most patients are ambulatory for most of the duration of the disease. Many patients recover without sequelae, but even those with X-ray evidence of significant deformities are usually symptom free until the onset of degenerative arthritis in the fifth and sixth decades.

**Complications:**   The disease process is usually more severe in girls. In general, the younger the age at onset, the less extensive the involvement; and the earlier treatment is initiated, the less likely the femoral head is to develop significant permanent deformities. The most typical sequelae include lack of appropriate growth in epiphyseal height, increased epiphyseal breadth, and alteration of the growth plate from linear to convex. These latter two cause coxa magna, decreased femoral neck length, and diminution of the neck-shaft angle, which in turn lead to functional coxa vara, with its potential for a painful pseudoarthrosis, and flattening of the femoral head often accompanied by flattening of the overlying acetabulum (coxa plana). Of these, all but coxa plana are part of the natural course of the condition.

With onset between ages six and nine years, the incidence of subsequent arthritis is 38%; and with onset after age 10 years, the incidence approaches 100%. In those children greater than six years old at onset with at least moderate involvement, surgical treatment has yielded good-to-fair results in 94%, with only 6% considered at-risk for developing early arthritis. In the nonoperative control group, only 66% had fair-to-good results, and 34% remained at significant risk.

Although many affected children are shorter than their sibs, many studies show catch-up growth during adolescence. In unilateral disease, however, leg length discrepancy may develop. In several large follow-up studies, patients were found to have a mild limp, minimal shortening, negligible pain, and minimal or no functional impairment. Eight percent needed arthroplasty in the fourth decade. By the fifth decade only 40% maintained good function. Another 40% had sought arthroplasty, which increased to 50% by the sixth decade. In a more recent study, 86% had functional hips at age 45 years.

**Associated Findings:**   Almost all affected children are shorter than their sibs; the average disparity is three inches in girls and one inch in boys. Ninety percent have a delayed bone age. These findings may be absent in familial cases. Many studies documented an increased incidence of genitourinary anomalies, including **Hernia, inguinal,** as well as a previous history of congenital hip dislocation. Some investigators believe that inadequate or very vigorous treatment of the original hip dislocation may interfere with the vascular supply to the femoral head. In familial cases there appears to be an increased incidence of genitourinary and/or congenital hip dislocation/subluxation in first-, second-, and third-degree relatives.

**Etiology:** Legg (1910) originally suggested trauma, but Perthes (1910) and subsequent investigators rejected this because <20% have an antecedent history of trauma or preceding synovitis. Generalized growth retardation with its disproportionate distal delay, as well as the recently reported lowered levels of somatomedin A, raise the question of hormonal influence. Levels of thyroid, growth, and other hormones are normal.

Genetic factors are unlikely to contribute significantly to sporadic cases or those that are truly unilateral, but may be important in familial cases. Most studies note an increased incidence among first degree relatives, especially sibs. Recurrence risks may vary from one to three percent for sibs, quickly dropping to the population risk for second- and third-degree relatives. Multifactorial inheritance alone, however, cannot explain this, since sibs are more frequently affected than parents and the recurrence risk does not increase with incidence in the less frequently affected sex (female).

Earlier reports of affected multigeneration families had suggested dominant inheritance, but many of these were later determined to have had bony dysplasias. Several investigators, however, have identified large kindreds, and associated findings that are compatible with dominant transmission.

**Pathogenesis:** An avascular, aseptic osteonecrosis of the femoral head secondary to one or more vascular insults that render at least some areas of the capital epiphysis and sometimes adjacent areas of the metaphysis ischemic. The cause(s) of the vascular interruption is not known and may be multiple or differ among individuals. Some investigators have postulated prenatal ischemia to the future growth plate. Thrombi in vessels supplying the epiphysis have been noted. Repeated vascular interruptions have created similar pathology experimentally in animals.

The pathologic changes occur in three tandem stages:

*Initial or condensation phase:* Following the initial ischemic insult, there is evidence of bone and marrow necrosis with sclerosis of the dead bone. This corresponds to the increased radiodensity. The patient is usually asymptomatic. Revascularization ensues, causing resorption of avascular bone. This often makes the subchondral area vulnerable to minor trauma, such as daily activity, that precipitates a subchondral fracture. This injury initiates a synovial reaction and often muscle spasm, causing a limp and/or pain.

*Fragmentation phase:* Collapse of bone adjacent to the fracture causes further ischemia and interrupts the structural stability of the capital epiphysis. Necrotic debris makes revascularization slow and irregular. Osteoblasts produce direct appositional bone formation on dead trabeculae, while osteoclasts resorb dead bone, allowing X-ray evidence of interdigitated radiodensity and radiolucency. At times the metaphysis is also involved. Distortion of the cartilaginous and bony matrix allows at least three separate pathologic processes within the femoral head: anteriolateral subluxation, posterior crumbling with distortion of the physis, and deformation of the femoral head. All subsequent complications arise from these pathologic changes.

*Regeneration phase:* Necrotic bone is gradually replaced by cancellous bone, and remineralization takes place. Remodeling of the femoral head and acetabulum begins here and continues until skeletal growth ceases.

**MIM No.:**  15060

**Sex Ratio:**  About M4:F1.

**Occurrence:** The incidence varies with race and geographic location. The condition is reported to be more frequent in Orientals, Eskimos, and Central Europeans, and rare in Australians, American Indians, Polynesians, and blacks. The incidence in Great Britain is 1:4,750 live births (1:3,000 males and 1:11,800 females) and in North America is 1:750 males and 1:3,700 females. Prevalence is thought to be 0.1–0.3%, but is exceedingly rare in Africa, with a prevalence of 1:550,000 in Nigeria, and only 0.45–1.7:100,000 in the United States.

**Risk of Recurrence for Patient's Sib:** For sporadic cases with unilateral disease, the risk is 1% for sibs and is .1% for second degree relatives. The risk for bilateral and/or familial cases was observed to be 2–3%, but may approach 50% in those families who appear to have dominant transmission. Often penetrance and expressivity in parents are unknown.

**Risk of Recurrence for Patient's Child:** Observed to be 2–3%. Most studies have not followed patients throughout childbearing years. Risk theoretically approaches 50% in families with suggestive dominant inheritance.

**Age of Detectability:** Rarely detected before age two years except in some familial cases. Most cases seen before age four years are mild clinically and on X-ray, and some cases are undoubtedly never recognized. Rarely diagnosed after age 10 years, and cases identified after age 12 years are all secondary to some systemic cause.

**Gene Mapping and Linkage:**  Unknown.

**Prevention:** None known. Genetic counseling indicated. Residual deformities of the femoral head are prevented or greatly minimized by timely therapeutic intervention.

**Treatment:** Decisions regarding therapy depend on the age of the child (treatment is rarely indicated in children less than four years of age), the sex (females usually require treatment), and the extent of avascularity. Serial X-rays that estimate the boundaries of involvement and monitor progression, coupled with arthrography to clarify joint status, guide therapeutic strategies. Bedrest and occasionally short-term traction is often all that is needed to eliminate pain and any inflammation as well as restore full range of motion within the hip. Older children and those with moderate to severe disease usually require additional treatment to center and contain the femoral head within the acetabulum. Several risk factors mandate such therapy: 1) any subluxation of the epiphysis, 2) shift of the growth plate from oblique to horizontal, 3) localized bone resorption in the lateral epiphysis (Cage sign), 4) lateral calcification of the epiphysis, and 5) any significant metaphyseal involvement. Containment of the head can sometimes be achieved using a Toronto abduction brace, but surgical approaches such as an innominate or a varus osteotomy may be necessary. Surgery often has the advantage of permitting earlier weight-bearing, an important factor in enhancing remodeling of the femoral head and acetabulum during the child's growth period.

**Prognosis:** Many patients who acquire the condition at a young age or show minimal pathology experience complete recovery with no sequelae. Since treatment is intended to prevent or diminish any residual deformity, the factors influencing prognosis for the remainder are similar to those governing therapy. If the femoral head is distorted >3 mm from the normal, it is at increased risk for degenerative arthritis. Even in those cases in which a significant residual deformity exists the risk for arthritis is low if onset is before age six years, because substantial remodeling occurs during growth periods. If onset is between ages six and nine years, the incidence of arthritis is 40%, but with an onset after age 10 years, almost 100% develop arthritis at some point. The presence of metaphyseal involvement or physeal changes usually portends poor growth and/or degenerative arthritis for that extremity. Otherwise, individuals enjoy a normal, pain-free life span with good functional capabilities.

**Detection of Carrier:** In possible familial cases, a positive family history for limps, leg length discrepancy, congenital hip dislocation, genitourinary anomalies, or early degenerative arthritis.

**References:**

Calve J: Sur une forme particuliere de pseudo-coxalgia. Rev Chir 1910; 30:54.

Legg AT: An obscure affection on the hip joint. Boston Med Surg J 1910; 162:202.

Perthes G: Uber arthritis deformans juvenilis. Dtsch Z Chir 1910; 107:111.

Katz JF (ed): Symposium: Legg-Calve-Perthes disease. Clin Orthop Rel Res 1980; 150:2–22. *
Gruebel Lee DM: Disorders of the hip. Philadelphia: J.B. Lippincott, 1983. * †
Katz JF: Legg-Calve-Perthes disease. New York: Praeger, 1984. †
McAndrew MP, Weinstein SL: A long-term follow-up of Legg-Calve-Perthes disease. J Bone Joint Surg 1984; 66(A):860–869.
Salter RB, Thompson GH: Legg-Calve-Perthes disease. J Bone Joint Surg 1984; 66(A):479–489. †

CA016 **Mary Esther Carlin**

**Hirschsprung agangliosis-albinism**
*See ALBINISM, WAARDENBURG TYPE-HIRSCHSPRUNG AGANGLIONOSIS*
**Hirschsprung disease**
*See COLON, AGANGLIONOSIS*

## HIRSCHSPRUNG DISEASE-CARDIAC DEFECT 3286

**Includes:**
Toes, polysyndactyly-Hirschsprung disease-cardiac defect
Ulnar polydactyly-Hirschsprung disease
Ventricular septal defect-Hirschsprung disease

**Excludes:**
**Colon, agangliosis** (0192)
**Hirschsprung disease-polydactyly-deafness** (3269)
**Waardenburg syndromes** (0997)

**Major Diagnostic Criteria:** The combination of Hirschsprung disease (see **Colon, agangliosis**), polydactyly, and cardiac defect.

**Clinical Findings:** In two affected boys; husky cry in infancy, cardiac defects (**Mitral valve stenosis** in both, **Ventricular septal defect** in one, **Mitral valve stenosis** and **Aorta, coarctation** in the other), Hirschsprung disease, phimosis, post-axial **Polydactyly**, and duplicate great toes.

**Complications:** Cardiac failure, complications of bowel surgery.

**Associated Findings:** None known.

**Etiology:** Probably autosomal or X-linked recessive inheritance.

**Pathogenesis:** Unknown.

**MIM No.:** 23575

**Sex Ratio:** M2:F0 (observed).

**Occurrence:** One family from Wales has been reported.

**Risk of Recurrence for Patient's Sib:**
See Part I, *Mendelian Inheritance.*

**Risk of Recurrence for Patient's Child:**
See Part I, *Mendelian Inheritance.*

**Age of Detectability:** At birth, although potentially prenatally by fetoscope or fetal ultrasound.

**Gene Mapping and Linkage:** Unknown.

**Prevention:** None known. Genetic counseling indicated.

**Treatment:** Surgical correction of the bowel and cardiac defects.

**Prognosis:** One child died at age two weeks, the other was 7 1/2 years with normal intellectual function at last report.

**Detection of Carrier:** Unknown.

**References:**
Laurence KM, et al.: Hirschsprung's disease associated with congenital heart malformation, broad big toes, and ulnar polydactyly in sibs: a case for fetoscopy. J Med Genet 1975; 12:334–338.

T0007 **Helga V. Toriello**

## HIRSCHSPRUNG DISEASE-MICROCEPHALY-COLOBOMA 3268

**Includes:**
Hurst syndrome
Neuronal migration, defective

**Excludes:**
**Albinism, Waardenburg type-Hirschsprung aganglionosis** (2823)
**Waardenburg syndromes** (0997)

**Major Diagnostic Criteria:** The combination of Hirschsprung disease with **Microcephaly**, minor facial anomalies, and coloboma.

**Clinical Findings:** In the three children described in detail, anomalies included low birthweight (1/3), growth failure (1/3), microcephaly (congenital in one, postnatal in two) iris coloboma (2/3), bulbous nose (3/3), highly arched palate (2/3), **Eye, hypertelorism** (1/3), prominent ears (3/3), tapering fingers (2/3), Hirschsprung disease (see **Colon, aganglionosis** (3/3), mental retardation (3/3), and CT scan findings consistent with defective neuronal migration (2/3). A fourth affected child, noted in the addendum, had **Corpus callosum agenesis** as well.

**Complications:** Unknown.

**Associated Findings:** None known.

**Etiology:** Autosomal recessive inheritance is suggested by the presence of two affected individuals in a highly inbred family.

**Pathogenesis:** The basic defect is thought to be related to defective neuronal migration.

**Sex Ratio:** M1:F1

**Occurrence:** Four affected children have been reported.

**Risk of Recurrence for Patient's Sib:**
See Part I, *Mendelian Inheritance.*

**Risk of Recurrence for Patient's Child:**
See Part I, *Mendelian Inheritance.*

**Age of Detectability:** At birth or during infancy by the presence of coloboma, microcephaly, and Hirschsprung disease.

**Gene Mapping and Linkage:** Unknown.

**Prevention:** None known. Genetic counseling indicated.

**Treatment:** Surgery for Hirschsprung disease.

**Prognosis:** Mental retardation is moderate; one child had a measured IQ of 50.

**Detection of Carrier:** Unknown.

**References:**
Hurst JA, et al.: Hirschsprung disease, microcephaly, and iris coloboma: a new syndrome of defective neuronal migration. J Med Genet 1988; 25:494–500.

T0007 **Helga V. Toriello**

**Hirschsprung disease-Ondine curse**
*See HYPOVENTILATION, CONGENITAL CENTRAL ALVEOLAR TYPE*
**Hirschsprung disease-pigmentary anomaly**
*See WAARDENBURG SYNDROMES*

## HIRSCHSPRUNG DISEASE-POLYDACTYLY-DEAFNESS 3269

**Includes:** Santos syndrome

**Excludes:**
**Albinism, Waardenburg type-Hirschsprung aganglionosis** (2823)
**Colon, aganglionosis** (0192)
**Hirschsprung disease-cardiac defect** (3286)
**Waardenburg syndromes** (0997)

**Major Diagnostic Criteria:** The combination of Hirschsprung disease (see **Colon, aganglionosis**, **Polydactyly**, renal agenesis, and deafness.

**Clinical Findings:** In the one affected child who has been reported in detail: **Eye, hypertelorism**, congenital sensorineural deafness, polydactyly, Hirschsprung disease, unilateral renal agenesis, and severe mental retardation. An older sister died at age two weeks following surgery for intestinal obstruction. She also had polydactyly.

**Complications:**  Unknown.

**Associated Findings:**  None known.

**Etiology:**  The presence of the condition in sibs of each sex, whose parents are consanguineous, suggests autosomal recessive inheritance.

**Pathogenesis:**  Unknown.

**Sex Ratio:**  M1:F1

**Occurrence:**  Reported in one family from the Azores.

**Risk of Recurrence for Patient's Sib:**
See Part I, *Mendelian Inheritance.*

**Risk of Recurrence for Patient's Child:**
See Part I, *Mendelian Inheritance.*

**Age of Detectability:**  Potentially prenatally by ultrasound evaluation, but only if polydactyly and/or renal agenesis are present.

**Gene Mapping and Linkage:**  Unknown.

**Prevention:**  None known. Genetic counseling indicated.

**Treatment:**  Surgery for Hirschsprung disease.

**Prognosis:**  If surgery is successful, life span is likely to be normal. However, severe mental retardation was present in the propositus.

**Detection of Carrier:**  Unknown.

**References:**
Santos H, et al.: Hirschsprung disease associated with polydactyly, unilateral renal agenesis, hypertelorism, and congenital deafness: a new autosomal recessive syndrome. J Med Genet 1988; 25:204–208.

T0007                                                **Helga V. Toriello**

**Hirsutism-gingival enlargement**
*See GINGIVAL FIBROMATOSIS-HYPERTRICHOSIS*
**Histidase deficiency**
*See HISTIDINEMIA*
**Histidine metabolism, disturbance of**
*See HISTIDINEMIA*

## HISTIDINEMIA                                                0472

**Includes:**
Histidase deficiency
Histidine metabolism, disturbance of
**Excludes:**
Histidinuria of pregnancy
**Phenylketonuria** (0808)

**Major Diagnostic Criteria:**  Persistent hyper-histidinemia. Persistent blood histidine values below 3 mg/dl are inconsistent with the diagnosis, unless absence of histidase has been proven. A false positive ferric chloride urine test for **Phenylketonuria** occurs.

**Clinical Findings:**  The biochemical aberrations can also be found in otherwise healthy people; these may represent the majority of homozygotes. Laboratory findings include positive urinary tests with ferric chloride or Phenistix. Increased concentration of histidine in plasma; values are generally above 6 mg/dl. Increased urinary output of histidine exceeding twice that of normal for comparable age.

Exaggerated response to an orally administered loading dose of 150 mg L-histidine per kg of body weight. The plasma peak at about two hours after ingestion of the dose should rise to values, about or generally above 15 mg/dl. The return to the baseline is generally delayed beyond the normal six hours after the administration of the dose.

Absence of histidase activity in the liver and the stratum corneum in most patients. Additional laboratory findings are persistently low glutamic acid and high α-alanine in biologic fluids, and the presence of imidazolepyruvic, imidazolelactic, and imidazoleacetic acids in the urine of the patients as shown by paper chromatography.

**Complications:**  While the literature recounts scholastic failure, emotional and behavior problems, speech impairment, and mild or moderate degree of mental retardation, these are "not higher than the frequency of these functional disorders in the nonhistidinemic population" (Scriver and Levy, 1983).

**Associated Findings:**  None known.

**Etiology:**  Autosomal recessive inheritance of enzyme defect. Heterogeneity exists.

**Pathogenesis:**  The lack of histidase activity causes histidine to be pushed through the subsidiary pathway of transamination or deamination to form imidazolepyruvic acid. The latter may then be reduced to imidazolelactic acid or converted to imidazoleacetic acid by decarboxylation. Imidazolepyruvic acid appears in abundance in urine.

**MIM No.:**  *23580

**Sex Ratio:**  M1:F1

**Occurrence:**  Estimated to be as high as 1:12,000 births. Calculated at 1:37,000 in Sweden on the basis of neonatal screening.

**Risk of Recurrence for Patient's Sib:**
See Part I, *Mendelian Inheritance.*

**Risk of Recurrence for Patient's Child:**
See Part I, *Mendelian Inheritance.*

**Age of Detectability:**  First week of life by blood histidine test or a histidase test of stratum corneum. Screening of newborns for histidinemia has been required by law in New York State since 1974.

**Gene Mapping and Linkage:**  HIS (histidase) has been tentatively mapped to 12.

**Prevention:**  None known. Genetic counseling indicated.

**Treatment:**  Dietary treatment is in the experimental stage.

**Prognosis:**  Normal life span.

**Detection of Carrier:**  LaDu's enzymic technique carried out on stratum corneum will identify the heterozygote. Stratum corneum can be conveniently obtained from the cuticles, the heel of the foot, and the toes. Administration of a loading dose of 150 mg/kg of histidine may also help to identify the carrier.

**References:**
Zannoni VG, LaDu BN: Determination of histidine, alpha-deaminase in human stratum corneum and its absence in histidinaemia. Biochem J 1963; 88:160.
Auerbach VH, et al.: Histidinemia: direct demonstration of absent histidine activity in liver and further observations on the histidinemia disorder. In Nyhan WL, ed: Amino acid metabolism and genetic variation. New York: McGraw-Hill Book Co, 1967:145.
Ghadimi H: Histidinemia: emerging clinical picture. In: Nyhan WL, ed: Heritable disorders of amino acid metabolism: patterns of clinical expression and genetic variation. New York: John Wiley & Sons, 1974 265.
Levy HL, et al.: Routine newborn screening for histidinemia: clinical and biochemical results. N Engl J Med 1974; 291:1214.
Anakura M, et al.: Histidinemia: classical and atypical form in siblings. Am J Dis Child 1975; 129:858.
Alm J, et al.: Histidinaemia in Sweden: report on a neonatal screening programme. Clin Genet 1981; 20:229.
Scriver CR, Levy HL: Histidinaemia Part I: reconciling retrospective and prospective findings. J Inherit Metab Dis 1983; 6:51–53.

GH000                                                **H. Ghadimi**

## HISTIDINURIA 2107

**Includes:** Renal histidinura

**Excludes:**
    **Hartnup disorder** (0453)
    **Histidinemia** (0472)

**Major Diagnostic Criteria:** All four known patients had CNS signs (mental retardation or myoclonic seizures). A selective hyperaminoaciduria comprising histidine alone, in the presence of normal plasma amino acid levels (and specifically so for histidine), identifies the condition. Intestinal absorption of histidine may also be impaired.

**Clinical Findings:** Renal histidinuria, in all reported patients (n=4, including two sibs), was identified during investigation of mental retardation or myoclonic seizures. Whether renal histidinuria can be asymptomatic is not known. Renal histidinuria seems not to have been reported from newborn urine screening programs.

**Complications:** May cause CNS disease.

**Associated Findings:** None known.

**Etiology:** Autosomal recessive inheritance.

**Pathogenesis:** Deficient activity of a specific membrane transport system for L-histidine in renal (and intestinal) epithelium would explain the findings: high renal clearance of histidine (indicating reabsorption <89% of filtered load) at a normal plasma histidine level; impaired plasma response to oral histidine load is found in some, but not all patients. CSF histidine is normal (in cases examined); urine histidine metabolites are normal.

**MIM No.:** *23583

**Sex Ratio:** Presumbably M1:F1

**Occurrence:** Four cases, two of which were sibs, have been reported.

**Risk of Recurrence for Patient's Sib:**
    See Part I, *Mendelian Inheritance.*

**Risk of Recurrence for Patient's Child:**
    See Part I, *Mendelian Inheritance.*

**Age of Detectability:** Presumably in the newborn period.

**Gene Mapping and Linkage:** Unknown.

**Prevention:** None known. Genetic counseling indicated.

**Treatment:** Unknown.

**Prognosis:** Unknown.

**Detection of Carrier:** Some parents apparently show attenuated intestinal absorption of histidine. No apparent increase of renal histidine clearance under endogenous conditions reported in parents.

**References:**
Holmgren G, et al.: Histidinemia and normo-histidinemic histidinuria. Acta Paediat Scand 1974; 63:220–224.
Sabater J, et al.: Histidinuria: a renal and intestinal histidine transport deficiency found in two mentally retarded children. Clin Genet 1976; 9:117–124.
Kamoun PP, et al.: Renal histidinuria. J Inherit Metab Dis 1981; 4:217–219.

SC050                                                        **Charles R. Scriver**

**Histiocytic dermatoarthritis, familial**
    *See DERMATOARTHRITIS, FAMILIAL HISTIOCYTIC*
**Histiocytosis, acute disseminated**
    *See LETTERER-SIWE DISEASE*
**Histiocytosis, proliferative**
    *See IMMUNODEFICIENCY, RETICULOENDOTHELIOSIS WITH EOSINOPHILIA*
**Histiocytosis, sea-blue**
    *See CHOLESTERYL ESTER STORAGE DISEASE*
**HLA-A histocompatibility type**
    *See RAGWEED POLLEN SENSITIVITY*
**HMG-CoA lyase deficiency**
    *See ACIDEMIA, 3-HYDROXY-3-METHYLGLUTARIC*

**Hodgkin disease, site-specific aggregations**
    *See CANCER, HODGKIN DISEASE, FAMILIAL*
**Hodgkin's disease**
    *See CANCER, HODGKIN DISEASE, FAMILIAL*
**Holmes heart**
    *See VENTRICLE, SEPTUM DEXTROPOSITION AND DOUBLE INLET LEFT VENTRICLE*
**Holmes-Gang syndrome**
    *See X-LINKED MENTAL RETARDATION-CRANIOFACIAL ABNORMALITIES-CLUB FOOT*
**Holocarboxylase synthetase deficiency**
    *See CARBOXYLASE DEFICIENCY, HOLOCARBOXYLASE DEFICIENCY TYPE*

## HOLOPROSENCEPHALY 0473

**Includes:**
    Arhinencephaly
    Cebocephaly
    Ethmocephaly
    Phenytoin, fetal effects of
    Premaxillary agenesis

**Excludes:**
    **Cyclopia** (0234)
    **Lip, median cleft of upper** (0595)

**Major Diagnostic Criteria:** Orbital hypotelorism with features of incomplete midline development (e.g., median or bilateral cleft lip, absent philtrum) and psychomotor retardation suggest the diagnosis. The demonstration of a single ventricle or incomplete development of cerebral lobes establishes the diagnosis. Although absent olfactory bulb and tracts are pathognomonic for the condition, this finding is usually only demonstrated at autopsy.

**Clinical Findings:** Holoprosencephaly is a series of malformations with cyclopia, median cleft lip and palate, and single ventricle representing the severe end of the spectrum; of moderate severity is orbital hypotelorism with a single-nostril nose and normal lip and palate, or with a flat nose and median cleft lip; the mild end of the spectrum is represented by a normal face, but absent olfactory bulb and tracts and a single maxillary incisor. Therefore, holoprosencephaly can be alobar, semilobar, or lobar. The degree of facial malformation is usually predictive of brain malformation. As a result, most affected people are severely retarded, although those with minor facial anomalies can have minimal handicap. Absence of the corpus callosum and endocrine abnormalities may also be part of the phenotype.

**Complications:** There have been reports with autopsy evidence of *in vivo* evidence of ACTH-adrenal axis failure. Other affected persons have had pitressin-responsive diabetes insipidus. Families have been reported in which two sibs with holoprosencephaly had a third sib with hypopituitarism, which suggests that hypo-

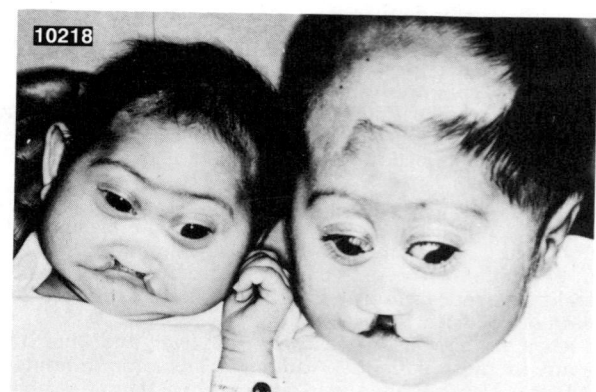

**0473**-10218: Premaxillary agenesis and ocular hypotelorism.

pituitarism may be a part of the holoprosencephaly phenotypic spectrum. Absence of facial bones, parotid glands, tongue, and muscles of mastication are also occasionally found, although rarely.

**Associated Findings:** Patients with a chromosome anomaly or a malformation syndrome have the extracranial anomalies of that syndrome.

**Etiology:** Although most cases of holoprosencephaly are sporadic, it is recognized that holoprosencephaly is a causally heterogeneous entity. As many as one-half of all cases are attributable to a chromosome anomaly, the most common of which is **Chromosome 13, trisomy 13.** Monogenic syndromes such as the **Meckel syndrome** have been reported as having holoprosencephaly as part of the phenotype. Furthermore, several families with apparent monogenic inheritance, either autosomal dominant or autosomal recessive, have been reported. Several environmental factors have been implicated as well, including viral infection (CMV), toxoplasmosis, and drugs such as phenytoin, retinoic acid, and alcohol. The incidence of holoprosencephaly in infants of diabetic mothers is estimated to be between 0.5 and one percent.

The clinical picture of holoprosencephaly can be viewed as a spectrum of facial anomalies, including cyclopia, ethmocephaly, and cebocephaly, since they all share similar cerebral malformations. The mildest end of the spectrum is considered to be hypotelorism with single central incisor. This view is further substantiated by reports of different combinations of these defects occurring in sibships, which is indicative of a common pathogenesis.

**Pathogenesis:** Holoprosencephaly is caused by a failure of the prosencephalon to cleave sagittally into the cerebral hemispheres, transversely into the telencephalon and diencephalon, and horizontally into the olfactory and optic bulbs.

**MIM No.:** *23610

**POS No.:** 3460

**CDC No.:** 742.260

**Sex Ratio:** M1:F3 for alobar holoprosencephaly; M1:F1, for the lobar form.

**Occurrence:** 6–12:100,000 in liveborns, 4:1,000 in embryos.

**Risk of Recurrence for Patient's Sib:**
See Part I, *Mendelian Inheritance.* Six percent for recurrence of sporadic, nonchromosomal holoprosencephaly. In families with holoprosencephaly in two generations, it is estimated that the risk to first degree relatives is 22.9% for holoprosencephaly and 34.3% for holoprosencephaly and other facial or CNS defects.

**Risk of Recurrence for Patient's Child:**
See Part I, *Mendelian Inheritance.*

**Age of Detectability:** Prenatally by ultrasound; at birth by clinical examination.

**Gene Mapping and Linkage:** Unknown.

**Prevention:** None known. Genetic counseling indicated.

**Treatment:** Treatment of seizures. Detection and treatment of hormonal deficiencies.

**Prognosis:** Most severely affected patients have died before six months of age. Survival beyond one year is rare, but survival into adulthood is possible for mildly affected individuals. Individuals with alobar and semilobar holoprosencephaly are severely mentally retarded. While a few individuals with lobar holoprosencephaly may have only mild to moderate mental retardation, most are also severely retarded.

**Detection of Carrier:** Unknown.

**References:**
DeMyer W: Holoprosencephaly. In Vinken PJ, Bruyn, DW, eds: Handbook of Clinical Neurology, vol 30. New York: North-Holland, 1977:431–478.
Campbell S, et al.: Ultrasound and fetoscopy in the early diagnosis of neural tube and other defects. symposium on the diagnosis and management of neural tube defects. R Coll Obstet Gynaecol 1979.
Cohen MM Jr.: An update on the holoprosencephalic disorders. J Pediatr 1982; 101:865–869. †
Barr M, et al.: Holoprosencephaly in infants of diabetic mothers. J Pediatr 1983; 102:565–568.
Benke PJ, Cohen MM Jr.: Recurrence of holoprosencephaly in families with a positive history. Clin Genet 1983; 24:324–328.
Saunders ES, et al.: What is the incidence of holoprosencephaly? J Med Genet 1984; 21:21–26.
Byrne PJ, et al.: Cyclopia and congenital cytomegalovirus infection. Am J Med Genet 1987; 28:61–65.
Cohen MM, Jr.: Perspectives on holoprosencephaly: part I. Epidemiology, genetics, and syndromology. Teratology 1989; 40:211–235.
Cohen MM, Jr.: Perspectives on holoprosencephaly: part III. Spectia, distinctions, continuities, and discontinuities. Am J Med Genet 1989; 34:271–288. *
Johnson VP: holoprosencephaly: a developmental field defect. Am J Med Genet 1989; 34:258–264.
Munke M: Clinical, cytogenetic, and molecular approaches to the genetic heterogeneity of holoprosencephaly. Am J Med Genet 1989; 34:237–245.

T0007          **Helga V. Toriello**

**Holoprosencephaly-agnathia**
*See AGNATHIA-HOLOPROSENCEPHALY*
**Holt-Oram syndrome**
*See HEART-HAND SYNDROME*

## HOMOCYSTINURIA        0474

**Includes:**
Cystathionine beta-synthase deficiency
Pyridoxine-responsive homocystinuria

**Excludes:**
**Anemia, pernicious congenital** (2656)
**Homocystinuria, N(5,10) methylene tetrahydrofolate deficiency type** (2404)
Homocystinuria-methylmalonic acidemia
**Marfan syndrome** (0630)
**Methylcobalamin deficiency** (2605)
N(5)-methyltetrahydrofolate homocysteine methyltransferase impairment
Transcobalamin deficiency

**Major Diagnostic Criteria:** Elevated urinary homocyst(e)ine with increased plasma methionine concentration. The presence of homocystine is suggested by a positive urinary cyanide-nitroprusside test, but diagnosis requires amino acid chromatography of urine and plasma. Without treatment, fasting plasma methionine concentrations may range from 0.15 to 2.0 $\mu$mol/ml (normally up to 0.03 $\mu$mol/ml) and plasma homocystine (normally not detectable) may be up to 0.2 $\mu$mol/ml. Plasma cyst(e)ine is decreased. Urinary excretion of homocyst(e)ine may exceed 1 mmol/day, and several unusual metabolites of homocysteine may be detected in the urine. The diagnosis can be confirmed by decreased cystathionine $\beta$-synthase activity in tissue from liver biopsy, in mitogen-stimulated lymphocytes, or in cultured fibroblasts.

**Clinical Findings:** One class of cystathionine $\beta$-synthase-deficient patients has a marked improvement of the biochemical

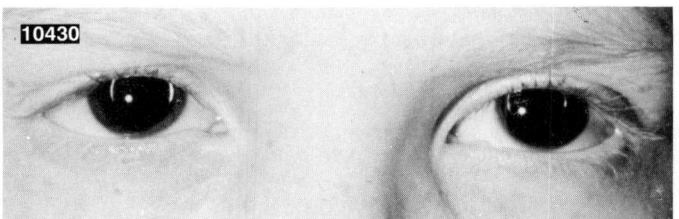

**0474A-**10430: Note lens dislocation.

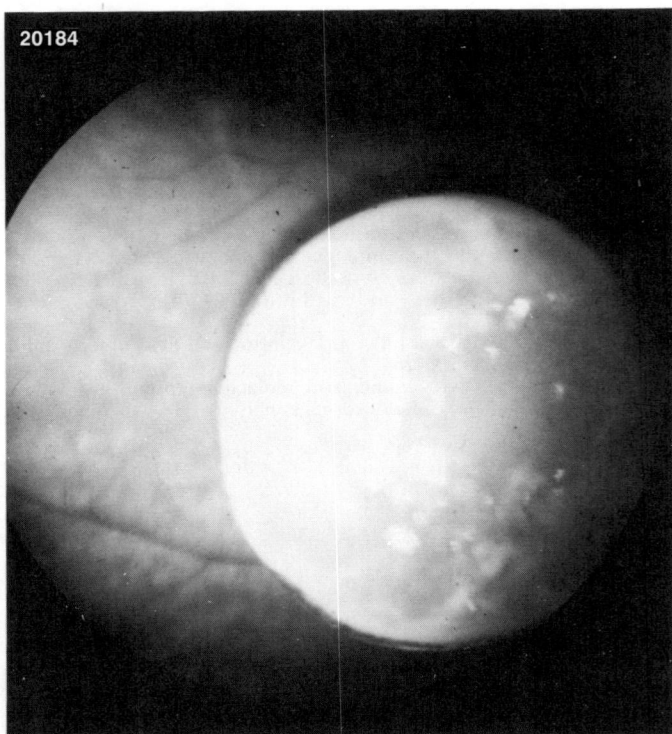

**0474B-20184:** Note downward dislocation of the lens in homocystinuria.

abnormalities following administration of pyridoxine (vitamin B₆). The clinical course of the disease is generally less severe in pyridoxine-responsive patients. Clinical features are present in four major systems, as outlined below.

1. *Eye:* Zonular fibers are thickened, and dislocation of the optic lens is a very characteristic finding. Iridodinesis may be observed. Myopia is common.

2. *Skeletal system:* Almost all untreated patients have abnormalities of the skeletal system. Dolichostenomelia and arachnodactyly may suggest Marfan syndrome. Other findings include genu valgum, pes cavus, pectus carinatum or excavatum, kyphoscoliosis, and dental malalignment. X-ray examination will demonstrate these skeletal abnormalities and, will commonly disclose osteoporosis, and sometimes will show biconcave vertebral bodies.

3. *Vascular system:* Thromboembolic events represent a significant risk factor for premature mortality. The basis of the accelerated thrombosis is still not well defined, and it may involve multiple mechanisms, including cytotoxic effects on the vascular endothelium, release of endothelial procoagulant, altered collagen and elastin structure, and increased adhesiveness of platelets. Arterial or venous occlusion may occur, and intravascular thrombosis may occur at any time in life, including infancy. Other vascular findings sometimes observed are malar flush and livedo reticularis.

4. *Central nervous system:* Between one third and three-fourths of untreated patients have mild or moderate mental retardation. The mental potential with early treatment is distinctly improved, particularly in the case of pyridoxine responders. Cerebrovascular thrombosis may obviously play a role in the neurologic symptoms of certain patients. Seizures may be evident and electroencephalographic abnormalities have been described, which may in certain cases reverse with treatment. A variety of psychiatric symptoms, including psychosis, may be associated.

**Complications:** Without treatment, ectopia lentis is found in about 55% of pyridoxine-responsive and about 82% of pyridoxine-

unresponsive cases by age 10 years. Associated complications include glaucoma, optic atrophy, and retinal detatchment. Some form of thromboembolic event occurs in 12 to 27% of untreated patients by age 15 years. Claudication, renovascular hypertension, abdominal angina, and stroke or ischemic cerebrovascular disease have resulted. Coronary artery disease appears to be less frequent. Surgery can be performed safely with precautions, although a number of patients have had fatal perioperative thrombotic complications. Fractures of bone are common in untreated patients. There has been a single report of hepatic toxicity associated with treatment using pyridoxal phosphate (but not pyridoxine hydrochloride) at 1000 mg/day.

**Associated Findings:**  None known.

**Etiology:**  Autosomal recessive inheritance.

**Pathogenesis:**  There appears to be considerable genetic heterogeneity among the lesions that produce cystathionine β-synthase deficiency. Approximately one-half of cases will have a biochemical response to high doses of pyridoxine, while there will be no effect in other cases. Residual cystathionine β-synthase in cultured fibroblasts derived from affected individuals varies widely with respect to enzymatic activity as does the amount of immunologically cross-reactive material. In certain cases alterations of the residual enzyme's heat stability, isoelectric point, or affinity for pyridoxal phosphate, serine, or homocysteine have been demonstrated. In general, it appears that the enzyme deficiencies arise from mutations in the structural gene, but cases of regulatory gene mutation are possible.

**MIM No.:**  *23620

**POS No.:**  3253

**Sex Ratio:**  M1:F1

**Occurrence:**  Programs that screen newborn infants based on blood methionine levels have been established in most parts of the world. The area of highest apparent incidence is Ireland, where approximately 1:60,000 infants have been detected. The yield in Japan has been about 1:146,000. Estimates from programs that screen newborn urine have given lower apparent prevalences. In light of several cases known to have been missed by mass screening programs of each type, it is likely that the true incidence is significantly higher.

**Risk of Recurrence for Patient's Sib:**
See Part I, *Mendelian Inheritance.*

**Risk of Recurrence for Patient's Child:**
See Part I, *Mendelian Inheritance.*

**Age of Detectability:**  The cystathionine β-synthase gene has recently been cloned, and it is anticipated that analysis of polymorphisms in affected kindreds will be of value, but as of the time of this writing, antenatal diagnosis has not been established. A few cases have been reported in which the diagnosis has correctly been excluded by enzymatic assay of amniocyte culture extracts. Newborn screening is generally reliable, but false-negative tests have been documented with both blood and urine tests. Variables leading to false-negative results may include reduced dietary methionine intake (as with breastmilk compared with proprietary formula) and high pyridoxine intake (as with certain programs of vitamin supplementation). Ascertainment on clinical grounds is often possible in early childhood.

**Gene Mapping and Linkage:**  CBS (cystathionine-beta-synthase) has been mapped to 21q22.3.

**Prevention:**  None known. Genetic counseling indicated.

**Treatment:**  It is important initially to determine whether a patient is responsive to pyridoxine. Doses of 100 to 500 mg/day or greater are given, and levels of plasma methionine, homocyst(e)ine and cyst(e)ine, and urinary homocystine should be followed over the course of a few weeks. Folic acid depletion has been noted in a number of cystathionine β-synthase-deficient patients, and the administration of pyridoxine may exacerbate the effect. Furthermore, the biochemical response to pyridoxine may be absent until after folate repletion. If responsiveness to pyridoxine is established, supplementation should be continued indefinitely.

Dietary management with low methionine intake may be of value if the response to pyridoxine is less than complete. The incidence of certain progressive complications appears to be reduced with dietary treatment. Supplementation with cystine may be of benefit. The diet must be adjusted in each patient individually so as to approach normal amino acid levels. Betaine (trimethylglycine) allows for remethylation of homocysteine by an alternate pathway. With betaine administration, a reduction of homocyst(e)ine and an increase of methionine are seen, and clinical improvement has been reported in numerous cases. The blood levels of methionine during betaine therapy should be monitored, because toxic effects are possible. Betaine is used for the most part in patients who are unresponsive to pyridoxine. Betaine may also improve the methionine tolerance in treated pyridoxine-responsive patients even when fasting plasma amino acid levels are normal, and it is possible that it should be considered as an additional measure in such patients.

Thrombotic complications appear to be reduced with metabolic control. Dipyridamole and low-dose aspirin may be useful adjuvants. Avoidance of agents that can promote thromboembolism, such as oral contraceptives, is probably prudent.

**Prognosis:** In untreated patients, the life span is markedly reduced because of thrombotic complications. The progress in treated pyridoxine-responsive patients can be markedly improved, and in untreated patients the course in those subsequently shown to be pyridoxine-responsive is generally less severe. Life span is expected to be normal in pyridoxine-responsive patients receiving therapy. Life span in pyridoxine-unresponsive patients will probably be reduced because of the difficulties of compliance and the generally suboptimal results of dietary therapy. However, evidence is accumulating that early treatment does improve prognosis.

**Detection of Carrier:** Cystathionine β-synthase activities in liver tissue or in fibroblast lines from obligate heterozygotes are lower than control activities but overlap is observed. A methionine load may be given, after which an elevated plasma peak concentration of total homocysteine is a fairly good parameter to discriminate heterozygotes. The potential exists in the near future for carrier detection by restriction fragment length polymorphisms in kindreds in which homozygotes have been detected. The issue of heterozygote detection without a family history of homocystinuria may have importance because of the suggestion that heterozygotes have an increased risk of thrombotic disease. In populations with premature peripheral and cerebrovascular obstructive arterial disease, there are reports of a disproportionate number with peak cysteine levels after methionine loads and fibroblast cystathionine β-synthase activities that fall in the range for obligate heterozygotes.

**Special Considerations:** Homocystinuria should be ruled out in all patients with features of **Marfan syndrome** or with nontraumatic ectopia lentis. The diagnosis must also be sought in all cases of unexplained thrombotic disease in infants or children.

At the time of diagnosis, it is important to distinguish cystathionine β-synthase deficiency from other causes of homocystinuria. The remethylation of homocysteine to methionine can be impaired by a deficiency of vitamin $B_{12}$, defective intestinal absorption of the $B_{12}$-intrinsic factor complex, deficiency of transcobalamin II, or a defect in the formation or availability of the coenzymatically active methyl-$B_{12}$. Remethylation will also be limited in cases of $N^{5,10}$-methylenetetrahydrofolate reductase deficiency because of reduced production of $N^5$-methyltetrahydrofolate. These defects of remethylation can be distinguished by a normal or decreased plasma methionine concentration in contrast to the situation in cystathionine β-synthase deficiency. Certain of the conditions that involve $B_{12}$ metabolism are also distinguished by an associated methylmalonic acidemia. The distinction is important, because treatment with a low methionine diet would be inappropriate and harmful in cases with remethylation defects.

**References:**

Boers GHJ, et al.: Heterozygosity for homocystinuria in premature peripheral and cerebral occlusive arterial disease. New Engl J Med 1985; 313:709–715.

Mudd SH, et al.: The natural history of homocystinuria due to cystathionine beta-deficiency. Am J Hum Genet 1985; 37:1–31.

Wilcken DEL, et al.: Homocystinuria due to cystathionine beta-synthase deficiency: the effects of betaine treatment in pyridoxine-responsive patients. Metabolism 1985; 34:1115–1121.

Kraus JP, et al.: Cloning and screening of nanogram amounts of immunopurified mRNAs: cDNA cloning and chromosomal mapping of cystathionine β-synthase and the β subunit of propionyl-CoA carboxylase. Proc Natl Acad Sci USA 1986; 83:2047–2051.

Abbott MH, et al.: Psychiatric manifestations of homocystinuria due to cystathionine beta-sythesis deficiency. Am J Med Genet 1987; 26:959–969.

Mudd SH, et al.: Disorders of transulfuration. In: Scriver C, et al., eds. The metabolic basis of inherited disease, 6th ed. New York: McGraw-Hill, 1989:693–734.*

BA063 **Bruce A. Barshop**

**Homocystinuria due to MTHFR deficiency**
*See HOMOCYSTINURIA, N(5,10) METHYLENE TETRAHYDROFOLATE DEFICIENCY TYPE*

## HOMOCYSTINURIA, N(5,10) METHYLENE TETRAHYDROFOLATE DEFICIENCY TYPE     2404

**Includes:**

Cystathioninuria due to MTHFR deficiency
Homocystinuria due to MTHFR deficiency
Methylenetetrahydrofolate reductase (MTHFR) deficiency
N(5,10) methylenetetrahydrofolate reductase deficiency

**Excludes:**

**Cystathioninuria** (0236)
Folate metabolism enzyme deficiencies, other
**Homocystinuria** (0474)
**Methylcobalamin deficiency** (2605)
Methylcobalamin, failure to accumulate
Vitamin B6 deficiency
Vitamin B12 deficiency

**Major Diagnostic Criteria:** **Homocystinuria**, homocystinemia, **Cystathioninuria**, low to normal blood methionine levels, enzyme deficiency confirmed in cultured fibroblasts, liver, lymphoblasts or leukocytes.

**Clinical Findings:** Neonatal encephalopathy, myopathy, developmental regression in first year of life, **Microcephaly**, seizures, apnea episodes, death in infancy, intravascular thromboses, dislocated lenses, peripheral neuropathy, and psychiatric manifestations. Varying degrees of severity appear to correlate best with varying degrees of enzymatic activity.

**Complications:** Neurologic abnormalities, mental retardation, vascular thromboses, collagen laxity, lens dislocations, and sudden death.

**Associated Findings:** Low plasma methionine.

**Etiology:** Autosomal recessive inheritance.

**Pathogenesis:** N(5,10) methylenetetrahydrofolate reductase is involved in the conversion of 5,10 methylene tetrahydrofolate to 5-methyltetrahydrofolate. 5-methyltetrahydrofolate is required for the conversion of homocysteine to methionine thus leading to the homocystinuria and cystathioninuria secondary to the conversion of homocysteine to cystathionine. Possibly a decrease in endogenous synthesis of methionine results in decreased synthesis of neurotransmitters such as serotonin and dopamine. Elevation of homocysteine results in connective tissue laxity and lens dislocation, perhaps due to homocysteine interfering with normal cross linking of collagen. Increased incidence of vascular thromboses may be secondary to direct endothelial damage.

**MIM No.:** *23625

**POS No.:** 3253

**Sex Ratio:** M1:F1

**Occurrence:** About two dozen cases have been documented in the literature. The most common of folate metabolism defects.

**Risk of Recurrence for Patient's Sib:**
See Part I, *Mendelian Inheritance.* Sibs have two-thirds chance of being a carrier.

**Risk of Recurrence for Patient's Child:**
See Part I, *Mendelian Inheritance.* No affected individuals are known to have reproduced.

**Age of Detectability:** In the neonatal period to the first decade of life. Prenatal diagnosis is possible using amniocentesis or chorionic villus biopsy.

**Gene Mapping and Linkage:** Unknown.

**Prevention:** None known. Genetic counseling indicated.

**Treatment:** No truly effective treatment is known. Oral folic acid, or folic acid B12, B6, methionine, and carnitine and betaine can help to to restore normal plasma methionine levels.

**Prognosis:** Unknown.

**Detection of Carrier:** Reduced activity, enzymes can be demonstrated in the fibroblasts of the parents of affected patients.

**References:**

Mudd SH, et al.: Homocystinuria associated with decreased methylenetetrahydrofolate reductase activity. Biochem Biophys Res Commun 1972; 46:905–912.
Shih VE, et al.: A new form of homocystinuria due to N(5,10) metholenetetrahydrofolate reductase deficiency. (Abstract) Pediatr Res 1972; 6:135 only.
Freeman JM, et al.: Folate-responsive homocystinuria and "schizophrenia": a defect in methylation due to deficient 5,10-methylenetetrahydrofolate reductase activity. New Engl J Med 1975; 292:491–496.
Wong PWK, et al.: Detection of homozygotes and heterozygotes with methylene tetrahydrofolate reductase deficiency. J Lab Clin Med 1977; 90:283–288.
Christensen E, Brandt NJ: Prenatal diagnosis of 5,10-methylenetetrahydrofolate reductase deficiency. (Letter) New Engl J Med 1985; 313:50–51.
Haan EA, et al.: 5,10-methylenetetrahydrofolate reductase deficiency: clinical and biochemical features of a further case. J Inherit Metab Dis 1985; 8:53–57.
Hyland K, et al.: Demyelination and decreased s-adenosyl methionine in 5,10-methyleletetrahydrofolate reductase deficiency. Neurology 1988; 38:459–462.
Rosenblatt DS: Inherited disorders of folate transport and metabolism. In: Scriver CR, et al, eds: The metabolic basis of inherited disease, 6th ed. New York: McGraw-Hill, 1989:2049–2064.

WI038                                                    **Susan C. Winter**

**Homocystinuria-megaloblastic anemia due to cobalamin defect**
*See METHYLCOBALAMIN DEFICIENCY*
**Homogentisic acid oxidase deficiency**
*See ALKAPTONURIA*
**Homogentisic aciduria**
*See ALKAPTONURIA*
**Homozygous dyschondrosteosis**
*See MESOMELIC DYSPLASIA, LANGER TYPE*
**Homozygous hypobetalipoproteinemia**
*See HYPOBETALIPOPROTEINEMIA*
**Homozygous protein C deficiency**
*See PROTEIN C DEFICIENCY*
**Homozygous sickle hemoglobinopathy**
*See ANEMIA, SICKLE CELL*
**Honey ear wax**
*See EAR, CERUMEN VARIATIONS*
**HOOD (hereditary onycho-osteo-dysplasia)**
*See NAIL-PATELLA SYNDROME*

## HOOFT DISEASE                                        2178

**Includes:**
Hypolipidemia-short stature-leukonychia
Leukonychia-short stature-hypolipidemia
Short stature-hypolipidemia-leukonychia

**Excludes:**
Erythematosquamous rashes
Short stature-leukonychia (other)

**Major Diagnostic Criteria:** Hypolipidemia, erythematosquamous rash, and short stature.

**Clinical Findings:** An erythematosquamous rash becomes evident toward the end of the first year of life, and poor growth is noticed at about the same time. Opaque leukonychia begins toward the end of the third year. The permanent incisors have dystrophic enamel. The hair is fine and brittle. Serum lipids are 384–465 mg/dl and serum cholesterol, 42–70 mg/dl.

**Complications:** Unknown.

**Associated Findings:** Slow development and hyperactivity. At age seven years, one sister had mental retardation, a mucoid macular dystrophy, an extinguished pattern on electroretinogram (ERG), and a pigmentary retinopathy consisting of an equatorial area of small grayish-yellow degenerative foci interspersed with pigment dots were present.

**Etiology:** Presumably autosomal recessive inheritance.

**Pathogenesis:** Unknown.

**MIM No.:** 23630

**Sex Ratio:** M0:F2 (observed).

**Occurrence:** One reported family with two sisters has been documented.

**Risk of Recurrence for Patient's Sib:**
See Part I, *Mendelian Inheritance.*

**Risk of Recurrence for Patient's Child:**
See Part I, *Mendelian Inheritance.*

**Age of Detectability:** In early childhood.

**Gene Mapping and Linkage:** Unknown.

**Prevention:** None known. Genetic counseling indicated.

**Treatment:** Unknown.

**Prognosis:** Unknown.

**Detection of Carrier:** Unknown.

**References:**

Hooft C, et al.: Familial hypolipidemia and retarded development without steatorrhea: another inborn error of metabolism? Helv Paediatr Acta 1962; 17:1–23.
François J: Ocular manifestations in certain congenital errors of metabolism. In: Symposium on surgical and medical management of congenital anomalies of the eye. Transactions of New Orleans Academy of Ophthalmology. St. Louis: C.V. Mosby, 1968:171–173.

TH017                                                    **T.F. Thurmon**

**Hopf disease**
*See ACROKERATOSIS VERRUCIFORMIS*

## HORNER SYNDROME                                      0475

**Includes:**
Miosis and partial ptosis
Oculopupillary syndrome
Oculosympathetic syndrome

**Excludes:** Acquired Horner syndrome

**Major Diagnostic Criteria:** Miosis and partial ptosis of the affected side.

**Clinical Findings:** The symptom-complex includes on the affected side: miosis, partial ptosis of the upper lid, anhidrosis. The first two signs are the most constant. Heterochromia iridis may be a part of the syndrome when the onset occurred before birth or within the first two years of life. The findings depend upon the site of interruption of the sympathetic nervous system between the hypothalamus and the orbit. Langham and Weinstein have proposed that pre- and postcervical ganglionic lesions in man can be differentiated by the presence or absence of supersensitivity of the affected eye to adrenergic amines applied topically. The absence of supersensitivity appears to be indicative of a preganglionic lesion of the sympathetic tract. In postganglionic lesions, sympathetic denervation supersensitivity of the pupil is due to the inability of the presynaptic endings to reabsorb catecholamines. The pupillary reaction to light and accommodation are maintained but may be diminished.

**Complications:** Alteration of tear secretion on the affected side, cataract formation, increase in the amplitude of accommodation, and glaucoma.

**Associated Findings:** Facial hemiatrophy.

**Etiology:** Autosomal dominant inheritance. An acquired form may result from neuroblastoma, thoracic surgery, or may follow an acute febrile illness.

**Pathogenesis:** Any interruption of the autonomic nervous system from the hypothalamus to the orbit.

**MIM No.:** *14300

**Sex Ratio:** M1:F1

**Occurrence:** At least 250 cases reported.

**Risk of Recurrence for Patient's Sib:**
See Part I, *Mendelian Inheritance.*

**Risk of Recurrence for Patient's Child:**
See Part I, *Mendelian Inheritance.*

**Age of Detectability:** At birth. Later in the acquired form.

**Gene Mapping and Linkage:** Unknown.

**Prevention:** None known. Genetic counseling indicated.

**Treatment:** Unknown.

**Prognosis:** Dependent upon associated findings.

**Detection of Carrier:** Clinical examination.

**Special Considerations:** Neuroblastoma of the upper chest and neck should be ruled out in infants and children presenting with Horner syndrome.

**References:**
Giles CL, Henderson JW: Horner's syndrome: an analysis of 216 cases. Am J Ophthalmol 1958; 46:289.
Langham ME, Weinstein GW: Horner's syndrome: ocular supersensitivity to adrenergic amines. Arch Ophthalmol 1967; 78:462.
Weinstein GW, Langham ME: Horner's syndrome and glaucoma: report of a case. Arch Ophthalmol 1969; 82:483.
Korczyn AD: Denervation supersensitivity in Horner's syndrome. Ophthalmologica. 1975; 170:313–319.
Woodruff G, et al.: Horner's syndrome in children. J Pediatr Ophthalmol Strabism 1988; 25:40–44.

RA004 **Elsa K. Rahn**

**Horseshoe kidneys**
*See KIDNEY, HORSESHOE*

## HOWEL-EVANS SYNDROME 3290

**Includes:**
Cancer of the esophagus-palmoplantar keratodermia
Palmoplantar keratodermia with carcinoma of esophagus
Tylosis with malignancy

**Excludes:**
Bazex syndrome
**Keratosis palmaris et plantaris of Unna-Thost (3264)**
**Skin** (other)

**Major Diagnostic Criteria:** Diffuse palmoplantar keratoderma with associated carcinoma of the esophagus.

**Clinical Findings:** The palmoplantar keratoderma is very similar to that see in **Keratosis palmaris et plantaris of Unna-Thost**. It consists of a dense homogeneous hyperkeratosis in a bilateral and symmetric distribution, limited to palms and soles (non-transgrediens). The only difference from **Keratosis palmaris et plantaris of Unna-Thost** is late onset, with the clinical findings in this condition usually becoming evident around the second decade of life. The age of onset of the esophageal cancer is around the fifth-to-sixth decade of life.

**Complications:** Unknown.

**Associated Findings:** Oral leukoplakia in one kindred, and squamous cell carcinoma in the tylotic skin in another kindred.

**Etiology:** Autosomal dominant inheritance.

**Pathogenesis:** Unknown.

**Sex Ratio:** Presumably M1:F1.

**Occurrence:** Unknown. A few kindreds have been reported.

**Risk of Recurrence for Patient's Sib:**
See Part I, *Mendelian Inheritance.*

**Risk of Recurrence for Patient's Child:**
See Part I, *Mendelian Inheritance.*

**Age of Detectability:** The keratoderma is usually evident after puberty, although occurrence at birth has been described. The cancer is usually detected later in life.

**Gene Mapping and Linkage:** Unknown.

**Prevention:** None known. Genetic counseling indicated. Periodic examination of the oral cavity and endoscopy of the esophagus is indicated in at-risk individuals.

**Treatment:** Unknown.

**Prognosis:** Unknown.

**Detection of Carrier:** Unknown.

**References:**
Howel-Evans W, et al.: Carcinoma of the esophagus with keratosis palmaris et plantaris (tylosis). Q J Med 1958; 27:413–429.*†
Shine I: Carcinoma of the esophagus with tylosis (keratosis palmaris et plantaris). Lancet 1966; I:951–953.
Harper PS, et al.: Carcinoma of the esophagus with tylosis. Q J Med 1970; 155:317–333.
Tyldesley WR: Oral leukoplakia associated with tylosis and esophageal carcinoma. J Oral Pathol 1974; 3:62–70.
Yesudian P, et al.: Genetic tylosis with malignancy: a study of a South Indian pedigree. Br J Derm 1980; 102:597–600.†

MI038 **Giuseppe Micali**

**Human growth hormone, dwarfism with high plasma immunoreactive**
*See DWARFISM, LARON*
**Human immunodeficiency virus (HIV), congenital infection**
*See FETAL ACQUIRED IMMUNE DEFICIENCY SYNDROME (AIDS) INFECTION*
**Human insulin Chicago**
*See DIABETES MELLITUS, MUTANT INSULIN TYPES*
**Human insulin Los Angeles**
*See DIABETES MELLITUS, MUTANT INSULIN TYPES*
**Human insulin Wakayama**
*See DIABETES MELLITUS, MUTANT INSULIN TYPES*
**Human T lymphotrophic virus (HTLV) III, congenital infection**
*See FETAL ACQUIRED IMMUNE DEFICIENCY SYNDROME (AIDS) INFECTION*

## HUMERO-RADIAL SYNOSTOSIS 0477

**Includes:**
Humero-radio-ulnar synostosis
Synostosis, humero-radial

**Excludes:**
**Acrocephalosyndactyly type V (2284)**
**Antley-Bixler syndrome (2125)**
Brachymesosymphalangism syndrome
**Femoral hypoplasia-unusual facies syndrome (2027)**
Humero-radial syostosis as a syndrome component
**Mietens-Weber syndrome (2013)**

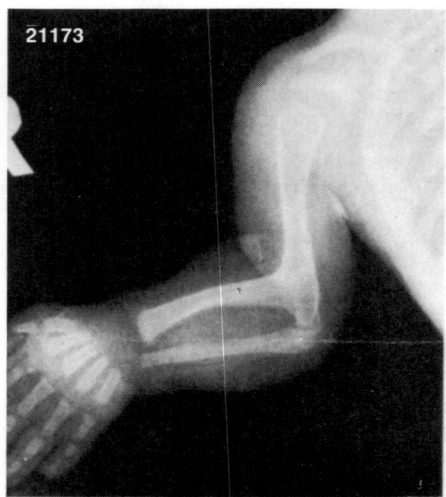

0477-21173:   Humeroradial synostosis.

Nail-patella syndrome (0704)
Radial-ulnar synostosis (0854)
Roberts syndrome (0875)
Synostosis, multiple synostosis syndrome (2312)

**Major Diagnostic Criteria:**   Decreased range of motion of elbow with X-ray evidence of fusion of humerus and radius.

**Clinical Findings:**   Flexion and extension at the elbow is severely reduced or absent. Familial cases are usually bilateral. Sporadic cases tend to be unilateral (65%) and to be associated with hypoplasia of the ulna and absent digits.

**Complications:**   Absent motion of the elbow.

**Associated Findings:**   In addition to *Excluded* syndromes above; hypoplastic patellae and nephropathy (one sibship); microphthalmia, iris coloboma (one sporadic case); microcephaly, occipital meningocele and mental retardation (one member of a sib pair); anosmia and Robin anomaly. The combination of *humero-radio-ulnar synostosis* has also been reported (Hersh et al, 1989; Ramer & Ladda, 1989).

**Etiology:**   Often sporadic. Autosomal recessive or possibly autosomal dominant inheritance.

**Pathogenesis:**   Unknown.

**MIM No.:**   *23640, 14305

**POS No.:**   3254

**Sex Ratio:**   M1:F1

**Occurrence:**   Undetermined but presumed rare.

**Risk of Recurrence for Patient's Sib:**
See Part I, *Mendelian Inheritance.*

**Risk of Recurrence for Patient's Child:**
See Part I, *Mendelian Inheritance.*

**Age of Detectability:**   At birth by examination and by X-ray after 1–2 months of age, when the intervening cartilage has ossified. Humeroradial synostosis in the Antley-Bixler syndrome has been detected by ultrasound in the second trimester of pregnancy.

**Gene Mapping and Linkage:**   Unknown.

**Prevention:**   None known. Genetic counseling indicated.

**Treatment:**   Surgery may be required to improve function.

**Prognosis:**   Normal life span predicted in the absence of associated abnormalities.

**Detection of Carrier:**   Unknown.

**References:**
Siwon P: Kongenitale, hereditare, doppelseitige Ankylosen der Ellenbogengelenke. Dtsch Z Chir 1928; 209:338–349.
Frostad H: Congenital ankylosis of the elbow joint. Acta Orthop Scand 1940; 11:296–306.
Frankel E: Humero-radial synostosis. Br J Surg 1942; 31:242–245.
Keutel J, et al.: Eine wahrscheinlich autosomal recessiv vererbte Skeletmissbildung mit Humeroradial synostose. Humangenetik 1970; 9:43–53.
Hunter AG, et al.: The genetics of and associated clinical findings in humero-radial synostosis. Clin Genet 1976; 9:470–478. *
Hersh JH, et al.: Humero-radio-ulnar synostosis: a new case and review. Am J Med Genet 1989; 33:170–171.
Ramer JC, Ladda RL: Humero-radial synostosis with ulnar defects in sibs. Am J Med Genet 1989; 33:176–179.

C0066                                                  **J. Michael Connor**

**Humero-radio-ulnar synostosis**
   *See HUMERO-RADIAL SYNOSTOSIS*
**Humeroperoneal neuromuscular disease**
   *See EMERY-DREIFUSS SYNDROME*
**Humerospinal dysostosis**
   *See DYSOSTOSIS, HUMEROSPINAL*
**Hunter oculo-encephalo-hepato-renal syndrome**
   *See OCULO-ENCEPHALO-HEPATO-RENAL SYNDROME*
**Hunter syndrome**
   *See MUCOPOLYSACCHARIDOSIS II*
**Hunter-Russell syndrome**
   *See FETAL METHYLMERCURY EFFECTS*
**Huntington chorea**
   *See HUNTINGTON DISEASE*

| **HUNTINGTON DISEASE** | **0478** |
| --- | --- |

**Includes:**
   Huntington chorea
   Progressive chorea

**Excludes:**
   **Acanthocytosis-neurologic defects** (2398)
   **Dentatorubropallidoluysian degeneration, hereditary** (3283)
   **Hallervorden-Spatz disease** (2526)
   **Hepatolenticular degeneration** (0469)
   **Lupus erythematosis, systemic** (2515)
   Paroxysmal choreoathetosis, familial
   Psychiatric disorders (others)
   Sydenham chorea
   **Torsion dystonia** (0957)
   **Tourette syndrome** (2305)

**Major Diagnostic Criteria:**   The age of onset, the progressive chorea and dementia are strongly suggestive of the diagnosis. However, the diagnosis cannot be established unless a positive family history is obtained. There is no specific diagnostic test. On CT scan the atrophy of the caudate nucleus may be demonstrable, particularly in advanced cases. However, caudate atrophy also occurs in other disorders such as neuroacanthocytosis and **Hallervorden-Spatz disease.**

**Clinical Findings:**   The cardinal features are chorea and dementia. The choreiform movements are rapid and involve the limbs, trunk and, face. The movements are constantly changing and are brought on or exaggerated by attempts at voluntary movement. They are not stereotyped. At times the movements are slower and twisting, and some patients have postural deformities suggestive of torsion dystonia.

The gait is clumsy and the patient often makes a shuffling, writhing, twisting movement of the body and arms when attempting to walk. The speech is likely to be indistinct, and the tongue and palate are involved in movement abnormalities.

The dementia appears independently of the movement disorders and in some families dementia is the prominent symptom. In others it appears months or years after the movement disorder has been present. Psychiatric symptoms often are a first manifestation of the dementia and emotional instability and paranoia may be the earliest signs of the disturbance in mentation.

The course is inexorably progressive, lasting 10–25 years. The age of onset is usually between ages 35 and 40. However, onset occurs as early as childhood and as late as 60–65.

There is a form in which the movement disorder is more one of rigidity, similar to Parkinsonism. This form is more likely to occur in younger children. Some patients with this rigid form subsequently develop the choreic manifestations as the disease progresses. The juvenile form is three to five times more likely to be inherited from the father rather than the mother.

It should be noted that children often present with progressive intellectual deterioration, seizures, and difficulties in speech. The movement disorder is less prominent, and a diagnosis in childhood may be dependent on obtaining a positive family history compatible with autosomal dominant inheritance.

**Complications:** In the advanced cases there are complications associated with being bedridden such as ulcerations of skin, pneumonia, and urinary tract infections. Cardiovascular failure and pneumonia are the usual causes of death.

**Associated Findings:** None known.

**Etiology:** Autosomal dominant inheritance.

**Pathogenesis:** The biochemical defect underlying this disease has not been determined. Pathologically, the brunt of the disease occurs in the basal ganglia and cerebral cortex. The caudate becomes shrunken and demyelinated and has a marked gliosis with a loss of neurons, particularly small ganglion cells. The cerebral cortex may show atrophy and loss of neurons, particularly in the 3rd and 5th layers.

**MIM No.:** *14310

**Sex Ratio:** M1:F1

**Occurrence:** Prevalence estimated at 1:18,000 as reported in England and Minnesota; 1:20,000 in Switzerland; 1:25,000 in Michigan but only 1:333,000 in Japan. The prevalence in African Blacks is lower than in Orientals.

**Risk of Recurrence for Patient's Sib:**
See Part I, *Mendelian Inheritance.*

**Risk of Recurrence for Patient's Child:**
See Part I, *Mendelian Inheritance.*

**Age of Detectability:** Usually 35 to 40 years, less commonly in childhood or after 50 years of age. The only diagnostic test for the disease in patients prior to the appearance of neurologic or psychiatric symptoms is based on DNA markers closely linked to the HD locus. The test requires information on the phenotype of the parents and at least one more relative. PET scanning may be helpful in presymptomatic diagnosis.

**Gene Mapping and Linkage:** HD (Huntington disease) has been mapped to 4pter-p16.3.

**Prevention:** None known. Genetic counseling indicated.

**Treatment:** There is no satisfactory treatment which will alter the inexorable progression of this disease. Some symptoms can be managed with appropriate drugs. Depression can be aided with antidepressants, incapacitating movements and behavioral problems with neuroleptics or reserpine. Unfortunately, prolonged use of neuroleptics can cause tardive dyskinesia as an additional movement disorder. Supportive nursing, and physical and speech therapy, can ameliorate the longterm consequences of neurological deterioration, bed sores, joint contractures, swallowing problems, and other complications.

**Prognosis:** Inexorable progression with death usually occuring during the second decade following onset. The childhood form progresses more rapidly, and has a shorter duration of disease before death.

**Detection of Carrier:** Unknown.

**Support Groups:**
CA; Santa Monica; Hereditary Disease Foundation
New York; The Huntington's Disease Society of America, Inc. (HDSA)
CANADA: Ontario; Cambridge; Huntington Society of Canada

**References:**
Hayden MR: Huntington's chorea. New York: Springer-Verlag, 1981.
Gusella JF, et al.: A polymorphic DNA marker genetically linked to Huntington's disease. Nature 1983; 306:234–238.
Folstein SE, et al.: Huntington disease in Maryland: clinical aspects of racial variation. Am J Hum Genet 1987; 41:168–179.
Mark JL: A parent's sex may affect gene expression. Science 1988; 239:352–353.
Brandt J, et al.: Presymptomatic diagnosis of delayed-onset disease with linked DNA markers: the experience in Huntington's disease. J Am Med Asso 1989; 261:3108–3114.
Morris MJ, et al.: Problems in genetic prediction for Huntington's disease. Lancet 1989; II:601–603.
Craufurd D, et al.: Uptake of presymptomatic predictive testing for Huntington's disease. Lancet 1989; II:603–605.

C0060                                              **P. Michael Conneally**

**Hurler syndrome**
*See MUCOPOLYSACCHARIDOSIS I-H*
**Hurler-Pfaundler syndrome**
*See MUCOPOLYSACCHARIDOSIS I-H*
**Hurler-Scheie syndrome**
*See MUCOPOLYSACCHARIDOSIS I-H*
**Hurst syndrome**
*See HIRSCHPRUNG DISEASE-MICROCEPHALY-COLOBOMA*
**Hutchinson incisors**
*See TEETH, ENAMEL HYPOPLASIA*
**Hutchinson-Gilford progeria syndrome**
*See PROGERIA*
**Hutchinson-Tay choroiditis**
*See OCULAR DRUSEN*
**Hutterite cataract**
*See CATARACT, HUTTERITE*
**Hutterite cerebro-osteo-nephrodysplasia**
*See CEREBRO-NEPHRO-OSTEODYSPLASIA, HUTTERITE TYPE*

---

**HUTTERITE SYNDROME, BOWEN-CONRADI TYPE**          **2422**

**Includes:** Bowen-Conradi Hutterite syndrome

**Excludes:**
**Cerebro-oculo-facio-skeletal syndrome** (0140)
**Chromosome 18, trisomy 18** (0160)
**Pena-Shokeir syndrome** (2080)

**Major Diagnostic Criteria:** Low birth weight, **Microcephaly**, characteristic dysmorphic appearance, and failure to thrive. Often mistaken for **Chromosome 18, trisomy 18**, but chromosomes are normal.

**Clinical Findings:** Low birth weight, OFC 31 cm or less, proud nose, micrognathia, limited extension of hips, vertical talus with rocker-bottom foot.

**Complications:** Breech presentation, **Hernia, inguinal**, undescended testes, developmental delay, poor sucking often requiring gavage feeding, failure to thrive, and pneumonia.

**Associated Findings:** Abnormal finger posture or **Camptodactyly**, congenital heart disease, cloudy corneas, renal anomalies **Kidney, horseshoe**, duplicated collecting system, CNS malformation (Dandy-Walker; absence of superior and inferior cerebellar vermis), hypoplasia of nails, and minor vertebral anomalies.

**Etiology:** Autosomal recessive inheritance. Recurrences have been documented in at least three sibships, with significant inbreeding in all cases. Most reported cases have been Hutterites.

**Pathogenesis:** Many of the findings could be secondary to a neurologic deficit. Breech presentation may have contributed to deformations present in some.

**MIM No.:** *21118

**POS No.:** 3812

**Sex Ratio:** M1:F1

**Occurrence:** About 20 cases have been recognized in Hutterites. May may be one of the most frequent autosomal recessive conditions affecting Hutterites.

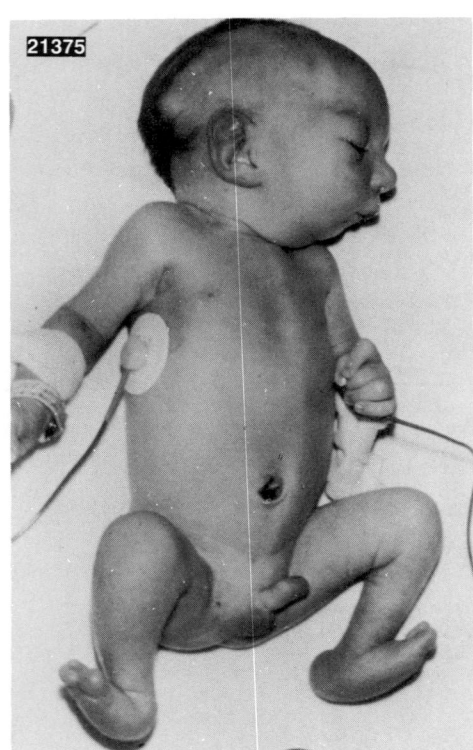

**2422-21375:** Note microcephaly and characteristic appearance resembling trisomy 18, prominent nose, micrognathia, and vertical talus with rocker-bottom feet.

**Risk of Recurrence for Patient's Sib:**
See Part I, *Mendelian Inheritance.*

**Risk of Recurrence for Patient's Child:**
See Part I, *Mendelian Inheritance.* Affected individuals are not expected to survive to reproduce.

**Age of Detectability:** At birth.

**Gene Mapping and Linkage:** Unknown.

**Prevention:** None known. Genetic counseling indicated.

**Treatment:** Supportive. Gastrostomy feeding has been required in some cases.

**Prognosis:** Lethal at an early age, despite aggressive management. The longest known survival has been 30.5 months.

**Detection of Carrier:** Unknown.

**References:**

Bowen P, Conradi GJ: Syndrome of skeletal and genitourinary anomalies with unusual facies and failure to thrive in Hutterite sibs. BD:OAS XII(6). New York: March of Dimes Birth Defects Foundation, 1976:101–108. * †

Hunter AGW, et al.: The Bowen-Conradi syndrome: a highly lethal autosomal recessive syndrome of microcephaly, micrognathia, low birth weight, and joint deformities. Am J Med Genet 1979; 3:269–279. * †

B0030                                          **Peter A. Bowen**

**Hyaline fibromas-gingival fibromatosis**
*See FIBROMATOSIS, JUVENILE HYALINE*
**Hyaline panneuropathy**
*See ALEXANDER DISEASE*
**Hyalinosis cutis et mucosae**
*See SKIN, LIPOID PROTEINOSIS*

**Hyalinosis, systemic (Ishikawa-Hori)**
*See FIBROMATOSIS, JUVENILE HYALINE*
**Hyaloid artery, persistence of**
*See EYE, VITREOUS, PERSISTENT HYPERPLASTIC PRIMARY*
**Hyaloideoretinal degeneration of Wagner**
*See RETINA, HYALOIDEORETINAL DEGENERATION OF WAGNER*
**Hyaloideotapetoretinal degeneration**
*See EYE, GOLDMANN-FAVRE DISEASE*
**Hydantoin anticonvulsants, fetal effects of**
*See FETAL HYDANTOIN SYNDROME*

## HYDATIDIFORM MOLE                                2400

**Includes:**
Gestational trophoblastic disease
Gestational trophoblastic neoplasm
Mole, hydatidiform

**Excludes:** Hydropic abortion

**Major Diagnostic Criteria:** In place of normal placental and fetal development, the conceptus is transformed completely (complete mole) or partly (partial mole) into a mass of vesicular villous structures resembling grapes.
A fetus is usually absent with complete moles, but frequently present with partial moles.

**Clinical Findings:** Molar pregnancy is suggested by vaginal bleeding, 97%; uterine enlargement greater than expected for dates, 51%; anemia, 54%; and ovarian theca-lutein cysts, 50%. Diagnosis is confirmed by marked elevation of serum β-hCG and ultrasound.

**Complications:** Ovarian theca-lutein cysts, 50%; local invasion, 13% (chorioadenoma destruens); metastasizing mole, 0.6–8.8%; choriocarcinoma. Toxemia, 27%; hyperemesis gravidarum, 26%; and thyrotoxicosis, 7%.

**Associated Findings:** Trophoblastic emboli, 2%.

**Etiology:** Complete hydatidiform moles result from abnormal fertilization events in which an empty ovum is fertilized either by two separate haploid sperms or by a single haploid sperm with immediate duplication of its 23 chromosomes. It has been suggested that 4.6% of women who have complete hydatidiform moles have balanced translocations. A partial hydatidiform mole is the result of a dispermic fertilization of a normal haploid ovum.

**Pathogenesis:** Complete moles result mainly from fertilization of an empty ovum (bearing no chromosomes) by a haploid sperm, with subsequent nuclear division without cytokinesis. This yields a 46,XX androgenetic conceptus that is homozygous.
Occasionally, dispermic fertilization of an empty ovum produces a complete mole. Such complete moles may have a 46,XX or 46,XY chromosomal constitution and are also androgenetic but heterozygous.
Partial moles are mostly triploid, occasionally tetraploid. The sex chromosome constitution of a partial mole may be XXX, XXY or XYY. These are composed of two-thirds paternal and one-third maternally-derived chromosomes (diandry).

**MIM No.:** 23109

**Sex Ratio:** Complete moles have a female karyotype, the majority 46,XX. Partial moles are triploid and may be 69,XXX, 69,XXY, or 69,XYY.

**Occurrence:** Complete moles occur in 1:173 to 1:2,500 pregnancies. The incidence of partial moles is unknown. The highest incidence is among Eurasian women, the lowest incidence is among Black women.

**Risk of Recurrence for Patient's Sib:** Twenty to forty fold increase in risk of recurrence for patient and/or sib(s).

**Risk of Recurrence for Patient's Child:** Unknown.

**Age of Detectability:** First or second trimester.

**Gene Mapping and Linkage:** Unknown.

**Prevention:** None known. Genetic counseling indicated.

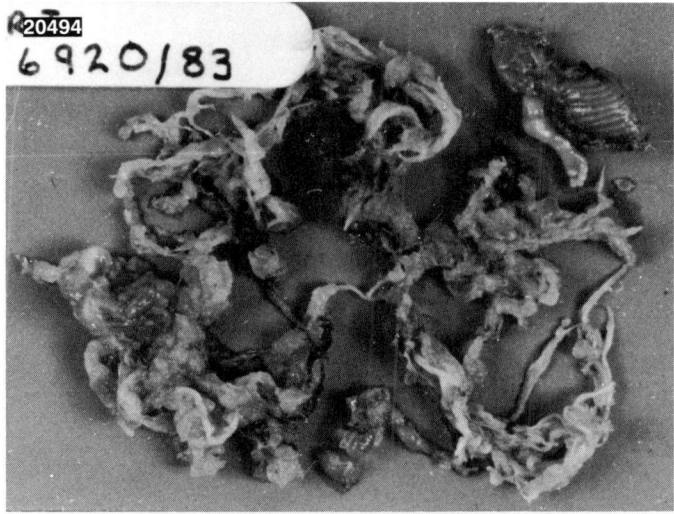

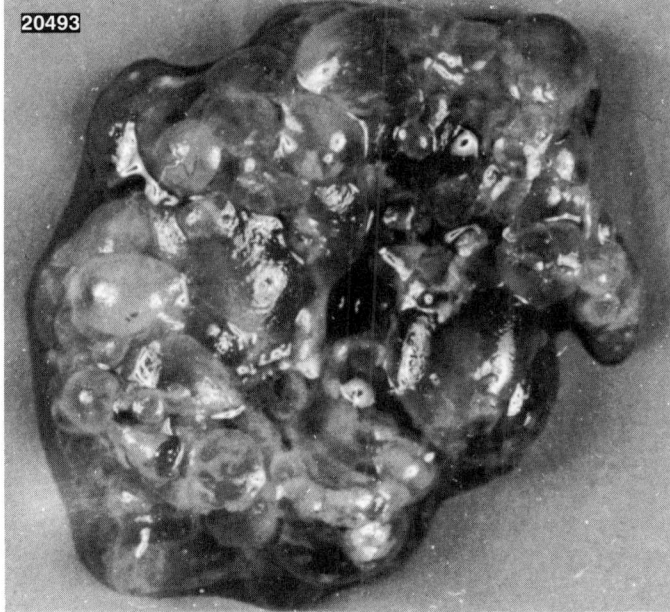

**2400-20494:** Hydatidiform mole; partial mole with macerated fetus. **20493:** Complete mole.

**Treatment:** Uterine evacuation, hysterectomy, or chemotherapy depending on clinicopathological stage of disease. Follow-up with serial estimations of serum β-hCG.

**Prognosis:** Spontaneous involution occurs in the majority of molar pregnancies. In these, pregnancy should be avoided during the one-to-two-year follow-up period.

Biologically, moles that are heterozygous are more aggressive than homozygous moles, so that karyotyping of the mole and both parents is an important facet of the laboratory investigation. Prognosis is also related to the serum β-hCG value, stage of the tumor at diagnosis, and other risk factors. These include pre-evacuation serum hCG > 100,000 mIU/ml; grade of trophoblastic activity; uterine size; theca-lutein cysts > 6 cm; maternal age > 40 years; hyperthyroidism; toxemia; trophoblastic embolization; and disseminated intravascular coagulation (DIC).

**Detection of Carrier:** The demonstration of a balanced translocation in some women who produce moles may be of predictive

value in due course, but no precise carrier state has been determined.

**Special Considerations:** The androgenetic concept of hydatidiform moles applies equally to the complete and partial varieties. The latter arise by diandry rather than digyny. Digyny apparently results in spontaneous abortion or a nonviable, malformed fetus without morphologic features of molar pregnancy.

Partial moles are usually of low-grade type with inconspicuous trophoblastic activity, by comparison with complete moles. They are associated with a lower incidence of sequelae, although some have shown troublesome persistence after evacuation and may require chemotherapy for their successful elimination.

**References:**
Vassilakos P, et al.: Hydatidiform mole: two entities. Am J Obstet Gynecol 1977; 127:167–170.
Jacobs PA, et al.: Mechanism of origin of complete hydatidiform moles. Nature 1980; 286:714–716.
Elston CW: Gestational tumours of trophoblast. In: Anthony PP, MacSween RNM, eds: Recent advances in histopathology, No. 11, Edinburgh: Churchill Livingstone, 1981:140–161.
Goldstein DP, Berkowitz RS: Gestational trophoblastic neoplasms. In: Friedman EA, ed: Major problems in obstetrics and gynecology. vol. 14. Philadelphia: WB Saunders, 1982.
Jacobs PA, et al.: Human triploidy: relationship between parental origin of the additional haploid complement and development of partial hydatidiform mole. Ann Hum Genet 1982; 46:223–231.
Gestational trophoblastic disease. Geneva: World Health Organization, 1983 (Technical Report Series 692).
Fisher RA, Lawler SD: Heterozygous complete hydatidiform moles: do they have a worse prognosis than homozygous complete moles? Lancet 1984; II:51.
Parrish SK: Hydatidiform mole and persistent trophoblastic disease in adolescents. J Pediatr 1986; 109:838–840.

M0036 **Gabriel Mortimer**

**Hydradenoma**
*See SCALP, CYLINDROMAS*
**Hydradenoma, nonpapillary hyalinizing**
*See SCALP, CYLINDROMAS*

## HYDRANENCEPHALY 0480

**Includes:** Schizencephaly with head enlargement

**Excludes:**
**Anencephaly** (0052)
**Fetal brain disruption sequence** (2254)
**Hydrocephaly** (0481)

**Major Diagnostic Criteria:** Diagnosis is suggested by transillumination that shows no cerebral tissue, but since this can occur in extreme **Hydrocephaly**, an angiogram or air study showing no cerebral wall is essential. An angiogram may demonstrate occlusion of the carotid arteries as they enter the cranium. Computerized tomography (CT) may show intact basal ganglia connected by a thin length of tissue to the cerebellum without a visible cerebral mantle.

**Clinical Findings:** Important features include an enlarged head at birth with large fontanel and a thin skull vault. Neurologic function may be assessed as "normal" with preservation of the Moro reflex, rooting, and sucking. Poor temperature control, increasing blindness, and loss of electrical activity on EEG may occur. Optic fundi show pale disks, but the optic nerve is present; pupillary light reflex is normal. The head transilluminates. On fontanel tap, cerebrospinal fluid (CSF) is obtained immediately upon puncture of the dura. The cerebral cortex is absent, although the skull or cranial meninges are intact; thalami are present as well as the choroid plexus, and the brain stem and optic nerves are intact.

**Complications:** Progressive head enlargement due to failure of CSF absorption.

**Associated Findings:** Seizures, poor hypothalamic control.

**Etiology:** Unknown.

**Pathogenesis:** Hydranencephaly may be due to an early fetal obstruction of the carotid vessels as they enter the cranial vault, with secondary degeneration of developing cerebral hemispheres. Those structures supplied by the basilar artery are spared including the basal portions of the temporal and occipital lobes, the hippocampi and basal nuclei, the brain stem and the cerebellum. Hydranencephaly differs from extreme porencephaly or hydrocephaly by the former's symmetry and the absence of large cystic cavities lined with ependyma.

**CDC No.:** 742.320

**Sex Ratio:** Presumably M1:F1.

**Occurrence:** Undetermined but presumed rare.

**Risk of Recurrence for Patient's Sib:** Unknown.

**Risk of Recurrence for Patient's Child:** Unknown.

**Age of Detectability:** At birth. Prenatal ultrasound shows fluid-filled fetal head, increased biparietal diameter, and incomplete falx formation.

**Gene Mapping and Linkage:** Unknown.

**Prevention:** None known. Genetic counseling indicated.

**Treatment:** A shunt operation is possible although the chances of survival are small.

**Prognosis:** Most infants die by the age of four months, although some live for years.

**Detection of Carrier:** Unknown.

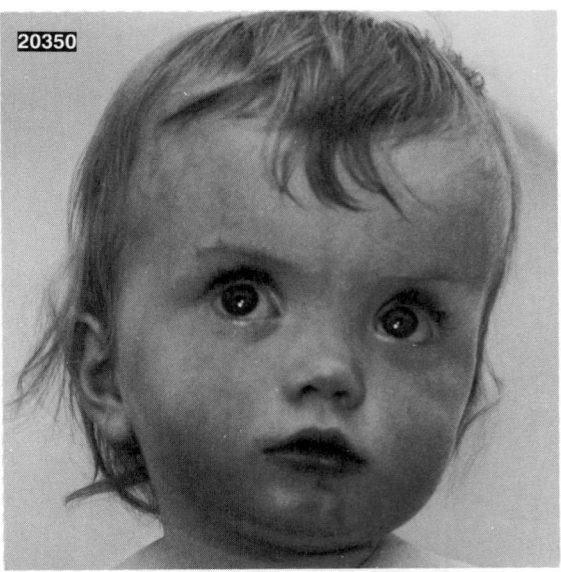

2936-20350: Note hypertelorism, epicanthal fold, low nasal bridge, anteverted nostrils and low-set ears.

**References:**
Hamby WB, et al.: Hydranencephaly: clinical diagnosis; presentation of 7 cases. Pediatrics 1950; 6:371.
Lorber J: Hydranencephaly with normal development. Dev Med Child Neurol 1965; 7:628.
Lee TG, Warren BH: Antenatal diagnosis of hydranencephaly by ultrasound: correlation with ventriculography and computed tomography. J Clin Ultrasound 1977; 5:271.
Aylward GP, et al.: Behavioral and neurological characteristics of a hydranencephalic infant. Dev Med Child Neurol 1978; 20:211–217.
Regec SP, Bernstine RL: Hydranencephaly in a twin gestation. Obstet Gynecol 1979; 54:369.
Sutton LN, et al.: Hydranencephaly versus maximal hydrocephalus: an important distinction. Neurosurgery 1980; 6:35–38.

SH007                                           **Kenneth Shapiro**

**Hydrocele**
  *See HERNIA, INGUINAL*
**Hydrocephalus**
  *See HYDROCEPHALY*
**Hydrocephalus-agyria-retinal dysplasia**
  *See WALKER-WARBURG SYNDROME*

## HYDROCEPHALUS-COSTOVERTEBRAL DYSPLASIA-SPRENGEL ANOMALY                    2936

**Includes:**
  Costovertebral dysplasia-hydrocephalus-Sprengel anomaly
  Sprengel anomaly-hydrocephalus-costovertebral dysplasia

**Excludes:**
  **Hydrocephaly** (0481)
  Intraventricular obstructive hydrocephalus, all varieties
  **Klippel-Feil anomaly** (2032)

**Major Diagnostic Criteria:** Communicating hydrocephalus, malformations of thoracic vertebrae, and sometimes the ribs, combined with Sprengel anomaly.

**Clinical Findings:** A family from western Norway has been reported in which a mother and all of her three daughters had various combinations of the following malformations and anomalies: spontaneously arrested communicating hydrocephalus, costovertebral dysplasias, Sprengel anomaly, **Eye, hypertelorism**, broad and low nasal bridge, anteverted nostrils, low-set ears, high-arched palate, prominent mandible, enamel hypoplasia, and

increased interspace between toes 1 and 2. All four had rib malformations; three had vertebral malformations and Sprengel anomaly. The mother and the youngest daughter had **Hydrocephaly**. One of the children had bilateral renal caliculi.

**Complications:** Kyphoscoliosis secondary to costovertebral dysplasias. Limitation of motion (elevation of ipsilateral arm, related to degree of scapular deformity). Gross and fine motor difficulties and mental impairment might occur secondary to hydrocephalus.

**Associated Findings:** None known.

**Etiology:** Probably autosomal dominant inheritance.

**Pathogenesis:** Unknown.

**MIM No.:** 14325

**POS No.:** 4218

**Sex Ratio:** Presumably M1:F1, M0:F4 observed.

**Occurrence:** The condition has been documented in one family from Norway.

**Risk of Recurrence for Patient's Sib:**
  See Part I, *Mendelian Inheritance.*

**Risk of Recurrence for Patient's Child:**
  See Part I, *Mendelian Inheritance.*

**Age of Detectability:** During infancy. Some cases may also be detected in late pregnancy.

**Gene Mapping and Linkage:** Unknown.

**Prevention:** None known. Genetic counseling indicated.

**Treatment:** Orthopedic measures for kyphoscoliosis. Shunt operations for hydrocephalus were not necessary in the Norwegian cases.

**Prognosis:** Good, with only moderate handicap.

**Detection of Carrier:** Unknown.

**References:**
Waaler PE, Aarskog D: Syndrome of hydrocephalus, costovertebral dysplasia and Sprengel anomaly with autosomal dominant inheritance. Neuropediatrics 1980; 11:291–297.

WA051                                          **Per Erik Waaler**

## HYDROCEPHALUS-HEART DEFECT-DENSE BONES, BEEMER TYPE                                         2786

**Includes:**
> Beemer lethal malformations syndrome
> Bones, dense-heart defects-hydrocephalus
> Heart defects-hydrocephalus-dense bones

**Excludes:**
> **Campomelic dysplasia** (0122)
> **Cerebro-hepato-renal syndrome** (0139)

**Major Diagnostic Criteria:** Dysmorphic facial features, **Hydrocephaly**, heart malformation, dense bones. Genital anomalies may be present.

**Clinical Findings:** Although gestation is uneventful, the clinical signs are present at birth. Birth weight has been between 10th and <3rd percentiles, length between the 50th and 5th percentiles, and skull circumference between the 60th and 50th percentiles. Severe asphyxia occurred after birth. Prominent features include a large anterior fontanelle with wide cranial sutures, a bulbous nose with broad nasal root and bridge, downward slanting palpebral fissures, deep folds under the eyes, and posteriorly angulated low-set ears. The ears may be malformed. The upper lip is thin with deep philtrum; and retrognathia may be present. **Heart, tetralogy of Fallot** with an open oval window and a double outlet right ventricle were present in one case each. Communicating **Hydrocephaly**, severe hypotonia, and irritability are present from birth. In males, the external genitalia may appear female, with enlarged clitoris and with testis embedded in labioscrotal fold.

The condition has a very severe course, with thrombocytopenia and leukocytosis without apparent infection or hypothermia.

**Complications:** Subarachnoid bleeding and death in the early weeks of life.

**Associated Findings:** None known.

**Etiology:** Possibly autosomal recessive or X-linked recessive inheritance. The two cases known are male sibs born of first cousin parents.

**Pathogenesis:** Biochemical studies in fibroblasts revealed a generalized loss of peroxisomal functions: impaired synthesis of plasmalogens with deficient activity of dihydroxyaceton phosphate-acyltransferase (DHAP-AT), defective peroxisomal beta ox-

idation system, and aberrant subcellular distribution of catalase. Although these biochemical findings resemble those found in **Cerebro-hepato-renal syndrome**, they are not identical, nor are the clinical features.

**MIM No.:** 20997

**POS No.:** 3644

**Sex Ratio:** M2:F0 (observed).

**Occurrence:** Two male sibs reported from The Netherlands.

**Risk of Recurrence for Patient's Sib:**
See Part I, *Mendelian Inheritance.*

**Risk of Recurrence for Patient's Child:**
See Part I, *Mendelian Inheritance.* Affected individuals are not expected to survive to reproduce.

**Age of Detectability:** At birth, or prenatally by DHAP-AT assay.

**Gene Mapping and Linkage:** Unknown.

**Prevention:** None known. Genetic counseling indicated.

**Treatment:** Symptomatic.

**Prognosis:** The condition has been fatal in early life.

**Detection of Carrier:** Unknown.

**References:**
Beemer FA, van Ertbruggen I: Peculiar facial appearance, hydrocephalus, double-outlet right ventricle, genital anomalies and dense bones with lethal outcome. Am J Med Genet 1984; 19:391–394. *

BE006                                              **Frits A. Beemer**

**Hydrocephalus-nephrosis-thin skin-blue sclera-growth defect**
*See NEPHROSIS-HYDROCEPHALUS-THIN SKIN-BLUE SCLERA-GROWTH DEFECT*

## HYDROCEPHALY                                                     0481

**Includes:**
> Aqueductal stenosis
> Atresia of foramina of Luschka and Magendie
> Dandy-Walker syndrome
> Hydrocephalus
> Obstructive hydrocephaly, extra- and intraventricular congenital
> Stenosis of aqueduct of Sylvius
> Ventriculomegaly

**Excludes:**
> **Achondroplasia** (0010)
> Acquired hydrocephaly due to tumor, infection
> **Encephalocele** (0343)
> **Hydranencephaly** (0480)
> **Meningomyelocele** (0693)
> **Mucopolysaccharidosis I-H** (0674)
> Subarachnoid hemorrhage

**Major Diagnostic Criteria:** Abnormal enlargement of the head due to ventricular dilation demonstrable by CT scan, echograph, or air studies.

**Clinical Findings:** An enlarged head either present at birth (30%) or detected during the first three months of life (50%); distended scalp veins; a large tense fontanel; and "sunsetting" of the pupils. The cerebrospinal fluid (CSF) is normal, as is the EEG. If the cortical mantle is extremely thin (1 cm), transillumination is positive. Pneumoencephalogram, or ventriculogram, shows enlarged ventricles with obstruction of air either within or outside the ventricle. CT scan will show ventricular enlargement but not the site of CSF obstruction.

**Complications:** Mental retardation, if untreated.

**Associated Findings:** **Meningomyelocele**, spina bifida cystica, **Encephalocele**, and **Klippel-Feil anomaly**, congenital heart disease, cleft lip/palate, neural tube defects.

**Etiology:** Genetically heterogeneous. Autosomal recessive inheritance for many cases, including those with atresia of foramina of

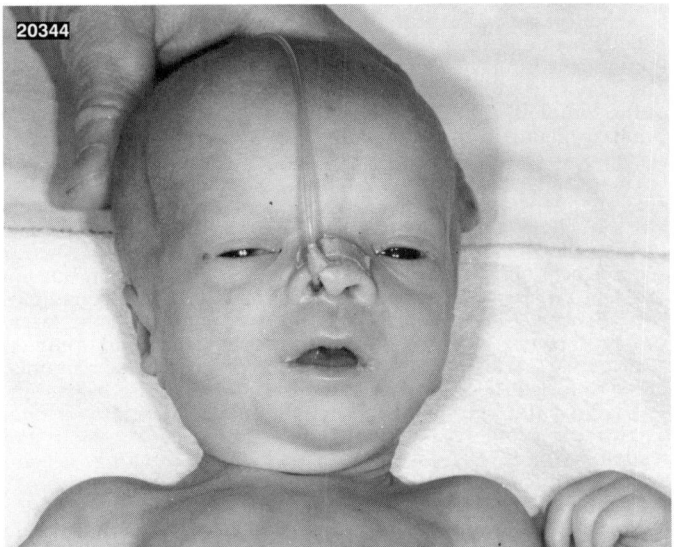

**2786-20344:** Newborn male; note bulbous nose with broad nasal bridge, downslanting palpebral fissures, and long upper lip.

Luschka and Magendie. X-linked recessive inheritance for congenital stenosis of aqueduct of Sylvius; in such instances the aqueduct is narrowed in its entire length, but most are stenotic at the inferior portion without ependymitis or gliosis. Possibly the syndrome of X-linked hydrocephalus comprises manifestations that are neither obligatory nor pathognomonic, and that the entire syndrome represents a genetically nonspecific set of secondary manifestations due to congenital obstructive hydrocephalus. Recent researchers have suggested that aqueductal stenosis, when present, is not the cause but the result of hydrocephaly (Willems et al, 1987). Teebi (1988) reported a case with apparent autosomal recessive inheritance.

**Pathogenesis:** All hydrocephaly is obstructive in that a normal amount of CSF is produced, but cannot be absorbed because of obstruction in the CSF pathways. Intraventricular obstruction occurs at the aqueduct of Sylvius or the outlets of the fourth ventricle. As fluid accumulates within the ventricle under increased pressure, the ependymal lining is disrupted; this allows CSF to pass into the periventricular white matter and causes myelin and axonal loss. The ventricles gradually increase in size, ultimately resulting in a thin mantle of brain containing chiefly cerebral gray matter. Blockage of the meninges or neurosinuses produces communicating hydrocephalus.

**MIM No.:** 22020, 23660, *30700

**CDC No.:** 742.3

**Sex Ratio:** M1:F1. M1:F<1 in aqueduct stenosis only.

**Occurrence:** 1:500–1500 live births.

**Risk of Recurrence for Patient's Sib:**
See Part I, *Mendelian Inheritance*. About 1–5% if not associated with a Mendelian disorder.

**Risk of Recurrence for Patient's Child:**
See Part I, *Mendelian Inheritance*. If hydrocephalic sib or maternal male relative, there is a 25% recurrence rate for each pregnancy and a 50% recurrence rate for each male fetus.

**Age of Detectability:** At birth: 30%; by first year: 80%. Small number detected in utero by ultrasonography, which shows dilated lateral ventricles, increased biparietal diameter, increased lateral ventricular width and lateral ventricular width to hemispheric dimension ratio, dilation of occipital horns of the ventricles. Also, may be detected by X-ray and elevated alpha-fetoprotein in maternal serum and amniotic fluid. X-linked aqueductal stenosis seen on X-ray as enlarged fetal head.

**Gene Mapping and Linkage:** HSAS (hydrocephalus, stenosis of the aqueduct of Sylvius) has been mapped to X.

**Prevention:** None known. Genetic counseling indicated.

**Treatment:** Surgical by-pass (shunt) carrying fluid from head into the vascular system, peritoneum, and other essential organs. The acquired varieties of hydrocephaly, i.e. tumor, infection, subarachnoid hemorrhage, or cyst, require a direct surgical approach to the obstructing lesion. While in utero diagnosis by ultrasound is possible, the efficacy of in utero shunting has not been demonstrated.

**Prognosis:** With shunt treatment, 80% of children reach five years of age; 80% of the survivors are normal or educable.

**Detection of Carrier:** Unknown.

**Support Groups:**
CA; San Diego; Hydrocephalus Parent Support Group
IL; Joliet; The National Hydrocephalus Foundation (NHF)
NY; Brooklyn; Guardians of Hydrocephalus Research Foundation
SWEDEN: Stockholm; International Federation for Hydrocephalus and Spina Bifida

**References:**
Johnson RT, Johnson KP: Hydrocephalus following viral infection: the pathology of aqueductal stenosis developing after experimental mumps virus infection. J Neuropathol Exp Neurol 1968; 27:591.
Gregory GA: Continuous positive airway pressure and hydrocephalus. Lancet 1973; 2:911.

Holmes LB, et al.: X-linked aqueductal stenosis. Clinical and neuropathological findings in two families. Pediatr 1973; 51:697–704.
Shurtleff DB, et al.: Follow-up comparison of hydrocephalus with and without myelomeningocele. J Neurosurg 1975; 3:61.
Halliday J, et al.: X-linked hydrocephalus: a survey of a 20 year period in Victoria, Australia. J Med Genet 1986; 23:23–31.
Caradi V, et al.: Prenatal diagnosis of X-linked hydrocephalus without aqueductal stenosis. J Med Genet 1987; 24:207–209.
Willems PJ, et al.: X-linked hydrocephalus. Am J Med Genet 1987; 27:921–928.
Varadi V, et al.: Heterogeneity and recurrence risk for congenital hydrocephalus (ventriculomegaly): a prospective study. Am J Med Genet 1988; 29:305–310.
Teebi A: Autosomal recessive nonsyndromal hydrocephalus. (Letter) Am J Med Genet 1988; 31:467–470.

SH007                                                **Kenneth Shapiro**

**Hydrocephaly-retinal nonattachment-falciform fold**
*See RETINAL FOLD*
**Hydrocephaly-thoracic dysplasia**
*See THORACIC DYSPLASIA-HYDROCEPHALUS*
**Hydrocytosis, hereditary**
*See ANEMIA, HEMOLYTIC, RED CELL MEMBRANE DEFECTS*

---

## HYDROLETHALUS SYNDROME                          2279

**Includes:** Salonen-Herva-Norio syndrome

**Excludes:**
Chromosome 13, trisomy 13 (0168)
Meckel syndrome (0634)

**Major Diagnostic Criteria:** Suspect hydrolethalus syndrome in a stillborn infant with **Hydrocephaly**, **Polydactyly**, and polyhydramnios.

**Clinical Findings:** The most constant anomaly is a severe hydrocephaly associated with a small mandible, polydactyly, clubfeet, a congenital heart defect, and abnormalities in the respiratory organs. Polyhydramnios is a constant finding and can be diagnosed by ultrasound from the 18th week of gestation. Premature birth is common, and most cases are stillborn, dying during delivery. Other than one patient reported living at more than five months of age, the longest survival time is two days; a B-twin born by elective cesarean section.

**Hydrocephaly** almost always occurs; few exceptions are known: one with anencephaly, and one with a normal cranial head circumference on which no autopsy or other brain examination was performed. The growth of the biparietal diameter begins usually before gestational week 20, and the midline structures of the brain, corpus callosum, and septum pellucidum are absent. The "keyhole" defect in the occipital bone is common, consisting of the foramen magnum and the midline defect dorsal to it. The pituitary gland is sometimes absent, and microphthalmia may occur.

The most striking facial anomaly is extreme micrognathia. The eyes are deep-set and small, the nose poorly formed and the ears low-set. Clefts and fissures in the upper and lower lip can occur. Limb malformations include postaxial **Polydactyly** in the hands and preaxial polydactyly in the feet, which are common but not constant findings. Additional postaxial toes have also sometimes been observed. Heart defects occur in over one-half of the cases. The type of defect varies, **Ventricular septal defect** and common atrioventricular canal are the most common; truncus communis, **Aortic arch, double**, and hypoplastic left heart have also been seen. The larynx, trachea, and/or bronchi are malformed in over one-half of the cases. Usually there is stenosis or atresia in the respiratory pathways. Incomplete lobulation of the lungs is common.

Cryptorchidism in males and bicornuate or duplicate uterus in females can occur. One or more accessory spleens and incomplete rotation of the gut can occur. Adrenal hypoplasia occurs in about one-third of cases, obviously secondary to the absence of the pituitary gland. Two cases have had hydronephrosis and one

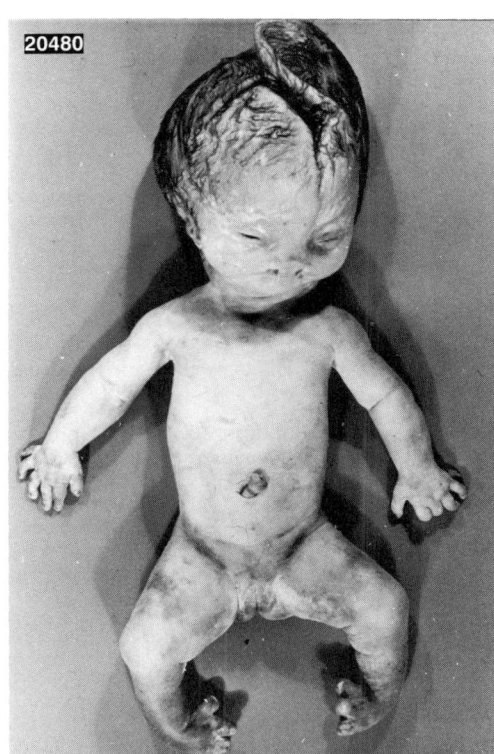

**2279A-20480:** A stillborn fetus with the hydrolethalis syndrome.

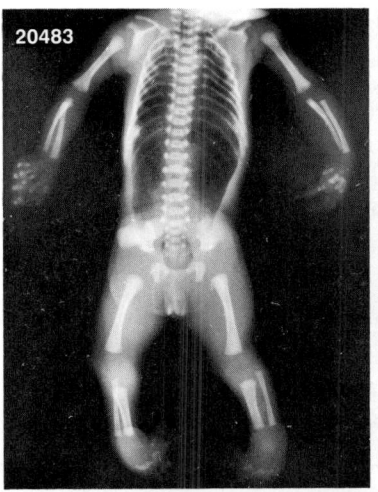
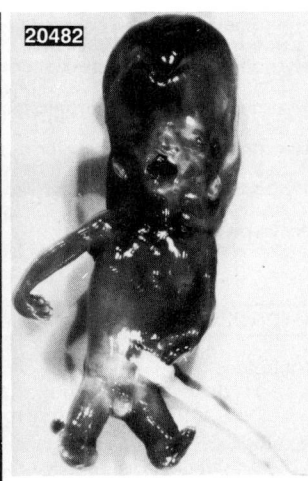
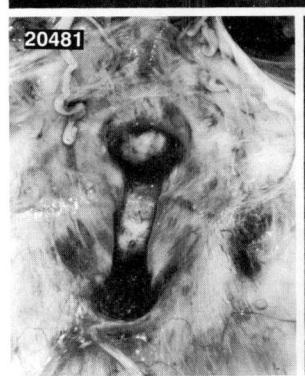
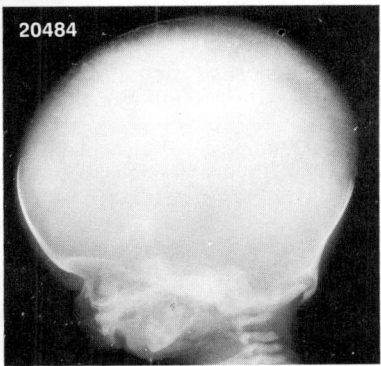

**2279B-20483:** X-ray shows bilateral hypoplasia of the tibiae in an affected infant. **20482:** Affected 20-week fetus. **20481:** Keyhole defect in the base of the skull. **20484.** Lateral view of the skull showing the bulging margins of the occipital bone with a defect.

case, a prenatally terminated fetus, had dysplastic, cystic, slightly enlarged kidneys.

X-ray findings include hydrocephaly of varying degrees, with a midline defect of the occipital bone and micrognathia, which have been found in all cases in which adequate X-rays were obtained. The upper limbs are most often short; postaxial polydactyly occurs in the hand. The lower limbs have hypoplastic tibiae, and in one case there was aplasia of both tibiae. A short tibia is usually associated with abnormalities of the respective bone ray, e.g., short first metatarsal bone, double hallux varus, and short hallux varus.

**Complications:** Severe hydrocephaly may make delivery difficult.

**Associated Findings:** Congenital diaphragmatic defect, **Cyclopia**, and **Omphalocele**.

**Etiology:** Autosomal recessive inheritance.

**Pathogenesis:** Unknown.

**MIM No.:** *23668

**POS No.:** 3567

**Sex Ratio:** M1:F1

**Occurrence:** 1:20,000 births in Finland. Over fifty cases have been documented (Aughton and Cassidy, 1987).

**Risk of Recurrence for Patient's Sib:**
See Part I, *Mendelian Inheritance.*

**Risk of Recurrence for Patient's Child:**
See Part I, *Mendelian Inheritance.*

**Age of Detectability:** Prenatal diagnosis by ultrasound from the 15th week of gestation is possible with early developing hydrocephaly and the absence of midline cerebral structures.

**Gene Mapping and Linkage:** Unknown.

**Prevention:** None known. Genetic counseling indicated.

**Treatment:** Unknown.

**Prognosis:** Poor; stillbirth or death soon after birth is the rule.

**Detection of Carrier:** Unknown.

**Special Considerations:** Some researchers, including R. Salonen and R. Herva who did much of the original work with this condition, feel that the cases published by Toriello & Bauserman (1985), Anyane-Yeboa et al (1987), and Aughton & Cassidy (1987) do not fullfill the criteria set for the hydrolethalus syndrome.

**References:**

Salonen R, et al.: The hydrolethalus syndrome: delineation of a "new" lethal malformation syndrome based on 28 patients. Clin Genet 1981; 19:321–330. *

Hartikainen-Sorri A-L, et al.: Prenatal detection of hydrolethalus syndrome. Prenat Diagn 1983; 3:219–224.

Herva R, Seppänen U: Roentgenologic findings of the hydrolethalus syndrome. Pediatr Radiol 1984; 14:41–43. *

Toriello HV, Bauserman SC: Bilateral pulmonary agenesis: association with the hydrolethalus syndrome and review of the literature from a developmental field perspective. Am J Med Genet 1985; 21:93–103.

Anyane-Yeboa K, et al.: Hydrolethalus (Salonen-Herva-Norio) syndrome: further clinicopathological delineations. Am J Med Genet 1987; 26:899–907.

Aughton DJ, Cassidy SB: Hydrolethalus syndrome: report of an apparent mild case, literature review, and differential diagnosis. Am J Med Genet 1987; 27:935–942.

HE036                                                                          **Riitta Herva**
SA037                                                                          **Riitta Salonen**

**Hydrometrocolpos (some causes)**
 *See HYMEN, IMPERFORATE*
**Hydrometrocolpos-postaxial polydactyly-congential heart anomalies**
 *See VAGINAL SEPTUM, TRANSVERSE*
**Hydronephrosis-dysmorphic facies, Ochoa type**
 *See UROFACIAL SYNDROME*
**Hydronephrosis-hydroureter-dysplastic bladder-grimacing facies**
 *See UROFACIAL SYNDROME*
**Hydronephrosis-oligodactyly**
 *See HAND, ULNAR AND FIBULAR RAY DEFICIENCY, WEYERS TYPE*
**Hydrops fetalis, idiopathic**
 *See HYDROPS FETALIS, NON-IMMUNE*

---

## HYDROPS FETALIS, NON-IMMUNE 2198

**Includes:**
 Hydrops fetalis, idiopathic
 Non-immune fetal hydrops
**Excludes:**
 **Angioedema, hereditary** (0054)
 Edema, congenital
 **Erythroblastosis fetalis** (3063)
 **Lymphedema I** (0614)

**Major Diagnostic Criteria:** Edema, anemia, and congestive heart failure at birth without any maternal-fetal hematologic incompatibility.

**Clinical Findings:** The sequence of events leading to the development of hydrops fetalis is not clear. At least three principal

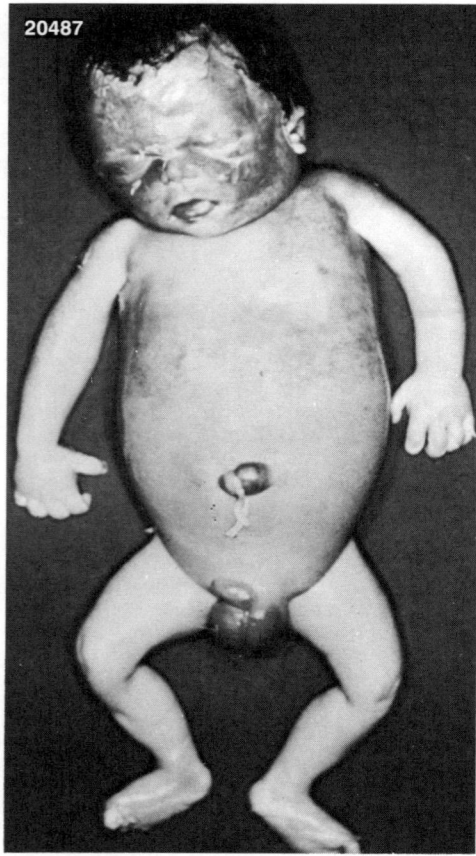

**2198-20487:** Hydrops fetalis, non-immune; note this stillborn 38-week fetus who shows abdominal distension and generalized edema.

factors appear to be involved: anemia, congestive heart failure, and decreased plasma colloid osmotic pressure.

Hydrops fetalis has a mortality rate in excess of 90%. It is idiopathic in about 60% of fetuses. Intrauterine diagnosis of hydrops by ultrasound may allow successful treatment and reversal in selected cases, but the majority die without an established causative diagnosis.

In nonimmunologic hydrops not due to isoimmunization the following changes occur: extreme pleural and peritoneal effusions with compression of abdominal and thoracic viscera, absence of hepatosplenomegaly, and absence of widespread erythropoiesis.

**Complications:** Death occurs in most cases. A few infants survive and develop normally.

**Associated Findings:** Depends on the individual cause of the hydrops.

**Etiology:** Usually it is idiopathic (60%), or from placental or maternal causes. The major causes include congenital heart defects (22%), chromosomal defects (14%), birth defect or malformation syndromes (12%), α-thalassemia (10%), twin-to-twin transfusion (8%), pulmonary defects (6%), and anatomic defects or congenital disorders (8%). The individual causes of nonimmune hydrops are many and varied (for a complete list see Holzgreve et al, 1984).

**Pathogenesis:** Excess fluid accumulation as the result of the precipitating condition. Some or all of the serous cavities may be affected, and generally there is edema of both the skin and the placenta.

**MIM No.:** 23675

**Sex Ratio:** M1:F1

**Occurrence:** Undetermined but presumed rare.

**Risk of Recurrence for Patient's Sib:** Unknown. Familial cases have been reported.

**Risk of Recurrence for Patient's Child:** Unknown.

**Age of Detectability:** Prenatally by ultrasound examination.

**Gene Mapping and Linkage:** Unknown.

**Prevention:** None known. May vary with specific etiology.

**Treatment:** Prenatal treatment can be instituted if the underlying disorder is amenable to treatment. Every attempt should be made to determine the etiology and a chromosome analysis as well as an ultrasound of the heart are indicated minimally.

**Prognosis:** Poor for survival; much better if the cause is found and is treatable, e.g. cardiac arrhythmia.

**Detection of Carrier:** Depends on the etiology. Possible if parents carry a defective gene, a translocated chromosome, or if the mother has an infection or maternal disease such as diabetes.

**References:**
Etches PC, et al.: Nonimmune hydrops fetalis: a report of 22 cases including three siblings. Pediatrics 1979; 64:326–332.
Machin GA: Differential diagnosis of hydrops fetalis. Am J Med Genet 1981; 9:341–350.
Schwartz SM, et al.: Idiopathic hydrops fetalis: report of 4 patients including 2 affected sibs. Am J Med Genet 1981; 8:59–66.
Holzgreve W, et al.: Investigation of nonimmune hydrops fetalis. Am J Obstet Gynecol 1984; 150:805–812.

GI005                          **Enid F. Gilbert-Barnes**

**Hydroxy methylglutaric aciduria**
 *See ACIDEMIA, 3-HYDROXY-3-METHYLGLUTARIC*
**Hydroxybutyric aciduria**
 *See ACIDEMIA, GAMMA-HYDROXYBUTYRIC*
**Hydroxylysine deficient collagen disease**
 *See EHLERS-DANLOS SYNDROME*

## HYDROXYPROLINEMIA 0482

**Includes:** Four-hydroxy-L-proline oxidase deficiency

**Excludes:** Bound hydroxyproline metabolism, disorders of

**Major Diagnostic Criteria:** Free hydroxyproline concentration in plasma 20–40 times above normal concentration of < 0.01 μmoles/ml. Free hydroxyproline excretion in urine is increased, but other amino acids are normal unless plasma concentration of hydroxyproline exceeds about 0.75 μmoles/ml; at this concentration, proline and glycine will be excreted in excess. Bound hydroxyproline excretion is normal.

**Clinical Findings:** A biochemical phenotype. No proven association with clinical disease. Condition reported in several pedigrees, some showing consanguinity.

**Complications:** Unknown.

**Associated Findings:** Mental retardation; possibly reflects ascertainment bias.

**Etiology:** Probably autosomal recessive inheritance of the enzyme defect.

**Pathogenesis:** "Hydroxyproline oxidase" deficiency. Source of *free* hydroxyproline is apparently normal collagen turnover. Collagen breakdown is not abnormal and excretion pattern of bound hydroxyproline is normal. The enzyme controlling the first step of free hydroxyproline oxidation in mammalian tissue has been proved to be independent of the enzyme controlling L-proline oxidation and degradation.

**MIM No.:** *23700

**Sex Ratio:** M1:F1

**Occurrence:** Estimated < 1:10,000,000.

**Risk of Recurrence for Patient's Sib:**
See Part I, *Mendelian Inheritance.*

**Risk of Recurrence for Patient's Child:**
See Part I, *Mendelian Inheritance.*

**Age of Detectability:** Presumably detectable in newborn.

**Gene Mapping and Linkage:** Unknown.

**Prevention:** None known. Genetic counseling indicated.

**Treatment:** Undetermined. Protein (gelatin) restriction of no use. Ascorbic acid depletion does not alter hydroxyprolinemia.

**Prognosis:** Unknown.

**Detection of Carrier:** Unknown.

**References:**
Efron ML, et al.: Hydroxyprolinemia. II: a rare metabolic disease due to a deficiency of the enzyme "hydroxyproline oxidase." New Engl J Med 1965; 272:1299–1309.
Pelkonen R, Kivirikko KI: Hydroxyprolinemia: an apparently harmless familial metabolic disorder. New Engl J Med 1970; 283:451–456.
Roesel RA, et al.: Hydroxyproline metabolism in two sisters with hydroxyprolinemia. Hum Hered 1979; 29:364–370.
Phang J and Scriver CR: Disorders of proline and hydroxyproline metabolism. In: Scriver CR, et al., eds: The metabolic basis of inherited disease, ed 6. New York: McGraw-Hill, 1989:577–598.

SC050 **Charles R. Scriver**

**Hygroma axillare**
*See CYSTIC HYGROMA*
**Hygroma cervicis**
*See NECK, CYSTIC HYGROMA, FETAL TYPE*
**Hygroma colli cysticum**
*See CYSTIC HYGROMA*

## HYMEN, IMPERFORATE 0483

**Includes:**
Hydrometrocolpos (some causes)
Imperforate hymen

**Excludes:**
Female pseudohermaphroditism (all forms)
Male pseudohermaphroditism (all forms)
Mullerian aplasia (0682)
Vaginal atresia (0984)

**Major Diagnostic Criteria:** Nonpatent hymen in a female (46,XX) with otherwise normal external and internal genitalia. Imperforate hymen should be distinguished from vaginal atresia. In the latter the lower portion of the vagina fails to form, and the nonpatent portion is too thick for simple incision.

**Clinical Findings:** In imperforate hymen the central portion of the hymen fails to develop its usual orifice. The external genitalia, vagina, cervix, uterus, fallopian tubes, and ovaries are otherwise normal for females. No somatic anomalies are present.

As a result of the absence of the hymenal orifice, mucus or blood may accumulate and hence may prevent outflow of menstrual fluid. Examination may reveal a bulging hymen, but usually no other abnormalities. Secondary sex development is otherwise normal.

**Complications:** Hydrocolpos or hydrometrocolpos.

**Associated Findings:** Usually none, although theoretically retention of blood could predispose to infection. Distention of uterus could also occur theoretically but this appears to be rare.

**Etiology:** Undetermined. Heritable tendencies have not been observed frequently. Not all cases are necessarily congenital, for some could represent adhesions of inflammatory origin.

**Pathogenesis:** Most investigators believe that the hymen arises from the urogenital sinus at the site at which the sinovaginal bulbs invaginate to form the caudal portion of the vagina; however, others believe that the hymen is a remnant of the urogenital membrane. Irrespective of origin, the hymen is ordinarily perforated after formation. Absence of perforation produces an imperforate hymen. Alternatively, postnatal inflammatory causes could sometimes lead to occlusion of a previously patent hymen.

**MIM No.:** 23710

**CDC No.:** 752.430

**Sex Ratio:** M0:F1

**Occurrence:** Undetermined, but relatively rare.

**Risk of Recurrence for Patient's Sib:** Undetermined, but apparently low.

**Risk of Recurrence for Patient's Child:** Undetermined, but apparently low.

**Age of Detectability:** Usually at puberty because of hydrometrocolpos. Occasionally at birth because of hydrocolpos.

**Gene Mapping and Linkage:** Unknown.

**Prevention:** None known. Genetic counseling indicated.

**Treatment:** Surgical evaluation and treatment is indicated. Cruciform incisions in central portion of hymen.

**Prognosis:** Normal life span; normal fertility.

**Detection of Carrier:** Unknown.

**References:**
McIlroy DM, Ward IV: Three cases of imperforate hymen occurring in one family. Proc R Soc Med 1930; 23:633–634.
Jones HW Jr, Scott WM: Hermaphroditism, genital anomalies, and related endocrine disorders, ed. 2. Baltimore: Williams & Wilkins Co, 1971:415–417.

SI018 **Joe Leigh Simpson**

**Hyper IgE, recurrent infection syndrome**
*See IMMUNODEFICIENCY, HYPER IgE TYPE*
**Hyper-2-oxoglutaric aciduria**
*See ACIDEMIA, 2-OXOGLUTARIC*

**Hyper-beta-carnosinemia**
See *CARNOSINEMIA*
**Hyper-IgM syndrome**
See *IMMUNODEFICIENCY, X-LINKED WITH HYPER IgM*
**Hyper-low density lipoproteinemia**
See *HYPERCHOLESTEREMIA*
**Hyperacetylation**
See *ACETYLATOR POLYMORPHISM*
**Hyperactive child syndrome**
See *ATTENTION-DEFICIT HYPERACTIVITY DISORDER (ADHD)*
**Hyperalaninemia**
See *HYPERBETA-ALANINEMIA*

---

## HYPERALDOSTERONISM, FAMILIAL GLUCOCORTICOID SUPPRESSIBLE                    0484

**Includes:**
 Aldosteronism, sensitive to dexamethasone
 Glucocorticoid-responsive hyperaldosteronism
 Nontumorous primary aldosteronism

**Excludes:**
 **Steroid 11 beta-hydroxylase deficiency** (0902)
 **Steroid 17 alpha-hydroxylase deficiency** (0903)
 Mineralocorticoid excess, syndrome of apparent
 Primary hyperaldosteronism (Conn syndrome)

**Major Diagnostic Criteria:** Must include hypokalemic alkalosis, hypertension, and hyperaldosteronism that are suppressed with glucocorticoids in the absence of a known enzyme block in adrenal steroid synthesis.

**Clinical Findings:** This is a familial disease characterized by hypertension, hypokalemic alkalosis, elevated aldosterone and suppressed renin. Polyuria has been reported. No specific enzyme defect has been identified from analysis of plasma and urinary steroids. **Steroid 17 alpha-hydroxylase deficiency** is readily excluded by finding normal or intermittently elevated 17-ketosteroids and 17-ketogenic steroids in the urine. **Steroid 11 beta-hydroxylase deficiency** is excluded by the lack of significant quantities of deoxycorticosterone (DOC) and 11-deoxycortisol (compound-S). Growth and sexual development are normal and reproductive capacity is unimpaired. The major concern is that patients may have hypertension late in life.

**Complications:** Persistent hypertension may lead to renovascular changes and poor suppression of elevated blood pressure by glucocorticoids. Hypertension may also predispose to early myocardial infarction or to cerebral hemorrhage. The sequelae of hypokalemia may also be present.

**Associated Findings:** Adrenal hyperplasia, similar to that seen in idiopathic aldosteronism, may be present.

**Etiology:** Probably autosomal dominant inheritance.

**Pathogenesis:** The hypertension, hypokalemia and low renin are due to the known effects of aldosterone. Suppressibility by glucocorticoids implies an enzyme defect, increased sensitivity to ACTH, or a related pituitary factor. None has been identified. The putative pituitary aldosterone-stimulating factor has not been found in this condition.

**MIM No.:** *10390

**Sex Ratio:** M1:F1

**Occurrence:** Undetermined but presumed rare.

**Risk of Recurrence for Patient's Sib:**
 See Part I, *Mendelian Inheritance.*

**Risk of Recurrence for Patient's Child:**
 See Part I, *Mendelian Inheritance.*

**Age of Detectability:** From childhood to adult life.

**Gene Mapping and Linkage:** Unknown.

**Prevention:** None known. Genetic counseling indicated.

**Treatment:** Treatment with glucocorticoids such as dexamethasone or prednisone reverses all the clinical findings. Several weeks of therapy may be required for reversal of hypertension. Spironolactone may be required in long-standing cases.

**Prognosis:** Excellent if treated before irreversible renovascular hypertension occurs.

**Detection of Carrier:** Unknown.

**Special Considerations:** This syndrome should be distinguished from the syndrome of apparent mineralocorticoid excess, characterized by hypertension, hypokalemia, low renin, and low aldosterone; with no evidence of overproduction of other mineralocorticoids. The hypertension of apparent mineralocorticoid excess responds to spironolactone. A defect in the peripheral metabolism of cortisol has been identified and proposed as the mechanism responsible for both hypertension and apparent mineralocorticoid excess.

**References:**
Giebink GS, et al.: A kindred with familial glucocorticoid-suppressible aldosteronism. J Clin Endocrinol Metab 1973; 36:715–723.
Ulick S, et al.: A syndrome of apparent mineralocorticoid excess associated with defects in the peripheral metabolism of cortisol. J Clin Endocrinol Metab 1979; 49:757–764.
Ganguly A, et al.: Anomalous postural aldosterone response in glucocorticoid-suppressible hyperaldosteronism. New Engl J Med 1981; 305:991–993.
Ganguly A, et al.: Genetic and pathophysiologic studies of a new kindred with glucocorticoid-suppressible hyperaldosteronism manifest in three generations. J Clin Endocrinol 1981; 53:1040–1046.
Mulrow PJ: Glucocorticoid-suppressible hyperaldosteronism: a clue to the missing hormone? New Engl J Med 1981; 305:1013–1014. *
Oberfield SE, et al.: Metabolic and blood pressure responses to hydrocortisone in the syndrome of apparent mineralocorticoid excess. J Clin Endocrinol Metab 1983; 56:332–339. *

SP004                                          **Mark A. Sperling**

---

## HYPERAMMONEMIA                                              1519

**Includes:** Urea cycle disorders

*Congenital hyperammonemia* refers to the urea cycle disorders **Carbamoyl phosphate synthetase deficiency**; **Ornithine transcarbamylase deficiency**; **Citrullinemia**; **Aciduria, argininosuccinic**; and **Argininemia**.

**Major Diagnostic Criteria:** Elevated levels of ammonium in plasma, usually in the range of 100–2,000 $\mu$M (normal, <50 $\mu$M). Among inborn errors of metabolism presenting in infancy, if hyperammonemia is associated with metabolic acidosis, it is likely to result from an organic acidemia or congenital lactic acidosis. These can be distinguished by measuring blood lactate levels and organic acids in urine. In urea cycle disorders, there is no metabolic acidosis; elevated citrulline levels are found in citrullinemia and argininosuccinic aciduria, and low to absent levels are found in CPS and OTC deficiencies. The latter two disorders should be distinguished by measuring orotic acid in urine. Specific enzyme determinations can be made in fibroblasts or leukocytes except for CPS and OTC, which must be measured in liver.

**Clinical Findings:** Hyperammonemia is manifested clinically by vomiting, lethargy, and neurologic impairment. In children it can result from a variety of inborn errors of metabolism, including urea cycle enzyme deficiencies, organic acidemias, congenital lactic acidosis, and dibasic aminoacidurias, as noted above. Hyperammonemia is also present in transient hyperammonemia of the newborn and in acquired disorders such as Reye syndrome, liver disease, and illness caused by various toxins and drugs.

 In the first week of life, the findings of poor suck, hypotonia, vomiting, lethargy, and grunting respirations, with or without seizures, should raise the possibility of hyperammonemia. During childhood, recurrent episodes of ataxia, vomiting, and lethargy should also raise concerns about hyperammonemia.

**Associated Findings:** Other inborn errors of metabolism that demonstrate hyperammonemia include **Acidemia, methylmalonic; Acidemia, propionic; Biotinidase deficiency; Carboxylase deficiency, holocarboxylase deficiency type; Acidemia, 3-ketothiolase deficiency; Acidemia, isovaleric; Acidemia, 3-hydroxy-3-methylglutaric; Acidemia,**

glutaric acidemia I; Acidemia, glutaric acidemia II, neonatal onset; Acidemia, ethylmalonic-adipic; Acyl-CoA dehydrogenase deficiency; Pyruvate dehydrogenase deficiency; Pyruvate carboxylase deficiency with lactic acidemia; Hyperdibasic aminoaciduria; and Hyperornithinemia-hyperammonemia-homocitrullinuria.

**Pathogenesis:** Ammonia is a metabolic toxin. Severe hyperammonemia (>500 $\mu$M) is associated with cerebral edema and cytotoxic changes in brain and liver. There is neuronal cellular swelling and the presence of Alzheimer type II astrocytes. The pathophysiology of ammonia toxicity, although unclear, has been ascribed to depletion of intermediates for enzyme metabolism, to cytotoxic effects on microtubular aggregates causing disruption of cellular integrity, and to neurotransmitter alterations. Other metabolic toxins in the various hyperammonemic disorders may also contribute to the pathogenesis.

**Occurrence:** Urea cycle disorders are found in 1:30,000 live births.

**Age of Detectability:** Children with complete enzyme deficiencies usually present with clinical symptoms in the first week of life. Partial deficiencies present later in childhood.

**Treatment:** Initial therapy involves elimination of protein, caloric supplements, and removal of ammonia by dialysis if the child is comatose. Long-term therapy depends on the underlying defect. In general, thereapy relies on protein restriction, cofactor therapy, and provision of alternative pathways of waste nitrogen excretion.

**Prognosis:** Depends on the individual disorder. Mortality remains high in children presenting with these disorders in the newborn period. This relates both to the severity of the disorder and to the frequent delay in its detection. There is a high incidence of mental retardation in survivors.

**References:**

Batshaw ML: Hyperammonemia. Curr Probl Pediatr 1984; 14:1–69.

Msall M, et al.: Neurologic outcome of children with inborn errors of urea synthesis. New Engl J Med 1984; 310:1500 only.

Robinson BH, Sherwood WG: Lactic acidemia. J Inherit Metab Dis 1984; 7(suppl 1):69–73.

Hudak ML, et al.: Differentiation of transient hyperammonemia of the newborn and urea cycle enzyme defects by clinical presentation. J Pediatr 1985; 107:712–719.

Tuchman M, Ulstrom RA: Organic acids in health and disease. Adv Pediatr 1985; 32:469–506.

Saheki T, et al.: Hereditary disorders of the urea cycle in man: biochemical and molecular approaches. Rev Physiol Biochem Pharmacol 1987; 108:21–68.

Brusilow J, Cox RP: Urea cycle enzymes. In: Scriver CR, et al, eds: The metabolic basis of inherited disease, 6th ed. New York: McGraw-Hill, 1989:629–670.

BA066                                                    **Mark L. Batshaw**

**Hyperammonemia due to ornithine transcarbamylase deficiency**
*See ORNITHINE TRANSCARBAMYLASE DEFICIENCY*
**Hyperammonemia III**
*See N-ACETYLGLUTAMATE SYNTHETASE DEFICIENCY*
**Hyperammonemia, congenital (some)**
*See CARBAMOYL PHOSPHATE SYNTHETASE DEFICIENCY*

---

## HYPERAPOBETALIPOPROTEINEMIA                           2394

**Includes:**
   Coronary disease, and hyperapobetalipoproteinemia
   Hyperlipidemia, familial combined
   Hypertriglyceridemia-coronary artery disease (some cases)

**Excludes:**
   **Hyperchylomicronemia** (0489)
   **Hyperlipoproteinemia, broad beta type** (0495)
   **Hyperlipoproteinemia V** (0501)

**Major Diagnostic Criteria:** An elevated plasma level of low-density lipoprotein (LDL) B protein and low ratio of LDL cholesterol to LDL B protein. These findings reflect an increased number of smaller, denser LDL particles.

**Clinical Findings:** The presence of hyperapo B in plasma can present in the first decade of life, but the expression may also be delayed until after age 20 years. The major clinical finding is the presence of coronary artery disease. The diagnosis of hyperapobetalipoproteinemia should be entertained in any patient with coronary artery disease before the age of 60 years who has a normal or near-normal level of plasma total and LDL cholesterol. The cholesterol levels can be normal or moderately elevated, and the triglyceride levels can be normal or moderately elevated. The common denominator is an elevated level of LDL B protein with a low ratio of LDL cholesterol to LDL B protein.

**Complications:** Coronary artery disease.

**Associated Findings:** Vertical ear creases have been found in some patients. In some families, the presence of pigmented irides and café-au-lait spots has been noted.

**Etiology:** Presumably autosomal dominant inheritance with variable expression, although autosomal recessive cases have been reported.

**Pathogenesis:** The current hypothesis indicates two metabolic defects: 1) an overproduction of apolipoprotein B and very-low-density lipoproteins (VLDL) in the liver; and 2) a defective clearance of chylomicrons, which are lipoprotein particles that transport triglyceride and cholesterol of dietary origin. An abnormality in the incorporation of free fatty acids into lipid esters in adipose tissue and fibroblasts in hyperapo B has been found.

**MIM No.:** *21025

**Sex Ratio:** About M1.5:F1.0

**Occurrence:** Has been found in about one-third of the patients with angiographically documented coronary disease, and in survivors of myocardial infarction. The prevalence in the general population is not known. Studies in families in Utah suggest three possible phenotypes: homozygous low, with a frequency of 73%; heterozygous, 25%, and homozygous high, 2%. Hyperapobetalipoproteinemia appears more frequent than the related *hyperlipidemia, familial combined* which Goldstein et al (1973) estimated to occur in approximately one percent of the general population, and in 12% of survivors of premature myocardial infarction.

**Risk of Recurrence for Patient's Sib:**
   See Part I, *Mendelian Inheritance.*

**Risk of Recurrence for Patient's Child:**
   See Part I, *Mendelian Inheritance.* One-third of the children of an affected parent are expected to be affected.

**Age of Detectability:** Usually evident between ages two and 20 years; however, the expression may be delayed.

**Gene Mapping and Linkage:** Unknown.

**Prevention:** None known. Genetic counseling indicated.

**Treatment:** A therapeutic diet low in total fat, saturated fat, and cholesterol. The use of a drug to decrease synthesis of VLDL in the liver, such as nicotinic acid, is often indicated.

**Prognosis:** Often associated with coronary artery disease.

**Detection of Carrier:** Examination of first degree relatives.

**Special Considerations:** Hyperapobetalipoproteinemia is most likely a heterogeneous group of disorders. The basis for the overproduction of apolipoprotein B and VLDL in the liver is not known. Possibilities include genetic defects in the regulation of apolipoprotein B production and the synthesis of mutant apolipoprotein B polypeptides, or the phenotype may be secondary to another abnormality in lipid metabolism that drives overproduction of apolipoprotein B. A defect in the incorporation of free fatty acids into lipid esters and adipose tissue has been proposed, possibly resulting in an increase in free fatty acids in the blood in the postprandial state, with enhanced uptake in the liver producing increased triglyceride synthesis and apolipoprotein B production. A relation between hyperapobetalipoproteinemia and *familial combined hyperlipidemia* is likely. The original description of familial combined hyperlipidemia did not include normolipidemic patients. Hyperapobetalipoproteinemia has also been found in a large Amish kindred with sitosterolemia. The simplest explanation for this observation is that there are two separate traits in the family, although a relation between the two syndromes has not been completely excluded.

**References:**
Sniderman A, et al.: The association of coronary atherosclerosis and hyperapobetalipoproteinemia (increased protein but normal cholesterol content in human plasma low density lipoprotein). Proc Natl Acad Sci USA 1980; 77:604–608.
Kwiterovich PO Jr, et al.: Hyperapobetalipoproteinemia in two families with xanthomas and phytosterolemia. Lancet 1981; I:466–469.
Sniderman A, et al.: Association of hyperapobetalipoproteinemia with endogenous hypertriglyceridemia and atherosclerosis. Ann Intern Med 1982; 97:833–839.
Kwiterovich PO Jr, Sniderman AS: Atherosclerosis and apoproteins B and apoA-I. Prev Med 1983; 12:815–834.
Teng B, et al.: Composition and distribution of low density lipoprotein fractions in hyperapobetalipoproteinemia, normolipidemia and familial hypercholesterolemia. Proc Natl Acad Sci 1983; 80:662–666.
Brunzell JD, et al.: Apoproteins B and A-1 and coronary artery disease in humans. Arteriosclerosis 1984; 4:79–83.
Sniderman AD, et al.: Familial aggregation and early expression of hyperapobetalipoproteinemia. Am J Cardiol 1985; 55:291–295.
Beaty TH, et al.: Genetic analysis of plasma sitosterol, apoprotein B, and lipoproteins in a large Amish pedigree with sitosterolemia. Am J Hum Genet 1986; 38:492–504.
Genest J, et al.: Hyperapobetalipoproteinemia: plasma lipoprotein responses to oral fat load. Arteriosclerosis 1986; 6:297–304.

KW001
SN006

**Peter O. Kwiterovich**
**Allan D. Sniderman**

**Hyperargininemia**
*See ARGININEMIA*
**Hyperbeta- and prebetalipoproteinemia**
*See HYPERLIPOPROTEINEMIA, BROAD BETA TYPE*

---

## HYPERBETA-ALANINEMIA 0486

**Includes:**
　　Alaninemia, hyperbeta
　　Hyperalaninemia

**Excludes:** Carnosinemia (0126)

**Major Diagnostic Criteria:** Persistent elevation of $\beta$-alanine in plasma above the normal level of 0.014 $\mu$moles/ml. Excessive urinary excretion of $\beta$-alanine, $\beta$-amino-iso-butyric acid ($\beta$AIB), and taurine. Presence of gamma-aminobutyric acid (GABA) in urine. Carnosine concentrations in urine and plasma are normal, but those in the tissues are excessive.

**Clinical Findings:** Symptoms included postnatal onset of somnolence, hypotonia, depressed reflexes, and intermittent seizures, which could not be controlled by the usual anticonvulsant medications. This fatal condition is identified so far in one infant. Fetal movements were thought to have been diminished. two other pregnancies had resulted in premature stillbirths in the 3rd trimester. $\beta$-Alanine was present in excessive amounts in plasma, CSF, and urine; the latter also contained $\beta$-aminoisobutyric acid and taurine in excessive amounts, directly proportional to the concentration of $\beta$-alanine. GABA was also present in urine, plasma, and CSF, independent of the $\beta$-alanine concentration. GABA concentration in postmortem brain tissue was greatly increased. At postmortem, brain and muscle contained $\beta$-alanine and carnosine in excess.

**Complications:** Seizures and inhibition of CNS function.

**Associated Findings:** None known.

**Etiology:** Probably autosomal recessive inheritance of the enzyme defect.

**Pathogenesis:** Deficiency of $\beta$-alanine transaminase suspected.

**MIM No.:** 23740

**Sex Ratio:** Presumably M1:F1.

**Occurrence:** Undetermined. One surviving case has been documented.

**Risk of Recurrence for Patient's Sib:**
See Part I, *Mendelian Inheritance.*

**Risk of Recurrence for Patient's Child:**
See Part I, *Mendelian Inheritance.*

**Age of Detectability:** Clinically in early newborn period; biochemical defect presumably also present at this time.

**Gene Mapping and Linkage:** Unknown.

**Prevention:** None known. Genetic counseling indicated.

**Treatment:** Large doses of pyridoxine may bring about biochemical and eventual clinical improvement, and this therapy should be attempted as early as possible in any future patient.

**Prognosis:** Likely to cause severe retardation in the few patients who survive.

**Detection of Carrier:** Unknown.

**Special Considerations:** Mechanism of hyper-$\beta$-aminoaciduria is combined overflow and competition, analogous to origin of iminoglycinuria in hyperprolinemia. The condition is of particular interest because of evidence of the following: 1) a membrane transport system with preference for $\beta$-amino compounds; 2) a significant metabolic pool of free $\beta$-alanine in man; 3) the bound $\beta$-alanine pool (carnosine) in man is equilibrated with the free pool; 4) impaired $\beta$-alanine metabolism in this case influences GABA metabolism; 5) carnosine and $\beta$-alanine in excess in brain interferes with cerebral function.

**References:**
Scriver CR, et al.: Hyper-beta-alaninemia associated with beta- aminoaciduria and gamma-aminobutyricaciduria, somnolence and seizures. New Engl J Med 1966; 274:635–643.
Scriver CR, et al.: Disorders of $\beta$-alanine and carnosine metabolism. In Stanbury JB, et al, eds: The metabolic basis of inherited disease, ed 5. New York, McGraw-Hill, 1983:570–585.

SC050

**Charles R. Scriver**

**Hyperbetalipoproteinemia**
*See HYPERCHOLESTEREMIA*

---

## HYPERBILIRUBINEMIA, CONJUGATED 3009

**Includes:**
　　Dubin-Johnson syndrome
　　Hepatic storage disease
　　Hyperbilirubinemia, type II
　　Hyperbilirubinemia, conjugated, type III
　　"Shunt" hyperbilirubinemia

**Excludes:**
　　**Hyperbilirubinemia, conjugated, Rotor type** (3237)
　　**Hyperbilirubinemia, transient familial neonatal** (3238)
　　**Hyperbilirubinemia, unconjugated** (0487)
　　**UDP-glucuronosyltransferase, severe deficiency type I** (0961)

**Major Diagnostic Criteria:** A chronic, benign, mild to moderate predominantly conjugated hyperbilirubinemia, due to congenital defect in hepatic excretion of bilirubin.

**Clinical Findings:** Usually asymptomatic mild icterus, with serum bilirubin concentrations of 2–5 mg/dl, but can be as high as 20 mg/dl. Rarely detected before puberty, although cases have been reported in neonates. Icterus is exacerbated by intercurrent illness, oral contraceptives, and pregnancy. Occasionally, mild constitutional complaints such as vague abdominal pains and weakness may occur. Pruritus is absent and physical examination is normal except for jaundice and occasional hepatosplenomegaly. Blood count, serum albumin, cholesterol, transaminases, alkaline phosphatase and prothrombin time are normal as are bile acid levels. Serum bilirubin can fluctuate, with frequent normal determinations. Oral cholecystography does not visualize the gall bladder. Grossly, the liver is black. Histology is normal except for accumulation of a dense pigment within lysosomes, which is thought to be a melanin derivative.

Computerized tomography of the liver reveals high attenuation values as compared with normal controls, although significant overlap exists.

Initial plasma disappearances of bilirubin sulfobromophthalein (BSP), indocyanine green (ICG), and [125I] rose bengal are normal. Plasma BSP concentration at 45 min is normal or slightly increased; however, at 90 min, there is a secondary rise in plasma BSP due to reflux of glutathione conjugated BSP from the liver cell into the circulation in 90% of patients. This pattern however does not distinguish Dubin-Johnson syndrome from other hepatobiliary disorders. Transport maximum is 10% of normal and the relative hepatic storage capacity is normal. A characteristic abnormality of porphyrin metabolism is that total urinary coproporphyrin excretion is normal, but over 80% is coproporphyrin I compared with less than 35% in normal individuals.

This condition should be differentiated from a rare idiopathic syndrome known as *"shunt"* hyperbilirubinemia which results in ineffective incorporation of heme into erythrocytes (Israels et al, 1959). The resulting increase in bilirubin production may lead to low grade unconjugated hyperbilirubinemia. Life-span of mature erythrocytes is normal in this condition. Shunt hyperbilirubinemia may run in families.

**Complications:** Unknown.

**Associated Findings:** Reversal of the coproporphyrin isomer I:III ratio in the urine, without a concomitant increase in the absolute excretion of coproporphyrin.

**Factor VII deficiency** is associated with the syndrome among Persian Jews.

**Etiology:** Autosomal recessive inheritance. Mutant Corriedale sheep and mutant albino rats are animal models.

**Pathogenesis:** Congenital decrease in hepatic transport of most organic anions including conjugated bilirubin, ICG, metanephrine glucuronide, and cholecystographic contrast medium (iopanoic acid). Bile salt excretion is normal.

**MIM No.:** *23750, 23755, *23780

**CDC No.:** 277.400

**Sex Ratio:** M1:F1

**Occurrence:** 1:1,300 among Persian Jews.

**Risk of Recurrence for Patient's Sib:**
See Part I, *Mendelian Inheritance.*

**Risk of Recurrence for Patient's Child:**
See Part I, *Mendelian Inheritance.*

**Age of Detectability:** Usually discovered after puberty and often is unmasked by contraceptives or pregnancy. Cases have also been reported in neonates.

**Gene Mapping and Linkage:** Unknown.

**Prevention:** None known. Reassurance is the goal of counseling.

**Treatment:** None required; oral contraceptives may be avoided.

**Prognosis:** This disorder is not harmful to health or life span.

**Detection of Carrier:** In heterozygotes, the total urinary coproporphyrin excretion is reduced by approximately 40%; the ratio of isomer I to isomer III is intermediate between results in control and affected patients.

**References:**
Dubin IN: Chronic idiopathic jaundice: a review of fifty cases. Am J Med 1958; 24:268–292.
Israels LG, et al.: Hyperbilirubinemia due to an alternate path of bilirubin production. Am J Med 1959; 27:693–697.
Schoenfield LJ, et al.: Studies of chronic idiopathic jaundice (Dubin-Johnson Syndrome): demonstration of hepatic excretory defect. Gastroenterology 1963; 44:101–111.
Cohen L, et al.: Pregnancy, oral contraceptives, and chronic familial jaundice with predominantly conjugated hyperbilirubinemia (Dubin-Johnson Syndrome). Gastroenterology 1972; 62:1182–1190.
Kondo T, et al.: Coproporphyrin isomers in Dubin-Johnson Syndrome. Gastroenterology 1976; 70:1117–1120.
Jansen PLM, et al.: Hereditary chronic conjugated hyperbilirubinemia in mutant rats caused by defective hepatic anion transport. Hepatology 1985; 5:573–579.
Chowdhury JR, et al.: Hereditary jaundice and disorders of

metabolism. In: Scriver CR, et al, eds: The metabolic basis of inherited disease, 6th ed. New York: McGraw-Hill, 1989:1367–1409. *

WA062
CH036

**Renata Wajsman**
**Jayanta Roy Chowdhury**

## HYPERBILIRUBINEMIA, CONJUGATED, ROTOR TYPE 3237

**Includes:**
Hepatic storage disease
Rotor type hyperbilirubinemia

**Excludes:**
**Hyperbilirubinemia, conjugated** (3009)
**Hyperbilirubinemia, transient familial neonatal** (3238)
**Hyperbilirubinemia, unconjugated** (0487)
**UDP-glucuronosyltransferase, severe deficiency type I** (0961)

**Major Diagnostic Criteria:** A benign, familial, conjugated hyperbilirubinemia characterized by greatly delayed plasma sulfobromophthalein disappearance and no increase in liver pigmentation.

**Clinical Findings:** Life-long mild jaundice, without pruritus, and an otherwise normal physical examination. Total serum bilirubin usually about 3–6 mg/dl, predominantly conjugated. Other blood tests are normal. The jaundice may fluctuate in intensity and increase in the presence of intercurrent infections. Cholecystograph visualizes the gall bladder and liver histology is normal without abnormal hepatic pigmentation. Sulfobromophthalein retention is abnormal (exceeds 25% after 45 min of intravenous injection) without a secondary rise of plasma levels. Serum bile acid levels are normal. Hepatic storage capacity is reduced by 75–90%, and transport maximum is reduced to 50% of normal.

Total urinary coproporphyrin excretion is 2.5–5 times greater than in controls, with approximately 65% being coproporphyrin I. This is probably due to reduced biliary excretion of coproporphyrins with concomitant increase in renal excretion.

**Complications:** Unknown.

**Associated Findings:** None known.

**Etiology:** Autosomal recessive inheritance.

**Pathogenesis:** Defect in hepatic uptake and storage of bilirubin; exact nature undetermined.

**MIM No.:** *23745

**CDC No.:** 277.400

**Sex Ratio:** M1:F1

**Occurrence:** Undetermined but presumed rare.

**Risk of Recurrence for Patient's Sib:**
See Part I, *Mendelian Inheritance.*

**Risk of Recurrence for Patient's Child:**
See Part I, *Mendelian Inheritance.*

**Age of Detectability:** Usually during childhood.

**Gene Mapping and Linkage:** Unknown.

**Prevention:** None known. Genetic counseling indicated.

**Treatment:** None required.

**Prognosis:** This disorder is not harmful to health or life span.

**Detection of Carrier:** Mildly abnormal sulfobromophthalein retention at 45 min, intermediate between that in affected patients and normal controls. Coproporphyrin excretory pattern is intermediate between that of controls and homozygotes.

**References:**
Rotor AB, et al.: Familial nonhemolytic jaundice with direct van den Bergh reaction. Acta Med Phil 1948; 5:37–49.
Wolkoff AW, et al.: Rotor's syndrome: a distinct heritable pathophysiologic entity. Am J Med 1976; 60:173–179.
Wolpert E, et al.: Abnormal sulfobromophthalein metabolism in Rotor's Syndrome and obligate heterozygotes. New Engl J Med 1977; 296:1099–1101.
Shimizu Y, et al.: Urinary coproporphyrin isomers in Rotor's Syndrome. a study in eight families. Hepatology 1981; 1:173–178.
Roy Chowdhury J, et al.: Hereditary jaundice and disorders of

bilirubin metabolism. In: Scriver CR, et al, eds: The metabolic basis of inherited disease, 6th ed. New York: McGraw-Hill, 1989:1367–1409. *

WA062
CH036

**Renata Wajsman**
**Jayanta Roy Chowdhury**

**Hyperbilirubinemia, conjugated, type III**
*See HYPERBILIRUBINEMIA, CONJUGATED*
**Hyperbilirubinemia, Crigler-Najjar type**
*See UDP-GLUCURONOSYLTRANSFERASE, SEVERE DEFICIENCY TYPE I*

## HYPERBILIRUBINEMIA, TRANSIENT FAMILIAL NEONATAL 3238

**Includes:** Lucey-Driscoll syndrome

**Excludes:**
**Hyperbilirubinemia, conjugated** (3009)
**Hyperbilirubinemia, conjugated, Rotor type** (3237)
**Hyperbilirubinemia, unconjugated** (0487)
**UDP-glucuronosyltransferase, severe deficiency type I** (0961)

**Major Diagnostic Criteria:** Transient unconjugated hyperbilirubinemia due to the presence of an inhibitor of bilirubin conjugation in the mother's serum.

**Clinical Findings:** Jaundice within the first four days of life with serum bilirubin peaking at 8.9 to 65 mg/dl within seven days. Kernicterus may occur. An unidentified inhibitor of UDP-glucuronyltransferase is found in the serum of mothers of the infants, unlike the hyperbilirubinemia associated with breast-feeding whose mothers are found to have an inhibitor of UDP-glucuronosyl transferase activity in the milk but not serum.

**Complications:** Kernicterus occurs occasionally if not treated, with possible neurological sequelae.

**Associated Findings:** None known.

**Etiology:** Some cases appear to be familial.

**Pathogenesis:** Presence of a steroidal substance (probably a progesterone) in the mother's serum that inhibits conjugation. Levels are 4–10 times higher than those in other pregnant mothers.

**MIM No.:** 23790

**CDC No.:** 277.400

**Sex Ratio:** M1:F1

**Occurrence:** Undetermined but presumed rare. At least 24 cases have been reported.

**Risk of Recurrence for Patient's Sib:** Unknown. In the known cases, all sibs have been affected.

**Risk of Recurrence for Patient's Child:** Unknown.

**Age of Detectability:** Within the first four days of life.

**Gene Mapping and Linkage:** Unknown.

**Prevention:** None known. Genetic counseling indicated.

**Treatment:** Exchange transfusion and phototherapy are recommended to prevent kernicterus. Patients should not receive drugs such as sulfonamides or warfarin that compete with bilirubin for albumin binding sites, thereby increasing the risk of kernicterus.

**Prognosis:** If treated adequately, the infants are subsequently normal.

**Detection of Carrier:** Unknown.

**Special Considerations:** This condition is clinically distinguished from jaundice observed in some breast-fed babies which is due to the presence of an inhibitor of UDP-glucuronosyltransferase in maternal milk, but not maternal serum.

**References:**
Lucey JF, et al.: Transient familial neonatal hyperbilirubinemia. Am J Dis Child 1960; 100:787–789.
Arias IM, et al.: Transient familial neonatal hyperbilirubinemia. J Clin Invest 1965; 44:1442–1450.

Hargreaeves T, Piper RF: Breast milk jaundice: effect of inhibitory breast milk and 3α,20β-pregnanediol on glucuronyl transferase. Arch Dis Child 1971; 46:195–198.

CH036
WA062

**Jayanta Roy Chowdhury**
**Renata Wajsman**

**Hyperbilirubinemia, type II**
*See HYPERBILIRUBINEMIA, CONJUGATED*

## HYPERBILIRUBINEMIA, UNCONJUGATED 0487

**Includes:**
Arias hyperbilirubinemia
Crigler-Najjar syndrome, type II
Gilbert syndrome
Hepatic dysfunction, constitutional
Jaundice, chronic benign
UDP-glucuronosyltransferase, severe deficiency type II

**Excludes:**
Chronic unconjugated hyperbilirubinemia after viral hepatitis
Compensated hemolytic states
**Hyperbilirubinemia, conjugated** (3009)
**Hyperbilirubinemia, conjugated, Rotor type** (3237)
**Hyperbilirubinemia, transient familial neonatal** (3238)
"Shunt" hyperbilirubinemia
**UDP-glucuronosyltransferase, severe deficiency type I** (0961)

**Major Diagnostic Criteria:** *Clinical:* Chronic, fluctuating, mild, unconjugated hyperbilirubinemia (serum bilirubin: 1.5 to 5.0 mg/dl) in an individual with normal serum transaminases, alkaline phosphatase activity, and bile salt concentration, and no evidence for a major degree of hemolysis or hepatic or splenic enlargement.
*Diagnostic tests:* 1) Caloric deprivation (40 kCal/24 hours): there is an exaggerated hyperbilirubinemic response to caloric deprivation. 2) Nicotinic acid: intravenous nicotinic acid administration results in an exaggerated hyperbilirubinemic response. Caloric deprivation and the nicotinic acid test are not completely diagnostic. 3) Analysis of bilirubin conjugates in bile: there is an increased proportion of bilirubin monoglucuronide in bile (greater than 30% of total bile pigments). 4) Liver biopsy: light microscopy reveals no abnormality. By electron microscopy, hypertrophy of the endoplasmic reticulum is observed in approximately one-half of the patients. Hepatic UDP-glucuronosyltransferase activity toward bilirubin in vitro is reduced, and there is delayed clearance of intravenously administered radiolabeled bilirubin. Liver biopsy is generally not required for the diagnosis of Gilbert syndrome.

**Clinical Findings:** Fluctuating unconjugated hyperbilirubinemia usually resulting in intermittent clinical jaundice. Physical examination is otherwise within normal limits. Hemolysis is not a part of the syndrome, but may coexist in some patients, resulting in higher serum bilirubin concentrations.

**Complications:** Kernicterus has occurred in the *UDP-glucuronosyltransferase, severe deficiency type II* form of unconjugated hyperbilirubinemia (Arias et al, 1969)

**Associated Findings:** None known.

**Etiology:** Autosomal dominant inheritance with variable expression. This condition is genetically and phenotypically heterogeneous. The Bolivian population of squirrel monkeys, a model for this condition, has higher fasting serum bilirubin levels compared with a closely related Brazilian population.

**Pathogenesis:** Reduced hepatic UDP-glucuronosyltransferase activity toward bilirubin is observed in all cases. Some patients also have defective hepatic uptake of bilirubin and other organic anions from serum.

**MIM No.:** *14350

**CDC No.:** 277.400

**Sex Ratio:** M1:F<1

**Occurrence:** Estimated 60:1,000.

**Risk of Recurrence for Patient's Sib:**
See Part I, *Mendelian Inheritance.*
**Risk of Recurrence for Patient's Child:**
See Part I, *Mendelian Inheritance.*
**Age of Detectability:** In the first three to four weeks of life, by persistent, mild, unconjugated hyperbilirubinemia.
**Gene Mapping and Linkage:** Unknown.
**Prevention:** This disorder is not harmful to health or longevity; prevention is not possible or necessary. Reassurance is the goal of counseling and medical management.
**Treatment:** Exposure to light reduces hyperbilirubinemia. Phenobarbital and corticosteroid administration ameliorates jaundice. Exchange transfusion, plasmapheresis, and phototherapy are occasionally needed during the neonatal period to prevent kernicterus in the *UDP-glucuronosyltransferase, severe deficiency type II* form of unconjugated hyperbilirubinemia. Usually, however, therapy is not required or recommended.
**Prognosis:** Usually only a cosmetic disorder.
**Detection of Carrier:** Unknown.

**References:**

Arias IM: Chronic unconjugated hyperbilirubinemia without overt signs of hemolysis in adolescents and adults. J Clin Invest 1962; 41:2233–2245.
Arias IM, et al.: Chronic nonhemolytic hyperbilirubinemia with hepatic glucuronyltransferase deficiency. Am J Med Genet 1969; 47:395–409.
Berk PD, et al.: Defective BSP clearance in patients with constitutional hepatic dysfunction (Gilbert's syndrome). Gastroenterology 1972; 63:472–481.
Dawson J, et al.: Gilbert's syndrome: evidence of morphological heterogeneity. Gut 20:848–853.
Reichen J: Familial unconjugated hyperbilirubinemia syndromes. Semin Liver Dis 1983; 3:24–35.
Chowdhury RJ, Arias IM: Disorders of bilirubin conjugation. In: Ostrow Jd, ed: Bile pigments and jaundice. New York: Marcel Dekker, 1986:317–332.

CH036                                                   **Jayanta Roy Chowdhury**

**Hypercalcemia, familial with nephrocalcinosis and indicanuria**
*See TRYPTOPHAN MALABSORPTION*
**Hypercalcemia-peculiar facies-supravalvular aortic stenosis**
*See WILLIAMS SYNDROME*
**Hypercalciuria, absorptive**
*See HYPERCALCIURIA, FAMILIAL IDIOPATHIC*

## HYPERCALCIURIA, FAMILIAL IDIOPATHIC          2302

**Includes:**
Hypercalciuria, absorptive
Hypercalciuria, renal
Rickets, hereditary hypophosphatemic with hypercalciuria (some)
**Excludes:**
Hyperparathyroidism, familial (0499)
Hyperoxaluria, primary
Renal tubular acidosis (0862)
Rickets, hereditary hypophosphatemic with hypercalciuria (HHRH) (3020)
**Major Diagnostic Criteria:** The formation of calcium-containing kidney stones or episodes of gross hematuria without detectable renal calculi; excessive excretion of urinary calcium ($> 4$ mg/kg of body weight per day), normal serum levels of calcium, and no acid-base disturbances.
**Clinical Findings:** Children less than 10 years of age usually have episodes of macroscopic hematuria without symptoms of flank pain, dysuria, edema, or hypertension. No evidence of urolithiasis is found on X-rays of the urinary tract. Long-term risk for eventual kidney stone formation is high. Older children and adults usually have symptomatic urolithiasis.
**Complications:** Related to urolithiasis: obstructive uropathy, urinary tract infection, and renal colic.

**Associated Findings:** Hyperphosphaturia, natriuresis.
**Etiology:** Familial aggregations suggest autosomal dominant inheritance, but heterogeneity also exists. Environmental factors, such as excessive sodium ingestion, may be responsible for some cases of hypercalciuria. Complete dietary history is recommended.
**Pathogenesis:** Three separate pathogenic mechanisms have been identified: 1) primary hyperabsorption of intestinal calcium, 2) a renal tubular defect in calcium reabsorption, and 3) a renal phosphorus leak leading to increased production of 1,25-dihydroxyvitamin D (see **Rickets, hereditary hypophosphatemic with hypercalciuria (HHRH)**. However, considerable overlap of biochemical features exists among all three pathogenic subtypes. Therefore, these subtypes may constitute a continuum arising from the same basic metabolic disturbance. Recent evidence suggests a defect in control of vitamin D metabolism as the primary pathogenic factor in many cases of familial hypercalciuria.
**MIM No.:** *14387
**Sex Ratio:** M4:F1
**Occurrence:** Estimated at 1.6:1,000 per year with a higher incidence in certain geographic regions (southeastern United States = 5:1,000).
**Risk of Recurrence for Patient's Sib:**
See Part I, *Mendelian Inheritance.*
**Risk of Recurrence for Patient's Child:**
See Part I, *Mendelian Inheritance.*
**Age of Detectability:** Varies from early childhood to adulthood. Peak incidence for urolithiasis is in the third decade of life.
**Gene Mapping and Linkage:** Unknown.
**Prevention:** None known. Genetic counseling indicated.
**Treatment:** Thiazide diuretics are highly effective in reducing urinary calcium and hematuria, and in decreasing the recurrence of calculi. Additional regimens include oral phosphate salts, high fluid intake, and dietary restriction of sodium or calcium.
**Prognosis:** Unknown.
**Detection of Carrier:** Unknown.
**Special Considerations:** An oral calcium loading test may be useful in diagnosis. In the renal subtype, secondary hyperparathyroidism and decreased bone mineralization may occur as a result of urinary calcium losses.

**References:**

Coe FL, et al.: Familial idiopathic hypercalciuria. New Engl J Med 1979; 300:337–400.
Sutton RAL: Disorders of renal calcium excretion. Kidney Int 1983; 23:665–673. *
Broadus AE, et al.: Evidence for disordered control of 1,25-dihydroxyvitamin D production in absorptive hypercalciuria. New Engl J Med 1984; 311:73–80.
Hymes LC, Warshaw BL: Idiopathic hypercalciuria: renal and absorptive subtypes in children. Am J Dis Child 1984; 138:176–180.
Smith CL: When should the stone patient be evaluated? Med Clin Am 1984; 68:455–459.
Hymes LC, Warshaw BL: Families of children with idiopathic hypercalciuria: evidence for the hormonal basis of familial hypercalciuria. Am J Dis Child 1985; 139:621–624.
Santos F, et al.: Idiopathic hypercalciuria in children: pathophysiologic considerations of renal and absorptive subtypes. J Pediatr 1987; 110:238–243.
Stapleton BF, et al.: Increased serum concentrations of 1,25(OH)2 vitamin D in children with fasting hypercalciuria. J Pediatr 1987; 110:234–237.

HY001                                                      **Leonard C. Hymes**

**Hypercalciuria, idiopathic (some forms)**
*See RICKETS, HEREDITARY HYPOPHOSPHATEMIC WITH HYPERCALCIURIA (HHRH)*
**Hypercalciuria, renal**
*See HYPERCALCIURIA, FAMILIAL IDIOPATHIC*
**Hypercalciuric rickets**
*See RICKETS, HEREDITARY HYPOPHOSPHATEMIC WITH HYPERCALCIURIA (HHRH)*
**Hypercementosis**
*See TEETH, ANKYLODONTIA, MULTIPLE HERITABLE TYPE*

# HYPERCHOLESTEROLEMIA                                    0488

**Includes:**
  Cholesterol, familial elevated
  Hyperbetalipoproteinemia
  Hypercholesteremic xanthomatosis
  Hyperlipidemia II
  Hyperlipoproteinemia II
  Hyper-low density lipoproteinemia
  LDL-receptor disorder
  Xanthoma tuberosum multiplex

**Excludes:**
  **Hypertriglyceridemia** (0500)
  **Hyperlipoproteinemia** (others)

**Major Diagnostic Criteria:** *Heterozygote:* In the absence of secondary causes of hyperlipidemia (e.g. liver disease, thyroid disease, renal disease), affected individuals have an elevated plasma cholesterol level with a normal or minimally elevated triglyceride level. Family analysis reveals evidence of vertical transmission. In addition, the diagnosis is virtually assured if xanthomas are present. Moreover, a specific biochemical test has been developed in which fibroblasts cultured from the skin of affected individuals are shown to have only one-half of their normal low-density lipoprotein (LDL) binding activity.

*Homozygote:* Affected individuals have greatly elevated plasma cholesterol levels (>600 mg/dl), approximately twice the values of heterozygotes in the same family. Family studies reveal heterozygous familial hypercholesterolemia in both parents. In addition, xanthomas appearing in the first decade of life and ischemic heart disease occurring usually in the second decade strongly suggest the diagnosis. Xanthomas of the planar variety are thought to be specific for this disease. Skin fibroblasts from these individuals show greatly diminished LDL binding (<10% of normal).

**Clinical Findings:** This disease has two distinct clinical phenotypes: individuals with heterozygous familial hypercholesterolemia have elevated cholesterol levels from birth. The mean cholesterol concentration in untreated adults is approximately 350 mg/dl. However, the cholesterol level for a given patient may be between 270 and 550 mg/dl. The elevation in plasma cholesterol is in the low density lipoprotein fraction. Heterozygotes usually display tendon xanthomas in the extensor tendons of the hands and Achilles tendons, and tuberous xanthomas at elbows and tibial tuberosities. These xanthomas start appearing in the second decade of life, and by the fourth decade, 90% of patients have this finding. Affected individuals may also have xanthelasmas and corneal arcus, although both of these occur in individuals with normal cholesterol levels. Premature coronary artery disease is commonly seen in this condition; the mean age of the first heart attack is in the 40s for affected men and in the 50s for affected women.

In the second clinical phenotype, individuals with homozygous familial hypercholesterolemia have greatly elevated cholesterol levels with reported values of 600 to 1,200 mg/dl. Xanthomas are more extensive in these individuals and include tendonous, tuberous and planar varieties. Xanthomas appear in the first decade of life. Affected individuals have accelerated coronary artery disease with the first myocardial infarction often occurring in the second decade of life. In addition, clinically significant aortic stenosis occurs frequently.

**Complications:** Coronary artery disease, arthritis and tendonitis in locations adjacent to xanthomas.

**Associated Findings:** Cholecystitis or cholelithiasis may have an increased incidence. Migratory arthritis is sometimes noted.

**Etiology:** Heterozygous form: autosomal dominant inheritance; Homozygous form: autosomal recessive inheritance.

**Pathogenesis:** A defect in the cell surface receptor that binds low density lipoprotein. A high-affinity receptor for LDL exists on the surface of cells of the body. A functional receptor permits efficient binding, internalization and degradation of LDL. In this process, exogenous cholesterol is introduced into the cell in such a way as to decrease the activity of the rate-limiting enzyme in cholesterol biosynthesis, stimulate esterification of free cholesterol, and diminish the number of LDL receptors on the cell surface. Fibroblasts from homozygotes with familial hypercholesterolemia have shown either no receptor activity (receptor negative) or less than 10% of normal receptor activity (receptor defective). Heterozygous fibroblasts have approximately 50% of normal LDL receptor activity. A few individuals with phenotypic homozygous familial hypercholesterolemia were found to have fibroblasts that bound LDL but did not internalize it. The lack of proper LDL binding or uptake by cells in the body leads to a decreased fractional catabolic rate of LDL. These particles build up to higher than normal concentrations in plasma and are eventually taken up by reticuloendothelial cells. When this occurs in the arterial wall, it results in the foam cell lesion characteristic of an early atherosclerotic plaque. Foam cells are also a central feature in the formation of the various xanthomas seen in this condition.

**MIM No.:** 14389, 14440

**Sex Ratio:** M1:F1

**Occurrence:** Heterozygotes: 1:500; homozygotes: 1:1,000,000. Gene frequency considerably increased in Lebanese and South Africans.

**Risk of Recurrence for Patient's Sib:**
  See Part I, *Mendelian Inheritance.*

**Risk of Recurrence for Patient's Child:**
  See Part I, *Mendelian Inheritance.*

**Age of Detectability:** *Heterozygotes:* In the first year of life by measuring cholesterol levels and evaluating the family. Diagnosis by measuring cholesterol levels in cord blood is controversial.
  *Homozygotes:* Prenatally in the second trimester by studying LDL receptors in amniotic fluid-derived cell cultures. At birth by measuring plasma cholesterol levels in cord blood.

**Gene Mapping and Linkage:** LDLR (low density lipoprotein receptor (familial hypercholesterolemia)) has been mapped to 19p13.

**Prevention:** None known. Genetic counseling indicated.

**Treatment:** *Heterozygotes:* Therapy is designed to lower plasma cholesterol levels to as close to 200 mg/dl as possible. Diet should be low in cholesterol and saturated fats. If this is sufficient to reduce the plasma cholesterol levels to below 240 mg/dl, the patient is kept on the diet alone. If levels remain above 240 mg/dl, various drugs either singly or in combination may be tried, including cholestyramine, nicotinic acid, gemfibrozil, or lovastatin.
  *Homozygotes:* These patients are generally resistant to the interventions that have helped heterozygotes. The most promising therapeutic modality currently appears to be pheresis therapy. The patient's plasma is removed by a continuous cell separator, and LDL is removed by affinity chromatography. The process is repeated approximately every 1–2 weeks and the patient's mean plasma cholesterol level is maintained at 250 mg/dl or less. Under this regime, homozygotes have shown regression of xanthomas and a lack of progression of cardiovascular disease.

**Prognosis:** First heart attacks of heterozygotes occur 25 to 30 years before unaffected individuals in the population. Lipid lowering has recently been shown to be of benefit in reducing coronary artery disease. The prognosis for homozygotes has improved with the advent of pheresis therapy, but it is too early to evaluate the long-term consequences of this approach.

**Detection of Carrier:** Heterozygous familial hypercholesterolemia is an autosomal dominant condition that can be detected in an individual by finding elevated plasma cholesterol levels and assessing cholesterol levels in family members.

**References:**
Levy RI, et al.: Dietary and drug treatment of primary hyperlipoproteinemia. Ann Intern Med 1972; 77:267.
Goldstein JL, Brown MS: The LDL receptor locus and the genetics of familial hypercholesterolemia. Ann Rev Genet 1979; 13:259.
King ME, et al.: Plasma exchange therapy for homozygous familial hypercholesterolemia. New Engl J Med 1980; 302:1457–1459.

Brown MS, Goldstein JL: A receptor-mediated pathway for cholesterol homeostasis. Science 1986; 232:34–47.

Hobbs HH, et al.: Deletion of the gene for the low-density-lipoprotein receptor in the majority of French Canadians with familial hypercholesterolemia. New Engl J Med 1987; 317:734–737.

Goldstein JL, Brown MS: Familial hypercholesterolemia. In: Scriver C, et al., eds: The metabolic basis of inherited disease, 6th ed. New York: McGraw-Hill, 1989:1215–1250.

BR010                                                    **Jan L. Breslow**

**Hypercholesteremic xanthomatosis**
  *See HYPERCHOLESTEREMIA*
**Hypercholesterolemia, familial with hyperlipemia**
  *See HYPERLIPOPROTEINEMIA, BROAD BETA TYPE*

---

## HYPERCHYLOMICRONEMIA                                    0489

**Includes:**
  Burger-Grutz syndrome
  Essential familial hyperlipemia
  Familial fat-induced hyperlipemia
  Familial hyperchylomicronemia
  Hyperlipoproteinemia I
  Lipase D deficiency
  Lipid, deficiency of
  Lipoprotein lipase deficiency, familial

**Excludes:   Hyperlipoproteinemia** (all other)

**Major Diagnostic Criteria:**   After an overnight fast of 10–12 hours, affected individuals on a normal fat-containing diet (25–40% of calories) still show chylomicrons in their plasma. (Chylomicrons are usually cleared from plasma within 4–6 hours after a fat-containing meal.) Chylomicrons are detected by the "refrigerator test". This is performed by placing the plasma in a narrow test tube and leaving it overnight at 4° C. The next morning, if chylomicrons are present, they will form a creamy layer at the top of the plasma. The presence of chylomicrons is also suggested by a band that stays at the origin on lipoprotein electrophoresis. In addition, if the plasma lipid analysis reveals severely elevated triglycerides with normal to only slightly elevated cholesterol levels (a triglyceride to cholesterol ratio of $\geq$ 10:1), chylomicrons are probably present. Lipoprotein analysis reveals low levels of the other lipoproteins, particularly high density lipoproteins (HDL). The diagnosis is supported by observing the disappearance of chylomicrons from fasting plasma after several days of intravenous or oral alimentation with a fat-free formula. Definitive diagnosis relies on documenting a primary deficiency of the activity of the enzyme lipoprotein lipase. There is no ideal way to measure this activity since it is normally absent from plasma and resides in endothelial cells in the capillaries of muscle and adipose tissue. However, intravenous heparin (60 IU/Kg) has been shown to elute this enzyme from its normal site in capillary beds. An enzyme assay of plasma 15 minutes after a heparin infusion for protamine inhibitable lipase activity reveals that affected patients have less than 10% of normal enzyme activity.

  Berger (1987) reported a variant case in which muscle lipaprotein lipase was essentially normal, although the enzyme in adipose tissue was markedly reduced.

**Clinical Findings:**   Some affected individuals have colic or splenomegaly in the first few weeks of life; others are quite asymptomatic and are detected during blood tests performed for other purposes. In general, individuals with this condition are asymptomatic, except for periodic attacks of abdominal pain associated with prostration, vomiting, and spasm of the abdominal wall. These episodes in some individuals can be quite frequent and disabling. Patients may intermittently develop eruptive xanthomas (small yellowish nodules on erythematous bases) and/or hepatosplenomegaly. Occasionally these individuals are found to have lipemia retinalis. These patients do not have tendinous, tuberous, or planar xanthomas, nor do they show signs of premature vascular disease, glucose intolerance, or hyperuricemia.

**Complications:**   In uncontrolled disease several complications may be present. Eruptive xanthomas may be sufficiently severe to cause cosmetic problems. Foam cells may be found in the bone marrow as well as the liver and spleen (to the point of causing hepatosplenomegaly). These are of no clinical consequence but may be confusing in a medical workup for other diseases. Episodes of abdominal pain may be associated with pancreatitis, which has been reported to be a fatal complication of this disease.

**Associated Findings:**   None known.

**Etiology:**   Autosomal recessive inheritance.

**Pathogenesis:**   Deficiency of lipoprotein lipase enzymatic activity. Chylomicrons are triglyceride-rich particles produced by the intestine after ingestion of dietary fat. These particles then travel in the lymph to the plasma in the capillary endothelium of muscle and adipose tissue where the enzyme lipoprotein lipase hydrolyzes most of their triglycerides. Defective enzymatic activity in these patients results in prolonged presence of chylomicrons in plasma. These particles are then taken up by the reticuloendothelial system, resulting in foam cell formation. The pathogenesis of the pancreatitis is unknown.

**MIM No.:**   *23860

**Sex Ratio:**   M1:F1

**Occurrence:**   Undetermined but presumed rare. Not associated with any ethnic group.

**Risk of Recurrence for Patient's Sib:**
  See Part I, *Mendelian Inheritance.*

**Risk of Recurrence for Patient's Child:**
  See Part I, *Mendelian Inheritance.*

**Age of Detectability:**   Severe hypertriglyceridemia and chylomicronemia in fasting plasma and deficient lipoprotein lipase activity in post-heparin plasma can be detected in the first few months of life.

**Gene Mapping and Linkage:**   LPL (lipoprotein lipase) has been provisionally mapped to 8p22.

**Prevention:**   None known. Genetic counseling indicated.

**Treatment:**   Plasma chylomicron levels can be reduced by a low-fat diet containing less than 15% of calories from long chain fatty acids. There is no need to restrict saturated fats as opposed to polyunsaturated fats or to limit carbohydrate intake. Dietary calories can be provided by medium chain triglycerides whose fatty acid moiety is not carried by chylomicrons. These measures reduce plasma triglyceride levels but do not normalize them. If triglycerides can be maintained at a concentration of less than 750 mg/dl, the eruptive xanthomas and episodes of abdominal pain should be controlled.

**Prognosis:**   A normal life span should be anticipated.

**Detection of Carrier:**   Unknown.

**Special Considerations:**   Severe hyperchylomicronemia can be seen in conditions with secondary deficiencies of lipoprotein lipase such as diabetic ketoacidosis. Other diseases that can mimic this condition are alcoholism with pancreatitis, systemic lupus erythematosus and the paraproteinemias.

**References:**

Levy RI, et al.: Dietary and drug treatment of primary hyperlipoproteinemia. Ann Intern Med 1972; 77:267.

Krauss RM, et al.: Selective measurement of two lipase activities in postheparin plasma from normal subjects and patients with hyperlipoproteinemia. J Clin Invest 1974; 54:1107.

Hoeg JM, et al.: Initial diagnosis of lipoprotein lipase deficiency in a 75-year-old man. Am J Med 1983; 75:889–892.

Berger GMB: An incomplete form of familial lipoprotein lipase deficiency presenting with type I hyperlipoproteinemia. Am J Clin Path 1987; 88:369–373.

Breslow JL: Familial disorders of high density lipoprotein metabolism. In: Scriver C, et al., eds: The metabolic basis of inherited disease, 6th ed. New York: McGraw-Hill, 1989:1251–1266.

BR010                                                    **Jan L. Breslow**

**Hyperchylomicronemia-lipoproteinemia, hyperprebeta**
  *See HYPERLIPOPROTEINEMIA V*
**Hypercortisolism (spontaneous) without Cushing syndrome**
  *See GLUCOCORTICOID RESISTANCE*

## HYPERCYSTINURIA 0490

**Includes:** Cystinuria without dibasic aminoaciduria

**Excludes:**
   Cystinosis (0238)
   Cystinuria (0239)
   Homocystinuria (0474)

**Major Diagnostic Criteria:** Positive urinary cyanide-nitroprusside test: markedly increased urinary content of cystine but not of lysine, arginine, or ornithine. No increase in cystine level of plasma.

**Clinical Findings:** Probably none; disorder has been described in only one family to date.

**Complications:** Unknown.

**Associated Findings:** Hypocalcemia and tetany due to familial hypoparathyroidism reported in one of two living siblings. A third sibling had died after an episode of hypocalcemic tetany.

**Etiology:** Probably autosomal recessive inheritance, since the affected children were of opposite gender.

**Pathogenesis:** Presumed to be due to a defect involving a cystine-specific carrier protein in renal tubules. Reabsorptive defect for cystine results in increased renal clearance (about 20 times normal).

**MIM No.:** 23820

**Sex Ratio:** Presumably M1:F1.

**Occurrence:** Reported in two siblings of unrelated parents.

**Risk of Recurrence for Patient's Sib:**
   See Part I, *Mendelian Inheritance*.

**Risk of Recurrence for Patient's Child:**
   See Part I, *Mendelian Inheritance*.

**Age of Detectability:** Unknown.

**Gene Mapping and Linkage:** Unknown.

**Prevention:** None known. Genetic counseling indicated.

**Treatment:** Unknown.

**Prognosis:** Probably normal life span.

**Detection of Carrier:** Parents of affected children excreted normal amounts of cystine in the urine.

**Special Considerations:** Defect significant since it indicates the probable presence of a renal tubular transport system exclusively for cystine, as well as the one shared with lysine, arginine, and ornithine. No data available about intestinal transport of cystine in the reported patients.

**References:**
Brodehl J, et al.: Isolierter Defekt der tubulären, Cystin-Rückresorption in einer Familie mit idiopathischem Hypoparathyroidismus. Klin Wochenschr 1967; 45:38–40.
Rosenberg LE, Scriver CR: Disorders of amino acid metabolism. In: Bondy PK, Rosenberg LE, eds: Diseases of metabolism, ed 7. Philadelphia: W.B. Saunders Co., 1974:465–653.

AM004                                    **Mary G. Ampola**

## HYPERDIBASIC AMINOACIDURIA 0491

**Includes:**
   Aciduria, hyperdibasic aminoaciduria
   Dibasic aminoaciduria II
   Hyperlysinuria with hyperammonemia
   Lysinuria, congenital
   Lysinuric protein intolerance

**Excludes:**
   Cystinuria (0239)
   Hyperlysinuria, isolated (2990)

**Major Diagnostic Criteria:** Hyperdibasic aminoaciduria occurs in two forms:
*Dibasic aminoaciduria I:* A rare form without hyperammonemia,
is incompletely recessive. It is clinically asymptomatic in heterozygotes manifesting hyperdibasic aminoaciduria involving the cationic amino acids, lysine, ornithine and arginine. Renal and intestinal transports of the free cationic amino acids are impaired and renal clearance values are above normal. Plasma values are normal. The homozygous form (putative. See Kihara et al, 1973) may cause mental retardation.
*Dibasic aminoaciduria II:* The Finnish form, know as lysinuric protein intolerance, is more prevalent, associated with hyperammonemia, and is completely recessive. It is not expressed (as hyperdibasic-aminoaciduria) in heterozygotes. The homozygous phenotype has impaired intestinal absorption of free and dipeptide-linked cationic amino acids; renal clearance values of free cationic amino acids are above normal.

**Clinical Findings:** *Dibasic aminoaciduria I:* Heterozygotes are asymptomatic. Homozygous phenotype may show mental retardation. Protein intolerance and hyperammonemia are absent.
*Dibasic aminoaciduria II:* The lysinuric protein intolerance phenotype occurs in the homozygote and includes failure to thrive, aversion to high protein diet, vomiting, hepato-splenomegaly, muscular hypotrophia and hypotonia, stupor and even coma; both associated with hyperammonemia and osteoporosis. Biochemical findings (in addition to hyperdibasic-aminoaciduria) include postpranidial hyperammonemia, orotic aciduria, and hyperferritinemia. Low plasma cationic amino acid values indicative findings. Clinical manifestations improve with citrulline feeding (0.5 mmole/g dietary protein).

**Complications:** *Dibasic aminoaciduria I:* Possibly mental retardation of unknown cause.
*Dibasic aminoaciduria II:* CNS signs with hyperammonemic episodes, osteoporosis, impaired somatic growth.

**Associated Findings:** *Dibasic aminoaciduria II:* Hyperammonemia and orotic aciduria after protein feeding. Plasma values of cationic amino acids are low or subnormal.

**Etiology:** Different genes are involved in the two disorders.
*Dibasic aminoaciduria I:* Autosomal incomplete recessive inheritance. The gene controls a cationic amino acid-selective carrier in the kidney and intestine.
*Dibasic aminoaciduria II:* Autosomal recessive inheritance. The gene controls a cationic amino acid carrier in the kidney and intestine that is different from the carrier involved in the *Type I* phenotype.

**Pathogenesis:** *Dibasic aminoaciduria I:* The involved carrier is probably located in brush border membranes of proximal nephron cells and the small intestine. Expression of mutation in the heterozygote (as hyperdibasicaminoaciduria) implies that the renal transport system is an important determinant of renal absorption in the normal phenotype. Location of the carrier "downstream", in proximal nephron, would explain the incomplete recessive phenotype.
*Dibasic aminoaciduria II:* There is indirect evidence that the involved carrier is located in the basolateral membrane of the proximal nephron cells, and direct evidence of this location in the small intestine. Intestinal absorption of cationic amino acids in free or dipeptide form is equally impaired, hence the hypoaminoacidemia. The transport defect, which involves different gene products and transport systems from those involved in *Type I*, is also expressed in plasma membrane of parenchymal cells (e.g. skin fibroblasts). Efflux of cationic amino acids from cell to extracellular fluid is impaired; a gene dose effect is observed (heterozygotes have half-normal trans-stimulated efflux). Findings imply that the basolateral membrane of epithelial cells and plasma membrane of parenchymal cells have homologous carriers for cationic amino acid. The transport defect, if expressed in hepatocytes, apparently impairs ammonia metabolism. The apparent involvement of hepatocyte leads to functional impairment of the urea cycle.

**MIM No.:** *22269, *22270

**Sex Ratio:** M1:F1

**Occurrence:** Approximately 1:60,000 live births for Type II in Finland; rarer elsewhere. Unknown for Type I.

**Risk of Recurrence for Patient's Sib:**
See Part I, *Mendelian Inheritance.*

**Risk of Recurrence for Patient's Child:**
See Part I, *Mendelian Inheritance.*

**Age of Detectability:** In infancy.

**Gene Mapping and Linkage:** Unknown.

**Prevention:** None known. Genetic counseling indicated.

**Treatment:** Protein intake suggested is <1.2–1.5 g/kg/day in type II. L-citrulline supplement, 0.5 mmol/g of dietary protein is considered beneficial; measurement of daily urinary orotic acid excretion is a useful tool in monitoring treatment. Lysine supplement apparently is without effect because of poor absorption. No treatment is indicated for Type I.

**Prognosis:** *Dibasic aminoaciduria I:* Heterozygotes are unaffected. Homozygotes may have impaired CNS development.
*Dibasic aminoaciduria II:* Guarded in the homozygous phenotype. Without treatment, life span may be shortened.

**Detection of Carrier:** *Dibasic aminoaciduria II:* Heterozygotes have hyperdibasic-aminoaciduria.
*Dibasic aminoaciduria II:* Silent heterozygote (for dibasic-aminoaciduria). Transport defect can be measured in fibroblasts.

**Special Considerations:** Two types of hyperdibasic aminoaciduria appear to exist. In the first type, dibasic aminoacid transport is defective in the renal tubule and in the intestine; the site of the defect in the epithelial cell is unknown, but it may be in the brush border. In the "Finnish" or LPI phenotype, the transport defect is located in basolateral plasma membrane of epithelium, and it may be shared by the plasma membrane of liver.

Impairment of the urea cycle, hyperammonemia, and protein intolerance are part of the picture, because the liver becomes deficient in the urea cycle intermediates, arginine and ornithine. Assuming two alleles or genes, they are expressed differently in quantitative and qualitative terms in the heterozygotes for the 2 traits.

**References:**
Whelan DT, Scriver CR: Hyperdibasicaminoaciduria: an inherited disorder of amino acid transport. Pediatr Res 1968; 2:525–534.
Oyanagi K, et al.: Congenital lysinuria: a new inherited transport disorder of dibasic amino acids. J Pediatr 1970; 77:259–266.
Kihara H, et al.: Hyperdibasicaminoaciduria in a mentally retarded homozygote with a peculiar response to phenothiazines. Pediatrics 1973; 51:223–229.
Awrich AE, et al: Hyperdibasicaminoaciduria, hyperammonemia, and growth retardation: treatment with arginine, lysine and citrulline. J Pediatr 1975; 87:731.
Simell O, et al.: Lysinuric protein intolerance. Am J Med 1975; 59:229–240.
Rajantie J, et al.: Lysinuric protein intolerance: a two-year trial of dietary supplementation therapy with citrulline and lysine. J Pediatr 1980; 97:927–932.
Rajantie J, et al.: Basolateral membrane transport defect for lysine in lysinuric protein intolerance. Lancet 1980; 1:1219.
Simell O, et al.: Lysinuric protein intolerance (LPI). In: Eriksson AW, et al, eds: Population structure and genetic disorders. New York: Academic Press, 1980; 633–636.
Smith D, et al.: Lysinuric-protein intolerance mutation is expressed in the plasma membrane of cultured skin fibroblasts. Proc Natl Acad Sci (USA) 1987; 84:7711–7715.

SC050
SI016

**Charles R. Scriver**
**Olli G. Simell**

---

**HYPEREKPLEXIA**           **3260**

**Includes:**
Hyperexplexia
Kok disease
Startle disease
Stiff-baby syndrome, hereditary
Stiff-man syndrome, congenital

**Excludes:**
**Epilepsy, reflex** (3239)
**Hallervorden-Spatz disease** (2526)
**Isaacs-Mertens syndrome** (3271)
**Jumping Frenchman of Maine** (3270)
**Myotonia congenita** (0701)

**Major Diagnostic Criteria:** Continuous muscular rigidity is present in the neonatal period. Older children and adults are less hypertonic, but display an exaggerated startle response to unexpected acoustic or tactile stimuli. Startling may be severe and accompanied by intense, generalized muscular rigidity and unchecked falling ("like a log") with resultant trauma. Electromyography (EMG), electroencephalography (EEG), cranial computed tomography, and muscle histology are normal.

**Clinical Findings:** Hypertonia is present at birth, and associated feeding difficulties and respiratory muscle spasm occasionally prove fatal. Congenitally dislocated hip may be present, and **Hernia, inguinal** and **Hernia, umbilical** (presumably due to sustained or paroxysmal elevation of intra-abdominal pressure) are common. Early gross motor delay is common, but mentation is normal, and "catch-up" motor development usually occurs by 24–36 months. An exaggerated startle response, although present in infants, is more obvious in older persons with minimal hypertonia. Children and adults typically display numerous facial scars from startle-induced falling. Nocturnal myoclonus is common. Cold, fatigue, and anxiety tend to exacerbate both the startle response and the continuous, mild rigidity experienced by many adults. Symptoms may fluctuate considerably from day to day, and may become milder or more severe with increasing age. Clonazepam produces sustained improvement without sedation in most, if not all, older patients. The neonatal experience with this agent, however, is limited.

After infancy, the neurologic examination is frequently normal, but stiffness or lack of fluidity of gait may be apparent, and tapping the nose may elicit excessive blepharospasm and head retraction.

Clinical variability is common, but penetrance is high in reported pedigrees. Sporadic patients with nonepileptic, startle-induced rigidity are sometimes encountered but are typically mentally retarded or have a history of anoxic brain injury. The diagnosis should be considered tentative when there are no affected relatives.

**Complications:** Skeletal fractures and intracranial hemorrhage may occur because of startle-induced falls. Congenitally dislocated hip and **Hernia, inguinal** may be seen in neonates. Neonatal death may occur due to apnea or aspiration.

**Associated Findings:** Occasional patients who also have epilepsy have been reported, but this relatively unusual association may be due to head trauma, and does not clearly exceed the incidence of epilepsy in the general population.

**Etiology:** Autosomal dominant inheritance with variable expressivity and nearly complete penetrance.

**Pathogenesis:** Unknown. An exaggerated long-loop reflex (a transcortical reflex arc) and high-amplitude somatosensory evoked potentials have been reported, suggesting a primary abnormality in the cerebral cortex. The striking resemblance of hyperekplexia to subconvulsive strychnine poisoning, however, suggests a defect in brainstem and spinal glycinergic transmission.

**MIM No.:** *14940, 18485

**Sex Ratio:** M1:F1

**Occurrence:** Undetermined but presumed rare; reported primarily in families of Northern European descent.

**Risk of Recurrence for Patient's Sib:**
See Part I, *Mendelian Inheritance.*

**Risk of Recurrence for Patient's Child:**
See Part I, *Mendelian Inheritance.*

**Age of Detectability:** Usually obvious at birth. Occasional patients, however, may not exhibit neonatal hypertonia and may not develop an exaggerated startle response until adolescence or young adulthood.

**Gene Mapping and Linkage:** Unknown.

**Prevention:** None known. Genetic counseling indicated.

**Treatment:** Clonazepam has produced dramatic and sustained amelioration of symptoms without sedation in almost all reported cases. Published experience with this drug during the neonatal period, however is limited. Other sedative-hypnotic agents (primarily barbiturates and other benzodiazepines) have not been consistently effective or have been poorly tolerated at therapeutic doses.

**Prognosis:** Neonatal mortality is probably less than 5–10%. Fatal complications in older patients are unusual. Many persons adapt to the illness and are employable full-time, even without treatment, despite occasional severe falls.

**Detection of Carrier:** A careful and thorough family history is essential to identify those who are minimally affected. Physical findings in mild cases may be subtle or absent.

**Special Considerations:** Electromyography of rigid muscles in neonates with hyperekplexia reveals continuous activity composed of normal-appearing motor units. Because muscular relaxation may not occur in this situation, true "spontaneous activity" may not be possible to evaluate. EEG reveals a normal background pattern, but muscle and eye movement artifacts occurring during a startle response may mimic epileptiform spikes. Additional electrodes (ocular and surface EMG) may aid in making the distinction.

**References:**
Suhren O, et al.: Hyperexplexia: a hereditary startle syndrome. J Neurol Sci 1966; 3:577–605.
Heller AH, Hallett M: Electrophysiological studies with the spastic mutant mouse. Brain Res 1982; 234:299–308.
Kurczynski TW: Hyperekplexia. Arch Neurol 1983; 40:246–248.
Markand ON, et al.: Familial Startle Disease (Hyperexplexia), electrophysiologic studies. Arch Neurol 1984; 41:71–74.
Ryan SG, et al.: Hereditary hyperexplexia: further delineation of the disease in a large pedigree. Ann Neurol 1988; 24:310 only.
Kelts KA, Harrison J: Hyperexplexia: effective treatment with clonazepam. Ann Neurol 1988; 24:309 only.
Nigro MA, Lim HC: Hyperexplexia: its role in sudden infant death. Ann Neurol 1989; 26:142 only.

RY001                                         **Stephen G. Ryan**

**Hyperexplexia**
  *See HYPEREKPLEXIA*
**Hyperextension of the knee**
  *See KNEE, GENU RECURVATUM*
**Hyperglycerolemia**
  *See GLYCEROL KINASE DEFICIENCY*
**Hyperglycinemia, idiopathic**
  *See HYPERGLYCINEMIA, NON-KETOTIC*
**Hyperglycinemia, ketotic**
  *See ACIDEMIA, PROPIONIC*

## HYPERGLYCINEMIA, NON-KETOTIC                    0492

**Includes:**
  Hyperglycinemia-hypooxaluria
  Hyperglycinemia, idiopathic
  Nonketotic hyperglycinemia
**Excludes:**
  **Glucoglycinuria** (0418)
  Glycinuria without hyperglycinemia
  **Acidemia, methylmalonic** (0658)
  **Acidemia, propionic** (0826)

**Major Diagnostic Criteria:** Onset of lethargy and seizures occurs in early infancy. Increased concentrations of glycine in the blood without recurrent ketoacidosis. Propionic and other organic acidemias should be excluded since patients with organic acidemia may present with severe illness and hyperglycinemia and there may be ketosis.

**Clinical Findings:** Onset of lethargy within the first days of life and convulsions at 3 days to 6 weeks. The patients described in detail developed severe mental retardation. Most have died in infancy without evidence of development. Those that have survived have shown little sign of intellectual development. Convulsions, especially myoclonic, are the rule. Hiccoughing may be prominent. The EEG is diffusely abnormal. It may show hypsarrhythmia or a burst-suppression pattern. Infants are usually hypotonic. Hypertonia develops later. There may be microcephaly or cerebral atrophy.

Plasma concentrations of glycine are distinctly elevated; a range of 5 to 11 mg/dl has been reported. Concentrations of glycine in the cerebrospinal fluid (CSF) are elevated. The ratio of the concentration of glycine in the CSF to that of the plasma is substantially higher in patients with nonketotic hyperglycinemia than in other hyperglycinemic patients. A mean ratio of 0.17 ± 0.09 has been reported in 12 patients, while in control individuals the ratio was 0.02. Urinary excretion of oxalate appears not to be a consistent characteristic of the disease.

A small number of patients has been described in whom a much milder, more indolent disease has been present, manifested only by mild mental retardation. In these individuals the ratio of glycine in the CSF to the plasma may be lower than in the classic form. We have also observed a patient whose course was that of a late infantile cerebral degenerative disease. Her CSF to plasma ratio of glycine was also lower than in the classic nonketotic hyperglycinemia.

**Complications:** Severe convulsive disorders and mental retardation.

**Associated Findings:** None known.

**Etiology:** Autosomal recessive inheritance.

**Pathogenesis:** Defective activity of the hepatic glycine cleavage enzyme system. This is a multicomponent system containing four enzyme proteins, designated: P-protein, H-protein, T-protein, and L-protein. Defects have been documented in individual patients in the P, H and T proteins.

**MIM No.:** *23830

**CDC No.:** 270.700

**Sex Ratio:** M1:F1

**Occurrence:** 1:12,000 in northern Finland. Probably lower but undetermined elsewhere.

**Risk of Recurrence for Patient's Sib:**
See Part I, *Mendelian Inheritance.*

**Risk of Recurrence for Patient's Child:**
See Part I, *Mendelian Inheritance.*

**Age of Detectability:** Within days of birth by quantitative assay of the plasma concentration of glycine.

**Gene Mapping and Linkage:** Unknown.

**Prevention:** None known. Genetic counseling indicated.

**Treatment:** Undetermined. Anticonvulsant medications have been used.

**Prognosis:** Most patients have died in infancy. Those who have survived have severe mental retardation.

**Detection of Carrier:** Unknown.

**References:**
Ando T, et al.: Metabolism of glycine in the nonketotic form of hyperglycinemia. Pediatr Res 1986; 2:254–263.
Ando T, et al.: Non-ketotic hyperglycinaemia in a family with an unusual phenotype. J Inherit Metab Dis 1978; 1:79–83.
Hiraga K, et al.: Defective glycine cleavage system in nonketotic hyperglycinemia: occurrence of a less active glycine decarboxylase and an abnormal aminomethyl carrier protein. J Clin Invest 1981; 68:525–534.
Hayasaka K, et al.: Nonketotic hyperglycinemia: two patients with primary defects pf P-protein and T-protein, respectively, in the glycine cleavage system. Pediatr Res 1983; 17:967–970.
Nyhan WL: Diagnostic recognition of genetic disease. Philadelphia: Lea & Febiger, 1987:85–95. *
Tada K, Hayasaka K: Non-ketotic hyperglycinaemia: clinical and biochemical aspects. Eur J Pediatr 1987; 146:221–227.

NY000            **William L. Nyhan**

**Hyperglycinemia-hypooxaluria**
*See HYPERGLYCINEMIA, NON-KETOTIC*
**Hyperglycinemia-ketoacidosis-leukopenia, type I**
*See ACIDEMIA, PROPIONIC*
**Hypergonadotropic hypogonadism**
*See KLINEFELTER SYNDROME*

## HYPERGONADOTROPIC HYPOGONADISM WITH CARDIOMYOPATHY    3195

**Includes:**
Cardiomyopathy, congestive-hypergonadotropic hypogonadism
Hypogonadism, hypergonadotropic-congestive cardiomyopathy

**Excludes:**
**Collagenoma, multiple cutaneous, familial** (3166)
**Gonadal dysgenesis, XX type** (0436)
**Hypogonadotropic hypogonadism** (2300)

**Major Diagnostic Criteria:** Ovarian dysgenesis and secondary hypergonadotropic hypogonadism with congestive cardiomyopathy.

**Clinical Findings:** History of adrenarche without thelarche or menarche. Very small breasts and scant pubic and axillary hair even after the age of 15 years. Evidence of ovarian dysgenesis and hypergonadotropic hypogonadism. The ovarian stroma with no oocytes. Karyotype: normal 46,XX.
Evidence of cardiovascular symptoms after the age of 20 years: dyspnea on exertion, orthopnea, paroxysmal nocturnal dyspnea. At that time chest X-ray reveals cardiomegaly and electrocardiogram is consistent with left ventricular hypertrophy. Radionuclide angiogram documents diffuse hypokinesia of all left ventricular segments. Echocardiography (M-mode and two-dimensional) shows a mildly dilated left ventricular cavity with concentric hypertrophy. Cardiac catheterization reveals a poorly contrasting left ventricle with normal coronary arteries. Endomyocardial biopsy shows myocardial hypertrophy with interstitial fibrosis.

**Complications:** The congestive cardiomyopathy may be complicated by refractory ventricular fibrillation causing the patient's demise.

**Associated Findings:** Ptosis of the eyelids.

**Etiology:** Possibly autosomal recessive inheritance.

**Pathogenesis:** Unknown.

**Sex Ratio:** M0:F2 (observed).

**Occurrence:** Two female siblings have been reported.

**Risk of Recurrence for Patient's Sib:**
See Part I, *Mendelian Inheritance*.

**Risk of Recurrence for Patient's Child:**
See Part I, *Mendelian Inheritance*.

**Age of Detectability:** After the age of 15 years.

**Gene Mapping and Linkage:** Unknown.

**Prevention:** None known. Genetic counseling indicated.

**Treatment:** Oral contraceptives and mammoplasty for menses and appearance of pubertal breasts. Diuretics, digoxin and, later, afterload-reducing agents for the cardiomyopathy.

**Prognosis:** One of the two sisters described died of refractory ventricular fibrillation at the age of 20 years.

**Detection of Carrier:** Unknown.

**References:**
Malouf J, et al.: Hypergonadotropic hypogonadism with congestive cardiomyopathy. Am J Med Genet 1985; 20:483–489.

DE030      **Vazken M. Der Kaloustian**
MA098          **Joe Malouf**

**Hypergonadotropic hypogonadism-partial skin appendages dysplasia**
*See HYPOGONADISM-PARTIAL ALOPECIA*
**Hyperhidrosis, gustatory**
*See SWEATING, GUSTATORY*

## HYPERHIDROSIS-PREMATURE GREYING-PREMOLAR APLASIA    0493

**Includes:**
Book syndrome
Hair greying-premolar aplasia-hyperhidrosis
Premolar aplasia-hyperhidrosis-canities

**Excludes:**
**Ectodermal dysplasia, Christ-Siemens-Touraine type** (0333)
**Hypodontia-nail dysgenesis** (0511)
**Werner syndrome** (0998)

**Major Diagnostic Criteria:** For single cases the presence of all three signs must be required. Otherwise diagnosis is aided by etiology and distribution of signs in affected family members.

**Clinical Findings:** These are based on 18 clinically examined patients from one pedigree: Premolar aplasia, confirmed in 17 patients (15 by X-rays and inconclusive in one due to unknown number of extractions). Lacking all 8 premolars 9:17. Lacking from 1–5 premolars 8:17. Hyperhidrosis occurred in 67% of the patients and was not seen in other members of the family. Premature hair greying (canities prematura) occurred in all patients.

**Complications:** Persistence of primary teeth until adult age in the premolar region and frequently backward dislocation of canines.

**Associated Findings:** None known.

**Etiology:** Autosomal dominant inheritance.

**Pathogenesis:** Unknown.

**MIM No.:** *11230

**POS No.:** 3041

**Sex Ratio:** M1:F1

**Occurrence:** Thirty-nine patients from one pedigree have been documented.

**Risk of Recurrence for Patient's Sib:**
See Part I, *Mendelian Inheritance*.

**Risk of Recurrence for Patient's Child:**
See Part I, *Mendelian Inheritance*.

**Age of Detectability:** Age of onset was from 6–10 years for 39%, from 11–20 years for 50% and from 21–23 years for 11%.

**Gene Mapping and Linkage:** Unknown.

**Prevention:** None known. Genetic counseling indicated.

**Treatment:** Dental prosthesis and orthodontic treatment may be necessary.

**Prognosis:** Excellent, with no significant consequences for the patient's health or life expectancy.

**Detection of Carrier:** Evidently there is complete penetrance in respect to premolar aplasia and premature hair greying in all heterozygotes.

**References:**
Böök JA: Clinical and genetical studies of hypodontia. I. Premolar aplasia, hyperhidrosis and canities prematura: a new hereditary syndrome in man. Am J Hum Genet 1950; 2:240–263. †
Böök JA, Modrzewska K, Rignell A: Hypodoncja w Zespole Ektrodermalnym Booka. Czas Stomat XXXIV:6:581–586.
Rignell A, et al.: Acta Univ Upsaliensis (abstracts of Uppsala dissertations from the faculty of medicine). 1981 #ISBN 91–506–0272–1. †

B0016                                                      **Jan A. Böök**

**Hyperimidodipeptiduria**
   *See PROLIDASE DEFICIENCY*
**Hyperimmunoglobulin E-recurrent infection syndrome**
   *See IMMUNODEFICIENCY, HYPER IgE TYPE*
**Hyperimmunoglobulinaemia D and periodic fever**
   *See FEVER, FAMILIAL MEDITERRANEAN (FMF)*
**Hyperkalemia-hyperchloremic acidosis-hypertension-hyporeninemia**
   *See ALDOSTERONE RESISTANCE*
**Hyperkalemic periodic paralysis**
   *See PARALYSIS, HYPERKALEMIC PERIODIC*
**Hyperkeratosis eccentrica**
   *See SKIN, POROKERATOSIS*
**Hyperkeratosis follicularis et parafollicularis in cutem penetrans**
   *See SKIN, KYRLE DISEASE*

## HYPERKERATOSIS PALMOPLANTARIS-PERIODONTOCLASIA                              0494

**Includes:**
   Papillon-Lefevre syndrome
   Parodontopathia acroectodermalis
   Periodontoclasia-hyperkeratosis palmoplantaris

**Excludes:**
   Keratosis palmoplantaris (all other)
   **Nails, pachyonychia congenita (0789)**
   **Werner syndrome (0998)**

**Major Diagnostic Criteria:** Hyperkeratosis of palms and soles with severe periodontal destruction (periodontoclasia) of both dentitions.

**Clinical Findings:** Hyperkeratosis of palms and soles. Severe periodontal destruction (periodontoclasia) of both primary and secondary dentition with consequent shedding of all teeth. Severe gingivostomatitis. Occasional ectopic calcification of the falx and increased susceptibility to infection.

**Complications:** Regional adenopathy and possible superimposed oral infections.

**Associated Findings:** Fragile nails, alopecia, cyst of eyelids in later life.

**Etiology:** Autosomal recessive inheritance.

**Pathogenesis:** Unknown.

**MIM No.:** *24500

**POS No.:** 3647

**Sex Ratio:** M1:F1

**Occurrence:** Approximately 1:1,000,000 general population.

**Risk of Recurrence for Patient's Sib:**
   See Part I, *Mendelian Inheritance.*

**Risk of Recurrence for Patient's Child:**
   See Part I, *Mendelian Inheritance.*

**Age of Detectability:** Suspected at birth on the basis of redness or hyperkeratosis palmoplantaris; positive diagnosis cannot be established until dental involvement, age 4 - 5 years.

**Gene Mapping and Linkage:** Unknown.

**Prevention:** None known. Genetic counseling indicated.

**Treatment:** Extraction of teeth and dental prosthesis. Oral retinoids have been used in the treatment of hyperkeratosis.

**Prognosis:** By age 5–6 years all of the primary teeth are lost. By age 13–14 all of the secondary teeth are lost. However, general health is not impaired.

**Detection of Carrier:** Unknown.

**References:**
Papillon MM, Lefèvre P: Deux cas de kératodermie palmaire et plantaire symétrique familiale (maladie de Meleda) chez le frère et la soeur. Coexistence dans le deux cas d'altérations dentaires graves. Bull Soc Franc Derm Syph 1924; 31:82–87.
Gorlin RJ, et al.: The syndrome of palmar-plantar hyperkeratosis and premature periodontal destruction of the teeth: a clinical and genetic analysis of the Papillon-Lefèvre syndrome. J Pediatr 1964; 65:895–908.
Giansanti JS, et al.: Palmar-plantar hyperkeratosis and concomitant periodontal destruction (Papillon-Lefèvre syndrome). Oral Surg 1973; 36:40–48.
Baghdady VS: Papillon-Lefevre syndrome: report of four cases. J Dent Chil 1982; 49:147–150.
Lyberg T: Immunological and metabolical studies in two siblings with Papillon-Lefevre syndrome. J Periodont Res 1982; 17:563–568.
Bravo-Piris J et al.: Papillon-Lefevre syndrome: report of a case treated with oral retinoid RO 10–9359. Dermatologica 1983; 166:97–103.

SE007                                                  **Heddie O. Sedano**

## HYPERKERATOSIS PALMOPLANTARIS-SPASTIC PARAPLEGIA-RETARDATION                              2828

**Includes:**
   Fitzsimmons syndrome
   Fitzsimmons-McLachlan-Gilbert syndrome
   Palmoplantar hyperkeratosis-spastic paraplegia-retardation
   Spastic paraplegia-palmoplantar hyperkeratosis-retardation
   X-linked mental retardation, Fitzsimmons type

**Excludes:**
   **Hyperkeratosis palmoplantaris-periodontoclasia (0494)**
   **Paraplegia, familial spastic (0295)**
   **Skin, Kyrle disease (0561)**
   **Sjogren-Larsson syndrome (2030)**
   **X-linked mental retardation, Fragile X syndrome (2073)**

**Major Diagnostic Criteria:** The combination of spastic paraplegia, palmoplantar hyperkeratosis, pes cavus deformity, and intellectual impairment.

**Clinical Findings:** Affected individuals are the result of normal pregnancies and have normal birth weight. However, developmental milestones are often delayed, and spasticity often appears by age two years. Palmoplantar hyperkeratosis develops later, having an onset between ages of five and 13 years, and may be more severe on the feet than on the hands. Physical anomalies in adults include a characteristic facial appearance of high forehead, frontal balding, and prominent nose; thickened nails; joint hyperextensibility; and pes cavus with clawed toes. Dysarthria may be severe, and ligamentous laxity with hyperextensibility of the fingers appears to be a constant feature. Height, weight, and head circumference are normal.

**Complications:** Thumb dislocations secondary to joint hypermobility.

**Associated Findings:** Two affected males had hypermetropic astigmatism; one also had left-side ptosis, nystagmus, and mild unilateral microphthalmia.

**Etiology:** Possibly X-linked recessive inheritance.

**Pathogenesis:** Unknown.

**MIM No.:** 30956

**POS No.:** 3596

**Sex Ratio:** Presumably M1:F0.

**Occurrence:** One family from England, with four affected brothers, has been documented.

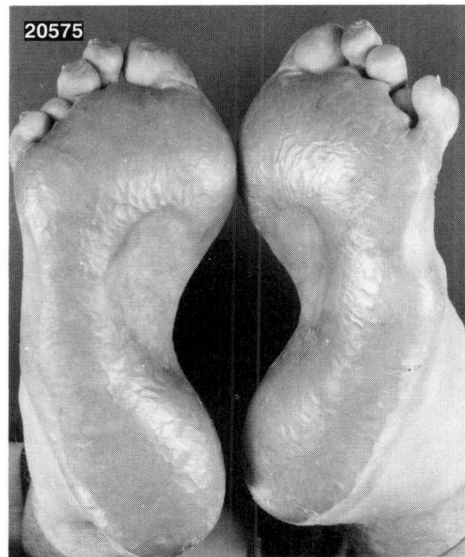

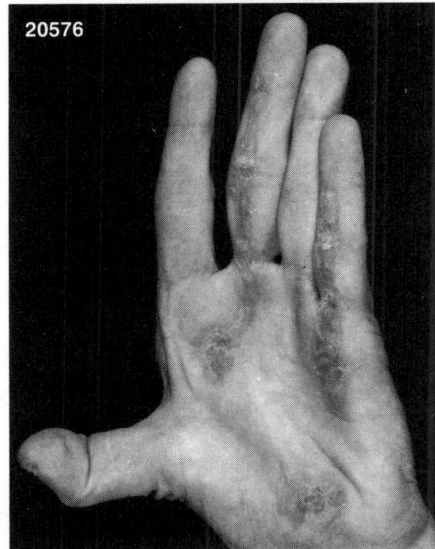

**2828**-20575: Severe generalized plantar hyperkeratosis in an affected male. 20576: Linear hyperkeratosis in the same subject; also demonstrates dislocatable thumb.

**Risk of Recurrence for Patient's Sib:**
See Part I, *Mendelian Inheritance.*

**Risk of Recurrence for Patient's Child:**
See Part I, *Mendelian Inheritance.*

**Age of Detectability:**  At one year of age by developmental delay and spasticity.

**Gene Mapping and Linkage:**  Unknown.

**Prevention:**  None known. Genetic counseling indicated.

**Treatment:**  Physiotherapy for gait disturbance. Cosmetic treatment for feet.

**Prognosis:**  Mental retardation to some degree is invariably present, with IQs in the range of 50–85. Life span appears unaffected.

**Detection of Carrier:**  The mother had some features of this condition, including a similar facial appearance, mild plantar hyperkeratosis, brisk lower limb reflexes, and slight clawing of the toes.

**References:**
Fitzsimmons JS, et al.: Four brothers with mental retardation, spastic paraplegia and palmoplantar hyperkeratosis: a new syndrome? Clin Genet 1983; 23:329–335.

FI022                                                   **J.S. Fitzsimmons**

**Hyperkeratosis-contracture syndrome**
    *See RESTRICTIVE DERMATOPATHY*
**Hyperkeratosis-corneal dystrophy-short stature-brachydactyly**
    *See CORNEO-DERMATO-OSSEOUS SYNDROME*
**Hyperkinetic syndrome**
    *See ATTENTION-DEFICIT HYPERACTIVITY DISORDER (ADHD)*
**Hyperkinetic-impulse disorder**
    *See ATTENTION-DEFICIT HYPERACTIVITY DISORDER (ADHD)*
**Hyperlipemia with familial hypercholesterolemic xanthoma**
    *See HYPERLIPOPROTEINEMIA, BROAD BETA TYPE*
**Hyperlipidemia II**
    *See HYPERCHOLESTEREMIA*
**Hyperlipidemia, familial combined**
    *See HYPERAPOBETALIPOPROTEINEMIA*
**Hyperlipoproteinemia I**
    *See HYPERCHYLOMICRONEMIA*
**Hyperlipoproteinemia II**
    *See HYPERCHOLESTEREMIA*
**Hyperlipoproteinemia III**
    *See HYPERLIPOPROTEINEMIA, BROAD BETA TYPE*
**Hyperlipoproteinemia IV**
    *See HYPERTRIGLYCERIDEMIA*

---

## HYPERLIPOPROTEINEMIA V                               0501

**Includes:**
    Hyperchylomicronemia-lipoproteinemia, hyperprebeta
    Hyperprebetalipoproteinemia and hyperchylomicronemia
    Lipoproteinemia-hyperchylomicronemia, hyperprebeta

**Excludes:**
    **Hyperchylomicronemia** (0489)
    **Hyperlipoproteinemia, broad beta type** (0495)
    **Hyperlipoproteinemia, combined** (0496)
    **Hypertriglyceridemia** (0500)

**Major Diagnostic Criteria:**  Affected individuals show chylomicrons in plasma obtained after an overnight fast of 10–12 hours. (Chylomicrons are usually cleared from plasma within 4–6 hours after a fat-containing meal.) In addition, very low density lipoprotein (VLDL) levels are elevated. Plasma placed in the refrigerator overnight shows a creamy layer on the top which contains chylomicrons, and a turbid infranatant indicative of severely elevated VLDL levels. Lipoprotein lipase measurements in post-heparin plasma reveal normal or low enzymatic activity.

**Clinical Findings:**  Patients have severely elevated triglyceride levels, often greater than 1000 mg/dl. The levels of low density lipoprotein (LDL) and high density lipoprotein (HDL) in these patients tend to be low. Many of the clinical findings in affected individuals are similar to those seen in **Hyperchylomicronemia**, including eruptive xanthomas, hepatosplenomegaly, abdominal pain and, occasionally, pancreatitis. Some of these patients have premature atherosclerotic vascular disease. In distinction from patients with familial lipoprotein lipase deficiency; glucose intolerance, hyperuricemia, and obesity are frequently present.

**Complications:**  In uncontrolled disease, eruptive xanthomas may cause cosmetic defects, foam cells in the liver and spleen may cause hepatosplenomegaly, and episodes of abdominal pain may be associated with pancreatitis.

**Associated Findings:**  None known.

**Etiology:**  Possibly autosomal dominant inheritance. Relatives have either normal, type IV (increased VLDL) or type V (increased VLDL and chylomicrons) hyperlipoproteinemia patterns.

**Pathogenesis:**  Undetermined. Post-heparin plasma reveals normal or low lipoprotein lipase activity. However, some activity is present and this helps distinguish this condition from familial lipoprotein lipase deficiency.

**MIM No.:** 14465

**Sex Ratio:** M1:F1

**Occurrence:** 1:1,000 adults in the general population.

**Risk of Recurrence for Patient's Sib:** Unknown.

**Risk of Recurrence for Patient's Child:** Unknown.

**Age of Detectability:** Expression is age related. Very few pediatric cases have been reported.

**Gene Mapping and Linkage:** Unknown.

**Prevention:** None known. Genetic counseling indicated.

**Treatment:** Severe hypertriglyceridemia (triglycerides >750 mg/dl) is associated with abdominal pain and pancreatitis, and can usually be controlled by weight reduction and mild dietary fat restriction. Restriction of alcohol consumption is helpful in certain individuals. If these measures fail, medical therapy with nicotinic acid can lower plasma triglyceride levels. However, this drug must be used cautiously since it may exacerbate glucose intolerance and hyperuricemia.

**Prognosis:** A normal life span should be anticipated.

**Detection of Carrier:** Unknown.

**References:**

Fredrickson DS, et al.: Fat transport in lipoproteins: an integrated approach to mechanisms and disorders. New Engl J Med 1967; 276:215–225.

Krauss RM, et al.: Selective measurement of two different triglyceride lipase activities in rat postheparin plasma. J Lipid Res 1973; 14:286.

Francois J, et al.: Genetic study of hyperlipoproteinaemia type IV and V. Clin Genet 1977; 12:202–207.

Greenberg BH, et al.: Primary type V hyperlipoproteinemia. Ann Intern Med 1977; 87:526.

Breslow JL: Familial disorders of high density lipoprotein metabolism. In: Scriver C, et al., eds: The metabolic basis of inherited disease, 6th ed. New York: McGraw-Hill, 1989:1251–1266.

BR010                                                          **Jan L. Breslow**

---

## HYPERLIPOPROTEINEMIA, BROAD BETA TYPE              0495

**Includes:**

Apolipoprotein E, deficiency or defect of
"Broad beta" disease
Carbohydrate-induced hyperlipemia
Familial dysbetalipoproteinemia
"Floating beta" disease
Hyperbeta- and prebetalipoproteinemia
Hypercholesterolemia, familial with hyperlipemia
Hyperlipemia with familial hypercholesterolemic xanthoma
Hyperlipoproteinemia III

**Excludes:**

Hypercholesteremia (0488)
Hyperlipoproteinemia (all others)

**Major Diagnostic Criteria:** Elevated plasma cholesterol and triglyceride levels are due to the accumulation in fasting plasma of lipoprotein particles not normally present in large amounts. These lipoprotein particles are intermediate density lipoproteins and chylomicron remnants. They have approximately equal amounts of cholesterol and triglycerides, and can sometimes be detected by finding a broad beta band on lipoprotein electrophoresis of whole plasma. However, a more reliable test is the ultracentrifugation of plasma at its own density and the subsequent demonstration of a floating beta migrating lipoprotein, so-called beta very low density lipoprotein (VLDL). This test is not ideal, since floating beta may not be present in all familial type III hyperlipoproteinemia patients, especially after treatment, and floating beta can occur in patients with other plasma lipid disorders. Another test that has been offered to help diagnose familial type III hyperlipoproteinemia is the finding of an elevated ratio of VLDL cholesterol to total triglycerides (> 0.3). In addition, recent studies have shown that

a particular form of one of the plasma apolipoproteins, apo E, is associated with type III hyperlipoproteinemia. Two-dimensional gel electrophoretic analysis of plasma apo E has revealed that it occurs in the population in six different phenotypes. These are determined by three alleles at a single genetic locus. Homozygosity for one of the alleles, E2, resulting in the apo E phenotype E2/2, is found in approximately 95% of individuals with type III hyperlipoproteinemia. This test may provide a specific biochemical marker that should greatly aid the clinical diagnosis of this disease.

**Clinical Findings:** Patients with familial type III hyperlipoproteinemia have elevated cholesterol and triglyceride levels. Affected individuals often show yellowish lipid deposits in the creases of the palms of the hands called xanthoma striata palmaris. In addition, eruptive and tuberous xanthomas are commonly seen. Xanthomas of the achilles tendons, extensor tendons of the hands, as well as xanthelasma and corneal arcus, do not often occur in familial type III hyperlipoproteinemia and are more characteristic of familial **Hypercholesteremia**. Coronary heart disease and peripheral vascular disease both occur commonly in familial type III hyperlipoproteinemia. Men tend to present in the fourth and women in the fifth decade of life with clinical symptoms of ischemic vascular disease. About one-half the patients with familial type III hyperlipoproteinemia have glucose intolerance and/or hyperuricemia. Obesity or hypothyroidism each have been shown to increase the expression of the disease.

**Complications:** Premature coronary artery disease. Peripheral vascular disease.

**Associated Findings:** None known.

**Etiology:** The association of the apo E phenotype E2/2, and homozygosity for the apo E allele E2, with familial type III hyperlipoproteinemia suggests autosomal recessive inheritance.

**Pathogenesis:** The intermediate density lipoproteins and chylomicron remnants that accumulate in the fasting plasma of familial type III hyperlipoproteinemia individuals is normally cleared very rapidly by the liver. Clearance of these particles is mediated through apo E. The apo E phenotype E2/2, present on the intermediate density lipoproteins and chylomicron remnants of familial type III hyperlipoproteinemia patients, is not recognized by hepatocyte receptors as well as apo E of the other phenotypes. In type III individuals, this leads to decreased clearance, accumulation of these cholesterol-rich particles in plasma, and the eventual formation of atherosclerotic disease and xanthomatosis. However, the gene frequency of the apo E allele, E2, is approximately 8–13%, which suggests that 1% of individuals have the apo E phenotype E2/2. Since familial type III hyperlipoproteinemia in its full clinical presentation is thought to occur much less frequently, it is certain that other genetic and/or environmental factors are important in the expression of this disease. It is already known that age, male sex, obesity, and thyroid status play a role; in addition, unknown factors are probably also involved.

**MIM No.:** 14450

**Sex Ratio:** M1:F<1

**Occurrence:** The complete clinical symptomatology, including extreme plasma lipid elevations, xanthomatosis, and ischemic vascular disease, is probably not more frequent than 1:2,000 to 1:10,000. However, the apo E phenotype E2/2 occurs in 1% of the population which may mean that a milder clinical state exists that may or may not have a significant component of premature vascular disease.

**Risk of Recurrence for Patient's Sib:**

See Part I, *Mendelian Inheritance.*

**Risk of Recurrence for Patient's Child:**

See Part I, *Mendelian Inheritance.* The carrier state of the apo E allele E2 is found in individuals with the apo E phenotypes E3/2 and E4/2. These apo E phenotypes occur commonly in the population, with frequencies of approximately 15% and 3%, respectively. If the spouse of an affected patient is a carrier, there is a 50% chance that a child will have the apo E phenotype E2/2. If the spouse is not a carrier, there is no chance of the child having the apo E phenotype E2/2. If the apo E phenotype of the spouse is unknown, there is approximately a 10% chance of a child having the apo E phenotype E2/2. The common occurrence of the carrier state of the apo E allele E2 appears to account for the cases of vertical transmission of familial type III hyperlipoproteinemia reported in the literature.

**Age of Detectability:** The apo E phenotype is a genetically determined marker and can be determined at any time of life. The expression of plasma lipid abnormalities, xanthomas, and ischemic vascular disease depends on many factors including age, male sex, obesity, thyroid status, and probably other as yet unknown genetic factors. Hyperlipidemia is not often seen before the third decade of life.

**Gene Mapping and Linkage:** The apo E gene has been mapped to human chromosome 19q13.

**Prevention:** None known. Genetic counseling indicated.

**Treatment:** Therapy is designed to lower plasma lipid levels. Initially, dietary management is attempted which includes weight reduction in the obese patient, and a low cholesterol, low saturated fat diet. Thyroid status should be checked and, if hypothyroidism is found, it should be treated. If these measures are insufficient to normalize plasma lipids, drug therapy with gemfibrozil or nicotinic acid should be attempted. Familial type III hyperlipoproteinemia is the most responsive to therapy of all the hyperlipoproteinemias. Appropriate therapy should result in normalization of plasma lipids, disappearance of xanthomas, and improvement of ischemic vascular disease.

**Prognosis:** Affected individuals develop ischemic vascular disease.

**Detection of Carrier:** Unknown.

**References:**
Fredrickson DS, et al.: Fat transport in lipoproteins: an integrated approach to mechanisms and disorders. New Engl J Med 1967; 276:34–42,94–103,148–156,215–225,273–281.
Morganroth J, et al.: The biochemical, clinical, and genetic features of type III hyperlipoproteinemia. Ann Intern Med 1975; 82:158–174.
Zannis VI, Breslow JL: Human VLDL apo E isoprotein polymorphism is explained by genetic variation and post-translational modification. Biochemistry 1981; 20:1033–1041.
Zannis VI, et al.: Human apolipoprotein E isoprotein patterns are genetically determined. Am J Hum Genet 1981; 33:11–24.
Scriver CR, et al, eds: The metabolic basis of inherited disease, 6th ed. New York: McGraw-Hill, 1989:

BR010

**Jan L. Breslow**

## HYPERLIPOPROTEINEMIA, COMBINED        0496

**Includes:** Multiple lipoprotein-type hyperlipidemia

**Excludes:**
    Hypercholesteremia (0488)
    Hyperlipoproteinemia V (0501)
    Hyperlipoproteinemia, broad beta type (0495)

**Major Diagnostic Criteria:** Family history and lipid analyses in family members are necessary to make this diagnosis in an individual with hyperlipidemia. Elevated levels of either cholesterol or triglycerides or both should be seen in approximately 50% of adult first degree relatives. The pattern in relatives does not have to be the same as in the propositus.

**Clinical Findings:** Patients with familial combined hyperlipidemia have elevated levels of either cholesterol or triglycerides or both. In a given individual, the pattern may change over time. Affected individuals have an increased incidence of coronary heart disease but do not develop tendon xanthomas. Affected patients may be obese, hyperinsulinemic, and glucose intolerant.

**Complications:** Premature coronary artery disease.

**Associated Findings:** Mild diabetes, hyperuricemia.

**Etiology:** Autosomal dominant inheritance.

**Pathogenesis:** At present, the basic defect in familial combined hyperlipidemia is not known and there is no specific genetic or biochemical marker for the disease. Fibroblasts from these individuals show normal low density lipoprotein (LDL) receptor activity. Post-heparin plasma reveals normal lipoprotein lipase activity and the apo E phenotypes are typical of those seen in the general population. An increased level of LDL apo B protein, with or without an increase in LDL cholesterol, is usually present. Metabolic studies show increased LDL apo B synthesis.

**MIM No.:** *14425

**Sex Ratio:** M1:F1

**Occurrence:** About 1–3:1,000 live births.

**Risk of Recurrence for Patient's Sib:**
    See Part I, *Mendelian Inheritance.*

**Risk of Recurrence for Patient's Child:**
    See Part I, *Mendelian Inheritance.*

**Age of Detectability:** Plasma lipid elevation is fully expressed in affected adult relatives, but less than 1:5 affected children show elevated lipid levels.

**Gene Mapping and Linkage:** Unknown.

**Prevention:** None known. Genetic counseling indicated.

**Treatment:** Therapy is designed mainly to lower plasma cholesterol levels to as close to 200 mg/dl as possible. Initially, this involves dietary management which includes weight reduction in the obese patient and a diet containing low cholesterol and saturated fat. If diet cannot consistently maintain plasma cholesterol levels below 240 mg/dl, drug treatment with nicotinic acid, gemfibrozil or lovastatin is indicated. Medical treatment of hypertriglyceridemia generally consists of recommending weight loss and carbohydrate restriction. Drug treatment of hypertriglyceridemia is currently controversial but nicotinic acid and gemfibrozil have been used successfully for this purpose in the past.

**Prognosis:** Individuals with familial combined hyperlipidemia develop premature coronary heart disease. It is hoped that through effective control of plasma lipid levels, especially cholesterol levels, this disease can be delayed.

**Detection of Carrier:** Unknown.

**References:**
Goldstein JL, et al.: Hyperlipidemia in coronary heart disease. Genetic analysis of lipid levels in 176 families and delineation of a new inherited disorder, combined hyperlipidemia. J Clin Invest 1973; 52:1533–1543.
Nikkila EA, Aro A: Family study of serum lipids and lipoproteins in coronary heart disease. Lancet 1973;I:954.
Rose HG, et al.: Inheritance of combined hyperlipoproteinemia: evidence for a new lipoprotein phenotype. Am J Med 1973; 54:148–160.
Kissebah AH, et al.: Low density lipoprotein metabolism in familial combined hyperlipidemia: mechanism of the multiple lipoprotein phenotypic expression. Arteriosclerosis 1984; 4:614–624.

BR010

**Jan L. Breslow**

## HYPERLYSINEMIA        0616

**Includes:**
    Lysine: alpha-ketoglutarate reductase deficiency
    Lysinemia, familial
    Saccharopine dehydrogenase deficiency
    Saccharopinuria

**Excludes:** Hyperlysinuria, isolated (2990)

**Major Diagnostic Criteria:** Persistent hyperlysinemia and hyperlysinuria; variant form has saccharopinuria; hyperpipecolatemia occasionally present. Hyperlysinemia and saccharopinuria both have deficient activity of the bifunctional enzyme alpha-aminoadipic semialdehyde synthase (AASS). The enzyme has two activities; lysine: ketoglutarate reductase and saccharopine dehydrogenase. The hyperlysinemia variant has less than 10% normal activity of AASS involving both functions. The saccharopinuria variant has no dehydrogenase activity but retains about one third normal reductase activity.

**Clinical Findings:** Prospective ascertainment by newborn screening indicates that hyperlysinemia and saccharopinuria variants are benign conditions. Another condition called congenital lysine intolerance has a clinical picture of ammonia intoxication; this manifestation is not observed in the hyperlysinemias. There is more hyperlysinuria than saccharopinuria in the hyperlysinemia variant; saccharopinuria is more prominent than hyperlysinuria in the saccharopinuria variant. There may be a combined hyperdibasic aminoaciduria, with overflow lysinuria and excess arginine and ornithine excretion by competition on the shared transport system.

**Complications:** Cases identified by newborn screening have not yet developed clinical complications.

**Associated Findings:** *Clinical:* The first reported cases had many associated findings, notably mental retardation, lax ligaments, eye findings, congenital malformations, etc. The cases were apparently identified retrospectively through these manifestations, therefore they constitute bias of ascertainment and the clinical findings are probably not related to hyperlysinemia, or the affected cases had another form of hyperlysinemia (e.g. congenital lysine intolerance).

*Metabolic:* Hyperpipecholatemia represents overflow of the lysine skeleton into the pipecholate pathway following removal of the α-amino group of lysine.

**Etiology:** Autosomal recessive inheritance.

**Pathogenesis:** Deficiency of a α-aminoadipic semialdehyde synthase (AASS). The enzyme is bifunctional and it possesses lysine ketoglutarate reductase and saccharopine dehydrogenase activities. The two activities are under control of a single locus and the enzyme is a homotetramer. The hyperlysinemia alleles confer 10% normal or less AASS activity; saccharopinuria alleles abolish dehydrogenase activity and leave about one third normal reductase activity.

**MIM No.:** *23870, 26870

**Sex Ratio:** M1:F1

**Occurrence:** About 2:1,000,000 births.

**Risk of Recurrence for Patient's Sib:**
See Part I, *Mendelian Inheritance.*

**Risk of Recurrence for Patient's Child:**
See Part I, *Mendelian Inheritance.*

**Age of Detectability:** Neonatal period by analysis of blood and urine.

**Gene Mapping and Linkage:** Unknown.

**Prevention:** None known. Genetic counseling indicated.

**Treatment:** Unknown.

**Prognosis:** Unknown.

**Detection of Carrier:** Unknown. Because the enzyme is a homotetramer, carriers may show deviant gene dosage effect with significantly less than 50% normal activity (negative allelic complementation effect).

**References:**
Colombo JP, et al.: Congenital lysine intolerance with periodic ammonia intoxication: a defect in L-lysine degradation. Metabolism 1967; 16:910–925.

Ghadimi H, Zischka R: Hyperlysinemia and lysine metabolism. In: Nyhan WL, ed: Amino acid metabolism and genetic variation. New York: McGraw-Hill, 1967:227–234.

Dancis J, et al.: The prognosis of hyperlysinemia: an interim report. Am J Hum Genet 1983; 35:438–442.

Markovitz PJ, et al.: Familial hyperlysinemias: Purification and characterization of the bifunctional aminoadipic semialdehyde synthase with lysine-ketoglutarate reductase and saccharopine dehydrogenase activities. J Biol Chem 1984; 259:11643.

Dancis J, Cox RP: Errors of lysine metabolism. In: Scriver CR, et al, eds: The metabolic basis of inherited disease, 6th ed. New York: McGraw-Hill, 1989:665–670.

SC050

**Charles R. Scriver**

**Hyperlysinuria with hyperammonemia**
*See HYPERDIBASIC AMINOACIDURIA*

## HYPERLYSINURIA, ISOLATED 2990

**Includes:**
 Lysine malabsorption syndrome
 Lysinuria-protein intolerance

**Excludes:**
 **Cystinuria** (0239)
 **Hyperdibasic aminoaciduria** (0491)
 **Hyperlysinemia** (0616)

**Major Diagnostic Criteria:** Hyperlysinuria (>130 mg/g creatine), normal (or low) plasma lysine, and high lysine renal clearance value (ml per min per 1.73 m²:>6.3, infants; >2.5, children; >2, adults). Normal values for other dibasic (cationic) amino acids (arginine ornithine) and for cystine. Evidence of impaired intestinal absorption of lysine by oral loading test. No hyperammonemia.

**Clinical Findings:** Possible ascertainment bias because the metabolic trait was found during investigation at age 21 months of a proposita with impaired mental and physical development. Clinical signs appeared and increased after the third month of life.

**Complications:** May cause CNS dysfunction.

**Associated Findings:** None known.

**Etiology:** Possibly autosomal recessive inheritance. Parents of the one known case were not related.

**Pathogenesis:** Deficient activity of a membrane transport system (possibly in brush-border) in renal tubule and small intestine; selective for lysine (and excluding arginine, ornithine, and cystine).

**MIM No.:** 24795

**Sex Ratio:** Presumably M1:F1.

**Occurrence:** One case has been documented in the literature.

**Risk of Recurrence for Patient's Sib:**
See Part I, *Mendelian Inheritance.*

**Risk of Recurrence for Patient's Child:**
See Part I, *Mendelian Inheritance.*

**Age of Detectability:** Presumably during the newborn period. No reports of cases identified by prospective newborn urine screening.

**Gene Mapping and Linkage:** Unknown.

**Prevention:** None known. Genetic counseling indicated.

**Treatment:** Unknown.

**Prognosis:** Unknown.

**Detection of Carrier:** Parents of proposita had normal urine lysine excretion values.

**References:**
Omura K, et al.: Lysine malabsorption syndrome: a new type of transport defect. Pediatrics 1987; 57:102–106.

SC050

**Charles R. Scriver**

**Hypernephroma**
*See CANCER, RENAL CELL CARCINOMA*
**Hyperodontia**
*See TEETH, SUPERNUMERARY*
**Hyperopia (bilateral) with marked difference between eyes**
*See EYE, ANISOMETROPIA*
**Hyperopia, unilateral**
*See EYE, ANISOMETROPIA*
**Hyperornithinemia with gyrate atrophy (HOGA)**
*See GYRATE ATROPHY OF THE CHOROID AND RETINA*

## HYPERORNITHINEMIA-HYPERAMMONEMIA-HOMOCITRULLINURIA 3169

**Includes:** HHH syndrome

**Excludes:**
> **Carbamoyl phosphate synthetase deficiency** (3022)
> **Gyrate atrophy of the choroid and retina** (0449)
> Homocitrullinuria of dietary origin
> Hyperammonemic syndromes (other)
> **Hyperdibasic aminoaciduria** (0491)
> Transient hyperammonemia of the newborn
> Urea cycle disorders, other

**Major Diagnostic Criteria:** The triad of high blood ammonia, increased blood ornithine, and the detection of urine homocitrulline in the absence of dietary source is essential for diagnosis. Orotic aciduria is common. The diagnosis can be confirmed by demonstrating failure of intact cultured cells to incorporate 14C from labelled ornithine into acid percipitable materials and normal activity of ornithine aminotransferase in cell extract or liver homogenate.

**Clinical Findings:** The most severely affected of the 30 known affected infants died of hyperammonemic coma at five days of age. Most patients developed symptoms in infancy. Clinical manifestations are related to hyperammonemia, i.e. protein intolerance, failure to thrive, developmental delay, seizures, and episodic lethargy. Retinopathy is notably absent. Ultrastructural changes in liver, lymphocytes, and fibroblast mitochondria have been described.

**Complications:** Intellectual deficit, seizures, tremor, and spastic paraparesis are common consequences.

**Associated Findings:** Low carbamylphosphate synthetase activity was found in one family.

**Etiology:** Autosomal recessive inheritance. The enzyme defect has not been identified.

**Pathogenesis:** Impairment of ornithine utilization by intact cells and decreased *in vitro* uptake of ornithine by mitochondrial preparation from patient tissues suggest that the defect is in the mitochondrial transport of ornithine. Such a defect results in functional deficiency of two mitochondrial enzymes; ornithine transcarbalylase and ornithine aminotransferase. The resulting hyperammonemia gives rise to brain damage and related clinical symptoms.

**MIM No.:** *23897

**Sex Ratio:** M1:F1

**Occurrence:** About 30 cases have been reported.

**Risk of Recurrence for Patient's Sib:**
> See Part I, *Mendelian Inheritance.*

**Risk of Recurrence for Patient's Child:**
> See Part I, *Mendelian Inheritance.*

**Age of Detectability:** Increased levels of blood ammonia and plasma ornithine, and urine homocitrulline, are detectable in the neonatal period, at least in severely affected patients. Prenatal diagnosis is possible using cultured amniocytes.

**Gene Mapping and Linkage:** HHH (hyperornithinemia-hyperammonemia-homocitrullinuria) has been tentatively mapped to 13q34.

**Prevention:** None known. Genetic counseling indicated.

**Treatment:** The goal of treatment is to lower ammonia accumulation in the body. Management is similar to that for urea cycle disorders. A protein restricted diet is prescribed. If needed, medication such as sodium benzoate, sodium phenylacetate and or sodium phenylbutyrate may be used to induce alternate pathways of nitrogen disposal. These drugs are still experimental in nature and may have side effects, especially in young infants. Oral ornithine supplement has been administered to a small number of patients on the assumption that high ornithine concentration may overcome the block in its mitochondrial transport. A lowering of the blood ammonia level was seen in some of these cases.

**Prognosis:** In untreated patients, developmental delay is likely, as well as the possible late complication of spastic paraparesis. Early treatment may improve the intellectual and neurological outcome.

**Detection of Carrier:** Unknown.

**Special Considerations:** Two women with the HHH syndrome have had uneventful pregnancies and have given birth to normal infants.

**References:**
Shih VE, et al: Hyperornithinemia, hyperammonemia, and homocitrullinuria: a new disorder of amino acid metabolism associated with myoclinic seizures and mental retardation. Am J Dis Child 1969; 117:83–92.
Gatfield PD, et al: Hyperornithinemia, hyperammonemia, and homocitrullinura associated with decreased carbamyl phosphate synthetase I activity. Pediat Res 1975; 9:488–497.
Hommes FA, et al: Decreased transport of ornithine across the inner mitochondrial membrane as a cause of hyperornithinemia. J Inherit Metab Dis 1982; 5:41–47.
Shih VE, et al: Defective ornithine metabolism in cultured skin fibroblasts from patients with the syndrome of hyperornithinemia, hyperammonemia and homocitrullinuria. Clin Chim Acta 1982; 118:149–157.
Gray RGF, et al: Studies on the pathway from ornithine to proline in cultured skin fibroblasts with reference to the defect in hyperornithinemia with hyperammonemia and homocitrullinuria. J Inherit Metab Dis 1983; 6:143–148.
Haust MD, Gordon BA: Possible pathogenetic mechanism in hyperornithinemia, hyperammonemia, and homocitrullinuria syndrome. BD:OAS XXIII(1). New York: March of Dimes Birth Defects Foundation Birth Defects, 1987:17–45.
Chadefaux B, et al.: Potential for the prenatal diagnosis of hyperornithinemia, hyperammonemia, and homocitrullinuria syndrome. (Letter) Am J Med Genet 1989; 32:264.

SH029                                                    **Vivian E. Shih**

**Hyperostoses of auditory canal**
> *See EAR, EXOSTOSES*

**Hyperostosis calvariae interna**
> *See HYPEROSTOSIS FRONTALIS INTERNA*

**Hyperostosis corticalis deformans juvenilis**
> *See OSTEOECTASIA*

**Hyperostosis corticalis generalisata**
> *See ENDOSTEAL HYPEROSTOSIS*

**Hyperostosis corticalis generalisata, benign Worth type**
> *See HYPEROSTOSIS, WORTH TYPE*

## HYPEROSTOSIS FRONTALIS INTERNA 0498

**Includes:**
> Endostosis cranii
> Hyperostosis calvariae interna
> Metabolic craniopathy
> Morgagni-Stewart-Morel syndrome

**Excludes:**
> Leontiasis ossea
> **Bone, Paget disease** (3081)

**Major Diagnostic Criteria:** X-ray evidence of hyperostosis of the inner table of the frontal bone. There is some doubt as to whether hyperostosis frontalis interna is more than a common benign anatomic peculiarity found in up to 12% of normal women. This lesion has been described in association with myotonic dystrophy, Crouzon disease and a variety of other disorders. It must be distinguished from leontiasis ossea, **Bone, Paget disease**, and the congenital anemias. Increased serum alkaline phosphatase levels have been found in about one-half of a group of affected females.

**Clinical Findings:** Hyperostosis of the inner table of the cranium confined primarily to the frontal or frontal-parietal areas. This anomaly has been reported in association with a variety of endocrine and neuropsychiatric disturbances such as obesity, virilization, gonadal disturbances, headache, epilepsy, and psychosis. These occur primarily in middle-aged and elderly women.

There is some question as to whether this variable constellation of abnormalities represents a true syndrome or is merely coincidental. X-rays reveal a bony proliferation of the inner table of the skull, with or without involvement of the diploë, confined primarily to the frontal bone. The outer table of the calvarium is uninvolved.

**Complications:** There is some controversy as to whether this endostosis can result in headache and endocrine imbalance or whether it is simply an incidental finding in middle-aged women and produces no symptoms.

**Associated Findings:** None known.

**Etiology:** The occurrence of this anomaly in multiple generations of several families suggests dominant inheritance, either sex-limited autosomal or X-linked transmission. No case of male-to-male transmission is known.

**Pathogenesis:** Since hyperostosis frontalis occurs almost twenty times as frequently in women with galactorrhea as in the general population, and since hyperprolactinemia was found in many of these cases, it is possible that such features as hirsutism, diabetes, and menstrual problems may be related to hyperprolactinemia.

**MIM No.:** 14480

**Sex Ratio:** M1:F9

**Occurrence:** Undetermined. Most frequent in women with galactorrhea.

**Risk of Recurrence for Patient's Sib:**
See Part I, *Mendelian Inheritance.*

**Risk of Recurrence for Patient's Child:**
See Part I, *Mendelian Inheritance.*

**Age of Detectability:** Usually found in middle-aged females, but it has been reported occasionally in adolescence.

**Gene Mapping and Linkage:** Unknown.

**Prevention:** None known. Genetic counseling indicated.

**Treatment:** Unknown.

**Prognosis:** Normal life span.

**Detection of Carrier:** Unknown.

**References:**
Moore S: Hyperostosis cranii (Stewart-Morel syndrome, metabolic craniopathy, Morgagni's syndrome, Stewart-Morel-Moore syndrome Ritvo, le syndrome de Morgagni-Morel). Springfield: Charles C. Thomas, 1964.
Perou, ML: Cranial hyperostosis, hyperostosis cranii or HC. Springfield: Charles C Thomas, 1964.
Rosatti P: Une famille atteinte d'hyperostose frontale interne (syndrome de Morgagni-Morel) a travers quatre generations successives. J Genet Hum 1972; 20:207–252.
Gegick CG et al.: Hyperostosis frontalis interna and hyperphosphatasemia. Ann Intern Med 1973; 79:71–75.
Pawlikowski M, Komorowski J: Hyperstosis frontalis, galactorrhoea/hyperprolactinaemia, and Stewart-Morel-Moore syndrome (letter). Lancet 1983; I:474 only.

B0025

**Zvi Borochowitz**
*David L. Rimoin*

**Hyperostosis generalisata with striations**
*See OSTEOPATHIA STRIATA-CRANIAL SCLEROSIS-MEGALENCEPHALY*

**Includes:**
    Bone dysplasia, Worth type hyperostosis
    Endosteal hyperostosis
    Hyperostosis corticalis generalisata, benign Worth type
    Osteosclerosis, autosomal dominant

**Excludes:**
    **Craniofacial dysostosis-diaphyseal hyperplasia** (0226)
    **Endosteal hyperostosis** (0497)
    **Osteomesopyknosis** (2695)
    **Osteopetrosis**

**Major Diagnostic Criteria:** Generalized bone dysplasia characterized by increased thickness and density of calvarium, mandible, clavicle, and diaphysis of tubular bones. Normal height.

**Clinical Findings:** Normal appearance until childhood, when facial features of high, flat forehead and square mandible develop. Increased incidence of dental problems in adult life.
    Normal stature and intelligence. Hyperostosis of the spine may lead to cervical or lower spinal root impingement. There is minimal progression of the bone pathology in adult life. Small excrescences along the cortex of the long bones may develop. No cranial nerve involvement has been reported.
    No metabolic abnormality of the bone is known. There is no increased tendency to fracture. Patients have reported difficulty swimming, presumably because of increased bone density. There is mild generalized joint stiffness.

**Complications:** Spinal root impingement syndromes. Adult tooth loss.

**Associated Findings:** **Palate, torus palatinus** is often present. Neurologic involvement was reported in one family (Perez-Vicente, 1987).

**Etiology:** Autosomal dominant inheritance.

**Pathogenesis:** Unknown.

**MIM No.:** *14475

**Sex Ratio:** M1:F1

**Occurrence:** At least seven kinships have been reported.

**Risk of Recurrence for Patient's Sib:**
    See Part I, *Mendelian Inheritance.*

**Risk of Recurrence for Patient's Child:**
    See Part I, *Mendelian Inheritance.*

**Age of Detectability:** In adolescence.

**Gene Mapping and Linkage:** Unknown.

**Prevention:** None known. Genetic counseling indicated.

**Treatment:** Decompression of spinal nerve roots.

**Prognosis:** Normal life span and intelligence.

**Detection of Carrier:** Unknown.

**References:**
Worth HM, Wollin DG: Hyperostosis corticalis generalisata congenita. J Can Assoc Radiol 1966; 17:67–74.
Beals RK: Endosteal hyperostosis. J Bone Joint Surg 1976; 58A:1172–1173. * †
Yasuda Y, et al.: Autosomal dominant osteosclerosis associated with familial spinal canal stenosis. Neurology 1986; 36:687–692.
Perez-Vicente JA, et al.: Autosomal dominant endosteal hyperostosis: report of a Spanish family with neurological involvement. Clin Genet 1987; 31:161–169.

BE047

**Rodney K. Beals**

## HYPERPARATHYROIDISM, FAMILIAL　　　　　0499

**Includes:**
　　Neonatal severe primary hyperparathyroidism (NSPH)
　　Parathyroid hyperplasia, hereditary

**Excludes:**
　　Hyperparathyroidism secondary to maternal
　　　　hypoparathyroidism
　　**Endocrine neoplasia** (all)

**Major Diagnostic Criteria:** Depending upon the duration of the disease: poor feeding, constipation, respiratory difficulty, failure to thrive, polydipsia, polyuria and hypotonia accompanied by hypercalcemia with elevated serum immunoreactive parathyroid hormone level. X-ray evidence of skeletal demineralization is a characteristic finding.

**Clinical Findings:** Common symptoms in the early weeks of life in the afflicted infants include poor feeding, constipation, respiratory difficulty, failure to thrive, unexplained anemia, hepatomegaly, splenomegaly, seizures, polydipsia, polyuria and hypotonia. In spite of generalized hypotonia, tendon reflexes may be exaggerated. Extreme hypercalcemia is common with peak serum calcium concentrations ranging between 15 and 30 mg/dl. Hypophosphatemia, hypercalcinuria, hyperphosphaturia, and aminoaciduria have been noted in most infants when appropriate measurements have been made. Skeletal X-rays reveal demineralization, subperiosteal resorption, and pathologic fractures. Serum alkaline phosphatase values are usually within normal range despite clear evidence of bone involvement. Renal calcinosis is a common finding.

**Complications:** Skeletal demineralization with pathologic fractures; renal calcinosis.

**Associated Findings:** Failure to thrive; hypotonia.

**Etiology:** Possibly autosomal recessive and/or autosomal dominant inheritance. Consanguinity has been noted. Some cases may represent early expression of the adult-onset form of dominant familial hyperparathyroidism, while others may result from homozygosity for the gene for hypocalcuric hypercalcemia.

**Pathogenesis:** The pathogenesis of parathyroid chief cell hyperplasia observed in this disorder is unknown.

**MIM No.:** 23920

**Sex Ratio:** M1:F1

**Occurrence:** Undetermined. Dozens of cases have been reported in the literature.

**Risk of Recurrence for Patient's Sib:**
　　See Part I, *Mendelian Inheritance.*

**Risk of Recurrence for Patient's Child:**
　　See Part I, *Mendelian Inheritance.*

**Age of Detectability:** In most infants the condition has been diagnosed by the age of four months.

**Gene Mapping and Linkage:** Unknown.

**Prevention:** None known. Genetic counseling indicated.

**Treatment:** Neonatal familial hyperparathyroidism is considered a surgical emergency requiring parathyroidectomy. Since recurrence has been observed in two infants following subtotal parathyroidectomy, the treatment of choice may be total parathyroidectomy.

　　Measures to combat hypercalcemia may be needed prior to surgery. Postoperative treatment of hypoparathyroidism requires vitamin D and calcium supplements.

**Prognosis:** If untreated, the disease progresses and death occurs in the early months of life.

**Detection of Carrier:** Heterozygotes may show asymptomatic hypercalcemia and elevated serum parathyroid hormone levels.

**References:**
Hillman DA, et al.: Neonatal familial primary hyperparathyroidism. New Engl J Med 1964; 270:483–490.

Goldbloom RB, et al.: Hereditary parathyroid hyperplasia: a surgical emergency of early infancy. Pediatrics 1972; 49:514–523.
Spiegel AM, et al.: Neonatal primary hyperparathyroidism with autosomal dominant inheritance. J Pediatr 1977; 90:269–272.
Marx SJ, et al.: An association between neonatal severe primary hyperparathyroidism and familial hypocalciuric hypercalcemia in three generations. New Engl J Med 1982; 306:257–264.
Marx SJ, et al.: Familial hypocalciuric hypercalcemia: mild expression in of the gene in heterozygotes and severe expression in homozygotes. Am J Med 1985; 78:15–22.

SC016　　　　　　　　　　　　　　**R. Neil Schimke**

**Hyperparathyroidism, hereditary (some cases)**
　　See *ENDOCRINE NEOPLASIA, MULTIPLE TYPE I*
**Hyperpepsinogenemic I duodenal ulcer**
　　See *PEPTIC ULCER DISEASES, NON-SYNDROMIC*
**Hyperphalangeal thumb**
　　See *THUMB, TRIPHALANGEAL*
**Hyperphalangism of thumbs-duplication of thumbs and big toes**
　　See *THUMB, TRIPHALANGEAL-DUPLICATED GREAT TOES*
**Hyperphalangy (symmetric)**
　　See *DIGITO-PALATAL SYNDROME, STEVENSON TYPE*
**Hyperphenylalaninemia**
　　See *PHENYLKETONURIA*
**Hyperphenylalaninemia due to abnormal biopterin metabolism**
　　See *DIHYDROPTERIDINE REDUCTASE DEFICIENCY*
　　also *BIOPTERIN SYNTHESIS DEFICIENCY*
**Hyperphenylalaninemia, mild**
　　See *FETAL EFFECTS FROM MATERNAL PKU*
**Hyperphosphatasemia tarda**
　　See *ENDOSTEAL HYPEROSTOSIS*
**Hyperphosphatasemia, chronic congenital idiopathic**
　　See *OSTEOECTASIA*
**Hyperpigmentation, familial progressive**
　　See *SKIN, HYPERPIGMENTATION, FAMILIAL*
　　also *SKIN, CUTANEOUS MELANOSIS, DIFFUSE*
**Hyperpigmentation-punctate palmoplantar keratoses-blistering**
　　See *EPIDERMOLYSIS BULLOSUM, TYPE I*
**Hyperpnea, episodic-abnormal eye movement-ataxia-retardation**
　　See *JOUBERT SYNDROME*
**Hyperprebetalipoproteinemia and hyperchylomicronemia**
　　See *HYPERLIPOPROTEINEMIA V*
**Hyperprebetalipoproteinemia, familial**
　　See *HYPERTRIGLYCERIDEMIA*
**Hyperproinsulinemia**
　　See *DIABETES MELLITUS, MUTANT INSULIN TYPES*

## HYPERPROLINEMIA　　　　　　　　　　0502

**Includes:**
　　Delta-1-pyrroline-5-carboxylate dehydrogenase deficiency
　　Hyperprolinemia type I
　　Hyperprolinemia type II
　　Proline oxidase deficiency

**Excludes:** N/A

**Major Diagnostic Criteria:** No clear clinical phenotype is yet proven; diagnosis is biochemical. Type I and type II hyperprolinemia result from different enzyme defects:

*Type I:* persistent elevation of plasma proline concentration above 5 mg/dl. Hyperaminoaciduria comprising proline (overflow), and glycine and hydroxyproline (competition) found when plasma proline concentration exceeds 8 mg/dl, about 0.70 $\mu$mole/ ml.

*Type II:* Same as type I, except proline concentration usually much higher (20–40 mg/dl). Urine contains δ-1-pyrroline-5-carboxylic acid (PC) and δ-1-pyrroline-3-hydroxy-5-carboxylate, the corresponding metabolite of hydroxyproline, as well as proline, glycine, and hydroxyproline.

**Clinical Findings:** A biochemical phenotype. No proven association with clinical disease, although identified frequently in pedigrees containing renal disease or convulsive disorders. The incidence in such pedigrees of subjects with disease but without hyperprolinemia, and the converse, as well as clear-cut examples of independent modes of inheritance of the familial disease trait and of hyperprolinemia, support the belief that hyperprolinemia and disease traits are incidentally associated.

**Complications:** Unknown.

**Associated Findings:** Possible convulsive disorders, renal disease. One patient was reported with a partial duplication of the short arm of chromosome 10, but the relationship of this finding to the condition is undetermined.

**Etiology:** Autosomal recessive inheritance for both types. The possibility of associated genes at different loci has not been ruled out as the basis for associated renal and CNS disease.

**Pathogenesis:** Type I: proline oxidase deficiency. Type II: δ-1-pyrroline-5-carboxylic acid dehydrogenase deficiency. Type II only is detectable in fibroblasts cultured from skin biopsy and in leukocytes. Any relationship to convulsive disorders and renal disease is unknown.

**MIM No.:** *23950, *23951

**Sex Ratio:** M1:F1

**Occurrence:** <1:20,000 live births; Over 20 families have been identified. Identified in Caucasians of Europe and North America, and also in the North American Indian.

**Risk of Recurrence for Patient's Sib:**
See Part I, *Mendelian Inheritance*.

**Risk of Recurrence for Patient's Child:**
See Part I, *Mendelian Inheritance*.

**Age of Detectability:** Presumably detectable in newborn.

**Gene Mapping and Linkage:** Unknown.

**Prevention:** None known. Genetic counseling indicated.

**Treatment:** None required. No effective way to restrict proline accumulation, nor proven benefit from such attempts.

**Prognosis:** Probably a benign trait, but association of type II with CNS manifestations cannot be ruled out.

**Detection of Carrier:** No consistent finding known; some type I heterozygotes manifest modest hyperprolinemia. Type II heterozygotes do not have hyperprolinemia.

**Special Considerations:** Two enzyme defects can cause the same trait, but PC-dehydrogenase deficiency is associated with greater hyperprolinemia than that caused by proline oxidase deficiency. The latter enzyme may be shared in hydroxyproline metabolism and account for evidence for impaired oxidation of the 2nd imino acid in type II hyperprolinemia.

Complex hyperaminoaciduria (proline, glycines and hydroxyproline) is of combined prerenal and renal origin. It does not appear unless plasma proline is sufficiently elevated (>8 mg/dl). Identification of this trait by detection of hyperaminoaciduria requires discrimination from renal iminoglycinuria.

**References:**
Schafer IA, et al.: Familial hyperprolinemia, cerebral dysfunction and renal anomalies occurring in a family with hereditary nephropathy and deafness. New Engl J Med 1962; 267:51–60.
Efron ML: Familial hyperprolinemia. Report of a second case, associated with congenital renal malformations, hereditary hematuria and mild mental retardation, with demonstration of an enzyme defect. New Engl J Med 1965; 272:1243–1254.
Valle DL, et al.: Type II hyperprolinemia: δ-1-pyrroline-5-carboxylic acid dehydrogenase deficiency in cultured skin fibroblasts and circulating lymphocytes. J Clin Invest 1976; 58:598–603.
Oyanagi K, et al.: Clinical, biochemical and enzymatic studies of type I hyperprolinemia associated with chromosomal abnormality. Tohoku J Exp Med 1987; 151:465–475.
Phang JM and Scriver CR: Disorders of proline and hydroxyproline metabolism. In: Scriver, CR, et al. eds: The metabolic basis of inherited disease, ed 6. New York: McGraw-Hill, 1989:577–598.

SC050                                          **Charles R. Scriver**

**Hyperprolinemia type I**
*See HYPERPROLINEMIA*
**Hyperprolinemia type II**
*See HYPERPROLINEMIA*

**Hypersarcosinemia**
*See SARCOSINEMIA*
**Hyperstat△, fetal effects**
*See FETAL EFFECTS FROM MATERNAL VASODILATOR*
**Hypertaurodontism**
*See TEETH, TAURODONTISM*
**Hypertelorism**
*See AARSKOG SYNDROME*
**Hypertelorism of eyes**
*See EYE, HYPERTELORISM*
**Hypertelorism-esophageal abnormality-hypospadias**
*See G SYNDROME*

## HYPERTELORISM-HYPOSPADIAS SYNDROME          0505

**Includes:**
BBB syndrome
Dystopia canthorum
Hypospadias-hypertelorism syndrome
Opitz oculo-genital-laryngeal syndrome
Telecanthus-hypospadias syndrome
Telecanthus with associated abnormalities

**Excludes:**
G syndrome (0401)
Hypospadias (0518)
Waardenburg syndromes (0997)

**Major Diagnostic Criteria:** A male with widely spaced inner canthi and hypospadias; or a female with telecanthus and affected male relatives.

**Clinical Findings:** At least 37 affected males have been documented. Recorded clinical findings include: wide-spaced inner canthi [telecanthus or apparent hypertelorism] (97%); hypospadias (97%); cranial asymmetry [plagiocephaly] (47%); mental retardation (43%); strabismus (37%); cryptorchidism (30%); congenital heart defects (25%); cleft lip and palate (23%) urinary tract abnormalities (19%); imperforate anus (5%).

Other findings are prominent nasal bridge, ear anomalies, laryngotracheal-esophageal cleft, multiple lipomas, flame nevi, bifid uvula, epicanthal folds, dermatoglyphic changes, diastasis recti and umbilical or inguinal herniae.

The affected males reported belong to 21 families; variable degrees of telecanthus are found in females in 16 of these families. One known obligate carrier female has an inner canthal distance within the normal range.

The name hypertelorism-hypospadias was chosen because it reflects the clinically most evident and common findings in affected males; however, not all affected individuals with wide-spaced inner canthi (telecanthus) have increased distance between the bony orbits (hypertelorism).

**Complications:** Urinary tract infections; amblyopia ex anopsia.

**Associated Findings:** Osteopenia and/or bone dysplasia (Krauss et al, 1985).

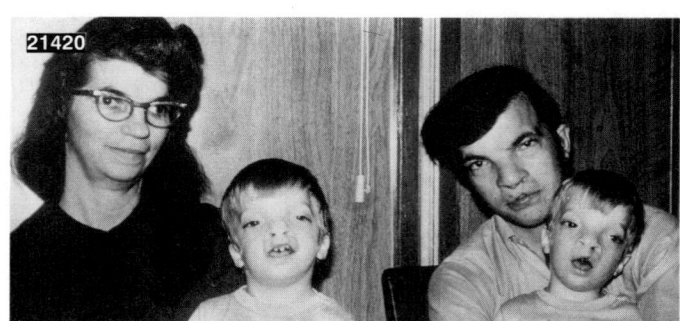

**0505A-21420:** The mother has telecanthus, her twin boys and their older brother have telecanthus and hypospadias.

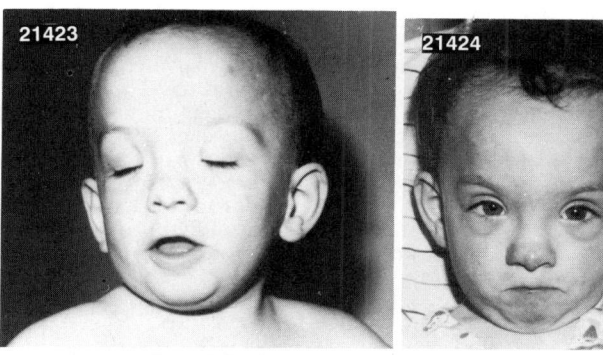

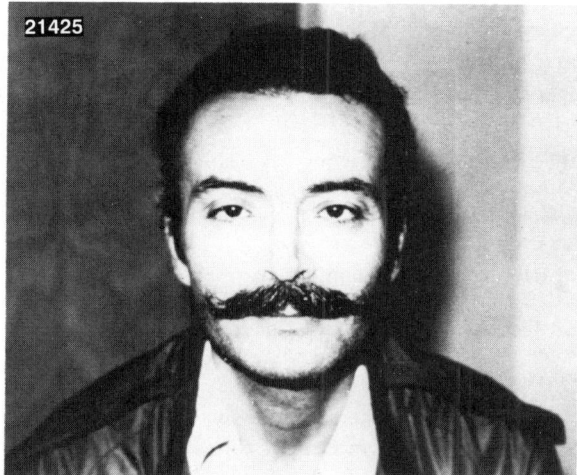

0505B-21423: Note the telecanthus, epicanthal folds and soft tissue mass at the tip of the nose in this 12-month-old male with characteristic facial and genital findings of BBB syndrome but with additional skeletal anomalies. 21424: Telecanthus is still evident at 19.5 months. 21425: Note the telecanthus in the father of the boy shown in 21423–24.

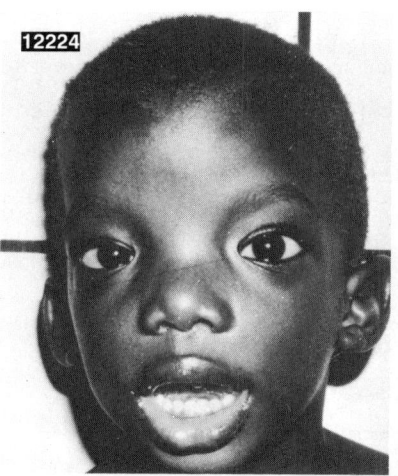

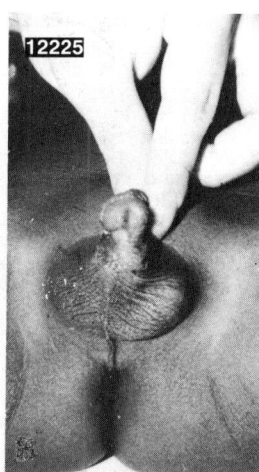

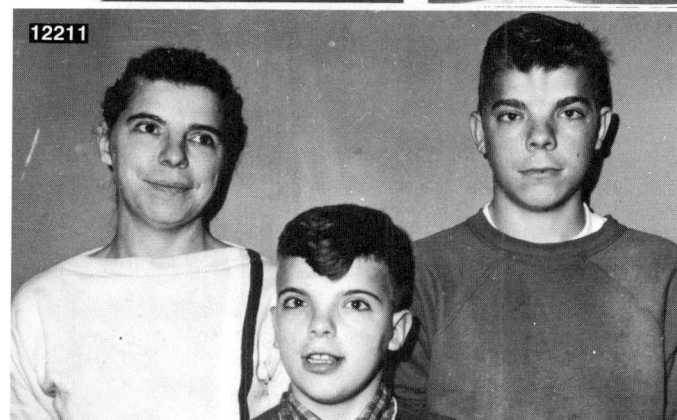

0505C-12224: Hypertelorism, epicanthal folds and esotropia. 12225: Glandular hypospadias. 12211: Affected mother and two affected sons; all have hypertelorism and prominent nasal bridge.

**Etiology:** Possibly autosomal dominant or X-linked inheritance. However, Stoll et al (1985) reported a father with hypertelorism and hypospadias who had a son with hypertelorism, hypospadias, heart defects and mental retardation, ruling out X-linkage in this family.

**Pathogenesis:** The most striking findings are midline defects, particularly of the craniofacial skeleton and the genital tubercle. Like-sexed twinning and midline facial clefts previously were reported associated in families. This condition seems to be associated with twinning more than can be expected by chance alone. Three affected individuals have been twins (2 pairs concordant and 1 pair discordant for the trait). A pathogenic relationship between the process of twinning and this syndrome may exist.

**MIM No.:** 31360

**POS No.:** 3258

**CDC No.:** 756.085, 752.600

**Sex Ratio:** M37:F31 (Observed, based on reported cases).

**Occurrence:** Undetermined; 37 affected males reported in 21 families, although unreported cases are know to exist.

**Risk of Recurrence for Patient's Sib:**
See Part I, *Mendelian Inheritance.*

**Risk of Recurrence for Patient's Child:**
See Part I, *Mendelian Inheritance.*

**Age of Detectability:** At birth by physical examination.

**Gene Mapping and Linkage:** Unknown.

**Prevention:** None known. Genetic counseling indicated.

**Treatment:** Repair of hypospadias and cleft palate, and appropriate therapy for associated birth defects.

**Prognosis:** Five affected males have died in infancy; no affected females are known to have died of the syndrome. Mental retardation occurred in one-half of affected males; no known mental retardation in the affected females. In general, the associated congenital anomalies are surgically correctable.

**Detection of Carrier:** Finding of isolated telecanthus in female.

**Special Considerations:** Because of the overlap in phenotypic features, some investigators have suggested that this condition and **G syndrome** may be variants of the same disorder. Sedano and Gorlin (1988) have proposed a joint name of *Opitz oculo-genital-laryngeal syndrome.*

**References:**
Christian JC, et al.: Familial telecanthus with associated congenital anomalies. BD:OAS;V(2). New York: March of Dimes Birth Defects Foundation, 1969:82–85.

Opitz JM, et al.: The BBB syndrome-familial telecanthus with associated congenital anomalies. BD:OAS;V(2). New York: March of Dimes Birth Defects Foundation, 1969:86–94.

Michaelis E, Mortier N: Association of hypertelorism and hypospadias: the BBB syndrome. Helv Paediatr Acta 1972; 27:575–581.

Cordero JF, Holmes LB: Phenotypic overlap in the BBB and G syndromes. Am J Med Genet 1978; 2:145–152.

Halal F, Farsky K: Coloboma-hypospadias. Am J Med Genet 1981; 8:53–57.

daSilva EO: The hypertelorism-hypospadias syndrome. Clin Genet 1983; 23:30–34.

Krauss CM, et al.: Syndrome of telecanthus, hypertelorism, strabismus, and pes cavus in father and son. Am J Med Genet 1985; 20:159–163.

Stoll C, et al.: Male-to-male transmission of the hypertelorism-hypospadias (BBB) syndrome. Am J Med Genet 1985; 20:221–225.

Sedano HO, Gorlin RJ: Opitz oculo-genital-laryngeal syndrome. (Letter) Am J Med Genet 1988; 30:847–849.

CH029                                                    **Joe C. Christian**

---

## HYPERTELORISM-MICROTIA-FACIAL CLEFT-CONDUCTIVE DEAFNESS                                0506

**Includes:**
> Bixler syndrome
> Clefting (facial)-hypertelorism-microtia-conductive deafness
> Deafness (conductive)-hypertelorism-microtia-facial clefting
> Hypertelorism-microtia-facial clefting (HMC) syndrome
> Microtia-facial clefting-hypertelorism

**Excludes:**
> **Hypertelorism-microtia-facial cleft-conductive deafness** (0506)
> **Face, median cleft face syndrome** (0635)
> **Oto-palato-digital syndrome, I** (0786)
> **Oto-palato-digital syndrome, II** (2258)

**Major Diagnostic Criteria:** Hypertelorism, microtia and cleft lip and palate.

**Clinical Findings:** Five patients from three families have been identified, among them a pair of identical twins, who have been described with hypertelorism, microtia, clefting and deafness. Hypertelorism and microtia with meatal atresia were found in

each case. Other findings include unilateral cleft lip and palate (4/5); microcephaly (2/5); syndactyly of 2nd and 3rd toes (4/5); shortening of the 5th finger (4/5); mandibular arch hypoplasia (5/5); flattened angle of mandible (5/5); broad nasal tip (3/5); bifid nose (1/5); microstomia (3/5); bilateral thenar hypoplasia (4/5); ectopic kidneys (3/5); congenital heart anomalies (3/5); and vertebral anomalies (4/5). Reduced body weight and size are noted in all. In two affected individuals polytomographic examination revealed hypoplasia of the auditory ossicles and normal vestibula, cochlea, semicircular canals and internal auditory canals bilaterally. Congenital heart and vertebral anomalies were seen in several family members.

**Complications:** Feeding problems and later speech difficulties if cleft palate is present. Recurrent ear, nasal and paranasal infections.

**Associated Findings:** Mental retardation.

**Etiology:** Autosomal recessive inheritance.

**Pathogenesis:** Unknown.

**MIM No.:** *23980

**POS No.:** 3259

**Sex Ratio:** M3:F2

**Occurrence:** Undetermined. Three reported families with five affected individuals.

**Risk of Recurrence for Patient's Sib:**
See Part I, *Mendelian Inheritance.*

**Risk of Recurrence for Patient's Child:**
See Part I, *Mendelian Inheritance.*

**Age of Detectability:** At birth.

**Gene Mapping and Linkage:** Unknown.

**Prevention:** None known. Genetic counseling indicated.

**Treatment:** Reconstructive surgery of the external auditory canal and auricle. Plastic surgery to repair cleft lip and palate. Hearing aid and special training when hearing impaired. Orthodontic treatment and speech therapy in cases of cleft palate.

**Prognosis:** Probably normal life span.

**Detection of Carrier:** Unknown.

**References:**
Bixler D, et al.: Hypertelorism, microtia and facial clefting. a newly described inherited syndrome. Am J Dis Child 1969; 118:495–498. *
Ionasescu V, Roberts RJ: Variant of Bixler syndrome. J Genet Hum 1974; 22:133–136.
Schweckendiek W, et al.: H.M.C. syndrome in identical twins. Hum Genet 1976; 33:315–318. †
Baraitser M: The hypertelorism microtia clefting syndrome. J Med Genet 1982; 19:387–388.

SH046                                                  **Kathleen Shaver**
                                                       *Cor W.R.J. Cremers*

**Hypertelorism-microtia-facial clefting (HMC) syndrome**
  *See* HYPERTELORISM-MICROTIA-FACIAL CLEFT-CONDUCTIVE DEAFNESS
**Hypertelorism-ulcer, peptic/hiatal hernia-cafe-au-lait-myopia**
  *See* GASTROCUTANEOUS SYNDROME
**Hypertension medication, fetal effects**
  *See* FETAL EFFECTS FROM MATERNAL VASODILATOR
**Hypertension, maternal treatment, fetal ACE inhibitors**
  *See* FETAL ANGIOTENSIN CONVERTING ENZYME (ACE) INHIBITION RENAL FAILURE
**Hypertension, maternal, and fetal developmental retardation**
  *See* FETAL DEVELOPMENTAL RETARDATION WITH MATERNAL HYPERTENSION
**Hypertensive congenital adrenal hyperplasia**
  *See* STEROID 17 ALPHA-HYDROXYLASE DEFICIENCY
**Hypertensive form of adrenal hyperplasia**
  *See* STEROID 11 BETA-HYDROXYLASE DEFICIENCY
**Hyperthermia of anesthesia**
  *See* MYOPATHY, MALIGNANT HYPERTHERMIA
**Hyperthermia, fetal effects from maternal**
  *See* FETAL EFFECTS FROM MATERNAL HYPERTHERMIA

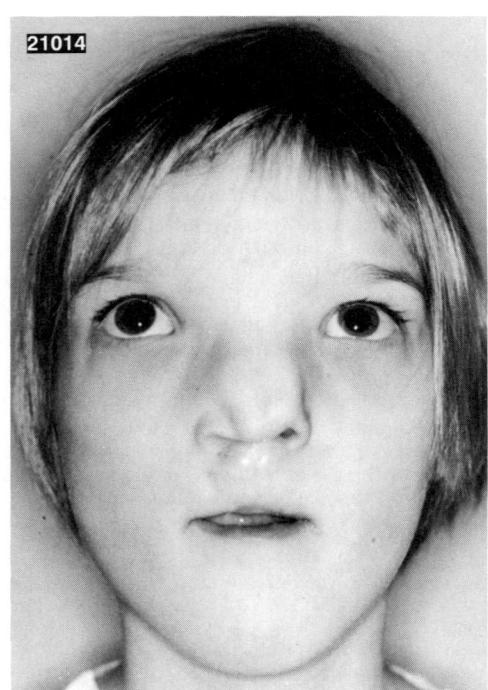

**0506-21014:** Affected girl with repaired cleft lip and palate, hypertelorism, and bifid nose.

**Hyperthyroidism**
*See THYROTOXICOSIS*
**Hypertrichosis lanuginosa, congenital**
*See HAIR, HYPERTRICHOSIS, LANUGINOSA*
**Hypertrichosis pinnae auris**
*See EAR, HAIRY*
**Hypertrichosis universalis**
*See HAIR, HYPERTRICHOSIS, LANUGINOSA*
**Hypertrichosis, congenital generalized**
*See HAIR, HYPERTRICHOSIS, X-LINKED*
**Hypertrichosis, fetal effect from maternal vasodilator**
*See FETAL EFFECTS FROM MATERNAL VASODILATOR*
**Hypertrichosis, X-linked**
*See HAIR, HYPERTRICHOSIS, X-LINKED*
**Hypertrichosis-gingival fibromatosis**
*See GINGIVAL FIBROMATOSIS-HYPERTRICHOSIS*
**Hypertrichosis-gingival fibromatosis-fibroadenomas of breasts**
*See GINGIVAL MULTIPLE HAMARTOMA SYNDROME*
**Hypertrichosis-midface retraction-X-ray and renal anomalies**
*See SCHINZEL-GIEDION SYNDROME*
**Hypertrichotic osteochondrodysplasia**
*See OSTEOCHONDRODYSPLASIA WITH HYPERTRICHOSIS*

---

## HYPERTRIGLYCERIDEMIA                      0500

**Includes:**

Carbohydrate-induced hyperlipemia
Hyperlipoproteinemia IV
Hyperprebetalipoproteinemia, familial
Lipoproteinemia-hyperprebeta

**Excludes:**
Hypercholesteremia (0488)
Hyperlipoproteinemia, broad beta type (0495)
Hyperlipoproteinemia V (0501)

**Major Diagnostic Criteria:** Family history including the demonstration of hypertriglyceridemia in approximately 50% of adult first degree relatives is necessary to make this diagnosis. At present, the basic defect in familial hypertriglyceridemia is not known, and there is no specific genetic or biochemical marker for the disease. Affected individuals may also have obesity, insulin resistance, fasting hyperinsulinemia, glucose intolerance, and hyperuricemia. Many individuals with hypertriglyceridemia have this condition on a nongenetic basis.

**Clinical Findings:** Patients with familial hypertriglyceridemia have elevated triglyceride levels typically in the range of 250 to 500 mg/dl. This is usually associated with diminished HDL cholesterol levels. Affected individuals have an increased incidence of coronary heart disease and perhaps peripheral vascular disease but do not develop xanthomas.

**Complications:** Premature coronary artery disease. Peripheral vascular disease.

**Associated Findings:** Possible relationship to diabetes and rheumatic manifestations.

**Etiology:** Autosomal dominant inheritance.

**Pathogenesis:** Undetermined. The major metabolic disturbance appears to be overproduction of triglycerides. Plasma triglyceride levels in some individuals with familial hypertriglyceridemia are very sensitive to carbohydrates in the diet. Postheparin plasma reveals normal lipoprotein lipase activity.

**MIM No.:** 14460, *14575

**Sex Ratio:** M1:F1

**Occurrence:** Probably on the order of 1–10:1000 live births.

**Risk of Recurrence for Patient's Sib:**
See Part I, *Mendelian Inheritance.*

**Risk of Recurrence for Patient's Child:**
See Part I, *Mendelian Inheritance.*

**Age of Detectability:** The plasma triglyceride elevation is fully expressed in affected adult relatives, but expression in children is incomplete.

**Gene Mapping and Linkage:** Unknown.

**Prevention:** None known. Genetic counseling indicated.

**Treatment:** Medical treatment generally consists of recommending weight loss and carbohydrate restriction. Drug treatment with gemfibrozil and nicotinic acid have been successfully used to lower triglyceride and raise HDL cholesterol levels.

**Prognosis:** May develop premature coronary or peripheral vascular disease. The benefit of therapies designed to lower plasma triglyceride and raise HDL cholesterol levels are not yet established.

**Detection of Carrier:** Unknown.

**References:**
Fredrickson DS, et al.: Fat transport in lipoproteins: an integrated approach to mechanisms and disorders. New Engl J Med 1967; 276:32,94,148,215,273.
Goldman JA, et al.: Musculoskeletal disorders associated with type IV hyperlipoproteinemia. Lancet 1972; II:449–452.
Levy RI, et al.: Dietary and drug treatment of primary hyperlipoproteinemia. Ann Intern Med 1972; 77:267.
Fredrickson DS, Levy RI: Familial hyperlipoproteinemia. In: Stanbury JB, et al., eds: The metabolic basis of inherited disease. ed. 5. New York: McGraw-Hill, 1982:545.
Karathanasis SK, et al.: Linkage of human apolipoproteins A-I and C-III genes. Nature 1983; 304:371–373.
Frederickson DS, Levy RI: Lipoprotein and lipid metabolism disorders. In: Scriver C, et al., eds: The metabolic basis of inherited disease, 6th ed. New York: McGraw-Hill, 1989:1129–1303.

BR010                                                     **Jan L. Breslow**

**Hypertriglyceridemia-coronary artery disease (some cases)**
*See HYPERAPOBETALIPOPROTEINEMIA*
**Hypertrophic ear lobes**
*See EAR LOBE, HYPERTROPHIC THICKENED*
**Hypertrophic interstitial neuropathy of Dejerine-Sottas**
*See DEJERINE-SOTTAS DISEASE*
**Hypertrophic osteoarthropathy, primary or idiopathic**
*See PACHYDERMOPERIOSTOSIS*
**Hypertrophic pyloric stenosis, congenital**
*See PYLORIC STENOSIS*
**Hypertrophy, unilateral**
*See HEMIHYPERTROPHY*
**Hyperuricemia, primary**
*See GOUT*
**Hyperuricemia, primary, familial**
*See GOUT*
**Hyperuricemia, X-linked primary**
*See LESCH-NYHAN SYNDROME*
**Hyperuricemia-deafness (sensorineural)-ataxia**
*See PHOSPHORIBOSYL PYROPHOSPHATE (PRPP) SYNTHETASE ABNORMALITY*

---

## HYPERVALINEMIA                            0509

**Includes:**
Valine transaminase deficiency
Valinemia

**Excludes:** Maple syrup urine disease (0628)

**Major Diagnostic Criteria:** Mental and growth retardation occur with vomiting and muscle weakness. Hypervalinemia is present with normal plasma levels of leucine and isoleucine. Ketoaciduria is not present. A deficiency in valine transamination is demonstrable in peripheral leukocytes.

**Clinical Findings:** Two families have been reported. A Japanese boy with mental and physical retardation, hyperkinesis, poor feeding and vomiting was noted to have hypervalinemia. A deficiency in valine transamination was demonstrated in peripheral leukocytes. A report from India describes two siblings, a boy and a girl, with mental and physical retardation, occasional vomiting, and muscular weakness. Plasma valine was greatly elevated in the children (150 μmoles/dl) and moderately elevated in parents (65 μmoles/dl). Enzymatic studies were not done.

**Complications:** In both reported families the diagnosis of hypervalinemia was made during diagnostic studies for retardation. A causal relation is therefore uncertain. In the Japanese child, vomiting stopped, weight gain began, and hyperkinesis was reduced following introduction of a low valine diet, suggesting that these symptoms were secondary to hypervalinemia.

**Associated Findings:** None known.

**Etiology:** Autosomal recessive inheritance. A specific valine transaminase is suggested by the observations.

**Pathogenesis:** The first step in the degradation of the branched chain amino acids is transamination to the respective keto acids. The next step, that of oxidative decarboxylation, is defective in **Maple syrup urine disease.** Experimental data have suggested that one transaminase is effective against the three branched chain amino acids. In contrast, the clinical entities of hypervalinemia and hyperleucine-isoleucinemia indicate that there are specific transaminases.

**MIM No.:** *27710

**Sex Ratio:** M1:F1

**Occurrence:** Three cases in two families have been reported.

**Risk of Recurrence for Patient's Sib:**
See Part I, *Mendelian Inheritance.*

**Risk of Recurrence for Patient's Child:**
See Part I, *Mendelian Inheritance.*

**Age of Detectability:** Enzymatic defect should be demonstrable at birth.

**Gene Mapping and Linkage:** Unknown.

**Prevention:** None known. Genetic counseling indicated.

**Treatment:** A low valine diet would be a rational approach. Its effectiveness in preventing retardation has not been confirmed, but it appears to relieve some of the associated symptoms.

**Prognosis:** Survival, at least for several years, is possible in the untreated child. Longer range studies have not been reported.

**Detection of Carrier:** Unknown.

**References:**
Wada Y, et al.: Idiopathic hypervalinemia: probably a new entity of inborn error of valine metabolism. Tohoku J Exp Med 1963; 81:46–55.
Wada Y: Idiopathic hypervalinemia: valine alpha-keto-acids in blood following an oral dose of valine. Tohoku J Exp Med 1965; 87:322–331.
Dancis J, et al.: Hypervalinemia: a defect in valine transamination. Pediatrics 1967; 39:813–817.
Jeune M, et al.: Hyperleucineisoleucinemia par defaut partial de transamination associée a une hyperprolinemie de type 2. Ann Pediat 1970; 17:349–363.
Reddi DS, et al.: A sibship with hypervalinemia. Hum Genet 1977; 39:139–142.

DA003                                               **Joseph Dancis**

**Hypervitaminosis A, fetal effects from**
*See FETAL RETINOID SYNDROME*
**Hypoacetylation**
*See ACETYLATOR POLYMORPHISM*
**Hypoadrenocorticism, familial**
*See ADRENAL HYPOPLASIA, CONGENITAL*
**Hypoadrenocorticism-hypoparathyroidism-superficial moniliasis**
*See POLYGLANDULAR AUTOIMMUNE SYNDROME*

## HYPOALPHALIPOPROTEINEMIA                                  3096

**Includes:**
AI apolipoprolipoprotein variants
Apolipoprolipoprotein A-I variants (3A, 3B, 3C)
Giessen (AI) apolipoprolipoprotein variants
Marburg (AI) apolipoprolipoprotein variants
Milano (AI) apolipoprolipoprotein variants

**Excludes:**
**Lecithin-cholesterol acyl transferase deficiency** (0580)
**Analphalipoproteinemia** (0048)
**Apolipoprotein A-I and C-III deficiency states** (3165)

**Major Diagnostic Criteria:** Plasma high density lipoproprotein (HDL) cholesterol levels below 35 mg/dl (mean approximately 25 mg/dl), and plasma apolipoprotein (apo) A-I levels below 100 mg/dl for all the disorders, and for apolipoprotein A-1 variants an abnormal isoelectric point is noted when apoA-I is subjected to isoelectric focusing (one abnormal and one normal band are noted because all affected subjects have been heterozygotes). For apoA-I (Milano) and apoA-I (Marburg) the charge difference was -1 compared to normal apoA-I while for other variants it was +1.

**Clinical Findings:** In hypoalphalipoproteinemia a clear association with premature coronary artery disease (CAD) prior to age 50 years as well as stroke has been reported. In the apoA-I Milano kindred no evidence of premature CAD was noted, and in the other apoA-I variants clinical features in probands and kindred members have not been clearly reported.

**Complications:** Accelerated atherosclerosis in hypoalphalipoproteinemia. No clear complications on other disorders.

**Associated Findings:** Plasma low density lipoprotein cholesterol and triglyceride values are generally normal in hypoalphalipoproteinemia, while in apoA-I Milano hypertriglyceridemia is often present.

**Etiology:** Autosomal dominant inheritance. The precise defect in hypoalphalipoproteinemia is not known, but the disorder has been associated with a Pst 1 restriction site polymorphism adjacent to the 3' end of the apoA-I gene. In the apoA-I variant states specific mutations in the apoA-I sequence have been reported. ApoA-I (Milano) is due to an arginine for cysteine substitution at residue 173, apoA-I (Marburg) is due to a deletion of lysine at residue 107, apoA-I (Giessen) is due to a proline for arginine substitution at residue 143, apoA-I (Munster 3A) is due to an aspartate for asparagine substitution at residue 103, apoA-I (Munster 3B) is due to a proline for arginine substitution at residue 4, while apoA-I (Munster 3C) is due to a proline for histidine substitution at residue 3. The mutation at residue 107 (apoA-I Marburg) results in a decreased ability of apoA-I to activate lecithin: cholesterol acyltransferase, the enzyme which esterifies cholesterol in plasma.

**Pathogenesis:** It has been reported that hypoalphalipoproteinemia is due to decreased apoA-I production, while in apoA-I (Milano) there is enhanced catabolism.

**MIM No.:** 10766, *10768, *10769, *10771

**Sex Ratio:** M1:F1

**Occurrence:** Hypoalphalipoproteinemia is a common disorder with an estimated frequency of 1:100, while the apoA-I variant states have only been reported for individual kindreds.

**Risk of Recurrence for Patient's Sib:**
See Part I, *Mendelian Inheritance.*

**Risk of Recurrence for Patient's Child:**
See Part I, *Mendelian Inheritance.*

**Age of Detectability:** Probably at birth by measurement of plasma HDL cholesterol and apoA-I levels.

**Gene Mapping and Linkage:** APOA1 (apolipoprotein A-I) has been mapped to 11q23-q24.
APOA4 (apolipoprotein A-IV) has been mapped to 11q23-qter.
APOC1 (apolipoprotein C-I) has been mapped to 19q13.2.
For some hypoalphalipoproteinemia kindreds and all apoA-I variant states, linkage has been established to abnormalities in the apoA-I, apoC-III, apoA-IV gene complex on the long arm of chromosome 11.

**Prevention:** None known. Genetic counseling indicated.

**Treatment:** For hypoalphalipoproteinemia, aggressive therapy of other risk factors for CAD if present such as hypertension, cigarette smoking, diabetes mellitus, and elevated LDL cholesterol, are indicated. Weight reduction in the overweight patient and a regular exercise program are also useful, as are medications such as niacin and gemfibrozil, to raise HDL cholesterol levels and hopefully decrease the risk of premature CAD.

**Prognosis:** Good. The incidence of premature CAD under age 55 years is high.

**Detection of Carrier:** For hypoalphalipoproteinemia, heterozygotes and homozygotes both appear to have HDL cholesterol and apoA-I values that are about 50% of normal, while for apoA-I variants only heterozygotes have been reported.

**References:**

Francheschini G, et al: A-I Milano apoprotein: decreased high density lipoprotein cholesterol with significant lipoprotein modifications and without significant atherosclerosis in an Italian family. J Clin Invest 1980; 66:892–900.

Weisgraber KH, et al: Apoprotein A-I Milano, isolation and characterization of a cysteine containing variant of the apoprotein A-I from human high density lipoprotein. J Clin Invest 1980; 66:901–909.

Vergani C, Bettale A: Familial hypoalphalipoproteinemia. Clin Chim Acta 1981; 114:45–52.

Ghiselli G, et al: Abnormal catabolism of apoA-I Milano. Clin Res 1982; 30:291A.

Menzel HJ, et al: Human apoprotein A-I polymorphism. J Biol Chem 1984; 259:3070–3076.

Rall SC Jr., et al: Abnormal lecithin: cholesterol acyltransferase activation by a human apolipoprotein variant in which a single lysine is deleted. J Biol Chem 1984; 259:10063–10070.

Schaefer EJ: Clinical, biochemical, and genetic features in familial disorders of high density lipoprotein deficiency. Arteriosclerosis 1984; 4:303–322.

Third JHLC, et al: Primary and familial hypoalphalipoproteinemia. Metabolism 1984; 33:136–146.

Ordovas JM, et al: Apolipoprotein A-I gene polymorphism associated with premature coronary artery and familial hypoalphalipoproteinemia. New Engl J Med 1986; 314:671–677.

SC065                            **Ernst J. Schaefer**
0R006                            **Jose M. Ordovas**

---

## HYPOBETALIPOPROTEINEMIA                  2386

**Includes:**

Acanthocytosis-hypobetalipoproteinemia
Beta-lipoprotein deficiency, congenital
Homozygous hypobetalipoproteinemia
Hypobetalipoproteinemia, familial
Primary hypobetalipoproteinemia

**Excludes:**

Abetalipoproteinemia (0002)
Hypobetalipoproteinemia, secondary
Hypobetalipoproteinemia-chylomicronemia, familial
Normotriglyceridemic abetalipoproteinemia

**Major Diagnostic Criteria:** *Heterozygotes*: Three criteria have been proposed: 1) decreased blood levels of low-density lipoproteins (LDL) and very-low-density lipoproteins (VLDL); 2) absence of diseases causing secondary hypobetalipoproteinemia; and 3) detection of similar abnormalities in first-degree relatives.

Blood cholesterol levels are generally decreased, and the plasma triglyceride concentration is usually less than 100 mg/dl. High-density lipoprotein (HDL) levels are usually normal.

*Homozygotes*: Profound hypocholesterolemia and hypotriglyceridemia with absence of LDL and VLDL. Distinction from abetalipoproteinemia is made by a study of the parents. In homozygous hypobetalipoproteinemia, each parent is heterozygous and has the chemical abnormalities described above. The parents of a patient with abetalipoproteinemia demonstrate no such abnormalities.

**Clinical Findings:** *Heterozygotes*: Patients heterozygous for hypobetalipoproteinemia are usually asymptomatic. Aversion to fatty foods is common in symptomatic patients. There is no evidence of fat malabsorption, acanthocytosis, or pigmentary retinal degeneration. Several subjects with neurologic disorders have been described. The neurologic picture generally is one of peripheral neuropathy and spinocerebellar degeneration without involvement of vision or hearing. One patient with psychomotor retardation, microcephaly, and seizures has been described. Neurologic dysfunction is not a constant feature of heterozygous hypobetalipoproteinemia. It is not at all clear why some patients

develop the neurologic disorder. Chemical studies show that blood cholesterol, triglyceride LDL, and VLDL levels are low. Apolipoprotein B is decreased.

*Homozygotes:* Patients with homozygous hypobetalipoproteinemia resemble those with **Abetalipoproteinemia**. They have fat malabsorption and accumulation of neutral fat in the epithelial cells of the intestinal mucosa. Acanthocytosis and pigmentary retinal degeneration have usually been present. Neurologic dysfunction, when present, is characterized by areflexia or hyporeflexia and mild peripheral neuropathy. These patients have milder neuromuscular dysfunction than patients with abetalipoproteinemia.

Blood cholesterol and triglyceride levels are profoundly decreased. There is no detectable LDL and VLDL, and apolipoprotein B is absent. Vitamin A and E levels are low, and hypoprothrombinemia is usually present. One report describes detection of apolipoprotein B in minute quantities in a homozygous patient.

**Complications:** Decreased sensitivity to local anesthetics has been noted. In the homozygotes, physical growth may be impaired because of malabsorption. Vitamin A and E levels are decreased, and supplementation with water-soluble forms may be necessary. Low serum LDL-cholesterol and normal HDL levels may be protective against coronary atherosclerosis.

**Associated Findings:** One patient with psychomotor retardation, **Microcephaly**, and seizures has been described.

**Etiology:** Autosomal dominant inheritance.

**Pathogenesis:** It is postulated that there is a decrease in the ability to synthesize apolipoprotein B-100 and B-48 with consequent decrease in LDL and VLDL levels. LDLs are the major cholesterol-carrying lipoproteins, and VLDLs are the major triglyceride carriers in plasma. Hence, levels of both the cholesterol and triglycerides are decreased. It is believed that decreased levels of fat-soluble vitamins (A, E, and K) may be responsible for at least part of the clinical picture.

**MIM No.:** 14595

**Sex Ratio:** M1:F1

**Occurrence:** Estimated at 3–10:10,000.

**Risk of Recurrence for Patient's Sib:**
See Part I, *Mendelian Inheritance.*

**Risk of Recurrence for Patient's Child:**
See Part I, *Mendelian Inheritance.*

**Age of Detectability:** Detectable by lipid analysis in childhood.

**Gene Mapping and Linkage:** Unknown.

**Prevention:** None known. Genetic counseling indicated.

**Treatment:** Treatment of asymptomatic heterozygote is not indicated. Only symptomatic heterozygotes and the affected homozygotes require treatment. Supplementation with vitamins A and E has been advocated. Hypoprothrombinemia is treated with vitamin K.

**Prognosis:** Low LDL-cholesterol and normal HDL levels may be protective against coronary atherosclerosis and may prolong life span in the heterozygotes.

**Detection of Carrier:** Measurement of LDL, VLDL, cholesterol, and triglycerides.

**Special Considerations:** There appears to be considerable variability in the neurologic disorder associated with hypobetalipoproteinemia. Vitamin E has been implicated in the pathogenesis even though vitamin E levels have been variable. Supplementary vitamins A, E, and K should be given when their levels are low or hypoprothrombinemia is present.

**References:**

Mars HN, et al.: Familial hypobetalipoproteinemia. Am J Med 1969; 46:886–900.

Aggerbeck LP, et al.: Hypobetalipoproteinemia: clinical and biochemical description of a new kindred with "Friedreich's ataxia." Neurology 1974; 24:1051–1063.

Cottrill C, et al.: Familial homozygous hypobetalipoproteinemia. Metabolism 1974; 23:779–791.

Malloy MJ, Kane JP: Hypolipidemia. Med Clin North Am 1982; 66:469–484.

Berger GMB, et al.: Apolipoprotein B detected in the plasma of a patient with homozygous hypobetalipoproteinemia: implications for aetiology. J Med Genet 1983; 20:189–195.

Parker CR Jr, et al: Endocrine changes during pregnancy in a patient with homozygous familial hypobetalipoproteinemia. New Engl J Med 1986; 314:557–560.

GA018                                                    **Bhuwan P. Garg**

**Hypobetalipoproteinemia, familial**
    *See HYPOBETALIPOPROTEINEMIA*
**Hypobetalipoproteinemia-apoprotein in intestinal cells**
    *See LIPID TRANSPORT DEFECT OF INTESTINE*
**Hypocalcemia-dwarfism-cortical thickening of tubular bones**
    *See TUBULAR STENOSIS*
**Hypocalcemic rickets, type IIa**
    *See RESISTANCE TO 1,25 DIHYDROXY VITAMIN D*
**Hypocalcemic, hypophosphatemic rickets with aminoaciduria**
    *See RESISTANCE TO 1,25 DIHYDROXY VITAMIN D*
    *also RICKETS, VITAMIN D-DEPENDENT, TYPE I*
**Hypoceruloplasminemia**
    *See HEPATOLENTICULAR DEGENERATION*

## HYPOCERULOPLASMINEMIA                                 3077

**Includes:**  Serum ceruloplasmin, low

**Excludes:**
    Copper retention
    Copper toxicosis, inherited
    **Hepatolenticular degeneration** (0469)
    Lenticular degeneration, progressive

**Major Diagnostic Criteria:**  Serum ceruloplasmin levels are below 21 mg/dl in males and below 23 mg/dl in females for this heterozygous, asymptomatic condition. Possible homozygotes in one reported family have a serum level below 1 mg/dl.

**Clinical Findings:**  There are no clinical findings in the heterozygous state. There are normal levels of serum and urine copper, no Kaiser-Fleischer rings, and no iron retention. Three presumably homozygous individuals have been reported; the oldest woman had retinal degeneration, blepharospasm, and iron deposition in the basal ganglia. A younger brother and sister had retinal degeneration and a region of high density in the basal ganglia, without neurologic symptoms. The son and daughter of the affected woman had diminished levels of ceruloplasmin.

**Complications:**  Unknown.

**Associated Findings:**  One family was identified during studies for hemochromatosis, but the affected individuals did not have hypoceruloplasminemia.

**Etiology:**  Autosomal dominant inheritance. Male-to-male transmission has been reported.

**Pathogenesis:**  In the heterozygous state, there is no pathologic consequence. In the homozygous condition, the absence of ceruloplasmin, which is also a ferroxidase, results in a disturbance of iron metabolism.

**MIM No.:**  *11770

**Sex Ratio:**  M1:F1

**Occurrence:**  Two small families and one large Utah kindred have been reported, with a total of 20 asymptomatic people with hypoceruloplasminemia. However, since this is a benign condition, any cases would be discovered serendipitously, and the occurrence is probably underestimated.

**Risk of Recurrence for Patient's Sib:**
    See Part I, *Mendelian Inheritance.*

**Risk of Recurrence for Patient's Child:**
    See Part I, *Mendelian Inheritance.*

**Age of Detectability:**  Ceruloplasmin levels are low in the neonate and increase rapidly during infancy, peaking above adult levels by ages 2–3 years. Then there is a steady decline in ceruloplasmin levels until age 12 years when adult levels are reached in female.

Male levels continue to decline somewhat. Therefore, for any age studied, age-matched controls are mandatory. Formulae are available for correction to adult levels.

**Gene Mapping and Linkage:**  CPP (ceruloplasmin pseudogene) has been mapped to 8q21.13-q23.1.
    CP (ceruloplasmin) has been mapped to 3q23-q25.

**Prevention:**  None known. Genetic counseling indicated. Since the condition is benign, prevention is not necessary.

**Treatment:**  No treatment is required.

**Prognosis:**  Excellent.

**Detection of Carrier:**  The carrier is the biochemically detected individual who has ceruloplasmin levels below 23 mg/dl.

**Special Considerations:**  A homozygous state is possible and has been reported.

**References:**
Cox DW: Factors influencing serum ceruloplasmin levels in normal individuals. J Lab Clin Med 1966; 68:893–904

Edwards CQ, et al.: Hereditary hypoceruloplasminemia. Clin Genet 1979; 15:311–316.

Weitkamp LR, et al.: Evidence for linkage between the loci for transferrin and ceruloplasmin in man. Ann Hum Genet 1983; 47:293–297.

Takahashi N, et al.: Single-chain structure of human ceruloplasmin: the complete amino acid sequence of the whole molecule. Proc Natl Acad Sci USA 1984; 81:390–394.

Yang F, et al.: Characterization, mapping, and expression of the human ceruloplasmin gene. Proc Natl Acad Sci USA 1986; 83:3257–3261.

Miyajima H, et al.: Familial apoceruloplasmin deficiency associated with blepharospasm and retinal degeneration. Neurology 1987; 37:761–767.

VI006                                                    **Jaclyn M. Vidgoff**

## HYPOCHONDROPLASIA                                     0510

**Includes:**  N/A

**Excludes:**
    **Achondroplasia** (0010)
    **Dwarfism** (other short-limbed)

**Major Diagnostic Criteria:**  Mild-to-moderate short-limb dwarfism with a combination of clinical and X-ray features qualitatively similar to **Achondroplasia**, but generally milder in expression.

**Clinical Findings:**  Both children and adults have small stature with disproportionately short limbs. Hands and feet are short and broad. The relative shortening of the limbs may be mild. Limitation of motion at the elbow is common. No trident hand deformity occurs. Fibulae are disproportionately long, and mild bowleg and heel varus deformities may be present. The head may be normal or large with the skull configuration tending to be brachycephalic with a prominent forehead. There is no depression of nasal bridge or other facial abnormality. Adult height is between 126–145 cm.

X-ray findings: Short ilia with less iliac crest flare than normal, but more than in achondroplasia. The femoral necks are usually short (frontal projection). Interpediculate distance is the same or narrows from L1 to L5 (frontal projection). This abnormality is not as marked as in achondroplasia and is usually not present in infants and young children. In most older children and adults, the backs of the lumbar bodies have a concave configuration, less marked than in achondroplasia. Pedicles are usually short (lateral projection).

Limbs are short, so the visual impression is that of mildly widened diaphyses and mildly flared metaphyses, both in long tubular bones and the bones of the hands and feet. Sites of muscle attachments are prominent. Ulnae are relatively short with prominence of ulnar styloid in adult. Square configuration of proximal tibial epiphysis and flare of adjacent metaphysis is found in the older child and adolescent. Distal fibulae are disproportionately long. In early childhood, there may be a shallow V-shaped indentation of distal femoral metaphysis, but, again not as marked

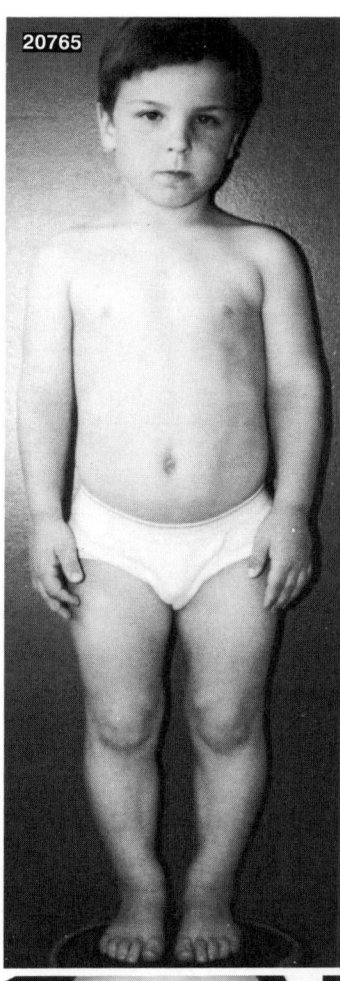
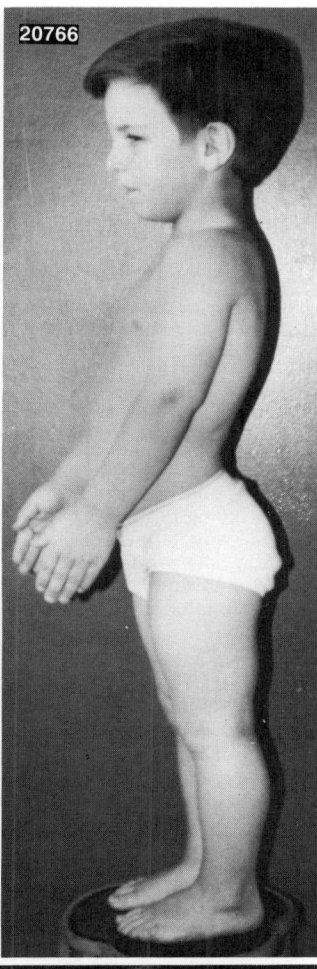
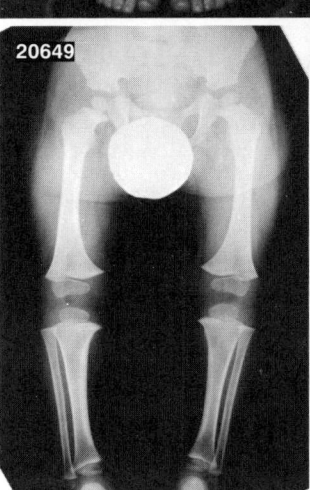
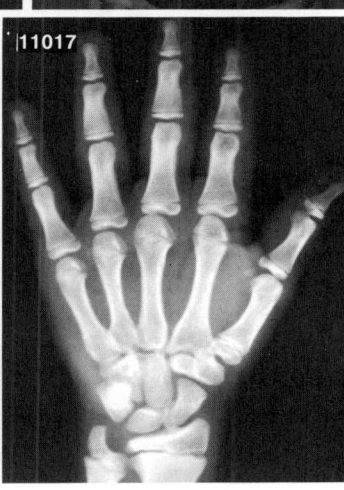

as in achondroplasia. This is a nonspecific change that occurs in other short-limb dwarf conditions. The skull X-rays are normal. No abnormal laboratory findings have been demonstrated.

Physical appearance and X-ray changes are qualitatively similar to those of achondroplasia, but they deviate from normal to a lesser degree. There is considerable variability in the severity of changes in hypochondroplasia in the severely involved hypochondroplastic. The differential diagnostic consideration is achondroplasia, and, in the mildly involved hypochondroplastic the differential diagnostic consideration is the small normal person. Individuals with the changes of both achondroplasia and hypochondroplasia have not been seen in the same family. Thus, the defect does not appear to represent mild achondroplasia, although severely affected hypochondroplasts have been so diagnosed in the past.

**Complications:** Spinal stenosis complications are rare. However, mild mental retardation has been reported to be higher than in the general population.

**Associated Findings:** None known.

**Etiology:** Autosomal dominant inheritance.

**Pathogenesis:** Relatively slow enchondral bone growth with normal membranous ossification.

**MIM No.:** 14600

**POS No.:** 3260

**Sex Ratio:** M1:F1

**Occurrence:** Undetermined. At least five kindreds have been documented, but it is felt that since the condition may be mild, it is probably not rare. It has been postulated that hypochondroplasia may represent an allele of the gene for achondroplasia. In mild cases, the disproportion may not be readily apparent without performing anthropometric measurements, and many patients have been considered at first to be proportionate and have received unnecessary endocrine evaluations.

**Risk of Recurrence for Patient's Sib:**
See Part I, *Mendelian Inheritance.*

**Risk of Recurrence for Patient's Child:**
See Part I, *Mendelian Inheritance.*

**Age of Detectability:** Mean birth length is decreased, but in sporadic cases the mild to moderate short stature may not be noticed until 4–6 years of age.

**Gene Mapping and Linkage:** Unknown.

**Prevention:** None known. Genetic counseling indicated.

**Treatment:** Osteotomies for significant bowleg deformity, laminectomy for symptomatic spinal stenosis, medical and surgical treatment for otitis media and complications. Cesarean section necessary for delivery in most affected pregnant women.

**Prognosis:** Normal life span.

**Detection of Carrier:** Unknown.

**References:**
Beals RK: Hypochondroplasia: a report of five kindreds. J Bone Joint Surg 1969; 51A:728–736.
Walker BA, et al.: Hypochondroplasia. Am J Dis Child 1971; 122:95–104.
Hall BD, Spranger J: Hypochondroplasia: clinical and radiological aspects in 39 cases. Radiology 1979; 133:95–100.
Sommer A, et al.: Achondroplasia-hypochondroplasia complex. Am J Med Genet 1987; 26:949–957.

B0025
LA006
LA016

Zvi Borochowitz
Ralph S. Lachman
Leonard O. Langer, Jr.

**0510**-20765–66: Hypochondroplasia; note short stature, short limbs with short broad hands, lordosis, and normal facies. 20649: Hypochondroplasia in a boy aged 2 years, 4 months; note small pelvis with square iliac wing, wide-appearing diaphysis of the long bones and flaring of the metaphyseal-epiphyseal junction. 11017: Generalized shortening of bones and long and curved ulna styloid.

**Hypochromic anemia, congenital**
*See ANEMIA, CONGENITAL SIDEROBLASTIC, NOT B(6) RESPONSIVE*
**Hypoctasia, primary**
*See LACTASE DEFICIENCY, PRIMARY*
**Hypodontia**
*See TEETH, ANODONTIA, PARTIAL OR COMPLETE*

**Hypodontia-mesoectodermal dysgenesis of iris and cornea**
*See RIEGER SYNDROME*
*also EYE, ANTERIOR SEGMENT DYSGENESIS*

## HYPODONTIA-NAIL DYSGENESIS 0511

**Includes:**
Nail dysgenesis and hypodontia
Tooth and nail syndrome

**Excludes:**
**Chondroectodermal dysplasia** (0156)
**Ectodermal dysplasia, Christ-Siemens-Touraine type** (0333)
**Ectodermal dysplasia, hidrotic** (0334)

**Major Diagnostic Criteria:** Congenitally missing teeth and history of slow growth of nails.

**Clinical Findings:** Children have congenitally missing teeth (from one to seldom more than 20) and a retardation in growth of nails best seen from birth to three years of age without other signs of anhidrotic ectodermal dysplasia. Nails are small, thin, and often spoon-shaped. Older children and adults frequently have normal fingernails, but small spoon-shaped toenails.

This is one cause of congenitally missing teeth that should be differentiated from the X-linked and autosomal recessive forms of anhidrotic or hypohidrotic ectodermal dysplasia, wherein missing teeth are common. **Ectodermal dysplasia, hidrotic** is common in French Canadians but is not accompanied by missing teeth. Hypoplasia of nails is frequently noted in retrospect by history of the mother not needing to trim the nails until the child is 18 to 24 months of age. Toenails are usually more severely affected than fingernails.

**Complications:** Possible loss of vertical face dimension due to loss of teeth, resulting in eversion of lips.

**Associated Findings:** Fine scalp hair (50%); eversion of lips (20%).

**Etiology:** Autosomal dominant inheritance with variable expressivity.

**Pathogenesis:** Undetermined. Gene probably acts on specialized ectodermal cells involved in formation of dental lamina and anlage of nails. Nails may be absent at birth, or so slow growing as to not require cutting until age 2–3 years. Primary and permanent teeth, or only permanent teeth, may be missing.

**MIM No.:** *18950

**POS No.:** 3261

**Sex Ratio:** M1:F1

**Occurrence:** Estimated 1–2:10,000. Over 10 kindreds documented in one year. Occurs with high frequency among Dutch Mennonites of Canada.

**Risk of Recurrence for Patient's Sib:**
See Part I, *Mendelian Inheritance.*

**Risk of Recurrence for Patient's Child:**
See Part I, *Mendelian Inheritance.*

**Age of Detectability:** May suspect disorder at birth when physical examination reveals absence of one or more toe or fingernails. Detection usually occurs at 4–5 years of age by noting absence of teeth and finding absent or hypoplastic nails. At 7 to 15 years of age, absence of permanent teeth and hypoplastic nails are more commonly observed.

**Gene Mapping and Linkage:** Unknown.

**Prevention:** None known. Genetic counseling indicated.

**Treatment:** Dental restoration.

**Prognosis:** No reduction of longevity or fitness noted in kindreds examined.

**Detection of Carrier:** Unknown.

**References:**
Witkop CJ Jr: Genetic disease of the oral cavity In: Tiecke RW, ed: Oral pathology. New York: McGraw-Hill, 1965:810–814. †
Hudson CD, Witkop CJ Jr: Autosomal dominant hypodontia with nail dysgenesis: report of twenty-nine cases in six families. Oral Surg 1975; 39:409–423. *

WI043     **Carl J. Witkop, Jr.**

**Hypogammaglobulinemia, familial**
*See IMMUNODEFICIENCY, COMMON VARIABLE TYPE*
**Hypogammaglobulinemia, X-linked**
*See IMMUNODEFICIENCY, AGAMMAGLOBULINEMIA, X-LINKED, INFANTILE*
**Hypogammaglobulinemia-retinal telangiectasia**
*See RETINAL TELANGIECTASIA-HYPOGAMMAGLOBULINEMIA*
**Hypogammaglobulinemia-thymoma syndrome**
*See AGAMMAGLOBULINEMIA-THYMOMA SYNDROME*
**Hypogenital dystrophy with diabetic tendency**
*See PRADER-WILLI SYNDROME*

## HYPOGLOSSIA-HYPODACTYLIA 0451

**Includes:**
Aglossia-adactylia syndrome
Aglossia congenita
Ankyloglossum superior syndrome
Glossopalatine ankylosis syndrome
Hanhart syndrome
Oromandibular limb hypoplasia
Peromelia-micrognathia

**Excludes:**
**Acheiropody** (2486)
**Amniotic bands syndrome** (0874)
**Charlie M syndrome** (2170)
**Diplegia, congenital facial** (0376)
**Ectrodactyly** (0336)
**Oro-cranio-digital** syndromes
**Splenogonadal fusion-limb defect** (3053)
**Yunis-Varon syndrome** (2405)

**Major Diagnostic Criteria:** Variable distal limb deficiency with micrognathia.

**Clinical Findings:** Variable distal limb deficiency, ranging from hypoplasia or absence of digits to severe peromelia, which may resemble amelia. Phocomelia (absence only of intercalary portions of the limb) does not occur. The limb defects are typically asymmetric. Micrognathia may be severe and associated with cleft palate, intraoral bands, or fusion of the temporomandibular joints. Hypodontia and anodontia, especially of maxillary incisors, occur frequently. Hypoglossia is variable in severity, and may not occur in all cases. True aglossia does not occur. Congenital cranial nerve palsies can be associated, most often of the sixth and seventh cranial nerves, occasionally the third, fifth, ninth, and twelfth cranial nerves.

**Complications:** *Newborn period:* Feeding problems due to oral anomalies, aggravated by coexisting cranial nerve palsies. One infant with hypoglossia-hypodactylia and concomitant cranial nerve palsies required mechanical ventilation because of central hypoventilation.
*After newborn period:* Motor handicaps resulting from limb deficiencies; speech impediment; occasional mental retardation.

**Associated Findings:** Splenogonadal fusion of the continuous type may occur. This may be manifested as an undescended testis or as a testicular mass. Porencephalic cyst, clubfoot, intestinal atresia with "apple-peel bowel," unilateral renal agenesis, imperforate anus, and mental retardation.

**Etiology:** Sporadic developmental disturbance with no conclusive reports of familial recurrence. Discordant monozygotic twins have been reported. A drug and/or teratogen influence has also been postulated.

**Pathogenesis:** Disruption of blood supply to "watershed" areas of the developing limb buds, Meckel cartilage, and tongue between the fifth and seventh weeks of embryonic development. Disruption may arise from thrombosis or embolus such as results from the in utero death of a co-twin or from hypoperfusion caused by drug-induced vasoconstriction or vascular stasis. A similar

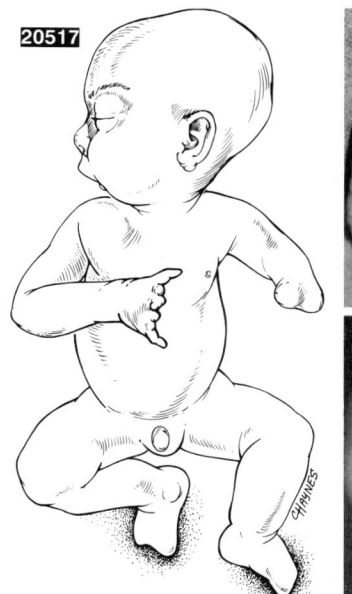

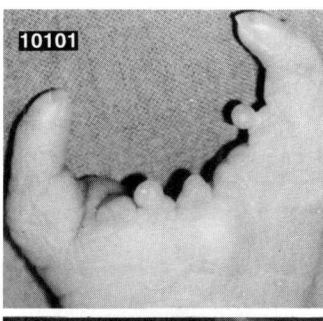

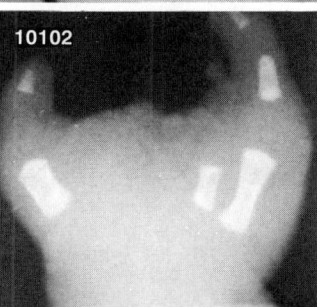

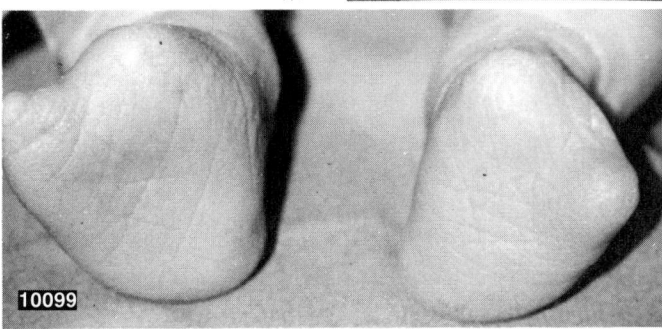

**0451-20517:** Variable limb deficiencies and micrognathia. **10099:** Deficiency of the anterior third of the feet. **10101:** Hypodactylia of the right hand with typical crab-type deformity. **10102:** X-ray demonstrating absence of most phalanges and some metacarpals.

spectrum of associated anomalies has been produced and studied in animal models.

**MIM No.:** 10330

**POS No.:** 3537

**CDC No.:** 750.110

**Sex Ratio:** M1:F1

**Occurrence:** <1:20,000 births.

**Risk of Recurrence for Patient's Sib:** Low (<1%).

**Risk of Recurrence for Patient's Child:** Low.

**Age of Detectability:** At birth. Potentially identifiable prenatally by ultrasound.

**Gene Mapping and Linkage:** Unknown.

**Prevention:** None known. Genetic counseling indicated.

**Treatment:** Plastic surgery, orthopedic surgery, limb prostheses, speech therapy, physical and occupational therapy.

**Prognosis:** With the exceptions noted above, the prognosis for health, life span, and intellectual development is good.

**Detection of Carrier:** Unknown.

**Special Considerations:** **Hypoglossia-hypodactylia**, Hanhart syndrome, Glossopalatine ankylosis syndrome, **Charlie M syndrome**, and Moebius syndrome are grouped together under the category of *Oromandibular-Limb Hypogenesis syndrome*. These are clearly overlapping conditions of unknown etiology. While we recognize that these may be variants of an environmentally (or other) induced spectrum of anomalies, the *Encyclopedia* has placed Hanhart syndrome and Glossopalatine ankylosis under the title **Hypoglossia-hypodactylia** and has separate articles on Moebius syndrome (**Diplegia, congenital facial**) and **Charlie M syndrome**.

**References:**

Hall BD: Aglossia-adactylia. BD:OAS;VII(7). New York: March of Dimes Birth Defects Foundation, 1971:233–236.

Herrmann J, et al.: Studies of malformation syndromes of man XXXXI B: nosologic studies in the Hanhart and the Möbius syndrome. Eur J Pediatr 1976; 122:19–55.

Johnson GF, Robinow M: Aglossia-adactylia. Radiology 1978; 128:127–132.

Van Allen MI, et al.: Expanded hypoglossia-hypodactylia spectra and its developmental pathology. Clin Res 1981; 29:133A.

Bokesoy I, et al.: Oromandibular limb hypogenesis/Hanhart's syndrome: possible drug influence on the malformation. Clin Genet 1983; 24:47–49.

Chandra Sekhar HK, et al.: Hanhart's syndrome with special reference to temporal bone findings. Ann Otol Rhinol Laryngol 1987; 96:309–314. †

FL001                                                        **David B. Flannery**

**Hypoglycemia with deficiency of glycogen synthetase in liver**
*See GLYCOGEN SYNTHETASE DEFICIENCY*

---

**HYPOGLYCEMIA, FAMILIAL NEONATAL**                         **0512**

**Includes:**

Hypoglycemia, leucine induced
Leucine-sensitive hypoglycemia of infancy, familial

**Excludes:**

Amino or organic acid metabolism, hereditary defects in
**Beckwith-Wiedemann syndrome (0104)**
Carbohydrate metabolism, hereditary defects in
Carnitine metabolism, hereditary defects in
Classic transient hypoglycemia
Early transitional neonatal hypoglycemia
Endocrine adenomatosis, familial
Glucagon deficiency, familial
Hormone deficiencies
Hyperammonemic states, hereditary defects in
Hyperinsulinism associated with islet cell insulinoma
Hyperinsulinism associated with nesidioblastosis, sporadic
Hypoglycemia, secondary transient neonatal
Hypoglycemia, idiopathic spontaneous
Urea synthesis, hereditary defects in

**Major Diagnostic Criteria:** Symptomatic and documented hypoglycemia usually occurs during the first two years of life. A family history of similar disease in sibs or relatives is helpful. Specific physical abnormalities are generally absent. Frequent and usually persistent low blood glucose levels occur before and after feeding, and are usually first detected because of generalized seizures. Serum insulin levels remain inappropriately high during hypoglycemia, although these need not be high in the absolute sense. Hypoglycemia is often severe and worsens with ingestion of foods high in protein or L-leucine content. Varying degrees of functional brain impairment are common when onset is in early infancy but gross malformations of the brain are absent. Spontaneous improvement from hypoglycemic tendency is noted over periods varying from 1–10 years. Adults are free of spontaneous hypoglycemia but may retain hyperreactivity to L-leucine as well as a tendency for hypoglycemia with moderate fasting. Pancreatic islet cell adenoma should be excluded although a variety of histopathology has included islet cell hyperplasia, absence of alpha cells, nesidioblastosis, and normal pancreatic histology at surgery or autopsy.

**Clinical Findings:** Convulsions (98%); onset in 1st year of life (98%); drowsiness, limpness, staring (98%); positive history in close relatives (98–100%); strabismus, alternating type (80%). Delayed mental development and/or prolonged unconscious if appropriate diagnosis is not made and treatment is delayed. First symptoms before age six months (51–80%); first symptoms after age six months (10–20%).

*Laboratory findings:* Absence of ketosis (100%); normal pituitary adrenocortical function (100%); absence of nonglucose sugars from blood and urine (100%); normal serum and urine amino acid patterns (100%); normal blood ammonia and liver function test (100%); normal glycemic response to glucagon or epinephrine (100%); low blood glucose during seizures (100%); low fasting blood glucose (95%); low serum levels of free fatty acids during hypoglycemia (100%); low serum levels of 3-hydroxybutyrate and acetoacetate during hypoglycemia (100%); normal urine organic acid levels (100%); persistance of detectable serum insulin levels when glucose levels are below 30 mg/dl (80–90%); hypoglycemic response to L-leucine during active phase (65%).

**Complications:** Mental retardation is found in 51–80% of cases if onset occurs during the first 6 months of life and 10–20% of cases if onset occurs after the first 6 months of life if the diagnosis and effective treatment are delayed following the onset of symptoms. The prognosis is excellent with prompt effective therapy even in severe cases with a very young age of onset. There is a tendency to convulsions, not associated with hypoglycemia, with a frequency similar to that for mental retardation as cited above. Strabismus, the alternating type, is very common during active hypoglycemia and occasionally persists. Ataxia from cerebellar dysfunction may be present during the active phase, but is rarely permanent. Spasticity is similarly present early and tends to improve with age, but may be permanent.

**Associated Findings:**

**Etiology:** Probably autosomal dominant inheritance. However, autosomal recessive inheritance appears to be associated with nesidioblastosis in at least seven such families confirmed histologically and clinically.

**Pathogenesis:** Nearly all patients appear to have leucine-induced hyperinsulinism when appropriately studied. The findings of beta cell hyperplasia, absence of alpha cells, and no pancreatic pathology cause uncertainty regarding the primary role of the pancreas. It may involve a basic abnormality at the ultrastructural level of cell-cell interaction within the islets. The general tendency to outgrow the clinical manifestations of the disease but persistence of subclinical abnormalities clouds the pathogenesis.

**MIM No.:** *24080

**CDC No.:** 251.200

**Sex Ratio:** M1:F1

**Occurrence:** Undetermined but presumed rare. Dominant form reported in Whites of northern European backround, and a Sephardic Jewish family. One Black family included among the seven kinships with documented autosomal recessive familial nesidioblastosis.

**Risk of Recurrence for Patient's Sib:**
See Part I, *Mendelian Inheritance.*

**Risk of Recurrence for Patient's Child:**
See Part I, *Mendelian Inheritance.*

**Age of Detectability:** From birth to 2 years of age, by plasma glucose determinations paired with serum insulin.

**Gene Mapping and Linkage:** Unknown.

**Prevention:** None known. Genetic counseling indicated.

**Treatment:** Maintenance of normoglycemia with intravenous glucose is essential during initial investigation. It may require up to 20 mg/kg/min or more in severe cases. Oral diazoxide 5–15 mg/kg/day is the treatment of choice but partial pancreatectomy is advisable promptly when drug therapy fails to completely control the hypoglycemia. Glucagon, ACTH, or corticosteroids may be

temporarily helpful. Somatostatin or glucagon combined with somatostatin are experimental but may be effective in stabilizing a poorly controlled patient prior to surgery. Supplemental treatment includes a diet high in calories and carbohydrates fed at frequent intervals around the clock. The dietary protein should be of high biological value but kept at the minimum level compatible with normal nutrition and distributed evenly throughout the day. Therapy with phenytoin has not been shown to be effective.

**Prognosis:** No evidence that life span is shortened, even if untreated.

**Detection of Carrier:** Unknown.

**Special Considerations:** Except for functioning islet cell adenoma, other causes of persistent hypoglycemia can be ruled out by appropriate studies. When an infant has no family history of hypoglycemia (such as when the first child affected in a family is studied) but otherwise fulfills all criteria, surgical exploration of the pancreas and partial pancreatectomy may be necessary for diagnosis and treatment. There is no other certain method of ruling out an islet cell adenoma. When other members of the family have neonatal hypoglycemia, the decision to perform pancreatic surgery must be based on the effectiveness of medical management. If complete elimination of hypoglycemia is not attained without unacceptable side effects, surgery should be undertaken promptly. Near complete pancreatectomy may be required in severe cases. Islet cell adenomata can be familial when associated with endocrine adenomatosis, but if other affected family members did not have adenomata, the decision to perform surgey would be based only on a need for therapy by partial pancreatectomy. The reported changes of pancreatic histology, other than adenoma, do not correlate with clinical response to surgery. Improvement of at least a temporary nature can be expected whether or not islet pathology is found. Occasionally the improvement is prolonged in such cases.

**References:**
Cochrane WA: Idiopathic infantile hypoglycemia and leucine sensitivity. Metabolism 1960; 9:386–399.
Ulstrom RA: Idiopathic spontaneous hypoglycemia. In: Linneweh F, ed: Erbliche stoffwechselkrankheiten. Munich: Urban and Schwarzenberg, 1962:225–234.
Sauls HS: Hypoglycemia in childhood. In: Kelley V, ed: Metabolic endocrine and genetic disorders of childhood. Hagerstown: Harper and Row 1974:703–704.
Schwartz SS, et al.: Familial nesidioblastosis: severe neonatal hypoglycemia in two families. J Pediatr 1979; 95:44–53.
Falkmer S, et al.: Significance of argyrophil parenchymal cells in the pancreatic islets in persistent neonatal hypoglycemia with hyperinsulism of familial type. Upsala J Med Sci 1981; 86:111–117.
Falkmer S, et al.: Immunohistochemical, morphometric and clinical studies of the pancreatic islets in infants with persistent neonatal hypoglycemia of familial type with hyperinsulinism and nesidioblastosis. ACTA Biol Med Germ 1981; 40:39–54.

UL001
S0013

**Robert A. Ulstrom**
**Joseph J. Sockalowsky**

**Hypoglycemia, glycerol-induced**
*See GLYCEROL INTOLERANCE SYNDROME*
**Hypoglycemia, leucine induced**
*See HYPOGLYCEMIA, FAMILIAL NEONATAL*
**Hypoglycemia, nonketotic and/or carnitine deficiency due to MCAD**
*See ACYL-CoA DEHYDROGENASE DEFICIENCY, MEDIUM CHAIN TYPE*
**Hypoglycemia, nonketotic, due to LCAD**
*See ACYL-CoA DEHYDROGENASE DEFICIENCY, LONG CHAIN TYPE*
**Hypoglycemic nonketotic dicarboxylic aciduria (some)**
*See VISCERA, FATTY METAMORPHOSIS*
**Hypogonadism, hypergonadotropic-congestive cardiomyopathy**
*See HYPERGONADOTROPIC HYPOGONADISM WITH CARDIOMYOPATHY*
**Hypogonadism-cataract-mental retardation-microcephaly**
*See MARTSOLF SYNDROME*
**Hypogonadism-deafness**
*See DEAFNESS-HYPOGONADISM*
**Hypogonadism-deafness-alopecia**
*See CRANDALL SYNDROME*

## HYPOGONADISM-DIABETES-ALOPECIA-DEAFNESS-RETARDATION-EKG ANOMALIES 2796

**Includes:** Diabetes-hypogonadism-alopecia-deafness-retardation-EKG anomalies

**Excludes:**
Alopecia-anosmia-deafness-hypogonadism, Johnson type (2765)
Alstrom syndrome (0041)
Bardet-Biedl syndrome (2363)
Crandall syndrome (3257)
Deafness-hypogonadism (2322)
Hypogonadism-partial alopecia (2797)
Kallmann syndrome (2301)
Laurence-Moon syndrome (0578)
Sohval-Soffer syndrome (3258)

**Major Diagnostic Criteria:** The combination of hypogonadism, diabetes mellitus, alopecia, deafness, mental retardation, and EKG abnormalities.

**Clinical Findings:** All individuals have had diabetes mellitus as demonstrated by low serum insulin levels. Scalp hair and eyebrows were sparse, without evidence of pili torti. EKG abnormalities consisted of T-wave flattening in four of five examined patients and S-T segment depression in two. Sensorineural deafness and mental retardation both ranged from mild to moderately severe.

Hypogonadism was present in all patients and was manifested as absence of breast tissue and sexual hair in women and eunuchoid proportions with moderate genital and sexual hair development in men. Testicular biopsy material demonstrated hypospermatogenesis and Leydig cell hypotrophy; laparotomy in females showed streak ovaries and hypoplastic uterus and fallopian tubes. Estradiol and testosterone levels were low in all patients. Cause of hypogonadism was determined to be hypogonadotrophic ovarian failure in two females, hypothalamic and ovarian failure in one female, and hypogonadotrophic testicular failure of hypothalamic origin in the males.

**Complications:** None. None of the patients have had diabetic nephropathy or retinopathy.

**Associated Findings:** None known.

**Etiology:** Autosomal recessive inheritance.

**Pathogenesis:** Unknown.

**MIM No.:** *24108

**POS No.:** 3612

**Sex Ratio:** M1:F1

**Occurrence:** Reported in six patients from two families in Saudi Arabia.

**Risk of Recurrence for Patient's Sib:**
See Part I, *Mendelian Inheritance.*

**Risk of Recurrence for Patient's Child:**
See Part I, *Mendelian Inheritance.*

**Age of Detectability:** Unknown. All patients were teens or adults when first examined.

**Gene Mapping and Linkage:** Unknown.

**Prevention:** None known. Genetic counseling indicated.

**Treatment:** Supportive.

**Prognosis:** Mental retardation ranged from mild to moderately severe. Life span appears unaffected.

**Detection of Carrier:** Unknown.

**References:**
Woodhouse NJY, Sakati NA: A syndrome of hypogonadism, alopecia, diabetes mellitus, mental retardation, deafness, and ECG abnormalities. J Med Genet 1983; 20:216–219.

T0007                                **Helga V. Toriello**

## HYPOGONADISM-PARTIAL ALOPECIA 2797

**Includes:**
Alopecia, partial-hypogonadism
Hypergonadotropic hypogonadism-partial skin appendages dysplasia

**Excludes:**
Alopecia-anosmia-deafness-hypogonadism, Johnson type (2765)
Gonadal dysgenesis, XX type (0436)
Hypogonadism-diabetes-alopecia-deafness-retardation-EKG anomalies (2796)
Sertoli cell-only syndrome (3163)

**Major Diagnostic Criteria:** Delayed puberty with **Hypogonadotropic hypogonadism** and bitemporal alopecia. In females, varying degrees of mullerian dysgenesis and gonadal dysgenesis. In males, manifestations of **Sertoli cell-only syndrome**.

**Clinical Findings:** In childhood, sparseness of scalp hair more in temporal regions is the presenting manifestation. By ages 15–20 years, there is sparseness of scalp hair and delayed puberty. Stature is usually average or above average with rather striking partial alopecia in that the scalp hair is thin and mostly located in the middle of the scalp in a mane-like configuration.

One male showed eunuchoid habitus, scant facial hair, normal penis, small and softish testes, and normal pubic and axillary hair. FSH levels were elevated but LH and testosterone levels were normal. This patient was azoospermic, and testicular biopsy material showed no germinal elements, but Sertoli and Leydig cells were present in adequate numbers.

Females showed average body build with eunuchoid proportions. Pubic and axillary hair were scant. They have small breasts and underdeveloped areolae, and they respond poorly to estrogen therapy with regard to breast size and not at all with regard to menses. Laparoscopy showed either no ovaries or a thin streak at the site of ovaries, with rudimentary uterus and fallopian tubes. Vaginas were normal. Intravenous pyelograms and bone age were normal. FSH and LH levels were elevated, and 17-β estradiol levels were quite low. Results of thyroid and adrenal function tests were normal.

Chromosomes were normal in males and females. Sweating and ability to detect scents were normal. Intelligence was normal.

**Complications:** Exaggerated lumbar lordosis and thoracic kyphosis. Lack of secondary sexual characteristics has caused some psychologic difficulties.

**Associated Findings:** Slightly diminished scholastic performance in one male and one female. Unilateral undescended testes in one male.

**Etiology:** Possibly autosomal recessive inheritance with intrafamilial variability in expression. Parental consanguinity was noted in two families.

**Pathogenesis:** Unknown.

**MIM No.:** 24109

**POS No.:** 4325

**Sex Ratio:** Presumably M1:F1. Observed figures showed a preponderance of females.

**Occurrence:** Two families have been documented. Probably more common in isolates and ethnic groups with a high rate of consanguinity.

**Risk of Recurrence for Patient's Sib:**
See Part I, *Mendelian Inheritance.*

**Risk of Recurrence for Patient's Child:**
See Part I, *Mendelian Inheritance.* Affected individuals are unable to reproduce.

**Age of Detectability:** During childhood. Confirmation by laparoscopy and hormonal profile. Testicular histopathology is diagnostic. Patients often presented in the late teens.

**Gene Mapping and Linkage:** Unknown.

**Prevention:** None known. Genetic counseling indicated.

**Treatment:** Cyclic estrogen therapy. Artificial mammoplasty in females. Possibly cosmetic hair substitution.

**Prognosis:** Probably normal for life span. Infertility.

**Detection of Carrier:** Unknown. Parents in the two families were apparently normal.

**Special Considerations:** Several hypogonadism syndromes have shown the association of alopecia, many of them being described from the Middle East. It is probable that some of the Middle East cases represent private syndromes, or that the gene frequencies of such disorders are relatively higher than in other parts of the world.

**References:**

Al-Awadi SA, et al.: Primary hypogonadism and partial alopecia in three sibs with Mullerian hypoplasia in the affected females. Am J Med Genet 1985; 22:619–622.

Teebi AS, et al.: Hypogonadotropic hypogonadism, mental retardation, obesity and minor skeletal abnormalities: another new autosomal recessive syndrome from the Middle East. Am J Med Genet 1986; 24:373–378.

AL030
FA015

**S. A. Al-Awadi**
**T. I. Farag**

---

## HYPOGONADOTROPIC HYPOGONADISM 2300

**Includes:**

Eunuchoidism, familial hypogonadotrophic
Fertile eunuch syndrome
Gonadotropin deficiency, familial idiopathic (FIGD)
Gonadotropin deficiency, isolated (one form)
LH deficiency, isolated

**Excludes:**

**Ataxia-hypogonadism syndrome** (0093)
Gonadal dysgenesis (all forms)
**Gonadotropin deficiencies** (0438)
**Kallmann syndrome** (2301)
**Klinefelter syndrome** (0556)

**Major Diagnostic Criteria:** Luteinizing hormone (LH) and follicle-stimulating hormone (FSH) levels of <5 mIU/ml.

**Clinical Findings:** LH and FSH levels are below the levels of clinical detection with current assay specificity. Biologic effects reflect the amount of total gonadotropin function, usually resulting in failure of the gonads to function and allow pubertal development. Although external and internal genitalia are well differentiated, normal secondary sexual development does not occur. Males have small testes that may be cryptorchid. External genitalia are small, with diminished pubic, axillary, and facial hair growth. Muscular development is less than expected for normal males, and the voice is not deepened. Females display a lack of breast development, and infantile vagina and uterus. Body proportions are eunuchoid in both sexes.

**Complications:** Lack of gonadal stimulation in both sexes results in failure of secondary sexual development and sterility.

Females exhibit estrogen deficiency syndrome, including vaginal atrophy with resultant dyspareunia, osteoporosis, hot flashes after initial estrogen replacement and sudden withdrawal.

**Associated Findings:** None known.

**Etiology:** Autosomal recessive inheritance.

**Pathogenesis:** Disordered gonadotropin releasing hormone (GNRH) signals to the pituitary results in absence of LH and FSH. This, in turn, results in failure of gonadal stimulation and therefore absence of the subsequent development stimulated by gonadal steroids, namely; secondary sex characteristics and reproductive processes.

**MIM No.:** 22720, 22830

**Sex Ratio:** M1:F1

**Occurrence:** Undetermined but presumed rare.

**Risk of Recurrence for Patient's Sib:**
See Part I, *Mendelian Inheritance.*

**Risk of Recurrence for Patient's Child:**
See Part I, *Mendelian Inheritance.*

**Age of Detectability:** During puberty.

**Gene Mapping and Linkage:** Unknown.

**Prevention:** None known. Genetic counseling indicated.

**Treatment:** Hormonal replacement to stimulate development and to maintain integrity of secondary sex characteristics and sexual function.

Gonadal steroid replacement is necessary for the initiation and maintenance of secondary sex characteristics in both males and females. Fertility may be achieved in both sexes by administration of pulsatile GNRH. Most patients are unresponsive to single-dose GNRH administration unless first primed by multiple doses. Human chorionic gonadotropin (hCG) injections in males and human menopausal gonadotropins (hMG) in females may also be used to stimulate gametogenesis. Clomiphene citrate is ineffective in the treatment of these patients.

**Prognosis:** Intelligence and life span are normal. Reproductive capability depends on the success of therapy to stimulate spermatogenesis or oogenesis.

**Detection of Carrier:** Unknown.

**Special Considerations:** *Isolated LH deficiency* (the *Fertile eunuch syndrome*) is a related but currently distinct entity. Several males have shown low LH but normal FSH levels. Predictably, they show spermatogenesis, but lack of completely normal secondary sexual development. A few individuals fulfilling this criteria have shown diminished FSH response to clomiphene, raising the possibility that fertile eunuch syndrome is a mildly expressed form of isolated gonadotropin deficiency. However, most authorities believe that the fertile eunuch syndrome is distinct. Isolated FSH deficiency has also been reported in a female.

**References:**

Le Marquand HS: Congenital hypogonadotrophic hypogonadism in five members of a family, three brothers and two sisters. Proc R Soc Med 1954; 47:442–446.

Ewer RW: Familial monotropic pituitary gonadotropin insufficiency. J Clin Endocrinol 1968; 28:783–788.

Faiman C, et al.: The 'fertile eunuch' syndrome: demonstration of isolated luteinizing hormone deficiency by radio-immuno-assay technique. Mayo Clin Proc 1986; 43:661–667.

Santen RJ, Paulsen CA: Hypogonadotropic eunuchoidism: gonadal responsiveness to exogenous gonadotropins. J Clin Endocrinol Metab 1973; 36:55–63.

Boyar RM, et al.: Clinical and laboratory heterogeneity in idiopathic hypogonadotropic hypogonadism. J Clin Endocrinol Metab 1976; 43:1268–1275.

Betend B, et al.: Familial idiopathic hypogonadotrophic hypogonadism. Acta Endocrinol (Copenh) 1977; 84:246–253.

Toledo SPA, et al.: Familial idiopathic gonadotropin deficiency: a hypothalamic form of hypogonadism. Am J Med Genet 1983; 15:405–416.

CA041

**Sandra Ann Carson**

**Hypogonadotropic hypogonadism with anosmia or hyposmia**
See KALLMANN SYNDROME
**Hypohidrosis-defective teeth-unusual dermatoglyphics**
See ECTODERMAL DYSPLASIA, BASAN TYPE
**Hypohidrosis-hypodontia-hypotrichosis**
See ECTODERMAL DYSPLASIA, CHRIST-SIEMENS-TOURAINE TYPE
**Hypohidrosis-onycholysis-enamel hypocalcification**
See AMELO-ONYCHO-HYPOHIDROTIC SYNDROME
**Hypokalemic alkalosis**
See BARTTER SYNDROME
**Hypokalemic periodic paralysis**
See PARALYSIS, HYPOKALEMIC PERIODIC
**Hypolipidemia-short stature-leukonychia**
See HOOFT DISEASE
**Hypomagnesemia (neonatal)-selective malabsorption of magnesium**
See HYPOMAGNESEMIA, PRIMARY
**Hypomagnesemia, isolated renal**
See HYPOMAGNESEMIA, PRIMARY

## HYPOMAGNESEMIA, PRIMARY      0514

**Includes:**

Hypomagnesemia, isolated renal
Hypomagnesemia (neonatal)-selective malabsorption of
    magnesium
Hypomagnesemia-secondary hypocalcemia
Hypomagnesemic tetany
Magnesium, defect in renal tubular transport of

**Excludes:**

Hypomagnesemia associated with GI and renal disorders
Transient hypomagnesemia of the newborn

**Major Diagnostic Criteria:** Seizures in early weeks of life due to hypomagnesemia, which is usually accompanied by secondary hypocalcemia. Other disorders, including transient neonatal hypomagnesemia, GI, and renal disorders must be excluded.

**Clinical Findings:** Tetany and convulsions in early weeks of life associated with hypomagnesemia and hypocalcemia. Serum inorganic phosphate is normal or somewhat increased. Hypoalbuminemia, anasarca, and diarrhea are occasional findings. Hypocalcemia and its symptoms are resistant to calcium and vitamin D therapy but respond well to magnesium treatment.

**Complications:** Convulsions, tetany, hypocalcemia, diarrhea, hypoalbuminemia.

**Associated Findings:** Possible psychomotor retardation as a result of repeated seizures.

**Etiology:** Reported cases suggest genetic heterogeneity with both autosomal and X-linked recessive forms of inheritance. A balanced translocation t(9;X)(q12;p22) was found in a microcephalic girl with dysmorphic facies.

**Pathogenesis:** Isolated defect in intestinal transport of magnesium. The hypocalcemia is due to impaired secretion of parathyroid hormone or impaired end-organ responsiveness to parathyroid hormone, each of which may result from the magnesium deficiency. The administration of magnesium corrects these abnormalities. The hypoalbuminemia has been attributed to impaired synthesis of albumin and/or to protein-losing enteropathy induced by magnesium deficiency.

**MIM No.:** *24825, *30760

**Sex Ratio:** M3:F1

**Occurrence:** About 35 cases reported since first described in 1968; ten in families.

**Risk of Recurrence for Patient's Sib:**
See Part I, *Mendelian Inheritance.*

**Risk of Recurrence for Patient's Child:**
See Part I, *Mendelian Inheritance.*

**Age of Detectability:** Usually in first three months of life.

**Gene Mapping and Linkage:** HOMG (hypomagnesemia, secondary hypocalcemia) has been provisionally mapped to X.

**Prevention:** None known. Genetic counseling indicated.

**Treatment:** Early recognition of affected infants and treatment with magnesium supplements.

**Prognosis:** Death may occur in untreated infants during early months of life. Somatic and intellectual development have been reported as normal after 12 years of treatment with magnesium supplements.

**Detection of Carrier:** Unknown.

**References:**

Suh SM, et al.: Pathogenesis of hypocalcemia in primary hypomagnesemia: normal end-organ responsiveness to parathyroid hormone, impaired parathyroid gland function. J Clin Invest 1973; 52:153–160.
Anast CS, et al.: Impaired release of parathyroid hormone in magnesium deficiency. Clin Endocrinol Metab 1976; 42:707–717.
Stromme JH, et al.: Familial hypomagnesemia: a follow-up examination of three patients after 9 and 12 years of treatment. Pediat Res 1981; 15:1134–1139.
Hennekam RCM, et al.: Primary hypomagnesemia: an autosomal recessive inherited disease. Lancet 1983; I:927 only.
Yamamoto T, et al.: Primary hypomagnesemia with secondary hypocalcemia: report of a case and review of the world literature. Magnesium 1985; 4:153–164.
Dudin KI, Teebi AS: Primary hypomagnesemia: a case report and literature review. Europ J Pediat 1987; 146:303–305.

CU013      **Floyd L. Culler**
HA076      **Alberto Hayek**

**Hypomagnesemia-secondary hypocalcemia**
*See HYPOMAGNESEMIA, PRIMARY*
**Hypomagnesemic tetany**
*See HYPOMAGNESEMIA, PRIMARY*

## HYPOMELANOSIS OF ITO      2264

**Includes:**

Incontinenti Pigmenti Achromians
Ito hypomelanosis
Seizures-skin lesions-mental retardation
Skin lesions-seizures-mental retardation

**Excludes:**

**Ectodermal dysplasia, Naegeli type** (0703)
**Incontinentia pigmenti** (0526)
Nevus Depigmentosus

**Major Diagnostic Criteria:** Skin lesions, seizures, and mental retardation.

**Clinical Findings:** Asymmetric, unilateral or bilateral areas of whorl-like hypopigmentation, occurring on any part of the body, except the scalp, palms or soles. During initial stages, there may be progression of these lesions so that many areas of skin are involved. With time there is a tendency for the area of hypopigmentation to darken. Histologic studies have revealed a decreased amount of melanin in the basal cell layer of the dermis, and decreased amounts of melanosomes in the melanocytes in the area of hypopigmentation. This may be associated with anomalies of other organ systems including the central nervous system (seizures, mental retardation) and eyes (strabismus, myopia, coloboma), as well as **Microcephaly** or **Megalencephaly**.

**Complications:** Unknown.

**Associated Findings:** Approximately 60% of cases have had associated anomalies. Mental retardation (19%) and seizures (17%) have been the most consistent associated findings. Decreased sweat response to pilocarpine over the areas of hypopigmentation has been observed. Various dental anomalies, including pointed extra cusps protruding from the palatal aspect of the crown of maxillary incisors, and irregularly formed coronal dentin, have been reported.

**Etiology:** Some patients may be mosaic for autosomal or X chromosome aneuploidy. Autosomal dominant inheritance has been suggested in some instances. This condition may prove to be a heterogeneous group of conditions whose only common feature is streaky hypopigmentation.

**Pathogenesis:** Unknown.

**MIM No.:** 14615

**POS No.:** 3525

**Sex Ratio:** M1:F2.

**Occurrence:** Undetermined. Because of the natural history of the hypopigmented areas, this disorder is probably under reported in older children and adult populations.

**Risk of Recurrence for Patient's Sib:**
See Part I, *Mendelian Inheritance.*

**Risk of Recurrence for Patient's Child:**
See Part I, *Mendelian Inheritance.*

**Age of Detectability:** As early as the neonatal period. More than 90% are detectable by childhood.

**Gene Mapping and Linkage:** A diversity of chromosomal rearrangements have been reported, with no consistent findings.

**Prevention:** None known. Genetic counseling indicated.

**Treatment:** Unknown.

**Prognosis:** Unknown.

**Detection of Carrier:** Possibly by use of the Wood's lamp for skin examination.

**Special Considerations:** This disorder has phenotypic overlap with **Incontinentia pigmenti** only in that both conditions are associated with signficant neural, ocular, dental and musculoskeletal anomalies. The pigmentary changes in Hypomelanosis of Ito have been described as being the reverse of that seen in incontinenti pigmenti. It is important to recognize that the pigmentary changes in Hypomelanosis of Ito are not preceded by a neonatal period of erythema and vesiculation, as in incontinenti pigmenti. Histology of the affected areas is different in the two disorders.

**References:**

Ito M: Incontinenti pigmenti achromians. a singular case of naevus depigmentosus systematicus bilateralis. Tohoku J Exp Med (Suppl) 1952; 55:57–59.

Jelinek JE, et al.: Hypomelanosis of Ito (Incontinenti pigmenti achromians). Arch Dermatol 1973; 107:596–601.

Schwartz MF, et al.: Hypomelanosis of Ito (incontinenti pigmenti achromians): a neurocuraneous syndrome. J Pediatr 1977; 90:236–240.

Happle R, Vakilzadeh F: Hamartomatous dental cusps in Hypomelanosis of Ito. Clin Genet 1982; 21:65–68.

Rosemberg S, et al.: Hypomelanosis of Ito: case report with involvement of the central nervous system and review of the literature. Neuropediatrics 1984; 15:52–55.

Bartholomew DW, et al.: Single maxillary central incisor and coloboma in hypomelanosis of Ito. Clin Genet 1987; 32:370–373.

Ritter CL, et al.: Chromosome mosaicism in hypomelanosis of Ito. Am J Med Genet 1990; 35:14–17.

CH034
SY000

**Philip F. Chance**
**Virginia P. Sybert**

**Hypomelia with Mullerian duct anomalies**
*See LIMB, UPPER HYPOPLASIA-MULLERIAN DUCT DEFECTS*

---

## HYPOPARATHYROIDISM, FAMILIAL                    0515

**Includes:** Hypoparathyroidism, X-linked neonatal

**Excludes:**
Hypoparathyroidism, juvenile and adult onset idiopathic
Hypoparathyroidism, maternal
**Immunodeficiency, thymic agenesis** (0943)

**Major Diagnostic Criteria:** Convulsions and other signs of tetany with hypocalcemia and hyperphosphatemia in the presence of low or undetectable serum immunoreactive parathyroid hormone level. Similar chemical findings may be observed in neonatal hypocalcemic tetany, but in contrast to idiopathic hypoparathyroidism, the chemical and clinical abnormalities in neonatal tetany are transient. Other hypocalcemic disorders, including renal insufficiency and pseudohypoparathyroidism, are characterized by elevated serum immunoreactive parathyroid hormone levels.

**Clinical Findings:** Convulsive seizures and increased neuromuscular irritability with signs and symptoms of tetany or its equivalent are prominent features of infantile hypoparathyroidism. The symptoms include muscle rigidity, laryngeal stridor, and carpopedal spasm. Hyperreflexia is common, and Chvostek and Trousseau signs frequently are positive. Diarrhea may be present and is secondary to hyperexcitability of gut muscles induced by hypocalcemia. Ocular manifestations include photophobia, blepharospasm, conjunctivitis, keratitis, corneal ulcerations, and lens opacity. Dental abnormalities, including aplasia or hypoplasia of teeth, may occur if hypoparathyroidism develops during the time that the teeth are being formed. Skeletal X-ray films usually reveal no significant changes from normal. Symmetric calcification of the cerebral basal ganglia may be observed. In some children there

may be signs of increased intracranial pressure; the underlying cause of this manifestation is poorly understood.

**Complications:** Impaired intellectual ability may occur in the presence of hypocalcemia and may improve with correction of serum calcium.

**Associated Findings:** None known.

**Etiology:** X-linked recessive inheritance.

**Pathogenesis:** Unknown.

**MIM No.:** *30770

**Sex Ratio:** M1:F0

**Occurrence:** At least three kindreds have been reported, including two from Missouri.

**Risk of Recurrence for Patient's Sib:**
See Part I, *Mendelian Inheritance.*

**Risk of Recurrence for Patient's Child:**
See Part I, *Mendelian Inheritance.*

**Age of Detectability:** During first year of life.

**Gene Mapping and Linkage:** HPT (hypoparathyroidism) has been provisionally mapped to Xq26-q27.

**Prevention:** None known. Genetic counseling indicated.

**Treatment:** Pharmacologic doses of vitamin D. Oral calcium supplements. Oral aluminium hydroxide. Antacids to bind phosphate in the gut.

**Prognosis:** If untreated, death may occur. With adequate treatment, the prognosis for life is good.

**Detection of Carrier:** Unknown.

**References:**

Peden VH: True idiopathic hypoparathyroidism as a sex-linked recessive trait. Am J Hum Genet 1960; 12:323–337.

Klein R, Haddow J: Hypoparathyroidism. In: Gardner LI, ed. Endocrine and genetic diseases of childhood and adolescence. 2nd ed. Philadelphia: W.B. Saunders, 1975:408.

Whyte MP, Weldon VV: Idiopathic hypoparathyroidism presenting with seizures during infancy. J Pediat 1981; 99:608–611.

SC016

**R. Neil Schimke**

**Hypoparathyroidism, resistant (ineffective) hormone**
*See PARATHYROID HORMONE RESISTANCE*
**Hypoparathyroidism, X-linked neonatal**
*See HYPOPARATHYROIDISM, FAMILIAL*
**Hypoparathyroidism-lymphedema-nephropathy**
*See LYMPHEDEMA-HYPOPARATHYROIDISM*
**Hypoparathyroidism-nephrosis-nerve deafness**
*See NEPHROSIS-NERVE DEAFNESS-HYPOPARATHYROIDISM,
BARAKAT TYPE*

---

## HYPOPHOSPHATASIA                    0516

**Includes:**
Alkaline phosphatase, liver/bone/kidney type
Phosphatase, liver alkaline
Phosphoethanolaminuria
Pseudohypophosphatasia

**Excludes:**
**Hypophosphatemia, non X-linked** (2040)
**Hypophosphatemia, X-linked** (0517)
**Skeletal dysplasia** (other)

**Major Diagnostic Criteria:** Very low alkaline phosphatase activity (total and tissue; non-specific bone/liver/kidney) in plasma (serum) at saturating concentration of substrate (16 mM) or, in pseudohypophosphatasia, reduced activity at low substrate concentration (4 mM), but normal total activity at saturating substrate concentration; phosphoethanolaminuria; radiographic and histologic rickets; osteomalacia in adults; histochemical evidence of low alkaline phosphatase activity in bone. Activities of intestinal and placental alkaline phosphatase, and circulating acid phosphatase are normal.

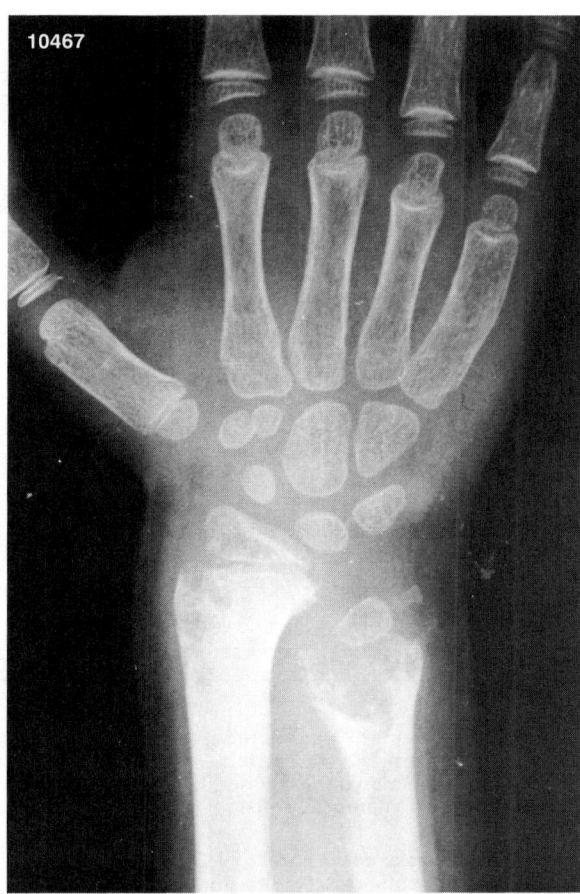

**0516**-10467: Coarse bony trabecular pattern in carpals, metacarpals, and phalanges. Irregular ossification of distal radius and ulna, and deep, cup-shaped defect of distal ulna with island of coarsely trabeculated bone.

**Clinical Findings:** Expression of major phenotype (inadequate mature bone formation) varies from intrauterine death (possibly the homozygous form), to modest handicap in childhood and adulthood (possibly the heterozygous form). Those affected with the severe congenital form may be stillborn or die from early respiratory insufficiency. Infantile cases have early failure to thrive, hypotonia, irritability, hypercalcemia, severe skeletal deformity, and and markedly deficient mineralization of metaphyses and margins of cranial bones. X-ray examination may show decreased mineralization of the skull, delayed closure of fontanels, and irregularly decreased metaphyseal mineralization. Rarely, nephrocalcinosis may present.

Spontaneous improvement has been observed in infancy. Bone lesions are least severe in the milder (heterozygotes) forms. Premature loss of deciduous teeth is characteristic. The skeletal findings include: craniosynostosis, bowed lower limbs (occasionally with overlying cutaneous dimpling), a small thorax with short ribs, and rachitic rosary deformity. Other findings include awkward gait, "poker-spine", and shortness of stature. Pseudofracture and pathologic fractures in adulthood may be the first findings. Diagnosis, in all forms, is confirmed by very low alkaline phosphatase activity and phosphoethanolaminuria.

**Complications:** Fractures and deformity; increased intracranial pressure (from craniostenosis); sequelae of chronic hypercalcemia.

**Associated Findings:** Secondary to craniostenosis if untreated.

**Etiology:** Autosomal recessive inheritance (possibly with modulators) is presumed for the lethal, congenital and early onset severe forms. Phenotypic variation within sibships, and the form presenting as pseudohypophosphatasia, suggests the existence of more than one allele. Later onset and mild forms are considered compatible with autosomal dominant inheritance.

**Pathogenesis:** Liver/bone/kidney/alkaline phosphatase deficiency is associated with a guanine to adenine transition in nucleotide 711 at the locus on chromosome 1. The mutation converts alanine 162 to threonine in the mature enzyme. The associated phenotype is a lethal form of hypophosphatasia.

The cause and pathogenesis of the phenotype have not been delineated in other forms of hypophosphatemia. The cardinal effects, in general, are: inadequate calcification of osteoid tissue, cleavage of inorganic pyrophosphate esters (including pyridoxal phosphate), and prerenal phosphoethanolaminuria.

**MIM No.:** *14630, *17176, *24150, *24151

**POS No.:** 3262

**Sex Ratio:** M1:F1

**Occurrence:** About 30 kindreds have been reported; about one-sixth of these from an inbred Hungarian village.

**Risk of Recurrence for Patient's Sib:**
See Part I, *Mendelian Inheritance.*

**Risk of Recurrence for Patient's Child:**
See Part I, *Mendelian Inheritance.*

**Age of Detectability:** At birth or prenatally. Intrauterine diagnosis of homozygotes is possible. Tissue non-specific alkaline phosphatase isozyme activity is very low in amniotic fluid, cultured amniocytes, and biopsied chorionic villous cells. Failure to visualize or poor visualization of fetal head on ultrasonography due to deficient bone mineralization is consistent with diagnosis of the severe phenotype. Long-chain triglycerides stimulate intestinal alkaline phosphatase activity, and cause plasma enzyme activity to rise. This response is intact in patients, indicating that intestinal alkaline phosphatase is present in hypophosphatasia.

**Gene Mapping and Linkage:** ALPL (alkaline phosphatase, liver/bone/kidney) has been mapped to 1p36.1-p34.

**Prevention:** None known. Genetic counseling indicated.

**Treatment:** There is no generally accepted therapy for the metabolic abnormality. Improved bone mineralization and transient increase of plasma alkaline phosphatase activity following repeated infusions of normal plasma has been reported by Whyte et al (1986) in a severely affected infant. This finding awaits confirmation. Hypercalcemia should be treated with a low calcium diet and steroids. Early surgical correction of craniosynostosis is important. Insertion of intramedullary rods can prevent fractures (Coe et al, 1986). Spontaneous improvement of the clinical course in some patients with severe phenotype make treatment evaluation difficult.

**Prognosis:** Varies from intrauterine death to a nearly symptomless course.

**Detection of Carrier:** About 60% of carriers can be recognized from elevation of urine and plasma phosphoethanolamine concentration. Liver disease, scurvy and hypothyroidism are also associated with elevated phosphoethanolaminuria. Depressed plasma alkaline phosphatase activity is a less reliable index, unless bone fraction is specified.

**References:**
Scriver CR, Cameron D: Pseudohypophosphatasia. New Engl J Med 1969; 281:604–606.
Eastman JR, Bixler D: Clinical laboratory and genetic investigations of hypophosphatasia: support for autosomal dominant inheritance with homozygous lethality. J Craniofac Genet Dev Biol 1983; 3:213–234.
Warren RC, et al.: First trimester diagnosis of hypophosphatasia with a monoclonal antibody to the liver/bone/kidney isoenzyme of alkaline phosphatase. Lancet 1985; II:856–858.
Whyte MP, et al.: Markedly increased circulating pyridoxal-5'-phosphate levels in hypophosphatasia. J Clin Invest 1985; 76:752–756.

Caswell AM, et al.: Normal activity of nucleoside triphosphate phosphatase in alkaline phosphatase-deficient fibroblasts from patients with infantile hypophosphatasia. J Clin Endocrinol Metab 1986; 63:1237.

Coe JD, et al.: Management of femoral fractures and pseudofractures in adult hypophosphatasia. J Bone Joint Surg (Am) 1986; 68:981–990.

Cole DE, et al.: Pseudohypophosphatasia. New Engl J Med 1986; 314:992–993.

Whyte MP, et al.: Infantile hypophosphatasia: normalization of circulating bone alkaline phosphatase activity followed by skeletal remineralization. J Pediatr 1986; 108:82–88.

Weiss MT, et al.; A missense mutation in the human liver/bone/kidney alkaline phosphatase gene causing a lethal form of hypophosphatemia. Proc Nat Acad Sci 1988; 85:7666–7669.

FR008                                 **Donald Fraser**
SC050                              **Charles R. Scriver**

## HYPOPHOSPHATEMIA, NON X-LINKED      2040

**Includes:** Bone disease, hypophosphatemic (HBD)

**Excludes:**
Hypophosphatemia, X-linked (0517)
**Rickets, hereditary hypophosphatemic with hypercalciuria (HHRH)** (3020)

**Major Diagnostic Criteria:** Chronic fasting age-specific hypophosphatemia unresponsive to vitamin D at the normal daily requirement. Normal serum calcium iPTH and 1,25-$(OH)_2D_3$ levels. Normal endogenous renal clearance of phosphate.

Renal clearance and fractional excretion of phosphate are normal under fasted conditions. Absolute TRP ($\mu$mole/100 ml GF) is below normal. TmP and TmP/GFR are below age-specific normal values. Renal responsiveness to PTH is present (vs. absent in **Hypophosphatemia, X-linked** males) but attenuated. These findings distinguish autosomal dominant and X-linked forms.

**Clinical Findings:** Despite hypophosphatemia (detectable in infancy), evidence of active rickets is minimal or absent. Genu varum in late infancy is the usual cause for presentation. Course trabeculation (osteomalacia) of long-bone shafts, sclerosis, and medial metaphyseal deformity of the distal femur are typical findings. Height is rarely below the third percentile. Serum alkaline phosphatase is only modestly or not elevated. Male to male transmission confirms autosomal dominant form of hypophosphatemia.

**Complications:** Rachitic lesions can occur during adolescence when linear growth is accelerated.

**Associated Findings:** None known.

**Etiology:** Autosomal dominant inheritance. Sporadic cases have been reported.

**Pathogenesis:** Deficient phosphate reabsorption in kidney. A transport system different from that affected in X-linked hypophosphatemia is apparently involved. Phosphate transport in erythrocytes is not abnormal.

**MIM No.:** 14635

**Sex Ratio:** M1:F1

**Occurrence:** Undetermined but apparently about 20% of that for **Hypophosphatemia, X-linked**, or .2–2:1,000,000 (average).

**Risk of Recurrence for Patient's Sib:**
See Part I, *Mendelian Inheritance.*

**Risk of Recurrence for Patient's Child:**
See Part I, *Mendelian Inheritance.*

**Age of Detectability:** In early infancy.

**Gene Mapping and Linkage:** Unknown.

**Prevention:** None known. Genetic counseling indicated.

**Treatment:** Renal transport defect and osteomalacia responsive to 1,25-$(OH)_2D_3$. Phosphate supplements usually not indicated.

**Prognosis:** No effect on life span. Deformities due to chronic hypophosphatemia are minimal in this condition.

**Detection of Carrier:** Overnight-fasted plasma phosphate concentration is below 95% confidence limit for age.

**Special Considerations:** Renal tubular reabsorption of phosphate in mammals apparently involves two different mechanisms (Dennis V, et al, Amer J Physiol, 1976). AD and XL mutations may be markers for gene loci that control the two mechanisms.

**References:**
Greenberg BG, et al.: The normal range of serum inorganic phosphorus and its utility as a discriminant in the diagnosis of congenital hypophosphatemia. J Clin Endocrinol Metab 1960; 20:364–379.

Dennis VW, et al.: Response of phosphate transport to parathyroid hormone in segments of rabbit nephron. Am J Physiol 1977; 233:F29–F38.

Scriver CR, et al.: Hypophosphatemic non-rachitic bone disease: an entity distinct from X-linked hypophosphatemia and the renal defect bone involvement and inheritance. Am J Med Genet 1977; 1:101–117.

Scriver CR, et al.: Autosomal hypophosphataemic bone disease responds to 1,25-(OH)2D3. Arch Dis Child 1981; 56:203–207.

SC050                              **Charles R. Scriver**

**Hypophosphatemia, type I (counterpart to mouse Hyp)**
*See HYPOPHOSPHATEMIA, X-LINKED*
**Hypophosphatemia, type II (counterpart to mouse Gyro)**
*See HYPOPHOSPHATEMIA, X-LINKED*

## HYPOPHOSPHATEMIA, X-LINKED      0517

**Includes:**
Hypophosphatemia, type I (counterpart to mouse Hyp)
Hypophosphatemia, type II (counterpart to mouse Gyro)
Hypophosphatemic vitamin D-resistant rickets
Rickets, familial vitamin D-resistant

**Excludes:**
**Hypophosphatemia, non X-linked** (2040)
Hypophosphatemic rickets with disorders of tubular function
Hypophosphatemic rickets with glycinuria; acidosis; glucosuria
**Rickets, hereditary hypophosphatemic with hypercalciuria (HHRH)** (3020)

**Major Diagnostic Criteria:** Age-dependent low concentration of inorganic phosphate in the plasma or serum in a fasting subject, the exclusion of other causes of hypophosphatemia, and osteomalacia or rickets. Failure to repair hypophosphatemia or the active rickets with amounts of vitamin D that would cure vitamin D-deficiency rickets and normal serum immunoreactive parathormone (iPTH) in serum of untreated patients.

**Clinical Findings:** Carriers of the gene have hypophosphatemia and depressed phosphate $T_m$ (or $T_mP/GFR$). Male hemizygotes have hypophosphatemia (low serum inorganic phosphorus) with active, "vitamin D-resistant" rickets in childhood, and short stature. Female heterozygotes have a range of abnormalities from asymptomatic hypophosphatemia, with no other clinical or chemical abnormalities, to florid rickets and short stature.

The hypophosphatemia is detectable shortly after birth; evidence of rickets appears later. Serum alkaline phosphatase is elevated when active rickets or osteomalacia is present. Serum calcium is usually normal or low normal. Serum immunoreactive PTH (iPTH) is normal or minimally elevated in untreated persons. Serum 1,25$(OH)_2D$ is normal (not elevated) in untreated persons. Associated X-ray findings include typical changes of active rickets (in childhood) and osteomalacia.

**Complications:** Rachitic deformities and short stature, particularly of lower limbs in childhood; limitation of motion at large joints (hips, knees, elbows) in adults, due to bony overgrowth at tendinous insertions. Acquired dolichocephaly.

**Associated Findings:** Attenuated renal synthesis of 1,25-$(OH)_2D_3$; plasma levels of hormone are inappropriately low for the degree of hypophosphatemia.

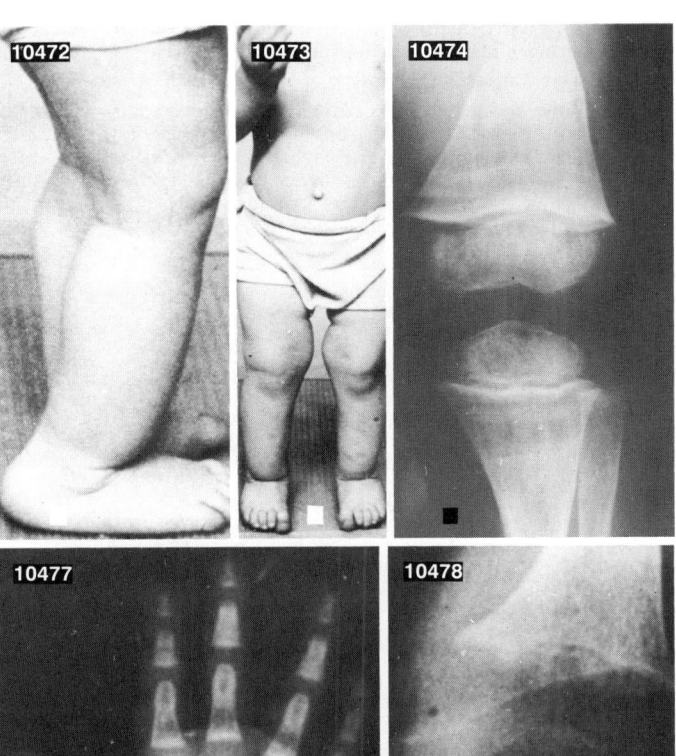

**0517-10472–73:** Marked anterior bowing of lower third of the tibias with minimal lateral bowing. **10474:** X-ray of knee prior to vitamin D therapy. **10477–78:** Severe active rickets.

**Etiology:** X-linked dominant inheritance. Two loci on the X chromosome may control renal phosphate transport. The murine genes are designated *Hyp* and *Gy*, and their putative human counterparts are designated hypophosphatemia (X-linked), types I and II respectively. Sporadic cases probably represent new mutations (estimated frequency; 1:200,000 genes per generation).

**Pathogenesis:** Recent evidence indicates that affected persons have an abnormal transepithelial transport system for reclamation of phosphate in kidney. The functional defect is located in the brush-border membrane and is selective for phosphate. "Negative reabsorption" of phosphate can occur at elevated levels of serum phosphate. Evidence exists both for and against a coexistent deficiency of transepithelial absorption of phosphate in the intestine. Phosphate entry into erythrocytes is not impaired.

**MIM No.:** *30780, 30781

**POS No.:** 3263

**Sex Ratio:** M1:F1

**Occurrence:** 1–10:1,000,000 live births. Several hundred cases have been reported.

**Risk of Recurrence for Patient's Sib:**
See Part I, *Mendelian Inheritance.*

**Risk of Recurrence for Patient's Child:**
See Part I, *Mendelian Inheritance.*

**Age of Detectability:** In early infancy.

**Gene Mapping and Linkage:** HYP (hypophosphatemia, vitamin D resistant rickets) has been mapped to Xp22.2-p22.1. HYP is between markers DXS41 and DXS43. Gy is linked to HYP in the mouse (< 1% cross over value).

**Prevention:** None known. Genetic counseling indicated.

**Treatment:** Early recognition of the affected infant improves the outcome. Early, continuous, and carefully monitored treatment with supplemental intake of inorganic phosphate (1–4 g per day every 4 hr x 5). $1,25-(OH)_2D_3$ is a useful adjunct to repair phosphate homeostasis and improve bone mineralization. Vitamin D hormone does not correct the primary renal defect. Corrective orthopedic surgery for existing limb deformities.

**Prognosis:** Life span probably not affected. Early and continuous phosphate treatment throughout the growth period can prevent deformities and impairment of linear growth.

**Detection of Carrier:** Low value (>2 SD below age-specific mean value) for inorganic phosphorus in fasting (morning) serum will identify the majority of carriers; measurement of $T_mP/GFR$ is recommended.

**Special Considerations:** In all patients with hypophosphatemia and rickets, other causes should be excluded, (e.g., **Renal tubular syndrome, Fanconi type**). There are rare instances of isolated renal glycosuria or glycinuria associated with what appears otherwise to be simple hypophosphatemic rickets; these may represent different genetic disorders or may be associated physiological findings. X-linked hypophosphatemia in the mouse is caused by mutations at two independent, closely-linked loci: *Hyp* and *Gy*. Mutation of the latter locus causes lesions of the cochlea and vestibular organ associated with deafness and movement disorder respectively. Sensorineural deafness and/or Meniere disease in human XLH patients may be the counterpart of the murine *Gy* mutation (Hypophosphatemia type II); Hypophosphatemia type I is the *Hyp* counterpart.

X-linked Hypophosphatemia should be distinguished from:

1.) **Hypophosphatemia, non X-linked** which has an equivalent degree of hypophosphatemia, a normal percent of tubular reabsorption of phosphate (% TRP) at the low endogenous filtered load, less severe bone disease, and a response to $1,25(OH)_2D_3$ with improved net reabsorption of phosphate.

2.) **Rickets, hereditary hypophosphatemic with hypercalciuria (HHRH)**, an autosomal recessive disease in which the serum $1,25(OH)_2D_3$ levels are elevated, there is impaired renal reabsorption of phosphate, and the heterozygote manifests hypercalciuria.

**References:**
Glorieux F, Scriver CR: Loss of a parathyroid hormone-sensitive component of phosphate transport in X-linked hypophosphatemia. Science 1972; 175:997–1000.
Glorieux F, et al.: Use of phosphate and vitamin D to prevent dwarfism and rickets in X-linked hypophosphatemia. New Engl J Med 1972; 287:481–487.
Tenenhouse HS, et al.: Renal handling of phosphate in vivo and in vitro by the X-linked hypophosphatemic male mouse: evidence for a defect in the brush border membrane. Kidney Int 1978; 14:236–244.
Costa T, et al.: X-linked hypophosphatemia: effect of calcitriol on renal handling of phosphate, serum phosphate, and bone mineralization. J Clin Endocrinol Metab 1981; 52:463–472.
Lyon M, et al.: The *Gy* mutation: another cause of X-linked hypophosphatemia in the mouse. Proc Natl Acad Sci (USA) 1986; 83:4899–4903.
Boneh A, et al.: Audiometric evidence for two forms of X-linked hypophosphatemia in humans. Am J Med Genet 1987; 27:997–1003.
Rasmussen H, Tenenhouse HS: Hypophosphatemias. Scriver CR, et

al, eds: The metabolic basis of inherited disease, 6th ed. New York: McGraw-Hill, 1989:2581–2604.

SC050                                                    **Charles R. Scriver**

**Hypophosphatemic D-resistant rickets**
 See HYPOPHOSPHATEMIA, X-LINKED
**Hypophosphatemic rickets with hypercalciuria**
 See RICKETS, HEREDITARY HYPOPHOSPHATEMIC WITH
  HYPERCALCIURIA (HHRH)
**Hypopigmentation**
 See ALBINOIDISM

## HYPOPIGMENTATION-IMMUNE DEFECT, GRISCELLI TYPE                                                   2360

**Includes:**
 Albinism and immunodeficiency
 Chediak-Higashi-like syndrome
 Griscelli syndrome
 Hypopigmentation-immunodeficiency disease
**Excludes:**
 **Albinism, oculocutaneous** (all types)
 **Albinoidism** (2359)
 **Chediak-Higashi syndrome** (0143)

**Major Diagnostic Criteria:** Silver-gray hair, normal or increased skin pigmentation, and repeated infections in a child in the absence of ocular features of albinism.

**Clinical Findings:** Clinical signs are manifest in the first year of life. The scalp hair, eyebrows, and eyelashes are silver-gray in color, and the skin is pale, normal, or mildly hyperpigmented. Ophthalmologic examination is normal, and nystagmus and photophobia are absent. Chronic diarrhea and repeated bacterial infection involving the respiratory tract, ear, lacrimal sac, or skin, associated with lymphadenopathy and hepatosplenomegaly, are characteristic. Episodic fevers are associated with an increase in hepatosplenomegaly, pancytopenia, and an increase in the silver color of the hair. These episodes do not always correlate with infections.

Large pigment clumps are present in the hair shafts, and the skin melanocytes are filled with mature melanosomes (pigment granules). Reduced numbers of dendrites on the melanocytes are associated with reduced transfer of melanosomes to surrounding keratinocytes. The white count is normal, but granulocytopenia is present. The bactericidal activity of polymorphonuclear cells and the circulating immunoglobulin levels are usually reduced or may be normal. Cellular immunity is abnormal, with an absence of in vivo (skin anergy) and in vitro response to a variety of antigens. B- and T-cell counts are normal. Phagocytosis of platelets and red blood cells is present in the liver and bone marrow, and serum from an affected individual promotes erythrophagocytosis *in vitro*.

**Complications:** Pneumonic and lung abscess.

**Associated Findings:** None known.

**Etiology:** Autosomal recessive inheritance.

**Pathogenesis:** The studies by Griscelli et al. (1978) suggest that a major part of the immune defect is the result of an abnormality in T helper cell function. The widespread immune and phagocytic changes suggest a primary membrane defect.

**MIM No.:** *21445

**Sex Ratio:** M1:F1

**Occurrence:** Three families have been reported in the literature.

**Risk of Recurrence for Patient's Sib:**
 See Part I, *Mendelian Inheritance.*

**Risk of Recurrence for Patient's Child:**
 See Part I, *Mendelian Inheritance.*

**Age of Detectability:** During the first three months of life.

**Gene Mapping and Linkage:** Unknown.

**Prevention:** None known. Genetic counseling indicated.

**Treatment:** Antibiotics for recurrent bacterial infections.

**Prognosis:** Early death or severe limitations secondary to recurrent pulmonary infections are expected.

**Detection of Carrier:** Unknown.

**Special Considerations:** Siccardi et al (1978) reported a boy with similar features; however, the boy's normal father had a similar abnormality in polymorphonuclear cell bactericidal activity, and the father, paternal grandfather, and paternal great-grandfather had silver hair. This appears to be a separate autosomal dominant condition.

**References:**
Griscelli C, et al.: A syndrome associating partial albinism and immunodeficiency. Am J Med 1978; 65:691–702.
Siccardi AG, et al.: A new familial defect in neutrophil bactericidal activity. Helv Pediatr Acta 1978; 33:401–412.
Brambilla E, et al.: Partial albinism and immunodeficiency: ultrastructural study of haemophagocytosis and bone marrow erythroblasts in one case. Pathol Res Pract 1980; 167:151–165.

KI007                                                    **Richard A. King**

**Hypopigmentation-immunodeficiency disease**
 See HYPOPIGMENTATION-IMMUNE DEFECT, GRISCELLI TYPE
**Hypopituitarism-imperforate anus-postaxial polydactyly**
 See HYPOTHALAMIC HAMARTOBLASTOMA SYNDROME,
  CONGENITAL
**Hypoplasia of inner ear**
 See EAR, INNER DYSPLASIAS
**Hypoplasia of iris with rudimentary root**
 See ANIRIDIA
**Hypoplasia of optic nerve**
 See OPTIC NERVE HYPOPLASIA
**Hypoplasia of the maxilla, primary familial**
 See MAXILLOFACIAL DYSOSTOSIS
**Hypoplasia, limb**
 See LIMB REDUCTION DEFECTS
**Hypoplasia, X-linked thymic epithelial type**
 See IMMUNODEFICIENCY, X-LINKED SEVERE COMBINED
**Hypoplasia/aplasia of tibia and/or ulna with split-hand/split foot**
 See TIBIAL HYPOPLASIA/APLASIA-ECTRODACTYLY
**Hypoplastic anemia, congenital**
 See ANEMIA, HYPOPLASTIC CONGENITAL
**Hypoplastic glomerulocystic kidney, familial**
 See KIDNEY, GLOMERULOCYSTIC
**Hypoproconvertinemia**
 See FACTOR VII DEFICIENCY

## HYPOPROTHROMBINEMIA                                          2679

**Includes:**
 Dysprothrombinemia
 Factor II deficiency
 Prothrombin
**Excludes:**
 Acquired factor II deficiency
 Acquired hypoprothrombinemia
 **Coagulation defect, familial multiple factors** (2674)
 Factor II inhibitors

**Major Diagnostic Criteria:** Rare congenital hemorrhagic disorder; prolonged prothrombin time and partial thromboplastin time; reduced plasma coagulant activity of Factor II (prothrombin).

**Clinical Findings:** Bleeding manifestations include ecchymoses, hematomas, epistaxis, menorrhagia, and excessive bleeding after surgical procedures. Patients with hypoprothrombinemia have reduced Factor II biologic activity and a similar reduction in immunologically detected prothrombin; in dysprothrombinemia the biologic activity is reduced, but normal amounts of prothrombin are detected by immunoassay. Homozygous patients have plasma Factor II activity levels between 1 and 25 units/dl.

**Complications:** Antibodies against Factor II as a consequence of treatment; death due to bleeding.

**Associated Findings:** None known.

**Etiology:** Autosomal recessive inheritance for congenital hypoprothrombinemia. Autosomal dominant inheritance for congenital dysprothrombinemia. Some affected individuals are genetic compounds.

**Pathogenesis:** Factor II is converted to thrombin in both the intrinsic and extrinsic coagulation pathways. Thrombin then converts fibrinogen to fibrin.

**MIM No.:** *17693

**Sex Ratio:** M1:F1

**Occurrence:** Fewer than 25 families have been detected with hypoprothrombinemia and fewer than 15 families with dysprothrombinemia.

**Risk of Recurrence for Patient's Sib:**
See Part I, *Mendelian Inheritance.*

**Risk of Recurrence for Patient's Child:**
See Part I, *Mendelian Inheritance.*

**Age of Detectability:** At birth.

**Gene Mapping and Linkage:** F2 (coagulation factor II (prothrombin)) has been provisionally mapped to 11p11-q12.
F2L (coagulation factor II (prothrombin)-like) has been tentatively mapped to Xpter-q25.

**Prevention:** None known. Genetic counseling indicated.

**Treatment:** Fresh or fresh-frozen plasma; prothrombin complex concentrates.

**Prognosis:** Normal life span.

**Detection of Carrier:** Heterozygotes have Factor II activity levels between 43 and 75 units/dl.

**References:**
Girolami A: The hereditary transmission of congenital "true" hypoprothrominemia. Br J Haematol 1971; 21:695–703.
Mammen EF: Congenital coagulation disorders. Semin Thromb Hemostas 1983; 9:13–16.
Rocha E, et al.: Prothrombin Segovia: a new congenital abnormality of prothrombin. Scand J Haemat 1986; 36:444–449.
Dumont M-D, et al.: Prothrombin Poissy: a new variant of human prothrombin. Brit J Haemat 1987; 66:239–243.
Valls-de-Ruiz M, et al.: Prothrombin "Medico City": an asymptomatic autosomal dominant prothrombin variant. Am J Hemat 1987; 24:229–240.

C0068                                            **James J. Corrigan**

**Hyposmia**
*See ANOSMIA, CONGENITAL*

---

## HYPOSPADIAS                                              0518

**Includes:** Hypospadias with or without chordee

**Excludes:**
 **Androgen insensitivity syndrome, incomplete** (0050)
 **Branchio-skeleto-genital syndrome** (0118)
 **Chromosome 4, monosomy 4p** (0164)
 **Chromosome mosaicism, 45x/46,XY type** (0173)
 Curvature of the penis
 Dystopia of the meatus
 **G syndrome** (0401)
 **Hermaphroditism, true** (0971)
 **Hypertelorism-hypospadias syndrome** (0505)
 **Oculo-cerebro-facial syndrome, Kaufman type** (2179)
 Penoscrotal transposition
 **Smith-Lemli-Opitz syndrome** (0891)
 **Steroid 3 beta-hydroxysteroid dehydrogenase deficiency** (0909)
 **Steroid 5 alpha-reductase deficiency** (3062)
 **Steroid 17 alpha-hydroxylase deficiency** (0903)
 **Steroid 17,20-desmolase deficiency** (0904)
 **Steroid 20–22 desmolase deficiency** (0907)
 Urethral fistula, congenital

**Major Diagnostic Criteria:** The presence of a urethral meatus at a location other than the tip of the glans penis in an otherwise normal boy. Foreskin is deficient on the ventral aspect of the penis.

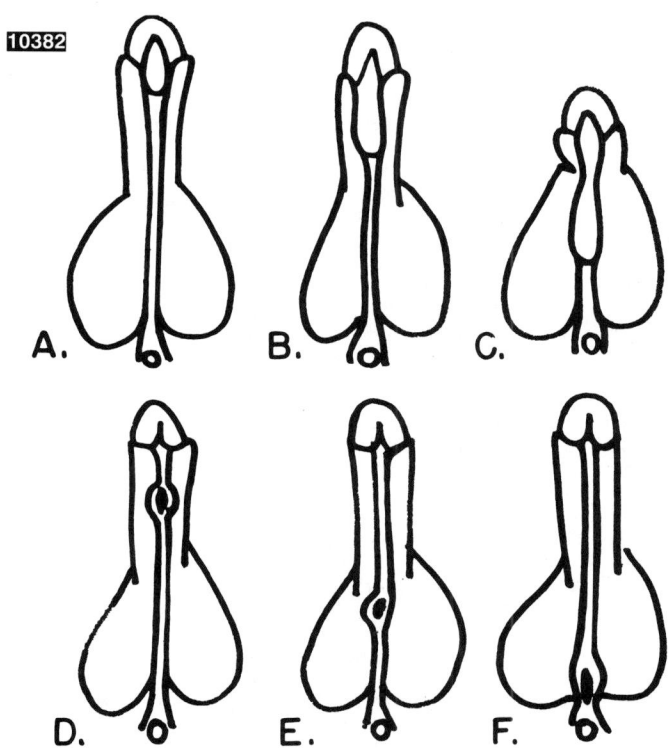

0518-10382: Schematic hypospadias. A) Glandular; B&C) peniglandular; D) penile; E) scrotal; F) perineal.

**Clinical Findings:** The hypospadic boy is readily recognized by physical examination. The urethral meatus is not at the tip of the glans penis. It is situated more proximally on the ventral aspect of the penis. In approximately one-half of the cases, there is associated chordee, which is the downward curvature of the glans penis with resultant penile deformity. Chordee can be cutaneous or fibrous, and is usually more severe as the meatus presents more proximally. The primary considerations are meatal location, control of voided stream, and ease of sexual intromission. Hypospadias can usually be classified by location of the meatus into coronal or glandular (60%), penile (15%), scrotal (20%), and perineal (3–5%). Eighty percent of hypospadic meati are distal to the penoscrotal junction.

**Complications:** Penile abnormalities (45%) as follows: chordee 35%, meatal stenosis 8%, microphallus, cobra head glans and bifid scrotum to a lesser degree. Cryptorchidism is found in 8–15%, hydrocele in 16% and congenital inguinal hernia in 8% of patients. Post-operative complications: urethrocutaneous fistula in 17%, urethral stricture in 6%, and psychological problems are reported in a majority of cases.

**Associated Findings:** Upper urinary tract abnormalities (2–12%): horseshoe kidney, renal ectopia, and duplication of ureters. There are many other system anomalies associated with hypospadias: cardiovascular amomalies, deafness, anal atresia, **Vater association**, hydrocephalus, omphalocele and neuromuscular abnormalities were all reported. These mostly belong to the syndromes or chromosomal abnormalities. Prematurity is four times as common in hypospadic patients as in the control group.

**Etiology:** In most cases the cause of the malformation is unknown. A polygenic mode of inheritance has been postulated. In some families with lesser degrees of hypospadias it is transmitted from father to son as autosomal dominant with sex limitation. Hypospadias may occur more often in males with earlier birth ranks. Testicular anomalies are reported present in 34% of the fathers of patients compared with 3% of the control fathers. Progestins are shown to cause hypospadias in animals and are implicated in humans.

**Pathogenesis:** The development of the phallus occurs between the seventh and sixteenth week of intrauterine life. At the early stage of development, the external genitalia are constituted by a genital tubercle and a urogenital groove that is limited by two urethral folds and laterally by labioscrotal swellings. The urethral folds may remain open forming labia minora in females, or they may fuse to form corpus spongiosum enclosing a phallic urethra.

In males, the urethral groove starts fusing in the pelvic region at about eight weeks of gestation, progressively bringing the urogenital ostium onto the phallus by the 14th week. The glans is the last portion of the normal urethra to close. If the urethral groove fails to fuse anywhere along its extent, hypospadias proximal to the glans results. The fusion of the urethral groove is brought about by the androgens produced by the fetal testes. Testosterone produced by the Leydig cells of the primary testes is bound to the specific target cells of the urogenital tubercle and sinus, and is converted to 5 α-dihydrotestosterone (5 α-DHT) by the microsomal enzyme, steroid D⁴ 5 α-reductase. 5 α-DHT is bound to a cytoplasmic receptor that induces differentiation of the male external genitalia.

Any failure of the testicular differentiation due to chromosomal imbalance, or in the synthesis of testosterone or its reduction to 5 α-DHT, causes progressive lack of virilization in phallic development resulting in variable degrees of hypospadias. Lack of androgen receptors as a cause of hypospadias in human males has also been described. Abnormal karyotypes were found in 7.5% of cases studied by Aarskog (1979).

Under normal conditions, the maternal hormones do not disturb organogenesis of the fetus. High doses of progesterone or 19-nor, 17 α-hydroxy progesterone, or low doses of synthetic progestational steroids administered to the mother during the pregnancy may interfere with urethral groove fusion. The available data may suggest that progestin exposure during the vulnerable period would double the incidence of hypospadias in predisposed fetuses (see **Fetal effects from maternal extrinsic androgens**).

**MIM No.:** 14645, 24175

**CDC No.:** 752.600

**Sex Ratio:** M10,000:F1

**Occurrence:** Incidence 0.8–8.2:1,000 live male births. Prevalence ranges from 50:100,000 to about 300:100,000. During recent years increasing incidence has been reported from England, Wales, Norway and Sweden. In the United States, the Centers for Disease Control reported an annual increase in the reported incidence of 3% per year from 1970 to 1975.

**Risk of Recurrence for Patient's Sib:** Bauer et al (1981) reported a 14% recurrence risk.

**Risk of Recurrence for Patient's Child:** Fathers were found to have hypospadias in 8% of cases.

**Age of Detectability:** At birth.

**Gene Mapping and Linkage:** Unknown.

**Prevention:** Avoidance of exposure to synthetic progesterone products during pregnancy. Genetic counseling when indicated.

**Treatment:** For lesion distal to the corona unassociated with chordee, surgery is not indicated . Otherwise surgical correction should be undertaken during the first year after the first 6 weeks of life, and completed by three years.

Advancement of urethra can be performed in a one stage operation in the majority of cases. More proximal lesions may require multi-stage repair. If microphallus is present, topical application of 3% testosterone should be considered. Psychological problems may require further counseling and therapy.

**Prognosis:** There is no shortening of life expectancy. The prognosis is good for uncomplicated milder cases.

**Detection of Carrier:** Unknown.

**Special Considerations:** It is important to differentiate cases of simple hypospadias of unknown etiology from hypospadias of a more complicated etiology: several genetic syndromes or chromosome abnormalities or male pseudohermaphroditism of various origin. The complexities of sex identification and assignment and management have made it imperative that a team approach be used in treatment of these known hypospadic patients. The team generally consists of a geneticist, pediatrician, endocrinologist, psychiatrist, and a reconstructive surgeon.

**References:**
Sweet RA, et al.: Study of the incidence of hypospadias in Rochester, MN, 1949–1970, and a case control comparison of possible etiologic factors. Mayo Clin Proc 1974; 49:52–58.
Aarskog D: Current concepts: maternal progestins as a possible cause of hypospadias. New Engl J Med 1979; 300:75–79.
Svenson J: Male hypospadias: 625 cases, associated malformations and possible etiological factors. Acta Paediatr Scan 1979; 68:587–592.
Bauer S, et al.: Genetic aspects of hypospadias. Urol Clin North Am 1981; 8:559–571.
Duckett JW: Hypospadias. In Walsh PC, et al, eds: Campbell's urology. Philadelphia: W.B. Saunders, 1985:1969–1999.
Frydman M, et al.: Uncomplicated familial hypospadias: evidence for autosomal recessive inheritance. Am J Med Genet 1985; 21:51–55.
Tsur M, et al.: Hypospadias in a consanguineous family (letter). Am J Med Genet 1987; 27:487–489.

BI012                      **Nesrin Bingol**
WA034            **Edward Wasserman**

**Hypospadias with or without chordee**
*See HYPOSPADIAS*
**Hypospadias-dysphagia syndrome**
*See G SYNDROME*
**Hypospadias-hypertelorism syndrome**
*See HYPERTELORISM-HYPOSPADIAS SYNDROME*
**Hypospadias-radial hypoplasia-triphalangeal thumbs-diastema**
*See RADIAL HYPOPLASIA-TRIPHALANGEAL THUMBS-HYPOSPADIAS-DIASTEMA*
**Hyposplenia, congenital isolated**
*See SPLEEN, CONGENITAL ISOLATED HYPOSPLENIA*
**Hypotaurodontism**
*See TEETH, TAURODONTISM*

---

## HYPOTHALAMIC HAMARTOBLASTOMA SYNDROME, CONGENITAL         2285

**Includes:**
> Hall-Pallister syndrome
> Hypopituitarism-imperforate anus-postaxial polydactyly
> Pallister-Hall syndrome

**Excludes:**
> **Chondroectodermal dysplasia** (0156)
> **Hydrolethalus syndrome** (2279)
> **Meckel syndrome** (0634)
> **Smith-Lemli-Opitz syndrome** (0891)
> **Vaginal septum, transverse** (0985)

**Major Diagnostic Criteria:** Hypothalamic hamartoblastoma or hamartoma is mandatory. Symptoms of hypopituitarism early in the perinatal period are persistent hypoglycemia, electrolyte abnormalities, and metabolic acidosis suggesting adrenocortical insufficiency; lethargy and jaundice suggesting hypothyroidism; and micropenis in males suggesting hypogonadism. Phenotypic features consist of small and posteriorly rotated ears, short nose with a flat nasal bridge, and long philtrum; microglossia, often associated with bifid epiglottis or laryngeal cleft; postaxial **Polydactyly** with nail hypoplasia; and imperforate or anteriorly placed anus.

**Clinical Findings:** Sixteen patients have been described. All except one treated survivor (age six years in 1990) were diagnosed at autopsy. Additional findings beyond the major diagnostic criteria may include natal teeth, buccal frenula, pes cavus, 2–3 **Syndactyly**, bilateral single transverse palmar creases, short neck, short limbs, dislocated hips, and spinal defects. Internal anomalies include pulmonary hypoplasia with abnormal lung segmen-

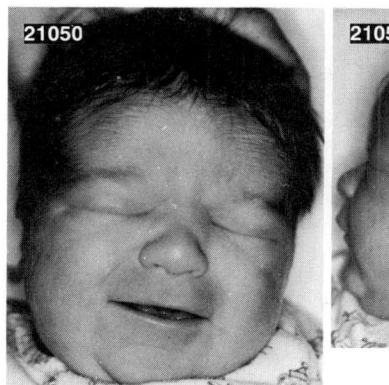
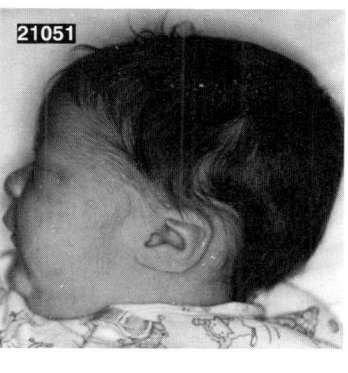
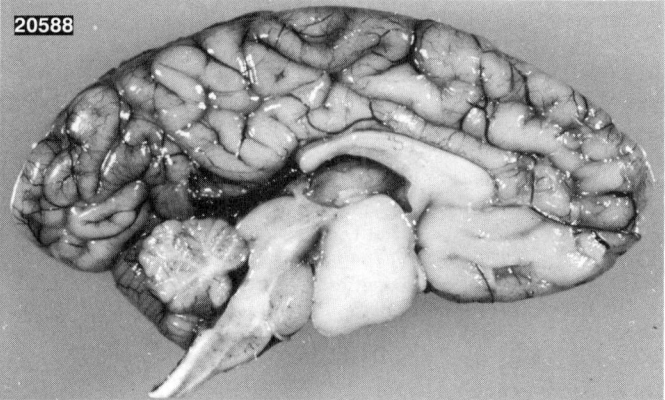

**2285A**-21050–51: Hypothalamic hamartoblastoma syndrome, congenital; note flat nasal bridge, short nose, posteriorly rotated simplified auricles. 20588: Hamartoblastoma is caudal to the brain stem and replaces the hypothalamus and its related nuclei.

tation, hypoplastic renal dysplasia with or without ectopia, and occasional heart defects. Males often present with microphallus and cryptorchidism. Chromosomes have been normal in patients tested.

**Complications:** Death in the perinatal period is probably due to untreated hypopituitarism. One other affected child was treated for hypopituitarism with thyroxine, hydrocortisone, and growth hormone. He died in his sleep at age 19 months, and the hypothalamic tumor was noted at autopsy. The only surviving child with this tumor was treated for hypopituitarism at birth, and

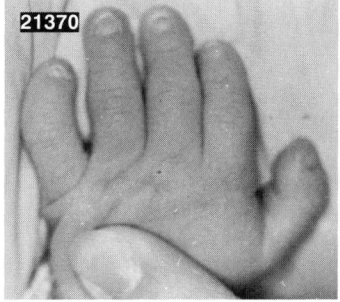
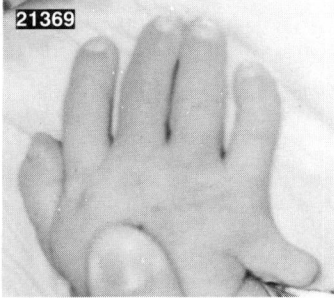

**2285B**-21369–70: Post-axial polydactyly of the left hand, bilateral clinodactyly of the fifth fingers and nail hypoplasia. The hand X-ray on the left showed a T-shaped fifth metacarpal.

her tumor was removed surgically at age one year because of the onset of **Hydrocephaly**. She had delayed development at age three years with no tumor recurrence. The prenatal consequence of this tumor appears to be disruption of the normal relationship between the pituitary gland and the hypothalamus, resulting in deficiencies of multiple pituitary hormones and an absence of the pituitary in some cases. In the single surviving patient, use of thyroid-stimulating hormone-releasing hormone and growth hormone-releasing hormone failed to result in release of their respective hormones, suggesting primary pituitary insufficiency. In children with treated hypopituitarism, increased intracranial pressure from the untreated tumor may lead to death in later infancy or early childhood.

**Associated Findings:** Most infants have been small at birth. Hydrocephaly has occurred prenatally, and hydrocephaly with seizures can develop postnatally, probably due to the space-occupying effects of the tumor. The tumor appears to grow at the same rate as surrounding brain tissue, with no apparent malignant potential, but increased intracranial pressure usually leads to death. Hypopituitarism occurs postnatally and must be treated promptly.

**Etiology:** Probably multifactorial.

**Pathogenesis:** The tumor is composed of small, dark cells resembling primitive, undifferentiated germinal cells. They appear to retain the potential to differentiate into relatively normal neural elements. Because of the associated malformations and tumor histology, it is suggested that this condition arises during the formation of the hypothalamic plate between 34 and 40 days gestation. The tumor is apparent on the inferior aspect of the hypothalamus, extending from the optic chiasma to the interpeduncular fossa. Clustering of cases in time and space suggests the possibility of a teratogenic cause, perhaps pesticides or herbicides applied during the spring in rural areas. There is one case of apparent familial recurrence in a maternal aunt, suggesting that genetic factors may also play a role. Chromosome studies have been normal.

**MIM No.:** 14651

**POS No.:** 3471

**Sex Ratio:** M11:F5 (observed).

**Occurrence:** Sixteen cases have been reported in the literature.

**Risk of Recurrence for Patient's Sib:**
See Part I, *Mendelian Inheritance.*

**Risk of Recurrence for Patient's Child:**
See Part I, *Mendelian Inheritance.*

**Age of Detectability:** Previously detected at autopsy. The condition has recently been detected at birth due to recognized symptoms of hypopituitarism.
Prenatal diagnosis is feasible based on 1) measurement of maternal estriol levels (decreased when fetal adrenals are hypoplastic); 2) prenatal ultrasound to detect fetal adrenal, renal, or brain alterations; and 3) measurement of disaccharidases in amniotic fluid (decreased with imperforate anus). Postnatal treatment can result in survival with early hormonal replacement therapy. Cranial CT or magnetic resonance imagery at regular intervals to monitor the tumor. Surgical removal of the tumor when space-occupying effects (i.e., hydrocephaly) become apparent, or visual apparatus is disturbed.

**Gene Mapping and Linkage:** Unknown.

**Prevention:** None known. Genetic counseling indicated.

**Treatment:** Unknown.

**Prognosis:** Unknown. The only survivor has delays in language and motor development evident at age six years (in 1990). There has been no recurrence of the tumor after surgical removal.

**Detection of Carrier:** Unknown.

**References:**
Clarren SK, et al.: Congenital hypothalamic hamartoblastoma, hypopituitarism, imperforate anus, and postaxial polydactyly: a new

syndrome? Neuropathological considerations. Am J Med Genet 1980; 7:75–83.

Hall JG, et al.: Congenital hypothalamic hamartoblastoma, hypopituitarism, imperforate anus, and postaxial polydactyly: a new syndrome? Clinical, causal, and pathogenic considerations. Am J Med Genet 1980; 7:47–74. †

Huff DS, Fernandes M: Two cases of congenital hypothalamic hamartoblastoma, polydactyly, and other congenital anomalies (Pallister-Hall syndrome). New Engl J Med 1982; 306:430–431.

Culler FL, Jones KL: Hypopituitarism in association with postaxial polydactyly. J Pediatr 1986; 104:881–884.

Graham JM Jr, et al.: A cluster of Pallister-Hall syndrome cases (congenital hypothalamic hamartoblastoma syndrome). Am J Med Genet 1986; 2(suppl):53–63. †

Iafolla K, et al.: Case report and delineation of the congenital hypothalamic hamartoblastoma syndrome (Pallister-Hall syndrome). Am J Med Genet 1989; 33:489–499. †

Pallister PD, et al.: Three additional cases of the congenital hypothalamic "hamartoblastoma" (Pallister-Hall) syndrome. Am J Med Genet 1989; 33:500–501.

GR000  
CH041

**John M. Graham, Jr.**  
**Catherine E. Charman**

**Hypothalamic hypothyroidism**  
*See THYROTROPIN DEFICIENCY, ISOLATED*  
**Hypothyroidism, congenital**  
*See THYROID, PEROXIDASE DEFECT*  
*also THYROTROPIN UNRESPONSIVENESS*  
*also THYROID, THYROGLOBULIN DEFECTS*  
**Hypothyroidism, congenital (some forms)**  
*See THYROID, IODIDE TRANSPORT DEFECT*  
*also THYROID, IODOTYROSINE DEIODINASE DEFICIENCY*  
**Hypotonia "floppy baby" syndrome**  
*See FETAL BENZODIAZEPINE EFFECTS*  
**Hypotonia-hypomentia-hypogonadism-obesity (HHHO)**  
*See PRADER-WILLI SYNDROME*  
**Hypotonia-obesity-prominent incisors**  
*See COHEN SYNDROME*  
**Hypotrichosis, congenital**  
*See HAIR, ATRICHIA CONGENITA*  
**Hypotrichosis, hereditary**  
*See HAIR, HYPOTRICHOSIS*  
**Hypotrichosis-retinopathy**  
*See RETINOPATHY-HYPOTRICHOSIS SYNDROME*  
**Hypouricemia-hypercalciuria-decreased bone density**  
*See RENAL HYPOURICEMIA* †

---

## HYPOVENTILATION, CONGENITAL CENTRAL ALVEOLAR TYPE     2606

**Includes:**
Autonomic control, congenital failure of
Autonomic nervous system dysfunction (congenital)
Congenital central hypoventilation syndrome (CCHS)
Hirschprung disease-Ondine curse
Ondine curse-Hirschprung disease

**Excludes:**
Colon, aganglionosis (0192)
Encephalopathy, necrotizing (0344)
Hypoventilation, secondary congenital central alveolar
Narcolepsy (3287)

**Major Diagnostic Criteria:** Cyanosis beginning shortly after birth, during periods of sleep. Normal respiratory function when awake. Increased ventilation after external stimulation. Reversibility of hypoxia and hypercapnia by assisted ventilation; absence of primary cardiac, pulmonary, thoracic, neuromuscular, or cerebral disease. Absence of ganglion cells in colon.

**Clinical Findings:** Episodes of cyanosis developing rapidly after birth without evidence of respiratory or cardiovascular disease. Respiration is normal while awake, but absent during non-REM sleep. Infants develop ileus and abdominal distension secondary to colonic distension because of the absence of ganglion cells from the terminal ileum to the rectum. Generalized muscle hypotonia. No other abnormalities have been noted and birth weight and

pregnancy histories have been unremarkable, although in two patients a lack of beat-to-beat variability in fetal heart tones was noted toward the end of pregnancy in two cases.

**Complications:** Hypoxia and hypercapnia during sleep with secondary cerebral changes if not treated. Possible right ventricular hypertrophy and pulmonary hypertension. Severe and abrupt decompensation, with upper airway infection.

**Associated Findings:** Total aganglionosis of the colon (see **Colon, aganglionosis**). Possible increased incidence of ganglioneuroblastomas.

**Etiology:** Possibly autosomal recessive inheritance, or autosomal dominant inheritance with incomplete penetrance. In one family two sisters were similarly affected. Another family was described with affected half siblings (male and female), related through their father. Consanguinity has not been noted.

**Pathogenesis:** Possible failure of chemoreceptors in the ventrolateral area of the medulla, or possibly a common defect of stem serotonergic cells (of neural crest origin).

**MIM No.:** *20988

**Sex Ratio:** Presumably M1:F1.

**Occurrence:** Nine cases of CCHS and total or partial aganglionosis of the colon have been documented. Five patients were Caucasian. The reported half sibs were Black. Race was not noted in the other cases.

**Risk of Recurrence for Patient's Sib:**
See Part I, *Mendelian Inheritance.*

**Risk of Recurrence for Patient's Child:**
See Part I, *Mendelian Inheritance.* Affected individuals are not expected to survive to reproduce.

**Age of Detectability:** Shortly after birth.

**Gene Mapping and Linkage:** Unknown.

**Prevention:** None known. Genetic counseling indicated.

**Treatment:** Mechanical ventilation/respirator care during sleep. Possible phrenic nerve pacing. Colostomy/ileostomy. Tracheostomy.

**Prognosis:** Patients usually die in early infancy, although the less severely affected half siblings are alive at two years 4 1/2 years of age. The 4 1/2 year-old patient now requires only ventilator support at night. Both she and her half brother have had colostomy closure at 20 months and 11 months respectively. These patients had short segment Hirschprung (see **Colon, aganglionosis**, whereas all other patients had total absence of ganglion cells in the colon. Both have developed cor pulmonale.

**Detection of Carrier:** Unknown.

**Support Groups:**
New York; Narcolepsy and Cataplexy Foundation of America
CA; Stanford; American Narcolepsy Association

**References:**
Haddad G, et al.: Congenital failure of autonomic control of ventilation, gastrointestinal motility and heart rate. Medicine 1978; 57:516–526.

Stern M, et al.: Total aganglionosis of the colon (Hirschsprung's disease) and total failure of automatic control of ventilation (Ondine's curse). Acta Paediatr Scand 1981; 70:121–124.

Guilleminault C, et al.: Congenital central alveolar hypoventilation syndrome in six infants. Pediatrics 1982; 70:684–694.

Peterson B, Tunnell S: Congenital central alveolar hypoventilation syndrome (CCHS) and Hirschsprung's megacolon (H.M.): report of a seventh case. Am J Hum Genet 1986; 39:75A only.

Hamilton J, Bodurtha J: Congenital central alveolar hypoventilation syndrome and Hirschsprung's disease in half sibs. J Med Genet 1989; 26:272–279.

TU003

**Sheila M. Tunnell**

**Hypoxanthine guanine phosphoribosyl transferase (HGPRT) deficiency**  
*See LESCH-NYHAN SYNDROME*  
**Hypoxanthine guanine phosphoribosyl transferase, deficiencies of**  
*See GOUT*

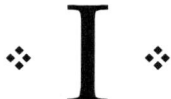

**I-cell disease**
 See *MUCOLIPIDOSIS II*
**Ibuprofen therapy; carnitine palmityl thransferase deficiency**
 See *MYOPATHY-METABOLIC, CARNITINE PALMITYL
 TRANSFERASE DEFICIENCY*
**Ibuprofen, fetal effects**
 See *FETAL EFFECTS OF NONSTEROIDAL ANTI-INFLAMMATORY
 DRUGS (NSAIDS)*
**Icelandic type amyloidosis**
 See *AMYLOIDOSIS, ICELANDIC TYPE*
**Ichthyosiform erythroderma with leukocyte vacuolization**
 See *STORAGE DISEASE, NEUTRAL LIPID TYPE*
**Ichthyosiform erythroderma, Brocq nonbullous form**
 See *ICHTHYOSIS, LAMELLAR RECESSIVE*
**Ichthyosiform erythroderma, non-bullous congenital**
 See *ICHTHYOSIS, CONGENITAL ERYTHRODERMIC*
**Ichthyosiform erythroderma, nonbullous, dominant form**
 See *ICHTHYOSIS, LAMELLAR DOMINANT*
**Ichthyosiform erythroderma-corneal involvement-deafness**
 See *ICHTHYOSIFORM ERYTHROKERATODERMA, ATYPICAL WITH
 DEAFNESS*

---

## ICHTHYOSIFORM ERYTHROKERATODERMA, ATYPICAL WITH DEAFNESS        2861

**Includes:**
 Burns syndrome
 Cornification, disorder of (one form)
 Deafness-ichthyosiform erythroderma
 Ichthyosiform erythroderma-corneal involvement-deafness
 Keratitis-Ichthyosis-Deafness (KID) syndrome
 Senter syndrome

**Excludes:**
 **Phytanic acid storage disease** (0810)
 **Skin, erythrokeratodermia, variable** (0361)
 **Skin, keratosis follicularis spinulosa decalvans** (2867)
 **Storage disease, neutral lipid type** (2859)

**Major Diagnostic Criteria:** A generalized disorder of cornification characterized by follicular hyperkeratosis and perioral furrowed plaques in conjunction with neurosensory deafness. Progressive neovascularizing keratitis develops in most patients.

**Clinical Findings:** The disorder of cornification in these patients is quite unique, and is characterized by 1) fixed keratotic plaques; 2) diffuse palmoplantar keratoderma; and 3) a generalized hyperkeratosis with prominent, follicular keratoses elsewhere on the body. The dermatosis presents at birth as erythematous, diffusely thickened skin that desquamates in the first week of life. Fixed, keratotic plaques, often with an erythematous base, are most common on the extremities and face, producing an aged or leonine appearance. Whereas most patients display generalized hyperkeratosis, skin thickening, and follicular prominence, in others, involvement may be limited to the face and extremities. Follicular hyperkeratosis may result in significant alopecia. The nails are hypoplastic or dystrophic, and teeth may be small and carious. The histopathology of the skin is characteristic but not diagnostic, demonstrating "basket-weave" hyperkeratosis.

Neurosensory deafness is nonprogressive and may be severe. Ocular involvement is characterized by keratoconjunctivitis, which progresses to neovascularization and pannus formation. Although keratitis commonly begins in infancy, the onset may be delayed until the second decade. Some patients develop recurrent skin infections, including multiple abscesses, atypical, granulomatous fungal infections, and recurrent deep tissue infections, e.g., pneumonia, otitis, and urinary tract infections. However, an immunologic basis for these lesions has not been established. Squamous cell carcinoma of the tongue has been reported.

**Complications:** Visual impairment due to progressive keratitis with scarring. The coexistence of deafness, which although nonprogressive may be severe, can add to the sensory handicap. Recurrent skin infections may lead to discomfort and disability. Recurrent pneumonia, otitis, and urinary tract infections may produce morbidity in some patients with this syndrome.

**Associated Findings:** Tight heel cords, 17%; impaired sweating, 13%. Other reported findings in single patients include cryptorchidism, hepatomegaly, pes cavus, **Hernia, inguinal**, neuropathy, and growth retardation.

**Etiology:** Most cases have been sporadic. A family with two affected sibs has been reported, suggesting possible autosomal recessive inheritance.

**Pathogenesis:** Unknown. Elevated serum steroid disulfate levels were reported in one patient.

**MIM No.:** 24215

**POS No.:** 3528

**CDC No.:** 757.197

**Sex Ratio:** F12:M10 (observed).

**Occurrence:** A recent literature review identified 23 cases from North America, Europe, and Vietnam.

**Risk of Recurrence for Patient's Sib:**
 See Part I, *Mendelian Inheritance.*

**Risk of Recurrence for Patient's Child:**
 See Part I, *Mendelian Inheritance.*

**Age of Detectability:** The skin is usually abnormal at birth, but the distinctive cutaneous phenotype may not become apparent until late in infancy. Deafness is congenital and nonprogressive. Keratitis usually begins in infancy, but onset may be delayed until adolescence.

**Gene Mapping and Linkage:** Unknown.

**Prevention:** None known. Genetic counseling indicated.

**Treatment:** Effective therapies for progressive keratitis are unknown. Cutaneous infections should be cultured and treated appropriately. Oral synthetic retinoids are considered experimental because of their toxicity.

**Prognosis:** Probably normal for life span. Intelligence is normal.

**Detection of Carrier:** Unknown.

**Support Groups:** San Francisco; Foundation for Ichthyosis and Related Skin Types (FIRST)

**References:**
Skinner BA, et al.: The keratitis, ichthyosis and deafness (KID) syndrome. Arch Dermatol 1981; 117:285–289. * †
Legrand J, et al.: Un syndrome rare oculo-auriculo-cutane (syndrome de Burns). J Fr Ophthalmol 1982; 5:441–445. †
Harms M, et al.: KID syndrome (keratitis, ichthyosis, and deafness) and chronic mucocutaneous candidiasis: case report and review of the literature. Pediatr Dermatol 1984; 2:1–7. *
Frieden IJ, Esterly NB: Selected genodermatoses in infants and children. Clin Dermatol 1985; 2:14–32. * †

WI013                                          **Mary L. Williams**

**Ichthyosiform erythryoderma, unilateral-ipsilateral malformations**
*See LIMB REDUCTION-ICHTHYOSIS*

## ICHTHYOSIFORM HYPERKERATOSIS, BULLOUS CONGENITAL                                    2852

**Includes:**
Bullous congenital ichthyosiform erythroderma
Bullous erythroderma ichthyosiformis congenita of Brocq
Bullous ichthyosis
Cornification, disorder of, bullous type (DOC 3)
Epidermolytic hyperkeratosis
Ichthyosis, bullous type
Ichthyosis congenita, wet type

**Excludes:**
Ichthyosiform erythroderma, non-bullous congenital
Ichthyosis congenita, dry type
**Ichthyosis hystrix, Curth-Macklin type** (2857)
**Nevus, epidermal nevus syndrome** (0593)

**Major Diagnostic Criteria:** Affected infants are born with widespread areas of blistered or denuded skin. After the newborn period, a severe, generalized hyperkeratosis ensues, that may be accentuated on palms and soles and around joints. Skin biopsy showing histological features of epidermolytic hyperkeratosis is required for the diagnosis, and excludes all other generalized disorders of cornification.

**Clinical Findings:** The newborn presents with widespread areas of denuded skin, resembling the infant with one of the severe mechano-bullous disorders (**Epidermolysis bullosum**). On careful examination, however, areas of hyperkeratosis may be present. After the neonatal period, as hyperkeratosis becomes prominent, the mechano-bullous component recedes; but focal blistering may continue, and bullae are most often induced by secondary infection rather than trauma. The scales are usually dark and warty, forming a ridged pattern which is particularly evident in the flexures. Verrucous hyperkeratoses in occluded areas become macerated and secondarily colonized by bacteria, producing a foul body odor. Scales may be shed in thick clumps of nearly full-thickness stratum corneum, leaving behind a pink, denuded, and often tender base. An underlying erythroderma is usually evident. Palmoplantar keratoderma is always present but varies in severity. Facial involvement may occur but without ectropion. Although the hair shaft itself is spared, severe scalp involvement results in "nit-like encasements" of hair shafts. Secondary nail dystrophy due to periungual inflammation is common.
Many patients have demonstrated limited and/or localized disease; in this cases, flexural involvement with the formation of spiney ridges is an important diagnostic sign. A wide range in the severity of disease expression occurs in this disorder, but most of this variability apparently is interfamilial rather than intrafamilial.
The skin biopsy distinguishes this disorder from any other generalized disorder of cornification. The epidermis is acanthotic, and the cells of the upper spinous and granular cell layers exhibit intracellular vacuolization; dense clumps of granular material that appear to be enlarged keratohyalin granules but in fact represent clumped keratin filaments; and dense, massive, hyperkeratosis. These features have been termed *epidermolytic hyperkeratosis*.

The histopathologic features of epidermolytic hyperkeratosis are not unique to this generalized disorder of cornification, but occur in such diverse settings as solitary acanthomas, epidermis overlying dermatofibromas, within epidermoid cyst walls, and as an incidental finding on oral mucosa. Furthermore, some kindreds with palmoplantar keratoderma exhibit the histology of epidermolytic hyperkeratosis, but are not at risk for this generalized disease. While epidermolytic hyperkeratosis observed in these other settings does not appear to be part of the phenotypic expression of bullous congenital ichthyosiform hyperkeratosis, there is still some uncertainty as to the relationship of epidermal nevi exhibiting this histopathologic feature and the present disorder.

**Complications:** The thick, macerated scales in intertriginous areas become heavily colonized with microorganisms resulting in foul body odor. Recurrent blisters on hands and feet may interfere with physical activities, as may thick keratoderma in these areas. Newborns with widespread areas of denuded skin are at high risk for sepsis and fluid/electrolyte imbalance.

**Associated Findings:** None known.

**Etiology:** Autosomal dominant inheritance with variability in expression, probably largely interfamilial. At least 50% of the cases reported in literature were sporadic, suggesting new mutations. The rare instances of more than one affected sibling of unaffected parents may represent instances of incomplete penetrance of a dominant trait; or of a phenotypically similar, recessively-inherited trait.

**Pathogenesis:** The underlying metabolic abnormality is undetermined. The epidermis is hyperproliferative. On electron microscopy, keratin filaments are clumped in lower epidermal cell layers and form ring-like perinuclear shells in upper spinous and granular cell layers. Intraepidermal vesiculation and clefting occurs as a result of loss of desmosomal attachment. Abnormal keratin profiles have been reported by two different groups, but the specific abnormality reported in each case was different, and these changes may represent a secondary disturbance of keratin synthesis consequent to epidermal hyperproliferation. Deficiency of lysosomal α-mannosidase in one patient with this disorder has been observed, but this finding awaits confirmation.

**MIM No.:** *11380, 14680

**CDC No.:** 757.190

**Sex Ratio:** Presumably M1:F1.

**Occurrence:** First recognized by Nikolsky in the late nineteenth century, numerous cases have been reported worldwide.

**Risk of Recurrence for Patient's Sib:**
See Part I, *Mendelian Inheritance*. Rare instances of more than two affected siblings with unaffected parents, suggest risk may be increased above general population in this setting.

**Risk of Recurrence for Patient's Child:**
See Part I, *Mendelian Inheritance*.

**Age of Detectability:** May be diagnosed *in utero* by fetal skin biopsy because the abnormal clumping of keratin filaments is expressed early in gestation (at least by 20 weeks). Because some amniotic fluid cells exhibit a similar clumped keratin pattern, it may be possible to diagnose this disorder by amniocentesis and examination of the sediment for abnormally cornified cells.

**Gene Mapping and Linkage:** Unknown.

**Prevention:** None known; genetic counseling is indicated.

**Treatment:** Careful attention to fluid and electrolyte balance in affected newborn and surveillance for sepsis. Topical keratolytic agents may be employed to remove thick scales, but are often poorly tolerated because of the blistering tendency of the skin. Systemic toxicity from absorption of these agents, especially corticosteroids and salicylates may occur. Blisters should be cultured and systemic antibiotic administered, because after the neonatal period these are often induced by bacterial infection, particulary *Staphylococcus aureus*. Use of antibacterial soap may improve body odor due to heavy bacterial colonization. Use of oral synthetic retinoids is controversial because of the significant toxicity of these agents, as well as their teratogenecity (see **Fetal retinoid syndrome**). Also, skin fragility with blisters may be exacerbated by retinoids.

**Prognosis:** Increased morbidity/mortality in neonatal period. Thereafter normal life span. Social adaptation may be impaired by severity of skin involvement. Intelligence is normal.

**Detection of Carrier:** By clinical examination.

**Special Considerations:** The term *epidermolytic hyperkeratosis* is in widespread use, because it emphasizes the distinctive skin histopathology in this generalized disorder of cornification, and permits distinction from all other such disorders. However, this histopathology may be seen in other clinical contexts, some of which are genetically transmitted (e.g. an autosomal dominant form of palmoplantar hyperkeratosis) and some of which are not (e.g. normal oral mucosa or over benign skin fibromas). With the exception of epidermal nevi with this histopathology, these other instances do not appear to be part of the phenotypic spectrum of this disorder.

Two reported instances of a father with an epidermal nevus that exhibited the histopathology of epidermolytic hyperkeratosis having an offspring with the generalized disorder of cornification may represent variable expression of the disorder or unrelated, chance occurrence. No instances are reported of the reverse; i.e., a parent with the generalized disorder of cornification with a child with partial expression (i.e., an epidermal nevus). Moreover, monozygotic twins have been discordant for epidermal nevi with epidermolytic hyperkeratosis.

While the histopathology is diagnostic, all features may not be equally well-developed in the fetus and neonate. Careful evaluation by electron microscopy is required looking for clumped keratin filaments, because the abnormal light microscopic features may not be well developed.

**Support Groups:** Raleigh, NC; Foundation for Ichthyosis and Related Skin Types (FIRST)

**References:**
Simpson JR: Congenital ichthyosiform erythroderma. Trans St Johns Hosp Derm Soc 1964; 50(New Series):53–104. *
Goldsmith LA: The ichthyosis. Prog Med Genet 1967; 1:185–240.
Holbrook KA, et al.: Epidermolytic hyperkeratosis: ultrastructure and biochemistry of skin and amniotic fluid cells from two affected fetuses and a newborn infant. J Invest Dermatol 1983; 80:222–227.
Lookingbill DP, et al.: Generalized epidermolytic hyperkeratosis in the child of a parent with nevus comedones. Arch Dermatol 1984; 120:223–226.
Eady RAJ, et al.: Prenatal diagnosis of bullous ichthyosiform erythroderma. J Med Genet 1986; 23:46–51.
Williams ML, Elias PM: Genetically transmitted, generalized disorders of cornification: the ichthyosis. Dermatologic Clinics 1987; 5:155–178. * †

WI013      **Mary L. Williams**

## ICHTHYOSIS      **1511**

**Includes:**
Collodian baby
Lamellar exfoliation of the newborn
Palmo-plantar keratodermas

The ichthyoses encompass a number of unrelated acquired and inherited disorders having in common the accumulation of visible scale on the skin surface. Ideally, the term *ichthyosis* should be replaced because of its derogatory connotations. The ichthyoses may be considered disorders of cornification, where cornification represents those processes leading to the production and maintenance of a normal stratum corneum. Scaling may result either from epidermal hyperproliferation resulting in excessive production of stratum corneum, often with features of incomplete cornification, or from abnormal retention of stratum corneum (i.e., failure to desquamate). The causes of acquired ichthyoses

and the number of genetically transmitted disorders are numerous. At present little is known about their pathogenesis; however, several of the genetic forms are known to be due to inborn errors of lipid metabolism, and among the causes of acquired ichthyosis are some cholesterol-lowering drugs and essential fatty acid deficiency. Because lipids are segregated to the intercellular spaces in stratum corneum, they are in a position to mediate cohesion and desquamation (for review, see Williams and Elias, 1986).

The genetic forms constitute a heterogeneous group exhibiting a wide range of severity of skin involvement, ranging from relatively mild, focal seasonal scaling to severe constrictive horny plates incompatible with life, as well as exhibiting a spectrum of organ system involvement, ranging from skin alone to severe multisystem disease (Goldsmith, 1976; Rand and Baden, 1983; Williams and Elias, 1987).

The clinical features of the individual inherited forms of ichthyosis are described elsewhere in individual articles. Most of the severe forms are evident at birth, and the milder forms usually become evident within the first year of life. However, age of onset is not invariably a reliable indicator of acquired vs. genetic causes; i.e., some genetic forms (e.g., **Phytanic acid storage disease**) may have delayed onset, and, conversely, neonates may be at particular risk for some of the acquired causes (e.g., essential fatty acid deficiency). Evaluation should include a detailed family history, including examination of family members, complete history and physical examination, and, in most instances, a skin biopsy. Usually the biopsy should be obtained from a well-developed area of scaling. Specific laboratory studies, such as examination of a peripheral blood smear, serum lipoprotein electrophoresis, and determination of serum phytanic acid level, may be required to establish or exclude a specific form of ichthyosis.

The appearance at birth of taut, shiny, inelastic, thickened skin with ectropion, eclabion, and fissures; the so-called *collodian baby*, because of the likeness to a film of dried collodian, is not specific to a single genetic disease but may occur in several disorders (Larreque et al, 1976). Most of these infants eventually can be classified as classic **Ichthyosis, lamellar**, congenital ichthyosiform erythroderma, or, in rare instances, another genetic form. However, in many instances, the disorder may resolve. This has been termed *lamellar exfoliation of the newborn* (Reed et al, 1972). Occurrence in sibs suggests that this may also be a genetic entity. The outcome of a collodian baby cannot be predicted, and a precise diagnosis may not be possible until the complete phenotype has developed.

The causes of acquired ichthyosis include xerosis (environmental dry skin), metabolic disorders such as renal insufficiency and hypothyroidism, nutritional deficiency due to malabsorption or essential fatty acid deficiency, and several drugs. In adults it is essential to rule out malignancy as the cause, particularly **Cancer, Hodgkin disease** and bronchogenic carcinoma (Polisky and Bronson, 1986).

Finally, the differential diagnosis of a given patient may include focal disorders of cornification, such as those primarily involving the palms and soles (*palmar-plantar keratodermas*), as well as other genetically determined scaling disorders such as **Darier disease** and **Skin, psoriasis vulgaris**, nongenetic disorders such as pityriasis rubra pilaris, unusual presentations of tinea infections or scabies infestations, and immunologic disorders such as graft vs. host disease.

**References:**
Reed WB, et al.: Lamellar ichthyosis of the newborn: a distinct clinical entity: its comparison to the other ichthyosiform erythrodermas. Arch Dermatol 1972; 105:394–399.
Goldsmith LA: The ichthyoses. Prog Med Genet 1976; 1:185–240.
Larreque M, et al.: Le bebe collodion evolution a propos de 29 cas. Ann Dermatol Syphiligr 1976; 103:31–54.
Rand RE, Baden HP: The ichthyoses: a review. J Am Acad Dermatol 1983; 8:285–305.
Polisky RB, Bronson DM: Acquired ichthyosis in a patient with adenocarcinoma of the breast. Cutis 1986; 38:359–360.
Williams ML, Elias PM: The ichthyoses. In: Theirs BH, Dobson RL,

eds: Pathogenesis of skin disease. New York: Churchill Livingstone, 1986:519–552.
Williams ML, Elias PM: Genetically transmitted, generalized disorders of cornification. The ichthyoses. Dermatol Clin 1987; 5:155–178.

WI013                               **Mary L. Williams**

**Ichthyosis congenita (some)**
*See ICHTHYOSIS, LAMELLAR RECESSIVE*
**Ichthyosis congenita fetalis**
*See ICHTHYOSIS, HARLEQUIN FETUS*
**Ichthyosis congenita gravis**
*See ICHTHYOSIS, HARLEQUIN FETUS*
**Ichthyosis congenita, wet type**
*See ICHTHYOSIFORM HYPERKERATOSIS, BULLOUS CONGENITAL*
**Ichthyosis follicularis**
*See SKIN, KERATOSIS FOLLICULARIS SPINULOSA DECALVANS*
**Ichthyosis hystrix gravior**
*See NEVUS, EPIDERMAL NEVUS SYNDROME*

## ICHTHYOSIS HYSTRIX, CURTH-MACKLIN TYPE     2857

**Includes:** Curth-Macklin syndrome
**Excludes:**
    **Ichthyosis** (other)
    **Nevus, epidermal nevus syndrome** (0593)

**Major Diagnostic Criteria:** Generalized or localized disorder of cornification with characteristic skin histopathology of keratin filaments amassed with perinuclear shells and with numerous binucleate keratinocytes.

**Clinical Findings:** In a large kindred reported by Curth and Macklin (1954), expression varied from palmoplantar hyperkeratosis and focal hyperkeratotic plaques on elbows, knees, and/or ankles, and in severely affected patients, dark, warty hyperkeratoses covering most of the body surface with an underlying erythroderma. Some family members exhibit a milder, generalized hyperkeratosis, clinically resembling **Ichthyosis vulgaris**, while others have had focal hyperkeratosis. Blisters do not occur. This disorder can be distinguished on light microscopy by the presence of numerous (10–30% of total) binucleate keratinocytes and on electron microscopy by the presence of continuous perinuclear shells of keratin filaments within spinous and granular cell layers. In contrast, in bullous congenital ichthyosiform hyperkeratosis, binucleate corneocytes are absent, intraepidermal vesiculation is prominent, and tonofilament clumps are evident ultrastructurally.

**Complications:** Severe palmoplantar hyperkeratosis may lead to functional impairment and formation of contractures.

**Associated Findings:** None known.

**Etiology:** Autosomal dominant inheritance with markedly variable expression.

**Pathogenesis:** Unknown.

**MIM No.:** *14659

**CDC No.:** 757.190

**Sex Ratio:** M1:F1

**Occurrence:** In addition to the large kindred from New York City reported by Curth and Macklin (1954), two sporadic cases from the United States and Finland have also been reported.

**Risk of Recurrence for Patient's Sib:**
See Part I, *Mendelian Inheritance.*

**Risk of Recurrence for Patient's Child:**
See Part I, *Mendelian Inheritance.*

**Age of Detectability:** At birth, for severely affected individuals.

**Gene Mapping and Linkage:** Unknown.

**Prevention:** None known. Genetic counseling indicated.

**Treatment:** Topical keratolytic agents (e.g., 5–10% lactic or glycolic acid in petrolatum) are the first line of therapy. Severely affected patients may respond to oral synthetic retinoids. However, in view of the known toxicity of these drugs, treatment should be considered on an individual basis.

**Prognosis:** Disease is persistent. Normal life span and intelligence.

**Detection of Carrier:** Clinical examination of the skin for elbow, knee, and palmoplantar hyperkeratoses.

**Special Considerations:** The term *ichthyosis hystrix* is subject to much confusion in the medical literature. Without the addition of an eponym, it is commonly used to indicate a bilaterally distributed epidermal nevus (i.e., focal warty hyperkeratoses distributed along the lines of cutaneous morphogenesis [the lines of Blashko]), often exhibiting the histopathology of epidermolytic hyperkeratoses. The genetic nature of these nevi is uncertain; identical twins may be discordant for these nevi, but two instances of transmission of bullous congenital ichthyosiform hyperkeratosis to offspring has been reported. These observations are suggestive of a somatic mutation that may on occasion affect the germ cell lines. These nevi can be distinguished from the Curth-Macklin type by the characteristic histopathology and ultrastructure. The dominant, ichthyosis hystrix gravior (porcupine man of Lambert; see **Nevus, epidermal nevus syndrome**) may be the same entity as the Curth-Macklin type; unfortunately, histopathology is unavailable to resolve this question.

**Support Groups:** San Francisco; Foundation for Ichthyosis and Related Skin Types (FIRST)

**References:**
Curth HO, Macklin MT: The genetic basis of various types of ichthyosis in a family group. Am J Hum Genet 1954; 6:371–381.
Pinkus H, Nagao S: A case of biphasic ichthyosiform dermatosis: light and electron microscopic study. Arch Klin Exp Dermatol 1970; 237:727–748.
Ollendorff-Curth H, et al.: Follow-up of a family group suffering from ichthyosis hystrix type Curth-Macklin. Humangenetik 1972; 17:37–48.
Kanerva L, et al.: Ichthyosis hystrix (Curth-Macklin): light and electron microscopic studies performed before and after etretinate treatment. Arch Dermatol 1984; 120:1218–1223.

WI013                               **Mary L. Williams**

**Ichthyosis nigricans**
*See ICHTHYOSIS, X-LINKED WITH STEROID SULFATASE DEFICIENCY*
**Ichthyosis simplex**
*See ICHTHYOSIS VULGARIS*

## ICHTHYOSIS VULGARIS     2534

**Includes:**
Ichthyosis, autosomal dominant
Ichthyosis simplex

**Excludes:**
    **Ichthyosis, lamellar dominant** (2854)
    **Ichthyosis, X-linked with steroid sulfatase deficiency** (2532)
    **Ichthyosis** (other)

**Major Diagnostic Criteria:** Widespread scaly skin, i.e., visible cracking of the stratum corneum. Histologically the stratum corneum is thickened, and, of diagnostic significance, the stratum granulosum is thin to absent. Steroid sulfatase activity and cholesterol sulfate levels in blood and scale are normal, thus excluding **Ichthyosis, X-linked with steroid sulfatase deficiency**.

**Clinical Findings:** Scaling usually is absent at birth but clinically apparent by age six months. The severity of scaling tends to diminish with "maturation" and aging. The scales tend to be fine, white, and adherent. Unlike patients with hyperkeratoses associated with hyperproliferation of the epidermis (e.g., **Skin, psoriasis vulgaris**, **Ichthyosis, lamellar**), patients with ichthyosis vulgaris do not leave a "trail" of scales around them. Scaling may lessen in the summer and worsen in the winter, but the seasonal variation is less prominent than it is in **Ichthyosis, X-linked with steroid sulfatase deficiency**. Scaling is more prominent at the calves, spares the neck, and may be associated with palmar hyperkeratosis. Palmar hyperlinearity may be prominent, but it is uncertain whether such hyperlinearity is specific for ichthyosis vulgaris or whether it is more a feature of the often-associated atopic dermatitis.

Although more severe cases of ichthyosis vulgaris are clincally obvious, and may even be confused with X-linked or even lamellar ichthyosis, milder cases may be difficult to differentiate from nonichthyotic "dry skin" present, for example, in patients with atopic dermatitis. The generally quoted incidence of 1:250 persons likely includes such milder cases. The incidence of scaling as severe as that in patients with X-linked ichthyosis doubtless is much lower-perhaps tenfold less-and one large survey of patients with ichthyosis (using clinical and pedigree data) noted an incidence of ichthyosis vulgaris twofold greater than that in X-linked ichthyosis, the latter being approximately 1:6,000 males. Reduction to absence of keratohyaline granules (in the epidermal stratum granulosum) is noted by light microscopy, but some have advocated the more rigorous diagnostic criterion of keratohyaline granule absence by electron microscopy. Reduced keratohyaline granules correlates with reduced amounts of the protein filaggrin and its precursor profilaggrin, but it is not known whether the reduction of that protein causes the scaling and whether the "genetic" abnormality is related directly to that protein (or to other components of the keratohyaline granule or to yet unknown gene products). The phenotype of reduced profilaggrin is maintained in keratinocyte culture.

**Complications:** Unknown.

**Associated Findings:** None known.

**Etiology:** Autosomal dominant inheritance.

**Pathogenesis:** Unknown.

**MIM No.:** *14670

**CDC No.:** 757.195

**Sex Ratio:** M1:F1

**Occurrence:** About 1:250, depending on the diagnostic criteria used.

**Risk of Recurrence for Patient's Sib:**
See Part I, *Mendelian Inheritance.*

**Risk of Recurrence for Patient's Child:**
See Part I, *Mendelian Inheritance.*

**Age of Detectability:** Usually clinically evident by age six months.

**Gene Mapping and Linkage:** Unknown.

**Prevention:** None known. Genetic counseling indicated.

**Treatment:** "Keratolytics" to reduce stratum corneum thickness and brittleness, e.g., topical agents containing salicylic acid, lactic acid, urea, or propylene glycol. Avoidance of soap.

**Prognosis:** Normal life span. Scaling tends to become less severe with maturation and aging.

**Detection of Carrier:** Clinical examination.

**Special Considerations:** Clinical heterogeneity probably exists. Some patients have mild "dry skin," and some have considerably more severe scaling. Probably the latter have more complete keratohyaline granule loss, but this finding may wane following successful topical treatment. Diagnostic criteria, especially for those with milder scaling, are now imprecise.

**Support Groups:** San Francisco; Foundation for Ichthyosis and Related Skin Types (FIRST)

**References:**
Wells RS, Kerr CB: Clinical features of autosomal dominant and sex-linked ichthyosis in an English population. Br Med J 1966; 1:97–950.
Fartasch M, et al.: Ultrastructural study of the occurrence of autosomal dominant ichthyosis vulgaris in atopic eczema. Arch Dermatol Res 1987; 279:270–272.
Fleckman P, et al.: Keratinocytes cultured from subjects with ichthyosis vulgaris are phenotypically abnormal. J Invest Dermatol 1987; 88:640–645.

EP005                                         **Ervin H. Epstein, Jr.**

**Ichthyosis, autosomal dominant**
*See ICHTHYOSIS VULGARIS*
**Ichthyosis, bullous type**
*See ICHTHYOSIFORM HYPERKERATOSIS, BULLOUS CONGENITAL*

## ICHTHYOSIS, CONGENITAL ERYTHRODERMIC            2855

**Includes:**
Collodion baby (some)
Cornification, disorder of, congenital erythrodermic type (DOC 5)
Ichthyosiform erythroderma, non-bullous congenital
Lamellar exfoliation of the newborn

**Excludes:**
Ichthyosis, harlequin fetus (2856)
Ichthyosis, lamellar dominant (2854)
Ichthyosis, lamellar recessive (2853)
Ichthyosis, linearis circumflexa (2858)
Ichthyosis vulgaris (2534)
Ichthyosis, X-linked with steroid sulfatase deficiency (2532)
Storage disease, neutral lipid type (2859)

**Major Diagnostic Criteria:** Generalized disorder of cornification affecting entire body surface, often with prominent erythroderma and fine white scales, and compatible histopathology. At birth, infants have collodion baby phenotype.

**Clinical Findings:** Affected infants are born with a taut, shiny encasement ("collodion membrane"). As this membrane is shed postnatally, an underlying erythroderma and generalized ichthyosis becomes apparent. As in **Ichthyosis, lamellar recessive,** generalized involvement is characteristic, including the face, palms/soles, and all of the flexures. Whereas, scales on the trunk, face and scalp are fine and whitish in color, scales on the extensor surfaces of the lower legs may be large, plate-like and dark in color. Severely affected patients exhibit an intense erythroderma and ectropion. Cicatricial alopecia may develop. Secondary nail dystrophies with thickening of the nail plate and ridging are common. The histopathology displays acanthosis, moderate hyperkeratosis, and usually focal or complete parakeratosis. Stratum corneum membrane regions stain with periodic acid-Schiff reagent.

**Complications:** Although there are no primary systemic manifestations, collodion babies have an increased incidence of premature birth with its attendant perinatal morbidity and mortality. Moreover, collodion babies are at risk for both sepsis and fluid and electrolyte imbalance, particularly hypernatremia, because of their abnormal skin barrier. In severely affected patients, skin tautness may not only produce ectropion and eclabion, and may also compromise the development of nasal and auricular cartilages. Patients may exhibit symptoms of heat intolerance, secondary to eccrine duct obstruction. Although most patients exhibit normal growth and development, mild growth retardation may occur in some severely erythrodermic patients.

**Associated Findings:** None known.

**Etiology:** Autosomal recessive inheritance with interfamilial and intrafamilial variability in disease expression.

**Pathogenesis:** Although the underlying cause is unknown, epidermal cell turnover rates are markedly increased, as in **Skin, psoriasis vulgaris.** Evidence for a primary abnormality in lipid metabolism derives from the observation of a marked increase in hydrocarbon (alkane) content in scales from these patients, which distinguishes this disorder from normals and **Ichthyosis, lamellar recessive.** However, the finding of elevated scale hydrocarbons is not entirely disease-specific, since they occur occasionally in patients with other disorders of cornification. Furthermore, the source of these hydrocarbons in epidermis is not known. Topically applied alkanes induce the hyperproliferative epidermis, suggesting a role in the pathogenesis of this disease.

**MIM No.:** *24210, *24230

**CDC No.:** 757.190

**Sex Ratio:** M1:F1.

**Occurrence:** On the order of 1:180,000. Cases are reported worldwide, without known ethnic predilection.

**Risk of Recurrence for Patient's Sib:**
See Part I, *Mendelian Inheritance*.

**Risk of Recurrence for Patient's Child:**
See Part I, *Mendelian Inheritance*.

**Age of Detectability:** At birth, as collodion baby.

**Gene Mapping and Linkage:** IC1 (ichthyosis 1, (autosomal recessive); congenital ichthyosiform erythroderma) is unassigned.

**Prevention:** None known. Genetic counseling indicated.

**Treatment:** Topical keratolytics (e.g. lactic or glycolic acids) are useful in removing scales but require continual applications. Topical retinoic acid cream may also be effective but is difficult to use. If topical salicylates are used, patients must be observed for signs of salicylism. Oral synthetic retinoids are effective but should be employed only after careful consideration of their long-term toxicity as well as teratogenicity (see **Fetal retinoid syndrome**).

**Prognosis:** Normal life span for those who survive the neonatal period. Some patients report improvement around puberty. Intelligence is normal.

**Detection of Carrier:** Unknown.

**Special Considerations:** *Collodion baby* should not be considered a disease entity, but a descriptive term for an infant born encased in a membranous-like covering, a phenotype that may be common to several disorders of cornification. In most patients (i.e. 2/3 or more), however, congenital erythrodermic ichthyosis is the underlying disorder. Some collodion babies progress to normal skin; they are diagnosed as *lamellar exfoliation of the newborn* in retrospect, which may represent a distinct, autosomal recessive disorder.

**Support Groups:** Raleigh, NC; Foundation for Ichthyosis and Related Skin Types (FIRST)

**References:**
Frost P, Van Scott EJ: Ichthyosiform dermatoses: classification based on anatomic and biometric observations. Arch Dermatol 1966; 94:113–126.
Reed WB, et al: Lamellar ichthyosis of the newborn, a distinct clinical entity: its comparison to the other ichthyosiform erythrodermas. Arch Dermatol 1972; 105:394–399.
Larregue M, et al: Le bebe collodion evolution a porpos de 29 cas. Ann Derm Syph (Paris) 1976; 103:31–54.
Williams ML, Elias PM: Elevated n-alkanes in congenital ichthyosiform erythroderma: phenotypic differentiation of two types of autosomal recessive ichthyosis. J Clin Invest 1984; 74:269–300.
Hazell M, Marks R: Clinical, histologic and cell kinetic discriminants between lamellar ichthyosis and non-bullous congenital ichthyosiform erythroderma. Arch Dermatol 1985; 121:489–493.
Williams ML, Elias PM: Heterogeneity in autosomal recessive ichthyosis: clinical and biochemical differentiation of lamellar ichthyosis and non-bullous congenital ichthyosiform erythroderma. Arch Dermatol 1985; 121:477–488. * †
Bernhardt M, Baden HP: Report of a family with an unusual expression of recessive ichthyosis: review of 42 cases. Arch Dermatol 1986; 122:420–433.

WI013                                              **Mary L. Williams**

## ICHTHYOSIS, HARLEQUIN FETUS                                    **2856**

**Includes:**
    Cornification, disorder of, harlequin type (DOC 6)
    Harlequin fetus ichthyosis
    Ichthyosis congenita fetalis
    Ichthyosis congenita gravis

**Excludes:**
    **Ichthyosis, congenital erythrodermic** (2855)
    **Ichthyosis, lamellar dominant** (2854)
    **Ichthyosis, lamellar recessive** (2853)

**Major Diagnostic Criteria:** Congenital onset of a severe generalized disorder of cornification composed of massive hyperkeratotic plates and resulting in severe eclabion, ectropion, and underdevelopment of cartilages and digits. Rare survivors from the perinatal period exhibit phenotype of severe generalized ichthyosiform erythroderma.

**Clinical Findings:** Affected infants are born with massive hyperkeratotic plates that produce grotesque facial features, with severe eclabion and ectropion and often deformities of other body parts, particularly the ears, hands, and feet. There are deep fissures between the hyperkeratotic plates. Many affected fetuses are stillborn, and most of the remaining do not survive more than a few days due to severe constriction of the chest and abdomen, resulting in compromised respiration and feeding. In the few instances in which patients have survived past the perinatal period, a severe generalized scaling disorder with erythroderma has occurred. Eclabion and ectropion improve, and further development of cartilaginous structures such as ears and nose takes place.

Skin biopsy material demonstrates massive orthohyperkeratosis, but diagnosis rests on the clinical phenotype in the newborn. Premature and excessive cornification occurs by at least 20 weeks *in utero*, and has been used successfully as a guide in prenatal diagnosis.

**Complications:** A high perinatal mortality is usually due to interference with vital functions produced by severe restrictive skin disease. Fissures between keratotic plates provide a portal of entry for microorganisms, placing newborns at high risk for sepsis. As in collodion babies, problems with fluid and electrolyte imbalance are likely. Deformities of hands and feet, such as mitten-like enclosures due to severe restrictive skin *in utero*, may require surgical correction in survivors. Casting for orthopedic procedures may result in reversion to restrictive skin plates, similar to those present at birth. Development of nose and ear cartilages may proceed in survivors, and ectropion and eclabion improves. However, symptomatic ectropion may require surgical correction.

**Associated Findings:** None known.

**Etiology:** Autosomal recessive inheritance.

**Pathogenesis:** Unknown. No consistent abnormalities in epidermal keratin or lipid composition have been recognized.

**MIM No.:** *24250

**CDC No.:** 757.100

**Sex Ratio:** M1:F1

**Occurrence:** On the order of 1:300,000. Established literature with no ethnic predilection.

**Risk of Recurrence for Patient's Sib:**
See Part I, *Mendelian Inheritance*.

**Risk of Recurrence for Patient's Child:**
See Part I, *Mendelian Inheritance*.

**Age of Detectability:** Prenatal diagnosis by fetoscopy or fetal skin biopsy has been successful after 20 weeks gestation. Electron microscopy of fetal skin demonstrates premature and excessive cornification.

**Gene Mapping and Linkage:** Unknown.

**Prevention:** None known. Genetic counseling indicated.

**Treatment:** Use of oral synthetic retinoids, e.g., etretinate, may be beneficial in liveborn infants to facilitate shedding of restrictive cornified plates. Use of these retinoids in older survivors is controversial because of long-term toxicity.

**Prognosis:** Until recently, this disorder was believed to be universally fatal in the perinatal period. One recent survivor suffered an unexpected crib death at age eight months. Other long-term survivors appear to have normal intelligence and life span.

**Detection of Carrier:** Unknown.

**Special Considerations:** Some authorities have included this disorder as part of the phenotypic spectrum of lamellar ichthyoses. However, the failure to observe overlapping phenotypes within kindreds suggests that these are genetically distinct disorders. An early report of an abnormal keratin pattern (cross $\beta$ configuration) has not been confirmed in subsequent studies. Abnormal keratin polypeptides have also been reported in two patients, but the specific abnormalities were not consistent. One patient with harlequin ichthyosis was suspected of having an abnormality in lipid metabolism, with prominent lipid vacuoles histologically and increased sterol ester content. It is possible that the harlequin ichthyosis phenotype may result from several different primary abnormalities of epidermal cornification.

**Support Groups:** Raleigh, NC; Foundation for Ichthyosis and Related Skin Types (FIRST)

**References:**

Goldsmith LA: The ichthyoses. Prog Med Genet 1976; 1:185–210. *
Buxman MM, et al.: Harlequin ichthyosis with epidermal lipid abnormality. Arch Dermatol 1979; 115:189–193.
Baden HP, et al.: Keratinization in the harlequin fetus. Arch Dermatol 1982; 118:14–18.
Lawler F, Peiris S: Harlequin fetus successfully treated with etretinate. Br J Dermatol 1985; 112:585–590. †
Williams ML, Elias PM: Genetically transmitted, generalized disorders of cornification: the ichthyoses. Dermatol Clin 1987; 5:165–178. * †

WI013 **Mary L. Williams**

---

## ICHTHYOSIS, LAMELLAR DOMINANT 2854

**Includes:**

Collodion baby (some)
Cornification, disorder of, lamellar dominant (DOC 6)
Ichthyosiform erythroderma, nonbullous, dominant form
Lamellar ichthyosis, autosomal dominant form
Lamellar ichthyosis, nonbullous congenital

**Excludes:**

**Ichthyosis, congenital erythrodermic** (2855)
**Ichthyosis, lamellar recessive** (2853)

**Major Diagnostic Criteria:** A generalized disorder of cornification with dominant pedigree and characteristic histopathology.

**Clinical Findings:** A kindred with a generalized disorder of cornification that phenotypically resembled **Ichthyosis, lamellar recessive** has been documented. Vertical transmission was documented over three generations, and consanguinity was absent. Skin involvement was evident at birth, with encasement in a collodion-like membrane. Thereafter, the entire body surface was involved with a large scale pattern, not as severe as is typical for **Ichthyosis, lamellar recessive**. Erythroderma was absent, as is common in **Ichthyosis, congenital erythrodermic**. Palmoplantar keratoderma was disproportionately severe in these patients, and may provide a useful phenotypic marker for this disorder. Ultrastructural histopathology may be diagnostic, because a prominent transitional zone is seen in the stratum corneum just overlying the stratum granulosum.

**Complications:** Unknown.

**Associated Findings:** None known.

**Etiology:** Presumably autosomal dominant inheritance.

**Pathogenesis:** Unknown.

**MIM No.:** 14675

---

**CDC No.:** 757.190

**Sex Ratio:** Presumably M1:F1; M1:F2 observed.

**Occurrence:** At least one kindred, with an affected grandfather, mother and daughter, has been reported in the literature.

**Risk of Recurrence for Patient's Sib:**
See Part I, *Mendelian Inheritance.*

**Risk of Recurrence for Patient's Child:**
See Part I, *Mendelian Inheritance.*

**Age of Detectability:** Clinically evident at birth as collodion baby.

**Gene Mapping and Linkage:** Unknown.

**Prevention:** None known. Genetic counseling indicated.

**Treatment:** Topical keratolytic agents to remove scale may improve appearance. Use of oral synthetic retinoids in generalized disorders of cornification is controversial because of long-term toxicity and teratogenecity (see **Fetal retinoid syndrome**).

**Prognosis:** Presumably normal life span and intelligence.

**Detection of Carrier:** By clinical examination.

**Support Groups:** San Francisco; Foundation for Ichthyosis and Related Skin Types (FIRST)

**References:**

Traupe H, et al.: Autosomal dominant lamellar ichthyosis: a new skin disorder. Clin Genet 1984; 26:457–461.
Kolde G, et al.: Autosomal-dominant lamellar ichthyosis: ultrastructural characteristics of a new type of congenital ichthyosis. Arch Dermatol Res 1985; 278:1–5.
Williams ML, Elias PM: Ichthyosis: genetic heterogeneity, genodermatoses, and genetic counseling. (Editorial) Arch Derm 1986; 122: 529–531.

WI013 **Mary L. Williams**

---

## ICHTHYOSIS, LAMELLAR RECESSIVE 2853

**Includes:**

Collodion fetus (some)
Cornification, disorders of, lamellar recessive (DOC 4)
Desquamation of the newborn
Ichthyosiform erythroderma, Brocq nonbullous form
Ichthyosis congenita (some)
Lamellar exfoliation of the newborn
Lamellar ichthyosis, classical

**Excludes:**

Ichthyosiform erythroderma, non-bullous congenital
**Ichthyosis, congenital erythrodermic** (2855)
Ichthyosis, erythrodermic, congenital
**Ichthyosis, harlequin fetus** (2856)
**Ichthyosis, lamellar dominant** (2854)
**Ichthyosis vulgaris** (2534)
**Ichthyosis** (other)

**Major Diagnostic Criteria:** Severe, life-long, generalized disorder of cornification with large dark plate-like scales and an underlying erythroderma, affecting the entire skin surface and producing facial tautness with ectropion, in association with compatible histopathology.

**Clinical Findings:** Generalized hyperkeratosis is evident from birth. The most striking clinical feature is that of large, dark, plate-like ("lamellar") scales. Most patients have an underlying erythroderma of variable intensity. Facial involvement results in significant ectropion. The scalp is involved, but hairs themselves are spared and alopecia does not occur. All flexures are involved as are palms and soles. The disorder is unremitting. Histopathology demonstrates massive orthohyperkeratosis with some acanthosis and papillomatosis; parakeratosis and features of epidermolytic hyperkeratosis are absent; the granular cell layers are well-developed.

**Complications:** Ectropion may result in corneal injury if uncorrected. Palmoplantar keratoderma may be severe enough to present some functional disability. Generally, the disorder is disfiguring but not physically disabling.

**Associated Findings:** None known.

**Etiology:** Autosomal recessive inheritance.

**Pathogenesis:** Unknown. Scale lipids are composed of an increased proportion of ceramides and free sterols, a pattern reminiscent of palmo-plantar stratum corneum. The epidermis is normoproliferative or only modestly hyperproliferative; excessive stratum corneum may be attributed primarily to stratum corneum retention.

**MIM No.:** *24210, *24230

**CDC No.:** 757.190

**Sex Ratio:** Presumably M1:F1.

**Occurrence:** On the order of <1:300,000. Cases of **Ichthyosis, congenital erythrodermic** are more common than this phenotype. The two disorders are separated by clinical, histological, histometric and biochemical differences. There appears to be little intrafamilial variability. No ethnic predilections are known.

**Risk of Recurrence for Patient's Sib:**
See Part I, *Mendelian Inheritance.*

**Risk of Recurrence for Patient's Child:**
See Part I, *Mendelian Inheritance.*

**Age of Detectability:** At birth. Prenatal diagnosis may be possible through fetoscopy and fetal skin biopsy with fetal skin showing excessive and premature cornification.

**Gene Mapping and Linkage:** IC1 (ichthyosis 1, (autosomal recessive); congenital ichthyosiform erythroderma) is unassigned.

**Prevention:** None known. Genetic counseling indicated.

**Treatment:** Topical keratolytics (e.g. lactic or glycolic acids) are useful in removing scales but require continual applications. Topical retinoic acid cream may also be effective but are difficult to use. If topical salicylates are used, patients must be observed for signs of salicylism. Oral synthetic retinoids are effective but should be employed only after careful consideration of their long-term toxicity as well as teratogenicity (see **Fetal retinoid syndrome**).

**Prognosis:** Normal life span. The skin disorder is unremitting and presents a significant cosmetic handicap which may impair psychosocial adaptation. Intelligence is normal.

**Detection of Carrier:** Unknown.

**Special Considerations:** For the first half of the 20th Century this disorder was commonly lumped together with **Ichthyosiform hyperkeratosis, bullous congenital** as *ichthyosis congenita*, dry and wet types, respectively, until the characteristic histopathology of epidermolytic hyperkeratosis and dominant inheritance pattern of **Ichthyosiform hyperkeratosis, bullous congenital** were generally appreciated.

**Support Groups:** Raleigh, NC; Foundation for Ichthyosis and Related Skin Types (FIRST)

**References:**
Frost P, Van Scott EJ: Ichthyosiform dermatoses. Classification based on anatomic and biometric observations. Arch Dermatol 1966; 94:113–126.
Williams ML, Elias PM: Elevated n-alkanes in congenital ichthyosiform erythrodermal: phenotypic differentiation of two types of autosomal recessive ichthyosis. J Clin Invest 1984; 74:269–300.
Hazell M, Marks R: Clinical, histologic and cell kinetic discriminants between lamellar ichthyosis and non-bullous congenital ichthyosiform erythroderma. Arch Dermatol 1985; 121:489–493. †
Williams ML, Elias PM: Heterogeneity in autosomal recessive ichthyosis: clinical and biochemical differentiation of lamellar ichthyosis and non-bullous congenital ichthyosiform erythroderma. Arch Dermatol 1985; 121:477–488. * †
Sybert VP, Holbrook KA: Prenatal diagnosis and screening. Dermatologic Clinics 1987; 5:17–41.

WI013

**Mary L. Williams**

---

## ICHTHYOSIS, LINEARIS CIRCUMFLEXA 2858

**Includes:**
Bamboo hair
Cornification, disorder of, Netherton type (DOC 9)
Hair, "bamboo"
Netherton syndrome

**Excludes:**
**Ichthyosis, lamellar recessive** (2853)
**Trichothiodystrophy** (2559)

**Major Diagnostic Criteria:** Affected individuals exhibit a distinctive disorder of cornification characterized by circinate lesions formed on either side by a free edge of scale ("double-edged" scale). Some patients may have a generalized hyperkeratosis resembling congenital erythrodermic ichthyosis. Scalp hairs are short and fragile due to structural defects of the hair shaft. Trichorrhexis invaginata, a ball-and-socket intussusception of the hair shaft, is diagnostic of this syndrome.

**Clinical Findings:** This disorder is characterized by the triad of 1) ichthyosis linearis circumflexa; 2) structural anomalies of the hair shaft, particularly trichorrhexis invaginata; and 3) an atopic diathesis. Ichthyosis linearis circumflexa refers to a generalized hyperkeratosis that, with desquamation, results in a circinate erythematous base with the pathognomonic "double-edged" scale along the margins. At birth, a generalized erythroderma or a collodion baby phenotype may be present. Later, the characteristic migratory, circinate plaques develop. Pruritis is variable but may be severe. Lichenification of the flexural surfaces may be present as a manifestation of the associated atopic dermatitis. The face, scalp, and eyebrows are often affected by dermatitis. Instead of the circinate pattern of ichthyosis linearis circumflexa, some patients phenotypically resemble **Ichthyosis, congenital erythrodermic**. Histopathologic examination is nondiagnostic, revealing features of both psoriasis and atopic dermatitis.

The characteristic hair shaft anomaly of Netherton syndrome is trichorrhexis invaginata, or bamboo hairs. Pili tori and trichorrhexis nodosa may also occur. These hair shaft anomalies result in fragile hairs that usually break off within a few inches of the scalp.

**Complications:** Pruritis may be severe, related to the atopic status. Anaphylactic reactions to foods may occur.

**Associated Findings:** The atopic diathesis in these patients manifests as either atopic dermatitis or asthma (see **Skin, atopy, familial**). Anaphylactic reactions to foods have been frequently observed, and marked elevation of serum IgE levels may be present. Other reported findings include a generalized aminoaciduria in up to one-half of patients, mild-to-severe mental retardation, and impaired cellular immunity.

**Etiology:** Autosomal recessive inheritance. The literature reflects a predominance of females, but well-documented cases in males and reports of consanguinity are most consistent with autosomal recessive inheritance.

**Pathogenesis:** Unknown. Bamboo hairs represent a ball-and-socket intussusception of the distal hair shaft into the proximal portion resulting from a defect in cornification of the internal root sheath.

**MIM No.:** *25650

**CDC No.:** 757.190

**Sex Ratio:** Presumably M1:F1; observed, M1:F2.

**Occurrence:** A few dozen cases have been documented.

**Risk of Recurrence for Patient's Sib:**
See Part I, *Mendelian Inheritance.*

**Risk of Recurrence for Patient's Child:**
See Part I, *Mendelian Inheritance.*

**Age of Detectability:** Usually at birth.

**Gene Mapping and Linkage:** Unknown.

**Prevention:** None known. Genetic counseling indicated.

**Treatment:** Avoidance of food allergens. Usual management for atopic dermatitis, if present. Some patients may respond to PUVA (psoralen plus UVA light). Retinoids and antimetabolites should be considered experimental.

**Prognosis:** Probably normal for life span.

**Detection of Carrier:** Unknown.

**Support Groups:** San Francisco; Foundation for Ichthyosis and Related Skin Types (FIRST)

**References:**

Altman J, Stroud J: Netherton's syndrome and ichthyosis linearis circumflexa: psoriasiform ichthyosis. Arch Dermatol 1969; 100:550–558. *

Hurwitz S, et al.: Reevaluation of ichthyosis and hair shaft abnormalities. Arch Dermatol 1971; 103:266–271. * †

Krafchik BR, Toole JWP: What is Netherton's syndrome? Int J Dermatol 1983; 22:459–462.

Caputo R, et al.: Netherton's syndrome in two adult brothers. Arch Dermatol 1984; 120:220–222.

WI013                                                       **Mary L. Williams**

## ICHTHYOSIS, X-LINKED WITH STEROID SULFATASE DEFICIENCY                                               2532

**Includes:**

Ichthyosis nigricans
Placental steroid sulfatase deficiency
Steroid sulfatase deficiency disease (SSDD)

**Excludes:**

**Ichthyosis vulgaris** (2534)
**Ichthyosis** (other)

**Major Diagnostic Criteria:** Widespread scaly skin, i.e., visible thickening and cracking of stratum corneum in a patient with a family history compatible with X-linked recessive inheritance. The diagnosis is confirmed by detecting an absence of steroid sulfatase activity with or without elevated quantities of its substrate cholesterol sulfate.

**Clinical Findings:** Scaling of skin usually becomes evident by age six months. The scales tend to be dark, adherent, and especially prominent on the lateral calves and (of diagnostic significance when prominent) on the sides of the neck: the typical appearance of a little boy with a dirty neck that soap cannot clean. The scaling is greatly reduced in the summer so that patients almost "moult" in the spring. In some sunny, moist climates (e.g., Southeast Asia, Central America) scaling may be nearly inapparent clinically all year long. Scaling tends to spare the palms and involve the cubital fossae, unlike that in ichthyosis vulgaris, in which the palms are often hyperkeratotic and the cubital fossae are spared. Scaling tends not to improve with advancing age. Even with careful attention to these clinical criteria, differentiation from ichthyosis vulgaris is often difficult, because scales sometimes may be rather lighter in color and less broadly distributed.

The stratum corneum is thickened and granular cells are present in normal numbers (cf. few to no granular cells in ichthyosis vulgaris) in skin biopsy material. Approximately 50% of patients and a smaller percentage of carriers have clinically inapparent corneal opacities detectable only by careful slit-lamp examinations. There is an increased incidence of delayed parturition, but the exact incidence is uncertain. Increased incidences of cryptorchidism and testicular carcinoma have been suggested.

Steroid sulfatase activity can be measured in scale, whole skin or epidermis, leukocytes, cultured fibroblasts, keratinocytes, and amniocytes. Elevated cholesterol sulfate can be measured in stratum corneum and blood. In blood, the cholesterol sulfate is "carried" on low-density lipoprotein (LDL). The sulfates impart an enhanced electronegativity to the LDLs that can be detected by enhanced LDL electromobility on serum lipoprotein electrophoresis.

**Complications:** Psychologic impairment due to embarassment at visible abnormality and fear of social ostracism.

**Associated Findings:** None known.

**Etiology:** X-linked recessive inheritance.

**Pathogenesis:** Approximately 90% of patients so far studied have deletions of most or all of the steroid sulfatase gene. The absence of steroid sulfatase catalytic activity at the periphery of the cells of the stratum corneum prevents the normal predesquamative desulfation of cholesterol sulfate to cholesterol. The intercellular cholesterol sulfate appears to act as a glue and prevents stratum corneum desquamation, leading to thickening and "cracking" of that layer.

**MIM No.:** *30810

**Sex Ratio:** M1:F0. However, one inbred family has been described in which three affected daughters were born to an affected male and a female who most likely was a carrier of the disease.

**Occurrence:** 1:4,000–6,000 males. Patients have been reported in all major ethnic groups.

**Risk of Recurrence for Patient's Sib:**
See Part I, *Mendelian Inheritance.*

**Risk of Recurrence for Patient's Child:**
See Part I, *Mendelian Inheritance.*

**Age of Detectability:** Clinically evident by age six months, although usually not at birth. Prenatal diagnosis can be made in the first trimester by detecting absence of steroid sulfatase enzyme activity in cultured amniocytes, elevated levels of the enzyme substrate dehydroepiandrosterone in amniotic fluid, or late in pregnancy by detection of abnormally low maternal urinary estriol. Gene deletion is likely to be detectable in chorionic villi.

**Gene Mapping and Linkage:** STS (steroid sulfatase (microsomal)) has been mapped to Xp22.32.

**Prevention:** None known. Genetic counseling indicated.

**Treatment:** "Keratolytics" to reduce stratum corneum thickness, e.g., topical agents containing salicylic acid, lactic acid, urea, or proplyene glycol. Avoidance of soap.

**Prognosis:** Normal life span.

**Detection of Carrier:** Peripheral blood leukocyte steroid sulfatase activity is lower in carriers than in normal women. In the 90% of families in which there are gene deletions, detection of a 50% reduction of steroid sulfatase gene sequences should be possible.

**Special Considerations:** The gene for steroid sulfatase is of particular interest in that it partially escapes X-inactivation (lyonization) and in that it is located in humans just proximal to the pseudoautosomal region (in mice it is located within the pseudoautosomal region). This location near the site of obligate crossing over between the X and Y chromosomes during male meiosis may be related to the very high incidence of gross deletions causing the enzyme deficiency. Rarely do patients have yet larger deletions and associated clinical abnormalities, including chondrodysplasia punctata. It is unclear whether the variably reported associated findings such as corneal opacities, cryptorchidism, and delayed onset of labor, are consequences of absent steroid sulfatase enzyme activity or are due to genomic deletions extending beyond the steroid sulfatase gene into adjacent regions of the X chromosome.

In the very rare multiple sulfatase deficiency, ichthyosis and increased cholesterol sulfate are associated with steroid sulfatase deficiency, but the enzymatic activity of many other sulfatases (e.g., arylsulfatases A and B) is also absent, and death occurs at an early age.

**Support Groups:** San Francisco; Foundation for Ichthyosis and Related Skin Types (FIRST)

**References:**

Wells RS, Kerr CB: Clinical features of autosomal dominant and sex-linked ichthyosis in an English population. Br Med J 1966; 1:947–950.

Shapiro LJ, et al.: X-linked ichthyosis due to steroid-sulphatase deficiency. Lancet 1978; I:70–72.

Shapiro LJ, et al.: Non-activation of a X-chromosome locus in man. Science 1979; 204:1224–1226.

Epstein EH Jr., et al.: X-linked ichthyosis: increased blood cholesterol sulfate and electrophoretic mobility of low-density lipoprotein. Science 1981; 214:659–660.

Williams ML, Elias PM: Stratum corneum lipids in disorders of cornification. J Clin Invest 1981; 68:1404–1410.

Bonifas JM, et al.: Cloning of a cDNA for steroid sulfatase. Frequent occurrence of gene deletions in patients with recessive X-chromosome-linked ichthyosis. Proc Natl Acad Sci USA 1987; 84:9248–9251.

Yen PH, et al.: Cloning and expression of steroid sulfatase cDNA and the frequent occurrence of deletions in STS deficiency: implications for X-Y interchange. Cell 1987; 49:443–454.

EP005                                                        **Ervin H. Epstein, Jr.**

## Ichthyosis-cataract
*See CATARACT-ICHTHYOSIS*

---

## ICHTHYOSIS-CHEEK-EYEBROW SYNDROME      3010

**Includes:**
     Cheek-eyebrow-ichthyosis syndrome
     Eyebrow-cheek-ichthyosis syndrome

**Excludes:** Ichthyosis (other)

**Major Diagnostic Criteria:** Ichthyosis vulgaris, prominent full cheeks until puberty, sparse lateral eyebrows, and other craniofacial and musculoskeletal anomalies.

**Clinical Findings:** *Craniofacial*: dysplastic ears (folded helices) (4/4), flat occiput (4/4), full cheeks until puberty (4/4), high-arched palate (4/4), prominent nose (4/4), sparse lateral eyebrows (4/4).
     *Musculoskeletal*: chest asymmetry (4/4), genu valgum (1/4), kyphoscoliosis (3/4), long fingers and toes (4/4), **Pectus carinatum** (1/4), **Pectus excavatum** (3/4), pes planus (4/4).
     *Skin*: Ichthyosis vulgaris (4/4), widely spaced nipples (3/4).

**Complications:** Unknown.

**Associated Findings:** None known.

**Etiology:** Autosomal dominant inheritance.

**Pathogenesis:** Unknown. The prominent full cheeks most probably represent excess adipose tissue in the buccal fat pad, which begins to diminish with the onset of puberty.

**MIM No.:** 14672

**POS No.:** 4277

**Sex Ratio:** Presumably M1:F1.

**Occurrence:** Reported in four generations of a Jewish Sephardic family from Israel.

**Risk of Recurrence for Patient's Sib:**
See Part I, *Mendelian Inheritance.*

**Risk of Recurrence for Patient's Child:**
See Part I, *Mendelian Inheritance.*

**Age of Detectability:** During infancy.

**Gene Mapping and Linkage:** Unknown.

**Prevention:** None known. Genetic counseling indicated.

**Treatment:** Supportive. Affected females may find the prominent cheeks disturbing during childhood and early teens, as they may be teased and accused of having the mumps.

**Prognosis:** Normal life span.

**Detection of Carrier:** Appears to be fully penetrant in the heterozygous state.

**Special Considerations:** The acronym *ICE*, sometimes used to describe this condition, has long been used as a descriptor for another distinct disorder; *Iridocorneal endothelial syndrome* (Yanoff, 1979). Use of acronyms, and this acronym in particular, is discouraged in favor of more complete terminology.

**Support Groups:** San Francisco; Foundation for Ichthyosis and Related Skin Types (FIRST)

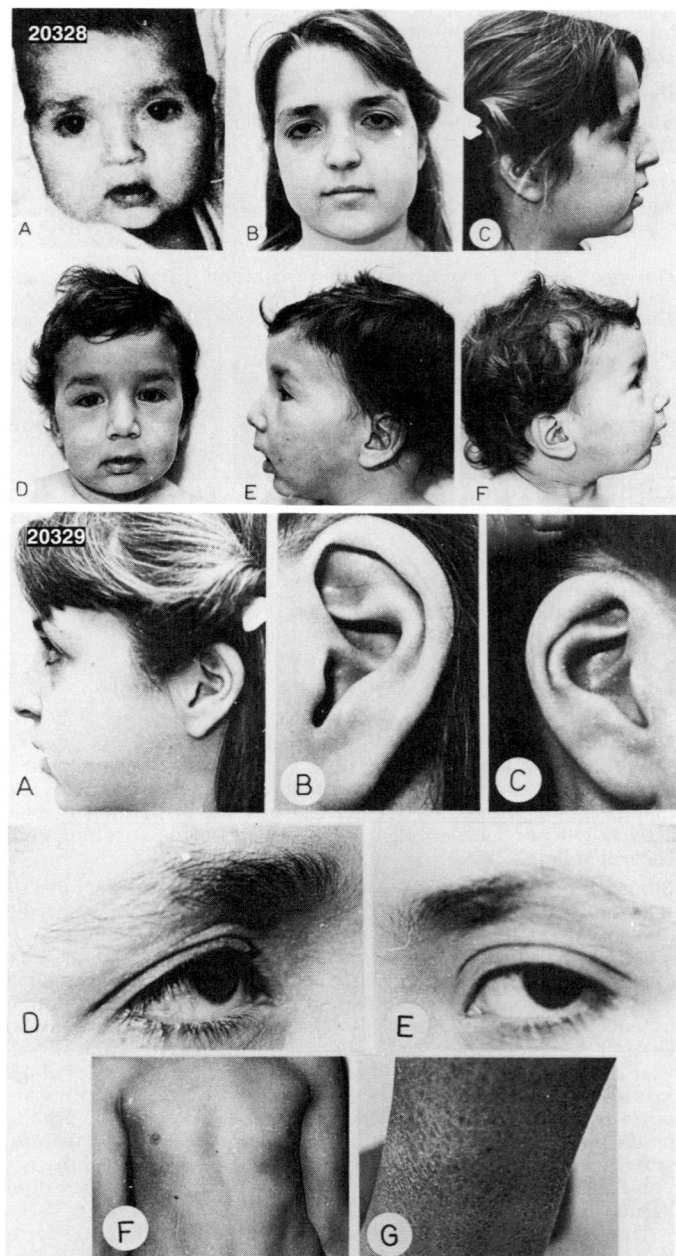

**3010-20328:** A–C) The prominent and full cheeks of the proband at the time of infancy and at age 11 years. D–F) The proband's affected brother at age 1 year and 8 months also with full cheeks and sparse lateral eyebrows. **20329:** Full cheek (A), folded helices (B,C), sparse lateral eyebrows (D,E), chest asymmetry with mild pectus excavatum (F), and icthyosis vulgaris involving the lower extremity (G) in the proband.

---

**References:**
Yanoff M: Iridocorneal endothelial syndrome: unification of a disease spectrum. Surv Ophthal 1979; 24:1–2.
Sidransky E, et al.: Ichthyosis-cheek-eyebrow (ICE) syndrome: a new autosomal dominant disorder. Clin Genet 1987; 31:137–142.

G0026                                                        **Richard M. Goodman**

## ICHTHYOSIS-COLOBOMA-HEART DEFECT-DEAFNESS-MENTAL RETARDATION 3214

**Includes:**
CHIME syndrome
Ichythyosiform dermatosis-neurologic/ophthalmologic abnormalities

**Excludes:**
**Charge association** (2124)
**Gingival fibromatosis-depigmentation-microphthalmia** (0413)
**Ichthyosiform erythrokeratoderma, atypical with deafness** (2861)
**Ichthyosis, linearis circumflexa** (2858)
Intrauterine exposure to aflatoxin B(1)
**Limb reduction-ichthyosis** (2019)
**Phytanic acid storage disease** (0810)
**Seizures-ichthyosis-mental retardation** (0741)
**Sjogren-Larsson syndrome** (2030)
**Skin, erythrokeratodermia, variable** (0361)
**Trichothiodystrophy** (2559)

**Major Diagnostic Criteria:** Bilateral retinal coloboma, migratory ichthyosiform dermatosis, normal to small "C" shaped ears with rolled helices, severe developmental delay, and congenital heart defect.

**Clinical Findings:** At birth, the children appear unusual with brachycephaly; one child had small head circumference and micrognathia. Length and weight are variable ranging from normal to less than the 3rd percentile. Retinal colobomas are usually readily apparent. True or apparent hypertelorism may be noted with epicanthal folds. Muscle tone is usually normal, but, in one child severe hypotonia occurred. Further investigation reveals congenital heart defects: **Heart, tetralogy of Fallot, Heart, transposition of great vessels,** and peripheral pulmonic stenosis. Respiratory distress may occur secondary to congestive heart failure. The

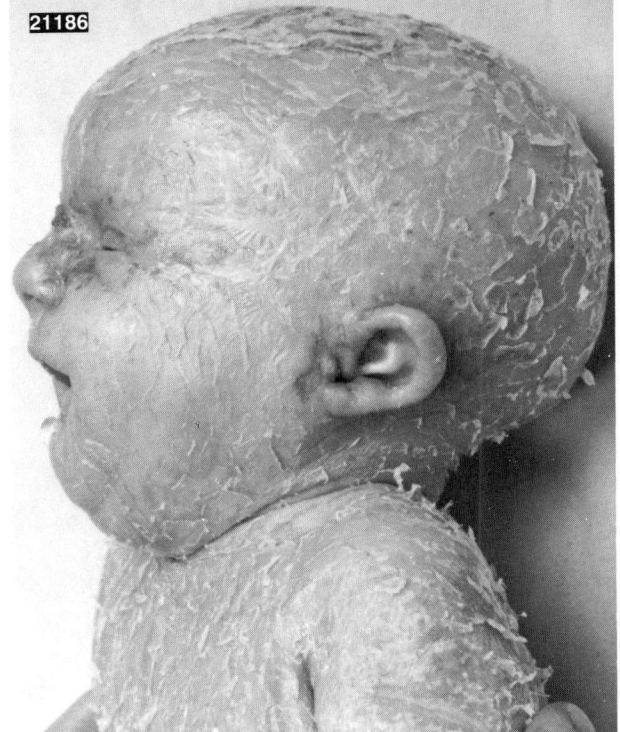

**3214B**-21186: Micrognathia, "C"-shaped ears with rolled helices, and the scaling of the transitory ichthyosiform rash.

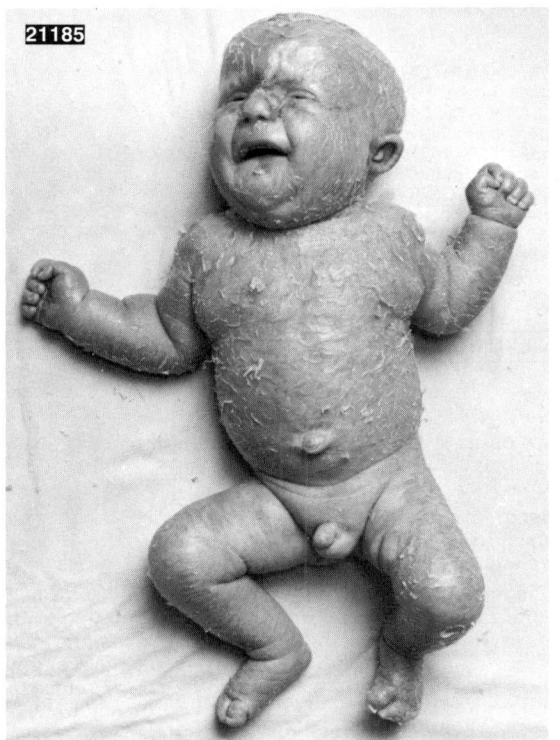

**3214A**-21185: Generalized distribution of the transient ichthyosiform dermatosis.

diagnosis may remain in doubt until the migratory ichthyosiform rash develops, usually by one week, but it may not appear until 4–6 weeks of life; persisting into late childhood. Developmental delay, hearing deficit and visual impairment are apparent from the outset. Seizures occur in early infancy. Dermatoglyphs show high percent of digital arches.

Chromosome analyses have been normal. No defects in immunoglobulin levels or cellular immunity have been detected.

**Complications:** Recurrent respiratory infections; otitis media; cutaneous infections and abscesses, contractures of digits and large joints, and failure to thrive with gastrointestinal reflux in one child.

**Associated Findings:** Dental anomalies; cleft palate (submucous cleft with bifid uvula); conductive hearing loss; bilateral inguinal hernias, undescended testes and umbilical hernias occurred in one neonate; one child had a large lipoma on the back and one had large bilateral lipomas in the pectoral-axillary areas.

**Etiology:** Presumably autosomal recessive inheritance.

**Pathogenesis:** Unknown.

**Sex Ratio:** M3:F1

**Occurrence:** Only four children (three reported and one by personal communication) are known in three unrelated families.

**Risk of Recurrence for Patient's Sib:**
See Part I, *Mendelian Inheritance.*

**Risk of Recurrence for Patient's Child:**
See Part I, *Mendelian Inheritance.*

**Age of Detectability:** Retinal coloboma, heart defect and ear anomalies are detected at birth or within a few days of life. Scaly skin changes may appear during the first week to month of life.

**Gene Mapping and Linkage:** Unknown.

**Prevention:** None known. Genetic counseling indicated.

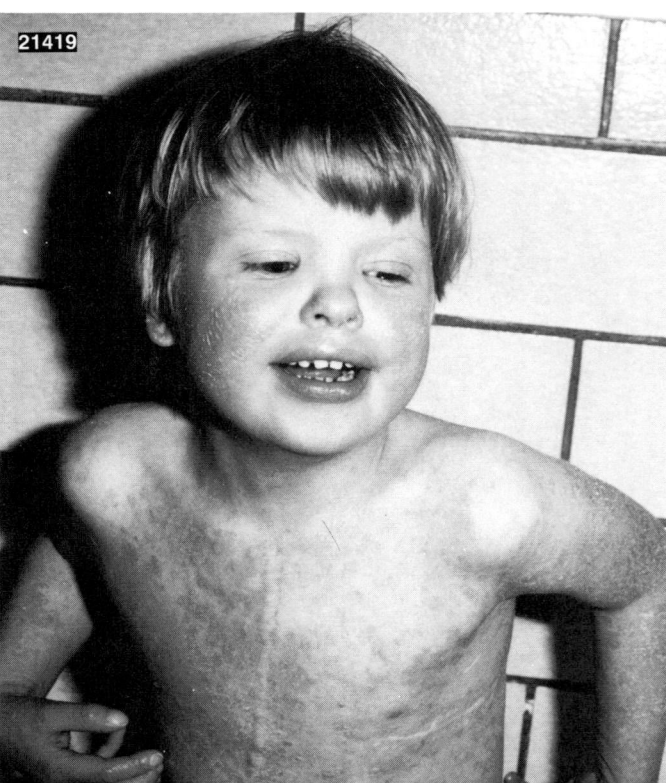

**3214C**-21419: Note unusual facies, generalized dermatitis and scar from heart surgery.

**Treatment:** Skin care is the major day-to-day problem. Warm baths followed by total body moisturizing preparations usually controls the scaling and erythroderma. Daily application of a topical steroid was highly effective in the most severely affected child. Keratolytic agents, uric acid and lactic acid preparations, are effective in removing scales and may be required daily. Gastro-esophageal reflux may require Nissan fundoplication and gastrostomy tube placement.

**Prognosis:** Mental retardation is severe. Two children at 4 and 6.5 years chronological age functioned at the 12 and 18 months levels respectively. Two other children at one year have shown little progress beyond 1–2 months level. Ichthyosis persists through childhood.

**Detection of Carrier:** Unknown.

**Special Considerations:** The acronym C.H.I.M.E. was drawn from "Coloboma, heart defect, ichthyosiform dermatosis, mental retardation, and ear anomalies" (CHIME).

**References:**
Zunich J, Kaye CI: New syndrome of congenital ichthyosis with neurologic abnormalities. Am J Med Genetics 1983; 15:331–333.
Zunich J, Kaye CI: Additional case report of new neuroectodermal syndrome (letter). Am J Med Genetics 1984; 17:707–710.
Zunich J, et al.: Congenital migratory ichthyosiform dermatosis with neurologic and ophthalmologic abnormalities. Arch Dermatol 1985; 121:1149–1156.
Zunich J, Kaye CI: Autosomal recessive transmission of new neuro-ectodermal syndrome. Pediatr Res 1988; 23:271A.

LA007
ZU000

**Roger L. Ladda**
**Janice Zunich**

**Ichthyosis-deafness-renal disease**
See DEAFNESS-HYPERPROLINURIA-ICHTHYOSIS
**Ichthyosis-epilepsy-oligophrenia**
See SEIZURES-ICHTHYOSIS-MENTAL RETARDATION
**Ichthyosis-erythema annulare centrifugum**
See SKIN, ERYTHROKERATODERMIA, VARIABLE
**Ichthyosis-hepatosplenomegaly-cerebellar degeneration**
See GIROUX-BARBEAU SYNDROME
**Ichthyosis-limb reduction**
See LIMB REDUCTION-ICHTHYOSIS
**Ichthyosis-neurologic disorder-hypogonadism**
See SEIZURES-ICHTHYOSIS-MENTAL RETARDATION
**Ichthyosis-oligophrenia-spasticity**
See SJOGREN-LARSSON SYNDROME
**Ichthyosis-skeletal bowing-cortical thickening-bone fragility**
See SKELETAL BOWING-CORTICAL THICKENING-BONE FRAGILITY-ICTHYOSIS
**Ichthyosis-trichothiodystrophy**
See TRICHOTHIODYSTROPHY
**Ichthyotic neutral lipid storage disease**
See STORAGE DISEASE, NEUTRAL LIPID TYPE
**Ichthyosiform dermatosis-neurologic/ophthalmologic abnormalities**
See ICHTHYOSIS-COLOBOMA-HEART DEFECT-DEAFNESS-MENTAL RETARDATION
**IDDM-MED syndrome**
See EPIPHYSEAL DYSPLASIA, MULTIPLE-DIABETES MELLITUS
**Idiopathic extrahepatic biliary atresia (EHBA)**
See BILIARY ATRESIA
**Idiopathic neutropenia, chronic benign**
See NEUTROPENIA, BENIGN FAMILIAL
**Idiopathic steatorrhea**
See GLUTEN-SENSITIVE ENTEROPATHY
**Idiopathic thrombocytopenic purpura**
See THROMBOCYTOPENIC PURPURA AND LIPID HISTIOCYTOSIS
**Idiopathic urticaria a-frigore (iUF)**
See COLD HYPERSENSITIVITY
**IgA constant heavy chain locus**
See SERUM ALLOTYPES, HUMAN
**IgA-Mangel**
See IMMUNOGLOBULIN A DEFICIENCY
**IgG heavy chain loci**
See SERUM ALLOTYPES, HUMAN
**IgG heavy chain locus**
See IMMUNODEFICIENCY, IgG SUBCLASS DEFICIENCIES
**Ileal B transport deficiency**
See VITAMIN B(12) MALABSORPTION
**Ileocolitis**
See INFLAMMATORY BOWEL DISEASE
**Iliac horns**
See NAIL-PATELLA SYNDROME
**IIIig-type growth hormone deficiency**
See GROWTH HORMONE DEFICIENCY, ISOLATED
**Illinois amyloidosis**
See AMYLOIDOSIS, ILLINOIS TYPE
**Imerslund-Grasbeck syndrome**
See VITAMIN B(12) MALABSORPTION
**Imidodipeptidase deficiency**
See PROLIDASE DEFICIENCY

---

**IMINOGLYCINURIA**                                                    **0520**

**Includes:**
DeVries hyperglycinuria
Glycinuria with or without oxalate urolithiasis
Iminoglycinuria type II
Renal iminoglycinuria

**Excludes:**
Hyperprolinemia (0502)
Iminoglycinuria of normal newborn

**Major Diagnostic Criteria:** The homozygotes have normal plasma concentration of proline, hydroxyproline (both imino acids), and glycine, as well as large amounts of imino acids and glycine in urine after 6 months of age. Heterozygotes have glycinuria exceeding 160 $\mu$mole/g total urinary nitrogen, or renal clearance exceeding 8.6 ml/min/1.73 $M^2$ in one type of heterozygote; the other (silent) type has normal glycine excretion.

**Clinical Findings:** No proven disease occurs with the trait that affects the common renal tubular reabsorptive mechanism for glycine, proline, and hydroxyproline. Its occasional association with seizures or mental retardation is probably fortuitous. Numerous healthy children and adults have now been recognized with selective impairment of cellular transport of proline, hydroxyproline, and glycine. Plasma levels of affected amino acids are normal. In homozygotes, net renal tubular reabsorption of proline, hydroxyproline, and glycine is about 80%, 80%, and 60%, respectively, of the normal amount. An intestinal transport defect restricted to the iminoglycine group of amino acids has also been identified in some, but not in all, pedigrees. Most heterozygotes have abnormal endogenous glycine reabsorption. Evidence for "silent" heterozygotes exists. On this basis, and on apparent evidence for heteroallelic homozygotes in some pedigrees, it is assumed that more than one mutant genotype determines the renal iminoglycinuric trait.

**Complications:** Unknown.

**Associated Findings:** None known.

**Etiology:** *Iminoglycinuria type I:* autosomal recessive inheritance. *Iminoglycinuria type II* (with or without oxalate urolithiasis): autosomal dominant inheritance.

**Pathogenesis:** Presumed deficiency of high-capacity, low-affinity, group-specific membrane transport system (protein or permease), in brush border membrane common to proline, hydroxyproline, and glycine.

**MIM No.:** 13850, *24260

**Sex Ratio:** M1:F1

**Occurrence:** About 1:17,000 live births for homozygous trait. *All* newborns have *normal* transient neonatal iminoglycinuria of a different mechanism.

**Risk of Recurrence for Patient's Sib:**
See Part I, *Mendelian Inheritance.*

**Risk of Recurrence for Patient's Child:**
See Part I, *Mendelian Inheritance.*

**Age of Detectability:** At birth.

**Gene Mapping and Linkage:** Unknown.

**Prevention:** None known. Genetic counseling indicated.

**Treatment:** Care for associated illnesses (if any).

**Prognosis:** Normal life span.

**Detection of Carrier:** Hyperglycinuria in one type of heterozygote.

**Special Considerations:** Renal iminoglycinuria is normally present in the newborn, reflecting ontogeny of independent transport systems for imino acids and for glycine and not controlled by the iminoglycinuria marker locus (Lasley and Scriver, 1979). Renal tubular conservation of imino acids and glycine approaches adult values by the 6th month of life in normal infants.

Evidence for more than one mutant genotype rests in the different forms of heterozygosity, the demonstration of an intestinal transport defect in some homozygotes, the failure to identify this feature in other homozygotes, and Mendelian evidence for genetic compounds.

**References:**
Rosenberg LE, et al.: Familial iminoglycinuria: an inborn error of renal tubular transport. New Engl J Med 1968; 278:1407–1413.
Scriver CR: Renal tubular transport of proline, hydroxyproline and glycine. III. Genetic basis for more than one mode of transport in human kidney. J Clin Invest 1968; 47:823–835.
Lasley L, Scriver CR: Ontogeny of amino acid reabsorption in human kidney: evidence from the homozygous infant with familial renal iminoglycinuria for multiple proline and glycine systems. Pediatr Res 1979; 13:65.
Scriver CR: Familial renal iminoglycinuria. In: Scriver CR, et al., eds: Metabolic basis of inherited disease, ed 6. New York: McGraw-Hill, 1989:2529–2538.

SC050                                           **Charles R. Scriver**

**Iminoglycinuria type II**
*See IMINOGLYCINURIA*

**Immotile cilia syndrome**
*See DEXTROCARDIA-BRONCHIECTASIS-SINUSITIS SYNDROME*
**Immune interferon deficiency**
*See INTERFERON DEFICIENCY*

## IMMUNODEFICIENCIES                          1508

Recent advances in immunology and molecular biology have been translated into improved understanding of the etiology and management of many disorders of the immune system. Immunodeficiencies constitute a wide spectrum of diseases with a diversity of underlying mechanisms of pathogenesis, ranging from arrest of development to infection with immunosuppressive etiologic agents. While it may be perceived that there has been a steady rise in the number of patients with a diagnosis of primary immune deficiency, it is unlikely that this reflects any change in the incidence of disease. More likely this is due to an increased awareness by the medical community of the possibility of immunodeficiency as well as improved methods of diagnosis.

What are some of the indications of underlying immunodeficiency disease? Recurrent infections, often due to opportunistic organisms, may be an early sign. It is difficult, however, to give specific examples of just what frequency may be cause for concern. Evidently what is needed is sufficient experience with a normal population to recognize the tremendous range of individual variability with regard to susceptibility to routine infections.

Familial clustering of immunodeficiencies may also assist in their diagnosis. Thus it is not uncommon to see families with several symptomatic members. While a single disease entity such as **Immunodeficiency, agammaglobulinemia, X-linked, infantile** may be scattered throughout a family, patterns of multiple, different syndromes are also not uncommon. It is prudent to consider a more extensive family evaluation when an index case is identified. Further, when a patient has been shown to express one immunodeficiency disorder, it is also recommended to look for other immunologic dysfunctions within that individual as several different immunodefiency syndromes may occur simultaneously or sequentially. One example of this is the increased incidence of atopy associated with immunodeficiencies. Another indication of immune deficiency is a familial tendency to fetal wastage or deaths in early childhood. These should indeed be specifically noted on taking the history. So-called cancer families or families with several members with malignant disease may also be associated with underlying immunodeficiency.

Several significant physical findings are often indicative of immunodeficiency disease. Many such patients have a paucity of peripheral lymphoid tissues including the absence of adenoids and/or tonsils. Occasionally immunodeficient patients may show evidence of growth retardation which may present initially as failure to thrive. This is not to be confused with dwarfism which may also be associated with immunodeficiency diseases. In response to frequent bouts of infection, patients may manifest hepatosplenomegaly. Certain immunodeficiencies may also be associated with specific dysmorphism such as the unique facies noted among patients with **Immunodeficiency, thymic agenesis**, or the bony abnormalities of the ribs found in **Immunodeficiency, severe combined** due to adenosine deaminase deficiency.

Treatment of immunodeficiencies has progressed remarkably. Numerous technical advancements have significantly reduced thier morbidity and mortality. Bone marrow transplantation has emerged as a recognized treatment modality. While at one time it was specifically restricted to closely related, major histocompatibility complex matched, donor-recipient pairs, successful transplantation across this barrier is now a reality. Elimination of mature, post-thymic T-lymphocytes from the donor marrow can significantly reduce the likelihood of serious graft-versus-host disease. Bone marrow transplantation has been successfully used to treat primary immunodeficiencies, a wide variety of hematologic and oncologic disorders, and some inborn errors of metabolism; additional applications are under consideration. Cellular engineering, as exemplified by bone marrow transplantation, may soon be complemented by the transfer of individual genes to replace defective ones in selected recipients. Recent preclinical studies have indicated that definitive treatment of severe combined immunodeficiency with adenosine deaminase deficiency may be achieved by the transfer of functional adenosine deaminase genes to the deficient recipient. We may soon bear witness to the first successful correction of a congenital defect by gene transplantation.

During the last several years a new class of immunotherapeutic agents have been identified, biological modifier substances. As their name implies these drugs are capable of modulating various biologic activities including immunologic functions. Several of these substances were first recognized to be the secretory products of various cells and were called cytokines; the secretory products of lymphocytes have been designated lymphokines. Included among these substances are interferons, interleukins, tumor necrosis factor, B-cell growth factor, supressor and helper factors, etc. The genes for many of these agents have been isolated and cloned and sufficient quantities of these substances have been produced by recombinant DNA technology for pharmacologic application. Biologic modifier substances are finding increasing application in the treatment of immunodeficiency and malignant disorders.

A mainstay in the treatment of humoral immunodeficiency diseases has been replacement therapy with intramuscular (IM) gamma globulin, resulting in significant improvements in morbidity and mortality among patients with humoral immunodeficiencies. Until recently gamma globulin replacement therapy has been limited by how much could be administered at any one time by the IM route. Many patients were thus inadequately treated. The recent development of gamma globulin preparations for intravenous administration have overcome the volume or dosage hurdle, resulting in improved patient management. Moreover this new form of gamma globulin has prompted exploration of its indications in other disease states such as the immune cytopenias and autoimmune syndromes.

Autoimmune diseases also constitute a large class of disorders due to dysfunction of immunoregulatory mechanisms and may occur together with immunodeficiency syndromes. The scientific advances described above have also impacted positively on the diagnosis and management of autoimmune conditions. Several laboratories have demonstrated that **Lupus erythematosus, systemic** is associated with a deficiency of suppressor T-cell functions. Attempts to treat this disorder by the administration of immunosuppressive lymphokines are currently under investigation. **Diabetes mellitus, insulin dependent type** is now thought to be an autoimmune disease. The development of a new generation of immunosuppressive drugs, such as cyclosporin A, has shown some promise in the treatment of this form of diabetes. While cyclosporin A is recognized to cause some serious adverse reactions, such as nephrotoxicity, newer related drugs with diminished side effects are currently under development. It is further likely that a seemingly unrelated array of disorders, including epilepsy, immune cytopenias, hemolytic anemia, myasthenia gravis, multiple sclerosis, pemphigoid, etc. may be responsive to immunomodulatory therapy. Reports of clinical trials are appearing regularly.

The acquired immunodeficiency syndrome (AIDS) is posing a major contemporary challenge to the health sciences. While the etiologic agent, the human immunodeficiency virus, has been characterized, a treatment for this devastating disease remains elusive. Many of the recent and forthcoming gains in our understanding and therapy of other immunologic diseases may have direct application to the AIDS epidemic. Thus it is hoped that the enthusiasm and successes of the disciplines of immunology and molecular biology achieved over the past several decades will also provide unique new treatments for some present day scurges.

SC039                                            **Stanley A. Schwartz**

**Immunodeficiency 5**
*See IMMUNODEFICIENCY, X-LINKED LYMPHOPROLIFERATIVE DISEASE*

## IMMUNODEFICIENCY WITH CENTROMERIC INSTABILITY                                      2520

**Includes:**
>   Centromeric instability-immunodeficiency
>   Chromosome 1, centromeric instability-immunodeficiency
>   Chromosome 9, centromeric instability-immunodeficiency
>   Chromosome 16, centromeric instability-immunodeficiency
>   Immunodeficiency-centromeric instability-facial anomalies (ICF)
>   Immunoglobulin deficiency-centromere instability

**Excludes:**
>   **Ataxia-telangiectasia** (0094)
>   **Bloom syndrome** (0112)
>   Chromosomal breakage syndromes, classical
>   **Chromosome instability, Nijmegen type** (2551)

**Major Diagnostic Criteria:** 1) Severe immunodeficiency including pronounced immunodeficiency and evidence for deficient cell-mediated deficiency; 2) developmental delay and facial abnormalities; and 3) instability of the centromeric regions of chromosomes 1, 9 and 16 resulting in multibranched configurations.

**Clinical Findings:** In the six patients reported; a series of variable immunodeficiencies, mild developmental delay, facial abnormalities including epicanthic folds, intestinal malabsorption, and severe failure to thrive was present in all.

All patients suffer from severe immunodeficiency associated with instability of the centromeric regions of chromosomes 1, 9 and 16, which results in multi-branched configurations.

**Complications:** Unknown.

**Associated Findings:** Pierre-Robin anomaly (micrognathia, cleft palate) in one patient. Internal malformations are poorly documented in the absence of autopsy data.

**Etiology:** Unknown.

**Pathogenesis:** None known.

**MIM No.:** 24286

**POS No.:** 4375

**Sex Ratio:** M3:F2

**Occurrence:** Six families have been reported, with affected sibs in two of the families.

**Risk of Recurrence for Patient's Sib:** Unknown.

**Risk of Recurrence for Patient's Child:** Unknown. Affected individuals are not expected to survive to reproduce.

**Age of Detectability:** First months of life by the finding of immunodeficiency, failure to thrive, developmental delay and the specific multibranched chromosomes 1, 9 and 16. In principle, prenatal diagnosis is feasible on fetal lymphocytes and amniocytes.

**Gene Mapping and Linkage:** See *Gene Map.*

**Prevention:** None known. Genetic counseling indicated.

**Treatment:** Symptomatic. Gammaglobulin replacement therapy and antibiotic treatment may reduce infections.

**Prognosis:** Long-term prognosis is poor. Three patients were last examined at five years of age and suffered from failure to

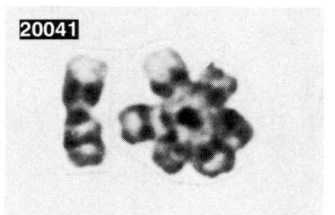
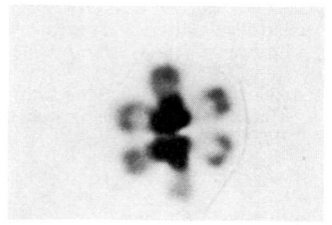

2520-20041:  G- and C-banding of centromeric instability.

thrive and recurrent infections. A fourth patient died at the age of 18 months.

**Detection of Carrier:** Unknown. Extensive chromosomal investigations of the parents of one child were normal.

**References:**
Hulten M: Selective somatic pairing and fragility at 1q12 in a boy with common variable immunodeficiency. Clin Genet 1978; 14:294 only.
Tiepolo L, et al.: Multibranched chromosomes 1, 9, and 16 in a patient with combined IgA and IgE deficiency. Hum Genet 1979; 51:127–137.
Fryns JP, et al.: Centromeric instability of chromosomes 1, 9, and 16 associated with combined immunodeficiency. Hum Genet 1981; 57:108–110. *
Howard PJ, et al.: Centromeric instability of chromosomes 1 and 16 with variable immune deficiency: a new syndrome. Clin Genet 1985; 27:501–505.
Valkova G, et al.: Centromeric instability of chromosomes 1, 9 and 16 with variable immune deficiency: support of a new syndrome. Clin Genet 1987; 31:119–124.
Turleau C, et al.: Multibranched chromosomes in the ICF syndrome: immunodeficiency, centromeric instability, and facial anomalies. Am J Med Genet 1989; 32:420–424. †

FR030                                                      **Jean-Pierre Fryns**

---

## IMMUNODEFICIENCY, ADENOSINE DEAMINASE DEFICIENCY                                         2196

**Includes:**
    ADA deficiency
    Adenosine aminohydrolase deficiency (ADA)
    Adenosine deaminase
    Severe combined immunodeficiency with ADA

**Excludes:** Nucleoside deaminase deficiencies, other

**Major Diagnostic Criteria:** Complete absence of adenosine deaminase (ADA) enzymatic activity in the appropriate assay. Lysed erythrocyte ADA activity may be tested in nontransfused patients, with confirmation by testing peripheral blood mononuclear cells, cultured fibroblasts or B-lymphocyte lines. Heterozygous carriers typically have enzyme activity detected at greater than two SD below normal. The gel method is often used for screening, but is not 100% sensitive. Assays that determine the conversion of adenosine to inosine (or to uric acid with addition of xanthine oxidase) are preferred.

**Clinical Findings:** Patients present with severe combined immunodeficiency (SCID), the prominent features of which are recurrent and severe infections, failure to thrive, and intestinal malabsorption. Of all SCID cases, approximately 20-30% have ADA deficiency as the underlying etiology. This subgroup may be identified clinically by the association of SCID with chondroosseous dysplasia, which is characterized on X-ray by prominent growth arrest lines, paucity of trabeculae, platyspondyly of the vertebral bodies, vertically shortened pelvis with squared ilia, and cupping of the anterior ends of the ribs. Growth plate histopathologic findings are diagnostic and include absence of transition from proliferating to hypertrophic cells, lack of organized columns of hypertrophic cells, and uninterrupted calcified cartilage formation. However, the ADA assay is both necessary and sufficient to confirm the diagnosis. Patients often show signs and symptoms in the first several months of life, but not until ages 4–12 months in 10–15%. The spectrum of severity may relate to small residual amounts of enzyme activity noted in peripheral blood mononuclear cells of those who manifest the disease at the later ages.

**Complications:** In addition to the complications of SCID, neurologic abnormalities may occur in 10% of patients. Resolution of neurologic manifestations is seen after therapeutic intervention that lowers circulating levels of adenosine and deoxyadenosine. Renal mesangial sclerosis and adrenal cortical fibrosis have also been reported.

**Associated Findings:** Bony abnormalities.

**Etiology:** Autosomal recessive inheritance.

**Pathogenesis:** ADA is a 35–42 kd polypeptide encoded by a single 32 kb locus on the long arm of chromosome 20. It also exists as a higher molecular weight form (280 kd) composed of two ADA molecules joined by a dimeric ADA complexing protein. Electrophoretic studies reveal a series of codominant allelic variants. Analysis of ADA-deficient cells with cDNA probes reveals intact mRNA, and in vitro translation of hybrid-selected mRNA leads to elaboration of appropriate molecular weight proteins that are only weakly immunoprecipitable and exhibit no enzymatic activity. Single point mutations, confirmed by restriction fragment length polymorphism, lead to single amino acid substitutions which appear to render the enzyme inactive and more susceptible to proteolytic degradation. ADA catalyzes the irreversible deamination of adenosine and 2'deoxyadenosine to inosine and 2' deoxyinosine, respectively. In the absence of ADA, phosphorylation to the respective ribo- and deoxyribonucleotides occurs. The accumulation of metabolites has various effects. Deoxyadenosine 5'triphosphate (dATP) appears to block DNA synthesis in mature B-cells by inhibiting ribonucleotide reductase. Deoxyadenosine (dAR) affects immature T-cells in the G0/Gl phase of the cell cycle and inhibits the expression of interleukin-2 receptors. T-cells appear to be very sensitive to dAR accumulation, becoming nonviable before significant phosphorylation to dATP has occurred. Immature murine B-cells are less sensitive in vitro to dAR than activated, complement receptor-bearing B-cells. Inactivation of S-adenosyl homocysteine hydrolase by dAR, depletion of phosphoribosylpyrophosphate, pyrimidine starvation, and depletion of NAD pools may all play a role in the cytotoxic events. Broadly speaking, these findings are consistent with the clinical presentation of profound T-cell but variable B-cell dysfunction.

**MIM No.:** *10270

**Sex Ratio:** M1:F1

**Occurrence:** Accounts for 20–30% of all patients with SCID, and half of the cases of autosomal recessive SCID. More than 20 cases have been documented. Noted in Blacks, West Indian and Mediterranean families.

**Risk of Recurrence for Patient's Sib:**
    See Part I, *Mendelian Inheritance.*

**Risk of Recurrence for Patient's Child:**
    See Part I, *Mendelian Inheritance.*

**Age of Detectability:** Prenatally by determination of ADA activity in cultured amniotic cells.

**Gene Mapping and Linkage:** ADA (adenosine deaminase) has been mapped to 20q13.11 or 20q13.2-qter.

**Prevention:** None known. Genetic counseling indicated.

**Treatment:** Repeated partial exchange transfusions with frozen irradiated RBCs every 2–4 weeks has been shown to ameliorate symptoms. However, immunologic function generally continues to deteriorate. Current therapy is haplo-identical or haplo-mismatched bone marrow transplantation. Retrovirus-mediated transfer of cloned human cDNA has been shown to correct ADA deficiency in vitro in cultured human T- and B-cell lines. ADA deficiency is considered to be the first candidate for attempting in vivo gene replacement therapy. Clinical and biochemical improvement has recently been demonstrated with intramuscular injections of polyethylene glycol-modified bovine adenosine deaminase.

**Prognosis:** Untreated patients rarely survive beyond age two years except in cases of partial ADA deficiency. With successful bone marrow transplantation, the prognosis is excellent.

**Detection of Carrier:** Heterozygotes can be detected with 90% accuracy using quantitative assays. Phenotypic studies of ADA showing lack of the expected genetic polymorphism consistent with inheritance of a "null" allele confirms that a family is at risk.

**Special Considerations:** Partial ADA deficiency has been described. Studies indicate that some may result from genetic compounds at the ADA locus. Similar clinical findings may also be found in **Immunodeficiency, nucleoside-phosphorylase deficiency,** and cytidine deaminase (CDA; cytidine aminohydrolase) deficiency has been described in association with immunologic deficiency.

## References:

Simmonds HA, et al.: Correlations between purine levels, clinical and immunological status in ADA deficiency. Adv Exp Med Biol 1985; 195(ptA):93.

Wortmann RL, et al.: Adenosine deaminase deficiency and chondroosseous dysplasia. Adv Exp Med Biol 1985; 195(ptA):81.

Hirschhorn R: Inherited enzyme deficiencies and immunodeficiency: adenosine deaminase (ADA) and purine nucleoside phosphorylase (PNP) deficiencies. Clin Immunol Immunopathol 1986; 40:157.

Kantoff PW, et al.: Correction of adenosine deaminase deficiency in cultured human T and B cells by retrovirus-mediated gene transfer. Proc Natl Acad Sci USA 1986; 83:6563.

Hirschhorn R, Ellenbogen A: Genetic heterogeneity in adenosine deaminase (ADA) deficiency: five different mutations in five new patients with partial ADA deficiency. Am J Hum Genet 1986; 38:13–25.

Hershfield MS, et al.: Treatment of adenosine deaminase deficiency with polyethylene glycol-modified adenosine deaminase. New Engl J Med 1987; 316:589–596.

SL002                                                     **Herbert B. Slade**

---

## IMMUNODEFICIENCY, AGAMMAGLOBULINEMIA, X-LINKED, INFANTILE                                          0027

**Includes:**
  Agammaglobulinemia, X-linked, infantile
  Bruton agammaglobulinemia
  Hypogammaglobulinemia, X-linked

**Excludes:**
  **Agammaglobulinemia-thymoma syndrome** (0944)
  Immunoglobulin G subclass deficiencies
  **Immunodeficiency, common variable type** (0521)
  **Immunodeficiency, X-linked severe combined** (0524)

**Major Diagnostic Criteria:**  Males with absent or severely diminished peripheral and intestinal lymphoid tissue, as demonstrable, for instance, by near absence of tonsils and adenoids. Histologically, plasma cells and germinal centers of lymphoid tissue are absent with or without antigenic stimulation. B-lymphocytes are absent. Absent or very diminished Ig and antibody response to administered antigens. The frequency and severity of bacterial infections increase starting toward the end of the first half-year of life, involving respiratory tract, sinuses, GI tract, and skin.

**Clinical Findings:**  Age of onset of manifestations is usually between 3 and 6 months in males; with repeated bouts of purulent conjunctivitis, otitis media, recurrent upper respiratory infections, bronchitis, and skin infections. Early sinusitis is frequent, and pneumonias begin during the first year of life, often leading to bronchiectasis. Recurrent episodes of septicemia may occur, and meningitis attacks may be seen repeatedly. There is a propensity to contract infectious hepatitis, which, not infrequently, becomes a fatal disease in these patients. Infections with echoviruses, especially those of the high-numbered types, can be devastating. Paralytic poliomyelitis, often associated with live vaccine administration, is unusually frequent. Varicella is another viral disease known to be more severe in these children both by recurrence and may be complicated by occasional accompanying pneumonia. Tonsillar and adenoid tissues are grosely deficient. X-rays reveal clouding of the sinuses with evident infection, obliteration, and destruction of the mastoid air cells, minimal hilar shadows, pulmonary infiltrates, segmental atelectasis, and areas of bronchiectasis, wasting of the tissues, and gaseous distention of the abdomen.

Laboratory findings reveal less than 100 mg% immunoglobulins (Ig), IgM and IgA are absent. IgG is normal at birth but drops to less than 100 mg% in the first 6 months. Peripheral blood is normal, but sometimes there is periodic neutropenia, transient eosinophilia, or monocytosis. B-lymphocytes are absent from the blood and lymphoid tissues. Bone marrow shows absence or severe paucity of plasma cells, but pre-B-lymphocytes recognized by appropriate surface markers and by cytoplasmic but not by surface Ig, are present in normal or near-normal numbers. Bacteriologic investigation of infections demonstrates recurrent diplococcus pneumonias, *Haemophilus influenzae*, meningococcus, streptococcus, and, after antibiotic therapy, usually *Pseudomonas*. ASOT remains negative in spite of documented streptococcal infections. Isoagglutinins are absent, and there is failure to respond to injected antigens such as DPT immunization with production of antibodies. Antibodies to pneumococcal antigens and *H. influenzae* are usually not found.

**Complications:**  Poor growth, clubbing of fingers and toes, erythema nodosum, potbelly, septicemias, bronchiectasis, pulmonary fibrosis and cor pulmonale, cholesteatoma, conductive hearing loss, anemia, diarrhea, hypocalcemia, protein-losing enteropathy, ulcerative colitis, regional enteritis.

**Associated Findings:**  Arthritis of the rheumatoid type in 20–40%, later a dermatomyositis-like illness, agranulocytosis, thrombocytopenia, autoimmune disease, malabsorption, amyloidosis. Persistent echovirus infection may lead to destructive CNS disease. These persistent virus infections may be accompanied by the dermatomyositis syndrome.

**Etiology:**  X-linked recessive inheritance.

**Pathogenesis:**  Pre-B cells fail to develop into B-lymphocytes. The inability to muster a humoral antibody response to pyogenic organisms, which surround the infant, leads to severe infections as soon as the maternal complement or immunoglobulins to the newborn are exhausted. Pneumococcus, *H. influenzae*, meningococcus, streptococcus, and *Pseudomonas aeruginosa* are the most successful invaders under these conditions, spreading from the natural portals of entry inward without effective host resistance. Thus recurrent and later chronic sinopulmonary disease is the outstanding clinical event, together with pyoderma, purulent conjunctivitis, and purulent otitis media. Further uncontrolled spread and dissemination are manifested by septicemias, meningitis, deep abscesses, osteomyelitis, and other parenchymatous pyogenic involvement. Progressive pulmonary impairment with bronchiectasis, fibrosis, and eventual right heart overload from increasing pulmonary vascular resistance are later sequelae. Intestinal involvement with diarrhea, protein-losing enteropathy, and development of regional enteritis and ulcerative colitis are probably consequences of the absence of plasma cells and lymphoid tissue aggregates normally responsible for host resistance in this area. The susceptibility to severe infectious hepatitis and recurrent varicella indicates that B-cell function or antibodies are involved in defense against these organisms. Long-range effects of the chronic infectious processes are physical underdevelopment, amyloidosis, and possible CNS damage. Survival beyond early childhood with the underlying deficiency makes the patient susceptible to rheumatoid arthritis, dermatomyositis-like illness, and autoimmune disease. The pathogenesis of these complications is not understood, but their occurrence in this pure antibody deficiency state indicates that cell-mediated immunity attributed to T-lymphocytes can be responsible for some of the manifestations of autoimmune disease. It has now been established that B-lymphocyte differentiation in these patients is arrested at the level of the pre-B-cell to B-cell differentiation step. Pre-B-cells are present in the marrow, but B-lymphocytes develop poorly or not at all and are not present in the blood.

**MIM No.:**  *30030

**Sex Ratio:**  M1:F0

**Occurrence:**  1:50,000 live births.

**Risk of Recurrence for Patient's Sib:**
  See Part I, *Mendelian Inheritance*. See Lau et al (1988).

**Risk of Recurrence for Patient's Child:**
  See Part I, *Mendelian Inheritance*. Affected individuals are not expected to survive to reproduce.

**Age of Detectability:**  Neonatal period by study of blood lymphocytes, bone marrow, or lymph node cells.

**Gene Mapping and Linkage:**  AGMX1 (agammaglobulinemia, X-linked 1 (Bruton)) has been mapped to Xq21.33-q22.

**Prevention:** None known. Genetic counseling indicated.

**Treatment:** IM immunoglobulin by injection, 0.6 cc/kg/month or 0.3 cc/kg/2 weeks, or plasma from hepatitis-free donors. Any of several preparations of gammaglobulin for intravenous administration given in doses suitable to maintaining the circulating gammaglobulin levels within the normal range of 700–1,300 mg/dl. Avoidance of exposure to infections; regular follow-up. Vigorous antibiotic therapy at earliest signs of infection.

**Prognosis:** Progressive sinopulmonary disease is occasionally a major problem. Untreated patients rarely survive infancy or early childhood. With good medical attention and preventive immunoglobulin therapy, outlook is much improved. Long-range survivors have now reached adulthood.

**Detection of Carrier:** RFLP markers have been used to identify carrier state and in early diagnosis (Schuurman et at, 1988).

**Special Considerations:** This defect has many clinical and laboratory features in common with **Immunodeficiency, common variable type.** However, the absence of B-cells in blood and the clear-cut defect in the humoral antibody-producing capacity without any thymic-mediated involvement makes it possible to distinguish clinically with the help of laboratory evidence. Lymphoreticular malignancy may be increased, although carcinoma and sarcoma are not known to be increased. This is an important prognostic consideration. Recent studies suggest that there may be two distinct and separate forms of X-linked infantile agammaglobulinemia.

**References:**
Good RA, et al.: Consideration of some questions asked by patients with an attempt at classification. In: BD:OAS 1968; IV(1):17.
Rosen FS, Janeway CA: Diagnosis and treatment of antibody deficiency syndromes. Postgrad Med 1968; 43:188.
Wollheim FA: Primary "acquired" hypogammaglobulinemia: genetic defect or acquired disease? In: 1968; IV(1):311.
Report of a WHO Scientific Group. Primary immunodeficiency diseases. In: 1983; XIX(3):345–360.
Report of a WHO Scientific Group. Primary immunodeficiency diseases 1. Introduction. In: Eibl MM, Rosen FS, eds: Primary immunodeficiency diseases. Amsterdam: Excerpta Medica, 1986;341–375.
Mensick, EJBM, et al.: Immunoglobulin heavy chain gene rearrangements in X-linked agammaglobulinemia. Eur J Immunol 1986; 110:963–967.
Schuurman RKB, et al.: Early diagnosis in X-linked agammaglobulinemia. Europ J Pediat 1988; 147:93–95.
Lau YL, et al.: Genetic prediction in X-linked agammaglobulinaemia. Am J Med Genet 1988; 31:437–448.
World Health Organization. Primary immunodeficiency diseases. Immunodeficiency Reviews 1989; 1:173–205.

G0023                                                                    **Robert A. Good**

---

## IMMUNODEFICIENCY, AGRANULOCYTOSIS, INFANTILE KOSTMANN TYPE                          2197

**Includes:**
    Agranulocytosis, infantile Kostmann type
    Kostmann syndrome
    Neutrophil differentiation factor

**Excludes:**
    Autoimmune neutropenia
    **Neutropenia, benign familial** (2215)
    **Neutropenia, cyclic** (0714)

**Major Diagnostic Criteria:** Persistent severe granulocytopenia, with an absolute neutrophil count less than 500 and often less than 200, is the hallmark of the disorder.

**Clinical Findings:** Affected infants appear normal, but they are either severely neutropenic at birth or become so in the neonatal period.

During the first few months of life these infants have severe infections. Initially, the infections usually involve the skin and mucosal surfaces, but all organ systems can be involved, with lymphadenitis, pneumonia, peritonitis, liver abscesses, and sep-

ticemia especially common. Infants who survive invariably develop subsequent serious infections. The prompt administration of broad-spectrum antibiotics has prolonged the survival of affected individuals, with survival to adolescence occasionally reported. Although recurrent bacterial infections begin during the first year of life, the other hematopoietic cell lines are not affected, and thus the total white count may be in the normal range because of lymphocytosis and monocytosis. Platelets are not affected, and although there may be an accompanying anemia of chronic illness, the red cell line is unaffected. Examination of the bone marrow shows markedly decreased numbers of mature granulocytes, with a predominance of vacuolated myelocytes and promyelocytes. There may be increased numbers of monocytes, eosinophils, plasma cells, and histiocytes.

**Complications:** One patient developed acute myelocytic leukemia at 14 years of age, which may indicate an increased susceptibility to neoplasia.

**Associated Findings:** None known.

**Etiology:** Autosomal recessive inheritance.

**Pathogenesis:** Unknown. Evidence obtained from bone marrow culture and from the results of bone marrow transplantation suggests that the cause is a defective stem cell. There are normal or even increased numbers of myeloid colony-forming cells in the marrow, but the maturation of the granulocytes is abnormal. These dysplastic cells either autolyze or are phagocytized by the macrophages in the marrow. Antineutrophil antibodies have not been implicated.

**MIM No.:** *20270

**Sex Ratio:** M1:F1

**Occurrence:** About 75 cases have been reported.

**Risk of Recurrence for Patient's Sib:**
    See Part I, *Mendelian Inheritance.*

**Risk of Recurrence for Patient's Child:**
    See Part I, *Mendelian Inheritance.*

**Age of Detectability:** Always within the first few months of life, but some have been neutropenic at birth.

**Gene Mapping and Linkage:** Unknown.

**Prevention:** None known. Genetic counseling indicated.

**Treatment:** Prompt administration of antibiotics at the first sign of infection has markedly prolonged the survival of affected individuals. For apparently localized infections, oral antibiotics can be tried, but if response is not prompt, parenteral broad-spectrum antibiotics (covering *Staphyloccocus aureus* and gram-negative enteritis) should be started. Prophylactic antibiotics, such as trimethoprim-sulfamethoxazole, have been advocated, but their efficacy has not been documented.

A more permanent therapeutic option is a bone marrow transplant from a compatible sib. With appropriate preconditioning with total body irradiation and cytotoxic drugs, engraftment has been accomplished with the establishment of normal granulocyte maturation. Granulocyte differentiation and subsequent development of circulating granulocytes has occurred following the subcutaneous administration of granulocyte-colony stimulating factor. The use of granulocytic colony stimulating factor should comprise the initial therapy.

**Prognosis:** In most of the early reports, the affected individuals died in infancy or early childhood. More recently, improvements in supportive care have led to survival into adolescence. The availability of a compatible sib offers the potential for cure by bone marrow transplant, although this procedure is certainly not without risk. A slight number of patients have developed acute leukemia. Amelioration of clinical infections has occurred in response to use of granulocyte-colony stimulating factor.

**Detection of Carrier:** Unknown.

**References:**
Kostmann R: Infantile genetic agranulocytosis: a review with presentation of ten new cases. Acta Paediatr Scand 1975; 64:362–368. *

Parmley RT, et al.: Congenital dysgranulocytopoietic neutropenia. Blood 1980; 56:465–475. *

Rappaport JM, et al.: Correction of infantile agranulocytosis by allogeneic bone marrow transplantation. Am J Med 1980; 68:605–609.

Lin CY, et al.: Infantile genetic agranulocytosis in three siblings. Med J Osaka Univ 1981; 31:111–116.

AX001            **Richard Axtell**
B0048          **Laurence A. Boxer**

**Immunodeficiency, C1r/C1s deficiency**
 *See COMPLEMENT COMPONENT 1, DEFICIENCY OF*
**Immunodeficiency, cartilage-hair hypoplasia**
 *See METAPHYSEAL CHONDRODYSPLASIA, TYPE McKUSICK*

---

## IMMUNODEFICIENCY, COMMON VARIABLE TYPE  0521

**Includes:**
 Agammaglobulinemia, acquired
 Agammaglobulinemia, adult
 Agammaglobulinemia, late-onset
 Hypogammaglobulinemia, familial
 Immunodeficiency, common varied
 Immunoglobulin deficiencies
 Late-onset immunoglobulin deficiency

**Excludes:**
 **Agammaglobulinemia-thymoma syndrome** (0944)
 IgA deficiency, selective
 **Immunodeficiency, agammaglobulinemia, X-linked, infantile** (0027)
 **Immunodeficiency, common variable type** (0521)
 **Immunodeficiency, X-linked severe combined** (0524)
 **Immunodeficiency, X-linked with hyper IgM** (2524)
 **Serum allotypes, human** (0476)
 **Transcobalamin II deficiency** (2624)
 Transient hypogammaglobulinemia of infancy

**Major Diagnostic Criteria:** Decreased concentration of all or some of the major immunoglobulins (IgG, IgA, IgM) in serum with nearly normal T-cell numbers and function. Conditions secondarily resulting in low serum immunoglobulins must be excluded; i.e. protein loss, drugs, malignancy, infection and **Transcobalamin II deficiency.**

**Clinical Findings:** Clinical symptoms and infective agents are very similar to those in **Immunodeficiency, agammaglobulinemia, X-linked, infantile,** but somewhat milder. Onset is usually after two years of age, most frequently in the second or third decade. Although occasional patients suffer remarkably few infections, recurrent or persistent sinopulmonary infeciton is the dominant clinical problem occurring in almost 90%. Patients suffer from pulmonary airway, parenchymal and pleural disease with 30–40% going on to develop serious pulmonary impairment (chronic bronchitis, bronchiectasis, interstitial fibrosis and panlobular emphysema). Chronic otitis media is frequent (30%). Gastrointestinal manifestations are found in up to 60% of patients and include chronic diarrhea, malabsorption or protein-losing enteropathy. Giardia lamblia infections occur in 35–65% and Clostridium difficile in 24%. There are decreased small bowel brush border enzyme activities and patchy histological abnormalities of the partial villous atrophy type.

It is likely that some changes are secondary to occult or proven infection. As many as 40% of patients will be anemic with pernicious anemia in approximately five percent. Cancer develops with a markedly increased incidence (5 to 13-fold) in the fifth and sixth decades of life. Stomach cancer is increased 50-fold and lymphoma 30-fold with an undue proportion of lymphomas occurring in female patients. The most common pathogens are high grade encapsulated bacteria but Mycoplasma and Ureaplasma have been identified as significant infectious agents. Echovirus meningoencephalitis and dermatomyositis occur infrequently compared with **Immunodeficiency, agammaglobulinemia, X-linked, infantile.** Patients are also at risk for developing vaccine-associated poliomyelitis.

There is considerable heterogeneity in laboratory findings with variability in numbers of circulating B-cells from nearly normal to very low. These B-cells do not differentiate into immunoglobulin producing plasma cells *in vivo* or *in vitro*. There is diversity with respect to the expression of surface membrane immunoglobulins, B-cell antigens and B-lymphocyte ecto-5'-nucleotidase activity. There are varying degrees of lymphopenia, T-cell subset imbalances and depression of blastogenic responses to mitogens. Laboratory findings may also vary with time in individual patients.

Careful study of family members is indicated and may reveal other antibody deficiency syndromes (especially IgA deficiency and immunoglobulin deficiency with increased IgM), autoimmune diseases and malignancies. This suggests wide intrafamilial variability in expression of a common defect.

**Complications:** Bronchiectasis, arthritis (7%), gastric carcinoma, lymphoreticular malignancy, cholelithiasis, lymphoid interstitial pneumonia, pseudolymphoma, amyloidosis, transfusion reactions, noncaseating granulomas of lungs, spleen, skin and liver. Echovirus and viral hepatitis infections are particularly troublesome.

**Associated Findings:** Intestinal nodular lymphoid hyperplasia, splenomegaly, thymoma, alopecia areata, autoimmune hemolytic anemia, neutropenia, sprue-like syndrome, gastric atrophy, achlorhydria, pernicious anemia, thyroid disease, and **Lupus erythematosus, systemic** occur.

**Etiology:** Autosomal recessive or dominant inheritance.

**Pathogenesis:** Progressive loss of humoral immune function due to a genetically determined abnormality of B-cell maturation into immunoglobulin-synthesizing and -secreting plasma cells. blocks occur at pre-B, B-cell, and plasma cell levels. Excessive T suppression of B-cell differentiation may be both primary and secondary and is potentially clinically significant if present. Failure of helper T-cell activity and enhanced suppressor activity of monocytes have been described. Autoantibodies to T- or B-cells may be present.

**MIM No.:** *24050, 14683, *14690, *14691, *14700, *14701, *14702, *14707, *14710, *14711, *14712, *14713, *14716, *14717, *14718, 14720

**Sex Ratio:** Presumably M1:F1, but some series report a male preponderance.

**Occurrence:** Sporadic and familial forms occur. True incidence is not known as detection is related to clinical index of suspicion but is less common than IgA deficiency.

**Risk of Recurrence for Patient's Sib:**
 See Part I, *Mendelian Inheritance.*

**Risk of Recurrence for Patient's Child:**
 See Part I, *Mendelian Inheritance.*

**Age of Detectability:** Onset is at any age but especially after the second decade.

**Gene Mapping and Linkage:** IGHA1 (immunoglobulin alpha 1) has been mapped to 14q32.33.

 IGHA2 (immunoglobulin alpha 2 (A2M marker)) has been mapped to 14q32.33.

 IGHJ (immunoglobulin heavy polypeptide, joining region) has been mapped to 14q32.3.

 IGHM (immunoglobulin mu) has been mapped to 14q32.33.

 IGHV (immunoglobulin heavy polypeptide, variable region (many genes)) has been mapped to 14q32.33.

 IGHG1 (immunoglobulin gamma 1 (Gm marker)) has been mapped to 14q32.33.

 IGHG2 (immunoglobulin gamma 2 (Gm marker)) has been mapped to 14q32.33.

 IGHG3 (immunoglobulin gamma 3 (Gm marker)) has been mapped to 14q32.33.

 IGHG4 (immunoglobulin gamma 4 (Gm marker)) has been mapped to 14q32.33.

 IGHEP1 (immunoglobulin epsilon pseudogene 1) has been mapped to 14q32.33.

 IGHD (immunoglobulin delta) has been mapped to 14q32.33.

 IGHE (immunoglobulin epsilon) has been mapped to 14q32.33.

IGKC (immunoglobulin kappa constant region) has been mapped to 2p12.

It is possible that the primary abnormalities may occur in genes which regulate immunoglobulin synthesis.

**Prevention:** None known. Genetic counseling indicated.

**Treatment:** Therapy involves replacement of IgG with intravenous immunoglobulin, 0.1–0.6 g/kg/month, with the total dose tailored to individual needs. The higher dose permits achievement of normal serum IgG levels and, in patients with significant sinopulmonary disease, it results in resolution of sinusitis, reduction in cough and improvement in pulmonary function tests. It is the treatment of choice for echovirus-caused meningoencephalitis and dermatomyositis. Adverse reactions to the administration of intravenous immunoglobulin can be prevented by prior administration of hydrocortisone. Specific infections should be treated aggressively with antimicrobial agents. Continous broad-spectrum antibiotics are often necessary. Cimetidine may reverse T suppressor activity, effecting increased serum IgG level and improved clinical status in some patients.

**Prognosis:** Guarded. There is increased mortality from all causes, but especially from late malignancies.

**Detection of Carrier:** Unknown.

**References:**
Wollheim FA: Inherited "acquired" hypogammaglobulinaemia. Lancet 1961; I:316–317.
Waldman TA, et al: Role of suppressor T cells in the pathogenesis of common variable hypogammaglobulinemia. Lancet 1974; II:609–613.
Hermans PE, et al: Idiopathic late-onset immunoglobulin deficiency. Am J Med 1976; 61:221–237.
Kinlen LJ, et al: Prospective study of cancer in patients with hypogammaglobulinaemia. Lancet 1985; I:263–266.
Roifman CM, et al: Benefit of intravenous IgG replacement in hypogammaglobulinemic patients with chronic sinopulmonary disease. Am J Med 1985; 79:171–174.
White WB, Ballow M: Modulation of suppressor-cell activity by cimetidine in patients with common variable hypogammaglobulinemia. New Engl J Med 1985; 312:198–202.
Watts WJ, et al: Respiratory dysfunction in patients with common variable hypogammaglobulinemia. Am Rev Respir Dis 1986; 134: 699–703.

RE030                                                    **Elena R. Reece**

**Immunodeficiency, common varied**
  *See IMMUNODEFICIENCY, COMMON VARIABLE TYPE*
**Immunodeficiency, complement component 3**
  *See COMPLEMENT COMPONENT 3, DEFICIENCY OF*
**Immunodeficiency, erythrophagocytic lymphohistiocytosis**
  *See LYMPHOHISTIOCYTOSIS, FAMILIAL ERYTHROPHAGOCYTIC*
**Immunodeficiency, functional C1q deficiency**
  *See COMPLEMENT COMPONENT 1, DEFICIENCY OF*
**Immunodeficiency, granulocyte glycoprotein deficiency**
  *See GRANULOCYTE GLYCOPROTEIN CD11/CD18 DEFICIENCY*

---

## IMMUNODEFICIENCY, HYPER IGE TYPE            2211

**Includes:**
  HIE syndrome
  Hyper IgE, recurrent infection syndrome
  Hyperimmunoglobulin E-recurrent infection syndrome
  Job syndrome

**Excludes:  Skin, atopy, familial** (3150)

**Major Diagnostic Criteria:** Severe and recurrent staphylococcal infections of the skin and lower respiratory tract from infancy. The diagnosis is confirmed by a history of recurrent furunculosis, staphylococcal pneumonia, and pneumatoceles. Affected individuals have a history of, or current, chronic pruritic dermatitis, with a rash that is not typical atopic eczema. Markedly elevated polyclonal serum IgE, and pronounced eosinophilia of blood and sputum, is found in all affected individuals.

**Clinical Findings:** Abscesses of the skin and/or lungs have occurred as early as the first day of life, but always begin during infancy and recur throughout life. The condition affects both males and females; members of successive generations within families have been afflicted. It has been reported in Blacks and Whites. In early life there is a predilection for furuncles to localize about the scalp, neck, and face: particularly around the eyes, where hordeolums and even lacrimal gland abscesses occur. Recurrent staphylococcal pneumonia, with resultant persistent pneumatoceles, is typically the major presenting problem. Pneumatocele formation is not seen to this extent in any other clinical condition, including **Granulomatous disease, chronic** (CGD) and **Cystic fibrosis**, where staphylococcal lung infections are common.

Surgical removal of lung cysts that persist for more than six months is usually necessary to prevent superinfection with *Haemophilus* influenzae or other gram-negative organisms or aspergilloma formation. Most have also had chronic or recurrent infections of the ears, sinuses, eyes, and oral mucosa. Fewer have had infections of joints, viscera, and blood. Sites that have usually been spared include the gastrointestinal and urinary tracts, the meninges, and the bones. Exceptions include two patients with cryptococcal meningitis and a rare patient with osteomyelitis. Infrequency of the latter in this condition contrasts with the high frequency of bone infections in CGD. *Staphylococcus aureus*, coagulase positive, has caused infections in all patients. *Candida albicans*, *Haemophilus* influenzae, pneumococci, and Group A streptococci have infected from one-fourth to one-half of patients. Miscellaneous gram-negative rods, *Aspergillus* and *Trichophyton* species, and other fungi, have been pathogens in some cases.

Serum IgE has been noted to rise rapidly during early infancy and is always significantly above the normal 95% confidence interval even when no dermatitis is present. Nevertheless, affected individuals have few or no respiratory allergic symptoms, and the pruritic rash often resembles seborrheic rather that atopic dermatitis in character as well as distribution. Skin testing for IgE-mediated hypersensitivity usually reveals multiple positive reactions to inhalant, food, and pollen allergens and to antigens from infectious agents. High titers of IgE antibodies to staphylococcal and candidal organisms have been detected by radioimmunoassay.

Serum concentrations of immunoglobulins other than IgE are usually normal, although IgD may also be elevated. However, patients usually have impaired anamnestic antibody responses to vaccine antigens, and responses to neoantigens are poor. Cell-mediated immune responses to ubiquitous antigens *in vivo* have been depressed in roughly one-half of patients studied. *In vitro* lymphocyte responses to mitogens have most often been normal, but are usually low to absent following specific antigen stimulation. In addition, responses to mononuclear cells from genetically different members of the patient's family are often low or nondetectable. Percentages and absolute numbers of B- and T-lymphocytes and subpopulations are usually normal, with no increase in IgE-bearing B-lymphocytes. Complement activity and levels of complement components are normal. Polymorphonuclear cell phagocytic and bactericidal functions are normal, as are chemiluminescence and nitroblue tetrazolium dye reduction following phagocytosis. Inconstant chemotactic abnormalities have been reported, but most often both polymorphonuclear and monocyte chemotaxis has been normal. The abscesses are filled with numerous polymorphonuclear cells, and the walls of lung cysts as well as the tissues are heavily infiltrated with eosinophils.

**Complications:** Superinfected persistent lung cysts are the most common complications, with eventual loss of lobes or of entire lungs if appropriate antibiotic and surgical treatments are not rendered. The second most common complication is cutaneous and other fungal infection. High dose multiple antibiotic therapy is required on a continuing basis. Aspergilloma formation in infected persistent pneumatoceles can lead to fatal hemoptysis. Cryptococcal meningitis and lymphomas have also been reported.

**Associated Findings:** Osteopenia is present in most patients, with no obvious defect of calcium or phosphorus metabolism, and is seemingly unrelated to the state of activity of the patient. Fractures of bones of the extremities or of the vertebral bodies are common. Coarse facial features are present in a majority, although the basis of this is undetermined. Craniosynostosis has also been reported (Hoger et al, 1985)

**Etiology:** Familial patterns have suggested autosomal dominant inheritance with incomplete penetrance. Autosomal recessive inheritance of the Job syndrome "variant" has been reported.

**Pathogenesis:** Disordered IgE regulation and defects in specific immunologic responsiveness are prominent abnormalities; neither is likely to be the primary biologic error.

**MIM No.:** 14706, *24370

**Sex Ratio:** M2:F1 is suggested by available data.

**Occurrence:** Undetermined. 23 cases were seen at one major United States referral center over a 15 year period.

**Risk of Recurrence for Patient's Sib:**
See Part I, *Mendelian Inheritance.*

**Risk of Recurrence for Patient's Child:**
See Part I, *Mendelian Inheritance.*

**Age of Detectability:** In early infancy.

**Gene Mapping and Linkage:** Unknown.

**Prevention:** None known. Genetic counseling indicated. Staphylococcal infections can be prevented by continuous prophylaxis with oral antistaphylococcal penicillins or cephalosporins, which should be initiated at time of diagnosis of the hyper-IgE syndrome.

**Treatment:** In addition to chronic antistaphylococcal antibiotic prophylaxis or therapy, thoracic surgery for persistent pneumatoceles is of utmost importance. Judicious use of other antibiotics or antifungals is indicated for superinfections. Incision and drainage of abscesses is frequently required if antistaphylococcal prophylaxis has not been employed.

**Prognosis:** If staphylococcal infections are prevented by prophylaxis with antistaphylococcal drugs from an early age, the prognosis is excellent. Many patients reach adulthood. If staphylococcal lung infections lead to persistent pneumatoceles, which become superinfected, death from extensive lung disease can occur at an early age. Extensive fungal superinfection also connotes a poor prognosis.

**Detection of Carrier:** Unknown.

**Special Considerations:** Some authors equate this condition with *Job Syndrome* (after "Satan...smote Job with sore boils from the sole of his foot unto his crown. Job 2:7). However, the latter condition was described in 1966 (a year before IgE was discovered) as one in which two red-haired, fair-skinned, nonallergic females with hyperextensible joints had "cold" abscesses. Few patients in the extensive series of hyper-IgE syndrome patients evaluated since 1966 have had red hair or hyperextensible joints. The limited published immunologic data on the two original "Job" patients (who reportedly were found several years later to have elevated serum IgE), and two others, makes it impossible to know whether there is any overlap between the Job and hyper-IgE syndromes. Chemotactic defects were suggested by a few investigators as a prominent feature of the hyper-IgE syndrome. However, numerous subsequent studies have shown this to be a rare and inconsistent defect, ruling out a primary role for chemotactic abnormalities in these patients' infection-susceptibility. Finally, a report from one laboratory stated that such patients have a deficiency in CD8+ T cells (T8+ or suppressor/cytotoxic subset). However, this has not be confirmed.

**References:**

Buckley RH, et al.: Extreme hyperimmunoglobulinemia E and undue susceptibility to infection. Pediatrics 1972; 49:59–70.
Merten DF, et al.: The hyperimmunoglobulinemia E syndrome: radiographic observations. Radiology 1979; 132:71–78.
Buckley RH, Sampson HA: The hyperimmunoglobulinemia E syndrome. In: Clinical immunology update. New York: Elsevier North-Holland, 1981.
Donabedian H, Gallin JI: The hyperimmunoglobulin E recurrent-infection (Job's) syndrome: a review of the NIH experience and the literature. Medicine 1983; 62:195–208.
Buckley RH: The hyper IgE Syndrome. In: Current therapy in allergy and immunology. Philadelphia: B.C. Decker (Mosby), 1984.
Hoger PH, et al.: Craniosynostosis in hyper-IgE-syndrome. Europ J Pediatr 1985; 144:414–417.

BU042                                    **Rebecca H. Buckley**

---

## IMMUNODEFICIENCY, IGG SUBCLASS DEFICIENCIES    2947

**Includes:**
Antibody deficiencies, partial
IgG heavy chain locus
Immunoglobulin Gm-1
Immunoglobulin Gm-2
Immunoglobulin Gm-3
Immunoglobulin Gm-4

**Excludes:**
**Immunodeficiency, agammaglobulinemia, X-linked, infantile** (0027)
**Immunodeficiency, combined variable hypogammaglobulinemia** (3105)
**Immunodeficiency, common variable type** (0521)
Immunodeficiency with increased IgM
**Immunoglobulin A deficiency** (0525)
Selective IgA deficiency
Selective IgM deficiency
**Serum allotypes, human** (0476)
Transient hypogammaglobulinemia of infancy

**Major Diagnostic Criteria:** Serum levels of one, two, or three IgG subclasses <2 SD below the mean for age. Clinical use of the designation is usually reserved for the finding of an inability to make expected antibody responses in a patient who is experiencing recurrent or chronic respiratory infections.

**Clinical Findings:** Clinical symptoms may begin at any age, although onset in infancy or early childhood is common. Patients reported to date have had symptoms localized to the respiratory tract. They most often experience recurrent pneumonia, sinusitis, and otitis media. Recurrent bronchitis and purulent rhinitis have also been reported in these patients. It is likely that IgG subclass deficiency can result in chronic respiratory tract symptoms as well.

Clinical variability is common. It is not clear why some patients with a given IgG subclass or antibody level experience severe symptoms while others with equivalent levels have mild symptoms. It has been suggested that in some patients there may be compensation through other host defense mechanisms.

In many children, IgG subclass deficiency may represent a maturational lag in development of immune function which will disappear with time. In other children and in adults, it may be a permanent, stable deficiency or it may be the precursor to the development of common variable immunodeficiency.

By definition, serum levels of one, two, or three IgG subclasses are <2 SD below mean for age. Patients with deficiency of IgG1 may have difficulty making antibody responses to protein antigens, while those with deficiency of IgG2 may have difficulty with certain polysaccharide antigens. Deficiencies of IgG2 and IgG4 often occur together. IgG2 and IgG2-IgG4 deficiencies have been associated with an IgA deficiency and may explain clinical symptoms in some patients previously thought to have only selective IgA deficiency. Total serum IgG is low usually only if IgG1 is low. A low IgG subclass level is usually associated with an abnormal antibody response in that or another IgG subclass. The latter finding and the documentation of other immune abnormalities in IgG subclass-deficient patients suggest that the low IgG subclass level is a marker of a more global immune abnormality. It should be noted that healthy individuals with a complete absence of one or more IgG subclasses have been reported.

**Complications:** Chronic otitis media, with hearing loss; chronic sinusitis; chronic bronchitis; reactive airway disease. Bronchiectasis occurs commonly in those patients who experience recurrent or chronic lower respiratory tract infections.

**Associated Findings:** Possibly defects in other arms of immunity.

**Etiology:** Possibly autosomal dominant inheritance.

**Pathogenesis:** Possibly related to inability to make certain V-D-J gene segment rearrangements or to make appropriate class switches to a particular C gene, limiting the antibody repertoire. This might occur because of gene deletion or for other as yet undefined reasons.

**MIM No.:** *14710, *14711, *14712, *14713

**Sex Ratio:** Presumably M1:F1.

**Occurrence:** Undetermined, but studies to date suggest that these may be the most common immunodeficiencies.

**Risk of Recurrence for Patient's Sib:** Unknown. Multiple affected sibs within a family have been reported.

**Risk of Recurrence for Patient's Child:** Unknown.

**Age of Detectability:** After clearance of the majority of maternal transplacentally acquired IgG, i.e., after ages 6–9 months.

**Gene Mapping and Linkage:** IGHG1 (immunoglobulin gamma 1 (Gm marker)) has been mapped to 14q32.33.

IGHG2 (immunoglobulin gamma 2 (Gm marker)) has been mapped to 14q32.33.

IGHG3 (immunoglobulin gamma 3 (Gm marker)) has been mapped to 14q32.33.

IGHG4 (immunoglobulin gamma 4 (Gm marker)) has been mapped to 14q32.33.

**Prevention:** None known. Genetic counseling indicated.

**Treatment:** Some patients may require only antibiotic therapy for acute infections; others, in addition, may benefit from prophylactic antibiotic coverage. Intramuscular gamma globulin has been administered to some patients with benefit, although incomplete resolution of symptoms may be seen because of limitations in dosage. Intravenous gamma globulin has appeared to be useful in eliminating symptoms. Although the optimum dosage has not been determined, it is likely that 300 mg/kg or more must be given about every three weeks. Regression of bronchiectasis has been seen after prolonged therapy with intravenous gamma globulin in high dosage.

**Prognosis:** Normal life span unless significant pulmonary compromise occurs because of recurrent or chronic lower respiratory tract infections.

**Detection of Carrier:** Unknown.

**Special Considerations:** The designation *IgG subclass deficiency* has inherent difficulties. Two and one-half percent of normal people will have a level of any given IgG subclass <2 SD below the mean for age. Also, the serum level of an IgG subclass is a poor predictor of IgG class antibody responses, especially in children. Thus, finding a low level of a subclass in a symptomatic patient does not necessarily indicate that this is the cause of the symptoms. Abnormal subclass-specific antibody responses have been demonstrated in patients who have normal serum levels of IgG subclasses yet experience symptoms identical to those with IgG subclass deficiencies.

It may be that finding a low level of an IgG subclass in an appropriate patient suggests the possibility of an immunodeficiency that may be limited to specific antibody responses or that may include other immune abnormalities. It is clear that finding normal levels of IgG or IgG subclasses does not rule out this possibility. On the other hand, finding a complete absence of one or more IgG subclasses may reflect a gene deletion that has no clinical significance.

In any event, diagnosis of immunodeficiency should rest on demonstration of lack of immune function. For IgG subclass deficiency, this currently should include lack of appropriate antibody responses. Thus, *partial antibody deficiency* may be a preferable term to describe this syndrome.

**References:**

Schur PH, et al.: Selective gamma-G globulin deficiencies in patients with recurrent pyogenic infections. New Engl J Med 1970; 283:631–634.

Oxelius V-A: Immunoglobulin G (IgG) subclasses and human disease. Am J Med (Suppl) 1984; 76:7–18.

Bjorkander J, et al.: Impaired lung function in patients with IgA deficiency and low levels of IgG2 or IgG3. New Engl J Med 1985; 313:7620–724.

Hanson LA, Oxelius V-A, eds: Proceedings of the First International Symposium on IgG Subclasses. Monogr Allergy, 1986; 20.

Smith TF: Immunodeficiency in chronic pediatric respiratory illness. Hosp Pract 1986; 21:143–158.

Heiner DC: Recognition and management of IgG subclass deficiencies. Pediatr Infect Dis J 1987; 6:235–238.

SM021                                          **Thomas F. Smith**

---

## IMMUNODEFICIENCY, MYELOPEROXIDASE DEFICIENCY TYPE                    2214

**Includes:** Myeloperoxidase deficiency

**Excludes:** **Granulomatous disease, chronic x-linked** (0443)

**Major Diagnostic Criteria:** The partial or total absence of myeloperoxidase from the azurophilic granules of neutrophils and monocytes. These phagocytes appear normal when stained with Wright's stain, but with a peroxidase stain, the normally strongly positive granules are either markedly decreased or totally absent. Eosinophils and basophils appear normal with Wright's stain and have normal amounts of peroxidase.

**Clinical Findings:** The disorder is usually discovered serendipitously by the new automated differential counters, which rely on peroxidase positivity to identify neutrophils. The patients are identified as being profoundly neutropenic by automated count, but they have normal numbers of neutrophils on standard Wright's stain. Those with either partial or complete myeloperoxidase deficiency generally have a very benign course, rarely displaying any increased susceptibility to infection. A few people with complete myeloperoxidase deficiency have exhibited increased susceptibility to candidal infections, but they have usually had an additional factor, such as diabetes mellitus, impairing their anticandidal defenses.

**Complications:** Unknown.

**Associated Findings:** None known.

**Etiology:** Originally thought to be straightforward autosomal recessive inheritance, but the recent identification of individuals with varying degrees of myeloperoxidase deficiency suggests that this is a recessive trait with variable expressivity.

**Pathogenesis:** Neutrophils of affected individuals have normal chemotaxis, normal phagocytosis, a normal respiratory burst, and normal degranulation, but bacterial killing is slower than normal, and candidal killing is markedly impaired. The degree of impairment is directly proportional to the quantitative deficiency of myeloperoxidase in the affected individual's neutrophils. Myeloperoxidase catalyzes the production of the hypochlorous ion, which is an important microbicidal agent.

The normal series of events following the engulfment of a pathogen begins with the occurrence of a respiratory burst, which results in the generation of superoxide by the following reaction: $NADPH + 2O_2 \rightarrow 2O_2^- + NADP^+ + H^+$. This superoxide then reacts with the hydronium ion in a reaction catalyzed by superoxide dismutase to form hydrogen peroxide.

$2O_2^- + 2H^+ \rightarrow H_2O_2 + O_2$ This hydrogen peroxide usually then reacts with a halide ion (such as chloride), and in the presence of myeloperoxidase a hypohalous anion (one of the principal microbicidal oxidants of phagocytes) is produced.

$H_2O_2 + Cl^- \rightarrow /myeloperoxidase\ OCl^- + H_2O$

Without myeloperoxidase, hypochlorous acid cannot be generated in significant quantities. Superoxide and hydrogen peroxide are only slightly microbicidal, and thus it is surprising that even individuals with complete myeloperoxidase deficiency have so few infections. Evidently, microbicial oxidants other than $OCl^-$ are generated by the respiratory burst because the bacteria are killed, and the respiratory burst is, if anything, prolonged in these individuals. The killing of phagocytized *Candida* is negligible (6%

of normal) in totally deficient individuals and moderately impaired in partially deficient individuals.

The low incidence of invasive candidal infections in these people reflects the presence of independent, probably cell-mediated mechanisms for destroying this pathogen.

**MIM No.:** *25460

**Sex Ratio:** M1:F1

**Occurrence:** Partial deficiency, 1:2,000; total deficiency, 1:4,000.

**Risk of Recurrence for Patient's Sib:**
See Part I, *Mendelian Inheritance*. Approximately 25% chance of being either partially or completely deficient.

**Risk of Recurrence for Patient's Child:**
See Part I, *Mendelian Inheritance*. Each child is at risk for being a carrier, but the uncertainty surrounding the mode of inheritance of this disorder makes such an estimation highly speculative.

**Age of Detectability:** From birth.

**Gene Mapping and Linkage:** MPO (myeloperoxidase) has been mapped to 17q21.3-q23.

**Prevention:** None known. Genetic counseling indicated.

**Treatment:** Parenteral antibiotics for serious infections. Early consideration of empiric antifungal therapy in clinically infected, myeloperoxidase-deficient individuals who fail to respond promptly to antibacterials; especially in the presence of **Diabetes mellitus**.

**Prognosis:** Vast majority of afflicted individuals appear to live full, unimpaired lives.

**Detection of Carrier:** Partially affected individuals can be detected by quantitatively assaying neutrophils for myeloperoxidase. The accuracy of such screening is hampered by the variable expressivity of the trait.

**References:**

Cech P, et al.: Hereditary myeloperoxidase deficiency. Blood 1979; 53:403–411.

Parry MF, et al.: Myeloperoxidase deficiency: prevalence and clinical significance. Ann Intern Med 1981; 95:293–301.

Larrocha C, et al.: Hereditary myeloperoxidase deficiency: study of 12 cases. Scand J Haematol 1982; 29:389–397.

Ross DW, Kaplow LS: Myeloperoxidase deficiency: increased sensitivity for immunocytochemical compared to cytochemical detection of enzyme. Arch Path Lab Med 1985; 109:1005–1006.

Murao S-I, et al.: Myeloperoxidase: a myeloid cell nuclear antigen with DNA-binding properties. Proc Nat Acad Sci 1988; 85:1232–1236.

Forehand JR, et al.: Inherited disorders of phagocyte killing. In: Scriver CR, et al, eds: The metabolic basis of inherited disease, 6th ed. New York: McGraw-Hill, 1989:2779–2801.

AX001
B0048

**Richard Axtell**
**Laurence A. Boxer**

## IMMUNODEFICIENCY, NEZELOF TYPE                    2216

**Includes:**
Alymphocytosis, pure
Combined immunodeficiency with immunoglobulins
Nezelof syndrome
Severe combined immunodeficiency, Nezelof type
Severe combined immunodeficiency, variant type
T-lymphocyte deficiency
Thymic aplasia
Thymic dysplasia with normal immunoglobulins

**Excludes:**
**Immunodeficiency, adenosine deaminase deficiency** (2196)
**Immunodeficiency, agammaglobulinemia, X-linked, infantile** (0027)
**Immunodeficiency, thymic agenesis** (0943)
**Immunodeficiency, Wiskott-Aldrich type** (0523)
**Metaphyseal chondrodysplasia, type Mckusick** (0653)

**Major Diagnostic Criteria:** Severe lymphopenia, diminished lymphoid tissue, and abnormal structure of the thymus are major findings in patients with Nezelof syndrome, as well as in patients with other forms of severe combined immunodeficiency syndromes (SCIDS). However, Nezelof syndrome can be differentiated from the other SCID subtypes by normal or increased levels of one or more of the major immunoglobulin classes. Antibody formation can be present, but it is often variable. Furthermore, plasma cells are present in the lymphoid tissue and gastrointestinal tract. In contrast to patients with Swiss-type agammaglobulinemia and other SCIDS such as ADA deficiency, the onset of symptoms can be delayed beyond six months of age, with a gradual course and survival beyond 4 years of age.

**Clinical Findings:** Nezelof syndrome is part of a spectrum of disorders that constitute SCIDS. As with all the clinical subtypes with severe combined immunodeficiency, patients with Nezelof syndrome have recurrent infections and failure to thrive, which often leads to early death. In Nezelof patients the onset of illness usually occurs at about six months of age. It is characterized by failure to thrive, chronic diarrhea, oral candidiasis, recurrent pulmonary infections, and recurrent skin infections. Of the infections, characteristic organisms include measles and varicella, gram-negative bacteria, and opportunistic organisms like *Pneumocystis carinii*. Patients may respond poorly or slowly to antibiotic therapy and other supportive measures. On physical examination, the failure to thrive may be a prominent sign. There is diminished lymphoid tissue such as the tonsils and peripheral lymph nodes, but there may also be hepatosplenomegaly. Aside from pyoderma, some patients may have an eczematoid-type rash.

On the chest X-ray there is usually absence of the thymic shadow. Recurrent or persistent lymphopenia (total lymphocyte count less than 2,000/mm$^3$) is present, and delayed skin hypersensitivity reactions to common antigens such as candida, tetanus, and mumps, are negative.

Serum levels of IgG, IgM, and IgA are normal or elevated. Occasionally there may be a partial deficiency of one of the immunoglobulin isotypes. In addition, patients may have markedly elevated levels of IgD, IgE, or both. Antibody responses are quite variable, but usually deficient. Some patients have preexisting natural antibodies, such as isohemagglutinins, which are naturally occurring antibodies to the ABO blood group antigens. Often patients have deficient antibody formation upon immunization with specific antigens. Autoantibodies have been reported in some patients. In vitro lymphocyte proliferative responses to mitogens are usually reduced or absent. However, lymphocyte proliferative responses in mixed lymphocyte culture in response to allogeneic cells can occur.

Pathologic findings are similar to those of other subtypes of SCIDS. There is diminished lymphoid tissue with abnormal architecture characterized by the absence of follicles and germinal centers. The thymus shows evidence of dysplasia, with predominantly epithelioid cells, rare lymphocytes, and absence of Hassall corpuscles. There is poor architectural demarcation between cortex and medulla. However, in contrast with the other SCID subtypes, plasma cells are present in lymph nodes, bone marrow, and the rectal mucosa.

**Complications:** As with other patients with severe deficiencies of cellular immunity, Nezelof patients are at risk for graft-vs.-host disease following the administration of viable allogeneic leukocytes by blood transfusion or by intrauterine maternal passage of lymphocytes through the placenta. Thus all blood products, including plasma, should be irradiated. Similarly, these patients are at risk for severe infection following immunization with live vaccines such as polio, bacillus Calmette-Guérin (BCG) or vaccinia. Therefore it is recommended that Nezelof patients, like patients with immunodeficiency disease, not receive any of the live viral or bacterial vaccines for immunizations.

**Associated Findings:** None known.

**Etiology:** Both autosomal recessive and X-linked recessive inheritance have been reported. There is a slight preponderance of affected males with Nezelof syndrome. In reviewing 34 cases of Nezelof syndrome, Lawlor et al (1974) found a suggestive or definitive family history either in sibs or a near relative in 55% of families.

**Pathogenesis:** Possibly a defect in lymphoid stem cell development and differentiation. However, the normal levels of immunoglobulins and plasma cells in the tissues suggest that there may have been some preexisting immunity, with attrition of immunologic function. Thus far, a biochemical or molecular abnormality has not been defined.

**MIM No.:** *24270

**Sex Ratio:** M1:F<1

**Occurrence:** About 50 cases have been described in the literature.

**Risk of Recurrence for Patient's Sib:**
See Part I, *Mendelian Inheritance.*

**Risk of Recurrence for Patient's Child:**
See Part I, *Mendelian Inheritance.*

**Age of Detectability:** In infancy.

**Gene Mapping and Linkage:** Unknown.

**Prevention:** None known. Genetic counseling indicated.

**Treatment:** Prompt, symptomatic treatment of infections is indicated. Bone marrow transplantation from a tissue-matched, compatible donor may be required.

**Prognosis:** Poor, unless a compatible donor is available for bone marrow transplantation.

**Detection of Carrier:** Unknown.

**References:**
Breton A, et al.: Lymphocytophisia avec dysgammaglobulinemie chez un nourrisson. Arch Fr Pediatr 1963; 20:131–139.
Nezelof C, et al.: L'hypoplasie héréditaire du thymus: sa place et sa responsabilité dans une observation d'aplasie lymphocytaire, normoplasmocytaire et normoglobulinemique du nourrisson. Arch Fr Pediatr 1964; 21:897–920.
Rothberg RM, ten Bensel RW: Thymic alymphoplasia with immunoglobulin synthesis. Am J Dis Child 1967; 113:639–648.
Nezelof C: Thymic dysplasia with normal immunoglobulins and immunologic deficiency: pure alymphocytosis. In: Good RA, ed: Immunologic deficiency diseases. New York: March of Dimes Birth Defects Foundation, 1968:104–112.
Lawlor GJ, Jr, et al.: The syndrome of cellular immunodeficiency with immunoglobulins. J Pediatr 1974; 84:183–192.
Rezza E, et al.: Familial lymphopenia with T lymphocyte defect. J Pediatr 1974; 84:178–182.

BA057                                                    **Mark Ballow**

---

## IMMUNODEFICIENCY, NUCLEOSIDE-PHOSPHORYLASE DEFICIENCY                                  0729

**Includes:**
Nucleoside-phosphorylase deficiency
Purine-nucleoside: orthophosphate ribosyltransferase

**Excludes: Immunodeficiency, adenosine deaminase deficiency** (2196)

**Major Diagnostic Criteria:** Absent to severely reduced red blood cell, lymphocyte, and fibroblast nucleoside-phosphorylase activity; defective cell-mediated immunity, with normal antibody-mediated immunity; and a history of recurrent infections consistent with immunodeficiency disease.

**Clinical Findings:** Patients may be asymptomatic for periods of several years. Initial manifestations usually include recurrent infection. Fatal varicella infection and progressive vaccinia following smallpox immunization have been reported. A fatal graft-versus-host reaction has been observed. Severe hemolytic anemia has been described in several patients. The oldest identified patient is over age 12 years, and continues to have recurrent infection. Immunologic studies have demonstrated normal B-cell immunity, with absent to severely depressed T-cell immunity. Although enzyme activity is absent at birth, immunologic function

may be normal, and it subsequently declines with age. Measurement of purine nucleosides in the urine and blood reveals increased amounts of inosine, deoxyinosine, guanosine, deoxyguanosine, and decreased amounts of uric acid. Orotic aciduria has been found in some patients. Treatment has included transfer factor, thymus transplantation, thymosin, deoxycytidine, and uridine given orally. In some patients partial reconstitution has been achieved. Infusions of radiated red blood cells as a possible source of enzyme has partially restored immunity in some patients. Patients should not be immunized with attenuated live viral vaccines or receive unirradiated blood products. Autoantibody and autoimmune disease has been described in several patients.

**Complications:** Unknown.

**Associated Findings:** Related to underlying immunodeficiency disease.

**Etiology:** Autosomal recessive inheritance.

**Pathogenesis:** Undetermined. Because a similar disorder, adenosine deaminase deficiency, also is associated with immunodeficiency disease, it is postulated that the purine salvage pathway is involved in some way in immunodeficiency disease. However, the mechanism whereby a deficiency of enzymes in this pathway results in immunodeficiency is unknown. Pyrimidine "starvation" secondary to the accumulation of adenine nucleotides or to elevated levels of cyclic nucleotides or deoxynucleotides might impair lymphocyte function. Alternatively, increased deoxynucleotides may also impair lymphocyte function by inhibiting ribonucleotide reductase. Inhibition of protein methylation may also occur.

**MIM No.:** *16405

**Sex Ratio:** Presumably M1:F1

**Occurrence:** Undetermined. Established literature.

**Risk of Recurrence for Patient's Sib:**
See Part I, *Mendelian Inheritance.*

**Risk of Recurrence for Patient's Child:**
See Part I, *Mendelian Inheritance.* All offspring are obligate carriers, but they are unlikely to manifest the disease as the frequency of the mutant gene appears to be low in the population.

**Age of Detectability:** At birth. Nucleoside-phosphorylase activity may be quantitated in fibroblasts; therefore the diagnosis can be made in utero.

**Gene Mapping and Linkage:** NP (nucleoside phosphorylase) has been mapped to 14q11.2.

**Prevention:** None known. Genetic counseling indicated.

**Treatment:** At present, nucleoside-phosphorylase cannot be replaced in the patient, either directly or by transfusion. Appropriate immunologic reconstitution for the defined immunodeficiency disease may modify or prevent recurrent infections. Bone marrow transplantation from an appropriate donor should correct the enzyme deficiency.

**Prognosis:** Guarded due to possible auto-antibody and autoimmune processes.

**Detection of Carrier:** By analysis of red blood cells for nucleoside-phosphorylase concentration; a carrier has approximately 50% normal concentration.

**References:**
Giblett ER, et al.: Nucleoside-phosphorylase deficiency in a child with severely defective T-cell immunity and normal B-cell immunity. Lancet 1975; I:1010–1013.
Cohen A, et al.: Abnormal purine metabolism and purine overproduction in a patient deficient in purine nucleoside phosphorylase. New Engl J Med 1976; 295:1449–1454.
Hirschhorn R: Defects of purine metabolism in immunodeficiency diseases. Prog Clin Immunol 1977; 3:67.
Ammann AJ: Immunological abnormalities in purine nucleoside phosphorylase deficiencies in enzyme defects and immune dysfunction. Ciba Found Symp 1979; 55.
Cowan MJ, et al.: Immunodeficiency syndromes associated with inherited metabolic disorders. Clin Haematol 1981; 10:139.

Capapella De Luca E, et al.: Prenatal exclusion of purine nucleoside phosphorylase deficiency. Eur J Pediatr 1986; 145:51–53.

Williams SR, et al.: A human purine nucleoside phosphorylase deficiency caused by a single base change. J Biol Chem 1987; 262:2332–2338.

WA022
AM003

**Diane W. Wara**
**Arthur J. Ammann**

## IMMUNODEFICIENCY, PLASMA-ASSOCIATED DEFECT OF PHAGOCYTOSIS    0812

**Includes:**

Complement C5 dysfunction
Leiners disease
Neonatal seborrheic dermatitis
Phagocytosis, plasma-related defect in

**Excludes:**  Complement deficiency, other

**Major Diagnostic Criteria:**  Demonstration in vitro of defective phagocytosis of yeast particles by normal polymorphonuclear leukocytes in the presence of serum or plasma from the patient. Correction of the opsonic defect by the addition of purified human C5 or mouse serum containing C5 ($D_{10}B_2$ old line) which also has C5 ($B_{10}D_2$). Commercial preparations of baker's yeast originally used for this assay have been substantially altered by manufacturers. Currently available preparations are closer to zymosan in cell surface, thereby making their opsonic dependency upon C5 less absolute than previously. The best preparations for the assay are from sources which have been maintained in long-term culture, rather than from retail outlets. Levels of complement components, including C5, are within normal limits.

**Clinical Findings:**  Severe infections recur shortly after birth accompanied by generalized seborrheic dermatitis with a marked inflammatory component, persistent diarrhea (usually associated with bacterial infection) that is resistant to antibiotic and dietary management, and an emaciated appearance.

It is of particular significance that the culture material shows almost exclusively gram-negative bacteria. *Staphylococcus aureus* is the only gram-positive organism seen with any frequency. Patients are likely to be markedly cachectic and show a generalized failure to thrive.

Common laboratory findings include neutrophilia, diffuse hyperglobulinemia, and elevated sedimentation rate. Despite treatment with systemic antibiotics, patients show little change in their clinical state.

**Complications:**  Disability, marked weakness, and death resulting from uncontrolled infection, usually by gram-negative bacteria.

**Associated Findings:**  None known.

**Etiology:**  Possibly autosomal recessive inheritance, although a dominant pattern has been reported in at least one family. In Leiner's (1908) series, twins contracted the disorder at six weeks of age, and both recovered after two months. In another family, two consecutive infants contracted the condition at age six weeks and died after several weeks. Leiner noted that the illness was limited almost exclusively to breast-fed infants.

**Pathogenesis:**  Dysfunction of the 5th component of complement (C5). The ability of patient's serum to enhance phagocytosis of yeast particles can be restored to normal by the addition of highly purified C5.

**MIM No.:**  17110

**Sex Ratio:**  M1:F1

**Occurrence:**  Some 57 cases were reported between 1902 and 1911. One kinship was reported in the 1960s.

**Risk of Recurrence for Patient's Sib:**
See Part I, *Mendelian Inheritance.*

**Risk of Recurrence for Patient's Child:**
See Part I, *Mendelian Inheritance.*

**Age of Detectability:**  At birth, by phagocytosis test.

**Gene Mapping and Linkage:**  Unknown.

**Prevention:**  None known. Genetic counseling indicated.

**Treatment:**  The only effective way to treat this disorder is by the infusion of fresh plasma or blood that contains adequate amounts of C5. Such therapy proved life-saving to two severely afflicted infants. The usual blood bank is not a satisfactory source of active C5; hence the requirement for fresh blood or plasma. Specific antibiotic therapy should be administered.

**Prognosis:**  Based on the experience of Leiner and subsequent families, the mortality rate is approximately 40%. Onset was generally under the age of one month, and duration of the illness varied from several weeks to several months. Fifteen of the original series of 43 infants (1902–1907), and three of the 14 infants in a later series (1907–1911) died. The use of plasma as a source of active C5 may be life-saving, and enable patients to eventually enjoy normal life expectancy. After two years of age, symptoms markedly decreased, hence the importance of early diagnosis and treatment.

**Detection of Carrier:**  The carrier state has been identified by phagocytic assay of yeast particles. However, these values have shown the carrier to be as low as the patient. Hence, the patient and clinically normal members of the family sharing the defect cannot be differentiated.

**Special Considerations:**  Although only a few children have been shown to have this defect, the implications of a humoral deficiency state causing impaired cellular function (such as phagocytosis) are important in understanding normal inflammation.

**References:**

Leiner C: Über erythrodermia desquamativa, eine eigenartige universelle Dermatose der Brustkinder. Arch Dermatol Syph 1908; 89:163–190.

Miller ME, et al.: A familial, plasma-associated defect of phagocytosis: a new cause of recurrent bacterial infections. Lancet 1968; II:60–63. *

Miller ME, Nilsson UR: A familial deficiency of the phagocytosis-enhancing activity of serum related to a dysfunction of the fifth component of complement (C5). New Engl J Med 1970; 282:354–358. *

Miller ME, Nilson UR: A major role of the fifth component of complement (C5) in the opsonization of yeast particles: partial dichotomy of function and immunochemical measurement. Clin Immunol and Immunopath 1974; 2:246–255.

Nilsson UR, et al.: A functional abnormality of the fifth component of complement (C5) from human serum of individuals with a familial opsonic defect. J Immunol 1974; 112:1164.

Miller ME, Ganges RG: Serum complement-like opsonic activities in human, animal, vegetable, and proprietary milks. Science 1977; 196:1115.

MI014

**Michael E. Miller**

## IMMUNODEFICIENCY, RETICULOENDOTHELIOSIS WITH EOSINOPHILIA    2688

**Includes:**

Cancer, reticulosis, familial histiocytic, Omenn type
Hemophagocytic reticulosis
Histiocytosis, proliferative
Immunodeficiency, severe combined, Omenn type
Omenn syndrome
Reticulosis, familial histiocytic

**Excludes:**

Graft-versus-host reaction
Histiocytic storage disorders
Histiocytosis, familial lipochromic
**Immunodeficiency, nucleoside-phosphorylase deficiency** (0729)
**Immunodeficiency, severe combined** (0522)
**Immunodeficiency, Wiskott-Aldrich type** (0523)
Langerhans cell histiocytosis
**Letterer-Siwe disease** (2181)
**Lymphohistiocytosis, familial erythrophagocytic** (2946)

**Metaphyseal chondrodysplasia with thymolymphopenia** (0655)
Viral-associated hemophagocytic syndromes

**Major Diagnostic Criteria:** Seborrhea-like dermatitis, desquamative erythroderma, eosinophilia, histiocytic lymphadenopathy, and hepatosplenomegaly arising in the early weeks of life and becoming fatal, without immunoreconstitution, within 4–6 months. Exclusion of infections and other histiocytic disorders. Affected sibs and parental consanguinity are commonly noted.

**Clinical Findings:** The first symptoms may appear within four weeks of birth and are predominantly cutaneous. Dry, reddened skin may have been present from birth, in retrospect, and progressive erythroderma and desquamation occur. Diarrhea, recurrent fevers, failure to thrive, lymphadenopathy, and progressive hepatosplenomegaly follow. Infections and inanition lead to a fatal outcome within 4–6 months if untreated and within 15 months even with aggressive therapy with cytotoxic agents, corticosteroids, and hyperalimentation. Use of matched allogeneic bone marrow transplantation has been reported from Texas Children's Hospital to normalize T-cell subsets, mitogen response, antigen response, and IgE, with freedom from serious infections for two years.

The distinctive hematologic abnormalities are eosinophilia, which may be quite marked, and combined immunodeficiency, with primary involvement of T-lymphocyte subsets. Immature T-cells appear in the peripheral blood, there is functional T-cell suppression of immunoglobulin production and reduction of B-cell populations, 5′-nucleotidase may be markedly deficient, and the T4:T8 ratio is decreased due to a decrease in T4 and an increase in T8. Cutaneous and lymph node biopsies show proliferative infiltration with histiocytes, immature T-cells, and eosinophils. Histologic examination of thymus at postmortem reveals severe atrophy with no Hassall corpuscles. Anemia is common. The clinical features and terminal lymphocyte depletion are suggestive of graft-versus-host disease, possibly intrauterine, in an immunocompromised patient; however, no evidence of cellular chimerism has been detected. Hyperlipidemia and hypofibrinogenemia may be found.

**Complications:** Life-threatening infections; chronic measles infection from vaccination with measles live virus vaccine; and terminal lymphoma, possibly related to treatments with transfer factor.

**Associated Findings:** None known.

**Etiology:** Autosomal recessive inheritance.

**Pathogenesis:** It is likely that the severe combined immunodeficiency is the underlying mechanism, but its cause is unknown. The autosomal recessive inheritance may be a clue to a primary enzyme deficiency, analogous to ADA and NP deficiencies, but none has been discovered. The deregulation and deficiency of T-cell suppressor subsets account for most of the immunologic abnormalities (including deficiency of B-cell-related 5′-nucleotidase and infectious complications. However, the eosinophilia and the histiocytic proliferation, hallmarks of the clinical disorder, are unexplained, and the prominent cutaneous involvement is unusual. A French child born in germ-free conditions and maintained in a sterile isolator developed skin involvement at day two and successively developed all expected clinical manifestations except that diarrhea appeared only after bacterial contamination.

**MIM No.:** *26770

**Sex Ratio:** M1:F1

**Occurrence:** One highly inbred Roman Catholic Irish-American kindred has accounted for at least 20 homozygotes, seen in more than a dozen medical centers in as many states. (Surnames were mostly Carroll, McDonald, Daley, Donahue, and Gregg.) However, it is clear that unrelated individual cases and multiple cases in unrelated families have occurred in the United States and other countries. Several authors suggest that the disorder is underdiagnosed, partly due to early death and largely due to nosologic confusion. An estimated 150 cases of familial erythrophagocytic lymphohistiocytosis, which may be different and/or heterogeneous, have been reported since 1952.

**Risk of Recurrence for Patient's Sib:**
See Part I, *Mendelian Inheritance.*

**Risk of Recurrence for Patient's Child:**
See Part I, *Mendelian Inheritance.* Affected individuals are not expected to survive to reproduce.

**Age of Detectability:** Clinically evident within 1–2 months after birth. Immunologic tests may be suggestive at birth or even *in utero.*

**Gene Mapping and Linkage:** Unknown.

**Prevention:** None known. Genetic counseling indicated.

**Treatment:** Appeared hopeless for many years. Now aggressive immunoreconstitution therapy, including bone marrow transplantation, may be effective, with nutritional support. Early diagnosis and treatment may be important to the outcome.

**Prognosis:** Uniformly fatal within six months without treatment; extension to at least 18 months with hyperalimentation and treatment of infections. Possibly curable with allogeneic bone marrow transplantation.

**Detection of Carrier:** Immunologic tests appear promising. Abnormal distribution of T4+ and T8+ cells in obligatory heterozygotes in a large kindred of affected persons suggests a phenotypic lymphocyte marker.

**Special Considerations:** Because of its recurrence risk and prospects for carrier detection and prenatal diagnosis, it is clinically important that this disorder be distinguished from other proliferative histiocytoses.

**Support Groups:** Atlanta; American Cancer Society

**References:**
Omenn GS: Familial reticuloendotheliosis with eosinophilia. New Engl J Med 1965; 273:427–432.
Ladisch S, et al.: Immunologic and clinical effects of repeated blood exchange in familial erythrophagocytic lympho-histiocytosis. Blood 1982; 60:814–821.
Fischer A, et al.: Heterogeneity of immunologic and enzymatic deficiencies in the familial reticuloendotheliosis syndrome. BD:OAS IXX. New York: March of Dimes Birth Defects Foundation, 1983: 317–319.
Karol RA, et al.: Imbalances of subsets of T lymphocytes in an inbred pedigree with Omenn's syndrome. Clin Immunol Immunopathol 1983; 27:412–427.
Gelfand EW, et al.: Absence of lymphocyte ecto-5′-nucleotidase in infants with reticuloendotheliosis and eosinophilia (Omenn's syndrome). Blood 1984; 63:1475–1480.
Hong R, et al.: Omenn disease: termination in lymphoma. Pediatr Pathol 1985; 3:143–154. †
Nemoto K, Ohnishi Y: Familial hemophagocytic reticulosis: clinicopathologic findings, and cytochemical, immunohistochemical and electron microscopic studies. Acta Path Jpn 1987; 37:1811–1812.
Junker AK, et al.: Clinical and immune recovery from Omenn syndrome after bone marrow transplantation. J Pediatr 1989; 114:596–600.

OM000

**Gilbert S. Omenn**

**IMMUNODEFICIENCY, SEVERE COMBINED**   **0522**

**Includes:**
Bare lymphocyte syndrome
Agammaglobulinemia, alymphocytotic type
Agammaglobulinemia, Swiss type
Aleukia, congenital
De Vaal disease
Gitlin syndrome
Hematopoietic hypoplasia, generalized
Immunodeficiency, severe dual system
Nonplasmatic thymic alymphoplasia or alymphocytosis
Reticular dysgenesis
Severe combined immunodeficiency (SCID) with leukopenia

Severe combined immunodeficiency-lack of HLA on lymphocytes

**Excludes:**
**Agammaglobulinemia-thymoma syndrome** (0944)
**Immunodeficiency, adenosine deaminase deficiency** (2196)
**Immunodeficiency, agammaglobulinemia, X-linked, infantile** (0027)
**Immunodeficiency, reticuloendotheliosis with eosinophilia** (2688)
**Immunodeficiency, thymic agenesis** (0943)
**Immunodeficiency, X-linked severe combined** (0524)

**Major Diagnostic Criteria:** In addition to the X-linked type of severe combined immunodeficieny (SCID), there are several autosomal recessive forms of this relatively heterogeneous class of SCID.

In the basic or *Swiss* type, lymphopenia (<1,000 lymphocytes per ml) is usually seen, as well as low numbers of mature T-lymphocytes. Levels of all immunoglobulin classes are low or absent, and no antibody formation is seen upon immunization. T- and B-lymphocyte functions are invariably low. In the *Bare lymphocyte* type, this is combined with a lack of expression of HLA antigens on some cells of hematopoietic origin. In the *Reticular dysgenesis* type, SCID is combined with leukopenia.

Growth and development of infants with severe combined immunodeficiency are generally normal for the first few months of life. Then, length and weight gain cease, and failure to thrive is seen. Intractable diarrhea and chronic or recurrent infections are common.

**Clinical Findings:** Laboratory findings include lymphopenia and low numbers of T-lymphocytes in circulation. The majority of circulating T-lymphocytes are usually not mature cells, but rather early or late thymocytes (often T10 positive). Mature T-lymphocytes in circulation are usually of maternal origin. Although most patients have low numbers of T- and B-lymphocytes, B-lymphocyte levels may be normal or elevated. The T4:T8 (T-helper to T-suppressor) cell ratio is generally normal. The lymphoproliferative response to mitogens or allogenic cells is decreased. Eosinophilia may be present in certain varieties of SCID. Delayed cutaneous anergy is seen.

All immunoglobulin levels are low. No antibody formation is seen following immunization.

The thymus gland, which may be normal in the X-linked form, is very small (≤2 g) and usually does not undergo normal descenaus. The thymus consists primarily of endodermal cells that have not become lymphoid. Hassall corpuscles are absent, as is corticomedullary distinction.

Depletion is seen in follicular and parafollicular areas of lymph nodes. The tonsils, adenoids, and Peyer patches are underdeveloped or absent.

In the *Bare lymphocyte* type, the failure of HLA expression leads to immunodeficiency affecting both cellular and humoral response to antigens. In the *Reticular dysgenesis*, or De Vaal type, the clinical and laboratory pictures are very similar to those of the more common Swiss type, plus the near absence of granulocytes. Bone marrow aspiration shows hypocellularity with very few lymphoid and granulocytic elements; the main cell type present is the erythroblast. Bone marrow promyelocytes are present, but few mature granulocytes are seen. However, normal erythropoietic and thrombopoietic cells, as well as macrophages in normal or elevated frequency, are present.

**Complications:** Infants may suffer from graft versus host disease (GVHD) due to maternal lymphocytes, resulting in the appearance of a morbilliform rash in the first few days of life. HLA-identical bone marrow transplantation (BMT) has been reported to result in donor lymphocytes cytotoxic for the maternal lymphocytes and in cessation of GVHD symptomology.

A similar GVHD may also result from the administration of nonirradiated blood or blood products. To prevent this GVHD, all blood and blood products should be irradiated at 3,000 to 6,000 R before transfusion to destroy any lymphocytes present.

Persistent oral thrush may be present throughout the neonatal period, with accompanying moniliasis of the larynx and skin.

Pneumonia is also commonly present, with tachypnea and hyperinflation of the lungs. The pneumonia is often interstitial, due to *Pneumocystis carinii*. Another common and potentially fatal cause of persistent pneumonia is parainfluenza virus, especially type III. Rous sarcoma virus pneumonia has also been reported in SCID patients.

Other common problems include intractable diarrhea; cutaneous bacterial infections, especially by *Pseudomonas aeruginosa*; and severe viral infections, including varicella, herpes group, vaccinia, measles, papovavirus, and enterovirus. Unusual viral infections, such as adenovirus hepatitis and necrotizing bronchitis, and parainfluenza type III pancreatitis have been reported. Vaccinations with live vaccines, such as bacille Calmette Guérin or polio, are often fatal.

**Associated Findings:** Patients may present with skin eruptions resembling **Letterer-Siwe disease**. Malignant reticuloendotheliosis (see **Lymphohistiocytosis, familial erythrophagocytic**) and noma, a necrotizing gingivostomatitis, have also been reported.

**Etiology:** Autosomal recessive inheritance.

**Pathogenesis:** The defect(s) involved may be in T-lymphocytes, stem cells, or the thymus. Thymic defect(s) may be intrathymic or due to abnormal embryogenesis of the thymic epithelium.

*Bare lymphocyte syndrome* has been interpreted as a pretranslational regulatory defect of expression in two genes (Sullivan et al, 1985).

*Reticular dysgenesis* probably is not in the multipotent hematopoietic stem cell, but in development of the myelomonocytic and lymphoid cells.

**MIM No.:** *20250, *20292, *26750

**CDC No.:** 279.200

**Sex Ratio:** M1:F1

**Occurrence:** About 1:500,000 live births in the general population, and 1:10,000 in first cousin matings.

**Risk of Recurrence for Patient's Sib:**
See Part I, *Mendelian Inheritance.*

**Risk of Recurrence for Patient's Child:**
See Part I, *Mendelian Inheritance.*

**Age of Detectability:** Prenatal diagnosis is possible. This diagnosis is usually performed in the mid-to-late second trimester (18–22 weeks gestation) using a microsample of pure fetal blood obtained at fetoscopy. Diagnostic criteria include lymphocyte count, total T-lymphocytes, T-lymphocyte subsets, and T-lymphocyte function. The latter is measured by response to mitogens such as phytohemagglutinin. Cell-mediated lympholysis with fetal lymphocytes is unreliable. B-lymphocyte levels may be normal or elevated. A source of error in these diagnoses is the presence of maternal lymphocytes, which may increase or normalize test results. Laboratory findings associated with SCID are present at birth, although complications do not generally begin to appear until the third month of life.

**Gene Mapping and Linkage:** Unknown.

**Prevention:** None known. Genetic counseling indicated.

**Treatment:** Successful treatment of SCID has been achieved predominantly with bone marrow transplantation (BMT). When HLA-identical marrow is not available, successful transplants may be performed using parental haploidentical marrow. In a 15-year retrospective study, HLA-matched BMT in SCID patients resulted in 68% disease-free survival, while T-lymphocyte-depleted HLA-mismatched BMT resulted in 57% disease-free survival. Although no preparative immunosuppression is needed in SCID patients prior to BMT, transplants may be impeded by nonimmune resistance. Also, SCID patients are highly susceptible to GVHD following HLA-mismatched BMT.

Other treatments that have been at least partially successful include fetal liver cell transplants, fetal thymus implants, and implants of fetal thymus epithelium. None of these treatments, however, have been as satisfactory as BMT. Treatment with thymic hormones has not proved beneficial.

The severe parainfluenza virus and RSV infections that are a common complication of SCID have been reported to be successfully treated with ribavirin.

**Prognosis:** Before the advent of BMT, prognosis was invariably poor, with death occurring in the first year of life. With BMT, prognosis is quite good.

*Reticular dysgenesis* is invariably fatal if untreated, with the longest survivor living 119 days. BMT is probably the treatment of choice.

**Detection of Carrier:** Unknown.

**Special Considerations:** An additional non-X-linked SCID is seen in **Immunodeficiency, reticuloendotheliosis with eosinophilia,** also known as Omenn syndrome.

**References:**

Buckley RH: Immunodeficiency. J Allergy Clin Immunol 1983; 72:627–641.

Rosen FS, et al.: The primary immunodeficiencies. New Engl J Med 1984; 311:300–310.

Roper M, et al.: Severe congenital leukopenia (reticular dysgenesis). Immunologic and morphologic characterizations of leukocytes. Am J Dis Child 1985; 139:832–835.

Sullivan KE, et al.: Molecular analysis of the bare lymphocyte syndrome. J Clin Invest 1985; 76:75–79.

Fisher A, et al.: Bone-marrow transplantation for immunodeficiencies and osteopetrosis: European survey, 1968–1985. Lancet 1986; II: 1080–1084.

Borzy MS: Prenatal diagnosis of immunodeficiency diseases. Curr Probl Dermatol 1987; 16:185–196.

Durandy A, et al.: Prenatal diagnosis of severe combined immunodeficiency with defective synthesis of HLA molecules. Prenatal Diag 1987; 7:27–34.

HA081
SC039

**Michael T. Halpern**
**Stanley A. Schwartz**

**Immunodeficiency, severe combined, Omenn type**
*See IMMUNODEFICIENCY, RETICULOENDOTHELIOSIS WITH EOSINOPHILIA*
**Immunodeficiency, severe dual system**
*See IMMUNODEFICIENCY, SEVERE COMBINED*

---

## IMMUNODEFICIENCY, THYMIC AGENESIS                    0943

**Includes:**

    DiGeorge anomaly
    DiGeorge syndrome
    Harrington syndrome
    Pharyngeal pouch syndrome
    Third and fourth pharyngeal pouch syndrome
    Thymic aplasia
    Thymic agenesis
    Thymus and parathyroids, congenital absence of the

**Excludes:**

    **Chromosome 10, monosomy 10p** (2457)
    **Immunodeficiency, agammaglobulinemia, X-linked, infantile** (0027)
    **Immunodeficiency, Nezelof type** (2216)
    **Immunodeficiency, severe combined** (0522)
    Reticular dysgenesis

**Major Diagnostic Criteria:** Congenital hypoparathyroidism, dysmorphic facies, absence of thymic shadow on X-ray, evidence of impaired cell-mediated immunity with decreased numbers of T-cells. Lymph nodes showing depletion in deep cortical areas with normal germinal centers.

**Clinical Findings:** Neonatal hypocalcemic tetany; dysmorphic facial features: hypertelorism, downward slant of eyes, shortened philtrum, low-set ears with notched pinnae and micrognathia; cardiac malformations mainly conotruncal and aortic arch anomalies. Shortened trachea with reduced number of cartilage rings has been described. There is an increased susceptibility to infection manifested by chronic rhinitis, recurrent pneumonia, abscesses and septicemia. Oral candidiasis and recurrent nonspecific diarrhea are common. Patients are weak, fail to thrive and prone to sudden death. Less common features include bifid uvula, esophageal atresia, hypothyroidism, urinary tract infections and nephrocalcinosis.

Laboratory findings: Hypocalcemia and hyperphosphatemia are usually present, with decreased levels of parathyroid hormone. However, this may be subclinical and may be detected by EDTA challenge. Hypocalcemia may also resolve with age. Immunologic evaluation reveals depressed cell-mediated immunity, as manifested by the following: failure to develop delayed hypersensitivity, absent or delayed homograft rejection, decreased numbers of lymphocytes, and impaired proliferative responses to mitogens, antigens and allogeneic cells. However, there have been instances when one or more of the above functions have been normal. Functions which are initially normal may later get depressed, and vice-versa. Depressed immunity on rare occasions can spontaneously recover. Lymphopenia may or may not be present. B-cell numbers (immunoglobulin bearing cells) are usually increased. Humoral immunity is intact, with normal levels of immunoglobulins and usually normal antibody response. The quality of antibodies may be poor. Complement components are normal. Lymph nodes show paucity of cells in deep cortical areas and well-developed germinal centers and plasma cells. Chest X-rays may show absence of thymic shadow.

**Complications:** Convulsions, recurrent infections, nephrocalcinosis.

**Associated Findings:** Anomalies of the great vessels of the heart, including **Heart, truncus arteriosus.**

**Etiology:** Thymic agenesis, as part of the DiGeorge anomaly, has multiple etiologies. There have been multiple reports of chromosome abnormalities, espically **Chromosome 10, monosomy 10p** and **Chromosome 22, monosomy 22q,** in association with DiGeorge anomaly. About 15% of patients will have chromosome abnormalities. Teratogenic exposures, especially alcohol (see **Fetal alcohol syndrome**) and retinoic acid (isotretinoin) or other vitamin A derivatives (see **Fetal retinoid syndrome**), have been reported to produce DiGeorge anomaly in humans. DiGeorge anomaly has also been reported in association with **Cerebro-hepato-renal syndrome.** In some families, DiGeorge anomaly appears to be inherited as an autosomal recessive or as an autosomal dominant condition without an obvious chromosome abnormality.

**Pathogenesis:** The absence of thymus and parathyroid glands has been attributed to a failure of embryonic differentiation of structures derived from the 3rd and 4th pharyngeal pouch endoderm and branchial cleft ectoderm.

Abnormal blood supply to the region of the third and fourth pharyngeal arches may play a role in the pathogenesis of DiGeorge anomaly. Experimentally DiGeorge anomaly may be produced in rodents by restriction of zinc intake to the dam during the crucial period of formation of the aortic arches, pharyngeal pouches, thymus and parathyroids. The syndrome also has been produced with all of its concomitants by administering a zinc chelating antibiotic to the mothers of developing rats at the critical time of formation of the aortic arches, pharyngeal pouches, parathyroid analgen and thymus analgen.

A study of the teratogenic effects of Fertilysin, bis(dichloroacetyl)diamine, on hamster embryos was undertaken for a comparison of Fertilysin induced malformations with the DiGeorge anomaly of human patients. In treated hamsters, malformations of the aortic arches were consistently produced. DiGeorge anomaly in humans has also been linked to alcohol; a major basis for zinc deficiency in humans.

DiGeorge anomaly has also been reported in association with retinoic acid (isotretinoin) teratogenicity. Vitamin A derivatives have been known to produce related defects in animals, and recently the teratogenic effect of retinoic acid has been shown experimentally to interfere with neural crest migration into the branchial arches.

**MIM No.:**  18840

**Sex Ratio:**  Presumably M1:F1.

**Occurrence:**  The birth prevalence of DiGeorge anomaly, including complete and partial cases, is estimated to be 1:20,000 births.

Specific risk factors, other then known teratogens such as alcohol or vitamin A derivatives, are undetermined.

**Risk of Recurrence for Patient's Sib:** Estimated at 2–4%.

**Risk of Recurrence for Patient's Child:** Unknown. May be as high as 50%.

**Age of Detectability:** In infancy. Prenatal chromosomal diagnosis for cases due to chromosome abnormality. Fetal echocardiography may detect associated congenital heart defects.

**Gene Mapping and Linkage:** DGCR (DiGeorge syndrome chromosome region) has been mapped to 22q11.21-q11.23.

Other genes important for branchial arch development appear to be located in the regions of chromosome 10p13 and chromosome 17p13.

**Prevention:** Avoidance of alcohol, retinoic acid, and vitamin A derivatives during pregnancy.

**Treatment:** *For hypoparathyroidism*: substitute function with parathyroid hormone, administer calcium, vitamin D. *For absent thymus*: transplant fetal thymus. Fetal thymus transplantation has completely or partially corrected the immunologic abnormality in the majority of the patients where this approach has been used. The recovery of immunological function was rapid in majority of the patients (from few hours to three weeks, to as long as four to five months). In one patient defect of precursor T-cells was found, along with absence of thymic tissue. Transplantation of two fetal thymuses failed to reconstitute the immune function in this patient with the DiGeorge anomaly.

Goldsobel et al (1987) have described an infant girl with DiGeorge anomaly who underwent successful bone marrow transplantation (BMT) at age 28 1/2 weeks. *In-vitro* incubation of this patient's peripheral blood lymphocytes with thymosin alpha-1 showed no increase in the number of T-cells on two occasions. A fetal thymus for transplantation was not available. The patient was given a bone marrow transplantation using a histocompatible brother as donor. The patient has had a good clinical and immunologic response to bone marrow transplant, with evidence of T-cell engraftment, improved B-cell function, and increased levels of serum, thymic hormone, and thymulin.

**Prognosis:** Usually failure to grow and develop normally. Neurologic impairment may result from neonatal seizures. Early death by infection is common. Cardiac anomalies, when severe, are a major cause of death. Survivors may be mentally retarded, especially if associated with an unbalanced chromosome abnormality. Long term survival may be complicated by Graves disease.

**Detection of Carrier:** Chromosome translocation may be detected in cases associated with a chromosome abnormality. Otherwise, undetermined.

**Special Considerations:** The defect of the thymus is often incomplete, and the clinical findings in the DiGeorge anomaly can be very variable. Normal function of thymic-dependent lymphocytes can be present at birth, but can deteriorate progressively. Circulating T-cells, however, are almost always decreased in number. Thymic dependent lymphoid function can rarely recover. The heterogeneity of the syndrome warrants individualization of each case. In the classic DiGeorge anomaly, the success of thymus grafts is unquestionable: six out of seven cases thus treated are living, whereas only 11 of 35 cases not transplanted are alive. Those surviving have been patients with only partial defects, often minimal, of thymus-dependent function. Chromosome analysis should be performed on all patients. Suspected patients should only be transfused with irradiated blood cells to prevent graft versus host disease.

**References:**

DiGeorge AM: Congenital absence of the thymus and its immunologic consequences: concurrence with congenital hypoparathyroidism. BD:OAS IV(1). White Plains: The National Foundation-March of Dimes, 1969:116–123.
Lischner HW: DiGeorge syndrome. J Pediatr 1972; 81:1042 only.
Conley ME, et al.: The Spectrum of DiGeorge syndrome. J Pediatr 1979; 94:883–890.
Pahwa S, et al.: Failure of immunologic reconstitution in a patient with

DiGeorge syndrome after fetal thymus transplantation. Clin Immunol Immunopathol 1979; 14:96–106.
Lammer EJ, Opitz JM: The DiGeorge Anomaly as a developmental field defect. Am J Med Genet 1986; 2(suppl.):113–127.
Goldsober AB, et al.: Bone marrow transplantation in DiGeorge syndrome. J Pediatr 1987; 111:40–44.
Pahwa R, Good RA: Immunologic deficiencies. In: Immunology essentials of surgical practice. Toledo-Rereyra L, ed: Littleton, MA: PSG Publishing, 1987:270.
Gidding SS, et al.: Unmasking of hypoparathyroidism in familial DiGeorge syndrome by challenge with disodium edetate. New Engl J Med 1988; 319:1589–1591.
Greenberg F, et al.: Cytogenetic findings in a prospective series of patients with DiGeorge anomaly. Am J Hum Genet 1988; 43:605–611.

PA046
PA005
GR011

Rajendra N. Pahwa
Savita Pahwa
Frank Greenberg

**Immunodeficiency, thymic agenesis from exposure to D-penicillamine**
See FETAL D-PENICILLAMINE SYNDROME
**Immunodeficiency, total C1q deficiency**
See COMPLEMENT COMPONENT 1, DEFICIENCY OF

---

## IMMUNODEFICIENCY, TUFTSIN DEFICIENCY TYPE 2217

**Includes:** Tuftsin deficiency

**Excludes:** Immunodeficiency (other)

**Major Diagnostic Criteria:** Patients with congenital tuftsin deficiency have repeated severe infections in childhood and repeated less severe infections in adulthood. These recurrent infections respond quite remarkably to injections of γ-globulin which carry sufficient quantity of tuftsin.

**Clinical Findings:** The biologic activity of the phagocytosis-stimulating tetrapeptide (Thr-Lys-Pro-Arg) tuftsin is highly specific. It stimulates the phagocytic activity of the blood polymorphonuclear leukocytes, as well as macrophages. A unique familial deficiency of the tetrapeptide has been detected. In such patients, infections occur with high frequency. These are most pronounced in childhood. Biochemical and symptomatic evidence can readily be obtained in one or more children. At least one parent of either sex shows clinical signs or laboratory evidence of defective phagocytosis. Recurring infections respond only temporarily to antibiotics. These include tonsillitis, pharyngitis, bronchitis, broncheolitis, pneumonitis, extensive skin infections, furunculosis (frequent in adults), extensive seborrheic dermatitis in children, lymph node infections that are purulent and draining, and occasionally septicemia.

Laboratory findings include absent tuftsin stimulation of phagocytosis, peptide extracts from patients are inhibitory to normal tuftsin activity, reduction on nitroblue tetrazolium tests below normal values, IgA, $IgG_{1-4}$ and IgM levels within normal limits, complement component C5 is normal quantitatively and functionally, complement component C3 is sometimes diminished (not unduly), polymorphonuclear leukocyte level not diagnostic (it can be low, normal, or increased), plasma opsonic activity to yeast particles normal, response to γ-globulin injection results in dramatically alleviated infection.

In every case of tuftsin deficiency that has been studied, an inhibitory peptide was readily demonstrable. In one patient, the peptide was isolated. Its structure is Thr-Glu-Pro-Arg, representing a replacement of lysine by glutamic acid residue. This was synthesized and proved to be an antagonist to tuftsin Thr-Lys-Pro-Arg.

**Complications:** The most severe complication in children is pneumococcus and staphylococcus pneumonia, infected eczematous skin, and purulent and draining lymph nodes.

**Associated Findings:** None known.

**Etiology:** Autosomal dominant inheritance.

**Pathogenesis:** A congenital mutation of tuftsin, where the triplets AAA or AAG that code for lysine are mutated to yield GAA or

GAG coding for glutamic acid residue. In the presence of the tuftsin mutant, the rate of phagocytosis remains very low and limits the defensive mechanism, particularly in early childhood.

**MIM No.:** 19115

**Sex Ratio:** Presumably M1:F1.

**Occurrence:** Unknown. Established literature. One New England study identified 20 cases.

**Risk of Recurrence for Patient's Sib:**
See Part I, *Mendelian Inheritance.*

**Risk of Recurrence for Patient's Child:**
See Part I, *Mendelian Inheritance.*

**Age of Detectability:** Early in infancy and childhood. May manifest itself during the first year of life.

**Gene Mapping and Linkage:** Unknown.

**Prevention:** None known. Genetic counseling indicated.

**Treatment:** Antibiotics along with γ-globulin.

**Prognosis:** Normal life span if treated early and survives childhood.

**Detection of Carrier:** Clinical history and laboratory examination show the presence in serum trypsin digest of inhibitory peptides to tuftsin activity. Radioimmunoassay shows false high values for tuftsin in serum. This is because the inhibitory peptides are tuftsin mutants that have a strong avidity for tuftsin receptor, about four times that of tuftsin. These false high values are diagnostic of the disease.

**References:**
Constantopoulos A, et al.: Tuftsin deficiency: a new syndrome with defective phagocytosis. J Pediatr 1972; 80:564–572.
Constantopoulos A, Najjar VA: Tuftsin deficiency syndrome. Acta Paediatr Scand 1973; 62:645–648.
Najjr VA: Tuftsin (Thr-Lsy-Pro-Arg): a natural activator of phagocytic cells with antibacterial and antineoplastic activity. In: Torrence PF, ed: Biological response modifiers. New York: Academic Press, 1985:141–169. *
Bump NJ, et al.: Isolation and subunit composition of tuftsin receptor. Proc Nat Acad Sci 1986; 83:7187–7191.

NA012                                                    **Victor Najjar**

## IMMUNODEFICIENCY, WISKOTT-ALDRICH TYPE          0523

**Includes:**
Aldrich syndrome
Eczema-thrombocytopenia-diarrhea-infection syndrome
Wiskott-Aldrich syndrome

**Excludes:**
**Immunodeficiency, X-linked severe combined** (0524)
**Thrombocytopenia-absent radius** (0941)

**Major Diagnostic Criteria:** Wiskott-Aldrich syndrome (WAS) is characterized by the triad of eczema, megakaryocytic thrombocytopenia, and recurrent infections. Levels of IgA and IgE are elevated, IgM is low to absent, and IgG level is variable.

**Clinical Findings:** Accompanying the abnormal immunoglobulin levels is an increase in the fractional catabolic rate for all immunoglobulin classes and for albumin, which is attributed to reticuloendothelial hyperplasia. All four IgG subclasses are generally within normal limits. Patients exhibit an early lack of response to polysaccharide antigens, resulting in the absence of isohemagglutinins. Paraproteins or monoclonal IgG, as well as restricted heterogeneity of immunoglobulins, may be present.

The ability to form specific antibody to antigen progressively declines, and anamnestic responses become decreased or absent.

T-lymphocyte number and function are usually normal at birth and show a progressive decline with age. Both the mixed lymphocyte reaction (MLR) and mitogen response normally become depressed. Lymphopenia is usually not evident until about age six years. T4 and T8 levels are both low, but the T4:T8 ratio is normal. Monocyte chemotactic defects may be present due to a lympho-

cyte product, which has been shown to render monocytes unresponsive to chemotactic stimuli *in vitro.*

There is a progressive loss of lymphoid elements normally in the thymus and in T-dependent areas of lymph nodes, spleen, and other peripheral lymphoid organs.

Microplatelets and thrombocytopenia are evident from birth. Platelets are approximately one-half the normal size and are rapidly catabolized. Megakaryocytes appear normal, although thrombopoiesis is depressed.

**Complications:** Due to variable thrombocytopenia, bleeding from the circumcision site or bloody diarrhea is often seen in the infant patient. Hemorrhagic syndromes may follow viral infections.

Recurrent infections are seen in the first year of life, often due to encapsulated bacteria, including pneumococcus. Common infections include otitis media, pneumonia, meningitis, and sepsis. As the patient grows older, infections due to *Pneumocystis carinii* and herpes-group viruses become more common. Hematemesis, melena, and chronic diarrhea are often seen.

Infants may have difficulty tolerating standard formulas made with intact protein, potentially resulting in malabsorption syndromes, but often tolerate elemental formulas. Difficulty in tolerating intact protein may persist beyond infancy.

Skin manifestations include thrombopenic purpura, petechiae, pyoderma, chronic viral warts, and intractable eczema.

**Associated Findings:** Increased incidence of malignant reticuloendotheliosis and lymphomas is seen in older patients, especially frequent are malignancies, particularly lymphomas that involve the CNS. Lymphomatoid granulomatosis has also been reported.

**Etiology:** X-linked recessive inheritance.

**Pathogenesis:** Patients appear to lack the 115 kD glycoprotein sialophorin on lymphocyte surface membranes and glycoprotein Ib on platelet surface membranes. This apparent absence may be due to an error in glycosylation, particularly of sialidation. Sialophorin is normally found on all thymocytes, CD4⁺ and CD8⁺ lymphocytes, and on a subpopulation of bone marrow cells and peripheral blood B-lymphocytes. Functional studies have suggested that sialophorin may play a role in activation of T-lymphocytes. Lymphocytes from WAS patients have also been reported to have fewer surface microvilli than did lymphocytes from normal individuals.

**MIM No.:** *30100

**Sex Ratio:** M1:F0

**Occurrence:** 1:250,000 male births.

**Risk of Recurrence for Patient's Sib:**
See Part I, *Mendelian Inheritance.*

**Risk of Recurrence for Patient's Child:**
See Part I, *Mendelian Inheritance.*

**Age of Detectability:** Fetal blood may be assessed for platelet number and size. Direct measurement of sialophorin may be possible. Phenotyping of fetal lymphocytes is not useful, because affected fetuses and infants initially have normal numbers of T- and B-lymphocytes. Recurrent infections and inability to produce antibody to polysaccharide antigens become evident within the first few years of life.

**Gene Mapping and Linkage:** WAS (Wiskott-Aldrich syndrome) has been mapped to Xp11.4-p11.21.

**Prevention:** None known. Genetic counseling indicated.

**Treatment:** The predominant treatment is bone marrow transplantation (BMT) following ablation of the recipient's marrow with busulfan or total body irradiation. In patients with advanced lymphoid depletion, BMT may be preformed without prior ablation. BMT is apparently curative for all symptoms with the exception of thrombocytopenia, which persists after transplantation. Cell-mediated lympholysis may also remain lower than normal following BMT. Treatment with transfer factor has not been proven to be beneficial.

Splenectomy may be useful in treating the thrombocytopenia. Synthetic steroids should not be used for eczema or thrombocytopenia, as they may further inhibit the patient's immune function. Topical corticosteroids may be administered.

**Prognosis:** Without appropriate treatment, survival beyond the teens is rare. The major cause of death is bleeding or infection, but malignancies account for 12% of deaths. With BMT, prognosis is good and even the complicating malignancies may be prevented.

**Detection of Carrier:** Obligate female carriers have an apparent preferential inactivation of the affected X chromosome in certain cell types. Detection is possible through metabolic stress of platelets.

**Special Considerations:** Immunodeficiencies in CBA/N mice are similar to those in WAS patients. Both exhibit X-linked inheritance and inability to produce antibody to polysaccharide antigens.

**References:**

Buckley RH: Immunodeficiency. J Allergy Clin Immunol 1983; 72:627–641.

Rosen FS, et al.: The primary immunodeficiencies. New Engl J Med 1984; 311:300–310. *

Saurat JH, et al.: Cutaneous symptoms in primary immunodeficiency. Curr Probl Dermatol 1985; 13:50–91.

Nahm MH, et al.: Patients with Wiskott-Aldrich syndrome have normal IgG$_2$ levels. J Immunol 1986; 137:3484–3487.

Borzy MS: Prenatal diagnosis of immunodeficiency diseases. Curr Probl Dermatol 1987; 16:185–296.

Mentzer SJ, et al.: Sialophorin, a surface sialoglycoprotein defective in the Wiskott-Aldrich syndrome, is involved in human T lymphocyte proliferation. J Exp Med 1987; 165:1383–1392.

Shapiro RS, et al.: Wiskott-Aldrich syndrome: detection of carrier state by metabolic stress of platelets. Lancet 1987; I:121–123.

HA081
SC039

**Michael T. Halpern**
**Stanley A. Schwartz**

## IMMUNODEFICIENCY, X-LINKED LYMPHOPROLIFERATIVE DISEASE

**2210**

**Includes:**

Duncan disease
Epstein-Barr virus-induced lymphoproliferative disease in males
Immunodeficiency 5
Infectious mononucleosis, susceptibility to
Lymphoproliferative disease, X-linked
Purtilo syndrome

**Excludes:**

**Granulomatous disease, chronic X-linked** (0443)
**Immunodeficiency, agammaglobulinemia, X-linked, infantile** (0027)
**Immunodeficiency, common variable type** (0521)
**Immunodeficiency, severe combined** (0522)
**Immunodeficiency, Wiskott-Aldrich type** (0523)
**Immunodeficiency, X-linked with hyper IgM** (2524)

**Major Diagnostic Criteria:** Following infection with Epstein-Barr virus (EBV), males with the X-linked lymphoproliferative syndrome (XLP) experience fatal infectious mononucleosis (two-thirds), acquire hypogammaglobulinemia (one-fifth), or malignant B-cell lymphoma (one-fifth). Maternally-related males show one or more of the three major phenotypes. The diagnosis is confirmed by demonstrating EBV genome in tissues and a failure to mount antibodies to EBV-specific antigens, especially EB nuclear antigen (EBNA).

**Clinical Findings:** Following infection with EBV, males with XLP most frequently develop life-threatening infectious mononucleosis. Approximately 50% of the males will succumb to infectious mononucleosis by ten years of age. Males surviving the primary EBV infection exhibit acquired hypogammaglobulinemia and/or malignant B-cell lymphoma, generally involving extranodal sites such as the ileocecal region. Young males with the infectious mononucleosis phenotype will show fever, lymphadenomegaly, hepatosplenomegaly, and evidence of liver or bone marrow damage. The peripheral blood shows atypical lymphocytosis,

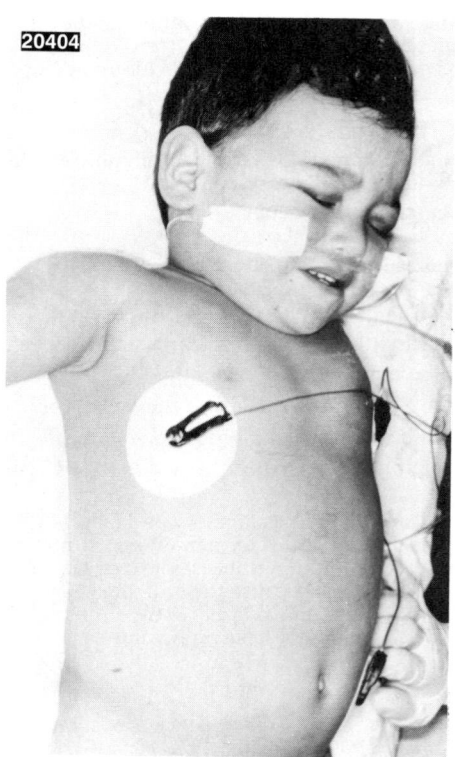

**2210A-20404:** Fulminant infectious mononucleosis in a 20-month old male. A rash, edema, lymphadenopathy, icterus and hepatosplenomegaly are evident.

especially plasmacytoid forms. Elevated transaminase enzymes and a polyclonal increase in immunoglobulin isotypes are found. The affected males fail to mount antibodies to EBV nuclear antigen. Critical to the diagnosis is identification of maternally related males with similar phenotypes.

The phenotypes can change from one type to another with time. This is likely due to defective immunoregulation of B-cell proliferation or alterations in immune function at various times. Invariably, XLP has been fatal by age 40 years.

Phenotypic variability occurs within a patient, among affected male family members, and between unrelated kindreds who are involved by the syndrome. Penetrance is generally complete. Immunologic and virologic examination for the phenotypes of all family members is essential. Thus far, no females have been affected; however, obligate carrier females of the XLP defect have often shown reactivated EBV infection, i.e., elevated antibodies in their sera to early antigen.

**Complications:** Massive liver failure associated with hemorrhage or hepatic coma. Also, suppression of bone marrow resulting in virus-associated hemophagocytic syndrome can lead to opportunistic infections by pyogenic agents. The thrombocytopenia these patients develop can lead to fatal hemorrhage. The patients acquiring hypogammaglobulinemia are also subject to opportunistic pyogenic infectious diseases unless they are given gamma-globulin replacement and prophylactic antibiotic therapy. Patients with malignant lymphoma show complications chiefly associated with the chemo- or radiotherapy given to these patients, i.e., opportunistic infections or hemorrhage due to depression of bone marrow.

**Associated Findings:** Congenital heart or central nervous system defects have occurred in a few affected males.

**Etiology:** X-linked recessive inheritance.

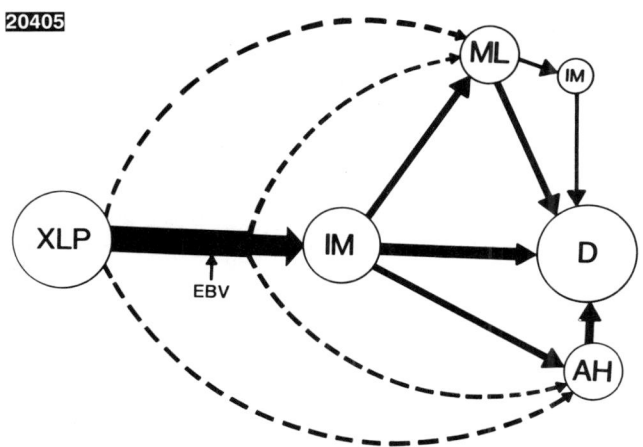

**20405**

**2210B-20405:** Natural history of the X-linked lymphoproliferative syndrome (XLP) after infection by Epstein-Barr virus (EBV), shown chronologically. Size of circles indicates relative number of patients thus far showing the various phenotypes, which include life-threatening or fatal infectious mononucleosis (IM) or malignant B cell lymphoma (ML), and acquired hypogammaglobulinemia (AH). Virtually 100% of the patients with XLP will manifest one of the three major phenotypes and the defect eventually leads to death (D). For example, infectious mononucleosis occurs at a median of 2.7 years; malignant lymphoma at 4.9 years; and acquired hypogammaglobulinemia at 6.9 years. Thickness of arrows indicates relative number of patients who subsequently develop various diseases shown. Broken arrows indicate hypothesized rare events that may occur.

**Pathogenesis:** Current theory postulates an inherited defect in T cells to recognize EBV viral antigens in infected B-cells. T-cells fail to control B-cell proliferation and function following infection by EBV. Tissue damage results from uncontrolled cytoxic cells and cytokines.

**MIM No.:** *30824

**Sex Ratio:** M1:F0. Very rare involvement of females is anticipated due to unequal lyonization of the normal X chromosome.

**Occurrence:** More than 220 patients from 56 kindreds have been registered in the XLP Registry. The affected kindreds have come from the United States, Canada, Great Britain, Scandinavia, France, West Germany, the Middle East, New Zealand and Australia.

**Risk of Recurrence for Patient's Sib:**
See Part I, *Mendelian Inheritance.*

**Risk of Recurrence for Patient's Child:**
See Part I, *Mendelian Inheritance.*

**Age of Detectability:** Usually clinically evident by ten years of age. The affected male is protected by maternally-derived antibodies to EBV for the initial four to six months of life. Defective switching from IgM to IgG antibody production on secondary intravenous challenge with bacteriophage ø0X174 has been detected. Moreover, IgG subclass deficiency prevails in most patients.

**Gene Mapping and Linkage:** LYP (lymphoproliferative syndrome) has been provisionally mapped to Xq25-q26.

**Prevention:** None known. Genetic counseling indicated. Early detection of affected males prior to EBV infection by RFLPs linkage analysis permits prophylactic therapy with gammaglobulin containing antibodies to EBV.

**Treatment:** Testing experimental therapy for the fulminant infectious mononucleosis phenotype is in progress using antiviral agents such as acyclovir and interferon-alpha. High dose intravenous gamma globulin is also recommended. Bone marrow transplantation can potentially reconstitute the immune defect. The individuals with the acquired hypogammaglobulinemia are given replacement immunoglobulin therapy and antibiotics prophylactically. Those developing malignant lymphoma are treated with conventional surgery, radiation therapy and chemotherapy. Care must be taken not to overtreat, as patients with the malignant lymphomas show good prognoses.

**Prognosis:** Fifty percent of the affected males die by age ten, and 100% by the end of the fourth decade. Approximately 15% of the patients in the Registry are surviving. Patients with hypogammaglobulinemia can maintain relatively normal lives with immunoglobulin replacement therapy. Invariably, patients develop fatal infectious mononucleosis or succumb to infections or hemorrhage.

**Detection of Carrier:** Pedigree analysis and elevated antibodies to EBV early antigen have been useful but not conclusive in identifying carriers of XLP. Restriction fragment length polymorphism linkage analyses reveals linkage with the DXS42 probe (LOD score 19.4 in seven families).

**Special Considerations:** The heterogeneity of clinical expression of XLP within an individual and a family must be kept in mind in making the diagnosis. Only a limited number of clinical laboratories are prepared to make the diagnosis.

Physicians are welcome to contact the XLP Registry for consultation in immunodeficiency, EBV detection, and Epstein-Barr virus-induced diseases by calling the University of Nebraska Medical Center, 42nd & Dewey Avenue, Omaha NE 48105, at (402) 559–4244.

**References:**
Purtilo DT, et al.: X-linked recessive progressive combined variable immunodeficiency (Duncan's disease). Lancet 1975; I:935–941.
Grierson H, Purtilo DT: Epstein-Barr virus infections in males with X-linked lymphoproliferative syndrome. Ann Intern Med 1987; 106: 538–545. *
Harrington DS, et al.: Malignant lymphoma in the X-linked lymphoproliferative syndrome. Cancer 1987; 59:1419–1429.
Skare JC, et al.: Mapping the X-linked lymphoproliferative syndrome. Proc Natl Acad Sci USA 1987; 84:2015–2018.
Purtilo DT, et al.: Detection of X-linked lymphoproliferative disease using molecular and immunovirologic markers. Am J Med 1989; 87:421–424.

PU007                                        **David T. Purtilo**

---

**IMMUNODEFICIENCY, X-LINKED SEVERE COMBINED**     **0524**

**Includes:**
    Agammaglobulinemia, X-linked recessive lymphopenic type
    Agammaglobulinemia, X-linked Swiss-type
    Alymphocytosis
    Alymphopenic immunologic deficiency, Gitlin form
    Dysplasia, congenital thymic type
    Hypoplasia, X-linked thymic epithelial type
    Immunodeficiency, X-linked severe dual system
    Immunologic deficiency, X-linked lymphopenic type
    Lymphocytophisis
    Lymphopenic hypogammaglobulinemia, X-linked recessive form
    Lymphopenia, X-linked, primary essential type
    Severe combined immunodeficiency, X-linked (SCIDX)
    Thymic alymphoplasia
    Thymic epithelial hypoplasia

**Excludes:**
    Achondroplasia-agammaglobulinemia
    **Agammaglobulinemia-thymoma syndrome** (0944)
    **Fetal Acquired Immune Deficiency Syndrome (AIDS) infection** (2497)
    **Immunodeficiency, adenosine deaminase deficiency** (2196)

**Immunodeficiency, agammaglobulinemia, X-linked, infantile** (0027)
Immunodeficiency, biotin-deficient type
**Immunodeficiency, severe combined** (0522)
**Immunodeficiency, thymic agenesis** (0943)
**Immunodeficiency, Wiskott-Aldrich type** (0523)
Nucleoside phosphorylase deficiency

**Major Diagnostic Criteria:** Male infant with recurrent severe infections, absent or low isohemagglutinins, absent or low T-cell levels, absent or low immunoglobulins, and positive Schick test following Diphtheria-Pertussis-Tetanus (DPT) immunization. There is no response to skin test antigens and a very low in vitro response to phytohemagglutinin (PHA) stimulation. Lateral X-ray views of oropharynx and retrosternum reveal absence of adenoid and thymic shadows, respectively. B-cell levels are usually elevated. Absence of plasma cells in bone marrow occurs. Without a positive family history of previous male infant deaths, X-linked recessive severe combined immunodeficiency (SCID) may not be distinguishable from autosomal recessive SCID.

**Clinical Findings:** Recurrent severe infections in a male child, including pneumonia, meningitis, otitis, pyoderma, moniliasis, sepsis, or diarrhea. Eczema, undue susceptibility to common viral diseases (e.g., varicella, morbilli), progressive vaccinia following smallpox vaccination, fatal generalized BCG reactions, absence of lymph nodes, small or absent tonsils, poor growth, furuncles, and a family history of male infant deaths.

**Complications:** Pneumonitis invariably occurs in these patients. The most common organisms that prove fatal are *Pseudomonas*, enterobacteria, cytomegalovirus, *Pneumocystis carinii*, and *Morbillivirus*. Deaths from varicella pneumonia have also been reported. Other infectious complications include meningitis, sepsis, chronic otitis media, moniliasis, and furunculosis. Chronic diarrhea and malabsorption secondary to fungal or parasitic infections may contribute to marked failure to thrive. Vaccination with any live virus can lead to uncontrollable reactions. Fatal reactions have also been reported following BCG vaccination. Fatal graft-versus-host reactions following fresh whole blood transfusions are among the most common causes of death in these infants who lack the ability to reject histoincompatible lymphocytes. Graft-versus-host disease (GVHD) occurs 7–25 days after transfusion, beginning with a coarse, maculopapular rash over the entire body, followed by diarrhea, hemolytic anemia, hepatosplenomegaly, progressive hepatitis, fever, pancytopenia, and death. A chronic form of GVHD, marked by scaling erythroderma, histiocytic infiltration in the nodes, and chronic diarrhea, may develop secondary to maternal-fetal transfusion or intrauterine transfusion for erythroblastosis fetalis.

**Associated Findings:** Malabsorption syndrome and lymphoid cancer.

**Etiology:** X-linked recessive inheritance.

**Pathogenesis:** Because both thymic-dependent (delayed hypersensitivity) and thymic-independent (circulating antibodies) systems are involved in this disease, an abnormality of the immunologic stem cell line was originally postulated. More recently, elevated B-cell levels and identification of immature non-E-rosetting T-cells (as identified by monoclonal antibodies against T-cells) suggest that other mechanisms may be responsible for the combined immunodeficiency in most patients. Despite these reservations, bone marrow transplantation totally corrects the immunodeficiency. During the first few months of life, these infants are partially protected by placentally transferred circulating antibodies. In the ensuing months, the immunoglobulin levels fall, as no new antibodies are being synthesized and the number of circulating lymphocytes decreases. With the failure of both immunologic systems, recurrent infections follow. On postmortem examination, both gross and microscopic abnormalities are found in the thymus, lymph nodes, spleen, and GI tract. These consist mainly of marked depletion of all lymphoid elements, especially lymphocytes and plasma cells.

**MIM No.:** *30040

**CDC No.:** 279.200

**Sex Ratio:** M1:F0

**Occurrence:** Less than 1:1,000,000 under one year of age. Seldom seen above two years of age. About 50 cases have been reported in the literature.

**Risk of Recurrence for Patient's Sib:**
See Part I, *Mendelian Inheritance.*

**Risk of Recurrence for Patient's Child:**
See Part I, *Mendelian Inheritance.*

**Age of Detectability:** At birth, by low T-cell levels, elevated B-cell levels, lymph node biopsy, low or absent lymphocyte responses to PHA, inability to reject skin grafts or to form antibody following antigenic stimulation (e.g., typhoid antigen), absent isohemagglutinins, and quantitative low or absent immunoglobulins. A positive family history should increase the index of suspicion.

**Gene Mapping and Linkage:** SCIDX1 (severe combined immunodeficiency, X-linked 1) has been mapped to Xq13-q21.1.

**Prevention:** None known. Genetic counseling indicated.

**Treatment:** Bone marrow transplantation provides an immunologically competent stem cell source from a donor who is histocompatible at the HLA-D/DR locus. If a histocompatible sibling is not available, other approaches can be considered, such as purging the bone marrow of unwanted cells using monoclonal antibodies or using fetal liver as a source of immunologically uncommitted stem cells.

For a number of years, gamma globulin replacement therapy and antibiotics, when necessary, have been used to support these patients. Although this regimen, coupled with good pulmonary hygiene, has probably prolonged the life span of these infants, few have survived beyond the second birthday.

Whenever whole blood transfusion becomes necessary in the treatment of these patients, care must be taken to minimize the number of viable histoincompatible lymphocytes in the transfusate in order to prevent GVHD. This can be accomplished by utilizing buffy-coat-poor blood or frozen red cells after irradiation with 3,000 rads.

**Prognosis:** Poor, if untreated. Good, if reconstituted by bone marrow transplantation from a histocompatible sib. If a "matched" sibling is not available, newer methods of purging the bone marrow of mature lymphoid cells using monoclonal antibodies have led to moderate success in transplanting bone marrow from a parent. The first recipient of a successful bone marrow transplant has required no further treatment and is completely healthy 20 years later.

**Detection of Carrier:** Possible through laboratory procedures (Puck et al, 1987)

**Special Considerations:** Patients with X-linked SCID do not always manifest as severe lymphopenia as do those infants with the autosomal recessive type. Lymphopenia is also occasionally missed when the total lymphocyte count alone is followed. Lymphopenia in these patients refers primarily to decreased numbers of circulating T-cells. B-cell levels are often elevated. The X-linked and autosomal recessive forms may differ on histologic examination of lymphoid tissues, the former group showing generally less severe depletion of lymphoid elements. Occasionally, normal lymphocyte counts are observed in these patients until relatively late in the course of their disease.

**References:**

Gitlin D, Craig JM: The thymus and other lymphoid tissues in congenital agammaglobulinemia. I. Thymic alymphoplasia and lymphocytic hypoplasia and their relation to infection. Pediatrics 1963; 32:517–530.

Gatti RA, et al.: Immunological reconstitution of sex-linked lymphopenic immunological deficiency. Lancet 1968; II:1366–1369.

Yount WJ, et al.: Immunoglobulin classes, IgG subclasses, Gm genetic markers, and Clq following bone marrow transplantation in X-linked combined immunodeficiency. J Pediatr 1974; 84:193–199.

Buckley RH, et al.: Correction of severe combined immunodeficiency by fetal liver cells. New Engl J Med 1976; 294:1076–1081.

Thomas ED: Current status of bone marrow transplantation. Transpl Proc 1985; 17:428–436.

Puck JM, et al.: Carrier detection in X-linked severe combined immunodeficiency based upon patters of X chromosome inactivation. J Clin Invest 1987; 79:1395–1400.

GA020                                         **Richard A. Gatti**

**Immunodeficiency, X-linked severe dual system**
*See IMMUNODEFICIENCY, X-LINKED SEVERE COMBINED*

## IMMUNODEFICIENCY, X-LINKED WITH HYPER IGM    2524

**Includes:**
   Agammaglobulinemia-beta-2 macroglobulinemia
   Antibody deficiency-beta-2 macroglobulinemia
   Dysgammaglobulinemia antibody deficiency syndrome
   Dysgammaglobulinemia, type I
   Dysgammaglobulinemia-deficient 7S and elevated 19S
      gammaglobulins
   Hyper-IgM syndrome
   Immunodeficiency-3

**Excludes:**
   **Ataxia-telangiectasia** (0094)
   Deficiencies of isolated immunoglobulin classes (e.g., IgA)
   **Fetal rubella syndrome** (0384)
   **Immunodeficiency, agammaglobulinemia, X-linked, infantile**
      (0027)
   **Immunodeficiency, common variable type** (0521)
   **Immunodeficiency, X-linked severe combined** (0524)
   Immunodeficiency, secondary or acquired
   **Immunoglobulin A deficiency** (0525)
   Waldenstrom macroglobulinemia

**Major Diagnostic Criteria:** Absent or severely diminished IgG, and IgA but IgM levels in excess of 300 mg/100 ml, plus an increased frequency and severity of bacterial infections, with onset during infancy or very early childhood.

Simple paper electrophoresis of serum to measure total gammaglobulins may appear falsely "normal" due to the large amount of IgM produced; therefore quantitative measurement of individual immunoglobulins (IgG, IgA, IgM) is necessary for diagnosis.

**Clinical Findings:** After age six months, when maternal IgG falls below protective levels, children are noted to have 1) serious persistent or recurrent bacterial infections with unusual frequency, including purulent rhinorrhea, conjunctivitis, otitis media, otitis externa, mastoiditis, sinusitis, facial cellulitis, tonsillitis, stomatitis, gingivitis, lymphadenitis, pneumonia, appendicitis, meningitis and sepsis; and 2) persistent monilial infections of the mouth and skin, and especially the diaper area, may be seen, possibly secondary to broad spectrum antibiotic use.

As early as age three months enlarged tonsils, lymph nodes, liver, and spleen are noted. Associated symptoms and signs may appear: 1) maculopapular rash of the scalp, face, or flexural surfaces; 2) chronic diarrhea/malabsorption; 3) failure to thrive (and possibly secondary developmental delay); 4) oral ulcers; 5) widespread verruca vulgaris; 6) bronchiectasis; 7) barrel chest deformity; 8) digital clubbing; 9) cyclic or persistent neutropenia; and 10) pancytopenia or mild hemolytic anemia possibly secondary to hypersplenism.

Arthritis and nephritis are less commonly reported. *Pneumocystis carinii* has repeatedly been demonstrated on autopsy. Other more commonly cultured organisms include *Haemophilus influenzae*, *Pseudomonas aeruginosa*, *Staphylococcus aureus*, *Streptococcus pneumoniae*, group A β-hemolytic *Streptococcus*, *Escherichia coli*, *Salmonella paratyphi* B, *Neisseria meningitidis*, and *Mycobacterium tuberculosis*.

Biopsied lymphoid tissues histologically demonstrate replacement of normal immunoglobulin-secreting cells with hypertrophied IgM-secreting plasmacytoid cells. Lymph node architecture is variable, ranging from diminished follicular size and number to normal or large follicles. Presence of germinal centers and plasma cells is also variable. Plasmacytoid cells showing specific immunofluorescence with labeled anti-IgM antiserum are described. In cases of malabsorption, small bowel biopsy material shows normal mucosa with lymphocytes, histiocytes, eosinophils, and plasma cells in the lamina propria.

**Complications:** Arthritis, acute nephritis, B-cell lymphoma of the GI tract especially in males presumed to have the X-linked variety.

**Associated Findings:** Bronchiectasis, hemolytic anemia, cyclic neutropenia with gingivitis, monilial infections of mucosal surfaces and skin, verruca vulgaris, malabsorption syndrome.

**Etiology:** X-linked or autosomal recessive inheritance, although in many cases a thorough study of the patient's family has not been reported and no affected relatives are known. Several immunologic defects could be postulated, among these: 1) intrinsic deficiency or absence of certain B-cell subclasses that could differentiate between IgA- and IgG-secreting plasma cells; 2) a block in B-cell differentiation between IgG- and IgA-secreting plasma cells (i.e., failure of the IgM and IgG "switch"); and 3) an additional nonisotype-specific T-cell-mediated suppression of Ig synthesis, in which IgM synthesis is least affected. Such a T-cell abnormality, reported in very few patients, may be inherited in the same way as the B-cell defect or may be a secondary phenomenon due to failure of further B-cell differentiation, causing an imbalance in cellular interactions and thereby leading to increased activity of suppressor T-cells.

**Pathogenesis:** Cellular immune defects are heterogeneous, with the majority of patients demonstrating an isolated intrinsic B-cell defect, whereas increased activity of T-suppressor cells is uncommon and probably represents assay variability. The phenotypic pattern of surface immunoglobulins on B-lymphocytes shows a large proportion expressing IgM and occasionally IgD. The quantity of IgM secreted by plasma cells is greater than normal. Cell mediated immunity appears intact. Blood group type O, although increased in prevalence in these patients, is not universal, nor is the expression of high levels of isohemagglutinins even in type O subjects. There have even been type O patients described with absence of isohemagglutinins.

**MIM No.:** *30823

**Sex Ratio:** M1:<1. Males far outnumber females. X-linked inheritance is believed to be much more common than autosomal recessive inheritance.

**Occurrence:** More than 25 cases have been reported in the literature.

**Risk of Recurrence for Patient's Sib:**
   See Part I, *Mendelian Inheritance.*

**Risk of Recurrence for Patient's Child:**
   See Part I, *Mendelian Inheritance.*

**Age of Detectability:** After six months of age.

**Gene Mapping and Linkage:** HIGM1 (hyper IgM syndrome) has been provisionally mapped to Xq24-q27.

**Prevention:** None known. Genetic counseling indicated.

**Treatment:** Therapeutic replacement with pooled gamma globulin, (single donor) plasma, or disaggregated intravenous gamma globulin; avoidance of exposure to infections; and regular medical follow-up. The use of hyperimmune immunoglobulin preparations (e.g., against tetanus, measles, or *Pseudomonas*) may be of value for patients exposed to these infections.

Vigorous antibiotic treatment at the earliest signs of infection, good pulmonary toilet and alternating courses of daily broad spectrum antibiotics in patients with bronchiectasis, nutritional counseling to meet increased metabolic demands of chronic infection, and treatment of malabsorption when present. Breast-fed infants are better protected than are formula-fed infants, particularly against the microbial flora from the intestinal tract of their own mothers. Attempts at permanent correction of the deficient functions by an allograft of immunocompetent tissues carry all the dangers of graft versus host reactions.

**Prognosis:** Assuming immunoglobulin replacement, appropriate use of antibiotics, and good medical follow-up, most patients survive to lead active, healthy lives; their life span thereafter is directly related to the presence and progression of bronchiectasis.

**Detection of Carrier:** Unknown.

**References:**
Kyong, CU, et al.: X-linked immunodeficiency with increased IgM: clinical, ethnic, and immunologic heterogeneity. Pediatr Res 1978; 12:1024–1026.
Brahmi Z, et al.: Immunologic studies of three family members with the immunodeficiency with hyper-IgM syndrome. J. Clin Immunol 1983; 3:127–134.
Levitt D, et al.: Hyper IgM immunodeficiency J Clin Invest 1983; 72:1650–1657.
Pascual-Salcedo D, et al.: Cellular basis of hyper IgM immunodeficiency. J Clin Lab Immunol 1983; 10:29–34.

GA024                                                    **Ellen Garibaldi**

**Immunodeficiency-3**
  See *IMMUNODEFICIENCY, X-LINKED WITH HYPER IgM*
**Immunodeficiency-centromeric instability-facial anomalies (ICF)**
  See *IMMUNODEFICIENCY WITH CENTROMERIC INSTABILITY*
**Immunodeficiency-microcephaly-malignancy**
  See *CHROMOSOME INSTABILITY, NIJMEGEN TYPE*
**Immunodeficiency-microencephaly-retardation-skeletal defects**
  See *MICROCEPHALY-RETARDATION-SKELETAL AND IMMUNE DEFECTS*
**Immunodeficiency-thymoma syndrome**
  See *AGAMMAGLOBULINEMIA-THYMOMA SYNDROME*

---

## IMMUNOGLOBULIN A DEFICIENCY                         0525

**Includes:**
  Dysgammaglobulinemia type IV
  Gamma-A-globulin, selective deficiency of
  IgA-Mangel
  Isolated IgA deficiency

**Excludes:**
  **Ataxia-telangiectasia** (0094)
  **Immunodeficiency, severe combined** (0522)
  **Immunodeficiency, X-linked severe combined** (0524)

**Major Diagnostic Criteria:** IgA in serum more than 3 SD below mean for age. IgA in secretions usually also is low; a few cases with IgA present in secretion.

**Clinical Findings:** None specific except those of associated defects when these are present. Other laboratory findings: 10% may have anti-IgA antibodies; not all of these can be explained as due to prior plasma or gammaglobulin therapy. Increased IgG, IgM, or more rarely, IgE is found. $IgG_2$ subclass deficiency may be present in 18% of IgA deficient subjects (see **Immunodeficiency, IgG subclass deficiencies**). These individuals may have more frequent sinopulmonary infections and are candidates for IM or IV gammaglobulin treatment if anti-IgA antibodies are lacking. High levels of antimilk antibodies (hemagglutinating and/or precipitating) are found in 50% and antibovidae antibodies in 40%. Circulating antigen-antibody complexes are found in the sera of 60% and dietary bovine milk antigens are involved in complex formation. Secretory component levels are normal; a rare lack of secretory component has been described, which results in a lack of IgA in secretions. A possible defect in interferon production by lymphocytes after mitogen stimulation has been identified in some patients with selective IgA deficiency. HLA-B8, -DR3, and a particular complotype are found in increased frequency in IgA deficiency.

**Complications:** Increased susceptibility to respiratory infections, atopic diseases, and GI disease (giardiasis).

**Associated Findings:** A number of associated defects are present, but whether they are commonly associated epiphenomena or derivative consequences is unknown. The following have been described: **Arthritis, rheumatoid, Lupus erythematosis, systemic**, thyroiditis, pernicious anemia, sprue syndrome, sarcoidosis, hepatic cirrhosis, "lupoid" hepatitis, dermatomyositis, pulmonary hemosiderosis, idiopathic Addison disease, **Sjogren syndrome**, Coombs positive hemolytic anemia, chronic granulomatous disease, scleroderma, regional enteritis, ulcerative colitis,

vitiligo, recurrent parotitis, idiopathic thrombocytopenic purpura, mental retardation, epilepsy (before treatment). Cancers of epithelial origin (gastric or pulmonary) may have an increased incidence. Three instances of IgA deficiency and angio-immunoblastic lymphadenopathy have been reported. A large family with IgA deficiency and correlated early onset chronic obstructive pulmonary disease has been reported. Partial IgA deficiency and circulating immune complexes were found in association with a severe and often fatal respiratory infection in 21/34 infants age four to 24 months.

**Etiology:** Occurs constantly as a part of congenital agammaglobulinemia syndromes, or unassociated with other immunologic defects. A familial autosomal form has been described. No definite chromosome abnormality has been identified. Since at least some IgA-bearing lymphocytes are present in most if not all cases, this may reflect the presence of an abnormality or suppression of cellular differentiation leading to an inability to secrete IgA, rather than a lack of a gene controlling the constant region of the α chain. This is compatible with the finding that the deficiency has been found to include both $IgA_1$ and $IgA_2$ subclasses in studied cases. An immature IgA B-cell (expressing surface IgM, IgD, and IgA) is present in peripheral blood, suggesting that IgA B-cell maturation is arrested at an early stage of differentiation.

Drug-induced IgA deficiency was reported in phenytoin (Dilantin) treated patients with epilepsy, and in a penicillamine treated patient with Wilson disease. The number of IgA-bearing B-lymphocytes was normal in both.

**Pathogenesis:** Perhaps related to local antibody deficiency, but many people with isolated IgA deficiency seem perfectly normal. Relation to associated diseases is unclear. Hammarstrom et al (1985) reported transferring IgA deficiency from an HLA-matched sib. doner in the course of successful treatment of aplastic anemia by bone marrow transplantation from this doner.

**MIM No.:** 13710

**Sex Ratio:** M1:F2

**Occurrence:** From 1–3:1000 in the normal population; higher in those with collagen diseases, and possibly higher in patients with some cancers.

**Risk of Recurrence for Patient's Sib:** Unknown.

**Risk of Recurrence for Patient's Child:** Unknown.

**Age of Detectability:** At year of age by immunoquantitation.

**Gene Mapping and Linkage:** Unknown.

**Prevention:** None known. Genetic counseling indicated.

**Treatment:** Supportive measures for chronic sinopulmonary infections; avoidance of gluten in **Gluten-sensitive enteropathy**, or lactose in those with lactose intolerance as indicated. Fresh plasma infusions in sprue syndrome and those with chronic respiratory infection may be of benefit, but severe anaphylactic transfusion reactions have occurred in patients lacking IgA and having anti-IgA. If blood transfusions are required, washed and packed cells are indicated.

**Prognosis:** That of the associated disease; in many cases compatible with normal longevity.

**Detection of Carrier:** Unknown.

**References:**
Vjas G, Fudenberg HH: Am(1)₁ the first genetic marker of human immunoglobulin A. Proc Natl Acad Sci USA 1969; 64:1211–1216.
Ammann AJ, Hong R: Selective IgA deficiency: presentation of 30 cases and a review of the literature. Medicine 1971; 50:223–236.
Van Loghem E: Familial occurrence of isolated IgA deficiency associated with antibodies to IgA: evidence against a structural gene defect. Eur J Immunol 1974; 4:57–60.
Koistinen J: Selective IgA deficiency in blood donors. Vox Sang 1975; 29:192–202.
Seager J, et al.: IgA deficiency, epilepsy, and phenytoin treatment. Lancet 1975; II:632–636.
Hjalmarson O, et al.: IgA deficiency during D-penicillamine treatment. Br Med J 1977;1:549.
Cunningham-Rundles C, et al.: Bovine antigens and the formation of circulating immune complexes in selective IgA deficiency. J Clin Invest 1979; 64:272–279.

Cunningham-Rundles C, et al.: Selective IgA and neoplasia. Vox Sang 1980; 38:61–67.

Conley ME, Cooper MD: Immature IgA B cells in IgA deficient patients. New Engl J Med 1981; 305:495–497.

Oxelius VA, et al.: IgG₂ subclass deficiency in selective IgA deficiency. New Engl J Med 1981; 304:1476–1477.

Hammarstrom L, Smith CIE: HLA-A, B, C and DR antigens in immunoglobulin A deficiency. Tissue Antigens 1983; 21:75–79.

Hammarstrom L, et al.: Transfer of IgA deficiency to a bone-marrow-grafted patient with aplastic anaemia. Lancet 1985; II:778–781.

G0023
CU006

**Robert A. Good**
**Charlotte Cunningham-Rundles**

**Immunoglobulin Am2**
*See SERUM ALLOTYPES, HUMAN*
**Immunoglobulin deficiencies**
*See IMMUNODEFICIENCY, COMMON VARIABLE TYPE*
**Immunoglobulin deficiency-centromere instability**
*See IMMUNODEFICIENCY WITH CENTROMERIC INSTABILITY*
**Immunoglobulin Gm-1**
*See IMMUNODEFICIENCY, IgG SUBCLASS DEFICIENCIES*
*also SERUM ALLOTYPES, HUMAN*
**Immunoglobulin Gm-2**
*See SERUM ALLOTYPES, HUMAN*
*also IMMUNODEFICIENCY, IgG SUBCLASS DEFICIENCIES*
**Immunoglobulin Gm-3**
*See IMMUNODEFICIENCY, IgG SUBCLASS DEFICIENCIES*
*also SERUM ALLOTYPES, HUMAN*
**Immunoglobulin Gm-4**
*See IMMUNODEFICIENCY, IgG SUBCLASS DEFICIENCIES*
**Immunoglobulin InV (Km)**
*See SERUM ALLOTYPES, HUMAN*
**Immunologic deficiency, X-linked lymphopenic type**
*See IMMUNODEFICIENCY, X-LINKED SEVERE COMBINED*
**Impacted teeth**
*See TEETH, IMPACTED*
**Imperforate anus, high and low**
*See ANORECTAL MALFORMATIONS*
**Imperforate anus-polydactyly syndrome**
*See VATER ASSOCIATION*
**Imperforate hymen**
*See HYMEN, IMPERFORATE*
**Incarcerated hernia**
*See HERNIA, INGUINAL*
**Incisor, single upper central**
*See TEETH, FUSED*
**Incisors (prominent)-obesity-hypotonia**
*See COHEN SYNDROME*
**Incisors, barrel-shape**
*See TEETH, INCISORS, SHOVEL-SHAPED*
**Incisors, mesiopalatal torsion of central**
*See TEETH, MESIOPALATAL TORSION OF CENTRAL INCISORS*
**Incisors, rotation of upper central**
*See TEETH, MESIOPALATAL TORSION OF CENTRAL INCISORS*
**Incisura mentalis types I, II, III, IV**
*See FACE, CHIN FISSURE*
**Inclusion cysts of the oral mucosa in the newborn**
*See MUCOSA, ORAL INCLUSION CYSTS OF THE NEWBORN*
**Incomplete feminizing testes syndrome**
*See ANDROGEN INSENSITIVITY SYNDROME, INCOMPLETE*
**Incomplete male pseudohermaphroditism, type 1 (Wilson & Goldstein)**
*See ANDROGEN INSENSITIVITY SYNDROME, INCOMPLETE*
**Incomplete testicular feminization syndrome**
*See ANDROGEN INSENSITIVITY SYNDROME, INCOMPLETE*
**Incontinenti Pigmenti Achromians**
*See HYPOMELANOSIS OF ITO*

## INCONTINENTIA PIGMENTI                     0526

**Includes:**
> Bloch-Siemens incontinentia pigmenti
> Bloch-Sulzberger syndrome
> Melanoblastosis cutis linearis
> Pigmented dermatosis, Siemens-Bloch type

**Excludes:**
> **Ectodermal dysplasia, Naegeli type** (0703)
> **Hypomelanosis of Ito** (2264)

**Major Diagnostic Criteria:**   Skin lesions, with or without alopecia, tooth anomalies.

**Clinical Findings:**   Characterized at birth or neonatal period by inflammation and bullae in females. The lesions are arranged in linear fashion and may come and go. They are then replaced by hypertrophic verrucous bands. Then a bizarre pattern of spattered or band-like hyperpigmentation appears mostly on the trunk but also on the scalp and limbs. The hyperpigmentation slowly fades and almost disappears by the third decade. The typical hyperpigmentation is usually preceded by inflammation and blisters. Alopecia of scalp, dental, ocular (vascular abnormalities of the retina and disorders of the retinal pigment epithelium), and osseous anomalies, deformities of ears, small stature, neurologic changes, and occasionally, mental retardation occurs.

**Complications:**   Convulsions, retrolental fibroplasia.

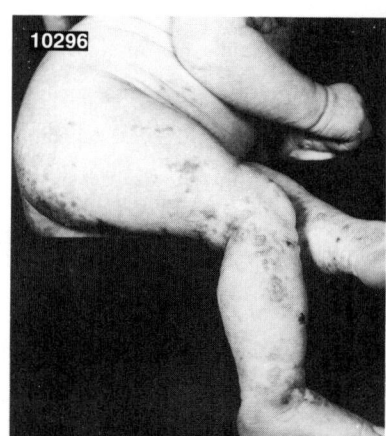
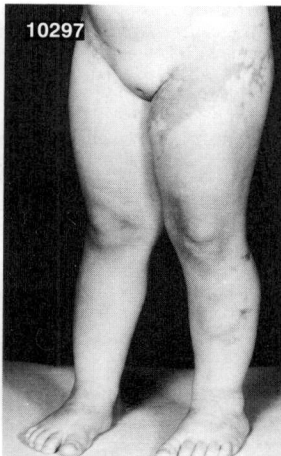
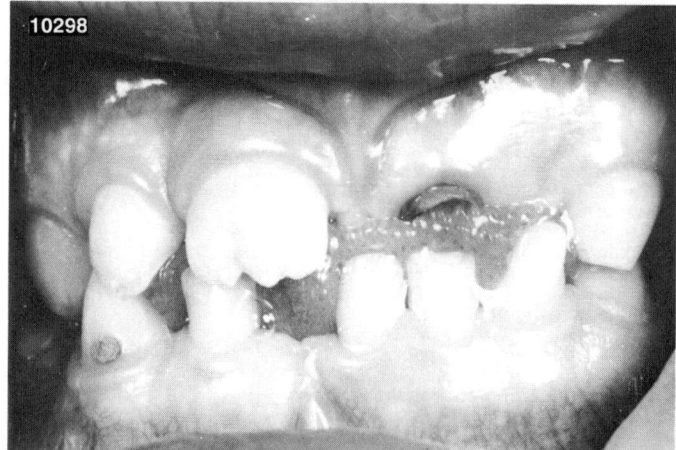

**0526**-10296:  Linear vesicles.  10297:  Spattered hyperpigmentation.  10298:  Dysplastic and conical teeth.

**Associated Findings:** Supernumerary tragi, chromosomal translocations, **Klinefelter syndrome**, extra ribs, and hemivertebrae.

**Etiology:** Presumably X-linked dominant inheritance, lethal in males.

**Pathogenesis:** Unknown.

**MIM No.:** *30830

**POS No.:** 3265

**CDC No.:** 757.350

**Sex Ratio:** M>0:F1

**Occurrence:** About 700 cases reported.

**Risk of Recurrence for Patient's Sib:**
See Part I, *Mendelian Inheritance*.

**Risk of Recurrence for Patient's Child:**
See Part I, *Mendelian Inheritance*.

**Age of Detectability:** In childhood.

**Gene Mapping and Linkage:** IP1 (incontinentia pigmenti 1) has been mapped to Xp11.21-cen.

**Prevention:** None known. Genetic counseling indicated.

**Treatment:** Unknown.

**Prognosis:** Normal life span. Some patients are mentally retarded. Disability may result from neurologic, ocular, osseous and other changes. Reproductive fitness somewhat impaired by major defects.

**Detection of Carrier:** Unknown.

**References:**
Carney RG: Incontinentia pigmenti: report of 5 cases and review of literature. Arch Dermatol Syph 1951; 64:126.
Carney RG, Carney RG Jr.: Incontinentia pigmenti. Arch Dermatol 1970; 102:157–162.
Carney RG Jr: Incontinentia pigmenti, a world statistical analysis. Arch Dermatol 1976; 112:535–542.
Wiklund DA, Weston WL: Incontinentia pigmenti: a four generation study. Arch Derm 1980; 116:701–703.
Wieacker P, et al.: X inactivation patterns in two syndromes with probable X-linked dominant, male lethal inheritance. Clin Genet 1985; 28:238–242.
Ormerod AD, et al.: Incontinentia pigmenti in a boy with Klinefelter's syndrome. J Med Genet 1987; 24:439–441.
Spallone A: Incontinentia pigmenti (Bloch-Sulzberger syndrome): seven case reports in one family. Brit J Ophthal 1987; 71:629–634.

CH034                                    **Philip F. Chance**

**Incontinentia pigmenti of Naegeli**
See ECTODERMAL DYSPLASIA, NAEGELI TYPE
**Index finger polydactyly**
See POLYDACTYLY
**Indiana type hereditary amyloidosis**
See AMYLOIDOSIS, INDIANA TYPE
**Indocin^, fetal effects**
See FETAL EFFECTS OF NONSTEROIDAL ANTI-INFLAMMATORY DRUGS (NSAIDS)
**Indomethacin, fetal effects**
See FETAL EFFECTS OF NONSTEROIDAL ANTI-INFLAMMATORY DRUGS (NSAIDS)
**Infant of diabetic mother (IDM)**
See FETAL EFFECTS FROM MATERNAL DIABETES
**Infant of gestational diabetic mother (IGDM)**
See FETAL EFFECTS FROM MATERNAL DIABETES
**Infantile cerebellar atrophy with retinal degeneration**
See OLIVOPONTOCEREBELLAR ATROPHY, DOMINANT WITH RETINAL DEGENERATION
**Infantile hemangioendothelioma**
See ORBITAL HEMANGIOMA
**Infantile malignant osteopetrosis**
See OSTEOPETROSIS, MALIGNANT RECESSIVE
**Infantile necrotizing encephalomyelopathy**
See ENCEPHALOPATHY, NECROTIZING
**Infantile paralysis**
See POLIO, SUSCEPTIBILITY TO
**Infantile phytanic acid storage disease**
See PHYTANIC ACID OXIDASE DEFICIENCY, INFANTILE TYPE

**Infantile polycystic disease (IPCD)**
See KIDNEY, POLYCYSTIC DISEASE, RECESSIVE
**Infantile polyposis**
See INTESTINAL POLYPOSIS, JUVENILE TYPE
**Infantile psychosis**
See AUTISM, INFANTILE
**Infarction defects in surviving monozygous twins**
See FETAL MONOZYGOUS MULTIPLE PREGNANCY DYSPLACENTATION EFFECTS
**Infection, Venezuelan equine encephalitis**
See FETAL VENEZUELAN EQUINE ENCEPHALITIS INFECTION
**Infections, recurrent severe**
See GRANULOCYTE GLYCOPROTEIN CD11/CD18 DEFICIENCY
**Infectious mononucleosis, susceptibility to**
See IMMUNODEFICIENCY, X-LINKED LYMPHOPROLIFERATIVE DISEASE
**Inferior vena cava, absent**
See VENA CAVA, ABSENT HEPATIC SEGMENT
**Inferior vena cava, absent hepatic segment**
See VENA CAVA, ABSENT HEPATIC SEGMENT
**Inflammation of the brain, skin and joints-infantile relapsing**
See INFLAMMATORY DISEASE, NEONATAL BATES-LORBER TYPE

**INFLAMMATORY BOWEL DISEASE**                    **2232**

**Includes:**

Crohn disease
Granulomatous colitis
Ileocolitis
Intestine, inflammatory bowel diseases
Regional enteritis/ileitis
Ulcerative colitis
Ulcerative proctitis

**Excludes:**

Colitis due to bacterial, fungal, viral, and protozoal agents
Colitis secondary to systemic disease
Diverticulitis
Drug or irradiation-induced colitis and proctitis
Ileocecal tuberculosis
Irritable bowel syndrome
Ischemic colitis
Pseudomembranous colitis

**Major Diagnostic Criteria:** The inflammatory bowel diseases (IBD) are chronic diseases characterized by inflammatory lesions of the large and small bowel. The clinical course is extremely variable, with unpredictable remissions and exacerbations and a wide range of local and systemic complications. Diagnosis is based on a combination of clinical, X-ray, and pathologic findings.

*Crohn disease:* No specific laboratory tests confirm this diagnosis. While classically affecting the small intestine, especially the terminal ileum, large bowel involvement is common as well, and the disease may involve any part of the gastrointestinal tract. Chronic clinical course includes fever, diarrhea, cramping abdominal pain, vomiting, and anemia. Perianal fissure, ulceration, or fistulas may be present at time of diagnosis. On X-ray, distribution of diseased bowel may be segmental. Common findings are strictures, fistulas, abdominal abscesses, and a characteristic "cobblestone" mucosal pattern in affected areas. Sigmoidoscopy findings may be normal, or show lumpy edema or areas of ulceration interspersed with normal areas. On biopsy, most tissue samples show granulomas.

*Ulcerative colitis:* There are no specific laboratory tests to confirm this diagnosis. The affected area is the large bowel. Common clinical manifestations include bloody rectal discharges, often with recurrent diarrhea, cramping lower abdominal pain, weight loss, and tenesmus. At onset, clinical symptoms may be mild or severe. Constipation may be present. Spontaneous remission and exacerbation of symptoms is characteristic. Diffuse inflammation of the rectal and sigmoid mucosa is seen on proctoscopy in the vast majority of patients. On X-ray, about one-half show involvement of the entire colon.

**Clinical Findings:** Symptoms at onset, as well as during the course of disease, are highly variable. Each patient's clinical course is characterized by distinct debilitating symptoms and complications. The chronic course will exacerbate and remit in such a variable way that some patients will have minimal social consequences from their disease, while others will require multiple hospitalizations, extensive surgery, and hyperalimentation.

**Complications:** Complications are numerous, involving virtually all organ systems. Included are skin lesions (aphthous ulcers of the mouth, pyoderma gangrenosum, erythema nodosum); eye lesions (conjunctivitis, iritis, and episcleritis); obstructive hydronephrosis, nephrolithiasis, venous thrombosis, hepatobiliary diseases (pericholangitis, primary sclerosing cholangitis, bile duct carcinoma, cholelithiasis, fatty infiltration of the liver, fibrosis, and cirrhosis of the liver); and musculoskeletal complications (peripheral arthritis, sacroiliitis, and **Ankylosing spondylitis**). Nutritional deficiencies are possible, secondary to decreased intestinal absorption, and growth retardation is seen in some cases with childhood onset. Both Crohn disease and ulcerative colitis patients have an increased risk for carcinomas of the gastrointestinal tract (2–3% of all IBD patients with duration of disease of 20 years or greater). Serious gastrointestinal complications include toxic megacolon, massive gastrointestinal bleeding, and strictures.

**Associated Findings:** Inflammatory bowel disease is found in increased frequency in two genetic syndromes: **Turner syndrome** and **Albinism, oculocutaneous, Hermansky-Pudlak type.** Four of 135 Turner syndrome patients (3%) in one series developed IBD (two Crohn and two ulcerative colitis). Hermansky-Pudlak syndrome, a tyrosine-positive albinism disorder, has a worldwide distribution. Puerto Rican patients with Hermansky-Pudlak syndrome have a high incidence of granulomatous colitis.

Patients with inflammatory bowel disease and either typical **Ankylosing spondylitis** (approximately 5% of cases) or sacroiliitis show an increased frequency of HLA-B27.

**Etiology:** Family studies demonstrate an increased family aggregation for both Crohn disease and ulcerative colitis. The etiology(s) appears to be complex, and Mendelian ratios are not observed in families. Crohn disease appears to be more strongly familial than does ulcerative colitis, and a higher monozygotic twin concordance rate has been reported for Crohn disease than for ulcerative colitis. Positive family history for IBD is reported to range from 14% to 30% in Crohn case series; for ulcerative colitis, the proportion of cases with a positive family history ranges from 6% to 8%. Some data suggest that early-onset IBD cases may have an increased incidence of affected second-degree relatives as well (in most series, the increased risk is mainly reported for first-degree relatives). Both Crohn disease and ulcerative colitis appear with increased frequency in relatives of probands with either disease, raising the possibility that these two diseases may be clinical variants of the same underlying disease process.

While environmental factors have been suggested as playing a role in the etiology of both Crohn disease and ulcerative colitis, experimental evidence is unclear at this time. Proposed environmental agents include dietary factors (most notably refined sugars, milk, dietary fiber, carrageenan) and microbial agents (most notably anaerobic bacteria, mycobacteria, and viral agents).

The basic underlying mechanisms in these diseases are unknown. The leading hypotheses are primary immunologic derangements consisting of either autoimmune or immune/toxin interactions.

**Pathogenesis:** The primary lesion is not yet known for either Crohn disease or ulcerative colitis.
*Crohn disease:* The early pathologic lesions are scattered superficial ulcers of the bowel. Also found are submucosal edema, lymphatic dilation, and transmural involvement of the bowel wall. Lymphatic involvement suggests a possible role of the immune system in the pathogenesis. Granulomas, found in most but not all Crohn patients, suggest a possible defect in host defenses against environmental agents (either chemical or biologic). Defects in cell-mediated immunity have been found, but these may be secondary to the disease process. Good animal models are not available.
*Ulcerative colitis:* The diffuse inflammatory reaction seen in the mucosa and submucosa of the colon suggests a possible reaction to cytotoxic agents. Increased plasma cells are found in the colon,

perhaps suggesting an immune reaction. Raised gut bacterial counts, also found in Crohn patients, raise the possibility of a viral or bacterial etiology, although no specific agent is clearly implicated. Other possibilities include an autoimmune etiology or specific immunologic defects originating in the bowel mucosa. It remains difficult to separate primary defects and those secondary to the disease process.

**CDC No.:** 751.880

**Sex Ratio:** M1:F0.8–1.6 in Crohn disease (increased in females with older age of onset).
M1:F1 in ulcerative colitis in many populations; slight female preponderance in others (mostly English, English-derived).

**Occurrence:** *Crohn disease:* 0.27–6.3:100,000 (lowest in Blacks, Asians; highest in northern Europeans, Ashkenazi Jews in Europe, United States).
*Ulcerative colitis:* 2–7:100,000 (highest in northern Europe).
Since 1950, the incidence of Crohn disease has steadily increased in most populations; this increase appears to be real. No such increase is seen for ulcerative colitis.

**Risk of Recurrence for Patient's Sib:** *Crohn disease:* 1:25. *Ulcerative colitis:* 1:50. *IBD total:* Ashkenazi Jew 1:40; non-Jewish 1:100.

**Risk of Recurrence for Patient's Child:** *Crohn disease:* 1:50. *Ulcerative colitis:* 1:150. *IBD total:* Ashkenazi Jew 1:40; Non-Jewish 1:100.
The sketchy data suggest that the empiric risk is very much a function of the specific population. All the above data are uncorrected for the age of the relative at risk Actual lifetime risks may be several fold higher, especially among offspring.

**Age of Detectability:** In infants (less than one year of age) through adulthood. Peak age of detection for Crohn disease is 20–29 years of age; ulcerative colitis at 60–80 years of age.

**Gene Mapping and Linkage:** A possible association between HLA-DR2 and ulcerative colitis in certain populations have been reported, and between HLA-DR4 and *Crohn disease* in the Japanese. There is also data implicating the involvement of the C3 locus on chromosome 19.

**Prevention:** None known. Genetic counseling indicated.

**Treatment:** Medical treatment is primarily symptomatic. Adrenal steroids, ACTH, and immunosuppressive drugs can be useful in controlling active disease in some patients. Sulfasalazine in maintenance doses has been successfully used in preventing relapses in some patients. Use of elemental diet and total parenteral nutrition may play a role in both maintenance and treatment. Surgery may be necessary for severe or debilitating disease in severe acute phases, or for complications.

**Prognosis:** *Crohn disease:* Even with current treatment, more than 50% of surgically treated, and 90% of medically treated cases, will have recurrent disease. Recurrence soon after resection surgery is a bad prognostic sign, as is extensive involvement of the small bowel.
*Ulcerative colitis:* Most severe episodes occur during the first year. Modern treatment has greatly improved the death rate due to acute attacks. Childhood and elderly onset have a worse prognosis than adulthood onset (3–5% mortality rate with good care). Risk for gastrointestinal cancer estimated to be increased 10- to 40-fold, with greatest risk to those with onset of colitis before age 30.

**Detection of Carrier:** Unknown.

**Special Considerations:** Crohn disease and ulcerative colitis may be the spectrum of one disease, with Crohn disease representing the more severe cases. Equally likely, there may be etiologic and genetic heterogeneity within each disease, with subtypes that may present as either disease.

**Support Groups:**
New York; National Foundation for Ileitis and Colitis
CANADA: BC; Burnaby; Northwestern Society of Intestinal Research

**References:**
Arulanantham K, et al.: The association of inflammatory bowel disease and Y chromosomal abnormality. Pediatrics 1980; 66:63–67.

Kirsner JB: Inflammatory bowel disease: clinical, etiologic, and genetic aspects. In: Rotter JI, Samloff IM, Rimoin DL, eds: The genetics and heterogeneity of common gastrointestinal disorders. New York: Academic Press, 1980:261–290.

Mayberry JF, Rhodes J: Epidemiological aspects of Crohn's disease: a review of the literature. Gut 1984; 25:886–899.

Weterman IT, Pena AS: Familial incidence of Crohn's disease in the Netherlands and a review of the literature. Gastroenterology 1984; 86:449–452.

McConnell RB: Genetic aspects of idiopathic inflammatory bowel disease. In: Kirsner JB, Shorter RG, eds: Inflammatory bowel disease, 3rd ed. Philadelphia: Lea & Febiger, 1988:87–95.

Roth M-P, et al.: Familial recurrence risks of inflammatory bowel disease in Ashkenazi Jews. Gastroenterology 1989; 96:1016–1020.

Shohat T, et al.: The genetics of inflammatory bowel disease. In: Gitnick G, ed: Inflammatory bowel disease: a physician's guide. New York: Igukiu-Shoin, 1989.

VA019

Constance M. Vadheim
*Jerome I. Rotter*

**Inflammatory disease, infantile multisystem**
*See INFLAMMATORY DISEASE, NEONATAL BATES-LORBER TYPE*

---

## INFLAMMATORY DISEASE, NEONATAL BATES-LORBER TYPE 2157

**Includes:**
Arthropathy-rash-uveitis-mental retardation
Bates syndrome
Epiphyseal damage with constitutional symptoms
Inflammation of the brain, skin and joints-infantile relapsing
Inflammatory disease, infantile multisystem
Inflammatory disease, neonatal onset multisystem
Lorber syndrome
Meningitis-polyarthritis-lymphadenitis-pulmonary hemosiderosis

**Excludes:**
**Arthritis, rheumatoid** (2517)
Infection (rubella, syphilis, toxoplasmosis, etc.)
**Lipogranulomatosis** (0598)
**Mucopolysaccharidosis**

**Major Diagnostic Criteria:** Features strongly suggestive of neonatal-onset, multisystem, inflammatory disease include evanescent

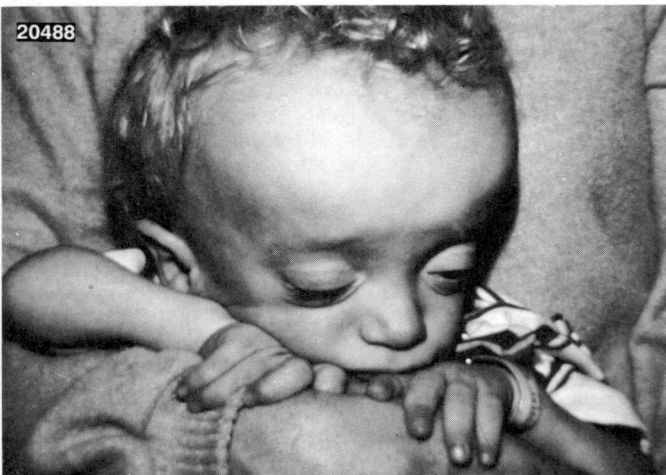

**2157A-20488:** Inflammatory disease, neonatal Bates-Lorber type; note subject age 18 months with frontal bossing, hydrocephalus, bony enlargement and arthritis of both elbows.

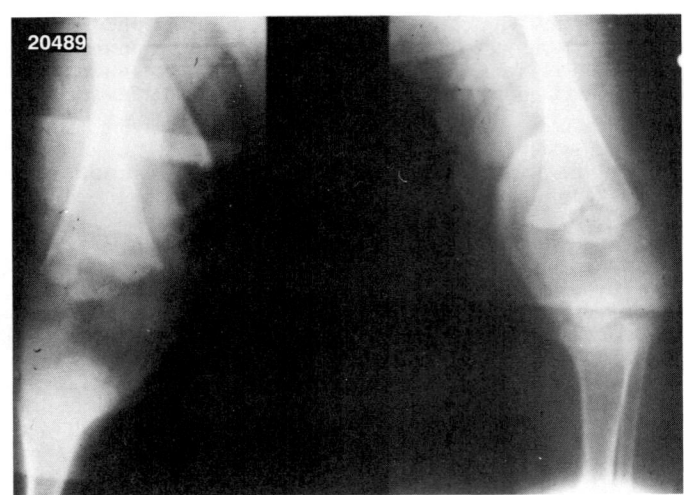

**2157B-20489:** X-ray of both knees at age 5 months; note soft tissue swelling, epiphyseal erosions of the distal femurs, and periosteal elevations surrounding the femoral metaphyses.

---

rash either similar to the eruption of systemic onset juvenile rheumatoid arthritis or to typical urticaria; persistent or intermittent episodes of fever resembling the pattern of systemic onset juvenile rheumatoid arthritis; reticuloendothelial involvement characterized by hepatosplenomegaly or generalized lymphadenopathy; progressive and destructive arthropathy; chronic central nervous system changes, which may include developmental delay, mental retardation, **Hydrocephaly** with persistent open fontanelle, non-bacterial meningitis, cerebral atrophy, and seizures; eye changes such as uveitis, vitreous inflammation, or papilledema. Laboratory changes are nonspecific, but a persistent anemia, leukocytosis, elevated erythrocyte sedimentation rate, and cerebrospinal fluid pleocytosis are usually present. X-ray findings of periosteal elevation, flared metaphyses and abnormal ossification are often seen.

**Clinical Findings:** The cutaneous findings, fever, lymphadenopathy, and hepatosplenomegaly start characteristically at birth or in the neonatal period. Of 13 patients, nine started at birth, one at two days, one at four months, and in one occurrence the age of onset was not recorded. Destructive arthropathy, then central nervous system and eye involvement usually develop during the first year. Clinical findings in 13 reported children consist of the following: 1. evanescent cutaneous eruption which may be urticarial in appearance or similar to the rash of systemic onset juvenile rheumatoid arthritis (all 13); 2. generalized lymphadenopathy but often very evident in the axillary and inguinal areas (all 13); 3. destructive, particularly bony, and progressive arthropathy involving multiple joints, but most frequently the elbows, wrists, knees, and ankles, and often leading to the formation of severe contractures with a subsequent significant physical disability (all 13); 4. fever suggestive of systemic onset juvenile rheumatoid arthritis persisting in cyclical fashion (12/13); 5. hepatosplenomegaly (9); 6. variable central nervous system abnormalities including persistently open fontanelle (11), hydrocephalus or increased head size (9), delayed developmental milestones (13), and seizures (6); feeding difficulties (4) with subsequent varying degrees of malnutrition, and secondary hearing loss also may be secondary to central nervous involvement; and 7. eye involvement consisting of uveitis (7), sometimes with vitreous inflammatory changes (2), papilledema (7), and optic atrophy (1).

Laboratory findings include a persistent and often severe anemia (usually hypochromic and microcytic) (9/9), an intermittent or persistent leukocytosis (13), and markedly increased sedimentation rate. Immunoglobulin G levels are often elevated (8/10), and antinuclear antibodies negative. Rheumatoid factor may be detected (1/4). Recurrent CSF pleocytosis (mononuclear cells predominantly) is seen (10/10). Low zinc and copper levels are reported in one child with prolonged malnutrition. Profound X-ray changes of periosteal reaction, abnormal epiphyseal ossification centers, and flared metaphyses.

**Complications:** Marked joint deformities frequently result in gait disturbance and progress to nonambulation.

Inflammatory eye changes may cause visual deficits. There is an apparent susceptibility to infections although measurements of immunologic function in selected cases are normal. One child developed fatal myelomonoblastic leukemia, implying that this may be a premalignant disorder, although this same patient two years previously had been treated with chlorambucil. Almost all patients have experienced some degree of failure to thrive, delayed developmental milestones, and mental retardation as a result of both poor nutrition and chronic inflammatory disease of the CNS (i.e., meningitis).

**Associated Findings:** **Omphalocele,** pulmonary hemosiderosis, psoriasis with possibly increased susceptibility to frequent and severe infectious diseases, or development of malignancy.

**Etiology:** Unknown.

**Pathogenesis:** Neonatal onset, vitreous inflammation, and early periosteal involvement suggest in utero infection, but a vigorous search to confirm this cause has not been successful. A relationship to psoriasis has been suggested because of biopsy findings in one patient and family history in two patients. Articular manifestations of psoriasis, however, are usually erosive and asymmetric, and chronic CNS inflammatory changes are not seen. The early onset of symptoms, accompanied by developmental delay and variable mental deficiency, is suggestive of progressive organ damage secondary to a metabolic storage disorder. Urinary screening for mucopolysaccharides and oligosaccharides, however, and fibroblast cultures for lysosomal hydrolase and neuroamidase activity in several patients, have yielded normal results; biopsy specimens have also not shown findings consistent with a storage process. Persistent inflammation of the skin and central nervous system suggest an ongoing immune response to sequestered antigens or antigenic fragments, or an inherited deficiency of one of the naturally occurring inhibitors of the inflammatory response.

**Sex Ratio:** M6:F7

**Occurrence:** 13 cases have been described in the literature.

**Risk of Recurrence for Patient's Sib:** Unknown. Two siblings of the opposite sex were affected in one family, but all other cases have been sporadic.

**Risk of Recurrence for Patient's Child:** There are no reports thus far of any patient having offspring.

**Age of Detectability:** The presence of maculopapular rash and hepatosplenomegaly at birth should alert the clinician to this disorder. Persistent fever, central nervous system changes, and destructive arthropathy usually follow within the first two to four months of life.

**Gene Mapping and Linkage:** Unknown.

**Prevention:** None known. Genetic counseling indicated.

**Treatment:** In most cases nonsteroidal anti-inflammatory agents or drugs, such as gold or penicillamine, are not very helpful. Corticosteroids are only partially successful in reducing systemic symptoms and improving joint function. Prompt recognition and treatment of infections is needed. A comprehensive program of joint conservation, if started early enough, will lessen the impact of severe joint contractures. Ocular inflammatory disease requires prompt therapy to prevent visual loss, and early audiologic testing is mandatory.

**Prognosis:** Of 13 patients reported thus far, three have died; causes were haemophilus influenzae pneumonia, necrotizing leukoencephalopathy, and myelomonoblastic leukemia. General clinical outcomes are varied. Severe joint deformities appear to persist, and some degree of mental retardation often occurs.

**Detection of Carrier:** Unknown.

**References:**

Lorber J: Syndrome for Diagnosis: dwarfing, persistently open fontanelle, recurrent meningitis, recurrent subdural effusions with temporary alternate-sided hemiplegia, high-tone deafness, visual defect with pseudo-papillaedema, slowing intellectual development, recurrent acute polyarthritis, erythema marginatum, splenomegaly, and iron-resistant hypochronic anemia. Proc R Soc Med 1973; 6:1070–1071.
Ansell BM: Rheumatic disorders in childhood. London, Butterworths, 1980:269–277. †
Prieur A, Griscelli C: Arthropathy with rash, chronic meningitis, eye lesions, and mental retardation. J Pediatr 1981; 99:79–83.
Hassink SG, Goldsmith DP: Neonatal onset multisystem inflammatory disease. Arthritis Rheum 1983; 26:668–673. * †
Goldsmith DP: The right stuff for a new syndrome. J Pediatr 1985; 106:441–443.
Yarom A, et al.: Infantile multisystem disease: a specific syndrome? J Pediatr 1985; 106:390–396. *

G0043        **Donald P. Goldsmith**

**Inflammatory disease, neonatal onset multisystem**
*See INFLAMMATORY DISEASE, NEONATAL BATES-LORBER TYPE*
**Inflammatory linear verrucous epidermal nevus (ILVEN)**
*See NEVUS, EPIDERMAL NEVUS SYNDROME*
**Inflammatory polyps**
*See INTESTINAL POLYPOSIS, JUVENILE TYPE*
**Infrahepatic interruption of inferior vena cava**
*See VENA CAVA, ABSENT HEPATIC SEGMENT*
**Inguinal hernia**
*See HERNIA, INGUINAL*
**INH (antituberculosis agent) inactivation**
*See NEUROPATHY, HERITABLE ISONIAZIDE TYPE (INH)*
**Inner ear, aplasia**
*See EAR, LABYRINTH APLASIA*
**Insulin receptor, defect in**
*See LEPRECHAUNISM*
**Insulin resistance, autosomal dominant type**
*See SKIN, ACANTHOSIS NIGRICANS*
**Insulin resistance, drug induced type**
*See SKIN, ACANTHOSIS NIGRICANS*
**Insulin resistance, familial severe**
*See LEPRECHAUNISM*
**Insulin-dependent diabetes mellitus (IDDM)**
*See DIABETES MELLITUS, INSULIN DEPENDENT TYPE*
**Insulin-like growth factor deficiency**
*See GROWTH DEFICIENCY, AFRICAN PYGMY TYPE*
**Insulins, structurally abnormal**
*See DIABETES MELLITUS, MUTANT INSULIN TYPES*
**Intercalary defects**
*See LIMB REDUCTION DEFECTS*

## INTERFERON DEFICIENCY      3090

**Includes:**
    Alpha-interferon deficiency
    Antiviral interferon deficiency
    Beta-interferon deficiency
    Fibroblast interferon deficiency
    Gamma-interferon deficiency
    Immune interferon deficiency
    Leukocyte interferon deficiency
    Lymphoblast interferon deficiency

**Excludes:**
    Antiviral antibody deficiency
    Cell-mediated immunity to viruses

**Major Diagnostic Criteria:** Decreased levels of one or more types of interferon (IFN) have been described in humans with various disorders, including tumors, leukemia, **Cancer, Hodgkin disease, familial**, chronic hepatitis B infection, the acquired immunodeficiency syndrome (AIDS), recurrent labial herpes, persistent Epstein-Barr virus infection, and congenital cytomegalovirus infection. It is not always possible to determine whether IFN deficiency is primary or secondary in these instances. A deficiency in IFN responsiveness also occurs in malnutrition, corticosteroid therapy, other forms of immunosuppression, and postrenal transplantation, strongly suggesting a secondary defect. Mice subjected to burn injury also have subnormal IFN responses.

IFN is not normally detected in tissue or serum, but is usually detectable during viral infections. Assays for IFN usually measure the inhibition of either virus production or viral cytopathic effect on cultured cell lines.

**Clinical Findings:** The consequences of IFN deficiency are thought to include 1) decreased resistance to viral infection, possibly due to decreased cellular synthesis of new mRNA and protein (IFN enhances the expression of classes I and II HLA molecules [histocompatibility antigens] on the surface of infected cells, making them more susceptible targets for cytotoxic lymphocytes); 2) decreased natural killer (NK) cell activity; and 3) decreased antibody synthesis.

Few if any of the specific defects in immunity described to date have been proven to be the result of a primary defect in IFN production, although several family studies suggest this may occur. Success in treating certain virus infections and malignancies with IFN suggests that it may play an important role in these disorders.

Alveolar macrophages and peripheral blood monocytes of newborns are more permissive of herpes simplex virus replication than are those of adults. This may be related to an inability of neonatal cells to produce PHA-induced gamma IFN. This inability diminishes until around age six months, when responses are similar to those of adults.

About 30% of patients with recurrent herpes labialis have low levels of IFN. Some children with frequent respiratory syncytial virus (RSV) infections also have low levels of IFN. In both instances, replacement therapy may be beneficial. Therapy with IFN also has been encouraging in some cases of hepatitis B infections and in hairy cell leukemia, Kaposi sarcoma, and renal cell carcinoma. Thus, the possibility of IFN deficiency should be considered in patients with these conditions as well as in persons who have other recurrent or persistent viral infections or as yet unstudied malignancies.

**Complications:** Interferon deficiency is presumed to cause an unusual susceptibility to infectious diseases and to malignant transformation in a variety of cells.

**Associated Findings:** IgA deficiency may be associated with IFN deficiency.

**Etiology:** Possibly autosomal dominant inheritance.

**Pathogenesis:** There are three major classes of IFN: alpha, beta, and gamma. They have different inducers, cell sources, amino acid sequences, physical properties, antigenicities, and genetic controls. Alpha-IFN is derived predominantly from B-lymphocytes. At least eight different polypeptides may have alpha-IFN activity. Both alpha- and beta-IFN are stable at pH 2.0. Beta-IFN is produced by fibroblasts. It is also comprised of a number of polypeptides that have a significant degree of homology with alpha-IFN molecules. Gamma-IFN (immune IFN) is derived from stimulated T lymphocytes. It may be induced by mitogens, bacterial or viral antigens, or allogeneic cells. It is labile at pH 2.0. A normal newborn infant can produce adequate amounts of alpha-IFN but not gamma IFN.

IFN is a potent regulator of NK activity and an enhancer of IgG antibody production. It also enhances IgE binding to basophils and chemical mediator release from basophils. Deficiency of IFN down-regulates these functions, making the host more susceptible to infections and malignancies.

**MIM No.:** *14757, *14762, *14764, *14766

**Sex Ratio:** Presumably M1:F1.

**Occurrence:** Undetermined despite established literature.

**Risk of Recurrence for Patient's Sib:**
See Part I, *Mendelian Inheritance.* Single gene defects are likely to cause only partial interferon deficiency. The effects of each defect are not well documented. Several affected patients have been reported to have sibs with low levels of alpha-IFN.

**Risk of Recurrence for Patient's Child:**
See Part I, *Mendelian Inheritance.* Probably slight.

**Age of Detectability:** Gamma-IFN deficiency is present in most infants for the first six months of life. Primary deficiency of IFN later in life is uncommon. Deficiency of IFN is often only one aspect of a more widely deranged metabolic state found in a variety of specific diseases.

**Gene Mapping and Linkage:** IFNA (interferon, alpha (leukocyte)) has been mapped to 9p22-p13.
IFNB1 (interferon, beta 1, fibroblast) has been mapped to 9p22.
IFNB3 (interferon, beta 3, fibroblast) has been mapped to 2p23-qter.
IFNG (interferon, gamma) has been mapped to 12q24.1.
IFNR (interferon production regulator) has been provisionally mapped to 16.
IL6 (interleukin 6) has been mapped to 7p21-p14.

**Prevention:** None known. Genetic counseling indicated. There is evidence that a nasal spray of alpha-IFN can inhibit rhinovirus infection in a significant number of household contacts.

**Treatment:** Should be directed toward replacement of the types of IFN that are deficient. Diseases treated to date include the following:
*Hairy cell leukemia (HCL):* Treatment with alpha-IFN results in decreased hairy cell infiltrates of the bone marrow. Seventy-five percent of HCL patients treated with alpha-IFN achieve sustained improvement in granulocyte, platelet, and hemoglobin levels. Immunity to infections improves, and the need for splenectomy and the mortality rate are reduced.
*Kaposi sarcoma in AIDS:* IFN has been reported to result in amelioration in approximately 40% of patients. However, there seems to be no augmentation of immunity to opportunistic infection in patients with AIDS.
*Non-Hodgkin lymphoma:* Treatment with alpha-IFN is frequently effective, especially in the early stages of the disease.
*Multiple myeloma, malignant melanoma, renal carcinoma, carcinoma of the bladder, and ovarian cancer:* Alpha-IFN is reported to be of benefit in a limited number of patients with these malignancies.
Alpha-IFN has been used prophylactically in organ and tissue transplants to inhibit cytomegalovirus infections. It may inhibit the activation of latent herpes simplex infections. It also may be of value in treating patients with chronic hepatitis B and in interrupting the cycle of recurrent respiratory syncytial virus infection in certain children.
*Complication of treatment:* A flu-like syndrome occurs in 80–90% of treated patients. It may include fever, chill, fatigue, headache, anorexia, nausea, vomiting, myalgia, arthralgia, low back pain, dry mouth, diarrhea, confusion, depression, hypotonia, skin rashes, hypotension, cardiac arrythmia, and central nervous system toxicity. These symptoms are dose-related and reversible.
Elevated liver enzymes (SGOT and SGPT) may be seen. Hematologic toxicity may result in mild thrombocytopenia and transient granulocytopenia.

**Prognosis:** Usually depends on the primary or associated disease.

**Detection of Carrier:** IFN assays on sibs and relatives may provide circumstantial evidence of a carrier state in parents of IFN-deficient children.

**Special Considerations:** The ramifications of IFN deficiency are not clear. IFN deficiency may be primary or secondary, may contribute to frequent or chronic infections and malignancies, and may play a role in a few autoimmune diseases. Defects in IFN genes and the molecules regulating their expression are poorly understood. Purified natural or recombinant IFN has been used with relative success in treating selected malignancies and viral infections.

**References:**
Isaacs D, et al.: Deficient production of leucocyte interferon (interferon-alpha) in vitro and in vivo in children with recurrent respiratory tract infections. Lancet 1981; II:950–952.
Naylor S, et al.: Human immune interferon gene is located on chromosome 12. J Exp Med 1983; 57:1020–1027.
Epstein L: Update on interferon. Immunol Allergy Pract 1985; 7:490–497. *

Spiegel R: INTRON A (interferon alfa-2b): clinical overview. Cancer Treat Rev 1985; 12:5–16. *

Taylor-Papadimitriou J: Interferons. Oxford: Oxford University Press, 1985.

Stites D, et al.: Basic and clinical immunology, ed 6. Norwalk, CT: Appleton and Lange, 1987. *

MA079

HE043

**Ghodsi Madani**
**Douglas C. Heiner**

**Intermediate (late-onset) cystinosis**
*See CYSTINOSIS*
**Intermediate filament, muscle type**
*See MYOPATHY OR CARDIOMYOPATHY DUE TO DESMIN DEFECT*
**Intermittent branched-chain ketonuria**
*See MAPLE SYRUP URINE DISEASE*
**Internal carotid artery aneurysm of middle ear**
*See EAR, ANEURYSM OF INTERNAL CAROTID ARTERY*
**Internal chondromatosis**
*See ENCHONDROMATOSIS*
**Interphalangeal skin creases, absent distal**
*See SKIN CREASES, ABSENT DISTAL INTERPHALANGEAL*
**Interstitial pyelonephritis, hereditary type**
*See NEPHRITIS-DEAFNESS (SENSORINEURAL), HEREDITARY TYPE*

## INTESTINAL ATRESIA OR STENOSIS                    0531

**Includes:**

Intestinal polyatresia syndrome, familial
Jejunoileal atresia and stenosis

**Excludes:**

**Colon, aganglionosis** (0192)
**Colon, atresia or stenosis** (0193)
**Duodenum, atresia or stenosis** (0300)
Gastric outlet obstruction, congenital
**Intestinal atresia, multiple** (2933)
**Intestinal ileus, isolated meconium ileus** (0545)

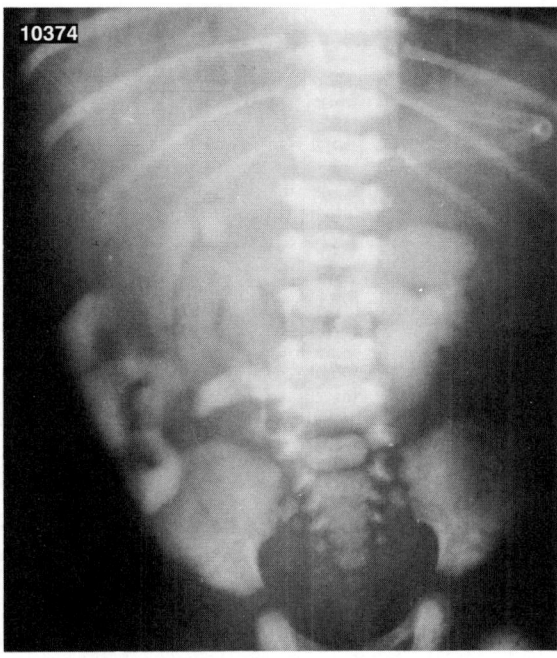

**0531-10374:** Abdomen in recumbent position. Note Levine tube in stomach; no air distal to stomach; multiple opacities with a calcium density in midabdomen.

**Jejunal atresia** (2934)
Meconium peritonitis
**Pancreas, annular** (0062)
**Pyloroduodenal atresia, hereditary** (2617)
**Pyloric stenosis** (0848)
Rotational abnormalities of the gastrointestinal tract
Other causes of neonatal intestinal obstruction (bands, hernias)

**Major Diagnostic Criteria:** Diagnosis of upper intestinal obstruction of the stomach, duodenum, and proximal jejunum rarely requires more than a plain upright X-ray film of the abdomen, demonstrating a double or triple bubble. Obstruction of the distal jejunum, ileum, and colon will require a barium enema following plain X-ray films of the abdomen. The barium study will help to demonstrate a mechanical obstruction or microcolon with proximal intestinal dilation, and will rule out an ileus, gastroenterocolitis of the newborn, or other lesions such as meconium ileus, meconium plug syndrome, or suggestion of Hirschsprung disease not requiring immediate surgery. An upper GI contrast study is necessary in older infants to demonstrate proximal stenosis of the gastrointestinal tract.

**Clinical Findings:** Vomiting is the most significant clinical finding in all forms of intestinal atresia or stenosis. The vomitus is usually bile stained except in gastric outlet obstruction, when it is clear or coffee-ground in nature. Increasing abdominal distention occurs with the more distal jejunoileal or colonic obstructions. Obstipation is a constant clinical feature; however, the neonate may pass an occasional small, gray, mucoid, pellet-sized stool. Classification of the jejunoileal intestinal atresias is as follows: type I, mucosal atresia with intact bowel and mesentery; type II, blind ends are separated by a fibrous cord; type IIIA, blind ends separated by a V-shaped mesenteric defect; type IIIB, "apple peel" atresia (see **Jejunal atresia**); and type IV, multiple atresias. A nearly similar classification exists for duodenal atresias.

Small intestine atresias occur in the jejunum (50%), the ileum (43%), and in both the ileum and jejunum, multiple points of atresia occur 7% of the time.

**Complications:** Dehydration and electrolyte imbalance occur without treatment within 12–48 hours. Aspiration, circulatory collapse, and intestinal perforation with peritonitis and sepsis will follow in a period of hours to several days.

**Associated Findings:** *Jejunoileal atresia and stenoses:* Low birth weight (30%); rotational abnormalities (10%); meconium peritonitis (12%); meconium ileus (10%); **Cystic fibrosis** (10–20%); multiple atresias (14%); **omphalocele** (5–10%); **gastroschisis** (10–15%).

*Colon atresias and stenoses:* Skeletal anomalies such as **Syndactyly, Polydactyly**, absent radius, and club foot are present. Ocular and cardiac anomalies have been noted, as well as abdominal wall defects such as **omphalocele, gastroschisis,** and vesicointestinal fissure.

**Etiology:** Undetermined, except in **Intestinal atresias, multiple** which is transmitted through autosomal recessive inheritance, and when part of another syndrome sych as **Cystic fibrosis**.

**Pathogenesis:** Intrauterine vascular accidents during the later gestational period are thought to occur jejunoileal atresia and stenosis, and colonic atresia and stenosis due to volvulus, intussusception, internal hernia, or constriction of the mesentery in a tight gastroschisis or omphalocele defect.

**MIM No.:**  *24315

**CDC No.:**  751.1

**Sex Ratio:**  M1:F1

**Occurrence:** Jejunoileal atresia and stenosis occurs in 1:1,000 to 1:5,000 live births throughout the world. It is more often reported in Western countries. Colon atresia and stenosis occurs 1:20,000 live births throughout the world.

**Risk of Recurrence for Patient's Sib:** Several reports have occurred in the literature with sibs affected; however, incidence is low.

**Risk of Recurrence for Patient's Child:** Risk of occurrence is low, but has been reported in several families.

**Age of Detectability:** All atresias and most stenoses present during the newborn period. The remaining 10–20% of stenoses occur before six months of age. Prenatal diagnosis has been performed (Morin et al, 1980).

**Gene Mapping and Linkage:** Unknown.

**Prevention:** None known. Genetic counseling indicated.

**Treatment:** Preoperative treatment includes fluid and electrolyte correction, nasogastric decompression, and temperature control and glucose and hyperbilirubinemia correction in the newborn. Surgical intervention with appropriate gastrointestinal anastomoses and intestinal decompression follows. Rather than performing an extensive intestinal resection in the proximal dilated bowel such as in jejunal atresia, a tapering procedure of the dilated intestine is performed. This conserves length and surface area of bowel for absorption and prevents short gut syndrome. This has resulted in earlier and improved intestinal motility and increased survival. This procedure is usually not necessary in ileal atresia. Usually 20–25 cm of the proximal dilated bowel can be sacrificed safely with a primary anastomosis. Postoperative care includes the necessary neonatal support and surveillance and parenteral and enteral alimentation. Parenteral alimentation may be prolonged in cases of short gut syndrome. Patients with ileal and jejunal atresia must be worked up for cystic fibrosis, since it will occur 10–20% of the time. Other treatment may be necessary for anomalies of other organ systems. The treatment of proximal colon atresia is resection and anastomsis. Distal atresia: diverting colostomy and at six months to one year, a primary anastomsis.

**Prognosis:** Excellent except in cases complicated by other complex malformation syndromes, or severe short gut. The distal atresia patients have a better prognosis than is the case in proximal atresia.

**Detection of Carrier:** Unknown.

**References:**
Recomb PP, Karplus M: Familial and hereditary intestinal atresia. Helv Paediatr Acta 1971; 26:561–564.
Melhem RE, et al.: Pyloroduodenal atresia. Pediatr Radiol 1975; 3:1–5.
Morin PR, et al.: Prenatal detection of intestinal obstruction: deficient amniotic fluid disaccharidases in affected fetuses. Clin Genet 1980; 18:217–222.
Blackburn WR, et al.: The familial intestinal poly-atresia syndrome (abstract). Proc Greenwood Genet Center 1983; 2:122–123.
Kirillova IA, et al.: Atresia, stenosis and duplication of the gastrointestinal tract. consideration of their origin. Acta Morphol Acad Sci Hung 1984; 32:9–21.
Grosfeld J: Jejunal atresia and stenosis. In: Welch K, et al.: Pediatric surgery, ed 4. Chicago: Year Book Medical Publishers, 1986, Chapter 85.
Philipport A: Atreasia, stenosis of colon. In: Welch K, et al.: Pediatric surgery, ed 4. Chicago: Year Book Medical Publishers, 1986:984–989.

BE049                               **Arthur S. Besser**

## INTESTINAL ATRESIAS, MULTIPLE              2933

**Includes:** Intestinal polyatresia syndrome (mucosal or septal variety)

**Excludes:**
Intestinal atresia or stenosis (0531)
Multiple atresias-foreshortened bowel-prematurity
Pyloroduodenal atresia, hereditary (2617)

**Major Diagnostic Criteria:** Multiple intestinal atresias that may involve the duodenum, jejunum, ileum, and rectum.

**Clinical Findings:** The pregnancy may be complicated by hydramnios. The condition is apparent in the neonatal period. The baby has continuous vomiting and usually does not pass meconium. On physical examination the only positive findings are a distended epigastric region, a scaphoid abdomen, and an empty anal canal. X-ray studies of the abdomen reveal a large solitary air bubble in the stomach, with no gas in the intestinal tract. Intraluminal calcifications may be demonstrable.

At laparotomy, the bowel from the duodenum to the rectum has a small caliber, is unused, and has multiple diaphragm-like septa, causing complete discontinuity of the intestinal lumen. In between the septa, there is intestinal lumen.

There is no loss of small bowel loops, no evidence of impairment of the vascular supply in the intact mesentery, and no volvulus, intussusception, internal hernias, or meconium ileus.

**Complications:** Because of the extensive pathologic lesions, surgery may have complications. With parenteral alimentation some cases may be managed successfully.

**Associated Findings:** None known.

**Etiology:** Autosomal recessive inheritance.

**Pathogenesis:** Unknown.

**MIM No.:** *24315

**CDC No.:** 751.100

**Sex Ratio:** M1:F1

**Occurrence:** Panethnic. Fewer than 50 patients with the hereditary type have been reported.

**Risk of Recurrence for Patient's Sib:**
See Part I, *Mendelian Inheritance*.

**Risk of Recurrence for Patient's Child:**
See Part I, *Mendelian Inheritance*.

**Age of Detectability:** During the neonatal period. Prenatal detection of intestinal obstruction is possible. The amniotic fluid disaccharidases are deficient when the fetus is affected. Results of low disaccharidase values are best followed by diagnostic ultrasound studies and, when necessary, amniography, for more certain delineation of the defect.

**Gene Mapping and Linkage:** Unknown.

**Prevention:** None known. Genetic counseling indicated.

**Treatment:** Surgical excision of septa with reestablishment of intestinal continuity.

**Prognosis:** Guarded.

**Detection of Carrier:** Unknown.

**Special Considerations:** In all cases of multiple-level intestinal atresia it is very important to keep the possibility of the hereditary type in mind, for proper counseling of the family and for a possible attempt at prenatal diagnosis during future pregnancies.

**References:**
Mishalany HG, Der Kaloustian VM: Familial multiple-level intestinal atresia: report of two siblings. J Pediatr 1971; 79:124 only.
Guttman FM, et al.: Multiple atresias and a new syndrome of hereditary multiple atresias involving the gastrointestinal tract from stomach to rectum. J Pediatr Surg 1973; 8:633–640.
Dallaire L, Perreault G: Hereditary multiple intestinal atresia: the clinical delineation of birth defects, XVI urinary system and others. Baltimore: Williams & Wilkins, 1974:259–264.
Milunsky A: Diagnosis of fetal abnormalities by ultrasound. In: Milunsky A, ed: Genetic disorders and the fetus, New York: Plenum, 1979:321–330.
Morin PR, et al.: Prenatal detection of intestinal obstruction: deficient amniotic fluid disaccharidases in affected fetuses. Clin Genet 1980; 18:217–222.
Blackburn WR, et al.: The familial intestinal poly-atresia syndrome. Proc Greenwood Genet Center 1983; 2:122–123.
Hauschild R: Familiäere Dunndarmatresie: genetik und humangenetische Beratung. Pediatr Grenzgeb 1983; 22:271–275.

DE030                          **Vazken M. Der Kaloustian**
MI039                              **Henry G. Mishalany**

## INTESTINAL DUPLICATION 0532

**Includes:**

Duplication of colon, external genitalia and lower urinary tract

Enteric cysts

Enterogenous cysts

Esophageal duplication (mediastinal cyst of foregut origin)

Neuroenteric cysts

Stomach-duodenum-small intestine-rectum, duplication of

**Excludes:**

Bronchogenic cysts

Bronchopulmonary foregut with gastric/esophageal communication

Esophageal cysts

Mesenteric or omental cysts

Other forms of mediastinal cysts of foregut origin

**Major Diagnostic Criteria:** Demonstration of cystic or communicating duplication of any intestinal structure. X-ray often leads to a presumptive diagnosis. Confirmation is surgical and by histopathology. There are two types of gastrointestinal duplications. One type is the completely enclosed or non-communicating form of duplication or cystic or spherical type. The other type is the communicating or cylindrical type. True duplications must contain gastrointestinal mucosa, but considerable heterotopia occurs.

**Clinical Findings:** Esophageal duplications present as posterior mediastinal masses which often produce dysphagia, dyspnea and chest pain. They may be seen on plain chest X-ray as a posterior mediastinal mass, often associated with vertebral anomalies. Intra-abdominal duplications most often present as a mass in the right lower quadrant. Abdominal pain, intestinal obstruction, perforation with peritonitis and failure to thrive are other common presentations.

Intra-abdominal duplications may be difficult to diagnose. Barium contrast studies, ultrasound, computerized tomography and nuclear magnetic resonance imaging are useful. Hemorrhage into the gastrointestinal tract may occur with communicating duplications which contain gastric mucosa and become ulcerated.

**Complications:** Gastrointestinal obstruction, hemorrhage, small bowel contamination syndrome, malabsorbtion, growth failure, meningitis (when communication with the central nervous system exists), torsion with mid-gut volvulus, perforation, and respiratory complications.

**Associated Findings:** Scoliosis and other vertebral abnormalities.

**Etiology:** Unknown.

**Pathogenesis:** There is support for several theories regarding the formation of intestinal duplication. Incomplete fission of the neuroenteric canal in early organogenesis could lead to duplications; a theory particularly applicable when communication between duplications and the central nervous system exists. Defective recanalization of the intestine later in gestation is the most commonly held theory for the pathogenesis of most duplications. Non-communicating diverticulae (intestinal cysts) often enlarge progressively because of secretion by the epithelial lining. Duplications often contain gastric mucosa capable of producing hydrochloric acid, which can produce ulceration of adjacent mucosa.

**CDC No.:** 751.810

**Sex Ratio:** M1:F1

**Occurrence:** 1:40,000–100,000 live births.

**Risk of Recurrence for Patient's Sib:** Unknown.

**Risk of Recurrence for Patient's Child:** Unknown.

**Age of Detectability:** Often in the newborn period or early infancy, but sometimes in older children or adults.

**Gene Mapping and Linkage:** Unknown.

**Prevention:** None known. Genetic counseling indicated.

**Treatment:** Treatment of esophageal duplications is surgical removal by easy separation of the cyst from the esophagus. Treatment of intra-abdominal duplications are divided into 1) simple excision and intestinal anastamosis in the smaller spherical type lesions; 2) simple excision of a rectal duplication; 3) marsupialization or internal drainage of a duodenal lesion; 4) excision of the common wall in the tubular type, especially near the terminal end of the duplication; and 5) mucosal stripping of the duplication when gastric mucosa is present. This latter procedure is preferred in extensive duplications rather than major bowel resections.

**Prognosis:** With treatment, no reduction of life span or function.

**Detection of Carrier:** Unknown.

**References:**

Holder T, Ashcraft K: Pediatric surgery. Philadelphia: W.B. Saunders, 1980.

Welsh K, et al.: Pediatric surgery, 4th ed. Chicago: Yearbook Medical Publishers, 1986.

BE049                                                    **Arthur S. Besser**

## INTESTINAL ENTEROKINASE DEFICIENCY 0533

**Includes:**

Enterokinase deficiency, primary

Enteropeptidase deficiency

**Excludes:**

Enterokinase deficiency, secondary

Pancreatic exocrine insufficiency, generalized

**Trypsinogen deficiency** (0973)

**Major Diagnostic Criteria:** Diarrhea and failure to thrive begin in early infancy. Normal small bowel histology with decreased enterokinase activity is diagnostic of primary enterokinase deficiency.

**Clinical Findings:** Patients present from early infancy with diarrhea (100%) and failure to thrive (100%). They will be found to excrete large amounts of fecal nitrogen. As a result of a negative nitrogen balance, hypoproteinemia and edema are usually apparent. Malnutrition may also result in failure of synthesis of pancreatic lipase and amylase, as well as intestinal disaccharidases, leading to generalized malabsorption of all nutrients. Steatorrhea and carbohydrate intolerance are clinically evident in this circumstance.

**Complications:** Protein malabsorption; malnutrition; failure to thrive (poor weight gain and short stature); hypoproteinemia; generalized pancreatic exocrine dysfunction secondary to malnutrition; intestinal disaccharidase deficiency secondary to malnutrition; and generalized malabsorption.

**Associated Findings:** Short stature.

**Etiology:** The finding of this abnormality in sibs, the offspring of unaffected parents, suggests possible autosomal recessive inheritance.

**Pathogenesis:** The pancreatic peptidases, trypsin, chymotrypsin, carboxypeptidase, and elastase, are secreted as proenzymes that require activation within the intestinal lumen. The peptidopeptidase of intestinal origin that initiates pancreatic propeptidase activation is enterokinase. In the absence of enterokinase, the rate of conversion of trypsinogen to trypsin is subnormal, resulting in concentrations of trypsin that are inadequate for protein hydrolysis, including activation of chymotrypsinogen, procarboxypeptidase, and proelastase. Lipase and amylase are secreted as functional enzymes not requiring activation. They are of normal activity in the patient with enterokinase deficiency.

**MIM No.:** *22620

**CDC No.:** 751.880

**Sex Ratio:** M1:F1

**Occurrence:** Less than a dozen cases have been reported.

**Risk of Recurrence for Patient's Sib:** Unknown.

**Risk of Recurrence for Patient's Child:** Unknown.

**Age of Detectability:** Early infancy.

**Gene Mapping and Linkage:** Unknown.

**Prevention:** None known. Genetic counseling indicated.

**Treatment:** Orally administered enterokinase or pancreatic extract normalizes intestinal function.

**Prognosis:** Excellent. Most patients have continued short stature, apparently from early severe malnutrition.

**Detection of Carrier:** Unknown.

**Special Considerations:** Study of pancreatic exocrine function is also diagnostic. In baseline and secretin-stimulated samples of duodenal aspirate, trypsinogen levels will be normal, but trypsin will be of low or absent activity. Trypsinogen may be activated to trypsin by incubation with enterokinase or trypsin (16-hour incubation at 4° C results in activation in some patients). The patient's duodenal fluid will have normal tryptic activity after incubation. Enterokinase activity may also be assayed by measuring the hydrolysis of artificial substrates (most recently gly-(Asp)$_4$-Lys-2 naphthylamide) after differentially inhibiting trypsin activity.

Histologic exam should also be performed since some patients with abnormal small bowel mucosa will have low levels of enterokinase activity.

The malnourished patient may have subnormal secretion of all pancreatic enzymes. Therefore, it is necessary to attain a state of adequate nutrition before pancreatic function studies are completed.

### References:

Tarlow MJ, et al.: Intestinal enterokinase deficiency: a newly recognized disorder of protein digestion. Arch Dis Child 1970; 45:651–655.

Haworth JC, et al.: Intestinal enterokinase deficiency occurrence in two sibs and age dependency of the clinical expression. Arch Dis Child 1975; 50:277–282.

Follett GF, MacDonald TH: Intestinal enterokinase deficiency. Acta Paediatr Scand 1976; 65:653–656.

Grant DAW, Hermon-Taylor J: Hydrolysis of artificial substrates by enterokinase and trypsin and the development of a sensitive specific assay for enterokinase in serum. Biochim Biophys Acta 1979; 567: 207.

Ghishan FK, et al.: Isolated congenital enterokinase deficiency: recent finding and a review of the literature. Gastroenterology 1983; 85:727–731.

WH007                                            **Peter F. Whitington**

---

## INTESTINAL HYPOPERISTALSIS, MEGACYSTIS-MICROCOLON TYPE                    2317

**Includes:**
   Berdon syndrome
   Megacystis-microcolon-intestinal hypoperistalsis syndrome
      (MMIHS)

**Excludes:**
   **Colon, aganglionosis** (0192)
   **Colon, duplication** (0194)
   **Intestinal atresia or stenosis** (0531)
   **Megacystis-megaduodenum syndrome** (2316)
   **Stomach, pyloric atresia** (0910)

**Major Diagnostic Criteria:** Megacystis, dilated small bowel, microcolon, and decreased or absent peristalsis with ganglion cells present.

**Clinical Findings:** Polyhydramnios occurs in approximately 25% of the cases. Length of gestation is usually term, and birth weight is within normal limits. Notable abdominal distention is present in the neonatal period. Vomiting is frequently encountered and is often with bile. Anatomic (organic) stenosis is absent. Ischemia of the bowel has been reported in a few cases. The proximal small bowel is usually dilated. Microcolon is a consistent finding. It may be malrotated and positioned entirely on the left side. Malfixation of the midgut occurs frequently, but volvulus is rare. Partial or complete absence of intestinal peristalsis, which is largely resis-

tant to treatment, is a constant finding. Reverse peristalsis has been demonstrated in some patients by retrograde passage of contrast medium.

The combined bowel length is frequently shortened to one-third of normal. Intestinal biopsies show mature ganglion cells in dilated and narrow segments of the intestine. Some patients have areas where the ganglion cells are absent or shrunken along with normal ganglion cells. Several patients have increased nerve fibers and mature ganglion cells. X-rays may show dilated air-filled, small intestine loops. The colon and/or rectum may not show gas. A ground glass appearance of the abdomen has been reported. The bladder is enlarged, frequently flaccid with thick walls, and without evidence of obstruction. As much as 700 ml of urine has been recovered by catheterization (usual amount 350–500 ml). Decompression of the bladder may relieve abdominal distention and result in a "prune belly" appearance. One-half of the cases had hydronephrosis. Seventy-five percent had tortuous, dilated ureters. Most did not have vesicoureteral reflux. After bladder drainage, the ureters returned to normal in three patients. Death usually occurs within the first year. There is a report of one person who has survived into adolescence.

**Complications:** Septicemia has been reported as the cause of death in several infants.

**Associated Findings:** The abdominal wall musculature in a few patients has been found to be thin and/or flaccid. A small **omphalocele** was present in two female infants. One patient was reported to have mild webbing of the neck. Cytogenetic studies were not mentioned in these reports. Another patient had an intra-abdominal testis, grade III/VI systolic ejection murmur and grade II/VI diastolic murmur of no clinical significance.

**Etiology:** Almost all cases have been sporadic. Autosomal recessive inheritance has been implied by one report of affected siblings. Another affected female had two healthy siblings and a sibling who died of "intestinal obstruction" at four days of age. An autopsy was not performed. The parents of another affected female were first cousins.

**Pathogenesis:** Prenatal transient anatomical and/or functional urinary tract obstruction has been considered. A female with a urachal remnant had two healthy brothers and a brother with **Prune-belly syndrome**. This report and intra-abdoninal testis in a reported male suggest a common pathogenesis. On the other hand, intestinal hypoperistalsis is a constant feature of this condition and rare in prune belly syndrome. Their different sex ratios also imply that the conditions are different. There are reports inferring that the urinary tract obstruction in this condition is secondary to the intestinal defect. It is not clear whether this is a primary neuropathy or myopathy.

**MIM No.:** *24921

**POS No.:** 3830

**CDC No.:** 751.880

**Sex Ratio:** M1:F6

**Occurrence:** A few dozen cases have been reported in the literature. Patients have been reported from the United States, Great Britain, Brazil, the Netherlands, India, Israel, Japan, and Polynesia.

**Risk of Recurrence for Patient's Sib:**
   See Part I, *Mendelian Inheritance*. Most cases of this usually fatal disorder have been sporadic, implying a low risk of recurrence. Two affected siblings and a consanguineous family suggests autosomal recessive inheritance.

**Risk of Recurrence for Patient's Child:**
   See Part I, *Mendelian Inheritance*. No patient is known to have reproduced.

**Age of Detectability:** May be suspected prenatally by sonographic evidence of cystic abdominal mass in the fetus. Involvement is readily apparent after birth.

**Gene Mapping and Linkage:** Unknown.

**Prevention:** None known. Genetic counseling indicated.

**Treatment:** Palliative surgery. Hyperalimentation is required. Parasympathomimetics, synthetic gastrointestinal stimulants, adrenergic blockers, and multiple gastrointestinal hormones have not been effective in inducing adequate bowel function. A cholinergic drug, bethanechol, did improve the peristalsis in one patient.

**Prognosis:** Poor; partial function of the urinary tract may appear after bladder drainage. The intestinal dysfunction does not appear to be amenable to treatment.

**Detection of Carrier:** Unknown.

**Special Considerations:** Megacystis is usually associated with oligohydramnios. The presence of polyhydramnios in 25% of the pregnancies with an affected fetus is probably due to the intestinal dysfunction. Prenatal volvulus could mimic this condition, while a normal bladder would exclude the diagnosis.

A manometric study of an affected infant documented a marked reduction of the number of total contractions of the stomach and duodenum. The mean amplitude of the contractions was notably diminished when compared to age-matched controls. Rhythmic contractions (type III) showed decreased amplitude and frequency. The findings in the smooth muscle layer are similar to those in **Megacystis-megaduodenum syndrome** (MMS). The gastrointestinal effects usually become evident in late childhood or early adolescence. It may be present neonatally. Megacystis and hydronephrosis may occur in MMS at varying ages. It has been suggested, however, that MMIHS and MMS are part of a spectrum, with the former representing the most severe manifestation.

**References:**

Berdon WE, et al.: Megacystis-microcolon-intestinal hypoperistalsis syndrome: a new cause of intestinal obstruction in the newborn: report of radiologic findings in five newborn girls. Am J Roentgenol Rad Ther Nucl Med 1976; 126:957–964.

Nelson LH, Reiff RH: Megacystis-microcolon-hypoperistalsis syndrome and anechoic areas in the fetal abdomen. Am J Obstet Gynecol 1982; 144:464–467.

Oliveira G, et al.: Megacystis-microcolon-intestinal hypoperistalsis syndrome in a newborn girl whose brother had prune belly syndrome: common pathogenesis? Pediatr Radiol 1983; 13:294–296.

Puri P, et al.: Megacystis-microcolon-intestinal hypoperistalsis syndrome: a visceral myopathy. J Ped Surg 1983; 18:64–69.

Redman JF, et al.: Megacystis-microcolon-intestinal hypoperistalsis syndrome: case report and review of the literature. J Urol 1984; 131:981–983.

Tomomasa T, et al.: Manometric study on the intestinal motility in a case of megacystis-microcolon-intestinal hypoperistalsis syndrome. J Pediatr Gastroenterol Nutr 1985; 4:307–310.

Winter RM, Knowles SAS: Megacystis-microcolon-intestinal hypoperistalsis syndrome: confirmation of autosomal recessive inheritance. J Med Genet 1986; 23:360–362.

HA069                 **James K. Hartsfield, Jr.**

## INTESTINAL ILEUS, ISOLATED MECONIUM ILEUS      0545

**Includes:**
Ileus, isolated meconium
Meconium ileus, isolated

**Excludes: Cystic fibrosis** (0237)

**Major Diagnostic Criteria:** Intestinal obstruction in a child with no evidence of cystic fibrosis but with X-rays and operative findings consistent with inspissated meconium.

**Clinical Findings:** Abdominal distention, bilious vomiting, and failure to pass meconium in neonates. Microcolon and terminal ileum obstructed by inspissated, sticky meconium.

**Complications:** Intestinal obstruction, perforation and meconium peritonitis.

**Associated Findings:** Microcolon, **Biliary atresia**, and **Niemann-Pick disease**.

**Etiology:** Unknown.

**Pathogenesis:** Presumed to be an abnormal form of meconium.

**CDC No.:** 759.870

**Sex Ratio:** M1:F1

**Occurrence:** Estimated 1:50,000 live births; five percent of all cases of meconium ileus.

**Risk of Recurrence for Patient's Sib:** Unknown.

**Risk of Recurrence for Patient's Child:** Unknown.

**Age of Detectability:** Prenatal ultrasonography shows multiple loops of distended bowel and calcification in fetal abdomen. At birth by X-ray and physical examination.

**Gene Mapping and Linkage:** Unknown.

**Prevention:** None known. Genetic counseling indicated.

**Treatment:** Gastrografin enemas or surgery with normal saline irrigations. Resection of bowel for perforation with some type of exteriorization.

**Prognosis:** Survival near 100% with appropriate treatment; no long-term consequences anticipated.

**Detection of Carrier:** Unknown.

**References:**

Olsen MM, et al.: The spectrum of meconium disease in infancy. J Pediatr Surg 1982; 17:479–481.

Carty H, Brereton RJ: The distended neonate. Clin Radiol 1983; 34:367–380.

Ein SH, et al.: Ileocaecal atresia. J Pediatr Surg 1985; 20:525–528.

Ein SH, et al.: Bowel perforation with nonoperative treatment of meconium ileus. J Pediatr Surg 1987; 22:146–147.

Goldstein RB, et al.; Sonographic diagnosis of meconium ileus in utero. J Ultrasoun Med 1987; 6:663–666.

Zamir O, et al.; Gastrointestinal perforations in the neonatal period. Am J Perinatol 1988; 5:131–133.

SE006                 **John H. Seashore**

## INTESTINAL LYMPHANGIECTASIA      0534

**Includes:**
Lymphangiectasia, intestinal
Protein-losing enteropathy with dilated intestinal lymphatics

**Excludes:**
**Lymphedema I** (0614)
**Lymphedema II** (0615)
Mesenteric neoplasms
Protein-losing enteropathy secondary to congestive heart failure

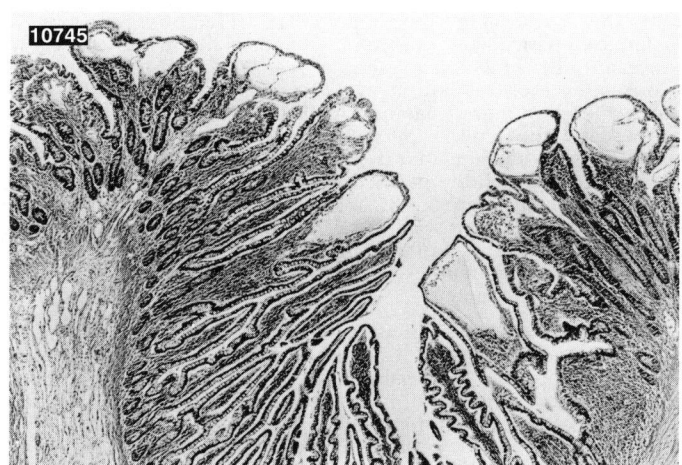

**0534**-10745: Intestinal biopsy; dilated lymphatic channels are present in mucosa and lamina propria.

Protein-losing enteropathy without dilated lymphatic channels
Whipple syndrome

**Major Diagnostic Criteria:** Dilated lymphatic channels of the small bowel, as demonstrated by peroral biopsy or laparotomy, is the hallmark morphologic lesion of this disorder and is required for its diagnosis.

The direct demonstration of gastrointestinal (GI) protein loss, hypoalbuminemia, hypogammaglobulinemia, lymphocytopenia, and generalized edema are also important diagnostic features. This syndrome should be differentiated from disorders in which the hypoproteinemia is secondary to decreased protein synthesis, or to accelerated endogenous protein catabolism by direct demonstration of excessive GI protein loss. The diagnosis can be made by determining the intestinal clearance of $\alpha$1-antitrypsin or by demonstrating increased fecal excretion of intravenously administered radiolabeled macromolecules such as $^{51}$Cr labeled serum proteins, $^{59}$Fe dextran, $^{95}$Nb albumin, or $^{131}$I PVP.

Other causes of protein-losing enteropathy with disorders of intestinal lymphatic channels, such as severe congestive heart failure, Whipple syndrome, or mesenteric malignancy, retroperitoneal fibrosis, and inflammatory processes should be ruled out.

**Clinical Findings:** Patients with intestinal lymphangiectasia have a generalized disorder of development of lymphatic channels with grossly dilated lymphatic vessels in the lamina propria of the small bowel demonstrable in all cases. The patients have edema that may be asymmetric (15%), and that may involve the macula, producing reversible blindness (7%). Chylous effusion is present at the onset or develops during the course of the disease in 45% of the patients. All patients have significant excessive loss of serum proteins into the GI tract through the disordered lymphatic channels. They have hypoalbuminemia (100%) and a marked reduction of IgG (97%). A significant but less marked reduction in the concentration of fibrinogen (30%), transferrin (50%), IgM (40%), and IgA (70%) is noted in many patients.

GI symptoms are usually mild, but may on occasion be entirely absent or severe. Diarrhea and steatorrhea (mild 60%, severe 20%), vomiting (15%), and abdominal pain (15%) are present in these patients. Carbohydrate absorption tests, including glucose, xylose, and lactose tolerance tests, are within normal limits in most of the patients studied. X-rays of the GI tract are completely negative in 20% of the patients. They show mild mucosal edema of the small bowel in 70% of the patients, and show significant segmentation and puddling of the barium in the remaining 10% of the patients. On biopsy of the small bowel, a dilatation of the lymphatic vessels of the lamina propria, the hallmark morphologic lesion of the disease, is revealed. Hypocalcemia and in some cases hypomagnesemia and tetany are present in 12% of the patients and are most common in those patients with steatorrhea. It is thought to be associated with malabsorption or loss of calcium into the GI tract. Lymphocytopenia (mean lymphocyte count 700 compared with 2400 in controls), secondary to the loss of lymphocytes into the bowel, is present in over 90% of the patients. As a consequence of this lymphocytopenia, 83% of the patients show skin anergy and are unable to manifest delayed hypersensitivity responses (tuberculin-type responses), and are unable to reject skin grafts from unrelated donors.

Less frequent findings include anemia and reduction in the serum concentration of fat soluble vitamins and $B_{12}$. Growth retardation (linear growth below 3rd%) is present in the majority of children with onset of edema and diarrhea within the first five years of life. It may be extreme in those patients with associated severe malabsorption.

**Complications:** Tuberculous infections and reticuloendothelial malignancies develop in 3–5% of the cases, possibly due to the lymphocytopenia and inability to make cellular immune responses. Chronic respiratory diseases (5–10%) associated with the disorder of delayed hypersensitivity and with abnormalities of lymphatics of the lungs. Intestinal obstruction due to adhesions occur especially in those patients with chylous ascites. Deficiency of fat-soluble vitamins, including vitamin K (20%), may cause hypoprothrombinemia.

**Associated Findings:** **Glaucoma, congenital** (3 in 75 cases); Peliosis hepatitis (2); Charcot-Marie-Tooth syndrome (2); **Heart, tetralogy of Fallot** (1); **Noonan syndrome** (2); **Hypobetalipoproteinemia** (2); and selective IgA deficiency (see **Immunoglobulin A deficiency**) (1).

**Etiology:** Possibly autosomal dominant inheritance. The majority of cases (over 75%) are, however, sporadic.

**Pathogenesis:** The basic defect appears to be a generalized disorder in lymphatic channel development with the most obvious disorder affecting small bowel lymphatics. As a consequence, serum proteins, lymphocytes, as well as lipids, iron, copper, and calcium are lost into the GI lumen. Hypoproteinemia results when the rate of protein loss and catabolism exceeds the body's capacity to synthesize the protein. The edema and effusions are due both to the extreme hypoproteinemia, and the generalized disorder of lymphatic channels. The abnormalities of the *in vivo* cellular (tuberculin-type) responses and the increased incidence in tuberculosis and reticuloendothelial neoplasms appear to be secondary to the lymphocytopenia that results from the loss of lymphocytes into the GI tract.

The hypocalcemia and malabsorption are due to an abnormality of absorption from the bowel, as well as loss of fat and calcium by direct loss of lymph into the bowel.

**MIM No.:** *15280

**CDC No.:** 751.880

**Sex Ratio:** M1:F1.34 (observed).

**Occurrence:** Approximately 300 cases have been reported; in Black, Oriental and Caucasian races.

**Risk of Recurrence for Patient's Sib:**
See Part I, *Mendelian Inheritance.* Most cases are sporadic.

**Risk of Recurrence for Patient's Child:**
See Part I, *Mendelian Inheritance.* Four cases of lymphedema in an offspring or parent of the proband have been reported. Otherwise, there are no reports of an affected individual in two generations. The patients have reproduced, although those patients with chylous ascites, or malabsorption and vitamin deficiency, may have reduced fertility.

**Age of Detectability:** Generalized edema, chylous effusions, asymmetric edema, diarrhea, or hypocalcemia may be the presenting symptom and is first detected at birth or in the first few weeks of life in 25% of the patients. In the remaining patients, the age of onset ranges to young adult life with, a mean age of onset of 10 years.

**Gene Mapping and Linkage:** Unknown.

**Prevention:** None known. Genetic counseling indicated.

**Treatment:** A very low-fat diet, or a diet in which medium-chain triglycerides are used in lieu of long-chain triglycerides, has been effective in significantly decreasing the hypoproteinemia, GI protein loss, edema, and diarrhea in approximately 50% of the patients. Such therapy has been of value in increasing the growth rate in children. In 5–10% of the cases, resection of a localized area of intestinal lymphangiectasia results in amelioration of the symptoms. There has been a reversal of the protein-losing enteropathy following corticosteroid therapy in some cases.

Diuretics are useful in reducing edema and effusions as well as in reversing blindness in the cases with macular edema. Other therapy, such as surgical relief of intestinal obstruction, or ligation of thoracic duct in patients with isolated chylothorax, may be indicated.

**Prognosis:** Life expectancy is somewhat shortened. In infancy, death may be related to extreme malabsorption, intestinal obstruction, or infections, especially in debilitated patients. Many cases, especially those with late onset, may be stable over periods from two to more than 40 years. No effect upon intelligence. Approximately 30% of the patients are unable to work because of extreme fatigue and weakness associated with the hypoproteinemia.

**Detection of Carrier:** Unknown.

**Special Considerations:** It should be emphasized that the primary features of this disorder, including edema, excessive GI protein loss, lymphocytopenia, and dilated lymphatics of the small intestine, may be seen in patients with Whipple syndrome, mesenteric tumors, or cardiac disorders, especially constrictive pericarditis. Significant care should be taken to rule out congestive failure in all patients with a tentative diagnosis of intestinal lymphangiectasia. The disorders of lymphocyte and protein metabolism are completely reversible in such patients when successful surgical or medical therapy of the cardiac disease is possible. In addition, corticosteroid therapy of patients with intestinal lymphangiectasia secondary to an inflammatory process may lead to remission of the protein losing enteropathy. It should be noted that patients with intestinal lymphangiectasia have skin anergy, and thus skin tests, such as the tuberculin skin test, cannot be used in the diagnosis of such chronic infectious disorders.

**References:**
Waldmann TA, et al.: The role of the gastrointestinal system in ''idiopathic hypoproteinemia.'' Gastroenterology 1961; 41:197–207.
Jeffries GH, et al.: Low-fat diet in intestinal lymphangiectasia: its effect on albumin metabolism. N Engl J Med 1964; 270:761–766.
Waldmann TA: Protein-losing enteropathy. Gastroenterology 1966; 50:422–443.
Murphy EA: Familial lymphatic dysplasia with intestinal lymphangiectasia. The clinical delineation of birth defects. BDOAS XIII. G.I. tract including liver and pancreas. Baltimore: Williams & Wilkins, 1972:180–181.
Weiden PL, et al.: Impaired lymphocyte transformation in intestinal lymphangiectasia: evidence for at least two functionally distinct lymphocyte populations in man. J Clin Invest 1972; 51:1319–1325.
Waldman TA: Protein-losing gastroenteropathies. In: Berk J, ed: Gastroenterology, vol. 3. Philadelphia: W.B. Saunders, 1985:1814–1834. *

WA007                                            **Thomas A. Waldmann**

**Intestinal monosaccharide intolerance**
   *See GLUCOSE-GALACTOSE MALABSORPTION*
**Intestinal neurofibromatosis**
   *See NEUROFIBROMATOSIS*
**Intestinal polyatresia syndrome (mucosal or septal variety)**
   *See INTESTINAL ATRESIAS, MULTIPLE*
**Intestinal polyatresia syndrome, familial**
   *See INTESTINAL ATRESIA OR STENOSIS*

---

| **INTESTINAL POLYPOSIS, JUVENILE TYPE** | **2259** |
|---|---|

**Includes:**
   Cystic polyps
   Hamartomatous polyps
   Infantile polyposis
   Inflammatory polyps
   Polyposis coli, juvenile type
   Polyposis, juvenile

**Excludes:**
   Common juvenile retention polyps
   **Intestinal polyposis (all)**

**Major Diagnostic Criteria:**  The presence of any polyps of the histologic type described in patients with a family history, or the occurrence of multiple such cystic polyps in any individual.

**Clinical Findings:**  The most common presenting findings are rectal bleeding (75%), prolapse of a polyp (15%), abdominal pain (15%), and diarrhea (9%). The majority of cases present in childhood, although adults are reported. The polyps are fragile and may be passed in the stool. Barium studies or colonoscopy usually reveals multiple pedunculated polyps up to 1cm in diameter in familial cases. Sporadic cases, without a family history of intestinal polyps, are without the associated risks for malignant degeneration and usually have solitary polyps.

The polyps have a smooth, round contour and are not fissured or lobulated, as are adenomatous polyps. On cut section, the polyps have multiple cystic spaces filled with mucin. The predominant histologic feature is increased supporting connective tissue, which contains cystically dilated tubules lined by normal epithelium. No muscularis mucosa is involved in the polyp stalk. Numerous inflammatory cells may be present. In some patients,

juvenile polyps with areas of focal adenomatous changes or carcinoma in situ have been identified.

The polyps may be distributed throughout the stomach, small intestine, and colon, although they are most frequently colonic.

**Complications:**  Thirteen of the 17 families reported through 1985 had some incidence of gastrointestinal, usually but not exclusively, colonic carcinoma. In nine families, the diagnosis of colonic cancer was made before 40 years of age. Thus, the risk for gastrointestinal malignancy is extremely great, approaching that of **Intestinal polyposis, type I.** This has been underestimated in the past, since the index cases are identified in childhood, and the malignancy usually occurs in adulthood. Intussusception, severe blood loss, intestinal obstruction, and malabsorption have been reported in children.

**Associated Findings:**  Failure to thrive, anemia, hypoproteinemia, and hypokalemia. Three families have been identified with cosegregation of pulmonary and CNS arteriovenous malformations, indicating a distinct subtype. **Megalencephaly** has been reported in at least two infants.

**Etiology:**  Autosomal dominant inheritance.

**Pathogenesis:**  Some polyps have developed atypical adenomatous features. These may show areas of malignant degeneration. Separate but coexisting adenomas are also reported in older children and adults. Transformation of juvenile polyps into adenomatous polyps has been suggested.

**MIM No.:**  *17490

**CDC No.:**  751.880

**Sex Ratio:**  M1:F1

**Occurrence:**  Seventeen families had been documented in the literature as of 1985.

**Risk of Recurrence for Patient's Sib:**
   See Part I, *Mendelian Inheritance.*

**Risk of Recurrence for Patient's Child:**
   See Part I, *Mendelian Inheritance.*

**Age of Detectability:**  Varies from nine months to adulthood.

**Gene Mapping and Linkage:**  Unknown.

**Prevention:**  None known. Genetic counseling indicated. Periodic colonic, and possibly gastric, examination is suggested for at-risk family members.

**Treatment:**  Excision biopsy of accessible lesions. Partial colectomy has been required for current bleeding or malignant degeneration. May require an early colectomy in infancy. Strong consideration should be given to prophylactic colectomy in early adulthood.

**Prognosis:**  Good, if bleeding is limited and malignant lesions do not develop. If untreated, the condition can be lethal. Polyps may persist into adulthood.

**Detection of Carrier:**  Air contrast barium enema in late childhood is recommended for at-risk family members.

**Special Considerations:**  Children without a family history of intestinal polyposis or intestinal cancer may frequently have solitary juvenile colonic polyps. These sporadic cases appear to lack the significant potential for GI malignancy that is present in familial cases or in individuals with many (>10) juvenile polyps.

**Support Groups:**  OH; Cleveland; Familial Polyposis Registry

**References:**
McColl I, et al.: Juvenile polyposis coli. Proc R Soc Med 1974; 57:896–897.
Cox KL, et al.: Hereditary generalized juvenile polyposis associated with pulmonary arteriovenous malformations. Gastroenterology 1980; 78:1566–1570.
Conte WJ, et al.: Juvenile gastrointestinal polyposis and arteriovenous malformations: heterogeneity within juvenile polyposis syndrome and a reassessment of cancer risk. Am J Hum Genet 1982; 34:69A.
Grotsky HW, et al.: Familial juvenile polyposis coli. Gastroenterology 1982; 82:494–501.
Jarvinen H, et al.: Familial juvenile polyposis coli: increased risk of colorectal cancer. Gut 1984; 25:792–800.

Ramaswamy G, et al.: Juvenile polyposis of the colon with atypical adenomatous change and carcinoma in situ. Dis Colon Rectum 1984; 27:393–398.
Grosfeld JL, West KW: Generalized juvenile polyposis coli: clinical management based on long-term observations. Arch Surg 1986; 121:530–534.

C0074
R0036

William J. Conte
Jerome I. Rotter

## INTESTINAL POLYPOSIS, TYPE I      0535

**Includes:**
Colon, familial polyposis
Adenomatous polyposis coli
Adenomatous polyposis, familial
Cancer, intestinal polyposis I
Polyposis, familial

**Excludes:**
Chromosome 5, monosomy 5q interstitial (2544)
Gingival multiple hamartoma syndrome (0412)
Intestinal polyposis, juvenile type (2259)
Intestinal polyposis, type II (2344)
Intestinal polyposis, type III (0536)

**Major Diagnostic Criteria:** The presence of 100 or more adenomatous colorectal polyps is diagnostic of familial polyposis coli. Fewer polyps or extraintestinal growths, together with a family history, is highly suggestive.

**Clinical Findings:** The great majority of individuals with familial polyposis coli are asymptomatic until colorectal cancer occurs. Adenomatous colorectal polyps begin to appear after age 10 years, with an average age of occurrence of 24.5 years. Although a small number of polyps may be seen early in the disease course, hundreds to many thousands of polyps (average approximately 1,000) are evident by the third or fourth decade. The colonic polyps are usually small (less than 0.5 cm), sessile, or early

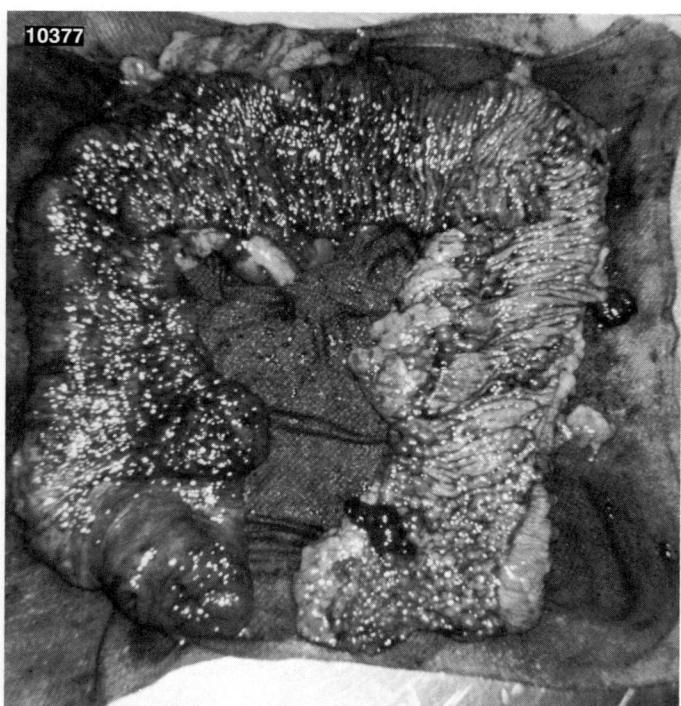

**0535-10377:** Multiple adenomatous polyps in colon specimen.

pedunculated tubular adenomas that "carpet" the colon. Villous histology is occasionally seen in polyps, and a pattern of fewer (scores to hundreds), larger, more pedunculated polyps has been described in many pedigrees.

Symptoms, including rectal bleeding, diarrhea, abdominal pain, and mucous discharge, begin at an average age of 33 years and are often indicative of colorectal cancer. The average age of cancer diagnosis is 39 years. All untreated individuals will eventually develop colorectal cancer.

Recent studies indicate that upper gastrointestinal polyps occur in **Intestinal polyposis, type I** as often as they are found in **Intestinal polyposis, type II**.

**Complications:** Colorectal cancer develops in 100% of untreated patients.

**Associated Findings:** Both desmoids and mesenteric fibromatosis have been reported in patients with familial polyposis coli.

**Etiology:** Autosomal dominant inheritance with complete penetrance.

**Pathogenesis:** Unknown.

**MIM No.:** *17510

**Sex Ratio:** M1:F1

**Occurrence:** 1:8300 births.

**Risk of Recurrence for Patient's Sib:**
See Part I, *Mendelian Inheritance.*

**Risk of Recurrence for Patient's Child:**
See Part I, *Mendelian Inheritance.*

**Age of Detectability:** Variable. Colonic polyposis may be seen in the second half of the first decade, and is often present in the second decade. DNA markers are now sufficiently accurate that highly probable diagnoses can be made at birth.

**Gene Mapping and Linkage:** APC (adenomatosis polyposis coli) has been mapped to 5q21-q22.

There is suggestive evidence that the APC locus regulates *c-myc* expression.

**Prevention:** None known. Genetic counseling indicated.

**Treatment:** Effective treatment depends on identification of affected individuals before cancer develops. Screening fiberoptic endoscopy of the colon should be done yearly, beginning at age 10 years, in all individuals at risk. Because polyps are equally distributed throughout the colon, flexible proctosigmoidoscopy is sufficient for screening. In occasional pedigrees where an excess of proximal colonic polyps and cancer is observed, yearly full colonoscopy may be necessary. Once polyps are detected, full colonoscopy should be performed every 6–12 months. Elective colectomy should be planned at the patient's earliest convienience once colonic polyposis is present. Numerous polyps, larger polyps, or villous histology make surgery more urgent. DNA markers may soon obviate the need for screening any but those with the mutant allele.

The optimal surgery is debated. Total colectomy with ileostomy or "ileoanal pull-through" eliminates the risk of colorectal cancer. Many centers have successfully used subtotal colectomy with careful follow-up for coagulation and removal of recurrent rectal polyps.

Screening intervals and treatment guidelines for upper gastrointestinal polyps are presently being developed. Initial upper GI endoscopy should be done once colonic polyps are detected. This should be repeated every 2–3 years until duodenal adenomatous polyps are found. One to two year examinations should then be done. The occurrance of large polyps or polyps with villous or moderately dysplastic histology should prompt consideration of endoscopic or surgical polyp removal.

Treatment of desmoids and mesenteric fibromatosis is a particular problem, since surgical dissection may stimulate their growth.

**Prognosis:** Good if colorectal cancer is prevented. Survival is somewhat decreased by duodenal cancer, abdominal desmoids and fibromatosis, but complete data are not available.

**Detection of Carrier:** There is no true "carrier" state, as all individuals with the mutant allele will eventually express the phenotype. DNA markers are now sufficiently accurate that highly probable diagnoses can be made at birth.

**Special Considerations:** The distinction from Gardner syndrome (see **Intestinal polyposis, type III**) is unclear. Hypotheses regarding the etiology of the two syndromes have included: 1) different mutations or deletions at the same chromosomal location, 2) variable expression of an identical gene defect, and 3) modifying genes separate from the APC locus.

**Support Groups:** OH; Cleveland; Familial Polyposis Registry

**References:**
Bussey HJR: Familial polyposis coli. Baltimore, Johns Hopkins Univ, Press, 1975. * †
Luk GD, Baylin SB: Ornithine decarboxylase as a biological marker in familial colonic polyposis. New Engl J Med 1984; 311:80–83.
Haggitt RC, Reid BJ: Hereditary gastrointestinal polyposis syndromes. Am J Surg Pathol 1986; 10:871–887. *
Klemmer S, et al.: Occurrence of desmoids in patients with familial adenomatous polyposis of the colon. Am J Med Genet 1987; 28:385–392.
Leppert M, et al.: The gene for familial polyposis coli maps to the long arm of chromosome 5. Science 1987; 238:1411–1413.
Quirke P, et al.: DNA aneuploidy and cell proliferation in familial adenomatous polyposis. Gut 1988; 29:603–607.
Erisman MD, et al.: Evidence that the familial adenomatous polyposis gene involved in a subset of colon cancers with a complementable defect in c-myc regulation. Proc Natl Acad Sci 1989; 86:4264–4268.
Tops CMJ, et al.: Presymptomatic diagnosis of familial adenomatous polyposis by bridging DNA markers. Lancet 1989; II:1361–1363.

BU036                             **Randall W. Burt**

## INTESTINAL POLYPOSIS, TYPE II      2344

**Includes:**
> Peutz-Jeghers syndrome
> Polyposis, intestinal, II

**Excludes:**
> **Gastrocutaneous syndrome** (2981)
> **Gingival fibromatosis-depigmentation-microphthalmia** (0413)
> **Gingival multiple hamartoma syndrome** (0412)
> **Intestinal polyposis, juvenile type** (2259)
> **Intestinal polyposis, type I** (0535)
> **Intestinal polyposis, type III** (0536)

**Major Diagnostic Criteria:** The presence of numerous pigmented spots on the lips and buccal mucosa, together with multiple gastrointestinal hamartomatous polyps, is diagnostic. The histopathology of the polyps is distinctive.

**Clinical Findings:** Abnormal mucocutaneous pigmentation occurs in infancy or childhood. It is described as multiple 1–5 mm melanotic macules which look like dark freckles but are unusual because of their location. They are most frequently seen on the lips and buccal mucosa but also occur on the face, forearms, palms, soles, digits, perianal area, and, rarely, on the intestinal mucosa. The pigmentation on the lips fades with age, making buccal mucosal pigmentation a more reliable finding in adults. Abnormal pigmentation is present in greater than 95% of affected individuals.

The clinically important feature of the disease is the occurrence of multiple hamartomatous polyps throughout the gastrointestinal tract. The polyps are histologically distinctive and vary in size from 1 mm to 4 cm. They occur in the ileum and jejunum in almost all patients, but they are also found in the rectum, colon, stomach, and duodenum. Polyps are rarely found in the nose, bronchi, renal pelvis, ureters, or bladder. Intestinal polyps usually become symptomatic from complications early in the third decade, although these may occur at a younger age. The average age of diagnosis is 22.5 years.

**Complications:** The most frequent complications arise secondary to larger polyps and include intestinal obstruction and intussus-

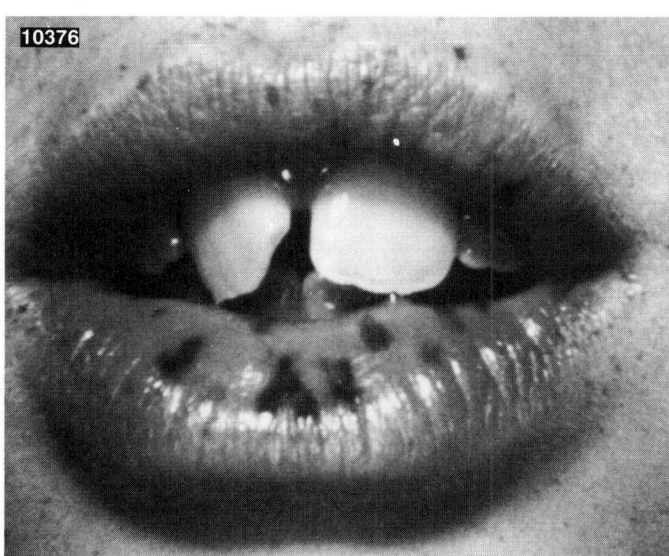

**2344-10376:** Lip pigmentation in intestinal polyposis II.

ception. These complications are heralded by the patient's complaining of severe recurrent colicky abdominal pain. Large polyps also commonly ulcerate and infarct, which results in gastrointestinal blood loss and anemia. Hematemesis may occur from gastric and duodenal polyps.

Recent evidence suggests a 2–13% risk of gastrointestinal cancer. The majority of cancers reported have been present in the stomach or duodenum of patients under the age of 40 years. Cancers also have been reported in the ileum, jejunum, and colon. Concomitant colonic adenomas were seen in the patients with colonic cancer, suggesting that the malignancies arose from these lesions. However, adenomatous change in the epithelium of the hamartomatous polyps has been observed. The estimated frequency of neoplastic change in polyps is 3–6%.

**Associated Findings:** Several extra-intestinal benign and malignant tumors, including breast carcinoma (often bilateral), cervical adenocarcinoma, and benign and malignant ovarian tumors occur. The benign ovarian tumors are "sex cord tumors with annular tubules." These are now considered a phenotypic characteristic of the disease, as they are present in almost all affected females. There is an association with testicular malignancy in males, and pancreatic cancer in both sexes. The overall occurrence of malignancy (gastrointestinal or extra-gastrointestinal) approaches 50%.

**Etiology:** Autosomal dominant inheritance with high penetrance.

**Pathogenesis:** Unknown.

**MIM No.:** *17520

**POS No.:** 3638

**CDC No.:** 759.600

**Sex Ratio:** M1:F1

**Occurrence:** Estimated at 1:120,000 births.

**Risk of Recurrence for Patient's Sib:**
See Part I, *Mendelian Inheritance.*

**Risk of Recurrence for Patient's Child:**
See Part I, *Mendelian Inheritance.*

**Age of Detectability:** Varies from early infancy if pigment spots are present in an individual at risk, to adulthood if melanin spots are absent or family history is not known.

**Gene Mapping and Linkage:** Unknown.

**Prevention:** None known. Genetic counseling indicated. It would be prudent to perform yearly occult stool testing, and flexible proctosigmoidoscopy every 3–5 years, beginning in the second decade, in at-risk individuals who have not developed symptoms. Regular breast and gynecologic screening should also be performed in affected individuals.

**Treatment:** Upper and lower gastrointestinal endoscopy with polypectomy and small bowel X-ray should be performed when any gastrointestinal symptoms develop in an individual who is at risk or who has typical orocutaneous pigmentation. Surgery is indicated for removal of symptomatic small bowel polyps or small bowel polyps larger than 1.5 cm. Intra-operative small bowel endoscopy should be performed when laparotomy becomes necessary, to remove all possible polyps. Upper and lower gastrointestinal endoscopy and small bowel X-ray should be repeated every 2–3 years once the diagnosis is made.

**Prognosis:** One study reported an actuarial survival identical to the general population (Linos et al, 1981), while another found it to be substantially decreased (Utsunomiya et al, 1975). In the latter study, 43% of deaths which occurred prior to age 30 resulted from complications of the polyposis, while 60% of deaths after that age were due to malignancy.

**Detection of Carrier:** Unknown.

**Support Groups:** OH; Cleveland; Familial Polyposis Registry

**References:**
Utsunomiya J, et al.: Peutz-Jeghers syndrome: its natural course and management. Johns Hopkins Med J 1975; 136:71–82. * †
Linos DH, et al.: Does Purtz-Jeghers syndrome predispose to gastrointestinal malignancy? Arch Surg 1981; 116:1182–1184.
Chen KTK: Female genital tract tumors in Peutz-Jeghers syndrome. Hum Pathol 1986; 17:858–861.
van Coevorden F, et al.: Combined endoscopic and surgical treatment in Peutz-Jeghers syndrome. Surg Gynecol Obstet 1986; 162:426–428.
Giardiello FM, et al.: Increased risk of cancer in the Peutz-Jeghers syndrome. New Engl J Med 1987; 316:1511–1514. *
Konishi F, et al.: Peutz-Jeghers polyposis associated with carcinoma of the digestive organs. Dis Colon Rectum 1987; 30:790–799.
Narita T, et al.: Peutz-Jeghers syndrome with adenomas and adenocarcinomas in colonic polyps. Am J Surg Path 1987; 11:76–81.
Foley TR, et al.: Peutz-Jeghers syndrome: a clinicopathologic survey of the "Harrisburg Family" with a 49-year follow-up. Gastroenterology 1988; 95:1535–1540. *

BU036

Randall W. Burt

## INTESTINAL POLYPOSIS, TYPE III  0536

**Includes:**
    Gardner syndrome
    Hallerman-Streiff syndrome
    Oldfield syndrome
    Polyposis, Gardner type

**Excludes:**
    Cancer, sebaceous gland tumor-mulitple visceral carcinoma (2743)
    Gastrocutaneous syndrome (2981)
    Gingival fibromatosis-depigmentation-microphthalmia (0413)
    Intestinal polyposis, juvenile type (2259)
    Intestinal polyposis, type I (0535)
    Intestinal polyposis, type II (2344)
    Turcot syndrome (2739)

**Major Diagnostic Criteria:** One hundred or more adenomatous colorectal polyps with extra-intestinal growths described below is diagnostic of Gardner syndrome. Fewer polyps or extraintestinal growths, together with a family history, is highly suggestive.

**Clinical Findings:** The colorectal polyposis and cancer occurrence in this disease is virtually identical to that in **Intestinal polyposis, type I**, except for a possible colonic pattern of fewer and larger polyps. The pattern of colonic polyp growth tends to be similar in individuals from the same pedigree.

In addition to colonic polyposis and cancer, individuals with this syndrome exhibit numerous benign extraintestinal growths.

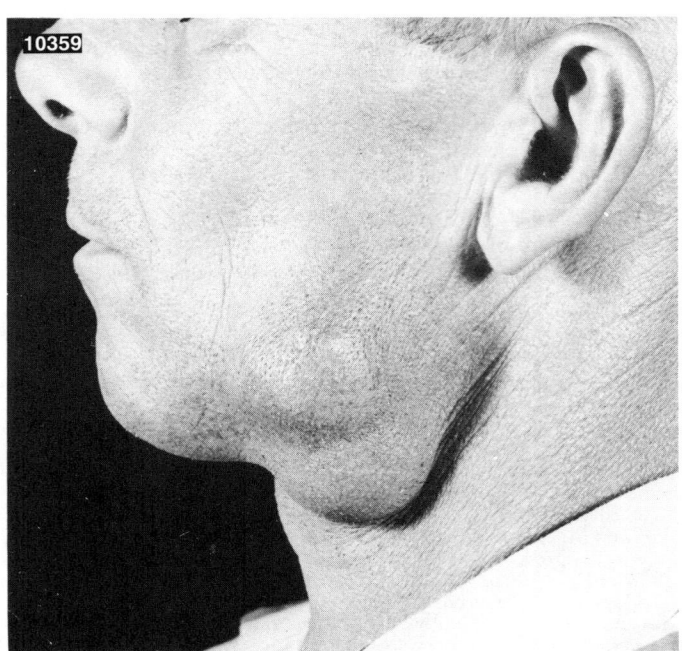

0536A-10359:  Osteoma of mandible.

These include osteomas, soft tissue tumors, and dental abnormalities. Osteomas are more commonly observed on the mandible and skull, but may occur on any bone. Soft tissue tumors include epidermoid cysts, sebaceous cysts, fibromas, and lipomas. Supernumerary teeth, unerupted teeth, and odontomas are the most common dental growth defects. The frequency of these benign growths is extremely variable, but usually consistent within a given pedigree. Members of some pedigrees exhibit most or all of

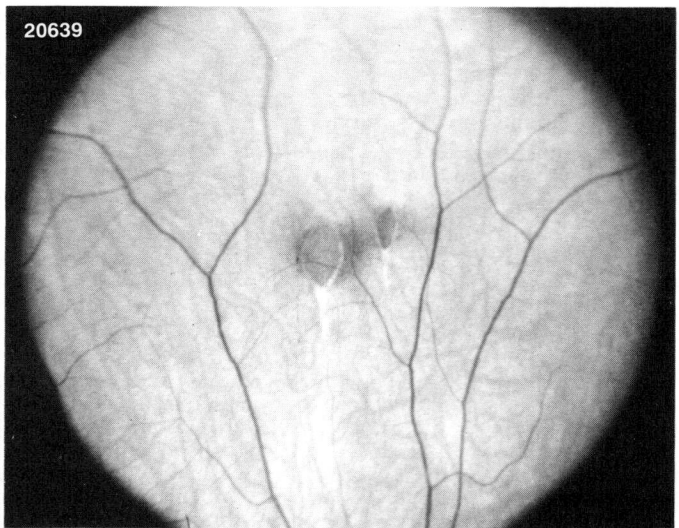

0536B-20639:  Intestinal polyposis, Gardner type. Two of a number of brown-black patches of congenital hypertrophy of the retinal pigment epithelium occurring in both eyes of a young male with Gardner Syndrome. The "snow shoe" or "comet-tail" points towards the posterior pole of the eye.

the growths, while only occasional benign lesions are observed in members of other pedigrees. The extraintestinal growths may occur years before colonic polyps are apparent.

Ocular features, particularly of the retina (see **Retina, congenital hypertrophy of retinal pigment epithelium** (CHRPE)) are very helpful in making this diagnosis. CHRPE is pedigree-specific, but is found in virtually all affected individuals in pedigrees in which it is present.

Dermoid tumors and mesenteric fibromatosis are frequent problems (up to 50% of the individuals in some pedigrees). Desmoids often occur postsurgically in the anterior abdominal wall, but may be seen prior to surgery and may occur in musculoaponeurotic structures throughout the body.

Gastric, duodenal, and small bowel polyps are a frequent finding. Gastric polyps are numerous small (1–5 mm) sessile hyperplastic polyps of the proximal stomach. They have little or no malignant potential, and occur in up to 50% of cases. Duodenal polyps are seen as numerous 1–5 mm adenomatous polyps and occur in up to 90% of patients. These appear to have some malignant potential, since duodenal cancer occurs in 3–12% of cases. Adenomatous polyps occasionally occur elsewhere in the small bowel, especially the terminal ileum, although cancer is rare outside of the duodenum. Upper gastrointestinal polyps seldom cause symptoms.

**Complications:** Colorectal cancer develops in all untreated patients at a relatively young age. Problems with extraintestinal manifestations are mainly cosmetic. Although desmoid tumors and mesenteric fibromatosis are benign, they may cause intestinal obstruction, and obstruction or compression of any adjacent structure.

**Associated Findings:** Cancers of many sites have been reported. The associations are probably coincidental, except for duodenal cancer, central nervous system cancer (see **Turcot syndrome**), and thyroid carcinoma.

**Etiology:** Autosomal dominant inheritance with virtually 100% penetrance. The frequency of extraintestinal manifestations is variable, but usually consistent within a pedigree.

**Pathogenesis:** Unknown.

**MIM No.:** *17530

**POS No.:** 3766

**CDC No.:** 759.630

**Sex Ratio:** M1:F1

**Occurrence:** 1:14,025 births.

**Risk of Recurrence for Patient's Sib:**
See Part I, *Mendelian Inheritance.*

**Risk of Recurrence for Patient's Child:**
See Part I, *Mendelian Inheritance.*

**Age of Detectability:** Colonic polyposis may be seen in the second half of the first decade, and is often present in the second decade. Extraintestinal manifestations are sometimes observed in the first few years of life. DNA markers are now sufficiently accurate that highly probable diagnoses can be made at birth.

**Gene Mapping and Linkage:** APC (adenomatosis polyposis coli) has been mapped to 5q21-q22.
Gardner syndrome shares the APC locus.

**Prevention:** None known. Genetic counseling indicated.

**Treatment:** Effective treatment depends upon identification of affected individuals before cancer develops. Screening fiberoptic endoscopy of the colon should be done yearly, beginning at ten years of age, in all individuals at risk. Because polyps are equally distributed throughout the colon, yearly flexible proctosigmoidoscopy is sufficient. In occasional pedigrees, where an excess of proximal colonic polyps and cancer is observed, yearly colonoscopy may be necessary. Once polyps are detected, full colonoscopy should be performed every 6–12 months. Elective colectomy should be planned at the patient's earliest convenience once colonic polyposis is present. Numerous polyps, larger polyps, or villous histology make surgery more urgent. DNA markers may

soon obviate the need for screening any but those with the mutant allele.

The optimal surgery is debated. Total colectomy with ileostomy or "ileoanal pull-through" eliminates the risk of colorectal cancer. Many centers have successfully used subtotal colectomy with careful follow-up for coagulation and removal of recurrent rectal polyps.

Screening intervals and treatment guidelines for upper gastrointestinal polyps are presently being developed. Initial upper GI endoscopy should be done once colonic polyps are detected. This should be repeated every 2–3 years until duodenal adenomatous polyps are found. One to two year examinations should then be done. The occurrence of large polyps or polyps with villous or moderately dysplastic histology should prompt consideration of endoscopic or surgical polyp removal.

Treatment of extraintestinal growths is cosmetic and symptomatic. Desmoids and mesenteric fibromatosis are particular problems, since surgical dissection may stimulate their growth.

**Prognosis:** Good if colorectal cancer is prevented. Survival is somewhat decreased by duodenal cancer, abdominal desmoids and fibromatosis, but complete data are not available.

**Detection of Carrier:** Carriers may exhibit congenital hypertrophy of the retinal pigment epithelium (CHRPE) (see **Retina, congenital hypertrophy of retinal pigment epithelium**) or other extracolonic manifestations before colonic polyposis develops. However, absence of these other manifestations does not exclude the gene (nonpenetrance in an obligate carrier). Ophthalmic examinations, as well as physical examination and regular proctoscopy, are recommended for at-risk individuals. DNA markers are now sufficiently accurate that highly probable diagnoses can be made at birth.

**Special Considerations:** The distinction from **Intestinal polyposis, type I** is unclear. Hypotheses regarding the etiology of these two syndromes have included: 1) different mutations or deletions at the same chromosomal location, 2) variable expression of an identical gene defect, and 3) modifying agents separate from the APC locus.

Several families have been described which exhibit adenomatous colonic polyposis and brain tumors. This has been termed **Turcot syndrome**. Predominant sebaceous cysts and polyposis coli have been referred to as *Oldfield syndrome*, which may be a variant of Gardner syndrome. Multiple cutaneous sebaceous neoplasms with or without keratoacanthomas in association with adenocarcinomas of the gastrointestinal tract is referred to as *Muir-Torre syndrome* (see **Cancer, sebaceous gland tumor-mulitple visceral carcinoma**). A case of Muir-Torre syndrome has been described in which multiple polyps of the colon were present.

**Support Groups:** OH; Cleveland; Familial Polyposis Registry

**References:**
Gardner EJ, et al.: Gastrointestinal polyposis: syndromes and genetic mechanisms. West J Med 1980; 132:488–499. †
Haggitt RC, Reid BJ: Hereditary gastrointestinal polyposis syndromes. Am J Surg Pathol 1986; 10:871–887. *
Burt RW, et al.: Villous adenoma of the duodenal papilla presenting as necrotizing pancreatitis in a patient with Gardner's syndrome. Gastroenterology 1987; 92:532–535. †
Sarre RG, et al.: Gastric and duodenal polyps in familial adenomatous polyposis: a prospective study of the nature and prevalence of upper gastrointestinal polyps. Gut 1987; 28:306–314.
Traboulsi EI, et al.: Prevalence and importance of pigmented ocular fundus lesions in Gardner's syndrome. New Engl J Med 1987; 316:661–667. †
Itoh H, et al.: Treatment of desmoid tumors in Gardner's syndrome: report of a case. Dis Colon Rectum 1988; 31:459–461.
Nakamura Y, et al.: Localization of the genetic defect in familial adenomatous polyposis within a region of chromosome 5. Am J Hum Genet 1988; 43:638–644.

BU036                                                  **Randall W. Burt**

**Intestinal polyposis-pigmentary changes of genitalia-megalencephaly**
*See OVERGROWTH, RUVALCABA-MYHRE-SMITH TYPE*

**Intestinal pseudo-obstruction-external ophthalmoplegia**
*See MUSCULAR DYSTROPHY, OCULO-GASTROINTESTINAL*

## INTESTINAL PSEUDO-OBSTRUCTION SYNDROMES    2330

**Includes:**
    Argyrophil myenteric plexus, deficiency of
    Gastric emptying disorders, idiopathic
    Megacolon, idiopathic
    Megacystis, idiopathic
    Megaduodenum, idiopathic
    Myopathy, visceral
    Pseudo-obstruction, chronic idiopathic intestinal, neuronal
      type
    Visceral neuropathy

**Excludes:**
    **Colon, aganglionosis** (0192)
    Endocrine disorders
    **Gluten-sensitive enteropathy** (0423)
    Intestinal pseudo-obstruction secondary to amyloidosis
    Intestinal pseudo-obstruction secondary to pharmacologic
      causes
    Muscle disease, primary
    Neurological disease, primary

**Major Diagnostic Criteria:** Signs and symptoms of chronic intestinal obstruction; no evidence of mechanical obstruction; no evidence of systemic etiologies; histologic evidence for involvement of smooth muscle or enteric nerves.

**Clinical Findings:** The clinical syndrome is characterized by chronically recurrent attacks suggestive of intestinal obstruction (defined clinically and by X-ray) in the absence of mechanical obstruction (established by appropriate X-ray, endoscopic, or surgical investigations) and in the absence of other recognized etiologies. This is a heterogeneous group of disorders.

In adults, a longstanding history of nonspecific symptoms suggestive of a gastrointestinal motility disorder (dysphagia, early satiety, constipation/diarrhea), or the presence of extraintestinal manifestations (megacystis, ophthalmoplegia), preceding the onset of acute symptoms is characteristic. In contrast, in neonates and infants, severe postprandial abdominal distension and obstruction are often the first manifestations of the disease. The most common symptoms in adults, despite different underlying pathologic lesions (visceral neuropathy, visceral myopathy), are abdominal pain and distension, early satiety, and diarrhea.

Positive findings on esophageal manometry (aperistalsis, incomplete relaxation of lower esophageal sphincter, gastric emptying studies (delayed for solids, variable for liquids), gastrointestinal manometry (usually a hypomotile pattern), and full-thickness biopsy with special silver stains of specimen are not mandatory for the diagnosis of intestinal pseudo-obstruction but allow the classification into visceral neuropathy or visceral myopathy; a more rational approach to management, including surgery; and the detection of asymptomatic but genetically affected relatives.

**Complications:** The presence and severity of complications depends on the age of the patient (infant vs. adult), primary site of involvement (proximal, distal, or entire GI tract), and degree of functional impairment. Malnutrition is common and can result from decreased food intake (operant conditioning to postprandial pain), maldigestion (impaired gastric dispersion of food), or malabsorption (bacterial overgrowth, sprue-like intestinal lesion, functional or surgical loss of absorptive capacity). In infants, failure to thrive or electrolyte and fluid imbalances are usually secondary to postprandial vomiting and diarrhea. Whereas gastroesophageal reflux appears to be rare in adults, reflux esophagitis and aspiration pneumonia occur in infants secondary to impaired gastroesophageal motility. Narcotic dependence may further compromise GI motility in adults with longstanding symptomatic disease.

**Associated Findings:** In visceral myopathy: megacystis, vesicoureteral reflux, ophthalmoplegia, ptosis, and small intestine diverticulosis. In visceral neuropathy: autonomic nervous system insufficiency, neurologic abnormalities (ataxia, dysarthria, abnormal pupillary reflexes, abnormal tendon reflexes, mental retardation), and basal ganglia calcification.

**Etiology:** Intestinal pseudo-obstruction is clearly due to a number of distinct genetic disorders, as both dominant, recessive, and sporadic families have been well described. In addition, different clinical associations have been noted, e.g., a specific pedigree with mental retardation and basal ganglia calcification. Finally, different pathology has been delineated in different pedigrees.

**Pathogenesis:** In kindreds with visceral myopathies, degenerative changes, and thinning of intestinal smooth muscle, preferentially of the longitudinal layers, have been described. Intestinal neurons were found to be normal. In kindreds with visceral neuropathies, special histologic techniques have revealed degenerative changes of myenteric plexus neurons, including pathognomonic intranuclear inclusions in one family. The intestinal smooth muscle was found to be normal.

**MIM No.:** *15531, *24318

**CDC No.:** 751.880

**Sex Ratio:** M1:F1

**Occurrence:** Several dozen kinships with inherited patterns have been documented.

**Risk of Recurrence for Patient's Sib:**
    See Part I, *Mendelian Inheritance.*

**Risk of Recurrence for Patient's Child:**
    See Part I, *Mendelian Inheritance.*

**Age of Detectability:** Clinical detectability is highly variable; usually in the second to fourth decade. Some sporadic cases are detectable in the neonatal period.

**Gene Mapping and Linkage:** Unknown.

**Prevention:** None known. Genetic counseling indicated.

**Treatment:** In mildly symptomatic cases, small frequent feedings and intake of prokinetic agents (metoclopramide, cisapride) may be useful. In severely affected cases, medical therapy is usually ineffective. Surgical interventions (gastrostomy tube, gastrointestinal resections) are useful only in selected cases resistant to conservative management. Long-term total parenteral nutrition is sometimes the only therapy.

**Prognosis:** Highly variable. Poor in patients with onset in infancy or with diffuse GI involvement.

**Detection of Carrier:** Gastric emptying studies and esophageal and gastrointestinal manometry may detect subclinically affected individuals.

**References:**
Byrne WJ, et al.: Chronic idiopathic intestinal pseudo-obstruction syndrome in children: clinical characteristics and prognosis. J Pediatr 1977; 90:585–589.
Schuffler MD, et al.: Chronic idiopathic intestinal pseudo-obstruction. a surgical approach. Ann Surg 1980; 192:752–761.
Schuffler MD, et al.: Chronic intestinal pseudo-obstruction: a report of 27 cases and review of the literature. Medicine 1981; 60:173–196.
Anuras S, et al.: A familial visceral myopathy with external ophthalmoplegia and autosomal recessive transmission. Gastroenterology 1983; 84:346–353.
Mayer EA, et al.: A familial visceral neuropathy with autosomal dominant transmission. Gastroenterology 1986; 91:1528–1536.
Faber J, et al.: Familial intestinal pseudoobstruction dominated by a progressive neurologic disease at a young age. Gastroenterology 1987; 92:786–790.
Mayer EA, et al.: Gastric emptying of a mixed solid-liquid meal in patients with chronic intestinal pseudo-obstruction. Diag Dis Sci 1987; 33:10–18.
Steiner I, et al.: Familial progressive neuronal disease and chronic idiopathic intestinal pseuoobstruction. Neurology 1987; 37:1046–1050.

Hyman PE, et al.: Antroduodenal motility in children with chronic intestinal pseuo-obstruction. J Pediatr 1988; 112:899–905.

MA081
R0036
Emeran A. Mayer
Jerome I. Rotter

**Intestinal pseudo-obstruction, idiopathic**
*See MEGACYSTIS-MEGADUODENUM SYNDROME*

## INTESTINAL ROTATION, INCOMPLETE 0537

**Includes:**
Malrotation
Malrotation of midgut
Nonrotation of midgut
Volvulus of midgut

**Excludes:**
**Duodenum, atresia or stenosis** (0300)
**Intestinal atresia or stenosis** (0531)

**Major Diagnostic Criteria:** X-ray demonstration of the anatomic abnormality, i.e., the cecum is not in the right lower quadrant, the small bowel is on the right side of the abdomen, and the colon tends to be on the left side of the abdomen. If the patient has undergone midgut volvulus, the duodenum may show complete obstruction and by barium enema the transverse colon may be obstructed.

**Clinical Findings:** Bile-stained emesis is the most frequent presenting symptom, indicating obstruction distal to the ampulla of Vater. The patient may have cyclic or recurrent vomiting, malabsorption of fat, and recurrent abdominal pain.

Any neonate who has the sudden onset of bile-stained emesis should have appropriate X-ray studies performed on an emergency basis because of the possibility of volvulus of the midgut, which may result in necrosis.

Malrotation is inherently associated with abdominal wall defects such as omphalocele and gastroschisis and with diaphragmatic hernia. The anomaly is evident at the time of surgical correction of these congenital anomalies.

If the patient has an anterior abdominal wall defect, the bowel has not gone through the normal phases of rotation. If the patient has a diaphragmatic hernia, the bowel resides in the thoracic cavity and therefore has not progressed through the normal stages of rotation. In the other patients who have neither an anterior abdominal wall defect nor a diaphragmatic hernia, the rotation of the bowel simply does not occur and there is no known rationale for the lack of rotation.

**Complications:** Midgut volvulus is the most serious complication. Other complications are malnutrition due to recurrent vomiting and the inability to absorb fats due to obstruction of the mesenteric lymphatics.

**Associated Findings:** Duodenal stenosis is rarely associated, and should be excluded at the time of surgical correction of the malrotation.

**Etiology:** Autosomal dominant inheritance has been demonstrated in two families. Most cases appear to be sporadic.

**Pathogenesis:** During embryonic development, the intestine grows at a more rapid rate than the celomic cavity. Part of the intestine develops in the base of the umbilical cord and in the normal sequence of events returns to the celomic cavity and simultaneously rotates in a counterclockwise direction around the superior mesenteric pedicle. Eventually the cecum and right colon are fixed to the posterior parietes. If the rotation does not proceed to completion, fixation of the right colon does not occur and the entire intestine is on a narrowed pedicle.

**MIM No.:** *19325

**CDC No.:** 751.490

**Sex Ratio:** Presumably M1:F1 (M2:F1 observed in one series).

**Occurrence:** Of asymptomatic patients having barium enemas, 0–2% have malrotation. One hundred fourteen patients operated on at the Children's Hospital of Los Angeles between 1937 and 1977 and 320 patient operated on at the Boston Children's Hospital through 1967 had malrotation.

**Risk of Recurrence for Patient's Sib:** Unknown.

**Risk of Recurrence for Patient's Child:** Unknown.

**Age of Detectability:** The majority of patients are diagnosed and treated in the first month of life.

**Gene Mapping and Linkage:** Unknown.

**Prevention:** None known. Genetic counseling indicated.

**Treatment:** The only effective therapy for this anomaly is surgical correction of the abnormally narrow mesenteric base by lysis of bands which traverse from the distal small bowel mesentery to the right posterior abdominal wall lateral to the duodenum. If volvulus is present, detorsion is performed prior to lysis of bands.

**Prognosis:** If the patient is operated on prior to vascular compromise of the small bowel, the prognosis is excellent. If the patient has progressed to necrosis of the entire small bowel and secondary shock, the prognosis is guarded.

**Detection of Carrier:** Unknown.

**Special Considerations:** If an infant feeds well during the early hours or days of life and has sudden onset of bile-stained emesis, midgut volvulus secondary to malrotation should be ruled out on an emergency basis. Observation with appropriate X-ray studies may allow the infant to progress to complete bowel necrosis before therapy is instituted.

**References:**
Stewart DR, et al.: Malrotation of the bowel in infants and children: a 15 year review. Surgery 1976; 79:716–720.
Andrassy RJ, Mahour GH: Malrotation of the midgut in infants and children: a 25-year review. Arch Surg 1981; 116:158–160.
Carmi R, et al.: Familial midgut anomalies: a spectrum of defects due to a single cause? Am J Med Genet 1981; 8:443–446.
Smith EI: Malrotation of the intestine. In: Welch K, et al., eds: Pediatric Surgery, ed 4, Vol 2. Chicago: Yearbook Medical, 1986: 882–895.

W0013
Morton M. Woolley

**Intestine, inflammatory bowel diseases**
*See INFLAMMATORY BOWEL DISEASE*
**Intimal fibrosis with fibromuscular dysplasia**
*See ARTERY, RENAL FIBROMUSCULAR DYSPLASIA*
**Intraadenoidal cysts**
*See NASOPHARYNGEAL CYSTS*
**Intraepithelial dyskeratosis**
*See MUCOSA (ORAL/EYE), INTRAEPITHELIAL DYSKERATOSIS, BENIGN*

## INTRAHEPATIC CHOLESTASIS OF PREGNANCY (ICP) 3278

**Includes:**
Cholestasis associated with oral contraceptive therapy
Cholestasis, intrahepatic, of pregnancy
Intrahepatic jaundice of pregnancy, recurrent
Obstetric hepatosis
Pregnancy-related cholestasis
Pruritus gravidarum
Recurrent intrahepatic cholestasis of pregnancy (RICP)

**Excludes:**
**Cholestasis, intrahepatic, recurrent, benign** (3276)
**Jaundice, intrahepatic cholestatic, Byler type** (2371)
Liver, acute fatty, of pregnancy
Preeclampsia/eclampsia associated liver dysfunction

**Major Diagnostic Criteria:** Jaundice or pruritus associated with elevated serum bile salts during pregnancy or with use of estrogen-containing oral contraceptives, and in the absence of biliary colic, fever or other manifestations of gallstone disease.

**Clinical Findings:** Patients usually present in the third trimester, but may become symptomatic as early as the second or third month of gestation. Pruritus is the most common initial complaint and can become intolerably severe in some. Fluctuating jaundice may also develop. Patients with a prior history of jaundice not associated with pregnancy or estrogen therapy are excluded from diagnosis. The disease usually recurs in multiparous women, but lack of symptoms during prior pregnancies does not preclude the diagnosis.

The liver may be enlarged and slightly tender. Hepatic histology is notable only for mild hepatocellular cholestasis. The gallbladder may appear distended by ultrasound, but there should be no evidence of biliary obstruction. There is a moderate increase in fasting serum bile acids, cholesterol, alkaline phosphatase, 5' nucleotidase and lipoprotein X. Serum gamma-glutamyl transpeptidase has been reported to be normal. Symptoms and biochemical abnormalities resolve within days after delivery.

**Complications:** Patients may develop vitamin K deficiency secondary to steatorrhea. The nutritional status of the mother and fetus may also be compromised by fat malabsorption. The incidence of stillbirths, premature deliveries and fetal distress among the offspring of affected mothers appears to be increased as compared to uncomplicated gestations.

**Associated Findings:** None known.

**Etiology:** Possibly an autosomal dominant trait that can be transmitted by phenotypically normal males.

**Pathogenesis:** ICP is speculated to be secondary to reduced inactivation of cholestatic steroid hormones, particularly estrogen. Exaggerated impairment of intravenous sulfobromophthalein clearance after low dose ethinyl estradiol administration has been demonstrated in males with a positive family history of this disorder.

**MIM No.:** 14748

**Sex Ratio:** M0:F1 (symptomatic patients are female by definition).

**Occurrence:** 1:1000–10,000 deliveries overall, 10 to 20 times higher prevalence in Scandinavian countries and Poland, highest incidence in Araucanian Indians of Chile where prevalence approaches 1:10 deliveries.

**Risk of Recurrence for Patient's Sib:**
See Part I, *Mendelian Inheritance.*

**Risk of Recurrence for Patient's Child:**
See Part I, *Mendelian Inheritance.*

**Age of Detectability:** Presumably after puberty.

**Gene Mapping and Linkage:** Unknown.

**Prevention:** None known. Genetic counseling indicated.

**Treatment:** Patients may show improvement in symptoms when treated with phenobarbital or cholesytramine. Cholestyramine does tend to aggravate fat malabsorption. Patients should also receive supplemental fat soluble vitamins, especially vitamin K.

**Prognosis:** Variable. The condition tends to recur in subsequent pregnancies. No associated residual liver dysfunction has been reported after the post-partum period.

**Detection of Carrier:** Male carriers may have impaired sulfobromophthalein clearance.

**References:**
Reyes H, et al.: Sulfobromophthalein clearance tests before and after ethinyl estradiol administration in women and men with familial history of intrahepatic cholestasis of pregnancy. Gastroenterology 1981; 81:226–231.
Reyes H: The enigma of intrahepatic cholestasis of pregnancy: lessons from Chile. Hepatology 1982; 2:87–96.
Holzbach RT, et al.: Familial recurrent intrahepatic cholestasis of pregnancy: a genetic study providing evidence for transmission of a sex-linked, dominant trait. Gastroenterology 1983; 85:175–179.
Riely CA: The liver in pregnancy. In: Schiff L, Schiff ER, eds: Diseases of the liver. Philadelphia: J.B. Lippincott, 1987:1059–1073.

AL037
FI035

**Estella M. Alonso**
**Mark Fishbein**

**Intrahepatic jaundice of pregnancy, recurrent**
*See INTRAHEPATIC CHOLESTASIS OF PREGNANCY (ICP)*

**Intraoral bands-cleft uvula**
See CLEFT PALATE-PERSISTENCE OF BUCCOPHARYNGEAL MEMBRANE
**Intraspinal lipomas**
See LIPOMENINGOCELE
**Intrauterine and neonatal enamel hypoplasia**
See TEETH, ENAMEL HYPOPLASIA
**Intrauterine death due to transplacental lead exposure**
See FETAL EFFECTS FROM MATERNAL LEAD EXPOSURE
**Intrauterine developmental retardation from fetal lead exposure**
See FETAL EFFECTS FROM MATERNAL LEAD EXPOSURE
**Intrauterine growth retardation**
See FETAL EFFECTS OF MATERNAL CIGARETTE SMOKING
**Intrauterine growth retardation (one type)**
See FETAL MONOZYGOUS MULTIPLE PREGNANCY DYSPLACENTATION EFFECTS
**Intrauterine growth retardation, and maternal hypertension**
See FETAL DEVELOPMENTAL RETARDATION WITH MATERNAL HYPERTENSION
**Intrauterine growth retardation-cutis laxa-hip dislocation**
See CUTIS LAXA-DELAYED DEVELOPMENT-LIGAMENTOUS LAXITY
**Intrauterine healed clefts**
See CLEFT LIP
**Intrauterine herpes simplex virus infection**
See FETAL HERPES SIMPLEX VIRUS INFECTION
**Intrauterine mortality in monozygous multiple pregnancies**
See FETAL MONOZYGOUS MULTIPLE PREGNANCY DYSPLACENTATION EFFECTS
**Intrinsic factor, abnormal**
See ANEMIA, PERNICIOUS CONGENITAL
**Inv (Km) antigens**
See SERUM ALLOTYPES, HUMAN
**Inversion of ventricles without reversal of arterial trunks**
See VENTRICLES, INVERTED WITHOUT TRANSPOSITION OF GREAT ARTERIES
**Inverted transposition of great arteries**
See VENTRICLES, INVERTED WITH TRANSPOSITION OF GREAT ARTERIES
**Iodide accumulation, transport or trapping defect**
See THYROID, IODIDE TRANSPORT DEFECT
**Iodide goiter**
See GOITER, GOITROGEN INDUCED
**Iodide peroxidase deficiency**
See THYROID, PEROXIDASE DEFECT
**Iodide transport defect, partial**
See THYROID, IODIDE TRANSPORT DEFECT
**Iodine deficiency, extrinsic, and fetal injury**
See CRETINISM, ENDEMIC, AND RELATED DISORDERS
**Iodotyrosine dehalogenase deficiency**
See THYROID, IODOTYROSINE DEIODINASE DEFICIENCY
**Iodotyrosine deiodinase deficiency, partial**
See THYROID, IODOTYROSINE DEIODINASE DEFICIENCY
**Iodotyrosine deiodinase deficiency, peripheral**
See THYROID, IODOTYROSINE DEIODINASE DEFICIENCY
**Iowa type amyloidosis**
See AMYLOIDOSIS, IOWA TYPE
**Ipsilateral vertebral artery from aortic arch**
See ARTERY, INDEPENDENT ORIGIN OF IPSILATERAL VERTEBRAL
**Iridocorneal mesodermal dysgenesis**
See EYE, ANTERIOR SEGMENT DYSGENESIS
**Iridogoniodysgenesis**
See EYE, ANTERIOR SEGMENT DYSGENESIS
**Iridogoniodysgenesis with somatic anomalies**
See RIEGER SYNDROME
**Iris coloboma, atypical**
See ANIRIDIA
**Iris coloboma-anal atresia**
See CAT EYE SYNDROME
**Iris, coloboma**
See EYE, MICROPHTHALMIA/COLOBOMA
**Iris, congenital absence**
See ANIRIDIA
**Iron overload disease**
See HEMOCHROMATOSIS, IDIOPATHIC
**Iron retention**
See HEMOCHROMATOSIS, IDIOPATHIC
**Iron-binding globulin deficiency**
See ATRANSFERRINEMIA
**Iron-loading anemia**
See ANEMIA, SIDEROBLASTIC

## ISAACS-MERTENS SYNDROME                    3271

**Includes:**
Continuous muscle fiber activity, hereditary
Neuromyotonia

**Excludes:**
**Hyperekplexia** (3260)
**Jumping Frenchman of Maine** (3270)
**Myotonia congenita** (0701)

**Major Diagnostic Criteria:** Myokymia (continuous, wormlike contractions of skeletal muscle), pseudomyotonia (difficulty relaxing after forceful grasp as in myotonia, but differing electrophysiologically), and persistent or intermittent abnormal postures of the hands and feet. Hyperhidrosis may also be present.

**Clinical Findings:** The disorder is quite variable clinically, but the term "Isaacs-Mertens syndrome" is often used in a strict sense to refer to patients who display isolated stiffness and myokymia, the electrophysiologic origin of which appears to be the terminal motor axon or its sprouts (as evidenced by abolition of the continuous motor unit activity by curare but not by peripheral nerve block or sleep). According to this definition, related syndromes with additional clinical features, such as peripheral neuropathy, muscle wasting, episodic titubation, and periodic ataxia, are excluded, as are disorders in which the myokymia is abolished by peripheral nerve block. Isaacs-Mertens syndrome in this narrow sense is usually sporadic, although apparent autosomal dominant inheritance has been described. The disorder is not typically accompanied by an abnormal startle response as in **Hyperekplexia**, and true myotonia is not present. Most reported patients have responded dramatically, although often not completely, to phenytoin or carbamazepine, but not to benzodiazepines (unlike **Hyperekplexia**). Calcium and phosphorus metabolism are normal, despite the presence of ischemia-induced carpopedal spasm (Trousseau's sign) in some patients.

**Complications:** Cyanosis from respiratory muscle stiffness, and fixed joint contractures, have been reported in severe cases.

**Associated Findings:** None known.

**Etiology:** Usually sporadic, although instances of apparent autosomal dominant inheritance have been described.

**Pathogenesis:** A defect in the terminal motor axonal membrane has been proposed but not proven.

**MIM No.:** 12102

**Sex Ratio:** M1:F1

**Occurrence:** The disorder has been reported in a variety of ethnic groups.

**Risk of Recurrence for Patient's Sib:**
See Part I, *Mendelian Inheritance.*

**Risk of Recurrence for Patient's Child:**
See Part I, *Mendelian Inheritance.*

**Age of Detectability:** Sometimes obvious at birth or in the first few months of life. However, signs and symptoms are often first apparent in the fourth or fifth decades.

**Gene Mapping and Linkage:** Unknown.

**Prevention:** None known. Genetic counseling indicated.

**Treatment:** Phenytoin and carbamazepine have both proven remarkably effective in most patients.

**Prognosis:** The clinical course is variable; some patients experience complete or partial remission, while others require lifelong treatment.

**Detection of Carrier:** A thorough family history and examination of first-degree relatives, possibly including electromyography, may occasionally identify mildly affected individuals.

**References:**
Isaacs H: A syndrome of continuous muscle fiber activity. J Neurol Neurosurg Psychiat 1961; 24:319–325.
Hanson PA, et al.: Contractures, continuous muscle discharges, and titubation. Ann Neurol 1977; 1:120–124.
Ashizawa T, et al.: A dominantly inherited syndrome with continuous motor neuron discharges. Ann Neurol 1983; 13:285–290.
McGuire SA, et al.: Hereditary continuous muscle fiber activity. Arch Neurol 1984; 41:395–396.
Rowland LP: Cramps, spasms and muscle stiffness. Rev Neurol 1985; 141:261–273.

RY001                                        **Stephen G. Ryan**

**Ischiopagus**
*See TWINS, CONJOINED*
**Isoimmune hemolytic disease of the newborn**
*See ERYTHROBLASTOSIS FETALIS*
**Isolated IgA deficiency**
*See IMMUNOGLOBULIN A DEFICIENCY*
**Isolated trypsinogen deficiency**
*See TRYPSINOGEN DEFICIENCY*
**Isolated TSH deficiency**
*See THYROTROPIN DEFICIENCY, ISOLATED*
**Isoleucine 33 amyloidosis**
*See AMYLOIDOSIS, ASHKENAZI TYPE*
**Isomaltase insufficiency**
*See SUCRASE-ISOMALTASE DEFICIENCY*
**Isomaltase-sucrase deficiency**
*See SUCRASE-ISOMALTASE DEFICIENCY*
**Isoniazid inactivation**
*See NEUROPATHY, HERITABLE ISONIAZIDE TYPE (INH)*
*also ACETYLATOR POLYMORPHISM*
**Isoniazid neuropathy**
*See NEUROPATHY, HERITABLE ISONIAZIDE TYPE (INH)*
**Isotretinoin, fetal effects of**
*See FETAL RETINOID SYNDROME*
**Isovaleric acid CoA dehydrogenase deficiency**
*See ACIDEMIA, ISOVALERIC*
**Isovaleric acidemia**
*See ACIDEMIA, ISOVALERIC*
**Israeli hereditary amyloidosis**
*See AMYLOIDOSIS, ASHKENAZI TYPE*
**Isthmic spondylolisthesis and spondylolysis**
*See SPINE, SPONDYLOLISTHESIS AND SPONDYLOLYSIS*
**Itching, hereditary localized**
*See PRURITUS, HEREDITARY LOCALIZED*
**Ito hypomelanosis**
*See HYPOMELANOSIS OF ITO*
**IVD deficiency**
*See ACIDEMIA, ISOVALERIC*
**Ivemark syndrome**
*See ASPLENIA SYNDROME*

## IVIC SYNDROME                              3043

**Includes:**
Deafness-radial hypoplasia-ophthalmoplegia-
thrombocytopenia
Oculo-oto-radial syndrome
Radial hypoplasia-deafness-ophthalmoplegia-
thrombocytopenia

**Excludes:**
**Aase-Smith syndrome** (3029)
**Heart-hand syndrome** (0455)
**Lacrimo-auriculo-dento-digital syndrome** (2180)
**Pancytopenia syndrome, Fanconi type** (2029)
**Radial-renal-ocular syndrome** (2643)
**Thrombocytopenia-absent radius** (0941)

**Major Diagnostic Criteria:** The combination of radial ray defects, congenital mixed-type hearing loss, and strabismus should distinguish this condition from other radial anomaly syndromes.

**Clinical Findings:** All affected individuals have some degree of upper limb anomaly affecting the radial ray, with thumb hypoplasia, triphalangism, or distal placement being the most common. The upper limb hypoplasia can also affect the forearm. Although lower limbs appear normal, retarded growth of the femora and spine occurs, leading to relatively short stature. X-ray evaluation demonstrates an abnormal first metacarpal (absent, short, or long); hypoplastic and sometimes fused carpal bones are also seen in at least one-half of the affected individuals. Proximal fusion of radius and ulna was also present in 4/22 individuals.

Extraocular muscle weakness is present in most affected individuals, with the medial and lateral recti being the most frequently and severely affected. Congenital mixed-type hearing loss is also almost always present, with greater loss in the higher frequencies (above 4,000 cps). Seven affected individuals had mild, incomplete bundle branch block of the heart. Thrombocytopenia and leukocytosis also occurred in some affected individuals. In addition, 3/25 had imperforate anus.

**Complications:** Strabismus secondary to extraocular muscle weakness.

**Associated Findings:** Present in one or two individuals were hypoplastic lateral incisors; ocular lens opacities; and unilateral ectopic kidney.

**Etiology:** Autosomal dominant inheritance.

**Pathogenesis:** Unknown. A defect in mesenchyme has been postulated.

**MIM No.:** *14775

**POS No.:** 3849

**Sex Ratio:** M1:F1

**Occurrence:** At least three families have been reported; one each from Venezuela, Italy, and Hungary.

**Risk of Recurrence for Patient's Sib:**
See Part I, *Mendelian Inheritance.*

**Risk of Recurrence for Patient's Child:**
See Part I, *Mendelian Inheritance.*

**Age of Detectability:** Prenatally if major limb defects are present, otherwise at birth.

**Gene Mapping and Linkage:** Unknown.

**Prevention:** None known. Genetic counseling indicated.

**Treatment:** Supportive; surgery for imperforate anus if indicated.

**Prognosis:** Intellectual development and growth are not impaired; life span is generally normal, with the oldest individual dying at age 110 years, although one affected individual died suddenly at age 3 1/2 years.

**Detection of Carrier:** Unknown.

**Special Considerations:** The acronym IVIC stands for Instituto Venezolano de Investigaciones Cientificas where Arias conducted his research.

**References:**

Arias S, et al.: The IVIC syndrome: a new autosomal dominant complex pleiotropic syndrome with radial ray hypoplasia, hearing impairment, internal ophthalmoplegia, and thrombocytopenia. Am J Med Genet 1980; 6:25–29. * †
Sammito V, et al.: IVIC syndrome: report of a second family. Am J Med Genet 1988; 29:875–881. †
Czeizel A, et al.: IVIC syndrome: report of a third family. (Letter) Am J Med Genet 1989; 33:282–283. †

T0007                                    **Helga V. Toriello**

**Ivory exostoses of ear canal**
*See EAR, EXOSTOSES*

# ❖ J ❖

**J. Chain**
See *LEUKEMIA, ACUTE LYMPHOCYTIC, FAMILIAL*
**Jabs syndrome**
See *GRANULOMATOSIS-POLYSYNOVITIS, FAMILIAL SYSTEMIC*
**Jackson-Weiss craniosynostosis**
See *CRANIOSYNOSTOSIS-FOOT DEFECTS, JACKSON-WEISS TYPE*
**Jacobs syndrome**
See *SYNOVITIS, FAMILIAL HYPERTROPHIC*
**Jacobsen syndrome**
See *ECTODERMAL DYSPLASIA, HIDROTIC*
also *CHROMOSOME 11, MONOSOMY 11q*
**Jadassohn linear nevus sebaceous syndrome**
See *NEVUS, EPIDERMAL NEVUS SYNDROME*
**Jadassohn-Lewandowsky syndrome**
See *NAILS, PACHYONYCHIA CONGENITA*
**Jaffe-Lichtenstein disease**
See *FIBROUS DYSPLASIA, MONOSTOTIC*
**Jansen metaphyseal dysostosis**
See *METAPHYSEAL CHONDRODYSPLASIA, TYPE JANSEN*
**Jansky-Bielchowsky disease (late infantile NCL or LINCL)**
See *NEURONAL CEROID-LIPOFUSCINOSES (NCL)*
**Jansky-Bielchowsky-Hagberg disease (late infantile variant of NCL)**
See *NEURONAL CEROID-LIPOFUSCINOSES (NCL)*
**Janz syndrome**
See *SEIZURES, MYOCLONIC, JUVENILE JANZ TYPE*
**Japanese-type hereditary amyloidosis**
See *AMYLOIDOSIS, TRANSTHYRETIN METHIONINE-30 TYPE*
**Jarcho-Levin syndrome**
See *SPONDYLOTHORACIC DYSPLASIA*
**Jaundice without bilirubin glucuronide in bile**
See *UDP-GLUCURONOSYLTRANSFERASE, SEVERE DEFICIENCY TYPE I*
**Jaundice, chronic benign**
See *HYPERBILIRUBINEMIA, UNCONJUGATED*

---

## JAUNDICE, INTRAHEPATIC CHOLESTATIC, BYLER TYPE      2371

**Includes:**
Byler disease (Amish kindred)
Cholestasis, progressive idiopathic
Fatal intrahepatic cholestasis
Progressive familial cholestasis

**Excludes:**
**Acidemia, Trihydroxycoprostanic** (3275)
**Bile ducts, interlobular, nonsyndromic paucity** (3277)
**Cholestasis, intrahepatic, recurrent, benign** (3276)
Hepatitis, neonatal, giant-cell type, nonprogressive
**Intrahepatic cholestasis of Pregnancy (ICP)** (3278)
Intrahepatic cholestasis, all other recognizable causes of
chronic

**Major Diagnostic Criteria:** Chronic, progressive cholestasis (as evidenced by jaundice, conjugated hyperbilirubinemia, pruritus, elevated serum bile salt concentration, hypercholesterolemia, and related signs and symptoms) without anatomic obstruction of extrahepatic biliary tract and without other recognizable causes.

**Clinical Findings:** The cholestasis is unremitting, although it may wax and wane in severity, and leads to progressive biliary cirrhosis. The onset of cholestasis is in the first year, usually in the first month, of life. Death due to hepatic failure or hepatocellular carcinoma occurs in the first or second decades. Usually hepatomegaly and often splenomegaly are present. Pruritus varies in severity; some affected patients exhibit cutaneous mutilation secondary to scratching. Serum bilirubin levels range from 3 to 10 mg/dl early in the course to over 30 mg/dl in the cirrhotic phase. Total serum bile salt concentration is usually between 100 and 200 $\mu$M (normal, <10). Hypercholesterolemia is usually mild, i.e., 250–400 mg/dl. Transaminases (ALT and AST) are elevated in the range of 150–500 U/liter and alkaline phosphatase in the range of 400–800 U/liter. Recent observations suggest that a low or normal level of gamma-glutamyl transpeptidase (GGTP), as opposed to high levels in most or all other cholestatic diseases, may be an important diagnostic finding in this disease. Liver biopsy material shows cellular and canalicular cholestasis; variable degrees of lobular disarray, giant cell transformation, and hepatocyte necrosis; and normal to moderately expanded portal areas with small or inapparent bile ducts (sometimes leading to misdiagnosis of a primary ductular hypoplasia syndrome). As the disease progresses, a pattern of micronodular biliary cirrhosis with marked pseudoductular proliferation is observed.

**Complications:** Cholestasis leads to submicellar concentrations of bile salts in bile, which results in a high incidence of cholescystolithiasis, and in the intestinal lumen, which causes malabsorption of fat and fat-soluble vitamins. All patients have moderate-to-severe growth failure, due to a number of factors: calorie malnutrition, vitamin D-deficient osteomalacia, anorexia secondary to abdominal discomfort, and probable effects of chronic cholestasis on metabolism and utilization of nutrients. Fat-soluble vitamin malabsorption can lead to deficiency states: vitamin D leads to osteomalacia, vitamin E to neuropathy, and vitamin K to prothrombin deficiency.
Cirrhosis with its many complications develops usually after 5–10 years. Hepatoma has developed in several patients in the first or second decades, and is a fatal complication.

**Associated Findings:** None known.

**Etiology:** Autosomal recessive inheritance.

**Pathogenesis:** Primary defect in bile formation leads to reduced bile flow (cholestasis) and retention of bile products. Retained bile products, particularly bile salts, cause hepatomegaly, elevated transaminases, hepatic fibrosis, and cirrhosis.

**MIM No.:** *21160

**CDC No.:** 751.880

**Sex Ratio:** M1:F1

**Occurrence:** About 75 cases have been reported, but the disease is probably underreported due to confusion with other cholestatic diseases and the absence of specific diagnostic criteria. Byler disease has been documented in the Old Order Amish, and in Greenland Eskimos.

**Risk of Recurrence for Patient's Sib:**
See Part I, *Mendelian Inheritance.*

**Risk of Recurrence for Patient's Child:**
See Part I, *Mendelian Inheritance.* To date no affected patients have reproduced. However, the advent of liver transplantation presents the possibility of doing so. In that case, the gene frequency and the risk for recurrence for the patient's child are probably very low, assuming absence of consanguinity.

**Age of Detectability:** Within the first week of life, if serum bile salt concentration is measured. Clinical detection may be delayed up to one year of age.

**Gene Mapping and Linkage:** Unknown.

**Prevention:** None known. Genetic counseling indicated.

**Treatment:** *Medical:* to increase bile flow: phenobarbital, rifampin; to reduce bile salt concentration: cholestyramine resin; to prevent vitamin deficiencies: supplemental vitamins D, E, and K and close monitoring of vitamin levels.
*Surgical:* liver transplantation.

**Prognosis:** All affected patients progress to cirrhosis.
Orthotopic homologous hepatic transplantation corrects the primary defect. However, some of the sequelae of chronic cholestasis, particularly bony abnormalities and neurologic deficits, are not reversible. The prevention of irreversible complications and the early detection of hepatoma improve the prognosis after transplantation.

**Detection of Carrier:** Unknown.

**References:**
Clayton RJ, et al.: Byler disease: fatal familial intrahepatic cholestasis in an Amish kindred. Am J Dis Child 1969; 117:112–124.
Ugarte N, Gonzales-Cruss F: Hepatoma in siblings with progressive familial cholestatic cirrhosis of childhood. Am J Clin Pathol 1981; 76:172–177.
Nakagawa M, et al.: Familial intrahepatic cholestasis associated with progressive neuromuscular disease and vitamin E deficiency. J Pediatr Gastro Nutr 1984; 3:385–389.
Nielsen I-M, et al.: Fatal familial cholestatic syndrome in Greenland Eskimo children. Acta Paediat Scand 1986; 75:1010–1016.

WH007                                            **Peter F. Whitington**

**Jaundice, prolonged obstructive**
See *ALPHA(1)-ANTITRYPSIN DEFICIENCY*
**Jaw excursion, limitation of**
See *CAMPTODACTYLY-TRISMUS SYNDROME*

## JAW, NEUROECTODERMAL PIGMENTED TUMOR                0711

**Includes:**
Heterotropic pigmented retinoblastoma
Melanotic ameloblastoma
Melanotic neuroectodermal tumor of infancy
Melanotic odontoma
Melanotic progonoma
Neuroectodermal pigmented tumor
Pigmented adamantinoma
Pigmented ameloblastoma
Pigmented epulis, congenital
Progonoma
Retinal anlage tumor
Retinal choristoma

**Excludes:**
Ameloblastoma
Oral melanoma
Oral nevi
**Teeth, epulis, congenital** (0360)

**Major Diagnostic Criteria:** Must be differentiated by microscopic examination. Nonencapsulated infiltrating tumor characterized by moderately vascularized fibrous connective tissue stroma, with tumor cells aggregated into alveolar spaces. Cells are cuboidal about alveolar periphery and decrease in size centrally. Nuclei are round, deeply basophilic, and surrounded by scanty cytoplasm. Pigment may be prominent or inconspicuous. Special stains dramatize presence of melanin pigment.

In view of the X-ray appearance of the irregular, ragged lytic lesion of bone and the clinical feature of rapid growth, care must be exercised to prevent an erroneous diagnosis of malignant neoplasm. Histopathologic examination should precede therapy whenever a pigmented neuroectodermal tumor of infancy is included in the differential diagnosis.

**Clinical Findings:** Nonulcerated, rapidly growing tumor in jaws of infants almost invariably less than one year of age. It locally destroys bone and displaces teeth. Most cases occur in the maxilla (80%), occasionally in the mandible (10%), both exhibiting midline predilection. Occasionally (10%) other sites are involved; including anterior fontanel, shoulder, and epididymis. High levels of urinary vanilmandelic acid excretion, which returned to normal upon removal of the tumor, were reported in two patients.

**Complications:** The natural history of untreated lesions is not known, however, disfigurement, displacement of associated teeth, and possible problem of impaired sucking, can occur.

**Associated Findings:** None known.

**Etiology:** Hypotheses include: *Neuroectodermal:* arises from cells of the neural crest that migrate to the site of tumor origin during embryogenesis. Identification of high urinary excretion of vanilmandelic acid, which falls to normal upon tumor removal, supports this hypothesis. *Odontogenic:* histogenic hypothesis. *Melanocarcinoma:* original concept, now discredited.

**Pathogenesis:** The tumor is often present at birth, and grows rapidly destroying bone locally, and displacing associated teeth.

**Sex Ratio:** M1:F1

**Occurrence:** Undetermined but presumed rare.

**Risk of Recurrence for Patient's Sib:** No increased risk reported.

**Risk of Recurrence for Patient's Child:** Unknown.

**Age of Detectability:** Often present at birth, almost invariably recognized during the first year of life.

**Gene Mapping and Linkage:** Unknown.

**Prevention:** None known. Genetic counseling indicated.

**Treatment:** Surgical removal indicated.

**Prognosis:** After surgical removal (slightly in excess of 10% have been irradiated as well), recurrence has occurred in 20% of the treated cases. Recurrences have been associated only with maxillary or mandibular examples of the tumor. Except for local surgical disfigurement, prognosis is excellent. A single incidence of malignant transformation has been noted.

**Detection of Carrier:** Unknown.

**References:**
Kerr DA, Pullon PA: A study of the pigmented tumors of jaws of infants (melanotic ameloblastoma, retinal anlage tumor, progonoma). Oral Surg 1964; 18:759.
Borello ED, Gorlin RJ: Melanotic neuroectodermal tumor of infancy - a neoplasm of neural crest origin: report of a case associated with high urinary excretion of vanilmandelic acid. Cancer 1966; 19:196.
Brekke JH, Gorlin RJ: Melanotic neuroectodermal tumor of infancy. J Oral Surg 1975; 33:858.
Dehner LP, et al.: Malignant melanotic neuroectodermal tumors of infancy. A clinical pathologic ultrastructural and tissue culture study. Cancer 1979; 43:1389.

R0039                                            **Nathaniel H. Rowe**
SA029                                            **John J. Sauk**

## JAW-WINKING SYNDROME     0548

**Includes:**
>Eyelid, winking upon movement of jaw
Marcus Gunn phenomenon
Maxillopalpebral synkinesis
Palpebromaxillary synergy, hereditary
Pterygoid-levator synkinesis
Ptosis, synkinetic
Synkinetic ptosis

**Excludes:**
>Marcus-Gunn phenomenon of the pupil
Reversed Marcus Gunn phenomenon
Winking-jaw phenomenon of Wartenberg

**Major Diagnostic Criteria:** Retraction of the upper eye lid upon movement of the jaw.

**Clinical Findings:** The classic Marcus Gunn syndrome, which is the most common, consists of unilateral ptosis at rest with elevation of the apparently paretic upper lid to a level higher than that of the other eye upon opening the mouth, or lateral movement of the lower jaw. Usually if the jaw is deviated to the affected side the ptosis increases, but if deviated to the opposite side maximal retraction occurs. Typically the ptosis recurs if the mouth is held open. Affected individuals habitually open the mouth when looking upwards. The phenomenon occurs more frequently on the left than the right. It rarely occurs bilaterally. Multiple variations of the classic syndrome have been described. Examples are retraction only with side-to-side motion of the jaw, or with masseter function, or with inspiration, or with eye movements.

**Complications:** Basically cosmetic.

**Associated Findings:** Amblyopia (50–60%), double elevatory palsy (25%), anisometropia (25–30%), and superior rectus muscle palsy (23%).

**Etiology:** Unknown except for those families in which an irregular autosomal dominant inheritance pattern exists. Multiple occurrences in the sibship of only one generation may represent autosomal recessive inheritance.

**Pathogenesis:** The pathogenesis has not been definitely established and many theories have been set forth. Anomalous connections or a reflex arc between the nuclei of the external pterygoid muscle (mesencephalic root $C_5$) and the levator palpebris ($C_3$) have been postulated. Antidromic nerve impulses and spread of stimulus rather than direct connection between nuclei also have been implicated.

**MIM No.:** 15460

**CDC No.:** 742.800

**Sex Ratio:** M1:F1

**Occurrence:** At least 200 cases have been documented. It has been estimated as the cause of 2–5% of congenital ptosis.

**Risk of Recurrence for Patient's Sib:**
>See Part I, *Mendelian Inheritance.*

**Risk of Recurrence for Patient's Child:**
>See Part I, *Mendelian Inheritance.*

**Age of Detectability:** Soon after birth, since the phenomenon is most noticeable during sucking.

**Gene Mapping and Linkage:** Unknown.

**Prevention:** None known. Genetic counseling indicated.

**Treatment:** Usually unwarranted. Some success has been reported with section of the motor root of the trigeminal nerve. More experience is available using the facial sling procedure involving sectioning the levator aponeurosis and using a fasciata sling to the brow musculature to produce voluntary lid control. Frequently, the identical procedure must be performed on the normal lid as well to produce a symmetrical result and acceptable appearance.

**Prognosis:** The condition usually grows slowly less noticeable with age.

**Detection of Carrier:** Unknown.

**References:**
Falls HF, et al.: Three cases of Marcus Gunn phenomenon in two generations. Am J Ophthalmol 1949; 32:53–59.
Duke-Elder S: System of ophthalmology. vol. 3, pt. 2. Congenital deformities. St. Louis: CV Mosby, 1963:900–902.
Kuder GG, Laws HW: Hereditary Marcus Gunn phenomenon. Can J Ophthalmol 1968; 3:97–105.
Bullock JD: Marcus-Gunn jaw-winking ptosis: classification and surgical management. J Pediat Ophthalmol Strab 1980; 17:375–379.
Doucet TW, Crawford JS: The quantification, natural course, and surgical results in 57 eyes with Marcus Gunn (jaw-winking) syndrome. Am J Ophthalmol 1981; 92:702–707.
Pratt SG, et al.: The Marcus Gunn phenomenon: a review of 71 cases. Ophthalmol 1984; 91:27–29.

DE034                    **Monte A. Del Monte**
BE026                 **Donald R. Bergsma**

**Jaws, intraosseous fibrous swelling**
*See CHERUBISM*
**Jaws/mouth (small or absent)-low set ears**
*See AGNATHIA-MICROSTOMIA-SYNOTIA*

## JEJUNAL ATRESIA     2934

**Includes:**
>Apple peel syndrome
Christmas tree syndrome

**Excludes:**
>Jejunal atresia, mucosal
Jejunal atresia, fibrous cord
Jejunal atresia with large, V-shaped defect in mesentery
**Pyloroduodenal atresia, hereditary** (2617)

**Major Diagnostic Criteria:** Complete high jejunal occlusion. The jejunum ends blindly in a dilated proximal loop, 3–4 cm beyond the ligament of Treitz.

**Clinical Findings:** Bilious vomiting, epigastric distention, and absence of stools in the neonatal period. Plain X-rays of the abdomen show a complete high jejunal occlusion. At laparotomy, the jejunum ends blindly in a dilated proximal loop. The bowel is incompletely rotated and is foreshortened, with a large mesenteric gap, precariously supplied in retrograde fashion by anastomotic arcades from a mesenteric artery.

**Complications:** If not corrected, the patient will die of starvation.

**Associated Findings:** None known.

**Etiology:** Autosomal recessive inheritance.

**Pathogenesis:** Unknown.

**MIM No.:** *24360

**CDC No.:** 751.190

**Sex Ratio:** M1:F1

**Occurrence:** At least 57 cases have been reported in the English literature.

**Risk of Recurrence for Patient's Sib:**
>See Part I, *Mendelian Inheritance.*

**Risk of Recurrence for Patient's Child:**
>See Part I, *Mendelian Inheritance.*

**Age of Detectability:** During the neonatal period. Prenatal detection of intestinal obstruction may be possible by testing the amniotic fluid disaccharidases, which are deficient in affected fetuses. Results of low disaccharidase values are best followed by diagnostic ultrasound studies and, when necessary, amniography for more certain delineation of the defect.

**Gene Mapping and Linkage:** Unknown.

**Prevention:** None known. Genetic counseling indicated.

**Treatment:** Surgical treatment is usually successful.

**Prognosis:** Good, in the majority of cases.

**Detection of Carrier:** Unknown.

**Special Considerations:** In all cases of jejunal atresia it is very important to keep the possibility of the hereditary type in mind, for proper counseling of the family. Thus, if a new child is born, the investigations can be done on time for proper and immediate surgical intervention, if necessary. This may be life-saving.

**References:**
Mishalany HG, Najjar FB: Familial jejunal atresia: three cases in one family. J Pediatr 1968; 73:753–755. *
Blyth HM, Dickson JAS: Apple peel syndrome (congenital intestinal atresia): a family study of seven index patients. J Med Genet 1969; 6:275–277.
Rickham PP, Karplus M: Familial and hereditary intestinal atresia. Helv Paediatr Acta 1971; 26:561–564.
Grosfeld JL: Jejunoileal atresia and stenosis. In: Welch KJ, et al., Pediatric surgery, ed 4. Chicago: Year Book Medical, 1986:838–848.
Seashore JH, et al.: Familial apple peel jejunal atresia: surgical, genetic, and radiographic aspects. Pediatrics 1987; 80:540–544.

DE030
MI039

**Vazken M. Der Kaloustian
Henry G. Mishalany**

**Jejunoileal atresia and stenosis**
*See INTESTINAL ATRESIA OR STENOSIS*
**Jervell syndrome**
*See CARDIO-AUDITORY SYNDROME*
**Jeune syndrome**
*See ASPHYXIATING THORACIC DYSPLASIA*
**Jewish amyloidosis**
*See AMYLOIDOSIS, ASHKENAZI TYPE*
**Job syndrome**
*See IMMUNODEFICIENCY, HYPER IgE TYPE*

## JOHANSON-BLIZZARD SYNDROME 2026

**Includes:**
Ectodermal dysplasia-exocrine pancreatic insufficiency
Malabsorption-ectodermal dysplasia-nasal alar hypoplasia
Nasal alar hypoplasia-hypothyroidism-pancreatic achylia-deafness

**Excludes:**
Cranio-carpo-tarsal dysplasia, whistling face type (0223)
Ectodermal dysplasias, without malabsorption, other
Oculo-dento-osseous dysplasia (0737)
Oculo-mandibulo-facial syndrome (0738)

**Major Diagnostic Criteria:** Abnormal craniofacies, including hypoplasia of the nasal alae, hypodontia, sparse hair; malabsorption due to exocrine pancreatic deficiency; and growth and psychomotor retardation.

**Clinical Findings:** The striking craniofacial features include absent or small alae nasi and short nose from base to tip, creating a beak-like appearance; midline scalp defects over the posterior and/or anterior fontanelles; nasolacrimo-cutaneous fistulae; maxillary hypoplasia; and microcephaly. Hypodontia and microdontia are common. Deciduous and permanent teeth that are present are small, conical, and widely spaced. Hair is sparse, coarse, and dry, with abnormal patterning. There is often an upsweep of frontal hair with extension of the hairline onto the sides of the forehead. Alopecia may be present over the vertex and/or occiput at former site of congenital scalp defects. Imperforate anus or anal stenosis is common. Occasional genito-urinary abnormalities include micropenis, large clitoris, double vagina or vulvar fistula, single urogenital orifice, and various grades of hydronephrosis.

During the first year, failure to thrive due to malabsorption is typical. Laboratory studies of stool and duodenal aspirate document a lipolytic, proteolytic, and amylolytic deficiency of the exocrine pancreas.

Hypotonia and neurosensory deafness are common. Bone age is delayed.

**Complications:** Respiratory infections appear to be common. Although most cases described have been mentally retarded, a few patients have been mentally normal.

**Associated Findings:** Asplenia; congenital heart defects including **Heart, transposition of great vessels**, **Pulmonary valve, atresia**, anomalous pulmonary venous return, common atrium, and hypothyroidism.

**Etiology:** Autosomal recessive inheritance. Sibship recurrence and consanguinity have been documented.

**Pathogenesis:** Karyotype is normal. Glucose tolerance curve is normal, suggesting normal islet cell function. Sweat chloride is also normal. With thorough studies, all exocrine pancreatic function is deficient. Normal amylase levels from duodenal aspirate is probably salivary in origin.

Autopsy has shown a small thyroid filled with colloid, complete replacement of the pancreas with adipose tissue, with few normal islets, and a brain with abnormal gyri formation and cortical neuronal organization, or structurally normal but small.

**MIM No.:** *24380

**POS No.:** 3269

**Sex Ratio:** Presumably M1:F1.

**Occurrence:** More than two dozen cases have been reported.

**Risk of Recurrence for Patient's Sib:**
See Part I, *Mendelian Inheritance.*

**Risk of Recurrence for Patient's Child:**
See Part I, *Mendelian Inheritance.* Possible infertility with delayed menarche was reported in one case.

**Age of Detectability:** At birth.

**Gene Mapping and Linkage:** Unknown.

**Prevention:** None known. Genetic counseling indicated.

**Treatment:** Replacement of pancreatic exocrine enzymes and thyroxine. Plastic reconstruction of the ala nasi has been described.

The severity of the imperforate anus or anal stenosis is variable, and may require an anoplasty or colostomy.

Medical treatment consists of a protein hydrolysate diet and oral pancreatin. The malabsorption syndrome of hypoproteinemic edema, chronic anemia, and slow weight gain responds to pancreatic enzyme replacement. Fat soluble vitamins should be monitored. However, the severe growth failure persists. The hypothyroidism, if present, may require more than the usual thyroxine dose because of associated poor intestinal absorption.

**Prognosis:** Shortened life expectancy because of failure to thrive, frequency of infection, and occasional cardiac defects.

**Detection of Carrier:** Unknown.

**References:**
Johanson AJ, Blizzard RM: A syndrome of congenital aplasia of the alae nasi, deafness, hypothyroidism, dwarfism, absent permanent teeth, and malabsorption. J Pediat 1971; 79:982–987. * †
Fox JW, et al.: Surgical correction of the absent nasal alae of the Johanson-Blizzard syndrome. Plast Reconstr Surg 1976; 57:484–486. †
Day DW, Israel JN: Johanson-Blizzard syndrome. BD:OAS VI(B). New York: March of Dimes Birth Defects Foundation, 1978:275–287. * †
Mardini MK, et al.: Johanson-Blizzard syndrome in a large inbred kindred with three involved members. Clin Genet 1978; 14:247–250.
Towne P, White M: Identity of two syndromes: proteolytic, lipolytic and amylolytic deficiency of the exocrine pancreas with congenital anomalies. Am J Dis Child 1981; 135:248–250. †
Zerres K, Holtgrave E-A: The Johanson-Blizzard syndrome: report of a new case with special reference to dentition and a review of the literature. Clin Genet 1986; 30:177–183. * †
Moeschler JB, et al.: The Johanson-Blizzard syndrome: a second report of full autopsy findings. Am J Med Genet 1987; 26:133–138.
Gould NS, et al.: Johanson-Blizzard syndrome: clinical and pathological findings in 2 sibs. Am J Med Genet 1989; 33:194–199. * †

J0010                                    **Virginia P. Johnson**

**Johnson neuroectodermal syndrome**
*See ALOPECIA-ANOSMIA-DEAFNESS-HYPOGONADISM, JOHNSON TYPE*
**Joint contractures-cleft palate-Dandy-Walker malformation**
*See AASE-SMITH SYNDROME*

**Joint defects with X-linked mental retardation**
  *See X-LINKED MENTAL RETARDATION-SKELETAL DYSPLASIA*
**Joint dislocations, multiple, lethal, Larsen-like**
  *See LARSEN SYNDROME, LETHAL TYPE*
**Joint dislocations-unusual facies-skeletal abnormalities**
  *See LARSEN SYNDROME*
**Joint dislocations-wormian bones-short stature**
  *See SHORT STATURE-WORMIAN BONES-JOINT DISLOCATIONS*
**Joint hyperextensibility-facial dysmorphia syndrome**
  *See FACIAL DYSMORPHIA-JOINT HYPEREXTENSIBILITY
    SYNDROME*
**Joint hypermobility-cutis laxa-retarded development**
  *See CUTIS LAXA-DELAYED DEVELOPMENT-LIGAMENTOUS LAXITY*
**Joint instability, familial**
  *See ARTICULAR HYPERMOBILITY, FAMILIAL*
**Joint laxity, Ehlers-Danlos syndrome**
  *See EHLERS-DANLOS SYNDROME*
**Joint laxity, familial**
  *See ARTICULAR HYPERMOBILITY, FAMILIAL*
**Joint laxity-retarded development-cutis laxa**
  *See CUTIS LAXA-DELAYED DEVELOPMENT-LIGAMENTOUS LAXITY*
**Joints, multiple congenital articular rigidities**
  *See ARTHROGRYPOSES*

---

## JOINTS, OSTEOCHONDRITIS DISSECANS         0774

**Includes:**
  Aseptic necrosis
  Epiphyseal osteochondritides
  Freiburg disease (head of second metatarsal)
  Juvenile osteochondritides
  Keinbock (carpal semilunar)
  Kohler disease (navicular)
  Legg-Calve-Perthes disease (capital femoral epiphysis)
  Osgood-Schlatter disease (tibial tubercle)
  Panner disease (capitellum of humerus)
  Perthes disease
  Scheuermann disease (vertebrae)
  Sever disease (os calcis)
  Sindig-Larsen-Johansson disease (patella)
  Thiemann disease (phalangeal epiphyses)

**Excludes:**
  Juvenile osteochondroses secondary to trauma or systemic
    disease
  **Epiphyseal dysplasia, multiple (0358)**

**Major Diagnostic Criteria:**  Characteristic clinical presentation, anatomical site, and X-ray appearance.

**Clinical Findings:**  May be asymptomatic or have pain, swelling, and/or limitation of motion.

**Complications:**  Unknown.

**Associated Findings:**  None known.

**Etiology:**  Mostly sporadic, of unknown etiology. A few by autosomal dominant inheritance.

**Pathogenesis:**  Unknown.

**MIM No.:**  *16580, 15060, 18144

**Sex Ratio:**  In the capital femoral epiphysis M4:F1; in the second metatarsal M1:F4; in the elbow M8:F1; in familial cases M1:F1.

**Occurrence:**  Incidence of Perthes disease 1:4,750 live births in South Wales. The osteochondritides are undetermined but presumed rare.

**Risk of Recurrence for Patient's Sib:**
  See Part I, *Mendelian Inheritance.* In the absence of a positive family history, empiric recurrence risks are low (under 1% in Perthes disease).

**Risk of Recurrence for Patient's Child:**
  See Part I, *Mendelian Inheritance.* In the absence of a positive family history, empiric recurrence risks are low (about 3% in Perthes disease).

**Age of Detectability:**  Tend to develop after the appearance of the bony epiphyseal nucleus, thus uncommon in infancy or after adolescence.

**Gene Mapping and Linkage:**  Unknown.

**Prevention:**  None known. Genetic counseling indicated.

**Treatment:**  Orthopedic intervention may be necessary.

**Prognosis:**  Normal life span. May leave some residual disability.

**Detection of Carrier:**  Unknown.

**Special Considerations:**  There is nosological overlap between osteochondritis dissecans and the other juvenile osteochondroses. Furthermore, the conditions in these categories are probably separate entities, each with its own specific pathogenesis. Abnormal development of epiphyses, especially the capital femoral epiphysis, which occurs in several skeletal dysplasias, may lead to problems in the differential diagnosis.

**References:**
Linden B: The incidence of osteochondritis dissecans in the condyles of the femur. Acta Orthop Scand 1976; 47:664–667.
Petrie PWF: Aetiology of osteochondritis dissecans: failure to establish a familial background. J Bone Joint Surg 1977; 59B:366–367.
Halal F, et al.: Dominant inheritance of Scheuermann's juvenile kyphosis. Am J Dis Child 1978; 132:1105–1107.
Andrew TA, et al.: Familial osteochondritis dissecans and dwarfism. Acta Orthop Scand 1981; 52:519–523.
Phillips HO, Grubb SA: Familial multiple osteochondritis dissecans. J Bone Joint Surg 1985; 67A:155–156.
Hall DJ: Genetic aspects of Perthe's disease: a critical review. Clin Orthop 1986; 209:100–114.

C0066                                   **J. Michael Connor**

**Joints, stiff-dwarfism-eye defects**
  *See DWARFISM-STIFF JOINTS*
**Jones syndrome**
  *See GINGIVAL FIBROMATOSIS-DEAFNESS, JONES TYPES*
**Jorgenson syndrome**
  *See ECTODERMAL DYSPLASIA, BASAN TYPE*
**Joseph disease**
  *See MACHADO-JOSEPH DISEASE*

---

## JOUBERT SYNDROME                         2908

**Includes:**
  Cerebellar parenchymal disorder, type IV
  Cerebellar vermis agenesis, familial
  Cerebellar vermis agenesis-neurologic abnormalities
  Cerebelloparenchymal disorder IV
  Chorioretinal coloboma-Joubert syndrome
  Hyperpnea, episodic-abnormal eye movement-ataxia-
    retardation
  Joubert-Boltshauser syndrome
  Kidneys, cystic-retinal aplasia-Joubert syndrome
  Polydactyly-Joubert syndrome
  Retinal aplasia-cystic kidneys-Joubert syndrome

**Excludes:**
  **Cerebellar agenesis (2011)**
  **Hydrocephaly (0481)**
  Mouth, wide-intermittent over breathing-mental retardation
  **Oro-palatal-digital syndrome, Varadi type (2368)**
  Tectocerebellar dysraphism, isolated-occipital encephalocele
  **Vermis agenesis (2106)**

**Major Diagnostic Criteria:**  Partial or complete absence of the cerebellar vermis is seen in all patients. Pneumoencephalography or CT scan shows an enlarged fourth ventricle communicating with a posterior fossa cyst and abnormally high positioning of the tentorium cerebelli. Alternating tachypnea and apnea, opsoclonus-like eye movements, hypotonia, and mental retardation are also important clinical features.

**Clinical Findings:**  Tachypnea, often likened to the "panting of a dog," in excess of 100 respirations/min, alternating with usually brief periods of apnea, is seen soon after birth. Although not usually associated with respiratory distress, cyanosis, bradycardia, and even death have been noted during the apneic phase. The abnormal respiratory pattern (which resembles cluster breathing and does not show the waxing and waning pattern of Cheyne-Stokes respiration) often subsides after several months. Tachypnea and apnea have been noted while both awake and asleep; tachypnea has been noted during both REM and non-REM sleep, but apnea seems to occur only in non-REM sleep. The opsoclonus-like eye movements may likewise subside, or may persist. Strabismus is frequent. Developmental delay and mental retardation tend to be profound, but two cases are described in which development reverted to normal. Truncal ataxia, as well as wide-based gait, dystonia, athetoid movements, and tongue protrusion are common.

**Complications:** Death associated with apneic episodes. Blindness. Seizures.

**Associated Findings:** Dysarthria has been noted in two cases. Retinal colobomas have been noted in eight cases (all male). **Retina, amaurosis congenita, Leber type** has occurred in six cases. Occipital neural tube defects, mostly **Meningocele**, were found in 13 cases.

Other CNS defects include agenesis of the corpus callosum, unsegmented midbrain tectum, brainstem dysplasia, heterotopias, polymicrogyria, and hypoplasia of the cerebellar hemispheres. Less common findings are seizures, hemifacial spasms, **Polydactyly, Syndactyly, Camptodactyly**, renal cysts, and club foot. No consistent pattern of facial dysmorphism has been described. A sibship with features of **Smith-Lemli-Opitz syndrome, Meckel syndrome**, and Joubert syndromes has been described (Casamassima et al, 1987).

**Etiology:** Autosomal recessive inheritance.

**Pathogenesis:** Abnormal fusion of the cerebellar plates at the tectum of the fourth ventricle has been postulated. As this process proceeds in a rostal to caudal direction, it is the inferoposterior portion of the cerebellar vermis that is absent in cases of partial agenesis. Secondary disruption of this fusion has also been postulated. The abnormal respiratory pattern may be due to lack of inhibition of the reticular activating system or to an accompanying brainstem dysplasia.

**MIM No.:** *21330

**POS No.:** 3593

**Sex Ratio:** M2.5:F1 observed.

**Occurrence:** More than 45 cases have been described in the literature.

**Risk of Recurrence for Patient's Sib:**
See Part I, *Mendelian Inheritance*.

**Risk of Recurrence for Patient's Child:**
See Part I, *Mendelian Inheritance*. No affected individuals are known to have reproduced.

**Age of Detectability:** During the neonatal period. At least one case of prenatal diagnosis has been accomplished by comparison of fetal cranial ultrasound to affected sibs' CT scans.

**Gene Mapping and Linkage:** Unknown.

**Prevention:** None known. Genetic counseling indicated.

**Treatment:** Symptomatic for apnea and seizures.

**Prognosis:** Death has occurred from ages less than one month to 4 1/2 years of age. Survivors tend to be profoundly retarded.

**Detection of Carrier:** Unknown.

**Special Considerations:** Agenesis of the vermis itself does not account for the clinical features, as isolated agenesis of the vermis is usually asymptomatic. A number of patients have been described who, in addition to the cerebellar defects and typical symptomatology, have other features which would suggest either variable expression in or heterogeniety of this disorder. Eight males with chorioretinal colobomas may represent a distinct, possibly X-linked recessive entity. Also, Joubert syndrome with retinal aplasia and cystic kidneys (King et al, 1984), Joubert syndrome with polydactyly (Egger et al, 1982), and the cases of Casamassima et al (1987), may represent distinct autosomal recessive conditions.

**References:**
Joubert M, et al.: Familial agenesis of the cerebellar vermis: a syndrome of episodic hyperpnea, abnormal eye movements, ataxia, and retardation. Neurology 1969; 19:813–825. *
Pfeiffer RA, et al.: Nosology of congenital non-progressive cerebellar ataxia. Neuropediatr 1974; 5:91–102.
Boltshauser E, et al.: Joubert syndrome: clinical and polygraphic observations in a further case. Neuropediatrics 1981; 12:181–191.
Egger J, et al.: Joubert-Boltshauser syndrome with polydactyly in siblings. J Neurol Neurosurg Psych 1982; 45: 737–739.
Aicardi J, et al.: Le syndrome de Joubert: a propos de cinq observations. Arch Fr Pediatr 1983; 40:625–629.
Campbell S, et al.: The prenatal diagnosis of Joubert's syndrome of familial agenesis of the cerebellar vermis. Prenatal Diagn 1984; 4:391–395.
King MD, et al.: Joubert's syndrome with retinal dysplasia: neonatal tachypnea as the clue to a genetic brain-eye malformation. Arch Dis Child 1984; 59:709–718. †
Casamassima AC, et al.: A new syndrome with features of the Smith-Lemli-Opitz and Meckel-Gruber syndromes in a sibship with cerebellar defects. Am J Med Genet 1987; 26:321–326.

CA035
PF001

**Anthony C. Casamassima**
**Rudolf A. Pfeiffer**

**Joubert syndrome with polydactyly**
*See ORO-PALATAL-DIGITAL SYNDROME, VARADI TYPE*
**Joubert-Boltshauser syndrome**
*See JOUBERT SYNDROME*
**Juberg-Hayward syndrome**
*See ORO-CRANIO-DIGITAL SYNDROME*
**Juberg-Hellman syndrome**
*See SEIZURES, IN FEMALES, JUBERG-HELLMAN TYPE*
**Juberg-Hirsch syndrome**
*See TELECANTHUS, HEREDITARY*
**Juberg-Holt type recessive multiple epiphyseal dysplasia tarda**
*See EPIPHYSEAL DYSPLASIA, MULTIPLE, RECESSIVE TARDA TYPE*
**Juberg-Marsidi mental retardation**
*See X-LINKED MENTAL RETARDATION-GROWTH-HEARING AND GENITAL DEFECTS*
**Jugular lymphatic obstruction sequence**
*See NECK, CYSTIC HYGROMA, FETAL TYPE*

---

**JUMPING FRENCHMAN OF MAINE**         **3270**

**Includes:**
   Latah
   Myriachit
   Ragin' Cajun
   Startle syndromes

**Excludes:**
   **Epilepsy** (all forms)
   **Hyperekplexia** (3260)

**Major Diagnostic Criteria:** Sudden commands to an affected individual cause excessive startling, often accompanied by jumping, swearing, and other complex behavioral phenomena.

**Clinical Findings:** The syndrome consists of an exaggerated startle response to sudden acoustic and tactile stimuli accompanied by complex behavioral phenomena, including echolalia, echopraxia, and "forced obedience." Echolalia is involuntary repetition of words, echopraxia is involuntary imitation of gestures, and forced obedience is the allegedly involuntary execution of commands. All of these phenomena are reported in "jumpers" when the stimulus (phrase, command, or gesture) is presented suddenly and forcefully.

Jumping Frenchman of Maine differs from **Hyperekplexia** in that neonatal rigidity is lacking and the startle response consists of jumping and running about excitedly rather than stiffness and unchecked falling.

**Complications:** Unknown.

**Associated Findings:** Shyness and ticklishness are described in some patients.

**Etiology:** Unknown.

**Pathogenesis:** It is speculated that "jumpers" may have a genetically determined exaggerated startle response, but that the complex behavioral phenomena are culturally or psychiatrically determined.

The condition may be psychiatric in origin. It displays apparently non-Mendelian familial clustering, and has been reported primarily in individuals from the Moosehead Lake region of Maine.

**MIM No.:** 24410

**Sex Ratio:** M1:F<1 (significantly more common in males).

**Occurrence:** Reported primarily in French-Canadian Lumberjacks from the Moosehead Lake region of Maine, although the reported "Ragin' Cajun" Frenchman of Louisiana (McFarling, 1988) is probably related. It has been argued that the disorder is also identical to *latah* and *myriachit* which are complex startle/behavioral syndromes seen in Malaysia and Siberia, respectively.

**Risk of Recurrence for Patient's Sib:** Unknown.

**Risk of Recurrence for Patient's Child:** Unknown.

**Age of Detectability:** Usually but not always apparent by late adolescence.

**Gene Mapping and Linkage:** Unknown.

**Prevention:** None known. Genetic counseling indicated.

**Treatment:** Sedative-hypnotic agents have not been effective. Change of occupation has been beneficial in some cases.

**Prognosis:** Symptoms generally diminish with age after the second or third decade.

**Detection of Carrier:** Unknown.

**References:**
Beard GM: Remarks upon jumpers or jumping Frenchman. J Nerv Ment Dis 1878; 5:526 only.
Stevens HF: Jumping Frenchmen of Maine. Arch Neurology 1966; 12:311–314.
Hardison JE: Are the Jumping Frenchmen of Maine goosey? J Amer Med Ass 1980; 244:70.
Sainte-Hilaire MH, et al.: Jumping Frenchmen of Maine. Neurology 1986; 36:1269–1271.
McFarling DA: "Ragin' Cajuns": the jumping Frenchman of Louisiana. Neurology 1988; 38(Suppl 1):361 only.

RY001                                    **Stephen G. Ryan**

**Junctional epidermolysis bullosa**
*See EPIDERMOLYSIS BULLOSUM, TYPE II*
**Juvenile diabetes mellitus, mild**
*See DIABETES MELLITUS, MATURITY ONSET OF THE YOUNG (MODY)*
**Juvenile diabetes mellitus-optic atrophy-deafness**
*See DIABETES (INSIPIDUS/MELLITUS)-OPTIC ATROPHY-DEAFNESS*
**Juvenile epithelial corneal dystrophy**
*See CORNEAL DYSTROPHY, JUVENILE EPITHELIAL, MEESMANN TYPE*
**Juvenile macular degeneration, hereditary**
*See RETINA, FUNDUS FLAVIMACULATUS*
**Juvenile myoclonic epilepsy (JME), Janz type**
*See SEIZURES, MYOCLONIC, JUVENILE JANZ TYPE*
**Juvenile or adolescent cystinosis**
*See CYSTINOSIS*
**Juvenile osteochondritides**
*See JOINTS, OSTEOCHONDRITIS DISSECANS*
**Juvenile osteoporosis**
*See OSTEOPOROSIS, JUVENILE IDIOPATHIC*
**Juvenile retinoschisis, X-linked**
*See RETINOSCHISIS*

# ⟡ K ⟡

## KABUKI MAKE-UP SYNDROME 2355

**Includes:**

    Niikawa-Kuroki syndrome
    Short stature-facial and skeletal defects-mental retardation
    Skeletal and facial defects-short stature-mental retardation

**Excludes:**

    **Aarskog syndrome** (0001)
    **Coffin-Lowry syndrome** (0190)
    **KBG syndrome** (0554)
    **Robinow syndrome** (0876)
    **Tricho-rhino-phalangeal syndrome, type II** (0967)
    **Weaver syndrome** (2036)

**Major Diagnostic Criteria:** The combination of unusual facial appearance (consisting of long palpebral fissures with eversion of lower palpebrae, highly arched, abnormal eyebrows; long, thick eyelashes; large ears; and depressed nasal tip) skeletal anomalies; abnormal dermatoglyphics, short stature and mental retardation.

**Clinical Findings:** Long palpebral fissures (100%) and eversion of the lateral one-third of the lower palpebra (98%) are the most characteristic features, being remniscent of the actor's make-up of Kabuki (a Japanese traditional play). Other craniofacial anomalies include sparse, arched eyebrows at their lateral half (88%), prominent, large and malformed ears (85%), depressed nasal tip (79%), short nasal septum (93%), high-arched or cleft palate (63%) and malocclusion of teeth (78%). The fifth fingers are short and incurved (89%). Thoraco-lumbar scoliosis (49%) with or without midline defects of the vertebral body such as sagittal clefts is not

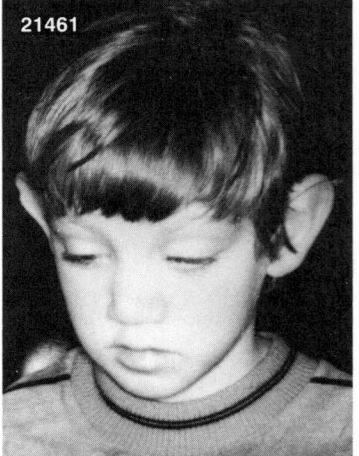

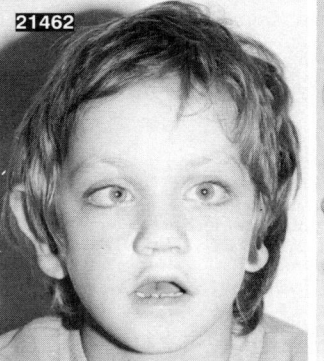
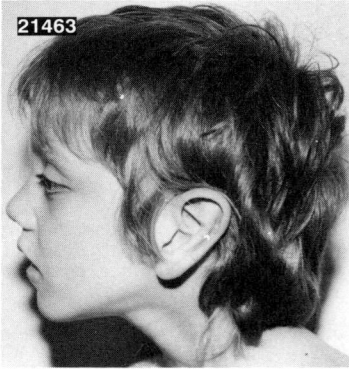

**2355B-21461–63:** Note large dysmorphic ears, prominent eyes, large nasal bridge, and broad nasal tip.

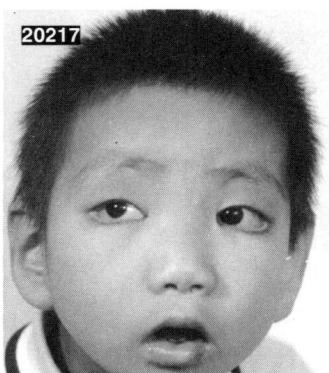
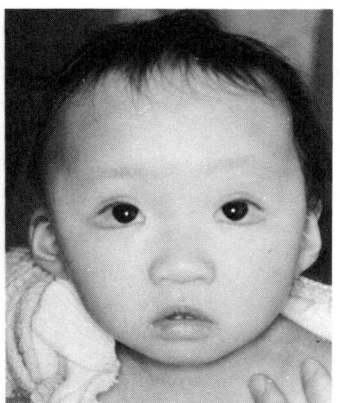

**2355A-20217:** Note the long palpebral fissures and everted lateral third of the lower eyelid reminiscent of the Kabuki actor's makeup.

uncommon. Growth deficiency (73%) usually appears postnatally. Average birth-length is 48.3 cm (49.1 cm after excluding the premature infants) and average birth-weight is 2,868 g (3,153 g and 2,943 g for male and female patients, respectively, excluding the premature). Short stature is evident by 1 year of age, most being at less than two SD below the mean. All patients are mildly to severely mentally retarded. Three-fourths of patients have the fingertip pad which is another characteristic feature. Dermatoglyphic findings include increasing ulnar loop patterns on the fingertip (63%), the absence of the digital triradius c or d (48%), and the presence of the interdigital triradius bc or cd and of hypothenar loops (70%).

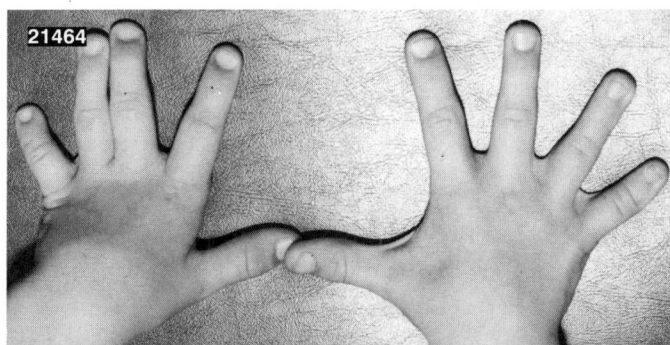

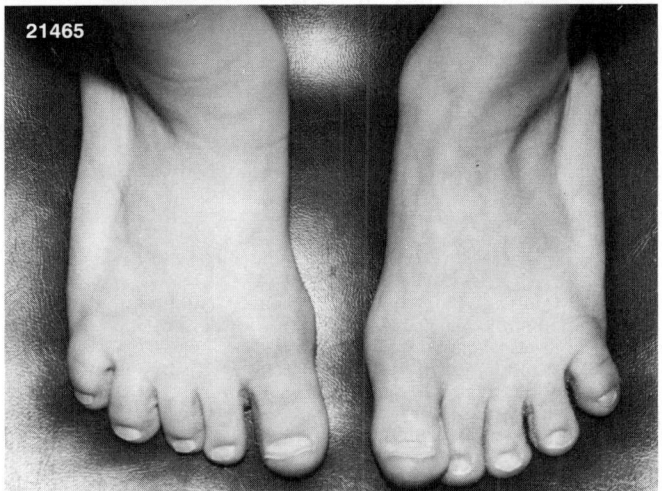

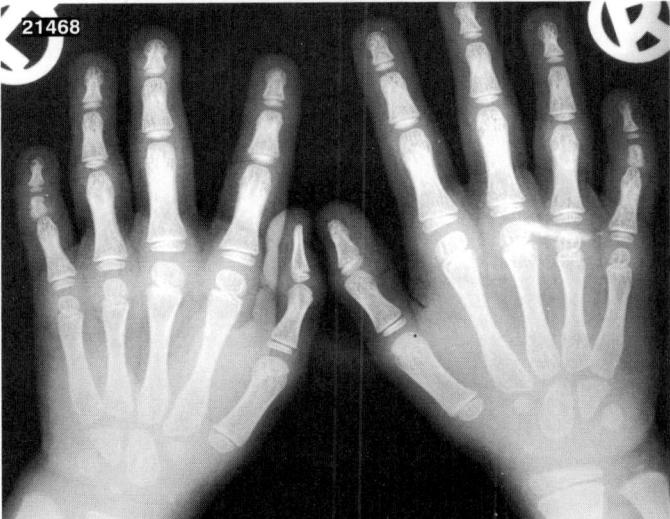

**2355C**-21464–65: Brachydactyly, syndactyly and broad short nails. 21468: X-ray shows brachydactyly, brachymesophalangy V and retarded bone age.

**Complications:** Susceptibility to upper respiratory infections or to otitis media in infancy (60%) followed sometimes by hearing impairment. Scoliosis usually develops with age.

**Associated Findings:** Precocious puberty (23%) in female infants, congenital heart diseases and great vessel anomalies (32%).

**Etiology:** Most cases have been sporadic. No parental consanguinity has been observed among 62 couples except for four cases. Parental ages are not higher than those of children in general population. There is no common history during pregnancy particular to every case such as radiation exposures, drug intakes, or infections. Karyotypes are normal in most patients, even with high-resolution bandings, except for three patients. One patient had inv(Y)(p11.2q11.23) and the other two had r(X)(p11.2q13) or r(Y)(p11.2q11.2). Niikawa et al (1988) speculated pseudoautosomal dominant inheritance. Halal et al (1989) reported a familial case suggestive of autosomal dominant inheritance.

**Pathogenesis:** Unknown. The fingertip pads, as observed in three-fourth of patients, have not previously been described in live born individuals and are the remnant of the fingerpads descernible in fetuses at the sixth week of gestation. Normally they begin to regress during the 10th and 12th weeks, to be gradually replaced by the primary dermal ridges that are formed between the 13th and 18th weeks. Therefore, the presence of the pads may reflect a developmental disturbance by the 18th week of gestation.

**MIM No.:** 14792

**POS No.:** 3541

**Sex Ratio:** M1:F1

**Occurrence:** More than 70 cases have been reported; 62 in Japan, three Canadians from one family, one each from Latin-American, Italian, and Germany, a Libyan Arab, and a United States citizen of English-Irish ancestry.

**Risk of Recurrence for Patient's Sib:**
See Part I, *Mendelian Inheritance.*

**Risk of Recurrence for Patient's Child:**
See Part I, *Mendelian Inheritance.*

**Age of Detectability:** At birth, by physical examination.

**Gene Mapping and Linkage:** KMS (Kabuki make-up syndrome) is unassigned.

**Prevention:** None known. Genetic counseling indicated.

**Treatment:** Orthopedic management may be indicated; physical therapy to prevent scoliosis. Detection and management of possible recurrent otitis.

**Prognosis:** Unknown.

**Detection of Carrier:** Unknown.

**References:**
Kuroki Y, et al.: A new malformation syndrome of long palpebral fissures, large ears, depressed nasal tip, and skeletal anomalies associated with postnatal dwarfism and mental retardation. J Pediatr 1981; 99:570–573.
Niikawa N, et al.: Kabuki make-up syndrome: a syndrome of mental retardation, unusual facies, large and protruding ears, and postnatal growth deficiency. J Pediatr 1981; 99:565–569. * †
Niikawa N, et al.: The dermatoglyphic pattern of the Kabuki make-up syndrome. Clin Genet 1982; 21:315–320.
Kaiser-Kupfer MI, et al.: The Niikawa-Kuroki (Kabuki make-up) syndrome in an American black. Am J Ophthalmol 1986; 102:667–668.
Niikawa N, et al.: Kabuki make-up (Niikawa-Kuroki) syndrome: a study of 62 patients. Am J Med Genet 1988; 31:565–589. *
Halal F, et al.: Autosomal dominant inheritance of the Kabuki make-up (Niikawa-Kuroki) syndrome. Am J Med Genet 1989; 33:376–381.

NI010                                                    **Norio Niikawa**

**Kahler disease**
*See CANCER, MULTIPLE MYELOMA*

## KALLMANN SYNDROME                                    2301

**Includes:**

DeMorsier dysplasia olfactogenitalis
Dysplasia olfactogenitalis of DeMorsier
Hypogonadotropic hypogonadism with anosmia or
    hyposmia
Olfactogenital dysplasia

**Excludes:**

**Ataxia-hypogonadism syndrome** (0093)
Gonadal dysgenesis (all forms)
**Gonadotropin deficiencies** (0438)
**Hypogonadotropic hypogonadism** (2300)
**Klinefelter syndrome** (0556)

**Major Diagnostic Criteria:** Luteinizing hormone (LH) and follicle-stimulating hormone (FSH) levels of <5 mIU/ml and anosmia or hyposmia.

**Clinical Findings:** LH and FSH levels are below the levels of clinical detection with current assay specificity. Biologic effects reflect the amount of total gonadotropin function and usually result in failure of the gonad to function and allow pubertal development. In addition, patients have decreased or absent ability to smell due to absent olfactory bulbs either unilaterally or bilaterally secondary to defective development of the rhinencephalon. Males may be cryptorchid.

In both sexes, somatic anomalies may exist.

**Complications:** Lack of gonadal stimulation in both sexes results in failure of secondary sexual development and sterility.

Females exhibit estrogen deficiency syndrome, including vaginal atrophy with resultant dyspareunia, osteoporosis, hot flashes after initial estrogen replacement and sudden withdrawal.

Cryptorchidism imposes the risk of decreased spermatogenesis and testicular tumors.

**Associated Findings:** Borderline normal intelligence; cleft lip and palate; hearing loss and deafness; renal anomalies, particularly unilateral agenesis; cardiac anomalies; diabetes mellitus; choanal atresia; short fourth metacarpal.

**Etiology:** Genetic heterogeneity. The disorder may be inherited differently in different families; thus, counseling will depend on presence or absence of other affected relatives and their relationship to the proband. Autosomal dominant, X-linked recessive, and autosomal recessive inheritance have all been observed. Relative proportions of the three modes are unknown. There is no evidence that different modes differ clinically.

**Pathogenesis:** Abnormal development of the rhinencephalon results in interference in the communication of the hypothalamus with the pituitary. Disordered gonadotropin releasing hormone (GNRH) signals to the pituitary result in absence of LH and FSH. In turn, this results in failure of gonadal stimulation and therefore absence of the subsequent development stimulated by gonadal steroids, namely, secondary sex characteristics and reproductive processes.

**MIM No.:** *14795, *24420, *30870

**POS No.:** 4216

**Sex Ratio:** M5:F1

**Occurrence:** 1:10,000 in males and 1:50,000 in females; prevalence is 1:25 hyposmic or anosmic patients and 1:30 46,XY individuals with hypogonadism.

**Risk of Recurrence for Patient's Sib:**

See Part I, *Mendelian Inheritance.* Varies with etiology. The disorder may be inherited differently in different families; thus, counseling depends on other affected relatives in the pedigree.

**Risk of Recurrence for Patient's Child:**

See Part I, *Mendelian Inheritance.* The disorder may be inherited differently in different families; thus counseling depends on other affected relatives in the pedigree. If no other relative is affected, risk could be as high as 50%.

**Age of Detectability:** During puberty, unless anosmia is diagnosed in childhood.

**Gene Mapping and Linkage:** KAL (Kallmann syndrome) has been mapped to Xp22.32.

Linkage to HLA has been excluded.

**Prevention:** None known. Genetic counseling indicated.

**Treatment:** Hormonal replacement to stimulate development and to maintain integrity of secondary sex characteristics and sexual function.

Gonadal steroid replacement is necessary for the initiation and maintenance of secondary sex characteristics and sexual function.

Fertility may be achieved in both sexes by administration of pulsatile GNRH. Most patients are unresponsive to single-dose GNRH administration unless first primed by multiple doses. Repeated hCG injections in males and hMG in females may also be used to stimulate gametogenesis. Clomiphene citrate is ineffective in treatment of these patients.

**Prognosis:** Life span is normal. Reproduction depends on the success of therapy to stimulate spermatogenesis or oogenesis.

**Detection of Carrier:** Unknown.

**References:**

Santen RJ, Paulsen CA: Hypogonadotropic eunuchoidism: clinical study of the mode of inheritance. J Clin Endocrinol 1973; 36:47–54.
Santen RJ, Paulsen CA: Hypogonadotropic eunuchoidism: gonadal responsiveness to exogenous gonadotropins. J Clin Endocrinol Metab 1973; 36:55–63.
Wegenke JD, et al.: Familial Kallmann syndrome with unilateral renal aplasia. Clin Genet 1975; 7:368–381.
Lieblich JM, et al.: Syndrome of anosmia with hypogonadotropic hypogonadism (Kallmann syndrome): clinical and laboratory studies in 23 cases. Am J Med 1982; 73:506–519.
White BJ, et al.: The syndrome of anosmia with hypogonadotropic hypogonadism: a genetic study of 18 new families and a review. Am J Med Genet 1983; 15:417–435.
Pawlowitzki IH, et al.: Estimating frequency of Kallmann syndrome among anosmic patients. Am J Med Genet 1987; 26:473–479.

CA041                                        **Sandra Ann Carson**

**Kanamycin, fetal effects**
*See FETAL AMINOGLYCOSIDE OTOTOXICITY*
**Kandori fleck retina**
*See RETINA, FLECKED KANDORI TYPE*
**Kanner disease**
*See AUTISM, INFANTILE*
**Kantrex△, fetal effects**
*See FETAL AMINOGLYCOSIDE OTOTOXICITY*
**Kaposi dermatosis**
*See XERODERMA PIGMENTOSUM*
**Kappa light chain of immunoglobulin**
*See SERUM ALLOTYPES, HUMAN*
**Kartagener syndrome**
*See DEXTROCARDIA-BRONCHIECTASIS-SINUSITIS SYNDROME*
**Kasabach-Merritt syndrome**
*See HEMANGIOMA-THROMBOCYTOPENIA SYNDROME*
**Kasabach-Merritt syndrome (some cases)**
*See HEMANGIOMAS OF THE HEAD AND NECK*
**Kaufman syndrome**
*See OCULO-CEREBRO-FACIAL SYNDROME, KAUFMAN TYPE*
**Kaufman-McKusick syndrome**
*See VAGINAL SEPTUM, TRANSVERSE*

## KBG SYNDROME                                        0554

**Includes:** Short stature-facial/skeletal anomalies-retardation-macrodontia

**Excludes:** Malformation-mental retardation syndromes (other)

**Major Diagnostic Criteria:** Rounded face, bow-shaped narrow lips, macrodontia, and broad eyebrows in a short, mentally retarded person combined, with X-ray abnormalities of ribs, vertebrae, hips, and hands.

**Clinical Findings:** Shows great variability in expression. Findings in the majority of patients include shortness of stature (below 3rd percentile), moderate mental retardation, biparietal prominence, brachycephaly, round face, telecanthus (75–90%), broad

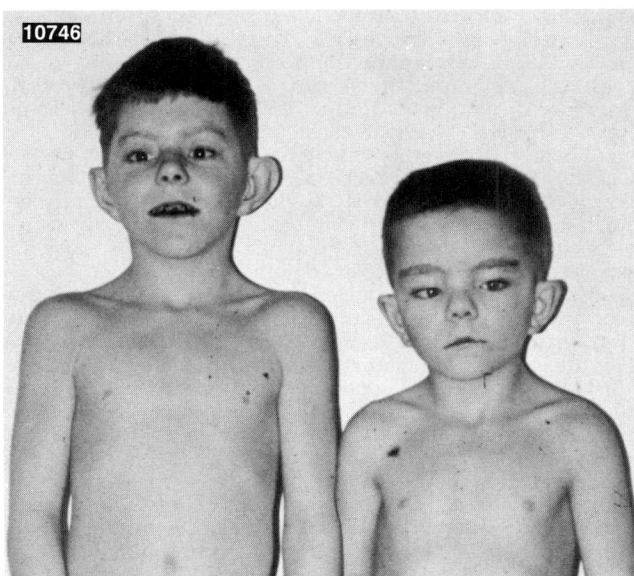

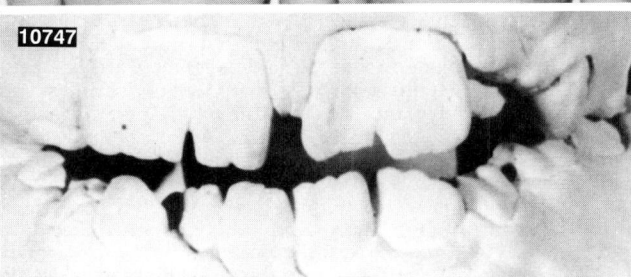

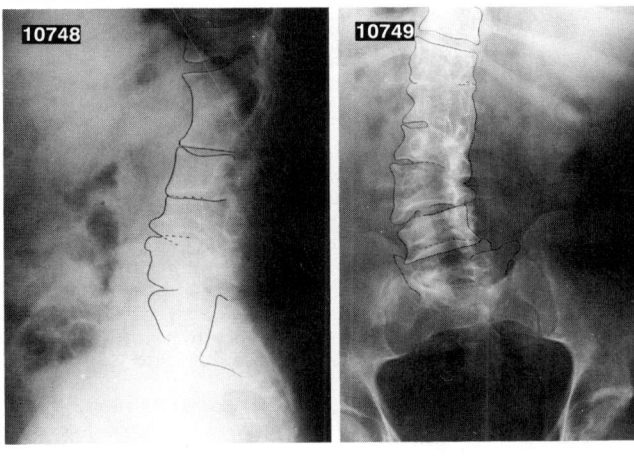

**0554-10746:** Characteristic round facies with bow-shaped lips and thick eyebrows with pectus excavatum. **10747:** Model of teeth shows macrodontia. **10748–49:** Block vertebrae from T12-L2, deformed and partially collapsed L3-5 vertebral bodies and short femoral necks.

eyebrows, short alveolar ridges, macrodontia, cervical ribs, abnormal vertebrae, short femoral necks, short tubular bones in hands, delayed bone age, syndactyly of toes 2–3, palmar distal axial triradius and simian crease. The EEG was abnormal in two cases investigated. Other significant low-frequency findings include pectus excavatum, hip dysplasia, hexadactyly, and hearing deficit.

**Complications:** Deformities and pain secondary to skeletal manifestations. Crowding and noneruption of teeth.

**Associated Findings:** None known.

**Etiology:** Autosomal dominant inheritance. There have been no instances to date of sibs born to unaffected parents. Sporadic cases may represent new mutations.

**Pathogenesis:** Undetermined. Many of the manifestations seem related to skeletal defects.

**MIM No.:** *14805

**POS No.:** 3270

**Sex Ratio:** Presumably M1:F1, although actual reports show a greater percentage of males.

**Occurrence:** At least five kindreds, with nine cases, have been reported.

**Risk of Recurrence for Patient's Sib:**
See Part I, *Mendelian Inheritance.*

**Risk of Recurrence for Patient's Child:**
See Part I, *Mendelian Inheritance.*

**Age of Detectability:** At birth.

**Gene Mapping and Linkage:** Unknown.

**Prevention:** None known. Genetic counseling indicated.

**Treatment:** Supportive and symptomatic; including especially orthopedic surgery for spine or hip problems, dental care, hearing aid, and speech therapy.

**Prognosis:** Apparently good for life span; dependent on degree of mental retardation and skeletal manifestations.

**Detection of Carrier:** Unknown.

**Special Considerations:** The designation KBG syndrome followed from John Opitz's practice of naming conditions after the initials of the affected families' surnames.

**References:**

Herrmann J, et al.: The KBG syndrome: a syndrome of short stature, characteristic facies, mental retardation, macrodontia and skeletal abnormalities. BD:OAS;XI(5). New York: National Foundation-March of Dimes, 1975:7–18.

Parloir C, et al.: Short stature, craniofacial dysmorphism and dento-skeletal abnormalities in a large kindred: a variant of KBG syndrome or a new mental retardation syndrome. Clin Genet 1977; 12:263–266.

Novembri A, et al.: K.B.G. syndrome: review of the literature and presentation of a case. Arch Put Chir Org Mo 1983; 33:423–430.

Fryns JP, Hospeslagh M: Mental retardation, short stature, minor skeletal anomalies, craniofacial dysmorphism and macrodontia in two sisters and their mother. Clin Genet 1984; 26:69–72.

Tollard I, et al.: Dento-maxillo-facial anomalies in the KBG syndrome. Minerva Stomatol 1984; 33:437–446.

GR021
HE023

**Arthur W. Grix**
**Jürgen Herrmann**

## KEARNS-SAYRE DISEASE 2070

**Includes:**
Kearns-Sayre syndrome, typical (KSS)
Kearns-Shy syndrome
Kiloh-Nevin dystrophy of the external ocular muscles
Mitochondrial cytopathy
Mitochondrial encephalomyopathy
Oculocraniosomatic neuromuscular disease
Ophthalmoplegia-pigmentary degeneration of retina-cardiomyopathy
Ophthalmoplegia plus syndrome
Partial Kearns-Sayre syndrome (PKSS)
Stephens syndrome (ophthalmoplegia-ataxia-peripheral neuropathy)

**Excludes:**
**Ataxia**
**Diplegia, congenital facial** (0376)
**Encephalopathy, necrotizing** (0344)

**Machado-Joseph disease** (2996)
**Muscular dystrophy, oculopharyngeal** (0692)
**Myopathy-metabolic, mitochondrial cytochrome C oxidase deficiency** (2707)
**Myopathy, myotubular** (0695)
Ocular myasthenia gravis
**Ophthalmoplegia, progressive external** (0752)
**Optic atrophy, Leber type** (0579)
Poliodystrophia cerebri progressiva

**Major Diagnostic Criteria:** Ophthalmoparesis, pigmentary retinal dystrophy, and cardiac conduction disorders are three major necessary clinical symptoms. Since age of onset varies from infancy to advanced adult years, other findings have been variably added through the years: cerebellar ataxia, proximal-axial muscle weakness, hearing loss, and/or vestibular dysfunction. Body undergrowth and polyglandular abnormalities include hypoparathyroid and hypothyroid states. The original laboratory finding of an increased CSF protein often includes abnormal plasma or CSF resting state lactate/pyruvate levels in 50%. Folic acid deficiency in CSF causes a high plasma:CSF ratio. Serum creatine kinase (CK) is normal in 75%, as are standard hematologic and urine examinations. Histologic, structural, or functional defects in mitochondria from muscle or fibroblasts may be identified without specific correlation to clinical findings, as well as many secondary biochemical effects in plasma and CSF, including amino acids and, in urine, organic acids. Plasma and tissue total and free carnitine may be altered. Phosphorus ($^{31}$P) magnetic resonance spectroscopy (MRS) in the noncarnitine forms of mitochondrial myopathy may show a reduced muscle energy state. Cerebral, cerebellar, and brainstem hypodense lesions occasionally suggesting vascular infarcts are seen by CT scanning, along with calcifications or hypodense lesions of the basal ganglia (50%). Reduced vision (40%) or optic atrophy may be observed as the condition progresses. Seizures are uncommon.

Electrophysiologic responses of retinal function (ERGs), visual-evoked potentials (VERs) with P100 latencies, somatosensory-evoked responses (SSERs), and muscle electromyograms (EMGs), as well as conduction velocities of peripheral motor and sensory nerves, may be altered. Specific saccadic velocity patterns in chronic progressive extraocular muscle paralysis (CPEO) by direct current electrooculogram (dc-EOG) may differentiate disorders of neurophthalmic motility. There is clinical evidence that peripheral neuropathy causes hyporeflexia and sensory loss in a few patients.

**Clinical Findings:** Often ptosis and extraocular motor abnormalities are the presenting symptom under age 20 years, and not infrequently under age five years, especially CPEO. Onset of an asymmetric ocular paresis preceded by ptosis then leads to total ophthalmoplegia without a pupillary defect in 90% of patients. A pigmentary retinopathy of fine, diffuse, granular character, centrally located, in some patients followed by CPEO, occurs over decades. Diminished visual acuity or night blindness occurs in 40% with rare corneal dystrophic opacities. Saccadic and smooth pursuit extraocular eye movements are restricted and slowed, causing a pendular opticokinetic nystagmus. Palatal and tongue movements may be limited, causing dysarthric speech and mild dysphagia accentuated by cerebellar involvement. Tongue bulk may be reduced, but fasciculations are not observed. Bilateral peripheral facial paralysis and sensorineural deafness may be evident initially in 54% of patients. Vestibular dysfunction occurs in one-third of patients. Temporal and masseter muscle bulk and strength are normal. Neck muscle strength reduction occurs especially in the flexor group, including the sternocleidomastoids, and may be detected early. The distribution of muscle involvement may be similar to **Muscular dystrophy, facio-scapulo-humeral**; **Muscular dystrophy, oculopharyngeal**; and **Diplegia, congenital facial**.

Facial sensation and corneal reflexes are intact. Occasionally abnormal facial (snout) and head-neck reflexes (head retraction) occur. Although myopathic extraocular muscle changes are observed, the structural changes in the central nervous system suggest that the pathogenesis of CPEO is of neurogenic origin. Proximal muscle paresis and hypotonia are seldom prominent initially. Weakness is proximal and especially axial. Upper extrem-

ities are involved first, then the shoulder-neck region, and later the proximal lower extremities, causing great difficulty in walking. Muscle bulk is symmetrically reduced, proximally early in life, suggesting a dysmorphic appearance as in a congenital myopathy (myotubular or centronuclear forms). The clinical findings are of a myopathic process without distal atrophy, fasciculations, or symptomatic or percussion myotonia, although myotonia and muscle hypertrophy have been observed. Motor function examination reveals cerebellar ataxia (40–70%), with truncal titubation, action tremors, occasionally "wing-beating," extremity dysmetria, dysdiadochokinesia, and extrapyramidal movements (chorea or dystonia) occurring singly or in combination.

Speech and gait slowly deteriorate with weakness as does coordination, limiting ambulation. A static or subtly progressive encephalopathy in children presents as mental retardation. Cognitive, intellectual, and behavioral deficiencies may be identified by history and neurologic and psychologic examination (40%). Intellectual function is normal (80%) in many. Sensory examination is most often normal. Reflexes are quite variable, with hypoactive responses and significant muscle weakness. Hyperactive reflexes, including bilateral Babinski signs, occur in the progressive disorder. Other systemic symptoms and signs are common, especially in partial Kearns-Sayre syndrome (PKSS). Cardiac conduction defects, including complete atrioventricular (AV) heart block appearing early, may remain asymptomatic for decades. Most patients are affected with serious cardiac involvement, including sudden death (in about two-thirds). The cardiomyopathy may be related to carnitine deficiency. Cardiac-related syncope is found in about one-half. Disordered endocrine system function may be polyglandular, including hypoparathyroidism, hypothyroidism, diabetes, pubertal delay, and hypercholesterolemia. Generalized seizures occur with hypocalcemia, but are not otherwise common (10%). A short stature observed in over two-thirds of patients occurs with delayed puberty in one-third.

In 1968 Drachman (see Berenberg et al, 1977) assembled these heterogeneous features of conditions surrounding progressive external ophthalmoplegia (PEO) into the *Ophthalmoplegia-Plus syndrome*. In 1975 Rowland suggested an eponym to recognize Kearns and Sayre (1958) and Daroff for their original clinical and pathologic findings of ophthalmoparesis and spongy degeneration in the brain. Descriptions of infantile, juvenile, and adult forms may relate to partial expression of typical KSS (TKSS). However, mild and moderate forms are not always progressive in family studies. The appellation *oculocraniosomatic syndrome* held only a brief popularity. In 1977 Berenberg et al attempted to resolve the complex issues of nosology in a careful analysis of 35 patients with "typical" Kearns-Sayre syndrome (TKSS), suggesting this eponym. Rowland later reaffirmed an "invariant triad": PEO, pigmentary retinopathy, and one additional finding of either heart block, a cerebellar syndrome, or a CSF protein over 100 mg/dl. Some authors add age of onset as a fourth criterion. While neuromuscular abnormalities occurred in other family members, there were no recorded instances of more than one "typical" KSS in any family.

Another review (see Petty et al, 1986) added 13 more patients with less restrictive major symptoms and accepted a positive family history that indicated a dominant mode of inheritance. The recognition of mitochondrial structural and functional defects associated with clinical and metabolic abnormalities with some response to treatment, including documented familial recurrence, may justify a "disease" concept.

**Complications:** The heterogeneous features of KSS, without a specific cause, accounts for the difficulty in separating primary from secondary complications. Several effects appear to be the result of the underlying disease process: Heart block with Stokes-Adams attacks occurs in 50% of patients. Conduction heart block accompanies cardiac muscle and conduction system mitochondrial abnormalities. One-half require cardiac pacemakers. Heart failure and cardiac arrest occur in one-third. One-third of affected patients die of cardiac complications. Proximal muscle weakness interferes with motor function, limiting ambulation as well as pulmonary function. Abrupt neurologic deterioration of sudden onset, especially in children, with coma and death may occur with or without cardiac findings. The therapeutic use of steroids potentiates this risk with a fatal ketotic or nonketotic metabolic acidosis and hyperglycemia. There appears to be an underlying unexplained CNS lactate-pyruvate metabolic defect in nonsteroid-treated patients as well. A separate or partial expression of an underlying mitochondrial defect associated with encephalopathy, lactic acidosis, and stroke-like episodes is known as the "MELAS" syndrome. Another syndrome with myoclonic seizures, optic atrophy, and sensory neural hearing loss, known as "Fukuhara disease" (MERRF), has similarities to KSS. There is also a characteristic pathologic cerebral, cerebellar, and brainstem spongiform encephalopathy in this group.

**Associated Findings:** The inclusion of many findings, possibly epiphenomena, in a less restrictive definition or "partial" expression of KSS may have utility, since the characteristic progressive systemic and neurologic deterioration alters clinical presentation at all ages. Many infrequent clinical and laboratory findings are of unknown significance. Some authors consider KSS to be merely a cluster of a more generic mitochondrial group of disorders and suggest that a rational classification on clinical grounds is not possible. Peripheral neuropathies are absent in typical KSS. Degenerative peripheral nerve demyelination (*Stephens syndrome*), and inclusions similar to Hirano bodies have been documented in less complete forms of KSS. Optic atrophy and optic neuritis have been reported. CPEO and parkinsonism, dementias, **Ataxia, Friedreich type**, **Machado-Joseph disease**, and Charcot-Marie-Tooth disease have been noted. Rarely hypoplastic anemias and renal dysfunction occur in children. Arachnodactyly, sternal deformities, high-arched palates, and myopia are rare dysmorphic features. Low CSF folate levels compared with plasma levels, resulting in a high plasma:CSF ratio, may be useful in diagnosis and as a guide to treatment. Folic acid deficiency rather than malabsorption may contribute to muscle carnitine reduction. Malabsorption in megaloblastic anemias is known to be associated with symptoms of mental retardation and calcification of the basal ganglia. Folic acid deficiencies may secondarily alter CSF neurotransmitters. Regional bilateral subcortical hypodense lesions in the thalamus, similar to those described in **Encephalopathy, necrotizing**, are associated with hypersomnia and altered nocturnal sleep patterns.

Histopathologic examination shows some muscle-fiber atrophy, and, on histochemical staining, a vacuolar myopathy with lipid or glycogen accumulation initially suggested a slow virus infection. Gomori trichrome stain shows abnormal structure or number of subsarcolemmal mitochondrial aggregations and paracrystalline inclusions identified as "ragged red fibers" (RRF) in type I fibers. This mitochondrial proliferation and the abnormalities in earlier reports suggested a "pleoconial" or "megaconial" myopathy. However, over 10% of myopathies demonstrate RRFs, while 5–25% of KSS muscle biopsy materials contain these abnormal aggregates. Intramitochondrial paracrystalline inclusions by electron microscopy are of unknown biochemical nature, and the pathophysiologic significance is undetermined. Similar structural abnormalities are found in cardiac muscle cells and in some cells of the conduction system. The role of mitochondria in brain is unknown. Skin and conjunctival biopsy may assist identification during life.

Low state III (to NAD- and FAD-linked substrates) respiration rates on polarographic studies and histochemically uncoupled respiration ($Mg^{2+}$-activated ATPase) suggest mitochondrial dysfunction with reduced glycolytic energy production. Reduced cytochrome oxidase (c, $aa_3$/b/cc1) and a decreased ratio of cytochrome oxidase/succinate-cytochrome c, normal monoamine oxidase, depend on the presence or absence of RRFs.

NADH-Coenzyme Q reductase may be low in muscle and fibroblasts. Mitochondrial metabolic malfunctions are variable and may affect complexes I, II, III, IV, or V (ATPase). Several malfunctions include muscle carnitine deficiency with normal plasma levels and reduced palmitoyl-CoA synthetase. Patients may also have normal cellular responses. Lactate and pyruvate elevations in plasma and CSF, with or without glucose loading, suggest a disorder of pyruvate utilization in the citric-acid cycle. Typically CSF protein is elevated over 100 mg/dl, while lower amounts may relate to partial disorders. Abnormalities in albumin, IgG, oligoclonal bands, and tau fractions with normal myelin basic protein are rarely reported. Muscular and humoral immunologic abnormalities and circulating immune complexes also are rarely observed.

**Etiology:** The decision to confine to TKSS three (occasionally four) clinical manifestations and to designate as partial forms or as separate syndromes the less consistent features is based on the state of knowledge regarding underlying etiology. Viral infections, immunologic disorders, and, more recently, metabolic defects of mitochondrial function have all been considered. Genetic issues are unclear. Some studies of TKSS found no families with more than one person with characteristic KSS, suggesting the pseudogenetic mechanisms of acquired disease and leading to the statement that there is no evidence of genetic abnormality or metabolic defect in this syndrome. Autosomal dominant inheritance has been observed in an only minimally less complete form of KSS, with 15 members of one family reported to be affected in two generations. Careful examinations of all family members have not always been achieved. The age differences of family members adds to the variable degree and number of clinical manifestations. Autosomal recessive inheritance, X-linked recessive inheritance, and an X-linked dominant inheritance have also been suggested.

The mitochondrial myopathies may be viewed as secondary to as yet unknown primary defects in different syndromes or as heterogeneous polygenetic syndromes. There is evidence for a disturbance of mitochondrial DNA (mtDNA) caused by defects of a mitochondrial genome and transmitted by maternal inheritance, with mitotic segregation accounting for mutual phenotypes.

**Pathogenesis:** The pathogeneses of TKSS and PKSS are unknown. Disorders of folic acid metabolism, confirmed in separate studies, and treatment responses to coenzymes, including coenzyme Q (CoQ), involved in the mitochondrial electron transport chain, along with the supplemental use of folic acid and carnitine, suggest basic metabolic mechanisms. Recent reports identify mitochondrial abnormalities associated with disordered metabolism of folic acid, mitochondrial enzymes, substrate, and transport defects. Functional and structural abnormalities in skeletal and cardiac muscle, liver, pancreas, and brain have been documented with a CNS spongy degeneration, especially in the brainstem. Abrupt neurologic deterioration may be an independent and sudden cause of death unrelated to cardiac failure.

**MIM No.:** 16510

**POS No.:** 3747

**Sex Ratio:** M1:F1

**Occurrence:** About 80 cases have been reported. No ethnic or demographic characteristics. Rare among the neuromusclar disorders. Needs consideration among conditions associated with congenital lactic acidoses, CPEO, and disorders of folic acid metabolism, although molecular mechanisms are not established. CT hypodense lesions and basal ganglion calcification especially with a pigmentary retinopathy are also suggestive.

**Risk of Recurrence for Patient's Sib:** No genetic risk known in TKSS, but probably as high as 1:2 (50%) if parent affected, as in some partial mitochondrial syndromes. There may be some unestablished risk if any family members in recent generations are affected.

**Risk of Recurrence for Patient's Child:** Depending on interpretation of complete and incomplete syndromes, may be as high as 1:2 for some, and probably no risk for others.

**Age of Detectability:** Infancy through adult years.

**Gene Mapping and Linkage:** Deletions of mtDNA have recently been identified (Zeviani et al, 1988).

**Prevention:** None known. Genetic counseling indicated.

**Treatment:** Folic acid (oral folinic acid) when the plasma or CSF folate ratio is low as determined by measurement of plasma or CSF folate ratios. Reduced muscle tissue carnitine to be supplemented by oral L-carnitine. The lactic-pyruvic acid abnormalities, resting or after oral glucose, may respond to the oral administration of CoQ. CSF protein may decrease as clinical improvement occurs. Cardiac pacemakers for conduction defects are essential. Tarsofrontalis surgical suspensions improve obstructed vision, but must be performed with extreme caution to avoid lagophthalmos and corneal exposure. Independent therapy for hypoparathyroidism, hypothyroidism, and diabetes may be required. Steroid use is to be carefully considered in view of the reports of steroid-associated acute neurologic deterioration with coma and death.

**Prognosis:** A progressive deterioration of all neuromuscular functions is expected without effective treatment. Limited physical function may require orthopedic equipment. Cardiac death may be avoidable by early studies of cardiac competence and use of a pacemaker. Acute neurologic deterioration occurs at any time, unprovoked and not related to cardiac status. Survival into adult years is likely with long-term supportive therapy.

**Detection of Carrier:** Carriers cannot be distinguished at this time. Careful examination of all family members, however, is warranted to delineate epidemiology.

**Special Considerations:** As in many neurologic conditions, there is an overlap among these disorders. Careful clinical, medical, and neurologic family examinations and comprehensive laboratory studies are appropriate. Confusion to date is largely related to the reports of individual families or patients in past decades studied by the then available procedures. DNA analysis may help separate the disorders. Magnetic resonance imaging (MRI) in early consideration of this diagnosis is potentially the most sensitive for spongy generalized or regional brain changes. Metabolic studies during and after acute illness should include electrolytes, plasma and urine organic acids, muscle and tissue biopsies for structural and functional mitochondrial abnormalities, CSF proteins, lactate-pyruvate, plasma and CSF folates, and carnitine. Clinical monitoring of supplemental therapies, including CoQ therapy, are needed in long-term care.

**References:**
Kearns TP, Sayre GP: Retinitis pigmentosa, external ophthalmoplegia, and complete heart block. Arch Ophthal 1958; 60:280–289.
Berenberg RA, et al.: Lumping or splitting? Ophthalmoplegia-Plus or Kearns-Sayre syndrome? Ann Neurol 1977; 1:37–54. *
Schnitzler ER, et al.: Familial Kearns-Sayre syndrome. Neurology 1979; 29:1172–1174.
Coulter DL, Allen RJ: Abrupt neurological deterioration in children with Kearns-Sayre syndrome. Arch Neurol 1981; 38:247–250.
Allen RJ, et al.: Kearns-Sayre syndrome with reduced plasma and cerebrospinal fluid folate. Ann Neurol 1983; 13:679–682.
Rowland LP: Molecular genetics, pseudogenetics, and clinical neurology. Neurology 1983; 33:1179–1195.
Arnold DL, et al.: Investigation of human mitochondrial myopathies by phosphorus magnetic resonance spectroscopy. Ann Neurol 1985; 18:189–196.
DiMauro S, et al.: Mitochondrial myopathies. Ann Neurol 1985; 17:521–528.
Ogasahara S, et al.: Improvement of abnormal pyruvate metabolism and cardiac conduction defects with coenzyme $Q_{10}$ in Kearns-Sayre syndrome. Neurology 1985; 35:372–377.
Petty RKH, et al.: The clinical features of mitochondrial myopathy. Brain 1986; 109:915–938. *
Holt IJ, et al.: Deletions of mitochondrial DNA in patients with mitochondrial myopathies. Nature 1988; 331:717–719.
Rowland LP, et al.: Kearns-Sayre syndrome in twins: lethal dominant mutation or acquired disease? Neurology 1988; 38:1399–1402.
Moraes CT, et al.: Mitochondrial DNA deletions in progressive external ophalmoplegia and Kearns-Sayre syndrome. New Engl J Med 1989; 320:1293–1299. *

AL028                              **Richard J. Allen**

**Kearns-Sayre syndrome, typical (KSS)**
  See KEARNS-SAYRE DISEASE
**Kearns-Shy syndrome**
  See KEARNS-SAYRE DISEASE
**Keinbock (carpal semilunar)**
  See JOINTS, OSTEOCHONDRITIS DISSECANS
**Keipert syndrome**
  See NASO-DIGITO-ACOUSTIC SYNDROME, KEIPERT TYPE
**Keipert-Fitzgerald-Danks syndrome**
  See NASO-DIGITO-ACOUSTIC SYNDROME, KEIPERT TYPE
**Kell blood group precursor substance**
  See ANEMIA, HEMOLYTIC, RED CELL MEMBRANE DEFECTS
**Kennedy disease**
  See SPINAL MUSCULAR ATROPHY
**Kennedy type spinal and bulbar muscular atrophy**
  See MUSCULAR ATROPHY, SPINAL AND BULBAR, X-LINKED KENNEDY TYPE
**Kennedy-Stefanis disease**
  See MUSCULAR ATROPHY, SPINAL AND BULBAR, X-LINKED KENNEDY TYPE
**Kenny disease**
  See TUBULAR STENOSIS
**Kenny-Caffey syndrome**
  See TUBULAR STENOSIS
**Keratansulfaturia**
  See MUCOPOLYSACCHARIDOSIS IV
**Keratitis-Ichthyosis-Deafness (KID) syndrome**
  See ICHTHYOSIFORM ERYTHROKERATODERMA, ATYPICAL WITH DEAFNESS
**Keratoatrophoderma, chronic progressive**
  See SKIN, POROKERATOSIS
**Keratocanthomas-cutaneous sebaceous tumors-other cancers**
  See CANCER, SEBACEOUS GLAND TUMOR-MULITPLE VISCERAL CARCINOMA
**Keratoconus**
  See EYE, KERATOCONUS
**Keratoderma, palmoplantar, Norrbotten recessive type**
  See KERATOSIS PALMARIS ET PLANTARIS OF UNNA-THOST
**Keratodermia palmoplantaris transgrediens**
  See MAL DE MELEDA
**Keratolysis exfoliativa congenita**
  See SKIN PEELING SYNDROME
**Keratolytic winter erythema**
  See SKIN, ERYTHROKERATOLYSIS HIEMALIS
**Keratomegalia**
  See CORNEA, MEGALOCORNEA
**Keratopachydermia-digital constrictions-deafness**
  See DEAFNESS-KERATOPACHYDERMIA-DIGITAL CONSTRICTIONS
**Keratopathy, band-shaped**
  See EYE, KERATOPATHY, BAND-SHAPED
**Keratosis follicularis**
  See DARIER DISEASE
**Keratosis follicularis serpiginosa**
  See SKIN, ELASTOSIS PERFORANS SERPIGINOSA
**Keratosis follicularis spinulosa decalvans cum ophiasi**
  See SKIN, KERATOSIS FOLLICULARIS SPINULOSA DECALVANS
**Keratosis follicularis-dwarfism-cerebral atrophy**
  See SHORT STATURE-CEREBRAL ATROPHY-KERATOSIS FOLLICULARIS, X-LINKED
**Keratosis of Greither**
  See KERATOSIS PALMARIS ET PLANTARIS OF UNNA-THOST

## KERATOSIS PALMARIS ET PLANTARIS OF UNNA-THOST                    3264

**Includes:**
  Epidermolytic hyperkeratosis
  Greither keratoderma
  Keratoderma, palmoplantar, Norrbotten recessive type
  Keratosis of Greither
  Palmo-plantar keratoderma, hereditary epidermolytic
  Palmo-plantar keratodermia, diffuse hereditary
  Thost-Unna disease
  Tylosis

**Excludes:**
  **Acrokeratoelastoidosis** (3068)
  **Howell Evans syndrome** (3290)
  **Hyperkeratosis palmoplantaris-periodontoclasia** (0494)
  **Mal de Meleda** (3289)

**Major Diagnostic Criteria:** Diffuse palmoplantar keratoderma without involvement of the dorsal surfaces of the hands and feet or distal sites.

**Clinical Findings:** Onset is usually evident after birth, and consists of slight thickening of the palms and soles. It is usually well-developed by the sixth to twelfth month and persists throughout life. The keratoderma is limited to either the palms, soles, or both; stopping abruptly at the lateral margins and often with an erythematous rim.

The skin lesions consists of a dense, homogenous hyperkeratosis with a whitish or yellow hue in a bilateral and symmetrical distribution.

Hyperhidrosis is present in most of the cases causing maceration and fissuring of the affected areas. The nails may be thickened, opaque, or curved. The hair and teeth are normal.

The histologic picture is not specific, consisting of hyperkeratosis, hypergranulosis, acanthosis, and a mild inflammatory infiltrate in the upper dermis.

Recently, many cases have been reported with the peculiar histologic feature of *epidermolytic hyperkeratosis*. At this time there is a debate whether this form, which is clinically indistinguishable from the Unna-Thost disease, is a separate entity.

**Complications:** Development of painful fissures as well as secondary dermatophyte infections have been frequently reported.

**Associated Findings:** Deafness has been reported in some kindred.

**Etiology:** Usually autosomal dominant inheritance, although a severe recessive form has been suggested.

**Pathogenesis:** Unknown.

**MIM No.:** *14840, 24485.

**Sex Ratio:** M1:F1

**Occurrence:** The incidence varies depending on geographic location, being 1:40,000 in Northern Ireland; 1:12,000 in Yugoslavia; and 1:200 in Northern Sweden.

**Risk of Recurrence for Patient's Sib:**
See Part I, *Mendelian Inheritance*.

**Risk of Recurrence for Patient's Child:**
See Part I, *Mendelian Inheritance*.

**Age of Detectability:** Usually shortly after birth.

**Gene Mapping and Linkage:** Unknown.

**Prevention:** None known. Genetic counseling indicated.

**Treatment:** Keratolytic agents can be useful to soften the hyperkeratotic skin. Recent studies have shown some effectiveness with oral synthetic retinoids.

**Prognosis:** Life span is not affected.

**Detection of Carrier:** Unknown.

**Special Considerations:** Some authors consider the recessive *Greither keratoderma* to be a distinct entity, which has the same clinical and histological features as Unna-Thost disease, but also involves the knees and elbows. Others, however, feel that this merely describes a severe variant of the Unna-Thost type of keratoderma.

**References:**
Unna PG: Uber das keratoma palmare et plantare ereditarium. Wochenschr Dermatol 1883; 10:231–274.
Kansky A, Arzensek J: Is palmoplantar keratoderma of Greither's type a separate nosologic entity? Dermatologica 1979; 158:244–248.
Bergfeld WF, et al.: The treatment of keratosis palmaris et plantaris with isotretinoin: a multicenter study. J Am Acad Dermatol 1982; 6:727–731.
Hatamochi A, et al.: Diffuse palmoplantar keratoderma with deafness. Arch Dermatol 1982; 118:605–607.
Camisa C, William H: Epidermolytic variant of hereditary palmoplantar keratoderma. Br J Dermatol 1985; 112:221–225.
Gamborg Neilsen P: Hereditary palmoplantar keratoderma in the northern most county of Sweden. Acta Derm Venereol (Stockh) 1985; 65:224–229.

MI038                                    **Giuseppe Micali**

**Keratosis palmoplantaris transgrediens**
See MAL DE MELEDA
**Keratosis palmoplantaris-corneal dystrophy**
See TYROSINEMIA II, OREGON TYPE
**Keratosis rubra figurata**
See SKIN, ERYTHROKERATODERMIA, VARIABLE

**Keratosis, focal palmoplantar and gingival**
See SKIN, HYPERKERATOSIS, FOCAL PALMOPLANTAR AND GINGIVAL
**Keto acid decarboxylase deficiency**
See MAPLE SYRUP URINE DISEASE
**Ketotic hyperglycinemia I**
See ACIDEMIA, PROPIONIC

## KEUTEL SYNDROME                                    0263

**Includes:**
Brachytelephalangy-peripheral pulmonary stenoses-deafness
Calcification of cartilages-brachytelephalangy-pulmonary stenosis
Deafness-peripheral pulmonary stenoses-brachytelephalangy
Pulmonary stenoses (peripheral)-brachytelephalangy-deafness

**Excludes:**
Chondrodysplasia punctata, X-linked dominant type (2730)
Heart, cor triatriatum (0204)
Fetal rubella syndrome (0384)
Pulmonary stenoses, familial multiple

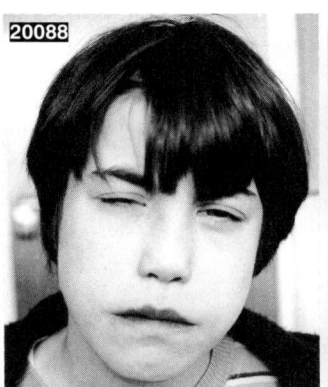
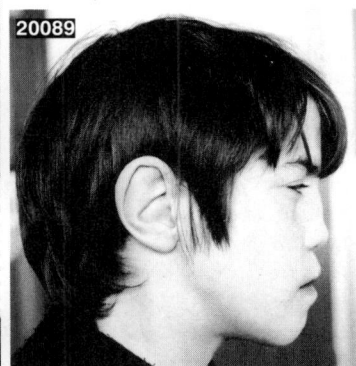
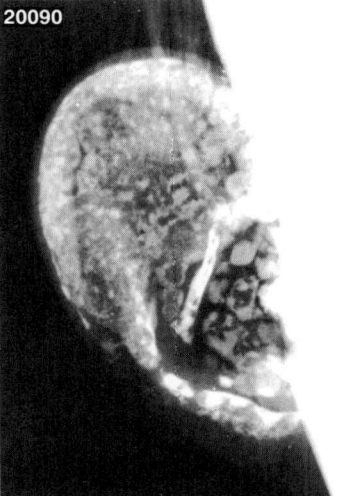

**0263**-20088: Characteristic dysmorphic facies with midface hypoplasia. 20089: Note small depressed nose and midface hypoplasia on lateral view of face. 20090: Cartilage calcifications in the ear.

**Major Diagnostic Criteria:** Brachytelephalangy, multiple peripheral pulmonary stenoses, mixed or conductive hearing loss, calcification of cartilage and typical craniofacial dysmorphism with small, depressed nose and midfacial hypoplasia.

**Clinical Findings:** Cormode et al. (1986) have summarized the clinical findings in the six reported patients. Two of these were sibs.

*Facies:* In one of the sibs, the face was described as coarse. In four other patients, the face was characteristic with midface hypoplasia, depressed nasal bridge, and small alae nasi.

*Hands and feet:* Brachytelephalangy was present in six of six patients. This includes short, malformed terminal phalanges, partial fusion of epiphyseal-metaphyseal joints, short nails, and interphalangeal webbing.

*Cartilage:* Widespread, diffuse calcifications throughout the nose, auricles, larynx, epiglottis, trachea, bronchial rings, and ribs were noted as early as age three years. Stippling of the epiphyses was seen as early as age 1.5 years. The ears especially were tough and showed perichondral and endochondral ossifications.

*Cardiovascular system:* Peripheral pulmonary artery stenoses, most frequently at the bifurcation of the pulmonary arteries, were present in three of six patients. One of these also had a ventricular septal defect (VSD).

*Hearing loss:* Mixed or conductive hearing loss was present in five of six patients, ranging from 30 to 70 db. Ossicular malformation was reported in one patient.

*Growth:* Delayed in the patient with VSD; normal in the other four patients for whom information was reported.

*Intellectual ability:* Mental retardation noted in two patients (one with VSD). Normal ability reported for three other patients.

*Respiratory system:* Chronic upper respiratory infections or wheezing noted in five of six patients.

**Complications:** Language delay secondary to hearing loss. Failure to thrive.

**Associated Findings:** Nasal speech possibly due to short palate, but without clefting.

**Etiology:** Probably autosomal recessive inheritance. Consanguinity noted in three of the five families reported.

**Pathogenesis:** Unknown.

**MIM No.:** *24515

**POS No.:** 3675

**Sex Ratio:** M1:F1

**Occurrence:** Six cases from five families have been reported.

**Risk of Recurrence for Patient's Sib:**
See Part I, *Mendelian Inheritance.*

**Risk of Recurrence for Patient's Child:**
See Part I, *Mendelian Inheritance.*

**Age of Detectability:** By X-ray in the first years of life.

**Gene Mapping and Linkage:** Unknown.

**Prevention:** None known. Genetic counseling indicated.

**Treatment:** Control of peripheral stenoses. Surgery as appropriate for cardiovascular defects. Amplification and speech and language therapy as needed for hearing loss. Educational intervention if intellectual impairment is present.

**Prognosis:** Apparently normal life span unless significant heart defect is present.

**Detection of Carrier:** No evidence of hearing loss or calcifications in obligate carriers.

**References:**
Keutel J, et al.: A new autosomal recessive syndrome: peripheral pulmonary stenoses, brachytelephalangism, neural hearing loss and abnormal cartilage calcifications-ossification. In: BD:OAS; VIII(5). New York: March of Dimes Birth Defects Foundation, 1972:60–68.
Say B, et al.: Unusual calcium deposition in cartilage associated with short stature and peculiar facial features: a case report. Pediatr Radiol 1973; 1:127–129.
Walbaum R, et al.: Le syndrome de Keutel. Ann Pediatr 1975; 51:461.

Temtamy S, McKusick V: The genetics of hand malformation. New York: Alan R. Liss, 1978:264.
Fryns JP, et al.: Calcification of cartilages, brachytelephalangy and peripheral pulmonary stenosis: confirmation of the Keutel syndrome. Eur J Pediatr 1984; 142:201–203.
Cormode EJ, et al.: Keutel syndrome: clinical report and literature review. Am J Med Genet, 1986; 24:289–294. * †

FR030
SM008

**Jean-Pierre Fryns**
**Shelley D. Smith**

**Kidney disease, autosomal recessive polycystic**
See *HEPATIC FIBROSIS, CONGENITAL*
**Kidney, adult polycystic disease of**
See *KIDNEY, POLYCYSTIC DISEASE, DOMINANT*
**Kidney, clear cell sarcoma**
See *CANCER, WILMS TUMOR*
**Kidney, congenital solitary**
See *RENAL AGENESIS, UNILATERAL*

## KIDNEY, GLOMERULOCYSTIC                                    3146

**Includes:**
Glomerular cysts
Glomerulocystic kidney
Glomerulocystic renal dysplasia
Hypoplastic glomerulocystic kidney, familial

**Excludes:**
**Kidney, polycystic disease, dominant** (0859)
**Kidney, polycystic disease, recessive** (2003)
**Meckel syndrome** (0634)
Tuberous sclerosis-cystic kidneys

**Major Diagnostic Criteria:** Glomerular cysts are usually discovered by examination of biopsy or postmortem specimens of kidney tissue obtained from patients with unexplained chronic renal failure or dysmorphic syndromes. The presence of glomerular cysts does not define or characterize any single disease entity, but may be found in several disparate conditions. The glomeruli may be small and primitive, and several small glomerular tufts may be seen within a large, dilated Bowman capsule. Proximal tubules may be dilated. Both kidneys are involved, and they may be large, normal, or small. The interstitium may be distorted and sclerosed.

Glomerulocystic kidney is characterized by the occurrence of chronic renal failure, small kidneys, absent renal papillae, and glomerular cysts. There are no major extrarenal malformations, and there is no associated hepatic fibrosis.

**Clinical Findings:** Familial hypoplastic glomerulocystic kidney disease presents with chronic renal failure during the first months of life. The renal function tends to be stable over several decades. Patients may fail to thrive. Two patients have had marked prognathism.

**Complications:** Chronic renal failure, hypertension, and failure to thrive.

**Associated Findings:** Glomerular cysts have also been seen in kidneys of patients with obstructive uropathy, **Chromosome 13, trisomy 13, Kidney, polycystic disease, dominant, Renal dysplasia-retinal aplasia, Loken-Senior type,** and in association with malformations of various organs.

**Etiology:** Presumably autosomal dominant inheritance. Glomerular cysts may also occur sporadically or in association with other defined syndromes that have dominant or recessive modes of inheritance.

**Pathogenesis:** Unknown.

**MIM No.:** 13792

**Sex Ratio:** M4:F8 (observed).

**Occurrence:** Twelve patients from four families have been documented in the literature.

**Risk of Recurrence for Patient's Sib:**
See Part I, *Mendelian Inheritance.*

**Risk of Recurrence for Patient's Child:**
See Part I, *Mendelian Inheritance.*

**Age of Detectability:** Patients can be detected when they present with chronic renal failure. Glomerulocystic kidneys have been detected *in utero* by ultrasonography at eight months gestation.

**Gene Mapping and Linkage:** Unknown.

**Prevention:** None known. Genetic counseling indicated.

**Treatment:** Chronic hemodialysis or continuous peritoneal dialysis. Renal transplantation.

**Prognosis:** All documented patients have survived but have mild-to-moderate, fairly stable or slowly progressive chronic renal failure.

**Detection of Carrier:** Unknown.

**References:**
Roos A: Polycystic kidney: report of a case studied by reconstruction. Am J Dis Child 1941; 61:116–127.
Rizzoni G, et al.: Familial hypoplastic glomerulocystic kidney: a new entity? Clin Nephrol 1982; 18:263–268.
Melnick SC, et al.: Cortical microcystic disease of the kidney with dominant inheritance: a previously undescribed syndrome. J Clin Pathol 1984; 37:494–499.
Fitch SJ, Stapleton FB: Ultrasonographic features of glomerulocystic disease in infancy: similarity to infantile polycystic kidney disease. Pediatr Radiol 1986; 16:400–402.
Barratt TM, et al.: Autosomal dominant hypoplastic glomerulocystic kidney disease. Am J Hum Genet 1987; 41:A45 only.

KA042                                    **Bernard S. Kaplan**

---

## KIDNEY, HORSESHOE                                    2004

**Includes:**
    Horseshoe kidneys
    Kidneys connected by a fibrous or parenchymatous
        isthmus

**Excludes:**
    Kidney, fusion anomalies of, other
    Kidney, true ectopic

**Major Diagnostic Criteria:** Physical examination may detect an abdominal mass. Urine examination may be normal or show pyuria, hematuria, proteinuria or positive bacterial cultures if infection or stones are present; excretory urography shows relatively low-lying kidneys, downward convergence of the renal axis, medially located and malrotated pelvis and high insertion of ureters from the anterior or lateral aspects of the kidney. Other confirmatory studies include retrograde pyelography, ultrasonography, or computed tomography.

**Clinical Findings:** Horseshoe kidney is the most common fusion anomaly of the kidneys. The kidneys are connected across the midline by a fibrous or parenchymatous isthmus which, in 40% of the patients, lies at the level of the fourth lumbar vertebra. In 95% of the cases the kidneys are joined at the lower pole. It is seen twice as often in males as in females. Approximately one-third of all patients are asymptomatic. Clinical symptoms are usually related to secondary complications such as infections, hydronephrosis, or calculus formation. The most common symptoms are abdominal or flank pain (approximately 33%), symptoms of urinary tract infection such as dysuria, hematuria, pyuria, and frequency (between 22–33%), renal calculi (approximately 20%), and palpable abdominal mass (approximately 5–10%). Ureteropelvic junction obstruction causing significant hydronephrosis is not uncommon; it is believed to be secondary to high insertion of the ureter in the renal pelvis, the abnormal course of the ureter and anomalous blood supply. The horseshoe kidney, even when asymptomatic, is frequently associated with other congenital anomalies. Boatman, et al reported that nearly one-third of 96 patients he studied had at least one other abnormality. The organ systems most commonly involved include: skeletal, cardiovascular, genitourinary, gastrointestinal, and central nervous systems. Horseshoe kidneys are frequently found in chromosomal abnor-

mality syndromes, e.g. **Turner syndrome** or **Chromosome 18, trisomy 18**. The clinical manifestations may be dominated by the associated anomalies of other organ systems. The diagnosis of horseshoe kidney is confirmed by excretory urography.

**Complications:** Most commonly related to malrotated renal pelvis causing urinary stasis, leading to infection and renal calculus. Ureteropelvic obstruction may cause hydronephrosis.

**Associated Findings:** The incidence of associated congenital anomalies in horseshoe kidney is high: approximately one-third of affected individuals have at least one other anomaly, which most frequently involves the cardiovascular system, the skeletal system, the central nervous system, or the genitourinary system. Genitourinary anomalies include ureteral duplication (10%); vesicoureteral reflux; in the male, hypospadias (4%); undescended testicles (4%); in the female, abnormalities of the vagina or uterus (7%). Central nervous system abnormalities include **Hydrocephaly**, **Meningomyelocele** or both as well as cerebral cortical atrophy and mental retardation. The cardiovascular anomalies, multiple and severe in nature, are varied and often lead to early death. The gastrointestinal findings include anorectal malformations, fistulas, a malrotated bowel, and **Meckel diverticulum**. Musculoskeletal anomalies include spina bifida, hip dislocation, webbed neck, **Polydactyly**, cleft lip, cleft palate, and clubfoot. Inguinal, umbilical and diaphragmatic hernias are also reported, as well as two patients with congenital deformity of the iris. Horseshoe kidney is seen in 60% of patients with **Turner syndrome** and 21% of patients with **Chromosome 18, trisomy 18**.

Renal cancer, **Cancer, renal cell carcinoma**, and **Cancer, Wilms tumor** are reported with higher incidence in association with horseshoe kidney. **Kidney, polycystic disease** has also been reported with horseshoe kidney.

**Etiology:** An embryologic abnormality which occurs between the fourth and sixth week of gestation. The exact cause is undetermined. Horseshoe kidney has been reported in identical twins, and among several siblings within the same family. Possibly the result of a genetic expression with a low penetrance.

**Pathogenesis:** Partial or complete fusion of the kidney results from failure of the metanephric cell mass to separate at the 5–8 mm. stage of embryogenesis; this occurs between 4–6 weeks of gestation, prior to renal rotation. Although the cause is unknown, it is theorized that deviation of the point of origin of the umbilical artery or other local mechanical factors may cause primary fusion by interfering with the normal upward growth of ureteral buds.

**CDC No.:** 753.320

**Sex Ratio:** M2:F1

**Occurrence:** 1:400–600 in the general population. Autopsy finding in 1:300 to 1:1000 autopsies. No particular ethnic distribution.

**Risk of Recurrence for Patient's Sib:** Presumably not significantly increased.

**Risk of Recurrence for Patient's Child:** Presumably not significantly increased.

**Age of Detectability:** Present at birth.

**Gene Mapping and Linkage:** Unknown.

**Prevention:** None known. Genetic counseling indicated.

**Treatment:** Asymptomatic horseshoe kidney requires no treatment. Urinary tract infection is treated with appropriate antibiotics. Complications such as ureteropelvic obstruction, hydronephrosis, and renal calculi may require surgical intervention.

**Prognosis:** Good for asymptomatic patients. Progression to renal failure is rare, and related to secondary complications. An increased incidence of renal cancer has been observed. If the horseshoe kidney is associated with other congenital anomalies, the severity of the involvement of other systems may determine the clinical course, and often lead to significant morbidity or early death.

**Detection of Carrier:** Unknown.

**Special Considerations:** The frequent association of horseshoe kidney with multiple congenital anomalies and certain chromosome abnormalities should prompt the physician to search for evidence of such association; and vice versa, a patient with birth defects should be investigated for the presence of horseshoe kidney.

**Support Groups:** New York; National Kidney Foundation

**References:**
Boatman DL, et al.: Congenital anomalies associated with horseshoe kidney. J Urol 1972; 107:205–207.
Perlmutter AD, et al.: Horseshoe kidney. In: Walsh PC, et al, eds: Campbell's urology, 5th ed, vol 2. Philadelphia: Saunders, 1986: 1686–1692.
Pitts WR, Muecke EC: Horseshoe kidneys: a 40 years experience. J Urol 1975; 113:743–746.
Kissane JM: Congenital malformations. In: Heptinstall RH, ed: Pathology of the kidney, 3rd ed., vol 1. Boston: Little, Brown, 1983:94–95.

SA008
BI012

**Inge Sagel**
**Nesrin Bingol**

## KIDNEY, MEDULLARY SPONGE KIDNEY          3019

**Includes:**
 Cystic dilation of renal collecting tubules
 Cystic disease of renal pyramids
 Medullary sponge kidney
 Precalyceal canalicular ectasia
 Sponge kidney
 Tubular ectasia

**Excludes:**
 **Kidney, nephronophthisis-medullary cystic desease** (3018)
 **Kidney, polycystic disease, dominant** (0859)
 **Kidney, polycystic disease, recessive** (2003)

**Major Diagnostic Criteria:** The patient is usually asymptomatic but may present with nephrolithiasis (80%), nephrocalcinosis, urinary tract infections, and hematuria. The combination of multiple pyramidal or calyceal calculi with cystic and ectatic medullary pyramidal changes on X-ray examination is diagnostic.

**Clinical Findings:** The patient is generally asymptomatic. Calculus formation and infection are usually responsible for the majority of symptoms: ureteral colic or loin pain (50–60%), nephrocalcinosis (40–60%), urinary tract infection and pyelonephritis (20–33%), and gross hematuria (10–30%). Few patients may be diagnosed incidentally on intravenous pyelogram (IVP) done to investigate a microscopic hematuria or pyuria, mild proteinuria, or enuresis. Hypertension is unusual. Progression to end-stage renal disease and death are rare, although a decrease in glomerular filtration rate (GFR) may be observed. Defective urinary solute-concentrating ability is present in the majority of patients; urinary dilution is unimpaired. Diagnosis is usually done by IVP. Renal ultrasound may show well-defined, highly echogenic pyramids due to multiple small cysts or pyramidal nephrocalcinosis.

**Complications:** Renal calculi (usually calcium phosphate, calcium oxalate, and ammonium magnesium phosphate); urinary tract infections; pyelonephritis; renal acidification and concentration defects; hematuria; absorptive (59%) and renal (18%) hypercalciuria; enhanced fractional excretion of sodium; interstitial nephritis; secondary renal failure; proteinuria; hyperuricemia.

**Associated Findings:** **Ehlers-Danlos syndrome, Hemihypertrophy,** congenital pyloric stenosis, adult polycystic kidney disease, pyeloureterocystitis cystica, renal ectopia and malrotation, **Kidney, horseshoe,** ureteral duplication, bifid ureter, calyceal diverticulae, megaureter, **Artery, renal fibromuscular dysplasia, Hyperparathyroidism,** parathyroid adenoma, distal renal tubular acidosis, **Meckel syndrome, Marfan syndrome,** hypokalemic paralysis, and **Gout.**

**Etiology:** Unknown. The disorder is considered to be a congenital abnormality. Most cases are sporadic, although the disease has been described in sibs and family members of successive generations.

**Pathogenesis:** Although the disease is considered to be a congenital abnormality, a variety of physical, chemical, and genetic factors may contribute to dysembryoplastic development. The most often-cited pathogenetic mechanism is dysplastic, cystic dilation of the first few generations of the metanephric duct arborizations within nephrogenic tissue early in embryonic development. This may represent a renal expression of more generalized abnormality of connective tissue.

**CDC No.:** 753.150

**Sex Ratio:** M1:F1

**Occurrence:** Incidence is estimated to be 1:1,000 to 1:5,000 cases in the population. The disease is reported to occur in 3.5–17% of stone formers. There is no racial preponderance.

**Risk of Recurrence for Patient's Sib:** Unknown.

**Risk of Recurrence for Patient's Child:** Unknown.

**Age of Detectability:** The disease usually presents in the fourth to fifth decade, although it has been observed at all ages.

**Gene Mapping and Linkage:** Unknown.

**Prevention:** None known. Genetic counseling indicated.

**Treatment:** Asymptomatic patients require no specific treatment except for yearly urinalysis. Treatment of symptomatic patients consists of high fluid intake and, when indicated, antibiotics. Renal calculi are managed conservatively. Urolithotomy and partial or total nephrectomy may be needed occasionally. Hypercalciuria may be treated with thiazides.

**Prognosis:** The course of uncomplicated medullary sponge kidney disease is benign and does not affect longevity. About 10% of symptomatic patients may have a poor long-term prognosis, urolithiasis, septicemia and renal failure.

**Detection of Carrier:** Unknown.

**Special Considerations:** *Medullary sponge kidney* should not be confused with **Kidney, nephronophthisis-medullary cystic desease** which is a distinctly different condition. The alternate terms of *precalyceal canalicular ectasia, cystic dilation of renal collecting tubules,* or *tubular ectasia* are more appropriate, but are not as widely accepted.

**Support Groups:** New York; National Kidney Foundation

**References:**
Morris RC, et al.: Medullary sponge kidney. Am J Med 1965; 38:883–892.
Kuiper JJ: Medullary sponge kidney. In: Gardner KD, ed: Cystic diseases of the kidney. New York: John Wiley & Sons, 1976:151–171. *
Backman U, et al.: Clinical and laboratory findings in patients with medullary sponge kidney. In: Smith LH, et al., eds: Urolithiasis: clinical and basic research. New York: Plenum, 1980:113–120.
O'Neill M, et al.: Metabolic evaluation of nephrolithiasis in patients with medullary sponge kidney. J Am Med Asso 1981; 245:1233–1236.
Yendt ER: Medullary sponge kidney and nephrolithiasis. New Engl J Med 1982; 306:1106–1107.

BA065

**Amin Y. Barakat**

## KIDNEY, NEPHRONOPHTHISIS-MEDULLARY CYSTIC DISEASE          3018

**Includes:**
 Cystic disease of the renal medulla
 Cysts of the renal medulla, congenital
 Fanconi nephronophthisis
 Kidney, uremic sponge
 Medullary cystic disease-nephronophthisis
 Medullary cystic kidney disease
 Microcystic disease of the renal medulla
 Nephritis, salt-losing
 Nephronophthisis, familial juvenile
 Nephronophthisis-medullary cystic disease
 Polycystic kidney disease, medullary type
 Renal medulla, familial disease
 Tubulointerstitial nephropathy, chronic idiopathic

**Excludes:**

> **Kidney, medullary sponge kidney** (3019)
> **Kidney, polycystic disease, dominant** (0859)
> **Kidney, polycystic disease, recessive** (2003)
> **Renal dysplasia-retinal aplasia, Loken-Senior type** (2687)

**Major Diagnostic Criteria:** Anemia, renal salt wasting, hyposthenuria, polyuria, scanty urinary abnormalities, and progressive renal failure. Histologic features consist of renal medullary or corticomedullary cysts (73%), relatively preserved glomeruli, interstitial fibrosis, and atrophied tubules.

**Clinical Findings:** The disease presents early in the second decade in the juvenile and sporadic types and late in the third decade in the adult type with polyuria, enuresis, and polydipsia (80%); normochromic, normocytic anemia (76%); azotemia (75%); renal sodium wasting (68%); weakness and pallor (60%); short stature in children (40%); hypertension (30%); abnormal bone metabolism and osteodystrophy (28%); asymptomatic relatives of patients (15%); and signs of azotemia (10%). Urinalysis may be normal in 32%; scanty urine findings (mild proteinuria, few blood cells, and an occasional cast) may be seen in 61% of patients.

**Complications:** Chronic renal failure.

**Associated Findings:** Eye changes consisting of **Retinitis pigmentosa**, tapetoretinal degeneration, and cataracts; **Bardet-Biedl syndrome**; red hair; **Kidney, horseshoe**; hepatic fibrosis; skeletal abnormalities; cerebellar ataxia, **Asphyxiating thoracic dysplasia**; **Ehlers-Danlos syndrome**.

**Etiology:** The evidence for two modes of inheritance suggests more than one etiology. Juvenile nephronophthisis by autosomal recessive inheritance; adult medullary cystic disease by autosomal dominant inheritance. Sporadic cases have been described.

**Pathogenesis:** Unknown. A nephrotoxic substance, probably the product of an inborn enzymatic defect and leading to early tubular dysfunction, has been suggested. An embryonal developmental anomaly in which the primary generation of uriniferous tubules do not undergo complete degeneration but persist as degenerating cysts; hypokalemia, and infection have been incriminated also in the pathogenesis of this disease. A primary defect in the renal tubular basement membrane of these patients has been described by Cohen and Hoyer (1986).

**MIM No.:** *17400, *25610,

**CDC No.:** 753.150, 753.140

**Sex Ratio:** M1:F1

**Occurrence:** Juvenile nephronophthisis occurs in about 1:50,000 births. Most reports describe affected Caucasians or do not mention race.

**Risk of Recurrence for Patient's Sib:**
See Part I, *Mendelian Inheritance*.

**Risk of Recurrence for Patient's Child:**
See Part I, *Mendelian Inheritance*.

**Age of Detectability:** In the early second decade in the juvenile and sporadic types and in late third decade in the adult type.

**Gene Mapping and Linkage:** Unknown.

**Prevention:** None known. Genetic counseling indicated.

**Treatment:** Chronic renal failure is treated symptomatically, eventually by renal transplantation. Changes of medullary cystic disease have not been observed in the transplanted kidney.

**Prognosis:** In untreated patients, death due to renal failure occurs in the second decade in the juvenile and sporadic types and in the fourth decade in the adult type.

**Detection of Carrier:** Asymptomatic family members of patients with nephronophthisis and tapetoretinal degeneration (see **Renal dysplasia-retinal aplasia, Loken-Senior type**) have been detected by electro-oculographic and retinographic studies.

**Special Considerations:** *Nephronophthisis* and *medullary cystic disease* are similar, clinically and histologically. However, the first is characterized by early onset, relatively longer course, and autosomal recessive inheritance; while in the second there is late onset, rapid progression, and autosomal dominant inheritance.

Most authors agree that these are very closely related entities and refer to them as the *nephronophthisis-medullary cystic disease complex*.

**Support Groups:** New York; National Kidney Foundation

**References:**

Gardner KD: Juvenile nephronophthisis and renal medullary cystic disease. In: Gardner KD, ed: Cystic disease of the kidney. New York: John Wiley & Sons, 1976:173–185. *
Chamberlin BC, et al.: Juvenile nephronophthisis and medullary cystic disease. Mayo Clin Proc 1977; 52:485–491.
Steele BT, et al.: Nephronophthisis. Am J Med 1980; 68:531–538.
Zerres K, et al.: Cystic kidneys: genetics, pathologic anatomy, clinical picture, and prenatal diagnosis. Hum Genet 1984; 68:104–135. *
Barakat AY, et al.: Nephronophthisis-medullary cystic disease. In: The kidney in genetic disease. Edinburgh: Churchill Livingstone, 1986: 30–32.
Cohen AH, Hoyer JR: Nephronophthisis: a primary tubular basement membrane defect. Lab Invest 1986; 55:564–572.

BA065

**Amin Y. Barakat**

---

## KIDNEY, POLYCYSTIC DISEASE, DOMINANT     0859

**Includes:**

> Adult polycystic kidney disease (APKD)
> Kidney, adult polycystic disease of
> Polycystic renal disease, adult type (Potter type III)
> Potter type III polycystic kidney disease
> Renal disease, polycystic adult type

**Excludes:**

> **Kidney, medullary sponge kidney** (3019)
> **Kidney, nephronophthisis-medullary cystic desease** (3018)
> **Kidney, polycystic disease, recessive** (2003)
> **Kidney, renal dysplasia, Potter type II** (3028)
> Medullary cystic disease
> Multilocular renal cysts
> **Nephrosis, congenital** (0709)
> Renal cortical cysts (Simple)

**Major Diagnostic Criteria:** Familial occurrence of bilateral flank masses with or without hypertension, proteinuria and/or hematuria. X-ray features are characteristic, and show large kidneys with lobulated margins and multiple cysts.

**Clinical Findings:** Dominant polycystic kidney disease occurs in both sexes and is characterized by progressive cystic enlargement of the kidneys, with eventual renal insufficiency. The vast majority of cases that become clinically apparent do so during the fourth decade. One-third of the individuals who have autosomal dominant polycystic kidney disease are asymptomatic. Fewer than 10% of cases present during the first decade of life. The entity occasionally presents in the newborn. Death from renal insufficiency usually occurs in the sixth decade of life in patients who have clinical manifestations, unless dialysis is instituted.

The presenting feature is often the feeling of abdominal fullness, discomfort, or pain. Bilateral abdominal masses may be detected on examination. Hypertension, proteinuria, hematuria, and headache are also important symptoms and signs. Pyuria and bacteriuria may be present. Loss of renal concentrating ability may be an early sign. Blood chemistries may be normal or may indicate renal impairment. Anemia is common, and polycythemia is observed occasionally. Some patients have ureteral colic resulting from passage of a blood clot from a ruptured cyst. Subarachnoid hemorrhage from a ruptured aneurysm can occur.

Diagnosis of polycystic disease may be confirmed by ultrasonography or intravenous pyelogram (IVP) which shows enlarged kidneys with lobulated margins. The cysts cause expansion of the renal cortex and displacement of the calyces. Occasionally, kidney size may be asymmetric or normal. In these instances nephrotomography may sometimes help define cysts as small as 1 cm in diameter. Ultrasound or computerized tomography (CT) scan may be able to define cysts that cannot be seen by nephrotomograms. Isotopic studies may be helpful to assess kidney size and contour. Ultrasound is a useful noninvasive technique to define cystic structures within the kidneys and to assess and follow kidney size.

**Complications:** Patients with polycystic kidney disease are prone to pyelonephritis (50- 75%) and arteriolar nephrosclerosis. Rupture of cysts and hemorrhage into cysts may occur. Renal colic due to renal calculi or blood clots are not infrequent. Renal calculi occur in 10–20% of patients. Compression of the ureter by the large kidney may lead to hydronephrosis.

Attacks of gout often precede symptoms of significant uremia. Approximately 8% of patients show a number of bone problems such as demineralization, trabeculation, and spontaneous fractures secondary to hyperparathyroidism.

Subarachnoid hemorrhage secondary to rupture of cerebral aneurysm occurs in 3–10% of patients.

The prevalence of neoplasms (carcinoma, sarcoma) in polycystic kidneys is a topic of controversy.

**Associated Findings:** Approximately one-third of patients with adult polycystic renal disease have one or more cysts of the liver. Cysts are found in the pancreas (10%), spleen, and lungs (5%); cysts of the ovary, endometrium, seminal vesicles, epididymis, bladder, and thyroid have been reported. Twenty-two percent of patients with polycystic kidney disease were found to have cerebral aneurysms on autopsy. Cardiovascular abnormalities such as dilatation of aortic root and annulus with aortic regurgitation and **Mitral valve prolapse** are found in 18% of patients. Echocardiogram may be a useful screening procedure.

**Etiology:** Autosomal dominant inheritance. In 25% of cases there is no family history of polycystic kidney disease; these are presumably new mutations.

**Pathogenesis:** Theories favor a developmental malformational abnormality; however, intrarenal obstruction may play a role. More recently, it has been suggested that a toxic or other intermediate factor may lead to cyst formation in a susceptible host. None of these theories is generally accepted. Cystic disease of kidneys may be induced in animals by intrauterine obstruction of ureters and by several chemicals including diphenylamine, diphenylthiazoles, lithium chloride, and corticosteroids.

In polycystic kidney disease, the kidney tissue is displaced by many cysts of varying size, which are scattered throughout the parenchyma; the cysts are dilated nephrons and collecting ducts. Cyst fluid composition indicates that the cyst walls are metabolically active; depending on whether they arise from proximal or distal nephron structures, the fluid composition resembles plasma or urine. The cystic structures slowly become more distended, gradually leading to gross enlargment of the kidneys and to progressive renal failure.

**MIM No.:** *17390

**CDC No.:** 753.120

**Sex Ratio:** M1:F1

**Occurrence:** Estimates for hospital populations generally range from between 1:3,000 to 1:5,000 patients. No ethnic group variation has been reported. Polycystic kidney disease is responsible for end-stage renal disease in the United States in 5%, and in Europe in 8%, of patients receiving renal dialysis.

**Risk of Recurrence for Patient's Sib:**
See Part I, *Mendelian Inheritance.*

**Risk of Recurrence for Patient's Child:**
See Part I, *Mendelian Inheritance.*

**Age of Detectability:** Usually after the fourth decade of life clinically, as early as 30 weeks gestation in utero by ultrasound. Prenatal diagnosis is possible by restriction fragment length polymorphism and linkage analysis of fetal DNA obtained by chorionic villus sampling.

**Gene Mapping and Linkage:** PKD1 (polycystic kidney disease 1 (autosomal dominant)) has been mapped to 16p13.

**Prevention:** None known. Genetic counseling indicated.

**Treatment:** Conservative management of renal insufficiency (protein-restricted diet, correction of electrolyte and acid-base imbalance, control of hypertension) and of cardiovascular compli-

cations and infection. Dialysis treatment and renal transplantation are needed for patients in end-stage renal failure.

**Prognosis:** The cystic conversion of renal parenchyma progresses, and uremia gradually develops. There are wide variations in the course of the disease. Some remain asymptomatic, while others have a slow progression of the disease. Once the renal function is impaired, most patients develop end-stage renal disease requiring dialysis within 3 years. Myocardial infarcts, congestive heart failure, and cerebral hemorrhage contribute significantly to mortality.

**Detection of Carrier:** In affected families urinalysis and ultrasound and/or IVP with nephrotomogram should be obtained on each family member to identify a carrier.

**Support Groups:**
MO; Kansas City; Polycystic Kidney Research (PKR) Foundation
NY; New York; National Kidney Foundation

**References:**
Kissane JM: Congenital malformations. In: Heptinstall RH, ed: Pathology of the kidney. Boston: Little Brown, 1974:3:89–93.
Danovitch GM: Clinical features and pathophysiology of polycystic kidney disease in man. In: Gardner KD Jr, ed: Cystic diseases of the kidney. New York: Wiley, 1976:125–150.
Baer JC, et al.: Age at clinical onset and at ultrasonographic detection of adult polycystic disease: data for genetic counseling. Am J Med Genet 1984; 18:45–53.
Reeder ST, et al.: A highly polymorphic DNA marker linked to adult polycystic kidney disease on chromosome 16. Nature 1985; 317:542–544.
Reeder ST, et al.: Prenatal diagnosis of autosomal dominant polycystic kidney disease with a DNA probe. Lancet 1986; II:6–7.
Sedman A, et al.: Autosomal dominant polycystic kidney disease in childhood: a longitudinal study. Kidney Int 1987; 31:1000–1005.

SA008      **Inge Sagel**
BI012      **Nesrin Bingol**
WA034      **Edward Wasserman**
KA042      **Bernard S. Kaplan**

## KIDNEY, POLYCYSTIC DISEASE, RECESSIVE      2003

**Includes:**
Cystic kidney, type I
Hepatic fibrosis, congenital
Infantile polycystic disease (IPCD)
Potter type I infantile polycystic kidney disease
Polycystic disease of infancy and childhood
Polycystic disease of the newborn
Renal-hepatic-pancreatic dysplasia (one form)

**Excludes:**
Kidney, polycystic disease, dominant (0859)
Kidney, renal dysplasia, Potter type II (3028)
Liver, congenital cystic dilatation of intrahepatic ducts (3155)
Renal cortical cysts
Renal cysts in hereditary syndromes
Renal medullary cysts

**Major Diagnostic Criteria:** Palpable enlarged kidneys in the infant are a prominent physical finding. Oligohydramnios sequence and "Potter face" ('squashed' nose, micrognathia, and large floppy low-set ears; resembling a face pressed against a window pane) may be present in the newborn. A family history of cystic kidney disease, or early death from kidney disease, or a history of oligohydramnios in the newborn suggest the diagnosis. Oliguria, anuria, proteinuria, pyuria and low specific gravity are found. Other laboratory data may indicate renal insufficiency. Excretory urography usually confirms the diagnosis, producing an irregularly mottled nephrogram and linear opacifications. It shows poor functioning in the newborn by the retention of the contrast medium within dilated collecting ducts. In older children uroradiographic findings are more variable. One may see variable renal enlargement and cyst formation. A characteristic finding is medullary tubular ductal ectasia. Ultrasonography and other radiographic techniques may be helpful in establishing the diagnosis. In an occasional patient, confirmation rests on kidney and especially liver biopsy.

**Clinical Findings:** Affects both the kidney and the liver. The clinical findings are age related and variable. Blyth and Ockenden characterized four subgroups according to age of onset and predominance of renal versus hepatic involvement.

*Perinatal*: Presentation at birth and with 90% of renal tubules dilated.

*Neonatal*: Presentation within the first month of life and with 60% of renal tubules dilated.

*Infantile*: Presentation between 3–6 months of age and with 25% of tubules dilated.

*Juvenile*: Presentation after the first year of life and less than 10% of tubules dilated.

The perinatal and neonatal forms of the disease are characterized by massive diffuse renal enlargement and oliguria. Many infants have the facial features of Potter syndrome and a history of oligohydramnios and dystocia. The abdomen is distended and the kidneys are palpable. Respiratory distress, apparently secondary to pulmonary hypoplasia, is common. Liver enlargement is variable. Hematuria is common. Death within the first few days of life is usually due to pulmonary rather than renal insufficiency.

The clinical picture in older children is more variable, with less severe initial renal enlargement, sometimes with progressive reduction in renal size with stabilization around 4–5 years. The kidneys are usually palpable. Renal insufficiency begins in early childhood, but its progression is very variable. Hypertension is almost always present, often leading to heart failure. Other nonspecific symptoms include nausea, abdominal pain, vomiting and growth retardation.

Hepatic involvement is always present, and is usually more pronounced in the older child, but rarely leads to functional impairment. The finding of marked hepatic fibrosis and portal hypertension with only mild renal involvement is referred to as congenital hepatic fibrosis. Hepatosplenomegaly and ascites may be present in these patients.

**Complications:** Hypertension is found in almost all patients and heart failure is common. Advancing renal insufficiency may lead to anemia and secondary hyperparathyroidism; this may result in skeletal involvement and growth failure. In patients with significant hepatic involvement, hepatocellular dysfunction and portal hypertension may be found. Hemorrhage from esophageal varices is not uncommon in these patients.

**Associated Findings:** Cystic lesions of the pancreas are occasionally found, but are asymptomatic. Hypoplasia rather than cystic changes are found in the lungs of newborns.

**Etiology:** Autosomal recessive inheritance.

**Pathogenesis:** The exact cause of cyst formation is not clear. Faulty embryologic development has been cited, but not proven. The association of characteristic cystic changes in the kidney and intrahepatic biliary system is suggestive of a generalized metabolic abnormality which affects both organs. A primary defect in the supporting structures of tubules and bile ducts, or a primary defect in the renal and biliary epithelium has also been suggested. None of these theories is proven or generally accepted. The kidneys are enlarged; more so in neonates than older children. The essential morphologic abnormality appears to be enlargement of the collecting tubules. Microdissections have shown a normal number of nephrons and other nephron structures, suggesting that the abnormality is acquired later in gestation. Although older children have less cystic dilatation than neonates, the fact that they have more peritubular fibrosis may be related to progressive tubular damage. It has been suggested that progressive tubular damage rather than cyst formation is responsible for progressive renal failure. The enlarged and fibrotic portal areas in the liver contain an increased number of bile ducts and periductal collagen; this abnormality leads to vascular obstruction and portal hypertension.

**MIM No.:** *26320

**POS No.:** 3368

**CDC No.:** 753.110

**Sex Ratio:** M1:F1

**Occurrence:** Estimated to be between 1:20,000 and 1:60,000.

**Risk of Recurrence for Patient's Sib:**
See Part I, *Mendelian Inheritance.*

**Risk of Recurrence for Patient's Child:**
See Part I, *Mendelian Inheritance.*

**Age of Detectability:** At birth for neonatal and perinatal form. Variable in older children. Prenatal detection is possible.

**Gene Mapping and Linkage:** Unknown.

**Prevention:** None known. Genetic counseling indicated.

**Treatment:** Medical therapy is supportive. Hypertension and heart failure may require antihypertensive drugs and digitalis. In end stage renal failure, hemodialysis and renal transplantation are indicated. Portal hypertansion, the principal hepatic complication, is currently treated by surgical portocaval shunt.

**Prognosis:** In the perinatal and neonatal form, death in the first few days or weeks of life often occurs, and is frequently related to pulmonary complications as well as renal failure. In older children, the course is variable as far as the development of renal insufficiency is concerned, although close to one-half now survive to at least 15 years of age. For those who survive their first year, the number alive at age 15 increases to 79%. Complications such as hypertension and heart failure contribute to mortality. In older children renal involvement is frequently mild and hepatic fibrosis dominates. Liver dysfunction is unusual; if portal hypertension exists, hemorrhage from esophageal varices may be a fatal complication.

**Detection of Carrier:** Unknown.

**Special Considerations:** There is marked clinical variability in this condition. While the disease is known to be transmitted as an autosomal recessive inheritance and the basic pathology in regard to cystic dilatation of renal collecting tubules and involvement of the intrahepatic biliary system is observed in all patients, the age of onset, the extent of renal and hepatic involvement and the rate of progression vary greatly.

The condition occurs in animals other than man; in goldfish (Grassius Auratus), mice (FWw strain), rats (Gunn strain) and rabbits.

Chronic administration of lithium chloride produced cystic kidneys in dogs.

**Support Groups:**
New York; National Kidney Foundation
MO; Kansas City; Polycystic Kidney Research (PKR) Foundation

**References:**
Blythe H, Ockenden BG: Polycystic disease of kidneys and liver presenting in childhood. J Med Genet 1971; 8:257.
Morin PR, et al.: Prenatal detection of the autosomal recessive type of polycystic kidney disease by trehalase assay in amniotic fluid. Prenatal diagn 1981; 1:75–79.
Zerres K, et al.: Cystic kidneys: genetics, pathologic anatomy, clinical picture and prenatal diagnosis. Hum Genet 1984; 68:104–135.
Bernstein J, et al.: Renal-hepatic-pancreatic dysplasia: a syndrome reconsidered. Am J Med Genet 1987; 26:391–403.
Kaariainen H: Polycystic kidney disease in children: a genetic and epidemiological study of 82 Finnish patients. J Med Genet 1987; 24:474–481.
Wirth B, et al.: Autosomal recessive and dominant forms of polycystic kidney disease are not allelic. Hum Genet 1987; 77:221–222.
Kaplan BS, et al.: Variable expression of autosomal recessive polycystic kidney disease and congenital hepatic fibrosis within a family. Am J Med Genet 1988; 29:639–647.
Kaplan BS, et al.: Autosomal recessive polycystic kidney disease. Pediatr Nephrol 1989; 3:43–49.

SA008                                    **Inge Sagel**
BI012                                  **Nesrin Bingol**
KA042                            **Bernard S. Kaplan**

## KIDNEY, POLYCYSTIC DISEASE-CATARACT-BLINDNESS                                                        3288

**Includes:**
Blindness-polycystic kidney disease-cataract
Cataract-polycystic kidney disease-blindness
Cystic kidney disease-cataract-blindness

**Excludes:**
**Cataract-renal tubular necrosis-encephalopathy, Crome type** (2162)
**Oculo-cerebro-renal syndrome** (0736)
**Renal dysplasia-retinal aplasia, Loken-Senior type** (2687)

**Major Diagnostic Criteria:** Congenital blindness, cystic kidney disease and cataracts.

**Clinical Findings:** Patients usually present with congenital blindness and renal disease mainly proteinuria. Hypertension, renal failure and findings suggestive of renal tubular disease may be present. Central cataracts, myopia and retinal dystrophy may also be present. Kidney abnormalities described include polycystic kidney disease, medullary cystic disease, pyramidal cysts, and microcystic renal dysplasia.

**Complications:** Chronic renal failure.

**Associated Findings:** Microcornia; retinal dysplasia, hypoplasia or aplasia; absence of ciliary body and nystagmus.

**Etiology:** Possibly autosomal recessive inheritance.

**Pathogenesis:** Possibly an antenatal dysgenetic process.

**MIM No.:** 26310

**Sex Ratio:** M1:F4 (observed).

**Occurrence:** Five cases have been documented in the literature.

**Risk of Recurrence for Patient's Sib:**
See Part I, *Mendelian Inheritance.*

**Risk of Recurrence for Patient's Child:**
See Part I, *Mendelian Inheritance.*

**Age of Detectability:** At any age. Congenital blindness may suggest the diagnosis.

**Gene Mapping and Linkage:** Unknown.

**Prevention:** None known. Genetic counseling indicated.

**Treatment:** Diagnosis and treatment of recurrent urinary tract infections and renal calculi help to prevent deterioration in renal function. The cataracts and chronic renal failure are treated as indicated.

**Prognosis:** Varies with the severity of the renal disease. Renal failure can occur in childhood.

**Detection of Carrier:** Unknown.

**Special Considerations:** Since polycystic kidney disease, medullary cystic disease, **Kidney, medullary sponge kidney**, and microcystic renal dysplasia have been described in patients with this syndrome, the term *cystic kidney disease* is more appropriate than "polycystic kidney" in the title.

**References:**
Fairley KF, et al.: Familial visual defects associated with polycystic kidney and medullary sponge kidney. Brit Med J 1963; 1:1060–1063.
Pierson M, et al.: Une curieuse association malformative congenitale et familiale atteignant l'oeil et le rein. J Genet Hum 1963; 12:184–213.

BA065                                                                      **Amin Y. Barakat**

**Kidney, renal cell carcinoma**
*See CANCER, RENAL CELL CARCINOMA*

## KIDNEY, RENAL DYSPLASIA, POTTER TYPE II                                      3028

**Includes:**
Cystic dysplasia
Cystic hydrocalicosis, congenital
Multicystic kidney, congenital unilateral
Multicystic renal dysplasia
Potter type II renal dysplasia

**Excludes:**
**Kidney, polycystic disease, dominant** (0859)
**Kidney, polycystic disease, recessive** (2003)
Renal dysplasia with primitive renal tubules

**Major Diagnostic Criteria:** The diagnosis of multicystic renal dysplasia should be suspected by the presence of multiple, irregular anechoic renal cysts in renal ultrasonographic examinations. Radionuclide renal scans demonstrate absence of blood flow and excretory function in affected kidneys. Histologic features include primitive epithelial ductal structures surrounded by fibrous tissue with islands of metaplastic, cartilage-scattered immature tubules, or glomeruli occasionally identified in otherwise disorganized mesenchyme.

**Clinical Findings:** Most patients are identified when an asymptomatic flank mass is palpated in the newborn nursery. Multicystic renal dysplasia is the most common unilateral flank mass in newborns and involves the left kidney more commonly than the right. Occasionally, multicystic renal dysplasia is bilateral and results in anuria and early death. The urinalysis is generally normal in neonates with unilateral multicystic renal dysplasia.

**Complications:** Rarely, hypertension may accompany unilateral multicystic renal dysplasia (Chen et al., 1985). Bilateral multicystic renal dysplasia results in pulmonary hypoplasia and shares the facial and cranial features of Potter syndrome.

**Associated Findings:** Obstruction of the contralateral kidney occurs in 30% of patients with unilateral multicystic renal dysplasia. Multicystic renal dysplasia is also frequently associated with ectopic kidney or **Kidney, horseshoe.** The ureter of a multicystic dysplastic kidney is usually not patent. Cystic dysplasia may be associated with cerebral malformation, including **Hydrocephaly, Polydactyly,** and hepatic dysgenesis (Simopoulos syndrome), Dandy-Walker malformation, **Meckel syndrome,** and Miranda syndrome. Biliary dysgenesis and multicystic renal dysplasia (usually bilateral) occurs in Meckle syndrome and in Jeune **Asphyxiating thoracic dysplasia.** Other syndromes that include bilateral multicystic renal dysplasia are **Asplenia syndrome, De Lange syndrome,** and **Short rib-polydactyly syndrome.**

**Etiology:** In most instances, multicystic renal dysplasia (particularly when unilateral) is sporadic. Rarely, bilateral multicystic renal dysplasia has been reported to occur in sibs, suggesting an autosomal recessive inheritance. Bernstein (1983) reports that renal ultrasonic examination of 51 family members of children with multicystic renal dysplasia revealed only one instance of cystic renal dysplasia; the one familial recurrence was a stillborn male infant with posterior urethral valves.

**Pathogenesis:** Osathanondh and Potter (1965) attributed multicystic renal dysplasia to inhibition of ampullary branching with failure to induce normal nephrogenesis in metanephric tissue. Bernstein (1971) proposed that most multicystic renal dysplasia is the result of injury following nephron induction and that the most plausible injury is ureteral obstruction.

**POS No.:** 3368

**Sex Ratio:** Presumably M1:F1, although some investigators report a male preponderance.

**Occurrence:** Unknown. There is no known racial difference, and incidence figures are not available.

**Risk of Recurrence for Patient's Sib:** Two percent (observed), although autosomal recessive inheritance (25%) has been suggested for some families with multiple affected sibs (Cole et al, 1976).

**Risk of Recurrence for Patient's Child:** Unknown. No instances of affected offspring have yet been reported.

**Age of Detectability:** During the third trimester.

**Gene Mapping and Linkage:** Unknown.

**Prevention:** None known. Genetic counseling indicated.

**Treatment:** Surgical removal of a unilateral multicystic renal dysplastic kidney may be required for abdominal discomfort, hypertension, or, rarely, infection.

**Prognosis:** Usually good.

**Detection of Carrier:** Unknown.

**Support Groups:** New York; National Kidney Foundation

**References:**
Osathanondh V, Potter EL: Pathogenesis of polycystic kidneys. Arch Pathol 1965; 77:459–512.
Bernstein J: The morphogenesis of renal parenchymal maldevelopment (renal dysplasia). Pediatr Clin North Am 1971; 18:395–407.
Cole BR, et al.: Bilateral renal dysplasia in three siblings: report of a survivor. Clin Nephrol 1976; 5:83–87.
Kissane JM: The morphology of renal cystic disease. In: Gardener KG, ed: Cystic diseases of the kidney. New York: John Wiley & Sons, 1976:31–63.
Bernstein J: Renal dysplasia: morphologic and family studies. In: Brodehl J, Ehrich JHH, eds: Pediatric nephrology. Berlin: Springer-Verlag, 1983:353–355.
Chen Y-H et al.: Neonatal hypertension from a unilateral multicystic dysplastic kidney. J Urol 1985; 133:664–665.

ST055 **F. Bruder Stapleton**

**Kidney, uremic sponge**
See KIDNEY, NEPHRONOPHTHISIS-MEDULLARY CYSTIC DESEASE
**Kidney-liver disease, adult type polycystic**
See LIVER, POLYCYSTIC AND MULTICYSTIC DISEASE, ADULT TYPE
**Kidneys connected by a fibrous or parenchymatous isthmus**
See KIDNEY, HORSESHOE
**Kidneys, absence of**
See RENAL AGENESIS, BILATERAL
**Kidneys, congenital bilateral absence of**
See RENAL AGENESIS, BILATERAL
**Kidneys, cystic-retinal aplasia-Joubert syndrome**
See JOUBERT SYNDROME
**Killian syndrome**
See PALLISTER-KILLIAN MOSAIC SYNDROME
**Kiloh-Nevin dystrophy of the external ocular muscles**
See KEARNS-SAYRE DISEASE
**Kindler-Weary syndrome**
See POIKILODERMA, HEREDITARY ACROKERATOTIC, KINDLER-WEARY TYPE

## KING SYNDROME 2492

**Includes:**
King-Denborough syndrome
Malignant hyperthermia-Noonan-like phenotype
Noonan-like phenotype-malignant hyperthermia

**Excludes:**
Kniest dysplasia (0557)
Muscular dystrophy, facio-scapulo-humeral (2049)
Myopathy, central core disease type (0134)
Myopathy, malignant hyperthermia (2710)
Noonan syndrome (0720)
Pterygium syndrome, multiple (2186)

**Major Diagnostic Criteria:** A Noonan-like phenotype and malignant hyperthermia. Absence of webbed neck, congenital heart defects and mental retardation, as well as presence of muscle weakness, differentiate King from **Noonan syndrome.** Its sporadic occurrence is another differentiating feature.

**Clinical Findings:** The most common major features are the Noonan-like facies, short stature, and episodes of malignant hyperthermia. Based on 11 reported patients, the approximate frequency of the clinical features is as follows: hyperthermia (11/11), short stature (9/11), transient delay of motor development (8/11), normal intelligence (11/11), muscle weakness (7/11), downward slant of palpebral fissures (7/11), ptosis (6/11), midface hypoplasia (9/11), micrognathia (11/11), low-set ears (7/11), **Pectus carinatum** (10/11), kyphoscoliosis and/or lordosis (11/11), and cryptorchidism (8/9).

The dysmorphic signs are usually apparent in early infancy. The short stature becomes evident in early childhood. The malignant hyperthermia is a pharmacogenetic feature which manifests when exposed to depolarizing skeletal muscle relaxants and/or volatile hydrocarbon anesthetics. End tidal carbon dioxide rises very early in the development of the hyperthermia and capnography during anesthesia appears useful for the early detection of this sign.

**Complications:** The life-threatening feature is the malignant hyperthermia. The muscle weakness is mild and appears to be non-progressive.

**Associated Findings:** Contractures have been reported in three of the 11 patients.

**Etiology:** While all cases have been sporadic, in four there was a family history of elevated serum creatine kinase (CK) levels in several relatives without the characteristic dysmorphic phenotypic features of the syndrome. Etiologic heterogeneity of the syndrome has been suggested by a family sibs with King-like phenotype, including hyperthermia. The parents in this family did not have any of the phenotypic features, and had normal CK levels.

**Pathogenesis:** The pathogenesis of the malignant hyperthermia appears similar to that of other malignant hyperthermias. Several studies of hyperthermias have implied disrupted intracellular calcium movement and enhanced calcium release, as well as tubular, mitochondrial, and sarcolemmal dysfunctions. Elevated levels and enhanced activity of phospholipase A in the muscles appear to represent another component of the pathogenetic mechanism. In another patient, CT scan of the extremities showed myopathic changes within certain muscle groups. The changes consisted of areas of degeneration and fatty infiltration. Thus CT scan of the extremities may be of diagnostic help.

**MIM No.:** *14560

**POS No.:** 4183

**Sex Ratio:** M5:F1

**Occurrence:** Fewer than a dozen cases have been documented.

**Risk of Recurrence for Patient's Sib:** If the syndrome is indeed sporadic, the risk should not be increased. In the families with elevated CK levels, the risk for malignant hyperthermia may be as high as 50%.

**Risk of Recurrence for Patient's Child:** Unknown.

**Age of Detectability:** Variable, but can be detected in infancy or whenever the malignant hyperthermia is encountered.

**Gene Mapping and Linkage:** Unknown.

**Prevention:** Capnography during anesthesia and prompt administration of dantrolene have already reduced the mortality of malignant hyperthermia from 70% to 10%. Muscle biopsy for a caffeine contracture test prior to anesthesia may detect a predisposition to hyperthermia. Elevated CK levels in relatives are found in only about 30% of those tested, making this a less reliable test. Exposure of platelet-rich plasma from patients with malignant hyperthermia to halothane produces a significant decrease in the platelet ATP pool compared to controls. Control patients who had hyperthermia, hyperkalemia, acidosis, or myopathy not related to malignant hyperthermia had nucleotide profiles that were indistinguishable from those of normal persons. Thus the platelet test appears to be specific for malignant hyperthermia. It can be done within 45 minutes and appears promising for the prevention of hyperthermia.

**Treatment:** Prompt administration of dantrolene for treatment of malignant hyperthermia is crucial. Physical therapy for the muscle weakness appears beneficial.

**Prognosis:** Shortened life span if fatal malignant hyperthermia occurs. If prevention or successful treatment of this feature occurs, there are no other clinical features in the syndrome expected to shorten the life span.

**Detection of Carrier:** Determination of CK levels in the families with sporadic King syndrome may detect relatives at risk for malignant hyperthermia.

**References:**
King JO, Denborough MA: Anesthetic-induced malignant hyper-pyrexia in children. J Pediatr 1973; 83:37–40.
McPherson EW, Taylor CA: The King syndrome: malignant hyper-thermia, myopathy, and multiple anomalies. Am J Med Genet 1981; 8:159–165.
Kousseff BG, Nichols P: A new autosomal recessive syndrome with Noonan-like phenotype, myopathy with congenital contractures and malignant hyperthermia. BD:OAS XXI(2). New York: March of Dimes Birth Defects Foundation, 1985:111–117.
Qazi QH, et al.: King syndrome with focal myopathic involvement demonstrated by C-T scan. Pediatr Res 1985; 19:329A.

K0018                                        **Boris G. Kousseff**

**King-Denborough syndrome**
  *See KING SYNDROME*
**Kinky hair disease**
  *See MENKES SYNDROME*
**Kirghizian dermato-osteolysis**
  *See DERMATO-OSTEOLYSIS, KIRGHIZIAN TYPE*
**Kitamura acropigmentatio reticularis**
  *See SKIN CREASES, RETICULATE PIGMENTED FLEXURES, DOWLING-DEGOS TYPE*
**Kjer optic atrophy**
  *See OPTIC ATROPHY, KJER TYPE*
**Klebcil△, fetal effects**
  *See FETAL AMINOGLYCOSIDE OTOTOXICITY*
**Kleeblattschadel craniosynostosis**
  *See CRANIOSYNOSTOSIS, KLEEBLATTSCHADEL TYPE*
**Klein-Waardenburg syndrome**
  *See WAARDENBURG SYNDROMES*

## KLINEFELTER SYNDROME                     0556

**Includes:**
  Chromosome XXY
  Hypergonadotropic hypogonadism
  Primary hypogonadism
  Seminiferous tubule dysgenesis
  True Klinefelter syndrome

**Excludes:**
  **Gonadotropin deficiencies** (0438)
  Hypogonadism (other forms)
  **Sertoli cell-only syndrome** (3163)

**Major Diagnostic Criteria:** X-chromatin-positive male with phenotypic male genitalia; small, firm testes; and karyotype usually 47,XXY, elevated serum; and urinary gonadotropins.

**Clinical Findings:** Most affected individuals appear normal as neonates and in early infancy, except when the testes are found to be significantly smaller than normal. As first described by Klinefelter, Reifenstein and Albright in 1942, the characteristic clinical features that become evident at adolescence are small atrophic testes, small penis, gynecomastia, incomplete virilization, variable eunuchoidism, and tendency to dull mentality. Tall stature occurs with the syndrome (an average 10 cm taller than XY males), and altered body proportions, i.e. low upper to lower segment ratio and span less than or equal to height.

The testes remain less than 2.5 cm in length even into adulthood and often less than 1.5 cm. Cryptorchidism, gynecomastia, and incomplete virilization occur in more than one-half of the cases. Plasma and urinary gonadotropins are increased. Plasma testosterone is often less than the normal range for men. Later disturbances of sexual function occur, i.e. complete infertility, impotence, and lack of libido.

The number of spermatogonia is decreased as early as infancy compared to normal 46,XY males of the same age. At and after puberty, progressive sclerosis and hyalinization of seminiferous

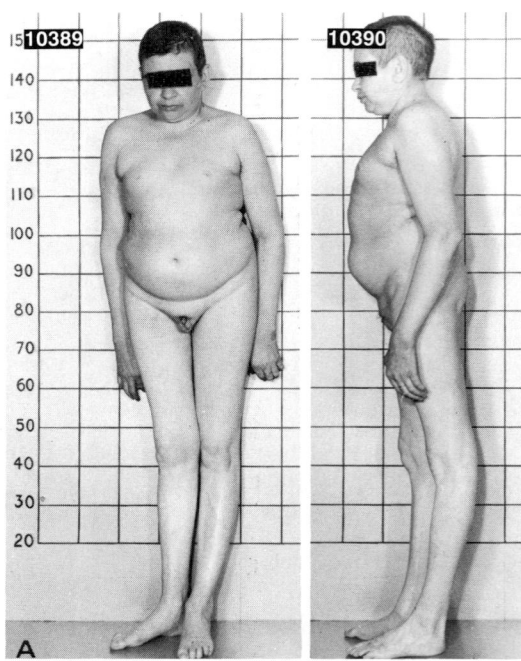

**0556-10389–90:** Tall stature with relatively long limbs and truncal obesity.

tubules leads to loss of germinal tissue with consequent secondary clumping ("nodular hyperplasia") of Leydig cells, which are ultimately also lost in a process of progressive fibrosis and atrophy.

Behavioral problems and personality disturbances are common in the syndrome but may not be evident until school age. The true frequency of such manifestations is unknown since patients with behavioral problems appear in treatment more frequently than those without.

**Complications:** Psychologic and psychiatric complications of a person with less than average intelligence, hypogonadism, and impotence. Vertebral collapse sometimes occurs secondary to osteoporosis. Increased predisposition to breast cancer has been reported in Klinefelter syndrome. Also, varicose veins appear to be more common in this syndrome.

**Associated Findings:** Multiple minor anomalies are common in the Klinefelter syndrome: brachycephalic skull configuration, at times with low nuchal hairline, minor defects of differentiation of auricles, clinodactyly of fifth fingers at times with only one flexion crease on that finger, simian creases and other variations of palmar crease patterns, decreased total ridge count of fingertip dermatoglyphic patterns, and increased incidence of hypothenar patterns with distal axial palmar triradius. Radioulnar synostosis occurs with increased incidence in this syndrome. In individuals with more complex sex chromosome aneuploidy (48,XXXY; 49XXXXY; 49,XXXYY, etc.) multiple somatic anomalies and mental retardation are common. Scoliosis during adolescence has been noted. Incidence of diabetes mellitus and thyroid dysfunction is increased in this syndrome.

**Etiology:** More complex meiotic nondisjunction in either parent results in 47,XXY, while mitotic nondisjunction after fertilization results in mosaicism, of which 46,XY/47,XXY is the most common.

**Pathogenesis:** Pathogenesis of seminiferous tubule dysgenesis is unknown. Eunuchoidism and other manifestations of hypogonadism presumably are due to progressive testicular sclerosis with loss of germinal and endocrine tissue.

About 2/3 of 47,XXY cases are of the $X^MX^MY$ type, 1/3 are

X^MX^PY, (M = maternal, P = paternal source). In the former group, increased maternal age supports the hypothesis of maternal meiotic nondisjunction; maternal age is not increased in the mosaic or X^MX^PY cases.

**MIM No.:** 23832, 25730

**POS No.:** 3107

**CDC No.:** 758.7

**Sex Ratio:** M1:F0

**Occurrence:** Buccal smear survey: incidence of males with X-chromatin: 1:590 live-born males (1:1250 to 1:110 live-born infants). Neonatal chromosome surveys: approximately 1:500 live-born males.

Prevalence estimated at 1:1000, primarily in the general Caucasian populations. In institutions for the mentally retarded; around 1:100 male patients.

Among populations of infertile men: 1:77 to 1:24 of all infertile men; 1:9 to 1:5 for men with high grades of infertility (i.e. azoospermia or sperm count less than 1 x 10^6/ml).

Among men in psychiatric institutions: 1:169.

**Risk of Recurrence for Patient's Sib:** Presumably not significantly increased.

**Risk of Recurrence for Patient's Child:** Only four fertile 46,XY/47,XXY mosaics are known; one child was a 47,XXY male; all other offspring were presumably normal. All 47,XXY patients are infertile.

**Age of Detectability:** Prenatally in the second trimester by amniocentesis and cytogenetic analysis of amniotic cells.

**Gene Mapping and Linkage:** HHG (hypergonadotropic hypogonadism) is ULG5.

**Prevention:** None known. Genetic counseling indicated.

**Treatment:** Treatment of hypogonadism. Supportive psychotherapy for emotional complications. Testosterone replacement therapy, beginning at age 11 to 12 years, is indicated to bring about adolescent development and prevent some of the features of adult Klinefelter syndrome. Depo-testosterone 50–100 mg every 3 weeks until adult dosage of 150–200 mg is achieved at age approximately 17 years.

**Prognosis:** Life span is presumably normal.

**Detection of Carrier:** Unknown.

**Special Considerations:** The patients with more complex sex chromosome aneuploidy (48,XXXY; 49,XXXXY; 48,XXYY; 49,XXXYY, etc.) are usually ascertained on the basis of mental retardation, generally with multiple anomalies. 47,XYY individuals do not have Klinefelter syndrome.

**References:**
Klinefelter HF, et al.: Syndrome characterized by gynecomastia, aspermatogenesis without aleydigism and increased secretion of follicle-stimulating hormone (gynecomastia). J Clin Endocrinol Metab 1942; 2:615.
Becker KL, et al.: Klinefelter's syndrome. Arch Intern Med 1966; 118:314.
Caldwell PD, Smith DW: The XXY syndrome in childhood detection and treatment. J Pediatr 1972; 80:250.
Laron Z: Klinefelter's syndrome: early diagnosis and treatment. Hosp Pract 1972; 7:135.
Williams RH, ed: Textbook of endocrinology. 6th ed. Philadelphia: W.B. Saunders, 1981.

BU007
HU010
SA024

**Bruce A. Buehler**
**Carol A. Huseman**
**Warren Sanger**

## KLIPPEL-FEIL ANOMALY 2032

**Includes:**
   Brevicollis, congenital
   Cervical vertebral fusion, congenital
   Klippel-Feil syndrome

**Excludes:**
   **Cervico-oculo-acoustic syndrome** (0142)
   **Eye, Duane retraction syndrome** (3180)
   **Spondylocostal dysplasia** (0896)
   **Spondylothoracic dysplasia** (0900)

**Major Diagnostic Criteria:** Congenital fusion of cervical vertebrae is the only constant sign, with typical patients presenting the clinical triad of short neck, limitation of head and neck movement, and low posterior hairline.

**Clinical Findings:** According to Feil's classification, there are three morphological types of vertebral fusion: *type I* is an extensive cervical and upper thoracic vertebral fusion; *type II* is a localized fusion of one or two pairs of cervical vertebrae, often accompanied by hemivertebrae and occipitoatlantal fusion; and *type III* is a combination of cervical and lower thoracic or lumbar fusion. Since

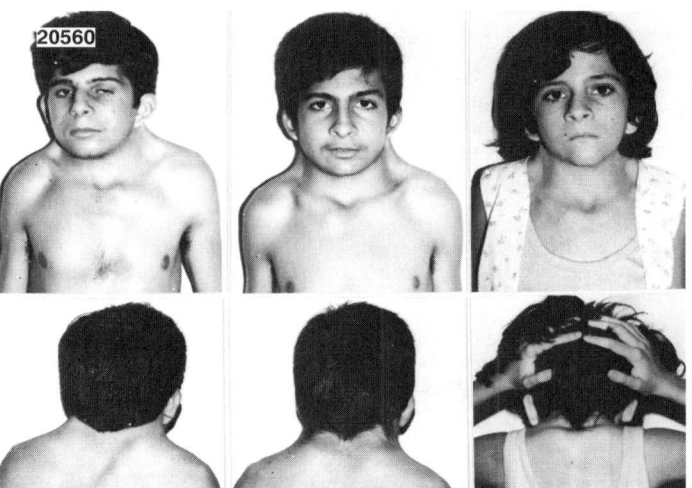

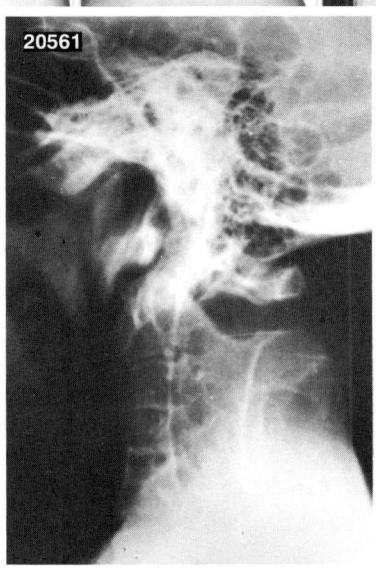

**2032**-20560: Note short neck and low posterior hairlines. 20561: Fusion of vertebrae C2-5.

this classification does not encompass all the reported cases of Klippel-Feil anomaly, a type IV fusion was recently proposed for patients with cervical, upper thoracic, lower thoracic and/or lumbar vertebral fusions. The classical cases of Klippel-Feil anomaly have a short webbed neck, limitation of head and neck, motion, and low posterior hairline. Usually, the neck motion is better preserved in the flexion and extension than in the lateral and rotational planes. Patients with the type II pattern of fusion, which is considered the most frequent and the less severe form, may have a normal or almost normal appearance.

A wide variety of anomalies has been associated with Klippel-Feil anomaly. Scoliosis or kyphoscoliosis is found in about 60% of the patients, and spina bifida occulta in 45%. Urinary anomalies also appear to be very frequent. The combined data of three large series showed that 55% of the patients (57/103) had urinary anomalies, one-half (29 cases) being **Renal agenesis, unilateral**. Other abnormalities include absence of both kidneys, renal dysgenesis or hypoplasia, ectopic kidney, horseshoe kidney, malrotation of kidney, absence of ureter, double collecting system, and hydronephrosis. Genital abnormalities are less frequent, but not uncommon; they are observed mostly in female patients and include absent vagina, absent or rudimentary uterus, absent or hypoplastic fallopian tube, and bicornuate uterus; **Hypospadias** and cryptorchidism are found in some male patients. Sprengel deformity, deafness (conductive, sensorineural, or mixed), and rib anomalies (mainly rib fusion) are found in 30% of the cases. Variable ocular defects (**Eye, microphthalmia/coloboma, Eyelid, ptosis, congenital, Eye, hypertelorism**, nystagmus, rectus palsy, and others), craniofacial asymmetry, fixed torticollis, and synkinesia (mirror movement) are observed in 20%; **Cleft palate** in 15%; and heart defects (mainly interventricular septal defects) in about 8%.

**Complications:** The most important complications are neurologic symptoms of cervical spinal cord injury (such as pain, easy fatigability, spasticity, hyperreflexia, paresthesia, hypesthesia, hemiparesis, and quadriplegia) as a consequence of occipitocervical instability. In many patients, these symptoms occur either spontaneously or after minor trauma. Sudden death after minor trauma has been reported. The complications are not directly derived from the fused cervical vertebrae, but result from adjacent unfused segments with the free joints becoming hypermobile and being subjected to an excessive stress, which can lead to a cervical instability and/or degenerative changes. A C2-C3 fusion with occipitalization of the atlas, for example, may lead to an atlantoaxial instability. The onset of these problems usually occurs between the second and third decades of life.

**Associated Findings:** **Meningocele, Encephalocele**, enlargement or narrowing of the cervical canal, **Brain, Arnold-Chiari malformation** basilar impression, **Syringomyelia, Cleft lip, Hydrocephaly, Microcephaly**, external ear anomalies, **Pectus carinatum, Pectus excavatum**, ectopic lungs, **Situs inversus viscerum**, enteric cysts and duplications, congenital megacolon, anal atresia, and upper extremity abnormalities. Short stature and mental retardation also were reported.

**Etiology:** Klippel-Feil anomaly appears to be etiologically heterogeneous. Most cases are sporadic. Environmental or multifactorial causes may be involved in many cases. In some families, an affected mother and daughter, father and daughter, and father and son have been described. In other families, including a large one with 12 cases, affected sibs of both sexes with normal consanguineous parents were reported. Based on these data, at least two single-gene forms of Klippel-Feil anomaly must be recognized: one autosomal dominant and the other autosomal recessive.

**Pathogenesis:** Congenital fusion of cervical vertebrae results from abnormal segmentation of the cervical somites between the fourth and eighth weeks of fetal life. A theory of vascular etiology has also been proposed (see **Poland syndrome**).

**MIM No.:** *11810, 14886, 14887, *14890, 21430

**POS No.:** 3274

**CDC No.:** 756.110

**Sex Ratio:** M1:F1.5 (approximately).

**Occurrence:** The reported incidence of about 1:40,000 live births which appears in the literature is probably an underestimate, since many mildly affected cases would not be diagnosed because of lack of significant symptoms.

**Risk of Recurrence for Patient's Sib:**
See Part I, *Mendelian Inheritance.*

**Risk of Recurrence for Patient's Child:**
See Part I, *Mendelian Inheritance.*

**Age of Detectability:** At birth.

**Gene Mapping and Linkage:** Unknown.

**Prevention:** None known. Genetic counseling indicated.

**Treatment:** Limited mostly to the complications and associated anomalies. In the presence of cervical spinal cord compression (usually due to cervical instability), decompression or stabilization surgical procedures are required. Patients with Klippel-Feil anomaly, especially those with extensive cervical synostosis, should be guided to avoid activities potentially harmful to the cervical spine. Corrective surgery of associated anomalies may be indicated; for example surgical correction of Sprengel deformity, in properly selected patients, may provide cosmetic and functional improvement.

**Prognosis:** Normal life span in the absence of serious complications and associated anomalies, especially renal abnormalities and scoliosis.

**Detection of Carrier:** Unknown.

**Special Considerations:** Klippel-Feil anomaly, with its wide constellation of associated anomalies, may represent a group of several related but distinct conditions, such as the **Cervico-oculo-acoustic syndrome** (which is virtually limited to females). Some female patients reported as having Klippel-Feil anomaly with associated deafness were possibly cases of **Cervico-oculo-acoustic syndrome**, and the mentioned excess of females with Klippel-Feil anomaly may not be realistic. The association of **Mullerian aplasia** with fused cervical vertebrae and other defects probably constitutes another distinct entity.

**References:**
Klippel M, Feil A: Un cas d'absence des vertébres cervicales avec cage thoracique remontant jusqu'á la base du crâne (cage thoracique cervicale). Nou Iconogr Saloet 1912; 25:223–250.
Gunderson CH, et al.: The Klippel-Feil syndrome: genetic and clinical reevaluation of cervical fusion. Medicine 1967; 46:491–512.
Hensinger RN, et al.: Klippel-Feil syndrome: a constellation of associated anomalies. J Bone Joint Surg 1974; 56A:1246–1253. *
Helmi C, Pruzansky S: Craniofacial and extracranial malformations in the Klippel-Feil syndrome. Cleft Palate J 1980; 17:65–88. †
da-Silva EO: Autosomal recessive Klippel-Feil syndrome. J Med Genet 1982; 19:130–134. *
Nagib MG, et al.: Identification and management of high-risk patients with Klippel-Feil syndrome. J Neurosurg 1984; 61:523–530.
Shaver KA, et al.: Deafness, facial asymmetry and Klippel-Feil syndrome in five generations. (Abstract) Am J Hum Genet 1986; 39:A81 only.

DA025                                    **Elias O. da-Silva**

**Klippel-Feil anomaly-deafness-abducens palsy**
*See CERVICO-OCULO-ACOUSTIC SYNDROME*
**Klippel-Feil syndrome**
*See KLIPPEL-FEIL ANOMALY*
**Klippel-Trenaunay-Weber syndrome (KTW)**
*See ANGIO-OSTEOHYPERTROPHY SYNDROME*

## KNEE, GENU RECURVATUM                            2938

**Includes:** Hyperextension of the knee

**Excludes:** Knee, dislocation

**Major Diagnostic Criteria:** Anterior overextension of the knee, generally present immediately after birth. Genu recurvatum may occur unilaterally, but is usually found bilaterally.

**Clinical Findings:** Hyperextension of the knee can be present as an isolated anomaly. In such circumstances the infants were generally constrained *in utero*, especially in full knee extension breech position, or confined to a bicorneate uterus. Other constraint-induced deformities of the legs and facies are often associated. Hyperextension of the knee may also occur because of primary malformations of ligament, bone and joint, or neuromuscular system. The overall physical examination and the gestational history will almost always suggest the deformational or malformational origin in this disorder.

**Complications:** When genu recurvatum is left untreated in the newborn period it may progress to dislocation of the knee, with secondary changes then occurring in the bones, ligaments, and muscles. Distortion of the distal femoral epiphysis and shortening or fibrosis of the quadriceps both occur frequently.

**Associated Findings:** Genu recurvatum of deformational origin is often associated with dislocated hip, plantar position of the forefoot, and flattening of the face. Infants with congenitally small patellas or the **Nail-patella syndrome** often have genu recurvatum or knee dislocations. Joint hyperextension and dislocations including the knee are seen in conditions of ligamentous laxity, such as the **Ehlers-Danlos syndrome**. **Meningomyelocele, Arthrogryposes**, and other intrinsic neuromuscular conditions can produce unusual muscle pull about the knee and hyperextension or dislocation.

**Etiology:** Heterogeneous, with both deformational and primary and secondary malformational causes.

**Pathogenesis:** The shape and growth of the knee, like any joint, is determined by a balanced interplay between intrinsic properties of bone and soft tissues and by extrinsic biomechanical forces. Intrinsic factors include the biochemical structure of the bones, their growth potential, and physical properties, while extrinsic factors include muscle pull and dynamic stress applied by the fetal confines.

**CDC No.:**   754.430

**Sex Ratio:**   M1:F1

**Occurrence:**   Estimated at 2:10,000 births.

**Risk of Recurrence for Patient's Sib:** Recurrence is unlikely when deformation occurred without evidence of a primary central nervous system process in the infant except when there is a maternal uterine process (like fibroids or a bicornate structure), which predisposes subsequent infants to constraint. When genu recurvatum is due to a primary or secondary malformation, specific risk recurrence for that causal disorder will apply.

**Risk of Recurrence for Patient's Child:** Recurrence is unlikely when deformation occurred without evidence of a primary central nervous system process in the infant except when there is a maternal uterine process (like fibroids or a bicornate structure), which predisposes subsequent infants to constraint. When genu recurvatum is due to a primary or secondary malformation, specific risk recurrence for that causal disorder will apply.

**Age of Detectability:**   Immediately after birth.

**Gene Mapping and Linkage:**   Unknown.

**Prevention:**   None known. Genetic counseling indicated.

**Treatment:** Genu recurvatum can be managed conservatively in the neonatal period with manipulation and mild pressure immobilization toward the normal joint position.

**Prognosis:** The prognosis for correction of genu recurvatum is fully dependent on the cause. Deformations of the knee should respond well to repositioning. Malformational hyperextension may respond to repositioning, but often requires surgery. In some cases of severe bony anomaly or neuromuscular imbalance, surgery may not be fully corrective or capable of preventing recurrence.

**Detection of Carrier:**   Unknown.

**References:**

Niebauer JT, King DE: Congenital dislocation of the knee. J Bone Joint Surg 1960; 42A:207–225.

Laurence M: Genu recurvatum congenitum. J Bone Joint Surg 1967; 49B:121–134.

Smith DW: Recognizable patterns of human deformation. Philadelphia: W.B. Saunders, 1981. †

CL006                                    **Sterling K. Clarren**

**Kniest disease**
*See KNIEST DYSPLASIA*

---

## KNIEST DYSPLASIA                                  0557

**Includes:**
   Dwarfism, metatropic, type II
   Kniest disease
   Metatropic dysplasia, type II
   Pseudometatropic dwarfism
   Swiss-cheese cartilage syndrome

**Excludes:**
   **Dwarfism, dyssegmental, Rolland-Desbuquois type** (2690)
   **Dwarfism, dyssegmental, Silverman-Handmaker type** (2935)
   **Metatropic dysplasia** (0656)
   **Mucopolysaccharidosis IV** (0678)
   **Spondyloepiphyseal dysplasia congenita** (0897)
   **Spondyloepiphyseal dysplasia, late** (0898)

**Major Diagnostic Criteria:** Disproportionate dwarfism with typical X-ray changes in the skeleton, frequently myopia and typical flat facies. Characteristic chondroosseous histopathology may be used to verify the diagnosis.

**Clinical Findings:** Disproportionate dwarfism and kyphoscoliosis associated with flat facies and prominent eyes, cleft palate, hearing loss, myopia, and limited joint motion. The skeletal abnormalities are recognizable at birth with shortening and deformity of the limbs and stiff joints. Marked lumbar lordosis and kyphoscoliosis develop in childhood resulting in disproportionate shortening of the trunk. Walking is delayed and difficult. The long bones are short and bowed and the joints appear enlarged. There is limitation of joint motion with pain, stiffness and flexion contractures of the major joints. The flexion contractures in the hips produce a characteristic stance. The fingers appear long and knobby, and flexion is limited resulting in an inability to form a fist. The face is flat and dish-shaped with prominent wide-set eyes, flat nasal bridge and a broad mouth. There is severe myopia which frequently leads to retinal detachment. Umbilical and inguinal herniae are common. Cleft palate may lead to chronic otitis media and both conductive and neurosensory hearing loss

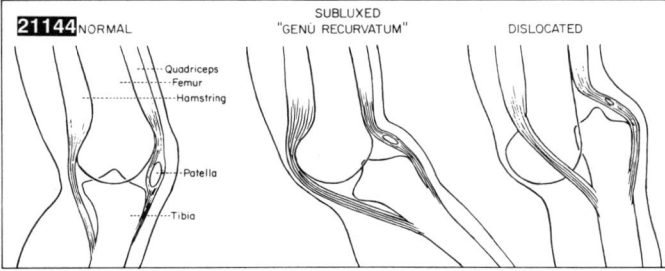

**2938-21144:** The subluxed knee is an intermediate pattern of anatomic distortion when compared to the normal or dislocated knee.

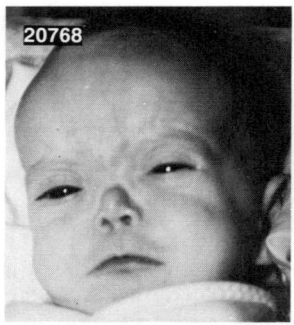
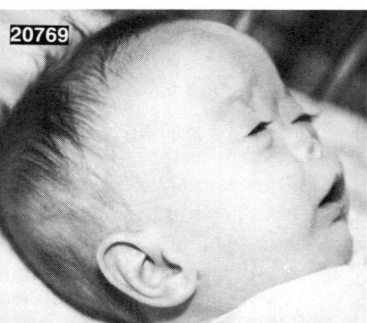
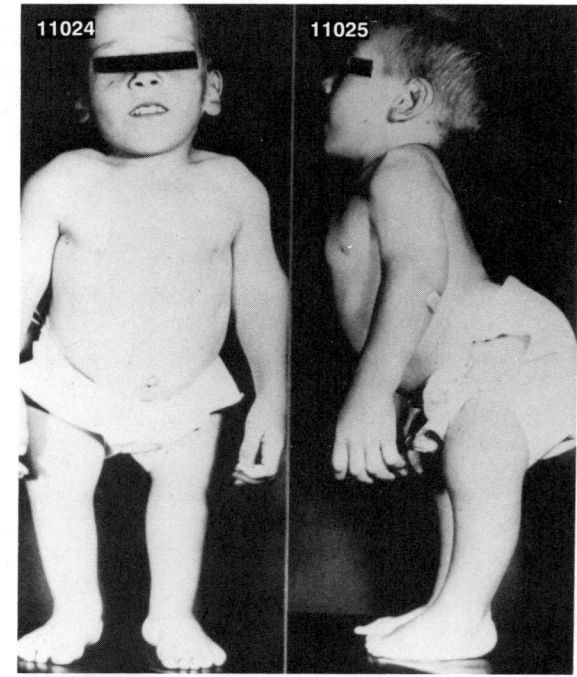
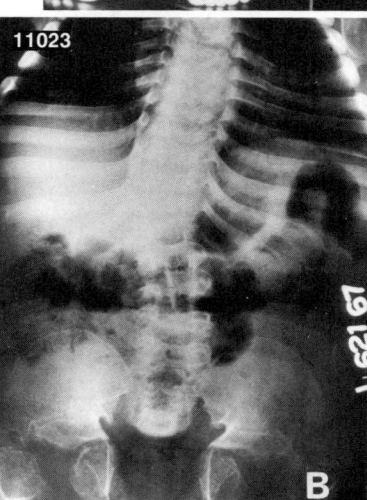
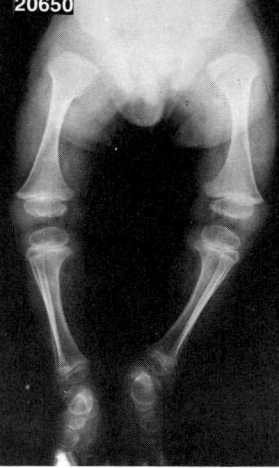

are common. Recurrent respiratory distress with tracheomalacia may occur in infancy. Motor milestones and speech development may be delayed, but intelligence usually is normal.

The characteristic X-ray abnormalities during the newborn period include dumbbell-shaped femora, hypoplastic pelvic bones, vertical clefts of the vertebrae, and platyspondyly. In infancy and childhood one sees a dessert-cup shaped pelvis, increased soft tissue densities around the joints, enlarged epiphyses, cloud-like calcifications near the epiphyseal plates, and flat elongated vertebral bodies with cloud-like calcifications. The bones of the hands are osteoporotic and show delay in formation of epiphyses; soft tissue swelling occurs near the joints. There are fragmented accessory ossification centers and joint spaces are narrowed. The femoral heads show a marked delay in ossification and may not appear until mid-childhood. In adult life, there is rhizomelic short stature but the cloud calcifications disappear after epiphyseal fusion. Hands show a bulbous enlargement of the ends of the short tubular bones, short thumb tufts, and a flat and squared appearance of the metacarpal-phalangeal joints.

**Complications:** Myopia may lead to retinal detachment. Shortened and deformed bones and limitation of joint motion may lead to severe orthopedic complications. Cleft palate may lead to speech impairment and chronic otitis media.

**Associated Findings:** Ocular findings include vitreoretinal degeneration, rhegmatogenous retinal detachment, dislocated lenses, and blepharoptosis.

**Etiology:** Presumably autosomal dominant inheritance.

**Pathogenesis:** The chondro-osseous histopathology is abnormal and distinctive. Resting cartilage contains large cells, a loosely woven matrix with irregular staining, and many "holes" which have been likened to "swiss-cheese cartilage." The growth plate contains hypercellular cartilage with ballooned chondrocytes and sparse matrix. The condition is characterized by an apparent abnormal processing of the C-propeptide of type II cartilage collagen, resulting in imperfect fibril assembly.

**MIM No.:** *15655

**POS No.:** 3272

**Sex Ratio:** M1:F1

**Occurrence:** Undetermined. Established literature.

**Risk of Recurrence for Patient's Sib:**
See Part I, *Mendelian Inheritance.*

**Risk of Recurrence for Patient's Child:**
See Part I, *Mendelian Inheritance.*

**Age of Detectability:** Prenatal diagnosis by ultrasound.

**Gene Mapping and Linkage:** Unknown.

**Prevention:** None known. Genetic counseling indicated.

**Treatment:** Orthopedic surgery for joint contractures, kyphoscoliosis, and epiphyseal dysplasia; repair of cleft palate, frequent regular ophthalmologic examinations for detection and prevention of retinal detachment.

**Prognosis:** Apparently normal for life.

**Detection of Carrier:** Unknown.

**Special Considerations:** This condition had been confused with **Metatropic dysplasia** in the past because of the similar dumbbell appearance of the long bones in the newborn. These disorders can be readily distinguished on the basis of skeletal X-rays and clinical features. Recently several distinct Kniest-like skeletal dysplasias have been reported which also appear to be autosomal recessive.

**References:**
Maroteaux P, Spranger J: La maladie de Kniest. Arch Fr Pediatr 1973; 30:735–750.
Rimoin DL, et al.: Metatropic dwarfism, the Kniest syndrome, and the pseudoachondroplastic dysplasias. Clin Orthop 1976; 114:70–82.
Sconyers SM, et al.: A distinct chondrodysplasia resembling Kniest dysplasia. J Pediatr 1983; 103:898–904.
Friede H, et al.: Craniofacial and mucopolysaccharide abnormalities in Kniest dysplasia. J Craniofac Genet Devel Biol 1985; 5:267–276.

**0557-20768–69:** Kniest dysplasia; note hypertelorism, flat facies, hemangioma on the glabella and low-set ears. **11024–25:** Note round facies; shortening of trunk and limbs. Pelvis and trunk are bent forward secondary to flexion contractures of the hip. **11023:** Moderately severe thoracolumbar scoliosis, decreased vertical diameter of ilia. **20650:** Lower limbs in a 1-year-old; note the short long bones, wide metaphyses, the large femoral distal epiphyses and the tibial proximal epiphyses contrasting with the femoral head which is not visible.

Maumenee IH, Traboulsi EI: The ocular findings in Kniest dysplasia. Am J Ophthal 1985; 100:155–160.

Poole AR, et al.: Kniest dysplasia is characterized by an apparent abnormal processing of the C-propeptide of type II cartilage collagen, resulting in imperfect fibril assembly. J Clin Invest 1988; 81:579–589.

B0025
LA006

**Zvi Borochowitz**
**Ralph S. Lachman**
*David L. Rimoin*

**Kniest, severe neonatal form**
*See KNIEST-LIKE DYSPLASIA*

## KNIEST-LIKE DYSPLASIA      2799

**Includes:**

Chondrodysplasia, Kniest-like
Chondrodysplasia, micromelic (misnomer)
Kniest-like dysplasia with pursed lips and ectopia lentis
Kniest, severe neonatal form
Skeletal dysplasia, Kniest-like

**Excludes:**

Dwarfism, dyssegmental, Rolland-Desbuquois type (2690)
Kniest dysplasia (0557)
Thanatophoric dysplasia (0940)
Thanatophoric dysplasia, Glasgow type (2821)

**Major Diagnostic Criteria:** Differentiation of this condition from other forms of neonatally lethal short-limbed dwarfisms is based on X-ray and histologic findings.

**Clinical Findings:** Both known cases were born prematurely, following a pregnancy complicated by hydramnios. Birth weights were normal, but birth lengths were at the 25th or less percentile, and head circumferences at or greater than the 90th percentile. The face was described as flat with wide-set-appearing eyes. **Cleft palate** was present in one, and an "unusual" pharynx in another. The ears were malformed and low set. Both infants also had severe rhizomelia, short neck, narrow thorax, talipes equinovarus, and edema. One had cardiac arrhythmia; the other had **Atrial septal defects** and **Ductus arteriosus, patent**.

X-ray findings included dumbbell-shaped long bones with flared, irregular metaphyses and markedly shortened diaphyses; platyspondyly with wide vertebral clefts; wide, shortened ribs; and hypoplastic ilia. Histologically, the cartilage was similar to the "Swiss-cheese" appearance described in **Kniest dysplasia**; however, there was also a "frayed" appearance to the matrix between chondrocytes. Ultrastructurally, the chondrocyte endoplasmic reticulum was not dilated as it is in Kniest dysplasia.

**Complications:** Pulmonary hypoplasia may be the result of small thoracic size. Hydrops may occur as a result of in utero cardiac arrhythmia.

**Associated Findings:** Pursed lips and ectopia lentis were reported in two siblings by Burton et al (1986). Upper limbs were normal, and histologic examination of bone did not show a Swiss cheese appearance.

**Etiology:** Possibly autosomal recessive inheritance.

**Pathogenesis:** Although this condition is a chondrodysplasia, the basic genetic defect is unknown. While the term "micromelic chondrodysplasia" has been applied to this group of disorders, the designation is generally considered inappropriate.

**MIM No.:** 24519

**POS No.:** 4510

**Sex Ratio:** Presumably M1:F1.

**Occurrence:** Reported in two sibs from California.

**Risk of Recurrence for Patient's Sib:**
See Part I, *Mendelian Inheritance.*

**Risk of Recurrence for Patient's Child:**
See Part I, *Mendelian Inheritance.*

**Age of Detectability:** At birth. Prenatal diagnosis by ultrasound may also be possible.

**Gene Mapping and Linkage:** Unknown.

**Prevention:** None known. Genetic counseling indicated.

**Treatment:** Unknown.

**Prognosis:** Both children died within one week of birth.

**Detection of Carrier:** Unknown.

**References:**

Stevenson RE: Micromelic chondrodysplasia: further evidence for autosomal recessive inheritance. Proc Greenwood Genet Center 1982; 1:52–57.

Sconyers SM, et al.: A distinct chondrodysplasia resembling Kniest dysplasia: clinical, roentgenographic, histologic, and ultrastructural findings. J Pediatr 1983; 103:898–904.

Burton BK, et al.: A new skeletal dysplasia: clinical, radiologic and pathologic findings. J Pediatr 1986; 109:642–648.

T0007      **Helga V. Toriello**

**Kniest-like dysplasia with pursed lips and ectopia lentis**
*See KNIEST-LIKE DYSPLASIA*

## KNUCKLE PADS-LEUKONYCHIA-DEAFNESS      0558

**Includes:**

Bart-Pumphrey syndrome
Deafness, knuckle pads and leukonychia
Knuckle pads-leukonychia-deafness, keratosis palmoplantaris
Leukonychia, knuckle pads and deafness

**Excludes:**

Deafness-keratopachydermia-digital constrictions (0259)
Deafness without appropriate cutaneous findings
Keratopachydermia-digital constriction-deafness
Knuckle pads without deafness
Nails, leukonychia (0589)

**Major Diagnostic Criteria:** Deafness, leukonychia (nails need not be dead white), and knuckle pads (thickened areas of skin over the knuckles).

**Clinical Findings:** Sensorineural deafness occurs in all cases but may require audiometric studies to confirm. Conductive hearing loss may be present in some cases. Increased whiteness of finger and toenails is seen in all cases studied. Knuckle pads are usually found and keratoderma palmare et plantare frequently occurs.

All patients have sensorineural loss, with the defect in the cochlea. Some patients have a superimposed conductive loss which may or may not be associated with structural abnormalities of the middle ear. Whether hearing loss may be progressive in some patients is not known. Keratoderma palmare et plantare is more commonly found in adults with the syndrome than in affected children.

**Complications:** Unknown.

**Associated Findings:** None known.

**Etiology:** Autosomal dominant inheritance with complete penetrance but variable expressivity.

**Pathogenesis:** Unknown.

**MIM No.:** *14920

**POS No.:** 4267

**Sex Ratio:** M1:F1

**Occurrence:** Two pedigrees have been reported. In addition, an isolated case with all the features of the syndrome has been reported; other members of the family had various abnormalities, but none was deaf.

**Risk of Recurrence for Patient's Sib:**
See Part I, *Mendelian Inheritance.*

**Risk of Recurrence for Patient's Child:**
See Part I, *Mendelian Inheritance.* Reproductive fitness probably unimpaired.

**Age of Detectability:** Hearing loss and knuckle pads can be first observed in infancy or early childhood. Leukonychia probably begins in early childhood.

**Gene Mapping and Linkage:** Unknown.

**Prevention:** None known. Genetic counseling indicated.

**Treatment:** That appropriate for the degree of hearing loss, including hearing aid and speech therapy.

**Prognosis:** Normal life span and intelligence.

**Detection of Carrier:** Unknown.

**References:**
Schwann J: Keratosis palmaris et plantaris cum surditate congenita et leuconychia totali unguium. Dermatologica 1963; 126:335–353.
Bart RS, Pumphrey RE: Knuckle pads, leukonychia and deafness: a dominantly inherited syndrome. New Engl J Med 1967; 276:202–207.
Konigsmark BW: Hereditary childhood hearing loss and integumentary system disease. J Pediatr 1972; 80:909–919.
Crosby EF, Vidurrizaga RH: Knuckle pads, leukonychia, deafness, and keratosis palmoplantaris: report of a family. Johns Hopkins Med J 1976; 139:90–92.
Paller A, Herbert AA: Knuckle pads in children. Am J Dis Child 1986; 140:915–917.

MI038                                          **Giuseppe Micali**

**Knuckle pads-leukonychia-deafness, keratosis palmoplantaris**
*See KNUCKLE PADS-LEUKONYCHIA-DEAFNESS*
**'Koala bear' faces**
*See CHONDRODYSPLASIA PUNCTATA, MILD SYMMETRIC TYPE*
**Koebberling-Dunnigan syndrome**
*See LIPODYSTROPHY, FAMILIAL LIMB AND TRUNK*
**Kohler disease (navicular)**
*See JOINTS, OSTEOCHONDRITIS DISSECANS*
**Kohlschutter syndrome**
*See AMELO-CEREBRO-HYPOHIDROTIC SYNDROME*
**Kohn-Romano syndrome**
*See BLEPHAROPTOSIS-BLEPHAROPHIMOSIS-EPICANTHUS INVERSUS-TELECANTHUS*
**Koilonychia, hereditary**
*See NAILS, KOILONYCHIA*
**Kok disease**
*See HYPEREKPLEXIA*
**Konigsmark syndrome**
*See DEAFNESS, DOMINANT LOW-FREQUENCY*
**Kopysc syndrome**
*See TRICHODENTAL DYSPLASIA WITH REFRACTIVE ERRORS*
**Kostmann syndrome**
*See IMMUNODEFICIENCY, AGRANULOCYTOSIS, INFANTILE KOSTMANN TYPE*
**Kousseff syndrome**
*See MENINGOCELE-CONOTRUNCAL HEART DEFECT, KOUSSEFF TYPE*
**Kozlova-Altschuler-Kravchenko syndrome**
*See DERMATO-OSTEOLYSIS, KIRGHIZIAN TYPE*
**Kozlowski chondrodysplasia, spondylometaphyseal**
*See SPONDYLOMETAPHYSEAL CHONDRODYSPLASIA, KOZLOWSKI TYPE*
**Krabbe disease**
*See LEUKODYSTROPHY, GLOBOID CELL TYPE*
**Kramer syndrome**
*See GINGIVAL FIBROMATOSIS-DEPIGMENTATION-MICROPHTHALMIA*
**Kranenburg syndrome**
*See OPTIC DISK PITS*
**Kufs disease**
*See NEURONAL CEROID-LIPOFUSCINOSES (NCL)*
**Kugelberg-Welander disease**
*See SPINAL MUSCULAR ATROPHY*

**Includes:** Arthrogryposis-like disorder

**Excludes:** Arthrogryposes (0088)

**Major Diagnostic Criteria:** Multiple joint contractures, often severely affecting the knees and ankles, with either atrophy or compensatory hypertrophy of associated muscle groups. Intelligence is normal. There is evidence for an autosomal recessive mode of inheritance.

**Clinical Findings:** Multiple joint contractures develop early with severe involvement of the knees and ankles and accompanying atrophy or compensatory hypertrophy of associated muscle groups. Gait is a duck-like waddle, or is accomplished by walking on the knees. Flexion contractures also are seen at the elbows but are less severe. Pigmented nevi and decreased corneal reflexes have been noted in several patients. Intelligence is normal. Laboratory studies, including serum muscle enzymes, calcium, and phosphorus measurements, and tests for urinary amino acids and mucopolysaccharides, are normal. Electromyography with nerve conduction velocities and muscle biopsies do not show any abnormalities; histochemical studies of frozen sections are also unremarkable. X-rays demonstrate hypoplasia of the first or second lumbar vertebral body, progressive elongation of the pedicles of the 5th lumbar vertebra, producing spondylolisthesis, cathedral chest, osteolytic areas in the outer clavicle and proximal humerus (particularly in children), and hypoplasia of the patella associated with knee contractures.

**Complications:** The patella, normally placed at birth, migrates proximally through attenuation elongation of the patella tendon, which becomes a yellowish, amorphous mass, blending into the retinaculum of the knee. The quadriceps femoris consistently migrates to the proximal one-third of the thigh. Equinus and planovalgus foot deformities commonly occur.

**Associated Findings:** None known.

**Etiology:** Probably autosomal recessive inheritance.

**Pathogenesis:** Kuskokwim syndrome is differentiated from **Arthrogryposes** by its mode of inheritance, lack of laboratory evidence of abnormalities of muscles or nerves around affected joints, and characteristic X-ray changes. Abnormal muscle attachment, predominantly involving the tendons of the extensor muscles which are under constant strain, is believed to be a primary defect.

**MIM No.:** *20820

**POS No.:** 4283

**Sex Ratio:** M1:F1

**Occurrence:** Less than 20 cases have been reported, all in Eskimos in the Kuskokwim River delta of southwestern Alaska. Cases are thinly distributed in this limited geographic area of isolated villages.

**Risk of Recurrence for Patient's Sib:**
See Part I, *Mendelian Inheritance.*

**Risk of Recurrence for Patient's Child:**
See Part I, *Mendelian Inheritance.*

**Age of Detectability:** At birth.

**Gene Mapping and Linkage:** Unknown.

**Prevention:** None known. Genetic counseling indicated.

**Treatment:** Advanced deformities are often treated with osteotomies and muscle transfer. Early treatment with selected casting and bracing with passive manipulation will circumvent some of the severe contractures seen in adults.

**Prognosis:** Normal for life span and intelligence; functional ambulation is variable.

**Detection of Carrier:** Unknown.

**References:**
Petajan JH, et al.: Arthrogryposis syndrome (Kuskokwim syndrome) in the Eskimo. J.A.M.A. 1969; 209:1481–1486.
Wright DG, Aase J: The Kuskokwim syndrome: an inherited form of

arthrogryposis in the Alaskan Eskimo. BD:OAS;V(3). New York: The National Foundation March of Dimes, 1969:91–95.

G0043 **Donald P. Goldsmith**

## KYPHOMELIC DYSPLASIA 2754

**Includes:**
Bowing, congenital, with short bones
Familial congenital bowing with short bones
Short-limbed campomelic syndrome, normocephalic type
Skeletal dysplasia, kyphomelic dysplasia

**Excludes:**
**Campomelic dysplasia** (0122)
**Cortical hyperostosis, infantile** (0221)
**Femoral hypoplasia-unusual facies syndrome** (2027)

**Major Diagnostic Criteria:** Dwarfism; predominant shortening and bowing of the femora, with metaphyseal abnormalities; skin dimples; and micrognathia.

**Clinical Findings:** Dwarfism with severely angulated, shortened femora are cardinal features. Other tubular bones are less affected. The trunk is shortened. Skin dimples are present and are located over the greater trochanters (100%). Restricted abductions and extension of the hip joints results in a waddling gait. The chest is narrow (100%) and may be deformed or flattened (60%), giving rise to respiratory distress in the neonate. Midfacial hypoplasia, a small anteverted nose, and micrognathia are clinical features that manifest early and revert to normality in mid-childhood.

On X-ray, all the long bones are bowed and broadened, especially the femora. Irregularity of the lower femoral metaphyses is usually present. The ribs are shortened with flared ends (100%), and absence of one pair of ribs sometimes occurs (40%). Platyspondyly (87%), underossification of the proximal tibial epiphyses (43%), hypoplastic fibulae and acetabulae, and sacral anomalies are less common findings.

**Complications:** Unknown.

**Associated Findings:** Small midfacial and eyelid hemangiomas are infrequently reported.

**Etiology:** Probable autosomal recessive inheritance as evidenced by the report of two sibs in two separate kindreds. Four of the eight known cases have been sporadic.

**Pathogenesis:** Unknown.

**MIM No.:** 21135

**POS No.:** 3930

**Sex Ratio:** M5:F1 (sex undetermined in two individuals).

**Occurrence:** Eight cases have been reported.

**Risk of Recurrence for Patient's Sib:**
See Part I, *Mendelian Inheritance.*

**Risk of Recurrence for Patient's Child:**
See Part I, *Mendelian Inheritance.*

**Age of Detectability:** At birth, or prenatally by ultrasound.

**Gene Mapping and Linkage:** Unknown.

**Prevention:** None known. Genetic counseling indicated.

**Treatment:** Orthopedic procedures to straighten limb bowing and aid hip joint mobility may be indicated.

**Prognosis:** Normal intelligence and life span.

**Detection of Carrier:** Unknown.

**Special Considerations:** Nosologic confusion between kyphomelic dysplasia and **Femoral hypoplasia-unusual facies syndrome** (FH-UFS) exists. FH-UFS can be diagnosed clinically in that the proximal portions of the femora are very hypoplastic. FH-UFS is sporadic, patients have persistent facial dysmorphology throughout life, and a history of maternal diabetes can often be obtained.

**References:**
Khajavi A, et al.: Heterogeneity in the campomelic syndromes: long- and short-bone varieties. Pediatr Radiol 1976; 120:641–647.

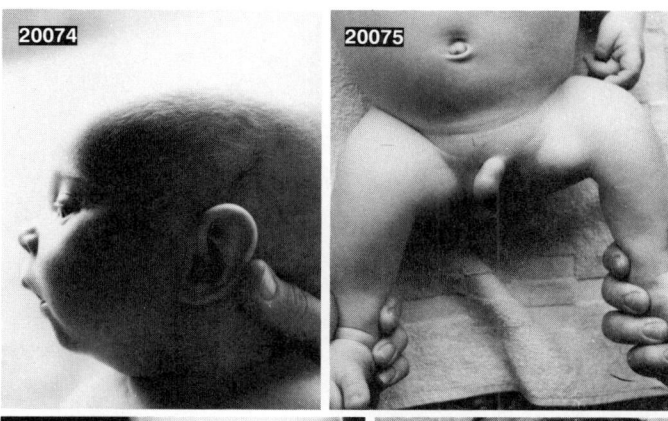
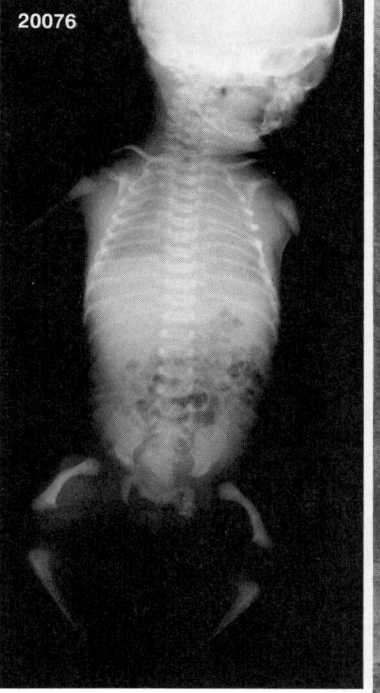
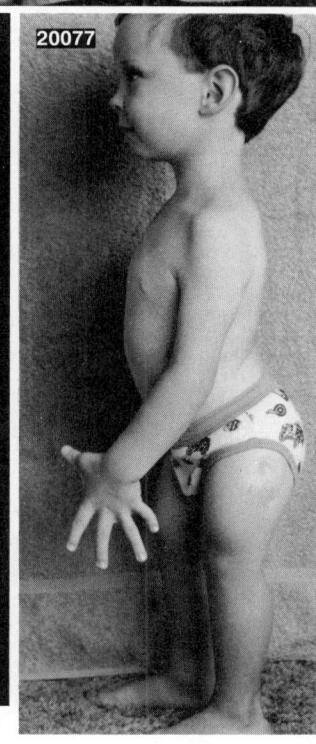

**2754-20074:** Note small upturned nose and micrognathia. **20075:** Short and bowed lower limbs. **20076:** Bowed femora, hypoplastic acetabulae, under-ossified pubic symphysis and abnormally segmented sacrum. **20077:** Note clinodactyly, lumbar lordosis and surgical scar over the trochanteric region in this 4-year-old boy.

Hall BD, Spranger JW: Familial congenital bowing with short bones. Pediatr Radiol 1979; 132:611–614.
Maclean RN, et al.: Skeletal dysplasia with short, angulated femora (kyphomelic dysplasia). Am J Med Genet 1983; 14:373–380. *
Viljoen D, Beighton P: Kyphomelic dysplasia-further delineation of the phenotype. Dysmorphol Clin Genet 1988; 1:136–141. †

VI005 **Denis L. Viljöen**

**Kyrle disease**
*See SKIN, KYRLE DISEASE*

# ❖ L ❖

**L-5-hydroxytryptophan induced scleroderma**
*See SCLERODERMA, FAMILIAL PROGRESSIVE*
**L-transposition with situs solitus**
*See VENTRICLES, INVERTED WITH TRANSPOSITION OF GREAT ARTERIES*
**L-xylulose reductase deficiency**
*See PENTOSURIA*
**L-xylulosuria**
*See PENTOSURIA*
**Laband syndrome**
*See GINGIVAL FIBROMATOSIS-DIGITAL ANOMALIES*
**Labile factor deficiency**
*See FACTOR V DEFICIENCY*
**Labyrinthine otosclerosis**
*See OTOSCLEROSIS*
**Labyrinthine otosclerosis-fixed stapes footplate**
*See OTOSCLEROSIS*

## LACRIMAL CANALICULUS ATRESIA                    0563

**Includes:**
    Lacrimal canaliculus with or without punctum absence
    Lacrimal canaliculus with or without punctum atresia

**Excludes:** Obstructed nasolacrimal duct at the valve of Hasner

**Major Diagnostic Criteria:** In cases of aplasia of the canaliculus there is coexistent aplasia of the punctum. In cases of aplasia of the punctum the canaliculus may be variably present.

**Clinical Findings:** Symptoms relate to epiphora (tearing) if the lower punctum or canaliculus is incompletely represented. Absence of the entire lacrimal drainage system may occur secondary to midline facial anomalies, such as cyclopia or arrhinencephaly, or to eyelid malformations, such as cryptophthalmos or colobomas.

**Complications:** Chronic epiphora.

**Associated Findings:** May be seen in **Ectrodactyly-ectodermal dysplasia-clefting syndrome** and **Branchial arch-premature aging syndrome.**

**Etiology:** Usually sporadic. Hereditary cases may be autosomal dominant with variable penetrance and expression.

**Pathogenesis:** Deficiency in outbudding of the superior end of the ectodermal core.

**MIM No.:** *14970

**CDC No.:** 743.640

**Sex Ratio:** M1:F1 in hereditary cases.

**Occurrence:** Undetermined.

**Risk of Recurrence for Patient's Sib:**
    See Part I, *Mendelian Inheritance.* Not all cases are hereditary.

**Risk of Recurrence for Patient's Child:**
    See Part I, *Mendelian Inheritance.* Not all cases are hereditary.

**Age of Detectability:** At birth.

**Gene Mapping and Linkage:** Unknown.

**Prevention:** None known. Genetic counseling indicated.

**Treatment:** Surgery. In cases with minimal disruption of the canaliculus or punctum, Quickert silicone intubation may prove sufficient. In cases with significant disruption conjunctivorhinostomy may prove necessary.

**Prognosis:** Good, following surgical correction.

**Detection of Carrier:** By examination.

**References:**
Lumbroso BD: On a case of congenital atresia of the lacrimal ducts with familial characteristics. Acta Genet Med Gemellol 1960; 9:290–295.
Waardenburg P, et al.: Genetics and ophthalmology, Vol 1. Oxford: Blackwell Scientific, 1961:293.
Werb A: The management of canalicular occlusion. Trans Ophthalmol Soc NZ 1976; 28:41.
Kohn R: Textbook of ophthalmic plastic and reconstructive surgery. Philadelphia: Lea & Febiger, 1988:261–262.

K0025                                                          **Roger Kohn**

**Lacrimal canaliculus with or without punctum absence**
*See LACRIMAL CANALICULUS ATRESIA*
**Lacrimal canaliculus with or without punctum atresia**
*See LACRIMAL CANALICULUS ATRESIA*
**Lacrimal gland, aberrant**
*See LACRIMAL GLAND, ECTOPIC*
**Lacrimal gland, congenital dislocation of**
*See LACRIMAL GLAND, ECTOPIC*

## LACRIMAL GLAND, ECTOPIC                    0564

**Includes:**
    Lacrimal gland, aberrant
    Lacrimal gland, congenital dislocation of

**Excludes:** Prolapse of normal lacrimal gland

**Major Diagnostic Criteria:** Presence of lacrimal gland tissue anywhere distant from its normal location in the lacrimal fossa.

**Clinical Findings:** Congenital lobulated fleshy tumor usually found beneath the conjunctiva near the limbus, at the lateral canthal region, or within the orbit distant from the lacrimal fossa. Intraocular involvement is rare. Lacrimal gland tissue, situated normally or ectopically, is subject to inflammatory or neoplastic changes; therefore, biopsy of symptomatic expanding lesion is indicated. Ectopic lacrimal gland tissue should be considered when evaluating intraocular or intraorbital mass.

**Complications:** Epibulbar lesions may distort the cornea or cause strabismus by impinging upon extraocular muscle. Intraorbital tumors may become symptomatic as a result of inflammation or neoplastic transformation. Computed tomographic scanning is useful to detect intraorbital involvement.

**Associated Findings:** Blepharochalasis, coloboma of the lids. Intraorbital vascular malformations.

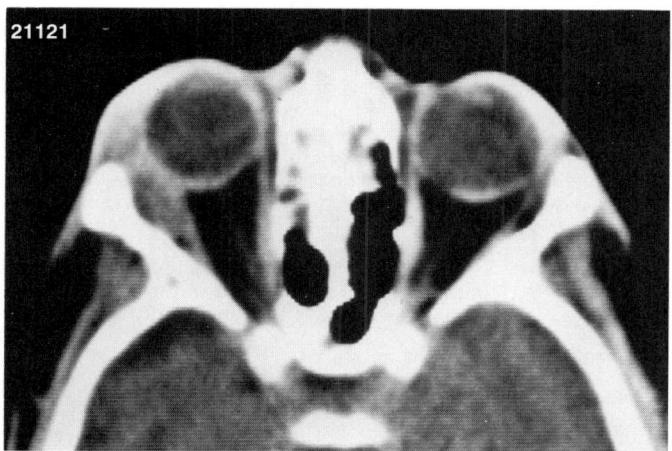

**0564A**-21121: Orbital CT scan (image viewed from below) shows ectopic lacrimal gland along the superotemporal aspect of the right orbit.

**Etiology:** Unknown.

**Pathogenesis:** Unknown.

**CDC No.:** 743.660

**Sex Ratio:** M1:F1

**Occurrence:** Undetermined but presumed rare.

**Risk of Recurrence for Patient's Sib:** Unknown.

**Risk of Recurrence for Patient's Child:** Unknown.

**Age of Detectability:** At birth.

**Gene Mapping and Linkage:** Unknown.

**Prevention:** None known. Genetic counseling indicated.

**Treatment:** Surgical removal for cosmesis and histologic confirmation of the diagnosis. When lesion distorts cornea, induces orbital inflammation, undergoes growth, or compromises intraocular structures, removal is indicated.

**Prognosis:** Good; no visual impairment occurs.

**Detection of Carrier:** Unknown.

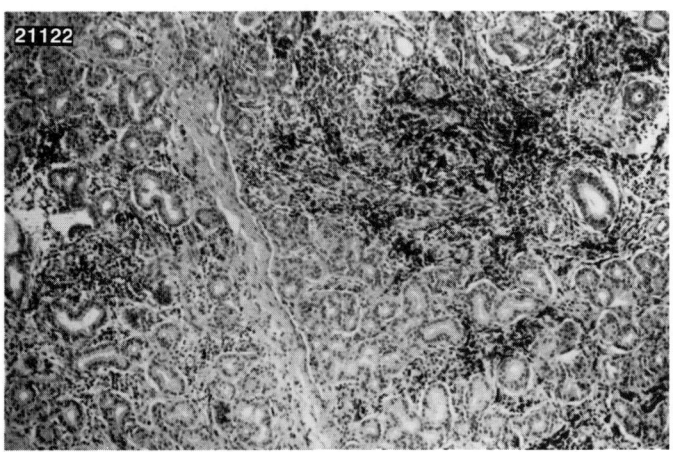

**0564B**-21122: Histopathologic specimen of orbital mass shows ectopic lacrimal gland infiltrated with inflammatory cells.

**References:**

Christiansen L, Anderson ED: Aberrant intraocular adenomata and epitheliazation of the anterior chamber. Arch Ophthalmol 1952; 48:19–29.

Green WR, Zimmerman LE: Ectopic lacrimal gland tissue: report of 8 cases with orbital involvement. Arch Ophthalmol 1967; 78:318–327.

Appel N, Som PM: Ectopic lacrimal gland tissue. J Comput Assist Tomogr 1982; 6:1010–1012.

Margo CE, et al.: Ectopic lacrimal gland tissue of the orbit and sclerosing dacryoadenitis. Ophthalmic Surg 1985; 16:178–181.

WE035                                    **Avery H. Weiss**

**Lacrimal passage ectasia**
*See LACRIMAL SAC FISTULA*
**Lacrimal puncta, absence of**
*See ALACRIMA-APTYALISM*

## LACRIMAL SAC FISTULA                              0565

**Includes:** Lacrimal passage ectasia

**Excludes:**
Lacrimal canaliculus atresia (0563)
Supernumerary puncta and canaliculi

**Major Diagnostic Criteria:** Abnormal opening (fistulous tract) from the lacrimal sac to the skin.

**Clinical Findings:** Lacrimal fistula present as a small opening at the inner canthus through which tears (sometimes purulent) drain. This is caused by an underlying obstruction at the nasolacrimal duct.

**Complications:** Dacryocystitis from the obstruction at the nasolacrimal duct.

**Associated Findings:** None known.

**Etiology:** Unknown.

**Pathogenesis:** Obstruction at the nasolacrimal duct.

**CDC No.:** 743.660

**Sex Ratio:** Presumably M1:F1

**Occurrence:** Undetermined. Somes estimates as high as 1:4,000 live births.

**Risk of Recurrence for Patient's Sib:** Low. Familial cases seldom reported.

**Risk of Recurrence for Patient's Child:** Low. Familial cases seldom reported.

**Age of Detectability:** At birth or during the neonatal period.

**Gene Mapping and Linkage:** Unknown.

**Prevention:** Resolution of the underlying obstruction at the nasolacrimal duct.

**Treatment:** Resolution of the underlying obstruction along with excision of the fistulous tract. Treatment of inflammation, if present.

**Prognosis:** Life span not reduced. Repeated inflammation may occur.

**Detection of Carrier:** Unknown.

**References:**

Masi A: Congenital fistula of the lacrimal sac. Arch Ophthalmol 1969; 81:701.

Kohn R: Textbook of ophthalmic plastic and reconstructive surgery. Philadelphia: Lea & Febiger, 1988:274.

K0025                                        **Roger Kohn**

**Lacrimal system, impatency of the**
*See NASOLACRIMAL DUCT OBSTRUCTION*

## LACRIMO-AURICULO-DENTO-DIGITAL SYNDROME    2180

**Includes:**

> LADD syndrome
> Levy-Hollister Syndrome
> Limb malformations-dento-digital syndrome

**Excludes:** Ectrodactyly-ectodermal dysplasia-clefting syndrome (0337)

**Major Diagnostic Criteria:** Upper limb malformations (most commonly radial defects) are a constant feature. Variable features include lacrimal malformations, small cupped ears, hearing loss, dental anomalies, absent salivary glands, aberrant dermal ridge patterns, and genitourinary anomalies.

**Clinical Findings:** Based on 12 individuals, upper limb malformations were present in 100%. The typical upper limb anomaly was a radial ray defect, with absent or hypoplastic radius and digitalization or hypoplasia of the thumb and second finger. Other upper limb anomalies included shortening of the radius and ulna, **Radial-ulnar synostosis**, triphalangeal thumb, preaxial polydactyly, duplication of the distal phalanx of the thumb, and **Syndactyly** of the second and third fingers, and clinodactyly of the fifth finger.

Although small, simple, cupped pinnae have been noted in 80% of affected patients, only 60% have a hearing loss. The hearing loss was of a mixed conductive and sensorineural nature. Audiometric studies in one family suggested otosclerosis or abnormalities of the ossicular chain. The pinnae were described as having a short helix and an underdeveloped antihelix.

Lacrimal malformations were present in 75% of affected individuals, and included nasolacrimal duct obstruction, hypoplasia or aplasia of the lacrimal puncta, and nasolacrimal duct fistulae.

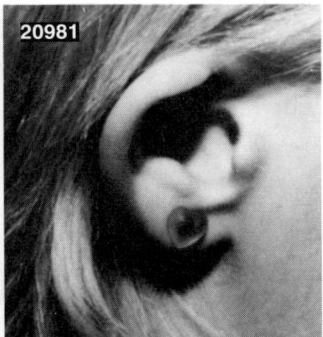

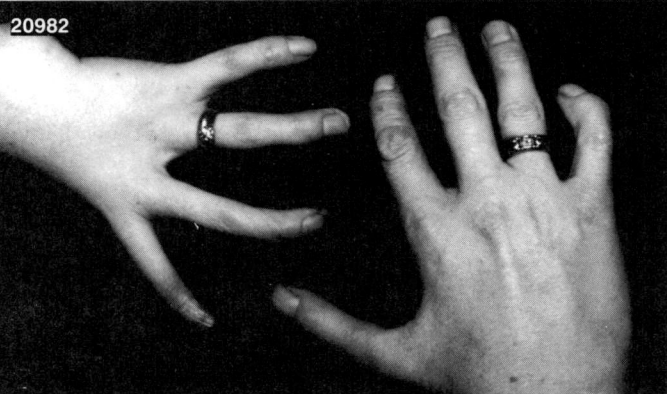

**2180-20980:** Lacrimo-auriculo-digital-dental syndrome; note the nasolacrimal duct fistula. **20981:** Small, cupped pinna. **20982:** Typical upper limb malformations; note the left radial aplasia and the hypoplastic thenar eminence, digitalized thumb, and fifth finger clinodactyly on the right.

Dental anomalies have been documented in 80% of patients and included hypodontia, enamel dysplasia with variations of premolar cusp patterns, peg-shaped maxillary lateral incisors, excessive wear patterns, tooth darkening, and enamel thinning, suggestive of a mild amelogenesis imperfecta-like defect.

Two (20%) of the patients described had unusual dermal ridge patterns with a predominance of low arch patterns. Two individuals previously described have had genitourinary malformations. One had **Renal agenesis, unilateral**, and the other had **Hypospadias** and nephrosclerosis.

**Complications:** Lacrimal malformations cause epiphora, chronic dacryocystitis, conjunctivitis, and keratoconjunctivitis. Renal anomalies may lead to hypertension and/or chronic renal disease.

**Associated Findings:** None known.

**Etiology:** Autosomal dominant inheritance.

**Pathogenesis:** Unknown.

**MIM No.:** *14973

**POS No.:** 3546

**Sex Ratio:** M1:F1

**Occurrence:** About a dozen cases have been described, most from Mexican-American and Caucasian-American populations.

**Risk of Recurrence for Patient's Sib:**
See Part I, *Mendelian Inheritance.*

**Risk of Recurrence for Patient's Child:**
See Part I, *Mendelian Inheritance.*

**Age of Detectability:** In infancy.

**Gene Mapping and Linkage:** Unknown.

**Prevention:** None known. Genetic counseling indicated.

**Treatment:** Ophthalmic surgery may be indicated to correct the lacrimal apparatus malformation and prevent further ophthalmologic complications. Regular dental care is indicated. Hearing aids may be successful in ameliorating the associated mixed hearing loss. Surgical correction of renal anomalies may also be indicated.

**Prognosis:** Normal for life span and intelligence.

**Detection of Carrier:** Unknown.

**Special Considerations:** All of the features of this syndrome have been reported as isolated genetically determined traits inherited in an autosomal dominant fashion. The radial ray defects characteristic of this disorder serve to distinguish it from **Ectrodactyly-ectodermal dysplasia-clefting syndrome**, in which digital anomalies consisting of a split hand and/or foot are found in conjunction with lacrimal, auricular, and dental anomalies.

**References:**

Levy WJ: Mesoectodermal dysplasia: a new combination of anomalies. Am J Ophthalmol 1967; 63:978–982.
Hollister D, et al.: The lacrimo-auriculo-dento-digital syndrome. J Pediatr 1973; 83:438–444. * †
Shiang EL, Holmes LB: The lacrimo-auriculo-dento-digital syndrome. Pediatrics 1977; 59:927–930. * †
Thompson E, et al.: Phenotypic variation in LADD syndrome. J Med Genet 1985; 22:382–385.
Wiedemann H-R, Drescher J: LADD syndrome: report of new cases and review of the clinical spectrum. Eur J Pediatr 1986; 144:579–582.
Kreutz JM, Hoyme HE: The Levy-Hollister syndrome. Pediatrics 1988; 82:96–99.

H0040

**H. Eugene Hoyme**

**Lactase deficiency, adult**
*See LACTASE DEFICIENCY, PRIMARY*

## LACTASE DEFICIENCY, CONGENITAL 0566

**Includes:**
    Alactasia, congenital
    Alactasia, early onset
    Disaccharide intolerance II
    Lactase insufficiency, hereditary

**Excludes:**
    **Glucose-galactose malabsorption** (0419)
    Lactase deficiency, acquired
    **Lactase deficiency, primary** (0567)
    Lactase deficiency, secondary
    **Lactose intolerance** (0569)
    Monosaccharide intolerance
    **Sucrase-isomaltase deficiency** (0920)

**Major Diagnostic Criteria:** Fermentative diarrhea from birth with lactose ingestion, and not with other carbohydrates. Deliberate feeding of measured dose of lactose yields flat serum glucose curve, abdominal discomfort, and explosive stool of pH below 5.0 containing reducing sugars. These findings do not occur on feeding glucose, galactose, or sucrose. If one is certain that the condition is hereditary, these criteria may suffice if the patient's condition precludes peroral biopsy. In all other instances, it is essential to demonstrate normal intestinal histology with decreased or absent lactase activity.

**Clinical Findings:** Symptoms of fermentative diarrhea (100%), and failure to thrive (100%), begin with initial ingestion of lactose (in human or cow's milk) at birth. Infants almost always have abdominal distention, suffer crampy abdominal pain, and vomit sporadically. They usually appear to be very hungry, despite diarrhea, unless the debilitating effects of secondary dehydration, acidosis, and inanition supervene. Diarrhea clears as soon as lactose is removed from the diet.

The stool is fluid and quite frothy from contained gas as it is passed, usually explosively. The pH of fresh stool is always below 5.0 if lactose has been ingested; such stool usually contains reducing sugars that can be identified as one or more of the following: lactose, glucose, and galactose. Lactosuria occurs in about one-third of the patients. Ingestion of a standard dose of lactose (1.5–2.0 g/kg or 45–60 g/m²) after an overnight fast is always associated with a flat 3-hour "tolerance curve" for serum glucose; the test dose almost universally produces clinical discomfort and explosive diarrhea during the 3-hour observation period. Accordingly, the oral loading test should be performed in a diarrhea-free period.

Hydrogen breath analysis, following the oral lactose dose, is a simple alternative. Samples of expired air are obtained before and at 30-minute intervals after administration of the lactose test dose. A rise of hydrogen excretion exceeding 20 parts per million above baseline is considered abnormal and indicates probable lactose malabsorption. Since the hydrogen is elaborated from colonic bacterial activity, false negative tests occur in patients taking oral antibiotics or in infants whose diarrhea stools are so acid that they inhibit hydrogen production by the flora. In many normal newborns, sufficient lactose reaches the colon in undigested form so as to give false positive tests by this method.

Peroral biopsy specimen of the upper small intestinal mucosa is histologically normal, but contains decreased β glycosidase (lactase) activity when compared with the activity of the maltose-, sucrose-, or isomaltose-digesting enzymes, or when assayed in relation to unit weight of tissue, or to protein content of the tissue.

**Complications:** Dehydration, electrolyte, and acid-base disturbance in almost all cases.

**Associated Findings:** Failure to thrive, or death, in all cases if correct diagnosis is not made or if treatment instituted early enough.

**Etiology:** Probably autosomal recessive inheritance.

**Pathogenesis:** Ingested lactose is not hydrolyzed to the component monosaccharides in the upper small intestine as in normal individuals, and therefore passes undigested to the colon. Here the disaccharide is hydrolyzed and fermented, and the resultant mixture contains two and three carbon volatile acids, glucose and galactose, and often some undigested lactose. The increase in osmolarity of the colonic contents induces net flux of water into the lumen. A combination of the irritant effect of excessive fermentation, increased colonic gas, and distension of the bowel walls by the increase in fluid results in explosive passage of the loose stool.

**MIM No.:** *22300

**Sex Ratio:** Presumably M1:F1

**Occurrence:** A relatively common disorder in Finland, with 16 of the approximately 35 patient reported representing 17 years of Finnish experience. Rarer outside of Finland.

**Risk of Recurrence for Patient's Sib:**
    See Part I, *Mendelian Inheritance.*

**Risk of Recurrence for Patient's Child:**
    See Part I, *Mendelian Inheritance.*

**Age of Detectability:** At birth, by lactose loading test and assay of enzymes in intestinal mucosal biopsy specimen.

**Gene Mapping and Linkage:** LCT (lactase) has been provisionally mapped to 2.

**Prevention:** None known. Genetic counseling indicated.

**Treatment:** Avoidance of lactose in the diet. This includes all forms of mammalian milk and milk products. Fluid and electrolyte support may be necessitated during the diarrhea, which results from upsets with lactose ingestion.

**Prognosis:** Current indications are for normal life span if patient is diagnosed and treated early. If not recognized in infancy, patients may die of severe inanition and electrolyte disturbances.

**Detection of Carrier:** Unknown.

**Special Considerations:** The condition must be distinguished from two closely allied conditions. Durant (1958) described, and others also reported, infants with diarrhea on ingestion of lactose. These patients additionally displayed excessive vomiting, lactosemia, lactosuria, other urinary sugars, aminoaciduria, or renal acidosis. Lactase activity was not studied in these patients and the outcomes varied from clearance of the intolerance to lactose to death in infancy (See **Lactose intolerance**). Infants may also develop transitory lactose intolerance in the course of acute diarrhea of presumed infectious origin. These infants also display lactosemia and lactosuria. Although confirmatory biopsy is not available in all cases, it is assumed that the defect in lactose absorption is secondary to temporary mucosal damage and secondary loss of enzyme activity, which returns to normal after a number of weeks or months on a lactose-free diet.

It is generally difficult to differentiate congenital lactase deficiency from secondary defects in the young infant. However, lactosemia, lactosuria, presence of other urinary sugars, histologically abnormal intestinal mucosal specimens, and development of tolerance to lactose after a period of its withdrawal from the diet all point away from the diagnosis of congenital lactase deficiency.

**References:**
Prader A, Auricchio S: Defects of intestinal disaccharide absorption. Annu Rev Med 1965; 16:345.
Davidson M: Disaccharide intolerance. Pediatr Clin North Am 1967; 14:93.
Hozel A: Sugar malabsorption and sugar intolerance in childhood. Proc R Soc Med 1968; 61:1095
Levin B. et al.: Congenital lactose malabsorption. Arch Dis Child 1970; 45:173.
Gray GM: Intestinal disaccharidase deficiencies and glucose-galactose malabsorption. In; Stanbury JB, et al, eds: The metabolic basis of inherited disease, 5th ed. New York: McGraw-Hill, 1983:1729.
Savilahti E, et al.: Congenital lactase deficiency. Arch Dis Child 1983; 58:246–252.
Semeneza G, Auricchio S: Small intestinal disaccharides. In: Scriver CR, et al, eds: The metabolic basis of inherited disease, 6th ed. New York: McGraw-Hill, 1989:2975–2992.

DA017                           **Murray Davidson**

## LACTASE DEFICIENCY, PRIMARY                    0567

**Includes:**
> Alactasia, late-onset
> Disaccharide intolerance III
> Hypoactasia, primary
> Lactase deficiency, adult
> Lactase insufficiency, noncongenital isolated
> Lactose intolerance, adult
> Racial lactase deficiency

**Excludes:**
> Lactase deficiency, acquired
> **Lactase deficiency, congenital** (0566)
> Lactase deficiency, secondary
> **Lactose intolerance** (0569)
> Monosaccharide intolerance
> **Sucrase-isomaltase deficiency** (0920)

**Major Diagnostic Criteria:** Patients must have a history of normal tolerance to mammalian milk in infancy with development of clinical intolerance to lactose-containing foods in later childhood or adult life. The discomfort, bloating, and fermentative diarrhea which occurs with lactose ingestion should be absent with other carbohydrates. Ingestion of a standard dose of lactose (1.5–2.0 g/kg or 45–60 g/m²) is always associated with a flat 3-hour "tolerance curve" for serum glucose; in some reports the clinical discomfort and explosive diarrhea, usually associated with the test among children with congenital lactase deficiency, was not observed at these doses among adults with primary lactase deficiency. However, feeding of 100 gm/m² produces symptoms more uniformly. The loose stools are pH below 5.0, and contain any or all of lactose, glucose and galactose. These findings do not occur on feeding glucose, galactose or sucrose.

Peroral biopsy is necessary to distinguish patients from those with secondary forms of insufficiency. Peroral biopsy specimen of the upper small intestinal mucosa is histologically normal, but it contains decreased β-glycosidase (lactase) activity when compared with the activity of the maltose, sucrose, or isomaltose digesting enzymes, or when assayed in relation to unit weight of tissue or to protein content of the tissue.

**Clinical Findings:** Ingestion of milk or other lactose-containing foods usually causes abdominal bloating, cramping, and sometimes diarrhea. The difficulty is absent in infants and appears in childhood or in adult life. Individuals with primary lactase deficiency are frequently asymptomatic, if it is their normal pattern not to ingest significant quantities of milk and milk products.

The syndrome has been reported from a number of laboratories to occur in Caucasian adults, as an explanation for "milk allergy." In the United States the adult deficiency is reported with increased frequency among Blacks and Orientals.

**Complications:** While dehydration, and electrolyte and acid base disturbances, as well as failure to thrive are theoretically possible in individuals with primary lactase deficiency (similar to those of individuals with congenital lactase deficiency), these are not reported. A combination of larger body size, less dependence on milk as an important dietary constituent, and less total diminution of lactase activity than in patients affected with congenital lactase deficiency may account for the differences in incidence of these complications.

**Associated Findings:** None known.

**Etiology:** Autosomal dominant inheritance. It is not clear if these are distinct infantile and adult lactases, or if lactose tolerance and intolerance represent differences in the regulation of a single locus.

**Pathogenesis:** Reduction in production of this enzyme with aging ultimately reduces lactase activity below a threshold level. From this time on, ingested lactose is not hydrolyzed to the component monosaccharides in the upper small intestine, as in normal individuals, and passes undigested to the colon. In this organ, the disaccharide is hydrolyzed and fermented and the resultant mixture contains two and three carbon volatile acids, glucose and galactose, and often some undigested lactose. The increase in osmolality of the colonic contents induces net flux of water to the lumen. A combination of the irritant effect of the excessive fermentation, increased colonic, gas and distention of the bowel wall by the increase in fluid, results in explosive passage of the loose stool.

**MIM No.:** *22310

**Sex Ratio:** Presumably M1:F1

**Occurrence:** Adult lactase deficiency affects 5–20% of whites and 70–75% of Blacks in North America. Other affected populations include American Indians (83–95%), Chinese (87%), and Thai (97%).

**Risk of Recurrence for Patient's Sib:**
> See Part I, *Mendelian Inheritance.*

**Risk of Recurrence for Patient's Child:**
> See Part I, *Mendelian Inheritance.*

**Age of Detectability:** Whereas lactose intolerance is usually first symptomatic in the teens in North American whites, it may become evident in younger children in other populations, and may appear in the first four years and even in the first six months in Africans. Not all lactase deficient individuals are lactose intolerant, and some classified as heterozygotes may be symptomatic. The condition appears to develop at approximately three years of age in populations in which more than one-half of the adults are affected.

**Gene Mapping and Linkage:** Unknown.

**Prevention:** None known. Genetic counseling indicated.

**Treatment:** Avoidance of lactose in the diet. This includes all forms of mammalian milk and milk products, unless they are pretreated *in vitro* with a commercially available lactase enzyme preparation. Small amounts of milk solids in foods may be tolerated by some patients. Patients and their physicians should be aware of the common use of lactose as the major component of most medicinal pills. Fluid and electrolyte support may be necessitated during the diarrheal activity that results from upsets with lactose ingestion.

**Prognosis:** Excellent for life and freedom from morbidity if lactose is avoided in the diet.

**Detection of Carrier:** Unknown.

**Special Considerations:** Secondary lactase deficiency may be differentiated from the primary defect by four distinguishing criteria: 1) Mucosal biopsy specimens from patients with primary lactase deficiency are normal on histologic examination but are distorted in accordance with the appropriate underlying condition among patients with secondary lactase deficiency. 2) In primary lactase deficiency, reduction of lactase activity in mucosal specimens is isolated, while in secondary deficiencies there is loss of activity of all disaccharidases. With ingestion of lactose, both groups would demonstrate flat serum glucose curves and GI intolerance. 3) However, lactosemia, lactosuria and presence of other urinary sugars are reported only with secondary deficiencies. 4) Development of tolerance to lactose after a period of its withdrawal from the diet, or after treatment for an underlying malabsorptive condition, precludes the diagnosis of primary lactase deficiency.

**References:**
Bayless TM, Rosensweig NS: A racial difference in incidence of lactase deficiency: a survey of milk intolerance and lactase deficiency in healthy adult males. J.A.M.A. 1966; 197:968–972.
Dahlqvist A, Lindquist B: Lactose intolerance and protein malnutrition. Acta Paediatr Scand 1971; 60:488.
Kretchmer N: Lactose and lactase: a historical perspective. Gastroenterology 1971; 61:805–813.
Ransome-Kuti O, et al.: A genetic study of lactose digestion in Nigerian families. Gastroenterology 1975; 68:431.
Welsh JD, et al.: Intestinal disaccharidase activities in relation to age, race, and mucosal damage. Gastroenterology 1978; 75:847.
Simoons FJ: Age of onset of lactose malabsorption. Pediatrics 1980; 66:646.
Ho MW, et al.: Lactase polymorphism in adult British natives. Am J Hum Genet 1982; 34:650–657.

Potter J, et al.: Human lactase and the molecular basis of lactase persistence. Biochem Genet 1985; 23:423–439.

DA017                                            **Murray Davidson**

**Lactase insufficiency, hereditary**
*See LACTASE DEFICIENCY, CONGENITAL*
**Lactase insufficiency, noncongenital isolated**
*See LACTASE DEFICIENCY, PRIMARY*
**Lactate dehydrogenase - A**
*See LACTATE DEHYDROGENASE ISOZYMES*
**Lactate dehydrogenase - B**
*See LACTATE DEHYDROGENASE ISOZYMES*
**Lactate dehydrogenase - C**
*See LACTATE DEHYDROGENASE ISOZYMES*
**Lactate dehydrogenase - K**
*See LACTATE DEHYDROGENASE ISOZYMES*

## LACTATE DEHYDROGENASE ISOZYMES                    0568

**Includes:**
   Lactate dehydrogenase - A
   Lactate dehydrogenase - B
   Lactate dehydrogenase - C
   Lactate dehydrogenase - K
   Nicotinamide adenine dinucleotide and oxidoreductase

**Excludes:** N/A

**Major Diagnostic Criteria:** Electrophoretic techniques are available for determining the isozyme composition of tissues and body fluids. In normal serum, lactate dehydrogenase (LDH) isozymes are present in the following proportions: LDH-2 > LDH-1 > LDH-3 > LDH-4 > LDH-5. A variety of diseases exhibit unique changes in serum isozyme patterns. LDH-1 is markedly increased in myocardial infarction, and LDH-5 in infectious hepatitis.

**Clinical Findings:** Abnormal elevation or depression of lactate dehydrogenase isozymes are associated with certain disease states but are not proven causes. Lactate dehydrogenase (LDH) is an enzyme of the Embden-Myerhoff pathway, which catalyzes the interconversion of pyruvate and lactate. Nicotinamide adenine dinucleotide (NAD) is a specific cofactor, NAD being formed during the reduction of pyruvate and reduced nicotinamide adenine dinucleotide (NADH) during the oxidation of lactate.

LDH exists in multiple molecular forms (isozymes) in the somatic and gametic tissues of many mammalian and avian species. Five molecular forms of LDH are present in human somatic tissues: LDH-1, LDH-2, LDH-3, LDH-4, and LDH-5. The type and amount of the molecular forms vary for each tissue. In adult human heart and kidney, the major forms are LDH-1, LDH-2 and LDH-3, whereas in adult human muscle and liver the dominant form is LDH-5. Multiple forms of LDH may exist in single cells. Thus hemolysates of thoroughly washed erythrocytes exhibit three isozymes, LDH-1, LDH-2, and LDH-3. A 6th isozymic form of LDH (LDH-X) appears in testis at the time of puberty. LDH-X is the predominant form of LDH in sperm.

The relative distribution of isozymes in each human tissue changes during development. In heart, for example, the pattern exhibited by adults is not attained until 3 years of age. In testis, the adult complement of isozymes appears at the time of puberty. Thus each tissue exhibits a unique profile of isozyme development.

A variety of diseases exhibit unique changes in serum isozyme patterns. LDH-1 is markedly increased in myocardial infarction, and LDH-5 in infectious hepatitis. Analysis of tissue isozyme patterns may also have diagnostic application. In chickens and humans a form of muscular dystrophy is associated with a failure of development of the adult isozyme pattern. Whether this abnormality is a primary or secondary event is unknown. These findings suggest that isozymic analyses may be helpful in determining at what period of development a metabolic abnormality occurs.

**Complications:** Unknown.

**Associated Findings:** A disturbed LDH pattern may indicate one of a variety of diseases e.g. myocardial infarction, infectious hepatitis, hemolytic disorders, meningitis and **Muscular dystrophy**.

**Etiology:** Autosomal dominant inheritance of isozymes. Discovery of polypeptide A and B variants in human and animal tissues, together with appropriate genetic studies, showed that the synthesis of A and B polypeptides is controlled by two separate nonallelic genes. Observations on pigeon testes have shown that the synthesis of the LDH-X subunit (C) is controlled by a 3rd genetic locus in the pigeon. The total complement of LDH isozymes can be explained on the basis of the activity of genes at three loci, A, B, and C, each being responsible for the synthesis of a corresponding polypeptide. The C locus, in contrast to the other loci, is not activated until pubescence in the male and remains inactive in the female.

**Pathogenesis:** Unknown.

**MIM No.:** *15000, *15010, *15015, 15016

**Sex Ratio:** For LDH-1, -2, -3, -4 and -5: M1:F1; for LDH-X: M1:F0

**Occurrence:** Each isozyme normally present at proper age and in appropriate tissue.

**Risk of Recurrence for Patient's Sib:**
   See Part I, *Mendelian Inheritance.*

**Risk of Recurrence for Patient's Child:**
   See Part I, *Mendelian Inheritance.*

**Age of Detectability:** Adult isozyme pattern in heart at age three, and LDH-X in testis at puberty.

**Gene Mapping and Linkage:** LDHA (lactate dehydrogenase A) has been mapped to 11p15.1-p14.
   LDHB (lactate dehydrogenase B) has been mapped to 12p12.2-p12.1.
   LDHC (lactate dehydrogenase C) has been provisionally mapped to 11.

**Prevention:** Not applicable.

**Treatment:** Not applicable.

**Prognosis:** Normal life span.

**Detection of Carrier:** Electrophoresis can determine LDH isozyme pattern.

**Special Considerations:** Molecular forms of lactate dehydrogenase (LDH) in heart and kidney are to a large extent different from those in muscle and liver. Each tissue exhibits characteristic changes of the isozyme patterns during development, and in at least one tissue, the testis, an entirely new isozyme appears at the time of puberty. Isozymic analysis of tissues and body fluids may aid in diagnosing certain diseases - myocardial infarction, infectious hepatitis, hemolytic disorders, meningitis, etc. Also further studies on the molecular heterogeneity of LDH, as well as other enzymes, will increase our understanding of the biochemical processes that accompany growth and development.

**References:**
Wroblewski F, Gregory KK: Lactic dehydrogenase isozymes and their distribution in normal tissues and plasma and in disease states. Ann NY Acad Sci 1961; 94:912–921.
Zinkham WH: Lactate dehydrogenase isozymes of testis and sperm: biological and biochemical properties and genetic control. Ann NY Acad Sci 1968; 151:598–609.
Mayeda K, et al.: Localization of the human lactate dehydrogenase B gene on the short arm of chromosome 12. Am J Hum Genet 1974; 26:59–64.
Francke U, Busby N: Assignments of the human genes for lactate dehydrogenase-A and thymidine kinase to specific chromosomal regions. Cytogenet Cell Genet 1975; 14:313–319.
Markert CH, et al.: Evolution of a gene. Science 1975; 189:102–114.
Anderson GR, Kovacik WP Jr: LDH (k), an unusual oxygen-sensitive lactate dehydrogenase expressed in human cancer. Proc Natl Acad Sci 1981; 78:3209–3213.
Benz C, et al.: Lactic dehydrogenase isozymes, 31P magnestic resonance spectroscopy, and in vitro antimitochondrial tumor toxicity with gossypol and rhodamine 123. J Clin Invest 1987; 79:517–523.

ZI000                                         **William H. Zinkham**

**Lactate dehydrogenase, M isozyme**
*See GLYCOGENOSES*
**Lactate transporter**
*See GLYCOGENOSES*
**Lactate transporter defect, myopathy due to**
*See ERYTHROCYTE, LACTATE TRANSPORTER DEFECT*
**Lactate transporter deficiency**
*See ERYTHROCYTE, LACTATE TRANSPORTER DEFECT*
**Lactate transporter myopathy, metabolic**
*See ERYTHROCYTE, LACTATE TRANSPORTER DEFECT*
**Lactic acidemia without hypoxemia**
*See PYRUVATE CARBOXYLASE DEFICIENCY WITH LACTIC
ACIDEMIA*
**Lactic acidosis**
*See MYOPATHY, MITOCHONDRIAL-ENCEPHALOPATHY-LACTIC
ACIDOSIS-STROKE*
**Lactic and pyruvic acidemia with carbohydrate sensitivity**
*See PYRUVATE DEHYDROGENASE DEFICIENCY*
**Lactic and pyruvic acidemia with episodic ataxia and weakness**
*See PYRUVATE DEHYDROGENASE DEFICIENCY*

---

## LACTOSE INTOLERANCE                                    0569

**Includes:**
> Gastrogen lactose intolerance
> Lactose intolerance with lactosuria, congenital
> Lactosuria, idiopathic

**Excludes:**
> Disaccharidase deficiency syndromes due to celiac disease
> **Lactase deficiency, congenital** (0566)
> Monosaccharide malabsorption
> Protein malnutrition (kwashiorkor)
> **Sucrase-isomaltase deficiency** (0920)

**Major Diagnostic Criteria:** Vomiting, failure to thrive, lactosuria, sucrosuria, and aminoaciduria. Lactose tolerance test results in a normal increase in blood glucose, but severe lactosuria appears. A normal glucose response to sucrose loading with sucrosuria is also seen.

In contrast, nolactosuria and sucrosuria occur when the lactose or the sucrose are given intraduodenally. Intestinal lactase and sucrase are normal.

Small intestinal biopsy shows a villous mucosa with slightly reduced height or a normal mucosa. Light and electron-microscopy of gastric mucosa from the fundus and corpus region are apparently normal. The morphology of the antral mucosa has not been studied. Lactose and sucrose are not normally found in the blood, and their presence may have toxic effects.

**Clinical Findings:** The disorder manifests soon after birth. Affected infants are characteristically critically ill, with vomiting and failure to thrive; diarrhea is uncommon. Dehydration develops quickly. Disacchariduria, aminoaciduria, and tubular acidosis indicate renal damage. Lactosuria is the most striking feature and can be profuse as long as milk intake persists. Pronounced sucrosuria may be also present on a diet rich in sucrose. The lactose and sucrose concentrations in urine are occasionally up to 100 times greater than normally found at this age.

The infant's general condition deteriorates rapidly and may be fatal unless lactose intake is curtailed. On a lactose-free diet, lactose intolerance disappears at 6 to 18 months after onset. Reintroduction of lactose in the diet before this period can be fatal.

**Complications:** Malnutrition; liver damage with bleeding tendency and renal damage are probably secondary phenomena caused by the disaccharides. Lactose malabsorption due to lactase deficiency can develop later in childhood.

**Associated Findings:** Pyloric stenosis and cataracts have been present in some infants.

**Etiology:** The cause of severe lactose intolerance is unknown. Familial incidence and consanguinity among the parents of the patients suggest a hereditary factor.

**Pathogenesis:** A gastrogenic origin of the disorder, with abnormal absorption of disaccharide likely; lactose passes through an abnormally permeable gastric mucosa and leading to lactosuria and sucrosuria. The gastric defect appears to be temporary.

**MIM No.:** 15022

**Sex Ratio:** M1:F1

**Occurrence:** More than 20 cases documented in the literature.

**Risk of Recurrence for Patient's Sib:** Unknown.

**Risk of Recurrence for Patient's Child:** Unknown.

**Age of Detectability:** First month of life.

**Gene Mapping and Linkage:** Unknown.

**Prevention:** None known. Genetic counseling indicated.

**Treatment:** In the acute phase, use of a formula free from disaccharides, or intraduodenal feeding with a disaccharide containing formula. Supportive measures such as intravenous fluid and electrolyte replacement are needed in infants with severe dehydration.

**Prognosis:** Timely removal of lactose from the feeding formula will assure recovery. Diet is well tolerated.

**Detection of Carrier:** Unknown.

**References:**
Durand P: Lattosuria idiopatica in una paziente con diarrea cronica ed acidosi. Minerva Pediatrica 1958; 10:706–711.
Durand P, et al.: Disorders due to intestinal defective carbohydrate digestion and absorption. New York: Grune and Stratton, 1964.
Russo G, et al.: Congenital lactose intolerance of gastrogen origin associated with cataracts. Acta Paediatr Scand 1974; 63:457–460.
Berg NO, et al.: A boy with severe infantile gastrogen lactose intolerance and acquired lactase deficiency. Acta Paediatr Scand 1979; 68:751–758.
Hirashima Y, et al.: Lactose intolerance associated with cataracts. Eur J Pediat 1979; 130:41–45.
Hoskova A, et al.: Severe lactose intolerance with lactosuria and vomiting. Arch Dis Child 1980; 55:304–316.

DU010                                                **Paolo Durand**

**Lactose intolerance with lactosuria, congenital**
*See LACTOSE INTOLERANCE*
**Lactose intolerance, adult**
*See LACTASE DEFICIENCY, PRIMARY*
**Lactosuria, idiopathic**
*See LACTOSE INTOLERANCE*
**LADD syndrome**
*See LACRIMO-AURICULO-DENTO-DIGITAL SYNDROME*
**Lafora body disease**
*See SEIZURES, PROGRESSIVE MYOCLONIC, LAFORA TYPE*
**Lafora disease**
*See SEIZURES, PROGRESSIVE MYOCLONIC, LAFORA TYPE*
**Lakuregebee**
*See ANEMIA, SICKLE CELL*
**LAMB syndrome**
*See NEVI-ATRIAL MYXOMA-MYXOID NEUROFIBROMAS-EPHELIDES*
**Lambdoid suture closure, premature**
*See CRANIOSYNOSTOSIS*
**Lambert type ichthyosis**
*See NEVUS, EPIDERMAL NEVUS SYNDROME*
**Lamellar cataract**
*See CATARACT, AUTOSOMAL DOMINANT CONGENITAL*
**Lamellar exfoliation of the newborn**
*See ICHTHYOSIS*
*also ICHTHYOSIS, LAMELLAR RECESSIVE*
*also ICHTHYOSIS, CONGENITAL ERYTHRODERMIC*
**Lamellar ichthyosis, autosomal dominant form**
*See ICHTHYOSIS, LAMELLAR DOMINANT*
**Lamellar ichthyosis, classical**
*See ICHTHYOSIS, LAMELLAR RECESSIVE*
**Lamellar ichthyosis, nonbullous congenital**
*See ICHTHYOSIS, LAMELLAR DOMINANT*
**Landouzy-Dejerine muscular dystrophy**
*See MUSCULAR DYSTROPHY, FACIO-SCAPULO-HUMERAL*
**Lane disease**
*See SKIN, PALMO-PLANTAR ERYTHEMA*
**Lange-Nielsen syndrome**
*See CARDIO-AUDITORY SYNDROME*
**Langer type mesomelic dwarfism**
*See MESOMELIC DYSPLASIA, LANGER TYPE*

**Langer-Giedion syndrome**
   See *TRICHO-RHINO-PHALANGEAL SYNDROME, TYPE II*
**Langer-Saldino achondrogenesis**
   See *ACHONDROGENESIS, LANGER-SALDINO TYPE*
**Language-induced epilepsy**
   See *EPILEPSY, REFLEX*
**Laron pituitary dwarfism**
   See *DWARFISM, LARON*

## LARSEN SYNDROME                                            0570

**Includes:**
   Desbuquois syndrome
   Joint dislocations-unusual facies-skeletal abnormalities
   Skeletal anomalies-joint dislocations-unusual facies

**Excludes:**
   **Arthrogryposes** (0088)
   **Larsen syndrome, lethal type** (2800)

**Major Diagnostic Criteria:** Flat facies with depressed nasal bridge, wide-spaced eyes, and prominent forehead; dislocations of multiple major joints and cylindrical, nontapering fingers with multiple carpal ossification centers.

**Clinical Findings:** Congenital joint dislocations, usually bilateral, involving the elbows, hips, and knees (typically anterior dislocation of the tibia or the femur); subluxation of the shoulders; cylindrical fingers; broad, spatulate thumbs; short metacarpals; a juxtacalcaneal accessory ossification center, short nails; equinovarus or valgus feet; unusual facies characterized by a prominent or bossed forehead, flat and depressed nasal bridge and wide-set eyes. Most affected individuals are mentally normal.

**Complications:** In early infancy decreased rigidity of the cartilage of the rib cage, epiglottis, arytenoid, and possibly trachea may cause respiratory difficulties.

**Associated Findings:** Congenital heart disease, cleft palate without cleft lip, **Hydrocephaly**, and abnormal spinal segmentation.

**Etiology:** Genetic heterogeneity is present, with both autosomal dominant and autosomal recessive inheritance reported. Differentiation between the two forms may be difficult, but the recessive form is generally more severe.

**Pathogenesis:** Undetermined. May be related to mesenchymal connective tissue.

**MIM No.:** *15025, *24560, 22188
**POS No.:** 3275
**CDC No.:** 755.810
**Sex Ratio:** M1:F1
**Occurrence:** Undetermined but presumed rare. Established literature.

**Risk of Recurrence for Patient's Sib:**
   See Part I, *Mendelian Inheritance.*

**Risk of Recurrence for Patient's Child:**
   See Part I, *Mendelian Inheritance.*

**Age of Detectability:** Usually at birth by physical examination, but mild cases may not be noticed until adulthood.

**Gene Mapping and Linkage:** Unknown.

**Prevention:** None known. Genetic counseling indicated.

**Treatment:** Early, intensive and continued orthopedic care.

**Prognosis:** Physically handicapped to a variable degree, depending on nature and extent of patient's condition and results of orthopedic surgery.

**Detection of Carrier:** Unknown.

**Special Considerations:** Cases of Larsen syndrome have been reported under other names, primarily centering on the striking knee deformities: genu recurvatum; congenital hyperextension and subluxation of the knee. *Desbuquois syndrome* is a possible variant in which supernumerary carpal ossification centers cause deviation of the fingers. This is discernible only during the first year or so of life, along with coronal clefts of the vertebrae (Beighton et al, 1988),

**References:**

Larsen LJ, et al.: Multiple congenital dislocations associated with characteristic facial abnormality. J Pediatr 1950; 37:574–581.
Latta RJ, et al.: Larsen's syndrome: a skeletal dysplasia with multiple joint dislocations and unusual facies. J Pediatr 1971; 78:291–298.
Steel HH, Kohl H: Multiple congenital dislocations associated with other skeletal anomalies (Larsen's syndrome) in three siblings. J Bone Joint Surg 1972; 54A:75–82.
Gorlin RJ, et al.: Syndromes of the head and neck. New York: McGraw-Hill, 1976.
de Nazar MM: Larsen's syndrome: Clinical and genetic aspects. J Genet Hum 1980; 28:83–88.
Houston CS, et al.: Separating Larsen's syndrome from the 'arthrogryposis basket'. J Canad Assoc Radiol 1981; 32:206–214.
Tsang MCK, et al.: Oral and craniofacial morphology of a patient with Larsen syndrome. J Craniofac Genet Dev Biol 1986; 6:357–362.
Beighton P, et al.: International nosology of heritable disorders of connective tissue, Berlin, 1986. Am J Med Genet 1988; 29:581–594.

MY001                                          **Terry L. Myers**

## LARSEN SYNDROME, LETHAL TYPE                              2800

**Includes:**
   Joint dislocations, multiple, lethal, Larsen-like
   Lethal, Larsen-like, multiple joint dislocations

**Excludes:** **Larsen syndrome** (0570)

**Major Diagnostic Criteria:** Multiple congenital dislocations of joints, severe short stature, cleft soft palate, skeletal abnormalities, abnormal dermal collagen bundles, pulmonary insufficiency due to laryngotracheomalacia and lung hypoplasia, and early death. X-rays confirm clinical impressions of joint dislocations and skeletal abnormalities. Histochemical and electron microscopy show abnormalities of cartilage matrix, collagen bundles of joint capsules, and hyaline cartilage of the trachea.

**Clinical Findings:** At birth, body length is short. A poor cry, severe hypotonia, and respiratory metabolic acidosis are present shortly after birth. Pulmonary insufficiency rapidly ensues due to laryngotracheomalacia and lung hypoplasia, leading to early death.

   Congenital dislocations may involve shoulders, hips, knees, ankles, elbows, and wrists. X-rays confirm the multiple dislocations and may, in addition, reveal hypoplasia of the fibulae and of the distal ends of the humeri, cervical kyphosis, coronal clefts of the lower lumbar vertebrae, small proximal tarsal bones, and talipes equinovarus. Rhizomelic shortening of the upper limbs may be present.

   Craniofacial features include a prominent forehead, large posterior fontanelle, flat nasal bridge, **Eye, hypertelorism**, cleft of soft

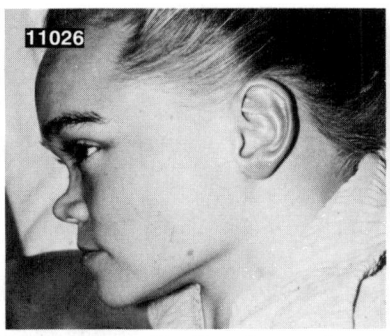
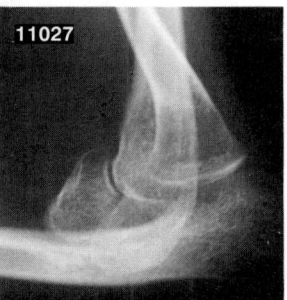

**0570-11026:** Profile shows depressed nasal bridge. **11027:** Lateral view of right elbow shows joint dislocation, underdeveloped bones and accessory ulnar ossicle.

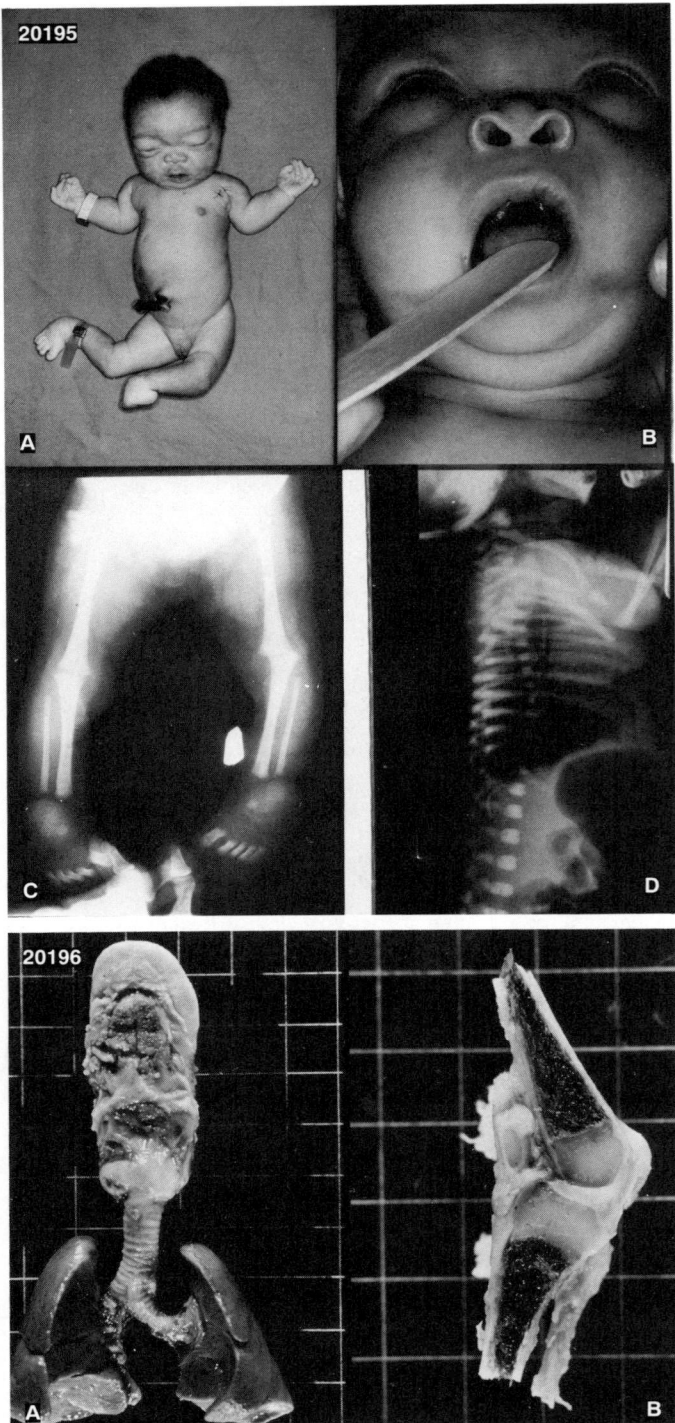

**2800-20195:** A) Gross view of a patient with Larsen syndrome, lethal type II. B) Close-up view of facial appearance and cleft palate. C) PA view of lower extremities, showing small proximal tarsal bones and hypoplasia of the fibulae. D) Lateral X-ray of lumbar spine showing coronal clefts of the lower lumbar vertebrae. **20196:** A) Gross view of the respiratory tract showing collapsed and soft trachea and hypoplastic lungs. B) Lateral view of the cross section of the knee showing thin fibrous ligament supporting the posterior aspect of the knee joint.

palate, small mouth, and low-set ears. In addition, short neck may be present due to an excess of subcutaneous tissue.

Dense, mature collagen bundles may be strikingly deficient, especially in the flexor aspects of the tendon sheath at the knees and shoulders. Dermal connective tissue, the matrix of tracheal and articular hyaline cartilages, and joint capsules may have abnormal histochemical properties; the dermal collagen bundles may appear broad and smudgy. Electron microscopic study may reveal loss of uniformity in the size of collagen fibers due to the presence of many small fibers in the hyaline cartilage of the trachea.

**Complications:** Pulmonary insufficiency due to laryngotracheomalacia and pulmonary hypoplasia is the main cause of death. Spinal instability due to vertebral anomalies may also be a cause of death.

**Associated Findings:** Signs and symptoms secondary to collagen dysmaturity.

**Etiology:** Probably autosomal recessive inheritance. Two reported cases have been sporadic with no family history.

**Pathogenesis:** Abnormal histochemical properties and morphologic findings of connective tissue fibers strongly suggest a disorder of connective tissue, possibly dysmaturity of collagen fibers with a predilection to joint capsules, tracheal cartilage, and possibly nasal cartilage. A striking deficiency of dense mature collagen bundles, especially in the flexor aspects of the tendon sheath at the knees and shoulders may be responsible for anterior dislocation of the tibia at the knee and lateral dislocation of the shoulder.

The significance of the decreased lysyl hydroxylase activity of cultured fibroblasts is unknown. However, the values are not in the range of lysyl hydroxylase deficiency that is seen in the type VI (ocular) **Ehlers-Danlos syndrome.**

**MIM No.:** 24565

**POS No.:** 3372

**CDC No.:** 755.810

**Sex Ratio:** Presumably M1:F1 (M0:F3 observed).

**Occurrence:** Three isolated females have been documented.

**Risk of Recurrence for Patient's Sib:**
See Part I, *Mendelian Inheritance.*

**Risk of Recurrence for Patient's Child:**
See Part I, *Mendelian Inheritance.*

**Age of Detectability:** At birth.

**Gene Mapping and Linkage:** Unknown.

**Prevention:** None known. Genetic counseling indicated.

**Treatment:** Symptomatic treatment for respiratory failure.

**Prognosis:** Death due to pulmonary insufficiency.

**Detection of Carrier:** Unknown.

**References:**
Chen H, et al.: A lethal, Larsen-like multiple joint dislocation syndrome. Am J Med Genet 1982; 13:149–161. †
Clayton-Smith J, Donnai D: A further patient with the lethal type of Larsen syndrome. J Med Genet 1988; 25:499–500.

CH015                                 **Harold Chen**

**Laryngeal abductor paralysis**
*See VOCAL CORD PARALYSIS*

## LARYNGEAL ABDUCTOR PARALYSIS-MENTAL RETARDATION 3045

**Includes:**
>  Plott syndrome
>  Vocal cord dysfunction, familial

**Excludes:** X-linked mental retardation (other)

**Major Diagnostic Criteria:** Inspiratory stridor due to laryngeal abductor paralysis is necessary to make the diagnosis.

**Clinical Findings:** All affected individuals have had inspiratory stridor from birth, with cyanosis occasionally occurring in the neonatal period. Subsequent growth and development are slow, with mental retardation being a constant finding. The facial expression is described as "blank," but with normal facial movement. Speech and swallowing difficulties also occur, suggesting involvment of ninth, tenth, and twelfth cranial nerves. The less severely affected individuals are described as clumsy, whereas the more severely affected individuals have hypotonia, severe cyanosis, and death.

**Complications:** Unknown.

**Associated Findings:** One boy also had optic atrophy and nystagmus.

**Etiology:** Presumably X-linked recessive inheritance.

**Pathogenesis:** Unknown. The cause of the laryngeal abductor defect is thought to be an abnormality of nucleus ambiguus function. However, the gene also apparently affects the brain in that retardation is also one of the findings.

**MIM No.:** 30885

**POS No.:** 4008

**Sex Ratio:** M7:F0 (observed).

**Occurrence:** Two families, both from North America, have been reported in detail.

**Risk of Recurrence for Patient's Sib:**
>  See Part I, *Mendelian Inheritance.*

**Risk of Recurrence for Patient's Child:**
>  See Part I, *Mendelian Inheritance.*

**Age of Detectability:** At birth, by inspiratory stridor.

**Gene Mapping and Linkage:** Unknown.

**Prevention:** None known. Genetic counseling indicated.

**Treatment:** Tracheostomy may be indicated.

**Prognosis:** Death occurred in the neonatal period in two individuals; mental retardation was present in all survivors, with measured IQs of 56–73.

**Detection of Carrier:** Unknown.

**References:**
Plott D: Congenital laryngeal-abductor paralysis due to nucleus ambiguus dysgenesis in three brothers. New Engl J Med 1964; 271:593–597.
Watters GV, Fitch N: Familial laryngeal abductor paralysis and psychomotor retardation. Clin Genet 1973; 4:429–433.

T0007            **Helga V. Toriello**

**Laryngeal aerocele**
*See LARYNGOCELE*
**Laryngeal and skeletal anomalies-motor and sensory neuropathy**
*See NEUROPATHY, CONGENITAL MOTOR & SENSORY-SKELETAL-LARYNGEAL DEFECTS*
**Laryngeal atresia, congenital**
*See LARYNX, ATRESIA*
**Laryngeal chondromalacia, congenital**
*See LARYNGOMALACIA*
**Laryngeal hernia**
*See LARYNGOCELE*
**Laryngeal mucocele**
*See LARYNGOCELE*
**Laryngeal papillomatosis, juvenile**
*See PAPILLOMA VIRUS, CONGENITAL INFECTION*

## LARYNGEAL PARALYSIS 3080

**Includes:**
>  Abductor vocal cord paralysis
>  Adductor vocal cord paralysis
>  Gerhardt syndrome
>  Plott syndrome
>  Vocal cord dysfunction

**Excludes:** Laryngeal abductor paralysis-mental retardation (3045)

**Major Diagnostic Criteria:** Laryngoscopy reveals bilateral adductor or abductor vocal cord paralysis, either partial or complete.

**Clinical Findings:** Hoarseness, usually since birth; however, it may develop later in life. The severity of hoarseness may be progressive throughout life. Laryngoscopy reveals bilateral adductor or abductor vocal cord paralysis, either partial or complete. Aspiration is not significant due to intact afferent laryngeal innervation.

**Complications:** Unknown.

**Associated Findings:** None known.

**Etiology:** Usually autosomal dominant inheritance, although X-linked recessive forms have been reported.

**Pathogenesis:** Unknown. No postmortem examinations have been performed on affected individuals. The cause of paralysis is probably neuronal, but may be due to a muscular abnormality of the adductor muscle itself (Mace et al., 1978).

**MIM No.:** *15026, *15027, 30885

**Sex Ratio:** Presumably M1:F1, but a male preponderance has been observed.

**Occurrence:** Some seven kinships have been reported.

**Risk of Recurrence for Patient's Sib:**
>  See Part I, *Mendelian Inheritance.*

**Risk of Recurrence for Patient's Child:**
>  See Part I, *Mendelian Inheritance.*

**Age of Detectability:** At birth, or when speech problems become apparent.

**Gene Mapping and Linkage:** Unknown.

**Prevention:** None known. Genetic counseling indicated.

**Treatment:** If aspiration becomes a problem, vocal cord medialization may be indicated.

**Prognosis:** Normal life span.

**Detection of Carrier:** Unknown.

**Special Considerations:** *Gerhardt syndrome* refers to an autosomal dominant form of laryngeal abductor paralysis, while *Plott syndrome* is an X-linked form of laryngeal abductor paralysis.

**References:**
Mace M, et al.: Autosomal dominantly inherited adductor laryngeal paralysis-a new syndrome with a suggestion of linkage to HLA. Clin Genet 1978; 14:265–270.
Morelli G, et al.: Familial laryngeal abductor paralysis with presumed autosomal dominant inheritance. Ann Otol Rhinol Laryngol 1982; 91:323–324.
Cunningham MJ, et al.: Familial vocal cord dysfunction. Pediatrics 1985; 76:750–753.

WI061           **Brian Wiatrak**
MY003           **Charles M. Myer III**

**Laryngeal pouch**
*See LARYNGOCELE*
**Laryngeal pyocele**
*See LARYNGOCELE*
**Laryngeal retention cyst**
*See EPIGLOTTIS, VALLECULAR CYST*
**Laryngeal stridor, congenital**
*See LARYNGOMALACIA*
**Laryngeal ventricle prolapse**
*See LARYNX, VENTRICLE PROLAPSE*

## LARYNGO-TRACHEO-ESOPHAGEAL CLEFT 0577

**Includes:**
Cleft larynx
Esophagotrachea, persistent
Larynx and trachea, congenital posterior cleft of
Tracheo-laryngo-esophageal cleft

**Excludes:** Tracheoesophageal fistula (0960)

**Major Diagnostic Criteria:** Direct endoscopic visualization of a congenital posterior cleft of the larynx and trachea with persistent esophagotrachea.

**Clinical Findings:** Symptoms depend on the size of the defect in the posterior laryngeal and tracheal wall. The most common finding is respiratory embarrassment with feeding; this includes cyanosis, choking, and aspiration. Additionally, abnormal voice, increased oral secretions, and stridor, predominantly expiratory due to aspirated oral secretions, are noted.

**Complications:** Repeated episodes of aspiration pneumonia and respiratory distress. Poor feeding results in nutritional deficiency and growth failure.

**Associated Findings:** Increased incidence of esophageal abnormalities, including atresia and various tracheoesophageal fistulas. Higher incidence of other tracheobronchial abnormalities.

**Etiology:** Unknown.

**Pathogenesis:** An arrest in the rostral advancement of the tracheoesophageal septum, which then prevents the dorsal fusion of the cricoid cartilages.

**POS No.:** 4341

**CDC No.:** 748.385, 748.390

**Sex Ratio:** M1:F1

**Occurrence:** Approximately 150 cases have been reported. However, four clefts were found in a series of 2,000 consecutive autopsies at a pediatric hospital.

**Risk of Recurrence for Patient's Sib:** Two instances of affected sibs have been reported.

**Risk of Recurrence for Patient's Child:** Unknown.

**Age of Detectability:** At birth.

**Gene Mapping and Linkage:** Unknown.

**Prevention:** None known. Genetic counseling indicated.

**Treatment:** Gastrostomy, tracheostomy, and surgical closure of defect have been successful when the lesion is limited to the cervical region.

**Prognosis:** Normal life span, intelligence, and function if surgical repair is successful.

**Detection of Carrier:** Unknown.

**References:**
Blumberg JB, et al.: Laryngotracheoesophageal cleft, the embryologic implications: review of the literature. Surgery 1965; 57:559–566.
Delahunty JE, Cherry J: Congenital laryngeal cleft. Ann Otol Rhinol Laryngol 1969; 78:96.
Imbrie JD, Doyle PJ: Laryngotracheoesophageal cleft: report of a case and review of the literature. Laryngoscope 1969; 79:1252–1274.
Cohen SR: Cleft larynx: a report of seven cases. Ann Otol 1975; 84:747–756.
Cotton RT, Schreiber JT: Management of laryngotracheoesophageal cleft. Ann Otol Rhinol Laryngol 1981; 90:401–405.

**R. Kirk Jackson**

## LARYNGOCELE 0575

**Includes:**
Diverticulum of larynx
Laryngeal aerocele
Laryngeal hernia
Laryngeal mucocele
Laryngeal pouch
Laryngeal pyocele
Laryngoceles: internal, external or combined
Ventricular cyst of larynx

**Excludes:**
Larynx, cysts (0572)
Larynx, ventricle prolapse (0573)

**Major Diagnostic Criteria:** A ventricular cystic mass or neck mass over the thyrohyoid membrane is the major clinical finding. Direct visualization by endoscopy establishes the diagnosis and rules out the possibility of a coexistent disease.

**Clinical Findings:** A cyst-like mass is present in the neck and laryngeal ventricle. The external component may enlarge with straining but decrease with rest; it may collapse with gentle pressure. This lesion arises as a saccular dilatation of the saccus or

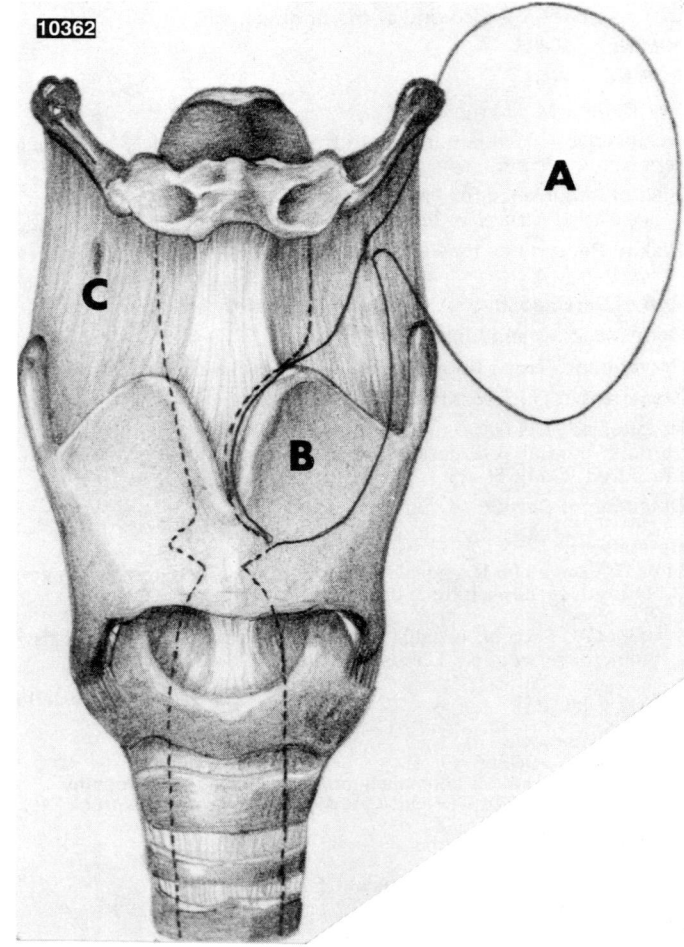

**0575-10362:** Laryngocele within larynx. External component (A) is connected with internal component (B) through thyrohyoid membrane at perforation of neurovascular bundle (C).

appendix of the laryngeal ventricle or the sinus of Morgagni. Herniation of mucosa occurs upward from the ventricle and lateral to the false vocal cord. This cystic mass remains within the interior of the larynx or passes through the thyrohyoid membrane at the perforation site of the neurovascular bundle (superior laryngeal nerve and vessels). Laryngoceles are subsequently classified by location as internal, external, or combined. Their classification by content is aerocele, pyocele, or mucocele.

The laryngeal appendix is larger in Caucasians than in other racial groups. In other primates it may extend into the neck, across the chest, and into the axilla. In the orangutan, a structure similar to a laryngocele is thought to be an air reservoir for use during climbing and phonation.

The clinical symptoms vary with the extent and location of the lesion. In one series, the initial symptoms were strider (90%), dyspnea (55%), feeding problems (50%), and coughing (20%). Seven of 20 children were premature, and five required ventilation for RDS. Emergency tracheotomy was needed in 20% of these cases.

The patient's voice may be normal, hoarse, or aphonic. A cystic swelling of the neck between the hyoid bone and the thyroid cartilage often occurs. Compression of the mass may produce gurgling and hissing in the throat (Bryce sign). The mass may also increase with straining and decrease with rest. Dysphagia and aspiration often develop with large lesions. Airway obstruction and asphyxiation are potential dangers. Small laryngoceles may be entirely asymptomatic.

The relationship between laryngoceles and laryngeal carcinoma has been studied by Micheau, et al (1978). Laryngoceles are found in approximately 2% of normal larynges; however, they may be found in 18% of laryngeal carcinoma specimens. It has been suggested that laryngeal carcinoma may play a role in the genesis of a laryngocele. Carcinoma may develop in laryngoceles in as many as 50% of patients. Pre-existing laryngoceles might provide a preferential site for tumor development.

**Complications:** Infection, hoarseness, aspiration, obstruction, and carcinoma of larynx may occur.

**Associated Findings:** None known.

**Etiology:** Undetermined. Subglottic cysts have resulted from the trauma of intubation.

**Pathogenesis:** Increased intraluminal laryngeal pressure in persons with congenitally large ventricular appendices are the major considerations in this disease. The laryngeal appendix becomes dilated with an increase in intraluminal pressure from straining, coughing, singing, glass blowing, and the playing of wind instruments. This dilated saccus (saccular cyst) then expands up into the false cord, or the aryepiglottic fold, or both; it passes into the neck through the perforation of the neurovascular bundle in the thyrohyoid ligament. These cysts are lined with ciliated respiratory epithelium that contain mucous-secreting glands. Varying degrees of inflammatory reactions occur in the wall of the cyst.

**CDC No.:** 748.300

**Sex Ratio:** M1:F1

**Occurrence:** Anout 200 cases have been documented.

**Risk of Recurrence for Patient's Sib:** Unknown.

**Risk of Recurrence for Patient's Child:** Unknown.

**Age of Detectability:** Mitchell (1987) reported the clinical findings of 20 patients with laryngeal cysts that were treated at the Hospital for Sick Children in London between 1969 and 1984. Forty percent of the cysts were apparent the first day of life, and 95% were discovered before six months of age.

**Gene Mapping and Linkage:** Unknown.

**Prevention:** None known. Genetic counseling indicated.

**Treatment:** In patients with a symptomatic laryngocele, a one-stage surgical excision of the lesion through an external incision may be necessary as well as a treatment of infections with antibiotics. Although incision and drainage should be avoided, they may be necessary with an acute infection. Tracheotomy may be necessary when airway obstruction or aspiration are problems.

Airway obstruction in children is a dangerous and life threat-ening situation. Booth and Birck (1981) report two infants, one with a saccular cyst and the other with a laryngocele, who presented with respiratory difficulty. Symptoms of both of these conditions are non-specific and can be confused with the symptoms of laryngomalacia. Early recognition and treatment is important because of the small airway. Surgical approach to laryngocele and large saccular cysts is usually by the external approach and tracheotomy. In infants, however, an endoscopic method of dealing with these conditions is preferred. Marsupialization of the dome and stripping of the cyst wall with laryngeal forceps is usually sufficient. The carbon dioxide laser may be useful in selected cases. Post-operatively, the endotracheal tube should be left in place approximately 72 hours to act as a stent.

**Prognosis:** With adequate treatment, the outlook for normal life span, intelligence, and functioning is good.

**Detection of Carrier:** Unknown.

**References:**
English GM, DeBlanc GB: Laryngocele: a case presenting with acute airway obstruction. Laryngoscope 1968; 78:386–398.
Harrison DFN: Saccular mucocele and laryngeal cancer. Arch Otolaryngol 1977; 103:232–234.
Holinger LD, et al.: Laryngocele and saccular cysts. Ann Otol Rhinol Laryngol. 1978; 87:675–685. *
Micheau C, et al.: Relationship between laryngoceles and laryngeal carcinomas. Laryngoscope 1978; 88:680–688.
Donegan JO, et al.: Internal laryngocele and saccular cysts in children. a comparative account of symptoms, diagnosis, and management. Ann Otol Rhinol Laryngol 1980; 89:409.
Booth JB, Birck HG: Operative treatment and postoperative management of saccular cyst and laryngocele. Arch Otolaryngol 1981; 107:500–502.
Baker HL, et al.: Manifestations and management of laryngoceles. Head Neck Surg 1982; 4:450–456. *
Mitchell DB: Cysts of the infant larynx. J Laryngol Otol 1987; 101:833–837.

EN002                                    **Gerald M. English**

**Laryngoceles: internal, external or combined**
*See LARYNGOCELE*

## LARYNGOMALACIA                                    0576

**Includes:**
  Croup, congenital
  Laryngeal chondromalacia, congenital
  Laryngeal stridor, congenital
  Larynx, congenital flaccid
  Stridor, congenital

**Excludes:**
  Croup (other)
  Laryngismus stridulous
  **Larynx, atresia (0571)**

**Major Diagnostic Criteria:** Persistent stuttering, inspiratory respirations with episodes of cyanosis, especially during feeding; neck, chest, and esophageal X-rays negative for possible thyroglossal duct cyst, tracheal compression, mediastinal mass, and vascular ring. Direct laryngoscopy shows fluttering arytenoids; curled or tubular epiglottis, and it demonstrates absence of other laryngeal or tracheal obstruction.

**Clinical Findings:** Stridorous, noisy, inspiratory crowing respirations, which may be associated with intermittent episodes of hypoxia and cyanosis, accompanied by indrawing at the suprasternal notch and epigastrium. Usually begins shortly after birth and increases in severity, lasting 6–18 months, then gradually subsides. Direct or flexible laryngoscopy shows flaccidity of all supraglottic structures; the epiglottis is often curled or tubular and soft, as are the arytenoids and aryepiglottic folds, which all flutter during inspiration. Cord motility is normal. Symptoms are often exacerbated during feeding, supine positioning, or agitation.

Exaggerated or persistent infantile features of the larynx, tubular longitudinal folding of the epiglottis, and inward rolling of the

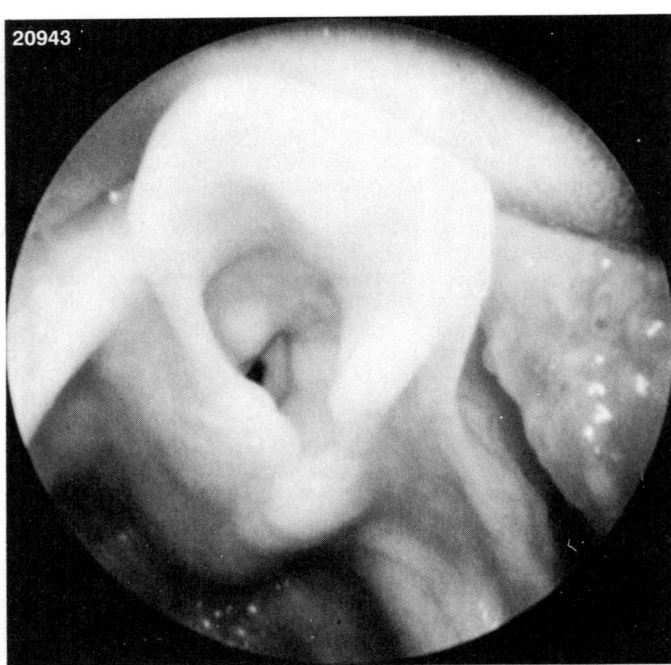

**0576**-20943: Laryngomalacia.

arytenoids and aryepiglottic folds have been recorded as postmortem findings. Histologically, edema and a slight increase in the lymphatic and polymorphonuclear cellular elements of the submucosa were found. Kelemen (1953) describes cartilages found to be about one-half the thickness of control specimens, and Shulman (1976) describes cartilages with unusual matrix staining.

**Complications:** Failure to gain weight, in severe cases. Pectus excavatum associated with the constant epigastric indrawing. Hypoxia and cyanosis may be found in addition to obstructive sleep apnea.

**Associated Findings:** Micrognathia, macroglossia.

**Etiology:** In one kindred, the mother of three affected sibs had respiratory problems in infancy, suggesting the possibility of autosomal dominant inheritance.

**Pathogenesis:** Unknown.

**MIM No.:** 15028

**CDC No.:** 748.300

**Sex Ratio:** M2:F1

**Occurrence:** Most common of congenital laryngeal anomalies, constituting 650 of a series of 866 laryngeal anomalies.

**Risk of Recurrence for Patient's Sib:** Unknown.

**Risk of Recurrence for Patient's Child:** Unknown.

**Age of Detectability:** At one to six months by direct or flexible laryngoscopy.

**Gene Mapping and Linkage:** Unknown.

**Prevention:** None known. Genetic counseling indicated.

**Treatment:** Interrupt feeding frequently to assist breathing; place infant in position of least obstruction. Surgical trimming of epiglottis and aryepiglottic folds may be effective in selective circumstances. Tracheotomy only in severe involvement.

**Prognosis:** Normal for life span, intelligence, and function.

**Detection of Carrier:** Unknown.

**Special Considerations:** Stridor is the auditory evidence of upper airway obstruction; therefore, laryngomalacia must be differentiated from all other causes of stridor in infants. Direct laryngoscopy usually shows a curled and flaccid epiglottis, with soft, edematous-appearing arytenoids that are drawn into the glottis with a fluttering appearance with each inspiration. The symptom is exaggerated when the infant is on its back and decreases in severity when the infant lies on its abdomen. The noise is increased with total relaxation, as during sleep, or with vigorous crying. Bronchoscopy often shows an associated, similar tracheo- and bronchomalacia.

**References:**
Schwartz L: Congenital laryngeal stridor (inspiratory laryngeal collapse): new theory as to its underlying cause and desirability of a change in terminology. Arch Otolaryngol 1944; 39:403.
Finlay HVL: Familial congenital stridor. Arch Dis Child 1949; 24:219.
Kelemen G: Congenital laryngeal stridor. Arch Otolaryngol 1953; 58:245.
Holinger PH, Brown WT: Congenital webs, cysts, laryngoceles and other anomalies of the larynx. Ann Otol Rhinol Laryngol 1967; 76:744.
Shulman JB, et al.: Familial laryngomalacia: a case report. Laryngoscope 1976; 86:84–91.
Belmont JR, Groundfast K: Congenital laryngeal stridor (laryngomalacia): etiologic factors and associated disorders. Ann Otol Rhinol Laryngol 1984; 93:430–437.

MY003                                              **Charles M. Myer III**

**Larynx and trachea, congenital posterior cleft of**
*See LARYNGO-TRACHEO-ESOPHAGEAL CLEFT*
**Larynx cancer**
*See CANCER, LUNG, FAMILIAL*

## LARYNX, ATRESIA                                      0571

**Includes:**
    Atresia of larynx, types I, II and III
    Glottic atresia
    Laryngeal atresia, congenital
    Stenosis at the conus elasticus

**Excludes:**
    **Laryngocele** (0575)
    **Laryngomalacia** (0576)
    **Larynx, cysts** (0572)
    **Larynx, web** (0574)

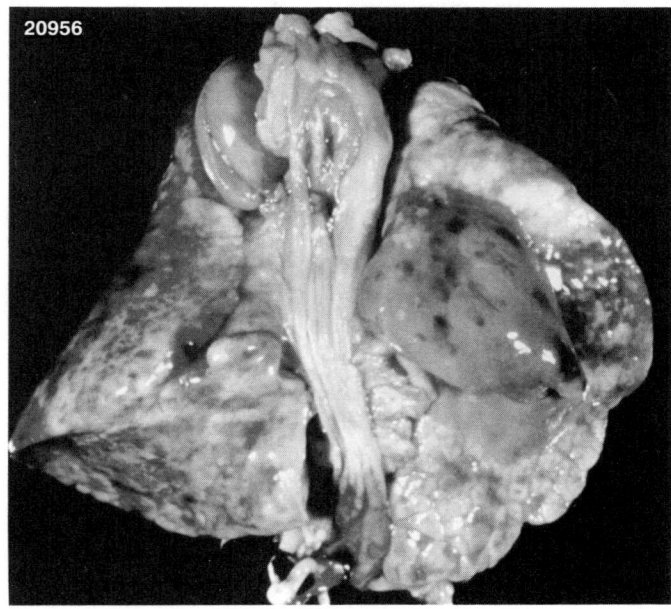

**0571**-20956: Laryngeal atresia.

**Subglottic stenosis** (0919)
**Tracheoesophageal fistula** (0960)

**Major Diagnostic Criteria:** Asphyxia neonatorum or stridor at birth, with complete or partial laryngeal obstruction.

**Clinical Findings:** Incompatible with life unless it is recognized immediately at birth and steps are taken at once to establish an airway. When the obstruction is incomplete, the signs and symptoms are related to the functioning diameter of the stenosed lumen. Marked respiratory effort without air exchange or stridor at birth, with or without cyanosis, depending on the severity of the stenosis, is the first sign of laryngeal obstruction.

Direct laryngoscopy will reveal a complete or partial membranous occlusion of the larynx. Smith and Bain (1965) distinguish three types of atresia:
Type I: supraglottic and infraglottic parts are atretic
Type II: atresia is infraglottic
Type III: atresia is glottic

**Complications:** The risk of neonatal death is extremely high with complete laryngeal atresia. In mild cases (i.e. stenosis or partial atresia) recurrent episodes of "croup" and repeated superimposed respiratory infections simulating laryngotracheobronchitis are common. Complications associated with tracheotomy in the newborn must also be considered. Chances of complications would be high in most instances because of the emergent nature of the situation should accidental decannulation occur.

**Associated Findings:** About one-half the cases reported in the literature had other potentially fatal malformations. Malformations include the CNS (hydrocephaly, malformations of the aqueduct); alimentary system (esophageal atresia, bronchoesophageal fistula, tracheoesophageal fistula and atresia); urogenital system (hypoplasia of kidney, hydroureter, urethral atresia, vesicovaginal fistula, bicornuate uterus), and skeletal system (varus deformity of feet, partial absence of cervical vertebrae, absence of radius, syndactyly).

**Etiology:** Presumably autosomal dominant inheritance.

**Pathogenesis:** The various types of atresia are the result of arrest of development. A chromosomal basis has also been suggested (Lewandowski and Yunis, 1977).

**MIM No.:** 15030

**CDC No.:** 748.300

**Sex Ratio:** Presumably M1:F1

**Occurrence:** Undetermined but presumed rare.

**Risk of Recurrence for Patient's Sib:**
See Part I, *Mendelian Inheritance.*

**Risk of Recurrence for Patient's Child:**
See Part I, *Mendelian Inheritance.*

**Age of Detectability:** At birth.

**Gene Mapping and Linkage:** Unknown.

**Prevention:** None known. Genetic counseling indicated.

**Treatment:** Establishment of immediate diagnosis and provision of immediate airway (i.e. tracheostomy). Treatment of secondary infections and stridor.

**Prognosis:** The vast majority of newborns with complete laryngeal atresia die because the condition is not recognized and not treated immediately or because of other life threatening anomalies. If the child survives the neonatal period, with proper surgical and medical treatment he or she will have a normal life span, unless the condition is complicated by serious associated malformations.

**Detection of Carrier:** Unknown.

**Special Considerations:** There is little doubt that atresia of the larynx is closely related to laryngeal webs, not only in its presenting signs and pathologic findings, but also in its mode of genesis. Most authors feel that the condition has not been recognized in many infants and, as webs are not uncommon, it is safe to assume that atresia too is no rarity. Baker and Savetsky (1966) believe that heredity is a factor in "congenital partial atresia of the larynx" (study includes laryngeal webs and other types of laryngeal

stenosis), as was demonstrated in a mother and her two children, all of whom had this entity.

**References:**
Smith II, Bain AD: Congenital atresia of the larynx. Ann Otol Rhinol Laryngol 1965; 74:338–349.
Baker DC Jr, Savetsky L: Congenital partial atresia of the larynx. Laryngoscope 1966; 78:616–620.
Holinger PH, Brown W: Congenital webs, cysts, laryngoceles and other anomalies of the larynx. Ann Otol Rhinol. Laryngol 1967; 76:744.
Jackson C: Anomalies of the larynx. In: Maloney WH, ed: Otolaryngology. vol. 4. Hagerstown: Harper & Row, 1969.
Holinger PH, et al.: Pediatric laryngology. Otolaryngol Clin North Am 1970; 3:625.
Lewandowski RC Jr, Yunis JJ. Phenotypic mapping in man. In: Yunis JJ, ed: New chromosomal syndromes. New York: Academic Press, 1977:369–394.

MY003                                          **Charles M. Myer III**

**Larynx, congenital flaccid**
*See LARYNGOMALACIA*

---

## LARYNX, CYSTS                                        0572

**Includes:**
Cysts, glottic
Cysts, saccular
**Excludes:**
Cysts, mucosal retention
**Laryngocele** (0575)
**Thyroglossal duct remnant** (0945)

**Major Diagnostic Criteria:** A cyst located in the larynx usually causing respiratory symptoms, which may result in feeding difficulties and an abnormal cry. A lateral X-ray of the neck may help with the diagnosis, but it is only made with certainty by direct laryngoscopy.

**Clinical Findings:** Saccular cysts of the larynx are non-air-containing, fluid-filled structures that do not communicate with the laryngeal lumen. They result from cystic distention of the laryngeal ventricle and lie beneath normal mucosa. They are usually sessile, but may be pedunculated. Most cysts are confined to the immediate area of the ventricular appendix. There are two types of cysts: 1) Anterior, which are located near the saccular orifice of the ventricle. They may bulge from deep within the ventricle and overhang the glottis. Some may be large enough to fill the entire ventricle. 2) Lateral cysts are typically located on the lateral wall of the supraglottic larynx or epiglottis. They may extend from the aryepiglottic fold and arytenoid downward to and including the ventricle, laterally into the pyriform sinus, or even through the thyrohyoid membrane into the neck.

Symptoms vary depending on the location, size, and age at presentation. In infants, respiratory distress, usually with inspiratory stridor, is the most common symptom because of the small size of the larynx. Cyanosis and use of the accessory muscles of respiration may be present. A change in the degree of obstruction can also occur with a change in head position. Dysphagia and an abnormal cry, which may be muffled, shrill, hoarse, feeble, or inaudible, are also common. Tracheostomy or endotracheal intubation is required for the severely compromised airway.

In an older child, hoarseness or a weak voice may be the presenting symptom.

**Complications:** Asphyxia at birth, respiratory distress, dysphagia, and an abnormal voice.

**Associated Findings:** Funnel chest may develop due to prolonged epigastric indrawing.

**Etiology:** Unknown.

**Pathogenesis:** Unknown. Several theories have been postulated; 1) a pinching off of some of the cells that normally form the appendix of the laryngeal ventricle, 2) failure of an epithelial cord of cells to hollow out between the fetal ventricle and laryngeal lumen, and 3) branchial derivation. Some investigators believe it need not be considered an actual malformation of the larynx, but simply a secondary disturbance in development.

**CDC No.:**  748.380

**Sex Ratio:**  M1:F4

**Occurrence:**  Undetermined but presumed rare.

**Risk of Recurrence for Patient's Sib:**  Unknown.

**Risk of Recurrence for Patient's Child:**  Unknown.

**Age of Detectability:**  At birth for severe cases causing symptoms; otherwise, at any age if symptoms occur and laryngeal examination is warranted.

**Gene Mapping and Linkage:**  Unknown.

**Prevention:**  None known. Genetic counseling indicated.

**Treatment:**  Aspiration under direct laryngoscopy. The cysts tend to recur and eventually may need to be unroofed and the frayed edges removed. Sometimes marsupialization is the initial procedure. Temporary tracheostomy may be required. Large cysts are treated by submucous resection through an external approach.

**Prognosis:**  A cyst causing complete obstruction at birth will result in death unless an airway is secured. Once cysts are diagnosed and treated, life spain is normal.

**Detection of Carrier:**  Unknown.

**Special Considerations:**  Ductal cysts form at any site in the larynx where there are mucous glands. This excludes only the gland-free area on the free edge of the true cords. Obstruction of the ducts, with retention of mucus and dilation of the glands, is thought to be the origin of these cysts.

Intralaryngeal true branchiogenic cysts and a thyroid cartilage foraminal cyst have been described in the literature.

Congenital cysts and laryngoceles have a similar development, but laryngoceles differ from congenital cysts in that they communicate with the lumen of the larynx and become clinically perceptible only when swollen by air forced into them or when filled with a collection of fluid.

**References:**

DeSanto LW, et al.: Cysts of the larynx: classification. Laryngoscope 1970; 80:145–176. *

Hollinger LD, et al.: Laryngocoele and saccular cysts. Ann Otol 1978; 87:675–685. †

Donegan JO, et al.: Internal laryngocele and saccular cysts in children. A comparative account of symptoms, diagnosis, and management. Ann Otol Rhinol Laryngol 1980; 89:409. *

Abramson AL, Zeilinski B: Congenital laryngeal saccular cyst of the newborn. Laryngoscope 1984; 94:1580–1582.

K0023
B0049

Frederick K. Kozak
Valerie L. Boswell

## LARYNX, VENTRICLE PROLAPSE                                   0573

**Includes:**
  Eversion of sacculus
  Eversion of ventricle
  Laryngeal ventricle prolapse
  Prolapse of laryngeal ventricle

**Excludes:**
  Chronic laryngitis
  Hyperplasia of larynx
  Laryngeal polyp
  **Laryngocele** (0575)
  Reinke edema

**Major Diagnostic Criteria:**  Intermittent hoarseness and a dry, irritating cough are produced by the prolapse of the ventricle. Direct laryngoscopic examination, manipulation of the mass to determine its site of origin, and biopsy to establish its histopathologic characteristics are necessary to establish the diagnosis.

**Clinical Findings:**  An irritating, nonproductive cough and intermittent hoarseness are the usual symptoms when a mass of prolapsed tissue extends onto the true vocal cords. The degree of hoarseness varies depending on the size of the mass. Pain is rare, and airway obstruction becomes a problem only after the mass reaches a size that occludes the glottic airway.

Idiopathic or true eversion of the ventricular mucosa is rare because this tissue is normally firmly attached to underlying structures. An associated disease that contributes to the development of saccular eversion should always be suspected. Eversion of the sacculus has been detected in persons from the 2nd to the 6th decades of life and is more common in men than in women. In one third of reported cases the lesion was bilateral, with the remainder of the cases divided nearly equally between the right and left sides of the larynx.

Examination reveals a smooth, pear-shaped, pale red mass, protruding from the ventricle onto the true vocal cord. This mass moves freely when palpated during direct laryngoscopy and can usually be pushed back into the ventricle. It should not be difficult to determine that the mass originates from the ventricle and not from the vocal cords. Aspiration during direct laryngoscopy may be required to distinguish this lesion from a cyst. Biopsies should be obtained to rule out possibility of a neoplasm.

**Complications:**  Neoplasms, recurrent airway obstruction, hoarseness, cough.

**Associated Findings:**  None known.

**Etiology:**  Undetermined. Infections of the larynx, cysts of the false vocal cord, aryepiglottic fold and ventricle, neoplasms of the larynx, chronic cough from pulmonary disease, and external laryngeal trauma have all been implicated. No known familial incidence exists. Seid, et al (1979), report that children may develop protrusion or prolapse of the laryngeal ventricle subsequent to endotracheal tube intubation. In these cases, the prolapsed ventricle caused airway obstruction necessitating tracheostomy. The prolapsed ventricle subsequently resolved and decannulation was possible.

**Pathogenesis:**  Eversion of the sacculus, or appendix of the ventricle, or a portion of the ventricular mucosa produces a mass that lies upon the true vocal cord. The prolapsed sacculus is lined with ciliated pseudostratified columnar epithelium resting on an intact basement membrane. Scott (1976) reports an anatomic study of 111 larynges from both sexes. He determined the dimensions of the laryngeal saccule and sinus, relative to the height and width of the larynx in the two sexes, and found pouches that were asymptomatic in two patients. The male saccule tended to be relatively shallower than the female.

**CDC No.:**  748.300

**Sex Ratio:**  M5:F1

**Occurrence:**  Undetermined.

**Risk of Recurrence for Patient's Sib:**  Unknown.

**Risk of Recurrence for Patient's Child:**  Unknown.

**Age of Detectability:**  Usually during early adulthood by indirect mirror examination of the larynx. Flexible laryngoscopy may allow earlier diagnosis in children.

**Gene Mapping and Linkage:**  Unknown.

**Prevention:**  None known. Genetic counseling indicated.

**Treatment:**  Surgical excision during direct laryngoscopy is recommended as well as appropriate treatment of associated diseases. Tracheostomy may be required when airway obstruction occurs or if there is excessive surgical trauma. An open surgical approach may be necessary in some cases.

**Prognosis:**  The prognosis is good when the mass is completely excised; however, any underlying disease may require more extensive therapy. In these patients the prognosis will depend on the success or failure of treatment for these disorders.

**Detection of Carrier:**  Unknown.

**References:**

Freedman AO: Diseases of the ventricle of Morgagni; with special references to pyocele of congenital air sac of ventricle. Arch Otolaryngol 1938; 28:329–343.

Scott GBD: A morphometric study of the laryngeal saccule and sinus. Clin Otolaryngol 1976; 1:115–122.

Seid AB, et al.: Protrusion of the laryngeal ventricle in a pediatric patient following nasotracheal tube intubation. Otolaryngol Head Neck Surg 1979; 87:199–202.

Barnes DR, et al.: Prolapse of the laryngeal ventricle. Otolaryngol Head Neck Surg 1980; 88:165–171. *

Canalis RF: Laryngeal ventricle. Ann Otol Rhinol Laryngol 1980; 89:184–187. *

Weissler MC, et al.: Laryngopyocele as a cause of airway obstruction. Laryngoscope 1985; 95:1345–1351.

EN002 **Gerald M. English**

## LARYNX, WEB 0574

**Includes:**
Glottic web
Subglottic web
Supraglottic web

**Excludes:**
Acquired webs of larynx
**Larynx, atresia (0571)**
**Subglottic stenosis (0919)**

**Major Diagnostic Criteria:** Diagnosis is based on the presence of a membranous web partially occluding the lumen in the supraglottic, glottic, or subglottic larynx. The diagnosis must be confirmed by direct laryngoscopy; indirect laryngoscopy may be used in those patients old enough to cooperate.

**Clinical Findings:** A laryngeal web or other laryngeal anomaly must be considered in a newborn with evidence of upper airway obstruction or dysphonia. Seventy-five percent of congenital laryngeal webs are present at birth. In the young child, this defect may go undetected until the cause of recurrent croup, tracheobronchitis, or pneumonia is sought. In adults or older children, hoarseness or dyspnea on exertion may be due to a laryngeal web.

The webs are usually grayish-white and glistening in appearance, but may be grayish-yellow or pink. Some of the reported webs have consisted of only a thin translucent membrane, but they are usually thin posteriorly and up to 1.5 cm thick anteriorly. Glottic webs are classified according to degree of occlusion of the lumen: type 1, 35% covering the anterior glottis, with the true vocal cords easily seen; type 2, 35–50% occlusion of the lumen, with the true vocal cords usually visible; type 3, 50–75% occlusion, with the vocal cords possibly visualized; type 4, 75–90% occlusion, with the vocal cords not seen. Type 3 is the most common type of glottic web. Subglottic webs may occur with or without cricoid involvement. Congenital interarytenoid fixation is included in the supraglottic web group.

Ninety-eight percent of all webs of the larynx are anterior, and 2% are posterior. The location and frequency of laryngeal webs are approximately: supraglottic 12.5%; glottic 75%; and subglottic, 12.5%.

Histologically, the superior surface of the web is lined by squamous epithelium, with the inferior surface covered by respiratory epithelium. The majority have a considerable mesodermal element of dense connective tissue, mucous glands, striated muscle, fat, and cartilage.

The severity of the symptoms is dependent upon the extent of the web. In infants, the most common signs, in the order of frequency, are aphonia, inspiratory and expiratory stridor, difficulty in feeding, and attacks of dyspnea. The most common symptoms in older children and adults are hoarseness; dyspnea on exertion or with respiratory tract infections; a weak, high-pitched voice, or easy tiring of the voice.

**Complications:** Minor manipulation of the airway or infections may lead to severe airway obstruction in patients with previously undetected webs.

**Associated Findings:** As many as 10–15% of individuals with laryngeal webs have other congenital anomalies, with one-third of these having associated abnormalities of the respiratory tract. The following anomalies have been reported: tetralogy of Fallot, ventricular septal defect, choanal atresia, bronchopulmonary dysplasia, cleft palate, bifid uvula and submucous cleft of the soft palate, tracheosophageal fistula, adherent lingual frenulum, ptosis of eyelids, preauricular sinus, subglottic hemangioma, subglottic stenosis, nevus flammeus, mental retardation, seizure disorders, syndactyly, and urogenital anomalies.

**Etiology:** Unknown.

**Pathogenesis:** Differentiation of the larynx occurs between the 4th and 10th weeks of gestation. In the development of the larynx there is epithelial fusion between the two sides, which is thought to dissolve at about the 10th week of gestation. A laryngeal web is the result of incomplete recannulization of the primitive larynx between the 7th and 8th weeks of gestation.

**CDC No.:** 748.2

**Sex Ratio:** M1:F1

**Occurrence:** Five percent of congenital anomalies of the larynx are webs. The overall occurrence of laryngeal webs is unknown.

**Risk of Recurrence for Patient's Sib:** Undetermined. Familial reports exist.

**Risk of Recurrence for Patient's Child:** Unknown.

**Age of Detectability:** At birth by direct laryngoscopy or later when symptoms present.

**Gene Mapping and Linkage:** Unknown.

**Prevention:** None known. Genetic counseling indicated.

**Treatment:** Treatment of a web is dependent upon its thickness, extent, and location. For severe airway compromise, establishment of an adequate airway by intubation or tracheostomy is required. Simple webs may respond to division with microsurgical scissors and repeated dilation with the bougienge. $CO_2$ laser techniques have recently been used, but long-term results are not available. Tracheostomy may or may not be required for extensive webs. The larger and thicker webs are amenable to external laryngofissure, in which the thyroid cartilage is divided in the midline, the larynx entered, and the web resected. Intralaryngeal stents or keels have been used to prevent restenosis in glottic webs.

Speech improvement is achieved, but restoration of normal speech is often not possible.

**Prognosis:** Normal life span if airway obstruction is adequately treated.

**Detection of Carrier:** Unknown.

**References:**
McHugh HE, Loch WE: Congenital webs of the larynx. Laryngoscope 1942; 52:43–65.

Cotton RT, Richardson MA: Congenital laryngeal anomalies. Otolaryngol Clin North Am 1981; 14:203–218.

Benjamin B: Congenital laryngeal webs. Ann Otol Rhinol Laryngol 1983; 92:317–326. †

Cohen S: Congenital glottic webs in children. A retrospective review of 51 patients. Ann Otol Rhinol Laryngol (Suppl) 1985; 121:2–16. * †

Hardingham M, Walsh-Waring GP: The treatment of a congenital laryngeal web. J Laryngol Otol 1985; 89:273–279.

B0049 **Valerie L. Boswell**
K0023 **Frederick K. Kozak**

**Latah**
*See JUMPING FRENCHMAN OF MAINE*
**Late fetal epidermal dysplasia, type II**
*See RESTRICTIVE DERMATOPATHY*
**Late-onset cystinosis**
*See CYSTINOSIS*
**Late-onset immunoglobulin deficiency**
*See IMMUNODEFICIENCY, COMMON VARIABLE TYPE*
**Lateral incisors, absence of**
*See TEETH, PEGGED OR ABSENT MAXILLARY LATERAL INCISOR*
**Lateral nasal proboscis**
*See NOSE, PROBOSCIS LATERALIS*
**Lattice corneal dystrophy**
*See CORNEAL DYSTROPHY, LATTICE TYPE*

## LAURENCE-MOON SYNDROME                                    0578

**Includes:** Laurence-Moon-Bardet-Biedl syndrome (some cases)

**Excludes:**
   **Acrocephalopolysyndactyly** (0013)
   **Alstrom syndrome** (0041)
   **Bardet-Biedl syndrome** (2363)
   **Biemond II syndrome** (2169)
   **Cohen syndrome** (2023)
   **Prader-Willi syndrome** (0823)
   Vasquez syndrome

**Major Diagnostic Criteria:** Hypogenitalism, mental retardation, retinitis pigmentosa, spastic paraplegia.

**Clinical Findings:** Hypogenitalism is present at birth but may not be noticed until later when normal genital growth is not observed. Postpubertal studies show hypogonadotrophic hypogonadism. Slow development, night blindness, mental retardation, and ataxic gait are noticed in turn during childhood. Ophthalmic examination then may show only retinal mottling due to thinning of the retina, leading to increased visibility of choroid. Retinal pigment accumulations are noticed peripherally in late childhood and gradually encroach on the central retina, accompanied by progressive optic atrophy. The ataxia slowly progresses to spastic paraplegia by early adulthood.

**Complications:** The retinitis pigmentosa leads to blindness. The mental defect is quite limiting, and the spastic paraplegia culminates in a bedridden state.

**Associated Findings:** None known.

**Etiology:** Presumably autosomal recessive inheritance.

**Pathogenesis:** Failure of normal embryologic development. The progressive nature suggests a metabolic error that interferes with development and continues after birth in some differentiated cells.

**MIM No.:** 24580

**POS No.:** 3113

**CDC No.:** 759.820

**Sex Ratio:** M1:F1

**Occurrence:** Presumably rare. Reportedly of increased frequency in the Arab population of Kuwait. The syndrome described by Laurence and Moon (1866) is a specific entity, while the syndrome described by Bardet and Biedl (see **Bardet-Biedl syndrome** is a different disorder. Shortly after the report of these two syndromes, the medical literature became confused, grouping many different disorders under the terms *Laurence-Moon-Biedl* syndrome or *Laurence-Moon-Bardet-Biedl* syndrome. Very few case descriptions truly fit into either the Bardet-Biedl syndrome or the Laurence-Moon syndrome. Most descriptions appear to represent either isolated cases or quite distinct syndromes rather than variants of either of the two classic syndromes. The **Bardet-Biedl syndrome** and the Laurence-Moon syndrome both breed true, as do several of the other disorders that have been grouped with them.

**Risk of Recurrence for Patient's Sib:**
   See Part I, *Mendelian Inheritance.*

**Risk of Recurrence for Patient's Child:**
   See Part I, *Mendelian Inheritance.* Most affected individuals are infertile.

**Age of Detectability:** Evident at birth, although definitive diagnosis is difficult until late childhood.

**Gene Mapping and Linkage:** Unknown.

**Prevention:** None known. Genetic counseling indicated.

**Treatment:** Unknown.

**Prognosis:** A deteriorating, handicapping condition due to mental retardation, progressive vision loss, and progressive spastic paraplegia.

**Detection of Carrier:** If genealogic studies identify the underlying cause as parental consanguinity stemming from membership in a small genetic isolate, normal relatives have as high as 50% chance of heterozygosity.

**Support Groups:** MD; Lexington Park; Laurence-Moon-Biedl Syndrome (LMBS) Support Network

**References:**
Laurence JZ, Moon RC: Four cases of retinitis pigmentosa occurring in the same family and accompanied by general imperfection of development. Ophthalmol Rev 1866; 2:32–41.
Roth AA: Familial eunuchoidism: the Laurence-Moon-Biedl syndrome. J Urol (Baltimore) 1947; 57:427–445.
Bowen P, et al.: The Laurence-Moon syndrome. Association with hypogonadotrophic hypogonadism and sex-chromosome aneuploidy. Arch Intern Med 1965; 116:598–604.
Schachat AP, Maumenee IH: The Bardet-Biedl syndrome and related disorders. Arch Ophthal 1982; 100:285–288.
Farag TI, Teebi AS: Bardet-Biedl and Lawrence-Moon syndromes in a mixed Arab population. Clin Genet 1988; 33:78–82.

TH017                                                      **T.F. Thurmon**
UR001                                                      **S.A. Ursin**

**Laurence-Moon-Bardet-Biedl syndrome (some cases)**
   *See LAURENCE-MOON SYNDROME*
**Laurence-Moon-Bardet-Biedl syndrome (some)**
   *See BARDET-BIEDL SYNDROME*
**Lawrence syndrome**
   *See LIPODYSTROPHY SYNDROME, BERARDINELLI TYPE*
**LCAT deficiency**
   *See LECITHIN-CHOLESTEROL ACYL TRANSFERASE DEFICIENCY*
   *also ANEMIA, HEMOLYTIC, RED CELL MEMBRANE DEFECTS*
**LDL-receptor disorder**
   *See HYPERCHOLESTEREMIA*
**Lead poisoning, susceptibility to**
   *See DELTA-AMINOLEVULINIC ACID DEHYDRASE DEFICIENCY*
**Lead, effects of postnatal exposure**
   *See FETAL EFFECTS FROM MATERNAL LEAD EXPOSURE*
**Lead, fetal effects from maternal exposure**
   *See FETAL EFFECTS FROM MATERNAL LEAD EXPOSURE*
**Leaky red cell syndrome**
   *See ANEMIA, HEMOLYTIC, RED CELL MEMBRANE DEFECTS*
**Leber hamartoma**
   *See LIVER, HAMARTOMA*
**Leber miliary aneurysms**
   *See RETINA, COATS DISEASE*
**Leber optic atrophy**
   *See OPTIC ATROPHY, LEBER TYPE*
**Lecithin-cholesterol acyl transferase (LCAT) deficiency**
   *See ANEMIA, HEMOLYTIC, RED CELL MEMBRANE DEFECTS*

## LECITHIN-CHOLESTEROL ACYL TRANSFERASE
## DEFICIENCY                                               0580

**Includes:**
   Alpha LCAT deficiency
   Alpha and beta LCAT deficiency
   Corneal opacities-dyslipoproteinemia
   Fish eye disease (obsolete; pejorative)
   LCAT deficiency
   Lecithin: cholesterol acyltransferase (LCAT) deficiency
   Norum disease
   Plasma cholesteryl ester deficiency, familial

**Excludes:**
   **Apolipoprotein A-I and C-III deficiency states** (3165)
   **Analphalipoproteinemia** (0048)
   **Cholesteryl ester storage disease** (0151)
   **Hypoalphalipoproteinemia** (3096)
   **Wolman disease** (1003)

**Major Diagnostic Criteria:** In familial lecithin:cholsterol acyltransferase (LCAT) deficiency, there is corneal opacities, proteinuria, and slight anemia, and a marked reduction in plasma cholesteryl esters and the activity of LCAT (both beta and alpha LCAT). In "fish eye disease", a variant of LCAT deficiency, marked corneal opacification, and deficiencies of HDL cholesterol and alpha LCAT activity are present.

**Clinical Findings:** In familial LCAT deficiency, marked changes in plasma lipids are invariable. All patients have low absolute and relative levels of cholesteryl esters, and increased levels of unesterified cholesterol. Plasma lecithin is increased and lysolecithin usually decreased. Most patients have increased levels of plasma triglycerides. Patients have low levels of high-density lipoproteins (HDL), and high levels of very-low-density lipoproteins (VLDL). Electron microscopy of lipoproteins reveals several abnormalities, the most frequent being disk-shaped HDL and the presence of chylomicron remnants in the VLDL fraction. Proteinuria, with late renal failure, is common. Several patients have died in renal failure. All patients have corneal opacities, and most have a slight normochromic anemia. There are no neurologic symptoms.

In "fish eye disease", there is a marked decrease in plasma HDL constituents, especially cholesterol esters, and also marked corneal opacification.

**Complications:** Disturbances in lipoprotein metabolism may give accelerated atherosclerosis. Cholesterol deposits in the kidney give rise to renal failure, which is the most severe complication. Corneal opacification affecting vision is a complication of both familial LCAT deficiency and "fish eye disease".

**Associated Findings:** None known.

**Etiology:** Autosomal recessive inheritance. Related disorders may exist because of a lack of LCAT or the presence of inhibitors of LCAT. Some patients have a very low level of normal LCAT, and others have a low level of abnormal LCAT.

**Pathogenesis:** LCAT has a role in normal cholesterol metabolism and turnover. One may therefore suggest that lack of the enzyme leads to decreased flux and transport of cholesterol from peripheral tissues to the liver. This may explain the increased unesterified cholesterol in the red blood cells and the accelerated atherosclerosis. A lack of LCAT may also cause cholesterol deposits in the glomerular tuft in the kidney, starting the events leading to renal failure. In familial LCAT deficiency there is decreased alpha and beta LCAT activity, while in "fish eye disease", only alpha LCAT activity is decreased.

**MIM No.:** *24590

**Sex Ratio:** M1:F1

**Occurrence:** Familial LCAT disease was first described in Norway, where most of the early patients were detected. Today patients are described in all parts of the world, including Japan and Germany, and more than 50 cases have been published. Alpha LCAT deficiency ("fish eye disease") has been described in several Swedish kindreds.

**Risk of Recurrence for Patient's Sib:**
See Part I, *Mendelian Inheritance.*

**Risk of Recurrence for Patient's Child:**
See Part I, *Mendelian Inheritance.*

**Age of Detectability:** The corneal opacities are usually detectable early in life. Proteinuria occurs usually from puberty. The enzyme defect is detectable from birth.

**Gene Mapping and Linkage:** LCAT (lecithin-cholesterol acyltransferase) has been mapped to 16q22.1.

**Prevention:** None known. Genetic counseling indicated.

**Treatment:** Dietetic to reduce plasma cholesterol. Secondary treatment of the renal failure may include kidney transplantation. No therapeutic effect has been obtained by infusions of purified enzyme or by transfusions of fresh plasma. Corneal transplantation can be used to treat the corneal opacification, but opacification can recur in the new cornea.

**Prognosis:** In familial LCAT deficiency, more than 50% of patients develop renal failure, which may lead to death. Some patients live into old age. In alpha LCAT deficiency, the prognosis is good except for the development of severe corneal opacification affecting vision.

**Detection of Carrier:** Heterozygotes have about 50% of the normal amount of LCAT. However, since the methods for detecting LCAT (both enzyme activity and enzyme protein) are somewhat difficult and uncertain, testing is normally confined to at-risk families.

**References:**
Norum KR, Gjone E: Familial lecithin:cholesterol acyltransferase deficiency: biochemical study of a new inborn error of metabolism. Scand J Clin Lab Invest 1967; 20:231–243.
Glomset JA: The plasma lecithin:cholesterol acyltransferase reaction. J Lipid Res 1968; 9:155–166.
Carlson LA, Philipson B: Fish eye disease: a new familial condition with massive corneal opacification and dyslipoproteinemia. Lancet 1979; II:921–923.
Norum KR: Familial lecithin:cholesterol acyltransferase deficiency. In: Miller NE, Miller GJ, eds: Clinical and metabolic aspects of high-density lipoproteins. New York: Elsevier Science Publisher, 1984: 297–324.
Carlson LA, Holmquist L: Evidence for deficiency of high density lipoprotein lecithin:cholesterol acyltransferase activity (alpha-LCAT) in fish eye disease. Acta Med Scand 1985; 218:189–196.
Norum KR, et al.: Familial lecithin:cholesterol acyltransferase deficiency, including fish eye disease. In: Scriver CR, et al, eds: The metabolic basis of inherited disease, 6th ed. New York: McGraw-Hill, 1989:1181–1194.

N0006    **Kaare R. Norum**

**Lecithin: cholesterol acyltransferase (LCAT) deficiency**
See *LECITHIN-CHOLESTEROL ACYL TRANSFERASE DEFICIENCY*
**Lefler-Wadsworth-Sidbury syndrome**
See *EYE, MACULAR DYSTROPHY, NORTH CAROLINA TYPE*
**Left atrial herniation**
See *HEART, PERICARDIUM AGENESIS*
**Left atrial myxoma**
See *MYXOMA, INTRACARDIAC*
**Left common carotid artery arising from innominate artery**
See *ARTERY, BRACHIOCEPHALIC AND CONTRALATERAL CAROTID, COMMON ORIGIN*
**Left coronary artery, anomalous origin from pulmonary artery**
See *ARTERY, CORONARY, ANOMALOUS ORIGIN FROM PULMONARY ARTERY*
**Left ventricle, double outlet**
See *VENTRICLE, DOUBLE OUTLET LEFT*
**Left ventricle, single papillary muscle**
See *VENTRICLE, SINGLE LEFT PAPILLARY MUSCLE*
**Left ventricular myxoma**
See *MYXOMA, INTRACARDIAC*
**Legg-Calve-Perthes disease (capital femoral epiphysis)**
See *HIP, OSTEONECROSIS, CAPITAL FEMORAL EPIPHYSIS*
**Legs, bowing of anterior-dwarfism**
See *SKELETAL DYSPLASIA, WEISMANN-NETTER-STUHL TYPE*
**Leiber sternal clefts and telangiectasia/hemangiomas**
See *STERNAL MALFORMATION-VASCULAR DYSPLASIA ASSOCIATION*
**Leigh disease**
See *ENCEPHALOPATHY, NECROTIZING*
**Leigh necrotizing encephalopathy (some cases)**
See *PYRUVATE CARBOXYLASE DEFICIENCY WITH LACTIC ACIDEMIA*
**Leigh syndrome (some cases)**
See *MYOPATHY-METABOLIC, MITOCHONDRIAL CYTOCHROME C OXIDASE DEFICIENCY*
**Leiners disease**
See *IMMUNODEFICIENCY, PLASMA-ASSOCIATED DEFECT OF PHAGOCYTOSIS*
**Leiomyomata, hereditary multiple, of skin**
See *SKIN, LEIOMYOMAS, MULTIPLE*
**Leiomyomata, multiple cutaneous**
See *SKIN, LEIOMYOMAS, MULTIPLE*
**Leiomyosarcoma**
See *CANCER, SOFT TISSUE SARCOMA*

## LENS AND PUPIL, ECTOPIC 0583

**Includes:** Pupil and lens, ectopic

**Excludes:** Lens, ectopic (0584)

**Major Diagnostic Criteria:** Dislocation of the pupil and lens.

**Clinical Findings:** Incomplete dislocation (subluxation) of both lenses with ectopic pupils is present at birth. Usually the lenses and pupils are displaced in opposite directions with the lenses most frequently displaced inferiorly. The direction may vary, however, and rare patients exhibit considerable asymmetry in the 2 eyes. The pupil is often oval or slit-shaped. Vision is often reduced and monocular diplopia may be present. Aphakic vision is sometimes seen. Transillumination of the iris is sometimes but not always present.

**Complications:** Aphakia, **Glaucoma, congenital**, retinal detachment.

**Associated Findings:** None known.

**Etiology:** Autosomal recessive inheritance.

**Pathogenesis:** Unknown.

**MIM No.:** *22520

**CDC No.:** 743.440

**Sex Ratio:** M1:F1

**Occurrence:** Undetermined but presumed rare.

**Risk of Recurrence for Patient's Sib:**
See Part I, *Mendelian Inheritance.*

**Risk of Recurrence for Patient's Child:**
See Part I, *Mendelian Inheritance.*

**Age of Detectability:** At birth.

**Gene Mapping and Linkage:** Unknown.

**Prevention:** None known. Genetic counseling indicated.

**Treatment:** Optical iridectomy or lens extraction may (rarely) be needed.

**Prognosis:** Normal life span, ocular prognosis dependent upon degree of defect.

**Detection of Carrier:** Unknown.

**References:**
Franceschetti A: Ectopia lentis et pupillae congenita als rezessives Erbleiden und ihre Manifestierung durch Konsanguinität. Klin Monatsbl Augenheilkd 1927; 78:351–362.

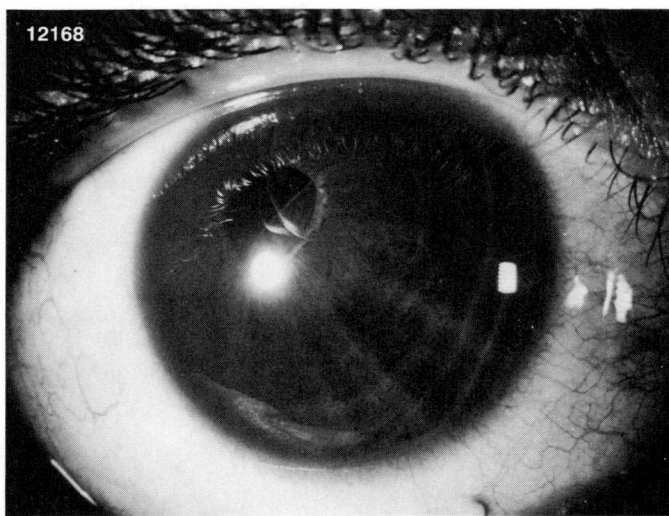

**0583-12168:** Ectopic lens and pupil.

Lueffers JA, et al.: Iris transillumination and variable expression in ectopic lens and pupil. Am J Ophthalmol 1977; 83:647–656.
Cross HE: Ectopic lens and pupil. Am J Ophthalmol 1979; 88:381–384. *

CR012

**Harold E. Cross**

**Lens opacities**
*See* CATARACTS
**Lens, aniridia**
*See* ANIRIDIA

## LENS, APHAKIA 0084

**Includes:** Aphakia

**Excludes:** Surgical aphakia

**Major Diagnostic Criteria:** Complete absence of the lens or presence of remnants.

**Clinical Findings:** Aphakia, or absence of the lens, may be divided into primary and secondary types. Primary aphakia is very rare and more serious than the secondary form because it is usually accompanied by gross malformations of the eye such as aplasia of the anterior segment, severe microphthalmia, or anophthalmia.

Secondary aphakia implies degeneration or rupture and absorption of the lens. This may occur without other eye disorders. Lens capsule remnants, often vascularized with fibrous tissue formation, are visualized along with ill-formed zonules within the pupil, which generally dilates poorly.

**Complications:** Visual impairment.

**Associated Findings:** Anterior segment anomalies, microphthalmia, anophthalmia, cataract in the opposite eye, facial malformations, retinal colobomas, nystagmus, congenital retinal folds, harelip, cleft palate, strabismus, and mental retardation; also seen in **Oculo-mandibulo-facial syndrome** and chromosomal aberrations.

**Etiology:** Undetermined. Possible intrauterine inflammation, teratogenic agents, or chromosomal abnormality. Occurs also in rats and pigs.

**Pathogenesis:** In primary aphakia an arrest or failure of development of the lens plate has been postulated. Secondary aphakia results from reabsorption of the lens. This may follow spontaneous rupture of an abnormally thin lens capsule or abnormality in either the surface ectoderm or lens fibers.

**CDC No.:** 743.300

**Sex Ratio:** Presumably M1:F1

**Occurrence:** Secondary more common than primary, but exact occurrence undetermined.

**Risk of Recurrence for Patient's Sib:** Unknown.

**Risk of Recurrence for Patient's Child:** Unknown.

**Age of Detectability:** Primary: at birth. Secondary: at birth or postnatally.

**Gene Mapping and Linkage:** Unknown.

**Prevention:** None known. Genetic counseling indicated.

**Treatment:** Correct refractive error whenever possible. Enucleation may be necessary if eye is grossly abnormal and cosmetically disfiguring. An oculoprothesis is inserted after enucleation.

**Prognosis:** Vision adequate-to-good in the presence of an otherwise normal eye. Vision guarded-to-poor dependent upon associated eye anomalies.

**Detection of Carrier:** Unknown.

**References:**
Mann I: Developmental abnormalities of the eye. Philadelphia: J.B. Lippincott, 1957:301–303.
Manschot WA: Primary congenital aphakia. Arch Ophthalmol 1963; 69:571.

Pratt JC, Richards RD: Bilateral secondary congenital aphakia. Arch Ophthalmol 1968; 80:420.

RA004

Elsa K. Rahn

## LENS, ECTOPIC                    0584

**Includes:**
Ectopia lentis, congenital
Ocular lens, dislocation of
Subluxation of lens

**Excludes:**
**Aciduria, sulfite oxidase deficiency** (0921)
**Homocystinuria** (0474)
**Lens and pupil, ectopic** (0583)
**Marfan syndrome** (0630)
**Spherophakia-brachymorphia syndrome** (0893)

**Major Diagnostic Criteria:** Dislocation of lens; if minimal, may require dilated slit-lamp biomicroscopy for diagnosis.

**Clinical Findings:** Isolated incomplete dislocation (subluxation) of the lens may be present at birth or occur later. The patient may have no symptoms or may complain of poor vision and monocular diplopia. Physical signs include iridodonesis, irregularly deep anterior chambers and uncorrected poor visual acuity in some cases. Bilateral dislocation is the rule. The lens is usually displaced upward and temporally.

**Complications: Glaucoma, congenital, cataract,** detached retina.

**Associated Findings: Cataract, Myopia, congenital,** astigmatism, **Aniridia,** persistent pupillary membrane, colobomas. Joint stiffness and dolichostenomelia have also been reported in one Black and one white family.

**Etiology:** Autosomal dominant inheritance. Most likely, heterogeneity exists with at least two recognizable disorders: simple ectopia lentis as a congenital, usually benign abnormality, and spontaneous late subluxation which is usually detected after the 3rd decade of life and often complicated by glaucoma.

**Pathogenesis:** Structural defect of lens zonules which may relate to persistence of the vascular tunic of the lens. Histologic studies show an absence of zonular fibers at the capsular attachments.

**MIM No.:** *12960

**CDC No.:** 743.330

**Sex Ratio:** M1:F1

**Occurrence:** Undetermined. Established literature.

**Risk of Recurrence for Patient's Sib:**
See Part I, *Mendelian Inheritance.*

**Risk of Recurrence for Patient's Child:**
See Part I, *Mendelian Inheritance.*

**Age of Detectability:** Usually at birth.

**Gene Mapping and Linkage:** Unknown.

**Prevention:** None known. Genetic counseling indicated.

**Treatment:** Optical iridectomy; cataract extraction when indicated.

**Prognosis:** Normal life span, ocular prognosis guarded.

**Detection of Carrier:** Unknown.

**References:**
Jaureguy BM, Hall JG: Isolated congenital ectopia lentis with autosomal dominant inheritance. Clin Genet 1979; 15:97–109. *
Nelson LB, Maumenee IH: Ectopic lentis: survey. Ophthalmology 1982; 27:143–160.
Stevenson RE, et al.: Dislocated lens, dolichostenomelia, and joint stiffness. Proc Greenwood Genet Center 1982; 1:16–22.

CR012

Harold E. Cross

## LENS, MICROSPHEROPHAKIA                    0663

**Includes:**
Microphakia and spherophakia, congenital
Microspherophakia

**Excludes:**
Acquired microphakia and spherophakia
**Spherophakia-brachymorphia syndrome** (0893)

**Major Diagnostic Criteria:** Small spherical lens within a dilated pupil.

**Clinical Findings:** Microphakia and spherophakia are usually concurrent. The lens has a smaller than normal diameter and is spherical in shape. The anterior-posterior measurement is increased and may cause the lens to protrude forward into the anterior chamber. This forward protrusion and close apposition of the lens to the iris may, in later life, result in glaucoma. Glaucoma in infancy is generally concomitant with abnormalities within the anterior chamber. The periphery of the lens is readily outlined with the pupil dilated. The zonules can also be visualized as radial strands between the pupillary and lens margins. Subluxation or luxation of the lens may occur from rupture of poorly developed, elongated and weakened zonules. Microspherophakia usually occurs bilaterally as an isolated phenomenon.

**Complications:** Myopia, cataract, glaucoma, subluxation or luxation of the lens.

**Associated Findings:** None known.

**Etiology:** Affected siblings and parental consanguinity suggest autosomal recessive inheritance of isolated defect. May be sporadic. When associated with other syndromes, it follows the inheritance mode of that symptom complex.

**Pathogenesis:** Arrest in development of the lens between the fifth or sixth fetal month. It has been postulated that an inadequate blood supply from the vascular tunic of the lens, or improper support secondary to faulty zonular development are possible mechanisms of pathogenesis.

**MIM No.:** 25175

**CDC No.:** 743.310

**Sex Ratio:** M1:F1

**Occurrence:** Undetermined, but literature over the past 70 years suggest that the condition is rare.

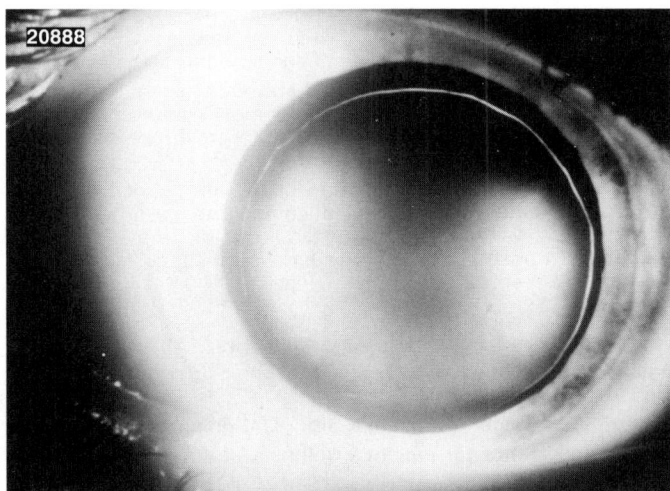

**0663-20888:** Spherophakia; note the edge of the lens is seen within the pupil.

**Risk of Recurrence for Patient's Sib:**
See Part I, *Mendelian Inheritance*.

**Risk of Recurrence for Patient's Child:**
See Part I, *Mendelian Inheritance*.

**Age of Detectability:** At birth.

**Gene Mapping and Linkage:** Unknown.

**Prevention:** None known. Genetic counseling indicated.

**Treatment:** Correction of existing refractive errors, usually myopia, due to the increased anterior-posterior diameter. Surgery is indicated if glaucoma occurs as a complication.

**Prognosis:** Generally good.

**Detection of Carrier:** Unknown.

**References:**
Waardenburg PJ, et al.: Genetics and ophthalmology. vol. 1. Springfield: Charles C Thomas, 1961.
Duke-Elder S: System of ophthalmology. vol. 3, part 2. Congenital deformities. London: Henry Kimpton, 1963:694.

RA004 **Elsa K. Rahn**

---

## LENTICONUS 0585

**Includes:** N/A

**Excludes:**
**Cornea, megalocornea** (0637)
**Eye, keratoconus** (0552)

**Major Diagnostic Criteria:** Protrusion of the anterior or posterior surface of the lens in either a conical (conus) or a spherical (globus) shape. Slit-lamp exam can confirm protruded lens surface.

**Clinical Findings:** The anterior variety usually presents as bilateral localized thickenings of the anterior lens cortex. The central lens may be clear. Although probably present at birth, the youngest described patient was 4 years old. The deformity may be progressive leading to further diminution of vision.

An oil globule appearance is characteristic of the posterior variety. Central high myopia is also found. On slit-lamp examination there is a ring reflex. This condition is usually unilateral. Visual acuity may be poor due to opacification of the posterior lens capsule. A remnant of the hyaloid artery is often seen attached.

**Complications:** Anterior polar cataracts may develop in anterior lenticonus, and posterior cateracts in posterior lenticonus.

**Associated Findings:** Posterior polar lens opacities are common (80%) concomitant features of posterior lentiglobus. Other associations include uveal colobomas, microphthalmos, lens colobomas, oxycephaly, deafness, hypertelorism and **Nephritis-deafness (sensorineural), hereditary type**. Associated defects are rare in anterior lenticonus, although it has been reported with **Fetal rubella syndrome** and a variety of forms of congenital cataract.

**Etiology:** Most cases are isolated, although rare families have been reported. Bilateral involvement is more common in familial cases. Both autosomal dominant and autosomal recessive inheritance have been reported.

**Pathogenesis:** Delayed separation of the lens vesicle from the surface epithelium in anterior lenticonus, and posterior hyaloid artery persistence with a weak posterior capsule or overgrowth of lens fibers in posterior lentiglobus have been suggested to be the mechanisms responsible for the defects.

**CDC No.:** 743.380

**Sex Ratio:** Lenticonus M1F<1; Lentiglobus M2:F3

**Occurrence:** Estimated at 1:100,000 births. Anterior lenticonus is rarer than posterior lentiglobus.

**Risk of Recurrence for Patient's Sib:** Unknown.

**Risk of Recurrence for Patient's Child:** Unknown.

**Age of Detectability:** At birth.

**Gene Mapping and Linkage:** Unknown.

**Prevention:** None known. Genetic counseling indicated.

**Treatment:** Lens extraction where indicated.

**Prognosis:** Life span normal; visual prognosis variable.

**Detection of Carrier:** Unknown.

**References:**
Howitt D, Hornblass A: Posterior lenticonus. Am J Ophthalmol 1968; 66:1133–1136.
Pollard ZF: Familial bilateral posterior lenticonus. Arch Ophthalmol 1983; 101:1238–1240.
Felt D, et al.: Infantile leucocoria caused by posterior lenticonus. Ann Ophthalmol 1984; 16:679–684.

CR012 **Harold E. Cross**

**Lenticular cataract**
*See CATARACT, AUTOSOMAL DOMINANT CONGENITAL*

---

## LENTIGINES SYNDROME, MULTIPLE 0586

**Includes:**
Cardiocutaneous syndrome
Cardiomyopathic lentiginosis
Generalized lentigo
Lentiginosis profusa syndrome
Leopard syndrome
Multiple lentigines syndrome
Progressive cardiomyopathic lentiginosis

**Excludes:**
**Mitral regurgitation-deafness-skeletal defects** (0667)
**Nevi-atrial myxoma-myxoid neurofibromas-ephelides** (2572)
**Noonan syndrome** (0720)
**Pulmonic stenosis-cafe-au-lait spots, Watson type** (2776)
Unilateral lentigo

**Major Diagnostic Criteria:** The diagnosis should be considered in a patient with some combination of multiple lentigines, EKG conduction defect, **Eye, hypertelorism, Pulmonary valve, stenosis,** growth retardation, sensorineural hearing loss, and genital defects.

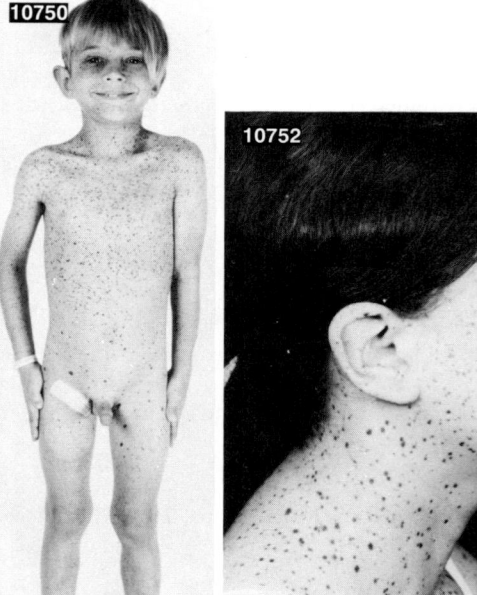

0586-10750–52: Multiple lentigines are present in a universal distribution.

**Clinical Findings:** The syndrome consists of multiple lentigines that are 2–8 mm in diameter and scattered over the face, scalp, neck, trunk, genitalia, upper limbs, palms and soles. They are sparser below the knees (ca. 80%) and the mucous membranes are spared; café "noir" spots occur in 20%. The lentigines may present at birth or during childhood and increase in number and darken with age. Biopsy of the lentigines reveals intracellular giant pigment granules similar to those found in neurofibromatosis. EKG abnormalities indicate axis deviations, unilateral or bilateral hypertrophy, and conduction abnormalities (prolonged P-R interval, hemiblock, bundle branch block, complete heart block) of varying severity in 60%. Other findings include ocular hypertelorism (ca. 25%); pulmonary stenosis, either valvular or infundibular (ca. 50%); aortic or mitral stenosis, obstructive cardiomyopathy (20%); abnormalities of the genitalia, such as cryptorchidism (ca. 15%); retardation of growth (ca. 35%) and sensorineural hearing loss (ca. 20%). Mild mental retardation has been noted in about 30% of cases, while oculomotor deficits occur in about 50%.

**Complications:** Sterility, if cryptorchidism is bilateral; speech difficulties.

**Associated Findings:** Other less common findings include triangular face with biparietal bossing, eyelid ptosis, delayed primary dentition, delayed puberty and various skeletal abnormalities such as kyphoscoliosis, **Pectus carinatum** or **Pectus excavatum**, winging of scapulae, and multiple granular cell myoblastomas.

**Etiology:** Autosomal dominant inheritance with variable expressivity.

**Pathogenesis:** Undetermined. Possibly a neurocristopathy.

**MIM No.:** *15110

**POS No.:** 3277

**Sex Ratio:** M1:F1

**Occurrence:** About 75 cases reported in the literature.

**Risk of Recurrence for Patient's Sib:**
See Part I, *Mendelian Inheritance.*

**Risk of Recurrence for Patient's Child:**
See Part I, *Mendelian Inheritance.* Affected males may have a somewhat reduced reproductive fitness due to cryptorchidism.

**Age of Detectability:** Four to 5 years of age, since lentigines usually become abundant by this time; possibly earlier if there is an involved sib.

**Gene Mapping and Linkage:** Unknown.

**Prevention:** None known. Genetic counseling indicated.

**Treatment:** Surgical correction of cryptorchidism and possibly of cardiac lesion.

**Prognosis:** Good, the pulmonary stenosis is rarely seriously disabling. Intellectual deficit occurs infrequently, and speech difficulties may be caused by deafness.

**Detection of Carrier:** Detailed examination will usually allow detection of affected individuals who do not have lentigines.

**References:**
Gorlin RJ, et al.: Multiple lentigines syndrome: complex comprising multiple lentigenes, electrocardiographic conduction abnormalities, ocular hypertelorism, pulmonary stenosis, abnormalities of genitalia, retardation of growth, sensorineural deafness and autosomal dominant hereditary pattern. Am J Dis Child 1969; 117:652–662.
Gorlin RJ, et al.: The LEOPARD (multiple lentigines) syndrome revisited. BD:OAS;VII(4). Baltimore: The Williams & Wilkins Co. for The National Foundation - March of Dimes, 1971:110–115.
Polani PE, Moynahan EJ: Progressive cardiopathic lentigines. Q J Med 1972; 41:205–225.
Seuanez H, et al.: Cardio-cutaneous syndrome (the "LEOPARD" syndrome): review of the literature and a new family. Clin Genet 1976; 9:266–276.
Voron DA, et al.: Multiple lentigines syndrome: case report and review of the literature. Am J Med 1976; 60:447–456.
Weiss LW, Zelickson AS: Giant melanosomes in multiple lentigines syndrome. Arch Dermatol 1977; 113:491–494.
St. John Sutton MG, et al.: Hypertrophic obstructive cardiomyopathy and lentiginosis: a little known neural ectodermal syndrome. Am J Cardiol 1981; 47:214–217.

G0038                                    **Robert J. Gorlin**

**Lentigines-peptic ulcer/hiatal hernia-hypertelorism-myopia**
*See GASTROCUTANEOUS SYNDROME*
**Lentiginosis profusa syndrome**
*See LENTIGINES SYNDROME, MULTIPLE*
**Lenz dysmorphogenetic syndrome**
*See LENZ MICROPHTHALMIA SYNDROME*
**Lenz dysplasia**
*See LENZ MICROPHTHALMIA SYNDROME*

## LENZ MICROPHTHALMIA SYNDROME                    3171

**Includes:**
Anophthalmos with associated anomalies
Lenz dysplasia
Lenz dysmorphogenetic syndrome
Microphthalmia with associated anomalies

**Excludes:**
**Charge association** (2124)
**Anophthalmia-limb defects, Waardenburg type** (2784)

**Major Diagnostic Criteria:** Microphthalmos is present in all cases. Other abnormalities include developmental retardation in 92% of cases, external ear abnormalities in 83% of cases, **Microcephaly** in 83% of cases, blepharoptosis (see **Eyelid, ptosis, congenital**) in 75% of cases, skeletal abnormalities in 67% of cases, dental abnormalities of number and position in 67% of cases, digital anomalies in 58% of cases, urogenital anomalies in 50% of cases and **Cleft lip/Cleft palate** abnormalities in one-third of patients.

**Clinical Findings:** The various congenital malformations associated with this syndrome are discovered at birth. The microphthalmos is usually bilateral and asymmetrical, colobomatous or non-colobomatous, and may even be extreme with clinical anophthalmia. The earlobes are usually large and protruding with thin hypoplastic antihelices, but may be small and hypoplastic. Teeth may be crowded or widely spaced. Skeletal abnormalities are most prominent in the thoracic cage, which is barrel-shaped

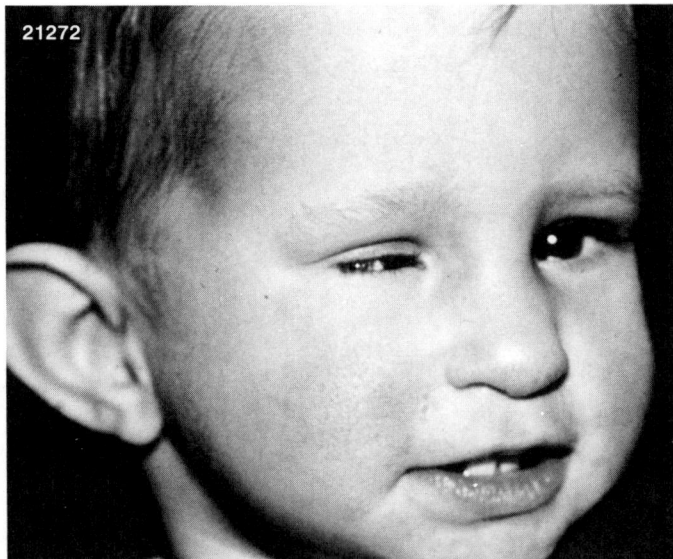

**3171-21272:** Three-year-old boy with the Lenz microphthalmia syndrome; note the bilateral microphthalmia more severe on the right, and the thin, anteverted protruding earlobes.

with kyphoscoliosis and occasional gibbus formation. Thinning of the lateral third of the clavicles is a particular finding in some patients. **Microcephaly** is present in a majority of patients, and developmental retardation ranging from mild to profound seems to be a universal finding. Digital anomalies, though found in only 58% of cases, are helpful in differentiating this syndrome from other malformation syndromes featuring microphthalmia; clinodactyly, **Camptodactyly**, and **Syndactyly** are most commonly observed, however thumb duplication has been noted in some patients. Clinically evident heart disease is not a feature of this syndrome, but autopsy on Lenz's original patient revealed a bicuspid arotic valve. Urogenital anomalies include cryptorchidism, renal hypoplasia and renal aplasia.

**Complications:** Retinal detachment has been observed in one patient.

**Associated Findings:** Cardiac anomalies, imperforate anus, hearing loss, spastic diplegia, sacral pits, webbed neck, and abnormal dermatoglyphs.

**Etiology:** X-linked recessive inheritance.

**Pathogenesis:** Unknown.

**MIM No.:** *30980

**POS No.:** 3277

**Sex Ratio:** M1:F0

**Occurrence:** Twelve documented cases have been reported.

**Risk of Recurrence for Patient's Sib:**
See Part I, *Mendelian Inheritance.*

**Risk of Recurrence for Patient's Child:**
See Part I, *Mendelian Inheritance.*

**Age of Detectability:** At birth. Fetal ultrasonography may detect major malformations in a fetus who has an affected sibling.

**Gene Mapping and Linkage:** MAA (microphthalmia or anophthalmia and associated anomalies) has been mapped to X.

**Prevention:** None known. Genetic counseling indicated.

**Treatment:** Surgical correction of malformations as indicated.

**Prognosis:** Good for life; poor for vision. Mental retardation is a universal finding, though mild in some cases.

**Detection of Carrier:** Carrier females may have digital anomalies, microcephaly and short stature.

**References:**
Lenz W: Recessivgeschlechtsgebundene mikrophtalmie mit multiplen Missbildunger. Z Kinderheilkd 1955; 77:384–390.
Hoefnagel D, et al: Heredofamilial bilateral anophthalmia. Arch Ophthalmol 1963; 69:760–764.
Goldberg MF, McKusick VA: X-linked colobomatous microphthalmos and other congenital anomalies: a disorder resembling Lenz's dysmorphogenetic syndrome. Am J Ophthalmol 1971; 71:1128–1133.
Traboulsi EI, et al: The Lenz microphthalmia syndrome. Am J Ophthalmol 1988; 105:40–45. * †

TR009 **Elias I. Traboulsi**

**Lenz-Majewski hyperostotic dwarfism**
*See CRANIODIAPHYSEAL DYSPLASIA, LENZ-MAJEWSKI TYPE*
**Leopard syndrome**
*See LENTIGINES SYNDROME, MULTIPLE*

---

| LEPRECHAUNISM | 0587 |
|---|---|

**Includes:**
Donohue syndrome
Insulin receptor, defect in
Insulin resistance, familial severe

**Excludes:**
Skin, acanthosis nigricans (0005)
Chromosome 8, trisomy 8 (0157)
Cockayne syndrome (0189)
Diabetes mellitus, maturity onset of the young (MODY) (2326)
Diabetes mellitus, non-insulin dependent type (2327)

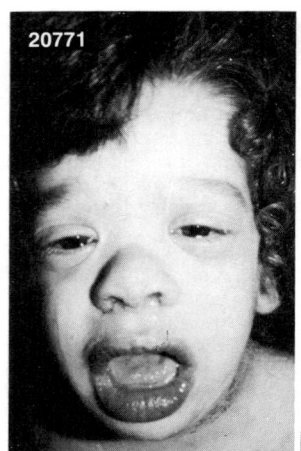
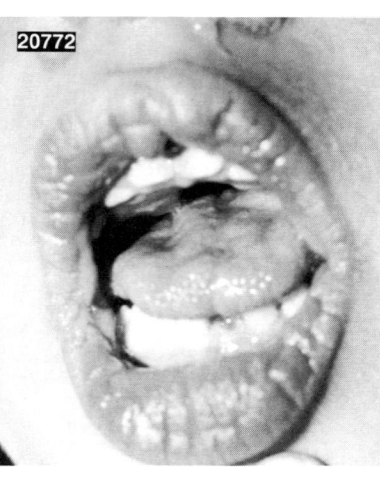

0587A-20771: Leprechaunism; note coarse facies with thick lips, coarse hair, hirsutism. 20772: Furrowed tongue and lips.

---

Lipodystrophy-coarse facies-acanthosis nigricans, Miescher type (2423)
Lipodystrophy, familial limb and trunk (2614)
Myotonic dystrophy (0702)
Skin, acanthosis nigricans (0005)

**Major Diagnostic Criteria:** A diagnosis of leprechaunism is made on the basis of clinical and laboratory findings. A presumptive clinical diagnosis of leprechaunism may be made if a newborn presents as small for gestational age with failure to thrive; elfin facies; thick lips; pachyderma; hirsutism; and relatively prominent breasts, hands, feet; **Skin, acanthosis nigricans**; and external genitalia. The clinical diagnosis is supported by the laboratory dem-

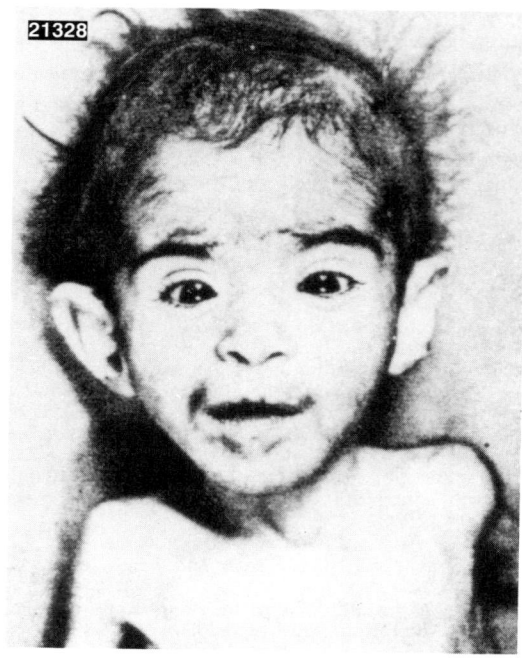

0587B-21328: Small face with prominent eyes, wide nostrils, large mouth, large ears, and hirsutism.

onstration of insulin resistance with hyperinsulinemia, fasting hypoglycemia, and postprandial hyperglycemia. Absence of antibodies to insulin and the insulin receptor is included. Pathohistology includes increased hepatic glycogen, hyperplasia of the endocrine pancreas, and ovarian cystic changes.

Laboratory diagnosis requires finding markedly decreased binding of insulin to the patient's cultured cells.

**Clinical Findings:** Leprechaunism is characterized by continued small stature; elfin facies, with a flat nasal bridge and flaring nostrils; thick lips; hirsutism; pachyderma, acanthosis nigricans; and breast enlargement. Because of small size, there is relative prominence of the clitoris and labia minora or penis, as well as ears, hands, and feet. There is a deficiency of subcutaneous tissue leading to the presence of excessive folding of the skin (pachyderma). Motor and mental retardation and severe failure to thrive are common sequelae.

Other less frequently noted features include **Microcephaly**, hypertelorism, high or narrowly arched palate, cardiac murmur, umbilical and inguinal herniae or diastasis recti, cryptorchidism, poor muscle tone, unusually large hands and feet, and delayed skeletal maturation.

**Complications:** Susceptibility to infection, hypoglycemia, early death.

**Associated Findings:** Intrauterine growth restriction.

**Etiology:** Autosomal recessive inheritance. Decreased-to-absent high-affinity insulin binding can be used as a genetic discriminant in cultured dermal fibroblasts. Several different mutant alleles involving the alpha subunit (insulin binding domain) of the insulin receptor gene have been identified.

**Pathogenesis:** A primary mutation in the insulin receptor gene results in decreased utilization of secreted insulin and end-organ resistance to insulin binding and signaling. The growth-promoting, embryologic effects of insulin are blunted, producing intrauterine growth restriction. Many different mutations with variably altered end-organ resistance are described. One mutation has absent insulin binding to the fibroblast insulin receptor with increased, noninsulin-responsive glucose transport. This may account for recurrent hypoglycemia in the presence of normal glycogen stores.

**MIM No.:** *24620

**POS No.:** 3278

**CDC No.:** 759.870

**Sex Ratio:** M1:F1

**Occurrence:** About 50 cases reported in the literature.

**Risk of Recurrence for Patient's Sib:**
See Part I, *Mendelian Inheritance.*

**Risk of Recurrence for Patient's Child:**
See Part I, *Mendelian Inheritance.* Most affected individuals do not survive to reproduce.

**Age of Detectability:** During early infancy. Prenatal monitoring using restriction fragment length polymorphism analysis of the insulin receptor gene is available.

**Gene Mapping and Linkage:** Mutations in the insulin receptor gene (19p13.2→13.3).

**Prevention:** None known. Genetic counseling indicated.

**Treatment:** Various complications, particularly infections and hypoglycemia, should be treated as indicated. Utilization of gastrostomy feedings has been of benefit in some cases.

**Prognosis:** Most classic patients have died in early childhood. A few, who are compound heterozygotes for two different alleles, survive childhood.

**Detection of Carrier:** By decreased insulin binding or DNA analysis if the exact mutation is known. Some severe mutations may be expressed in the heterozygote as **Diabetes mellitus, non-insulin dependent type**. Type A insulin resistance with acanthosis nigricans has been associated with mutations in the insulin receptor gene. Insulin binding may be normal in these patients.

**References:**
D'Ercole AJ, et al.: Leprechaunism: studies of the relationship among hyperinsulinism, insulin resistance, and growth retardation. J Clin Endocrinol Metab 1979; 48:495.
Elsas LJ, et al.: Leprechaunism: an inherited defect in insulin-receptor interaction. In: Wapnir RA, ed: Congenital metabolic diseases: diagnosis and treatment. New York: Marcel Dekker, 1985:301–334.
Elsas LJ, et al.: Leprechaunism: an inherited defect in a high-affinity insulin receptor. Am J Hum Genet 1985; 37:73–88.
Yang-Feng TL, et al.: Gene for human insulin receptor: localization to site on chromosome 19 involved in pre-β cell leukemia. Science 1985; 228:728–730.
Cantani A, et al.: A rare polydysmorphic syndrome: leprechaunism - review of 49 cases reported in the literature. Ann Genet 1987; 30:221–227.
Elsas LJ, Longo N: Impaired insulin binding and excess glucose transport in fibroblasts from a patient with leprechaunism. Enzyme 1987; 38:184–193.
Endo F, et al.: Structural analysis of normal and mutant insulin receptors in fibroblasts cultured from families with leprechaunism. Am J Hum Genet 1987; 4:102–106.
Elsas LJ, et al.: Comparison of the insulin receptor gene and insulin binding in families with severe insulin resistance. Trans Asso Am Phys 1988; CI:137–148.
Kadowaki T, et al.: Two mutant alleles of the insulin receptor gene in a patient with extreme insulin resistance. Science 1988; 240:787–790.
Kahn CR, Goldstein BJ: Molecular defects in insulin action. Science 1989; 245:13–14.
Taira M, et al: Human diabetes associated with deletion of the tyrosine kinase domain of the insulin receptor. Science 1989; 245:63–65.

EL009                                    **Louis J. Elsas, II**

## LERI PLEONOSTEOSIS SYNDROME                2102

**Includes:** Pleonosteosis

**Excludes:**
**Dyschondrosteosis** (0308)
**Mucopolysaccharidosis**

**Major Diagnostic Criteria:** Limitation of joint movement and flexion contractures of interphalangeal joints.

**Clinical Findings:** Broad, deformed, thumbs and great toes; short stature; and flattened facies. Enlargement of the posterior neural arches of the cervical vertebrae has been reported as a significant diagnostic X-ray finding.

**Complications:** Cervical cord compression due to stenosis of the cervical canal has been reported. Carpal tunnel compression of the median nerve and Morton metatarsalgia have also been reported.

**Associated Findings:** Blepharophimosis and microcornea have been reported.

**Etiology:** Autosomal dominant inheritance with variable expression.

**Pathogenesis:** Unknown.

**MIM No.:** *15120

**POS No.:** 3615

**Sex Ratio:** M1:F1

**Occurrence:** Over 20 cases have been reported.

**Risk of Recurrence for Patient's Sib:**
See Part I, *Mendelian Inheritance.*

**Risk of Recurrence for Patient's Child:**
See Part I, *Mendelian Inheritance.*

**Age of Detectability:** In early childhood.

**Gene Mapping and Linkage:** Unknown.

**Prevention:** None known. Genetic counseling indicated.

**Treatment:** Conservative, symptomatic treatment in most cases.

**Prognosis:** Normal intelligence and life span.

**Detection of Carrier:** Possibly on the basis of X-ray changes.

**References:**

Leri A: Une maladie congenitale et hereditaire de l'ossification: la pleonosteose familiale. Bull Soc Med Paris 1921; 45:1228.

Watson-Jones R: Leri's pleonosteosis, carpal tunnel compression of the median nerves and Morton's metatarsalgia. J Bone Joint Surg 1949; 31B:560–571.

Rukavina JG, et al.: Leri's pleonosteosis: a study of a family with a review of the literature. J Bone Joint Surg 1959; 41A:397–408.

Hilton RC, Wentzel J: Leri's pleonosteosis. Q J Med 1980; 49:419–429.

Friedman M, et al.: Leri's pleonosteosis. Brit J Radiol 1981; 54:517–518.

Metcalfe RA, Butler P: Spinal cord compression in Leri's pleonosteosis. Brit J Radiol 1985; 58:1117–1119.

GR011                                            **Frank Greenberg**

**Leri-Weill disease**
  *See DYSCHONDROSTEOSIS*
**Leroy disease**
  *See MUCOLIPIDOSIS II*

---

## LESCH-NYHAN SYNDROME                                      0588

**Includes:**
  Hyperuricemia, X-linked primary
  Hypoxanthine guanine phosphoribosyl transferase (HGPRT) deficiency
  Uric acid metabolism-central nervous system disorder

**Excludes:**
  **Adenine phospho-ribosyl-transferase (APRT) deficiency** (3104)
  **Gout** (0441)
  HGPRT, partial variants of

**Major Diagnostic Criteria:** Patients with complete absence of hypoxanthine guanine phosphoribosyl transferase (HGPRT) activity with resulting hyperuricemia (see **Gout**) and evidence of cerebral dysfunction; choreoathetosis, **Cerebral palsy**, mental retardation, and self-mutilation.

**Clinical Findings:** Patients appear normal at birth but develop progressive choreoathetosis and spastic cerebral palsy. Mental

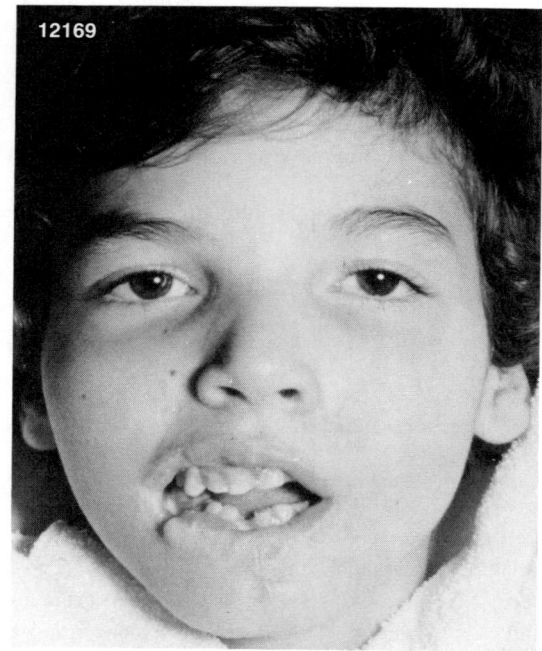

**0588**-12169: Lesch-Nyhan syndrome. Note self-mutilation of lips.

retardation and motor defects are such that these patients do not walk and few can sit without assistance. They are characterized by bizarre aggressive behavior; its most prominent manifestation is self-mutilation, usually by biting. In addition to the features relevant to the nervous system, these patients have all the clinical findings of gout, including hyperuricemia, hematuria, crystalluria, urinary tract stones, nephropathy, tophi, and acute arthritis. Mild anemia may be encountered and megaloblasts are occasionally seen in the marrow.

**Complications:** Nephropathy; renal failure; athetoid dysphagia is extreme and vomiting is prominent; thus these patients are hard to feed. They may die of inanition or aspiration and pneumonia, as well as of renal failure.

**Associated Findings:** None known.

**Etiology:** X-linked recessive inheritance.

**Pathogenesis:** Absence of hypoxanthine guanine phosphoribosyl transferase (HGPRT) activity. The manner in which this leads to the cerebral manifestations of the disease is unknown.

**MIM No.:** *30800

**POS No.:** 3279

**Sex Ratio:** M1:F0

**Occurrence:** About 1:100,000 births.

**Risk of Recurrence for Patient's Sib:**
  See Part I, *Mendelian Inheritance.*

**Risk of Recurrence for Patient's Child:**
  See Part I, *Mendelian Inheritance.*

**Age of Detectability:** At birth; it is now possible to detect prior to birth by assay of the enzyme in cultured cells obtained by amniocentesis. Gibbs et al (1984) have reported the use of chorionic villus biopsy and employed enzyme assay to diagnose Lesch-Nyhan syndrome in the first trimester.

**Gene Mapping and Linkage:** HPRT (hypoxanthine phosphoribosyltransferase) has been mapped to Xq26.

**Prevention:** None known. Genetic counseling indicated.

**Treatment:** As for gout, Allopurinol is excellent therapy for the management of hyperuricemia. It will prevent all of those manifestations of this disease that are direct consequences of elevated concentrations of uric acid. It does not prevent or alleviate the cerebral manifestations. Appropriate restraint binding of hands or elbows to prevent mutilation of hands is necessary.

**Prognosis:** In the absence of allopurinol most patients have died under five years of age. A few long survivors have lived to 20 years.

**Detection of Carrier:** Culture of fibroblasts from the skin and cloning have yielded two populations of cells from the maternal heterozygote. One population has normal enzyme activity and the other is completely deficient like the patient's. This identifies the carrier and is consistent with the Lyon hypothesis. Hair follicles are also largely clonal and they are the most practical method for the detection of the heterozygote by analysis of the enzyme activity in hair roots. The blood cannot be used for this purpose as the blood of the maternal carrier of this disease is always normal.

**References:**

Lesch M, Nyhan WL: A familial disorder of uric acid metabolism and central nervous system function. Am J Med 1964; 36:561–570. *

Bland J, ed: Proceedings of the seminars on the Lesch-Nyhan syndrome. Fed Proc 1968; 27:1019–1112.

Christie R, et al.: Lesch-Nyhan disease: clinical experience with nineteen patients. Develop Med Child Neurol 1982; 24:293–306.

Gibbs DA et al.: First trimester diagnosis of Lesch-Nyhan syndrome. Lancet 1984; 2:1180–1183.

Gibbs RA, Caskey CT: Identification and localization of mutations of the Lesch-Nyhan locus by ribonuclease A cleavage. Science 1987; 236:303–305.

Nyhan WL: Diagnostic recognition of genetic disease. Philadelphia: Lea & Febiger, 1987:1–8. *

NY000                                            **William L. Nyhan**

**Lethal congenital contracture syndrome**
*See CONTRACTURES, CONGENITAL LETHAL FINNISH TYPE*
**Lethal multiple pterygium syndrome**
*See PTERYGIUM SYNDROME, MULTIPLE LETHAL*
**Lethal osteopetrosis**
*See OSTEOPETROSIS, MALIGNANT RECESSIVE*
**Lethal, Larsen-like, multiple joint dislocations**
*See LARSEN SYNDROME, LETHAL TYPE*

## LETTERER-SIWE DISEASE 2181

**Includes:**
    Histiocytosis, acute disseminated
    Reticuloendotheliosis, nonlipoid
    Reticulosis, familial histiocytic

**Excludes:**
    Eosinophilic granuloma of bone
    Hand-Schuler-Christian disease
    **Immunodeficiency, reticuloendotheliosis with eosinophilia**
    (2688)

**Major Diagnostic Criteria:** 1) Onset in first year of life; 2) skin lesions, although variable in nature, often of the scalp; 3) organomegaly of liver and spleen; 4) adenopathy; and 5) pulmonary infiltration. The microscopic picture of the lesions shows a nodular or spreading infiltration containing numerous large histiocytes.

**Clinical Findings:** 1) Onset of signs in first year of life; 2) diffuse, papulous eruption of a vesicular nature; 3) scaly and petechial dermatitis, particularly on the forehead and trunk; 4) moist, denuded involvement in intertriginous areas; 5) seborrheic eruption of scalp and in ear canals; 6) stomatitis; 7) pulmonic infiltrations; 8) general adenopathy; 9) hepatomegaly; 10) splenomegaly; 11) fever; and 12) lytic osseous lesions, often of the cranium. Laboratory studies show only the nonspecific effects to be expected from the organ or tissue involvement. Anemia is common, and leukocytosis may occur.

**Complications:** General exhaustion, toxemia, bone marrow depletion, septicemia, and **Diabetes insipidus**.

**Associated Findings:** None known.

**Etiology:** Autosomal recessive inheritance with reduced (7/8ths) penetrance.

**Pathogenesis:** Progressive granulomatous process.

**MIM No.:** *24640

**Sex Ratio:** M1:F1

**Occurrence:** Extensive literature. No geographic predilection. One study found over 50 deaths per year in the United States from this condition.

**Risk of Recurrence for Patient's Sib:**
    See Part I, *Mendelian Inheritance*.

**Risk of Recurrence for Patient's Child:**
    See Part I, *Mendelian Inheritance*.

**Age of Detectability:** Within the first year of life.

**Gene Mapping and Linkage:** Unknown.

**Prevention:** None known. Genetic counseling indicated.

**Treatment:** None specific except for pitressin in the event of diabetes insipidus. Radiotherapy may affect individual bone lesions, skin eruptions, and large lymph nodes.

**Prognosis:** Fatal outcome when general process becomes advanced. Spontaneous recovery has been reported.

**Detection of Carrier:** Unknown.

**Special Considerations:** This or a similar disorder was reported by Kloepfer et al (1972) in an inbred triracial group in Louisiana known as the "Redbones".

**References:**
Schoeck VW, et al.: Familial occurrence of Letterer-Siwe disease. Pediatrics 1963; 32:1055–1063.
Juberg RC, et al.: Genetic determination of acute disseminated histiocytosis X (Letterer-Siwe syndrome). Pediatrics 1970; 45:753–765. * †

Kloepfer HW, et al.: Fulminating disseminated histiocytosis simulating Letterer-Siwe disease. BD:OAS VIII(3). New York: March of Dimes Birth Defects Foundation, 1972:112–114.
Frisell E, et al.: Familial occurrence of histiocytosis. Clin Genet 1977; 11:163–170.

JU000                                        **Richard C. Juberg**

**Leucine metabolism, defect in**
    *See ACIDEMIA, 3-HYDROXY-3-METHYLGLUTARIC*
**Leucine-sensitive hypoglycemia of infancy, familial**
    *See HYPOGLYCEMIA, FAMILIAL NEONATAL*

## LEUKEMIA, ACUTE LYMPHOCYTIC, FAMILIAL 3073

**Includes:**
    Acute lymphocytic leukemia (ALL)
    J. Chain
    Lymphocytic leukemia, cell type-childhood acute

**Excludes:** Cytogenetic and other syndromes that predispose to leukemia

**Major Diagnostic Criteria:** Two or more first-degree relatives with childhood (onset under age 15 years) acute lymphocytic leukemia.

**Clinical Findings:** Although the annual age-adjusted incidence of childhood leukemia is low (40 cases of leukemia per one million children under age 15 years), this malignancy accounts for 30% of childhood cancer. In Western countries, incidence rates of acute lymphocytic leukemia (ALL) are three times higher than those for acute nonlymphocytic leukemia (ANLL) among children, although ANLL comprises a substantially higher proportion of childhood leukemia in Japanese and other Asian children of all ages. Despite the relatively rare occurrence, familial childhood leukemia, particularly ALL, has been recognized for several decades. Familial aggregation of a number of types has been described, including a 20–25% concordance for ALL among identical twins following occurrence in one member of the pair; significantly increased risk of ALL among sibs of an affected child; and association with a number of congenital conditions characterized by chromosomal abnormalities and other hereditary disorders.

The clinical symptoms and course are usually indistinguishable from nonfamilial ALL of childhood, with the exception of the often striking similarity of age of onset (within a few months and usually in infancy) and age at death for concordant ALL in identical twins. Although four immunologic subtypes have become widely recognized since the advent of immunologic and enzymatic phenotyping in the 1970s, use of standardized immunophenotyping techniques has only recently become widespread. Separate examination of postulated risk factors by leukemia histologic cell type (ALL vs. ANLL) has only recently begun to occur in reports of epidemiologic studies, and the new immunologic subgroups have not been used in such studies.

**Complications:** Similar to sporadic childhood ALL, familial childhood ALL usually causes death by infection or hemorrhage. In the last couple of decades, survivorship has greatly improved due to increasingly effective combination chemotherapy and treatment prophylaxis with chemotherapy and radiation specifically directed at the central nervous system.

**Associated Findings:** None known.

**Etiology:** A number of postulated genetic, immunologic, and environmental factors have been identified. Clinical reports have implicated familial and nonfamilial congenital chromosomal abnormalities (including the Philadelphia or Ph[1] chromosome, inv(11)(p15q13), ring chromosomes, and others). Unlike the associations of **Retinoblastoma** and some cases of **Cancer, Wilms tumor** with specific constitutional chromosome abnormalities, no one specific chromosome deletion or other abnormality has been exclusively linked with childhood ALL, although **Chromosome 21, trisomy 21** has been associated with an increased risk of childhood ALL. Two large U.S. death certificate studies of 4,670 and 10,390 leukemia cases demonstrated a concordance of 20 to 25% for ALL among identical (probably monozygotic) twins. A similar study in England and Wales failed to identify any concordant pairs among 5,763 with childhood cancer (numbers of leukemia deaths not separately reported).

An excess risk of childhood leukemia has been observed among children with several hereditary conditions characterized by a tendency to chromosomal abnormalities or breaks, including **Chromosome 21, trisomy 21** (risk of leukemia of both major histologic types estimated as 1:74), **Bloom syndrome** (risk estimated as 1:8 before age 26 years), **Ataxia-telangiectasia** (1:8 before age 25 years), and **Pancytopenia syndrome, Fanconi type** (1:12 before age 21 years). Due to the rare nature of virtually all of the above conditions and the lack of population-based studies, the cumulative risk of subsequent childhood leukemia among subjects with each of these rare conditions represents an estimate, based on literature review.

As further evidence of a possible genetic basis of childhood ALL, aggregation of childhood leukemia in sibships can be demonstrated when the sample size is large enough (>1,000 sibs). A fourfold excess risk has been estimated from at least one large population-based study. Acute leukemia may also aggregate among sibs in families with other heritable leukemia-prone disorders, such as Bloom, Fanconi, and so forth. Thus, if leukemia occurs among two or more sibs, cytogenetic and immunologic tests should be undertaken within the family. The affected cases should also be studied in detail to determine if the morphology or natural history of childhood ALL in these families differs from usual. HLA studies suggest that the genetic background of patients with ALL may have restricted heterogeneity; there appears to be an increased occurrence of haplotype sharing in parents of patients with ALL. HLA genotypes of patients with ALL and those with acute myelocytic leukemia have been found more frequently than the expected 25% among their sibs. Although the HLA antigen types A2 and B12 have been associated in some reports with childhood ALL, these findings are not consistent, nor are associations with specific haplotypes.

There have been reports of familial childhood ALL occurring in families with many consanguineous marriages. One group of investigators has suggested that closer degrees of consanguinity are associated with leukemia onset at younger ages. Childhood leukemia has been occasionally linked with occurrence of congenital anomalies in case mothers. Although some investigators attribute multiple occurrences of ALL in a sibship to a rare recessive gene with high penetrance, such occurrences are extremely rare, and other investigators have discounted the likelihood of a homozygous recessive mechanism.

A number of studies examining immunologic characteristics of first-degree relatives of patients with ALL have shown a variety of differences between family members of cases and controls. Mothers of children with leukemia have been reported to have a significantly lower number of monocytes, higher levels of gamma globulin, IgA, IgG, and IgM; both fathers and mothers have been found to have higher numbers of basophils. Some investigators have noted a history of an increased occurrence of autoimmune disorders, including **Arthritis, rheumatoid**, **Thyrotoxicosis**, Hashimoto thyroiditis, rheumatic fever, and other conditions among parents of patients compared with parents of controls, although these findings have not been consistent. Several studies have indicated that parents of patients have suffered an excess of serious or life-threatening infections compared with parents of controls. Atopy has also inconsistently been reported more commonly among parents of patients. The inconsistency of these findings may reflect small numbers, selected case groups, and differences between studies in types of controls. Nevertheless, there is some support for the observation that there may be an underlying immune system dysfunction among a proportion of mothers, and possibly fathers, of childhood ALL patients. Further studies of immunologic function ought to be undertaken among parents of patients compared with those of parents of controls within the context of large-scale, population-based, case-control studies of childhood ALL.

It is interesting to note that **Chromosome 21, trisomy 21**, associated with an excess risk of ALL, is also characterized by a number of immunologic abnormalities, including increased levels of IgG, elevated numbers of basophils, and decreased IgM, as well as a decreased response for delayed hypersensitivity to bacterial and viral antigens and a decreased response to phytohemagglutinin. Several maternal reproductive and pregnancy-related disorders have been linked to ALL, including higher birth weight, birth order (first), and maternal age (older), although these findings have not been consistent across studies. Postnatal exposure to high levels of ionizing radiation and prenatal exposure to diagnostic ionizing radiation are the most consistently demonstrated associations. A number of parental occupational exposures have also been implicated, although findings have been inconsistent and specific exposures not isolated. Childhood environmental exposures and medically related conditions have also been implicated, including pesticides, certain viral disorders (particularly varicella during fetal development; see **Fetal effects from varicella-zoster**), and use of chloramphenicol.

Among the several non-random chromosomal translocations associated with childhood ALL are t(q;22) (q34;q11) found in six percent of cases (primarily pre-B and B-cell precursors, ALL and T-ALL); t(4;11) (q21;q23) linked with five percent of childhood cases, particularly non-T, non-B ALL; t(1;19) (q23;p13.3) associated with pre-B ALL; t(11;14) (p13;q13) found in T-ALL , and three translocations unique to B-ALL including t(8;14) (q24;q32), t(2;8) (p11–13;q24), and t(8;22) (q24;q11).

**Pathogenesis:** The cause(s) of familial childhood ALL are unknown, although interactions of underlying genetic or immunogenetic disorders with a number of environmental variables is probable. Some familial cases appear to be associated with various chromosomal abnormalities, others with heritable disorders characterized by increased chromosomal abnormalities or breakage. The relationship of familial ALL to the apparently increased haplotype sharing among parents or to underlying immunologic dysfunction among mothers, and perhaps fathers, requires further study. The basis of the high concordance rate for leukemia in identical twins under age six years seems to be intrauterine transfusion (via placental anastomosis; see **Fetal monozygous multiple pregnancy dysplacentation effects**) of leukemia cells from one fetus to the co-twin.

**MIM No.:** *14779

**Sex Ratio:** M1.3:F1.0. There appears to be no difference in the sex ratio of familial ALL cases compared with the sex ratio of sporadic cases.

**Occurrence:** Although concordance among identical twins is 20–25% overall, and certain rare disorders are associated with an exceptionally high subsequent risk of childhood leukemia, a relatively small fraction of childhood ALL cases are familial. Data are not available to quantify prevalence or incidence of familial ALL.

**Risk of Recurrence for Patient's Sib:**
See Part I, *Mendelian Inheritance*. Surveys have suggested a fourfold excess risk.

**Risk of Recurrence for Patient's Child:**
See Part I, *Mendelian Inheritance*.

**Age of Detectability:** Virtually all cases among identical twins are diagnosed before ten years of age.

**Gene Mapping and Linkage:** IGJ (immunoglobulin J polypeptide) has been provisionally mapped to 4q21.

**Prevention:** Data from the United Kingdom and from the Connecticut Tumor Registry suggest an increase in childhood ALL over the last four decades. The underlying reasons for this rise in incidence are not known. Epidemiologic studies have failed to identify consistently major environmental risk factors other than postnatal exposure to high levels of ionizing radiation and prenatal exposure to diagnostic ionizing radiation. Children with **Chromosome 21, trisomy 21** or a number of other rare heritable disorders and sibs of affected persons are at increased risk, and genetic counseling may be of benefit to parents of such children.

**Treatment:** As with non-familial ALL.

**Prognosis:** As with non-familial ALL.

**Detection of Carrier:** Unknown.

**Support Groups:** New York; Leukemia Society of America

**References:**

Vidabaek A: Heredity in human leukemia and its relation to cancer: a genetic and clinical study of 209 probands. London: HK Lewis and Co., 1947.

Miller RW: Down's syndrome (mongolism), other congenital malformations and cancers among sibs of leukemic children. New Engl J Med 1963; 268:393–401.

MacMahon B, Levy MA: Prenatal origin of childhood leukemia: evidence from twins. New Engl J Med 1964; 270:1082–1085.

Miller RW: Relation between cancer and congenital defects: an epidemiologic evaluation. JNCI 1968; 40:1079–1085. *

Zuelzer WW, Cox DE: Genetic aspects of leukemia. Semin Hematol 1969; 6:228–249.

Miller RW: Deaths from childhood leukemia and solid tumors among twins and other sibs in the United States, 1960–1967. JNCI 1971; 46:203–209. *

Gunz GW, et al.: Familial leukemia: a study of 909 families. Scand J Haematol 1975; 15:117–131. *

Koshland ME: The coming of age of the immunoglobulin J chain. Ann Rev Immun 1985; 3:425–453.

Pendergrass TW: Epidemiology of acute lymphoblastic leukemia. Semin Oncol 1985; 12:80–91.

Max EE, et al.: Human J chain gene: chromosomal localization and associated restriction fragment length polymorphisms. Proc Nat Acad Sci 1986; 83:5592–5596.

Neglia JP, Robison LL: Epidemiology of childhood acute leukemias. Pediatr Clin N Am 1988; 35:675–692.

LI029                                                              **Martha S. Linet**

**Leukemia, chronic granulocytic**
 *See LEUKEMIA, CHRONIC MYELOID (CML)*
**Leukemia, chronic lymphatic**
 *See LEUKEMIA/LYMPHOMA, B-CELL*
**Leukemia, chronic lymphatic type II**
 *See LEUKEMIA/LYMPHOMA, B-CELL*
**Leukemia, chronic lymphatic, type 2**
 *See LYMPHOMA, NON-HODGKIN*

## LEUKEMIA, CHRONIC MYELOID (CML)                    3092

**Includes:**
 Breakpoint cluster region-1
 Granulocytic leukemia, chronic
 Leukemia, chronic granulocytic

**Excludes:**
 Erythroleukemia
 **Gaucher disease** (0406)
 Leukemoid reaction
 Myelofibrosis
 Polycythemia vera
 Thrombocytopenia, primary

**Major Diagnostic Criteria:** Bone marrow is hyperplastic. There is an increased number of immature granulocytes. The ratio of granulocytes/erythrocytes is 10–50:1 rather than 2–5:1, as seen in the normal bone marrow. In nearly all cases, the Philadelphia (Ph) chromosome has been found cytogenetically in the granulocytes. In a blood film from CML cases, there is granulocytic leukocytosis. The white count is elevated (avg. 200,000/dl with a range of 15,000/dl to 600,000/dl). The platelet count is above 450,000/dl in about 50% of the cases.

**Clinical Findings:** The basic abnormality is granulocytic leukocytosis. The blood film gives a picture of granulocytes in all stages of differentiation but which appear to be morphologically normal. The composition of the granulocytes found in the blood are 50% neutrophils, 22% myelocytes, less than 10% are promyelocytes and blast cells, and the eosinophils and basophils are less than 5%. The mature neutorphils appear to function normally. There is an associated anemia that is normocytic and normochromic, having an average hemoglobin level of 9–12 g/dl. The platelets are

functionally and morphologically abnormal. The metabolic rate is increased in CML cases, leading to weight loss, fever and increased sweating. Occasionally the bone marrow and spleen presents with lipid-containing histocytes resembling those observed in **Gaucher disease**.

The level of glucocerebrosidase is elevated in CML cases rather than deficient, as is observed in **Gaucher disease**. The level of uric acid is elevated in untreated CML cases. Neutrophil alkaline phosphatase is markedly decreased in CML cases. There is a considerable elevation of serum vitamin $B_{12}$ and serum lactic dehydrogenase in CML cases. During the chronic phase, hepatosplenomegaly is often observed, but lymphadenopathy is rare. The presence of lymphadenopathy should alert one to the involvement of the disease to the terminal stage or an extramedullary myeloblastoma.

**Complications:** The terminal phase of CML could present either as a "myeloproliferative acceleration" or as a "blastic transformation." This phase can occur at any point during the chronic phase of the disease. The "myeloproliferative acceleration" leads to a progressive leukocytosis. The disease becomes refractory to previously effective treatment. In approximately 33% of the cases, myelofibrosis occurs. There is an increased basophilia at the terminal phase. During the terminal phase, there is weakness due to progressive anemia, weight loss and an increase in pain due to splenomegaly. In the "blastic transformation" approximately 30–40% of the cells in the bone marrow are blasts which may be lymphoid or myeloid in origin, but the presence of anemia and thrombocytopenia are also necessary for this diagnosis. The lymphatic cells are differentiated by their cytoplasmic TdT (terminal deoxynucleotidyl transferase) expression. These patients respond to chemotherapy effective for lymphoid leukemias.

Approximately 50% of the CML cases at this phase will have cytogenetic abnormalities, especially aneuploidy, usually being trisomic for chromosomes 1, 8, 17, isochromosome of the long arm of chromosome 17, or an additional Ph chromosome.

**Associated Findings:** None known.

**Etiology:** An increased incidence of CML has been observed after exposure to significant amounts of ionizing radiation.

**Pathogenesis:** Considered to be a neoplastic disease of the pluripotent stem cell in the bone marrow.

**MIM No.:** *15141

**Sex Ratio:** M1:F<1

**Occurrence:** CML is rarely found in children; only about 1–3% of childhood leukemias are CML. The median age is 40–45 years for CML. About 20% of all the leukemias in the Western countries are CML.

**Risk of Recurrence for Patient's Sib:** Unknown.

**Risk of Recurrence for Patient's Child:** Unknown.

**Age of Detectability:** At any age.

**Gene Mapping and Linkage:** BCR (breakpoint cluster region) has been mapped to 22q11.

Nearly all CML cases have the Ph chromosome present in their hemopoietic cells. By using glucose-6-phosphate dehydrogenase isozyme analyses, the clonal nature of the cells containing the Ph chromosome has been demonstrated. The neoplastic cells most probably derived from a Ph chromosome containing pluripotential stem cell. The consistent chromosomal translocation associated with CML is t(9;22)(q34;q11), which results in the Ph chromosome. The c-abl oncogene which is located at 9q34 is translocated to chromosome 22q11 when the t(9;22) occurs. The breakpoint on chromosome 22 is clustered around a 5.8 kb region identified as the "breakpoint cluster region" (bcr). This bcr-abl fusion gene is expressed at the transcriptional level, giving rise to a fusion mRNA of 8 kb in size, and also at the translational level, giving rise to a fusion bcr-abl protein of 210 kd. The role of this fusion protein is unknown. Occasionally a Ph negative CML case appears, but at the molecular level there is a rearrangement at 22q11 at the location of bcr; thus these cases contain a masked Ph chromosome.

**Prevention:** None known. Genetic counseling indicated.

**Treatment:** The chronic phase of the disease can be controlled by oral chemotherapeutic drugs such as hydroxyurea or busulfan. This treatment is stopped once the white cell count drops to 10,000/dl. New therapeutic trials with high dose chemotherapy and autologous bone marrow or allogenic bone marrow transplantation for curative approaches are being analyzed.

**Prognosis:** The median survival time after the diagnosis ranges from 36 months to four years for the chronic phase. In the terminal phase, the median survival time is about 2–3 months. A white cell count of less than 100,000/mm$^3$, the presence of less than 1% myeloblasts and erythroid precursors in the peripheral blood and the absence of hepatosplenomegaly are good prognostic indicators, with median survival time of approximately 60 months.

**Detection of Carrier:** Unknown.

**Support Groups:** New York; Leukemia Society of America

**References:**

Williams WJ, et al: Hematology, ed. 3. New York: McGraw-Hill, 1983. *
Yunis JJ: The chromosomal basis of human neoplasia. Science 1983; 221:227–236.
Reich PR: Hematology, ed. 2. Boston: Little, Brown & Co, 1984. †
DeVita VT Jr, et al: Cancer: principles and practice of oncology, ed. 2. Philadelphia: J.B. Lippincott Co, 1985. †
Haluska FG, et al: Oncogene activation by chromosome translocation in human malignancy. Ann Rev Genet 1987; 21:321–345. *

L0016
CR024

**Elaine Louie
Carlo M. Croce**

---

## LEUKEMIA/LYMPHOMA, B-CELL                                3097

**Includes:**

    B-cell chronic lymphocytic leukemia
    B-cell prolymphocytic leukemia
    Follicular lymphoma
    Leukemia, chronic lymphatic
    Leukemia, chronic lymphatic type II
    Lymphoma, B-cell
    Non-Hodgkin lymphoma of B-cell type
    Oncogene B-cell leukemia
    Small cell lymphocytic lymphoma

**Excludes:**

    **Leukemia/lymphoma, T-cell (3095)**
    **Lymphoma, non-Hodgkin (3107)**

**Major Diagnostic Criteria:** In B-cell chronic lymphocytic leukemia (CLL), there is peripheral lymphocytosis, lymphoadenopathy and, splenomegaly. Minimal requirements leading to this diagnosis are the presence of 40% or greater lymphocytosis in the bone marrow and an absolute lymphocytosis of greater than 15,000/dl. The B-cells in CLL have a restricted Ig class, IgG subclass and light chain type. Distinction between lymphocytic leukemia and lymphocytic lymphoma is based mainly on the distribution of the abnormal B-cells.

**Clinical Findings:** In chronic lymphocytic leukemia there is an accumulation and proliferation of abnormal, relatively immature B-cells in the bone marrow, lymph nodes and spleen. There is a generalized lymphadenopathy, and 75% of the cases have splenomegaly. Normocytic and normochromic anemia and/or enlarged lymph nodes are also present. The peripheral lymphocytes are uniformly small cells with condensed nuclei. Surface immunoglobulin of a specific light chain and heavy chain isotype identifies the clonal nature of the neoplastic B-cells. B-cells are functionally abnormal, leading to an immunodeficiency state. Prolymphocytic leukemia of B-cells is considered to be a rare variant of B-cell chronic lymphocytic leukemia, with an increased expression of membrane immunoglobulin. There is massive splenomegaly, while lymphoadenopathy is minimal. The total peripheral lymphocyte count is greater than 100 x 10$^9$/L. In small cell lymphocytic leukemia, there is a diffuse growth pattern in the lymph nodes. The majority of the cells are similar to those seen in chronic lymphocytic leukemia. These lymphomas are considered

to be the solid tumor counterpart of chronic lymphocytic leukemia.

**Complications:** There is an increased risk of all types of infections due to the impaired immune state of the patient. The final stage can lead to a refractory anemia, splenomegaly, leukemic cells replacing the bone marrow and hypogammaglobulinemia which leads to fatal septicemia. Rarely is a blastic stage seen in chronic lymphocytic leukemias.

**Associated Findings:** There is an increased risk in developing other cancers such as skin cancer, melenoma, sarcoma and lung cancer.

**Etiology:** There is a tendency of closely-related persons to have CLL, but no well-defined mode of inheritance has been found.

**Pathogenesis:** A clonal proliferation of neoplastic B-cells at a relatively immature stage in differentiation.

**MIM No.:** *15140, *15143

**Sex Ratio:** M3:F1

**Occurrence:** This is the commonest leukemia in Western countries. The median age is 60 years, and it occurs in adults older than 30 years. Chronic lymphocytic leukemia is rare in Japan.

**Risk of Recurrence for Patient's Sib:** There appears to be a slight increase in risk for patient's sib.

**Risk of Recurrence for Patient's Child:** There appears to be a slight increase in risk for patient's child.

**Age of Detectability:** At any age.

**Gene Mapping and Linkage:** BCL1 (B cell CLL/lymphoma 1) has been mapped to 11q13.3.

    BCL2 (B cell CLL/lymphoma 2) has been mapped to 18q21.3.

    In 10% of B-cell chronic lymphocytic leukemias, the leukemic cells carry t(11;14)(q13;q32). This translocation is present in certain small cell lymphomas as well. The translocation involves the immunoglobulin heavy chain locus and a putative oncogene on chromosome 11 called bcl-1 (B-cell leukemia/lymphoma 1). The breakpoints on the chromosome is clustered around the 5' ends of the joining regions (J region) of the immunoglobulin heavy chain locus. The clustering of the breakpoint on chromosome 14 occurs near sequences involved in the normal V-D-J rearrangement seen during normal B-cell differentiation. This association has suggested that the translocation observed in the leukemia may represent an aberrant V-D-J joining event.

**Prevention:** None known. Genetic counseling indicated.

**Treatment:** Intensive therapy is rarely used because of the advanced age of the patients and the indolent nature of the disease. The symptomatic enlarged lymph node is treated effectively with involved field radiation therapy. For systemic treatment, steroids and alkylating agents such as chlorambucil have been employed.

**Prognosis:** The median survival time is greater than 70 months if anemia or thrombocytopenia is absent. Patients who present with thrombocytopenia in addition to anemia, splenomegaly, and lymphadenopathy have a median survival time of less than 2 years.

**Detection of Carrier:** Unknown.

**Support Groups:** New York; Leukemia Society of America

**References:**

Williams WJ, et al: Hematology, ed 3. New York: McGraw-Hill 1983. *
Yunis JJ: The chromosomal basis of human neoplasia. Science 1983; 221:227–236.
Reich PR: Hematology, ed 2. Boston: Little, Brown & Co, 1984. †
DeVita VT Jr., et al: Cancer: principles and practice of oncology, ed 2. Philadelphia: J.B. Lippincott Co, 1985. †
Milo JV, et al: Relationship between chronic lymphocytic leukemia and prolymphocytic leukemia. J Haematol 1986; 3:377–387.
Chenevix-Trench G: The molecular genetics of human non-Hodgkin's lymphoma. Cancer Genet Cytogenet 1987; 27:191–213.
Haluska FG, et al: Oncogene activation by chromosome translocation in human malignancy. Ann Rev Genet 1987; 21:321–345. *

L0016
CR024

**Elaine Louie
Carlo M. Croce**

## LEUKEMIA/LYMPHOMA, T-CELL      3095

**Includes:**
    Cutaneous T-cell lymphomas
    Diffuse T-cell lymphoma
    Mycosis fungoides
    Non-Hodgkin lymphoma of T-cell type
    Sezary syndrome
    T-cell antigen receptor, alpha subunit (TCRA)
    T-cell chronic lymphocytic leukemia
    T-cell leukemia/lymphoma, adult
    T-cell prolymphocytic leukemia

**Excludes:**
    **Leukemia/lymphoma, B cell** (3097)
    **Lymphoma, non-Hodgkin** (3107)

**Major Diagnostic Criteria:** In adult T-cell chronic lymphocytic leukemia, there is erythroderma, hepatosplenomegaly and neurological involvement. The neoplastic cells are negative for surface immunoglobulin but instead have the mature T-cell phenotype. Characteristically the cells are large and have convoluted nuclei. The deep paracortex of the lymph nodes and the skin is infiltrated by these T-cells. In *cutaneous T-cell lymphomas* (*Mycosis fungoides* and *Sezary syndrome*), the skin (both epidermis and upper dermis) is infiltrated by T lymphocytes. During the later stages of this disease there is also systemic organ involvement. The neoplastic cells are pleiomorphic, their nuclei are highly convoluted, and they have the phenotype of T-cells.

**Clinical Findings:** The patient presents with hepatosplenomegaly, neutropenia and skin infiltration, but not with lymphadenopathy. Leukemic cells are positive for T-cell surface antigens, negative for surface immunoglobulin, and they form rosettes with sheep red blood cells. The karyotype in the leukemic cells is usually aneuploid. Adult T-cell leukemia/lymphoma have been associated with HTLV-1 (human T-cell leukemia/lymphoma virus-1). The leukemic cells have surface antigens of mature immunocompetent T-cells. There is infiltration of the skin by these T-cells, hypercalcemia, lymphadenopathy and hepatosplenomegaly. The cells are large and pleiomorphic. The T-cells are usually OKT-4 positive with a high density of T-cell receptors, but they function abnormally.

**Complications:** In T-cell leukemias, involvement of the central nervous system is characteristic.

**Associated Findings:** None known.

**Etiology:** Adult T-cell leukemia/lymphoma is associated with HTLV-1 but no etiological factors have been identified.

**Pathogenesis:** An uncontrolled expansion of monoclonal T-cells.

**MIM No.:** *18688

**Sex Ratio:** M1:F<1

**Occurrence:** Adult T-cell leukemia/lymphoma is endemic to certain regions of Japan and the Caribbean. Both of these diseases are rare in developed countries. *Cutaneous T-cell lymphoma* is not very common, having a rate of 2–3 cases per million in the United States. Usually it occurs in patients 30 years or older; it rarely occurs in patients less than 30 years.

**Risk of Recurrence for Patient's Sib:** Unknown.

**Risk of Recurrence for Patient's Child:** Unknown.

**Age of Detectability:** At any age.

**Gene Mapping and Linkage:** TCRA (T cell receptor, alpha (V,D,J,C)) has been mapped to 14q11.2.
    TAL1 (T cell acute lymphoblastic leukemia 1) has been mapped to 11p15.
    Some T-cell leukemias and lymphomas exhibit specific nonrandom chromosomal traslocations which frequently involve 14q11, where the alpha and delta chains of the T-cell receptor are located. The most frequent chromosomal abnormalities are inversions -- inv(14) -- and translocations -- t(14;14)(q11;q32), t(8;14)(q24;q11), t(10;14)(q24;q11), or t(11;14)(p13;q11). The T-cell receptor genes are organized in a similar manner to the immunoglobulin genes, and during normal cellular differentiation the gene undergoes rearrangement at the DNA level in a manner similar to the immunoglobulin loci. Putative oncogenes have been hypothesized to exist at or near the site of the breakpoint on chromosomes 14q32, 11p13 and 10q24, called *tcl*-1, *tcl*-2 and *tcl*- 3, respectively (T-cell leukemia/lymphoma-1, -2 and -3). In the case of the t(8;14)(q24;11), the T-cell alpha locus on chromosome 14 translocates into the 3' end of the proto-oncogene c-*myc* locus on chromosome 8. Thus, the T-cell receptor alpha locus is split between the Vα and Jα regions, and the c-*myc* locus remains intact.

    The question of whether c-*myc* is deregulated in cells containing the t(8;14) has been approached using somatic cell hybrids. These experiments demonstrate that only the translocated intact c-*myc* locus is expressed, which suggests that the T-cell receptor alpha locus can activate the transcription of a juxtaposed oncogene *in cis*. The inv(14) and other translocations specific for T-cell leukemias and lymphomas may have the T-cell receptor loci activate *in cis* a newly-juxtaposed gene in the vicinity of the chromosomal breakpoint. It should be noted that the T-cell receptor beta chain locus and T-cell receptor gamma chain locus which maps to chromosome 7q35 and 7p13, respectively, are also sites of chromosomal translocations in T-cell leukemias and lymphomas but at a lesser frequency than 14q11.

**Prevention:** None known. Genetic counseling indicated.

**Treatment:** The T-cell leukemias and lymphomas do not respond well to therapy. Therapy is usually palliative using radiotherapy or combination chemotherapy. In cutaneous T-cell lymphoma, application of nitrogen mustard, combined ultraviolet A light and psoralen therapy, whole body irradiation with an electron beam, or systemic chemotherapy are often used to control the skin lesions that arise from this disease.

**Prognosis:** Survival time is less than one year.

**Detection of Carrier:** Unknown.

**Support Groups:** New York; Leukemia Society of America

**References:**
Williams WJ, et al: Hematology, ed. 3. New York: McGraw-Hill, 1983. *
Yunis JJ: The chromosomal basis of human neoplasia. Science 1983; 221:227–236.
Reich PR: Hematology, ed. 2. Boston: Little, Brown & Co, 1984. †
DeVita VT Jr, et al: Cancer: principles and practive of oncology, ed. 2. Philadelphia: J.B. Lippincott Co, 1985. †
Chenevix-Trench G: The molecular genetics of human non-Hodgkin's lymphoma. Cancer Genet Cytogenet 1987; 27:191–213.
Haluska FG, et al: Oncogene activation by chromosome translocation in human malignancy. Ann Rev Genet 1987; 21:321–345. *

L0016                            **Elaine Louie**
CR024                        **Carlo M. Croce**

**Leukocyte adherence deficiency**
    *See GRANULOCYTE GLYCOPROTEIN CD11/CD18 DEFICIENCY*
**Leukocyte interferon deficiency**
    *See INTERFERON DEFICIENCY*

## LEUKOCYTE, MAY-HEGGLIN ANOMALY 2681

**Includes:**
  May-Hegglin anomaly
  Megathrombocytopenia
  Nephritis-megathrombocytopenia-deafness
  Platelet, May-Hegglin anomaly
  Thrombocytopenia-Dohle bodies in neutrophils

**Excludes:**
  Alder anomaly
  **Chediak-Higashi syndrome** (0143)
  Dohle bodies, transient, from infections or chemotherapy
  **Nephritis-deafness (sensorineural), hereditary type** (0708)
  Toxic granulation of neutrophils

**Major Diagnostic Criteria:** The presence of bizarre giant platelets in the circulation and basophilic inclusions (Döhle bodies) within a large portion of the granulocytes (neutrophils, eosinophils, and basophils) and in occasional monocytes. These inclusions are large (2–5 $\mu$m) RNA-containing granules located in the cytoplasm (usually one per cell) which stain sky blue with Wright stain. Under the electron microscope the Döhle bodies are spindle-shaped and consist of linear arrays of 7–10 nm filaments. Approximately 50% of the reported patients have had platelet counts of <75,000/mm³, sometimes associated with a mild bleeding tendency. The survival time and function of the platelets are normal. Döhle bodies caused by infection can appear transiently in neutrophils but are not associated with giant platelets.

**Clinical Findings:** Mild hemorrhagic manifestations have been the only specific clinical problem encountered. In a review of all 89 documented cases in the literature by Godwin and Ginsburg (1974), 43% had features of abnormal bleeding, including recurrent epistaxis, easy bruisability, gingival bleeding, menorrhagia, and excessive bleeding following dental extraction, tonsillectomy, or trauma. This bleeding tendency was associated with a platelet count of <75,000/mm³ in 86% of the symptomatic patients. The remaining patients cited in this review were entirely asymptomatic. No increased incidence of bacterial or fungal infections due to the granulocyte inclusions has been reported.

There is some variability in the expression of the morphologic and thrombocytopenic manifestations of the disorder. Even within a given family, not all members will necessarily have thrombocytopenia and some will have transitory decreases in the platelet count. Similarly, the percentage of granulocytes containing Döhle bodies can vary within a family and can be as low as <10%.

**Complications:** Severe bleeding can potentially occur in those patients with the lowest platelet counts.

**Associated Findings:** Hereditary nephritis and deafness associated with the May-Hegglin anomaly.

**Etiology:** Autosomal dominant inheritance.

**Pathogenesis:** The defect responsible for the formation of the Döhle bodies is unknown, although the finding that cytotoxic drugs can also cause this abnormality suggests that a metabolic disorder could be responsible. The giant platelets are thought to arise from abnormal maturation and fragmentation of normal-appearing megakaryocytes in the bone marrow. The reason for this abnormality or how it relates to the granulocyte inclusions is unknown.

**MIM No.:** *15510

**Sex Ratio:** M1:F1

**Occurrence:** In their 1974 report, Godwin and Ginsburg were able to find 83 patients reported in the literature of whom 22 belonged to a single kinship.

**Risk of Recurrence for Patient's Sib:**
  See Part I, *Mendelian Inheritance.*

**Risk of Recurrence for Patient's Child:**
  See Part I, *Mendelian Inheritance.*

**Age of Detectability:** During infancy. In one report, a child was diagnosed at age five months.

**Gene Mapping and Linkage:** Unknown.

**Prevention:** None known. Genetic counseling indicated.

**Treatment:** Patients with severe thrombocytopenia may require platelet transfusions for surgical procedures or severe trauma.

**Prognosis:** Normal life span.

**Detection of Carrier:** Due to the dominant mode of inheritance, carriers exhibit the May-Hegglin anomaly.

**Special Considerations:** This condition is distinct from Alport syndrome associated with macrothrombocytopenia (Peterson et al, 1985), and Döhle bodies and leukemia (Goudsmit et al, 1971).

**References:**
Oski FA, et al.: Leukocytic inclusions-Döhle bodies-associated with platelet abnormality (the May-Hegglin anomaly): report of a family and review of the literature. Blood 1962; 20:657–667. *
Jordan SW, Larsen WE: Ultrastructural studies of the May-Hegglin anomaly. Blood 1965; 25:921–932. †
Goudsmit R, et al.: Dohle bodies and acute myeloblastic leukemia in one family: a new familial disorder. Brit J Haemat 1971; 20:557–562.
Cawley JC, Hayhoe FGJ: The inclusions of the May-Hegglin anomaly and Döhle bodies of infection: an ultrastructural comparison. Br J Haematol 1972; 22:491–496. †
Godwin HA, Ginsburg AD: May-Hegglin anomaly: a defect in megakaryocyte fragmentation? Br J Haematol 1974; 26:117–128. *
Brivet F, et al.: Hereditary nephritis associated with May-Hegglin anomaly. Nephron 1981; 29:59–62. †
Peterson L, et al.: Fechtner syndrome: a variant of Alport's syndrome with leukocyte inclusions and macrothrombocytopenia. Blood 1985; 65:397–406. †

CU012                                    **John T. Curnutte**

**Leukocytes, granulation anomaly of**
  *See CHEDIAK-HIGASHI SYNDROME*
**Leukoderma acquisitum centrifugum of Sutton**
  *See SKIN, VITILIGO*
**Leukoderma, primary**
  *See SKIN, VITILIGO*

## LEUKODYSTROPHY, ADULT-ONSET PROGRESSIVE DOMINANT TYPE 2975

**Includes:** Adult-onset leukodystrophy, hereditary

**Excludes:**
  **Adrenoleukodystrophy, X-linked** (2533)
  **Brain, spongy degeneration** (0115)
  **Cerebro-hepato-renal syndrome** (0139)
  **Leukodystrophy, globoid cell type** (0415)
  **Metachromatic leukodystrophies** (0651)
  **Multiple sclerosis, familial** (2598)
  Multiple systems atrophies: Shy-Drager syndrome
  **Olivopontocerebellar atrophy**
  **Pelizaeus-Merzbacher syndrome** (0803)

**Major Diagnostic Criteria:** Steadily progressive symptoms of cerebellar, pyramidal, and autonomic nervous system dysfunction with onset in the early thirties to late forties. Leg pain, weakness, postural hypotension, neurogenic bladder, rectal incontinence, progressive loss of balance, spasticity, and slurred speech are accompanied by little or no mental deterioration. Death occurs within 15–25 years. X-ray findings show symmetric decrease in white matter density.

**Clinical Findings:** Of the two kindreds reported, one is of Irish and the other of Scots-Irish origin. The clinical picture is that of an adult-onset (ranging from early fourth to late fifth decade), slowly progressive multisystem nondementing neurologic disorder that, in some aspects, resembles multiple sclerosis. The most common initial symptoms include lower extremity pain, weakness, gait disturbance, vertigo, loss of fine motor control, orthostatic hypotension, and lower back pain. As the disease progresses, affected individuals often have slurred speech, diaphoresis, intermittent rigidity, spasticity, paraplegia, bladder and bowel incontinence, and impotence. Personality and orientation remain intact, but patients are usually bedridden prior to death. The immediate cause of death is most frequently bronchopneumonia or "stroke."

Cranial CT scans and magnetic resonance imaging have shown symmetric atrophy of white matter in affected individuals and in at least one presymptomatic affected woman whose mother was affected.

Pathologic studies of the brains of some of the affected individuals revealed white matter degeneration of the cerebral hemispheres and cerebellum. There was little involvement of the internal capsule, brainstem, and cervical cord and no involvement of the subcortical tracts. Microscopic examination showed spongiform leukoencephalopathy with no gliosis, inflammation, or storage.

Laboratory findings include theta activity showing on EEG in three affected family members, abnormalities of central conduction on somatosensory evoked potentials, which evolved over a period of two years in the presymptomatic daughter of the affected mother mentioned above, abnormal brainstem evoked auditory response, and abnormal visual evoked response. Laboratory testing for known metabolic diseases has been repeatedly uninformative.

**Complications:** Postural hypotension is usually associated with severe vertigo. Progression of symptoms leads to increasing disability through incontinence, spasticity, and inability to walk. Patients are usually bedridden prior to death and require 24-hour nursing care.

**Associated Findings:** None known. The clinical picture is relatively consistent, and affected individuals in both kindreds have had remarkably similar clinical courses. A personality change was described in one of the patients, but it is more probable that it was caused by frustration and emotional reaction to the disease.

**Etiology:** Autosomal dominant inheritance. In each kindred there are at least four consecutive generations of affected individuals. While the families described have been referred to as having **Pelizaeus-Merzbacher syndrome**, their condition does not cause dementia.

**Pathogenesis:** A demyelinating process is suspected, and symmetric white matter degeneration has been documented through imaging as well as at autopsy.

**MIM No.:** *16950

**Sex Ratio:** M1:F1

**Occurrence:** Two kinships have been documented. Extensive efforts have not resulted in the discovery of a common ancestor of the two families, although the possibility has not been completely ruled out. The families are of Irish and Scots-Irish origin. Two other families, one American and the other German, were reported previously with a disorder that had a similar clinical course to that described here; however, the patients also deteriorated intellectually, so it is unclear whether all four kindreds have the same disorder.

**Risk of Recurrence for Patient's Sib:**
See Part I, *Mendelian Inheritance*.

**Risk of Recurrence for Patient's Child:**
See Part I, *Mendelian Inheritance*.

**Age of Detectability:** Ranges from the early thirties to late forties, although presymptomatic identification of affected individuals may be possible through imaging or electrophysiologic techniques. No prenatal detection known. It is possible that presymptomatic individuals could be identified (if they desire) with imaging or electrophysiologic techniques.

**Gene Mapping and Linkage:** Unknown.

**Prevention:** None known. Genetic counseling indicated.

**Treatment:** Symptomatic only. Emotional support for patients and families similar to that available to families with **Huntington disease**.

**Prognosis:** The clinical course is slowly progressive; death occurs usually within 10–25 years of onset of symptoms and follows a period of severe disability.

**Detection of Carrier:** Unknown.

**Support Groups:** IL; Sycamore; United Leukodystrophy Foundation

**References:**
Eldridge R, et al.: Hereditary adult-onset leukodystrophy simulating chronic progressive multiple sclerosis. New Engl J Med 1984; 331:948–953.
Laxova R, et al.: A new autosomal dominant adult onset progressive leukodystrophy. Am J Hum Genet 1985; 37:A65.

LA033                                                    **Renata Laxova**

**Leukodystrophy, Alexander disease**
*See ALEXANDER DISEASE*

## LEUKODYSTROPHY, GLOBOID CELL TYPE                    0415

**Includes:**
   Galactosylceramidase deficiency
   Galactosylceramide beta-galactosidase deficiency
   Globoid cell leukodystrophy
   Krabbe disease
   Psychosine lipidosis

**Excludes:**
   **Adrenoleukodystrophy, X-linked** (2533)
   **Alexander disease** (2712)
   **Brain, spongy degeneration** (0115)
   **Encephalopathy, necrotizing** (0344)
   **Metachromatic leukodystrophies** (0651)
   **Paraplegia, familial spastic** (0295)
   **Phytanic acid oxidase deficiency, infantile type** (2278)
   Sudanophilic leukodystrophy

**Major Diagnostic Criteria:** Definitive antemortem diagnosis can be established only by profound deficiency of galactosylceramidase activity in serum, leukocytes, fibroblasts, cultured amniotic fluid cells, chorionic villi, and solid tissues. Diagnosis should be suspected in infants with early hyperirritability, rapidly progressive neurologic signs, particularly of the white matter, and elevated spinal fluid protein. Postmortem examination of the central nervous system can also provide the definite diagnosis. The white matter is almost completely devoid of myelin, which is replaced by severe astrocytic gliosis and the unique, multinucleated, PAS-positive globoid cells.

**Clinical Findings:** The onset of clinical symptoms in typical cases is between ages 3 and 6 months. Rarely, the clinical onset can be immediately after birth. The initial symptoms are usually vague and nonspecific, such as episodic fever of unknown origin, hyperirritability, and hypersensitivity to external stimuli. Vomiting and feeding difficulty with or without seizures may occur as initial clinical symptoms. Rapidly progressive severe mental and motor deterioration follows. Neurologic signs are largely referrable to the central white matter and to the peripheral nerves. There is marked hypertonicity with extended and crossed legs, flexed arms, and opisthotonus. Tendon reflexes are hyperactive. Cherry red spots have been reported. Optic atrophy and sluggish pupillary reflexes are common. Toward the terminal stage, the patients are often blind, deaf, decerebrate, and have no contact with the surroundings. The early hyperactive reflexes are replaced by diminished or absent reflexes. Because of their severity, clinical signs of the white matter lesions often overshadow signs of the pathologically less-involved gray matter. Signs of peripheral nervous system involvement, such as reduced nerve conduction velocity, are almost always present except in the very early stages of the disease.

Radiologic findings can trace the evolution of the disease. At first, discrete and symmetric dense areas on CT are found in deep gray matter of the cerebral hemispheres, thalamus, posterior limb of the internal capsule, quadrigeminal plate and cerebellum, and also in the periventricular and capsular white matter. MRI shows decreased T1 values with normal or slilghtly decreased T2 values in white matter of the centrum semiovale. Later, both CT and MRI show diffuse reduction in gray matter and, more profoundly, in the white matter mass.The spinal fluid protein is highly elevated from the early stages. Systemic organs are usually not affected. Typically patients die before two years of age.

However, the exceedingly rare, late-onset form of the disease shows more variable clinical features and is probably heterogeneous genetically. The clinical onset can be in late infancy, childhood, or even later. Visual impairment due to cortical blindness and optic atrophy, spasticity with pyramidal signs, and difficulty walking are common manifestations. Clinical signs of peripheral nervous system involvement are not obvious. The spinal fluid protein is normal or only slightly elevated. Clinical diagnosis of the late-onset form is difficult to impossible without galactosylceramidase assays.

**Complications:** Blindness, deafness, spasticity (early), difficulty feeding, contracture of the limbs, decerebration.

**Associated Findings:** Macrocephaly, **Hydrocephaly**, infantile spasms.

**Etiology:** Autosomal recessive inheritance of deficient activity of galactosylceramidase.

**Pathogenesis:** The affected enzyme, galactosylceramidase, normally hydrolyzes galactosylceramide, which is quantitatively almost exclusively localized in the myelin sheath. This explains the highly restricted pathology to the myelin-containing tissues. The plausible hypothesis concerning the biochemical pathogenesis of the disease postulates that a toxic side-product of the involved metabolic pathway causes destruction of the myelin-forming cells, the oligodendrocytes in the CNS, and the Schwann cells in the PNS (the psychosine hypothesis). Galactosylsphingosine (psychosine) can be formed as a by-product of galactosylceramide synthesis. It is also a substrate for galactosylceramidase. Patients with this disease therefore cannot catabolize galactosylsphingosine. Psychosine is highly cytotoxic and destroys the cells in which it accumulates due to the genetic defect. Because galactosylceramide is almost exclusively localized in myelin, the above events take place only in the myelin-generating cells, resulting in the destruction of the oligodendrocytes and Schwann cells.

**MIM No.:** *24520

**Sex Ratio:** M1:F1

**Occurrence:** The disease is pan-ethnic, and the geographic distribution is widespread. The incidence appears to be higher in the Scandinavian countries. An incidence of 2–4:100,000 births has been reported for Sweden, and the calculated figure for Japan was 2–3 per 1 million births. Incidence in most other countries is probably closer to that in Japan. An exceedingly high frequency of 6:1,000 births was recently reported for a large inbred Druze isolate in Israel.

**Risk of Recurrence for Patient's Sib:**
See Part I, *Mendelian Inheritance.*

**Risk of Recurrence for Patient's Child:**
See Part I, *Mendelian Inheritance.* Few affected individuals survive to reproduce.

**Age of Detectability:** Definitive diagnosis is possible at 7–8 weeks of gestation by the galactosylceramidase assay on biopsied chorionic villi and several weeks later by the same assay on cultured amniotic fluid cells. The enzyme assay can also establish the diagnosis at any age after birth.

**Gene Mapping and Linkage:** GALC (galactosylceramidase) has been provisionally mapped to 17.

**Prevention:** None known. Genetic counseling indicated.

**Treatment:** No effective treatment is known.

**Prognosis:** A vast majority of patients die within 2–3 years of birth. Patients with the late-onset form are exceedingly rare, and only a few have been reported to survive into their teens.

**Detection of Carrier:** Carrier detection is possible by galactosylceramidase assays on leukocytes, serum, or cultured fibroblasts. No large-scale statistical data are available concerning the accuracy of carrier detection. A zone of uncertainty of ±10% would seem to be a reasonable estimate of the reliability.

**Special Considerations:** A genetic deficiency of galactosylceramidase is known to occur in other mammalian species, including the dog, mouse, and sheep. They all exhibit clinical and pathologic features similar to those of the human disease. The dog model was used extensively for research of this disease, but it is no longer available on a regular basis. The more recently discovered mouse model (the twitcher mutant) has been increasingly popular as a research tool. Transplantation of normal bone marrow to affected mice has been shown to prolong the life span of the hosts from the usual 30–40 days to over 100 days, although it did not prevent or arrest the disease process.

**Support Groups:** IL; Sycamore; United Leukodystrophy Foundation (ULF)

**References:**
Krabbe K: A new familial infantile form of diffuse brain-sclerosis. Brain 1916; 39:74–114.
Suzuki K, Suzuki Y: Globoid cell leucodystrophy (Krabbe's disease): deficiency of galactocerebroside β-galactosidase. Proc Natl Acad Sci USA 1970; 66:302–309.
Loonen MCB, et al.: Late-onset globoid cell leucodystrophy. Neuropediatrics 1985; 16:137–142.
Harzer K, et al.: Prenatal enzymatic diagnosis and exclusion of Krabbe's disease (globoid-call leukodystrophy) using chorionic villi in five risk pregnancies. Hum Genet 1987; 77:342–344.
Suzuki K, Suzuki Y: Galactosylceramide lipidosis: globoid cell leukodystrophy (Krabbe's disease). In: Scrivner CR, et al., eds: The metabolic basis of inherited disease, ed 6. New York: McGraw-Hill, 1989:1699–1720.

SU021                                                  **Kunihiko Suzuki**

**Leukodystrophy, sudanophilic**
*See PELIZAEUS-MERZBACHER SYNDROME*
**Leukokeratosis, hereditary mucosal**
*See MUCOSA, WHITE FOLDED DYSPLASIA*
**Leukomelanoderma-hypodontia-hypotrichosis-retardation**
*See BERLIN SYNDROME*
**Leukomelanoderma-infantilism-retardation-hypodontia-hypotrichosis**
*See BERLIN SYNDROME*
**Leukonychia totalis**
*See ULCER-LEUKONYCHIA-GALLSTONES*
*also NAILS, LEUKONYCHIA*
**Leukonychia, knuckle pads and deafness**
*See KNUCKLE PADS-LEUKONYCHIA-DEAFNESS*
**Leukonychia-short stature-hypolipidemia**
*See HOOFT DISEASE*
**Leukonychia-ulcer-gallstones**
*See ULCER-LEUKONYCHIA-GALLSTONES*
**Leung syndrome**
*See MICROCEPHALY-LYMPHEDEMA*
**Levin syndrome**
*See CRANIO-ECTODERMAL DYSPLASIA*
**Levine-Critchley syndrome**
*See ACANTHOCYTOSIS-NEUROLOGIC DEFECTS*
**Levy-Hollister Syndrome**
*See LACRIMO-AURICULO-DENTO-DIGITAL SYNDROME*
**Leyden-Moebius muscular dystrophy**
*See MUSCULAR DYSTROPHY, LIMB-GIRDLE*
**Leydig cell agenesis**
*See LEYDIG CELL HYPOPLASIA*
**Leydig cell differentiation, abnormality of**
*See LEYDIG CELL HYPOPLASIA*
**Leydig cell hypofunction**
*See LEYDIG CELL HYPOPLASIA*
**Leydig cell hypogenesis**
*See LEYDIG CELL HYPOPLASIA*

## LEYDIG CELL HYPOPLASIA      2298

**Includes:**
Gonadotropin unresponsiveness
Leydig cell agenesis
Leydig cell differentiation, abnormality of
Leydig cell hypofunction
Leydig cell hypogenesis

**Excludes:**
**Agonadia** (0029)
**Androgen insensitivity syndrome, incomplete** (0050)
**Anorchia** (0068)
**Gonadal dysgenesis, XY type** (0437)
**Gonadotropin deficiencies** (0438)
**Hermaphroditism, true** (0971)
**Hypogonadotropic hypogonadism** (2300)
**Kallmann syndrome** (2301)
**Steroid 5 alpha-reductase deficiency** (3062)
**Steroid 3 beta-hydroxysteroid dehydrogenase deficiency** (0909)
**Steroid 17 alpha-hydroxylase deficiency** (0903)
**Steroid 17-ketosteroid reductase deficiency** (2299)
**Steroid 17,20-desmolase deficiency** (0904)
**Steroid 20–22 desmolase deficiency** (0907)

**Major Diagnostic Criteria:** Absence or severe reduction in Leydig cells in 46,XY individuals.

**Clinical Findings:** In Leydig cell hypoplasia the primary defect involves absence or hypoplasia of Leydig cells.

Affected individuals show female or ambiguous external genitalia despite their normal male chromosomal complement. Sometimes the clitoris may be normal for females, with the urethra located in the normal position for the female. In most affected individuals, however, labial fusion exists and a urogenital sinus is present. Sometimes the single perineal orifice leads anteriorly to the bladder and posteriorly to a (vaginal) pouching. In other cases separate perineal orifices lead to both the urethra and a blindly ending vagina. Testes are similar in size to that of normal testes and typically are palpable at the inguinal canal. Spermatogenesis to the stage of spermatocytes is demonstrable. The interstitial area contains few if any completely mature Leydig cells. Epididymides and vasa deferentia are usually present. As would be predicted for 46,XY individuals, no female internal organs are present. Specifically, the uterus and fallopian tubes are absent.

Testosterone is low despite elevated FSH and LH levels. Administration of human chorionic gonadotropin (hCG) does not increase testosterone production. Secondary sexual development thus does not occur. Somatic anomalies do not coexist.

**Complications:** Lack of testosterone results in genital differentiation inappropriate for the genetic sex. Lack of hormonal secretion at puberty further results in inadequate secondary sexual development. Eventually, osteoporosis and other signs of estrogen deficiencies occur.

**Associated Findings:** None known.

**Etiology:** Possibly autosomal recessive inheritance, based on 1) one family with affected multiple sibs and 2) observations of parental consanguinity. Other etiologies are not excluded.

**Pathogenesis:** Absence or early destruction of Leydig cells results in lack of testosterone synthesis by fetal testes. Androgen-dependent steps in differentiation are thus inhibited, either partially or completely. Embryonic differentiation not dependent on testosterone or its derivatives remains undisturbed. The actual mechanism responsible for hypoplasia of Leydig cells remains uncertain. It could be secondary to abnormalities in trophic hormones or it could involve Leydig cell differentiation per se.

**MIM No.:** 23344

**Sex Ratio:** M1:F0

**Occurrence:** Fewer than a dozen cases have been reported.

**Risk of Recurrence for Patient's Sib:**
See Part I, *Mendelian Inheritance.* In as much as this condition is male-limited, risk is 1:8 for any sib, or 1:4 for male sibs. However, X-linked recessive inheritance is not excluded.

**Risk of Recurrence for Patient's Child:** Affected individuals are sterile.

**Age of Detectability:** Usually at birth. Cases with female external genitalia may not be detected until puberty.

**Gene Mapping and Linkage:** Unknown.

**Prevention:** None known. Genetic counseling indicated.

**Treatment:** Reconstructive surgery is applicable to assure female sex of rearing and sexual adaptation. Administration of sex steroids to prevent osteoporosis and to enhance secondary sexual development and function.

**Prognosis:** Intelligence and life span are probably normal, assuming proper hormonal treatment. Fertility is not possible, but secondary sexual development can be achieved with hormones. Reconstructive surgery can enhance sexual adaptation.

**Detection of Carrier:** Unknown.

**References:**
Berthezene F, et al.: Leydig-cell agenesis: a cause of male pseudohermaphroditism. New Engl J Med 1976; 295:969–972.
Perez-Palacios G, et al.: Inherited male pseudohermaphroditism due to gonadotropin unresponsiveness. Acta Endocrinol 1981; 98:148–155.
Lee PA, et al.: Leydig cell hypofunction resulting in male pseudohermaphroditism. Fertil Steril 1982; 37:675–679.
Rogers RM, et al.: Leydig cell hypogenesis: a rare cause of male pseudohermaphroditism and a pathological model for the understanding of normal sexual differentiation. J Urol 1982; 128:1325–1329.
El-Awady MK, et al.: Familial Leydig cell hypoplasia as a cause of male pseudohermaphroditism. Hum Hered 1987; 37:36–40.
Saldenha PH, et al.: A clinico-genetic investigation of Leydig cell hypoplasia. Am J Med Genet 1987; 26:337–344.

SI018      **Joe Leigh Simpson**

**LFA-1 (CD11a/CD18) deficiency**
*See GRANULOCYTE GLYCOPROTEIN CD11/CD18 DEFICIENCY*
**LH deficiency, isolated**
*See HYPOGONADOTROPIC HYPOGONADISM*
**Li-Fraumeni syndrome (some cases)**
*See CANCER, BREAST, FAMILIAL*
**Librium^, fetal effects**
*See FETAL BENZODIAZEPINE EFFECTS*
**Lichen acuminatus**
*See SKIN, PITYRIASIS RUBRA PILARIS*
**Lichen ruber acuminatus**
*See SKIN, PITYRIASIS RUBRA PILARIS*

## LIDDLE SYNDROME      0590

**Includes:**
Nephropathy, potassium-losing with low aldosterone
Potassium-losing nephropathy with low aldosterone
Pseudoaldosteronism

**Excludes:** Hypokalemic alkalosis-renal potassium loss-hyperaldosteronism

**Major Diagnostic Criteria:** Polydipsia, polyuria and hypertension secondary to a potassium-losing nephropathy with subnormal-to-low aldosterone secretion.

**Clinical Findings:** Hypokalemic alkalosis, hypertension, and renal potassium wasting of as much as 80 mEq of K+ daily. Growth is unaffected. Polydipsia, polyuria, and an inability to concentrate urine are also present. In contrast to expectations, aldosterone secretion is low and does not increase with sodium deprivation even when potassium stores are repleted. Neither spironolactone, that which blocks the renal tubular effects of aldosterone, nor a drug (SU9055) that blocks aldosterone biosynthesis, modifies the renal loss of electrolytes. Renin levels are normal or high, which differs from the situation in primary hyperaldosteronism where renin levels are low. There is a satisfactory renal response to ammonium chloride, acetezolamide, and exogenous aldosterone. Renal function appears normal apart from the potassium loss.

Triamterene, which blocks renal tubular exchange of potassium for sodium, is effective; it corrects the high blood pressure, hypokalemic alkalosis, and the increasing sodium excretion.

**Complications:** Related to the degree of hypokalemia.

**Associated Findings:** None known.

**Etiology:** Probably autosomal dominant inheritance.

**Pathogenesis:** Presumably related to membrane transport of sodium at the renal tubular level, perhaps reflecting a generalized membrane defect affecting other tissues and sites.

**MIM No.:** 17720

**Sex Ratio:** M1:F1

**Occurrence:** Undetermined but presumed rare.

**Risk of Recurrence for Patient's Sib:**
See Part I, *Mendelian Inheritance.*

**Risk of Recurrence for Patient's Child:**
See Part I, *Mendelian Inheritance.*

**Age of Detectability:** From birth.

**Gene Mapping and Linkage:** Unknown.

**Prevention:** None known. Genetic counseling indicated.

**Treatment:** Triamterene is effective in correcting blood pressure, potassium loss and alkalosis. This therapy should be maintained since the clinical findings return on discontinuation of treatment.

**Prognosis:** The prognosis appears normal for life span if treated.

**Detection of Carrier:** Unknown.

**References:**
Liddle CW, et al.: A familial renal disorder simulating primary aldosteronism but with negligible aldosterone secretion. In: Baulieu EE, Robel P, eds: Aldosterone, a symposium. Oxford: Blackwell Scientific, 1964:353–368.
Aarskog D, et al.: Hypertension and hypokalemic alkalosis associated with underproduction of aldosterone. Pediatrics 1967; 39:884–890.
Gardner JD, et al.: Abnormal membrane sodium transport in Liddle's syndrome. J Clin Invest 1971; 50:2253–2258.
Hyman PE, et al.: Liddle syndrome. J Pediatr 1979; 95:77–78.
Levine LB, et al.: Hypertension in childhood. In: Lavin N, ed: Manual of endocrinology and metabolism. Boston: Little Brown, 1986:169.

SP004                                              **Mark A. Sperling**

**Ligamentous laxity-cutis laxa-delayed development**
*See CUTIS LAXA-DELAYED DEVELOPMENT-LIGAMENTOUS LAXITY*
**Light, sensitivity to**
*See PORPHYRIA, PROTOPORPHYRIA*
**Ligneous conjunctivitis**
*See EYE, LIGNEOUS CONJUNCTIVITIS*

## LIMB AND SCALP DEFECTS, ADAMS-OLIVER TYPE          0459

**Includes:**
  Absence defects of limbs, scalp, and skull
  Adams-Oliver syndrome
  Amniotic bands complex
  Aplasia cutis congenita-terminal, transverse defects of limbs
  Hemimelia-scalp skull defects
  Scalp defect-ectrodactyly
  Scalp, skull, and limbs; absence defect of Adams-Oliver

**Excludes:**
  Ectrodactyly (0336)
  Ectrodactyly-ectodermal dysplasia-clefting syndrome (0337)
  Skin, localized absence of (0608)
  Tibial hypoplasia/aplasia-ectrodactyly (2388)

**Major Diagnostic Criteria:** Terminal transverse defects (TTD) of hands, and sometimes feet, with skull and scalp defects.

**Clinical Findings:** Central skull and scalp defects present at birth, such as denuded ulcerated area or areas on the vertex of the scalp associated with underlying bony defects of the skull. The scalp defect ranges from 2.5mm by 5mm to 7cm by 9cm. The skull and scalp defects usually heal spontaneously and completely in the first few months of life. In a few cases, plastic surgery was required. The limb deformity affects one or more limbs and varies from aphalangia, adactylia or acheiria, and apodia, to transverse hemimelia. Usually the feet are more severely affected. The terminal phalanges are sometimes short. Association of the congenital scalp defect and post-axial **Polydactyly** A has been described in two cases. Cutis marmorata and markedly dilated and tortuous scalp veins are also found.

**Complications:** Dilated and tortuous scalp veins, which can be injured in cases of head trauma. Scalp defects may lead to infection.

**Associated Findings:** Congenital heart defects, club feet, cryptorchidism, cleft lip.

**Etiology:** Probably autosomal dominant inheritance with complete penetrance and variable expression. Some observations suggest reduced penetrance. Reports suggestive of autosomal recessive inheritance were made. Almost one-half of the reported cases have been sporadic.

**Pathogenesis:** Aplasia cutis congenita (ACC) is also observed in cases of congenital ring constrictions, in epidermolysis bullosa, in focal dermal hypoplasia, in **Chromosome 13, trisomy 13**, and in cases of deletion of chromosome four. These findings illustrate the etiologic heterogeneity of skull and scalp defects of which ACC associated with TTD represents a distinct genetic entity. TTD is not simply inherited except in the rare acheiropody trait. The finding of ACC in patients with TTD, not associated with congenital ring constrictions, is a useful clue to inheritance. The cutis marmorata could be part of the syndrome and could be interpreted as a pleiotropic effect of the mutant gene.

Some observers have suggested that the TTD results from *constricting* or *amniotic bands.* While this general concept has been in and out of favor (Gellis, 1977), it has been used to explain a wide range of fetal "amputation" malformations (Pauli et al, 1985).

**MIM No.:** *10030, 21710

**POS No.:** 3250

**CDC No.:** 756.080

**Sex Ratio:** M1:F1

**Occurrence:** Thirty-eight cases have been reported in the literature of which 19 were familial and 19 sporadic.

**Risk of Recurrence for Patient's Sib:**
See Part I, *Mendelian Inheritance.*

**Risk of Recurrence for Patient's Child:**
See Part I, *Mendelian Inheritance.*

**Age of Detectability:** At birth.

**Gene Mapping and Linkage:** Unknown.

**Prevention:** None known. Genetic counseling indicated.

**Treatment:** Plastic surgery to scalp, if required, and appropriate surgery and/or prosthesis for limbs. Helmet for head when engaged in physical activities if marked dilation of scalp veins is present.

**Prognosis:** Normal life span and intelligence. Variable for function.

**Detection of Carrier:** Unknown.

**References:**
Adams FH, Oliver CP: Hereditary deformities in man due to arrested development. J Hered 1945; 36:3–7.
Scribanu N, Temtamy SA: Syndrome of aplasia cutis congenita with terminal transverse defects of limbs. J Pediatr 1975; 87:79–82. †
Gellis SS: Constrictive bands in the human. BD:OAS;XIII(1). New York: March of Dimes Birth Defects Foundation, 1977:259–268.
McMurray BR, et al.: Hereditary aplasia cutis congenita and associated defects: three instances in one family and a survey of reported cases. Clin Pediatr 1977; 16:610–614.
Bonafede RP, Beighton P: Autosomal dominant inheritance of scalp defects with ectrodactyly. Am J Med Genet 1979; 3:35–41.
Shapiro SD, Escobedo MK: Terminal transverse defects with aplasia

cutis congenita (Adams-Oliver syndrome). BD:OAS;XXI(2). New York: March of Dimes Birth Defects Foundation, 1985:135–142.
Pauli RM, et al.: Familial recurrence of terminal transverse defects of the arm. Clin Genet 1985; 27:555–563.
Sybert VP: Aplasia cutis congenita: a report of 12 new families and review of the literature. Pediatr Dermatol 1985; 3:1–14. * †
Fryns JP: Congenital scalp defects with distal limb reduction anomalies. J Med Genet 1987; 24:493–496.
Kuster W, et al.: Congenital scalp defects with distal limb anomalies (Adams-Oliver syndrome): report of ten cases and review of the literature. Am J Med Genet 1988; 31:99–115.

SC052                                            **Nina Scribanu**
GU008                                    **Alan E. Guttmacher**

**Limb anomalies (upper)-Waardenburg syndrome**
*See WAARDENBURG SYNDROMES*

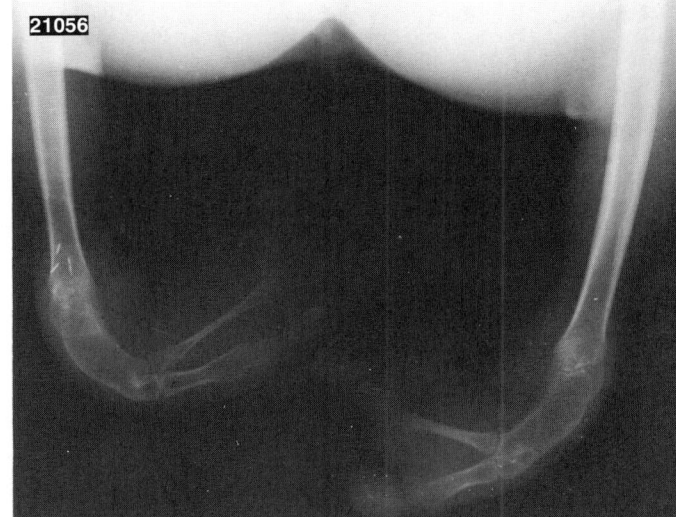

21056

---

## LIMB DEFECT WITH ABSENT ULNA/FIBULA          2822

**Includes:**
> Fibular and ulnar absence with severe limb deficiency
> Limb deficiency-thoracic dystrophy-unusual facies
> Ulnar and fibular absence with severe limb deficiency

**Excludes:**
> **Fibula, congenital absence of** (2229)
> **Mesomelic dysplasia, Reinhardt-Pfeiffer type** (0648)
> **Roberts syndrome** (0875)

**Major Diagnostic Criteria:**  Absent ulnae and fibulae, hypoplastic femora, absence of some ulnar and foot rays. Minor facial abnormalities with thoracic and pelvic dystrophy.

**Clinical Findings:**  Defects are evident at birth with severe deficiency of the four limbs, less severe in the upper limbs. Elbow joints have not functioned, with contracture deformities at the site with absent ulna and some ulnar rays in both hands. Absence defects are variable. Nails are absent or vestigial. The lower limbs are useless, and the appendages very short, consisting of one deformed long bone (tibia) and rudimentary or absent femora with some tarsal bones and foot rays. The anomalies in both lower limbs are also variable. The patients' facies are unusual and looked different from their parents and normal sibs. Facies are elongated with a broad nasal bridge and bulbous nose, epicanthic folds, and broad necks. Development and intelligence is normal.

**Complications:**  Thoracic dystrophy with barrel-shaped chest and prominent sternum, thoracic kyphosis, lumbar lordosis, and marked pelvic deformities. Patients tend to be shy.

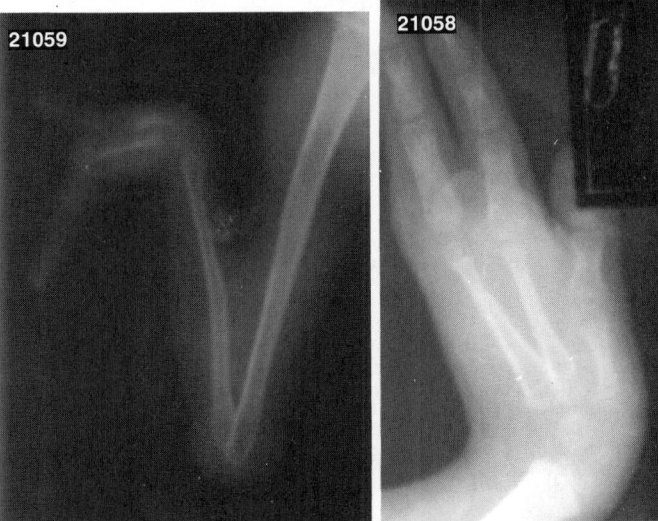

21059                                            21058

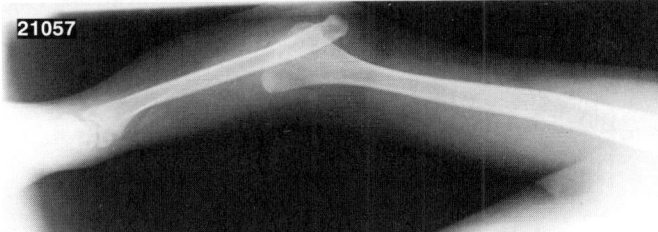

21057

**2822B-**21056-59:  Note the degree and severity of the absence defects in these limbs.

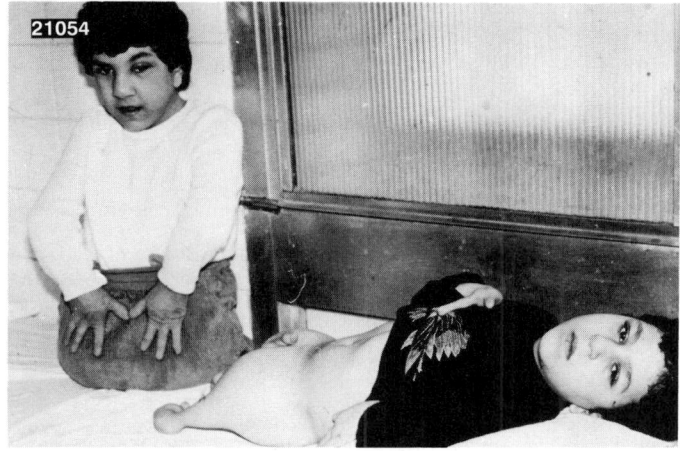

21054

**2822A-**21054:  Severe lower limb deficiencies with milder upper limb defects and mildly dysmorphic facies.

**Associated Findings:**  None known.

**Etiology:**  Probable autosomal recessive inheritance, based on parental consanguinity and affected sibs of both sexes. Expression is variable.

**Pathogenesis:**  Unknown.

**MIM No.:**  27682

**POS No.:**  3294

**Sex Ratio:**  Presumably M1:F1.

**Occurrence:** A brother and sister of consanguineous Palestinian Arab parents have been documented, and at least two other Jewish patients have been reported. A similar phenotype restricted to the lower limbs has been reported in a man from the endogamous Malay community of Cape Town (a relative of a patient with rhizomelic dysplasia reported in Viljoen et al, 1987). This is *not* a private syndrome and may be diagnosed in isolates with a high rate of intermarriage.

**Risk of Recurrence for Patient's Sib:**
See Part I, *Mendelian Inheritance.*

**Risk of Recurrence for Patient's Child:**
See Part I, *Mendelian Inheritance.*

**Age of Detectability:** Clinically evident at birth. Prenatal diagnosis is feasible by ultrasonography which can be performed in the second trimester.

**Gene Mapping and Linkage:** Unknown.

**Prevention:** None known. Genetic counseling indicated.

**Treatment:** Rehabilitation and physical therapy, artificial limbs.

**Prognosis:** Probably normal for life span. Physical handicaps lead to a change in life-style. Intelligence is normal.

**Detection of Carrier:** Unknown.

**References:**
Pfeiffer RA: Bectrag Zur erblichen Verkuerzung von Ulna und Fibula. In: Wiedemann HR, ed: Dysostosen. Stuttgart: Gustav Fischer Verlag, 1966.
Langer LO Jr: Mesomelic dwarfism of the hypoplastic ulna, fibula, mandible type. Radiology 1967; 89:654–660.
Al-Awadi SA, et al.: Profound limb deficiency, thoracic dystrophy, unusual facies, and normal intelligence: a new syndrome. J Med Genet 1985; 22:36–38.
Viljoen D, et al.: Familial rhizomelic dysplasia: phenotypic variation or heterogeneity? Am J Med Genet 1987; 62:941–947.

AL030     **S. A. Al-Awadi**
TE012     **Ahmad S. Teebi**

**Limb deficiency-splenogonadal fusion**
*See SPLENOGONADAL FUSION-LIMB DEFECT*
**Limb deficiency-thoracic dystrophy-unusual facies**
*See LIMB DEFECT WITH ABSENT ULNA/FIBULA*
**Limb malformations-dento-digital syndrome**
*See LACRIMO-AURICULO-DENTO-DIGITAL SYNDROME*

## LIMB REDUCTION DEFECTS     3285

**Includes:**
Amelia
Amputation, congenital
Central ray defects
Dysmelia
Hemimelia
Hypoplasia, limb
Intercalary defects
Limb, absence of
Micromelia
Phocomelia
Reduction defects of limb
Terminal longitudinal defects
Terminal transverse defects

**Excludes:**
**Amniotic bands syndrome (ADAM complex)** (0874)
**Hand, radial club hand** (2409)
**Hand, ulnar and fibular ray deficiency, Weyers type** (2292)
**Hand, ulnar drift** (2410)
**Poland syndrome** (0813)
**Skeletal dysplasia**
**Thrombocytopenia-absent radius** (0941)
Limb defects, syndromes with (other)

**Major Diagnostic Criteria:** Complete or partial absence of a limb bone or bones.

**Clinical Findings:** Limb reduction defects are heterogeneous defects that range from mild absence of a limb bone to total absence of the limb (amelia). Several classifications systems exist but none has gained universal acceptance. In general, defects can be divided into *amelia*, i.e. total absence of a limb, or *meromelia*, i.e. partial absence of a limb. Partial absence is further classified as being either terminal or intercalary. A *terminal defect* is characterized by partial or total absence of limb bones distal from the defect named, i.e. no normal parts exist distal to the defect. An *intercalary defect* consists of partial or total absence of the proximal or distal segments of a limb with significant or relatively normal distal parts. The distal parts need not be completely normal.

Defects are further subclassified as *transverse*, i.e. the defect extends across the total width of the limb, or *longitudinal*, i.e. the defect occurs lengthwise along the limb. If known, the precise missing bone is included in the classification.

*Hypoplasia* is a term used to describe a generalized reduction in limb size when the defect can not easily be identified more specifically. *Central ray defects* are used to describe defects of the 2, 3 and 4th phalanges. *Phocomelia* is used to describe limbs with relatively normal distal parts and absent or nearly absent proximal and medial parts.

Terminal transverse defects are more common than transverse longitudinal defects. Seventy-five percent of limb defects involve the upper limb, 25% the lower limb. There is no evidence of a predilection for a particular side.

**Complications:** Vary with the site and extent of the defect.

**Associated Findings:** About half of affected individuals have other defects, usually in the muscular skeletal system, e.g. **Foot, congenital clubfoot,** dislocated hip, and congenital contracture. Other systems that may have associated congenital defects include the cardiovascular system, the gastrointestinal system, and the genitourinary system.

**Etiology:** Unknown. Probably heterogeneous. A vascular accident is also a possible etiology.

**Pathogenesis:** Unknown.

**Sex Ratio:** M>1:F1.

**Occurrence:** 5.97:10,000 live births (1:1,692 live births) in British Columbia.

**Risk of Recurrence for Patient's Sib:** Unknown. In the British Columbia study, 6.5% had another family member with a limb defect.

**Risk of Recurrence for Patient's Child:** Unknown.

**Age of Detectability:** By ultrasound examination at 16 weeks gestation. Most are apparent at birth or within the first year of life.

**Gene Mapping and Linkage:** Unknown.

**Prevention:** None known. Genetic counseling indicated.

**Treatment:** Orthopedic, rehabilitative, and reconstructive therapy is indicated depending on the nature and extent of the defect.

**Prognosis:** Death occurs in 12.9–20% within the first year of life, but of these, 85% had additional defects. Overall prognosis depends on the size and location of the defect.

**Detection of Carrier:** Unknown.

**References:**
Frantz CH, O'Rahilly R: Congenital skeletal limb deficiency. J Bone Joint Surg 1961; 430A:1202–1224.
Henkel L, et al.: Dysmelia: a classification and a pattern of malformation in a group of congenital defects of the limbs. J Bone Joint Surg 1969; 51B:399–414.
Smith ESO, et al.: An epidemiological study of congenital reduction deformities of the limbs. Br J Prev Soc Med 1977; 31:39–41.
Kallen B, et al.: Infants with congenital limb reduction registered in the Swedish register of congenital malformations. Teratology 1984; 29:73–85.
Froster-Iskenius, UG, Baird P: Limb reductions defects in over one million consecutive livebirths. Teratology 1989; 39:127–135.

BU032     **Mary Louise Buyse**

## LIMB REDUCTION-ICHTHYOSIS    2019

**Includes:**
CHILD syndrome
Ectromelia, unilateral-psoriasis-CNS anomalies
Hemidysplasia-ichthyosis, congenital
Ichthyosiform erythryoderma, unilateral-ipsilateral
    malformations
Ichthyosis-limb reduction
Limbs, absence deformity of-ichthyosiform erythryoderma

**Excludes:**
**Chondrodysplasia punctata**
**Incontinentia pigmenti** (0526)
**Nevus, epidermal nevus syndrome** (0593)

**Major Diagnostic Criteria:** Unilateral skin erythema and scaling, with ipsilateral limb defects.

**Clinical Findings:** All affected individuals have unilateral ichthyosiform erythroderma affecting the trunk and limbs, but generally sparing the face. The nails are often hyperkeratotic, and alopecia occasionally occurs on the same side. Ipsilateral limb anomalies, ranging from hypoplastic phalanges and metacarpals to absent limbs, are also a constant finding. Skeletal hypoplasia of the trunk and head also occur, but less consistently. Ipsilateral visceral anomalies are also common, and include unilateral brain hypoplasia, cardiac defects, unilateral renal agenesis, and unilateral lung hypoplasia. Punctate calcification of the cartilage on X-rays disappears by two years of age. Histologic examination has shown acanthotic epidermis with thickened, parakeratotic stratum corneum, and a broadened or absent granular layer. In 20 affected individuals, the right side was affected in 14, and the left in six. A few individuals also had skin lesions, skeletal anomalies, and/or visceral defects on the contralateral side.

**Complications:** Scoliosis may occur as a result of either limb asymmetry or vertebral defects. Mild mental retardation, presumably secondary to unilateral brain hypoplasia, has also been reported.

**Associated Findings:** **Cleft lip**, bilateral mild hearing loss, **Hernia, umbilical**, **Hydrocephaly**, and **Meningomyelocele** have each been reported as occasional findings.

**Etiology:** Possibly X-linked dominant inheritance.

**Pathogenesis:** The basic gene defect is unknown. Lyonization is unable to account for the unilateral distribution of anomalies without invoking an auxiliary hypothesis.

**MIM No.:** 30805

**POS No.:** 3457

**CDC No.:** 755.2

**Sex Ratio:** M1:F28

**Occurrence:** At least 29 cases from different parts of the world have been described.

**Risk of Recurrence for Patient's Sib:**
See Part I, *Mendelian Inheritance.*

**Risk of Recurrence for Patient's Child:**
See Part I, *Mendelian Inheritance.*

**Age of Detectability:** At birth, by the presence of limb defects. Severe limb defects may also be detectable in utero by ultrasound. Skin defects are usually present at or soon after birth, but may not appear until later.

**Gene Mapping and Linkage:** Unknown.

**Prevention:** None known. Genetic counseling indicated.

**Treatment:** Topical skin ointment occasionally improves the skin condition; orthopedic treatment may also be indicated.

**Prognosis:** If visceral anomalies are not present, then life span is not affected. Intellectual development is usually normal, although mild mental retardation has also been reported. The skin condition can improve, or alternatively can improve and worsen.

**Detection of Carrier:** Unknown.

**References:**
Cullen SI, et al.: Congenital unilateral ichthyosiform erythroderma. Arch Dermatol 1969; 99:724–729. †
Tang TT, McCreadie SR: Congenital hemidysplasia with ichthyosis. BD:OAS X(5). New York: March of Dimes Birth Defects Foundation, 1974::257–260.
Happle R, et al.: The CHILD syndrome. Europ J Pediatr 1980; 134:27–33. *
Wettke-Schafer R, Kantner G: X-linked dominant inherited diseases with lethality in hemizygous males. Hum Genet 1983; 64:1–23.
Hebert AA, et al.: The CHILD syndrome: histologic and ultrastructural studies. Arch Derm 1987; 123:503–509.

T0007                                    **Helga V. Toriello**

## LIMB REDUCTION-MENTAL RETARDATION    3128

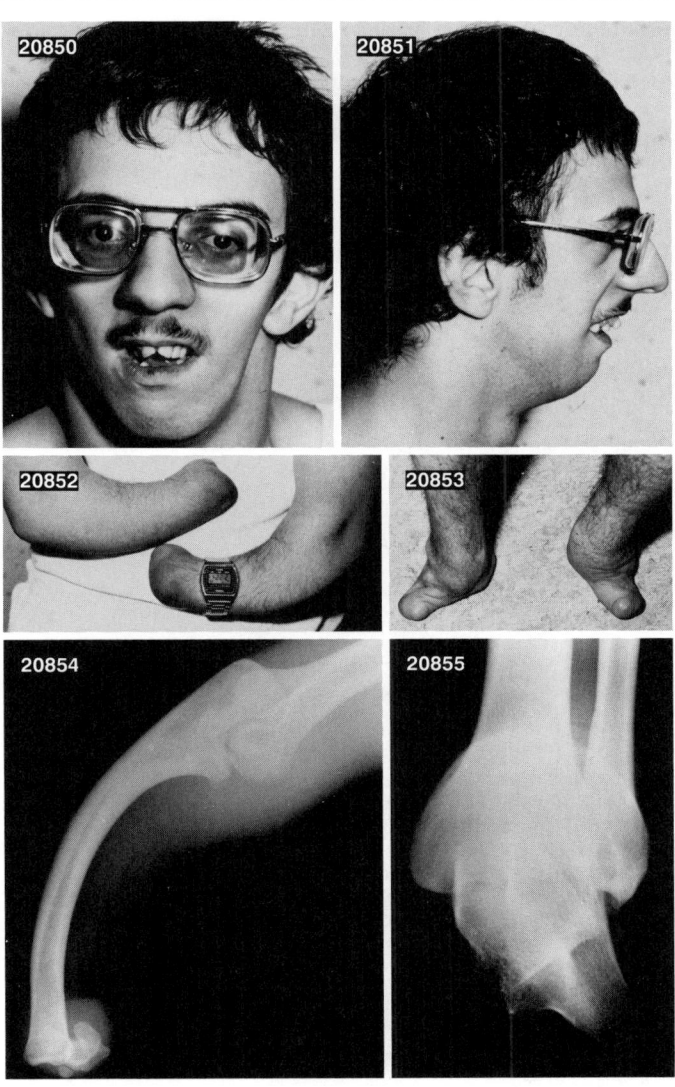

**3128**-20850–51: Limb reduction-mental retardation; note midface hypoplasia and micrognathia. **20852–53:** Severe transverse limb defects of the upper and lower limbs. **20854:** Note absent radius, hypoplastic distal ulna, and four rudimentary carpal bones. **20855:** Synostosis of the rudimentary calcaneus and talus.

**Includes:** Mental retardation-limb deficiency

**Excludes:** Hypoglossia-hypodactylia (0451)

**Major Diagnostic Criteria:** The combination of transverse limb reduction defect, oral anomalies, and mental retardation.

**Clinical Findings:** In the reported sibs (one male, one female), both had limb anomalies of all extremities, with the limb defects resembling transverse terminal defects, but actually being a paraxial radial/preaxial limb defect. In addition, both had maxillary hypoplasia, micrognathia, small mouth with highly arched palate, normal tongue, and mild-to-moderate mental retardation. One sib also had myopia and oligomeganephronia; the other also had short stature.

**Complications:** Unknown.

**Associated Findings:** None known.

**Etiology:** Possibly autosomal recessive inheritance.

**Pathogenesis:** Unknown.

**Sex Ratio:** M1:F1

**Occurrence:** Documented in one pair of Greek sibs.

**Risk of Recurrence for Patient's Sib:**
See Part I, *Mendelian Inheritance.*

**Risk of Recurrence for Patient's Child:**
See Part I, *Mendelian Inheritance.*

**Age of Detectability:** At birth, although prenatal diagnosis using ultrasound may be possible.

**Gene Mapping and Linkage:** Unknown.

**Prevention:** None known. Genetic counseling indicated.

**Treatment:** Orthopedic intervention for the limb defects.

**Prognosis:** Mental retardation is variable, being mild in one sib and moderate in the other. Life span is presumably normal.

**Detection of Carrier:** Unknown.

**References:**
Buttiens M, Fryns JP: Apparently new autosomal recessive syndrome of mental retardation, distal limb deficiencies, oral involvement, and possible renal defect. Am J Med Genet 1987; 27:651–660.

T0007                                            **Helga V. Toriello**

**Limb, absence of**
*See LIMB REDUCTION DEFECTS*

---

## LIMB, REDUCTION DEFORMITIES OF UPPER LIMBS          2885

**Includes:** Bone aplasias-hypoplasias of the upper extremities

**Excludes:** Acheiropody (2486)

**Major Diagnostic Criteria:** Multiple, extensive, and variable reduction deformities of the upper limbs.

**Clinical Findings:** Unilateral amelia; unilateral amelia with bidactyly; modification of the configuration of the articular elements of the shoulder and elbow, bowed humerus, aplasia of radius (with associated defects such as a short, thick, and bent ulna), absence of some carpal bones, absence of the first radial ray and manus vara; hypoplasia of the humerus, whose remaining part (with irregular contours) is disarticulated from the glenoid fossa, aplasia of the radius, bowed ulna, absence of some carpal bones, absence of first and second radial rays, and manus vara; hypoplasia of both clavicles and scapulas, absence of the glenoid fossae, unilateral amelia, presence of a rounded prominence constituted of soft tissues; unilateral amelia with the presence of only one finger with two phalanges, and some bones without precise X-ray characteristics.

**Complications:** The highly mutilating nature of this anomaly may affect social life and marriage.

**Associated Findings:** None known.

**Etiology:** Reduction deformities of the limbs are generally sporadic and due to unknown etiology. However, a minority of them

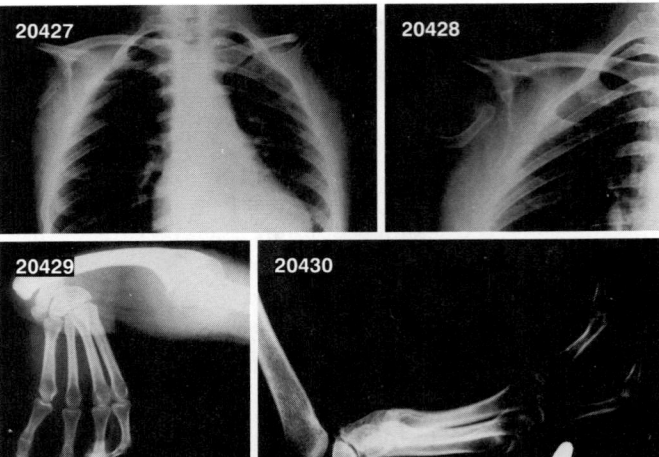

**2885-20427:** X-ray of an affected woman; note total absence of the left arm and a few remaining bones of the right arm (see fig. 20428). **20428:** Detail of the remaining left arm of an affected woman. **20429:** Right forearm and hand of an affected man; note absence of radius; short, thick, and bent ulna; absence of five carpal bones and of the first radial ray; and manus vara. **20430:** Left forearm and hand of the man shown in fig. 20429; note the absence of first and second radial rays, and manus vara among other defects.

---

are due to either autosomal dominant or autosomal recessive inheritance.

**Pathogenesis:** Unknown.

**Sex Ratio:** Presumably M1:F1.

**Occurrence:** One Brazilian kindred with two men and two women belonging to three sibships has been reported in the literature.

**Risk of Recurrence for Patient's Sib:**
See Part I, *Mendelian Inheritance.* Recurrence risk ranges from a low of zero to 25–50% for reduction deformities in general.

**Risk of Recurrence for Patient's Child:**
See Part I, *Mendelian Inheritance.*

**Age of Detectability:** At birth, or prenatally by ultrasound.

**Gene Mapping and Linkage:** Unknown.

**Prevention:** None known. Genetic counseling indicated.

**Treatment:** Orthopedic care as indicated.

**Prognosis:** Normal for life span and reproduction. Three of the four affected individuals married and had children.

**Detection of Carrier:** A heterozygote was born with aplasia of the right thumb and the corresponding metacarpal.

**References:**
Birch-Jensen A: Congenital deformities of the upper extremities. Copenhagen: Ejnar Munksgaard, 1949.
Freire-Maia N, et al.: Hereditary bone aplasias and hypoplasias of the extremities. Acta Genet Stat Med 1959; 9:33–40.
Freire-Maia N, Freire-Maia A: Multiple congenital abnormalities. Lancet 1964; I:113–114.
Freire-Maia N, Freire-Maia A: Recurrence risks of bone aplasias and hypoplasias of the extremities. Acta Genet Stat Med 1967; 17:418–421.
Freire-Maia N, Azevedo JBC: Skeletal limb deficiencies. Lancet 1968; II:1296 only.
Freire-Maia N: Congenital skeletal limb deficiencies: a general view. BD:OAS V(3). New York: March of Dimes Birth Defects Foundation, 1969:7–13.

Freire-Maia N: A heterozygote expression of a "recessive" gene? Hum Hered 1975; 25:302–304.

FR033                                                    **Newton Freire-Maia**

## LIMB, UPPER HYPOPLASIA-MULLERIAN DUCT DEFECTS                                              2932

**Includes:**
>    Hypomelia with Mullerian duct anomalies
>    Limb-uterus syndrome
>    Mullerian duct defects-upper limb hypoplasia
>    Uterus-limb syndrome

**Excludes:**
>    **Acro-renal-mandibular syndrome** (2778)
>    **Aredyld syndrome** (2785)
>    Camptobrachydactyly
>    Cryptophthalmos
>    **Ectrodactyly-ectodermal dysplasia-clefting syndrome** (0337)
>    **Hand-foot-genital syndrome** (2570)
>    **Meckel syndrome** (0634)
>    **Renal-genital-middle ear anomalies** (0860)
>    **Vaginal septum, transverse** (0985)

**Major Diagnostic Criteria:** Upper limb hypoplasia with Müllerian duct anomalies.

**Clinical Findings:** The association of upper limb anomalies with genital defects was described in five members of a French Canadian family. Two of the three affected women had upper limb anomalies and Müllerian duct defects, and one had only a Müllerian duct anomaly. The two affected males had both upper limb or acral malformation, and one had a genital anomaly (micropenis). Limb anomalies varied in expression from postaxial **Polydactyly**, to ectrodactyly (ulnar ray defect), to severe upper limb hypoplasia with split hand. Genital anomalies varied from a complete duplication of the uterus and vagina in two individuals, to only a vaginal septum in one female.

All affected individuals examined had a distal loop in the hallucal area, two had a hypothenar pattern, and one had distal axial triradii.

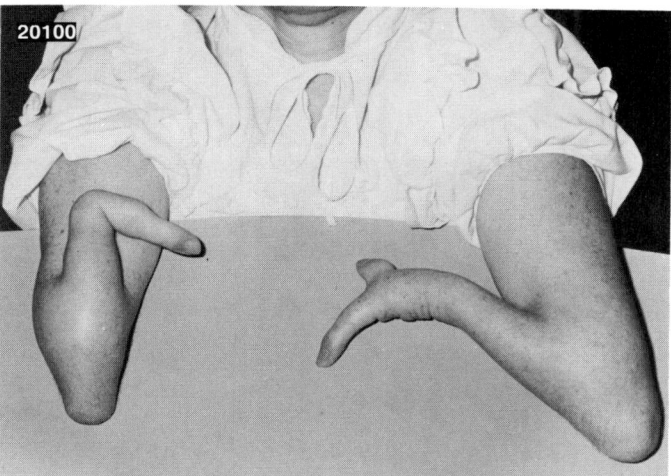

**2932-20100:** The hypoplastic forearms are tightly flexed over the arms. On the right, she has one digit with fixed radial deviation and on the left she has a split hand with a thumb and one other digit.

**Complications:** The two individuals with split hand had hypoplastic forearms. The latter were tightly flexed over the arms, allowing very little passive and active extension.

**Associated Findings:** Bilateral mild tubular ectasia in one individual. Hypothyroidic goiter in one affected female and euthyroidic goiter in another.

**Etiology:** Probably autosomal dominant inheritance with variable expressivity.

**Pathogenesis:** Unknown.

**MIM No.:** 14616

**POS No.:** 3896

**CDC No.:** 755.2

**Sex Ratio:** Presumably M1:F1 (M2:F3 observed).

**Occurrence:** Reported in five members of three generations of a French Canadian family.

**Risk of Recurrence for Patient's Sib:**
See Part I, *Mendelian Inheritance.*

**Risk of Recurrence for Patient's Child:**
See Part I, *Mendelian Inheritance.*

**Age of Detectability:** At birth. Prenatal diagnosis of limb anomalies is possible by ultrasonography.

**Gene Mapping and Linkage:** Unknown.

**Prevention:** None known. Genetic counseling indicated.

**Treatment:** Prosthetic replacement of severely malformed limbs.

**Prognosis:** Normal life span.

**Detection of Carrier:** Gynecologic examination of female relatives for evidence of the trait (vaginal or uterine septum), since Müllerian duct anomaly can be present without limb defects.

**References:**
Halal F: A new syndrome of severe upper limb hypoplasia and Müllerian duct anomalies. Am J Med Genet 1986; 24:119–126.

HA074                                                        **Fahed Halal**

**Limb-blood syndrome**
>    *See WT SYNDROME*
**Limb-face syndrome (one form)**
>    *See CHARLIE M SYNDROME*
**Limb-girdle muscular dystrophy**
>    *See MUSCULAR DYSTROPHY, LIMB-GIRDLE*

## LIMB-OTO-CARDIAC SYNDROME                                          0592

**Includes:**
>    Cardiac-limb-oto syndrome
>    Facioauriculoradial dysplasia
>    Oto-limb-cardiac syndrome
>    Phocomelia-ectrodactyly-oto-sinus arrhythmia syndrome

**Excludes:**
>    **Fetal thalidomide syndrome** (0386)
>    **Heart-hand syndrome** (0455)
>    **Acrofacial dysostosis, Nager type** (2167)

**Major Diagnostic Criteria:** Hypoplasia of upper limbs, malformed external ear, conduction deafness, vertebral anomalies.

**Clinical Findings:** Dysmorphic facial features include mid-face hypoplasia, a long philtrum, and flattened nasal bridge. Hypoplasia of the upper limbs, sinus arrhythmia, malformed external ears, profound conduction deafness, and vertebral anomalies have been reported in two families. The malformation of the upper limbs is characterized by the absence of the radius, hypoplasia of the humerus, and metacarpophalangeal hypoplasia. Lumbar vertebral abnormalities and fibular hypoplasia have been variably present. Short stature was present in two instances. Malformation of the middle ear was characterized by the absence of the incus and stapes and an aplasia of the oval window.

**Complications:** Unknown.

**Associated Findings:** None known.

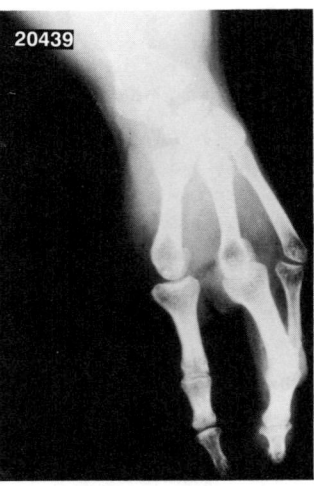

0592-20440: Hypoplasia of the upper limbs. 20439: Absent carpals, metacarpals, and digits.

**Etiology:** Presumably autosomal dominant inheritance.

**Pathogenesis:** Unknown.

**MIM No.:** 17148

**POS No.:** 3280

**Sex Ratio:** M2:F3

**Occurrence:** Two reported families with two affected males, a father and son, and three females (two sisters and one daughter).

**Risk of Recurrence for Patient's Sib:**
See Part I, *Mendelian Inheritance.*

**Risk of Recurrence for Patient's Child:**
See Part I, *Mendelian Inheritance.*

**Age of Detectability:** Limb anomalies may be detectable by ultrasound or fetoscope prenatally; otherwise at birth.

**Gene Mapping and Linkage:** Unknown.

**Prevention:** None known. Genetic counseling indicated.

**Treatment:** Surgery. Because of the absence of the oval window, reconstructive middle ear surgery was impossible in these cases. Arrhythmias reported in some cases may be normal sinus arrhythmias.

**Prognosis:** Probably normal life span; intelligence is normal.

**Detection of Carrier:** Unknown.

**References:**
Stoll C, et al.: L'association phocomélie-ectrodactylie, malformations des oreilles avec surdité, arythmie sinusale: constitue-t-elle un nouveau syndrome héréditaire? Arch Fr Pediatr 1974; 31:669–680.
Harding AE, et al.: Autosomal asymmetric radial dysplasia, dysmorphic facies, and conductive hearing loss (facioauriculoradial dysplasia). J Med Genet 1982; 19:110–115.

MU020

**Jeff Murray**
*Cor W.R.J. Cremers*

**Limb-uterus syndrome**
*See LIMB, UPPER HYPOPLASIA-MULLERIAN DUCT DEFECTS*
**Limbal dermoid**
*See OCULAR DERMOIDS*
**Limbs and trunk, familial lipodystrophy of**
*See LIPODYSTROPHY, FAMILIAL LIMB AND TRUNK*
**Limbs, absence deformity of-ichthyosiform erythryoderma**
*See LIMB REDUCTION-ICHTHYOSIS*
**Limbs, deformities of long bones-cleft lip/palate**
*See ROBERTS SYNDROME*
**Limbs, duplicated**
*See LIMBS, SUPERNUMERARY*

**Limbs, ectopic**
*See LIMBS, SUPERNUMERARY*

## LIMBS, SUPERNUMERARY      2494

**Includes:**
    Limbs, duplicated
    Limbs, ectopic
    Twins, parasitic conjoined without spinal columns

**Excludes:**
    Spinal tail
    **Twins, conjoined** (0202)

**Major Diagnostic Criteria:** An extra limb, including all tissue layers, long bones with an intercalated joint, and a terminal digital structure, in the absence of duplication of the spinal column.

**Clinical Findings:** The most common situation, conjoined twins with duplications of the spinal cord, is excluded as representing a complete central duplication. Otherwise, extra limbs are unusual, but can be seen in several situations: 1) So-called "parasitic conjoined twins" which typically involve bilateral (although not always symmetrical) limbs on both sides of the midline, but lack any indications of a head or spinal column. 2) Duplicated limbs, which are unilateral and in situ. They may be relatively complete, polydactylous, or abortive with only a few digits. There is no duplication of spinal elements. 3) True ectopic limbs, which are single midline posterior structures. Again, they may be relatively complete or terminally abortive or polydactylous.

**Complications:** Those due to mechanical problems from the physical presence of the extra limb(s).

**Associated Findings:** Other midline problems are common. Heart and spinal anomalies, and teratomatous structures ranging

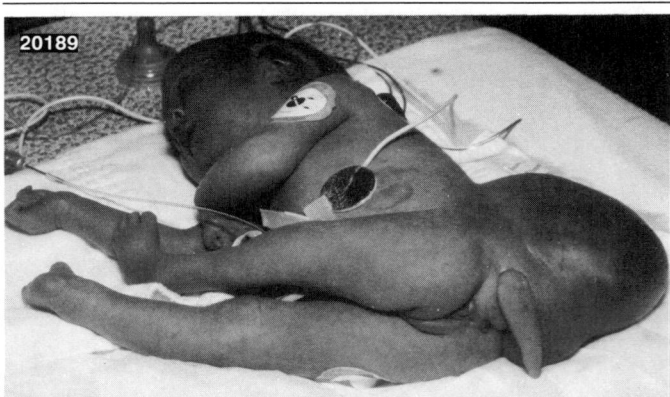

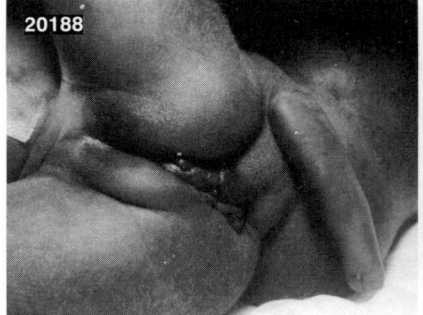
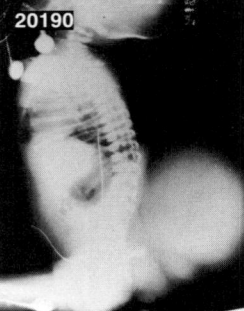

2494-20189: The additional limb is attached to the myelomeningocele sac. 20188: Additional limb and duplication of the external genitalia. 20190: X-ray view of the third limb and the myelomeningocele sac.

from dermoid cysts to malignant teratomas can be seen, mostly with types 2 and 3.

**Etiology:** Unknown. Maternal trauma has been suggested, but is unproved. Factors predisposing to duplications or midline disruptions may be involved.

**Pathogenesis:** For parasitic conjoined twins, duplication of the Wolffian ridges has been suggested. However, the origins of the bilaterality of these structures is difficult to understand under this hypothesis. A spectrum including "typical" conjoined twins is possible, but it is likely that these are pathogenetically different. Duplications in situ often are found with vertebral defects and may represent the induction of a second limb bud near the site of the first. True ectopic limbs are difficult to explain with any variant of normal embryology. Their invariable midline location suggests a pathogenetic relationship that somehow involves this area. A case of formed digits with nails, phalanges, and metacarpals within a sacrococcygeal teratoma is instructive; nerves to the digits came from the sacral nerves of the host. Teratomas are certainly capable of full differentiation given the proper circumstances. Rarely, this may occur in situ, perhaps with an atypical inductive stimulus supplied by a disrupted spinal cord.

**Sex Ratio:** Undetermined but presumably M1:F1.

**Occurrence:** Undetermined but presumed rare.

**Risk of Recurrence for Patient's Sib:** Unknown, but there are no reported familial cases.

**Risk of Recurrence for Patient's Child:** Unknown.

**Age of Detectability:** Presumably prenatally by ultrasound, although interpretation would probably be very difficult.

**Gene Mapping and Linkage:** Unknown.

**Prevention:** None known. Genetic counseling indicated.

**Treatment:** Surgical removal and repair of the primary anomaly and of any associated problems. Awareness of possible malignant teratoma.

**Prognosis:** Depends on associated anomalies. Reports of unoperated cases indicate that long-term survival and good overall function are possible, although obviously psychosocial difficulties can be great.

**Detection of Carrier:** Unknown.

**Special Considerations:** These are rare and poorly characterized anomalies about which little is certain. The relationship to other teratologia, such as conjoined twins and midline "tails", is unknown. Any cases should be well studied anatomically and reported if possible.

A possible mouse model for these anomalies is the semidominant mutant, Disorganization. This gene causes a wide range of anomalies, including limb duplications and hamartomas. The latter often resembled limbs and digits. Extra limbs can be seen, usually close to normal limbs, but limb-like projections can be found elsewhere, particularly on the ventral abdomen.

**References:**
Nicholson GW: A sacro-coccygeal teratoma with three metacarpal bones and digits. Guy's Hosp Rep 1937; 87:46.
Hummel KP: Developmental anomalies in mice resulting from action of the gene, disorganization, a semi-dominant lethal. Pediatrics 1959; 23:212.
Stephens TD, et al.: Parasitic conjoined twins, two cases, and their relation to limb morphogenesis. Teratology 1982; 26:115.
Saul RA, Stevenson RE: Limb amputation/autotransplantation: follow-up. Proc Greenwood Genet Cen 1985; 4:78.

LU001                                    **Mark Lubinsky**

**Limit dextrinosis**
See GLYCOGENOSIS, TYPE III
**Lindau disease**
See VON HIPPEL-LINDAU SYNDROME
**Linear nevus sebaceous syndrome**
See NEVUS, EPIDERMAL NEVUS SYNDROME
**Linear porokeratosis**
See SKIN, POROKERATOSIS
**Linear sebaceous nevus syndrome**
See NEVUS, EPIDERMAL NEVUS SYNDROME
**Linear sebaceous nevus-mental retardation-seizures**
See PROTEUS SYNDROME
**Lingua fissurata types I, II, and III**
See TONGUE, FISSURED
**Lingua plicata**
See TONGUE, GEOGRAPHIC
**Lingual thyroid**
See THYROGLOSSAL DUCT REMNANT
**Lip pits or mounds and cleft lip or palate**
See CLEFT LIP/PALATE-LIP PITS OR MOUNDS

**LIP, CHEILITIS GLANDULARIS** 0144

**Includes:**
Baelz syndrome
Cheilitis glandularis apostematosa
Lip, enlargement of lower

**Excludes:**
**Blepharochalasis-double lip-nontoxic goiter** (0111)
Cheilitis exfolitiva
**Cheilitis granulomatosa, Melkersson-Rosenthal type** (2083)

**Major Diagnostic Criteria:** Enlargement of lower lip, increased secretion of mucus, vesicle-like lesions, or palpable enlargement of mucous glands.

**Clinical Findings:** There is enlargement of the lower lip and increased secretion of mucus on the lower lip, resulting in a wet, sticky lip; collection of mucus in dilated mucous ducts beneath the mucosa gives vesicle-like cystic lesions; there is protrusion and eversion of the lower lip; and nodular enlargement of mucous glands of the lip can be detected by palpation. All of these features are present in the well-developed stage, but earlier changes consist of enlargement of the lower lip and excess mucous secretion with or without vesicle-like lesions.

**Complications:** Mucous cyst (mucocele) formation is due to traumatic rupture of mucous ducts, and this complication is common. In Caucasians, 18–35% of patients reported with cheilitis glandularis have developed squamous cell carcinoma. This complication is due presumably to protrusion of the lip, making it susceptible to solar radiation and other irritations such as smoking. Secondary bacterial infection may occur with fistula formation.

**Associated Findings:** None known.

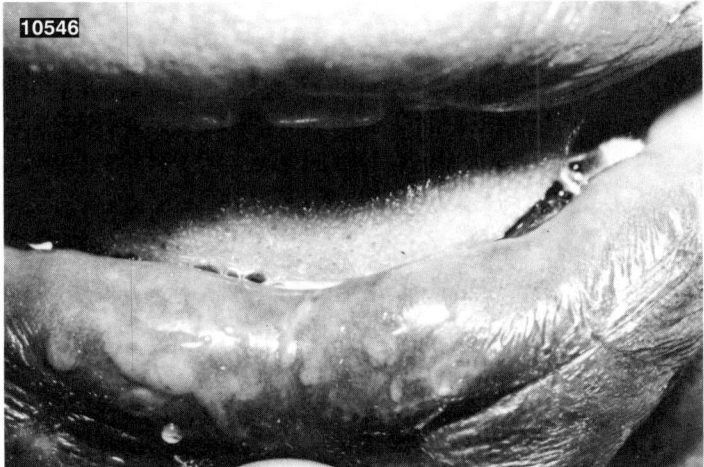

0144-10546: Cheilitis glandularis.

**Etiology:** Possibly autosomal dominant inheritance. The majority of patients with cheilitis glandularis recognized in the past have not been reported as having a hereditary form of the disease.

**Pathogenesis:** The gross structural defect in the fully developed condition includes enlargement of lower lip two to four times normal size, enlargement of mucous glands up to 12 mm in size, dilation of the mucous ducts in the mucosa or submucosa, a marked hypertrophy of the mucous glands, chronic inflammation involving the stroma of the mucous glands consisting mainly of plasma cells and fibrosis, and edema of the stroma. It is probable that the glandular hypertrophy with increased mucous secretion occurs as the initial change, with secondary changes of partial obstruction resulting in dilatation of ducts and inflammation.

**MIM No.:** 11833

**CDC No.:** 750.270

**Sex Ratio:** Presumably M1:F1 (males predominate in reported cases).

**Occurrence:** Over one hundred cases reported.

**Risk of Recurrence for Patient's Sib:**
See Part I, *Mendelian Inheritance.*

**Risk of Recurrence for Patient's Child:**
See Part I, *Mendelian Inheritance.*

**Age of Detectability:** Usually between 5 and 10 years by enlargement of lower lip, increased mucous secretion of lip, and vesicle-like lesions.

**Gene Mapping and Linkage:** Unknown.

**Prevention:** None known. Genetic counseling indicated.

**Treatment:** Partial excision of the lower lip with removal of enlarged mucous glands. This will prevent complications and give a cosmetically and functionally satisfactory result.

**Prognosis:** If treated, there is minimal morbidity and normal life span. If untreated, complications may cause moderate morbidity, and if squamous cell carcinoma develops and is not treated, death may occur.

**Detection of Carrier:** Unknown.

**References:**
Doku HC, et al.: Cheilitis glandularis. Oral Surg 1965; 20:563–571.
Weir TW, Johnson WC: Cheilitis glandularis. Arch Dermatol 1971; 103:433–437.
Rada DC, et al.: Cheilitis glandularis: a disorder of ductal ectasia. J Dermatol Surg Oncol 1985; 11:4:372–375.

J0009                                            **Waine C. Johnson**

**Lip, cleft**
*See CLEFT LIP*

---

## LIP, DOUBLE                                            0594

**Includes:**
Duplicate labiale
Lip, double upper or lower
Midline maxillary double lip

**Excludes:**
**Blepharochalasis-double lip-nontoxic goiter** (0111)
**Lip, cheilitis glandularis** (0144)
**Lip, pits or mounds** (0596)
Macrocheilia

**Major Diagnostic Criteria:** The appearance of two vermilion borders of the upper or lower lip when smiling in a patient without blepharochalasis and nontoxic thyroid enlargement.

**Clinical Findings:** The vermilion border of the lip is divided into two parts by a transverse furrow (horizontal sulcus) so that the inner portion of the lip, the pars villosa, sags below the outer portion, the pars glabra. When the lip is drawn tightly across the teeth in smiling, it gives the impression of two vermilion margins of the lip and two masses of hyperplastic tissue on either side of the midline. In most cases only the upper lip is involved, but

deformity is bilateral and involves the upper lip alone; rarely both upper and lower lips show the deformity. Unilateral and midline deformities have been described.

**Complications:** May be of cosmetic concern to the patient.

**Associated Findings:** May occur as one sign of **Blepharochalasis-double lip-nontoxic goiter**.

**Etiology:** Most cases are sporadic, has been observed in sibs, and autosomal dominant inheritance has been suggested.

**Pathogenesis:** The defect has ben ascribable to displacement of the orbicularis oris fibers because of hypertrophy of the mucous gland ducts and submucous tissues, resulting in the herniation of submucosa. Endocrine and allergic factors have been postulated.

**CDC No.:** 750.270

**Sex Ratio:** M1:F1

**Occurrence:** Chileans, 1:480; Caucasians in Utah in the United States, 1:200. Overall incidence data is, however, undetermined, and is not assumed to be as high as that shown for Chile and Utah.

**Risk of Recurrence for Patient's Sib:** Unknown.

**Risk of Recurrence for Patient's Child:** Unknown.

**Age of Detectability:** Usually during infancy.

**Gene Mapping and Linkage:** Unknown.

**Prevention:** None known. Genetic counseling indicated.

**Treatment:** Surgery.

**Prognosis:** Of cosmetic concern only; general health is not impaired.

**Detection of Carrier:** Unknown.

**References:**
Guerrero-Santos J, Altamirano JT: The use of W-plasty for correction of double lip deformity. Plast Reconstr Surg 1967; 39:478–481.
Witkop CJ Jr: The face and oral structures. In: Rubin A, ed: Handbook of congenital malformations. Philadelphia: W.B. Saunders, 1967: 103–139.
Rintala AE: Congenital double lip and Ascher syndrome: II. Relationship to the lower lip sinus syndrome. Br J Plast Surg 1981; 34:31–34.
Lamster IB: Mucosal reduction for correction of a maxillary double lip. Oral Surg 1983; 55:457–458.

BL002                                            **Will Blackburn**

**Lip, double upper or lower**
*See LIP, DOUBLE*
**Lip, double-blepharochalasis-goiter**
*See BLEPHAROCHALASIS-DOUBLE LIP-NONTOXIC GOITER*
**Lip, enlargement of lower**
*See LIP, CHEILITIS GLANDULARIS*
**Lip, indentations of upper**
*See CLEFT LIP*

---

## LIP, MEDIAN CLEFT OF UPPER                                            0595

**Includes:**
Median cleft of upper lip
True median cleft

**Excludes:**
**Agnathia-holoprosencephaly** (2780)
Cebocephaly
**Chondroectodermal dysplasia** (0156)
**Face, median cleft face syndrome** (0635)
**Oro-facio-digital syndrome** (all)

**Major Diagnostic Criteria:** Midline cleft of the upper lip.

**Clinical Findings:** Midline cleft of the upper lip.

**Complications:** Unknown.

**Associated Findings:** Midline cleft of the upper lip may be present alone, or in association with **Face, median cleft face syndrome**.

**Etiology:** Unknown.

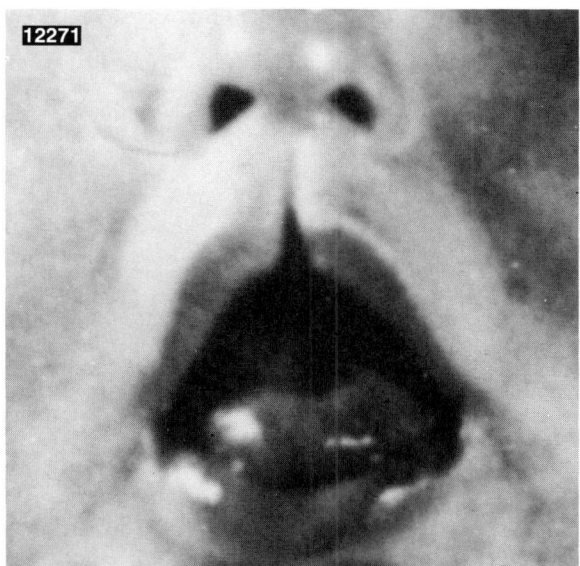

0595-12271: Median cleft of upper lip.

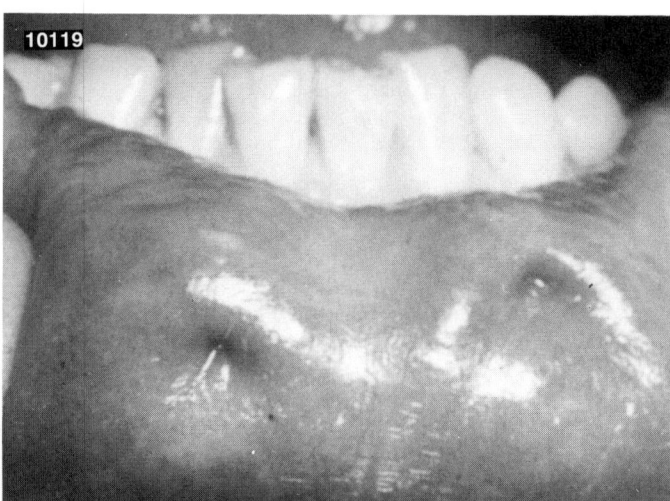

0596-10119: Lower lip pits.

**Pathogenesis:** Midline mesenchymal filling defect with persistent infranasal furrow.

**Sex Ratio:** Presumably M1:F1

**Occurrence:** Undetermined but presumed rare.

**Risk of Recurrence for Patient's Sib:** Unknown.

**Risk of Recurrence for Patient's Child:** Unknown.

**Age of Detectability:** At birth.

**Gene Mapping and Linkage:** Unknown.

**Prevention:** None known. Genetic counseling indicated.

**Treatment:** Surgical closure of the cleft.

**Prognosis:** Full recovery following surgery.

**Detection of Carrier:** Unknown.

**References:**

Millard DR, Williams S: Median lip clefts of the upper lip. Plast & Reconstr Surg 1968; 42:4–14. *

Lehman JA, Cuddapah S: The true hare lip: a case report. Cleft Palate J 1974; 11:497–498. †

Nakamuna J, et al.: True median cleft of the upper lip associated with three pedunculated club-shaped skin masses. Plast Reconst Surg 1985; 75:727–731.

J0027

**Ronald J. Jorgenson**
*Hermine M. Pashayan*

## LIP, PITS OR MOUNDS                    0596

**Includes:**
> Commissural lip pits (isolated trait)
> Paramedian pits of lower lip (isolated trait)
> Pits of upper lip

**Excludes:**
> **Cleft lip/palate-filiform fusion of eyelids** (0176)
> **Cleft lip/palate-lip pits or mounds** (0177)
> **Oro-facio-digital syndrome** (0770)
> **Pterygium syndrome, popliteal** (0818)

**Major Diagnostic Criteria:** Presence of pits on the vermilion border of lips.

**Clinical Findings:** *Commissural lip pits* are small openings or fistulas on the lip vermilion at the angles of the lips. They are either bilateral or unilateral. The pits do not cause any discomfort or cosmetic problems.

*Paramedian pits of the lower lip* are usually bilateral, or occasionally unilateral, fistulas located lateral to the midline on the vermilion border of the lower lip. The openings may be minute but occur in the center of a mound of lip tissue; they may be openings of fistulas 10 to 15 mm deep, which excrete mucous. Rarely, a single centrally located pit may be present.

*Pits of the upper lip* are exceedingly rare and are usually unilateral openings on the vermilion border.

While kindreds are known in which individuals have had only paramedian lip pits, in general, these are not extensive kindreds. Kindreds more fully documented have individuals with clefts of lip and palate. For this reason, individuals or families with paramedian pits should be viewed as also having a high risk for clefts of lip or palate.

**Complications:** Rarely, infection may occur.

**Associated Findings:** Commissural lip pits are associated with aural sinuses (auricular pits) in 4% of cases. Paramedian lip pits are associated with cleft lip/palate syndromes, cleft lip or palate and filiform fusion of eyelids, and with popliteal pterygium syndrome. Pits of upper lip are associated with cysts in line of fusion of premaxilla and maxillary processes.

**Etiology:** *Commissural lip pits:* No genetic study has been published but there are reports of familial occurrence suggesting autosomal dominant transmission (father and son, mother and two sons, father and two daughters, mother, son and daughter, and transmission through three generations).

*Paramedian pits of the lower lip:* Reported in kindreds showing autosomal dominant transmission, and with no known relative with cleft lip/palate. However, data are still insufficient to say with certainty whether this occurs as an isolated trait or whether it is always part of the cleft lip or palate and lip pits syndromes. Shprintzen et al (1980) observed penetrance to be 100%.

*Pits of the upper lip:* Probably of nongenetic origin.

**Pathogenesis:** *Commissural lip pits* originate from epithelial rests in the line of the embryonal furrow between maxillary and mandibular processes.

*Paramedian pits of the lower lip* originate as vestigial remnants of the "lateral sulci" appearing in the embryonic mandible at the 7.5–12.5 mm long stage.

*Pits of the upper lip* are due to failure of complete fusion of premaxilla and maxillary processes.

**MIM No.:** 12050, 15163

**CDC No.:** 750.260

**Sex Ratio:** *Commissural lip pits:* M1:F1 in Caucasians, American blacks, and North American Indians (Chippewa).
*Paramedian pits of the lower lip:* M1:F1 in Caucasians.
*Pits of the upper lip:* Undetermined.

**Occurrence:** *Commissural lip pits:* Caucasians: 1:500 to 1:83; American blacks: 1:48; North American Indians (Chippewa): 1:110.
*Paramedian pits of the lower lip:* Undetermined.

**Risk of Recurrence for Patient's Sib:** Unknown.

**Risk of Recurrence for Patient's Child:** Unknown.

**Age of Detectability:** At birth.

**Gene Mapping and Linkage:** Unknown.

**Prevention:** None known. Genetic counseling indicated.

**Treatment:** *Commissural lip pits:* No treatment necessary. *Paramedian pits of the lower lip:* Plastic surgery. *Pits of the upper lip:* Surgical excision.

**Prognosis:** Normal for life span and intelligence when an isolated trait.

**Detection of Carrier:** Unknown.

**References:**

Everett FG, Wescott WB: Commissural lip pits. Oral Surg 1961; 14:202–209.
Witkop CJ: Genetic diseases in the oral cavity. In: Tiecke RW, ed: Oral pathology. New York: McGraw-Hill, 1965:786–843.
Baker BR: Pits of the lip commissures in caucasoid males. Oral Surg 1966; 21:56–60.
Cervenka J, et al.: The syndrome of pits of the lower lip and cleft lip and/or palate: genetic considerations. Am J Hum Genet 1967; 19:416–432.
Fenner von W, v der Leyen, U-E: Über die kongenitale Oberlippenfistel. Dtsch Zahnaerztl Z 1969; 24:963–968.
Shprintzen RJ, et al.: The penetrance and variable expression of the Van der Woude syndrome. Implications for genetic counseling. Cleft Palate J 1980; 17:52–57.

CE003                                                      **Jaroslav Červenka**

**LIPA deficiency**
*See CHOLESTERYL ESTER STORAGE DISEASE*
**Lipa deficiency**
*See WOLMAN DISEASE*
**Lipase D deficiency**
*See HYPERCHYLOMICRONEMIA*

## LIPASE, CONGENITAL ABSENCE OF PANCREATIC          0597

**Includes:**
    Pancreatic lipase deficiency, congenital
    Pancreatic lipase deficiency, congenital isolated

**Excludes:**
    Co-lipase deficiency
    Lipase/co-lipase deficiency, isolated congenital
    Pancreatic exocrine insufficiency, generalized

**Major Diagnostic Criteria:** Steatorrhea is the only significant clinical finding. Basal and secretin-stimulated pancreatic juices are deficient in lipase activity. Peptidase, amylase and co-lipase activities are normal. Absent lipase has recently been demonstrated by an immunologic technique which improves specificity.

**Clinical Findings:** Steatorrhea is the only significant clinical finding. All patients have had the onset of oily, slightly foul stools in early infancy. The oil separates from the bulk movement and will solidify at room temperature. Soiling of clothing with oil is common.

Normal growth and development is the rule. Abdominal distention is unusual. Basal and secretin-stimulated pancreatic juices obtained by peroral duodenal intubation are found to contain normal activities of peptidase and amylase but to be deficient in lipase. Lipase assays are reliable only if performed by experienced investigators. Reproducibility is marginal, and incubation condi-

tions are critical. Newer immunologic assay provides improved specificity.

Co-lipase is necessary for optimal function of lipase in the conditions present in the intestinal lumen. In vivo, co-lipase deficiency could masquerade as lipase deficiency. Recently a patient with deficiencies of both lipase and co-lipase has been described.

**Complications:** Steatorrhea.

**Associated Findings:** None known.

**Etiology:** Autosomal recessive inheritance.

**Pathogenesis:** Pancreatic lipase is essential for optimal fat absorption. Hydrolysis of triglycerides to $\alpha$-fatty acids and $\beta$-monoglycerides occurs at the surface of emulsified fat globules by the action of pancreatic lipase in the presence of bile salts and co-lipase. In the absence of lipase, limited hydrolysis occurs as a result of the action of gastric lipolytic activity and pancreatic esterase. The coefficient of fat absorption in the lipase deficient patient is 50–80%.

**MIM No.:** *24660

**Sex Ratio:** M3:F1 (observed in four cases in which sex was reported)

**Occurrence:** Fewer than 20 cases have been documented.

**Risk of Recurrence for Patient's Sib:**
    See Part I, *Mendelian Inheritance.*

**Risk of Recurrence for Patient's Child:**
    See Part I, *Mendelian Inheritance.*

**Age of Detectability:** In infancy.

**Gene Mapping and Linkage:** Unknown.

**Prevention:** None known. Genetic counseling indicated.

**Treatment:** Treatment with orally administered pancreatic enzyme replacement improves fat absorption but does not usually normalize function. Dietary fat restriction is necessary to abolish steatorrhea. Medium-chain triglycerides may be used as a fat substitute when needed for nutrition in the infant.

**Prognosis:** Excellent.

**Detection of Carrier:** Unknown.

**References:**

Sheldon W: Congenital pancreatic lipase deficiency. Arch Dis Child 1964; 39:268–271.
Figarella C, et al.: Congenital pancreatic lipase deficiency. J Pediatr 1980; 96:412–416.
Ghishan FK, et al.: Isolated congenital lipase-colipase deficiency. Gastroenterology 1984; 86:1580–1582.

WH007                                              **Peter F. Whitington**

**Lipid histiocytosis of spleen**
*See THROMBOCYTOPENIC PURPURA AND LIPID HISTIOCYTOSIS*

## LIPID TRANSPORT DEFECT OF INTESTINE          3226

**Includes:**
    Anderson disease
    Apoprotein in intestinal cells-hypobetalipoproteinemia
    Chylomicron retention disease
    Hypobetalipoproteinemia-apoprotein in intestinal cells
    Intestine, lipid transport defect

**Excludes:**
    Abetalipoproteinemia (0002)
    Hypobetalipoproteinemia (2386)
    Normotriglyceridemic abetalipoproteinemia

**Major Diagnostic Criteria:** Failure of enterocytes to secrete chylomicrons in response to the absorption of dietary lipid. In contrast to abetalipoproteinemia in which enterocyte apo B is reduced or absent in the face of cellular steatosis, fasting enterocytes in this disorder reveal increased apo B immunostaining in association with accumulation of intracellular lipid droplets. Apo B-48 and associated chylomicrons of intestinal origin are not detectable in plasma after fat-feeding. Plasma triglyceride levels are within the normal range, but the total plasma cholesterol concentration is reduced. Plasma lipoprotein isolation reveals increased VLDL cholesterol and decreased LDL and HDL cholesterol. The plasma apo B level is mildly reduced and is present exclusively as the larger liver-derived apo B-100 form.

**Clinical Findings:**  Diarrhea and failure to thrive associated with fat malabsorption with onset usually in the first year of life are the prominent clinical features of this disorder. Neurologic and ophthalmologic findings typical of **Abetalipoproteinemia** are usually absent or very mild in this disease. Atypical retinitis pigmentosa has not been described, although mild subclinical retinal electrophysiologic abnormalities may occur. As in abetalipoproteinemia, these findings, when present, may be secondary to vitamin E deficiency. Acanthocytosis of circulating red blood cells, a diagnostic feature of abetalipoproteinemia, is absent. If treated with dietary long chain fat restriction supplemented with essential and medium chain fatty acids and fat-soluble vitamins, growth has been reported to normalize, and neurologic symptoms, if present, may improve or resolve.

**Complications:**  If untreated, diarrhea and steatorrhea with associated growth failure will persist. Mild neurologic and ophthalmologic dysfunction, if present, may persist in the untreated patient.

**Associated Findings:**  None known.

**Etiology:**  Autosomal recessive inheritance. Since intestinal synthesis of apo B and uptake and esterification of long chain fatty acids appear to be unimpaired in in vitro studies, a defect in the final assembly and secretion of chylomicrons has been proposed. Whether the enterocyte secretory block is at the pre- or post-Golgi level is controversial at present. A defect in glycosylation of apo B has been observed in jejunal explants.

**Pathogenesis:**  Unknown.

**MIM No.:**  24670

**Sex Ratio:**  M11:F5

**Occurrence:**  Sixteen well-described cases have been reported in the literature.

**Risk of Recurrence for Patient's Sib:**
See Part I, *Mendelian Inheritance.*

**Risk of Recurrence for Patient's Child:**
See Part I, *Mendelian Inheritance.*

**Age of Detectability:**  Many patients reported with symptoms in the first month of life.

**Gene Mapping and Linkage:**  Unknown.

**Prevention:**  None known. Genetic counseling indicated.

**Treatment:**  Restriction of long chain dietary fat and supplementation of essential and medium chain fats and fat soluble vitamins, particularly vitamin E.

**Prognosis:**  Long-term follow-up into adulthood has not been reported. However, since response to treatment is usually favorable, long term prognosis is probably good.

**Detection of Carrier:**  Unknown.

**References:**
Anderson CM, et al.: Unusual causes of steatorrhea in infancy and childhood. Med J Aust 1961; 2:617–622.
Bouma M-E, et al.: Hypobetalipoproteinemia with accumulation of an apoprotein B-like protein in intestinal cells: immunoenzymatic and biochemical characterization of seven cases of Anderson's disease. J Clin Invest 1986; 78:398–410.
Levy E, et al.: Intestinal apo B synthesis, lipids, and lipoproteins in chylomicron retention disease. J Lipid Res 1987; 28:1263–1274.
Roy CC, et al.: Malabsorption, hypocholesterolemia, and fat-filled enterocytes with increased intestinal apo B. Gastroenterology 1987; 92:390–399.
Bouma M-E, Infante R: Chylomicron retention disease. Gastroenterology 1988; 94:554–556.

**Dennis D. Black**

**Lipid, deficiency of**
See HYPERCHYLOMICRONEMIA
**Lipid-storage myopathy secondary to SCAD**
See ACYL-CoA DEHYDROGENASE DEFICIENCY, SHORT CHAIN TYPE
**Lipidosis, late infantile systemic**
See G(M1)-GANGLIOSIDOSIS, TYPE 2
**Lipidosis, sulfatide**
See METACHROMATIC LEUKODYSTROPHIES
**Lipidosis-thrombocytopenia-angiomata of the spleen**
See THROMBOCYTOPENIC PURPURA AND LIPID HISTIOCYTOSIS
**Lipoatrophic diabetes with dominant transmission, familial**
See LIPODYSTROPHY, FAMILIAL LIMB AND TRUNK
**Lipoatrophic diabetes, congenital**
See LIPODYSTROPHY SYNDROME, BERARDINELLI TYPE
**Lipodermoid**
See EYE, DERMOLIPOMA

## LIPODYSTROPHY SYNDROME, BERARDINELLI TYPE        2038

**Includes:**
> Berardinelli-Seip syndrome
> Gigantism, acromegaloid-lipodystrophy
> Lawrence syndrome
> Lipoatrophic diabetes, congenital
> Seip syndrome
> Total lipodystrophy-acromegaloid gigantism

**Excludes:**
> **De Lange syndrome** (0242)
> Diabetes, insulin-resistant with acanthosis nigricans
> **Leprechaunism** (0587)
> **Lipodystrophy, familial limb and trunk** (2614)
> Partial lipodystrophy syndromes

**Major Diagnostic Criteria:**  The diagnosis is made clinically, based upon growth characteristics, physical features, and laboratory data. The index findings are absence of clinically apparent adipose tissue and hepatomegaly. Patients are tall and thin as infants and children, with advanced dental and skeletal maturation. However, their ultimate height potential is limited. Insulin-resistant, non-ketotic diabetes mellitus with hyperlipidemia develops with age and supports the diagnosis.

**Clinical Findings:**  Affected patients have abundant, often curly scalp hair and a gaunt, triangular face. Skin pigmentation is increased, generalized hypertrichosis may be found, and acanthosis nigricans may be present in the axillae, groin, or other intertriginous regions. Significant hepatomegaly is usually present, and splenomegaly and genitomegaly are frequent findings. Muscles and veins are prominent, and abdominal distension with umbilical herniation is common. Stature is increased in childhood but may be decreased in adults; the extremities may appear enlarged. Weight is normal but is usually low in relation to height. Skeletal maturation is advanced for chronologic age and for height age in childhood. X-ray features can include sclerotic and angiomatous lesions of the long bones and hands, and cardiomegaly. Laboratory findings include hyperglycemia, hypercholesterolemia, hypertriglyceridemia, hyperinsulinemia, and hyperglucagonemia. Liver function tests are often abnormal. Other endocrine investigations have not shown consistent abnormalities.

**Complications:**  Patients develop the typical microvascular manifestations of chronic diabetes mellitus, as well as premature atherosclerosis. Fatty infiltration of the liver may evolve into overt cirrhosis, with portal hypertension and gastrointestinal hemorrhage.

**Associated Findings:**  Protracted vomiting with failure to thrive in infancy has been reported. Renal involvement manifests with proteinuria or frank nephrotic syndrome. The central nervous system can be affected, and findings can include dilated ventricles and mental retardation. Polycystic ovaries and oligomenorrhea have been described. Corneal opacities may be found.

**Etiology:**  Although total lipodystrophy is a heterogeneous condition, there is a high incidence of parental consanguinity in the

BIRTH   1 YEAR   2 YEARS   5 YEARS

7 YEARS   16 YEARS   18 YEARS

**2038**-20613: Lipodystrophy, Berardinelli type; note the development of a gaunt, triangular facial appearance in these serial photographs of an affected subject.

families of patients with the congenital form, strongly suggesting autosomal recessive inheritance. At present, this causation should be ascribed only to patients with features of the classical phenotype present at birth.

**Pathogenesis:** Patients are hypermetabolic with increased fat catabolism, markedly decreased fat storage, and fatty infiltration of the liver. Hypothalamic dysfunction has been postulated, but structural lesions are not usually demonstrable. Hyperglycemia and hyperinsulinemia are present without insulin antibodies; in some patients, decreased binding by insulin receptors has been noted. The receptor defect appears to be heterogeneous even within the group of patients with the congenital form. The number of fat cells in adipose tissue is probably normal, but intracellular fat deposits are markedly reduced. Muscular prominence is partly due to reduced subcutaneous fat, but there may be an element of primary muscular hypertrophy or hyperplasia with excess glycogen deposition as well. The pathogenesis and natural history of liver and cardiac involvement are not well understood.

**MIM No.:** *26970

**POS No.:** 3439

**Sex Ratio:** M1:F1 in the congenital form; M1:F2–3 in the acquired form.

**Occurrence:** Undetermined but presumed rare. Established literature. No particular ethnic group, with the possible exception of the Portuguese, appears to be at additional risk.

**Risk of Recurrence for Patient's Sib:**
See Part I, *Mendelian Inheritance.*

**Risk of Recurrence for Patient's Child:**
See Part I, *Mendelian Inheritance.*

**Age of Detectability:** At birth for the congenital form.

**Gene Mapping and Linkage:** Unknown.

**Prevention:** None known. Genetic counseling indicated.

**Treatment:** Without a clear understanding of the pathogenesis of the syndrome(s) of total lipodystrophy, treatment has been symptomatic, empirical, and largely unsatisfactory. The treatment of the diabetic syndrome and its related lipemia is made difficult by profound resistance to exogenous insulin observed in many patients. Fortunately, ketoacidosis is infrequent. Salutory effects of a neuroleptic diphenylbutylpiperidine, (pimozide), have been reported in a few patients but have not been sustained at puberty. Improvement in some of the characteristic endocrine and metabolic abnormalities has been noted with short-term caloric restric-

tion but this approach is obviously impractical in gaunt, undernourished patients. Recently, improvement has been reported in one patient during eucaloric feeding with medium-chain triglycerides substituted for dietary long-chain fatty acids. The efficacy of medium chain triglyceride feeding has not been examined in other patients.

**Prognosis:** Patients have a shortened life expectancy as a result of inanition, premature atherosclerosis, gastrointestinal hemorrhage secondary to cirrhosis, and the development of microvascular complications of diabetes mellitus.

**Detection of Carrier:** Unknown.

**Special Considerations:** The lipodystrophies as a group are quite heterogeneous with respect to age of onset, degree of involvement, and associated findings. The above discussion is limited to one subset of these conditions, namely that which is total, involving all body regions. Although clinical features were present at birth in the patients described by Berardinelli (1954) and Seip (1959), many of the somatic clues to the diagnosis and abnormal laboratory findings evolve with age, and a period of observation may be necessary to reach a secure diagnosis. Lawrence (1946) originally described a form of total lipodystrophy that differs in its later onset (often following a systemic illness or infection) and absence of reported parental consanguinity. This suggests different causation for these closely related conditions, but, because of significant clinical similarities they must currently be classified together.

**Support Groups:** New York; American Diabetes Association

**References:**

Lawrence RD: Lipodystrophy and hepatomegaly with diabetes, lipaemia, and other metabolic disturbances. Lancet 1946; I:724–731, 733–775.

Berardinelli W: An undiagnosed endocrinometabolic syndrome: report of two cases. J Clin Endocr 1954; 14:193–204. * †

Seip M: Lipodystrophy and gigantism with associated endocrine manifestation. Acta Paediat 1959; 48:555–574.

Senior B, Gellis SS: The syndromes of total lipodystrophy and of partial lipodystrophy. Pediatrics 1964; 33:593–612. *

Rossini AA, Cahill GF Jr: Lipoatrophic diabetes. In: DeGroot LJ, ed: Endocrinology. New York: Grune & Stratton, 1979:1093–1098.

Wachslicht-Rodbard H, et al.: Heterogeneity of the insulin-receptor interaction in lipoatrophic diabetes. J Clin Endocrinol Metab 1981; 52:416–425.

Wilson DE, et al.: Eucaloric substitution of medium chain triglycerides for dietary long-chain fatty acids in acquired total lipodystrophy: effects on hyperlipoproteinemia and endogenous insulin resistance. J Clin Endocrinol Metab 1983; 57:517–523.

J0012
WI060

**John P. Johnson**
**Dana E. Wilson**

## LIPODYSTROPHY, FAMILIAL LIMB AND TRUNK      2614

**Includes:**
Dunnigan syndrome
Koebberling-Dunnigan syndrome
Limbs and trunk, familial lipodystrophy of
Lipodystrophy, reverse partial
Lipoatrophic diabetes with dominant transmission, familial
Partial lipodystrophy-lipoatrophic diabetes-hyperlipidemia

**Excludes:**
Barraquer-Simons disease
Diabetes, acquired lipoatrophic
Fetthals
Launois-Bensaude adenolipomatosis
Lipoatrophic diabetes, congenital
Lipoatrophy secondary to insulin hypersensitivity, acquired
Lipodystrophy, cephalo-thoracic
Lipodystrophy, partial with familial C3 deficiency
**Lipodystrophy-rieger anomaly-short stature-diabetes** (2834)
**Lipodystrophy syndrome, Berardinelli type** (2038)
**Nevi-atrial myxoma-myxoid neurofibromas-ephelides** (2572)

**Major Diagnostic Criteria:** Partial lipodystrophy involving the limbs (which may extend to the trunk), diabetes mellitus, and hyperlipidemia.

**Clinical Findings:** Females have been described with diabetes commencing in the first or second decade, symmetric atrophy of fat in the arms and legs, preservation of subcutaneous fat over the neck, face and shoulders. Muscle bulk and power may resemble masculine body habitus and true muscular hypertrophy has been reported. Lean, muscular limbs with apparent fat accumulation around the neck, shoulders, and face may simulate the appearance of **Nevi-atrial myxoma-myxoid neurofibromas-ephelides. Hyperlipoproteinemia** Type IIb, III or IV, as well as hyperuricemia, have been reported. Associated skin lesions include tuberoeruptive xanthomata over the elbows and knees, acanthosis nigricans in the axillae, and thin skin with increased visibility of subcutaneous veins. Hepatosplenomegaly does not occur to the extent seen in acquired total lipodystrophy.

**Complications:** Diabetic microangiopathic retinopathy and peripheral vascular disease.

**Associated Findings:** None known.

**Etiology:** Autosomal dominant inheritance with sex limitation. One male patient was reported by Burn and Baraitser (1986). The predominance of female patients has been attributed to the more extensive distribution of fat in females, but X-linked dominant inheritance with lethality in hemizygous males has also been suggested.

**Pathogenesis:** Unknown.

**MIM No.:** *15166

**POS No.:** 3439

**Sex Ratio:** M<1:F1.

**Occurrence:** Several sibships and at least one isolated case has been reported.

**Risk of Recurrence for Patient's Sib:**
See Part I, *Mendelian Inheritance.*

**Risk of Recurrence for Patient's Child:**
See Part I, *Mendelian Inheritance.*

**Age of Detectability:** Late childhood or early adult life. Lipodystrophy usually appears at puberty.

**Gene Mapping and Linkage:** Unknown.

**Prevention:** None known. Genetic counseling indicated.

**Treatment:** Insulin as indicated for diabetes. Insulin resistance requiring high dosage, as seen in total acquired lipodystrophy, is rare.

**Prognosis:** Lipodystrophy is not reversible in affected areas. Otherwise, prognosis is that of the associated diabetes, and is generally good.

**Detection of Carrier:** Unknown.

**Support Groups:** New York; American Diabetes Association. NJ; Elizabeth; National Lipid Diseases Foundation

**References:**
Dunnigan MG, et al.: Familial lipoatrophic diabetes with dominant transmission: a new syndrome. Quart J Med 1974; 43:33–48.
Kobberling J, et al.: Lipodystrophy of the extremities: a dominantly inherited syndrome associated with lipoatrophic diabetes. Humangenetik 1975; 29:111–120.
Wettke-Schafer R, Kantner G: X-linked dominant inherited diseases with lethality in hemizygous males. Hum Genet 1983; 64:1–23.
Burn J, Baraitser M: Partial lipoatrophy with insulin resistant diabetes and hyperlipiaemia (Dunnigan's syndrome). J Med Genet 1986; 23:128–130.
Kobberling J, Dunnigan MG: Familial partial lipodystrophy: two types of an X linked dominant syndrome, lethal in the homizygous state. J Med Genet 1986; 23:120–127.

LE050                                   **Raymond M. Lewkonia**

**Lipodystrophy, reverse partial**
*See LIPODYSTROPHY, FAMILIAL LIMB AND TRUNK*

## LIPODYSTROPHY-COARSE FACIES-ACANTHOSIS NIGRICANS, MIESCHER TYPE                 **2423**

**Includes:**
   Bloch-Miescher syndrome
   Mendenhall syndrome
   Miescher syndrome
   Rabson-Mendenhall syndrome

**Excludes:**
   Insulin resistance-acanthosis nigricans, types A and B (Kahn)
   **Leprechaunism** (0587)
   **Lipodystrophy syndrome, Berardinelli type** (2038)
   **Lipodystrophy** (others)

**Major Diagnostic Criteria:** Lipodystrophy, coarse facies, dental anomalies, acanthosis nigricans, and lanugo-type hypertrichosis. An additional and important feature is insulin-resistant diabetes.

**Clinical Findings:** The earliest manifestation, typically present at birth or shortly thereafter, is an augmented pigmentation, which later in childhood develops into acanthosis nigricans with typical localization (neck; nape; and axillary, inguinal, and genital regions). In the severe form, acanthosis nigricans is complicated by multiple skin tags. Premature dentition also occurs in the first months of life. Longitudinal growth and bone maturation can be temporarily accelerated; however, some of the patients showed a slight growth retardation. Mental retardation is *not* present. In addition, the patients are dysmorphic, and in the severe form of the disorder lipatrophy develops. These described characteristics cause children and youth to appear older than the corresponding chronologic age.

Further characteristics are coarse facies with prominent upper and lower jaw, full lips, and relatively large ears. Irregular and supernumerary, often carious, teeth are striking and can be abnormally large (macrodontia). The tongue is furrowed. A lanugo-type hypertrichosis is seen early in life, and scalp hair is often abundant. On the other hand, females in early adulthood may have alopecia. Hands and feet may be short and plump, with thickened nails. A prominent abdomen and enlarged phallus (especially in females) can occur.

During childhood or later in youth, a mild diabetes with only slight tendency toward ketosis may develop. The basal plasma insulin concentration can increase 100-fold. Examination of the insulin receptors shows a pathologic diminished binding capacity. Although the total number of the receptors is normal, there appears to be a complete absence of receptors with high affinity. Additional characteristics in females are menstrual disorders (oligomenorrhea or amenorrhea) and reduced fertility.

There is strikingly variable expression of clinical manifestations, not only interfamilial but also among patients of the same sibship.

**Complications:** Patients are prone to benign tumors in the thyroid gland and to polycystic ovaries. Even in childhood, recurrent gastric and duodenal ulcers can appear. The diabetes leads to diminished resistance against possibly fatal infections. Late complications of the diabetes, such as retinopathy or neuropathy, have been documented.

**Associated Findings:** A pathogenetically obscure hyperplasia of the pineal body was demonstrated in some patients at autopsy.

**Etiology:** Autosomal recessive inheritance with variable expression.

**Pathogenesis:** There is no current theory to explain all the manifestations of this homozygous autosomal recessive gene, but hyperinsulinism per se (in different types of insulin-resistant diabetes) apparently leads to characteristics such as lipodystrophy, acanthosis nigricans, hypertrichosis, polycystic ovaries, and reduced fertility.

**MIM No.:** *26219, *24309

**POS No.:** 3741

**Sex Ratio:** M1:F1

**Occurrence:** Possibly a dozen or more cases, under various designations, have been reported in the literature.

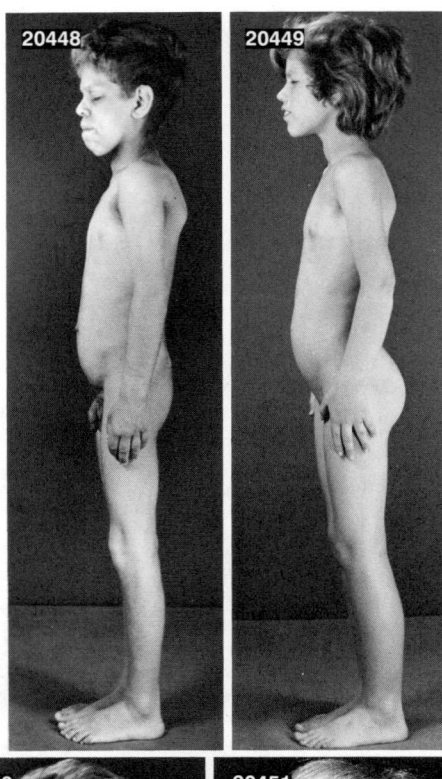

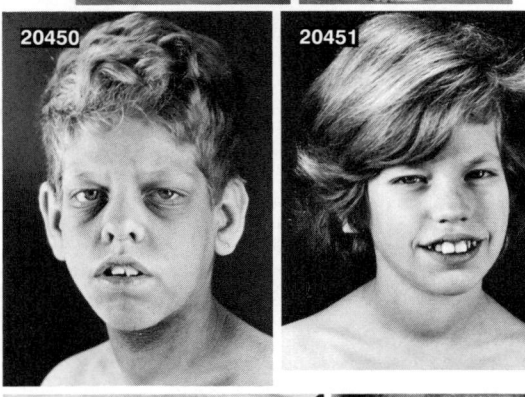

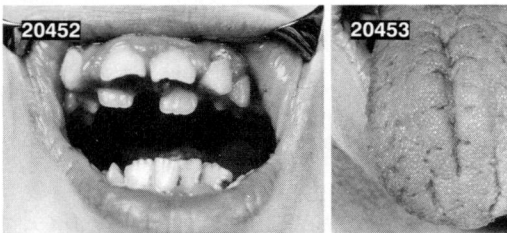

**2423**-20448–20453: Characteristics in a pair of sibs with variably expressed lipodystrophy, Miescher type. The boy is 13.5 years old, the girl 11.5 years old. 20448–49: Note lipodystrophy and hypertrichosis, more pronounced in the brother. 20450–51: Coarse facial features; note also acanthosis nigricans, macrodontia, and abundant scalp hair. 20452: Note large, supernumerary (double row), and carious teeth in the male patient. 20453: Furrowed tongue in the male patient.

**Risk of Recurrence for Patient's Sib:**
See Part I, *Mendelian Inheritance.*

**Risk of Recurrence for Patient's Child:**
See Part I, *Mendelian Inheritance.*

**Age of Detectability:** During the first year of life.

**Gene Mapping and Linkage:** Unknown.

**Prevention:** None known. Genetic counseling indicated.

**Treatment:** Treatment of the diabetes is only possible with high doses of insulin and therefore is hardly practicable. A therapy with biguanides can be successful, because it leads to an increased number of insulin receptors. Further treatment is symptomatic and is confined to surgical procedures in cases of recurrent gastric or duodenal ulcers and to orthodontic measures. In the case of hirsutism, cosmetic measures are indicated.

**Prognosis:** Life span may be diminished by later complications of diabetes, but precise data are not available. On the other hand, there are several reports on partial remission of the disorder; diabetes and acanthosis nigricans tend to improve in adulthood. Affected women showed reduced fertility, but pregnancies are possible.

**Detection of Carrier:** Clinical examination to detect those who are only mildly affected.

**Special Considerations:** The extraordinary complexity of this syndrome may be the cause for the correspondingly large number of different designations in the literature. This has led to considerable difficulties in nosologic classification. The early reports on the same pair of sibs by Bloch in 1920 and by Miescher in 1921, both in German, remained largely unknown in the English literature. It was not until about 30 years later that Mendenhall (1950) and Rabson and Mendenhall (1956) described three typically affected sibs in the American literature. Since then there have been a number of publications in the American but also in the European literature, most of which have been cited by Wiedemann et al (1985).

Since about the mid-1970s, insulin-resistant diabetes has gained special attention. For example, Kahn et al (1976) described types A and B of insulin-resistant diabetes with acanthosis nigricans. Whereas type A shares several of the characteristics with the above mentioned syndrome but is probably a different disorder, type B is an immunologic disorder with circulating antibodies to the insulin receptors. The type A literature, however, came to include reports by Rüdiger et al (1981) and further by Rüdiger et al (1983) concerning the same sibship. They described three adult sibs with mild diabetes, acanthosis nigricans, dental anomalies, dystrophy, mild acral hypertrophy, and excessively elevated fasting plasma insulin levels. Insulin binding was defective as a result of a complete lack of receptors with high affinity. Two of these patients (then children) had been described by Wiedemann et al. (1968) in the German pediatric literature. Comparable receptor studies such as those by Rüdiger et al. have been done by several authors, e.g. Taylor et al (1981). An exact interpretation of these results seems still to be controversial (Taylor, 1982).

Lastly, there are some striking parallels between this syndrome and **Leprechaunism** in respect to nosology. However, these are distinct entities.

**References:**
Rabson SM, Mendenhall EN: Familial hypertrophy of pineal body, hyperplasia of adrenal cortex and diabetes mellitus. Am J Clin Pathol 1956; 26:283–290.
Kahn CR, et al.: The syndromes of insulin resistance and acanthosis nigricans: insulin-receptor disorders in man. New Engl J Med 1976; 294:739–745.
Rüdiger HW, et al.: Insulin resistant diabetes mellitus due to a genetic defect of the insulin receptor. Jerusalem: Sixth Int Cong Hum Genet, 1981:255.
Taylor SI, et al.: Decreased insulin binding in cultured lymphocytes from two patients with extreme insulin resistance. J Clin Endocrinol Metab 1982; 54:919–930.
Rüdiger HW, et al.: Familial insulin-resistant diabetes secondary to an affinity defect of the insulin receptor. Hum Genet 1983; 64:407–411. *

Wiedemann HR, et al.: An atlas of characteristic syndromes: a visual aid to diagnosis, ed 2. London: Wolfe Medical Publications, 1985. * †

ME008
WI003

**Peter Meinecke**
**Hans-Rudolf Wiedemann**

## LIPODYSTROPHY-RIEGER ANOMALY-SHORT STATURE-DIABETES                    2834

**Includes:**
  Aarskog lipodystrophy syndrome
  Diabetes-Rieger anomaly-lipodystrophy-short stature
  Rieger anomaly-lipodystrophy-short stature-diabetes
  Short stature-Rieger anomaly-lipodystrophy-diabetes

**Excludes:**
  **Aarskog syndrome** (0001)
  **Lipodystrophy, familial limb and trunk** (2614)
  **Lipodystrophy syndrome, Berardinelli type** (2038)
  Lipodystrophy, partial sporadic
  **Short syndrome** (2098)

**Major Diagnostic Criteria:** Facial lipodystrophy, Rieger anomaly, and short stature.

**Clinical Findings:** Lipodystrophy is present from infancy, affecting the face and limited areas of the buttocks and without progression. In the one known family, the condition was present in a grandfather, two of his daughters, and the propositus, son of one of the daughters. All affected persons had short stature and Rieger anomaly. Additional features were retarded bone age, delayed puberty, midface hypoplasia, large anteverted ears, hypospadias, and hypotrichosis. The propositus developed diabetes mellitus at age 14 years, his mother at age 39 years, and the maternal aunt had glucose intolerance at age 55 years.

**Complications:** Unknown.

**Associated Findings:** None known.

**Etiology:** Probably autosomal dominant inheritance.

**Pathogenesis:** Unknown.

**MIM No.:** 15168

**POS No.:** 3496

**Sex Ratio:** M1:F1

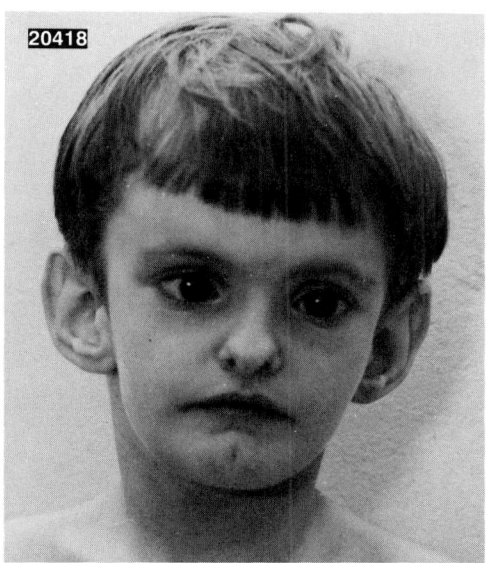

**2834-20418:** Note paucity of facial fat, deep-set eyes, pinched nose, wide mouth and large ears.

**Occurrence:** One family from the Lofoten Islands of Norway has been reported in which four persons in three generations were affected.

**Risk of Recurrence for Patient's Sib:**
  See Part I, *Mendelian Inheritance.*

**Risk of Recurrence for Patient's Child:**
  See Part I, *Mendelian Inheritance.*

**Age of Detectability:** During infancy or early childhood.

**Gene Mapping and Linkage:** Unknown.

**Prevention:** None known. Genetic counseling indicated.

**Treatment:** Treatment of the possible manifestation of diabetes mellitus.

**Prognosis:** Bone age is delayed, and growth might continue into the late teenage years. Puberty is delayed but otherwise normal. The ultimate prognosis depends on the development of diabetic complications.

**Detection of Carrier:** Unknown.

**References:**
Gorlin RJ: A selected miscellany. In: BD:OAS XI(2). New York: March of Dimes Birth Defects Foundation, 1975:46–48.
Sensenbrenner JA, et al.: A low birth weight syndrome? Rieger syndrome. In: BD:OAS XI(2). New York: March of Dimes Birth Defects Foundation, 1975:423–426.
Aarskog D, et al.: Autosomal dominant partial lipodystrophy associated with Rieger anomaly, short stature, and insulinopenic diabetes. Am J Med Genet 1983; 15:29–38.
Köbberling J, Dunnigan MG: Familial partial lipodystrophy: two types of an X-linked dominant syndrome, lethal in the hemizygous state. J Med Genet 1986; 23:120–127.

AA002                                                **Dagfinn Aarskog**

**Lipoglycoproteinosis**
  *See SKIN, LIPOID PROTEINOSIS*

## LIPOGRANULOMATOSIS                                                    0598

**Includes:**
  Ceramidase deficiency
  Ceramide deficiency
  Disseminated lipogranulomatosis
  Farber disease

**Excludes:**
  **Arthritis, rheumatoid** (2517)
  Histiocytosis
  Lipoid dermatoarthritis
  Sarcoid arthritis

**Major Diagnostic Criteria:** The hallmark of this syndrome is the clinical triad of discrete lumpy masses over the wrists and ankles, combined with joint deformities and hoarseness. Diagnosis is confirmed by demonstrating deficient activity of acid ceramidase. Biopsy lesion material shows foam cells that contain characteristic inclusions and infiltration by histiocytes, lymphocytes, and fibroblasts.

**Clinical Findings:** Typical cases develop normally for the first weeks or months, until parents note that movement of fingers, wrists, or ankles may be painful, that these joints are tender, and that there are subcutaneous nodules near these joints or over pressure points. A second and nearly constant feature is that the child's cry is hoarse. The nodules enlarge, and the joint deformities progress. There is difficulty in feeding and swallowing, progressive inanition, intermittent fever, and respiratory disturbances due to pulmonary infiltrates that may cause death during the first year. The liver is enlarged in about one-fourth of the cases. Central nervous system function is relatively intact, but may be difficult to assess due to the severe systemic illness. One-third of the patients have peripheral nerve involvement, evidenced by diminished or absent deep tendon reflexes and signs of denervation in neurometric studies. The retina may show

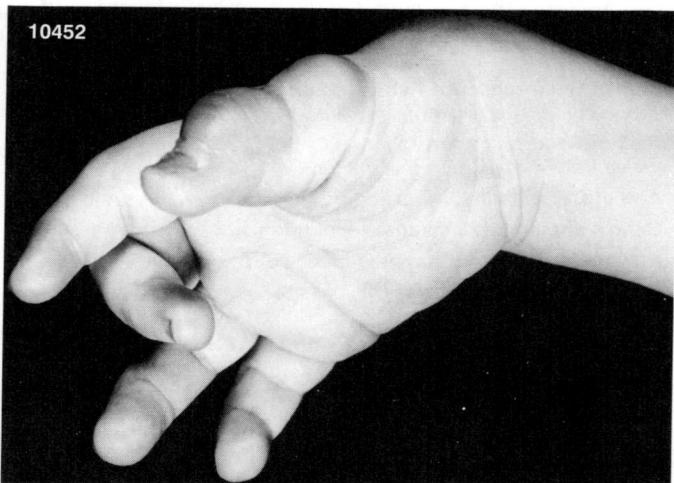

10452

**0598-10452:** Lipogranulomatosis of hand.

diffuse grayish opacification about the foveola, with a cherry-red spot.

Several variant forms are now recognized. These include a mild variant in which four patients are in stable condition in their second or third decade. They show moderate arthropathy, subcutaneous nodules, hoarseness, and moderate psychomotor retardation. They appear free of pulmonary or hepatic disease. Intermediate degrees of involvement are shown by children 4–10 years old who have severe arthropathy and prominent nodules, as well as seizures and signs of CNS involvement but no lung involvement. Two other variants have been described recently. In three children the presenting signs were hepatosplenomegaly and osteolytic lesions during the first few weeks of life, leading to the diagnosis of malignant histiocytosis. Subcutaneous nodules were absent in one patient and not prominent in the other two. In the other variant form the presenting signs were progressive psychomotor retardation and retinal cherry-red spots. Subcutaneous nodules and hoarseness were present but mild.

Laboratory diagnosis depends on demonstration of deficient acid ceramidase activity in leukocytes or cultured skin fibroblasts and on evidence of ceramide storage by biochemical or microscopic techniques. Abnormally high ceramide levels may be present in urine, but some cases have failed to show this. Biochemical assays of nodule biopsy material show high levels of ceramide (up to 30% of total lipids). Under the electron microscope these nodules show characteristic inclusions, which have been referred to as *Farber bodies.*

Momoi et al (1982) have proposed that N-(1-14C) lauroylsphingosine may be a better substrate for the diagnosis of Farber disease than N-(1-14C) oleoylsphingosine. A different and valuable approach to the enzymatic diagnosis of Farber disease has been provided by Kudoh and Wenger (1982). These investigators incubated cultured skin fibroblasts with [14C] stearic acid-labeled cerebroside sulfate and measured its rate of degradation. Cells from Farber disease patients had a deficient capacity (15% of control) to degrade the ceramide that is formed from cerebroside-sulfate.

**Complications:** The laryngeal involvement may lead to difficulties with breathing and swallowing. Pulmonary infiltrates due to alveolar lipid infiltrates cause respiratory insufficiency and are difficult to distinguish from pneumonia. The nodules and joint involvement cause discomfort and limit mobility and well-being. The osteolytic lesions may cause hypercalcemia. Neurologic involvement may cause seizures, ataxia, weakness, and dementia.

**Associated Findings:** None known.

**Etiology:** Autosomal recessive inheritance.

**Pathogenesis:** The defective function of acid ceramidase leads to tissue accumulation of ceramide within lysosomes. This causes cell damage and an inflammatory response manifest by nodule formation and arthropathy. Ceramides have important roles (water barrier) in skin and form the "core" of gangliosides and sphingoglycolipids. Impaired capacity to degrade this "core" leads to its accumulation in the nervous system.

**MIM No.:** *22800

**POS No.:** 3436

**Sex Ratio:** M1:F1

**Occurrence:** Thirty-eight cases have been reported or identified. High incidence of consanguinity in parents. No predilection in any particular group.

**Risk of Recurrence for Patient's Sib:**
See Part I, *Mendelian Inheritance.*

**Risk of Recurrence for Patient's Child:**
See Part I, *Mendelian Inheritance.* No affected individuals are known to have reproduced.

**Age of Detectability:** In typical cases, signs and symptoms permit strong clinical suspicion during the first few months of life, and this can be confirmed by laboratory studies. Prenatal diagnosis has been made by demonstrating deficient activity of acid ceramidase in cultured amniocytes.

**Gene Mapping and Linkage:** Unknown.

**Prevention:** None known. Genetic counseling indicated.

**Treatment:** Tracheostomy may be required for airway obstruction. In mildly involved older patients unsightly nodules may be removed by plastic surgery. Other therapies are symptomatic. The more mildly involved Farber disease patients may be candidates for bone marrow transplantation. Enzymatically competent circulating bone marrow-derived cells may be able to clear the unmetabolized ceramide that appears to be the cause of the disabling nodules and infiltrates. The relatively mild or absent CNS involvement would also favor such an approach. Up to now this procedure has not been used in any Farber disease patients. In the severely ill young children with pulmonary involvement the procedure would be extremely hazardous.

**Prognosis:** The patients with typical Farber disease usually die before age two years due to pulmonary involvement, sometimes with general inanition. A second group of somewhat more mildly involved patients live to ages 5–10 years. These patients appear not to have lung involvement and succumb to the combination of joint involvement and progressive neurologic disease.

The most mildly involved patients appear in relatively stable condition in their teens or early adulthood. This group has been defined only recently, and information about the long-term outlook is lacking.

**Detection of Carrier:** Carriers have approximately 50% of normal acid ceramidase activity in leukocytes or cultured skin fibroblasts. The enzyme assay requires a synthetic substrate that is not commercially available and must be performed under carefully controlled conditions in a laboratory that has experience with the procedure.

**Support Groups:** NJ; Elizabeth; National Lipid Diseases Foundation

**References:**

Farber S, et al : Lipogranulomatosis: a new lipo-glyco-protein storage disease. J Mt Sinai Hosp 1957; 24:816.

Crocker AC, et al.: The "lipogranulomatosis" syndrome; review with report of patient showing milder involvement. In: Aronson SM, Volk BW, eds: Inborn disorders of sphingolipid metabolism. Oxford: Pergamon, 1967:485.

Dulaney JT, Moser HW: Farber's disease (lipogranulomatosis). In Glew RH, Peters SP, eds: Practical enzymology of the sphingolipidoses. New York: Alan R. Liss, Inc., 1977:283–296.

Fenson AH, et al.: Prenatal diagnosis of Farber's disease. Lancet 1979; II:990–992.

Kudoh T, Wenger DA: Diagnosis of metachromatic leukodystrophy, Krabbe disease, and Farber disease after uptake of fatty acid-labeled cerebroside sulfate into cultured skin fibroblasts. J Clin Invest 1982; 70:89–97.

Momoi T, et al.: Substrate-specificities of acid and alkaline ceramidases in fibroblasts from patients with Farber disease and controls. Biochem J 1982; 205:419–425.

Antonarakis S, et al.: Phenotypic variability in siblings with Farber disease. J Pediatr 1984; 104:406–409.

Moser HW, et al.: Ceramidase deficiency: Farber lipogranulomatosis. In: Scriver CR, et al., eds: The metabolic basis of inherited disease, ed 6. New York: McGraw-Hill, 1989:1645–1654.

M0038 **Hugo Moser**

**Lipoid adrenal hyperplasia with male pseudohermaphroditism**
*See STEROID 20-22 DESMOLASE DEFICIENCY*

## LIPOMAS, FAMILIAL SYMMETRIC 0600

**Includes:**
   Lipomas, multiple circumscribed
   Lipomatosis, multiple familial

**Excludes:**
   Adiposis dolorosa
   Launois-Bensaude syndrome
   Lipomatosis, multiple symmetric
   Lipomatosis, benign diffuse symmetric
   **Neck/face, lipomatosis (0601)**

**Major Diagnostic Criteria:** Presence of multiple encapsulated subcutaneous lipomas spread over the extremities and torso in association with a positive family history.

**Clinical Findings:** Multiple lipomas may be present anywhere on the torso or extremities in a symmetric pattern. Generally, they have developed by the third or fourth decade. They gradually increase in size and number and may be associated with pain during the growth phase. The number of lipomas may range from a few up to several hundred. They are generally less than 5 cm in size. Rarely, spontaneous regression occurs.

**Complications:** Pain or neurologic symptoms related to nerve compression; cosmetic deformity.

**Associated Findings:** Multiple telangiectases or angiomas, multiple endocrine abnormalities, diaphyseal aclasis, hyperkeratosis of the palms and soles, hypercholesterolemia.

**Etiology:** Autosomal dominant inheritance.

**Pathogenesis:** Unknown.

**MIM No.:** *15190

**CDC No.:** 214.800

**Sex Ratio:** M2:F1 (the higher proportion of males is unexplained).

**Occurrence:** Several large kindreds have been reported.

**Risk of Recurrence for Patient's Sib:**
   See Part I, *Mendelian Inheritance.*

**Risk of Recurrence for Patient's Child:**
   See Part I, *Mendelian Inheritance.*

**Age of Detectability:** The lipomas usually begin in early adulthood but have been described as early as age nine years.

**Gene Mapping and Linkage:** Unknown.

**Prevention:** None known. Genetic counseling indicated.

**Treatment:** Excision if lipomas are causing pain or nerve compression and for cosmetic indications.

**Prognosis:** Normal for life span and intelligence.

**Detection of Carrier:** Examination for evidence of lipomas in family members.

**Special Considerations:** Some lipomas may follow the course of peripheral nerves but do not appear to arise from the neural sheath. Inheritance may be difficult to assess. The disorder may have variable severity within a given family, the lipomas may not present until after age 35 years. Unrelated, solitary lipomas are not an uncommon finding in the general population. Multiple lipomas may occur in the GI tract, but do not appear to have a familial tendency and are most likely unrelated to this disorder. Benign

diffuse symmetric lipomatosis may be differentiated from this disorder by the presence of unencapsulated subcutaneous symmetric fat deposits on the trunk and neck, in a typical horse collar distribution, as well as deep accumulations of adipose tissue. It has been reported that chromosomal abnormalities, often involving chromosome 12, in the region (q13-q14), are found in some lipomas. However, no such association has yet been made with the lipomas of this disorder.

**References:**
Kurzweg FT, Spencer R: Familial multiple lipomatosis. Am J Surg 1951; 82:762–765.
Osment LS: Cutaneous lipomas and lipomatosis. Surg Gynecol Obstet 1968; 127:129–132.
Rabbiosi G, et al.: Familial multiple lipomatosis. Acta Dermatol Venereol 1977; 57:265–267.
Mandahl N, et al.: Lipomas have characteristic structural chromosomal rearrangements of 12q13-q14. Int J Cancer 1987; 39:685–688.

FI032 **Janice Finkelstein**
JA014 **Ethylin Wang Jabs**

**Lipomas, multiple circumscribed**
   *See LIPOMAS, FAMILIAL SYMMETRIC*
**Lipomatosis of face and neck**
   *See NECK/FACE, LIPOMATOSIS*
**Lipomatosis of pancreas, congenital**
   *See SHWACHMAN SYNDROME*
**Lipomatosis, benign symmetric**
   *See NECK/FACE, LIPOMATOSIS*
**Lipomatosis, multiple familial**
   *See LIPOMAS, FAMILIAL SYMMETRIC*
**Lipomatosis-angiomatosis-macrencephalia**
   *See OVERGROWTH, BANNAYAN TYPE*
**Lipomembranous osteodystrophy**
   *See OSTEODYSPLASIA, LIPOMEMBRANOUS POLYCYSTIC-DEMENTIA*

## LIPOMENINGOCELE 0602

**Includes:**
   Cauda equina lipoma
   Intraspinal lipomas
   Lumbosacral lipoma
   Spinal dysraphism syndrome

**Excludes:**
   Dermal sinus tract
   **Meningomyelocele (0693)**

**Major Diagnostic Criteria:** A visible mass present over the vertebral column, accompanied by spina bifida occulta and widening of interpedicular distances, is the usual presentation. Myelogram will show widened subarachnoid space, with filling defect of lipoma, at termination of spinal cord.

**Clinical Findings:** A skin-covered mass in the lumbosacral region is noted at birth. This mass may have an associated angioma or tuft of hair. Neurologic function is normal for legs and sphincters, or there may be minor deficits. X-rays indicate the presence of a spina bifida. As the child grows, scoliosis and neurologic loss may occur, as they do in diastematomyelia. Asymmetry of the lower extremities may be present. In some cases lipomeningocele has been associated with cloacal exstrophy.

**Complications:** Progressive neurologic and sphincter loss; progressive orthopedic deformity.

**Associated Findings:** Minor dysraphic changes in spinal cord, i.e. enlarged central canal.

**Etiology:** Unknown.

**Pathogenesis:** Displaced or heterotopic adipose tissue.

**Sex Ratio:** M1:F>1

**Occurrence:** Unknown.

**Risk of Recurrence for Patient's Sib:** Varies with ethnic group and geographic location. In the range of 2–6%.

**Risk of Recurrence for Patient's Child:** Varies with ethnic group and geographic location. In the range of 2–6%.

**Age of Detectability:** At birth.

**Gene Mapping and Linkage:** Unknown.

**Prevention:** None known. Genetic counseling indicated.

**Treatment:** An exploration and excision of lipomatous tissue, particularly the tissue connecting the skin mass to the cord, so that the spinal cord may ascend with growth. Neurologic loss can be stabilized by surgery and may possibly be prevented by early surgery.

**Prognosis:** Good.

**Detection of Carrier:** Unknown.

**References:**

Dubowitz V, et al.: Lipoma of the cauda equina. Arch Dis Child 1965; 40:207.

James CCM, Lassman L: Spina bifida occulta. New York: Grune & Stratton, 1981.

SH007                                        **Kenneth Shapiro**

**Lipomucopolysaccharidosis**
  *See MUCOLIPIDOSIS I*
**Lipoprotein deficiency, familial high-density**
  *See ANALPHALIPOPROTEINEMIA*
**Lipoprotein lipase deficiency, familial**
  *See HYPERCHYLOMICRONEMIA*
**Lipoproteinemia-hyperchylomicronemia, hyperprebeta**
  *See HYPERLIPOPROTEINEMIA V*
**Lipoproteinemia-hyperprebeta**
  *See HYPERTRIGLYCERIDEMIA*
**Lipoproteinosis**
  *See SKIN, LIPOID PROTEINOSIS*
**Liposarcoma**
  *See CANCER, SOFT TISSUE SARCOMA*
**Lips, thick-oral mucosa**
  *See ACROMEGALOID FACIAL APPEARANCE SYNDROME*
**Lisinopril, possible fetal effects**
  *See FETAL ANGIOTENSIN CONVERTING ENZYME (ACE) INHIBITION RENAL FAILURE*
**Lissencephaly sequence**
  *See LISSENCEPHALY SYNDROME*

## LISSENCEPHALY SYNDROME                    0603

**Includes:**

> Chromosome 17, deletion 17p13
> Chromosome 17, monosomy 17p13
> Lissencephaly sequence
> Miller-Dieker syndrome
> Norman-Roberts syndrome

**Excludes:**

> **Brain, schizencephaly (3001)**
> **Fetal retinoid syndrome (2261)**
> **Neu-laxova syndrome (2092)**
> **Walker-Warburg syndrome (2869)**

**Major Diagnostic Criteria:** Lissencephaly (smooth brain) with absence of the gyri (agyria) or pachygyria. The appearance of the brain on CT scan is that of a figure eight with failure of opercularization. There is a wide cortical mantle and posterior enlargement of the ventricles (colpocephaly). This is combined with characteristic facial features and monosomy for the distal portion of the short arm of chromosome 17 in most of the cases studied.

**Clinical Findings:** *Prenatal*: polyhydramnios, decreased fetal movement.

*Perinatal*: low Apgar score, prolonged jaundice, low birth weight.

*Brain*: lissencephaly, heterotopias, colpocephaly, ventricular enlargement, hypoplasia of the corpus callosum, midline calcifications.

*Neurologic function*: profound mental retardation, early hypotonia, subsequent hypertonia, poor feeding, seizures, decreased spontaneous activity.

*Head*: congenital microcephaly, bitemporal hollowing, high forehead, prominent occiput.

*Face*: broad nasal bridge with epicanthal folds, upturned nares, malformed and/or malpositioned ears, abnormal irides, tortuous fundal vessels, micrognathia, long thin upper lip, late eruption of primary teeth, prominent palatine ridges. There is sometimes an unusual vertical wrinkling of the forehead.

*Other*: abnormal palmar creases, clinodactyly, camptodactyly, polydactyly, cryptorchidism, inguinal hernia, sacral dimple, rudimentary tail, congenital heart defects, other visceral defects.

**Complications:** Failure to thrive, apneic and cyanotic spells, and infantile spasms with hypsarrhythmia. Seizures may be refractory to anticonvulsant drugs, ACTH, or steroids.

**Associated Findings:** Duodenal atresia, urinary tract abnormalities.

**Etiology:** Most patients who have been adequately studied have monosomy of the distal short arm of chromosome 17. These chromosome deletions arise as de novo terminal deletions, inherited or de novo unbalanced translocations involving 17p, or unbalanced inversions of chromosome 17. However, there are some patients who have normal prophase chromosome studies. Whether these cases represent submicroscopic deletions of 17p or a phenocopy is currently unknown.

The Miller-Dieker lissencephaly/monosomy 17p13 syndrome is one of several conditions with type I lissencephaly. Type I lissencephaly is defined as agyria with or without pachygyria in conjunction with a wide cortical mantle and minimal or no hydrocephalus. A form of type I lissencephaly with sloping forehead and other facial features was described in a consanguineous family and is distinct from the Miller-Dieker type. This condition has been designated the Norman-Roberts syndrome and is felt to be autosomal recessive. Some cases of type I lissencephaly are not associated with monosomy 17p13 or with the features of Miller-Dieker syndrome or the Norman-Roberts syndrome. These cases have been described as having isolated lissencephaly sequence, which is of unknown etiology.

Patients with lissencephaly can be categorized into one of the

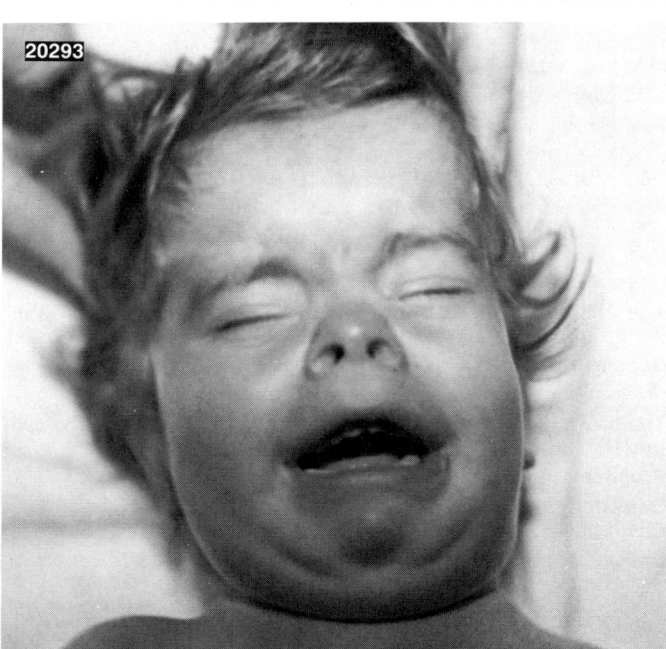

**0603A-20293:** Lissencephaly syndrome; note wrinkling of the forehead, broad nasal bridge, anteverted nares, long, thin upper lip, and low-set ears.

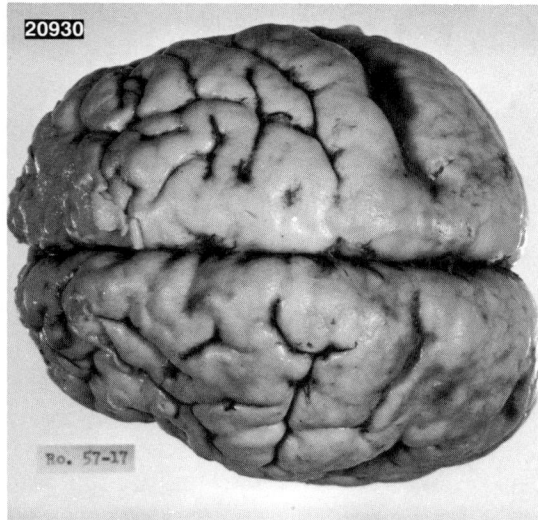

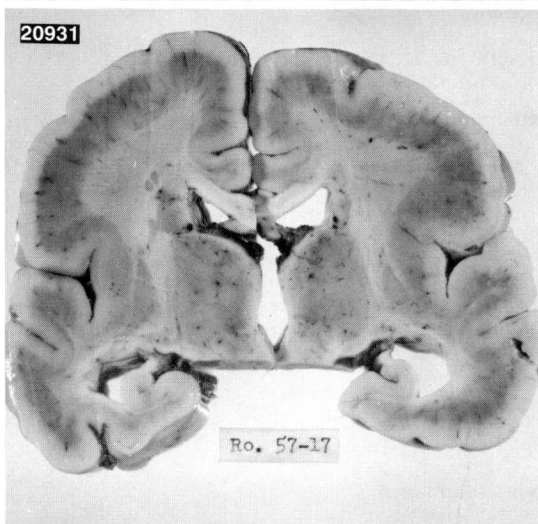

**0603B**-20930: Cerebral hemispheres, top view; there is a simple, convolutional pattern formed by broad gyri. 20931: Coronal section through both hemispheres shows reduction in the number of sulci and convolutions.

above conditions based on clinical, X-ray, and cytogenetic findings. Unless a chromosomal etiology can be found, couples should probably be given a recurrence risk as high as 25% for an autosomal recessive condition.

**Pathogenesis:** Lissencephaly appears to be due to defect in neuronal migration with four rather than six layers in the cortex.

**MIM No.:** *24720

**POS No.:** 3134

**CDC No.:** 742.240

**Sex Ratio:** M8:F18

**Occurrence:** About a dozen kinships, as well as sporadic cases, have been reported.

**Risk of Recurrence for Patient's Sib:**
See Part I, *Mendelian Inheritance*. Probably low if de novo deletion or translocation. As high as 25% if caused by inherited translocation from one parent or if chromosome studies are normal.

**Risk of Recurrence for Patient's Child:**
See Part I, *Mendelian Inheritance*. Affected individuals are not expected to survive to reproduce.

**Age of Detectability:** Monosomy 17p13 can be detected prenatally by amniocentesis or chorionic villus sampling. Otherwise, it is usually detected postnatally based on clinical features and CT scan appearance.

**Gene Mapping and Linkage:** MDCR (Miller-Dieker syndrome chromosome region) has been mapped to 17p13.3.

**Prevention:** None known. Genetic counseling indicated.

**Treatment:** Supportive.

**Prognosis:** Patients are usually severely mentally retarded and have a reduced life span. Most affected children die by five years of age.

**Detection of Carrier:** Chromosome analysis.

**References:**
Jones KL, et al.: The Miller-Dieker syndrome. Pediatrics 1980; 66:277–281. * †
Dobyns WB, et al.: Miller-Dieker syndrome: lissencephaly and monosomy 17p. J Pediatr 1983; 102:552–558. * †
Dobyns WB, et al.: Syndromes with lissencephaly. I: Miller-Dieker and Norman-Roberts syndromes and isolated lissencephaly. Am J Med Genet 1984; 18:509–526. * †
Stratton RF, et al.: New chromosomal syndromes: Miller-Dieker syndrome and monosomy 17p13. Hum Genet 1984; 67:193–200. * †
Greenberg F, et al.: Familial Miller-Dieker syndrome associated with pericentric inversion of chromosome 17. Am J Med Genet 1986; 23:853–859.

GR011                                          **Frank Greenberg**

**Lissencephaly syndrome II**
See WALKER-WARBURG SYNDROME
**Lithium induced goiter**
See GOITER, GOITROGEN INDUCED
**Lithium, fetal effects**
See FETAL LITHIUM EFFECTS
also TRICUSPID VALVE, EBSTEIN ANOMALY
**Lithobid∧ induced goiter**
See GOITER, GOITROGEN INDUCED
**Lithobid∧, fetal effects**
See TRICUSPID VALVE, EBSTEIN ANOMALY
also FETAL LITHIUM EFFECTS
**Lithone∧ induced goiter**
See GOITER, GOITROGEN INDUCED
**Lithone∧, fetal effects**
See FETAL LITHIUM EFFECTS
also TRICUSPID VALVE, EBSTEIN ANOMALY
**Livedo reticularis**
See CUTIS MARMORATA
**Liver cholesteryl ester storage**
See CHOLESTERYL ESTER STORAGE DISEASE
**Liver cyst, solitary but multilocular**
See LIVER, CYST, SOLITARY
**Liver disease-erythrohepatic protoporphyria**
See PORPHYRIA, PROTOPORPHYRIA
**Liver disease-neuronal degeneration of childhood**
See ALPERS DISEASE
**Liver fibrosis and cirrhosis, adult**
See ALPHA(1)-ANTITRYPSIN DEFICIENCY
**Liver glycerol kinase deficiency-hypertriglyceridemia**
See GLYCEROL KINASE DEFICIENCY
**Liver glycerol kinase deficiency-pseudohypertriglyceridemia**
See GLYCEROL KINASE DEFICIENCY
**Liver phosphorylase deficiency**
See GLYCOGENOSIS, TYPE VI
**Liver phosphorylase kinase deficiency**
See GLYCOGENOSIS, TYPE IXa

## LIVER, ACCESSORY LOBE 0467

**Includes:**
    Accessory hepatic lobes
    Hepatic lobes, accessory
    Hepatic lobes anomalous

**Excludes:** Liver anomalies (other)

**Major Diagnostic Criteria:** Evidence of additional hepatic lobe.

**Clinical Findings:** The lobes of the liver may vary in size and shape with either one being absent, or there may be more than two. The Reidel lobe is a tongue-like downward projection of liver tissue from the right lobe. This may resemble a large or mobile right kidney and rarely causes concern as a possible hepatic neoplasm.

Accessory lobes are not uncommonly seen in cases of anterior abdominal wall defects (i.e. omphalocele), where liver tissue may project through the defect.

**Complications:** Unknown.

**Associated Findings:** Omphalocele.

**Etiology:** Unknown.

**Pathogenesis:** Unknown.

**CDC No.:** 751.620

**Sex Ratio:** Presumably M1:F1.

**Occurrence:** Unknown.

**Risk of Recurrence for Patient's Sib:** Unknown.

**Risk of Recurrence for Patient's Child:** Unknown.

**Age of Detectability:** Unknown.

**Gene Mapping and Linkage:** Unknown.

**Prevention:** None known. Genetic counseling indicated.

**Treatment:** Unknown.

**Prognosis:** Unknown.

**Detection of Carrier:** Unknown.

**References:**
Abernathy J: Account of two instances of uncommon formation of the viscera of the human body. Philos Trans Royal Soc London [Biol] 1793; 83:59–66.

GR022                                                   **Jay L. Grosfeld**
CL007                                          **H. William Clatworthy, Jr.**

## LIVER, AGENESIS 0463

**Includes:** Hepatic agenesis

**Excludes:** Biliary atresia (0110)

**Major Diagnostic Criteria:** Complete absence of liver.

**Clinical Findings:** Agenesis of the liver is incompatible with life. This finding has been reported in stillborn fetuses, usually in association with other severe anomalies.

**Complications:** Unknown.

**Associated Findings:** None known.

**Etiology:** Failure of development of hepatic bud from foregut; causes unknown.

**Pathogenesis:** Unknown.

**CDC No.:** 751.600

**Sex Ratio:** Presumably M1:F1.

**Occurrence:** Unknown.

**Risk of Recurrence for Patient's Sib:** Unknown.

**Risk of Recurrence for Patient's Child:** Unknown.

**Age of Detectability:** In stillborn.

**Gene Mapping and Linkage:** Unknown.

**Prevention:** Unknown.

**Treatment:** Unknown.

**Prognosis:** Incompatible with life.

**Detection of Carrier:** Unknown.

**Support Groups:**
    NJ; Cedar Grove; American Liver Foundation
    NJ; Maplewood; The Children's Liver Foundation, Inc.

**References:**
Weichert RF, 3rd, et al.: Atrophy of the right lobe of the liver: case report and review of the syndromes associated with atrophy or agenesis of the liver. Am Surg 1970; 36:667–673.

GR022                                                   **Jay L. Grosfeld**
CL007                                          **H. William Clatworthy, Jr.**

## LIVER, ARTERIAL ANOMALIES 0464

**Includes:** Hepatic arterial anomalies

**Excludes:**
    Liver, hemangiomatosis (0466)
    Liver, venous anomalies (0468)

**Major Diagnostic Criteria:** Direct visualization either by angiography or at operation.

**Clinical Findings:** The common hepatic artery arises from the celiac axis and bifurcates into a right and left hepatic artery in the great majority of cases. The right hepatic artery divides into anterior and posterior segmental branches and the left hepatic artery into the medial and lateral branches to supply their appropriate lobes and segments.

In 17% of people, the right hepatic artery arises in an aberrant fashion from the superior mesenteric artery. In 14–23% of cases, the left hepatic artery originates directly from the left gastric artery. The recognition of these aberrant vessels is of great importance during the performance of hepatobiliary or gastric operations.

**Complications:** Unknown.

**Associated Findings:** None known.

**Etiology:** Unknown.

**Pathogenesis:** Unknown.

**CDC No.:** 751.620

**Sex Ratio:** Presumably M1:F1

**Occurrence:** Unknown.

**Risk of Recurrence for Patient's Sib:** Unknown.

**Risk of Recurrence for Patient's Child:** Unknown.

**Age of Detectability:** Unknown.

**Gene Mapping and Linkage:** Unknown.

**Prevention:** Unknown.

**Treatment:** Unknown.

**Prognosis:** Unknown.

**Detection of Carrier:** Unknown.

**References:**
Michels N: The hepatic, cystic and retroduodenal arteries and their relation to the biliary ducts. Ann Surg 1951; 133:503.
Michels N: Blood supply and the anatomy of the upper abdominal organs. Philadelphia: J.B. Lippincott, 1955.

GR022                                                   **Jay L. Grosfeld**
CL007                                          **H. William Clatworthy, Jr.**

## LIVER, CONGENITAL CYSTIC DILATATION OF INTRAHEPATIC DUCTS                                    3155

**Includes:**
Caroli disease
Nonobstructive dilation of the intrahepatic biliary tree

**Excludes:**
**Bile duct choledochal cyst** (0149)
**Cystic fibrosis** (0237)
Hepatic cyst, isolated primary
**Kidney, polycystic disease, recessive** (2003)

**Major Diagnostic Criteria:**  Demonstration of fusiform, saccular, or cystic dilation of intrahepatic bile ducts in the absence of obstruction and portal fibrosis.

**Clinical Findings:**  Patients present at any age with fever and right upper quadrant pain. These symptoms usually result from cholangitis, which frequently complicates this condition. The symptom may also result from acute obstruction from stones, which may form in ducts. Hepatomegaly and jaundice are infrequent. Transaminases are usually normal, whereas alkaline phosphates and gamma-glutamyltranspeptidase levels are elevated.

Ultrasound and computed tomography of the liver will reveal multiple enlarged ducts or cystic structures. Cholangiogram, either percutaneous transhepatic or endoscopic retrograde, will demonstrate the typical ductular dilation. Filling defects represent intraductal stones.

**Complications:**  Cholangitis results from stagnation of bile. Infection can cause acute febrile episodes and worsening of liver function. Hepatic abcess can result. Liver failure is infrequent, and can be treated with orthotopic hepatic transplantation. Cholangiocarcinoma occurs at increased frequency.

**Associated Findings:**  Occasional patients will have renal lesions as in congenital hepatic fibrosis (see **Kidney, polycystic disease, recessive**). **Bile duct choledochal cyst** has also been reported.

**Etiology:**  Sporadic; no known familial incidence.

**Pathogenesis:**  During early organogenesis, when ductular elements are proliferating, an uncontrolled overproliferation of cellular elements may occur. During subsequent canalization, redundant ductular epithelium results in dilated or cystic ducts.

**MIM No.:**  *26320

**Sex Ratio:**  M1:F1

**Occurrence:**  Fewer than 50 cases have been documented.

**Risk of Recurrence for Patient's Sib:**  Presumably not increased.

**Risk of Recurrence for Patient's Child:**  Presumably not increased.

**Age of Detectability:**  Clinically, from infancy to old age.

**Gene Mapping and Linkage:**  Unknown.

**Prevention:**  None known. Genetic counseling indicated.

**Treatment:**  Acute episodes of cholangitis are treated with intravenous antibiotics. Acute obstructions are managed by surgical drainage. If one lobe is particularly involved, partial hepatectomy may be performed. Orthotopic liver transplantation is curative.

**Prognosis:**  Variable. Recurrent cholangitis can result in rapid progression to liver failure.

**Detection of Carrier:**  Unknown.

**References:**
Caroli J, et al.: La dilatation polykystique congenitale desvoies biliares intra-hepatiques: essai de classification. Sem Hop Paris 1958; 34:128–135.
Murray-Lyon IM, et al.: Non-obstructive dilatation of the intrahepatic biliary tree with cholangitis. Q J Med 1972; 41:477–489.
Hermansen MC, et al.: Caroli disease: the diagnosis approach. J Pediatr 1979; 94:879–882.
Thung SN, Gerber MA: Caroli's disease: a rarely recognized entity. Arch Pathol Lab Med 1979; 103:650–652.
Fagundes-Nato U, et al.: Caroli's disease in childhood: report of two new cases. J Pediatr Gastro Nutr 1983; 2:708–711.

WH007                                    **Peter F. Whitington**

## LIVER, CYST, SOLITARY                                    0465

**Includes:**
Cysts, solitary liver
Hepatic cyst, nonparasitic
Hepatic cyst, solitary
Hepatic cyst, unilocular
Liver cyst, solitary but multilocular

**Excludes:**
**Bile duct choledochal cyst** (0149)
**Liver, hamartoma** (0604)
**Liver, hepatic fibrosis, congenital** (0605)
Parasitic cysts

**Major Diagnostic Criteria:**  A mass in right upper quadrant makes solitary hepatic cyst a possible diagnosis.

**Clinical Findings:**  Solitary hepatic cysts are unilocular (90%) or multilocular (10%), and are usually located in the anteroinferior margin of the right lobe. While most of these cysts are slow growing and asymptomatic, pain and the presence of a mass are common findings. Pain may be due to distention of the liver capsule, resulting from torsion of a pedunculated cyst, or hemorrhage into the cyst. A solitary hepatic cyst is occasionally seen associated with abdominal wall defect (omphalocele). Ultrasonography, radioisotopic scintiscans, and CAT scan may be useful diagnostic adjuncts.

**Complications:**  Torsion of a pedunculated tumor, hemorrhage, infection, and rarely, portal hypertension.

**Associated Findings:**  Strangulation due to torsion of a pedunculated lesion, rupture and hemorrhage into the abdominal cavity, and rarely, development of portal hypertension with bleeding varices.

**Etiology:**  Undetermined. It is thought that these cysts arise from aberrant bile ducts obstructed as a result of congenital malformation.

**Pathogenesis:**  The solitary hepatic cyst is non-calcified and lined with an inner layer of cuboidal epithelial cells or a dense fibrous layer. The outer layer often contains portions of bile duct remnants. The cyst has low internal tension and fluid that contains albumin, cholesterol, mucin, and epithelial elements. Infection, hemorrhage into, and torsion of the cysts may occur.

**CDC No.:**  751.610

**Sex Ratio:**  M1:F4

**Occurrence:**  1:1000 autopsies.

**Risk of Recurrence for Patient's Sib:**  Not demonstrably increased.

**Risk of Recurrence for Patient's Child:**  Not demonstrably increased.

**Age of Detectability:**  The majority of these cysts are asymptomatic and usually do not become apparent until the fourth or fifth decade or are incidental findings at necropsy studies. Solitary hepatic cysts (nonparasitic) are rarely observed in childhood. Although often asymptomatic throughout life, the cyst is potentially dangerous.

**Gene Mapping and Linkage:**  Unknown.

**Prevention:**  None known. Genetic counseling indicated.

**Treatment:**  Simple excision of the cyst is the treatment of choice when possible, with internal drainage as an alternative. Under certain conditions, hepatic lobectomy may be required. Marsupialization is an alternative for non-resectable lesions as the cyst secretions can be absorbed by the peritoneum. However, if a biliary radical enters the cyst, marsupialization should be avoided because it may result in persistent bile drainage and the risk of biliary peritonitis.

**Prognosis:** Good. Many remain asymptomatic throughout life and are noted only as an autopsy finding. Others are usually amenable to operative extirpation. Overall mortality rate due to the cyst is 2.4–5.0%, related perhaps to portal hypertension and its complications.

**Detection of Carrier:** Unknown.

**References:**
Henson SW Jr, et al.: Benign tumors of the liver. III. Solitary cysts. Surg Gynecol Obstet 1956; 103:607.
Clark DD, et al.: Solitary hepatic cysts. Surgery 1967; 61:687.
Longmire WP Jr. Hepatic surgery: trauma, tumors and cysts. Ann Surg 1965; 161:1.

GR022                                                    **Jay L. Grosfeld**
CL007                                          **H. William Clatworthy, Jr.**

**Liver, diffuse capillary or cavernous hemangioma of**
*See LIVER, HEMANGIOMATOSIS*

## LIVER, HAMARTOMA                                          0604

**Includes:**
    Cystic hamartoma of liver
    Hamartoma of liver
    Hepatic hamartoma
    Leber hamartoma
    Mesenchymal hamartoma of liver

**Excludes:**
    Hepatic adenoma
    Hepatic nodular hyperplasia
    **Liver, cyst, solitary** (0465)
    **Liver, hemangiomatosis** (0466)

**Major Diagnostic Criteria:** Large, asymptomatic, right-upper quadrant mass in an infant. Actual histologic evaluation is necessary for a final diagnosis.

**Clinical Findings:** Mesenchymal hamartoma of the liver is a rare benign tumor of infancy that is usually asymptomatic, except for the presence of a mass. Most are located in the right lobe of the liver; in one-third of the cases the mass is on a pedicle. These tumors may be exceptionally large and may occupy much of the peritoneal cavity.† They are more common in patients with hemihypertrophy.

**Complications:** Respiratory embarrassment from diaphragmatic elevation due to large mass; rarely, torsion of tumor on pedicle.

**Associated Findings:** None known.

**Etiology:** Unknown.

**Pathogenesis:** The tumor is composed of collagenous tissue thought to arise from primitive mesenchyme and small cystic areas having distorted hepatic tissue components. Grossly, the lesion appears as a reddish-brown, firm, elastic tumor that is solitary and spherical. It is quite large, weighing between 1,500–3,000 gm. There are two types: one in which loose collagenous fibrous stroma predominate, and one in which multiple small cysts predominate. The cyst walls may be of bile duct or lymphangiomatous origin. Smaller cysts have a single layer of lining cells, while larger cysts are usually devoid of lining cells.

**CDC No.:** 751.620

**Sex Ratio:** Presumably M1:F1.

**Occurrence:** Undetermined but presumed rare.

**Risk of Recurrence for Patient's Sib:** Unknown.

**Risk of Recurrence for Patient's Child:** Unknown.

**Age of Detectability:** Usually detected within the first two years of life.

**Gene Mapping and Linkage:** Unknown.

**Prevention:** None known. Genetic counseling indicated.

**Treatment:** The therapy of choice for mesenchymal hamartoma of the liver is surgical resection. This is simple if a pedicle is present (1/3 of cases), since it is not necessary to resect beyond the tumor into normal liver when the diagnosis can be established at the time of operation. When such a distinction cannot be made, hepatic lobectomy is indicated.

**Prognosis:** Excellent when resection is possible.

**Detection of Carrier:** Unknown.

**Special Considerations:** Mesenchymal hamartoma of the liver is an interesting congenital lesion that only recently has been appreciated as an entity. This lesion should be differentiated from hemangiomatosis (which is a more diffuse lesion with skin components and heart failure) and from solitary cysts and polycystic disease of the liver. It is important to separate this entity from true hepatic adenomas and focal nodular hyperplasia. True hepatic adenomas are very rare; they and consist of normal-appearing or atypical liver cells arranged in cords and, occasionally, forming bile ducts. Portal triads and central veins are absent. Hepatic adenomas are usually solitary and occur in otherwise normal livers. Focal nodular hyperplasia is a "tumor-like" condition that is seen with regeneration following liver injury. The cause of this disorder is unknown; however, some type of injury to the liver and interference with and diminution of the blood supply has been suggested. Many of these tumors and conditions have a strikingly similar gross appearance, so differentiation by appearance alone is unreliable, and careful microscopic analysis is important.

**References:**
Edmondson HA: Differential diagnosis of tumors and tumor-like lesions of the liver in infancy and childhood. Am J Dis Child 1956; 91:168–186.
Ishida M, et al.: Mesenchymal hamartoma of the liver. Ann Surg 1966; 164:175–182.

GR022                                                    **Jay L. Grosfeld**
CL007                                          **H. William Clatworthy, Jr.**

## LIVER, HEMANGIOMATOSIS                                    0466

**Includes:**
    Liver, diffuse capillary or cavernous hemangioma of
    Hepatic hemangiomatosis
    Hepatic infantile hemangioendothelioma

**Excludes:**
    **Liver, hamartoma** (0604)
    Solitary hepatic hemangioma

**Major Diagnostic Criteria:** Consider hepatic hemangiomatosis in any infant in the first six months of life with hepatomegaly, congestive heart failure, and cutaneous hemangiomas. Confirm with hepatic scintiscan and celiac angiogram.

**Clinical Findings:** Hepatic hemangiomatosis of infancy is usually seen with the triad of progressive hepatomegaly (100%), congestive heart failure (93%), and multiple cutaneous hemangiomas (86%). These lesions attain their maximum growth rate in the first six months of life. Due to their immense size, they may trap platelets causing thrombocytopenia, produce arteriovenous shunting leading to cardiac failure, or may cause symptoms by compressing adjacent viscera. Hepatic hemangiomatosis is a diffuse process usually involving the entire organ. A wide pulse pressure, bounding peripheral pulses, and a systolic bruit and thrill over the liver can usually be observed. Jaundice is rare and ascites has not been observed. Dilutional anemia may be noted as a result of compensatory expansion of plasma volume. Flat-plate and erect abdominal X-rays may show an enlarged liver shadow. Hepatic scintiscan will show a large filling defect. Celiac angiogram shows a characteristic arteriovenous blush within the liver with a large celiac axis and hepatic artery. A decrease in the circumference of the abdominal aorta beyond the celiac axis consistent with the diversion of blood flow through the liver is also seen. Computerized axial tomography may be a useful diagnostic aid.

**Complications:** Thrombocytopenia due to platelet trapping, congestive heart failure due to arteriovenous shunting, hemorrhage due to rupture of hemangioma.

**Associated Findings:** Multiple cutaneous hemangiomas.

**Etiology:** These tumors represent a congenital vascular malformation composed of endothelial-lined channels of capillary size and are very cellular. Capillary hemangiomas usually involve the skin, but may be of multicentric origin, which helps explain occurrence in the liver.

**Pathogenesis:** The pathophysiology of hepatic hemangiomatosis includes a wide-open conduit between the hepatic artery and veins. The arteriovenous (A-V) fistula increases the venous return to the heart, and raises the cardiac output with subsequent increase in right atrial pressure as congestive failure occurs. The severity of the symptoms corresponds to the natural history of the tumor and its growth pattern.

**CDC No.:** 751.620

**Sex Ratio:** M1:F2

**Occurrence:** Unknown.

**Risk of Recurrence for Patient's Sib:** Unknown.

**Risk of Recurrence for Patient's Child:** Unknown.

**Age of Detectability:** Usually within the first six months of life.

**Gene Mapping and Linkage:** Unknown.

**Prevention:** None known. Genetic counseling indicated.

**Treatment:** Corticosteroid therapy, radiation, and hepatic-artery ligation have all been employed with some degree of success. Transangiographic catheter embolization with gel-foam has been occasionally successful. Steroids are also useful if thrombocytopenia is present. Congestive heart failure develops within six weeks of birth in 50% of cases. The failure of digitalis and diuretics in the past makes other avenues of therapy a most important consideration. Since the liver is diffusely involved by hemangioendothelioma, hepatic lobectomy is also an ineffective form of treatment.

Steroids have caused noticeable regression of hemangioma within two weeks of therapy. Although the mechanism of steroid therapy is unknown, it is suggested that the rapidly proliferating endothelium in the hemangioma is sensitive to circulating steroids. The frequency of response to steroids has not been documented.

Although radiotherapy is a somewhat controversial method of therapy, occasional reports of its effectiveness have been recorded. Catheter embolization may be useful.

Hepatic-artery ligation has been successfully employed when accomplished proximal to the collateral branches so that obliteration of all arterial inflow is prevented.

All of these adjuncts to therapy hopefully are employed to "buy time" until spontaneous involution and shrinkage of the tumor occurs.

Digitalis derivatives and diuretics alone do not improve most infants in failure because of the large A-V shunts.

**Prognosis:** Mortality is greater than 90% if diuretics or digitalis alone are employed. In all fatal cases, death occurs within six months of birth during the rapid growth of the lesion and prior to spontaneous involution.

**Detection of Carrier:** Unknown.

**References:**
DeLorimier AA, et al.: Hepatic-artery ligation for hepatic hemangiomatosis. New Engl J Med 1967; 277:333.
Fost NC, Esterly, NB: Successful treatment of juvenile hemangiomas with prednisone. J Pediatr 1968; 72:351.
Goldberg SJ, Fonkalsrud EW: Successful treatment of hepatic hemangioma with corticosteroids. J.A.M.A. 1969; 208:2473.
Larcher V, et al.: Hepatic artery ligation in hepatic hemangioma. Arch Dis Child 1981; 56:7.

GR022
CL007

**Jay L. Grosfeld**
**H. William Clatworthy, Jr.**

## LIVER, POLYCYSTIC AND MULTICYSTIC DISEASE, ADULT TYPE     3201

**Includes:**
> Hepatic (liver) cysts
> Kidney-liver disease, adult type polycystic
> Multiple autosomal dominant liver-kidney cystic disease

**Excludes:**
> Hepatic cysts, secondary and infectious
> **Kidney, polycystic adult type** (0859)
> **Kidney, polycystic disease infantile potter type I** (2003)
> **Kidney, renal dysplasia, Potter type II** (3028)
> **Liver, congenital cystic dilatation of intrahepatic ducts** (3155)
> **Liver, cyst, solitary** (0465)
> **Liver, hepatic fibrosis, congenital** (0605)

**Major Diagnostic Criteria:** Demonstration by ultrasound or computerized tomography of multiple cysts in the liver and/or kidney in an individual with positive family history.

**Clinical Findings:** The peak age of detection is about 50 years. There is usually no liver dysfunction, and the lesions are often found at autopsy. About one-half of patients have symptoms, which include dull pain, a sense of fullness and a mass in the right upper abdominal quadrant. Fifty to 70 percent of patients will have coexistant polycystic kidneys, and about one-sixth of all patients will be seen first for renal symptoms, particularly hypertension.

Any of the newer imaging techniques, which include ultrasound, computerized X-ray tomography and nuclear magnetic resonance imaging, can be used to demonstrate multiple cysts in the liver and kidneys. The number of cysts vary from fewer than ten to many hundreds. Cysts vary in size from <1 to >12 cm. diameter.

The cysts are filled with thin, straw-colored fluid, *not* bile. Bile-filled cysts are biliary in origin and communicate with functional bile ducts, which is an important differentiation from polycystic disease. Pathologic examination reveals a thin cuboidal lining of uncertain origin. About a third of cases will have associated von Meyenberg complexes, which are thought to originate from biliary epithelium.

**Complications:** Significant complications are rare. Portal hypertension with esophageal varices have been reported. Post-traumatic rupture with bleeding and infection also occur.

**Associated Findings:** Fifty to seventy percent have polycystic kidneys; 4:70 in one series had intracranial arterial aneurysms; occasional cysts in other glandular organs and lungs; rarely intestinal duplication.

**Etiology:** Autosomal dominant inheritance.

**Pathogenesis:** The cell or tissue origin of the cysts is uncertain. The presence of many organic anions and proteins in the fluid suggests that transport of solutes into the cyst space drives the accumulation of fluid. Bile salts do not enter the space, which suggests that these cysts do not communicate with or share the functions of the excretory system of the liver.

**MIM No.:** 17405

**CDC No.:** 751.610

**Sex Ratio:** M1:F1

**Occurrence:** Undetermined. 1:687 autopsies in Michigan, and 29 cases in the surgical pathology files of the Mayo Clinic from 1907–1954, suggest the probable frequency.

**Risk of Recurrence for Patient's Sib:**
See Part I, *Mendelian Inheritance.*

**Risk of Recurrence for Patient's Child:**
See Part I, *Mendelian Inheritance.*

**Age of Detectability:** As early as first decade, usually during the fifth and sixth decades.

**Gene Mapping and Linkage:** Unknown.

**Prevention:** None known. Genetic counseling indicated.

**Treatment:** Excisional therapy is impractical and often impossible because of the diffuse hepatic involvement. Aspiration and incision have the disadvantage of high recurrence. More permanent relief can be obtained by internal drainage if the cysts can be fenestrated to communicate with the liver surface. Instances of polycystic disease that are asymptomatic need no treatment. Portal hypertension, when present, can be treated with conventional medical and surgical techniques. Rarely orthotopic liver transplantation will be required for management.

**Prognosis:** Usually excellent, with polycystic disease of the liver having no impact on longevity. Associated findings, particularly renal disease, may produce significant morbidity.

**Detection of Carrier:** Possibly by ultrasound of the liver and kidneys.

**Support Groups:**
  MO; Kansas City; Polycystic Kidney Research (PKR) Foundation
  NY; New York; National Kidney Foundation

**References:**
Melnick PJ: Polycystic liver. Arch Pathol 1955; 59:162–172.
Henson SW, et al.: Benign tumors of the liver: polycystic disease of surgical significance. Surg Gynecol Obstet 1957; 104:63–67.
Fisher J, et al.: Polycystic liver disease: studies on the mechanisms of cyst fluid formation. Gastroenterology 1974; 66:423–428.
Luoma PV, et al.: Low high-density lipoprotein and reduced antipyrine metabolism in members of a family with polycystic liver disease. Scand J Gastroent 1980; 15:869–873.
Berrebi G, et al.: Autosomal dominant polycystic liver disease: a second family. Clin Genet 1982; 21:342–347.
Karhunen PJ, Tenhu M: Adult polycystic liver and kidney diseases are separate entities. Clin Genet 1986; 30:29–37.

WH007                                      **Peter F. Whitington**

**Liver, steatosis of**
*See VISCERA, FATTY METAMORPHOSIS*

## LIVER, TRANSPOSITION                                 0606

**Includes:**
  Hepatic situs inversus
  Transposition of liver

**Excludes:** N/A

**Major Diagnostic Criteria:** The liver is found in the left side of the abdomen.

**Clinical Findings:** Mirror-image transposition places the liver on the left side, rather than its usual right-upper-quadrant position. Abdominal situs inversus may be complete or partial and is usually associated with dextrocardia. This anomaly should be suspected if the abdominal X-ray shows the gastric air bubble on the right.

**Complications:** Unknown.

**Associated Findings:** Findings are related to associated congenital malformations: congenital heart disease (tetralogy of Fallot, transposition of great vessels, pulmonic stenosis) and intra-abdominal anomalies (duodenal atresia or stenosis, incomplete bowel fixation prone to midgut volvulus), preduodenal portal vein, biliary atresia, asplenia, polysplenia syndrome, and Kartagener triad of bronchitis, sinusitis, and situs inversus.

**Etiology:** Unknown.

**Pathogenesis:** Related to presence of associated malformations.

**CDC No.:** 751.620

**Sex Ratio:** M1.5:F1

**Occurrence:** Undetermined. 1:11,000 in an X-ray survey.

**Risk of Recurrence for Patient's Sib:** Undetermined, but is more common in sibs of patients with situs inversus.

**Risk of Recurrence for Patient's Child:** Unknown.

**Age of Detectability:** Some 46% are detected in the first month of life.

**Gene Mapping and Linkage:** Unknown.

**Prevention:** None known. Genetic counseling indicated.

**Treatment:** Operations are often required for associated correctable intraabdominal anomalies such as duodenal atresia, biliary atresia, etc. Because of situs inversus, the abdominal incision should be placed in the proper location. The frequent association of cardiovascular and GI anomalies must be emphasized in these infants. Individuals in whom dextrocardia is observed should be carefully evaluated for a heart lesion, and, in addition, they should have X-ray studies of the abdomen for possible abdominal manifestations of situs inversus. Similarly, in the newborn with intestinal obstruction, the presence of dextrocardia on chest X-ray should alert the surgeon to place the incision on the appropriate side of the abdomen. In regard to the liver itself, biliary atresia has been reported in approximately 8% of the cases of situs inversus. The prognosis of the biliary atresia is not altered by the left-sided hepatic position.

**Prognosis:** This depends on the presence and severity of associated anomalies of the cardiovascular and GI systems, in which case mortality may be greater than 50%.

**Detection of Carrier:** Unknown.

**References:**
Merklin RJ, et al.: Situs inversus and cardiac defects: a study of 111 cases of reversed asymmetry. J Thorac Cardiovasc Surg 1963; 45:334–342.
Fonkalsrud EW, et al.: Abdominal manifestations of situs inversus in infants and children. Arch Surg 1966; 92:791–795.

GR022                                      **Jay L. Grosfeld**
CL007                            **H. William Clatworthy, Jr.**

## LIVER, VENOUS ANOMALIES                              0468

**Includes:**
  Anterior duodenal portal vein
  Cavernous transformation of portal vein
  Hepatic venous anomalies
  Portal-vein atresia
  Preduodenal portal vein
  Total anomalous hepatic venous return

**Excludes:**
  **Liver, arterial anomalies** (0464)
  **Liver, hemangiomatosis** (0466)

**Major Diagnostic Criteria:** Specific criteria vary by type of anomaly.

**Clinical Findings:** *Preduodenal portal vein* is a rare congenital anomaly that occurs when the embryonic caudal branch persists between 2 primitive vitelline veins while the middle and cephalic branches atrophy, placing the portal vein anterior to the pancreas and duodenum. Preduodenal portal vein is of surgical significance since it may readily cause difficulties in operations involving the duodenum and biliary tract. Its presence should be observed and care taken not to divide it inadvertently.

*Portal-vein atresia:* excessive obliteration of the fetal umbilical vein and ductus venosus may lead to involvement of the portal vein resulting in atresia or stenosis. The atresia may involve the whole extent of the vein or may be localized to the portion just proximal to its division into its 2 main branches in the porta hepatis.

*Cavernous transformation of portal vein:* controversy exists whether this anomaly represented by spongy trabeculated venous lakes involving the portal vein is an angiomatous tumor or a result of portal vein thrombosis with recanalization and compensatory enlargement of collateral capillaries and veins. This is frequently associated with portal hypertension, splenomegaly, and bleeding esophageal varices.

*Other hepatic vein anomalies:* rarely, the portal vein may enter directly into the vena cava by-passing the liver or may enter directly into the right atrium. Duplication of the portal vein has been seen, but is quite rare.

In certain cases of total anomalous hepatic venous return, the pulmonary veins may drain directly into the portal vein or the ductus venosus. The pulmonary plexus drains into a common channel closely associated with the esophagus, and pierces the diaphragm entering the portal venous system. Eighty-three percent of these cases occur in male infants.

**Complications:**  Unknown.

**Associated Findings:  Biliary atresia**, situs inversus, complete bowel rotation, dextrocardia, and most frequently, **Duodenum, atresia or stenosis** are associated with preduodenal portal vein. Portal hypertension, splenomegaly, and rarely, variceal hemorrhage may be associated with portal-vein atresia or cavernous transformation of portal vein.

**Etiology:**  Unknown.

**Pathogenesis:**  Unknown.

**CDC No.:**  747.480

**Sex Ratio:**  Presumably M1:F1.

**Occurrence:**  Unknown.

**Risk of Recurrence for Patient's Sib:**  Unknown.

**Risk of Recurrence for Patient's Child:**  Unknown.

**Age of Detectability:**  Unknown.

**Gene Mapping and Linkage:**  Unknown.

**Prevention:**  None known. Genetic counseling indicated.

**Treatment:**  Unknown.

**Prognosis:**  Unknown.

**Detection of Carrier:**  Unknown.

**References:**
Boles ET Jr, et al.: Preduodenal portal vein. Pediatrics 1961; 28:805.
Marks C: Developmental basis of the portal venous system. Am J Surg 1969; 117:671.
Rudolph AM: Hepatic and ductus venosus blood flows during fetal life. Hepatology 1983; 2:254–258.
Whitington PF: Portal hypertension in children. Pediatr Ann 1985; 14:494–499.
Abramson SJ, et al.: Biliary atresia and noncardiac polysplenic syndromes and surgical considerations. Radiology 1987; 163:377.
McCarten K, Tule R: Preduodenal portal vein: venography, ultrasonography, and review of the literature. Ann Radiol 1978; 21:155.

GR022                                          **Jay L. Grosfeld**
CL007                               **H. William Clatworthy, Jr.**

**Liver-kidney disease, infantile polycystic**
  *See HEPATIC FIBROSIS, CONGENITAL*
**Liver-kidney, polycystic disease, autosomal recessive type**
  *See HEPATIC FIBROSIS, CONGENITAL*
**Lobar adenomatosis, lung, congenital**
  *See LUNG, CONGENITAL LOBAR ADENOMATOSIS*
**Lobar atrophy**
  *See PICK DISEASE OF THE BRAIN*
**Lobar emphysema, infantile**
  *See LUNG, EMPHYSEMA CONGENITAL LOBAR*
**Lobar tension emphysema in infancy**
  *See LUNG, EMPHYSEMA CONGENITAL LOBAR*
**Lobe of lung, aberrant**
  *See LUNG, ABERRANT LOBE*
**Lobe, ear, absent**
  *See EAR, LOBE, ABSENT*
**Lobodontia**
  *See TEETH, LOBODONTIA*
**Lobstein syndrome**
  *See OSTEOGENESIS IMPERFECTA*
**Lobster claw deformity**
  *See ECTRODACTYLY*
**Localized absence of skin**
  *See SKIN, LOCALIZED ABSENCE OF*
**Loken-Senior syndrome**
  *See RENAL DYSPLASIA-RETINAL APLASIA, LOKEN-SENIOR TYPE*
**Long QT syndrome (one form)**
  *See CARDIO-AUDITORY SYNDROME*

**Long QT syndrome without deafness**
  *See ARRHYTHMIA, WITH LONG QT INTERVAL WITHOUT DEAFNESS*
**Long-chain acyl-CoA dehydrogenase deficiency (LCAD)**
  *See ACYL-CoA DEHYDROGENASE DEFICIENCY, LONG CHAIN TYPE*
**Loniten^, fetal effects**
  *See FETAL EFFECTS FROM MATERNAL VASODILATOR*
**Lorazelam, fetal effects**
  *See FETAL BENZODIAZEPINE EFFECTS*
**Lorber syndrome**
  *See INFLAMMATORY DISEASE, NEONATAL BATES-LORBER TYPE*
**Lou Gehrig's disease**
  *See AMYOTROPHIC LATERAL SCLEROSIS*
  *also AMYOTROPHIC LATERAL SCLEROSIS, FAMILIAL ADULT AND JUVENILE TYPES*
**Louis-Barr syndrome**
  *See ATAXIA-TELANGIECTASIA*
**Low sinus venosus type defect**
  *See ATRIAL SEPTAL DEFECTS*
**Low-set ear**
  *See EAR, LOW-SET*
**Lowe syndrome**
  *See OCULO-CEREBRO-RENAL SYNDROME*
**Lowry syndrome**
  *See CRANIOSYNOSTOSIS-FIBULAR APLASIA, LOWRY TYPE*
**Lubs syndrome**
  *See ANDROGEN INSENSITIVITY SYNDROME, INCOMPLETE*
**Lucey-Driscoll syndrome**
  *See HYPERBILIRUBINEMIA, TRANSIENT FAMILIAL NEONATAL*
**Luder-Sheldon syndrome**
  *See RENAL TUBULAR SYNDROME, FANCONI TYPE*
**Luetic disease**
  *See FETAL SYPHILIS SYNDROME*
**Lumbosacral lipoma**
  *See LIPOMENINGOCELE*
**Lung cancer**
  *See CANCER, LUNG, FAMILIAL*
**Lung disease, familial chronic obstructive**
  *See ALPHA(1)-ANTITRYPSIN DEFICIENCY*

---

**LUNG, ABERRANT LOBE**                                    **0611**

**Includes:**
   Accessory lung arising from bronchial tree, esophagus, and stomach
   Accessory lung with foregut communication
   Bronchus, aberrant
   Esophageal lobe of the lung
   Lobe of lung, aberrant
   Tracheal lobe of the lung

**Excludes:**
   Accessory lobe(s) caused by accessory fissures
   Azygous lobe of the lung
   **Lung, lobe sequestration** (0612)
   Subcardiac lobe of the lung

**Major Diagnostic Criteria:**  Demonstration of aberrant bronchus originating from trachea or esophagus.

**Clinical Findings:**  *Aberrant lobe* generally refers to either a tracheal or esophageal lobe. Tracheal lobe is associated with an aberrant or extra bronchus arising from the lateral wall of the trachea. Patients usually present by age five years. About 50% present with recurrent pneumonia. Stridor is another frequent clinical sign. At least two cases have occurred in children with **Chromosome 21, trisomy 21**. There is an increased incidence of associated malformations (vide infra).

*Esophageal lobe* refers to the abnormal origin of a mainstem bronchus from the esophagus. Therefore, there is no ventilation of the involved lung. Blood supply is from the pulmonary artery.

**Complications:**  Infection and hemorrhage.

**Associated Findings:**  In one series 14/18 cases of tracheal lobe had associated malformations. Five patients had hypoplastic, fused, or extra ribs. Two patients had **Chromosome 21, trisomy 21**, one with associated duodenal web. **Klippel-Feil anomaly**, tracheoesophageal fistula, **Larynx, web**, omphalocele, and **Ventricular septal defect** were also reported in individual patients.

**Etiology:** Unknown.

**Pathogenesis:** The theory suggests a failure of regression of extra tracheal buds during embryogenesis of the foregut. Another theory is local disruption of normal embryogenesis, with the high incidence of associated malformation cited as supporting evidence.

**CDC No.:** 748.690

**Sex Ratio:** M1:F1

**Occurrence:** Undetermined. Established literature.

**Risk of Recurrence for Patient's Sib:** Unknown.

**Risk of Recurrence for Patient's Child:** Unknown.

**Age of Detectability:** At birth. Depending on symptoms, child may present during infancy, childhood, or, less commonly, adulthood.

**Gene Mapping and Linkage:** Unknown.

**Prevention:** None known. Genetic counseling indicated.

**Treatment:** Surgery is indicated in symptomatic cases. Lobectomy, or segmental resection in some cases, removes the aberrant lobe.

**Prognosis:** Normal. In one series surgery (lobectomy in all but one case) was performed in 10/18 patients.

**Detection of Carrier:** Unknown.

**Special Considerations:** The differentiation of esophageal lobe from **Lung, lobe sequestration** is important. The latter does not frequently involve the entire lung, and the trachea branches normally. The arterial supply in sequestration is anomalous, arising from the descending or, rarely, abdominal aorta.

**Support Groups:** New York; American Lung Association

**References:**
Young LW: Anomalous apical bronchus of the right upper lobe. Am J Dis Child 1980; 134:615–616.
Lacina S, et al.: Esophageal lung with cardiac abnormalities. Chest 1981; 79:468–470.
McLaughlin FJ, et al.: Tracheal bronchus: association with respiratory morbidity in childhood. J Pediatr 1985; 106:751–755.

BI009                                    **Robert M. Bilenker**

## LUNG, BRONCHOGENIC CYST                                    2702

**Includes:** Bronchogenic cyst

**Excludes:**
  **Lung, aberrant lobe** (0611)
  **Lung, congenital lobar adenomatosis** (2501)
  Lung, extralobar sequestration
  Lung, intralobar sequestration
  **Lung, lobe sequestration** (0612)

**Major Diagnostic Criteria:** Extrapulmonary unilobular cystic lesion adherent to left main stem bronchus or carina.

**Clinical Findings:** Infants with obstructing bronchogenic cysts present with symptoms of moderate or severe respiratory distress and clinical signs such as wheezing, stridor, and cyanosis. Chest X-ray may show emphysema or severe obstructive atelectasis with a mediastinal shift. Bronchoscopy is thought to be too dangerous and is usually not recommended. Barium swallow will suggest the preoperative diagnosis. In the rare instance of a juxtadiaphragmatic lesion, evaluation of the lower thorax and upper abdomen with computed tomography (CT) to diagnose a "dumbell" bronchogenic cyst is of value. CT is a standard part of evaluation of lung cysts.

**Complications:** Infection in the cyst or adjacent atelectatic lung segments. Rhabdomyosarcoma arising in the wall of a bronchogenic cyst has been reported twice.

**Associated Findings:** None known.

**Etiology:** Undetermined. In view of associated malignancy, Krous and Sexaur (1981) recommend screening family members.

**Pathogenesis:** Abnormal diverticulum of a lung bud in the fifth week of gestation. The cyst is lined by ciliated columnar epithelium and has a fibrous tissue wall with nests of cartilage and sometimes bronchial glands. The cyst does not have its own blood supply. Distal structures, such as alveoli, do not form.

**CDC No.:** 748.480

**Sex Ratio:** M1:F1

**Occurrence:** Undetermined but presumed rare.

**Risk of Recurrence for Patient's Sib:** Unknown.

**Risk of Recurrence for Patient's Child:** Unknown.

**Age of Detectability:** Most cases are detected from the neonatal period to childhood. Age at presentation depends on location, size, and symptoms.

**Gene Mapping and Linkage:** Unknown.

**Prevention:** None known. Genetic counseling indicated.

**Treatment:** Surgical removal is the only effective treatment and is almost always indicated.

**Prognosis:** Excellent for complete recovery.

**Detection of Carrier:** Unknown.

**Support Groups:** New York; American Lung Association

**References:**
Crawford TJ, Cahill JL: The surgical treatment of pulmonary cystic disorders in infancy and childhood. J Pediatr Surg 1971; 6:251–255.
Krous HF, Sexauer CL: Embryonal rhabdomyosarcoma arising within a congenital bronchogenic cyst in a child. J Pediatr Surg 1981; 16:506–508.
Amendola MA, et al.: Transdiaphragmatic bronchopulmonary foregut anomaly: "dumbell" bronchogenic cyst. Am J Radiol 1982; 138:1165–1167.
Mendelson DS, et al.: Bronchogenic cysts with high CT numbers. Am J Radiol 1983; 149:463–465.

BI009                                    **Robert M. Bilenker**

## LUNG, CONGENITAL LOBAR ADENOMATOSIS                         2501

**Includes:**
  Cystic adenomatoid dysplasia of the lung
  Cystic adenomatoid malformation of the lung
  Lobar adenomatosis, lung, congenital

**Excludes:**
  Bronchiectasis
  Bronchopulmonary dysplasia
  Bullous emphysema
  **Diaphragmatic hernia** (0289)
  **Lung, bronchogenic cyst** (2702)
  **Lung, emphysema congenital lobar** (2703)
  **Lung, lobe sequestration** (0612)
  Lymphangiectasia, congenital pulmonary
  Mesothelial cysts
  Pneumatocele
  Pneumothorax

**Major Diagnostic Criteria:** In the neonatal period, a classical X-ray pattern of a cystic mass with a mediastinal shift is the key to the diagnosis.

**Clinical Findings:** In the neonatal period, respiratory distress, characterized by tachypnea and cyanosis. Chest X-rays show an expansible multicystic lesion with shift of the mediastinum toward the contralateral side. Because the condition has been reported in preterm hydropic stillborns (Aslam et al, 1970), sonar examination should be added to the prenatal diagnostic tools and carried out in all pregnancies complicated by hydramnios (Oster and Fortune, 1978).

**Complications:** Respiratory failure following progressive respiratory distress in the neonatal period, or persistent and recurrent

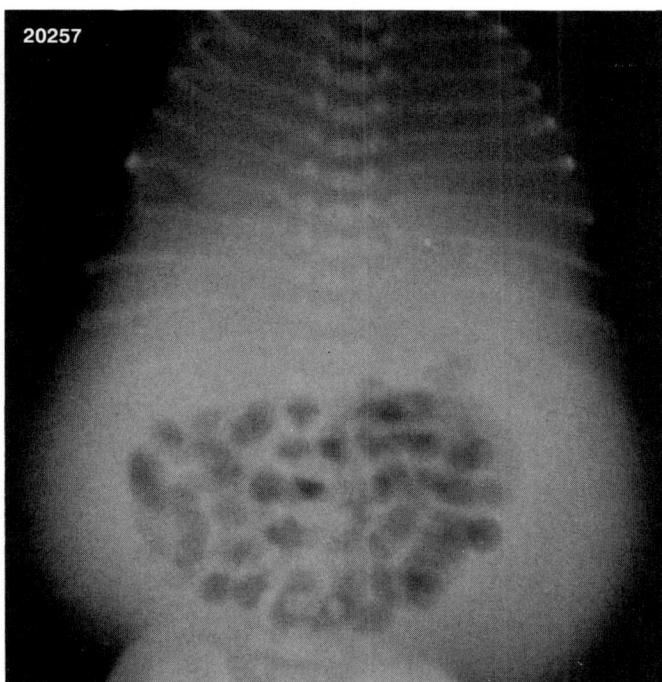

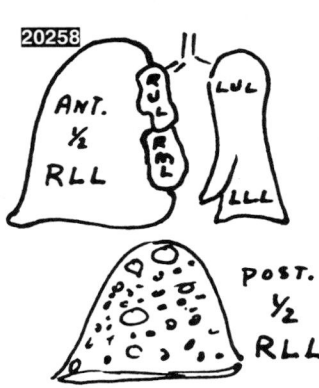

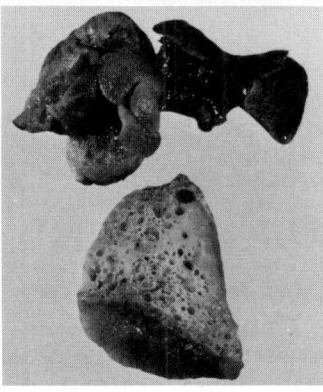

**2501-20257:** X-ray of the chest and abdomen showing right lower lobe cystic mass and ascites. **20258:** Pathological specimens of the lungs and an artist's drawing of the cystic adenomatoid malformation of the right lower lobe of the lung.

pneumonic processes in the affected segment of the lung in the older child.

**Associated Findings:** Compression of the heart and vena cava by the mass may result in fetal hydrops (Elhassani and Webb, 1984). **Pectus excavatum** occurred in four of 32 patients reported by Wolf et al (1980). Other overall associated anomalies were present in 26% of the infants described by Stoker et al (1970). Such anomalies include **Renal agenesis, bilateral** or dysgenesis and **Diaphragmatic hernia.**

**Etiology:** Unknown.

**Pathogenesis:** Cystic, solid, or mixed masses typically involving one pulmonary lobe. According to the histologic appearance of the lesion, three classes are recognized: *type I* is characterized by multiple large cysts; *type II*, by smaller and more numerous cysts; and *type III*, by a bulky, firm mass with evenly spaced small cysts (Stoker et al, 1978).

**CDC No.:** 748.580

**Sex Ratio:** M1:F1

**Occurrence:** About 150 cases have been reported in the literature.

**Risk of Recurrence for Patient's Sib:** Presumably not increased.

**Risk of Recurrence for Patient's Child:** Presumably not increased.

**Age of Detectability:** Although the majority of patients develop respiratory distress in the first week of life, the condition may be overlooked in asymptomatic children.

**Gene Mapping and Linkage:** Unknown.

**Prevention:** None known. Genetic counseling indicated.

**Treatment:** Surgical resection of the involved area of the lung.

**Prognosis:** Unknown.

**Detection of Carrier:** Unknown.

**Support Groups:** New York; American Lung Association

**References:**
Aslam PA, et al.: Congenital cystic adenomatoid malformation of the lung. J Am Med Asso 1970; 212:622–624.
Stoker JT, et al.: Congenital cystic adenomatoid malformation of the lung: classification and morphological spectrum. Hum Pathol 1977; 8:156–171.
Ostor AG, Fortune DW: Congenital cystic adenomatoid malformation of the lung. Am J Clin Pathol 1978; 70:595–604.
Stoker JT, et al.: Cystic and congenital lung disease in the newborn. Perspect Pediatr Pathol 1978; 4:93–154.
Wolf SA, et al.: Cystic adenomatoid dysplasia of the lung. J Pediatr Surg 1980; 15:925–930.
Avitabile IM, et al.: Congenital cystic adenomatoid malformations of the lung in adults. Am J Surg Pathol 1984; 8:193–202.
Elhassani SB, Webb CM: Right lower lobe congenital adenomatosis of the lung with anasarca. J Calif Perinat Assoc 1984; 4:59–60.

EL013                                                   **Sami B. Elhassani**

---

## LUNG, EMPHYSEMA CONGENITAL LOBAR          2703

**Includes:**
   Emphysema, congenital lobar
   Emphysema, localized congenital
   Lobar emphysema, infantile
   Lobar tension emphysema in infancy

**Excludes:**
   Atelectasis with compensatory emphysema
   Lung cyst, congenital
   Mucous plug, isolated

**Major Diagnostic Criteria:** Hyperinflated, emphysematous lung lobe with persistence of lung markings (vessels) seen on chest X-ray.

**Clinical Findings:** Affected infants present with respiratory distress of variable severity precipitated by crying, feeding, or respiratory infection. Left upper lobe is most often involved, followed by right middle lobe. The thoracic wall over the involved lobe(s) may be prominent, with hyperresonance on percussion and decreased breath sounds. Apical beat may be shifted away from the involved side. Chest X-ray shows the hyperinflated lobe with mediastinum displaced away from the affected side. Differential diagnosis often includes pneumothorax, pneumatocele, and congenital lung cyst. These disorders, however, all have absent lung markings in involved areas on X-ray.

**Complications:** Infection. Pneumothorax is rare.

**Associated Findings:** Cardiac defects present in a higher percentage (14% in one series) of cases in this disease than in other congenital cystic disorders of the lungs. Most often found are **Ventricular septal defect** and **Ductus arteriosus, patent. Pectus excavatum** deformities have been related to presence of congenital localized emphysema (CLE). Approximately 70% have some degree of segmental **Bronchomalacia.**

**Etiology:** Unknown. Sporadic in the vast majority of cases. Possible autosomal recessive inheritance has been reported twice, and dominant transmission once.

**Pathogenesis:** CLE is the result of several possible pathogenetic mechanisms. Lesion is most often attributed to deficient bronchial cartilage in the affected main stem bronchus. This causes endobronchial proliferation of mucous membrane, with subsequent obstruction, or extrinsic compression of a bronchus by an anomalous vessel. In 50% of cases no cause is demonstrated. In these cases an alveolar wall defect in quality, quantity, or distribution of collagen or elastin has been theorized.

**MIM No.:** 13071

**CDC No.:** 748.580

**Sex Ratio:** M1:F1

**Occurrence:** Undetermined but presumed rare.

**Risk of Recurrence for Patient's Sib:**
See Part I, *Mendelian Inheritance.*

**Risk of Recurrence for Patient's Child:**
See Part I, *Mendelian Inheritance.*

**Age of Detectability:** During the newborn period.

**Gene Mapping and Linkage:** Unknown.

**Prevention:** None known. Genetic counseling indicated.

**Treatment:** Lobectomy is generally advocated with excellent results. Segmental resection may be curative in some cases.

**Prognosis:** Excellent in almost all cases.

**Detection of Carrier:** Unknown.

**Support Groups:** New York; American Lung Association

**References:**
DeMuth GR, Sloan H: Congenital lobar emphysema: long term effects and sequelae in treatment cases. Surgery 1961; 59:601–607.
Hendren WH, McKee DM: Lobar emphysema of infancy. J Pediatr Surg 1966; 1:24–39.
Eigen H, et al.: Congenital lobar emphysema: long term evaluation of surgically conservatively treated children. Am Rev Respir Dis 1976; 113:823–831.
Wall MA, et al.: Congenital lobar emphysema in a mother and daughter. Pediatrics 1982; 70:131–133.

BI009                                                   **Robert M. Bilenker**

**Lung, hypoplastic-systemic arterial supply-venous drainage**
*See SCIMITAR SYNDROME*

## LUNG, LOBE SEQUESTRATION                              0612

**Includes:**
    Aortic pulmonary lobe
    Pulmonary sequestration, extralobar
    Pulmonary sequestration, intralobar

**Excludes:** N/A

**Major Diagnostic Criteria:** Extralobar sequestration is a nonfunctional pulmonary tissue mass with its own pleural covering and systemic blood supply, often associated with bronchial or gastrointestinal malformations, presenting in the thoracic or, rarely, the retroperitoneal cavity.

Intralobar sequestration is found as a mass within an existing lobe of the lung, consisting of nonfunctional pulmonary tissue not connected to the tracheobronchial tree and commonly receiving its own systemic blood supply.

**Clinical Findings:** Findings vary depending on the type of sequestration. Extralobar lesions present earlier, with approximately one-half found at less than age one year. Earlier age at discovery is often associated with other malformations. Approximately one-half of intralobar sequestrations are initially diagnosed in adults. Patients present with infection from contiguous or hematogenous spread. A mass is seen on X-ray with further information available from computed tomographic (CT) scanning. Aor-

tography may be used to demonstrate the aberrant systemic blood supply in either form of the disorder.

Establishing the diagnosis has been enhanced with CT scanning supplemented by selective angiography to demonstrate aberrant vascular supply and drainage.

**Complications:** Infection is frequent in intralobar but is unusual in extralobar (own pleural sac); hemorrhage is rare in both types.

**Associated Findings:** Diaphragmatic hernia may be associated on the ipsilateral, usually left, side with extralobar lesions. Foregut duplication, fistulous connection, aberrant pancreatic tissue, bronchial isomerism, and congestive heart failure have been reported with intralobar sequestration.

**Etiology:** Unknown.

**Pathogenesis:** There are two general theories of aberrant development. First, accessory budding from lung buds or from distal esophagus (in cases of bronchoesophageal fistula). Timing of the budding determines the type of sequestration. Early accessory budding causes intralobar sequestration and late accessory budding extralobar sequestration. The second theory is persistence of a pulmonary branch of the dorsal aorta predominating when the pulmary artery fails to vascularize the periphery of the lower lobe.

**CDC No.:** 748.520

**Sex Ratio:** Intralobar, M1:F1; extralobar, M4:F1

**Occurrence:** Less than 10% of congenital pulmonary malformations. General incidence not known.

**Risk of Recurrence for Patient's Sib:** Unknown.

**Risk of Recurrence for Patient's Child:** Unknown.

**Age of Detectability:** From birth onward for both types. One-half of extralobar lesions found before age one year. One-half of intralobar lesions are found in adults.

**Gene Mapping and Linkage:** Unknown.

**Prevention:** None known. Genetic counseling indicated.

**Treatment:** Lobectomy for intralobar lesions. Segmental resection for extralobar lesions, with medical and surgical treatment for associated findings as indicated.

**Prognosis:** Normal.

**Detection of Carrier:** Unknown.

**Support Groups:** New York; American Lung Association

**References:**
Smith RA: A theory of the origin of intralobar sequestration of lung. 1956; Thorax 11:10–24.
de Parades CG, et al.: Pulmonary sequestration in infants and children: a 20 year experience and review of the literature. J Pediatr Surg 1970; 5:136–147.
Lilly JR, et al.: Segmental lung resection in the first year of life. Ann Thorac Surg 1976; 22:16–22.

BI009                                                   **Robert M. Bilenker**

**Lung, unilobular-polydactyly-sex reversal-renal hypoplasia**
*See SMITH-LEMLI-OPITZ SYNDROME, TYPE II*
**Lupus erythematosis, neonatal, arrhythmia from**
*See ARRHYTHMIA, FROM MATERNAL AUTOIMMUNE DISEASE, CONGENITAL*

## LUPUS ERYTHEMATOSUS, SYSTEMIC                        2515

**Includes:** Systemic lupus erythematosis (SLE)

**Excludes:**
    Complement component 1, deficiency of (3210)
    Discoid lupus erythematosus
    Drug-induced lupus
    Mixed connective tissue disease
    Subacute cutaneous lupus erythematosus

**Major Diagnostic Criteria:** Revised criteria for the classification of systemic lupus erythematosus (SLE) have been established by the American Rheumatism Association (Tan et al, 1982). A person is said to have SLE if any four or more of the following 11 criteria are present serially or simultaneously during any time period: malar rash, discoid rash, photosensitivity, oral ulcers, arthritis, serositis, renal disorder, neurologic disorder, hematologic disorder, immunologic disorder, and the presence of antinuclear antibody.

**Clinical Findings:** Systemic lupus erythematosus (SLE) is a systemic connective tissue disease with marked and varied immunologic abnormalities. Systemic symptoms include fever, weight loss, and fatigue. The majority (85%) of affected individuals have cutaneous lesions, the most common being an erythematous butterfly rash of the face and a maculopapular rash that develops on exposed surfaces after exposure to sunlight. Alopecia is common (67%). Joint involvement with arthritis, arthralgia, and myalgia is the most common manifestation of SLE. Nonerosive arthritis associated with pain on motion, swelling, or effusion is common (75%). The arthritis is symmetric and commonly involves the proximal interphalangeal, metacarpophalangeal, knee, and wrist joints, with less involvement of the ankle, elbow, hip, and distal interphalangeal joints. Clinically evident renal disease is present in approximately 50% of individuals with SLE, while the majority (>90%) have immunopathologic changes on renal biopsy. Focal (mild) proliferative, diffuse (severe) proliferative, or membranous and mesangial (minimal) lupus nephritis can occur. Serosal involvement leads to clinically evident cardiac and pulmonary changes, the most common of which are pericarditis (25%), pleurisy (46%), and pleural effusion (40%). Nervous system involvement may be central or peripheral, as with a peripheral neuropathy. Central nervous involvement may lead to psychiatric

abnormalities, seizures, long tract signs, and cranial nerve abnormalities.

Nearly all affected individuals have hematologic changes, including anemia of chronic disease, leukopenia with an absolute lymphopenia, and a mild thrombocytopenia. Hemolytic anemia with reticulocytosis and severe thrombocytopenia are infrequent. The eye, liver, and gastrointestinal tract can be involved.

SLE is an autoimmune disease in which antibodies are directed against a variety of nuclear, cytoplasmic, and cell membrane self-antigens. No antibody is specific for SLE. The fluorescent antinuclear antibody test has been the established screening test for SLE, since most affected individuals will have one or more of these antibodies, but the lack of specificity has reduced its usefulness. Antibodies directed against specific antibodies, including native DNA (positive in 80%) and the Sm nuclear antigen (positive in less than 50%), are more confirmatory. Reduced hemolytic complement ($CH_{50}$) levels and hypergammaglobulinemia are found with active disease.

**Complications:** These depend on the organ system involved. For example, severe renal involvement may lead to acute or chronic renal failure. Treatment with steroids and cytotoxic agents can lead to other complications such as opportunistic infections. Pregnancy in a woman with SLE leads to special problems, both for the mother and the child. Pregnancy may exacerbate the activity of the disease, and the fetus can develop neonatal lupus erythematosus, presenting as skin lesions and/or congenital heart block. Transplacental transfer of maternal autoantibodies directed

**Table 2515-1** Revised Criteria for Lupus Erythematosus, Systemic (SLE)

| Criterion | Definition |
|---|---|
| Malar rash | Fixed erythema, flat or raised, over the malar eminences, tending to spare nasolabial folds. |
| Discoid rash | Erythematous raised patches with adherent keratotic scaling and follicular plugging; atrophic scarring may occur in older lesions. |
| Photosensitivity | Skin rash as a result of unusual reaction to sunlight, by patient history or physician observation. |
| Oral ulcers | Oral or nasopharyngeal ulceration, usually painless, observed by physician. |
| Arthritis | Nonerosive arthritis involving two or more peripheral joints, characterized by tenderness, swelling, or effusion. |
| Serositis | 1. Pleuritis—Convincing history of pleuritic pain or rub heard by a physician or evidence of pleural effusion. *or* 2. Pericarditis—Documented by ECG or rub or evidence of pericardial effusion. |
| Renal disorder | 1. Persistent proteinuria greater than 0.5 g per day of greater than 3+ if quantitation not performed. *or* 2. Cellular casts—May be red cell, hemoglobin, granular, tubular, or mixed. |
| Neurologic disorder | 1. Seizures—In the absence of offending drugs or known metabolic derangements (e.g., uremia, ketoacidosis, or electrolyte imbalance). *or* 2. Psychosis—In the absence of offending drugs or known metabolic derangements (e.g., uremia, ketoacidosis, or electrolyte imbalance). |
| Hematologic Disorder | 1. Hemolytic anemia—With reticulocytosis. *or* 2. Leukopenia—Less than 4,000/mm³ total on two or more occasions. *or* 3. Lymphopenia—Less than 1,500/mm³ on two or more occasions. *or* 4. Thrombocytopenia—Less than 100,000/mm³ in the absence of offending drugs. |
| Immunologic disorder | 1. Positive LE cell preparation. *or* 2. Anti-DNA—Antibody to native DNA in abnormal titer. *or* 3. Anti-Sm—Presence of antibody to Sm nuclear antigen. *or* 4. False-positive serologic test for syphilis known to be positive for at least 6 months and confirmed by *Treponema pallidum* immobilization or fluorescent treponemal antibody absorption test. |
| Antinuclear antibody | An abnormal titer of antinuclear antibody by immunofluorescence or an equivalent assay at any point in time and in the absence of drugs known to be associated with "drug-induced lupus" syndrome |

SOURCE: Tan EM, Cohen AS, Fries JF, et al; The 1982 revised classification of SLE. *Arthritis Rheum* 25:1271, 1982. Reprinted from ARTHRITIS AND RHEUMATISM Journal, copyright 1982. Used by permission of the American College of Rheumatology.

against the SS-A (Ro) antigen is thought to be the responsible mechanism for neonatal lupus.

**Associated Findings:** Spontaneous abortion, premature birth, and newborns who are small for gestational age are more common with maternal SLE.

**Etiology:** Undetermined. Probably multifactorial with genetic, environmental and endocrine factors playing some part. The genetic susceptibility is related to histocompatibility antigens, complement, and immunoglobulin allotypes by unknown mechanisms.

Approximately 1–2% of the first-degree relatives of an affected individual have SLE, and the frequency of those with antinuclear antibodies and hypergammaglobulinemia is greater. Impressive pedigrees with many affected members have been published. Concordance for SLE in monozygotic twins is approximately 50–70%. Rare inherited deficiencies of C2, C1q, C1r, C1s, C4, C5, C8, and C1 esterase inhibitor are associated with the development of SLE, the most common being a deficiency of C2. The frequencies of HLA-B8, HLA-DR3, and HLA-DR2 are increased in affected individuals when compared with a control population. The C4A null allele is in linkage disequilibrium with HLA-B8 and HLA-DR3 and is found in excess in SLE. Family studies to determine haplotype sharing and linkage between HLA and a possible SLE susceptibility gene (or genes) are inconclusive. An association between SLE and the immunoglobulin (Gm) allotypes has been established, and studies have suggested an interaction between Gm and HLA that is important in the genetic predisposition to lupus nephritis.

**Pathogenesis:** SLE is probably not a single disease but a syndrome. Genetic, hormonal, and environmental factors (e.g. sunlight, drugs, infections) all seem to play a role. The occurrence of a variety of autoantibodies, the presence of circulating immune complexes, demonstration of immune complexes in affected organs, and consumption of complement suggest that the clinical manifestations of the disease is mediated by immune complexes. However, it is not clear whether the primary defect is with the uncontrolled function of B-cells or with defects in T-cell regulation of B-cells.

**MIM No.:** 15270

**Sex Ratio:** M1:F3 in children, increasing to M1:F8–9 in young adults (aged 20–30 years) and falling to M1:F3 after ages 40–50 years. The altered sex ratio and the fact that SLE has been described in **Klinefelter syndrome** suggest that hormone balance may be important in the development of SLE.

**Occurrence:** Worldwide. Annual incidence is 6–7:100,000 for low-risk populations and up to 35:100,000 for high-risk populations. SLE is three times more common in American Blacks and Orientals than in American Caucasians. Certain Amerindian tribes (Sioux, Crow, Arapahoe) have a high incidence.

**Risk of Recurrence for Patient's Sib:**
See Part I, *Mendelian Inheritance.*

**Risk of Recurrence for Patient's Child:**
See Part I, *Mendelian Inheritance.*

**Age of Detectability:** Usually clinically evident by ages 20–30 years of age. Neonatal lupus can be a complication of maternal SLE.

**Gene Mapping and Linkage:** Unknown.

**Prevention:** None known. Genetic counseling indicated. Detection of a slow acetylator phenotype may be helpful in predicting an increased susceptibility to drug-induced SLE.

**Treatment:** Variable, depending on the systems involved and the severity of the condition. Nonsteroidal anti-inflammatory drugs, hydroxychloroquin, steroids, and cytotoxic agents have been used.

**Prognosis:** Dependent on the organ systems involved. Genetic factors do not clearly predict severity of disease or prognosis.

**Detection of Carrier:** Unknown. Autoantibodies are common in healthy relatives of an affected individual and do not identify those individuals who will develop clinical disease.

**Special Considerations:** It is unlikely that SLE is a single disease; rather, it is a genetically heterogeneous group of disorders with a common phenotype. The component responsible for the genetic susceptibility will differ from family to family, as will the responsible environmental component(s).

Many of the immunologic, genetic, and hormonal factors in this disease have been studied extensively in the murine counterpart of human SLE (NZB/NZW $F_1$ mice).

**Support Groups:**
New York; Systemic Lupus Erythematosus Foundation
CA; Torrance; American Lupus Society
CA; Van Nuys; National Lupus Erythematosus Foundation
DC; Washington; The Lupus Foundation of America

**References:**
Block SR, et al.: Studies of twins with systemic lupus erythematosus: a review of the literature and presentation of 12 additional sets. Am J Med 1975; 59:533–552.
Russell AS: Genetic factors in systemic lupus erythematosus. Semin Arthritis Rheu 1981; 10:255–263.
Tan EM, et al.: The 1982 revised criteria for the classification of systemic lupus erythematosus. Arthritis Rheum 1982; 25:1271–1277.
Rothfield N: Clinical features of systemic lupus erythematosus. In: Kelley WN, et al, eds: Textbook of rheumatology, ed 2. Philadelphia: W.B. Saunders, 1985:1070–1097.
Agnello V: Lupus diseases associated with hereditary and acquired deficiencies of complement. Springer Semin Immunopathol 1986; 9:161–178.
Howard PF, et al.: Relationship between C4 null genes, HLA-D region antigens, and genetic susceptibility to systemic lupus erythematosus in Caucasian and black Americans. Am J Med 1986; 81:187–193.
Mintz G, et al.: Prospective study of pregnancy in systemic lupus erythematosus. Results of a multidisciplinary approach. J Rheumatol 1986; 13:732–739.
Stenszky V, et al.: Interplay of immunoglobulin G heavy chain markers (Gm) and HLA in predisposing to systemic lupus nephritis. J Immunogenet 1986; 13:11–17.
McCune AB, et al.: Maternal and fetal outcome in neonatal lupus erythematosus. Ann Intern Med 1987; 106:518–523.
Greer JM, Panush RS: Incomplete lupus erythematosus. Arch Intern Med 1989; 149:2473–2476.

KI007                                      **Richard A. King**

**Luteinizing hormone (LH), deficiency of**
*See GONADOTROPIN DEFICIENCIES*
**Luteinizing hormone-releasing hormone (LHRH) deficiency-ataxia**
*See ATAXIA-HYPOGONADISM SYNDROME*
**Lyme borreliosis**
*See FETAL EFFECTS FROM LYME DISEASE*
**Lyme disease**
*See FETAL EFFECTS FROM LYME DISEASE*
**Lymphadenopathy associated virus (LAV) congenital infection**
*See FETAL ACQUIRED IMMUNE DEFICIENCY SYNDROME (AIDS) INFECTION*
**Lymphangiectasia, intestinal**
*See INTESTINAL LYMPHANGIECTASIA*
**Lymphangioma of alveolar ridges**
*See ALVEOLAR RIDGES, LYMPHANGIOMA*
**Lymphangioma of mesentery**
*See MESENTERIC CYSTS*
**Lymphangioma of salivary gland**
*See SALIVARY GLAND LYMPHANGIOMA*
**Lymphangioma, cavernous**
*See CYSTIC HYGROMA*
**Lymphangioma, cystic**
*See CYSTIC HYGROMA*
**Lymphangioma, multifocal**
*See CYSTIC HYGROMA*
**Lymphatic cyst of mesentery**
*See MESENTERIC CYSTS*
**Lymphedema forme tarde**
*See LYMPHEDEMA II*

# LYMPHEDEMA I                                                    0614

**Includes:**
 Edema (vs. Lymphedema)
 Lymphedema, congenital hereditary
 Lymphedema, early-onset
 Microcephaly-lymphedema-normal intelligence
 Milroy disease
 Nonne-Milroy type hereditary lymphedema

**Excludes:**
 Acquired lymphedema (post radiation, surgical, infectious)
 **Lymphedema II** (0615)
 **Lymphedema-hypoparathyroidism** (2801)

**Major Diagnostic Criteria:** Usually present at birth; a firm or brawny edema usually of the lower extremity, distal to Poupart's ligament. May be generalized to the leg or limited to portions of a foot or toes.

Lymphedema and "edema" are not the same and should not be confused (Watts, 1985).

**Clinical Findings:** Congenital hereditary lymphedema is one of two principal types of chronic hereditary lymphedema (see **Lymphedema II**) This form is equivalent to that originally described by Milroy, earlier and independently by Nonne. Milroy's valuable 35 year follow up (1928) of his original family discussed and distinguished the possibly variant form now known as Meige disease, or late-onset chronic hereditary lymphedema. Schroeder and Helweg-Larsen (qua Schroeder infra) (1950) considered these as variants of one process. The paper marking the modern era of study is that of (Esterly, 1965), which contains a still useful review of earlier reports. Esterly distinguished the two types. There are differences in manifestation, other than the age of effective clinical onset, which suggest some value in continuing to consider chronic hereditary lymphedema as having two subtypes, pending further studies. Nevertheless, the overlap is such that classification of the various lymphedema can not be done simply or with certainty.

In most forms of lymphedema, the edema pits with ease (Esterly, 1965) and shows diurnal fluctuation, with lessening at night (Schroeder and Helweg-Larsen, 1950). The swelling is neither painful or tender (Milroy, 1928). Temperature differences of skin surface may be found. A high tissue fluid flow rate has been demonstrated, possibly explaining Esterly's observation of tachycardia in an adult with congenital hereditary lymphedema. While usually found in the legs, clinically and pathologically significant cases occur with isolated arm involvement (Merrick, et al. 1971).

Under the designation of "primary lymphedema" (Dale, 1985) reported four anatomic subtypes according to lymphographic findings:
*Distal hypoplasia*: a reduced number and/or size of lymph channels.
*Proximal hypoplasia*: vessels and nodes too small or too few in groins and pelvis. This is associated with dilated and tortuous, numerous distal vessels.
*Distal and proximal hypoplasia*: a combination of the above.
*Hyperplasia*: large, numerous, dilated, and tortuous vessels in leg, groin or pelvis with or without megalymphatics. The latter are usually unilateral whereas hyperplasia is often bilateral.

Generally, systemic pathophysiologic manifestations have been absent or not well documented. Hypotonia is often seen in the congenital form.

In making a diagnosis in an infant, other forms of extremity enlargement, such as in hemihypertrophy, would need to be distinguished. In adults with apparent congenital lymphedema, local causes of lymphatic obstruction would need to be ruled out, such as postinfectious states, radiation fibrosis, metastatic or primary tumor in regional lymph nodes, or after surgical interruption as in mastectomy.

**Complications:** Poor healing of the tissues following minor trauma would seem to be a possibility but the literature is silent on this. Milroy cited Hope and French as describing acute "attacks" characterized by shivering, emesis, onset of pain over the lymphedema, tachycardia, fever, tachypnea, and an acute redness, added

swelling, and increased tenderness too painful to attempt pitting. Milroy pointed out that none of his cases ever showed this peculiar finding. Subsequent literature has failed to comment on the matter. The attacks were self limited and never fatal, points which, given the era of the report by Hope and French (1907), would seem to rule out superimposed infection.

A significant longer term complication is the occurrence of malignant disease within the involved extremity. This has been mainly lymphangiosarcoma (Dubin, et al 1974); Merrick, et al 1971) but squamous (epidermoid) carcinoma has also been described (Epstein and Mendelsohn, 1984). In three cited cases the interval between diagnosis of the lymphedema and the appearance of tumor was 52 years for lymphangiosarcoma in an arm showing congenital lymphedema, 53 years for squamous carcinoma of the foot of the leg with congenital lymphedema, and 28 years for another case of lymphangiosarcoma following on lymphedema first diagnosed at age 6 months. Both sarcomas were fatal, with survival post diagnosis of 30 and 9 months respectively. A larger series indicated a 50% mortality rate within 24 months after diagnosis of lymphangiosarcoma (Woodward, et al 1972). A man with squamous carcinoma had nonhealing ulcers 15 and 10 years earlier treated by excision and skin grafting, to no avail.

**Associated Findings:** Most lesions are isolated findings. Recently, however associated syndromes with other heritable conditions have been described. The most consistent has been the combination of microcephaly and lymphedema with normal intelligence (Robinow et al, 1970; Crowe & Dickerman, 1986; Leung, 1985, 1987; Meinecke, 1987) (see also **Microcephaly-lymphedema**). Intestinal lymphangiectasis (Vardy, et al 1975) and extradural cysts (Chynn, 1981) have been described in association with lymphedema I. When distichiasis occurs with primary lymphedema the latter is of the bilateral hyperplastic type (Dale, 1987) (see also **Distichiasis-lymphedema syndrome**).

**Etiology:** Autosomal dominant inheritance with variable expressivity approaching 50%. Father to son inheritance has been reported.

**Pathogenesis:** There is usually a slow, asymptomatic progression in the severity of the edema with age. Attempts to visualize lymphatics in involved areas have been unsuccessful. For this reason, the edema appears to be due to a defect in the development of lymphatic drainage rather than increased filtration, which may be secondary to edema of any type.

**MIM No.:** *15310

**CDC No.:** 757.000

**Sex Ratio:** M1:F3 (Dale, 1985) to M1:F1 (Esterly, 1965; sequential generations) or M1:F2 (Esterly; skipped generations). There is nonuniform passage by sex.

**Occurrence:** Estimated 1:6,000. Association with microcephaly is expected in 1–2:50,000.

**Risk of Recurrence for Patient's Sib:**
 See Part I, *Mendelian Inheritance*. About 10% risk by the time the sibling is five years older than when the proband was first diagnosed. The risk to siblings of a male proband is about 50% greater than for a female proband.

**Risk of Recurrence for Patient's Child:**
 See Part I, *Mendelian Inheritance*. About 10% risk by the time the sibling is five years older than when the proband was first diagnosed. The risk to siblings of a male proband is about 50% greater than for a female proband.

**Age of Detectability:** At birth. Lymphedema II is usually diagnosed around puberty, while lymphedema diagnosed after age 30 is most likely acquired.

**Gene Mapping and Linkage:** Unknown.

**Prevention:** None known. Genetic counseling indicated.

**Treatment:** Resection of subcutaneous tissues with subsequent skin autografts have been performed with variable results. Diuretics and bed rest are partially and temporarily effective. Chronic lymphedema is primarily a cosmetic handicap. The potential complications of a proposed therapy should be evaluated accordingly. Reports of lymphangiosarcoma indicate that attempts to reduce the lesions by radiotherapy are contraindicated because of enhanced risk of carcinogenesis.

**Prognosis:** Normal life span and intelligence. Some degree of disability may result from edema of lower limbs. Many members of the Omaha family studied by Milroy were prominent in public and professional life. Malignant transformation, especially into vascular sarcoma, is a grave complication with a very poor prognosis thereafter.

**Detection of Carrier:** By clinical examination. Strong familial penetrance warrants close observation of apparently unaffected relatives (Esterly, 1965; Leung, 1985; Opitz, 1986).

**Support Groups:** MA; Cambridge; National Lymphatic and Venous Diseases

### References:

Hope WB, French H: Persistant hereditary oedema of the legs with acute exacerbations: Milroy's disease. Quart J Med 1907–08; 1:312–330.

Milroy WF: Chronic hereditary edema: Milroy's disease. J Am Med Assoc 1928; 91:1172–1175.

Schroeder E, Helweg-Larson HF: Congenital hereditary lymphedema (Nonne-Milroy-Meige's disease). Acta Med Scand 1950; 137:198.

Esterly JR: Congenital hereditary lymphoedema. J Med Genet 1965; 2:93–98.

Merrick TA, et al.: Lymphangiosarcoma of a congenitally lymphedematous arm. Arch Pathol 1971; 91:365–371.

Woodward AH, et al.: Lymphangiosarcoma arising in chronic lymphedematous extremities. Cancer 1972; 30:562–572.

Dubin HV, et al.: Lymphangiosarcoma and congenital lymphedema of the extremity. Arch Dermatol 1974; 110:608–614.

Vardy AH, et al.: Lymphangiosarcoma arising in chronic lymphedematous extremities. Cancer 1972; 30:562–572.

Chynn K: Congenital spinal extradural cyst in two siblings. Clin Genet 1981; 20:25–27.

Epstein JI, Mendelsohn G: Squamous carcinoma of the foot arising in association with long-standing verrucous hyperplasia in a patient with congenital lymphedema. Cancer 1984; 54:943–947.

Leung AK: Dominantly inherited syndrome of microcephaly and congenital lymphedema. Clin Genet 1985; 27:611–612.

Watts GT: Lymphedema (non-pitting) and simple (pitting) edema are different. Lancet 1985; II:1414–1415.

Crowe CA, Dickerman LH: A genetic association between microcephaly and lymphedema. Am J Med Genet 1986; 24:131–135.

Opitz JM: On congenital edema. (Editorial) Am J Med Genet 1986; 24:127–129.

Dale RF: Primary lymphedema when found with distichiasis is of the type defined as bilateral by lymphograph. J Med Genet 1987; 24:170–171.

Leung AKC: Dominantly inhherited syndrome of microcephaly and congenital lymphedema with normal intelligence. (Letter) Am J Med Genet 1987; 26:231 only.

Meinecke P: A genetic association between microcephaly and lymphedema. (Letter) Am J Med Genet 1987; 26:233 only.

SH054
ES003

**Douglas R. Shanklin**
**John R. Esterly**

## LYMPHEDEMA II                                              0615

### Includes:
Lymphedema forme tarde
Lymphedema, idiopathic
Lymphedema, late-onset
Lymphedema praecox
Lymphedema, primary non-inflammatory
Lymphedema with multiple congenital malformations
Lymphedema with onset after childhood, familial
Meige type lymphedema
Yellow nail syndrome with familial late-onset lymphedema

### Excludes:
Distichiasis-lymphedema syndrome (2039)
Lymphangiosarcoma in chronic lymphedema of the lower limb
Lymphedema of the Turner or Bonnevie-Ullrich syndrome

Lymphedema I (0614)
Lymphedema-hypoparathyroidism (2801)
Secondary lymphedema from multiple causes
Tumorigenic lymphedema

**Major Diagnostic Criteria:** The diagnosis is clinical, with onset of limb edema occuring between the second and fifth decade. A positive family history is helpful and all forms of secondary lymphedema should be ruled out. If the edema presents after the age of 40 years, an underlying malignant lesion should be suspected.

Lymphangiographic studies can be helpful in considering the differential diagnosis and, in cases of idiopathic lymphedema, these may show aplasia, hypoplasia, or dilated lymph trunks.

**Clinical Findings:** Late-onset lymphedema II may make its appearance as early as the teens, but the most common time of onset is between ages 20 and 40 years. Upper and lower limbs may be involved, but in the vast majority of cases it is the lower limbs that are affected. In one series of 131 cases only five patients had upper limb involvement. Bilateral lower limb lymphedema occurred in approximately half of those cases with lower limb involvement. The degree of involvement can be quite variable and may be so minimal as to go undetected, or, in contrast, it may be so extensive that ambulation is a problem. Since there is no specific laboratory test to diagnose this form of lymphedema, it becomes imperative that all causes of secondary lymphedema be excluded. Namely, such processes as infection, postphlebitic lymphedema, postlymphangitic lymphedema, and neoplasia should be excluded. In general, other genetic abnormalities have not been associated with the hereditary form of late-onset lymphedema II. However, in 1966 Wells described a family with affected members showing dystrophic yellow nails and lymphedema involving both lower limbs and, occasionally, the hands and face. Whether these two findings are related or represent a coincidental occurrence is not known.

Recently, a three-year-old male child was reported with congenital lymphedema of the hands and feet and having other skeletal and facial deformities: macrocephaly, frontal bossing, depressed nasal bridge, anteverted nares and a high-arched palate.

**Complications:** The most common complication is single or recurrent episodes of lymphangitis or cellulitis, and these may lead to ulceration. Trichophytosis has been found in approximately 10% of the cases. Lymphangiosarcoma may develop, but this occurs in less than 1% of the cases.

**Associated Findings:** Cleft palate. Possibly yellow, dystrophic nails.

**Etiology:** Most forms are sporadic, or by autosomal dominant inheritance.

**Pathogenesis:** Undetermined. Anatomically, there seems to be a hypoplasia of the lymphatic system in all genetic forms of lymphedema.

**MIM No.:** *15320, 15330

**CDC No.:** 757.000

**Sex Ratio:** Typically M1:F1. However, it is M1:F10 in lymphedema praecox and lymphedema forme tarde.

**Occurrence:** About a half-dozen kindreds reported with inherited forms. Primary types are more common than the genetic.

**Risk of Recurrence for Patient's Sib:**
See Part I, *Mendelian Inheritance.*

**Risk of Recurrence for Patient's Child:**
See Part I, *Mendelian Inheritance.*

**Age of Detectability:** Late-onset lymphedema II, around puberty. Yellow nail syndrome with lymphedema, middle age. Primary form, detectable between the ages of 10 and 40 years, most common between 20 and 30 years.

**Gene Mapping and Linkage:** Unknown.

**Prevention:** None known. Genetic counseling indicated.

**Treatment:** Either type of edema may partially respond to a pararubber bandage or an elastic stocking. Some patients have been reported to have had a reduction of the edema with the use of a diuretic. When the lymphedema is severe and uncontrollable, surgery may be indicated.

**Prognosis:** The lymphedema per se does not alter the normal life span or intelligence. However, complications such as lymphangitis or the development of lymphangiosarcoma may result in an early death. If the edema is extreme with an unsightly appearance, problems in ambulation, coupled with various emotional difficulties, are usually present.

**Detection of Carrier:** Unknown.

**Support Groups:** MA; Cambridge; National Lymphatic and Venous Diseases

**References:**
Goodman RM: Familial lymphedema of the Meige's type. Am J Med 1962; 32:651–656.
Schirger A, et al.: Idiopathic lymphedema: review of 131 cases. JAMA 1962; 182:14–22.
Samman PD, White WF: The "yellow nail" syndrome. Brit J Derm 1964; 76:153–157.
Wells GC: Yellow nail syndrome: with familial primary hypoplasia of lymphatics, manifest late in life. Proc R Soc Med 1966; 59:447 only.
Wheeler ES, et al.: Familial lymphedema praecox: Meige's disease. Plast Reconst Surg 1981; 67:362–364.
Figueroa AA, et al.: Meige disease (familial lymphedema praecox) and cleft palate: report of a family and review of the literature. Cleft Palate J 1983; 20:151–157.
Herbert FA, Bowen PA: Hereditary late-onset lymphedema with pleural effusion and laryngeal edema. Arch Int Med 1983; 143:913–915.

G0026                                    **Richard M. Goodman**

**Lymphedema praecox**
*See LYMPHEDEMA II*
**Lymphedema with multiple congenital malformations**
*See LYMPHEDEMA II*
**Lymphedema with onset after childhood, familial**
*See LYMPHEDEMA II*
**Lymphedema, congenital hereditary**
*See LYMPHEDEMA I*
**Lymphedema, early-onset**
*See LYMPHEDEMA I*
**Lymphedema, idiopathic**
*See LYMPHEDEMA II*
**Lymphedema, late-onset**
*See LYMPHEDEMA II*
**Lymphedema, primary non-inflammatory**
*See LYMPHEDEMA II*
**Lymphedema-distichiasis**
*See DISTICHIASIS-LYMPHEDEMA SYNDROME*

## LYMPHEDEMA-HYPOPARATHYROIDISM                    2801

**Includes:**
    Hypoparathyroidism-lymphedema-nephropathy
    Nephropathy-hypoparathyroidism-lymphedema
**Excludes:**
    **Noonan syndrome** (0720)
    **Parathyroid hormone resistance** (0830)

**Major Diagnostic Criteria:** The combination of congenital lymphedema, hypoparathyroidism, nephropathy, mitral valve prolapse, and brachytelephalangy.

**Clinical Findings:** Each of the documented cases had a history of developing lymphedema soon after birth. They also had short stature; dry, thickened skin; and an unusual facial appearance consisting of medial eyebrow flare, broad nasal bridge, telecanthus, and hypertrichosis of the face and forehead; **Mitral valve prolapse**; **Brachydactyly**; and increased carrying angle. One boy also had cataracts at age 19 years and ptosis. Laboratory studies indicated both nephropathy and hypoparathyroidism in that hemoglobin, calcium, phosphate, magnesium, serum creatinine, parathyroid hormone, and blood urea nitrogen levels were all abnormal. Intravenous pyelogram demonstrated small, inade-

quately functioning kidneys in each sib. Chest X-rays indicated that pulmonary lymphangiectasia was also likely to be present.

**Complications:** Hypertension and cellulitis each occurred as a complication.

**Associated Findings:** None known.

**Etiology:** Possibly autosomal recessive or X-linked inheritance.

**Pathogenesis:** Unknown.

**MIM No.:** 24741

**POS No.:** 3599

**Sex Ratio:** M2:F0 (observed).

**Occurrence:** Reported in two adult male sibs in the United States.

**Risk of Recurrence for Patient's Sib:**
    See Part I, *Mendelian Inheritance.*

**Risk of Recurrence for Patient's Child:**
    See Part I, *Mendelian Inheritance.*

**Age of Detectability:** Soon after birth by the development of lymphedema.

**Gene Mapping and Linkage:** Unknown.

**Prevention:** None known. Genetic counseling indicated.

**Treatment:** Renal transplantation may be indicated. Vitamin D and calcium carbonate for hypoparathyroidism, penicillin V or other antibiotics for cellulitis, and propranolol and methyldopa for hypertension are all possible treatments for the symptoms.

**Prognosis:** Intellectual development appears to be normal; life span may be shortened because of renal failure.

**Detection of Carrier:** Unknown.

**Support Groups:** MA; Cambridge; National Lymphatic and Venous Diseases

**References:**
Dahlberg PJ, et al.: Autosomal or X-linked recessive syndrome of congenital lymphedema, hypoparathyroidism, nephropathy, prolapsing mitral valve, and brachytelephalangy. Am J Med Genet 1983; 16:99–104.

T0007                                    **Helga V. Toriello**

**Lymphedema-microcephaly**
*See MICROCEPHALY-LYMPHEDEMA*
**Lymphoblast interferon deficiency**
*See INTERFERON DEFICIENCY*
**Lymphocytes, natural killer, defect in**
*See CHEDIAK-HIGASHI SYNDROME*
**Lymphocytic leukemia, cell type-childhood acute**
*See LEUKEMIA, ACUTE LYMPHOCYTIC, FAMILIAL*
**Lymphocytophisis**
*See IMMUNODEFICIENCY, X-LINKED SEVERE COMBINED*

## LYMPHOHISTIOCYTOSIS, FAMILIAL ERYTHROPHAGOCYTIC                    2946

**Includes:**
    Erythrophagocytic lymphohistiocytosis, familial
    Familial hemophagocytic lymphohistiocytosis
    Immunodeficiency, erythrophagocytic lymphohistiocytosis
    Reticulosis, familial histocytic
**Excludes:**
    Histiocytosis X
    **Immunodeficiency, reticuloendotheliosis with eosinophilia** (2688)
    Langerhans cell histiocytosis
    Malignant histiocytosis
    Viral-associated hemophagocytic syndrome

**Major Diagnostic Criteria:** In the absence of an infectious etiology, the diagnosis is supported by lymphohistiocytic infiltration of lymph nodes and other tissues. The diagnosis is strongly supported by a positive family history of the disease. Care must be taken to exclude other similar diseases by histopathologic evaluation of biopsy specimens.

**Clinical Findings:** Familial erythrophagocytic lymphohistiocytosis (FEL) is a systemic disease that commonly presents with irritability, recurrent fevers, hepatosplenomegaly, and failure to thrive.

Laboratory findings may include abnormal liver function tests, hypofibrinogenemia, anemia, and intermittent leukopenia and thrombocytopenia. Hyperlipidemia (of types I, IV, and V) is a characteristic finding. Familial erythophagocytic lymphohistiocytosis is characterized by an immunologic deficiency syndrome that includes defects in both humoral and cellular immunity and a plasma inhibitor of immune function. Defects in humoral immunity include low natural antibody titers, low titers to antigens to which patients had previously been immunized, and poor responses to polysaccharide antigens. Cellular defects include defective T-cell cytotoxic function, monocyte antibody-dependent cellular cytotoxicity, and antigen-specific lymphocyte proliferative responses. Associated with the hyperlipidemia in FEL is plasma-mediated suppression of normal cellular immune responses in vitro.

Clinical onset may occur any time within the first several years of life, and the course thereafter is usually relentlessly progressive, culminating rapidly in death usually caused by infection.

**Complications:** Seizures and cortical blindness may result secondary to central nervous system involvement. The infections that frequently are the ultimate cause of death may be secondary to the immunodeficiency.

**Associated Findings:** None known.

**Etiology:** Autosomal recessive inheritance.

**Pathogenesis:** One hypothesis suggests that the expression of a primary genetic defect is triggered by an environmental stimulus (e.g., an infection or an unknown antigen) that results in the lymphohistiocytosis seen on histopathologic examination of affected tissues. The abnormal immune response contributes to the ultimate death by infection.

**MIM No.:** *26770

**Sex Ratio:** M1:F1

**Occurrence:** Approximately 150 cases have been reported since the initial description by Farquhar & Claireaux in 1952.

**Risk of Recurrence for Patient's Sib:**
See Part I, *Mendelian Inheritance.*

**Risk of Recurrence for Patient's Child:**
See Part I, *Mendelian Inheritance.* Affected individuals are not expected to survive to reproduce.

**Age of Detectability:** Only upon the onset of clinical symptoms, which may occur from the neonatal period on. The latest documented onset is age five years.

**Gene Mapping and Linkage:** Unknown.

**Prevention:** None known. Genetic counseling indicated.

**Treatment:** Treatment remains experimental and has included cytotoxic chemotherapy, repeated plasmaphereses remove immunosuppresive activity and thereby ameliorate the defective immune responses, and bone marrow transplantation.

**Prognosis:** Ultimately fatal, usually within months of the onset of clinical symptoms, which is between birth and age five years.

**Detection of Carrier:** Unknown.

**Special Considerations:** It is extremely important to differentiate familial erythrophagocytic lymphohistiocytosis from several other clinically similar syndromes, which have markedly different prognoses and treatment approaches. These are Langerhans cell histiocytosis (characterized by Birbeck granules seen in the lesional cells by electron microscopy), malignant histiocytosis, which has clearly malignant morphologic characteristics, and the viral-associated hemophagocytic syndrome, which can be expected to resolve in most cases if immunosuppressive therapy is avoided.

**References:**
Farquhar JW, Claireaux AE: Familial haemophagocytic reticulosis. Arch Dis Child 1952; 27:519–525.
Ladisch S, et al.: Immunodeficiency in familial erythrophagocytic lymphohistiocytosis. Lancet 1978; I:581–583.
Ladisch S, et al.: Immunologic and clinical effects of repeated blood exchange in familial erythrophagocytic lympho-histiocytosis. Blood 1982; 60:814–821.
Janka GE: Familial hemophagocytic lymphohitiocytosis. Eur J Pediatr 1983; 140:221–230.

LA039                                    **Stephan K. Ladisch**

**Lymphoma, B-cell**
*See LEUKEMIA/LYMPHOMA, B-CELL*

## LYMPHOMA, BURKITT TYPE                               3089

**Includes:**
>    African Burkitt lymphoma
>    Burkitt-like lymphoma
>    Diffuse undifferentiated lymphoma
>    Endemic Burkitt lymphoma
>    Non-African Burkitt lymphoma
>    Non-Hodgkin lymphoma of the B-cell type
>    Protooncogene homologous to myelocytomatosis virus
>    Small non-cleaved cell lymphoma
>    Sporadic Burkitt lymphoma
>    Transformation gene:ONC:MYC

**Excludes:**
>    **Fetal toxoplasmosis syndrome** (0387)
>    Lymph node hyperplasia
>    **Lymphoma, non-Hodgkin** (3107)
>    Lymphoma, pleiomorphic variant

**Major Diagnostic Criteria:** *African Burkitt lymphoma* may present with either the involvement of the mandible, maxilla, or with bulky masses within the abdomen. The non-African *Burkitt lymphoma* presents in the ileocecal area of the gastrointestinal tract or in the cervical nodes. Frequently, there is involvement of the lymphatic system, while this is rare in African Burkitt lymphoma. The neoplastic B-cells in the lymph nodes have uniform sized nuclei with prominent nucleoli, and the cytoplasm is more baosophilic. Frequent mitotic figures are present, and when there are macrophages present, it gives the lymph node biopsy a "starry sky" appearance. The use of imprint preparations helps in distinguishing this type of lymphoma from lymphoblastic types. Immunological studies have demonstrated the presence of membrane and cytoplasmic monoclonal immunoglobulin in the abnormal B-cells.

**Clinical Findings:** An association has been found between *African Burkitt lymphoma* and Epstein-Barr virus (EVB), but this association is rare in non-African Burkitt lymphoma. *Burkitt lymphoma* is a very aggressive neoplasma. Frequently, the bone marrow and central nervous system also becomes involved. An increase in serum lactic dehydrogenase, uric acid, and antibodies to EBV early antigen are observed. These increases correlate with the stage and are indicators of the prognosis of the disease.

**Complications:** Obstruction in the respiratory, urinary and gastrointestinal tracts due to enlarged lymph nodes is a frequent complication. Hyperuricemia and lactic acidosis are common.

**Associated Findings:** None known.

**Etiology:** An association with EBV, but no other etiological factors have been identified.

**Pathogenesis:** A solid neoplasm of the B-cell of the immune system.

**MIM No.:** *19008

**Sex Ratio:** M1:F<1 in both the African and non-African Burkitt lymphomas.

**Occurrence:** *African Burkitt lymphoma* is a childhood disease found endemically in tropical Africa and New Guinea. In the non-African Burkitt lymphoma, there is a wider age range (up to 35 years). A higher mean age exists in non-African Burkitt versus African Burkitt lymphoma (11 versus 7 years).

**Risk of Recurrence for Patient's Sib:** Presumably not increased.

**Risk of Recurrence for Patient's Child:** Presumably not increased.

**Age of Detectability:** At any age.

**Gene Mapping and Linkage:** MYC (avian myelocytomatosis viral (v-myc) oncogene homolog) has been mapped to 8q24.

Approximately 75% of Burkitt lymphomas, independent of whether they are African or non-African types, carry the typical t(8;14) chromosomal translocation. The variant t(8;22) and t(2;8) translocations are present in 16% and 9% of Burkitt lymphomas, respectively. Recently, it has been shown that the immunoglobulin loci are involved in these translocations. It involves either chromosomes 14q32, 22q11 or 2p12 where immunoglobulin heavy chain locus (IgH), immunoglobulin light chain lambda or kappa loci are mapped, respectively, and the protooncogene c-myc is located on chromosome 8q24. In the t(8;14) (q24;q32), the breakpoints on both chromosomes 8 and 14 are very heterogeneous. Breakpoints in the IqH locus have been found within the $D_H$ segments, upstream of the $S\mu$ region and also within the $S\mu$ region, $S\gamma$ region and $S\alpha$ region. In the variant translocations, the breakpoints may occur within the Vk or Jk segments on chromosome 2 or 5' of $C\delta$ on chromosome 22. Breakpoints on chromosome 8 may occur far 5' of c-myc, immediately upstream of the first exon of c-myc or within the first intron when the translocation occurs with chromosome 14. When the translocation occurs with either chromosome 2 or 22, the breakpoint on chromosome 8 occurs at variable distances 3' of the c-myc coding regions. The cellular event which appears to be of primary importance to Burkitt lymphoma is the loss of ability to regulate c-myc expression. Various hypotheses have been suggested: trans-acting control of c-myc expression is interrupted; the feedback control by the c-myc gene itself is interrupted; an increased stability in mRNA transcripts from translocated genes; an escape from translational suppression due to translocation; importance of nucleotide changes in the non-coding or coding region of c-myc; and finally, cis-acting enhancer or enhancer-like elements of the Ig loci which are brought in by the translocation act upon c-myc. Most of these hypotheses have evidence supporting them based on experiments performed on cell lines derived from Burkitt lymphoma, but rarely has fresh biopsy material been used. It should be noted that the molecular complexity underlying the Burkitt lymphoma translocation may be indicative that more than one hypothesis is necessary to explain the phenomenon of constitutive expression of c-myc in Burkitt lymphoma at levels similar to those seen in proliferating but normal cells.

**Prevention:** None known.

**Treatment:** This condition is highly sensitive to chemotherapeutic drugs such as cyclophosphamide. Intermittent high dose cyclophosphamide in combination with high dose glucocorticoids, vincristine, methotrexate and central nervous system prophylaxis with chemotherapy or ratiotherapy has been found to be effective.

**Prognosis:** Over 50% of the cases survive up to two years.

**Detection of Carrier:** Unknown.

**Support Groups:** Atlanta; American Cancer Society

**References:**
Williams WJ, et al: Hematology, ed. 3. New York: McGraw-Hill, 1983. *
Yunis JJ: The chromosomal basis of human neoplasia. Science 1983; 221:227–236.
Reich PR: Hematology, ed. 2. Boston: Little, Brown & Co, 1984. †
DeVitta VT Jr, et al: Cancer: principles and practice of oncology, ed. 2. Philadelphia: JB Lippincott Co, 1985. †
Chenevix-Trench G: The molecular genetics of human non-Hodgkin's lymphoma. Cancer Genet Cytogenet 1987; 27:191–213.
Haluska FG, et al: Oncogene activation by chromosome translocation in human malignancy. Ann Rev Genet 1987; 21:321–345. *

L0016
CR024

**Elaine Louie**
**Carlo M. Croce**

**Includes:**
Follicular lymphoma
Follicular small cleaved lymphoma
Follicular mixed small cleaved and large cell lymphoma
Follicular large cell lymphoma
Leukemia, chronic lymphatic, type 2
Oncogene B-cell leukemia-2

**Excludes:** Lymphoma (other)

**Major Diagnostic Criteria:** Follicular small cleaved lymphoma presents with a follicular growth pattern on the lymph nodes. The cells are small, have an irregular, angular-shaped nuclei with a small nucleoli. The frequency of mitotic figures is low. Follicular mixed small cleaved and large cell lymphoma is similar to follicular small cleaved lymphoma. But an even mixture of two cell types, centrocytes and centroblasts, small germinal center cells and large germinal center cells, respectively, are present. Follicular large cell lymphoma has a majority of large germinal center cells (centroblasts), and the follicular pattern of growth becomes diffuse in the lymph node.

**Clinical Findings:** These lymphomas originate from a corresponding B-cell type found in the normal germinal center follicles of lymph nodes. The abnormal cells have monoclonal surface IgM and complement receptors, as is also present in their normal counterparts. These abnormal B-cells can circulate throughout the blood, lymphatic tissue and bone marrow, leading to peripheral areas of adenopathy. Abdominal involvement is observed in greater than 60% of the cases. The abdominal nodes most often involved are the mesenteric, portal, para-aortic and celiac ones. The affected lymph node will lose its normal architecture and show a diffuse pattern. Greater than 60% of the cases will also have bone marrow involvement, and approximately 90% will have the retroperitoneal nodes involved upon lymphangiography. Follicular lymphomas are composed of three types: the small cleaved cell type which represents 20% of all non-Hodgkin lymphomas; the mixed small and large cell types which represent another 20% of all non-Hodgkin lymphomas; and the large cell type which represents only 3–10% of all non-Hodgkin lymphomas.

**Complications:** About two-thirds of the patients with follicular lymphoma will proceed to diffuse large cell lymphoma.

**Associated Findings:** None known.

**Etiology:** Unknown.

**Pathogenesis:** A solid neoplasm involving the B-cells characteristically found in the germinal center follicles of lymph nodes.

**MIM No.:** *15143

**Sex Ratio:** M1:F1

**Occurrence:** Unknown. Primarily found in the middle-aged and elderly population.

**Risk of Recurrence for Patient's Sib:** Unknown.

**Risk of Recurrence for Patient's Child:** Unknown.

**Age of Detectability:** At any age, but usually at or after middle age.

**Gene Mapping and Linkage:** BCL2 (B cell CLL/lymphoma 2) has been mapped to 18q21.3.

A consistent chromosomal translocation, the t(14;18)(q34;q21), is associated with follicular lymphoma in approximately 80–90% of the cases. The molecular cloning and analysis of a number of these translocations have revealed that the breakpoint on chromosome 14 is clustered tightly 5'of the $J_H$ segments of the immunoglobulin heavy chain locus located on chrosegments of the immunoglobulin heavy chain locus located on chrosegments of the immunoglobulin heavy chain locus located on chromosome 14q32. On chromosome 18, in 60–70% of the translocations the breakpoint interupts a 100 base pair region immediately 3' of the gene that is involved, and less frequently the breakpoint occurs further 3' downstream from the gene or 5' of the first exon of the gene. The gene, a putative oncogene, on chromosome 18 has been disegnated as *bcl*-2 (B-cell leukemia/lymphoma-2). The *bcl*-2 gene is composed of 2 exons and is expressed in several B-cell lines, but the highest levels occur in cells carrying the t(18;14). Three different size mRNA transcripts have been found (.5, 5.5 and 3.5 kb). These mRNAs are generated by either differential splicing or polyadenylation. The 8.5 and 5.5 kb mRNA give rise to a protein of 239 amino acids, and the 3.5 kb mRNA gives rise to a protein 205 amino acids long, called bcl-2 α and bcl-2 β, respectively. The function of these two proteins is unknown. As yet, the function of the bcl-2 gene in normal B-cells or in follicular lymphoma is unknown.

**Prevention:** None known.

**Treatment:** Careful staging of the disease is necessary before any therapy is given. Radiation therapy is used to manage localized disease. The more aggressive lymphoma, follicular lymphoma of the large cell type, requires the use of chemotherapeutic drugs such as a combination of cyclophosphamide, vincristine, methotrexate and Prednisone. Current treatment protocols that include high dose chemotherapy with autologous bone marrow transplantation are in progress.

**Prognosis:** Follicular lymphoma is usually an indolent disease. A good prognosis exists for the patient if there is a greater amount of nodularity in comparison to the amount of diffuse pattern in the lymph nodes.

**Detection of Carrier:** Unknown.

**Support Groups:** Atlanta; American Cancer Society

**References:**
Williams WJ, et al: Hematology, ed 3. New York: McGraw-Hill, 1983. *
Yunis JJ: The chromosomal basis of human neoplasia. Science 1983; 221:227–236.
Reich PR: Hematology, ed 2. Boston: Little, Brown & Co, 1984. †
DeVita VT Jr., et al: Cancer: principles and practice of Oncology, ed 2. Philadelphia: J.B. Lippincott Co, 1985. †
Chenevix-Trench G: The molecular genetics of human non-Hodgkin's lymphoma. Cancer Genet Cytogenet 1987; 27:191–213.
Haluska FG, et al: Oncogene activation by chromosome translocation in human malignancy. Annual Review of Genetics 1987; 21:321–345. *

L0016
CR024

**Elaine Louie**
**Carlo M. Croce**

**Lymphopenia, X-linked, primary essential type**
See IMMUNODEFICIENCY, X-LINKED SEVERE COMBINED
**Lymphopenia-agammaglobulinemia-dwarfism**
See METAPHYSEAL CHONDRODYSPLASIA, TYPE McKUSICK
**Lymphopenic agammaglobulinemia-short limbed dwarfism**
See METAPHYSEAL CHONDRODYSPLASIA WITH THYMOLYMPHOPENIA
**Lymphopenic hypogammaglobulinemia, X-linked recessive form**
See IMMUNODEFICIENCY, X-LINKED SEVERE COMBINED
**Lymphoproliferative disease, X-linked**
See IMMUNODEFICIENCY, X-LINKED LYMPHOPROLIFERATIVE DISEASE
**Lynch syndrome II (some cases)**
See CANCER, BREAST, FAMILIAL
**Lynch syndrome II (some)**
See CANCER, GASTRIC FAMILIAL
**Lynch syndromes I and II**
See CANCER, SEBACEOUS GLAND TUMOR-MULITPLE VISCERAL CARCINOMA
**Lysine malabsorption syndrome**
See HYPERLYSINURIA, ISOLATED
**Lysine: alpha-ketoglutarate reductase deficiency**
See HYPERLYSINEMIA
**Lysinemia, familial**
See HYPERLYSINEMIA
**Lysinuria, congenital**
See HYPERDIBASIC AMINOACIDURIA
**Lysinuria-protein intolerance**
See HYPERLYSINURIA, ISOLATED
**Lysinuric protein intolerance**
See HYPERDIBASIC AMINOACIDURIA
**Lysis of type I fibers, familial**
See MYOPATHY, FAMILIAL LYSIS OF TYPE I FIBERS

**Lysosomal acid lipase deficiency**
See WOLMAN DISEASE
also CHOLESTERYL ESTER STORAGE DISEASE
**Lysosomal alpha-1,4 glucosidase, late onset**
See GLYCOGENOSIS, TYPE IIb
**Lysosomal alpha-D-mannosidase deficiency**
See MANNOSIDOSIS
**Lysosomal alpha-mannosidase A and B deficiencies**
See MANNOSIDOSIS
**Lysosomal glucosidase deficiency**
See GLYCOGENOSIS, TYPE IIa
**Lysosomal glycogen storage disease limited to the heart**
See GLYCOGENOSIS, TYPE IId
**Lysosomal glycogen storage disease without acid maltase deficiency**
See GLYCOGENOSIS, TYPE IIc
**Lysyl oxidase**
See EHLERS-DANLOS SYNDROME
**Lytico-bodig**
See AMYOTROPHIC LATERAL SCLEROSIS, GUAM TYPE

# ❖ M ❖

**Machado disease**
*See MACHADO-JOSEPH DISEASE*

---

## MACHADO-JOSEPH DISEASE           2996

**Includes:**
    Azorean neurologic disease (pejorative)
    Joseph disease
    Machado disease
    Motor system degeneration, autosomal dominant
    Neurological disease, Machado-Joseph type
    Nigrospinodentatal degeneration with nuclear
       ophthalmoplegia
    Spinopontine atrophy
    Striatonigral degeneration, autosomal dominant

**Excludes:**
    **Dentatorubropallidoluysian degeneration, hereditary** (3283)
    **Olivopontocerebellar atrophy**
    Striatonigral degeneration, nongenetic

**Major Diagnostic Criteria:** Cerebellar ataxia, pyramidal signs, and progressive external ophthalmoplegia (PEO). Dystonia, contraction fasciculations of the face and tongue, and bulging eyes are very specific signs.

**Clinical Findings:** Onset is always with an unsteady gait. Cerebellar signs, PEO, and fasciculation-like movements (after contraction of the periorbital and perioral muscles and tongue) are virtually always present. Other findings may vary.

*Type 1 - 14.7% of cases*: Patients with an earlier onset who tend to develop a marked dystonic-rigid extrapyramidal syndrome. *Type 2 - 45.0% of cases*: In these intermediate cases, cerebellar and pyramidal signs dominate.

*Type 3 - 40.3% of cases*: Tend to show striking peripheral amyotrophies and (on occasion) mild sensory loss and to have a later onset.

Different types may be seen in sibs. Mental deterioration is typically absent. CNS involvement is highly variable; structures most often involved include the substantia nigra, dentate, pontine, and motor cranial nerve nuclei, anterior horn cells, Clarke columns, and spinal root ganglia. Bulbar olives are always spared.

**Complications:** Pulmonary infections (the major cause of death).

**Associated Findings:** Diabetes and hyperuricemia have been described.

**Etiology:** Autosomal dominant inheritance.

**Pathogenesis:** Unknown.

**MIM No.:** *10915

**Sex Ratio:** M1.16:F1. The slight preponderance of males may reflect preferential ascertainment.

**Occurrence:** Found mostly in the Azores Islands (1:3,900) and in people of Azorean extraction in the United States (1:6,000) and Canada; also found in non-Azorean Portuguese, United States Blacks, Japanese, Indians, Italians, French, Brazilians, Spanish,

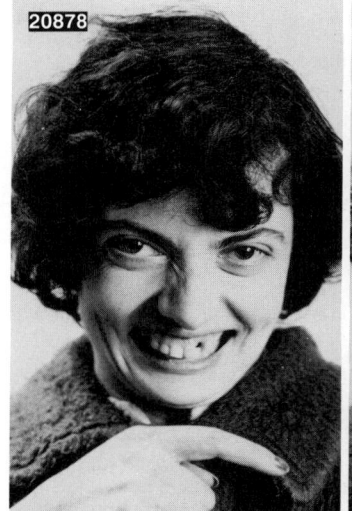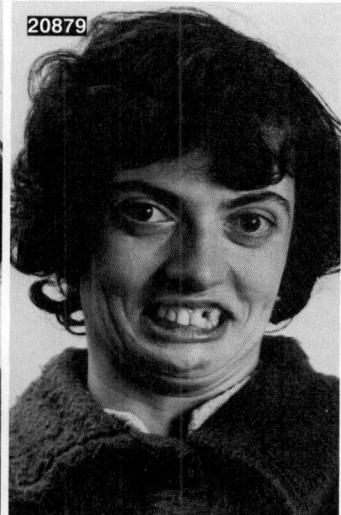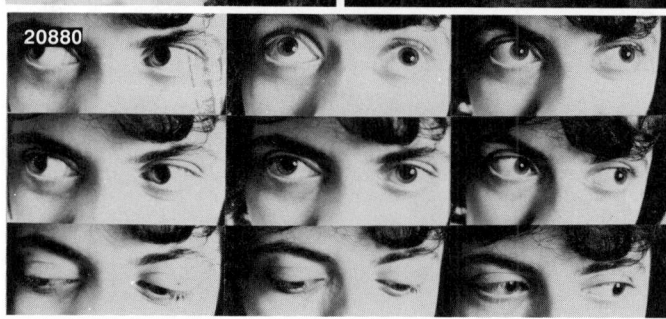

**2996**-20878–79: Machado-Joseph disease; note dystonic posturing in a woman with subphenotype 1. **20880**: Progressive external ophthalmoplegia. This is a constant finding that first affects the gaze upwards, then horizontally, and later downwards. Typical bulging, injected eyes are also evident.

---

Russian, and Chinese. Close to one thousand cases have been documented.

**Risk of Recurrence for Patient's Sib:**
    See Part I, *Mendelian Inheritance*. Penetrance is virtually complete by the eighth decade. Age-dependent correction based on 377 patients: about 40% risk at age 31, 20% at age 48, and 10% at age 55 years.

**Risk of Recurrence for Patient's Child:**
See Part I, *Mendelian Inheritance.*

**Age of Detectability:** Range, 1–73 years; mean, 37.44 years; SD, 14.10 years.

**Gene Mapping and Linkage:** MJD (Machado-Joseph disease) is unassigned.

Unconclusive (loose linkage with PGM1 on chromosome 1 has been reported, but not confirmed).

**Prevention:** None known. Genetic counseling indicated.

**Treatment:** None known to affect progression or prognosis.

**Prognosis:** Variable (most serious in type 1, better in type 3), though poor in general. The typical patient will be confined to a wheel-chair within a few years, and later bedridden; death occurs 15–20 years (on average) after onset.

**Detection of Carrier:** Unknown.

**Special Considerations:** Two cases of presumed homozygotes, with extreme phenotype and early age of onset (six and eight years) have been reported. Rare asymptomatic heterozygotes (as old as age 90) have been documented.

**Support Groups:** CA; Livermore (Box 2550); International Joseph Diseases Foundation, Inc.

**References:**

Nakano KK, et al.: Machado disease: an hereditary ataxia in Portuguese emigrants to Massachusetts. Neurology 1972; 22:49–55.

Woods BT, Schaumburg HH: Nigro-spino-dentatal degeneration with nuclear ophthalmoplegia. In: Vinken PJ, Bruyn G, eds: Handbook of clinical neurology, vol 22. Amsterdam: North Holland, 1975:157–176.

Rosenberg RN, et al.: Autosomal dominant striatonigral degeneration: a clinical, pathologic, and biochemical study of a new genetic disorder. Neurology 1976; 26:703–714.

Coutinho P, Andrade C: Autosomal dominant system degeneration in Portuguese families of the Azores Islands: a new genetic disorder involving cerebellar, pyramidal, extrapyramidal and spinal cord motor functions. Neurology 1978; 28:703–709.

Rosenberg RN, et al.: Joseph's disease: an autosomal dominant neurological disease in the Portuguese of the United States and the Azores Islands. In: Kark RAP, et al., eds: Advances in neurology 21 (The inherited ataxias). New York: Raven, 1978:33–57.

Lima L, Coutinho P: Clinical criteria for diagnosis of Machado-Joseph disease: report of a non-Azorean Portuguese family. Neurology 1980; 30:319–322.

Coutinho P, et al.: The pathology of Machado-Joseph disease: report of a possible homozygous case. Acta Neuropathol (Berlin) 1982; 58:48–54.

Barbeau A, et al.: The natural history of Machado-Joseph disease: an analysis of 138 personally examined cases. Can J Neurol Sci 1984; 11:510–525.

Fowler HL: Machado-Joseph-Azorean disease: a ten-year study. Arch Neurol 1984; 41:921–925.

Sequeiros J, Murphy EA: Age of onset and genetic counseling in Machado-Joseph disease. Am J Hum Genet 1984; 36:126S.

Myers SM, et al.: Machado-Joseph disease: linkage analysis between the loci for the disease and 18 protein markers. Cytogenet Cell Genet 1986; 43:226–228.

Sequeiros J, Suite NDA: Spinopontine atrophy disputed as a separate entity: the first description of Machado-Joseph disease. Neurology 1986; 36:1408.

SE020
C0069

**Jorge Sequeiros**
**Paula Coutinho**

**Macrocephaly**
*See MEGALENCEPHALY*
**Macrocephaly, benign familial**
*See MEGALENCEPHALY*
**Macrocephaly-diffuse hamartomas**
*See OVERGROWTH, BANNAYAN TYPE*
**Macrocephaly-hemangioma**
*See OVERGROWTH, MACROCEPHALY-HEMANGIOMA, RILEY-SMITH TYPE*
**Macrocephaly-multiple lipomas-hemangiomata**
*See OVERGROWTH, BANNAYAN TYPE*

**Macrocephaly-pseudopapilledema-multiple hemangiomata**
*See OVERGROWTH, MACROCEPHALY-HEMANGIOMA, RILEY-SMITH TYPE*
**Macroencephaly**
*See MEGALENCEPHALY*
**Macrogenitosomia praecox**
*See STEROID 21-HYDROXYLASE DEFICIENCY*

---

## MACROGLOSSIA            0618

**Includes:**
>  Muscular macroglossia
>  Tongue gigantism
>  Tongue, isolated congenital enlarged
>  Tongue, large and protruding

**Excludes:**
>  **Amyloidosis**
>  **Beckwith-Wiedemann syndrome** (0104)
>  **Chromosome 21, trisomy 21** (0171)
>  **Glycogenosis, type IIa** (0011)
>  Hypothyroidism, congenital
>  **Mucolipidosis**
>  **Mucopolysaccharidosis**
>  **Neurofibromatosis** (0712)

**Major Diagnostic Criteria:** An excessively large and protruding tongue.

**Clinical Findings:** At birth, large and protruding tongue causing stridor, transient cyanosis, and feeding difficulties. From early infancy, there may be mouth breathing with later articulation difficulties, tongue interposition between the teeth during daytime, snoring, indentations along the tongue border, retruded maxillary incisors, and a class III molar relationship (Angle classification).

**Complications:** Macroglossia secondary to hemangioma, lymphangioma, or neurofibroma can involve the tongue and the floor of the mouth and can extend to contiguous structures in the neck and oral area. If the macroglossia persists until the age of five years, such problems as malocclusion, open bite, drooling, and difficulty with speech are encountered. Occasionally superficial ulcerations may appear and become infected, specifically in hemangiomatous and lymphangiomatous macroglossia. Psychosocial impact due to large and protruding tongue.

**Associated Findings:** None known.

**Etiology:** Two kinships with 18 cases have been reported with autosomal dominant inheritance. All other cases appear sporadic or in association with syndromes.

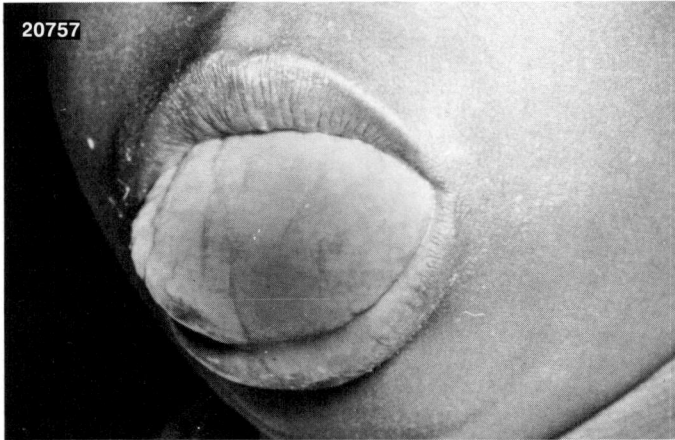

0618A-20757: Tongue, macroglossia.

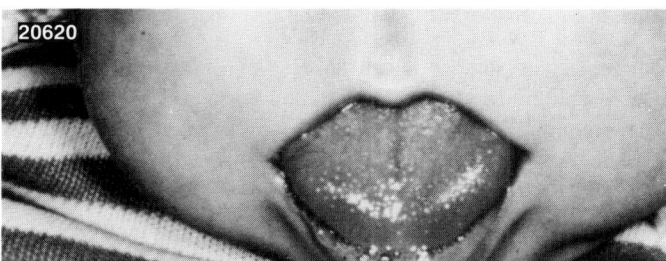

**0618B-20620:** Tongue, macroglossia.

**Pathogenesis:** Depends upon the type of macroglossia. Hemangiomatous and lymphangiomatous macroglossia result from hamartomatous overgrowth of vascular and lymphatic tissue, respectively. Hypertrophy of muscle fibers is noted in muscular macroglossia.

**MIM No.:** *15363

**CDC No.:** 750.120

**Sex Ratio:** Presumably M1:F1.

**Occurrence:** Two kindreds with inherited form have been reported.

**Risk of Recurrence for Patient's Sib:**
See Part I, *Mendelian Inheritance.*

**Risk of Recurrence for Patient's Child:**
See Part I, *Mendelian Inheritance.*

**Age of Detectability:** At birth.

**Gene Mapping and Linkage:** Unknown.

**Prevention:** None known. Genetic counseling indicated.

**Treatment:** Early surgical treatment should be avoided, as sometimes with facial growth, the tongue fits inside the mouth. If by the age of four or five years the macroglossia causes malocclusion, open bite, drooling, and interferes with social acceptance, surgical reduction can be carried out. This usually means marginal wedge excision sometimes accompanied by an anterior wedge excision.

**Prognosis:** Life expectance is unimpaired in uncomplicated cases.

**Detection of Carrier:** Unknown.

**Special Considerations:** Macroglossia as a mendelian trait should be distinguished from syndromes with associated anomalies, mainly those with autosomal dominant inheritance. The genetic basis for other forms of uncomplicated macroglossia, such as those due to hamartomatous overgrowth of vascular and lymphatic tissue, remains undetermined.

**References:**
Warkany J: Congenital malformations. Notes and comments. Chicago: Year Book Medical Publishers, 1971:662–663.
Massengill R, Pickrell K: Surgical correction of macroglossia. Pediatrics 1978; 61:485–488.
Kharbanda OP, et al.: Isolated true macroglossia. J Ind Med Assoc 1984; 82:29–30.
Rizer FM, et al.: Macroglossia: etiologic considerations and management techniques. Int J Ped Otorhinolaryngol 1985; 8:225–236. *
Reynoso MC, et al.: Autosomal dominant macroglossia in two unrelated families. Hum Genet 1986; 74:200–202.

RE027      **Martha Celina Reynoso**
CA011      **José María Cantú**
J0027      **Ronald J. Jorgenson**

**Macroglossia-omphalocele-visceromegaly syndrome**
*See BECKWITH-WIEDEMANN SYNDROME*
**Macrosomia associated with polydactyly and craniosynostosis**
*See ACROCEPHALOPOLYDACTYLOUS DYSPLASIA*
**Macrostomia**
*See FACIAL CLEFT, LATERAL*

**Macrostomia-ablepharon**
*See ABLEPHARON-MACROSTOMIA*
**Macrothrombopathia-deafness-nephritis**
*See DEAFNESS-NEPHRITIS-MACROTHROMBOPATHIA*
**Macrotia**
*See EAR, MACROTIA*

## MACULAR COLOBOMA-BRACHYDACTYLY      0621

**Includes:**
Apical dystrophy
Brachydactyly and macular coloboma
Sorsby syndrome

**Excludes:**
**Brachydactyly** (0114)
**Fetal toxoplasmosis syndrome** (0387)

**Major Diagnostic Criteria:** Congenital macular coloboma and demonstration of digital malformation.

**Clinical Findings:** Characterized by 1) bilateral pigmented macular colobomata of 5 to 6 DD by 3 to 4 DD, with the larger diameter horizontally placed, and 2) an apical dystrophy of hands and feet. The latter consists of rudimentary nails on the index finger of each hand and hallux of each foot, plus an abnormal appearance of the terminal part of the thumb and big toe, which varies from extreme broadness to complete bifurcation. X-rays reveal diminution or actual suppression of the second phalanx of the little finger, a variable bifurcation of the terminal phalanx of thumb and hallux, with a considerable atrophy of all terminal phalanges of both hands and feet. Absence of the small toe is a variable feature.

**Complications:** Horizontal pendular nystagmus and decreased visual acuity (maximally 10/200 corrected).

**Associated Findings:** None known.

**Etiology:** Possibly autosomal dominant inheritance.

**Pathogenesis:** Unknown.

**MIM No.:** 12040

**Sex Ratio:** M1:F1

**Occurrence:** One family has been described.

**Risk of Recurrence for Patient's Sib:**
See Part I, *Mendelian Inheritance.*

**Risk of Recurrence for Patient's Child:**
See Part I, *Mendelian Inheritance.*

**Age of Detectability:** Neonatal period.

**Gene Mapping and Linkage:** Unknown.

**Prevention:** None known. Genetic counseling indicated.

**Treatment:** Unknown.

**Prognosis:** Normal for life span and intelligence. Visual acuity is in the legally blind range.

**Detection of Carrier:** Unknown.

**References:**
Sorsby A: Congenital coloboma of the macula, together with an account of the familial occurrence of bilateral macular coloboma in association with apical dystrophy of hands and feet. Br J Ophthalmol 1935; 19:65–90.
Smith RD, et al.: Congenital macular colobomas and short-limb skeletal dysplasia. Am J Med Genet 1980; 5:365–371.

MA054      **Irene H. Maumenee**

**Macular corneal dystrophy**
*See CORNEAL DYSTROPHY, MACULAR TYPE*
**Macular degeneration and fundus flavimaculatus**
*See RETINA, FUNDUS FLAVIMACULATUS*
**Macular degeneration, polymorphic vitelliruptive**
*See RETINA, MACULAR DEGENERATION, VITELLIRUPTIVE*
**Macular dystrophy, atypical vitelliform**
*See RETINA, MACULAR DEGENERATION, VITELLIRUPTIVE*
**Macular pseudocysts**
*See RETINA, MACULAR DEGENERATION, VITELLIRUPTIVE*

**Madarosis**
  *See EYELID, MADAROSIS*
**Madelung deformity**
  *See DYSCHONDROSTEOSIS*
**Madelung disease**
  *See NECK/FACE, LIPOMATOSIS*
**Maffucci syndrome**
  *See ENCHONDROMATOSIS AND HEMANGIOMAS*
**Magnesium, defect in renal tubular transport of**
  *See HYPOMAGNESEMIA, PRIMARY*
**Magnocellular nevus**
  *See OPTIC DISK, MELANOCYTOMA*
**Majewski short rib-polydactyly syndrome**
  *See SHORT RIB-POLYDACTYLY SYNDROME, TYPE II*
**Major affective disorders**
  *See MOOD AND THOUGHT DISORDERS*

---

## MAL DE MELEDA                                   3289

**Includes:**
  Keratodermia palmoplantaris transgrediens
  Keratosis palmoplantaris transgrediens
  Meleda disease
  Mljet disease
  Siemens disease

**Excludes:**
  **Howel Evans syndrome** (3290)
  **Keratosis palmaris et plantaris of Unna-Thost** (3264)
  **Skin** (other)

**Major Diagnostic Criteria:** Diffuse, progressive palmoplantar keratoderma with involvement of the dorsal surfaces (transgrediens).

**Clinical Findings:** Onset is usually evident after birth and consists of palmoplantar erythema followed by hyperkeratosis and thickening. The disease is usually well developed by the second-to-third year of life. With time, the thickening of the skin extends to the dorsal surfaces of the hand and feet, including fingers and toes. In some patients, especially in those reported in geographic areas other than the Island of Meleda, the erythema may persist.

Gradually, the hyperkeratosis becomes progressive involving the wrists, forearms, and knees. The trunk and the axillary region are rarely involved. Some patients may show a non-keratotic perioral erythema.

The skin lesions consist of yellow brown hyperkeratotic plaques, in a symmetrical and bilateral distribution. Sometimes the hyperkeratotic lesions may be isolated, resembling lichenoid plaques.

Marked hyperkeratosis with malodor is present in almost all cases. The nails are always affected, presenting longitudinal striae, koilonychia, pachyonychia, and onychogryphosis. Brachyphalangia of the fingers has been reported. Hair and teeth are unaffected. Histology shows marked hyperkeratosis, acanthosis, hypergranulosis and moderate perivascular chronic inflammatory infiltration.

**Complications:** Development of painful fissures as well as constriction bands of the distal phalanx has been described.

**Associated Findings:** **Macroglossia**, lingua plicata, partial **Syndactyly**, and in males hair growth over the thenar area and the sole, have been reported.

**Etiology:** Autosomal recessive inheritance.

**Pathogenesis:** Unknown.

**MIM No.:** *24830

**Sex Ratio:** M1:F1

**Occurrence:** Mal de Meleda received its name from the Dalmatian island of Mljet (Yugoslavia) where it was originally observed. In the past, most of the cases described were originally from that region. In the past two decades, many cases have been reported in different countries.

**Risk of Recurrence for Patient's Sib:**
  See Part I, *Mendelian Inheritance.*

**Risk of Recurrence for Patient's Child:**
  See Part I, *Mendelian Inheritance.*

**Age of Detectability:** Usually shortly after birth.

**Gene Mapping and Linkage:** Unknown.

**Prevention:** None known. Genetic counseling indicated.

**Treatment:** Keratolytic agents may be helpful to soften the hyperkeratosis. The oral synthetic retinoids have been used successfully for the relief of significant discomfort.

**Prognosis:** The disease persists throughout life. Life span is not affected.

**Detection of Carrier:** Unknown.

**References:**
Kogoj FR; Die Krankheit von Mljet (Mal de Meleda). Acta Derm Venereol (Stock) 1934; 15:264–299.
Schnyder UW, et al.: La Maladie de Meleda autochtone. Ann Derm Syph Paris 1969; 96:517–530.*†
Reed ML, et al.: Mal de Meleda treated with 13-cis-retinoid acid. Arch Derm 1979; 115:605–608.
Jee SH, et al.: Report of a family with Mal de Meleda in Taiwan. Dermatologica 1985; 171:30–37.
Salomon T: Hairgrowth over thenar and the sole in Mal de Meleda (Mljet disease). Acta Derm Venereol 1985; 65:352–353.†

MI038                                        **Giuseppe Micali**

**Malabsorption of vitamin B(12) (two types)**
  *See VITAMIN B(12) MALABSORPTION*
**Malabsorption, methionine**
  *See METHIONINE MALABSORPTION*
**Malabsorption-ectodermal dysplasia-nasal alar hypoplasia**
  *See JOHANSON-BLIZZARD SYNDROME*
**Maladie de Gelineau**
  *See NARCOLEPSY*
**Malaria, susceptibility to vivax malaria**
  *See MALARIA, VIVAX, SUSCEPTIBILITY TO*

---

## MALARIA, VIVAX, SUSCEPTIBILITY TO          3065

**Includes:**
  Duffy blood group positive
  Benign tertian malaria
  Plasmodium vivax malaria
  Haemamoeba vivax malaria
  Malaria, susceptibility to vivax malaria

**Excludes:** Malaria, susceptibility to other types

**Major Diagnostic Criteria:** All individuals with erythrocytic Duffy antigens Fy$^a$ and or Fy$^b$ are susceptible to vivax malaria. The presence of vivax malaria is unequivocally diagnosed by the identification of characteristic species-specific morphologic features of schizonts and gametocytes in erythrocytes from thin and thick peripheral blood smears stained with Romanowsky type stains. Paroxysms of fever and chills occurring every 48 hours are indicative of *P. vivax* malaria.

**Clinical Findings:** Duffy factor has no known ill effects on erythrocytic morphology or physiology. When vivax malaria does occur, classical paroxysms of fever, chills and sweating occur at intervals of 48 hours. These are the most prominent features. However, myalgia, anorexia and nausea are commonly associated. Developing immunity alters the classical findings to produce irregular fever and chills. Anemia, leukopenia and thrombocytopenia commonly occur. Thick or thin peripheral blood smears will show schizonts in synchronous development depending on when the blood sample is taken. Urine may contain protein indicative of immune complex deposition in glomerulus. The presence of hemoglobinuria is indicative of excessive hemolysis with elevated direct and indirect serum bilirubin.

**Complications:** Duffy factor alone has no untoward effects. In vivax malaria, anemia is commonly seen. Death is seldom seen in vivax malaria.

**Associated Findings:** None known.

**Etiology:** Autosomal condominant inheritance: Duffy alleles, Fᵃ, Fyᵇ.

**Pathogenesis:** Duffy factor (Fyᵃ or Fyᵇ) on red blood cell membranes acts as ligand for receptor on *P. vivax* merozoites (trophozoites) to allow entry into erythrocytes and parasitization. Development of schizonts in erythrocytes leads to destruction of these cells. The Duffy Fy⁴ antigen does not seem to act as a ligand as all Fy(a-b-) erythrocytes are positive for Fy⁴ antigen but refractory to *P. vivax* infection.

**MIM No.:** *11070

**Sex Ratio:** M1:F1

**Occurrence:** Fyᵃ and Fyᵇ alleles are found throughout the world. In whites, the gene frequencies are: Fyᵃ 0.425; Fyᵇ 0.557; and Fy 0.002. The less defined Fyˣ has a frequency of 0.016. Fyᵃ is very frequent in Southeast Asia, Korea, Japan, Melanesia and Micronesia. However, the gene frequencies in Blacks are: Fyᵃ 0.0646; Fyᵇ 0.1130; and Fy 0.8224.

**Risk of Recurrence for Patient's Sib:**
See Part I, *Mendelian Inheritance.*

**Risk of Recurrence for Patient's Child:**
See Part I, *Mendelian Inheritance.*

**Age of Detectability:** Fyᵃ and Fyᵇ antigens are found in red blood cells in fetuses from six weeks onwards and well-developed at birth. The course of Fy⁴ antigen development is undetermined.

**Gene Mapping and Linkage:** FY (Duffy blood group) has been mapped to 1q21-q25.
Duffy factor was first blood group system to be localized on an autosome. Duffy group is linked to uncoiler-1 (1qh); an inherited visible deformity of the lone arm of autosome no. 1, close the centromere. Close linkage of Duffy system with "congenital zonular, pulverulent cataract" was determined by higher mathematics and computer analysis. Linkage of Fy with amylase, pancreatic (AmP) and amylase, salivary (AmS) was identified in 1972.

**Prevention:** None known. Genetic counseling indicated. Prevention of vivax malaria by chemoprophylaxis is possible with chloroquine in endemic areas. Additional prevention by personal strategies to reduce exposure to potentially infective anopheline mosquito bites.

**Treatment:** None needed for Duffy factor. Treatment of vivax malaria with chloroquine and primaquine.

**Prognosis:** Life span not affected.

**Detection of Carrier:** Duffy factor, Fyᵃ and or Fyᵇ detected by erythrocyte agglutination assays using anti-Fyᵃ and anti-Fyᵇ antibodies.

**References:**
Sanger R, et al: The Duffy blood groups in New York Negroes: the phenotype Fy (a-b-). Brit J Haematol 1958; 1:370–374. *
Renwick JH, Lawler SD: Probable linkage between a congenital cataract locus and the Duffy blood group locus. Ann Hum Genet 1963; 27:67–84.
Donahue RP, et al: Probably assignment of the Duffy blood group locus to chromosome 1 in man. Proc Natl Acad Sci USA 1968; 61:949–955. *
Kamaryt J, et al: Possible linkage between uncoiler chromosome Un 1 and amylase polymorphism Amy 2 loci. Humangenetik 1971; 11:218–220.
Benzad O, et al: A new anti-erythrocyte antibody in the Duffy system: anti-Fy⁴. Vox Sang 1973; 24:337–342.
Merritt AD, et al: Human amylase loci: genetic linkage with the Duffy blood group locus and assignment to linkage group 1. Am J Hum Genet 1973; 25:523–538.
Race RR, Sanger R: Blood Groups in Man, ed. 6. Oxford, Blackwell, 1975.
Miller LH, et al: The resistance factor to Plasmodium vivax in blacks: the Duffy-blood-group genotype, FyFy. New Engl J Med 1976; 295:302–304. *
Mourant AE, et al: The distribution of the human blood groups and other polymorphisms, ed. 2. London: Oxford University Press, 1976.

HI014              **Gene I. Higashi**

**Malattia levantinese**
*See OCULAR DRUSEN*
**Malaysian-Melanesian elliptocytosis**
*See ELLIPTOCYTOSIS*
**Male hypogonadism-mental retardation-skeletal anomalies**
*See SHOVAL-SOFFER SYNDROME*
**Male pattern baldness**
*See HAIR, BALDNESS, COMMON*
**Male pseudo-precocious puberty**
*See STEROID 21-HYDROXYLASE DEFICIENCY*
**Male pseudohermaphroditism due to 17-KSR deficiency**
*See STEROID 17-KETOSTEROID REDUCTASE DEFICIENCY*
**Male pseudohermaphroditism due to 5 alpha reductase deficiency**
*See STEROID 5 ALPHA-REDUCTASE DEFICIENCY*
**Male Turner syndrome**
*See NOONAN SYNDROME*
**Malignant acanthosis nigricans (AN)**
*See SKIN, ACANTHOSIS NIGRICANS*
**Malignant congenital osteopetrosis**
*See OSTEOPETROSIS, MALIGNANT RECESSIVE*
**Malignant fibrous histiocytoma**
*See CANCER, SOFT TISSUE SARCOMA*
**Malignant hyperpyrexia**
*See MYOPATHY, MALIGNANT HYPERTHERMIA*
**Malignant hyperthermia**
*See MYOPATHY, MALIGNANT HYPERTHERMIA*
**Malignant hyperthermia-Noonan-like phenotype**
*See KING SYNDROME*
**Malignant melanoma**
*See CANCER, MALIGNANT MELANOMA, FAMILIAL*
**Malignant melanoma, site-specific aggregation of**
*See CANCER, MALIGNANT MELANOMA, FAMILIAL*
**Malignant rhabdoid tumor of the kidney (MRTK)**
*See CANCER, WILMS TUMOR*
**Maloschisis**
*See FACIAL CLEFT, OBLIQUE*
**Malpuech facial clefting syndrome**
*See FACIAL CLEFTING SYNDROME, GYPSY TYPE*
**Malrotation**
*See INTESTINAL ROTATION, INCOMPLETE*
**Malrotation of midgut**
*See INTESTINAL ROTATION, INCOMPLETE*
**Mammary gland tissue without nipple or areola**
*See BREAST, POLYTHELIA*
**Mammary glands, complete supernumerary**
*See BREAST, POLYTHELIA*
**Mammary-ulnar syndrome**
*See ULNAR-MAMMARY SYNDROME*

## MANDIBLE, TORUS MANDIBULARIS     0958

**Includes:**
Mandibular enlargement
Torus mandibular

**Excludes:** N/A

**Major Diagnostic Criteria:** A bony swelling that interrupts the smooth curvature of the lingual surface of the mandible.

**Clinical Findings:** An enlargement of bone on the lingual surface of the mandible above the mylohyoid line and usually opposite the cuspid and premolar teeth. They may have single or multiple lobes.

**Complications:** Only if swelling grows so large as to interfere with mastication or the wearing of a denture.

**Associated Findings:** None known.

**Etiology:** Autosomal dominant inheritance with variable expression and incomplete penetrance according to sex. It has been suggested that this condition is due to the same gene responsible for **Palate, torus palatinus.**

**Pathogenesis:** Unknown.

**MIM No.:** *18970

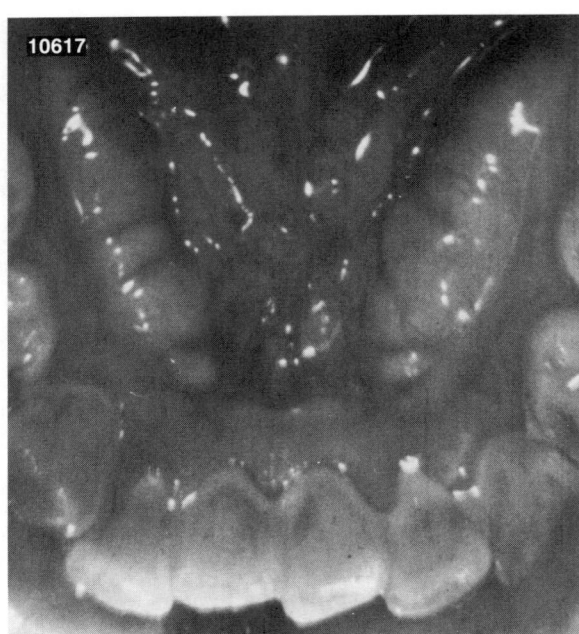

**0958-10617:** Torus mandibularis.

**CDC No.:** 750.280

**Sex Ratio:** M0.7:F1

**Occurrence:** United States whites: 1:13 over 15 years of age; United States Blacks: 1:9; Chileans: 1:2,000; Peruvians: 1:290; American Indians: 1:7; Eskimos: 1:2.5; Aleuts: 1:1.7.

**Risk of Recurrence for Patient's Sib:**
See Part I, *Mendelian Inheritance.* If parent is affected, about 1:3 for sons and 1:2 for daughters. Negligible for all sibs if patient is the result of a fresh mutation.

**Risk of Recurrence for Patient's Child:**
See Part I, *Mendelian Inheritance.* About 1:3 for sons (assuming 70% penetrance in males), and about 1:2 for daughters. These figures exclude children under 15 years of age.

**Age of Detectability:** Usually by 15 years of age.

**Gene Mapping and Linkage:** Unknown.

**Prevention:** None known. Genetic counseling indicated.

**Treatment:** Surgical removal, if interfering with oral functions.

**Prognosis:** Excellent. Does not recur after removal.

**Detection of Carrier:** By clinical examination of first degree relatives.

**References:**
Suzuki M, Sakai T: A familial study of torus palatinus and torus mandibularis. Am J Phys Anthropol 1960; 18:263–272.
Austin JE, et al.: Palatal and mandibular tori in the Negro. NY Dent J 1965; 31:187.
Johnson CC, et al.: Torus mandibularis: a genetic study. Am J Hum Genet 1965; 17:433–439.
Axelsson G, Hedegard B: Torus mandibularis among Icelanders. Am J Phys Anthropol 1981; 54:383–389.

J0011                                          **Clinton C. Johnson**

**Mandibular cleft, median**
*See CLEFTS, LOWER MEDIAN LIP, MANDIBLE AND TONGUE*
**Mandibular enlargement**
*See MANDIBLE, TORUS MANDIBULARIS*

## MANDIBULAR PROGNATHISM                                    0626

**Includes:**
    Hapsburg jaw
    Progenie
    Prognathism, mandibular
    Skeletal malocclusion, class III

**Excludes:**
    Dental malocclusion, class III
    Maxillary retrognathism

**Major Diagnostic Criteria:** Overgrowth of the mandible.

**Clinical Findings:** With overgrowth of the mandible, the lower teeth are carried forward and interdigitate more anteriorly than normal with the upper teeth. This is a Class III relationship and is usually judged on the basis of molar interdigitation. The chin protrudes and the lower lip assumes a pouting configuration in mandibular prognathism. The angle between the ascending portion of the condyle and the body of the mandible is more obtuse than usual.

**Complications:** Dental malocclusion.

**Associated Findings:** None known.

**Etiology:** Multifactorial, autosomal dominant inheritance.

**Pathogenesis:** Besides an inherent discrepancy of mandibular growth, a number of factors contribute to mandibular prognathism. Enlarged tonsils and nasal obstruction may interfere with normal breathing and lead to abnormal posture of the mandible and subsequently to prognathism. Trauma, irregular eruption or loss of teeth, and endocrine disturbances may also lead to mandibular prognathism.

**MIM No.:** *17670

**Sex Ratio:** M1.5:F1

**Occurrence:** 1:25 to 1:50.

**Risk of Recurrence for Patient's Sib:** 10% for sisters, 20% for brothers.

**Risk of Recurrence for Patient's Child:** 20 to 25%.

**Age of Detectability:** Mandibular prognathism is rarely evident at birth, but becomes obvious with eruption of the teeth. Some cases are progressive.

**Gene Mapping and Linkage:** Unknown.

**Prevention:** None known. Genetic counseling indicated.

**Treatment:** Orthodontics may suffice for mild cases, but orthognathic surgery is needed in some.

**Prognosis:** Normal life span.

**Detection of Carrier:** Unknown.

**Special Considerations:** Mandibular prognathism was transmitted through several generations of the European Hapsburg royal family. It has also been observed in at least one Black family. The condition is a feature of the XXY, XXXY, and XXXXY syndromes, progressing as the number of X chromosomes increases. Nevertheless, the trait is not X-linked.

**References:**
Stiles KA, Luke JE: The inheritance of malocclusion due to mandibular prognathism. J Hered 1953; 44:241–245.
Horowitz SL, et al.: Craniofacial relationships in mandibular prognathism. Arch Oral Biol 1969; 14:121–131.
Litton SF, et al.: A genetic study of class III malocclusion. Am J Orthod 1970; 58:565–577. *

J0027                                          **Ronald J. Jorgenson**

**Mandibular-acro-renal syndrome**
*See ACRO-RENAL-MANDIBULAR SYNDROME*
**Mandibulo-facial-oculo syndrome**
*See OCULO-MANDIBULO-FACIAL SYNDROME*
**Mandibulo-melic dwarfism with corneal clouding**
*See OPHTHALMO-MANDIBULO-MELIC DWARFISM*

# MANDIBULOACRAL DYSPLASIA          **2082**

**Includes:**
> Acromandibular dysplasia
> Craniomandibular dermatodysostosis

**Excludes:**
> **Cleidocranial dysplasia** (0185)
> **Hajdu-Cheney syndrome** (2022)
> **Pyknodysostosis** (0846)

**Major Diagnostic Criteria:** The combination of micrognathia, atrophic skin, joint limitation, and hypoplastic terminal phalanges.

**Clinical Findings:** Birth weight and length are normal. Facial changes often do not appear until after infancy. Clinical findings in 11 reported cases include micrognathia (11/11); short, broad terminal phalanges (11/11); atrophic skin (10/11); protruding eyes (7/11); decreased amount of subcutaneous fat on extremities (6/11); increased facial fat (6/11); brown skin mottling (6/11); beaked nose (6/11); dysplastic, brittle nails (5/11); short stature (5/11); hardening of subcutaneous tissue (5/11); and scanty hair (4/11).

X-ray findings have included hypoplastic distal phalanges, thought to be acroosteolysis (11/11); widening of cranial sutures (10/11); absent or hypoplastic clavicles (10/11); wormian bone in sutures (9/11); coxa valga (7/11); hypoplastic ramus of the mandible (5/11); and narrow chest (5/11).

**Complications:** Complications have included joint limitation secondary to skin defect; and dental crowding and respiratory obstruction secondary to the micrognathia.

**Associated Findings:** Findings present in only one or two affected individuals have included increased subcutaneous fat on the trunk (2/11); cortical sclerosis of the long bones on X-ray (2/11); delayed onset of puberty (2/11); highly arched palate (1/11); relative macrocephaly (1/11); scoliosis (1/11); and deformed medial condyles on X-ray (1/11).

**Etiology:** Autosomal recessive inheritance.

**Pathogenesis:** The tissues involved are mainly of mesodermal origin, although the basic defect is unknown.

**MIM No.:** *24837

**POS No.:** 3161

**Sex Ratio:** Presumably M1:F1 (M8:F3 observed).

**Occurrence:** At least nine reported families; five of which are Italian (possibly due to a founder effect).

**Risk of Recurrence for Patient's Sib:**
> See Part I, *Mendelian Inheritance.*

**Risk of Recurrence for Patient's Child:**
> See Part I, *Mendelian Inheritance.*

**Age of Detectability:** The somatic changes usually occur by the age of 6–7 years, although one child was diagnosed at 18 months of age.

**Gene Mapping and Linkage:** Unknown.

**Prevention:** None known. Genetic counseling indicated.

**Treatment:** Orthopedic management may be indicated.

**Prognosis:** Life span and intellect are apparently not impaired. The oldest reported patient was 37 years of age, and was healthy at the time of the report. It is unknown whether males are fertile; one affected female has reproduced, and, of ten pregnancies, five resulted in spontaneous abortions.

**Detection of Carrier:** Unknown.

**References:**
Young LW, et al: New syndrome manifested by mandibular hypoplasia, acro-osteolysis, stiff joints, and cutaneous atrophy (mandibulacral dysplasia) in two unrelated boys. BD:OAS VII(7). New York: March of Dimes Birth Defects Foundation, 1971:291–297.

Danks DM, et al: Craniomandibular dermatodysostosis. BD:OAS X(12). New York: March of Dimes Birth Defects Foundation, 1974: 99–105.

Welsh O: Study of a family with a new progeroid syndrome. BD:OAS XI(5). New York: March of Dimes Birth Defects Foundation, 1975: 25–38.

Palotta R, Morgese G: Mandibuloacral dysplasia: a rare progeroid syndrome. Clin Genet 1984; 26:133–138. *

Tenconi R et al. Another Italian family with mandibuloacral dysplasia: why does it seem more frequent in Italy? Am J Med Genet 1986; 24:357–364. * †

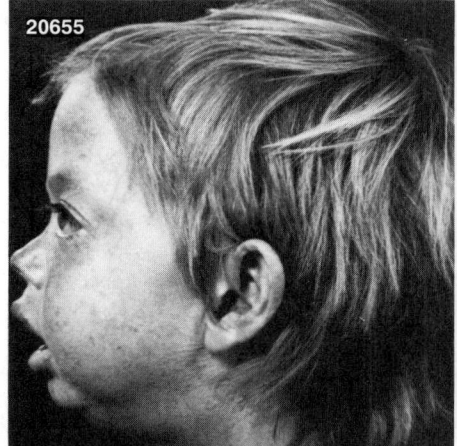
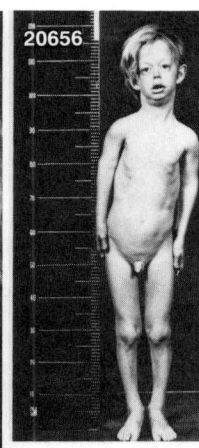
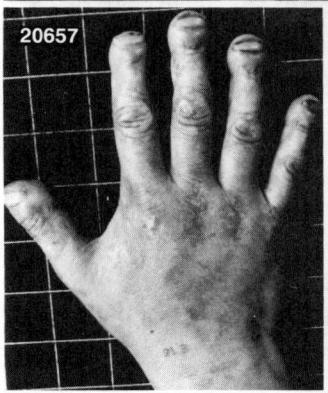
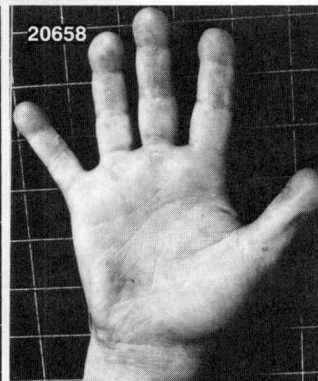
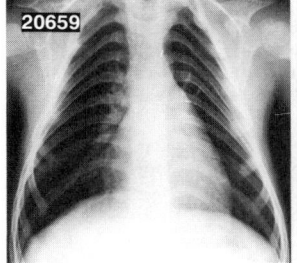
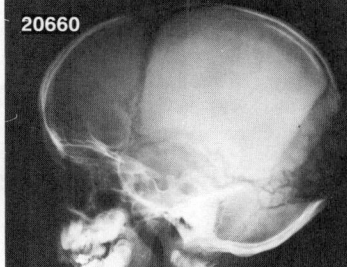

**2082-20655–56:** Mandibuloacral dysplasia in subject aged 8 years; note micrognathia, prominent eyes and increased buccal fat with short stature, proximal arm shortening, chest wall deformity, scarring and atrophy of the skin, abnormal pigmentation. **20657–58:** Note short distal phalanges and scarring with abnormal pigmentation. The larger scars on the hands are at sites of spontaneous subcutaneous calcification followed by extrusion of the calcified lump. **20659:** Chest X-ray shows rib-cage abnormality and absent clavicles. **20660:** Skull X-ray shows greatly delayed closure of the sutures and multiple wormian bones.

**Helga V. Toriello**

## MANDIBULOFACIAL DYSOSTOSIS                                    0627

**Includes:**
> Dysostosis mandibulofacial
> Franceschetti-Klein syndrome
> Treacher Collins syndrome
> Treacher Collins-Franceschetti syndrome

**Excludes:**
> Achard syndrome
> **Acrofacial dysostosis, Nager type** (2167)
> **Cervico-oculo-acoustic syndrome** (0142)
> **Mandibulofacial dysostosis, Treacher Collins type, recessive** (2802)
> **Oculo-auriculo-vertebral anomaly** (0735)

**Major Diagnostic Criteria:** Findings include microtia, hearing loss, midface hypoplasia, downward slant of palpebral fissures, colobomata of lower lids, and micrognathia.

**Clinical Findings:** Downward slant of palpebral fissures (89%); malar hypoplasia (81%); micrognathia (78%); lower lid coloboma (69%); partial or total absence of lower eyelashes medial to the coloboma (53%); microtia (77%); external ear canal defect (36%); conductive hearing loss (40%); cleft palate (35%); projection of scalp hair onto lateral cheek (26%).

An affected person may be misdiagnosed as being mentally retarded because of an associated severe hearing loss. Respiratory and/or feeding problems may be present in the neonatal period because of severe micrognathia. In such cases obstructive sleep apnea may be a persistent problem in the older infant and young child.

**Complications:** Unknown.

**Associated Findings:** Microphthalmia (very rare), macrostomia, choanal atresia, blind fistulas, and skin tags between the auricle and the angle of mouth.

**Etiology:** Autosomal dominant inheritance with high penetrance and variable expressivity. About half of the cases represent fresh mutations, some of which have been found to be associated with advanced paternal age. An excess of affected offspring from affected females and of normal offspring from affected males has been reported. For a recessive form of this condition, see **Mandibulofacial dysostosis, Treacher Collins type, recessive**.

**Pathogenesis:** Balestrazzi et al (1983) reported a girl with a de novo balanced translocation and decreased level of hexosaminidase. The malformations produced in mice by isotretinoin have

been suggested as a model by Sulik et al (1987). Lungarotti et al (1987) speculated on a maternal hyposensitivity to vitamin A.

**MIM No.:**  *15450

**POS No.:**  3283

**CDC No.:**  756.045

**Sex Ratio:**  M1:F1

**Occurrence:**  Undetermined. Several large multi-generation kindreds have been documentaed.

**Risk of Recurrence for Patient's Sib:**
See Part I, *Mendelian Inheritance.*

**Risk of Recurrence for Patient's Child:**
See Part I, *Mendelian Inheritance.*

**Age of Detectability:**  At birth, by physical examination. Prenatal diagnosis has been accomplished by ultrasound.

**Gene Mapping and Linkage:**  Unknown.

**Prevention:**  None known. Genetic counseling indicated.

**Treatment:**  Orthodontic and surgical correction of the facial deformities. Hearing aids at an early age if hearing loss is present.

**Prognosis:**  Good when hearing loss is diagnosed and treated early. In rare cases where severe micrognathia leads to respiratory problems or sleep apnea, serious consideration to tracheotomy should be given.

**Detection of Carrier:**  Unknown.

**Special Considerations:**  One name for this condition is drawn from the author of the original paper; Dr. E. Treacher Collins who first described cases in the Transactions of the Ophthalmology Society of the United Kingdom in 1933. The frequent practice of hyphenating the name is, therefore, incorrect.

**Support Group:**  NH; Concord; (P.O. Box 5) Treacher Collins Foundation

**References:**
Franceschetti A, Klein D: Mandibulo-facial dysostosis: new hereditary syndrome. Acta Ophthalmol 1949; 27:141–224.
Roven S, et al.: Mandibulofacial dysostosis: a family study of five generation. J Pediat 1964; 65:215–221.
Frazen L, et al.: Mandibulo-facial dysostosis (Treacher-Collins syndrome). Am J Dis Child 1967; 113:405–410.
Herring SW, et al.: Anatomical abnormalities in mandibulofacial dysostosis. Am J Med Genet 1979; 3:225–259.
Balestrazzi P, et al.: Franceschetti syndrome in a child with a de novo balanced translocation (5;13)(q11;p11) and significant decrease of hexosaminidase B. Hum Genet 1983; 64:305–308.
Crane JP, Beaver HA: Midtrimester sonographic diagnosis of mandibulofacial dysostosis. Am J Med Genet 1986; 25:251–255.
Lungarotti MS, et al.: Multiple congenital anomalies associated with apparently normal maternal intake of vitamin A. Am J Med Genet 1987; 27:245–248.
Sulik KK, et al.: Mandibulofacial dysostosis (Treacher Collins syndrome): a new proposal for its pathogenesis. Am J Med Genet 1987; 27:359–372.
Kay ED, Kay CN: Dysmorphogenesis of the mandible, zygoma, and middle ear ossicles in hemifacial microsomia and mandibulofacial dysostosis. Am J Med Genet 1989; 32:27–31.

J0027                                    **Ronald J. Jorgenson**
                                         *Hermine M. Pashayan*

**Mandibulofacial dysostosis, recessive type**
*See MANDIBULOFACIAL DYSOSTOSIS, TREACHER COLLINS TYPE, RECESSIVE*

**0627**-12204–05: Microtia, downward slanting palpebral fissures, and maxillary hypoplasia.

## MANDIBULOFACIAL DYSOSTOSIS, TREACHER COLLINS TYPE, RECESSIVE 2802

**Includes:**

Mandibulofacial dysostosis, recessive type
Treacher Collins mandibulofacial dysostosis, recessive type

**Excludes:** Mandibulofacial dysostosis (0627)

**Major Diagnostic Criteria:** The combination of down-slanting palpebral fissures, lower lid coloboma, absent eyelashes, malar hypoplasia, malformed ears, deafness, and absence of a positive family history.

**Clinical Findings:** The clinical findings are the same as in **Mandibulofacial dysostosis**, autosomal dominant type, and consist of down-slanting palpebral fissures, lower lid colobomas, absent eyelashes, malar and mandibular hypoplasia, malformed ears, auditory canal narrowing or stenosis, conductive deafness, cleft hard palate, cleft soft palate and projection of scalp hair onto the lateral cheek.

**Complications:** Delayed speech development secondary to conductive hearing loss.

**Associated Findings:** None known.

**Etiology:** Presumably autosomal recessive inheritance.

**Pathogenesis:** The basic defect is thought to be an abnormality of the first and second branchial arch placodes.

It has been suggested by Reynolds et al (1986) that mandibulofacial dysostosis is a developmental field defect and can therefore have several causes. If this is so, then it would not be unusual to find both an autosomal recessive and autosomal dominant form of the same condition. However, germinal mosaicism could also explain the occurrence of affected sibs to normal parents.

**MIM No.:** 24839

**POS No.:** 3283

**2802-21040:** Proband has downward slanting palpebral fissures, lower lid coloboma, malar hypoplasia, and abnormal pinnae.

**CDC No.:** 756.045

**Sex Ratio:** M1:F1

**Occurrence:** Reported in sibs in a Hutterite population. There are eight other reports of affected sibs born to apparently unaffected parents from different parts of the world.

**Risk of Recurrence for Patient's Sib:**
See Part I, *Mendelian Inheritance.*

**Risk of Recurrence for Patient's Child:**
See Part I, *Mendelian Inheritance.*

**Age of Detectability:** At birth by physical examination.

**Gene Mapping and Linkage:** Unknown.

**Prevention:** None known. Genetic counseling indicated.

**Treatment:** Hearing loss can be treated with hearing aids.

**Prognosis:** Intellectual development, growth, and life span are normal.

**Detection of Carrier:** Unknown.

**Special Considerations:** Gonadal mosaicism for autosomal dominant mandibulofacial dysostosis (Treacher Collins) could also account for the findings described above.

**References:**

Lowry RB, et al.: Mandibulofacial dysostosis in Hutterite sibs: a possible recessive trait. Am J Med Genet 1985; 22:501–512.
Reynolds JF, et al.: A new autosomal dominant acrofacial dysostosis syndrome. Am J Med Genet 1986; Suppl 2:143–150.

T0007 **Helga V. Toriello**

**Mandibulofacial dysostosis, Treacher Collins type-limb anomalies**
*See ACROFACIAL DYSOSTOSIS, NAGER TYPE*
**Manic-depressive (bipolar) disorders**
*See MOOD AND THOUGHT DISORDERS*
**Mannen-Balcom syndrome**
*See SARCOIDOSIS*

## MANNOSIDOSIS 2079

**Includes:**

Alpha-mannosidosis
Lysosomal alpha-mannosidase A and B deficiencies
Lysosomal alpha-D-mannosidase deficiency
Mannosidosis, type I
Mannosidosis, type II

**Excludes:** N/A

**Major Diagnostic Criteria:** Psychomotor retardation, coarse facies resembling that of the Hurler syndrome, dysostosis multiplex, hepatosplenomegaly, hearing loss, and recurrent infections. Confirmation of the diagnosis is made by demonstration of deficiency of alpha-mannosidase A and B activities in plasma, leukocytes, or cultured skin fibroblasts assayed at the appropriate acidic pH.

**Clinical Findings:** The more severe infantile phenotype is referred to as type I, characterized by severe disease with hepatosplenomegaly, severe recurrent infections, and early death, usually between three and 10 years of age. Type II patients have a milder, or juvenile-adult, phenotype, which is characterized by hearing loss, mental retardation, milder dysostosis multiplex, and survival into adulthood.

Clinical findings that can be seen in either phenotype include psychomotor retardation, a coarse facies, hernias, lenticular or corneal opacities, and hepatosplenomegaly. Hearing loss is particularly prominent in type II patients. The skeletal dysplasia includes thickening of the calvaria, abnormalities of the vertebral bodies, gibbus deformity, and bony abnormalities of the metacarpals. The vertebral bodies are prominently involved and can be ovoid, flat, hypoplastic, or recessed with anteroinferior beaking. The skeletal abnormalities are more severe in type I patients.

Laboratory findings include vacuolated lymphocytes in the peripheral blood, storage cells ("foamy macrophages") in the bone marrow, and the accumulation of mannose-rich oligosaccharides in the urine and in neural and visceral tissues. Decreased serum IgG and a shortened PR interval on EKG have been reported.

**Complications:** The recurrent infections seen in affected patients are felt to be due to abnormalities of neutrophil function. Studies in one type I patient revealed depressed chemotactic responsiveness, delayed phagocytosis of bacteria, and decreased response of lymphocytes to phytohemagglutinin. Hearing loss may lead to speech and language delay.

**Associated Findings:** **Megalencephaly**, muscular hypotonia, and tall stature.

**Etiology:** Autosomal recessive inheritance of a deficiency of acidic alpha-mannosidase A and B.

**Pathogenesis:** Deficiency of lysosomal acidic alpha-mannosidase A and B activities results in the lysosomal accumulation of mannose-rich oligosaccharides in neural and visceral tissues. This lysosomal storage results in the clinical abnormalities seen.

**MIM No.:** *24850

**Sex Ratio:** M1:F1

**Occurrence:** Over 75 cases have been reported in the literature.

**Risk of Recurrence for Patient's Sib:**
See Part I, *Mendelian Inheritance.*

**Risk of Recurrence for Patient's Child:**
See Part I, *Mendelian Inheritance.*

**Age of Detectability:** Can be detected clinically in the first year of life, or prenatally. Confirmation of diagnosis can be made by enzyme assay in plasma, leukocytes, or cultured fibroblasts.

**Gene Mapping and Linkage:** MANB (mannosidase, alpha B, lysosomal) has been mapped to 19cen-q13.1.

**Prevention:** None known. Genetic counseling indicated.

**Treatment:** No means presently available for correction of the enzymatic defect or for stimulation of residual enzyme activity.

**Prognosis:** Patients with type I disease usually die in childhood, often between three and 10 years of age. Patients with type II disease survive into adulthood.

**Detection of Carrier:** The enzymatic identification of heterozygotes has been difficult. The ratio of alpha-mannosidase to total beta-hexosaminidase activities at pH 4.4 has been used in heterozygote detection, but does not always discriminate heterozygotes. Multiple determinations of acidic alpha-mannosidase activity in several different sources may be required.

**References:**
Öckerman PA: A generalized storage disorder resembling Hurler's syndrome. Lancet 1967; II:239–241.
Masson PK, et al.: Mannosidosis: detection of the disease and of heterozygotes using serum and leukocytes. Biochem Biophys Res Commun 1974; 56:296–303.
Desnick RJ, et al.: Mannosidosis: clinical, morphologic, immunologic, and biochemical studies. Pediatr Res 1976; 10:985–996.
Poenaru L, et al.: Antenatal diagnosis in three pregnancies at risk for mannosidosis. Clin Genet 1979; 16:428–432.
Spranger J, et al.: The radiographic features of mannosidosis. Radiology 1976; 119:401–407.
Montgomery TR, et al.: Mannosidosis in an adult. Johns Hopkins Med J 1982; 151:113–117.
Press OW, et al.: Pancytopenia in mannosidosis. Arch Int Med 1983; 143:1266–1268.
Warner TG, et al.: Alpha-mannosidosis: analysis of urinary oligosaccharides with high performance liquid chromatography and diagnosis of a case with unusually mild presentation. Clin Genet 1984; 25:248–255.

IR000                                                      **Mira Irons**

**Mannosidosis, type I**
*See MANNOSIDOSIS*
**Mannosidosis, type II**
*See MANNOSIDOSIS*
**Map-dot-fingerprint corneal dystrophy**
*See CORNEAL DYSTROPHY, RECURRENT EROSIVE*

## MAPLE SYRUP URINE DISEASE                                 0628

**Includes:**
>     Branched-chain alpha-keto acid dehydrogenase deficiency
>     Branched-chain ketoaciduria
>     Branched-chain ketonuria
>     Intermittent branched-chain ketonuria
>     Keto acid decarboxylase deficiency
>     Thiamine-responsive MSUD

**Excludes:** Hypervalinemia (0509)

**Major Diagnostic Criteria:** Elevation of the branched-chain amino acids (BCAA), leucine, isoleucine, and valine, and/or the respective keto acids (BCKA) in blood and in urine is almost diagnostic. The presence of alloisoleucine, not normally detectable in blood, is an important diagnostic aid. The diagnosis is confirmed by demonstrating a reduction in BCKA decarboxylase activity in leukocytes or cultured skin fibroblasts. Screening programs of newborn infants to detect serum elevations of BCAA exist in many states and in Europe.

In the mildest variants, the plasma BCAA may be normal during asymptomatic periods. The enzymatic deficiency is always demonstrable.

**Clinical Findings:** The "classical" or most severe type of MSUD causes symptoms with onset during the first week of life. These are poor feeding, vomiting, shrill cry, lethargy, convulsions, coma, and possibly death. The only specific sign is that of a maple syrup-like odor in urine and other secretions. The untreated child that survives is neurologically damaged.

Many variants have been described and classified according to symptomatology (classic, intermediate, intermittent). A more useful approach to clinical classification derives from the tolerance to dietary BCAA. In the classic form, the ability to degrade the BCAA is extremely limited, so dietary intake may not far exceed the maintenance and growth requirements without symptoms. As a result, a purified amino acids diet is required. With greater dietary tolerance, symptoms may be delayed and more subtle. Limitation of protein intake without amino acid supplements may be adequate. In the mildest variants, patients may tolerate a normal diet without elevations in the BCAA or BCKA. They are at risk of "decompensating" either unpredictably or with acute infections or surgery, at which time plasma BCAA and BCKA increase, neurological symptoms appear, and death may occur.

A thiamine-responsive type of MSUD has been reported. Thiamine is a cofactor in the first step of the oxidative-decarboxylase series of reactions.

**Complications:** Unknown.

**Associated Findings:** Acidosis, hypoglycemia.

**Etiology:** Autosomal recessive inheritance involving a mutation of the decarboxylase of the three BCKA.

**Pathogenesis:** The first two steps in the degradation of the BCAA, leucine, isoleucine, and valine are transamination to the respective keto acids followed by oxidative-decarboxylation to isovaleric acid, 2-methylbutyric acid and isobutyric acid. Two inborn errors of metabolism, hypervalinemia and hyperleucine-isoleucinemia, suggest that there are two specific transaminases. The evidence is that one decarboxylase is effective against the three BCKA. The many clinical variants, which reproduce within families, indicate a variety of enzymatic mutations.

The acute and chronic consequences of MSUD can be avoided by controlling the intake of BCAA, making it clear that the cause of the symptoms is the elevation of the BCAA and their metabolites. Clinical and experimental studies suggest that ketoisocaproic acid (keto-leucine) is the most "toxic" of the metabolites. The compound causing the maple syrup odor has not been identified but appears to be related to isoleucine.

**MIM No.:** *24860

**POS No.:** 3784

**CDC No.:** 270.300

**Sex Ratio:** M1:F1

**Occurrence:** Reported variously as 1:125,000 to 1:300,000 live births. Described in many ethnic groups and in many geographic locations.

**Risk of Recurrence for Patient's Sib:**
See Part I, *Mendelian Inheritance.*

**Risk of Recurrence for Patient's Child:**
See Part I, *Mendelian Inheritance.*

**Age of Detectability:** The enzyme defect is demonstrable at any age, including antepartum. Increased concentrations of BCAA and BCKA become evident in severe cases within the first few days of life.

**Gene Mapping and Linkage:** Unknown.

**Prevention:** None known. Genetic counseling indicated.

**Treatment:** Dietary therapy with control of BCAA intake to meet nutritional requirements and not exceed tolerance. In the severe form of the disease, diagnosis must be made very early in life, and dietary treatment must be started promptly if neurological sequelae are to be avoided. Early diagnosis has been facilitated by screening programs. In the acutely decompensated case, intravenous fluids, reduction of protein intake, and peritoneal dialysis may be life-saving. Dietary care must be maintained for life. Thiamine has been reported to lower BCAA levels in some of the mildly affected cases but has not succeeded in replacing dietary control.

**Prognosis:** Very poor if untreated. Death occurs almost invariably before the end of the second year. With careful dietary control, normal growth and development are possible.

**Detection of Carrier:** Unknown. There is a great deal of genetic heterogeneity.

**Special Considerations:** Dihydrolipoyl dehydrogenase deficiency (E3) may also be associated with elevated levels of BCAA and BCKA. This is accompanied by a massive lactic aciduria and some elevation of ketoglutarate excretion.

**Support Groups:** IN; Goshen; Maple Syrup Urine Disease Support Group (Joyce Brubacher 24806 SR 119, Zip 46526)

**References:**
Dancis J, et al.: Enzyme activity in classical and variant forms of maple syrup urine disease. J Pediatr 1972; 81:312–320.
Wendel IJ, Cloussen U: Antenatal diagnosis of maple-syrup-urine disease. Lancet 1979; 1:161–162.
Chuang DT, et al.: Activities of branched-chain 2-oxo acid dehydrogenase and its components in skin fibroblasts from normal and classical maple syrup urine disease subjects. Biochem J 1981; 200: 59–67.
Chuang DT, et al.: Biochemical basis of thiamin-responsive maple syrup urine disease. Trans Asso Am Phys 1982; 95:196–204.
Duran M, Wadman SK: Thiamine-responsive inborn errors of metabolism. J Inherit Metab Dis 1985; 8(suppl. 1):70–75.
Snyderman SE: Maple syrup urine disease. In: Wapnir RA, ed: Congenital metabolic diseases. New York: Marcel Dekker, 1985:153–168.
Snyderman SE: Newborn screening for maple syrup urine disease. J Pediatr 1985; 107:259–261.

SN005                    **Selma Snyderman**
DA003                    **Joseph Dancis**

**Marble bone disease**
*See OSTEOPETROSIS, BENIGN DOMINANT*
*also OSTEOPETROSIS, MALIGNANT RECESSIVE*
**Marble brain disease**
*See OSTEOPETROSIS, MALIGNANT RECESSIVE*
*also RENAL TUBULAR ACIDOSIS-OSTEOPETROSIS SYNDROME*
**Marble skin**
*See CUTIS MARMORATA*
**Marbling effect of newborn skin**
*See CUTIS MARMORATA*
**Marburg (Al) apolipoprolipoprotein variants**
*See HYPOALPHALIPOPROTEINEMIA*
**Marcus Gunn phenomenon**
*See JAW-WINKING SYNDROME*

## MARDEN-WALKER SYNDROME          0629

**Includes:** Connective tissue disorder, Marden-Walker type

**Excludes:** Chondrodystrophic myotonia, Schwartz-Jampel type (0155)

**Major Diagnostic Criteria:** Distinctive facies consisting of blepharophimosis, flat nasal bridge, micrognathia, fixed facial expression, cleft or high-arched palate, low-set ears, joint contractures, reduced muscle mass, psychomotor and growth retardation.

**Clinical Findings:** Micrognathia, ptosis, hypertelorism, and muscle hypotonia are common. Microcephaly is often present, but the head circumference was increased in a few newborn and in one 5 year old. There may be heart, genitourinary, or bony abnormalities. Deep tendon reflexes may be decreased or absent.

Electromyography is usually abnormal. There may be myopathic changes in the form of many small-amplitude, short-duration motor unit potentials. Muscle biopsy specimens usually show that some fibers (types I and II) are reduced in size. Electron microscopy of muscle material from one patient showed replacement of myofibrils by glycogen particles and massive subsarcolemmal accumulation of glycogen. There was also subsarcolemmal accumulation of vesicular profiles and invasion by macrophages.

Pneumocephalogram in one case showed enlarged cisterna magna, medullary cistern, fourth ventricle, and suprapineal recess. Ventriculography in another infant showed moderate dilation of the lateral ventricles and basal cisterns and widening of the cerebral sulci.

**Complications:** Kyphosis, scoliosis, pectus excavatum or carinatum, and osteoporosis may be due to joint and muscle abnormalities.

**Associated Findings:** Preauricular tag, small mouth, short neck, low hairline, abnormal eyelashes, microphthalmos, Zollinger-Ellison syndrome, pyloric stenosis, duodenal bands, and pancreatic insufficiency have been reported.

**Etiology:** Autosomal recessive inheritance.

**Pathogenesis:** The abnormal muscles may be secondary to CNS abnormalities.

**MIM No.:** *24870

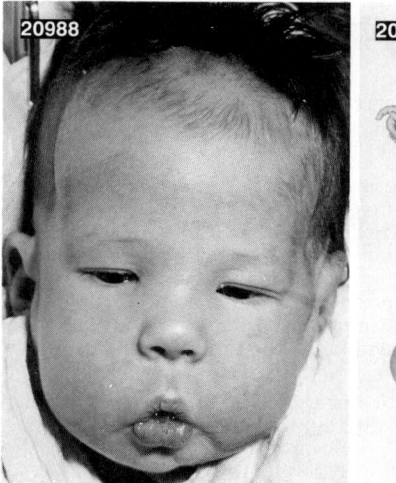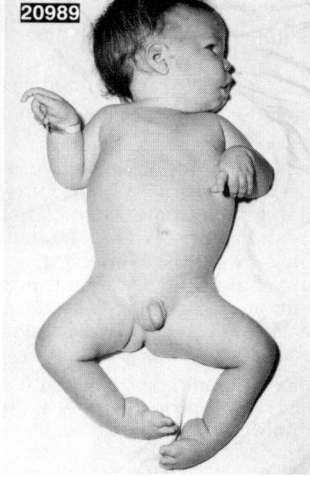

**0629-20988:** Marden-Walker syndrome; facies at birth includes blepharophimosis, small, pursed mouth with everted lower lip and sagging cheeks. **20989:** Congenital contractures and preauricular tags.

**POS No.:** 3284

**Sex Ratio:** M11:F3 (observed).

**Occurrence:** About twenty cases reported in the literature.

**Risk of Recurrence for Patient's Sib:**
See Part I, *Mendelian Inheritance*.

**Risk of Recurrence for Patient's Child:**
See Part I, *Mendelian Inheritance*.

**Age of Detectability:** Newborn period.

**Gene Mapping and Linkage:** Unknown.

**Prevention:** None known. Genetic counseling indicated.

**Treatment:** Supportive.

**Prognosis:** Severe psychomotor and growth retardation, with one exception reported as having normal intelligence.

**Detection of Carrier:** Unknown.

**Special Considerations:** Two reports of microphthalmos suggest that it is important to study the eyes, because microphthalmos may be the cause of blepharophimosis and also may indicate early disturbance in brain development.

**References:**
Younessian S, Amman F: Deux cas de malformations cranio-faciales: microphthalmie ("nanisme oculo-palpebral") avec dysostose craniofaciale et status dysraphique; 2. Dysmorphie mandibulo-oculofaciale (syndrome d'Hallermann-Streiff). Ophthalmologica 1964; 147:108–117.
Marden PM, Walker WA: A new generalized connective tissue syndrome. Am J Dis Child 1966; 112:225–228. *
Fitch N, et al.: Congenital blepharophimosis, joint contractures, and muscular hypotonia. Neurology 1971; 21:1214–1220.
King CR, Magenis E: The Marden-Walker syndrome. J Med Genet 1978; 15:366–369.
Abe K, et al.: Zollinger-Ellison syndrome with Marden-Walker syndrome. Am J Dis Child 1979; 133:735–738.
Ferguson SD, et al.: Congenital myopathy with oculo-facial and skeletal abnormalities. Dev Med Child Neurol 1981; 23:237–242.
Howard FM, Rowlandson P: Two brothers with the Marden-Walker syndrome: case report and review. J Med Genet 1981; 18:50–53.
Jaatoul NY, et al.: The Marden-Walker syndrome. Am J Med Genet 1982; 11:259–271. †
Gossage D, et al.: A 26-month-old child with Marden-Walker syndrome and pyloric stenosis. Am J Med Genet 1987; 26:915–919.

FI020
MA030

**Naomi Fitch**
**Philip Marden**

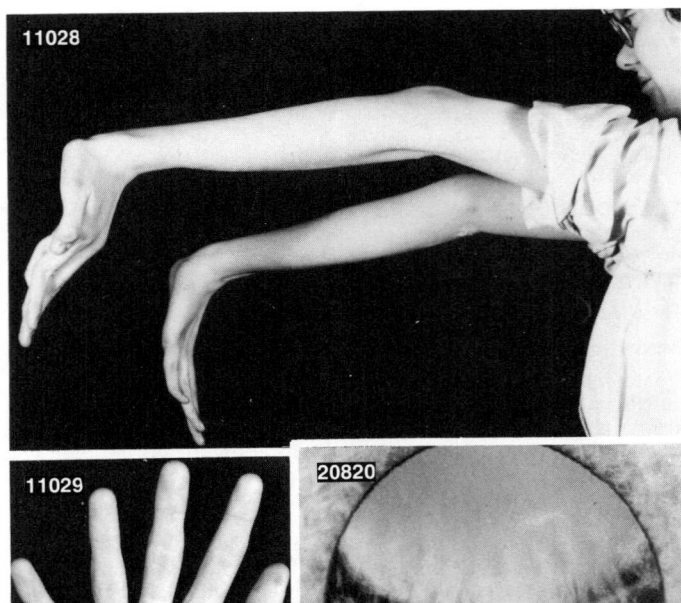

0630-11028: Joint hyperextensibility and long arms. 11029: Arachnodactyly. 20820: Upward dislocation of the lens.

---

## MARFAN SYNDROME                                    0630

**Includes:**
Marfanoid hypermobility syndrome
Contractural arachnodactyly (some cases)

**Excludes:** Homocystinuria (0474)

**Major Diagnostic Criteria:** Arachnodactyly, dolichostenomelia, scoliosis, anterior chest deformity, ectopia lentis, dilatation of the ascending aorta. When a first-degree relative has documented Marfan syndrome, characteristic features must be present in two organ systems; when the family history is negative, three systems must be affected. More diagnostic weight is given to features uncommon in the general population (ectopia lentis, aortic dilation, aortic dissection, and dural ectasia) than to common abnormalities (e.g., tall stature, myopia, and mitral valve prolapse). No laboratory test is available for definitive diagnosis.

**Clinical Findings:** Skeletal features include tall stature, arachnodactyly, dolichostenomelia, highly arched palate, vertebral column deformity (scoliosis, thoracic lordosis), and deformity of the anterior chest. Joints may be hypermobile or congenitally contracted. The ocular features are ectopia lentis in 50–60%, myopia, flattening of the cornea and retinal detachment, the latter most likely when the lens has been removed. Spontaneous pneumothorax occurs in about 5%. The cardiovascular features are progressive dilation of the ascending aorta and mitral valve prolapse.

Other features include ectasia of the dura, especially in the lumbosacral region, striae atrophicae, inguinal hernias, reduced subcutaneous tissue and muscle hypoplasia, and neuropsychologic problems, especially attention deficit disorder and verbal performance discrepancy on cognitive function tests.

**Complications:** Joint instability, severe thoracic deformity and restrictive lung disease, loss of vision, aortic regurgitation, mitral regurgitation, aortic dissection, sudden death, bacterial endocarditis, learning disability. Without treatment, life span reduced by 30–50% on average.

**Associated Findings:** None known.

**Etiology:** Autosomal dominant inheritance with complete penetrance but highly variable expression; undoubtedly genetically heterogeneous.

**Pathogenesis:** A recently discovered glycoprotein, fibrillin, which is a major component of microfibrils, may be the common pathogenetic link among the pleiotropic manifestations.

**MIM No.:** *15470, 15474, 15475

**POS No.:** 3285

**CDC No.:** 759.860

**Sex Ratio:** M1:F1

**Occurrence:** Prevalence at least 1:10,000 in most populations.

**Risk of Recurrence for Patient's Sib:**
See Part I, *Mendelian Inheritance*.

**Risk of Recurrence for Patient's Child:**
See Part I, *Mendelian Inheritance*.

**Age of Detectability:** Usually apparent clinically in infancy if suspected, but often not detected until second or third decade.

**Gene Mapping and Linkage:** MFS (Marfan syndrome) is unassigned.

Studies using blood group markers, serum protein polymorphisms, and candidate gene probes for procollagens (alpha1(I), alpha2(I), alpha1(II), and alpha1(III)) and elastin have excluded close linkage.

**Prevention:** None known. Genetic counseling indicated.

**Treatment:** Chronic treatment with a beta-adrenergic blocking drug (atenolol or propranolol) retards the rate of aortic dilation and the occurrence of dissection; treatment should be started before the aorta is widely dilated. Replacement of the aortic root with a valved conduit should be strongly considered whenever the ascending aortic diameter reaches 60 mm regardless of symptoms. Early detection and bracing of scoliosis may prevent severe deformity. In females, early induction of puberty with hormones can avert excessive height and possibly retard scoliosis. Correction of anterior chest deformity should be delayed until near skeletal maturity unless cardiopulmonary compromise is present. Early ophthalmologic evaluation is essential to correct visual acuity and to prevent amblyopia. Removal of the lens should be avoided. Spontaneous pneumothorax tends to recur unless the apical bleb is resected. Antibiotic prophylaxis for endocarditis should be recommended. Physical activity should be restricted: no body contact sports, exertion at maximal capacity, isometric exercise, or heavy weight lifting.

**Prognosis:** Markedly variable; infants have died from severe aortic or mitral regurgitation, whereas some patients have survived into the eighth decade. The average age of death in a retrospective series of patients who died before 1970 was the fourth decade for males and the fifth decade for females; when a cause of death could be ascribed, aortic complications accounted for over 90%.

**Detection of Carrier:** N/A

**Support Groups:** NY; Port Washington; National Marfan Foundation

**References:**
Pyeritz RE, McKusick VA: The Marfan syndrome: diagnosis and management. New Engl J Med 1979; 300:772–777.
Pyeritz RE, Wappel MA: Mitral valve dysfunction in the Marfan syndrome. Am J Med 1983; 74:797–807.
Sisk HE, et al.: The Marfan syndrome in early childhood: analysis of 15 patients diagnosed at less than 4 years of age. Am J Cardiol 1983; 52:353–358.
Gott VL, et al.: Surgical treatment of aneurysm of the ascending aorta in the Marfan syndrome: result of composite repair in 50 patients. New Engl J Med 1986; 314:1070–1074.
Beighton P, et al.: International nosology of heritable disorders of connective tissue, Berlin, 1986. Am J Med Genet 1988; 29:581–594.
Hofman KJ, et al.: Marfan syndrome: neuropsychologic aspects. Am J Med Genet 1988; 31:331–338.
Pyeritz RE, et al.: Dural ectasia is a common feature of the Marfan syndrome. Am J Hum Genet 1988; 43:726–732.
Hollister DW, et al.: Marfan syndrome: abnormalities of the microfibrillar fiber array detected by immunohistopatholgic studies. (Abstract) Am J Med Genet 1989; 32:244 only.
Pyeritz RE: Effectiveness of beta-adrenergic blockade in the Marfan syndrome: experience over 10 years. (Abstract) Am J Med Genet 1989; 32:245 only.
Pyeritz RE, ed: Conference report: first international symposium on the Marfan syndrome. Am J Med Genet 1989; 32:233–238.

PY000                                    **Reed E. Pyeritz**

**Marfanoid habitus and X-linked mental retardation**
  See X-LINKED MENTAL RETARDATION, MARFANOID HABITUS TYPE
**Marfanoid hypermobility syndrome**
  See MARFAN SYNDROME
**Marfanoid mental retardation syndrome**
  See FACIO-NEURO-SKELETAL SYNDROME
**Marie Unna type hypotrichosis**
  See HAIR, HYPOTRICHOSIS
**Marie-Sainton disease**
  See CLEIDOCRANIAL DYSPLASIA
**Marie-Strumpell spondylitis**
  See ANKYLOSING SPONDYLITIS
**Marinesco-Garland syndrome**
  See MARINESCO-SJOGREN SYNDROME

## MARINESCO-SJOGREN SYNDROME                2031

**Includes:**
  Ataxia, hereditary cerebellar-childhood cataracts
  Cerebello-lental degeneration with mental retardation
  Oligophrenic cerebello-lental degeneration
  Marinesco-Garland syndrome
  Marinesco-Sjogren-Garland syndrome
  Marinesco-Sjogren syndrome-hypergonadotropic hypogonadism
  Marinesco-Sjogren syndrome-myopathy
  Marinesco-Sjogren syndrome-neuropathy
  Moravcsik-Marinesco-Sjogren syndrome
  Myopathy-Marinesco-Sjogren syndrome

**Excludes:**
  **Ataxia, Friedreich type** (2714)
  **Oculo-cerebro-renal syndrome** (0736)
  **Sjogren syndrome** (2101)

**Major Diagnostic Criteria:** Cerebellar ataxia, hypotonia, mental subnormality, cataracts in infancy or childhood, myopathy, hypergonadotropic hypogonadism, and skeletal defects.

**Clinical Findings:** The most common reported features are cataracts in infancy or childhood, cerebellar ataxia, and mental retardation. Dysarthria, nystagmus, and squint are also common. The most prominent clinical features are cerebellar ataxia (100%), cataracts (100%), nystagmus (90%), dysarthria (90%), mental retardation (85%), squint (65%), myopathy (50%), hypotonia (50%), spasticity (35%), microcephaly (30%), contractures (30%), short stature (30%), skeletal defects (30%), and hypergonadotropic hypogonadism (20%).

The clinical course is characteristic. At birth, the cardinal feature is hypotonia. Affected infants have normal lenses and subsequently develop cataracts (mainly nuclear). In infancy, cerebellar ataxia, delayed psychomotor development, and bilateral cataracts become apparent. Biochemical and histologic evidence of myopathy are present in infancy. Muscle weakness is progressive, and although most patients are ambulatory during childhood, by adulthood most need wheelchairs. The signs of cerebellar ataxia are clearcut. Some patients also have a Babinski sign, which may later dissipate. Puberty is delayed, and hypergonadotropic hypogonadism is common. In the teens, skeletal deformations become evident. A bulging sternum with or without scoliosis is most common. Scoliosis can be severe and has been successfully treated surgically. Asymmetric and variable shortening of metacarpals and metatarsals are common. Most patients stabilize in their late twenties, some with signs of end-stage muscle disease. Limb motion is barely possible against gravity, and serum creatinine kinase returns to normal. Most adults are able to walk with crutches, although there are patients who may be less severely affected. IQ is generally between 60 and 70.

Additional clinical features include short stature; pes planovalgus valgoplanus; long, slender limbs; and increased carrying angle in adults. These features may reflect the combination of muscle weakness and sexual infantilism. Skeletal defects seen include scoliosis; bulging sternum; variable-symmetric shortening of the metacarpals (44%), metatarsals (67%), and phalanges; gracile long bones (71%); cubitus valgus (67%); and coxa valga (50%). The percentages shown have been reported to shift significantly between patient populations.

Computerized tomography (CT) and magnetic resonance imaging (MRI) may show cerebellar hypoplasia, particularly of the vermis. Supratentorial abnormalities have occasionally been found and may be incidental; cerebral atrophy and agenesis of the corpus callosum have been observed. Muscle biopsy, even of young children, reveals marked variation of myofiber size, internalization of nuclei, focal myofibril degeneration and regeneration. Electron micrographs demonstrate subsarcolemmal accumulation of membranous inclusions and abnormally enlarged and distorted mitochondria separating the myofibrils. Peripheral nerve biopsies have generally been uninformative, but some investigators have found nerve conduction studies to be suggestive of a neuropathic component.

**Complications:** Weakness is severe, and most patients need wheelchairs. Visual acuity problems are common.

**Associated Findings:** Hypotrichosis and cryptorchidism have been occasionally noted, and some have reported signs of peripheral neuropathy. Seizures are reported in occasional patients and unaffected relatives.

**Etiology:** Autosomal recessive inheritance.

**Pathogenesis:** Electron microscopic studies have shown enlarged lysosomes with inclusion bodies in fibroblasts. This may represent a type of lysosomal storage disease.

**MIM No.:** *24880

**POS No.:** 3438

**Sex Ratio:** M1:F1

**Occurrence:** Over 100 cases have been documented. There appears to be an increased frequency in Scandinavia, Italy, and in a tri-racial isolated population in Mobile and Washington counties in southern Alabama in the United States.

**Risk of Recurrence for Patient's Sib:**
See Part I, *Mendelian Inheritance.*

**Risk of Recurrence for Patient's Child:**
See Part I, *Mendelian Inheritance.* Many patients suffer from hypogonadism and do not reproduce.

**Age of Detectability:** At birth or in infancy. Prenatal examination of the posterior fossa may reveal cerebellar hypoplasia.

**Gene Mapping and Linkage:** MSS (Marinesco-Sjogren syndrome) is ULG5.

**Prevention:** None known. Genetic counseling indicated.

**Treatment:** Treatment for individual clinical problems as they occur, including resection of cataracts, correction of scoliosis and other orthopedic problems, special education, and orthopedic appliances as needed.

**Prognosis:** Life span is normal or may be slightly shortened. Complications from progressive scoliosis, myopathy, immobilization, weakness, and visual loss may be significant.

**Detection of Carrier:** Unknown.

**Special Considerations:** Only a few of the reported patients have had detailed electrophysiologic, electron microscopic, nerve, muscle, and skin biopsy studies. These studies have suggested lysosomal storage in fibroblasts (Walker et al, 1985) and segmental demyelination in peripheral nerves (Hakamada et al, 1981). Thus further studies are warranted, particularly in homozygotes and obligate carriers.

In 1904, Moravcsik described this syndrome a quarter century prior to Marinesco in 1931. Occasional investigators have elicited signs suggestive of peripheral neuropathy, but peripheral nerve biopsies have been generally normal. The presence of Babinski signs, with subsequent reversal, were noted, and may relate to the occasional presence of calcifications in the upper cervical cord and brain stem. Such signs may be sequelae of inflammatory events in these sites. Streak ovaries and testicular tubular atrophy have been documented in a few patients.

Six of 17 patients from one kindred underwent muscle biopsies. Active myopathy was evident at the ages of 1.5, two, 21, 24, and 29 years, while one patient had end stage myopathy at the age of 26 years. Elevated serum CK and myopathic EMGs appear to be the rule. These changes may be present at birth. Signs of abnormal mitochondrial morphology were noted, and may provide a clue to pathogenesis. Clinical variability was extensive, and one 45 year old patient remained ambulatory.

**References:**
Todorov A: Le syndrome de Marinesco-Sjögren: premiere etude anatomo-clinique thesis. Geneva: Editions Medicine et Hygiene, 1964.

Ron MA, Pearce J: Marinesco-Sjögren-Garland syndrome with unusual features. J Neurol Sci 1971; 13:175–179.
Skre H, Berg K: Linkage studies on the Marinesco-Sjögren syndrome and hypergonadotropic hypogonadism. Clin Genet 1977; 11:57–66.
Hakamada S, et al.: Peripheral neuropathy in Marinesco-Sjögren syndrome. Brain Dev 1981; 3:403–406.
Walker PD, et al.: Marinesco-Sjögren syndrome: evidence for a lysosomal storage disorder. Neurology 1985; 35:415–419.
Superneau DW, et al.: Myopathy in Marinesco-Sjogren syndrome. Eur Neurol 1987; 26:8–16.

K0018
WE029

**Boris G. Kousseff**
**W. Wertelecki**

**Marinesco-Sjogren syndrome-hypergonadotropic hypogonadism**
*See MARINESCO-SJOGREN SYNDROME*
**Marinesco-Sjogren syndrome-myopathy**
*See MARINESCO-SJOGREN SYNDROME*
**Marinesco-Sjogren syndrome-neuropathy**
*See MARINESCO-SJOGREN SYNDROME*
**Marinesco-Sjogren-Garland syndrome**
*See MARINESCO-SJOGREN SYNDROME*
**Maroteaux rhizomelic dysplasia**
*See OMODYSPLASIA*
**Maroteaux-Lamy syndrome**
*See MUCOPOLYSACCHARIDOSIS VI*
**Maroteaux-Martinelli-Campailla acromesomelic dysplasia**
*See ACROMESOMELIC DYSPLASIA, MAROTEAUX-MARTINELLI-CAMPAILLA TYPE*
**Marshall syndrome**
*See DEAFNESS-MYOPIA-CATARACT-SADDLE NOSE, MARSHALL TYPE*
**Marshall syndrome, accelerated skeletal maturation type**
*See MARSHALL-SMITH SYNDROME*

## MARSHALL-SMITH SYNDROME                    2193

**Includes:**
Accelerated skeletal maturation syndrome
Marshall syndrome, accelerated skeletal maturation type
Shurtleff syndrome
Skeletal maturation (fast)-dysmorphic facies-failure to thrive

**Excludes:**
**Cebebral gigantism** (0137)
**Deafness-myopia-cataract-saddle nose, Marshall type** (0261)
**Weaver syndrome** (2036)

**Major Diagnostic Criteria:** The syndrome should be suspected in infants or children with early overgrowth but subsequent growth failure, dysmorphic facial features, chronic pulmonary disease, and advanced skeletal maturation ("bone age").

**Clinical Findings:** The most frequent dysmorphic facial findings in 14 reported patients include prominent eyes (13), low nasal bridge (13), upturned nose (11), micrognathia (11), prominent forehead (10), metopic suture ridging (7), and blue sclerae (7). Hypertrichosis (8) and **Hernia, umbilical** (7) are also consistent features.

Respiratory complications are a major component of this syndrome. Anatomical abnormalities of the respiratory tract include choanal atresia or stenosis. **Laryngomalacia**, and unusual laryngeal positioning causing intubation to be difficult. Functional consequences include stridor, lingual airway obstruction, and chronic neck hyperextension as a compensatory posture to maintain airway patency. Recurrent aspiration, atelectasis, hemorrhagic pneumonia, and pulmonary hypertension are serious pulmonary sequelae.

X-ray features are helpful and essential for diagnosis of the syndrome. These include increased skull radiodensity; craniofacial disproportion with predominance of the cranial vault; slender tubular bones; wide, bullet-shaped proximal and middle phalanges of the hand; and a striking advancement of bone age beyond 2 SDs above the mean for the patient's age. At birth, the bone age often exceeds that normal for a two year old.

**Complications:** Most of the reported patients have developed respiratory distress in the first few months of life and have required extensive hospitalization. Attempts to maintain an open airway, including tracheostomy, suturing of the tongue to the lip, and fixing the mandible to the hyoid bone, have generally been unsuccessful. Failure to thrive is an accompanying problem at least partly due to the respiratory symptomatology. Birth weight is average, length average is at the 90th percentile, and head circumference is at the 75th percentile. Thereafter, weight gain is significantly below normal with length often maintained in the normal range.

Development is significantly retarded. Central nervous system complications, such as intracranial hemorrhage and hydrocephalus, contribute to this problem. Eleven of the 14 cases have died in the first two years of life due to pulmonary and central nervous system debilitation. Reported weights at death have been far below the third percentile for age, lengths have been in the third to tenth percentile, and head circumference has been at the third percentile.

**Associated Findings:** Occasional findings include sagittal or metopic synostosis; **Hydrocephaly**; low-set, large, and/or dysplastic ears; hypo- or hypertelorism with up- or downslanting palpebral fissures; megacornea; small nose; long philtrum; high palate; long thin hands and feet; **Camptodactyly**; low-set thumbs; clinodactyly; prominent heels; deep foot creases; narrow thorax; scoliosis; cryptorchidism; hydronephrosis; **Omphalocele**; and congenital heart disease.

**Etiology:** Unknown. Karyotypes and standard metabolic studies are normal. There are 16 unaffected siblings to the 14 reported cases. One mother was treated with thyroxine and another, addicted to heroin, was withdrawn on methadone during pregnancy. There have been no other significant maternal complications of pregnancy, and mean parental age is within the normal range (mother 25.4, father 30.1). Autopsy findings have been unrevealing.

**Pathogenesis:** The pulmonary problems appear to derive primarily from respiratory obstruction with both congenital and functional components as described above. Aspiration, with resulting chemical and superimposed bacterial pneumonia, is a common problem. This may be further complicated by congenital heart defects (**Atrial septal defects, Ductus arteriosus, patent**), and a frequent end result is right heart failure with pulmonary hypertension.

One patient demonstrated a deficiency in absolute number of T cells as well as in the suppressor T-cell fraction. The significance of this finding is unknown. Reported immunoglobulin levels have been normal, and thymic hypoplasia in one patient was felt to be a secondary finding. The contribution of subtle immunodeficiency to the pulmonary pathology is therefore undetermined.

**POS No.:** 3316

**Sex Ratio:** M1:F1

**Occurrence:** Some 14 cases have been documented.

**Risk of Recurrence for Patient's Sib:** Unknown.

**Risk of Recurrence for Patient's Child:** Unknown.

**Age of Detectability:** At birth.

**Gene Mapping and Linkage:** Unknown.

**Prevention:** None known. Genetic counseling indicated.

**Treatment:** Supportive care for respiratory distress and pulmonary infection is required. In one case, tracheostomy was beneficial, though this procedure and other methods of maintaining the airway were not successful in other patients.

**Prognosis:** Eleven of the 14 patients have died at reported ages of seven days to 20 months. The living patients were aged nine months, 30 months, and three years when described. All of the patients have exhibited significant development retardation, though the patient treated successfully with tracheostomy was subsequently showing improvement at age 30 months.

**Detection of Carrier:** Unknown.

**Special Considerations:** Careful attention to airway anatomy and function both pre- and postmortem may contribute to the understanding of this disorder. Likewise, investigation of im-

mune function would be helpful to determine the incidence and significance of immunodeficiency.

**References:**

Marshall R, et al.: Syndrome of accelerated skeletal maturation and relative failure to thrive: a newly recognized clinical growth disorder. J Pediatr 1971; 78:95–101.

Fitch N: The syndromes of Marshall and Weaver. J Med Genet 1980; 17:174–178. *

LaPenna R, Folger GM Jr: Extreme upper airway obstruction with the Marshall syndrome. Clin Pediatr 1982; 21:507–510.

Johnson JP, et al.: Marshall-Smith syndrome: two case reports and a review of pulmonary manifestations. Pediatrics 1983; 71:219–223. * †

J0012 **John P. Johnson**

**Martin-Bell X-linked mental retardation**
See X-LINKED MENTAL RETARDATION, FRAGILE X SYNDROME

## MARTSOLF SYNDROME 2556

**Includes:**

Cataract-mental retardation-hypogonadism-microcephaly
Hypogonadism-cataract-mental retardation-microcephaly

**Excludes:**

**Borjeson-Forssman-Lehmann syndrome** (2272)
**Cohen syndrome** (2023)
**Retinopathy-microcephaly-mental retardation** (2846)

**Major Diagnostic Criteria:** Cataracts, mental retardation, hypergonadotropic hypogonadism, and microcephaly.

**Clinical Findings:** In 50% or more of the cases, the following physical and laboratory findings were evident: cataracts developing between ages two months and 14 years, severe mental retardation, hypergonadotropic hypogonadism, short stature, **Microcephaly**, brachycephaly, premature aged appearance, maxillary retrusion, malaligned teeth, broad and flat sternum, broad fingertips, lax finger joints, short palms, abnormal finger and palm ratios, lumbar lordosis, and talipes valgus.

In less than one-half of the cases, the following clinical and laboratory findings were evident: short philtrum, furrowed tongue, pouting lower lip, sparse facial hair, low posterior hairline, prominent nipples, ulnar deviation of fingers 2 and 3, excess palmar creases, abnormal toenails, hypotelorism, short ulna, prognathism, delayed bone age, and cardiopathy.

Extensive biochemical, metabolic, X-ray, and enzymatic laboratory tests did not show any specific findings except for elevated FSH and LH levels, and relatively low testosterone, delayed bone age, and pneumoencephalographic evidence of cerebral atrophy. Chromosome studies were normal. Cases described by Mikati et al (1985) are distinctly different due to the absence of cataracts and the presence of genua valga and cubiti valgi.

**Complications:** Visual problems secondary to the presence of cataracts, as well as lenticular opacification from residual pupillary membranes that were present from previous cataract aspirations. Secondary orthopedic problems may develop from the marked lordosis. Dental hygiene and orthodontic problems are expected because of the malaligned and crowded teeth in conjunction with the prognathism.

**Associated Findings:** None known.

**Etiology:** Although the majority of reported patients to date have been males, autosomal recessive inheritance is suggested by consanguinity in the initial cases, possible consanguinity in subsequent cases, and the occurrence in females.

**Pathogenesis:** Unknown.

**MIM No.:** 21272

**POS No.:** 3497

**Sex Ratio:** Presumably, M1:F1; (M7:F2 observed).

**Occurrence:** Nine cases have been observed; two Polish Jews, two Sephardic Jews, one in nonspecified non-Jewish population, two Dutch-Belgian, and two Pakistanian.

**2556-20391–92:** Two brothers with Martsolf syndrome; note prominent antitragus, mild maxillary hypoplasia, short philtrum, pouting lower lip, and sparse facial hair. The brother on the left has an opacity in the right eye. **20393:** Lateral view shows maxillary hypoplasia, prominent nipples and increased lumbar lordosis. **20394:** Note the bulbous fingertips and mild distal clinodactyly of several fingers. **20395:** Skull X-ray marked for cephalometric analysis; note maxillary hypoplasia and relative prognathism.

**Risk of Recurrence for Patient's Sib:**
See Part I, *Mendelian Inheritance.*

**Risk of Recurrence for Patient's Child:**
See Part I, *Mendelian Inheritance.* There is no reported case of affected individuals reproducing. With the small testicles and the hypogonadism, decreased fertility is expected.

**Age of Detectability:** The disorder is usually clinically evident by ages 10–20 years, but developmental retardation and the cataracts may be present earlier during childhood.

**Gene Mapping and Linkage:** Unknown.

**Prevention:** None known. Genetic counseling indicated.

**Treatment:** Special education programs, cataract removal, dental care, and general supportive measures as indicated.

**Prognosis:** Severe mental retardation, but life span is normal.

**Detection of Carrier:** Unknown.

**Special Considerations:** The cases reported by Mikati et al (1985) are similar but do not have cataracts and do have genua valga and cubiti valgi, and are therefore considered a different condition.

**References:**
Cuendet JF, et al.: Association de cataracte congenitale et d'oligophrenie. Bull Mem Soc Fr Ophtalmol 1976; 87:164–168.
Martsolf JT, et al.: Severe mental retardation, cataracts, short stature, and primary hypogonadism in two brothers. Am J Med Genet 1978; 1:291–299.
Mikati MA, et al.: Microcephaly, hypergonadotropic hypogonadism, short stature, and minor anomalies: a new syndrome. Am J Med Genet 1985; 22:599–608.
Sanchez JM, et al.: Two brothers with Martsolf's syndrome. J Med Genet 1985; 22:308–310.
Hennekam RCM, et al.: Martsolf syndrome in a brother and sister: clinical features and pattern of inheritance. Europ J Pediatr 1988; 147:539–543.
Strisciuglo P, et al.: Martsolf's syndrome in a non-Jewish boy. J Med Genet 1988; 25:267–269.
Harbord MG, et al.: Microcephaly, mental retardation, cataracts, and hypogonadism in sibs: Martsolf's syndrome. J Med Genet 1989; 26:397–406.

MA043                                      **John T. Martsolf**

**Mason type diabetes**
*See DIABETES MELLITUS, MATURITY ONSET OF THE YOUNG (MODY)*
**Mast cell disease**
*See URTICARIA PIGMENTOSA (UP)*
**Mastocytosis**
*See URTICARIA PIGMENTOSA (UP)*
**Maternal hyperphenylalaninemia**
*See FETAL EFFECTS FROM MATERNAL PKU*
**Maternal hyperthermia, fetal effects from**
*See FETAL EFFECTS FROM MATERNAL HYPERTHERMIA*
**Maternal phenylketonuria**
*See FETAL EFFECTS FROM MATERNAL PKU*
**Maturity-onset diabetes of the young (MODY)**
*See DIABETES MELLITUS, MATURITY ONSET OF THE YOUNG (MODY)*
**Maturity-onset type hyperglycemia of the young (MOHY)**
*See DIABETES MELLITUS, MATURITY ONSET OF THE YOUNG (MODY)*
**Maumenee congenital corneal edema**
*See CORNEAL DYSTROPHY, ENDOTHELIAL, CONGENITAL HEREDITARY*
**Maumenee corneal dystrophy**
*See CORNEAL DYSTROPHY, ENDOTHELIAL, CONGENITAL HEREDITARY*

---

**MAXILLA, MEDIAN ALVEOLAR CLEFT**          **0631**

**Includes:** Cleft, maxillary median alveolar

**Excludes:**
**Lip, median cleft of upper** (0595)
Maxillary bone, failure of formation of premaxillary portion

**Major Diagnostic Criteria:** X-ray evidence of a cleft in the premaxilla that measures at least 2 mm. The maxillary incisors must be or must have been present.

**Clinical Findings:** X-ray evidence of a cleft in the midline of the premaxillary portion of the maxilla. There may be a diastema between the central incisors. A divergence of the roots of the central incisors may be present.

**Complications:** Orthodontic movement of the maxillary central incisors could cause the loss of teeth because of lack of bone support.

**Associated Findings:** None known.

**Etiology:** Postulated by Stout and Collett (1969) to be entrapment of epithelial nests which prevents fusion of the center of calcification of the premaxilla.

**Pathogenesis:** Failure of fusion of the primary ossification center of the premaxilla during early embryonic development.

**Sex Ratio:** Undetermined. M0:F5 observed.

**Occurrence:** Undetermined but presumed rare.

**Risk of Recurrence for Patient's Sib:** Unknown.

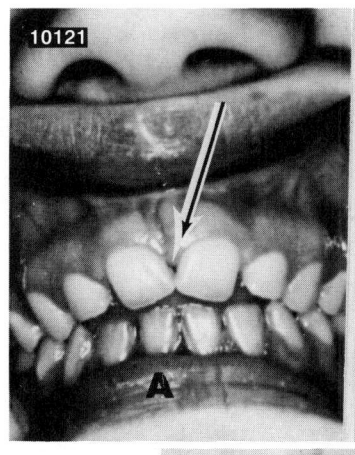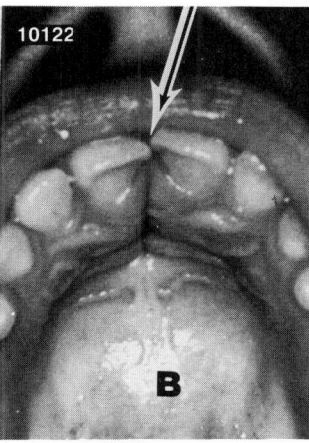

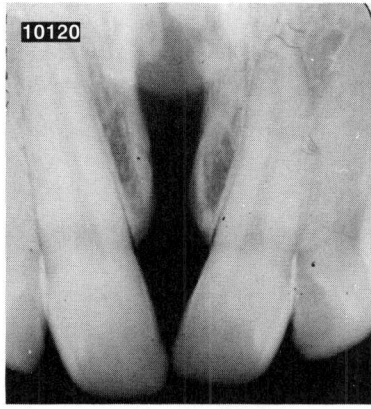

**0631**-10121: Maxillary median alveolar cleft. 10122: Intraoral view of cleft. 10120: Periapical X-ray of maxillary median alveolar cleft.

**Risk of Recurrence for Patient's Child:** Unknown.

**Age of Detectability:** Earliest reported case detected at seven years on routine X-ray examination. This condition can now be diagnosed only when all four maxillary incisors are present, indicating that there has been at least primary formation of the premaxillary portion of the maxilla.

**Gene Mapping and Linkage:** Unknown.

**Prevention:** None known.

**Treatment:** None indicated. Orthodontic movement is not recommended.

**Prognosis:** Normal life span and function.

**Detection of Carrier:** Unknown.

**References:**
Gier RE, Fast TB: Median maxillary anterior alveolar cleft: case reports and discussion. Oral Surg 1967; 24:496–502.
Miller AS, et al.: Median maxillary anterior cleft: report of three cases. J Am Dent Assoc 1969; 79:896–897.
Stout FW, Collett WK: Etiology and incidence of median maxillary anterior alveolar cleft. Oral Surg 1969; 28:66–72.

GI004                                              **Ronald E. Gier**

**Maxillary hypoplasia-metaphyseal dysplasia-brachydactyly**
  *See METAPHYSEAL DYSPLASIA-MAXILLARY HYPOPLASIA-BRACHYDACTYLY*
**Maxillary incisor, single central**
  *See TEETH, FUSED*

**Maxillary lateral incisor, hypodontia of**
  *See TEETH, PEGGED OR ABSENT MAXILLARY LATERAL INCISOR*
**Maxillary lateral incisor, pegged or missing**
  *See TEETH, PEGGED OR ABSENT MAXILLARY LATERAL INCISOR*

## MAXILLOFACIAL DYSOSTOSIS                         2512

**Includes:** Hypoplasia of the maxilla, primary familial
**Excludes:**
  **Acrodysostosis** (0016)
  **Acrofacial dysostosis** (0017)
  **Mandibulofacial dysostosis** (0627)

**Major Diagnostic Criteria:** All reported patients have presented with maxillary hypoplasia, delayed development of speech and language skills with dysarthria in the absence of hearing loss, and normal or near-normal intelligence.

**Clinical Findings:** The most consistent malformations seen in maxillofacial dysostosis include anteroposterior shortening of the maxilla, occasionally resulting in a relative mandibular prognathism; downslanting palpebral fissures; minor malformations of the auricles; and severely delayed onset of speech, with poor vocabulary development and poorly connected discourse, as well as nonfluent and inarticulate speech, including prolonged hesitations, vowel and consonant substitutions, omissions, and distortions.
  Other clinical findings include flat occiput, maxillary hypoplasia, flat nasal bridge, narrow beaked nose, ptosis of eyelids, nystagmus, strabismus, **Pectus excavatum**, and hypoplastic nipples.
  Cephalometric analysis confirms a small anterior cranial fossae and a decreased anteroposterior size of the maxilla.

**Complications:** Unknown.

**Associated Findings:** Most of these patients have had normal or near-normal intelligence; however, because of their speech difficulties, teachers and school officials have thought them to be mentally retarded.

**Etiology:** Autosomal dominant inheritance.

**Pathogenesis:** A genetic disorder that induces branchial arch developmental delay. This delay also affects the neuronal pathways connecting Brocca and Wernicke areas in the brain, producing a clinical condition similar to conduction aphasia.

**MIM No.:** *15500

**POS No.:** 3921

**Sex Ratio:** M1:F1

**Occurrence:** About a dozen cases have been reported.

**Risk of Recurrence for Patient's Sib:**
  See Part I, *Mendelian Inheritance.*

**Risk of Recurrence for Patient's Child:**
  See Part I, *Mendelian Inheritance.*

**Age of Detectability:** At birth, with affected individuals showing maxillary hypoplasia and eye and ear anomalies.

**Gene Mapping and Linkage:** Unknown.

**Prevention:** None known. Genetic counseling indicated.

**Treatment:** If the facial malformations are severe, plastic reconstructive surgery and orthodontic treatment may be helpful. It is important not to interfere with growth centers, because this syndrome's facial features improve with age, giving a close to normal profile in adulthood. The patients seen by Melnick and Eastman (1977) and by Escobar et al (1977) all responded positively to speech therapy.

**Prognosis:** Speech developmental delay, which may hamper intellectual achievement and school progress. Life span does not seem to be impaired.

**Detection of Carrier:** Clinical examination.

**References:**
Villaret M, Desoille H: L'hypoplasie primitive familiale du maxillaire superieur. Ann Med 1932; 32:378–381.

Peters A, Hovels O: Die Dysostosis maxillo-facialis, eine erbliche, typische Fehlbildung des 1. Visceralbogens Z Menschl Vererb. Konstitutionsl 1960; 35:434–444.

Escobar V, et al.: Maxillofacial dysostosis. J Med Genet 1977; 14:355–358.

Melnick M, Eastman JR: Autosomal dominant maxillofacial dysostosis. BD:OAS XII(3B). New York: March of Dimes Birth Defects Foundation, 1977:39–44.

ES000 **Victor Escobar**

**Maxillonasal dysostosis**
*See MAXILLONASAL DYSPLASIA, BINDER TYPE*

## MAXILLONASAL DYSPLASIA, BINDER TYPE 2235

**Includes:**
> Binder syndrome
> Maxillonasal dysostosis
> Nasomaxillary hypoplasia
> Nasomaxillovertebral syndrome

**Excludes:**
> **Aarskog syndrome** (0001)
> **Chondrodysplasia**
> **Deafness-myopia-cataract-saddle nose, Marshall type** (0261)
> **Fetal warfarin syndrome** (0389)
> **Robinow syndrome** (0876)
> Syphilis, congenital

**Major Diagnostic Criteria:** Collapsed nasal pyramid lacking cartilaginous support; short nose with a flat bridge; acute nasolabial angle; short and hypoplastic columella; hypoplastic alar cartilages; and atrophic nasal mucosa with normal sense of smell. X-ray findings including hypoplasia of the frontal process of the maxilla with absence of the anterior nasal spine, thinness of the alveolar bone labial to the maxillary incisors, and obtuse nasofrontal angle and obtuse gonial angle.

**Clinical Findings:** The face is characterized by nasomaxillary hypoplasia with a flat nose, absence of the nasal septum, short columella, and hypoplastic perialar areas. The external nares may have a "cat's ear" shape or "half moon" appearance. The sense of smell and intelligence are normal. Dental findings usually include an Angle Class III malocclusion with proclination of the maxillary incisors.

X-ray findings include Class III facial skeletal pattern with a retrognathic maxilla, absence of the anterior nasal spine, thinness of the alveolar bone labial to the maxillary incisors, obtuse nasofrontal angle, acute nasolabial angle, and obtuse gonial angle. Less frequent findings include abnormalities of the cervical spine (53%).

**Complications:** Frequent upper respiratory infections; psychosocial consequences of unusual facial appearance.

**Associated Findings:** Neonatal respiratory distress; labiomaxillary cleft.

**Etiology:** Both sporadic and inherited (dominant and recessive) cases have been described. Maxillonasal dysplasia also occurs as a finding in several syndromes.

**Pathogenesis:** A defect in cartilage development during weeks five to six has been proposed as the mechanism for the simultaneous occurrence of anomalies in the cervical spine and maxillonasal complex.

**MIM No.:** 15505

**POS No.:** 3330

**Sex Ratio:** Presumably M1:F1.

**Occurrence:** Over 100 cases have been reported in the literature.

**Risk of Recurrence for Patient's Sib:** If the patient represents a new occurrence in the family, the risk to the sib is near zero. However, given inheritance patterns in some families, a careful family history is needed before assigning risk figures.

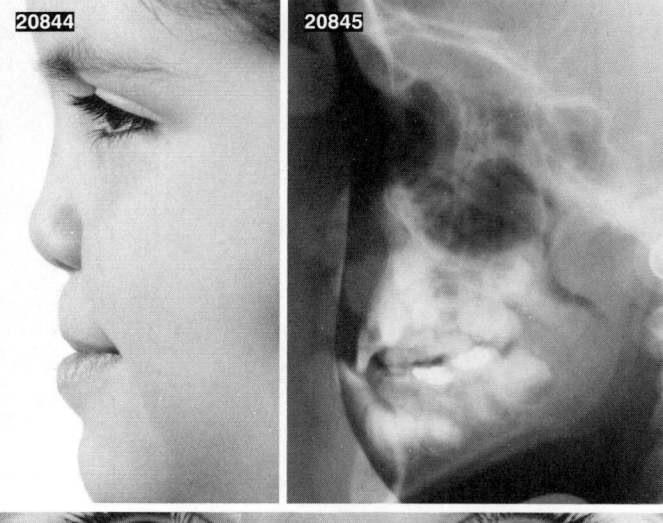
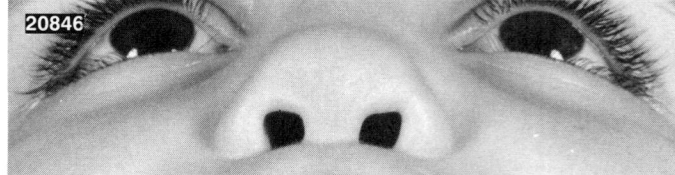
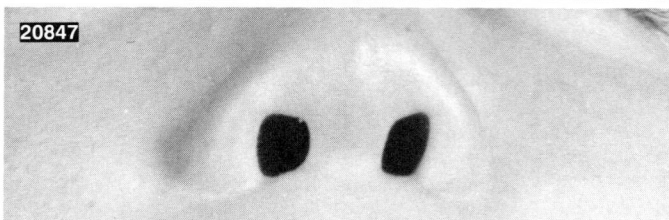
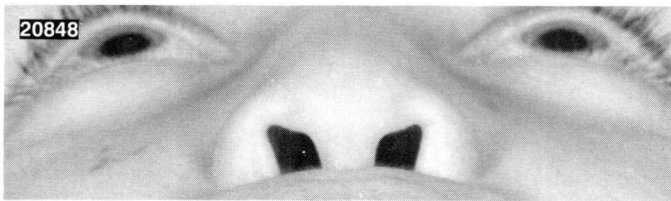
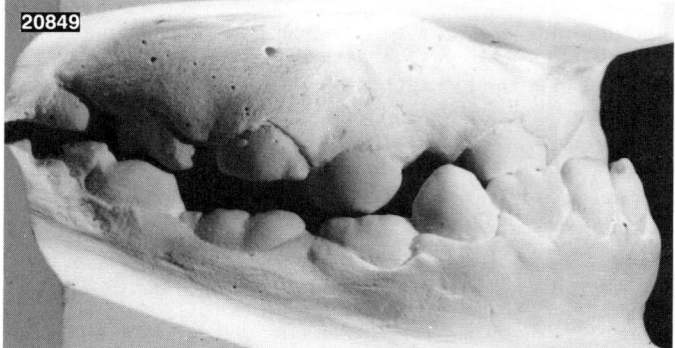

**2235-20844:** Maxillonasal dysplasia, Binder type; note characteristic facial profile. **20845:** X-ray shows the bony dysplasia in the maxilla and the nasal bones. **20846–48:** Note different nasal shapes seen in maxillonasal dysplasia. **20849:** Dental cast shows the relative positions of the maxilla and the mandible.

**Risk of Recurrence for Patient's Child:** Recent reports suggest autosomal dominant inheritance with variable expression in some families. If so, the risk to the child may be as high as 1:2.

**Age of Detectability:** At birth.

**Gene Mapping and Linkage:** Unknown.

**Prevention:** None known. Genetic counseling indicated.

**Treatment:** Nasal bone grafts, surgical and/or orthopedic maxillary advancement, orthodontic and/or prosthodontic treatment.

**Prognosis:** Good.

**Detection of Carrier:** Unknown.

**Special Considerations:** Maxillonasal dysplasia is a finding, not a diagnosis, and therefore is likely to be heterogeneous.

**References:**
Binder KH: Dysostosis maxillo-nasalis, ein arinencephaler Missbildungskomplex. Deutsch Zahnaerztl A 1962; 17:438–444.

Munro IR, et al.: Maxillonasal dysplasia (Binder's syndrome). Plast Reconstr Surg 1979; 63:657–663.

Delair J, et al.: Clinical and radiologic aspects of maxillonasal dysostosis (Binder syndrome). Head Neck Surg 1980; 3:105–122. *

Resche F, et al.: Craniospinal and cervicospinal malformations associated with maxillonasal dysostosis (Binder syndrome). Head Neck Surg 1980; 3:123–131.

Gross-Kieselstein E, et al.: Familial variant of maxillonasal dysplasia? J Craniofacial Genetics and Developmental Biology 1986; 6:331–334.

Horswell BB, et al.: Maxillonasal dysplasia (Binder's syndrome): a critical review and case study. J Oral Maxillofac Surg 1987; 45:114–122. *

EV002
H0058

Carla A Evans
Lili K. Horton

**Maxillopalpebral synkinesis**
*See JAW-WINKING SYNDROME*
**May-Hegglin anomaly**
*See LEUKOCYTE, MAY-HEGGLIN ANOMALY*
**Mayer-Rokitansky-Kuster (MRK) anomaly**
*See MULLERIAN APLASIA*
**McArdle disease**
*See GLYCOGENOSIS, TYPE V*
**McCune-Albright syndrome**
*See FIBROUS DYSPLASIA, POLYOSTOTIC*

## MCDONOUGH SYNDROME 0632

**Includes:** Noonan-like McDonough syndrome

**Excludes:**
> **Noonan syndrome** (0720)
> **Turner syndrome** (0977)

**Major Diagnostic Criteria:** The combination of mental retardation, short stature, kyphoscoliosis, pectus carinatum/excavatum, cardiac defect, diastasis recti, cryptorchidism, and a possibly altered facial appearance.

**Clinical Findings:** Only two families have been reported; features present in affected individuals of both families include short stature (third to 25th percentile), mental retardation, synophrys, strabismus, malocclusion, anteverted auricles, kyphoscoliosis, **Pectus carinatum** or **Pectus excavatum**, cardiac defect (including **Atrial septal defects** or **Ventricular septal defect** with pulmonic stenosis and aortic stenosis), diastasis recti, and cryptorchidism. Further delineation of the phenotype is difficult, however, since in each family, unaffected family members shared some of the variant features with affected individuals. In the first reported family (Neuhauser and Opitz, 1975), additional features included upslanting palpebral fissures, grooved tongue, micrognathia, single transverse palmar crease, hypoplastic toenails, and clinodactyly. In the second reported family (Garcia-Sagredo et al, 1984), features included sparse or bristly hair, apparent **Eye, hypertelorism**, ptosis, large nose, short philtrum, and prognathism. In one family, one affected individual had an XXY karyotype apparently inherited from his XY/XXY father; in the second family a

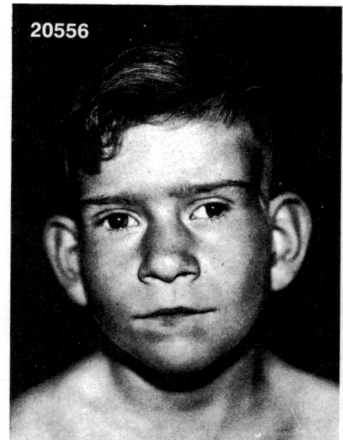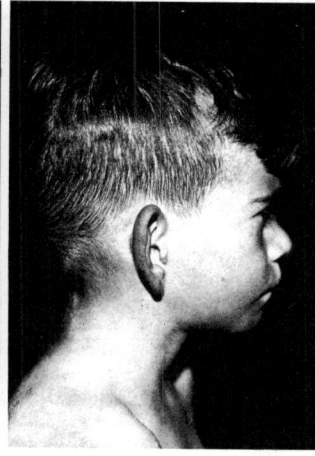

**0632-20556:** McDonough syndrome; note anteverted auricles, upward slanting palpebral fissures and synophrys in this boy who also had a 47, XYY chromosome constitution.

balanced X;20 translocation was found in one affected child and his mother.

**Complications:** Heart failure, scoliosis.

**Associated Findings:** None known.

**Etiology:** Possibly autosomal recessive inheritance.

**Pathogenesis:** Unknown.

**MIM No.:** 24895

**POS No.:** 3286

**Sex Ratio:** Presumably M1:F1

**Occurrence:** Two families have been reported; one from the United States and one from Spain.

**Risk of Recurrence for Patient's Sib:**
> See Part I, *Mendelian Inheritance.*

**Risk of Recurrence for Patient's Child:**
> See Part I, *Mendelian Inheritance.*

**Age of Detectability:** Soon after birth by the presence of the cardiac defect.

**Gene Mapping and Linkage:** Unknown.

**Prevention:** None known. Genetic counseling indicated.

**Treatment:** Treatment of the kyphoscoliosis may be indicated, as well as surgical correction of the cardiac defect and cryptorchidism.

**Prognosis:** All affected individuals have been mentally retarded, with IQs between 47 and 71. Prognosis is undetermined, although life span should be normal.

**Detection of Carrier:** Unknown.

**References:**
Neuhauser G, Opitz JM: Studies of malformation syndromes in man. XXXX: multiple congenital anomalies/mental retardation syndrome or variant familial developmental pattern; differential diagnosis and description of the McDonough syndrome (with XXY son from XY/XXY father). Z Kinderheilkd 1975; 120:231–242.

Garcia-Sagredo JM, et al.: Mentally retarded siblings with congenital heart defect, peculiar facies and cryptorchidism in the male: possible McDonough syndrome with coincidental (X;20) translocation. Clin Genet 1984; 26:117–124.

T0007
NE012

Helga V. Toriello
Gerhard Neuhäuser

**McKusick-Kaufman syndrome**
*See VAGINAL SEPTUM, TRANSVERSE*

**McLeod phenotype**
*See ANEMIA, HEMOLYTIC, RED CELL MEMBRANE DEFECTS*

---

## MECKEL DIVERTICULUM                              0633

**Includes:**
Omphalomesenteric duct
Vitelline duct, remnant

**Excludes:** Intestinal duplication (0532)

**Major Diagnostic Criteria:** Positive diagnosis can only be made by the gross anatomic findings made at operation or autopsy. The diverticulum can vary in size, both in diameter and length, and arises from the antimesenteric border of the ileum, usually within 100 cm of the ileocecal valve (90%). Ectopic gastric or pancreatic tissue is present in approximately two-thirds of the diverticula; the lesion presents most frequently in the pediatric age group with massive gastrointestinal hemorrhage, and in the older patients with inflammation or intestinal obstruction.

**Clinical Findings:** Asymptomatic, except if a complication occurs. Fifteen percent to 20% become symptomatic, and the rest are asymptomatic. The presenting symptoms are related to the complication and include, in the pediatric age group, hemorrhage, intestinal obstruction, inflammation (simulating appendicitis), peritonitis, and umbilical drainage. Rarely, carcinoma can arise in a Meckel diverticulum. Hemorrhage results from a peptic ulcer in the diverticulum or in the adjacent ileum and is associated with gastric mucosa in the diverticulum. Intestinal obstruction can result from congenital bands, either mesodiverticular or omphalomesenteric, previous inflammatory adhesion, intussusception (ileo-ileo with the diverticulum as the lead point), and from the incarceration of the diverticulum in a hernia: the so-called Littre hernia. Inflammation is related to obstruction of the mouth of the diverticulum, as in appendicitis, or in association with a foreign body such as a fish-bone stuck in the diverticulum. Perforation results from diverticulitis or from perforation of an ulcer. Umbilical drainage results from an omphalomesenteric duct sinus or fistula. The sinus may present only as an umbilical polyp of intestinal mucosa. Very rarely, the diverticulum can be demonstrated by ordinary X-ray examinations, such as a small bowel series or a barium enema with reflux into the ileum. A 99 m$_{Tc}$-pertechnetate scan of the abdomen may demonstrate a Meckel diverticulum by showing gastric mucosa, present in 50% of symptomatic diverticula. Asymptomatic diverticula are usually found incidentally at celiotomy for some other reason. Symptomatic patients usually present with one of the four following condition: an omphalomesenteric duct remnant recognized as such on examination of the umbilicus; an acute surgical abdomen of uncertain origin, but signifying inflammation with peritonitis or obstruction of the small bowel; gross rectal bleeding, or intermittent abdominal pain. Sixty percent of symptomatic diverticula present in childhood, and 50% manifest in the first three years of life. Of the symptomatic patients, 75% are male.

**Complications:** Hemorrhage (40%), obstruction (25%), inflammation (23%), perforation (5%), or umbilical discharge (5%). The above percentages are for the pediatric age group; older patients present more commonly with obstruction and inflammation.

**Associated Findings:** There is an increased incidence of a Meckel diverticulum in children born with a major malformation of the umbilicus, alimentary tract, and nervous and cardiovascular systems (in descending order of frequency). For omphalocele and gastroschisis the association is 25%; for esophageal atresia it is 12%.

**Etiology:** Unknown.

**Pathogenesis:** Meckel diverticulum, or its variants, develops as a gross structural defect of the yolk sac, vitelline duct and/or omphalomesenteric duct, which are a normal structures of the 5–9 mm embryo. At this stage (the end of the fifth week), the yolk stalk or vitelline duct constricts and separates from the intestine and disappears. A persistence of the yolk stalk appears in several forms. The stalk may remain patent and continuous, forming an umbilical-intestinal fistula. It may be patent at the outer end, producing a sinus. A cyst will form if the central portion is patent. Most commonly, a blind pouch occurs on the ileum, free in the abdomen except for its attachment to the ileum or sometimes connected to the umbilicus by a fibrous band. The diverticulum is a true diverticulum showing all layers of the intestinal wall. Some diverticula contain gastric mucosa or pancreatic tissue. One of the vitelline arteries persists as a branch of the terminal superior mesenteric artery to form the arterial blood supply to the diverticulum. The other vitelline artery can form a mesodiverticular band.

**CDC No.:** 751.010

**Sex Ratio:** M1:F1

**Occurrence:** 1:60 live births.

**Risk of Recurrence for Patient's Sib:** Unknown.

**Risk of Recurrence for Patient's Child:** Unknown.

**Age of Detectability:** By complications that occur more commonly before the age of three years (50%), but can occur at any age.

**Gene Mapping and Linkage:** Unknown.

**Prevention:** None known. Genetic counseling indicated.

**Treatment:** Excision of the diverticulum by means of a wedge diverticulectomy is the usual surgical treatment. In certain complications of a Meckel diverticulum, such as obstruction or bleeding from an ileal ulcer, it may be necessary to do an ileal resection and ileo-ileal anastomosis. An incidental resection of a Meckel diverticulum at the time of laparotomy may be done to prevent the subsequent complications of the diverticulum if good surgical judgment calls for its removal. Elective resection may be considered advisable if there are atypical features, such as abnormal bands or attachments, or heterotopic tissue, noted on inspection and palpation of the diverticulum. The evidence of heterotopic tissue is indirect and consists of mucosal or submucosal nodules, evidence of inflammation, and serosal scarring and adhesions. Other risk factors for future symptoms are age of the patient and length of the diverticulum. The younger the patient, the more likely he or she is to be symptomatic. And the longer diverticula are more symptomatic than the shorter ones; 2 cm is the critical differential point. The diameter and the position of the diverticulum are not factors significant for future symptoms. It is estimated that 5% of incidentally found Meckel diverticula lead to symptoms during a lifetime.

**Prognosis:** Excellent with recovery from surgical treatment. Most deaths occur from a delayed recognition of a perforation and obstruction in infants.

**Detection of Carrier:** Unknown.

**Special Considerations:** In the newborn there occurs a distinct form of the anomaly, known as giant Meckel diverticulum. This type of diverticulum can measure 4–8 cm in diameter, and presents as a palpable or viable abdominal mass and as intestinal obstruction. Surgical resection is urgently required to relieve the obstruction.

**References:**
Kiesewetter WB: Meckel's diverticulum in children. Arch Surg 1957; 75:914–919.
Craft AW, et al.: Giant Meckel's diverticulum causing intestinal obstruction of newborn. J Pediatr Surg 1976; 11:1037–1038.
Simms MH, Corkery JJ: Meckel diverticulum: association with congenital malformation and the significance of atypical morphology. Br J Surg 1980; 67:216–219.
Williams RS: Management of Meckel's diverticulum. Br J Surg 1981; 68:477–480.
Cooney DR, et al.: The abdominal technetium scan (a decade of experience). J Pediatr Surg 1982; 17:611–619.
Mackey WC, Dineen P: A fifty year experience with Meckel's diverticulum. Surg Gynec Obstet 1983; 153:56–64.

J0013                                                    **Paul W. Johnston**

## MECKEL SYNDROME 0634

**Includes:**
  Dysencephalia splanchnocystica
  Gruber syndrome
  Meckel-Gruber syndrome

**Excludes:**
  **Chromosome 13, trisomy 13** (0168)
  **Oculo-encephalo-hepato-renal syndrome** (3242)
  **Smith-Lemli-Opitz syndrome** (0891)

**Major Diagnostic Criteria:** Cystic dysplasia of the kidneys with fibrotic changes of the liver, occipital encephalocele, or some other CNS malformation plus other frequently seen anomalies such as polydactyly, cleft lip and/or palate, microcephaly, small or ambiguous genitalia.

**Clinical Findings:** Microcephaly is commonly associated with occipital encephalocele. On occasion there may be hydrocephaly or anencephaly. The facies is described as Potter-like, especially in cases with severe oligohydramnios. Facial characteristics include a

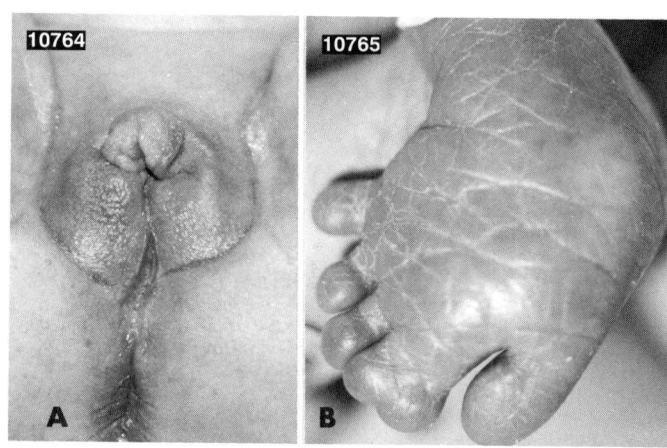

**0634B-**10764: Hypoplastic phallus with dorsal prepuce, urethral opening at base of phallus, and fusion of labioscrotal swellings. 10765: Short 1st toe, postaxial hexadactyly, complete cutaneous syndactyly of 2nd and 3rd toes, and severe valgus deformity.

shape that is broad and round, low sloping forehead, broad cheeks, small chin, hypertelorism, upslanted palpebral fissures, broad flattened nose, wide mouth, full lips, and low-set ears. The neck is often short. Other associated craniofacial malformations include microphthalmia, colobomata, cataracts, cleft lip and more commonly cleft palate, natal teeth, small lobulated or cleft tongue with or without papillomatous processes, and buccal frenula.

Renal dysplasia is almost always bilateral. Both kidneys are usually grossly enlarged, but on occasion slightly enlarged, normal, or smaller than normal. Kidneys usually have macroscopic cysts. On histologic examination they invariably show cystic

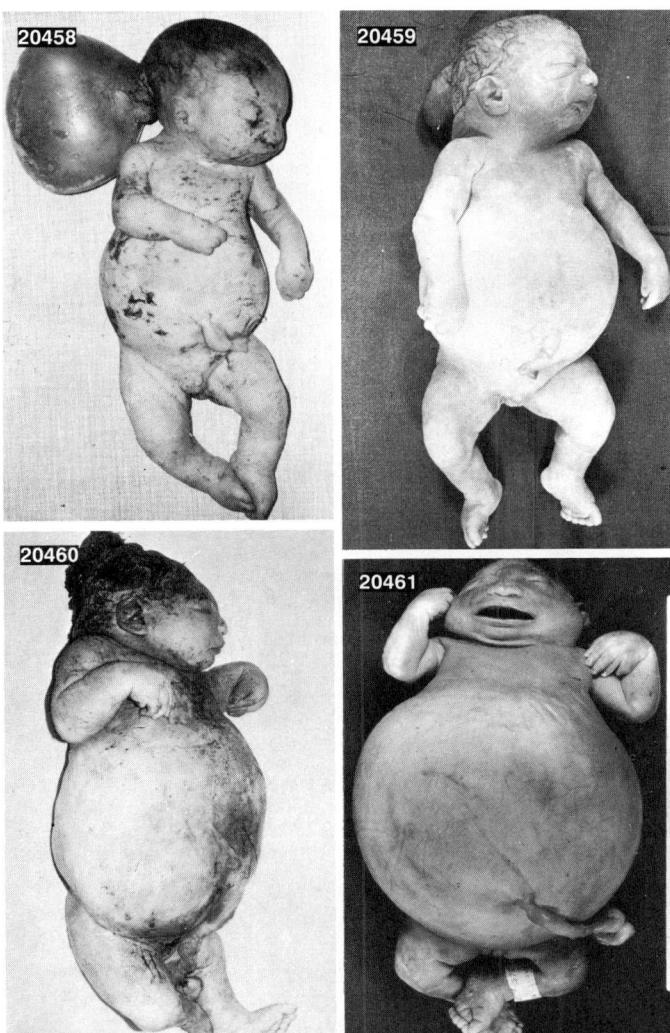

**0634A-**20458–61: Meckel syndrome; note occipital encephalocele, polydactyly, and abdominal enlargement from megacystic kidneys.

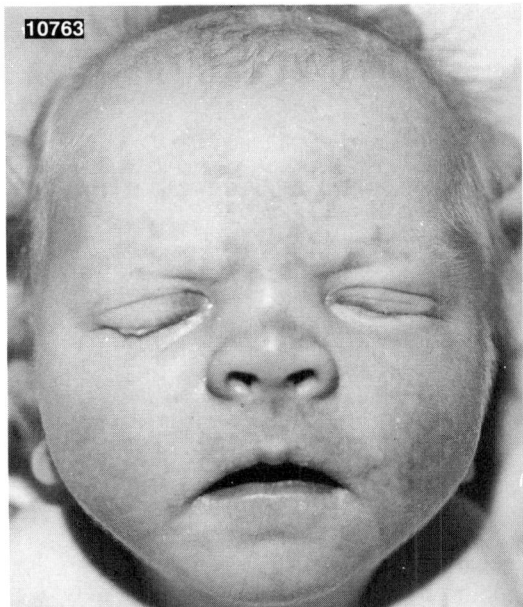

**0634C-**10763: Facial features include overlapping eyelids, capillary hemangiomas on forehead, bridge and top of the nose; downturned corners of the mouth.

dysplastic changes with very little normal parenchyma. Anomalies of the urinary tract are common, including hypoplastic ureters, hypoplastic bladder, bladder not connected to the urethra, or an absent urethra.

CNS malformations are varied, with occipital encephalocele being the most common. Occipital holes are found in the skull, which may be connected by an occipitoschisis with the foramen magnum. The encephalocele is usually accompanied by microcephaly, and on occasion, hydrocephaly. There are various grades of aplasia/hypoplasia of the cerebrum, cerebellum, and olfactory lobes and microencephaly.

Limb malformations are also common. Polydactyly is present in the vast majority of cases, such that previous reports required minimal criteria to include two out of three features: occipital encephalocele, cystic kidneys, and polydactyly. One or two extra digits are present postaxially, almost always bilaterally on both hands and feet. There may be partial or total syndactyly involving fingers and toes. Ulnar deviation of the hands and clubfeet are also common. Short limbs have been described. Genital anomalies are also a common feature. Ambiguous genitalia often turn out to be cases of male pseudohermaphroditism with testes or 46,XY karyotype. Both testes and ovaries have been, rarely, found.

Other internal organ defects include cardiac, gastrointestinal, and pulmonary abnormalities. The liver is usually too large for gestational age, up to twice the normal size. Microscopic cysts are often present. Bile ducts may be dilated, and the gall bladder may be absent. Microscopically, the liver shows fibrosis of the portal areas with ductal proliferation and dilation of the liver. Heart anomalies consist of atrial septal defect, **Ventricular septal defect**, and other complex malformations. There may be an accessory spleen, absent spleen, splenomegaly, and absent or hypoplastic adrenals. Hypoplasia of the lungs is common, assumed to be secondary to the enlarged abdomen and oligohydramnnios.

All cases are stillborn or die within a few hours after birth, due to renal insufficiency, with or without pulmonary or cardiac complications. A long term survival of one week is reported with death due to renal failure.

**Complications:** Breech presentation is frequent. Caesarean section is common because of hydrocephaly, abnormal fetal position or fetal distress. Oligohydramnios is also common.

**Associated Findings:** None known.

**Etiology:** Autosomal recessive inheritance.

**Pathogenesis:** Unknown.

**MIM No.:** *24900

**POS No.:** 3287

**CDC No.:** 759.890

**Sex Ratio:** M1:F1

**Occurrence:** Found world-wide, but particularly prevalent in Finland (1:9,000 births), among the Tatars of the Soviet Union, and among Gujarati Indians.

**Risk of Recurrence for Patient's Sib:**
See Part I, *Mendelian Inheritance.*

**Risk of Recurrence for Patient's Child:**
See Part I, *Mendelian Inheritance.* Affected individuals are not expected to survive to reproduce.

**Age of Detectability:** Prenatal diagnosis using ultrasonography and alpha fetoprotein determination is well documented. The condition is often suspected because of a previous affected sibling. Sonography often detects the occipital encephalocele or cystic dysplastic kidneys. Maternal serum and amniotic fluid alpha fetoprotein is often elevated from the associated encephalocele or anencephaly. These findings are present in midtrimester. The syndrome is also diagnosable at birth.

**Gene Mapping and Linkage:** Unknown.

**Prevention:** None known. Genetic counseling indicated.

**Treatment:** Unknown.

**Prognosis:** Invariably fatal within the first hours or days of life.

**Detection of Carrier:** Unknown.

**Special Considerations:** This condition is named after Johann Friedrich Meckel who first described it in 1822. G.B. Gruber, who termed the condition dysencephalia splanchnocystica, published his findings in 1934. In 1984, the American Journal of Medical Genetics devoted much of its volume 18 to the proceedings of a Meckel symposium organized by John M. Opitz on the bicentennial of Meckel's death.

**References:**
Opitz JM, Howe JJ: The Meckel syndrome (dysencephalia splanchnocystica, the Gruber syndrome). BD:OAS V(2). New York: The National Foundation-March of Dimes, 1969:167–179.
Meckel S, Passarge E: Encephalocele, polycystic kidneys and polydactyly as an autosomal recessive trait simulating certain other disorders: the Meckel syndrome. Ann Genet 1971; 14:97–103.
Hsia YE, et al.: Genetics of the Meckel syndrome (dysencephalia splanchnocystica). Pediatrics 1971; 48:237–247.
Johnson VP, et al.: Prenatal diagnosis of Meckel syndrome: case reports and literature review. Am J Med Genet 1984; 18:699–711.
Salonen R: The Meckel syndrome: clinicopathologic findings in 67 patients. Am J Med Genet 1984; 18:671–689.
Rapola J, Salonen R: Visceral anomalies in the Meckel syndrome. Teratology 1985; 31:193–201.

J0010                                    **Virginia P. Johnson**

**Meckel-Gruber syndrome**
*See MECKEL SYNDROME*
**Meconium ileus, isolated**
*See INTESTINAL ILEUS, ISOLATED MECONIUM ILEUS*
**MED-IDDM syndrome**
*See EPIPHYSEAL DYSPLASIA, MULTIPLE-DIABETES MELLITUS*
**Medial coronary sclerosis of infancy**
*See ARTERY, CORONARY CALCINOSIS*
**Medial fibroplasia**
*See ARTERY, RENAL FIBROMUSCULAR DYSPLASIA*
**Median cleft face syndrome**
*See FACE, MEDIAN CLEFT FACE SYNDROME*
**Median cleft of upper lip**
*See LIP, MEDIAN CLEFT OF UPPER*
**Median clefts of lower lip, mandible and tongue**
*See CLEFTS, LOWER MEDIAN LIP, MANDIBLE AND TONGUE*
**Median incisal diastema**
*See TEETH, DIASTEMA, MEDIAN INCISAL*
**Median rhomboid glossitis**
*See GLOSSITIS, MEDIAN RHOMBOID*
**Mediterranean anemia**
*See THALASSEMIA*
**Mediterranean fever, familial (FMF)**
*See FEVER, FAMILIAL MEDITERRANEAN (FMF)*
**Medium-chain acyl-CoA dehydrogenase deficiency (MCAD)**
*See ACYL-CoA DEHYDROGENASE DEFICIENCY, MEDIUM CHAIN TYPE*
**Medullary cystic disease-nephronophthisis**
*See KIDNEY, NEPHRONOPHTHISIS-MEDULLARY CYSTIC DESEASE*
**Medullary cystic kidney disease**
*See KIDNEY, NEPHRONOPHTHISIS-MEDULLARY CYSTIC DESEASE*
**Medullary sponge kidney**
*See KIDNEY, MEDULLARY SPONGE KIDNEY*
**Medullary thyroid carcinoma and pheochromocytoma syndrome**
*See ENDOCRINE NEOPLASIA, MULTIPLE TYPE II*
**Medullary thyroid carcinoma syndrome (most cases)**
*See ENDOCRINE NEOPLASIA, MULTIPLE TYPE II*
**Medulloblastoma**
*See CNS NEOPLASMS*
**Meesmann corneal dystrophy**
*See CORNEAL DYSTROPHY, JUVENILE EPITHELIAL, MEESMANN TYPE*
**Mefenamic acid, fetal effects**
*See FETAL EFFECTS OF NONSTEROIDAL ANTI-INFLAMMATORY DRUGS (NSAIDS)*
**Megacolon, aganglionic**
*See COLON, AGANGLIONOSIS*
**Megacolon, idiopathic**
*See INTESTINAL PSEUDO-OBSTRUCTION SYNDROMES*
**Megacystis, idiopathic**
*See INTESTINAL PSEUDO-OBSTRUCTION SYNDROMES*

## MEGACYSTIS-MEGADUODENUM SYNDROME 2316

**Includes:**
Intestinal pseudo-obstruction, idiopathic
Megaduodenum-megacysts syndrome
Visceral myopathy, familial
Visceral myopathy, hereditary hollow

**Excludes:**
**Colon, aganglionosis** (0192)
**Colon, atresia or stenosis** (0193)
**Colon, duplication** (0194)
**Duodenum, atresia or stenosis** (0300)
**Intestinal atresia or stenosis** (0531)
**Intestinal hypoperistalsis, megacystis-microcolon type** (2317)
**Pyloric stenosis** (0848)
**Stomach, pyloric atresia** (0910)

**Major Diagnostic Criteria:** Familial megaduodenum and/or megacystis without evidence of organic obstruction in the gastrointestinal or urinary tracts. Intestinal activity is intermittently abnormal with reverse peristalsis. The severity of the symptoms is variable.

**Clinical Findings:** May present as intermittent abdominal pain with constipation or diarrhea. Vomiting is a common sign. The abdomen is distended. The esophagus may show aperistalsis or other disturbance of motility. The esophagus, stomach, colon, or small bowel may be dilated. Symptoms are progressive and may remit and relapse. Hydronephrosis secondary to a neurogenic bladder with reflux has been reported. Examination of the bladder has revealed a thickening of the wall with fibrosis. Some patients have a normal number and appearance of ganglion cells, while others have shown hyperplasia or a decrease in the number of ganglion cells.

**Complications:** Malnutrition and weight loss may lead to death.

**Associated Findings:** The smooth muscle of the iris (pupillary sphincter) may be involved, as evidenced by mydriasis.

**Etiology:** Autosomal dominant inheritance. There are also pedigrees with similar clinical findings consistent with X-linked and autosomal recessive inheritance, even though most show dominant inheritance. Sporadic cases have also been reported.

**Pathogenesis:** Histologic studies of families with apparent autosomal dominant inheritance found normal number and appearance of ganglion cells and smooth muscle fibers. Reports of patients with decreased number of ganglion cells and nerve fibers by silver stain indicated a neuronal disorder. Another group of patients had fiber loss, degeneration, and fibrosis of the longitudinal intestinal muscle layer. The circular muscle layer may be similarly affected. Silver staining produced no evidence of ganglion cell or nerve fiber involvement; thus, a primary myopathy was considered. It may be due to alteration in contractile protein synthesis. Neuronal and smooth muscle abnormalities have been reported in one patient. Manometric studies showed a decrease in the total contractual activity of the bowel, including rhythmic short and propulsive (type III) waves.

**MIM No.:** *15531

**POS No.:** 4259

**Sex Ratio:** Unknown. A predominance of affected females was reported in one family without clear male-to-male transmission, suggesting heterogeneity with X-linked inheritance as a possibility.

**Occurrence:** Over 100 cases have been reported, including patients of German, Italian, and American-Black extraction.

**Risk of Recurrence for Patient's Sib:**
See Part I, *Mendelian Inheritance.*

**Risk of Recurrence for Patient's Child:**
See Part I, *Mendelian Inheritance.*

**Age of Detectability:** The gastrointestinal symptoms of the condition usually become manifest by late childhood or early adolescence, even though occurrence in middle age has been reported. The signs and symptoms may be progressive. The urinary tract is surprisingly asymptomatic, despite the underlying anomalies; it may become symptomatic, however, at varying ages.

**Gene Mapping and Linkage:** Unknown.

**Prevention:** None known. Genetic counseling indicated.

**Treatment:** Chronic abdominal pain and nausea may be assuaged by bed rest, intravenous fluids, and analgesics. Nasogastric suction and hyperalimentation may be used to treat the episodes of hypoperistalsis. Surgery may be of help in a few patients. Ileo-colic anastomosis has been of temporary benefit. Laparotomy may determine whether or not an anatomic obstruction exists in the proband; resection is not necessary. Further laparotomies may not be necessary in other affected family members. If bacterial overgrowth contributes to the abdominal distention, antibiotics may be helpful. Persistence of the hypoperistalsis requires hyperalimentation.

**Prognosis:** Growth and development do not appear to be significantly affected. Life span does not appear to be shortened, except in acute severe cases.

**Detection of Carrier:** Asymptomatic family members should be examined, especially for silent megaduodenum or renal abnormalities.

**Special Considerations:** Intestinal pseudo-obstruction can occur either as a primary or as a secondary condition. It may be due to **Scleroderma**, **Amyloidosis**, **Myotonic dystrophy**, or Chagas disease. Tricyclic antidepressants and phenothiazine may cause intestinal pseudo-obstruction. Patients without underlying disease are considered to have the heterogeneous "chronic idiopathic intestinal pseudo-obstruction" (CIIP), due to sporadic or familial *visceral neuropathy or myopathy*. The lack of an underlying condition, and the evidence of autosomal dominant mode of inheritance, are indicative of megacystis microcolon syndrome, which appears to be the most common cause of primary chronic intestinal pseudo-obstruction.

**References:**
Law DH, Ten Eyck EA: Familial megaduodenum and megacystis. Am J Med 1962; 33:911–922.
Faulk DL, et al.: A familial visceral myopathy. Ann Intern Med 1978; 89:600–606.
Roy AD, et al.: Idiopathic intestinal pseudo-obstruction: a familial visceral neuropathy. Clin Gen 1980; 18:291–297.
Schuffler MD, et al.: Chronic intestinal pseudo-obstruction: a report of 27 cases and review of the literature. Medicine 1981; 60:173–196. *
Mitros FA, et al.: Pathologic features of familial visceral myopathy. Hum Pathol 1982; 13:825–833.
Smout AJPM, et al.: Chronic idiopathic intestinal pseudo-obstruction: coexistence of smooth muscle and neuronal abnormalities. Dig Dis Sci 1985; 30:282–287.

HA069                                      **James K. Hartsfield, Jr.**

**Megacystis-microcolon-intestinal hypoperistalsis syndrome (MMIHS)**
*See INTESTINAL HYPOPERISTALSIS, MEGACYSTIS-MICROCOLON TYPE*
**Megadontia**
*See TEETH, MACRODONTIA*
**Megaduodenum, idiopathic**
*See INTESTINAL PSEUDO-OBSTRUCTION SYNDROMES*
**Megaduodenum-megacysts syndrome**
*See MEGACYSTIS-MEGADUODENUM SYNDROME* .
**Megaepiphyseal dwarfism**
*See OTO-SPONDYLO-MEGAEPIPHYSEAL DYSPLASIA*
**Megaesophagus**
*See ESOPHAGUS, ACHALASIA*
**Megakaryocytopenia-radius aplasia**
*See THROMBOCYTOPENIA-ABSENT RADIUS*

## MEGALENCEPHALY 2319

**Includes:**
Macrocephaly
Macrocephaly, benign familial
Macroencephaly
Megalobarencephaly
Megalocephaly

**Excludes:**
Brain edema
**Cebebral gigantism** (0137)
**CNS Neoplasms**(0188)
**Hydrocephaly** (0481)
Megalencephaly due to metabolic causes
Specific syndromes with anatomic megalencephaly

**Major Diagnostic Criteria:** The patient must have an occipitofrontal circumference (OFC) greater than 2 SD above the mean, and normal-sized or slightly enlarged but not enlarging ventricles, with no evidence of a metabolic cause for megalencephaly.

**Clinical Findings:** The question of megalencephaly arises when the patient's OFC exceeds 2 SD above the mean. It may be present at birth or discovered first as the head increases too rapidly after birth. If the patient has no neurologic deficits, the diagnosis is benign (and often familial) anatomic megalencephaly, or the patient may have any neurologic manifestation of a congenitally abnormal brain, such as retardation, seizures, or any variety of motor signs from hypotonia to spasticity. Although some megalencephalic infants have a normal birth weight, many have a birthweight in the 4,000–5,000g range. Some infants, as they grow, will become huge in stature, but many also have a dwarfed stature.

In spite of the increasing head size, the infant usually does not show symptoms and signs of increased intracranial pressure in the form of vomiting, or bulging fontanelle, but some may have a slight separation of skull sutures. The development of megalencephalic infants with neurologic deficits will fall behind the normal time table, but will not show a developmental peak followed by retrogression, which would characterize metabolic megalencephaly, increasing **Hydrocephaly**, or other lesions that progressively impair neurologic function.

**Complications:** Learning disabilities, mental retardation, seizures.

**Associated Findings:** A variety of mostly minor skeletal or visceral dysplasias may occur with megalencephaly. These include abnormal head shape, single palmar creases, ambiguous genitalia, heterotropia, and either gigantism or dwarfism.

**Etiology:** Usually autosomal dominant inheritance, in contrast to the metabolic megalencephalies, which tend to have an autosomal recessive pattern. No consistent chromosomal error is reported. In many instances, no genetic pattern is apparent. No exogenous teratogens are known to cause megalencephaly in man.

**Pathogenesis:** The enlarged brain has cells that are too large or too numerous. Whether this overgrowth in size or number affects neuronal and glial elements equally is unknown. While many large brains have a normal surface, some of the larger brains have distinct disorders of the gyral pattern. Some will show neuronal heterotopias and other evidence of a disturbance in the migration of neuroblasts from the periventricular proliferative zone to the cerebral surface. These patients will have severe impairment of mental and motor functions. No consistent biochemical error is known.

**MIM No.:** 24800

**CDC No.:** 742.400

**Sex Ratio:** M4:F1

**Occurrence:** Undetermined but presumed uncommon.

**Risk of Recurrence for Patient's Sib:**
See Part I, *Mendelian Inheritance.*

**Risk of Recurrence for Patient's Child:**
See Part I, *Mendelian Inheritance.*

**Age of Detectability:** Neonatal period or early infancy.

**Gene Mapping and Linkage:** Unknown.

**Prevention:** None known. Genetic counseling indicated.

**Treatment:** Unknown.

**Prognosis:** Depends on the functional capacity of the patient's brain.

**Detection of Carrier:** Measurement of OFC.

**Special Considerations:** The term, *megalocephaly* refers to any head with an excessive occipitofrontal circumference, without regard to the case or brain size. While some use the term *megalocephaly* or *macrocephaly* to describe megalencephaly, we urge all to use the most specific term possible. Also, it is wise not to interchange the terms, as a large head may contain a large brain as in megalencephaly; a dilated cerebrum as in **Hydrocephaly**; a small cerebrum (*micrencephaly*); or no cerebrum as in severe **Hydranencephaly**. *Macrocephaly* and its antonym, *microcephaly* refer only to the size of the cranium itself, while megalencephaly and its antonym, *micrencephaly* refer to an abnormal brain size. All of these quantitative terms denote size without regard to cause.

Major problems in differential diagnosis include how to classify the patient with a small body and an OFC that may remain within the upper border of normal, but is disproportionately large, or those huge-framed individuals who occupy the upper reaches of the normal distribution curve whose large head and brain merely reflect extremes of normal variation (these individuals have benign (asymptomatic) familial megalencephaly. When the diagnosis of megalencephaly is considered, the OFC of all available family members should be measured and any neurologic deficits that may exist should be determined. Whenever the suspicion arises of a neurologic deficit in a patient with megalencephaly, a CT or MRI scan should be ordered. If the patient has neurologic retrogression, a scan and a full workup for lysosomal enzyme defects and a metabolic type of megalencephaly may be necessary. Patients with benign familial anatomic megalencephaly have normal karyotypes.

**References:**
Portnoy HD, Croissant PD: Megalencephaly in infants and children: the possible role of increased dural sinus pressure. Arch Neurol 1978; 35:306–316.
Lorber J, Priestley BL: Children with large heads: a practical approach to diagnosis in 557 children, with special reference to 109 children with megalencephaly. Dev Med Child Neurol 1981; 23:494–504.
Lewis BA, et al.: Language and motor findings in benign megalencephaly. Ann Neurol 1983; 14:364 only.
Gooskens RH, et al.: Cerebrospinal fluid dynamics and cerebrospinal fluid infusion in children: clinical application of lumbar cerebrospinal fluid infusion in children with macrocephaly and normal growth rate of the head circumference. Neuropediatrics 1985; 16:121–125.
Alvarez LA, et al.: Idiopathic external hydrocephalus: natural history and relationship to benign familial macrocephaly. Pediatrics 1986; 77:901–907.
DeMyer W: Megalencephaly: types, clinical syndromes, and management. Pediatr Neurol 1986; 2:321–328.

DE007 **William DeMyer**

**Megalencephaly-cranial sclerosis-osteopathia striata**
*See OSTEOPATHIA STRIATA-CRANIAL SCLEROSIS-MEGALENCEPHALY*
**Megalencephaly-intestinal polyposis-pigmentary changes of genitali**
*See OVERGROWTH, RUVALCABA-MYHRE-SMITH TYPE*
**Megalobarencephaly**
*See MEGALENCEPHALY*
**Megalocephaly**
*See MEGALENCEPHALY*
**Megalocornea**
*See CORNEA, MEGALOCORNEA*

## MEGALOCORNEA-MENTAL RETARDATION SYNDROME      0638

**Includes:**
    Cerebral palsy, hypotonic-seizures-megalocornia
    MMR syndrome
    Seizures-hypotonic cerebral palsy-megalocornea-mental
      retardation

**Excludes:**   Marfan syndrome (0630)

**Major Diagnostic Criteria:** Megalocornea, short stature, and mental retardation.

**Clinical Findings:** Short stature and mental retardation of moderate-to-severe range. Hypotonic cerebral palsy consisting of delayed motor development, muscular hypotonia, and ataxia was present in most affected persons. Choreoathetotic movements were seen occasionally. Epileptic seizures occurred in most patients and EEG anomalies with generalized or focal discharges were noted. Megalocornea was present in all children, with a corneal diameter greater than 12–15 mm and accompanied by deep anterior chamber (anterior megalophthalmus), iris hypoplasia, and iridodonesis. Most patients were microcephalic from birth. Minor anomalies of the face included prominent forehead, telecanthus, epicanthus, and micrognathia.

**Complications:** Glaucoma, cataracts.

**Associated Findings:** None known.

**0638-20558:** Megalocornea-mental retardation syndrome; note megalocornea, prominent forehead, telecanthus, epicanthal folds and micrognathia in these affected siblings.

**Etiology:** Autosomal recessive inheritance.

**Pathogenesis:** Unknown.

**MIM No.:** *24931

**POS No.:** 3734

**Sex Ratio:** M1:F1

**Occurrence:** The syndrome has been observed in two boys and one girl of non-consanguineous parents, and in at least eight sporadic cases.

**Risk of Recurrence for Patient's Sib:**
    See Part I, *Mendelian Inheritance.*

**Risk of Recurrence for Patient's Child:**
    See Part I, *Mendelian Inheritance.*

**Age of Detectability:** Infancy or early childhood.

**Gene Mapping and Linkage:** Unknown.

**Prevention:** None known. Genetic counseling indicated.

**Treatment:** Early treatment of increased intraocular pressure and cataracts; physiotherapy and anticonvulsant medication.

**Prognosis:** Many patients are severely retarded.

**Detection of Carrier:** Unknown.

**References:**
Frank Y, et al.: Megalocornea associated with multiple skeletal anomalies-new genetic syndrome. J Genet Hum 1973; 21:67–72.
Neuhäuser G, et al.: Syndrome of mental retardation, seizures, hypotonic cerebral palsy and megalocorneae, recessively inherited. Z Kinderheilk 1975; 120:1–18.
Schmidt R, Rapin I: The syndrome of mental retardation and megalocornea. Am J Hum Genet 1981; 33:90A.
Del Giudice E, et al.; Megalocornea and mental retardation syndrome: two new cases. Am J Med Genet 1987; 26:417–420.
Gronbech-Jensen M: Megalocornea and mental retardation syndrome: a new case. Am J Med Genet 1989; 32:468–469.

NE012                     **Gerhard Neuhäuser**

**Megathrombocytopenia**
    *See LEUKOCYTE, MAY-HEGGLIN ANOMALY*
**Meige type lymphedema**
    *See LYMPHEDEMA II*
**Meischer cheilitis (oligosymptomatic forms)**
    *See CHEILITIS GRANULOMATOSA, MELKERSSON-ROSENTHAL TYPE*
**Melanesian ovalocytosis**
    *See ELLIPTOCYTOSIS*
**Melanin formation, reduction or absence**
    *See ALBINISM*
**Melanoblastosis cutis linearis**
    *See INCONTINENTIA PIGMENTI*
**Melanocytic nevus, congenital**
    *See NEVUS, CONGENITAL NEVOMELANOCYTIC*
**Melanocytic nevus, giant congenital**
    *See NEVUS, CONGENITAL NEVOMELANOCYTIC*
**Melanocytic nevus, small congenital**
    *See NEVUS, CONGENITAL NEVOMELANOCYTIC*
**Melanocytoma, optic disk**
    *See OPTIC DISK, MELANOCYTOMA*
**Melanoderma, familial generalized**
    *See SKIN, CUTANEOUS MELANOSIS, DIFFUSE*
**Melanodermic leukodystrophy**
    *See ADRENOLEUKODYSTROPHY, X-LINKED*
**Melanoleucoderma**
    *See BERLIN SYNDROME*
**Melanoma, benign of optic nerve head**
    *See OPTIC DISK, MELANOCYTOMA*
**Melanophoric nevus**
    *See ECTODERMAL DYSPLASIA, NAEGELI TYPE*
**Melanosis oculi, congenital**
    *See EYE, MELANOSIS OCULI, CONGENITAL*
**Melanosis retinae**
    *See RETINA, GROUPED HYPERTROPHY OF RETINAL PIGMENT EPITHELIUM*
**Melanosis retinae, congenital grouped**
    *See RETINA, GROUPED HYPERTROPHY OF RETINAL PIGMENT EPITHELIUM*

**Melanosis, neurocutaneous**
  See NEUROCUTANEOUS MELANOSIS
**Melanosis, universal**
  See SKIN, HYPERPIGMENTATION, FAMILIAL
**Melanotic ameloblastoma**
  See JAW, NEUROECTODERMAL PIGMENTED TUMOR
**Melanotic neuroectodermal tumor of infancy**
  See JAW, NEUROECTODERMAL PIGMENTED TUMOR
**Melanotic odontoma**
  See JAW, NEUROECTODERMAL PIGMENTED TUMOR
**Melanotic progonoma**
  See JAW, NEUROECTODERMAL PIGMENTED TUMOR
**MELAS**
  See MYOPATHY, MITOCHONDRIAL-ENCEPHALOPATHY-LACTIC
    ACIDOSIS-STROKE
**Meleda disease**
  See MAL DE MELEDA
**Melkersson-Rosenthal syndrome**
  See CHEILITIS GRANULOMATOSA, MELKERSSON-ROSENTHAL
    TYPE
**Melnick-Fraser syndrome**
  See BRANCHIO-OTO-RENAL DYSPLASIA
**Melnick-Needles osteodysplasty**
  See OSTEODYSPLASTY

## MELORHEOSTOSIS                                            0641

**Includes:**
  Flowing hyperostosis
  Melorheostosis Leri
  Osteosis eburnisans monomelica
**Excludes:**
  **Diaphyseal dysplasia** (0290)
  **Endosteal hyperostosis** (0497)

**Major Diagnostic Criteria:** This rare unilateral hyperostosis causes pain and joint stiffness and is diagnosed from the typical X-ray changes resembling melting wax dripping down from the side of a candle.

**Clinical Findings:** This disorder is a rare form of hyperostosis, which has a linear distribution along the major axis of the long

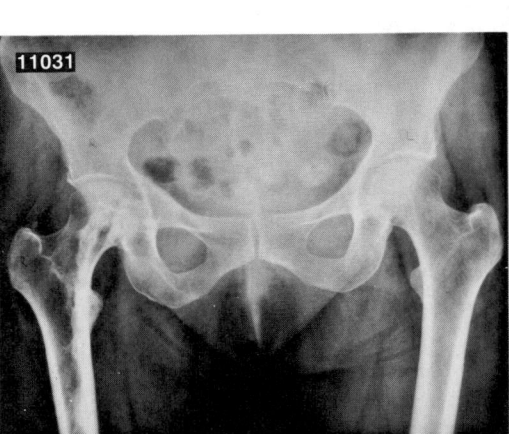

bones. On X-ray, the hyperostosis resembles melting wax dripping down the side of a candle, hence the term, melorheostosis, from the Greek words *melos* (member) and *rhein* (flow). The disease is almost always unilateral in its distribution, and usually affects a single limb. It is usually first detected in childhood or young adulthood, but it has been diagnosed at birth because of deformities of the fingers. Patients usually present because of progressive pain, stiffness, and limitation of motion, or deformity such as contractures of the fingers. The pain ranges from a dull to sharp ache; it is not constant, and is often aggravated by activity. The overlying skin is often normal in appearance, but may be tense, shiny, or erythematous. Linear scleroderma has been described. The subcutaneous tissues are often indurated and edematous, and the overlying muscles may be atrophic and weak. The adjacent joints may be intermittently warm and swollen with eventual limitation of joint motion due to soft tissue fibrosis. The affected limb may be shorter or, less commonly, longer. It usually appears larger in circumference, and may be angulated or curved.

X-rays reveal the typical molten wax appearance, with streaked sclerotic thickening of the side of the long bone. This irregular linear opacity runs along the major axis of the long bone, and may extend from one bone to an adjacent bone. The limb girdle is usually involved as well. The sclerosis may extend into the epiphyseal regions as streaks, but the articular areas are usually unaffected. The hyperostosis may not be prominent in infancy or childhood, but becomes more apparent with age.

Biopsies of affected sclerotic bones have revealed irregularly arranged Haversian systems, with dense thickened trabeculae and occasional islands of cartilage. Cellular fibrotic tissue is seen in the marrow spaces. Fibrosis of the subcutaneous tissues and skeletal muscle atrophy have been described. Degenerative, inflammatory, and obliterative changes have been noted in the surrounding blood vessels.

**Complications:** This disorder can lead to painful limitation of motion and weakness of the affected limb, as well as fibrous contractures of the adjacent joints.

**Associated Findings:** Some reports have described associated disorders such as scleroderma, **Neurofibromatosis**, lymphedema, hemangioma, vascular nevus, and A-V aneurysms, and localized osteopecilia.

**Etiology:** Possibly autosomal dominant inheritance.

**Pathogenesis:** Approximation of the anatomical distribution to the sclerotomes suggests a major, if not primary, role for the sensory nerve.

**MIM No.:** 15595

**Sex Ratio:** M1:F1

**Occurrence:** Unknown.

**Risk of Recurrence for Patient's Sib:** Undetermined. All cases to date have been sporadic.

**Risk of Recurrence for Patient's Child:** Unknown.

**Age of Detectability:** From birth by medical imaging. Usually not diagnosed until late childhood or early adulthood, when a limb is X-rayed because of pain symptoms or joint immobility.

**Gene Mapping and Linkage:** Unknown.

**Prevention:** None known. Genetic counseling indicated.

**Treatment:** Orthopedic procedures to prevent or correct limb deformities.

**Prognosis:** Apparently normal for life span. The pain and disability are usually progressive.

**Detection of Carrier:** Unknown.

**References:**
Morris JM, et al.: Melorheostosis. J Bone Joint Surg [Am] 1963; 45A:1191–1206.
Patrick JH: Melorheostosis associated with arteriovenous aneurysm of the left arm and trunk. J Bone Joint Surg [Br] 1969; 51B:126–129.

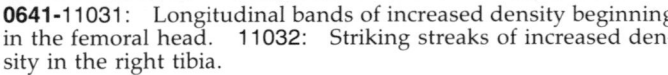

**0641-11031:** Longitudinal bands of increased density beginning in the femoral head.   **11032:** Striking streaks of increased density in the right tibia.

Murry RO, McCredi E: Melorheosteosis and the sclerotomes: a radiological correlation. Skeletal Radiol 1979; 4:57–71.

B0025          **Zvi Borochowitz**
*David L. Rimoin*

**Melorheostosis Leri**
  *See MELORHEOSTOSIS*
**Meltzer-Franklin syndrome**
  *See CRYOGLOBULINEMIA*
**Membranous cataract**
  *See CATARACT, AUTOSOMAL DOMINANT CONGENITAL*
**Membranous choanal atresia, anterior**
  *See NOSE, ANTERIOR ATRESIA*
**Membranous choanal atresia, posterior**
  *See NOSE, POSTERIOR ATRESIA*
**Membranous conjunctivitis**
  *See EYE, LIGNEOUS CONJUNCTIVITIS*
**Membranous lipodystrophy**
  *See OSTEODYSPLASIA, LIPOMEMBRANOUS POLYCYSTIC-DEMENTIA*
**Membranous septal defect**
  *See VENTRICULAR SEPTAL DEFECT*
**Membranous subaortic stenosis**
  *See HEART, SUBAORTIC STENOSIS, FIBROUS*
**MEN II syndrome**
  *See ENDOCRINE NEOPLASIA, MULTIPLE TYPE II*
**MEN IIa syndrome**
  *See ENDOCRINE NEOPLASIA, MULTIPLE TYPE II*
**MEN IIb syndrome**
  *See ENDOCRINE NEOPLASIA, MULTIPLE TYPE III*
**Mendenhall syndrome**
  *See LIPODYSTROPHY-COARSE FACIES-ACANTHOSIS NIGRICANS, MIESCHER TYPE*
**Mendes da Costa syndrome**
  *See SKIN, ERYTHROKERATODERMIA, VARIABLE*
**Meningeal capillary angiomatosis**
  *See STURGE-WEBER SYNDROME*
**Meningitis-polyarthritis-lymphadenitis-pulmonary hemosiderosis**
  *See INFLAMMATORY DISEASE, NEONATAL BATES-LORBER TYPE*

## MENINGOCELE      0642

**Includes:**
  Cranial meningoceles
  Neural-tube defect
  Spina bifida cystica without neurologic deficit

**Excludes:**
  **Encephalocele** (0343)
  **Lipomeningocele** (0602)
  **Meningomyelocele** (0693)
  Myelorachischisis
  **Schisis association** (2249)
  Spina bifida occulta

**Major Diagnostic Criteria:** Translucent skin mass over the vertebral column or cranium, with spina bifida and widening of interpedicular distance seen on X-ray.

**Clinical Findings:** Most commonly seen in the lumbar area, a skin-covered mass of soft tissue occurs either over the midline of the back or slightly off to one side of the midline. Herniation of the meninges can occur over the midline of the cervical spine and cranium. In the latter location they are called cranial meningoceles. The overlying skin may have an angiomatous or hairy patch. There is no paralysis or sensory loss. The head circumference is normal; hydrocephaly rarely is associated. On X-ray, spina bifida underlies the mass.

**Complications:** Breakdown of the skin covering. Rarely, nerve roots are trapped in the sac, causing leg weakness.

**Associated Findings:** May be a component of many other syndromes.

**Etiology:** Polygenic.

**Pathogenesis:** Failure of complete midline fusion of the vertebral arches, with cystic distention of the meninges, but without neural tissue in the sac. Gardner's (1968) theory is based upon the existence of hydrocephalus and hydromyelia as a normal condition in early embryonic life: a result of fluid first secreted by the neural epithelium and then by the choroid plexus. By preventing the normal circulation of cerebrospinal fluid, the delay or failure of permeation of the roof of the fourth ventricle will produce all grades of anomalies seen in the dysraphic states. A meningocele results when the internal hydromyelia becomes external; the expanding subarachnoid space then bulges beneath cutaneous ectoderm impeding, at the same time, proper mesodermal closure.

**POS No.:** 3720

**Sex Ratio:** M1:F1

**Occurrence:** Estimated 1:20,000 live births.

**Risk of Recurrence for Patient's Sib:** Depends on ethnic group and geographic location. Can vary between 2–6%, as in other neural tube defects.

**Risk of Recurrence for Patient's Child:** Depends on ethnic group and geographic location. Can vary between 2–6%, as in other neural tube defects.

**Age of Detectability:** Prenatally in second trimester by amniography, fetoscopy and, ultrasonography, which shows a U-shaped deformity of the fetal spine, with a sonolucent area.

**Gene Mapping and Linkage:** Unknown.

**Prevention:** Mulinare et al (1988) have presented data showing that preconceptional use of multivitamins can reduced the risk of neural tube defects.

**Treatment:** Repair of cystic mass during first year of life.

**Prognosis:** Good.

**Detection of Carrier:** Unknown.

**Support Groups:**
  MD; Rockville; Spina Bifida Association of America (SBAA)
  CANADA: Manitoba; Winnipeg; Spina Bifida Association of Canada
  SWEDEN: Stockholm; International Federation for Hydrocephalus and Spina Bifida

**References:**
Gardner WJ: Myelocele: rupture of the neural tube? Clin Neurosurg 1968; 15:57.
Shulman K, Shapiro K: Defects of closure of the neural plate. In: Rudolph A, ed: Pediatrics. 16th ed. New York: Appleton-Century-Crofts, 1977:1757.
Mulinare J, et al.: Periconceptional use of multivitamins and the occurrence of neural tube defects. JAMA 1988; 260:3141–3145.
Mills JL, et al.: The absence of a relationship between the periconceptional use of vitamins and neural-tube defects. New Engl J Med 1989; 321:430–435.

SH007        **Kenneth Shapiro**

**Meningocele, anterior sacral**
  *See TERATOMA, PRESACRAL-SACRAL DYSGENESIS*

## MENINGOCELE-CONOTRUNCAL HEART DEFECT, KOUSSEFF TYPE      2266

**Includes:**
  Sacral meningocele-conotruncal heart defects-head/neck anomalies
  Kousseff syndrome

**Excludes:**
  **Heart, transposition of great vessels** (0962)
  **Heart, truncus arteriosus** (0972)
  **Hydrocephaly** (0481)
  **Meningocele** (0642)
  **Meningomyelocele** (0693)
  **Schisis association** (2249)

**Major Diagnostic Criteria:** Characteristic head and neck anomalies, conotruncal heart defects, and sacral meningoceles.

**Clinical Findings:** Findings in four known cases included depressed nasal tip (1), retrognathia (4) short neck/excess neck skin (3), minimally low-set ears (4); conotruncal cardiac defects (3); sacral **Meningocele** / **Meningomyelocele** (4); unilateral renal agenesis (1).

Birth weight, length, and occipito-frontal circumference are all normal.

**Complications:** **Hydrocephaly** occurred in three cases, seizures in one case.

**Associated Findings:** None known.

**Etiology:** The occurrence of this syndrome is sibs of each sex is strongly suggestive of autosomal recessive inheritance.

**Pathogenesis:** Unknown.

**MIM No.:** 24521

**POS No.:** 3172

**Sex Ratio:** M3:F1 (observed).

**Occurrence:** Undetermined. May account for as much as 1% of spina bifida cases. Four cases have been reported.

**Risk of Recurrence for Patient's Sib:**
See Part I, *Mendelian Inheritance.*

**Risk of Recurrence for Patient's Child:**
See Part I, *Mendelian Inheritance.*

**Age of Detectability:** At birth by physical examination. In the one case in which prenatal diagnosis was attempted, serum alpha feto-protein levels were normal; amniotic alpha feto-protein levels were slightly elevated. An increased number of rapidly adhering cells were also observed from the amniotic sample. Ultrasound at 15, 17, and 22 weeks did not detect any defects (although this infant was subsequently found to be affected).

**Gene Mapping and Linkage:** Unknown.

**Prevention:** None known. Genetic counseling indicated.

**Treatment:** When indicated, surgical repair of the cardiac and sacral defects; shunting for the **Hydrocephaly**.

**Prognosis:** Unknown.

**Detection of Carrier:** Unknown.

**Support Groups:**
MD; Rockville; Spina Bifida Association of America (SBAA)
CANADA: Manitoba; Winnipeg; Spina Bifida Association of Canada
SWEDEN: Stockholm; International Federation for Hydrocephalus and Spina Bifida

**References:**
Kousseff BG: Sacral meningocele with conotruncal heart defects: a possible autosomal recessive trait. Pediatrics 1984; 74:395–398. *
Toriello HV, et al.: Autosomal recessive syndrome of sacral and contruncal developmental field defects (Kousseff syndrome). Am J Med Genet. 1985; 22:357–360. †

T0007                                          Helga V. Toriello

## MENINGOMYELOCELE                                          0693

**Includes:**
Myelomeningocele
Myeloschisis
Neural-tube defect
Spina bifida cystica with paralysis
Valproic acid, fetal effects

**Excludes:**
**Hydrocephaly** (0481)
**Lipomeningocele** (0602)
**Meningocele** (0642)

**Major Diagnostic Criteria:** Midline spinal defect with neurologic deficit.

**Clinical Findings:** A visible sac or epithelial defect over the spine, caudal to the level of the lesion in which nerve tissue can be seen,

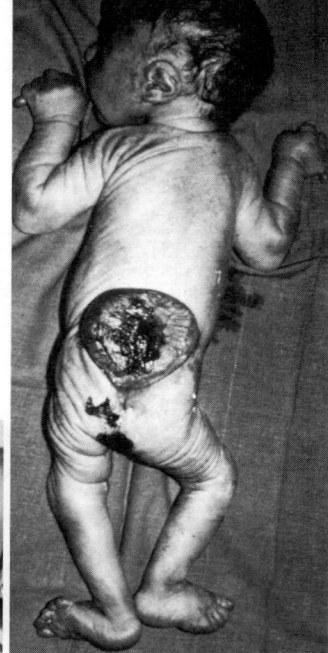

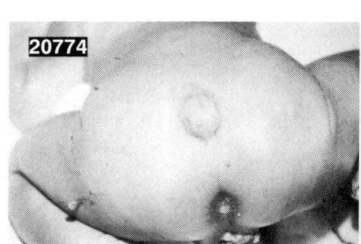

0693-20774: Meningomyelocele, small lumbar-sacral meningomyelocele. 20775: Lumbar meningomyelocele.

and associated with neurologic deficit. The surface lesion varies from one that is almost completely skin covered to a fully exposed lower spinal cord and cauda equina. In myeloschisis, the paravertebral muscle mass is also exposed. Neurologic loss is generally of the lower motor neuron type, with absent reflexes and segmental sensory loss. However, spotty sensory deficit may be seen. Bowel and bladder sphincter loss is usual. Myelomeningocele occurs most frequently in the lumbosacral area followed by the cervical area. An enlarged head indicating hydrocephaly associated with the Arnold-Chiari malformation is often found.

**Complications:** *Nervous system*: Hydrocephalus is present in about 90% of patients secondary to the **Brain, Arnold-Chiari malformation**. Lower cranial nerve abnormalities and long tract signs also may complicate the Arnold-Chiari malformation. Mental retardation is noted in about 10% of children.
*Urologic*: Neurogenic bladder may be complicated by recurrent urinary tract infection or hydronephrosis. Urinary incontinence is usually found.
*Orthopedic*: Foot, knee, and/or hip deformities may be found, depending upon the level of the spinal cord defect. Scoliosis develops frequently.

**Associated Findings:** Structural GU anomalies and, less frequently, cardiac, craniofacial, and limb anomalies.

**Etiology:** Multifactorial. Nutritional factors may play a role. Some children with **Chromosome 18, trisomy 18** have neural tube defects. Recent data suggest maternal exposure to valproic acid may cause this defect (see **Fetal valproate syndrome**).

**Pathogenesis:** Failure of neural tube closure at four weeks gestation or later. Cleft formation and cord splitting due to central cord distention with overgrowth of neural elements.

**POS No.:** 3720

**CDC No.:** 741

**Sex Ratio:** M1:F>1. Slightly more common in females.

**Occurrence:** 1:500 to 1:2,000 live births. Spina bifida occured in 4.3:10,000 live births in the United States in 1987. There is wide geographic and ethnic variation, and "epidemics" have been well documented. The condition is associated with low socioeconomic status; the rate in Appalachia is more than twice the United States national average, and the rate in rural China is about nine times that in the United States.

**Risk of Recurrence for Patient's Sib:** 2–5% depending on family history, ethnic group, and geographic location.

**Risk of Recurrence for Patient's Child:** 2–5% depending on family history, ethnic group, and geographic location.

**Age of Detectability:** Prenatally in second trimester by amniography, fetoscopy, and ultrasonography; which show a U-shaped deformity of fetal spine with a sonolucent area. In the amniotic fluid, there are elevated levels of alpha-fetoprotein (AFP), and acetylcholinesterase, as well as other substances. AFP is elevated in maternal serum.

**Gene Mapping and Linkage:** Unknown.

**Prevention:** Recent research suggests a possible relationship between maternal nutrition or vitamin deficiency and neural tube defects (Mulinare et al, 1988).

**Treatment:** Repair of open defects to prevent meningitis and loss of neural function. Treatment of hydrocephaly. Treatment of urologic, orthopedic, and CNS complications.

**Prognosis:** Good in patients with minimal neurologic defects without hydrocephaly. Prognosis in others varies with extent of lesion and presence of complications. The number of children surviving with spina bifida is increasing. Of about 13,600 American children born with the condition between 1980 and 1987, an estimated 9,800 were alive in 1987.

**Detection of Carrier:** Unknown.

**Support Groups:**
MD; Rockville; Spina Bifida Association of America (SBAA)
CANADA: Manitoba; Winnipeg; Spina Bifida Association of Canada
SWEDEN: Stockholm; International Federation for Hydrocephalus and Spina Bifida

**References:**
Holmes LB, et al.: Etiologic heterogenicity of neural tube defects. New Engl J Med 1976; 294:365.
Black PM: Selective treatment of infants with myelomeningocele. Neurosurgery 1979; 5:334.
Colgan MT: The child with spina bifida. Am J Dis Child 1981; 135:854.
Toriello HV, Higgins JV: Occurrence of neural tube defects among first-, second-, and third-degree relatives of probands: results of a United States study. Am J Med Genet 1983; 15:601.
Mulinare J, et al.: Periconceptional use of multivitamins and the occurrence of neural tube defects. JAMA 1988; 260:3141–3145.
Mills JL, et al.: The absence of a relationship between the preconceptional use of vitamins and neural-tube defects. New Engl J Med 1989; 321; 430–435.
Milunsky A, et al.: Multi-vitamin/folic acid supplementation in early pregnancy reduces the prevalence of neural tube defects. J Am Med Asso 1989; 262:2847–2852.

SH007                                       **Kenneth Shapiro**
BA039                             **Louis E. Bartoshesky**

---

## MENKES SYNDROME                     0643

**Includes:**
Copper transport disease
Kinky hair disease
Sex-linked neurodegenerative disease associated with monilethrix
Steely hair disease
Trichopoliodystrophy
X-linked copper malabsorption

**Excludes:**
Aciduria, argininosuccinic (0087)

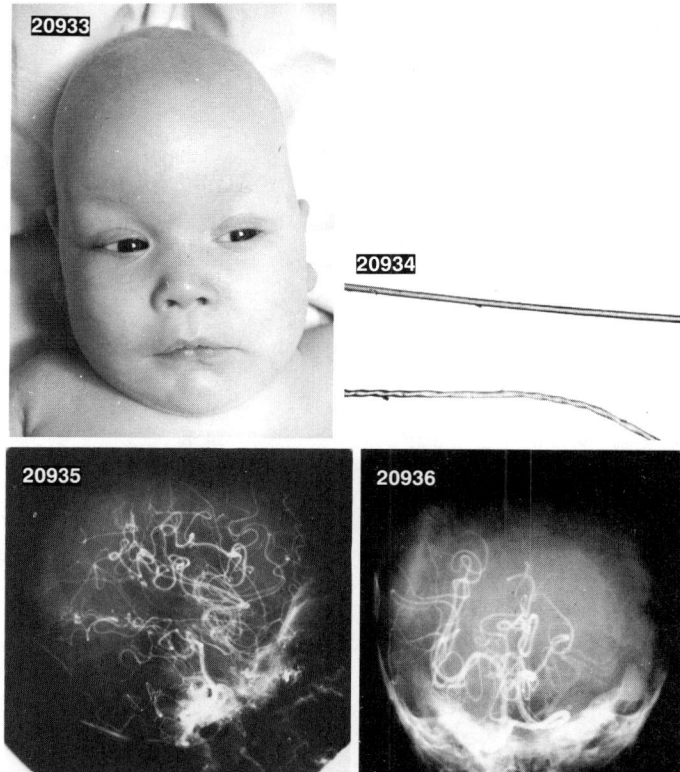

**0643A-20933:** Menkes syndrome; note the cherubic appearance of the face and the sparse, brittle scalp hair and lashes. **20934:** Spiral, twisted microscopic appearance of the scalp hair (lower) from the child shown in 20933 compared with a straight, normal hair (upper). **20935:** Lateral view of cerebral arteriogram showing tortuous, winding vessels. **20936:** Vertebral cerebral arteriogram shows tortuous vessels.

---

Biotinidase deficiency (2591)
Nutritional copper deficiency

**Major Diagnostic Criteria:** Male sex, abnormal hair, seizures, developmental retardation, low serum copper and ceruloplasmin, abnormalities as they appear on X-rays and EEG.

The relatively unique clinical feature of Menkes syndrome is the coarse, colorless, sparse, friable secondary scalp hair, with variable microscopic abnormalities, of which pili torti (twisting of the shaft) is most common, but also including monilethrix (variations in diameter) or trichorrhexis nodosa (fragmentation).

Seizures are the most common initial symptom and have a peak incidence at age 3 months. After age five months the EEG pattern often resembles hypsarrhythmia. The typical facial appearance has been described as cherubic with pudgy cheeks, irregular eyebrows, micrognathia, and expressionless facies. The course is progressively fatal and is characterized by developmental failure or regression. Bone changes may lead to the misdiagnosis of child abuse.

Average birth weight is 2,660 grams. Neuropathological findings consist of widespread cortical neuronal loss, demyelination and gliosis of the white matter, and profound reduction of all elements of the cerebellum.

**Clinical Findings:** Percentages calculated from review by French (1977), N=37.
*Clinical findings:* Progressively fatal course (100%); male sex [X-linked inheritance] (100%); seizures (95%); abnormal secondary hair (94%); developmental regression or failure after earlier devel-

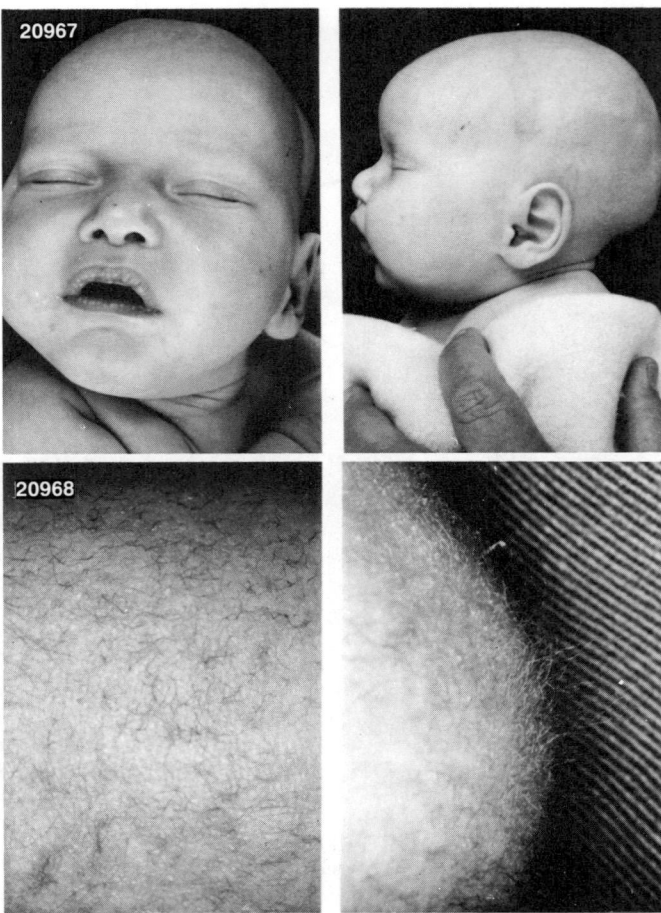

**0643B-20967:** Menkes syndrome; note sparse, fine, brittle hair and decreased eyebrows and eyelashes. **20968:** Close-up of sparse, brittle, wiry hair which is depigmented and lacks lustre. The short stubbles of broken hair are characteristic.

opmental progress (81%); abnormal muscle tone [hyperreflexia and spasticity most common - 38%] (68%); prematurity [gestational age 34–37 weeks] (55%); terminal or intermittent respiratory infections (49%); micrognathia (46%); thermal instability [intermittent or persistent] (43%); oral abnormalities [high-arched palate, failure or delay of tooth eruption] (32%); microcephaly [less than second percentile] (32%); abnormal neonatal adaptation [depressed Apgar, meconium staining, lethargy, respiratory problems, feeding problems, thermal instability] (30%); weight less than third percentile (30%); variable congenital malformations [pectus excavatum, talipes, hernias, undescended testes, etc.] (30%); intracranial subdural fluid collections and/or membranes (22%); neonatal icterus (19%); gastrointestinal symptoms [emesis, gastroenteritis, feeding difficulty] (19%); abnormal skull or facial shape [asymmetry, bossing, etc.] (16%); neuro-ophthalmic deficits [disc pallor; dysplastic optic disks; horizontal nystagmus; episodic, rapid, vertical eye movements; nystagmoid eye movements] (16%); survival past age two years (12%); neonatal-onset developmental failure (11%); and growth failure (common but percentage undetermined).

*Other findings:* Low serum copper (100%); low serum ceruloplasmin (97%); abnormal EEG at some time during life (97%); tortuous, abnormal cerebral arteries [based on 6 of 7 cases with cerebral angiograms] (86%); metaphyseal spurring or fractures [with or without periosteal thickening or new bone formation (19/24)] (80%); long bone metaphyseal cupping or anterior rib end flaring [based on 20 of 27 patients X-rayed] (80%). Additional findings for which percentages are unknown include abnormal visual evoked responses; abnormal electroretinogram; tortuous systemic arteries; anemia, usually hypochromic; wormian bones; bladder diverticuli; hydroureters, and ureteric reflux.

**Complications:** Developmental failure or regression, death.

**Associated Findings:** Seborrheic dermatitis (16%), simian creases (15%), pyogenic leptomeningitis (8%), macrocephaly, neonatal occurrence of "kinky hair" (one reported case) or "steely, depigmented hair" (2 cases), early infancy vascular collapse (one reported case).

**Etiology:** X-linked inheritance of copper malabsorption.

**Pathogenesis:** Evidence suggests that the basic defect in Menkes syndrome is a selective defect in tissue uptake or retention of copper, or abnormal copper transport. This concept is supported by an incomplete gastrointestinal absorption defect (10–25% of normal) when patients are given oral $^{67}Cu$, while duodenal biopsies have shown increased copper concentration. Intravenous copper therapy can normalize serum copper levels but not brain copper levels. In spite of hypocupremia in untreated patients, erythrocyte copper concentration is normal. This is in contrast to normal children with nutritional copper deficiency in whom erythrocyte copper is depleted. The findings of characteristic hair abnormalities, elevated blood copper and ceruloplasmin, decreased hepatic copper levels, and increased urinary copper excretion in two newborns with Menkes syndrome who subsequently had a decrease in blood copper levels is further evidence for the presence of adequate transplacental copper transport combined with in utero selective deficits of copper transport, or tissue uptake or retention. These selective defects may account for the failure of simple parenteral copper therapy.

Most of the clinical and laboratory deficits are postulated to be caused by dysfunction of the numerous copper-dependent enzyme systems. These enzyme systems are involved in connective tissue synthesis and cross linkage (lysyoxidase), melanin synthesis (tyrosinase), catabolism of superoxide (superoxide dismutase), neurotransmitter synthesis (dopamine-β-hydroxylase), nicotinic acid synthesis (hepatic tryptophan pyrollase), and mitochondrial function (cytochrome c oxidase). Hypoceruloplasminemia may lead to deficient ferroxidase activity and may disrupt ascorbic acid oxidation.

**MIM No.:** *30940

**POS No.:** 3290

**CDC No.:** 759.870

**Sex Ratio:** M1:F0

**Occurrence:** Incidence in Australia 29:1,000,000. Less than 40 cases documented in the literature.

**Risk of Recurrence for Patient's Sib:**
See Part I, *Mendelian Inheritance.*

**Risk of Recurrence for Patient's Child:**
See Part I, *Mendelian Inheritance.* Affected individuals are not expected to survive to reproduce.

**Age of Detectability:** Prenatally by amniotic fibroblast copper incorporation studies, or at birth by finding elevated serum copper and ceruloplasmin, decreased hepatic copper levels, increased urinary copper excretion.

**Gene Mapping and Linkage:** MNK (Menkes syndrome) has been mapped to Xcen-q13.

**Prevention:** None known. Genetic counseling indicated.

**Treatment:** Administration of parenteral copper or oral copper chelated to trisodium nitrilotriacetate or histidine has resulted in increased ceruloplasmin levels and normal blood and liver copper levels, but the copper level in the brain has remained low. There is currently no effective treatment; however, copper therapy may improve seizure control (Grover et al, 1982). To be successful, initiation of therapy in utero may be required. Treatment of complications includes anticonvulsants for seizures, drainage for subdural fluid collections, antibiotics for meningitis, and iron for iron-deficiency anemia.

**Prognosis:** Death usually occurs within two years and is commonly associated with pneumonia.

**Detection of Carrier:** Mothers or sisters of some boys with Menkes syndrome have had microscopic hair abnormalities. Scanning electron microscopy of the hair may aid carrier identification. If hair abnormalities are not present, there is no reliable method of carrier detection. The sister of a Black American boy had mottled skin. Fibroblast copper concentration has been elevated in all tested children with Menkes syndrome. Fibroblast copper concentration was elevated in one of two possible maternal heterozygotes; however, in another study, two presumed heterozygote mothers had copper concentration values indistinguishable from controls.

**Special Considerations:** The concept of allelic variation with differing manifestations or genetic heterogeneity is supported by cases of Menkes disease with a milder course (Procopis et al, 1981).

A disorder of copper metabolism with X-linked inheritance was studied by Haas et al (1981) in two brothers. The boys were thought to have a disorder distinct from Menkes syndrome because of several features unlike the typical Menkes profile; i.e., prolonged survival, hypotonia, choreoathetosis, and the absence of hair, skin, facial, or bony changes. However, the possibility that these cases represent an allelic variant of Menkes is strengthened by several factors: hair changes become less prominent with age in untreated Menkes syndrome; hair abnormalities (pili torti) present by scanning electron microscope may not be discernible by light microscope (Taylor and Green, 1981); cases occur with hypotonia (Grover et al, 1979); and finally, the presence of choreoathetosis in the patients of Haas et al may be due to their long survival (choreoathetosis in their patients was not commented on until the ages of two and nine years). DNA linkage studies may clarify these issues.

**Support Groups:** VA; Dumfries; Wilson's Disease Association

**References:**

Danks DM, et al.: Menkes' kinky hair syndrome; an inherited defect in copper absorption with widespread effects. Pediatrics 1972; 50:188–201.

Horn N: Copper incorporation studies on cultured cells for prenatal diagnosis of Menkes' disease. Lancet 1976; I:1156–1158.

French JH: X-chromosome-linked copper malabsorption. In: Vinken PJ, Bruyn GW, eds: Handbook of clinical neurology. vol. 29. Amsterdam: North Holland Publishing, 1977:279–309.

Grover WD, et al.: Clinical and biochemical aspects of tricho-poliodystrophy. Ann Neurol 1979; 5:65–71.

Haas RH, et al.: An X-linked disease of the nervous system with disordered copper metabolism and features differing from Menkes disease. Neurology 1981; 31:852–859.

Procopis P, et al.: A mild form of Menkes steely hair syndrome. J Pediatr 1981; 98:97–99.

Taylor CJ, Green SH: Menkes's syndrome (trichopoliodystrophy): use of a scanning electron microscope in diagnosis and carrier identification. Develop Med Child Neurol 1981; 23:361–368.

Grover WD, et al.: A defect in catecholamine metabolism in kinky-hair disease. Ann Neurol 1982; 12:263–266.

Kuivaniemi H, et al.: Type IX Ehlers-Danlos syndrome and Menkes syndrome: the decrease in lysyl oxidase activity is associated with a corresponding deficiency in the enzyme protein. Am J Hum Genet 1985; 37:798–808.

Leone A, et al.: Menkes' disease: abnormal metallothionein gene regulation in response to copper. Cell 1985; 40:301–309.

Moore CM, Howell RR: Ectodermal manifestations in Menkes disease. Clin Genet 1985; 28:532–540.

Tonnesen T, et al.: Measurement of copper in chorionic villi for first trimester diagnosis of Menkes disease (letter) Lancet 1985; I:1038–1039.

Beighton P, et al.: International nosology of heritable disorders of connective tissue, Berlin, 1986. Am J Med Genet 1988; 29:581–594.

Danks DM: The mild form of Menkes disease: progress report on the original case. Am J Med Genet 1988; 30:859–864.

KA008
DS000

**Raymond S. Kandt**
**Bernard D'Souza**

Menotropin, ovulation induction trisomy
  *See OVULATION INDUCTION TRISOMY*
Mental deficiency-epilepsy-endocrine disorders
  *See BORJESON-FORSSMAN-LEHMANN SYNDROME*
Mental retardation syndrome, Mietens-Weber type
  *See MIETENS-WEBER SYNDROME*
Mental retardation, ACD type
  *See ALOPECIA-SKELETAL ANOMALIES-SHORT STATURE-MENTAL RETARDATION*
Mental retardation, Buenes Aires type
  *See MUTCHINICK SYNDROME*
Mental retardation, from extrinsically caused iodine disorder
  *See CRETINISM, ENDEMIC, AND RELATED DISORDERS*

---

**MENTAL RETARDATION, HEMOGLOBIN H RELATED**     **3103**

**Includes:**
  Chromosome 16, interstitial deletions at alpha-globin loci
  Hemoglobin H disease-mental retardation-multiple anomalies

**Excludes:**
  Alpha-thalassemia, silent carrier and trait forms of Hemoglobin H disease without mental retardation

**Major Diagnostic Criteria:** Developmental delay and hemoglobin H disease with or without congenital anomalies.

**Clinical Findings:** The mental retardation is moderate to severe, with reported IQ scores ranging from 76 to <50. Congenital anomalies and features reported in over one-half of cases include hypotonia, **Microcephaly**, telecanthus, onset of seizures in childhood, foot deformity, and cryptorchidism. One child also had **Hypospadias** and **Ductus arteriosus, patent**. In the one reported female patient, no associated congenital anomalies were noted.

In all reported cases studied by DNA analysis, one parent had a normal alpha-globin genotype ($\alpha\alpha/\alpha\alpha$) while the other was heterozygous for alpha-thalassemia 2 ($-\alpha/\alpha\alpha$). This is different from the usual form of hemoglobin H disease in which offspring result from matings between alpha-thal 2 and alpha-thal 1 heterozygotes ($[-\alpha/\alpha\alpha]$ X $[-/\alpha\alpha]$). All karyotypes performed were normal.

**Complications:** Unknown.

**Associated Findings:** None known.

**Etiology:** Hemoglobin H-related mental retardation appears to be a sporadic event arising from matings between an alpha-thalassemic and a non-alpha-thalassemic parent. Thus, it may result from *de novo* interstitial deletions of portions of chromosome 16 contiguous to and including the alpha-globin loci.

**Pathogenesis:** The effect of this hypothesized acquired abnormality of chromosome 16 is unclear. It has been proposed that this disorder may result from intrauterine anoxia secondary to deficient alpha-globin synthesis in the fetus, but this seems unlikely since the association is not reported in the Oriental and Mediterranean populations where familial hemoglobin H disease is relatively more common.

**MIM No.:** 14175

**Sex Ratio:** M4:F1 (observed).

**Occurrence:** Hemoglobin H-related mental retardation has been reported in four unrelated male children and one female child of Northern European origin. Hemoglobin H disease is a form of alpha-thalassemia that usually occurs in persons of Oriental or Mediterranean origin and only rarely in Northern Europeans. As a rule, affected individuals are the offspring of matings between alpha-thal 2 and alpha-thal 1 heterozygotes ($[-\alpha/\alpha\alpha]$ X $[-/\alpha\alpha]$). Patients with hemoglobin H and mental retardation are unusual, not only for their Northern European background but also because each had one parent without alpha-thalassemia. Restriction endonuclease mapping demonstrated one child to be ($-/-\alpha$) from a de novo cis deletion on the paternally derived chromosome 16 paired with the single alpha-globin gene inherited from the mother. While this child had the genotype typically seen in Oriental and Mediterranean populations affected with hemoglobin H disease, two other patients evaluated by restriction endonuclease mapping showed no deletion in either the affected children or the parents, indicating they had nondeletion forms of the disease ($\alpha\alpha^T/\alpha^T\alpha^T$). In these three patients a spontaneous mutation or unequal crossing-over event affecting alpha-globin gene expression is implied since at least one parent does not have alpha-thalassemia. The effects of these mutations on contiguous gene(s) may cause the associated mental retardation and congenital anomalies.

**Risk of Recurrence for Patient's Sib:** Unknown. *De novo* deletions implied.

**Risk of Recurrence for Patient's Child:** Unknown. *De novo* deletions implied.

**Age of Detectability:** During infancy.

**Gene Mapping and Linkage:** Presumably the affected gene(s) are contiguous with the alpha-globin loci on chromosome 16.

**Prevention:** None known. Genetic counseling indicated.

**Treatment:** Management of clinical symptoms as indicated.

**Prognosis:** All affected individuals have had moderate-to-severe mental retardation. Life span is undetermined.

**Detection of Carrier:** Unknown.

**References:**

Ronisch P, Kleihauer E: Alpha-thalassamie mit HbH und Hb Bart's in einer deutschen familie. Klin Wochenschr 1967; 45:1193–1200.
Borochovitz D, et al.: Hemoglobin-H disease in association with multiple congenital abnormalities. Clin Pediatr 1970; 9:432–435.
Phillips JA III, et al.: Unequal crossing-over: a common basis of single alpha-globin genes in Asians and American blacks with hemoglobin-H disease. Blood 1980; 55:1066–1069.
Weatherall DJ, et al.: Hemoglobin H disease and mental retardation: a new syndrome or a remarkable coincidence? New Engl J Med 1981; 305:607–612. †
Schmickel RD: Contiguous gene syndromes: a component of recognizable syndromes. J Pediat 1986; 109:231–241.

ST056
PH003

**Stephen M. Strakowski**
**John A. Phillips, III**

**Mental retardation, Smith-Fineman-Myers type**
*See SMITH-FINEMAN-MYERS SYNDROME*
**Mental retardation, X-linked-marXq28**
*See X-LINKED MENTAL RETARDATION, FRAGILE X SYNDROME*
**Mental retardation-alopecia**
*See ALOPECIA-MENTAL RETARDATION*
**Mental retardation-alopecia-skeletal anomalies-short stature**
*See ALOPECIA-SKELETAL ANOMALIES-SHORT STATURE-MENTAL RETARDATION*
**Mental retardation-aplasia-shuffling gait-adducted thumbs (MASA)**
*See X-LINKED MENTAL RETARDATION-CLASPED THUMB*
**Mental retardation-ears (malformed)-deafness**
*See DEAFNESS-MALFORMED EARS-MENTAL RETARDATION*
**Mental retardation-growth/hearing/genetal defects, X-linked**
*See X-LINKED MENTAL RETARDATION-GROWTH-HEARING AND GENITAL DEFECTS*

## MENTAL RETARDATION-HEART DEFECTS-BLEPHAROPHIMOSIS  3132

**Includes:**
Blepharophimosis-blepharoptosis-heart defects-mental retardation
Heart defects-blepharophimosis-mental retardation
Ohdo-Madokoro-Hayakawa syndrome

**Excludes:**
**Blepharoptosis-blepharophimosis-epicanthus inversus-telecanthus (2103)**
**Marden-Walker syndrome (0629)**
**Mutchinick syndrome (3274)**

**Major Diagnostic Criteria:** The combination of blepharophimosis, ptosis, hypoplastic teeth, cardiac defect, and mental retardation.

**Clinical Findings:** In the three reported girls, blepharophimosis and ptosis were present at birth. One girl had an **Atrial septal defect**, and another had a **Ventricular septal defect** (in neither case was the diagnosis made at birth). Other anomalies also became apparent with age, including small, conical teeth; amblyopia; and mental retardation.

**Complications:** Unknown.

**Associated Findings:** Microphthalmia (1/3); narrow ear canals (1/3); and mild short stature (2/3).

**Etiology:** Possibly autosomal recessive or autosomal dominant inheritance with reduced penetrance, or a small chromosome rearrangement.

**Pathogenesis:** Unknown.

**MIM No.:** 24962

**POS No.:** 3875

**Sex Ratio:** M0:F3 (observed).

**Occurrence:** One family from Japan with two female sibs and an affected cousin has been documented.

**Risk of Recurrence for Patient's Sib:** Unknown. May be as high as 50%.

**Risk of Recurrence for Patient's Child:** Unknown. May be as high as 50%.

**Age of Detectability:** At birth, by the presence of blepharophimosis and ptosis.

**Gene Mapping and Linkage:** Unknown.

**Prevention:** None known. Genetic counseling indicated.

**Treatment:** Cosmetic surgery for the blepharophimosis and ptosis; corrective lens for amblyopia.

**Prognosis:** Mental retardation is severe, with IQs of 37–42 in the three reported girls. Life span is undetermined, although unlikely to be impaired to a significant degree.

**Detection of Carrier:** Unknown.

**References:**

Ohdo S, et al.: Mental retardation associated with congenital heart disease, blepharoptosis, and hypoplastic teeth. J Med Genet 1986; 23:242–244.

T0007

**Helga V. Toriello**

**Mental retardation-limb deficiency**
*See LIMB REDUCTION-MENTAL RETARDATION*
**Mental retardation-osteodystrophy, Ruvalcaba type**
*See OSTEODYSTROPHY-MENTAL RETARDATION, RUVALCABA TYPE*
**Mental retardation-retinopathy-microcephaly**
*See RETINOPATHY-MICROCEPHALY-MENTAL RETARDATION*
**Mental retardation-seizures-adenoma sebaceum**
*See TUBEROUS SCLEROSIS*
**Mental retardation-sexual maturity (delayed)-short stature**
*See SHORT STATURE-MENTAL RETARDATION-DELAYED SEXUAL MATURITY*
**Mental retardation-spondyloepiphyseal dysplasia**
*See SPONDYLOEPIPHYSEAL DYSPLASIA-MENTAL RETARDATION*
**Mental retardation-unusual facies-intrauterine growth retardation**
*See DWARFISM-DYSMORPHIC FACIES-RETARDATION, PITT TYPE*
**Mental retardation-xeroderma pigmentosum**
*See XERODERMA PIGMENTOSUM-MENTAL RETARDATION*
**Mephenytoin, fetal effects of**
*See FETAL HYDANTOIN SYNDROME*
**Meretoja-type amyloidosis**
*See AMYLOIDOSIS, FINNISH TYPE*
**MERRF**
*See MYOCLONIC EPILEPSY-RAGGED RED FIBERS*
**Merten-Singleton syndrome**
*See SINGLETON-MERTEN SYNDROME*
**Mesangial sclerosis, diffuse renal-ocular abnormalities**
*See RENAL MESANGIAL SCLEROSIS-EYE DEFECTS*
**Mesantoin^, fetal effects of**
*See FETAL HYDANTOIN SYNDROME*
**Mesenchymal dysplasie of Puretic**
*See FIBROMATOSIS, JUVENILE HYALINE*
**Mesenchymal hamartoma of liver**
*See LIVER, HAMARTOMA*

## MESENTERIC CYSTS 0645

**Includes:**
    Cystic hygroma of mesentery
    Lymphangioma of mesentery
    Lymphatic cyst of mesentery

**Excludes:** Intestinal duplication (0532)

**Major Diagnostic Criteria:** A cystic mass in the mesentery, which does not share a wall with the intestine, has no muscular lining of its wall, and has an alkaline content.

**Clinical Findings:** Presenting complaints may include an abdominal mass, pain, partial or complete intestinal obstruction, or fever of unknown etiology. They may appear alone or in combination.

**Complications:** Infection, rupture, intestinal obstruction.

**Associated Findings:** None known.

**Etiology:** Unknown.

**Pathogenesis:** Anomaly of the lymphatic tissue in the mesentery, with obstructed lymphatics and cyst formation.

**Sex Ratio:** M1:F1

**Occurrence:** 8:820,000 admissions at Mayo Clinic; 3:12,425 admissions at Children's Hospital, Los Angeles.

**Risk of Recurrence for Patient's Sib:** Unknown.

**Risk of Recurrence for Patient's Child:** Unknown.

**Age of Detectability:** Any age; 25% occur in first decade.

**Gene Mapping and Linkage:** Unknown.

**Prevention:** None known.

**Treatment:** Resection of the cyst from the mesentery, with or without adjacent bowel, depending on the blood supply to the cyst. Marsupialization of cyst generally results in recurrence or ascites.

**Prognosis:** Excellent for complete recovery with resection.

**Detection of Carrier:** Unknown.

**References:**
Colodny AH: Mesenteric and omental cysts. In: Welch KJ, et al, eds: Pediatric surgery, 4th ed, vol 2. Chicago: Year Book Medical Publishers, 1986:921–925.

SE006                               **John H. Seashore**

**Mesiodens**
    *See TEETH, SUPERNUMERARY*
**Mesiodens-cataract syndrome**
    *See CATARACTS-OTO-DENTAL DEFECTS*
**Mesiolabial rotation of upper central incisors**
    *See TEETH, MESIOPALATAL TORSION OF CENTRAL INCISORS*
**Mesiopalatal rotation of upper central incisors**
    *See TEETH, MESIOPALATAL TORSION OF CENTRAL INCISORS*
**Mesoaxial hexadactyly-cardiac malformation**
    *See HEART-HAND SYNDROME IV*
**Mesodermal dysmorphodystrophy, brachymorphic type, congenital**
    *See SPHEROPHAKIA-BRACHYMORPHIA SYNDROME*
**Mesoectodermal dysgenesis of anterior segment**
    *See EYE, ANTERIOR SEGMENT DYSGENESIS*
**Mesoectodermal dysgenesis of iris and cornea**
    *See EYE, ANTERIOR SEGMENT DYSGENESIS*
**Mesoectodermal dysplasia**
    *See CHONDROECTODERMAL DYSPLASIA*
**Mesomelic dwarfism of Campailla and Martinelli**
    *See ACROMESOMELIC DYSPLASIA, CAMPAILLA-MARTINELLI TYPE*
**Mesomelic dwarfism of hypoplastic tibia and radius**
    *See MESOMELIC DYSPLASIA, WERNER TYPE*
**Mesomelic dwarfism-Madelung deformity**
    *See DYSCHONDROSTEOSIS*
**Mesomelic dwarfism, hypoplastic ulna, fibula, and mandible type**
    *See MESOMELIC DYSPLASIA, LANGER TYPE*

## MESOMELIC DYSPLASIA, LANGER TYPE 0646

**Includes:**
    Homozygous dyschondrosteosis
    Langer type mesomelic dwarfism
    Mesomelic dwarfism, hypoplastic ulna, fibula, and
        mandible type

**Excludes:**
    Acrodysostosis (0016)
    Acromesomelic dysplasias
    Chondroectodermal dysplasia (0156)
    Dyschondrosteosis (0308)
    Mesomelic dysplasia (other)
    Robinow syndrome (0876)

**Major Diagnostic Criteria:** Severe dwarfism, with shortening maximal in the radius and tibia, both of which are curved, and aplasia or severe hypoplasia of the ulna and fibula.

**Clinical Findings:** Disproportionate dwarfism with shortening of the forearms and lower legs is characteristic. Adult height seldom exceeds 130 cm. Movement at the elbows is restricted in extension, as is pronation and supination of the forearms. Increase in lumbar lordosis is present, and the mandible is variably hypoplastic. The hands and feet are displaced laterally, and mild brachydactyly may be a feature. By X-ray, severe hypoplasia or aplasia of the ulna and fibula is present with bowing. The radius is short, thick, and laterally curved, while the tibia is usually straight but foreshortened. Apart from the lumbar lordosis, the remainder of the skeleton is normal.

**Complications:** Unknown.

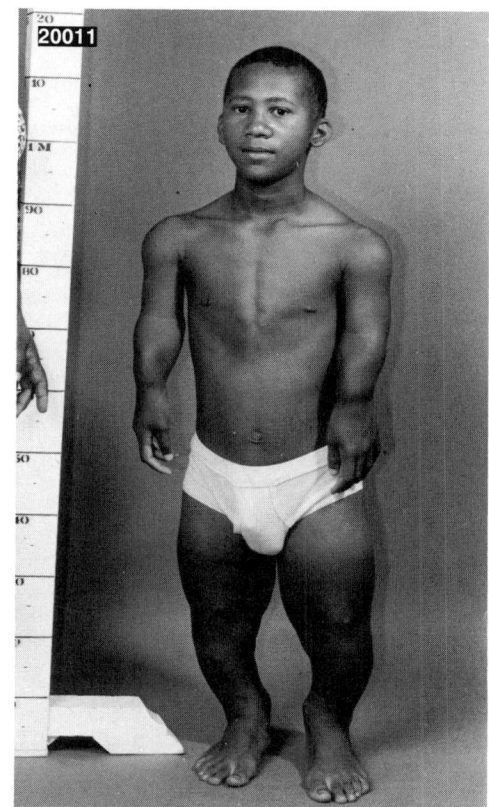

**0646-20011:** Note 16-year-old male with disproportionate short stature and short limbs with marked shortening of the middle segment of the limbs.

**Associated Findings:** None known.

**Etiology:** Presumably autosomal recessive inheritance. The homozygous state is expressed as mesomelic dysplasia, and the heterozygote state manifests as **Dyschondrosteosis**.

**Pathogenesis:** Unknown.

**MIM No.:** 24970

**POS No.:** 3292

**Sex Ratio:** M1:F1

**Occurrence:** About ten kindreds have been documented.

**Risk of Recurrence for Patient's Sib:**
See Part I, *Mendelian Inheritance*. Fifty percent for **Dyschondrosteosis**.

**Risk of Recurrence for Patient's Child:**
See Part I, *Mendelian Inheritance*. One-hundred percent for dyschondrosteosis.

**Age of Detectability:** At birth. Ultrasonographic prenatal detection may be possible.

**Gene Mapping and Linkage:** Unknown.

**Prevention:** None known. Genetic counseling indicated.

**Treatment:** Orthopedic procedures and physiotherapy can relieve the ulnar deviation of the hands.

**Prognosis:** Normal intelligence and life span.

**Detection of Carrier:** Clinical and X-ray examination of the forearms will enable detection of **Dyschondrosteosis** and is recommended for the spouse of a patient with this condition.

**Special Considerations:** Evidence for **Dyschondrosteosis** representing the heterozygous state of this condition has been forthcoming from several sources (see Fryns and van der Bergh, 1979; Goldblatt et al, 1987). It is possible that the mandibular manifestation is a syndromic component of Langer mesomelic dysplasia.

**References:**
Langer LO: Mesomelic dwarfism of the hypoplastic ulna, fibula, mandible type. Radiology 1967; 89:654–660.
Kaitila II, et al.: Mesomelic skeletal dysplasias. Clin Orthop 1976; 114:94–103. *
Fryns JP, van der Berghe H: Langer type of mesomelic dwarfism as the possible homozygous expression of dyschondrosteosis. Hum Genet 1979; 46:21–27.
Goldblatt J, et al.: Heterozygous manifestations of Langer mesomelic dysplasia. Clin Genet 1987; 31:19–24. †
Evans MI, et al.: Prenatal diagnosis and fetal pathology of Langer mesomelic dwarfism. Am J Med Genet 1988; 31:915–920.

VI005                                    **Denis L. Viljöen**

---

## MESOMELIC DYSPLASIA, NIEVERGELT TYPE          0647

**Includes:** Nievergelt syndrome

**Excludes:**
**Acrodysostosis** (0016)
**Acromesomelic dysplasia**
**Chondroectodermal dysplasia** (0156)
**Dyschondrosteosis** (0308)
**Mesomelic dysplasia**
**Robinow syndrome** (0876)

**Major Diagnostic Criteria:** Mesomelic shortening of the limbs, with a rhomboid appearance of the tibia and fibula on X-ray.
Restricted mobility of the elbows due to radioulnar luxation or subluxation of the redial head.

**Clinical Findings:** Moderate to severe disproportionate dwarfism occurs in which there exists specific deformities of the radius, ulna, tibia and fibula. Physical examination reveals bony protuberances with cutaneous dimples present at both medial and lateral aspects of the lower legs. Moderate valgus deformity is present at the knees. Atypical club feet with prominent equinovarous deformity may be present. Extension at the elbows and supination of the forearms are moderately limited, and the hands

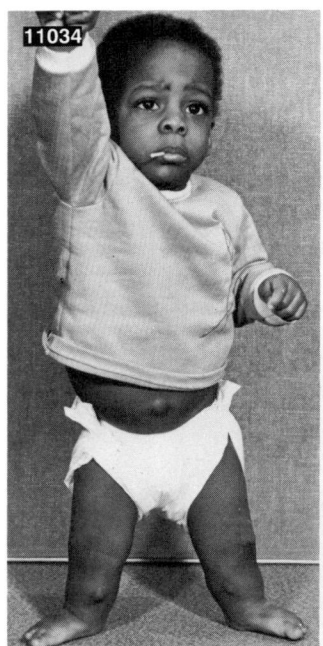
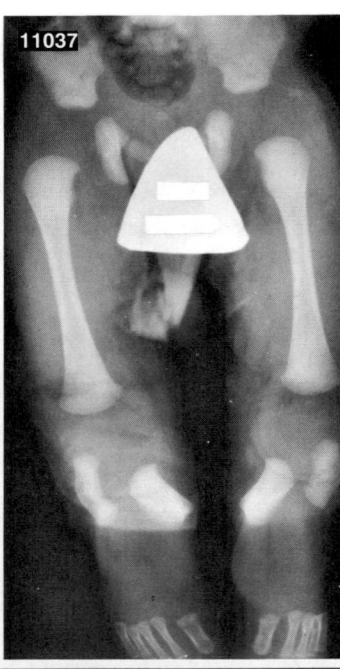
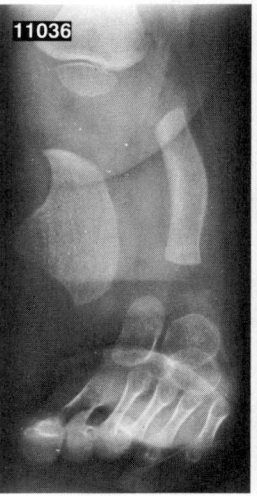
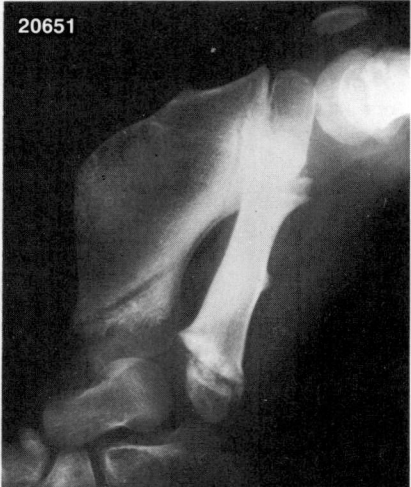

**0647-11034:** Note bilateral medial protuberances of the underlying tibial apices at age 2 years. **11037:** X-ray of pelvis and lower limbs in neonatal period; note normal variant "strip defect" in pubic rami and lack of ossification of talis and calcanei. **11036:** Tibial profile at 2 years; note the triangular configuration and vertically oriented "post-growth arrest" type lines suggesting sidewards growth. **20651:** Short tibia and fibula and triangular configuration of the tibia in a 7-year-old.

---

deviate medially at the wrists. Adult height is reported to be 135–147 cm and intelligence is normal.

X-ray findings are very specific. The middle segment bones, especially the tibia and fibula, are rhomboid in appearance. The proximal head of the radius and often the ulna are dislocated and may be synostotic. Metatarsal synostosis is common. The growth plates of the tibia and fibula are severely slanted. There is considerable clinical variability.

**Complications:** Walking is delayed.

**Associated Findings:** None known.

**Etiology:** Autosomal dominant inheritance with variable expressivity. Sporadic cases have been reported.

**Pathogenesis:** The severely disturbed development of the tubular bones, with anomalous slanting of the growth plates in the middle segment of the limbs, results in marked growth retardation and deformity of the bones.

**MIM No.:** *16340

**POS No.:** 3293

**Sex Ratio:** M1:F1

**Occurrence:** Several kindreds, as well as sporadic cases, have been reported.

**Risk of Recurrence for Patient's Sib:**
See Part I, *Mendelian Inheritance*.

**Risk of Recurrence for Patient's Child:**
See Part I, *Mendelian Inheritance*.

**Age of Detectability:** At birth.

**Gene Mapping and Linkage:** Unknown.

**Prevention:** None known. Genetic counseling indicated.

**Treatment:** Orthopedic surgery and physiotherapy for correction of the atypical clubfeet and possibly of the malaligned growth plates of the tibia and fibula.

**Prognosis:** Normal life span with orthopedic problems.

**Detection of Carrier:** Unknown.

**References:**

Nievergelt K: Positiver Vaterschaftsnachweis auf Grund erblicher Missbildungen der Extremitäten. Arch Julius Klaus-Stiftung Vererbungsforsch 1944; 19:157 only.

Solonen KA, Sulamaa M: Nievergelt syndrome and its treatment: a case report. Ann Chir Gynaecol Fenn 1958; 47:142–147.

Spranger, et al.: Bone Dysplasias. W. B. Saunders, 1974:222–223.

Young LW, Wood BP: Nievergelt syndrome (mesomelic dwarfism-type Nievergelt). BD:OAS X(5). Miami: Symposia Specialists for The National Foundation-March of Dimes, 1974:81–86.

Hess OM, et al.: Familiaerer mesomeler Kleinwuchs (Nievergelt-syndrom). Schweiz Med Wschr 1978; 108:1202–1206.

KA004
GR044

**Ilkka I. Kaitila**
**Gisele A. Greenhaw**

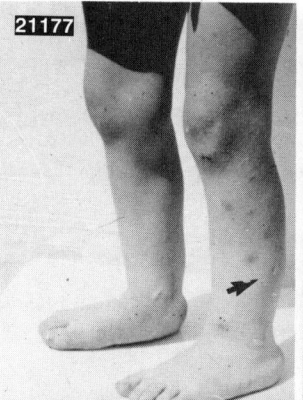
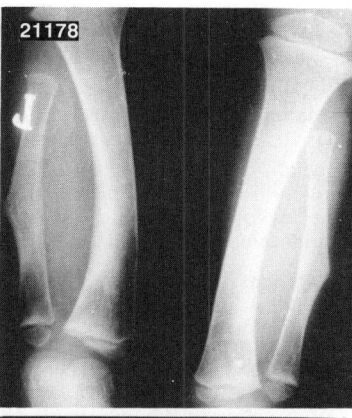
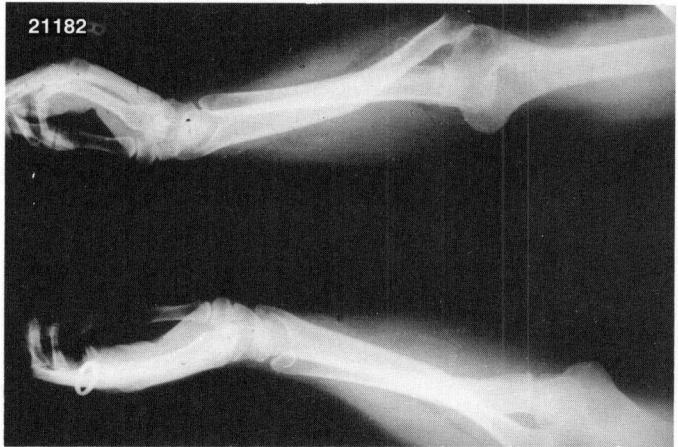

**0648-21177:** Typical dimple above the curvature of the fibula (see arrow). **21178:** Short, triangular fibula. **21182:** Bowed radius, dysplastic distal ulna and subluxed elbow.

## MESOMELIC DYSPLASIA, REINHARDT-PFEIFFER TYPE 0648

**Includes:**
Reinhardt-Pfeiffer mesomelic dysostosis
Ulna and fibula, hypoplasia of

**Excludes:**
**Dyschondrosteosis** (0308)
**Mesomelic dysplasia** (other)
**Skeletal dysplasia, boomerang dysplasia** (2522)

**Major Diagnostic Criteria:** Hypoplasia of ulna and fibula in the absence of constant skeletal dysplasia elsewhere.

**Clinical Findings:** In the presence of a mildly retarded body stature, there are normal upper arms and legs while lower arms and legs are shortened symmetrically. Pro- and supination of the arms are diminished. The ulna is short and broad. The radius is bowed anteriorly and radially; the radial head is dislocated in the same directions. Usually, a radioulnar joint is not formed; the bones do not touch. There is a fork-like abnormality of the wrist. Slight deformations of elbows and dislocations of carpal bones appear to be secondary. In 12 of 14 patients the abnormalities of the lower arm are as severe as those of the lower leg; in the remaining two, the lower arm is more severely affected. The fibula is hypoplastic, the fibular head does not reach the tibial head, but is displaced dorsally. In the middle part of the tibial diaphysis there is a triangular exostosis, pointing laterally. The distal part of the fibular bone is also hypoplastic; the fibulotalar joint may be missing. The middle-third part of the fibula is broad and anteriorly angulated, leading to a skin identation with a central dark brown pigmentation. Deformations of knee joint and tarsus are secondary. There may be severe valgus feet with more or less marked talus and calcaneus changes on X-ray.

**Complications:** The radial bowing may become more severe during growth; a slight valgus deformity of the tibia may also develop.

**Associated Findings:** One quarter of the patients had -5D myopia and strabismus.

**Etiology:** Probably autosomal dominant inheritance with full penetrance and very variable expression.

**Pathogenesis:** Unknown.

**MIM No.:** 19140

**POS No.:** 3294

**Sex Ratio:** M1:F2.7.

**Occurrence:** Fifteen cases known; fourteen in Western Germany, one in France.

**Risk of Recurrence for Patient's Sib:**
See Part I, *Mendelian Inheritance*.

**Risk of Recurrence for Patient's Child:**
See Part I, *Mendelian Inheritance*.

**Age of Detectability:** May be present at birth. Detection by prenatal ultrasound may be possible.

**Gene Mapping and Linkage:** Unknown.

**Prevention:** None known. Genetic counseling indicated.

**Treatment:** Orthopedic treatment for triangular angulation of the lower leg.

**Prognosis:** Normal life span. Occasionally patients do have difficulties in ambulation.

**Detection of Carrier:** Careful clinical and X-ray examination of all relatives will help indicate those who are minimally affected.

**Special Considerations:** It has been suggested that this disorder is allelic to **Dyschondrosteosis**. The absence of major radial and tibial dysplasias makes it possible to differentiate this condition from **Mesomelic dysplasia, Nievergelt type**.

**References:**
Pfeiffer RA: Beitrag zur erblichen Verkuerzung von Ulna und Fibula. In: Wiedemann H-R, ed: Dysostosen. Stuttgart: Gustav Fischer Verlag, 1966.
Reinhardt K, Pfeiffer RA: Ulno-fibulare Dysplasie. Eine autosomal-dominant vererbte Mikromesomelie aehnlich dem Nievergeltsyndrom. Fortschr Rontgenstr 1967; 107:379–391. * †
Maroteaux P, Spranger J: Essai de classification des chondrodysplasies a predominance mesomelique. Arch Fr Pediatr 1977; 34:945–958.
Lewin SO, Opitz JM: Fibular a/hypoplasia: review and documentation of the fibular developmental field. Am J Med Genet 1986; (Suppl 2):215–238. *

BE006                                          **Frits A. Beemer**

**Mesomelic dysplasia, type Robinow**
*See ROBINOW SYNDROME*

---

## MESOMELIC DYSPLASIA, WERNER TYPE                          0649

**Includes:**
    Eaton-McKusick syndrome
    Femoral duplication
    Mesomelic dwarfism of hypoplastic tibia and radius
    Tibia, absece of, with polydactyly
    Tibia, bilateral aplasia of with polydactyly and absent
      thumbs
    Tibia, hypoplasia of, with polydactyly

**Excludes:**
    **Acrodysostosis** (0016)
    **Acromesomelic dysplasia**
    **Chondroectodermal dysplasia** (0156)
    **Dyschondrosteosis** (0308)
    **Mesomelic dysplasia**
    **Robinow syndrome** (0876)
    **Tibial hypoplasia/aplasia-ectrodactyly** (2388)
    Tibia, unilateral aplasia of with polydactyly and absent
      thumbs

**Major Diagnostic Criteria:** Absent or hypoplastic tibia bilaterally with **Polydactyly** and absent thumbs.

**Clinical Findings:** Dwarfism that is due to marked shortening of the lower legs. In most cases, there is aplasia or severe hypoplasia of the tibia. There may be preaxial polydactyly of hands and feet and all digits may be triphalangial. The forearms are usually normal, but the carpal bones may be fused; range of movement is limited at the wrists. There may be pedunculated postminimi.

On X-ray, the tibia is rudimentary or totally absent and has no growth plates. The proximal head of the fibula is posteriorly and laterally dislocated and lies lateral to the middle shaft of the femur. The distal end of the fibula extends down to the lateral side of the foot. The patellae are hypoplastic. The bones in the ankle are deformed, and the number of metatarsals and phalanges is increased. In the hand, even the extra fingers appear normal, with three phalanges and normal metacarpal bones. There are no thumbs.

**Complications:** Those associated with orthopedic problems. Walking is delayed.

**Associated Findings:** Generally, no other associated defects have been described. However, there is one report of an infant born with absent tibias, preaxial polydactyly of the feet and

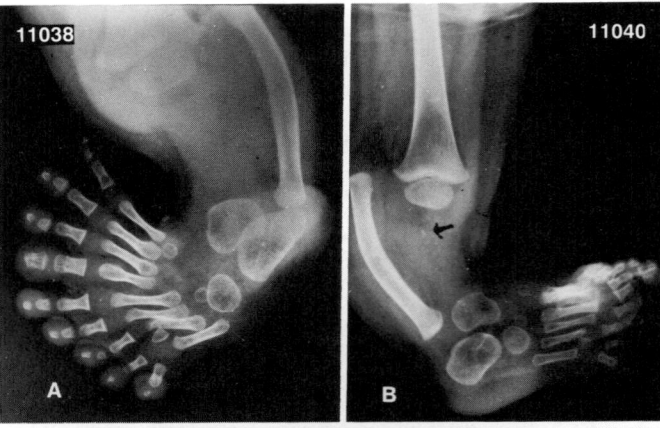

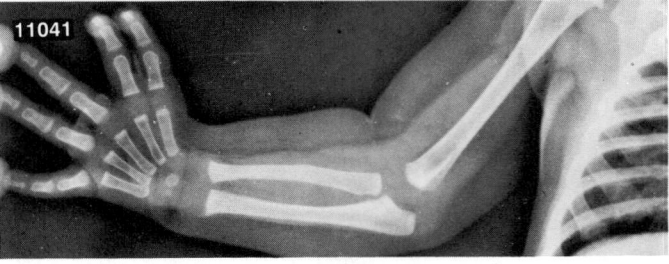

**0649-11038:** Preaxial polydactyly with 4th toe from medial aspect appearing as the hallux; postaxial polydactyly with a trapezoidal 8th metatarsal.    **11040:** Absent tibia with rudimentary calcified proximal remnant; bowed and dislocated fibula.    **11041:** Digitalized thumb with syndactyly of the 1st and 2nd digits.

---

normal thumbs who had multiple other congenital malformations, including **Cleft lip**, **Ventricular septal defect**, micrognathia, and wormian bones. Another report describes a child with **Polydactyly**, tibial dysplasia, **Ventricular septal defect**, and **Colon, aganglionosis**.

**Etiology:** Autosomal dominant inheritance with marked variability in phenotypic expression.

**Pathogenesis:** The short stature presumably results from the absence of growth plates of the tibia. The cause of the digital anomalies is unknown.

**MIM No.:** *15623, *18877, 18874

**POS No.:** 3295

**Sex Ratio:** M1:F1

**Occurrence:** Undetermined but presumed rare. The variability of this condition makes definitive diagnosis difficult.

At least six kindreds have been described with variable presentation in family members. For example, the father of two identically affected daughters with severly hypoplastic tibias and with polydactyly and absent thumbs had identical manifestations in his hands whereas his tibiae were completely normal. In another kindred, a father and two sons had varying degrees of tibial and radial hypoplasia without polydactyly.

**Risk of Recurrence for Patient's Sib:**
See Part I, *Mendelian Inheritance*.

**Risk of Recurrence for Patient's Child:**
See Part I, *Mendelian Inheritance*.

**Age of Detectability:** At birth. Prenatal diagnosis by ultrasound may be possible.

**Gene Mapping and Linkage:** Unknown.

**Prevention:** None known. Genetic counseling indicated.

**Treatment:** Orthopedic surgery to remove the supernumerary digits may be recommended to improve upper extremity function.

In cases of complete tibial agenesis, disarticulation at the knee with prosthetic replacement has been advocated to give the best functional result. In cases of partial tibia absence, transfer of the fibula into the tibial remnant can be considered.

**Prognosis:** Normal life span.

**Detection of Carrier:** Clinical and X-ray examination.

**References:**
Werner P: Ueber einen seltenen Fall von Zwergwuchs. Arch Gynakol 1915; 104:278–300.
Eaton GO, McKusick VA: A seemingly unique polydactyly-syndactyly syndrome in four persons in three generations. BD:OAS V(3). New York: March of Dimes Birth Defects Foundation, 1969:221–225.
Pashayan H, et al.: Bilateral aplasia of the tibia, polydactyly and absent thumbs in father and daughter. J Bone Joint Surg [Br] 1971; 53:495–499.
Ho CH, et al.: Congenital malformations: Cleft palate, congenital heart disease, absent tibia and polydactyly. Am J Dis Child 1975; 129:714–716.
LeRoy JG, et al.: Dominant mesomelic dwarfism of the hypoplastic tibia, radius type. Clin Genet 1975; 7:280–286.
Tetamy S, McKusick VA: The genetics of hand malformations. New York: Alan R. Liss, 1978.
Hall CM: Werner's mesomelic dysplasia with ventricular septal defect and Hirschsprung's disease. Ped Radiol 1981; 10:247–249.
Lamb PW, et al.: Five-fingered hand associated with partial or complete tibial absence and pre-axial polydactyly. J Bone Joint Surg 1983; 65:60–63.
Canun S, et al.: Absent tibia, triphalangeal thumbs and polydactyly: description of a family and prenatal diagnosis. Clin Genet 1984; 25:182–186.
Cordeiro I, Maroteaux HS: Congenital absence of the tibae and thumbs with polydactyly. Ann de Genet 1986; 29:275–277.
Al-Awadi SA, et al.: Hypoplastic tibiae with postaxial polysyndactyly: a new dominant syndrome. J Med Genet 1987; 23:367–372.
Bodurtha J, et al.: Femoral duplication: a case report. Am J Med Genet 1989; 33:165–169.
Kohn G, et al.: Aplasia of the tibia with bifurcation of the femur and ectrodactyly. Am J Med Genet 1989; 33:172–175.
Pavone L, et al.: Two rare developmental defects of the lower limbs with confirmation of the Lewin and Opitz hypothesis on the fibular and tibial developmental fields. Am J Med Genet 1989; 33:161–164.

KA004
GR044

**Ilkka I. Kaitila**
**Gisele A. Greenhaw**

**Mesotaurodontism**
*See TEETH, TAURODONTISM*
**Mesothelial cysts-squamous metaplasia**
*See SPLEEN, CYSTS*
**Metabolic craniopathy**
*See HYPEROSTOSIS FRONTALIS INTERNA*
**Metacarpal 4-5 fusion**
*See SYNDACTYLY*

## METACHONDROMATOSIS                           0650

**Includes:** N/A

**Excludes:**
   Enchondromatosis (0345)
   Exostoses, multiple cartilaginous (0685)

**Major Diagnostic Criteria:** Both exostoses and enchondromata in the same patient. This disorder must be distinguished from both **exostoses, multiple cartilaginous** and **enchondromatosis**. The presence of both lesions in the same patient, and the fact that the exostoses point toward the epiphyses, frequently occurring in the hands, are differentiating features of this disorder.

**Clinical Findings:** Exostotic lesions occur in the hands and long bones of a person who is unusually short. In contrast to multiple exostoses, the osteochondromata point toward the joint. Furthermore, they frequently regress and may disappear. Both exostoses and enchondromata are seen on X-rays. The exostoses frequently involve the hands, as well as the long bones, and the enchondro-

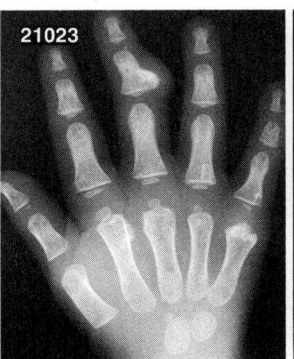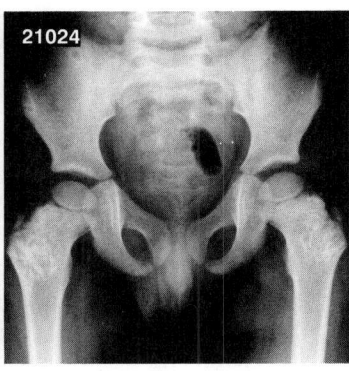

**0650-21023–24:** Metachondromatosis; note exostoses and enchondromata.

mata are in various growth plates. The spine may have irregular vertebral end plates.

**Complications:** Short stature secondary to enchondromata in the growth plates of the long bones. Deformity and limitation of function of fingers due to exostoses.

**Associated Findings:** None known.

**Etiology:** Presumably autosomal dominant inheritance.

**Pathogenesis:** Iliac crest biopsy has demonstrated typical lobulated enchondromata. The exostoses are histopathologically indistinguishable from both solitary and multiple exostoses.

**MIM No.:** 15625

**POS No.:** 4015

**Sex Ratio:** Presumably M1:F1.

**Occurrence:** About 20 cases documented.

**Risk of Recurrence for Patient's Sib:**
   See Part I, *Mendelian Inheritance.*

**Risk of Recurrence for Patient's Child:**
   See Part I, *Mendelian Inheritance.*

**Age of Detectability:** Infancy to early childhood.

**Gene Mapping and Linkage:** Unknown.

**Prevention:** None known. Genetic counseling indicated.

**Treatment:** Orthopedic surgery to remove exostoses if they produce pain, deformity, or limitation of function.

**Prognosis:** Undetermined. No malignancies have been reported.

**Detection of Carrier:** Unknown.

**References:**
Maroteaux P: La metachondromatose. Z Kinderheilk 1971; 109:246–261.
Lachman RS, et al.: Metachondromatosis. BD:OAS X(9). Miami: Symposia Specialists for The National Foundation-March of Dimes, 1974:171–178.
Kennedy LA: Metachondromatosis. Radiology 1983; 148:117–118.
Bassett GS, Cowell HR: Metachondromatosis: report of four cases. J Bone Joint Surg 1985; 67A:811–814.

B0025
LA006

**Zvi Borochowitz**
**Ralph S. Lachman**

**Metachromatic form of diffuse cerebral sclerosis**
*See METACHROMATIC LEUKODYSTROPHIES*

## METACHROMATIC LEUKODYSTROPHIES 0651

### Includes:

Arsacerebroside sulfatase deficiency
Arylsulfatase A deficiency
Cerebral sclerosis, degenerative diffuse, Scholz type
Cerebroside sulfatidosis
Lipidosis, sulfatide
Metachromatic form of diffuse cerebral sclerosis
Multiple sulfatase deficiency
Pseudo-arylsulfatase A deficiency
Sulfatide lipidosis
Sulfatidosis, juvenile, Austin type (some forms)

### Excludes:

**Leukodystrophy, globoid cell type** (0415)
Leukodystrophy, sudanophilic type
**Pelizaeus-Merzbacher syndrome** (0803)
Other leukodystrophies of nervous system

**Major Diagnostic Criteria:** The three known clinical forms are named for their usual age of presentation. In the late infantile form, affected children usually present in the second year of life with delayed development and progressive weakness. The juvenile form usually presents later with ataxia and progressive gait involvement. In the adult form, dementia is progressive, and there is evidence of basal ganglial or long tract involvement. All may be suspected on the basis of the clinical picture plus increased CSF protein, prolonged nerve conduction times, or the demonstration of metachromatic material in a peripheral nerve biopsy. In all forms of the disease, the diagnosis is established by demonstration of the enzymatic defect in white cells or skin fibroblasts. MRI and CT scans may direct attention to distinct degenerative changes in white matter. These are more diffuse in younger patients, and multifocal in older patients.

**Clinical Findings:** The three clinical forms of metachromatic leukodystrophy (MLD) are late infantile, juvenile, and adult:
*Late infantile metachromatic leukodystrophy*: the child is usually normal until approximately 12–16 months of life. Early symptoms and signs include delayed motor development, particularly in terms of the lower limbs, followed by a progressive loss of the ability to walk. With a genu recurvatum, the child then regresses to hanging onto objects to stand. Following these symptoms, there is involvement of the upper limbs. Some patients may show nystagmus. By the age of 2 or 2 1/2 years, the patient is unable to pull himself to a sitting position, has dysarthria, is hypotonic, and may have difficulty with swallowing. Since both the central and peripheral nervous systems are involved, the child may have spasticity and hyperreflexia or hypotonicity and hyporeflexia. At times, there are combinations of both the decreased reflexes in the lower limbs and increased reflexes in the upper limbs. Eventually the child loses speech, and it is difficult to tell if the child is in contact with his surroundings. However, prior to the loss of speech, intellect seems to be relatively preserved, and seizures are an uncommon phenomenon. There may be involvement of the retina with optic atrophy or retinal changes.
*Juvenile metachromatic leukodystrophy*: is more likely to present as ataxia. There is then progressive involvement of gait and a slower progression than seen in the late infantile form.
*Adult metachromatic leukodystrophy*: presents as a dementia or an involvement of basal ganglia and long-tract findings. The progression is one of increasing dementia, often with behavioral disturbance.
Arylsulfatase A screening tests are useful, but the finding of "low" arylsulfatase A activity per se does not suffice to make a diagnosis of MLD. The demonstration of a cerebroside sulfatase deficiency and of increased sulfatide excretion in urine are much more specific tests.

**Complications:** Progressive loss of motor function, aspiration pneumonia, urinary tract infections, and a bedridden patient.

**Associated Findings:** None known.

**Etiology:** Autosomal recessive inheritance and possibly X-linked inheritance.

**Pathogenesis:** The basic defect is a failure to split sulfatide (the sulfate ester of galactocerebroside). The enzymatic defect is the lack of activity of the lysosomal enzyme, cerebroside sulfatase. Rarely, an activator protein is defective.
Sulfatide catabolism is abnormally slow. The defective cerebroside sulfatase activity causes a widespread increase in sulfatides, notably in the brain, peripheral nerves, and gallbladder. Associated with the sulfatide accumulation is the progressive breakdown of membranes of the myelin sheath, which contains abnormal amounts of sulfatide.

**MIM No.:** 25000, *25010, 25020, 30270, *27220

**POS No.:** 3775

**Sex Ratio:** M1:F1

**Occurrence:** 1:40,000–50,000 births in northern Sweden.

**Risk of Recurrence for Patient's Sib:**
See Part I, *Mendelian Inheritance.*

**Risk of Recurrence for Patient's Child:**
See Part I, *Mendelian Inheritance.* Late infantile and juvenile forms are lethal prior to reproductive age.

**Age of Detectability:** In utero by demonstration of the enzymatic defect in amniotic cells, as well as at birth from leukocytes or from skin fibroblasts.

**Gene Mapping and Linkage:** ARSA (arylsulfatase A) has been mapped to 22q13.31-qter.

**Prevention:** None known. Genetic counseling indicated.

**Treatment:** Supportive as indicated.

**Prognosis:** Late infantile form: death 2–4 years after diagnosis. Juvenile form: death 4–6 years after diagnosis. Adult form unknown.

**Detection of Carrier:** The heterozygote can be detected by enzymatic assay of leukocytes or skin fibroblasts using the arylsulfatase assay. Carriers have 40–60% of the activity of control patients.

**Special Considerations:** In a special form of this disease, multiple sulfatase deficiency (MLD), a variant of *sulfatidosis, juvenile, Austin type*; a condition which combines the enzyme deficiency and phenotypic features of several other conditions (Kihara, 1982), not only do sulfatides accumulate, but also sulfated steroids, sulfated mucopolysaccharides, and gangliosides in cerebral cortex. The accumulated sulfated mucopolysaccharide resembles heparan sulfate. These patients have skeletal abnormalities, ichthyosis and deafness. They also show a distinctive granulation abnormality in their leukocytes and have a deficiency not only of sulfatase A, but also of sulfatase B and sulfatase C.
A "pseudodeficiency" allele at the arylsulfatase A locus has been delineated by Schaap et al (1981). Otherwise healthy relatives of MLD patients may show ARSA levels in the range with MLD patients, but cultured fibroblasts from such relatives catabolize cerebroside sulfate; fibroblasts from MLD patients do not.

### References:

Schaap T, et al.; The genetics of the aryl sulfatase A locus. Am J Hum Genet 1981; 33:531–539.
Kihara H: Genetic heterogeneity in metachromatic leukodystrophy. Am J Hum Genet 1982; 34:171–181.
Skomer C, et al.: Metachromatic leukodystrophy (MLD). XV: adult MLD with focal lesions by computed tomograph. Arch Neurol 1983; 40:354–355.
McKhann G: Metachromatic leukodystrophy: clinical and enzymic parameters. Neuropediatrics 1984; 15(suppl):4–10.
Farrell K, et al.: Pseudoarylsulfatase-A deficiency in the neurologically impaired patient. Can J Neurol Sci 1985; 12:274–277.
Waltz G, et al.: Adult metachromatic leukodystrophy: value of computed tomographic scanning and magnetic resonance imaging of the brain. Arch Neurol 1987; 44:225–227.
Austin J: Metachromatic leukodystrophy. In: Rowland L, ed: Merritt's textbook of neurology, 8th ed. Philadelphia: Lea and Febiger, 1988. *
Kolodny E: Metachromatic leukodystrophy and multiple sulfatase

deficiency. In: Scriver CR, et al, eds: The metabolic basis of inherited disease, 6th ed. New York: McGraw-Hill, 1989:1721–1750.

AU002
K0010

**James H. Austin**
**Edwin H. Kolodny**

## METAPHYSEAL CHONDRODYSPLASIA WITH THYMOLYMPHOPENIA                    0655

**Includes:**

Achondroplasia, so-called, and Swiss-type
  agammaglobulinemia
Adenosine deaminase deficiency
Agammaglobulinemia, variant form of Swiss type
Dwarfism-immunodeficiency, Swiss type
Immunodeficiency, Swiss type-dwarfism
Lymphopenic agammaglobulinemia-short limbed dwarfism
Metaphyseal dysostosis with Swiss type
  agammaglobulinemia

**Excludes:**

**Hypoparathyroidism**
**Metaphyseal chondrodysplasia** (other)
Metaphyseal osteochondrodystrophies
**Rickets**
Swiss type agammaglobulinemia without bone disease
Other immunologic conditions

**Major Diagnostic Criteria:**  Recurrent, severe infections in a child with ectodermal dysplasia, absence of thymic-dependent and thymic-independent lymphoid tissue, and metaphyseal chondrodysplasia.

**Clinical Findings:**  At birth, short-limbed short stature, and ectodermal dysplasia; cutis laxa, scalp alopecia; ichthyosiform dermatosis. Within weeks, failure to thrive and recurrent bacterial, fungal and viral infections. Severe combined immune deficiency (lymphopenia, total or selective immunoglobulin deficiency). On X-ray, metaphyseal chondrodysplasia, pelvic dysplasia (flat acetabulae); flaring of the anterior ends of the ribs, osteoporosis; absent tonsils, adenoids, and thymus. Accumulation of toxic metabolites can disturb neurologic functions.

**Complications:**  Recurrent severe infections.

**Associated Findings:**  Lymphopenia with none of the B-cells and T-cell surface markers. After maternal antibodies are cleared, hypogammaglobulinemia, and negative skin test reactions to infectious and chemical agents. Very low or immeasurable levels of adenosine deaminase.

**Etiology:**  Presumably autosomal recessive inheritance; one-third of severe combined immunodeficiency cases are inherited as a recessive trait caused by adenosine deaminase deficiency.

**Pathogenesis:**  A deficiency of adenosine deaminase leads to accumulation of adenosine in the cells and disruption of cellular proliferation of lymphoid and cartilage tissues.

**MIM No.:**  20090

**POS No.:**  3299

**CDC No.:**  756.450

**Sex Ratio:**  M1:F1

**Occurrence:**  About 50 families have been identified.

**Risk of Recurrence for Patient's Sib:**
  See Part I, *Mendelian Inheritance.*

**Risk of Recurrence for Patient's Child:**
  See Part I, *Mendelian Inheritance.* No probands have survived to reproduce.

**Age of Detectability:**  Deficient adenosine deaminase activity in cultured amniotic fluid cells or chorionic villus biopsy; in neonatal period with appropriate methods.

**Gene Mapping and Linkage:**  Unknown.

**Prevention:**  None known. Genetic counseling indicated.

**Treatment:**  Bone marrow transplantation can result in complete immune reconstitution. Enzyme replacement therapy may improve function.

**Prognosis:**  Death in infancy, unless protective measures are taken.

**Detection of Carrier:**  Carriers have about one-half the normal levels of erythrocyte adenosine deaminase.

**References:**
Alexander WJ, Dunbar JS: Unusual bone changes in thymic alymphoplasia. Ann Radiol [Paris] 1968; 11:389–394.
Gatti RA, et al.: Hereditary lymphopenic agammaglobulinemia associated with a distinctive form of short-limbed dwarfism and ectodermal dysplasia. J Pediatr 1969; 75:675–684.
Sutcliffe J, Stanley P: Metaphyseal chondrodysplasias. Progr Pediatr Radiol 1973; 4:250–269.
Meuwissen HJ, et al.: Combined immunodeficiency disease associated with adenosine deaminase deficiency. J Pediatr 1975; 86:169–181. * †
Spranger JW: Metaphyseal chondrodysplasia. Postgrad Med J 1977; 53:480–486.
Young LW, et al.: Severe combined immunodeficiency associated with adenosine deaminase deficiency. Am J Dis Child 1978; 132:621–622.
Kredich NM, Hershfield MS: Immunodeficiency disease caused by adenosine deaminase deficiency and purine nucleoside phosphorylase deficiency. In: Scriver CR, et al, eds: The metabolic basis of inherited disease, 6th ed. New York: McGraw-Hill, 1989:1045–1076.

K0021

**K.S. Kozlowski**

## METAPHYSEAL CHONDRODYSPLASIA, TYPE JANSEN    0652

**Includes:**

Jansen metaphyseal dysostosis
Murk Jansen metaphyseal chondrodysplasia

**Excludes:**

**Enchondromatosis** (0345)
**Enchondromatosis and hemangiomas** (0346)
**Hypophosphatasia** (0516)

**Major Diagnostic Criteria:**  Dwarfism and peculiar facies, with severe metaphyseal chondrodysplasia.

**Clinical Findings:**  Progressive, short-limb dwarfism with contractural deformities of the joints and expansion of the ends of the long bones. Adult height about 120 cm. Facies are dysmorphic. Often elevated serum calcium levels. Diagnostic X-ray findings: severe, generalized metaphyseal changes. The metaphyses are expanded and irregularly mottled (an expression of severely disorganized enchondral ossification). The short tubular bones show marked cupping. Additional characteristic findings include shortening of the diaphyses and progressive sclerosis; particularly of the base of the skull. Minor spinal and epiphyseal changes may also be noted.

**Complications:**  Severe, early progressive osteoarthritic changes, kyphoscoliosis.

**Associated Findings:**  None known.

**Etiology:**  Autosomal dominant inheritance.

**Pathogenesis:**  Disorganized metaphyseal ossification with presence of irregular masses of abnormal cartilage in the metaphyseal regions.

**MIM No.:**  *15640

**POS No.:**  3296

**CDC No.:**  756.450

**Sex Ratio:**  M1:F1

**Occurrence:**  About 20 verified cases have been reported.

**Risk of Recurrence for Patient's Sib:**
  See Part I, *Mendelian Inheritance.*

**Risk of Recurrence for Patient's Child:**
  See Part I, *Mendelian Inheritance.*

**Age of Detectability:**  In infancy, by X-ray.

**Gene Mapping and Linkage:**  Unknown.

**Prevention:** None known. Genetic counseling indicated.

**Treatment:** Physiotherapy; orthopedic treatment. It is important to distinguish this disorder from metabolic disorders, especially rickets, as in presence of hypercalcemia, vitamin D therapy may be harmful.

**Prognosis:** Normal life span.

**Detection of Carrier:** Unknown.

**References:**

Jansen M: Über atypische chondrodystrophie (achondroplasie) und über eine noch nicht beschriebene angeborene wachstumsstörung des knochensystems: metaphysäre dysostose. Z Orthop Chir 1934; 61:253–286.

Ozonoff MB: Metaphyseal dysostosis of Jansen. Radiology 1969; 93:1047–1050.

De Haas WHD, et al.: Metaphyseal dysostosis. A late follow-up of the first reported case. J Bone Joint Surg 1969; 51B:290–299.

Sutcliffe J, Stanley P: Metaphyseal chondrodysplasias. Prog Pediatr Radiol 1973; 4:250–269.

Holthusen W, et al.: The skull in metaphyseal chondrodysplasia, type Jansen. Pediatr Radiol 1975; 3:137–144. †

Silverthorn KG, et al.: Murk Jansen's metaphyseal chondrodysplasia with long term follow-up. Pediatr Radiol 1987; 17:119–123. *

K0021                                                          **K.S. Kozlowski**

## METAPHYSEAL CHONDRODYSPLASIA, TYPE MCKUSICK                                            0653

**Includes:**

Agammaglobulinemia-lymphopenia-dwarfism
Cartilage-hair hypoplasia
Dwarfism-lymphopenia-agammaglobulinemia
Immunodeficiency, cartilage-hair hypoplasia
Lymphopenia-agammaglobulinemia-dwarfism

**Excludes:**

**Dyschondrosteosis** (0308)
**Hypochondroplasia** (0510)
**Hypophosphatasia** (0516)
Hypophosphatemic rickets and other types of "renal rickets"
**Immunodeficiency, adenosine deaminase deficiency** (2196)
**Shwachman syndrome** (0885)

**Major Diagnostic Criteria:** Short-limb dwarfism with fine sparse hair. Metaphyseal chondrodysplasia with predominant peripheral involvement. Cellular immunodeficiency may be noted, particularly a marked impairment of T-cell function due to an intrinsic defect in cell proliferation.

**Clinical Findings:** Progressive short-limb dwarfism with predominant peripheral involvement. Fine, sparse, usually light-colored hair, eyebrows, and lashes, otherwise normal head and skull. Adult height about 120 cm. Characteristic X-ray findings include metaphyseal chondrodysplasia with predominant hand, foot, and knee involvement; cupping of the anterior ends of the ribs and little change in the proximal femoral and humeral metaphyses. There is considerable variability of expressivity, not only in X-ray findings but in possible associated cellular immunodeficiency.

**Complications:** Early osteoarthritic changes. Equinovarus deformity of the feet subsequent to overgrowth of the fibula.

**Associated Findings:** Malabsorption, Hirschsprung disease and impaired cellular immunity with chronic neutro- and lymphopenia sometimes reported. Varicella, anemia, and various malignancies have been reported, as have dental anomalies.

**Etiology:** Autosomal recessive inheritance.

**Pathogenesis:** Relation between ectodermal and bone defects, immunodeficiency, and associated diseases is unclear.

**MIM No.:**   *25025

**POS No.:**   3061

**CDC No.:**   756.450

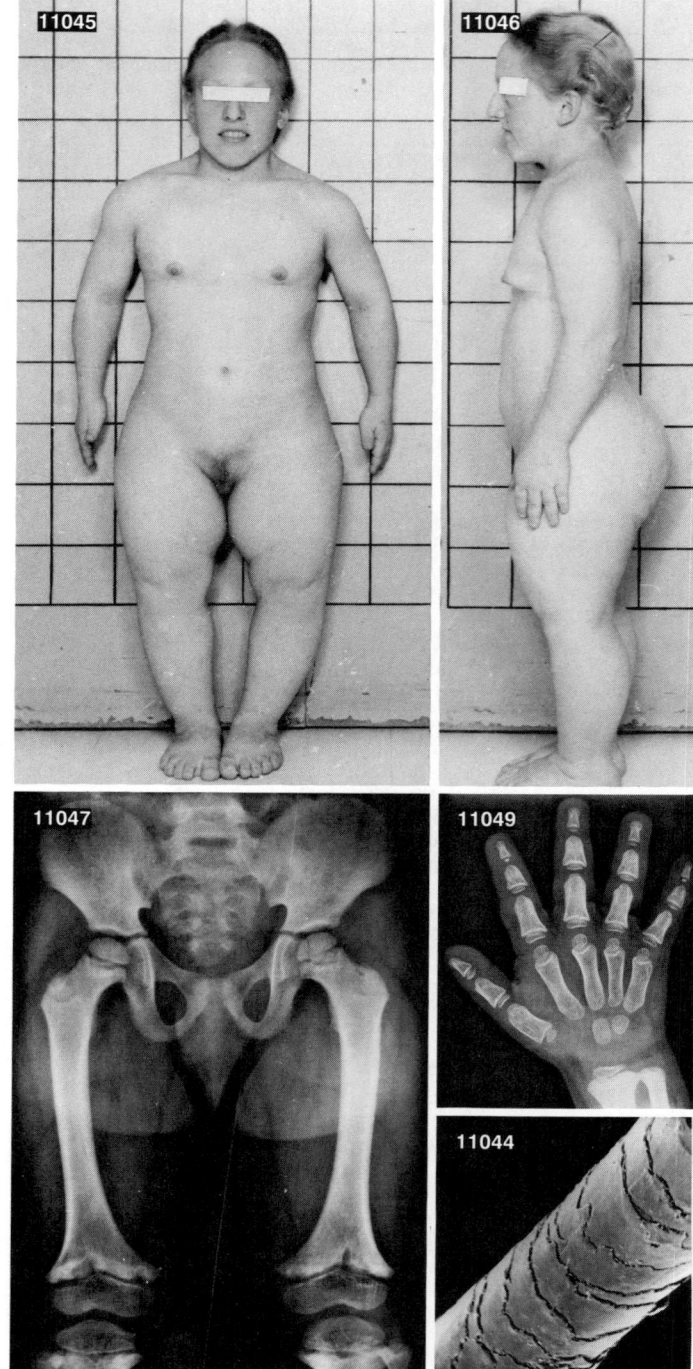

**0653-11045–46:** Mild bowing of the femurs and tibiae, excessively long fibulae, and sparse, short blond hair which has never been cut. **11047:** Long bones are short with flared ends; metaphyseal zones of provisional calcification are scalloped and irregular but of normal density. **11049:** Carpal ossification is delayed; phalanges are relatively wide with mild metaphyseal cupping. **11044:** Scanning electron micrograph of hair.

**Sex Ratio:** M1:F1

**Occurrence:** With exception of some inbred groups, presumed rare. 170:100,000 among Amish population in the United States. Increased gene frequency in some areas in Finland.

**Risk of Recurrence for Patient's Sib:**
See Part I, *Mendelian Inheritance.*

**Risk of Recurrence for Patient's Child:**
See Part I, *Mendelian Inheritance.*

**Age of Detectability:** Sometimes in infancy, usually early preschool age.

**Gene Mapping and Linkage:** Unknown.

**Prevention:** None known. Genetic counseling indicated.

**Treatment:** Physiotherapy; orthopedic treatment. Affected individuals should avoid smallpox vaccinations and be guarded against all viral infections. Leukocyte interferon has been proposed as a treatment for patients who also have varicella. Serial transfusions and steroids have been used in cases with associated congenital anemia.

**Prognosis:** Usually a normal life span if treated. One patient with severe combined immunodeficiency died despite thymus transplantation.

**Detection of Carrier:** Unknown.

**References:**
McKusick VA, et al.: Dwarfism in the Amish. II. Cartilage-hair hypoplasia. Bull Johns Hopkins Hosp 1965; 116:285–326. * †
Lux SE, et al.: Chronic neutropenia and abnormal cellular immunity in cartilage-hair hypoplasia. New Engl J Med 1970; 282:231–236.
Ray HC, Dorst JP: Cartilage-hair hypoplasia. Prog Pediatr Radiol 1973; 4:270–298.
Kartila I, Perheentupa J: Cartilage-hair hypoplasia (CHH). In: Eriksson AW, et al., eds: Population structure and genetic disorders. New York: Academic Press, 1980:588–591.
Harris RE, et al.: Cartilage-hair hypoplasia, defective T-cell function, and Diamond-Blackfan anemia in an Amish child. Am J Med Genet 1981; 8:291–297.
Polmar SH, Pierce GF: Cartilage-hair hypoplasia: immunological aspects and their clinical implications. Clin Immunol Immunopathol 1986; 40:87–93.

K0021
WI024

K.S. Kozlowski
Golder N. Wilson

## METAPHYSEAL CHONDRODYSPLASIA, TYPE SCHMID    0654

**Includes:** Schmid metaphyseal dysostosis

**Excludes:**
**Dyschondrosteosis** (0308)
**Hypochondroplasia** (0510)
**Hypophosphatasia** (0516)
Hypophosphatemic rickets and other types of "renal" rickets

**Major Diagnostic Criteria:** Moderate shortening of stature, normal head circumference, and bowed legs. Bony changes of moderately severe metaphyseal chondrodysplasia are found in X-rays, which show expanded cupped metaphyses and disorganized metaphyseal ossification.

**Clinical Findings:** Moderate, progressive shortening of stature with bowed legs and waddling gait. Adult height is about 140 cm. Characteristic X-ray findings show expanded, cupped metaphyses with disorganized metaphyseal ossification. There is often coxa vara and genu varum deformity of the hips, and cupping of the anterior ends of the ribs. The density and texture of the bones is normal (an important differential diagnostic sign with all forms of rickets). The spinal, epiphyseal, and diaphyseal changes are minimal. The skull is normal.

**Complications:** Coxa and genua vara; early progressive osteoarthritis.

**Associated Findings:** None known.

**Etiology:** Autosomal dominant inheritance.

**Pathogenesis:** Disorganized metaphyseal ossification, biochemical defect not defined.

**MIM No.:** *15650

**POS No.:** 3298

**CDC No.:** 756.450

**Sex Ratio:** M1:F1

**Occurrence:** Several large kindreds have been documented.

**Risk of Recurrence for Patient's Sib:**
See Part I, *Mendelian Inheritance.*

**Risk of Recurrence for Patient's Child:**
See Part I, *Mendelian Inheritance.*

**Age of Detectability:** Early preschool age.

**Gene Mapping and Linkage:** Unknown.

**Prevention:** None known. Genetic counseling indicated.

**Treatment:** Physiotherapy; orthopedic treatment. It is important to distinguish this disorder from metabolic diseases, especially rickets, as vitamin D therapy is unnecessary and may be harmful.

**Prognosis:** Normal life span.

**Detection of Carrier:** Unknown.

**References:**
Schmid F: Beitrag zur Dysostosis enchondralis metaphysarea. Monatsschr Kinderheilkd 1949; 97:393–397.
Rosenbloom AL, Smith DW: The natural history of metaphyseal dysostosis. J Pediatr 1965; 66:857–868.
Sutcliffe J, Stanley P: Metaphyseal chondrodysplasias. Prog Pediatr Radiol 1973; 4:250–269.
Beluffi G, et al.: Metaphyseal dysplasia type Schmid: Early X-ray detection and evolution with time. Ann Radiol 1983; 26:237–243. * †

K0021

K.S. Kozlowski

**Metaphyseal dysostosis with Swiss type agammaglobulinemia**
*See METAPHYSEAL CHONDRODYSPLASIA WITH THYMOLYMPHOPENIA*

## METAPHYSEAL DYSOSTOSIS-DEAFNESS    0250

**Includes:**
Deafness-metaphyseal dysostosis
Metaphyseal dysostosis-mental retardation-conductive deafness
Skeletal dysplasia-deafness

**Excludes:**
**Metaphyseal chondrodysplasia** (other)
Other disorders associated with metaphyseal dysostosis

**Major Diagnostic Criteria:** Metaphyseal dysostosis, conductive hearing loss, and mental retardation.

**Clinical Findings:** A kindred has been reported in which all three sibs were found to have short-limbed dwarfism, metaphyseal dysostosis, conductive hearing loss, and mild mental retardation. The parents were fourth cousins. The skeletal disorder can be classified as "metaphyseal dysostosis," since the major lesions consist of widening and fragmentation of the metaphyses of the long bones with relative sparing of the skull, spine, and epiphyses. Coxa vara, genua vara, scoliosis, or lumbar lordosis were noted. The feet and hands were short and broad, and the fingers were loose-jointed. Two sibs were hyperopic and had alternating esotropia. Anterior polar cataract was present in one sib. Polytomography revealed bilateral low placement of the ossicles in all three sibs. There was a striking upward angulation of the internal auditory canals. Audiologic examination in the three boys demonstrated a moderate bilateral conductive hearing deficit.

**Complications:** Unknown.

**Associated Findings:** None known.

**Etiology:** Autosomal recessive inheritance.

**Pathogenesis:** Unknown.

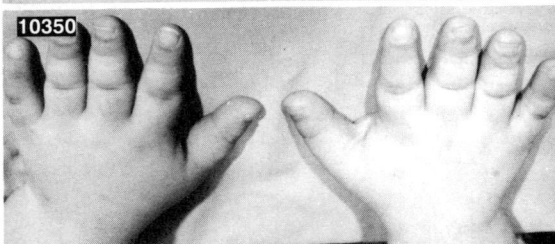

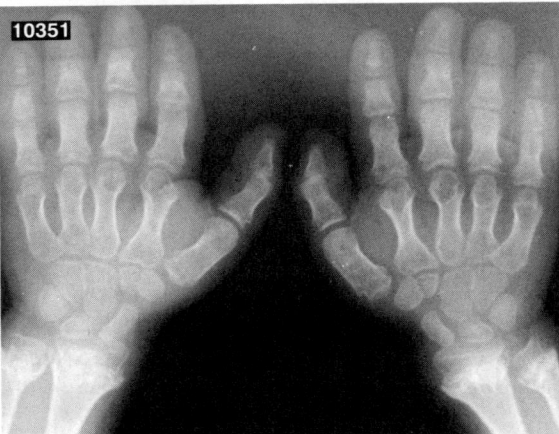

**0250-10348:** Short stature, coxa vara, genua vara and scoliosis in two brothers. **10350:** Short, stubby hands with squared-off nails. **10351:** Short tubular bones with widened metaphyses.

**MIM No.:** 25042

**POS No.:** 3194

**Sex Ratio:** M3:F0 (observed)

**Occurrence:** One reported family with three affected sibs.

**Risk of Recurrence for Patient's Sib:**
See Part I, *Mendelian Inheritance.*

**Risk of Recurrence for Patient's Child:**
See Part I, *Mendelian Inheritance.*

**Age of Detectability:** Early childhood.

**Gene Mapping and Linkage:** Unknown.

**Prevention:** None known. Genetic counseling indicated.

**Treatment:** Orthopedic therapy and a hearing aid may be useful.

**Prognosis:** Probably normal life span.

**Detection of Carrier:** Unknown.

**References:**
Rimoin DL, McAlister WH: Metaphyseal dysostosis, conductive hearing loss, and mental retardation: a recessively inherited syndrome. In: BD:OAS; VII(4). Baltimore: Williams & Wilkins, for The National Foundation-March of Dimes, 1971:116–122.

MU020

**Jeff Murray**
*Cor W.R.J. Cremers*

**Metaphyseal dysostosis-mental retardation-conductive deafness**
*See METAPHYSEAL DYSOSTOSIS-DEAFNESS*
**Metaphyseal dysplasia**
*See PYLE DISEASE*

## METAPHYSEAL DYSPLASIA-MAXILLARY HYPOPLASIA-BRACHYDACTYLY    2768

**Includes:**
Brachydactyly-maxillary hypoplasia-metaphyseal dysplasia
Maxillary hypoplasia-metaphyseal dysplasia-brachydactyly

**Excludes:**
**Cranio-diaphyseal dysplasia** (0224)
**Craniometaphyseal dysplasia** (0228)
**Diaphyseal dysplasia** (0290)
**Dysosteosclerosis** (0310)
**Frontometaphyseal dysplasia** (0394)
**Oculo-dento-osseous dysplasia** (0737)
**Pyle disease** (0847)

**Major Diagnostic Criteria:** Metaphyseal dysplasia with maxillary hypoplasia and **Brachydactyly.**

**Clinical Findings:** Metaphyseal flaring, a constant finding in affected individuals, is symmetric and mild. It is most obvious in the proximal humeri, distal femora, and proximal tibiae. Aside from a few wormian bones and mild hyperostosis of the inner frontoparietal area of the skull in some affected persons, the cranium was normal. Changes in the spine varied from severe osteoporosis with several spontaneous fractures and platyspondyly to no abnormalities. The majority of affected individuals (4/6) were short.

Facial changes of small head circumference (proportionate to short stature), beaked nose or high nasal bridge, short philtrum, thin lips, maxillary hypoplasia with relative prognathism, and yellow dystrophic deciduous and permanent teeth with dental extraction in adolescence were present in most affected individuals. A part of the maxillary hypoplasia may be secondary to early loss of teeth. There was a suggestion of mild hypoplasia of the malar bones in at least one affected individual.

Acral anomalies were present in (4/5) affected individuals with available hand X-rays (the index patient did not have hand anomalies). These consisted of severe bilateral shortness of metacarpal 5 with or without shortness of the middle phalanx of fingers 2 and 5. The Poznanski hand pattern profile failed to show any other significant changes in the hand bones of affected persons.

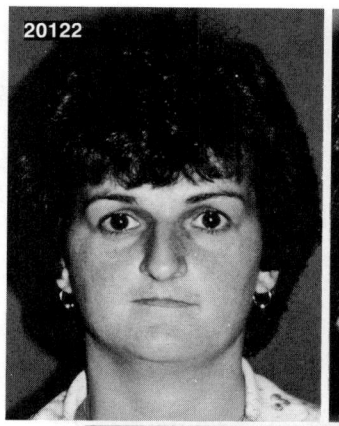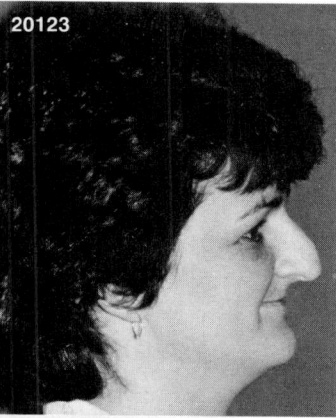
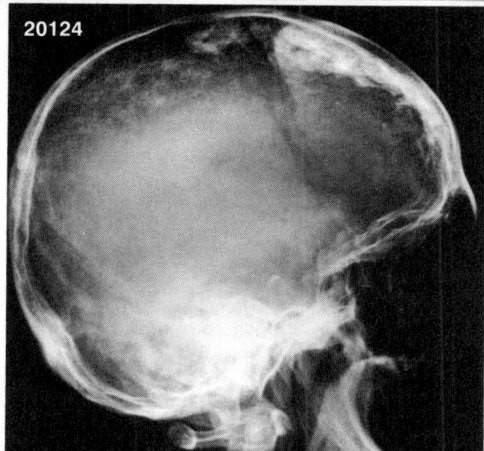
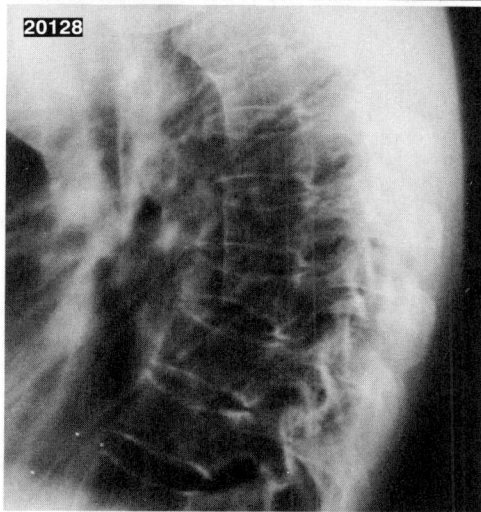

**2768**-20122–20123: Note beaked nose, short philtrum, thin lips, and maxillary hypoplasia with relative prognathism. 20124: Mild hyperostosis of inner frontal and parietal areas of the skull. 20128: Platyspondyly, multiple spontaneous small vertebral fractures, and osteoporosis of the spine.

**Complications:** Spontaneous fractures of the vertebrae, severe back pain, the need for dental extraction at adolescence.
**Associated Findings:** Mild **Camptodactyly** of DIP joints of fifth fingers in one affected female.

**Etiology:** Possibly autosomal dominant inheritance with variable expression.

**Pathogenesis:** Unknown. Serum levels of calcium; phosphorus; alkaline phosphatase; vitamin D; 25(OH) vitamin D; 24,25(OH)$_2$ vitamin D; 1,25(OH)$_2$ vitamin D; and parathormone were normal in two affected individuals.

**MIM No.:** 15651
**POS No.:** 3947
**CDC No.:** 756.450
**Sex Ratio:** Presumably M1:F1.
**Occurrence:** Reported in four generations of a French Canadian family.
**Risk of Recurrence for Patient's Sib:** See Part I, *Mendelian Inheritance.*
**Risk of Recurrence for Patient's Child:** See Part I, *Mendelian Inheritance.*
**Age of Detectability:** The youngest patient was diagnosed five years of age. X-ray manifestations could probably be present at an earlier age.
**Gene Mapping and Linkage:** Unknown.
**Prevention:** None known. Genetic counseling indicated.
**Treatment:** Physiotherapy. Orthopedic intervention if necessary. Avoid competitive sports to decrease the risk of fractures.
**Prognosis:** Normal life span.
**Detection of Carrier:** By skeletal survey.

**References:**
Halal F, et al.: Metaphyseal dysplasia with maxillary hypoplasia and brachydactyly. Am J Med Genet 1982; 13:71–79.

HA074 **Fahed Halal**

**Metaphyseal dysplasia-pancreatic hypoplasia-marrow dysfunction**
*See SHWACHMAN SYNDROME*
**Metatarsus adductus**
*See FOOT, CONGENITAL CLUBFOOT*
**Metatarsus varus**
*See FOOT, CONGENITAL CLUBFOOT*
**Metatarsus varus, type I**
*See FOOT, METATARSUS VARUS*
**Metatropic dwarfism**
*See METATROPIC DYSPLASIA*

## METATROPIC DYSPLASIA 0656

**Includes:**
Chondrodystrophy, hyperplastic form
Dwarfism, metatropic
Metatropic dwarfism

**Excludes:**
**Achondroplasia** (0010)
**Asphyxiating thoracic dysplasia** (0091)
**Kniest dysplasia** (0557)
**Mucopolysaccharidosis IV** (0678)

**Major Diagnostic Criteria:** Skeletal dysplasia with tongue-like flattening of the vertebral bodies, short ribs, progressing kyphoscoliosis, crescent-like iliac wings, osseous hyperplasia of the trochanteric region and the metaphyses of the tubular bones, irregular metaphyses and epiphyses, normal cranial vault and viscerocranium, and dysplastic skull base.

**Clinical Findings:** In infancy, long narrow thorax and relatively short limbs; rapidly progressing kyphoscoliosis. In later infancy and childhood, reversion of body proportions, with development of short-spine dwarfism. On X-ray, severe spondyloepimetaphyseal dysplasia of the skeleton.

**Complications:** Severe progressive kyphoscoliosis, and early arthroses.

**Associated Findings:** None known.

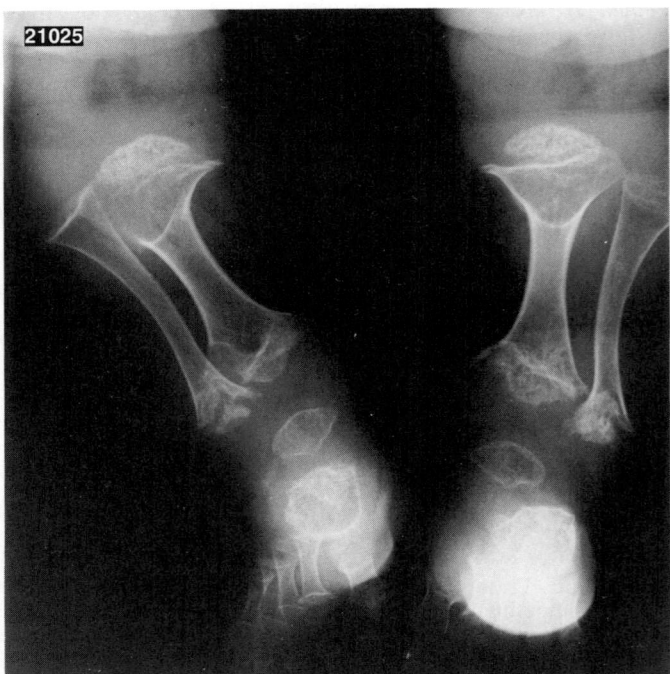

**0656-21025:** Metatropic dysplasia; note short long bones and osseous hyperplasia.

**Etiology:** Both autosomal dominant and autosomal recessive inheritance has been reported.

**Pathogenesis:** Presumed shortening of the tubular bones with irregular metaphyseal and epiphyseal ossification. Irregular arrangement of bone trabeculae, which contain islands of cartilage. Endochondral ossification processes are grossly reduced in quantity. Boden et al (1987), after study of bone samples, concluded that there had been an uncoupling of endochondral and perichondral growth, which explained the dumbbell-shaped changes in the metaphysis.

**MIM No.:** *25060

**POS No.:** 3300

**CDC No.:** 756.446

**Sex Ratio:** M1:F1

**Occurrence:** Undetermined but presumed rare.

**Risk of Recurrence for Patient's Sib:**
See Part I, *Mendelian Inheritance.*

**Risk of Recurrence for Patient's Child:**
See Part I, *Mendelian Inheritance.*

**Age of Detectability:** At birth, by X-ray, especially lateral view of the spine.

**Gene Mapping and Linkage:** Unknown.

**Prevention:** None known. Genetic counseling indicated.

**Treatment:** Intensive orthopedic care to prevent kyphoscoliosis and secondary positional defects.

**Prognosis:** Guarded, because of incapacitating physical deformities. Death frequently occurs in early infancy. Surviving patients may reach at least their third decade of life. Ultimate body height between 110 and 120 cm.

**Detection of Carrier:** Unknown.

**Special Considerations:** Cases of "hyperplastic chondrodystrophy" of the older literature probably had metatropic dwarfism. There exist one or more closely related, though ill-defined, conditions (pseudometatropic dwarfism) necessitating the obser-

vance of rigid diagnostic criteria. No criteria are available to distinguish the autosomal recessive from the autosomal dominant form.

**References:**

Maroteaux P, et al.: Der metatropische Zwergwuchs. Arch Kinderheilkd 1966; 173:211–226.

Spranger J, et al.: Bone dysplasias. Philadelphia: W.B. Saunders, Co., 1974.

Beck MM: Heterogeneity of metatropic dysplasia. Eur J Pediatr 1983; 140:231–237.

Boden SD, et al.: Metatropic dwarfism: uncoupling of endochondral and perichondral growth. J Bone Joint Surg 1987; 69A:174–184.

SP007                                    **Jürgen W. Spranger**

**Metatropic dysplasia, type II**
*See KNIEST DYSPLASIA*
**Methemoglobin reductase deficiency**
*See METHEMOGLOBINEMIA, NADH-DEPENDENT DIAPHORASE DEFICIENCY*

## METHEMOGLOBINEMIA, NADH-DEPENDENT DIAPHORASE DEFICIENCY                               2682

**Includes:**
Diaphorase deficiency
Methemoglobin reductase deficiency
NADH cytochrome b5 reductase deficiency

**Excludes:**
Cytochrome b5, deficiency of
**Glucose-6-phosphate dehydrogenase deficiency** (0420)
Hb M and other hemoglobin variants that produce cyanosis
NADPH-dependent methemoglobin reductase deficiency
Toxic methemoglobinemia

**Major Diagnostic Criteria:** Increased levels of methemoglobin (ferrihemoglobin) in the erythrocytes (typically between 10 and 40%) with NADH-dependent diaphorase activity of less than 20% of normal.

**Clinical Findings:** Affected individuals characteristically exhibit cyanosis, which is apparent at birth or shortly afterward, with an absence of demonstrable cardiac or pulmonary disease. The abnormality is ordinarily not accompanied by accelerated hemolysis or other hematologic changes; however, mild erythrocytosis has been observed in some affected individuals. The disorder has a characteristically benign course (but see below). Affected women have not experienced adverse obstetric events. Three clinical phenotypes of NADPH-dependent diaphorase deficiency have been described:

*Type I:* The abnormality is apparently confined to the erythrocytes and has benign methemoglobinemia as its only clinical abnormality. Most known individuals with NADPH-dependent diaphorase deficiency fall within this group.

*Type II:* Represents a more generalized abnormality in which the enzyme deficiency involves the leukocytes, platelets, fibroblasts, and other tissues. In addition to methemoglobinemia, affected individuals exhibit severe progressive encephalopathy with neurologic abnormalities, **Microcephaly,** and retardation. Approximately 10% of individuals with NADPH-dependent diaphorase deficiency are estimated to have this severe syndrome.

*Type III:* Associated with a deficiency of NADH-dependent diaphorase demonstrable in platelets and leukocytes as well as erythrocytes, but apparently not in other tissues. Affected individuals in the two reported families with this type did not exhibit any neurologic abnormalities.

**Complications:** Individuals with this enzyme deficiency are presumed to be at increased risk of developing toxic methemoglobinemia following exposure to drugs and chemicals that are known to produce methemoglobinemia in normal persons; care to prevent exposure to these agents is therefore advised. Levels of methemoglobin greater than 25% may produce mild fatigue and dyspnea. Cosmetic consequences of the accompanying cyanosis may also sometimes result in psychologic difficulties.

**Associated Findings:** None known.

**Etiology:** Autosomal recessive inheritance.

**Pathogenesis:** The NADH-dependent diaphorase is the physiologically active methemoglobin reductase in the erythrocytes, and in normal individuals it functions to maintain methemoglobin levels of less than 1%. The enzyme catalyzes the reduction of methemoglobin (ferrihemoglobin), which is incapable of binding oxygen, to the deoxyferrohemoglobin form. NADH and cytochrome $b_5$ are necessary cofactors, with the diaphorase functioning to catalyze the transfer of electrons from NADH to the cytochrome $b_5$. Cytochrome $b_5$ appears to reduce methemoglobin by a nonenzymatic mechanism. A deficiency of cytochrome $b_5$ has also been shown to produce congenital methemoglobinemia.

**MIM No.:** *25080

**Sex Ratio:** M1:F1

**Occurrence:** Numerous electrophoretic variants, deficiency forms, and stability variants have been described. The occurrence of affected homozygous or compound-heterozygous individuals with cyanosis is undetermined but nevertheless presumed rare.

**Risk of Recurrence for Patient's Sib:**
See Part I, *Mendelian Inheritance.*

**Risk of Recurrence for Patient's Child:**
See Part I, *Mendelian Inheritance.*

**Age of Detectability:** Junien et al. (1981) have reported successful prenatal diagnosis of the severe type II syndrome by measurement of cytochrome $b_5$ reductase activity in amniocytes.

**Gene Mapping and Linkage:** DIA1 (diaphorase (NADH) (cytochrome b-5 reductase)) has been mapped to 22q13.31-qter.

**Prevention:** None known. Genetic counseling indicated.

**Treatment:** Cosmetic improvement of the accompanying cyanosis may be achieved by treatment with methylene blue (100–300 mg/day), ascorbic acid (0.5 g/day), or riboflavin (20 mg/day). No effective treatment is known for the encephalopathic manifestations of the type II syndrome.

**Prognosis:** *Types I and III:* normal growth, development, and life span. *Type II:* severe and progressive neurologic dysfunction, poor growth, and mental retardation, often with a fatal outcome during infancy or childhood.

**Detection of Carrier:** Carriers of deficiency variants with altered electrophoretic mobility are readily identified by electrophoretic diaphorase analysis of red cell lysates. Enzyme activity in heterozygous carriers is approximately one-half of normal.

**References:**
Jaffe ER, et al.: Hereditary methemoglobinemia with and without mental retardation: a study of three families. Am J Med 1966; 41:42–55.
Hsieh H-S, Jaffe ER: Electrophoretic and functional variants of NADH-methemoglobin reductase in hereditary methemoglobinemia. J Clin Invest 1971; 50:196–202.
Jaffe ER, Hsieh H-S: DPNH-methemoglobin reductase deficiency and hereditary methemoglobinemia. Semin Hematol 1971; 8:417–437.
McAlpine PJ, et al.: Is the DIA-1 locus linked to the P blood group locus? Cytogenet Cell Genet 1978; 22:629–632.
Junien C, et al.: Prenatal diagnosis of congenital enzymopenic methaemoglobinaemia with mental retardation due to generalized cytochrome $b_5$ reductase deficiency: first report of two cases. Prenatal Diagn 1981; 1:17–24.
Hegesh E, et al.: Congenital methemoglobinemia with a deficiency of cytochrome $b_5$. New Engl J Med 1986; 314:757–761.

H0024                                          **George R. Honig**

**Methimazole, fetal effects, scalp and urachal**
*See FETAL EFFECTS FROM METHIMAZOLE AND CARBIMAZOLE*
**Methionine 111 amyloidosis**
*See AMYLOIDOSIS, DANISH CARDIAC TYPE*
**Methionine 30 amyloidosis**
*See AMYLOIDOSIS, TRANSTHYRETIN METHIONINE-30 TYPE*

## METHIONINE MALABSORPTION                    0657

**Includes:**
  Malabsorption, methionine
  Oast-house urine disease
  Smith-Strang disease

**Excludes:** Hartnup disorder (0453)

**Major Diagnostic Criteria:** This rare condition is associated with convulsions, mental retardation, and a sweet odor of body fluids in a child with fair hair and blue eyes. Diagnosis is suspected by detection of increased $\alpha$-hydroxybutyric acid in urine and feces in amounts related to methionine intake.

**Clinical Findings:** Mental retardation with normal physical development. Clinical findings included white hair, blue eyes, convulsions, intermittent diarrhea, and an intermittent sweet odor to the urine and the patient. The level of dietary intake of protein determined the presence or absence of intestinal symptoms, seizures, and odor; a high protein intake provoked symptoms.

Alpha-hydroxybutyric acid is found in urine and feces in amounts related to the methionine intake. This compound is believed to account for the peculiar odor. Its formation occurs in the intestine from bacterial degradation of methionine. Methionine excretion is increased in feces but not in the urine under usual endogenous conditions. Oral loading with methionine increases fecal excretion of many amino acids; loading with branched-chain compounds does not affect methionine excretion.

**Complications:** Diarrhea, seizures, and mental retardation seem related to metabolic disorder; whether they are incidental findings cannot be ruled out, but this seems unlikely.

**Associated Findings:** None known.

**Etiology:** Autosomal recessive inheritance.

**Pathogenesis:** Proposed deficiency of specific intestinal membrane transport system for L-methionine.

**MIM No.:** *25090

**Sex Ratio:** Presumably M1:F1.

**Occurrence:** Two or three families reported in the literature, including English and Belgian cases.

**Risk of Recurrence for Patient's Sib:**
See Part I, *Mendelian Inheritance.*

**Risk of Recurrence for Patient's Child:**
See Part I, *Mendelian Inheritance.*

**Age of Detectability:** Presumably at birth.

**Gene Mapping and Linkage:** Unknown.

**Prevention:** None known. Genetic counseling indicated.

**Treatment:** Low methionine intake, e.g., low animal protein or soy protein diet, improves symptoms and EEG.

**Prognosis:** Unknown.

**Detection of Carrier:** Evidence for partial intestinal transport defect.

**Special Considerations:** The Belgian male proband was the youngest of 12 children. Both parents showed partial trait. Smith and Strang's (1958) female infant with "oasthouse" odor had similar appearance and clinical symptoms. Her urine contained $\alpha$-hydroxybutyric acid, but phenylpyruvic acid was also present, plus many hydroxy-, keto-, and amino acids. She is the only case of "oasthouse urine syndrome" reported to date, but probably similar to a case reported by Hooft et al. (1968).

**References:**
Jepson JB, et al.: An inborn error of metabolism with urinary excretion of hydroxyacids, ketoacids, and aminoacids (Letter). Lancet 1958; II:1334–1335.
Smith AJ, Strang LB: An inborn error of metabolism with the urinary excretion of alpha-hydroxy-butyric acid and phenylpyruvic acid. Arch Dis Child 1958; 33:109–113.

Hooft C, et al.: Further investigations in the methionine malabsorption syndrome. Helv Paediatr Acta 1968; 23:334–349.

SC050                                              **Charles R. Scriver**

**Methotrexate, fetal effects of**
*See FETAL AMINOPTERIN SYNDROME*

## METHYLCOBALAMIN DEFICIENCY                          2605

**Includes:**
 Anemia, megaloblastic-homocystinuria
 B(12) responsive homocystinuria without methylmalonic
  aciduria
 Cobalamin E disease (cb1E)
 Cobalamin G disease (cb1G)
 Homocystinuria-megaloblastic anemia due to cobalamin
  defect

**Excludes:**
 B(12) responsive homocystinuria with methylmalonic
  aciduria
 **Cobalamin C disease (cb1C)**
 **Cobalamin D disease (cb1D)**
 **Homocystinuria** (0474)
 Methylene-tetrahydrofolate reductase deficiency

**Major Diagnostic Criteria:** Homocystinuria with normal organic acid quantitation, megaloblastic anemia with normal serum $B_{12}$, folate, and orotic acid levels. Biochemical assay documenting failure of production of methylcobalamin.

**Clinical Findings:** Feeding difficulties, developmental delay, seizures, megaloblastic anemia, cortical atrophy, and **Microcephaly**.

**Complications:** Mental retardation, seizure disorders, failure to thrive, infections, cerebral atrophy, and death.

**Associated Findings:** None known.

**Etiology:** Autosomal recessive inheritance.

**Pathogenesis:** Inborn error of metabolism.

**MIM No.:** *23627

**Sex Ratio:** Cobalamin E: M5:F0 observed; Cobalamin G: M3:F4 observed.

**Occurrence:** Twelve cases have been documented in the literature.

**Risk of Recurrence for Patient's Sib:**
 See Part I, *Mendelian Inheritance.*

**Risk of Recurrence for Patient's Child:**
 See Part I, *Mendelian Inheritance.*

**Age of Detectability:** At birth, or by prenatal diagnosis by measurement of $B_{12}$ distribution and methyl-tetrahydrofolate incorporation in amniocytes.

**Gene Mapping and Linkage:** Unknown.

**Prevention:** None known. Genetic counseling indicated.

**Treatment:** Pharmacologic doses of hydroxycobalamin. Two patients have been maintained with cyanocobalamin, but in others, response to cyanocobalamin has been poor. Methylcobalamin, betaine, and folinic acid have been used. Prenatal treatment of an affected fetus has been reported.

**Prognosis:** Appears to be good if treatment is begun early. The anemia has been easier to correct than the neurologic manifestations.

**Detection of Carrier:** Unknown.

**Special Considerations:** Heterogeneity exists among patients with methylcobalamin deficiency. At present, two complementation groups have been demonstrated. This implies that there are multiple mutations capable of producing methylcobalamin deficiency, which may not be allelic. Methionine synthase has been localized to chromosome 1 using human-hamster hybrids; the relationship to the cb1E and cb1G loci is not clear.

**References:**
Rosenblatt DS, et al.: Altered vitamin B12 metabolism in fibroblasts from a patient with megaloblastic anemia and homocystinuria due to a new defect in methionine biosynthesis. J Clin Invest 1984; 74:2149–2156.
Schuh S, et al.: Homocystinuria and megaloblastic anemia responsive to vitamin B-12 therapy. New Engl J Med 1984; 310:686–690. *
Rosenblatt DS, et al.: Prenatal vitamin B-12 therapy of a fetus with methylcobalamin deficiency (cobalamin E disease). Lancet 1985; I:1127–1129.
Rosenblatt DS, et al.: Vitamin B-12 responsive homocystinuria and megaloblastic anemia: heterogeneity in methylcobalamin deficiency. Am J Med Genet 1987; 26:377–383.
Tuchman M, et al.: Vitamin B-12 responsive megaloblastic anemia, homocystinuria, and transient methylmalonic aciduria in cb1E disease. J Pediatr 1988; 113:1052–1056.
Watkins D, Rosenblatt DS: Genetic heterogeneity among patients with methylcobalamin deficiency. J Clin Invest 1988; 81:1690–1694. * (cb1G)

FL001                                         **David B. Flannery**
WA053                                            **David Watkins**
R0052                                       **David S. Rosenblatt**

**Methylenetetrahydrofolate reductase (MTHFR) deficiency**
 *See HOMOCYSTINURIA, N(5,10) METHYLENE TETRAHYDROFOLATE DEFICIENCY TYPE*
**Methylmalonic acidemia**
 *See ACIDEMIA, METHYLMALONIC*
**Methylmalonic aciduria**
 *See ACIDEMIA, METHYLMALONIC*
**Methylmalonic aciduria due to B release defect**
 *See VITAMIN B(12) LYSOSOMAL TRANSPORT DEFECT*
**Methylmercury, organic, fetal effects of**
 *See FETAL METHYLMERCURY EFFECTS*
**Mevalonate kinase deficiency**
 *See ACIDEMIA, MEVALONIC*
**Mevalonic aciduria**
 *See ACIDEMIA, MEVALONIC*
**Mexican cardiomelic dysplasia**
 *See HEART-HAND SYNDROME IV*
**Michail-Matsoukas-Theodorou-Rubinstein-Taybi syndrome**
 *See RUBINSTEIN-TAYBI BROAD THUMB-HALLUX SYNDROME*
**Michel malformation of inner ear**
 *See EAR, LABYRINTH APLASIA*

## MICHELIN TIRE BABY SYNDROME                          2642

**Includes:**
 Skin creases, multiple benign circumferential of the limbs
 Skin, generalized folded with an underlying lipomatous
  nevus

**Excludes:**
 **Amniotic bands syndrome** (0874)
 **Cutis verticus gyrata** (2295)
 **Deafness-keratopachydermia-digital constrictions** (0259)
 Disruption complex
 Skin, generalized folded in short-limb dwarfism

**Major Diagnostic Criteria:** Generalized symmetric folding of skin around arms, legs, and trunk without symptoms of strangulation.

**Clinical Findings:** Multiple benign ring-shaped skin creases on all extremities, fingers, toes, and the trunk without amputations or limb deformities.

**Complications:** Unknown.

**Associated Findings:** Findings in only one affected individual each: such minor anomalies as epicanthic folds, upward-slanting palpebral fissures, hypertelorism, median **Cleft palate**, neuroblastoma; micrognathia, malformed ears, ureteroceles; febrile convulsions; slight mental retardation; left hemihypertrophy; and idiopathic scarring of the skin. Underlying lipomatous nevus and a median cleft were observed in two patients.

**Etiology:** Autosomal dominant inheritance. Heterogeneity may exist.

**Pathogenesis:** Unknown.

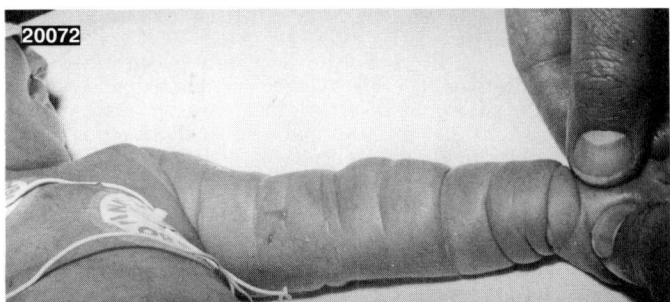

**2642-20072:** Note the multiple, irregular ring-shaped skin creases on the arm of this 6-day-old infant.

**MIM No.:** *15661

**POS No.:** 4404

**Sex Ratio:** M8:F7 (observed).

**Occurrence:** Several sibships have been reported. Wiedemann (1987) pointed out that the condition appears in a bronze representation on the door of the cathedral of Hildesheim in northwestern Germany.

**Risk of Recurrence for Patient's Sib:**
See Part I, *Mendelian Inheritance.*

**Risk of Recurrence for Patient's Child:**
See Part I, *Mendelian Inheritance.*

**Age of Detectability:** At birth by physical examination.

**Gene Mapping and Linkage:** Unknown.

**Prevention:** None known. Genetic counseling indicated.

**Treatment:** Unknown.

**Prognosis:** In all familial cases, the circular skin alterations almost disappeared in later life.

**Detection of Carrier:** Unknown.

**References:**
Ross CM: Generalized folded skin with an underlying lipomatous nevus. Arch Dermatol 1969; 100:320–323.
Gardner EW, et al.: Folded skin associated with underlying nevus lipomatous. Arch Dermatol 1979; 115:978–979.
Wallach D, et al.: Naevus musculaire généralisé avec aspect clinique de ''Bébé Michelin.'' Arch Dermatol Venereol 1980; 107:923–927.
Burgdorf WH, et al.: Folded skin with scarring: Michelin tire baby syndrome? J Am Acad Dermatol 1982; 7:90–93.
Kunze J, et al.: A new genetic disorder: autosomal-dominant multiple benign ring-shaped skin creases. Eur J Pediatr 1982; 138:301–303.
Niikawa N, et al.: The ''Michelin tire baby'' syndrome: an autosomal dominant trait. (Letter) Am J Med Genet 1985; 22:637–638.
Kunze J: The ''Michelin tire baby syndrome'': an autosomal-dominant trait. Am J Med Genet 1986; 25:169 only.
Niikawa N, et al.: Letter to the editor: response to Dr. Kunze. Am J Med Genet 1986; 25:171 only.
Wiedemann H-R: Multiple benign circumferential skin creases on limbs: a congenital anomaly existing from the begining of mankind. (Letter) Am J Med Genet 1987; 28:225–226.

KU008                                    **Jürgen Kunze**

**Microcephalic primordial dwarfism**
*See SECKEL SYNDROME*
**Microcephalic primordial dwarfism, type II**
*See DWARFISM, OSTEODYSPLASTIC PRIMORDIAL, MAJEWSKI-RANKE TYPE*

---

## MICROCEPHALY                                    0659

**Includes:** Microencephaly

**Excludes:**
Congenital diplegia with small head
Cranial sutures, premature closure of
**Fetal cytomegalovirus syndrome** (0381)
**Fetal rubella syndrome** (0384)
**Fetal toxoplasmosis syndrome** (0387)
**Microcephaly, autosomal recessive with normal intelligence** (2838)
**Microcephaly, isolated autosomal dominant type** (2334)
**Microcephaly** (other)
Relative microcephaly associated with cerebral lesions of infancy

**Major Diagnostic Criteria:** Head circumference is very small; in infancy, normal open sutures are seen on X-ray. Mental retardation is usually present.

**Clinical Findings:** A heterogeneous state in which head circumference is smaller than 2 SD below the mean for age. A narrow, sloping forehead, often with a flat occiput. Varying degrees of mental retardation occur, although severe amentia is the most common. In infancy, X-rays show that the cranial sutures are open. Skull thickness may be normal or increased. EEG is frequently normal. Seizures are present in a small percentage of affected individuals. Care must be taken to distinguish microcephaly secondary to degenerative brain disorders from microcephaly as a primary inherited disorder.

**Complications:** Mental retardation.

**Associated Findings:** Cataracts, short stature.

**Etiology:** Usually autosomal recessive inheritance. This condition may follow a degenerative brain disorder, birth trauma, intrauterine infection, or exposure to X-rays in utero. Rarely, autosomal dominant inheritance is reported (see **Microcephaly, isolated autosomal dominant type**).

**Pathogenesis:** Microcephaly is the result of failure of normal growth of the brain. The brain may show various abnormalities of sulcation and gyration, or an essentially normal pattern.

**MIM No.:** *25120

**POS No.:** 3301

**CDC No.:** 742.100

**Sex Ratio:** Presumably M1:F1

**Occurrence:** 1:250,000 based on Netherlands studies.

**Risk of Recurrence for Patient's Sib:**
See Part I, *Mendelian Inheritance.*

**Risk of Recurrence for Patient's Child:**
See Part I, *Mendelian Inheritance.*

**Age of Detectability:** In infancy. Ultrasound shows abnormal fetal head growth rate, fetal chest and abdominal diameters greater than biparietal diameter, biparietal diameter and head area greater than 3 SD below mean, no midline fetal brain echo, oligohydramnios.

**Gene Mapping and Linkage:** Unknown.

**Prevention:** None known. Genetic counseling indicated.

**Treatment:** Unknown.

**Prognosis:** Varies with degree of mental retardation.

**Detection of Carrier:** Unknown.

*The author wishes to thank Kenneth Shulman for his contribution to a previous version of this article.*

**References:**
Cowie V: The genetics and sub-classification of microcephaly. J Ment Defic Res 1960; 4:42–47.
Qazi QH, Reed TE: A possible major contribution to mental retardation in the general population by the gene for microcephaly. Clin Genet 1975; 7:85.

Haslam RHA, Smith DW: Autosomal dominant microcephaly. J Pediatr 1979; 95:701–705.

Ramirez ML, et al.: Silent microcephaly. Clin Genet 1983; 23:281–286.

Tolmie JL, et al.: Microcephaly: genetic counseling and antenatal diagnosis after the birth of an affected child. Am J Med Genet 1987; 27:583–594.

SH007                                          **Kenneth Shapiro**

## MICROCEPHALY WITH CHORIORETINOPATHY          2333

**Includes:**
> Chorioretinopathy-congenital microcephaly
> Pseudotoxoplasmosis syndrome

**Excludes:**
> **Craniosynostosis** (0230)
> **Fetal cytomegalovirus syndrome** (0381)
> **Fetal rubella syndrome** (0384)
> **Fetal toxoplasmosis syndrome** (0387)
> **Microcephaly** (0659)
> Microcephaly in other syndromes
> Relative microcephaly associated with cerebral lesions of infancy

**Major Diagnostic Criteria:** Congenital microcephaly and chorioretinal degeneration.

**Clinical Findings:** Congenital microcephaly; chorioretinal dysplasia with retinal pigmentation and a progressive visual deficiency evident during childhood; choroidal and optic atrophy; embryonic remnants, pale optic disks, and cataracts sometimes with microphthalmia; nystagmus; delayed psychomotor development; and variable degrees of mental deficiency. Normal intelligence is also found in affected individuals.

X-ray studies show that all the cranial diameters are diminished. There may be craniofacial disproportion without calcifications or closed sutures. The EEG suggests encephalodysplasia. Serologic studies for toxoplasmosis, rubella, cytomegalovirus, and herpes infection are negative.

This is a distinct microcephaly consistently accompanied by chorioretinal dysplasia. There is widely variable expressivity in patients with the autosomal dominant form ranging from normocephaly to microcephaly, from normal eyes to chorioretinal dysplasia, and from normal intelligence to mental retardation.

**Complications:** Decreased visual acuity. Mental retardation probably due to microcephaly.

**Associated Findings:** In the autosomal recessive form, early nanosomy, **Cutis marmorata**, nystagmus, and severe neurologic problems can also be found. Embryonic remnants, mainly persistence of primary vitreous, may be present in both autosomal dominant and recessive forms.

**Etiology:** Autosomal dominant or autosomal recessive inheritance.

**Pathogenesis:** Unknown.

**MIM No.:** 15659, *25127

**POS No.:** 3240

**Sex Ratio:** M1:F1

**Occurrence:** Reported in eight kinships and a Mennonite sect.

**Risk of Recurrence for Patient's Sib:**
See Part I, *Mendelian Inheritance.*

**Risk of Recurrence for Patient's Child:**
See Part I, *Mendelian Inheritance.*

**Age of Detectability:** At birth.

**Gene Mapping and Linkage:** Unknown.

**Prevention:** None known. Genetic counseling indicated. Given the similarity between chorioretinopathy and toxoplasmosis, at-risk individuals should be managed with care (Daffos et al, 1988).

**Treatment:** Surgery, as needed, for ophthalmologic abnormalities.

**Prognosis:** Normal life span.

**Detection of Carrier:** Unknown.

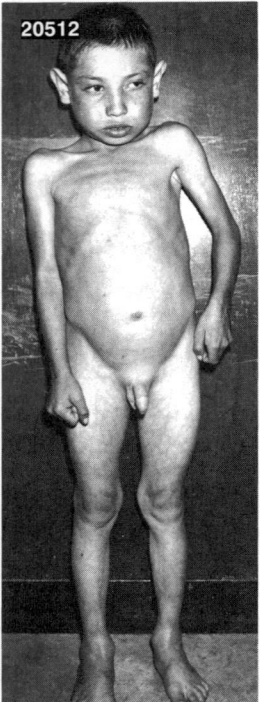

**References:**

McKusick VA, et al.: Chorioretinopathy with hereditary microcephaly. Arch Ophthalmol 1966; 75:597–600. †

Schmidt B, et al.: Ein mikrozephalie-syndrom mit atypischer tapetoretinaler Degeneration bei 3 Geschwister. Klin Mbnatsbl Augenheilkd 1968; 150:188–196.

Cantú JM, et al.: Autosomal recessive microcephaly associated with chorioretinopathy. Hum Genet 1977; 36:243–247. *

Alzial C, et al.: Microcephalie "vraie" avec dysplasie chorioétinienne a hérédité dominante. Ann Genet (Paris) 1980; 23:91–94. * †

Tenconi R, et al.: Chorio-retinal dysplasia, microcephaly and mental retardation: an autosomal dominant syndrome. Clin Genet 1981; 20:347–351.

Parke JT, et al.: A syndrome of microcephaly and retinal pigmentary abnormalities without mental retardation in a family with coincidental autosomal dominant hyperreflexia. Am J Med Genet 1984; 17:585–594.

Daffos F, et al.: Prenatal management of 746 pregnancies at risk for congenital toxoplasmosis. New Engl J Med 1988; 318:271–275.

CR023                                    **Diana García-Cruz**
CA011                                    **José María Cantú**

**2333-20512:** Note microcephaly, short stature, cutis marmorata in this boy with chorioretinal degeneration.

**Microcephaly without mental retardation**
*See MICROCEPHALY, ISOLATED AUTOSOMAL DOMINANT TYPE*

## MICROCEPHALY, AUTOSOMAL RECESSIVE WITH NORMAL INTELLIGENCE                           2838

**Includes:**  Microcephaly, nonsyndromal with normal intelligence

**Excludes:**
> Chromosome instability, Nijmegen type (2551)
> Dwarfism, microcephalic primordial with cataracts (2584)
> Microcephaly (0659)
> Microcephaly, familial with normal intelligence
> Microcephaly, isolated autosomal dominant type (2334)
> Seckel syndrome (0881)

**Major Diagnostic Criteria:**  Microcephaly significantly below the third percentile for age, peculiar facies, normal stature or stature at the lower limit of normal, and normal psychomotor development and intelligence.

**Clinical Findings:**  At birth, head circumference is small (between 30 and 32 cm) but with normal length and body weight. Affected persons show a low receding forehead with normal scalp hair, unlike patients with autosomal recessive "true" microcephaly, whose foreheads incline acutely and scalp may be excessively furrowed. Facial features also include prominent eyes with an upward slant, epicanthic folds, long and straight nose, high nasal bridge, widely spaced teeth with or without malocclusion, and receding chin. Affected individuals often reach normal developmental milestones with no clinical evidence of immunodeficiency. There is no neurologic deficit. Data indicate that none had mental retardation, often with fairly good scholastic performance but were not "clever" compared to their normal sibs. Only one had borderline intelligence.

Interfamilial variability is minimal. Careful examination of parents is essential to rule out the possibility of **Microcephaly, isolated autosomal dominant type**. The condition must be distinguished from that with immunodeficiency and risk for lymphoreticular malignancies (see **Chromosome instability, Nijmegen type**). In both of these conditions, the facies are similar.

**Complications:**  Affected individuals are usually "shy" and lack self-confidence. A sporadic case 1 1/2 years of age was hyperactive.

**Associated Findings:**  None known.

**Etiology:**  Probably autosomal recessive inheritance. All known sibships with affected individuals have consanguineous parents.

**Pathogenesis:**  Unknown.

**MIM No.:**  *25126

**Sex Ratio:**  Presumably M1:F1; M2:F1 observed.

**Occurrence:**  Ten cases have been reported; a kindred with eight affected individuals, and two sporadic cases.

**Risk of Recurrence for Patient's Sib:**
See Part I, *Mendelian Inheritance*. Observed frequency is 30 percent.

**Risk of Recurrence for Patient's Child:**
See Part I, *Mendelian Inheritance*.

**Age of Detectability:**  Usually clinically evident at birth. Confirmation by age 1–2 years when adequate intelligence testing can be performed. IQ is around 100.

**Gene Mapping and Linkage:**  Unknown.

**Prevention:**  None known. Genetic counseling indicated.

**Treatment:**  Assurance of patients and parents of this condition's benign nature. Special attention to those with borderline intelligence.

**Prognosis:**  Out of ten patients reported, two died in early life during the early 1970s in areas with limited medical care, one with postmeasles bronchopneumonia and the other with leukemia. Two patients lived for 60 and 65 years and had normal reproductive lives. No physical handicaps. In general, life span and function are probably normal.

**Detection of Carrier:**  Unknown.

**Special Considerations:**  Though allelism is not exluded between this entity and **Chromosome instability, Nijmegen type**, genetic heterogeneity remains a possibility in the patients with microcephaly and normal intelligence in general, which includes in addition to these two autosomal recessive types, **Microcephaly, isolated autosomal dominant type** and **Seckel syndrome**.

**References:**
Teebi AS, et al.: Autosomal recessive nonsyndromal microcephaly with normal intelligence. Am J Med Genet 1987; 26:355–359.

TE012                                         **Ahmad S. Teebi**

## MICROCEPHALY, ISOLATED AUTOSOMAL DOMINANT TYPE                                 2334

**Includes:**
> Microcephaly without mental retardation
> Silent microcephaly

**Excludes:**
> Microcephaly with mental retardation
> Microcephaly, all other forms
> "True" microcephaly

**Major Diagnostic Criteria:**  A cephalic circumference below the third percentile or 2 SD below the mean for the corresponding age and sex, with normal skull by X-ray studies, and average intelligence.

**Clinical Findings:**  Microcephaly as the sole trait can be recognized by the occipitofrontoal circumference (OFC) below the third percentile. The facies are not dysmorphic and are proportional to the small head. Normal stature, behavior, and scholastic performance are the rule. Neurologic and psychometric evaluations, and X-rays of the skull, are also normal.

**Complications:**  Unknown.

**Associated Findings:**  Short stature was reported in a Black family (Burton, 1981).

**Etiology:**  Autosomal dominant inheritance.

**Pathogenesis:**  Unknown.

**MIM No.:**  *15658

**POS No.:**  3600

**Sex Ratio:**  M1:F2 (observed).

**Occurrence:**  Over a dozen kinships have been documented, including several Italian families and at least one Black family.

**Risk of Recurrence for Patient's Sib:**
See Part I, *Mendelian Inheritance*.

**Risk of Recurrence for Patient's Child:**
See Part I, *Mendelian Inheritance*.

**Age of Detectability:**  Usually at birth.

**Gene Mapping and Linkage:**  Unknown.

**Prevention:**  None known. Genetic counseling indicated.

**Treatment:**  Unknown.

**Prognosis:**  Good for life span and intelligence.

**Detection of Carrier:**  Unknown.

**References:**
Burton BK: Dominant inheritance of microcephaly with short stature. Clin Genet 1981; 20:25–27.
Ramírez ML, et al.: Silent microcephaly: a distinct autosomal dominant trait. Clin Genet 1983; 23:281–286.
Rossi LN, et al.: Autosomal dominant microcephaly without mental retardation. Am J Dis Child 1987; 141:655–659.

RA021                                     **Maria Lourdes Ramírez**
CA011                                         **José María Cantú**

**Microcephaly, nonsyndromal with normal intelligence**
> *See* MICROCEPHALY, AUTOSOMAL RECESSIVE WITH NORMAL INTELLIGENCE
**Microcephaly, X-linked**
> *See* X-LINKED MENTAL RETARDATION-GROWTH-HEARING AND GENITAL DEFECTS

**Microcephaly-albinism-digital defects**
 *See ALBINISM-MICROCEPHALY-DIGITAL DEFECTS*
**Microcephaly-branchial arch, X-linked**
 *See BRANCHIAL ARCH SYNDROME, X-LINKED*
**Microcephaly-chemotactic defect-transient hypogammaglobulinemia**
 *See MICROCEPHALY-RETARDATION-SKELETAL AND IMMUNE DEFECTS*
**Microcephaly-growth/mental retardation-unusual facies-cleft palate**
 *See WEAVER-WILLIAMS SYNDROME*

## MICROCEPHALY-HIATUS HERNIA-NEPHROSIS, GALLOWAY TYPE                                    2755

**Includes:**
 Galloway syndrome
 Hiatus hernia-microcephaly-nephrosis, Galloway type
 Nephrosis-microcephaly-hiatus hernia, Galloway type

**Excludes:**
 **Hernia, hiatal** (0471)
 **Microcephaly** (0659)
 **Nephrosis, congenital** (0709)
 **Nephrosis, familial type** (0710)

**Major Diagnostic Criteria:** **Microcephaly** is evident at birth. **Hernia, hiatal** may be suspected because of recurrent vomiting, and confirmed by X-ray studies. Nephrotic syndrome appears within a few days to two years after birth.

**Clinical Findings:** Pregnancies were uneventful, and birth weights ranged between 2,240 and 3,100 g. Striking **Microcephaly** was observed at birth associated with a peculiarly shaped head with narrow and receding forehead, flat occiput, and flat vertex. Head size grew very little with age. Skull X-rays showed asymmetry and secondary craniosynostosis but no calcifications. Neurologic observations included poor head control; marked generalized hypotonia; lack of interest in surroundings; nonexistence of purposeful movements of eyes, hands, and feet; absence of any motor development even at age three years; and profound psychomotor retardation. Neck retraction episodes and seizures were common.

Recurrent and sometimes projectile vomiting episodes began very early, leading to suspicion of hiatus hernia, which was confirmed by contrast X-ray studies in three of five patients.

Proteinuria associated with microscopic hematuria was noted as early as the first week of life in two patients, but was delayed until age two years in one. These findings, along with periorbital and dependent edema, hypoalbuminemia, and anemia were consistent with the diagnosis of the nephrotic syndrome. There was no associated aminoaciduria.

Autopsy information is available on three of five patients reported to date. Brain weights were considerably smaller than that expected for age. In one patient microscopic studies showed lack of cortical stratification, hypomyelination of the brainstem and the spinal cord, complete absence of the internal granular layer of the cerebellum and dentate gyrus within the hippocampal formation, and hypoplasia of the olivary nuclei. Kidneys were large; histologic observations included hypercellularity, microcystic dysplasia, and focal glomerulosclerosis. In one patient the biopsy findings were interpreted as being similar to those observed in the "Finnish-type" nephrotic syndrome. Hiatus hernia was not seen at autopsy in two patients, although it had been demonstrated premortem by X-ray.

**Complications:** Severe psychomotor retardation, hypotonia, failure to thrive, massive edema, hypoalbuminemia, and early death due to renal failure.

**Associated Findings:** Large floppy ears (low and posteriorly set), micrognathia, high-arched palate, **Eye, hypertelorism**, calcifications in intervertebral disk, failure of cleavage of anterior chamber of the eye, and optic atrophy.

**Etiology:** Autosomal recessive inheritance.

**Pathogenesis:** Unknown.

**MIM No.:** *25130

**POS No.:** 3985

**Sex Ratio:** M1:F1

**Occurrence:** Five patients have been reported in three families; two Caucasian and one Black American.

**Risk of Recurrence for Patient's Sib:**
 See Part I, *Mendelian Inheritance.*

**Risk of Recurrence for Patient's Child:**
 See Part I, *Mendelian Inheritance.* Affected individuals are not expected to survive to reproduce.

**Age of Detectability:** Of the three obligatory features of the syndrome, small head with peculiar shape is readily evident at birth. Hiatus hernia may be suspected in the first weeks because of recurrent vomiting. Onset of nephrosis may be delayed for several months.

**Gene Mapping and Linkage:** Unknown.

**Prevention:** None known. Genetic counseling indicated.

**Treatment:** Supportive for seizures and nephrotic syndrome. The hiatus hernia could be treated surgically.

**Prognosis:** All reported patients have died between ages two weeks and three years. Severe psychomotor retardation is the rule.

**Detection of Carrier:** Unknown.

**References:**
Galloway WH, Mowat AP: Congenital microcephaly with hiatus hernia and nephrotic syndrome in two sibs. J Med Genet 1968; 5:319–321. *
Shapiro LR, et al.: Congenital microcephaly, hiatus hernia and nephrotic syndrome: an autosomal recessive syndrome. BD:OAS XII(5). New York: March of Dimes Birth Defects Foundation, 1976: 275–278. †
Qazi QH, et al.: Galloway syndrome in a black infant. Pediatr Res 1985; 19:252A.
Roos RAC, et al.: Congenital microcephaly, infantile spasms, psychomotor retardation, and nephrotic syndrome in two sibs. Europ J Pediat 1987; 146:532–536.
Kozlowski PB, et al.: Brain morphology in the Galloway syndrome. Clin Neuropathol 1989; 8:85–91.

QA000                                                    **Qutub H. Qazi**

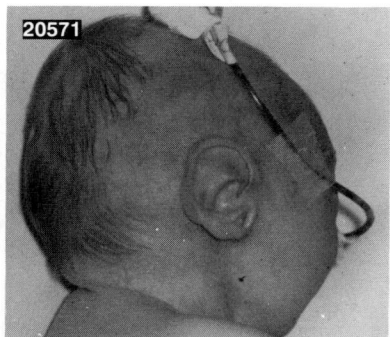
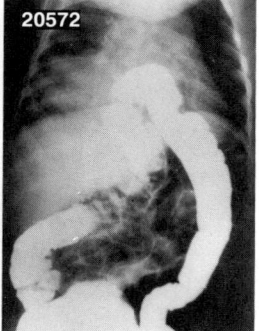

**2755**-20571: Large floppy ears and microcephaly.   20572: Hiatal hernia of the colon.

**Microcephaly-immunodeficiency-lymphoreticular malignancy**
 *See CHROMOSOME INSTABILITY, NIJMEGEN TYPE*

## MICROCEPHALY-LYMPHEDEMA 2639

**Includes:**
> Leung syndrome
> Lymphedema-microcephaly

**Excludes:**
> **Distichiasis-lymphedema syndrome** (2039)
> **Fabry disease** (0373)
> **Lymphedema I** (0614)
> **Microcephaly** (0659)

**Major Diagnostic Criteria:** The combination of congenital **Microcephaly** and **Lymphedema** of the lower limbs in the absence of other findings.

**Clinical Findings:** Affected individuals have congenital **Microcephaly** (OC ≥2 SD below the mean) and congenital lymphedema of the lower limbs. The lymphedema apparently disappears with age, although the propositus in one reported family still had pitting edema of the feet at age one year, and an affected individual in another family had intermittent swelling of feet and legs his entire life. Minor facial anomalies, including epicanthal folds, flat nasal bridge, micrognathia, and prominent ear helix can also be present. These minor anomalies have been termed the "congenital lymphedema face" by Opitz (1986).

**Complications:** Unknown.

**Associated Findings:** None known.

**Etiology:** Probably autosomal dominant inheritance.

**Pathogenesis:** Unknown.

**MIM No.:** *15295

**POS No.:** 3754

**Sex Ratio:** M1:F1

**Occurrence:** Four generations of one Canadian family of Chinese ethnic origin, and at least two members of a second family, have been reported.

**Risk of Recurrence for Patient's Sib:**
> See Part I, *Mendelian Inheritance.*

**Risk of Recurrence for Patient's Child:**
> See Part I, *Mendelian Inheritance.*

**Age of Detectability:** At birth, although prenatal diagnosis by ultrasound may be possible.

**Gene Mapping and Linkage:** Unknown.

**Prevention:** None known. Genetic counseling indicated.

**Treatment:** Unknown.

**Prognosis:** Life span and intellect are not affected.

**Detection of Carrier:** Unknown.

**References:**
Leung AKC: Dominantly inherited syndrome of microcephaly and congenital lymphedema. Clin Genet 1985; 27:611–612.
Crowe CA, Dickerman LH: A genetic association between microcephaly and lymphedema. Am J Med Genet 1986; 24:131–135.
Opitz JM: On congenital lymphedema. (Editorial) Am J Med Genet 1986; 24:127–129.
Leung AKC: Dominantly inherited syndrome of microcephaly and congenital lymphedema with normal intelligence. (Letter) Am J Med Genet 1987; 26:231 only.

T0007                      **Helga V. Toriello**

**Microcephaly-lymphedema-normal intelligence**
> *See LYMPHEDEMA I*

**Microcephaly-mental retardation-retinopathy**
> *See RETINOPATHY-MICROCEPHALY-MENTAL RETARDATION*

**Microcephaly-microphthalmia-falciform retinal folds**
> *See RETINAL FOLD*

**Microcephaly-multiple congenital anomalies**
> *See CEREBRO-OCULO-FACIO-SKELETAL SYNDROME*

**Microcephaly-nephrosis-hiatal hernia**
> *See NEPHROSIS-HYDROCEPHALUS-THIN SKIN-BLUE SCLERA-GROWTH DEFECT*

## MICROCEPHALY-RETARDATION-SKELETAL AND IMMUNE DEFECTS 3131

**Includes:**
> Immunodeficiency-microencephaly-retardation-skeletal defects
> Microcephaly-chemotactic defect-transient hypogammaglobulinemia
> Say-Barber-Miller syndrome

**Excludes:**
> **Dwarfism, osteodysplastic primordial, Majewski-Ranke type** (2582)
> **Dwarfism, osteodysplastic primordial, Majewski-Winter type** (2581)

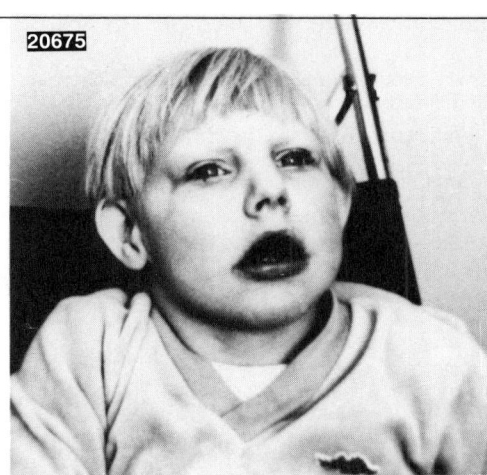

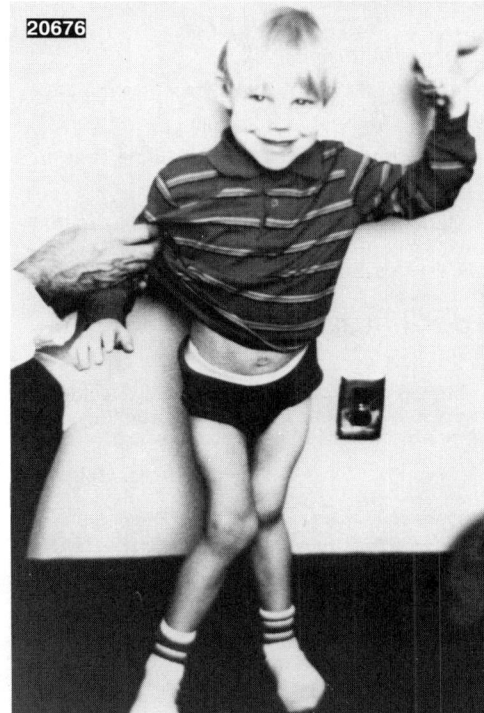

**3131**-20675: Microcephaly-retardation-skeletal and immune defects; note affected proband at 6 years of age. Craniofacial features include sloping forehead, prominent beaked nose, prominent ears, and micrognathia. **20676:** Affected sib at age 4 years; note similar craniofacial features, dislocated hip, and decreased subcutaneous fat. Both boys had retinitis pigmentosa.

**Immunodeficiency, thymic agenesis** (0943)
**Oculo-mandibulo-facial syndrome** (0738)
**Seckel syndrome** (0881)

**Major Diagnostic Criteria:** The combination of hypogammaglob-ulinemia, **Microcephaly**, growth delay, skeletal anomalies, and hypogenitalism.

**Clinical Findings:** The reported affected sibs both had normal birth weights, with postnatal growth deficiency. Craniofacial features included **Microcephaly**, sloping forehead, prominent beaked nose with a high nasal bridge, highly arched palate, micrognathia, and large protruding ears. Other anomalies included small genitalia, scoliosis, hypoplastic patellae, decreased subcutaneous fat. Frequent respiratory infections and eczema affected both boys. Immune deficiency was characterized by transient hypogammaglobulinemia, with defective chemotaxis. Mental retardation was severe in the older boy and mild in the younger boy.

**Complications:** Frequent respiratory infections, herpes, eczema, and otitis media secondary to the immune defect.

**Associated Findings:** In one of the children, craniosynostosis of the left coronal suture, posterior aspect of the sagittal sutures, hypodontia, anal stenosis, and hip dislocation.

**Etiology:** Presumbably either autosomal or X-linked recessive inheritance.

**Pathogenesis:** Unknown.

**MIM No.:** 25124

**POS No.:** 3899

**Sex Ratio:** M2:F0 observed.

**Occurrence:** One family with two affected male sibs has been reported.

**Risk of Recurrence for Patient's Sib:**
See Part I, *Mendelian Inheritance.*

**Risk of Recurrence for Patient's Child:**
See Part I, *Mendelian Inheritance.*

**Age of Detectability:** At birth, by physical examination.

**Gene Mapping and Linkage:** Unknown.

**Prevention:** None known. Genetic counseling indicated.

**Treatment:** Symptomatic.

**Prognosis:** Mental retardation is progressive in that development becomes more delayed over time. Life span is undetermined; the oldest boy was aged 6.5 years at the time of the last report.

**Detection of Carrier:** Unknown.

**References:**
Say B, et al.: Microcephaly, short stature, and developmental delay associated with a chemotactic defect and transient hypogammaglob-ulinemia in two brothers. J Med Gent 1986; 23:355–359.

T0007                                                    **Helga V. Toriello**

**Microcephaly-syndactyly-mental retardation, Filippi type**
*See SYNDACTYLY-MICROCEPHALY-MENTAL RETARDATION, FILIPPI TYPE*
**Microcephaly-vitreoretinal dysplasia**
*See NORRIE DISEASE*
**Microcornea-cataract**
*See CATARACT-MICROCORNEA SYNDROME*
**Microcystic disease of the renal medulla**
*See KIDNEY, NEPHRONOPHTHISIS-MEDULLARY CYSTIC DESEASE*
**Microcystic dystrophy**
*See CORNEAL DYSTROPHY, RECURRENT EROSIVE*
**Microcystic renal disease**
*See NEPHROSIS, CONGENITAL*
**Microcythemia**
*See THALASSEMIA*
**Microdontia**
*See TEETH, MICRODONTIA*

**Microdontia, generalized**
*See TEETH, AMELOGENESIS IMPERFECTA*
**Microencephaly**
*See MICROCEPHALY*
**Microepiphyseal dysplasia**
*See EPIPHYSEAL DYSPLASIA, MULTIPLE RIBBING TYPE*
**Microgastria**
*See STOMACH, HYPOPLASIA*
**Micrognathia-cleidocranial dysplasia**
*See YUNIS-VARON SYNDROME*
**Micrognathia-glossoptosis-cleft palate**
*See CLEFT PALATE-MICROGNATHIA-GLOSSOPTOSIS*
**Micrognathia-limb deficiency-splenogonadal fusion**
*See SPLENOGONADAL FUSION-LIMB DEFECT*
**Microgyria**
*See BRAIN, MICROPOLYGYRIA*
**Micromelia**
*See LIMB REDUCTION DEFECTS*
**Micromelia (lethal)-spondylocostal dysostosis-skeletal anomalies**
*See SPONDYLOCOSTAL DYSOSTOSIS-VISCERAL DEFECTS-DANDY WALKER CYST*
**Micromesomelia, Campailla-Martinelli**
*See ACROMESOMELIC DYSPLASIA, CAMPAILLA-MARTINELLI TYPE*
**Micropenis, isolated**
*See ANDROGEN INSENSITIVITY (RESISTANCE), MINIMAL*
**Microphakia and spherophakia, congenital**
*See LENS, MICROSPHEROPHAKIA*
**Microphthalmia with associated anomalies**
*See LENZ MICROPHTHALMIA SYNDROME*
**Microphthalmia, colobomatous isolated**
*See EYE, MICROPHTHALMIA/COLOBOMA*
**Microphthalmia-cataract**
*See CATARACT, POLAR AND CAPSULAR*
**Microphthalmia-gingival fibromatosis-depigmentation**
*See GINGIVAL FIBROMATOSIS-DEPIGMENTATION-MICROPHTHALMIA*
**Microplasmin**
*See PLASMINOGEN DEFECTS*
**Micropolygyria**
*See BRAIN, MICROPOLYGYRIA*
**Micropolygyria-muscular dystrophy**
*See MUSCULAR DYSTROPHY, CONGENITAL WITH MENTAL RETARDATION*
**Microspherophakia**
*See LENS, MICROSPHEROPHAKIA*
**Microstomia-agnathia-synotia**
*See AGNATHIA-MICROSTOMIA-SYNOTIA*
**Microtia from exposure to retinoids**
*See FETAL RETINOID SYNDROME*
**Microtia-atresia**
*See EAR, MICROTIA-ATRESIA*
**Microtia-facial clefting-hypertelorism**
*See HYPERTELORISM-MICROTIA-FACIAL CLEFT-CONDUCTIVE DEAFNESS*
**Microtia-meatal atresia-conductive deafness**
*See EAR, MICROTIA-ATRESIA*
**Microvillus atrophy, congenital**
*See MICROVILLUS INCLUSION DISEASE*

---

**MICROVILLUS INCLUSION DISEASE**                        **3222**

**Includes:**
Brush border, congenital disorganization of
Diarrhea with hypoplastic microvillus atrophy
Davidson disease
Enteropathy, familial
Microvillus atrophy, congenital

**Excludes:**
Autoimmune enteropathies and hypersensitivity
**Diarrhea, congenital chloride** (0148)
Enteropathy, infectious or post-infectious

**Major Diagnostic Criteria:** Typically, severe secretory diarrhea in these infants begins shortly after birth, no later than one week of age.

The initial small bowel biopsy shows hypoplastic microvillus atrophy with abnormal surface enterocytes lacking brush border definition and showing vacuolation of apical cytoplasm. Transmission electron microscopy (essential for confirmation of diagno-

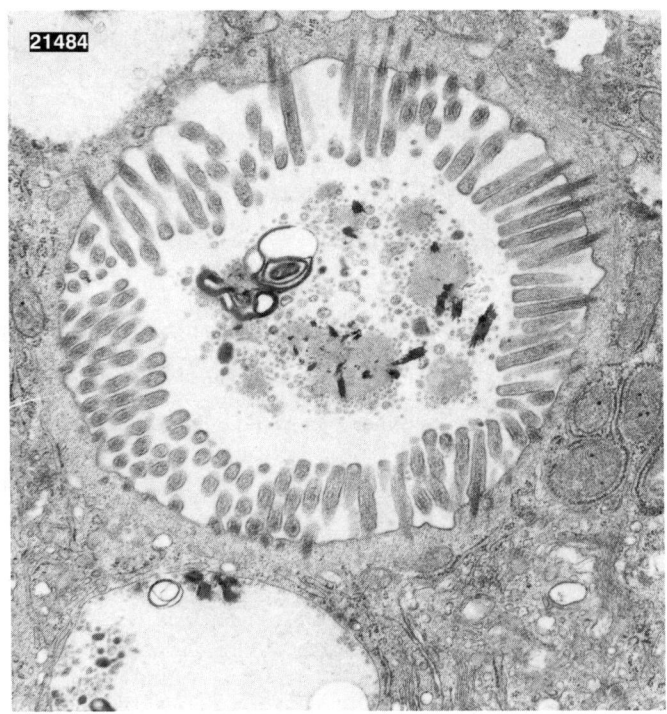

**3222-21484:** Electron microscopic appearance of small bowel enterocyte in microvillus inclusion disease. Microvillus inclusion with inwardly facing brush border microvilli. Core filaments and the terminal web appear to be well developed. The lumen of the inclusion has an aggregate of small vesicles, patches of moderately electron-dense floccular material, and myelin-like figures.

sis) shows a combination of the following three diagnostic features, confined mainly to the surface enterocytes: 1) absent or sparse and disorganized microvilli on apical membrane; 2) intracytoplasmic, cyst-like inclusions ("microvillus inclusions") enclosed by well-formed brush border microvilli (microvillus inclusions are seen only in some cells); and 3) numerous pleomorphic vesicular inclusion bodies, lined by a single limiting membrane, which may sometimes show an occasional microvillus, and containing floccular to homogeneous material of moderate to high electron density. The inclusions do not appear to be phagosomes, as originally proposed, because they are bound by only one membrane (that of the brush border) and because acid phosphatase, a lysosomal marker, has not been localized in larger vesicular bodies or microvillus inclusions.

Rectal (colonic) biopsies appear normal by light microscopy, but on electron microscopy the apical cytoplasm of proximal colonocytes contains microvillus inclusions similar to those in the small intestine as well as numerous clear vesicular bodies.

**Clinical Findings:** Severe watery diarrhea with stool volumes usually more than 80 ml/kg/d beginning during the first week of life results from impaired absorption across the enterocyte brush border. Stools are similar in electrolyte composition to normal small intestinal juice (Na > 75 mM, K < 30 mM). Affected infants tolerate less than 10 cal/kg/day of enteral feeding.

The small intestine of all patients shows diffuse villus atrophy, crypt hypoplasia, and normal or decreased numbers of inflammatory cells in the lamina propria. An abnormal distribution of periodic acid-schiff positive material in in apical cytoplasm of proximal enterocytes is in contrast to normal PAS staining which is confined to the brush border membrane (glycocalyx). Several lines of evidence suggest that this material represents intracytoplasmic sequestration of glycocalyx material.

Electron microscopy confirms the lack of well formed brush border microvilli and provides further evidence that microvillus

inclusions are unlikely to form by surface invaginations of apical membrane. The most severe ultrastructural changes are confined to proximal (most mature) enterocytes; mid and upper crypt cells may show early changes, whereas immature crypt cells, goblet, Paneth and enteroendocrine cells show no abnormalities. A similar pattern of cellular involvement is observed in colonic (rectal) mucosa.

**Complications:** Severe dehydration and acidosis result from fluid and electrolyte loss. Malnutrition is usually responsive only to total parenteral nutrition, which can be complicated by catheter-related septicemia and hepatobillary disease. Growth delay is also a problem.

**Associated Findings:** None known. Maternal polyhydramnios is not usually observed.

**Etiology:** Four families have now been described in which more than one sibling was affected. Sex of the affected siblings has been different. Because the disease is lethal, the pattern conforms best to autosomal recessive inheritance.

**Pathogenesis:** The possible pathogenic mechanisms proposed include: 1) a defect in crypt cell maturation; 2) a disorder of cytoskeletal proteins, namely myosin; and 3) an inborn error of intracellular vesicular transport leading to abnormal assembly of the microvillus membrane on the inner surface of intracytoplasmic vesicles rather than at the apical cell surface. Similar aberrant assembly of the brush border has been induced in experimental models in rodents by administration of colchicine or in human fetal intestinal organ cultures by adding cytochalasin.

**Sex Ratio:** Presumably M1:F1.

**Occurrence:** A total of 15 infants with this condition have been described. During a six year period at a large children's hospital, of the eight infants diagnosed with severe congenital watery diarrhea, six had microvillus inclusion disease. Patients with this condition have now been described in Canada, Great Britain, France, and the United States. Some patients reported were originally from the Middle East (Lebanon, Eqypt).

**Risk of Recurrence for Patient's Sib:**
See Part I, *Mendelian Inheritance.*

**Risk of Recurrence for Patient's Child:**
See Part I, *Mendelian Inheritance.*

**Age of Detectability:** Days 1–3 of life, on rectal biopsy examined by electron microscopy.

**Gene Mapping and Linkage:** Unknown.

**Prevention:** None known. Genetic counseling indicated.

**Treatment:** Typically, massive amounts of intravenous electrolytes are required for replacement (e.g., Na, 25 mEq/kg/day). Total parenteral nutrition is required. Attempts to stimulate small bowel growth with human colostrum, glucocorticoids, pentagastrin, and epidermal growth factor have not been successful. In one patient, a reduction in stool output from 250 to 180 ml/kg/day occurred in response to twice-daily injections of the long-acting somatostatin analogue octreotide. Subtotal enterectomy to alleviate and stabilize the massive fluid losses has not been tried. Multiorgan transplant including liver and bowel in one patient was not successful (R. Jaffe, personal communication).

**Prognosis:** All patients described to date except one have died before their second birthday.

**Detection of Carrier:** Unknown.

**Special Considerations:** Heterogeneity may exist. A single patient, presenting after two months of life with microvillus inclusions in small intestinal and rectal biopsies, experienced a milder clinical course (Carruthers et al, 1986).

**References:**
Davidson GP, et al.: Familial enteropathy: a syndrome of protracted diarrhea from birth, failure to thrive, and hypoplastic villus atrophy. Gastroenterology 1978; 75:783–790. *
Phillips AD, et al.: Congenital microvillous atrophy: specific diagnostic features. Arch Dis Child 1985; 60:135–140. †
Carruthers L, et al.: Disorders of the cytoskeleton of the enterocyte. Clinics in Gastroenterology 1986; 15:105–120. * †

Drumm B, et al.: Urogastrone/epidermal growth factor in treatment of congenital microvillous atrophy. Lancet 1988; I:111–112.
Lake BD, et al.: Microvillus inclusion disease: specific diagnostoc features shown by alkaline phosphatase histochemistry. J Clin Pathol 1988; 41:880–882.
Cutz E, et al.: Microvillus inclusion disease: an inherited defect of brush-border assembly and differentiation. New Engl J Med 1989; 320:646–651. * †

RH005
CU015

**J. Marc Rhoads**
**Ernest Cutz**

**Middle ear aneurysm of internal carotid artery**
*See EAR, ANEURYSM OF INTERNAL CAROTID ARTERY*
**Middle ear malformations with hearing loss**
*See EAR, OSSICLE AND MIDDLE EAR MALFORMATIONS*
**Midface retraction-X-ray and renal anomalies-hypertrichosis**
*See SCHINZEL-GIEDION SYNDROME*
**Midface nerve loss, hereditary**
*See DEAFNESS (SENSORINEURAL), MIDFREQUENCY*
**Midfrequency sensorineural deafness**
*See DEAFNESS (SENSORINEURAL), MIDFREQUENCY*
**Midline defects**
*See SCHISIS ASSOCIATION*
**Midline diastema**
*See TEETH, DIASTEMA, MEDIAN INCISAL*
**Midline maxillary double lip**
*See LIP, DOUBLE*
**Midsystolic click-late systolic murmur syndrome**
*See MITRAL VALVE PROLAPSE*
**Miescher elastoma**
*See SKIN, ELASTOSIS PERFORANS SERPIGINOSA*
**Miescher syndrome**
*See LIPODYSTROPHY-COARSE FACIES-ACANTHOSIS NIGRICANS, MIESCHER TYPE*

## MIETENS-WEBER SYNDROME 2013

**Includes:** Mental retardation syndrome, Mietens-Weber type
**Excludes:**
Arachnodactyly, contractural Beals type (0085)
Arthrogryposes (0088)

**Major Diagnostic Criteria:** The combination of mental retardation, eye findings (e.g., corneal opacity, nystagmus), and upper limb anomalies (flexion contractures of the elbow, short radius, and ulna).

**Clinical Findings:** The clinical findings in the six reported cases were corneal opacity (6); nystagmus, horizontal and rotational (6); strabismus (6); small, pointed nose (6); short radius and ulna with elongated humerus (6); flexion contractures of the elbows (6); pes valgus planus (5); short stature (5); mental retardation (IQ 70–80) (6); and clinodactyly (4).

Anomalies noted on X-ray include dislocated radial head (5), absence of epiphysis of the radial head (3), and hypoplastic upper third of the radius (1).

The growth failure seems to be progressive, in that the youngest child had a normal length at five months of age. The corneal opacities and elbow contractures are likely congenital.

**Complications:** Blindness secondary to corneal opacity.

**Associated Findings:** Low birth weight, microphthalmia, hip dislocation, and small testes were each noted in one or two of the affected children.

**Etiology:** Affected siblings of normal, consanguineous parents suggest autosomal recessive inheritance.

**Pathogenesis:** Unknown.

**MIM No.:** 24960

**POS No.:** 3317

**Sex Ratio:** M1:F3 (observed in the four reported cases).

**Occurrence:** One family with four affected children, and two sporadic cases, have been reported.

**Risk of Recurrence for Patient's Sib:**
See Part I, *Mendelian Inheritance.*

**Risk of Recurrence for Patient's Child:**
See Part I, *Mendelian Inheritance.*

**Age of Detectability:** At birth, by physical examination.

**Gene Mapping and Linkage:** Unknown.

**Prevention:** None known. Genetic counseling indicated.

**Treatment:** Unknown.

**Prognosis:** All affected individuals have been retarded (IQ 70–80); Life span seems unaffected.

**Detection of Carrier:** Unknown.

**References:**
Mietens C, Weber H: A syndrome characterized by corneal opacity, nystagmus, flexion contractures of the elbows, growth failure, and mental retardation. J Pediatr 1966; 69:624–629.
Carnevale A, Ruiz Garcia FJ: Sindrome de Mietens-Weber: descripcion de un nuevo caso. Rev Invest Clin (Medico) 1976; 28:347–351.
Nagano A, et al.: Mietens' syndrome. Arch Orthop Unfall-Chir 1977; 89:81–86.

T0007

**Helga V. Toriello**

**Migeon syndrome**
*See ADRENOCORTICAL UNRESPONSIVENESS TO ACTH, HEREDITARY*

## MIGRAINE 3223

**Includes:**
Basilar migraine
Benign exertional headache
Benign sexual headache
Classic migraine
Coital headache
Common migraine
Childhood migraine
Exertional headache, benign
Headache, benign exertional
Headache, benign sexual
Headache, migraine
Migraine, familial hemiplegic
Migraine, complicated
Ophthalmoplegic migraine
Sexual headache, benign
Transformational migraine
Transient migraine accompaniments

**Excludes:**
Headache, cluster
Headache secondary to structural, metabolic, or infectious disease
Headache, tension

**Major Diagnostic Criteria:** Since 1962, the report of the Ad Hoc Committee on the Classification of Headache has served as the basis for the diagnostic criteria for migraine. Presently, the classification and diagnostic criteria for headache (and migraine) are undergoing transition, with a new but preliminary international classification currently being circulated. The following represent consensus opinion with respect to diagnostic criteria.

*Migraine without aura* (formerly "common migraine") is an idiopathic, chronic, recurring head pain disorder, with each attack lasting 4–72 hours (untreated or unsuccessfully treated) or longer, and separated by pain-free intervals. Features typical of migraine include unilateral or bilateral discomfort with a pulsating quality and moderate to severe intensity; nausea and/or vomiting; photophobia and/or phonophobia; aggravation by physical activity; and absence of an organic cause for headache.

*Migraine with aura* (formerly "classic migraine") is an idiopathic, chronic, recurring headache disorder which is manifested by headache episodes preceded by neurological symptoms unequivocally localizable to the cerebral cortex or brainstem. The neurological symptoms develop over 15–20 minutes, usually lasting less than 60 minutes. Headache, nausea, photophobia, and other symptoms generally follow the neurological (aura) symptoms directly or after an interval of less than one hour. Neurological and physical examinations do not suggest the presence of organic disease.

*Familial hemiplegic migraine* is a variant of migraine (with aura), the primary neurological symptom being hemiparesis in which at least one first degree relative has identical attacks.

*Basilar migraine* is a migraine (with aura) variant originating in the brainstem or from both occipital lobes, and may include symptoms of dysarthria, vertigo, tinnitus, ataxia, decreased consciousness, and bilateral neurological symptoms.

*Ophthalmoplegic migraine* is a migraine (with aura) variant with paresis of one or more ocular cranial nerves.

*Transformational migraine* is a pattern of migraine which reflects the evolutive or transformational transition seen in some patients with migraine, in which intermittent migraine (without aura) episodes evolve to a daily or almost daily pattern. Mild to moderate pain occurs on a daily basis and paroxysmal (episodic) more intense attacks (fulfilling migraine without aura criteria) develop less often. It is believed that over one-half of those who have this transformational syndrome have accompanying depression and sleep disturbances.

*Transient migraine accompaniments* are neurological symptoms (usually visual) in the absence of headache, occurring periodically and which first develop after age 50.

*Benign sexual headache* consists of three patterns of headache which may occur in association with sexual exertion or masturbation. The most common pattern occurs in about 70% of reported cases, beginning shortly before or after orgasm. This consists of a high-intensity pain, usually frontal or occipital in location, and may have an explosive or throbbing quality, lasting for a few minutes to several hours.

A second pattern, occurring in about 25% of cases, begins early in the course of intercourse, is occipital or diffuse in location, and has a dull, aching quality which intensifies at the time of orgasm. The form occurring least often is an occipital headache present when the patient is standing, and is often associated with nausea and vomiting. A low CSF pressure has been considered a probable cause, perhaps occurring as a consequence of a dural tear from exertion during sexual activity. No consistent biological factor has been identified as a cause for these headache phenomena, but a relationship to migraine or mechanical alteration of the CSF dynamics has been postulated. Aneurysm, intracranial mass lesion, or structural abnormality must be ruled out. Treatment consists of a variety of drugs, many of which are useful in migraine, including beta adrenergic blockade and indomethacin treatment.

**Clinical Findings:** Migraine may begin at any time in life, with over 21% of patients reporting the first headache prior to age 10 and over 50% of patients before age 20. Later life onset (after age 40) is noted in up to 8% of patients. Although it is assumed that migraine attacks will cease over the course of years, little data can confirm this belief. Periodic and recurring episodes may span the entire lifetime of some patients, cease permanently after childhood or at some other milestone (hormonal, etc.), or return after a period of remission, decades after the last attack.

Though not all attacks of migraine are associated with headache, most migraine episodes, by diagnostic criteria, reflect episodic attacks of head pain accompanied by one or more symptoms, including, but not limited to, neurological events; nausea and vomiting (87% and 56% respectively); sensitivity to light and/or sound (82%); visual disturbances (36%); paresthesias (33%); lightheadedness (72%); and dizziness (33%). Autonomic disturbances, i.e., vasomotor changes and edema, and mental and mood disturbances are common.

In women, migraine attacks are often influenced by various hormonal milestones, including menarche, menstruation, pregnancy, and menopause. The use of oral contraceptives, exogenous estrogen, or other hormonal manipulations usually adversely affect the course.

The location of pain is variable, as is the intensity. Some attacks are characterized by occipital (neck pain) discomfort, but most have a hemicranial or transcranial expression. Facial pain can occur during migraine.

Throughout the years of vulnerability, the pattern and frequency of attacks may be influenced by hypothalamic (chronobiological) factors which alone or in conjunction with external provoking factors (activating, precipitating factors) incite the onset of the attack. Among the well known migraine activating events are dietary factors, head trauma, stress and anxiety, hormonal fluctuation, sleep cycles, weather changes, physical exertion, and others.

The natural history of migraine is variable. Current attention focuses upon the transformational, evolutive phenomenon in which periodic migraine events evolve to a daily or almost daily pain pattern. Cervical/occipital, and/or frontal pain occurs on a daily basis, and episodic, intense, "typical" migraine attacks develop periodically.

Currently available diagnostic tests are normal in migraine, and the diagnosis rests upon the absence of other identifiable causes for head pain.

Childhood migraine, the most common of the recurring headaches in childhood, affects males more than females and is usually characterized by briefer attacks (than in adults), with prominent GI symptoms, sleep disturbance, and a generally favorable prognosis, particularly for males. Migraine "equivalents" (symptoms of migraine in the absence of headache in children) include episodic vertigo, dizziness, abdominal pain and cyclical vomiting, and episodic mood disturbance. Typical adult-type migraine attacks are also common in children.

**Complications:** Complications of migraine are of two forms: iatrogenic (treatment-related) and natural (physiological) attributed to the disease process itself.

Iatrogenic complications reflect the consequences of excessive treatment with a variety of pharmacological agents. These include GI, liver, and renal disturbances secondary to excessive use of mixed analgesic preparations; addictive disease resulting from dependency upon narcotic analgesics or addicting tranquilizers; and vascular complications arising from excessing use of ergotamine tartrate and other vasoconstrictive preparations.

The natural risks of migraine include the persistence of hemiplegic, aphasic, hemianopic, and retinal sequelae of individual migraine (with aura) attacks. When persistent, it is called *complicated migraine*. Though rare, numerous examples are documented in the literature. It is currently believed that complicated migraine may result from nonischemic impairment of brain rather than from occlusive, ischemic disease. Recently, several cases of brain hemorrhage during migraine have been reported, though a certain linkage between acute migraine and hemorrhage into the brain is yet to be confirmed.

Many migraine sufferers experience accompanying depression and sleep disturbance, which may reflect the primary factors related to the pathogenesis of the illness.

**Associated Findings:** Few associated findings have been confirmed, although a higher than expected incidence of depression and sleep disturbance has been tentatively noted in transformational migraine. Moreover, 60% of migraineurs report motion sickness (sometimes severe) during early childhood, and over 60% of adult migraine patients report unrelated episodes of motion sickness from time to time, compared to 11% of controls. Migraine occurs with a higher-than-chance frequency in children with primary familial dyslipoproteinemia. **Raynaud disease** and labile hypertension are also noted in many migraine sufferers and may be related to autonomic disturbances.

**Etiology:** Autosomal dominant inheritance with incomplete penetrance. In familial hemiplegic migraine; autosomal dominant inheritance. A family history of migraine is obtained in 60–91% of patients with migraine.

**Pathogenesis:** Attitudes regarding the pathogenesis of migraine are currently in transition and dispute. Traditional considerations had focused upon overactive vasomotor systems, resulting in excessive cranial and extracranial vascular responses. The most favored current concept suggests that migraine is caused by a central (brain) disturbance involving neurotransmission (serotonergic and monoaminergic) within the upper brainstem and diencephalic pathways.

**MIM No.:** 15730

**Sex Ratio:** In childhood, boys and girls seem equally affected (perhaps slightly more males than females). In adults, the male-to-female ratio is M1:F7.5.

**Occurrence:** Because precise diagnostic criteria for migraine and its classification are not universally agreed upon, determinations of actual incidence and prevalence are varied and remain uncertain. The most reliable current data on recent prevalence in the Western world is 30% of women between the ages of 21 and 34 (declining to 10% in those 75 years or older) and 17% of men (declining to 5% in those 75 years or older). Approximately 40% of individuals in the United States and Europe have reported severe headaches at some point in their lives. No apparent relationship exists between migraine and intelligence, social class, race, or educational background. It may be higher in the United States and Europe than in China and rural Ecuador.

**Risk of Recurrence for Patient's Sib:**
See Part I, *Mendelian Inheritance.*

**Risk of Recurrence for Patient's Child:**
See Part I, *Mendelian Inheritance.*

**Age of Detectability:** Migraine has been reported in two and three year-olds. Between 20% and 35% of children with headache are under five years of age when symptoms begin. Over 90% of all patients with migraine have experienced their first attack before the age of 40.

**Gene Mapping and Linkage:** Unknown.

**Prevention:** None known. Genetic counseling indicated.

**Treatment:** The treatment of migraine consists of non-medical and medical interventions. *Non-medical therapies* include avoidance of provoking factors, biofeedback and stress management techniques, improving general health and leisure aspects of life, and regulating day-to-day routines such as time of retiring and arising each day and taking meals. *Pharmacological techniques* address both acute attacks and prevention of recurring attacks. Acute attacks are treated with a variety of agents, including analgesics, specific migraine preparations (such as ergotamine tartrate, dihydroergotamine, etc.), nonsteroidal anti-inflammatory drugs (NSAID), hypnotics, and tranquilizers.

Preventive therapy for recurring attacks employs a long list of pharmacological agents, including β-adrenergic blocking agents, calcium channel antagonists, methysergide, antidepressants, nonsteroidal anti-inflammatory agents (NSAID), and many others.

It is believed that most effective agents act through a mechanism involving central serotonergic or mono-aminergic pathways.

**Prognosis:** Variable. In its natural untreated state, migraine will vary in intensity and frequency throughout the life span, with periods of remission and exacerbation. Cyclical patterns are noted. With treatment, the natural history is not altered, but control of recurring episodes of pain can be achieved in over 75% of those treated.

**Detection of Carrier:** The diagnosis is established through delineation of the history and the exclusion of organic disease.

**Special Considerations:** The concepts and perspectives on migraine are changing rapidly. Many respected authorities now believe that most chronic recurring headaches, with the possible exception of cluster headache and its variants, are actual variations of migraine. Central (brain) disturbances are now believed to be the primary pathogenetic process, and reactions of blood vessels and muscles are secondary events or epiphenomena. The periodicity of migraine may be determined by hypothalamic, chronobiological influences. The vulnerability to migraine is though to result primarily from a genetically-determined disturbance, either activated or in some cases acquired from ''perturbation'' of critical brain regions.

Among the external factors which may ''perturb'' or influence migraine are: mild to moderate head trauma, prolonged emotional duress, metabolic or infectious illness, or neuronal stimulation from pathological processes along the course of the fifth cranial nerve. The most effective treatments appear to influence central mechanisms rather than extracranial targets as has traditionally been assumed. Comprehensive outpatient and special hospital treatment units (the first of its kind in Ann Arbor, Michigan, in 1978) have been developed to address the most resistent cases.

**References:**
Allan W: Inheritance of migraine. Arch Intern Med 1928; 42:590–599.
Goodell H, et al.: The familial occurrence of migraine headache: a study of heredity. Arch Neurol Psychiat 1954; 72:325–334.
Refsum S: Genetic aspects of migraine. In: Vinken PJ, Bruyn GW, eds: Handbook of Clinical Neurology, Vol. 5. Amsterdam: North Holland Publishing, 1968:258–270.
Paulson GW, Klawans HL: Benign orgasmic cephalgia. Headache 1974; 13:181–187.
Lance, JW: Mechanism and management of headache, 4th ed. Boston: Butterworth, 1982.
Saper JR: Headache disorders: current concepts and treatment strategies. Boston: Wright-PSG Medical Publishers, 1983. *
Johns DR: Benign sexual headache within a family. Arch Neurol 1986; 43:1158–1160.
Saper JR: Changing perspectives in headache treatment. Clin J Pain 1986; 2:19–28.
Waters WE: Headache (series in clinical epidemiology). London: Croom Helm, 1986.
Saper JR: Drug treatment of headache: changing concepts and treatment strategies. Semin Neurol 1987; 7:178–191.
Raskin NH: Headache. New York: Churchill-Livingstone, 1988. *

SA047                                                          **Joel R. Saper**

**Migraine, complicated**
*See MIGRAINE*
**Migraine, familial hemiplegic**
*See MIGRAINE*
**Mikulicz disease**
*See PAROTITIS, PUNCTATE*
**Mikulicz syndrome**
*See SJOGREN SYNDROME*
**Milano (AI) apolipoprolipoprotein variants**
*See HYPOALPHALIPOPROTEINEMIA*
**Miller syndrome**
*See ACROFACIAL DYSOSTOSIS, POSTAXIAL TYPE*
**Miller-Dieker syndrome**
*See LISSENCEPHALY SYNDROME*
**Milroy disease**
*See LYMPHEDEMA I*
**Minamata disease**
*See FETAL METHYLMERCURY EFFECTS*
**Mineralocorticoid-receptor deficiency**
*See ALDOSTERONE RESISTANCE*
**Minimal pigment albinism**
*See ALBINISM, OCULOCUTANEOUS, MINIMAL PIGMENT TYPE*
**Minkowski-Chauffard syndrome**
*See SPHEROCYTOSIS*
**Minkowski-Chauffard syndrome (obsolete)**
*See ANEMIA, HEMOLYTIC, RED CELL MEMBRANE DEFECTS*
**Minoxidil, fetal effects**
*See FETAL EFFECTS FROM MATERNAL VASODILATOR*
**Miosis and partial ptosis**
*See HORNER SYNDROME*
**Mirhosseini-Holmes-Walton syndrome**
*See RETINOPATHY-MICROCEPHALY-MENTAL RETARDATION*
**Mitochondrial acetoacetyl-CoA thiolase deficiency**
*See ACIDEMIA, 3-KETOTHIOLASE DEFICIENCY*
**Mitochondrial ALDH deficiency**
*See ALCOHOL INTOLERANCE*
**Mitochondrial cytopathy**
*See KEARNS-SAYRE DISEASE*
*also OPHTHALMOPLEGIA, PROGRESSIVE EXTERNAL*
**Mitochondrial encephalomyopathy**
*See KEARNS-SAYRE DISEASE*
**Mitochondrial myopathy**
*See MYOPATHY, MITOCHONDRIAL-ENCEPHALOPATHY-LACTIC ACIDOSIS-STROKE*
*also MYOPATHY, METABOLIC*
**Mitochondrial myopathy due to cytochrome C oxidase deficiency**
*See MYOPATHY-METABOLIC, MITOCHONDRIAL CYTOCHROME C OXIDASE DEFICIENCY*

**Mitral insufficiency due to isolated clefts of the valve leaflets**
*See MITRAL VALVE INSUFFICIENCY*
**Mitral regurgitation, congenital**
*See MITRAL VALVE INSUFFICIENCY*

## MITRAL REGURGITATION-DEAFNESS-SKELETAL DEFECTS 0667

**Includes:**
   Deafness-mitral regurgitation-skeletal malformations
   Skeletal malformations-heart disease-conductive hearing
      loss

**Excludes:**
   **Arthro-ophthalmopathy, hereditary, progressive, Stickler type**
      (0090)
   **Lentigines syndrome, multiple** (0586)
   **Mitral valve prolapse** (0668)
   Pulmonic stenosis-deafness

**Major Diagnostic Criteria:** Conductive hearing loss, mitral regurgitation, and osseous abnormalities.

**Clinical Findings:** Three relatives have been described with conductive hearing loss, mitral regurgitation, and osseous abnormalities. All three were of short stature and normal intelligence, had similar facies, and prominent freckling over the face and shoulders. External auditory canals were narrow and oblique; middle ear exploration in two cases revealed a fixed footplate. Audiograms prior to surgery demonstrated a conductive hearing loss with normal cochlear function. X-rays showed varying degrees of fusion of the cervical vertebrae, carpal and tarsal bones; the phalanges appeared shortened. All had mild degrees of mitral regurgitation of unclear cause; whether mitral stenosis was also present was not addressed. The EKG showed an incomplete right-bundle branch block and cardiac catheterization showed normal hemodynamics. Karyotypes were normal.

**Complications:** Language delay may result from the hearing loss. The long-term course of the mitral valve abnormality is undetermined.

**Associated Findings:** One child had a left exotropia. A high-arched palate and crowded dentition were present. The thyroid was palpable in each case, but thyroid function studies were normal.

**Etiology:** Presumably autosomal dominant inheritance with variable expression.

**Pathogenesis:** Unknown.

**MIM No.:** 15780

**POS No.:** 3303

**Sex Ratio:** Undetermined. All three reported cases were female.

**Occurrence:** Undetermined; three cases reported.

**Risk of Recurrence for Patient's Sib:**
   See Part I, *Mendelian Inheritance.*

**Risk of Recurrence for Patient's Child:**
   See Part I, *Mendelian Inheritance.*

**Age of Detectability:** Theoretically diagnosable at birth by physical examination and audiogram. The murmur and conductive hearing loss may easily be missed on initial examination and newborn audiometric screening.

**Gene Mapping and Linkage:** Unknown.

**Prevention:** None known. Genetic counseling indicated.

**Treatment:** Middle ear surgery may improve hearing, although amplification may be necessary prior to surgery. Cardiac surgery could correct severe valvular problems.

**Prognosis:** Good.

**Detection of Carrier:** Unknown.

**References:**
Forney WR, et al.: Congenital heart disease, deafness and skeletal malformations: a new syndrome? J Pediatr 1966; 68:14–26.

PY000                                          **Reed E Pyeritz**

## MITRAL VALVE ATRESIA 0665

**Includes:** Atresia, mitral valve

**Excludes:**
   Mitral atresia associated with other major cardiac anomalies

**Major Diagnostic Criteria:** Clinical presentation varies depending on the anatomical features but may include cyanosis, systolic murmur or congestive heart failure. Echocardiography is suggestive with selective left atrial angiocardiography being diagnostic. Ventriculography will delineate the associated anatomic abnormalities.

**Clinical Findings:** Mitral atresia is represented by a complete fusion of the mitral valve leaflets with no entry into the left ventricle. The left ventricle is almost always hypoplastic with a small cavity. The left atrium is similarly reduced in size. The communication between the atria is usually a patent foramen ovale rather than a defect of the secundum or primum variety. The atrial septum is rarely (<10%) intact and, under these circumstances, entry into the right side of the heart is via a levocardinal vein. The hemodynamic alterations are dependent on the presence or absence of pulmonary stenosis and the size of the atrial communication. Oxygenated blood in this malformation returns from the lungs into the left atrium and then passes into the right atrium via the foramen ovale or atrial defect to mix with the caval return. Following right ventricular filling, both great arteries receive blood: the pulmonary artery from the right ventricle, and the aorta through a VSD and the LV, or through a patent ductus arteriosus. The size of the aorta and pulmonary artery reflects the proportion of right ventricular output directed into each major vessel as determined by pulmonary and systemic vascular resistances.

The age of presentation and clinical picture depend largely on the size of the atrial patency and the status of pulmonary blood flow. In those patients with diminished pulmonary blood flow, ie associated pulmonary stenosis, cyanosis is the main finding. Auscultation in this group reveals a harsh systolic ejection murmur along the left sternal border secondary to pulmonary outflow tract obstruction. There is a single second heart sound. Signs of congestive heart failure are not present. In the group with augmented pulmonary blood flow or pulmonary venous obstruction, congestive heart failure is the dominant feature. Tachypnea and hepatomegaly are then the chief presenting findings along with nonspecific murmurs. On occasion, a continuous murmur has been described along the left upper sternal margin secondary to flow from the high pressure left atrium to the lower pressure right atrium.

No specific X-ray picture has been described, and the findings vary according to the hemodynamic alterations present. In patients with increased pulmonary blood flow, cardiac enlargement with prominent pulmonary vascular markings is seen. If the size of the atrial communication is small, a predominantly pulmonary venous obstructive pattern will be noted. When pulmonary stenosis is present, the heart is usually of normal size and the vascularity of the lungs diminished. In cases with associated transposition of the great arteries, a narrow cardiac base has been observed.

The EKG commonly shows right axis deviation, right atrial enlargement and severe right ventricular hypertrophy. The latter is associated with a QR pattern in the right precordial leads.

The echocardiogram shows absence of the mitral leaflet motion pattern, a variable-sized left atrium and a dilated right ventricle, exaggerated tricuspid motion, a slit-like or absent left ventricular cavity and, generally, a hypoplastic aortic root in the anterior-posterior and superior-inferior echocardiographic axes. The echocardiogram, when all of the above are noted, is definitive in this diagnosis. (See also **Aortic valve atresia**).

Cardiac catheterization with selective left atrial angiocardiography is crucial for the confirmation of the diagnosis. A left-to-right shunt is usually present at the atrial level. The right ventricular and pulmonary artery pressures are elevated to systemic levels in the absence of pulmonary stenosis. The left atrial pressure is variably increased, depending on the size of the left atrial communication and the magnitude of the pulmonary blood flow. Large prominent a waves are generally found. When a large opening exists, the pressures in both atria tend to be equal. Injection of contrast material into the left atrium will show a direct passage of the contrast media into the right atrium, right ventricle, and then simultaneous opacification of both great arteries. Right ventricular injection may also be helpful in the delineation of the origin of the great arteries and the presence or absence of pulmonary stenosis.

**Complications:** Death is usually secondary to congestive heart failure or hypoxemia.

**Associated Findings:** **Aorta, coarctation** or **Aortic arch interruption, Heart, transposition of great vessels,** and **Ventricular septal defect** or single ventricle; a high incidence (40%) of noncardiac malformations has been reported. They are of wide variety, including horseshoe kidney, ectopic pancreas, and **Cleft lip**.

**Etiology:** Unknown.

**Pathogenesis:** Congenital mitral atresia is due to fusion of left AV primordia at an early age. It has also been suggested by some authors that premature closure of the foramen ovale in utero is the primary event and the consequent hemodynamic changes result in the left ventricular underdevelopment.

**CDC No.:** 746.505

**Sex Ratio:** M1:F>1

**Occurrence:** 5:1,000 cases of autopsied congenital heart disease.

**Risk of Recurrence for Patient's Sib:** 1:50 (2%) for each sibling to be affected.

**Risk of Recurrence for Patient's Child:** Affected individuals are not expected to survive to reproduce.

**Age of Detectability:** From birth, by cardiac catheterization and selective angiocardiography.

**Gene Mapping and Linkage:** Unknown.

**Prevention:** None known. Genetic counseling indicated.

**Treatment:** If the patient is in congestive heart failure, digitalis, diuretics, etc should be promptly instituted. Pulmonary artery banding is frequently required. In children with decreased pulmonary blood flow, an appropriate aorticopulmonary shunt is necessary. Attempt should be made during cardiac catheterization to enlarge the atrial septum using the balloon atrial septostomy technique as this is often a site of obstruction.

**Prognosis:** The overall prognosis is poor. In selective cases, palliation with pulmonary artery banding and atrial septostomies as well as systemic pulmonary artery shunts can lead to long-term survival.

**Detection of Carrier:** Unknown.

**References:**
Meyer RA, Kaplan S: Echocardiography in the diagnosis of hypoplasia of the left or right ventricles in the neonate. Circulation 1972; 46:55–65.
Baylen BG, Criley JM: Diseases of the mitral valve. In: Adams FH, Emmanouilides GC, eds: Heart disease in infants, children, and adolescents. Baltimore: Williams & Wilkins, 1983:516–526.

**James J. Nora**

## MITRAL VALVE INSUFFICIENCY 0666

**Includes:**
Chordae tendineae, anomalous shortened
Heart, arcade formation of the leaflets and chordae
Heart, shortened or defective valve tissue
Mitral insufficiency due to isolated clefts of the valve leaflets
Mitral regurgitation, congenital
Mitral valve, double orifice

**Excludes:**
Endocardial cushion defects, partial or complete
Mitral insufficiency, acquired
Mitral insufficiency associated with metabolic defects
Mitral insufficiency secondary to anomalous left coronary artery
**Mitral valve prolapse (0668)**
Rheumatic mitral insufficiency

**Major Diagnostic Criteria:** Auscultation of a harsh holosystolic murmur at the cardiac apex with radiation to the axilla and back indicates the presence of mitral insufficiency. Echocardiography using two-dimensional and pulsed Doppler is the diagnostic modality of choice to confirm the diagnosis. Cardiac catheterization is frequently needed to assess the severity of insufficiency.

**Clinical Findings:** The presentation of mitral insufficiency is extremely variable due to the multiple etiologies of this disorder. It is also complicated by the high frequency of other associated cardiac defects. An isolated lesion of the mitral valve may consist of single or multiple clefts in the anterior or posterior leaflet. Shortening of the chordae tendineae with abnormalities of the papillary muscles also results in varying degrees of mitral insufficiency. Occasionally these form an "arcade" type appearance to the anterior leaflet. As isolated defects these lesions are extremely rare. More commonly these defects occur in association with other cardiac defects. In these circumstances, the finding of mitral insufficiency may be obscured by the coexisting lesions.

Secondary mitral insufficiency may also result in the presence of normal valve anatomy. Idiopathic hypertrophic obstructive cardiomyopathy has resulted in mitral insufficiency in severe cases. Anomalous origin of the left coronary artery from the pulmonary artery frequently results in left ventricular and papillary muscle dysfunction with resultant mitral insufficiency. Various metabolic disorders result in degeneration of the mitral valve and subsequent insufficiency. Most common of these are **Marfan syndrome** and **Mucopolysaccharidosis** types I and II. Myxomatous degeneration of valve tissue, and rarely cardiac tumor, are also causes of mitral insufficiency.

The age of presentation may range from early infancy to late adulthood. The clinical findings and age of presentation will vary with the severity of the insufficiency and presence of associated defects. The patient may present with an asymptomatic murmur in cases of mild insufficiency. In severe cases, a history of easy fatigue, poor growth, or respiratory abnormalities may be elicited. In isolated mitral insufficiency, apical activity is increased. A palpable apical thrill may also be present. A high frequency harsh holosystolic murmur is audible with radiation to the axilla and back. The split of the second heart sound will be narrowed with an increased pulmonic component in the presence of significant pulmonary hypertension. With severe insufficiency, a low pitched diastolic rumble (Carey-Coombs murmur) may be heard. The electrocardiogram in the presence of significant mitral insufficiency shows left ventricular hypertrophy and left atrial enlargement. Chest X-ray shows left ventricular and left atrial enlargement. In the presence of severe insufficiency, pulmonary vascular markings are also increased. Echocardiography is a useful diagnostic modality to diagnose mitral insufficiency. Clefts and abnormalities of the chordae are visualized well with two-dimensional echocardiography. Parasternal short axis views will show clefts in both anterior and posterior mitral valve leaflets. This view also allows visualization of the papillary muscle size and location. Parasternal long axis and especially the apical four-chamber views allow evaluation of the chordal structure and attachments. These views may show valve tissue prolapse into the left atrium. Doppler echocardiography is very sensitive in identifying the presence of insufficiency. Mapping of the regurgitant jet with Doppler in the apical four-chamber and parasternal long view has been used to estimate the degree of severity from mitral insufficiency. This is limited by the angle of the Doppler beam and remains only a qualitative estimate of the severity of the insufficiency. Color Doppler may be found to be more useful for this purpose but remains unvalidated at this time. Cardiac catheterization is therefore indicated when the degree of mitral insufficiency is uncertain. Direct measurement of the left atrial pressure and left ventricular angiography are used to establish the severity of the mitral insufficiency. High pulmonary artery capillary wedge pressures with large V waves are usually present in cases of mitral insufficiency. Because prominent V waves can occur in the absence of significant mitral insufficiency, direct measurement of the left atrial pressure pattern is preferable. Pulmonary arterial pressure may also be elevated in the face of severe insufficiency with left ventricular failure. Left ventricular angiography will show systolic regurgitation of contrast into the left atrium and depending upon the severity, into the pulmonary veins as well. The degree of left atrial and ventricular dilation and the rapidity of clearing of the dye from the left atrium is used to evaluate the severity of the insufficiency.

**Complications:** Severe, chronic mitral insufficiency will result in left ventricular volume overload and left ventricular failure. Pulmonary venous congestion results in pulmonary hypertension and right heart failure. Infective endocarditis may occur. This risk is greatest in very abnormal valves with some degree of concomitant mitral stenosis.

**Associated Findings:** Mitral insufficiency presents only rarely as an isolated defect. It is seen with other cardiac defects especially secundum atrial septal defect, **Ductus arteriosus, patent, Aortic valve stenosis**, and **Aorta, coarctation**. Mitral regurgitation has been reported in association with **Turner syndrome**. Secondary mitral regurgitation occurs with idiopathic hypertrophic cardiomyopathy and anomalous origin of the left coronary artery from the pulmonary artery. Mitral insufficiency is also seen in connective tissue disorders such as **Marfan syndrome** and various **Mucopolysaccharidosis**.

**Etiology:** Probably multifactorial inheritance.

**Pathogenesis:** An isolated cleft probably represents a form of **Heart, endocardial cushion defects**, despite the absence of other components normally seen in endocardial cushion type defects.

**MIM No.:** 12100

**CDC No.:** 746.600

**Sex Ratio:** Presumably M1:F1

**Occurrence:** Less than 1:1,000

**Risk of Recurrence for Patient's Sib:** Unknown.

**Risk of Recurrence for Patient's Child:** Unknown. Presumably in the range of two to five percent.

**Age of Detectability:** From birth with two-dimensional and pulsed Doppler echocardiography.

**Gene Mapping and Linkage:** Unknown.

**Prevention:** None known. Genetic counseling indicated.

**Treatment:** In infants and children, treatment should be conservative with attempts to avoid surgical intervention if possible. Valvuloplasty is surgical procedure of choice in children. Valve replacement may be necessary in severe cases, especially in adults and adolescents.

**Prognosis:** Variable depending upon etiology and associated lesions. Excellent surgical results in older children can be obtained with valvuloplasty or replacement. Management of infants and young children remains difficult with a high mortality.

**Detection of Carrier:** Unknown.

**References:**
Titus JL: Congenital malformations of the mitral and aortic valves and related structures. Dis Chest 1969; 55:358–367.

Friedensohn A, et al.: An unusual form of mitral insufficiency accompanying atrial septal defect. Clin Cardiol 1979; 2:158–161.
Baylen BG, Criley MJ: Diseases of the mitral valve. In: Adams FM, Emmanoulides GC, eds: Moss's heart disease in infants, children and adolescents. 3rd ed. Baltimore: Williams & Wilkins, 1983:516–526. *
Segni ED, et al.: Isolated cleft mitral valve: a variety of congenital mitral regurgitation identified by 2-dimensional echocardiography. Am J Cardiol 1983; 51:927–931.
Barth CW, et al.: Mitral valve cleft without cardiac septal defect causing severe mitral regurgitation but allowing long survival. Am J Cardiol 1985; 55:1229–1231.

PA045
BR014                                    **Stephen M. Paridon**
                                         **J. Timothy Bricker**

## MITRAL VALVE PROLAPSE                              0668

**Includes:**
  Balloon or billowing mitral valve
  Barlow syndrome
  Click-murmur syndrome
  Floppy mitral valve
  Midsystolic click-late systolic murmur syndrome
  Mitral valve regurgitation, familial

**Excludes:**
  **Heart, endocardial cushion defects** (0347)
  Rheumatic and other acquired types of mitral valve insufficiency

**Major Diagnostic Criteria:** An apical midsystolic click, particularly if it is followed by a late systolic murmur of mitral insufficiency, suggests the diagnosis. Echocardiography can be diagnostic in the mitral valve prolapse syndrome by demonstrating the displacement of the mitral leaflets above the mitral anulus. Selective left ventricular angiocardiography may be used to confirm the diagnosis and to establish the degree of valvar insufficiency.

**Clinical Findings:** An aneurysmal protrusion of the posterior or anterior mitral valve leaflet, or both, into the left atrium, usually late in ventricular contraction. Patients with isolated mitral valve prolapse are asymptomatic, or complain of mild exercise intolerance or vague chest pain. Upon physical examination there is an apical midsystolic click or a late systolic murmur of mitral valve insufficiency. Both auscultatory findings are highly influenced by postural changes and often can only be detected in the left reclining or upright position. Chest X-rays usually are normal, but thoracic skeletal anomalies are common: "straight back," scoliosis or pectus excavatum. The EKG may show an indeterminate or left QRS axis and, particularly, biphasic or negative T waves in leads aVF or III.

Mitral valve prolapse sometimes is associated with atrial septal defects of the ostium secundum or sinus venosus type. These patients have all the clinical and radiologic findings of an atrial septal defect. In addition, an apical click or a late systolic murmur of mitral insufficiency may be present. When an ASD coexists, the EKG shows right ventricular hypertrophy and sometimes an indeterminate QRS axis or mild left axis deviation. Abnormal T waves in leads aVF or III may be found.

The M-mode echocardiogram can support the clinical diagnosis of a prolapsing mitral valve by demonstrating an abrupt posterior dip in late systole. Pansystolic "hammock" type displacement of the mitral leaflets is sometimes seen but can be a technical artifact. Two-D echocardiography using multiple views can also demonstrate the abnormal prolapse motion of either leaflet in systole. Strict diagnostic criteria should be used to avoid overdiagnosis.

Selective left ventriculography will confirm the prolapsing of the valve leaflets into the left atrium during ventricular contraction. In some instances there is a mild-to-moderate degree of mitral valve insufficiency. Frequently, the left ventricle will show an asymmetric contraction with a convex bulging in the mid-aspect of the anterolateral wall, or a localized protrusion of the posteroinferior wall into the left ventricular cavity ("ballerina" slipper configuration).

**Complications:** Little is known about the natural history of a congenital prolapsing mitral valve identified in childhood. Adults, however, have been found to have significant complications as a result of similarly malformed atrioventricular valves. Dysfunction of the mitral apparatus may produce insufficiency that, once established, may become progressively worse. Infective endocarditis has been reported even when the valve is competent. In rare instances, sudden death is presumably caused by significant cardiac arrhythmias, mostly of ventricular origin.

**Associated Findings:** Findings include other congenital heart defects, particularly **Atrial septal defects** of the ostium secundum or sinus venosus type, as well as thoracic skeletal anomalies ("straight back" syndrome, scoliosis and **Pectus excavatum**. Similarly, malformed mitral valves have been reported in both **Marfan syndrome** and **Ehlers-Danlos syndrome**.

**Etiology:** The majority of cases are sporadic. Several families have been described with autosomal dominant inheritance, with increased expression among females.

**Pathogenesis:** Myxomatous-type degeneration of the valve leaflets, or stretching of the mitral annulus resulting in disjunction between the atrium and ventricle.

**MIM No.:** *15770

**Sex Ratio:** M1:F2

**Occurrence:** Undetermined, but mitral valve prolapse may be the most commonly diagnosed cardiac valvar abnormality.

**Risk of Recurrence for Patient's Sib:**
See Part I, *Mendelian Inheritance.*

**Risk of Recurrence for Patient's Child:**
See Part I, *Mendelian Inheritance.* Depends on etiology; low recurrence risk in most cases.

**Age of Detectability:** From infancy, with echocardiography or selective angiocardiography.

**Gene Mapping and Linkage:** Unknown.

**Prevention:** None known. Genetic counseling indicated.

**Treatment:** The susceptibility of these patients to bacterial endocarditis warrants prophylactic antibiotics for dental or surgical procedures. Antiarrhythmic therapy for symptomatic patients with signs of ventricular irritability may be required. Mitral valve annuloplasty or replacement may be necessary in case of severe insufficiency.

**Prognosis:** Good, particularly during childhood and adolescence.

**Detection of Carrier:** Unknown.

**References:**
Barlow JB, et al.: Late systolic murmurs and non-ejection ("mid-late") systolic clicks: an analysis of 90 patients. Brit Heart J 1968; 30:203–218. *
Rizzon P, et al.: Familial syndrome of midsystolic click and late systolic murmur. Br Heart J 1973; 35:245–259.
Victorica BE, et al.: Ostium secundum atrial septal defect associated with balloon mitral valve in children. Am J Cardiol 1974; 33:668–673.
Salomon J, et al.: Thoracic skeletal abnormalities in idiopathic mitral valve prolapse. Am J Cardiol 1975; 36:32–36.
Sahn DJ, et al.: Echocardiographic spectrum of mitral valve motion in children with and without mitral valve prolapse. Am J Cardiol 1977; 39:422–431.
Jeresaty RM: Mitral valve prolapse. New York: Raven Press, 1979. *
Venkatesh A, et al.: Mitral valve prolapse in anxiety neurosis (panic disorder). Am Heart J 1980; 100:302–305.
Malcolm AD: Mitral valve prolapse associated with other disorders: casual coincidence, common link, or fundamental genetic disturbance. Brit Heart J 1985; 53:353–362.
Hutchins GM, et al.: The association of floppy mitral valve with disjunction of the mitral annulus fibrosus. New Eng J Med 1986; 314:535–541.

VI001                                    **Benjamin E. Victorica**

**Mitral valve regurgitation, familial**
*See MITRAL VALVE PROLAPSE*

## MITRAL VALVE STENOSIS                                    0669

**Includes:**
Parachute mitral valve
Supramitral ring

**Excludes:**
Lutembacher syndrome
Rheumatic and other forms of acquired mitral stenosis
**Scimitar syndrome** (0879)
**Ventricle, endocardial fibroelastosis of left ventricle** (0348)
**Ventricle, endocardial fibroelastosis of right ventricle** (0349)

**Major Diagnostic Criteria:** The presence on auscultation of loud first and second heart sounds accompanied by a low pitched apical diastolic murmur in an infant or child exhibiting signs or symptoms of congestive heart failure should raise the possibility of congenital mitral stenosis. Echocardiography and cardiac catheterization establish the diagnosis.

**Clinical Findings:** The anatomic findings in congenital mitral stenosis are variable and may include one or more of the following: thickened, rolled valve leaflets; shortened, thickened chordae tendineae; fused chordae; partial obliteration of interchordal spaces by fibrous tissue; abnormal or underdeveloped papillary muscles. Occasionally a double orifice of the mitral valve may be associated with stenosis. In the parachute mitral valve, the chordae (usually shortened and thickened) insert into one papillary muscle. Accummulation of connective tissue in a circumferential ring arising from the atrial insertions of the mitral valve leaflets may encroach on the mitral orifice producing obstruction. The left atrium in all forms of significant obstruction is enlarged, often with evidence of wall thickening and fibroelastosis. Dilatation and hypertrophy of the right ventricle and atrium are present in varying degrees depending on the severity of obstruction to left ventricular inflow.

Obstruction to flow across the mitral valve results in elevation of left atrial pulmonary venous, capillary and arterial pressures with pulmonary hypertension. The right ventricle hypertrophies and, with long standing mitral stenosis, may fail. In severe mitral stenosis, cardiac output may be diminished.

The age at which symptoms develop varies with the degree of stenosis and with the presence and type of associated cardiac defects. Infants often present with recurrent pulmonary infections, poor growth and tachypnea. Other symptoms include diaphoresis and dyspnea with feeds, chronic cough and irritability. Cyanosis is usually a late finding. Older children present with exertional dyspnea, fatigue and orthopnea. Syncope, hemoptysis and aphonia occur rarely. Symptoms tend to occur earlier in patients with associated cardiac anomalies.

On physical examination, pulses are normal except with severe stenosis. A right ventricular impulse is often palpable at the left sternal border. The first heart sound is loud. The second sound is narrowly split with a loud pulmonary component. In most patients, a low pitched, long diastolic murmur is audible at the apex, often with a presystolic component. Fifteen percent of patients have no murmur. An opening snap may be heard, but is not common. When right heart failure is present, jugular venous pulsations and hepatomegaly may be evident. Other physical findings may be present with associated cardiac anomalies.

Mild to marked cardiomegaly is evident on chest X-ray. There is often left atrial enlargement, pulmonary venous congestion (ranging from redistribution of flow to Kerley B lines), a prominent pulmonary trunk, and right-sided cardiac enlargement.

The electrocardiogram usually demonstrates a frontal plane QRS axis between $+90°$ and $+150°$. Right ventricular hypertrophy, left atrial enlargement and sometimes right atrial enlargement are evident. The presence of left ventricular hypertrophy suggests an additional cardiac defect.

M-mode echocardiography may show qualitative abnormalities of mitral stenosis. Anterior (instead of posterior) diastolic motion of the posterior mitral leaflet, decreased E-F slope, absent A wave, and left atrial enlargement are the typical findings, but M-mode is unreliable in assessing either the severity or the site of stenosis. Two-dimensional echocardiography may be helpful in determining the site and type as well as the severity of obstruction. Evaluation of the supravalvar region may reveal a supramitral ring, while views of the valve and subvalve regions may reveal abnormal papillary muscle anatomy and parachute mitral valve. The severity of stenosis can be evaluated by estimating the valve orifice area and by measuring the maximal transmitral inflow velocity by Doppler interrogation. In addition, two-dimensional echocardiography may reveal associated cardiac defects.

At cardiac catheterization, pulmonary artery and capillary wedge pressures are elevated. The left atrial mean as well as A wave pressures are also elevated with a diastolic pressure gradient between the left atrium and left ventricle. Cineangiography demonstrates left atrial enlargement and may show delayed emptying of the left atrium with dilated pulmonary veins. Thickened leaflets with decreased mobility may be seen with valve stenosis, or an hourglass left ventricular filling defect may be seen with parachute mitral valve.

**Complications:** Pulmonary hypertension with pulmonary vascular disease may develop, leading to right heart failure. Death occurs due to severe congestive heart failure or recurrent pulmonary infections.

**Associated Findings:** Congenital mitral stenosis occurs uncommonly as an isolated defect. It often occurs in association with obstructive lesions of the aorta and aortic valve. Shone syndrome or complex includes four potentially obstructive left-sided anomalies that have a tendency to coexist: parachute mitral valve, supravalvular ring of the left atrium, subaortic stenosis and **Aorta, coarctation**. Other anomalies associated with congenital mitral stenosis include patent ductus arteriosus, **Ventricular septal defect, Heart, tetralogy of Fallot, Heart, transposition of great vessels**, and double outlet right ventricle.

**Etiology:** Unknown.

**Pathogenesis:** The pathogenesis varies with the type of stenosis present. Abnormal development of any of the major components of the valve (leaflets, chordae tendineae, papillary muscles, annulus) may produce obstruction to left ventricular inflow).

**MIM No.:** 12100

**CDC No.:** 746.500

**Sex Ratio:** M1.5–2.2:F1

**Occurrence:** 6–12:1,000 cases of autopsied congenital heart disease; 2–4:1,000 cases in clinical series.

**Risk of Recurrence for Patient's Sib:** Unknown.

**Risk of Recurrence for Patient's Child:** Unknown.

**Age of Detectability:** From birth, with echocardiography and cardiac catheterization.

**Gene Mapping and Linkage:** Unknown.

**Prevention:** None known. Genetic counseling indicated.

**Treatment:** Medical treatment with diuretics and digoxin may be effective in patients with mild to moderate stenosis. Intractable congestive heart failure, pulmonary edema or systemic pulmonary hypertension are indications for surgery, mitral valvotomy or mitral valve replacement (or resection of supravalvar tissue in supramitral ring).

**Prognosis:** The prognosis depends on the severity of the obstruction and the nature of associated cardiac defects. The median age at death varies with the type of obstruction: parachute mitral valve: 9 11/12 years; supramitral ring: 5 6/12 years; typical congenital mitral valve stenosis: 6 months. Fifty-three percent of all patients live to age 10, 42% of those managed medically and 56% of the surgical patients.

**Detection of Carrier:** Unknown.

**References:**
Shone JD, et al.: The developmental complex of "parachute mitral valve", supravalvular ring of left atrium, subaortic stenosis, and coarctation of aorta. Am J Cardiol 1963; 11:714–725.
Van der Horst RL, Hastreiter AR: Congenital mitral stenosis. Am J Cardiol 1967; 20:773–783.
Collins-Nakai RL, et al.: Congenital mitral stenosis. a review of 20 years' experience. Circulation 1977;56:1039–1047.
Baylen BG, Criley JM: Diseases of the mitral valve. In: Adams FH, Emmanoulides OC, eds: Heart disease in infants, children and adolescents. Baltimore: Williams & Wilkins, 1983:516–526. *
Grenadier E, et al.: Two-dimensioanl echo Doppler study of congenital disorders of the mitral valve. Am Heart J 1984; 107:319–325.
Vitarelli A, et al.: Echocardiographic assessment of congenital mitral stenosis. Am Heart J 1984; 108:523–531.
Kveselis DA, et al.: Balloon angioplasty for congenital and rheumatic mitral stenosis. Am J Cardiol 1986; 57:348–350.

BR014
TA007

**J. Timothy Bricker**
**Lloyd Tani**

**Mitral valve, double orifice**
*See MITRAL VALVE INSUFFICIENCY*
**Microvillus atrophy, congenital**
*See MICROVILLUS INCLUSION DISEASE*
**Mixed central and peripheral neurofibromas**
*See NEUROFIBROMATOSIS*
**Mixed cryoglobulinemia, familial**
*See CRYOGLOBULINEMIA*
**Mixed cyst on head or neck**
*See NECK/HEAD, DERMOID CYST OR TERATOMA*
**Mixed hemangioma**
*See HEMANGIOMAS OF THE HEAD AND NECK*
**Mixed porphyria**
*See PORPHYRIA, VARIEGATE*
**Mljet disease**
*See MAL DE MELEDA*
**MMR syndrome**
*See MEGALOCORNEA-MENTAL RETARDATION SYNDROME*
**Mo1 (CD11b/CD18) deficiency**
*See GRANULOCYTE GLYCOPROTEIN CD11/CD18 DEFICIENCY*
**Moebius syndrome**
*See DIPLEGIA, CONGENITAL FACIAL*
**Mohr syndrome**
*See ORO-FACIO-DIGITAL SYNDROME, MOHR TYPE*
**Mohr-Majewski syndrome**
*See SHORT RIB-POLYDACTYLY SYNDROME, TYPE II*
**Molar roots, pyramidal-juvenile glaucoma-unusual upper lip**
*See DENTO-FACIO-SKELETAL DEFECTS, ACKERMAN TYPE*
**Molars, reincluded**
*See TEETH, MOLAR REINCLUSION*
**Mole, hydatidiform**
*See HYDATIDIFORM MOLE*

## MOLYBDENUM CO-FACTOR DEFICIENCY　　　　2412

**Includes:**
  Sulfite oxidase/xanthine dehydrogenase/aldehyde oxidase
    deficiency
  Xanthine dehydrogenase/sulfite oxidase/aldehyde oxidase
    deficiency
  Aldehyde oxidase/sulfite oxidase/xanthine dehydrogenase
    deficiency

**Excludes:** Aciduria, sulfite oxidase deficiency (0921)

**Major Diagnostic Criteria:** Facial dysmorphia, encephalopathy with **Microcephaly**, hypertonia with hypertonic seizures, bilateral ocular lens dislocation. Low serum uric acid. Low urinary uric acid with increased urinary S-sulfo-cysteine. Urinary sulfite thiosulfate taurine, xanthine, and hypoxanthine are also elevated. Sulfate excretion is diminished.

**Clinical Findings:** This condition generally presents in the first or second week of life but one case has been reported as late as five years of age. The findings are similar to those of **Aciduria, sulfite oxidase deficiency**, probably because this is the most important enzyme defect in that condition. The patients present with dysmorphic features, psychomotor retardation, extensive neurologic dysfunction, and seizures. Dislocation of the ocular lens may not be present in the first few weeks of life, but generally appears by the third month.

**Complications:** Progressive cerebral dysfunction and death.

**Associated Findings:** None known.

**Etiology:** Autosomal recessive inheritance.

**Pathogenesis:** There is a deficiency of a molybdenum containing cofactor. An unusual pterin is also found in this cofactor. The absence of this cofactor leads to a deficiency of the enzymes sulfite oxidase (sulfite-oxygen oxido reductase E.C. 1.8.2.1) and xanthine oxidase (E.C. 1.2.3.2).

**MIM No.:** *25215

**Sex Ratio:** M1:F1

**Occurrence:** About 15 cases cases have been reported in the literature.

**Risk of Recurrence for Patient's Sib:**
See Part I, *Mendelian Inheritance.*

**Risk of Recurrence for Patient's Child:**
See Part I, *Mendelian Inheritance.* Affected individuals are not expected to survive to reproduce.

**Age of Detectability:** As early as the first day of life, or by amniocentesis. The amniocentesis fluid is analysed for S-sulfocysteine and amniotic cells analysed for sulfite oxidase.

**Gene Mapping and Linkage:** Unknown.

**Prevention:** None known. Genetic counseling indicated.

**Treatment:** Unknown.

**Prognosis:** Most patients die within one year of diagnosis, although one was reported alive at five years of age.

**Detection of Carrier:** Unknown.

**References:**
Duran M, et al.: Combined deficiency of xanthine oxidase and sulfite oxidase: a defect of molybdenum metabolism or transport. J Inherit Metab Dis 1978; 1:175.
Johnson JL, et al.: Characterization of the molybdenum cofactor of sulfite oxidase, xanthine oxidase and nitrate reductase. J Biol Chem 1980; 255:1783.
Wadman SK, et al.: Absence of hepatic molybdenum cofactor: an inborn error of metabolism leading to a combined deficiency of sulfite oxidase and xanthine dehydrogenase. J Inherit Metab Dis 1983; 6(Suppl 1):78.
Desjacques P, et al.: Combined deficiency of xanthine and sulfite oxidase: diagnosis of a new case followed by an antenatal diagnosis. J Inherit Metab Dis 1985; 8(Suppl 2):117.
Roth A, et al.: Anatomo-pathological findings in a case of combined deficiency of sulfite oxidase and xanthine oxidase with a defect of molybdenum cofactor. Virchows Arch [Pathol Anat] 1985; 405:379.
Roesel RA, et al.: Combined xanthine and sulphite oxidase defect due to a deficiency of molybdenum cofactor. J Inherit Metab Dis 1986; 9:343–347.
Johnson JL, Wadman SK: Molybdenum cofactor deficiency. In: Scriver CR, et al, eds: The metabolic basis of inherited disease, 6th ed. New York: McGraw-Hill, 1989:1463–1477.

CR006                                                          **John C. Crawhill**

**Mondini-Alexander malformation of inner ear**
*See EAR, INNER DYSPLASIAS*
**Mongolian spot**
*See SKIN, CUTANEOUS MELANOSIS: MONGOLIAN SPOT*
**Mongolism (obsolete/pejorative)**
*See CHROMOSOME 21, TRISOMY 21*
**Monilethrix hair**
*See HAIR, MONILETHRIX*
**Moniliasis, familial**
*See POLYGLANDULAR AUTOIMMUNE SYNDROME*
**Monodactyly**
*See ECTRODACTYLY*
**Monodermoma of head or neck**
*See NECK/HEAD, DERMOID CYST OR TERATOMA*
**Mononeuritis, Familial recurrent**
*See NEUROPATHY, HEREDITARY WITH PRESSURE PALSIES*
**Monostotic cortical fibrous dysplasia**
*See OSTEOFIBROUS DYSPLASIA OF TIBIA AND FIBULA*
**Monozygotic co-twin, fetal effects of vascular obstruction**
*See FETAL BRAIN DISRUPTION SEQUENCE*
**Monozygotic twins, conjoined**
*See TWINS, CONJOINED*

## MOOD AND THOUGHT DISORDERS                              1532

**Includes:**
- Affective personality disorders
- Bipolar affective disorder
- Depressive disorders
- Manic-depressive (bipolar) disorders
- Major affective disorders
- Panic disorder
- Schizophrenic disorders

**Excludes:**
- **Attention-deficit hyperactivity disorder (ADHD)** (3240)
- **Autism, infantile** (2128)
- Neurologically determined behavioral disorders (other)
- **Tourette syndrome** (2305)

**Major Diagnostic Criteria:** Major affective disorders are characterized by a significant disturbance in mood: depressed or excited/elated (manic). Schizophrenic disorders are characterized by some combination of impaired thought processes, disturbed thought content, disturbed perceptual processes (e.g. hallucinations), and flattened or inappropriate emotional tone.

**Clinical Findings:** Major affective disorders display a high degree of phenotypic variability, even within a given family. In addition to the spectrum of classic bipolar and unipolar manic-depressive disorders, certain types of personality disorders, anxiety disorders, and eating disorders also aggregate in affective disorder families and respond to affective disorder medications. Onset of symptomatology can occur at any age and symptoms can change or progress from mild to severe over time. A cyclical pattern of episodes is frequent and may follow the seasons.

Manic symptomatology may include: elated, excited or irritable mood; increased activity and decreased sleep; expanded "flight of ideas" and rapid, pressured talking; and over-inflated grandiosity with impulsive acting-out (e.g. buying sprees). Manic episodes may be of psychotic proportions (e.g. grandiose delusions).

A severe depression may include depressed mood and a loss of interest or pleasure in life's activities; depressive ideation with excessive self-reproach or guilt; thoughts of death or suicide; fatigue; diminished concentration; and vegetative signs and symptoms such as disturbed sleep, appetite, psychosomatic, or psychomotor activity. Again, episodes can be psychotic.

Schizoaffective disorders display, in addition to the affective components discussed above, a disorder of thought. The schizoaffective diagnosis is genetically heterogeneous, present in schizophrenic families as well as affective disorder families.

Schizophrenic symptomatology is classified as positive or negative. Negative symptoms can include a poverty of thought and speech, flattened affect, and psychomotor retardation or catatonia. Hallucinations, delusions, bizarre or inappropriate affect, and excited behavior are examples of positive symptoms. Onset may be sudden or insidious. Onset occurs at any age and peaks in early adulthood.

**Complications:** Self-destructive behaviors. Impaired adaptation to life.

**Associated Findings:** None known.

**Etiology:** Major affective disorders and schizophrenia probably consist of a collection of disorders with heterogeneous etiologies. Genetics as well as environmental factors and development play etiological roles.

**Pathogenesis:** Dysregulations of numerous neuroendocrine, circadian, neurotransmitter and neuropeptidergic systems have been demonstrated in some patients with major affective disorders. Catecholaminergic hypotheses have been intensely pursued, in part, because of the known interactions of antidepressant medications with catecholaminergic systems.

Dysfunctional dopaminergic systems are implicated in the pathogenesis of schizophrenia. Most antipsychotic medications are potent dopamine antagonists.

**MIM No.:** *12548, *30920, 18150, 16787

**Sex Ratio:** M1:F1 for bipolar disorders and schizophrenia. M1:F2 for major depression.

**Occurrence:** Bipolar disorder prevalence ranges from 0.5 to 1.2% of the general population. Lifetime prevalence rates for major depression in males range from 3% to 10%; females 6% to 20%. The lifetime prevalence of schizophrenia is approximately 1%.

**Risk of Recurrence for Patient's Sib:**
See Part I, *Mendelian Inheritance*. Major affective disorders and schizophrenia often display reduced penetrance.

**Risk of Recurrence for Patient's Child:**
See Part I, *Mendelian Inheritance*. Major affective disorders and schizophrenia often display reduced penetrance.

**Age of Detectability:** May be diagnosed at any age. Most frequently detected after puberty for bipolar disorders and after late adolescence for schizophrenia. Behavioral manifestations of affective disorder are being increasingly recognized in childhood.

**Gene Mapping and Linkage:** MAFD1 (major affective disorder 1) has been mapped to 11p15.5 [in one Old Order Amish family only.] Subsequent studies on this same family have demonstrated insignificant mild positive linkage to the 11p15.5 probes (Barinaga, 1989)].

MAFD2 (major affective disorder 2) has been mapped to Xq27-q28 [in some families].

SCZD2 (schizophrenia disorder 2) is unassigned.

BDM (behavior disorder modifier) has been provisionally mapped to X.

While there have been recent attempts to gene map mood and personality variables, most have provided interesting but inconclusive findings.

**Prevention:** None known. Genetic counseling indicated.

**Treatment:** A variety of psychopharmacological interventions are successful in the treatment of major affective illness (e.g. antidepressants, lithium carbonate) and schizophrenia (e.g. dopamine blocking neuroleptics). Electroconvulsive treatment is beneficial in certain cases of major depression. Psychotherapy is beneficial in many cases.

**Prognosis:** Extremely variable.

**Detection of Carrier:** Clinical assessment.

**Support Groups:**
VA; Alexandria; National Mental Health Association
DC; Washington; National Alliance for the Mentally Ill

**References:**
DeLong GR: Lithium carbonate treatment of select behavior disorders in children suggesting manic-depressive illness. J Pediat 1978; 93:689–694.
Weissman MM, et al.: Family-genetic studies of psychiatric disorders. Arch Gen Psychiatry 1986; 43:1104–1116.
Baron M, et al.: Genetic linkage between X-chromosome markers and bipolar affective illness. Nature 1987; 326:289–292.
Egeland JA, et al.: Bipolar affective disorders linked to DNA markers on chromosome 11. Nature 1987; 325:783–787.
Hodgkinson S, et al.: Molecular genetic evidence for heterogeneity in manic depression. Nature 1987; 325:805–806.
Diagnostic and Statistical Manual of Mental Disorders - Revised (DSM-III-R) APA Press, 1988.
Kennedy JL, et al.: Evidence against linkage of schizophrenia to markers on chromosome 5 in a northern Swedish pedigree. Nature 1988; 336:167–170.
Sherrington R, et al.: Localization of a susceptibility locus for schizophrenia on chromosome 5. Nature 1988; 336:164–167.
Barinaga M: Manic depression gene put in limbo. Science 1989; 246:886–887.
Weissman MM, et al.: Suicidal ideation and suicide attempts in panic disorder and attacks. New Engl J Med 1989; 321:1209–1214.

LE057                                **James E. Lee**

**Moore-Federman syndrome**
*See DWARFISM-STIFF JOINTS*
**Moravcsik-Marinesco-Sjogren syndrome**
*See MARINESCO-SJOGREN SYNDROME*

**Moreno syndrome**
*See CRANIO-FRONTO-NASAL DYSPLASIA*
**Morgagni-Stewart-Morel syndrome**
*See HYPEROSTOSIS FRONTALIS INTERNA*
**Morning glory disc anomaly**
*See OPTIC DISC, MORNING GLORY ANOMALY*
**Morquio syndrome**
*See MUCOPOLYSACCHARIDOSIS IV*
**Morquio-Ullrich syndrome**
*See MUCOPOLYSACCHARIDOSIS IV*
**Mosaic gonadal dysgenesis**
*See CHROMOSOME MOSAICISM, 45,X/46,XY TYPE*
**Mosaic Turner syndrome**
*See TURNER SYNDROME*
**Motor and sensory neuropathy, hereditary type II**
*See NEUROPATHY, HEREDITARY MOTOR AND SENSORY, TYPE II*
**Motor and sensory neuropathy, type I**
*See NEUROPATHY, HEREDITARY MOTOR AND SENSORY, TYPE I*
**Motor and sensory neuropathy, X-linked**
*See NEUROPATHY, HEREDITARY MOTOR AND SENSORY, TYPE I*
**Motor neuron disease, juvenile and adult**
*See AMYOTROPHIC LATERAL SCLEROSIS*
*also AMYOTROPHIC LATERAL SCLEROSIS, FAMILIAL ADULT AND JUVENILE TYPES*
**Motor system degeneration, autosomal dominant**
*See MACHADO-JOSEPH DISEASE*
**Motrin^, fetal effects**
*See FETAL EFFECTS OF NONSTEROIDAL ANTI-INFLAMMATORY DRUGS (NSAIDS)*
**Mouth, dryness from salivary gland dysfunction**
*See SALIVARY GLAND, AGENESIS*
**Mouth, inability to open completely-camptodactyly**
*See CAMPTODACTYLY-TRISMUS SYNDROME*
**Moynahan alopecia syndrome**
*See ALOPECIA-EPILEPSY-OLIGOPHRENIA, MOYNAHAN TYPE*
**Mozart ear**
*See EAR, MOZART TYPE*
**Muckle-Wells syndrome**
*See URTICARIA-DEAFNESS-AMYLOIDOSIS*
**Mucocutaneous lentigines-myxomas-multiple blue nevi**
*See NEVI-ATRIAL MYXOMA-MYXOID NEUROFIBROMAS-EPHELIDES*

---

**MUCOLIPIDOSIS I**                         **0671**

**Includes:**
Cherry-red spot-myoclonus syndrome
Glycoprotein neuraminidase, deficiency of
Lipomucopolysaccharidosis
Myoclonus syndrome-cherry red spot
Neuraminidase deficiency
Sialidase deficiency
Sialidosis

**Excludes:**
**Dentatorubropallidoluysian degeneration, hereditary** (3283)
**Mucolipidosis II** (0672)
**Mucolipidosis III** (0673)
**Mucopolysaccharidosis**

**Major Diagnostic Criteria:** The primary means of diagnosis is the demonstration of an isolated deficiency of the lysosomal enzyme neuraminidase (sialidase), which can be accomplished in peripheral leukocytes or cultured fibroblasts. Other lysosomal enzymes need to be shown to be at normal levels to exclude the diagnosis of mucolipidosis (ML) II or III. In all three forms of ML, there is an increased urinary excretion of bound sialic acid that can be used as a simple screening test. If excessive urinary bound-sialic acid is found, measurement of serum hexosaminidase will give normal results in ML I and markedly elevated levels in ML II and III.

**Clinical Findings:** Lysosomal storage diseases are noted for a series of phenotypes associated with deficiency of the same enzyme; this is carried to the extreme in ML I in which, in general, the disease in each family appears to result in a distinct phenotype. Lowden and O'Brien (1979) have suggested two major categories, defined as dysmorphic and nondysmorphic sialidosis; *Hurler-like* and *non-Hurler-like* are more descriptive designations.

The Hurler-like forms of ML I occur as infantile (death between ages one and six years) and childhood (a slower progressing

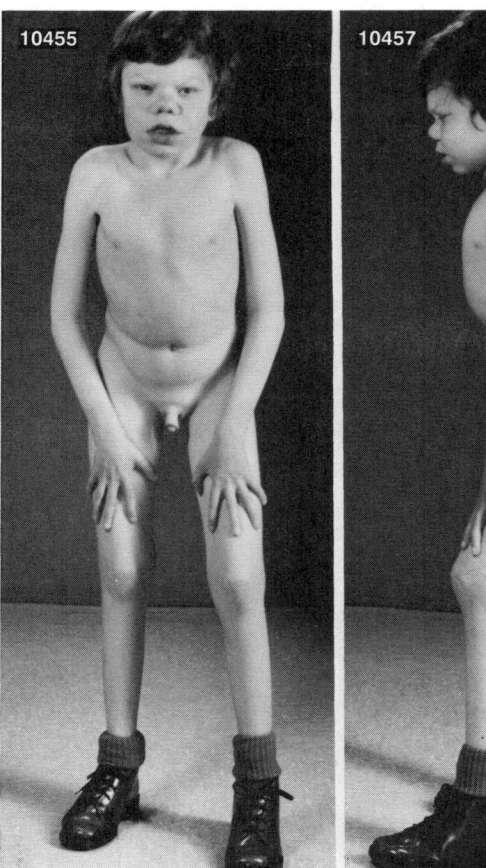

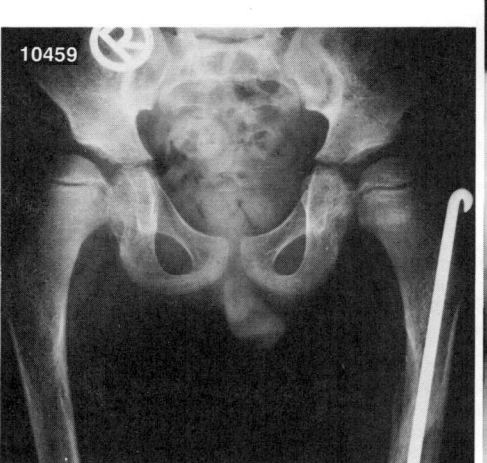

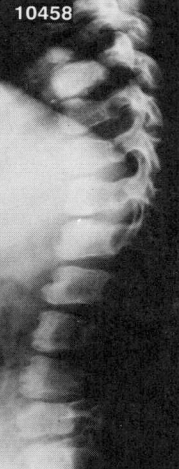

**0671**-10455–57: Stature is short due to shortened and deformed trunk. 10459: Mild hypoplasia of basilar portion of ilia. Subluxed femoral heads, small epiphyses, and necks in valgus position. Note the pathologic fracture in the left femoral shaft. 10458: Vertebral bodies are rounded and dorsally wedged. There are hook-shaped deformities of L1-L4.

disorder with survival into young adulthood) types. As implied by the term *Hurler-like*, the disorder involves multiple organ systems with skeletal, ocular, CNS, and visceral manifestations. The infantile form may be as clinically striking as ML II (I-cell disease) with coarse facies, severe skeletal contractures, marked hepatosplenomegaly, and an early onset of mental decline. Early deaths have occurred secondary to renal, hepatic, and cardiac complications. The childhood form was the first form described clinically and was designated *ML I* by Spranger et al. (1977).

The non-Hurler-like form of ML I is better known as the *cherry-red spot myoclonus syndrome* with an onset in the late teen or early adult years. It follows a slowly progressive course thereafter. A cherry-red spot of the macula may be seen with several forms of childhood lysosomal storage diseases, but it is virtually unique in adulthood to ML I.

**Complications:** The multisystem involvement of ML I leads to a preponderance of clinical manifestations varying with individual patients from renal, hepatic, or cardiac failure in infantile forms to skeletal and mental decline dominating childhood forms. The adult forms are compatible with reasonably good health, while slow mental regression occurs over a number of years.

**Associated Findings:** While one organ system pathology may dominate the course of individual patients, this occurs against the background of a progressive, multisystem disease.

**Etiology:** Autosomal recessive inheritance for mutations at the structural gene locus for neuraminidase. The different phenotypes occur as the result of combinations of different mutant neuraminidase alleles.

**Pathogenesis:** The accumulation of sialic acid-rich oligosaccharides in many tissues leads to local cell death and dysfunction. The phenotypic difference among individual patients apparently reflects differences in residual enzyme activity and accumulation of different compounds, depending on the age of the patient and the kinetics of the mutant enzyme toward its natural substrates.

**MIM No.:** *25240, *25655

**POS No.:** 3305

**Sex Ratio:** M1:F1

**Occurrence:** Collectively, the mutations resulting in the varying forms of ML I lead to an incidence of roughly 1:250,000

**Risk of Recurrence for Patient's Sib:**
See Part I, *Mendelian Inheritance.*

**Risk of Recurrence for Patient's Child:**
See Part I, *Mendelian Inheritance.* No recorded instances of reproduction by an affected individual, but dependent on frequency of carrier state, which is presumably low.

**Age of Detectability:** The infantile form may be clinically apparent in the newborn, whereas the other forms vary with the cherry red spot-myoclonus syndrome not apparent clinically until early adulthood. The biochemical abnormality can be detected at any age, including assays of cultured amniotic fluid cells and chorionic villi.

**Gene Mapping and Linkage:** NEU (neuraminidase) has been inconsistently mapped to 10pter-q23 or 6.

**Prevention:** None known. Genetic counseling indicated.

**Treatment:** As with all lysosomal diseases, no specific therapy exists, and symptomatic care of the patient and support of the family are important.

**Prognosis:** Varies with individual cases, and the course must be established by follow-up of individual patients.

**Detection of Carrier:** By enzyme assay in peripheral leukocytes, but overlap between carriers and noncarriers is observed.

**Support Groups:** NJ; Elizabeth; National Lipid Diseases Foundation

**References:**
Spranger JW, et al.: Lipomucopolysaccharidose. Z Kinderheilkd 1968; 103:285–306.
Spranger JW, Wiedemann HR: The genetic mucolipidoses: diagnosis and differential diagnosis. Humangenetik 1970; 9:113–139.

Kelly TE, Graetz GS: Isolated acid neuraminidase deficiency: a distinct lysosomal storage disease. Am J Med Genet 1977; 1:31–46. †

Spranger JW, et al.: Mucolipidosis I-a sialidosis. Am J Med Genet 1977; 1:21–29.

O'Brien JS: Neuraminidase deficiency in the cherry red spot-myoclonus syndrome. Biochem Biophys Res Commun 1977; 79:1136–1140.

Lowden JA, O'Brien JS: Sialidosis: a review of human neuraminidase deficiency. Am J Hum Genet 1979; 31:1–18.

Kelly TE, et al.: Mucolipidosis I (acid neuraminidase deficiency): three cases and delineation of the variability of the phenotype. Am J Dis Child 1981; 135:703–708.

Young ID, et al.: Neuraminidase deficiency: case report and review of the phenotype. J Med Genet 1987; 24:283–290.

KE012                                                    **Thaddeus E. Kelly**

---

## MUCOLIPIDOSIS II                                        0672

**Includes:**
> I-cell disease
> Leroy disease
> N-acetylglucosamine-1-phosphotransferase deficiency

**Excludes:**
> **Fucosidosis** (0398)
> **G(M1)-gangliosidosis, type 1** (0431)
> **G(M1)-gangliosidosis, type 2** (0432)
> **Mannosidosis** (2079)
> **Mucolipidosis III** (0673)
> **Mucolipidosis** (other)
> **Mucopolysaccharidosis**

**Major Diagnostic Criteria:** The clinical presentation includes a pseudo-Hurler phenotype with an absence of urinary excretion of mucopolysaccharides. Clinical findings include coarse facies, severe skeletal changes including kyphoscoliosis, lumbar gibbus, anterior vertebral breaking and wedging, wide ribs, and joint contractures. Cardiomegaly and congestive heart failure are common and may be present at birth. Serum levels of a variety of lysosomal acid hydrolases are elevated; these include beta-N-acetylhexosaminidase and arylsulfatase A, iduronate sulfatase, glycosidases, and the like. There is a corresponding deficiency of these enzymes in cultured fibroblasts. Some cells do not show this deficiency (leukocytes) or show it minimally (nerve cells and hepatocytes). Prominent phase-dense inclusion bodies are present in cultured fibroblasts. In trophoblasts, the enzyme most conspicuously deficient is beta-galactosidase.

**Clinical Findings:** Pseudo-Hurler phenotype with growth and psychomotor retardation. Cardiomegaly, congestive heart failure, and respiratory infections are potentially lethal complications. Hepatomegaly is also exaggerated by heart failure. Corneal clouding may be present, but this is not generally a prominent feature that can aid early diagnosis. The skin is tight and puffy; this can be very dramatic around the eyes. Gum hyperplasia may also be striking. Clinical onset is quite early, and most patients have obvious problems by six months of age.

**Complications:** Congestive heart failure, orthopedic deformities, and psychomotor retardation.

**Associated Findings:** Frequent respiratory infections.

**Etiology:** Autosomal recessive inheritance.

**Pathogenesis:** There is an absence or deficiency of N-acetyl-glucosamine phosphotransferase. In the absence of this enzyme, the acid hydrolases that are intended for the lysosomes lack the recognition marker, mannose-6-phosphate. The enzymes are secreted instead of being trapped within the lysosome. Ordinarily, these acid hydrolases are further "processed" in the lysosomes. Because they are not trapped in this organelle, the resultant secreted acid hydrolases differ from the "normal, trapped" lysosomal enzymes.

**MIM No.:** *25250

**POS No.:** 3306

**Sex Ratio:** M1:F1

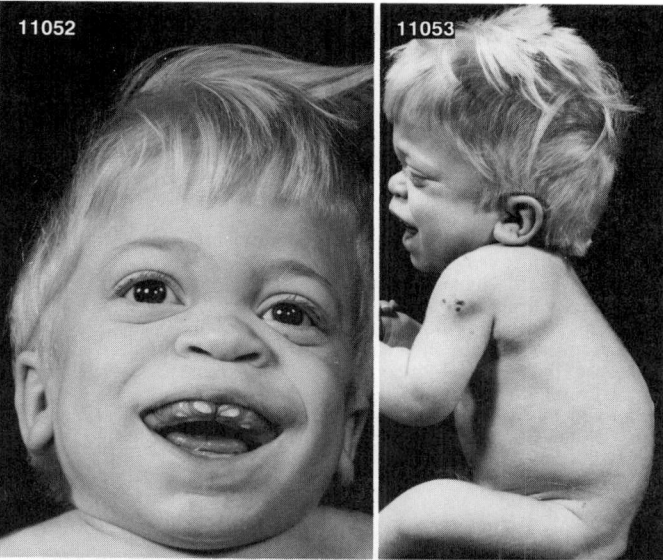

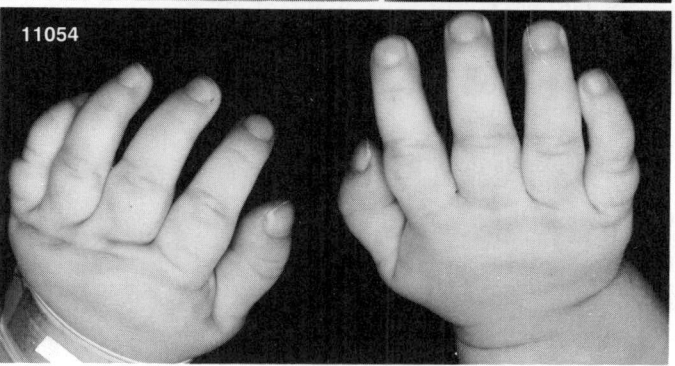

0672-11052–53: Coarse facies with proptotic eyes; open, wide mouth; hyperplastic gingiva; abundant hair; scaphocephaly and gibbus. 11054: Short digits and the beginning of a claw-hand deformity.

---

**Occurrence:** More than 30 reported cases; many from Japan.

**Risk of Recurrence for Patient's Sib:**
See Part I, *Mendelian Inheritance.*

**Risk of Recurrence for Patient's Child:**
See Part I, *Mendelian Inheritance.* Affected individuals are not expected to survive to reproduce.

**Age of Detectability:** Clinically, in early infancy. Prenatal diagnosis can be made from amniocytes obtained by conventional amniocentesis and from trophoblasts at 10 weeks menstrual (8 weeks embryonic) age.

**Gene Mapping and Linkage:** GNPTA (UDP-N-acetylgluco.-lysosomal-enzyme N-acetylglucosaminephosphotrans.) has been provisionally mapped to 4q21-q23.

**Prevention:** None known. Genetic counseling indicated.

**Treatment:** Supportive therapy.

**Prognosis:** Usually death by five years of age.

**Detection of Carrier:** No reproducible abnormalities have been identified in heterozygotes.

**Support Groups:** NJ; Elizabeth; National Lipid Diseases Foundation

**References:**

Sly WS and Fischer HD: The phosphomannosyl recognition system for intracellular and intercellular transport of lysosomal enzymes. J Cell Biochem 1982; 18:67–85.

Whelan DT, et al.: Mucolipidosis II: the clinical, radiological and biochemical features in three cases. Clin Genet 1983; 24:90–96.

Okada S, et al.: I-cell disease: clinical studies of 21 Japanese cases. Clin Genet 1985; 28:207–215.

Kornfeld S: Trafficking of lysosomal enzymes in normal and disease states. J Clin Invest 1986; 77:1–6.

Herzog V, et al.: Thyroglobulin, the major and obligatory exportable protein of thyroid follicle cells, carries the lysosomal recognition marker mannose-6-phosphate. EMBO J 1987; 6:555–560.

Ben-Yoseph Y, et al.: First trimester prenatal evaluation for I-cell desease by N-acetyl-glucosamine 1-phosphototransferase assay. Clin Genet 1988; 33:38–43.

Nolan CM, Sly WS: I-cell disease and pseudo-Hurler polydystrophy. In: Scriver CR, et al, eds: The metabolic basis of inherited disease, 6th ed. New York: McGraw-Hill, 1989:1589–1602.

AM001                                    **R. Stephan S. Amato**

## MUCOLIPIDOSIS III                                    0673

**Includes:**

Pseudo-Hurler polydystrophia
Pseudopolysystrophy

**Excludes:**

**Mucolipidosis II** (0672)
**Mucopolysaccharidosis**

**Major Diagnostic Criteria:** Early onset of painless joint stiffness and decreased mobility, short stature, some coarseness of the facial features suggesting a mild mucopolysaccharidosis, mild mental retardation, no excess urinary acid mucopolysaccharides, and X-ray evidence of dysostosis multiplex. Ten to twenty-fold elevations (compared to intracellular fibroblast levels) of beta-

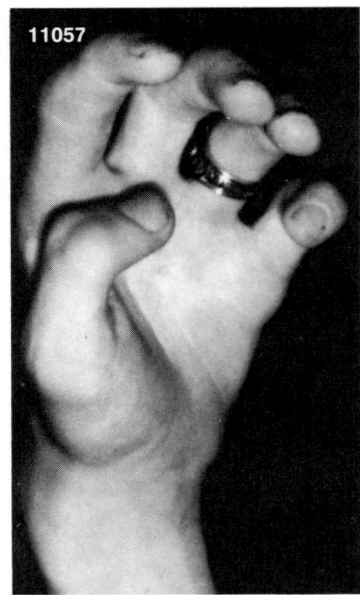

**0673B**-11057:   Joint contractures.

hexosaminidase, iduronate sulfatase, and aryl-sulfatase A are found in plasma (as they are in I-cell disease).

**Clinical Findings:**   Early childhood onset of joint stiffness; limitation of mobility is slowly progressive but seems to become stationary after puberty. Other characteristics are corneal opacities detected by slit-lamp examination; short stature with short trunk

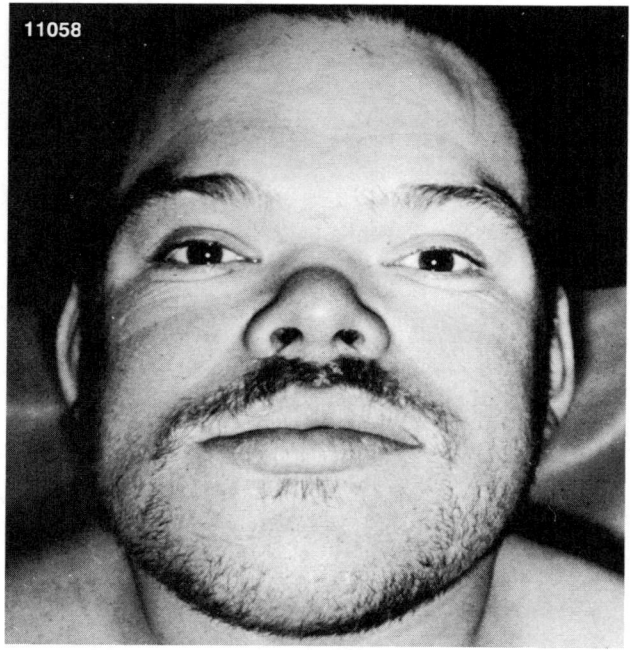

**0673A**-11058:   Note coarse facial features.

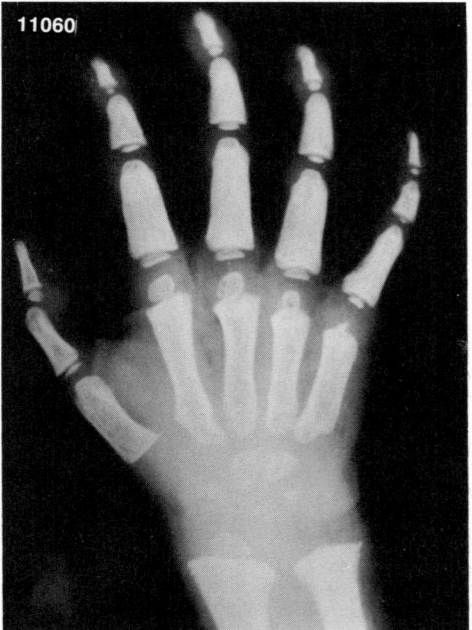

**0673C**-11060:   X-ray at age 7 years shows rather mild Hurler-like changes of the hand skeleton: reduction of carpal space, misshaped metacarpals, expanded diaphyses of proximal and middle phalanges, and hypoplastic distal phalanges.

and relatively long extremities; and mild mental retardation in some patients. Liver and spleen are usually not enlarged. The urinary excretion of acid mucopolysaccharides is normal; that of sialyloligosaccharides is excessive. Skin fibroblast cultures are metachromatic; the I-cell phenomenon is found too. Peripheral leukocytes are normal in light microscopic appearance, although they have a deficiency of the enzyme. Vacuolated plasma cells are found in the bone marrow. X-ray of the skeleton shows abnormalities that resemble milder forms of the mucopolysaccharidoses, except for severe pelvic dysplasia; vertebral anomalies are common. There is generalized osteoporosis.

**Complications:** Easy fatigability. Congestive heart failure may occur. Carpal tunnel compression is occasional.

**Associated Findings:** Aortic valvular disease, carpal tunnel compression.

**Etiology:** Autosomal recessive inheritance. Deficiency of UDP-N-acetylglucosamine-1-phosphotransferase.

**Pathogenesis:** The primary deficiency of mucolipidosis (ML) III is in UDP-N-acetylglucosamine-1-phosphatotransferase. In normal fibroblasts, acid hydrolases are glycosylated and phosphorylated. UDP-N-acetylglucosamine phosphatase brings the phosphate to the oligosaccharide chain of the lysosomal enzymes. Subsequently, the glucosamine is removed and leaves the phosphate attached to the mannose. This acts like a recognition marker that finds the receptor in the endoplasmic reticulum or Golgi apparatus and drives the enzyme to the lysosome. There the enzymes acquire their mature form by limited proteolysis. Normally, very little of the enzymes is secreted outside of the cell, and they can be recovered by endocytosis. In ML III, the partial lack of phosphorylation deprives acid hydrolases of the recognition marker, and they are secreted after additional carbohydrate modifications (sialization). They cannot be taken up by endocytosis and thus remain in the extracellular spaces or in the serum, increasing their concentration to the levels previously noted.

**MIM No.:** *25260

**POS No.:** 3307

**Sex Ratio:** M1:F1

**Occurrence:** A few dozen cases have been documented, including four original French cases (Maroteaux and Lamy, 1966), and two Cape Coloured cases.

**Risk of Recurrence for Patient's Sib:**
See Part I, *Mendelian Inheritance.*

**Risk of Recurrence for Patient's Child:**
See Part I, *Mendelian Inheritance.*

**Age of Detectability:** Joint stiffness has been noted as early as 13 months, but usually manifests itself after the second year of life. Prenatal diagnosis is possible by measuring the levels of lysosomal enzymes, especially hexosaminidases, in the amniotic fluid and in the amniocytes and by the analysis of the specific enzyme UDP-N-acetylglucosamine-1-phosphotransferase.

**Gene Mapping and Linkage:** GNPTA (UDP-N-acetylglucosamine-lysosomal-enzyme N-acetylglucosaminephosphotransferase) has been provisionally mapped to 4q21-q23.

**Prevention:** None known. Genetic counseling indicated.

**Treatment:** Symptomatic.

**Prognosis:** Joint stiffness typically is evident by age 2–4 years. This can cause a significant handicap for the adult. Progressive destruction of the hip joints results in the most disabling problems for these individuals by late teens. Mental retardation, if present, is mild and not progressive. Survival to age 50 years is known, but there is little information available on the course of the disease in adulthood.

**Detection of Carrier:** Heterozygote detection has been reported using [32P]UDP-G1cNAc and 3H or 14C labeled UDP-G1cNAc as the donor substrate for the UDP-N-acetylglucosamine-1-phosphotransferase. These reports show some overlap between the activity ranges of presumed heterozygotes and normals.

**Special Considerations:** The finding of three different complementation groups in fibroblasts suggests the heterogeneous nature of ML III and could be due to either allelic variation in the expression of defects in a single gene, or mutations in distinct genes. Varki et al (1981) found that fibroblasts from two sibs with ML III had normal enzyme activity when measured with the assay using alpha methyl-mannose as acceptor, but a low activity when assayed with endogenous acceptor. The diagnosis of the condition is made by recognition of the clinical and developmental signs previously noted, by the highly elevated levels of lysosomal enzymes in serum, and by the demonstration of the deficiency of the enzyme UDP-N-acetylglucosamine-1-phosphotransferase.

**Support Groups:** NJ; Elizabeth; National Lipid Diseases Foundation

**References:**
Maroteaux P, Lamy M: La pseudo-polydystrophie de Hurler. Presse Med 1966; 74:2889–2892.
Reitman ML, et al.: Fibroblast from patients with I-cell disease and pseudo-Hurler polydystrophy are deficient in uridine 5'-diphosphate-N-acetylglucosamine: glycoprotein N-acetylglucosaminylphosphotransferase activity. J Clin Invest 1981; 67:1574–1578.
Varki AP, et al.: Identification of a variant of mucolipidosis III: a catalytically active N-acetylglucosaminyl-phosphotransferase that fails to phosphorylate lysosomal enzymes. Proc Natl Acad Sci USA 1981; 78:7773–7777.
Neufeld EF, McKusick VA: Mucolipidosis III. In: Stanbury JB, et al., eds: The metabolic basis of inherited disease. 5th ed. New York: McGraw-Hill, 1983.
Little LE, et al.: Heterogeneity of N-acetylglucosmine 1-phosphotransferse within mucoloipidosis III. J Biol Chem 1986; 261:733–735.
Traboulsi EI, Maumenee IH: Ophthalmologic findings in mucolipidosis III (pseudo-Hurler polydystrophy). Am J Ophthal 1986; 102:592–597.
Mueller OT, et al.: Chromosomal assignment of N-acetylglucosaminylphospho-transferase, the lysosomal hydrolase trageting enzyme deficient in mucolipodosis II and III. (Abstract) Cytogenet Cell Genet HGM9, 1987.
Nolan CM, Sly WS: I-cell disease and pseudo-Hurler polydystrophy. In: Scriver CR, et al, eds: The metabolic basis of inherited disease, 6th ed. New York: McGraw-Hill, 1989:1589–1602.

TR008                                    **Carlos J. Trujillo-Botero**

---

## MUCOLIPIDOSIS IV                      2251

**Includes:**
Ganglioside neuraminidase deficiency
Ganglioside sialidase deficiency
Neuraminidase deficiency

**Excludes:**
**Mucolipidosis** (other)
**Mucopolysaccharidosis**
**Niemann-Pick disease** (0717)

**Major Diagnostic Criteria:** Corneal clouding; slowly progressive neurologic degeneration with mental retardation; normal urinary mucopolysaccharides; cytoplasmic inclusions seen with electron microscopy (EM) in conjunctival biopsies, skin fibroblasts, and cultured amniotic fluid cells. Skeletal changes and hepatosplenomegaly are usually absent.

**Clinical Findings:** Corneal opacities, slowly progressive pyramidal tract signs with hypotonia and extrapyramidal involvement. Corneal opacities were reported in 100% of cases, but may vary with age in the same patient. Visual acuity was diminished, sometimes profoundly, and an abnormal electroretinogram (ERG) was found in one-half. Strabismus was noted in 7%. Facial coarsening was subtle, but milder cases have been reported.

Bone marrow and leukocytes were normal. Electron microscopy (EM) of skin biopsies and/or conjunctiva were abnormal in all cases and showed both single membrane-bound granular inclusions and lamellar concentric bodies. These were also noted in cultured fibroblasts, amniocytes, and in liver, muscle, and brain. All phospholipids were increased in liver, skin fibroblasts, and urine, and only phosphatidylcholine in brain. Lysobisphosphatidic acid (LBPA) was markedly increased in these tissues, but was the only lipid stored in muscle. A mild increase in gangliosides has been reported in urine, brain white matter, and cultured fibroblasts.

**Complications:** Photophobia associated with corneal clouding and diminished visual acuity.

**Associated Findings:** None known.

**Etiology:** Autosomal recessive inheritance.

**Pathogenesis:** A partial ganglioside sialidase deficiency has been found in cultured fibroblasts. Whether this is the primary enzyme defect is doubtful. Increased phospholipids have now been reported in urine (2/6) and fibroblasts (5/6) from six unrelated patients. The nature of a putative defect in lysosomal membrane turnover remains undetermined.

**MIM No.:** *25265

**POS No.:** 3548

**Sex Ratio:** M11:F6 (observed).

**Occurrence:** Prevalence <1:100,000. About 20 cases, including three pairs of siblings, have been reported: eight in Ashkenazi Jews and nine in non-Jewish families.

**Risk of Recurrence for Patient's Sib:**
See Part I, *Mendelian Inheritance*.

**Risk of Recurrence for Patient's Child:**
See Part I, *Mendelian Inheritance*.

**Age of Detectability:** From one to two months of age; or prenatally from study of cultured fibroblasts.

**Gene Mapping and Linkage:** Unknown.

**Prevention:** None known. Genetic counseling indicated.

**Treatment:** A corneal graft was attempted without success in one case.

**Prognosis:** Age of oldest known patient is in the mid-twenties.

**Detection of Carrier:** Unknown.

**Support Groups:**
NY; Moncey; The Children's Association for Research on Mucolipidosis IV
NJ; Elizabeth; National Lipid Diseases Foundation

**References:**
Tellez-Nagel I, et al.: Mucolipidosis IV: clinical, ultrastructural, histochemical and chemical studies of a case, including a brain biopsy. Arch Neurol 1976; 33:828–835.
Philippart M, et al.: Mucolipidosis IV: a phospholipidosis. Trans Am Soc Neurochem 1980; 11:72.
Caimi L, et al.: Mucolipidosis IV: a sialolipidosis due to ganglioside sialidase deficiency. J Inherit Metab Dis 1982; 5:218–224.
Crandall BF, et al.: Mucolipidosis IV. Am J Med Genet 1982; 12:301–308. *
Lake BD, et al.: A mild variant of mucolipidosis type 4 (ML4). BD:OAS (XVIII(6). New York: March of Dimes Birth Defects Foundation, 1982:391–404.
Riedel KG, et al.: Ocular abnormalities in mucolipidosis IV. Am J Ophthal 1985; 99:125–136.
Amir N, et al.: Mucolipidosis type IV: clinical spectrum and natural history. Pediatrics 1987; 79:953–959.
Ornoy A, et al.: Early prenatal diagnosis of mucolipidosis IV. (Letter) Am J Med Genet 1987; 27:983–985.
Bargal R, et al.: Phospholipids accumulation in mucolipidosis IV cultured fibroblasts. J Inherit Metab Dis 1988; 11:144–150.
O'Brien JS: Beta-galactosidase deficiency. In: Scriver CR, et al, eds: The metabolic basis of inherited disease, 6th ed. New York: McGraw-Hill, 1989:1797–1806.

CR018
PH000

**Barbara Crandall**
**Michel Philippart**

**Mucopolysaccharidosis (MPS) III, types A, B, C and D**
*See MUCOPOLYSACCHARIDOSIS III*
**Mucopolysaccharidosis (MPS) IV, types A and B**
*See MUCOPOLYSACCHARIDOSIS IV*
**Mucopolysaccharidosis F**
*See FUCOSIDOSIS*

---

## MUCOPOLYSACCHARIDOSIS I-H      0674

**Includes:**
Alpha-L-iduronidase deficiency
Gargoylism (obsolete/pejorative)
Hurler syndrome
Hurler-Pfaundler syndrome
Hurler-Scheie syndrome
Mucopolysaccharidosis I-H/I-S compound

**Excludes:**
G(M1)-gangliosidosis, type 1 (0431)
Mucolipidosis II (0672)
Mucolipidosis III (0673)
Mucopolysaccharidosis (other)

**Major Diagnostic Criteria:** Coarse facies, corneal clouding, joint contractures and hepatosplenomegaly. Excess mucopolysacchariduria occurs, but for confirmation, laboratory studies must demonstrate either 1) deficient α-L-iduronidase in leukocytes or fibroblasts, or 2) abnormal sulfate incorporation and degradation by cultured fibroblasts which can be "corrected" by addition of "Hurler factor." Metachromatic staining of fibroblasts and leukocyte inclusions are non-specific findings.

**Clinical Findings:** Normal appearance at birth but may have excessive birth weight. In early months of life, onset of progressive coarsening of facial features, depressed nasal bridge, corneal clouding, hepatosplenomegaly, joint stiffness, and thoracolumbar kyphosis. Other constant features seen by age two years include inguinal or umbilical herniae; abundance of fine body hair, particularly over extensor areas and back; enlarged and scaphoid head; large tongue and lips; small, widely spaced teeth; mucoid rhinorrhea; noisy respiration; and limitation of joint mobility, especially at phalanges, elbows, shoulders, and hips. Later signs include cardiac murmurs, deafness, blindness, and short stature. Growth is normal or excessive during first year, with decline thereafter. Short stature is apparent by three years. Motor and mental development reach a peak before two years and deteriorate thereafter.

X-ray findings include scaphocephaly; "shoe-shaped" and enlarged sella; diaphyseal widening of tubular bones, most pro-

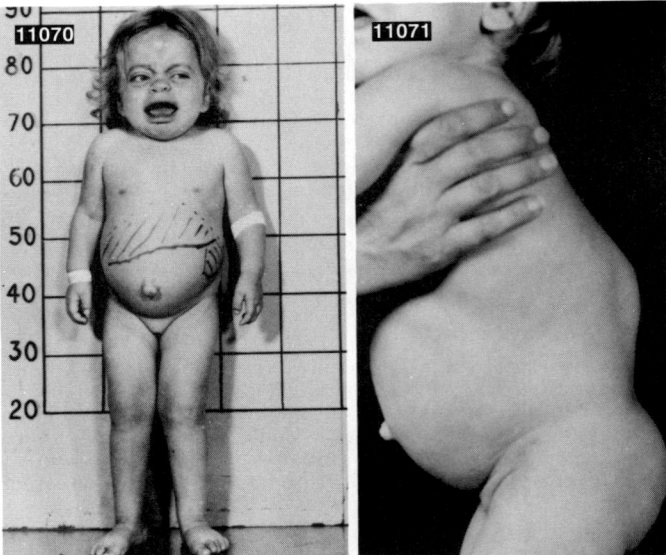

**0674-11070:** Coarse facial features and hepatosplenomegaly are evident in this young child. **11071:** Umbilical hernia, protruding abdomen and gibbus.

nounced in upper limbs; expansion of shaft of the ribs; and anterior beaking of the vertebrae.

Laboratory findings include mucopolysacchariduria, with excessive excretion of dermatan sulfate and heparan sulfate. Deficiency of the lysosomal enzyme, α-L-iduronidase is demonstrable in fibroblasts or leukocytes. Fibroblasts have abnormal sulfate kinetics in culture, incorporating excessive sulfate from the media and failing to normally degrade sulfated mucopolysaccharide when grown in sulfate-deficient media. Leukocytes and fibroblasts show metachromatic staining granules.

**Complications:** Loss of vision because of corneal clouding and retinal degeneration; mental deterioration because of deposits in CNS and hydrocephaly; cardiac decompensation from mucopolysaccharide deposits in intima of coronary vessels and valves; deafness; skeletal incapacitation because of joint limitation; and death, usually from cardiorespiratory decompensation.

**Associated Findings:** None known.

**Etiology:** Autosomal recessive inheritance.

**Pathogenesis:** The Hurler features develop because of progressive deposition of acid mucopolysaccharide (AMPS) in various tissues. Deficient function of α-L-iduronidase, an enzyme responsible for degradation of AMPS underlies this condition.

**MIM No.:** *25280

**POS No.:** 3308

**CDC No.:** 277.510

**Sex Ratio:** M1:F1

**Occurrence:** Incidence probably about 1:100,000 live births; described in Caucasians, Orientals, and Blacks. Prevalence less because of early death.

**Risk of Recurrence for Patient's Sib:**
See Part I, *Mendelian Inheritance.*

**Risk of Recurrence for Patient's Child:**
See Part I, *Mendelian Inheritance.* Affected individuals are not expected to survive to reproduce.

**Age of Detectability:** At 10 weeks gestation, by iduronidase assay of chorionic villi. Clinically detectable in the first year of life.

**Gene Mapping and Linkage:** IDUA (iduronidase, alpha-L-) has been provisionally mapped to 22pter-q11.

**Prevention:** None known. Genetic counseling indicated.

**Treatment:** Curative therapy is not available. Surgical correction of joint contractures, corneal transplantation, and cardiac valvular replacement do not give lasting benefits. Umbilical and inguinal hernias often require surgical correction but may recur. None of these surgical measures impede mucopolysaccharide deposition or progressive deterioration. Physical therapy and special education, with attention to deafness, visual difficulties, and physical handicaps, are necessary. Enzyme replacement therapies have shown no clinical benefits to date. Bone marrow transplanation is now being evaluated.

**Prognosis:** Physical and mental deterioration leads to death before age 10 years in most patients. Death results from pneumonia or cardiac decompensation.

**Detection of Carrier:** The heterozygote can be identified by assay of α-L-iduronidase in leukocytes, and in cultured fibroblasts.

**Special Considerations:** In the truest sense, the mucopolysaccharidoses are storage diseases. The signs are progressive, developing parallel to the accumulation of tissue mucopolysaccharide. In addition to the seven generally acknowledged types of mucopolysaccharidoses (MPS), occasional patients are seen in whom the combination of clinical, X-ray, and laboratory findings prevent easy classification.

MPS I (I-H) and MPS V (I-S) have deficiency of the same enzyme, α-L-iduronidase; hence the suggestion that they are allelic conditions. In keeping with this hypothesis, a group of patients has been identified with iduronidase deficiency who have intermediate clinical features. These patients, thought to have one Hurler mutant gene and 1 Scheie mutant gene, have the onset of signs between ages one and two years, normal or near normal

intelligence, and intermediate progression of signs. The oldest patient is in her 20s. This condition has been termed *Hurler-Scheie compound* or *Mucopolysaccharidoses I-H/I-S compound.*

Other patients with intermediate phenotypes may represent the homozygous state for a third mutation of the iduronidase gene.

**Support Groups:**
NY; Hicksville; National Mucopolysaccharidoses (MPS) Society CANADA: Manitoba; Flin Flon Society for Mucopolysaccharide Diseases

**References:**
Maroteaux P, Lamy M: Hurler's disease, Morquio's disease and related mucopolysaccharidoses. J Pediatr 1965; 67:312–322.
Leroy JG, Crocker AC: Clinical definition of the Hurler-Hunter phenotypes. Am J Dis Child 1966; 112:518–530.
McKusick VA: Heritable disorders of connective tissue, 4th ed. St. Louis: C.V. Mosby Co., 1972.
Pennock CA, Barnes IC: Review article: the mucopolysaccharides. J Med Genet 1976; 13:169–181.
Stevenson RE, et al.: The iduronidase deficient mucopolysaccharidoses: clinical and roentgenographic features. Pediatrics 1976; 57:111–122. * †
Roubicek M, et al.: The clinical spectrum of alpha-L-iduronidase deficiency. Am J Med Genet 1985; 20:471–481.
Whitley CB, et al.: A nonpathologic allele (I-W) for low alpha-L-iduronidase enzyme activity via-a-vis prenatal diagnosis of Herler syndrome. Am J Med Genet 1987; 28:233–243.
Schuchman EH, Desnick RJ: Mucopolysaccharidosis type I subtypes: presence of immunologically cross-reactive material and in vitro enhancement of the residual alpha-L-iduronidase activities. J Clin Invest 1988; 81:98–105.
Neufeld EF, Muenzer J: The mucopolysaccharidoses. In: Scriver CR, et al., eds: The metabolic basis of inherited disease, ed 6. New York: McGraw-Hill, 1989:1565–1588.

ST021                                              **Roger E. Stevenson**

**Mucopolysaccharidosis I-H/I-S compound**
*See MUCOPOLYSACCHARIDOSIS I-H*

---

**MUCOPOLYSACCHARIDOSIS I-S**                                    **0675**

**Includes:**
Mucopolysaccharidosis V
Scheie syndrome

**Excludes:**
G(M1)-gangliosidosis, type 1 (0431)
G(M1)-gangliosidosis, type 2 (0432)
Mucolipidosis III (0673)
Mucopolysaccharidosis (other)

**Major Diagnostic Criteria:** Corneal clouding, mild or absent intellectual impairment, variable but generally mild somatic features plus mucopolysacchariduria plus 1) specific abnormal sulfate kinetics in fibroblast culture, or 2) deficiency of α-L-iduronidase activity in fibroblasts or leukocytes. The distinction from the severe mucopolysaccharidosis (MPS) I-H, and the moderately severe MPS I-H/I-S compound is clinical; all three types having the same laboratory findings.

**Clinical Findings:** Corneal clouding and herniae may be present at birth or soon thereafter; otherwise, signs of mucopolysaccharide disease are absent during infancy. By early school age, joint stiffness with limitation of phalanges, elbows, and shoulders. Genu valgum is the rule. Cardiac murmurs, often aortic in origin, appear; corneal clouding, retinal degeneration, and skeletal involvement increase; auditory and visual acuity decrease, and carpal tunnel signs and psychotic episodes may develop; hepatosplenomegaly, mental retardation, and stunting of growth are not features. Hurler-like features, if present at all, are mild.

X-ray findings include mild changes of dysostosis multiplex. Laboratory findings include excessive heparan sulfate and dermatan sulfate excretion in the urine; fibroblasts and leukocyte inclusions may stain metachromatically; leukocytes and fibroblasts have deficient α-L-iduronidase activity.

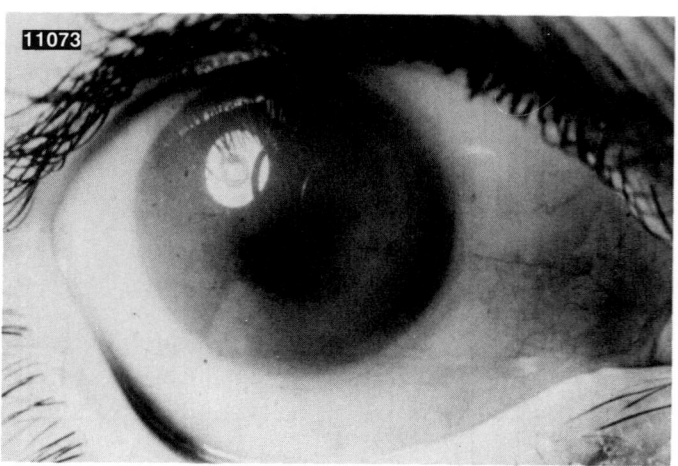

11073

0675-11073: Diffuse corneal clouding involving the entire stroma.

**Complications:** Aortic regurgitation, carpal tunnel syndrome, blindness from corneal clouding and retinal degeneration, hearing loss, and psychotic episodes.

**Associated Findings:** Unknown.

**Etiology:** Autosomal recessive inheritance.

**Pathogenesis:** Deficiency of α-L-iduronidase, one of the lysosomal enzymes responsible for mucopolysaccharide degradation, leading to deposition of acid mucopolysaccharide in soft tissues and interruption of normal bone development.

**MIM No.:** *25280

**POS No.:** 3312

**Sex Ratio:** M1:F1

**Occurrence:** Undetermined, but presumed rare.

**Risk of Recurrence for Patient's Sib:**
See Part I, *Mendelian Inheritance.*

**Risk of Recurrence for Patient's Child:**
See Part I, *Mendelian Inheritance.*

**Age of Detectability:** At 10 weeks gestation, by assay of α-L-iduronidase using chorionic villi.

**Gene Mapping and Linkage:** IDUA (iduronidase, alpha-L-) has been provisionally mapped to 22pter-q11.

**Prevention:** None known. Genetic counseling indicated.

**Treatment:** Curative treatment is not available. Surgical correction of hernias, joint contractures, and carpal tunnel compression is beneficial. Corneal transplantation has provided at least temporary benefit. Physical therapy for joint contractures, hearing aids, and medical or surgical management of aortic valve disease may be necessary.

**Prognosis:** The few patients reported have survived into adulthood.

**Detection of Carrier:** Carriers have intermediate levels of α-L-iduronidase in leukocytes and cultured fibroblasts.

**Special Considerations:** Scheie syndrome is considered allelic to Hurler syndrome because both lack α-L-iduronidase.

**Support Groups:**
NY; Hicksville; National Mucopolysaccharidoses (MPS) Society
CANADA: Manitoba; Flin Flon Society for Mucopolysaccharide Diseases

**References:**
Scheie HG, et al.: A newly recognized forme fruste of Hurler's disease (gargoylism). Am J Ophthalmol. 1962; 53:753–769.
Wiesmann UN, Neufeld EF: Scheie and Hurler syndromes: apparent identity of the biochemical defect. Science 1970; 169:72–74.
McKusick VA, et al.: Allelism, nonallelism and genetic compounds among the mucopolysaccharidoses. Lancet 1972; I:993–996.
Stevenson RE, et al.: The iduronidase-deficient mucopolysaccharidoses: clinical and roentgenographic features. Pediatrics 1976; 57: 111–122. * †
McKusick VA, et al.: The mucopolysaccharide storage diseases. In: Stanbury JB, et al, eds: Metabolic basis of inherited disease, 4th ed. New York: McGraw-Hill, 1978:1282–1307. * †
Neufeld EF, Muenzer J: The mucopolysaccharidoses. In: Scriver CR, et al, eds: The metabolic basis of inherited disease, 6th ed. New York: McGraw-Hill, 1989:1565–1588.

ST021                                      **Roger E. Stevenson**

## MUCOPOLYSACCHARIDOSIS II                          0676

**Includes:**
Hunter syndrome
Mucopolysaccharidosis II, types A and B
Sulfatidosis, juvenile, Austin type (Some forms)
Sulfo-iduronate sulfatase deficiency

**Excludes:**
G(M1)-gangliosidosis, type 1 (0431)
G(M1)-gangliosidosis, type 2 (0432)
Mannosidosis (2079)
Mucolipidosis
Mucopolysaccharidosis (other)

**Major Diagnostic Criteria:** Affected males have normal or impaired intellect, clear corneas, hernias, hepatosplenomegaly, skin nodules, progressive stiffening of joints, thickening of skin, coarsening of facies, and mucopolysacchariduria. Diagnosis can be confirmed by cultured fibroblasts, corrected by Hunter factor, or demonstration of sulfoiduronate sulfatase deficiency in fibroblasts, serum, or leukocytes.

**Clinical Findings:** Appearance is normal at birth with normal or excessive growth during first 1–2 years. During infancy few clinical signs occur except for respiratory symptoms (noisy breathing from upper airway obstruction, recurrent rhinorrhea), large scaphoid head, and herniae (inguinal and umbilical). Coarsening of facial features, with thickening of the nostrils, lips, and tongue; joint stiffness, growth failure, excessive growth of fine body hair, and hepatosplenomegaly become obvious at about age two years and progress in severity. Thick skin, short neck, widely spaced teeth, hearing loss of some degree, and papilledema are commonly present; nodular skin lesions on the arms or posterior chest wall, retinal pigmentation, mild pectus excavatum, pes cavus, mucoid diarrhea and seizures are less common. The spine is straight; corneas are clear grossly; and intellect may be normal, but with a tendency to disruptive, destructive behavior. Mentation, valvular and coronary heart disease, hearing, and joint mobility slowly deteriorate.

Two more or less distinctive types of mucopolysaccharidosis (MPS) II are recognized clinically: in the "mild form" (MPS II-B) mentation may be normal, and deterioration of mental function only slowly progressive; in the "severe form" (MPS II-A) profound mental retardation becomes obvious by late childhood. Other clinical features may be the same, but with slower progression in the "mild form." With rare exception, the subtypes "breed true" within a family.

X-ray findings include scaphoid skull, enlarged sella with anterior excavation, skeletal findings of dysostosis multiplex, minimal vertebral changes, and precocious osteoarthritis of femoral head.

Laboratory findings include acid mucopolysacchariduria with excessive excretion of dermatan sulfate and heparan sulfate; leukocytes and fibroblasts are deficient in the enzyme sulfoiduronate sulfatase; metachromatic staining of leukocyte granules and fibroblasts; cultured fibroblasts accumulate sulfated mucopolysaccharides at an enhanced rate and can be "corrected" with purified

Hunter factor or with fibroblast secretion from non-Hunter individuals.

**Complications:** Coronary and valvular cardiac disease from AMPS deposition, myelopathy due to meningeal thickening, hydrocephaly, progressive hearing loss, immobilization by joint contractures, and degenerative hip disease.

**Associated Findings:** None known.

**Etiology:** Usually X-linked recessive inheritance. The possibility of a rare autosomal recessive form has not been excluded, but may represent cases of *sulfatidosis, juvenile, Austin type* (Burch et al, 1986).

**Pathogenesis:** Accumulation of acid mucopolysaccharide in tissues underlies most of the observed clinical features. The block in mucopolysaccharide metabolism has been shown to be a deficiency of the enzyme sulfoiduronate sulfatase.

**MIM No.:** *30990, *27220

**POS No.:** 3309

**Sex Ratio:** M1:F0. Females have rarely been affected, the presumed result of nonrandom lyonisation or selection for cells whose active X chromosome bore the mutant (Hunter) gene.

**Occurrence:** Estimated 1:100,000 live births in Caucasians, blacks, Orientals, and American Indians. Prevalence lower than birth frequency because of early death, particularly in severe type.

**Risk of Recurrence for Patient's Sib:**
See Part I, *Mendelian Inheritance.*

**Risk of Recurrence for Patient's Child:**
See Part I, *Mendelian Inheritance.*

**Age of Detectability:** At 9–11 weeks gestation, by studies of chorionic villous samples. Karyotypic analysis should accompany such tests to confirm sex of fetus.

**Gene Mapping and Linkage:** IDS (iduronate 2-sulfatase (Hunter syndrome)) has been mapped to Xq27.3-q28.

**Prevention:** None known. Genetic counseling indicated.

**Treatment:** No curative treatment is available. Attempts at enzyme replacement with plasma or leukocyte infusions have not produced definite benefits. Supportive measures include hearing devices, physical therapy, and special education. Surgical correction of hernias, joint contractures, myelopathy, carpal tunnel syndrome, and hydrocephaly may become necessary.

**Prognosis:** Compatible with survival to adult life. However, the majority of patients with the severe subtype (MPS II-A) die prior to age 20 years of cardiac decompensation, pulmonary infection, or neurologic complications. Several patients with the mild subtype (MPS II-B) have survived beyond age 60 years, and a number have reproduced.

**Detection of Carrier:** May be identified by enzyme assay or sulfate incorporation studies of fibroblasts. Utilizing cloning techniques, two cell lines, one with the mucopolysaccharide abnormality and the other normal, can be discerned. Carrier identification may also be made by demonstrating a mosaic pattern of enzyme activity in the hair bulbs and, in many cases, by reduced enzyme activity in serum.

**Special Considerations:** Individuals with MPS I and MPS II excrete the same acid mucopolysaccharides qualitatively and quantitatively; yet they are quite distinct genetically and clinically. MPS II has all the features of MPS I; but to a remarkably milder degree, the corneal changes can be seen only with the slit-lamp; intellect may be normal, at least initially; the skeletal changes are less severe, and outlook for longevity is greater. The mild and severe subtypes of MPS II both lack the same enzyme; hence they are probably allelic conditions.

*Sulfatidosis, juvenile, Austin type* is an autosomal recessive disorder which combines features of metachromatic leukodystrophy and mucopolysaccharidosis. The condition combines the enzyme deficiency and phenotypic features of a number of other conditions (Burch et al, 1986).

**Support Groups:**
NY; Hicksville; National Mucopolysaccharidoses (MPS) Society

CANADA: Manitoba; Flin Flon Society for Mucopolysaccharide Diseases

**References:**
Leroy JG, Crocker AC: Clinical definition of the Hurler-Hunter phenotypes. Am J Dis Child 1966; 112:518–530. * †
Erickson R, et al.: Biochemical differentiation of two forms of mucopolysaccharidosis II (Hunter's disease). Am J Hum Genet 1972; 24:26A.
McKusick VA: Heritable disorders of connective tissue. ed. 4. St. Louis: CV Mosby, 1972. * †
Bach G, et al.: The defect in the Hunter syndrome: deficiency of sulfoiduronate sulfatase. Proc Natl Acad Sci 1973; 70:2134–2138.
Yatziv D, et al.: Mild and severe Hunter syndrome (MPS II) within the same sibships. Clin Genet 1977; 11:319–326.
Hobolth N, Pedersen C: Six cases of a mild form of the Hunter syndrome in five generations: three affected males with progeny. Clin Genet 1978; 13:121 only.
Tonnesen T, et al.: Diagnosis of Hunter's syndrome carriers: radioactive sulphate incorporation into fibroblasts in the presence of fructose 1-phosphate. Hum Genet 1982; 60:167–171.
Zlotogora J, et al.: Hunter syndrome among Ashkenazi Jews in Israel; evidence for prenatal selection favoring the Hunter allele. Hum Genet 1985; 71:329–332.
Burch M, et al.: Multiple sulphatase deficiency presenting at birth. Clin Genet 1986; 30:409–415.

ST021                                             **Roger E. Stevenson**

**Mucopolysaccharidosis II, types A and B**
*See MUCOPOLYSACCHARIDOSIS II*

---

## MUCOPOLYSACCHARIDOSIS III                          0677

**Includes:**

Acetyl CoA:alpha-glucosaminide N-acetyltransferase deficiency
Heparan sulfate sulfatase deficiency
Mucopolysaccharidosis (MPS) III, types A, B, C and D
N-acetyl-alpha-D-glucosaminidase deficiency
N-acetylglucosamine-6-sulfate sulfatase deficiency
Polydystrophia oligophrenia
Sanfilippo syndrome

**Excludes:**
G(M1)-gangliosidosis, type 2 (0432)
Mucolipidosis
Mucopolysaccharidosis (others)

**Major Diagnostic Criteria:** Severe mental deterioration, mild Hurler-like somatic defects, and the urinary excretion of heparan sulfate alone are findings sufficient for the diagnosis of MPS III. Metachromatic staining is non-specific. Confirmatory enzyme assay or sulfate kinetic studies on cultured fibroblasts are necessary to distinguish the four types currently delineated.

**Clinical Findings:** Normal appearance at birth, initial developmental milestones normal. Slowing of development, usually obvious within one to two years, may not become apparent until early school age. Mental and motor development reach a peak by early school age, followed by behavioral disturbances and dramatic intellectual decline. Mental and motor skills are lost, and the often agitated, demented patient becomes bedridden. Growth is minimally affected, the head enlarged, hirsutism present. The mild coarsening of facial features, limitation of joint mobility, and hepatosplenomegaly never become prominent features. Deafness, although hard to evaluate, is thought to occur. Corneal clouding and cardiac abnormalities are not to be expected, although both have been seen in individual patients. The A, B, C, and D subtypes are not clinically separable but can be distinguished by enzymatic assays.

All bone changes on X-ray, except for the skull, are similar but milder than in MPS I. The calvarium is remarkably thickened, and sellar enlargement is not pronounced.

Laboratory findings show urinary excretion of heparan sulfate. Sanfilippo A, the more common of the subtypes, lacks heparan

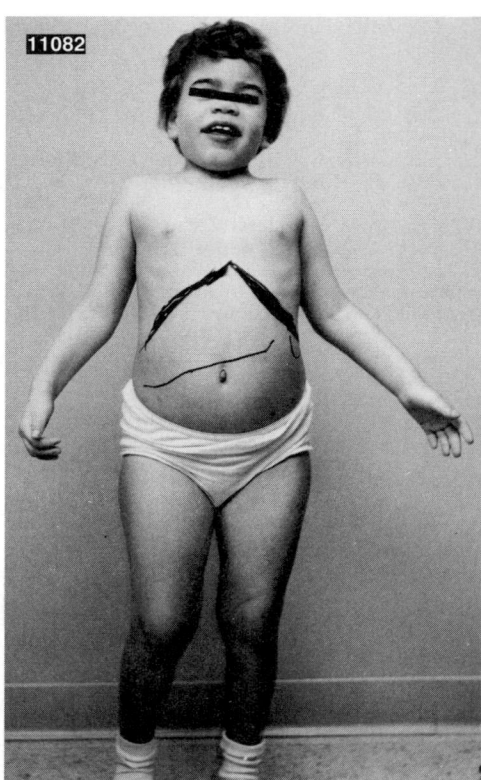

**0677**-11082:  MPS III; note mild coarsening of facial features, hepatosplenomegaly.

**Treatment:**  No curative treatment is available. Attempts at enzyme replacement therapy have produced no clinical benefits.

**Prognosis:**  Death in bedridden, severely demented state by age 20. Few survivors to age 30.

**Detection of Carrier:**  Intermediate enzyme levels in asymptomatic carriers.

**Special Considerations:**  MPS III carries the grave prognosis of severe CNS involvement but is largely spared the pronounced skeletal, corneal, and visceral involvement of the other mucopolysaccharidoses. The four subtypes presently known, although identical clinically, are separable biochemically.

**Support Groups:**
   NY; Hicksville; National Mucopolysaccharidoses (MPS) Society
   CANADA: Manitoba; Flin Flon Society for Mucopolysaccharide Diseases

**References:**
Sanfilippo SJ, et al.: Mental retardation associated with acid mucopolysacchariduria (heparitin sulfate type). J Pediatr 1963; 63:837–838.
Maroteaux P, Lamy M: Hurler's disease, and related mucopolysaccharidoses. J Pediatr 1965; 67:312–322.
Andria G, et al.: Sanfilippo B syndrome (MPS III B): mild and severe forms within the same sibship. Clin Genet 1979; 15:500–504.
Bartsocas C, et al.: Sanfilippo type C disease: clinical findings in four patients with a new variant of mucopolysaccharidosis III. Eur J Pediatr 1979; 130:251–258.
Kresse H, et al.: Sanfilippo disease type D: deficiency of N-acetylglucosamine-6-sulfate sulfatase required for heparan sulfate degradation. Proc Natl Acad Sci USA 1980; 77:6822–6826.
van de Kamp JJP, et al.: Genetic heterogeneity and clinical variability in the Sanfilippo syndrome (types A, B, and C). Clin Genet 1981; 20:152–160. * †
Beratis NG, et al.: Sanfilippo disease in Greece. Clin Genet 1986; 29:129–132.
Kaplan P, Wolfe LS: Sanfilippo syndrome type D. J Pediatr 1987; 110:267–271.

ST021                                        **Roger E. Stevenson**

sulfate sulfatase; Sanfilippo B lacks N-acetyl-α-glucosaminidase; Sanfilippo C lacks acetyl CoA:α-glucosaminide N-acetyltransferase; Sanfilippo D lacks N-acetyl-α-glucosamine-6-sulfate sulfatase. Fibroblasts and lymphocyte granules stain metachromatically.

**Complications:**  Severe mental deterioration.

**Associated Findings:**  None known.

**Etiology:**  Autosomal recessive inheritance.

**Pathogenesis:**  An enzymatic error in degradation of acid mucopolysaccharide underlies each subtype. Unlike the enzymes in the A, B, and D subtypes, the enzyme in Sanfilippo C is not hydrolytic but transfers an acetyl group from acetyl CoA to the free amino portion of a glucosamine residue.

**MIM No.:**  *25290, *25292, *25293, *25294

**POS No.:**  3310

**Sex Ratio:**  M1:F1

**Occurrence:**  About 1:25,000. Sanfilippo A is the more common subtype. Prevalence less than incidence because of early death.

**Risk of Recurrence for Patient's Sib:**
   See Part I, *Mendelian Inheritance*.

**Risk of Recurrence for Patient's Child:**
   See Part I, *Mendelian Inheritance*. Affected individuals are not expected to survive to reproduce.

**Age of Detectability:**  At 10 weeks gestation by enzyme assay of chorionic villi.

**Gene Mapping and Linkage:**  GNS (N-acetylglucosamine-6-sulfatase (Sanfilippo disease IIID)) has been provisionally mapped to 12q14.

**Prevention:**  None known. Genetic counseling indicated.

## MUCOPOLYSACCHARIDOSIS IV                              0678

**Includes:**
   Brailsford syndrome
   Chondroosteodystrophy
   Galactosamine-6-sulfatase deficiency
   Keratansulfaturia
   Morquio syndrome
   Morquio-Üllrich syndrome
   Mucopolysaccharidosis (MPS) IV, types A and B

**Excludes:**
   Beta-galactosidase deficiency
   Dwarfism, other forms of short-trunk
   **G(M1)-gangliosidosis, type 1** (0431)
   **Mucolipidosis**
   **Mucopolysaccharidosis** (other)

**Major Diagnostic Criteria:**  Short-trunk dwarfism with normal intellect, cloudy corneas, and lax joints, plus pathognomonic X-ray findings and keratansulfaturia. Confirmation by enzyme assay (6-sulfate sulfatase).

**Clinical Findings:**  The normal intrauterine growth and development continues during the early postnatal months. By age 18 months, growth retardation and skeletal changes (genu valgum, flaring of lower ribs, kyphoscoliosis) become obvious. Intellectual development proceeds at a normal pace and may remain relatively normal despite progressive somatic changes: marked growth retardation, diffuse steamy corneal clouding, prominent lower face, enamel hypoplasia in deciduous and secondary teeth, short neck, pectus carinatum, exaggerated lumbar lordosis, laxity and subluxation of joints (e.g. wrists), and flat feet. Hearing loss present in many patients, and cardiac signs (aortic insufficiency) are found in a minority.

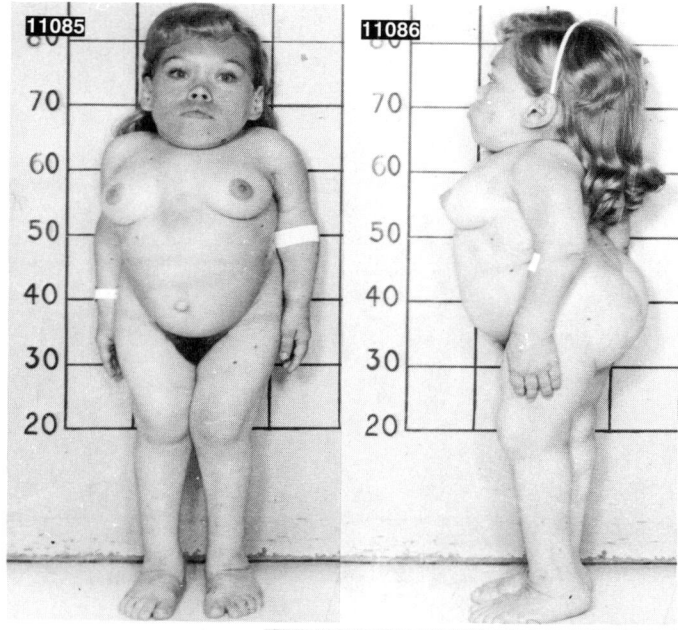

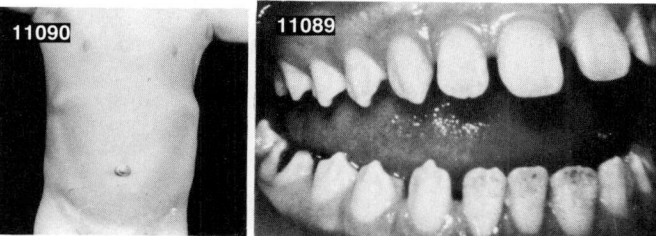

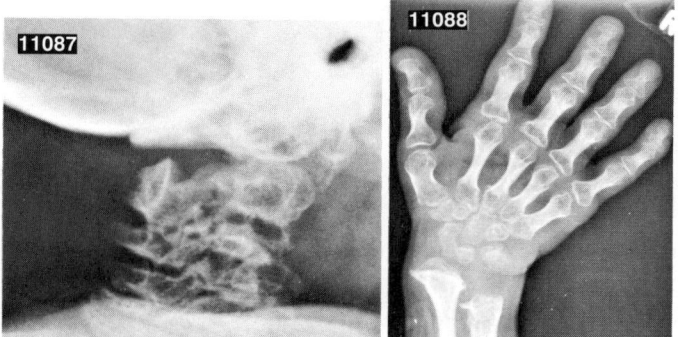

**0678**-11085—86: Prominent lower face, short neck, short-trunk dwarfism and skeletal deformities. 11090: Young male showing flaring of the lower ribs. 11089: Enamel hypoplasia. 11087: Cervical spine shows rudimentary dens and the atlas closely applied to the occiput. 11088: Small, extremely irregular carpals; short ulna and ulnar deviation; short metacarpals and phalanges with wide ends but well constructed shafts.

X-ray findings predate clinical abnormalities and progressively worsen. Vertebral flattening with central anterior projections occurs in the thoracic area, and hook-shaped projections are found in the lumbar area. The odontoid is hypoplastic. Other findings include increased intervertebral spaces, delayed ossification centers, irregular epiphyses, proximal pointing of metacarpals, wide ribs and generalized osteoporosis. A normal skull is present.

Laboratory findings include keratansulfaturia, with normal or increased total urinary AMPS excretion. Deficiency of N-acetyl-galactosamine-6-sulfate sulfatase is demonstrated in cultured fibroblasts. Granular inclusions are found in a small percentage of granulocytes.

Clinically similar but milder findings have been found in several patients with β-galactosidase deficiency. This condition has been designated as MPS IV-B to distinguish it from sulfate sulfatase deficiency, which is designated MPS IV-A . The enzyme defect(s) are yet to be identified in other patients who have mild features, with or without keratansulfaturia.

**Complications:** Neurologic signs from spinal cord and nerve root compression, hearing loss, aortic regurgitation, and compensatory hyperpnea. Atlantoaxial subluxation due to aplasia of the odontoid and ligamentous laxity may lead to acute or chronic neurologic signs. Weakness in the legs usually results, and paraplegia is frequent.

**Associated Findings:** None known.

**Etiology:** Autosomal recessive inheritance.

**Pathogenesis:** In MPS IV-A, a deficiency of n-acetyl-galactosamine-6-sulfate sulfatase leads to lysosomal accumulation of keratan sulfate in susceptible tissues. In MPS IV-B, a deficiency of β-galactosidase underlies the abnormal tissue storage of mucopolysaccharide.

**MIM No.:** *25300, 25301

**POS No.:** 3311

**Sex Ratio:** M1:F1

**Occurrence:** Probably <1:100,000.

**Risk of Recurrence for Patient's Sib:**
See Part I, *Mendelian Inheritance.*

**Risk of Recurrence for Patient's Child:**
See Part I, *Mendelian Inheritance.* Few patients have reproduced. Offspring would be obligate carriers.

**Age of Detectability:** Prenatally by enzyme assay of amniocyte culture or chorionic villi in both types; postnatally prior to one year of age by X-ray changes and keratansulfate excretion.

**Gene Mapping and Linkage:** The locus for the enzyme N-acetyl-galactosamine-6-sulfate sulfatase is not known; the β-galactosidase locus is on chromosome 3.

**Prevention:** None known. Genetic counseling indicated.

**Treatment:** No curative therapy is available. Surgical correction of herniae; upper cervical spinal fusion to avert or remedy spinal cord compression. Corneal transplantation not helpful, cardiac valve replacement not appropriate. Physical therapy and hearing aids may be helpful.

**Prognosis:** May survive to early adulthood; many die prior to age 20 years from cardiac or neurologic complications. Few survive to an advanced age. Greater longevity is seen in less severely affected individuals.

**Detection of Carrier:** Unknown.

**Special Considerations:** Designation of Morquio disease as a mucopolysaccharidosis is based on urinary excretion of keratansulfate. Excessive keratansulfaturia may occur in the absence of elevated total urinary mucopolysaccharides. Keratansulfaturia may decrease or disappear entirely in older patients. Study of the kinetics of sulfate metabolism has not been useful in the diagnosis of MPS IV. At least two subtypes exist: the classic form described above, and a type with less severe features without excessive mucopolysacchariduria. Additionally, a group of patients with very mild clinical features and keratansulfaturia and β-galactosidase deficiency have been designated MPS IV-B.

A three-part set of articles by Nelson and colleages, published in volume 33 of Clinical Genetics (1988, pages 111–130), was devoted to the issue of heterogeneity in Morquio disease.

**Support Groups:**
NY; Hicksville; National Mucopolysaccharidoses (MPS) Society
CANADA: Manitoba; Flin Flon Society for Mucopolysaccharide Diseases

**References:**
Langer LO Jr, Carey LS: The roentgenographic features of the KS mucopolysaccharidosis of Morquio (Morquio-Brailsford' disease). Am J Roentgenol Radium Ther Nucl Med 1966; 97:1–20.

Arbisser AI, et al.: Morquio-like syndrome with beta-galactosidase deficiency and normal hexosamine sulfatase activity: mucopolysaccharidosis IV B. Am J Med Genet 1977; 1:195–205.

Groebe H, et al.: Morquio syndrome (mucopolysaccharidosis IV-B) associated with beta-galactosidase deficiency: report of two cases. Am J Hum Genet 1980; 32:258–272.

Holzgreve W, et al.: Morquio syndrome: clinical findings in 11 patients with MPS IV A and 2 patients with MPS IV B. Hum Genet 1981; 57:360–365. * †

Yuen M, Fensom AH: Diagnosis of classic Morquio's disease. J Inherit Metab Dis 1985; 8:80–86.

ST021                                    **Roger E. Stevenson**

## Mucopolysaccharidosis V
*See MUCOPOLYSACCHARIDOSIS I-S*

---

## MUCOPOLYSACCHARIDOSIS VI                          0679

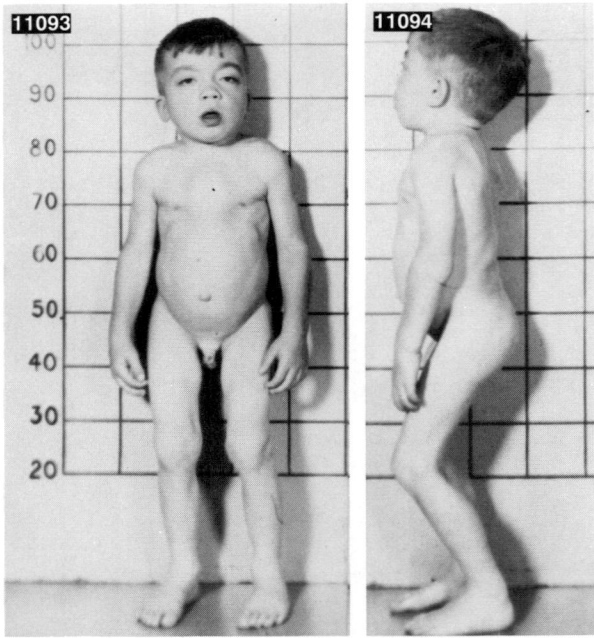

**Includes:**
> Arylsulfatase B deficiency
> Maroteaux-Lamy syndrome

**Excludes:**
> **G(M1)-gangliosidosis, type 1** (0431)
> **Mucolipidosis**
> **Mucopolysaccharidosis** (other)

**Major Diagnostic Criteria:** Severe Hurler-like somatic features, such as growth retardation, cloudy corneas, coarse facies, joint contractures, hepatosplenomegaly, and kyphosis develop progressively in early childhood. Intelligence is normal. Laboratory findings include urinary dermatan sulfate excess, arylsulfatase B deficiency, and abnormal sulfate kinetics in cultured fibroblasts.

**Clinical Findings:** Normal appearance at birth. Mental development is normal or nearly so. Growth retardation is noted by two to three years. Progressive clouding of corneas, hearing loss, joint stiffness, coarsening of facial features with thick nostrils and lips, are obvious by early school age. Hepatosplenomegaly, lumbar kyphosis, genu valgum, herniae, carpal tunnel, cervical spinal cord compression, and hip dysplasia also occur. Mild, intermediate, and severe forms of this condition exist.

X-rays show calvaria with greatly enlarged sella, fragmented epiphyses, mild flattening of vertebrae with anterior wedging of lumbar vertebrae, and expanded ribs.

Laboratory findings include urinary excretion of dermatan sulfate, and metachromatic staining of fibroblasts and leukocyte inclusions. Fibroblasts and leukocytes have deficient arylsulfatase B (N-acetylgalactosamine-4-sulfatase) activity.

**Complications:** Visual loss, progressive hearing loss, cardiac and respiratory decompensation, hydrocephaly, cervical spinal cord compression from atlantoaxial subluxation or thickened dura.

**Associated Findings:** None known.

**Etiology:** Autosomal recessive inheritance.

**Pathogenesis:** Deficiency of arylsulfatase B prevents normal lysosomal degradation of mucopolysaccharide, allowing accumulation of AMPS in soft tissues, and disruption of bone development.

**MIM No.:** *25320

**POS No.:** 3313

**Sex Ratio:** M1:F1

**Occurrence:** Undetermed but presumed rare. Prevalence less than incidence because of early death.

**Risk of Recurrence for Patient's Sib:**
> See Part I, *Mendelian Inheritance.*

**Risk of Recurrence for Patient's Child:**
> See Part I, *Mendelian Inheritance.* Pregnancy has occurred in several females.

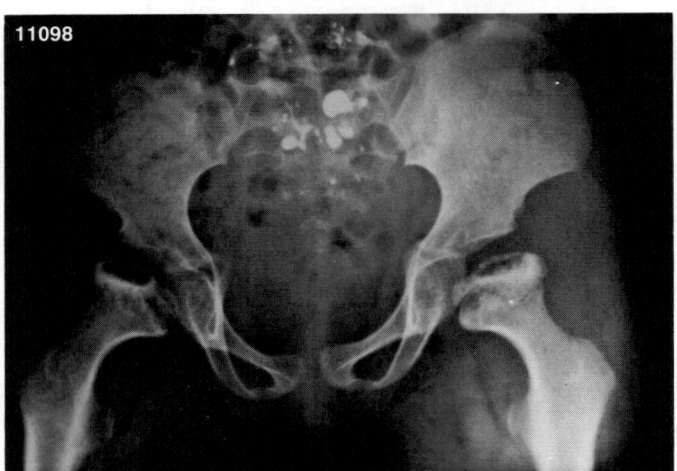

**0679**-11093–94: Short stature, coarse facies, protruding tongue, short neck, deformed chest and semicrouching stance. **11098:** Flat femoral capital epiphyses with large, cyst-like radiolucencies; surrounding sclerosis; narrow necks; gracile pelvic bones; oblique acetabular roofs.

---

**Age of Detectability:** At 10 weeks gestation by study of chorionic villi.

**Gene Mapping and Linkage:** ARSB (arylsulfatase B) has been mapped to 5p11-q13.

**Prevention:** None known. Genetic counseling indicated.

**Treatment:** Curative therapy is not available. Surgical correction of herniae, joint contractures, cardiac valves, carpal tunnel compression, hydrocephaly, and cervical spinal cord compression benefit patients. Physical therapy and hearing devices may be helpful.

**Prognosis:** Death prior to 20 years, generally of cardiorespiratory complications in the severe subtype. Patients with the mild subtype are productive and intelligent in mid-adult life, but can develop significant myelopathy or cardiovascular problems.

**Detection of Carrier:** Possible by enzyme (arylsulfatase B) assay of leukocytes or cultured fibroblasts.

**Special Considerations:** There appears to be a milder form that is less common than the classic form described above. One patient with the mild subtype and normal stature has been reported. Sulfate incorporation, "correction" studies, and enzyme analysis, indicate the two subtypes to be allelic. Intermediate forms may represent compound conditions.

**Support Groups:**
NY; Hicksville; National Mucopolysaccharidoses (MPS) Society
CANADA: Manitoba; Flin Flon Society for Mucopolysaccharide Diseases

**References:**
Maroteaux P, Lamy M: Hurler's disease, Morquio's disease, and related mucopolysaccharidoses. J Pediatr 1965; 67:312–323.
McKusick VA: Heritable disorders of connective tissue, 4th ed. St. Louis: C.V. Mosby, 1972. * †
Beratis NG, et al.: Arylsulfatase B deficiency in Maroteaux-Lamy syndrome: cellular studies and carrier identification. Pediatr Res 1975; 9:475–480.
Levy LA, et al.: Ultrastructures of Reilly bodies (metachromatic granules) in the Maroteaux-Lamy syndrome (mucopolysaccharidosis VI): a histochemical study. Am J Clin Pathol 1980; 73:416–422.
Saul RA, et al.: Atypical presentation with normal stature in Maroteaux- Lamy syndrome (MPS VI). Proc Greenwood Genet Ctr 1984; 3:49–52.
Black SH, et al.: Maroteaux-Lamy syndrome in a large consanguineous kindred: biochemical and immunological studies. Am J Med Genet 1986; 25:273–279.

ST021
SA030

**Roger E. Stevenson**
**Robert A. Saul**

---

## MUCOPOLYSACCHARIDOSIS VII                    0680

**Includes:**
Beta-glucuronidase deficiency
GUSB deficiency
Sly syndrome

**Excludes:**
**Aspartylglucosaminuria** (2042)
**Fucosidosis** (0398)
**Mannosidosis** (2079)
**Mucolipidosis**
**Mucopolysaccharidosis** (others)

**Major Diagnostic Criteria:** At least two phenotypes may be present. One has early onset of coarse facies, hepatosplenomegaly, corneal clouding, and other features consistent with the Hurler phenotype. Onset of this first form has been reported in the second decade of life. The other form begins in the second decade with mild skeletal abnormalities, corneal opacities, aortic regurgitation, and normal growth and mentation. Hepatosplenomegaly is not present. Diagnosis is established by demonstrating β-glucuronidase deficiency in tissues, fibroblasts, leukocytes, or serum. Although a mucopolysaccharidosis (MPS) screen is usually positive, no diagnostic pattern of MPS excretion has been identified.

**Clinical Findings:** The clinical description is based on the first 20 described cases of MPS VII. Although this disease is not yet well defined, two major groups appear to be emerging. Some patients (13 cases) have had clinical signs at birth or within the first years of life. These patients exhibit coarsened facies, hepatosplenomegaly, corneal clouding, frequent respiratory infections, umbilical or additional inguinal herniae, leukocyte inclusions, short stature, and developmental retardation. Three of these patients were affected at birth. Non-immune hydrops fetalis has been reported in two patients. The X-ray features of the early-onset form include moderate-to-severe bony abnormalities with J-shaped sella, vertebral beaking and broadening of the tubular bones (dysostosis multiplex). A second form, presenting in the second decade of life, has been recognized in six cases. In these

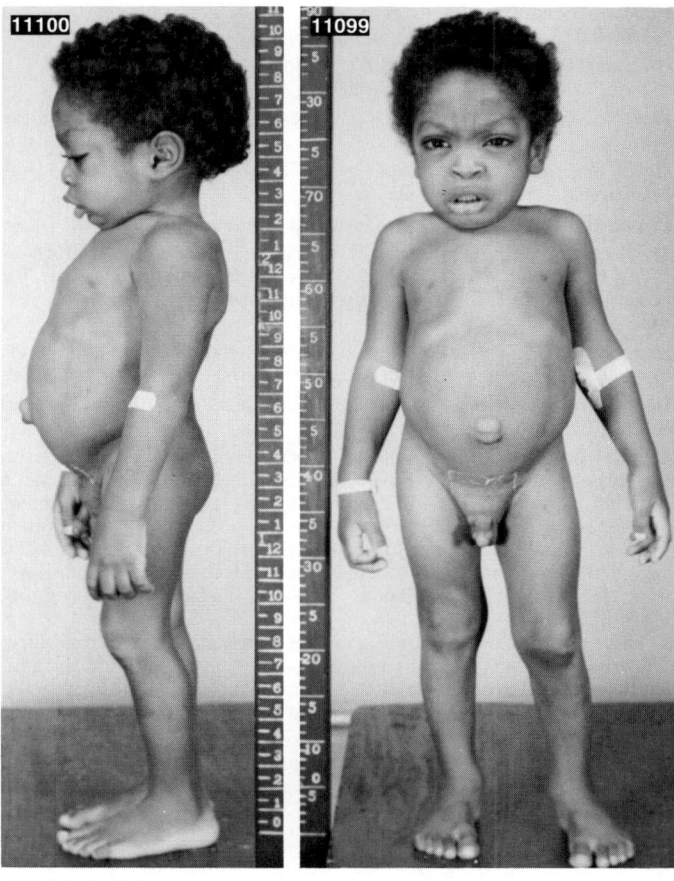

**0680A-**11099–11100: Short stature, coarse facial features, abdominal protuberance from hepatosplenomegaly, chest configuration including pigeon breast and flared ribs and umbilical hernia are present by age 3 years. By his late teens his main problems were orthopedic including kyphoscoliosis, odontoid hypoplasia and progressive hip deformity. His mental retardation has been moderate but non-progressive.

---

patients, mild bony changes, little facial coarsening, normal growth and mentation, and no hepatosplenomegaly is seen. Fibromuscular dysplasia with aortic regurgitation was noted in one case.

A final reported case that does not fit well into the above two classifications was noted to have somatic features much like the early-onset form but presented at 13 years of age.

**Complications:** Moderate mental retardation in early onset cases; orthopedic problems include joint contractures and spinal malformations. Severe aortic infiltration results in fibromuscular dysplasia and aortic regurgitation.

**Associated Findings:** Frequent respiratory illnesses and dislocated hips.

**Etiology:** Autosomal recessive inheritance.

**Pathogenesis:** Absence of lysosomal enzyme β-glucuronidase in all tissues examined and storage of mucopolysaccharides in various organs. The clinical variability is not yet explained.

**MIM No.:** *25322

**POS No.:** 3314

**Sex Ratio:** M8:F12 (observed).

**Occurrence:** At least 20 cases reported to date.

**Risk of Recurrence for Patient's Sib:**
See Part I, *Mendelian Inheritance.*

**Risk of Recurrence for Patient's Child:**
See Part I, *Mendelian Inheritance.*

**Age of Detectability:** At 10 weeks gestation by study of chorionic villi.

**Gene Mapping and Linkage:** GUSB (glucuronidase, beta) has been mapped to 7q21.2-q22.

**Prevention:** None known. Genetic counseling indicated.

**Treatment:** Prenatal diagnosis; enzyme replacement therapy is being investigated but is not yet feasible. Surgical procedures for correction of herniae, and orthopedic, ophthalmologic, and cardiac problems.

**Prognosis:** The disease course exhibits marked variability and, as such, accurate prediction of the prognosis is not yet possible.

**Detection of Carrier:** Possible by fibroblasts or leukocyte assays for β-glucuronidase activity.

**Special Considerations:** Mucopolysaccharidosis VII differs from the other mucopolysaccharidoses in that it was defined as a biochemical entity as quickly as it was clinically recognized. Subsequent cases, therefore, were identified on biochemical grounds and not on the basis of clinical findings. It has been suggested that the clinical forms represent allelic disorders; however, the genetic and molecular basis for phenotypic heterogeneity is unknown.

Two siblings were found to have marked clinical variability. Cultured fibroblasts from four early-onset cases showed antigenically cross-reactive material to β-glucuronidase. All four showed different titration patterns suggesting even further heterogeneity.

**Support Groups:**
NY; Hicksville; National Mucopolysaccharidoses (MPS) Society
CANADA: Manitoba; Flin Flon Society for Mucopolysaccharide Diseases

**References:**
Sly WS, et al.: Beta-glucuronidase deficiency: report of clinical, radiologic and biochemical features of a new mucopolysaccharidosis. J Pediatr 1973; 82:249–257. †
Beaudet AL, et al.: Variation in the phenotypic expression of β-glucuronidase deficiency. J Pediatr 1975; 86:388–394.

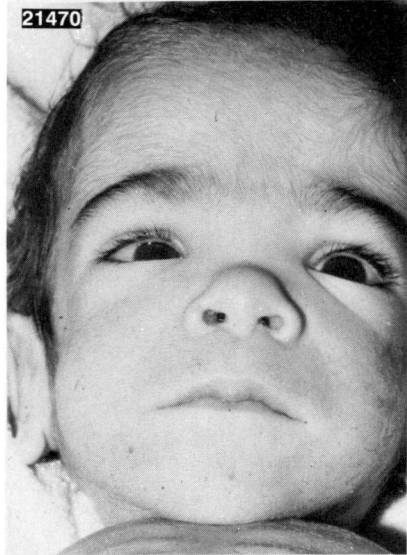

**0680B**-21470: Coarsening of the facies in this affected 7-month-old.

Francke U: The human gene for beta glucuronidase is on chromosome 7. Am J Hum Genet 1976; 28:357–362.
Bell CE Jr, et al.: Human beta-glucuronidase deficiency mucopolysaccharidosis: identification of cross-reactive antigen in cultured fibroblasts of deficient patients by enzyme immunoassay. J Clin Invest 1977; 59:97–105.
Hoyme HE, et al.: Presentation of mucopolysaccharidosis VII (beta-glucuronidase deficiency) in infancy. J Med Genet 1981; 18:237–239.
Lee JES, et al.: Beta-glucuronidase deficiency: a heterogeneous mucopolysacchiridosis. Am J Dis Child 1985; 139:57–59. *
Neufeld EF, Muenzer J: The mucopolysaccharidoses. In: Scriver CR, et al, eds: The metabolic basis of inherited disease, 6th ed. New York: McGraw-Hill, 1989:1565–1588.

AL006                                                  **Kirk Aleck**

**Mucopolysaccharidosis, 'focal'**
*See GELEOPHYSIC DWARFISM*

---

## MUCOSA (ORAL/EYE), INTRAEPITHELIAL DYSKERATOSIS, BENIGN                          0538

**Includes:**
Benign intraepithelial dyskeratosis
Dyskeratosis, intraepithelial
Intraepithelial dyskeratosis

**Excludes:**
**Dermal hypoplasia, focal** (0281)
**Dyskeratosis congenita** (2024)
Focal epithelial hyperplasia of oral mucosa
Leukoplakia
Mucosa, white folded dysplasia
**Nails, pachyonychia congenita** (0789)
**Skin, vitiligo** (0993)

**Major Diagnostic Criteria:** Perilimbal gelatinous plaques on a hyperemic bulbar conjunctiva with white shaggy lesions of oral mucosa occurs. Diagnosis is made on Papanicolaou-stained smear, with compatible history or tissue section.

**Clinical Findings:** Affected persons have white, soft shaggy lesions of oral mucosa. Gelatinous perilimbal plaques occur in the bulbar conjunctiva with a hyperemic base. Temporary blindness occurs in summer in about one-fourth of cases due to vernal exacerbation and autumnal remissions. Vascularization of cornea with loss of vision results by the fifth to sixth decade. Occasional involvement occurs in the lid conjunctiva with white plaques. X-ray findings are normal. Exfoliative cytologic smears of oral and eye lesions stained with Papanicolaou stain are characterized by two types of cells: elongated waxy orangeophilic cells (resembling the grains of keratosis follicularis) and a cell-within-cell body consisting of a central abnormal cell and a normal appearing epithelial cell that surrounds it. Central cell is dyskeratotic, orangeophilic with abnormal nucleus. The surrounding cell appears normal but with an eccentric nucleus and refractile hyaline membrane separating normal cells from the central cell. Histologic characteristics show a thickened stratum spinosum containing many dyskeratotic waxy appearing cells with elongated nuclei and cell-within-cell dyskeratotic bodies. No basal lacuna or inflammation occurs in the lamina propria, but dilated vessels may occur.

**Complications:** Temporary blindness in about one-fourth of cases in summer. Vascularization of cornea in late adulthood with loss of vision.

**Associated Findings:** None known.

**Etiology:** Autosomal dominant inheritance with moderate variation in expressivity. The severity of manifestation of the eye lesion possibly depends on the response to unknown environmental factors. This may explain the vernal exacerbations and autumnal remissions.

**Pathogenesis:** Primary protein defect is unknown. However, by analogy with the fact that identical cellular lesions can be produced experimentally in man by use of agents affecting nucleic acid integrity (X-radiation, methotrexate, 5-fluorouracil) the gene

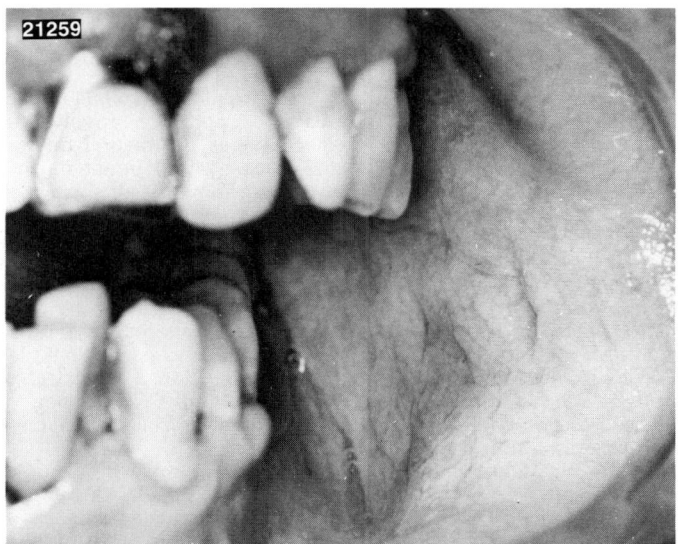

**0538**-21259: Intraepithelial dyskeratosis affecting the buccal mucosa is a soft non-indurated white lesion which accompanies similar white gelatenous lesions of the sclera with prominent underlying vascular dilation. The presence of the eye lesions differentiates the oral lesions from leukoplakia, white folded dysplasia of the mucosa, leukoedema and lichen planus.

defect appears to result in nucleic acid damage to epithelial cell nuclei. These damaged cells are then surrounded by normal epithelial cells and exfoliated. Electron microscopic features show degenerated cell surrounded by a more normal-appearing epithelial cell. Included cell shows dense bundles of tonofibrils and nuclear fragments.

**MIM No.:** *12760

**Sex Ratio:** M1:F1

**Occurrence:** Only three large kindreds are known. Among "Haliwa" (from Halifax and Warren counties) Indians of North Carolina, however, 1:52.

**Risk of Recurrence for Patient's Sib:**
See Part I, *Mendelian Inheritance.*

**Risk of Recurrence for Patient's Child:**
See Part I, *Mendelian Inheritance.*

**Age of Detectability:** By visual examination most cases detected by one year of age. Confirmed by exfoliative cytology or biopsy.

**Gene Mapping and Linkage:** Unknown.

**Prevention:** None known. Genetic counseling indicated.

**Treatment:** Avoidance of sunlight and dust reduces the severity of eye lesions.

**Prognosis:** No reduced longevity. Lesion does not appear to predispose to neoplastic change. Blindness from vascularization of cornea in fifth to sixth decade occurs in about 50% of affected persons.

**Detection of Carrier:** Unknown.

**Special Considerations:** Must be differentiated from white folded dysplasia of mucosa, especially if such patients also have pterygia, and histologically from keratosis follicularis, which shows basilar clefting absent in benign intraepithelial dyskeratosis. Cortisone eye drops temporarily reduce the hyperemia of conjunctivae but do not alter the basic lesion. Penetrating keratoplasty may benefit corneal opacification.

**References:**
Von Sallmann L, Paton D: Hereditary benign intraepithelial dyskeratosis. I. Ocular manifestations. Arch Ophthalmol 1960; 63:421–429.
Witkop CJ Jr, et al.: Hereditary benign intraepithelial dyskeratosis. II. Oral manifestations and hereditary transmission. Arch Pathol 1960; 70:696–711. *
Sadeghi EM, Witkop CJ Jr: Ultrastructural study of hereditary benign intraepithelial dyskeratosis. Oral Surg 1977; 44:567–577.
Reed JW, et al.: Corneal manifestations of hereditary benign intraepithelial dyskeratosis. Arch Ophthalmol 1979; 97:297–300. †

WI043                                        **Carl J. Witkop, Jr.**

---

## MUCOSA, ORAL INCLUSION CYSTS OF THE NEWBORN          3236

**Includes:**
>    Bohn nodules
>    Cysts, inclusion of the oral mucosa of the newborn
>    Dental lamina cyst
>    Epstein pearls
>    Gingival cyst of the newborn
>    Inclusion cysts of the oral mucosa in the newborn

**Excludes:**
>    **Alveolar ridges, lymphangioma** (0613)
>    Eruption cysts
>    **Teeth, natal or neonatal** (0933)

**Major Diagnostic Criteria:** White nodules located in the mucosa overlying the alveolar ridges or hard palate.

**Clinical Findings:** Inclusion cysts generally present as multiple, small, 1–3 mm diameter, white-yellow, raised, firm mucosal nodules on the palate or alveolar ridges. Most are inconspicuous. Occasionally a solitary inclusion cyst is observed. Palatal cysts ("Epstein's pearls" and "Bohn's nodules") are more common than alveolar ridge cysts. Dental lamina cysts are more common in the anterior aspects of the maxilla or mandible.

All three entities represent epithelial inclusion cysts of the oral mucosa. Histologically they are all true cysts lined by a thin layer of stratified squamous epithelium surrounding a keratin-filled lumen.

Inclusion cysts are asymptomatic and, generally, do not cause discomfort. They rupture spontaneously and usually exfoliate within the first weeks to three months of age. Occasionally they present and/or persist later in infancy or childhood.

**Complications:** These cysts exfoliate spontaneously and do not interfere with tooth eruption.

**Associated Findings:** Inclusion cysts of the oral mucosa in the newborn have been observed in stillborns (80%), and in infants with congenital anomalies including **Cleft lip** and **Cleft palate** (58%).

**Etiology:** Gingival cysts of the newborn (dental lamina cyst) arise from postfunctional dental lamina epithelium and are found on the crest, buccal and lingual surfaces of the maxillary and mandibular alveolar ridges.

*Epstein pearls* are found only in the midline of the hard palate and are thought to represent entrapped epithelial remnants in the line of fusion of the palate during embryological development.

*Bohn nodules* were originally described on the hard and soft palate arising from epithelial remnants of the developing salivary glands. In the literature, Bohn nodules also refer to epithelial inclusion cysts of the buccal and lingual aspects of the maxillary and mandibular alveolar ridges and probably represent, in this location, dental lamina cysts arising from postfunctional dental lamina or, less likely, ectopic remnants of salivary gland ductal epithelium.

**Pathogenesis:** During embryogenesis ectoderm forms the oral epithelium that covers the palatal processes and also differentiates into dental lamina and salivary gland primordia. Entrapped epithelium may degenerate or persist between the lines of palatal fusion. Following odontogenesis, remnants of dental lamina may degenerate or persist. Persistent epithelial rests may undergo cystic degeneration resulting in inclusion cysts of the oral mucosa.

**Sex Ratio:** M1:F1

**Occurrence:** 76.8% of Caucasian babies. 62.0% of black babies.

**Risk of Recurrence for Patient's Sib:** Unknown.

**Risk of Recurrence for Patient's Child:** Unknown.

**Age of Detectability:** May be present at birth. Often appear and spontaneously exfoliate, usually within the first three months of life.

**Gene Mapping and Linkage:** Unknown.

**Prevention:** None known. Genetic counseling indicated.

**Treatment:** None necessary. The inclusion cysts enlarge and rupture when in contact with the oral mucosal epithelium. Healing occurs rapidly.

**Prognosis:** Excellent.

**Detection of Carrier:** Unknown.

**References:**
Fromm A: Epstein's pearls, Bohn's nodules and inclusion-cysts of the oral cavity. J Dent Child 1967; 34:275–287.
Maher WP, et al.: Etiology and vascularization of dental lamina cysts. Oral Surg 1970; 29:590–597.
Cohen RL: Clinical perspectives on premature tooth eruption and cyst formation in neonates. Pediatric Dermatol 1984; 1:301–306.
Gilhar A, et al.: Gingival cysts of the newborn. Int J Dermatol 1988; 27:261–262.

ZU002                                                 **Susan L. Zunt**

## MUCOSA, WHITE FOLDED DYSPLASIA                     **0681**

**Includes:**
    Leukokeratosis, hereditary mucosal
    White folded dysplasia of mucosa
    White sponge nevus of Cannon

**Excludes:**
    **Dermal hypoplasia, focal** (0281)
    **Dyskeratosis congenita** (2024)
    Focal epithelial hyperplasia of oral mucosa
    **Mucosa (oral/eye), intraepithelial dyskeratosis, benign** (0538)
    Leukoedema
    Leukoplakia
    Oral epithelial nevus of Cooke
    **Nails, pachyonychia congenita** (0789)

**Major Diagnostic Criteria:** A congenital, soft, white, folded hyperplastic lesion occurs in the mucosa of the oral, and possibly

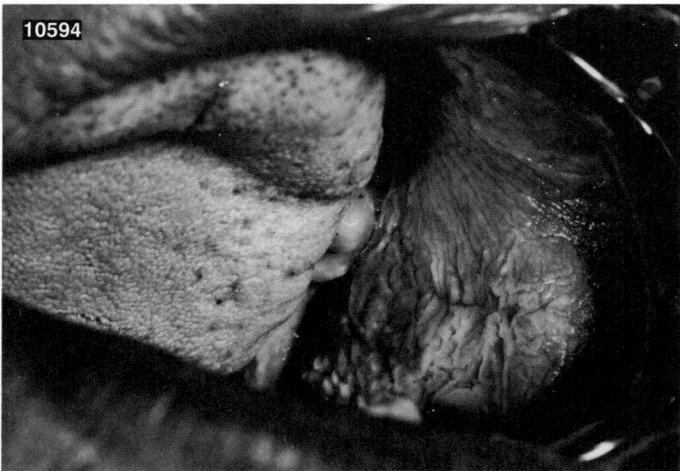

**0681**-10594: Mucosa, white folded dysplasia.

vagina, rectum and nasal cavities. No eye involvement is present. There may be a history of similar mucosal lesions in other family members.

**Clinical Findings:** Congenital, asymptomatic, white, folded, soft, hyperplastic mucosal lesions are reported to involve the following mucosal sites in the percentages given: oral mucosa (100%); vaginal mucosa (60%); anal mucosa (40%); penile mucosa (30%); and nasal mucosa (10%). It is not known if all sites listed were examined in all cases.

There are no X-ray changes. Cytologic smears (Papanicolaou stain) show that the majority of mucosal cells contain a perinuclear or cytoplasmic condensation in the cytoplasm (by electron microscopy, tonofibrils) that stain intensely (hematoxylin & eosin, and Papanicolaou). Tissue sections demonstrate hyperplasia of prickle-cell layer, moderate acanthosis, and intracellular edema which give a "chicken wire" appearance to the section. Perinuclear or cytoplasmic condensations are best seen on Papanicolaou or Periodic acid-Schiff stains, and show little or no change in lamina propria or submucosa.

Must be differentiated from leukoedema, which is acquired, usually found in debilitated conditions, and usually not folded; from leukoplakia, which is acquired, not congenital and usually is a firm hard lesion of the mucosa. (Any patient with atypical vaginal "leukoplakia" should be examined for lesions at other mucosal sites, as a possible example of this condition, and radical therapy should be avoided.) Must also be differentiated from focal hyperplasia of oral mucosa, which is the same color as the adjacent normal mucosa and histologically shows only increased thickness of the epithelial cell layer.

This condition must also be differentiated from intraepithelial dyskeratosis, which has perilimbal gelatinous plaques of the bulbar conjunctivae, and from oral epithelial nevus of Cooke which is not familial and histologically has a basket weave pattern of the superficial cornified layer, and a granular layer absent in normal oral mucosa. Diagnosis of this condition can be made on smears which show the perinuclear or cytoplasmic condensations, giving this disease the designation of the "spotted cell disease." Distribution of cytoplasmic condensation is the opposite of that seen in pemphigus, which has a perinuclear halo and peripheral cytoplasmic condensation.

**Complications:** Iatrogenic effects resulting from surgical or X-ray therapy for supposed precancerous lesion, when treatment was initiated while the lesion was mistaken for leukoplakia, especially in response to vaginal involvement.

**Associated Findings:** None known.

**Etiology:** Autosomal dominant inheritance.

**Pathogenesis:** An intracellular lesion with alterations in the cytoplasmic distribution of tonofibrils in epithelial cells.

**MIM No.:** *19390

**Sex Ratio:** M1:F1

**Occurrence:** Over 100 reported cases.

**Risk of Recurrence for Patient's Sib:**
    See Part I, *Mendelian Inheritance.*

**Risk of Recurrence for Patient's Child:**
    See Part I, *Mendelian Inheritance.*

**Age of Detectability:** Diagnosed in neonatal period by visual examination confirmed by cytologic or histologic examination. Most cases are not diagnosed until late childhood.

**Gene Mapping and Linkage:** Unknown.

**Prevention:** None known. Genetic counseling indicated.

**Treatment:** Undetermined. Stripping and other surgical procedures, especially for vaginal and penile lesions, should be avoided. There is no indication that this is a precancerous lesion.

**Prognosis:** Excellent. Does not predispose to malignant disease. There is no demonstrable reduction in reproductive fitness or longevity. The main complications result when lesions are treated by surgery or radiation on the basis of a mistaken diagnosis.

**Detection of Carrier:** Unknown.

References:

Zegarelli EV, et al.: Familial white folded dysplasia of the mucous membranes. Arch Dermatol 1959; 80:59–65.

Witkop CJ Jr, Gorlin RJ: Four hereditary mucosal syndromes: comparative histology and exfoliative cytology of Darier-White's disease, hereditary benign intraepithelial dyskeratosis, white sponge nevus, and pachyonychia congenita. Arch Dermatol 1961; 84:762–771. *

Browne WG, et al.: White sponge naevus of the mucosa: clinical and linkage data. Ann Hum Genet 1969; 32:271–282.

Whitten JB: The electron microscopic examination of congenital keratoses of the oral mucous membranes. I. White sponge nevus. Oral Surg 1970; 29:69–84.

Jorgenson RJ, Levin S: White sponge nevus. Arch Dermatol 1981; 117:73–76.

WI043                                         **Carl J. Witkop, Jr.**

**Mucosal neuroma syndrome**
  *See ENDOCRINE NEOPLASIA, MULTIPLE TYPE III*
**Mucosulfatidosis**
  *See SULFATASE DEFICIENCY, MULTIPLE*
**Mucoviscidosis**
  *See CYSTIC FIBROSIS*
**Muir-Torre (MT) syndrome**
  *See CANCER, SEBACEOUS GLAND TUMOR-MULITPLE VISCERAL CARCINOMA*
**Mulberry molars**
  *See TEETH, ENAMEL HYPOPLASIA*
**Mulibrey nanism**
  *See DWARFISM, MULIBREY TYPE*

---

## MÜLLERIAN APLASIA                                    0682

**Includes:**

  Mayer-Rokitansky-Kuster (MRK) anomaly
  Mullerian duct failure
  Rokitansky-Kuster-Hauser syndrome
  Rokitansky sequence
  Uterus, congenital absence of
  Vagina, congenital absence of
  Vaginal atresia
  Von Mayer-Rokitansky-Kuster anomaly

**Excludes:**

  **Androgen insensitivity syndrome, complete** (0049)
  **Mullerian fusion, incomplete** (0684)
  **Spinal cord, neurenteric cyst** (0894)
  Transverse vaginal septum, incomplete

**Major Diagnostic Criteria:** Congenital absence of the uterus in a 46,XX individual with normal ovarian development and normal female external genitalia. Müllerian remnants or fallopian tubes may persist.

**Clinical Findings:** Individuals with Müllerian aplasia show normal sexual development, except for absence of Müllerian derivatives; thus, fallopian tubes, uterine corpus, uterine cervix, and the upper portion of the vagina are absent. Often fibromuscular remnants or even rudimentary fallopian tubes persist. The external genitalia are those of a normal female. The hymen is intact, but the vagina ends blindly. At puberty, normal female secondary sexual development occurs, including breast enlargement, pubic and axillary hair, and an appropriate increase in the size of external genitalia. The presenting symptom is most often primary amenorrhea. Pelvic examination at puberty reveals a blindly ending vaginal pouch, usually 4–5 cm long, but occasionally no more than 1–2 cm long. Ovaries are normal; sex steroid levels are normal, and plasma gonadotropin levels respond appropriately to normal feedback control. Urologic anomalies are associated with Müllerian aplasia more frequently than expected; the most frequent are unilateral renal aplasia, pelvic kidney, and renal ectopia. The frequency of certain skeletal abnormalities, particularly vertebral abnormalities, is increased.

**Complications:** Lack of adequate vaginal length may cause difficulties with coitus; infertility.

**Associated Findings:** Renal and vertebral anomalies.

**Etiology:** Cytogenetic studies are normal, and no teratogenic factors have been demonstrated. There are several reports of multiple affected sibs. Recurrence risk is very low, despite Shokeir's (1978) suggestion that this may be a sex-limited autosomal dominant disorder. Multifactorial inheritance is more likely.

**Pathogenesis:** The Müllerian ducts differentiate into the fallopian tubes, uterus, uterine cervix, and upper portion of the vagina. The lower portion of the vagina is derived from invaginations of the urogenital sinus. Thus, the phenotype observed in these individuals can be explained completely by absence or aplasia of Müllerian ducts. Cramer et al (1987) have suggested that maternal deficiency of glactose-1-phosphate uridyl transferase may be a factor in the pathogenesis.

**MIM No.:**  15833, 27700

**Sex Ratio:**  M0:F1

**Occurrence:** About 20% of women with primary amenorrhea have Müllerian aplasia, which is a more common explanation for "absence of uterus" than complete **Androgen insensitivity syndrome, complete.**

**Risk of Recurrence for Patient's Sib:** Probably 1–2%.

**Risk of Recurrence for Patient's Child:** All affected individuals are infertile.

**Age of Detectability:** At puberty, on the basis of primary amenorrhea.

**Gene Mapping and Linkage:** Unknown.

**Prevention:** None known. Genetic counseling indicated.

**Treatment:** Construction of artificial vagina may be necessary, but often dilators and other nonsurgical methods can produce normal vaginal depth. Hormonal therapy is not necessary, nor is laparotomy or laparoscopy necessary to confirm the diagnosis.

**Prognosis:** Presumably normal life span, unless renal abnormalities are severe.

**Detection of Carrier:** Unknown.

**Special Considerations:** In many affected individuals there persist rudimentary Müllerian structures--relatively undifferentiated fibromuscular elements, rudimentary fallopian tubes, or, occasionally, a small uterine-like structure. If such Müllerian remnants persist, many investigators apply the term Rokitansky-Küster-Hauser syndrome. It seems likely that Müllerian aplasia and the Rokitansky-Küster-Hauser syndrome represent the same entity.

A separate group of individuals show absence of the lower portion of the vagina. The caudal portion is replaced by 2–3 cm of fibrous tissue, superior to which lie a well-differentiated upper vagina, uterine cervix, uterine corpus, and fallopian tubes. These individuals have vaginal atresia.

A phenotypic female with normal secondary sexual development, but without a uterus, has either Müllerian aplasia or complete androgen insensitivity (testicular feminization). These two disorders are readily distinguished by cytogenetic studies, with the former being more common.

References:

Jones HW Jr, Mermut S: Familial occurrence of congenital absence of the vagina. Am J Obstet Gynecol 1972; 114:1100–1106.

Simpson JL: Disorders of sexual differentiation: Etiology and clinical delineation. New York: Academic Press, 1976:342–345.

Sarto GE, Simpson JL: Abnormalities of the Müllerian and Wolffian duct systems. BD:OAS XIV(6c) New York: Alan R. Liss, Inc for The National Foundation-March of Dimes, 1978:37–54.

Shokeir MHK: Disorders of sexual differentiation: etiology and clinical delineation. BD:OAS XIV(6c). New York: Alan R. Liss, Inc for The National Foundation-March of Dimes, 1978:147–165.

Carson SA, et al.: Heritable aspects of uterine anomalies: genetic analysis of Müllerian aplasia. Fertil Steril 1983; 40:86–90.

Jones HW Jr, Rock JA: Reparative and constructive surgery of the female generative tract. Baltimore: Williams & Wilkins, 1983; 146–158.

Cramer DW, et al.: Mullerian aplasia associated with maternal deficiency of glactose-1-phosphate uridyl transferase. Fertil Steril 1987; 47:930–934.

Opitz JM: Vaginal atresia in hereditary renal adysplasia. (Editorial) Am J Med Genet 1987; 26:873–876.

Pavanello R deC M, et al.: Relationship between Mayer-Rokitansky-Kuster (MRK) anomaly and hereditary renal adysplasia (HRA). Am J Med Genet 1988; 29:845–849.

SI018 **Joe Leigh Simpson**

## MÜLLERIAN DERIVATIVES IN MALES, PERSISTENT    0683

**Includes:**

> Hernia uteri inguinale syndrome
> Mullerian inhibitor factor, deficiency of
> Oviducts in males, persistence of
> Pseudohermaphroditism, male internal
> Persistent oviduct syndrome
> Tubular male pseudohermaphroditism
> Uterine hernia syndrome
> Uterine inguinal hernia syndrome

**Excludes:**

> **Chromosome mosaicism, 45x/46,XY type** (0173)
> **Hermaphroditism, true** (0971)
> Male pseudohermaphroditism, all other forms of

**Major Diagnostic Criteria:** 46,XY individual, with normal male external genitalia and testes, who has a uterus and fallopian tubes.

**Clinical Findings:** A uterus and fallopian tubes are present in otherwise normal males. Affected individuals have normal male external genitalia, normal Wolffian derivatives (vasa deferentia, epididymides, and seminal vesicles), and usually anatomically normal testes. No somatic anomalies are present. At puberty virilization occurs. Endocrine studies produce results expected of a normal male. The disorder is often detected because the uterus and fallopian tubes prolapse into an inguinal hernia; thus, these patients are often said to have the uterine inguinal hernia syndrome. However, many affected individuals do not have inguinal herniae.

**Complications:** Herniation of the uterus and fallopian tubes into the inguinal canal; neoplastic transformation of cryptorchid testes.

**Associated Findings:** Infertility.

**Etiology:** Probably X-linked recessive inheritance, based upon one report of affected maternal half-sibs. Sex-limited autosomal recessive inheritance is also possible.

**Pathogenesis:** Undetermined. Müllerian derivatives presumably fail to regress, either because of failure of the fetal testes to elaborate anti-Müllerian hormone (AMH) or because of the inability of the Müllerian ducts to the AMH. If the disorder is X-linked recessive, location of the locus for AMH on an autosome (19p13.3) suggests that pathogenesis involves not synthesis of AMH, but perhaps a receptor.

**MIM No.:** *26155

**Sex Ratio:** M1:F0

**Occurrence:** Undetermined and presumably rare. Many cases may remain undetected.

**Risk of Recurrence for Patient's Sib:**

> See Part I, *Mendelian Inheritance*.

**Risk of Recurrence for Patient's Child:**

> See Part I, *Mendelian Inheritance*.

**Age of Detectability:** Usually after puberty or later in life, when herniation occurs.

**Gene Mapping and Linkage:** AMH (anti-Müllerian hormone) has been provisionally mapped to 19p13.3.

**Prevention:** None known. Genetic counseling indicated.

**Treatment:** Inguinal herniorrhaphy. Uterus and fallopian tubes should be removed if discovered. Orchiopexy may be necessary if testes are intra-abdominal.

**Prognosis:** Presumably normal life span, provided neoplastic transformation does not occur.

**Detection of Carrier:** Unknown.

**References:**

Armendares S, et al.: Two male sibs with uterus and fallopian tubes: a rare probably inherited disorder. Clin Genet 1973; 4:291–296.

Brook CGD, et al.: Familial occurrence of persistent Müllerian structures in otherwise normal males. Br Med J 1973; 1:771–773.

Sloan WR, Walsh PC: Familial persistent Müllerian duct syndrome. J Urol 1976; 115:459–461.

Malamayaman D, et al.: Male pseudohermaphroditism with persistent Müllerian and Wolffian structures complicated by intra-abnormal seminoma. Urology 1984; 24:67–69.

Naguib KK, et al.: Familial uterine hernia syndrome: report of an Arab family with four affected males. Am J Med Genet 1989; 33:180–181.

SI018 **Joe Leigh Simpson**

**Mullerian duct defects-upper limb hypoplasia**
 *See LIMB, UPPER HYPOPLASIA-MULLERIAN DUCT DEFECTS*
**Mullerian duct failure**
 *See MULLERIAN APLASIA*
**Mullerian duct-renal-cervicothoracic and upper limb defects**
 *See MURCS ASSOCIATION*

## MÜLLERIAN FUSION, INCOMPLETE    0684

**Includes:**

> Arcuate uterus
> Bicornuate uterus
> "Double uterus" (misnomer)
> Rudimentary uterine horn
> Uterus arcuatus
> Uterus bicornus
> Uterus bicornus unicollis
> Uterus bilocularis
> Uterus bipartitus
> Uterus didelphys
> Uterus pseudodidelphys
> Uterus subseptus
> Uterus unicornus

**Excludes:**

> **Hymen, imperforate** (0483)
> **Mullerian aplasia** (0682)
> True duplication of Müllerian ducts
> **Vaginal septum, transverse** (0985)

**Major Diagnostic Criteria:** Broadening and medial depression of the superior portion of the uterine septum (arcuate uterus) or more severe fusion defects in a 46,XX individual with normal ovarian and external genital development. Diagnosis should be confirmed by X-ray studies, or by hysteroscopic or laparoscopic visualization.

**Clinical Findings:** Failure of fusion of the paired Müllerian ducts results in two hemiuteri; each hemiuterus has a single fallopian tube. Sometimes one Müllerian duct fails to contribute to the definitive uterus or produces only a rudimentary horn. The extent of Müllerian fusion may vary from slight broadening and medial depression of the superior portion of the uterine septum (arcuate uterus) to completely separated hemiuteri with separate cervices, vaginas, and perineal orifices. The most frequent types of incomplete Müllerian fusion include uterine arcuatus, uterus unicornus (absence of one uterine horn), uterus septus (persistence of the entire uterine septum), uterus bicornis unicollis (two hemiuteri, each leading to the same cervix), and uterus bicornis bicollis (two hemiuteri, each leading to separate cervices). Vaginal septa and paired perineal orifices are relatively uncommon.

The external genitalia usually are normal, but a vaginal septum may be present. Ovarian development and puberty are normal.

**Complications:** A rudimentary uterine horn may retain blood, produce pain, and possibly rupture. Pregnancy in a rudimentary uterine horn may lead to uterine rupture or missed abortion.

Pregnancies may be complicated by an increase in the incidences of second trimester abortion and premature labor. Malpresentations are not uncommon. Following delivery, the placenta may fail to separate readily from the uterus.

**Associated Findings:** Urologic anomalies may occur ipsilateral to a rudimentry or absent uterine horn. Incomplete Müllerian fusion may be present in the **Meckel syndrome, Ectrodactyly-ectodermal dysplasia-clefting syndrome**, and the **Hand-foot-genital syndrome**.

**Etiology:** Reported familial aggregates have included several kindreds with multiple affected sibs, and several kindreds in which both mother and daughter were affected. Only one formal study has been conducted, with low recurrence risks (3%) for female sibs most consistent with polygenic or multifactorial etiology.

**Pathogenesis:** The Müllerian ducts are originally paired organs that fuse and subsequently canalize to form the upper vagina, uterus, and fallopian tubes. Failure of fusion or canalization results in uterine septa or hemiuteri, each associated with no more than one fallopian tube. More extensive failure of fusion results in persistence of vaginal septa.

**MIM No.:** 19200, 19205

**Sex Ratio:** F1:M0

**Occurrence:** About 1:1,000 females, although very minor uterine anomalies have been claimed in as many as 2–3% of women whose uteri are examined immediately following delivery. A relatively high proportion of the latter have uterus arcuatus or uterus subseptus.

**Risk of Recurrence for Patient's Sib:** Estimated at 1–5%.

**Risk of Recurrence for Patient's Child:** Estimated at 1–5%.

**Age of Detectability:** Variable. Retention of menstrual blood in rudimentary horns may produce symptoms shortly after puberty, but affected individuals are usually detected at a later age because of recurrent second trimester abortions, abnormal uterine contour during labor, or other intrapartum or postpartum abnormalities. Many affected individuals are probably never detected, particularly those with uterus arcuatus or uterus subseptus.

**Gene Mapping and Linkage:** Unknown.

**Prevention:** None known. Genetic counseling indicated.

**Treatment:** Many patients with hemiuteri or septal defects have normal pregnancies and require no treatment. Extirpation of a rudimentary uterine horn may be necessary. Reunification of paired hemiuteri or removal of a septum may permit full-term pregnancy; however, in general, surgery should not be undertaken unless the patient has had a least one second trimester abortion.

**Prognosis:** Normal life span, provided rupture of a uterine horn does not lead to life-threatening complications.

**Detection of Carrier:** Unknown.

**Special Considerations:** Incomplete Müllerian fusion should be distinguished from true Müllerian duplication, an anomaly that probably results from division of one or both Müllerian ducts early in embryogenesis. Such individuals have two separate uteri, each of which may have two fallopian tubes.

Several unusual clinical situations may result from the presence of a rudimentary horn. Menstrual blood may be retained, producing a pelvic mass and pelvic pain. Pregnancy occurring in a rudimentary tube that communicates with the uterus may terminate in uterine rupture or missed abortion; the latter may lead to lithopedian formation. A canal between hemiuteri may exist, even if a septum extends to the cervix or if two cervices are present. A vaginal septum bulging with blood from a rudimentary horn may obscure the cervix, mimicking Müllerian aplasia.

**References:**
Jones HW Jr, Wheeless CR: Salvage of the reproductive potential of women with anomalous development of the Müllerian ducts: 1868–1968–2068. Am J Obstet Gynecol 1969; 104:348–364.
Simpson JL: Disorders of sexual differentiation: etiology and clinical delineation. New York: Academic Press, 1976:351–354.
Wiersma AF, et al.: Uterine anomalies associated with unilateral renal agenesis. Obstet Gynecol 1976; 47:654–657.
Jones HW Jr, Rock JA: Reparative and constructive surgery of the female generative tract. Baltimore: Williams & Wilkins, 1983:164–185.
Verp MS, et al.: Heritable aspects of Müllerian anomalies. I. Three familial aggregates with Müllerian fusion anomalies. Fertil Steril 1983; 40:80–85.
Elias S, et al.: Genetic studies in incomplete Müllerian fusion. Obstet Gynecol 1984; 63:276–279.

SI018                                    **Joe Leigh Simpson**

**Mullerian inhibitor factor, deficiency of**
*See MULLERIAN DERIVATIVES IN MALES, PERSISTENT*
**Multicentric osteolysis**
*See OSTEOLYSIS, ESSENTIAL*
**Multicentric osteolysis with recessive transmission**
*See OSTEOLYSIS, RECESSIVE CARPAL-TARSAL*
**Multicentric osteosarcoma**
*See OSTEOSARCOMA*
**Multicystic kidney, congenital unilateral**
*See KIDNEY, RENAL DYSPLASIA, POTTER TYPE II*
**Multicystic renal dysplasia**
*See KIDNEY, RENAL DYSPLASIA, POTTER TYPE II*
**Multiple Acyl-CoA Dehydrogenation (MAD) disorders, mild variants**
*See ACIDEMIA, ETHYLMALONIC-ADIPIC*
**Multiple acyl-CoA dehydrogenation deficiency (MADD)**
*See ACIDEMIA, GLUTARIC ACIDEMIA II*
**Multiple acyl-CoA dehydrogenation deficiency, severe variants**
*See ACIDEMIA, GLUTARIC ACIDEMIA II*
**Multiple autosomal dominant liver-kidney cystic disease**
*See LIVER, POLYCYSTIC AND MULTICYSTIC DISEASE, ADULT TYPE*
**Multiple carboxylase deficiency, infantile**
*See BIOTINIDASE DEFICIENCY*
**Multiple carboxylase deficiency, juvenile-onset**
*See BIOTINIDASE DEFICIENCY*
**Multiple carboxylase deficiency, late-onset**
*See BIOTINIDASE DEFICIENCY*
**Multiple carboxylase deficiency, neonatal or early onset form**
*See CARBOXYLASE DEFICIENCY, HOLOCARBOXYLASE DEFICIENCY TYPE*
**Multiple cartilaginous exostoses**
*See EXOSTOSES, MULTIPLE CARTILAGINOUS*
**Multiple cysts anomaly, abnormal karyotype other than 45,X**
*See FETAL MULTIPLE CYSTS ANOMALY*
**Multiple enchondromatosis**
*See ENCHONDROMATOSIS*
**Multiple epiphyseal dysplasia, flat epiphyses type**
*See EPIPHYSEAL DYSPLASIA, MULTIPLE RIBBING TYPE*
**Multiple epiphyseal dysplasia, mild**
*See EPIPHYSEAL DYSPLASIA, MULTIPLE RIBBING TYPE*
**Multiple exostoses**
*See EXOSTOSES, MULTIPLE CARTILAGINOUS*
**Multiple hamartoma syndrome**
*See GINGIVAL MULTIPLE HAMARTOMA SYNDROME*
**Multiple hemangiomata-macrocephaly-pseudopapilledema**
*See OVERGROWTH, MACROCEPHALY-HEMANGIOMA, RILEY-SMITH TYPE*
**Multiple lentigines syndrome**
*See LENTIGINES SYNDROME, MULTIPLE*
**Multiple lipoprotein-type hyperlipidemia**
*See HYPERLIPOPROTEINEMIA, COMBINED*
**Multiple myeloma**
*See CANCER, MULTIPLE MYELOMA*

---

**MULTIPLE SCLEROSIS, FAMILIAL**                    **2598**

**Includes:**
"Creeping paralysis" (obsolete, pejorative)
Demyelinating disease
Disseminated sclerosis

**Excludes:**
**Adrenoleukodystrophy, X-linked** (2533)
**Alexander disease** (2712)
**Amyotrophic lateral sclerosis** (2067)
Behcet syndrome
Brainstem neoplasms-arteriovenous malformations-infections
Cerebral arteritis
Degenerative neurological disorders
**Encephalopathy, necrotizing** (0344)
**Leukodystrophy**

Lupus erythematosus, neuropsychiatric forms
Meningovascular syphilis
**Olivopontocerebellar atrophy**

**Major Diagnostic Criteria:** 1) demonstration of lesions reflecting mainly white matter dysfunction disseminated in time and space; 2) objective abnormalities on neurologic examination; 3) either two clear-cut episodes of significant worsening, each lasting over 24 hours and separated by at least one month, or slow progression of the same pattern over a minimum of six months; 4) determination by an appropriately experienced physician that no other disease process better explains the signs and symptoms.

Tests to aid in the diagnosis include evoked potentials, computed tomography (CT scan), magnetic resonance imaging (MRI), and analysis of cerebrospinal fluid (CSF) to identify abnormalities such as oligoclonal banding and an increased gamma globulin fraction in the total protein.

**Clinical Findings:** Within families, there is great variability in symptoms, age at onset, and disease course, even among close relatives such as siblings, parents, and children. In a series of 742 patients, the most common initial symptoms were motor symptoms (52%), sensory symptoms in limbs or face (32%), optic neuritis (14%), brainstem symptoms such as vertigo and diplopia (9%), gait disturbance (10%), bladder disturbance (2%), l'hermitte sign (1%), acute transverse myelitis (1%), and pain (1%). Ninety percent of patients were monosymptomatic at onset; 10% were polysymptomatic.

**Complications:** Sensory problems such as numbness or tingling, optic neuritis, diplopia, l'hermitte sign (sudden electric-like shocks extending down the spine upon flexion of the head), motor weakness (acute or chronic), bladder and/or bowel disturbances, acute transverse myelitis, vertigo, cerebellar ataxia of a limb, nonspecific gait disturbance, slurred speech, and pain. Fatigue can make daily living extremely difficult. Cognitive changes may occur late in the disease course.

**Associated Findings:** Iritis, ocular venous sheathing, and depression are frequently experienced by patients and require appropriate treatment. Recent data indicate that the suicide rate among patients is higher compared with that for the age-matched general population.

**Etiology:** Not definitively established. Heredity appears to play an important role in disease susceptibility. At a critical age, perhaps puberty, it has been suggested that in a genetically susceptible individual there may be infection by an environmental agent, e.g., a virus, that either becomes latent or initiates a cyclic immune regulatory defect. During an incubation period postulated to last from 5–20 years, repeated challenges to the immune system may result in the development of an autoimmune process. Subsequent to this, an environmental trigger, such as infection or trauma, or an endogenous trigger such as stress or other disease, may result in the first major episode of demyelination and clinically evident disease.

**Pathogenesis:** It is generally considered that multiple sclerosis exclusively affects the central nervous system (CNS). It was previously believed that indications of peripheral nerve involvement were secondary to the CNS pathology or incidental. However, there is growing evidence that distal demyelination may be present in the peripheral nervous system.

The individual plaques or lesions are characterized by demyelination with relative preservation of the axon. It is unclear whether the destruction of the myelin represents a primary attack against normal myelin or is secondary to previously injured and/or abnormal myelin. The earliest lesions are probably inflammatory. As the plaques age and develop, the amount of inflammation decreases and gliosis begins. With time, there is less axonal preservation, and eventually there is demyelination of entire tracts secondary to axonal loss. Plaques occur most often in the optic nerves, spinal cord, and cerebral hemispheres. In chronic cases, eventually there will be very few areas of central nervous system white matter that are not involved. Demyelination is often symmetric. Many plaques are apparently neurologically asymptomatic.

**MIM No.:** 12620, *16950

**Sex Ratio:** Ranges from M1:F1.5 to M1:F2

**Occurrence:** Varies with ethnic group and geographic location. Most frequent among Caucasians of central and northern European ancestry. Areas of high prevalence (at least 50:100,000 population) include northern and central Europe, northern North America, New Zealand, Japan, and parts of southern Australia. In well-documented series, 20% of patients have at least one other relative affected.

**Risk of Recurrence for Patient's Sib:** The risks given below are age-corrected, lifetime risks. The risk for brothers of female patients is 2.27±0.71%, and for sisters is 5.65±1.10%. The risk for brothers of male patients is 4.15±1.28%, and for sisters is 3.46±1.14%. These rates are computed on the British Columbia population with a prevalence of 1:1,000 population. The concordance rate for monozygotic twins is 25.9%, compared with a rate of 2.3% for dizygotic twins.

**Risk of Recurrence for Patient's Child:** The risk for children of female patients is 2.58±1.14%. The risk for children of male patients is 2.47±1.72%. These rates are for the British Columbia population with a prevalence of 1:1,000 population. There appears to be a greatly reduced father-son concordance rate, controlling for the observed sex ratio in the condition. Mother-daughter, mother-son, and father-daughter concordance rates are as expected, controling for the sex ratio.

**Age of Detectability:** Onset ranges from 10–60 years of age, with the majority having onset between 20–40 years of age.

**Gene Mapping and Linkage:** Reportedly a multiple sclerosis susceptibility gene exists in the HLA complex in linkage disequilibrium with HLA-D (Francis et al, 1987).

**Prevention:** None known. Genetic counseling indicated.

**Treatment:** Adrenocorticotropic hormone (ACTH) or corticosteroids are used when acute relapses produce disabling symptoms. Due to their relative ease of administration, oral steroids such as prednisone may be preferable to intravenous ACTH. Long-term steroid treatment should be avoided for patients following a remitting and relapsing course or for patients with chronic progressive disease. Bed rest is recommended only when fatigue is a significant factor in the relapse. In patients with chronic progressive disease, immunosuppressive agents may be effective. Specific symptoms such as spasticity, bladder and bowel problems, pain, and excessive fatigue may be treated on an individual basis.

**Prognosis:** The course of the disease is highly variable. At opposite extremes are a benign course, which occurs in 4–20% of cases, and a malignant course with death within five years of onset, which occurs in approximately 3% of cases. About 18% of patients have chronic progressive disease from the onset. The majority of patients initially undergo episodes of relapses and remissions, and the average length of time that patients follow this pattern is 6.8 years, after which the disease commonly becomes chronic progressive. Five and 11 years after onset, 30% and 50% of patients, respectively, are in a chronically progressive phase of their illness.

There are no fully reliable prognostic indicators, although age at onset and severity after five years may give some indication about the future course. Females with early onset of sensory symptoms, optic neuritis, or vertigo may have a relatively good prognosis. Conversely, males with late-onset disease who have significant pyramidal or cerebellar signs and symptoms either at onset or early in the disease seem to have a relatively poor prognosis. Gait disorder at onset also appears to be a poor prognostic sign for both sexes.

In terms of life expectancy, 90% of patients are alive 10 years after disease onset; about 75% at 20 years; and approximately 68% at 25 years. In general, there appears to be a significant increase in mortality 10–15 years after the onset of clinical disease.

**Detection of Carrier:** Unknown.

**Support Groups:** New York; National Multiple Sclerosis Society

**References:**
Antel JP, ed: Symposium on multiple sclerosis. Neurol Clin 1983; 1:571–785.
Paty DW, et al.: The diagnosis of multiple sclerosis. New York: Thieme-Stratton, 1984. *
Matthews WB, et al.: McAlpine's multiple sclerosis. New York: Churchill Livingstone, 1985. *
Ebers GC, et al.: A population-based study of multiple sclerosis in twins. New Engl J Med 1986; 315:1638–1642.
Hashimoto SA, Paty DW: Multiple sclerosis. Disease-a-Month 1986; 32:518–589.
Francis DA, et al.: HLA genetic determinants in familial MS: a study from the Grampian region of Scotland. Tissue Antigens 1987; 29:7–12.
Sadovnick AD, et al.: Multiple sclerosis: updated risks for relatives. Am J Med Genet 1988; 29:533–541.

BA011                        **Patricia A. Baird**
SA043                     **Adele D. Sadovnick**

**Multiple sulfatase deficiency**
*See METACHROMATIC LEUKODYSTROPHIES*
**Multisynostotic osteodysgenesis-long bone fractures**
*See ANTLEY-BIXLER SYNDROME*

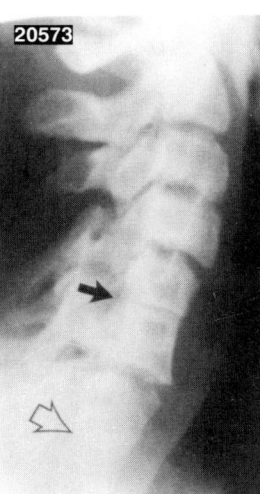
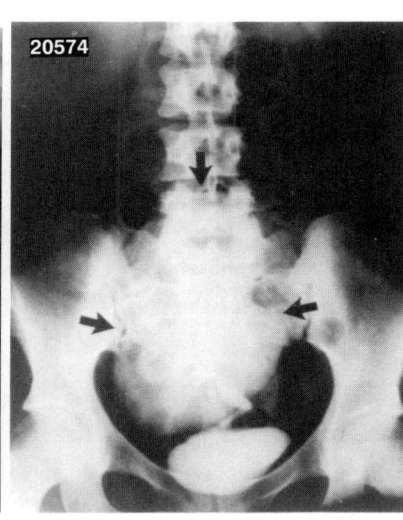

**2406-20573:** Complete and incomplete asymptomatic fusions of the cervical vertebrae. **20574:** Solitary pelvic kidney demonstrated by intravenous pyelography.

## MURCS ASSOCIATION           2406

**Includes:** Mullerian duct-renal-cervicothoracic and upper limb defects

**Excludes:**
    **Klippel-Feil anomaly** (2032)
    **Mullerian aplasia** (0682)
    **Noonan syndrome** (0720)
    **Renal agenesis, bilateral** (0856)
    **Renal agenesis, unilateral** (0857)
    **Turner syndrome** (0977)
    **Vater association** (0987)

**Major Diagnostic Criteria:** Cervicothoracic vertebrae, rib, and/or upper limb malformations in association with uterovaginal anomalies and renal agenesis and/or ectopy.

**Clinical Findings:** The usual clinical presentation occurs in young adult females with primary amenorrhea, vaginal agenesis, and short stature but with normal development of secondary sexual characteristics. Diagnosis of the MURCS association can be established by identification of the Rokitansky sequence (96%) in association with renal agenesis and/or ectopy (88%) and dysmorphic cervicothoracic vertebrae (80%) and/or rib or upper limb abnormalities, and a normal female karyotype (46,XX).

**Complications:** Urinary tract infection, obstruction, or failure; growth deficiency (adult stature is usually less than 152 cm).

**Associated Findings:** Moderate occurrence: Sprengel scapular anomaly. Infrequent occurrence: deafness, dysmorphic ears, facial asymmetry, cleft lip and/or palate, micrognathia, hemifacial microsomia, and gastrointestinal anomalies.

**Etiology:** Has occurred sporadically in otherwise normal families.

**Pathogenesis:** A hypothesis has been proposed that attributes the major components of the MURCS Association to an alteration of the blastema of the lower cervical and upper thoracic somites, arm buds, and pronephric ducts, all of which have an intimate spatial inter-relationship late in the fourth embryonic week.

**POS No.:** 3535

**Sex Ratio:** M0:F1 (Sex-limited).

**Occurrence:** About 40 cases have been reported.

**Risk of Recurrence for Patient's Sib:** Presumably not significantly increased.

**Risk of Recurrence for Patient's Child:** Probands are infertile.

**Age of Detectability:** Shortly after puberty.

**Gene Mapping and Linkage:** Unknown.

**Prevention:** None known. Genetic counseling indicated.

**Treatment:** Corrective surgery for genitourinary and limb complications. Medical management of renal complications.

**Prognosis:** Normal for life span unless renal complications are severe. Affected individuals are infertile, intelligence is not affected.

**Detection of Carrier:** Unknown.

**Special Considerations:** MURCS is an acronym for Müllerian duct (MU); Renal (R); Cervicothoracic vertebrae, rib and upper limb (CS) anomalies.

**References:**
Duncan PA, et al.: The MURCS Association: müllerian duct aplasia, renal aplasia, and cervicothoracic somite dysplasia. J Pediatr 1979; 95:399–402. *
Duncan PA, Shapiro LR: MURCS and VATER associations: vertebral and genitourinary malformations with distinct embryologic pathogenetic mechanisms. Teratology 1979; 19:24A only.
Winer-Muram HT, et al.: The concurrence of facioauriculovertebral spectrum and the Rokitansky syndrome. Am J Obstet Gynecol 1984; 149:569–570.
Greene RA, et al.: MURCS association with additional congenital anomalies. Hum Pathol 1986; 17:88–91.
Lo Iudice G, et al.: The MURCS association: clinical, radiological, endocrinological and familial data in a 40-year-old patient. Minerva Endocrinol 1986; 11:205–209.
Jones KL: Smith's recognizable patterns of human malformation, 4rd ed. Philadelphia: W.B. Saunders Company, 1988:604–605.

DU003                       **Peter A. Duncan**
SH009                  **Lawrence R. Shapiro**

**Murk Jansen metaphyseal chondrodysplasia**
*See METAPHYSEAL CHONDRODYSPLASIA, TYPE JANSEN*
**Murray syndrome**
*See FIBROMATOSIS, JUVENILE HYALINE*
**Murray-Puretic syndrome**
*See FIBROMATOSIS, JUVENILE HYALINE*
**Murray-Puretic-Drescher syndrome**
*See FIBROMATOSIS, JUVENILE HYALINE*
**Muscle adenosine monophosphate (AMP) deaminase deficiency**
*See MYOPATHY-METABOLIC, MYOADENYLATE DEAMINASE DEFICIENCY*

**Muscle adenylate deaminase deficiency**
See MYOPATHY-METABOLIC, MYOADENYLATE DEAMINASE DEFICIENCY
**Muscle atrophy-contractures-oculomotor apraxia**
See CONTRACTURES-MUSCLE ATROPHY-OCULOMOTOR APRAXIA
**Muscle atrophy-mental retardation, X-linked-contractures-apraxia**
See X-LINKED MENTAL RETARDATION-MUSCLE ATROPHY-CONTRACTURES-APRAXIA
**Muscle carnitine deficiency**
See MYOPATHY-METABOLIC, CARNITINE DEFICIENCY, PRIMARY AND SECONDARY
**Muscle glycogen phosphorylase deficiency**
See GLYCOGENOSIS, TYPE V
**Muscle phosphofructokinase deficiency**
See GLYCOGENOSIS, TYPE VII

## MUSCLE WASTING OF HANDS-SENSORINEURAL DEAFNESS 0450

**Includes:**
Arthrogryposis-like hand anomaly-sensorineural deafness
Deafness, sensorineural-hand muscle wasting
Hands, muscle wasting-sensorineural deafness

**Excludes:**
**Arthrogryposes** (isolated or with syndromes)
**Cranio-carpo-tarsal dysplasia, whistling face type** (0223)
Hand anomalies associated with dwarfism
**Synostosis, multiple synostosis syndrome** (2312)

**Major Diagnostic Criteria:** Congenital flexion contractures and atrophy of thenar, hypothenar and, interosseous muscles in a patient with congenital sensorineural hearing loss and normal joints by X-ray are characteristic of the condition.

**Clinical Findings:** Familial congenital bilateral or unilateral sensorineural hearing losses of varying degrees. A congenital hand abnormality is seen in both non-hearing and deaf patients. There are congenital flexion contractures of the digits and wasting of the thenar, hypothenar, and interosseous muscles which is nonprogressive. Flexion creases over the interphalangeal joints are absent. Active and passive flexion and extension of the fingers is limited. Some of the fingers may show ulnar deviation. There may be muscle weakness, most marked in the distribution of the ulnar nerve. There is no pain; there are no other neurologic deficits; nerve conduction studies and electromyography are normal. Dermatoglyphics show a striking vertical orientation of the palmar digital lines. X-rays in both adults and children show normal joints. Petrous pyramid polytomography, electronystagmography, and various laboratory tests (CBC, urinalysis, serum electrolytes, BUN, blood glucose, serum glutamic oxalic transaminase, aldolase, CPK, urine and plasma amino acid screening, urine mucopolysaccharide screening, EKG, and karyotype) are normal.

**Complications:** Failure to acquire speech and language in a patient with profound hearing loss. Articulation errors and poor school progress occur in patients with lesser degrees of hearing loss.

**Associated Findings:** Limitation of motion of other joints has been seen. These include the wrist, toes, forearm pronation and supination, and elbow extension. Clubfoot, acetabular dysplasia, coxa vera may also be present.

**Etiology:** Autosomal dominant inheritance with complete penetrance but variable expressivity.

**Pathogenesis:** Unknown.

**MIM No.:** 10820

**POS No.:** 3486

**Sex Ratio:** M1:F1

**Occurrence:** Undetermined. One reported kindred had 12 affected persons in five generations.

**Risk of Recurrence for Patient's Sib:**
See Part I, *Mendelian Inheritance.*

**Risk of Recurrence for Patient's Child:**
See Part I, *Mendelian Inheritance.*

**Age of Detectability:** The hand abnormality is detectable at birth and if bilateral, the hearing loss may be detected at birth also, unless the loss is mild. A unilateral loss may escape detection for years.

**Gene Mapping and Linkage:** Unknown.

**Prevention:** None known. Genetic counseling indicated.

**Treatment:** Hearing loss, if significant, should be treated by hearing aids and special speech training. Less severe losses may be managed by preferential seating in school, lip-reading training, and the use of hearing conservation (regular otologic and audiologic checkups, avoidance of acoustic trauma, and ototoxic drugs). Mumps immunization might be desirable in susceptible patients with unilateral hearing loss. Physical therapy may be of benefit in patients with more severe contractures. An infant with the characteristic hand abnormality should have audiometric evaluation and periodic follow-up to rule out hearing loss. The hearing loss is the only potential serious disability, as the hand abnormality seems not to hinder patients in their daily activities and occupations.

**Prognosis:** Normal for life expectancy and intelligence. There is some evidence to suggest that the inner ears in these patients may be more susceptible to injury from febrile illnesses.

**Detection of Carrier:** Unknown.

**References:**
Stewart J, Bergstrom L: Familial hand abnormality and sensori-neural deafness: new syndrome. J Pediatr 1971; 78:102–110.
Akbarnia BA, et al.: Familial arthrogrypotic-like hand abnormality and sensorineural deafness. Am J Dis Child 1979; 133:403–405.
Martinon F, et al.: Sindrome de Stewart y Bergstrom: anales españoles de pediatria. 1979; 12:549–552.
Drachman DB, Banker BQ: Arthrogryposis multiplex congenita. Arch Neurol 1961; 5:77–93.

BE028

**LaVonne Bergstrom**
*Janet M. Stewart*

**Muscle wasting-deafness-vitiligo**
See DEAFNESS-VITILIGO-MUSCLE WASTING
**Muscle weakness**
See SINGLETON-MERTEN SYNDROME

## MUSCLE-EYE-BRAIN SYNDROME 3047

**Includes:**
Brain-muscle-eye syndrome
Eye-muscle-brain syndrome

**Excludes:** Facio-neuro-skeletal syndrome (2339)

**Major Diagnostic Criteria:** The combination of severe hypotonia, mental retardation, and visual failure is sufficient to suggest the diagnosis.

**Clinical Findings:** Abnormal findings are confined to muscle, eye, and brain. Muscular anomalies present in all include severe early hypotonia and subsequently retarded motor development and reduced or absent deep tendon reflexes. Diagnostic studies in all patients indicated myopathic EMG, elevated serum CK, and histologic features of muscular dystrophy. Eye anomalies include visual failure in all affected children, with myopia described as severe in 10/14 and mild in 4/14; in addition, glaucoma (8/11), optic disk hypoplasia or pallor (7/10), and retinal hypoplasia (9/10) have also been described. The brain anomalies are mental retardation and slight spasticity (14/14), mild **Hydrocephaly** (7/11), and myoclonic jerks or convulsions (6/11). Abnormal electroencephalograms were found in children thus investigated.

**Complications:** Unknown.

**Associated Findings:** None known.

**Etiology:** Autosomal recessive inheritance.

**Pathogenesis:** Unknown.

**MIM No.:** *25328

**POS No.:** 3589

**Sex Ratio:** M1:F1

**Occurrence:** Some 14 affected individuals have been reported, all from Finland.

**Risk of Recurrence for Patient's Sib:**
See Part I, *Mendelian Inheritance.*

**Risk of Recurrence for Patient's Child:**
See Part I, *Mendelian Inheritance.*

**Age of Detectability:** Soon after birth by the presence of severe hypotonia.

**Gene Mapping and Linkage:** Unknown.

**Prevention:** None known. Genetic counseling indicated.

**Treatment:** Treatment of glaucoma as indicated; regular physiotherapy may also be useful.

**Prognosis:** Mental retardation is a constant finding; prognosis for life span is unknown.

**Detection of Carrier:** Unknown.

**References:**
Raitta C, et al.: Ophthalmological findings in a new syndrome with muscle, eye and brain involvement. Acta Ophthalmol (Copenh) 1978; 56:465–472.
Santavuori P, Leisti J: Muscle, eye and brain disease (MEB). In: Eriksson AW, et al., eds: Population structure and genetic disorders. New York: Academic, 1980:647–651.

T0007                                                    **Helga V. Toriello**

**Muscular atrophy, adult spinal**
*See SPINAL MUSCULAR ATROPHY*
**Muscular atrophy, juvenile spinal**
*See SPINAL MUSCULAR ATROPHY*
**Muscular atrophy, progressive**
*See AMYOTROPHIC LATERAL SCLEROSIS, FAMILIAL ADULT AND JUVENILE TYPES*
*also AMYOTROPHIC LATERAL SCLEROSIS*

---

## MUSCULAR ATROPHY, SPINAL AND BULBAR, X-LINKED KENNEDY TYPE                    2493

**Includes:**
Bulbospinal muscular atrophy, X-linked
Calves, hypertrophy of-spinal muscular atrophy
Kennedy type spinal and bulbar muscular atrophy
Kennedy-Stefanis disease
Spinal muscular atrophy-hypertrophy of the calves
X-linked adult onset spinobulbar muscular atrophy
X-linked adult spinal muscular atrophy

**Excludes:**
**Adrenoleukodystrophy, X-linked** (2533)
**Spinal muscular atrophy** (0895)

**Major Diagnostic Criteria:** Facial, bulbar, and spinal proximal muscle atrophy with fasiculations; especially around the lips, chin, and tongue. Cramps, tremor, sexual dysfunction, and gynecomastia are common findings. The age of onset ranges from 15–59 years of age. The inheritance pattern is X-linked recessive.

**Clinical Findings:** Based on over 50 patients: onset age > 15 years (100%); facial weakness (75%); bulbar symptoms (75%); muscle fasiculations (90%); gynecomastia (50%); sexual dysfunction (75%); X-linked family history (95%).

**Complications:** Slow progression of muscular disease. Although patients have normal sexual function prior to onset of the disease, they develop decreased libido and impotence after onset. In addition, sperm production diminishes with decreasing fertility as the disease progresses.

**Associated Findings:** None known.

**Etiology:** X-linked inheritance.

**Pathogenesis:** There appears to be some overlap with X-linked adrenomyeloneuropathy (see **Adrenoleukodystrophy, X-linked**), which is associated with abnormalities in long chain fatty acid metabolism and peroxisomal dysfunction.

**MIM No.:** *31320

**Sex Ratio:** M1:F0

**Occurrence:** Over 50 cases have been reported. Represents about 3% of all spinal muscular atrophy patients in one center.

**Risk of Recurrence for Patient's Sib:**
See Part I, *Mendelian Inheritance.*

**Risk of Recurrence for Patient's Child:**
See Part I, *Mendelian Inheritance.*

**Age of Detectability:** Usually in adulthood.

**Gene Mapping and Linkage:** SBMA (spinal and bulbar muscular atrophy (Kennedy disease)) has been mapped to Xq13-q22.

**Prevention:** None known. Genetic counseling indicated.

**Treatment:** Supportive.

**Prognosis:** Life span and intelligence are not affected.

**Detection of Carrier:** Unknown.

**References:**
Kennedy WR, et al.: Progressive proximal spinal and bulbar muscular atrophy of late onset, a sex-linked recessive trait. Neurology (Minneap) 1968; 18:671–680.
Papapetropoulos T, Panayotopoulos CP: X-linked spinal and bulbar muscular atrophy of late onset (Kennedy-Stefanis disease?). Eur Neurol 1981; 20:485–488.
Hausmanova-Petrusewicz I, et al.: X-linked adult form of spinal muscular atrophy. J Neurol 1983; 229:175–188.
Fischbeck KH, et al.: X-linked neuropathy: gene localization with DNA probes. Annals Neurol 1986; 20:527–532.
Mukai E, Yasuma T: A pedigree with protanopia and bulbospinal muscular atrophy. Neurology 1987; 37:1019–1021.

GR011                                                    **Frank Greenberg**

**Muscular atrophy, spinal, intermediate type**
*See SPINAL MUSCULAR ATROPHY*
**Muscular atrophy-mental retardation, X-linked**
*See X-LINKED MENTAL RETARDATION-MUSCULAR WEAKNESS-AWKWARD GAIT*
**Muscular central core disease**
*See MYOPATHY, CENTRAL CORE DISEASE TYPE*
**Muscular dystrophy**
*See MYOPATHIES*
**Muscular dystrophy (Duchenne type)-glycerol kinase deficiency**
*See GLYCEROL KINASE DEFICIENCY*
**Muscular dystrophy I**
*See MUSCULAR DYSTROPHY, LIMB-GIRDLE*
**Muscular dystrophy without central nervous system damage**
*See MUSCULAR DYSTROPHY, CONGENITAL WITH ARTHROGRYPOSIS*

---

## MUSCULAR DYSTROPHY, ADULT PSEUDOHYPERTROPHIC                    0687

**Includes:**
Becker muscular dystrophy
Muscular dystrophy, benign X-linked recessive
Muscular dystrophy, pseudohypertrophic adult type

**Excludes:**
**Muscular dystrophy, autosomal recessive pseudohypertrophic** (0688)
**Muscular dystrophy, childhood pseudohypertrophic** (0689)
**Muscular dystrophy, limb-girdle** (0691)

**Major Diagnostic Criteria:** Pelvic muscle weakness accompanied by pseudohypertrophy of the calf muscles. Onset is in late childhood, followed by a slow progressive course, allowing the patients to reach adult age. Highly elevated serum creatine kinase. Positive family history.

**Clinical Findings:** This disease was identified by the German geneticist Becker. Weakness is first apparent in the proximal muscles of the lower extremities and usually manifests itself by difficulty in running, rising from the floor, or climbing stairs. The age of onset in about 75% of the patients is between four and 19 years of age, with a mean age of 12 years. The patients are almost always able to walk until at least the age of 16 and this has been used as the differentiating point between the diagnosis of adult and childhood pseudohypertrophic muscular dystrophy. Of 144 patients with adult type, only 28.5% were confined to a wheelchair, 60.4% were alive and mobile at the time of the investigations, and 11.1% died while still ambulatory.

Neurologic evaluation shows waddling gait, with increased lordosis, and positive Gowers and Trendelenburg signs. There is mild to moderate atrophy and weakness of the gluteals, iliopsoas, tibialis anterior, supraspinati, infraspinati, serratus anterior, and sternocleidomastoids. Other muscles such as pectoralis, biceps, and brachioradialis show only very mild atrophy and weakness. Marked pseudohypertrophy of the calves is present in all patients. The Achilles tendons are contracted bilaterally and cannot be dorsiflexed beyond neutral position. Deep tendon reflexes are usually present or decreased.

Serum creatine kinase is highly elevated, with values of 10,000 to 20,000 IU (normal 50–200 IU). The creatine kinase isozymes show a 90–97% predominance of MM and MB isozymes. The electromyogram usually demonstrates a pattern of short duration, small amplitude, polyphasic potentials with some fibrillation potentials. Nerve conduction velocities are normal. Muscle biopsy reveals marked random variation in fiber size (many atrophic and some hypertrophic fibers), internal displacement of nuclei, split fibers, necrosis, phagocytosis, regeneration and endomysial fibrosis. According to some observers, about half the biopsies demonstrate neurogenic atrophy or denervation atrophy in addition to myopathic changes. However, some of the "neurogenic changes," such as fiber type grouping, could be caused by muscle

fiber splitting. The EKG may be abnormal (right ventricular or combined ventricular hypertrophy) in 46% of patients.

**Complications:** Congestive heart failure secondary to cardiomyopathy may be present. Wheelchair confinement occurs in about one-third of the patients, when in an advanced stage of the disease.

**Associated Findings:** Unknown.

**Etiology:** X-linked recessive inheritance. Becker muscular dystrophy (BMD) described here, and Duchenne muscular dystrophy (DMD) (See **Muscular dystrophy, childhood pseudohypertrophic**) are allelic disorders. Affected males may represent new mutations (one-third of BMD cases). The DMD/BMD gene has been cloned and its protein product, called *dystrophin*, has been identified. Mutations involving the dystrophin gene are 60–70% intragenic deletions. Several studies have tried to explain the phenotypical characteristics of DMD (severe muscular dystrophy with less than 2% of normal dystrophin) and BMD (mild muscular dystrophy with qualitative abnormality of dystrophin; larger or smaller protein) by the location and/or size of the deletion and the mutation's effect on translational reading frame. Medori et al (1989) have suggested that deletions at the 5' end of the gene are associated with BMD while those in the central portion are associated with DMD. By contrast, Baumbach et al (1989) conclude that the size and location of the deletion does not account for differences between DMD and BMD.

Monaco et al (1988) and Hoffman (1988) suggest that the effect of the mutation on translational reading frame may account for the differences between DMD and BMD. BMD deletions remove nucleotides in exact multiples of three so that the reading frame (three nucleotides for each amino acid) is preserved. DMD deletions were found to remove an odd number of nucleotides, which shift the reading frame and make the remaining message beyond the site of the mutation meaningless. However, a later study by Malhotra et al (1988) showed exceptions to this rule, with deletions in some BMD patients producing shifts in the reading frame similar to those found in DMD patients. A significant number of DMD/BMD families (30–40%) have no detectable deletions, and must be studied by RFLP linkage.

**Pathogenesis:** Dystrophin is associated with sarcolemma of skeletal muscle. The abnormality of dystrophin may account for the increased permeability of sarcolemma resulting in high levels of serum creatine kinase in BMD patients.

**MIM No.:** *31020

**Sex Ratio:** M1:F0

**Occurrence:** In a 12-year prospective study in the Campania region of southern Italy, the incidence of Becker adult pseudohypertrophic muscular dystrophy was found 3.2:100,000, which is one-seventh the incidence of **Muscular dystrophy, childhood pseudohypertrophic** in the same region.

**Risk of Recurrence for Patient's Sib:**
See Part I, *Mendelian Inheritance.*

**Risk of Recurrence for Patient's Child:**
See Part I, *Mendelian Inheritance.*

**Age of Detectability:** Prenatal diagnosis relies on dystrophin cDNA probes for deletion identification in the male fetus, and on genetic linkage between the Becker gene and DNA intragenic markers. The condition can be diagnosed clinically at between four and 19 years of age.

**Gene Mapping and Linkage:** DMD (muscular dystrophy, Duchenne and Becker types) has been mapped to Xp21.3-p21.1.

**Prevention:** None known. Genetic counseling indicated.

**Treatment:** Physical therapy to prevent contractures (stretching exercises). Appropriate orthoses (braces) may be helpful. Treatment of congestive heart failure secondary to cardiomyopathy usually induces only a short improvement.

**Prognosis:** Decreased life expectancy to 30–55 years. For function, progressive decrease in muscular strength and difficulty in ambulation. Almost one-third of patients need a wheelchair in the last ten years of life.

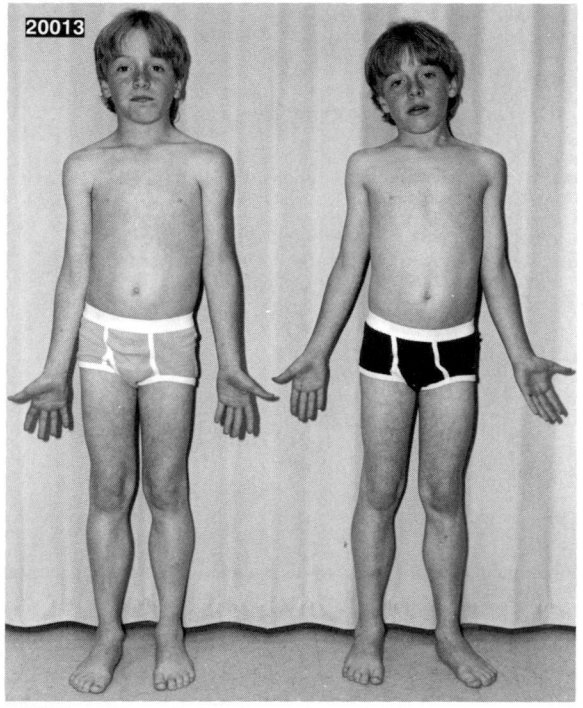

**0687-20013:** The twin patients (propositi) at 12 years of age show identical phenotype. Significant calves pseudohypertrophy is present in both.

**Detection of Carrier:** Based on both serum creatine kinase (elevated in 50% of carriers), dystrophin cDNA probes for deletion identification (Darras et al, 1988), and linkage between Becker locus and cloned DNA markers mapped in the area of Xp21.

**Support Groups:**

New York; Muscular Dystrophy Association (MDA)
ENGLAND: London; Muscular Dystrophy Group of Great Britain

**References:**
Becker PE: Two new families of benign sex linked recessive muscular dystrophy. Rev Can Biol 1962; 21:551–556.
Bradley WG, et al.: Becker type muscular dystrophy. Muscle Nerve 1978; 1:111–132. *
Nigro G, et al.: Prospective study of X-linked progressive muscular dystrophy in Campania. Muscle Nerve 1983; 6:253–262.
Kunkel LM, et al.: Analysis of deletions in DNA from patients with Becker and Duchenne muscular dystrophy. Nature 1986; 323:73–77.
Darras BT, et al.: Direct method for prenatal diagnosis and carrier detection in Duchenne/Becker muscular dystrophy using the entire dystrophin cDNA. Am J Med Genet 1988; 29:713–726.
Hoffman EP: Characterization of dystrophin in muscle biopsy specimen from patients with Duchenne's or Becker's muscular dystrophy. New Engl J Med 1988; 318:1363–1368.
Ionasescu V, et al.: Becker muscular dystrophy: recombinant DNA studies in identical twins. Muscle Nerve 1988; 11:287–290.
Malhotra SB, et al.: Frame shift deletions in patients with Duchenne and Becker muscular dystrophy. Science 1988; 242:755–759.
Monaco AP, et al.: An explanation of the phenotypic differences between patients bearing partial deletions of the DMD locus. Genomics 1988; 2:90–95.
Baumbach LL, et al.: Molecular and clinical correlation of deletions leading to Duchenne and Becker muscular dystrophies. Neurology 1989; 39:465–474.
Medori R, et al.: Genetic abnormalities in Duchenne and Becker dystrophies: clinical correlations. Neurology 1989; 39:461–465.

I0000                                    **Victor V. Ionasescu**

---

## MUSCULAR DYSTROPHY, AUTOSOMAL RECESSIVE PSEUDOHYPERTROPHIC                                    **0688**

**Includes:**
Duchenne-like autosomal recessive muscular dystrophy
Pseudohypertrophic muscular dystrophy

**Excludes:**
**Muscular dystrophy, adult pseudohypertrophic** (0687)
**Muscular dystrophy, childhood pseudohypertrophic** (0689)

**Major Diagnostic Criteria:** Occurrs in both male and female children, with progressive proximal weakness and atrophy of the legs, hypertrophy of the calf muscles, high serum creatine kinase, and dystrophic alterations confirmed on muscle biopsy.

**Clinical Findings:** Onset before five years of age, with pelvic muscle weakness, pseudohypertrophy of the calves, and contractures of Achilles tendons in both boys and girls, or only in girls. Progression of the disease is variable, usually slower with ability to walk until adult age. However, a severe form has been reported in Tunisia, where wheelchair confinement with flexion contractures occur between ages 10 and 20 years. Cardiac involvement with congestive heart failure is common in advanced cases. Intellectual functions are normal.

The serum creatine kinase activity is markedly high in the first stages of the disease. There is a necrotic regenerative pattern shown on muscle biopsy. Electromyography shows short duration, small amplitude, multiphasic potentials. Chromosomal studies show normal findings.

**Complications:** Hip-girdle weakness may contribute to accidents.

**Associated Findings:** None known.

**Etiology:** Autosomal recessive inheritance, often associated with consanguinity in the parents. The 28 kindreds from Tunisia included 45 pairs of parents with dystrophic children. Seventy-six percent of the parental pairs were closely consanguineous, compared with consanguinity rates of 16–23% in the general population.

**Pathogenesis:** Undetermined. The progressive deterioration of the proximal muscles of the extremities resembles limb-girdle muscular dystrophy. Laboratory studies (serum creatine kinase, electromyography, and muscle biopsy) are not helpful in the differential diagnosis.

**MIM No.:** *25370

**Sex Ratio:** M1:F1

**Occurrence:** Most frequent in Tunisia and Sudan. Ninty-three cases have been reported in Tunisia, and 15 in the Sudan.

**Risk of Recurrence for Patient's Sib:**
See Part I, *Mendelian Inheritance.*

**Risk of Recurrence for Patient's Child:**
See Part I, *Mendelian Inheritance.*

**Age of Detectability:** Varies from three to 15 years.

**Gene Mapping and Linkage:** Unknown.

**Prevention:** None known. Genetic counseling indicated.

**Treatment:** Physical therapy for prevention of contractures, and orthopedic surgery for correction of scoliosis.

**Prognosis:** Guarded because of cardiac involvement and possible severe motor handicap.

**Detection of Carrier:** Unknown.

**Support Groups:**

New York; Muscular Dystrophy Association (MDA)
ENGLAND: London; Muscular Dystrophy Group of Great Britain

**References:**
Ionasescu V, Zellweger H: Duchenne muscular dystrophy in young girls? Acta Neurol Scand 1974; 50:619–630.
Ben Hamida M, et al.: Severe childhood muscular dystrophy affecting both sexes and frequent in Tunisia. Muscle Nerve 1983; 6:469–480.
Salih M, et al.: Severe autosomal recessive muscular dystrophy in an extended Sudanese kindred. Dev Med Child Neurol 1983; 25:43–52.
Somer H, et al.: Duchenne-like muscular dystrophy in two sisters with normal karyotypes: evidence for autosomal recessive inheritance. Clin Genet 1985; 28:151–156.

I0000                                    **Victor V. Ionasescu**

---

**Muscular dystrophy, benign X-linked recessive**
*See MUSCULAR DYSTROPHY, ADULT PSEUDOHYPERTROPHIC*

---

## MUSCULAR DYSTROPHY, CHILDHOOD PSEUDOHYPERTROPHIC                                    **0689**

**Includes:**
Childhood pseudohypertrophic muscular dystrophy
Duchenne muscular dystrophy
Muscular dystrophy, classic X-linked recessive
Muscular dystrophy, pseudohypertrophic progressive, Duchenne type
Progressive muscular dystrophy of childhood

**Excludes:**
**Glycerol kinase deficiency** (2310)
**Muscular dystrophy, adult pseudohypertrophic** (0687)
**Muscular dystrophy, autosomal recessive pseudohypertrophic** (0688)
**Muscular dystrophy** (other)

**Major Diagnostic Criteria:** Pelvic weakness and atrophy accompanied by pseudohypertrophy of the calves and tight heelcords in a male child, manifested between 3–5 years of age; highly elevated serum creatine kinase.

**Clinical Findings:** While most newborn boys who inherit Duchenne muscular dystrophy (DMD) do not show clinical evidence of the disease during infancy, a more or less pronounced hypotonia is noticeable in others. Some children remain symptom free for a number of years, whereas others acquire the milestones of motor development at a slow pace; they walk late and fall frequently. At about the age of 3–5 years, weakness of the pelvic muscles is obvious in all cases. Squatting and climbing stairs are difficult; running and jumping are impossible. The patient shows a waddling gait, with increased lordosis on his toes. Neurologic evaluation at this stage reveals positive Gowers and Trendelenburg signs related to weakness of gluteus maximus and gluteus medius, respectively. Neck flexors (sternocleidomastoids) and back muscles (rhomboids, lower trapezius, latissimus dorsi) are also weak. Enlargement of the calves (pseudohypertrophy, i.e. related to fibrous tissue and fat infiltration) and Achilles tendon contractures are other early findings. Weakness of the shoulder girdle and arms follows, but distal muscles are preserved for a longer period of time. Deep tendon reflexes become depressed or absent.

Between nine and 14 years of age, DMD patients cease to ambulate. Various contractures of iliopsoas, hamstrings, forearm flexors, and finger flexors, and severe pes equinovarus develop in many patients. Severe paralytic thoracolumbar scoliosis becomes prominent. The arms, thighs, and pectoral muscles become atrophic. Intercostals become weak, and the lungs are hypoventilated and easily infected, causing pneumonia and bronchopneumonia. Death occurs between ages 20 and 25 years in 90% of the patients.

The disease process of DMD is not limited to skeletal musculature; the heart muscle is affected as well (cardiomyopathy), and death due to congestive heart failure is common. About one third of the DMD patients are mentally subnormal. Verbal IQ seems to be particularly affected, and many patients have reading problems. The overall IQ is between 70 and 85. The mental retardation is static and does not progress with the muscle involvement. Some DMD patients are of normal or even superior intelligence. Behavioral abnormalities, such as stubbornness, negativism, and selective mutism, are also reported.

Laboratory tests that are of value include the serum creatine kinase (CK), the electrocardiogram (EKG), electromyogram (EMG), and muscle biopsy. Elevated levels of CK are always seen in the early stages of the illness; reaching 10,000–40,000 IU (normal 50–200 IU). There is no well documented case of a patient with a normal CK during the first year of life who later develops DMD; thus, a normal CK is strong presumptive evidence against the possibility of the disease. As the illness progresses, the levels of CK fall, although they never attain normal values. The CK remains in the hundreds even in the patient who is severely disabled and in a wheelchair. Abnormalities in the EKG are common in DMD in the neighborhood of 70–90%. There are tall, right precordial R waves and deep limb lead and precordial Q waves. Arrhythmias and persistent tachycardias have been noted in patients with DMD. Many different explanations have been postulated for all of these EKG changes, but none has been entirely satisfactory. Correlation of EKG, echocardiogram and autopsy studies of the heart demonstrated replacement fibrosis of the wall of the left ventricle.

Electromyography shows small polyphasic potentials and increased recruitment of motor units. In the advanced stages, there may be additional changes such as fibrillations.

The muscle biopsy is characteristic, even early in the disease. There is increased fibrosis. Most of the fibers are circular rather than the usual polygonal shape. There is evidence of necrosis and phagocytosis and, in particular, small groups of basophilic fibers. Often large circular fibers demonstrating very dark staining, the so-called "opaque" hypercontracted fibers are present. Many type 2C or undifferentiated fibers are noted, often leading to poor separation into type 1 and type 2 fibers with the routine ATPase stains. Dystrophin evaluation (by immunoblotting or by immunofluorescence) demonstrates absence of the protein in the muscle biopsy.

**Complications:** Congestive heart failure secondary to cardiomyopathy; thoracolumbar scoliosis secondary to weakness of back muscles; and respiratory failure secondary to pulmonary hypoventilation and intercostal muscle weakness.

**Associated Findings:** Mild mental retardation with learning disability, particularly dyslexia.

**Etiology:** Usually X-linked recessive inheritance. The entire 14kb cDNA of the DMD gene has been cloned (Koenig et al, 1987) and its protein product, called *dystrophin*, has been identified (Hoffman et al, 1987). Mutations involving the dystrophin gene can cause either severe DMD or the milder allelic form such as Becker Muscular Dystrophy (BMD) (see **Muscular dystrophy, adult pseudohypertrophic**). Affected males may represent new mutations (one-third of the DMD cases). The majority of mutations (60–70%) are intragenic deletions clustered in a region near the center of the gene, or less frequently near the 5' end. There have been several reports (about 10% of cases) of germ line mosaicism in mothers of sons with DMD deletions. Therefore, it is possible that the mother could have two populations of ova; only one population carrying the deletion. No detectable deletions have been found in 30–40% of DMD families, and these must studied by RFLP linkage analysis using intragenic DNA markers. Other genetic defects in DMD include duplications which are seen in six percent (Den Dunnen et al, 1989), and insertions.

An estimated 6.8% of DMD cases are thought to be autosomal recessive (Zatz et al, 1989). The possibility of an autosomal DMD mutation should be suspected when the cytogenetic and molecular genetic (deletions, RFLP linkage analysis) screenings are negative, and when dystrophin evaluation of the muscle biopsy demonstrates normal size and abundance by immunoblotting (Francke et al, 1989).

**Pathogenesis:** Dystrophin protein is localized in the sarcolemma of human muscle (Zubrzycka-Gaarn et al, 1988), and the absence of dystrophin in the sarcolemma could explain the leakage of soluble sarcoplasmic enzymes, such as creatine kinase, in the serum of DMD affected individuals. The transcript of the DMD gene and the amino terminal of the encoded protein differ in brain and muscle. This difference may account for the mental retardation which is present only in 30% of DMD patients (Nudel et al, 1989).

**MIM No.:** *31020

**Sex Ratio:** M1:F>0. There are unusual situations in which DMD is expressed in females: manifesting heterozygotes, females with X chromosomal abnormalities, and in autosomal recessive DMD. Cytogenetic evaluations should be made of all female DMD patients.

**Occurrence:** Incidence varies between 1:1,700 and 1:7,700 live born boys. The average incidence for the United States, Japan, and Australia is 1:3,300 live born boys. In a 12-year prospective study in the Campania region of Southern Italy, the incidence of DMD was 21.7:100,000 live births. DMD monozygotic twins with deletion of the dystrophin gene have been reported (Ionasescu et al, 1989).

**Risk of Recurrence for Patient's Sib:**
See Part I, *Mendelian Inheritance.*

**Risk of Recurrence for Patient's Child:**
See Part I, *Mendelian Inheritance.* DMD patients are usually infertile. There is only one case report in the literature of a DMD patient who fathered a normal son.

**Age of Detectability:** Prenatal diagnosis is preceded by fetal sex determination. Prenatal diagnosis uses dystrophin cDNA probes for deletion identification and genetic linkage between intragenic DNA markers and the DMD gene. The condition can be recognized clinically between two and six years of age.

**Gene Mapping and Linkage:** DMD (muscular dystrophy, Duchenne and Becker types) has been mapped to Xp21.3-p21.1.

**Prevention:** None known. Genetic counseling indicated.

**Treatment:** Physical therapy to prevent contractures (stretching exercises). Night splints may be helpful for a limited period of time. Surgical treatment of scoliosis will help prevent severe restrictive lung syndrome. Management of end-stage respiratory failure is based on overnight mouth intermittent positive pressure. Life expectancy is improved following treatment, and in one patient death occurred at 30 instead of 20 years. Treatment of congestive heart failure using digitalis and diuretics produces only mediocre results.

**Prognosis:** Invariably fatal, usually by age 20. For function, progressive decline in muscular capability with wheelchair confinement by age 10–12.

**Detection of Carrier:** Based on both serum CK (elevated in 60% of carriers), dystrophin cDNA probes for screening of deletions, and linkage between DMD locus and cloned genomic DNA sequences mapped on the short arm of the X chromosome.

**Support Groups:**

New York; Muscular Dystrophy Association (MDA)

ENGLAND: London; Muscular Dystrophy Group of Great Britain

**References:**

Monaco AP, et al.: Detection of deletions spanning the Duchenne muscular dystrophy locus using a tightly linked DNA segment. Nature 1985; 316:842–845.

Heitmancik JF, et al.: Carrier diagnosis of Duchenne muscular dystrophy using restriction fragment length polymorphisms. Neurology 1986; 86:1553–1562.

Kunkel LM, et al.: Analysis of deletions in DNA from patients with Becker and Duchenne muscular dystrophy. Nature 1986; 322:73–77. *

Hoffman EP, et al.: Dystrophin: the protein product of the Duchenne muscular dystrophy locus. Cell 1987; 51:919–928.

Koenig M, et al.: Complete cloning of the Duchenne muscular dystrophy (DMD) cDNA and preliminary genomic organization of the DMD gene in normal and affected individuals. Cell 1987; 50:509–517.

Darras BT, et al.: Direct method for prenatal diagnosis and carrier detection in Duchenne/Becker muscular dystrophy using the entire dystrophin cDNA. Am J Med Genet 1988; 29:713–726.

Zubrzycka-Gaarn EK, et al.: The Duchenne muscular dystrophy gene product is localized in sarcolemma of human muscle. Nature 1988; 333:466–469.

LeRoy BS, et al.: Identification of carriers of Duchenne muscular dystrophy: value of molecular analysis. Am J Med Genet 1988; 31:709–721.

Den Dunnen JT, et al.: Topography of the Duchenne Muscular Dystrophy (DMD) gene: FIGE and cDNA analysis of 194 cases reveals 115 deletions and 13 duplications. Am J Hum Genet 1989; 45:835–847.

Francke U, et al.: Brother/sister pairs affected with early onset, progressive muscular dystrophy: molecular studies reveal etiologic heterogeneity. Am J Hum Genet 1989; 45:63–72.

Ionasescu V, et al.: Duchenne muscular dystrophy in monozygotic twins: deletion of 5' fragments of the gene. Am J Med Genet 1989; 33:113–116.

Nudel V, et al.: Duchenne muscular dystrophy gene product is not identical in muscle and brain. Nature 1989; 337:76–78.

Zatz M, et al.: Estimate of the proportion of Duchenne muscular dystrophy with autosomal recessive inheritance. Am J Med Genet 1989; 32:407–410.

I0000                                        **Victor V. Ionasescu**

**Muscular dystrophy, classic X-linked recessive**
*See MUSCULAR DYSTROPHY, CHILDHOOD PSEUDOHYPERTROPHIC*

## MUSCULAR DYSTROPHY, CONGENITAL WITH ARTHROGRYPOSIS                                       2706

**Includes:**

Arthrogryposis multiplex congenita-muscle involvement
Atonic sclerotic muscular dystrophy, Ullrich type
Muscular dystrophy without central nervous system damage
Myosclerosis, Lowenthal type

**Excludes:** Myopathies, congenital, with characteristic pathology

**Major Diagnostic Criteria:** Affected infants are usually hypotonic and weak at birth. Many display multiple joint contractures. Mental development is usually normal. The disease is nonprogressive.

**Clinical Findings:** The infants show generalized muscular weakness, more severe proximally than distally. Facial, neck, and chest muscles are variably involved, and extraocular muscles are spared. The tendon reflexes are usually depressed or absent. Contractures of the joints, particularly of the elbows, hips, knees, and ankles, occur at birth. During the course of the illness, there is very little loss of functions already gained. The patients have normal intelligence and do well in school. These children may adapt without difficulty to braces or devices such as "stand in" tables, which will allow them to stand. Some patients develop kyphoscoliosis as they grow older.

The laboratory findings are the same as in other muscular dystrophies. Serum creatine kinase is usually mildly increased. The EMG is abnormal, revealing brief, small-amplitude, low-duration, polyphasic potentials. Fibrillation potentials are usually not detected. Muscle biopsy shows increased fibrosis with random variability in the size of the muscle fibers. There is often type 1 fiber predominance, as there is in many other congenital muscle diseases. Necrosis of single muscle fibers is usually not detected. Ultrastructural changes serve only to amplify the above muscle alterations.

**Complications:** Paralytic kyphoscoliosis can become a troublesome problem. Respiratory infections are common.

**Associated Findings:** Dysmorphic features such as high-arched palate, deformed chest, and posterior displacement of the calcaneum have been noted.

**Etiology:** Autosomal recessive inheritance has been reported in several kindreds. In a series of 24 children with congenital muscular dystrophy, there were three sets of affected sibs, including two sisters, a brother and sister, and one set of female twins. Sporadic cases have also been reported.

**Pathogenesis:** The abundance of collagen and its structural appearance suggested that an abnormality of collagen synthesis is basic to this disease.

**MIM No.:**  *25390, 25560

**Sex Ratio:**  M1:F1

**Occurrence:** About a half-dozen kindreds have been reported.

**Risk of Recurrence for Patient's Sib:**
See Part I, *Mendelian Inheritance.*

**Risk of Recurrence for Patient's Child:**
See Part I, *Mendelian Inheritance.*

**Age of Detectability:** During the first three years of life. Prenatal ultrasound diagnosis may show absence or decreased movement of the extremities (Baty et al, 1988; Gorczyca et al, 1989).

**Gene Mapping and Linkage:**  Unknown.

**Prevention:**  None known. Genetic counseling indicated.

**Treatment:** Symptomatic and supportive, based on physiotherapy and orthopedic surgery for correction of contractures.

**Prognosis:** Kyphoscoliosis and recurrent upper respiratory infections may generate high mortality.

**Detection of Carrier:**  Unknown.

**Support Groups:**  New York; Muscular Dystrophy Association (MDA)

**References:**

Banker BQ, et al.: Arthrogryposis multiplex due to congenital muscular dystrophy. Brain 1957; 80:319–334.

Fidzianska A, et al.: Congenital muscular dystrophy: a collagen formative disease? J Neurol Sci 1982; 55:79–86.

McMenamin JB, et al.: Congenital muscular dystrophy: a clinicopathologic report of 24 cases. J Pediatr 1982; 100:692–697.

Banker BQ: Congenital muscular dystrophy. In: Engel AG, Banker BQ, eds: Myology, vol 2. New York: McGraw-Hill, 1986:1367–1382. †

Socol ML, et al.: Prenatal diagnosis of congenital muscular dystrophy producing arthrogryposis. (Letter) New Engl J Med 1986; 313: 1230 only.

Baty BJ, et al.: Prenatal diagnosis of distal arthrogryposis. Am J Med Genet 1988; 29:501–510.

Gorczyca DP, et al.: Arthrogryposis multiplex congenita: prenatal ultrasonographic diagnosis. J Clin Ultrasound 1989; 17:40–44.

I0000                                                              **Victor V. Ionasescu**

**Muscular dystrophy, congenital with central nervous involvement**
*See MUSCULAR DYSTROPHY, CONGENITAL WITH MENTAL RETARDATION*

## MUSCULAR DYSTROPHY, CONGENITAL WITH MENTAL RETARDATION                                                    2705

**Includes:**
    Cerebromuscular dystrophy, Fukuyama type
    Fukuyama disease
    Muscular dystrophy, congenital with central nervous
        involvement
    Micropolygyria-muscular dystrophy

**Excludes:   Myopathies** (other)

**Major Diagnostic Criteria:**   Onset before nine months of age, with generalized muscle weakness, hypotonia, and mental retardation. Many patients have seizures. More than 95% are Japanese. Electroencephalogram (EEG) and CT scan of the head show abnormalities. Muscle biopsy and electromyography (EMG) reveal myopathic alterations.

**Clinical Findings:**   Mothers are often aware that fetal movements of affected infants are diminished. The children are born floppy, suck and swallow poorly, and have a weak cry. A funnel chest is noted in about 30% of patients. Weakness is generalized, but proximal muscles are affected more than distal muscles. Facial and neck weakness is also present. Mild contractures at knees and elbows are often reported early or develop by age three. Hip dislocations are not uncommon. Tendon reflexes are decreased or absent. Affected children are severely mentally retarded, the development of speech is affected, and many children have seizures; either grand mal or petit mal. Few of the children learn to walk and most lead a passive existence and die by ten years of age.

Laboratory studies demonstrate elevation of the serum creatine kinase (CK), lactic dehydrogenase, and glutamic oxaloacetic transaminase. After the age of six, these values begin to decline. The EEG shows a diffuse and marked decrease in the frequency of brain waves and abnormal focal paroxysmal discharges of spikes mostly in the frontoparietal zones. CT scan of the head reveals poor cortical gyral development as well as prominent sylvian fissures. The lateral ventricles are dilated and there is an increased lucency of the cerebral white matter particularly in the periventricular areas. The findings are consistent with such developmental defects as pachygyria and polymicrogyria. The EMG demonstrates a myopathic pattern consisting of low-amplitude, short-duration motor units and no spontaneous discharges. Muscle biopsy shows marked variation in the size of the fibers, and all are embedded in fibrous tissue, (endomysial and perimysial fibrosis). There is no remarkable change in the fiber types, although occasional type 1 predominance and numerous type 2 C fibers are noted. The cortex is thick and the sulci are shallow or absent (lissencephaly). In many cases, there is micropolygyria and agyria with distortion of the architecture of both the cerebral and cerebellar cortices. The changes are in general dysplastic.

**Complications:**   Status epilepticus occurs occasionally and may result in death.

**Associated Findings:**   Myocardial fibrosis was reported in one case.

**Etiology:**   Autosomal recessive inheritance, with high rates of consanguinity in the parents of the patients, was reported by a genetic study in Japan on 153 families with 186 cases. Consanguineous marriage of the parents was found in 41 families (26.80%). Inbreeding coefficients in the patients was 10 times higher than in the general population. No single parent of the patients was affected. Recurrence among sibs was frequent: nine out of 41 sibs in offspring of related parents and 18 out of 110 sibs

in offspring of unrelated parents were affected. The segregation ratio was 23.91–27.08% in offspring of related parents and 10.00–22.94% in offspring of unrelated parents. These values are not significantly different from the 25% expected for autosomal recessive mode of inheritance. Two twin pairs were part of the analyzed sample of patients, of which one male twin pair was identical. Sporadic cases were not significantly more numerous than expected. All these data indicate that the disorder is caused by homozygosity of an autosomal recessive gene.

**Pathogenesis:**   Undetermined. The major changes in the central nervous system represent an arrest in the migration and differentiation of neurons early in the course of fetal development. This defect is expressed as **Microcephaly**, polymicrogyria, pachygria, lissencephaly and heterotopias. The occurrence of lissencephaly and polymicrogyria in siblings suggests that the underlying defect in the migration and differentiation of neurons is transmitted genetically. The disorder of muscle is characterized by an active degeneration of the muscle fibers. The fact that both systems are involved would indicate that the genetic factor responsible for the brain developmental defect is also responsible for the active progressive degeneration of muscle. A pleiotropic gene accounting for the lesions of muscle and central nervous system was postulated.

Follow-up studies of CT scan of the head revealed that the cerebral white matter low density areas were most apparent around the age of one year, and decreased or disappeared at 2–3 years of age. From these observations, delayed myelination was suspected for the pathogenesis of the low density areas (Yoshioka & Saiwai, 1988).

**MIM No.:**   *25380

**Sex Ratio:**   M1.1:F1

**Occurrence:**   This condition been almost completely confined to Japan, where it reaches relative high frequency. Recently, several Caucasian patients were also reported. Frequency of the gene in Japan was estimated to be 5.2 to 9.7 x 10$^{-3}$ and frequency of the patients 6.9–11.9 x 10$^{-5}$. In Japan the ratio of **Muscular dystrophy, childhood pseudohypertrophic** to Fukuyama congenital muscular dystropy is 2.1:1. Mutation rate was estimated to be 6.9 - 11.0 x 10$^{-5}$.

**Risk of Recurrence for Patient's Sib:**
    See Part I, *Mendelian Inheritance.*

**Risk of Recurrence for Patient's Child:**
    See Part I, *Mendelian Inheritance.*

**Age of Detectability:**   During infancy.

**Gene Mapping and Linkage:**   Unknown.

**Prevention:**   None known. Genetic counseling indicated.

**Treatment:**   Anticonvulsants are necessary to control the seizures. Physiotherapy is helpful in preventing contractures. In infants with aqueductal obstruction, shunt procedures may be necessary to prevent the progressive enlargement of the ventricular system.

**Prognosis:**   Guarded; short life expectancy.

**Detection of Carrier:**   Unknown.

**References:**
Dambaka M, et al.: Cerebro-oculo-muscular syndrome: variant of Fijuyama congenital cerebro-muscular dystrophy. Clin Neuropath 1982; 1:93–98.
Nonaka I, et al.: Muscle histochemistry in congenital muscular dystrophy with central nervous system involvement. Muscle Nerve 1982; 5:102–106.
Fukuyama Y, Ohsawa M: A genetic study of the Fukuyama type of congenital muscular dystrophy. Brain Dev 1984; 6:373–390.
Takada K, et al.: Cortical dysplasia in congenital muscular dystrophy with central nervous system involvement (Fukuyama type). J Neuropath Exp Neurol 1984; 43:395–407.
Miura K, Shirasawa H: Congenital muscular dystrophy of the Fukuyama type (FCMD) with severe myocardial fibrosis. Acta Path Jpn 1987; 37:1823–1835.
Yoshioka M, Saiwai S: Congenital muscular dystrophy (Fukuyama

type): changes in the white matter low density on CT. Brain Dev 1988; 10:41–44.

I0000                                                     **Victor V. Ionasescu**

## MUSCULAR DYSTROPHY, DISTAL                            0690

**Includes:**
Distal muscular dystrophy
Gowers form of dystrophy
Muscular dystrophy, late distal hereditary
Myopathy, late distal hereditary
Swedish type distal myopathy
Welander type of muscular dystrophy

**Excludes:**
Charcot-Marie-Tooth disease
**Neuropathy, hereditary motor and sensory**
Distal spinal muscular atrophy
**Myopathy, malignant hyperthermia** (2710)
**Myopathy, myotubular** (0695)
**Myopathy, nemaline** (0696)
**Myotonic dystrophy** (0702)

**Major Diagnostic Criteria:** Weakness of distal limb muscles. Electromyogram and muscle biopsy consistent with myopathy. Positive family history.

**Clinical Findings:** *Autosomal dominant form (Welander)*: Onset is in late adult life (usually after age 40). The initial symptoms are clumsiness and weakness of hand movements, such as fastening buttons, handling needles, or typing. Slow progression, with weakness spreading proximally to the forearm, whereas the leg muscles are spared or involved later. Weakness of foot extensors, steppage gait, and twisting of ankles, were present initially in only nine of 249 patients. The deep tendon reflexes are relatively preserved in the early stage of the disease, but become decreased or absent after many years. Sensation is not impaired, in contrast to **Neuropathy, hereditary motor and sensory**. The disorder does not shorten life expectancy.
*Autosomal recessive form*: Onset is in early adult life. The involvement of distal leg muscles is first noticed with weakness and atrophy of peroneal muscles and subsequent rapid progression to thigh and hand muscles. Neurologic evaluation may include absent Achilles and patellar reflexes in a few patients, but the majority have intact deep tendon reflexes. Cardiomyopathy may occur.
Laboratory studies in distal muscular dystrophy show moderate to striking elevation of serum creatine kinase. Electromyographic studies are compatible with myopathy; e.g. brief duration, small amplitude, and abundant motor unit potentials. No myotonic discharges are recorded. Motor and sensory nerve conductions are normal in both arms and legs. Muscle biopsy is characterized by marked variation in fiber size with frequent splitting, occasional degenerating fibers with secondary vacuolar degenerations, necrotic fibers with associated phagocytosis, numerous internal nuclei, and occasional basophilic fibers. These histologic features are characteristic for muscular dystrophy.

**Complications:** Unknown.

**Associated Findings:** None known.

**Etiology:** The autosomal dominant form of inheritance is variable in expression. The autosomal recessive form may appear to be sporadic when only one person is affected in a small family.

**Pathogenesis:** Unknown.

**MIM No.:** *16050

**Sex Ratio:** M1:F1

**Occurrence:** The autosomal dominant (Welander) form is frequent in Sweden, where 249 affected persons distributed in 72 kindreds were originally reported. The trait had 80% penetrance in males and 69% penetrance in females. The autosomal recessive form has been reported in the United States, Italy, and Japan. The exact incidence is not known.

**Risk of Recurrence for Patient's Sib:**
See Part I, *Mendelian Inheritance.*

**Risk of Recurrence for Patient's Child:**
See Part I, *Mendelian Inheritance.*

**Age of Detectability:** Between 30–40 years of age.

**Gene Mapping and Linkage:** Unknown.

**Prevention:** None known. Genetic counseling indicated.

**Treatment:** There is no specific treatment. Patients with distal leg weakness can be helped with bilateral ankle-foot orthoses. Molded polypropylene orthoses are usually the most successful.

**Prognosis:** Good for life, but guarded for ambulation in autosomal recessive form.

**Detection of Carrier:** Examination of relatives for evidence of the trait.

**Support Groups:**
New York; Muscular Dystrophy Association (MDA)
ENGLAND: London; Muscular Dystrophy Group of Great Britain

**References:**
Eastrom L: Histochemical and histopathological changes in skeletal muscle in late-onset hereditary distal myopathy. J Neurol Sci 1975; 26:147–157. *
Markesbery WR, et al.: Distal myopathy: electron microscopic and histochemical studies. Neurology 1977; 27:727–735. *
Matsubara S, Tanabe H: Hereditary distal myopathy with filamentous inclusions. Acta Neurol Scand 1982; 65:363–365.
Scoppetta C, et al.: Distal muscular dystrophy with autosomal recessive inheritance. Muscle Nerve 1984; 7:478–481.

I0000                                                     **Victor V. Ionasescu**

## MUSCULAR DYSTROPHY, FACIO-SCAPULO-HUMERAL       2049

**Includes:**
Facio-scapulo-humeral dystrophy
Facio-scapulo-humeral dystrophy, infantile
Landouzy-Dejerine muscular dystrophy

**Excludes:**
Myopathies with facial muscle weakness, other congenital
**Myopathy, central core disease type** (0134)
**Myopathy, myotubular** (0695)
**Myopathy, nemaline** (0696)
**Myotonic dystrophy** (0702)
**Spinal muscular atrophy** (0895)

**Major Diagnostic Criteria:** Facial and scapular muscle weakness is apparent clinically. The diagnosis is confirmed by EMG evidence of a myopathy and histologic evidence of dystrophy (phagocytosis, necrosis, internal nuclei in about 20% of fibers). Serum creatinine phosphokinase may be elevated.

**Clinical Findings:** Clinical signs may manifest anytime in the first two decades of life. Facial weakness is the earliest sign and produces difficulty in activities such as blowing or puckering the lips. As the facial muscle weakness progresses, by adolescence there may be a characteristic mask-like facial expression with horizontal movement of lips during an effort to smile and an inability to close the eyes during sleep.
An early clinical sign of shoulder girdle involvement is the inability to lift the arms and hands above the head. The neck and the scapular muscles become weak and wasted with relative sparing of deltoid muscles. Further involvement of the shoulder girdle is characterized by progressive loss of function. Some affected individuals are unable to raise their arms to eye level because of their inability to fixate the scapula. Wrist-drop may occur. The dystrophy may also involve the hip girdle muscles. The more severely affected individuals are unable to walk because of hip-girdle muscle weakness. Muscle involvement may be asymmetric.
Clinical variability is common; the muscle weakness may be moderately or very slowly progressive, or it may even be static

with involvement of a few muscles. Penetrance is generally complete, although there may be wide intrafamilial variability in clinical expression of the trait. For example, in a single kindred there may be an individual with profound weakness requiring a wheelchair, while facial weakness may be the only manifestation in another relative. Careful examination of all family members is essential. *A severe, early onset form* of facioscapulohumeral dystrophy has been described. Clinical expression is evident in infancy, and it progresses rapidly, leading to profound muscle weakness requiring the use of a wheelchair by age ten. This severe infantile type disease has been described in families where one parent might have only minimal facial weakness (Bailey, 1986).

**Complications:** Lordosis, foot drop and gait abnormalities are sometimes seen. Muscle weakness can make some activities of daily living difficult. For example, combing the hair may be difficult or impossible. Hip girdle weakness may contribute to accidents. Heart muscle involvement and congestive heart failure are rare.

**Associated Findings:** Sensorineural hearing loss is found in 5–15%. Fitzsimmons et al (1987) noted retinal capillary abnormalities, and suggested that capillary anomalies may play a role in the pathogenesis of the disease.

**Etiology:** Autosomal dominant inheritance with variability in expression. Heterogeneity may exist. An autosomal recessive variant of facioscapulohumeral dystrophy has been postulated, but this condition could be a variant of **Muscular dystrophy, limb-girdle** involving the facial muscles.

**Pathogenesis:** Current theory postulates a defect in the muscle membrane, possibly related to capillary anomalies.

**MIM No.:** *15890

**POS No.:** 3229

**Sex Ratio:** M1:F1

**Occurrence:** In general, this muscular dystrophy is less common than the Duchenne type. However, the incidence varies with ethnic group and geographic location. There are high incidences in southern Germany and in Utah, presumably from a few large affected kindreds. Mutations are thought to be rare. The mutation rate was estimated to be between $4.7 \times 10^{-6}$ and $5 \times 10^{-7}$. The prevalence was estimated by Morton (1959) to be 2:1,000,000, but this may be an underestimate.

**Risk of Recurrence for Patient's Sib:**
See Part I, *Mendelian Inheritance.*

**Risk of Recurrence for Patient's Child:**
See Part I, *Mendelian Inheritance.*

**Age of Detectability:** Usually clinically evident by 10–20 years of age; however, it may be present as early as the first year of life.

**Gene Mapping and Linkage:** FMD (facioscapulohumeral muscular dystrophy) has been tentatively mapped to unassigned.

**Prevention:** None known. Genetic counseling indicated.

**Treatment:** Physical therapy to prevent contractures. Appropriate orthoses may be helpful depending upon disability. Surgical fixation of scapula allows use of the proximal muscles of upper extremities.

**Prognosis:** Normal life expectancy in 98%. Physical handicaps leading to a change in lifestyle occurs in about 5–10%. Intelligence is normal.

**Detection of Carrier:** Careful clinical muscle examination and history for all relatives will help indicate those who are minimally affected.

**Support Groups:**
New York; Muscular Dystrophy Association (MDA)
ENGLAND: London; Muscular Dystrophy Group of Great Britain

**References:**
Morton NE, Chung CS: Formal genetics of muscular dystrophy. Am J Med Genet 1959; 11:360–379.
Carroll JH, Brooke MH: Infantile facioscapulohumeral dystrophy. In:

Serratrice G, Roux H, eds: Peroneal atrophies and related disorders. New York: Masson USA, 1979.
Ionasescu V, Zellweger H: Genetics in neurology. New York: Raven Press, 1983:412–413.
Bailey RO, et al.: Infantile facioscapulohumeral muscular dystrophy: new observations. Acta Neurol Scand 1986; 74:51–58.
Bodensteiner JB, Schochet SS: Facioscapulohumeral muscular dystrophy: the choice of a biopsy site. Muscle Nerve 1986; 9:544–547.
Brooke MH: A clinician's view of neuromuscular diseases, 2nd ed. Baltimore: Williams & Wilkins, 1986:158–170.
Fitzsimmons RB, et al.: Retinal vascular abnormalities in facioscapulohumeral muscular dystrophy: a general association with genetic and therapeutic implications. Brain 1987; 110:631–648.

RU013                                                    **Barry S. Russman**

**Muscular dystrophy, late distal hereditary**
*See MUSCULAR DYSTROPHY, DISTAL*

## MUSCULAR DYSTROPHY, LIMB-GIRDLE                0691

**Includes:**
Erb muscular dystrophy
Leyden-Moebius muscular dystrophy
Limb-girdle muscular dystrophy
Muscular dystrophy I
Pelvofemoral muscular dystrophy

**Excludes:**
**Glycogenosis, type IIb** (2873)
**Muscular dystrophy, adult pseudohypertrophic** (0687)
**Muscular dystrophy, childhood pseudohypertrophic** (0689)
**Muscular dystrophy, facio-scapulo-humeral** (2049)
**Myopathy** (others)
**Spinal muscular atrophy** (0895)

**Major Diagnostic Criteria:** Onset in second decade. Findings include weakness of proximal muscles in hip and shoulder area; "myopathic" electromyogram; muscle biopsy consistent with a "dystrophy" pattern (phagocytosis, split fibers, internal nuclei), and elevation of serum creatine kinase.

**Clinical Findings:** Patient first complains of difficulty climbing stairs; will use railing during this activity. In some cases, primary complaint will be difficulty holding hands above head. Onset of symptoms typically begins in the second decade of life, but the patient may not seek medical help until the third decade. Physical findings include weakness of proximal leg muscles and shoulder muscles; the biceps and brachioradialis muscles are weaker than the triceps muscle. Pseudohypertrophy of calf muscles is seen in 20% of patients. Serum creatine kinase is mildly elevated, but may be normal. Twenty percent of the patients will develop severe, intractable low back pain.

**Complications:** Low back pain, rarely contractures.

**Associated Findings:** Heart failure, which may occur late in the course of the disease (10%).

**Etiology:** Usually autosomal recessive inheritance; there have been few reports of an autosomal dominant transmission with complete penetrance and partial expression.

**Pathogenesis:** Presumably a defect of muscle membrane.

**MIM No.:** *25360

**Sex Ratio:** M1:F1

**Occurrence:** There is a high occurrence of this condition in the Amish community of Indiana. Studies (Jackson, 1961) traced this to descendents from Swiss Canton (Berne).
With new techniques of muscle biopsy analysis, specifically histochemical staining, it is anticipated that this category of muscular dystrophy will become less frequent. For the present, an individual who has proximal weakness of extremities and no facial weakness, with a complete muscle biopsy analysis showing necrosis, internal nuclei, and split fibers may, be placed in this category. With a totally negative family history, including physical examination and CPK testing, it may be difficult to exclude

**Muscular dystrophy, adult pseudohypertrophic** (Becker) in male patients except on the basis of X chromosome genetic linkage.

**Risk of Recurrence for Patient's Sib:**
See Part I, *Mendelian Inheritance.*

**Risk of Recurrence for Patient's Child:**
See Part I, *Mendelian Inheritance.*

**Age of Detectability:** Clinically, at 10–25 years of age.

**Gene Mapping and Linkage:** LGMD2 (limb girdle muscular dystrophy 2 (autosomal recessive)) is unassigned.

**Prevention:** None known. Genetic counseling indicated.

**Treatment:** Physical therapy to minimize contractures and use of orthoses as indicated.

**Prognosis:** Normal life span. May need wheelchair eventually. Occasionally, onset may be later than usual, with rapid progression leading to wheelchair over a three year period of time.

**Detection of Carrier:** Unknown.

**Support Groups:**
New York; Muscular Dystrophy Association (MDA)
ENGLAND: London; Muscular Dystrophy Group of Great Britain

**References:**
Jackson CE, Carey JH: Progressive muscular dystrophy: autosomal recessive type. Pediatrics 1961; 28:77–84.
DeCoster W, et al.: A late autosomal dominant form of limb-girdle muscular dystrophy. Neurology 1974; 12:159–172.
Cöers C, Telerman-Toppet N: Differential diagnosis of limb-girdle muscular dystrophy and spinal muscular atrophy. Neurology 1979; 29:957–972.
Fowler WM, Nayak NN: Slowly progressive proximal weakness: limb-girdle syndromes. Arch Phys Med Rehabil 1983; 64:527–538.
Yates JRW, Emery AEH: A population study of adult onset limb-girdle muscular dystrophy. J Med Genet 1985; 22:250–257.
Chutkow JG, et al.: Adult-onset autosomal dominant limb-girdle muscular dystrophy. Ann Neurol 1986; 20:240–248.
Norman A, et al.: Distinction of Becker from limb-girdle muscular dystrophy by means of dystrophin cDNA probes. Lancet 1989; I:466–468.

RU013                                    **Barry S. Russman**

---

## MUSCULAR DYSTROPHY, OCULO-GASTROINTESTINAL    2016

**Includes:**
Intestinal pseudo obstruction-external ophthalmoplegia
Muscular dystrophy, oculogastrointestinal
Oculogastrointestinal muscular dystrophy
Ophthalmoplegia-intestinal pseudo-obstruction
Visceral myopathy-external ophthalmoplegia

**Excludes:**
**Kearns-Sayre disease** (2070)
**Ophthalmoplegia, progressive external** (0752)
**Muscular dystrophy, oculopharyngeal** (0692)

**Major Diagnostic Criteria:** Ptosis, external ophthalmoplegia, and progressive intestinal pseudo-obstruction leading to malnutrition. Autosomal recessive inheritance.

**Clinical Findings:** The clinical syndrome becomes apparent between childhood and age 50 years, and is manifested by ptosis and external ophthalmoplegia followed by gastrointestinal symptoms. The latter include postprandial abdominal distension and pain, chronic diarrhea, malnutrition with severe weight loss and rarely, nausea and vomiting. Physical evaluation shows peristaltic waves visible over the abdominal wall, hyperactive bowel sounds, mild-to-moderate proximal limb muscle weakness and atrophy, ptosis and external ophthalmoplegia. Peripheral facial weakness, peripheral neuropathy with distal weakness, hypesthesia and decreased deep tendon reflexes may also occur. Heterogeneity of the disease is suggested by the presence of two clinical forms. The childhood onset of the disease has a rapid progression with death before age 30 years.

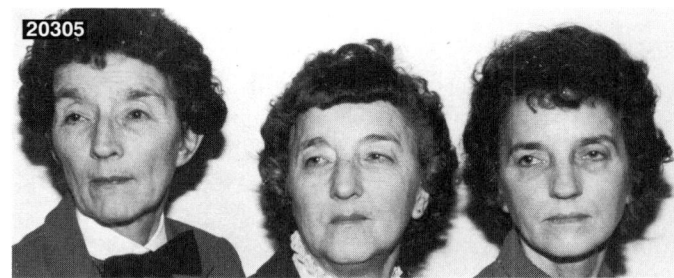

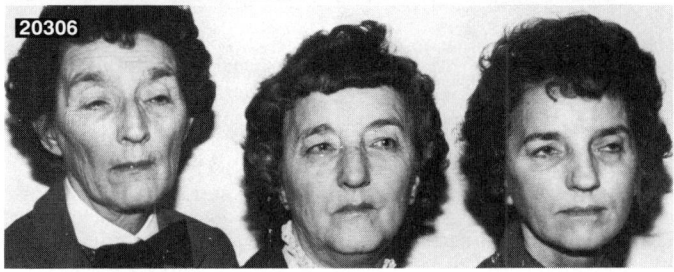

**2016A-20305:** Note marked limitation of eye movements and ptosis in extreme right gaze.   **20306:** Limitation in extreme left gaze.

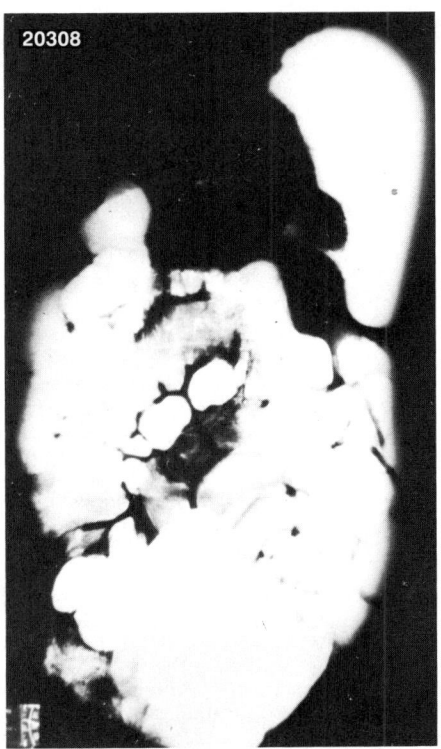

**2016B-20308:** Upper gastrointestinal X-ray shows presence of barium in the stomach after 8 h, jejunal dilatation and jejunal diverticula.

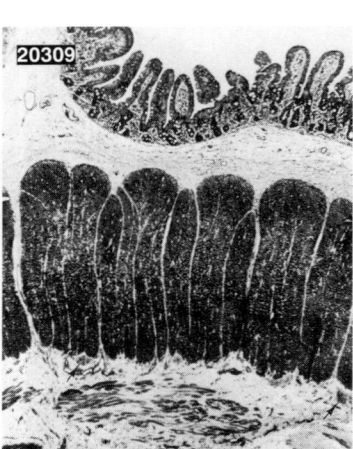
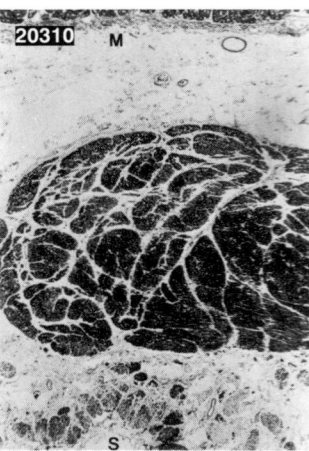

**2016C-20309:** Full thickness section of the stomach shows muscle atrophy and fibrosis affecting the more external muscle bundles located near the serosa (S); the mucosa, including muscularis mucosa (M) appears to be intact. Trichrome stain, original magnification × 20. **20310:** Section of jejunum reveals severe atrophy of the longitudinal muscle layer while circular muscle layer is intact. The atrophic muscle fibers are replaced by connective tissue. Trichrome stain, original magnification × 25.

The late adult-onset type (around age 50 years) has a mild course. Upper gastrointestinal X-rays shows delayed gastric emptying, jejunal dilation, and diverticulosis. Autopsy pathologic studies in two cases showed primary myopathic lesions of the smooth muscle of the stomach and intestine with severe atrophy and fibrosis, while the neurogenic structures (myenteric plexus and vagus nerves) were intact. Jejunal mucosal biopsy showed preserved villus architecture, without inflammatory changes. Absorption tests for fat, protein, carbohydrate, folic acid and vitamin $B_{12}$ are normal. Mild-to-moderate myopathic changes are seen in the biopsy of proximal limb muscles and include variability of fiber size, atrophic fibers of both types I and II and several "moth-eaten" fibers. A neurogenic component of the disease was documented only in one case and consisted of demyelinating and axonal peripheral neuropathy as well as spongiform degeneration of the posterior columns.

**Complications:** Intestinal pseudo-obstruction was present in 56% of cases as the result of severe smooth muscle myopathic involvement of both stomach and jejunum.

**Associated Findings:** Prolapse of the mitral valve in one case.

**Etiology:** Autosomal recessive inheritance has been suggested. The disease was originally described in three sibships of an inbred kindred of German extraction. Three of four affected persons were products of consanguineous marriages and the proportion of diseased sibs approached 25%, consistent with autosomal recessive inheritance. The father of the proposita had ptosis and died of spontaneous rupture of the esophagus. This may be an example of pseudodominance. The second reported family had three diseased sisters with unaffected, nonconsanguineous parents and four unaffected sibs.

**Pathogenesis:** Biochemical studies of contractile proteins (myosin, actin and tropomyosin) in the fresh and cultured smooth muscle cells of one patient obtained at the time of gastrectomy showed a 50–75% decrease in the synthesis of different contractile proteins. Turnover of contractile proteins and synthesis and turnover of collagen showed normal values. The reduction in synthesis of contractile proteins may account for the weak peristalsis, and be a factor in the pathogenesis of the intestinal pseudo-obstruction.

**MIM No.:** 27732

**POS No.:** 3996

**Sex Ratio:** M1:F6

**Occurrence:** Undetermined. Seven cases in two families have been reported.

**Risk of Recurrence for Patient's Sib:**
See Part I, *Mendelian Inheritance.*

**Risk of Recurrence for Patient's Child:**
See Part I, *Mendelian Inheritance.*

**Age of Detectability:** Varies from childhood to late adulthood.

**Gene Mapping and Linkage:** Unknown.

**Prevention:** None known. Genetic counseling indicated.

**Treatment:** No specific treatment is available. Surgical treatment (partial gastrectomy and gastrojejunostomy) was tried unsuccessfully in one case.

**Prognosis:** Good for life span only in the late adult-onset type. Guarded prognosis in the early-onset type, where life expectancy may be significantly reduced.

**Detection of Carrier:** Unknown.

**Support Groups:** New York; Muscular Dystrophy Association (MDA)

**References:**
Ionasescu VV: Oculogastrointestinal muscular dystrophy. Am J Med Genet 1983; 15:103–112. *
Ionasescu VV, et al.: Inherited ophthalmoplegia with intestinal pseudo-obstruction. J Neurol Sci 1983; 59:215–228. †
Ionasescu VV, et al.: Late onset oculogastrointestinal muscular dystrophy. Am J Med Genet 1984; 18:781–788.

I0000                                   **Victor V. Ionasescu**

**Muscular dystrophy, oculogastrointestinal**
*See MUSCULAR DYSTROPHY, OCULO-GASTROINTESTINAL*

---

## MUSCULAR DYSTROPHY, OCULOPHARYNGEAL          0692

**Includes:**
Oculopharyngeal muscular dystrophy
Oculopharyngeal myopathy
Pharyngeal muscular dystrophy

**Excludes:**
Bulbar weakness and ptosis, other causes of
**Muscular dystrophy** (other)
Myasthenia gravis
**Myotonic dystrophy** (0702)

**Major Diagnostic Criteria:** Adult onset of ptosis and pharyngeal muscle weakness, along with a positive family history of this condition, or a muscle biopsy disclosing myopathic or dystrophic features, with rimmed vacuoles and intra-nuclear filamentous inclusion.

**Clinical Findings:** Late-onset bilateral ptosis of the eyelids and progressive dysphagia. The onset of weakness of those involved muscle groups may occur anywhere from the fourth to eighth decades. There may be progressive ptosis, necessitating correction of the ptotic defect. Dysphagia often proves to be progressive with increasing difficulty in handling solid foods and eventually in handling fluids. After being present for 1–2 decades in the above mentioned muscle groups, mild evidence of proximal muscle weakness develops in the shoulder and pelvic girdles.

There are no definitive laboratory tests aside from muscle biopsies that are helpful in this condition. Serum enzymes, such as creatine kinase (CK), are invariably normal or only mildly elevated. Electromyography of the involved muscles may disclose a "myopathic pattern", but this type of study is rarely done.

**Complications:** Aspiration pneumonitis or other problems associated with serious swallowing difficulty may supervene at any time, especially late in the course of the disease.

**Associated Findings:** **Ophthalmoplegia**, **Retinitis pigmentosa**, and distal wasting.

**Etiology:** Autosomal dominant inheritance.

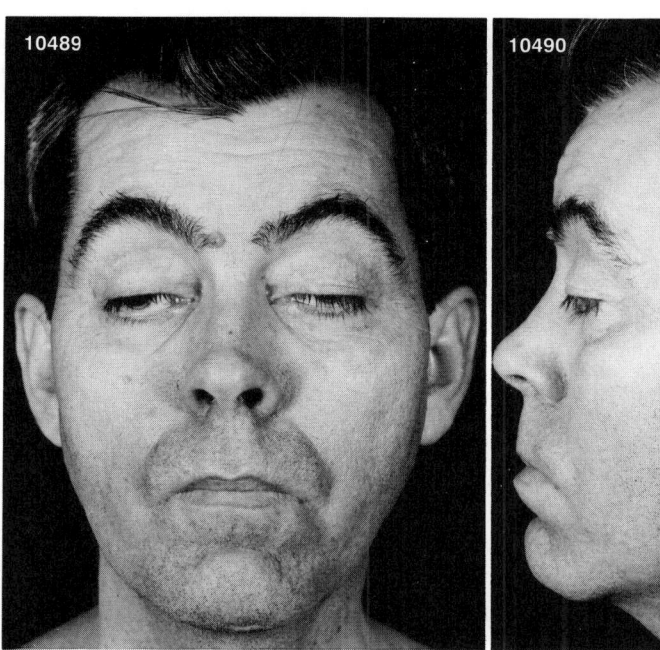

**0692-10489–90:** Muscular weakness produces bilateral ptosis and an expressionless face.

**Pathogenesis:** Progressive deterioration of the muscle fibers.

**MIM No.:** *16430

**POS No.:** 4328

**Sex Ratio:** M1:F1

**Occurrence:** Undetermined. Many affected individuals are of French Canadian descent, and can be traced to one common ancestor who landed in Quebec in 1634. Also reported in Melanesian and Swiss families.

**Risk of Recurrence for Patient's Sib:**
See Part I, *Mendelian Inheritance.*

**Risk of Recurrence for Patient's Child:**
See Part I, *Mendelian Inheritance.*

**Age of Detectability:** Clinically, by the third to fifth decade of life.

**Gene Mapping and Linkage:** Unknown.

**Prevention:** None known. Genetic counseling indicated.

**Treatment:** Supportive measures, such as eyelid crutches to overcome ptotic defect. Operative partial correction of ptosis. Careful nursing and other management to avoid spillover aspiration pneumonitis from dysphagia.

**Prognosis:** Generally good for life span unless the patient develops aspiration pneumonia associated with the dysphagia problem.

**Detection of Carrier:** Unknown.

**Support Groups:**
New York; Muscular Dystrophy Association (MDA)
ENGLAND: London; Muscular Dystrophy Group of Great Britain

**References:**
Victor M, et al.: Oculopharyngeal muscular dystrophy: a familial disease of late life characterized by dysphagia and progressive ptosis of the eyelids. New Engl J Med 1962; 267:1267–1272. *
Murphy SF, Drachman DB: The oculopharyngeal syndrome. JAMA 1968; 203:1003–1008.
Morgan-Hughes JA, Mair WGP: Atypical muscle mitochondria in oculo-skeletal myopathy. Brain 1973; 96:215–224.

Schmitt HP, Krause KH: An autopsy study of a familial oculopharyngeal muscular dystrophy (OPMD) with distal spread and neurogenic involvement. Muscle Nerve 1981; 4:296–305.
Fukuhara N, et al.: Oculopharyngeal muscular dystrophy and distal myopathy. Acta Neurol Scand 1982; 65:458–467.
Scrimgeour EM, Mastaglia FL: Oculopharyngeal and distal myopathy. Am J Med Genet 1984; 17:763–771.

I0000             **Victor V. Ionasescu**
                                   *Walter G. Bradley*

**Muscular dystrophy, pseudohypertrophic adult type**
See *MUSCULAR DYSTROPHY, ADULT PSEUDOHYPERTROPHIC*
**Muscular dystrophy, pseudohypertrophic progressive, Duchenne type**
See *MUSCULAR DYSTROPHY, CHILDHOOD PSEUDOHYPERTROPHIC*
**Muscular dystrophy, tardive with contractures**
See *EMERY-DREIFUSS SYNDROME*
**Muscular dystrophy-cataract-hypogonadism**
See *MYOPATHY-CATARACT-GONADAL DYSGENESIS*
**Muscular dystrophy-cerebroocular dysplasia**
See *WALKER-WARBURG SYNDROME*
**Muscular dystropy-muscular shortening**
See *HAUPTMANN-THANHAUSER SYNDROME*
**Muscular macroglossia**
See *MACROGLOSSIA*
**Muscular septum, defects in various portions of**
See *VENTRICULAR SEPTAL DEFECT*
**Muscular shortening and dystrophy**
See *HAUPTMANN-THANHAUSER SYNDROME*
**Muscular subaortic stenosis**
See *HEART, SUBAORTIC STENOSIS, MUSCULAR*
**Muscular torticollis**
See *TORTICOLLIS*
**Musculo-skeletal-oto-oculo syndrome**
See *OTO-OCULO-MUSCULO-SKELETAL SYNDROME*
**Musicogenic epilepsy**
See *EPILEPSY, REFLEX*

---

**MUTCHINICK SYNDROME**                     **3274**

**Includes:** Mental retardation, Buenes Aires type

**Excludes:**
    **Dwarfism, osteodysplastic primordial, Majewski-Winter type** (2581)
    **Seckel syndrome** (0881)

**Major Diagnostic Criteria:** The combination of short stature, **Microcephaly**, facial anomalies, mental retardation, and mild cardiac and renal anomalies.

**Clinical Findings:** Both of the female sibs in which this condition has been reported had marked short stature, microcephaly, **Eye, hypertelorism**, downslanting palpebral fissures, long and curly eyelashes, broad nose with prominent nasal bridge, wide downturned mouth, highly arched palate, malocclusion, prognathism, large ears, clinodactyly, hyperconvex thumb nails, spasticity, and mental retardation. Both girls had dilation of one or both renal calyces; rotated right kidney was present in one, and dilated right ureter was present in the other as well. Both girls also had **Atrial septal defects**, although one also had right bundle branch block and valvular pulmonic stenosis. Light blonde hair, blue irides, and photophobia were also present in both, which is unusual given the ethnic origin of these children.

**Complications:** Unknown.

**Associated Findings:** None known.

**Etiology:** The presence of consanguinity in the parents suggests that autosomal recessive inheritance is most likely.

**Pathogenesis:** The basic defect is unknown, although a melanin defect as a part of the pleiotropic effect of the gene was suggested by the authors.

**MIM No.:** 24963

**Sex Ratio:** M1:F1

**Occurrence:** One family from Argentina has been described.

**Risk of Recurrence for Patient's Sib:**
See Part I, *Mendelian Inheritance.*

**Risk of Recurrence for Patient's Child:**
See Part I, *Mendelian Inheritance.*

**Age of Detectability:** At birth, by physical examination.

**Gene Mapping and Linkage:** Unknown.

**Prevention:** None known. Genetic counseling indicated.

**Treatment:** Supportive.

**Prognosis:** Mental retardation is present, and the IQ in one child was 42. Life span is unknown since both girls were under the age of eight years at the time of the report.

**Detection of Carrier:** Unknown.

**References:**
Mutchinick O: A syndrome of mental and physical retardation, speech disorders, and peculiar facies in two sisters. J Med Genet 1972; 9:60–63.

T0007                                    **Helga V. Toriello**

**Mutilating keratoderma**
*See DEAFNESS-KERATOPACHYDERMIA-DIGITAL CONSTRICTIONS*
**Myasthenia gravis, familial infantile**
*See MYASTHENIC SYNDROME, FAMILIAL INFANTILE TYPE*
**Myasthenia, familial infantile**
*See MYASTHENIC SYNDROME, FAMILIAL INFANTILE TYPE*

## MYASTHENIC SYNDROME, CONGENITAL SLOW CHANNEL TYPE                           2912

**Includes:** Slow-channel syndrome

**Excludes:**
Autoimmune myasthenia gravis
**Diplegia, congenital facial** (0376)
**Kearns-Sayre disease** (2070)
Lambert-Eaton myasthenic syndrome
**Muscular dystrophy, facio-scapulo-humeral** (2049)
**Muscular dystrophy, limb-girdle** (0691)
**Myasthenic syndrome, familial infantile type** (2913)
Myasthenic syndromes, acquired
Myasthenic syndromes, other
**Myotonic dystrophy** (0702)
**Syringomyelia** (0924)

**Major Diagnostic Criteria:** Abnormal fatigability on exertion; variable weakness of cranial, limb, and trunk muscles; EMG evidence of a repetitive compound muscle action potential evoked by a single nerve stimulus in all rested muscles; abnormally prolonged duration of end-plate potentials and miniature end-plate potentials in all muscles; reduced amplitude of miniature end-plate potentials and a decremental EMG response at 2-Hz stimulation in some muscles.

Acetylcholinesterase activity is intact at all motor end-plates. In clinically affected muscles, the findings include 1) focal degeneration of the junctional folds with concomitant loss of the acetylcholine receptor at the end-plates; 2) degenerative changes in the muscle fibers, most severe near the end-plates; and 3) variable muscle fiber atrophy.

**Clinical Findings:** Weakness and abnormal fatigability occur in all cases. However, the age of onset, the initial and eventual pattern of muscle involvement, the rate of progression, and the degree of weakness and fatigability may vary from case to case. The disease may present in infancy, childhood, or adulthood. In some patients the disease progresses gradually. In others, it progresses intermittently, remaining stationary for years or decades between periods of worsening. The typical clinical findings consist of selectively severe involvement of cervical, scapular, and finger extensor muscles; mild-to-moderate ptosis and limitation of ocular movements with only occasional diplopia; and variable involvement of masticatory, facial, and other upper extremity, respiratory, and trunk muscles. In some patients the lower limbs are spared or are less severely affected than the upper ones. The

clinically affected muscles are weak and atrophic and fatigue abnormally. The weakness and fatigability can fluctuate, but not as rapidly as in acquired autoimmune myasthenia gravis. The deep tendon reflexes are usually normal, but can be reduced in severely affected limbs. The edrophonium test is negative or gives ambiguous results.

Anticholinesterase drugs are either ineffective or provide only slight subjective improvement. The serum creatine kinase level is normal. Tests for circulating antibodies against the acetylcholine receptor are negative.

Differential diagnoses include **Diplegia, congenital facial**, peripheral neuropathy, radial nerve palsy, motor neuron disease, **Syringomyelia**, **Kearns-Sayre disease**, **Muscular dystrophy, limb-girdle**, **Muscular dystrophy, facio-scapulo-humeral**, and **Myotonic dystrophy**. After careful assessment of the clinical and EMG features, each of the above entities can be excluded. Light microscopic muscle biopsy findings may suggest a primary myopathy or neuropathy. However, the concentration of vacuoles and tubular aggregates near the end-plates should suggest the possibility of neuromuscular transmission defect. Electron microscopic studies reveal structural alterations in postsynaptic regions of end-plates in clinically affected muscles.

**Complications:** Feeding difficulty from masticatory or pharyngeal muscle weakness; difficulty in holding the head erect; degenerative changes of the cervical spine from abnormal posture; scoliosis and lordosis. Limb muscle weakness makes activities of daily living difficult.

**Associated Findings:** None known.

**Etiology:** Autosomal dominant inheritance with variable expression. Sporadic cases, possibly from new mutations, can also occur.

**Pathogenesis:** Current theory postulates abnormally slow closure (and hence prolonged opening) of the acetylcholine receptor ion channel at the motor end-plate. This results in an abnormal influx of cations, including calcium, into the junctional folds and into the nearby muscle fiber regions. Degeneration of the junctional folds results in acetylcholine receptor loss and a defect in neuromuscular transmission. Degeneration of the muscle fibers results in a permanent myopathy.

**MIM No.:** 25420

**Sex Ratio:** M1:F1

**Occurrence:** Eight cases have been reported in the literature. Encountered much less frequently than acquired autoimmune myasthenic disorders, such as myasthenia gravis or the Lambert-Eaton myasthenic syndrome.

**Risk of Recurrence for Patient's Sib:**
See Part I, *Mendelian Inheritance.*

**Risk of Recurrence for Patient's Child:**
See Part I, *Mendelian Inheritance.*

**Age of Detectability:** EMG abnormalities are probably present from birth in all cases. Weakness and abnormal fatigability begin in infancy, childhood, or adulthood.

**Gene Mapping and Linkage:** Unknown.

**Prevention:** None known. Genetic counseling indicated.

**Treatment:** Appropriate orthoses may be helpful depending on disability. Anticholinesterase medications are ineffective.

**Prognosis:** Life span is probably not affected. Physical handicaps leading to changes in life style occurred in all affected patients observed to date.

**Detection of Carrier:** Careful EMG studies to detect a repetitive evoked compound muscle action potential evoked by a single nerve stimulus in well rested muscles will identify affected patients even before the onset of abnormal weakness or fatigability.

**Support Groups:**
New York; Myasthenia Gravis Foundation (MGF)
New York; Muscular Dystrophy Association (MDA)

**References:**
Engel AG, et al.: A newly recognized congenital myasthenic syndrome attributed to a prolonged open time of the acetylcholine-induced ion channel. Ann Neurol 1982; 11:553–569.
Engel AG: Myasthenic syndromes. In: Engel AG, Banker BQ, eds: Myology. New York: McGraw-Hill, 1986:1955–1990.
Oosterhuis HJGH, et al.: The slow channel syndrome: two new cases. Brain 1987; 110:1161–1179.

EN005                                        **Andrew G. Engel**

---

## MYASTHENIC SYNDROME, FAMILIAL INFANTILE TYPE    2913

**Includes:**
    Acetylcholine receptor, defect in
    Myasthenia gravis, familial infantile
    Myasthenia, familial infantile

**Excludes:**
    Lambert-Eaton myasthenic syndrome
    Myasthenia gravis, autoimmune
    **Myasthenic syndrome, congenital slow channel type** (2912)
    Myasthenic syndromes, acquired
    Myasthenic syndromes, other

**Major Diagnostic Criteria:** Intermittent myasthenic symptoms from birth associated with crises provoked by stress or fever. A decremental EMG response at 2-Hz stimulation is present only in clinically weak muscles. Weakness can be induced in some, but not all, muscles by exercise or by repetitive indirect stimulation at 10 Hz for a few minutes. The EMG decrement, when present, can be corrected by edrophonium. Tests for antibodies to the acetylcholine receptor are negative. *In vitro* microelectrode studies of neuromuscular transmission demonstrate a normal amplitude of the miniature end-plate potential (MEPP) in rested muscles, but the MEPPs become abnormally small after a 5-minute stimulation at 10 Hz. Ultrastructural studies of the end-plates reveal no abnormalities of the postsynaptic region, and normal amounts of the acetylcholine receptor are present on the junctional folds.

**Clinical Findings:** The typical history is one of fluctuating ptosis from birth; feeding difficulty during infancy; secondary respiratory infections; easy fatigability on exertion; and episodic crises of increased weakness, hypoventilation, or apnea precipitated by crying, vomiting, or fever. The apnea can cause sudden death during infancy or can lead to anoxic brain injury. Between crises the patients appear unaffected or show minimal weakness of cranial or limb muscles. Weakness can be induced by exercise even between crises. The crises decrease in frequency and the symptoms may improve with age.

**Complications:** Sudden death or anoxic brain injury from intermittent episodes of apnea are the most serious complications. Secondary respiratory infections can result from respiratory muscle weakness, and the infection and fever can further worsen the defect of neuromuscular transmission. Abnormal fatigability on exertion can make activities of daily living difficult.

**Associated Findings:** None known.

**Etiology:** Autosomal recessive inheritance.

**Pathogenesis:** Current theory postulates a defect in the resynthesis of acetylcholine in the motor nerve terminal or a defect in the packaging of acetylcholine into the synaptic vesicles.

**MIM No.:** *25421

**Sex Ratio:** M1:F1

**Occurrence:** Fewer than 50 cases have been described to date. The disease is encountered much less frequently than acquired autoimmune myasthenic disorders, such as autoimmune myasthenia gravis or the Lambert-Eaton myasthenic syndrome.

**Risk of Recurrence for Patient's Sib:**
    See Part I, *Mendelian Inheritance.*

**Risk of Recurrence for Patient's Child:**
    See Part I, *Mendelian Inheritance.*

**Age of Detectability:** EMG abnormalities in clinically affected muscles are present from the neonatal period. The symptoms typically present during the neonatal period and occur intermittently thereafter.

**Gene Mapping and Linkage:** Unknown.

**Prevention:** None known. Genetic counseling indicated.

**Treatment:** The muscle weakness, when present, responds well to small or modest doses of anticholinesterase drugs. Some patients are asymptomatic or have only minimal weakness except during crises and require anticholinesterase drugs on an emergency basis only. Parents of affected children must be indoctrinated to anticipate sudden worsening of the weakness and possible apnea with febrile illnesses, excitement, or overexertion. The parents also must be familiar with the use of a hand-assisted ventilatory device and should be able to administer appropriate doses of prostigmine intramuscularly during crises. Patients with a febrile illness and a previous history of crisis should be hospitalized for close observation and ventilatory support as needed.

**Prognosis:** Guarded because of the possibility of sudden death or anoxic brain damage from episodes of apnea.

**Detection of Carrier:** Unknown.

**Special Considerations:** The clinical features of this syndrome have been described in the literature under the rubric of "familial infantile myasthenia." It was recognized as a distinct entity, however, when the autoimmune origin of acquired myasthenia gravis was established and when electrophysiologic and morphologic studies revealed the unique features of this congenital myasthenic syndrome. The differential diagnosis includes autoimmune myasthenia gravis and other congenital myasthenic syndromes. The distinction from autoimmune myasthenia gravis may be difficult if the family history is negative. Although the acetylcholine receptor antibody test is consistently negative in the congenital syndrome, it also can be negative in autoimmune myasthenia gravis, and both disorders respond to anticholinesterase drugs. Careful EMG studies may distinguish between the two entities, but in some patients in vitro studies of neuromuscular transmission and ultrastructural and cytochemical studies of the end-plate are required to clarify the diagnosis.

**Support Groups:** New York; Myasthenia Gravis Foundation (MGF)

**References:**
Hart Z, et al.: A congenital, familial, myasthenic syndrome caused by a presynaptic defect of transmitter resynthesis or mobilization. Neurology 1979; 29:556–557.
Robertson WC, et al.: Familial infantile myasthenia. Arch Neurol 1980; 37:117–119.
Engel AG: Myasthenic syndromes. In: Engel AG, Banker BQ, eds: Myology. New York: McGraw-Hill, 1986:1955–1990.
Mora M, et al.: Synaptic vesicle abnormality in familial infantile myasthenia. Neurology 1987; 37:206–214.

EN005                                        **Andrew G. Engel**

---

**Mycosis fungoides**
    *See LEUKEMIA/LYMPHOMA, T-CELL*
**Mydriasis, congenital**
    *See EYE, IRIDOPLEGIA, FAMILIAL*
**Myelo-Optico neuropathy, subacute**
    *See NEUROPATHY, MYELO-OPTICO, SUBACUTE TYPE*
**Myeloma, multiple**
    *See CANCER, MULTIPLE MYELOMA*
**Myelomatosis**
    *See CANCER, MULTIPLE MYELOMA*
**Myelomeningocele**
    *See MENINGOMYELOCELE*
**Myeloperoxidase deficiency**
    *See IMMUNODEFICIENCY, MYELOPEROXIDASE DEFICIENCY TYPE*
**Myeloschisis**
    *See MENINGOMYELOCELE*
**Myhre syndrome**
    *See GROWTH-MENTAL DEFICIENCY, MYHRE TYPE*

**Myoadenylate deaminase deficiency, myopathy due to**
*See MYOPATHY-METABOLIC, MYOADENYLATE DEAMINASE DEFICIENCY*

**Myocardial hypertrophy-endocardial fibroelastosis**
*See VENTRICLE, ENDOCARDIAL FIBROELASTOSIS OF LEFT VENTRICLE*

**Myoclonic epilepsy, benign**
*See SEIZURES, MYOCLONIC, JUVENILE JANZ TYPE*

---

## MYOCLONIC EPILEPSY-RAGGED RED FIBERS　　　　3225

**Includes:**

Epilepsy, myoclonic-ragged red fibers
MERRF
Ragged red fibers-myoclonic epilepsy

**Excludes:**

**Dentatorubropallidoluysian degeneration, hereditary** (3283)
**Kearns-Sayre disease** (2070)
**Myopathy, mitochondrial-encephalopathy-lactic acidosis-stroke** (3224)
**Myopathy** (other mitochondrial)

**Major Diagnostic Criteria:** Myoclonus, generalized, or myoclonic seizures; ataxia; and myopathy.

**Clinical Findings:** Onset of the disease is before age 20 with myoclonus, which is usually the presenting symptom. Cerebellar ataxia, muscle weakness and generalized or myoclonic seizures are the subsequent symptoms. The disease is frequently familial. These patients were originally described as having a combination of "dyssynergia cerebellaris myoclonica" (Ramsay-Hunt syndrome) and mitochondrial myopathy. The individual clinical features of the disease worsen over time for all patients. However, mildly affected patients have not become moderately affected and moderately affected patients have not become severely affected.

Serum lactate and pyruvate may be elevated. Muscle biopsy reveals an excessive number of structurally abnormal mitochondria on electron microscopy, and numerous ragged red fibers on light microscopy. Conventional EEG findings are highly variable, with generalized epileptiform discharges and a background of slow waves. Very high-amplitude visual and somatosensory evoked responses are also reported. Post mortem examination reveals spongy degeneration of the brain.

**Complications:** Spasticity, hypoventilation.

**Associated Findings:** Sensorineural hearing loss, vestibular dysfunction.

**Etiology:** MERRF syndrome is a maternally inherited mitochondrial disease, like **Myopathy, mitochondrial-encephalopathy-lactic acidosis-stroke** and **Myopathy-metabolic, mitochondrial cytochrome C oxidase deficiency**.

**Pathogenesis:** A mitochondrial enzymatic defect is postulated.

**Sex Ratio:** M1:F1

**Occurrence:** Undetermined but presumed rare.

**Risk of Recurrence for Patient's Sib:** One hundred percent, if the mother is affected.

**Risk of Recurrence for Patient's Child:** If the mother is affected, 100%. The children of an affected male are not at risk.

**Age of Detectability:** Usually between 10 and 20 years of age.

**Gene Mapping and Linkage:** Unknown.

**Prevention:** None known. Genetic counseling indicated.

**Treatment:** Symptomatic treatment of seizures and deafness.

**Prognosis:** Guarded.

**Detection of Carrier:** Unknown.

**References:**

Fukuhara N: Myoclonus epilepsy and mitochondrial myopathy. In: Scarlato G, Cerri C, eds: Mitochondrial pathology in muscle diseases. Padova: Piccini Medical Books, 1983:88–110.
Di Mauro S, et al.: Mitochondrial myopathies. Ann Neurol 1985; 17:521–528.

Rosing HS, et al.: Maternally inherited mitochondrial myopathy and myoclonic epilepsy. Ann Neurol 1985; 17:228–237.
Wallace DC, et al.: Familial mitochondrial encephalopathy myoclonic epilepsy and ragged red fibers. Cell 1988; 55:601–610.

I0000　　　　　　　　　　　　　　　　**Victor V. Ionasescu**

**Myoclonus epilepsy with Lafora bodies progressive**
*See SEIZURES, PROGRESSIVE MYOCLONIC, LAFORA TYPE*

**Myoclonus epilepsy, Unverricht-Lundborg type**
*See SEIZURES, PROGRESSIVE MYOCLONIC, UNVERRICHT-LUNDBORG TYPE*

**Myoclonus syndrome-cherry red spot**
*See MUCOLIPIDOSIS I*

**Myogenic stiff ptosis**
*See EYELID, PTOSIS, CONGENITAL*

**Myoglobinuria, idiopathic recurrent**
*See MYOPATHY-METABOLIC, CARNITINE PALMITYL TRANSFERASE DEFICIENCY*

**Myopathic ophthalmoplegia externa**
*See OPHTHALMOPLEGIA, PROGRESSIVE EXTERNAL*

---

## MYOPATHIES　　　　1500

**Includes:**

"Floppy infant"
Muscular dystrophy

The term *myopathy* designates a primary abnormality of muscle in contrast to denervation atrophy in which muscle fiber, lacking innervation, is secondarily affected. Any attempt to understand the many diverse types of myopathies requires that they be classified into several well-defined clinical and pathologic groups.

The *muscular dystrophies* denote a group of inherited progressive degenerations of muscle without known cause. The particular type of dystrophy is determined by the distribution of the weakness and atrophy, age of onset, associated features, and mode of genetic transmission. As a group, the dystrophies demonstrate a constellation of pathologic alterations characteristic of a primary disease of muscle: striking variation in fiber diameter, prominence of centrally placed nuclei, increase in endomysial connective tissue, and degeneration and loss of muscle fibers. More specifically, in the **Muscular dystrophy, childhood pseudohypertrophic / Muscular dystrophy, adult pseudohypertrophic** type of dystrophy, a muscle membrane defect can be detected (Mokri & Engel, 1975).

In *myotonic* dystrophy, centrally placed nuclei, ringbinden, sacroplasmic masses, and often an increased number of intrafusal muscle fibers are characteristic. In **Muscular dystrophy, oculopharyngeal**, rimmed vacuoles can be detected by histochemical and electron microscope techniques. Intranuclear inclusions consisting of tubular filaments that form tangles or palisades can also be observed in muscle fibers (Tomé & Fardeau, 1980).

In contrast to the muscular dystrophies, the *congenital myopathies* are relatively nonprogressive disorders, and possess a number of common characteristics. In most, a clear pattern of inheritance has been defined. Muscular weakness and thinness, the chief clinical manifestations, usually but not always have their onset early in life. Often the clinical presentation is in infancy, with generalized hypotonia and associated weakness (the "floppy infant"). The weakness is symmetric and usually affects the limb-girdle musculature and proximal limb muscles, although in some infants the weakness may be generalized. Certain congenital myopathies are characterized by particular somatic abnormalities, e.g., **Myopathy, myotubular** with ptosis, and **Myopathy, nemaline** with dysmorphic features such as scoliosis, elongated facies, and high-arched palate.

In all congenital myopathies, the deep tendon reflexes are usually decreased or absent. The concentration of serum creatine kinase is usually not elevated, or if it is, the increase is mild in degree. The electromyogram shows short-duration, small-amplitude, polyphasic motor unit potentials. Motor nerve conduction velocities are normal. All of the diseases within this group have distinguishing, but not necessarily specific, morphologic features. Since diagnosis of these disorders cannot be made with confidence on clinical grounds alone, an accurate method of diagnosis is the muscle biopsy and, more specifically, the application of histochemical and electron microscope techniques.

The study of conventional paraffin-embedded material may disclose no alterations or only nonspecific changes. The use of histochemical and ultrastructural methods provides information about the general histologic pattern of the muscle as well as the individual fiber types as defined by their histochemical reactions, distribution, and selective involvement.

The *mitochondrial myopathies* often present as congenital myopathies, but in addition have an often detectable metabolic abnormality. Abnormalities of mitochondrial metabolism are uncommon but are important features of myopathy and of certain diseases that involve systems other than muscle. The mitochondrial myopathies exhibit prominent and selective alterations in the mitochondrial number, activity, and fine structure. The ragged red fibers and intramitochondrial crystalloid inclusions as detected by electron microscopy characterize most of the mitochondrial myopathies.

The *metabolic myopathies* constitute a vast category of muscle diseases characterized by deviations in anabolic and catabolic biochemical reactions. These encompass such groups of disease as the periodic paralyses (see **Paralysis**), disorders of carbohydrate metabolism (see **Glycogenosis**), **Myopathy, malignant hyperthermia**, toxic myopathies, nutritional deficiencies, and diseases associated with myoglobinuria.

The *endocrine myopathies* form a discrete category of muscle disease, the result of the dysfunction of an endocrine gland.

In the *lipid storage myopathies*, abnormal amounts of lipid accumulate in muscle and constitute the predominant pathologic alteration. Triglycerides are abundant in the lipid deposits. The carnitine deficiency syndromes, in which there is insufficient intracellular free carnitine for either transport of long-chain fatty acids into mitochondria, or for modulation of the intramitochondrial coenzyme A/acyl-coenzyme A ratio, are usually included in the lipid myopathy group (Engel, 1986).

**References:**
Mokri B, Engel AG: Duchenne dystrophy: electron microscopic findings pointing to a basic or early abnormality in the plasma membrane of the muscle fiber. Neurology 1975; 25:1111–1120.
Tomé FMS, Fardeau M: Nuclear inclusions in oculopharyngeal dystrophy. Acta Neuropathol 1980; 49:85–87.
Ionasescu V, Zellweger H: Genetics in neurology. New York: Raven Press, 1983.
Engel AG: Carnitine deficiency syndromes and lipid storage myopathies. In: Engel AG, Banker BQ, eds: Myology. New York: McGraw-Hill, 1986:1663–1696.
Harper PS: The muscular dystrophies. In: Scriver CR, et al, eds: The metabolic basis of inherited disease, 6th ed. New York: McGraw-Hill, 1989:2868–2903. *

BA060                                      **Betty Q. Banker**

**Myopathy (metabolic), lactate transporter defect**
*See ERYTHROCYTE, LACTATE TRANSPORTER DEFECT*
**Myopathy (vacuolar) with glycogen**
*See GLYCOGENOSIS, TYPE IIc*

---

## MYOPATHY OR CARDIOMYOPATHY DUE TO DESMIN DEFECT                                         3072

**Includes:**

Cardiomyopathy due to desmin defect
Desmin defect
Intermediate filament, muscle type
Myopathy with Mallory body-like inclusions
Myopathy with sarcoplamic bodies and intermediate filaments

**Excludes:  Myopathy** (other)

**Major Diagnostic Criteria:**  Nonspecific clinical symptoms of myopathy with variable localization of weakness and atrophy. Diagnosis is confirmed by morphologic and immunohistologic study of muscle biopsies, which show storage of intermediate filaments containing desmin (DES).

**Clinical Findings:**  This disease is very heterogeneous, with three clinical forms: 1) *Distal myopathy with late onset* starts around age 40 years with weakness of the thenar muscles and the hand flexors. It has a more severe course than **Muscular dystrophy, distal.** 2) *Congenital proximal myopathy* is characterized by weakness of facial, shoulder, and pelvic muscles and kyphoscoliosis. Two of four patients developed pulmonary hypertension and cardiac insufficiency from which they died within one year at ages 11 and 13 years. 3) *Cardiomyopathy* is manifested by complete atrioventricular block requiring implantation of a pacemaker. Concentric and obstructive ventricular hypertrophy are also present.

Laboratory findings include normal or myopathic electromyogram, moderately elevated serum creatine kinase, and abnormal electrocardiogram. Muscle biopsy shows myopathic appearance with considerable variation in fiber diameter, multiple central nuclei, fiber splitting, fibrosis, and stored intermediate filaments. In addition, inclusions composed of granular material and intermediate filaments, rich in DES, can be demonstrated by immunofluorescence studies in all three clinical forms.

**Complications:**  Congestive heart failure.

**Associated Findings:**  None known.

**Etiology:**  Autosomal dominant inheritance in the distal myopathy type. The other two clinical types could follow autosomal recessive inheritance.

**Pathogenesis:**  DES is the muscle-specific subunit of the intermediate filaments. The onset of DES expression during muscle development and the redistribution of DES from free cytoplasmic filaments to the Z disk during the formation of myofibrils suggest a role for this gene in muscle differentiation. Accumulation of DES and lack of contractile activity have been reported in muscular dysgenesis by Tassin et al (1988). An increase of phosphorylated DES (three-fold) and DES isovariants (6 vs 3) have been documented by muscle protein electrophoresis and DES-specific antibodies in four cases with autosomal dominant desmin distal myopathy (Rappaport et al, 1988). Their studies suggest that post-translational events affect, in this condition, both the polymerization and the amount of DES intermediate filaments.

**MIM No.:**  *12566

**CDC No.:**  756.880

**Sex Ratio:**  M1:F1

**Occurrence:**  Undetermined. One kindred (Goebel et al, 1980) has been extensively studied.

**Risk of Recurrence for Patient's Sib:**
See Part I, *Mendelian Inheritance.*

**Risk of Recurrence for Patient's Child:**
See Part I, *Mendelian Inheritance.*

**Age of Detectability:**  From birth to age 40 years.

**Gene Mapping and Linkage:**  DES (desmin) has been provisionally mapped to 2.

**Prevention:**  None known. Genetic counseling indicated.

**Treatment:**  Pacemaker implantation is recommended in complete atrioventricular block. Congestive heart failure should be treated by standard procedures.

**Prognosis:**  Variable, depending upon specific symptoms; in particular cardiac involvement can lead to sudden death by acute congestive heart failure (Goebel et al, 1980).

**Detection of Carrier:**  Unknown.

**References:**
Edstrom L, et al.: A new type of hereditary distal myopathy with characteristic sarcoplasmic bodies and intermediate (skeletin) filaments. J Neurol Sci 1980; 47:171–190.
Goebel HH, et al.: A form of congenital muscular dystrophy. Brain Dev 1980; 2:387–400.
Porte A, et al.: Unusual familial cardiomyopathy with storage of intermediate filaments in the cardiac muscular cells. Virchows Arch [Pathol Anat] 1980; 386:43–58.

Stoeckel ME, et al.: An unusual familial cardiomyopathy characterized by aberrant accumulations of desmin-type intermediate filaments. Virchows Arch [Pathol Anat] 1981; 393:53–60.

Fidzianska A, et al.: Mallory body-like inclusions in a hereditary congenital neuromuscular disease. Muscle Nerve 1983; 6:195–200.

Quax W, et al.: The human desmin and vimentin genes are located on different chromosomes. Gene 1985; 38:189–196.

Rappaport L, et al.: Storage of phosphorylated desmin in a familial myopathy. FEBS Lett 1988; 231:421–425.

Tassin AM, et al.: Unusual organization of desmin intermediate filaments in muscular dysgenesis and tetrodotoxin-treated myotubes. Dev Biol 1988; 129:37–47.

I0000                                          **Victor V. Ionasescu**

**Myopathy with Mallory body-like inclusions**
*See MYOPATHY OR CARDIOMYOPATHY DUE TO DESMIN DEFECT*
**Myopathy with sarcoplamic bodies and intermediate filaments**
*See MYOPATHY OR CARDIOMYOPATHY DUE TO DESMIN DEFECT*
**Myopathy with storage of glycoproteins and glycosaminoglycans**
*See MYOPATHY-METABOLIC, GLYCOPROTEIN-GLYCOSAMINOGLYCANS STORAGE TYPE*

## MYOPATHY, CENTRAL CORE DISEASE TYPE          0134

**Includes:**
    Central core disease of muscle (CCD)
    Muscular central core disease
    Shy-Magee disease

**Excludes:**
    **Muscular dystrophy, childhood pseudohypertrophic** (0689)
    **Myopathy, myotubular** (0695)
    **Myopathy, nemaline** (0696)

**Major Diagnostic Criteria:**    Nonprogressive or slowly progressive weakness and hypotonia since birth. Family history is positive. Muscle biopsy has well-demarcated cores within most of the muscle fibers.

**Clinical Findings:**    The onset is noted at or shortly after birth. The patient is floppy, weak, and attains motor milestones slowly. Running and jumping are often impossible. The weakness is diffuse but more prominent in the pelvic muscles. Mild weakness of the face and neck muscles may also be seen. The deep tendon reflexes are normal. Skeletal deformities are not uncommon; hip dislocations and kyphoscoliosis are more frequent. In adult life the patients are often slender and short statured but without any focal muscle atrophy. Serum creatine kinase is not elevated.

Electromyography shows nonspecific findings. The muscle biopsy is strikingly abnormal. The center of most of the fibers contains an area that is unreactive with oxidative enzyme histochemistry. With succinic dehydrogenase and nicotinamide adenine dinucleotide dehydrogenase (NADH), the absence of oxidative enzyme activity in the core contrasts sharply with the normal activity in the surrounding muscle fiber. The lack of activity in the core reflects the absence of mitochondria as proven by electron microscopy. On the "unstructured" cores, the absence of phosphorylase activity correlates with the decrease in glycogen. With the ATPase reaction, the reactivity of the central cores is either decreased or on occasion increased. The term "structured cores" indicates the maintenance of a very precise pattern of cross striation with clear retention of A-, I- and Z-banding. In the "unstructured" cores, the A, I and Z bands can still be traced across the cores, but they are markedly disrupted. The number of cores in the biopsies varies widely, from changes affecting 100% of the fibers to those affecting fewer than 20%. Deeply situated fibers contain more cores than superficial ones. Central cores and type 1 fiber predominance are conjoined in the disease.

**Complications:**    Malignant hyperthermia should always be considered in a patient about to undergo surgery. In vitro muscle contraction studies with caffeine and halothane identify those susceptible to malignant hyperthermia.

**Associated Findings:**    Hip dislocation, kyphoscoliosis and other skeletal malformations.

**Etiology:**    Autosomal dominant inheritance in most cases. Five different sibships in three generations of the original family were affected. There have been reports of sporadic cases as well.

**Pathogenesis:**    There are multiple metabolic deficiencies including oxidative enzymes and phosphorylase within the central cores because of the absence of mitochondria. It is possible that the central core morphologic change may be nonspecific and may occur with other types of myopathy in addition to the specific entity to which the name central core disease can be applied. It has been suggested that core formation may be the result of protein synthesis disturbance in the fetal stage of myogenesis. The similar appearance of central cores and target fibers has given rise to the hypothesis that an abnormality of innervation early in the development of muscle is responsible for central core disease. The relation of central cores to type 1 fiber predominance is still unexplained.

**MIM No.:**    *11700
**CDC No.:**    756.880
**Sex Ratio:**    M1:F1
**Occurrence:**    Undetermined. Established literature.
**Risk of Recurrence for Patient's Sib:**
    See Part I, *Mendelian Inheritance.*
**Risk of Recurrence for Patient's Child:**
    See Part I, *Mendelian Inheritance.*
**Age of Detectability:**    Usually within the first year of life.
**Gene Mapping and Linkage:**    Unknown.
**Prevention:**    None known. Genetic counseling indicated.
**Treatment:**    Most patients are so mildly handicapped that no treatment is necessary.
**Prognosis:**    Life expectancy is normal. The disease is non-progressive and is not severely limiting.
**Detection of Carrier:**    Careful clinical muscle evaluation is useful for carrier detection. However, there are documented central core cases by muscle biopsy where the neurologic examinations was normal.

**References:**
Shy GM, Magee KR: A new congenital non-progressive myopathy. Brain 1956; 79:610–621. *
Ionasescu VV: Miopatie congenite. Prospettive in Pediatria 1975; 5:305–315.
Radu H, et al.: Focal abnormalities in mitochondrial distribution in muscle. Acta Neuropathal (Berl) 1977; 39:25–31.
Frank JP, et al.: Central core disease and malignant hyperthermia syndrome. Ann Neurol 1980; 7:11–17.
Gamstorp I: Non-dystrophic myogenic myopathies with onset in infancy or childhood: a review of some congenital syndromes. Acta Paediatr Scand 1982; 71:881–886. *
Fidzianska A, et al.: Is central core disease with structural core a fetal defect? J Neurol 1984; 231:212–219.

I0000                                          **Victor V. Ionasescu**

## MYOPATHY, DISPROPORTIONATE FIBER TYPE I          2056

**Includes:**    Fiber-type disproportion myopathy

**Excludes:**
    **Facio-neuro-skeletal syndrome** (2339)
    Hypotonia, benign congenital
    **Muscular dystrophy** (congenital forms)

**Major Diagnostic Criteria:**    The diagnosis can only be made by muscle biopsy using histochemical staining (ATPase reaction) and histographic analysis. Type I fibers are smallest. The largest fibers are Type II. The difference between the mean fiber diameters of the largest and smallest fiber type is always greater than 12% of the value of the mean diameter of the largest fiber type. The variability coefficient (Standard deviation x 1,000 divided by mean fiber diameter) is less than 250 for the largest fibers. Type I fiber predominance is frequently found.

**Clinical Findings:** Hypotonia and weakness from birth, delayed acquisition of motor milestones (without mental retardation). Hypoflexia or areflexia, highly arched palate, dislocated hips, normal CK, normal or equivocal EMG, normal MNCV.

**Complications:** Death secondary to respiratory failure/paralysis, kyphoscoliosis.

**Associated Findings:** Ophthalmoplegia (see **Eye, fibrosis of the extraocular muscles, generalized**).

**Etiology:** Autosomal recessive inheritance, although sporadic cases have been reported and heterogeneity is likely.

**Pathogenesis:** Unknown. May be neurogenic.

**MIM No.:** *25531

**CDC No.:** 756.880

**Sex Ratio:** Presumably M1:F1.

**Occurrence:** Undetermined but presumably rare.

**Risk of Recurrence for Patient's Sib:** Unknown.

**Risk of Recurrence for Patient's Child:** Unknown.

**Age of Detectability:** In infancy, from muscle using the criteria of Dubowitz (1985).

**Gene Mapping and Linkage:** Unknown.

**Prevention:** None known. Genetic counseling indicated.

**Treatment:** Symptomatic, for muscle weakness.

**Prognosis:** Unknown.

**Detection of Carrier:** Unknown.

**References:**

Cavanagh NPC, et al.: Congenital fibre type disproportion myopathy: a histological diagnosis with an uncertain clinical outlook. Arch Dis Child 1979; 54:735–743.

Clancy RR, et al.: Clinical variability in congenital fiber type disproportion. J Neurol Sci 1980; 46:257–266.

Dubowitz V: Muscle biopsy: a practical approach. Philadelphia: W.B. Saunders, 1985:460–462.

Brooke MH: A clinician's view of neuromuscular disease, 2nd ed. Baltimore: Williams and Wilkins, 1986:355–359.

Jaffe M, et al.: Familial congenital fiber type disproportion (CFTD) with an autosomal recessive inheritance. Clin Genet 1988; 33:33–37.

HA015                                                          **Jerome S. Haller**

---

## MYOPATHY, FAMILIAL LYSIS OF TYPE I FIBERS       2059

**Includes:** Lysis of type I fibers, familial

**Excludes:** **Myopathy** (others)

**Major Diagnostic Criteria:** A nonprogressive proximal weakness is present from early infancy. The affected children are slow to pass their motor milestones. Serum creatine kinase may be elevated (2/3). A muscle biopsy, which is essential to establish the diagnosis, and must include histochemical and electron microscopic studies. Nerve conduction studies are normal (1/1). Electromyography may reveal a myopathic pattern (1/2) or may be normal.

**Clinical Findings:** Affected children are inactive, weak, and hypotonic from birth; they pass their motor milestones very slowly. The weakness is generalized and symmetric and is most marked in the proximal limb muscles. A lumbar lordosis may develop early in life (2/3). The affected muscles are thinned.

**Complications:** Lumbar lordosis may be observed when the child begins to ambulate.

**Associated Findings:** The sternocleidomastoid and trapezius muscles may be absent (1/3).

**Etiology:** Probably autosomal recessive inheritance.

**Pathogenesis:** The pathologic features of the muscle biopsy specimen are similar in each case (3/3). The diameter of the muscle fibers is either normal or small, and the muscle fibers tend to cluster into these two groups. The cytoplasm of the smaller fibers is divided into a central area containing myofibrils with striations and a peripheral zone that lacks organized contractile substance and appears homogenized. The larger fibers are identified histochemically as type II and the smaller ones as type I. In the involved type I fibers the peripheral zones contain no oxidative enzyme activity, but the myosin ATPase activity is intense. The electron microscopic study of these affected type I fibers demonstrates an absence of myofibrils at the periphery. In such zones, the sarcoplasm consists of a fine granular matrix containing nuclei, scattered mitochondria, and dense granules resembling glycogen. There is an abrupt transition to the more central areas of the muscle fiber where the myofibrils are normal. The structure of the type 2 fibers is normal. It has been postulated that the myofibrils in the peripheral zones of the type I fibers have been lysed.

**MIM No.:** 25516

**CDC No.:** 756.880

**Sex Ratio:** Presumably M1:F1 (M1:F2 observed).

**Occurrence:** Two reports, covering three cases, have appeared in the literature. In one family, two of six sibs were clinically affected.

**Risk of Recurrence for Patient's Sib:**
See Part I, *Mendelian Inheritance*. In a family of six sibs, two children (a boy and a girl) were affected. The parents are said to be normal, although there are no descriptions of their examination. The parents have not been subjected to muscle biopsy or to serum creatine kinase testing.

**Risk of Recurrence for Patient's Child:**
See Part I, *Mendelian Inheritance*.

**Age of Detectability:** The proximal weakness is discovered when the child begins to ambulate.

**Gene Mapping and Linkage:** Unknown.

**Prevention:** None known. Genetic counseling indicated.

**Treatment:** Prevention of the accentuation of the lordosis.

**Prognosis:** This disorder appears to be a nonprogressive congenital myopathy.

**Detection of Carrier:** Unknown.

**References:**

Cancilla PA, et al.: Familial myopathy with probable lysis of myofibrils in type 1 fibers. Neurology 1971; 21:579–585.

Sahgal V, Sahgal S: A new congenital myopathy: a morphological, cytochemical and histochemical study. Acta Neuropathol 1977; 37:225–230.

Banker BQ: The congenital myopathies In: Engel AG, Banker BQ, eds: Myology. New York: McGraw-Hill, 1986:1570.

BA060                                                          **Betty Q. Banker**

**Myopathy, late distal hereditary**
See MUSCULAR DYSTROPHY, DISTAL
**Myopathy, lipid storage (one form)**
See OVERGROWTH, RUVALCABA-MYHRE-SMITH TYPE

---

## MYOPATHY, MALIGNANT HYPERTHERMIA       2710

**Includes:**
Anesthesia, malignant hyperthermia susceptibility
Duchenne muscular dystrophy (atypical cases)
Hyperthermia of anesthesia
Malignant hyperpyrexia
Malignant hyperthermia
Sudden infant death syndrome (SIDS), one theory of

**Excludes:**
Hyperthermia associated with hypercalcemia
Hyperthermia associated with hyperthyroidism
Hyperthermia associated with polymyositis

**Major Diagnostic Criteria:** The diagnosis is suspected whenever tachycardia, muscle rigidity, hyperthermia, and metabolic acidosis develop during or after general anesthesia induced by volatile hydrocarbon anesthetics (halothane) and depolarizing muscle relaxants (succinylcholine). Pre-existing neuromuscular disorder and, in particular, a hereditary myopathy are important diagnostic indicators.

**Clinical Findings:** The characteristic features appear during or shortly after general anesthesia. Masseter spasm may be the only sign; tachycardia (tachyarrythmia), however, is the most common presenting sign and is the forerunner of the forthcoming disaster of hyperthermia, muscle rigidity, and respiratory and metabolic (lactic) acidosis with profound derangement of calcium, potassium, phosphate, and glucose metabolism within the muscle fiber. Rhabdomyolysis with markedly elevated serum creatine kinase (CK) and myoglobin levels and the infrequent disseminated intravascular coagulation are late features. These two features usually indicate a delay in diagnosis and management of the malignant hyperthermia and the preceding myopathy. A history of previous uneventful anesthesia is present in 30% of the patients.

**Complications:** Cardiac arrest and disseminated intravascular coagulopathy cause the 10% mortality of malignant hyperthermia (down from 70% in the 1970s; early diagnosis and dantrolene therapy are responsible for the reduced mortality).

**Associated Findings:** Those of the pre-existing myopathy or syndrome. Malignant hyperthermia also occurs more frequently with surgery for ptosis, strabismus, dislocations, and herniorrhaphies. Pre-existing conditions include central core disease of muscle, **Muscular dystrophy, childhood pseudohypertrophic, Kniest dysplasia, King syndrome, Myotonia congenita**, Evans myopathy, and Barnes muscular dystrophy.

**Etiology:** Usually autosomal dominant inheritance, although cases reflect the heterogeneity of malignant hyperthermia. Families with "isolated" malignant hyperthermia also have demonstrated autosomal dominant inheritance by showing elevated serum CK in several unaffected relatives. **King syndrome** is a sporadic condition, and the sibs with **Noonan syndrome**-like phenotype and contractures imply autosomal recessive inheritance. **Muscular dystrophy, childhood pseudohypertrophic** is an X-linked recessive trait.

**Pathogenesis:** Malignant hyperthermia is among the best examples of pharmacogenetic disorders. The administration of the anesthetic is necessary for the hypermetabolic state to occur. The skeletal muscle fiber appears to be the site of the primary defect. In addition to the aberrant intracellular calcium metabolism that leads to muscle contractures with catabolic generation of heat, tubular, mitochondrial, and sarcolemmal dysfunctions have also been suggested in some studies; and enhanced activity of phospholipase A has been encountered. The abnormal calcium uptake into the mitochondria leads to uncoupled phosphorylation with a low ATP/ADP ratio. The latter spurs heat production, increases the permeability of the muscle membrane, and diminishes the activity of the calcium pump of the sarcoplasmic reticulum. Extremely stable low-energy myosin-actin complexes (rigor complexes) cause the muscle rigidity.

**MIM No.:**  *14560

**POS No.:**  4183

**CDC No.:**  756.880

**Sex Ratio:**  Presumably M1:F1 for the families with "isolated" malignant hyperthermia.

**Occurrence:**  In the United States, accepted incidence figures for malignant hyperthermia are 1:14,000 pediatric anesthesias and 1:40,000 adult anesthesias. These figures may represent underestimates; based on paradoxical increases in masseter tone following succinylcholine administration, the incidence in pediatric anesthesias may be as high as 1:100

**Risk of Recurrence for Patient's Sib:**
See Part I, *Mendelian Inheritance*. Depends on the etiology of the pre-existing condition; thus, it varies from 0–50%.

**Risk of Recurrence for Patient's Child:**
See Part I, *Mendelian Inheritance*. Depends on the etiology of the pre-existing condition.

**Age of Detectability:**  Whenever the malignant hyperthermia is encountered. The susceptibility of a particular individual in a family could be determined in advance by *in vitro* testing of the contractibility of skeletal muscle fibers exposed to halothane or caffeine. The testing requires a muscle biopsy and a specialized laboratory, and it is not yet a part of standard medical care.

**Gene Mapping and Linkage:**  Unknown.

**Prevention:**  Determination of malignant hyperthermia susceptibility prior to surgery appears to be the best prevention. CK determinations are the simplest and least reliable testing for malignant hyperthermia susceptibility. *In vitro* muscle fiber response to halothane provides the highest yield (88%). The suggested platelet ATP pool assay appears to be promising, but it requires further testing. Capnography during anesthesia appears to be reliable for the early diagnosis and treatment of malignant hyperthermia. It is based on the early rise of end tidal carbon dioxide in the development of the hyperthermia. According to some reports, oral prophylaxis with dantrolene is an effective preventive measure.

**Treatment:**  Intravenous dantrolene 2.5 mg/kg (mean dose) is life-saving. Intensive symptomatic treatment is also necessary.

**Prognosis:**  The prognosis of malignant hyperthermia has been improved considerably by dantrolene treatment. The mortality rate has been reduced from 70 to 10%. Thus, the long-term prognosis equals that of the underlying pre-existing myopathy or syndrome.

**Detection of Carrier:**  As for the pre-existing conditions. A CT scan of the extremities of patients with **King syndrome** may detect areas of degeneration and fatty infiltration within the muscles.

**Special Considerations:**  The hyperthermia in **Muscular dystrophy, childhood pseudohypertrophic** appears to be somewhat different from the malignant hyperthermia of the other myopathies and syndromes. Bradycardia, instead of tachycardia, is the usual presenting sign, and temperature elevations are rare and small. Rigidity is hardly encountered. Whenever administered, dantrolene did not alter the course of the metabolic catastrophe in these patients. Thus, the anesthetic reactions in this condition may not be a true malignant hyperthermia.

The association of malignant hyperthermia and sudden infant death syndrome (SIDS) is unclear. It is probably not coincidental that five of 15 parents of SIDS victims had muscle membrane dysfunction, despite normal CK levels and muscle electron microscopy. In addition, pathologic findings in the bowel of victims of SIDS have shown similarity to those of heat stroke.

**Support Groups:**  CT; Darien; Malignant Hyperthemia Association of the United States (MHAUS)

**References:**
Guedel AE: Inhalation anesthesia, ed 2. New York: McMillan, 1951: 110.

Karpati G, Watters GV: Adverse anesthetic reactions in Duchenne dystrophy. In: Angelini C, et al., eds: Muscular dystrophy research: advances and new trends. International Congress Series No. 527. Amsterdam: Excerpta Medica, 1980:206–217.

Denborough MA, et al.: Malignant hyperpyrexia and sudden infant death. Lancet 1982; II:1068–1069.

Ording H, et al.: Investigation of malignant hyperthermia in Denmark and Sweden. Br J Anaesth 1984; 56:1183–1190.

Willner J: Malignant hyperthermia. Pediatr Ann 1984; 13:128–132.

Kousseff BG, Nichols P: A new autosomal recessive syndrome with Noonan-like phenotype, myopathy with congenital contractures and malignant hyperthermia. BD:OAS XXI(2). New York: March of Dimes Birth Defects Foundation, 1985:111–117.

Steenson AJ, Torkelson RD: King's syndrome with malignant hyperthermia: potential outpatient risks. Am J Dis Child 1987; 141:271–273.

K0018 **Boris G. Kousseff**

**Myopathy, mitochondrial-cataract**
*See MYOPATHY-CATARACT-GONADAL DYSGENESIS*

## MYOPATHY, MITOCHONDRIAL-ENCEPHALOPATHY-LACTIC ACIDOSIS-STROKE                                    3224

**Includes:**

Encephalopathy-lactic acidosis-mitochondrial myopathy
Lactic acidosis-mitochondrial myopathy-encephalopathy
MELAS
Strokelike episodes

**Excludes:**

**Brain, spongy degeneration** (0115)
**Kearns-Sayre disease** (2070)
**Myoclonic epilepsy-ragged red fibers** (3225)
**Myopathy** (other mitochondrial)

**Major Diagnostic Criteria:**  Patients are usually normal at birth and during the first years of life, then they show stunted growth, episodic vomiting with symptoms of MELAS (seizures, hemiparesis, etc) beginning between ages three and 11 years. Significant cerebellar dysfunction and interictal myoclonus are absent, allowing clinical differential diagnosis from **Myoclonic epilepsy-ragged red fibers**. Heart block, ophthalmoplegia, and retinal pigmentary changes are not found, in contrast to **Kearns-Sayre disease**.

**Clinical Findings:**  Lactate is elevated in the blood and/or cerebrospinal fluid, with values above 4 $\mu$m/l. Activities of pyruvate carboxylase and pyruvate dehydrogenase enzyme were reported normal in cultured skin fibroblasts, except in one case (Monnens et al, 1975). Two cases of MELAS syndrome showed NADH-coenzyme Q reductase deficiency (Kobayashi et al, 1987). In all cases, muscle biopsy studies demonstrated ragged red fibers indicative of mitochondrial dysfunction. Computerized axial tomography of the brain revealed low density areas of the cortex and basal ganglia. Post mortem examination showed spongy degeneration of the brain.

**Complications:**  Dementia was reported in many patients.

**Associated Findings:**  Neurosensory hearing loss.

**Etiology:**  The hereditary transmission of MELAS syndrome, as in other primary mitochondrial diseases, is non-Mendelian and based on maternal inheritance. At least two pairs of affected siblings have been reported.

**Pathogenesis:**  It is postulated that MELAS syndrome is related to disturbed energy supply of the brain and muscle caused by a mitochondrial enzyme defect and lactate toxicity. High levels of lactate destroy neurons and cause vessel proliferation or intimal abnormalities of tissues.

**CDC No.:**  756.880

**Sex Ratio:**  M1:F1

**Occurrence:**  Undetermined but presumed rare.

**Risk of Recurrence for Patient's Sib:**  One hundred percent, if the mother is affected.

**Risk of Recurrence for Patient's Child:**  If the mother is affected, 100%. An affected mother would pass the disease to all her children, but only her daughters would transmit the trait to subsequent generations. The children of an affected male are not at risk.

**Age of Detectability:**  Usually between three and 11 years of age.

**Gene Mapping and Linkage:**  Unknown.

**Prevention:**  None known. Genetic counseling indicated.

**Treatment:**  Symptomatic treatment of seizures, hemiparesis, and deafness.

**Prognosis:**  Guarded.

**Detection of Carrier:**  Unknown.

**References:**

Monnens L, et al.: A metabolic myopathy associated with chronic lactic acidemia, growth failure and nerve deafness. J Pediatric 1975; 86:983–986.
Pavlakis SG, et al.: Mitochondrial myopathy, encephalopathy, lactic acidosis and strokelike episodes: a distinctive clinical syndrome. Ann Neurol 1984; 16:481–488.
Cohen SR: Why does the brain make lactate? J Theor Biol 1985; 112:429–432.
Di Mauro S, et al.: Mitochondrial myopathies. Ann Neurol 1985; 17:521–528.
Kobayashi M, et al.: Two cases of NADH-coenzyme Q reductase deficiency: relationships to MELAS syndrome. J Pediatr 1987; 110: 223–227.

I0000                                              **Victor V. Ionassescu**

## MYOPATHY, MYOGLOBINURIA-ABNORMAL GLYCOLOSIS, HEREDITARY TYPE                                    2058

**Includes:**

Lactic acidosis-myopathy
Myopathy-lactic acidosis

**Excludes:**

**Glycogen storage disease**
Lactic acidosis, chronic
**Paralysis, hypokalemic periodic** (0795)
Paroxysmal myoglobinuria

**Major Diagnostic Criteria:**  Elevated serum lactate and pyruvate with exercise. Muscle biopsy during acute phase shows necrotic fibers and degeneration. In the chronic phase degeneration appears to be complete. No evidence of fatty replacement, increased connective tissue, or glycogen accumulation within muscle fibers.

**Clinical Findings:**  Fatigue, dyspnea, and tachycardia with slight to moderate exercise pain, tenderness, weakness of exercised muscles, hypertrophied calves, nausea, vomiting with complaints beginning in childhood, dark urine present during acute episodes of extreme weakness and severe muscle pain (myoglobinuria).

**Complications:**  Periods of muscle weakness requiring prolonged bed rest for recovery.

**Associated Findings:**  Sideroblastic anemia.

**Etiology:**  Autosomal recessive inheritance.

**Pathogenesis:**  Unknown.

**MIM No.:**  *25515

**CDC No.:**  756.880

**Sex Ratio:**  Presumably M1:F1.

**Occurrence:**  Fourteen patients from five Swedish families (two with consanguinity) have been described. Two brothers with the same or similar condition have since been reported.

**Risk of Recurrence for Patient's Sib:**
See Part I, *Mendelian Inheritance.*

**Risk of Recurrence for Patient's Child:**
See Part I, *Mendelian Inheritance.*

**Age of Detectability:**  Several patients have been identified in their teens.

**Gene Mapping and Linkage:**  Unknown.

**Prevention:**  None known. Genetic counseling indicated.

**Treatment:**  Symptomatic.

**Prognosis:**  Unknown.

**Detection of Carrier:**  Calf hypertrophy has been found in healthy relatives and sibs in 1:5 affected families.

**References:**

Larsson LE, et al.: Hereditary metabolic myopathy with myoglobinuria due to abnormal glycolysis. J Neurol Neurosurg Psychiat 1964; 27:361–380.
Linderholm H, et al.: Hereditary abnormal muscle metabolism with hyperkinetic circulation during exercise. Acta Med Scand 1969; 185:153–166.
Rawles JM, Weller RO: Familial association of metabolic myopathy, lactic acidosis and sideroblastic anemia. Am J Med 1974; 56:891–897.

HA015                                              **Jerome S. Haller**

## MYOPATHY, MYOTUBULAR      0695

**Includes:**
> Centronuclear myopathy
> Myotubular myopathy
> Myotubular myopathy, X-linked

**Excludes:** Myopathy (others)

**Major Diagnostic Criteria:** Early childhood onset with weakness of extraocular, facial, neck, and limb musculature, and a slow progressive course. Genetic heterogeneity is present; characteristic histopathology consists of predominance of atrophic type I fibers, most of them containing centrally placed nuclei.

**Clinical Findings:** There are three types of the disease:

*Congenital type with an autosomal recessive inheritance* is characterized by respiratory distress in the newborn period. Dysmorphic features such as elongated, thin facies and high-arched palate are often present. Ptosis, strabismus, facial weakness, weak crying and sucking, weakness, and atrophy of sternocleidomastoids and of the extremities are the main symptoms. The muscular weakness is diffuse but more severe in a proximal distribution. Speech is often nasal in quality. Talipes equinovarus deformity becomes apparent after the child begins to walk. The deep tendon reflexes are depressed or absent; sensation is entirely normal. In the first 12 years of life, there is usually a slow progression of the weakness and often scoliosis, accentuated lordosis, and winging of the scapulae appear. By adolescence or early adult life, many patients are confined to a wheelchair. Approximately 18% develop seizures which are well controlled by antiepileptic medication.

*Congenital X-linked recessive type* has similar symptoms to the autosomal recessive phenotype, but is more severe, with high mortality in infancy. Respiratory distress due to weakness of respiratory muscles is usually the main symptom. The affected infants are weak and hypotonic with poor cry, sucking, and coughing; weak neck muscles, and an inability to swallow. Bilateral ptosis, facial diplegia, and limitation of eye movements have been observed in some infants. Deep tendon reflexes are absent but the infant's response to painful stimuli is normal. Maternal polyhydramnios is often noted, and a history of abortions and neonatal death of males is frequent. Cardiomyopathy has also been reported.

*Autosomal dominant type* has its onset between the first and third decades. The muscular weakness shows limb-girdle distribution with slow progressivity. In addition, the weakness may involve facial musculature, but not ocular or pharyngeal muscles. All patients have increasing difficulty in walking, and are eventually confined only in a mother and daughter.

The diagnosis of centronuclear myopathy types can be made only based on the histologic features of the muscle biopsy. Alterations are present in all muscles. The central position of muscle nuclei, which constitutes the common major feature, can be evaluated by hematoxylin and eosin or Gomori trichrome stain in at least 50% of the muscle fibers. The nuclei are usually surrounded by a clear halo. There are usually two populations of muscle fibers: atrophic type 1 fibers and normal type 2 fibers. Usually the type 1 fibers predominate. The perinuclear halo may lack enzymatic activity and myofibrils. Clusters of mitochondria, lipopigments, glycogen, autophagic vacuoles, rough endoplasmic reticulum, and Golgi complexes are frequently observed in the perinuclear central zone. Post mortem examination of the central and peripheral nervous system in the autosomal recessive and X-linked recessive types showed no abnormalities. Serum creatine kinase level revealed either normal or slightly elevated levels. Electromyographic studies were considered "myopathic" in three reports with brief, small amplitude, polyphasic motor potentials.

**Complications:** Aspiration pneumonitis, secondary to respiratory distress; congestive heart failure, secondary to cardiomyopathy.

**Associated Findings:** Epilepsy.

**Etiology:** Three forms; with autosomal recessive, X-linked recessive, or autosomal dominant inheritance.

**Pathogenesis:** The primary defect appears to be in the muscle fiber but its nature is unknown.

**MIM No.:** *16015, 25520, *31040

**CDC No.:** 756.880

**Sex Ratio:** M1:F1.5 in autosomal recessive form; M2:F1 in autosomal dominant form, and M1:F0 in X-linked recessive form.

**Occurrence:** The autosomal recessive form has been described in many parts of the world. In contrast to the other congenital myopathies, there appears to be a higher incidence of involvement of Blacks (seven families reported). The original family of X-linked recessive form described the disorder in five affected males belonging to four sibships connected through females who in two instances showed partial manifestations consistent with carrier state on muscle biopsy. The original pedigree of the autosomal dominant form had sixteen affected members in five generations of a large family. The exact incidence of the disease is not known in any of its three forms.

**Risk of Recurrence for Patient's Sib:**
> See Part I, *Mendelian Inheritance.*

**Risk of Recurrence for Patient's Child:**
> See Part I, *Mendelian Inheritance.*

**Age of Detectability:** Age one year or less for the autosomal recessive and X-linked recessive form; 10–30 years for the autosomal dominant form.

**Gene Mapping and Linkage:** MTM1 (myotubular myopathy 1) has been provisionally mapped to Xq27-q28.

**Prevention:** None known. Genetic counseling indicated.

**Treatment:** Focused on the respiratory distress syndrome in the autosomal recessive and X-linked recessive forms, with poor results. Antiepileptic medication is used successfully when seizures appear. Supportive treatment with stretching exercises and wheelchair confinement is recommended in the autosomal dominant form.

**Prognosis:** Very poor in the X-linked recessive form. Most of the patients die in infancy due to the severe weakness of the intercostals and of the diaphragm. the prognosis is fair in the other two forms.

**Detection of Carrier:** Possible only in the X-linked recessive form by muscle biopsy.

**References:**
Spiro AJ, et al.: Myotubular myopathy. Arch Neurol 1966; 14:1–14.*
Schochet SS, et al.: Centronuclear myopathy: disease entity or a syndrome? J Neurol Sci 1972; 16:215–228. *
Bruyland M, et al.: Neonatal myotubular myopathy with a probable X-linked inheritance: observations on a new family with a review of the literature. J Neurol 1984; 231:220–222.
Goebel HH, et al.: Centronuclear myopathy with special consideration of the adult form. Eur Neurol 1984; 23:425–434.
Torres CF, et al.: Severe neonatal centronuclear myopathy with autosomal dominant inheritance. Arch Neurol 1985; 42:1011–1014.
Keppen LD, et al.: X-linked myotubular myopathy: intrafamilial variability and normal muscle biopsy in a heterozygous female. Clin Genet 1987; 32:95–99.

10000                     **Victor V. Ionasescu**

## MYOPATHY, NEMALINE      0696

**Includes:**
> Nemaline myopathy
> Rod body myopathy

**Excludes:** Myopathy (others)

**Major Diagnostic Criteria:** Weakness, hypotonia, and dysmorphic features; usually congenital onset and nonprogressive or slowly progressive course. Muscle biopsy with appropriate stains shows nemaline rods.

**Clinical Findings:** There are three clinical types:
*Congenital nonprogressive or slowly progressive myopathy* is the

most common type. Clinical signs and symptoms become apparent in infancy and include mild weakness and hypotonia. The weakness is greater in proximal than in distal muscles. Some children have only delayed motor milestones. In others there is involvement of muscles innervated by cranial nerves, particularly the facial and masticatory muscles. The eye muscles are usually spared. The deep tendon reflexes are decreased or absent. The extremities appear slender due to muscle underdevelopment. Dysmorphic features are often present and include elongated face, small jaw, and narrow and highly arched palate. Skeletal malformations, i.e. kyphosis, lordosis, pes cavus, and talipes equinovarus, are sometimes present.

*Congenital rapidly fatal myopathy.* Infants with this form display severe intercostal and diaphragmatic weakness superimposed on generalized weakness and muscular hypotonia with little spontaneous motor activity. Deep tendon reflexes and Moro response are absent. The infants are often cyanotic and require respiratory assistance. Accumulation of pharyngeal secretions, and feeding difficulties with aspiration, result in frequent bouts of pneumonia and death usually in the first year of life.

*Adult onset myopathy* is characterized by scapuloperoneal weakness with significant foot-drop. Dysmorphic features are usually absent. Cardiomyopathy has been reported as a prominent feature and may be the cause of sudden death. Otherwise, this form has a slow progression.

Laboratory studies are noncontributory except for muscle biopsy. Only rarely is the serum creatine kinase elevated. Electromyography shows brief duration, small amplitude, and abundant polyphasic motor unit potentials. The muscle biopsy (Bouin or Zenker fixation and phosphotungstic acid hematoxylin staining) shows nemaline rods which measure 1 to 7 $\mu$m in length and 0.3 to 3 $\mu$m in width. Their distribution is random with a tendency to cluster in subsarcolemmal and paranuclear locations. Most patients also have type 1 fiber predominance (up to 90% of fibers), while type 2 fibers are sparse or absent. There is often type 1 fiber atrophy, particularly in the congenital types. The electron microscopic features consist of the accumulation of nemaline bodies and enlargement and streaming of the Z disks. The rods are contiguous with thin filaments and display periodic lines parallel and perpendicular to their long axis.

**Complications:** Congestive heart failure secondary to cardiomyopathy, and recurrent pneumonia secondary to weakness of respiratory muscles.

**Associated Findings:** Mandibular hypoplasia, high-arched palate, kyphoscoliosis, pes cavus, talipes equinovarus.

**Etiology:** Autosomal dominant inheritance with incomplete penetrance in most cases. The disorder has been well documented in successive generations. The lack of transmission from father to son has been emphasized, and the possibility of an X-linked dominant form has been raised. Autosomal recessive inheritance has been claimed in two families based on the finding that both parents of each index patient had rods, and an increased number of fibers with central nuclei; a presumed heterozygote manifestation.

**Pathogenesis:** Nemaline rods are thought to originate from the Z disks. Experiments in which electron microscopic studies were combined with biochemical and immunological techniques suggested that a major component of the nemaline rods was alpha-actinin. Desmin, another structural protein of muscle, accumulates at the periphery of the Z disk as well as of nemaline rods. The total amount of muscle alpha-actinin in two patients with congenital nemaline myopathy was increased two-to-three fold. Abnormalities in the light-chain composition of fast myosin, such as absence of LC3F and markedly decreased levels of LC2F and LC1F, were also reported in the muscle of some patients with this illness. There was also evidence of dipeptidyl-peptidase I deficiency, a protease that may participate in post-translational modification of proteins that are to be assembled into Z lines or, alternatively, in the disassembly and degradation of Z-line material.

**MIM No.:** *16180, *25603

**CDC No.:** 756.880

**Sex Ratio:** M1:F>1. The vast majority of patients are female.

**Occurrence:** Occurs worldwide. The exact incidence and prevalence are not known.

**Risk of Recurrence for Patient's Sib:**
See Part I, *Mendelian Inheritance.*

**Risk of Recurrence for Patient's Child:**
See Part I, *Mendelian Inheritance.*

**Age of Detectability:** Clinically, at early childhood or young adult age.

**Gene Mapping and Linkage:** Unknown.

**Prevention:** None known. Genetic counseling indicated.

**Treatment:** Respiratory assistance in congenital types. Treatment of congestive heart failure in severe cardiomyopathy. Physical therapy using ankle-foot orthosis for the foot-drop.

**Prognosis:** Guarded for both life span and muscle functions in congenital types. Physical handicaps in adult onset form leading to a change in life style occurs in about 5–10%.

**Detection of Carrier:** Based on muscle biopsy of the close relatives who are at risk for carrying the gene. The presence of nemaline rods has been described in carriers.

**References:**
Shy GM, et al.: Nemaline myopathy: a new congenital myopathy. Brain 1963; 86:793–810. *
Afifi AK, et al.: Congenital nonprogressive myopathy: central core

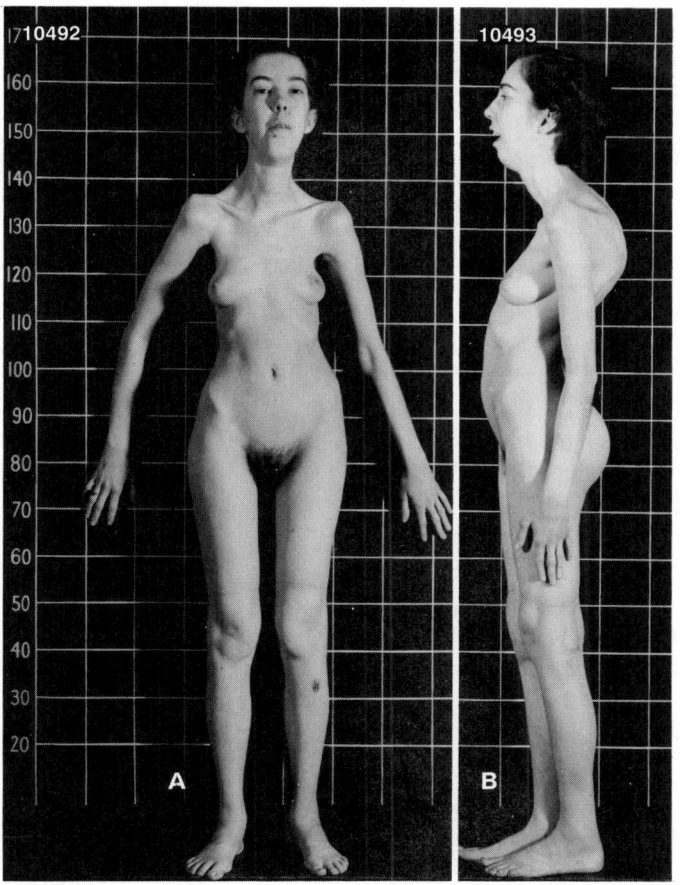

**0696**-10492: Expressionless facies, muscle loss and extremely narrow thorax. 10493: Marked kyphosis and lordosis.

disease and nemaline myopathy in one family. Neurology 1965; 15:371–381.

Kondo K, Yuasa T: Genetics of congenital nemaline myopathy. Muscle Nerve 1980; 3:308–315. *

Jennekens FGI, et al.: Congenital nemaline myopathy I: defective organization of alpha-actinin is restricted to muscle. Muscle Nerve 1983; 6:61–68.

Meier C, et al.: Nemaline myopathy appearing in adults as cardiomyopathy. Arch Neurol 1984; 41:443–445.

Stauber WT, et al.: Nemaline myopathy: evidence of dipeptidyl peptidase I deficiency. Arch Neurol 1986; 43:39–41.

Schmalbruch H, et al.: Early fetal nemaline myopathy: case report and a review. Dev Med Child Neurol 1987; 29:800–804.

I0000                                                    **Victor V. Ionasescu**

### Myopathy, recessive phosphorylase kinase deficiency
*See GLYCOGENOSIS, TYPE IXb*

## MYOPATHY, REDUCING BODY                               2062

**Includes:** Reducing body myopathy

**Excludes:** Myopathy (other congenital)

**Major Diagnostic Criteria:** Affected infants have hypotonia and delayed motor milestones but normal intelligence. Progressive weakness involves both proximal and distal muscles. Muscle biopsy reveals characteristic alterations (reducing bodies).

**Clinical Findings:** Affected infants are weak and hypotonic very early in life. Facial weakness, ptosis, and multijoint contractures may be present. Weakness of the intercostals is severe and results in frequent pneumonias. In some children, death has resulted from pulmonary disease and cardiac failure, but in others the course has been more benign. Five cases have been described thus far. Muscle biopsy material shows distinctive inclusions (intracytoplasmic bodies). These are nonreactive for oxidative enzymes and ATPase, but are able to reduce nitroblue tetrazolium directly when mediated by menandione, hence the suggested name of *reducing body myopathy*. The inclusions are also rich in sulfhydryl groups and contain RNA and glycogen. The electron microscopy is characteristic, the inclusions being round or oval shaped and often in close proximity to a nucleus but separate from it under the sarcolemma. They are composed of closely packed, variably shaped, and moderately basophilic particles measuring 12–16 nm in diameter. The majority of muscle fibers are otherwise normal in structure apart from occasional nonspecific necrotic changes.

The serum CK level was normal in four children and elevated in only one. EMG studies revealed short polyphasic potentials, motor and sensory nerve conduction velocities were normal.

**Complications:** Pneumonias and congestive heart failure.

**Associated Findings:** None known.

**Etiology:** The disorder has been sporadic except for one family in which two sibs were affected. This suggests autosomal recessive inheritance.

**Pathogenesis:** A partial biochemical characterization of the reducing bodies was done in one patient. Two abnormal proteins of molecular weights of 62,000 and 53,000 were identified. It has been suggested that the reducing bodies have either ribosomal or myofibrillary origin.

**CDC No.:** 756.880

**Sex Ratio:** M1:F1

**Occurrence:** Undetermined but presumed rare.

**Risk of Recurrence for Patient's Sib:**
See Part I, *Mendelian Inheritance*. Most cases are sporadic.

**Risk of Recurrence for Patient's Child:**
See Part I, *Mendelian Inheritance*. No affected individuals have reached reproductive age.

**Age of Detectability:** Within the first four years of age.

**Gene Mapping and Linkage:** Unknown.

**Prevention:** None known. Genetic counseling indicated.

**Treatment:** The complications (pneumonias and congestive heart failure) should be treated.

**Prognosis:** Guarded.

**Detection of Carrier:** Unknown.

**References:**
Brooke MH, Neville HE: Reducing body myopathy. Neurology 1972; 22:829–840.

Dubowitz V, Brooke MH: Muscle biopsy: a modern approach. London: W.B. Saunders, 1973:351 only.

Tome FHS, Fardeau M: Congenital myopathy with "reducing bodies" in muscle fibers. Acta Neuropathol 1975; 31:207–217.

Carpenter S, et al.: New observations in reducing body myopathy. Neurology 1985; 35:207–217.

I0000                                                    **Victor V. Ionasescu**

## MYOPATHY, SARCOTUBULAR                               2063

**Includes:** Sarcotubular myopathy

**Excludes:**
    Muscular dystrophy
    Myopathy (other congenital)

**Major Diagnostic Criteria:** A nonprogressive proximal weakness is apparent early in life. The electromyogram may be normal (1/2) or may show a myopathic pattern (1/2). Motor and sensory nerve velocities are normal (2/2). Serum creatine kinase may be normal or elevated (1/2). Muscle biopsy is essential to establish the diagnosis. The myopathy is characterized by a structural alteration of the sarcotubular system. This vacuolar change selectively affects the type II muscle fibers.

**Clinical Findings:** The muscular weakness dates from infancy. Intrauterine movements may be reduced. When the child begins to walk, a proximal weakness is recognized by a waddling gait and difficulty in climbing stairs and rising from a chair. It becomes obvious by the end of the first decade that the child has a symmetric proximal weakness of both upper and lower extremities, with involvement of the flexors of the neck and facial muscles. The muscles of the chest may also be weak and the cough may be feeble. The bulk of the affected muscles is reduced, and the tendon reflexes are hypoactive (1/2). The weakness does not appear to progress.

**Complications:** Unknown.

**Associated Findings:** None known.

**Etiology:** Probably autosomal recessive inheritance, although a sex-linked recessive trait cannot be excluded.

**Pathogenesis:** When electron cytochemical markers for the transverse tubules and the sarcoplasmic reticulum were applied to biopsied muscle material, the transverse tubules were visualized as displaying a close topographic relationship to the small vacuoles in that they abutted at their periphery or projected into the interior. In addition, the limiting membranes of the vacuoles reacted for sarcoplasmic reticulum-associated ATPase. For these reasons, the disorder is regarded as a segmental vacuolation resulting from the alteration of the sarcotubular system, particularly of the type II muscle fibers.

**MIM No.:** 26895

**CDC No.:** 756.880

**Sex Ratio:** Unknown. Two males have been reported.

**Occurrence:** Two brothers from an inbred Hutterite colony have been reported.

**Risk of Recurrence for Patient's Sib:**
See Part I, *Mendelian Inheritance*. Two brothers are affected in a sibship of nine boys and one girl. The parents are Hutterites and are third cousins. Members of two previous generations were not known to have muscle disease.

**Risk of Recurrence for Patient's Child:**
See Part I, *Mendelian Inheritance*.

**Age of Detectability:** The proximal weakness can be detected when the child begins to stand and to walk.

**Gene Mapping and Linkage:** Unknown.

**Prevention:** None known. Genetic counseling indicated.

**Treatment:** Avoid excessive exercise and fatigue.

**Prognosis:** This disorder appears to run a nonprogressive course and to represent a congenital myopathy.

**Detection of Carrier:** Unknown.

**References:**

Jerusalem F, et al.: Sarcotubular myopathy: a newly recognized, benign, congenital, familial muscle disease. Neurology 1973; 23:897–906.

Engel AG: Myopathy, sarcotubular In: Myrianthopoulas NC, ed: Handbook of clinical neurology. Neurogenetic directory, Vol 43, Pt 2. Amsterdam: Elsevier/North-Holland, 1982:120–121, 129–130.

Carpenter S, Karpati G: Pathology of skeletal muscle. New York: Churchill Livingstone, 1984:336–342.

BA060                                             **Betty Q. Banker**

**Myopathy, visceral**
*See INTESTINAL PSEUDO-OBSTRUCTION SYNDROMES*

## MYOPATHY-CATARACT-GONADAL DYSGENESIS          2052

**Includes:**

Cataracts-gonadal dysgenesis-myopathy, familial congenital type

Gonadal dysgenesis-cataracts-myopathy, familial congenital type

Muscular dystrophy-cataract-hypogonadism

Myopathy-cataract-hypogonadism

Myopathy, mitochondrial-cataract

**Excludes:**

**Kearns-Sayre disease** (2070)
**Myotonic dystrophy** (0702)
**Myopathy** (others)

**Major Diagnostic Criteria:** Myopathy, gonadal dysgenesis, and cataracts begin in infancy or early childhood. Electromyogram (EMG), muscle biopsy, gonadotropin, and hormone findings are confirmatory.

**Clinical Findings:** *Myopathy*: nonprogressive hypotonia, weakness, myopathic facies, and hyporeflexia are present from infancy. Ataxia, myotonia, fasciculations, and spasticity are not found. EMG findings show the pattern of myopathy. Muscle biopsy shows variations in fiber diameter, increased amounts of endomysial connective tissue and no inflammatory cells.

*Cataracts* appear in early childhood. Ptosis, esotropia, and myopia also occur.

*Gonadal dysgenesis*: Male and female siblings have been reported by Bassoe (1956), each with hypergonadotropic hypogonadism. The female was 139 cm tall. She had primary amenorrhea, minimal breast development, and scant pubic hair. Her uterus was small and her ovaries fibrous. Gonadotropins were elevated, estrogen decreased. Microscopic examination of the ovaries showed no primary follicles and increased fibrous tissue. The male was 158 cm tall with scant pubic hair, small, soft testes, and a small prostate. Testicular biopsy showed increased hyaline and fibrous tissue, a thick fibrous capsule, clusters of Leydig cells and few Sertoli cells.

IQ appears to be normal.

**Complications:** Joint contractures, gross motor developmental delay, blindness, short stature, predisposition to respiratory illness.

**Associated Findings:** Cubitus valgus, short fourth metatarsal, mild osteoporosis.

**Etiology:** Both autosomal recessive and autosomal dominant inheritance has been suggested.

**Pathogenesis:** Involvement of skeletal muscle, gonads, lens, and skeletal system suggests a generalized early gestational effect. The biochemical defect is undetermined.

**MIM No.:** 16055, 25400, 25517

**POS No.:** 3926

**CDC No.:** 756.880

**Sex Ratio:** Presumably M1:F1.

**Occurrence:** Undetermined but presumed rare. One large kindred has been documented in Norway.

**Risk of Recurrence for Patient's Sib:**
See Part I, *Mendelian Inheritance.*

**Risk of Recurrence for Patient's Child:**
See Part I, *Mendelian Inheritance.* Affected individuals appear to be sterile.

**Age of Detectability:** In infancy.

**Gene Mapping and Linkage:** Unknown.

**Prevention:** None known. Genetic counseling indicated.

**Treatment:** Physical therapy, treatment of respiratory complications, cataract surgery. Replacement of gonadal hormones at age of puberty may be useful in producing secondary sexual characteristics.

**Prognosis:** Good for survival. Myopathy is apparently not progressive.

**Detection of Carrier:** Unknown.

**Special Considerations:** Hereditary myopathy, oligophrenia, cataract, skeletal abnormalities, and hypergonadotropic hypogonadism described in a Swedish family (Lundberg, 1974) differs in that this condition is marked by moderate to severe mental retardation, pyramidal tract involvement, and substantial skeletal deformation and malformation. A myotubular myopathy with cataract (Hawkes and Absolon, 1975) and a familial mitochondrial myopathy with cataract (Pepin et al, 1980) have also been described, and each of these could be distinct entities.

**References:**

Bassoe HH: Familial congenital muscular dystrophy with gonadal dysgenesis. J Clin Endocrinol 1956; 16:1614–1620.

Lundberg PO: Hereditary myopathy oligophrenia, cataract, skeletal abnormalities, and hypergonadotropic hypogonadism. Eur Neurol 1973; 10:261–280.

Lundberg PO: Hereditary myopathy, oligophrenia, cataract, skeletal abnormalities and hypergonadotropic hypogonadism: a new syndrome. Acta Genet Med Gemellol 1974; 23:245–247.

Hawkes CH, Absolon MJ: Myotubular myopathy associated with cataract and electrical myotonia. J Neurol Neurosurg Psychiatry 1975; 38:761–770.

Pepin B, et al.: Familial mitochondrial myopathy with cataract. J Neurol Sci 1980; 45:191–197.

BA039                                      **Louis E. Bartoshesky**

**Myopathy-cataract-hypogonadism**
*See MYOPATHY-CATARACT-GONADAL DYSGENESIS*
**Myopathy-hemolysis**
*See GLYCOGENOSIS, TYPE VII*
**Myopathy-lactic acidosis**
*See MYOPATHY, MYOGLOBINURIA-ABNORMAL GLYCOLOSIS, HEREDITARY TYPE*
**Myopathy-Marinesco-Sjogren syndrome**
*See MARINESCO-SJOGREN SYNDROME*
**Myopathy-metabolic, acid maltase deficiency, infant onset**
*See GLYCOGENOSIS, TYPE IIa*
**Myopathy-metabolic, acid maltase deficiency, late onset**
*See GLYCOGENOSIS, TYPE IIb*
**Myopathy-metabolic, brancher disease**
*See GLYCOGENOSIS, TYPE IV*

## MYOPATHY-METABOLIC, CARNITINE DEFICIENCY, PRIMARY AND SECONDARY                    0124

**Includes:**
    Carnitine deficiency, myopathic
    Carnitine deficiency, primary
    Carnitine deficiency, secondary
    Carnitine deficiency, systemic
    Muscle carnitine deficiency
    Renal reabsorption of carnitine, defect in

**Excludes:**
    Cardiomyopathy (other)
    Dicarboxylic aciduria (other)
    Lipid myopathy (other)
    Mitochondrial myopathies (other)
    **Myopathy-metabolic, carnitine palmityl transferase deficiency**
    (0125)
    **Viscera, fatty metamorphosis** (0990)

**Major Diagnostic Criteria:** Failure to thrive, generalized muscle weakness, hepatomegaly, cardiomyopathy, lowered plasma carnitine levels, lowered muscle carnitine levels, dicarboxylic aciduria, elevated free fatty acids.

**Clinical Findings:** The clinical picture of L-carnitine deficiency has been evolving since its first description in 1973. Presentation may be primarily myopathic with progressive muscle weakness, myalgias, delayed gross motor development, cardiomyopathy, and biopsy showing lipid myopathy. Systemic signs and symptoms include failure to thrive, recurrent infections, acute Reye-like encephalopathy, and hepatic toxicity with elevated hepatic enzymes, elevated ammonia, hypoglycemia, and lack of ketosis. Dicarboxylic aciduria results from extra mitochondrial oxidation of fats.

**Complications:** Progressive muscle weakness, cardiomyopathy, hepatic dysfunction, failure to thrive, and hepatic encephalopathy.

**Associated Findings:** Elevated ammonia, liver enzymes, free fatty acids and dicarboxylic aciduria.

**Etiology:** Etiology of the deficiency is heterogeneous. The distinction between primary muscle carnitine deficiency with normal plasma, but low muscle carnitine levels and systemic carnitine deficiency where levels are low in both muscle and plasma may be accurate, or may just represent varying severities of the same disorder. Muscle deficiency may be due to an autosomal recessive inherited defect of active transport. The systemic deficiency is usually secondary to another metabolic disorder (liver disease, prolonged parenteral nutrition, poor generalized nutrition or chronic illness). Renal loss secondary to an isolated autosomal recessive renal reabsorption defect of carnitine generalized renal Fanconi syndrome, or increased loss during dialysis can also lead to deficiency. Many inherited organic acidurias result in increase loss of esterified carnitines in the urine.

**Pathogenesis:** The primary function of L-carnitine is transport of long chain fatty acids across the inner mitochondrial membrane, thus delivering the fatty acids for beta oxidation. There is active transport of L-carnitine into muscle and 98% of the total body L-carnitine is found in muscle. L-carnitine is synthesized from lysine and methionine mainly in the liver and dietary sources include red meats and dairy products. 99% of the L-carnitine loss is via urine and there is active reabsorption of filtered carnitine (>95% filtered). L-carnitine exists in both a free form and an acyl carnitine esterified form. In normal humans, the esters account for 10–20% of the total carnitine measurement in plasma.

Deficiency of L-carnitine results in the failure of delivery of long chain fatty acids for beta oxidation. Since cardiac muscle and skeletal muscle rely heavily on oxidation of fatty acids for energy supply, deficiency of L-carnitine results in muscular weakness, cardiomyopathy and lipid storage.

**MIM No.:** *21214, *21216

**CDC No.:** 756.880

**Sex Ratio:** M>1:F1

**Occurrence:** Depends on etiology. High with renal Fanconi syndrome, certain organic acidurias, stress states such as illness or starvation, and for infants on total parenteral nutrition. Particular risk is associated with neonates because of poor synthetic capabilities.

Secondary deficiency is more common than once suspected. Certainly highest among pediatric patients presenting with muscle weakness, failure to thrive, hepatic dysfunction, or cardiomyopathy.

**Risk of Recurrence for Patient's Sib:**
See Part I, *Mendelian Inheritance.*

**Risk of Recurrence for Patient's Child:**
See Part I, *Mendelian Inheritance.* May be increased in offspring of mothers who are carnitine deficient.

**Age of Detectability:** Newborn period through maturity.

**Gene Mapping and Linkage:** Unknown.

**Prevention:** Supplementation with oral L-carnitine in patients at high risk such as infants on total parenteral nutrition, renal disease states with renal Fanconi syndrome, organic acidurias, or stress states such as pregnancy, chronic illness.

**Treatment:** Once deficiency occurs, oral L-carnitine therapy at 50–200 mg/kg/day p.o. divided q4-q12h daily. IV L-carnitine also available.

**Prognosis:** Depends on etiology and treatment. If treated, symptomatic improvement begins shortly after beginning therapy. If primary disease state is under control, complete recovery while being maintained on therapy should be expected. If untreated, progressive muscle weakness, cardiomyopathy and hepatic dysfunction leads to premature death.

**Detection of Carrier:** Unknown.

**References:**
Engel AG, Angelini C: Carnitine deficiency of human skeletal muscle with associated lipid storage myopathy: a new syndrome. Science 1973; 179:899.
Cruse RP, et al.: Familial systemic carnitine deficiency. Arch Neurol 1984; 41:301–305.
Engel AG, Rebouche CJ: Carnitine metabolism and inborn errors. J Inherit Metab Dis 1984; 7(Suppl):38–43.
Etzioni A, et al.: Systemic carnitine deficiency exacerbated by a strict vegitarian diet. Arch Dis Child 1984; 59:177–179.
Matsuishi T, et al.: Successful carnitine treatment in two siblings having lipid storage myopathy with hypertrophic cardiomyopathy. Neuropediatrics 1985; 16:6–12.
Treem WR, et al: Primary carnitine deficiency due to a failure of carnitine transport in kidney, muscle, and fibroblasts. New Engl J Med 1988; 319:1331–1336.

WI038                                                              **Susan C. Winter**

## MYOPATHY-METABOLIC, CARNITINE PALMITYL TRANSFERASE DEFICIENCY                    0125

**Includes:**
    Carnitine palmityl-transferase-A(I) deficiency
    Carnitine palmityl-transferase-B(II) deficiency
    Hepatic carnitine palmitoyl transferase deficiency (some)
    Ibuprofen therapy with carnitine palmityl transferase
      deficiency
    Myoglobinuria, idiopathic recurrent

**Excludes:**
    Myoglobinuria following exertion
    Myopathies (other)

**Major Diagnostic Criteria:** Muscle cramps and myoglobinuria after exercise, fasting, or high fat diets. Hypoglycemia with low plasma ketone bodies. Family history of similar problems. Enzymatic assay of carnitine palmityl transferase A or B deficient in muscle, liver, leukocytes, platelets, lymphoblasts, or fibroblasts.

**Clinical Findings:** Muscle cramping and myoglobinuria with onset in late childhood or teenage years and being precipitated by strenuous exercise, fasting, or high fat diet. One set of eight-month-old sisters have been described presenting with hypogycemia and lack of ketosis and total absence of this enzyme activity in the liver. Partial deficiency of carnitine palmityl transferase A deficiency has been described with rhabdomyolysis after ibuprofen therapy. This was reported in a 45-year-old woman who developed muscle weakness and tenderness with rhabdomyolysis and respiratory failure after initiation of ibuprofen therapy. Muscle carnitine palmityl transferanse-a deficiency was diagnosed, and persisted after stopping ibuprofen therapy.

**Complications:** Potential acute renal tubular necrosis secondary to massive myoglobinuria, fibrosis of muscle following repeat attacks, carnitine deficiency.

**Associated Findings:** On at least two occasions, reduced levels of carnitine acetyl transferase has been found associated with carnitine palmityl transferase deficiency.

**Etiology:** Probable autosomal recessive inheritance resulting in partial enzyme deficiency or X-linked recessive inheritance.

**Pathogenesis:** Carnitine palmityl transferase occurs in two isoenzymatic forms. Carnitine palmityl transferase-A is located on the cytosol side of the inner mitochondrial membrane and carnitine palmityl transferase-II is located in the matrix side of the same inner mitochondrial membrane. Deficiency of both enzymes have been described and it is still uncertain as to whether these represent the same or different genetic entities. Evidence points to separate genetic control for these enzymes. There are likely three acyl transferases: a short chain acyl transferase, a C14–16 carnitine palmityl transferase, and a C6–10 octanoyl transferase. **Acyl-CoA dehydrogenase deficiency, short chain type** and **Acyl-CoA dehydrogenase deficiency, medium chain** have been reported.

The carnitine palmityl transferases A and B are involved in transport of C14–16 long chain fatty acyl carnitine esters from the outer surface of the inner mitochondrial membrane to the matrix of the inner mitochondrial membrane. Reduced activity of this enzyme results in reduced palmityl CoA delivered to the inner mitochondrial matrix and this reduced beta oxidation. Therefore, during states which require increased energy production such as fasting or excessive exercise, muscle breakdown and myoglobinuria occurs. In complete absence of the enzyme, hypoglycemia, and lack of ketosis is seen.

**MIM No.:** *25511, *25512

**CDC No.:** 756.880

**Sex Ratio:** M10:F1

**Occurrence:** Rare, but at least 30 cases reported.

**Risk of Recurrence for Patient's Sib:**
See Part I, *Mendelian Inheritance.*

**Risk of Recurrence for Patient's Child:**
See Part I, *Mendelian Inheritance.*

**Age of Detectability:** Generally early teens to early 20's--as early as infancy. Biochemical measurements could be done shortly after birth and should demonstrate deficiency.

**Gene Mapping and Linkage:** Unknown.

**Prevention:** None known. Genetic counseling indicated.

**Treatment:** High carbohydrate, low fat diet, and avoiding fasting and excessive exercise, and carnitine supplementation.

**Prognosis:** Unknown.

**Detection of Carrier:** Enzymatic studies have been done on muscle, liver, fibroblasts, thrombocytes, and leukocytes.

**References:**
Engel WK, et al.: A skeletal-muscle disorder associated with intermittent symptoms and a possible defect of lipid metabolism. New Engl J Med 1970; 282:697.
DiMauro S, DiMauro PM: Muscle carnitine palmityltransferase deficiency and myoglobinuria. Science 1973; 182:929.
Bougneres PF, et al.: Fasting hypoglycemia resulting from hepatic carnitine palmitoyl transferase deficiency. J Pedaitr 1981; 98:742–746.
Bremer J: Carnitine--metabolism function. Physiol Rev 1983; 63(4).
Coates PM, et al.: Detection of medium-chain acyl CoA dehydrogenase deficiency in leukocytes. Pediatr Res 1983; 17:288A.
Trevisan CP, et al.: Myoglobinuria and carnitine palmityl transferase deficiency: studies with malonyl CoA suggests absence of only CPT. Neurology 1984; 34:3538–3546.
Turnbull DM, et al.: Short-chain acyl-CoA dehydrogenase deficiency associated with a lipid-storage myopathy and secondary carnitine deficiency. New Engl J Med 1985; 311:1232–1236.
Ross NS, Hoppel CL: Partial muscle carnitine palmityltransferase-A deficiency. J Am Med Assoc 1987; 257:62–65.

WI038                                    **Susan C. Winter**

---

## MYOPATHY-METABOLIC, GLYCOPROTEIN-GLYCOSAMINOGLYCANS STORAGE TYPE                    2868

**Includes:**
>   Glycoprotein-glycosaminoglycan storage myopathy
>   Myopathy with storage of glycoproteins and
>     glycosaminoglycans
>   Polysaccharide storage cardioskeletal myopathy

**Excludes:** Glycogen storage myopathies (other)

**Major Diagnostic Criteria:** Cardioskeletal myopathy with variable onset of weakness and progression. Storage of glycoproteins and glycosaminoglycans can be demonstrated in muscle biopsy and cultured fibroblasts by histochemical and biochemical procedures. Positive family history.

**Clinical Findings:** Of the five known patients, the first was a women who had slow progressive weakness of the legs manifested at age 21 years and who died at age 31 years with severe involvement of both striated and heart muscle. Eight members of her family, both males and females in two generations, died at an early age from conditions vaguely referred to as pneumonia and heart disease. The most striking histologic abnormality was the infiltration of cardiac and skeletal muscle with a basophilic substance that appeared to be a neutral mucopolysaccharide. The second patient was a 19-year-old man who developed an acute nonobstructive cardiomyopathy with fatal heart failure in one month. His two brothers and sister had died of unidentified heart disease. Chemical analyses of the striated muscle showed low glycogen content and storage of glycosaminoglycans.

The third patient, a 13-year-old male, developed progressive weakness and atrophy of pelvic muscles with enlargement of the calves and diminished deep tendon reflexes. The heart was not affected. Biochemical studies showed accumulation of glycosaminoglycans in both fibrillar structures and intermyofibrillar spaces. The synthesis of glycosaminoglycans was found to be increased. The last two patients (mother and daughter, ages 28 and five years) manifested moderate weakness and atrophy of facial and shoulder muscles with congenital onset and mild progression. The heart was normal. Serum creatine kinase was elevated only in the child. Muscle biopsy material from both patients revealed vacuolar myopathy with storage of granular material. Muscle glycogen values were low-normal, and glycolytic enzymes were normal. Storage of granular material was also identified in fibroblasts that were weakly periodic acid-Schiff-positive, stained metachromatically with toluidine blue, and orthochromatically with alcian blue. Repeated biochemical studies of cultured fibroblasts identified excessive storage of glycoproteins and glycosaminoglycans. The uptake of $^3$H-glucosamine in cultured fibroblasts was 1.7–3.4 times greater in the patients than in control individuals, while the rate of turnover of the radioisotope was normal.

**Complications:** Unknown.

**Associated Findings:** None known.

**Etiology:** Presumably autosomal dominant inheritance with variability in expression, although the family of patient No. 2 suggested recessive inheritance.

**Pathogenesis:** Possibly excessive synthesis of glycoproteins and glycosaminoglycans. The specific defect in the synthesis of mucopolysaccharides is undetermined.

**MIM No.:** 16057

**CDC No.:** 756.880

**Sex Ratio:** M1:F1

**Occurrence:** Five cases have been documented.

**Risk of Recurrence for Patient's Sib:**
See Part I, *Mendelian Inheritance.*

**Risk of Recurrence for Patient's Child:**
See Part I, *Mendelian Inheritance.*

**Age of Detectability:** Between childhood and adulthood.

**Gene Mapping and Linkage:** Unknown.

**Prevention:** None known. Genetic counseling indicated.

**Treatment:** Unknown.

**Prognosis:** Good, except in cases with cardiomyopathy, which can limit life span.

**Detection of Carrier:** Unknown.

**References:**

Holmes JM, et al.: A myopathy presenting in adult life with features suggestive of glycogen storage disease. J Neurol Neurosurg Psychiatry 1960; 23:302–311.
Karpati G, et al.: Peculiar polysaccharide accumulation in muscle in a case of cardioskeletal myopathy. Neurology 1969; 19:553–564.
Radu H, et al.: A new metabolic disorder: myopathy with glycosamino (sialo) glycans accumulation. Eur Neurol 1974; 12:209–225.
Ionasescu VV, et al.: Inherited metabolic myopathy with storage of glycoproteins and glycosaminoglycans. Am J Med Genet 1984; 18:333–343.

I0000                                                        **Victor V. Ionasescu**

---

## MYOPATHY-METABOLIC, MITOCHONDRIAL CYTOCHROME C OXIDASE DEFICIENCY          **2707**

**Includes:**
Complex IV deficiency of the mitochondrial respiratory chain
Cytochrome c oxidase deficiency
de Toni-Fanconi-Debre syndrome (some cases)
Leigh syndrome (some cases)
Mitochondrial myopathy due to cytochrome c oxidase deficiency

**Excludes:**
Encephalopathy, necrotizing (0344)
Myopathy (other mitochondrial)

**Major Diagnostic Criteria:** The most common clinical presentation is severe generalized myopathy, beginning soon after birth and causing respiratory insufficiency, cardiomyopathy, and death before age one year. Lactic acidosis is severe and represents an important diagnostic feature.

**Clinical Findings:** Clinical phenotypes fall into two main groups, one in which myopathy is the predominant or exclusive manifestation, and another in which brain dysfunction predominates.
Fatal infantile mitochondrial myopathy includes generalized weakness of striated muscles and heart, renal dysfunction (de Toni-Fanconi-Debre syndrome), and lactic acidosis. Only a few patients were overtly weak at birth. In the others, poor cry, difficult sucking and swallowing, and floppiness became apparent after 3–4 weeks of life. Few patients had bilateral ptosis. The respiratory insufficiency related to intercostals and diaphragm weakness required assisted ventilation and caused death before age 4–8 months. In contrast to this dramatic clinical picture, a few patients showed benign infantile mitochondrial myopathy characterized by spontaneous recovery to normal motor function by age two or three years.
Muscle biopsy studies demonstrate ragged-red fibers and ultrastructural alterations of the mitochondria. There is markedly decreased cytochrome c oxidase activity (COX) in crude muscle extracts and histochemically at the level of the ragged-red fibers (Reichmann et al, 1988). Muscle biopsy and serum lactate returned to normal in benign infantile mitochondrial myopathy.
Of the second group of disorders, dominated by involvement of the central nervous system, **Encephalopathy, necrotizing** (Leigh syndrome) is the most common finding. This devastating encephalopathy is characterized clinically by psychomotor retardation, cranial nerve dysfunction, respiratory abnormalities, and seizures. The characteristic neuropathologic alterations are focal, symmetric, necrotic lesions affecting mostly the brainstem. Microscopically, these "spongiform" lesions show demyelination, vascular proliferation, and astrocytosis. Slowly progressive mitochondrial encephalomyopathy characterized by adult onset, weakness and atrophy of limb muscles, sensorineural hearing loss, and complex partial seizures was recently reported in a 52-year-old man. Biochemical studies showed only partial COX deficiency in crude muscle extracts and in isolated mitochondria (44 and 30% of normal, respectively).

**Complications:** Congestive heart failure and respiratory failure frequently occur in the fatal infantile form.

**Associated Findings:** Endocrine involvement (hypothyroidism, hypogonadism) was reported by Doriguzzi et al (1989).

**Etiology:** The hereditary transmission of COX deficiency, as in other primary mitochondrial diseases, is nonmendelian and based on maternal inheritance. The mitochondrion has its own DNA (mtDNA) and its own transcription and translation apparatuses. The mtDNA encodes only about 12 polypeptides, and nuclear DNA controls the synthesis of 90% of all mitochondrial proteins. These include six subunits of complex I of the respiratory chain, the apoprotein of cytochrome b, the three larger subunits of COX (complex IV), and one subunit of ATPase (complex V). In the formation of the zygote, almost all the mitochondria are contributed by the ovum. Therefore, mtDNA is transmitted by maternal inheritance in a "vertical" nonmendelian fashion. In mammalian tissues, COX is composed of 13 different subunits. The complexity of the enzyme structure most likely accounts for the clinical heterogeneity of COX deficiency.

**Pathogenesis:** The essential properties of the COX enzyme are electron transport and proton translocation. These functions are related to the three larger subunits (I-III), which are encoded by mtDNA. The function of the nuclearly encoded subunits is uncertain, but it has been suggested that they have a regulatory role and confer tissue specificity to COX. The clinical heterogeneity of COX deficiency is accompanied by biochemical heterogeneity. The enzyme defect may be localized to one tissue only (striated muscle) or expand to several other tissues (heart, liver, kidney, brain, fibroblasts). In Leigh syndrome (see **Encephalopathy, necrotizing**), COX deficiency appears to be generalized.
The clinical and biochemical heterogeneity of COX deficiency suggests that different genetic defects are involved. Further studies are needed to determine these defects at the molecular level.

**MIM No.:** *22011

**CDC No.:** 756.880

**Sex Ratio:** M1:F1

**Occurrence:** Over a dozen cases have been documented in the literature.

**Risk of Recurrence for Patient's Sib:** 1:1 (100%).

**Risk of Recurrence for Patient's Child:** If the mother is affected, 100%. An affected mother would pass the disease to all her children, but only her daughters would transmit the trait to subsequent generations. There is no risk of recurrence for the children of an affected male.

**Age of Detectability:** Varies between infancy (most cases detected at that age) and adulthood. COX deficiency is present in cultured fibroblasts in Leigh syndrome, which may provide a useful tool for prenatal diagnosis.

**Gene Mapping and Linkage:** Unknown.

**Prevention:** None known. Genetic counseling indicated.

**Treatment:** Symptomatic (congestive heart failure and respiratory insufficiency).

**Prognosis:** Guarded in the severe forms with the total COX deficiency, but good in benign infantile mitochondrial myopathy.

**Detection of Carrier:** Unknown.

## References:

Morgan-Hughes JA, et al.: Mitochondrial encephalomyopathies: biochemical studies in two cases revealing defects in the respiratory chain. Brain 1982; 105:553–582.

Di Mauro S, et al.: Mitochondrial myopathies. Ann Neurol 1985; 17:521–528.

Di Mauro S, et al.: Metabolic myopathies. Am J Med Genet 1986; 25:635–651.

Glerum M, et al.: Abnormal kinetic behavior of cytochrome oxidase in a case of Leigh disease. Am J Hum Genet 1987; 41:584–593.

Zeviani M, et al.: Benign reversible muscle cytochrome c oxidase deficiency: a second case. Neurology 1987; 37:64–67.

Reichmann C, et al.: Enzyme activity measured in single muscle fibers in partial cytochrome c oxidase deficiency. Neurology 1988; 38:244–249.

Doriguzzi C, et al.: Endocrine involvement in mitochondrial encephalomyopathy with partial cytochrome c oxidase deficiency. J Neurol Neurosurg Psychiatry 1989; 52:122–125.

I0000                                                    **Victor V. Ionasescu**

## MYOPATHY-METABOLIC, MYOADENYLATE DEAMINASE DEFICIENCY                              2709

## Includes:

Muscle adenosine monophosphate (AMP) deaminase deficiency
Muscle adenylate deaminase deficiency
Myoadenylate deaminase deficiency, myopathy due to

**Excludes:** Myopathy-metabolic (other)

**Major Diagnostic Criteria:** 1) Failure of blood ammonia to increase, despite an adequate lactate increase, on an ischemic forearm exercise test; 2) absence of histoenzymatic staining for adenylate deaminase on a frozen muscle biopsy despite adequate controls; 3) quantitative biochemical assay demonstrating less than 10% normal mean specific activity levels of adenylate deaminase in a properly prepared muscle homogenate.

**Clinical Findings:** A small proportion of patients manifest infantile hypotonia, which may be marked during the neonatal period, especially in premature infants. The deep tendon reflexes are normal, and the hypotonia regresses gradually and is rarely a problem after childhood. Most patients develop symptoms of exercise intolerance only in adulthood or middle age, with various combinations of muscle cramping and aching, easy fatigue, and slowly progressive weakness that is never incapacitating. About one-third of cases may have an elevated serum creatine kinase level (perhaps 10 times, but not 100 times, the upper normal limit) and sometimes a nonspecifically abnormal EMG. There are no neurologic signs other than muscle weakness and tenderness. Easy fatigue may suggest myasthenia gravis, but the eye muscles are not involved and the fatigue never progresses to paresis. The tenderness and myalgia may suggest polymyositis, while the lack of impressive objective findings may suggest neurasthenia. The enzyme deficiency, unaccompanied by other neuromuscular abnormalities, is not a severe or dangerous disease, and some patients never manifest symptoms.

**Complications:** Affected patients may have a somewhat increased risk of exercise-induced rhabdomyolysis and malignant hyperthermia susceptibility, but this is still uncertain.

**Associated Findings:** About one-half of the cases occur in association with other neuromuscular disease, which may be of any type and is then the determining factor in treatment and prognosis. Of this group, about one-half probably represent coincidental association with primary myoadenylate deaminase deficiency, while the other one-half are myoadenylate deaminase heterozygotes whose enzyme level has been depleted to the deficient category secondarily by the associated disease process ("secondary" cases).

**Etiology:** Autosomal recessive inheritance.

**Pathogenesis:** During heavy exercise adenylate deaminase within the muscle cell contributes to 1) ameliorating acidosis, 2) maximizing the ATP/ADP ratio, and 3) maintaining adequate levels of Krebs cycle intermediates and carbohydrate fuels. Its absence results in inefficient muscular contraction and metabolism during prolonged heavy exertion.

**MIM No.:** *25475

**CDC No.:** 756.880

**Sex Ratio:** M1:F1

**Occurrence:** Prevalence in the general population is unknown. In the muscle biopsy population, the frequency of new cases is about 1.0% primary cases plus 0.5% secondary cases. The frequency of carriers is estimated to be 10–15% of muscle biopsies.

**Risk of Recurrence for Patient's Sib:**
See Part I, *Mendelian Inheritance.*

**Risk of Recurrence for Patient's Child:**
See Part I, *Mendelian Inheritance.* Less than 1:40, assuming carrier incidence in the general population is less than 10%.

**Age of Detectability:** At any age by surgical or needle muscle biopsy, if frozen properly.

**Gene Mapping and Linkage:** Unknown.

**Prevention:** None known. Genetic counseling indicated.

**Treatment:** The disease is not serious enough to warrant the danger of side effects from long-term analgesic treatment. No drug has been proved to increase muscular performance, although oral ribose has been claimed to benefit a few affected individuals. Counseling the patient to make the necessary psychologic adjustments is probably the most important therapy, along with reassurance.

**Prognosis:** Normal muscle function and life span are to be expected. In cases with associated neuromuscular disease, the latter will determine the prognosis.

**Detection of Carrier:** Quantitative biochemical assay of a muscle homogenate can be used to evaluate carrier status. The problem is rendered difficult by 1) variation of enzyme levels from muscle to muscle and within a given muscle by the fiber type distribution encountered, and 2) requirement for specific solution conditions to maintain maximal activity for this enzyme.

**Special Considerations:** The enzyme level may drop markedly in severe muscle disease of any kind, causing difficulty in separating primary and secondary deficiency states. There is controversy regarding symptomaticity and therapy of both deficient and carrier states.

## References:

Fishbein WN, et al.: Myoadenylate deaminase deficiency: a new disease of muscle. Science 1978; 200:545–548.

Fishbein WN, et al.: Levels of adenylate deaminase, adenylate kinase, and creatine kinase in frozen muscle biopsies relative to type 1/type 2 fiber distribution: evidence for a carrier state of myoadenylate deaminase deficiency. Ann Neurol 1984; 15:271–277.

Sabina RL, et al.: Myoadenylate deaminase deficiency: functional and metabolic abnormalities associated with disruption of the purine nucleotide cycle. J Clin Invest 1984; 73:720–730.

Fishbein WN: Myoadenylate deaminase deficiency: inherited and acquired forms. Biochem Med 1985; 33; 158–169. *

Fishbein WN: Myoadenylate deaminase deficiency. In: Engel AG, Banker BQ, eds: Myology, ed 1. New York: McGraw-Hill, 1986; 1745–1762. *

Zöllner N, et al.: Myoadenylate deaminase deficiency: successful symptomatic therapy by high dose oral administration of ribose. Klin Wochenschr 1986; 64:1281–1290.

Sabina RL, et al.: Myoadenylate deaminase deficiency. In: Scriver CR, et al, eds: The metabolic basis of inherited disease, 6th ed. New York: McGraw-Hill, 1989:1077–1084. *

FI028                                                    **William Fishbein**

**Myophosphorylase deficiency**
*See GLYCOGENOSIS, TYPE V*
**Myopia**
*See MYOPIA, CONGENITAL*
**Myopia (bilateral) with marked difference between eyes**
*See EYE, ANISOMETROPIA*

**Myopia (high-grade)-nightblindness**
*See NIGHTBLINDNESS, CONGENITAL STATIONARY, AUTOSOMAL RECESSIVE*
**Myopia severe infantile**
*See MYOPIA, CONGENITAL*

## MYOPIA, CONGENITAL                                   0699

**Includes:**

Myopia severe infantile
Myopia

**Excludes:**

**Retina, amaurosis congenita, Leber type** (0043)
**Retinopathy of prematurity** (0872)
Myopia secondary to forceps corneal injury
Myopia with myelinated nerve fibers and anisometropic amblyopia
**Myopia** (in other syndromes)

**Major Diagnostic Criteria:** Myopia of -5D or more in a child of 6 years of age or less who has a history of assuming nearsighted mannerisms before age 1 year.

**Clinical Findings:** Myopia at or shortly after birth which persists. A positive family history often alerts the parents to watch for mannerisms of nearsightedness which may be confirmed by retinoscopy after cyclopegia and ophthalmoscopy. The average age at diagnosis is 3 years. Congenital myopia may remain relatively stationary and shows no gender predilection; however, some patients, especially those with a positive family history of myopia, will increase their refractive errors up to -8D. Other patients will show a mild to moderate decrease in their myopia. The average amount of myopia is approximately -8.00 diopters. Visual acuity may be correctable to 20/30 or better; however, typically the visual acuity ranges between 20/50 and 20/60. Not infrequently, strabismus is present also. Fundus changes occur in 50% of cases and include posterior sclerectasia, juxtapapillary choroidal crescents, tilted optic nerve head, tigroid choroidal mottling, pigment thinning, and vitreous syneresis and condensations. Nystagmus is seen in 3–9% of cases.

**Complications:** Decreased (uncorrected) visual acuity, retinal detachment.

**Associated Findings: Retinopathy of prematurity, Marfan syndrome, Osteogenesis imperfecta, Chromosome 21, trisomy 21, Eye, keratoconus, Arthro-ophthalmopathy, hereditary, progressive, Stickler type, Spondyloepiphyseal dysplasia congenita, Myopathy, malignant hyperthermia,** and other syndromes.

**Etiology:** Heterogeneity exists; myopia is probably multifactorial. These disorders are usually autosomal dominant, but autosomal recessive inheritance has been argued in cases of consanguineous matings (Karlsson, 1975); at least one X-linked pedigree has been reported (Bartsocas and Kastrantas, 1981).

**Pathogenesis:** It has been postulated that increased axial length might be related to delayed scleral condensation during embryonic life with resultant stretching of the posterior pole under normal intraocular tension. Contributing factors include corneal curvature and lens structure and position. More recent theories (Kolata, 1985) have drawn on animal models, and it has even been suggested that nearsightedness may be an adaptation to changing environmental demands.

**MIM No.:** *16070, 25550, 31046

**Sex Ratio:** M1:F1

**Occurrence:** High myopia in newborn populations has a prevalence of about 2%.

**Risk of Recurrence for Patient's Sib:**
See Part I, *Mendelian Inheritance.*

**Risk of Recurrence for Patient's Child:**
See Part I, *Mendelian Inheritance.*

**Age of Detectability:** Congenital myopia can be detected as early as infancy, usually before age 3, Prevalence of myopia and other reductions in visual acuity tend to increase with age.

**Gene Mapping and Linkage:** Unknown.

**Prevention:** None known. Genetic counseling indicated.

**Treatment:** Correction of refractive error with appropriate lenses, as early as feasible. Avoidance of physically injurious, athletic, or occupational activities is recommended to prevent retinal detachment.

**Prognosis:** Favorable, since most cases of myopia are stationary. Visually guarded if myopia is progressive or if retinal detachment develops.

**Detection of Carrier:** Unknown.

**References:**
Curtin BJ: The pathogenesis of congenital myopia: a study of 66 cases. Arch Ophthalmol 1963;69:166–173.
Hiatt R, et al: Clinical evaluation of congenital myopia. Arch Ophthalmol 1965;74:31–35.
Karlsson JL: Evidence for recessive inheritance of myopia. Clin Genet 1975;7:197–202.
Bartsocas CS, Kastrantas AD: X-linked form of myopia. Hum Hered 1981;31:199–200.
Curtin BJ: The Myopias. Harper and Row, Publishers, Inc. 1985.*
Kolata G: What causes nearsightedness? Science 1985;229:1249–1250.

RA004                                                    **Elsa K. Rahn**

**Myopia, unilateral**
*See EYE, ANISOMETROPIA*
**Myopia-cataract-saddle nose-hypertelorism-short stature-deafness**
*See DEAFNESS-MYOPIA-CATARACT-SADDLE NOSE, MARSHALL TYPE*
**Myopia-cochlear deafness-intellectual impairment**
*See DEAFNESS-MYOPIA*
**Myopia-external ophthalmoplegia**
*See OPHTHALMOPLEGIA EXTERNA-MYOPIA*
**Myopia-hearing loss**
*See DEAFNESS-MYOPIA*
**Myopia-nightblindness, X-linked**
*See NIGHTBLINDNESS, CONGENITAL STATIONARY, X-LINKED RECESSIVE*
**Myosclerosis, Lowenthal type**
*See MUSCULAR DYSTROPHY, CONGENITAL WITH ARTHROGRYPOSIS*

## MYOSITIS OSSIFICANS PROGRESSIVA                       0700

**Includes:** Fibrodysplasia ossificans progressiva

**Excludes:** Localized posttraumatic myositis ossificans

**Major Diagnostic Criteria:** Progressive, widespread ectopic ossification of many muscles, microdactyly (monophalangeal digit) of the great toe and of the thumb, exostoses, broad neck of the femur, abnormal teeth, absence of the two upper incisors, hypogenitalism, baldness of the scalp, absence of lobules of the ears, deafness.

**Clinical Findings:** Onset in the first decade of life, with firm, warm, and tender subcutaneous masses around the back of the neck and shoulders. Masses progressively shrink and become bony hard in consistency. Muscles of the back, abdominal wall, chest, and extremities are gradually involved. Usually severe restriction of movement of the shoulders and spine occurs by age 10 years. The hips are involved by age 20 years, and most patients are confined to a wheelchair by age 30 years.

Muscle biopsy material shows hemorrhage, inflammation, and proliferation of collagen in the muscle fascia and dermis. New cartilage and bone formation circumscribe and infiltrate the altered tissues, mimicking a fibroma or fibrosarcoma. Eventually columns and plates of bone replace tendons, fascia, ligaments, and muscle.

**Complications:** Wheelchair confinement occurs in most patients during the advanced stage of the disease.

**Associated Findings:** Pathologic fractures, absence of the lobules of the ears, and mild mental retardation.

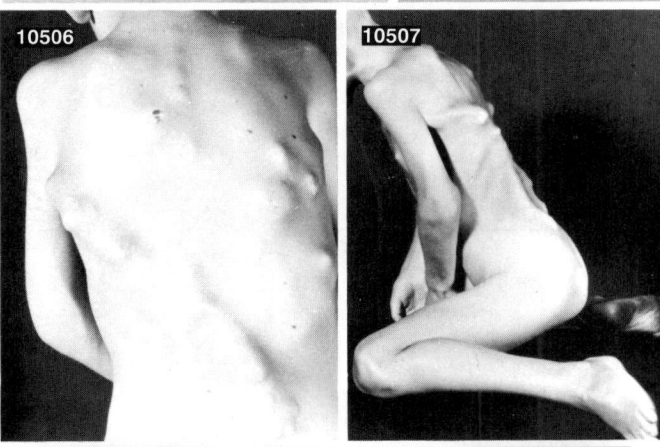

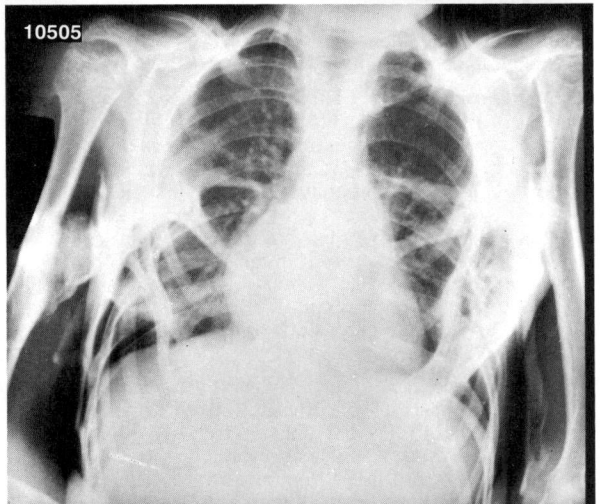

**Etiology:** Autosomal dominant inheritance is postulated based on several instances of parent-to-child transmission, including father-to-son. The disease has complete penetrance but variable expression as shown by some parents who manifest only a skeletal malformation (shortened or monophalangic big toe). Two sets of affected monozygotic twins were reported. Mutation rate is estimated at 1.8 per million gametes per generation. A parental age effect has been noted in sporadic cases.

**Pathogenesis:** Appears to be excessive proliferation and turn-over of collagen with new bone formation.

**MIM No.:** *13510

**POS No.:** 3233

**Sex Ratio:** M1:F1

**Occurrence:** Prevalence of 0.61:1,000,000 was found in Great Britain. About 500 cases have been reported in the literature.

**Risk of Recurrence for Patient's Sib:**
See Part I, *Mendelian Inheritance.*

**Risk of Recurrence for Patient's Child:**
See Part I, *Mendelian Inheritance.*

**Age of Detectability:** Usually within the first decade of life.

**Gene Mapping and Linkage:** Unknown.

**Prevention:** None known. Genetic counseling indicated.

**Treatment:** Beneficial effects have been reported in some patients with disodium ethane 1-hydroxy-1, 1-diphosphate (EHDP) in doses of 20 mg/kg of body weight per day. However, progression of the disability in most patients was not influenced by this treatment.

**Prognosis:** Life span is shortened. The disease is progressive, and severe motor handicap develops after age 30 years. Death occurs around age 40 years.

**Detection of Carrier:** Unknown.

**References:**
Bland JH, et al.: Myositis ossificans progressiva. Arch Intern Med 1973; 132:209–212.
Connor JM, Evans DAP: Fibrodysplasia ossificans progressiva: the clinical features and natural history of 34 patients. J Bone Joint Surg 1982; 64B:76–83.
Connor JM, Evans DAP: Genetic aspects of fibrodysplasia ossificans progressiva. J Med Genet 1982; 19:35–39.

10000                                          **Victor V. Ionasescu**

**Myotonia atrophica**
*See MYOTONIC DYSTROPHY*

---

**MYOTONIA CONGENITA**                                    **0701**

**Includes:**
Becker generalized myotonia
Myotonia, generalized
Thomsen congenital myotonia

**Excludes:**
**Chondrodystrophic myotonia**
**Myotonic dystrophy** (0702)
**Paralysis, hyperkalemic periodic** (0794)
**Paramyotonia congenita** (0796)

**Major Diagnostic Criteria:** Dominant congenital myotonia (Thomsen) is characterized by myotonia from infancy and lack of clinical progression. Recessive generalized myotonia (Becker) starts after the age of three years and the clinical course is often progressive.

**Clinical Findings:** *Dominant congenital myotonia* was described by Thomsen (1876) in his own family. No special muscle groups are involved at first, but later the myotonia produces most symptoms in hands, legs, and eyelids. There is marked variation in severity of myotonia among family members, with males more affected than females. Cold is an aggravating factor, and myotonic symptoms improve after movements of a muscle group. Difficulty with speech, chewing, and swallowing, and transient double vision,

**0700**-10508–09:  Characteristic posture with stiff spine and arms held close to his sides.    10506–07:  Bony ridges and nodules are evident along the entire length of the back.  10505:  Bony bridges are present between the humerus and the rib cage bilaterally.

are features that result from myotonia of laryngeal, pharyngeal, and ocular muscles. Muscle hypertrophy is frequent, although less marked than in the recessive from. Neurologic evaluation shows normal muscle strength or minimal weakness. Percussion myotonia is obvious, and unlike myotonic dystrophy, it can usually be elicited in many muscle groups as well as in the hands and tongue. A few patients with Thomsen disease, including Thomsen's own son, were considered as malingerers because of their athletic appearance and good muscle strength. One patient was a football player, and his slow, stiff movements related to myotonia were misinterpreted by his coach as "laziness." The patients show no cataracts or any other systemic features of myotonic dystrophy (frontal baldness, diabetes mellitus, testicular atrophy). There is no cardiomyopathy and no smooth muscle involvement.

*Recessive generalized myotonia* (Becker) is progressive during childhood, beginning in the legs after age three years. Myotonic symptoms may sometimes become severe and mimic rigidity. Muscle hypertrophy can be striking and is more marked than in the dominant form. Neurologic evaluation may detect weakness in addition to myotonia, and this may cause confusion with myotonic dystrophy. Often the nomenclature itself seems confusing. Infants with congenital myotonic dystrophy do not have significant myotonia but have other features such as severe hypotonia and weakness, muscle hypoplasia, and frequent mental retardation. Their mothers are almost always affected.

*Electrical myotonia* is not influenced by cold, in contrast to *paramyotonia*, in which the prolonged cold state induces electrical silence, with absence of muscle action potentials. Serum creatine kinase is normal or only slightly elevated. Muscle histology is essentially normal, and mild myopathic changes are reported rarely in the recessive type; e.g. increased internal nuclei and lack of 2B muscle fibers with myosin ATPase staining. Similarly, ultrastructural changes are few with no obvious changes in the transverse tubular system, sarcolemma, or sarcoplasmic reticulum.

**Complications:** Unknown.

**Associated Findings:** None known.

**Etiology:** Thomsen congenital myotonia by autosomal dominant inheritance. The disease occurs over multiple generations, usually without skips, although exceptions were reported. Becker generalized myotonia by autosomal recessive inheritance. This condition is characterized by the occurrence of multiple affected sibs with normal but possibly consanguinous parents. Isolated cases have been reported. This recessive form accounts for two-thirds of all sporadic cases.

**Pathogenesis:** Electrophysiological studies show a decrease in the number of Cl-1 channels, which accounts for most of the symptoms of myotonia congenita. An additional abnormality of Na$^+$ channel activation has also been also postulated. Fatty acid composition of muscle phospholipids has been reported in recessive generalized myotonia (Becker, 1977). The arachidonic acid (C20:4), oleic acid (C18:1) and linoleic acid (C18:2) levels were significantly decreased; the eicosadienoic (C20:2) and eicosatrienoic acid (C20:3) levels were significantly increased, thus establishing a distinction from the autosomal dominant form (Thomsen).

**MIM No.:** *16080, *25570

**Sex Ratio:** M1:F1

**Occurrence:** The frequency of dominant myotonic congenita (Thomsen) in the Federal Republic of Germany is about 4.4: 1,000,000. The frequency of recessive generalized myotonia (Becker) in the same country is about 2:1,000,000.

**Risk of Recurrence for Patient's Sib:**
See Part I, *Mendelian Inheritance.*

**Risk of Recurrence for Patient's Child:**
See Part I, *Mendelian Inheritance.*

**Age of Detectability:** Early childhood to adult age, based on clinical and electromyographic signs of myotonia.

**Gene Mapping and Linkage:** Unknown.

**Prevention:** None known. Genetic counseling indicated.

**Treatment:** Unlike patients with myotonic dystrophy, the patients with myotonia congenita suffer the effects of myotonia. Some beneficial effects were obtained with 300 mg quinine sulfate ( X 3/day) and diphenylhydantoin (Dilantin) (100 mg X 3/day).

**Prognosis:** Generally excellent for life in Thomsen disease. The patients with recessive generalized myotonia show normal life expectancy, but mild to moderate weakness of proximal limb muscles, in addition to myotonia.

**Detection of Carrier:** Possibly by electromyography (myotonic discharges) in some asymptomatic cases.

**References:**
Becker PE: Myotonia congenita and syndromes associated with myotonia. Topics in human genetics. vol. III. Stuttgart: Georg Thieme, 1977. *
Kuhn E, et al.: The autosomal recessive (Becker) form of myotonia congenita. Muscle Nerve 1979; 2:109–117.
Bryant SH: Physical basis of myotonia. In: Schottland DL, ed: Disorders of the motor unit. New York: John Wiley, 1982:381–389.
Subramony SH, et al.: Distinguishing paramyotonia congenita and myotonia congenita by electromyography. Muscle Nerve 1983; 6:374–379.
Sun SF, Streib EW: Autosomal recessive generalized myotonia. Muscle Nerve 1983; 6:143–148.
Ricker K: Myotonia, paramyotonia and periodic paralysis. In: Struppler A, Weindl A, eds: Electromyography and evoked potentials. New York: Springer Verlag, 1985:239–245.

10000

Victor V. Ionasescu

**Myotonia congenita intermittens**
*See PARAMYOTONIA CONGENITA*
**Myotonia, generalized**
*See MYOTONIA CONGENITA*

---

**MYOTONIC DYSTROPHY** 0702

**Includes:**
    Dystrophia myotonica
    Myotonia atrophica
    Steinert disease

**Excludes:**
    **Chondrodystrophic myotonia**
    **Muscular dystrophy, distal** (0690)
    **Myopathy** (other)
    **Myotonia congenita** (0701)
    **Paralysis, hyperkalemic periodic** (0794)
    **Paramyotonia congenita** (0796)

**Major Diagnostic Criteria:** *Late onset myotonic dystrophy*: weakness and atrophy of temporalis, facial, neck, oropharyngeal muscles and distal muscles of the extremities. Percussion and voluntary myotonia, cataracts, cardiac involvement, mental retardation, testicular atrophy, and behavior problems. Electromyography shows myotonic discharges and myopathic alterations. Positive family history with autosomal dominant inheritance.

*Congenital myotonic dystrophy*: myotonic mother, hydramnios in late pregnancy, reduced fetal movements, bilateral facial weakness, hypotonia, neonatal respiratory distress, feeding difficulties, multiple joint contractures with talipes equinus, and mental retardation.

**Clinical Findings:** *Late onset myotonic dystrophy*: skeletal muscle involvement consists of a combination of muscular weakness, atrophy, and myotonia. The former two symptoms develop in selected muscle groups, such as facial, oropharyngeal muscles, temporalis, masseter, neck flexors and distal muscles of both upper and lower extremities. Finger muscles (flexors, adductors, and abductors), wrist extensors, as well as foot extensors, are often weak; the latter resulting in foot drop, steppage gait, and Achilles tendon contractures. Deep tendon reflexes are present initially, then diminished and even abolished as the disease

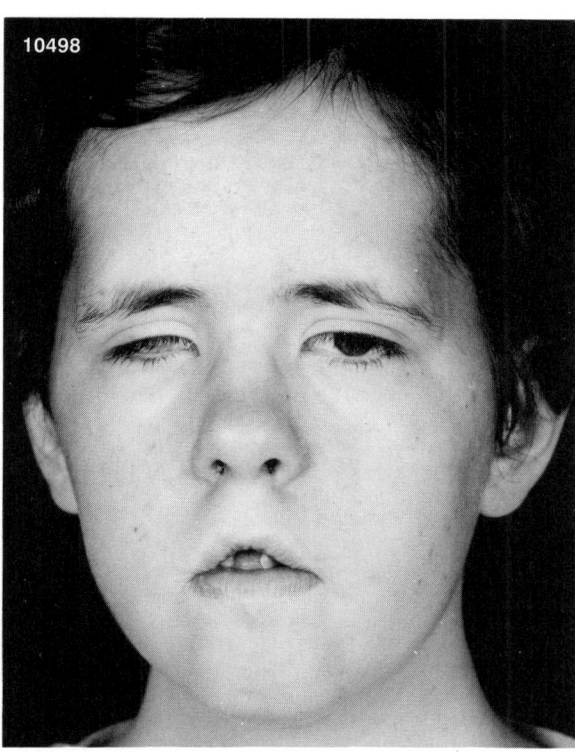

0702-10498: Note expressionless face, ptosis, and corneal opacification OD.

progresses. Deterioration of the condition is insidious, and major incapacitation requiring wheelchair is rarely seen.

Facial diplegia causes a flat and sagging face and, in association with the hollow temples (atrophy of temporalis), a sad and lugubrious expression of the patients. The mouth is frequently kept open, shaped like an inverted V (also called *shark mouth*). Atrophy of the sternocleidomastoid muscles is pronounced; on palpation they often feel like thin, fibrous strands. The neck is thin, the head is bent forward, and kyphosis of the cervical spine may develop. Involvement of the oropharyngeal muscles is recognized by dysphagia and nasal regurgitation. Defective speech (dysarthria) may be a leading symptom and is due to palatal and pharyngeal weakness. Swallowing is altered as well; food particles accumulate and stagnate in the hypopharynx, creating a persistent hazard of food aspiration. Some patients complain of persistent cough and recurrent bronchitis.

Myotonia is usually not as marked as in Thomsen disease (see **Myotonia congenita**). It is limited to some muscles, e.g. hand (thenar muscles) and tongue. Myotonia rarely causes a grave handicap, and most patients interpret it as "stiffness" aggravated by cold. Myotonia is thus a sign that has to be actively sought, and failure to do so is the most common reason for the misdiagnosis of myotonic dystrophy. If a firm grip is followed by the instruction to let go rapidly, this will usually detect active (voluntary) myotonia, while firm percussion of the thenar eminence will show the characteristic delayed relaxation.

Electromyography should always be done. It is valuable when the myotonia is equivocal or absent clinically and the diagnosis is in doubt. The test shows excessive insertional activity and myotonic potentials (discharges). These repetitive potentials wax and wane both in frequency and amplitude and eventually decline, giving a highly distinctive pattern, even more so on auditory recordings ("dive-bomber sound"). Myopathic changes may also be present in the form of short duration, low amplitude, abundant polyphasic potentials.

Muscle biopsy shows central nuclei, often occurring in long chains. Ringed fibers (Ringbinden) are common, being present in at least 70% of biopsies. Ultrastructural studies show sarcoplasmic masses, scattered bundles of myofilaments, free ribosomes and tubular aggregates. Fiber splitting, necrosis, and phagocytosis are less common than in other dystrophies. Histograms demonstrate type 1 fiber atrophy, variation in fiber size, and an enlargement of type 2 muscle fibers. Muscle spindles show an increased number of intrafusal fibers. Serum creatine kinase level is normal or slightly elevated.

Cardiac involvement is common, and present in up to 90% of the patients. Conduction defects (first degree heart block), atrial flutter, other arrhythmias, and mitral valve prolapse are the most frequent cardiac signs. One of our patients with atrial flutter developed cerebral embolism. Cardiomyopathy causing sudden death or congestive heart failure is rare, but can occur at anytime. Postmortem studies of the heart showed atrophy of myocardial fibers, nuclear changes, and replacement of degenerated myofibers by fat and fibrous tissues.

Smooth muscles of various organs, notably upper and lower gastrointestinal tract, gallbladder, and urinary excretory pathways, are affected in some patients with myotonic dystrophy. Achalasia, gastroparesis, constipation, dilatation of the colon with megacolon, gallstones, dysuria, and urinary retention are the clinical syndromes related to smooth muscle pathology.

Lenticular opacities, either iridescent dust or cataracts, are identified by slit-lamp examination in almost every case. The cataracts originate more often in the posterior pole, yet can arise from the anterior pole of the lens as well. It has been proven that apparently unrelated families could be linked by relatives displaying cataracts alone. Other ocular symptoms are ocular hypotonia, ptosis, extraocular weakness, and retinal degenerations (peripheral or macular), with alterations shown on electroretinogram.

Respiratory pathology consists in diaphragmatic and, to a lesser extent, intercostal involvement underlying the chronic alveolar hypoventilation and respiratory distress. Additional respiratory problems include aspiration pneumonia and bronchiectases, while postanesthetic respiratory failure is a serious hazard.

Endocrine disorders include hypogonadism with testicular atrophy due to primary tubular degeneration. Male infertility is a frequent complaint. Overt diabetes is not common even though hyperinsulinism is seen in most patients. Sometimes abnormalities of growth hormone and other pituitary functions may develop. Skin involvement is limited to premature frontal baldness, more pronounced in males than in females. Skeletal abnormalities include cranial hyperostoses, large sinuses, small sella turcica, clubfoot (congenital cases), scoliosis (uncommon), and thin ribs (congenital cases). Severe mental retardation is present in the affected infants. Adults usually show mild mental deterioration. Other signs consistent with central nervous involvement include hypersomnia, which can occur in the absence of detectable respiratory involvement. Some affected individuals were noted to display lack of social responsibility, and they may drop out of work long before physical incapacitation; their social and economic status declines significantly. However, structural changes in the brain are not prominent, even in congenital cases, although CAT scans have shown generalized atrophy and ventricular dilation in some cases.

*Congenital myotonic dystrophy*: Facial weakness, usually bilateral, is present in over 85% of the cases, and is accompanied by masseter weakness. In older children the immobile facies and open mouth are equally characteristic. Involvement of respiratory muscles is probably the major cause of mortality in affected infants. Hypoplasia of the diaphragm and intercostals was documented histologically, and is responsible for the elevation of the diaphragm and thin ribs. The pulmonary immaturity resulting from reduced intrauterine respiratory action aggravates the respiratory distress caused by primary weakness. Talipes equinus occurs in 50% of the cases and illustrates the selective failure of foot extensors and evertors in utero. A small proportion of patients show other joint contractures, mimicking generalized arthrogryposis. Hypotonia is present in most affected infants, but may disappear within weeks. Myotonia is usually absent, becoming obvious clinically between ages 3–10 years. Motor delay is present in all cases and often improves strikingly during childhood. They may walk unsupported. Mental retardation appears to be present from birth, is static, and usually moderate in degree; IQ levels less than 40 were not reported.

Other symptoms of congenital myotonic dystrophy are swallowing and speech difficulties related to palatal, pharyngeal, and esophageal involvement, as well as strabismus and colonic dilatation. The in utero muscle involvement is manifested by poor fetal movements and hydramnios, the latter being caused by impaired fetal swallowing.

**Complications:**  Malignant hyperthermia was reported in several patients after general anesthesia; halothane, succinylcholine, and thiopental represent particular risks. It has been suggested that local anesthesia be used whenever feasible, and to withhold general anesthesia whenever possible.

**Associated Findings:**  Hernia, undescended testes, congenital hip dislocation, congenital heart defect, and **Hydrocephaly** have been reported in congenital myotonic dystrophy.

**Etiology:**  Autosomal dominant inheritance. The mutant gene is pleiotropic, its expressivity varies, and its penetrance is not always complete. However, in all cases in which both parents were examined, definite signs of the disease are present in one parent. For this reason the mutation rate has been estimated near zero. The recommendation is to base genetic counseling on a case being transmitted as an autosomal dominant trait, even when it is not possible to verify.

The most remarkable phenomenon in the genetics of myotonic dystrophy is the occurrence of congenital myotonic dystrophy exclusively in the offspring of affected mothers.

Anticipation, i.e., earlier onset in more recent generations, has been described in myotonic dystrophy. Anticipation may be an artifact of ascertainment.

**Pathogenesis:**  Myotonia can be defined electrophysiologically as an abnormal tendency of the muscle membrane to discharge trains of repetitive action potentials in response to a voluntary contraction or to direct electrical or mechanical stimulation. This altered excitability persists following alpha-tubocurarine or nerve block. Three different theories on the pathogenesis of late onset myotonic dystrophy have been proposed:

*Circulating myotonic factors* based on the demonstration that cholesterol-lowering agents such as diazocholesterol were associated with muscle cramping and electrical evidence of myotonia. These chemical compounds appear to change the permeability of the membrane and to cause a decrease in chloride conductivity. The intracellular $Na^+$ concentration in muscle is also abnormally increased, and this leads to an abnormal $Na^+$ channel function;

*Missing neural trophic factors* theory claims that the muscle membrane in myotonic dystrophy exhibits some of the changes of denervation. However, the involvement of peripheral nerves is rarely significant, according to recent studies. In addition, the widespread tissue alterations in myotonic dystrophy represents evidence against neural trophic factors. It is hard to accept that cardiac, smooth muscle, bone, endocrine glands, lens, and gammaglobulin abnormalities are secondary effects to impaired neural function.

*Primary membrane defect* theory relies on experimental and clinical data suggesting that human myotonic disorders represent genetically induced primary alterations in the structure and function of cellular membranes. Studies using endogenous protein kinase have shown a significant decrease in phosphorylation of the protein from the red cells and muscle membrane in myotonic dystrophy. It seems unlikely that an alteration in protein kinase represents the primary defect. It is assumed that the altered phosphorylation is related to an unidentified abnormality of a lipid-lipid or lipid-protein complex present in the structure of membranes. Thus, the primary defect of myotonic dystrophy is still unknown. The cloning of the abnormal gene located on chromosome 19 in the near future will allow in vitro translation of the gene product and clarify the pathogenesis of late onset myotonic dystrophy.

The causative factors underlying congenital myotonic dystrophy remain entirely unknown. In all cases of congenital myotonic dystrophy the mother is the affected parent (adult form). Thus, a maternal factor of some type is necessary for the pathogenesis of the disease. An environmental rather than genetic factor was claimed, but this is not likely. No cases of transient congenital myotonic dystrophy were reported as in congenital myasthenia gravis, and affected infants developed progressive myotonia and muscle weakness, indicating that the myotonic dystrophy gene is necessary; finally, at least 50% of children in sibships appear to be entirely normal.

**MIM No.:**  *16090

**POS No.:**  3193

**Sex Ratio:**  M1:F1

**Occurrence:**  The incidence of the disease varies from 1.2: 1,000,000 in England, to 2.4:1,000,000 in Northern Ireland, and 5:1,000,000 in Switzerland. The latter incidence is probably accurate for most European and American populations. Myotonic dystrophy has proved to be the most common adult muscular dystrophy in most of the populations studied, and no racial group is exempt.

**Risk of Recurrence for Patient's Sib:**
  See Part I, *Mendelian Inheritance.*

**Risk of Recurrence for Patient's Child:**
  See Part I, *Mendelian Inheritance.* A number of studies have shown reduced fertility in both sexes to around 75% of normal, although the data are contradictory.

**Age of Detectability:**  Prenatal diagnosis using linkage with ApoC2 and LDR 152 (D19519) in combination with ultrasonography for hydramnios detection characteristic of congenital form. Clinically, from birth to one year of age for congenital form, 10–20 years of age for the adult form.

**Gene Mapping and Linkage:**  DM (dystrophia myotonia) has been mapped to 19q13.2-q13.3.

**Prevention:**  None known. Genetic counseling indicated.

**Treatment:**  Myotonia is usually mild and does not require antimyotonic drugs. Physical therapy and orthopedic measures are helpful in correcting the equinus and other muscle contractures. Surgical resection of advanced cataracts and an external cardiac pacemaker for patients with atrioventricular blocks are also recommended. Myotonic patients should avoid general anesthesia with halothane and succinylcholine because of the risk of developing malignant hyperthermia.

**Prognosis:**  Good for life span, and activity for many years after clinical onset. Sudden death may occur due to cardiac arrythmias.

**Detection of Carrier:**  Based on clinical evaluation, electromyography, ophthalmologic evaluation (slit-lamp, intraocular pressure, electroretinography), and genetic linkage with ApoC2 and LDR 152 (D19519).

**References:**

Zellweger H, Ionasescu V: Myotonic dystrophy and its differential diagnosis. Acta Neurol Scand 1973; 49(suppl 55):1–28.

Harper P: Myotonic dystrophy. Philadelphia: W.B. Saunders, 1979. *

Nowak TV, et al.: Gastrointestinal manifestations of muscular dystrophies. Gastroenterology 1982; 82:800–810.

Roses AD: Myotonic muscular dystrophy from clinical description to molecular genetics. Arch Intern Med 1985; 45:1487–1492.

Jamal GA, et al.: Myotonic dystrophy: a reassessment by conventional and more recently introduced neurophysiological techniques. Brain 1986; 109:1279–1296.

Spaans, F, et al.: Myotonic dystrophy associated with hereditary motor and sensory neuropathy. Brain 1986; 109:1149–1168.

Bartlett RJ, et al.: A new probe for the diagnosis of myotonic muscular dystrophy. Science 1987; 235:1648–1650.

I0000                                              **Victor V. Ionasescu**

**Myotonic myopathy-dwarfism-chondrodystrophy-eye/face anomalies**
  *See CHONDRODYSTROPHIC MYOTONIA, SCHWARTZ-JAMPEL TYPE*
**Myotubular myopathy**
  *See MYOPATHY, MYOTUBULAR*

**Myotubular myopathy, X-linked**
*See MYOPATHY, MYOTUBULAR*
**Myriachit**
*See JUMPING FRENCHMAN OF MAINE*
**Mysoline, fetal effects of**
*See FETAL PRIMIDONE EMBRYOPATHY*
**Myxedematous endemic cretinism**
*See CRETINISM, ENDEMIC, AND RELATED DISORDERS*

---

## MYXOMA, INTRACARDIAC                              2160

**Includes:**
    Atrial, myxoma
    Biatrial myxoma with atrial septal defect
    Left atrial myxoma
    Left ventricular myxoma
    Right atrial myxoma
    Right ventricular myxoma

**Excludes:**
    Fibroma
    **Nevi-atrial myxoma-myxoid neurofibromas-ephelides** (2572)
    Rhabdomyoma
    Sarcoma
    Tumors, other intracardiac

**Major Diagnostic Criteria:** Echocardiographic, angiocardiographic, or necropsy evidence of myxoma.

**Clinical Findings:** Congestive heart failure; systolic and or diastolic murmurs; arrhythmias; tachycardia; in presence of infection, febrile episodes and bacteremia; EKG evidence of chamber enlargement and various types of heart block; X-ray evidence of cardiomegaly; echocardiographic evidence of mass lesion; angiocardiographic evidence of intracardiac mass. Undiagnosed patients may have infective endocarditis, embolic phenomena (particularly stroke), and symptoms compatible with rheumatic fever.

**Complications:** Infective endocarditis, cerebral vascular accidents, and other manifestations of embolism. Prolapse and incompetence of the mitral and pulmonary valves.

**Associated Findings:** Atrial septal defects, Mitral valve prolapse.

**Etiology:** Possibly autosomal recessive inheritance. Most cases appear to be sporadic, but familial cases have been reported. These include four siblings whose parents were unaffected, and a mother and all three of her sons. Both autosomal recessive and dominant modes of inheritance have been considered. Multifactorial inheritance cannot be ruled out on the basis of the limited number of familial cases studied so far. An environmental relationship to rheumatic fever, as seen in two families, requires further evaluation.

**Pathogenesis:** Apparently neoplastic.

**MIM No.:** *25596

**Sex Ratio:** M1:F1

**Occurrence:** Undetermined; about 1:12,000 autopsied cases.

**Risk of Recurrence for Patient's Sib:**
See Part I, *Mendelian Inheritance*. Most cases are sporadic.

**Risk of Recurrence for Patient's Child:**
See Part I, *Mendelian Inheritance*.

**Age of Detectability:** Patients become symptomatic in late childhood or in adult life. The lesions could probably be detected earlier by echocardiographic examination of first-degree relatives.

**Gene Mapping and Linkage:** Unknown.

**Prevention:** None known. Genetic counseling indicated.

**Treatment:** Surgical excision. Antibacterial therapy for infective endocarditis.

**Prognosis:** Guarded. The earlier the intervention, the better the outlook, although recurrences are not uncommon.

**Detection of Carrier:** Echocardiography for preclinical cases and asymptomatic relatives.

**Support Groups:** Dallas; American Heart Association

**References:**
Lortscher RH, et al.: Left atrial myxoma presenting as rheumatic fever. Chest 1974; 66:302–303.
Farah MG: Familial atrial myxoma. Ann Intern Med 1975; 83:358–360. *
Grauer K, Grauer MC: Familial atrial myxoma with bilateral recurrence. Heart Lung 1983; 12:600–602.
Dewald GW, et al.: Chromosomally abnormal clones and nonrandom telomeric translocations in cardiac myxomas. Mayo Clin Proc 1987; 62:558–567.

N0003                         **James J. Nora**

**Myxoma-adrenocortical dysplasia syndrome**
*See NEVI-ATRIAL MYXOMA-MYXOID NEUROFIBROMAS-EPHELIDES*
**Myxomas-spotty pigmentation-endocrine overactivity**
*See NEVI-ATRIAL MYXOMA-MYXOID NEUROFIBROMAS-EPHELIDES*

# ❖ N ❖

N(5,10) methylenetetrahydrofolate reductase deficiency
*See HOMOCYSTINURIA, N(5,10) METHYLENE
TETRAHYDROFOLATE DEFICIENCY TYPE*
N-acetyl-alpha-D-glucosaminidase deficiency
*See MUCOPOLYSACCHARIDOSIS III*
N-acetylglucosamine-1-phosphotransferase deficiency
*See MUCOLIPIDOSIS II*
N-acetylglucosamine-6-sulfate sulfatase deficiency
*See MUCOPOLYSACCHARIDOSIS III*

## N-ACETYLGLUTAMATE SYNTHETASE DEFICIENCY          3170

**Includes:**
Hyperammonemia III
AGA deficiency
NAGS deficiency

**Excludes:**
**Carbamoyl phosphate synthetase deficiency** (3022)
**Hyperornithinemia-hyperammonemia-homocitrullinuria** (3169)
**Ornithine transcarbamylase deficiency** (3023)
Transient hyperammonemia of the newborn

**Major Diagnostic Criteria:**  Elevated levels of ammonium in plasma, decreased plasma citrulline and urinary orotate, normal organic acids, deficient activity of N-acetylglutamate synthetase in liver.

**Clinical Findings:**  Episodes of ataxia, vomiting, lethargy/coma, hyperpnea, hypotonicity associated with hyperammonemia.

**Complications:**  The one surviving patient is mentally retarded.

**Associated Findings:**  None known.

**Etiology:**  Presumably autosomal recessive inheritance.

**Pathogenesis:**  N-acetylglutamate is a known activator of the first enzyme in the urea cycle, carbamylphosphate synthetase (the enzyme deficient in hyperammonemia II). Its formation from glutamate and acetyl CoA is catalyzed in the liver by mitochondrial N-acetylglutamate synthetase. In the absence of N-acetylglutamate, activity of carbamylphosphate synthetase is approximately 5% of normal. Thus, the mechanism of hyperammonemia in this disorder is a secondary deficiency of carbamylphosphate synthetase induced by deficient activity of N-acetylglutamate synthetase.

**MIM No.:**  23731

**Sex Ratio:**  M1:F1

**Occurrence:**  One affected family has been described in which one infant survived with treatment and two of his sibs died without treatment during the newborn period.

**Risk of Recurrence for Patient's Sib:**
See Part I, *Mendelian Inheritance.*

**Risk of Recurrence for Patient's Child:**
See Part I, *Mendelian Inheritance.* The one patient described has not reached reproductive age. The risk is likely to be low.

**Age of Detectability:**  At birth by appropriate assays. However, detection in a previously unaffected family is likely to occur only when the child becomes symptomatic.

**Gene Mapping and Linkage:**  Unknown.

**Prevention:**  None known. Genetic counseling indicated.

**Treatment:**  Nitrogen restriction plus supplements with carbamyl glutamate (a congener of N-acetyl glutamate), arginine, sodium benzoate, and sodium phenylacetate.

**Prognosis:**  Guarded. Affected individuals are at risk for recurrent episodes of hyperammonemia associated with dietary indescretions or intercurrent infections.

**Detection of Carrier:**  Unknown.

**References:**
Bachmann C, et al: N-acetylglutamate synthetase deficiency: diagnosis, clinical observations and treatment. Adv Exp Med Biol 1981; 153:39–46.

BA066                                              **Mark L. Batshaw**

N-acetylneuraminic acid storage disease
*See SIALIC ACID STORAGE DISEASE, INFANTILE TYPE*
N-acetylneuraminic acid storage disease, infantile (one form)
*See SALLA DISEASE*
N-acetyltransferase polymorphism
*See NEUROPATHY, HERITABLE ISONIAZIDE TYPE (INH)*
NADH cytochrome b5 reductase deficiency
*See METHEMOGLOBINEMIA, NADH-DEPENDENT DIAPHORASE
DEFICIENCY*
Naegeli syndrome
*See ECTODERMAL DYSPLASIA, NAEGELI TYPE*
Naegeli-Franceschetti-Jadassohn syndrome
*See ECTODERMAL DYSPLASIA, NAEGELI TYPE*
Nager acrofacial dystosis
*See ACROFACIAL DYSOSTOSIS, NAGER TYPE*
NAGS deficiency
*See N-ACETYLGLUTAMATE SYNTHETASE DEFICIENCY*
Nail absent
*See NAILS, ANONYCHIA, HEREDITARY*
Nail dysgenesis and hypodontia
*See HYPODONTIA-NAIL DYSGENESIS*
Nail dysplasia-curly hair-ankyloblepharon syndrome
*See CHANDS*
Nail dystrophy and sensorineural deafness
*See DEAFNESS-ONYCHODYSTROPHY*
Nail-hair-bone-tooth dysplasia
*See TRICHO-DENTO-OSSEOUS SYNDROME*

## NAIL-PATELLA SYNDROME 0704

**Includes:**
Anonychia-onychodystrophy
Arthroosteoonychodysplasia
Fong disease
HOOD (hereditary onycho-osteo-dysplasia)
Iliac horns
Onychoosteodysplasia
Turner-Kieser syndrome

**Excludes:**  Turner syndrome (0977)

**Major Diagnostic Criteria:**  Hypoplastic nails and hypoplastic patella.

**Clinical Findings:**  Dysplasia of the nails, absent or hypoplastic patellae, abnormality of the elbows interfering with supination, pronation or extension, and iliac horns. The nails of both hands and feet may be affected; most frequently those of the index and middle fingers and thumb. Hypoplasia, narrowness, and splitting of the nails are the usual findings. Triangular lunulae, sharp and distally pointed at apex, may be present. The patella may be small, tripartite, polygonal, or absent; lateral dislocation of the patella occurs. Iliac horns are seen, arising from the posterior ilium, and if present are pathognomonic for this entity. There may be webbing of the elbow, preventing full extension. Nephropathy occurs in some 30% of patients and may be either glomerulonephritic or nephrotic in type. Scoliosis occasionally occurs.

**Complications:**  Subluxation of the knee, genu varum, early onset osteoarthritis of the knee. Lateral dislocation of the patella may complicate walking, especially down the stairs. The elbow may subluxate. The nephropathy, although usually benign, may cause death at an early age.

**Associated Findings:**  Deformity of sternum, spina bifida occulta, bilateral first rib hypoplasia, shoulder anomalies, anomalies of pectoralis minor, triceps and biceps, hyperostosis frontalis interna, clinodactyly of fifth finger, partial symphalangism of distal interphalangeal joints, hypothyroidism and goiter, mental retardation, cataracts, microcornea, microphthalmia, calcaneal and valgus foot deformities.

**Etiology:**  Autosomal dominant inheritance with variable expressivity.

**Pathogenesis:**  Electron microscopic studies have shown many collagen fibrils in thickened basement membranes and in mesangial matrix of otherwise normal glomeruli, the presence of which is unrelated to demonstrable symptomatic alterations of renal function.

**MIM No.:**  *16120, 10700

**POS No.:**  3331

**CDC No.:**  756.830

**Sex Ratio:**  M1:F1

**Occurrence:**  Undetermined; established literature.

**Risk of Recurrence for Patient's Sib:**
See Part I, *Mendelian Inheritance.*

**Risk of Recurrence for Patient's Child:**
See Part I, *Mendelian Inheritance.*

**Age of Detectability:**  At birth, on the basis of nail defects.

**Gene Mapping and Linkage:**  NPS1 (nail patella syndrome 1) has been mapped to 9q34.

**Prevention:**  None known. Genetic counseling indicated.

**Treatment:**  Orthopedic treatment for problems arising in the knee or elbow. Patients should be repeatedly assessed for renal abnormalities.

**Prognosis:**  The renal complications have caused death as early as eight years of age. About eight percent of patients died of renal disease.

**Detection of Carrier:**  Unknown.

**Special Considerations:**  *Anonychia-onychodystrophy* (Timerman et al, 1969) shows many of the nail characteristics of this syndrome but without the associated manifestations.

**References:**
Lucas GL, Opitz JM: The nail-patella syndrome. J Pediatr 1966; 68:273–288. * †
Timerman I, et al.: Dominant anonychia and onychodystrophy. J Med Genet 1969; 6:105–106.
Bennett WM, et al.: The nephropathy of the nail-patella syndrome. Am J Med 1973; 54:304–319 *
Garces MA, et al.: Hereditary onchyo-osteo-dysplasia (HOOD syndrome): report of two cases. Skeletal Radiol 1982; 8:55–58.
Yakish SD, Fu FH: Long term follow-up of the treatment of a family with nail-patella syndrome. J Pediatr Orthop 1983; 3:360–363.
Green ST, Natarajan S: Bilateral first-rib hypoplasia: a new feature of the nail-patella syndrome. Dermatologica 1986; 172:323–325. †

ZA000                                              **Elaine H. Zackai**

**Nails (abnormal)-deafness-retardation-seizures-dermatoglyphics**
*See DEAFNESS-ONYCHO-OSTEO-DYSTROPHY-RETARDATION-SEIZURES (DOORS)*
**Nails (hypoplastic)-neutropenia-onychorrhexis**
*See ONYCHO-TRICHODYSPLASIA-NEUTROPENIA*
**Nails, absence of, congenital**
*See NAILS, ANONYCHIA, HEREDITARY*

## NAILS, ANONYCHIA, HEREDITARY 0066

**Includes:**
Anonychia
Nail absent
Nails, absence of, congenital
Onychial dysplasia, hereditary

**Excludes:**
Ectrodactyly-anonychia (0065)
Epidermolysis bullosum, type III (2562)
Nail-patella syndrome (0704)

**Major Diagnostic Criteria:**  Partial or total absence of nails.

**Clinical Findings:**  Characterized by various abnormalities of finger- or toenails and phalanges including complete absence of nail, rudimentary nail matrix at proximal or lateral edge of nail bed, large pointed lunulae, longitudinal furrowing, and thinning or thickening of nail plate. Usually symmetric. May be present at birth or may develop at a later age. Nail beds are present. X-ray

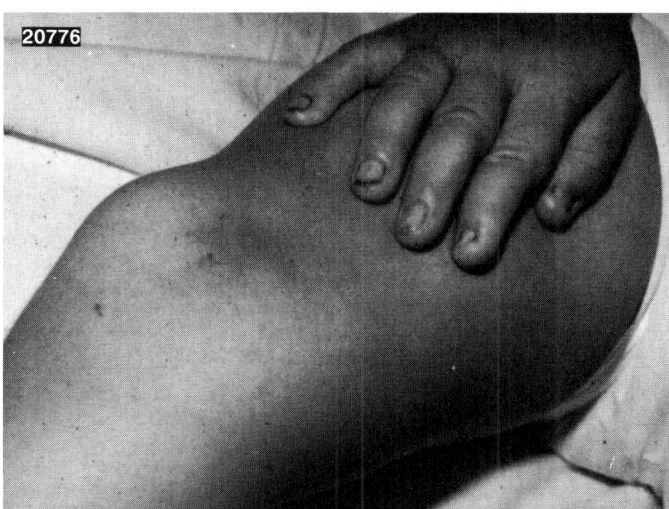

20776

0704-20776:  Nail-patella syndrome; note thin, dysplastic nails and dent on the knee due to the absent patella.

studies occasionally show tapering and spatulation of distal phalanges and shortening of phalanges and metacarpal bones.

**Complications:** Unknown.

**Associated Findings:** Dental anomalies, aplasia or hypoplasia of upper lateral incisors, spaced teeth, and lack of some molars have been reported. Lymphedema was present in one case.

**Etiology:** Both autosomal dominant and autosomal recessive inheritance have been reported.

**Pathogenesis:** Unknown.

**MIM No.:** *20680

**CDC No.:** 757.500

**Sex Ratio:** Presumably M1:F1

**Occurrence:** Rare.

**Risk of Recurrence for Patient's Sib:**
See Part I, *Mendelian Inheritance.*

**Risk of Recurrence for Patient's Child:**
See Part I, *Mendelian Inheritance.*

**Age of Detectability:** At birth or later.

**Gene Mapping and Linkage:** Unknown.

**Prevention:** None known. Genetic counseling indicated.

**Treatment:** Unknown.

**Prognosis:** No impact on life span or intelligence.

**Detection of Carrier:** Unknown.

**References:**
Cockayne EA: Abnormalities of the nails. In: Inherited abnormalities of the skin and its appendages. London: Oxford University Press, 1933:265–268.
Littman A, Levin S: Anonychia as a recessive autosomal trait in man. J Invest Dermatol 1964; 42:177–178.
Maisels DO: Anonychia in association with lymphoedema. Br J Plast Surg 1966; 19:37–42.
Hopsu-Hava VK, Jensen CT: Anonychia congenita. Arch Derm 1973; 107:752–753.
Freire-Maia N, Pinheiro M: Recessive anonychia totalis and dominant aplasia (or hypoplasia) of upper lateral incisors in the same kindred. J Med Genet 1979; 16:45–48.

MI038                                        **Giuseppe Micali**

## NAILS, KOILONYCHIA                                  0559

**Includes:**
Koilonychia, hereditary
Spoon nails

**Excludes:** Secondary koilonychia

**Major Diagnostic Criteria:** Concavity of the fingernails. The toenails are commonly concave in normal children and therefore unimportant unless the fingernails are also involved.

**Clinical Findings:** Concave nail shape with everted edges and thinning of the nail. The thumb is almost always affected; the toenails are involved in over 50%. Not all the nails are involved in each patient. Occasionally, a wide fissure is seen in the center of the nail in addition to spooning. The trait is rarely associated with monilethrix, palmar hyperkeratosis, steatocystoma multiplex, or **Nail-patella syndrome**.

**Complications:** Unknown.

**Associated Findings:** None known.

**Etiology:** Autosomal dominant inheritance with a high degree of penetrance, and variable expressivity in degree of nail involvement. The great majority of isolated cases of koilonychia are not hereditary, but rather traumatic or secondary to a large number of medical disorders.

**Pathogenesis:** Unknown.

**MIM No.:** *14930

**CDC No.:** 757.520

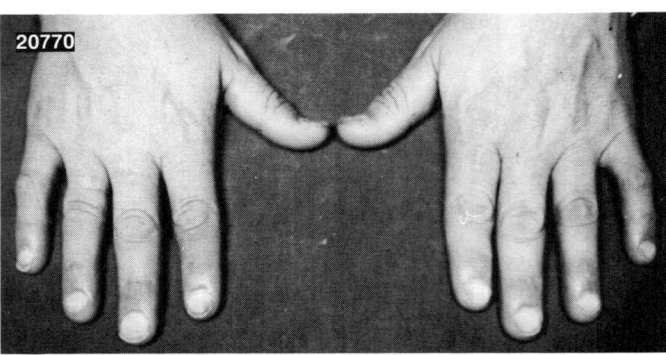

0559-20770:   Nails, koilnychia.

**Sex Ratio:** M1:F1

**Occurrence:** Six kindreds reported in the literature, including 16 cases over five generations in the family reported by Hellier (1950).

**Risk of Recurrence for Patient's Sib:**
See Part I, *Mendelian Inheritance.*

**Risk of Recurrence for Patient's Child:**
See Part I, *Mendelian Inheritance.*

**Age of Detectability:** At birth or early childhood.

**Gene Mapping and Linkage:** Unknown.

**Prevention:** None known. Genetic counseling indicated.

**Treatment:** Occasionally a deformed toenail that causes discomfort is permanently destroyed surgically.

**Prognosis:** Normal for life span, intelligence and function.

**Detection of Carrier:** Unknown.

**References:**
Hellier FF: Hereditary koilonychia. Br J Dermatol 1950; 62:213–214.
Stone OJ, Maberry JD: Spoon nails and clubbing: review and possible structural mechanisms. Tex State J Med 1965; 61:620–627.
Bergeron JR, Stone OJ: Koilonychia: a report of familial spoon nails. Arch Dermatol 1967; 95:351–353.
Bumpers RD, Bishop ME: Familial koilonychia: a current case history. Arch Derm 1980; 116:845–846.
Stone OJ: Clubbing and koilonychia. Dermatologic Clinics 1985; 3:485–490.

ST030                                        **Orville J. Stone**

## NAILS, LEUKONYCHIA                                  0589

**Includes:** Leukonychia totalis

**Excludes:** Leukonychia, punctate

**Major Diagnostic Criteria:** White discoloration of the nails.

**Clinical Findings:** A whitish discoloration of the nails is present, either as a single, broad, or transverse band, one or more narrow bands, a large white area, or a completely white nail. Either the nails of the fingers, toes, or both may be involved. The nails are not brittle or frayed. Nail thickness appears to be average, and no grooves or other irregularities are observed.

**Complications:** Unknown.

**Associated Findings:** Reported association with leukotrichia, total alopecia, extensive vitiligo, multiple sebaceous cysts, and renal calculi.

**Etiology:** Autosomal dominant inheritance.

**Pathogenesis:** Two major theories propose that the white color is due to opacity of the nail plate. One theory holds that abnormal keratinization of the nail plate is sufficient to cause the opacity, while the other postulates that air must be present within the nail plate.

**MIM No.:** *15160

**CDC No.:** 757.530

**Sex Ratio:** Estimated M1:F1.5

**Occurrence:** Several kindreds reported in the literature.

**Risk of Recurrence for Patient's Sib:**
See Part I, *Mendelian Inheritance.*

**Risk of Recurrence for Patient's Child:**
See Part I, *Mendelian Inheritance.*

**Age of Detectability:** At birth.

**Gene Mapping and Linkage:** Unknown.

**Prevention:** None known. Genetic counseling indicated.

**Treatment:** Unknown.

**Prognosis:** Normal life span.

**Detection of Carrier:** Unknown.

**References:**

Medansky RS, Fox JM: Hereditary leukonychia totalis. Arch Dermatol 1960; 82:412–414.
Albright SD III, Wheeler CE Jr: Leukonychia: total and partial leukonychia in a single family with a review of the literature. Arch Dermatol 1964; 90:392.
Bushkell LL, Gorlin RJ: Leukonychia totalis, multiple sebaceous cysts, and renal calculi. Arch Derm 1975; 111:899–901.

ME005                                     **Roland S. Medansky**

## NAILS, PACHYONYCHIA CONGENITA                     0789

**Includes:**
    Jadassohn-Lewandowsky syndrome
    Pachyonychia congenita
    Pachyonychia ichthyosiforme
    Pachyonychia neonatorum
    Polykeratosis congenita

**Excludes:**
    **Dyskeratosis congenita** (2024)
    Onychauxis
    Onychogryphosis
    **Pachyonychia congenita-steatocystoma multiplex** (2905)

**Major Diagnostic Criteria:** Hypertrophy of the nail bed and nail plate, usually involving all 20 digits and associated with other defects. The nails are red to yellow to brown in color and compressed laterally. The diagnosis may be confirmed by a biopsy specimen of the nail unit that reveals epidermal hyperplasia with acanthosis, hyperkeratosis, and focal parakeratosis. There is noted atypical individual cell keratinization of the Malpighian layer cells, which have highly eosinophilic cytoplasm.

**Clinical Findings:** Nail units are abnormal. These patients have palmar and plantar hyperhidrosis with symmetric focal hyperkeratosis. Follicular hyperkeratosis of the trunk with mildly ichthyosiform skin and hyperpigmentation have occurred. Bullae;

ulcerations; leukokeratosis of the tongue (scalloped) and oral mucous membranes, resembling leukoplakia; and verrucous lesions over the extensor areas as well as buttocks and popliteal fossae have been reported. Cataracts and corneal dyskeratosis involve the eyes. Steatocystoma multiplex, oral herpes simplex, elevated serum copper and iron, and increased urinary excretion of hexoseamine and hydroxyproline are other associations.

**Complications:** Unknown.

**Associated Findings:** Natal and carious teeth with early loss (before age 30 years), other dental anomalies, dry dystrophic alopecia, short stature, mental retardation, epidermolysis bullosa, osteomas, respiratory involvement, and intestinal diverticuli have been reported.

**Etiology:** Usually autosomal dominant inheritance with incomplete penetrance. An autosomal recessive variant has been reported.

**Pathogenesis:** Unknown.

**MIM No.:** *16720, 26013

**POS No.:** 4181

**CDC No.:** 757.516

**Sex Ratio:** Presumably M1:F1.

**Occurrence:** Several large kindreds have been documented. More frequent among Jewish and Slavic males.

**Risk of Recurrence for Patient's Sib:**
See Part I, *Mendelian Inheritance.*

**Risk of Recurrence for Patient's Child:**
See Part I, *Mendelian Inheritance.*

**Age of Detectability:** Clinically, at about 3–5 months of age, except for natal teeth.

**Gene Mapping and Linkage:** Unknown.

**Prevention:** None known. Genetic counseling indicated.

**Treatment:** Surgical resection of the nail unit with possible matricectomy. Specific and symptomatic therapy for associated defects. Intralesional corticosteroids to the nail unit has been suggested to be a beneficial though inconsistent form of therapy.

**Prognosis:** Normal life span unless some of the more serious associated defects are present. Patients usually adapt well to the disorder.

**Detection of Carrier:** Examination of relatives for evidence of the trait.

**References:**

Chong-Hai T, Rajagopalan K: Pachyonychia congenita with recessive inheritance. Arch Dermatol 1977; 113:685–687.
Zaias N: The nail in health and disease. New York: SP Medical and Scientific Books, 1980.
Franzot J, et al.: Pachyonychia congenita. Dermatologica 1981; 160: 462–472.
Stieglitz JB, Centerwall WR: Pachyonychia congenita: a seventeen-member, four generation pedigree with unusual respiratory and dental involvement. Am J Med Genet 1983; 14:21–28.
Baran R, Dawber RPR: Diseases of the nails and their management. Oxford: Blackwell Scientific, 1984.
Sivasundram A, et al.: Pachyonychia congenita. Int J Dermatol 1985; 24:179–180.

SC060                                     **Richard K. Scher**

**Nails, pachyonychia congenita, Jackson-Lawler type**
    *See PACHYONYCHIA CONGENITA-STEATOCYSTOMA MULTIPLEX*
**Naito-Oyanagi disease**
    *See DENTATORUBROPALLIDOLUYSIAN DEGENERATION,
    HEREDITARY*
**Nakajo nodular erythema with digital changes**
    *See DIGITAL DEFECTS-NODULAR ERYTHEMA-EMACIATION,
    NAKAJO TYPE*
**Nakajo syndrome**
    *See DIGITAL DEFECTS-NODULAR ERYTHEMA-EMACIATION,
    NAKAJO TYPE*
**Namaqualand hip dysplasia**
    *See HIP, DYSPLASIA, NAMAQUALAND TYPE*

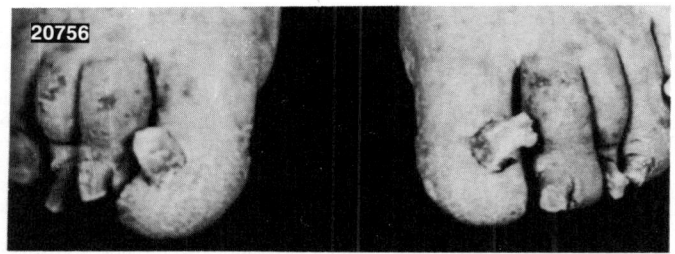

**0789-20756:** Nails, pachyonychia congenita; note "horn nails."

**NAME syndrome**
  *See NEVI-ATRIAL MYXOMA-MYXOID NEUROFIBROMAS-EPHELIDES*
**Nance deafness**
  *See DEAFNESS WITH PERILYMPHATIC GUSHER*
**Nance-Horan syndrome**
  *See CATARACTS-OTO-DENTAL DEFECTS*
**Nance-Insley syndrome**
  *See OTO-SPONDYLO-MEGAEPIPHYSEAL DYSPLASIA*
  *also CHONDRODYSTROPHY-SENSORINEURAL DEAFNESS, NANCE-INSLEY TYPE*
**Nance-Sweeney syndrome**
  *See CHONDRODYSTROPHY-SENSORINEURAL DEAFNESS, NANCE-INSLEY TYPE*
**Nanocephalic dwarf**
  *See SECKEL SYNDROME*
**Nape nevus**
  *See NEVUS FLAMMEUS*
**Naprosyn^, fetal effects**
  *See FETAL EFFECTS OF NONSTEROIDAL ANTI-INFLAMMATORY DRUGS (NSAIDS)*
**Naproxen, fetal effects**
  *See FETAL EFFECTS OF NONSTEROIDAL ANTI-INFLAMMATORY DRUGS (NSAIDS)*

## NARCOLEPSY                                            3287

**Includes:**
  Cataplexy
  Maladie de Gelineau
  Narcoleptic syndrome
  Sleep disorder

**Excludes:**
  Apnea, obstructive sleep
  Encephalitis
  Epilepsy
  Hypersomnia, essential
  Hypoventilation, congenital central alveolar type (2606)
  Klein-Levin hibernation syndrome
  Myoclonus
  Tremor-duodenal ulcer syndrome (0963)

**Major Diagnostic Criteria:** Chronic daytime somnolence, unavoidable daytime napping, *cataplexy*. Symptoms may also include sleep paralysis and hypnagogic hallucinations. Polygraphic testing with nocturnal recording, followed by daytime multiple sleep latency testing, will find short sleep latencies at each nap; frequent occurrence of REM sleep at sleep onset, rather than at a later time during sleep; and nocturnal disrupted sleep.

**Clinical Findings:** The first symptoms often develop near puberty. The peak age of reported symptoms is between 15–25 years of age, but narcolepsy and other symptoms have been noted at 5–6 years, and a second, smaller peak of onset has been noted between 35–45 years, near menopause in women.

Excessive daytime somnolence and irresistible sleep episodes usually occur as the first symptoms, either independently or associated with one or more other symptoms. They are enhanced by high temperature, indoor activity, and idleness. Symptoms may abate with time but never phase out completely. Attacks of *cataplexy* (an abrupt, reversible decrease or loss of muscle tone, most frequently elicited by strong emotions such as anger or laughter) generally appear in conjunction with abnormal episodes of sleep, but may occur as much as 20 years later. They occasionally, but seldom, occur before the abnormal sleep episodes, in which case they are a major source of difficulty in diagnosis. Episodes can vary in frequency from a few during the subject's entire lifetime to one or several per day.

Hypnagogic hallucinations and sleep paralysis do not affect all subjects and are often transitory. Disturbed nocturnal sleep seldom occurs in the first stages and generally builds up with age.

**Complications:** Narcolepsy leads to a variety of complications such as driving or machine accidents; difficulties at work resulting in disability, forced retirement or job dismissal; impotence; and depression.

**Associated Findings:** Sleep apnea is found in ten percent of narcoleptic subjects. Periodic leg movement (PLM) syndrome is also found frequently with the condition. The idea of an association between narcolepsy and **Multiple sclerosis** is conceptually interesting, as both conditions have been hypothesized as possible immune disorders, but the association has not been demonstrated.

**Etiology:** Multifactorial inheritance strongly influenced by environmental factors. In very limited studies with monozygotic twins, the twins of narcoleptic subjects had an incidence of narcolepsy 6–18 times higher than that of the general population. However, several elderly monozygotic twins have been proven discordant for narcolepsy. The major histocompatibility complex (MHC) antigen HLA-DR2 has been linked to the condition. All known Japanese narcoleptic subjects are HLA-DR2 positive and, secondarily, have the antigen DQw6. Caucasians and Blacks present DR2-negative isolated and familial cases; as many as nine percent of unrelated North American Caucasians with narcolepsy are predicted to be DR2 negative. In more recent studies, a separate gene, *canarc-1*, has been found to be the determinant of the condition in certain dogs. It is postulated that this gene's human analogue is a second genetic factor in the occurence of narcolepsy in humans.

**Pathogenesis:** Unknown. Special circumstances such as an abrupt change of sleep-wake schedule and/or a severe psychological stress (e.g. death of a relative, divorce) precede the occurence of the first symptom in half of the cases.

**MIM No.:** *16140

**Sex Ratio:** M1:F<1

**Occurrence:** In the San Francisco Bay Area its occurence has been calculated at 0.05%, and in the Los Angeles area at 0.067%. Its prevalence is estimated to be between 0.02 and 0.08% in North American Caucasions.

**Risk of Recurrence for Patient's Sib:**
  See Part I, *Mendelian Inheritance*. A frequency of narcolepsy among first-degree relatives has been calculated at 0.9%.

**Risk of Recurrence for Patient's Child:**
  See Part I, *Mendelian Inheritance*. A frequency of narcolepsy among first-degree relatives has been calculated at 0.9%. There was no abnormal dominance of a subgroup (i.e. parents, siblings, or children).

**Age of Detectability:** Age at onset varies from childhood to the fifth decade, with a peak in the second decade. Signs may be visible as early as 2–3 years of age.

**Gene Mapping and Linkage:** HLA-DR2 is located on the small arm of the 6th chromosome. The location of canarc-1 is unknown. It is not linked to the major histocompatibility complex.

**Prevention:** None known. Genetic counseling indicated.

**Treatment:** Many symptoms will respond to drug therapy. Central nervous system stimulants, especially amphetamines, are effective against excessive daytime somnolence. Tricyclic medications such as protriptyline and clomipramine are often used in the treatment of cataplexy, sleep paralysis, and hypnagogic hallucinations.

Short daytime naps will also help the subject maintain alertness during the day; in fact, it has not been established that stimulant medications are more effective than this simple treatment. Also important for narcoleptic subjects are support groups. Narcolepsy is often poorly understood, and its victims may find rejection from families and other social entities.

**Prognosis:** Normal life span.

**Detection of Carrier:** Examination of relatives for evidence of the trait. However, presence of DR2 DQw6 is neither sufficient nor necessary for the development of narcolepsy.

**References:**
Guilleminault C, et al., eds: Narcolepsy. New York: Spectrum Publications, 1976.
Honda Y, Juji T, eds: HLA in Narcolepsy. Berlin-Heidelberg: Springer-Verlag, 1978

Guilleminault C, et eal.: Familial Patterns of Narcolepsy. Lancet 1989; II:1376–1379.

GU010                                    **Christian Guilleminault**

**Narcoleptic syndrome**
*See NARCOLEPSY*
**Nasal agenesis**
*See NOSE, TURBINATE DEFORMITY*
**Nasal alar hypoplasia-hypothyroidism-pancreatic achylia-deafness**
*See JOHANSON-BLIZZARD SYNDROME*
**Nasal atresia, posterior-lymphedema**
*See NOSE, CHOANAL ATRESIA-LYMPHEDEMA*
**Nasal crease**
*See NOSE, TRANSVERSE GROOVE*
**Nasal dermoids**
*See NECK/HEAD, DERMOID CYST OR TERATOMA*
**Nasal duplication**
*See NOSE, DUPLICATION*
**Nasal fundus ectasia**
*See OPTIC DISK, TILTED*
**Nasal glioma**
*See NOSE, GLIOMA*
**Nasal groove, familial transverse**
*See NOSE, TRANSVERSE GROOVE*
**Nasal groove, transverse**
*See NOSE, TRANSVERSE GROOVE*
**Nasal hypoplasia-peripheral dysostosis-mental retardation**
*See ACRODYSOSTOSIS*
**Nasal septum, absence of**
*See NOSE/NASAL SEPTUM DEFECTS*
**Nasal septum, subluxed or dislocated**
*See NOSE, DISLOCATED NASAL SEPTUM*
**Nasal stripe, transverse**
*See NOSE, TRANSVERSE GROOVE*
**Nasal-fronto-faciodysplasia**
*See FRONTO-FACIO-NASAL DYSPLASIA*
**Naso-blepharo-facial syndrome**
*See BLEPHARO-NASO-FACIAL SYNDROME*

---

## NASO-DIGITO-ACOUSTIC SYNDROME, KEIPERT TYPE        2085

**Includes:**
Deafness-digito-naso syndrome, Keipert type
Digito-naso-acoustic syndrome, Keipert type
Keipert-Fitzgerald-Danks syndrome
Keipert syndrome

**Excludes:**
**Acrocephalosyndactyly type V** (2284)
**Polysyndactyly-dysmorphic craniofacies, Greig type** (2925)
**Rubinstein-Taybi broad thumb-hallux syndrome** (0119)

**Major Diagnostic Criteria:**  A combination of most of the seven characteristic clinical features should be present for diagnosis.

**Clinical Findings:**  1. Normal height and weight.
2. Characteristic craniofacial features including a large head circumference ( 98%), broad face, mildly down-slanted palpebral fissures, broad and high nasal bridge, upturned and prominent nasal alae, large rounded columella, protruding upper lip with a marked cupid's bow configuration, straight lower lip, and open mouth.
3. Intra-oral features of a double upper alveolar margin, narrow and widely spaced teeth, and narrow palate.
4. Unilateral or bilateral severe sensorineural hearing loss.
5. Short and broad distal phalanges of the thumbs, the first, second and third fingers and all of the toes. Clinodactyly and brachydactyly of the fifth fingers. No radial deviations of thumbs were present but a slight tibial deviation of 1st, 2nd, and 3rd toes was present.
6. Neurologic impairment including mental deficiency (present in one out of the two cases).
7. X-ray findings included broad short terminal phalanges, one sib had bifid terminal phalanges in both index index fingers. In the halluces of both patients, the proximal phalanges were short and the terminal phalanges were to the anterior cranial fossa, slender

long bones and coxa valga. Pneumoencephalography had shown mild communicating hydrocephalus in one case.

**Complications:**  Speech delay due to hearing loss, as well as to the global developmental delay.

**Associated Findings:**  None known.

**Etiology:**  Most probably X-linked recessive inheritance, based on affected male siblings and affected maternally related male cousins.

**Pathogenesis:**  Unknown.

**MIM No.:**  25598

**POS No.:**  3047

**Sex Ratio:**  M2:F0 (observed).

**Occurrence:**  Two pedigrees have been documented.

**Risk of Recurrence for Patient's Sib:**
See Part I, *Mendelian Inheritance.*

**Risk of Recurrence for Patient's Child:**
See Part I, *Mendelian Inheritance.*

**Age of Detectability:**  At birth or in the first year of life.

**Gene Mapping and Linkage:**  Unknown.

**Prevention:**  None known. Genetic counseling indicated.

**Treatment:**  Speech therapy if indicated, hearing aid, as well as referral to special developmental and educational program.

**Prognosis:**  Life span probably not reduced.

**Detection of Carrier:**  Unknown.

**References:**
Keipert JA, et al.: A new syndrome of broad terminal phalanges and facial abnormalities. Aust Paediatr J 1973; 9:10–13.

G0003                                            **Mahin Golabi**

**Naso-maxillary cleft**
*See FACIAL CLEFT, OBLIQUE*
**Naso-ocular cleft**
*See FACIAL CLEFT, OBLIQUE*

---

## NASOLACRIMAL DUCT OBSTRUCTION        0705

**Includes:**
Dacryostenosis, congenital
Lacrimal system, impatency of the
Nasolacrimal duct, occlusion
Tear duct, blocked

**Excludes:**
Eyelid abnormalities (other)
**Glaucoma, congenital** (0414)

**Major Diagnostic Criteria:**  Epiphora with or without a mucoid or purulent discharge is apparent after the first week of life. Regurgitation of mucus or pus through the lacrimal punctum when digital pressure is applied to the lacrimal sac localizes the obstruction to the nasal end of the nasolacrimal duct. Definitive diagnosis is made through attempt at irrigation of the system through one canaliculus and recovery of fluid through the opposite punctum.

**Clinical Findings:**  Presenting signs and symptoms are variable and become evident after the first week of life. Epiphora may be the only symptom, however, it is usually accompanied by a mucoid or purulent discharge. The eyelids are often matted when the infant wakes up. The finding of reflux of muco-purulent material when pressure is applied to the lacrimal sac confirms the diagnosis. The conjunctiva is not injected.
Signs and symptoms may be intermittent or continuous persisting for weeks or months. An upper respiratory tract infection may exacerbate the symptoms. Spontaneous resolution of an obstructed nasolacrimal duct can be expected in up to 90% of cases by twelve months of age.

**Complications:**  Acute and chronic dacryocystitis.

**Associated Findings:** Other defects of the lacrimal drainage system such as stenosis or occlusion of the puncta and/or canaliculi, and mucocoele of the lacrimal sac. It is a common finding in a number of syndromes and malformations of the head, and is a major manifestation of the **Lacrimo-auriculo-dento-digital syndrome**.

**Etiology:** Undetermined. Some reports of autosomal dominant inheritance exist when nasolacrimal duct impatency coexists with atresia of the lacrimal puncta or canaliculi.

**Pathogenesis:** The lacrimal drainage system develops from a core of surface ectodermal cells buried in facial neuroectoderm in a cleft between the maxillary process and lateral nasal process. Outbuddings originate from its upper end to form the canaliculi. A rod of epithelial cells grows upwards to become continuous with the main cord of buried ectodermal cells. At 3 months of gestation, canalization of the passages (puncta, canaliculi, lacrimal sac, and nasolacrimal duct) begins at the upper end and proceeds downwards. At birth, the entire system is patent except the nasal end of the nasolacrimal duct, which may be occluded by a membrane composed of nasal mucosa and the epithelium lining the nasolacrimal duct. The membrane disappears either shortly before or a few weeks after birth. Persistence of the membrane produces the characteristic signs and symptoms of nasolacrimal duct obstruction.

**MIM No.:** *14970

**Sex Ratio:** Presumably M1:F1.

**Occurrence:** Between 2–6% of newborns.

**Risk of Recurrence for Patient's Sib:** Unknown.

**Risk of Recurrence for Patient's Child:** Unknown.

**Age of Detectability:** After the first week of life.

**Gene Mapping and Linkage:** Unknown.

**Prevention:** None known. Genetic counseling indicated.

**Treatment:** Conservative medical management is initially suggested as the method of treatment. The parents are instructed to massage the lacrimal sac and to apply a topical antibiotic ointment if there is purulence.

Lacrimal probing and irrigation are effective means of treating obstructed nasolacrimal ducts. The timing of the initial probing is controversial. Some ophthalmologists advocate probing without sedation or general anesthesia between 3–6 months of age if the signs do not resolve with medical therapy. Others recommend a probing under general anesthesia at 12–13 months as up 90% of cases are expected to improve spontaneously by that age. A second probing should be done in failed cases before considering a silicone intubation of the lacrimal system or a dacryocystorhinostomy.

**Prognosis:** Excellent.

**Detection of Carrier:** Unknown.

**References:**
Veirs ER: Lacrimal disorders diagnosis and treatment. St. Louis, CV Mosby, 1976; 1–53. *
Petersen RA, Robb RM: The natural course of congenital obstruction of the nasolacrimal duct. J Pediat Ophthalmol Strabismus 1978; 15:246–250.
Kushner BJ: Congenital nasolacrimal system obstruction. Arch Ophthalmol 1982; 100:597–600.
Baker JD: Treatment of congenital nasolacrimal duct obstruction. J Pediat Ophthalmol Strabismus 1985; 22:34–5.
Paul TO: Medical management of congenital nasolacrimal duct obstruction. J Pediat Ophthalmol Strabismus 1985; 22:68–70.
Katowitz JA, Welsh MG: Timing of initial probing and irrigation in congenital nasolacrimal duct obstruction. Ophthalmology 1987; 94:698–705. *

P0024                                                    **Robert C. Polomeno**

**Nasolacrimal duct, occlusion**
*See NASOLACRIMAL DUCT OBSTRUCTION*
**Nasomaxillary hypoplasia**
*See MAXILLONASAL DYSPLASIA, BINDER TYPE*
**Nasomaxillovertebral syndrome**
*See MAXILLONASAL DYSPLASIA, BINDER TYPE*

---

## NASOPALPEBRAL LIPOMA-COLOBOMA SYNDROME        3049

**Includes:**
    Coloboma-nasopalpebral lipoma syndrome
    Palpebral coloboma-lipoma syndrome
    Penchaszadeh-Velasquez-Arwillagi syndrome

**Excludes:**
    **Face, median cleft face syndrome** (0635)
    **Oculo-auriculo-vertebral anomaly** (0735)

**Major Diagnostic Criteria:** Nasopalpebral lipomas, upper and lower lid colobomas, telecanthus, maxillary hypoplasia.

**Clinical Findings:** Anomalies are limited to the face and head. The facial appearance, in six described individuals, consists of broad forehead (6/6); widow's peak (6/6); telecanthus (6/6); laterally displaced outer canthi (5/6); normal interorbital distance (6/6); upper and lower lid colobomas (6/6); sparse, maldirected eyebrows (6/6); misplaced (5/6) or absent (1/6) upper lacrimal punctae; misplaced (1/6) or absent (1/6) lower lacrimal punctae; nasopalpebral lipomas (6/6); abnormal eyelashes (6/6); and midface hypoplasia (6/6).

**Complications:** Divergent strabismus and exotropia secondary to inner canthal lipomas; conjunctival hyperemia and corneal opacities secondary to chronic corneal exposure.

**Associated Findings:** Open metopic suture was reported in one affected individual.

**Etiology:** Autosomal dominant inheritance, based upon the presence of the condition in three generations, with male-to-male transmission.

**Pathogenesis:** Unknown. A defect in adipose tissue differentiation or neural crest cell migration has been postulated.

**MIM No.:** *16773

**POS No.:** 3542

**Sex Ratio:** M1:F1

**Occurrence:** Eight members, from three generations, of one family from Venezuela have been documented.

**Risk of Recurrence for Patient's Sib:**
    See Part I, *Mendelian Inheritance*.

**Risk of Recurrence for Patient's Child:**
    See Part I, *Mendelian Inheritance*.

**Age of Detectability:** At birth by the presence of lipomas and colobomas.

**Gene Mapping and Linkage:** Unknown.

**Prevention:** None known. Genetic counseling indicated.

**Treatment:** Supportive for the ocular defects; cosmetic surgery may also be indicated.

**Prognosis:** Affected individuals have had normal growth, intellectual development, and life span.

**Detection of Carrier:** Unknown.

**References:**
Penchaszadeh VB, The nasopalpebral lipoma-coloboma syndrome: a new autosomal dominant dysplasia-malformation syndrome with congenital nasopalpebral lipomas, eyelid colobomas, telecanthus, and maxillary hypoplasia. Am J Med Genet 1982; 11:397–410.

T0007                                                    **Helga V. Toriello**

**Nasopharyngeal atresia**
*See NOSE, NASOPHARYNGEAL STENOSIS*

## NASOPHARYNGEAL CYSTS                                 0706

**Includes:**
Branchial cleft cysts, Bailey type IV
Cysts of the nasopharynx, congenital
Extra-adenoidal cysts
Intra-adenoidal cysts

**Excludes:**
Cysts of seromucinous glands with occluded excretory ducts
Interstitial pseudocysts, no epithelium, due to tissue edema
Intra-adenoidal pseudocyst secondary to incomplete adenoidectomy
Pseudocyst secondary to inflammation of fascial envelope
Sealed over crypt secondary to repeated inflammatory episodes

**Major Diagnostic Criteria:** With the extra-adenoidal cyst, the excised velum of tissue theoretically should show appropriate epithelial coverings on both surfaces, but careful pathologic examinations are rarely carried out in such cases. The true branchial cyst is lateral and often bilateral. Lesions lacking an inner epithelial lining are merely pseudocysts. In as much as the pharyngeal tubercle may hide the essential lesion, direct nasopharyngeal examination is desirable.

**Clinical Findings:** Symptoms include purulent postnasal discharge not coming through the choanae. Aching pain high in the throat or at the base of the skull, with a feeling of pressure or fullness, periodically relieved by evacuation of secretion.

*Intra-adenoidal cysts* derive from the medial pharyngeal recess. An elliptical opening on the nether surface of the adenoid, axis anteroposterior, lying in the midline, differing from the usual crypt opening in that it is more regular. Usually there is no special swelling, but pus and debris may be extruded on suction or pressure in the untreated state.

*Extra-adenoidal cysts* located deep to the pharyngobasilar fascia are derived from bursa pharyngea embryonalis (midline). They will not be diagnosed in children until the adenoid is removed, but, in the adult, they may be seen caudal to the lowermost extent of any adenoid present. Usually no swelling is seen in the nasopharynx, but there is a small hole in the midline, slightly rostral to the pharyngeal tubercle. In the untreated state, this hole may be surrounded by a cuff of granular, inflamed mucosa. It may exude pus intermittently. The hole usually leads to a small cavity, separated from the general nasopharyngeal space by a thin velum of tissue. In rare instances, the space in question can enlarge caudally to the level of the epiglottis. Indentation of the basiocciput has been described but must be quite rare.

*Branchial cleft cysts, Bailey type IV* are derived from first and dorsal portion of second pharyngeal pouch. They are often paired, and are present on the lateral aspects of the nasopharyngeal wall. The branchial nature is not easy to establish. Cystic nature may be established by injection of radiopaque material, but this may deceive. Lateral location and bilaterality strongly suggest branchial origin. Pathologic findings are more cogent.

It is of the utmost importance to evaluate sinonasal disease as a cause of symptoms. This can only be done with reasonable certainty by careful clinical examination supplemented by X-ray study of the sinuses.

**Complications:** Chronic or subacute bronchitis; chronic blepharoconjunctivitis; subacute or chronic otitis media, sometimes with conductive hearing loss. Rarely, paranasal sinusitis; fever, and recurring pharyngitis.

**Associated Findings:** None known.

**Etiology:** Unknown.

**Pathogenesis:** The true bursa pharyngea is due to the inductive effect of chorda mesoderm on the pharyngeal epithelium in the fornix region where the bundles of pharyngobasilar fascia do not commingle to form a barrier, as they do more anteriorly, to the extrusion of pharyngeal entoderm.

Intra-adenoidal midline cysts may be due to such an embryonic disturbance of the median pharyngeal recess which, precedes

development of the pharyngeal tonsil itself, but the products of which may be incorporated within the adenoid.

Branchial cleft cysts arise here, as elsewhere, but much more rarely. They are prone to remain intramural (Bailey type IV) and not to migrate into the neck.

**Sex Ratio:** Presumably M1:F1.

**Occurrence:** Undetermined but presumed rare.

**Risk of Recurrence for Patient's Sib:** Unknown.

**Risk of Recurrence for Patient's Child:** Unknown.

**Age of Detectability:** Nasopharyngeal cysts are discovered either at the time of adenoid or adenotonsil surgery in childhood; or, less commonly, in adults on careful investigation of postnasal pus which cannot be demonstrated to come from the nose or paranasal sinuses.

**Gene Mapping and Linkage:** Unknown.

**Prevention:** None known. Genetic counseling indicated.

**Treatment:** *Intra-adenoidal cyst* is cured by a thorough adenoidectomy under direct visual control, whether it is of true bursal origin or not.

*Extra-adenoidal cyst* is usually cured by marsupialization or saucerization.

*Branchial cleft cysts* are best treated by excision under direct vision.

Aspiration and injection of sclerosing agents or marsupialization temporize only, and recurrence may be expected.

**Prognosis:** Normal for life span and intelligence; functionally good in all types with proper treatment.

**Detection of Carrier:** Unknown.

**References:**
Taylor JNS, Burwell RG: Branchiogenic nasopharyngeal cysts. J Laryngol Otol 1954; 68:677.
Wilson CP: A case of bilateral congenital sinuses of the nasopharynx. Acta Otolaryngol (Stockh) 1957; 48:76.
Wilson CP: Observations on the surgery of the nasopharynx. Ann Otol Rhinol Laryngol 1957; 66:5.
Guggenheim P: Cysts of the nasopharynx. Laryngoscope 1967; 77:2147–2168.
Toomly JM: Cysts and tumors of the pharynx. In: Paparella MM, Shumrick DA, eds: Otolaryngology, vol 3. Philadelphia: W.B. Saunders, 1980:2323–2324.
Michaels L: Normal anatomy and histology; adenoids; infections; developmental lesions. In: Ear, nose and throat histopathology. New York: Springer-Verlag, 1987:242.

AU005                                       **Thomas Aufdemorte**

**Nasopharyngeal stenosis**
*See NOSE, NASOPHARYNGEAL STENOSIS*
**Nasopharyngeal teratomas**
*See NECK/HEAD, DERMOID CYST OR TERATOMA*
**Nasu-Hakola disease**
*See OSTEODYSPLASIA, LIPOMEMBRANOUS POLYCYSTIC-DEMENTIA*
**Nathalie syndrome**
*See OTO-OCULO-MUSCULO-SKELETAL SYNDROME*
**Naumoff type short-rib polydactyly syndrome**
*See SHORT RIB-POLYDACTYLY SYNDROME, VERMA-NAUMOFF TYPE*

## NECK, BRANCHIAL CLEFT, CYSTS OR SINUSES          0117

**Includes:**
Branchial cleft fistula
Cervical cyst or sinus
Pharyngeal cyst or fistula

**Excludes:**
**Branchio-oto-renal dysplasia** (2224)
Cavernous hemangioma of neck
Cervical adenopathy
**Laryngocele** (0575)
Neck/head, dermoid cyst or teratoma (0283)

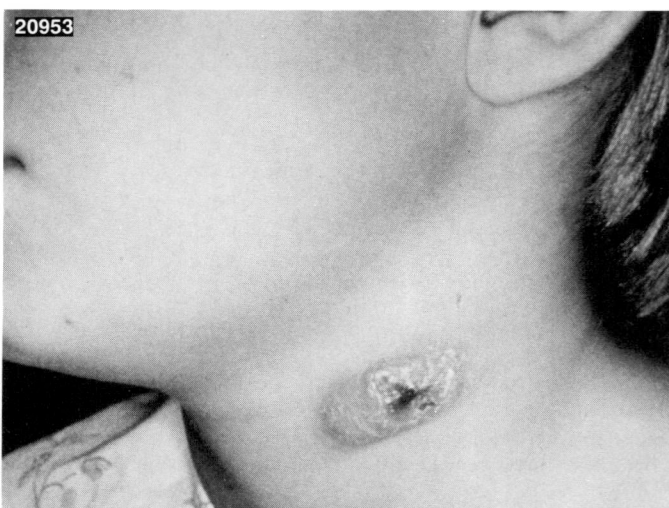

**0117A-20953:** Branchial cleft sinus (infected).

Pharyngocele
Solitary lymph cysts
Thymic cyst
**Thyroglossal duct remnant** (0945)
Thyroid cyst

**Major Diagnostic Criteria:** Histopathologic examination of a cystic mass or sinus medial to the sternocleidomastoid muscle.

**Clinical Findings:** Either a cyst or a sinus or both can result from abnormal development of the pharyngeal pouches or cervical sinus. These lesions generally appear along the anterior border of the sternocleidomastoid muscle or medial to this muscle. They may also be in the periauricular region.

The branchial cyst is a slowly enlarging, painless mass in the head and neck region that may be present at birth. Pressure and a sense of fullness in the neck with mild dysphagia and hoarseness are frequent symptoms. Children with large cysts may have stridorous breathing and cyanosis. Uncomplicated cysts are characteristically soft, mobile, and transparent when transilluminated. The cyst may vary in size, increasing with infection and decreasing as infection subsides. Neck injuries may cause the cyst to become enlarged, tense, and painful.

Small cysts may be difficult to palpate, particularly those lying medial to the sternocleidomastoid muscle. These may be detected by having the patient push his chin firmly against the examiner's palm. Needle aspiration yields a mucoid material.

A typical sinus has an external opening at the junction of the lower third and upper two-thirds of the sternocleidomastoid muscle. This small pinpoint opening may not be noticed until mucoid material or food particles pass from it. Symptoms of vagal irritation, such as cough, hoarseness, pallor, bradycardia, sweating, and faintness have been elicited by probing the sinus. Persistent cough, drainage into the pharynx, and pain from repeated infections of the external openings are unusual symptoms of a cervical sinus. X-ray examination after injecting the sinus with radiopaque oil reveals a typical smooth-walled tract. A cyst may develop at any point along the sinus tract.

**Complications:** Upper airway obstruction, dysphagia, aspiration, infection of cyst or sinus, malignant tumor formation.

**Associated Findings:** None known.

**Etiology:** Autosomal dominant inheritance. Widstrom et al. (1980) found a 36% positive family history for complete fistulae from the second cleft or pouch and a 10% positive family history with regard to the external sinus. There is no evidence of heredity being associated with lateral neck cysts.

**Pathogenesis:** Pharyngeal pouches and branchial grooves are present for only a short time during embryonic life. Epithelial rests, incomplete closure of the branchial grooves, rupture of the closing membranes between the pharyngeal pouches and branchial grooves, and persistence of the cervical sinus are thought to be responsible for these abnormalities. The constant relationship between the cyst or sinus and anatomic structures normally formed by the branchial apparatus substantiates this concept.

The question has been raised, do branchial cysts arise from cystic degeneration of cervical lymph nodes? Schewitsch, et al. (1980) presented a series of 82 cysts and sinuses. None of their patients had other developmental abnormalities. All of the cysts contained abundant lymphoid tissue without sinusoids. Lymph nodes were present but separated from the cyst wall by thin, fibrous layers. Histology of the cysts showed columnar ciliated epithelium, consistent with a branchiogenic origin. The authors conclude that it is unlikely that cervical cysts originate from salivary inclusions or lymph nodes. Their data support the classic theory that the majority of lateral cervical cysts originate from embryonic entrapment of epithelial tissue.

**MIM No.:** *11360

**CDC No.:** 239.200

**Sex Ratio:** M3:F1

**Occurrence:** These are relatively common abnormalities. The occurrence rate is unknown, partly because they may not be apparent until later life.

**Risk of Recurrence for Patient's Sib:**
See Part I, *Mendelian Inheritance.*

**Risk of Recurrence for Patient's Child:**
See Part I, *Mendelian Inheritance.*

**Age of Detectability:** From birth through adulthood, depending on the occurrence of symptoms and clinical findings.

**Gene Mapping and Linkage:** Unknown.

**Prevention:** None known. Genetic counseling indicated.

**Treatment:** Total excision of the cyst and sinus tract will give the patient a complete cure. Stepladder incisions may be indicated to remove the entire sinus tract. When the sinus originates from the tonsillar fossa, a tonsillectomy must be performed to ensure complete excision of the tract. Facial nerve exploration and preservation is necessary for all lesions around the ear.

**Prognosis:** Normal life span unless rare malignancy occurs.

**Detection of Carrier:** Unknown.

**Special Considerations:** The knowledge of embryologic development and related anatomy is essential for understanding branchial cysts and sinuses. There are two types of lateral neck lesions that share the name branchial. One group of cysts are located anterior

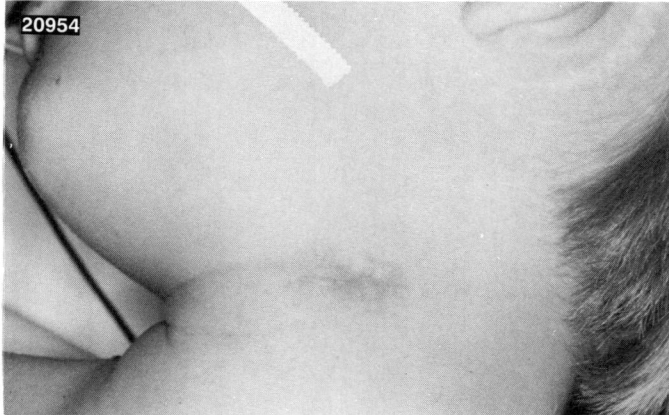

**0117B-20954:** Branchial cleft sinus.

to the upper part of the sternocleidomastoid muscle. The others are tube-like lesions that open into the skin of the neck. They may be either fistulae with openings at both ends or sinuses with one open end. Howie and Proops (1982) examined 57 lesions that were located in the lateral neck, including cysts, sinuses and fistulae. The lesions fell into two well-defined groups and one miscellaneous group. The first included 46 cysts that presented as a swelling in the neck behind the angle of the mandible and anterior to the junction of the upper third and lower two-thirds of the sternocleidomastoid muscle. In group two, there were four congenital lesions, which were characterized with an opening into the skin of the neck at the anterior border of the sternocleidomastoid. There were seven miscellaneous lesions that had unique features.

*A first branchial cleft fistula* will be located entirely above the hyoid bone, with its upper end opening into the external auditory canal. The tract is superficial to the mandible and passes through the parotid gland. It may lie deep or superficial to the facial nerve. The lesion may be seen in the periauricular region in the anterior neck.

*The second arch sinus* begins in the tonsillar fossa. It extends between the internal and external carotid arteries above and superficial to the hypoglossal nerve, glossopharyngeal nerve, and stylopharyngeus muscle. The sinus opens onto the skin along the anterior border of the sternocleidomastoid muscle. The junction of the lower and middle thirds of the muscle is the most common site for this opening. The second arch sinus is the most common of these abnormalities.

A sinus formed from *the third branchial cleft* opens in the same cutaneous region as the second branchial sinus. This tract passes deep to the platysma muscle along the sheath of the common carotid artery, but extends behind the internal carotid artery. The tract is superficial to the vagus nerve and crosses the hypoglossal nerve, but does not ascend above the glossopharyngeal nerve or stylopharyngeus muscle. The internal opening is in the pyriform sinus.

Cysts or sinuses of *the fourth branchial cleft* are theoretically possible, but very few have been reported. The tract would pass below the aorta on the left and the subclavian artery on the right; it ascends into the neck and empties into the upper esophagus after crossing the hypoglossal nerve. Downey and Ward (1969) have described a mediastinal cyst that they believe originated from a fourth branchial cleft. That cyst was lined with squamous and transitional epithelium with islands of lymphoid tissue in its wall. Shugar and Healy (1980) report a patient with the fourth branchial cleft anomaly. This tract extended under the clavicle near the subclavian vessels. Others believe that perithyroidal abscesses occur secondary to infection of a fourth branchial cleft, cyst, or sinus. Contamination is thought to occur from a connection to the apex of the pyriform sinus. This may be demonstrated by a barium esophagram obtained during a quiescent period.

**References:**

Downey WL, Ward PH: Branchial cleft cysts in the mediastinum. Arch Otolaryngol 1969; 89:762–765. *

Schewitsch I, et al.: Cysts and sinuses of the lateral head and neck. J Otolaryngol 1980; 9:1–6.

Shugar MA, Healy GB: The fourth branchial cleft anomaly. Head Neck Surg 1980; 3:72–75.

Widstrom A, et al.: Aspects on the lateral fistulae and cysts of the neck. J Otolaryngol 1980; 9:291–296.

Chandler JR, Mitchell B: Branchial cleft cysts, sinuses, and fistulas. Otolaryngol Clin North Am 1981; 14:175–186.

Howie AJ, Proops DW: The definition of branchial cysts, sinuses and fistulae. Clin Otolaryngol 1982; 7:51–57.

Albers GD: Congenital sinuses and fistulas of the neck and pharynx. In: English FM, ed: Otolaryngology, ch. 12. Philadelphia: Harper & Row, 1988. *

**Gerald M. English**

## NECK, CYSTIC HYGROMA, FETAL TYPE  2252

**Includes:**
    Cystic hygroma of the neck (posterior)
    Hygroma cervicis
    Jugular lymphatic obstruction sequence
    Nuchal lymphangioma
    Pterygium colli
    Turner syndrome phenotype

**Excludes:**
    **Cystic hygroma** (3284)
    **Encephalocele** (0343)
    **Hydrops fetalis, non-immune** (2198)
    Lymphangiomatous malformations localized to other body areas

**Major Diagnostic Criteria:** A mass on the fetal posterolateral cervical area.

**Clinical Findings:** A septated, fluid-filled mass or masses occupying the posterolateral cervical area without communication to the brain or to an underlying defect of the fetal skull. Survivors may exhibit redundant nuchal skin or neck webbing.

Failure of the jugular lymphatic sacs to establish venous communication during fetal development leads to massive enlargement of these sacs in the posterolateral cervical areas. The enlarging masses may rotate the axis of the developing auricle posteriorly and elevate the lower pinna. Late communication of the sacs with the internal jugular vein may be manifest by redundancy of posterior nuchal skin or a webbed neck in adult life. Complete obstruction of lymphatic drainage usually results in generalized fetal edema and ascites (hydrops fetalis). The establishment of late or alternative lymphatic drainage may be manifest in survivors by limb edema. Complex cardiac malformations are frequent in affected fetuses, even in cases with euploid chromosome karyotypes (3/10 index cases) or deficient migration of cephalic neural crest cells.

**Complications:** It has been suggested that intrathoracic distention of lymphatic channels or deficient migration of cephalic neural crest cells in early fetal life might interfere with development of the aortic arch and conotruncal region. **Diaphragmatic hernia** (2/10) has been attributed to the same mechanism.

**Associated Findings:** None known.

**Etiology:** The majority of cases are associated with **Turner syndrome** (45,X or 45,X mosaic chromosome constitution). This malformation sequence or its postnatal consequences, nuchal skin

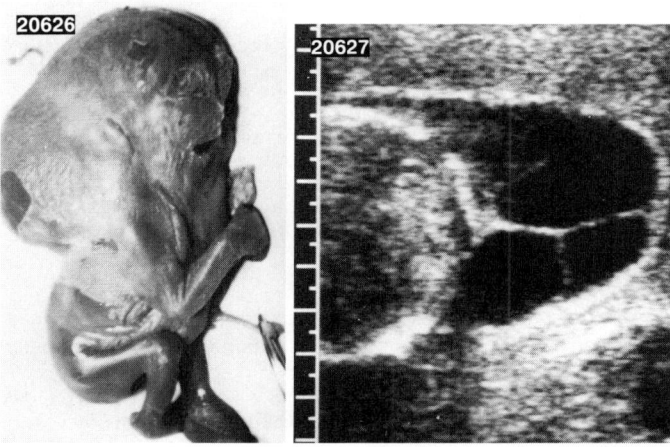

**2252A-20626:** One of two affected sibs with cystic hygroma. **20627:** Ultrasound study of nuchal cystic hygroma with typical septations; fetal head is to the left.

**2252B-20949:** Cystic hygroma on the right side of this CAT scan.

redundancy and neck webbing, has also been described in association with **Pterygium syndrome, multiple, Roberts syndrome** (tetraphocomelia), **Asplenia syndrome, Noonan syndrome, Fetal alcohol syndrome,** 46,XY gonadal dysgenesis, and chromosomal aneuploidy: +13, +18, +21, +22, 13q-, 18p-, +11p/22q, t6q/12q.

**Pathogenesis:** Nuchal cystic hygroma is the clinical consequence of delay or absence of the communication that normally develops between the jugular lymph sacs and the internal jugular veins at approximately 40 days gestation. In the course of normal development, the sacs become the terminal portions of the right lymphatic duct and the thoracic duct. The obstructed jugular lymph sacs dilate along the path of least resistance in the posterior and lateral cervical areas, tethered posteromedially by the nuchal ligament and bounded anteriorly by the sternomastoid muscle. The dilated sacs result in the characteristic septated mass or masses, divided posteriorly by the nuchal ligament. Generalized hypoplasia of major lymphatic trunks usually results in fetal edema, ascites, and pleural and pericardial effusions. The absence of fetal hydrops may help to differentiate cystic hygroma associated with a euploid karyotype from that found in cases of Turner syndrome. Localized lymphatic dilatation or tissue edema during early development may lead to the complications noted above.

**MIM No.:** 25735

**CDC No.:** 239.200, 744.900

**Sex Ratio:** M<1:F1. The vast majority are phenotypically female.

**Occurrence:** 1:875 spontaneous abortions; 1:200 spontaneous abortions with crown-rump length (CRL) > 30 mm.

**Risk of Recurrence for Patient's Sib:** Depends on associated disorders. If phenotypic male and/or euploid chromosome karyotype noted, autosomal recessive inheritance should be considered (25%).

**Risk of Recurrence for Patient's Child:** Undetermined. Affected individuals generally do not survive to reproduce.

**Age of Detectability:** By ultrasound examination at 16 weeks' gestation.

**Gene Mapping and Linkage:** Unknown.

**Prevention:** None known. Genetic counseling indicated.

**Treatment:** Unknown.

**Prognosis:** Generally lethal in utero when accompanied by hydrops. Prognosis for survivors will depend on etiology of the malformation sequence.

**Detection of Carrier:** By karyotype in instances of unbalanced translocation.

**References:**

Graham JM Jr, Smith DW: Dominantly inherited pterygium colli. J Pediatr 1981; 98:664–665.
Cowchock FS, et al.: Not all cystic hygromas occur in the Ullrich-Turner syndrome. Am J Med Genet 1982; 12:327–331. †
Chervenak FA, et al.: Fetal cystic hygroma: cause and natural history. New Engl J Med 1983; 309:822–825. *
Byrne J, et al.: The significance of cystic hygroma in fetuses. Hum Pathol 1984; 15:61–67. †
Miyabara S, et al.: Significance of cardiovascular malformations in cystic hygroma. Am J Med Genet 1989; 34:489–501. †

C0061

**Susan Cowchock**

**Neck, limber-mental retardation**
*See X-LINKED MENTAL RETARDATION-MUSCULAR WEAKNESS-AWKWARD GAIT*

## NECK/FACE, LIPOMATOSIS 0601

**Includes:**
Adenolipomatosis
Cervical lipomatosis, familial benign
Face, diffuse symmetric lipomatosis of
Lipomatosis, benign symmetric
Lipomatosis of face and neck
Madelung disease
Tongue, Pleomorphic lipoma

**Excludes:**
**Lipomas, familial symmetric** (0600)
**Neurofibromatosis** (0712)
**Parotitis, punctate** (0799)
**Stiff skin syndrome** (2629)

**Major Diagnostic Criteria:** Symmetric masses in the head and neck region. These masses are clinically and pathologically identical with lipoma.

**Clinical Findings:** Symmetric fatty growths may involve the neck, parotid area, occipital area, and, in some instances, both the neck and axilla. When the neck, axillary, and orbital regions are affected this condition has been called adenolipomatosis, although lymph nodes are not involved. Telangiectasis and hypertrophy of bone or muscle may accompany the fatty growths. This disorder may be confused with neurofibromatosis. Some cases are associated with an elevated blood cholesterol. Onset is usually in adulthood. In most cases the masses are painless. They remain quiescent for many years but suddenly may enlarge. The major disabilities are cosmetic and respiratory obstruction from lipoma in the neck. Pleomorphic lipoma of the tongue has also been described, and its bulk creates speech impairment. In 145 cases of oral lipoma, 19% were found in the tongue.

**Complications:** Upper respiratory obstruction.

**Associated Findings:** Hyperuricemia, diabetes mellitus, elevated plasma triglyceride levels, type 4 lipoprotein pattern, somatic, autonomic and peripheral neuropathy, and renal tubular acidosis. Chemical analysis of the lipoma shows that the neck lipoma contains more lipid than in the buttock and that 39% of the lipid is triglyceride as compared with 3% in other body locations.

**Etiology:** Undetermined. Affected individuals frequently have a history of alcohol abuse. Possibly autosomal dominant inheritance.

**Pathogenesis:** This condition is probably only one manifestation of several varieties of hereditary fatty tumors that can involve almost any area of the body. It is not certain now that tumors of the face and neck are a separate entity. This presentation may occur sporadically.

**MIM No.:** 15180

**Sex Ratio:** M<1:F1

**Occurrence:** About 200 cases cases have documented in the literature.

**Risk of Recurrence for Patient's Sib:**
See Part I, *Mendelian Inheritance.*

**Risk of Recurrence for Patient's Child:**
See Part I, *Mendelian Inheritance.*

**Age of Detectability:** Tumors usually become clinically evident after the second decade.

**Gene Mapping and Linkage:** Unknown.

**Prevention:** None known. Genetic counseling indicated.

**Treatment:** Surgical removal is the only effective method to obtain tissue for diagnosis, to improve appearance, and to relieve airway obstruction. The lipoma infiltrates and and readily recurs, so debulking, rather than total excision, should be performed.

**Prognosis:** Normal for life span.

**Detection of Carrier:** Unknown.

**References:**
Pack GT, Ariel IM: Tumors of adipose tissue. In: Tumors of the soft somatic tissues; a clinical treatise. New York: Hoeber-Harper, 1958: 343–365.
McKusick VA: Familial benign cervical lipomatosis. In: Medical genetics, 1961. J Chronic Dis 1962; 15:417–572.
Argenta LC, et al.: Benign symmetrical lipomatosis (Madelung's disease). Head Neck Surg 1981; 3:240–241.
Stevenson RE, et al.: Symmetrical lipomatosis associated with stiff skin and systemic manifestations in four generations. Proc Greenwood Genet Center 1984; 3:56–64.
Enzi G, et al.: Sensory, motor and autonomic neuropathy in patients with multiple symetric lipomatosis. Medicine 1985; 64:388–393.
Gallou L, et al.: Pleomorphic lipoma of the tongue: case report and literature review. J Otolaryngol (Can.) 1986; 15:313–316.

BE028                                         LaVonne Bergstrom

## NECK/HEAD, DERMOID CYST OR TERATOMA          0283

**Includes:**
Bidermoma of head or neck
Cervical teratomas
Dermoid cyst or teratoma of head or neck
Dermoids of the head and neck
Embryoma of head or neck
Epignathus
Hairy cyst on head or neck
Mixed cyst on head or neck
Monodermoma of head or neck
Nasal dermoids
Nasopharyngeal teratomas
Teratoid tumor of head or neck
Teratomas of the orbit
Tridermoma of head or neck

**Excludes:**
Inclusion cysts of head or neck lined with squamous epithelium
**Neck, branchial cleft, cysts or sinuses** (0117)
Preauricular tags and cysts
**Salivary gland, mixed tumor** (0878)
**Thyroglossal duct remnant** (0945)
**Thyroid, dysgenesis** (0946)
Other congenital head and neck tumors

**Major Diagnostic Criteria:** A tumor, cyst, or sinus opening in the head or neck areas. Histopathologic study is necessary to establish the diagnosis.

**Clinical Findings:** Dermoid cysts or teratomas of the head and neck occur almost exclusively in infants and young children. A review of 103 dermoid cysts of the head and neck revealed the following;

**Dermoid Cysts of Head and Neck by Site**

| Site | No. of Patients | % |
|---|---|---|
| Nose | 13 | 12.6 |
| Orbit | 51 | 49.5 |
| Floor of mouth, submental,submaxillary | 24 | 23.3 |
| Occipital, frontal, lip, neck, soft palate | 15 | 14.6 |

The signs and symptoms depend on the size and location of the tumor.

*Nasal dermoids* are usually detected shortly after birth. A small midline pit or depression on the bridge of the nose with hair protruding from it may be the only abnormality. This pit represents the opening of a sinus tract that may extend between the nasal bones into the cribriform plate or nasal septum. A CT scan of the skull and facial bones is essential, and injection of the tract with a radiopaque substance before this examination may be helpful in establishing the extent of the sinus tract. Nasal obstruction and rhinorrhea may be present.

*Teratomas of the orbit* may be associated with a unilateral exophthalmos and some degree of microphthalmos. The patient with a teratoma is usually born with a mass behind the eye, whereas the dermoid cyst may not become apparent until later in life. Orbital teratomas may extend through defects in the orbit or skull into the anterior cranial fossa, middle cranial fossa, temporal fossa, or nasal cavity. Clinical findings will depend upon the size and extensions of the tumor.

*Dermoid cysts* of the floor of the mouth are congenital inclusion cysts that form along the lines of embryologic fusion. They usually become manifest during the second and third decade of life. These cysts, while characteristically midline, may also be in the lateral neck. Evidence indicates that both midline and lateral dermoid cysts are of common origin and frequently have attachments to the midline of the hyoid bone or mandible. This attachment to the midline may be epithelialized, and failure to follow the tract and excise it completely will result in recurrence.

*Cervical teratomas* are rare after the age of one year. Equally distributed between the two sexes, most of these tumors are present at birth. A mass in the neck is the usual presentation. Acute respiratory symptoms of stridor, apnea, and cyanosis result from compression or deviation of the trachea. Dysphagia may arise from esophageal compression. Cystic lymphangioma, congenital goiter, branchial cleft cysts, and thyroglossal duct cysts must be considered in the differential diagnosis. These tumors, measuring between 5 and 12 cm, are usually unilateral and quite large. The medial border may extend across the anterior midline in close relation to the thyroid gland and trachea. They may be solid, multiloculated or cystic. The skin overlying the tumor is moveable. The mass may grow to a considerable size, causing cosmetic deformities. X-ray examination of the neck mass may reveal areas of calcification within the tumor. A CT scan should be obtained before excision to assess tumor extent.

*Nasopharyngeal teratomas* are present at birth and occur in females six times as often as in males. These tumors may be either pedunculated or sessile. Airway obstruction, cough, rhinorrhea, and a nasal or nasopharyngeal tumor are the most common findings. These tumors may be associated with deformities of the skull such as anencephaly, hemicrania, or fissures of the palate.

**Complications:** Airway obstruction, rhinitis and sinusitis, epistaxis, meningitis, cosmetic deformities, exophthalmos, decreased vision, malignant degeneration.

**Associated Findings:** The orbital, nasal, and nasopharyngeal teratomas may be associated with cranial defects. Cervical teratomas are not associated with these or other defects.

**Etiology:** Undetermined. This condition is believed to arise from embryonal disturbances of development. A growth disturbance of the primary axis (the notochord and contiguous structures from Hensen node in the early embryo) has been proposed.

**Pathogenesis:** There is no sharp delineation between dermoid cysts and simple congenital inclusion cysts. As the cyst enlarges and the patient grows, the lesion may migrate away from its primary location. Dermoid cysts may contain a small percentage of mesodermal elements in addition to predominant dermal elements. Teratomas are much more complex tumors, and their structure varies greatly according to the variety of tissues they contain. Usually they are cystic and the skin-lined cavities contain sebaceous material. The cavities not lined with skin contain mucoid or watery secretions. Skin, hair, bone, cartilage, and teeth may be recognized on gross examination. Microscopically, the tissues within these tumors vary considerably. Skin, hair follicles, sebaceous glands, and sweat glands are common. Respiratory epithelium, intestinal epithelium, nervous tissue, cartilage, bone, and nonstriated muscle are present in varying proportions. Liver, lung, thyroid, and renal tissues are uncommon. Teeth are found in a few tumors. These components are arranged in a chaotic fashion, but they closely resemble their normal counterparts. The benign teratoma and dermoid cyst are usually easy to recognize.

**CDC No.:** 239.200

**Sex Ratio:** Nasal dermoid: Slight male preponderance
Orbital dermoid or teratoma: M1:F1
Cervical dermoid or teratoma: M1:F1
Nasopharyngeal teratoma: M1:F6

**Occurrence:** Unknown.

**Risk of Recurrence for Patient's Sib:** Unknown.

**Risk of Recurrence for Patient's Child:** Unknown.

**Age of Detectability:** Oral: prenatal ultrasonography shows mass attached to fetal head. Hydramnios is also present. Nasal: at birth. Orbital dermoid: childhood. Orbital teratoma: at birth. Cervical: prenatal ultrasonography shows displaced fetal head associated with a large mass. Hydramnios is also present. Nasopharyngeal: at birth.

**Gene Mapping and Linkage:** Unknown.

**Prevention:** None known. Genetic counseling indicated.

**Treatment:** Complete surgical excision is required to prevent recurrences and other complications. Combined ophthalmologic, neurosurgical, and otolaryngologic operations may be needed to successfully treat the orbital tumors. Cervical tumors are usually encapsulated in fibrous tissue, which makes complete surgical excision possible.

Tracheostomy, an extraoral feeding route, antibiotics, and reconstructive procedures for cosmetic deformities may be necessary.

**Prognosis:** A normal life span can be expected when the tumor is completely excised. Malignant degeneration is rare, except in cases of nasopharyngeal teratoma.

**Detection of Carrier:** Unknown.

**References:**
Dekelboum AM: Teratoma of the nasopharynx in the newborn. Otolaryngol Head Neck Surg 1979; 87:628–634.
Leveque H, et al.: Dermoid cysts of the floor of the mouth and lateral neck. Laryngoscope 1979; 89:296–305.
McCaffrey TV, et al.: Dermoid cysts of the nose: review of 21 cases. Otolaryngol Head Neck Surg 1979; 87:52–59.
Hughes GB, et al.: Management of the congenital midline nasal mass: a review. Head Neck Surg 1980; 2:222–233.
Tobey DN, Mangham C: Malignant cervical teratomas. Otolaryngol Head Neck Surg 1980; 88:215–217.
English GM: Embryology and anomalies of the mouth and throat. In: English GM, ed: Otolaryngology. Ch. 5. Philadelphia: Harper & Row, 1983. *

EN002                                   **Gerald M. English**

**Neck/head, hemangiomas**
See HEMANGIOMAS OF THE HEAD AND NECK
**Necrosis of the capital femoral epiphysis-primary coxa plana**
See HIP, OSTEONECROSIS, CAPITAL FEMORAL EPIPHYSIS
**Nemaline myopathy**
See MYOPATHY, NEMALINE
**Neonatal nephrosis**
See NEPHROSIS, CONGENITAL
**Neonatal osseous dysplasia I**
See SKELETAL DYSPLASIA, DE LA CHAPELLE TYPE
**Neonatal seborrheic dermatitis**
See IMMUNODEFICIENCY, PLASMA-ASSOCIATED DEFECT OF PHAGOCYTOSIS
**Neonatal severe primary hyperparathyroidism (NSPH)**
See HYPERPARATHYROIDISM, FAMILIAL
**Neoplasms of CNS**
See CNS NEOPLASMS
**Nephritis, salt-losing**
See KIDNEY, NEPHRONOPHTHISIS-MEDULLARY CYSTIC DESEASE

## NEPHRITIS-DEAFNESS (SENSORINEURAL), HEREDITARY TYPE                     0708

**Includes:**
Alport syndrome
Alport syndrome-like hereditary nephritis
Deafness-nephritis
Fechtner syndrome
Hearing loss-nephritis
Interstitial pyelonephritis, hereditary type
Nephropathy-deafness, hereditary type

**Excludes:**
Deafness-diverticulitis-neuropathy (0265)
Hematuria, benign familial
Kidney, nephronophthisis-medullary cystic desease (3018)
Nephritis (hereditary) without deafness
Nephropathy-deafness-hyperparathyroidism
Nephrosis, familial type (0710)

**Major Diagnostic Criteria:** Hematuria (100%) and proteinuria (70%-80%), at times variable, with sensorineural hearing loss in patient, parent, or sibs, and family history of other members with nephritis, deafness, or both. Renal function may be normal or decreased. Electron microscopy may show patchy glomerular basement membrane thickening and thinning, or thickening and splitting of the basement membrane thought to be pathognomonic for Alport syndrome.

**Clinical Findings:** When first recognized, it may present with variable hematuria, proteinuria, and occasional pyuria. Initial renal function is usually normal, but progressive deterioration occurs, resulting in renal failure in males by the second or third decade, with a more benign course in females. Abnormal tubular function is rarely seen, and urinary tract infection is unusual. Urinary findings consist of gross or microscopic hematuria; proteinuria; and hyaline, granular, and cellular casts. Renal biopsy in younger children shows thin, irregular basement membrane, which may be due to persistence of fetal or neonatal capillary basement membrane. Diffuse or focal thickening and splitting of the basement membrane predominates in older children and adults.

Bilateral sensorineural hearing loss is present in about half the patients. It may develop within the first few years of life, is more common in males, and is slowly progressive. Audiometric studies show high-tone sensorineural hearing loss with recruitment, high SISI scores, absent tone decay, and type II Bekesy tracings typical of cochlear pathology. Hearing loss and renal involvement may occur separately in affected family members.

Ocular defects occur in about 15% of patients and include anterior or posterior lenticonus, spherophakia, congenital cataracts, and macular or peripheral flecks.

Thrombocytopenia, hypoparathyroidism, polyneuropathy, thyroid antibodies, prolinuria, and ichthyosis have also been described.

The *Fechtner* variant of Alport syndrome is characterized by renal disease, hearing loss, cataracts, and the May Hegglin anomaly (giant platelets, thrombocytopenia, and white blood cell inclusions).

**Complications:**  Those of chronic renal disease.

**Associated Findings:**  Hearing loss in 40–60%; ocular defects in 15%; thrombocytopenia, hypoparathyroidism, polyneuropathy, and ichthyosis in less than 10%.

**Etiology:**  X-linked inheritance with greater severity in males. Some pedigrees have suggested autosomal dominant inheritance. Autosomal recessive transmission has also been reported, though not so well established. The *Fechtner* variant is autosomal dominant with variable expressivity.

**Pathogenesis:**  Unknown. Renal pathology is variable even among members of the same family. Earliest alteration is thickening of glomerular basement membrane. Abnormal antigenicity of the basement membrane has been reported. In some individuals, the histologic pattern is similar to glomerulonephritis; in others, there is periglomerular fibrosis with tubular atrophy and interstitial infiltrates resembling pyelonephritis. Foam cells, although not limited to Alport syndrome, are frequently seen in later stages of disease. The initial renal lesions are mild and tend to progress slowly. Immunofluorescence is negative. Temporal bone histologic findings are inconsistent; atrophy of the organ of Corti and hyalinization and thinning of the tectorial membrane have been described.

**MIM No.:**  *10420, 20378, *30105

**CDC No.:**  759.870

**Sex Ratio:**  M1:F2 unless autosomal; then M1:F1

**Occurrence:**  Accounts for an estimated one-sixth of familial glomerular disease.

**Risk of Recurrence for Patient's Sib:**
See Part I, *Mendelian Inheritance.*

**Risk of Recurrence for Patient's Child:**
See Part I, *Mendelian Inheritance.*

**Age of Detectability:**  As early as the first few weeks of life, by intermittent albuminuria and microscopic hematuria. It might be possible to detect the thrombocytopenia and giant platelets of the *Fechtner* variant through fetal blood sampling.

**Gene Mapping and Linkage:**  ATS (Alport syndrome) has been mapped to Xq21.3-q24.

**Prevention:**  None known. Genetic counseling indicated.

**Treatment:**  Peritoneal or hemodialysis in cases of renal failure. Kidney transplantation has been successful in many patients.

**Prognosis:**  Males have a poor outlook, with death from uremia likely before age 30 and often during adolescence. The condition in females is variable but usually benign, though renal abnormalities persist. While quite uncommon, death from renal failure may occur in females.

**Detection of Carrier:**  Presence of either nephritis or sensorineural deafness with a history of other affected family members.

**Special Considerations:**  An autosomal recessive syndrome of nephropathy, deafness, and hyperparathyroidism has been described in several members of a consangineous Pakistani family (Edwards et al, 1989). The hematuria and proteinuria found in Alport syndrome were, however, lacking.

**References:**
Myers GJ, Tyler HR: The etiology of deafness in Alport's syndrome. Arch Otolaryngol 1972; 96:333–340.
Gubler M, et al.: Alport's syndrome: report of 58 cases and review of the literature. Am J Med 1981; 70:493–505. * †
Yosikawa N, et al.: Glomerular basal lamina in hereditary nephritis. J Pathol 1981; 135:199–209.
Drayna D, et al.: Genetic mapping of human X chromosome by using RFLPs. Proc Natl Acad Sci USA 1984; 81:2836–2839.

Hasstedt SJ, et al.: Genetic heterogeneity among kindreds with Alport syndrome. Am J Hum Genet 1986; 38:940–953.
Melvin T, et al.: Amyloid P component is not present in the glomerular basement membrane in Alport-type hereditary nephritis. Am J Path 1986; 125:460–464.
Yoshikawa N, et al.: Nonfamilial hematuria associated with glomerular basement membrane alterations charcteristic of hereditary nephritis. J Pediatr 1987; 111:519–524.
Flinter F, et al.: Genetics of classic Alport's syndrome. Lancet 1988; 2:1005–1007. *
Gershoni-Baruch R, et al.: Fechtner syndrome: clinical and genetic aspects. Am J Med Genet 1988; 31:357–367. †
Edwards BD, et al.: A new syndrome of autosomal recessive nephropathy, deafness, and hyperparathyroidism. J Med Genet 1989; 26: 289–293.

BA041                                               **Harold N. Bass**

**Nephritis-deafness-macrothrombopathia**
 *See DEAFNESS-NEPHRITIS-MACROTHROMBOPATHIA*
**Nephritis-megathrombocytopenia-deafness**
 *See LEUKOCYTE, MAY-HEGGLIN ANOMALY*
**Nephroblastoma**
 *See CANCER, WILMS TUMOR*
**Nephroblastomatosis**
 *See CANCER, WILMS TUMOR*
**Nephrogenic diabetes insipidus**
 *See DIABETES INSIPIDUS, VASOPRESSIN RESISTANT TYPES I AND II*
**Nephronophthisis, familial juvenile**
 *See KIDNEY, NEPHRONOPHTHISIS-MEDULLARY CYSTIC DESEASE*
**Nephronophthisis-medullary cystic disease**
 *See KIDNEY, NEPHRONOPHTHISIS-MEDULLARY CYSTIC DESEASE*
**Nephronophtisis-associated ocular anomalies, familial juvenile**
 *See RENAL DYSPLASIA-RETINAL APLASIA, LOKEN-SENIOR TYPE*
**Nephronophtisis-congenital hepatic**
 *See HEPATIC FIBROSIS, CONGENITAL*
**Nephropathic cystinosis**
 *See CYSTINOSIS*
**Nephropathy-deafness, hereditary type**
 *See NEPHRITIS-DEAFNESS (SENSORINEURAL), HEREDITARY TYPE*
**Nephropathy-diabetes-deafness-photomyoclonus**
 *See DEAFNESS-DIABETES-PHOTOMYOCLONUS-NEPHROPATHY*
**Nephropathy-hypoparathyroidism-lymphedema**
 *See LYMPHEDEMA-HYPOPARATHYROIDISM*
**Nephropathy-pseudohermaphroditism-Wilms tumor**
 *See WILMS TUMOR-PSEUDOHERMAPHRODITISM-GLOMERULOPATHY, DENYS-DRASH TYPE*

## NEPHROSIS, CONGENITAL                              0709

**Includes:**
  Finnish nephrosis
  Microcystic renal disease
  Neonatal nephrosis
  Nephrosis, infantile
  Pulmonic stenosis-congenital nephrosis

**Excludes:**
  Nephrosis, congenital-diffuse mesangial sclerosis
  **Nephrosis, familial type** (0710)
  Nephrotic syndrome, hereditary late
  Nephropathies (other)

**Major Diagnostic Criteria:**  Edema, hypoproteinemia, hypoalbuminemia, and proteinuria at birth or shortly thereafter. Onset occurs before the age of four months. Tests are negative for syphilis, malaria, mercury, toxoplasma and cytomegalovirus. Renal biopsy shows cystic dilatation of proximal tubules in cortex.

**Clinical Findings:**  Newborns present with edema, abdominal distention, hypoproteinemia, hypoalbuminemia, and proteinuria. Occasionally the edema is absent at birth, but shortly thereafter it becomes generalized, severe, and persistent. Congenital nephrosis may be suspected when the placenta is large and heavy (25–40% of the weight of the infant) and the infant has a low birth weight. Respiratory distress is often seen in the postnatal period. Laboratory findings consist of proteinuria; hypoproteinemia with serum protein of 2.5–3.7 g/dl; low serum albumin of 0.4–0.9 g/dl. Serum cholesterol may be lower than 200 mg initially, but in most cases, this value varies between 200–400 mg with tendency to rise as high as 800 mg. Many infants die within the first year as a result of infection and, rarely, as the result of renal failure.

**Complications:**  Electrolyte imbalance, infections, renal failure, retardation of growth and development, and coagulation abnormalities.

**Associated Findings:**  Hypothyroidism, pyloric stenosis, and gastroesophageal reflux. One family reported by Fournier et al (1963) had a combination of pulmonary stenosis and congenital nephrosis in the four affected children.

**Etiology:**  Autosomal recessive inheritance. In nearly one-third of the marriages, consanguinity has been noted.

**Pathogenesis:**  Hypothesized inborn error of metabolism that leads to faulty structure of glomerular basal lamina. Decreased heparan sulfate-rich anionic sites have been demonstrated in the lamina rara externa of the glomerular basement membrane. Loss of negatively charged sites may lead to penetration of basement membrane by proteins.

**MIM No.:**  *25630, 26560

**Sex Ratio:**  M1:F1

**Occurrence:**  In Finland, the incidence is 1:10,000 live births. Elsewhere, the incidence is undetermined. Prevalence is undetermined but the greatest number of cases have been reported from Finland and areas outside of Finland where there is a large aggregation of people of Finnish extraction.

**Risk of Recurrence for Patient's Sib:**
See Part I, *Mendelian Inheritance.*

**Risk of Recurrence for Patient's Child:**
See Part I, *Mendelian Inheritance.* Affected individuals are not expected to survive to reproduce.

**Age of Detectability:**  At birth or shortly thereafter, by clinical picture. Prenatal detection is available, since mothers at risk of bearing a child with congenital nephrosis have been noted to have markedly elevated alpha-fetoprotein in their own sera and amniotic fluid starting from the 15th week of gestation.

**Gene Mapping and Linkage:**  Unknown.

**Prevention:**  None known. Genetic counseling indicated.

**Treatment:**  Steroid and other immunosuppressive drugs are of no demonstrated value. Successful renal transplantations have been reported. Adequate therapy for infections is necessary.

**Prognosis:**  Very poor without renal transplantation. No recurrences in transplanted kidney. Without transplantation, most succumb within first year of life.

**Detection of Carrier:**  Unknown.

**References:**

Fournier A, et al.: Syndromes nephrotiques familiaux: syndrome nephrotigue associe a une cardiopathie congenitale chez quatre soeurs. Pediatrie 1963; 18; 677–685.

Hoyer JR, et al.: The nephrotic syndrome of infancy: clinical, morphological and immunological studies of four infants. Pediatrics 1967; 40:233–246.

Hoyer JR, et al.: Successful renal transplantation in 3 children with congenital nephrotic syndrome. Lancet 1973; I:1410–1412.

Aula P, et al.: Prenatal diagnosis of congenital nephrosis in 23 high-risk families. Am J Dis Child 1978; 132:984–987.

Rapola J, Hallman N: A.F.P and congenital nephrosis, Finnish type. Lancet 1979; I:274–275.

Risteli L, et al.: Slow accumulation of basement membrane collagen in kidney cortex in congenital nephrotic syndrome Lancet 1982; I:712–714.

Vernier RL, et al: Heparan sulfate-rich anionic sites in the human glomerular basement membrane: decreased concentration in congenital nephrotic syndrome. New Engl J Med 1983; 309:1001–1009. *

Mahan JD, et al.: Congenital nephrotic syndrome: evolution of medical management and results of renal transplantation. J Pediatr 1984; 105:549–557. *

M0035                                                          **Donald I. Moel**

---

## NEPHROSIS, FAMILIAL TYPE                                      0710

**Includes:**
Nephrotic syndrome occurring postnatally, familial
Nephrotic syndrome-focal glomerular sclerosis

**Excludes:**
**Nephritis-deafness (sensorineural), hereditary type** (0708)
Nephritis, other types of hereditary
**Nephrosis, congenital** (0709)
**Nephrosis-nerve deafness-hypoparathyroidism, Barakat type** (3026)

**Major Diagnostic Criteria:**  Edema, hypoproteinemia, hypercholesterolemia, and proteinuria. Renal biopsy may reveal findings of minimal change disease, membranoproliferative glomerulonephritis, mesangial sclerosis, and IgM nephropathy. A family history of nephrosis helps to confirm the diagnosis.

**Clinical Findings:**  Onset of familial nephrosis, with the insidious onset of edema, is similar to all types of nephrosis. Anasarca is not present at birth but may appear as early as two months of age. There may be a history of an upper respiratory infection prior to the onset of edema. With increasing edema, there is often history of a decrease in urinary output. Physical examination reveals generalized edema, at times including ascites. Hypertension and hematuria are generally absent at onset. Laboratory studies reveal severe-to-moderate proteinuria, hypoproteinemia, hypercholesterolemia, normal BUN, and no marked reduction in creatinine clearance at onset. Recently, low or absent immunoglobulin levels have been reported in this syndrome. Absence of protective immunoglobulins may contribute to the observed high rate of sepsis in affected infants. Serum complement levels are normal. It is not until the same type of nephrosis develops in a sib that one becomes aware this this is a familial form of nephrosis. Familial nerve deafness is not associated with this form of renal disease and, if present, suggests **Nephritis-deafness (sensorineural), hereditary type** (Alport syndrome).

The course may follow two patterns of response to steroid therapy and outcome. In one group, steroid therapy produces little or no improvement, and death from infection or renal failure ultimately results. Alternatively, the patient responds to steroids, with evidence of complete remission; thereafter the patient may have one or more relapses that respond to steroid therapy, but eventually there is complete recovery. The pattern of response in the second involved member of the family usually follows a course similar to that of the first affected sib.

**Complications:**  Extremely low immunoglobulin levels may predispose the newborn to sepsis. For those who do not respond to steroids, infection or renal failure may be the cause of death. For those who are steroid-responsive, the clinical course may be relatively uncomplicated.

**Associated Findings:**  None known.

**Etiology:**  Undetermined. Autosomal recessive inheritance seems likely.

**Pathogenesis:**  Unknown.

**MIM No.:**  25635

**Sex Ratio:**  M1:F<1

**Occurrence:**  Undetermined. Established literature.

**Risk of Recurrence for Patient's Sib:**
See Part I, *Mendelian Inheritance.*

**Risk of Recurrence for Patient's Child:**
See Part I, *Mendelian Inheritance.*

**Age of Detectability:**  Anytime after the age of two months.

**Gene Mapping and Linkage:**  Unknown.

**Prevention:**  None known. Genetic counseling indicated.

**Treatment:**  Steroid therapy, antibiotics.

**Prognosis:**  The prognosis is favorable for those patients who are steroid-responsive. If there is no response to steroid therapy, the prognosis is unfavorable.

**Detection of Carrier:**  Unknown.

**Special Considerations:** The pathologic findings vary and do not provide a means to distinguish this form of the nephrotic syndrome from nonfamilial forms. Some may show no abnormalities on routine light microscopy of the kidney; however, on electron microscopy, there is fusion of the foot processes (so-called minimal change). In others, the microscopic features are those of membranous glomerulonephritis, with or without lobular nephritis or focal sclerosing glomerulonephritis. The form with minimal change renal pathology is the steroid-responsive form; with a good outlook for ultimate recovery.

**References:**

Moncrieff M, et al.: The familial nephrotic syndrome: a clinicopathological study. Clin Nephrol 1973; 1:220–229. *
White R: The familial nephrotic syndrome: a European study. Clin Nephrol 1973; 1:215–219.
Bader P, et al.: Familial nephrotic syndrome. Am J Med 1974; 56:34–43. *
Naruse T, et al.: Familial nephrotic syndrome with focal glomerular sclerosis. Am J Med Sci 1980; 280:109–113.
Chandra M, et al.: Familial nephrotic syndrome and focal segmental glomerulosclerosis. J Pediatr 1981; 98:556–560.
Tejani A, et al.: Familial focal segmental glomerulosclerosis. Int J Ped Nephrol 1983; 4:231–234.
Harris HW, et al.: Altered immunoglobulin status in congenital nephrotic syndrome. Clin Nephrol 1986; 25:308–313.

LI022                                    **David A. Link**

**Nephrosis, infantile**
*See NEPHROSIS, CONGENITAL*
**Nephrosis-deafness-digital anomalies**
*See NEPHROSIS-HYDROCEPHALUS-THIN SKIN-BLUE SCLERA-GROWTH DEFECT*

## NEPHROSIS-DEAFNESS-URINARY TRACT AND DIGITAL DEFECTS                    3122

**Includes:**
Braun-Bayer syndrome
Deafness-nephrosis-urinary tract and digital defects
Digital defects-nephrosis-deafness urinary tract defects
Urinary tract and digital defects-nephrosis-deafness

**Excludes:**
**Deafness-nephritis-macrothrombopathia** (3046)
**Nephrosis-nerve deafness-hypoparathyroidism, Barakat type** (3026)
**Renal tubular acidosis** (0862)

**Major Diagnostic Criteria:** Familial nephrosis, familial deafness, congenital urinary tract abnormalities, digital defects.

**Clinical Findings:** Nephrotic syndrome, conductive and sometimes perceptive deafness, urinary tract abnormalities (ureterovesical and bladder neck obstruction, duplication of collecting system, hydronephrosis), digital abnormalities (short and bifid distal phalanges of thumbs and big toes), bifurcation of the uvula.

**Complications:** Hydronephrosis, pyelonephritis.

**Associated Findings:** Allergic manifestations with bronchial asthma.

**Etiology:** Presumably either autosomal recessive or X-linked dominant inheritance.

**Pathogenesis:** Unknown.

**MIM No.:** 25620

**POS No.:** 4340

**Sex Ratio:** M5:F0 (observed).

**Occurrence:** Five brothers have been reported in the literature.

**Risk of Recurrence for Patient's Sib:**
See Part I, *Mendelian Inheritance.*

**Risk of Recurrence for Patient's Child:**
See Part I, *Mendelian Inheritance.*

**Age of Detectability:** Most patients have been diagnosed before age two years.

**Gene Mapping and Linkage:** Unknown.

**Prevention:** None known. Genetic counseling indicated.

**Treatment:** As per the respective manifestations.

**Prognosis:** No follow-up of the known affected individuals has been reported.

**Detection of Carrier:** The deafness and digital anomalies in one brother and the isolated nephrosis in another may represent a variable expression of the same gene.

**References:**

Braun FC, Jr., Bayer JF: Familial nephrosis associated with deafness and congenital urinary tract anomalies in siblings. J Pediatr 1962; 60:33–41.

BA065                                 **Amin Y. Barakat**

## NEPHROSIS-HYDROCEPHALUS-THIN SKIN-BLUE SCLERA-GROWTH DEFECT                    2187

**Includes:**
Ehlers-Danlos, type IV (possible form)
Growth defect-hydrocephalus-nephrosis-thin skin-blue sclera
Hydrocephalus-nephrosis-thin skin-blue sclera-growth defect
Microcephaly-nephrosis-hiatal hernia
Nephrosis-deafness-digital anomalies
Sclera (blue)-hydrocephalus-nephrosis-thin skin-growth defect
Skin (thin)-hydrocephalus-nephrosis-blue sclera-growth defect

**Excludes:**
**Ehlers-Danlos syndrome** (0338)
**Microcephaly-hiatus hernia-nephrosis, Galloway type** (2755)
**Nephrosis-deafness-urinary tract and digital defects** (3122)

**Major Diagnostic Criteria:** Infantile nephrosis; **Hydrocephaly**; thin, transparent skin.

**Clinical Findings:** Based on two brothers: nephrosis, hydrocephaly, thin skin, blue sclera, growth delay, recurrent infections, and T-cell dysfunction. In addition, both brothers had distinctive facial features, including frontal prominence, narrow midface, thin upper lip, and small ears.

**Complications:** Both children developed renal failure and died by age three years.

**Associated Findings:** Recurrent otitis media.

**Etiology:** Possible autosomal or X-linked recessive inheritance.

**Pathogenesis:** Possible collagen defect.

**POS No.:** 3846

**Sex Ratio:** M2:F0 (observed).

**Occurrence:** Reported in two brothers of one family.

**Risk of Recurrence for Patient's Sib:**
See Part I, *Mendelian Inheritance.*

**Risk of Recurrence for Patient's Child:**
See Part I, *Mendelian Inheritance.* No affected individuals have survived to reproduce.

**Age of Detectability:** Usually at birth. Prenatal detection theoretically possible in at-risk pregnancies if hydrocephaly or polyhydramnios is detected by ultrasound.

**Gene Mapping and Linkage:** Unknown.

**Prevention:** None known. Genetic counseling indicated.

**Treatment:** Nephrosis has not been responsive to steroids.

**Prognosis:** Death in both sibs by three years of age. Otherwise, normal development.

**Detection of Carrier:** Unknown.

**Special Considerations:** Another two male sibs with nephrosis and neuronal heterotopias (and hydrocephalus in one) were reported by Palm et al. (1986). It is uncertain whether these sibs had the same disorder, since there was no mention of thin skin, blue sclera or similar facial features in the clinical description.

**References:**
Daentl DL, et al.: Familial nephrosis, hydrocephalus, thin skin, blue sclerae syndrome: clinical, structural, and biochemical studies. BD:OAS XIV(6B). New York: March of Dimes Birth Defects Foundation, 1978:315–339.
Palm L, et al.: Nephrosis and disturbances of neuronal migration in male siblings - a new hereditary disorder? Arch Dis Child 1986; 61:545–548.
Beighton P, et al.: International nosology of heritable disorders of connective tissue, Berlin, 1986. Am J Med Genet 1988; 29:581–594.

GR011                                                      **Frank Greenberg**

**Nephrosis-microcephaly-hiatus hernia, Galloway type**
 *See MICROCEPHALY-HIATUS HERNIA-NEPHROSIS, GALLOWAY TYPE*

---

## NEPHROSIS-NERVE DEAFNESS-HYPOPARATHYROIDISM, BARAKAT TYPE        3026

**Includes:**
 Barakat syndrome
 Deafness (nerve)-nephrosis-hypoparathyroidism
 Hypoparathyroidism-nephrosis-nerve deafness
**Excludes:**
 **Immunodeficiency, thymic agenesis** (0943)
 **Nephritis-deafness (sensorineural), hereditary type** (0708)
**Major Diagnostic Criteria:** Steroid-resistant nephrotic syndrome, bilateral nerve deafness, hypoparathyroidism.

**Clinical Findings:** Asymptomatic proteinuria progressing to nephrotic syndrome, severe bilateral nerve deafness, edema, vomiting, lethargy.

**Complications:** Chronic renal failure, nephrocalcinosis.

**Associated Findings:** Absent or hypoplastic parathyroid glands.

**Etiology:** Probably autosomal recessive or X-linked inheritance.

**Pathogenesis:** Unknown.

**MIM No.:** 25634

**POS No.:** 3821

**Sex Ratio:** M4:F0 observed.

**Occurrence:** Reported in four brothers, two of whom were twins.

**Risk of Recurrence for Patient's Sib:**
 See Part I, *Mendelian Inheritance.*

**Risk of Recurrence for Patient's Child:**
 See Part I, *Mendelian Inheritance.*

**Age of Detectability:** During early childhood.

**Gene Mapping and Linkage:** Unknown.

**Prevention:** None known. Genetic counseling indicated.

**Treatment:** Unknown. Kidney transplantation was not attempted.

**Prognosis:** All four patients died with uremia before eight years of age.

**Detection of Carrier:** Unknown.

**References:**
Barakat AY, et al.: Familial nephrosis, nerve deafness, and hypoparathyroidism. J Pediatr 1977; 91:61–64.

BA065                                                    **Amin Y. Barakat**

**Nephrotic syndrome occurring postnatally, familial**
 *See NEPHROSIS, FAMILIAL TYPE*

**Nephrotic syndrome-focal glomerular sclerosis**
 *See NEPHROSIS, FAMILIAL TYPE*
**Nerve malformations of middle ear**
 *See EAR, OSSICLE AND MIDDLE EAR MALFORMATIONS*
**Nerve trunk palsies, familial**
 *See NEUROPATHY, HEREDITARY WITH PRESSURE PALSIES*
**Nervous system endemic cretinism**
 *See CRETINISM, ENDEMIC, AND RELATED DISORDERS*
**Netherton syndrome**
 *See ICHTHYOSIS, LINEARIS CIRCUMFLEXA*
**Netilmycin, fetal effects**
 *See FETAL AMINOGLYCOSIDE OTOTOXICITY*
**Netromycin^, fetal effects**
 *See FETAL AMINOGLYCOSIDE OTOTOXICITY*
**Nettleship-Falls ocular albinism**
 *See ALBINISM, OCULAR*
**Neu syndrome**
 *See NEU-LAXOVA SYNDROME*

---

## NEU-LAXOVA SYNDROME        2092

**Includes:** Neu syndrome

**Excludes:**
 Cerebral-arthro digital syndrome
 **Cerebro-oculo-facio-skeletal syndrome** (0140)
 **Lissencephaly syndrome** (0603)
 **Pena-Shokeir syndrome** (2080)
 **Pterygium syndrome, multiple lethal** (2274)

**Major Diagnostic Criteria:** Should be considered in an infant who is stillborn or dies shortly after birth who has the major features of intrauterine growth retardation, generalized edema, limb contractures, and abnormalities in central nervous system development. Icthyotic-like skin changes are also common.

**Clinical Findings:** *Pregnancy:* Frequent polyhydramnios (12/14). Third trimester ultrasound abnormalities have included hydramnios, scalp edema, hydrothorax, microcephaly, and growth retardation. *Delivery:* Term (11/14). Short umbilical cord in at least six cases. *Survival:* Stillborn (7/14). 6/14 died within hours. The longest survivor was seven weeks of age.
*Physical examination and growth parameters:* Affected infants have usually demonstrated extremely low birth weights, lengths, and head circumferences. Reduction in head circumference is, however, the most striking and uniform finding. Head circumferences at term have ranged from 20–26.5 cm. Head circumference may, however, be artifactually increased due to the presence of massive scalp edema. One infant had demonstrated macrocephaly in association with a midline cleft and probable hydranencephaly (Povýšilová, et al (1976).
*Craniofacial findings:* Sloping forehead and hypertelorism are described in over one-half the cases. Nasal bridge is described as broad and prominent. Eyes have frequently been abnormal. Prominent protuberant eyes with retracted, apparently absent lids and ectropion have been noted in five cases, cataracts in three, and microphthalmia in two. Micrognathia is common, and short neck was specifically noted in eight cases.
*Limbs:* The limbs frequently have shown contractures of the major joints; a few cases had webbing at the knees and elbows. Fingers are frequently described as overlapping, particularly in those without severe hand edema. Rocker bottom feet are described in several cases. Alteration in palmar creases and camptodactyly and clinodactyly of digits has been noted. Partial syndactyly of fingers and toes have been described in five cases. Hands inflated like yellow rubber gloves have been described in five cases. As seen on pathologic examination, this massive swelling is apparently due to deposition of excessive fat, in addition to the presence of edema fluid.
*Skin:* Generalized edema of the skin has been a uniform finding in all cases, but the severity has varied dramatically. Myxomatous connective tissue has been noted on sections of subcutaneous tissue in two patients; this is an unusual pathologic finding that may be helpful in the diagnosis of this syndrome. The abnormal deposition of fat described pathologically in a few cases may also be helpful diagnostically. The skin has frequently been described

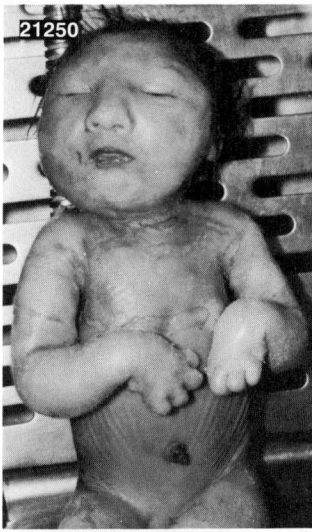
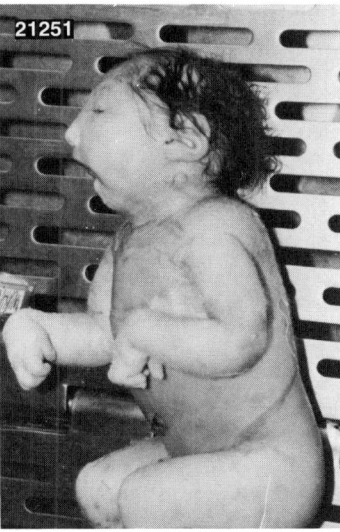
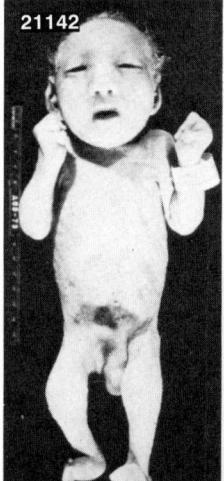
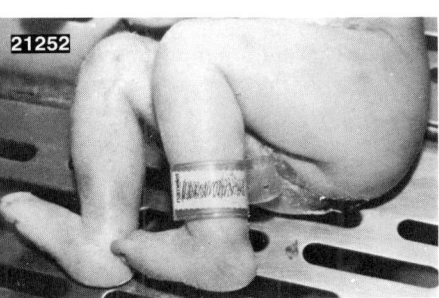

**2092**-21250–52, 21142: Micrognathia, dysmorphic facies, limb contractures, prominent nasal bridge, sloping forehead, unusual auricles, and edema.

as abnormal, either thin, lemon-colored and scaly; tight, shiny with collodion-like appearance; or ichthyotic. Peeling of the skin and desquamation of the skin in sheets has been a frequent observation. No detailed pathologic examinations of skin have been performed.

*X-Ray findings:* The skeletal X-rays have generally shown mild undermineralization of the skeleton. Flat acetabular roofs and dysplastic ilia have been noted. Spina bifida occulta at L-5 and S-1 was noted in one case. Intrauterine fractures reported in two cases.

**Complications:** Lethal.

**Associated Findings:** Large ventral hernia (1), micropenis (1), and hypoplastic genitalia (2).

*Autopsy findings:* A neuropathological examinations was performed in nine cases. Hypoplastic cerebellum has been documented in eight, and the absence of the corpus callosum in four. Lissencephaly has been noted in five cases. Several cases have noted dilated lateral ventricles and/or polymicrogyria. Histologic examinations have revealed a thinned cerebral cortex. Other abnormalities at autopsy have included lung hypoplasia, abnor-

mal fetal lobulation of the kidneys, nephroptosis, and gross underdevelopment of skeletal muscle.

**Etiology:** Autosomal recessive inheritance is presumed on the basis of recurrence in four sibships. Consanguinity has been noted in four reported families.

**Pathogenesis:** Unknown. No detailed biochemical evaluations of these infants have been performed. It is unlikely that this syndrome is due to a single problem in central nervous system development.

**MIM No.:** *25652

**POS No.:** 3326

**Sex Ratio:** Presumably M1:F1.

**Occurrence:** About 16 cases have been reported. May be underdiagnosed because of early lethality. Death prior to delivery may also make confirmation of the diagnosis impossible. Three literature reports of Pakistani families (Laxova, 1972, Mueller, 1983) suggests that this gene may be relatively frequent in that population. One family was of Asian-Indian extraction.

**Risk of Recurrence for Patient's Sib:**
See Part I, *Mendelian Inheritance.*

**Risk of Recurrence for Patient's Child:**
See Part I, *Mendelian Inheritance.*

**Age of Detectability:** In utero detection by ultrasound should be possible by the latter half of second trimester, the syndrome is otherwise identified at birth.

**Gene Mapping and Linkage:** Unknown.

**Prevention:** None known. Genetic counseling indicated.

**Treatment:** Unknown.

**Prognosis:** Lethal.

**Detection of Carrier:** Unknown.

**References:**
Neu RL, et al.: A lethal syndrome of microcephaly with multiple congenital anomalies in three siblings. Pediatrics 1971; 47:610–612.
Laxova R, et al.: A further example of a lethal autosomal recessive condition in sibs. J Ment Defic Res 1972: 16:139–143.
Povyšilová V, et al.: Letální syndrom mnohočetných malformací u tří sourozenc°u. Ces Pediat 1976; 31:190–194.
Lazjuk GI, et al.: The Neu-Laxova syndrome: a distinct entity. Am J Med Genet 1979; 3:261–267.
Scott C, et al.: Comments on the Neu-Laxova syndrome and the CAD complex. Am J Med Genet 1981; 9:165–175.
Winter RM, et al.: Syndromes of microcephaly, microphthalmia, cataracts and joint contractures. J Med Genet 1981; 18:129–133.
Curry CJR: Further comments on the Neu-Laxova syndrome. Am J Med Genet 1982; 13:441–444.
Fitch N, et al.: The Neu-Laxova syndrome: comments on syndrome identification. Am J Med Genet 1982; 13:445–452.
Karimi-Nejad MH, et al.: Neu-Laxova syndrome: report of a case and comments. Am J Med Genet 1987; 28:17–23.
Muller LM, et al.: A case of the Neu-Laxova syndrome: prenatal ultrasonographic monitoring in the third trimester and the histopathological findings. Am J Med Genet 1987; 26:421–429.
Ostrovskaya TI, Lazjuk GI: Cerebral abnormalities in the Neu-Laxova syndrome. Am J Med Genet 1988; 30:747–756.

CU009                                                       **Cynthia J.R. Curry**

**Neural crest, syndrome of**
*See NEUROPATHY, CONGENITAL SENSORY WITH ANHIDROSIS*
**Neural deafness, recessive early-onset**
*See DEAFNESS (SENSORINEURAL), RECESSIVE EARLY-ONSET*
**Neural tube defects (some)**
*See SCHISIS ASSOCIATION*
**Neural tube defects, X-linked**
*See ANENCEPHALY*
**Neural-tube defect**
*See MENINGOMYELOCELE*
*also MENINGOCELE*
**Neuralgic amyotrophy, familial**
*See NEUROPATHY, HEREDITARY RECURRENT BRACHIAL*
**Neuralgic amyotrophy-brachial predilection, familial**
*See NEUROPATHY, HEREDITARY RECURRENT BRACHIAL*

**Neuraminidase deficiency**
 *See MUCOLIPIDOSIS I*
 *also MUCOLIPIDOSIS IV*
**Neuraminidase deficiency with beta-galactosidase deficiency**
 *See GALACTOSIALIDOSIS*
**Neuraminidase/beta-galactosidase expression**
 *See GALACTOSIALIDOSIS*
**Neurenteric cyst**
 *See ESOPHAGUS, DUPLICATION*
**Neurenteric cyst of spinal cord**
 *See SPINAL CORD, NEURENTERIC CYST*
**Neuritis with brachial predilection, heredo-familial**
 *See NEUROPATHY, HEREDITARY RECURRENT BRACHIAL*
**Neuritis, peripheral with isoniazid**
 *See NEUROPATHY, HERITABLE ISONIAZIDE TYPE (INH)*

## NEURO-FACIO-DIGITO-RENAL SYNDROME — 2897

**Includes:** NFDR syndrome

**Excludes:** FG syndrome, Opitz-Kaveggia type (0754)

**Major Diagnostic Criteria:** Limb malformations, renal agenesis, high and prominent forehead, vertical groove on tip of nose, ear abnormalities, **Megalencephaly**, hypotonia, mental retardation, and abnormal EEG.

**Clinical Findings:** Long thumbs with unilateral triphalangism, broad halluces, flat feet, valgus hips, winging of scapulae, hyperextensible elbows, protruding abdomen, small testes, mandibular prognathism, intrauterine growth retardation, shortness of stature, disproportionately great OFC (see **Megalencephaly**), unilateral renal agenesis, hypotonia, mental retardation, abnormal EEG, high and prominent forehead, vertical groove on tip of nose, frontal upsweep of hairline, bilateral alternating exotropia, epicanthal folds.

**Complications:** Poor school performance.

**Associated Findings:** None known.

**Etiology:** Autosomal recessive or possibly X-linked recessive inheritances.

**Pathogenesis:** Unknown.

**MIM No.:** 25669

**POS No.:** 4336

**Sex Ratio:** M2:F0 (observed).

**Occurrence:** Two Brazilian brothers have been reported.

**Risk of Recurrence for Patient's Sib:**
 See Part I, *Mendelian Inheritance.*

**Risk of Recurrence for Patient's Child:**
 See Part I, *Mendelian Inheritance.*

**Age of Detectability:** At birth, by physical examination.

**Gene Mapping and Linkage:** Unknown.

**Prevention:** None known. Genetic counseling indicated.

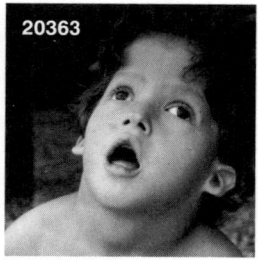 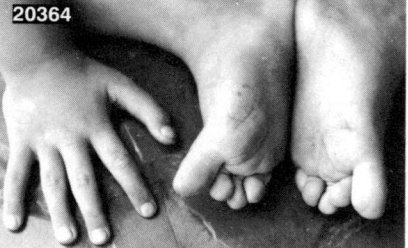

**2897**-20363: Mouth-breathing facies, small and abnormal auricles, exotropia, vertical groove on tip of the nose and frontal upsweep of the hairline. 20364: Large halluces and long thumb.

**Treatment:** Early special education; special medical care mainly in case of problems with the solitary kidney.

**Prognosis:** Probably normal life span with good medical care.

**Detection of Carrier:** Unknown.

**References:**
Freire-Maia N, et al.: The neurofaciodigitorenal (NFDR) syndrome. Am J Med Genet 1982; 11:329–336.

FR033           **Newton Freire-Maia**

**Neuro-facio-skeletal syndrome**
 *See FACIO-NEURO-SKELETAL SYNDROME*
**Neuroacanthocytosis**
 *See ACANTHOCYTOSIS-NEUROLOGIC DEFECTS*

## NEUROAXONAL DYSTROPHY, INFANTILE — 2701

**Includes:** Seitelberger disease

**Excludes:**
 **Alpha-N-acetylgalactosaminidase deficiency** (3254)
 **Brain, spongy degeneration** (0115)
 **Encephalopathy, necrotizing** (0344)
 **Hallervorden-Spatz disease** (2526)
 **Metachromatic leukodystrophies** (0651)
 Neuroaxonal dystrophy, secondary
 **Pelizaeus-Merzbacher syndrome** (0803)

**Major Diagnostic Criteria:** The disease can be suspected in an initially normal infant who first exhibits slowing and/or arrest of development, followed by deterioration, with marked hypotonia and visual and auditory impairment, usually unaccompanied by seizures. Confirmation requires demonstration of axonal spheroids either in the brain or via a muscle, skin, or conjunctival biopsy that includes peripheral nerve endings. The electromyo-

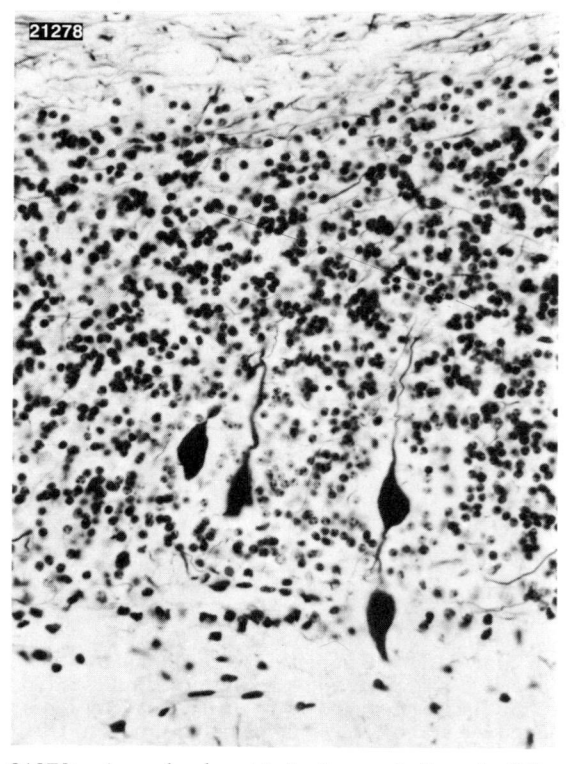

**2701**-21278: Axonal spheroids in the cerebellum (×400).

gram (EMG) may show denervation changes with normal nerve conduction. Electroretinogram (ERG) findings are normal, but there is a decreased or absent visual envoked response.

**Clinical Findings:** The most common manifestation is a slowing and/or arrest of development, or a disturbance in gait, between the ages of six months and two years of age, in a previously healthy child. The degree of hypotonia is striking, and may suggest a myopathy, although the children may eventually become spastic. Pyramidal tract signs with upgoing toes and hyperreflexia are characteristic, although reflexes may be decreased due to the marked hypotonia and weakness. Visual impairment is early and significant, and characterized by strabismus, pendular nystagmus, dysconjugate eye movement, and decreased vision with optic atrophy. Hearing and response to tactile stimulation are also impaired.

The clinical course is one of progressive dementia and decerebration, with death before 10 years of age. The central, peripheral, and often autonomic systems are involved. Axonal spheroids are not specific to neuroaxonal dystrophy, and it is the combined clinical and overall pathologic distribution that is diagnostic. The spheroid bodies are widespread in the CNS, especially in the cortex, spinal cord, brainstem, basal ganglia, and peripheral nerve endings in the skin, neuromuscular junctions, and conjunctiva. Atrophy is prominent in the cerebellum, optic pathways, pyramidal tracts, brainstem nuclei, and inferior olivary bodies; there is marked gliosis, especially in the cerebral hemispheres.

**Complications:** The progressive neurologic deterioration with inanition increases the susceptibility to respiratory disease and aspiration which are commonly the immediate cause of death.

**Associated Findings:** None known.

**Etiology:** Autosomal recessive inheritance with very little intrafamilial variation in expression.

**Pathogenesis:** Undetermined in most cases, but the axonal dystrophy is probably primary. Schindler et al (1989) detected a deficiency of α-N-acetylgalactosamidase in two affected brothers, but the results in eight unrelated patients were normal.

**MIM No.:** *25660

**Sex Ratio:** M1:F1

**Occurrence:** Fewer than 100 cases have been reported. Patients have been reported from most European countries, Israel, the United States, Canada, and Japan.

**Risk of Recurrence for Patient's Sib:**
See Part I, *Mendelian Inheritance.*

**Risk of Recurrence for Patient's Child:**
See Part I, *Mendelian Inheritance.* Affected individuals are not expected to survive to reproduce.

**Age of Detectability:** The typical infantile case shows clinical signs between the ages of six months to two years. A few cases with either earlier or later onset have been reported. The earliest age at which axonal spheroids might be seen on biopsy of peripheral nerve endings is undetermined.

**Gene Mapping and Linkage:** Unknown.

**Prevention:** None known. Genetic counseling indicated.

**Treatment:** Supportive.

**Prognosis:** Life expectancy is less than ten years, and death usually occurs about five years from onset.

**Detection of Carrier:** Unknown.

**Special Considerations:** Several children of both sexes have been reported with prenatal or connatal onset of axonal dystrophy. These children have displayed a rapidly lethal course, with more frequent seizures and less pathologic involvement of the cerebellum. Two male sibs with prenatal onset of neuroaxonal dystrophy manifested a dry peripheral gangrene at two months of age that resulted in autoamputation of the toes and distal fingertips. X-linked recessive inheritance cannot be ruled out for these cases.

**References:**
Jellinger K: Neuroaxonal dystrophy: its natural history and related disorders. In: Zimmerman HM, ed: Progress in neuropathology, Vol 2. New York: Grune and Stratton, 1973:129–180. *
Aicardi J, Castelein P: Infantile neuroaxonal dystrophy. Brain 1979; 102:727–748. *
Janota I: Neuroaxonal dystrophy in the neonate. Acta Neuropathol 1979; 46:151–154.
Hunter AGW, et al.: Neuroaxonal dystrophy presenting with neonatal dysmorphic features, early onset of peripheral gangrene, and a rapidly lethal course. Am J Med Genet 1987; 28:171–180.
Ramaekers VT, et al.: Diagnostic difficulties in infantile neuroaxonal dystrophy: a clinicopathological study of eight cases. Neuropediatrics 1987; 18:170–175.
Schindler D, et al.: Neuroaxonal dystrophy due to lysosomal α-N-acetylgalactosaminidase deficiency. New Engl J Med 1989; 320:1735–1740.

HU008                                        **Alasdair G.W. Hunter**

**Neuroaxonal dystrophy, infantile (one form)**
*See ALPHA-N-ACETYLGALACTOSAMINIDASE DEFICIENCY*
**Neuroaxonal dystrophy, late-infantile**
*See HALLERVORDEN-SPATZ DISEASE*
**Neuroblastoma and related lesions (all types)**
*See CANCER, NEUROBLASTOMA*
**Neuroblastoma, adult**
*See CANCER, EWING SARCOMA*
**Neurocutaneous melanosis**
*See SKIN, NEUROCUTANEOUS MELANOSIS*

---

**NEUROCUTANEOUS MELANOSIS**                 **2014**

**Includes:**
Melanosis, neurocutaneous
Skin, neurocutaneous melanosis

**Excludes:**
**Jaw, neuroectodermal pigmented tumor** (0711)
Melanosis coli
Melanotic neuroectodermal tumor of the brain during infancy
**Skin, cutaneous melanosis, diffuse** (2309)
**Skin, hyperpigmentation, familial** (2362)

**Major Diagnostic Criteria:** Congenital giant or multiple melanocytic nevi associated with leptomeningeal melanosis. The skin lesions should be benign, and there should be no presence of malignant melanoma in other organs to assure that the leptomeningeal melanoma is an independent lesion.

**Clinical Findings:** The skin lesions are characterized by single or multiple giant hairy pigmented nevi, usually assuming a "cape" or "bathing suit" distribution. The multiple large pigmented nevi are usually less common. Both types of lesions represent cosmetic problems. CNS involvement consists of a marked infiltration and pigmentation of melanin-containing cells of the leptomeninges at the base of the brain and over the brainstem. On most of the patients studied the areas frequently affected included the pons, medulla, cerebellum, cerebral peduncles, interpeduncular fossae, and the inferior surfaces of the frontal, temporal, and occipital lobes. A diffuse pigmentation and thickening of the full length of the spinal cord meninges is present in 20% of the cases. A variety of neurologic features may be present depending on the site and the extent of the primary leptomeningeal tumor. These may include epilepsy, psychiatric disturbances, meningeal hemorrhage, cranial nerve palsies, subdural hemorrhage, and intracranial hemorrhage. The first presentation of this disorder, usually occurring during early life, is often the development of hydrocephalus secondary to obstruction of the cerebrospinal fluid (CSF) circulation either at the fourth ventricular outlets or within the basal subarachnoid cisterns. Although the CSF may be normal, the CSF protein content is commonly elevated and glucose concentration decreased. Cytologic examination may show the presence of melanin-containing cells.

**Complications:** Melanoma and death.

**Associated Findings:** Progressive **Syringomyelia** has been reported. Seizures, mental retardation, and **Hydrocephaly** have also been reported.

**Etiology:** Possibly autosomal recessive inheritance.

**Pathogenesis:** Melanocytes are known to exist normally in the epidermis, hair bulb, uveal tract, retina, and leptomeninges. In these areas they commonly reach sufficient numbers to enable pigmentation to be observed microscopically. Neurocutaneous melanosis is thought to be due to an excessive accumulation of melanin-producing cells in a local or diffuse distribution within both the skin and the leptomeninges. Ultrastructural studies of pigment cells in nevi and meningeal melanosis have shown a marked similarity of cellular structures consistent with a neural crest origin for pigment cells.

Ferris et al (1987) have suggested that this condition could be a consequence of one or more somatic mutations which would result in prenatal lethality if they occurred in the germ line cells.

**MIM No.:** 24940

**POS No.:** 3757

**Sex Ratio:** Presumably M1:F1.

**Occurrence:** Undetermined but presumably rare.

**Risk of Recurrence for Patient's Sib:**
See Part I, *Mendelian Inheritance.*

**Risk of Recurrence for Patient's Child:**
See Part I, *Mendelian Inheritance.*

**Age of Detectability:** In the first decade of life.

**Gene Mapping and Linkage:** Unknown.

**Prevention:** None known. Genetic counseling indicated.

**Treatment:** Skin lesions can be removed by a plastic surgeon and replaced by a flap or by using skin expanders. Treating hydrocephalus with shunting procedures helps to prevent the dissemination of melanoma; this procedure has only been palliative. There is no effective treatment for primary malignant leptomeningeal melanosis.

**Prognosis:** Death often usually occurs in early childhood, often as a result of malignant degeneration or occlusion of the ventricular outflow areas.

**Detection of Carrier:** Unknown.

**References:**
Reed WB, et al.: Giant pigmented nevi, melanoma, and leptomeningeal melanocytosis: a clinical and histopathological study. Arch Dermatol 1965; 91:100–119.
Lamas E, et al.: Neurocutaneous melanosis: report of a case and review of the literature. Acta Neurochir (Wien) 1977; 36:93–105.
Leaney BJ, et al.: Neurocutaneous melanosis with hydrocephalus and syringomyelia: a case report. J Neurosurg 1985; 62:148–52.
Yu HS, et al.: Neurocutaneous melanosis: electron microscopic comparison of the pigmented melanocytic nevi of skin and meningeal melanosis. J Dermatol (Tokio) 1985; 12:267–276.
Ferris MK, et al.: Neurocutaneous melanosis syndrome. (Abstract) Am J Hum Genet 1987; 41:A57 only.

MI038
M0040

**Giuseppe Micali**
**David M. Mosher**

**Neuroectodermal melanolysosomal disease**
*See NEUROECTODERMAL MELANOLYSOSOMAL SYNDROME*

## NEUROECTODERMAL MELANOLYSOSOMAL SYNDROME 2361

**Includes:**
Hair (silver)-psychomotor and developmental retardation
Neuroectodermal melanolysosomal disease

**Excludes:**
**Albinism** (all types)
**Albinism, cutaneous** (0031)
**Albinism, oculocutaneous, Hermansky-Pudlak type** (0033)
**Albinoidism** (2359)
**Chediak-Higashi syndrome** (0143)
**Gingival fibromatosis-depigmentation-microphthalmia** (0413)
**Hypopigmentation-immune defect, Griscelli type** (2360)

**Major Diagnostic Criteria:** A striking silver-leaden color of the hair, severe congenital hypotonia, and hypoactive deep tendon reflexes. All known patients have profound psychomotor retardation and hypopigmented skin, with normal growth. The lesions are static and do not suggest a degenerative disorder of the CNS.

Melanin is organized in clumps inside the hair shafts, in both the peripheral and central areas of the hair. Melanosomes are abnormal and have irregular shapes; most of them are incompletely melanized. Some of them have bizarre forms, with fiber in concentric arrangements.

Skin and bone marrow cells show abnormal, round granules that have variable electron density and variable texture of their matrix; they appear to follow a pattern of maturation from a diffuse matrix to a granular one. The "mature granules" are excreted and found in the extracellular space. These granules appear to be derived from lysosomes. Cultured fibroblasts show a prominent Golgi apparatus. These granules show a strongly positive reaction when stained with periodic acid-Schiff, mildly intense with Fontana, and slightly positive with oil red O. They are negative when stained with luxol fast blue, alkaline phosphatase, peroxidase, tyrosinase, and oil red O after extraction with cold acetone, hot acetic acid, or toluidine blue.

Patients do not have visceromegaly, and all signs and symptoms are confined to derivatives of the neuroectoderm.

**Clinical Findings:** The condition is usually suspected when the infant fails to progress and has a history of congenital hypotonia. The next sign to appear is the lightly colored hair, which progresses to be silver-leaden. The psychomotor retardation is so severe that these infants never speak, sit, or reach any of the developmental milestones completed by normal children aged two years.

There is no special tendency to develop infectious disease, and affected individuals do well regarding common diseases.

When exposed to sunlight, skin shows some degree of tanning. Affected individuals do not show evidence of being blind or deaf. Some patients show severe myopia, signs of myopic degeneration with elongated papillae, normal macula, and normal pigmentation of the fundus.

With age, patients show the consequences of profound hypotonia (probably of prenatal onset), most noticeable in the face, with signs of being hypotonic and "mouth breathers." The chest is flat as a consequence of the almost complete absence of voluntary muscular movements. The joints become stiff and their range of movement limited.

The oldest patient known at last examination was aged 10 years, and she still did not have any type of interaction with those around her.

**Complications:** The complications seen in these patients can be divided into two major groups: 1) those due to the profound mental retardation, and 2) those due to the severe motor impairment. Patients are completely dependent on others to fulfill their basic needs. The most complex activity shown by one of the patients was to smile.

The consequences of hypotonia and the almost complete absence of voluntary movements are the other source of complications in this condition. The midface is hypoplastic, with crowded teeth and narrow palate; patients are "mouth breathers." The chest is flat, and patients develop respiratory infections that are

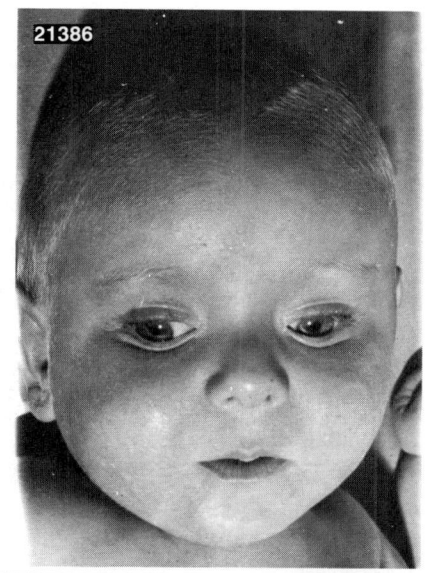

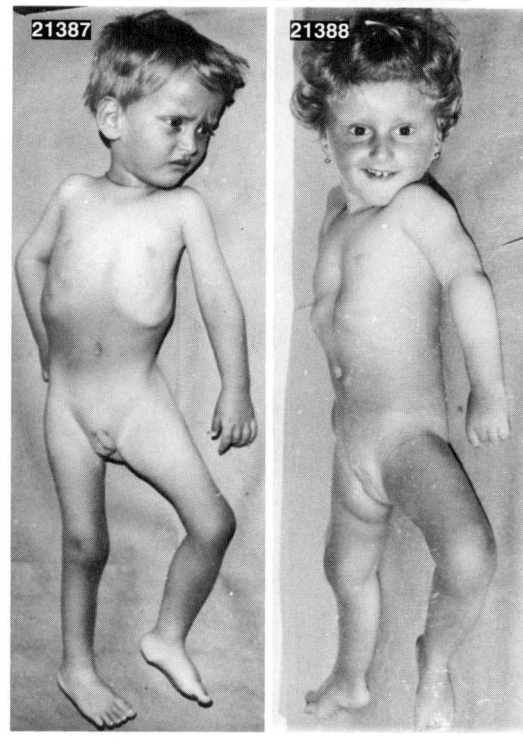

**2361A**-21386:  This young affected infant has a normal appearance and light-colored hair.    21387:  This older affected boy has reduced muscle mass and generalized hypotonia.    21388:  This affected girl shows the hypotonic posture and reduced muscle mass. Her smile is the most advanced developmental milestone that she reached.

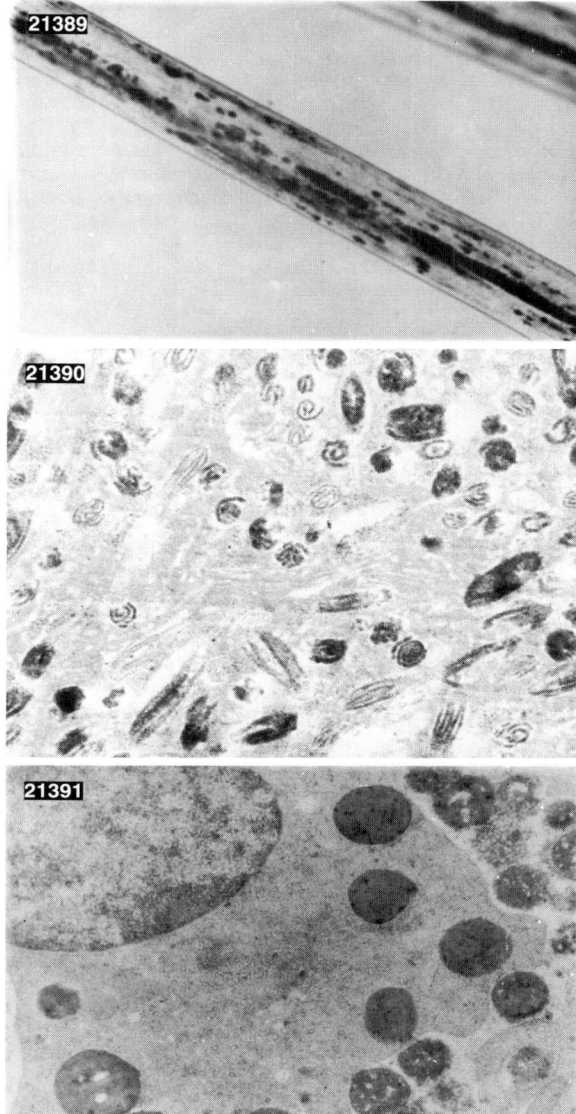

**2361B**-21389:  Microscopic view of a shaft of hair showing the characteristic marked clumping of the melanin in the peripheral and central areas of the hair. This pigment distribution changes the refraction and absorption of light and produces the silver leaden color characteristic of the hair.    21390:  Electron micrograph of a melanocyte from the skin shows the different types of melanosomes. All of the melanosomes are incompletely melanized; the matrix is incompletely formed and disorganized in many of them.    21391:  Electron micrograph of a bone marrow histiocyte contains large round granules with variable electron density and variable texture of the matrix, which varies from very homogenous inside the cells to granulated in the extracellular space. The granules appear to be secreted by the cell; fibroblasts have similar granulations.

more difficult to treat than in normal children. It is necessary to provide physical and occupational therapy. Other complications include plagiocephaly, micrognathia, and respiratory **Pectus excavatum**.

**Associated Findings:**  Absence of upward-slanted palpebral fissures, small hypoplastic nose, upper central incisors, hyperpig-

mented enamel and hypertrophic gingiva, bilateral cryptorchidism, and hypoplastic scrotum.

**Etiology:**  Autosomal recessive inheritance, having pleiotropic effects in different tissues, as demonstrated by segregation analysis in the affected families.

**Pathogenesis:** The phenotypic characteristics of the condition appear to be the pleiotropic effects of an autosomal recessive gene that preferentially affects the neuroectoderm and some of the tissues derived from it. The hypomelanization of the skin and the lysosomal inclusions in fibroblasts, lymphocytes, and bone marrow cells can be considered autophenes. The severe CNS dysfunction could represent relational pleiotropy. This gene alters the formation of melanosomes and the synthesis of melanin and allows for the fibroblasts and bone marrow cells to produce abnormal lysosomal granules that appear to be related to the formation of the melanosomes.

Possibly the CNS dysfunction is produced by an abnormal neuromelanin as a primary or secondary defect. In the second case it may be related to the dopaminergic system. This possibility is supported by the histochemical similarity of the granules with ceroid and lipofuscin.

**MIM No.:** *25671

**Sex Ratio:** M1:F1

**Occurrence:** Four families have been documented, including an inbred Columbian kindred.

**Risk of Recurrence for Patient's Sib:**
See Part I, *Mendelian Inheritance.*

**Risk of Recurrence for Patient's Child:**
See Part I, *Mendelian Inheritance.* Reproduction does not appear to be possible given the profound mental retardation of the patients.

**Age of Detectability:** At birth or in early childhood.

**Gene Mapping and Linkage:** Unknown.

**Prevention:** None known. Genetic counseling indicated.

**Treatment:** Patients benefit from the types of therapy usually used for profound mental retardation and psychomotor developmental delay.

**Prognosis:** For those affected, the prognosis is the same as for profoundly mentally retarded individuals. Most do not survive into their teen-age years.

**Detection of Carrier:** Unknown.

**References:**
Elejalde BR, et al.: Neuro-ectodermal melanolysosomal disease: an autosomal recessive pigment mutation in man. Am J Hum Genet 1977; 29:39A only.
Elejalde BR, et al.: Mutations affecting pigmentation in man: neuro-ectodermal melanolysosomal disease. Am J Hum Genet 1979; 3:65–80.

EL002
EL014

**B. Rafael Elejalde**
**Maria Mercedes de Elejalde**

**Neuroectodermal pigmented tumor**
*See JAW, NEUROECTODERMAL PIGMENTED TUMOR*

---

**NEUROECTODERMAL SYNDROME, FLYNN-AIRD TYPE  2173**

**Includes:** Flynn-Aird syndrome

**Excludes:**
**Cockayne syndrome** (0189)
**Myotonic dystrophy** (0702)
**Phytanic acid storage disease** (0810)
**Werner syndrome** (0998)

**Major Diagnostic Criteria:** The combination of deafness, neurologic involvement, and skin and bone defects should suggest the diagnosis.

**Clinical Findings:** This syndrome has only been described in one family, in which 15 members were affected. Sensorineural deafness was usually the first manifestation of the disorder, which developed in the latter part of the first or the second decade. Other early findings included myopia; ataxia; severe, peripheral neuritic pain; and joint stiffness.

Although severe myopia was the most common ocular finding,

cataracts and retinitis pigmentosa also occurred. Epilepsy consisting of episodes of aphasia, blurring of vision, and facial and limb numbness and parasthesia occurred in one third of affected individuals. Although intelligence was unimpaired, change of affect occurred. Another neurologic manifestation was peripheral neuritis, which usually preceded muscular wasting, ataxia, neuritic pain, and joint stiffness. These findings occurred in half of the affected individuals. Skin atrophy and dental caries are other common manifestations. A few individuals developed diabetes (2/15), goiter (4/15), or defective steroid production (2/15).

Most routine laboratory studies have been normal, although in a few cases, elevated cerebrospinal fluid was found following a spinal tap. X-rays have demonstrated increased bone density and cystic areas, particularly of the pelvis. Kyphosis has also been noted in a few individuals. Skin biopsies showed atrophic changes, including generalized hyalinization, sparseness of hair follicles, and marked hyperkeratosis. Autopsies on five individuals were available and demonstrated cardiac and brain involvement in four, adrenal enlargement or cortical atrophy in three, and enlarged thyroid and/or basophilic hyperplasia of the pituitary in two.

**Complications:** Blindness, osteoporosis, debility, skin ulcers, and kyphoscoliosis have been reported.

**Associated Findings:** None known.

**Etiology:** Autosomal dominant inheritance with apparently complete penetrance, but variable expressivity.

**Pathogenesis:** An enzymatic defect has been suggested, but not identified.

**MIM No.:** *13630

**POS No.:** 3437

**Sex Ratio:** M1:F1

**Occurrence:** Described in 15 members of one family in North America.

**Risk of Recurrence for Patient's Sib:**
See Part I, *Mendelian Inheritance.*

**Risk of Recurrence for Patient's Child:**
See Part I, *Mendelian Inheritance.*

**Age of Detectability:** By the second decade of life.

**Gene Mapping and Linkage:** Unknown.

**Prevention:** None known. Genetic counseling indicated.

**Treatment:** Supportive.

**Prognosis:** Life span and intelligence appear unimpaired, although many affected individuals become disabled.

**Detection of Carrier:** Unknown.

**References:**
Flynn A, Aird RB: A neuroectodermal syndrome of dominant inheritance. J Neurol Sci 1965; 2:161–182. * †

T0007

**Helga V. Toriello**

**Neuroectodermal syndrome, Johnson type**
*See ALOPECIA-ANOSMIA-DEAFNESS-HYPOGONADISM, JOHNSON TYPE*
**Neuroenteric cysts**
*See INTESTINAL DUPLICATION*
**Neuroepithelioma**
*See CANCER, EWING SARCOMA*
**Neuroepithelioma adenoids**
*See SCALP, CYLINDROMAS*

# NEUROFIBROMATOSIS 0712

**Includes:**
Intestinal neurofibromatosis
Mixed central and peripheral neurofibromas
Neurofibromatosis-pheochromocytoma-duodenal carcinoid
 syndrome
NF-1
von Recklinghausen disease

**Excludes:**
**Acoustic neuromata** (0012)
Phakomatoses (other)
**Pulmonic stenosis-café-au-lait spots, Watson type** (2776)
**Tuberous sclerosis** (0975)

**Major Diagnostic Criteria:** Inclusive criteria include two or more of the following: > 5 café-au-lait spots (standarized criteria vary), with or without intertriginous freckling; multiple discrete neurofibromas or at least one plexiform neurofibroma; iris Lisch nodules; optic pathway glioma; a distinctive bone lesion, such as sphenoid wing dysplasia or tibial pseudarthrosis; a definitely affected first degree relative.

**Clinical Findings:** Café-au-lait spots and/or axillary freckling may be present at birth. Café-au-lait spots tend to increase in number and size as the child gets older. The diagnosis must be considered if multiple café-au-lait spots are found at any age. The patient's skin color tends to be darker than that of unaffected family members, and freckling becomes more widespread, preferentially involving skin-fold areas. Cutaneous and subcutaneous neurofibromas most usually develop in the second decade, often associated with puberty. They are found on all body segments, but tend

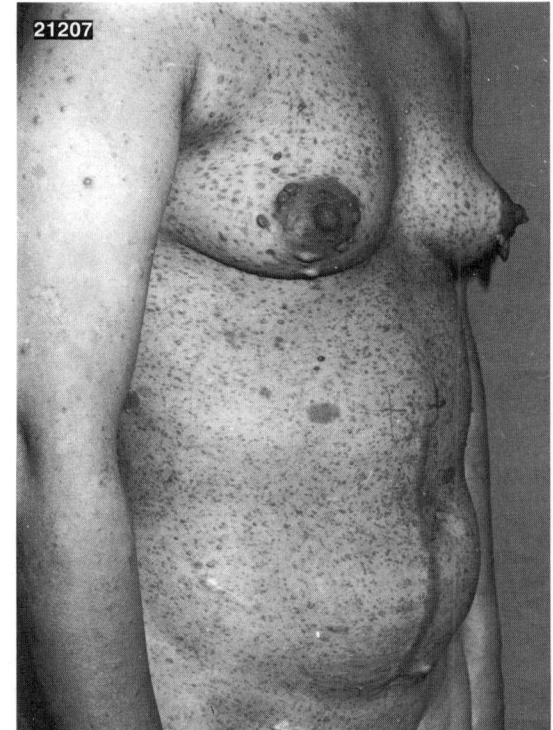

**0712B-21207:** Multiple neurofibromas and café au lait spots.

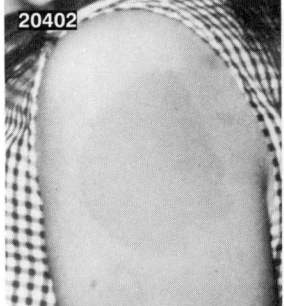
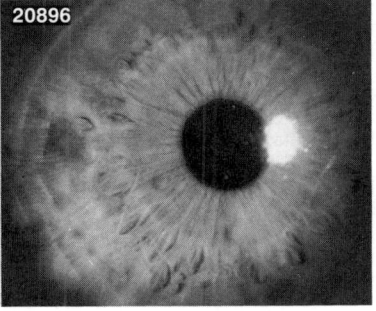

**0712A-20401–20779:** Cutaneous neurofibromas. 20402: Café au lait spot. 20896: Lisch nodules.

to be most numerous on the trunk. Cutaneous neurofibromas may be sessile or pedunculated, and they increase in size with age. Congenital plexiform neurofibromas, with or without overlying hyperpigmentation, may also occur anywhere on the body, and progressive growth is typical, sometimes leading to segmental hypertrophy. Pruritus not infrequently is associated with growing neurofibromas. Paraspinal, mediastinal, and retroperitoneal neurofibromas may cause serious problems. Malignant degeneration to a neurofibrosaracoma probably occurs with a frequency of about 6%, but is very rare before the end of the first decade. Iris Lisch nodules are present in at least 90% of patients over the age of six years, and they increase in number with age; they cause no clinical impairment, but they are very useful for diagnostic purposes. Optic pathway gliomas may occur in upwards of 15% of patients. Astrocytomas may be seen in other intracranial sites as well. Acoustic neuromas do not occur in this disorder. Congenital glaucoma may occur in as many as 1% of patients. A variety of skeletal dysplasias may be seen, including sphenoid wing dysplasia, vertebral dysplasia, and pseudarthrosis, which usually involves the tibia and/or fibula on one side. Scoliosis, with or without cervical-thoracic kyphosis, occurs in at least 5% to 10% of patients. Short stature and macrocephaly are very common. There is a modest excess of seizures of all types, and an even larger number of patients have an asymptomatically abnormal EEG. Hydrocephalus or asymptomatic cerebral ventricular dilation may occur in several percent of patients. Mental retardation may be slightly increased in frequency, but at least 40% of patients have learning disabilities, often associated with speech defects and nonspecific incoordination. Blood vessel involvement, primarily a vascular dysplasia, is seen in all major and medium-sized arteries, particularly those of the brain, the gastrointestinal tract, and the kidneys. The latter may lead to renovascular hypertension. Hypertension may also result from a pheochromocytoma. Biopsies of café-au-lait spots or of tumors merely confirm the nature of the lesion: they do not establish the diagnosis.

Several variations of neurofibromatosis have been described

(Riccardi & Eichner, 1986). The classic von Recklinghausen type, described above, has been designated type 1 (*NF-1*). **Acoustic neuromata**, or familial acoustic neuromas, have been designated type 2 (NF-2). A *mixed central and peripheral neurofibromas* has been designated type 3 (NF-3).

In NF-2, bilateral acoustic neuromas, posterior fossa and upper cervical meningiomas, and spinal/paraspinal neurofibromas are characteristic features. Iris Lisch nodules, which occur in close to two-thirds of NF-1 cases, do not occur in NF-2, and optic gliomas have not been reported. CNS tumors appear in the second or third decade and advance rapidly, resulting, unlike NF-1, in a shortened lifespan.

A variant or atypical form has been designated type 4 (NF-4). This is a heterogeneous group, and is distinguished chiefly on the basis of prognosis. Once again, the iris Lisch nodules, characteristic of NF-1, are usually absent.

Familial *intestinal neurofibromatosis* may share the features of NF-1, or may consist simply of multiple intestinal neurofibromatosis without the cutaneous features of NF-1. This rare variation has occurred in sporadic cases or, as with all neurofibromatosis, in an inherited dominant pattern.

A few cases (less than 10) of a *neurofibromatosis-pheochromocytoma-duodenal carcinoid syndrome* have also been reported, as well as a similar number of cases with a neurofibromatosis-Noonan phenotype (See **Noonan syndrome**). Unless otherwise qualified, however, the term neurofibromatosis refers to the classic von Recklinghausen NF-1.

**Complications:** Blindness may result from optic pathway gliomas. Spinal cord compression may result from paraspinal neurofibromas, vertebral dysplasia and/or severe kyphoscoliosis. Vascular compromise may lead to cerebral or cerebellar infarcts, abdominal angina, or renovascular hypertension. Gastrointestinal neurofibromas may lead to gastrointestinal hemorrhage. A pheochromocytoma may lead to hypertension and death. Death may also result from a neurofibrosarcoma. Pseudarthroses may require amputation proximal to the lesion. Cosmetic disfigurement from facial neurofibromas is common.

**Associated Findings:** Hyperganglionosis of the large bowel, mimicking **Colon, aganglionosis**. Premature or delayed puberty. **Glaucoma, congenital.** A major psychosocial burden is often seen among patients with NF-1.

**Etiology:** Autosomal dominant inheritance.

**Pathogenesis:** Unknown.

**MIM No.:** *16220, *16222, 16224, 16226, 16227.

**POS No.:** 3332

**CDC No.:** 237.700

**Sex Ratio:** M1:F1

**Occurrence:** Prevalence about 1:3000. No ethnic differences are noted. There are an estimated 80,000 affected individuals in the United States alone.

**Risk of Recurrence for Patient's Sib:**
See Part I, *Mendelian Inheritance.*

**Risk of Recurrence for Patient's Child:**
See Part I, *Mendelian Inheritance.*

**Age of Detectability:** Often at birth, almost always by the end of the first year, and always by five years of age.

**Gene Mapping and Linkage:** NF1 (neurofibromatosis 1 (von Recklinghausen disease, Watson disease)) has been mapped to 17q11.2.

**Prevention:** None known. Genetic counseling indicated.

**Treatment:** For enlarging or otherwise problematic neurofibromas, surgery is standard treatment; likewise for neurofibrosarcomas, although adjuvant chemotherapy and/or radiation therapy may be used. For optic pathway gliomas, close observation or radiation therapy are standard, though chemotherapy occasionally may have a place. Reparative surgery may be attempted for pseudarthrosis, though amputation is often required. Placement of a Harrington rod or alternative internal fixation procedures are standard for severe or progressive kyphoscoliosis.

**Prognosis:** Seventy-five percent of patients probably develop at least a moderate level of severity by 30 years of age, but prognosis depends on the presence of the various complications and associated features.

**Detection of Carrier:** Unknown.

**Special Considerations:** The Neurofibromatosis Institute, Inc., 715 Bison Drive, Houston, Texas 77079, provides a variety of print and computer-based information services regarding neurofibromatosis (NFormation), including electronic mail, resource identification, over 2,000 NF-related references, annotated bibliographies, an NF-patient database, and an expert system. The Institute, in conjunction with Karger Publishing Co., also produces the journal, *Neurofibromatosis*. NFormation is available online at 713/558-9908.

**Support Groups:**
New York; The National Neurofibromatosis Foundation (NF) Marland (Washington, D.C. area); Neurofibromatosis, Inc.
AUSTRALIA: NSW; Riverwood; The Neurofibromatosis Association of Australia

**References:**
Schenkein I, et al.: Increased nerve-growth-stimulating activity in disseminated neurofibromatosis. New Engl J Med 1974; 292:1134–1136.
Bader JL, Miller RW: Neurofibromatosis and childhood leukemia. J Pediatr 1978; 92:925–929.
Kanter WR, et al.: Central neurofibromatosis with bilateral acoustic neuroma: genetic, clinical and biochemical distinctions from peripheral neurofibromatosis. Neurology 1980; 30:851–859.
Riccardi VM, Mulvihill JJ: Neurofibromatosis (von Recklinghausen's disease). In: Advances in neurology, vol. 29. New York: Raven Press, 1981.
Riccardi VM: Von Recklinghausen neurofibromatosis. New Engl J Med 1981; 305:1617–1626.
Riccardi VM, et al.: The pathophysiology of neurofibromatosis. Am J Med Genet 1984; 18:169–176.
Zehavi C, et al.: Iris (Lisch) nodules in neurofibromatosis. Clin Genet 1986; 29:51–55.
Riccardi VM, Eichner JE: Neurofibromatosis: phenotype, natural history and pathogenesis. Baltimore, Johns Hopkins University Press, 1986.
Rubenstein AE, et al.: Neurofibromatosis. Ann New York Acad Sci 1986; 486:1–414.
Fountain JW, et al.: Physical mapping of a translocation breakpoint in neurofibromatosis. Science 1989; 244:1085–1088.

RI000                                   **Vincent M. Riccardi**

**Neurofibromatosis 2**
*See ACOUSTIC NEUROMATA*
**Neurofibromatosis-Noonan syndrome**
*See NOONAN SYNDROME*
**Neurofibromatosis-pheochromocytoma-duodenal carcinoid syndrome**
*See NEUROFIBROMATOSIS*
**Neurofilaments (accumulation)-polyneuropathy**
*See NEUROPATHY, GIANT AXONAL*
**Neurogenic flaccid ptosis**
*See EYELID, PTOSIS, CONGENITAL*
**Neurological disease, Machado-Joseph type**
*See MACHADO-JOSEPH DISEASE*
**Neuromata, mucosal-endocrine tumors**
*See ENDOCRINE NEOPLASIA, MULTIPLE TYPE III*
**Neuromyotonia**
*See ISAACS-MERTENS SYNDROME*

## NEURONAL CEROID-LIPOFUSCINOSES (NCL)  0713

**Includes:**
Amaurotic familial idiocy
Batten disease
Batten-Mayou disease
Batten-Vogt syndrome
Cerebromacular degeneration, familial
Haltia-Santavuori disease (infantile NCL or INCL)
Jansky-Bielchowsky disease (late infantile NCL or LINCL)
Jansky-Bielchowsky-Hagberg disease (late infantile variant of NCL)
Kufs disease
Spielmeyer-Vogt disease (juvenile NCL or JNCL)
Spielmeyer-Sjogren disease (juvenile NCL)

**Excludes:**
**Alpers disease** (3261)
**Alzheimer disease, familial** (2354)
**Cerebro-hepato-renal syndrome** (0139)
**Dentatorubropallidoluuysian degeneration, hereditary** (3283)
**Hallervorden-Spatz disease** (2526)
**Huntington disease** (0478)
Juvenile metachromatic leukodystrophy
**Mucolipidosis I** (0671)
**Neuroaxonal dystrophy**
Neuronal sphingolipidoses
**Phytanic acid storage disease** (0810)
**Seizures, progressive myoclonic, Lafora type** (2601)
**Seizures, progressive myoclonic, Unverricht-Lundborg type** (2602)
Subacute sclerosing panencephalitis

**Major Diagnostic Criteria:** The neuronal ceroid-lipofuscinoses (NCL) are characterised by progressive motor and cognitive decline, seizures, visual loss due to pigmentary retinal degeneration and the storage of autofluorescent lipopigment in the central nervous system, other organs and skin. The four types are differentiated on the basis of age of onset, temporal relation of visual loss to neurologic deterioration, seizures and electron microscopy of the storage material. A subdivision into infantile (*Haltia-Santavuori*), late-infantile (*Jansky-Bielchowsky*), juvenile (*Spielmeyer-Vogt*), and adult (*Kufs*) is in use. There is overlap between the different types in some patients, especially between late infantile and juvenile symptomatology and pathology.

**Clinical Findings:** In the *infantile* form, microcephaly, seizures, ataxia, visual impairment with a retinal dystrophy and rapidly progressive developmental delay appear before age 18 months. Seizures common at the beginning disappear by the second year of life. The electroencephalogram (EEG), initially disorganized becomes flat by the end of the second year. The electroretinogram shows progressive decrease in amplitude then abolition. The visual evoked response (VER) is usually flat. CT scan or MRI reveals generalized atrophy and a skull X-ray will show a thickened calvarium. Intralysosomal granular osmiophilic deposits have been found in conjunctival, skin, muscle, or rectal biopsies and brain. They are absent from bone marrow.
In the *late infantile* form, ataxia, seizures (grand mal and myoclonic) and intellectual decline begin between ages 2–4 years and precede retinal degeneration. The EEG shows bursts of diffuse synchronous slow waves. The ERG becomes flat and there is increased amplitude of the VER. CT scan and MRI reveal cerebral and cerebellar atrophy. Intralysosomal curvilinear bodies and occasional fingerprint-like inclusions are seen in conjunctival, skin, muscle, rectal and bone marrow biopsies and brain.
In *juvenile NCL*, pigmentary retinopathy occurs between the ages of 4–10 years. Cognitive decline and seizures (predominantly myoclonic) follow. Some patients show extrapyramidal and cerebellar signs. CT scan or MRI shows thinning of the cortical mantle and MRI shows loss of white matter. Intralysosomal fingerprint-like inclusions associated with curvilinear bodies are seen in conjunctiva, skin, muscle, rectal or bone marrow biopsies and brain and buffy coat preparations.
The clinical findings in *Kufs* disease begin early in the third

decade of life and may take the form of cognitive decline and psychotic or motor disturbance. Extrapyramidal signs such as facial dyskinesias and rigidity can be associated. Rarely patients have seizures (myoclonic) and ocular symptoms are notably absent. Brain biopsy is the only definitive way to make the diagnosis and usually granular osmiophilic deposits are seen by electron microscopy.
Elevated urine sediment didohols are a nonspecific finding common to all types.

**Complications:** Intractable seizures and incapacitating myoclonus are severely debilitating and death occurs from intercurrent illness such as pneumonia.

**Associated Findings:** **Microcephaly** in the infantile and late infantile variant. Mixed seizure disorder in the late infantile and juvenile types. Behavior problems in the late infantile and juvenile types, and psychiatric disorders in the adult form.

**Etiology:** Autosomal recessive inheritance. Rare families with autosomal dominantly inherited Kufs disease are described.

**Pathogenesis:** Pathology suggests a lysosomal storage disease. Brains accumulate large amounts of dolichol oligosaccharides suggesting NCL could be due to faulty glycosylation of proteins. Cathepsin H, a protease, is claimed to be deficient in some late infantile cases.

**MIM No.:** *25673, 20450, *20420, *20430, *16235

**POS No.:** 3333

**Sex Ratio:** M1:F1

**Occurrence:** Three hundred and sixty children in the United States are registered with the Batten Disease Support and Research Association, most with the juvenile or late infantile form. The incidence of infantile NCL in Finland is 1:13000.

**Risk of Recurrence for Patient's Sib:**
See Part I, *Mendelian Inheritance.*

**Risk of Recurrence for Patient's Child:**
See Part I, *Mendelian Inheritance.*

**Age of Detectability:** Ages at which symptoms first occur are *infantile form*, within the first year of life; *late-infantile*, by three years of age; *juvenile*, between 7–12 years; *adult form*, in the late teens to early 30s. Prenatal diagnosis was accomplished in the sib of a patient with the late-infantile form by electron microscopic examination of amniotic fluid cells.

**Gene Mapping and Linkage:** BTS (Batten disease) has been provisionally mapped to 16.

**Prevention:** None known. Genetic counseling indicated.

**Treatment:** Undetermined for the underlying condition. General supportive care and anticonvulsants are the mainstay of therapy. Neuroleptics for behavior disturbances and anti-Parkinsonian drugs are used when indicated. Antioxidants such as vitamin E and C and selenium have been tried and have not been of great benefit to most patients.

**Prognosis:** Patients with INCL die in early childhood. Patients with LINCL die in the first decade of life or early teenage years. Patients with JNCL live into their twenties. In Kufs disease the course is slowly progressive and patients may survive into late middle age.

**Detection of Carrier:** Unknown.

**Special Considerations:** Metabolic disease with known enzymatic defects must be ruled out in infants and children. It is conjectural whether these diseases are separate entities or due to genetic defects that are different but occurring at the same gene locus (i.e. allelic variants). The late infantile and juvenile forms are more similar than the others, and intermediate forms are recognized (suggesting compound heterozygous status).

**Support Groups:**
San Francisco; The Children's Brain Diseases Foundation for Research
NY; Brooklyn; Myoclonus Families United
WA; Spanaway; Batten Disease Support and Research Association

**References:**
Zeman W, et al.: The neuronal ceroid lipofuscinoses. In: Handbook of clinical neurology, leukodystrophies and poliodystrophies, vol. 10 Amsterdam, North Holland, 1970:588–679. * †
Zeman W: Studies in the neuronal ceroid-lipofuscinoses. Presidential address. J Neuropathol Exp Neurol 1974; 33:1–12.
Boustany R-M, et al.: Clinical classification of neuronal ceroid-lipofuscinoses subtypes. Am J Med Genet 1988; 5(suppl):47–58.
Boustany R-M, et al.: The neuronal ceroid-lipofuscinoses: a review. Rev Neurol 1989; 142:105–110.

B0053
H0057
TR009

**Rose Mary N. Boustany**
**John H. Holtkamp**
**Elias I. Traboulsi**

**Neuronal degeneration of childhood-liver disease, progressive**
*See ALPERS DISEASE*
**Neuronal migration, defective**
*See HIRSCHPRUNG DISEASE-MICROCEPHALY-COLOBOMA*
**Neuronopathy, sensorimotor-agenesis of the corpus callosum**
*See CORPUS CALLOSUM AGENESIS-SENSORIMOTOR NEUROPATHY, FAMILIAL*
**Neuropathy with liability to pressure palsies, recurrent familial**
*See NEUROPATHY, HEREDITARY WITH PRESSURE PALSIES*

## NEUROPATHY, CONGENITAL MOTOR & SENSORY-SKELETAL-LARYNGEAL DEFECTS 3013

**Includes:**
    Charcot-Marie-Tooth disease with skeletal and laryngeal anomalies
    Laryngeal and skeletal anomalies-motor and sensory neuropathy
    Skeletal and laryngeal anomalies-motor and sensory neuropathy

**Excludes:**
    **Neuropathy, hereditary motor and sensory, type II** (2105)
    Charcot-Marie-Tooth disease, other

**Major Diagnostic Criteria:** Neuronal type of motor and sensory neuropathy with prenatal onset. At birth, laryngeal stridor or laryngomalacia, as well as dysmorphic features.

**Clinical Findings:** A single family with the father and two sons affected has been reported. The two sons presented flexion contractures at birth. All three had delayed motor development, walking after ages 2–4 years, with a widebased and clumsy gait and frequent falls. The course was slowly progressive, and the father's gait improved after surgical lengthening of the Achilles tendons. In adulthood, the picture was that of Charcot-Marie-Tooth disease with atrophy and weakness of peroneal, hand, and feet muscles, pes cavus, absent tendon reflexes, and distal sensory loss. Electromyography revealed a denervation pattern, and motor nerve conduction velocity was normal. Microscopic examination of sural nerves showed loss of predominantly large, myelinated nerve fibers, and demyelinization. One patient had laryngomalacia, and two presented laryngeal stridor in the first months of life.

All three patients showed the following dysmorphic features: high-arched palate, short neck, narrow shoulders, dorsal kyphosis, and protruding chest.

**Complications:** Unknown.

**Associated Findings:** None known.

**Etiology:** Presumably autosomal dominant inheritance.

**Pathogenesis:** Unknown. A widespread neurologic disorder affecting lower motor neuron axons could explain all findings.

**Sex Ratio:** Presumably M1:F1; M3:F0 observed.

**Occurrence:** One family with an affected father and two sons has been reported.

**Risk of Recurrence for Patient's Sib:**
    See Part I, *Mendelian Inheritance.*

**Risk of Recurrence for Patient's Child:**
    See Part I, *Mendelian Inheritance.*

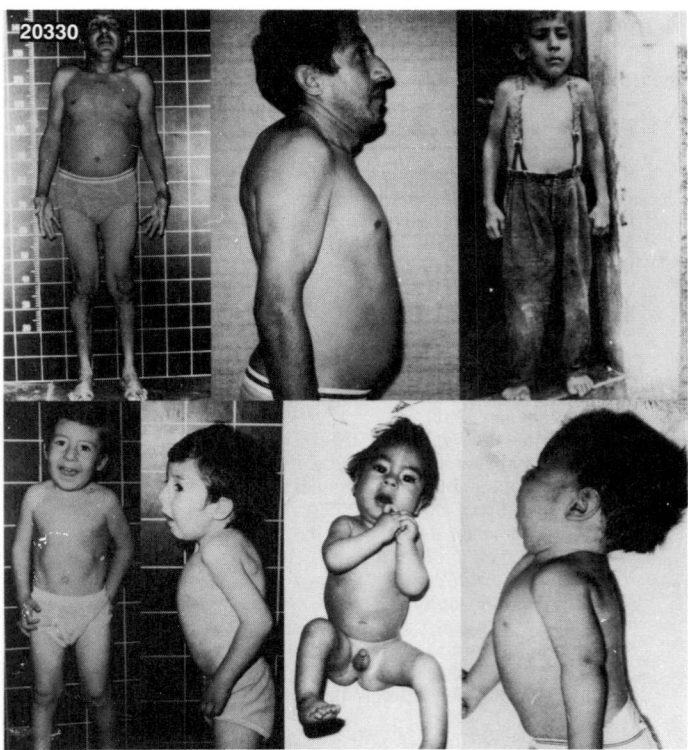

3013-20330: The reported family showing the dysmorphic features. Note the early development of claw hand and late appearance of peroneal atrophy.

**Age of Detectability:** At birth when flexion contractures are present; otherwise, during the first years of life.

**Gene Mapping and Linkage:** Unknown.

**Prevention:** None known. Genetic counseling indicated.

**Treatment:** Physical therapy reversed most flexion contractures. In one case **Foot, talipes equinovarus (TEV)** required surgery. Surgical lengthening of the Achilles tendon improved the gait in one patient.

**Prognosis:** Presumably normal life span. The gait disturbance may restrict life-style alternatives.

**Detection of Carrier:** Unknown.

**References:**
Ruíz C, et al.: A distinct motor and sensory neuropathy (neuronal type) with dysmorphic features in a father and two sons: a variant of Charcot-Marie-Tooth disease. Clin Genet 1987; 31:109–113.

RU019
CA011

**Carlos Ruíz**
**José María Cantú**

## NEUROPATHY, CONGENITAL SENSORY WITH ANHIDROSIS 2390

**Includes:**
    Analgesia, familial
    Dysautonomia, type II, familial
    Hereditary sensory and autonomic neuropathy IV (HSAN-IV)
    Neural crest, syndrome of
    Pain, insensitivity to, with anhidrosis of Swanson (congenital)

**Excludes:**
    Biemond congenital and familial analgesia

**Dysautonomia I, Riley-Day type** (0307)
**Lesch-Nyhan syndrome** (0588)
**Neuropathy, hereditary motor and sensory, type II** (2105)
Neuropathy, nonprogressive sensory radicular

**Major Diagnostic Criteria:**  Impaired perception of pain and temperature with normal tactile perception. Autonomic dysfunction manifested by neurogenic anhidrosis, recurrent unexplained fever, vasomotor instability, abnormal intradermal histamine test, self-mutilation, and mental retardation.

**Clinical Findings:**  Clinical findings manifest in the first year of life. Recurrent unexplained fever, blotching, and irritability are some of the earliest manifestations of this disorder. Other features diagnosable early are insensitivity to pain, which is generalized, truncal anhidrosis, and pupillary hypersensitivity to methacholine chloride. Self-mutilation of the tongue, lips, and extremities (fingers) starts as soon as the incisor teeth erupt. Fungiform papillae are present, in contrast to **Dysautonomia I, Riley-Day type** in which fungiform papillae are absent. The skin is parchment-like, especially on the extremities. There is lack of development of erythematous flare on the intradermal histamine test. Deep tendon reflexes are decreased, and the perception of temperature seems to be decreased. The perception of light touch is preserved, as is that of touch. Electroencephalogram and serum catecholamine levels are normal. Hypotonia is a constant feature of the disease. The patient usually functions cognitively in the moderately retarded range and has delayed motor development. Clinical variability is uncommon, and expression is complete.

**Complications:**  Severe lacerations of the tongue and lips, edentulation, scarred excoriations of the fingers, and corneal opacities can be seen due to self-mutilation behavior. Failure to thrive has been reported. Orthopedic complications usually include repeated episodes of osteomyelitis, fractures, and dislocated and neuropathic joints.

**Associated Findings:**  Hyperactive behavior.

**Etiology:**  Autosomal recessive inheritance.

**Pathogenesis:**  Neuropathologic findings show that the brain is normal except for the absence of small neurons in the dorsal ganglia, lack of small fibers in the dorsal roots, absence of the Lissauer tract, and reduction in size of the spinal tract of the trigeminal nerve and its paucity of small fibers. Peripheral (sural) nerve biopsy reveals an almost total absence of nonmyelinated axons and a marked decrease in myelinated axons. Fiber diameters showed an abnormal distribution and an absence of large diameter, and diminution of the number of small myelinated axons.

**MIM No.:**  *25680, 21030

**Sex Ratio:**  M1:F1

**Occurrence:**  About two dozen cases have been reported in the literature.

**Risk of Recurrence for Patient's Sib:**
See Part I, *Mendelian Inheritance.*

**Risk of Recurrence for Patient's Child:**
See Part I, *Mendelian Inheritance.*

**Age of Detectability:**  In early infancy.

**Gene Mapping and Linkage:**  Unknown.

**Prevention:**  None known. Genetic counseling indicated.

**Treatment:**  None available for the basic manifestations of the disorder. The infections and orthopedic and ophthalmic complications should be managed appropriately. Plastic surgery on the severely lacerated lower lip of one of the patients with this disorder has been attempted without success due to the continuing self-mutilating behavior.

**Prognosis:**  Guarded, due to the complications, especially the frequent bouts of osteomyelitis. There is not enough information concerning the natural history of this disorder to comment on the life span of the patients.

**Detection of Carrier:**  Unknown.

**Special Considerations:**  *Familial analgesia* has also been described by Biemond (1955) and Freytag and Lindenberg (1967).

**Support Groups:**  New York; The Dysautonomia Foundation, Inc.

**References:**
Biemond A: Investigations of the brain in a case of congenital and familial analgesia. Proc 11th Intern Cong Neuropath, London, September, 1955.
Swanson AG, et al.: Anatomic changes in congenital insensitivity to pain. Arch Neurol 1965; 12:11–18.
Swanson AG: Congenital insensitivity to pain with anhidrosis: a unique syndrome in two male siblings. Arch Neurol 1963; 8:299–306.
Pinsky L, DiGeorge AM: Congenital familial sensory neuropathy with anhidrosis. J Pediatr 1966; 68:1–13. †
Freytag E, Lindenberg R: Neuropathologic findings in patients of a hospital for the mentally deficient: a survey of 359 cases. Johns Hopkins Med J 1967; 121:379–392.
Scribanu N, Grover-Johnson N: Atypical nerve histology in a case of congenital sensory neuropathy with anydrosis. Neurology 1982; 32:A184.
Dyck PJ, et al.: Not "indifference to pain" but varieties of hereditary sensory and autonomic neuropathy. Brain 1983; 106:373–390.
Axelrod FB, Pearson J: Congenital sensory neuropathies. Am J Dis Child 1984; 138. *
Donaghy M, et al.: Hereditary sensory neuropathy with neurotrophic keratitis. Brain 1987; 110:563–583.

SC052                                                    **Nina Scribanu**

**Neuropathy, dominantly inherited hypertrophic**
*See NEUROPATHY, HEREDITARY MOTOR AND SENSORY, TYPE I*

---

## NEUROPATHY, GIANT AXONAL                              3140

**Includes:**
> Giant axonal neuropathy (GAN)
> Neurofilaments (accumulation)-polyneuropathy
> Polyneuropathy-accumulation of neurofilaments

**Excludes:**
> **Ataxia, Friedreich type** (2714)
> **Dejerine-Sottas disease** (2054)
> **Phytanic acid storage disease** (0810)

**Major Diagnostic Criteria:**  Distal symmetric progressive weakness and sensory loss, cerebellar syndrome, bilateral Babinski sign, kinky hair, normal mental activity, onset at ages 2–3 years. Sural nerve biopsy shows characteristic accumulation of neurofilaments.

**Clinical Findings:**  Onset of polyneuropathy in children at toddler age. Distal weakness and atrophy are accompanied by areflexia and impairment in perceiving touch, position sense, and vibration. Central nervous system involvement, including cerebellar ataxia and corticospinal tract signs with bilateral extensor plantar responses. Tightly curled hair is a common feature.

Light microscopic evaluation of sural nerve biopsy reveals abnormally large masses corresponding to axons that are segmentally enlarged to enormous proportions. Ultrastructurally, axons are distended by masses of tightly woven neurofilaments. Neurofilament masses often begin at a node of Ranvier, and paranodal retraction of myelin can be noticed. Axonal organelles, including mitochondria and vesicles of smooth endoplasmic reticulum, are displaced into a subaxolemmal disposition. The protein composition of neurofilaments that accumulate in this disorder is not appreciably altered.

**Complications:**  Severe distal weakness and cerebellar ataxia lead to wheelchair confinement after several years of progression.

**Associated Findings:**  Distal renal tubular acidosis manifested by metabolic acidosis was reported in one case. Other atypical associations include bilateral vocal cord paralysis due to involvement of laryngeal nerves, skeletal abnormalities (thoracic kyphoscoliosis, **Pectus carinatum**, coxa valga, pes planovalgus), and **Ichthyosis**.

**Etiology:** Usually autosomal recessive inheritance, although an autosomal dominant form with onset during infancy or childhood, and a congenital form, have also been reported. Parental consanguinity and affected sibs have been reported in several families.

**Pathogenesis:** One hypothesis assumes a metabolic block of neurofilament transport along axons. A second hypothesis, based on experimental GAN in rats treated with 2,5-hexanedione, claims an acceleration of neurofilament transport (Monaco et al, 1985). Griffin & Watson (1988) also report fast axonal transport through giant axonal swellings in experimental hexacarbon neuropathy.

**MIM No.:** *25685

**Sex Ratio:** M1:F1

**Occurrence:** Approximately 20 cases have been reported worldwide.

**Risk of Recurrence for Patient's Sib:**
See Part I, *Mendelian Inheritance.*

**Risk of Recurrence for Patient's Child:**
See Part I, *Mendelian Inheritance.*

**Age of Detectability:** Age two to seven years. One congenital case has also been reported.

**Gene Mapping and Linkage:** Unknown.

**Prevention:** None known. Genetic counseling indicated.

**Treatment:** Unknown.

**Prognosis:** Guarded. The disease has a slow progression, over at least ten years in most cases.

**Detection of Carrier:** Unknown.

**References:**

Dooley JM, et al.: Clinical progression of giant-axonal neuropathy over a twelve year period. Can J Neurol Sci 1981; 8:321–323.

Duncan ID, et al.: Inherited canine giant axonal neuropathy. Muscle Nerve 1981; 4:223–227.

Ionasescu V, et al.: Giant axonal neuropathy: normal protein composition of neurofilaments. J Neurol Neurosurg Psychiatry 1983; 46:551–554. *

Ionasescu V, Zellweger H: Genetics in neurology. New York: Raven, 1983:386–389. †

Kinney RB, et al.: Congenital giant axonal neuropathy. Arch Pathol Lab Med 1985; 109:636–641. *

Monaco S, et al.: Giant axonal neuropathy: acceleration of neurofilament transport in optic axons. Proc Natl Acad Sci USA 1985; 82:920–924.

Griffin JW, Watson DF: Axonal transport in neurological disease. Ann Neurol 1988; 23:3–13.

I0000                                                          **Victor V. Ionasescu**

---

## NEUROPATHY, HEREDITARY MOTOR AND SENSORY, TYPE I                                                                    2104

**Includes:**
Charcot-Marie-Tooth disease, hypertrophic (some cases)
Charcot-Marie-Tooth disease, slow nerve conduction type
Charcot-Marie-Tooth peroneal muscular atrophy
Foot, claw-absent tendon jerks
Friedreich disease, abortive type
Motor and sensory neuropathy, type I
Motor and sensory neuropathy, X-linked
Neuropathy, dominantly inherited hypertrophic
Peroneal muscular atrophy, axonal type
Peroneal muscular atrophy, hypertrophic
Roussy-Levy syndrome

**Excludes:**
**Abetalipoproteinemia** (0002)
**Ataxia, Friedreich type** (2714)
Charcot-Marie-Tooth disease, sporadic
**Dejerine-Sottas disease** (2054)
**Muscular dystrophy, distal** (0690)
**Neuropathy, hereditary motor and sensory, type II** (2105)

**Phytanic acid storage disease** (0810)
**Spinal muscular atrophy** (0895)

**Major Diagnostic Criteria:** Peroneal muscle weakness and wasting, pes cavus, significantly decreased median nerve conduction velocity and a family history of one or more of these signs.

**Clinical Findings:** Foot deformities (pes cavus) and scoliosis appear in early childhood. Difficulties in walking and running become prominent in the second decade, while the small muscles of the hand atrophy. As the weakness and atrophy of those small muscles progress, a claw-like hand results. Atrophy of the leg and lower third of the thigh leads to the typical stork leg or inverted champagne bottle appearance.

One fourth of affected persons have palpably enlarged ulnar, radial, peroneal, or posterior auricular nerves. Sensory disturbances are not as severe as the motor deficit. Nerve conduction velocity is strikingly diminished early in life. Sensory nerve action potentials are of long latency if they are elicitable at all.

**Complications:** The disease is slowly progressive, with moderate ambulation disability and disordered fine motor skills.

**Associated Findings:** Autonomic changes of decreased sweating in the legs, decreased tear production, and orthostatic hypotension may occur. In some patients an apparent ataxia of lower limbs and tremulousness of the upper extremities is present.

**Etiology:** Autosomal dominant, autosomal recessive, and X-linked recessive inheritance have all been reported in various kindreds. Sporadic cases have also been reported. There is extreme variability of expression. Dyck (1984) maintains that kinships suggestive of autosomal recessive inheritance probably represent the partial expression of a dominant trait. In support of dominant inheritance, intensive evaluation by a neurologist, including assessment of nerve conduction, has demonstrated abnormalities consistent with type I neuropathy in the parents of some sporadic cases, as well as those thought to be autosomal recessive.

**Pathogenesis:** The process is essentially one of selective and restricted motor, and to a lesser extent, sensory nerve segmental demyelination. Onion bulb formation and areas of demyelination are prominent in sural nerve biopsies. A biochemical basis for this disorder is unknown.

**MIM No.:** *11820, *11822, *18080, *21440, *30280

**Sex Ratio:** M1:F1

**Occurrence:** Prevalence in western Norway is 36:100,000 for the autosomal dominant form, 1.4:100,000 for the autsomal recessive form, and 3.6:100,000 for the X-linked recessive form. In Newcastle-upon-Tyne, England, 4.7:100,000 for the autosomal dominant form.

**Risk of Recurrence for Patient's Sib:**
See Part I, *Mendelian Inheritance.*

**Risk of Recurrence for Patient's Child:**
See Part I, *Mendelian Inheritance.*

**Age of Detectability:** In a recognized family, it is common to have children diagnosed in the first decade of life. Index cases, however, usually come to medical attention in the second decade.

**Gene Mapping and Linkage:** CMT1 (Charcot-Marie-Tooth neuropathy 1) has been mapped to 1q.
CMT2 (Charcot-Marie-Tooth neuropathy 2) has been mapped to 17p13.1-q12.
CMTX (Charcot-Marie-Tooth neuropathy, X-linked) has been mapped to Xq11-q13.

**Prevention:** None known. Genetic counseling indicated.

**Treatment:** Supportive for the selected weaknesses and sensory deficits.

**Prognosis:** Variable. Life span is probably not reduced.

**Detection of Carrier:** The variability of expression in this dominant disorder is extreme. However, mildly affected parents and siblings may show unappreciated skeletal deformities (hammer toes, pes cavus, scoliosis). Median nerve conduction velocities in apparently unaffected parents and other relatives is a reasonably accurate test of the sub-clinical state. In such instances, median nerve conduction velocity will be less than 40 m/sec.

**Special Considerations:** Although the condition is generally recognized by the second decade of life, a number of children have become clinically affected in infancy. The additional signs of gait ataxia and upper extremity tremor, originally described as a separate entity (the *Roussy-Levy syndrome*, also known as *familial claw-foot with absent tendon jerks* and *abortive type Friedreich disease*), may occur in otherwise typical families.

**Support Groups:**
Philadelphia; National Foundation for Peroneal Muscular Atrophy
CANADA: Ontario; St. Catharines; Charcot-Marie-Tooth (CMT) International

**References:**
Buchthal F, Behse F: Peroneal muscular atrophy (PMA) and related disorders. Brain 1977; 100:41–66.
Davis CJF, et al.: The peroneal muscular atrophy syndrome: clinical, genetic and electrophysiologic findings and classification. J Genet Hum 1978; 26:311–349.
Harding AE, Thomas PK: The clinical features of hereditary motor and sensory neuropathy types I and II. Brain 1980; 103:259–280. *
Dyck PJ, et al., eds: Peripheral neuropathy, 2nd ed. Philadelphia: W.B. Saunders, 1984. * †
Hogan-Dann, CM, et al.: Polyneuropathy following vincristine therapy in two patients with Charcot-Marie-Tooth syndrome. J Am Med Asso 1984; 252:2862–2863.
Rozear MP, et al.: Hereditary motor sensory neuropathy, X-linked: a half century follow-up. Neurology 1987; 37:1460–1465. †
Vance JM, et al.: Linkage of Charcot-Marie-Tooth neuropathy type 1a to chromosome 17. Exp Neurol 1989; 104:186–189.

CR011      **Carl J. Crosley**

## NEUROPATHY, HEREDITARY MOTOR AND SENSORY, TYPE II    2105

**Includes:**
Axonal type Charcot-Marie-Tooth disease
Charcot-Marie-Tooth disease, neuronal (some cases)
Motor and sensory neuropathy, hereditary type II
Peroneal muscular atrophy, neuronal

**Excludes:**
Abetalipoproteinemia (0002)
Ataxia, Friedreich type (2714)
Dejerine-Sottas disease (2054)
Muscular dystrophy, distal (0690)
Neuropathy, hereditary motor and sensory, type I (2104)
Phytanic acid storage disease (0810)
Spinal muscular atrophy (0895)

**Major Diagnostic Criteria:** Peroneal muscular atrophy, pes cavus, evidence of denervation on electromyography, and mildly decreased median nerve conduction velocity with a family history of one or all of these signs.

**Clinical Findings:** The onset of weakness is later in this disorder than in **Neuropathy, hereditary motor and sensory, type I** (NHMS I). The peak onset is in the second and third decade with some individuals affected as late as the sixth or seventh decade. Distal weakness of the upper limbs occurs in only 50% of affected persons. Lower limb weakness, on the other hand, tends to be as severe, if not more so, than in NHMS I. Tendon reflexes are only moderately depressed. Muscle atrophy and the characteristic lower extremity deformities (stork leg, pes cavus) remain prominent. Sensory loss (vibration and position sense) is mild. Nerve conduction velocity is abnormal but significantly faster than in NHMS I. The median nerve conduction velocity is greater than 40 m/sec. Nerves are not hypertrophic.

**Complications:** This disease is very slowly progressive. The onset occasionally may be as late as the sixth or seventh decade. Disability is largely the consequence of leg weakness.

**Associated Findings:** Tremor of the upper extremities and gait ataxia may be present, but are uncommon findings.

**Etiology:** Autosomal dominant inheritance.

**Pathogenesis:** The biopsies of sural nerves reveal loss of large fibers with only occasional segments of demyelination and onion bulb formation. The biochemical basis of this disorder is unknown.

**MIM No.:** *11821

**Sex Ratio:** Presumably M1:F1.

**Occurrence:** Approximately 25% of all peroneal muscular atrophy is thought to be of the type II variety, implying a prevalence of 1–10:100,000.

**Risk of Recurrence for Patient's Sib:**
See Part I, *Mendelian Inheritance.*

**Risk of Recurrence for Patient's Child:**
See Part I, *Mendelian Inheritance.*

**Age of Detectability:** In the first decade of life in 20% of the cases.

**Gene Mapping and Linkage:** Unknown.

**Prevention:** None known. Genetic counseling indicated.

**Treatment:** Largely supportive for complications resulting from progressive leg weakness.

**Prognosis:** Variable but generally good.

**Detection of Carrier:** Since nerve conduction velocities may be only mildly depressed, the appreciation of subtle deformities or weakness is essential in recognizing an affected individual.

**Support Groups:**
Philadelphia; National Foundation for Peroneal Muscular Atrophy
CANADA: Ontario; St. Catharines; Charcot-Marie-Tooth (CMT) International

**References:**
Buchthal F, Behse F: Peroneal muscular atrophy (PMA) and related disorders. Brain 1977; 100:41–66.
Davis CJF, et al.: The peroneal muscular atrophy syndrome. J Genet Hum 1978; 26:311–349.
Harding AE, Thomas PK: The clinical features of hereditary motor and sensory neuropathy types I and II. Brain 1980; 103:259–280. *
Dyck PJ, et al., eds: Peripheral neuropathy, 2nd ed. Philadelphia: W.B. Saunders, 1984.
Berciano J, et al.: Hereditary motor and sensory neuropathy type II: clinicopathological study of a family. Brain 1986; 109:897–914.

CR011      **Carl J. Crosley**

## NEUROPATHY, HEREDITARY RECURRENT BRACHIAL    2071

**Includes:**
Brachial neuritis, recurrent familial
Brachial neuropathy, familial
Brachial plexopathy, hereditary
Brachial plexus neuropathy, heredo-familial
Neuralgic amyotrophy, familial
Neuralgic amyotrophy-brachial predilection, familial
Neuritis with brachial predilection, heredo-familial

**Excludes:**
Neuropathy, hereditary with pressure palsies (2108)
Sporadic brachial neuropathies

**Major Diagnostic Criteria:** Familial recurrent attacks of weakness of the shoulder girdle muscles occur unilaterally or asymmetrically in both arms. Symptoms are frequently preceded by pain and followed by amyotrophy. Early childhood onset and tomaculous (ie, focal thickening of myelin) neuropathy on biopsy are also very characteristic of the condition.

**Clinical Findings:** Attacks of pain in one arm lasting several days or weeks, followed by the relatively rapid onset of weakness and atrophy of some of the proximal muscles of that arm. The pain often subsides with the onset of the weakness, and in some cases may not occur at all. There may be some sensory loss. The opposite arm may also be asymmetrically involved.

The distribution of the weakness corresponds to that of a nerve, nerve root or plexus, usually proximal. Other peripheral nerve trunks, cranial or autonomic nerves may be involved.

Functional recovery occurs within months, although long-standing residual weakness and atrophy may ensue. The intervals between recurrences may vary from months to years. There is a tendency for attacks to start in early childhood.

Precipitant factors are infections, pregnancy, parturition and, perhaps, strenuous exhertion. Other relapses occur without obvious cause.

Congenital dysmorphology has been described: hypotelorism, small stature, epicanthic folds, facial asymmetry, syndactyly of second-third toes, cleft palate.

Nerve conduction study / electromyogram (NCS/EMG) shows a somewhat patchy sensorimotor polyneuropathy of axonal type, more severe in arm nerves. In some occasions the findings are minor. Sural or radial nerve biopsy shows segmental demyelination-remyelination, with sausage-shaped focal thickenings of myelin (tomaculous neuropathy). These findings are not pathognomonic, and may be absent.

**Complications:** Permanent arm weakness after one or several attacks may ensue.

**Associated Findings:** Facial paresis was reported in one case.

**Etiology:** Autosomal dominant inheritance with variable penetrance.

**Pathogenesis:** Unknown.

**MIM No.:** *16210

**Sex Ratio:** M1:F1

**Occurrence:** Less than two dozen families have been reported.

**Risk of Recurrence for Patient's Sib:**
See Part I, *Mendelian Inheritance.*

**Risk of Recurrence for Patient's Child:**
See Part I, *Mendelian Inheritance.*

**Age of Detectability:** The first attack usually occurs in early childhood.

**Gene Mapping and Linkage:** Unknown.

**Prevention:** None known. Genetic counseling indicated.

**Treatment:** Prevention of precipitant factors. During the attack: rest, analgesics and physiotherapy. The usefulness of corticosteroids is still controversial. If paralysis develops, physiotherapy.

**Prognosis:** Unknown.

**Detection of Carrier:** Unknown.

**Special Considerations:** The sporadic form of the disease is far more frequent than the familial form. In the sporadic form there is a male predominance, the first attack is not during childhood, there is less tendency to relapses and there are no congenital stigmata. Tomaculae have not been described in the nerve biopsy of sporadic cases. Tomaculous neuropathy and electrically detected generalized neuropathy point to related pathological mechanisms for the familial recurrent brachial neuropathy and **Neuropathy, hereditary with pressure palsies**.

**References:**
Geiger LR, et al.: Familial neuralgic amytrophy. report of three families with review of the literature. Brain 1974; 97:87–102.
Madrid R, Bradley WG: The pathology of neuropathies with focal thickening of the myelin sheath (tomaculous neuropathy). J Neurol Sci 1975; 25:415–448.
Dunn HG, et al.: Heredofamilial brachial plexus neuropathy (hereditary neuralgic amytrophy with brachial predilection) in childhood. Dev Med Child Neurol 1978; 20:28–46.
Airaksinen EM, et al.: Hereditary recurrent brachial plexus neuropathy with dysmorphic features. Acta Neurol Scand 1985; 71:309–316.
Phillips, LH, II: Familial long thoracic nerve palsy: a manifestation of brachial plexus neuropathy. Neurology 1986; 36:1251–1253.

M0016

**Jesus S. Mora**
*Walter G. Bradley*

---

## NEUROPATHY, HEREDITARY WITH PRESSURE PALSIES 2108

**Includes:**
> Compression syndrome of peripheral nerves, hereditary
> Mononeuritis, Familial recurrent
> Nerve trunk palsies, familial
> Neuropathy with liability to pressure palsies, recurrent familial
> Polyneuropathy, familial recurrent
> Pressure palsies (hereditary) and neuropathy
> Tomaculous neuropathy

**Excludes:**
> Neuralgic amyotrophy with brachial plexus predilection
> **Neuropathy, hereditary recurrent brachial** (2071)

**Major Diagnostic Criteria:** Familial recurrent mononeuropathy or multiple neuropathy, with symptoms triggered by compression or stretching of the nerves, and tomaculous neuropathy in the nerve morphology.

**Clinical Findings:** Mononeuropathy or multiple neuropathy, with wide variation in symptoms, ranging from paresthesiae, numbness or absent DTR's, to paralysis and objective sensory disturbances. These are triggered by compression or stretching of the nerve trunks, even slightly.

Most frequently affected are peroneal, ulnar, radial and median nerves. Musculocutaneous, axillary, long thoracic, suprascapular, femoral, sciatic, facial or trigeminal nerves are less frequently affected.

Triggering factors include using scissors, knitting, leaning on elbows, squatting, kneeling or crossing legs, wearing tight shoes, etc.

There is recovery within days, weeks or months. Recurrence in the same or in other areas may occur, sometimes leaving permanent damage.

Nerve conduction study/electromyogram (NCS/EMG) shows signs of entrapment neuropathies and peripheral neuropathy. Muscle biopsy shows neurogenic amyotrophy. Teased-nerve studies show sausage-like swellings of the myelin sheaths and extensive demyelination-remyelination, even in non-symptomatic nerves ("tomaculous neuropathy"). These findings are not pathognomonic.

**Complications:** Permanent nerve trunk damage after one or several recurrences.

**Associated Findings:** None known.

**Etiology:** Autosomal dominant inheritance with variable expression.

**Pathogenesis:** Probable biochemical defect related to the process of myelination. The defect produces lability of the myelin sheath of the peripheral nerves to pressure or stretch. There is aberration of the myelin sheath formation with redundant loops and abnormal irregular thickenings. The remyelination after demyelination is also abnormal.

**MIM No.:** *16250

**Sex Ratio:** M1:F1

**Occurrence:** About 40 families have been described in the literature.

**Risk of Recurrence for Patient's Sib:**
See Part I, *Mendelian Inheritance.*

**Risk of Recurrence for Patient's Child:**
See Part I, *Mendelian Inheritance.*

**Age of Detectability:** Onset varies from four to 67 years of age, but occurs mostly between age 20 and 45.

**Gene Mapping and Linkage:** Unknown.

**Prevention:** None known. Genetic counseling indicated.

**Treatment:** Prevention of the triggering factors; physical therapy if paralysis develops.

**Prognosis:** Most of the episodes are followed by a good recovery. Some, however, may leave a more permanent deficit.

**Detection of Carrier:** Unknown.

**Special Considerations:** The microscopic abnormalities (tomaculae) and the electrophysiologically detected generalized neuropathy are also features of **Neuropathy, hereditary recurrent brachial**. In this condition pain is a frequent feature, and compression is not a specific triggering factor.

**References:**

De Jong JGY: Over families met hereditaire disposities tot het optreden van neuriteden, gecorreleerd met migraine. Psychiatr Neurol Med Psychol Beih 1947; 50:60–77.

Behse F, et al.: Hereditary neuropathy with liability to pressure palsies: electrophysiological and histopathological aspects. Brain 1972; 95:777–794.

Madrid R, Bradley WG: The pathology of neuropathies with focal thickening of the myelin sheath (tomaculous neuropathy): studies on the formation of the abnormal myelin sheath. J Neurol Sci 1975; 25:415–448.

Debruyne J, et al.: Hereditary pressure-sensitive neuropathy. J Neurol Sci 1980; 47:385–394.

Sellman MS, Mayer RF: Conduction block in hereditary neuropathy with susceptibility to pressure palsies. Muscle Nerve 1987; 10:621–625.

M0016 **Jesus S. Mora**
*Walter G. Bradley*

## NEUROPATHY, HERITABLE ISONIAZIDE TYPE (INH) 2044

**Includes:**

    Acetylator phenotype, slow
    INH (antituberculosis agent) inactivation
    Isoniazid inactivation
    Isoniazid neuropathy
    N-acetyltransferase polymorphism
    Neuritis, peripheral with isoniazid
    Pyridoxine deficiency induced by isonizid therapy
    Tuberculosis, INH inactivation peripheral neuropathy

**Excludes:**

    **Acetylator polymorphism** (0007)
    Ethionamide neuropathy
    Hydralazine neuropathy
    Neuropathy induced by pyridoxine deficiency
    Nutritional neuropathy

**Major Diagnostic Criteria:** In patients receiving the antituberculosis agent INH, the clinical history and examination are compatible with peripheral neuropathy. Serum pyridoxine levels may be low. These patients demonstrate a genetic phenotype for metabolizing INH slowly.

**Clinical Findings:** Symptoms include numbness, tingling, or the sensation of "pins and needles" initially in the toes and spreading proximally in a symmetric fashion. There are complaints of muscle aching and soreness, calf tenderness and sometimes burning pain in the skin or muscles. Occasionally, loss of balance, weakness in the legs, and loss of sleep occur.

Examination shows impaired superficial sensation in the legs and weakness of toe movements. Foot plantar and dorsiflexion weakness may be found later or in the more severely affected patients. Dysesthesias in response to contact stimuli are common. Reflexes are decreased at the ankles and occasionally at the knees.

Laboratory findings may show low serum pyridoxine levels. Biochemical evidence of pyridoxine deficiency is indicated by increased urinary excretion of xanthurenic acid or N-methylnicotinamide following tryptophan loading. Slow acetylation of INH and several other drugs can be demonstrated by half-life determinations of plasma INH. A more convenient means of detecting the presence of the slow acetylator phenotype measures the ratio of monoacetyldapsone to dapsone.

**Complications:** A gradually evolving, predominantly sensory greater than motor neuropathy without rapid deterioration occurs if INH is continued without pyridoxine replacement.

**Associated Findings:** Seizures, altered behavior (hyperactivity), and dermatologic changes may occur in children with INH-induced pyridoxine deficiency.

**Etiology:** Autosomal recessive inheritance.

**Pathogenesis:** Two separate genetic polymorphisms for drug metabolism by acetylation utilizing N-acetyltransferase exist (slow and fast acetylators). The slow acetylation phenotype is autosomal recessive. Acetylation is the first stage of metabolism of INH. INH interferes with pyridoxine metabolism, with increased urinary excretion of pyridoxine. Patients with the slow acetylator phenotype taking INH are more prone to develop pyridoxine deficiency coincident with the peripheral neuropathy. Patients who are fast acetylators may also develop a similar peripheral neuropathy after taking large doses of INH for an extended time period (see **Acetylator polymorphism**).

Light and electron microscopic examinations of sural nerves demonstrate degenerative axonal changes indistinguishable from wallerian degeneration. Both myelinated and unmyelinated fibers are affected. INH is known to enter the endoneurium readily, but the exact mechanism of injury and its relationship to pyridoxine deficiency is unknown.

**MIM No.:** *24340

**Sex Ratio:** M1:F1. However, in a study of Swedish men over age 65 years, the ability to acetylate INH decreased as compared with younger men. No similar pattern was found in women.

**Occurrence:** Undetermined. There is a higher incidence of rapid acetylators among the Japanese than among Europeans. In patients receiving INH 3–5 mg/kg/day, clinical pyridoxine deficiency is reported in 2% of the cases and approximately six months are necessary for clinical manifestations to occur. At 6 mg/kg/day, 10% of patients developed symptoms, often within 3–5 weeks. At 20 mg/kg/day, 40% of patients developed neuropathy.

**Risk of Recurrence for Patient's Sib:**
See Part I, *Mendelian Inheritance*.

**Risk of Recurrence for Patient's Child:**
See Part I, *Mendelian Inheritance*.

**Age of Detectability:** Well-documented in adults, and has been reported in an 11-month-old infant.

**Gene Mapping and Linkage:** Unknown.

**Prevention:** The onset of neuropathy varies with dosage and length of therapy. Pyridoxine 150–450 mg daily given in conjunction with INH prevents development of this neuropathy.

**Treatment:** Early discontinuation of INH when possible will resolve the symptoms, although when treatment was continued for more than a week after the first symptoms appeared, only slight recovery occurred over months.

Pyridoxine supplementation will prevent the development of neuropathy, but has little effect on the speed of recovery.

**Prognosis:** The neuropathy shows gradual resolution after discontinuation of INH. Except in severely affected patients, recovery is virtually complete but may be delayed for months.

**Detection of Carrier:** Slow versus rapid inactivators of INH may be determined by half-life determinations of INH. Other methods of detection include dapsone loading with measurement of the ratio of monoacetyldapsone to dapsone. These screening methods demonstrate a bimodal distribution for ability to acetylate both fast and slow. Some investigators suggest that an intermediate heterozygote state also exists.

**Special Considerations:** Several other drugs are metabolized by the same enzyme system used for acetylation. These include procainamide, hydralazine, sulfamethazine, some sulfonamides, phenelzine, dapsone, and some carcinogenic arylamines. The variability in their metabolism may account for some differences in the incidence of toxic responses to these drugs.

**References:**

Gammon GD, et al.: Neural toxicity in tuberculous patients treated with isoniazid (isonicotinic acid hydrazide). Arch Neurol Psychiatry 1964; 70:64–69.

Carr K, et al.: Simultaneous analysis of dapsone and monoacetyldapsone employing high performance liquid chromatography: a rapid method for determination of acetylator phenotype. Br J Clin Pharmacol 1978; 6:421–427.

Cavanagh JB: The "dying back" process: a common denominator in many naturally occurring and toxic neuropathies. Arch Pathol Lab Med 1979; 103:659–664.

Clark DWJ: Genetically determined variability in acetylation and oxidation: therapeutic implications. Drugs 1985; 29:342–375.

Paulsen O, Nilsson LG: Distribution of acetylator phenotype in relation to age and sex in Swedish patients. Eur J Clin Pharmacol 1985; 28:311–315.

Pellock JM, et al.: Pyridoxine deficiency in children treated with isoniazid. Chest 1985; 87:658–661.

Nhachi CFB: Polymorphic acetylation of sulphamethazine in a Zimbabwe population. J Med Genet 1988; 25:29–31.

MA075          **Janice M. Massey**
H0056          **Kenneth W. Holmes**

**Neuropathy, motor sensory, hereditary**
*See DEJERINE-SOTTAS DISEASE*

---

## NEUROPATHY, MYELO-OPTICO, SUBACUTE TYPE          2047

**Includes:**

> Clioquinol induced subacute myelo-optico neuropathy
> Myelo-optico neuropathy, subacute
> Quinoform induced subacute myelo-optico neuropathy (SMON)
> Subacute myelo-optico neuropathy (SMON)

**Excludes:**

> Benign myalgic encephalomyelitis (Iceland disease)
> Cervical spondylosis
> Encephalomyelitis and viral meningomyelitis
> Guillain-Barre syndrome
> **Multiple sclerosis, familial** (2598)
> Neuromyelitis optica (Devic disease)
> Neurosyphilis
> **Porphyria**
> Subacute combined degeneration of the cord
> Toxic neuropathies, other

**Major Diagnostic Criteria:** A characteristic prodromal abdominal disorder, leading to an ascending bilateral sensory disturbance, typically preceded by a history of abdominal complaints treated by clioquinol. Cardinal symptoms include 1) abdominal symptoms as a prodrome, typically preceded by treatment with clioquinol, and 2) neurologic sensory symptoms, often ascending. Other major signs include impaired deep sensation and weakness in the legs, occasional bilateral visual impairment, mental status changes, greenish discoloration of the tongue and feces, sphincter disturbances, protracted course, no significant blood abnormalities (but often increased glucose or amylase), no significant CSF findings except occasional increased protein, and only rare occurrence in children.

**Clinical Findings:** There is often a recent history of mild GI upset treated with clioquinol. Two to four weeks after clioquinol is given, a separate abdominal prodrome occurs, followed by the onset of neurologic manifestations. Severe abdominal pains, abdominal fullness, and constipation are seen in 70% of the patients and typically last less than two weeks. Fifty percent of the patients have greenish discoloration of the tongue, with elongation of the filiform papillae due to clioquinol-iron complex deposition. Green stool is reported in 8% of patients.

Onset of neurologic dysfunction occurs over several days to about two weeks. Initial symptoms include paresthesias of the feet (72%), numbness and fatigue of the legs (25%), paresthesias of the hands (2%), and blurred vision (1%). There is then an ascending progression of the paresthesias in a bilateral, symmetric fashion. Examination shows normal mental status; decreased visual acuity (27%); motor weakness (50–73%), more prominent in the lower extremities, dermatomal levels below which sensation is lost typically at T10 or lower, with virtually all patients showing sensory loss (light touch, pinprick, and vibration); and variable

deep tendon reflexes. Seventy-five percent of patients have a sensory ataxic gait. Bladder problems occur in 15–20%. Rare cases have unconsciousness, convulsions, or palatal myoclonus. Autonomic disturbances include cold feelings in the feet (68%), edema of the legs and feet (39%), dyshidrosis (36%), and urinary frequency (26%). Following the acute stage, the disease usually takes a chronic course, with symptomatic fluctuation over many months.

Laboratory evaluation shows normal blood chemistries and nonspecific abnormalities (7%). A few patients have shown increased sedimentation rates, C-reactive protein, rheumatoid factor, and SGOT and SGPT levels. Blood sugar and serum amylase are frequently elevated in the initial stages of the disease. Immunoglobulin levels are elevated in 48%, with IgG levels higher than IgA or IgM. The CSF is usually normal, but may show increased protein (10%). Skin biopsy material often shows atrophy of all skin layers. EEG shows bursts of theta activity in 32% of the patients. Slowed motor nerve conduction velocities in the lower extremities are seen in 28–31% of patients. Electromyography of the anterior tibialis occasionally shows fibrillations and positive waves (16–21%) or a decreased interference pattern (37–52%). Sural nerve biopsy shows axonal swelling, demyelination, fibrous proliferation of interstitial tissue, and proliferation of Schwann cells. Axonal degeneration in a "dying back" pattern at 10–14 days after onset is found more prominently than demyelinating changes. Pathologic specimens of the spinal cord show symmetric lesions of the posterior tracts from the sacral to the cervical regions with axonal disruption. The lumbosacral area shows demyelination and gliosis of a secondary degenerative character. There is disintegration of the inner ganglion cells of the retina and bilateral symmetric degeneration throughout almost the entire length of the optic nerve, chiasm, and tract.

**Complications:** Persistent sensory, abdominal, and visual disturbances are common. Gait problems are also frequent.

**Associated Findings:** A past history of gastrointestinal diseases (including peptic ulcer disease, hepatitis, and chronic diarrhea), tuberculosis, renal disease, or gynecologic diseases is frequent. Allergic diseases are found in 30–58% of all patients. A history of laparotomy was found in 48% of patients. Appendectomy was eight times as frequent as in the general population.

**Etiology:** Treatment with quinoform (clioquinol, or 5-chloro-7-iodo-8-hydroxyquinoline) for abdominal discomfort or for *acrodermatitis enteropathica* (a heritable disorder of zinc deficiency, see Gordon et al, 1981) is the most important etiologic factor. The disorder is reproduced by administering quinoform to animals. Although there is a vast amount of epidemiologic data supporting quinoform as the cause of SMON, 4% of patients with clinical SMON have no history of quinoform use. There is no known etiology in these patients, other than for some cases of misdiagnosis. Although the "Inoue-Melnick virus," which has been isolated from the CSF and stool in some patients with SMON and causes a paraplegia in mice, has been raised as a possible cause of SMON, no evidence for any infectious transmission to primates has been found. The pathology in Inoue-Melnick virus mice is not similar to SMON. It is interesting to note that various strains of the Inoue-Melnick virus have been isolated from **Multiple sclerosis** patients in the United States.

**Pathogenesis:** The toxic effect of clioquinol is not known. Based on the similarity of the disease to subacute combined degeneration of the cord, a possible effect on vitamin $B_{12}$ has been considered. A chelation effect of clioquinol on Co (II) has been proposed to possibly interfere with electron transport in the mitochondria.

It is unclear why the disease was so prevalent in Japan, and not in other countries where clioquinol was also used. The Japanese have had more exposure to metals via environmental pollution than inhabitants of most other countries. Clioquinol can increase the penetration of metallic cations through cellular membranes by forming lipophilic metal chelates, and it has been suggested that the accumulation of these metals in the nervous system may cause the toxicity. There are many similarities between SMON and metal toxicities.

There are also pathologic similarities to phenothiazine toxicity, suggesting abnormal metabolism of nicotinic acid.

The possibility of a metabolic error in amino acid metabolism has been considered based on some similarities of SMON to the megaloneuropathies seen in hepatocerebral diseases associated with increased blood amino acid levels, aminoaciduria, and impaired CSF and urine ceruloplasmin metabolism. No such metabolic error has been discovered in SMON.

**MIM No.:** *20110

**Sex Ratio:** M1:F1.8

**Occurrence:** Undetermined but presumed rare at present. At its peak in 1970 the incidence was 125:100,000 women and 60:100,000 men in Nagoya, Japan, and 35:100,000 women and 18:100,000 men in all of Japan. Nearly 10,000 cases were reported by the early 1970s, but very few since the side-effects of the involved medications have become well known.

**Risk of Recurrence for Patient's Sib:** Minimal unless also given clioquinol.

**Risk of Recurrence for Patient's Child:** Minimal unless also given clioquinol.

**Age of Detectability:** The age of onset usually ranges from nine to 81 years, with the youngest patient having been six months old. Only 0.3% of patients are less than 10 years old.

**Gene Mapping and Linkage:** N/A

**Prevention:** The Japanese government officially banned the sale of clioquinol in September 1970.

**Treatment:** Discontinue clioquinol. General health care, psychologic care to deal with the disability, physical therapy, occupational therapy, and rehabilitation are useful as needed. Treatments proposed for the neurologic and abdominal symptoms have included steroids (methylprednisolone, 30–60 mg/day with taper over months; ACTH), intravenous vitamin $B_{12}$, pantothenic acid (100–500 mg/day), acupuncture, and hyperbaric oxygen. Warm water lavage often gives symptomatic relief of abdominal complaints. Oral cinnarizine, indomethacin, and imipramine have been reported to decrease dysesthesias.

**Prognosis:** On follow-up 1.5 to 10 years after onset of symptoms, 6% are cured, one-half to three-fourths are significantly improved, one-third are minimally improved, and 3–6% are dead. The death rates over the 10 years after onset are about twice as high as those for the corresponding age group. Motor recovery is generally very good, but sensory recovery tends to be poor. Chronic abdominal symptoms are present in 50–60%. There is usually no improvement of visual symptoms if optic atrophy is present. Milder visual disturbances improve in 33–49% of patients. A relapse has been reported in 17% of patients, but is related to clioquinol readministration. Fourteen percent need assistance with acts of daily living, and 10% remain unable to walk or unable to walk without an aid. Sixty-five percent returned to work within 12 months.

**Detection of Carrier:** Unknown.

**References:**

Kono R: Introductory review of subacute myelo-optico-neuropathy (SMON) and its studies done by the SMON research commission. Jpn J Med Sci Biol 1975; 28:1–21.

Sobue I, et al.: Prognosis of SMON patients. Jpn J Med Sci Biol 1975; 28:203–217.

Shiraki H: Neuropathological aspects of the etiopathogenesis of subacute myelo-optico-neuropathy (SMON). In: Vinken PJ, Bruyn GW, eds: Handbook of clinical neurology, vol. 37. New York: North Holland, 1978:141–197.

Sobue I: Clinical aspects of subacute myelo-optico-neuropathy (SMON). In: Vinken PJ, Bruyn GW, eds: Handbook of clinical neurology, vol. 37. New York: North Holland, 1978:115–139.

Gordon EF, et al.: Zinc metabolism: basic, clinical, and behavioral aspects. J Pediatr 1981; 99:341–349.

H0056
MA075

**Kenneth W. Holmes**
**Janice M. Massey**

---

**Neuropathy-deafness-diverticulitis**
 *See DEAFNESS-DIVERTICULITIS-NEUROPATHY*
**Neuroretinopathy, optic Leber type**
 *See OPTIC ATROPHY, LEBER TYPE*
**Neurovisceral lipidosis, familial**
 *See G(M1)-GANGLIOSIDOSIS, TYPE 1*
**Neutral 17-beta-hydroxysteroid oxidoreductase deficiency**
 *See STEROID 17-KETOSTEROID REDUCTASE DEFICIENCY*
**Neutral lipid storage disease with ichthyosis**
 *See STORAGE DISEASE, NEUTRAL LIPID TYPE*

---

## NEUTROPENIA, BENIGN FAMILIAL                              2215

**Includes:**

 Idiopathic neutropenia, chronic benign
 Neutropenia, ethnic benign

**Excludes:**

 Autoimmune neutropenia
 **Immunodeficiency, agranulocytosis, infantile Kostmann type** (2197)

**Major Diagnostic Criteria:** Absolute neutropenia with an absolute neutrophil count ranging from 300 to 1,500 cells/ml with no identifiable cause (such as malignancy, drugs, toxins, or connective tissue disease). There may be an accompanying overall leukopenia, but this is not a constant feature. There is no anemia and no thrombocytopenia, and generally there are normal numbers of monocytes, eosinophils, and basophils. Neutrophil morphology is normal.

**Clinical Findings:** Affected individuals are usually identified serendipitously following routine blood screening. They generally do not display any increased susceptibility to infection, although in some individuals occasional stomatitis and gingivitis are reported. The neutropenia is persistent and not cyclic.

**Complications:** Unknown.

**Associated Findings:** None known.

**Etiology:** Autosomal dominant and autosomal recessive inheritance has been reported. Sporadic cases do occur.

**Pathogenesis:** Appears to be in the release of neutrophils from the marrow storage pool. Examination of the bone marrow reveals normal cellularity, a normal myeloid to erythroid ratio, and normal maturation of the myeloid cells right up to mature granulocytes. Marrow culture shows normal or, more often, increased numbers of granulocyte colony-forming cells. Therefore this probably is not a stem cell defect. The administration of endotoxin or corticosteroids, both potent stimuli of granulocyte egress from the marrow storage pool, to these individuals results in an increase in their absolute neutrophil count, but the increment is significantly less than that seen in non-neutropenic controls. Studies with $^{32}P$-labeled granulocytes do not support either increased margination or increased destruction of the granulocytes as the cause of the neutropenia. The exact nature of this defect in neutrophil release from the bone marrow is not known.

**MIM No.:** *16270

**Sex Ratio:** M1:F1

**Occurrence:** About 20 kinships identified involving well over 100 cases. Most common in Yemenite Jews and American, West Indian, and African Blacks. The true incidence of this condition is unknown because of the mild nature of the defect.

**Risk of Recurrence for Patient's Sib:**
 See Part I, *Mendelian Inheritance.*

**Risk of Recurrence for Patient's Child:**
 See Part I, *Mendelian Inheritance.*

**Age of Detectability:** In early childhood.

**Gene Mapping and Linkage:** Unknown.

**Prevention:** None known. Genetic counseling indicated.

**Treatment:** None necessary. In particular, corticosteroids, splenectomy, and prophylactic antibiotics are not indicated.

**Prognosis:** Affected individuals appear to live full, unimpaired lives.

**Detection of Carrier:** Unknown.

**References:**

Cutting HO, et al.: Familial benign chronic neutropenia. Ann Intern Med 1964; 61:876–887. *
Mason BA, et al.: Marrow granulocyte reserves in black Americans. Am J Med 1979; 67:201–205.
Schneider M, et al.: Evaluation of bone marrow granulocyte reserves in neutropenic and nonneutropenic Yemenite Jews. Isr J Med Sci 1982; 18:671–674.
Schoenfeld Y, et al.: The mechanism of benign hereditary neutropenia. Arch Intern Med 1982; 142:797–799.
Berrebi A, et al.: Leukopenia in Ethiopian Jews. (Letter) New Engl J Med 1987; 316:549 only.

AX001
B0048

**Richard Axtell**
**Laurence A. Boxer**

---

## NEUTROPENIA, CYCLIC                                        0714

**Includes:**
Cyclic neutropenia
Periodic neutropenia

**Excludes:**
**Angioedema, hereditary** (0054)
**Fever, familial mediterranean (FMF)** (2161)
Thrombocytopenia, Periodic

**Major Diagnostic Criteria:** Regularly recurrent episodes of profound neutropenia at specific intervals as determined by repeated differential counts.

**Clinical Findings:** The oscillations of neutrophil counts in cyclic neutropenia have a periodicity of approximately 21 days and are consistent from patient to patient. The peripheral blood neutrophil count is severely depressed and in some cases reaches 0/mm³. Symptoms are minimal when the neutrophil count is greater than 500/mm³. During the neutropenic period, patients may have aphthous stomatitis, fever, malaise, occasional cutaneous and subcutaneous infections and cervical adenopathy. Mild splenomegaly is occasionaly observed. The neutrophil counts in the recovery phase attain normal levels in some patients, while in others neutrophil counts remain below normal values.

**Complications:** Skin infections, chronic gingivitis, abscesses, and oral mucosal ulcers are common. Episodes of recurrent boils, otitis media, cervical adenitis, bronchitis, and pneumonia have been reported.

**Associated Findings:** Abdominal pain, diarrhea, arthralgia, headache, depression, septicemia, furunculosis, cellulitis, infection of superficial cuts or abrasions with or without lymphangitis. Cyclic neutropenia has also been associated with coincident conditions such as agammaglobulinemia, diabetes insipidus, pancreatic insufficiency, and lymphosarcoma.

**Etiology:** Possibly autosomal dominant inheritance. May be transferred through bone marrow transplantation (Krance et al, 1982).

**Pathogenesis:** Peripheral blood neutropenia is always preceded by lower numbers of neutrophil precursors in the bone marrow. Periods of severe neutropenia are also regularly associated with an absolute monocytosis. At the nadir early myeloid precursors in the absence of mature neutrophils may be found in circulation. The disease appears to be due to damage to marrow cells or to a defect in their feedback control mechanisms, the cycle being an expression of deranged control.

**MIM No.:** 16280

**Sex Ratio:** M1:F1. A slight preponderance of males has been observed (Wright et al, 1981).

**Occurrence:** Less than 1:100,000

**Risk of Recurrence for Patient's Sib:**
See Part I, *Mendelian Inheritance.* About one in three patients have a sib, parent, or child affected with the disease.

**Risk of Recurrence for Patient's Child:**
See Part I, *Mendelian Inheritance.*

**Age of Detectability:** From birth through childhood.

**Gene Mapping and Linkage:** Unknown.

**Prevention:** None known. Genetic counseling indicated.

**Treatment:** Timely recognition and prompt treatment of serious infections. Avoidance of activities that cause minor injuries. Careful oral and dental care. Although there is as yet no therapeutic cure for the disease, clinical and hemotologic improvements have been achieved following administration of ACTH, corticosteroids, testosterone, staphylococcal vaccine, and infusion of normal plasma or plasma from a volunteer given typhoid vaccine. Recent studies indicated that lithium carbonate might be an effective and safe therapy. Bone marrow transplantation may provide a definitive cure. Temporary improvement has been associated with neutrophil transfusions.

**Prognosis:** Although chronic morbidity is characteristic, life-threatening complications are not unusual. Growth, onset of puberty, and intellectual development are normal. Some patients experience a symptom-free state of nearly 2–6 months duration with no spontaneous changes in neutrophil cycling, suggesting a long-term evolution toward milder recurrent illness.

**Detection of Carrier:** Unknown.

**Special Considerations:** There is a naturally occurring animal model of cyclic neutropenia in gray collie dogs. In humans, a secondary dip in neutrophil counts about 10–14 days after the period of maximum neutropenia has also been reported. Cycling of other blood elements, such as platelets, eosinophils, monocytes, and reticulocytes, may also be apparent. The presence of reciprocal cycling of T8 lymphocytes has been observed.

**References:**

Wright DG, et al.: Human cyclic neutropenia: clinical review and long term follow-up of patients. Medicine 1981; 60:1–13.
Krance RA, et al.: Human cyclic neutropenia transferred by allogenic bone marrow grafting. Blood 1982; 60:1263–1266.
Verma DS, et al.: Cyclic neutropenia and T lymphocyte suppression of granulopoiesis: abrogation of the neutropenic cycles by lithium carbonate. Leuk Res 1982; 6:567–576.
Smith JG, et al.: Cyclical neutropenia and T8 lymphocyte mediated stimulation of granulopoiesis. Br J Haematol 1985; 60:481–489.

NA013

**Madhavan P. N. Nair**

**Neutropenia, ethnic benign**
*See NEUTROPENIA, BENIGN FAMILIAL*
**Neutropenia-onychotrichodysplasia**
*See ONYCHO-TRICHODYSPLASIA-NEUTROPENIA*
**Neutrophil differentiation factor**
*See IMMUNODEFICIENCY, AGRANULOCYTOSIS, INFANTILE KOSTMANN TYPE*
**Nevi flammei**
*See NEVUS FLAMMEUS*

---

## NEVI-ATRIAL MYXOMA-MYXOID NEUROFIBROMAS-EPHELIDES                                        2572

**Includes:**
Adrenocortical nodular dysplasia-Cushing syndrome-cardiac myxomas
Carney complex
Carney Syndrome
Cushing disease-atrial myxoma-pigmentation
Cushing syndrome, familial
Endocrine overactivity-spotty pigmentation-myxomas
LAMB syndrome
Mucocutaneous lentigines-myxomas-multiple blue nevi
Myxoma-adrenocortical dysplasia syndrome
Myxomas-spotty pigmentation-endocrine overactivity
NAME syndrome
Pigmented lesions-myxoid neurofibromas-atrial myxoma
Pigmentation (spotty)-myxomas-endocrine overactivity

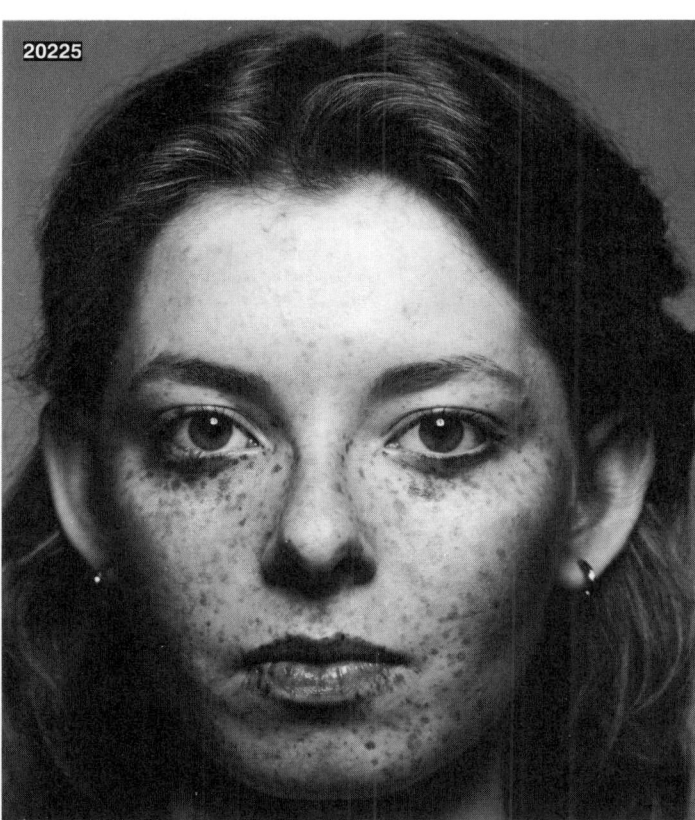

20225

2572-20225:  Multiple, non-elevated black-brown spots on face, vermilion border of lips and right upper eyelid. There is a nodule, three times recurrent and histologically a myxoma, on the right-lower eyelid.

**Excludes:**
Intestinal polyposis, type II (2344)
Lentigines syndrome, multiple (0586)

**Major Diagnostic Criteria:**  Myxoma(s) of the heart, skin, and breast; mucocutaneous lentiginosis and multiple blue nevi; Cushing syndrome, acromegaly or gigantism, and sexual precocity.

**Clinical Findings:**  The cardiac myxoma(s) occur in young patients (mean age, 24 years), tend to be multicentric (45%), and often affect multiple chambers (38%). The cutaneous myxoma(s), often an asymptomatic opalescent papule, typically affects the ears, eyelids, and nipples. Mammary myxoid fibroadenoma(s) tend to be multicentric and bilateral. Lentigines characteristically occur on the face, including the vermilion border of the lips (but infrequently affect the buccal mucosa), the conjunctiva, the trunk and limbs, and the genitalia, especially in the female. The blue nevi have a widespread distribution and are often multiple. Cushing syndrome is due to autonomous adrenocortical overactivity that is caused by a rare bilateral adrenocortical pathology, variously termed *microradular adrenal disease, primary adrenocortical nodular dysplasia,* and *primary pigmented nodular adrenocortical disease.* The adrenal disorder is unusual in that the total adrenal weight is often normal or less than normal, both adrenal glands being studded with small (<4 mm) black or brown nodules set in an atrophic extranodular cortex. Acromegaly or gigantism is due to a growth hormone-producing pituitary adenoma. Testicular tumors (large-cell calcifying Sertoli cell tumor, Leydig cell tumor, and adrenocortical rest tumor) are bilateral and multicentric and may be associated with sexual precocity (40% of males). Calcifying

melanotic schwannomas, sometimes multicentric, occur in superficial (skin) and deep locations and are usually asymptomatic.

**Complications:**  Acute ischemic phenomena, especially hemiplegia, result from embolization of fragments of cardiac myxoma, a lesion that also may cause acute and chronic heart failure. Morbidity results from multiple operations to excise cardiac myxomas. Partial deafness due to blockage of the external auditory canal by cutaneous myxoma. Osteoporosis due to Cushing syndrome. Growth failure due to Cushing syndrome, testicular tumors, or both.

**Associated Findings:**  None known.

**Etiology:**  Autosomal dominant inheritance with variable expression.

**Pathogenesis:**  Unknown.

**MIM No.:**  *16098

**POS No.:**  4335

**Sex Ratio:**  M1:F1

**Occurrence:**  Has been reported in North America, Europe, Australia, New Zealand, and Japan. The number of affected Jewish families appears to be disproportionately high.

**Risk of Recurrence for Patient's Sib:**
See Part I, *Mendelian Inheritance.*

**Risk of Recurrence for Patient's Child:**
See Part I, *Mendelian Inheritance.*

**Age of Detectability:**  Usually clinically evident by ages 10–20 years. May be present as early as the first year of life.

**Gene Mapping and Linkage:**  Unknown.

**Prevention:**  None known. Genetic counseling indicated.

**Treatment:**  Surgery for excision of myxomas, most importantly cardiac myxoma, keeping in mind that multiple cardiac chambers may be affected. Skin myxomas may need to be excised for diagnostic or cosmetic reasons. Disfiguring lentigines and blue nevi may need to be removed for similar reasons. Bilateral adrenalectomy cures the Cushing syndrome (the Nelson syndrome has not occurred following such surgery). Treatment of the testicular tumors should be conservative; no tumor has yet metastasized. Tumors causing sexual precocity need to be eradicated. The pituitary adenoma is best treated by transphenoidal hypophysectomy. Calcifying melanotic schwannomas are treated by surgical excision.

**Prognosis:**  Long-term outlook is unknown. It may ultimately be found to depend largely on the results of multiple surgical procedures to control multiple episodes of cardiac myxoma. Several patients have had three cardiac operations for removal of recurrent (more likely multicentric) myxomas. About 25% of the patients have died of cardiac myxoma.

**Detection of Carrier:**  Careful clinical examination and history of first-degree relatives together with echocardiogram and study of adrenocortical function.

**Special Considerations:**  The oldest living affected patient (a member of an affected family who has mucocutaneous lentiginosis only) is aged 67 years. The cardiac myxoma has presented as early as age six years and as late as age 58 years (in a patient who was asymptomatic). Abnormalities of steroid metabolism may be present without the clinical features of the Cushing syndrome.

**Support Groups:**  Atlanta; American Cancer Society

**References:**
Atherton DJ, et al.: A syndrome of various cutaneous pigmented lesions, myxoid neurofibromata and atrial myxoma: the NAME syndrome. Br J Dermatol 1980; 103:421–429.
Rhodes AR, et al.: Mucocutaneous lentigines, cardiomucocutaneous myxomas, and multiple blue nevi: the "LAMB" syndrome. J Am Acad Dermatol 1984; 10:72–82.
Carney JA, et al.: The complex of myxomas, spotty pigmentation, and endocrine overactivity. Medicine 1985; 64:270–283.
Carney JA, et al.: Dominant inheritance of the complex of myxomas, spotty pigmentation, and endocrine overactivity. Mayo Clin Proc 1986; 61:165–172.

Vidaillet HJ, Jr: "Syndrome myxoma": a subset of patients with cardiac myxoma associated with pigmented skin lesions and peripheral and endocrine neoplasms. Brit Heart J 1986; 57:247–255.

Cook CA, et al.: Mucocutaneous pigmented spots and oral myxomas: the oral manifestations of the complex of myxomas, spotty pigmentation, and endocrine overactivity. Oral Surg, Oral Med, Oral Path 1987; 63:175–183.

Danoff A, et al.: Adrenocortical micronodular dysplasia, cardiac myxomas, lentigines, and spindle cell tumors: report of a kindred. Arch Intern Med 1987; 147:443–448.

Kennedy RH, et al.: Ocular pigmented spots and eyelid myxomas. Am J Ophthal 1987; 104:533–538.

Carney JA: Psammomatous melanotic schwannoma. Modern Pathol 1988; 1:15A.

CA042                                                    **J. A. Carney**

## NEVO SYNDROME                                              3273

**Includes:** Overgrowth-congenital edema-positional defects of the feet

**Excludes:** Cebebral gigantism (0137)

**Major Diagnostic Criteria:** The combination of overgrowth with congenital edema and positional defects of the feet.

**Clinical Findings:** Three affected children (two sibs and their cousin) from an inbred family have been described. Anomalies include excessive birth length (97th centile) (3/3), hypotonia (3/3), congenital edema (2/3), congenital dorsiflexion of the feet (2/3), calcaneovalgus (1/3), dolichocephaly (2/3), highly arched, narrow palate (2/3), large, low-set ears (3/3), kyphosis (3/3), cryptorchidism (2/2 males), clinodactyly (1/3), tapering digits (2/3), single transverse palmar crease (1/3), and advanced bone age (2/3).

**Complications:** Unknown.

**Associated Findings:** One child had severe mental retardation, one child developed postnatal **Hydrocephaly**.

**Etiology:** The presence of the condition in sibs born to consanguineous parents and their double first cousin suggests autosomal recessive inheritance.

**Pathogenesis:** Unknown.

**MIM No.:** *11755

**Sex Ratio:** M1:F1

**Occurrence:** Documented in one family from Israel.

**Risk of Recurrence for Patient's Sib:**
See Part I, *Mendelian Inheritance.*

**Risk of Recurrence for Patient's Child:**
See Part I, *Mendelian Inheritance.*

**Age of Detectability:** At birth by excessive length and edema.

**Gene Mapping and Linkage:** Unknown.

**Prevention:** None known. Genetic counseling indicated.

**Treatment:** Supportive.

**Prognosis:** Variable, in that one child died at one month of complications from **Hydrocephaly** (postnatal). Of the two surviving children, one had normal intelligence and one was mentally retarded.

**Detection of Carrier:** Unknown.

**Special Considerations:** Although the authors suggested a diagnosis of **Cebebral gigantism** for these children, both the mode of inheritance and the presence of congenital edema, dorsiflexion of the feet, severe kyphosis and normal head circumference are not consistent with such a diagnosis.

**References:**
Nevo S, et al.: Evidence for autosomal recessive inheritance in cerebral gigantism. J Med Genet 1974; 11:158–165.

T0007                                            **Helga V. Toriello**

**Nevocellular nevus, congenital**
*See NEVUS, CONGENITAL NEVOMELANOCYTIC*

## NEVOID BASAL CELL CARCINOMA SYNDROME           0101

**Includes:**
  Basal cell nevi
  Basal cell nevus syndrome
  Carcinoma, nevoid basal cell syndrome
  Fifth phacomatosis
  Gorlin-Goltz syndrome
  Nevus, basal cell nevus syndrome

**Excludes:**
  Achrochordons
  Epithelioma adenoides cysticum
  Follicular atrophoderma-hypotrichosis-face and head anhidrosis

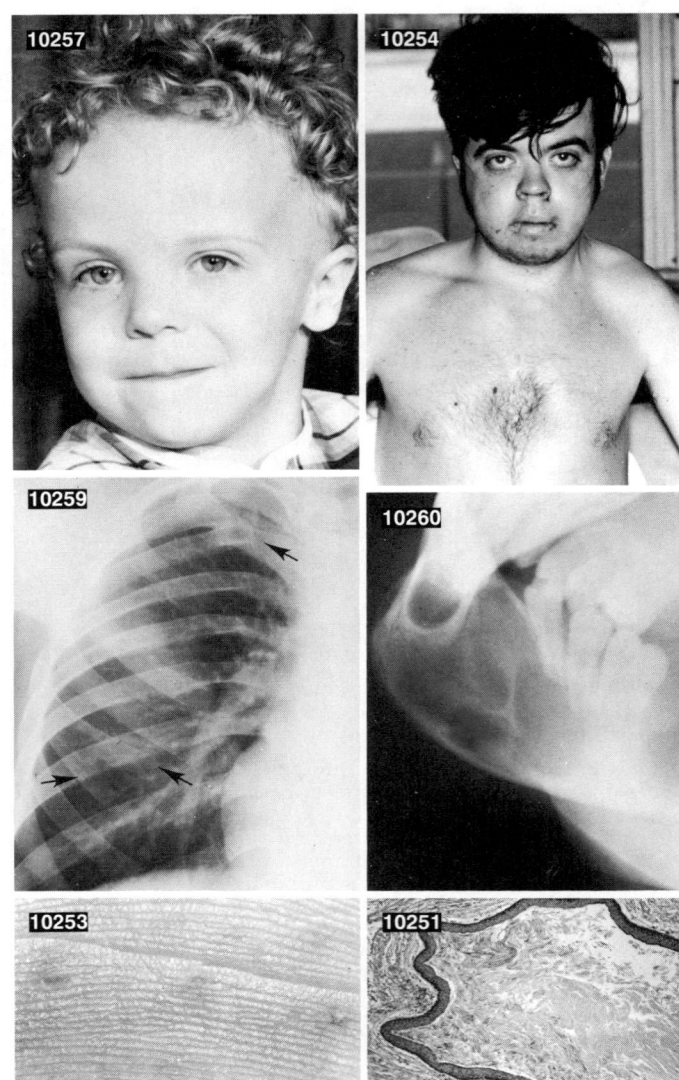

0101-10257: Young affected male with hypertelorism, strabismus, and craniofacial disproportion. 10254: Older male shows macrocephaly, pectus excavatum, hypertelorism and sunken eyes. 10259: Chest X-ray shows posterior fusion of ribs 3 and 4 and anterior bifurcation of rib 5. 10260: Jaw cysts. 10253: Palmar pits. 10251: Keratocyst of the jaw; note thin epithelial layer with parakeratinazation.

Linear basal cell nevus
Multiple nevocytic or melanocytic nevi
**Neurofibromatosis** (0712)
**Nevus, epidermal nevus syndrome** (0593)
Non-nevus multiple basal cell carcinomas

**Major Diagnostic Criteria:**  Multiple basal cell carcinomas with an early age at onset, epithelium-lined cysts of mandible and maxilla with unique daughter cysts, distinctive pits of the hands and feet, a variety of congenital skeletal anomalies, and ectopic calcification. In the absence of a positive family history, any two major components may be sufficient for diagnosis. With a positive family history, any of the major or a combination of several minor anomalies reflects expression of the syndrome.

**Clinical Findings:**  *Cutaneous:* Multiple basal cell carcinomas (75%); pits of hands and feet (65%); cutaneous keratocysts, numerous milia (20–40%); ectopic calcification of basal cell (?%); carcinomas and subcutaneous tissues (?%).

*Osseous:* Jaw cysts (mandibular and maxillary) (80%); sellar bridging (75%); vertebral anomalies (spina bifida occulta, scoliosis) (65%); rib anomalies (bifidness, splaying, synostoses) (60%); subcortical cystic changes (long bones and phalanges) (45%); brachymetacarpalism (30%); Sprengel deformity (5%); defective dentition (?%); frontal and biparietal bossing (?%); mandibular prognathism (?%).

*Neurologic:* Calcification of the falx cerebri (lamellar pattern), tentorium cerebelli, and petroclinoid ligaments (80%); mental aberration, retardation (1–10%); EEG changes (non-specific), various neurological defects (?%); medulloblastoma (50% have onset before age 2 years) (1–5%).

*Ophthalmologic:* Hypertelorism, dystopia canthorum (25–50%); strabismus (25%); congenital blindness (colobomas, cataracts, glaucoma) (5–10%).

*Reproductive:* Ovarian fibromas (?%); hypogonadism (?%), ovarian cysts and fibromas; ovarian adenocarcinoma and fibrosarcoma.

*Miscellaneous:* Lymphatic mesenteric cysts; squamous cell carcinoma of jaw cyst; subconjunctival cysts of eyelids; fibrosarcoma of jaw (radiation-induced following radiation treatment for jaw cysts).

Syndrome may have variable or delayed expressivity. X-rays of skull, mandible, maxilla, ribs, vertebrae, and hands may be helpful in identifying the syndrome, particularly in children, before the basal cell carcinomas become manifest.

**Complications:**  Loss of one or both eyes from basal cell carcinomas of lids and canthi; destruction of skin, scalp, subcutaneous tissue, cartilage, bone, nose, ears, etc. from infiltrating basal cell carcinomas; infection of jaw cysts, with swelling and pain from enlarging jaw cysts, resulting in loss and malposition of teeth; strangulation of mesenteric cyst; death from infiltrating basal cell carcinomas intracranially with or without infection; erosion of sizable blood vessels; or, rarely, metastasis. Death from medulloblastoma, fibrosarcoma, ovarian adenocarcinoma, or squamous cell carcinoma.

Radiation-induced basal cell carcinomas appear as early as 6 months to 3 years after irradiation. Radiation appears to increase the incidence of those tumors that would spontaneously occur in affected individuals. A few female syndrome survivors of medulloblastoma treated with ionizing irradiation have developed multiple ovarian fibrosarcomas and ovarian fibroma.

**Associated Findings:**  None known.

**Etiology:**  Autosomal dominant inheritance with high penetrance of gene (97%) and variable expressivity.

**Pathogenesis:**  Unknown.

**MIM No.:**  *10940

**POS No.:**  3527

**Sex Ratio:**  M1:F1

**Occurrence:**  Over 300 cases reported in the past decade.

**Risk of Recurrence for Patient's Sib:**
See Part I, *Mendelian Inheritance.*

**Risk of Recurrence for Patient's Child:**
See Part I, *Mendelian Inheritance.*

**Age of Detectability:**  At birth, by skeletal anomalies; in childhood, by jaw cysts, defective dentition, skeletal anomalies, or medulloblastoma. In early adult life, by multiple basal cell carcinomas, jaw cysts, pits of hands and feet, skeletal defects of development, and ectopic calcification.

**Gene Mapping and Linkage:**  NBCCS (nevoid basal cell carcinoma syndrome) has been tentatively mapped to 1p.

**Prevention:**  None known. Genetic counseling indicated.

**Treatment:**  Basal cell carcinomas rarely exhibit aggressive biological behavior before puberty. Treatment, therefore, is usually unnecessary until after puberty unless growth of one or several tumors is noted. An exception are children who have received ionizing irradiation for medulloblastoma or other reasons. Radiation-induced tumors appear 6 months to 3 years following treatment. Prevention of problem lesions is desirable by treating nevoid basal cell carcinomas early in their growth phase with surgical excision or open removal using curettage and electrosurgery. Tumors of the eyelids, periorbital and nasomalar areas, and near orifices such as the ear canal should be removed as they appear. Frequent follow-up visits are needed if tumor growth and new tumor development are occurring. Administration of systemic retinoids for retarding tumor growth, preventing new lesions, or treating aggressive lesions, though promising, is still under study and is not practical with available retinoids. Avoid irradiation therapy of tumors as well as modalities not highly curative, e.g., dermabrasion and, 5-fluorouracil.

*Other therapy:* Cryotherapy of tumors; the Mohs method of excision for problem tumors is very useful. The future value of photoradiation, interferon, and newer retinoids is uncertain.

**Prognosis:**  Generally good for an average life span, but variable depending on location and invasiveness of the basal cell carcinomas and the less common tumors.

**Detection of Carrier:**  Anthropometrics of skull identifies carriers in 85–90% of cases.

**References:**

Howell JB, Caro MR: The basal cell nevus: its relationship to multiple cutaneous cancers and associated anomalies of development. Arch Dermatol 1959; 79:67–80.
Gorlin RJ, et al.: Multiple basal cell nevi syndrome: an analysis of a syndrome consisting of multiple nevoid basal-cell carcinoma, jaw cysts, skeletal anomalies, medulloblastoma and hyporesponsiveness to parathormone. Cancer 1965; 18:89.
Berlin NI, et al.: Basal cell nevus syndrome. Ann Intern Med 1966; 64:403–421.
Anderson DE, et al.: The nevoid basal cell carcinoma syndrome. Am J Hum Genet 1967; 19:12.
Howell JB, Anderson DE: The nevoid basal cell carcinoma syndrome. In: Andrade R, ed: Cancer of the skin. Philadelphia: W.B. Saunders, 1976:883–898.
Howell JB: The roots of the nevoid basal cell carcinoma syndrome. Clin Exp Dermatol 1980; 5:337–348.
Howell JB, Anderson DE: Commentary: the nevoid basal cell carcinoma syndrome. Arch Dermatol 1982; 118:824–826.
Levine DJ, et al.: Familial subconjunctival epithelial cysts associated with nevoid basal cell carcinoma syndrome. Arch Dermatol 1987; 123:23–24.

H0050
AN017

**James B. Howell
David E. Anderson**

**Nevoid pigmentation of the retina**
*See RETINA, GROUPED HYPERTROPHY OF RETINAL PIGMENT EPITHELIUM*
**Nevomelanocytic nevus, congenital**
*See NEVUS, CONGENITAL NEVOMELANOCYTIC*
**Nevus anemicus**
*See SKIN, VITILIGO*

## NEVUS FLAMMEUS                                           0715

**Includes:**
"Angel's kiss"
"Birthmark" (obsolete)
Capillary hemangioma
Capillary nevus
Erythema nuchae
Nape nevus
Nevi flammei
Nevus flammeus of nape of neck
Nevus planus
Nevus simplex
"Pressure marks" (obsolete)
Port-wine stain
Salmon patch
"Stork bite" mark
Unna nevus

**Excludes:** Hemangiomas of the head and neck (2514)

**Major Diagnostic Criteria:** Vascular skin lesions.

**Clinical Findings:** Nevus flammeus can be divided into two categories: the salmon patch and the port-wine stain. Salmon patches are commonly seen on the nape of the neck, occiput, forehead, glabella, and eyelids. On the forehead and glabella, they usually have a tornado-funnel shape, with the apex pointing downward. Salmon patches of the eyelids, forehead, and glabella generally disappear by the end of the first year of life. A considerable number of those on the occiput and nape of the neck, however, persist.

Port-wine stains consist of pink macules varying in size from one to many centimeters. They can occur anywhere on the body but have a special predilection for the face. The lesion is generally unilateral, and it often approximates a dermatomal pattern. Although both salmon patches and port-wine stains show the same histologic features, ectasia of blood vessels in the superficial dermis without vascular proliferation, port-wine stains do not disappear. With increasing age the vessels become more ectatio and more engorged with erythrocytes. Clinically, a darkening in color and a nodular, "cobblestone" appearance of the skin surface is observed.

**Complications:** Unknown.

**Associated Findings:** Glaucoma, phocomelia, **Chromosome 13, trisomy 13, Chromosome 4, monosomy 4p, Beckwith-Wiedemann syndrome,** underlying arteriovenous communication, and possibly congenital heart disease.

Approximately 5% of port-wine stains may be associated with a cavernous hemangioma involving deep dermis, subcutaneous tissue, and even muscle. In some patients, especially those in whom the "cobblestone" pattern is pronounced, there may occur some blood vessel and stromal proliferation.

**Etiology:** Probably autosomal dominant inheritance, but the high prevalence of salmon patches precludes a definite conclusion regarding these lesions. Nevi flammei of trunk and limbs have also been reported to follow irregularly dominant patterns.

**Pathogenesis:** Arterial, venous, and capillary circulation of the skin arises from a primitive, pluripotential capillary network. During fetal development certain portions of this network are normally resorbed. Failure or incomplete resorption is thought to result in nevus flammeus.

In their development, appearance, and distribution, nevi flammei may be under neural influences. Phocomelic "thalidomide babies" and infants with various chromosome anomalies have exhibited facial nevi flammei. Rarely, nevi flammei first appear following exposure to intense cold or other physical injury.

It is not known why progressive ectasia of blood vessel walls occurs in port-wine stains. Direct immunofluorescent studies of three major components of blood vessel walls (collagenous basement membrane, fibronectin, and Factor VIII) have shown no differences in the distribution or amount of these materials in either port-wine stains and normal skin. One explanation for these findings is that proteins are antigenically normal but non-

functional. Another possibility may be that the progressive ectasia is not due to an intrinsic abnormality of the vessel itself, but rather to the supporting connective tissue of the dermis.

**MIM No.:** *16310

**CDC No.:** 757.380

**Sex Ratio:** M1:F1 for most types. M>1:F1 in Cobb syndrome.

**Occurrence:** Salmon patch in over 40% of neonates (i.e. "normal anatomic variants"). Port-wine stains found in 0.3% of 1,058 newborns (80% white). Nape nevi persist in about 30% of adults. Lower figures reported in Blacks, but lesions are less visible.

**Risk of Recurrence for Patient's Sib:**
See Part I, *Mendelian Inheritance.*

**Risk of Recurrence for Patient's Child:**
See Part I, *Mendelian Inheritance.*

**Age of Detectability:** Usually in the neonatal period.

**Gene Mapping and Linkage:** Unknown.

**Prevention:** None known. Genetic counseling indicated.

**Treatment:** Salmon patches are generally not treated.

Treatment of port-wine stains has included cosmetic coverage, excision and graft, laser beam, $CO_2$ ice, electrodesiccation, tattooing, and various forms of radiotherapy. Both argon and $CO_2$ laser have been used, but most clinical experience to date has centered on the argon laser. Results have been fair to good, although advances in this technology offer promise (Tan et al, 1989). Excision and grafting, cryotherapy, electrodessication, dermabrasion, and therapeutic tatoo have been used with inconsistent success. Radiotherapy (thorium X, grenz ray, radiophosphorus) has, for the most part, been abandoned. Special opaque cosmetics have been developed for the express purpose of concealing port-wine stains and similar disfiguring lesions, and the use of these cosmetics should be encouraged.

**Prognosis:** Normal for life span, intelligence, and function when changes are limited to the skin.

**Detection of Carrier:** Unknown.

**Special Considerations:** The theory that salmon patches are caused by trauma directly to the lesional area has been dispelled; the expression "pressure marks" and "birthmark" should no longer be used.

Salmon patches are trivial lesions unassociated with other vascular malformations. Port-wine stains, on the other hand, may portend an underlying vascular anomaly, the most serious of which is **Sturge-Weber syndrome.** A number of other eponymic syndromes have been described in which vascular anomalies of the eyes and central nervous system have been inconsistently associated with nevus flammeus. These syndromes are thought by some to be variations of the Sturge-Weber syndrome. Tissue hypertrophy may accompany nevi flammei of the limbs (see **Angio-osteohypertrophy syndrome**), genitalia, lips, and other sites.

**References:**
Jacobs AH, Walton RG: The incidence of birthmarks in the neonate. Pediatrics 1976; 58:218–222.
Finley JL, et al.: Immunofluorescent staining with antibodies to factor VIII, fibronectin, and collagenous basement membrane protein in normal human skin and port-wine stains. Arch Dermatol 1982; 118:971–975.
Jacobs AH: Vascular nevi. Pediatr Clin North Am 1983; 30:465–482.
Buecker JW, et al.: Histology of port-wine stain treated with carbon dioxide laser. J Am Acad Dermatol 1984; 10:1014–1019.
Finley JL, et al.: Argon laser-port-wine stain interaction. Arch Dermatol 1984; 120:613–619.
Finley JL, et al.: Port-wine stains. Arch Dermatol 1984; 120:1453–1455.
Merlob P, Reisner SH: Familial nevus flammeus of the forehead and unna's nevus. Clin Genetics 1985; 27:165–166.
Tan OT, et al.: Treatment of children with port-wine stains using the flashlamp-pulsed tunable dye laser. New Engl J Med 1989; 320:416–421.

SE014                                                    **Victor J. Selmanowitz**
PE018                                                    **Frederick A. Pereira**

**Nevus flammeus of nape of neck**
*See NEVUS FLAMMEUS*
**Nevus fuscoceruleus ophthalmomaxillaris**
*See NEVUS OF OTA*

## NEVUS OF OTA 0716

**Includes:**
Dermal melanocytosis
Nevus fuscoceruleus ophthalmomaxillaris
Oculocutaneous melanosis
Oculocutaneous pigmentation syndrome
Oculodermal melanocytosis

**Excludes:**
Conjuctival melanosis
Malignant melanoma
Melanocytoma
Mongolian spot
**Nevus, blue rubber bleb nevus syndrome** (0113)
Ocular melanosis
**Optic disk, melanocytoma** (0639)
Precancerous melanosis

**Major Diagnostic Criteria:** Nevus of Ota is a benign, macular or slightly raised, indistinctly marginated discoloration of the face in the region of innervation of the first and second divisions of the trigeminal nerve. The color of the lesion varies from tan to brown, black, slate-blue, or purple.

**Clinical Findings:** About one-half of cases of nevus of Ota become apparent in the first year of life. Other cases develop later, and onset or exacerbation during puberty or pregnancy is common. Ninety-five percent of cases are unilateral. Nevus of Ota is associated with ipsilateral ocular hyperpigmentation in one-half to two-thirds of affected patients. Scleral involvement is most common, but hyperpigmentation of the cornea, conjunctiva, uveal tract, optic disk, optic nerve, orbital soft tissue, or periosteum of the bony orbit may occur. Heterochromia of the iris has also been observed. The dermal discoloration may extend beyond the immediate region of the eye to the temple, forehead, cheek, or nose. Pigmentation of the tympanic membrane, palate, and oral or nasal mucosa is commonly associated with nevus of Ota.

Histologically, the nevus of Ota resembles the **Nevus, blue rubber bleb nevus syndrome** and **Skin, cutaneous melanosis: Mongolian spot**. The dermis of affected skin contains heavily pigmented melanocytes with a fusiform, dendritic, or stellate shape.

**Complications:** A predisposition to development of malignant melanoma (as high as 23% among severe cases) appears to exist with nevus of Ota.

**Associated Findings:** Persistent mongolian spots on the buttocks or back occasionally are found in adults with nevus of Ota, especially if bilateral. Blue nevi may occur within the nevus of Ota or at neighboring sites. Glaucoma, angiomas, bony anomalies, and neurologic problems have rarely been reported in association with nevus of Ota and may represent coincidental observations.

**Etiology:** Undetermined. Familial cases are uncommon.

**Pathogenesis:** Unknown.

**CDC No.:** 757.380

**Sex Ratio:** M1:F4, but this may reflect a greater likelihood for females to consult a physician because of a cosmetic lesion on the face.

**Occurrence:** Undetermed presumably uncommon; more frequent among Orientals (0.2–0.8%) and Blacks than among whites.

**Risk of Recurrence for Patient's Sib:** Presumably small.

**Risk of Recurrence for Patient's Child:** Presumably small.

**Age of Detectability:** The lesion appears in the first year of life in about one-half of cases, and during childhood, adolescence, or early adulthood in the other one-half.

**Gene Mapping and Linkage:** Unknown.

**Prevention:** None known. Genetic counseling indicated.

**Treatment:** Cosmesis.

**Prognosis:** Nevus of Ota is generally only a cosmetic problem. The lesion is permanent, but may become lighter or darker with aging or hormonal changes.

**Detection of Carrier:** Unknown.

**References:**
Kopf AW, Weidman AI: Nevus of Ota. Arch Dermatol 1956; 85:195–208.
Mishima Y, Mevorah B: Nevus Ota and nevus Ito in American Negroes. J Invest Dermatol 1961; 36:133–154.
Hagler WS, Brown CC: Malignant melanoma of the orbit arising in a nevus of Ota. Transact Am Acad Ophthalmol 1966; 70:817–822.
Hidano A, et al.: Natural history of nevus of Ota. Arch Derm 1967; 95:187–195.
Guérin JC, Daudon-Conteaux R: Le naevus de Ota. Arch Ophtalmol (Paris) 1974; 34:359–384.

FR017 **J.M. Friedman**

**Nevus planus**
*See NEVUS FLAMMEUS*
**Nevus sebaceus of Jadassohn**
*See NEVUS, EPIDERMAL NEVUS SYNDROME*
**Nevus simplex**
*See NEVUS FLAMMEUS*
**Nevus varicosus osteohypertrophicus**
*See ANGIO-OSTEOHYPERTROPHY SYNDROME*
**Nevus, basal cell nevus syndrome**
*See NEVOID BASAL CELL CARCINOMA SYNDROME*

## NEVUS, BLUE RUBBER BLEB NEVUS SYNDROME 0113

**Includes:**
Bean syndrome
Blue rubber bleb nevus of skin and gastrointestinal tract
Hemangiomatosis, generalized cavernous
Hamartoma, venous

**Excludes:**
**Enchondromatosis and hemangiomas** (0346)
**Fabry disease** (0373)
Multiple hemangiomatosis
Solitary cavernous hemangioma
**Telangiectasia, osler hemorrhagic** (2021)

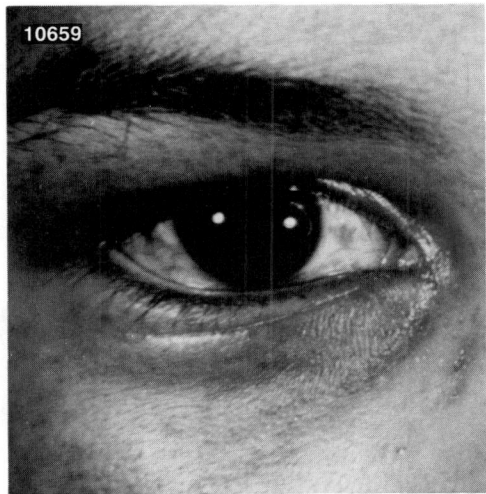

**0716**-10659: Nevus of Ota.

**Major Diagnostic Criteria:** Multiple hemangiomas of the skin are present. The hemangiomas range in size from 0.1 to 5.0 cm, are bluish in color, and are characterized by easy compressibility.

**Clinical Findings:** Multiple cavernous hemangiomas are present in the skin (100%), GI tract (90%), and are less frequently reported to occur in the subcutaneous tissue, mucous membranes, lungs, liver, skeletal muscle, thyroid, brain, spinal cord, meninges, cranial bones, spleen, heart, and kidney. The hemangiomas are 0.2–4 cm in diameter and are bluish to purplish-red to black in color. They are rumpled in appearance when partially emptied by squeezing and slowly refill when pressure is released. Bleeding is common.

**Complications:** Serious spontaneous GI bleeding and anemia occur frequently. Spontaneous bleeding of the skin lesions is rare, but they may bleed from injury. The skin lesions may produce serious cosmetic problems. Lesions of the soles may interfere with walking. Oozing, irritation, and offensive odor from involvement of the genital area and perianal area may occur.

**Associated Findings:** Meningioma, medulloblastoma, osteoma, syringomyelia, and cysts of many organs have been reported.

**Etiology:** Autosomal dominant inheritance. Numerous multi-generation pedigrees have been reported. Sporadic cases may represent new dominant mutations or phenocopies.

**Pathogenesis:** Microscopically the lesions are thin-walled and filled with blood, with the walls resembling those of veins. Sweat glands are often closely related to vascular lesions.

**MIM No.:** *11220

**POS No.:** 4229

**CDC No.:** 757.380

**Sex Ratio:** Presumably M1:F1

**Occurrence:** Rare, but reported in various races.

**Risk of Recurrence for Patient's Sib:**
See Part I, *Mendelian Inheritance.*

**Risk of Recurrence for Patient's Child:**
See Part I, *Mendelian Inheritance.*

**Age of Detectability:** Lesions are usually present at birth.

**Gene Mapping and Linkage:** Unknown.

**Prevention:** None known. Genetic counseling indicated.

**Treatment:** Most troublesome skin lesions may be excised. Anemia due to bleeding from GI lesions should be treated as needed. Carbon dioxide laser treatment has been reported to be effective. Argon laser therapy may also be useful.

**Prognosis:** Life span may be normal, or patients may die in early adult life from associated conditions or from internal hemorrhage.

**Detection of Carrier:** Unknown.

*The author is indebted to J. Sidney Rice, who authored an earlier version of this article.*

**References:**
Jaffe RH: Multiple hemangiomas of skin and of internal organs. Arch Pathol 1929; 7:44.
Rice JS, Fischer DS: Blue rubber bleb nevus syndrome: generalized cavernous hemangiomatosis or venous hamartoma with medulloblastoma of the cerebellum; case report and review of the literature. Arch Dermatol 1962; 86:503–511.
Morris SJ, et al.: Blue rubber bleb nevus syndrome. JAMA 1978; 239:1887.
McCauley RGK, et al.: Blue rubber bleb nevus syndrome. Radiology 1979; 133:375–377.
Olsen TG, et al.: Laser surgery for blue rubber bleb nevus. Arch Dermatol 1979; 115:81–82.
Munkvad M: Blue rubber bleb nevus syndrome. Dermatologica 1983; 167:307–309.
Satya-Murti S, et al.: Central nervous system involvement in blue-rubber-bleb-nevus syndrome. Arch Neurol 1986; 43:1184–1186.

**Virginia P. Sybert**

---

**Includes:**

> Giant pigmented hairy nevus (GPHN)
> Hairy melanocytic nevus, giant congenital
> Melanocytic nevus, congenital
> Melanocytic nevus, giant congenital
> Melanocytic nevus, small congenital
> Nevocellular nevus, congenital
> Nevomelanocytic nevus, congenital

**Excludes:**

> **Nevus, epidermal nevus syndrome** (0593)
> Non-nevomelanocytic congenital nevi

**Major Diagnostic Criteria:** A congenital nevomelanocytic nevus is a collection of nevus cells in the skin, first apparent at birth.

**Clinical Findings:** Lesions may be diagnosed on the basis of gross morphology and parental history. Nevomelanocytic nevi are round or oval plaques, pigmented one or more shades or brown, distorting the skin surface by accentuated skin markings or follicles when examined using tangential light, having fine speckling of pigment when examined using bright light and 10X hand lens magnification of the mineral-oil covered lesion surface. Excessive hair may or may not be present. The definition of small is a lesion that can be excised easily and the defect closed primarily without the use of flaps or grafts. Giant is a subset of large, occupying a major portion of a major anatomic site.

**Complications:** Giant congenital nevomelanocytic nevi have a risk of cutaneous melanoma approaching 10% over a lifetime. Of those giant congenital nevomelanocytic nevi developing cutaneous melanoma, about half the cases are diagnosed in the first three to five years of life. Giant nevi may be the precursor for 0.1% of cutaneous melanomas.

The risk of melanoma associated with small varieties of congenital nevomelanocytic nevi has been estimated to be as high as 5% by age 60 years. Up to 15% of melanomas are alleged to have developed in a small congenital nevus; 2.6% to 8.1% of melanomas may show evidence of a dermal nevus having one or more "congenital" features, in contiguity with the tumor. Although there appears to be a definite risk of melanoma associated with small congenital nevi, the exact magnitude of the risk is regarded as controversial.

**Associated Findings:** Possibly ear deformities, preauricular appendages, angiomas, and other skin anomalies, according to one study.

**Etiology:** Possibly autosomal dominant inheritance, in some cases.

**Pathogenesis:** Presumed dysplasia of neural crest-derived melanoblasts.

**MIM No.:** 13755, *15560

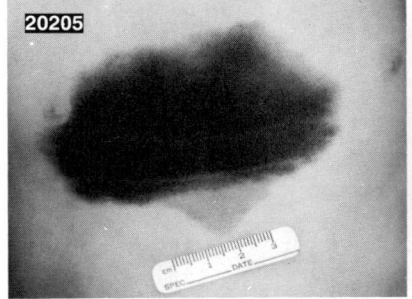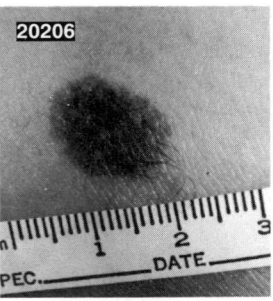

**2165-20205:** Relatively large congenital nevus on the anterior torso of a 10-month-old male. **20206:** Small congenital nevus which is uniformly pigmented medium brown with well-demarcated smooth borders and coarse dark hairs on the surface.

**CDC No.:** 757.380

**Sex Ratio:** M1:F1

**Occurrence:** One percent of newborns for small lesions, 1:20,000 newborns for lesions ≥9.9 cm in greatest diameter; 1:500,000 newborns for giant lesions.

**Risk of Recurrence for Patient's Sib:** Increased, but exact risk not known.

**Risk of Recurrence for Patient's Child:** Increased, but exact risk not known.

**Age of Detectability:** At birth.

**Gene Mapping and Linkage:** CMM (cutaneous malignant melanoma/dysplastic nevus) has been provisionally mapped to 1p36.

**Prevention:** None known. Genetic counseling indicated.

**Treatment:** Because of the increased risk of melanoma associated with congenital nevomelanocytic nevi (regardless of size), all such lesions should be evaluated for excision. Melanoma associated with very large lesions may occur even in the first several years of life, so prophylactic excision should be considered early. Melanoma associated with small congenital nevi usually does not occur until after 12 years. Excision of small congenital nevi may be delayed until local anesthesia can be used at the end of the first decade of life, as long as the lesion maintains a benign appearance and lends itself to photographic follow-up. Atypical-appearing nevomelanocytic nevi should be evaluated for immediate excision.

The management of small congenital nevi is considered controversial. Ascertainment of congenital nevomelanocytic nevi in contiguity with cutaneous melanoma has been based on history and histology. Neither of these methods of ascertainment is perfect. The management of congenital nevomelanocytic nevi needs to be individualized. In general, there seems to be little justification for recommending lifetime follow-up for lesions that can be excised easily. The risk of melanoma associated with large lesions is less controversial, but such lesions are more difficult to excise.

**Prognosis:** Unknown.

**Detection of Carrier:** Unknown.

**References:**

Trozak DJ, et al.: Metastatic melanoma in prepubertal children. Pediatrics 1975; 55:191–204.

Walton RG, et al.: Pigmented lesions in newborn infants. Br J Dermatol 1976; 95:389–396.

Lorentzen M, et al.: The incidence of malignant transformation in giant pigmented nevi. Scand J Plast Reconstr Surg 1977; 11:163–167.

Alper J, et al.: Birthmarks with serious medical significance: nevocellular nevi, sebaceous nevi, and multiple cafe au lait spots. J Pediatr 1979; 95:696–700.

Castilla EE, et al.: Epidemiology of pigmented naevi: incidence rates and relative frequency. Br J Dermatol 1981; 104:307–315.

Castilla EE, et al.: Epidemiology of pigmented naevi: risk factors. Br J Dermatol 1981; 104:421–427.

Rhodes AR, et al.: Non-epidermal origin of malignant melanoma associated with giant congenital nevocellular nevi. Plast Reconstr Surg 1981; 67:782–790.

Rhodes AR, et al.: Familial aggregation of small congenital nevomelanocytic nevi. Am J Med Genet 1985; 22:315–326.

Rhodes AR: Neoplasms: benign neoplasms, hyperplasias, and dysplasias of melanocytes. In: Fitzpatrick TB, et al., eds: Dermatology in General Medicine, ed. 3. New York: McGraw Hill, 1987: 902–915.

RH003

**Arthur R. Rhodes**

## NEVUS, EPIDERMAL NEVUS SYNDROME                0593

**Includes:**
 Epidermal nevus syndrome
 Ichthyosis hystrix gravior
 Inflammatory linear verrucous epidermal nevus (ILVEN)
 Jadassohn linear nevus sebaceous syndrome
 Lambert type ichthyosis
 Linear nevus sebaceous syndrome
 Linear sebaceous nevus syndrome
 Nevus sebaceus of Jadassohn
 "Porcupine man"
 Sebaceous nevus syndrome

**Excludes:**
 **Angio-osteohypertrophy syndrome** (0055)
 **Ichthyosis** (all generalized forms)
 **Ichthyosis hystrix, Curth-Macklin type** (2857)
 **Incontinentia pigmenti** (0526)
 **Limb reduction-ichthyosis** (2019)
 **Nevus, congenital melanocytic** (2165)
 **Proteus syndrome** (2382)

**Major Diagnostic Criteria:** At birth or soon after, alopecia with absent or primitive hair follicles and numerous small hypoplastic sebaceous glands with hyperpigmentation and hyperkeratosis. Lesions are usually on the scalp, in the para-midfacial area, from the forehead down into the nasal area. These tend to be linear in distribution, and may also affect the trunk and limbs. At puberty, the lesions become verrucous with hyperplastic sebaceous glands, and tumors may develop. The condition may be associated with

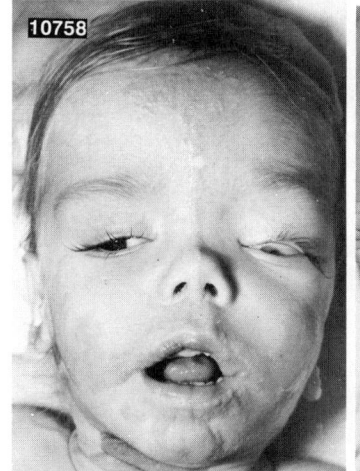
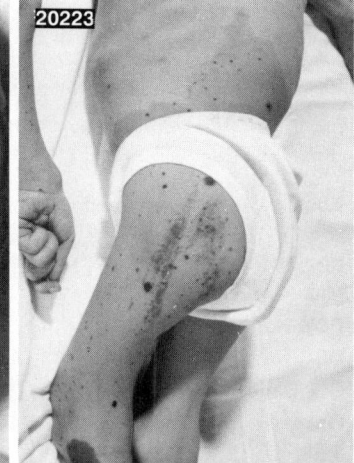
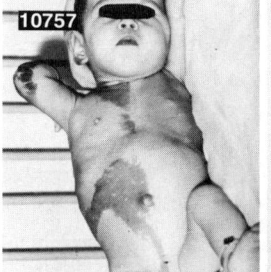
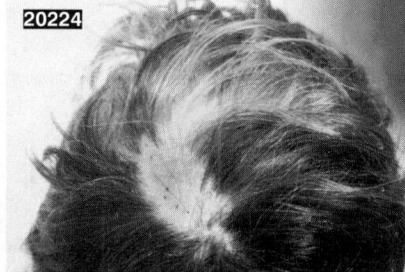

**0593-10758:** Facial distribution of epidermal nevus. **20223:** Linear distribution on the trunk and leg. **10757:** Note the asymmetry and linear distribution of the skin lesions. **20224:** Orange lesion of the scalp in an area of alopecia.

bony anomalies, ocular anomalies, central nervous system dysfunction, or nevoid anomalies.

**Clinical Findings:** The first stage consists of alopecia with absent or primitive hair follicles and numerous small hypoplastic sebaceous glands with hyperpigmentation and hyperkeratosis. One or more of the five major types of epidermal nevi may appear (dark, velvety patches; raised warty streaks; scaly streaks on segments of the body; polyp-like masses arranged in a linear manner; or an orange, bald, velvety mass covering part of the scalp, face, eyes, and nose). Lesions often involve the midfacial area, from the forehead down into the nasal area. These tend to be linear in distribution, and may also affect the trunk and limbs. The skin lesions usually progress after birth, altering their size, thickness, and severity with growth and stabilization at age 15–20 years. The lesions tend to become verrucous, and early surgical removal should be considered since there is a risk of tumor; especially basal cell epithelioma.

Other findings can include: epidermal nevus (60%); mental retardation (40%); seizures (33%); skeletal anomalies (70%), including bony hypertrophy; cysts, kyphosis, and scoliosis (28%); ankle, and foot deformities (15%); and ocular abnormalities (33%); including dermolipoid.

Periods of unpredictable rapid growth of the lesions have been reported. Onset of seizures, in cases with central nervous system involvement, has been between two months and two years of age. Intelligence ranges from normal to severe mental retardation.

Inflammatory linear verrucous epidermal nevus (ILVEN) is a related but possibly distinct condition (Hamm and Happle, 1986).

**Complications:** Oral and ocular involvement with the nevus; severe social and learning problems; with hypertrophic changes, functional problems of walking and using hands may develop. Buying clothes becomes more difficult. Cerebrovascular accidents may be a major problem.

**Associated Findings: Hemihypertrophy; Cancer, Wilms tumor;** vitamin D-resistant rickets; vascular defects of skin, bone, brain, and kidney.

Specific ocular findings can include cloudy cornea, coloboma of the eyelid, iris and choroid, esotropia, and lipodermoid of the conjunctiva. Other reported anomalies include asymmetric cortical atrophy, **Hydrocephaly, Aorta, coarctation, Ventricular septal defect,** hypoplastic teeth, renal hamartomata, and nephroblastoma.

**Etiology:** Undetermined. Some pedigrees (about two-thirds) suggest autosomal dominant inheritance.

**Pathogenesis:** Unknown.

**MIM No.:** 16320, *14660

**POS No.:** 3215

**CDC No.:** 757.380

**Sex Ratio:** M1:F1

**Occurrence:** Undetermined. About 450 cases have been reported among whites, Blacks, Indians, Orientals, and Hispanics.

**Risk of Recurrence for Patient's Sib:** Unknown. Available data suggest about a 1% risk.

**Risk of Recurrence for Patient's Child:** Unknown.

**Age of Detectability:** For most patients, at birth.

**Gene Mapping and Linkage:** Unknown.

**Prevention:** None known. Genetic counseling indicated.

**Treatment:** Surgical removal of a large lesion is often not possible or does not improve the appearance. Smaller lesions may be surgically removed. Topically, 5–10% lactic acid in 50% aqueous solution of propylene glycol helps somewhat. Propylene glycol absorbed in quantity may be nephrotoxic and caution is advised. Lubricants help somewhat. Topical retinoic acid solution is helpful. Orally administered 13-cis-retinoic acid may help in some patients, but it has many unwanted side effects and its use for this purpose is experimental at this time. Involvement of bones, eyes, and other organs may require attention.

**Prognosis:** Longevity is occasionally affected because of the relatively high incidence of associated malignancies. (e.g., malignant astrocytoma). In most instances, however, longevity is unaffected. Functional impairment varies with the extent to which the central nervous system, vascular system, kidneys, and skeleton are involved.

**Detection of Carrier:** Undetermined. Bianchine (1970) reported seizures and/or mental deficiency without skin lesions in first degree relatives of one patient.

**Special Considerations:** Opinions are divided as to the overlap between this condition and several related disorders. One good example is the famous Lambert pedigree *ichthyosis hystrix gravior*, sometimes called the "porcupine man", discussed in some detail by Anton-Lamprecht (1978).

**References:**
Solomon LM, et al.: The epidermal nevus syndrome. Arch Dermatol 1968; 97:273–285.
Bianchine JW: The nevus sebaceus of Jadassohn: a neurocutaneous syndrome and a potentially premalignant lesion. Am J Dis Child 1970; 120:223–228.
Lansky LL, et al.: Linear sebaceous nevus syndrome. Am J Dis Child 1972; 123:587–590.
Anton-Lamprecht I: Electron microscope in the early diagnosis of genetic disorders of the skin. Dermatologica 1978; 157:65–85.
Leonidas JC, et al.: Radiographic features of the linear sebaceous syndrome. Am J Roentgenol 1979; 132:277–279.
Monk BE, Vollum DI: Familial naevus sebaceus. J Royal Soc Med 1982; 75:660–661.
Hamm H, Happle R: Inflammatory linear verrucous epidermal nevus (ILVEN) in a mother and her daughter. Am J Med Genet 1986; 24:685–690.
Baker RS, et al.: Neurologic complications of the epidermal nevus syndrome. Arch Neurol 1987; 44:227–232.
Rogers M, et al.: Epidermal nevi and the epidermal nevus syndrome: a review of 131 cases. J Am Acad Derm 1989; 20:476–488.

S0009                                    **Lawrence M. Solomon**

**Nezelof syndrome**
    *See IMMUNODEFICIENCY, NEZELOF TYPE*
**NF-1**
    *See NEUROFIBROMATOSIS*
**NFDR syndrome**
    *See NEURO-FACIO-DIGITO-RENAL SYNDROME*
**Nicotinamide adenine dinucleotide and oxidoreductase**
    *See LACTATE DEHYDROGENASE ISOZYMES*

---

**NIEMANN-PICK DISEASE**                              **0717**

**Includes:**
    Niemann-Pick disease with cholesterol esterification block
    Nova Scotian type Niemann-Pick disease
    Sea-blue histiocyte disease
    Sphingomyelin lipidosis
    Sphingomyelinase deficiency

**Excludes:**
    Gaucher disease (0406)
    G(M1)-gangliosidosis, type 1 (0431)
    G(M2)-gangliosidosis with hexosaminidase A deficiency (0434)
    Wolman disease (1003)

**Major Diagnostic Criteria:** Enlargement of liver or spleen; presence of foam cells in bone marrow, liver, or spleen; demonstration of abnormal intracellular accumulation of sphingomyelin, and a negative search for other situations that may produce secondary formation of similar foam cells.

**Clinical Findings:** The term "Niemann-Pick disease" is applied to five phenotypes that have areas of clinical and genetic difference but a presumed biochemical relationship:
    *Group A:* Acute neuronopathic form.
    *Group B:* Chronic form without nervous system involvement.
    *Group C:* Chronic neuronopathic form.
    *Group D:* Nova Scotia variant.

*Group E:* Adult non-neuronopathic form.

Enlargement of the spleen and liver is common to all Groups and is usually quite notable, while lymphadenopathy is not prominent. The hematologic effects of the spenomegaly ("hypersplenism") are common, but are less intense than in **Gaucher disease**. Pulmonary infiltration is characteristic in the circumstances in which organomegaly is of high order and growth impairment is of varying degree. All forms except the remarkable "adult" type (Group B) have increasingly serious neurologic involvement, including developmental delay and arrest followed by general functional deterioration. Occasional patients have seizures, and the older children may show ataxia or other cerebellar signs. Cherry-red macular changes are noted in some of the patients, especially the younger ones. Occasional children develop small papular or nodular skin xanthomas, which are apparently not secondary to hyperlipidemia, the latter being seen only in Group A and B patients. It is usual to find vacuolization of some of the lymphocytes in the peripheral blood. The diagnosis can be made by recognition of a large foamy cell in the bone marrow. Electron microscopic studies show cytoplasmic lipid inclusions consisting of concentric laminar bodies.

A sixth form, sometimes called Group F, has been identified in populations of Spanish background. This group is distinguished, in part, by sea-blue or foamy histiocytes. At present, it is not clear if this is a unique form of Niemann-Pick, a specific condition sometimes called *Sea-blue histiocyte disease*, or a variation of Groups A, B, or C Niemann-Pick disease.

**Complications:** Chronic nutritional failure eventually ensues, as well as progressive debility and mental retardation (except in Group B patients). Bronchopneumonia occurs in the terminal patients, as does anemia and ascites. Hepatic failure has been described in Group B.

**Associated Findings:** Prolonged jaundice of moderate degree in the first 6 months of life is reported in about one-quarter of the patients and is of unknown significance.

**Etiology:** Autosomal recessive inheritance.

**Pathogenesis:** Specific sphingomyelinase deficiency has been identified in the tissues, cultured fibroblasts, and white blood cells of patients from Group A and B. In Group C the exact enzymatic defect is not known; recent works seem to demonstrate that the impairment of sphingomyelin metabolism is not the primary defect, the sphingomyelin levels are normal in most of the tissues, and there is accumulation of cholesterol, which could be responsible for the inhibition of sphingomyelin degradation. Pentchev et al (1984) found Group C cell lines to differ from Group A and B in that Group C showed a major block in cholesterol esterification. Somatic cell hybridization experiments suggest that the defect in Group C is under separate genetic control from that in Groups A and B. Group D might represent an allelic form of the Group C gene.

It appears reasonable to assume that local tissue sphingomyelin accumulation can be adequately explained on the basis of the lysosomal enzyme insufficiency. An explanation is also needed, however, for the simultaneous cholesterol increase in tissues, unless, as Brady (1983) has suggested, a specific intermolecular complex (of cholesterol and sphingomyelin) is formed. The specific origin of the CNS defect is incompletely understood. Only in Group A patients is there a cortical increase in sphingomyelin, per se, and in Group B patients (with the same enzymopathy) the brain is normal.

**MIM No.:** *25720, *25722, *25725, 26960

**POS No.:** 3334

**Sex Ratio:** M1:F1

**Occurrence:** Several hundred cases reported. About 80% of Group A patients, which account for about 85% of all Niemann-Pick cases, are of Ashkenazi Jewish ancestry. The carrier rate among Jews is about 1:100. Group D is usually found among decendents of a 17th Century French Acadian couple from Yarmouth county, Nova Scotia.

**Risk of Recurrence for Patient's Sib:**
See Part I, *Mendelian Inheritance.*

**Risk of Recurrence for Patient's Child:**
See Part I, *Mendelian Inheritance.* A number of persons with Group B involvement are now known to have had normal children.

**Age of Detectability:** Prenatal diagnosis is possible for Groups A and B patients. Hepatosplenomegaly is detectable after age 2–3 months, and developmental delays are detectable shortly thereafter. Group C and D patients often have prolonged jaundice in the early months of life.

**Gene Mapping and Linkage:** SMPD1 (sphingomyelin phosphodiesterase 1, acid lysosomal) has been provisionally mapped to 17.

**Prevention:** None known. Genetic counseling indicated.

**Treatment:** No specific therapy is known. Supportive treatment is important for the child and family. This includes assistance in feeding, control of infection, anticonvulsants where needed, transfusion, or splenectomy.

**Prognosis:** Group A patients present the so-called classic picture, with onset of symptoms in early infancy, marked organomegaly, rapidly advancing CNS handicaps, and death by three years of age. Group B patients show the same massive sphingomyelin accumulation in the liver and spleen, and the pulmonary changes, as seen in the classically involved infants (Group A), but the nervous system is not affected. Although these patients survive into adulthood, they may not live a normal life span because of complications from visceral lipid storage. Group C patients show a pattern now being identified with reasonable frequency, characterized by developmental slowing beginning in late infancy, moderate chemical changes, enlargement of the liver and spleen, and gradual debilitation leading to death by 3 to 9 years of age. Group D involvement has been found most notably in persons of French-Canadian ancestry from Nova Scotia, with neurologic difficulties in mid-childhood (including cerebellar and athetoid symptoms), and survival until 12–20 years of age. Group E occurs in adults with moderate hepatosplenomegaly and no neurologic signs. Some of these could be a late onset variant of Group C.

**Detection of Carrier:** Parents and uninvolved sibs have no known clinical handicaps. The level of sphingomyelinase activity in the white blood cells and cultured fibroblasts from Group A and B is significantly reduced.

**Special Considerations:** A new classification system proposed by Spence and Callahan (1989) is expected to replace the old A-E classifications.

*The author is indebted to Allen C. Crocker for his contributions to an earlier version of this article.*

**References:**

Fried K, et al.: Biochemical, genetic and ultrastructural study of a family with sea-blue histiocyte syndrome: chronic and non-neuropathic Niemann-Pick disease. Europ J Clin Invest 1978; 8:249–253.

Walton DS, et al: Ocular manifestations of group A Niemann-Pick disease. Am J Ophthal 1978; 85:174–180. †

Winsor EJT, Welch JP: Genetic and demographic aspects of Nova Scotia Niemann-Pick disease (type D). Am J Hum Genet 1978; 30:530–538.

Wenger DA, et al.: Niemann-Pick disease type B: prenatal diagnosis and enzymatic and chemical studies on fetal brain and liver. Am J Hum Genet 1981; 33:337–344.

Pentchev PG, et al.: A genetic storage disorder in BALB/C mice with a metabolic block in esterification of exogenous cholesterol. J Biol Chem 1984; 259:5784–5791.

Palmer M, et al.: Niemann-Pick disease, type C: ocular, histopathologic and electron microscopic studies. Arch Ophthal 1985; 103:817–822. †

Levade T, Salvayre R, Douste-Blazy: Sphingomyelinases and Niemann-Pick disease. J Clin Chem Clin Biochem 1986; 24:205–220.

Maciejko D, Tylky-Szymanska A: Clinical and biochemical diagnostics of Niemann-Pick Disease. Klin Padiat 1986; 198:103–106.

Spence MW, Callahan JW: Sphingomyelin-cholesterol lipidosis: the Niemann-Pick group of diseases. In: Scriver CR, et al, eds: The metabolic basis of inherited disease, 6th ed. New York: McGraw-Hill, 1989:1655–1676.

TR008                                                    **Carlos J. Trujillo-Botero**

**Niemann-Pick disease with cholesterol esterification block**
*See NIEMANN-PICK DISEASE*
**Nievergelt syndrome**
*See MESOMELIC DYSPLASIA, NIEVERGELT TYPE*
**Nightblindness (congenital stationary) with normal fundus**
*See NIGHTBLINDNESS, CONGENITAL STATIONARY, AUTOSOMAL DOMINANT*

---

## NIGHTBLINDNESS, CONGENITAL STATIONARY, AUTOSOMAL DOMINANT                3205

**Includes:**
> Hemeralopia
> Nightblindness (congenital stationary) with normal fundus
> Nougaret disease

**Excludes:**
> Nightblindness with myopia
> **Nightblindness, congenital stationary, X-linked recessive** (0718)
> **Nightblindness, congenital stationary, autosomal recessive** (3204)
> **Nightblindness, Oguchi type** (0740)

**Major Diagnostic Criteria:**  Infantile onset, nonprogressive nightblindness with normal visual acuity, visual fields, and fundus. There is generally a positive family history. Electrophysiologic testing is diagnostic with a diminished ERG and an abnormal EOG. The ERG shows a very reduced photopic response without any scotopic increment.

**Clinical Findings:**  Infantile onset nightblindness of a nonprogressive nature. Visual acuity is normal as are the visual fields and color vision. The paradoxical (Flynn-Barricks) pupil response may occur. Funduscopically the disc, macula, retinal vessels and periphery are normal. The ERG shows a very reduced photopic response without scotopic increment. The initial 'a' wave is attenuated and there is an absence of the large 'b' wave response. In affected patients, the EOG is abnormal with a marked reduction in the EOG light rise.

**Complications:**  Unknown.

**Associated Findings:**  **Syndactyly** has been reported in one family member of a five generation pedigree.

**Etiology:**  Autosomal dominant inheritance.

**Pathogenesis:**  Apparently a result of a defect in neural transmission. The defect may lie at the level of the inner segment of the photoreceptors. Histology has been shown to be normal (except for slightly weak staining with Mac Mannus staining of the outer segments of the photorecptors.) Rhodopsin metabolism is normal.

**MIM No.:**  *16350

**Sex Ratio:**  M1:F1

**Occurrence:**  Several hundred cases have been documented, including Blacks, since Cunier (1838) first identified the condition among decendants of Jean Nougaret, a French butcher.

**Risk of Recurrence for Patient's Sib:**
> See Part I, *Mendelian Inheritance*.

**Risk of Recurrence for Patient's Child:**
> See Part I, *Mendelian Inheritance*.

**Age of Detectability:**  Correlation of history, clinical findings, and electrophysiologic testing allow early diagnosis.

**Gene Mapping and Linkage:**  Unknown.

**Prevention:**  None known. Genetic counseling indicated.

**Treatment:**  Unknown.

**Prognosis:**  This is a nonprogressive disorder. Visual acuity remains stable.

**Detection of Carrier:**  Unknown.

**Special Considerations:**  It must be noted that patients may have either of two types of ERG response and the response is not specific to a particular hereditary pattern, although a "Nougaret type" ERG response refers to one in which there is a reduced photopic response and no scotopic increment.

**References:**
Cunier F: Historie d'une hemeralopie hereditaire du puis deux siecles dans une famille de al commune de Vendemian pres Montpellier. Annales de la societe de medicin de Gaand 1838; 4:385–395.
Nettleship E: A history of congenital stationary nightblindness in nine consecutive generations. Trans Ophthalmol Soc U.K. 1907; 27:269–293.
Carr RE: Congenital stationary nightblindness. Trans Am Ophthalmol Soc 1974; 82:448–487.

AL031                                                   **Deborah Alcorn**
MA054                                               **Irene H. Maumenee**

---

## NIGHTBLINDNESS, CONGENITAL STATIONARY, AUTOSOMAL RECESSIVE                3204

**Includes:**
> Myopia (high-grade)-nightblindness
> Nightblindness-high-grade myopia
> Stationary nightblindness with normal fundus, congenital

**Excludes:**
> **Nightblindness, congenital stationary, autosomal dominant** (3205)
> **Nightblindness, congenital stationary, X-linked recessive** (0718)
> **Nightblindness, Oguchi type** (0740)
> **Retina, amaurosis congenita, Leber type** (0043)
> **Retina, fundus albipunctatus** (0399)

**Major Diagnostic Criteria:**  Infantile onset, nonprogressive nightblindness. Most have normal visual acuity, but it may be diminished secondary to myopic changes. Most patients demonstrate a "negative" type ERG. Dark adaptation testing shows a bipartite curve with very slight adaptation of the rod system and the cone level is above the threshold.

**Clinical Findings:**  Infantile onset nightblindness, nonprogressive. Visual acuity is normal as are the visual fields and color vision. The paradoxical (Flynn-Barricks) pupil always occurs. Funduscopically the disc, macula, retinal vessels, and periphery are normal unless there is associated myopia. ERG findings may be of two types. The first shows a reduced photopic response with any scotopic increment. In these patients the EOG is abnormal with a marked reduction in the light rise. The second type shows a "negative" ERG in which the 'a' wave is normal to increased in size and the positive 'b' wave is absent or markedly reduced. EOG in this second group shows a normal light rise.

**Complications:**  Patients may be at increased risk of rhegmatogenous retinal detachments, associated with the myopia.

**Associated Findings:**  None known.

**Etiology:**  Autosomal recessive inheritance.

**Pathogenesis:**  It has been shown that the rods have a normal density of pigment and that following bleaching, rod pigment regenerates normally, and manifest a normal 'a' wave on ERG testing. All of the above indicate that the rod outer segments are functioning. But the 'b' wave is markedly reduced and therefore it has been suggested that the defect may lie in the neural transmission from the photoreceptor terminals to bipolar cells.

**MIM No.:**  *25727

**Sex Ratio:**  M1:F1

**Occurrence:**  Undetermined but presumably rare.

**Risk of Recurrence for Patient's Sib:**
> See Part I, *Mendelian Inheritance*.

**Risk of Recurrence for Patient's Child:**
> See Part I, *Mendelian Inheritance*.

**Age of Detectability:**  Correlation of history, clinical findings, and electrophysiologic testing allows early diagnosis.

**Gene Mapping and Linkage:**  Unknown.

**Prevention:**  None known. Genetic counseling indicated.

**Treatment:**  Unknown.

**Prognosis:** This is a stationary disease and visual acuity should remain stable.

**Detection of Carrier:** Unknown.

**Special Considerations:** In the cases of autosomal recessive CSNB with associated myopia, the patients may also have poor vision, strabismus, and nystagmus as seen in **Nightblindness, congenital stationary, X-linked recessive**. These patients are at increased risk of retinal detachments. They will also demonstrate a "negative" type ERG response and have a normal EOG.

**References:**

Gassler VJ: Ueber eine bis jetzt nicht bekannte recessive Verknuepfung von hochgradiger Myopie mit angeborener Hemaralopie. Arch Klaus Stift Vererbungoforsch 1925; 1:259–272.

Der Kaloustian VM, Baghdassarian SA: The autosomal recessive variety of congenital stationary night blindness with myopia. J Med Genet 1972; 9:67–69.

Carr RE: Congenital stationary nightblindness. Trans Am Ophthalmol Soc 1974; 72:448–487.

Weleber RG, Tongue AC: Congenital stationary night blindness presenting as Leber's congenital amaurosis. Arch Ophthal 1987; 105: 360–365.

AL031
MA054

**Deborah Alcorn**
**Irene H. Maumenee**

## NIGHTBLINDNESS, CONGENITAL STATIONARY, X-LINKED RECESSIVE      0718

**Includes:**

    Hemeralopia-myopia, X-linked
    Myopia-nightblindness, X-linked
    Stationary nightblindness with high myopia congenital

**Excludes:**

    **Forsius-Eriksson syndrome** (3183)
    **Retina, fundus albipunctatus** (0399)
    **Nightblindness, congenital stationary, autosomal dominant** (3205)
    **Nightblindness, congenital stationary, autosomal recessive** (3204)
    **Nightblindness, Oguchi type** (0740)

**Major Diagnostic Criteria:** Infantile onset nonprogressive nyctalopia, nystagmus, and moderate to severe myopia. Corrected visual acuity is usually reduced and mild nystagmus may persist lifelong. The fundus is normal except for myopic changes. The ERG is characterized by small or absent oscillatory potentials and a "negative" ERG with a large "a" and a small "b" wave.

**Clinical Findings:** The nightblindness is congenital and stationary. Visual acuity is usually subnormal, and may vary from 20/20 to 3/200 among patients. The degree of myopia ranges from -2.00 D to -20.00 D. Patients with subnormal vision usually have associated horizontal nystagmus and strabismus is common. The visual fields are normal or reveal defects consistent with the degree of myopia. Color vision is usually normal, although slight abnormalities may be seen as a tritan axis on Farnsworth-Munsell 100 hue testing. The anterior segment examination is normal, although the paradoxical (Feynn-Barricks) pupil occurs in younger individuals. The fundus demonstrates myopic changes of the posterior pole of variable severity. This includes peripapillary choroidal atrophy, temporal disc pallor, or tilted disc. ERG testing after dark adaptation shows a large "a" wave with a distinctive squared-off appearance and a small "b" wave. This results in a "negative" ERG. There are identical peak times of the dark and light adapted responses. The oscillatory potentials under photopic testing are very small or absent. Dark adaptation testing reveals a delayed rod-cone break with an elevated cone and rod threshold. The EOG shows a normal light rise. The disease is stationary and visual acuity does not deteriorate. There may be an increase in the amount of myopia, particularly in those patients with a high degree of myopia at a young age.

It has been shown that the ERG pattern of congenital stationary nightblindness is not specific to any particular hereditary pattern.

**Complications:** Related to myopia, but without an increased frequency of retinal detachment compared to other patients with high myopia.

**Associated Findings:** None known.

**Etiology:** X-linked inheritance.

**Pathogenesis:** Because of the findings of a normal EOG and a normal "a" wave on ERG testing, the outer retinal layers are presumed to be normal. The abnormal "b" wave, originating from the bipolar cell regions suggests an abnormality in neural transmission. Both the rod and cone systems are affected. Rhodopsin kinetics are normal.

**MIM No.:** *31050

**Sex Ratio:** M1:F0

**Occurrence:** Undetermined but presumed rare.

**Risk of Recurrence for Patient's Sib:**
See Part I, *Mendelian Inheritance.*

**Risk of Recurrence for Patient's Child:**
See Part I, *Mendelian Inheritance.*

**Age of Detectability:** Congenital onset of nyctalopia with nonprogression of disease. Correlation of history, clinical findings, and electrophysiologic studies permits an early diagnosis.

**Gene Mapping and Linkage:** CSNB1 (congenital stationary night blindness 1) has been mapped to Xp21.1-p11.23.

**Prevention:** None known. Genetic counseling indicated.

**Treatment:** No effective treatment known except to accurately correct the refractive error (myopia).

**Prognosis:** Visual acuity usually remains stable, but with increasing degree of myopia with age, particularly those patients with high myopia at a young age. The visual function may actually improve with age. The nightblindness remains stationary.

**Detection of Carrier:** Carrier females have normal visual acuity, visual fields, and color vision. Their ERGs show a selective reduction in the amplitude of oscillatory potentials, but with peak time of each of the oscillatory potentials being normal.

**References:**

Morton AS: Two cases of hereditary congenital night blindness without visible fundus change. Trans Opthal Soc U.K. 1893;13:147–150.

Francois J, DeRouck A: Sex-linked myopic chorioretinal heredodegeneration. Am J Ophthal 1965;60:670–678.

Merin S, et al: Syndrome of congenital high myopia with nyctalopia. Am J Ophthalmol 1970;70:541–547.

Carr RE: Congenital stationary nightblindness. Trans Am Ophthalmol Soc 1974;72:448–487.

AL031
MA054

**Deborah Alcorn**
**Irene H. Maumenee**

## NIGHTBLINDNESS, OGUCHI TYPE      0740

**Includes:** Oguchi disease types 1, 2A and 2B

**Excludes:**

    Cone dystrophy, X-linked late onset
    **Nightblindness** (other)
    **Retina, fundus albipunctatus** (0399)

**Major Diagnostic Criteria:** Abnormal fundus discoloration in patient with nightblindness with characteristic disappearance of discoloration and occurrence of secondary dark-adaptation after prolonged period in the dark.

**Clinical Findings:** This form of stationary nightblindness is associated with a peculiar discoloration of the fundus, which, with prolonged dark-adaptation, will usually lead to a disappearance of the abnormal fundus coloration and marked improvement or normalization of subjective dark-adaptation. The coloration is described as grey or yellow and may be homogenous or streaky in appearance. The abnormal coloration may be found throughout the entire eyegrounds, only in the midperipheral area or mainly in the posterior eyegrounds. The abnormal zones of coloration are brilliant with more pronounced reflexes than normal. The underlying choroid is usually invisible under areas of abnormal coloration and it may be difficult to distinguish retinal veins from retinal arterioles in such areas.

Patients with Oguchi disease have been divided into two major types. Most patients fall into type 1 and are characterized by the occurrence of secondary or rod dark-adaptation after a sufficient period of time in the dark. The final threshold may be normal or elevated. With time in the dark, the abnormal fundus discoloration disappears. This latter event is known as Mizuo phenomenon. Patients with type 2 show no secondary or rod dark-adaptation. These patients have less striking abnormal fundus coloration than those classified as type 1. Some of these patients, type 2A, show Mizuo phenomenon, whereas others, type 2B, do not.

The disorder is stationary. Although some patients have been reported to have mild color defects and some visual field constriction, there is usually no other impairment of vision associated with the disease. The ERG shows a normal cone response. The rod response after several minutes of dark adaptation is grossly abnormal with mainly an A wave seen. Even after the patient is allowed to achieve a secondary dark adaptation and the Mizuo phenomenon, the ERG has been reported as abnormal by some investigators but a normal scotopic response to a single flash of light has been reported. The EOG is normal, reflection densitometry and rhodopsin kinetics are normal as is fluorescein angiography. The disorder is most likely one of neural transmission rather than a structural rod abnormality.

**Complications:** Unknown.

**Associated Findings:** None known.

**Etiology:** Autosomal recessive inheritance.

**Pathogenesis:** In two reports, light microscopy showed an abnormal number of cones, many of them larger than normal, in the posterior eyegrounds. Many of these cones were arranged in double rows and contained vesicular spaces between them. In addition there was an abnormal positioning of the cone nuclei, many lying outside of the external limiting membrane. Also, an extra layer with a syncytial structure and strongly pigmented was described between the photoreceptors and the true pigment epithelium. The pigment epithelium cells had dense and shrunken nuclei. However, in a recent histologic examination the extra layer was not detected. Although displaced cone nuclei were seen, the authors noted that in controls without Oguchi disease cone nuclei could sometimes be detected beyond the external limiting membrane. A nodular bulging of the inner side of the pigment epithelium was noted in some areas. This bulging was due to aggregates of fuchsin granules. These same granules were also seen to an abnormal degree among the rods and cones. In areas the pigment epithelium showed thinning and irregularities in cellular structure in many sites.

**MIM No.:** *25810

**Sex Ratio:** M1:F1

**Occurrence:** Undetermined. Has been reported in all races, but most patients were Japanese.

**Risk of Recurrence for Patient's Sib:**
See Part I, *Mendelian Inheritance.*

**Risk of Recurrence for Patient's Child:**
See Part I, *Mendelian Inheritance.*

**Age of Detectability:** When able to respond to necessary testing.

**Gene Mapping and Linkage:** Unknown.

**Prevention:** None known. Genetic counseling indicated.

**Treatment:** Unknown.

**Prognosis:** Normal life span.

**Detection of Carrier:** Unknown.

*The authors are indebted to the late Alex E. Krill for his contributions to an earlier version of this article.*

**References:**

Franīçois J, et al.: La maladie d'Oguchi. Ophthalmologica 1956; 131:1–40.

Carr RE, Gouras P: Oguchi's disease. Arch Ophthalmol 1965; 73:646–656.

Carr RE, Ripps H: Rhodopsin kinetics and rod adaptation in Oguchi's disease. Invest Ophthalmol 1967; 6:426–436.

Yamanaka M: Histologic study of Oquchi's disease: its relationship to pigmentary degeneration of the retina. Am J Ophthalmol 1969; 68:19–26.

Gouras P: Electroretinography: some basic principles. Invest Ophthalmol 1970; 9:557–569.

Gass JDM: Oguchi disease. Stereoscopic atlas of macular diseases. St. Louis: C.V. Mosby, 1987:270–271.

Remler B: New findings in Oguchi's disease. Klin Monatsbl Augenheilkd 1988; 192:239–243.

W0003                                                        **Mitchel L. Wolf**
BE026                                                      **Donald R. Bergsma**

**Nightblindness-high-grade myopia**
See NIGHTBLINDNESS, CONGENITAL STATIONARY, AUTOSOMAL RECESSIVE

**Nigrospinodentatal degeneration with nuclear ophthalmoplegia**
See MACHADO-JOSEPH DISEASE

**Niikawa-Kuroki syndrome**
See KABUKI MAKE-UP SYNDROME

**Nijmegen chromosome breakage syndrome**
See CHROMOSOME INSTABILITY, NIJMEGEN TYPE

**Nipple, congenital absence**
See BREAST, AMASTIA

**Nipples, accessory**
See BREAST, POLYTHELIA

**Nipples, supernumerary nipples**
See BREAST, POLYTHELIA

**Noack syndrome**
See ACROCEPHALOSYNDACTYLY TYPE V
also ACROCEPHALOPOLYSYNDACTYLY

**Nodular erythema-digital changes**
See DIGITAL DEFECTS-NODULAR ERYTHEMA-EMACIATION, NAKAJO TYPE

**Non-African Burkitt lymphoma**
See LYMPHOMA, BURKITT TYPE

**Non-Hodgkin lymphoma of T-cell type**
See LEUKEMIA/LYMPHOMA, T-CELL

**Non-Hodgkin lymphoma of the B-cell type**
See LYMPHOMA, BURKITT TYPE

**Non-Hodgkin lymphoma of B-cell type**
See LEUKEMIA/LYMPHOMA, B-CELL

**Non-immune fetal hydrops**
See HYDROPS FETALIS, NON-IMMUNE

**Non-insulin dependent diabetes mellitus (NIDDM)**
See DIABETES MELLITUS, NON-INSULIN DEPENDENT TYPE

**Non-insulin-dependent diabetes of the young (NIDDY)**
See DIABETES MELLITUS, MATURITY ONSET OF THE YOUNG (MODY)

**Nondisjunction**
See CHROMOSOME 18, TRISOMY 18

**Nonketotic hyperglycinemia**
See HYPERGLYCINEMIA, NON-KETOTIC

**Nonne-Milroy type hereditary lymphedema**
See LYMPHEDEMA I

**Nonobstructive dilation of the intrahepatic biliary tree**
See LIVER, CONGENITAL CYSTIC DILATATION OF INTRAHEPATIC DUCTS

**Nonopalescent opalescent dentine**
See TEETH, DENTIN DYSPLASIA, RADICULAR

**Nonplasmatic thymic alymphoplasia or alymphocytosis**
See IMMUNODEFICIENCY, SEVERE COMBINED

**Nonpolyposis colerectal cancer, hereditary Lynch syndromes**
See CANCER, COLORECTAL

**Nonrotation of midgut**
See INTESTINAL ROTATION, INCOMPLETE

**Nonsteroidal synthetic estrogens, fetal effects**
See FETAL DIETHYLSTILBESTROL (DES) EFFECTS

**Nontropical sprue**
See GLUTEN-SENSITIVE ENTEROPATHY

**Nontumorous primary aldosteronism**
See HYPERALDOSTERONISM, FAMILIAL GLUCOCORTICOID SUPPRESSIBLE

## NOONAN SYNDROME               0720

**Includes:**
- Female pseudo-Turner syndrome
- Female Turner syndrome with normal XX karyotype
- Male Turner syndrome
- Neurofibromatosis-Noonan syndrome
- Noonan-neurofibromatosis syndrome
- Pterygium colli syndrome
- Status Bonnevie-Ullrich
- Turner phenotype with normal karyotype
- Turner syndrome, familial
- Ullrich-Noonan syndrome
- Ullrich syndrome
- XX-XY Turner phenotype

**Excludes:**
- **Fetal primidone syndrome** (2982)
- **Klippel-Feil anomaly** (2032)
- **Lentigines syndrome, multiple** (0586)
- **Pterygium syndrome, multiple** (2186)
- **Pulmonic stenosis-cafe-au-lait spots, Watson type** (2776)
- **Turner syndrome** (0977)

**Major Diagnostic Criteria:** The Noonan syndrome must be delineated at the clinical level. Cardinal features include congenital heart disease, particularly valvular pulmonary stenosis, mild mental retardation, short stature, broad or webbed neck, a peculiar chest deformity with pectus carinatum superiorly and pectus excavatum inferiorly, and characteristic facies that alter predictably with age to produce a discrete but changing phenotype.

**Clinical Findings:** Craniofacial dysmorphism is manifest in the newborn period, when the main features are hypertelorism with down-slanting palpebral fissures (95%), low-set posteriorly-rotated ears with a thick helix (90%), a deeply-grooved philtrum

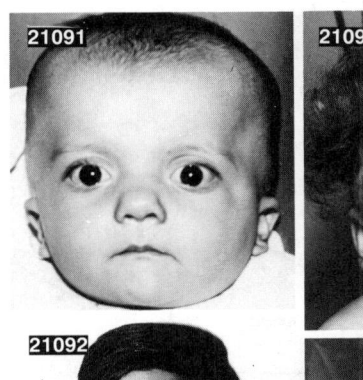
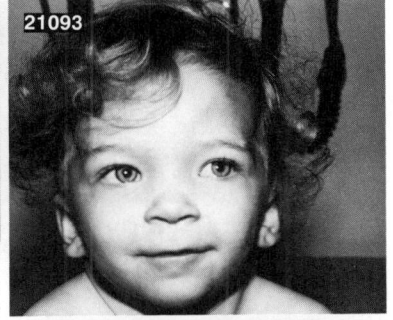
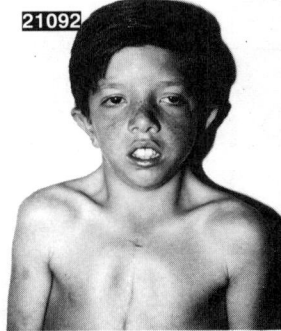
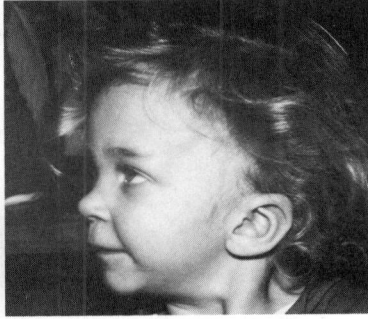

**0720-21091:** Infant with prominent eyes, hypertelorism, depressed nasal bridge and wide nasal base. **21092:** Adolescent male with triangular facies, coarse facial features, webbed neck and pectus deformity. **21093:** Face of a young child with Noonan syndrome; note the posteriorly angulated ears with a thickened helix.

with high wide peaks of the vermilion border of the upper lip (95%), high-arched palate (45%), micrognathia (25%), and excess nuchal skin with a low posterior hairline (55%). There is a consistent predictable change in phenotype with age. In infancy, the head appears relatively large with turricephaly, prominent eyes with level palpebral fissures, hypertelorism, and thick-hooded eyelids or ptosis. The nose has a depressed root, wide base, and bulbous tip. In later childhood, the face often appears coarse or myopathic. With increasing age the contour of the face becomes more triangular. The neck lengthens, accentuating the webbing or prominent trapezius (90%). In the adolescent, the eyes are less prominent, the nose has a pinched root, thinner higher bridge, and wide base. In the older adult, there are prominent nasolabial folds, a high anterior hairline, and transparent wrinkled skin. Hair may be wispy in the infant, but often is curly or woolly in the older child and adolescent. Strikingly blue or blue-green irides, diamond-shaped arched eyebrows, and low-set posteriorly-rotated ears with a thick helix are frequently present.

Birth weight is generally normal (40%), but may be falsely elevated by the presence of subcutaneous edema. Failure to thrive in infancy is common (40%). Prepubertal growth often parallels the third percentile (60%), with a relatively normal growth velocity. The pubertal growth spurt may be reduced or absent. Bone age is delayed in up to 20% of cases. Cryptorchidism, commonly bilateral, occurs in 60% of affected males, and may lead to deficient spermatogenesis. However, normal virilization at puberty, with subsequent fertility, has been documented in males. In females, puberty may be normal or delayed, and fertility is generally unimpaired.

Congenital heart defects occur in approximately 66% of patients. Common lesions include **Pulmonary valve, stenosis** (50%), **Atrial septal defects** (10%), and asymmetric septal hypertrophy (10%). Electrocardiograph typically shows left axis deviation (33%) despite the fact that most cardiac lesions involve the right side of the heart.

A characteristic pectus deformity is seen (70%) with pectus carinatum superiorly and pectus excavatum inferiorly. Other skeletal anomalies include cubitus valgus (50%), clinobrachydactyly with blunt fingertips (30%), vertebral/sternal anomalies (25%), and dental malocclusion (35%).

IQ ranges between 64 and 127, with a median of 102. Mild mental retardation is seen in up to 33% of cases, and motor developmental delay is found in 25% of patients. Language delay (20%) may be secondary to perceptual motor disabilities (15%), mild hearing loss (12%), or articulation abnormalities (72%).

Various bleeding anomalies, including **Factor XI deficiency**, **Von Willebrand disease**, and platelet dysfunction, are documented (20%). Congenital lymphatic abnormalities (20%) may cause general or peripheral lymphedema, pulmonary or intestinal lymphangiectasia, hydrops fetalis, and cystic hygroma. Neonatal peripheral edema is common and may be associated with an increased total fingertip ridge count.

Wide intrafamilial variability in clinical expression is common. The phenotype, particularly in adults, may be extremely subtle. Careful examination of all first-degree relatives is essential, with a review of serial photographs, searching for the discrete change in phenotype.

**Complications:** In males, inadequate secondary sexual development and sterility may be associated with deficient spermatogenesis secondary to earlier cryptorchidism. Congestive heart failure or pulmonary complications resulting from the cardiac defect may occur.

**Associated Findings:** Various skin manifestations include café-au-lait patches (10%), pigmented nevi (25%), and lentigines (2%). Several patients with **Neurofibromatosis** and the Noonan phenotype are reported. Malignant hyperthermia is seen with the Noonan phenotype (see **King syndrome**).

**Etiology:** Autosomal dominant inheritance with variability in expression. Direct transmission from parent to child is documented in 30–75% of cases. "Sporadic" cases are thought to represent new dominant mutations. Maternal transmission of the gene is three times more common than paternal transmission.

This is probably attributable to the frequent occurrence of cryptorchidism and consequent male infertility.

**Pathogenesis:** One current hypothesis implicates lymphedema in the development of the Noonan phenotype. Disruption of normal tissue migration of organ placement by lymphedema may explain pterygium colli, cryptorchidism, wide-spaced nipples, low-set posteriorly-rotated ears, hypertelorism, abnormal dermatoglyphics, and congenital heart defects. The cause of lymphedema is unknown and is likely to be heterogeneous.

**MIM No.:** *16395, 16229

**POS No.:** 3335

**CDC No.:** 759.800

**Sex Ratio:** M1:F1

**Occurrence:** Incidence has been estimated to be between 1:1,000 and 1:2,500 live births.

**Risk of Recurrence for Patient's Sib:**
See Part I, *Mendelian Inheritance.*

**Risk of Recurrence for Patient's Child:**
See Part I, *Mendelian Inheritance.*

**Age of Detectability:** Clinically evident at birth. Prenatal detection of cystic hygroma and/or edema with ultrasound is possible in some cases.

**Gene Mapping and Linkage:** Unknown.

**Prevention:** None known. Genetic counseling indicated.

**Treatment:** Speech therapy is valuable for the child with language delay and/or articulation abnormalities. Cardiac surgery and orchidopexy may be indicated. Abnormal coagulation, when present, may require therapy.

**Prognosis:** Life expectancy is probably normal in those individuals without severe congenital heart disease or profound failure to thrive.

**Detection of Carrier:** Careful clinical examination of all first-degree relatives is essential to identify those who are minimally affected. Review of serial photographs will help to document the change in phenotype. Electrocardiogram and echocardiogram provide additional information when clinical examination is ambiguous.

**Special Considerations:** Preference for the term Noonan syndrome should avoid the confusing use of the *Turner* and *Ullrich* eponyms. While patients with Noonan syndrome, both male and female, share some phenotypic features with females with Turner syndrome, the absence of a detectable chromosome abnormality, the familial nature of Noonan syndrome, and careful clinical examination should allow differentiation of the two conditions.

No characteristic cytogenetic, biochemical, or metabolic abnormality has been detected. Several patients are reported with Noonan syndrome and trimethylaminuria or a fishy odor to the urine, in association with platelet dysfunction.

Lymphatic obstruction has been shown to cause left heart defects in a canine model. Lymphatic obstruction could similarly reduce right-sided cardiac blood flow and cause pulmonary stenosis.

The association between Noonan syndrome and **Neurofibromatosis** reported in several cases, remains controversial. Both neurofibromatosis and Noonan syndrome are common conditions with variable expression. The two conditions share some manifestations: short stature, learning disabilities or mild mental retardation, scoliosis or other skeletal abnormalities, and pulmonary stenosis. All cases of *neurofibromatosis-Noonan syndrome* until now appear to be sporadic. The presence of increased paternal age in some cases is suggestive of a new dominant mutation. Although occasional patients with neurofibromatosis may have a Noonan-like phenotype and although Noonan syndrome patients are predisposed to neural crest dysplasias (café-au-lait spots, multiple pigmented moles, tumors originating from neural tissue), it seems likely that the cases with neurofibromatosis-Noonan syndrome (or "Noonan-neurofibromatosis") have a separate "new" neurocristopathy.

**References:**
Noonan JA, Ehmke DA: Associated noncardiac malformations in children with congenital heart disease. J Pediatr 1963; 63:468–470.
Allanson JE, et al.: Noonan phenotype associated with neurofibromatosis. Am J Med Genet 1985; 21:457–462.
Allanson JE, et al.: Noonan syndrome: the changing phenotype. Am J Med Genet 1985; 21:507–514. †
Opitz JM, Weaver DD: The neurofibromatosis-Noonan syndrome. Am J Med Genet 1985; 21:477–490.
Mendez HMM, Opitz JM: Noonan syndrome: a review. Am J Med Genet 1985; 21:493–506. *
Allanson JE: Noonan syndrome. J Med Genet 1987; 24:9–13. * †
Witt DR, et al.: Lymphedema in Noonan syndrome: clues to pathogenesis and prenatal diagnosis and review of the literature. Am J Med Genet 1987; 27:841–856.
Witt DR, et al. Bleeding diathesis in Noonan syndrome. Am J Med Genet 1988; 31:305–317.

AL010                                              **Judith E. Allanson**

**Noonan-like McDonough syndrome**
*See McDONOUGH SYNDROME*
**Noonan-like phenotype-malignant hyperthermia**
*See KING SYNDROME*
**Noonan-neurofibromatosis syndrome**
*See NOONAN SYNDROME*
**Norman-Roberts syndrome**
*See LISSENCEPHALY SYNDROME*
**Normokalemic periodic paralysis**
*See PARALYSIS, NORMOKALEMIC PERIODIC*
**Normopepsinogenemic I duodenal ulcer**
*See PEPTIC ULCER DISEASES, NON-SYNDROMIC*
**Norrbottnian Gaucher disease**
*See GAUCHER DISEASE*

## NORRIE DISEASE                                          0721

**Includes:**
Atrophia bulborum hereditaria
Episkopi blindness
Microcephaly-vitreoretinal dysplasia
Oculo-acoustic cerebral degeneration, congenital progressive
Pseudoglioma of the retina, congenital, bilateral, X-linked
Vitreoretinal dysplasia, X-linked

**Excludes:**
**Chromosome 13, trisomy 13** (0168)
Encephaloretinal dysplasia
**Retinal dysplasia** (0866)
**Eye, vitreous, persistent hyperplastic primary** (0994)

**Major Diagnostic Criteria:** Recessive X-linked dysplasia of the retina existing bilaterally in boys blind from birth.

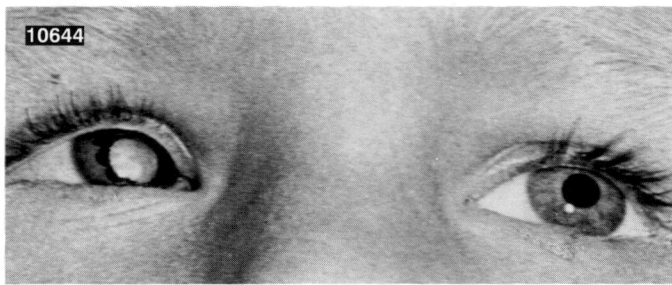

0721-10644: The right eye is deep-set. There is a white mass— not a cataract—behind the lens. This is the totally detached retina with hemorrhages and vascular hyperplasia. The left eye is artificial. This eye was removed due to suspicion of retinoblastoma.

**Clinical Findings:** The typical presenting sign is bilateral white pupillary reflexes (leukocoria) in micro-ophthalmic eyes evident at birth or shortly afterward. The anterior chamber is shallow, and the pupil is commonly dilated with no light reflex.

Posterior synechia, ectropion of the iris pigment fringe, and a hypoplastic iris usually are present. A gray membrane or gray-yellow opaque vascularized mass, which may be hemorrhagic, is apparent behind the lens. Elongated ciliary processes are often visible, and, in cases in which the fundus can be seen, retinal folds, retinal detachment, and pseudotumor formations may be observed. The affected patients are totally blind from birth. The lens and cornea are initially clear; however, both typically become opaque with time. Phthisis bulbi is the usual end result and typically occurs by age 10 years. Many of the observed patients become mentally retarded (25–40%) and severe deafness (25–35%) frequently develops later in life.

**Complications:** *Developmental:* mental retardation, sensorineural deafness.

*Secondary:* complicated cataract, retinal detachment, corneal opacities, secondary glaucoma, band keratopathy, phthisis bulbi.

**Associated Findings:** Microencephaly, cryptorchidism, hypogonadism, increased susceptibility to infection, growth disturbances.

**Etiology:** X-linked recessive inheritance.

**Pathogenesis:** Unknown.

**MIM No.:** *31060

**POS No.:** 3336

**Sex Ratio:** M1:F0. Homozygous affected females may occur.

**Occurrence:** About 100 cases from over a dozen kindreds have been reported in the literature, including a Greek family living in Episkopi, Cyprus.

**Risk of Recurrence for Patient's Sib:**
See Part I, *Mendelian Inheritance.*

**Risk of Recurrence for Patient's Child:**
See Part I, *Mendelian Inheritance.*

**Age of Detectability:** At birth. Prenatal diagnosis in utero by chorion villus biopsy is possible. Prenatal exclusion has also been accomplished using flanking DNA markers (Gal et al, 1988)

**Gene Mapping and Linkage:** NDP (Norrie disease (pseudoglioma)) has been mapped to Xp11.4-p11.3.

**Prevention:** None known. Genetic counseling indicated.

**Treatment:** Early surgical intervention consisting of cataract extraction, vitrectomy, and retinal detachment repair have been attempted. These procedures may prevent phthisis bulbi, but they will not improve vision.

Sound amplification and rehabilitation for hearing loss and appropriate treatment for each specific associated defect.

**Prognosis:** Irreversibly blind from birth.

**Detection of Carrier:** Chromosomal analysis; pedigree analysis to determine obligate heterozygotes.

**Special Considerations:** The ocular picture of Norrie disease is somewhat similar to the retinal dysplasia that occurs in **Chromosome 13, trisomy 13** and in other conditions. It is distinguished by the absence of other systemic abnormalities, by the concomitant mental retardation and deafness, and by the X-linked recessive mode of inheritance. *Pseudoglioma* is a clinical term describing a number of conditions that produce a white reflex or amaurotic "cat's eye reflex" in the pupil. Reese has grouped these conditions as "leukocoria" which may be produced by developmental abnormalities such as persistent hyperplastic primary vitreous, retinal dysplasia, congenital retinal folds, or by inflammatory conditions such as metastatic endophthalmitis, larval granulomatosis, and toxoplasmosis. Leukocoria may also be present in children with retinopathy of prematurity (retrolental fibroplasia and retinoblastoma.)

The psychiatric and otologic components of this syndrome are never congenital. If mental retardation begins early (age 3–4 years), the afflicted patient is more likely to be severely retarded.

Electrocochleography and brain stem-evoked responses reveal that the hearing loss is primarily of cochlear origin. A varient of Norrie disease with the typical stigmata and associated microcephaly has been well described (Moreira-Filho and Neustein, 1979).

**References:**

Warburg M: Norrie's disease: a congenital progressive oculo-acousti-cocerebral degeneration. Acta Ophthalmol 1966; 89:1–47.

Apple DJ, et al.: Ocular histopathology of Norrie's disease. Am J Ophthalmol 1974; 78:196–203.

Parving A, et al.: Electrophysiological study of Norrie's disease. Audiology 1978; 17:293–298.

Moreira-Filho CA, Neustein I: A presumptive new variant of Norrie's disease. J Med Genet 1979; 16:125–128.

de laChapelle A, et al.: Norrie disease caused by a gene deletion allowing carrier detection and prenatal diagnosis. Clin Genet 1985; 28:317–320.

Gal A, et al.: Submicroscopic interstitial deletion of the X chromosome explains a complex genetic syndrome dominated by Norrie disease. Cytogenet Cell Genet 1986; 42:219–224.

Gal A, et al.: Prenatal exclusion of Norrie disease with flanking DNA markers. Am J Med Genet 1988; 31:449–453.

Zhu D, et al.: Microdeletion in the X-chromosome and prenatal diagnosis in a family with Norrie Disease. Am J Med Genet 1989; 33:485–488.

EL007

HA068

WE038

**Robert M. Ellsworth**
**Barrett G. Haik**
**Robert A. Weiss**

**North Carolina macular dystrophy (NCMD)**
*See EYE, MACULAR DYSTROPHY, NORTH CAROLINA TYPE*
**Norum disease**
*See ANEMIA, HEMOLYTIC, RED CELL MEMBRANE DEFECTS*
*also LECITHIN-CHOLESTEROL ACYL TRANSFERASE DEFICIENCY*
**Nose, absence of**
*See NOSE/NASAL SEPTUM DEFECTS*
**Nose, absence of half**
*See NOSE/NASAL SEPTUM DEFECTS*

---

## NOSE, ANTERIOR ATRESIA  0723

**Includes:**
    Anterior nasal atresia
    Atresia, nasal anterior
    Atresia of anterior nares
    Bony choanal atresia, anterior
    Choanal atresia, anterior
    Membranous choanal atresia, anterior
    Stenosis of anterior nares

**Excludes:**
    Nose and nasal septum defects
    **Nose, nasopharyngeal stenosis** (0707)
    **Nose, posterior atresia** (0727)

**Major Diagnostic Criteria:** Bony or membranous atresia of the anterior nares, with underdeveloped nostril. Anterior nasal atresia can be differentiated from half-nose by the presence of posterior choanae on examination of the nasopharynx, absence of purulent dacryocystitis, and presence of a partial nasal chamber and paranasal sinuses on X-ray examination.

**Clinical Findings:** A narrowing or stenosis of the anterior nares, usually unilateral, and either membranous or bony. The newborn may have respiratory distress when not crying if the lesion is bilateral. The nasolacrimal duct is present and normal, but X-ray examination may show lack of anterior ethmoid and maxillary sinuses. Computerized tomography will help to delineate the abnormality.

**Complications:** When bilateral, possible respiratory distress of the newborn.

**Associated Findings:** None known.

**Etiology:** Unknown.

**Pathogenesis:** The anterior nares are closed by epithelial plugs from the second to sixth month of intrauterine life. Failure of absorption of these plugs results in anterior atresia or stenosis of varying degrees.

**CDC No.:** 748.000

**Sex Ratio:** Presumably M1:F1

**Occurrence:** Undetermined but presumed rare.

**Risk of Recurrence for Patient's Sib:** Unknown.

**Risk of Recurrence for Patient's Child:** Unknown.

**Age of Detectability:** At birth.

**Gene Mapping and Linkage:** Unknown.

**Prevention:** None known. Genetic counseling indicated.

**Treatment:** Reconstructive surgery can be performed to provide an epithelial lined nasal cavity with cosmetically acceptable nostrils. This can be done through either a sublabial or a transnasal approach.

**Prognosis:** Good for life span, intelligence, and function, unless bilateral and associated with respiratory distress that is not recognized and not corrected.

**Detection of Carrier:** Unknown.

**References:**
Ballenger JJ: Diseases of the nose, throat and ear. Philadelphia: Lea & Febiger, 1969.
Maloney WH, ed: Otolaryngology, vol. 3. Hagerstown: Harper & Row, 1969.
Brown OE, et al.: Congenital piriform aperture stenosis in children. Larynoscope 1988; 99:86–91.

MY003                                    Charles M. Myer III

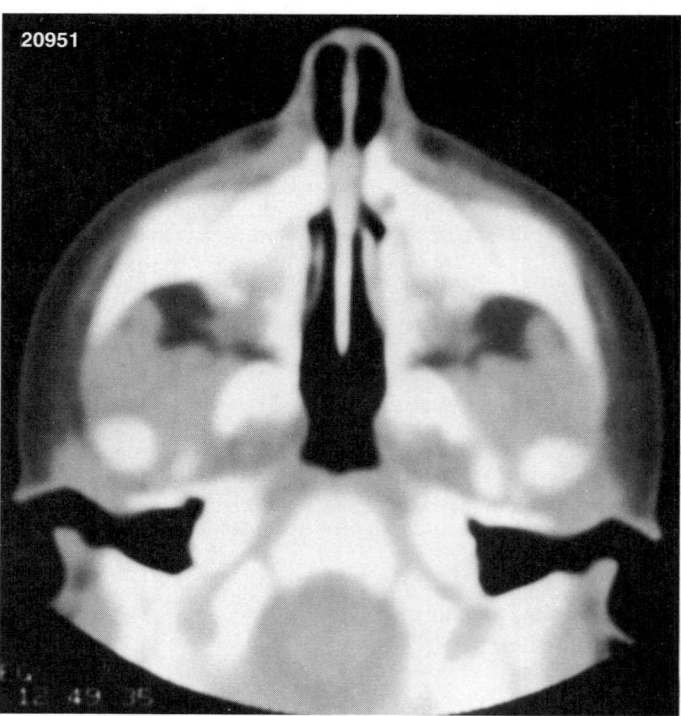

2718-20951: Anterior nasal stenosis as seen on CT scan.

---

## NOSE, ANTERIOR STENOSIS                        2718

**Includes:** Anterior nasal stenosis

**Excludes:**
Choanal atresia
**Nose, anterior stenosis** (2718)
**Nose, bifid** (0724)
**Nose, dislocated nasal septum** (2719)

**Major Diagnostic Criteria:** The affected infant presents with cyanosis and respiratory distress. On examination of the nose there is a hard bony mass presenting from the lateral nasal wall within the anterior nares, along with a narrowed nasal airway.

**Clinical Findings:** Infants with anterior nasal stenosis present with nasal airway obstruction, and may have a cyclic pattern of cyanosis relieved by crying (similar to infants with bilateral posterior choanal atresia or stenosis).

Nasal examination reveals a hard bony mass protruding medially at the area of the lumen vestibuli. The nasal airway is narrowed to 1–2 mm. It is frequently impossible to pass a small catheter through the nose.

Infants are obligate nasal breathers for a variable period of time; hence, a risk of nasal airway obstruction exists. Since the effects of this lesion are similar to those of bilateral posterior choanal atresia, sudden death due to an inadequate oral airway may result. Nasal airway obstruction may contribute to development of a "long face" syndrome.

**Complications:** Surgical complications include tooth bud damage, damage to nasolacrimal apparatus, maxillary sinus damage, and maldevelopment of the midface.

**Associated Findings:** None known.

**Etiology:** Unknown.

**Pathogenesis:** Unknown.

**CDC No.:** 748.000

**Sex Ratio:** Undetermined but presumably M1:F1.

**Occurrence:** Overall frequency < 1%.

**Risk of Recurrence for Patient's Sib:** Unknown.

**Risk of Recurrence for Patient's Child:** Unknown.

**Age of Detectability:** At birth.

**Gene Mapping and Linkage:** Unknown.

**Prevention:** None known.

**Treatment:** Sublateral resection of the bony stenosis.

**Prognosis:** Good.

**Detection of Carrier:** Unknown.

**References:**
Shetty R: Nasal pyramid surgery for correction of bony inlet stenosis. J Laryngol Otol 1977; 91:201–208.
Sprinkle PM, Sponck FT: Congenital malformations of the nose and paranasal sinuses. In: Bluestone CD, Stool SE, eds: Pediatric otolaryngology. Philadelphia: W.B. Saunders, 1983:769–779.

MY003                                    Charles M. Myer III
OR005                                        Peter Orobello

---

## NOSE, BIFID                                    0724

**Includes:**
Bifid nose
"Doggennose"
Nose, congenital median fissure of
Nose, median cleft of

**Excludes:**
**Encephalocele** (0343)
**Eye, hypertelorism** (0504)
**Face, median cleft face syndrome** (0635)
**Nose/nasal septum defects** (0722)
**Nose, duplication** (0725)

**Major Diagnostic Criteria:** Vertical midline cleft of the nose.

**Clinical Findings:** The tip and dorsum of the nose are divided by a vertical central sulcus of variable width, resulting in a broad and flat nose. The columella is broad and short, separating abnormally shaped nostrils. The septum may be duplicated, and the nasal bones may be normal or excessively broad. Computerized tomography is helpful in determining presence of the choanal atresia or associated abnormalities of the skull and sinuses.

**Complications:** Bifid nose is almost always found in association with hypertelorism, a real or illusory increase in interpupillary distance, and can be associated with other congenital midline defects of the face, such as cranium bifidum occultum (32%), median cleft lip (16%), and triad of bifid nose, cranium bifidum occultum, and cleft lip (12%). Incidence of severe mental retardation is 8%, and of borderline retardation, 12%.

**Associated Findings:** None known.

**Etiology:** Autosomal dominant and recessive inheritance has been reported in a few pedigrees. Three of 25 patients with bifid nose had ancestors with hypertelorism without bifid nose. One reported patient with a bifid nose had a normal twin.

**Pathogenesis:** In the five-week embryo the medial nasal processes are widely separated by the frontal process. Normally, the frontal process grows upward and away from the lower face, and the paired medial nasal processes grow toward the midline, over the frontal process to form the mesodermal structures of the midface. Failure of these processes to merge or failure of obliteration of ectodermal remnants may result in midline clefts of the nose.

**MIM No.:** 10974, 21040

**CDC No.:** 748.120

**Sex Ratio:** M1:F1

**Occurrence:** 1:1,000 congenital defects of the face. Over 140 cases have been reported in the literature.

**Risk of Recurrence for Patient's Sib:**
See Part I, *Mendelian Inheritance.*

**Risk of Recurrence for Patient's Child:**
See Part I, *Mendelian Inheritance.*

**Age of Detectability:** At birth.

**Gene Mapping and Linkage:** Unknown.

**Prevention:** None known. Genetic counseling indicated.

**Treatment:** Plastic surgical procedure to remove excess midline tissue and approximate nostrils. Use of flaps or skin grafts may be necessary to fill cleft defect.

**Prognosis:** Normal for life span, intelligence, and function if an isolated defect.

**Detection of Carrier:** Unknown.

**References:**
Boo-Chai K: The bifid nose; with a report of 3 cases in siblings. Plast Reconstr Surg 1965; 36:626–628.
Baibak G, Bromberg BE: Congenital midline defects of the midface. Cleft Palate J 1966; 3:392–401.
DeMyer W: The median cleft face syndrome: differential diagnosis of cranium bifidum occultum, hypertelorism, and median cleft nose, lip and palate. Neurology 1967; 17:961–971.
Kawamotod HK: The kaleidoscopic world of rare craniofacial clefts. Clinics in Plastic Surg 1976; 3:529–571, 533–534, 542–549.
Anyane-Yeboa K, et al.: Dominant inheritance of bifid nose. Am J Med Genet 1984; 17:561–563.
Miles JH, Smith V: Dominant bifid nose syndrome in four generations. (Abstract). Am J Hum Genet 1985; 37:A69.

BE028                                    **LaVonne Bergstrom**

---

## NOSE, CHOANAL ATRESIA-LYMPHEDEMA          2597

**Includes:**
   Atresia choanal posterior-lymphedema
   Atresia of posterior nares-lymphedema
   Bony choanal atresia, posterior-lymphedema
   Choanal atresia, posterior-lymphedema
   Lymphedema-choanal atresia
   Nasal atresia, posterior-lymphedema

**Excludes:**
   **Brachydactyly** (0114)
   **Charge association** (2124)
   **Lymphedema I** (0614)
   **Lymphedema II** (0615)
   Lymphedema, early onset
   Lymphedema, other
   **Nose, anterior atresia** (0723)
   **Nose, nasopharyngeal stenosis** (0707)
   **Nose, posterior atresia** (0727)

**Major Diagnostic Criteria:** Congenital bilateral posterior choanal atresia (PCA) detected soon after birth; onset of lymphedema of the lower extremities occurs after age two years.

**Clinical Findings:** Acute respiratory distress with cyanosis and struggling develops soon after birth due to atresia of the posterior nares, suspected by inability to pass a catheter in the oral pharynx and confirmed by lateral X-rays of the nasopharynx with radiopaque dye in the anterior portion of the nose. Infant is unable to nurse because of breathing difficulty.

Chronic, pitting edema is first noticed around the dorsal aspects of feet and ankles after the second birthday and progresses gradually upwards to involve the lower leg. The upper limb and thigh involvement may not be observed until ten years of age. The overlying skin appears shiny, but is otherwise normal. Older children have complained of tiredness during usual physical activities. The degree of involvement can be quite variable from individual to individual, and from side to side.

All causes of secondary lymphedema should be excluded. Lymphangiographic and Doppler studies may show aplasia, hypoplasia, or dilated lymph trunks. A history of PCA during the newborn period may be helpful in establishing the relationship between the two conditions. Physical growth is the normal range (height and weight between 5th and 45th percentiles); development and intelligence are normal.

**Complications:** Bilateral PCA causes serious breathing difficulty and may result in death unless an oral airway is established and surgical correction is carried out. Difficulties in nursing will result in failure to thrive. If the condition goes unrecognized and the infant suffers chronic hypoxia, intelligence and function may be affected. Although primarily a cosmetic and psychosocial handicap, the severe edema is likely to affect walking and movements.

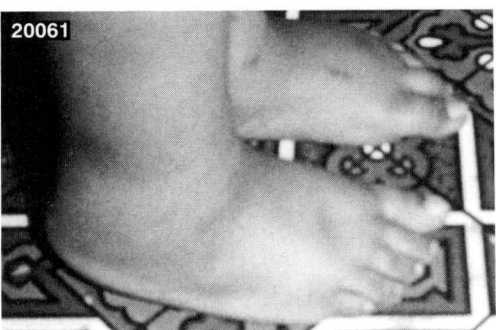

**2597-20061:** Note edema in both feet and lower legs. The edema is pitting type.

In addition, it may lead to recurrent episodes of lymphangitis or cellulitis, and to ulceration.

**Associated Findings:**  Mild **Pectus excavatum** (5/5), highly arched palate (4/5), radial loop patterns on fourth fingertips (3/5), and relatively large head size (70–98th percentile) (4/5).

**Etiology:**  Autosomal recessive inheritance.

**Pathogenesis:**  The pathogenesis of PCA appears to be the failure of the bucconasal membrane to rupture between the 35th and 39th days of fetal life; persistent tissue is then carried posteriorly and vertically as the face develops. In 85% of the cases, the atresia is bony and is commonly located 1–2 mm anterior to the posterior edge of the hard palate.

Pathogenesis of lymphedema is largely unknown. The edema is likely due to a defect in the development of the lymphatic drainage associated with the congenital hypoplasia of the lymphatic system. The combined syndrome was observed in a large kindred in which several consanguinous marriages had taken place. The existence of tightly linked recessive genes for PCA and lymphedema in this an inbred kindred may explain concurrence of the two conditions. All children with PCA have already developed the edema.

**POS No.:**  4265

**Sex Ratio:**  M1:F1

**Occurrence:**  Observed in two generations of three sibships of one large kindred.

**Risk of Recurrence for Patient's Sib:**
See Part I, *Mendelian Inheritance.*

**Risk of Recurrence for Patient's Child:**
See Part I, *Mendelian Inheritance.*

**Age of Detectability:**  Soon after birth because of respiratory difficulty and cyanosis. Lymphedema is detectable after the second birthday.

**Gene Mapping and Linkage:**  Unknown.

**Prevention:**  None known. Genetic counseling indicated.

**Treatment:**  Early recognition of the PCA; establishing and maintaining an oral airway until surgery. Surgical correction can be performed intranasally during the newborn period, or transpalatally after the age of six months. Lymphedema is difficult to manage and treat. Partial and/or temporary response has been reported by administration of diuretics, bed rest, and use of a pararubber bandage or an elastic stocking. In severe and uncontrollable edema, resection of subcutaneous tissues with subsequent skin autografts may be performed. Supportive therapy for psychosocial problems may be needed.

**Prognosis:**  Apparently normal for life span and intelligence once the PCA is surgically corrected. The prognosis for lymphedema is dictated by its severity and response to available treatment modalities.

**Detection of Carrier:**  Unknown.

**References:**
Qazi QH, et al.: Inheritance of posterior choanal atresia. Am J Med Genet 1982; 13:413–416.
Sheikh TM, et al.: Posterior choanal atresia lymphedema association in a kindred. Pediatr Res 1986; 20:272A. *

QA000                                                      **Qutub H. Qazi**

**Nose, congenital median fissure of**
*See NOSE, BIFID*

---

## NOSE, DISLOCATED NASAL SEPTUM                    2719

**Includes:**
Dislocation of the nasal septum
Nasal septum, subluxed or dislocated
Subluxed nasal septum, congenital

**Excludes:**
Choanal atresia
**Nose, anterior stenosis** (2718)
Turbinate defect

**Major Diagnostic Criteria:**  Outward deviation of the nose to one side, accompanied by leaning of the columella and a loss of nasal tip stability.

**Clinical Findings:**  Outward deviation of the nose to one side, leaning of the columella, loss of nasal tip stability, flattening of the nasal aperture on the side of dislocation, and diminished movement of the ala on the same side during inspiration.

**Complications:**  Nasal obstruction, external deformity, risk of septal hematoma, and increased risk of upper and lower respiratory tract infections later in life.

**Associated Findings:**  None known.

**Etiology:**  Usually intrauterine pressure and strain, primarily during the first stage of labor in primipara.

**Pathogenesis:**  The left occipitoanterior presentation results in a more frequent deviation to the right. Significant nasal trauma is possible any time after the fourth month of gestation and is subject to the pressure of intrauterine growths or fetal limbs.

**CDC No.:**  754.020

**Sex Ratio:**  Undetermined but presumably M1:F1.

**Occurrence:**  Overall frequency of < 1%.

**Risk of Recurrence for Patient's Sib:**  Unknown.

**Risk of Recurrence for Patient's Child:**  Unknown.

**Age of Detectability:**  At birth.

**Gene Mapping and Linkage:**  Unknown.

**Prevention:**  None known.

**Treatment:**  Manual reduction of septal cartilage into the septal groove within the first three days of life.

**Prognosis:**  Once septal reduction has been performed, there is usually good stability.

**Detection of Carrier:**  Unknown.

**References:**
Gray L: The deviated nasal septum. J Laryngol Otol 1965; 79:567–575.
Jazbi B: Subluxation of the nasal septum in the newborn: etiology, diagnosis and treatment. Otol Clin North Am 1977; 10:125–138.
Sprinkle PM, Sponck FT: Congenital malformations of the nose and paranasal sinuses. In: Bluestone CD, Stool SE, eds: Pediatric otolaryngology. Philadelphia: W.B. Saunders, 1983:769–779.

MY003                                              **Charles M. Myer III**
OR005                                                   **Peter Orobello**

---

## NOSE, DUPLICATION                                0725

**Includes:**  Nasal duplication

**Excludes:**
**Amniotic bands syndrome** (0874)
**Nose/nasal septum defects** (0722)
**Nose, bifid** (0724)
Supernumerary nostrils

**Major Diagnostic Criteria:**  Two distinct and complete noses, each with two nostrils, two nasal cavities, a nasal septum, and alar cartilages.

**Clinical Findings:**  In the newborn with nasal duplication, preliminary inspection reveals what appears to be a bifid nose with two well-developed nostrils; however, in addition, there exist between the nares two small sinus openings that, on careful examination, prove to be definite nostrils leading into separate nasal cavities. As the child grows, these openings develop into unmistakable nostrils with obvious alar cartilages. Finally, with further development, two separate and complete noses become distinctly evident. Although the small mesial nostrils usually open into definite nasal cavities separate from the lateral, larger nasal cavities, the former spaces may be nothing more than blind pouches without a posterior opening. However, the lateral nasal cavities may extend through choanae into the nasopharynx. X-rays are difficult to interpret but do reveal an indeterminate nasal defect.

**Complications:** Mild to moderate hypertelorism. The medially-placed nares and nasal chambers are smaller than the lateral ones, and may be patent or stenotic. Respiratory distress at birth, and excessive nasal discharge, may lead to exhaustion and interfere with sleeping and sucking.

**Associated Findings:** Muecke's (1923) patient had tiny, round depressions on the medial aspect of the root of each nose that Muecke speculated were lacrymal fissures. Ethmoid masses have been reported. One case was reported with a supplementary anterior cerebral lobe. A second complete nose, with or without duplication of the maxilla and/or orbits/eyes, is sometimes found in more severely affected cases of facial duplication.

**Etiology:** Possibly errors in cell duplication or reproduction.

**Pathogenesis:** From nasal embryology, one can assume that various forms of bifid nose, median clefts of the upper lip, notches in the nostrils, dermoid cysts, sinuses, and other ectodermal inclusions on the bridge of the nose are the result of arrested development of the frontonasal process (especially the globular processes) and the olfactory sacs.

Although it seems apparent that failure of the nasal laminae to consolidate into a single nasal septum is the cause of a bifid nose, it is most difficult to understand the faulty embryologic processes that initiate the formation of two noses with four nostrils and four nasal cavities. One can theorize that some irregularity in the evolution of the two olfactory placodes causes them to bring forth four olfactory pits, all in a horizontal plane, rather than two; such an anomaly would alter the developmental pattern of the medial nasal process. If such were the case, it would tend to explain why the lateral nostrils are larger and more normal in size than are the mesial nostrils, since the lateral nasal processes have not been involved in the developmental defect. Furthermore, it is possible that the two medial olfactory pits probably form olfactory sacs, which are interposed between the two nasal laminae. These sacs, which become medial nasal cavities, thus prevent the laminae from fusing into one nasal septum; instead, they stay divided and form two septa. With the presence of two septa, four nostrils, and four nasal cavities, the developmental anomaly goes on to form two separate noses.

**CDC No.:** 748.110

**Sex Ratio:** M1:F2 (observed).

**Occurrence:** About ten cases reported in the literature.

**Risk of Recurrence for Patient's Sib:** Unknown.

**Risk of Recurrence for Patient's Child:** Unknown.

**Age of Detectability:** At birth.

**Gene Mapping and Linkage:** Unknown.

**Prevention:** None known. Genetic counseling indicated.

**Treatment:** Surgical rectification of the deformity. The correction of nasal duplication requires three or four surgical procedures several years apart.

**Prognosis:** Normal for life span and intelligence.

**Detection of Carrier:** Unknown.

**References:**
Muecke FF, Souttar HS: Double nose. Proc R Soc Med 1924; 17:8–9.
Erich JB: Nasal duplication: report of case of patient with two noses. Plast Reconstr Surg 1962; 29:159–166.
Ghosh P, et al.: Double nose. J Laryngol Otolaryngol 1971; 85:963–969. †

Mazzola RF: Congenital malformations in the frontonasal area. Clin Plast Surg 1976; 3:573–609. * †
Barr M, Jr: Facial duplication: case review and embryogenesis. Teratology 1982; 25:152–159. *

ER001          **John B. Erich**
EV002          **Carla A. Evans**

**Nose, ear, digital anomalies-gingival fibromatosis**
  *See GINGIVAL FIBROMATOSIS-DIGITAL ANOMALIES*
**Nose, flattened tip and depressed bridge (some)**
  *See CHONDRODYSPLASIA PUNCTATA, MILD SYMMETRIC TYPE*

## NOSE, GLIOMA                                              0726

**Includes:**
  Encephalochoristoma nasofrontalis
  Glioma, nasal
  Nasal glioma

**Excludes:**
  **Neck/head, dermoid cyst or teratoma** (0283)
  **Encephalocele** (0343)
  Hemangioma of nose
  **Meningocele** (0642)
  Nasal neurofibroma
  Nasal polyps

**Major Diagnostic Criteria:** A unilateral intra- or extranasal mass present at birth, producing a broad nasal bridge and wide-set eyes is the characteristic clinical picture. Sixty percent of nasal gliomas are extranasal, 30% are intranasal, and 10% are combined in location. Nasal gliomas have no fluid connection with the subarachnoid space. If, with straining or crying, the mass pulsates or increases in size, a spinal fluid communication may exist, and then a meningocele or an encephalocele must be ruled out. Biopsy of the mass with histopathologic study will help establish the diagnosis, but this should be delayed until appropriate X-ray studies have been performed and one is prepared definitively to excise the mass.

**Clinical Findings:** These congenital neurogenic tumors are often located externally at the nasal bridge; however, they can present as an intranasal or nasopharyngeal tumor. A combination of locations rarely will be evident. A nasal bridge that is broader in width and eyes that are more widely separated than normal suggest an intranasal tumor. The external tumor is raised and usually covered with intact skin. These tumors, ranging from 1 to 5 cm in diameter, are firm, mobile, round, and smooth. Color varies from pink to red.

Intranasal tumors are located high in the nasal cavity, but they may extend down to the anterior nares. These tumors appear to arise from above the middle turbinate or olfactory fissure; they should not be confused with nasal polyps. They are usually unilateral and cause airway obstruction.

Nasal gliomas are benign in clinical behavior. They rarely enlarge, and recurrence after complete excision is rare. Communication between the tumor and the anterior cranial fossa is not present in true nasal glioma, although a fibrous stalk is present about 20% of the time.

**Complications:** Nasal cosmetic deformities, rhinitis, meningitis, encephalitis, sinusitis, nasal obstruction, cerebrospinal fluid rhinorrhea, epistaxis, anosmia.

**Associated Findings:** Meningocele, encephalocele.

**Etiology:** Unknown.

**Pathogenesis:** Tumors probably arise from congenital malformations of the nose, the base of the skull, and CNS in the region of the foramen cecum. Glial tissue is separated from the CNS and remains outside the calvaria. These abnormalities result from developmental defects in the frontal, nasal, ethmoid, or sphenoid bones of the skull. Tumors composed of CNS tissues arise from such defects. Nasal gliomas contain glial tissues, are separated from the brain, and are occasionally connected to the base of the skull with a fibrous stalk. Nasal gliomas per se have no fluid connection with the CNS and hence contain no spinal fluid that circulates between the tumors and the subarachnoid space.

**CDC No.:** 748.180

**Sex Ratio:** M3:F1

**Occurrence:** Undetermined but presumed rare.

**Risk of Recurrence for Patient's Sib:** Unknown.

**Risk of Recurrence for Patient's Child:** Unknown.

**Age of Detectability:** At birth or soon after.

**Gene Mapping and Linkage:** Unknown.

**Prevention:** None known. Genetic counseling indicated.

**Treatment:** Complete surgical excision usually results in a cure. Intracranial communication must be ruled out before excising the tumor. If there is an intracranial connection, an intracranial excision should be performed before the external nasal mass is excised. Antibiotics for infections and rhinoplasty for nasal deformities may be necessary.

**Prognosis:** Good, when total excision is performed.

**Detection of Carrier:** Unknown.

**Special Considerations:** X-ray examination, including polytomography of the base of the skull and CT scans will often reveal a defect in the calvaria when a fluid communication does exist. The mass can be "tapped" with a needle to determine the presence of spinal fluid, but careful aseptic techniques must be used to avoid subsequent infections. When spinal fluid is present in the tumor, air or dye contrast studies of the CNS should be performed. The presence or absence of fluid communication must be determined before considering surgical therapy.

Encephaloceles may be difficult to differentiate from nasal gliomas, although they are quite different in structure. The encephalocele contains an ependyma-lined space filled with cerebrospinal fluid that communicates with the ventricles of the brain. Glial and fibrous tissues are present beneath the ependymal lining. A biopsy from the wall of such a tumor may not reveal the true nature of this tumor. A defect in the base of the skull on X-ray examination helps make this diagnosis. These tumors pulsate and increase in size when the infant strains or cries.

Meningoceles are rare and consist of meninges that herniate through a developmental defect in the cranium. They have clinical characteristics similar to those of the encephalocele. There are two types of meningocele that occur about the nose. The sphenopharyngeal dehiscence involves the sphenoid or ethmoid bones with a tumor presenting in the orbit, nasal cavity, nasopharynx, or medial to the ramus of the mandible. An intranasal (sincipital) dehiscence involves the cribriform plate, with a tumor either in the nasal cavity or externally at the medial canthus of the eye, or in the orbit.

**References:**
Black BK, Smith DE: Nasal glioma: two cases with recurrence. Arch Neurol Psychiatry 1950; 64:614–630.
Proctor B, Proctor C: Congenital lesions of the head and neck. Otolaryngol Clin North Am 1970; 3:221–248. *
Karma P, et al.: Nasal gliomas. A review and report of two cases. Laryngoscope 1977; 87:1169–1179.
Gorenstein A, et al.: Nasal gliomas. Arch Otolaryngol 1980; 106:536–540.
Hughes GB, et al.: Management of the congenital midline nasal mass: a review. Head Neck Surg 1980; 2:222–223.
Whitaker SR, et al.: Nasal glioma. Arch Otolaryngol 1981; 107:550–554. *
Bradley PJ, Singh SD: Nasal glioma. J Laryngol Otol 1985; 99:247–252.

EN002                                            **Gerald M. English**

## NOSE, GRANULOSIS RUBRA NASI                                    0444

**Includes:** Granulosis rubra nasi
**Excludes:**
   Acne rosacea
   Acne vulgaris
   **Lupus erythematosis, systemic** (2515)
   Lupus vulgaris
   Perioral dermatitis
   Other causes of erythema

**Major Diagnostic Criteria:** Hyperhidrosis of the nose. Erythema of the tip of the nose, which may extend to the rest of the nose.

**Clinical Findings:** Hyperhidrosis of the nose may be the first symptom. Erythema of the nasal tip, possibly the remainder of the nose, and sometimes migrating to involve the cheeks, upper lid and chin, is a reliable feature. Pinpoint to pinhead-sized dark red papules are scattered irregularly on the erythematous base associated with sweat droplets. Vesicles and small cystic lesions have been described. The nose feels cold to the touch, and there may be slight itching without other local symptoms. Volar hyperhidrosis and poor peripheral circulation are associated. Histopathologically, there is dilation of dermal blood and lymphatic vessels. There is perivascular infiltration, including mast cells and dilation of sweat ducts. The connective tissue, epidermis, and pilosebaceous elements are normal. Laboratory and X-ray findings are unremarkable.

The majority of patients are children, six months to 10 years of age. A few adult patients have been reported. The disease process commonly resolves at puberty.

**Complications:** Unknown.

**Associated Findings:** None known.

**Etiology:** Both autosomal recessive and dominant inheritance have been suggested.

**Pathogenesis:** Endocrinopathy, vasomotor disturbances in the form of sympathetic dysfunction, and a form of sweat retention are hypothesized causes.

**MIM No.:** 13900

**CDC No.:** 748.180

**Sex Ratio:** M1:F1

**Occurrence:** Unknown. At least one large kindred has been documented.

**Risk of Recurrence for Patient's Sib:**
   See Part I, *Mendelian Inheritance.*

**Risk of Recurrence for Patient's Child:**
   See Part I, *Mendelian Inheritance.*

**Age of Detectability:** Six months to 10 years.

**Gene Mapping and Linkage:** Unknown.

**Prevention:** None known. Genetic counseling indicated.

**Treatment:** No known effective therapy.

**Prognosis:** Excellent, with normal life span. Disease process usually resolves at puberty, but may persist indefinitely.

**Detection of Carrier:** Unknown.

**References:**
Binazzi M: Ulteriori relievi su di una osservazione di granulosis rubra nasi ereditaria. Rass Dermatol Sif 1958; 11:23–26.
Allen AC: The skin, ed 2, New York: Grune and Stratton, 1967.
Aram H, Mohagheghi AP: Granulosis rubra nasi. Cutis 1972; 10:463–464. *

HU015                                            **Richard Hubbell**
MY003                                            **Charles M. Myer III**

**Nose, half, plus proboscis**
*See NOSE/NASAL SEPTUM DEFECTS*
**Nose, median cleft of**
*See NOSE, BIFID*

## NOSE, NASOPHARYNGEAL STENOSIS 0707

**Includes:**
Nasopharyngeal atresia
Nasopharyngeal stenosis

**Excludes:**
**Nose, anterior atresia** (0723)
**Nose, posterior atresia** (0727)

**Major Diagnostic Criteria:** Complete or incomplete attachment of the soft palate to the posterior nasopharynx. Nasopharyngeal stenosis should be considered in the newborn with obstruction of the nasal airway without choanal atresia.

**Clinical Findings:** The posterior soft palate and posterior nasopharynx are connected by a thin membrane. Although respiratory distress in the newborn with a complete membrane would be expected, it has not been reported. The patients do have excessive nasal discharge.

**Complications:** Reduced nasal airway proportional to the amount of obstruction produced by the membrane. Nasal discharge due to impaired flow of the nasal mucous into the pharynx.

**Associated Findings:** Shallow nasopharynx reported in about one-half of cases.

**Etiology:** Undetermined. One case of congenital syphilitic nasopharyngeal stenosis has been reported.

**Pathogenesis:** Undetermined. Incomplete rupture of buccopharyngeal membrane has been proposed; however, this is questionable since the buccopharyngeal membrane is thought to rupture prior to fusion of the lateral palatal processes to form the soft palate, and the buccopharyngeal membrane should not be attached to the posterior nasopharynx.

**CDC No.:** 748.180

**Sex Ratio:** Presumably M1:F1. Sex reported in only two cases, both of which were female.

**Occurrence:** Undetermined but presumed rare.

**Risk of Recurrence for Patient's Sib:** No known increase of risk.

**Risk of Recurrence for Patient's Child:** No known increase of risk.

**Age of Detectability:** At birth, by palpation between the soft palate and posterior pharyngeal wall.

**Gene Mapping and Linkage:** Unknown.

**Prevention:** None known.

**Treatment:** The cases of membranous connection between the palate and pharynx have responded to blunt penetration of the membrane followed by a digital dilation without recurrence of the stenosis. If a cicatricial stenosis or thick membrane is encountered, it can be treated with a seton suture or by mucosal flaps.

Although respiratory difficulties have not been reported, they would be expected in cases of complete or severe obstruction of the nasopharynx. This should be treated with an oral airway pending definitive treatment of the stenosis.

While membranous occlusion of the nasopharynx will respond to simple penetration and dilation of the stenotic segment, cicatricial stenosis will almost surely recur with this form of therapy.

**Prognosis:** *Treated:* Membranous stenosis: excellent prognosis for permanent establishment of a nasal airway. Cicatricial stenosis tends to recur; however, permanent establishment of a nasal airway has been accomplished with the seton procedure and with mucosal flaps.

*Untreated:* Death may result from complete or severe nasopharyngeal stenosis because the newborn does not breathe through his mouth except, when crying or gasping for air.

**Detection of Carrier:** Unknown.

**References:**
MacKenty JE: Nasopharyngeal atresia. Arch Otolaryngol 1927; 6:1–27.
Stevenson EW: Cicatricial stenosis of the nasopharynx. Laryngoscope 1969; 79:2035–2067.
Cotton RT: Nasopharyngeal stenosis. Arch Otolaryngol 1985; 111:146–148.

MY003      **Charles M. Myer III**

## NOSE, POSTERIOR ATRESIA 0727

**Includes:**
Atresia choanal posterior
Atresia of posterior nares
Bony choanal atresia, posterior
Choanal atresia, posterior
Membranous choanal atresia, posterior
Posterior nasal atresia

**Excludes:**
**Nose, nasopharyngeal stenosis** (0707)
**Nose, anterior atresia** (0723)

**Major Diagnostic Criteria:** Obstruction to nasal breathing due to posterior choanal atresia. A lateral X-ray of the head will demonstrate radiopaque dye in the nasal cavities and air in the unoccluded nasopharynx behind the obstructing membrane. Computerized tomography and MRI scanning are helpful diagnostic procedures. The inability to pass nasal catheters through the nose a distance of 32 mm will confirm the diagnosis.

**Clinical Findings:** The newborn infant develops acute respiratory distress every time he or she attempts to breathe quietly with the mouth closed because most newborns are obligatory nasal breathers. Cyanosis, struggling, exhaustion, and death can occur

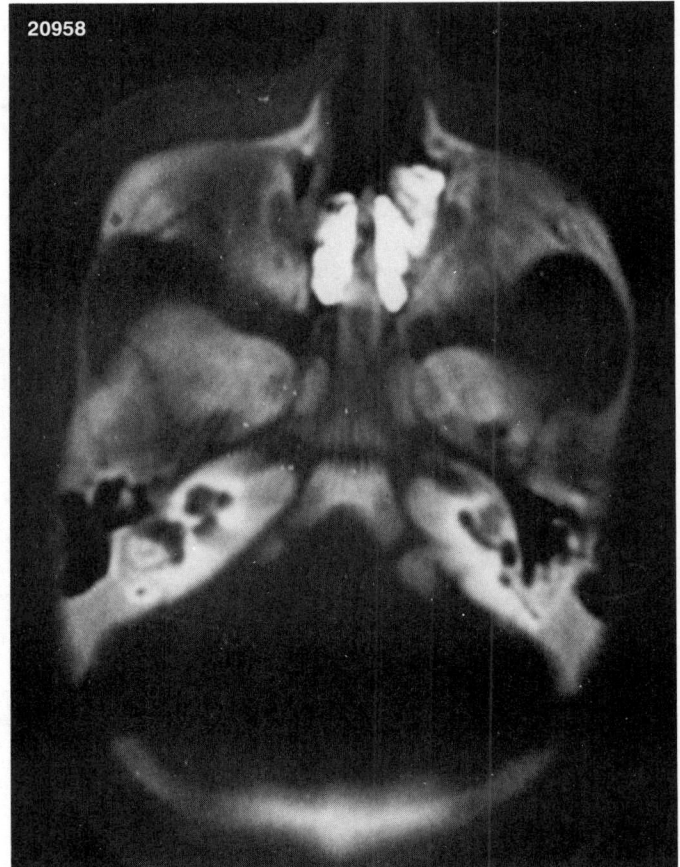

**0727-20958:** Choanal atresia.

unless an oral airway is obtained. When crying, the infant does well because the mouth is open. The newborn normally tends to breathe with the mouth closed. Nursing becomes a problem as the infant frequently has to stop feeding to gasp for breath.

A catheter cannot be passed into the oropharynx. If the airways are cleaned and decongested, an obstructing membrane may be seen in the depths of the nostril posteriorly, with a dimple in the center. Lateral X-rays of the head, with radiopaque dye injected into the nares, will demonstrate the soft tissue obstruction between the dye and the air in the nasopharynx. A computerized tomographic (CT) scan offers the most complete X-ray assessment of the problem.

**Complications:** Death may occur unless an oral airway is immediately placed and maintained.

**Associated Findings:** Cardiac defects (25%), branchial arch abnormalities (21%), abnormalities of pinna (15%), microcephaly (15%), micrognathia (15%), miscellaneous palatal abnormalities (15%), nasopharyngeal abnormalities (15%), mandibulofacial dysostosis (11%), cleft palate (10%), conductive or mixed hearing loss (3.5–7%), digital abnormalities (7%), miscellaneous tongue abnormalities (7%), cleft lip and palate (4%), tracheoesophageal fistula (3%), cervical meningocele, cleidocranial dysplasia, hiatus hernia, diaphragmatic hernia, oxycephaly, hypertelorism, facial cleft, absent nasal septum, imperforate anus, hydronephrosis, facial nerve paralysis, mental retardation, absent spleen, ileal atresia, cerebral agenesis, micropenis, coloboma. A feature of **Charge association**, it has also been observed in **Mandibulofacial dysostosis**.

Twenty-five percent of cases have a single minor associated abnormality; 25% have a single major associated abnormality, and 50% have multiple associated abnormalities. In unilateral choanal atresia, 45% have associated anomalies. In bilateral choanal atresia, 60% have associated anomalies. Sex incidence of associated anomalies: M2:F1.

**Etiology:** Presumably multifactorial.

**Pathogenesis:** Failure of complete excavation of the nasal cavities as they form (failure of rupture of buccopharyngeal membranes).

**MIM No.:** 21480

**CDC No.:** 748.000

**Sex Ratio:** M1:F2

**Occurrence:** Incidence 1:5,000 live births. Prevalence 1:4,000 to 1:8,000 in the general population.

**Risk of Recurrence for Patient's Sib:** Unknown.

**Risk of Recurrence for Patient's Child:** Unknown.

**Age of Detectability:** At birth by lack of a nasal airway causing acute respiratory distress with the mouth closed.

**Gene Mapping and Linkage:** Unknown.

**Prevention:** None known. Genetic counseling indicated.

**Treatment:** If the condition is bilateral, then an oral airway must be maintained until the bilateral choanal atresia is surgically corrected. The correction may be made immediately after birth by the intranasal or transpalatal route.

The application of modern otologic techniques, including micro instrumentation and the operating microscope, allow safe surgical correction with a relatively minor operative procedure in the first few days of life. Nonreactive silastic tubes maintain the patency of the corrected defect until re-epithelialization occurs and simultaneously allows for a patent airway.

**Prognosis:** Normal for life span, intelligence, and function if no life-threatening associated finding exists and if the infant survives the first days or weeks of life when he or she tends to breathe entirely through the nose. Death occurring in the first days of life usually is from acute respiratory obstruction.

**Detection of Carrier:** Unknown.

**References:**
Baker MC: Congenital atresia of posterior nares. Arch Otolaryngol 1953; 58:431–434.

Singleton GT, Hardcastle B: Congenital choanal atresia. Arch Otolaryngol 1968; 87:620–625.

Evans JNG, MacLachlan RF: Choanal atresia. J Laryngol 1971; 85:903–929.

Feuerstein S, et al.: Transnasal correction of choanal atreasia. Head Neck Surg 1980; 3:97–104.

Maniglia AJ, Goodwin WJ: Congenital choanal atresia. Otolaryngol Clin North Am 1981; 14:167–173.

Qazi Q, et al.: Inheritance of posterior choanal atresia. Am J Med Genet 1982; 13:413–416.

Greenberg F: Choanal atresia and athelia: methimazole teratogenicity or a new syndrome? Am J Med Genet 1987; 28:931–934.

HA032 **B. Hardcastle**

---

## NOSE, PROBOSCIS LATERALIS 0824

**Includes:**
Proboscis lateral
Lateral nasal proboscis
Arrhinencephalia unilateralis
Tubular nostril congenital

**Excludes:**
Nose, bifid (0724)
Nose/nasal septum defects (0722)

**Major Diagnostic Criteria:** A pendulous soft tissue tube resembling, as described in the literature, a "little elephant trunk" is attached at the medial orbit-nasal bridge area.

**Clinical Findings:** While usually a unilateral condition (90%), bilateral and midline cases have been reported. The unilateral cases are almost evenly divided between right and left sides of the face. A typical proboscis measures 20–40 mm in length and 10–15 mm in diameter. It may have a distal opening about 1 mm in size and is usually, but not always, blind. Heminasal aplasia commonly occurs on the side of the proboscis (90%). Eye defects, especially coloboma of the iris or eyelid, occur in nearly all individuals.

**Complications:** Abnormalities of the eye and its adnexa or the nasal wall are likely to cause disturbances in vision and handling of secretions.

**Associated Findings:** The adjacent nasal wall malformation may range from a soft tissue deficiency to absence of ipsilateral frontal and maxillary sinus, nasolacrimal apparatus, vomer, lateral nasal wall and nasal bone. Ophthalmic findings include coloboma of eyelid or iris, microphthalmia or anophthalmia, cystic degeneration of the optic nerve, cyclopean eye, and choroidal cleft.

Other associated findings are cleft lip/palate (20%); absence of the lateral incisor, vomer, premaxilla; and absence or diminution of the cribriform plate, olfactory bulb, and olfactory tract.

**Etiology:** Undetermined, but probably results from a defect in the anterior portion of the early neural crest and plate. Proboscis lateralis and microphthalmos has been produced in chicks with microlaser irratiation to anterior neural crest region.

**Pathogenesis:** Occurrence of proboscii may be related to facial clefting. The tube can be attached at various points along line of embryonic fusion between anterior maxillary process and frontonasal process. Imperfect mesodermal proliferation and epidermal breakdown produces a tube-like structure arising at frontonasal region.

**CDC No.:** 748.185

**Sex Ratio:** M2:F1

**Occurrence:** Approximately 40 cases reported.

**Risk of Recurrence for Patient's Sib:** Not increased.

**Risk of Recurrence for Patient's Child:** Not increased.

**Age of Detectability:** Proboscis lateralis has been detected in the fetus by sonography, but is usually noted at birth.

**Gene Mapping and Linkage:** Unknown.

**Prevention:** None known. Genetic counseling indicated.

**Treatment:** The nasal anomaly requires a surgical construction utilizing the proboscis when a tissue deficiency exists in the nasal wall. The plastic surgical procedure is usually staged. An early repair that improves esthetic appearance may promote more normal psychological development, but is more difficult to plan and execute due to the influences of growth on size and structure of the constructed nose.

Especially in heminasal aplasia, it is important to retain the proboscis so that adequate local tissue will be available for surgical procedures.

**Prognosis:** Unless severe cranial base and cerebral anomalies are present, a normal life span is expected.

**Detection of Carrier:** Unknown.

**References:**
Rontal M, et al: Proboscis lateralis: case report and embryologic analysis. Laryngoscope 1977; 87:996–1005. †
Lieuw Kie Song SH, et al.: Median faciocerebral anomalies in chick embryos resulting from local destruction of the anteriormost parts of the early neural plate and neural crest. Acta Morph Neerl Scand 1980; 18:231–252.
Wang S, et al.: Proboscis lateralis, microphthalmos, and cystic degeneration of the optic nerve. Ann Opthal 1983; 15:756–758.
Boo-Chai K: The proboscis lateralis-a 14-year follow-up. Plast Reconstr Surg 1985; 75:569–577.

EV002                                                    **Carla A. Evans**

## NOSE, TRANSVERSE GROOVE                              0728

**Includes:**
 Nasal crease
 Nasal groove, familial transverse
 Nasal groove, transverse
 Nasal stripe, transverse

**Excludes:** Nose (other)

**Major Diagnostic Criteria:** A horizontal red depression or groove 1–3 mm wide and about 1 mm deep, located just caudad to the ala nasi.

**Clinical Findings:** A horizontal red depression or groove 1–3 mm wide and about 1 mm deep, located just caudad to the ala nasi has been observed in two affected families.

**Complications:** Unknown.

**Associated Findings:** Otosclerosis, hyperlaxity of the joints, severe dental caries.

**Etiology:** Autosomal dominant inheritance with variable penetrance.

**Pathogenesis:** Unknown.

**MIM No.:** *16150

**CDC No.:** 748.180

**Sex Ratio:** M1:F1

**Occurrence:** Documented in two kindreds.

**Risk of Recurrence for Patient's Sib:**
 See Part I, *Mendelian Inheritance.*

**Risk of Recurrence for Patient's Child:**
 See Part I, *Mendelian Inheritance.*

**Age of Detectability:** Becomes prominent in childhood, at which time it may have a rose color.

**Gene Mapping and Linkage:** Unknown.

**Prevention:** None known. Genetic counseling indicated.

**Treatment:** Not necessary.

**Prognosis:** Normal for life span, intelligence, and function; the groove disappears after puberty.

**Detection of Carrier:** Unknown.

**References:**
Anderson PC: Familial transverse nasal groove. Arch Dermatol 1961; 84:316–317.

Pierre ER, Teneyck FD: Hereditary hyperpigmentation anomalies in blacks. J Hered 1974; 65:157–159.

MY003                                                **Charles M. Myer III**

## NOSE, TURBINATE DEFORMITY                            2720

**Includes:**
 Nasal agenesis
 Turbinate deformity

**Excludes:**
 Choanal atresia
 **Nose, anterior stenosis** (2718)
 **Nose, bifid** (0724)
 **Nose, dislocated nasal septum** (2719)
 **Nose/nasal septum defects** (0722)

**Major Diagnostic Criteria:** The inferior or middle turbinate may acquire a rounded, bulbous appearance, causing airway obstruction.

**Clinical Findings:** There is extra space in one nasal cavity due to long standing septal deviation. Both bone and mucosal elements may be involved, and hypertrophy to fill the larger nasal cavity.

**Complications:** Nasal obstruction, and turbinate invasion by ethmoid air cells.

**Associated Findings:** None known.

**Etiology:** Unknown.

**Pathogenesis:** Whether the turbinate enlargement causes the septum to be deformed or the turbinate enlarges to fill the space created by the septal deformity is unknown.

**CDC No.:** 748.180

**Sex Ratio:** Undetermined but presumably M1:F1.

**Occurrence:** Ethmoid invasion of the middle turbinate is found in 12% of adults.

**Risk of Recurrence for Patient's Sib:** Unknown.

**Risk of Recurrence for Patient's Child:** Unknown.

**Age of Detectability:** During childhood.

**Gene Mapping and Linkage:** Unknown.

**Prevention:** It is undetermined whether repair of septal dislocation will prevent this deformity.

**Treatment:** It is controversial whether turbinate enlargement in children should be treated at all. Septal repair and surgical reduction procedure of turbinate (cautery vs. turbinectomy) is sometimes performed.

**Prognosis:** Good for function with treatment.

**Detection of Carrier:** Unknown.

**References:**
Sprinkle PM, Sponck FT: Congenital malformations of the nose and paranasal sinuses. In: Bluestone CD, Stool SE, eds: Pediatric otolaryngology. Philadelphia: W.B. Saunders, 1983:769–779.

MY003                                                **Charles M. Myer III**
0R005                                                    **Peter Orobello**

## NOSE/NASAL SEPTUM DEFECTS                            0722

**Includes:**
 Dermoid cysts of nose of both skin and dural origin
 Nasal septum, absence of
 Nose, absence of
 Nose, absence of half
 Nose, half, plus proboscis
 Persistent frontonasal process
 "Potato" nose
 Triple nares

**Excludes:**
 Nasal deformities secondary to cleft lip or cleft palate

**Nose, abnormalities of growth of the maxillary processes**
**Nose, anterior atresia** (0723)
**Nose, bifid** (0724)
**Nose, duplication** (0725)

**Major Diagnostic Criteria:** Evidence of a nasal defect other than bifid nose or nasal duplication.

**Clinical Findings:** The degree of nasal deformity can vary from a small notch in one ala to total absence of the nose. The minor abnormalities are much more frequent.

**Complications:** Total nasal obstruction may be associated with asphyxia at birth. Intermediate degrees of nasal obstruction may also lead to a higher incidence of acquired ear disease. Speech defects are occasionally present. Psychologic problems occur due to the cosmetic deformity.

**Associated Findings:** Hypertelorism and abnormal location of the anterior fontanel are frequently seen with major deformities of the nose and are probably directly related to an abnormality of development of the frontonasal process.

**Etiology:** Some cases appear to be inherited.

**Pathogenesis:** The external nose and nasal septum are derived from a prolongation of the frontonasal process together with an infolding which produces the nasal septum. Unequal growth of the two sides of the nasal septum or excessive infolding of the septal portion without fusion of the 2 parts can account for the majority of the abnormalities of the nose and septum. The unusual inclusion dermoids of dural origin can be accounted for by dural extensions which have become included in the frontonasal process as it grows out from the anterior cranium.

**MIM No.:** 16400

**Sex Ratio:** M1:F1

**Occurrence:** Undetermined but presumed rare.

**Risk of Recurrence for Patient's Sib:** Unknown.

**Risk of Recurrence for Patient's Child:** Unknown.

**Age of Detectability:** At birth.

**Gene Mapping and Linkage:** Unknown.

**Prevention:** None known. Genetic counseling indicated.

**Treatment:** Operative repair of defect or reconstruction is indicated if either functional or cosmetic problems are present.

**Prognosis:** Generally good except for cases with total nasal obstruction occurring at birth when asphyxia may lead to death, or brain damage. Newborn infants are obligate nose breathers and temporary measures to keep the mouth open should be used until definitive surgery can be performed, including use of an oral airway.

**Detection of Carrier:** Unknown.

**References:**
Badrawy R: Mid-line congenital anomalies of the nose. J Laryngol Otol 1967; 81:419.
Toriello HV, et al.: Familial occurrence of a developmental defect of the medial nasal process. Am J Med Genet 1985; 21:131–135.

MY003                                    **Charles M. Myer III**

**Nougaret disease**
*See NIGHTBLINDNESS, CONGENITAL STATIONARY, AUTOSOMAL DOMINANT*
**Nova Scotian type Niemann-Pick disease**
*See NIEMANN-PICK DISEASE*
**Nuchal lymphangioma**
*See NECK, CYSTIC HYGROMA, FETAL TYPE*
**Nuclear cataract**
*See CATARACT, AUTOSOMAL DOMINANT CONGENITAL*
*also CATARACT, COPPOCK*
**Nuclear facial palsy**
*See PALSY, CONGENITAL FACIAL*
**Nuclear hypoplasia congenital (6th and 7th cranial nerves)**
*See DIPLEGIA, CONGENITAL FACIAL*
**Nucleoside-phosphorylase deficiency**
*See IMMUNODEFICIENCY, NUCLEOSIDE-PHOSPHORYLASE DEFICIENCY*

**Nuidudui**
*See ANEMIA, SICKLE CELL*
**Nyssen-van Bogaert syndrome**
*See OPTICO-COCHLEO-DENTATE DEGENERATION*
**Nystagmus-brachydactyly-cerebellar ataxia syndrome**
*See BIEMOND I SYNDROME*

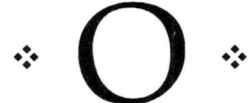

Oast-house urine disease
  See METHIONINE MALABSORPTION
Obesity-hypotonia-prominent incisors
  See COHEN SYNDROME
Obstetric hepatosis
  See INTRAHEPATIC CHOLESTASIS OF PREGNANCY (ICP)
Obstructing muscular bands of the right ventricle
  See VENTRICLE, DOUBLE CHAMBERED RIGHT
Obstruction within the right ventricular body
  See VENTRICLE, DOUBLE CHAMBERED RIGHT
Obstructive hydrocephaly, extra- and intraventricular congenital
  See HYDROCEPHALY

## OCCIPITAL HORN SYNDROME                          3219

**Includes:**
  Cutis laxa, X-linked
  Ehlers-Danlos syndrome IX (obsolete)

**Excludes:**
  **Ehlers-Danlos syndrome** (0338)
  **Menkes syndrome** (0643)

**Major Diagnostic Criteria:** *Clinical:* Skin lax and mildly hyperextensible, hypermobile digits, and bony protuberances of the occiput.

*Biochemical:* Moderate increase in serum copper and ceruloplasmin levels. Excess of copper and increased $^{64}$Cu accumulation, attached to metallothionein, in cultured fibroblasts. Lysyl oxidase deficiency.

The nosology of occipital horn syndrome (OHS) has been complicated; initially the condition was designated X-linked Cutis laxa and thereafter it was termed ''Ehlers-Danlos syndrome type IX''. Recently it has been established that OHS is due to a defect in copper metabolism and the OHS is now grouped with other disorders of copper transport.

**Clinical Findings:** The skin of the affected males is lax or mildly hyperextensible. Digits are hypermobile, while the elbows and knees have limitation of extension due to abnormalities of bone modelling. Bony protuberances of the occiput, known as occipital horns, which present as bony nubbins in the first decade are an important diagnostic indicator.

Other skeletal stigmata include short clavicles, carpal bone coalescences and osteomalacia.

Diverticulae of the bladder may rupture spontaneously. Chronic diarrhea and postural hypotension are inconsistent features.

*X-ray findings:* occipital exostoses, clavicles short and thickened at horny distal ends. Micturating cystogram confirms bladder diverticulae. Other changes are variable.

**Complications:** Limitation of extension of knees and elbows; bladder rupture; **Hernia, inguinal.**

**Associated Findings:** None known.

**Etiology:** X-linked recessive inheritance.

**Pathogenesis:** Disorder of copper transport. Decreased activity of lysyl oxidase, the extracellular copper enzyme that initiates crosslinking of collagen and elastin. Corresponding to this decreased activity is a deficiency in the enzyme protein.

**MIM No.:** *30415

**Sex Ratio:** M1:F0

**Occurrence:** Undetermined but presumed rare, with no specific geographical grouping.

**Risk of Recurrence for Patient's Sib:**
  See Part I, *Mendelian Inheritance.*

**Risk of Recurrence for Patient's Child:**
  See Part I, *Mendelian Inheritance.*

**Age of Detectability:** In the first decade of life.

**Gene Mapping and Linkage:** LOX (lysyl oxidase; ?cutis laxa-X; ?Ehlers-Danlos V) has been provisionally mapped to X.

**Prevention:** None known. Genetic counseling indicated.

**Treatment:** Parenteral copper administration seems unlikely to remedy the low lysyl oxidase activity.

**Prognosis:** Life span is not significantly reduced.

**Detection of Carrier:** Unknown.

**Special Considerations:** The designation of this disorder as occipital horn syndrome, and the discontinuation of the use of the terms ''EDS IX'' or ''XL Cutis Laxa'', was formalized at the Workshop for the Nosology of Inherited Connective Tissue Disorders in Berlin in 1986 (Beighton et al, 1988).

**References:**
Byers PH, et al.: X-linked cutis laxa. New Engl J Med 1980; 303:61–65.
Sartons DJ, et al.: Type IX Ehlers-Danlos syndrome. Radiology 1984; 152:665–670.
Kuivaniemi H, et al.: Type IX Ehlers-Danlos syndrome and Menkes syndrome: the decrease in lysyl oxidase activity is associated with a corresponding deficiency in the enzyme protein. Am J Hum Genet 1985; 37:798–808.
Beighton P, et al.: International Nosology of Heritable Disorders of Connective Tissue, Berlin, 1986. Am J Med Genet 1988; 29:581–594.

WI055                                      **Ingrid M. Winship**

Occipito-facial-cervico-thoracic-abdomino-digital dysplasia
  See SPONDYLOTHORACIC DYSPLASIA
Ochoa syndrome
  See UROFACIAL SYNDROME
Ochronosis
  See ALKAPTONURIA
Ochronotic arthritis
  See ALKAPTONURIA
Octanoyl-CoA or general acyl-CoA dehydrogenase deficiency
  See ACYL-CoA DEHYDROGENASE DEFICIENCY, MEDIUM CHAIN
    TYPE
Ocular albinism
  See ALBINISM
  also ALBINISM, OCULAR, AUTOSOMAL RECESSIVE TYPE
  also ALBINISM, OCULAR

**Ocular albinism, Forsius-Eriksson type**
  *See FORSIUS-ERIKSSON SYNDROME*
**Ocular albinism-sensorineural deafness (OASD)**
  *See ALBINISM, OCULAR-LATE-ONSET-SENSORINEURAL
  DEAFNESS, X-LINKED*
**Ocular and facial anomalies-proteinuria-deafness**
  *See FACIO-OCULO-ACOUSTIC-RENAL SYNDROME (FOAR
  SYNDROME)*
**Ocular coloboma-imperforate anus-preauricular appendages**
  *See CAT EYE SYNDROME*

## OCULAR DERMOIDS                                              0591

**Includes:**
  Conjunctival dermoid
  Dermoid of the cornea
  Epibulbar dermoid
  Eyelid tumor
  Limbal dermoid

**Excludes:**
  **Eye, dermolipoma** (0284)
  **Orbital and periorbital dermoid cysts** (0761)

**Major Diagnostic Criteria:**  Congenital tumor composed of choristomatous tissues usually located at the limbus.

**Clinical Findings:**  Solid or cystic, whitish mass located at the limbus, or upon the sclera, conjunctiva, or, rarely, the cornea. Usually single lesion involves one eye and remains stationary. Mattos, et al have reported five members of a three generation pedigree with bilateral annular limbal dermoids. Tumors are covered by stratified squamous epithelium with epidermal appendages, and may contain various well differentiated choristomatous tissues such as fat, smooth muscles or skeletal muscles, brain, teeth, cartilage, or bone.

**Complications:**  If tumor encroaches upon cornea it may cause astigmatism, lipid deposits, or obstruct the visual axis. Extension into anterior chamber through a scleral defect may cause glaucoma.

**Associated Findings:**  **Mandibulofacial dysostosis**, Goldenhar syndrome, **Proteus syndrome**, preauricular appendages, **Eyelid, coloboma**, and **Nevus, epidermal nevus syndrome**.

**Etiology:**  Unknown.

**Pathogenesis:**  Unknown.

**Sex Ratio:**  Presumably M1:F1

**Occurrence:**  Undetermined but presumably rare.

**Risk of Recurrence for Patient's Sib:**  Unknown.

**Risk of Recurrence for Patient's Child:**  Unknown.

**Age of Detectability:**  At birth.

**Gene Mapping and Linkage:**  Unknown.

**Prevention:**  None known. Genetic counseling indicated.

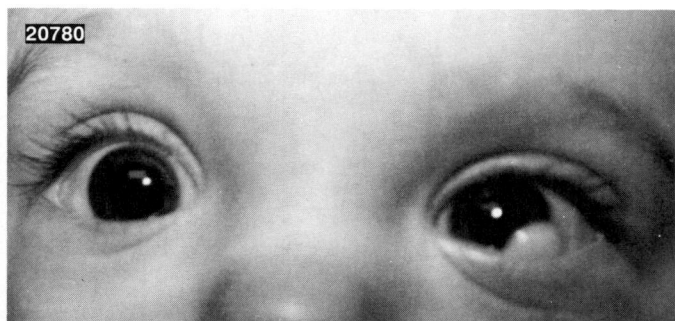

**0591A**-20780:  Ocular dermoid OS.

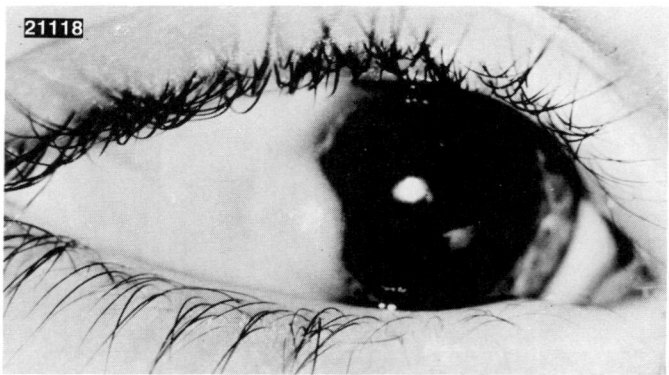

**0591B**-21118:  Dermoid along the inferotemporal limbus.

**Treatment:**  Excision. Caution is necessary during surgical excision since dermoid may be associated with area of thinned sclera (staphyloma).

**Prognosis:**  Benign tumor. Unless dermoid involves cornea, visual function is normal.

**Detection of Carrier:**  Unknown.

**References:**
Duke-Elder S: System of ophthalmology, vol. 3, Pt 2. Congenital deformities. St. Louis: CV Mosby, 1963:820–826.
Schultze RR: Limbal dermoid tumor with intraocular extension. Arch Ophthalmol 1966; 75:803–805.
Benjamin SJ, Allen HF: Classification for limbal dermoid, choristomatous and branchial arch anomalies. Arch Ophthalmol 1972; 87:305–314.
Hutchinson DS, et al.: Ectopic brain tissue in a limbal dermoid associated with a scleral staphyloma. Am J Ophthalmol 1973; 76:984–986.
Mattos J, et al.: Ring dermoid syndrome. Arch Ophthalmol 1980; 98:1059–1061.

WE035                                              **Avery H. Weiss**

## OCULAR DRUSEN                                              0734

**Includes:**
  Colloid bodies, familial
  Doyne honeycombed retinal degeneration
  Drusen, ocular
  Drusen of Bruch membrane
  Hutchinson-Tay choroiditis
  Malattia levantinese

**Excludes:**
  Drusen secondary to disease of choroid
  **Retina, fundus albipunctatus** (0399)
  **Retina, fundus flavimaculatus** (0400)
  Giant drusen of optic disk

**Major Diagnostic Criteria:**  Drusen beginning in the third or fourth decade with no evidence of other choroidal disease. Detection in more than one member of family helps to confirm the diagnosis.

**Clinical Findings:**  The eyegrounds are characterized by deep yellowish lesions usually round or oval in configuration and varying in size from small, dot-like to larger foci about four times the caliber of the first order retinal arterioles. They may have pigment flecks in the center or around their borders, and frequently show secondary changes such as calcification. The lesions are usually of greatest concentration in the posterior polar region. They are frequently present in the periphery and are sometimes widespread over most of the retina. These lesions may become

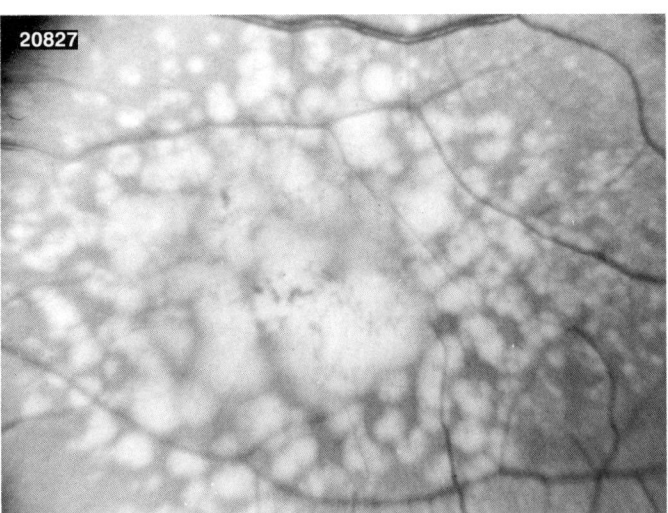

0734-20827: Retina, drusen.

confluent, particularly in or near the macular area into well-defined cloverleaf shapes or multilevel plaques. With fluorescein angiography, the lesions are well defined and overwhelmingly of distinct round shape with little tendency for confluence. These deposits are usually first seen in the third decade or first half of the fourth decade of life.

White or yellowish plaques may be seen in the macula and numerous clusters of drusen elsewhere. Secondary macular degeneration occurs frequently in the last stage. Not all cases follow the typical sequence. There is considerable variation in the ophthalmoscopic appearance even within the same family.

Visual acuity is affected when drusen appear in the fovea. The loss is often moderate with vision maintained at 20/30 to 20/60. However, widespread macular degeneration can occur either with extensive drusen or serous retinal detachment.

Peripheral vision remains good but central scotomas are present when macular degeneration supervenes. Dark adaptation may be mildly abnormal but the ERG is normal. The EOG was initially reported as severely affected but recent data do not support those claims and most patients have a normal EOG.

**Complications:**  Macular degeneration.

**Associated Findings:**  None known.

**Etiology:**  Autosomal dominant inheritance, with occasional reports of autosomal recessive inheritance.

**Pathogenesis:**  These deposits are hyaline excrescences in the cuticular portion of Bruch membrane--numerous discrete, round, fluorescent spots of varying size which far outnumber the drusen seen with the ophthalmoscope and are compatible with a diffuse pigment epithelium alteration. Pigment epithelium changes may be seen even in areas where there are no drusen, suggesting a widespread disturbance of the pigment epithelium in this condition. The drusen probably represent a secretion of the abnormal pigment epithelium.

**MIM No.:**  *12660, 12670

**Sex Ratio:**  M1:F1

**Occurrence:**  More than a dozen kindreds have been well documented since Doyne (1899) first described the condition at the turn of the century, with many of them tracing their history back to the area around Oxford, England, and possibly to a common ancestor.

**Risk of Recurrence for Patient's Sib:**
See Part I, *Mendelian Inheritance.*

**Risk of Recurrence for Patient's Child:**
See Part I, *Mendelian Inheritance.*

**Age of Detectability:**  Usually between 25–35 years of age.

**Gene Mapping and Linkage:**  Unknown.

**Prevention:**  None known. Genetic counseling indicated.

**Treatment:**  Unknown.

**Prognosis:**  Normal life span with frequent minimal reduction of vision in later life. Occasional moderate to severe reduction of vision.

**Detection of Carrier:**  Clinical examination.

**Special Considerations:**  Drusen may be secondary to numerous diseases of the choroid and are frequently noted in patients over 60 years of age on this basis. Melanoma of the choroid is a frequent cause of secondary drusen in younger patients.

**Retina, fundus flavimaculatus** and **Retina, fundus albipunctatus** are both of autosomal recessive inheritance. Fluorescein characteristics particularly distinguish fundus flavimaculatus from drusen. The lesions of fundus albipunctatus are white or yellow-white, uniform, dot-like, discrete and are usually present over most of the fundus with greatest density in the midperiphery. Their size usually corresponds to a 2nd order arteriole. The early lesions of drusen may be confused with the typical lesions of fundus albipunctatus. Drusen, however, are eventually characterized by variability in size, shape, color and a tendency to confluence. The ERG and dark adaptation are always affected in fundus albipunctatus but these tests are normal in drusen.

**References:**
Doyne RW: A peculiar condition of choroiditis occuring in several members of the same family. Trans Ophthal Soc UK 1899; 19:71 only.
Krill AE, Klein BA: Flecked retina syndrome. Arch Ophthalmol 1965; 74:496–508.
Ernest JT, Krill AE: Fluorescein studies in flavimaculatus and drusen. Am J Ophthalmol 1966; 62:1–6.
Pearce WG: Doyne's honeycomb retinal degeneration: clinical and genetic features. Br J Ophthalmol 1968; 52:73–78.
Deutman AF, Janse LMAA: Dominantly inherited drusen of Bruch's membrane. Brit J Ophthal 1970; 54:373–382.
Fishman GA, et al.: The electrooculogram in diffuse (familial) drusen. Arch Ophthalmol 1971; 92:231–233.

W0003 **Mitchel L. Wolf**

**Ocular fibrosis syndrome, congenital**
*See EYE, FIBROSIS OF THE EXTRAOCULAR MUSCLES, GENERALIZED*
**Ocular hypertelorism**
*See EYE, HYPERTELORISM*
**Ocular lens, dislocation of**
*See LENS, ECTOPIC*
**Ocular lymphangioma**
*See ORBITAL AND PERIORBITAL LYMPHANGIOMA*
**Ocular melanocytosis, congenital**
*See EYE, MELANOSIS OCULI, CONGENITAL*

## OCULAR MOTOR APRAXIA, COGAN CONGENITAL TYPE 0191

**Includes:**  Cogan ocular motor apraxia, congenital

**Excludes:**  Ataxia-telangiectasia (0094)

**Major Diagnostic Criteria:**  Failure of normal ocular fixation and head thrusting; retention of normal vertical eye movements. The possibility of blindness should be excluded by normal response on measurement of visual evoked response.

**Clinical Findings:**  Congenital ocular motor apraxia is a defect in the horizontal eye movements involved in voluntary gaze and in the fast phase of both vestibular and optokinetic nystagmus. The pursuit movements are usually normal.

Compensatory head thrusts on attempting to fixate an object to either side is the most obvious clinical sign. Being unable to initiate the eye movement readily, the infant or child rotates the head toward the object of regard. But, due to the associated defect in initiating the fast phase of the vestibular response, the eyes show a contraversive deviation during the rotation. This head thrust is highly characteristic of the clinical presentation. Also characteristic is the maintained deviation of the eyes when the patient is rotated about a vertical axis.

In contrast to the defect in voluntary eye movement, the patient makes normal random movements of the eyes when not alerted to make a voluntary fixation. Also, contrasting with the defect of horizontal gaze are the normal vertical movements for all parameters of gaze.

The head thrusts are usually noted at 3–4 months of age when the infant begins to hold his head erect. Prior to this, the failure to fixate an object may be misinterpreted as indicating blindness or cerebral palsy. General development is typically normal, but the child tends to be clumsy in sports and to be a poor reader in the first few years of school. The signs and symptoms progressively improve during childhood and are not known to cause any functional deficit in adult life.

Similar head thrusts and defects of the vestibular and optokinetic reflexes are seen with **ataxia telangiectasia** and possibly with other defects of the saccadic system, but, unlike congenital ocular motor apraxia, these involve the vertical as well as the horizontal eye movements.

**Complications:** Children are reported to be clumsy and are poor readers in the first few years of school.

**Associated Findings:** A similar ocular motor syndrome occurs frequently in **Gaucher disease** (type III), occasionally in patients with congenital defects of the midbrain, and rarely in infants with tumors of the pontocerebellar region (two cases). Two cases have been reported with brain tumors in the posterior fossa. Several cases have been reported with midline structural defects of the brain or with vermal aplasia of the cerebellum.

**Etiology:** Autosomal recessive inheritance. Several familial cases have been documented, including one family of apparent dominant transmission, and one occurrence in identical twins. Most cases occur sporadically unaccompanied by other abnormalities.

**Pathogenesis:** Unknown.

**MIM No.:** *21650

**Sex Ratio:** M2:F1

**Occurrence:** Some fifty cases documented.

**Risk of Recurrence for Patient's Sib:**
See Part I, *Mendelian Inheritance.*

**Risk of Recurrence for Patient's Child:**
See Part I, *Mendelian Inheritance.*

**Age of Detectability:** In infancy.

**Gene Mapping and Linkage:** Unknown.

**Prevention:** None known. Genetic counseling indicated.

**Treatment:** Unknown.

**Prognosis:** Symptoms progressively improve during the first two decades of life and are not known to cause any functional deficit in the adult.

**Detection of Carrier:** Unknown.

**References:**
Cogan DG: A type of congenital ocular motor apraxia presenting jerky head movements. Trans Am Acad Ophthalmol Otolaryngol 1952; 56:853–862.
Vassella F, et al.: Cogan's congenital ocular motor apraxia in two successive generations. Dev Med Child Neurol 1972; 14:788–796.
Zee DS, et al.: Congenital ocular motor apraxia. Brain 1977; 100:581–599.
Cogan DG, et al.: A long-term follow-up of congenital ocular motor apraxia. Neuro-ophthalmol 1980; 1:145–147.
Cogan DG, et al.: Notes on congenital ocular motor apraxia: associated anomalies. In: Glaser J, ed: Neuro-ophthalmology. St. Louis: C.V. Mosby, 1980:171–179.
Zaret CR, et al.: Congenital ocular motor apraxia and brain stem tumor. Arch Ophthalmol 1980; 98:328–330.
Gittinger JW, Sokol S: The visual-evoked potential in the diagnosis of congenital ocular motor apraxia. Am J Ophthalmol 1982; 93:700–703.

C0004                                    **David G. Cogan**

**Ocular myopathy**
*See OPHTHALMOPLEGIA, PROGRESSIVE EXTERNAL*
**Ocular retraction syndrome**
*See EYE, DUANE RETRACTION SYNDROME*
**Ocular-scoliotic type Ehlers-Danlos syndrome**
*See EHLERS-DANLOS SYNDROME*
**Oculo-acoustic cerebral degeneration, congenital progressive**
*See NORRIE DISEASE*

## OCULO-AURICULO-VERTEBRAL ANOMALY     0735

**Includes:**
Facio-auriculo-vertebral spectrum
First and second branchial arch syndrome
Goldenhar syndrome
Goldenhar-Gorlin syndrome
Hemifacial microsomia

**Excludes:**
Acrofacial dysostosis, Nager type (2167)
Acrofacial dysostosis, postaxial type (2126)
Anus-hand-ear syndrome (0072)
Branchio-oto-renal dysplasia (2224)
Charge association (2124)

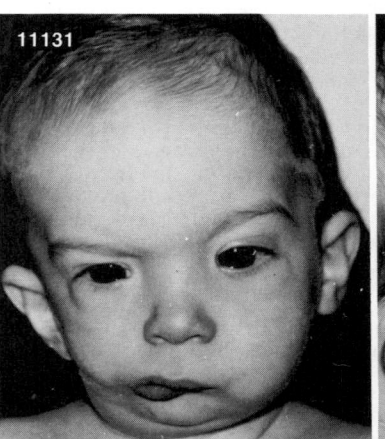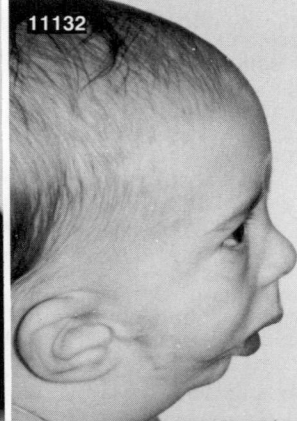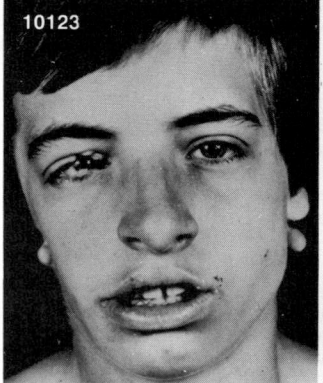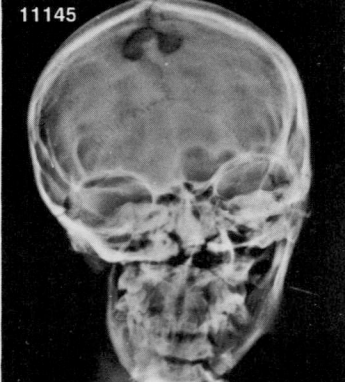

**0735-11131–32:** Facial asymmetry secondary to hemifacial microsomia. **10123:** Coloboma of upper eyelid, abnormal auricles and unilateral facial hypoplasia. **11145:** X-ray demonstrates right-sided hypoplasia of the face and right mandible.

**Hemifacial atrophy, progressive** (2615)
**Mandibulofacial dysostosis** (0627)
**Mandibulo-facial dysostosis, Treacher-Collins type, recessive** (2802)
**MURCS association** (2406)
**Oro-facio-digital syndrome**
**Vater association** (0987)

**Major Diagnostic Criteria:** External ear malformations with associated middle ear anomalies and conductive hearing loss, macrostomia, mandibular hypoplasia, epibulbar dermoids or lipodermoids, and/or anomalies of the cervical spine. X-ray may be required to detect vertebral anomalies and facial asymmetry. Microtia or preauricular tags may represent the most mild expression of the defect in some families.

**Clinical Findings:** Variability of expression is characteristic of oculo-auriculo-vertebral dysplasia (OAV). Ten to 33% of patients have bilateral facial involvement. The disorder is nearly always more severe on one side. The right side is involved more severely in over 60% of patients. Marked facial asymmetry is present in 20% of patients; some degree of asymmetry is evident in 65%. The asymmetry may not be apparent in the infant or young child but is usually evident by age four years.

The maxillary, temporal, and malar bones on the more severely involved side may be small and flattened. The mandibular ramus and condyle may be hypoplastic or absent. Reduced pneumatization of the mastoid region may be observed.

At least 35% of patients with agenesis of the mandibular ramus have associated macrostomia; i.e., lateral facial cleft, usually of a mild degree. The macrostomia is almost always unilateral and on the more severely affected side. There may be associated agenesis of the parotid gland. Intraorally, the palate and tongue muscles may be unilaterally hypoplastic.

Malformation of the external ear may vary from anotia to a mildly dysmorphic ear. Approximately one-third of cases show bilateral ear involvement. Preauricular tags of skin and cartilage are common and may occur anywhere from the tragus to the angle of the mouth. Preauricular sinuses may be present. Narrow or atretic external auditory canals may be observed. Small auricles with normal architecture may occasionally be seen. Conductive and, less frequently, sensorineural hearing loss occurs in the majority of patients because of hypoplasia or agenesis of ossicles, aberrant facial nerves, and abnormalities of the eustachian tube.

Blepharophimosis, or narrowing of the palpebral fissure, occurs in 10% of patients. Anophthalmia or microphthalmia has been described, as have retinal abnormalities. Epibulbar tumors (dermoids, lipodermoids) are found in 35% of patients; they appear as solid, yellow or pink ovoid masses up to 10mm in diameter. Bilateral lesions may occur. Vision may be impaired.

Cervical vertebral fusions occur in 20–25% of patients, and **Klippel-Feil anomaly** has occasionally been observed. Platybasia and occipitalization of the atlas is found in about 30% of patients.

**Complications:** Infants may be small for gestational age and may have feeding difficulties because of associated cleft lip and/or cleft palate or an anatomically narrow pharyngeal airway. Obstructive sleep apnea has been described.

Significant visual impairment may be present because of epibulbar tumors or anophthalmia/microphthalmia. Removal of epibulbar tumors can lead to scar formation with resultant leukoma.

Velopharyngeal insufficiency has been reported unassociated with cleft palate.

**Associated Findings:** Cranial defects consisting of plagiocephaly, microcephaly, skull defects, or intracranial dermoid cysts have been reported. Occipital encephalocele has been noted. Mental retardation occurs in 5–15% of the patients, and those with cranial defects are at higher risk. Unilateral or bilateral cleft lip and/or palate occurs in 7–15% of patients. Cleft palate is twice as common as cleft lip with or without cleft palate. Pulmonary anomalies, ranging in severity from incomplete lobulation to unilateral agenesis, have been reported. A variety of kidney abnormalities have been reported, including absent kidney, double ureter, ectopia, hydronephrosis, and hydroureter.

Congenital heart disease occurs with increased frequency; reported incidence figures range from 5 to 58%. Although no single cardiac lesion is characteristic, **Ventricular septal defect** and **Heart, tetralogy of Fallot** appear to be the most common.

A wide variety of skeletal abnormalities have been reported, affecting 30% of patients. Spina bifida, anomalous vertebrae, scoliosis, and anomalous ribs are relatively common. Talipes equinovarus has been reported in 20%. Limb anomalies may affect approximately 10% of patients. Radial limb anomalies may include aplasia of the radius and/or thumb or a bifid or digitalized thumb.

**Etiology:** There are multiple reports of familial cases, with widely varying expression between affected family members. Patterns of inheritance are consistent with autosomal dominant, autosomal recessive, and multifactorial inheritance. Several aberrant karyotypes have been reported.

**Pathogenesis:** May be related to abnormal neural crest cell morphology and subsequent malformation of the derivatives of the first and second visceral arches. Vascular abnormalities during embryogenesis have produced branchial arch anomalies in animals. Jongbloet (1987) suggested a theory of "overripeness ovopathy".

**MIM No.:** 14140, 16421, 25770

**POS No.:** 3339

**CDC No.:** 756.060

**Sex Ratio:** M3:F2

**Occurrence:** Grabb (1965) observed 1:5,600 births in the Midwest of the United States. Another study recorded 1:26,500 live births in a prospective study of United States newborns. No other population differences have been reported.

**Risk of Recurrence for Patient's Sib:** Empiric recurrence risk is 2–3%.

**Risk of Recurrence for Patient's Child:** Unknown.

**Age of Detectability:** At birth, based on clinical features. Mandibular hypoplasia may be masked by overlying soft tissue, but usually becomes apparent by age four years. Audiologic evaluation at an early age can detect hearing loss. High-resolution ultrasound may be used for prenatal detection of severe ear malformations, mandibular hypoplasia, facial clefts, and other skeletal abnormalities. Prenatal chromosome analysis may be helpful in some instances.

**Gene Mapping and Linkage:** Unknown.

**Prevention:** Avoidance of exposure to known teratogens.

**Treatment:** Detect and manage associated conductive hearing loss early in life. Repair facial clefts by age six months when possible. Speech therapy is often required. Orthodontic and dental care to correct malocclusion and other dental anomalies. Plastic surgery may improve the facial appearance. Surgical gastrostomy may be required for treatment of feeding problem. Other manifestations should be treated appropriately.

**Prognosis:** Varies with etiology and associated malformations. For those patients with no associated chromosomal anomalies or other severe associated malformations, life span is normal. Five to 15% have reduced intelligence. Some patients may develop emotional problems secondary to their facial defects.

**Detection of Carrier:** Careful evaluation of first degree relatives will help to identify individuals with mild facial manifestations of the condition and other extracranial anomalies.

**Special Considerations:** Originally, the term *hemifacial microsomia* was used do denote unilateral microtia, macrostomia, and failure of the formation of mandibular ramus and condyle. *Goldenhar syndrome* referred to a variant characterized by vertebral anomalies, most often hemivertebrae, and epibulbar dermoids. *First arch syndrome* and *First and second branchial arch syndrome* were also used, but implied that involvement was limited to facial structures.

As evidence emerged that each of these individual terms referred to variations within a single phenotypically variable and etiologically heterogeneous condition, which showed a wide range of clinical expression, Gorlin et al (1963) evolved the term *Oculo-auriculo-vertebral dysplasia* to describe the overall condition and its variants. Since forms of the condition may exists without "dysplasia" in the strict sense, the term "anomaly" has been substituted.

Within families, the spectrum of severity may range from severe microtia with significant mandibular involvement, to a unilateral ear tag. X-ray studies may be required to demonstrate a mildly hypoplastic mandible. Because of this wide range of expression, the numbers of alternative diagnoses with overlapping features becomes very extensive.

### References:
Gorlin RJ, et al.: Oculoariculovertebral dysplasia. J Pediatr 1963; 63:991–999.
Grabb WC: The first and second branchial arch syndrome. Plast Reconstr Surg 1965; 36:485–508.
Rollnick BR, Kaye CI: Hemifacial microsomia and variants: pedigree data. Am J Med Genet 1983; 15:233–253.
Tenconi R, Hall BD: Hemifacial microsomia: phenotypic classification, clinical implications and genetic aspects. In: Harvold EP, ed: Treatment of hemifacial microsomia. New York: Alan R. Liss, 1983:39–49.
Mansour AM, et al.: Ocular findings in the facioauriculovertebral sequence (Goldenhar-Gorlin syndrome). Am J Ophthalmol 1985; 100:555–559.
Boles DJ, et al.: Goldenhar complex in discordant monozygotic twins: a case report and review of the literature. Am J Med Genet 1987; 28:103–109.
Jongbloet PH: Goldenhar syndrome and overlapping dysplasias, in vitro fertilization and ovopathy. J Med Genet 1987; 24:616–620.
Rollnick BR, et al.: Oculoauriculovertebral dysplasia and variants: phenotypic characteristics of 294 patients. Am J Med Genet 1987; 26:361–375.
Kay ED, Kay CN: Dysmorphogenesis of the mandible, zygoma, and middle ear ossicles in hemifacial microsomia and mandibulofacial dysostosis. Am J Med Genet 1989; 32:27–31.

R0016
KA029

**Beverly R. Rollnick**
**Celia I. Kaye**

## OCULO-CEREBRO-CUTANEOUS SYNDROME 2752

### Includes:
Delleman-Oorthuys syndrome
Orbital cyst-cerebral and focal dermal malformations

### Excludes:
**Dermal hypoplasia, focal** (0281)
**Oculo-auriculo-vertebral anomaly** (0735)

**Major Diagnostic Criteria:** Orbital cysts in association with cerebral malformations, skin tags, and focal dermal regions of aplasia or hypoplasia. A computed tomographic scan or magnetic resonance image of the brain may be needed to document central nervous system malformations.

**Clinical Findings:** Clinical signs are recognized at birth. All patients exhibit orbital cysts, some of which (2/5) may be bilateral. Some of the orbital cysts may be filled with hamartomas containing distorted ocular structures including dysplastic rosettes of retinal neuroepithelium, as well as primitive tissue resembling brain. Other ophthalmic defects include eyelid colobomas (3/5), microphthalmos (4/5), and a persistent hyaloid artery (1/5).
Cerebral defects include multiple porencephalic cysts (4/4) and agenesis of the corpus callosum (3/4) which may been seen on X-ray. Mental retardation (4/5) and seizures (5/5) are common. These abnormalities may be unilateral or bilateral.
Skin tags are found in all infants in the periorbital and preauricular region. Multiple focal aplastic, hypoplastic, or punched-out skin lesions, also found in all children, are concentrated on the head and trunk but may be found anywhere on the body.
Other findings include skull defects and anomalies of the skeletal system, hands, feet, and genitalia. Generalized body asymmetry may occur (3/5) in association with both unilateral and bilateral orbital cysts.

**Complications:** Unknown.
**Associated Findings:** None known.

**Etiology:** Presumably sporadic, or possibly by autosomal dominant inheritance with variable expressivity or the result of an autosomal "dominant" lethal gene surviving by mosaicism (Happle, 1987).

**Pathogenesis:** The ocular involvement is possibly related to failure of the embryonic optic fissure and related structures to close during early development. There is no explanation for the systemic manifestations of the syndrome.

**MIM No.:** 16418

**POS No.:** 3506

**Sex Ratio:** M3:F2

**Occurrence:** Five cases have been reported in the literature; four of Dutch ancestry.

**Risk of Recurrence for Patient's Sib:** Unknown.

**Risk of Recurrence for Patient's Child:** Unknown.

**Age of Detectability:** At birth.

**Gene Mapping and Linkage:** Unknown.

**Prevention:** None known. Genetic counseling indicated.

**Treatment:** Surgical removal of the orbital cysts and hamartomas with cosmetic reconstruction is usually necessary. Anticonvulsant medication for seizures. Shunting procedures may be needed for **Hydrocephaly**.

**Prognosis:** Life span is undetermined. One child died at age two years from cerebral complications.

**Detection of Carrier:** Unknown.

### References:
Delleman JW, et al: Orbital cyst in addition to congenital cerebral and focal dermal malformations: a new entity? Clin Genet 1981; 19:191–198. * †
Delleman JW, et al: Orbital cyst in addition of congenital cerebral and focal dermal malformations: a new entity. Clin Genet 1984; 25:470–472. †
Ferguson JW, et al: Ocular, cerebral, and cutaneous malformations: confirmation of an association. Clin Genet 1984; 25:464–469.
Wilson RD, et al: Oculocerebrocutaneous syndrome. Am J Ophthalmol 1985; 99:142–148. * †
Happle R: Lethal genes surviving by mosaicism: a possible explanation for sporadic birth defects involving the skin. J Am Acad Dermatol 1987; 16:899–906.

ST057
CH037

**Gerald G. Striph**
**Fred C. Chu**

## OCULO-CEREBRO-FACIAL SYNDROME, KAUFMAN TYPE 2179

### Includes:
Cerebro-oculo-facial syndrome
Facial-oculo-cerebro syndrome
Kaufman syndrome

### Excludes:
**Cerebro-oculo-facio-skeletal syndrome** (0140)
**Heart-Hand syndrome IV** (3272)
**Oculo-dento-osseous dysplasia** (0737)
**Oculo-mandibulo-facial syndrome** (0738)

**Major Diagnostic Criteria:** The concomitant involvement of CNS (mental retardation, **Microcephaly**), eye (e.g., optic atrophy, microcornea), and mandibular arch (micrognathia, preauricular tags) is strongly suggestive of the diagnosis.

**Clinical Findings:** In three siblings on whom physical examinations were done and two other unrelated cases, the findings included: **Microcephaly** (5); sparse eyebrows (3); upslanting palpebral fissures (5); telecanthus (2); epicanthal folds (2); blepharophimosis or ptosis (2); microcornea (4); nystagmus (2); exotropia (1); amblyopia (1); strabismus (3); myopia (4); flat philtrum (2); highly arched palate (3); poorly formed teeth (4); micrognathia (4); preauricular tags (3); small, lowset ears (1); lordosis (2); large clitoris (1); joint contractures (2); edema of extremities (1); cutis

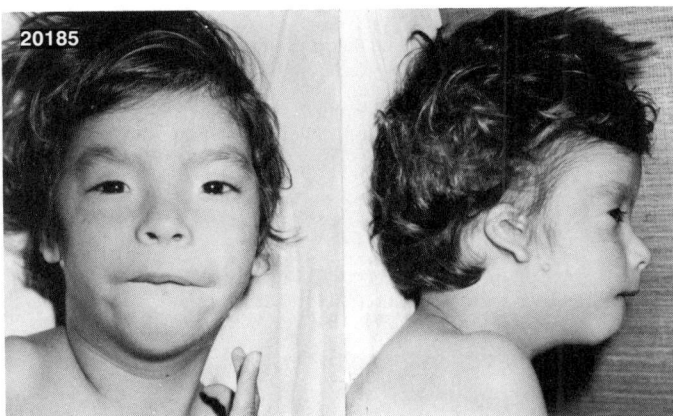

2179-20185: Note long narrow face, sparse eyebrows, mild blepharophimosis, epicanthal folds, telecanthus, large mouth with thin lips, poorly defined philtrum, bilateral skin tags, and micrognathia.

laxa (1); mental retardation (4); decreased muscle tone (3); respiratory difficulties in the newborn period (3); seizures (1); and choreiform movements (2).

**Complications:** Unknown.

**Associated Findings:** None known.

**Etiology:** Autosomal recessive inheritance.

**Pathogenesis:** Unknown.

**MIM No.:** *24445

**POS No.:** 3029

**Sex Ratio:** M2:F3 (observed in the five reported cases).

**Occurrence:** Four cases in one North American family of seven siblings, and two sporadic cases, have been reported.

**Risk of Recurrence for Patient's Sib:**
See Part I, *Mendelian Inheritance.*

**Risk of Recurrence for Patient's Child:**
See Part I, *Mendelian Inheritance.*

**Age of Detectability:** At birth, by physical examination.

**Gene Mapping and Linkage:** Unknown.

**Prevention:** None known. Genetic counseling indicated.

**Treatment:** Correction of ocular anomalies may be indicated.

**Prognosis:** Mental retardation is moderate to severe, lifespan is apparently not affected.

**Detection of Carrier:** Unknown.

**References:**
Kaufman RL, et al.: An oculocerebrofacial syndrome. BD:OAS VII(1). New York: March of Dimes Birth Defects Foundation, 1971:135–138.
Jurenka SB, Evans J: Kaufman oculocerebrofacial syndrome: case report. Am J Med Genet 1979; 3:15–19.
Garcia-Cruz D, et al.: Kaufman oculocerebrofacial syndrome: a corroborative report. Dysmorph Clin Genet 1988; 1:152–154.

T0007                                                          **Helga V. Toriello**

## OCULO-CEREBRO-RENAL SYNDROME                              0736

**Includes:**
  Cerebro-oculo-renal syndrome
  Lowe syndrome
  Renal-oculo-cerebro syndrome

**Excludes:**
  **Kidney, polycystic disease-cataract-blindness** (3288)
  **Renal tubular syndrome, Fanconi type** (0864)

**Major Diagnostic Criteria:** Bilateral cataracts at birth, physical and mental retardation, and hypotonia in a male child are the clinical hallmarks. Evidence of renal tubular dysfunction includes some or all of the following: generalized renal hyperaminoaciduria; "tubular" proteinuria (soluble with heat after initial precipitation with 20% sulfosalicylic acid) comprising $\beta$-globulins; low $T_m$ glucosuria; high renal clearance of inorganic phosphate with hypophosphatemia; renal tubular acidosis with impaired bicarbonate conservation; defect in $H^+$ secretion and ammonia production.

**Clinical Findings:** The complete phenotype is expressed uniformly in males only and is characterized by dense to mature cataracts (100%); glaucoma with or without buphthalmos, corneal scarring, or superficial granulations (50%); enophthalmos; growth failure; mental retardation; hypotonia at birth; reduced or absent deep tendon reflexes; metabolic acidosis; generalized hyperaminoaciduria; and tubular proteinuria after early infancy. Hypophosphatemic rickets appears as a later manifestation in about one-half the untreated patients. Bilateral cryptorchidism is common.

The tubular dysfunction increases in severity with age; its manifestations are thought to be minimal at birth, although only

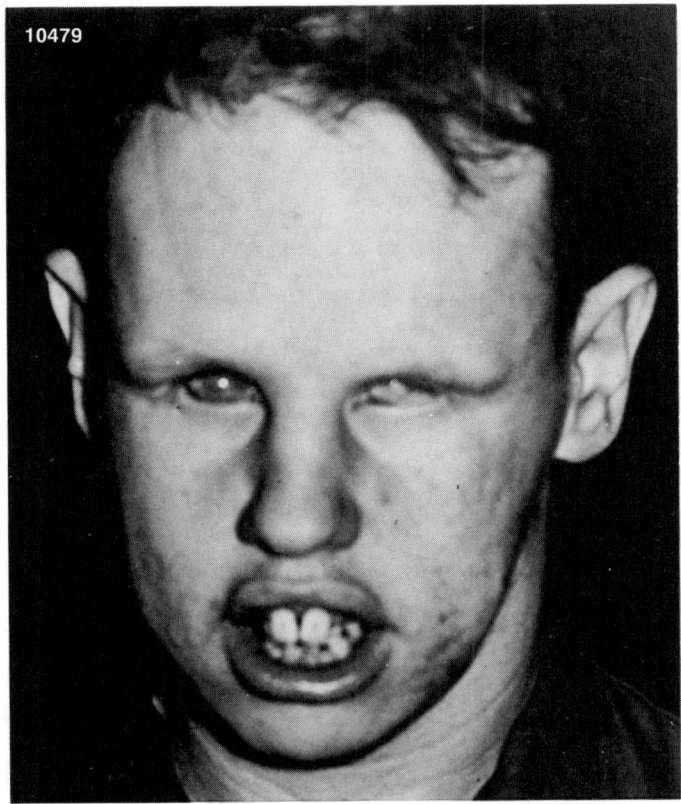

0736-10479: Cataracts, corneal scarring and enophthalmos are present in this 23-year-old mentally retarded male.

a few patients have yet been studied from birth onward. Rickets and/or osteomalacia are secondary to hypophosphatemia. Progresssive glomerular and interstitial fibrosis have been reported.

Histologic examination of eyes reveals warty excrescences and defects of the capsule of microphakic lenses. It has been postulated that the glaucoma is secondary to the small lens pulling on the ciliary body centrally, and thus preventing normal anterior chamber angle cleavage.

**Complications:** In untreated patients, renal tubular dysfunction appears during early infancy; failure to offset the latter is followed by predictable complications.

**Associated Findings:** Unknown.

**Etiology:** X-linked recessive inheritance.

**Pathogenesis:** It is presumed that all features are related to an undefined derangement of metabolism. The condition is expressed prenatally; a cataract-like lesion has been described in a male fetus (24th week) at risk; patients are born with cataracts. Deficient γ-glutamyl transpeptidase activity is not substantiated.

Reduced sulfation of glycosaminoglycans has been studied in several laboratories anticipating an abnormality in this condition. Recent studies of the synthesis of proteoglycans and glycosaminoglycans revealed marked variation in the rate of synthesis in normal and mutant cultures, but no significant difference in the two phenotypes. The authors (Harper et al, 1987) concluded that Lowe syndrome fibroblasts do not express a defect in sulfation of glycosaminoglycans or in the synthesis of proteoglycans.

**MIM No.:** *30900

**POS No.:** 3340

**Sex Ratio:** M1:F0

**Occurrence:** Undetermined. Established literature.

**Risk of Recurrence for Patient's Sib:**
See Part I, *Mendelian Inheritance.*

**Risk of Recurrence for Patient's Child:**
See Part I, *Mendelian Inheritance.*

**Age of Detectability:** At birth for cataracts; three to six months for tubular manifestations.

**Gene Mapping and Linkage:** OCRL (oculocerebrorenal syndrome of Lowe) has been mapped to Xq25-q26.1.

**Prevention:** None known. Genetic counseling indicated.

**Treatment:** Early treatment and good clinical home care reduce the phenotypic impact of the mutation; metabolic treatment includes correction of acidosis, hypophosphatemia, and other manifestations of tubulopathy. Care of ocular manifestations as indicated.

**Prognosis:** Poor for normal lifestyle, development, and longevity. All patients have loss of vision. Without treatment, the majority die in their first decade; a few survive into adolescence or beyond. Life span is increased by early diagnosis and symptomatic treatment.

**Detection of Carrier:** A study of the correlation between lecticular opacities and DNA haplotypes, using polymorphic markers in the region Xq24-q26, showed that carriers can be detected by slit lamp. Females at risk who have >100 opacities in the equatorial area of *both* lenses can be considered carriers (Wadelius et al., 1989).

**Support Groups:** IN; West Lafayette; Lowe's Syndrome Association

**References:**
Abbassi V, et al.: Oculo-cerebro-renal syndrome: a review. Am J Dis Child 1968; 115:145–168.
Witzleben CL, et al.: Progressive morphologic renal changes in the oculo-cerebro-renal syndrome of Lowe. Am J Med 1968; 44:319–324.
Gardner RJM, Brown N: Lowe's syndrome: identification of carriers by lens examination. J Med Genet 1976; 13:449–464.
Manz F, et al.: Renal transport of amino acids in children with oculocerebrorenal syndrome. Helv Paediatr Acta 1978; 33:37–44.
Hodgson SV, et al.: A balanced de novo X/autosome translocation in a girl with manifestations of Lowe syndrome. Am J Med Genet 1986; 23:837–847.
Tripathi R, et al.: Lowe's syndrome. BD:OAS XVIII(6). New York: March of Dimes Birth Defects Foundation, 1986:629–644.
Harper GS, et al.: Proteoglycan synthesis in normal and Lowe syndrome fibroblasts. J Biol Chem 1987; 262:5637–5643.
Wadelius C, et al.: Lowe-oculocerebral syndrome: DNA-based linkage of the gene Xq24-q26 using tightly linked flanking markers and the correlation to lens examination in carrier diagnosis. Am J Hum Genet 1989; 44:241–247.

SC050 **Charles R. Scriver**

**Oculo-cervico-acoustic syndrome**
*See CERVICO-OCULO-ACOUSTIC SYNDROME*
**Oculo-cranio-somatic neuromuscular disease with ragged-red fibers**
*See OPHTHALMOPLEGIA, PROGRESSIVE EXTERNAL*
**Oculo-dento-digital dysplasia**
*See OCULO-DENTO-OSSEOUS DYSPLASIA*

# OCULO-DENTO-OSSEOUS DYSPLASIA                0737

**Includes:**
> Dento-oculo-osseous dysplasia
> Oculo-dento-digital dysplasia
> ODD syndrome
> Osseous-oculo-dento dysplasia

**Excludes:**
> **Acrocephalosyndactyly type III** (0229)
> Microcornea
> **Oro-cranio-digital syndrome** (0769)
> **Teeth, amelogenesis imperfecta** (0046)

**Major Diagnostic Criteria:** Characteristic facies, consisting of thin nose, hypoplastic alae and narrow nostrils, microcornea, and syndactyly of the fourth and fifth fingers.

**Clinical Findings:** Head circumference may be somewhat reduced. Characteristic facies exhibiting thin nose with hypoplastic alae and thin, anteverted nostrils, microcornea, soft tissue syndactyly, and camptodactyly of fourth and fifth fingers (rarely the third); less often second, third, and fourth toes are involved; hypoplasia of enamel and microdontia. The fifth fingers may only exhibit clinodactyly in some patients. There may be associated epicanthal folds, strabismus, short narrow palpebral fissures, and various other eye findings such as secondary glaucoma, persistence of pupillary membranes, and optic atrophy. The iris appears porous, and the frill may overide the pupillary rim. The lip and/or palate are cleft in a few cases. The hair may be dry and lusterless and grows very slowly. Frequent skeletal alterations include thickened mandible, metaphyseal widening of long bones, lack of formation of middle phalanges of toes, and hypoplasia of middle phalanx of fifth fingers.

There may be a less common autosomal recessive form of this condition. Affected patients are more severly affected; marked cranial hyperostosis, massive mandibular overgrowth, gross clavicular widening, blindness, microphthalmia, calcification of basal ganglia, cataracts, cleft lip-palate, spastic quadriplegia, and persistence of primary vitreous have been reported.

**Complications:** Blindness may result.

**Associated Findings:** None known.

**Etiology:** Autosomal dominant inheritance. New mutations represent about one-half of the new cases. Paternal age appears to be a factor in new mutations. Genetic heterogeneity has been suggested.

**Pathogenesis:** Unknown.

**MIM No.:** *16420

**POS No.:** 3341

**Sex Ratio:** M1:F1

**Occurrence:** About 85 cases have been documented in the literature.

**Risk of Recurrence for Patient's Sib:**
See Part I, *Mendelian Inheritance.*

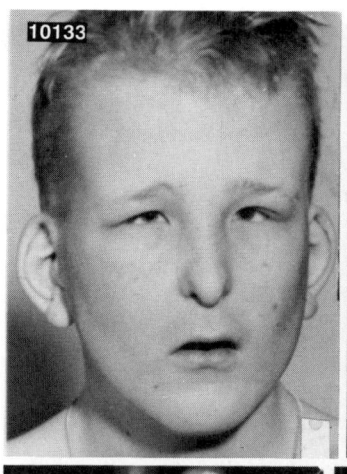
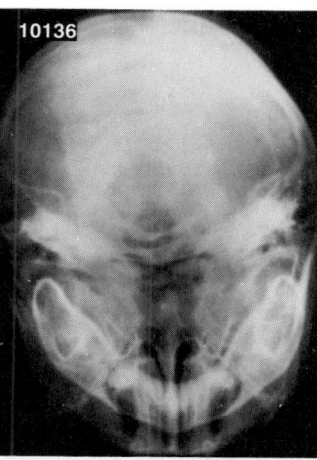
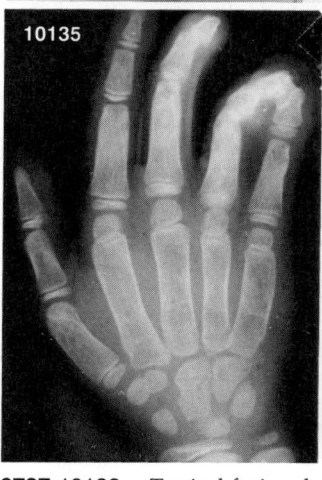
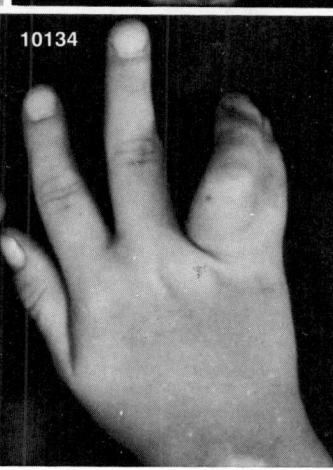

**0737**-10133: Typical facies characterized by pinched nose, small mouth, and overlapping upper lip. 10136: X-ray shows thickened mandible. 10134–35: Typical 4-5 syndactyly with ulnar deviation of the involved fingers. Note the lack of modeling; tiny, cube-shaped middle phalanges in the involved digits; and terminal bony syndactyly.

**Risk of Recurrence for Patient's Child:**
See Part I, *Mendelian Inheritance.*

**Age of Detectability:** At birth.

**Gene Mapping and Linkage:** Unknown.

**Prevention:** None known. Genetic counseling indicated.

**Treatment:** Surgical correction of syndactyly, crowning of teeth.

**Prognosis:** Good. No reduction in lifespan.

**Detection of Carrier:** Unknown.

**References:**
Reisner SH, et al.: Oculodentodigital dysplasia. Am J Dis Child 1969; 118:600–607.
Dudgeon J, Chisolm IA: Oculo-dento-digital dysplasia. Trans Ophthalmol Soc UK 1974; 94:203–210.
Fára M, et al.: Oculodentodigital dysplasia. Acta Clin Plast (Praha) 1977; 19:110–114.
Beighton P, et al.: Oculo-dento-osseous dysplasia: heterogeneity or variable expression? Clin Genet 1979; 16:169–177.
Judisch GF, et al.: Oculodentodigital dysplasia: four new reports and a literature review. Arch Ophthalmol 1979; 97:878–884.
Patton MA, Lawrence KM: Three new cases of oculodentodigital

(ODD) syndrome: development of the facial phenotype. J Med Genet 1985; 22:386–389.

G0038                                                      **Robert J. Gorlin**

## OCULO-ENCEPHALO-HEPATO-RENAL SYNDROME            3242

**Includes:**
COACH syndrome
Hepatic fibrosis-polycystic kidneys-colobomata
Hunter oculo-encephalo-hepato-renal syndrome
Thompson-Baraitser syndrome

**Excludes:**
**Joubert syndrome** (2908)
**Meckel syndrome** (0634)

**Major Diagnostic Criteria:** Congenital ataxia with cerebellar vermis hypo/aplasia, coloboma, and hepatic fibrosis.

**Clinical Findings:** Clinical delineation is based on seven known patients. At birth, coloboma of variable size (6/6), occipital encephalocele (1/7), and postaxial **Polydactyly** (1/7) may be present. Neurologic findings include marked hypotonia (3/4), and tachypnea (4/4) observed since the first weeks, and are related to vermis malformation in 4/4 cases who had CT scan. Ataxia (6/6) and psychomotor retardation (7/7) are obvious before one year of age. Mental retardation (6/6) and some degree of spasticity (3/6) are observed later. Hepatomegaly due to fibrocirrhosis occurs between 1–6 years of age (7/7). Kidney involvement includes small subcapsular or tubular cysts (2/3), interstitial fibrosis (1/3), proximal tubular acidosis, kidney hypoplasia, and slight functional impairment. Dysmorphic features include flat, round facies, **Eye, hypertelorism**, mild ptosis, upturned nose, macrostomia, and small chin, somewhat reminiscent of **Smith-Lemli-Opitz syndrome**.

**Complications:** Life-threatening esophageal bleeding of infantile onset.

**Associated Findings:** None known.

**Etiology:** Autosomal recessive inheritance. The condition has been reported in three pairs of sibs, one with consanguineous parents.

**Pathogenesis:** Unknown.

**Sex Ratio:** M1:F1

**Occurrence:** Seven cases have been reported from Europe and United States.

**Risk of Recurrence for Patient's Sib:**
See Part I, *Mendelian Inheritance.*

**Risk of Recurrence for Patient's Child:**
See Part I, *Mendelian Inheritance.*

**Age of Detectability:** During infancy.

**Gene Mapping and Linkage:** Unknown.

**Prevention:** None known. Genetic counseling indicated.

**Treatment:** Portal shunting may be required during childhood.

**Prognosis:** Survival beyond age 20 years is likely if portal hypertension is successfully managed.

**Detection of Carrier:** Unknown.

**Special Considerations:** The acronym COACH (Cerebellar vermis hypo/aplasia, Oligophrenia, congenital Ataxia, Coloboma, Hepatic fibrocirrhosis) has been proposed.
Nosology of this syndrome is unclear. Clinical overlap does exist with syndromes such as **Smith-Lemli-Opitz syndrome, type II** and **Meckel syndrome**. The original patients with oculo-encephalo-hepato-renal syndrome (Hunter et al. 1974; Thompson et al. 1986) had slight differences (spasticity, lack of renal fibrosis) from the three children reported by Verloes & Lambotte (1989).

**References:**
Hunter AGW, et al.: Hepatic fibrosis, polycystic kydneys, colobomata and encephalopathy in siblings. Clin Genet 1974; 6:82–89.
Thompson E, Baraitser M: An autosomal recessive mental retardation syndrome. Am J Med Genet 1986; 24:151–158.

Verloes A, Lambotte C: Further delineation of a syndrome of cerebellar vermis hypo/aplasia, oligophrenia, congenital ataxia, coloboma and hepatic fibrosis. Am J Med Genet 1989; 32:227–232.

VE010

**A. Verloes**

## OCULO-FACIAL SYNDROME, BENCZE TYPE      2364

**Includes:**
    Bencze syndrome
    Facial-oculo syndrome
    Hemifacial hyperplasia with strabismus (HFH)

**Excludes:**
    **Hemifacial atrophy, progressive** (2615)
    **Hemihypertrophy** (0458)
    **Oculo-auriculo-vertebral anomaly** (0735)

**Major Diagnostic Criteria:** Facial asymmetry, esotropia, and amblyopia with normal intelligence.

**Clinical Findings:** The most consistent finding is facial asymmetry, affecting soft tissue and bone, but not the eyeball. Teeth are often larger on the larger half of the face, although there is no evidence that they erupt sooner than those on the smaller half. Esotropia is a common finding; often, but not always, it affects the eye on the smaller side of the face. The palpebral fissure of the smaller side is often upslanting and narrow. Submucous cleft palate occurred in one-half of the members of one reported family. Intellectual development appears normal.

**Complications:** If strabismus is untreated, amblyopia may result. Malocclusion is a common complication of the asymmetry.

**Associated Findings:** One affected male had growth deficiency, mild mental retardation, primary telecanthus, mild thoracolumbar scoliosis, and hyperextensible knees; these were thought to be unrelated to the primary defect.

**Etiology:** Autosomal dominant inheritance.

**Pathogenesis:** Unknown.

**MIM No.:** *14135

**POS No.:** 3492

**Sex Ratio:** M1:F1

**Occurrence:** Two kinships have been reported.

**Risk of Recurrence for Patient's Sib:**
See Part I, *Mendelian Inheritance.*

**Risk of Recurrence for Patient's Child:**
See Part I, *Mendelian Inheritance.*

**Age of Detectability:** In early childhood.

**Gene Mapping and Linkage:** Unknown.

**Prevention:** None known. Genetic counseling indicated.

**Treatment:** Orthodontic and/or dental treatment may be indicated. Correction of strabismus is also indicated.

**Prognosis:** Life span and intelligence are normal.

**Detection of Carrier:** Unknown.

**References:**
Bencze J, et al.: Dominant inheritance of hemifacial hyperplasia associated with strabismus. Oral Surg 1973; 35:489–501.
Kurnit D, et al.: An autosomal dominantly inherited syndrome of facial asymmetry, esotropia, amblyopia, and submucous cleft palate (Bencze syndrome). Clin Genet 1979; 16:301–304. * †

T0007

**Helga V. Toriello**

**Oculo-mandibulo dyscephaly**
*See OCULO-MANDIBULO-FACIAL SYNDROME*

## OCULO-MANDIBULO-FACIAL SYNDROME      0738

**Includes:**
    Dyscephaly with congenital cataract and hypotrichosis
    Facial-oculo-mandibulo syndrome
    Francois dyscephalic syndrome
    Hallermann-Streiff syndrome
    Mandibulo-facial-oculo syndrome
    Oculo-mandibulo dyscephaly

**Excludes:**
    **Chondroectodermal dysplasia** (0156)
    **Cleidocranial dysplasia** (0185)
    **Dermo-chondro-corneal dystrophy, Francois type** (0282)
    **Mandibulofacial dysostosis** (0627)
    **Oculo-dento-osseous dysplasia** (0737)
    **Progeria** (0825)
    **Pyknodysostosis** (0846)
    **Seckel syndrome** (0881)

**Major Diagnostic Criteria:** Proportionate dwarfism, normal mentation, congenital cataracts, microphthalmia, dyscephaly with mandibular and nasal cartilage hypoplasia, hypotrichosis, cutaneous atrophy limited to scalp and nose, and dental anomalies.

**Clinical Findings:** Dyscephaly is the most constant feature. Brachycephaly, microcephaly, frontal bossing, and disproportionately small face with a narrow nose are common features. Parietal and occipital bossing may be present. The rami of the mandible are hypoplastic, with their condylar heads being displaced anteriorly.

Dental anomalies, hypotrichosis, and cataracts are constant features. There may be natal teeth, hypodontia, malformed teeth, enamel dysplasia, or malocclusion. Other intraoral features include abnormally high palatal vault, microglossia or macroglossia, glossoptosis, and microstomia. The hypotrichosis is most common and most pronounced over the scalp, but also involves the eyelashes and eyebrows, beard, and axillary and pubic hair. Cataracts are always bilateral and complete. Micropthalmia is commonly reported. Other ocular defects include nystagmus, strabismus, blue sclerae, and in descending order of frequency, various defects of the fundus, conjunctiva, cornea, and iris.

Atrophy of the facial skin is common. The skin over the nose is thin, dry, smooth, and covered by telangiectasias. Other reported skin defects include vitiligo, nevi, and ichthyosis.

Feeding and respiratory difficulties are common during infancy, and can be fatal. Visual acuity is frequently decreased. Mentation is usually within normal limits.

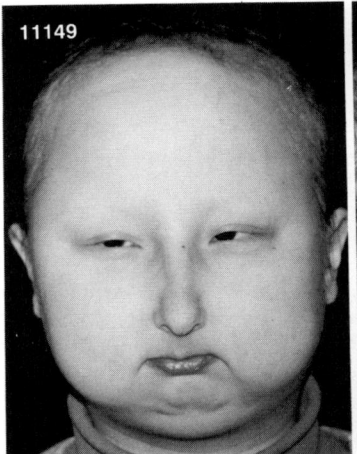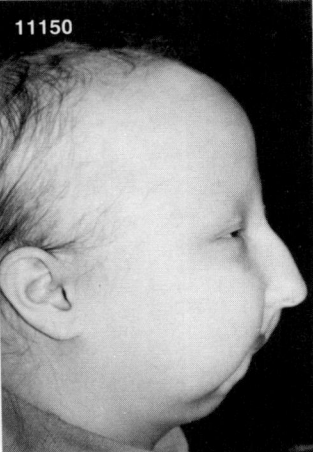

0738-11149–50: Hypotrichosis, narrow, beaked nose; small mandible and microphthalmia.

**Complications:** Vitiligo, respiratory and feeding difficulties in infancy, blindness, psychological disturbances, and deafness.

**Associated Findings:** A few instances of death in childhood from pulmonary infection have been recorded.

**Etiology:** The mode of transmission is unclear. Although most cases reported are sporadic, an equal sex ratio of affected persons, parental consanguinity (7% of cases), and several pairs of affected sibs suggest autosomal recessive inheritance. However, at least three multigenerational families, one with male-to-male transmission, have been reported.

**Pathogenesis:** Undetermined. Developmental defect early in embryonic life (perhaps as early as the fifth week). A defect of elastin has been reported, and glycoprotein metabolism has been suggested to be abnormal.

**MIM No.:** 23410

**POS No.:** 3342

**CDC No.:** 756.046

**Sex Ratio:** M1:F1

**Occurrence:** More than 150 cases reported.

**Risk of Recurrence for Patient's Sib:**
See Part I, *Mendelian Inheritance.*

**Risk of Recurrence for Patient's Child:**
See Part I, *Mendelian Inheritance.* Reproductive fitness is greatly reduced.

**Age of Detectability:** Within first year of life.

**Gene Mapping and Linkage:** Unknown.

**Prevention:** None known. Genetic counseling indicated.

**Treatment:** Tracheostomy in cases of severe respiratory distress.

**Prognosis:** Average life span is undetermined.

**Detection of Carrier:** Unknown.

**References:**

Franqis J: A new syndrome: dyscephalia with bird face and dental anomalies, nanism, hypotrichosis, cutaneous atrophy, microphthalmia, and congenital cataract. Arch Ophthalmol 1958; 60:842–862. *

Steele RW, Bass JW: Hallermann-Streiff syndrome: clinical and prognostic considerations. Am J Dis Child 1970; 120:462–465. * †

Imamura S, et al.: Hallermann-Streiff syndrome. Dermatologica 1980; 160:354–357.

Franqis J: Francois' dyscephalic syndrome. Birth Defects 1982; 18:595–619. *

Slootweg PJ, Huber J: Dento-alveolar abnormalities in oculomandibulodyscephaly (Hallermann-Streiff syndrome). J Oral Path 1984; 13:147–154.

J0027                                          **Ronald J. Jorgenson**

---

## OCULO-OSTEO-CUTANEOUS SYNDROME, TOUMAALA-HAAPANEN TYPE                                                    **2078**

**Includes:**
Anodontia-hypotrichosis syndrome
Brachymetapody-anodontia-hypotrichosis-albinoidism
Toumaala-Haapanen syndrome

**Excludes:**
**Brachydactyly** (0114)
**Ectodermal dysplasia, hidrotic** (0334)
**Parathormone resistance** (0830)

**Major Diagnostic Criteria:** A combination of ocular, cutaneous and skeletal anomalies should be present to suspect the diagnosis. Ocular anomalies include convergent strabismus, myopia, nystagmus, lenticular opacities, foveal hypoplasia. Cutaneous anomalies include scanty hair and hypopigmentation. Skeletal anomalies include short stature, small maxilla and short metacarpals and metatarsals (3–5). Congenital edentia is also a consistent finding.

**Clinical Findings:** In three reported cases, short stature (3); light, relatively inelastic skin (3); hypotrichosis (3); short skull A-P

diameter (3); antimongoloid slant of the palpebral fissures (3); hypoplastic tarsus (3); strabismus (3); nystagmus (3); lenticular opacities (3); foveal hypoplasia (3); high myopia (3); distichiasis (3); small maxilla (3); edentia (3); prominent mandible (3); hypoplastic genitalia (2); short fingers and toes (especially 3–5) (3); normal great toes and thumbs (3); congenital palmar hyperkeratosis (1).

**Complications:** Poor vision and possible blindness were the only complications noticed.

**Associated Findings:** None known.

**Etiology:** Possibly autosomal recessive inheritance.

**Pathogenesis:** Unknown. Although several findings are consistent with an ectodermal dysplasia, others are more likely attributable to a mesodermal defect. Skin biopsies were normal.

**MIM No.:** 21137

**POS No.:** 3044

**Sex Ratio:** M1:F2 (in the three observed siblings).

**Occurrence:** One family from northeast Finland has been documented.

**Risk of Recurrence for Patient's Sib:**
See Part I, *Mendelian Inheritance.*

**Risk of Recurrence for Patient's Child:**
See Part I, *Mendelian Inheritance.*

**Age of Detectability:** At birth, by physical examination.

**Gene Mapping and Linkage:** Unknown.

**Prevention:** None known. Genetic counseling indicated.

**Treatment:** Correction of vision problems, as indicated.

**Prognosis:** Life span is apparently normal; one affected individual was described as intellectually normal. Nothing is known about the intelligence of the other two affected individuals.

**Detection of Carrier:** Unknown.

**References:**

Tuomaala P, Haapanen E: Three siblings with similar anomalies in the eyes, bones and skin. Acta Ophthalmol 1968; 46:365–371.

T0007                                          **Helga V. Toriello**

---

## OCULO-OTO-NASAL MALFORMATIONS WITH OSTEO-ONYCHO DYSPLASIA                                                  **2188**

**Includes:** Osteo-onycho dysplasia and oculo-oto-nasal defects

**Excludes:** **Oculo-cerebro-facial syndrome, Kaufman type** (2179)

**Major Diagnostic Criteria:** Ptosis, prominent midface, large ears, large penis, dystrophic nails, large first and second toes.

**Clinical Findings:** Facial findings include ptosis, absence of medial eyebrows and eyelashes, hypertelorism, prominent midface, and receding chin. The ears are large, low-set, and have simply formed pinnae. The penis is large, with hypospadias. The nails are dystrophic with longitudinal ridges. Some are partially absent. The first and second toes are broad and large. X-rays show enlargement of the lateral part of the clavicle, resorption of some of the tufts of the terminal phalanges, broadened epiphyses of long bones, poorly formed acetabulum, and synostoses of the tarsals and metacarpals.

**Complications:** Unknown.

**Associated Findings:** None known.

**Etiology:** Possibly autosomal recessive inheritance.

**Pathogenesis:** Unknown.

**Sex Ratio:** The only reported case was male.

**Occurrence:** One case has been reported.

**Risk of Recurrence for Patient's Sib:** Unknown.

**Risk of Recurrence for Patient's Child:** Probably negligible.

**Age of Detectability:** At birth.

**Gene Mapping and Linkage:** Unknown.

**Prevention:** None known. Genetic counseling indicated.

**Treatment:** Unknown.

**Prognosis:** Unknown.

**Detection of Carrier:** Unknown.

**References:**
Leiba S, et al.: Oculootonasal malformations associated with osteoony-chodysplasia. BD:OAS XI(2). New York: March of Dimes Birth Defects Foundation, 1975:67–73.

TH017                                    **T.F. Thurmon**
UR001                                    **S.A. Ursin**

**Oculo-oto-radial syndrome**
  *See IVIC SYNDROME*
**Oculo-palatal-cerebral dwarfism**
  *See DWARFISM, OCULO-PALATO-CEREBRAL TYPE*

---

## OCULO-RENO-CEREBELLAR SYNDROME                3050

**Includes:**
  Cerebellar-oculo-renal syndrome
  Renal-oculo-cerebellar syndrome

**Excludes:**
  Cerebellar granular layer, isolated absence of
  **Oculo-cerebro-renal syndrome** (0736)
  **Nephritis**
  Nephronophthisis, juvenile
  **Retinopathy-hypotrichosis syndrome** (2627)

**Major Diagnostic Criteria:** A progressive condition that leads to early dementia and choreoathetosis, accompanied by tapetoretinal degeneration, spastic diplegia, and a glomerulopathy. A single autopsied case had absence of the cerebellar granular layer.

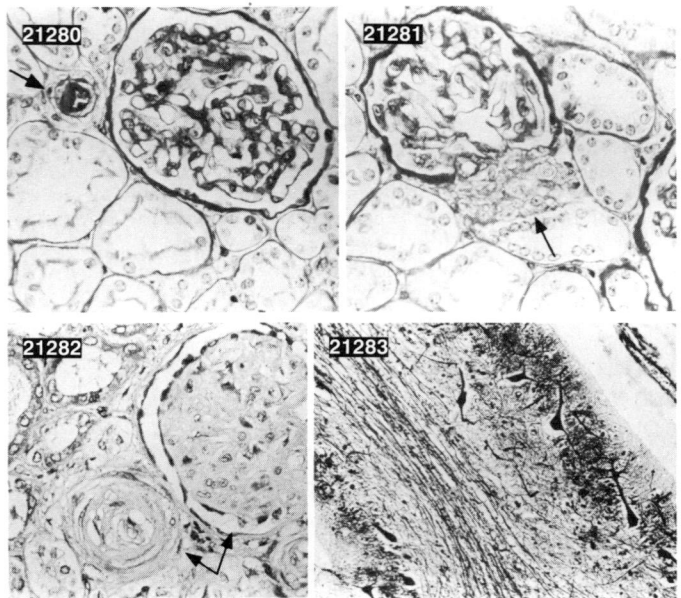

3050B-21280: Section from renal biopsy showing glomerulus in deep cortex with mild thickening of the basement membrane and PAS-positive material in an adjacent arteriole. 21281: Juxtaglomerular prominence seen in renal biopsy section. 21282: Completely sclerosed glomerulus and "onion skin" appearance in the adjacent arteriole. 21283: Silver-stain preparation from cerebellum showing lack of granular layer, disorganization of the Purkinje cells; and normal orientation of underlying axons.

---

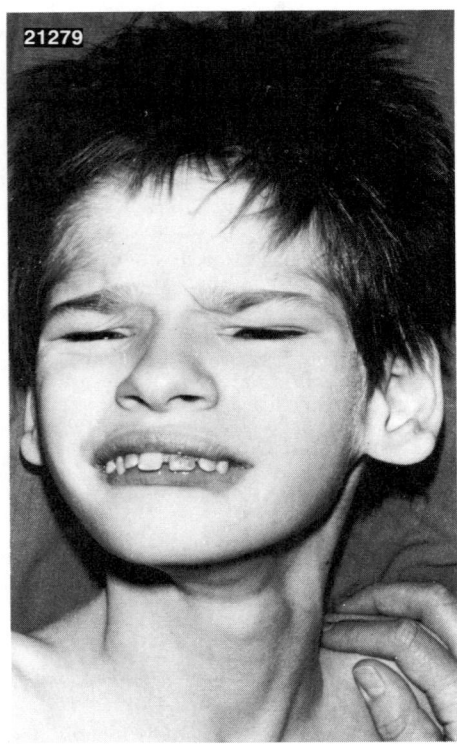

3050A-21279: Note large mouth and prominent ears; in profile the nose has a "ski-jump" shape.

**Clinical Findings:** By history, affected children had some very early development, but quickly (within 1–3 months) deteriorated to become profoundly demented. Choreoathetoid movement was an early sign, later accompanied by spastic diplegia, but with continued joint hyperextensibility. Death occurred within the first two decades from renal failure, which was due to a progressive glomerulopathy, with pathologic findings similar to segmental or focal hyalinosis. A severe progressive tapetoretinal degeneration was accompanied by dramatic hypoplasia of the retinal vasculature, which reached the point where retinal vessels were no longer clinically visible. There was hypoplasia of the cerebellum, which on light microscopy showed absence of granular cells in the internal granular layer, a reduced thickness of the molecular layer, and disoriented, displaced Purkinje cells with infrequent axons and occasional asteroid bodies.

Proteinuria was an early sign of the renal impairment, and the typical renal pathology of focal/segmental hyalinosis was seen in biopsy material. Periglomerular asteroids often contained a thick, PAS-positive basement membrane or hyaline deposits. Presumably imaging techniques now available would demonstrate the cerebellar hypoplasia.

**Complications:** Profound retardation, progressive visual impairment and blindness, progressive renal failure, and death.

**Associated Findings:** **Microcephaly**, strabismus, and cataracts were variable features. An unusual facial appearance that differed from other family members may simply have reflected poor muscle bulk and tone.

**Etiology:** Autosomal recessive inheritance.

**Pathogenesis:** Unknown. Some signs could result from progressive small vessel disease, as seen in the kidney and eye.

**MIM No.:** *25797

**POS No.:** 3995

**Sex Ratio:** M1:F1; M3:F2 observed.

**Occurrence:** Five members of one Mennonite family from Manitoba, Canada, have been reported.

**Risk of Recurrence for Patient's Sib:**
See Part I, *Mendelian Inheritance.*

**Risk of Recurrence for Patient's Child:**
See Part I, *Mendelian Inheritance.* Affected individuals are not expected to survive to reproduce.

**Age of Detectability:** Signs of delay are apparent within the first few months. The earliest age of appearance of renal and visual signs is unknown but is within the first decade (one child died at age seven years), and cerebellar pathology is probably also early (possibly during infancy).

**Gene Mapping and Linkage:** Unknown.

**Prevention:** None known. Genetic counseling indicated.

**Treatment:** Supportive care for child and family.

**Prognosis:** Profound dementia and early death from renal disease.

**Detection of Carrier:** Unknown.

**References:**
Hunter AGW, et al.: Absence of the cerebellar granular layer, mental retardation, tapetoretinal degeneration, and progressive glomerulopathy: an autosomal recessive oculo-renal-cerebellar syndrome. Am J Med Genet 1982; 11:383–395.

HU008                     **Alasdair G.W. Hunter**

**Oculocerebral syndrome with hypopigmentation**
*See GINGIVAL FIBROMATOSIS-DEPIGMENTATION-MICROPHTHALMIA*
**Oculocraniodental syndrome**
*See ACROCEPHALOSYNDACTYLY TYPE III*
**Oculocraniosomatic neuromuscular disease**
*See KEARNS-SAYRE DISEASE*
**Oculocraniosomatic syndrome**
*See OPHTHALMOPLEGIA, PROGRESSIVE EXTERNAL*
**Oculocutaneous albinism**
*See ALBINISM*
**Oculocutaneous albinoidism**
*See ALBINOIDISM*
**Oculocutaneous melanosis**
*See NEVUS OF OTA*
**Oculocutaneous pigmentation syndrome**
*See NEVUS OF OTA*
**Oculocutaneous tyrosinemia or tyrosinosis**
*See TYROSINEMIA II, OREGON TYPE*
**Oculodermal melanocytosis**
*See NEVUS OF OTA*
**Oculogastrointestinal muscular dystrophy**
*See MUSCULAR DYSTROPHY, OCULO-GASTROINTESTINAL*
**Oculoleptomeningeal type amyloidosis**
*See AMYLOIDOSIS, OHIO TYPE*
**Oculomotor apraxia-contractures-muscle atrophy**
*See CONTRACTURES-MUSCLE ATROPHY-OCULOMOTOR APRAXIA*
**Oculopharyngeal muscular dystrophy**
*See MUSCULAR DYSTROPHY, OCULOPHARYNGEAL*
**Oculopharyngeal myopathy**
*See MUSCULAR DYSTROPHY, OCULOPHARYNGEAL*
**Oculopupillary syndrome**
*See HORNER SYNDROME*
**Oculosympathetic syndrome**
*See HORNER SYNDROME*
**ODD syndrome**
*See OCULO-DENTO-OSSEOUS DYSPLASIA*

## ODONTO-ONYCHODERMAL DYSPLASIA      **2618**

**Includes:** Ectodermal dysplasia, odonto-onychodermal dysplasia type

**Excludes:** Odonto-onychodysplasia-alopecia (2890)

**Major Diagnostic Criteria:** Erythema, atrophy, and scalings on cheeks, nose, upper lip, chin, and forehead. Diffuse erythema and mild-to-moderate hyperkeratosis, fissuring, and hyperhidrosis of palms and soles. Dry and sometimes sparse scalp hair. Abnormal and missing teeth. Peg-shaped or conical maxillary central incisors. Thickening of toenails.

**Clinical Findings:** The disease is apparent early in childhood. There are ill-defined patches of erythema, atrophy, and scaliness on cheeks, nose, upper lip, and, to a lesser extent, on the chin and forehead. Cherry-red spots and telangiectases can be seen over the cheeks and nose. The skin is generally dry and scaly. Scalp hair is dry and may be sparse. The palms have diffuse erythema with mild-to-moderate hyperkeratosis and fissuring. The soles are similarly affected, but to a lesser extent. In addition, there is hyperhidrosis of the palms and soles and thickening of the nails of the big toes. The nipples and areolae are normal.

Oral examination may reveal a class I occlusion with severe overbite. Panorex film of the teeth may show peg-shaped or conical maxillary central incisors with a large diastema. The deciduous teeth have a marked erosion of their occlusal surfaces.

The X-ray survey of the axial skeleton shows no abnormalities. In particular, there is no fusion of the metacarpals and no evidence of **Polydactyly.**

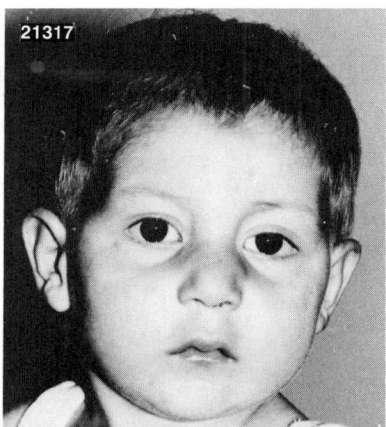

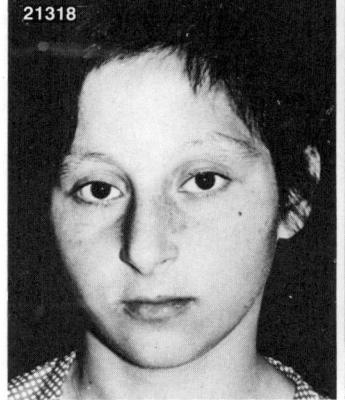
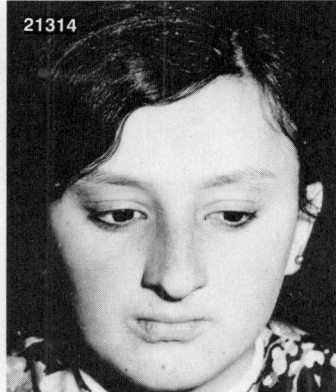

**2618A-**21317, 18, 14: Note facial erythema, sparse hair and eyebrows.

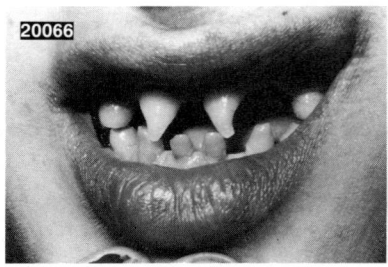
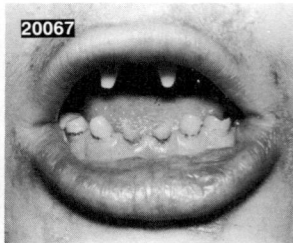
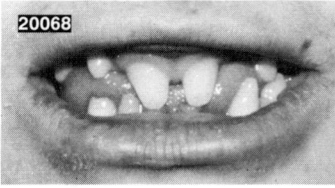
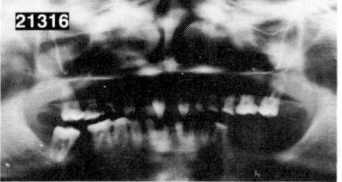

**2618B**-20066–68: Note the range of dental defects. 21316: Panorex film of hypoplastic teeth.

The audiogram documents normal hearing.

Biopsy from the skin of the face may demonstrate basket-weave hyperkeratosis and spotty parakeratosis, irregular acanthosis alternating with atrophy, and effacement of the rete ridges. The basal cell layer is preserved. The dermis may show basophilic degeneration, compatible with solar-elastosis, and dilated blood

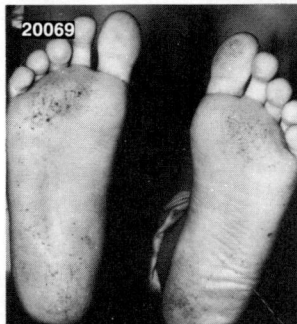
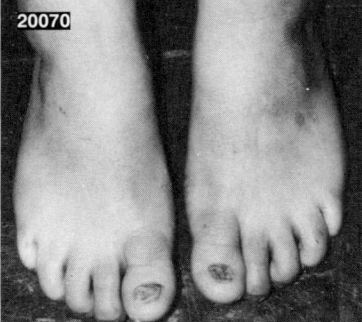

**2618C**-21323: Note the moderate hyperkeratosis and fissuring of the palms. 20069: Hyperkeratosis and fissuring of the soles. 20070: Irregular and thickened first toenails.

vessels. The sebaceous glands may be decreased in size and number, and the eccrine glands appear normal.

Biopsy from the sole shows hyperkeratosis, irregular hypergranulosis, and mild acanthosis in the epidermis. The dermis is unremarkable.

**Complications:** The abormalities of the teeth interfere with a comfortable chewing process.

**Associated Findings:** Recurrent ear discharges.

**Etiology:** Probably autosomal recessive inheritance. Parents of the affected individuals (five males and two females) are normal and first cousins, and the segregation ratio in the reported families is 7:24 (close to 0.25).

**Pathogenesis:** Freire-Maia (1971, 1977) suggested that in order to classify disorders as ectodermal dysplasias, they should have at least two of the following disturbances: 1) trichodysplasia, 2) dental defects, 3) onychodysplasia, and 4) dyshidrosis (group A) or at least one of the above plus at least one other ectodermal defect (group B). Odonto-onychodermal dysplasia belongs to the 1–2–3–4 subgroup of group A. Solomon and Keuer (1980) have reserved the term *ectodermal dysplasia* for conditions that 1) are congenital; 2) have diffuse involvement of the epidermis, and at least one of the following: hair, sebaceous glands, eccrine glands, nail, mucosa, or teeth; and 3) are not progressive. Odonto-onychodermal dysplasia is also an ectodermal dysplasia according to these criteria.

**MIM No.:** 25798

**POS No.:** 3609

**Sex Ratio:** M5:F2 (observed).

**Occurrence:** Seven cases from two Lebanese Moslem Shiite families have been observed.

**Risk of Recurrence for Patient's Sib:**
See Part I, *Mendelian Inheritance.*

**Risk of Recurrence for Patient's Child:**
See Part I, *Mendelian Inheritance.*

**Age of Detectability:** Usually clinically diagnosable by age 1.5 years, when the abnormalities of the teeth become evident.

**Gene Mapping and Linkage:** Unknown.

**Prevention:** None known. Genetic counseling indicated.

**Treatment:** Symptomatic care for the skin lesions and orthodontic treatment.

**Prognosis:** Normal life span.

**Detection of Carrier:** Unknown.

**References:**
Freire-Maia N: Ectodermal dysplasias. Hum Hered 1971; 21:309–312.
Freire-Maia N: Ectodermal dysplasias revisited. Acta Genet Med Gemellol 1977; 26:121–131.
Solomon LM, Keuer EJ: The ectodermal dysplasias: problems of classification and some newer syndromes. Arch Dermatol 1980; 116:1295–1299.
Pinheiro M, et al.: A previously undescribed condition, tricho-odonto-onycho-dermal syndrome: a review of the tricho-odonto-onychial subgroup of ectodermal dysplasias. Br J Dermatol 1981; 105:371–382.
Fadhil M, et al.: Odonto-onychodermal dysplasia: a previously apparently undescribed ectodermal dysplasia. Am J Med Genet 1983; 14:335–346.

DE030                    **Vazken M. Der Kaloustian**

## ODONTO-ONYCHODYSPLASIA-ALOPECIA 2890

**Includes:**
Alopecia-odonto-onychodysplasia
Ectodermal dysplasia, odonto-onychodysplasia-alopecia
type

**Excludes:**
Ectodermal dysplasia, Christ-Siemens-Touraine type (0333)
Ectodermal dysplasia, hidrotic (0334)
Odonto-onychodermal dysplasia (2618)
Tricho-dermodysplasia-dental defects (2903)
Tricho-odonto-onychial dysplasia (2889)

**Major Diagnostic Criteria:** Trichodysplasia, dental anomalies, and onychodysplasia.

**Clinical Findings:** Almost total alopecia; sparse, thin, brittle, and slow-growing hair at the occipital and temporal regions; scanty

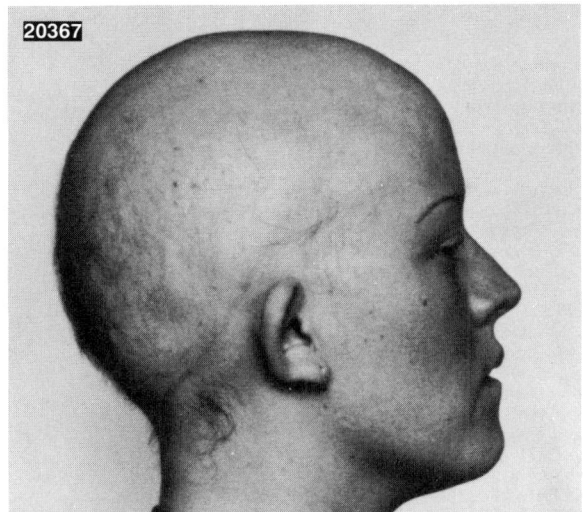

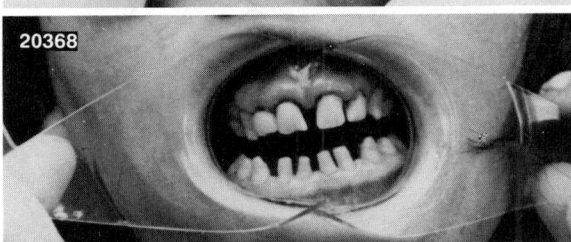

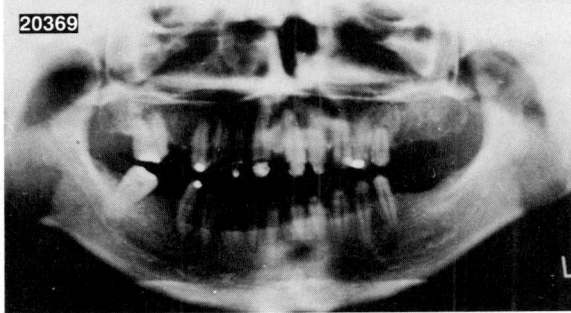

**2890-20367:** Odonto-onychodysplasia-alopecia; note anteverted auricles, absent eyebrows that are pencilled in, and alopecia with sparse hair at the base of the skull. **20368:** The apparently normal upper incisors are capped. **20369:** Orthopantomogram showing dental alterations.

eyebrows and lashes; absent axillary and pubic hair; hypodontia of both dentitions; enamel hypoplasia; microdontia; widely spaced and abnormally shaped teeth; dystrophic finger- and toenails with subungual corneal layer; sparse café-au-lait spots; irregular outlines of areolae; hypertrophied Montgomery glands; extranumerary nipples; palmoplantar keratosis; toe syndactyly; flat feet; anteverted auricles; recurrent atrophic rhinitis and external otitis; cysts of both ovaries; uterine fibroma; uterine retroversion; unilateral deviation of the lacrimal duct; dermatoglyphic changes; transpalmar creases.

**Complications:** Psychologic problems due to hair and dental alterations.

**Associated Findings:** None known.

**Etiology:** Probably autosomal recessive inheritance. Parental consanguinity is probable.

**Pathogenesis:** Defective formation of several derivatives of the embryonic ectoderm suggests that this condition must be classified as an ectodermal dysplasia.

**Sex Ratio:** Presumably M1:F1; M0:F2 observed.

**Occurrence:** Reported in two Caucasian Brazilian sisters; the only children of a probably consanguineous, normal couple.

**Risk of Recurrence for Patient's Sib:**
See Part I, *Mendelian Inheritance.*

**Risk of Recurrence for Patient's Child:**
See Part I, *Mendelian Inheritance.*

**Age of Detectability:** During childhood, by physical examination.

**Gene Mapping and Linkage:** Unknown.

**Prevention:** None known. Genetic counseling indicated.

**Treatment:** Prosthetic replacement and orthodontic treatment; wigs are cosmetically and psychologically helpful; surgery for uterine fibroma.

**Prognosis:** Normal for life span.

**Detection of Carrier:** Unknown.

**References:**
Pinheiro M, et al.: Odontoonychodysplasia with alopecia: a new pure ectodermal dysplasia with probable autosomal recessive inheritance. Am J Med Genet 1985; 20:197–202.

PI008                      **Marta Pinheiro**

**Odonto-onychohypohidrotic dysplasia with midline scalp defect**
*See ECTODERMAL DYSPLASIA-ADRENAL CYST*
**Odonto-trichomelic hypohidrotic dysplasia**
*See ODONTO-TRICHOMELIC SYNDROME*

## ODONTO-TRICHOMELIC SYNDROME 2887

**Includes:**
Cleft lip-tetramelia-deformed ears-ectodermal dysplasia
Ectodermal dysplasia, tetramelic
Freire-Maia syndrome
Odonto-trichomelic hypohidrotic dysplasia
Tetramelic deficiencies-ectodermal dysplasia-deformed ears

**Excludes:** Ectrodactyly-ectodermal dysplasia-clefting syndrome (0337)

**Major Diagnostic Criteria:** Extensive tetramelic deficiencies, severe hypotrichosis, abnormal dentition, and deformed auricles.

**Clinical Findings:** Extensive deficiencies of the four limbs associated with dermatoglyphic abnormalities; hypotrichosis; small, conical, and widely spaced teeth; persistence of deciduous teeth; hypodontia; large, thin, protruding, and deformed auricles; hypoplastic areolae and nipples; thin, dry, and shiny skin; abnormalities of tyrosine and/or tryptophane metabolism; growth retardation; cleft lip; and EEG and EKG abnormalities.

**Complications:** Unknown.

**Associated Findings:** Hypoplastic nails.

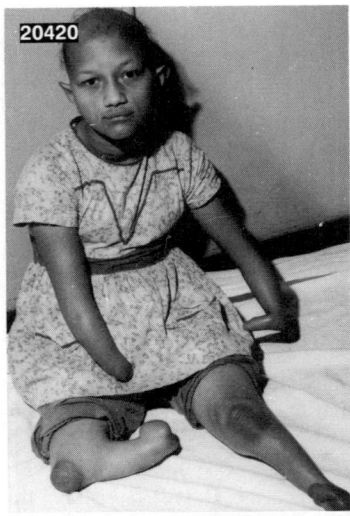
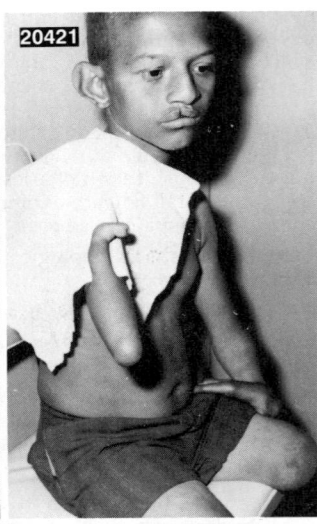
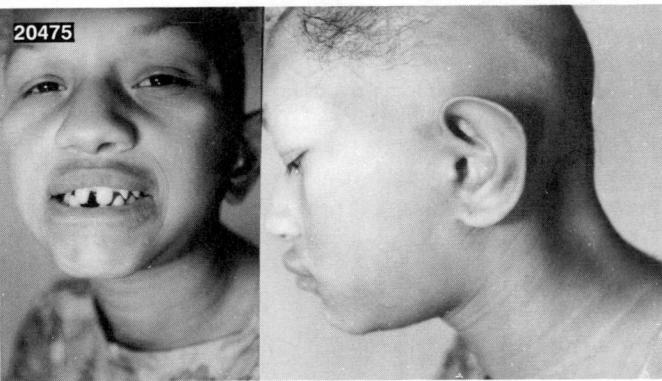

**2887-20420:** Affected girl at age 12 years; note hypotrichosis, abnormal auricles, and extensive tetramelic reductions. **20421:** Affected boy at age 14 years, note hypotrichosis, abnormal auricle, incomplete left cleft lip and extensive tetramelic reductions. The reduction deformity of the left leg is identical to that of the right leg. **20475:** Affected female at 12 years of age; note extensive hypotrichosis, abnormal auricle, dental alterations and unusual number of wrinkles.

**Etiology:** Probably autosomal recessive inheritance. The two sibships thus far investigated have normal parents. In one instance the parents were possibly consanguineous, while in the other they are first cousins.

**Pathogenesis:** Unknown.

**MIM No.:** 27340

**POS No.:** 3355

**Sex Ratio:** Presumably M1:F1; M3:F2 observed.

**Occurrence:** Four of eight siblings in one Caucasian Brazilian family, and one of three siblings in a Caucasian Italian family, have been reported in the literature.

**Risk of Recurrence for Patient's Sib:**
See Part I, *Mendelian Inheritance.*

**Risk of Recurrence for Patient's Child:**
See Part I, *Mendelian Inheritance.*

**Age of Detectability:** At birth, on the basis of physical findings.

**Gene Mapping and Linkage:** Unknown.

**Prevention:** None known. Genetic counseling indicated.

**Treatment:** Orthopedic services. Plastic surgery and use of wigs and dental prostheses are cosmetically and psychologically helpful.

**Prognosis:** Normal for life span.

**Detection of Carrier:** Unknown.

**References:**

Chautard EA, Freire-Maia N: Dermatoglyphic analysis in a highly mutilating syndrome. Acta Genet Med Gemellol 1970; 3:421–424. †

Freire-Maia N: A newly recognized genetic syndrome of tetramelic deficiencies, ectodermal dysplasia, deformed ears, and other abnormalities. Am J Hum Genet 1970; 22:370–377. * †

Freire-Maia N, et al.: A new malformation syndrome? Lancet 1970; I:840–841. †

Cat I, et al.: Odontotrichomelic hypohidrotic dysplasia: a clinical reappraisal. Hum Hered 1972; 22:91–95.

Pinheiro M, Freire-Maia N: EEC and odontotrichomelic syndromes. Clin Genet 1980; 17:363–364.

Pavone L, et al.: A case of the Freire-Maia odontotrichomelic syndrome: nosology with EEC syndrome. Am J Med Genet 1989; 33:190–193. †

FR033            **Newton Freire-Maia**

**Odontoblastic dysplasia, focal**
See TEETH, ODONTOBLASTIC DYSPLASIA, FOCAL
**Odontodysplasia**
See TEETH, ODONTODYSPLASIA
**Odontogenesis imperfecta**
See TEETH, ODONTODYSPLASIA
**Odontogenic dysplasia**
See TEETH, ODONTODYSPLASIA
**Oguchi disease types 1, 2A and 2B**
See NIGHTBLINDNESS, OGUCHI TYPE
**Ohdo-Hirayama-Terawaki syndrome**
See ECTODERMAL DYSPLASIA-ECTRODACTYLY-MACULAR DYSTROPHY
**Ohdo-Madokoro-Hayakawa syndrome**
See MENTAL RETARDATION-HEART DEFECTS-BLEPHAROPHIMOSIS
**Ohio type amyloidosis**
See AMYLOIDOSIS, OHIO TYPE
**Oily ear wax**
See EAR, CERUMEN VARIATIONS
**Okihiro syndrome**
See RADIAL-RENAL-OCULAR SYNDROME
also EYE, DUANE RETRACTION SYNDROME
**Oldfield syndrome**
See INTESTINAL POLYPOSIS, TYPE III
**Olfaction loss, congenital**
See ANOSMIA, CONGENITAL
**Olfactogenital dysplasia**
See KALLMANN SYNDROME
**Oligoazoospermia, idiopathic**
See ANDROGEN INSENSITIVITY (RESISTANCE), MINIMAL
**Oligodactyly-hydronephrosis**
See HAND, ULNAR AND FIBULAR RAY DEFICIENCY, WEYERS TYPE
**Oligodontia, isolated**
See TEETH, ANODONTIA, PARTIAL OR COMPLETE
**Oligodontia-cleft lip/palate-syndactyly-hair defects**
See CLEFT LIP/PALATE-OLIGODONTIA-SYNDACTYLY-HAIR DEFECTS
**Oligohydramnios, fetal, with NSAID exposure**
See FETAL EFFECTS OF NONSTEROIDAL ANTI-INFLAMMATORY DRUGS (NSAIDS)
**Oligophrenia phenylpyruvica**
See PHENYLKETONURIA
also FETAL EFFECTS FROM MATERNAL PKU
**Oligophrenia-aniridia-cerebellar ataxia**
See ANIRIDIA-CEREBELLAR ATAXIA-MENTAL DEFICIENCY
**Oligophrenia-cochlear deafness-myopia**
See DEAFNESS-MYOPIA
**Oligophrenia-epilepsy-ichthyosis syndrome**
See SEIZURES-ICHTHYOSIS-MENTAL RETARDATION
**Oligophrenia-gingival fibromatosis-depigmentation-microphthalmia**
See GINGIVAL FIBROMATOSIS-DEPIGMENTATION-MICROPHTHALMIA
**Oligophrenia-ichthyosis-spasticity**
See SJOGREN-LARSSON SYNDROME

**Oligophrenic cerebello-lental degeneration**
   See MARINESCO-SJOGREN SYNDROME
**Oliguria, neonatal, with NSAID exposure**
   See FETAL EFFECTS OF NONSTEROIDAL ANTI-INFLAMMATORY
      DRUGS (NSAIDS)
**Oliver-MacFarlane syndrome**
   See TRICHOMEGALY-RETARDATION-DWARFISM-RETINAL
      PIGMENTARY DEGENERATION
**Olivopontocerebellar atrophy I**
   See OLIVOPONTOCEREBELLAR ATROPHY, DOMINANT MENZEL
      TYPE
**Olivopontocerebellar atrophy II**
   See OLIVOPONTOCEREBELLAR ATROPHY, RECESSIVE FICKLER-
      WINKLER TYPE
**Olivopontocerebellar atrophy III (OPCA type III)**
   See OLIVOPONTOCEREBELLAR ATROPHY, DOMINANT WITH
      RETINAL DEGENERATION
**Olivopontocerebellar atrophy IV**
   See OLIVOPONTOCEREBELLAR ATROPHY, DOMINANT SCHUT-
      HAYMAKER TYPE
**Olivopontocerebellar atrophy V**
   See OLIVOPONTOCEREBELLAR ATROPHY, DOMINANT WITH
      OPHTHALMOPLEGIA

---

## OLIVOPONTOCEREBELLAR ATROPHY, DOMINANT MENZEL TYPE
**0742**

**Includes:**
   Olivopontocerebellar atrophy I
   OPCA I

**Excludes:**
   **Olivopontocerebellar atrophy, dominant Schut-Haymaker type**
      **(0743)**
   **Olivopontocerebellar atrophy** (others)

**Major Diagnostic Criteria:**  Adult life onset of progressive ataxia, computed tomography of the brain indicating olivopontocerebellar atrophy (OPCA), and evidence of autosomal dominant transmission.

**Clinical Findings:**  Onset in the second to fifth decades of life, (usually about 30 years of age), of a slowly progressive unsteadiness of gait, and later of all limbs. There is progressive dysarthria with scanning speech, tremors, involuntary movements, often of choreiform type, and sensory impairment. Later, upper motor neuron signs with extensor plantar responses may develop.

There is moderate variability in some of the signs of this disease. Some cases may have no apparent sensory loss. Some patients may show weakness due to lower motor neuronal loss, while others have normal strength.

**Complications:**  Patients become bedridden and debilitated.

**Associated Findings:**  None known.

**Etiology:**  Autosomal dominant inheritance. Penetrance appears complete, but age of onset is variable.

**Pathogenesis:**  The brain shows the changes of OPCA with sparing of the cerebellar vermis, marked loss of cerebellar Purkinje cells, and less striking granule cell loss in the remainder of the cerebellum. The dentate nucleus is usually involved, and there is decreased size of the superior cerebellar peduncles and cerebellar white matter. The basis pontis is small, with loss of transverse fibers and fiber loss in the middle cerebellar peduncles. There is marked neuronal loss in the inferior olivary nuclei. The substantia nigra also frequently shows neuronal loss. In most cases the spinal cord shows loss of fibers in the posterior funiculus, spinocerebellar tracts, and, on occasion, in the pyramidal tracts. Sometimes neuronal loss is found in the posterior horns, Clarke column, or anterior horns. Clues to the biochemical origin of this disease are provided by studies in other inherited ataxias that demonstrate deficiencies in pyruvate dehydrogenase and mitochondrial enzymes.

**MIM No.:**  *16440

**Sex Ratio:**  M1:F1

**Occurrence:**  Although only a few families with this particular variant have been described in the United States, the combined prevalence of the dominantly inherited forms of OPCA is estimated to be 1:31,250.

**Risk of Recurrence for Patient's Sib:**
   See Part I, *Mendelian Inheritance.*

**Risk of Recurrence for Patient's Child:**
   See Part I, *Mendelian Inheritance.*

**Age of Detectability:**  At about age 30 years when onset of symptoms occurs.

**Gene Mapping and Linkage:**  SCA1 (spinal cerebellar ataxia (olivopontocerebellar ataxia)) has been mapped to 6p24-p21.3.

**Prevention:**  None known. Genetic counseling indicated.

**Treatment:**  The evidence for pyruvic dehydrogenase deficiency has led to the use of cholinergic agonists (physostigmine and lecithin) with some efficacy. However, supportive personal and family therapy remain the mainstay of treatment.

**Prognosis:**  Patients may die in their fourth to seventh decades of life, usually of debilitation and pneumonia.

**Detection of Carrier:**  In some families, HLA typing may be helpful in carrier identification, but only after an index case has been discovered.

**References:**
Menzel P: Beitrag Zur Kenntniss der hereditaeren Ataxie und Kleinhirnatrophie. Arch Psychiatr Nervenkr 1890; 22:160–190.
Konigsmark BW, Weiner LP: The olivopontocerebellar atrophies: a review. Medicine 1970; 49:227–242. *
Skre H: Spino-cerebellar ataxia in western Norway. Clin Genet 1974; 6:265–288.
Jackson JF, et al: Spinocerebellar ataxia and HLA linkage: risk prediction by HLA typing. New Engl J Med 1977; 296:1138–1141. *
Rodriguez-Budelli M, et al.: Action of physostigmine on inherited ataxia. In: Kark RAP, et al, eds: The inherited ataxias. New York: Raven Press, 1978:195–202.
Gilman S, et al.: Disorders of the cerebellum. Philadelphia: F.A. Davis, 1981.
Stumpf DA, et al.: Mitochondrial malic enzyme deficiency in Friedreich's ataxia. Ann Neurol 1981; 10:283 only.
Sorbi S, et al.: Abnormal platelet glutamate dehydrogenase activity and activation in dominant and nondominant olivopontocerebellar atrophy. Ann Neurol 1986; 19:239–245.

CR011                                                    **Carl J. Crosley**

---

## OLIVOPONTOCEREBELLAR ATROPHY, DOMINANT SCHUT-HAYMAKER TYPE
**0743**

**Includes:**
   Olivopontocerebellar atrophy IV
   OPCA IV

**Excludes:**
   **Olivopontocerebellar atrophy, dominant Menzel type** (0742)
   **Olivopontocerebellar atrophy** (other)

**Major Diagnostic Criteria:**  Adult life onset of cerebellar ataxia and variable upper motor neuron signs; computed tomography of the brain or autopsy findings of olivopontocerebellar atrophy (OPCA) with variable anterior horn cell and spinocerebellar tract loss, and loss of neurons in 9th, 10th and 12th cranial nerves. Evidence of autosomal dominant transmission helps to confirm the diagnosis.

**Clinical Findings:**  Onset between about 17 and 35 years of age of a slowly progressive cerebellar ataxia. Tendon reflexes vary from completely absent to hyperactive. Plantar responses are flexor in most cases, but extensor in a few. Muscle tone varies from minimal to marked rigidity. Sensation varies from normal to moderate loss of position and pain sensation. Some cases may show clinical signs of **Ataxia, Friedreich type**, with absent deep tendon reflexes and mild coordination defect; others may show more prominent cerebellar ataxia, with variable deep tendon reflexes and moderate coordination disturbances, and some will show prominent pyramidal signs suggesting spastic quadriplegia.

Of all the olivopontocerebellar degenerations, this disease shows the greatest variation in clinical signs and pathologic changes. Schut and Haymaker (1951), who reported 42 affected persons in one kindred, divided the clinical types in this family into three groups: Friedreich ataxia type, cerebellar ataxia type, and spastic paraplegia type. The pathologic findings showed a similar variation, with a variable degree of severity of involvement of different structures.

**Complications:** Patients become incapacitated and bedridden.

**Associated Findings:** None known.

**Etiology:** Autosomal dominant inheritance with complete penetrance.

**Pathogenesis:** The brain shows the changes of OPCA with moderate-to-severe cerebellar atrophy and cerebellar cortical cell loss. Most severely affected in all cases are the inferior olivary nuclei, restiform bodies, brachium conjunctivum, cerebellum, and 12th nerves. There is marked neuronal and fiber loss in the inferior olivary nuclei. The basis pontis shows some variation from case to case with moderate atrophy in some cases and no changes in others. In the brainstem, neuronal loss varies in the 9th, 10th and 12th cranial nerves and substantia nigra. The white matter of the spinal cord varies from normal to severe fiber loss in the posterior funiculus and spinocerebellar tracts. The anterior motor horn cells may be normal or may show moderate loss. Clues to the biochemical origin of this disease are provided by studies in other inherited ataxias that demonstrate deficiencies in pyruvate dehydrogenase and mitochondrial malic enzyme.

**MIM No.:** *16460

**Sex Ratio:** M1:F1

**Occurrence:** In one western European population, 1:300,000.

**Risk of Recurrence for Patient's Sib:**
See Part I, *Mendelian Inheritance*.

**Risk of Recurrence for Patient's Child:**
See Part I, *Mendelian Inheritance*.

**Age of Detectability:** At about age 25 years.

**Gene Mapping and Linkage:** Unknown.

**Prevention:** None known. Genetic counseling indicated.

**Treatment:** The evidence for pyruvic dehydrogenase deficiency has led to the use of cholinergic agonists (physostigmine and lecithin) with some efficacy. However, supportive personal and family therapy remain the mainstay of treatment.

**Prognosis:** Patients die about 15 years after onset, usually of debilitation and infection.

**Detection of Carrier:** In some families, HLA typing may be helpful in carrier identification, but only after an index case has been discovered.

**References:**
Schut JW, Haymaker W: Hereditary ataxia: pathologic study of five cases of common ancestry. J Neuropathol Clin Neurol 1951; 1:183–213.
Konigsmark BW, Weiner LP: The olivopontocerebellar atrophies: a review. Medicine 1970; 49:227–242. *
Skre H: Spino-cerevellar ataxia in western Norway. Clin Genet 1974; 6:265–288.
Jackson JF, et al.: Spino-cerebellar ataxia and HLA linkage: risk prediction by HLA typing. New Engl J Med 1977; 296:1138–1141.
Rodriguez-Budelli M, et al.: Action of physostigmine on inherited ataxia. In: Kark RAP, et al, eds: The inherited ataxias. New York: Raven Press, 1978:195–202.
Gilman S, et al.: Disorders of the cerebellum. Philadelphia: F.A. Davis, 1981.
Stumpf DA, et al.: Mitochondrial malic enzyme deficiency in Friedreich's ataxia. Ann Neurol 1981; 10:283 only.

**Carl J. Crosley**

## OLIVOPONTOCEREBELLAR ATROPHY, DOMINANT WITH OPHTHALMOPLEGIA 0744

**Includes:**
Cerebelloolivary degeneration-rigidity and dementia
Olivopontocerebellar atrophy V
Olivopontocerebellar atrophy-dementia-extrapyramidal signs
OPCA V

**Excludes:** Olivopontocerebellar atrophy (other)

**Major Diagnostic Criteria:** Adult life onset of progressive ataxia, tremor, rigidity, ophthalmoplegia, and severe mental deterioration. Computed tomography of the brain, or autopsy findings, of olivopontocerebellar atrophy (OPCA), and cerebral cortical atrophy. Evidence of autosomal dominant transmission helps to confirm the diagnosis.

**Clinical Findings:** Adult onset of progressive ataxia, dysarthria, rigidity, tremor, and mental deterioration. Patients may be diagnosed as having Parkinson disease when the rigidity and tremor are prominent. Walking, writing, and speech generally become difficult. Patients in their third decade of life show mental deterioration, with disorientation to time and place, and are only able to follow simple commands. Dysarthria is characterized by a high-pitched scanning voice. Eye movements become involved first with paresis of upward and lateral gaze and then complete external ophthalmoplegia. Marked rigidity and coarse resting and intention tremor become evident.

**Complications:** Patients become bedridden and debilitated.

**Associated Findings:** None known.

**Etiology:** Autosomal dominant inheritance with complete penetrance.

**Pathogenesis:** The gross brain is small, ranging from 700 to 1200g. There is OPCA, as well as cerebral cortical atrophy. There is a severe loss of neurons in the inferior olivary nuclei, the basis pontis, and the cerebellar cortex. In the spinal cord there is loss of posterior funiculus fibers. The substantia nigra shows marked neuronal loss, and there is a mild neuronal loss in the globus pallidus, caudate nuclei, and cerebral cortex. Clues to the biochemical origin of this disease are provided by studies in other inherited ataxias that demonstrated deficiencies in pyruvate dehydrogenase and mitochondrial malic enzyme.

**MIM No.:** *16470

**Sex Ratio:** M1:F1

**Occurrence:** While there are only a few kindreds reported in detail with this specific variant, the combined prevalence of the dominantly inherited forms of OPCA is estimated to be 1:31,250.

**Risk of Recurrence for Patient's Sib:**
See Part I, *Mendelian Inheritance*.

**Risk of Recurrence for Patient's Child:**
See Part I, *Mendelian Inheritance*.

**Age of Detectability:** At about age 20 years.

**Gene Mapping and Linkage:** Unknown. A single family has been described in whom HLA typing has accurately predicted the presence of ataxia. More tentative evidence is available in another family in which linkage between glyoxalase and spino-cerebellar degeneration is suggested.

**Prevention:** None known. Genetic counseling indicated.

**Treatment:** Supportive therapy for ataxia, and for the mental deterioration and disorientation.

**Prognosis:** Affected persons die about 10 years after onset of symptoms, usually from debility and infection.

**Detection of Carrier:** In some families, HLA typing may be helpful in carrier identification, but only after an index case has been discovered.

**Special Considerations:** This disease differs clinically from the other OPCAs because of the marked mental deterioration, and pathologically because of the marked brain atrophy with olivopontocerebellar degeneration and cerebral cortical neuronal loss.

Some patients have been diagnosed as having Parkinson disease because of prominent rigidity and tremor. Heterogeneity within and among reported families, both clinically and pathologically, has been observed.

**References:**
Konigsmark BW, Lipton HL: Dominant olivopontocerebellar atrophy with dementia and extrapyramidal signs: report of a family through three generations. BD:OAS VII(1). Baltimore: Williams & Wilkins for The National Foundation March of Dimes, 1971:178–202. *
Skre H: Spino-cerebellar ataxia in western Norway. Clin Genet 1974; 6:265–288.
Jackson JF, et al.: Spino-cerebellar ataxia and HLA linkage. N Engl J Med. 1977; 296:1138–1141.
Rodriguez-Budelli M, et al.: Action of physostigmine on inherited ataxia. In: Kark RAP, et al, eds: The inherited ataxias. New York: Raven Press, 1978:195–202. *
Gilman S, et al.: Disorders of the cerebellum. Philadelphia: F.A. Davis, 1981.
Stumpf DA, et al.: Mitochondrial malic enzyme deficiency in Friedreich's ataxia. Ann Neurol 1981; 10:283 only.

CR011                                                          **Carl J. Crosley**

## OLIVOPONTOCEREBELLAR ATROPHY, DOMINANT WITH RETINAL DEGENERATION                              0745

**Includes:**
Cerebellar-macular abiotrophy
Infantile cerebellar atrophy with retinal degeneration
Olivopontocerebellar atrophy III (OPCA type III)
OPCA III
Retinal dystrophy associated with spinocerebellar ataxia

**Excludes:**
**Cerebro-hepato-renal syndrome** (0139)
**Neuronal ceroid-lipofuscinoses (NCL)** (0713)
**Olivopontocerebellar atrophy** (other)
**Phytanic acid oxidase deficiency, infantile type** (2278)

**Major Diagnostic Criteria:**  Infancy or adult onset of ataxia, dysarthria and tremor; progressive visual loss, beginning about the same time as the ataxia and involving the macula and then remainder of the retina; evidence of autosomal dominant transmission, and computed tomography of the brain or neuropathologic findings of OPCA.

**Clinical Findings:**  This disease is characterized by a remarkably variable age of onset of cerebellar ataxia and retinal dystrophy. The disease may show first signs from the age of one year to over 50 years of age; however, the usual age of onset is about 20 years. The syndrome is characterized by a progressive visual loss, ataxia and tremor. Clinically, eye signs are prominent with an unusual retinal pigmentary dystrophy and sometimes with ophthalmoplegia and nystagmus. When the disease begins in infancy, retinal involvement is diffuse with fine pigmentary changes in the macula and fundus periphery. When symptoms begin in adulthood, retinal changes typically remain restricted to the macula and take the form of a bull's eye lesion with mild pigmentary changes. Geographic atrophy of the retinal pigment epithelium and visual loss is much more severe and rapidly progressive when the disease has its onset in infancy. Cerebellar ataxia involving the limbs and speech begins about the same time as the retinal changes. The ataxia and rigidity progress leading to confinement in bed about 10 years after onset. The syndrome in infancy is characterized by tremor, ataxia, retinal dystrophy weakness, and early death.

**Complications:**  Affected persons become bedridden, with death usually resulting from infection.

**Associated Findings:**  None known.

**Etiology:**  Autosomal dominant inheritance. Penetrance is complete, with variability in age of onset and rate of progression.

**Pathogenesis:**  The changes of olivopontocerebellar (OPCA) atrophy are seen grossly and histologically. Cerebellar Purkinje cells are markedly decreased in numbers, particularly in the vermis, while granule cells are relatively preserved. There is also moderate loss of substantia nigra neurons. In early cases, the retina shows marked loss of rods and cones outer segments with preservation of bipolar cells and ganglion cells. The choriocapillaris is normal. The retinal pigment epithelium is variably pigmented. The pathology seems to start in the central retina and spreads to involve the periphery. With advanced disease, there is neuronal dropout in other retinal layers. The optic nerve is generally normal in appearance and color.

Clues to the biochemical origin of these diseases have been provided by studies demonstrating deficiencies in pyruvate dehydrogenase and by other studies recording mitochondrial malic enzyme deficiencies in patients with various inherited ataxias.

**MIM No.:**  *16450

**Sex Ratio:**  M1:F1

**Occurrence:**  Only a few kindreds affected with this disease have been described in the United States. The prevalence of dominantly inherited OPCA is estimated to be 1:31,250.

**Risk of Recurrence for Patient's Sib:**
See Part I, *Mendelian Inheritance.*

**Risk of Recurrence for Patient's Child:**
See Part I, *Mendelian Inheritance.*

**Age of Detectability:**  Highly variable, usually at about 20 years of age.

**Gene Mapping and Linkage:**  Unknown.

**Prevention:**  None known. Genetic counseling indicated.

**Treatment:**  Supportive.

**Prognosis:**  Affected persons generally die of debilitation and infection about 15 years after onset.

**Detection of Carrier:**  There is no known method for the identification of asymptomatic carriers.

**Special Considerations:**  In one family studied, two sibs died of this disease before the diagnosis was made in the affected father, who had only minimal retinal changes. Clinically this disease generally shows more rigidity than the other types of OPCA, and ophthalmoplegia is a prominent feature.

**References:**
Carpenter S, Schumacher GA: Familial infantile cerebellar atrophy associated with retinal degeneration. Arch Neurol 1966; 14:82–94.
Weiner LP, et al.: Herediatary olivopontocerebellar atrophy with retinal degeneration: report of a family through six generations. Arch Neurol 1967; 16:364–376.
Skre H: Spino-cerebellar ataxia in western Norway. Clin Genet 1974; 6:265.
Ryan SJ, et al.: Olivopontocerebellar degeneration: clinicopathologic correlation of the associated retinopathy. Arch Ophthalmol 1975; 93:169–172.
deJong PTVM, et al.: Olivopontocerebellar atrophy with visual disturbances: an ophthalmologic investigation into four generations. Ophthalmology 1980; 87:793–804.
Stumpf DA, et al.: Mitochondrial malic enzyme deficiency in Friedreich's ataxia. Ann Neurol 1981; 10:287.
Harding AE: The clinical features and classification of the late onset autosomal dominant cerebellar ataxia: a study of 11 families including descendants of the Drero family of Walworth. Brain 1982; 105:1–28.
Harding AE: Classification of the hereditary ataxias and paraplegia. Lancet 1983; 1:1151–1154.

CR011                                                          **Carl J. Crosley**

## OLIVOPONTOCEREBELLAR ATROPHY, LATE-ONSET     0746

**Includes:** N/A

**Excludes:**
   Holmes cerebelloolivary atrophy
   Marie ataxia
   **Olivopontocerebellar atrophy** (other)

**Major Diagnostic Criteria:** Onset in adult life of progressive ataxia, tremor, and dysarthria with olivopontocerebellar atrophy (OPCA) as demonstrated by computed tomography of the brain or by autopsy.

**Clinical Findings:** Onset is in the fifth or sixth decades of life, with a progressive cerebellar ataxia of the limbs and trunk, slowness of voluntary movements, scanning speech, nystagmus, and tremor of the head and trunk. In some cases, Parkinsonian signs are prominent, with rigidity, tremor, bradykinesia, and immobile facies. Urinary incontinence and other frontal lobe signs will occur occasionally. Reflexes are usually normal, although there may be loss of knee and ankle jerks or an extensor plantar response.

**Complications:** Patients become incapacitated in 5–10 years.

**Associated Findings:** None known.

**Etiology:** Undetermined. May be **Olivopontocerebellar atrophy, recessive Fickler-Winkler type** with very late expressivity. Other etiologic possibilities include toxic factors or a specific deficiency.

**Pathogenesis:** There may be neuronal loss in the cerebellar dentate nuclei or substantia nigra. The spinal cord and cerebral cortex are minimally affected. Clues to the biochemical origin of this disorder are provided by studies in other inherited ataxias that demonstrate deficiencies in pyruvate dehydrogenase and mitochondrial malic enzyme.

**Sex Ratio:** M1:F1

**Occurrence:** The prevalence of **Olivopontocerebellar atrophy, recessive Fickler-Winkler type**, of which this may or may not be a subset, was determined to be 1.2:100,000 in one western European population.

**Risk of Recurrence for Patient's Sib:**
   See Part I, *Mendelian Inheritance.*

**Risk of Recurrence for Patient's Child:**
   See Part I, *Mendelian Inheritance.*

**Age of Detectability:** Onset of symptoms at about age 45 years.

**Gene Mapping and Linkage:** Unknown.

**Prevention:** None known. Genetic counseling indicated.

**Treatment:** Recognition that defects in pyruvate oxidation result in inhibition of the synthesis of acetylcholine has led to the use of cholinergic agonists (physostigmine and lecithin) with some efficacy. However, supportive personal and family therapy remain the mainstay of treatment.

**Prognosis:** Slow progression, with incapacitation in 5–10 years, and death due to debility and infection about five years later.

**Detection of Carrier:** In some families, HLA typing may be helpful in carrier identification, but only after an index case has been discovered.

**References:**
Jackson JF, et al.: Spino-cerebellar ataxia and HLA linkage. New Engl J Med 1977; 296:1138–1141. *
Rodriguez-Budelli M, et al.: Action of physostigmine on inherited ataxia. In: Kark RAP, et al, eds: The inherited ataxias. New York: Raven Press, 1978:195–202.
Skre H: Spino-cerebellar ataxia in western Norway. Clin Genet 1974; 6:265–288. *
Gilman S, et al.: Disorders of the cerebellum. Philadelphia: F.A. Davis, 1981.
Stumpf DA, et al.: Mitochondrial malic enzyme deficiency in Friedreich's ataxia. Ann Neurol 1981; 10:283 only.

CR011                                      **Carl J. Crosley**

## OLIVOPONTOCEREBELLAR ATROPHY, RECESSIVE FICKLER-WINKLER TYPE     0747

**Includes:**
   Fickler-Winkler olivopontocerebellar atrophy
   Olivopontocerebellar atrophy II
   OPCA II

**Excludes:** **Olivopontocerebellar atrophy** (other)

**Major Diagnostic Criteria:** Progressive cerebellar ataxia and dysarthria, computed tomography of the brain or autopsy findings of olivopontocerebellar atrophy, and evidence of autosomal recessive transmission.

**Clinical Findings:** Variable age of onset, between about seven and 50 years of age, of a slowly progressive cerebellar ataxia, head tremor, and dysarthria, with scanning speech. There are no choreiform movements; strength and sensation are normal.

The age of onset generally is younger than that of **Olivopontocerebellar atrophy, dominant Menzel type**, and there is no sensory loss or involuntary movements.

**Complications:** Patients gradually become bedridden and debilitated.

**Associated Findings:** None known.

**Etiology:** Autosomal recessive inheritance. Penetrance appears to be complete.

**Pathogenesis:** Clues to the biochemical origin of this disease are provided by studies in other inherited ataxias that demonstrate deficiencies in pyruvate dehydrogenase and mitochondrial malic enzyme.

**MIM No.:** *25830

**Sex Ratio:** M1:F1

**Occurrence:** Although Fickler and Winkler reported only two sibs with this condition, Skre (1974) has documented nine families with autosomal recessive OPCA. The prevalence of autosomal recessive OPCA has been reported to be 1.2:100,000 in a western European population.

**Risk of Recurrence for Patient's Sib:**
   See Part I, *Mendelian Inheritance.*

**Risk of Recurrence for Patient's Child:**
   See Part I, *Mendelian Inheritance.*

**Age of Detectability:** At onset of symptoms, from about age 7–50 years.

**Gene Mapping and Linkage:** Unknown.

**Prevention:** None known. Genetic counseling indicated.

**Treatment:** Recognition that defects in pyruvic oxidation result in inhibition of the synthesis of acetylcholine has led to the use of cholinergic agonists (physostigmine and lecithin) with some efficacy. However, supportive personal and family therapy remain the mainstay of treatment.

**Prognosis:** Affected persons die from 5–15 years after onset, usually of debilitation and infection.

**Detection of Carrier:** In some families, HLA typing may be helpful in carrier identification, but only after an index case has been discovered.

**References:**
Winkler C: A case of olivo-pontine cerebellar atrophy and our conceptions of neo and palaeocerebellum. Schweiz Arch Neurol Neurochir Psychiatr 1923; 13:684–702.
Konigsmark BW, Weiner LP: The olivopontocerebellar atrophies: a review. Medicine 1970; 49:227–240.
Skre H: Spino-cerebellar ataxia in western Norway. Clin Genet. 1974; 6:265–288.
Jackson JF, et al.: Spino-cerebellar ataxia and HLA linkage. New Engl J Med 1977; 296:1138–1141.
Rodriguez-Budelli M, et al.: Action of physostigmine on inherited ataxia. In: Kark RAP, et al, eds: The inherited ataxias. New York: Raven Press, 1978:195–202.
Gilman S, et al.: Disorders of the cerebellum. Philadelphia: F.A. Davis, 1981.

Stumpf DA, et al.: Mitochondrial malic enzyme deficiency in Friedreich's ataxia. Ann Neurol 1981; 10:283 only.

CR011                                                    **Carl J. Crosley**

**Olivopontocerebellar atrophy-dementia-extrapyramidal signs**
*See OLIVOPONTOCEREBELLAR ATROPHY, DOMINANT WITH OPHTHALMOPLEGIA*
**Ollier syndrome**
*See ENCHONDROMATOSIS*
**Omenn syndrome**
*See IMMUNODEFICIENCY, RETICULOENDOTHELIOSIS WITH EOSINOPHILIA*

## OMODYSPLASIA                                                    3280

**Includes:**
Dwarfism, omodysplasia
Maroteaux rhizomelic dysplasia
Rhizomelic dysplasia, familial
Viljoen rhizomelic dysplasia

**Excludes:**
Humerus varus
**Rhizomelic syndrome, Urbach type** (2816)
**Robinow syndrome** (0876)

**Major Diagnostic Criteria:** Short humerus with a defect of growth of the distal end of the humerus and upper radio-ulnar diastasis.

**Clinical Findings:** Recognized at birth on the basis of shortened humeri; flexion and extension of the elbow are limited. Craniofacial morphology is characterized by a small but broadened nose, depressed nasal bridge, and a long philtrum. This upper limb anomaly can be isolated, but in some cases a severe micromelic dwarfism, with short and stubby femora and restricted motions of the hips and knees, is also present.

On X-ray, the diaphysis of the humerus is twisted, so that the distal end appears *en profil*. The condyle is hypoplastic and laterally everted. The radial head is dislocated anteriorly and laterally. There is a diastasis of the proximal end of the radius and ulna. If the lower limbs are involved, the diaphyses of the femora are short, broadened and twisted, and the tibiae and fibulae are short and thick.

**Complications:** In cases with severe micromelic dwarfism, patients may die shortly after birth.

**Associated Findings:** Congenital heart defects.

**Etiology:** Autosomal dominant inheritance has been observed in a family without shortness of the lower limbs. In the family reported by Viljoen et al (1987), recessive inheritance was suggested.

**Pathogenesis:** Unknown.

**Sex Ratio:** Presumably M1:F1.

**Occurrence:** Fewer than ten cases have been reported in the literature.

**Risk of Recurrence for Patient's Sib:**
See Part I, *Mendelian Inheritance.*

**Risk of Recurrence for Patient's Child:**
See Part I, *Mendelian Inheritance.*

**Age of Detectability:** At birth on the basis of shortened humeri, or possibly prenatally by fetal ultrasound.

**Gene Mapping and Linkage:** Unknown.

**Prevention:** None known. Genetic counseling indicated.

**Treatment:** Unknown.

**Prognosis:** The defect in the growth of the lower limbs may result in severe dwarfism. Intelligence is unaffected.

**Detection of Carrier:** Unknown.

**References:**
Vallee L, et al.: Syndrome de Robinow à transmission dominante. Arch Fr Pédiatr 1982; 39:447–448.

Viljoen D, et al.: Familial rhizomelic dysplasia: phenotype variation or heterogeneity. Am J Med Genet 1987; 26:941–947.
Maroteaux P, et al.: Omodysplasia. Am J Med Genet 1989; 32:371–375.

MA034                                                **Pierre Maroteaux**

## OMPHALOCELE                                                    0748

**Includes:**
Celosomia
Herniation into the umbilical cord
Umbilical cord hernia

**Excludes:**
**Gastroschisis** (0405)
**Hernia, umbilical** (2575)
**Omphalomesenteric duct anomalies** (2574)
**Schisis association** (2249)
Umbilical cord, large

**Major Diagnostic Criteria:** A transparent sac covering the umbilical ring, with the umbilical cord inserted onto the sac rather than the abdominal wall. Ultrasonography offers antenatal diagnosis of anterior abdominal wall defects, including omphalocele and gastroschisis.

**Clinical Findings:** Intra-abdominal viscera herniate the umbilical cord. The mass is not covered with peritoneum, fascia, muscles, or skin. The size of an omphalocele depends on the amount of the abdominal viscera herniated into the amniotic sac surrounding the umbilical cord.

**Complications:** Infection, dehydration, and trauma or vascular compromise to the herniated abdominal viscera may occur; prenatal as well as postnatal rupture of the covering sac.

**Associated Findings:** Associated anomalies occur in 67% of patients with omphalocele (Rickham et al, 1978). Such anomalies include those in the cardiovascular, genitourinary, and central nervous systems. Of special importance is the diagnosis of **Beckwith-Wiedemann syndrome** (omphalocele, macroglossia, and gigantism) because of the associated intractable hypoglycemia due to pancreatic hyperplasia.

**Etiology:** Unknown. Autosomal dominant and X-linked inheritance have been reported.

**Pathogenesis:** Failure of migration and fusion of the two lateral embryonic folds of the anterior abdominal wall. Central herniation of the contents of the abdomen through the umbilical ring into a transparent sac composed of amnion and peritoneum with Wharton's jelly between them.

**MIM No.:** 16475, 31098

**CDC No.:** 756.700

**Sex Ratio:** M1:F1

**Occurrence:** 1:4,000 births.

**Risk of Recurrence for Patient's Sib:** Unknown.

**Risk of Recurrence for Patient's Child:** Unknown.

**Age of Detectability:** At birth.

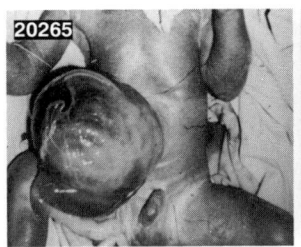 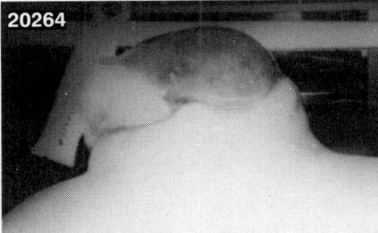

**0748-20265–64:** The transparent sac of the omphalocele covers the abdominal viscera.

**Gene Mapping and Linkage:** Unknown.

**Prevention:** None known. Genetic counseling indicated.

**Treatment:** Surgical closure, either primary or staged using silicone rubber parasthesis.

**Prognosis:** With early recognition and successful repair, survival in 50–60% of cases. Most deaths due to associated anomalies.

**Detection of Carrier:** Unknown.

**References:**

Rickham PP, et al.: Neonatal surgery. London: Butterworth & Co, 1978.

Seashore JH: Congenital abdominal wall defects. Clinics in Perinatology 1978; 5:61–78.

Havalad S, et al.: Familial occurrence of omphalocele suggesting sex-linked inheritance. Arch Dis Child 1979; 54:142–151.

DiLiberti JH: Familial omphalocele: analysis of risk factors and case report. Am J Med Genet 1982; 13:263–268.

Lurie IW, Ilyina HG: Familial omphalocele and recurrent risk. (Letter) Am J Med Genet 1984; 17:541–543.

SE006                                                     **John H. Seashore**

**Omphalocele with hypoplasia of pharynx and larynx**
  *See PHARYNX/LARYNX HYPOPLASIA-OMPHALOCELE, SHPRINTZEN-GOLDBERG TYPE*
**Omphalocele-cleft palate**
  *See CLEFT PALATE-OMPHALOCELE*
**Omphalocele-exstrophy-imperforate anus-spina bifida (OEIS)**
  *See EXSTROPHY OF CLOACA SEQUENCE*
**Omphalocele-pharynx/larynx hypoplasia, Shprintzen-Goldberg type**
  *See PHARYNX/LARYNX HYPOPLASIA-OMPHALOCELE, SHPRINTZEN-GOLDBERG TYPE*
**Omphalocele-visceromegaly-macroglossia syndrome**
  *See BECKWITH-WIEDEMANN SYNDROME*
**Omphalomesenteric duct**
  *See MECKEL DIVERTICULUM*

---

## OMPHALOMESENTERIC DUCT ANOMALIES                    2574

**Includes:**

Enteroumbilical fistula
Meckel diverticulum
Omphalomesenteric duct cyst
Omphalomesenteric sinus
Patent omphalomesenteric duct
Umbilical polyp
Vitelline cyst
Vitelline duct anomalies

**Excludes:**

Angiomyxomas
Hemangiomas
**Teratomas** (2919)
Umbilical cord, large
Umbilical cord, tumors
Umbilical cysts
**Urachal anomalies** (2573)

**Major Diagnostic Criteria:** A visible or palpable umbilical mass with or without a discharge. The type of lesion may be outlined by injecting contrast material into the sinus.

**Clinical Findings:** *Patent omphalomesenteric duct*: fecal discharge from the umbilicus or the umbilical stump coupled with visualization of the fistulous tract following injection of a radio-opaque material.
*Omphalomesenteric sinus*: presents as a pouting mucous membrane projecting from the base of the umbilical wall and draining mucoid discharge.
*Umbilical polyp*: a bright red nodule with no demonstrable orifice or sinus tract.
*Vitelline cyst*: a palpable cystic mass buried superficially beneath the umbilicus.
**Meckel diverticulum**: the most common symptom is abdominal pain accompanied by sudden profuse rectal bleeding. Intussus-

ception occurs as the presenting problem in 25% of individuals with **Meckel diverticulum**.

**Complications:** Early and definitive diagnosis of the type of lesion is desirable because of the potential hazards of infection, injury, dehydration, and small bowel obstruction or perforation.

**Associated Findings:** None known.

**Etiology:** Aberrant development of the yolk sac coupled with an abnormal closure of the omphalomesenteric duct.

**Pathogenesis:** The wall in the nonobliterated vitelline duct may be lined by cuboidal or columnar epithelium with gastrointestinal differentiation with or without mucous production.

**CDC No.:** 751.000

**Sex Ratio:** M4:F1 for omphalomesenteric duct cyst
  M8:F1 for complete patency of the duct
  M6:F1 for cutaneous remnants of the duct

**Occurrence:** Varies according to the type of malformation. A completely patent omphalomesenteric duct is rare, occurring in 6.7:100,000 population.

**Risk of Recurrence for Patient's Sib:** Probably not increased.

**Risk of Recurrence for Patient's Child:** Probably not increased.

**Age of Detectability:** At birth or in the first year of life. Asymptomatic lesions may be discovered accidentally during abdominal operation or at autopsy.

**Gene Mapping and Linkage:** Unknown.

**Prevention:** None known. Genetic counseling indicated.

**Treatment:** Surgical excision of patent omphalomesenteric, omphalomesenteric duct cyst, or sinus and prompt treatment of symptomatic **Meckel diverticulum** is advisable. In the absence of a sinus tract, the treatment of choice of an umbilical polyp is cauterization.

**Prognosis:** Unknown.

**Detection of Carrier:** Unknown.

**References:**

Brown KL, Glover DM: Persistent omphalomesenteric duct. Am J Surg 1952; 83:680–685.

EL013                                                   **Sami B. Elhassani**

**Omphalomesenteric duct cyst**
  *See OMPHALOMESENTERIC DUCT ANOMALIES*
**Omphalomesenteric sinus**
  *See OMPHALOMESENTERIC DUCT ANOMALIES*
**Omphalopagus**
  *See TWINS, CONJOINED*
**Oncogene B-cell leukemia**
  *See LEUKEMIA/LYMPHOMA, B-CELL*
**Oncogene B-cell leukemia-2**
  *See LYMPHOMA, NON-HODGKIN*
**Ondine curse-Hirschprung disease**
  *See HYPOVENTILATION, CONGENITAL CENTRAL ALVEOLAR TYPE*
**Onion bulb neuropathy**
  *See DEJERINE-SOTTAS DISEASE*
**Onychial dysplasia, hereditary**
  *See NAILS, ANONYCHIA, HEREDITARY*
**Onycho-osteo dystrophy-deafness**
  *See DEAFNESS-TRIPHALANGEAL THUMBS-ONYCHODYSTROPHY*

---

## ONYCHO-TRICHODYSPLASIA-NEUTROPENIA                   2331

**Includes:**

Nails (hypoplastic)-neutropenia-onychorrhexis
Neutropenia-onychotrichodysplasia
Onychotrichodysplasia-chronic neutropenia-mild mental retardation
Tricho-onycho-dysplasia-neutropenia

**Excludes:**

**Ectodermal dysplasia, Christ-Siemens-Touraine type** (0333)
**Ectodermal dysplasia, hidrotic** (0334)
**Ectodermal dysplasia** (other)

**Immunodeficiency, agranulocytosis, infantile Kostmann type**
(2197)
Nail dysplasia
Nails, hypoplastic
**Nails, pachyonychia congenita** (0789)
**Nail-patella syndrome** (0704)
**Nails, koilonychia** (0559)
**Neutropenia, benign familial** (2215)

**Major Diagnostic Criteria:** Neutropenia, trichorrhexis, hypoplastic nails.

**Clinical Findings:** The scalp and body hair is scanty, fine, dry, lusterless, short, curly, and sparse. Other characteristic findings are mild keratosis follicularis, hypoplastic nails, onychorrhexis, and koilonychia.

White blood cell counts show neutropenia (neutrophil counts range from 502 to 2,633/μl) and monocytosis (ranging from 1% to 6%). Immunoglobulin levels (IgA, IgG, and IgM), immune response to vaccination with common antigens, antistreptolysins, and C-reactive protein are normal. Responses to coccidioidin and histoplasmin are negative. Microscopic studies of the hair, eyebrows, and eyelashes show trichorrhexis.

**Complications:** Recurrent infections, i.e., conjunctivitis, tonsillitis, sinusitis, otitis, vaginitis, and cystitis.

**Associated Findings:** Verhage et al (1987) has suggested that the mild mental retardation (IQ ranges from 62 to normal), observed in most cases, may be a result of repeated infestions.

**Etiology:** Autosomal recessive inheritance.

**Pathogenesis:** Neutropenia is probably present from birth, leading to increased susceptibility to infections.

**MIM No.:** *25836

**POS No.:** 3490

**Sex Ratio:** M1:F3 (observed)

**Occurrence:** About a half-dozen cases have been reported.

**Risk of Recurrence for Patient's Sib:**
See Part I, *Mendelian Inheritance.*

**Risk of Recurrence for Patient's Child:**
See Part I, *Mendelian Inheritance.*

**Age of Detectability:** At birth.

**Gene Mapping and Linkage:** Unknown.

**Prevention:** None known. Genetic counseling indicated.

**Treatment:** Symptomatic.

**Prognosis:** One affected child died from acute meningitis. Two other affected individuals were alive beyond 20 years of age.

**Detection of Carrier:** Unknown.

**References:**
Cantú JM, et al.: Syndrome of onychotrichodysplasia with chronic neutropenia in an infant from consanguineous parents. BD:OAS XI(2). New York: March of Dimes Birth Defects Foundation, 1975: 63–66.
Hernández A, et al.: Autosomal recessive onychotrichodysplasia, chronic neutropenia and mild mental retardation: delineation of the syndrome. Clin Genet 1979; 15:147–152. *
Corona-Rivera E, et al.: Further delineation of the onycho-trichodysplasia, chronic neutropenia and mild retardation syndrome. (Abstract) Sixth Int Cong Hum Genet, Jerusalem 1981:267.
Verhage J, et al.: A patient with onychotrichodysplasia, neutropenia, and normal intelligence. Clin Genet 1987; 31:374–380.

HE039
CA011

**Alejandro Hernández
José María Cantú**

**Onycho-trichodysplasia-xeroderma**
*See TRICHO-ONYCHODYSPLASIA-XERODERMA*
**Onychodystrophy-conical teeth-hearing loss**
*See ONYCHODYSTROPHY-CONIFORM TEETH-SENSORINEURAL HEARING LOSS*

## ONYCHODYSTROPHY-CONIFORM TEETH-SENSORINEURAL HEARING LOSS — 2034

**Includes:**
Deafness-onychodystrophy, dominant form
Ectodermal dysplasia-hearing loss (sensorineural)-digital defects
Onychodystrophy-conical teeth-hearing loss
Robinson ectodermal dysplasia-deafness
Teeth (coniform)-onychodystrophy-deafness

**Excludes:**
**Chondroectodermal dysplasia** (0156)
**Deafness-onychodystrophy** (0252)
**Ectodermal dysplasia, hidrotic** (0334)

**Major Diagnostic Criteria:** The combination of nail dystrophy, missing and/or conical teeth, and sensorineural hearing loss and, in some cases, polydactyly and/or syndactyly.

**Clinical Findings:** This condition has only been reported in four individuals in a single family, and is considered a hidrotic ectodermal dysplasia. Affected individuals all have sensorineural hearing loss, which is more severe in the higher tones. The nails are small and dystrophic, with furrows and cracks. All individuals had delayed dentition, partial anodontia, and conical teeth, affecting both primary and secondary dentition. One individual had unilateral post-axial polydactyly of the hand, and another had unilateral syndactyly of toes 1 and 2, and 3 and 4. Laboratory investigations showed elevated sweat chloride and sodium.

**Complications:** Unknown.

**Associated Findings:** None known.

**Etiology:** Autosomal dominant inheritance, probably with a high degree of penetrance.

**Pathogenesis:** An ectodermal dysplasia seems most likely, although no specific defect has been identified.

**MIM No.:** *12448

**Sex Ratio:** M1:F1

**Occurrence:** Documented in a five members across three generations of one family.

**Risk of Recurrence for Patient's Sib:**
See Part I, *Mendelian Inheritance.*

**Risk of Recurrence for Patient's Child:**
See Part I, *Mendelian Inheritance.*

**Age of Detectability:** At birth, by the presence of polydactyly, syndactyly, or nail defects.

**Gene Mapping and Linkage:** Unknown.

**Prevention:** None known. Genetic counseling indicated.

**Treatment:** Orthodontic treatment for anodontia or hypodontia is indicated; appropriate schooling for deafness.

**Prognosis:** Life span and intellect appear normal.

**Detection of Carrier:** Unknown.

**References:**
Robinson GC, et al.: Familial ectodermal dysplasia with sensorineural deafness and other anomalies. Pediatrics 1962; 30:797–802. *

T0007

**Helga V. Toriello**

**Onychodystrophy-deafness**
*See DEAFNESS-ONYCHODYSTROPHY*
**Onychodystrophy-digital malformation-deafness**
*See DEAFNESS-TRIPHALANGEAL THUMBS-ONYCHODYSTROPHY*
**Onycholysis-hypohidrosis-enamel hypocalcification**
*See AMELO-ONYCHO-HYPOHIDROTIC SYNDROME*
**Onychoosteodysplasia**
*See NAIL-PATELLA SYNDROME*
**Onychotrichodysplasia-chronic neutropenia-mild mental retardation**
*See ONYCHO-TRICHODYSPLASIA-NEUTROPENIA*
**Opalescent dentin**
*See TEETH, DENTINOGENESIS IMPERFECTA*

**OPCA I**
  *See OLIVOPONTOCEREBELLAR ATROPHY, DOMINANT MENZEL TYPE*
**OPCA IV**
  *See OLIVOPONTOCEREBELLAR ATROPHY, DOMINANT SCHUT-HAYMAKER TYPE*
**OPCA V**
  *See OLIVOPONTOCEREBELLAR ATROPHY, DOMINANT WITH OPHTHALMOPLEGIA*
**Ophiasis**
  *See HAIR, ALOPECIA AREATA*
**Ophthalmo-acromelic syndrome**
  *See ANOPHTHALMIA-LIMB ANOMALIES*
**Ophthalmo-mandibulo-melic dwarfism**
  *See DWARFISM (SHORT LIMBED)-PETERS ANOMALY OF THE EYE*

---

## OPHTHALMO-MANDIBULO-MELIC DWARFISM          3259

**Includes:**
  Dwarfism, ophthalmo-mandibulo-melic
  Mandibulo-melic dwarfism with corneal clouding
  Pillay syndrome

**Excludes:**
  **Dwarfism (short limbed)-Peters anomaly of the eye** (2812)
  **Eye, anterior segment dysgenesis** (0439)
  **Fetal alcohol syndrome** (0379)
  **Walker-Warburg syndrome** (2869)

**Major Diagnostic Criteria:** Mesomelic dwarfism with bowed radius and short ulna. Congenital corneal clouding. Micrognathia, obtuse jaw angle, temporomandibular joint fusion.

**Clinical Findings:** Bowed forearms due to radial bowing and marked shortening of ulna. Corneal clouding due to **Eye, anterior segment dysgenesis**. Relative shortening of tibia and fibula.

**Complications:** Visual loss from corneal opacities.

**Associated Findings:** Pupillary membrane.

**Etiology:** Autosomal dominant inheritance.

**Pathogenesis:** Unknown.

**MIM No.:** *16490

**Sex Ratio:** M1:F1

**Occurrence:** Pillay described a father with an affected daughter and son (1964). Another possible case in a female who underwent corneal transplantation has been observed. The histology revealed Peters anomaly (see **Eye, anterior segment dysgenesis**).

**Risk of Recurrence for Patient's Sib:**
  See Part I, *Mendelian Inheritance.*

**Risk of Recurrence for Patient's Child:**
  See Part I, *Mendelian Inheritance.*

**Age of Detectability:** At birth.

**Gene Mapping and Linkage:** Unknown.

**Prevention:** None known. Genetic counseling indicated.

**Treatment:** Early management of ocular conditions to promote normal visual development.

**Prognosis:** Guarded for vision. Severe short stature.

**Detection of Carrier:** Unknown.

**References:**
Pillay, VK: Ophthalmo-mandibulo-melic dysplasia: a hereditary syndrome. J Bone Joint Surg 1964; 46A:858–862.

KI021                                                    **Jane D. Kivlin**

**Ophthalmoarthropathy**
  *See ARTHRO-OPHTHALMOPATHY, HEREDITARY, PROGRESSIVE, STICKLER TYPE*

---

## OPHTHALMOPLEGIA EXTERNA-MYOPIA          0750

**Includes:**
  External ophthalmoplegia-myopia
  Myopia-external ophthalmoplegia

**Excludes:**
  **Eyelid, ptosis, congenital** (0834)
  Ocular myasthenia gravis
  **Ophthalmoplegia, familial static** (0751)
  **Ophthalmoplegia, progressive external** (0752)
  Ophthalmoplegia secondary to generalized myopathy or neuropathy

**Major Diagnostic Criteria:** Clinical diagnosis based upon limited mobility of extraocular muscles (external ophthalmoplegia) at birth and high myopia.

**Clinical Findings:** Although congenital, external ophthalmoplegia is difficult to detect in the newborn period; bilateral blepharoptosis is the most obvious sign. Ocular excursions are severely limited in all directions of gaze, vertical more than horizontal. High myopia is prevalent. The pupil is frequently eccentric. Examination of the fundi shows thinning of the choroid and retina, owing to high myopia.

**Complications:** The major ophthalmological complications are macular degeneration with visual loss and increased incidence of retinal detachment due to the high myopia. Some patients have strabismus. Moderate to severe blepharoptosis causes hyperextension of the neck which explains abnormal head posture and musculoskeletal strain.

**Associated Findings:** Systemic findings include absent knee and ankle jerks, spina bifida, scoliosis, dental malocclusion, cardiac defects, and hernia.

**Etiology:** X-linked recessive inheritance.

**Pathogenesis:** Thought to be due to dysgenesis of extraocular muscle, although mitochondrial cytopathies have not been excluded.

**MIM No.:** *31100

**Sex Ratio:** M1:F0

**Occurrence:** One pedigree from Argentina has been described (Salleras and Ortiz de Zarate, 1950) and reviewed again in a 15-year follow-up (Ortiz de Zarate, 1966).

**Risk of Recurrence for Patient's Sib:**
  See Part I, *Mendelian Inheritance.*

**Risk of Recurrence for Patient's Child:**
  See Part I, *Mendelian Inheritance.*

**Age of Detectability:** Soon after birth.

**Gene Mapping and Linkage:** OPEM (ophthalmoplegia, external, with myopia) has been provisionally mapped to X.

**Prevention:** None known. Genetic counseling indicated.

**Treatment:** Ptosis surgery is indicated for visual deprivation or chin-up head posture. Eye muscle surgery is not beneficial to those with their eyes aligned in primary position but, may be to those with strabismus or both eyes fixed in downgaze.

**Prognosis:** Life expectancy is dependent upon the severity of the associated findings.

**Detection of Carrier:** Female carriers have absent knee and ankle jerks.

**References:**
Salleras A, Ortiz de Zarate JC: Recessive sex-linked inheritance of external ophthalmoplegia and myopia coincident with other dysplasias. Br J Ophthalmol 1950; 34:662–667.
Ortiz de Zarate JC: Recessive sex-linked inheritance of congenital ophthalmoplegia and myopia coincident with other dysplasias: a reappraisal after 15 years. Br J Ophthalmol 1966; 50:606–607.

WE035                                                    **Avery H. Weiss**

**Ophthalmoplegia plus syndrome**
See KEARNS-SAYRE DISEASE
also OPHTHALMOPLEGIA, PROGRESSIVE EXTERNAL
**Ophthalmoplegia totalis**
See OPHTHALMOPLEGIA, FAMILIAL STATIC
**Ophthalmoplegia, chronic progressive external**
See OPHTHALMOPLEGIA, PROGRESSIVE EXTERNAL
**Ophthalmoplegia, congenital**
See EYE, FIBROSIS OF THE EXTRAOCULAR MUSCLES,
GENERALIZED

## OPHTHALMOPLEGIA, FAMILIAL STATIC　　　　0751

**Includes:**
External ophthalmoplegia congenita
Ophthalmoplegia, hereditary congenital nonprogressive
Ophthalmoplegia totalis

**Excludes:**
**Eye, fibrosis of the extraocular muscles, generalized** (3185)
Ocular myasthenia gravis, congenital
**Ophthalmoplegia externa-myopia** (0750)
**Ophthalmoplegia, progressive external** (0752)
Ophthalmoplegia secondary to generalized myopathy or
neuropathy
**Ophthalmoplegia, total with ptosis and miosis** (0753)

**Major Diagnostic Criteria:** Clinical diagnosis based upon limited mobility of extraocular muscles (external ophthalmoplegia) from birth.

**Clinical Findings:** Congenital external ophthalmoplegia presents with bilateral ptosis and limitation of ocular excursions in all directions of gaze. Clinical variability is common. Ptosis is the only manifestation in some cases, while ptosis and complete external ophthalmoplegia are evident in others. Ocular alignment is usually normal in primary gaze due to the symmetrical involvement. Various abnormalities of the pupillary response are described; pupillary constriction to accomodative stimuli is sometimes decreased while the response to light stimuli is usually normal. Visual acuity is normal (except for those with strabismic amblyopia). Examination of the anterior and posterior segments is normal. Familial static ophthalmoplegia is one type of congenital external ophthalmoplegia, but there are other types with different associated manifestations and different patterns of inheritance. Also, the condition should be distinguished from *fibrosis of the extraocular muscles* (Harley, et al, 1978).

**Complications:** Bilateral ptosis, or hypodeviation of both eyes, causes compensatory hyperextension of the neck and musculoskeletal strain. Strabismus occurs in some cases. Amblyopia may complicate strabismus or severe ptosis in infancy.

**Associated Findings:** None known.

**Etiology:** Autosomal dominant inheritance with variable expression. Rarely, autosomal recessive inheritance.

**Pathogenesis:** A few histopathological studies have shown atrophy of muscle associated with variable amounts of fibrous tissue. Metabolic defects, such as mitochondrial cytopathies, have not been excluded.

**MIM No.:** *16500

**Sex Ratio:** M1:F1

**Occurrence:** Several kinships have been documented, including one Sicilian family.

**Risk of Recurrence for Patient's Sib:**
See Part I, *Mendelian Inheritance.*

**Risk of Recurrence for Patient's Child:**
See Part I, *Mendelian Inheritance.*

**Age of Detectability:** Soon after birth.

**Gene Mapping and Linkage:** Unknown.

**Prevention:** None known. Genetic counseling indicated.

**Treatment:** Surgical treatment of ptosis is indicated predominantly for abnormal head posture, and to prevent deprivation amblyopia in infant. Eye muscle surgery does not correct the limited ocular motility, and is recommended only for ocular misalignment (strabismus) or deviation of both eyes downwards in primary gaze.

**Prognosis:** Normal life span. Vision is usually normal.

**Detection of Carrier:** Examination of relatives for evidence of ptosis and external ophthalmoplegia.

**References:**
Holmes WJ: Hereditary congenital ophthalmoplegia. Am J Ophthalmol 1956; 28:23–30.
Lees F: Congenital static familial ophthalmoplegia. J Neurol Neurosurg Psych 1960; 23:46–51. *
Mace JW, et al.: Congenital hereditary nonprogressive external ophthalmoplegia. Am J Dis Child 1971; 122:261–263.
Harley RD, et al.: Congenital fibrosis of the extraocular muscles. J Pediat Ophthal 1978; 15:346–358.
Mollica F, et al.: Variabilite intrafamiliale de l'ophthalmologie externe congenitale: etude d'une famille sicilienne. J Hum Genet 1980; 28:23–30.

WE035　　　　　　　　　　　　　**Avery H. Weiss**

**Ophthalmoplegia, hereditary congenital nonprogressive**
See OPHTHALMOPLEGIA, FAMILIAL STATIC

## OPHTHALMOPLEGIA, PROGRESSIVE EXTERNAL　　　0752

**Includes:**
Abiotrophic ophthalmoplegia externa
Extraocular muscular dystrophy, progressive
Mitochondrial cytopathy
Myopathic ophthalmoplegia externa
Oculo-cranio-somatic neuromuscular disease with ragged-red fibers
Ocular myopathy
Oculocraniosomatic syndrome
Ophthalmoplegia, chronic progressive external
Ophthalmoplegia-pigmentary dystrophy of retina-cardiomyopathy
Ophthalmoplegia plus syndrome
Ophthalmoplegia, progressive external, recessive
Ophthalmoplegia, progressive external, with ragged-red fibers

**Excludes:**
**Abetalipoproteinemia** (0002)
**Diplegia, congenital facial** (0376)
**Eye, fibrosis of the extraocular muscles, generalized** (3185)
**Eyelid, ptosis, congenital** (0834)
**Kearns-Sayre disease** (2070)
**Muscular dystrophy, oculopharyngeal** (0692)
Ocular myasthenia gravis
**Ophthalmoplegia externa-myopia** (0750)
**Ophthalmoplegia, familial static** (0751)
Ophthalmoplegia secondary to generalized myopathy or neuropathy
Ophthalmoplegia secondary to thyroid disease
**Ophthalmoplegia, total with ptosis and miosis** (0753)
**Phytanic acid storage disease** (0810)

**Major Diagnostic Criteria:** Differentiation from other causes of ptosis and ophthalmoplegia is necessary. Myasthenia gravis is diagnosed by a characteristic response to anticholinesterases or the presence of antiacetylcholine receptor antibody. Ptosis also occurs with sympathetic lesions (see **Horner syndrome**), oculomotor nerve lesions, and after head trauma; but these causes are seldom confused with progressive external ophthalmoplegia.

Isolated ptosis does occur. Such cases are not considered *formes frustes* of progressive external ophthalmoplegia. **Muscular dystrophy, oculopharyngeal** presents with bilateral ptosis, which does not usually involve eye movement disorders, and swallowing difficulties; it is most prevalent among elderly French-Canadians. Rarely, ophthalmoplegia occurs with other neuromuscular diseases (Type I muscle fiber hypotrophy and central nuclei, myotonic atrophy, and even isolated case reports of polymyositis and **Spinal muscular atrophy**).

The presence of characteristic abnormalities on skeletal muscle biopsy strongly supports the diagnosis. These consist of accumulations of abnormal mitochondria subsarcolemmally, and lipids diffusely, in histochemical Type I muscle fibers. On light microscopy, after modified Masson trichrome staining, these are described as ragged-red fibers. By electron microscopy, the mitochondria have whorled lamellae, paracrystalline inclusions, and are of abnormal size. The mitochondrial abnormalities are also found in the liver, sweat glands, and brain. Ocular muscle biopsies are more difficult to interpret, since some ragged-red fibers are a normal constituent. Rarely, otherwise typical cases of progressive external ophthalmoplegia lacking ragged-red fibers on skeletal muscle biopsy are reported. Autopsied cases of progressive external ophthalmoplegia have shown both normal ocular motor nuclei and a spongiform encephalopathy.

**Clinical Findings:** A bilateral, often asymmetrical, ptosis presents at any age. This is followed by the insidious, usually asymptomatic, onset of ophthalmoplegia. Downward gaze may be relatively spared as compared to lateral and upward gaze. Before the ophthalmoplegia becomes complete, normally rapid eye movements are slowed. Orbicularis weakness is regularly associated; pupillary reactions remain normal in most cases.

**Complications:** Visual difficulties occur when the ptosis occludes the pupillary axis. Affected individuals often develop a chin elevation-backward head tilt in an attempt to compensate. The most serious complications of progressive external ophthalmoplegia arise from its associated disorders.

**Associated Findings:** Progressive external ophthalmoplegia has been reported with endocrine abnormalities (diabetes mellitus, hypoparathyroidism, thyroid disease, hyperaldosteronism, and hypogonadism), other neuromuscular abnormalities (small stature, weakness, intellectual deterioration, ataxia, spasticity, retinal degeneration, abnormal electroencephalogram, and increased cerebrospinal fluid protein), and cardiac defects (heart block, Wolff-Parkinson-White syndrome, cardiomyopathy).

Considerable debate has centered around whether particular combinations of these numerous associations represent separable nosological entities. The combination of heart block, retinal pigmentary degeneration and progressive external ophthalmoplegia is referred to as the **Kearns-Sayre disease**. A familial ophthalmoplegia with ataxia and amyotrophy is sometimes called the *Stephens syndrome* (see **Kearns-Sayre disease**). A variant of progressive external ophthalmoplegia occurs in **Abetalipoproteinemia** (*Bassen-Kornsweig*).

**Etiology:** Possibly autosomal dominant inheritance, or rarely autosomal recessive inheritance.

**Pathogenesis:** A history of meningitis-encephalitis in sporadically occurring cases of the **Kearns-Sayre disease** variant, and the similarity of the central nervous system pathology to the spongiform encephalopathy of *Creutzfeldt-Jacob disease* has led some authors to suggest the possibility of a slow virus infection, but this is unsupported by animal inoculations. Whitaker et al (1987), upon restudy of the pituitary from one of Kearns and Sayre's cases, concluded that the patient actually had **Laurence-Moon syndrome**.

There is a disagreement as to whether the ophthalmoplegia is primarily neurogenic or myogenic in origin. The regular association of neuropathological alterations argues for the former; the experimental production of morphological changes resembling ragged-red fibers in animal muscle perfused with metabolic poisons may support the latter.

**MIM No.:** 16510, 16513, 25845

**Sex Ratio:** M1:F1

**Occurrence:** About 30 kinships documented in the literature.

**Risk of Recurrence for Patient's Sib:**
See Part I, *Mendelian Inheritance.*

**Risk of Recurrence for Patient's Child:**
See Part I, *Mendelian Inheritance.*

**Age of Detectability:** Infancy to old age; most commonly in second decade of life.

**Gene Mapping and Linkage:** Unknown.

**Prevention:** None known. Genetic counseling indicated.

**Treatment:** Surgical treatment of strabismus is rarely indicated. Ptosis surgery should be approached with great caution because of the risk of exposure keratitis postoperatively. Ptosis crutch spectacles are occasionally tolerated.

Treatment of the associated disorders is important. Several cases of sudden death in patients with cardiac conduction defects are reported; pacemaker insertion is indicated when heart block is present. Death from hyperglycemic acidotic coma has been reported following administration of oral prednisone. Early studies of metabolic therapy with coenzyme $Q_{10}$ have been promising, with improvement of EKG abnormalities and neurologic symptoms.

**Prognosis:** Progressive external ophthalmoplegia is compatible with a normal lifespan. In patients with retinal pigmentary degeneration, the visual prognosis is better than in the usual **Retinitis pigmentosa**. Children with the **Kearns-Sayre disease** variant have a poor prognosis, with progression of weakness, intellectual deterioration, visual loss, and death from cardiac complications or intercurrent infection.

**Detection of Carrier:** Unknown.

**References:**
Drachman DA: Ophthalmoplegia plus: the neurodegenerative disorders associated with progressive external ophthalmoplegia. Arch Neurol 1968; 18:654–674.
Daroff RB: Chronic progressive external ophthalmoplegia. Arch Ophthalmol 1969; 82:845–851.
Butler IJ, Gadoth N: Kearns-Sayre syndrome: a review of a multisystem disorder of children and young adults. Arch Intern Med 1976; 136:1290–1293.
Berenberg RA, et al.: Lumping or splitting? Ophthalmoplegia plus or Kearns-Sayre syndrome. Ann Neurol 1977; 1:37–54.
Ringel SP, et al.: Extraocular muscle biopsy in chronic progressive external ophthalmoplegia. Ann Neurol 1979; 6:326–341.
Eagle RC, Jr., et al.: The atypical pigmentary retinopathy of Kearns-Sayre: a light and electron microscope study. Ophthalmology 1982; 89:1433–1440.
Egger J, Wilson J: Mitochondrial inheritance in a mitochondrially mediated disease. New Engl J Med 1983; 309:142–146.
Mitsumoto H, et al.: Chronic progressive external ophthalmoplegia: clinical, morphologic, and biochemical studies. Neurology 1983; 33:452–461.
Ogasahara S, et al.: Improvement of abnormal pyruvate metabolism and cardiac conduction defect with coenzyme Q(10) in Kearns-Sayre syndrome. Neurology 1985; 35:372–377.
Whitaker MD, et al.: The pituitary gland in the Lawrence-Moon syndrome. Mayo Clin Proc 1987; 62:216–222.

DE034                   **Monte A. Del Monte**
BE026                   **Donald R. Bergsma**

**Ophthalmoplegia, progressive external, recessive**
*See OPHTHALMOPLEGIA, PROGRESSIVE EXTERNAL*
**Ophthalmoplegia, progressive external, with ragged-red fibers**
*See OPHTHALMOPLEGIA, PROGRESSIVE EXTERNAL*

## OPHTHALMOPLEGIA, TOTAL WITH PTOSIS AND MIOSIS 0753

**Includes:** Ptosis and miosis with ophthalmoplegia totalis

**Excludes:**
**Eyelid, ptosis, congenital** (0834)
Ocular myasthenia gravis, congenital
**Ophthalmoplegia externa-myopia** (0750)
**Ophthalmoplegia, familial static** (0751)
**Ophthalmoplegia, progressive external** (0752)
Ophthalmoplegia secondary to generalized myopathy or neuropathy

**Major Diagnostic Criteria:** Clinical diagnosis based upon the presence of external and internal ophthalmoplegia (total ophthalmoplegia), blepharoptosis, and pupillary miosis.

**Clinical Findings:** Bilateral blepharoptosis and limitation of ocular movement in all directions of gaze (external ophthalmoplegia) are noted soon after birth. Pupillary miosis is present. Pupillary constriction in response to light and accomodative stimuli are decreased (internal ophthalmoplegia). Visual acuity and examination of the anterior and posterior segments are normal.

**Complications:** Blepharoptosis causes affected patients to hyperextend the neck, leading to abnormal head posture and musculoskeletal strain. Strabismus and deprivation amblyopia can occur in infants.

**Associated Findings:** None known.

**Etiology:** Autosomal recessive inheritance.

**Pathogenesis:** Congenital ophthalmoplegias are thought to be due to dysgenesis of extraocular muscle, although metabolic disorders, such as mitochondrial cytopathies, have not been excluded.

**MIM No.:** *25840

**Sex Ratio:** M1:F1

**Occurrence:** Two families have been described.

**Risk of Recurrence for Patient's Sib:**
See Part I, *Mendelian Inheritance.*

**Risk of Recurrence for Patient's Child:**
See Part I, *Mendelian Inheritance.*

**Age of Detectability:** Clinically evident in infancy.

**Gene Mapping and Linkage:** Unknown.

**Prevention:** None known. Genetic counseling indicated.

**Treatment:** Ptosis surgery is indicated when upper eyelid obstructs visual axis and induces chin-up head posture. Eye muscle surgery is not beneficial to those with eyes aligned in the primary position, but may be beneficial to those with strabismus, or those with both eyes fixed in downgaze.

**Prognosis:** Normal life span.

**Detection of Carrier:** Examination of relatives for evidence of the trait.

**References:**
Francois J: Heredity in ophthalmology. St Louis: C.V. Mosby, 1961:242 only.
Waardenberg PJ: Genetics and ophthalmology, vol 2. Springfield: Charles C Thomas, 1963:78 only.

WE035                                    **Avery H. Weiss**

**Ophthalmoplegia-intestinal pseudo-obstruction**
*See MUSCULAR DYSTROPHY, OCULO-GASTROINTESTINAL*
**Ophthalmoplegia-pigmentary degeneration of retina-cardiomyopathy**
*See KEARNS-SAYRE DISEASE*
**Ophthalmoplegia-pigmentary dystrophy of retina-cardiomyopathy**
*See OPHTHALMOPLEGIA, PROGRESSIVE EXTERNAL*
**Ophthalmoplegic migraine**
*See MIGRAINE*
**Opitz G-syndrome**
*See G SYNDROME*
**Opitz oculo-genital-laryngeal syndrome**
*See HYPERTELORISM-HYPOSPADIAS SYNDROME*
**Opitz oculo-genito-laryngeal syndrome**
*See G SYNDROME*
**Opitz trigonocephaly syndrome**
*See C SYNDROME*
**Opitz-Frias syndrome**
*See G SYNDROME*
**Opitz-Kaveggia FG syndrome**
*See FG SYNDROME, OPITZ-KAVEGGIA TYPE*
**Opitz-Pallister-Herrmann syndrome**
*See HERRMANN-PALLISTER-OPITZ SYNDROME*

## OPSISMODYSPLASIA 2240

**Includes:**
Chondrodysplasia secondary to chondroosseous transformation defect
Skeletal dysplasia, opsismodysplasia

**Excludes:**
**Achondroplasia** (0010)
**Asphyxiating thoracic dysplasia** (0091)
**Spondyloepiphyseal dysplasia congenita** (0897)

**Major Diagnostic Criteria:** Micromelia, very retarded bone maturation, marked shortness of the bones of the hands and feet, concave metaphyses, and thin lamellar vertebral bodies.

**Clinical Findings:** Opsismodysplasia is recognized at birth on the basis of micromelia and facial abnormalities. Hands and feet are notably short and stocky with clubby fingers. Hypotonia is striking. The craniofacial morphology is characterized by frontal bossing, large fontanelles, and short nose, with a flattened root contrasting with the length of the upper lip. The upper part of the auricle deviates outward and the helix pattern is abnormal.

On X-ray, the retardation in ossification is very striking. The height of the vertebral bodies is very much reduced. The iliac bones have a square appearance. The diaphyses of the long bones are short, and the metaphyses are irregular and enlarged. The

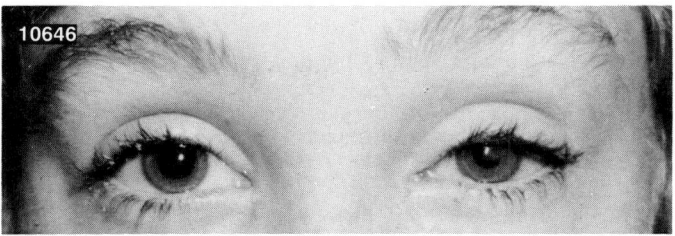

**0753-10646:** Ptosis and miosis OS; acute ulcer of the left cornea produces haziness.

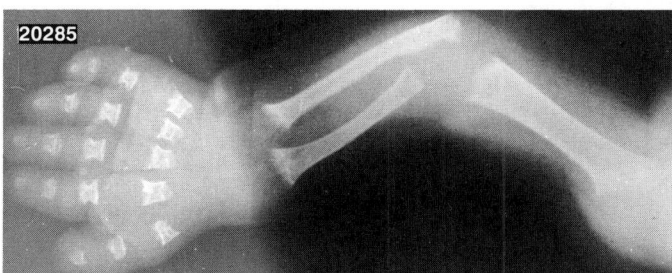

**2240-20285:** Opsismodysplasia, hand and arm X-ray of a 15-month-old male; note short hand bones with cup-shaped deformation of the metaphyses and retarded ossification.

appearance of the hand bones is typical and their extreme shortness is associated with a cup-shaped deformation of the epiphyseal and nonepiphyseal ends of the metaphyses.

**Complications:** Severe dwarfism and a particular susceptibility to respiratory infections. Most patients died in the first three years of life.

**Associated Findings:** None known.

**Etiology:** Autosomal recessive inheritance.

**Pathogenesis:** The most striking abnormality of the growth cartilage is the wide and irregular hypertrophic zone. This provides a strong immunologic reaction for type I collagen, which is shown by gel electrophoresis analysis. It may be that the abnormal calcification and bone induction observed in these patients result because cells secreted predominantly type I collagen instead of type II.

**MIM No.:** 25848

**POS No.:** 3649

**Sex Ratio:** Presumably M1:F1.

**Occurrence:** Less than a dozen cases have been reported.

**Risk of Recurrence for Patient's Sib:**
See Part I, *Mendelian Inheritance.*

**Risk of Recurrence for Patient's Child:**
See Part I, *Mendelian Inheritance.* Few affected individuals survive to reproduce.

**Age of Detectability:** In the newborn period, by X-ray study.

**Gene Mapping and Linkage:** Unknown.

**Prevention:** None known. Genetic counseling indicated.

**Treatment:** Treatment of respiratory infection or distress.

**Prognosis:** Usually fatal during infancy.

**Detection of Carrier:** Unknown.

**References:**
Zonana J, et al.: A unique chondrodysplasia secondary to a defect in chondroosseous transformation. BD:OAS XIII(3D). New York: March of Dimes Birth Defects Foundation, 1973:155–163.
Maroteaux P, et al.: Opsismodysplasia: a new type of chondrodysplasia with predominant involvement of the bones of the hand and the vertebrae. Am J Med Genet 1984; 19:171–182. *

MA034                                    **Pierre Maroteaux**

---

## OPTIC ATROPHY, INFANTILE HEREDOFAMILIAL                    0755

**Includes:**
Atrophy, optic
Behr syndrome (complicated optic atrophy)

**Excludes:**
**Optic atrophy, Kjer type** (3069)
**Optic atrophy, Leber type** (0579)
Optic atrophy of metabolic, degenerative, and demyelinating causes
Optic atrophy of inflammatory and toxic causes
Optic nerve anomalies, congenital

**Major Diagnostic Criteria:** Hereditary optic atrophy may occur with or without associated neurologic or systemic signs. Inheritance pattern and degree of visual impairment vary.

**Clinical Findings:** The recessive type of congenital optic atrophy is extremely rare. Profound visual loss, occurring early in life, causes nystagmus and allows detection during the first year of life. Visual loss is stationary without associated neurologic or systemic signs. Dominant optic atrophy is the most common hereditary form. Visual acuity ranges between 20/30 and 20/200, pallor is often limited to the temporal segment of the nerve, and the color defect is blue-yellow rather than red-green. Visual field defects are central or paracentral and nystagmus is typically absent. Usually presents between 1–8 years of age with no associated neurologic or systemic signs. Mental retardation and

sensorineural hearing loss can occur (see, also, **Optic atrophy, Kjer type**).

Because the normal newborn optic nerve is often pale, fundus examination is suboptimal, and it is difficult to diagnose optic atrophy within the first year of life. Anomalous optic nerve development, ocular albinism, and congenital cone-rod dysfunction, are more common causes of visual loss and nystagmus in this age group and need to be carefully excluded by detailed ocular examination and visual electro-physiologic testing (electroretinogram, visual evoked response).

**Complications:** Visual acuity reduction and loss of visual field. Neurologic and systemic complications vary with the associated conditions.

**Associated Findings:** Hereditary optic atrophy can be associated with a variety of neurologic or systemic signs, including congenital deafness, **Diabetes (insipidus/mellitus)-optic atrophy-deafness** (DIDMOAD), **Ataxia, Friedreich type**, Marie's ataxia, Charcot-Marie-Tooth disease, or various combinations of pyramidal tract signs, mental retardation, urinary incontinence, and pes cavus (Behr syndrome).

**Etiology:** Possibly autosomal recessive inheritance.

**Pathogenesis:** Undetermined. Muscle biopsy material has disclosed extensive collections of "cylindrical spiral structures" like myelin figures or onion-skin lesions.

**MIM No.:** 21000

**Sex Ratio:** Presumably M1:F1

**Occurrence:** Several kinships documented in a literature which extends back to the turn of the century.

**Risk of Recurrence for Patient's Sib:**
See Part I, *Mendelian Inheritance.*

**Risk of Recurrence for Patient's Child:**
See Part I, *Mendelian Inheritance.*

**Age of Detectability:** At birth, or in the first decade of life.

**Gene Mapping and Linkage:** Unknown.

**Prevention:** None known. Genetic counseling indicated.

**Treatment:** Appropriate vision aids

**Prognosis:** Vision is in the range of 20/200.

**Detection of Carrier:** Clinical examination of first degree relatives.

**References:**
Glaser J: Heredofamilial disorders of the optic nerve. In: Goldberg M, ed: Genetic and metabolic eye disease. Boston: Little, Brown, 1974.
Hoyt CS: Autosomal dominant optic atrophy: a spectrum of disability. Ophthalmology 1980; 87:245–251.
Miller, et al.: Clinical neuro-ophthalmology, vol. 1: The hereditary optic neuropathies. Baltimore: Williams & Wilkins, 1982.
Thomas PK, et al.: Behr's syndrome: a family exhibiting pseudodominant inheritance. J Neurol Sc 1984; 64:137–148.

WE035                                    **Avery H. Weiss**

**Optic atrophy, juvenile (infantile), dominant**
*See OPTIC ATROPHY, KJER TYPE*

---

## OPTIC ATROPHY, KJER TYPE                    3069

**Includes:**
Kjer optic atrophy
Optic atrophy, juvenile (infantile), dominant

**Excludes:**
**Deafness-optic nerve atrophy, progressive** (0253)
**Diabetes (insipidus/mellitus)-optic atrophy-deafness** (0550)
**Optic atrophy, infantile heredofamilial** (0755)
**Optic atrophy, Leber type** (0579)

**Major Diagnostic Criteria:** Bilateral visual loss with insidious onset usually appears before ten years of age. Central or cecocentral scotomata are present on visual field testing. Tritan dyschromatopsia or severe generalized dyschromatopsia including blue-yellow axes is typical. Temporal optic disk pallor is evident in every patient. Visual evoked responses may be reduced in amplitude and have a prolonged latency even in the presence of good visual acuity.

**Clinical Findings:** Clinical onset is often undefinable and symptoms can be present as early as age two years; the majority of patients are affected by age twenty years. Visual loss is slowly progressive with visual acuities, even in adulthood, varying widely from 20/25 to less than 20/400. Visual loss is bilateral but may be asymmetric. Both interfamilial and intrafamilial variation in acuity and attendant dyschromatopsia have been reported.

A characteristic central or cecocentral scotoma of variable density is present on visual field testing. Other visual field abnormalities include paracentral scotomas, pericecal enlargement, and depression of isopters in the temporal field, simulating bitemporal hemianopsia, although generally the peripheral field is intact. A tritan color defect is characteristic, at times coexisting with a non-specific red-green dyschromatopsia. Neither the severity or the type of dyschromatopsia necessarily relate directly to either visual acuity or duration of disease. Ophthalmoscopically, temporal optic pallor is evident, with neuroretinal rim defects visible on monochromatic examination, which appear to be characteristic (although not unique) of this disease.

The nasal three-fourths of the optic nerve is either uninvolved, or diffusely pale, but invariably less severely affected than the papillomacular nerve fiber bundle insertion. Pupillary light reflexes may be slightly diminished with reduced visual acuity and paradoxical pupils (constriction to an ''off'' response) have been documented. Electroretinography and dark adaptation studies are normal. Nystagmus is only rarely present, eg, when acuity is extremely poor and early in life. Neurologic examinations are normal.

**Complications:** Reduced visual acuity to levels ranging from 20/25 to less or equal to 20/400. Various color vision defects, always including the tritan axis.

**Associated Findings:** None known.

**Etiology:** Autosomal dominant inheritance with almost complete penetrance but variable expressivity.

**Pathogenesis:** The optic atrophy in this disease appears to be due to a primary degeneration of the ganglion cell layer in the retina with ascending optic atrophy. Histopathology has shown atrophy of the retinal ganglion cell layer and gliosis of the optic nerve. The optic nerves, optic chiasm, and optic tracts show an increased content of collagen tissue and a decreased number of neurofibrils and myelin sheaths. In the lateral geniculate body, extensive loss of ganglion cells has been seen. There are no changes in the calcarine cortex.

**MIM No.:** *16550

**Sex Ratio:** M1:F1

**Occurrence:** Undetermined. Several large kindreds have been reported; some 200 cases examined by Kjer alone.

**Risk of Recurrence for Patient's Sib:**
See Part I, *Mendelian Inheritance.*

**Risk of Recurrence for Patient's Child:**
See Part I, *Mendelian Inheritance.*

**Age of Detectability:** During the first decade of life in severe cases. Some mildly expressed individual may escape detection until adulthood, when a severely affected sibling or offspring mandates complete family screening. No congenital case has been documented.

**Gene Mapping and Linkage:** OPA1 (optic atrophy (autosomal dominant)) is unassigned.

One gene for this disease may be located on chromosome 2 (linkage with Kidd blood group, lod score 2.0 at 0 = 0.18) (Kivlin et al., 1984).

**Prevention:** None known. Genetic counseling indicated.

**Treatment:** Unknown.

**Prognosis:** The overall prognosis is unpredictable with final visual acuity ranging from 20/25 to 20/400. None of the 200 individuals examined by Kjer had vision reduced to hand motions or light perception levels.

**Detection of Carrier:** Prolonged latency of visual evoked responses precedes visual loss and theoretically may be used to detect affected individuals. Careful ophthalmoscopy and standardized color screening is probably more efficient.

**Special Considerations:** The differential diagnosis of Kjer optic atrophy includes other entitites presenting with insidious reduction of visual acuity and central or cecocentral scotomas, such as nutritional amblyopia, toxic optic neuropathy, demyelinating disease, mistaken oversight of hereditary macular dystrophies, and other hereditary optic atrophies. The separation of Kjer optic atrophy from other hereditary atrophies should be based on detailed family history, careful examination of family members, clinical presentation and course, color-vision testing, and absence of neurosensory hearing impairment.

**References:**
Kjer P: Infantile optic atrophy with dominant mode of inheritance: a clinical and genetic study of 29 Danish families. Acta Ophthalmol (suppl) 1959; 54:1–146. *
Kline LB, Glaser JS: Dominant optic atrophy: the clinical profile. Arch Ophthalmol 1979; 97:1680–1686. *
Kjer et al.: Histopathology of eye, optic nerve and brain in a case of dominant optic atrophy. Acta Ophthalmol 1983; 61:300–312.
Kivlin JD, et al.: Optic atrophy possibly linked to the Kidd blood group locus. (Abstract) Cytogenet Cell Genet 1984; 37:512 only.

CH042
TR009

**Georgia A. Chrousos**
**Elias I. Traboulsi**

## OPTIC ATROPHY, LEBER TYPE                                    0579

**Includes:**
Leber optic atrophy
Neuroretinopathy, optic Leber type

**Excludes:**
**Optic atrophy, infantile heredofamilial** (0755)
**Retina, amaurosis congenita, Leber type** (0043)

**Major Diagnostic Criteria:** Central visual loss, optic atrophy.

**Clinical Findings:** Sudden loss of central vision occurs in the second and third decades of life. The loss of central vision, which is usually bilateral, progresses rapidly. Elevation of the optic disk and swelling of nerve fiber bundles may be observed. Headaches may accompany the onset of visual loss. Progressive optic atrophy ensues, leaving a flat pale disk. The visual fields show large dense central scotomas.

**Complications:** Unknown.

**Associated Findings:** None known.

**Etiology:** The disorder, with male preponderance, has been considered X-linked recessive, but does not conform to rigid Mendelian rules. There is absence of transmission through males, and passage occurs from the female to most of her offspring.

**Pathogenesis:** Older theories included: an infective agent, especially a slow virus; failure to detoxify cyanide; and opticochiasmatic arachnoidal adhesions. Recently, however, Wallace et al. (1988) discovered a characteristic mitochondrial DNA mutation that encodes a histidine instead of an arginine in a respiratory protein.

**MIM No.:** 30890

**Sex Ratio:** Undetermined; 84.8% of European cases, but only 59.1% of Japanese cases, are male.

**Occurrence:** Undetermined; extensive literature.

**Risk of Recurrence for Patient's Sib:** Maternal transmission.

**Risk of Recurrence for Patient's Child:** Maternal transmission.

**Age of Detectability:** Typically in the late teens to middle 20s, but the range is from 5–65 years.

**Gene Mapping and Linkage:** Unknown.

**Prevention:** None known. Genetic counseling indicated.

**Treatment:** Unconfirmed approaches include the use of hydroxycobalamin, and lysis of opticochiasmatic arachnoidal adhesions. Metabolic therapies that increase cellular respiratory metabolism have been proposed.

**Prognosis:** Progressive visual loss.

**Detection of Carrier:** Neuro-ophthalmologic testing has revealed abnormalities of color discrimination in asymptomatic individuals thought to be at risk by pedigree analysis.

**References:**

Livingstone IR, et al.: Leber's optic neuropathy: clinical and visual evoked response studies in asymptomatic and symptomatic members of a 4-generation family. Br J Ophthalmol 1980; 64:751–757.

Nikoskelainen E, et al.: Ophthalmoscopic findings in Leber's hereditary optic neuropathy. Arch Ophthalmol 1983; 101:1059–1068.

Nikoskelainen E: New aspects of genetic etiology and the clinical puzzle of Leber's disease. Neurology 1984; 34:1482–1484.

Novotny EJ, Jr., et al.: Leber's disease and dystonia: a mitochondrial disease. Neurology 1986; 36:1053–1060.

Nikoskelainen EK, et al.: Leber's hereditary optic neuroretinopathy, a maternally inherited disease: a genealogic study in four pedigrees. Arch Ophthal 1987; 105:665–671.

Wallace DC, et al.: Mitochondrial DNA mutation associated with Leber's hereditary optic neuropathy. Science 1988; 242:1427–1430.

CH034

**Philip F. Chance**
*Morton E. Smith*

**Optic atrophy-deafness, progressive**
*See DEAFNESS-OPTIC NERVE ATROPHY, PROGRESSIVE*
**Optic atrophy-juvenile diabetes-deafness**
*See DIABETES (INSIPIDUS/MELLITUS)-OPTIC ATROPHY-DEAFNESS*
**Optic atrophy-nerve deafness-distal neurogenic amyotrophy**
*See DEAFNESS-POLYNEUROPATHY-OPTIC ATROPHY*

| **OPTIC DISK, MORNING GLORY ANOMALY** | **3158** |
|---|---|

**Includes:**
Handmann disk anomaly
Morning glory disk anomaly

**Excludes:**
Optic disk pits (0756)
Uveoretinal coloboma, typical

**Major Diagnostic Criteria:** An excavated, funnel-shaped but anomalously large optic nerve head with white glial elements at its center, surrounded by a variably pigmented and elevated annulus of subretinal tissues.

**Clinical Findings:** Strabismus, especially exotropia, is the presenting sign in 40–50% of cases, usually in the first two years of life. Poor vision in the affected eye leads to the detection of older patients. Occasionally a white or altered pupillary reflex from the enlarged optic nerve leads to eye examination and diagnosis.

Ophthalmoscopic findings vary with the degree of dysplasia, excavation, central glial proliferation, sheathing of retinal vessels, pigmentation of the surrounding annulus, and neuroretinal dysplasia. Visual acuity ranges from 20/100 to poor light perception, although rarely good visual acuity has been reported.

**Complications:** Poor visual acuity probably results from dysplasia of both the neural retina and the optic nerve. Strabismic amblyopia also contributes. Retinal detachment occurs in one-third of reported cases and is thought to be due to cerebrospinal fluid leakage into the subretinal space via a communication through either an anomalous nerve or its dural sheaths. Results of surgical repair of retinal detachment are poor.

**Associated Findings:** Common ocular findings in the same eye include retinal detachment, strabismus, hyaloid remnants, and **Retinal dysplasia**. Rare findings include **Cataracts**, epiretinal membranes, ciliary body cysts, vitreous cysts, pupillary membrane remnants, microphthalmos (see **Eye, microphthalmia/coloboma**), and rarely **Aniridia**.

Rare associations in the fellow eye are retinal vascular tortuos-

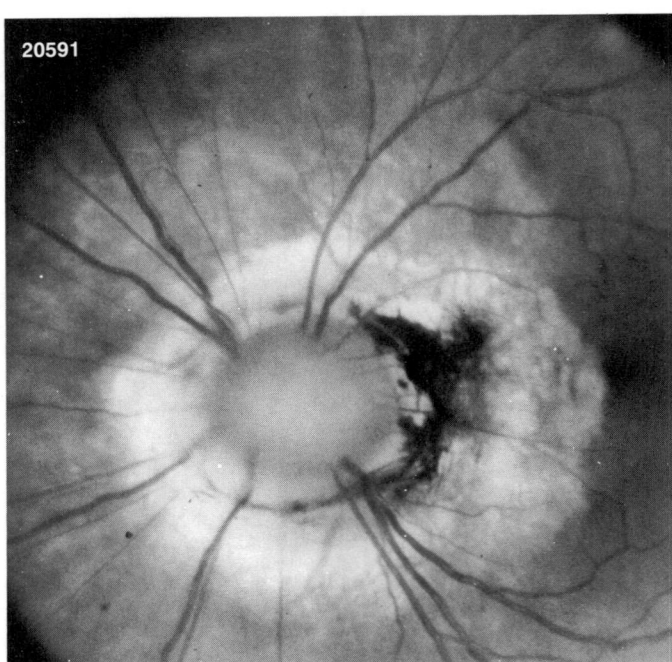

20591

**3158-20591:** Classical "morning glory" configuration of optic nerve head. Note enlarged excavated nerve head, central patch of gliotic tissue and peripapillary pigmented annulus. Retinal vessels, derived from central retinal artery, leave disk at its edge and run a straight course to the periphery of the fundus.

ity, **Optic disk pits**, microphthalmos, **Eye, anterior segment dysgenesis**, **Eye, Duane retraction syndrome**, and persistent pupillary membrane remnants. Various craniofacial anomalies include **Eye, hypertelorism**, basal (and other) **Encephalocele**, **Corpus callosum agenesis**, and **Cleft lip** and/or **Cleft palate** (occasionally occult).

**Etiology:** Unknown.

**Pathogenesis:** Defective formation of posterior sclera and lamina cribrosa with herniation of disk tissue and cone formation. Neuroectodermal layers in the area may be secondarily involved. Hyaloid system may fail to resolve completely resulting in presence of remnants at the center of the disk. The findings of an optic pit in the fellow eye of two unrelated patients in the literature, and the similar mechanism of retinal detachment in both anomalies suggest that these two malformations may share common pathogenetic mechanisms. The association with various midline brain and craniofacial defects suggests an early embryologic defect in fusion.

**CDC No.:** 743.520

**Sex Ratio:** M1:F1. Some authors have suggested a slight female predominance.

**Occurrence:** More than 70 cases have been reported in the literature.

**Risk of Recurrence for Patient's Sib:** Isolated defect; recurrence risk not increased.

**Risk of Recurrence for Patient's Child:** Presumably not increased.

**Age of Detectability:** During infancy or early childhood. Occasionally cases may go undetected until adulthood.

**Gene Mapping and Linkage:** Unknown.

**Prevention:** None known. Genetic counseling indicated.

**Treatment:** Correction of strabismus for cosmesis. Amblyopia therapy is generally unrewarding. Surgical treatment of associated retinal detachment is usually unsatisfactory, however successful reattachment has been reported. Spontaneous reattachment has also occurred.

**Prognosis:** Most reported patients have had poor visual outcomes. This should not preclude all efforts toward amblyopia therapy and retinal reattachment surgery.

**Detection of Carrier:** Unknown.

**Special Considerations:** Consider this diagnosis in infants presenting with total retinal detachment. Midline cranial defects, especially basal encephaloceles should be sought with non-invasive scanning; nasal masses have been biopsied and found to contain brain tissue.

**References:**

Handman M: Erbliche, vermutlich angeborene zentrale gliose Entartunk des Sehnerven mit besonderer Beteilgung der Zentralgefasse. Klin Monatsbl Augenheilkd 1929; 83:145–152.

Kindler P: Morning glory syndrome: unusual congenital optic disk anomaly. Am J Ophthalmol 1970; 69:376–384.

Steinkuller PG: The morning glory disk anomaly: case report and literature review. J Pediatr Ophthalmol Strabismus 1980; 17:81–87.

Koenig SB, et al.: The morning glory syndrome associated with sphenoidal encephalocele. Ophthalmology 1982; 89:1368–1373.

Dempster AG, et al.: The "morning glory syndrome": a mesodermal defect? Ophthalmologica 1983; 187:222–230.

Chang S, et al.: Treatment of total retinal detachment in morning glory syndrome. Am J Ophthalmol 1984; 97:596–600.

Traboulsi EI, O'Neill JF: The spectrum in the morphology of the so-called "morning glory disc anomaly". J Pediatr Ophthalmol Strabism 1988; 25:93–98. †

TR009                                                    **Elias I. Traboulsi**

**Optic disk holes**
*See OPTIC DISK PITS*

---

## OPTIC DISK PITS                                          0756

**Includes:**
> Kranenburg syndrome
> Optic disk, crater-like cavities in
> Optic disk holes

**Excludes:**
> Ocular colobomas
> **Optic nerve hypoplasia** (0758)

**Major Diagnostic Criteria:** Sharp-edged pits in the optic disk.

**Clinical Findings:** The pits occur typically as oval depressions in the optic disk. They are usually one-eighth to one disk diameter in size, with sharp edges and of varying depth (approximately 1.5–20 diopters; average 2–7 diopters). They usually occur in the lower temporal quadrant of the disk; the floor may be covered with a soft gray tissue or may be heavily pigmented. The pits are single and unilateral in the majority (95%) of cases, but bilateral pits and multiple pits in the same disk do occur. The pit may have a partial or total overlying membrane, obscuring view of its true dimensions. The arrangement of the retinal vessels is usually not disturbed, but, in some cases, branches of the central retinal vessels or opticociliary veins descend into it and occasionally cilioretinal arteries emerge from it.

Symptoms may be absent, but frequently there is enlargement of the blind spot or sector defects in the visual field. If the maculopapillary bundle is involved, acuity may be diminished and a partial or complete paracentral or central scotoma may be present. In about 30% of these cases, associated fluid accumulation in the macula and serous detachment of the sensory retina is observed. The fluid appears to originate from either the cerebrospinal fluid or vitreous and passes from the nervehead to the macula.

**Complications:** *Developmental:* true colobomas of the optic disk, retina, or choroid; abnormalities of the retinal vasculature; peripapillary subretinal neovascularization.

*Secondary:* serous macular detachment, now believed to be due

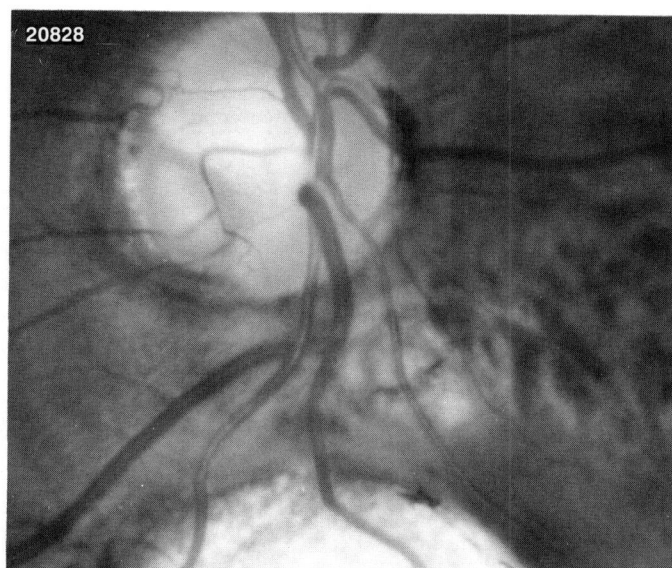

**0756-20828:** Optic disk pit with coloboma of retina and choroid.

to Schisis-like separation of the internal retinal layers and secondary macular detachment after formation of the outer layer macular hole (Lincoff et al, 1988).

**Associated Findings:** None known.

**Etiology:** Unknown.

**Pathogenesis:** A developmental defect of the optic nerve head. During differentiation of the primitive epithelial papilla, the pluripotential neuroepithelial cells of the walls of the optic vesicle may form atypical transparent retinal tissue instead of neuroglial supporting tissue at about the 15-mm stage. Some investigators believe that optic disk pits may represent atypical colobomas secondary to incomplete fusion of the embryonic fissure (the opening along the inferior aspect of the optic cup and optic stalk).

**CDC No.:** 743.520

**Sex Ratio:** M1:F1

**Occurrence:** Undetermined.

**Risk of Recurrence for Patient's Sib:** Unknown.

**Risk of Recurrence for Patient's Child:** Unknown.

**Age of Detectability:** The pit in the optic nerve is present at birth, but the related macular lesion occurs later, usually during the second or third decade of life.

**Gene Mapping and Linkage:** Unknown.

**Prevention:** None known. Genetic counseling indicated.

**Treatment:** The use of photocoagulation to the temporal margin of the optic disk adjacent to the pits remains controversial, but appears to speed resorption of subretinal fluid in some cases. This form of treatment may result in visual field defects and, therefore, is considered only after a significant delay, when there has been ample opportunity for spontaneous resorption.

**Prognosis:** Good, except in cases with secondary degenerative macular lesions, in which central acuity is lost. In a relatively large series of cases, the vision was good in 40% of cases, diminished but useful in 35%, and seriously diminished in 25%. Some investigators believe that photocoagulation can positively alter the long-term prognosis of this disease.

**Detection of Carrier:** Unknown.

**Special Considerations:** An acquired form may exist, and enlargement of pits has been noted; however, these observations are probably secondary to movement, thinning, or loss of an overlying glial veil that previously obscured visualization of the pit.

This condition has been confused with low-tension glaucoma and other causes of optic atrophy, especially when associated visual field defects exist. Careful stereoscopic ophthalmoscopy should allow this differentiation.

There is a rare association between optic pits and other optic nerve anomalies with midline defects, such as basal encephalocele and **Corpus callosum agenesis**. Therefore, it is appropriate to perform computed tomography (CT) or magnetic resonance imaging (MRI) studies, even if midline facial defects (hypertelorism, broad-based flat nose, cleft lip, cleft palate, or cleft face) are not present.

**References:**
Weithe T: Ein Fall von angeborener Difformitat der Sehnervenpapille. Arch Augenheilkd 1882; 11:14–19.
Kranenburg EW: Crater-like holes in the optic disc and central serous retinopathy. Arch Ophthalmol 1960; 64:912.
Sugar HS: Congenital pits in the optic disk. Am J Ophthalmol 1967; 63:298.
Gass JDM: Serous detachment of the macula secondary to pit of the optic nerve head. Am J Ophthalmol 1969; 67:821–841.
Brown GC, et al.: Congenital pits of the optic nerve-head: II: clinical studies in humans. Ophthalmology 1980; 87:51–65.
Alexander TA, Billson FA: Vitrectomy and photocoagulation in the management of serous detachment associated with optic nerve pits. Aust J Ophthalmol 1984; 12:139–142.
Borodic GE, et al.: Peripapillary subretinal neovascularization and serous macular detachment association with congenital optic nerve pits. Arch Ophthalmol 1984; 102:229–231.
Lincoff H, et al.: Retinoschisis associated with optic nerve pits. Arch Ophthalmol 1988; 106:61–67. *

EL007
HA068
WE038

Robert M. Ellsworth
Barrett G. Haik
Robert A. Weiss

**Optic disk, crater-like cavities in**
*See OPTIC DISK PITS*
**Optic disk, crescent, congenital**
*See OPTIC DISK, TILTED*
**Optic disk, dysversion of**
*See OPTIC DISK, TILTED*
**Optic disk, melanocytoma**
*See OPTIC DISK, MELANOCYTOMA*

---

## OPTIC DISK, MELANOCYTOMA                    0639

**Includes:**
    Magnocellular nevus
    Melanocytoma, optic disk
    Melanoma, benign of optic nerve head
    Optic disk, melanocytoma
    Optic disk, pigmentation of, congenital

**Excludes:**
    **Eye, melanosis oculi, congenital** (0640)
    Melanosis oculi, acquired

**Major Diagnostic Criteria:**  Grey, or more often jet-black, discolorations of the optic nerve head, rarely more than 1–2 mm in height.

**Clinical Findings:**  Grey or black tumor of the optic disk usually less than two disk diameters in size with extension into the adjacent retina giving the lesion a feathered margin. More common in Negroes and other heavily pigmented non-Caucasians. Visual acuity is normal, and visual fields usually normal except for enlargement of blind spot. Most tumors remain stationary, but growth can occur, and histologic transformation to melanoma has presented (Zimmerman, 1975). Sometimes melanocytoma may appear in the uveal tract and rarely the conjunctiva or sclera.

**Complications:**  Glaucoma can occur if there is extensive tumor in the posterior pole or when there is diffuse uveal involvement. Visual loss can occur if optic disk tumors cause optic atrophy or

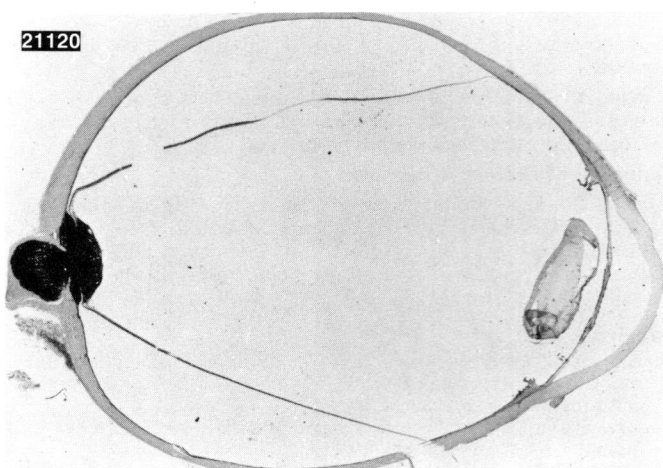

**0639-21120:**  Histopathologic specimen shows whole globe with extensive optic disk melanocytoma.

---

associated choroidal involvement extends into the macula. Although these tumors can be locally invasive, there are no reports of orbital extension or metastases.

**Associated Findings:**  Choroidal nevi, melanocytosis of the meninges, retinal pigment epithelial hypertrophy.

**Etiology:**  Unknown.

**Pathogenesis:**  This lesion is considered to be hamartomatous or progonomatous rather than neoplastic and can probably be regarded as atavistic, comparable with the tumor-like pigment formation in the optic nerve of certain subhuman species.

**CDC No.:**  743.520

**Sex Ratio:**  M1:F>1

**Occurrence:**  Undetermined but presumed rare

**Risk of Recurrence for Patient's Sib:**  Unknown.

**Risk of Recurrence for Patient's Child:**  Unknown.

**Age of Detectability:**  At birth

**Gene Mapping and Linkage:**  Unknown.

**Prevention:**  None known.

**Treatment:**  Unknown.

**Prognosis:**  Excellent; visual impairment is unusual and no threat to life.

**Detection of Carrier:**  Unknown.

**Special Considerations:**  This lesion is a benign pigmented tumor involving the optic disk and needs to be distinguished from choroidal melanoma invading the nerve. Similarly, melanocytomas of uveal tract, sclera and conjunctiva need to be distinguished from malignant melanoma.

**References:**
Zimmerman LE, Garron LK: Melanocytoma of the optic disk. Int Ophthalmol Clinic 1962; 2:431–440.
Zimmerman LE, Spindle A: Melanoma emerging from a melanocytoma of the optic disc. Read before the Verhoeff Society Meeting, Washington, D.C., April 14–15, 1975.
Joffe L, Shields JA: Clinical and follow-up studies of melanocytoma of the optic disc. Ophthalmology 1979; 86:1067–1083.
Lee JS, Smith RE, Minckler DS: Scleral melanocytoma. Ophthalmology 1982; 89:178–182.
Croxatto JO, et al.: Angle closure glaucoma as initial manifestation of melanocytoma of the optic disc. Ophthalmology 1983; 90:830–834.
Frangieh GT, et al.: Melanocytoma of the ciliary body: presentation of

four cases and review of nineteen reports. Surv Ophthalmol 1985; 29:328–334. *

WE035                                                    Avery H. Weiss

**Optic disk, pigmentation of, congenital**
*See OPTIC DISK, MELANOCYTOMA*
**Optic disk, situs inversus of**
*See OPTIC DISK, TILTED*

---

## OPTIC DISK, TILTED                                    0757

**Includes:**
> Conus, congenital
> Fuch coloboma
> Nasal fundus ectasia
> Optic disk, crescent, congenital
> Optic disk, dysversion of
> Optic disk, situs inversus of

**Excludes:**
> Coloboma of optic nerve
> Optic nerve, congenital pit of

**Major Diagnostic Criteria:** Tilted appearance of disk with D-shaped scleral opening; congenital peripapillary crescent (conus); oblique direction of major retinal vessels; myopic astigmatism; inferonasal thinning of the choroid and retinal pigment epithelium; relative superotemporal field depression (or other field defects).

**Clinical Findings:** Normally the excavation in the optic disk is directed toward the lens or is tilted slightly temporally in the direction of the macula. In a "tilted disk," the disk is tilted in another direction, usually nasally or inferiorly. The disk appears abnormally D-shaped, and the central retinal vessels stream out in the direction of the tilt. The condition is bilateral in 80% of cases, and typical crescents appear in the direction of the tilt (nasally, 60%; infero-temporally, 28%; and inferiorly, 12%). Hypopigmentation and decreased nerve fiber density are noted in the inferonasal fundus of most patients. B-scan ultrasonography and histopathology may reveal a local ectasia in this area. An A-scan may demonstrate an increase in the dural diameter of the optic nerve. The condition is often associated with a major refractive error, usually (90%) myopia and astigmatism at an oblique axis. Temporal depression (usually superotemporal) of the visual field is most common; however, altitudinal defects, arcuate scotomas, and bizarre defects have been noted in the visual field. The field defect does not change with time and often slopes across the vertical meridian.

**Complications:** *Developmental:* refractive errors, usually myopic with oblique astigmatism.
*Secondary:* occasionally amblyopia in unilateral cases secondary to anisometropia.

**Associated Findings:** Oxycephaly, corneal opacities, ectopia of the macula, cilioretinal arteries, strabismus, and early open angle glaucoma are rarely associated.

**Etiology:** Unknown.

**Pathogenesis:** Developmental, possibly involving an anomalous insertion of the optic stalk into the optic vesicle, misdirection of retinal ganglion cell fibers, and anomalous closure of the embryonic fissure. Considered by some to be a form of optic nerve hypoplasia; however, none of the midline defects often associated with optic nerve hypoplasia are present. Mechanical compression of the optic nerve fibers or abnormalities in vascularization of the nerve during development may also contribute to the pathogenesis of this condition. Visual field defects may be related to ectasia of the posterior portion of the globe with or without hypoplasia of the optic nerve, retina, and choroid.

**CDC No.:** 743.520

**Sex Ratio:** M1:F1

**Occurrence:** Undetermined.

**Risk of Recurrence for Patient's Sib:** Unknown.

**Risk of Recurrence for Patient's Child:** Unknown.

**Age of Detectability:** At birth.

**Gene Mapping and Linkage:** Unknown.

**Prevention:** None known. Genetic counseling indicated.

**Treatment:** Unknown.

**Prognosis:** Field defects do not progress.

**Detection of Carrier:** Unknown.

**Special Considerations:** The often encountered bitemporal depression on visual field testing seen in this condition must be differentiated from that of a chiasmal lesion. In chiasmal lesions, the field defect tends to respect the midline and end in a sharp edge, which in the early stages does not cross into the nasal field. In contrast, with a tilted disk, rather than a distinct midline step, there is sloping of the temporal defect. In addition, patients with tilted optic disks do not demonstrate red hemianopsia (particularly when tested centrally) as is evident in chiasmal lesions. In some patients with tilted disks, the visual fields improve with refractive correction. The anatomic abnormalities of the tilted disk often are confused with papilledema, and may lead to unnecessary neurodiagnostic studies.

**References:**
Rucker CW: Bitemporal defects in visual fields resulting from developmental anomalies of optic discs. Arch Ophthalmol 1946; 35:546.
Graham M, Wakefield G: Bitemporal visual field defects associated with anomalies of the optic disc. Br J Ophthalmol 1973; 57:307.
Young SE, et al.: The tilted disc syndrome. Am J Ophthalmol 1976; 82:16.
Dorrel D: The tilted disc. Br J Ophthalmol 1978; 62:16.
Brown G, Tasman W: Congenital anomalies of the optic disc. New York: Grune & Stratton, 1983.
Guiffre G: Hypothesis on the pathogenesis of the papillary dysversion syndrome. J Fr Ophthalmol 1985; 8:565–572.
Singh J: Echographic features of tilted optic disc. Ann Ophthalmol 1985; 17:382–383.

EL007                                          Robert M. Ellsworth
HA068                                              Barrett G. Haik
WE038                                            Robert A. Weiss

**Optic glioma, orbital**
*See ORBITAL NERVE GLIOMA*

---

## OPTIC NERVE HYPOPLASIA                                0758

**Includes:**
> Hypoplasia of optic nerve
> Optic nerve, partial absence of
> Quinine, fetal effects of
> Sulfonamides, fetal effects of

**Excludes:** Optic nerve aplasia

**Major Diagnostic Criteria:** Ophthalmoscopic appearance in conjunction with reduced vision.

**Clinical Findings:** Hypoplasia of the optic nerve is not uncommon, and may be unilateral or bilateral in equal frequency. It is more often found with other anomalies than as an isolated entity. The optic nerve appears small, pale, and misshapen. It may have a greyish or brownish-black pigment crescent on the temporal side, a deep physiologic cup, a peripapillary cuff, or may appear mottled throughout. The foveolar reflex may be absent. The retinal vasculature is normal or tortuous. The visual acuity, if diminished in the affected eye, is proportionate to the severity of the hypoplastic disk with or without strabismus on the same side. Visual field defects, and on X-ray, a small optic foramen has been noted on the involved side.

**Complications:** Unknown.

**Associated Findings:** Microphthalmia, nystagmus, partial fourth or sixth nerve palsies, dacryostenosis, cyclopia, anencephaly, hydrocephaly, orbital encephalomeningocele, ptosis, blepharophimosis, hypopituitarism, and agenesis of the septum pellucidum (*DeMorsier syndrome*, see **Kallmann syndrome**); deafness, and anomalies of the urinary and skeletal systems. The majority of patients with unilateral or segmental optic nerve hypoplasia have no accompanying abnormalities.

**Etiology:** A familial tendency has been observed in bilateral cases, suggesting autosomal dominant inheritance. Maternal diabetes causing an adverse intrauterine environment may also be a cause.

**Pathogenesis:** Embryologic defect of differentiation in the ganglion cell layer. Some of the optic nerve fibers fail to develop and reach the disk, but mesoderm has invaginated the optic stalk, and retinal vessels exist. Teratogenic substances, for example drugs such as quinine and possibly sulfonamides, have been implicated if taken during the early weeks of gestation.

**MIM No.:** 16555

**CDC No.:** 743.520

**Sex Ratio:** Presumably M1:Fl

**Occurrence:** Undetermined but presumed rare. More common when found in association with hypopituitarism.

**Risk of Recurrence for Patient's Sib:**
See Part I, *Mendelian Inheritance.*

**Risk of Recurrence for Patient's Child:**
See Part I, *Mendelian Inheritance.*

**Age of Detectability:** In infancy, by ophthalmoscopic examination.

**Gene Mapping and Linkage:** Unknown.

**Prevention:** None known. Genetic counseling indicated.

**Treatment:** Unknown.

**Prognosis:** Visual prognosis dependent upon degree of severity of the hypoplasia and associated anomalies.

**Detection of Carrier:** Clinical examination of first degree relatives.

**References:**
Whinery RD, Blodi FC: Hypoplasia of the optic nerve: a clinical and histopathologic correlation. Trans Am Acad Ophthalmol Otolaryngol 1963; 67:733–738.
Helveston EM: Unilateral hypoplasia of the optic nerve. Arch Ophthalmol 1966; 76:195–196.
Ewald RA: Unilateral hypoplasia of the optic nerve. Am J Ophthalmol 1967; 63:763–767.
Hackenbrauch Y, et al.: Familial bilateral optic nerve hypoplasia. Am J Ophthalmol 1975; 79:314–320.
Patel H, et al.: Optic nerve hypoplasia with hypopituitarism. Am J Dis Child 1975; 129:175–180.
Petersen RA, Walton DS: Optic nerve hypoplasia with good visual acuity and visual field defects. Arch Ophthalmol 1977; 95:254–258.
Lambert SR, et al.: Optic nerve hypoplasia. Surv Ophthalmol 1987; 32:1–9.

RA004                                    **Elsa K. Rahn**

**Optic nerve, partial absence of**
*See OPTIC NERVE HYPOPLASIA*
**Optic-septo dysplasia**
*See SEPTO-OPTIC DYSPLASIA*

---

**OPTICO-COCHLEO-DENTATE DEGENERATION        0759**

**Includes:** Nyssen-van Bogaert syndrome
**Excludes:**
**Deafness-optic nerve atrophy, progressive** (0253)
**Deafness-polyneuropathy-optic atrophy** (0268)
**G(M2)-gangliosidosis**
**Huntington disease** (0478)
**Pelizaeus-Merzbacher syndrome** (0803)
**Major Diagnostic Criteria:** Optic atrophy, sensorineural deafness, and spastic quadriplegia.

**Clinical Findings:** Most reported cases have presented before age one, and all by early childhood. The disorder presents with motor disturbances in early-onset cases; poor head control, decreased lower limb use, inability to sit or stand, flexion contractures of the legs, and kyphoscoliosis are seen. Spastic quadriplegia developed progressively with marked involvement of lower limbs in late-onset cases; ataxic gait, intention tremor with spasticity, and cerebellar myoclonus were present. Tendon stretch reflexes were hyperactive or absent. All patients have a thin, wasted appearance, with disuse atrophy. Progressive blindness caused by optic atrophy is frequent. In two cases, nystagmus was seen before age one year. All developed progressive sensorineural deafness caused by atrophy of the acoustic nerve nucleus, most within the first decade of life. Eight patients never developed speech. Neuropathologic lesions included atrophy and demyelination of the primary optic and cochlear pathways, atrophy of the nerve cells of dorsal and ventral cochlear nuclei, disseminated nerve cell loss of the dentate nucleus, degeneration of the medial lemnisci and, in some cases, of the pyramidal tracts. Nonspecific parenchymal losses (diffuse cortical nerve cell loss producing brain atrophy) and alteration of blood vessels may be seen. It appears that the severity of the disorder, head circumference, level of mental functioning, and degree of neuronal loss correlate with the age of onset.

**Complications:** Microcephaly, speech disturbances, mental retardation.

**Associated Findings:** In late-onset cases, deafness and blindness may cause psychologic isolation, which may give rise to affective disturbances. Intercurrent infections.

**Etiology:** Autosomal recessive inheritance with variability of expressivity. This syndrome represents a nosologic entity, but genetic heterogeneity is possible.

**Pathogenesis:** Unknown.

**MIM No.:** *25870

**Sex Ratio:** M7:F5 (observed).

**Occurrence:** Twelve cases have been recorded; two or more sibs have been involved in each family.

**Risk of Recurrence for Patient's Sib:**
See Part I, *Mendelian Inheritance.*

**Risk of Recurrence for Patient's Child:**
See Part I, *Mendelian Inheritance.*

**Age of Detectability:** Most often in early infancy.

**Gene Mapping and Linkage:** Unknown.

**Prevention:** None known. Genetic counseling indicated.

**Treatment:** Physical therapy, positioning to prevent decubitus ulcers.

**Prognosis:** Progression varies and may be very rapid or slow, 80% of deaths have occurred before puberty. Onset of vision loss usually precedes the onset of hearing loss.

**Detection of Carrier:** Unknown.

**References:**
Müller J, Zeman W: Dégénérescence systématisée optico-cochléo-dentelée. Acta Neuropathol (Berl) 1965; 5:26–39.
Zeman W: Dégénérescence systématisée optico-cochléo-dentelée. Handbook Clin Neurol 1975; 21:535 only.
Konigsmark BW, Gorlin RJ: Genetic and metabolic deafness. Philadelphia: W.B. Saunders, 1976.

MI029                                    **Joyce Mitchell**
                                         *Cor W.R.J. Cremers*

## ORAL DERMOIDS                                    0760

**Includes:**
Cyst, developmental
Cyst, dysontogenetic
Cyst, epidermoid
Cyst, teratoid
Cystic teratoma
Dermoids, oral
Teratoma

**Excludes:**
**Neck, Branchial cleft, cysts or sinuses** (0117)
Cellulitis of the floor of the mouth
Cystic hygroma
Ranula
**Thyroglossal duct remnant** (0945)

**Major Diagnostic Criteria:** An elevation of the floor of the mouth, or a slight fullness in the submental area, usually eliciting the complaint of a "fullness" of the floor of the mouth which interferes with speaking or eating.

**Clinical Findings:** Dermoids present as sublingual masses and are located either above or below the mylohyoid muscle, usually in the midline. They may occasionally be on one side only. When below the mylohyoid muscle, they will present as pendulous, submental masses beneath the mandible.

Oral dermoids generally feel "dough-like," but may feel cystic, depending on the consistency of the contents, which may vary from a cheesy, sebaceous-like substance to a more liquefied material. They may contain hair, nails, and keratin, and may contain pus when secondarily infected.

These lesions vary in weight from 1 gram to several hundred grams, and may vary from a small pea-sized growth to the size of a grapefruit. Fistulous tracts may develop, opening either intraorally into the floor of the mouth, or extraorally into the skin beneath the chin.

Dermoids may undergo malignant degeneration and metastasize to lymph nodes.

A classification of dysontogenetic cysts of the floor of the mouth based upon embryology and histopathology has been presented by Meyer (1955) as follows:

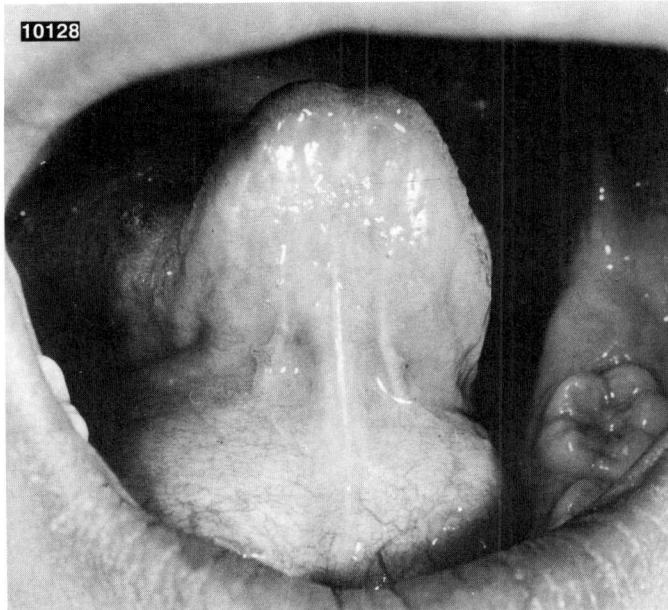

**0760**-10128:   Sublingual oral dermoid.

*Epidermoid*: An epithelial-lined cavity surrounded by a capsule with no skin appendages; this is a simple-type lesion with embryologic ectodermal elements.

*Dermoid*: An epithelial-lined cavity with 1) skin appendages of hair, hair follicles, sebaceous glands, sweat glands, and 2) connective tissue, fat tissue, etc. This is a compound-type of cyst with ectodermal and mesodermal derivatives.

*Teratoid*: An epithelial-lined cavity with the following elements present in the capsule: 1) skin appendages including hair follicles, sebaceous glands, keratin, etc., 2) connective tissue derivatives such as fibers, bone, muscle, blood vessels, etc., and 3) respiratory and GI tissues. This is a complex cyst with derivatives of all three embryonic tissues of ectoderm, mesoderm and endoderm.

The term dermoid cyst is, unfortunately, frequently used as a synonym for benign cystic teratoma. That the same name is applied justifiably to unrelated sequestration cysts makes separation of the two types of lesions difficult.

**Complications:** Interference with speaking, eating or breathing; disfigurement; secondary infection with or without cellulitis; fistulae.

**Associated Findings:** None known.

**Etiology:** Unknown.

**Pathogenesis:** The majority of the oral dermoids are developmental cysts derived from epithelial rests enclaved during the midline closure of the bilateral mandibular (first) and hyoid (second) branchial arches. Some of these dermoid cysts may possibly be formed by remnants of the tuberculum impar of His, which together with the lateral processes from the inner surface of each mandibular arch form the body of the tongue and the floor of the mouth. These developments take place during the third and fourth weeks of embryonic life.

The growth of these cysts may be either gradual or sudden. It is suggested that the development of oral dermoids occurs during the period of increased activity of epithelial tissues, such as sweat glands or hair, which fill the lumen of the cyst. This increased growth activity coincides with the ages of 15–35 years, when most of these lesions become clinically evident.

**Sex Ratio:** M1:F1

**Occurrence:** Over 200 cases reported in the world literature. Of 1,495 dermoid cysts at Mayo Clinic (1910–1935), 103 (6.94%) were in the head and neck and of these only 24, or 0.6%, were in the floor of the mouth. There is no known predilection for race or ethnic group.

**Risk of Recurrence for Patient's Sib:** Unknown.

**Risk of Recurrence for Patient's Child:** Unknown.

**Age of Detectability:** Clinically, from birth on. Most come to clinical attention at age 15–35 years.

**Gene Mapping and Linkage:** Unknown.

**Prevention:** None known. Genetic counseling indicated.

**Treatment:** Either intraoral or extraoral surgical removal, depending on the position of the dermoid in relation to the mylohyoid muscle. Those lying between the mylohyoid muscle and oral mucous membrane (sublingual) are best removed by an intraoral approach, while those lying between the mylohyoid muscle and platysma muscle are approached through an extraoral or skin incision.

**Prognosis:** Excellent, if the tumor is surgically removed in its entirety. If the lesion is incompletely removed, the remaining epithelial cells may proliferate to form a new lesion. Dermoids may undergo malignant degeneration and may even metastasize to lymph nodes, and, therefore, should be completely removed when first diagnosed.

**Detection of Carrier:** Unknown.

**References:**
New GB, Erich JB: Dermoid cysts of the head and neck. Surg Gynecol Obstet 1937; 65:48–55.
Meyer I: Dermoid cysts (dermoids) of the floor of the mouth. Oral Surg 1955; 8:1149–1164.

Howell CJ: The sublingual dermoid cyst: report of five cases and a review of the literature. Oral Surg Med Oral Pathol 1985; 59:578–580.

ME028                                                    Irving Meyer

**Oral-facial-digital syndrome**
  *See ORO-FACIO-DIGITAL SYNDROME I*
**Oral-facial-digital syndrome II**
  *See ORO-FACIO-DIGITAL SYNDROME, MOHR TYPE*
**Oral-facial-digital syndrome IV**
  *See ORO-FACIO-DIGITAL SYNDROME, BARAITSER-BURN TYPE*
**Oral-facial-digital syndrome V**
  *See ORO-FACIO-DIGITAL SYNDROME, THURSTON TYPE*

## ORBITAL AND PERIORBITAL DERMOID CYSTS          0761

**Includes:** Dermoid cysts, orbital and periorbital

**Excludes:**
  Corneal dermoid
  **Eye, dermolipoma** (0284)
  Limbal dermoid
  Orbital cyst-microphthalmia, congenital

**Major Diagnostic Criteria:** Periorbital dermoids are diagnosed clinically on the basis of circumscribed subcutaneous tumors located near the orbital rim and present since birth. Orbital dermoids present as expanding masses within the orbit that displace the globe. CT scan shows their cystic nature. Histopathological examination shows an encapsulated tumor with stratified squamous epithelium and skin appendages in its wall and desquamated keratin and hair shafts within its lumen.

**Clinical Findings:** Although congenital, periorbital dermoids become clinically apparent as they enlarge between one and three years of age. They appear as firm circumscribed masses, ranging from 0.5 to 1.5cm, located usually along the superotemporal rim of the orbit and less frequently along the nasal rim. In general, they are attached to the underlying bone but not the overlying skin. Skull X-rays show a concave depression of bone underlying the tumor. Orbital dermoids are less frequent and often go undetected until adulthood. As they enlarge, dermoids displace the globe or restrict its movement. Orbital CT scan is necessary to delineate its size, and position. The cystic appearance of dermoids on CT scan helps to distinguish it from other orbital tumors.

**Complications:** Spontaneous rupture or incomplete excision of the tumor incites acute and sometimes chronic inflammation in or around the orbit. As dermoids enlarge, they can cause significant displacement of the globe.

**Associated Findings:** None known.

**Etiology:** Sporadic.

**Pathogenesis:** Recent evidence indicates that most of the mesenchymal tissues of the eye and the orbit are derived from neural crest cells. As a consequence of abnormal cellular interactions with the overlying ectoderm, these ectodermal tumors develop beneath the skin.

**Sex Ratio:** Presumably M1:F1.

**Occurrence:** Comprise nearly 40% of orbital tumors of childhood.

**Risk of Recurrence for Patient's Sib:** Probably not increased.

**Risk of Recurrence for Patient's Child:** Probably not increased.

**Age of Detectability:** Although present at birth, periorbital dermoids usually manifest between one and three years of age as they enlarge, while orbital dermoids usually manifest in adulthood.

**Gene Mapping and Linkage:** Unknown.

**Prevention:** None known. Genetic counseling indicated.

**Treatment:** Surgical excision. The tumor should be excised intact to avoid release of cystic contents which leads to inflammation within surrounding tissues. Orbital CT scan is necessary in orbital dermoids, and some periorbital dermoids, to delineate their extent of involvement.

**Prognosis:** Dermoids are benign with no malignant potential.

**Detection of Carrier:** Unknown.

**Special Considerations:** In adults, so called "giant" dermoid cysts can be equal to or greater in size than the globe. Such lesions can be mistaken for lacrimal gland tumors. Excision of these is technically difficult.

**References:**
Duke-Elder S: System of ophthalmology, vol 3, part 2, Congenital deformities. London: Henry Kimptom, 1964:956–963.
Reese AB: Hamartomas, progonomas, choristomas, miscellaneous tumors and tumefactions. In: Reese AB, ed: Tumors of the eye. New York: Harper and Row, 1976:15:416–417.
Iliff WJ, Green WR: Orbital tumors in children. In: Jakobiec FA, ed: Ocular and adnexal tumors. Birmingham: Aesculapius 1978:47:673–675.
Nevares RL, et al.: Ocular dermoids. Plast Reconstr Surg 1989; 82:959–964.

WE035                                              Avery H. Weiss

## ORBITAL AND PERIORBITAL LYMPHANGIOMA          0765

**Includes:**
  Capillary lymphangiomas of orbit
  Cavernous lymphangiomas of orbit
  Cystic lymphangiomas of orbit
  Ocular lymphangioma

**Excludes:**
  Arteriovenous malformations
  Capillary hemangioma, orbital
  Cavernous hemangioma, orbital
  Venous varix of the orbit

**Major Diagnostic Criteria:** The tumor appears as a cystic mass of the eyelid, conjunctiva, or orbit. On histopathological examination, lymphangiomas are comprised of flattened endothelial cells without surrounding smooth muscle or pericytes, which distinguishes them from hemangiomas and venous varices.

**Clinical Findings:** These tumors may occur in the eyelid, conjunctiva, or orbit. Jones (1978) reported the following distributions for location of 61 lymphangiomas: lid, conjunctiva, and face (18%); conjunctiva only (35%); and orbit only (47%). When visible, they appear as a bluish cystic mass. Orbital tumors cause progressive proptosis that increases with an upper respiratory infection or Valsalva maneuver. Spontaneous hemorrhage into a lymphangioma, so-called "chocolate cyst", may cause subconjunctival hemorrhage or increasing proptosis. Orbital echography shows multiple irregular echos intermixed with cystic spaces. Orbital CT scan shows nonenhancing diffusely infiltrating mass with expansion of the orbit in some cases.

**Complications:** Expansion of orbital lymphangioma may displace the globe, restrict ocular motility, and cause optic atrophy.
  Acute hemorrhage into such tumors can be an emergency if vascular perfusion to the optic nerve or retina is compromised. Cellulitis within a facial lymphangioma can spread to the orbit.

**Associated Findings:** Occasionally associated with similar tumors elsewhere: face, oropharynx, and paranasal sinuses.

**Etiology:** Unknown.

**Pathogenesis:** Since the orbit, unlike the eyelid and conjunctiva, does not normally contain lymphatic tissue, the origin of lymphangiomas is not established. Lymphangiomas may arise from primordial cells destined to become endothelial cells that remain isolated and fail to interconnect with arteries or veins.

**Sex Ratio:** M1:F1

**Occurrence:** Lymphangiomas were found in 2.8% of 358 children with orbital tumors.

**Risk of Recurrence for Patient's Sib:** Unknown.

**Risk of Recurrence for Patient's Child:** Unknown.

**Age of Detectability:** Lymphangiomas of the eyelid and conjunctiva can present at any time in the child or adult.

**Gene Mapping and Linkage:** Unknown.

**Prevention:** None known. Genetic counseling indicated.

**Treatment:** Surgical excision of symptomatic tumors is treatment of choice. As they diffusely infiltrate surrounding tissues, excision from the eyelid and orbit are seldom complete. There is no proven role for radiation therapy or use of sclerosing agents.

**Prognosis:** In the absence of complications, there is no impairment of visual function.

**Detection of Carrier:** Unknown.

**References:**

Jones IS, Desjardins L: Management of orbital neurofibromatosis and lymphangiomas. In: Jakobiec FA, ed: Ocular and adnexal tumors. Birmingham: Aesculapius, 1978:50:735–740.

Iliff WJ, et al.: Orbital lymphangiomas. Ophthalmology 1979; 86:914–929.

Jakobiec FA, Jones IS: Vascular tumors, malformations and degenerations. In: Duane TD, ed: Clinical ophthalmology. Philadelphia: Harper and Row, 1986.

Rootman J, et al.: Orbital-adnexal lymphangiomas: a spectrum of hemodynamically isolated vascular hamartomas. Ophthalmology 1986; 93:1558–1570.

WE035                                                    **Avery H. Weiss**

## ORBITAL CEPHALOCELES                              0762

**Includes:**

    Encephalocele, orbital
    Orbital encephalocele
    Orbital hydrocephalocele
    Orbital meningocele

**Excludes:**

    Basal encephaloceles to nasal or nasopharyngeal
        passageways
    Encephaloceles, nonsphenoidal, nonethmoidal
    Posttraumatic pseudomeningocele

**Major Diagnostic Criteria:** True cephaloceles have specific constituents derived from remnant protrusions of encephalic tissues from within the cranial vault. They may contain meningeal or cerebral tissues or both. There may or may not be any identifiable connecting remnant through the optic foreamen or at fusion lines of facial or orbital bones.

Orbital cephaloceles are one of three types of basal encephalo-

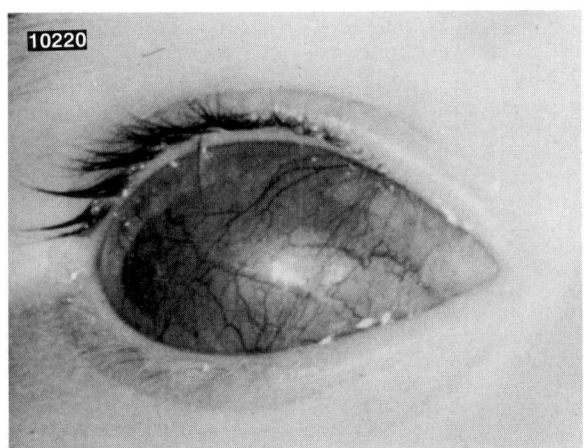

**0762**-10220: Encephalocele in orbit.

celes in which the meninges and brain substance in varied amounts protrude through the sphenoid and sometimes the ethmoid bones: 1) sphenopharyngeal (seen in the nasopharynx), 2) transethmoidal and sphenoethmoidal (seen in the nose), and 3) sphenorbital (seen in the orbit). The literature uses the term *encephalocele* to cover all varieties of tissue components, but the protrusion should be named according to the tissues within. If only meningeal membranes are present, then the term *orbital meningocele* is used; if neural tissue is present, then *orbital encephalocele* is used; and if cerebrospinal fluid is included, it is an *orbital hydrocephalocele*.

**Clinical Findings:** The orbit is distorted, most often by a protrusion of the eye, usually with displacement downward and outward. The mass appears cystic and may be fluctuant or pulsatile. Pressure may produce an oculocardiac reflex. Proptosis is often progressive and may increase transiently upon straining, sneezing, or coughing. Bony defects may show on X-ray or computed tomography (CT) scan. Orbital echography will demonstrate the density and complexity of the lesion.

There are two types by location and site of origin of orbital cephaloceles: 1) an *anterior* group arising from the nasofrontal or anterior part of the orbit, and 2) a less frequent *posterior* group arising from the middle cerebral fossa with protrusion through the optic foramen or the sphenoid bone. Clinically, the differential diagnosis includes other swellings of the orbit, such as specific tumors, pseudotumors, and other anomalies. Pulsatile exophthalmos may result from defects in the bony orbit without encephalocele. The pathological differential diagnosis includes hemangioma and teratoma. Hemangiomas are farily common in brain, meningeal, and cephalic tissues, and their hypervascularity and connective tissue patterns can be confused with cephalocele. Spontaneous regression of hemangioma has been noted, but this is unlikely in cephalocele. Teratoma is less common, perhaps 10–20% as frequent, and is harder to distinguish, in part because some cephaloceles have solid areas and some teratomas are cystic and would be indistinguishable from cephaloceles, were it not for tissues of other germ layers. Nasofrontal glioma is a known entity, possibly different from encephalocele, but since some cases have a transcranial connection (Younun and Coode, 1986) these lesions may well be simply points along a developmental spectrum. The connecting pathway between the orbit and the intracranial space has great potential for complex lesions, including cephalocele. This is shown by a unique case of combined orbital-intracranial teratoma (Garden and McManis, 1986).

**Complications:** Papilledema, compressive optic atrophy, oculomotor palsies, pits, colobomas and other dysplasias of the optic disk, and megalopapilla.

**Associated Findings:** Acrocephaly, microphthalmos, anophthalmia, uveoretinal colobomas, **Optic disk, morning glory anomaly,** and atresia of the lacrimal passages. **Corpus callosum agenesis** is occasionally associated. May be a feature of other complex malformation syndromes.

**Etiology:** Undetermined. Familial and ethnic patterns have been noted.

**Pathogenesis:** Unknown.

**Sex Ratio:** From M5:F7 to M1:F3.

**Occurrence:** Estimated at 1:80,000 to 1:400,000 births.

**Risk of Recurrence for Patient's Sib:** Unknown.

**Risk of Recurrence for Patient's Child:** Unknown.

**Age of Detectability:** Early life; may be present *in utero*, allowing possible detection by prenatal ultrasound.

**Gene Mapping and Linkage:** Unknown.

**Prevention:** None known. Genetic counseling indicated.

**Treatment:** Surgical removal of the tumefaction with effort at salvage of the eye is the only useful treatment, and may require sealing of the deep orbital bony defect(s). Decompression rather than removal has the risk of leaving behind teratomatous tissues with malignant potential (Garden and McManis, 1986).

**Prognosis:** Moderately good in isolated cases; poor when part of multiple malformations of the brain and head. Salvage of functional vision is possible only rarely.

**Detection of Carrier:** Unknown.

**References:**

Cook GR, Knobloch WH: Autosomal recessive vitreoretinopathy and encephaloceles. Am J Ophthalmol 1982; 94:18–25.
Koenig SB, et al.: The morning glory syndrome associated with sphenoidal encephalocele. Ophthalmology 1982; 89:1368–1373.
van Nouhuys E: Autosomal recessive vitreoretinopathy and encephaloceles. Am J Ophthalmol 1982; 94:820.
Ferguson JW, et al.: Ocular, cerebral and cutaneous malformations: confirmation of an association. Clin Genet 1984; 25:464–469.
Shields JA, et al.: Classification and incidence of space-occupying lesions of the orbit. Arch Ophthalmol 1984; 102:1606–1611.
Grossniklaus HE, et al.: Childhood orbital pseudotumor. Ann Ophthalmol 1985; 17:372–377.
Mamalis N, et al.: Congenital orbital teratoma: a review and report of two cases. Surv Ophthalmol 1985; 30:41–46.
Garden JW, McManis J: Congenital orbital-intracranial teratoma with subsequent malignancy: case report. Br J Ophthalmol 1986; 70:111–113.
Younus M, Coode PE: Nasal glioma and encephalocele: two separate entities. J Neurosurg 1986; 64:516–519.

ES003
SH054

John R. Esterly
Douglas R. Shanklin

**Orbital cyst-cerebral and focal dermal malformations**
*See OCULO-CEREBRO-CUTANEOUS SYNDROME*
**Orbital encephalocele**
*See ORBITAL CEPHALOCELES*

## ORBITAL HEMANGIOMA 0764

**Includes:**
Cellular hemangioma of infancy
Hemangioma of eye lids and orbit
Infantile hemangioendothelioma

**Excludes:** Orbital lymphangioma

**Major Diagnostic Criteria:** Hemangioma of the ocular adnexae.

**Clinical Findings:** These are the most common orbital tumors in children. Any portion of the ocular adnexae may be involved. They present as a soft compressible purplish mass often palpable through the lids or conjunctiva and may produce unilateral exophthalmos. There might be an increase in tumor volume or depth of bluish discoloration when the child cries. Around 25% have coexisting nonophthalmic strawberry marks. Visual acuity may be unaltered or the tumor might press on the optic nerve, leading to papilledema and optic atrophy.

**Complications:** Visual defects secondary to papilledema. Occlusion of the eye by the tumor, or induced refractive errors due to its impingement on the eye, can cause amblyopia. Occasionally they cause strabismus by interfering with muscle action. Thrombocytopenia due to entrapment of platelets within the capillary hemangioma can lead to bleeding. The tumor may also ulcerate and become necrosed.

**Associated Findings:** Occasionally there are hemangiomas elsewhere in the body. Typically there are no associated retinal or intraocular malformations.

**Etiology:** Unknown.

**Pathogenesis:** The lesion is considered to be a congenital hamartoma.

**Sex Ratio:** M1:F2

**Occurrence:** In 1% to 2% of newborn children.

**Risk of Recurrence for Patient's Sib:** Unknown.

**Risk of Recurrence for Patient's Child:** Unknown.

**Age of Detectability:** About one-third of lid and orbital hemangiomas are evident at birth, and 95% are recognized by six months of age.

**Gene Mapping and Linkage:** Unknown.

**Prevention:** None known. Genetic counseling indicated.

**Treatment:** The overwhelming majority of these lesions will spontaneously subside within the first few years of life. The mainstay of management is directed primarily toward correction of associated refractive errors, and vigorous treatment of amblyopia if tumor causes eyelid to occlude pupillary axis. If a lesion is so extensive as to threaten vision, a trial of therapy with systemic corticosteroids should be considered. Direct injections of corticosteroids into the lesion have also been effective in provoking involution of the hemangioma. Low doses of radiotherapy might also be beneficial. Surgery is sometimes necessary.

**Prognosis:** Normal for life and intelligence; vision might be decreased due to amblyopia.

**Detection of Carrier:** Unknown.

**Special Considerations:** It is important to distinguish the orbital hemangiomas from the port wine stain or **Nevus flammeus**. This is a flat vascular malformation that represents telangiectasia, not a true angioma. When this lesion occurs on the eyelids it may be part of the **Sturge-Weber syndrome**.

**References:**

de Venecia G, Lobeck CC: Successful treatment of eyelid hemangioma with prednisone. Arch Ophthalmol 1970; 84:98.
Jakobiec FA: Ocular and adnexal tumors. Birmingham: Aesculapius, 1978.
Kushner BJ: Local steroid therapy in adnexal hemangioma. Ann Ophthalmol 1979; 11:1005.
Nicholson DH, Green RW: Pediatric ocular tumors. Masson, 1981.
Crawford JS, Morin JD: The eye in childhood. Grune & Stratton, 1983.

MU026

Michelle Munoz
*Morton E. Smith*

**Orbital hydrocephalocele**
*See ORBITAL CEPHALOCELES*
**Orbital meningocele**
*See ORBITAL CEPHALOCELES*

## ORBITAL NERVE GLIOMA 0763

**Includes:**
Glioma, of optic nerve
Optic glioma, orbital

**Excludes:** Meningioma of the optic nerve

**Major Diagnostic Criteria:** Optic nerve glioma is diagnosed clinically on the basis of visual loss, proptosis, or optic atrophy associated with X-ray evidence of optic nerve tumor. Disk swelling is rarely observed. Histopathologically, optic nerve glioma is a pilocytic astrocytoma of the juvenile type. In most cases, the astrocytomas belong to grade I group due to absence of histologic features indicative of infiltration or spread.

**Clinical Findings:** Tumors of the optic nerve are uncommon. Optic glioma is the most prevalent tumor arising in the optic nerve. Approximately 85% are present in childhood before 15 years of age. Patients present with visual loss, proptosis, and disk atrophy and swelling. With chronic compression, optic atrophy, and rarely optociliary shunt veins may occur. Visual fields show constriction of peripheral field with depression or scotoma of central field. Some tumors are confined to the orbital segment of the nerve but a substantial proportion extend intracranially. Thin-section computed tomography (CT) scan of the orbit, or magnetic resonance imaging (MRI), shows fusiform swelling of the nerve. CT scan or MRI studies of the brain with detailed views of optic canal, chiasm, optic tracts, and surrounding structures are necessary to define intracranial extension. Adults with optic gliomas may present with visual loss that is rapidly progressive and disk swelling with superimposed vascular occlusion. In this group, the tumor is very aggressive and frequently invades the CNS leading to death.

**Complications:** Progressive enlargement of the orbital segment of the nerve causes increasing visual loss, proptosis, restricted ocular motility, and pressure on the posterior aspect of the globe. Primary involvement or extension into the chiasmal region can disturb hypothalamic and pituitary function, raise intracranial pressure, induce seizures, and invade surrounding structures causing variable neurological impairment and even death.

**Associated Findings:** Among all individuals with **Neurofibromatosis**, gliomas of the anterior visual pathways occur in the CT and MRI studies of 15%.

**Etiology:** Usually sporadic, except when associated with **Neurofibromatosis**.

**Pathogenesis:** Unknown.

**Sex Ratio:** M1:F>1

**Occurrence:** In large series of orbital tumors not biased by neurosurgical or pathological referral basis, optic nerve glioma comprises 1.6 to 5.6% of orbital tumors in childhood.

**Risk of Recurrence for Patient's Sib:**
See Part I, *Mendelian Inheritance.*

**Risk of Recurrence for Patient's Child:**
See Part I, *Mendelian Inheritance.*

**Age of Detectability:** Usually by the second decade of life.

**Gene Mapping and Linkage:** Unknown.

**Prevention:** None known. Genetic counseling indicated.

**Treatment:** Treatment is controversial. Some authors view glioma as a benign tumor with self-limited pattern of growth. Surgical excision is recommended only if tumor growth and severe visual loss is documented. Others view optic nerve glioma as a malignant astrocytoma with invasive potential; thus aggressive surgical excision is advised to prevent intracranial extension.

**Prognosis:** Gliomas which remain confined to the optic nerve have a good prognosis whether excised or not. Gliomas which extend into the chiasm or other intracranial structures may respond to chemotherapy or irradiation, but some tumors continue to grow resulting in death. Visual morbidity varies with the severity of optic nerve involvement.

**Detection of Carrier:** Clinical examination of first degree relatives.

**Special Considerations:** The presence of nystagmus strongly suggests chiasmal involvement and less likely optic nerve involvement bilaterally. Numerous reports have noted spasmus nutans, an acquired benign condition, is frequently confused with chiasmal glioma in young children. Since there are no other ocular or CNS abnormalities in spasmus nutans, the distinction is made on clinical grounds or by brain CT or MRI scan.

**References:**
Hoyt W, Baghdassarian S: Optic glioma of childhood: natural history and rationale for conservative treatment. Br J Ophthalmol 1969; 53:793–798.

Hoyt WF, et al.: Malignant optic glioma of adulthood. Brain 1973; 96:121–132.

Yanoff M, et al.: Juvenile pilocytic astrocytoma ("Glioma") of optic nerve: clinicopathologic study of sixty-three cases. In: Jakobiec FA, ed: Ocular and adnexal tumors. Birmingham: Aesculapius 1978:685–707.

Riccardi VM: von Recklinghausen neurofibromatosis. New Engl J Med 1981; 305:1617–1627.

Rush JA, et al.: Optic glioma: long-term follow-up of 85 histopathologically verified cases. Ophthalmology 1982; 89:1213–1219.

Imes RK, Hoyt WF: Childhood chiasmal gliomas: update on the fate of patients in the 1969 San Francisco Study. Br J Ophthalmol 1986; 70:179–182.

Alvord EC, Lofton S: Gliomas of the optic nerve or chiasm: outcome by patient's age, tumor, site and treatment. J Neurosurg 1988; 68:85–98.

WE035                                                     **Avery H. Weiss**

**Orbital teratoma**
*See EYE, ORBITAL TERATOMA, CONGENITAL*

**Orbitopagus parasiticus**
*See EYE, ORBITAL TERATOMA, CONGENITAL*
**'Oregon type' tyrosinosis**
*See TYROSINEMIA II, OREGON TYPE*
**Orengua**
*See ANEMIA, SICKLE CELL*
**Organoid nevus syndrome**
*See PROTEUS SYNDROME*
**Organomercurials (phenyl and alkylmercury), fetal effects**
*See FETAL METHYLMERCURY EFFECTS*
**Ornithine carbamoyl transferase deficiency**
*See ORNITHINE TRANSCARBAMYLASE DEFICIENCY*
**Ornithine ketoacid aminotransferase deficiency**
*See GYRATE ATROPHY OF THE CHOROID AND RETINA*

---

## ORNITHINE TRANSCARBAMYLASE DEFICIENCY          3023

**Includes:**
Hyperammonemia due to ornithine transcarbamylase deficiency
Ornithine carbamoyl transferase deficiency
Valproate sensitivity

**Excludes:**
**Aciduria, argininosuccinic** (0087)
**Argininemia** (0086)
**Carbamoyl phosphate synthetase deficiency** (3022)
**Citrullinemia** (0174)
**Hyperdibasic aminoaciduria** (0491)
**Hyperornithinemia-hyperammonemia-homocitrullinuria** (3169)
Lactic acidosis, congenital
**N-acetylglutamate synthetase deficiency** (3170)
Organic acidemias
Reye syndrome
Transient hyperammonemia of the newborn
Transient hyperammonemia of the newborn

**Major Diagnostic Criteria:** In most hemizygous affected males, coma associated with hyperammonemia (plasma ammonium >500 $\mu$M, normal <50 $\mu$M) occurs in the first three days of life. However, some males have first developed symptoms in later childhood and may have clinical findings similar to symptomatic female heterozygotes. Some ten percent of heterozygous females are symptomatic. In symptomatic heterozygotes, recurrent episodes of ataxia, migraine-like headaches, vomiting, lethargy, and coma with elevated plasma ammonium levels (>100 $\mu$M) and low serum urea nitrogen levels occur. Plasma amino acids show low levels of citrulline (absent or trace levels in the neonatal onset form of the disorder) distinguishing it from citrullinemia and argininosuccinic aciduria, in which citrulline levels are high. Plasma arginine level is low, in contrast to that in argininemia, in which arginine level is elevated. Plasma glutamine and alanine levels are elevated. Urinary orotic acid excretion is high, distinguishing this disorder from carbamyl phosphate synthetase deficiency, in which urinary orotic acid excretion is low. Organic acids and dibasic amino acids are not found in the urine. A definitive diagnosis can be made by measuring activity of ornithine transcarbamylase in liver, duodenal, or rectal tissue. The enzyme is not expressed in fibroblasts or leukocytes.

**Clinical Findings:** Hemizygous males generally present with respiratory distress, poor feeding, hypotonia, progressive lethargy, and coma within the first three days of life. Untreated, there is universal mortality. Approximately one-half survive following treatment with hemodialysis/peritoneal dialysis. Pulmonary and gastrointestinal hemorrhages have been reported. Girls with partial deficiencies have recurrent episodes of vomiting, hyperactivity, lethargy, and coma, occurring from early childhood and often associated with protein loads or intercurrent illnesses.

**Complications:** In children with neonatal-onset hyperammonemic coma lasting longer than 48 hours, there is a high incidence of cortical atrophy associated with mental retardation and other developmental disabilities. Despite treatment, affected children are at risk for future episodes of coma, which may cause further brain damage or death.

**Associated Findings:** Chronic anorexia, food avoidance.

**Etiology:** X-linked dominant inheritance.

**Pathogenesis:** Ornithine transcarbamylase deficiency is caused by a deficiency of the mitochondrial urea cycle enzyme ornithine transcarbamylase. Ornithine transcarbamylase is the second enzyme in the urea cycle. Deficient activity leads to an accumulation of ammonium in blood and brain, especially following a protein load or an intercurrent infection. Ammonia is a neurotoxin. Additionally, there may be alterations in brain energy and neurotransmitter metabolism induced by prolonged hyperammonemic coma that result in brain damage. Alzheimer type II cells have been found in the brain.

**MIM No.:** *31125

**Sex Ratio:** M1:F1 (manifestations vary by sex).

**Occurrence:** About 1:30,000. More than 100 cases have been reported.

**Risk of Recurrence for Patient's Sib:**
See Part I, *Mendelian Inheritance.*

**Risk of Recurrence for Patient's Child:**
See Part I, *Mendelian Inheritance.*

**Age of Detectability:** In the neonatal period for affected males and later in childhood, generally ages 2–4 years, in females. Prenatal detection by RFLP is possible in about 85% of affected families. Prospective treatment is possible for at-risk infants from birth.

**Gene Mapping and Linkage:** OTC (ornithine carbamoyltransferase) has been mapped to Xp21.1.

**Prevention:** None known. Genetic counseling indicated.

**Treatment:** Treatment involves combining protein restriction with the induction of alternate pathways of nitrogen waste excretion. This is accomplished using a protein-restricted diet supplemented with essential amino acids (including citrulline) and providing sodium benzoate and sodium phenylacetate. Liver transplant has been performed in two affected males.

**Prognosis:** The few affected children who have been treated prospectively from birth, because of a previously affected sib, have done better developmentally than those rescued from hyperammonemic coma. The majority of children who have suffered neonatal hyperammonemic coma are mentally retarded. Symptomatic female heterozygotes have a better prognosis, depending on maintaining adequate control of plasma ammonium levels. Life span is uncertain because of the risk of intercurrent hyperammonemic episodes.

**Detection of Carrier:** Carrier detection has been done using protein tolerance tests or allopurinol tests and then measuring urinary excretion of orotic acid or other pyrimidines. RFLP has also been useful in carrier detection of informed families.

**References:**
Hokanson JT, et al.: Carrier detection in ornithine transcarbamylase deficiency. J Pediatr 1978; 93:75–78.
Bachmann C, Colombo JP: Diagnostic value of orotic acid excretion in heritable disorders of the urea cycle and in hyperammonemia due to organic aciduria. Eur J Pediatr 1980; 134:109–113.
Zimmermann A, et al.: Ultrastructural pathology in congenital defects of the urea cycle: ornithine transcarbamylase and carbamyl phosphate synthetase deficiency. Virchows Arch Pathol 1981; 393:321.
Batshaw ML, et al.: Treatment of inborn errors of urea synthesis: activation of alternative pathways of waste nitrogen synthesis and excretion. New Engl J Med 1982; 306:1387–1392. *
Batshaw ML: Hyperammonemia. Curr Prob Pediatr 1984; 16:1–69. *
Msall M, et al.: Neurologic outcome of children with inborn errors of urea synthesis. New Engl J Med 1984; 310:1500–1505. *
Fox J, et al.: Prenatal diagnosis of ornithine transcarbamylase deficiency with use of DNA polymorphisms. New Engl J Med 1986; 315:1205–1208.
Rowe PC, et al.: Natural history of symptomatic partial ornithine transcarbamylase deficiency. New Engl J Med 1986; 314:541–547.
Schwartz M, et al.: Detection and exclusion of carriers of ornithine transcarbamylase deficiency by RFLP analysis. Clin Genet 1986; 29:449–452.
Brusilow SW: Urea cycle disorders and other hereditary hyperammonemic syndromes. In: Scriver CR, et al, eds: The metabolic basis of inherited disease, 6th ed. New York: McGraw-Hill, 1989:629–664. *
Spence JE, et al.: Prenatal diagnosis and heterozygote detection by DNA analysis in ornithine transcarbamylase deficiency. J Pediatr 1989; 114:582–588.

BA066

**Mark L. Batshaw**

**Ornithine-delta-aminotransferase deficiency**
*See GYRATE ATROPHY OF THE CHOROID AND RETINA*
**Ornithinemia with gyrate atrophy of the choroid & retina**
*See GYRATE ATROPHY OF THE CHOROID AND RETINA*

## ORO-CRANIO-DIGITAL SYNDROME 0769

**Includes:**
Cleft lip/palate-abnormal thumbs-microcephaly
Cranio-oro-digital syndrome
Digital-oro-cranio syndrome
Juberg-Hayward syndrome

**Excludes:**
**Acrocephalosyndactyly type III** (0229)
**Oculo-dento-osseous dysplasia** (0737)
**Oro-facio-digital syndrome** (see all)
**Oto-palato-digital syndrome** (see all)

**Major Diagnostic Criteria:** For an isolated case: bilateral or unilateral cleft lip, cleft palate, or occult cleft of the lip; microcephaly; anomaly of the thumbs such as hypoplasia, distal placement, or inflexibility; anomaly of the toes such as mediodorsal curvature or syndactyly. Fewer criteria apparently are needed, once the syndrome is recognized in a sibship.

**Clinical Findings:** Mediodorsal curvature of the fourth toes (4/5); minimal syndactyly of the second and third toes (4/5); growth

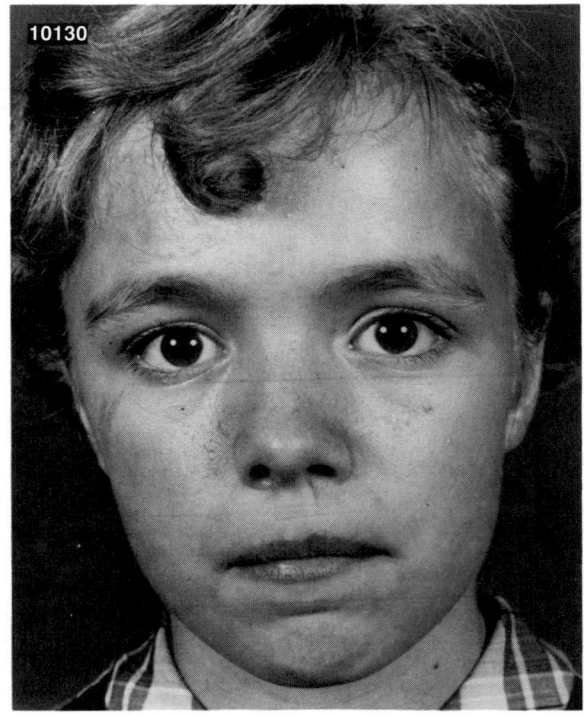

**0769A-**10130: Occult cleft lip, left edge of philtrum, and wide nasal septum.

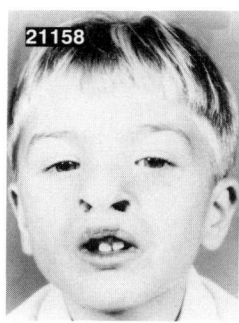
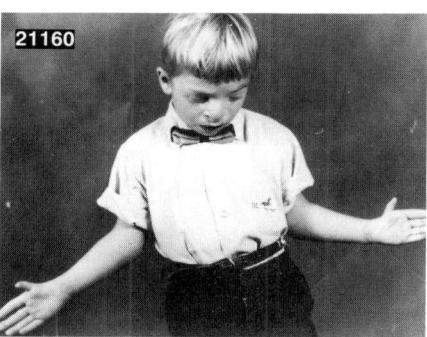
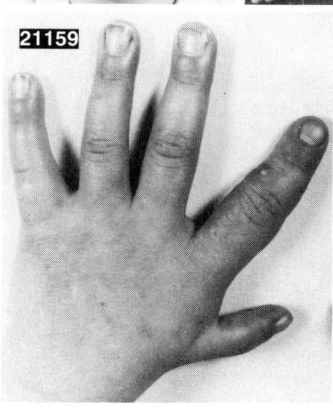
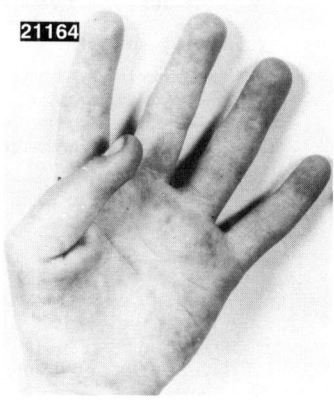

**0769B-21158:** Propositus at age five years; note repaired cleft lip and ptosis. **21160:** Incomplete extension at both elbows. **21159:** Hypoplasia and distal displacement of the thumb. **21164:** Interphalangeal inflexibility of the thumb is bilateral in this affected sib.

retardation (3/5); microcephaly (3/5); hypoplasia and inflexibility of thumbs (3/5); low birthweight (3/5); dislocation and shortening of radii (2/5); cleft lip or palate (2/5); mental retardation (1/5); and occult cleft lip (1/5).

**Complications:** Speech defect will accompany cleft palate defect. Difficulty in upper extremity range of motion occurs with dislocation and shortening of the radii.

**Associated Findings:** Absence of pituitary fossa (reported in one isolated female).

**Etiology:** Possibly autosomal recessive inheritance.

**Pathogenesis:** Unknown.

**MIM No.:** 21610

**POS No.:** 3138

**Sex Ratio:** M2:F3 (observed in one sibship).

**Occurrence:** One sibship of five, and two isolated cases, have been reported.

**Risk of Recurrence for Patient's Sib:**
See Part I, *Mendelian Inheritance.*

**Risk of Recurrence for Patient's Child:**
See Part I, *Mendelian Inheritance.*

**Age of Detectability:** During neonatal period, by clinical examination.

**Gene Mapping and Linkage:** Unknown.

**Prevention:** None known. Genetic counseling indicated.

**Treatment:** Plastic and orthopedic operative procedures, speech correction, physical therapy.

**Prognosis:** Probably normal life expectancy.

**Detection of Carrier:** Undetermined. Parents of the one reported sibship were phenotypically normal.

**References:**
Juberg, RC, Hayward JR: A new familial syndrome of oral, cranial, and digital anomalies. J Pediatr 1969; 74:755–762. * †
Nevin NC, et al.: A case of orocraniodigital (Juberg-Hayward) syndrome. J Med Genet 1981; 18:478–480.
Kingston HM, et al.: Orocraniodigital (Juberg-Hayward) syndrome with growth hormone deficiency. Arch Dis Child 1982; 57:790–792.

JU000 **Richard C. Juberg**

**Oro-digito-facial dysostosis**
*See ORO-FACIO-DIGITAL SYNDROME I*

---

### ORO-FACIO-DIGITAL SYNDROME I 0770

**Includes:**
Gorlin-Psaume syndrome
Oral-facial-digital syndrome
Oro-facio-digital syndrome I (OFD I)
Oro-digito-facial dysostosis
Papillon-Leage syndrome
Psaume syndrome

**Excludes:** Oro-facio-digital syndrome (all others)

**Major Diagnostic Criteria:** Patients are all females (except in the case of **Klinefelter syndrome**) with multiple hyperplastic frenula, multilobulated tongue, broad nasal root, evanescent facial milia, and digital anomalies (brachydactyly, clinodactyly).

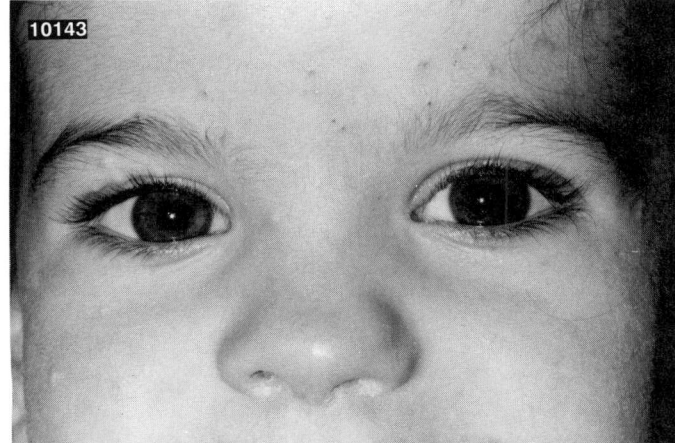
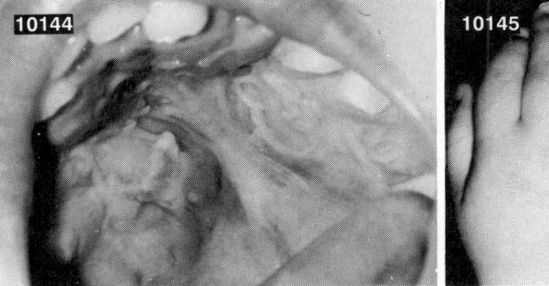
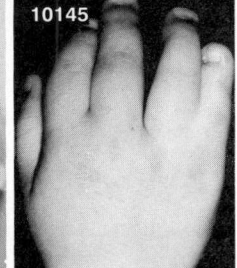

**0770-10143:** Milia, dystopia canthorum and asymmetric alar cartilages. **10144:** Bizarre clefting of the palate. **10145:** Brachydactyly and partial soft-tissue syndactyly of the 4th and 5th digits.

**Clinical Findings:** Hyperplastic frenula (ca. 75%); tongue cleft into two or more lobes (ca. 80%); hamartoma of tongue (40%); cleft palate (35%); median cleft of upper lip (35%); dystopia canthorum (30%); hypoplasia of malar bone (25%); clinodactyly, brachydactyly or syndactyly (60%); duplicated hallux (unilateral) (25%); mental retardation (40%); hypoplastic alar cartilages (35%); alopecia (30%); and evanescent facial milia (35%).

**Complications:** Unknown.

**Associated Findings:** Various cerebral abnormalities (10%); coarse dry hair (15%); polycystic kidney (15%); agenesis of lower lateral incisor teeth (20%); supernumerary teeth (20%); ankyloglossia (10%); grooved anterior alveolar process of mandible (10%); and lateral grooving of maxillary alveolar process (10%).

**Etiology:** X-linked dominant inheritance, lethal in male. Segregation analysis has shown some female lethality in lyonized heterozygotes.

**Pathogenesis:** Unknown.

**MIM No.:** *31120

**POS No.:** 3347

**CDC No.:** 759.800

**Sex Ratio:** M0:F1

**Occurrence:** Possibly 1:50,000 live births. Over 200 cases reported.

**Risk of Recurrence for Patient's Sib:**
See Part I, *Mendelian Inheritance.* If male receives mutant gene from mother, the pregnancy is not completed.

**Risk of Recurrence for Patient's Child:**
See Part I, *Mendelian Inheritance.* Fifty percent if a daughter; zero if a son. Hence there is a M1:F2 ratio in all offspring of affected females. The overall ratio of affected to unaffected offspring of affected mothers is 1:2.

**Age of Detectability:** At birth.

**Gene Mapping and Linkage:** OFD1 (oral-facial-digital syndrome I) is X.

**Prevention:** None known. Genetic counseling indicated.

**Treatment:** Plastic surgery for correctible defects.

**Prognosis:** Normal life span, with average IQ about 70. Functional limitations primarily due to mental retardation.

**Detection of Carrier:** Clinical examination of first degree relatives.

**References:**
Gorlin RJ, Psaume J: Orodigitofacial dysostosis: a new syndrome, a study of 22 cases. J Pediatr 1962; 61:520–530.
Fuhrmann W, et al.: Das oro-facio-digitale Syndrom: zugleich eine Diskussion der Erbgänge mit geschlechtsbegrenztem Letaleffekt. Humangenetik 1966; 2:133–164.
Gorlin RJ: The oral-facial-digital (OFD) syndrome. Cutis 1968; 4:1345–1349.
Melnick M, Shields ED: Orofaciodigital syndrome, type I: a phenotype and genetic analysis. Oral Surg 1975; 40:599–610.
Wood BP, et al.: Cerebral abnormalities in the oral-facial-digital syndrome. Pediatr Radiol 1975; 3:130–136.
Townes PL, et al.: Further heterogeneity of the oral-facial-digital syndrome. Am J Dis Child 1976; 130:548–554.
Towfighi J, et al.: Neuropathology of oro-facial-digital syndrome. Arch Path Lab Med 1985; 109:642–646.
Donnai D, et al.: Familial orofaciodigital syndrome type I presenting as adult polycystic disease. J Med Genet 1987; 24:84–87.

G0038        **Robert J. Gorlin**

**Oro-facio-digital syndrome I (OFD I)**
*See ORO-FACIO-DIGITAL SYNDROME I*
**Oro-facio-digital syndrome II (OFD II)**
*See ORO-FACIO-DIGITAL SYNDROME, MOHR TYPE*
**Oro-facio-digital syndrome III**
*See ORO-FACIO-DIGITAL SYNDROME, SUGARMAN TYPE*
**Oro-facio-digital syndrome IV**
*See ORO-FACIO-DIGITAL SYNDROME, BARAITSER-BURN TYPE*

**Oro-facio-digital syndrome V**
*See ORO-FACIO-DIGITAL SYNDROME, THURSTON TYPE*
**Oro-facio-digital syndrome VI**
*See ORO-PALATAL-DIGITAL SYNDROME, VARADI TYPE*
**Oro-facio-digital syndrome VII**
*See ORO-FACIO-DIGITAL SYNDROME, WHELAN TYPE*

## ORO-FACIO-DIGITAL SYNDROME, BARAITSER-BURN TYPE     2585

**Includes:**
Digital-oro-facio syndrome
Facio-digital-oro syndrome
Oral-facial-digital syndrome IV
Oro-facio-digital syndrome IV

**Excludes:**
Chondroectodermal dysplasia (0156)
Oro-facio-digital syndrome, Mohr type (0771)
Oro-facio-digital syndrome (others)
Short rib-polydactyly syndrome, type II (0883)

**Major Diagnostic Criteria:** The combination of tibial defects with oral, facial, and digital anomalies.

**Clinical Findings:** Facial anomalies include broad nasal root and/or tip, hypertelorism or telecanthus, micrognathia, and low-set ears. Oral anomalies are similar to those reported for other oro-facio-digital syndromes, and include midline cleft lip, cleft or highly arched palate, bifid uvula, oral frenulae, and lingual hamartoma. Absent or supernumerary teeth are occasionally found. Pre- and/or post-axial **Polydactyly** is found in most, but not all cases. **Syndactyly**, clinodactyly, and brachydactyly are sometimes present. However, all cases (and thus the reason for inclusion in this category) have had some degree of tibial dysplasia, ranging from pseudoarthrosis to metaphyseal flaring on X-ray. Short stature, conductive deafness, **Pectus carinatum** or **Pectus excavatum** and clubfoot occasionally occur. Mental retardation can be present, but is not a consistent finding.

**Complications:** Unknown.

**Associated Findings:** None known.

**Etiology:** Possibly autosomal recessive inheritance.

**Pathogenesis:** Unknown.

**MIM No.:** 25886

**POS No.:** 3147

**CDC No.:** 759.800

**Sex Ratio:** M1:F1

**Occurrence:** Undetermined but presumed rare. Many cases were originally described as **Oro-facio-digital syndrome, Mohr type** or a Mohr-Majewski compound (see **Short rib-polydactyly syndrome, type II**). Cases from different parts of the world have been described.

**Risk of Recurrence for Patient's Sib:**
See Part I, *Mendelian Inheritance.*

**Risk of Recurrence for Patient's Child:**
See Part I, *Mendelian Inheritance.*

**Age of Detectability:** At birth, although prenatal ultrasound may detect severe tibial defects.

**Gene Mapping and Linkage:** Unknown.

**Prevention:** None known. Genetic counseling indicated.

**Treatment:** Orthopedic treatment may be indicated.

**Prognosis:** Life span appears unimpaired; mental retardation, when present, can be mild to severe.

**Detection of Carrier:** Unknown.

**Special Considerations:** Further heterogeneity within this category may be possible, in that some individuals have rather severe limb defects and mental retardation, whereas others have short long bones and normal intellect. There appears to be consistency within families regarding the severity of the condition.

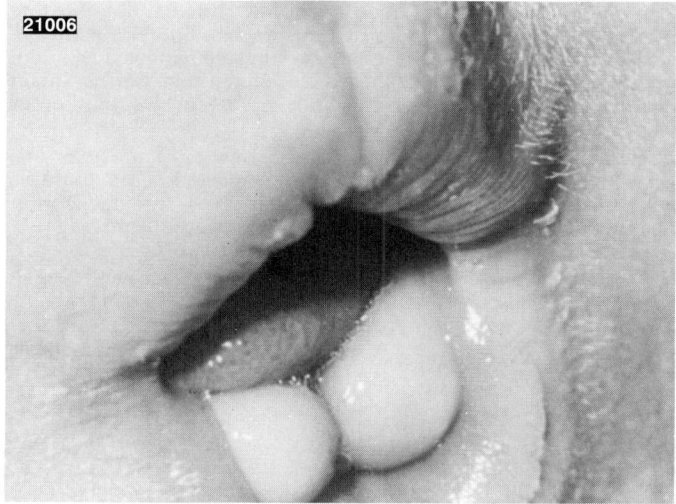

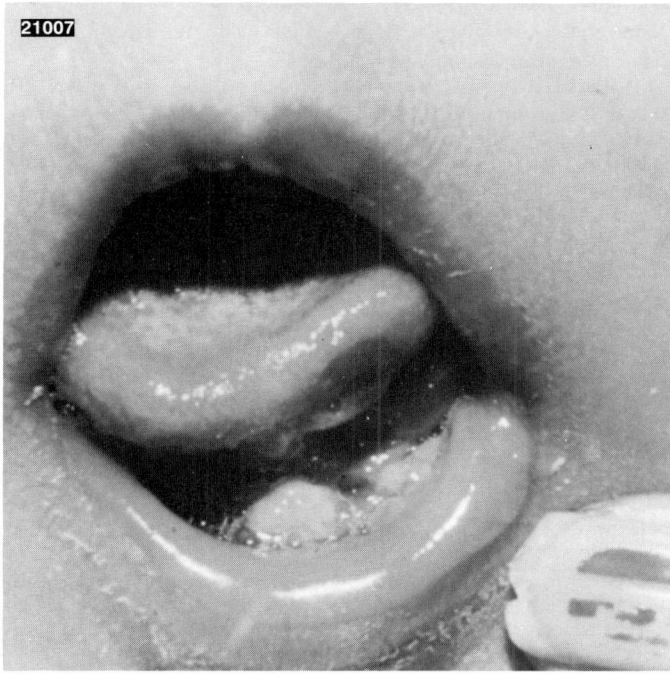

**2585A**-21006–07: Sublingual hamartomas.

**References:**

Baraitser M, et al.: A female infant with features of Mohr and Majewski syndromes: variable expression, a genetic compound, or a distinct entity? J Med Genet 1983; 20:65–67.

Burn J, et al.: Orofacial digital syndrome with mesomelic limb shortening. J Med Genet 1984; 21:189–192. * †

Fenton OM, Watt-Smith SR: The spectrum of the oro-facial digital syndrome. Br J Plast Surg 1985; 38:532–539.

Baraitser M: The orofaciodigital (OFD) syndromes. J Med Genet 1986; 23:116–119.

Nevin NC, Thomas PS: Orofaciodigital syndrome type IV: report of a patient. Am J Med Genet 1989; 32:151–154. †

T0007                                    **Helga V. Toriello**

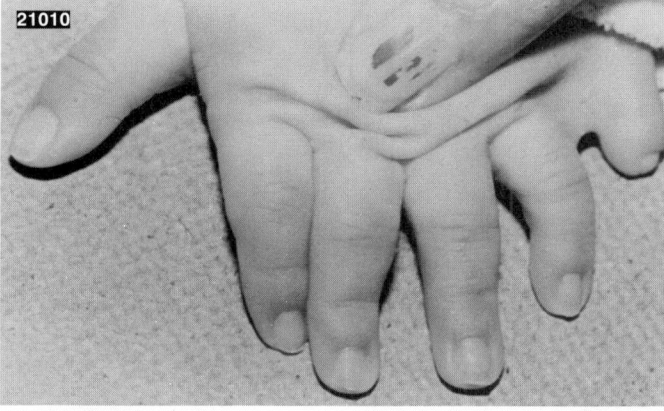

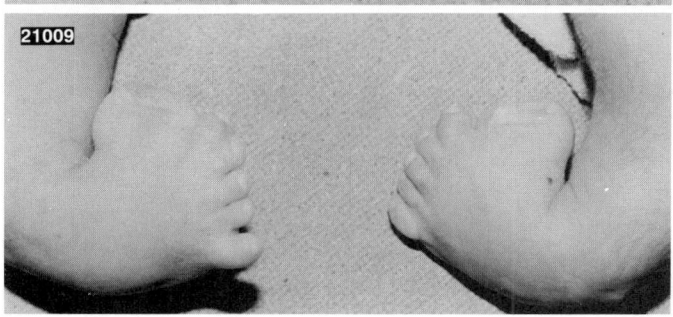

**2585B**-21010: Post-axial polydactyly. 21009: Pre- and post-axial polydactyly.

## ORO-FACIO-DIGITAL SYNDROME, MOHR TYPE          0771

**Includes:**
 Mohr syndrome
 Oral-facial-digital syndrome II
 Oro-facio-digital syndrome II (OFD II)

**Excludes:**
 **Acrocallosal syndrome, Schinzel type** (2263)
 **Asphyxiating thoracic dysplasia** (0091)
 **Chondroectodermal dysplasia** (0156)
 **Oro-facio-digital syndrome** (type I and others)
 **Short rib-polydactyly syndrome, type II** (0883)

**Major Diagnostic Criteria:** Oral manifestations include lingual or sublingual hamartomatous nodules with or without a lobate tongue, hypodontia, hyperplastic frenula, pseudocleft of the upper lip, broad nasal bridge, broad or bifid nasal tip, zygomatic hypoplasia and hypoplasia of the body of the mandible, and polysyndactyly.

**Clinical Findings:** The cleft upper lip may be severe or so mild as to be considered a "pseudocleft." The upper lip may appear to be tethered by the hypertrophied midline frenula. Multiple lateral frenula are present less frequently. A midline cleft of the lower alveolar ridge may also be present and may be severe enough to require bone grafting. Hypodontia involving the central lower incisors is common. Other dental abnormalities may include absence of other teeth, small malformed teeth, and dental malocclusion related to the mandibular defects.

On X-ray, there is hypoplasia of the body of the mandible, and clinically there is often micrognathia. Less frequently there is prognathism because of marked midface hypoplasia. The nasal root and tip are broad, and the tip may be bifid but without a true cleft. True hypertelorism occurs rarely if at all, but dystopia canthorum may be present.

The most characteristic digital abnormality is duplication of the

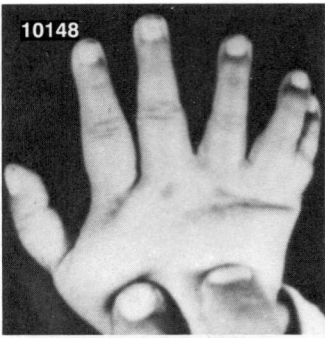
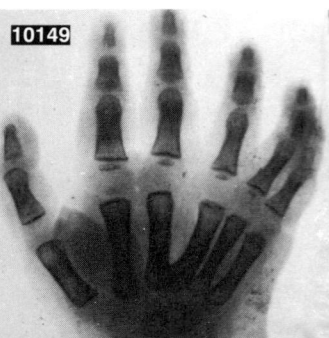
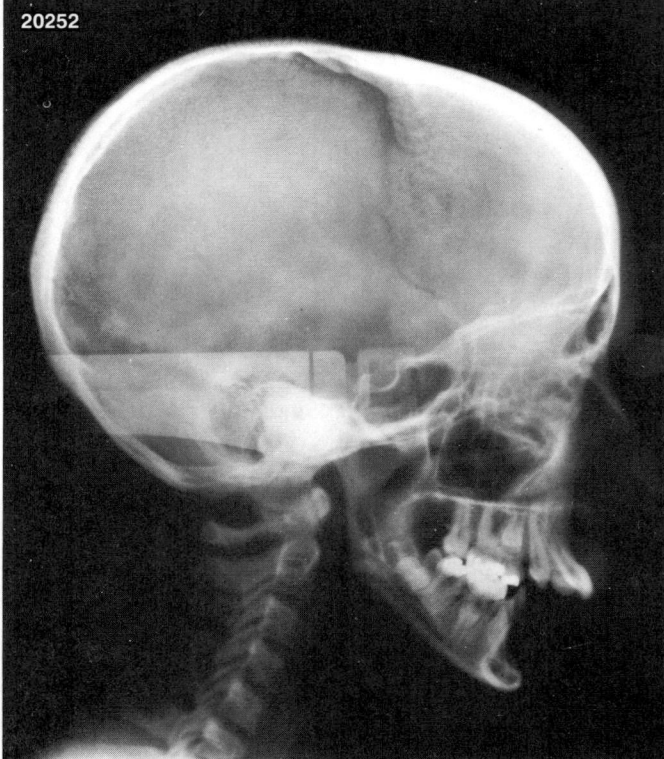

**0771-10148–49:** Postaxial polydactyly. **20252:** Lateral skull X-ray shows hypoplasia of the body of the mandible.

hallux; almost always bilateral. Although usually clinically obvious, hallucal defects may be demonstrated in other cases on X-ray as broad first metatarsals and notching of the distal phalanx. Duplication of the medial cuneiform and navicular bones may be present. Polydactyly and syndactyly of other digits are frequently present; the average number of fingers per hand in one selected series of patients was 5.8 (post-axial polydactyly was more common than pre-axial) and of toes was 6.0 (pre-axial more common than post-axial). Up to seven digits may be present on each hand or foot. Syndactyly may involve the extra digits, fingers 3–4 or 4–5, or toes 2–3 or 1–7. In addition, fifth finger clinodactyly and brachydactyly may be present. Mild short stature and mesomelic shortening of extremities, especially of the tibia, may be present. X-rays may show metaphyseal flaring and irregularity of the tibia. Metaphyseal and sometimes epiphyseal abnormalities of the radius are less frequently observed. Some patients have equinovarus deformities.

Moderately severe conductive hearing loss may be present, and in one case it was related to a malformed incus that did not articulate with the stapes. No patient has had complete hearing loss. Intellect ranges from normal to significant subnormality. In several families, intellect seems to be similar in affected sibs, but severity in general cannot be predicted because stillbirths, infant deaths, and prolonged survival with good outcome may occur within a single sibship.

**Complications:** There is an increased frequency of stillbirths. Infant deaths related to respiratory problems and failure to thrive may occur, but other infants thrive. In survivors, mental subnormality and hearing loss are the major medical problems.

The lobate tongue and hamartomatous nodules infrequently interfere with speech development, but usually do not impair speech, respirations or feeding.

**Associated Findings:** None known.

**Etiology:** Autosomal recessive inheritance.

**Pathogenesis:** Unknown.

**MIM No.:** *25210

**POS No.:** 3348

**CDC No.:** 759.800

**Sex Ratio:** M1:F1

**Occurrence:** About 25 cases have been documented.

**Risk of Recurrence for Patient's Sib:**
See Part I, *Mendelian Inheritance.*

**Risk of Recurrence for Patient's Child:**
See Part I, *Mendelian Inheritance.*

**Age of Detectability:** At birth. Prenatal diagnosis has not been reported, but an affected fetus could potentially be detected by ultrasound on the basis of polydactyly.

**Gene Mapping and Linkage:** Unknown.

**Prevention:** None known. Genetic counseling indicated.

**Treatment:** Surgical correction of cleft lip and palate, polysyndactyly, and, if warranted, lingual abnormalities. Hearing aids are helpful for patients with conductive hearing deficits. Mandibular and dental procedures may alleviate dental malocclusion and improve cosmetic appearance. Clubfoot deformity may respond to casting.

**Prognosis:** An increased frequency of stillbirths and infant deaths. In survivors, outcome is mainly determined by intellectual status.

**Detection of Carrier:** By clinical examination, and X-rays of mandible and feet.

**Special Considerations:** Misdiagnosis may account for some of the clinical heterogenity with regard to presence or absence of structural central nervous system malformations, severe limb defects, and renal abnormalities. Alternatively, these features may represent a more severe clinical spectrum of this condition.

Although many patients with this condition have mild mesomelic shortening of the tibia, some researchers have designated patients with more severe limb defects as having **Oro-facio-digital syndrome, Baraitser-Burn type**. Others maintain that these patients simply have a more severe form of **Oro-facio-digital syndrome, Mohr type**, and also classify patients with tibial pseudoarthroses as having the Mohr type. It has even been suggested that **Short rib-polydactyly syndrome, type II** ("Majewski") represents a severe spectrum of the Mohr type, but it is nevertheless reasonable to maintain for the moment that this uniformly severe and lethal disorder is a distinct clinical entity. Whether or not some of these disorders are allelic is undetermined.

Some consider patients with central nervous system abnormalities such as Dandy-Walker malformation, porencephalic cysts and agenesis of the corpus callosum to have Mohr type OFD. However, some of these patients may have **Joubert syndrome** or some other distinct condition. It is difficult to definitely categorize some of these patients because of overlapping clinical features. Similarly, some patients with renal hypoplasia or aplasia have overlapping features with Mohr OFD, and it is not clear if these patients have a separate disorder.

Finally, some have suggested that **Acrocallosal syndrome, Schin-**

**zel type** is a related genetic entity with an additional loss of the corpus callosum.

**References:**

Mohr O: A hereditary sublethal syndrome in man. Avh Norske Videnskad Oslo 1941; 14:1–18.

Rimoin DL, Edgerton MT: Genetic and clinical heterogeneity in the oral-facial-digital syndromes. J Pediatr 1967; 71:94–102. *

Haumont D, Pelc S: The Mohr syndrome: are there two variants? Clin Genet 1983; 24:41–46.

Anneren G, et al.: Oro-facio-digital syndromes I and II: radiological methods for diagnosis and the clinical variations. Clin Genet 1984; 26:178–182.

Michels VV, et al.: Polysyndactyly in the orofacial digital syndrome, Type II. J Clin Dysmorphol 1985; 3:2–9.

Baraitser M: The orofacial digital (OFD) syndromes. J Med Genet 1986; 23:116–119. *

Silengo MC, et al.: Oro-facial-digital syndrome II: transition type between the Mohr and the Majewski syndromes: report of 2 new cases. Clin Genet 1987; 31:331–336.

MI002                                               **Virginia V. Michels**

## ORO-FACIO-DIGITAL SYNDROME, SUGARMAN TYPE     3058

**Includes:**

    Digital-oro-facio syndrome III
    Facio-oro-digital syndrome III
    Oro-facio-digital syndrome III
    Sugarman syndrome

**Excludes:**

    **Bardet-Biedl syndrome** (2363)
    **Oro-facio-digital syndrome** (other)

**Major Diagnostic Criteria:** The combination of oral, facial, and digital anomalies with see-saw winking or myoclonic jerks affecting the ocular area is necessary to make the diagnosis.

**Clinical Findings:** Phenotypic features include lobed tongue with hamartomas, malocclusion and supernumerary teeth, bifid uvula, postaxial **Polydactyly** of hands and feet, **Pectus excavatum**, short sternum, kyphosis, and mental retardation. One child had see-saw winking of the eyelids, one had blepharospasm, and three had myoclonic jerks of the eyelids and extraocular muscles.

**Complications:** Unknown.

**Associated Findings:** None known.

**Etiology:** Autosomal recessive inheritance.

**Pathogenesis:** Unknown.

**MIM No.:** *25885

**POS No.:** 3098

**Sex Ratio:** M1:F1

**Occurrence:** Five patients in two families have been reported, both from the United States.

**Risk of Recurrence for Patient's Sib:**
    See Part I, *Mendelian Inheritance*.

**Risk of Recurrence for Patient's Child:**
    See Part I, *Mendelian Inheritance*.

**Age of Detectability:** At birth, although prenatal diagnosis using ultrasound may also be useful.

**Gene Mapping and Linkage:** Unknown.

**Prevention:** None known. Genetic counseling indicated.

**Treatment:** Unknown.

**Prognosis:** Mental retardation has been severe in all cases; life span is unknown.

**Detection of Carrier:** Unknown.

**Special Considerations:** Three of the five cited cases of this condition consist of two brothers and a sister observed (unpublished) by Victor McKusick, for whom other diagnoses have been suggested.

**References:**

Sugarman GI, et al.: See-saw winking in a familial oral-facial-digital syndrome. Clin Genet 1971; 2:248–254.

T0007                                           **Helga V. Toriello**

## ORO-FACIO-DIGITAL SYNDROME, THURSTON TYPE     2592

**Includes:**

    Cleft lip-polydactyly
    Oral-facial-digital syndrome V
    Oro-facio-digital syndrome V
    Polydactyly, postaxial-median cleft of upper lip
    Thurston syndrome

**Excludes:**

    **Cleft lip** (0178)
    **Oro-facio-digital syndrome** (others)
    **Polydactyly** (0814)

**Major Diagnostic Criteria:** The combination of median **Cleft lip** and **Polydactyly** without other anomalies confirms the diagnosis.

**Clinical Findings:** The only anomalies consist of median **Cleft lip** and **Polydactyly** of hands and/or feet, which can be unilateral or bilateral. Polydactyly is usually post-axial, and six or seven digits may be present.

**Complications:** Unknown.

**Associated Findings:** None known.

**Etiology:** Possibly autosomal recessive inheritance.

**Pathogenesis:** Unknown.

**MIM No.:** 17430

**POS No.:** 3870

**CDC No.:** 759.800

**Sex Ratio:** M1:F1

**Occurrence:** Undetermined but presumed rare. All cases have been of Indian ethnic origin.

**Risk of Recurrence for Patient's Sib:**
    See Part I, *Mendelian Inheritance*.

**Risk of Recurrence for Patient's Child:**
    See Part I, *Mendelian Inheritance*.

**Age of Detectability:** At birth by the presence of the cleft lip and/or polydactyly.

**Gene Mapping and Linkage:** Unknown.

**Prevention:** None known. Genetic counseling indicated.

**Treatment:** Repair of the cleft lip. Removal of the extra digits for cosmetic reasons may also be considered.

**Prognosis:** Life span and intelligence are normal.

**Detection of Carrier:** Unknown.

**References:**

Thurston EO: A case of median hare-lip associated with other malformations. Lancet 1909; II:996–997.

Chowdhury J: A study of five siblings with median cleft lips and polydactyly. Trans 6th Cong Plast Reconstr Surg Paris, 1975:208–211.

Khoo CT, Saad MN: Median cleft of the upper lip in association with bilateral hexadactyly and accessory toes. Plast Reconstr Surg 1980; 33:407–409.

Gopalakrishna A, Thatte RL: Median cleft lip associated with bimanual hexadactyly and bilateral accessory toes: another case. Br J Plast Surg 1982; 35:354–355. †

T0007                                           **Helga V. Toriello**

## ORO-FACIO-DIGITAL SYNDROME, WHELAN TYPE    2586

**Includes:**
Digital-facio-oro syndrome
Facio-oro-digital syndrome
Oro-facio-digital syndrome VII
Whelan syndrome

**Excludes:**
Oculo-auriculo-vertebral anomaly (0735)
Oro-facio-digital syndrome (other)

**Major Diagnostic Criteria:** Facial asymmetry, unilateral pseudo-cleft lip, and hydronephrosis, in addition to oral anomalies and clinodactyly.

**Clinical Findings:** In a reported mother and daughter; apparent hypertelorism, pseudocleft upper lip, highly arched palate, lobed tongue, and facial asymmetry. The daughter also had unilateral preauricular tags and low-set ears. Both had clinodactyly, but no other digital anomalies, and hydronephrosis.

**Complications:** Renal complications secondary to hydronephrosis.

**Associated Findings:** None known.

**Etiology:** Possibly X-linked or autosomal dominant inheritance.

**Pathogenesis:** Unknown.

**CDC No.:** 759.800

**Sex Ratio:** M0:F2 (observed).

**Occurrence:** Reported in a mother and daughter.

**Risk of Recurrence for Patient's Sib:**
See Part I, *Mendelian Inheritance.*

**Risk of Recurrence for Patient's Child:**
See Part I, *Mendelian Inheritance.*

**Age of Detectability:** At birth.

**Gene Mapping and Linkage:** Unknown.

**Prevention:** None known. Genetic counseling indicated.

**Treatment:** Appropriate treatment for hydronephrosis is indicated.

**Prognosis:** Mental retardation is mild to minimal; life span appears unimpaired.

**Detection of Carrier:** Unknown.

**Special Considerations:** This case was reported as an example of Oro-facio-digital syndrome I; however, the presence of some findings in both mother and daughter, but not in other cases of OFD I syndrome, suggests, albeit tentatively, that this may be a distinct condition.

**References:**
Whelan DT, et al.: The oro-facial-digital syndrome. Clin Genet 1975; 8:205–212.

T0007                                              **Helga V. Toriello**

**Oro-ocular cleft**
*See FACIAL CLEFT, OBLIQUE*

## ORO-PALATAL-DIGITAL SYNDROME, VARADI TYPE    2368

**Includes:**
Digital-oro-palatal syndrome
Joubert syndrome with polydactyly
Oro-facio-digital syndrome VI
Palatal-digital-oro syndrome
Polydactyly-cleft lip/palate/lingual lump-psychomotor
  retardation
Varadi-Papp syndrome

**Excludes:**
Joubert syndrome (2908)
Oro-facio-digital syndrome, Mohr type (0771)
Oro-facio-digital syndrome (others)

**Major Diagnostic Criteria:** Oral, facial, digital (OFD) and cerebellar anomalies.

**Clinical Findings:** Facial features consist of hypertelorism, epicanthal folds, broad nasal tip, **Cleft palate**, and posteriorly rotated, low-set ears. Oral frenulae, lingual nodules, cleft or highly arched palate are the oral findings. Postaxial polydactyly, clinodactyly, and syndactyly affect the hands; on X-ray, a bifid metacarpal has been noted in all cases. The feet can have pre- or postaxial polydactyly. Cerebellar defects range from features of the Dandy-Walker malformation to hypoplasia of the vermis. Severe mental retardation is a constant finding; growth delay, hypotonia, and deafness also occur.

**Complications:** Motor incoordination and speech delay are likely secondary to the cerebellar defects.

**Associated Findings:** Findings reported in one case only include arhinencephaly, **Aortic valve stenosis**, **Aorta, coarctation**, and **Renal agenesis, unilateral**.

**Etiology:** Possibly autosomal recessive inheritance.

**Pathogenesis:** Unknown.

**MIM No.:** 27717

**Sex Ratio:** M1:F1

**Occurrence:** Undetermined but presumed rare. Cases have been reported from different areas of the world.

**Risk of Recurrence for Patient's Sib:**
See Part I, *Mendelian Inheritance.*

**Risk of Recurrence for Patient's Child:**
See Part I, *Mendelian Inheritance.*

**Age of Detectability:** At birth, although prenatal diagnosis by ultrasound may be possible.

**Gene Mapping and Linkage:** Unknown.

**Prevention:** None known. Genetic counseling indicated.

**Treatment:** Supportive.

**Prognosis:** Mental retardation is severe; life span is unknown. Some cases have died in infancy.

**Detection of Carrier:** Unknown.

**References:**
Varadi V, et al.: Syndrome of polydactyly, cleft lip/palate or lingual lump, and psychomotor retardation in endogamic gypsies. J Med Genet 1980; 17:119–122. †
Haumont D, Pelc SC: The Mohr syndrome: are there two variants? Clin Genet 1983; 24:41–46.
Mattei JF, Ayme S: Syndrome of polydactyly, cleft lip, lingual hamartomas, renal hypoplasia, hearing loss, and psychomotor retardation: variant of the Mohr syndrome or a new syndrome? J Med Genet 1983; 20:433–435. * †

T0007                                              **Helga V. Toriello**

**Oromandibular limb hypoplasia**
*See HYPOGLOSSIA-HYPODACTYLIA*
**Oromandibular-limb hypogenesis syndrome**
*See DIPLEGIA, CONGENITAL FACIAL*
**Orotate phosphoribosyltransferase-omp decarboxylase deficiency**
*See ACIDEMIA, OROTIC*
**Orotic acidemia**
*See ACIDEMIA, OROTIC*
**Orotic aciduria**
*See ACIDEMIA, OROTIC*
**Orotidylic decarboxylase deficiency**
*See ACIDEMIA, OROTIC*
**Orotidylic pyrophosphorylase-orotidylic decarboxylase deficiency**
*See ACIDEMIA, OROTIC*
**Orthochromatic leukodystrophy**
*See ADRENOLEUKODYSTROPHY, X-LINKED*
**Osgood-Schlatter disease (tibial tubercle)**
*See JOINTS, OSTEOCHONDRITIS DISSECANS*
**Osler disease**
*See TELANGIECTASIA, OSLER HEMORRHAGIC*
**Osler-Weber-Rendu disease**
*See TELANGIECTASIA, OSLER HEMORRHAGIC*

**Osseous-oculo-dento dysplasia**
*See OCULO-DENTO-OSSEOUS DYSPLASIA*
**Ossicle malformations**
*See EAR, OSSICLE AND MIDDLE EAR MALFORMATIONS*
**Ossicles, malformed and conductive hearing loss**
*See EAR, MICROTIA-ATRESIA*
**Ossifying fibroma of the long bones**
*See OSTEOFIBROUS DYSPLASIA OF TIBIA AND FIBULA*
**Osteitis deformans**
*See BONE, PAGET DISEASE*
**Osteo-onycho dysplasia and oculo-oto-nasal defects**
*See OCULO-OTO-NASAL MALFORMATIONS WITH OSTEO-ONYCHO DYSPLASIA*
**Osteoarthropathy, hypertrophic**
*See PACHYDERMOPERIOSTOSIS*
**Osteochondritis deformans juvenilis**
*See HIP, OSTEONECROSIS, CAPITAL FEMORAL EPIPHYSIS*

## OSTEOCHONDRODYSPLASIA WITH HYPERTRICHOSIS    2332

**Includes:** Hypertrichotic osteochondrodysplasia

**Excludes:**
 Gingival fibromatosis-hypertrichosis (0410)
 Hair, hypertrichosis, lanuginosa (0507)
 Hair, hypertrichosis, X-linked (2314)
 Hypertrichosis, acquired
 Hypertrichosis, other forms of familial localized
 Localized hypertrichosis, sporadic or associated with spina bifida

**Major Diagnostic Criteria:** Excessive generalized hairiness at birth with macrosomy, typical facial appearance, and X-ray findings that include narrow thorax, cardiomegaly, wide ribs, platyspondyly, hypoplastic ischiopubic branches, bilateral coxa valga, "Erlenmeyer flask" long-bone appearance, wide distal phalanx of the first toes, and generalized osteopenia.

**Clinical Findings:** Excessive hairiness occurs practically all over the body, except the palms, soles, and mucous membranes. Coarse facial features; abundant and curly eyelashes; epicanthal folds; flattened, broad nasal bridge; small nose with hypoplastic alae nasi (in younger patients); anteverted nostrils; long philtrum; prominent mouth; short neck; narrow shoulders and thorax; cardiomegaly; some patients with confirmed cardiopathy (**Ductus arteriosus, patent, Aortic valve stenosis**); **Hernia, umbilical**; short hands; clinodactyly of the fifth fingers; and short, wide thumbs and first toes.

Typical X-ray findings: narrow thorax, global cardiomegaly, wide ribs, platyspondyly, irregularities on the articular surfaces of the vertebral bodies (in oldest patients), vertebral bodies with an ovoid shape (in youngest patients), hypoplastic ischiopubic branches, small obturator foramen, bilateral coxa valga, enlarged medullary canal, long bones with an "Erlenmeyer flask" appearance, thick and bright cortical margins, generalized osteopenia, bands of growth arrest, shortness of the distal phalanx of the first fingers, short and wide distal phalanx of the first toe and delayed bone age.

This is a distinct osteochondrodysplasia with congenital hypertrichosis. The physical appearance in some patients during early infancy may erroneously suggest hypothyroidism. The typical abnormal skeletal findings are easily distinguishable from other skeletal dysplasias.

**Complications:** Psychosocial impact from the physical appearance.

**Associated Findings:** Some patients may have dental anomalies and, rarely, gingival hyperplasia. Hepatomegaly of unknown cause was observed in one patient, and mild mental deficiency in another.

**Etiology:** Although no parental consanguinity can be found in any family, the presence of affected males and females from healthy parents and its occurrence in sibs suggest autosomal recessive inheritance.

**Pathogenesis:** Unknown.

**MIM No.:** 23985

**POS No.:** 3941

**CDC No.:** 756.580

**Sex Ratio:** M1:F1

**Occurrence:** Seven cases have been observed from three families.

**Risk of Recurrence for Patient's Sib:**
 See Part I, *Mendelian Inheritance.*

**Risk of Recurrence for Patient's Child:**
 See Part I, *Mendelian Inheritance.*

**Age of Detectability:** At birth.

**Gene Mapping and Linkage:** Unknown.

**Prevention:** None known. Genetic counseling indicated.

**Treatment:** Cosmetic treatment of the hair by depilatory applications, shaving, diathermy, radiation, or bleaching.

**Prognosis:** Normal life span, no functional impairment, and normal intelligence.

**Detection of Carrier:** Unknown.

**References:**
Cantú JM, et al.: A distinct osteochondrodysplasia with hypertrichosis: individualization of a probable autosomal recessive entity. Hum Genet 1982; 60:36–41. * †

CA011
CR023

**José María Cantú**
**Diana García-Cruz**

**Osteochondroma of the distal femoral epiphysis**
*See DYSPLASIA EPIPHYSEALIS HEMIMELICA*
**Osteochondroma, intra-articular of the astragalus**
*See DYSPLASIA EPIPHYSEALIS HEMIMELICA*
**Osteochondromatosis**
*See ENCHONDROMATOSIS*
**Osteodermatopoikilosis**
*See OSTEOPOIKILOSIS*
**Osteodysgenesis, multisynostotic, with fractures**
*See ANTLEY-BIXLER SYNDROME*
**Osteodysplasia enostotica**
*See OSTEOPOIKILOSIS*
**Osteodysplasia with acro-osteolysis, hereditary**
*See HAJDU-CHENEY SYNDROME*
**Osteodysplasia, auricular**
*See AURICULO-OSTEODYSPLASIA*

## OSTEODYSPLASIA, LIPOMEMBRANOUS POLYCYSTIC-DEMENTIA    2227

**Includes:**
 Brain-bone-fat disease
 Dementia (progressive)-lipomembranous polycystic osteodysplasia
 Lipomembranous osteodystrophy
 Membranous lipodystrophy
 Nasu-Hakola disease
 Polycystic lipomembranous osteodysplasia-leukoencephalopathy

**Excludes:**
 Alzheimer disease, familial (2354)
 Fibrous dysplasia, monostotic (0390)
 Fibrous dysplasia, polyostotic (0391)
 Gaucher disease (0406)
 Hallervorden-Spatz disease (2526)
 Wolman disease (1003)

**Major Diagnostic Criteria:** Pain and tenderness in wrists, ankles or knees of a young adult with X-ray evidence of pathologic fractures; with onset in the fourth or fifth decade of dementia, neurologic defects and seizures.

**Clinical Findings:** Infancy and childhood are usually unremarkable but the young adult has onset of pain and tenderness in ankles, wrists or knees with X-ray evidence of pathologic fractures. Bone biopsy shows yellow gelatinous substance with markedly abnormal fat cell histology. Also, in adulthood, there is onset of slowly progressive dementia typically beginning in the fourth or fifth decade. Dementia is often accompanied by frontal lobe signs, confabulation, euphoria, upper motor neuron signs, and there is also adult onset of generalized seizures. CT brain scan shows evidence of cerebral cortical atrophy and calcification in the basal ganglia. Pathologic fractures, progressive dementia and generalized seizures occur in almost every patient. Death occurs in a vegetative state with poorly controlled seizures and aspiration pneumonia, typically in the fifth decade. The EEG may show typical symmetrical, synchronous, episodic 6–8 Hz activity with diffuse slow wave activity.

**Complications:**  Severe dementia; vegetative state.

**Associated Findings:**  Two patients have been described with associated megacolon and paralytic ileus. One patient also had chronic myelogenous leukemia. Senile plaques and neurofibrillary tangles were found in the cortex of a single 48-year-old-man, but have not been found in other patients. Myoclonic twitches have been reported in some cases.

**Etiology:**  Autosomal recessive inheritance, with affected siblings and unaffected parents.

**Pathogenesis:**  No specific metabolic or chemical abnormality has been found. Histologic changes have been noted in fat cells throughout the body, including tissue from the bone cysts and subcutaneous fat. Fat cell membranes are markedly convoluted, and lipid vesicles may accumulate in the extracellular space. The jelly-like material in the bone cysts is PAS positive, suggesting a glycoprotein structure. Arteries, including those in the basal ganglia, have been abnormal with poorly developed tunica media, abnormal elastica exterma, and interna with thickened intima. Arterioles may be completely blocked and calcified. The brain shows generally normal gray matter with atrophy and marked gliosis of subcortical white matter, compatible with a leukodystrophy. One autopsied Japanese case demonstrated a sudanophilic leukodystrophy with an increase in brain free fatty acids and a decrease in unsaturated fatty acids.

**MIM No.:**  *22177

**POS No.:**  4262

**Sex Ratio:**  M1:F1

**Occurrence:**  At least 55 cases from 16 kinships have been reported. Most cases have been reported from Finland, Sweden, and Japan.

**Risk of Recurrence for Patient's Sib:**
See Part I, *Mendelian Inheritance.*

**Risk of Recurrence for Patient's Child:**
See Part I, *Mendelian Inheritance.*

**Age of Detectability:**  No specific test, but earliest abnormality may be bone cysts noted on careful X-ray examination in adolescence or young adulthood.

**Gene Mapping and Linkage:**  Unknown.

**Prevention:**  None known. Genetic counseling indicated.

**Treatment:**  Symptomatic as needed. Seizures should be treated with long-term anticonvulsant therapy.

**Prognosis:**  Poor. Death typically in the fifth decade following a five to 20 year course of increasing pathologic fractures, initially mild psychiatric symptoms progressing to a severe dementia, poorly controlled seizures, and end-stage vegetative neurologic state.

**Detection of Carrier:**  Unknown.

**Special Considerations:**  The slowly progressive presenile dementia can be confused with **Alzheimer disease, familial,** but can be distinguished from Alzheimer's by the presence of polycystic bone disease, calcification of the basal ganglia on CT scan, and sometimes, a history of affected sibs. The cystic bone lesions must be distinguished from the nonspecific and more common X-ray diagnosis of fibrous dysplasia. X-rays of wrists and ankles should probably be obtained in all cases of unexplained presenile dementia. Biopsy of bone cysts in suspicious cases may provide valuable diagnostic information.

**References:**
Hakola HPA: Neuropsychiatric and genetic aspects of a new hereditary disease characterized by progressive dementia and lipomembranous polycystic osteodysplasia. Acta Psychiatry Scand (Suppl) 1972; 232:1–171. *
Hakola HPA, Iivanainen M: A new hereditary disease with progressive dementia and polycystic osteodysplasia: neuroradiological analysis of seven cases. Neuroradiology 1973; 6:162–168.
Nasu T, et al.: A lipid metabolic disease: 'membranous lipodystrophy' an autopsy case demoonstrating peculiar membrane-structures composed of lipid in bone and bone marrow and various adipose tissues. Acta Pathol Jpn 1973; 23:539–558.
Tanaka J: Leukoencephalopathic alteration in membranous lipodystrophy. Acta Neuropathol (Berl) 1980; 50:193–197.
Matsushita M, et al.: Nasu-Hakola's disease (membraneous lipodystrophy). Acta Neuropathol (Berl) 1981; 54:89–93.
Bird TD, et al.: Lipomembranous polycystic osteodysplasia (brain, bone, and fat disease): a genetic cause of presenile dementia. Neurology 1983; 33:81–86. *

BI019

**Thomas D. Bird**

**Osteodysplasias**
*See DWARFISM*
**Osteodysplastic primordial dwarfism, type II**
*See DWARFISM, OSTEODYSPLASTIC PRIMORDIAL, MAJEWSKI-RANKE TYPE*
**Osteodysplastic primordial dwarfism, type IV**
*See DWARFISM, MICROCEPHALIC PRIMORDIAL WITH CATARACTS*
**Osteodysplastic primordial dwarfism, types I and III**
*See DWARFISM, OSTEODYSPLASTIC PRIMORDIAL, MAJEWSKI-WINTER TYPE*

## OSTEODYSPLASTICA GERODERMIA, BAMATTER TYPE     2099

**Includes:**
Bamatter syndrome
Geroderma osteodysplastica hereditaria (GOH)
Gerodermia osteodysplastica
Walt Disney dwarfism

**Excludes:**
**Cockayne syndrome** (0189)
**Cutis laxa** (0233)
**Cutis laxa-growth defect, De Barsy type** (2138)
**Ehlers-Danlos syndrome** (0338)
**Werner syndrome** (0998)

**Major Diagnostic Criteria:**  A combination of lax, wrinkled skin; aged appearance; osteoporosis; and joint laxity.

**Clinical Findings:**  In 17 affected individuals, the findings have included lax, wrinkled skin from birth (17); joint hyperextensibility (17); short stature (8); brachycephaly (7); prominent forehead (10); ptosis of upper eyelids (7); microcornea (3); malar flushing (5); malar flattening (8); down-turned corners of the mouth (7); narrow and/or highly arched palate (13); dental malocclusion (12); mandibular hypoplasia (9); narrow chest (4); kyphosis plus scoliosis (11); winged scapulae (10); **Hernia, inguinal** (4); dislocated hips (14); minor hand anomalies (8); flat feet (14); increased lambdoid wormian bones (6); vertebral compression (14); osteoporosis (16).

The skin shows lack of normal recoil, although there is no abnormality with scar formation, nor is skin fragility or bruisability increased. Laboratory studies which have been done, and found to be normal, include blood and urine metabolic studies, creatinine phosphokinase levels, thyroxine levels, electromyography, nerve conduction studies, EEG, EKG, and chromosome studies. In some patients skin biopsies have been interpreted as normal. However, in others excessive fragmentation of collagen fibers was noted, and in one, elastic fibers were found to be underdeveloped as well. On X-ray, osteoporosis is most marked in the vertebrae. Bone age has been normal.

**Complications:**  Fractures following minimal trauma are common.

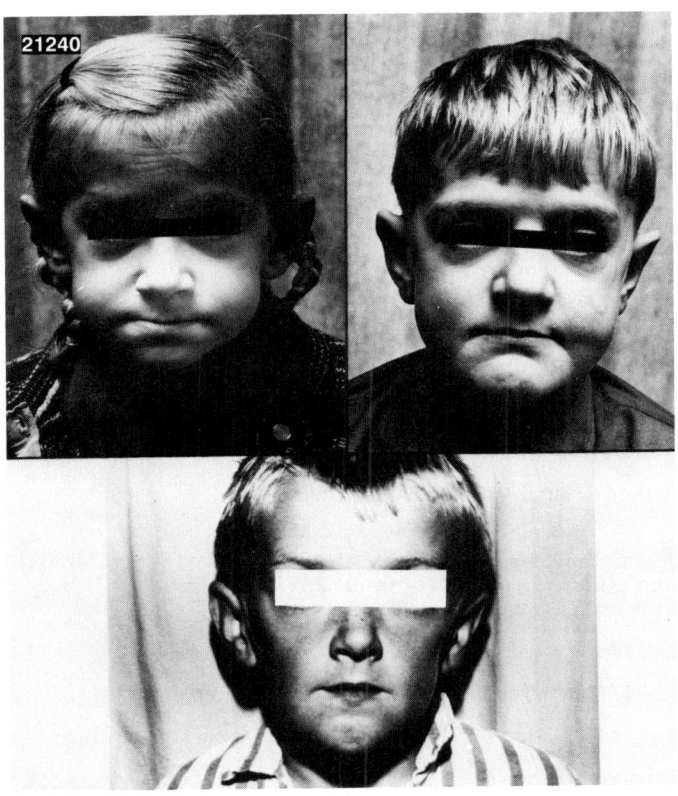

**2099A**-21240: Note prominent forehead, ptosis, malar flush and flattening, downturned corners of the mouth and small chin.

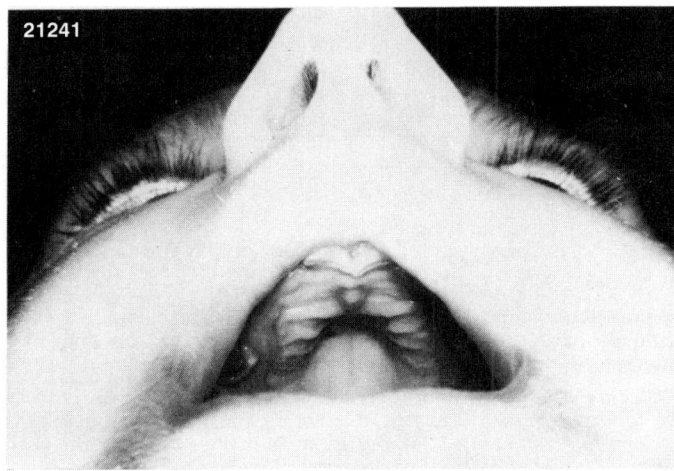

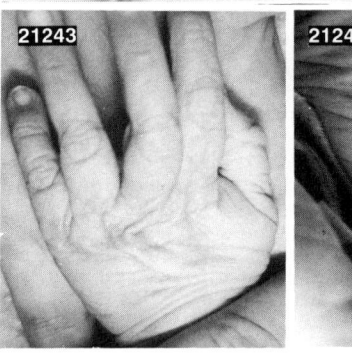

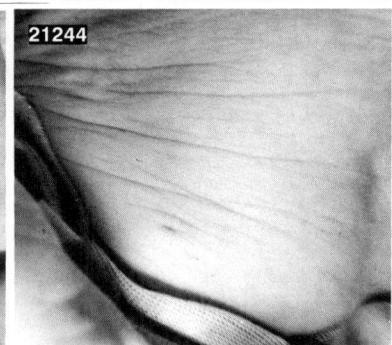

**2099C**-21241: Narrow and highly arched palate. 21243: Lax and wrinkled skin is seen in this child's hand. 21244: Lax and wrinkled abdominal skin.

**Associated Findings:** Reported in only one or two affected individuals were exophthalmos, iris heterochromia, premature arcus senilis, strabismus, **Tongue, geographic**, inverted nipples, cryptorchidism, simian crease, hyperconvex nails, small sella turcica, and absent left pisiform bone.

**Etiology:** Autosomal recessive inheritance.

**Pathogenesis:** Unknown. Both ectodermal and mesodermal derivatives are involved.

**MIM No.:** *23107

**POS No.:** 3243

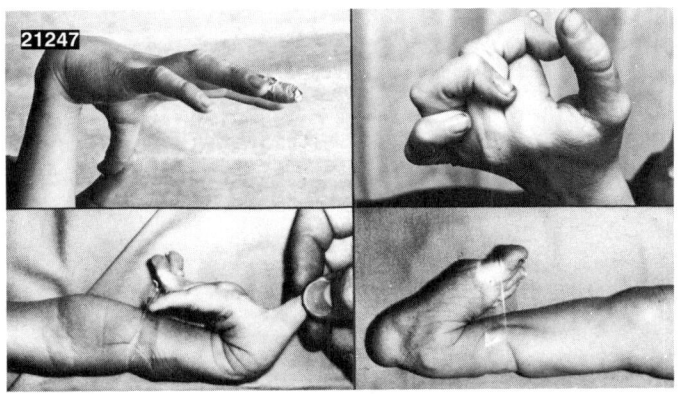

**2099B**-21247: Note joint hyperextensibility.

**Sex Ratio:** M1:F1

**Occurrence:** Reported in four kinships plus isolated cases.

**Risk of Recurrence for Patient's Sib:**
See Part I, *Mendelian Inheritance*.

**Risk of Recurrence for Patient's Child:**
See Part I, *Mendelian Inheritance*.

**Age of Detectability:** At birth, by physical examination.

**Gene Mapping and Linkage:** Unknown.

**Prevention:** None known. Genetic counseling indicated.

**Treatment:** If indicated, treatment for hip dislocation, and prevention of excessive trauma to minimize fracture incidence.

**Prognosis:** Life span appears normal, and intelligence is usually not impaired, although one patient had an IQ of 68.

**Detection of Carrier:** Unknown.

**References:**
Bamatter F, et al.: Gerodermie osteodysplastique hereditaire. Ann Pediatr 1950; 174:126–127
Boreux G: La gerodermie osteodysplastie. J Genet Hum 1969; 17:137–178
Hunter AGW, et al.: Geroderma osteodysplastica: a report of two affeted families. Hum Genet 1978; 40:311–325.
Lisker R, et al.: Geroderma osteodysplastica hereditaria: report of three affected brothers and a literature review. Am J Med Genet 1979; 3:389–395
Suter H, et al.: Geroderma osteodysplastica hereditaria (GOH) in a girl. In: Papadatos CT, Bartsocas CS, eds: Skeletal dysplasias. New York: Alan R. Liss, 1982:327–329.
Hall BD: Geroderma osteodysplastica: a rare autosomal recessive

connective tissue disorder with either variability or heterogeneity or both. Proc Greenwood Genet Center 1983; 2:101–102.

T0007                                        **Helga V. Toriello**

## OSTEODYSPLASTY                                        0775

**Includes:**
Melnick-Needles osteodysplasty
Osteodysplasty, precocious, of Danks-Mayne-Kozlowski

**Excludes:** N/A

**Major Diagnostic Criteria:** Generalized bone dysplasia characterized primarily by cortical irregularity, shortening, bowing, and metaphyseal flaring of the long bones.

**Clinical Findings:** In addition to the unusual cortical irregularity of the long bones, this rare skeletal dysplasia is identified by a ribbon-like appearance of the ribs, an increase in height with anterior concavity of the vertebral bodies, pelvic contracture, sternal abnormalities, delayed closure of the anterior fontanel, sclerosis at the base of the skull, and scoliosis. Facial dysmorphia consisting of exophthalmos, hypertelorism, micrognathia, dental malocclusion, and full cheeks are prominent features. Adults have only mildly reduced stature, normal intelligence, no increase in bone fragility, normal serum chemistries, and a normal life expectancy. At least four cases of affected males born to mothers with osteodysplasty have been reported, but all died in utero or immediately after birth. In addition to micrognathia, exophthalmos, thin calvaria, and severe long bone, rib, and clavicular irregularity and bowing, these males were growth retarded, had hypoplastic thoraces, abdominal wall defects, and abnormalities in their renal collecting systems.

**Complications:** Gait disturbances, osteoarthritis of the hips, predisposition to urinary tract infections, and difficulty in childbirth secondary to contracted pelvis.

**Associated Findings:** Vesico-ureteral reflux, congenital heart disease.

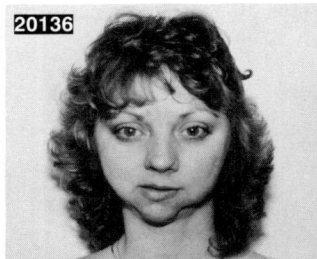
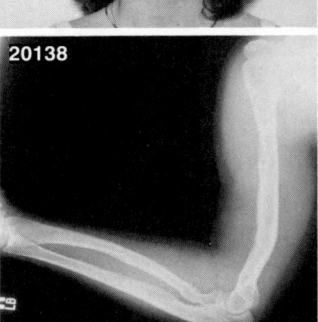
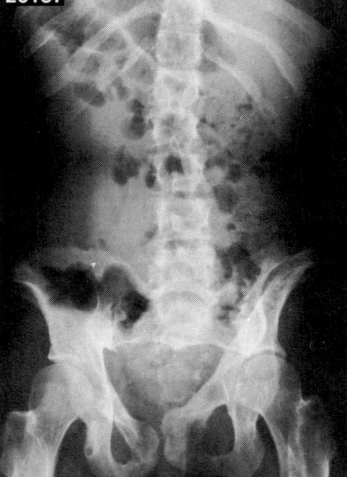

**0775-20136:** Note hypertelorism, micrognathia and full cheeks. **20137:** Ribbon-like ribs, increased height of vertebral bodies and contracted pelvis. **20138:** Unusual cortical irregularity of the long bones.

**Etiology:** Usually X-linked dominant inheritance with lethality in hemizygous males. Autosomal dominant and autosomal recessive (ter Haar et al, 1982) inheritance have also been suggested.

**Pathogenesis:** Unknown.

**MIM No.:** *30935, 24942, 25927

**POS No.:** 3354

**CDC No.:** 756.580

**Sex Ratio:** M0:F1. All viable individuals are female. Males usually die *in-utero* or immediately after birth.

**Occurrence:** Unknown. At least 30 viable individuals have been reported, all female. Four males with malformations incompatible with life have been identified.

**Risk of Recurrence for Patient's Sib:**
See Part I, *Mendelian Inheritance.*

**Risk of Recurrence for Patient's Child:**
See Part I, *Mendelian Inheritance.*

**Age of Detectability:** At birth, by physical and X-ray examination. Affected males have been recognized *in utero* by ultrasound in the early second trimester.

**Gene Mapping and Linkage:** Unknown.

**Prevention:** None known. Genetic counseling indicated.

**Treatment:** Appropriate dental and orthopedic management.

**Prognosis:** Females have normal life span in most cases, and normal intelligence. Affected males have malformations incompatible with life.

**Detection of Carrier:** Unknown.

**Special Considerations:** This condition is very similar to *Osteodysplasty, precocious, of Dank-Mayne-Kozlowski* (1974). Three patients with this condition, two being siblings of Albanian extraction, were reported with a generalized disturbance of modeling of the long and tubular bones and pelvis, with severe hypoplasia of the bones of the fingers and toes. All three died before reaching their first birthday.

**References:**
Melnick JC, Needles CF: An undiagnosed bone dysplasia: a two family study of four generations and three generations. Am J Roentgen 1966; 98:39–48.
Maroteaux P, et al.: L'osteodysplastie (syndrome de Melnick et de Needles). Presse Med 1968; 76:715–718.
Danks DM, et al.: Precocious autosomal recessive type of osteodysplasty. BD:OAS X(12). New York: March of Dimes Birth Defects Foundation, 1974:124–127.
Gorlin RJ, Knier J: X-linked or autosomal dominant lethal in the male inheritance of the Melnick-Needles (osteodysplasty) syndrome? a reappraisal. Am J Med Genet 1982; 13:465–467. *
ter Haar B, et al.: Melnick-Needles syndrome: indication for an autosomal recessive form. Am J Med Genet 1982; 13:469–477.
von Oeyen P, et al.: Omphalocele and multiple severe congenital anomalies associated with osteodysplasty (Melnick-Needles syndrome). Am J Med Genet 1982; 13:453–463.
Donnenfeld AE, et al.: Melnick-Needles syndrome in males: a lethal multiple congenital anomalies syndrome. Am J Med Genet 1987; 27:159–173.

D0025                                        **Alan E. Donnenfeld**
ZA000                                        **Elaine H. Zackai**

**Osteodysplasty, precocious, of Danks-Mayne-Kozlowski**
*See OSTEODYSPLASTY*
**Osteodystrophy-mental retardation**
*See OSTEODYSTROPHY-MENTAL RETARDATION, RUVALCABA TYPE*

## OSTEODYSTROPHY-MENTAL RETARDATION, RUVALCABA TYPE 2076

**Includes:**
 Mental retardation-osteodystrophy, Ruvalcaba type
 Osteodystrophy-mental retardation
 Ruvalcaba syndrome

**Excludes:**
 **Oculo-mandibulo-facial syndrome** (0738)
 **Tricho-rhino-phalangeal syndrome, type I** (0966)
 **Tricho-rhino-phalangeal syndrome, type II** (0967)

**Major Diagnostic Criteria:** The combination of mental retardation, postnatal growth failure, characteristic facies, hypoplastic skin lesions, and skeletal anomalies.

**Clinical Findings:** Prenatal growth is normal, whereas postnatal growth failure occurs. Clinical findings in 11 evaluated individuals include mental retardation (6); short stature (8); delayed adolescence (5); **Microcephaly** (3); down-slanting palpebral fissures (5); narrow, small nose (9); down-turned mouth (5); narrow maxilla (9); low-set ears (1); **Pectus carinatum** (5); narrow trunk (6); scoliosis (6); kyphosis (5); abnormal kidney position (2); **Hernia, inguinal** (2); undescended testes (2); hypoplastic genitalia (5); joint limitation (3); prominent elbows (2); short limbs (6); short hands (9); proximal thumbs (4) clinodactyly (6); small feet (7); small toes (7); enlarged areola (2); and hypoplastic skin lesions (3).

 X-ray findings include spine osteochondritis (4); fusion of scaphoid and lunate (2); short metacarpals (6); short phalanges (4); short metatarsals (6); cone-shaped epiphyses (2).

**Complications:** Unknown.

**Associated Findings:** One individual had low frontal hairline with a white forelock, and broad great toe with valgus defect. Craniosynostosis and cardiac defects were reported in three generations of a family by Hunter et al (1977). Another boy had an apparently balanced 13;14 translocation which he inherited from his apparently unaffected father.

**Etiology:** Probably autosomal dominant inheritance with reduced penetrance and variable expressivity.

**Pathogenesis:** Unknown. Growth hormone levels, thyroid studies, metabolic studies, calcium, phosphorus, alkaline phosphatase, immunoglobulins, cortisol, uric acid, and banded karyotype have all been normal.

**MIM No.:** 18087

**POS No.:** 3131

**Sex Ratio:** M1:F1

**Occurrence:** Sixteen cases have been reported from Europe, Japan, and North America.

**Risk of Recurrence for Patient's Sib:**
 See Part I, *Mendelian Inheritance.*

**Risk of Recurrence for Patient's Child:**
 See Part I, *Mendelian Inheritance.*

**Age of Detectability:** At birth by physical examination.

**Gene Mapping and Linkage:** Unknown.

**Prevention:** None known. Genetic counseling indicated.

**Treatment:** Unknown.

**Prognosis:** Mental retardation can occur as part of the phenotype; life span is normal.

**Detection of Carrier:** Unknown.

**References:**
Ruvalcaba RHA, et al.: A new familial syndrome with osseous dysplasia and mental deficiency. J Pediatr 1971; 79:450–455.
Hunter AGW, et al.: A "new" syndrome of mental retardation with characteristic facies and brachyphalangy. J Med Genet 1977; 14:430–437
Geormaneanu M, et al.: Veberein "neus syndrome" in verbindung mit familiaerer translokation 13/14. Klin Paediat 1978; 190:500–506.
Sugio Y, Kajii T: Ruvalcaba syndrome: autosomal dominant inheritance. Am J Med Genet 1984; 19:741–753. * †

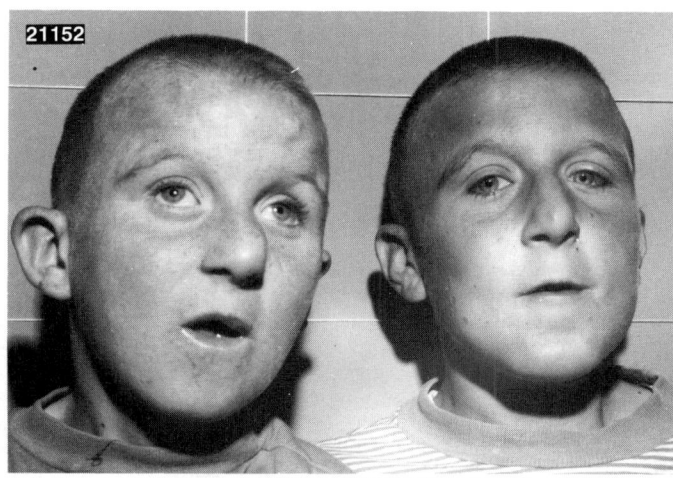

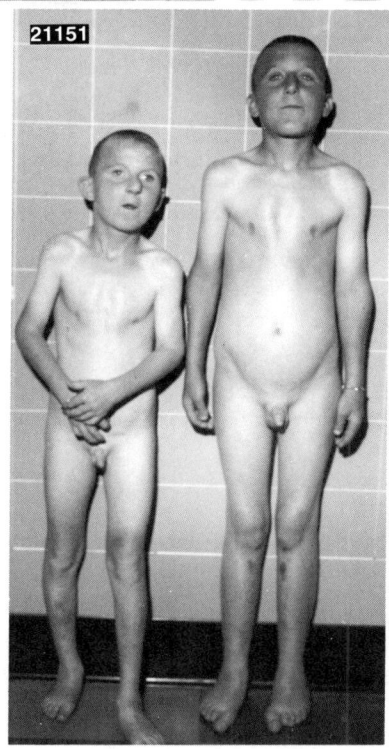

**2076-21152:** Two brothers with microcephaly, downslanting palpebral fissures, small alae nasi, small mouth, thin lips with downturned corners, and low-set ears. **21151:** Short stature, microcephaly, unusual facies, narrow trunk, pectus carinatum, small genitalia, and prominent elbows.

Bianchi E, et al.: Ruvalcaba syndrome: a case report. Europ J Pediatr 1984; 142:301–303.
Hunter A: Ruvalcaba syndrome. (Letter) Am J Med Genet 1985; 21:785–786.

T0007

**Helga V. Toriello**

## OSTEOECTASIA                                              0776

**Includes:**
Bone, excessive turnover
Chronic osteopathy with hyperphosphatasia
Hyperostosis corticalis deformans juvenilis
Hyperphosphatasemia, chronic congenital idiopathic
Osteoectasia with macrocranium (with hyperphosphatasia)
Paget disease, juvenile

**Excludes:**
**Cortical hyperostosis, infantile** (0221)
**Hyperostosis, Worth type** (2691)

**Major Diagnostic Criteria:** Calvarial thickening; demineralization and expansion of the tubular bones; and elevated alkaline phosphatase.

**Clinical Findings:** Small stature; large skull, progressive bowing of the legs and arms with pain, tenderness, and muscular weakness; tendency to bone fractures. X-rays show a thickened calvaria, with loss of normal bone structure and changes reminiscent of Paget disease; generalized demineralization; expansion and bowing of the long bones, and widening of the short tubular bones. In some patients and some sites, there is dissolution of the normal cortical architecture of the tubular bones.

Laboratory findings include an elevated activity of serum alkaline and acid phosphatase, and of serum aminopeptidase. Uric acid levels are increased in serum and urine. There is an elevation of the urinary peptide-bound hydroxyproline.

**Complications:** Angioid streaks of the retina, macular atrophy, vascular hypertension. Hearing deficit and optic atrophy due to continued new bone formation at the skull base.

**Associated Findings:** None known.

**Etiology:** Autosomal recessive inheritance with considerable variability of expression.

**Pathogenesis:** Excessive bone turnover, which leads to decreased amounts of mature lamellar bone. The defect is possibly related to a defective production or action of calcitonin.

**MIM No.:** *23900

**CDC No.:** 756.580

**Sex Ratio:** M1:F1

**Occurrence:** Over thirty cases have been documented.

**Risk of Recurrence for Patient's Sib:**
See Part I, *Mendelian Inheritance.*

**Risk of Recurrence for Patient's Child:**
See Part I, *Mendelian Inheritance.*

**Age of Detectability:** Between the third and eighteenth month of life.

**Gene Mapping and Linkage:** Unknown.

**Prevention:** None known. Genetic counseling indicated.

**Treatment:** Long-term treatment with calcitonin seems to be highly effective. Surgical correction of bone deformities; removal of excessive bone compressing the optic nerves, if necessary.

**Prognosis:** Untreated, most patients are severely deformed and incapacitated by the age of 14 years. Vascular hypertension may lead to cerebrovascular accidents and death.

**Detection of Carrier:** Undetermined. Possibly through serum phosphatases.

**References:**
Caffey J: Familial hyperphosphatasemia with ateliosis and hypermetabolism of growing membranous bone. Progr Pediatr Radiol 1973; 4:438–468.
Iancu TC, et al.: Chronic familial hyperphosphatasemia. Radiology 1978; 129:669–676.
Dunn V, et al.: Familial hyperphosphatasemia: diagnosis in early infancy and response to human calcitonin therapy. Am J Roentgen 1979; 132:541–545.

SP007                                    **Jürgen W. Spranger**

---

**Osteoectasia with macrocranium (with hyperphosphatasia)**
*See OSTEOECTASIA*

## OSTEOFIBROUS DYSPLASIA OF TIBIA AND FIBULA        2502

**Includes:**
Monostotic cortical fibrous dysplasia
Ossifying fibroma of the long bones
Osteogenic fibroma

**Excludes:**
**Fibrous dysplasia, monostotic** (0390)
**Fibrous dysplasia, polyostotic** (0391)
**Neurofibromatosis** (0712)

**Major Diagnostic Criteria:** *Clinical:* isolated, unilateral bowing of the leg associated with a painless mass. *Radiologic:* localized diaphyseal enlargement; intracortical radiolucence, with thinning of the external cortex and sclerosis of the medullary surface; and narrowing of the medullary canal. *Histopathologic:* fibrous tissue surrounding bone trabeculae lined by osteoblasts; "zonal" architecture.

**Clinical Findings:** Isolated bowing of the leg, usually in its middle one-third, but occasionally in the distal one-third; the bowing is usually anterior. A painless mass is generally apparent. A pathologic fracture may occur, and rarely pseudoarthrosis may develop. A lesion may heal spontaneously or be slowly progressive. Relapse after surgical treatment is frequent. The presence of other findings, particularly patchy skin hyperpigmentation anywhere on the body or additional sites of osseous abnormalities, should suggest an alternative diagnosis.

**Complications:** Relapse after surgical treatment; permanent bowing deformity; and, rarely, pseudoarthrosis.

**Associated Findings:** Possibly the histologic presence of an adamantinoma.

**Etiology:** Unknown.

**Pathogenesis:** Unknown.

**CDC No.:** 756.580

**Sex Ratio:** M1:F<1

**Occurrence:** About 100 cases have been reported.

**Risk of Recurrence for Patient's Sib:** Presumably very low.

**Risk of Recurrence for Patient's Child:** Unknown.

**Age of Detectability:** During the first decade of life.

**Gene Mapping and Linkage:** Unknown.

**Prevention:** None known. Genetic counseling indicated.

**Treatment:** If minor, close observation. Otherwise, curettage or other surgical techniques to limit or remove the lesion, although relapse is frequent after curettage. In general, surgery is restricted to patients more than five years of age who have extensive lesions.

**Prognosis:** Generally good, but variable, depending on the presence of complications as noted above.

**Detection of Carrier:** Unknown.

**References:**
Campanacci M: Osteofibrous dysplasia of long bones: a new clinical entity. Ital J Orthop Traumatol 1976; 2:221–237.
Capusten BM, et al.: Osteofibrous dysplasia. J Can Assoc Radiol 1980; 31:50–53.
Campanacci M, Laus M: Osteofibrous dysplasia of the tibia and fibula. J Bone Joint Surg 1981; 63:367.
Campbell CJ, Hawk T: A variant of fibrous dysplasia (osteofibrous dysplasia). J Bone Joint Surg 1982; 64:231–236.
Nakashima Y, et al.: Osteofibrous dysplasia (ossifying fibroma of long bones): A study of 12 cases. Cancer 1983; 52:909–914.
Sissons HA, et al.: Ossifying fibroma of bone: report of two cases. Bull Hosp Joint Dis Orthop Inst 1983; 43:1–14.
Alguacil-Garcia A, et al.: Osteofibrous dysplasia (ossifying fibroma) of the tibia and fibula and adamantinoma: a case report. Am J Clin Pathol 1984; 82:470–474.

Kerr R: Radiologic case study: osteofibrous dysplasia. Orthopedics 1987; 10:1085–1089.

RI000                                                     **Vincent M. Riccardi**

## OSTEOGENESIS IMPERFECTA                             0777

**Includes:**
  Lobstein syndrome
  Osteogenesis imperfecta congenita, neonatal lethal
  Osteogenesis imperfecta congenita-microcephaly-cataracts
  Osteogenesis imperfecta, lethal preinatal
  Osteogenesis imperfecta, progressively deforming, normal sclerae
  Osteogenesis imperfecta tarda
  Osteogenesis imperfecta-blue sclerae
  Osteogenesis imperfecta-normal sclerae
  Osteogenesis imperfecta-opalescent teeth
  Osteogenesis imperfecta-opalescent teeth-Wormian bones
  Vrolik disease

**Excludes:**
  **Hypophosphatasia** (0516)
  **Osteoporosis, juvenile idiopathic** (0782)
  **Osteoporosis-pseudoglioma syndrome** (0783)

**Major Diagnostic Criteria:** Skeletal fractures with minimal trauma and/or evidence of osteopenia and/or blue sclerae; typical X-ray changes or otosclerosis. Considerable heterogeneity exists in phenotype and in genetic transmission.

**Clinical Findings:** Osteogenesis imperfecta (OI) is a descriptive term applied to a group of multisystem diseases involving the skeletal, ocular, cutaneous, otologic, dental and vascular tissues, with the greatest morbidity arising from the skeletal manifestations. The spectrum of severity varies considerably. Patients range from those with severe neonatal onset characterized by multiple intrauterine fractures of the limbs and ribs, soft membranous cranium, and usually neonatal death from intracranial hemorrhage or respiratory distress; to those manifesting only a slight tendency toward, or no history at all of bone fractures, but with blue sclerae or mild deafness. The current nomenclature divides OI into four major types (Beighton 1988) with type I and IV subdivided according to presence or absence of opalescent dentin (see **Teeth, dentinogenesis imperfecta**) (Silence 1988) and type II

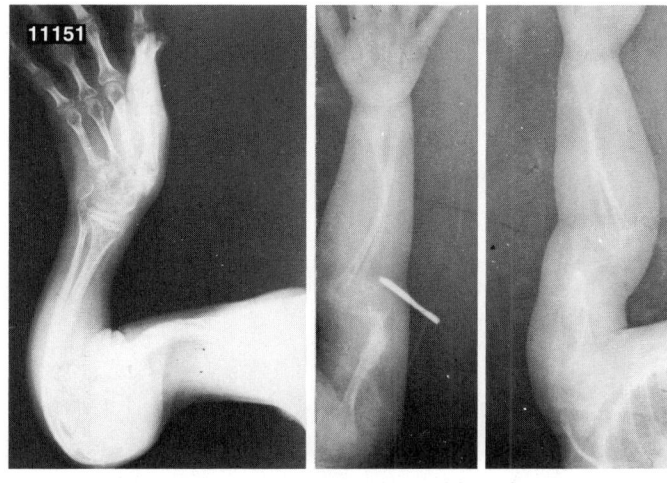

**0777B-11151:** Note thin, severely bowed long bones.

subdivided into 3 sub-groups on the basis of X-ray findings in the long bones and ribs (Thompson et al. 1987). The majority of cases can be encompassed by one of these eight types.

*OI type I:* The classic syndrome of dominantly inherited OI with distinctly blue-gray sclerae. It is further subdivided into families with normal teeth (OI type I, group A), and families with opalescent dentin (OI type I, group B). The dental involvement

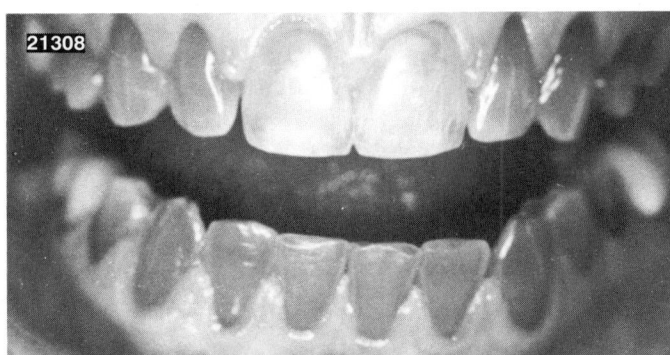

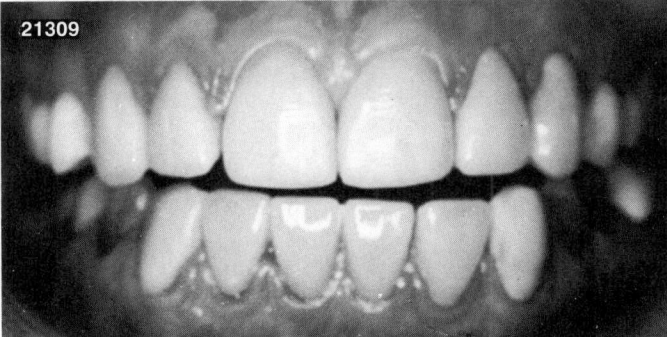

**0777C-21308:** Teeth of a woman with type IB osteogenesis imperfecta; note the good formation of the teeth despite the hypoplasia of the dentin with translucency of the teeth.   **21309:** Same woman as shown in **21308** after dental lamination of all teeth; note the untreated mandibular premolars.

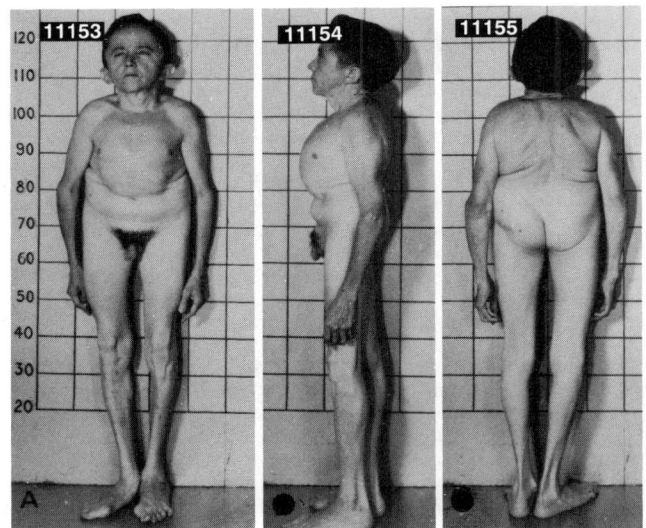

**0777A-11153–55:** Note short barrel-shaped chest and short neck.

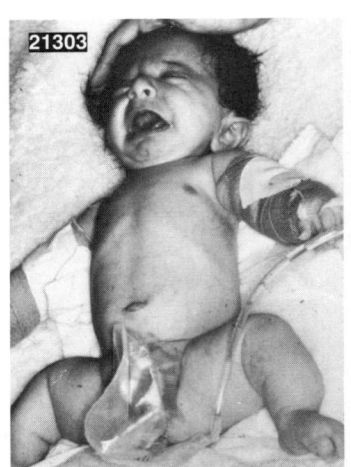

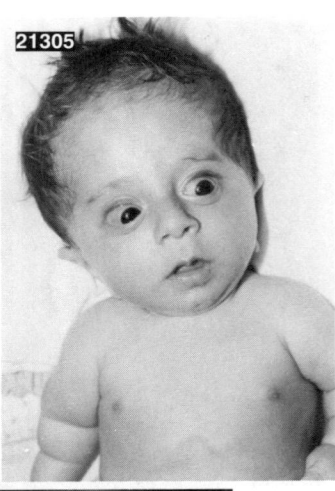

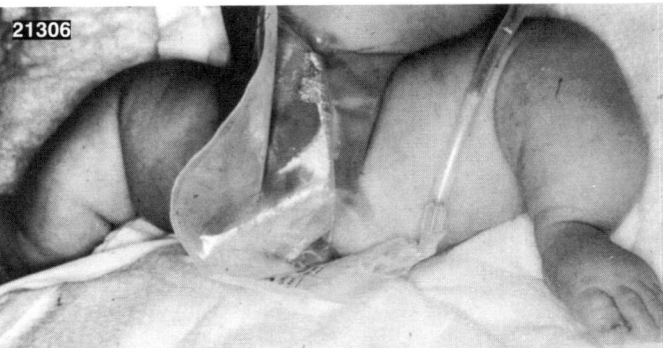

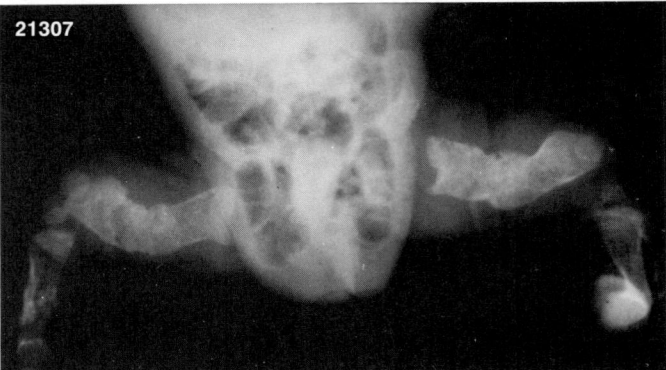

**0777E-21306:** Neonate with phenotypic OI type II with short and bowed lower limbs. **21307:** X-ray shows multiple fractures and crumpled appearance of the long bones, which are shortened and deformed. Note also the poorly ossified callus and deformed, heart-shaped pelvis.

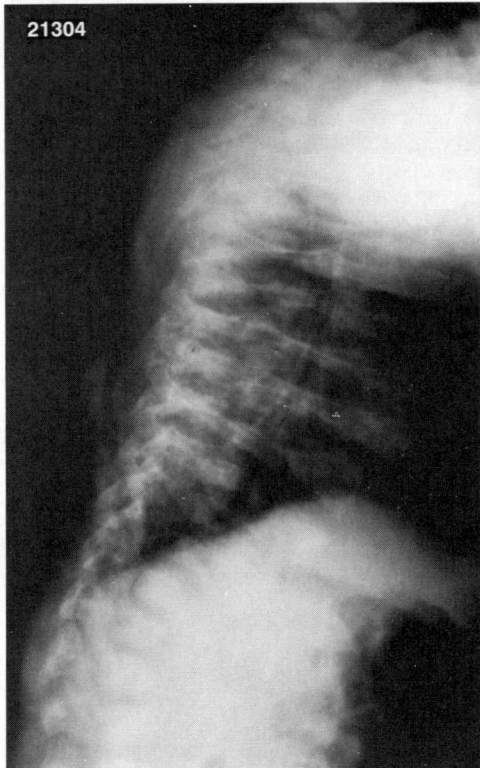

**0777D-21303:** Male infant with osteogenesis type II; note short and deformed limbs from congenital fractures. **21305:** Round facies with prominent eyes and blue sclerae; note the short limbs with excessive skin folds secondary to multiple healed fractures. **21304:** Lateral spine of a neonate with OI type II shows osteoporotic platyspondyly with vertebrae resembling those of a fish (fish spine) and thin ribs.

can be highly variable, and these sub-categories are not always clear-cut. Some 10% of individuals in these families present with fractures at birth. The majority of affected persons have their first fractures before five years of age; other persons may have no fractures during childhood or adult life. In all affected persons the sclerae are distinctly blue-gray and remain so throughout life. The hearing impairment is predominantly conductive and is due to sclerosis and deformity of the ossicles, but in some cases mixed conductive and sensory hearing impairment occurs, with high frequency loss. While these patients have a high fracture frequency, bowing and curvature deformity of long bones and spine are usually mild. Although kyphosis and loss of skeletal height with age are frequent findings, only a few affected adults develop severe scoliosis. In families with opalescent dentin (group B), the teeth appear yellow-brown in color; they are easily cracked or worn. X-rays of these teeth show constricted corono-radicular junctions. X-rays also indicate that the predominant feature throughout the skeleton is osteopenia, with deformity of the spine and long bones in some cases. Wormian bones are seen in the skull of the majority of individuals with OI type I. Biochemical studies show a quantitative defect in the production of type I procollagen. Linkage has been demonstrated to COL I A1 by RFLP analysis.

*OI type II:* This syndrome, characterized by extreme bone fragility, leads to intrauterine fractures and either stillbirth or neonatal death. Considerable clinical heterogeneity exists. Three subgroups can be defined by X-ray (Sillence et al. 1984, Thompson et al. 1987). Type II group A shows broad crumpled femora with continuous rib beading on, X-ray; group B has broad crumpled femora but minimal or no rib fractures; and group C has thin femora with fractures and thin ribs with extensive fracturing. Biochemical studies in group A patients show a marked reduction in type I collagen synthesis. Collagen protein and gene studies show defects which for the most part are heterozygous deletions:

   (a) COL I A1 glycine 988 → cysteine (Steinmann et al. 1988)

   (b) COL I A1 glycine 664 → arginine (Bateman et al. 1988)

A few patients with type II OI have demonstrated a marked diversity of specific defects; however, all lead to a decrease in type I collagen or a structurally abnormal type I collagen. The nature of the defects often suggest new dominant mutations, thus genetic heterogeneity is likely.

*OI type III:* This group is probably heterogeneous, but in each case inheritance is autosomal recessive (by definition). These individuals frequently survive the newborn period, i.e. in these cases the disease is not generally lethal; their X-rays lack the continuously beading ribs and crumpled long bones that are seen in the OI type II cases in the newborn period. However, in some instances there is overlap of OI type III cases with OI type II. Survivors have severe short stature and with age develop progressive deformities of long bones and spine. The sclerae, although bluish at birth, become progressively less blue with age, and are usually white by late childhood. In the third and fourth decades there is a high mortality from cardiorespiratory failure. Biochemical studies in one instance show decreased collagen synthesis due to mutation affecting transcription of the alpha 2 chain of type I collagen (Nicholls et al. 1984).

*OI type IV:* The major characteristic of this dominantly inherited form of OI is normal sclerae. Although at birth the sclerae of affected individuals are bluish, they become progressively less blue with age; by adolescence, they have a normal hue. This group can be further subdivided into families with normal teeth (OI type IV group A) and families with opalescent dentin (OI type IV group B). The onset of fractures frequently occurs in the newborn period although some affected persons show only the congenital bowing of the long bones and have no subsequent fractures; they appear to improve with age. As in OI type III progressive kyphoscoliosis may occur in adult life. Available biochemical data suggest that structural alterations in the alpha 2(I) chain of type I collagen may be the underlying mechanism in some affected families.

**Complications:** In addition to those mentioned above, other complications include tendon sprains, tendon avulsion, increased capillary fragility, subcutaneous hemorrhage, peri-operative malignant hyperthermia, and neurologic dysfunction due to platybasia.

**Associated Findings:** Elastosis perforans (rarely).

**Etiology:** Osteogenesis imperfecta appears to be clinically and genetically very heterogeneous. The classic syndrome (OI type I) is by far the most prevalent form of OI in most populations.

The vast majority of sporadic cases appear to be inherited in an autosomal dominant manner from the previous generation, or represent new dominant mutations. When parents are consanguineous and clinically normal, autosomal recessive inheritance should be suspected.

**Pathogenesis:** In view of the clinical and genetic heterogeneity, it is clear that OI must be pathogenetically heterogeneous. As the manifestations include abnormality of the skeleton, eye, and skin, the OI disorders must represent generalized defects in connective tissue.

Available data indicates marked heterogeneity at the biochemical level in OI type II. However, the defects appear to reduce the amount of type I collagen or to produce a structurally abnormal type I collagen. Fewer patients with the other types of OI have been studied, but structural or functional defects of the constituent chains of type I collagen are suspected.

An absence of secretion of the alpha 2(I) collagen by cultured fibroblasts in one patient with an autosomal recessive non-lethal form of OI (OI type III) has been reported. In this patient $\alpha_2$ (I) collagen is not recoverable from tissues, and structural collagen presumably consists of $\alpha_1$ (I) trimers.

**MIM No.:** *16620, *16621, *16622, 16623, 16624, *25940, 25941, *25942, *12015, *12016

**POS No.:** 3349

**CDC No.:** 756.500

**Sex Ratio:** M1:F1

**Occurrence:** Based on an Australian study, the incidence of OI type I is 3.5:100,000 live births; and of type II is 1.6:100,000 live births. Prevalence of OI type I was calculated at 3.4:100,000 population. OI type III is common in the black population of South Africa, where more than 80 cases have been documented.

**Risk of Recurrence for Patient's Sib:**
See Part I, *Mendelian Inheritance.* If there is no consanguinity, and neither parent has evidence of the disorder (i.e. blue sclerae and excessive fractures), then the risk is generally small unless the patient has the severe perinatal lethal OI type II group B or OI type II group C.

Where X-ray changes are of OI type II group B, a recurrence risk of 8% can be given. Similarly with OI type II group C a risk of 25%. When X-ray studies are not available in severe lethal OI, a British study suggests a recurrence risk of 6%. (Thompson et al, 1987).

**Risk of Recurrence for Patient's Child:**
See Part I, *Mendelian Inheritance.*

**Age of Detectability:** Because of clinical variability, detection may range from birth through adulthood. Prenatal diagnosis of OI type II has been accomplished using ultrasonography. In addition, biochemical studies on cultured amniotic cells have been employed to confirm a decreased type I collagen secretion in recurrence of OI type II. Chorion villus specimens can be investigated for over-modification of lysine residues in pregnancies at risk for OI type II where study of fibroblasts from a previous affected have shown this abnormality. Ultrasound studies may be used in conjunction with X-ray studies to screen pregnancies at risk for severe forms of OI type III. However, no measure of reliability can yet be placed on such studies.

**Gene Mapping and Linkage:** OI4 (osteogenesis imperfecta type IV) has been provisionally mapped to 7q21.3-q22.1.

COL1A1 (collagen, type I, alpha 1) has been mapped to 17q21.3-q22.

COL1A2 (collagen, type I, alpha 2) has been mapped to 7q21.3-q22.1.

**Prevention:** None known. Genetic counseling indicated.

**Treatment:** Oral magnesium oxide, calcitonin, sodium fluoride, and vitamin C have been suggested to be potentially useful therapeutic agents; however, definite improvement of clinical symptoms with any of these treatments is yet to be documented. Immobilization should be avoided. Careful alignment of fractures may reduce residual deformity. Multiple fragmentation and intramedullary rodding may be useful in some patients in stabilizing a long bone subject to recurrent fractures and in correcting the deformity. Selective spinal fusion has been reported to be useful in stabilizing spinal curvature (scoliosis).

Because of hormonal effects, pregnancy may be deleterious to severely affected females. An increase in fracture frequency may occur, and hearing may deteriorate. Cesarean section is usually indicated.

**Prognosis:** Dependent upon type of OI. Ranges from death in perinatal period to normal life span with little if any morbidity.

**Detection of Carrier:** There is a wide range of expressivity within families showing autosomal dominant inheritance. An affected member may demonstrate only blue sclerae, while sibs or offspring may demonstrate the full manifestations of the disorder. At present no biochemical test is available to routinely distinguish carriers; however if a specific collagen biochemical defect is known in a patient, carrier testing may be possible.

**Support Groups:**
DC; Washington; Osteogenesis Imperfecta National Capital Area
PA; West Chester; American Brittle Bone Society (ABBS)
NH; Manchester; Osteogenesis Imperfecta Foundation (OIF)

**References:**
Paterson CR, et al.: Heterogeneity in osteogenesis imperfecta type I. J Med Genet 1983; 20:203–205.
Paterson CR, et al.: Osteogenesis imperfecta with dominant inheritance and normal sclerae. J Bone Joint Surg 1983; 65B:35–39.
Nicholls et al.: The clinical features of homozygous $\alpha$2(I) collagen deficient Osteogenesis Imperfecta. J Med Genet 1984; 21:257–262.
Sillence DO, et al.: Osteogenesis imperfecta type II: delineation of the phenotype with reference to genetic heterogeneity. Am J Med Genet 1984; 17:407–423.
Beighton P, Versfeld GA: On the paradoxically high relative preva-

lence of osteogenesis imperfects type III in the Black population of South Africa. Clin Genet 1985; 27:398–404.

Byers PH, Bonadio JF: The molecular basis of clinical heterogeneity in osteogenesis imperfecta: mutations in type I collagen genes have different effects on collagen processing. In: Lloyd JK, Scriver CR, eds: Genetics and metabolic disease in pediatrics. London: Butterworths, 1985:56–90.

Sillence DO, et al: Osteogenesis imperfecta type III: delineation of the phenotype with special reference to genetic heterogeneity. Am J Med Genet 1986; 23:821–832.

Thompson EM, et al.: Recurrence risks and prognosis in severe sporadic osteogenesis imperfecta. J Med Genet 1987; 24:390–405.

Tsipouras P, et al.: Prenatal prediction of osteogenesis imperfecta type IV: exclusion of inheritance using a collagen gene probe. J Med Genet 1987; 24:406–409.

Bateman JF, et al.: BIochemical heterogeneity of type I collagen mutations in Osteogenesis Imperfecta. Ann New York Acad Sci 1988; 543:95–105.

Beighton P, et al.: International nosology of heritable disorders of connective tissue. Am J Med Genet 1988; 29:581–594.

Sillence DO: Osteogenesis imperfecta: nosology and genetics. Ann New York Acad Sci 1988; 543:1–15.

Steinmann B, et al.: Imperfecta collagenesis in Osteogenesis Imperfecta. Ann New York Acad Sci 1988; 543;47–61.

SI009          **David Sillence**
BA021          **Kristine K. Barlow**

**Osteogenesis imperfecta congenita, neonatal lethal**
*See OSTEOGENESIS IMPERFECTA*

**Osteogenesis imperfecta congenita-microcephaly-cataracts**
*See OSTEOGENESIS IMPERFECTA*

**Osteogenesis imperfecta tarda**
*See OSTEOGENESIS IMPERFECTA*

**Osteogenesis imperfecta, lethal preinatal**
*See OSTEOGENESIS IMPERFECTA*

**Osteogenesis imperfecta, ocular form**
*See OSTEOPOROSIS-PSEUDOGLIOMA SYNDROME*

**Osteogenesis imperfecta, possible variant**
*See SHORT STATURE-WORMIAN BONES-JOINT DISLOCATIONS*

**Osteogenesis imperfecta, progressively deforming, normal sclerae**
*See OSTEOGENESIS IMPERFECTA*

**Osteogenesis imperfecta-blue sclerae**
*See OSTEOGENESIS IMPERFECTA*

**Osteogenesis imperfecta-normal sclerae**
*See OSTEOGENESIS IMPERFECTA*

**Osteogenesis imperfecta-opalescent teeth**
*See OSTEOGENESIS IMPERFECTA*

**Osteogenesis imperfecta-opalescent teeth-Wormian bones**
*See OSTEOGENESIS IMPERFECTA*

**Osteogenic fibroma**
*See OSTEOFIBROUS DYSPLASIA OF TIBIA AND FIBULA*

**Osteogenic sarcoma**
*See OSTEOSARCOMA*

**Osteoglophonic dwarfism**
*See OSTEOGLOPHONIC DYSPLASIA*

---

| OSTEOGLOPHONIC DYSPLASIA | 2571 |
|---|---|

**Includes:**  Osteoglophonic dwarfism

**Excludes:**
   **Craniofacial dysostosis** (0225)
   **Craniometaphyseal dysplasia** (0228)
   **Hypophosphatasia** (0516)
   **Skeletal dysplasia** (others)

**Major Diagnostic Criteria:**  Dwarfism, gross craniofacial abnormalities and characteristic metaphyseal lucencies on X-ray.

**Clinical Findings:**  Rhizomelic dwarfism and limb malalignment are associated with frontal prominence, hypertelorism and massive mandibular prognathism. The palate is high, the teeth are maldeveloped and the nostrils are anteverted. Developmental milestones are delayed, due to the skeletal problems, but intelligence is normal. There are no visceral ramifications.

On X-ray the skull is scaphocephalic, due to sagittal stenosis, with gross frontal bossing. Cystic changes are present in the mandibular ramus, and the teeth may remain unerupted. In the

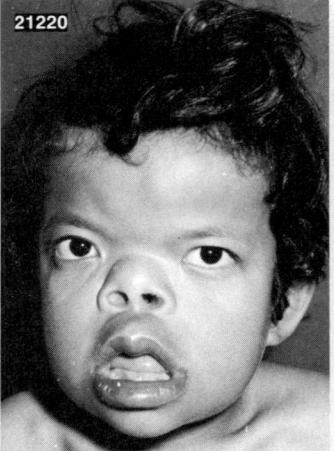
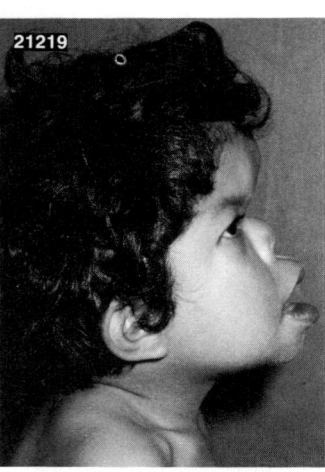

**2571A**-21219–20:  Affected 12-year-old girl with hypertelorism, mandibular prognathism, depressed nasal bridge and bossing of the forehead.

---

spine, platyspondyly with anterior projection of the vertebral bodies is a striking feature. The ribs and clavicles are normal, but the pelvis is distorted, with radiolucent areas in the ilia. The long bones show gross undermodeling, with generalized osteoporosis, cortical thinning and loss of the normal trabecular pattern. Lucent patches throughout the metaphyses, especially in the distal femora and proximal tibiae, produce a hollowed out appearance. The tubular bones of the extremities are short and broad, with dysplastic epiphyseal ossification centers.

**Complications:  Craniosynostosis** may produce severe facial abnormalities. Dental maleruption may be troublesome. The narrow nasal passages predispose to recurrent upper respiratory infections. Gait is impaired due to the skeletal abnormalities.

**Associated Findings:**  None known.

**Etiology:**  Possibly autosomal dominant inheritance, although most cases have been sporadic.

**Pathogenesis:**  Unknown.

**MIM No.:**  16625

**POS No.:**  4004

**CDC No.:**  756.580

**Sex Ratio:**  M1:F1

**Occurrence:**  Six patients have been reported in the United Kingdom and United States, and another affected female infant is known in Portugal.

**Risk of Recurrence for Patient's Sib:**
   See Part I, *Mendelian Inheritance.*

**Risk of Recurrence for Patient's Child:**
   See Part I, *Mendelian Inheritance.*

**Age of Detectability:**  At birth.

**Gene Mapping and Linkage:**  Unknown.

**Prevention:**  None known. Genetic counseling indicated.

**Treatment:**  Craniotomy in infancy may diminish craniofacial distortion. Orthodontic measures may be necessary for dental maldevelopment.

**Prognosis:**  Intelligence and general health are normal. Dwarfism is severe, and the facial appearance is grotesque.

**Detection of Carrier:**  Unknown.

**References:**
Fairbank T: An atlas of general affections of the skeleton. Edinburgh: Livingstone, 1959.

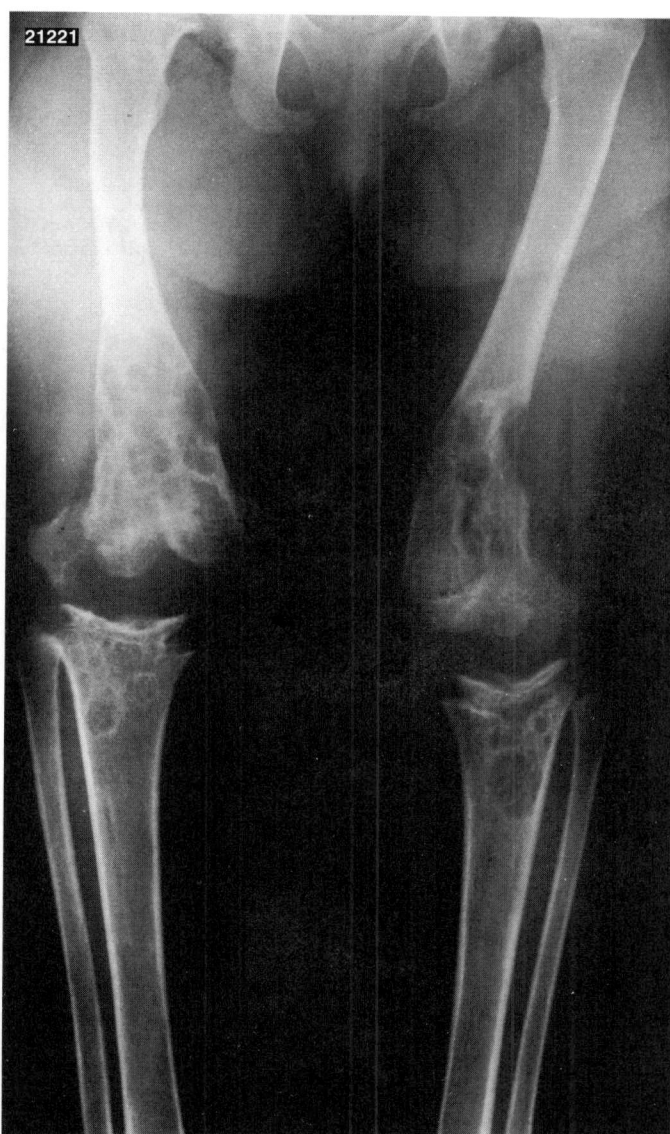

**2571B-21221:** A-P view of the legs of an affected girl aged 12 years; note multiple irregular lucent areas in the metaphyses.

Keats TE, et al.: Craniofacial dysostosis with fibrous metaphyseal defects. Am J. Roentgenol 1975; 124:271–275.

Beighton P, et al.: Osteoglophonic dwarfism. Pediatr Radiol 1980; 10:46–50. * †

Kelley RI, et al.: Osteoglophonic dwarfism in two generations. J Med Genet 1983; 20:436–440.

BE008                                                    **Peter Beighton**

## OSTEOLYSIS                                              1521

Osteolysis is a general term referring to the appearance on X-ray of intense, focal resorption of bone. The resorption may be either focal and segmental or focal and generalized. The term osteolysis is used to distinguish focal bone resorption from generalized osteopenia, and it should be used to express an X-ray finding rather than a specific disease process.

Osteolysis can be caused by a myriad of disorders such as osteomyelitis, tuberculosis, granulomatous bone disease, stress fractures, benign or malignant primary bone tumors, multiple myeloma, leukemia, mast cell disease, histiocytosis, metastatic carcinoma, metabolic disorders (such as brown tumors of hyperthyroidism or the lytic phase of **Bone, Paget disease**), extreme pressure on bone, periarticular inflammation, inflammatory arthropathies, reflex sympathetic dystrophy, transient regional osteoporosis, migratory osteolysis, the lytic phase of osteonecrosis, focal denervation (pseudomyelomatous osteopenia), or several specific and extremely rare genetic conditions such as **Osteopoikilosis; Fibromatosis, juvenile hyaline; Pyknodysostosis; Winchester syndrome**; or **Osteolysis, carpal-tarsal and chronic progressive glomerulopathy**.

In light of the myriad causes of osteolysis, the age of onset can vary widely from prenatal to beyond the tenth decade of life, and it has no sex predilection. Depending on the cause, the condition may be either painless or painful. The treatment of the condition is essentially the treatment of the underlying condition, if known.

KA033                                                    **Frederick S. Kaplan**

## OSTEOLYSIS, CARPAL-TARSAL AND CHRONIC PROGRESSIVE GLOMERULOPATHY          0128

**Includes:**
> Carpal-tarsal osteolysis-chronic progressive glomerulopathy
> Essential osteolysis-nephropathy
> Gorham osteolysis
> Osteolysis, essential hereditary, of carpal bones-nephropathy
> Osteolysis-proteinuria
> Proteinuria-osteolysis

**Excludes:**
> **Acro-osteolysis, dominant type** (0021)
> **Arthritis, rheumatoid** (2517)
> Conorenal syndrome
> **Hajdu-Cheney syndrome** (2022)
> Osteoarthropathy of Schinz and Furtwaengler
> **Osteolysis, essential** (2596)
> **Osteolysis, recessive carpal-tarsal** (0129)
> Various aseptic necrosis syndromes

**Major Diagnostic Criteria:** Osteolysis of carpal and tarsal bones associated with moderate-to-marked involvement of adjacent tubular bones, proteinuria, and microscopic hematuria.

**Clinical Findings:** Osteolysis of carpal and tarsal bones begins in the first decade, usually before age 5 years. It may occur without symptoms or may be accompanied by tenderness, swelling, and painful limitation of motion of ankle or wrist. As a rule, osteolysis is bilaterally symmetric and progresses slowly to complete dissolution of carpal and tarsal bones. Adjacent tubular bones are shortened with marked tapering, resembling a "sucked-candy" appearance on X-ray. Progressive shortening of the forearms is noted, and lytic involvement of the elbow leads to loss of mobility and function. Cortical thinning of the nonaxial tubular bones also becomes evident. Other nonprogressive skeletal defects have been associated with this syndrome.

Progressive proteinuria with onset at about the end of the first decade, associated with microscopic hematuria, is found. Azotemia is usually manifested by the late second early third decade; nonoliguric renal insufficiency (with the nephrotic syndrome) rapidly progresses to frank renal failure and death.

Pathologic examination of affected wrists has revealed replacement of bone and cartilage by fibrofatty tissue, and a notable lack of inflammatory response or vascular or hemangiomatous changes. Arrest of endochondral bone formation and areas of fibrocartilaginous metaplasia have been observed. Both percutaneous biopsy and autopsy specimens of kidney have demonstrated a proliferative glomerulopathy with epithelial crescent formation and numerous hyalinized glomeruli. Unusual neovascularization of glomeruli by capillary ingrowths from the Bowman capsule have been observed. Immunopathologic studies show some IgM in unsclerosed segments of glomeruli.

Laboratory evaluations early in the course of this syndrome are normal; erythrocyte sedimentation rate, latex fixation, and LE preparations are normal. Somewhat later, proteinuria and hematuria are found; and, finally, the chemical finding of uremia and massive proteinuria becomes manifest.

**Complications:** Painful limitation of motion of affected areas with progressive dysfunction due to loss of bone and resultant deformity (volar subluxation of hands, flexion contractures of elbows and pes cavum). Marked muscle atrophy without neurologic deficit is presumably due to loss of bony insertions. Progressive chronic renal insufficiency results in death in the late second to third decade.

**Associated Findings:** None known.

**Etiology:** Autosomal dominant inheritance. Monocentric massive osteolysis (Gorham and Stout, 1955) appears to be non-Mendelian.

**Pathogenesis:** Unknown.

**MIM No.:** *16630

**POS No.:** 3053

**CDC No.:** 756.580

**Sex Ratio:** Presumably M1:F1

**Occurrence:** Undetermined. Extensive literature.

**Risk of Recurrence for Patient's Sib:**
See Part I, *Mendelian Inheritance.*

**Risk of Recurrence for Patient's Child:**
See Part I, *Mendelian Inheritance.*

**Age of Detectability:** First decade of life.

**Gene Mapping and Linkage:** Unknown.

**Prevention:** None known. Genetic counseling indicated.

**Treatment:** Symptomatic treatment with mild analgesics for wrist and ankle pain. Supportive therapy for chronic renal failure. There is no reported experience with immunosuppressive agents.

**Prognosis:** Death from uremia in late second to early third decades. Function is variable depending on degree and extent of osteolysis.

**Detection of Carrier:** Unknown.

**Special Considerations:** Whether carpal-tarsal osteolysis without glomerulopathy and with extensive lytic involvement of adjacent tubular bones and elbow joints is a separate entity is not clear. This syndrome is easily distinguished from **Osteolysis, recessive carpal-tarpal** by the above criteria and by the notable osteoporosis, cortical thinning, and especially increased caliber of phalanges and metacarpals found in the recessive syndrome. The syndrome is easily distinguished from the various acro-osteolysis syndromes and aseptic necrosis syndromes by distribution of the lesions. The lack of acute phase reactants, systemic illness, and inflammatory reaction in biopsy material distinguishes this syndrome from rheumatoid arthritis. The lack of generalized joint stiffness and other skeletal disorders separates this syndrome from the osteoarthropathy of Schinz and Furtwaengler.

**References:**
Gorham LW, Stout AP: Massive osteolysis. J Bone Joint Surg 1955; 37A:985–1004.
Marie J, et al.: Acro-osteolyse essentielle compliquée d'insuffisance renal d'evolution fatale. Presse Med 1963; 71:249–252.
Shurtleff DB, et al.: Hereditary osteolysis with hypertension and nephropathy. JAMA 1964; 188:363–368.
Lagier R, Rutishauser E: Osteoarticular changes in a case of essential osteolysis. J Bone Joint Surg 1965; 47B:339–353. *
Torg JS, Steel HH: Essential osteolysis with nephropathy. J Bone Joint Surg 1968; 50A:1629–1638.
Counahan, R et al.: Multifocal osteolysis with nephropathy. Arch Dis Child 1976; 51:717–719. *
Hardegger F, et al.: The syndrome of idiopathic osteolysis: classification, review, and case report. J Bone Joint Surg 1985; 67B:89–93.

B0025

**Zvi Borochowitz**
*David L. Rimoin*

## Osteolysis, distal-short stature-characteristic facies
*See OSTEOLYSIS, ESSENTIAL*

## OSTEOLYSIS, ESSENTIAL 2596

**Includes:**
Acroosteolysis
Acroosteolysis-osteoporosis-skull and mandible changes
Arthrodentoosteodysplasia
Cheney syndrome
Essential carpotarsal osteolysis
Multicentric osteolysis
Osteolysis, distal-short stature-characteristic facies
Osteolysis, idiopathic
Osteolysis, idiopathic multicentric
Osteolysis, idiopathic phalangeal

**Excludes:**
Acroosteolysis, secondary
Acroosteolysis-neurologic deficit
**Hajdu-Cheney syndrome** (2022)
**Osteolysis, carpal-tarsal and chronic progressive glomerulopathy** (0128)
**Osteolysis, recessive carpal-tarsal** (0129)

**Major Diagnostic Criteria:** X-ray demonstration of osteolytic destruction of clinically affected bones.

**Clinical Findings:** In all types of idiopathic osteolyses, osteolytic bone changes result in variable degrees of disability. The osteolytic process starts in early infancy and is characterized by arthritis-like episodes with pain and swellings of the affected bones. Concomitant atrophy of the muscles and flexion contractures progressively become evident in most patients. In all of the subtypes of essential osteolyses, the osteolytic destruction is more or less diffuse and not exclusively restricted to one or another bone segment. All patients have characteristc facial changes

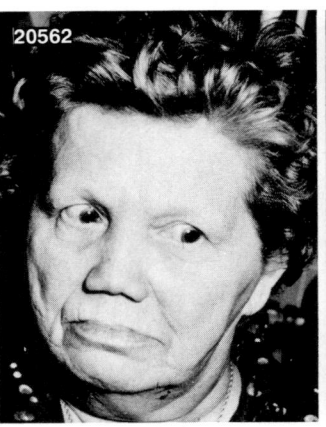
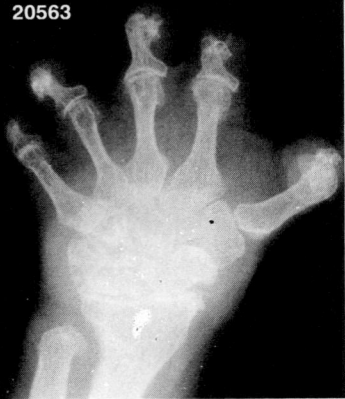

**2596-20562:** Characteristic facial changes: maxillary hypoplasia, relative exophthalmos, and broad nasal tip. **20563:** Note destruction of the distal phalanges of all fingers.

consisting of maxillary hypoplasia, relative exophthalmos, and broad nasal tip.

**Complications:** Unknown.

**Associated Findings:** Associated renal abnormalities and hypertension have been documented. Whereas in most patients the renal symptoms are limited to a fluctuating proteinuria and an abnormal cell count, in a few patients death occurred about the age of 20 years from renal failure with histologic lesions resembling chronic glomerulonephritis. Corneal opacities were reported in at least four patients.

**Etiology:** Different forms of idiopathic osteolysis have been differentiated on the basis of clinical, X-ray, and genetic criteria. *Idiopathic multicentric osteolysis* has been reported as an autosomal dominant condition. At least three apparently distinct types of acro-osteolysis have been delineated, each with autosomal dominant inheritance: *essential carpotarsal osteolysis*, **Hajdu-Cheney syndrome**, and *idiopathic acroosteolysis* of the phalanges. A few examples of probable autosomal recessive types of essential osteolysis have been reported. For all types of essential osteolysis, the etiology remains obscure.

**Pathogenesis:** Vascular and immunological disturbances have been considered, but biopsy and necropsy studies have failed to provide definite clue as to the nature of the disorder.

**MIM No.:** *10250, 25961

**CDC No.:** 756.580

**Sex Ratio:** M1:F1

**Occurrence:** Undetermined but presumed rare.

**Risk of Recurrence for Patient's Sib:**
See Part I, *Mendelian Inheritance.*

**Risk of Recurrence for Patient's Child:**
See Part I, *Mendelian Inheritance.*

**Age of Detectability:** The osteolytic process usually starts in early childhood and is slowly progressive. Facial changes become evident after puberty.

**Gene Mapping and Linkage:** Unknown.

**Prevention:** None known. Genetic counseling indicated.

**Treatment:** In addition to supportive treatment, sympathectomy has been performed in some patients, with inconsistent results. Treatment of hypertension and renal insufficiency, if present.

**Prognosis:** The osteolytic changes start in early childhood and are slowly progressive, resulting in functional disability, muscular atrophy, and joint contractures. Life span prognosis is generally good, except in patients with renal involvement.

**Detection of Carrier:** Unknown.

**References:**

Joseph R, et al.: Acro-ostéolyse idiopathique familiale. Ann Pediatr 1959; 35:622–629.

Spranger J, et al.: Bone dysplasias: an atlas of constitutional disorders of skeletal development. Stuttgart: Gustav Fischer Verlag 1974: 209–218. *

Beals RK, Bird CB: Carpal and tarsal osteolysis. J Bone Joint Surg 1975; 57A:681–686.

Bennett WM, et al.: Nephropathy of idiopathic multicentric osteolysis. Nephron 1980; 25:134–138.

Petit P, Fryns JP: Distal osteolysis, short stature, mental retardation, and characteristic facial appearance: delineation of an autosomal recessive subtype of essential osteolysis. Am J Med Genet 1986; 25:537–541. †

Osterberg PH, et al.: Familial expansile osteolysis: a new dysplasia. J Bone Joint Surg 1988; 70:255–260.

Barr RJ, et al.: Idiopathic multicentric osteolysis: report of two new cases and a review of the literature. Am J Med Genet 1989; 32:556 only.

FR030                                                    **Jean-Pierre Fryns**

**Osteolysis, idiopathic multicentric**
*See OSTEOPOIKILOSIS*
**Osteolysis, idiopathic**
*See OSTEOLYSIS, ESSENTIAL*

**Osteolysis, idiopathic multicentric**
*See OSTEOLYSIS, ESSENTIAL*
**Osteolysis, idiopathic phalangeal**
*See OSTEOLYSIS, ESSENTIAL*

---

## OSTEOLYSIS, RECESSIVE CARPAL-TARSAL     0129

**Includes:**
　　Carpal-tarsal osteolysis, recessive
　　Multicentric osteolysis with recessive transmission

**Excludes:**
　　**Acro-osteolysis** (all forms)
　　**Arthritis, rheumatoid** (2517)
　　Aseptic necrosis in other syndromes
　　Gorham disease
　　**Hajdu-Cheney syndrome** (2022)
　　Osteoarthropathy of Schinz and Furtwaengler
　　**Osteolysis, carpal-tarsal and chronic progressive glomerulopathy** (0128)
　　**Osteolysis, essential** (2596)
　　Osteolysis with dominant transmission, idiopathic hereditary
　　**Winchester syndrome** (1000)

**Major Diagnostic Criteria:** Flexion contractures of the knees, hips, and elbows; fusiform enlargement of the digits; and the absence of systemic renal and neurological defects. X-rays show collapse and resorption of carpal and tarsal bones, and appendicular osteopenia, cortical thinning, and an increased diameter of long and tubular bones. Evidence of autosomal recessive inheritance is helpful.

**Clinical Findings:** A single pedigree with three young affected members has been described. Beginning in early childhood, onset of a progressive osteolysis of the carpal and tarsal bones occurs, usually accompanied by swelling, tenderness, and painful limitation of motion of the affected area. Fusiform swelling of the fingers may be observed, with deformity of the proximal interphalangeal joints. In at least one patient, nontender subcutaneous nodules on knees, feet, elbows, and fingers were observed, and "hyperpigmented and erythematous" skin lesions were noted.

X-rays prior to the onset of osteolysis demonstrate decreased mineralization of the hand bones and increased caliber of phalanges, metacarpals, and long tubular bones of the upper limbs with thinning of cortical bone. Osteolysis of carpal and tarsal bones is usually bilaterally symmetric but may be unilateral. In the most advanced case (age 10 years), complete loss of all carpal bones and extensive lysis of tarsal bones was found with increased caliber, osteoporosis, and cortical thinning of nonaxial tubular bones. The phalanges demonstrated focal areas of resorption. There was a notable lack of metacarpal erosion or resorption of long tubular bone with the exception of the distal epiphyses of the radius and ulna.

Length discrepancies of a limb may develop, apparently secondary to involvement of epiphyses of long tubular bones. In addition to the deformities due to bony loss at the wrist and ankle, flexion contractures of elbows and knees and deformities of metacarpophalangeal and interphalangeal joints gradually develop.

Biopsy of a metacarpal bone demonstrated only osteopenia; the subcutaneous nodules showed only normal fibrofatty tissue, and the hyperpigmented skin lesions demonstrated normal histology.

Laboratory studies in a 7-year-old boy revealed increased erythrocyte sedimentation rate (ESR) and +1 latex fixation; all other blood and urine studies were normal.

The original family as described by Torg and Steel (1968) is thought to demonstrate an autosomal recessively transmitted trait as there was consanguinity and expression in one generation only with 3/6 children affected.

**Complications:** Limb length discrepancies and contractures at multiple small and large joints may occur. Painful joint limitation may compromise function as does deformity secondary to bony loss (volar subluxation of the hand and pes cavum).

**Associated Findings:** None known.

**Etiology:** The pattern is consistent with either autosomal recessive or X-linked recessive inheritance.

**Pathogenesis:** Unknown.

**MIM No.:** 25960

**CDC No.:** 756.580

**Sex Ratio:** M3:F0 Observed.

**Occurrence:** One family reported.

**Risk of Recurrence for Patient's Sib:**
See Part I, *Mendelian Inheritance*.

**Risk of Recurrence for Patient's Child:**
See Part I, *Mendelian Inheritance*.

**Age of Detectability:** Two to six years by clinical and X-ray examinations.

**Gene Mapping and Linkage:** Unknown.

**Prevention:** None known. Genetic counseling indicated.

**Treatment:** Orthopedic care may be appropriate for specific developmental deformities, but the lifelong natural history of the untreated condition is not known, and the potential benefits of orthopedic modalities such as casting, bracing, physical therapy medication, and/or surgery can only be surmized.

**Prognosis:** Unknown for life span (oldest reported patient reached at least early teens), apparently normal for intelligence, variable for function, but probably poor for hand and foot function depending on degree and extent of osteolysis.

**Detection of Carrier:** Unknown.

**Special Considerations:** The various aseptic necrosis syndromes and acro-osteolysis syndromes are distinguished by the distribution and extent of the lesions. Subcutaneous nodules, elevated ESR, swelling and tenderness, and a positive latex fixation may suggest **Arthritis, rheumatoid**, but biopsy materials fail to reveal the characteristic pathologic changes. The lack of generalized joint stiffness and other skeletal disorders separates this syndrome from the osteoarthropathy of Schinz and Furtwaengler. Lack of corneal opacity, coarse face, and generalized osteoporosis distinguish this from **Winchester syndrome**.

Several other conditions involving idiopathic osteolysis are known. These include Gorham disease (massive osteolysis or disappearing bone disease) in which generalized intraosseous hemangiomatosis has been described; essential multifocal osteolysis with nephropathy, a progressive nonfamilial disorder characterized by carpo-tarsal osteolysis and progressive nephropathy; and idiopathic hereditary osteolysis with dominant transmission but without nephropathy, a disorder in which an inherent vascular abnormality has been hypothesized.

Advances in the cellular biology of bone modeling and remodeling, along with specific noncollagenous protein markers of bone metabolism and undercalcified processing of bone biopsy specimens following dynamic tetracycline labeling hold promise of bringing a more basic understanding to these complex but related disorders.

**References:**
Abell JM, Badgley CE: Disappearing bone disease. JAMA 1961; 177: 771.

Halliday DR, et al.: Massive osteolysis and angiomatosis. Radiology 1964; 82:637.

Shurtleff DB, et al.: Hereditary osteolysis with hypertension and nephropathy JAMA 1964; 188:363.

Torg JS, Steel HH: Essential osteolysis with nephropathy: case report of an unusual syndrome. J Bone Joint Surg 1968; 50A:1629.

Torg JS, et al.: Hereditary multicentric osteolysis with recessive transmission: a new syndrome. J Pediatr 1969; 75:243–252.

Kohler E, et al.: Hereditary osteolysis. Radiology 1973; 108:99.

KA033
B0025

**Frederick S. Kaplan**
**Zvi Borochowitz**
*David L. Rimoin*

**Osteolysis-proteinuria**
See *OSTEOLYSIS, CARPAL-TARSAL AND CHRONIC PROGRESSIVE GLOMERULOPATHY*

**Osteolysis. essential hereditary, of carpal bones-nephropathy**
See *OSTEOLYSIS, CARPAL-TARSAL AND CHRONIC PROGRESSIVE GLOMERULOPATHY*

**Osteomata, multiple compact**
See *EAR, EXOSTOSES*

**Osteomesopycnose**
See *OSTEOMESOPYKNOSIS*

## OSTEOMESOPYKNOSIS 2695

**Includes:**
Axial osteosclerosis
Osteomesopycnose

**Excludes:**
**Craniometaphyseal dysplasia** (0228)
**Dysosteosclerosis** (0310)
Osteomalacia, atypical axial
**Osteopetrosis, benign dominant** (0779)
**Pyknodysostosis** (0846)

**Major Diagnostic Criteria:** X-rays show osteosclerosis localized to the axial spine, the pelvis, and the proximal part of the long bones.

**Clinical Findings:** Osteomesopycnosis is usually discovered because of chronic lower back pain. Sometimes, the patient is asymptomatic and is diagnosed on incidental X-rays or because of a genetic analysis of his family. Physical examination is normal, except for tenderness in the back or moderate dorsal kyphosis.

X-ray examination reveals the increased bone density in the vertebral bodies, the pelvis, and the proximal part of the femora. Sclerosis does not involve the skull, clavicles, ribs, hands, feet, or tubular bones other than the proximal part of the femora. Inconstantly the height of the vertebral bodies may be slightly reduced with an ovalar form. A "sandwich" appearance can develop with the densification of the upper and lower plates or more in homogenous patches of osteosclerosis. A radiolucent defect has been described in the proximal part of the femur in three patients.

**Complications:** The severe complications of osteopetrosis are absent.

**Associated Findings:** Tubular acidosis and abnormal aminoaciduria were reported in one case.

**Etiology:** Probably autosomal dominant inheritance.

**Pathogenesis:** Unknown.

**MIM No.:** 16645

**POS No.:** 4457

**CDC No.:** 756.580

**Sex Ratio:** M1:F1

**Occurrence:** At least six kinships have been reported.

**Risk of Recurrence for Patient's Sib:**
See Part I, *Mendelian Inheritance*.

**Risk of Recurrence for Patient's Child:**
See Part I, *Mendelian Inheritance*.

**Age of Detectability:** During adolescence or in the young adult for chronic lower back pain.

**Gene Mapping and Linkage:** Unknown.

**Prevention:** None known. Genetic counseling indicated.

**Treatment:** Physiotherapy.

**Prognosis:** Functional impairment is possible. Should be clearly distinguished from **Osteopetrosis, benign dominant** because of their different prognoses.

**Detection of Carrier:** Examination of relatives for evidence of vertebral anomalies.

**References:**
Simon D, et al.: Une ostéosclérose axiale de transmission dominante autosomique: une nouvelle entité? Rev Rhum 1979; 46:375–382.

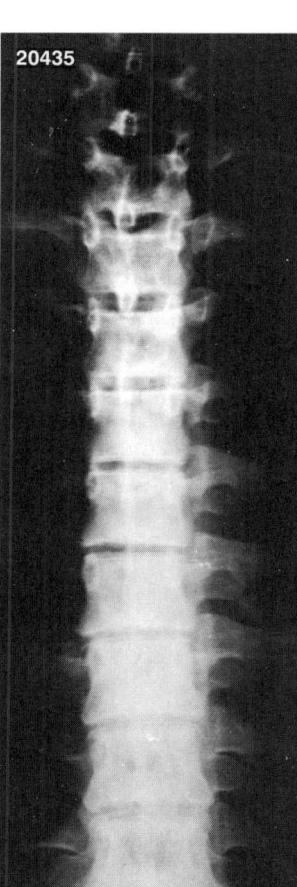

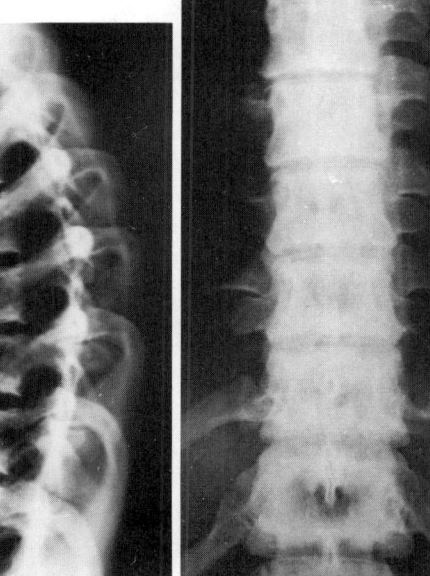

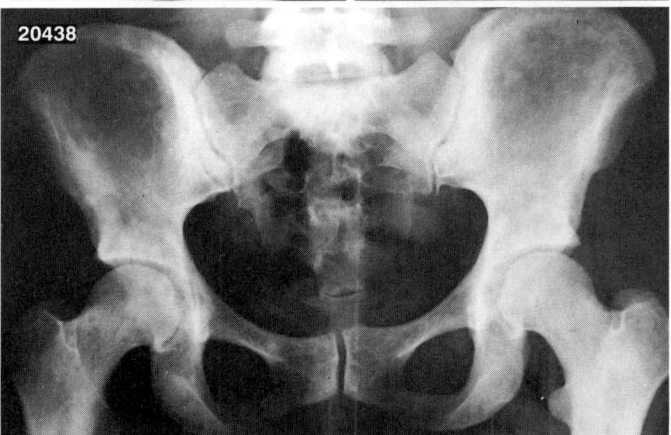

**2695**-20284: Sclerosis of vertebral bodies. 20435: Increased density of the upper and lower vertebral plates; these changes are similar to those seen in osteopetrosis except in osteomesopycnosis the long bones are normal except for the proximal femur. 20438: Sclerosis in the pelvis.

Maroteaux P: L'ostéomésopycnose: une nouvelle affection conden-sante de transmission dominante autosomique. Arch Fr Pédiatr 1980; 37:153–157. *

Stoll CG, et al.: Osteomesopyknosis: an autosomal dominant osteo-sclerosis. Am J Med Genet 1981; 8:349–353.

Maroteaux P, et al.: Four recently described osteochondrodysplasias. In: Papadatos CJ, Bartsocas CS, eds: Skeletal dysplasias. New York: Alan R. Liss, 1982:345–350.

Proschek R, et al.: Osteomesopyknosis: case report. J Bone Joint Surg 1985; 67A:652–653.

Griffith TM, et al.: Osteomesopyknosis benign axial osteosclerosis. Br J Radiol 1988; 61:951–953.

Delcambre B, et al.: Osteomesopyknosis: report of two new cases. Skeletal Radiol 1989; 18:21–24.

MA034                                                                  **Pierre Maroteaux**

**Osteopathia hyperostotica scleroticans multiplex infantilis**
*See DIAPHYSEAL DYSPLASIA*

---

## OSTEOPATHIA STRIATA                                                  0778

**Includes:**
Osteopathia striata with pigmentary dermopathy-white forelock
Voorhoeve disease

**Excludes:**
**Osteopathia striata-cranial sclerosis** (2237)
**Osteopoikilosis** (0781)

**Major Diagnostic Criteria:** The typical X-ray appearance of longi-tudinal striations of osteosclorosis in the long bones.

**Clinical Findings:** Patients with striated bony lesions have been reported with dermatofibrosis lenticularis, and in families with osteopoikilosis.

X-rays show longitudinal striations in the long bones, beginning at the epiphyseal line and most prominently in the metaphyses. Irregular fan-like striations are seen in the ilium. Increased bone density has been reported in the skull and ribs. Thickening of the cranial vault, with projection of dense bone from the inner table, and obliteration of the sinuses has been observed, but this condition may be a separate entity. No abnormal laboratory results have been reported. Unilateral involvement has been reported.

**Complications:** Conductive deafness has been reported in two cases, probably resulting from the narrow auditory canals, fixation of the ossicular chain, and loss of mastoid air cells.

**Associated Findings:** Reduced intelligence has been reported in two patients, cleft palate in two cases, and premature cortical cataracts have been reported in one patient. Dermatofibrosis lenticularis has also been reported. Osteopathis striata is fre-quently seen in **Dermal hypoplasia, focal**. Associated X-ray findings include small areas of translucency in the metaphysis, localized thinning of the cortex, and small exostoses.

**Etiology:** Undetermined. An X-linked variant with dermopathy and white forelock has been described.

**Pathogenesis:** Pathology has been reported to be similar to **Osteopetrosis** in involved areas, with loss of lamellar structure due to the obliteration of canaliculi. The pathogenesis is unknown, although similar lesions have been produced in mice by inhibition of resorption of metaphyseal spongiosa with estrogens.

**MIM No.:** 31128

**POS No.:** 3795

**CDC No.:** 756.580

**Sex Ratio:** Presumably M1:F1, except in X-linked instances.

**Occurrence:** Over a dozen cases documented, plus three sisters reported with X-linked variant.

**Risk of Recurrence for Patient's Sib:** Unknown.

**Risk of Recurrence for Patient's Child:** Unknown.

**Age of Detectability:** Usually detected in adults as an incidental X-ray finding, although it is probably detectable in childhood, and severe cases may be detected prenatally.

**Gene Mapping and Linkage:** Unknown.

**Prevention:** None known. Genetic counseling indicated.

**Treatment:** Hearing aid and surgical mobilization of the ossicles may be necessary for accompanying deafness.

**Prognosis:** Normal for life span, probably normal for intelligence and function, except for possible loss of hearing or sight.

**Detection of Carrier:** Unknown.

**References:**

Hurt RL: Osteopathia striata-Voorhoeve's disease; report of a case presenting the features of osteopathia striata and osteopetrosis. J Bone Joint Surg 1953; 35B:89.

Walker BA: Osteopathia striata with cataracts and deafness. BD:OAS V(4). White Plains: The National Foundation-March of Dimes, 1969:295–297.

Larregue M, et al.: L'osteopathie striee, symptome radiologique de l'hypoplasie dermique en aires. Ann Radiol 1972; 15:287–295.

Horan FT, Beighton PH: Osteopathia striata with cranial sclerosis: an autosomal dominant entity. Clin Genet 1978; 13:201–206.

Whyte MP, Murphy WA: Osteopathia striata associated with familial dermopathy and white forelock: evidence for postnatal development of osteopathia striata. Am J Med Genet 1980; 5:227–234.

Coutina H, et al.: Familial osteopathia striata with cranial condensation. Pediatr Radiol 1981; 11:87–90.

LA006

Ralph S. Lachman

**Osteopathia striata with pigmentary dermopathy-white forelock**
*See OSTEOPATHIA STRIATA*

---

## OSTEOPATHIA STRIATA-CRANIAL SCLEROSIS-MEGALENCEPHALY      2237

**Includes:**
    Cranial sclerosis-osteopathia striata-macrocephaly
    Hyperostosis generalisata with striations
    Megalencephaly-cranial sclerosis-osteopathia striata

**Excludes:**
    Cranial sclerosis (others)
    **Dermal hypoplasia, focal** (0281)
    **Osteopathia striata** (0778)

**Major Diagnostic Criteria:** **Osteopathia striata**, non-progressive **Megalencephaly** (head circumference paralleling the normal curve), and progressive cranial sclerosis.

**Clinical Findings:** **Megalencephaly** with prominant forehead, hypoplastic orbital ridges, and moderate **Eye, hypertelorism.**

X-ray features: longitudinal striations of tubular bones and pelvis, progressive sclerosis of cranial bones, gradual development of generalized hyperostosis.

**Complications:** Neurosensory deafness, facial nerve palsy.

**Associated Findings:** **Cleft palate**, mental retardation.

**Etiology:** Autosomal dominant inheritance with high penetrance but variable expressivity.

**Pathogenesis:** Osteopathia striata has been attributed to persistence of the fetal pattern of bone trabeculation.

**MIM No.:** *16650

**POS No.:** 4249

**CDC No.:** 756.580

**Sex Ratio:** Presumably M1:F1, but current observed M1:F2.

**Occurrence:** About 25 cases have been reported.

**Risk of Recurrence for Patient's Sib:**
    See Part I, *Mendelian Inheritance.*

**Risk of Recurrence for Patient's Child:**
    See Part I, *Mendelian Inheritance.*

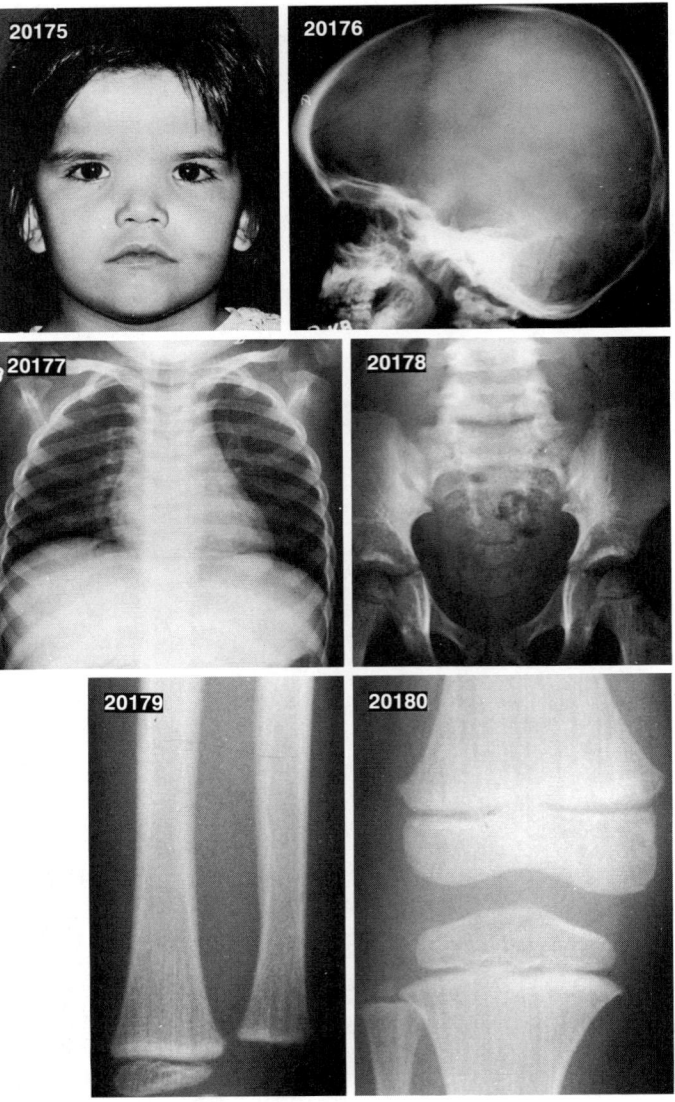

**2237-20175:** Note prominent forehead, hypertelorism, telecanthus and hypoplastic orbital ridges. **20176:** Lateral skull X-ray shows craniomegaly, thickened frontal bone, sclerosis of the skull base, poor mastoid pneumatization and lack of sinus aeration. **20177:** Chest X-ray shows generalized hyperostosis with widening of the ribs. **20178:** Longitudinal striations appear in the proximal femora and central ilia. **20179:** Striations appear in the distal ulna and radius. **20180:** Striations in distal femora and proximal tibia. There is no cortical thickening, periosteal new bone formation or defective tubular modeling.

---

**Age of Detectability:** Usually in infancy or childhood. One familial case was diagnosed prenatally by ultrasonography.

**Gene Mapping and Linkage:** Unknown.

**Prevention:** None known. Genetic counseling indicated.

**Treatment:** Unknown.

**Prognosis:** Hyperostosis, usually progressive, is in some cases stationary. Life span is normal. No functional impairment except for rare cases with facial palsy or neurosensory deafness.

**Detection of Carrier:** Skeletal X-rays may detect previously unsuspected heterozygotes.

**Special Considerations:** The triad of osteopathia striata, macrocephaly, and cranial sclerosis was first delineated in 1978 by Horan and Beighton. Classification of several earlier published cases of osteopathia striata combined with **Osteopoikilosis** or with generalized osteosclerosis and medullary expansion remains uncertain.

**References:**
Horan FT, Beighton PH: Osteopathia striata with cranial sclerosis: an autosomal dominant entity. Clin Genet 1978; 13:201–206. * †
Winter RM, et al.: Osteopathia striata with cranial sclerosis: highly variable expression within a family including cleft palate in two neonatal cases. Clin Genet 1980; 18:462–474.
Robinow M, Unger F: Syndrome of osteopathia striata, macrocephaly, and cranial sclerosis. Am J Dis Child 1984; 138:821–823. * †

R0004                                              **Meinhard Robinow**

**Osteopathic childhood osteoporosis**
  See OSTEOPOROSIS, JUVENILE IDIOPATHIC
**Osteoperiostosis, secondary hypertrophic with pernio**
  See DIGITAL DEFECTS-NODULAR ERYTHEMA-EMACIATION, NAKAJO TYPE
**Osteopetrosis tardia**
  See OSTEOPETROSIS, BENIGN DOMINANT
**Osteopetrosis with late manifestation**
  See OSTEOPETROSIS, BENIGN DOMINANT
**Osteopetrosis, benign adult form of**
  See OSTEOPETROSIS, BENIGN DOMINANT

---

## OSTEOPETROSIS, BENIGN DOMINANT                     0779

**Includes:**
  Albers-Schonberg disease
  Marble bone disease
  Osteopetrosis, benign adult form of
  Osteopetrosis, dominant
  Osteopetrosis tardia
  Osteopetrosis with late manifestation
  Osteosclerosis fragilis generalisata

**Excludes:**
  **Craniometaphyseal dysplasia** (0228)
  **Diaphyseal dysplasia** (0290)
  **Dysosteosclerosis** (0310)
  Hyperostosis generalisata
  Leontiasis ossea
  **Osteopetrosis** (other)
  **Osteopoikilosis** (0781)
  **Pyknodysostosis** (0846)

**Major Diagnostic Criteria:** The clinical features are variable. X-rays shows pathologic fractures, dental abscesses, and cranial hyperostosis later in life. Serum chemistry shows elevated acid phosphatase levels in some cases.

**Clinical Findings:** Clinically the disorder is detected later in life, usually in adolescence, and sometimes upon routine X-ray of the chest. It is characterized by a generalized sclerosis of the bone, with marked variability in its clinical manifestations.

Close to 50% of patients are asymptomatic and are diagnosed on incidental X-rays or because of genetic analysis of their family due to a more severely affected relative. The most common problem in this disorder is pathologic fractures; 40% of reported cases had a history of fractures. About 10% have osteomyelitis of the mandible. Dental abscesses are frequent.

Bone pain, primarily of the lumbar spine, occurs in 20% of patients. The cranial hyperostosis may result in cranial nerve palsies which have been described in 16% of cases. The nerves most commonly affected are the 2nd, 3rd, and 7th cranial nerves, resulting in optic atrophy, extraocular muscle palsies, and facial palsy. Frontal bossing, exophthalmos, or facial palsies may result in a peculiar facial appearance. There is marked intrafamilial variability in the clinical features of this disorder, and nonpenetrance has been described. Hepatosplenomegaly and severe anemia are usually not features of the dominant form of osteopetro-

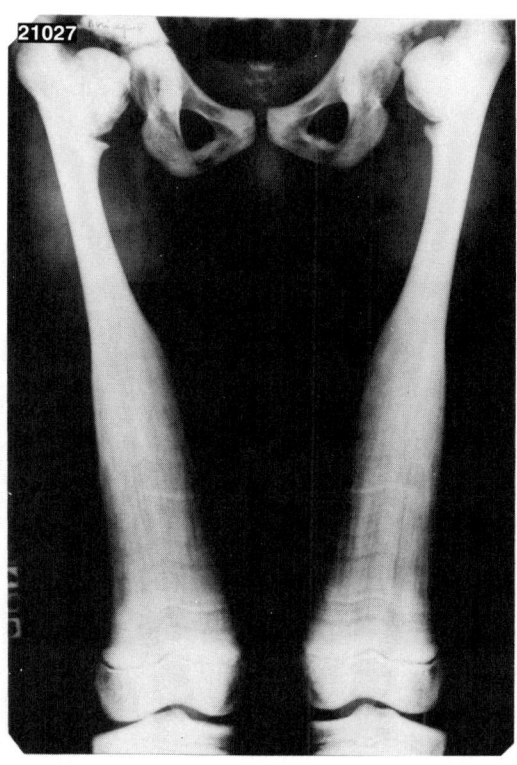

**0779A**-21027:  Osteopetrosis, autosomal dominant; note generalized sclerosis and parallel radiolucent striations in the metaphyseal region.

---

sis. Elevated serum acid phosphatase levels have been found in almost all reported cases, but other serum chemistries and calcium balance studies have been normal.

Skeletal X-rays reveal a generalized sclerotic process. The earliest features are an increase in the density of the diaphyseal regions of the growing bone, with parallel radiolucent striations in the metaphyseal regions. The vertebral bodies may develop a "sandwich" appearance, with sclerosis of the upper and lower plates and an intervening less dense appearance. The tubular bones, especially the metacarpals, may show a "bone within a bone" appearance. The skull is thickened and dense, especially at the base. The sinuses decrease in size and even disappear.

Histologic examination of the affected bones shows absence of a true medullary cavity with noncalcified hyaline cartilage remnants scattered diffusely within the bone. The bone itself is made up primarily of Haversian systems with scanty fibrillar composition. Foci of osteoblastic and osteoclastic activity can be seen.

**Complications:** Teeth are affected by dental abscesses and osteomyelitis. Pathologic fractures occur following minor trauma.

**Associated Findings:** Cranial nerve palsy, strabismus.

**Etiology:** Autosomal dominant inheritance with variable expressivity. Could be non-penetrant.

**Pathogenesis:** Of several hypotheses, the most favored is defective resorption of primary spongiosa by abnormal osteoclasts, which results in increased osseous density.

**MIM No.:** *16660

**CDC No.:** 756.540

**Sex Ratio:** M1:F1

**Occurrence:** About 1:100,000, based on data from Brazil.

**Risk of Recurrence for Patient's Sib:**
  See Part I, *Mendelian Inheritance.*

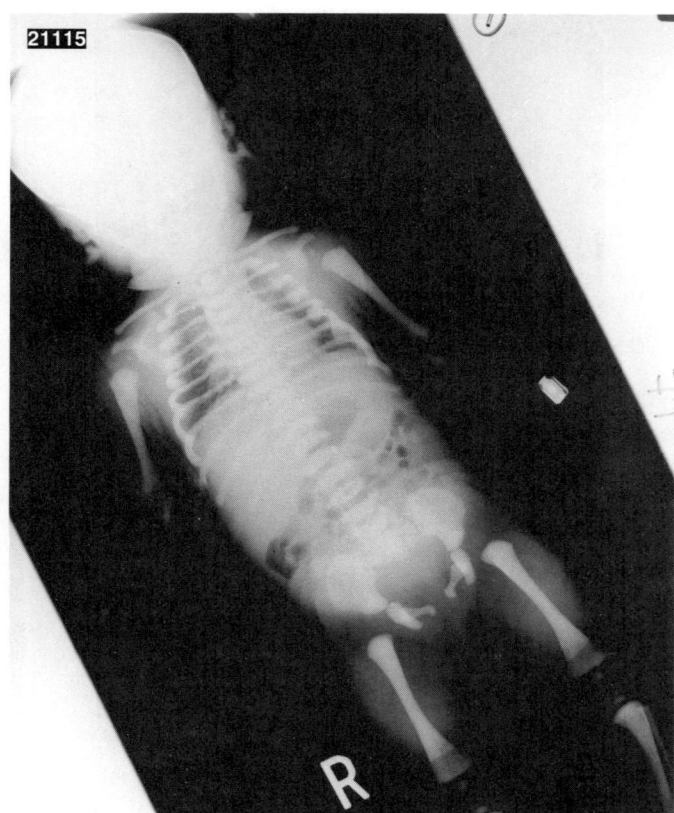

0779B-21115: X-ray of an infant shows increased bone density.

**Risk of Recurrence for Patient's Child:**
See Part I, *Mendelian Inheritance.*

**Age of Detectability:** Clinically not remarkable within the first several years of life, but could be detected early by skeletal X-rays. It is often not diagnosed until adolescence or adulthood.

**Gene Mapping and Linkage:** Unknown.

**Prevention:** None known. Genetic counseling indicated.

**Treatment:** Successful use of calcitriol has been reported. Calcitriol is a metabolite of vitamin D with a bone-resorbing effect.

**Prognosis:** Life span is not affected.

**Detection of Carrier:** Unknown.

**Special Considerations:** This disorder is distinct from the congenital malignant form of the disease, both clinically and genetically. Severe anemia and hepatosplenomegaly are not features of this dominant disorder. Any adolescent or adult with the X-ray features of osteopetrosis will almost certainly have the dominant form of the disease. This disease must be differentiated from the other forms of skeletal sclerosis such as fluorosis, heavy metal intoxication, **Craniometaphyseal dysplasia**, **Osteopoikilosis**, Camurati-Engelmann disease, **Cranio-diaphyseal dysplasia**, Schwarz-Lélek syndrome, **Endosteal hyperostosis**, **Sclerosteosis**, and **Pyknodysostosis**.

**Support Groups:** PA; West Chester; American Brittle Bone Society (ABBS)

**References:**
Ghormley RK: A case of congenital osteosclerosis. Bull Johns Hopkins Hosp 1922; 33:444–446.
Welford NP: Facial paralysis associated with osteopetrosis (marble bones). J Pediatr 1959; 55:67–72.
Salzano FM: Osteopetrosis: review of dominant cases and frequency in a Brazilian state. Acta Genet Med Gemellol (Roma) 1961; 10:353–358.
Johnston CC Jr, et al.: Osteopetrosis. Medicine 1968; 47:149–167. *
Beighton P, et al.: A review of the osteopetroses. Postgrad Med J 1977; 53:507–515.
Key L, et al.: Treatment of congenital osteopetrosis with high dose calcitrol. New Engl J Med 1984; 310:409–415.

CE003

Jaroslav Červenka
David L. Rimoin
David W. Hollister

**Osteopetrosis, dominant**
*See OSTEOPETROSIS, BENIGN DOMINANT*
**Osteopetrosis, intermediate type**
*See OSTEOPETROSIS, MILD RECESSIVE*

## OSTEOPETROSIS, MALIGNANT RECESSIVE     0780

**Includes:**
    Albers-Schonberg disease
    Carbonic anhydrase II deficiency
    Guibaud-Vainsel syndrome
    Infantile malignant osteopetrosis
    Lethal osteopetrosis
    Malignant congenital osteopetrosis
    Marble bone disease
    Marble brain disease
    Osteopetrosis-renal tubular acidosis

**Excludes:**
    **Craniometaphyseal dysplasia** (0228)
    **Diaphyseal dysplasia** (0290)
    **Dysosteosclerosis** (0310)
    **Osteopetrosis** (other)
    **Osteopoikilosis** (0781)

**Major Diagnostic Criteria:** Skeletal X-rays show sclerosis of all bones. Serum chemistry sometimes shows hypocalcemia and hyperphosphatemia. Clinically, early onset of deafness, blindness, severe anemia, hepatosplenomegaly, facial paralysis, and macrocephaly is observed.

**Clinical Findings:** Dense brittle bones, macrocephaly, progressive deafness and blindness, hepatosplenomegaly, and severe anemia beginning in early infancy or in utero. Affected children may be stillborn or exhibit failure to thrive; they may die in infancy

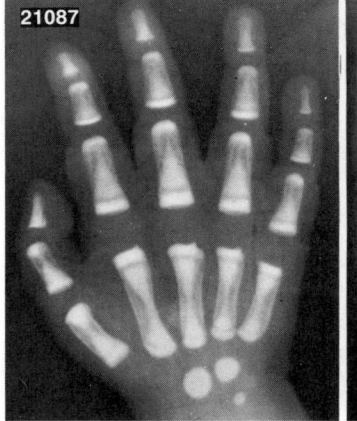
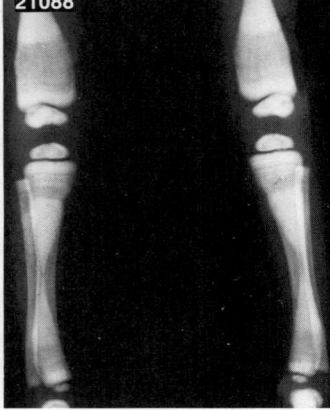

0780-21087: Hand X-ray shows the "bone within a bone" appearance in the tubular bones. 21088: The long bones are undermodelled and the lower femoral metaphyses have a club-shaped configuration. The bones show regions of lucency and increased density.

or early childhood. The osteosclerotic process impinges on the marrow cavity, resulting in severe anemia and pancytopenia with extramedullary hematopoiesis producing hepatosplenomegaly and lymphadenopathy, often with nucleated red blood cells in the peripheral blood (myeloid metaplasia). Cranial sclerosis may result in macrocephaly and hydrocephaly, as well as impingement on the cranial nerve foramina, leading to blindness with optic or retinal atrophy, deafness, facial palsies, and strabismus. Dentition may be delayed and severe dental caries has been reported. Growth and developmental retardation are common, but intelligence is normal in over 75% of cases. The sclerotic skeletal system predisposes to pathologic fractures and osteomyelitis. Serum chemistry is usually normal, although hypocalcemia and hyperphosphatemia may be detected and tetany has been described.

Skeletal X-rays reveal uniformly dense sclerotic bones, with associated metaphyseal splaying and clubbing. The medullary canals and trabecular patterns are obliterated. Radiolucent streaks appear in the long bone metaphyses, while the epiphyses are sclerotic but of normal contour. The skull is thickened, particularly at the base, with narrowing of the cranial foramina. The mastoids and paranasal sinuses are poorly aerated. The metacarpals and metatarsals may appear block-shaped, with a "bone in bone" appearance, and there may be partial aplasia of the distal phalanges. The vertebrae are of normal shape, but the ribs appear flared.

Histologic examination of bone reveals obliteration of the medullary cavity by a lattice-like network of hyaline cartilage surrounded by thick bone that exhibits a paucity of fibrils. Foci of osteoblastic and osteoclastic activity can be seen.

**Complications:** Cranial nerve palsies and facial paralysis, deafness, strabismus, nystagmus, blindness, anemia, failure to thrive, and short life span.

**Associated Findings:** A possible form in which osteoclasts are markedly reduced was reported by El Khazen et al (1986) and designated *lethal osteopetrosis*.

**Etiology:** Autosomal recessive inheritance.

**Pathogenesis:** Several hypotheses have been proposed. It appears likely that the abnormality of osteoclasts leads to the disease. Dysfunctioning osteoclasts then fail in resorption of primary spongiosa.

**MIM No.:** *25970, *25973, 25972

**POS No.:** 3374

**CDC No.:** 756.540

**Sex Ratio:** M1:F1

**Occurrence:** Less than 100 cases have been reported. A high frequency has been observed in Costa Rica.

**Risk of Recurrence for Patient's Sib:**
See Part I, *Mendelian Inheritance*.

**Risk of Recurrence for Patient's Child:**
See Part I, *Mendelian Inheritance*. Affected individuals are not expected to survive to reproduce.

**Age of Detectability:** Usually at birth. Prenatal diagnosis is made by X-ray, revealing a generalized sclerotic skeletal system.

**Gene Mapping and Linkage:** Unknown.

**Prevention:** None known. Genetic counseling indicated.

**Treatment:** Steroid therapy has been reported to be of some value, and an increasing experience with bone marrow transplantation has demonstrated that the disease can be greatly ameliorated.

**Prognosis:** Survival past the age of 20 years is rare. Death in infancy or childhood is usually due to anemia or secondary infection.

**Detection of Carrier:** Unknown.

**Special Considerations:** The eponym *Albers-Schonberg disease* is usually reserved for the benign dominant form of this disorder (see **Osteopetrosis, benign dominant**).

Autosomal recessive osteopetrosis with renal tubular acidosis, also known as *carbonic anhydrase II deficiency, Guibaud-Vainsel syndrome* and *marble brain disease* (Sly et al, 1985) is a separate entity. Affected individuals have reduced intelligence, short stature, pancytopenia, basal ganglion calcification, renal tubular acidosis, and deficiency of carbonic anhydrase II in erythrocytes. This is a severe form of osteopetrosis, with early onset.

**Support Groups:** PA; West Chester; American Brittle Bone Society (ABBS)

**References:**

Moe PJ, Skjaeveland A: Therapeutic studies in osteopetrosis. Acta Paediatr Scand 1969; 58:593–600.

Loria-Cortés R, et al.: Osteopetrosis in children: a report of 26 cases. J Pediatr 1977; 91:43–47. *

Beighton P, Cremin BJ: Sclerosing bone dysplasias. New York: Springer Verlag, 1980. *

Coccia PF, et al.: Successful bone-marrow transplantation for infantile malignant osteopetrosis. New Engl J Med 1980; 302:701–708.

Sorrel M, et al.: Marrow transplantation for juvenile osteopetrosis. Am J Med 1981; 70:1280–1287.

Sieff CA, et al.: Allogeneic bone-marrow transplantation in infantile malignant osteopetrosis. Lancet 1983; I:437–441.

Sly WS, et al.: Carbonic anhydrase II deficiency in 12 families with the autosomal recessive syndrome of osteopetrosis with renal tubular acidosis and cerebral calcification. New Engl J Med 1985; 313:139–145.

El Khazen N, et al.: Lethal osteopetrosis with multiple fractures in utero. Am J Med Genet 1986; 23:811–819.

Fischer A, et al.: Bone-marrow transplantation for immunodeficiencies and osteopetrosis: European survey 1968–1985. Lancet 1986; II:1080–1084.

Bollerslev J: Osteopetrosis: a genetic and epidemiologic study. Clin Genet 1987; 31:86–90.

CE003

**Jaroslav Červenka**
*David L. Rimoin*
*David W. Hollister*

---

## OSTEOPETROSIS, MILD RECESSIVE     2253

**Includes:** Osteopetrosis, intermediate type

**Excludes:**
   **Osteopetrosis, benign dominant** (0779)
   **Osteopetrosis, malignant recessive** (0780)
   **Renal tubular acidosis-osteopetrosis syndrome** (3086)

**Major Diagnostic Criteria:** Characteristic X-ray changes, including sclerosis of the cranial base, generally increased bone density, sclerosis of the vertebral end plates, and transverse bands and poor diaphyseal modeling of the long bones. Pedigree consistent with autosomal recessive inheritance.

**Clinical Findings:** Physical findings include relative or absolute short stature, with increased upper/lower segment ratio and decreased arm span. Mandibular prognathism may also be a feature, along with dental abnormalities. Patients have often been asymptomatic in childhood, except for increased susceptibility to fractures or mandibular osteomyelitis. The X-ray changes are probably present from early childhood. Clinical manifestations are much milder than in **Osteopetrosis, malignant recessive**.

**Complications:** Osteomyelitis, especially mandibular actinomycosis; mild anemia due to marrow encroachment, with compensatory extramedullary hematopoiesis; impacted teeth; fractures.

**Associated Findings:** Midface hypoplasia was thought to be part of the syndrome in one family. Acid or alkaline phosphatase was elevated in some patients.

**Etiology:** Autosomal recessive inheritance.

**Pathogenesis:** Unknown.

**MIM No.:** 25971

**CDC No.:** 756.540

**Sex Ratio:** M12:F6 (observed).

**Occurrence:** About 20 cases have been documented.

**Risk of Recurrence for Patient's Sib:**
See Part I, *Mendelian Inheritance*.

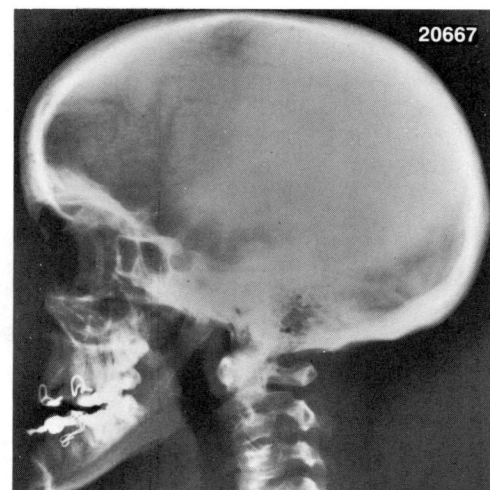

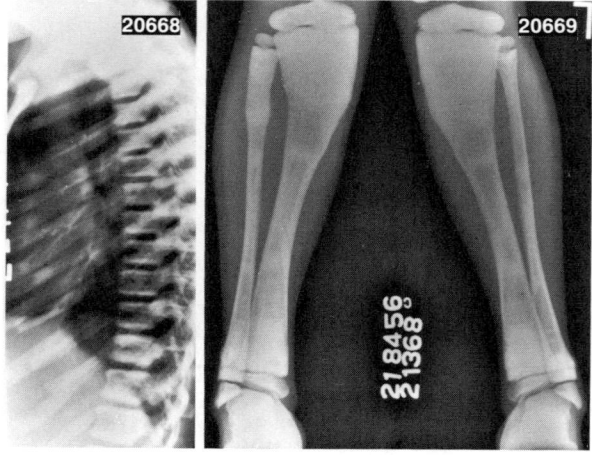

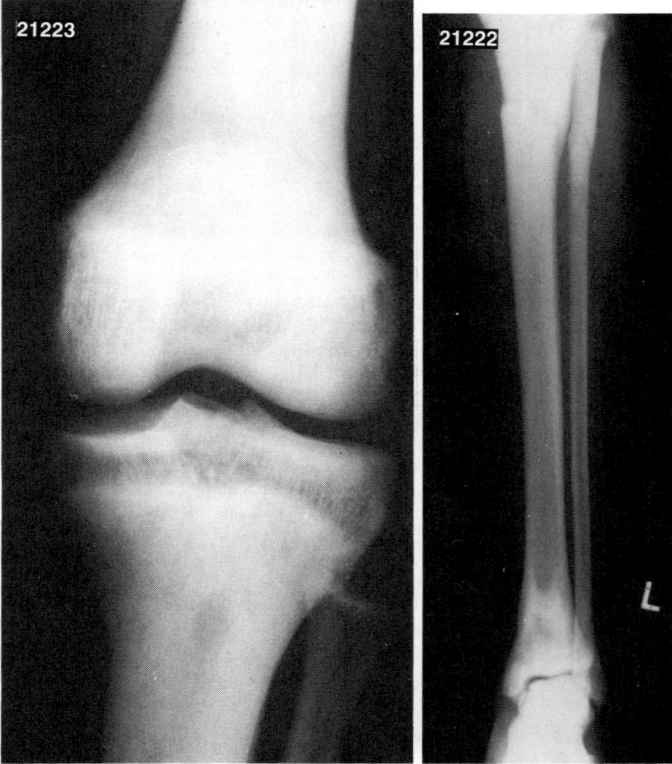

**2253B**-21223: The bones are brittle with a propensity to fracture. 21222: The tubular bones are sclerotic but their external contours are undisturbed. Note the transverse fracture of the tibia and fibula.

**2253A**-20667: Osteoporosis, mild autosomal recessive type; note lateral view of the skull shows marked thickening of the base. The cranium also shows increased bone density and there is mid-face hypoplasia. 20668: Lateral view of the spine shows increased density at the ends of the vertebral bodies ("rugger-jersey" appearance), and widening and increased density of the ribs. 20669: AP view of the lower legs shows generalized increased density of bone with horizontal areas of greater and lesser density, widening of the metaphyses, and deformation of the shaft of the long bones.

**Support Groups:** PA; West Chester; American Brittle Bone Society (ABBS)

**References:**
Trias A, Fery A: Osteopetrosis in adults. Rev Chir Orthop 1974; 60:593–606.
Beighton P, et al.: Osteopetrosis in South Africa. S Afr Med J 1979; 55:659–665.
Horton WA, et al.: Osteopetrosis: further heterogeneity. J Pediatr 1980; 97:580–585.
Kahler SG, et al.: A mild autosomal recessive form of osteopetrosis. Am J Med Genet 1984; 17:451–464. * †

KA002                             **Stephen G. Kahler**

**Osteopetrosis-renal tubular acidosis**
*See OSTEOPETROSIS, MALIGNANT RECESSIVE*
**Osteopetrosis-renal tubular acidosis-cerebral calcification**
*See RENAL TUBULAR ACIDOSIS-OSTEOPETROSIS SYNDROME*

---

**OSTEOPOIKILOSIS**                                **0781**

**Includes:**
    Buscke-Ollendorf syndrome
    Dermatoosteopoikilosis
    Disseminated dermatofibrosis-osteopoikilosis
    Osteodermatopoikilosis
    Osteodysplasia enostotica
    Osteolysis, idiopathic multicentric
    "Spotted bones"
**Excludes:**
    **Chondrodysplasia punctata, X-linked dominant type (2730)**

---

**Risk of Recurrence for Patient's Child:**
See Part I, *Mendelian Inheritance.*

**Age of Detectability:** In childhood.

**Gene Mapping and Linkage:** Unknown.

**Prevention:** None known. Genetic counseling indicated.

**Treatment:** No specific treatment known. Osteomyelitis must be treated early and vigorously. Mandibular actinomycosis may be fatal, but it has been treated successfully with long-term penicillin augmented with hyperbaric oxygen. Dental abnormalities, fractures, and cranial nerve compression (optic, facial, and acoustic) may occur and require treatment.

**Prognosis:** Good for health and life span.

**Detection of Carrier:** Unknown.

Osteoblastic metastases
**Osteopetrosis, benign dominant** (0779)
Osteosclerosis of other etiologies

**Major Diagnostic Criteria:** Typical grain-to-pea size densities on X-rays.

**Clinical Findings:** This disorder is usually discovered accidently, by X-ray. The typical appearance is oval or round densities, oriented in longitudinal directions, and most abundant in the pelvis and shoulder girdles and in the epiphyses and metaphyses of the long bones. The skull is rarely involved. Although the round densities are rarely seen in the diaphyses, the distinct parallel lines of density extending from the epiphyseal line down into the diaphyses, as seen in osteopathia striata, may be found in patients with osteopoikilosis or in their relatives. This has led some observers to consider them as the same process. Dermatofibrosis lenticularis is the skin manifestation of the disorder, occurring in over 50% of patients with X-ray changes. These are raised, yellowish lesions, which may coalesce and form stripes. The common locations are the buttocks, thighs, back, and abdominal skin, but not the face. The skin lesions have been reported without the X-ray changes in families with osteopoikilosis. The eponym "Buscke-Ollendorf" is applied to the syndromic association of the bone and skin abnormalities.

**Complications:** Keloids.

**Associated Findings:** Fibrous nodules of the peritoneal lining. Associations that have been reported but may not be real are short stature, diabetes, cleft lip, scleroderma, palmar and plantar keratosis, subcutaneous fibrous nodules, and hyperostosis frontalis interna. Osteopoikilosis is usually innocuous, but a single report of the development of osteosarcoma may have serious implications. Spinal canal stenosis and basal cell nevus syndrome have also been recognized in persons with osteopoikilosis. The significance of these inter-relationships is undetermined.

**Etiology:** Autosomal dominant inheritance with incomplete penetrance. Skipped generations are common. The skin lesions and bony lesions may occur separately in the same family.

**Pathogenesis:** Appears to be a spotty hyperplasia of collagen in the corium and bone matrix. The bony lesions are due to a thickening of the trabecular spongiosa.

**MIM No.:** *16670

**CDC No.:** 756.560

**Sex Ratio:** Presumably M1:F1, although males are more frequently detected because they more frequently have X-rays for trauma, etc.

**Occurrence:** 1:20,000 X-rays in a German survey (Jonaseh, 1955).

**Risk of Recurrence for Patient's Sib:**
See Part I, *Mendelian Inheritance.*

**Risk of Recurrence for Patient's Child:**
See Part I, *Mendelian Inheritance.*

**Age of Detectability:** At birth, but has been detected prenatally.

**Gene Mapping and Linkage:** Unknown.

**Prevention:** None known. Genetic counseling indicated.

**Treatment:** Unknown.

**Prognosis:** Normal for life span, intelligence, and function.

**Detection of Carrier:** Unknown.

**References:**
Busch KFB: Familial disseminated osteosclerosis. Acta Radiol (Stockh) 1937; 18:693–714.
Danielsen L, et al.: Osteopoikilosis associated with dermatofibrosis lenticularis disseminata. Arch Dermatol 1969; 100:465–470.
Mindell ER, et al.: Osteosarcoma associated with osteopoikilosis: case report. J Bone Joint Surg (Am) 1978; 60:406 only.
Weisz GM: Lumbar spinal canal stenosis in osteopoikilosis. Clin Orthopaed 1982; 166:89–92.
Blinder G, et al.: Widespread osteolytic lesions of the long bones in the basal cell nevus syndrome. Skel Radiol 1984; 12:196–198.
Lagier R, et al.: Osteopoikilosis: a radiological and pathological study. Skel Radiol 1984; 11:161–168.
Verbov J, et al.: Disseminated dermatofibrosis osteopoikilosis. Clin Exper Derm 1986; 11:17–26.
Carnevale A, et al.: Idiopathic multicentric osteolysis with facial anomalies and nephropathy. Am J Med Genet 1987; 26:877–886.

BE008                                              **Peter Beighton**

---

## OSTEOPOROSIS, JUVENILE IDIOPATHIC                    0782

**Includes:**
Juvenile osteoporosis
Osteopathic childhood osteoporosis

**Excludes:**
**Osteogenesis imperfecta** (0777)
Osteoporosis secondary to any identifiable cause

**Major Diagnostic Criteria:** Fractures follow minor trauma in a previously normal child or adolescent who has no signs or family history of osteogenesis imperfecta. X-rays show diminished bone density in the absence of any defined underlying disease.

**Clinical Findings:** Juvenile osteoporosis is a disease of childhood and adolescence exhibiting marked clinical variability. The disease usually begins in the peripubertal period (age 8–13 years), but several younger cases (age 3–8 years) have been reported, and the disorder has been documented in at least one adult. The affected individuals are clinically normal, as are their X-rays, until the onset of fractures following minor trauma. The fractures usually occur in the vertebrae, but long bone fractures are also common. Metabolic studies indicate negative calcium balance, but serum calcium, phosphorus, and alkaline-phosphatases are often normal. Calcitriol (1,25 dihydroxycholecalciferol) deficiency has been documented in one case. X-rays typically show marked diminution in bone density. The disease can persist for many years, but usually remits, or markedly improves, within five years. Even after remission, severe sequelae due to spinal cord compression, malaligned long bones, and pseudoarthroses can persist. It has not been determined if these patients have an increased propensity for senile osteoporosis.

**Complications:** Bony deformities secondary to fractures lead to decreased height, kyphosis, protuberant sternum and malalignment of long bones, and pseudoarthroses.

**Associated Findings:** None known.

**Etiology:** Possibly autosomal recessive inheritance, but a clear inheritance pattern has not been established. This condition might not represent a single entity, but rather a heterogeneous group of disorders with a common clinical appearance. Dent (1969) has emphasized that the younger onset group (3–8 years) may comprise a distinct entity called *osteopathic childhood osteoporosis.*

**Pathogenesis:** Undetermined. Calcitriol deficiency and negative calcium balance have been documented.

**MIM No.:** 25975

**CDC No.:** 756.580

**Sex Ratio:** M1:F1

**Occurrence:** About 50 cases reported. Mild cases may go unrecognized.

**Risk of Recurrence for Patient's Sib:**
See Part I, *Mendelian Inheritance.*

**Risk of Recurrence for Patient's Child:**
See Part I, *Mendelian Inheritance.*

**Age of Detectability:** Early childhood to adulthood.

**Gene Mapping and Linkage:** Unknown.

**Prevention:** None known. Genetic counseling indicated.

**Treatment:** Avoidance of any activity that might cause fractures or exacerbate old fractures is recommended. Calcitriol was reported as helpful in one patient.

**Prognosis:** Normal life span and intelligence. Spontaneous remission is usual, but long standing cases have had severe residual damage.

**Detection of Carrier:** Unknown.

**Support Groups:** PA; Marshallton; American Brittle Bone Society

**References:**
Dent CE, Friedman M: Idiopathic juvenile osteoporosis. Q J Med 1965; 34:177–210. *
Dent CE: Idiopathic juvenile osteoporosis. BD:OAS V(4). New York: The National Foundation-March of Dimes, 1969:134–147. *
Marder HK, et al.: Calcitriol deficiency in idiopathic juvenile osteoporosis. Am J Dis Child 1982; 136:914–917.

AL006                                           **Kirk Aleck**

### Osteoporosis-ocular pseudoglioma
*See OSTEOPOROSIS-PSEUDOGLIOMA SYNDROME*

## OSTEOPOROSIS-PSEUDOGLIOMA SYNDROME          0783

**Includes:**
  Blindness (pseudogliomatous)-osteoporosis-mild mental retardation
  Osteogenesis imperfecta, ocular form
  Osteoporosis-ocular pseudoglioma

**Excludes:**
  **Osteogenesis imperfecta** (0777)
  **Osteoporosis** (all other forms)

**Major Diagnostic Criteria:** Blindness from "pseudogliomatous" retinal detachment causing phthisis bulbi; osteoporosis; fractures from minor accidents and deformities; and mild mental retardation.

**Clinical Findings:** Blindness in infancy is probably due to "pseudogliomatous" retinal detachment or from fetal uveitis, resulting in microphthalmia, phthisis bulbi, corneal opacity, and cataracts; calcification of the lens may occur. Osteoporosis of variable severity is manifested at age 2–3 years, sometimes resulting in incapacitating deformities secondary to multiple fractures from minor trauma. Vertebral deformities result in a short trunk. Ligaments are lax. Microcephaly and macular hypotonia are present in some. Mental retardation when present usually is of mild-to-borderline degree (special verbal abilities are occasionally seen, e.g. idiot savant). Hearing is usually normal. X-ray findings include osteoporosis, thin cortex, and coarse trabecular structure of long bones; spontaneous fractures, bowing of limbs, metaphyseal cysts, codfish vertebrae, and wormian bones.

**Complications:** Blindness, deformities, physical handicap, and mental deficiency.

**Associated Findings:** **Ventricular septal defect**.

**Etiology:** Autosomal recessive inheritance.

**Pathogenesis:** Unknown.

**MIM No.:** *25977

**POS No.:** 3711

**CDC No.:** 756.580

**Sex Ratio:** M1:F1

**Occurrence:** About a dozen families have been documented. May be more frequent in Mediterranean countries.

**Risk of Recurrence for Patient's Sib:**
  See Part I, *Mendelian Inheritance*.

**Risk of Recurrence for Patient's Child:**
  See Part I, *Mendelian Inheritance*.

**Age of Detectability:** Infancy (blindness) and early childhood (fractures and osteoporosis).

**Gene Mapping and Linkage:** Unknown.

**Prevention:** None known. Genetic counseling indicated.

**Treatment:** Treatment of osteoporosis; care for fractures and deformities. Prevention of retinal detachment in patients at risk.

**Prognosis:** Osteoporosis may progress during childhood; stabilization usually occurs after childhood.

**Detection of Carrier:** Incomplete manifestation of the syndrome may be seen in heterozygotes.

**Special Considerations:** "Pseudoglioma" is a nonspecific term; usually retinal detachment is the cause of blindness. The syndrome is probably a connective tissue dysplasia primarily involving eyes, bones, and ligaments. Biochemical findings reported from some cases include hypercalcinuria and hydroxyprolinuria as nonspecific secondary manifestations of osteoporosis. A decreased rate of bone formation and an increased rate of bone resorption have been shown by microautoradiographic studies.

**Support Groups:** PA; Marshallton; American Brittle Bone Society

**References:**
Bianchine JW, Murdoch JL: Juvenile osteoporosis (?) in a boy with bilateral enucleation of the eyes for pseudoglioma. BD:OAS V(4). New York: The National Foundation-March of Dimes, 1969:225–226.
Neuhäuser G, et al.: Autosomal recessive syndrome of pseudogliomatous blindness, osteoporosis and mild mental retardation. Clin Genet 1976; 9:324–332.
Bartsocas CS, et al.: Syndrome of osteoporosis with pseudoglioma. Ann Genet 1982; 25:61–62.
Frontali M, et al.: Osteoporosis-pseudoglioma syndrome: report of three affected siblings and a review. Am J Med Genet 1985; 22:35–47.
Beighton P, et al.: The ocular form of osteogenesis imperfecta. Clin Genet 1986; 28:69–75.
Teebi AS, et al.: Osteoporosis-pseudoglioma syndrome with congenital heart disease. J Med Genet 1988; 25:32–36.

NE012                                     **Gerhard Neuhäuser**

## OSTEOSARCOMA                                 3101

**Includes:**
  Cancer, osteosarcoma
  Multicentric osteosarcoma
  Osteogenic sarcoma
  Periosteal osteosarcoma
  Telangiectatic osteosarcoma

**Excludes:**
  **Bone, Paget disease** (3081)
  Dedifferentiated chondrosarcoma
  Low-grade osteosarcoma
  Malignant fibrous-histiocytoma
  Parosteal osteosarcoma

**Major Diagnostic Criteria:** Pain and a tender mass are present usually at the metaphyseal end of a long bone. X-rays reveal a destructive lesion of bone and a soft tissue mass, often mineralized. Alkaline phosphatase level may be elevated. Histology

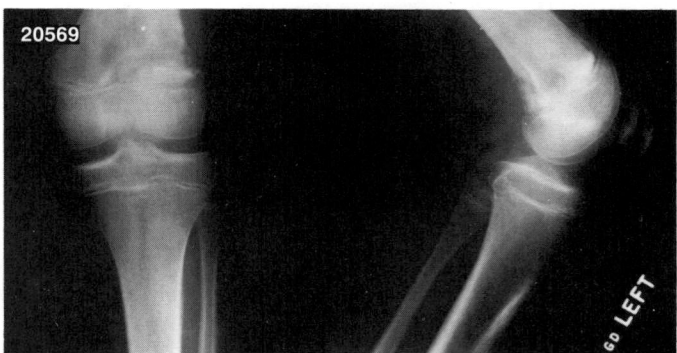

**3101-20569:** AP and lateral views of a typical osteosarcoma of the distal femur showing a poorly defined destructive lesion in the metaphysis. The cortex has been transgressed and there is a soft tissue mass which is partially mineralized. A Codman's triangle is evident.

shows a highly pleomorphic sarcoma with tumor bone production.

**Clinical Findings:** Osteosarcoma is a rare malignant neoplasm of bone occurring most frequently in the second decade of life. It usually presents as a painful mass of one or several months duration, located most commonly about the knee or shoulder. There is often a history of trauma that is not considered etiologic. The symptoms are progressive and the soft tissue mass may grow to large proportions, or a pathological fracture of the involved bone may occur if treatment is not instituted. Without treatment, patients would die of metastatic disease (most commonly pulmonary), and even with local treatment (amputation or radiation) of the primary disease, 80–90% will develop metastatic disease, suggesting that micrometastases are present in most patients at presentation.

The metaphyses of the long bones are the sites most frequently involved, but any bone may be affected. The distal femur is the most common site, followed by the proximal tibia (approximately 50% occur about the knee), proximal humerus, and femur. X-rays show a poorly defined destructive lesion of bone, which may be purely lytic or extremely blastic, but is usually a combination of both. The lesion is not marginated and usually transgresses the cortex of the bone to involve the adjacent soft tissues. The soft tissue component is variably mineralized, sometimes producing vertical striations: the so-called starburst appearance. An incomplete periosteal reaction (Codman triangle) is seen at the periphery of the lesion, but this is not specific for osteosarcoma. Computed tomograms and magnetic resonance images show the intramedullary and soft tissue extent more precisely than do plane X-rays and are useful in planning surgical approaches. Radionuclide bone scans show uptake in the area of involvement and are needed to exclude bony metastases.

There are no laboratory blood tests specific for osteosarcoma, although the alkaline phosphatase may be elevated, and patients with serum lactic dehydrogenase elevations were shown in one study to have a less favorable prognosis.

The diagnosis is made by biopsy of the lesion. Histologic findings are variable and may contain areas of fibrosarcomatous and chondrosarcomatous change, but the presence of a highly pleomorphic stroma producing tumor osteoid or bone is diagnostic.

**Complications:** Metastases, primarily to the lung, occur within two years in patients receiving local treatment only. Other bones are the second most common site for metastatic disease, and other organs, such as the brain, heart, and liver, are involved as a late, terminal event. Locally, if untreated, the large soft tissue mass may fungate through the skin, and a pathologic fracture may develop in the involved bone.

**Associated Findings:** Adults with **Bone, Paget disease** have a 5–10% incidence of osteosarcoma. Osteosarcoma has been reported in association with other congenital diseases and bone dysplasias such as **Enchondromatosis, Enchondromatosis and hemangiomas, Exostoses, multiple cartilaginous,** and **Osteogenesis imperfecta.** Some patients with osteosarcoma have been found to have abnormal glucose metabolism.

**Etiology:** There is no established inheritance of classic osteosarcoma; however, autosomal recessive inheritance has been suggested in several families with multiple cases of osteosarcomas, and sets of sibs with osteosarcoma have been reported. Among patients with **Retinoblastoma,** the incidence of osteosarcoma is increased 500 times above the incidence in other groups.

**Pathogenesis:** An association with growth is presumed because the peak incidence is during the adolescent growth spurt, and the most frequent locations are in the skeletal areas of most rapid growth. Similarly, in dogs, osteosarcoma occurs predominantly in large breeds (Great Danes, Saint Bernards, and German shepherds). Ionizing radiation to bone and thorium derivative administration is associated with the subsequent development of osteosarcoma. Viruses have been shown to cause osteosarcoma in some experimental animal systems, but not in humans.

**MIM No.:** 25950

**Sex Ratio:** During preadolescent years, M1:F1; overall, M1.6:F1.

**Occurrence:** Among patients <20 years old in the United States: 3.36:1,000,000 whites; 2.88:1,000,000 Blacks. Higher incidence in United Kingdom due to Paget disease. There is an initial peak incidence of occurrence during the adolescent years, followed by a second peak later in life (fifth and sixth decades) due to osteosarcomas in **Bone, Paget disease** and radiation-associated sarcomas.

**Risk of Recurrence for Patient's Sib:**
See Part I, *Mendelian Inheritance.* At least 16 sets of sibs with osteosarcoma have been reported.

**Risk of Recurrence for Patient's Child:** Unknown.

**Age of Detectability:** Rare under age five years, but case reports of patients as young as age two years have been reported.

**Gene Mapping and Linkage:** OSRC (osteosarcoma) has been DISCONTINUED.

**Prevention:** None known. Genetic counseling indicated. Avoidance of irradiation and thorium derivatives is encouraged.

**Treatment:** Wide or radical resection of the primary tumor is necessary to achieve local control. Traditionally this has been accomplished by amputation, but recent efforts at limb-preserving resection and reconstruction seem to provide equivalent disase control and adequate function. Recent randomized studies confirm the benefit of multiagent chemotherapy in improving the disease-free survival in patients without detectable metastases at diagnosis.

**Prognosis:** With adequate surgical control of the primary and adjuvant chemotherapy, disease-free survival figures of 50–70% at five years and an overall survival of 70–80% have been reported from several cancer centers.

**Detection of Carrier:** Unknown.

**Special Considerations:** Osteosarcoma, although rare, has a considerable impact because of its highly malignant nature and occurrence during the adolescent years. Great strides have been made in treatment with adjuvant chemotherapy, but controversy exists regarding the timing of surgery and chemotherapy. Preliminary evidence suggests that preoperative administration ("neoadjuvant chemotherapy") may be beneficial because it treats micrometastatic disease earlier, identifies "responders" (those who demonstrate nearly complete necrosis of the tumor after treatment), allows for the possibility of tailoring postoperative therapy for those who do not respond, and may make surgical resection easier and safer.

Other efforts are being directed toward identifying markers to predict prognosis and response to therapy, such as DNA aneuploidy and labeling index. Further informations regarding genetic markers (such as the deletion of the Rb locus) will add to the understanding of the disease and hopefully to improved treatment outcomes. Finally, much effort is being directed toward means of reconstruction following limb-sparing procedures and in evaluating the functional results of these procedures relative to amputation.

**Support Groups:** New York; American Cancer Society

**References:**
Colyer RA: Osteogenic sarcoma in siblings. Johns Hopkins Med J 1979; 145:131–135.
Bode U, Levine AS: The biology and management of osteosarcoma. In: Levine A, ed: Cancer in the young. New York: Masson, 1982:575–602.
Goorin AM, et al.: Osteosarcoma: fifteen years later. New Engl J Med 1985; 313:1637–1643.
Friend, SH, et al.: A human DNA segment with properties of the gene that predisposes to retinoblastoma and osteosarcoma. Nature 1986; 323:643–646.
Link MP et al.: The effect of adjuvant chemotherapy on relapse-free survival in patients with osteosarcoma of the extremity. New Engl J Med 1986; 314:1600–1606.
Dahlin DC: Osteosarcoma. In: Dahlin DC, ed: Bone tumors. Springfield, Il: Charles C. Thomas, 1987:226–260.

GE020      **Mark C. Gebhardt**

Osteosarcoma, retinoblastoma-related
  See RETINOBLASTOMA
Osteosclerosis fragilis generalisata
  See OSTEOPETROSIS, BENIGN DOMINANT
Osteosclerosis, autosomal dominant
  See HYPEROSTOSIS, WORTH TYPE
Osteosclerosis-ichthyosis-fractures
  See SKELETAL BOWING-CORTICAL THICKENING-BONE FRAGILITY-
    ICTHYOSIS
Osteosclerosis-platyspondyly
  See DYSOSTEOSCLEROSIS
Osteosis eburnisans monomelica
  See MELORHEOSTOSIS
Ostertag type amyloidosis, familial
  See AMYLOIDOSIS, FAMILIAL VISCERAL
Ostium primum atrial septal defect, persistent ostium primum
  See HEART, ENDOCARDIAL CUSHION DEFECTS
'Ostrich-footed' tribe
  See ECTRODACTYLY
Oto-branchio-renal dysplasia
  See BRANCHIO-OTO-RENAL DYSPLASIA
Oto-branchio-ureteral syndrome
  See BRANCHIO-OTO-URETERAL SYNDROME

---

## OTO-DENTAL DYSPLASIA                                  0784

**Includes:**

  Dental-oto dysplasia
  Globodontia-high frequency hearing loss
  Otodental syndrome

**Excludes:**

  **Teeth, macrodontia** (0617)
  Molarization of premolar teeth

**Major Diagnostic Criteria:** Large, globe-shaped molar teeth occur with sensorineural hearing loss.

**Clinical Findings:** Large, globe-shaped tooth crowns occur in both dentitions affecting the canine teeth and teeth posterior to the canines. Some affected persons have only the molar teeth involved. The incisor teeth are spared and are of normal size and shape. Over one-half have one or more congenitally missing premolars, or the premolars may be small. Age of onset of hearing loss varies from birth to third and fourth decade. The sensorineural hearing loss is high frequency and moderate to profound (50 db or greater hearing loss). Persons with only isolated hearing loss have transmitted the full syndrome. Data from one kindred show 30/37 had the full syndrome, 3/37 had globodontia only and 4/37 had only hearing loss. The last two had offspring affected with both defects. Local spots of yellow hypomature enamel have been noted in those with large teeth. Duplication of pulp chambers in molar teeth is seen on X-ray.

**Complications:** Malocclusion, full-face appearance, long philtrum, delayed eruption of teeth, and impacted teeth.

**Associated Findings:** Some families have shown thin enamel with large interrod spaces.

**Etiology:** Autosomal dominant inheritance. Patients within affected kindreds with isolated hearing loss have had offspring with the complete syndrome. High frequency hearing loss is common and can be due to a number of other genetic and environmental causes. Thus within kindreds, isolated hearing loss may indicate incomplete expression of the gene, but also may not indicate those bearing the gene.

**Pathogenesis:** Abnormal tooth form appears to be result of massive development of each tooth mamelon, or twinning-fusion of tooth germ.

**MIM No.:** *16675

**Sex Ratio:** M1:F1

**Occurrence:** At least eight kindreds with 62 affected members have been reported.

**Risk of Recurrence for Patient's Sib:**
  See Part I, *Mendelian Inheritance.*

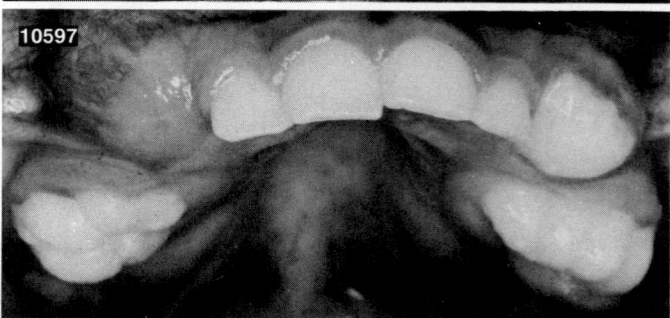

0784-10596–97:   Abnormally large and globular-shaped molars.

---

**Risk of Recurrence for Patient's Child:**
  See Part I, *Mendelian Inheritance.*

**Age of Detectability:** At time of eruption of posterior primary teeth, 18 months-2 years of age.

**Gene Mapping and Linkage:** Unknown.

**Prevention:** None known. Genetic counseling indicated.

**Treatment:** Orthodontic treatment with selected tooth extraction. Hearing aids.

**Prognosis:** Does not appear to affect longevity. Hearing loss may be progressive, and eventually involve conversational frequencies.

**Detection of Carrier:** Examination of first degree relatives.

**References:**

Levin LS, et al.: Otodental dysplasia: a new ectodermal dysplasia. Clin Genet 1975; 8:136–144. *
Witkop CJ Jr, et al.: Globodontia in the otodental syndrome. Oral Surg 1976; 41:472–483. †
Cook RA, et al.: Otodental dysplasia: a five year study. Ear Head 1981; 2:90–94.

WI043                                                    **Carl J. Witkop, Jr.**
LE028                                                    **L. Stefan Levin**

Oto-facio-cervical syndrome
  See BRANCHIO-OTO-RENAL DYSPLASIA
Oto-limb-cardiac syndrome
  See LIMB-OTO-CARDIAC SYNDROME

## OTO-OCULO-MUSCULO-SKELETAL SYNDROME     0785

**Includes:**
    Cataract-deafness-musculo-skeletal defects
    Deafness-cataract-muscular atrophy-skeletal defects
    Musculo-skeletal-oto-oculo syndrome
    Nathalie syndrome

**Excludes:** Deafness and cataract in other syndromes

**Major Diagnostic Criteria:** Early childhood deafness, cataract, muscular atrophy, EKG abnormalities.

**Clinical Findings:** This syndrome was reported in four of seven sibs (Cremers, 1975), one of which was named Nathalie. Early childhood (2–10 years) deafness was present in 4/4, cataract in 4/4, spinal muscular atrophy in 3/4, skeletal defects (osteochondrosis) in 3/4, retardation of growth in 3/4, EKG abnormalities in 4/4 and underdeveloped sexual characteristics in 2/4. The proposita suffered intermittently from regular and very frequent palpitations of the heart. The EKG showed ventricular extrasystoles, possibly multifocal in origin, or supraventricular extrasystoles with an aberrant intraventricular conduction. The proposita died during an attack of these palpitations.
    Sensorineural hearing loss (slopes from a 25–60 dB loss at 250 Hz to a 100 dB loss at 4000 Hz - nonprogressive in 3/4 cases) was diagnosed at the age of 5 in 3/4 and by the age of 4 in 1/4. X-rays of the temporal bones in the proposita were normal. Vestibular function examined in 2/4 was normal.

**Complications:** Death secondary to extrasystoles.

**Associated Findings:** Enuresis, nocturia in some cases and some family members, albuminuria in one case.

**Etiology:** Presumably autosomal recessive inheritance.

**Pathogenesis:** Unknown.

**MIM No.:** 25599

**POS No.:** 3351

**Sex Ratio:** Presumably M1:F1 (M1:F3 observed)

**Occurrence:** Four affected sibs reported.

**Risk of Recurrence for Patient's Sib:**
    See Part I, *Mendelian Inheritance.*

**Risk of Recurrence for Patient's Child:**
    See Part I, *Mendelian Inheritance.*

**Age of Detectability:** In the first years of life.

**Gene Mapping and Linkage:** Unknown.

**Prevention:** None known. Genetic counseling indicated.

**Treatment:** Special education for deafness. Lens discission for cataract, and orthopedic treatment of skeletal defects. Medication for extrasystoles.

**Prognosis:** Possibly diminished life span due to cardiac rhythm disturbances.

**Detection of Carrier:** Unknown.

**References:**
Cremers CWRJ, et al.: The Nathalie syndrome: a new hereditary syndrome. Clin Genet 1975; 8:330–340.

MI029

**Joyce Mitchell**
*Cor W.R.J. Cremers*

## OTO-ONYCHO-PERONEAL SYNDROME     2810

**Includes:**
    Anonychia-fibular dysplasia
    Fibula dysplasia-anonychia-abnormal ears

**Excludes:**
    **Craniosynostosis-fibular aplasia, lowry type** (2184)
    **Fibula, congenital absence of** (2229)
    **Nails, anonychia, hereditary** (0066)
    **Pterygium syndrome, popliteal** (0818)
    **Skeletal dysplasia, Fuhrmann type** (2696)

**Major Diagnostic Criteria:** Dysplasia of the fibula associated with anonychia of several medial fingers and toes. Abnormally shaped ears with missing lobules are also possibly characteristic.

**Clinical Findings:** Craniofacial dysmorphy with dolichocephaly; flared temporal areas; depressed nose; epicanthal folds; strabismus; large, floppy, peculiarly shaped ears; and hypoplastic lobules. Nails are missing on the first and second fingers and toes, partially absent and replaced by a cutaneous fold on the third, and hypoplastic folds on the other digits. The fibulae are either hypoplastic or absent. There are contractures of the hips, knees, and ankle joints with pes calcaneovalgus position. Mental retardation is moderate. One child died unexpectedly after an attack of respiratory asphyxia. Similar episodes and rare general fits have been noted in the surviving child in whom optic atrophy has also been noted.

**Complications:** Episodic asphyxia.

**Associated Findings:** Difficulty walking, even with orthopedic aid.

**Etiology:** Autosomal recessive inheritance has been proposed on the basis of possibly remote consanguinity.

**Pathogenesis:** Unknown.

**MIM No.:** 25978

**POS No.:** 3582

**Sex Ratio:** Presumably M1:F1; M2:F0 observed.

**Occurrence:** The condition has been documented in two brothers.

**Risk of Recurrence for Patient's Sib:**
    See Part I, *Mendelian Inheritance.*

**Risk of Recurrence for Patient's Child:**
    See Part I, *Mendelian Inheritance.*

**Age of Detectability:** Prenatally by ultrasound of the fibulae, or at birth.

**Gene Mapping and Linkage:** Unknown.

**Prevention:** None known. Genetic counseling indicated.

**Treatment:** Orthopedic treatment as necessary, but has proven of limited benefit.

**Prognosis:** Probably poor because of attacks of asphyxia, motor handicap, and mental retardation.

**Detection of Carrier:** Unknown.

**References:**
Pfeiffer RA: The oto-onycho-peroneal syndrome: a probably new genetic entity. Eur J Pediatr 1982; 138:317–320.

PF001

**Rudolf A. Pfeiffer**

## OTO-PALATO-DIGITAL SYNDROME, I 0786

**Includes:**
Digito-oto-palatal syndrome
Palato-oto-digital syndrome

**Excludes:**
Cleft palate-flattened facies-multiple congenital dislocations
**Larsen syndrome** (0570)
**Oro-cranio-digital syndrome** (0769)
**Oto-palato-digital syndrome, II** (2258)

**Major Diagnostic Criteria:** Cleft palate, downward slant of palpebral fissures, severe conductive hearing loss, and shortness of the terminal phalanges.

**Clinical Findings:** Cleft palate, downward slant of palpebral fissures, conductive hearing loss, short halluces, clinodactyly and variable syndactyly of other toes, flattened and short terminal phalanges, subluxation of head of radius, and broad nasal bridge giving pugilistic facial appearance.

X-ray findings include frontal and occipital bossing and thickening giving, the skull a mushroom-like appearance. The base of the skull is thick; the facial bones are hypoplastic, and the paranasal sinuses and mastoids are poorly pneumatized. The mandibular plane angle is increased, and the clivus or base sphenoid tends to be more vertical. There is lack of normal flare of ilia, mild coxa valga, secondary ossification centers of proximal second metacarpal, and second and third metatarsals, which fuse with the cuneiform bones, producing paddle-shaped structures. Intertarsal fusion is common.

Abnormalities of the ossicles and chronic serous otitis media are frequently noted.

**Complications:** Speech development is slow; this may be related to bilateral conductive hearing loss.

**Associated Findings:** Scoliosis.

**Etiology:** X-linked recessive inheritance, with variable expression in females.

**Pathogenesis:** Unknown.

**MIM No.:** *31130

**POS No.:** 3352

**Sex Ratio:** M1:F0

**Occurrence:** About 30 cases documented in the literature.

**Risk of Recurrence for Patient's Sib:**
See Part I, *Mendelian Inheritance.*

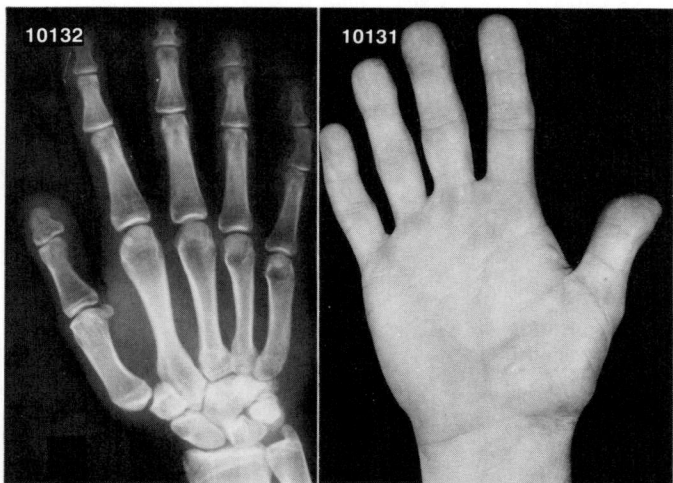

**0786A-10132–31:** Short distal phalanges of thumb and digits 3 and 4, and fusion of hamate and capitate bones.

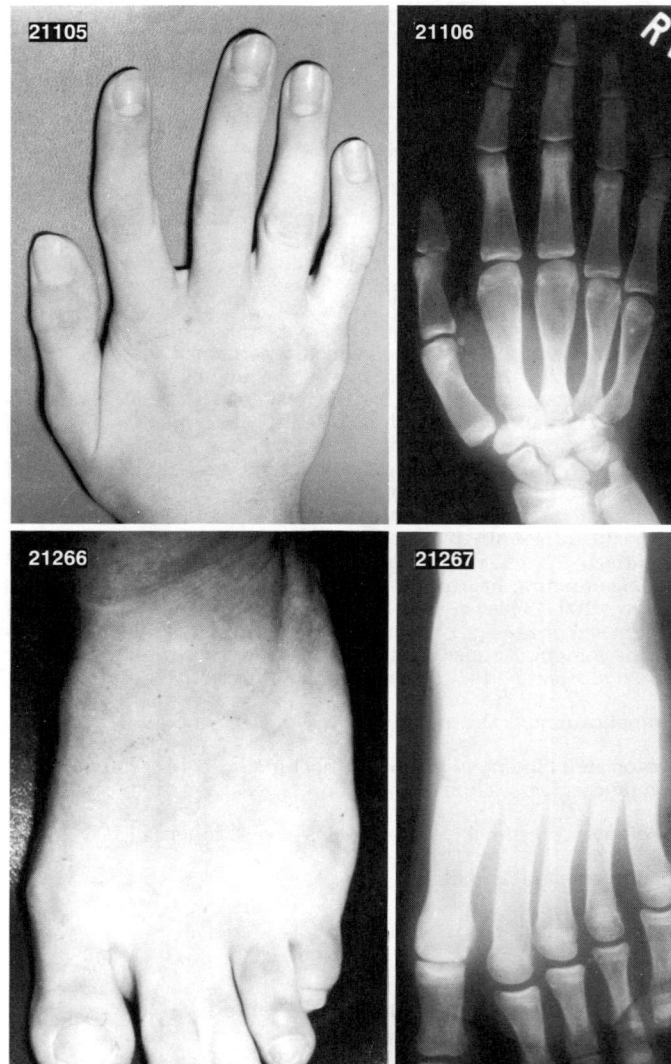

**0786B-21105–06:** Short distal phalanges and characteristic flask-shaped metacarpals in an affected female. **21266–67:** Tree frog toes, shortened great toe and distal phalanges in the toes of an affected female.

**Risk of Recurrence for Patient's Child:**
See Part I, *Mendelian Inheritance.*

**Age of Detectability:** At birth.

**Gene Mapping and Linkage:** OPD (otopalatodigital syndrome) has been provisionally mapped to X.

**Prevention:** None known. Genetic counseling indicated.

**Treatment:** Repair of cleft palate. Treatment of hearing loss has been limited, with variable improvement. No therapy is needed for the abnormalities of hands or feet.

**Prognosis:** Good, except for deafness.

**Detection of Carrier:** Facial features in the female heterozygote are variable. Most constant is overhanging brow with prominent supraorbital ridges, depressed nasal bridge, and flat midface.

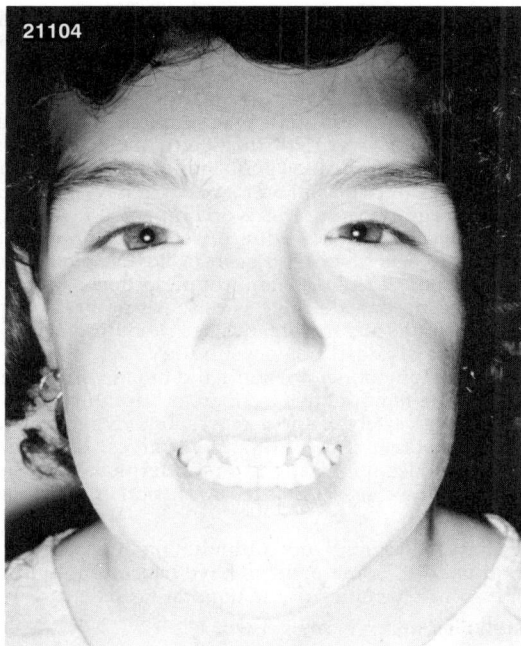

0786C-21104: Note hypertelorism and telecanthus, and down-slanting palpebral fissures in an affected female.

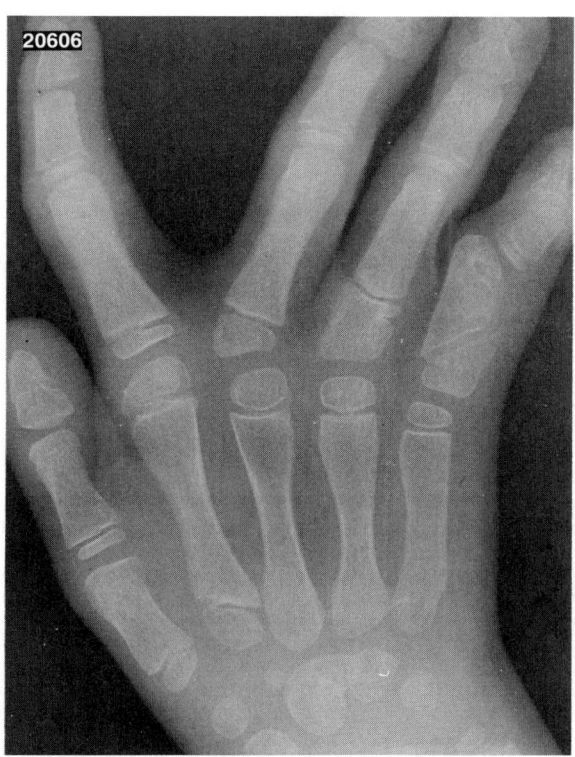

2258-20606: Oto-palato-digital syndrome, type II; note transverse capitate bone and extra bone in the capitate-hamate complex in this 5-year-old subject. The first metacarpal is short and there is digital deviation.

Other skeletal alterations are variable. Females have a higher frequency of greater multangular-navicular fusion.

**References:**

Dudding B, et al.: The otopalato-digital syndrome: a new symptom-complex consisting of deafness, dwarfism, cleft palate, characteristic facies, and a generalized bone dysplasia. Am J Dis Child 1967; 113:214–221.

Gall JC Jr, et al.: Oto-palato-digital syndrome. Comparison of clinical and radiographic manifestations in males and females. Am J Hum Genet 1972; 24:24–36.

Gorlin RJ, et al.: The oto-palato-digital syndrome in females: heterozygous expression of an X-linked trait. Oral Surg 1973; 35:218–224.

Poznanski AK, et al.: The hand in the oto-palato-digital syndrome. Ann Radiol 1973; 16:203–206.

Kozlowski K, et al.: Oto-palato-digital syndrome with severe x-ray changes in two half brothers. Pediatr Radiol 1977; 6:97–103.

Pazzaglia UE, Beluffi G: Oto-palato-digital syndrome in four generations of a large family. Clin Genet 1986; 30:338–344.

G0038                                                      **Robert J. Gorlin**

| OTO-PALATO-DIGITAL SYNDROME, II | 2258 |
|---|---|

**Includes:**

Andre syndrome
Cranio-oro-digital syndrome
Digital-oto-palato syndrome
Facio-palato-osseous syndrome
Palato-digital-oto syndrome

**Excludes:**

**Frontometaphyseal dysplasia** (0394)
**Oto-palato-digital syndrome, I** (0786)
**Cleft palate-dysmorphic facies-digital defects, Martsolf type** (2579)

**Major Diagnostic Criteria:** Typical facies with broad forehead, hypertelorism, apparently low-set ears, downward obliquity of palpebral fissures, flattened nose bridge, microstomia, microg-nathia and **Cleft palate**, fingers overlapping and flexed, short thumbs and short big toes, curved long bones in forearm and legs at birth, short first metacarpal, wide proximal phalanges 2–4 in the hand and clinodactyly of fingers 2 and 4, short or absent metatarsal, proximal phalanx and distal phalanx in big toe. Other metatarsals and middle toe phalanges may be short or absent.

**Clinical Findings:** The newborn infant usually has a large anterior fontanelle, wide sutures, low-set ears, prominent forehead, antimongoloid slant, flattened bridge of nose, micrognathia, cleft palate, flexed overlapping fingers, and short thumbs and big toes.

X-ray findings include small facial bones, small mandible with obtuse angle, dense long bones at birth, and curved long bones in arms and legs. The fibula may be small or absent, elbow and sometimes the wrist dislocated or subluxated, and ribs may be short and wavy. The vertebral bodies and acetabula are flat. The first metacarpal is short; the proximal phalanges 2–4 in the hand are wide and there is clinodactyly of fingers 2 and 4. Foot abnormalities include short or absent metatarsal 1, short or absent metatarsals 2 and 5, and short or absent proximal phalanges 1 and 5. The distal phalanx of the big toe is short or absent.

The neonatal period is usually complicated by respiratory and feeding difficulties, and six of the nine known patients died in infancy. Those who survived had bilateral conductive hearing loss. One was severely mentally retarded, and one had normal intelligence; there is no information on the mental status of the third case. The capitate bone is transverse, and an extra bone in the capitate-hamate complex may be present. The osteosclerosis, with the exception of the skull, tends to disappear, as does the long bone curvature.

**Complications:** Unknown.

**Associated Findings:** None known.

**Etiology:** X-linked semidominant inheritance.

**Pathogenesis:** Undetermined. Chondro-osseous histopathology is normal.

**MIM No.:** 30412

**POS No.:** 3710

**Sex Ratio:** M9:F0 (observed).

**Occurrence:** Nine cases, all male, have been described.

**Risk of Recurrence for Patient's Sib:**
See Part I, *Mendelian Inheritance.*

**Risk of Recurrence for Patient's Child:**
See Part I, *Mendelian Inheritance.*

**Age of Detectability:** In the newborn period.

**Gene Mapping and Linkage:** OPD (otopalatodigital syndrome) has been provisionally mapped to X.

**Prevention:** None known. Genetic counseling indicated.

**Treatment:** Repair of cleft palate.

**Prognosis:** May be mentally retarded.

**Detection of Carrier:** The mothers of two of the patients described by André et al. (1981) had broad facies, midline frontal bossing, downward slant of palpebral fissures, flattened noses, hypertelorism, and low-set ears. Both had hyperostosis frontalis interna, hypoplastic mandibles, and a narrow pelvis. The mother of patient 3 had a normal face, but the same X-ray anomalies. In addition, she had had an operation for conductive deafness when it was noticed that the stapes was ankylosed and crudely formed, there was a knuckle in the descending branch of the incus, and the right stapedial arch was completely closed. The sister of patient 2 had the same dysmorphic face and a cleft palate. The mother of the boys described by Fitch et al. (1976) had a highly arched palate, bifid uvula, and clinodactyly fingers 3–5. Her mother had a cleft palate. The mother of the infant described by Kaplan and Maroteaux (1984) had polydactyly of the hands and feet, and the mother of the infants described by Brewster et al. (1985) had mild frontal bossing and downslanting palpebral fissures.

**References:**
Fitch N, et al.: A familial syndrome of cranial, facial, oral and limb anomalies. Clin Genet 1976; 10:226–231.
Kozlowski K, et al: Oto-palato-digital syndrome with severe X-ray changes in two half brothers. Pediatr Radiol 1977; 6:97–102. *
André M, et al.: Abnormal facies, cleft palate and generalized dysostosis: a lethal X-linked syndrome. J Pediatr 1981; 98:747–752. †
Fitch N, et al.: The oto-palato-digital syndrome, proposed type II. Am J Med Genet 1983; 15:655–664. *
Kaplan J, Maroteaux P: Syndrome oto-palato-digital de Type II. Ann Gent 1984; 27:79–82.
Brewster TG, et al.: Oto-palato-digital type II: an X-linked skeletal dysplasia. Am J Med Gent 1985; 20:249–254.

FI020                                                          **Naomi Fitch**

**Oto-spondylo-megaepiphyseal dysplasia**
*See CHONDRODYSTROPHY-SENSORINEURAL DEAFNESS, NANCE-INSLEY TYPE*

## OTO-SPONDYLO-MEGAEPIPHYSEAL DYSPLASIA          2304

**Includes:**
Chondrodystrophy-sensorineural deafness
Megaepiphyseal dwarfism
Nance-Insley syndrome

**Excludes:**
**Arthro-ophthalmopathy, hereditary, progressive, Stickler type** (0090)
**Arthro-ophthalmopathy, Weissenbacher-Zweymuller variant** (2424)
**Deafness-myopia-cataract-saddle nose, Marshall type** (0261)
**Kniest dysplasia** (0557)
**Metatropic dysplasia** (0656)
**Oto-palato-digital syndrome, I** (0786)
**Oto-palato-digital syndrome, II** (2258)

**Major Diagnostic Criteria:** Short-limbed skeletal dysplasia with large epiphyses, sensorineural hearing loss, and platyspondyly.

**Clinical Findings:** Most patients have shown prenatal onset of short-limbed disproportionate short stature, although some demonstrate the disproportion with overall height remaining in the normal range. The facies are distinctive, with severely depressed nasal bridge and an upturned "snubbed" nose, retrognathia, **Cleft palate**, and malar hypoplasia. Some patients have had epicanthal folds. Sensorineural hearing loss is accompanied in some patients by a conductive hearing loss due to recurrent otitis media. No severe visual defects have been seen. Mild **Camptodactyly** of the hands is present. Kyphosis and hyperlordosis are common. During the second decade there is onset of progressive contractures of the major joints. Intelligence has been normal in all except one patient who also had homocystinuria.

On X-ray, the long bones are short and broad with flaring of the metaphyses. The femora are described as "dumb-bell shaped" in some cases. The vertebrae show platyspondyly, coronal clefts in the lumbar vertebrae, and molding deformities. Large epiphyses at the knees, ankles, elbows, and first interphalangeal joints are the hallmark of the disease. Progressive fusion of the carpal bones has been noted.

**Complications:** Progressive joint limitation and pain are seen in the second decade. Some patients have had osteophytic changes in the spine or deformities of the femoral heads.

**Associated Findings:** None known.

**Etiology:** Autosomal recessive inheritance.

**Pathogenesis:** Unknown.

**MIM No.:** *21515

**POS No.:** 3630

**Sex Ratio:** M1:F1

**Occurrence:** Two or three kindreds have been reported.

**Risk of Recurrence for Patient's Sib:**
See Part I, *Mendelian Inheritance.*

**Risk of Recurrence for Patient's Child:**
See Part I, *Mendelian Inheritance.*

**Age of Detectability:** At birth.

**Gene Mapping and Linkage:** Unknown.

**Prevention:** None known. Genetic counseling indicated.

**Treatment:** Orthopedic surgery as indicated.

**Prognosis:** Normal life span.

**Detection of Carrier:** Unknown.

**Special Considerations:** The patients described appear to have the same clinical entity. Without a defined etiology, however, genetic heterogeneity cannot be excluded.

**Support Groups:**
MA; Quincy; Prescription Parents, Inc.
CANADA: Ontario; Toronto; Canadian Cleft Lip and Palate Family Association

**References:**
Nance WE, Sweeney A: A recessively inherited chondrodystrophy. BD:OAS VI(4). New York: March of Dimes Birth Defects Foundation, 1970:25–27.
Gorlin RJ, et al.: Megaepiphyseal dwarfism. J Pediatr 1973; 83:633–635.
Insley J, Astley R: A bone dysplasia with deafness. Br J Radiol 1974; 47:244–251.
Giedion A, et al.: Oto-spondylo-megaepiphyseal dysplasia (OSMED). Helv Paediatr Acta 1982; 37:361–380.
Miny P, Lenz W: Autosomal recessive deafness with skeletal dysplasia and facial appearance of Marshall syndrome. Am J Med Genet 1985; 21:317–324.
Salinas C, et al.: Bone dysplasia, deafness and cleft palate syndrome. (Abstract) 7th Int Cong Hum Genet, Berlin, 1986; 1:259 only.

H0025                                                          **O.J. Hood**
H0033                                                 **William A. Horton**

**Otocephaly**
*See AGNATHIA-MICROSTOMIA-SYNOTIA*
**Otodental syndrome**
*See OTO-DENTAL DYSPLASIA*

## OTOSCLEROSIS                            0787

**Includes:**
    Labyrinthine otosclerosis
    Labyrinthine otosclerosis-fixed stapes footplate

**Excludes:**
    Hearing loss, postinflammatory conductive
    Ossicular fixation, congenital
    **Osteogenesis imperfecta** (0777)
    Stapes fixation due to Paget osteitis deformans
    Tympanosclerosis

**Major Diagnostic Criteria:** Progressive conductive or mixed hearing loss in a young or middle-aged adult without evidence of other middle ear disease. Clinical onset prior to age six years has rarely been reported.

**Clinical Findings:** With otosclerosis there is a slowly progressive conductive or mixed hearing loss of insidious onset unrelated to inflammatory middle ear findings. Approximately 75% of cases are bilateral. The patient may describe a history of hearing better in noisy situations ("paracusis Willisiani"). Tinnitus is a frequent complaint and is usually a low-frequency type sometimes accompanied by an audible pulse. Vertigo is found in about 5–8% of patients with otosclerosis.

The tympanic membranes are normal at inspection, and their mobility is unaltered. There may be a pink flush seen through the eardrum caused by increased vascularity of the mucosa over the otosclerotic focus on the promontory of the middle ear ("Schwartze sign"). This sign is believed to be correlated with increased vascularity in the mucosa of the promontory overlying the focus, and is believed to signify an "active" focus. An "inactive" focus is thought to be a healed area of otosclerosis and grossly appears whiter than the surrounding normal area. Audiometry reveals a conductive hearing loss of varying severity, which is initially more marked in the lower frequencies, but as the lesion progresses with increased stapes fixation, all frequencies are affected. Middle ear impedance is increased as measured by an acoustic bridge. Labyrinthine or cochlear otosclerosis results in a sensorineural hearing loss. This may or may not be accompanied by a conductive component. The pathology is not clear but seems to be related to destruction of the endosteal membrane of the cochlea adjacent to the spiral ligament. X-ray examination by high-resolution computerized tomography is generally not necessary clinically, but may be helpful in distinguishing otosclerotic stapes fixation from other acquired ossicular fixation or in identifying otosclerotic invasion of the cochlea in a patient with an associated sensorineural loss.

At surgery the stapes footplate is found to be partially or completely fixed to the otic capsule by an otosclerotic focus. This most commonly occurs at the anterior footplate, but it can be at any other location; it may be circumscribed, or the lesion may obliterate the oval window niche.

**Complications:** Labyrinthine or cochlear otosclerosis has been suspected to be a cause of severe sensorineural hearing loss. There has been evidence that sensorineural hearing losses are not increased in otosclerosis compared to the normal population, but there is a small percentage of these patients who show a severe progressive sensorineural hearing loss long before presbycusis could be assumed to be an explanation.

**Associated Findings:** Vestibular disturbances are more common in patients with otosclerosis than in the general population. There is a statistically significant correlation with the ability to taste phenylthiocarbamide, but the significance of this is unknown.

**Etiology:** Autosomal dominant inheritance with incomplete penetrance, estimated at between 25 to 40%, depending on the series studied.

**Pathogenesis:** Otosclerosis is a focal, progressive replacement of the endochondral bone of the otic capsule with abnormal bone, which has the microscopic appearance of healing fibrous bone, but which is normally calcified. The site of predilection is the otic capsule anterior to the stapes footplate, and the process progresses to involve the stapes footplate and fix it to the surrounding bone. The pathogenesis of the sensorineural hearing loss is not yet completely understood.

**MIM No.:** *16680

**Sex Ratio:** M1:F1

**Occurrence:** Clinical otosclerosis is 1:330 in the White population, about 1:3,300 in the Black population, and estimated to be 1:33,000 in the Oriental. Series of temporal bone specimens which show histologic otosclerosis, not necessarily with hearing loss, have shown the histologic changes to be present in 1:14 to 1:10 of white subjects studied in the United States, and approximately 1:100 in Blacks.

**Risk of Recurrence for Patient's Sib:**
See Part I, *Mendelian Inheritance*. If only one parent is affected, 1:5 to 1:8 depending on expressivity.

**Risk of Recurrence for Patient's Child:**
See Part I, *Mendelian Inheritance*. If mate is not affected, 1:5 to 1:8.

**Age of Detectability:** A conductive hearing loss is first seen at age 11–15 years in 10% of cases, progressing to 50% at age 21–25 years, and reaching 100% at age 40 years. Earlier detectability could possibly be achieved with temporal bone tomograms in the absence of clinical findings, but the significance of this in terms of morbidity is unclear.

**Gene Mapping and Linkage:** Unknown.

**Prevention:** None known. Genetic counseling indicated.

**Treatment:** Stapedectomy to restore hearing in those with a conductive loss secondary to otosclerosis has been highly developed and is generally very successful. The most common procedure is removal of the fixed stapes from the oval window and replacement with a wire or Teflon prosthesis. The oval window is cleaned of otosclerotic bone and covered with Gelfoam^, fat, or vein and the prosthesis is placed between the incus and this new membrane. Improvement in hearing occurs in approximately 90+%, with an incidence of surgical complications of about 3%. Sodium fluoride has been used orally to treat cochlear otosclerosis, but the treatment is controversial.

**Prognosis:** Normal for life span and intelligence.

**Detection of Carrier:** Unknown.

**References:**
Kelemen G, Linthicum FH Jr: Labyrinthine otosclerosis. Acta Otolaryngol [suppl] (Stockh) 1969; 253:1–12.
Morrison AW, Bundey SE: The inheritance of otosclerosis. J Laryngol Otol 1970; 84:921–932.
Johnsson LG, et al.: Cochlear and vestibular lesions in capsular otosclerosis as seen in microdissection. Ann Otol Rhinol Laryngol (Suppl) 1978; 87:48:1–40.
Schaap T, Gapany-Gapanavicius B: The genetics of otosclerosis. I. Distorted sex ratio. Am J Hum Genet 1978; 30:59–64. *
Schuknecht HF, Jones DD: Stapedectomy postmortem findings. Ann Otol Rhinol Laryngol (Suppl 88) 1979; 55:1–43.
Vollrath M, Schreiner C: Influence of argon laser stapedectomy on cochlear potentials. Acta Oto Laryngologica (suppl) 1982; 385:1–31.

BE028                                      **LaVonne Bergstrom**

**Oudtshoorn skin**
*See SKIN, ERYTHROKERATOLYSIS HIEMALIS*
**Ovalocytoses, Malaysian-Melanesian type**
*See ELLIPTOCYTOSIS*
**Ovalocytosis, hereditary**
*See ELLIPTOCYTOSIS*
**Ovarian dysgenesis, familial**
*See GONADAL DYSGENESIS, XX TYPE*
**Ovarian dysgenesis-sensorineural deafness**
*See PERRAULT SYNDROME*
**Overgrowth disorder, hemihypertrophy**
*See HEMIHYPERTROPHY*

## OVERGROWTH, BANNAYAN TYPE                    2381

**Includes:**

Bannayan-Zonana syndrome
Lipomatosis-angiomatosis-macrencephalia
Macrocephaly-diffuse hamartomas
Macrocephaly-multiple lipomas-hemangiomata
Protean gigantism, Bannayan type
Zonana syndrome

**Excludes:**

**Angio-osteohypertrophy syndrome** (0055)
Chromosome abnormalities
**Cutis marmorata** (2296)
Disseminated hemangiomatosis
**Neurofibromatosis** (0712)
**Overgrowth, macrocephaly-hemangioma, Riley-Smith type** (2192)
**Overgrowth, Ruvalcaba-Myhre-Smith type** (2120)
**Proteus syndrome** (2382)

**Major Diagnostic Criteria:** The diagnosis is based on **Megalencephaly** with normal ventricles and mesodermal multiple hamartomas. Motor, speech, and coordination delays are common and transient. Intelligence is usually within the average range. Computerized tomographic (CT) head scan is necessary to confirm the normal size of the ventricles. Familial occurrence is also of help to the diagnosis.

**Clinical Findings:** The **Megalencephaly** is present at birth, with head circumference at least 2 SD above the mean. Hamartomas may be apparent at that time; these usually manifest in infancy or early childhood. The majority of the tumors are subcutaneous lipomas. Some may show elements of lymphangioma and/or hemangioma. Spontaneous regression of these tumors may occur. Congenital macrosomia may be present. Periods of decelerated growth and occasional transient failure to thrive have been reported. Ultimate height is within normal range. Other nonspecific signs delineate further the phenotype.

In the fewer than 20 reported patients, the approximate frequency of the clinical features is: **Megalencephaly** (18/18), accelerated fetal growth (5/9), decelerated postnatal growth (10/10), lipomas (14/18), hemangiomas (8/18), lymphangioma (2/18), other tumors (3/18), motor delay (9/12), speech delay (10/18), adult motor dysfunction (4/5), mental retardation (3/18), seizures (3/18), strabismus/amblyopia (3/18), obliquity of palpebral fissures (7/13), high palate (6/10), joint hyperextensibility (5/10), **Pectus excavatum** (2/10), hypotonia (2/10) and drooling (4/10). Clinical variability appears to exist. First degree relatives should have genetic evaluation to detect minimally affected individuals.

**Complications:** Localization, size, and structure of the hamartomas may lead to space occupying symptomatology particularly within the central nervous system. Manifestations of the infrequent arteriovenous malformations may also complicate the clinical picture.

**Associated Findings:** Follicular cell carcinoma of the thyroid was found in one patient; it is not clear whether or not the carcinoma was causally related to the syndrome. Meningoepithelial meningioma has also been reported in one patient and angioleiomyoma in another. One patient with *de novo* translocation, t(Y;19), had a similar phenotype to that of Bannayan syndrome.

**Etiology:** Autosomal dominant inheritance with variable expressivity.

**Pathogenesis:** One of the mesodermal phakomatoses. The pathogenesis probably represents a genetically determined interference with the differentiation, migration, and interaction of the mesodermal cells within the affected organs. Dysregulated paracrine growth factor may play a critical role in pathogenesis.

**MIM No.:** *15348

**POS No.:** 3556

**Sex Ratio:** M4:F1

**Occurrence:** Reported in about 15 kinships, including an American Black family. As with most other hamartoses, the syndrome is most likely underdiagnosed.

**Risk of Recurrence for Patient's Sib:** See Part I, *Mendelian Inheritance.*

**Risk of Recurrence for Patient's Child:** See Part I, *Mendelian Inheritance.*

**Age of Detectability:** **Megalencephaly** is present at birth. Prenatal diagnosis is theoretically possible. The hamartomas become apparent in infancy or later.

**Gene Mapping and Linkage:** Unknown.

**Prevention:** None known. Genetic counseling indicated.

**Treatment:** The usually noninvasive hamartomas are amenable to surgery.

**Prognosis:** Normal life span is presumed.

**Detection of Carrier:** Detailed diagnostic evaluation of the first degree relatives may detect minimally affected individuals.

**Special Considerations:** Bannayan syndrome appears to be the same as Zonana syndrome. However, other proposals to unify various overgrowth syndromes into a single entity are considered premature at this time.

**References:**

Bannayan GA: Lipomatosis, angiomatosis and macrencephalia. Arch Pathol 1971; 92:1–5.
Zonana J, et al.: Macrocephaly with multiple lipomas and hemangiomas. J Pediatr 1976; 89:600–603.
Higginbottom MC, Schultz C: The Bannayan syndrome: an autosomal dominant disorder consisting of macrocephaly, lipomas, hemangiomas, and risk of intracranial tumors. Pediatrics 1982; 69:632–634.
Miles JH, et al.: Macrocephaly with hamartomas: Bannayan-Zonana syndrome. Am J Med Genet 1984; 19:225–234.
Israel JN: 19/Y translocation in a patient with features of Zonana syndrome. Am J Hum Genet 1985; 37:A60.
Saul RA, Stevenson RE: Bannayan syndrome and Ruvalcaba-Myhre-Smith syndrome discrete entities? Proc Greenwood Genet Center 1986; 5:3–7.
Kousseff BG, Madan S: The phakomatoses - an hypothesis: paracrine growth regulation disorders? Dysmorph Clin Genet 1988; 2:76–90.

K0018                                    **Boris G. Kousseff**

**Overgrowth, encephalo-cranio-cutaneous lipomatosis type**
*See PROTEUS SYNDROME*
**Overgrowth, Golabi-Rosen type**
*See SIMPSON-GOLABI-BEHMEL SYNDROME*

## OVERGROWTH, MACROCEPHALY-HEMANGIOMA, RILEY-SMITH TYPE                    2192

**Includes:**

Bannayan-Riley-Ruvalcaba syndrome
Macrocephaly-hemangioma
Macrocephaly-pseudopapilledema-multiple hemangiomata
Multiple hemangiomata-macrocephaly-pseudopapilledema
Pseudopapilledema-macrocephaly-multiple hemangiomata
Riley-Smith syndrome

**Excludes:**

**Enchondromatosis and hemangiomas** (0346)
**Hemangioma-thrombocytopenia syndrome** (0456)
Macrocephaly, benign familial
**Overgrowth, Bannayan type** (2381)
**Sturge-Weber syndrome** (0915)
**Von Hippel-Lindau syndrome** (0995)

**Major Diagnostic Criteria:** The combination of **Microcephaly**, pseudopapilledema, and multiple hemangiomata are strongly suggestive of the diagnosis. If the family history is positive, then one of the above features is sufficient to make the diagnosis.

**Clinical Findings:** In the five reported and two subsequently identified affected individuals, the following clinical features were observed: congenital macrocephaly (7); pseudopapilledema (6);

cutaneous and/or subcutaneous hemangiomata (4); and frequent respiratory infections (4).

The only significant X-ray finding has been increased thickness of the cranial bones. Chest X-rays have revealed minimal pulmonary fibrosis in three affected individuals. Histologic studies of nodules have been characteristic for hemangiomata. Ophthalmologic findings have been consistent with pseudopapilledema (blurred disk margins). Metabolic and hematologic studies, pneumoencephalograms, electroencephalograms, and electrocardiograms have all been normal.

**Complications:** Posttraumatic bleeding of the hemangiomata and bronchopneumonia have been reported.

**Associated Findings:** One affected individual also had a **Tracheoesophageal fistula.**

**Etiology:** The presence of the syndrome in four generations of a single family is strongly suggestive of autosomal dominant inheritance.

**Pathogenesis:** Unknown.

**MIM No.:** 15350

**Sex Ratio:** M3:F4 (in the seven known cases).

**Occurrence:** A mother and sibs in one family have been reported.

**Risk of Recurrence for Patient's Sib:**
See Part I, *Mendelian Inheritance.*

**Risk of Recurrence for Patient's Child:**
See Part I, *Mendelian Inheritance.*

**Age of Detectability:** Macrocephaly is present at birth, whereas the hemangiomata were congenital in two cases and appeared after the age of three years in two cases.

**Gene Mapping and Linkage:** Unknown.

**Prevention:** None known. Genetic counseling indicated.

**Treatment:** Unknown.

**Prognosis:** Vision and intellect are unimpaired. Life span appears to be normal.

**Detection of Carrier:** A large head size may be the only obvious finding. A funduscopic exam is necessary to detect pseudopapilledema.

**Special Considerations:** Although Cohen suggested that this condition is the same as the **Overgrowth, Bannayan type** and **Overgrowth, Ruvalcaba-Myhre-Smith type** syndromes, based on a paper published by Dvir et al in 1988, Di Liberti suggested, in a companion letter, that appropriate research needs to be done before these conditions be "lumped" into a *Bannayan-Riley-Ruvalcaba syndrome.* It is possible that the condition Dvir et al is describing, which included macrocephaly, hamartomas, pseudopapilledema and macropenia as phenotypic features, could be a distinct, albeit pathogenetically related, syndrome.

**References:**
Riley HD, et al.: Macrocephaly, pseudopapilledema and multiple hemangiomata. Pediatrics 1960; 26:293–300.
Dvir M, et al.: Heredofamilial syndrome of mesodermal hamartomas, macrocephaly, and pseudopapilledema. Pediatrics 1988; 81:287–290.
Cohen MM Jr.: Bannayan-Riley-Ruvalcaba syndrome: renaming three formerly recognized syndromes as one etiologic entity. (Letter) Am J Med Genet 1990; 35:291.
Di Liberti JH: Comments on Dr. Cohen's letter. (Letter) Am J Med Genet 1990; 35:292.

T0007
RI018

Helga V. Toriello
Harris D. Riley

**Overgrowth, Proteus type**
*See PROTEUS SYNDROME*

## OVERGROWTH, RUVALCABA-MYHRE-SMITH TYPE    2120

**Includes:**
  Genitalia, pigmentary changes-megalencephaly-intestinal polyposis
  Intestinal polyposis-pigmentary changes of genitalia-megalencephaly
  Megalencephaly-intestinal polyposis-pigmentary changes of genitalia
  Myopathy, lipid storage (one form)
  Ruvalcaba-Myhre-Smith syndrome

**Excludes:**
  **Overgrowth, Bannayan type** (2381)
  **Cebebral gigantism** (0137)
  **Overgrowth, macrocephaly-hemangioma, Riley-Smith type** (2192)

**Major Diagnostic Criteria:** Clinical findings include megalencephaly, hypotonia or developmental delay, normal stature, pigmented macules on the penis, prominent Schwalbe's lines and corneal nerves, hamartomatous intestinal polyps, lipid storage myopathy, and lipomas or angiolipomas.

**Clinical Findings:** **Megalencephaly** is often present at birth, and the head circumference remains large (≥97th percentile) throughout life. The CT scan is always normal except for the increased head size. Hypotonia (90%) is a common problem in childhood but appears to improve with age. Signs of proximal muscle weakness may be present in the pre-school child. Mental retardation is found in some affected patients but normal intellect has been observed in several. Pigmented macules on the glans and shaft of the penis (80%) are first noted between infancy and adulthood. Similar lesions may be found on other parts of the body. Hamartomatous intestinal polyps (<20%) may produce intestinal bleeding or intussusception and have been found in early childhood through adulthood. Prominent Schwalbe's lines and corneal nerves (50%) do not appear to cause clinical problems.

An unusual lipid storage myopathy is often present (≥50% in children), even in asymptomatic patients. The EMG may be abnormal without clinical signs of myopathy, and no signs of deterioration have been observed. Serum CPK activity is normal. In spite of a high mean birth weight (4,120 g), growth rates are normal and adult stature is average.

**Complications:** Anemia, intestinal bleeding, and intussusception occur secondary to hamartomatous polyps.

**Associated Findings:** Acanthosis nigricans, mucoepidermoid carcinoma of the parotid, lipoma, **Pectus excavatum**, accessory nipples, diabetes mellitus, epilepsy.

**Etiology:** Possibly autosomal dominant inheritance.

**Pathogenesis:** Unknown.

**MIM No.:** 18089

**POS No.:** 3526

**Sex Ratio:** Presumably M1:F1, although a disproportionate number of males have been observed.

**Occurrence:** A dozen or so cases have been reported in the literature.

**Risk of Recurrence for Patient's Sib:**
See Part I, *Mendelian Inheritance.*

**Risk of Recurrence for Patient's Child:**
See Part I, *Mendelian Inheritance.*

**Age of Detectability:** At birth.

**Gene Mapping and Linkage:** Unknown.

**Prevention:** None known. Genetic counseling indicated.

**Treatment:** Unknown.

**Prognosis:** Variable. One patient was severely retarded, but intellectual performance in others has varied through the normal range, at least in childhood. Most known patients have done well in follow-up, although the lipomas may grow quite large and cause cosmetic problems. The myopathy does not appear to be progressive and has not caused problems beyond mid-childhood.

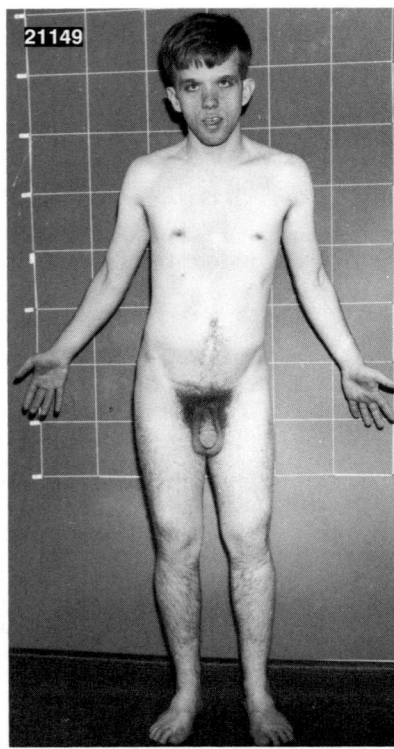

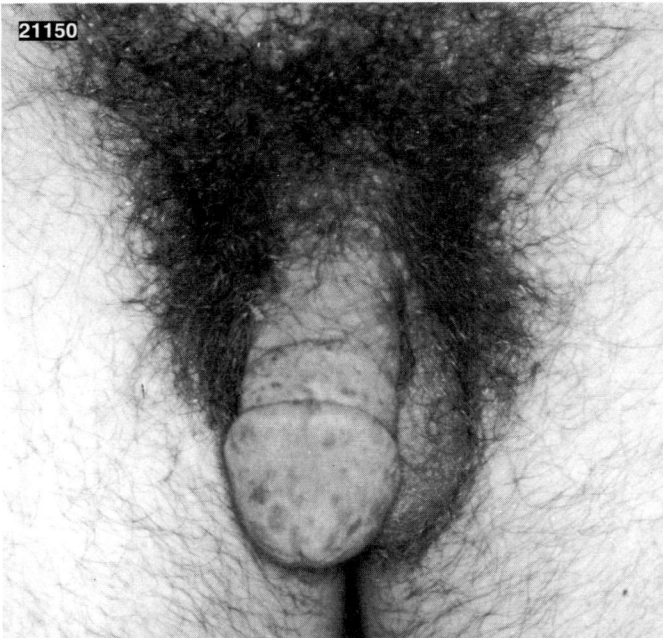

**2120**-21149: Macrocephaly, supernumerary nipple, and scar from early colectomy. 21150: Tan macular lesions on the glans and shaft of the penis.

One adult patient continues to have difficulties caused by intestinal polyps. Life span appears to be normal.

**Detection of Carrier:** Megalencephaly or prominent Schwalbe's lines may be the only manifestations in some individuals.

**Special Considerations:** This disorder has similarities to **Overgrowth, Bannayan type** and other reported conditions which feature macrocephaly and hamartoma. Available data do not permit differentiation between a single allele-variable expression model or multiple genotypes (see **Overgrowth, macrocephaly-hemangioma, Riley-Smith type**).

**References:**

Ruvalcaba RHA, et al.: Sotos syndrome with intestinal polyposis and pigmentary changes of the genitalia. Clin Genet 1980; 18:413–416. * †

Di Liberti JH, et al.: The Ruvalcaba-Myhre-Smith syndrome: a case with probable dominant inheritance and additional manifestations. Am J Med Genet 1983; 15:491–496. * †

Di Liberti JH, et al.: A new lipid storage myopathy in the the Ruvalcaba-Myhre-Smith syndrome. Am J Med Genet 1984; 18:163–167. †

Gretzula JC, et al.: Ruvalcaba-Myhre-Smith syndrome. Pediatr Dermatol 1988; 5:28–32. †

Halal F, Silver K: Slowly progressive macrocephaly with hamartomas: a new syndrome? Am J Med Genet 1989; 33:182–185. †

DI001                                                     **John H. Di Liberti**

**Overgrowth-congenital edema-positional defects of the feet**
*See NEVO SYNDROME*
**Overgrowth-mental retardation syndrome, X-linked**
*See SIMPSON-GOLABI-BEHMEL SYNDROME*

---

**OVERGROWTH-RENAL HAMARTOMA, PERLMAN TYPE    2241**

**Includes:**
  Fetal ascites-macrosomia-Wilms tumor
  Hamartoma and nephroblastomatosis
  Perlman syndrome
  Renal hamartoma syndrome
  Renal hamartomas-nephroblastomatosis-fetal gigantism

**Excludes:**
  **Beckwith-Wiedemann syndrome** (0104)
  **Hemihypertrophy** (0458)

**Major Diagnostic Criteria:** Macrosomia at birth; unusual facial appearance; distended abdomen; hypoglycemia.

**Clinical Findings:** Macrosomia at birth; unusual facial appearance characterized by upsweep of anterior hairline, apparent enophthalmos, hypoplastic bridge of nose, inverted "V" shape of the upper lip, micrognathia; prominent, bifid xiphisternum; distended abdomen; cryptorchidism in males; and hypoglycemia.

**Complications:** Cancer, **Wilms tumor**; hypoglycemic coma; developmental delay.

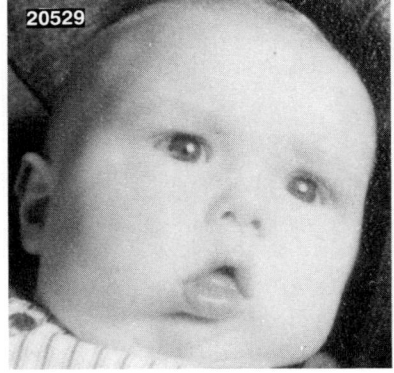
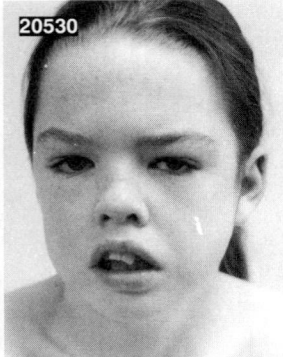

**2241**-20529–30: Perlman syndrome; note these 2 affected sibs at ages 6 months and 12 years respectively. The inverted "v" shaped upper lip is characteristic.

**Associated Findings:** Polyhydramnios; fetal ascites.

**Etiology:** Autosomal recessive inheritance.

**Pathogenesis:** It has been suggested that a defect in a gene regulating cell proliferation during embryonic and fetal life causes macrosomia with minor anomalies, hyperplasia of the endocrine pancreas and renal dysplasia with nephroblastomatosis. Macrosomia regresses during postnatal life, with ensuing developmental delay and so probably does the pancreatic hyperplasia, although hypoglycemia can be a persistent complication and hypoglycemic coma a possible cause of death. The kidney dysplasia, on the other hand, has a strong tendency to develop into a Wilms tumor.

**MIM No.:** *26700

**POS No.:** 3648

**Sex Ratio:** M1:F1

**Occurrence:** Ten patients, of both sexes, have been described from three families, one of Jewish Yemenite origin (six affected sibs) and another Caucasian (two affected sibs). Origin of the third family (two patients) was not stated. Parents were healthy, and consanguineous in the Jewish family.

**Risk of Recurrence for Patient's Sib:**
See Part I, *Mendelian Inheritance.*

**Risk of Recurrence for Patient's Child:**
See Part I, *Mendelian Inheritance.* There are no reports of an affected individual having reproduced.

**Age of Detectability:** At birth. Prenatal diagnosis may be possible.

**Gene Mapping and Linkage:** Dao et al (1987) studied chromosome 11 p markers in a bilateral Wilms tumor from a patient with this condition and found the same loss of 11p DNA sequences found in non-syndromal cases of **Cancer, Wilms tumor.** Genetic differences between the two tumors indicated that they developed independently, and were the results of different genetic events.

**Prevention:** None known. Genetic counseling indicated.

**Treatment:** Surgical excision of Wilms tumor, followed by chemo- and radiotherapy as indicated.

**Prognosis:** Most affected individuals so far described died in the neonatal period. At least one survivor was reported at age 14 years, with some psychomotor retardation. Early diagnosis may lead to effective treatment of the kidney dysplasia through appropriate chemotherapy, and of the developmental delay through adequate correction of the hypoglycemia.

**Detection of Carrier:** Unknown.

**References:**
Liban E, Kozenitsky I: Metanephric hamartomas and nephroblastomatosis in siblings. Cancer 1970; 25:885–888.
Perlman M, et al.: Renal hamartomas and nephroblastomatosis with fetal gigantism: a familial syndrome. J Pediatr 1973; 83:414–418.
Perlman M, et al.: Syndrome of fetal gigantism, renal hamartomas, and nephroblastomatosis with Wilms tumor. Cancer 1975; 35:1212–1217.
Neri G, et al.: The Perlman syndrome: familial renal dysplasia with Wilms tumor, fetal gigantism and multiple congenital anomalies. Am J Med Genet 1984; 19:195–207. †
Greenberg F, et al.: The Perlman familial nephroblastomatosis syndrome. Am J Med Genet 1986; 24:101–110. †
Perlman M: Perlman syndrome: familial renal dysplasia with Wilms tumor, fetal gigantism, and multiple congenital anomalies. Am J Med Genet 1986; 25:793–795. †
Dao DD, et al.: Genetic mechanisms of tumor-specific loss in 11p DNA sequences in Wilms tumor. Am J Hum Genet 1987; 41:202–217.
Greenberg F, et al.: Expanding the spectrum of the Perlman syndrome. Am J Med Genet 1988; 29:773–776.

NE019                                    **Giovanni Neri**

**Oviducts in males, persistence of**
*See MULLERIAN DERIVATIVES IN MALES, PERSISTENT*

## OVULATION INDUCTION TRISOMY                    2993

**Includes:**
> Chlomaphen, ovulation induction trisomy
> Chromosome, ovulation induction trisomy
> Clomid^, ovulation induction trisomy
> Clomiphene ovulation induction trisomy
> Menotropin, ovulation induction trisomy
> Trisomy, ovulation induction

**Excludes:**
> **Chromosome** (other)
> **Fetal effects** (other)

**Major Diagnostic Criteria:** Trisomy with ovulation induction.

**Clinical Findings:** Oakley and Flynt (1972) reported six **Chromosome 21, trisomy 21** cases among 2,239 infants in the new drug investigations for ovulation-inducing agents (five following clomiphene, one following menotropin administration). This was 2.5 times the expected number. A further suggestion of association between trisomy and ovulation induction was found in the data of Boue et al (1975) on karyotyped spontaneous abortions. The ratio of trisomies to normal karyotypes was 3.5 times as high in spontaneous abortions following ovulation-inducing agent administration as in controls.

A total of 30 trisomy births following clomiphene ovulation induction are known to the Food and Drug Administration (FDA). Twenty of the cases were **Chromosome 21, trisomy 21**; two were **Chromosome 18, trisomy 18** (or trisomy 17); four were **Chromosome 13, trisomy 13** (or trisomy 14 or 15); two were **Chromosome 8, trisomy 8**; and two were unspecified trisomies. Five cases occurred among 2,082 investigational patients (included in Oakley and Flynt's data). Ten cases occurred among 3,815 exposed pregnancies in other cohorts in the scientific literature. Both the numerator and the denominator in the latter data may be undercounted: the numerator because some cases were not followed-up long enough to identify trisomy cases and the exposure denominator because some of the numerous small cohorts not having abnormalities were unpublished. Although maternal age is not given in some of these reports, available information indicates that the age of ovulation induction is not sufficiently elevated to be a substantial confounding factor. Fifteen other isolated case reports of trisomy births with maternal clomiphene exposure submitted to the FDA include 12 from the United States and three from other countries.

The possible association has also been examined in case control studies because of adequate maternal recall for ovulation induction and good definition of cases. However, the case control data available to date, limited to about 400 cases of **Chromosome 21, trisomy 21**, do not show an association. This discrepancy between the cohort and case control data could be due to mothers avoiding trisomy births on the basis of antenatal testing.

**Complications:** Unknown.

**Associated Findings:** None known.

**Etiology:** Maternal nondisjunction associated either with fertility problems for which ovulation-inducing agents are given, or with the agents themselves.

**Pathogenesis:** Unknown. Infertility problems in the mother could be a factor.

**Sex Ratio:** Presumably M1:F1.

**Occurrence:** Unlikely to exceed one trisomy birth in 300 exposures.

**Risk of Recurrence for Patient's Sib:** Unknown.

**Risk of Recurrence for Patient's Child:** Unknown.

**Age of Detectability:** At birth, or by amniocentesis.

**Gene Mapping and Linkage:** Unknown.

**Prevention:** An association, if present, does not mean the agent caused the defect. However, a practical clinical question, regardless of cause, is whether risk is sufficiently high to justify the hazard of amniocentesis in subfertile women strongly desiring a child.

**Treatment:** Unknown.

**Prognosis:**  Unknown.

**Detection of Carrier:**  Unknown.

**References:**

Oakley GP, Flynt GO: Increased prevalence of Down's syndrome (mongolism) among offspring of women treated with ovulation-inducing agents. (Abstract) Teratology 1972; 5:264 only.

Boue J, et al.: Retrospective and prospective studies of 1,500 karyotyped spontaneous human abortions. Teratology 1975; 14:11–26.

Merrill National Laboratories: Pregnancy outcome of humans following Clomid (clomiphene citrate USP) with summary of information of reported possible neural related anomalies of offspring. NDA 15–131, October 14, 1980.

Rosa FW: Ovulation induction trisomy. Food and Drug Administration ADR Highlight, 1981, No. 20.

Kurachi K, et al.: Congenital malformation of newborn infants after clomipene induced ovulation. Fertil Steril 1983; 40:187–189.

Wramsby H, et al.: Chromosome analysis of human oocytes recovered from preovulatory follicles in stimulated cycles. New Engl J Med 1987; 316:121–124.

R0018                                               **Franz W. Rosa**

**Owren parahemophilia**
  See FACTOR V DEFICIENCY

**'Ox eye' (buphthalmos)**
  See GLAUCOMA, CONGENITAL

**Oxazepam, fetal effects of**
  See FETAL BENZODIAZEPINE EFFECTS

**Oxycephally**
  See CRANIOSYNOSTOSIS

# ❖ P ❖

P450 side-chain cleavage enzyme, deficiency of
*See STEROID 20-22 DESMOLASE DEFICIENCY*
P450C11B1, deficiency of
*See STEROID 11 BETA-HYDROXYLASE DEFICIENCY*

## PACHYDERMOPERIOSTOSIS                                    0788

**Includes:**
   Hypertrophic osteoarthropathy, primary or idiopathic
   Osteoarthropathy, hypertrophic
   Rosenfeld-Kloepfer syndrome
   Touraine-Solente-Gole syndrome

**Excludes:**
   Pulmonary hypertrophic osteoarthropathy
   Thyroid acropachy

**Major Diagnostic Criteria:**  The presence of at least two of the three major abnormalities; clubbing, periostosis, cutis gyrata; in an individual with a negative family history and no sign of a predisposing lesion (e.g. bronchogenic carcinoma), or the presence of one of these major lesions in a close relative of a typical case.

**Clinical Findings:**  Clubbing of the fingers and toes; periosteal new bone formation, especially over the distal ends of the long bones; coarse facial features with thickening, furrowing, and excessive oiliness of the skin of the face and forehead; cutis verticis gyrata (often appearing in the early teenage years); hyperhidrosis of the hands and feet and occasional intermittent swelling or pain in the large joints. X-rays reveal irregular subperiosteal ossification over the long bones, primarily at the distal ends and most pronounced at the insertion of tendons and ligaments. There is marked variability in expressivity, the disorder being more severe in males than in females.

A combination of pubertal onset, male predominance, feminine hair distribution, increased estrogen excretion, and decreased serum sodium with increased aldosterone excretion suggests an endocrinologic disturbance.

**Complications:**  Ptosis due to hypertrophy of the eyelids, skeletal pain secondary to periostosis, and seborrheic dermatitis and secondary folliculitis associated with large and open skin pores.

**Associated Findings:**  A severe duodenal ulcer presented in an affected individual at the third decade of life.

**Etiology:**  Presumably autosomal dominant inheritance with marked variability in expression. Usually more severe in males.

**Pathogenesis:**  This syndrome usually appears around puberty, slowly progresses for about 10 years, and is self-limited thereafter. Periostosis and clubbing may be related to an autonomic nervous system defect, since there is a decrease in peripheral blood flow, and vagal resection has been reported to improve joint swelling.

**MIM No.:**  16710

**POS No.:**  3369

**Sex Ratio:**  M7:F1 observed among reported cases, but possibly related to increased severity of the disease in males.

**Occurrence:**  Undetermined but presumed rare.

**Risk of Recurrence for Patient's Sib:**
   See Part I, *Mendelian Inheritance.*

**Risk of Recurrence for Patient's Child:**
   See Part I, *Mendelian Inheritance.*

**Age of Detectability:**  In childhood or adolescence, by clinical features.

**Gene Mapping and Linkage:**  Unknown.

**Prevention:**  None known. Genetic counseling indicated.

**Treatment:**  Plastic surgery to improve facial appearance. Vagotomy is reported to relieve skeletal pain and swelling.

**Prognosis:**  Normal life span.

**Detection of Carrier:**  Skeletal X-rays may detect periosteal new bone formation in otherwise unaffected female relatives.

**Special Considerations:**  It is important to distinguish this disorder from secondary hypertrophic osteoarthropathy, as the latter condition may be associated with a treatable primary lesion (e.g. bronchogenic carcinoma, bronchiectasis, ulcerative colitis). A full clinical examination for a primary lesion must be performed on all sporadic cases of pachydermoperiostosis, as the diagnosis of this genetic disorder in isolated cases can only be made by exclusion.

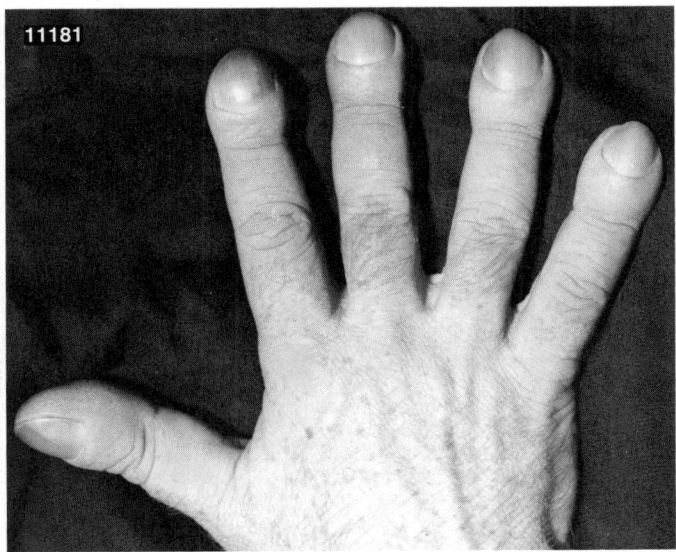

**0788**-11181:  Diffuse enlargement of fingers with clubbing producing drumstick appearance.

The unequal sex ratio is probably due to the variable expression of this dominant trait, which is much more severe in males. The phenotypic expression of this trait in females may be limited to asymptomatic periosteal new bone formation, and these individuals would go undetected unless skeletal X-rays were obtained.

The *Rosenfeld-Kloepfer syndrome* (Rosenthal & Kloepfer, 1962) is usually considered to be a variant of pachydermoperiostosis. This autosomal dominant condition is characterized by acromegaloid features, prominence of the frontal bone, cutis verticus gyrata, and corneal leukoma.

*The authors are indebted to Sonja A. Rasmussen and Jaime L. Frias for their contributions to this article.*

**References:**

Rosenthal JW, Kloepfer HW: An acromegaloid, cutis verticis gyrata, corneal leukoma syndrome. Arch Ophthalmol 1962; 68:722–726.

Vogl A, Goldfischer S: Pachydermoperiostosis: primary or idiopathic hypertrophic osteoarthropathy. Am J Med 1962; 33:166–187.

Rimoin DL: Pachydermoperiostosis (idiopathic clubbing and periostosis): genetic and physiologic considerations. New Engl J Med 1965; 272:923–931.

Hambrick GW Jr, Carter BM: Pachydermoperiostosis: Touraine-Solente-Golé syndrome. Arch Dermtol 1966; 94:594–608.

Hedayati H, et al.: Acrolysis in pachydermoperiostosis (primary or idiopathic hypertrophic osteoarthropothy). Arch Intern Med 1980; 140:1087–1088.

Shiu Kum Lana, et al.: Pachydermoperiostosis, hypertrophic gastropathy, and peptic ulcer. Gastroenterology 1983; 84:834–839.

B0025                                    **Zvi Borochowitz**
                                         *David L. Rimoin*

**Pachyonychia congenita**
  *See NAILS, PACHYONYCHIA CONGENITA*
**Pachyonychia congenita, Jackson-Lawler type**
  *See PACHYONYCHIA CONGENITA-STEATOCYSTOMA MULTIPLEX*

---

## PACHYONYCHIA CONGENITA-STEATOCYSTOMA MULTIPLEX                                    2905

**Includes:**
  Nails, pachyonychia congenita, Jackson-Lawler type
  Pachyonychia congenita, Jackson-Lawler type
  Steatocystoma-pachyonychia congenita

**Excludes:**
  **Dyskeratosis congenita** (2024)
  Keratoderma of palms and soles
  **Nails, pachyonychia congenita** (0789)
  Steatocystoma multiplex, isolated

**Major Diagnostic Criteria:** Milia in infancy, supernumerary teeth, subcutaneous cysts, and thickened nails that are almost impossible to cut.

**Clinical Findings:** The disease affects the nails and skin. Clinical signs, especially milia and neonatal teeth, may be present at birth. The former disappears in childhood. Deformed nails appear shortly after birth. The free edge of the nail is raised in a thick, horny mass, while the base is normal. Finger- and toenails may have to be cut with a hacksaw. Subcutaneous cysts that are painful, enlarge, become infected, and discharge pus are common. Other skin manifestations include hyperhidrosis, bullae, follicular keratoses, ichthyosis, and acne conglobata. Skin lesions may be scattered to almost confluent. The soles of the feet are hyperkeratotic and painful, and there is hyperhidrosis of both palms and soles. Corneal dystrophy may be present. Pachyonychia congenita may occur as an isolated condition or with various skin and oral lesions. There is obviously much heterogeneity.

**Complications:** Infection of the cysts. Psychologic problems due to the cosmetic effects.

**Associated Findings:** None known.

**Etiology:** Autosomal dominant inheritance.

**Pathogenesis:** The cysts appear to be hamartomas.

**MIM No.:** 16721

**Sex Ratio:** Presumably M1:F1.

**Occurrence:** About 20 cases have been documented in the literature.

**Risk of Recurrence for Patient's Sib:**
  See Part I, *Mendelian Inheritance.*

**Risk of Recurrence for Patient's Child:**
  See Part I, *Mendelian Inheritance.*

**Age of Detectability:** At birth.

**Gene Mapping and Linkage:** Unknown.

**Prevention:** None known. Genetic counseling indicated.

**Treatment:** Symptomatic. Antibiotics as needed for infection.

**Prognosis:** Apparently consistent with normal life span. Scarring after spontaneous evacuation of skin lesions.

**Detection of Carrier:** By clinical examination.

**Special Considerations:** Gorlin et al (1976) discuss the distinction between this Jackson-Lawler form of pachyonychia congenita and the Jadassohn-Lewandowsky form (see **Nails, pachyonychia congenita**).

**References:**

Jackson ADM, Lawler SD: Pachyonychia congenita: a report of six cases in one family, with a note on linkage data. Ann Eugen 1951; 16:142–146.

Vineyard WR, Scott RA: Steatocystoma multiplex with pachyonychia congenita: eight cases in four generations. Arch Dermatol 1961; 84:824–827.

Gorlin RJ, et al.: Syndromes of the head and neck, ed 2. New York: McGraw-Hill, 1976:600–603.

Hodes ME, Norins AL: Pachyonychia congenita and steatocystoma multiplex. Clin Genet 1977; 11:359–364.

Hurwitz S: Clinical pediatric dermatology. Philadelphia: W.B. Saunders, 1981:183.

H0003                                    **M.E. Hodes**
N0008                                    **A.L. Norins**

**Pachyonychia ichthyosiforme**
  *See NAILS, PACHYONYCHIA CONGENITA*
**Pachyonychia neonatorum**
  *See NAILS, PACHYONYCHIA CONGENITA*
**Paget disease**
  *See BONE, PAGET DISEASE*
**Paget disease, juvenile**
  *See OSTEOECTASIA*
**Pagon syndrome**
  *See WALKER-WARBURG SYNDROME*
**Pain, insensitivity to, with anhidrosis of Swanson (congenital)**
  *See NEUROPATHY, CONGENITAL SENSORY WITH ANHIDROSIS*
**Palatal incompetence, congenital**
  *See PALATOPHARYNGEAL INCOMPETENCE*
**Palatal-digital-oro syndrome**
  *See ORO-PALATAL-DIGITAL SYNDROME, VARADI TYPE*
**Palate enlargement**
  *See PALATE, TORUS PALATINUS*
**Palate, cleft, occult submucous**
  *See PALATOPHARYNGEAL INCOMPETENCE*
**Palate, cleft, submucous with a bifid uvula**
  *See CLEFT PALATE*
**Palate, congenital short**
  *See PALATOPHARYNGEAL INCOMPETENCE*

## PALATE, FISTULA                                                    0790

**Includes:**  Fistula of palate

**Excludes:**
Median palatal fistula and cyst
Nasoalveolar fistula and cyst

**Major Diagnostic Criteria:**  Small openings in anterior pillars at the junction of the soft palate and pharynx.

**Clinical Findings:**  Bilateral or unilateral fistulas at junction of soft palate and pharynx in the anterior pillars without cicatrization.

**Complications:**  Unknown.

**Associated Findings:**  Absence or hypoplasia of one or both palatine tonsils, preauricular fistulas, deafness and strabismus.

**Etiology:**  Unknown.

**Pathogenesis:**  Maldevelopment of the second branchial pouch occurs with failure of complete obliteration of the pouch. The resultant fistulas are lined by stratified squamous epithelium, with lymphoid tissue adjacent.

**Sex Ratio:**  Presumably M1:F1.

**Occurrence:**  Undetermined but presumed rare.

**Risk of Recurrence for Patient's Sib:**  Unknown.

**Risk of Recurrence for Patient's Child:**  Unknown.

**Age of Detectability:**  At birth, by visual examination.

**Gene Mapping and Linkage:**  Unknown.

**Prevention:**  None known. Genetic counseling indicated.

**Treatment:**  Unknown.

**Prognosis:**  Excellent.

**Detection of Carrier:**  Unknown.

**References:**
Claiborne JH Jr: Hiatus in the anterior pillar of the fauces of the right side with congenital absence of tonsil on either side. Am J Med Sci 1885; 89:490–491.
Miller AS, et al.: Lateral soft palate fistula. Arch Otolaryngol 1970; 91:200.
Gorlin RJ, et al.: Syndromes of the head and neck. 2nd ed. New York: McGraw-Hill, 1976.
Saito T: Congenital fistulas of the cleft and palate. J Jap Cleft Palate Asso 1982; 7:189–193.

JI001                                                        **Jan E. Jirásek**

## PALATE, TORUS PALATINUS                                            0959

**Includes:**
Palate enlargement
Torus palatinus

**Excludes:**  N/A

**Major Diagnostic Criteria:**  A rounded elevation in the midline of the palate, with a smooth edge.

**Clinical Findings:**  A slowly growing enlargement of bone on the hard palate at the junction of the midpalatal suture usually covered with normal appearing mucosa. These can be single or lobulated, and show remarkable variation in morphology (flat, spindle, nodular).

**Complications:**  Complications occur only if the palatal elevations grow so large as to interfere with mastication, speech, or the fitting of a denture.

**Associated Findings:**  None known.

**Etiology:**  Probably autosomal dominant inheritance with variable expressivity and penetrance close to 85%, although X-linked dominant inheritance has also been proposed, and there is also evidence also for multifactorial inheritance. There is no evidence of sporadic cases. Suzuki and Sakai (1960) have suggested this condition is due to the same gene as that responsible for **Mandible, torus mandibularis**.

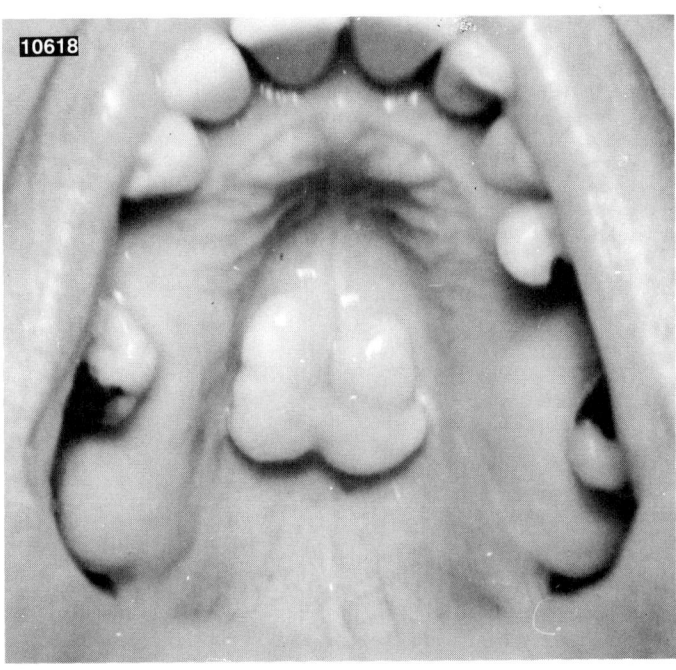

0959-10618:  Torus palatinus.

**Pathogenesis:**  Gradual enlargement of bone in the region of the midpalatal suture.

**MIM No.:**  *18970

**Sex Ratio:**  Estimated M1:F2 in Caucasians; M3:F1 American Indians.

**Occurrence:**  Incidence 1:5 in a midwestern United States Caucasian population. Prevalence 1:50 children.

**Risk of Recurrence for Patient's Sib:**
See Part I, *Mendelian Inheritance.*

**Risk of Recurrence for Patient's Child:**
See Part I, *Mendelian Inheritance.*

**Age of Detectability:**  Occasionally seen in children, but usually apparent by puberty.

**Gene Mapping and Linkage:**  Unknown.

**Prevention:**  None known. Genetic counseling indicated.

**Treatment:**  Surgical removal, if interfering with oral function or placement of denture.

**Prognosis:**  Excellent.

**Detection of Carrier:**  By clinical examination of first degree relatives.

**References:**
Kolos S, et al.: The occurrence of torus palatinus and torus mandibularis in 2,478 dental patients. Oral Surg 1953; 6:1134.
Suzuki M, Sakai T: A familial study of torus palatinus and torus mandibularis. Am J Phys Anthrop 1960; 18:263–272.
Gould AW: An investigation of the inheritance of torus palatinus and torus mandibularis. J Dent Res 1964; 43:159.
Gorlin RJ: Developmental anomalies of the face and oral structures. In: Gorlin RJ, Goldman HM, eds: Thoma's oral pathology, ed 6. vol. 1. St. Louis: C.V. Mosby, 1970:21.
King DR, Moore GE: The prevalence of torus palatinus. J Oral Med 1971; 26:113.
Barbujani G, et al.: Torus palatinus: a segregation analysis. Hum Hered 1986; 36:317–325.

J0011                                                    **Clinton C. Johnson**

**Palato-digital-oto syndrome**
  *See* OTO-PALATO-DIGITAL SYNDROME, II
**Palato-oto-digital syndrome**
  *See* OTO-PALATO-DIGITAL SYNDROME, I

## PALATOPHARYNGEAL INCOMPETENCE                2118

**Includes:**
  Cleft palate, occult submucous
  Palatal incompetence, congenital
  Palate, congenital short
  Palate, cleft, occult submucous
  Rhinolalia
  Speech, hypernasal
  Velopharyngeal incompetence
  Velopharyngeal insufficiency

**Excludes:  Cleft palate** (0180)

**Major Diagnostic Criteria:** An abnormal resonance of speech in the nasal cavity as a result of a failure of closure of the palato-pharyngeal (velopharyngeal) orifice during phonation. The nasal resonance is variable from person to person depending partly upon the size of the palato-pharyngeal opening during speech as well as other vocal tract dynamics. Occasionally, abnormal speech may be accompanied by nasal regurgitation of food or fluids during deglutition, but this is a relatively rare occurrence. Frequently, nasal resonance is accompanied by audible nasal air flow (nasal turbulence, or "snorting").

**Clinical Findings:** Palatal-pharyngeal gaps are most easily diagnosed and recognized by motion picture fluoroscopic studies of the palato-pharyngeal orifice during speech, or by direct nasal endoscopy. A variety of other procedures, such as nasal airflow studies, may be helpful in confirming the presence of abnormal nasal resonance, but the final determination of the degree of abnormality of the speech symptom depends most heavily upon a thorough speech evaluation. Palato-pharyngeal incompetence may be related to any disorder of the palate, pharynx, or nervous system (central or peripheral), including structural anomalies, neuromuscular disease, and anomalies of the CNS. Palato-pharyngeal incompetence is a nonspecific finding symptomatic of a broad range of disorders; it is not characterized by any particular set of physical findings (such as short stature, reduced head size, etc.). The relative frequency of palato-pharyngeal incompetence rank-ordered by pathogenesis is probably as follows:
  1. cleft palate, submucous cleft palate, occult submucous cleft palate.
  2. trauma or degenerative disease of the CNS.
  3. CNS malformations.
  4. neuromuscular disease or peripheral nerve damage.
  5. iatrogenic (usually a complication of adenotonsillectomy).

**Complications:** Developmental problems occur because proper functioning of the palato-pharyngeal valve is necessary for the acquisition of normal speech and articulation. Many individuals with palato-pharyngeal incompetence develop compensatory errors in their speech patterns. This often makes their speech entirely unintelligible and may give the appearance of significant language delay at ages one to two years due to the inability to decode their utterances. Patients with palato-pharyngeal incompetence also often develop facial grimaces in their efforts to constrict the abnormal nasal air flow at the nostrils.

Some patients may tend to avoid speech or speaking situations because of the secondary psychological complications of poor intelligiblity.

**Associated Findings:** Bifid uvula, highly arched palate, dental anomalies (especially in the area of the lateral incisors, cuspids, and bicuspids), notching of the maxillary alveolus, conductive hearing loss with recurrent middle ear effusions, **Microcephaly**, small stature, congenital heart disease, auricular anomalies, and orbital hypertelorism. Such associated findings may be related to the large number of malformation syndromes with palato-pharyngeal incompetence as a feature.

**Etiology:** Unknown.

**Pathogenesis:** Occurs in association with multiple types of anomalies and syndromes. Etiologically, three types of anomalies can cause palato-pharyngeal incompetence: structural anomalies of the palate and pharynx, neuromuscular disorders, and CNS anomalies.

Structural anomalies of the palate and pharynx may include abnormal insertions of the palatal muscles, missing muscle groups in the palate, excessively large pharynx, asymmetry of the palate and/or pharynx, and abnormal structural relationships between the palate and pharynx. As such, palato-pharyngeal incompetence can occur in a variety of disorders with multiple pathogeneses, such as **Mandibulofacial dysostosis**, **Acrofacial dysostosis, Nager type**, **Oto-palato-digital syndrome, I**, and **Chromosome 21, trisomy 21**.

Neuromuscular disorders are frequently first expressed by speech abnormalities such as hypernasality indicative of palato-pharyngeal incompetence. Many of the muscular dystrophies have associated palato-pharyngeal incompetence, most particularly **Myotonic dystrophy**. Palato-pharyngeal incompetence is also a frequent finding in **Neurofibromatosis**.

CNS anomalies, both malformations and deformations, frequently result in palato-pharyngeal incompetence. Hypernasality is associated with the Arnold-Chiari deformation, among others. Any disorder with involvement of the motor cortex and upper pyramidal tracts may result in palato-pharyngeal incompetence.

**MIM No.:**  16750

**CDC No.:**  750.210

**Sex Ratio:**  M1:F1

**Occurrence:**  Prevalence more than 1:1,000.

**Risk of Recurrence for Patient's Sib:**
  See Part I, *Mendelian Inheritance*. If an isolated trait, the risk may be as high as 50%. Otherwise the risk is that of the condition with which the palato-pharyngeal incompetence is associated.

**Risk of Recurrence for Patient's Child:**
  See Part I, *Mendelian Inheritance*.

**Age of Detectability:**  With the onset of speech (approximately 10–18 months of age).

**Gene Mapping and Linkage:**  Unknown.

**Prevention:**  None known. Genetic counseling indicated.

**Treatment:**  Depending on etiology, may be surgical reconstruction of the palate and/or pharynx, prosthetic augmentation of the palato-pharyngeal orifice, or speech therapy.

**Prognosis:**  With treatment, prognosis for normal speech is excellent.

**Detection of Carrier:**  Unknown.

**Special Considerations:** Because of the multiple etiologies of palato-pharyngeal incompetence, some potentially serious, it is extremely important to determine the reason for this common disorder in each individual case. For example, surgical correction of palato-pharyngeal incompetence is usually performed without complication in most instances. However, such surgery could prove to be hazardous in patients with **Myotonic dystrophy** because of the risk of malignant hyperthermia under anesthesia, or in patients with **Mandibulofacial dysostosis** because of the risk of obstructive apnea postoperatively. Furthermore, because this disorder may be the first noticeable symptom of a variety of syndromes, its source must be delineated to provide appropriate counseling (both genetic and treatment). The first clinically evident symptom of **Cleft lip/palate-lip pits or mounds**, for example, is often palato-pharyngeal incompetence. This is also true for such conditions as **Velo-cardio-facial syndrome** and **Neurofibromatosis**. Therefore, this disorder must be regarded in a broader context than simply speech impairment.

**References:**
Peterson-Falzone S, Pruzansky S: Cleft palate and congenital palatopharyngeal incompetency in mandibulofacial dysostosis: frequency and problems in treatment. Cleft Palate J 1976; 13:354–360.
Luce EA, et al.: Velopharyngeal insufficiency in hemifacial microsomia. Plast Reconstr Surg 1977; 60:602–606.

Pollack MA, et al.: Velopharyngeal insufficiency: the neurologic perspective. Dev Med Child Neurol 1979; 21:194–201. *

Lewin ML, et al.: Velopharyngeal insufficiency due to hypoplasia of the musculus uvulae and occult submucous cleft palate. Plast Reconstr Surg 1980; 65:585–591. * †

Andres R, et al.: Dominant inheritance of velopharyngeal incompetence. Clin Genet 1981; 19:443–447.

Pollack MA, Shprintzen RJ: Velopharyngeal insufficiency in neurofibromatosis. Int J Pediatr Otorhinolaryngol 1981; 3:257–262.

Williams MA, et al.: Adenoid hypopladia in the velo-cardio-facial syndrome. J Craniofac Genet Devel Biol 1987; 7:23–26.

SH040                                                    **Robert J. Shprintzen**

**Pallister mosaic syndrome**
  *See PALLISTER-KILLIAN MOSAIC SYNDROME*
**Pallister syndrome**
  *See ULNAR-MAMMARY SYNDROME*
**Pallister-Hall syndrome**
  *See HYPOTHALAMIC HAMARTOBLASTOMA SYNDROME,*
    *CONGENITAL*
**Pallister-Herrmann-Opitz syndrome**
  *See HERRMANN-PALLISTER-OPITZ SYNDROME*

---

## PALLISTER-KILLIAN MOSAIC SYNDROME          2189

**Includes:**
  Chromosome 12, isochromosome 12p mosaicism
  Killian syndrome
  Pallister mosaic syndrome
  Teschler-Nicola/Killian syndrome

**Excludes:**
  **Chromosome 12, partial trisomy 12p** (2130)
  Chromosome 21, mosaic tetrasomy 21
  **Hypomelanosis of Ito** (2264)

**Major Diagnostic Criteria:** Affected newborn infants are profoundly hypotonic with sparsity of scalp hair, especially bitemporally, and a prominent forehead. There is coarsening of facial features over time. Blood chromosomes are usually normal. Analysis of fibroblast chromosomes shows mosaicism for an isochromosome of 12p.

**Clinical Findings:** Clinical signs are evident at birth with profound hypotonia, distinct facial appearance, and sparsity of scalp hair, especially bitemporally. Birth weight is within the normal range. Craniofacial manifestations include "coarse" face with prominent high forehead, normal head circumference, hypertelorism, epicanthal folds, flat bridge of nose, highly arched palate, and abnormal ears. Most affected individuals have a generalized pigmentary dysplasia, which may vary from sparse hypopigmented macules to an incontinentia pigmenti-like pattern. Pigmentary changes may be evident only with a Woods lamp in some individuals. Many have accessory nipples.

In infancy the facial appearance becomes more "coarse," hypotonia persists, cognitive delays are obvious, and seizures may occur. Contractures may also develop, and strabismus is common. Cranial CT scan abnormalities were found in 10/15 tested, with cerebral atrophy being the most common finding.

Of the three adult patients, two are severely retarded, bedridden, have seizures and severe contractures of limbs, and lack speech and all self-help skills. The third adult is healthy, ambulatory, and has no contractures but is profoundly retarded, nonverbal, has seizures, and lacks self-help skills.

**Complications:** **Laryngomalacia** may cause respiratory problems in the newborn period. Gastroesophageal reflux and poor feeding may be secondary to hypotonia. Contractures (2/3) and cataracts (2/3) may develop in adulthood.

**Associated Findings:** Congenital heart defects (3/33), **Diaphragmatic hernia** (3/33), sensorineural hearing loss (3/33), imperforate anus (2/33).

**Etiology:** Tetrasomy for chromosome 12p. All cases have been sporadic. There is no significant pattern of advanced parental age, and there is no history of recurrent fetal wastage in their families.

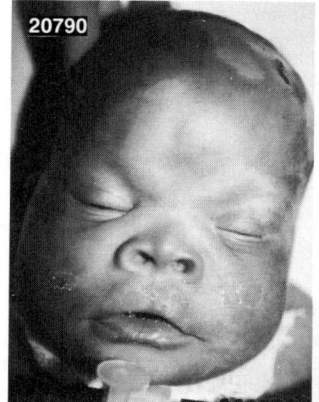
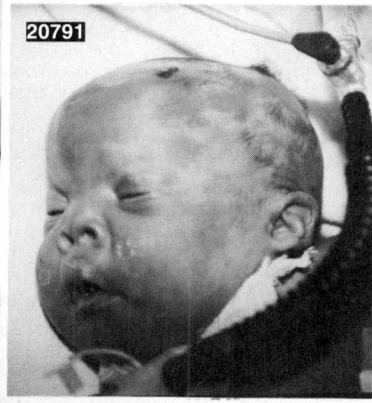
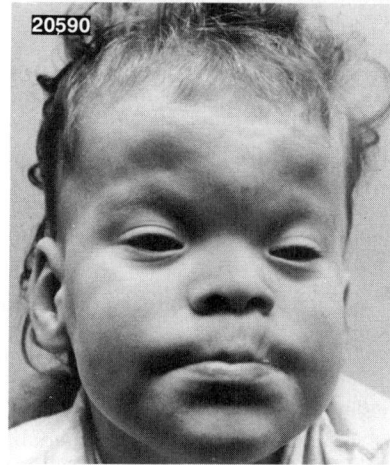

**2189**-20790–91: Pallister-Killian mosaic syndrome in an infant; note epicanthal folds, upward slanted palpebral fissures, anteverted nares, flat nasal bridge and prominent cheeks.  20590: Facial coarsening, high forehead and flat nasal bridge. There is now hair in the area where frontal balding occurs in infancy.

---

**Pathogenesis:** Unknown.

**POS No.:** 3800

**Sex Ratio:** M1:F1

**Occurrence:** More than 30 cases have been reported.

**Risk of Recurrence for Patient's Sib:** Low. All cases are sporadic.

**Risk of Recurrence for Patient's Child:** Unknown. No affected individuals are known to have reproduced.

**Age of Detectability:** At birth. Has been detected prenatally in amniocytes.

**Gene Mapping and Linkage:** See *Gene Map.*

**Prevention:** None known. Genetic counseling indicated.

**Treatment:** Unknown.

**Prognosis:** Athough early death does occur, oldest patients are in their 40s. Severe mental retardation is common, but some children are attending special education classes. Contractures may develop with time.

**Detection of Carrier:** Unknown.

**References:**
Pallister PD, et al.: The Pallister mosaic syndrome. BD:OAS XIII(3B). New York: March of Dimes Birth Defects Foundation, 1977:103–110.
Teschler-Nicola M, Killian W: Case report 72. Synd Ident 1981; 7:6–7.
Reynolds JF, et al.: Isochromosome 12p mosaicism (Pallister mosaic

aneuploidy or Pallister-Killian syndrome): report of 11 cases. Am J Med Genet 1987; 27:257–274. * †

Warburton D, et al.: Mosaic tetrasomy 12p: four new cases, and confirmation of the chromosomal origin of the supernumerary chromosome in one of the original Pallister-mosaic syndrome cases. Am J Med Genet 1987; 27:275–283.

RE029                                              **James F. Reynolds**

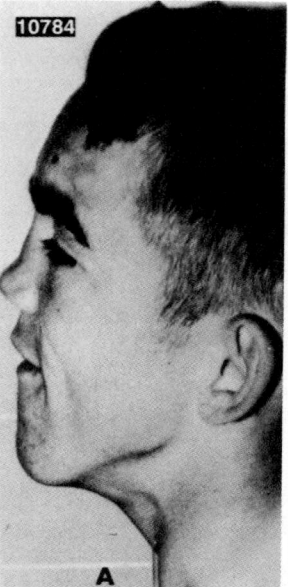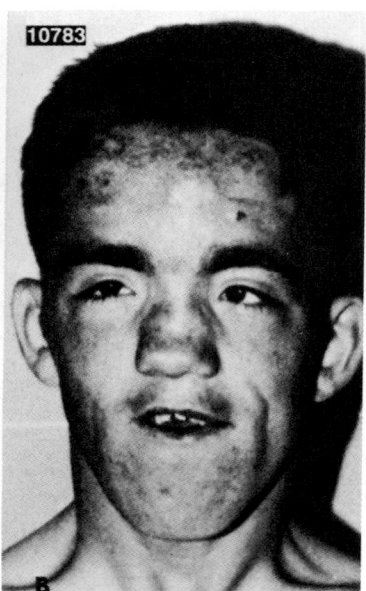

## PALLISTER-W SYNDROME                                    0791

**Includes:** W Syndrome

**Excludes:** Oto-palato-digital syndrome

**Major Diagnostic Criteria:** Mental retardation, some manifestations of a median oral cleft, the characteristic facial appearance, and mild skeletal abnormalities of the upper limbs. Patients present very much like the **Oto-palato-digital syndrome**, but without the characteristic hand and foot manifestations.

**Clinical Findings:** Presently the syndrome is defined on the basis of two male sibs having a malformation-mental retardation syndrome with the following features: moderate mental retardation, grand mal seizures, tremor, mild spasticity, an incomplete median cleft in the palate and upper lip, broad tip of nose, broad and flat maxilla, telecanthus, alternating esotropia, and high forehead. Skeletal abnormalities in the upper limbs included cubitus valgus, shortness of the ulnae, bowing of the radii, and clinocamptodactyly. One patient had pes cavus; the other had metatarsus varus and pes planus.

**Complications:** Broad uvula, absent incisors, and nasal speech secondary to oral cleft; antimongoloid slant of palpebral fissures secondary to hypoplastic maxillae; anterior cowlick secondary to high forehead. Injury secondary to seizures and mental retardation.

**Associated Findings:** Prematurity.

**Etiology:** Probably X-linked recessive inheritance (with some expression in female heterozygotes), or possibly autosomal dominant inheritance (with manifestations expressed more severely in males than in females).

**Pathogenesis:** A number of the facial manifestations can be related to incomplete median clefting.

**MIM No.:** 31145

**POS No.:** 3357

**Sex Ratio:** Presumably M1:F1 (2 brothers had severe symptoms, their mother and sister had mild manifestations).

**Occurrence:** One family consisting of two brothers, their mother, and a sister has been documented. The sister has since produced a severely affected son.

**Risk of Recurrence for Patient's Sib:**
See Part I, *Mendelian Inheritance.*

**Risk of Recurrence for Patient's Child:**
See Part I, *Mendelian Inheritance.*

**Age of Detectability:** At birth.

**Gene Mapping and Linkage:** Unknown.

**Prevention:** None known. Genetic counseling indicated.

**Treatment:** Cleft palate care and repair, correction of strabismus, orthopedic surgery. Special education, speech therapy, seizure control.

**Prognosis:** Survival into adulthood.

**Detection of Carrier:** Carrier females may show mild craniofacial manifestations.

**References:**
Pallister PD, et al.: The W syndrome. BD:OAS X(7). Miami: Symposia Specialists for The National Foundation-March of Dimes. 1974:51–60.

PA010                                          **Philip D. Pallister**
HE023                                          **Jürgen Herrmann**

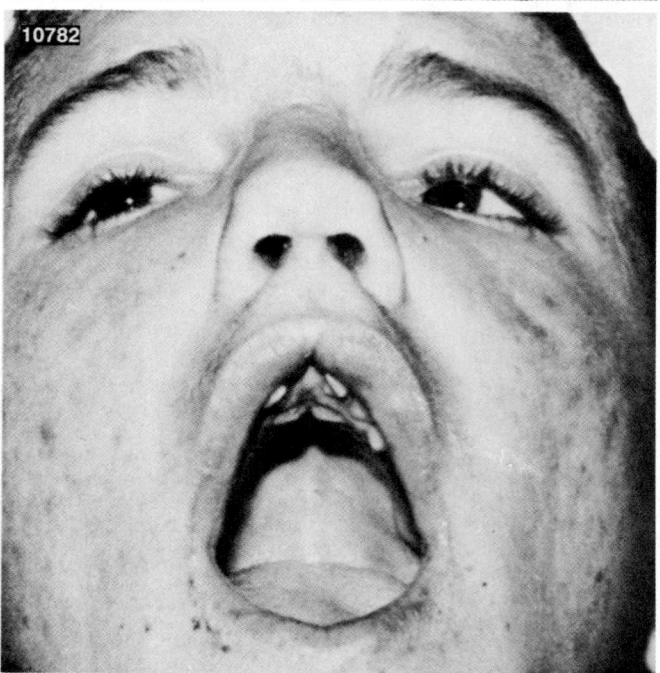

**0791-10784–83:** Characteristic facies shows broad nasal tip, broad maxilla, telecanthus, broad forehead and long chin. **10782:** Incomplete median cleft of the palate and upper lip.

**Palm, single line**
   *See SKIN CREASE, SINGLE PALMAR*
**Palmar clinodactyly**
   *See CAMPTODACTYLY*
**Palmar crease, single transverse**
   *See SKIN CREASE, SINGLE PALMAR*
**Palmar fibromatosis**
   *See CONTRACTURE, DUPUYTREN*
**Palmityl-CoA dehydrogenase deficiency**
   *See ACYL-CoA DEHYDROGENASE DEFICIENCY, LONG CHAIN TYPE*

**Palmo-plantar erythema**
*See SKIN, PALMO-PLANTAR ERYTHEMA*
**Palmo-plantar keratoderma, hereditary epidermolytic**
*See KERATOSIS PALMARIS ET PLANTARIS OF UNNA-THOST*
**Palmo-plantar keratodermas**
*See ICHTHYOSIS*
**Palmo-plantar keratodermia with carcinoma of esophagus**
*See HOWEL EVANS SYNDROME*
**Palmo-plantar keratodermia, diffuse hereditary**
*See KERATOSIS PALMARIS ET PLANTARIS OF UNNA-THOST*
**Palmoplantar hyperkeratosis-gingival hyperkeratosis**
*See SKIN, HYPERKERATOSIS, FOCAL PALMOPLANTAR AND GINGIVAL*
**Palmoplantar hyperkeratosis-reticular pigmentation**
*See ECTODERMAL DYSPLASIA, NAEGELI TYPE*
**Palmoplantar hyperkeratosis-spastic paraplegia-retardation**
*See HYPERKERATOSIS PALMOPLANTARIS-SPASTIC PARAPLEGIA-RETARDATION*
**Palpebral coloboma-lipoma syndrome**
*See NASOPALPEBRAL LIPOMA-COLOBOMA SYNDROME*
**Palpebromaxillary synergy, hereditary**
*See JAW-WINKING SYNDROME*

## PALSY, CONGENITAL FACIAL     0377

**Includes:**
Facial palsy, congenital partial
Facial palsy, congenital unilateral or bilateral
Facial paralysis, familial congenital peripheral
Nuclear facial palsy

**Excludes:**
Agenesis of facial musculature
Bell palsy, sporadic cases of
Facial palsy as part of a complex malformation syndrome
Facial palsy due to birth trauma or application of forceps
**Palsy, late-onset facial, familial** (0378)

**Major Diagnostic Criteria:** Bilateral (occasionally unilateral) peripheral palsy present from birth and not caused by trauma. Electrodiagnostic tests will show denervation as differentiated from muscular agenesis. Petrous pyramid polytomography may show middle ear anomalies or an aberrant course of the facial nerve canal.

**Clinical Findings:** Peripheral facial palsy is present at birth and is usually bilateral. Some pedigrees have been described in which each affected member was involved unilaterally and on the same side. History and physical findings are negative for birth trauma and, unlike most cases due to obstetric forceps pressure, no degree of recovery has been reported. In most instances no other neurologic deficits can be found, although in some families scattered members have shown associated homolateral ptosis or nystagmus or strabismus. In some instances associated congenital conductive hearing loss due to middle ear malformations has been reported, but these appeared to be sporadic. Various laboratory tests may be helpful in differential diagnosis, prognosis and in determining whether therapy might be beneficial in some instances. However, for therapy to have optimum results, evaluation should be carried out at about 7–14 days of age. Four tests have been found useful: the facial nerve excitability test, the strength-duration or intensity-duration test (recorded graphically), electromyography, and facial muscle biopsy in selected cases. Acoustic middle ear reflex (stapedius reflex) testing may help establish the site of lesion but needs to be combined with audiologic evaluation, probably including brainstem auditory evoked response testing, so that the level of hearing and type of hearing loss (if one exists) may be documented. The facial nerve-excitability test is most useful in unilateral cases where the response between the normal and abnormal side can be compared. In neurapraxia (physiologic or conductive block), there will be no difference in excitability between the normal and abnormal nerve. In partial denervation, the involved nerve will require more intensity of stimulation to evoke a response. In both of these instances, recovery can be anticipated and a good prognosis given but confirmation should be obtained using strength-duration testing. This test is of no value if performed before the 14th day

*after onset of paralysis.* However, the time of onset of paralysis in congenital cases is unknown. Therefore, it might be worthwhile trying the test before the 14th day of life. In total denervation no response to facial nerve-excitability stimulation is seen. Accordingly, this test is useful for both unilateral and bilateral facial weakness. Strength-duration curves are confirmatory. Facial nerve-excitability and strength-duration tests are best carried out in the infant under light general anesthesia which can then be deepened for definitive surgery, should this prove advisable. Electromyography and stapedius reflex testing should be done without anesthetic, although sedation may be required. In the absence of muscle potentials of any kind, specific muscle biopsy might be advisable in some instances to rule out absence of muscle fibers. The stapedius reflex will be absent in lesions proximal to the takeoff of the main trunk of the facial nerve as it descends through the mastoid. If hearing loss is also present, it is important to measure acoustic impedance to see if an associated anomaly of the middle ear ossicles may exist. Instances of partial facial palsy have been reported in which only the lower half of the face was paralyzed. The stapedius reflex was also impaired but taste and lacrimation were unimpaired. This was believed to be a partial nuclear lesion, not cortical. Petrous pyramid computerized tomography may delineate the anatomy of the facial nerve canal in the temporal bone and is a useful adjunct to diagnosis and therapy. It should be remembered, however, that the facial nerve may not be in the fallopian canal.

**Complications:** Corneal drying and ulceration could occur if the eye is unable to be closed sufficiently. Most patients, however, have an adequate eye closure. Eventually, denervated muscles undergo atrophy and fibrosis, and if the defect is unilateral, pulling of the opposite facial muscles will make the asymmetry even more noticeable. Bilateral involvement of the buccinator muscles may make feeding of the newborn infant very difficult but children and adults compensate for this.

**Associated Findings:** Middle ear anomalies, usually of second branchial arch origin but sometimes involving first arch structures, may be associated without mandibulofacial anomalies. Associated deficits of other cranial nerves have been reported in a few patients. Isolated absence or abnormality of the ramus mandibularus of the facial nerve associated with cardiac defects has been reported but this appears to be a separate entity. Congenital facial palsy may be found in a variety of syndromes.

**Etiology:** Autosomal dominant inheritance with high penetrance. It is possible that idiopathic, sporadic cases of congenital facial palsy are representative of autosomal dominance with variable penetrance. In congenital unilateral facial palsy, partial agenesis of the motor nucleus of the seventh cranial nerve has been found at autopsy. If hypoplasia of the facial nerve is found combined with middle ear anomalies, a nongenetic cause for branchial arch malformation may exist. Thalidomide ingestion by the mother during pregnancy may cause facial nerve agenesis.

**Pathogenesis:** The pathogenesis is unknown except that in instances of bony compression of the facial nerve within the temporal bone, it is believed the blood supply to the nerve is compromised. Wide variations in the anatomy of the facial nerve and the fallopian canal are known to occur. Hypoplasia and "hyperplasia" of the nerve have been reported. The facial nerve lies encased in a bony canal which may be abnormally narrow and compress the nerve. Narrowing at the stylomastoid foramen has been reported. Secondary edema may cause further decrease of the blood supply with death of the nerve fibers. There is some experimental evidence that ischemia of the facial nerve causes paralysis.

**MIM No.:** 13410

**Sex Ratio:** M1:F1

**Occurrence:** Several kindreds have been documented.

**Risk of Recurrence for Patient's Sib:**
See Part I, *Mendelian Inheritance.*

**Risk of Recurrence for Patient's Child:**
See Part I, *Mendelian Inheritance.*

**Age of Detectability:** At birth. In unilateral cases the facial asymmetry is obvious. Bilateral cases may go unrecognized for a prolonged time. Detection is by physical examination and confirmation is by electrodiagnostic testing.

**Gene Mapping and Linkage:** Unknown.

**Prevention:** None known. Genetic counseling indicated.

**Treatment:** Surgical decompression of the facial nerve in the temporal bone may be useful in early cases. This technique has been used so seldom in such ideal cases that its success cannot be assessed. Later, plastic and reconstructive procedures, such as fascial slings and reinnervation of the facial musculature using other nearby motor nerves, might be done. Reinnervation of already atrophic or fibrotic muscles is hopeless, and electromyography should be done before attempting any such procedure. If the patient has inadequate eye closure, tarsorrhaphy should be performed and the patient given safety glasses as additional protection. Tube feeding, gavage, or feeding with a syringe may be necessary in the bilaterally affected infant who cannot suck. Gastrostomy may be indicated in extreme cases. Surgical correction of associated middle ear anomalies that have caused conductive hearing loss may be feasible. In inoperable cases a hearing aid should be prescribed if the hearing loss is bilateral.

**Prognosis:** Normal for life span and intelligence. For function, no recovery can be anticipated without therapy. With therapy, variable degrees of recovery may be possible.

**Detection of Carrier:** Unknown.

**Special Considerations:** Physicians caring for these infants need to be aware that a more sophisticated approach to the problem than mere observation is now available. Facial paralysis is a major disability, and every attempt should be made to diagnose and, if possible, treat it early. Middle ear anomalies may be present in some instances, causing maximum conductive hearing loss. Audiometry should be done early to rule out this possibility, and appropriate habilitation should be begun. In many cases the etiology or pathogenesis remain unknown because either a ''wait-and-see'' or a hopeless attitude is taken by parents or physician. Very few patients have electrodiagnostic studies made shortly after birth, and even fewer patients have surgical exploration and decompression of the facial nerve as it courses through the temporal bone.

**References:**

Skyberg D, Van der Hagen CB: Congenital hereditary unilateral facial palsy in four generations. Acta Paediatr Scand 1965; 159(suppl):77–79.

Rubin A: Handbook of congenital malformations. Philadelphia: WB Saunders, 1967.

Cayler CG: Cardiofacial syndrome: congenital heart disease and facial weakness. Arch Dis Child 1969; 44:69–75.

McHugh HE, et al.: Facial paralysis and muscle agenesis in the newborn. Arch Otolaryngol 1969; 89:131–143.

Bergstrom L, Baker B: Syndromes associated with congenital facial paralysis. Otolaryngol Head Neck Surg 1981; 89:336–342.

BE028                                   **LaVonne Bergstrom**

**Palsy, double elevator**
*See EYELID, PTOSIS, CONGENITAL*

---

**PALSY, LATE-ONSET FACIAL, FAMILIAL**                **0378**

**Includes:**
   Bell palsy, single or recurrent episodes of
   Facial palsy, familial recurrent peripheral
   Facial palsy, late-onset

**Excludes:**
   Bell palsy, sporadic cases of
   **Cheilitis granulomatosa, Melkersson-Rosenthal type** (2083)
   **Fetal effects from Lyme disease** (3212)
   **Palsy, congenital facial** (0377)

**Major Diagnostic Criteria:** Typical peripheral facial palsy not present at birth, often recurrent; occurring in a family or kindred.

**Clinical Findings:** Inability to move the ipsilateral muscles of the face or close the eye. Decreased salivary secretion of the submaxillary gland, decreased tearing of the eye, diminished or absent stapedius reflex, impaired taste sensation on the ipsilateral side may be present.

Affected persons may show one or repeated episodes of peripheral facial palsy. Family history for more than one generation reveals an increased incidence of Bell palsy among family members. One survey found such an incidence to be nine times greater in the families of patients with Bell palsy as compared to the families of control patients. The same study showed that the episodes of Bell palsy in families could not be associated with exogenous factors, such as viral outbreaks. Although in one family several members had repeated episodes of facial palsy associated with upper respiratory and ear infections. Disorders such as diabetes or hypertension do not seem to be associated with an increased incidence of familial facial palsy.

There is a tendency for episodes of recurrent Bell palsy to recur on the same side, suggesting an anatomic variation as a factor in etiology. Usually the palsy clears spontaneously. However, in some instances nerve excitability may be lost; and in those instances the nerve would not be expected to recover without treatment. Pain, when it occurs, is a poor prognostic sign and also suggests the need for urgent surgical intervention. Jepson reported the following findings for facial nerve lesions at different levels:

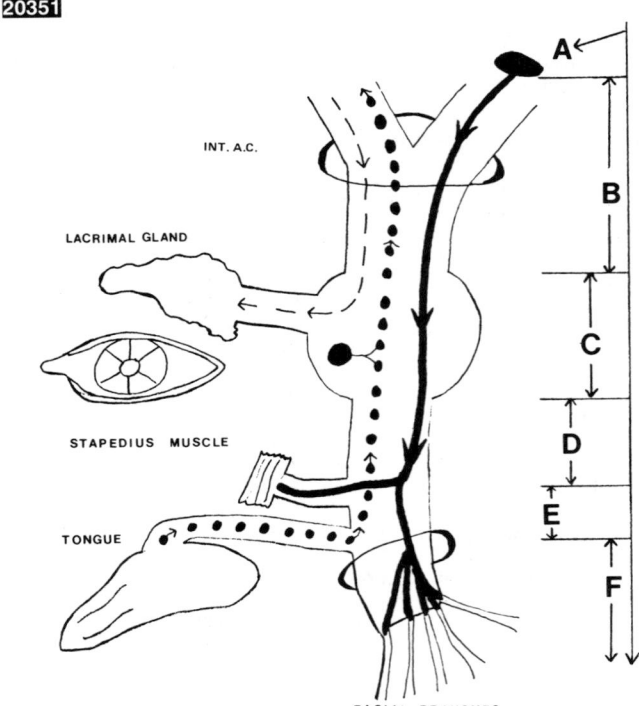

20351

**0378-20351:** Schematic drawing of the facial nerve restricted to motor, gustatory (via chorda tympani nerve), and lacrimal (via greater superficial petrosal nerve) branches. INT. A. C. = internal auditory canal. A, seventh (facial) nerve nucleus; B, suprageniculate; C, geniculate ganglion; D, suprastapedial; E, infrastapedial; F, infrachordal.

## Facial Nerve Lesions by Level

| Regional Diagnosis | Taste | Lacrimation | Stapedius Reflex |
|---|---|---|---|
| Nuclear | + | + | - |
| Suprageniculate | +/- | - | - |
| Transgeniculate | - | - | - |
| Suprastapedial | - | + | - |
| Infrastapedial | - | + | + |
| Infrachordal | + | + | + |

**Complications:** The nerve may fail to recover causing permanent paralysis. This may occur in 10–25% of cases. There is some evidence that recovery is less after repeated episodes of facial palsy. Corneal drying and ulceration may occur if there is inadequate eye closure.

**Associated Findings:** None known.

**Etiology:** Autosomal dominant inheritance with reduced penetrance. There may also be instances of autosomal recessive inheritance. Hypersensitivity to cold or to horse serum has been associated with increased susceptibility to facial paralysis in experimental animals.

**Pathogenesis:** Unknown.

**MIM No.:** *13420

**Sex Ratio:** M1:F1

**Occurrence:** Undetermined. At least a dozen kindreds have been documented.

**Risk of Recurrence for Patient's Sib:**
See Part I, *Mendelian Inheritance*.

**Risk of Recurrence for Patient's Child:**
See Part I, *Mendelian Inheritance*.

**Age of Detectability:** When it first occurs, usually in adults.

**Gene Mapping and Linkage:** Unknown.

**Prevention:** None known. Genetic counseling indicated.

**Treatment:** If nerve excitability remains equal to that of the normal side, a conduction block exists. Nerve conduction should be tested twice daily for up to two weeks to be certain denervation is not occurring. Probably no therapy is needed in these cases but if the palsy persists more than a few weeks, massage, local heat and electrical stimulation of the facial muscles to minimize atrophy and fibrosis may be beneficial.

If denervation occurs and if other neurologic deficits or a systemic cause are not present, immediate surgical decompression of the nerve throughout its course in the temporal bone seems to be of benefit. This should be done as soon as denervation becomes apparent. However, it may be of some benefit even after a prolonged period of denervation. In late cases, anastomosis of the facial nerve with another nerve, excision of an involved segment and grafting have been proposed. To minimize deformity, facial slings may be created to support the sagging paralyzed side of the face.

If coverage of the eye is inadequate, temporary or permanent tarsorrhaphy should be done.

Other medical treatments have been proposed. These include the administration of steroids, vasodilating drugs and stellate ganglion block. However, their efficacy seems to approximate the spontaneous recovery rate.

**Prognosis:** Normal for life span and intelligence. Spontaneous recovery of nerve function occurs in 75–90% of cases. In some cases recovery is partial, resulting in synkinesis or only partial movement.

**Detection of Carrier:** Unknown.

**Special Considerations:** Careful electrodiagnostic testing and neurologic examination of patients are essential for accurate diagnosis and rational therapy.

**References:**
Danforth HB. Familial Bell's palsy. Ann Otol Rhinol Laryng. 1964; 73:179–183.
McGovern FH. A review of the experimental aspects of Bell's palsy. Laryngoscope. 1968; 78:324.
DeSanto LW, Schubert HA. Bell's palsy: ten cases in a family. Arch Otolaryngol. 1969; 89:700–702.
Sullivan JA, et al. Management of Bell's palsy. Arch Otolaryngol. 1969; 89:144.
Auerbach SH, Depiero TJ, Mejlszenkier J. Familial recurrent peripheral facial palsy: observations of the pediatric population. Arch Neurol. 1981; 38:463–464.
Markby DP: Lyme disease facial palsy: differentiation from Bell's palsy. Br Med J 1989; 299:605–606.

BE028                                              **LaVonne Bergstrom**

## PALSY, PROGRESSIVE BULBAR OF CHILDHOOD      2045

**Includes:**
Brown-Vialetto-Van Leare syndrome
Bulbopontine paralysis, chronic-deafness
Fazio-Londe disease
Progressive bulbar palsy associated with neural deafness (PBPND)
Progressive bulbar palsy of childhood (PBPC)

**Excludes:**
**Amyotrophic lateral sclerosis, familial adult and juvenile types** (2069)
Amyotrophy in multisystem disease
**Arthrogryposes** (0088)
**G(M2)-gangliosidosis with hexosaminidase A deficiency** (0434)
Motor neuron disorders due to other causes
Poliomyelitis and other viral encephalitides
**Spinal muscular atrophy** (0895)

**Major Diagnostic Criteria:** Progressive paralysis of cranial nerve innervated muscles with or without upper motor neuron signs. EMG evidence of a diffuse neuropathic process in the absence of neuromuscular junction defect and exclusion of an infectious or neoplastic lesion helps to make the diagnosis of PBPC.

**Clinical Findings:** PBPC is probably not a single entity, and its symptomatology of progressive paralysis of cranial nerve innervated muscles is a common signature of different etiologic agents. Less than 20 cases of Fazio-Londe disease have been published. PBPC most frequently manifests as unilateral facial paralysis, followed in frequency by dysarthria associated with facial weakness, dysphagia and difficulty with chewing, palpebral ptosis, and palatal weakness. Progression to involve other cranial nerve innervated muscle occurs over a period of months or years. The facial nerve is affected in all cases, followed in frequency by the hypoglossal, vagus, trigeminal, spinal accessory, abducens, oculomotor, cochlear, and glossopharyngeal. Corticospinal tract involvement has been reported but may be rare. The disease may progress relentlessly to the patient's death in as short as nine months, or it may have a slower evolution with plateaus and the patient may live for more than eight years.

There are 20 cases of Brown-Vialetto-Van Leare (PBPND) disease (chronic bulbopontine paralysis with deafness) described in the world literature. Four autopsy reports are available. Clinical PBPND resembles Fazio-Londe disease except for sensorineural deafness (eighth nerve involvement) and usually, though not always, a more indolent course and a much more variable age of onset. Corticospinal tract involvement may be present.

PBPC must be diagnosed after the common causes of bulbar palsy in childhood are excluded. These include astrocytomas of the brain stem or extramedullary tumors, progressive myopathies, vascular malformations and congenital anomalies, cranial polyneuritis, brain stem encephalitis, myasthenia gravis or pseudobulbar palsy associated with perinatal hypoxia. Neuroimaging techniques, together with EMG examination, CSF examination, and antiacetylcholine receptor antibody titers usually help to differentiate these entities.

**Complications:** Muscle weakness interferes with basic functions of life, such as sucking of milk, breathing, and speaking. Motor milestones gained may be lost. Scoliosis develops in the more chronic cases. Hearing loss poses a problem in appropriate communication.

**Associated Findings:** **Retinitis pigmentosa** has been reported.

**Etiology:** Usually autosomal recessive inheritance. Patients with giant axonal neuropathy have been reported to have findings of PBPC. Nosologically, some cases with upper motor neuron findings and without extraocular muscle weakness may be diagnosed as juvenile-onset **Amyotrophic lateral sclerosis**, and others may be form-frustes of **Spinal muscular atrophy**. Dominant, recessive, and sporadic patterns of inheritance have been described in PBPC.

**Pathogenesis:** Degeneration of motor neurons of cranial nerve nuclei and sometimes spinal motor neurons. Corticospinal and spinocerebellar tracts may also be involved. The ventral portion of the cochlear nuclei shows severe neuronal loss in PBPND.

**MIM No.:** *21150

**Sex Ratio:** M1:F1

**Occurrence:** About 40 cases have been described in the literature.

**Risk of Recurrence for Patient's Sib:**
See Part I, *Mendelian Inheritance.*

**Risk of Recurrence for Patient's Child:**
See Part I, *Mendelian Inheritance.*

**Age of Detectability:** In Fazio-Londe disease, age of detectability may vary from one to 12 years, and in juvenile-onset disorder it may be even later. In PBPND, age of onset of sensorineural hearing defect may occur simultaneously with other bulbar and spinal symptoms or it may be separated from them by as many as three years. Sensorineural deafness may be present as early as the first year of life or as late as three years. In PBPND patients onset is before the age of 10 years.

**Gene Mapping and Linkage:** Unknown.

**Prevention:** None known. Genetic counseling indicated.

**Treatment:** Appropriate measures to ensure feeding. Respiration may have to be supported depending on the severity of involvement. A tracheostomy may help breathing in patients with vocal cord paralysis. Physical therapy measures for range of motion exercises to prevent contractions is indicated.

**Prognosis:** Some patients die within a year of onset of symptoms. Others may live longer, with long plateaus in the progression of illness.

**Detection of Carrier:** Unknown.

**References:**
Gomez MR: Progressive bulbar paralysis of childhood. In: Vinken PJ, Bruyn GW, eds: Handbook of clinical neurology. Amsterdam: North-Holland, 1975:103–109.
Latbrisseau A, et al.: Generalized giant axonal neuropathy: a case with features of Fazio-Londe disease. Neuropaediatrie 1979; 1:76–86.
Gallai V, et al.: Ponto-bulbar palsy with deafness (Brown-Vialetto-Van Leare syndrome). J Neurol Sci 1981; 50:259–275.
Albers JW, et al.: Juvenile progressive bulbar palsy: clinical and electrodiagnostic findings. Arch Neurol 1983; 40:351–353.

SI032                                           **Teepu Siddique**

## PANCREAS, ANNULAR                                     0062

**Includes:**
Annular pancreas
Pancreas, malrotation of

**Excludes:** **Duodenum, atresia or stenosis (0300)**

**Major Diagnostic Criteria:** Intestinal obstruction with a "double bubble" gas pattern by X-ray, and demonstration of a collar of pancreas surrounding the duodenum at laparotomy.

**Clinical Findings:** All grades of obstruction ranging from complete duodenal obstruction in the neonate, associated with maternal hydramnios and with bile-stained vomiting, to intermittent

vomiting and failure to thrive. Nonobstructing forms may be found at operation or autopsy without symptoms.

**Complications:** Defective pancreatic drainage with pancreatitis later in life; occasional stasis ulcer of the duodenum with perforation into the annular pancreas; failure to thrive, secondary to occasional vomiting.

**Associated Findings:** **Chromosome 21, trisomy 21** occurs in 20–30% of patients with annular pancrease; anomalies in other organs in 40–50% of cases (Merrill and Raffensperger, 1976).

**Etiology:** Possibly autosomal dominant inheritance.

**Pathogenesis:** There are several versions of basic incomplete rotation of the dorsal and ventral anlagen of the pancreas so that portions of the pancreas remain on both sides of the second portion of the duodenum. The exact mode of formation of the defect is not known; perhaps several different variations in rotation may result in annular rings of the pancreas and various grades of obstruction. Several investigators believe that the obstruction when present is due to a stenosis of the duodenum and that there is no true constriction by the surrounding pancreas.

**MIM No.:** 16775

**CDC No.:** 751.720

**Sex Ratio:** Presumably M1:F1

**Occurrence:** 1:10,000 live births.

**Risk of Recurrence for Patient's Sib:**
See Part I, *Mendelian Inheritance.*

**Risk of Recurrence for Patient's Child:**
See Part I, *Mendelian Inheritance.*

**Age of Detectability:** At birth.

**Gene Mapping and Linkage:** Unknown.

**Prevention:** None known. Genetic counseling indicated.

**Treatment:** Duodenojejunostomy or duodenoduodenostomy should be performed. Cutting into pancreatic substance is dangerous, since it may produce a pancreatic fistula.

**Prognosis:** Excellent for relief of obstruction. There is normal life expectancy. Rarely, pancreatitis or biliary tract disease may occur in later life. Mortality is usually due to associated anomalies.

**Detection of Carrier:** Unknown.

**References:**
Merrill JR, Raffensperger JG: Pediatric annular pancreas: twenty year's experience. J Pediatr Surg 1976; 11:921–925.
Jackson LG, Apostolides P: Autosomal dominant inheritance of annular pancreas. Am J Med Genet 1978; 1:319–321.
MacFadyen UM, Young ID: Annular pancreas in mother and son (letter). Am J Med Genet 1987; 27:987–988.

SE006                                           **John H. Seashore**

**Pancreas, malrotation of**
*See PANCREAS, ANNULAR*
**Pancreatic acinar carcinoma**
*See CANCER, PANCREAS, FAMILIAL ADENOCARCINOMA OF*
**Pancreatic cancer**
*See CANCER, PANCREAS, FAMILIAL ADENOCARCINOMA OF*
**Pancreatic fibrosis**
*See CYSTIC FIBROSIS*
**Pancreatic hypoplasia-marrow dysfunction-metaphyseal dysplasia**
*See SHWACHMAN SYNDROME*
**Pancreatic insufficiency-growth failure-ectodermal dysplasia**
*See DONLAN SYNDROME*
**Pancreatic lipase deficiency, congenital**
*See LIPASE, CONGENITAL ABSENCE OF PANCREATIC*
**Pancreatic lipase deficiency, congenital isolated**
*See LIPASE, CONGENITAL ABSENCE OF PANCREATIC*
**Pancreatitis, familial**
*See PANCREATITIS, HEREDITARY*

## PANCREATITIS, HEREDITARY 0793

**Includes:** Pancreatitis, familial

**Excludes:**
Cystic fibrosis (0237)
Pancreatitis, acute idiopathic
Pancreatitis associated with hyperlipidemia or
hyperparathyroidism

**Major Diagnostic Criteria:** Increased serum amylase and lipase during the acute phase of illness are diagnostic features of pancreatitis. Increased urinary amylase-to-creatinine clearance ratio helps confirm serum values, and should be performed when possible. Some patients will not have elevated enzyme tests, particularly those with advanced disease.

Calcifications distributed throughout the pancreas, especially if apparent in childhood, strongly suggest hereditary pancreatitis.

The diagnosis can be made if there is documentation of repeated episodes of acute pancreatitis and a family history of similar illness. Analysis of serum lipoproteins and evaluation of parathyroid function are necessary to exclude familial hyperlipidemia and hyperparathyroidism.

**Clinical Findings:** Hereditary pancreatitis presents with episodes of recurrent epigastric or abdominal pain that may radiate through to the back and subscapular area. The pain is often initiated by a large fatty or spicy meal. The attack progresses to maximal intensity in 24–48 hours and abates in four days to several weeks. Nausea and vomiting frequently accompany the pain and may result in serum electrolyte disturbances. Serum and urinary amylase and lipase will be elevated during the active phase. The attacks of acute pancreatitis are separated by symptom-free periods of days to years in duration. During the symptom-free periods there will be no disturbance in serum amylase and lipase.

In time, the repeated episodes of pancreatitis result in pancreatic fibrosis, with exocrine insufficiency (30–50%) or glucose intolerance (30%). Pancreatic exocrine insufficiency produces steatorrhea in most instances, but subclinical disease may be diagnosed by measurement of the pancreatic peptidases or lipase obtained at duodenal intubation. Secretin stimulation may provide another degree of discrimination of exocrine function.

Pancreatic calcifications observed on abdominal X-ray are of diagnostic importance. Some patients (50%) will exhibit coarse, rounded calcifications in the head of the pancreas. Linear distribution is consistent with the anatomic finding of calcifications in the major pancreatic ducts. CT scanning improves the sensitivity for detecting pancreatic calcifications.

Involvement of multiple family members has been documented in all series.

**Complications:** Acute dehydration and serum electrolyte disturbances (common in acute attacks); pancreatic exocrine insufficiency (often with steatorrhea); pancreatic endocrine insufficiency (glucose intolerance); pancreatic carcinoma (25%); portal or splenic vein thrombosis (rare); acute hemorrhagic pancreatitis (with or without hemorrhagic pleural and peritoneal effusions) (rare); and pancreatic pseudocyst.

**Associated Findings:** Aminoaciduria (cystine and lysine) has been documented in two families. Abnormal sweat electrolytes have been found in one family.

**Etiology:** Autosomal dominant inheritance with variable expressivity.

**Pathogenesis:** Unknown.

**MIM No.:** *16780

**CDC No.:** 751.780

**Sex Ratio:** M1:F1

**Occurrence:** About 400 known or suspected cases have been reported.

**Risk of Recurrence for Patient's Sib:**
See Part I, *Mendelian Inheritance.*

**Risk of Recurrence for Patient's Child:**
See Part I, *Mendelian Inheritance.*

**Age of Detectability:** The majority of cases have their onset in childhood, often in infancy.

**Gene Mapping and Linkage:** Unknown.

**Prevention:** None known. Genetic counseling indicated.

**Treatment:** Supportive measures during acute attacks include restorative and maintenance intravenous fluids and electrolytes, nothing orally, nasogastric suction; and narcotic pain medication. Enzyme replacement and a low-fat diet for pancreatic exocrine insufficiency. Appropriate measures for control of glucose intolerance.

**Prognosis:** Life expectancy is generally normal, if acute attacks are managed appropriately and if pancreatic carcinoma is not a complicating factor.

**Detection of Carrier:** Asymptomatic parents of affected individuals have been shown to have abnormalities in pancreatic exocrine function.

**References:**
Gross JB, et al.: Hereditary pancreatitis: description of a fifth kindred and summary of clinical features. Am J Med 1962; 33:358–364.
Kattwinkel J, et al.: Hereditary pancreatitis: three new kindreds and a critical review of the literature. Pediatrics 1973; 51:55–69.
Girard RM, et al.: Hereditary pancreatitis: report of an affected Canadian kindred and review of the disease. Can Med Asso J 1981; 125:576–580.
Dalton-Clark HJ, et al.: Familial chronic calcific pancreatitis: a family study. Br J Surg 1985; 72:307–308.

WH007                                    **Peter F. Whitington**

## PANCYTOPENIA SYNDROME, FANCONI TYPE 2029

**Includes:**
Estren-Dameshek variant of Fanconi anemia
Fanconi anemia, I
Fanconi pancytopenia, type I

**Excludes:**
Anemia, hypoplastic congenital (0051)
Anemia, hypoplastic-triphalangeal thumbs, Aase-Smith type (2028)
Bloom syndrome (0112)
Dyskeratosis congenita (2024)
Thrombocytopenia-absent radius (0941)
Thrombocytopenia-multiple malformations-neurologic dysfunction
WT syndrome (3145)

**Major Diagnostic Criteria:** Progressive pancytopenia and spontaneous chromosome breakage, which worsens after exposure to bifunctional alkylating agents. Multiple congenital anomalies may occur, including low birth weight, abnormal skin pigmentation, skeletal deformities, kidney malformations, and hypogonadism. Variation in number and severity of anomalies precludes diagnosis on clinical grounds alone. Clinical diagnosis must be confirmed cytogenetically.

**Clinical Findings:** The usual symptoms relate to anemia or thrombocytopenia. Most affected children present with pallor, fatigue, bleeding, or easy bruisability. The history reveals that the child was small for gestational age and had congenital anomalies. Review of 155 patients with Fanconi anemia showed that 76% of probands had hyperpigmentation, café-au-lait spots, or both; 65% were of small stature for age; 40% had thumb anomalies (aplasia, hypoplasia, supernumerary); 30% were microcephalic, 31% had renal anomalies (including absent kidney, duplication of the kidney or collecting system, renal ectopia, or a horseshoe kidney); 28% had other skeletal malformations (most commonly of the skull, spine, and extremities), 23% had strabismus; 20% hyperreflexia; 19% microophthalmia; 18% mental retardation; 12% ear anomalies or deafness; and 7% congenital heart disease. Absence of congenital anomalies, however, does not rule out a diagnosis of Fanconi anemia. In a study of 44 affected siblings of probands,

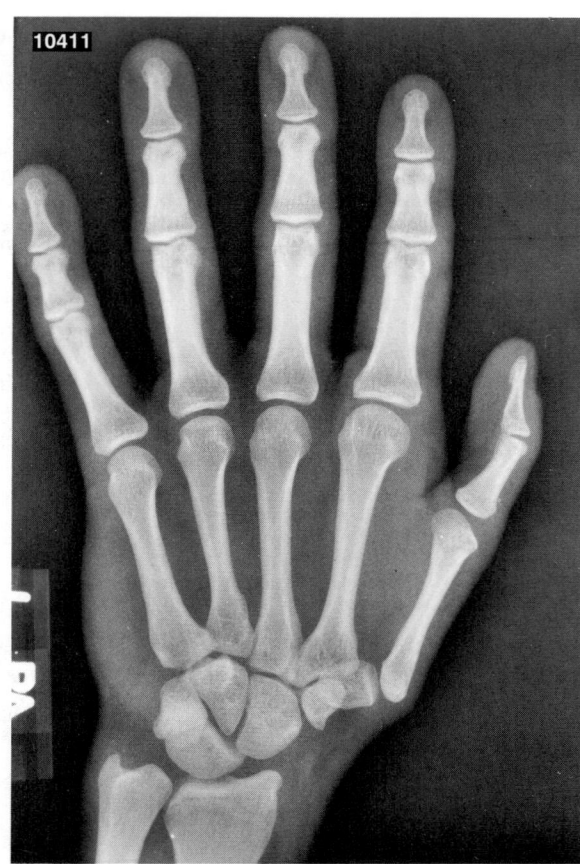

**2029**-10411: Hypoplastic 1st metacarpal and phalanges of thumb; absent navicular.

25% had no dysmorphic features. There may be wide clinical variability, even within families.

Anemia characteristically develops in early to mid-childhood. Laboratory findings may include macrocytosis, mild poikilocytosis, mild anisocytosis, leukopenia, thrombocytopenia, and reticulocytopenia. The stressed hypocellular bone marrow will produce erythrocytes with fetal-like qualities (expressing i surface antigen and containing fetal hemoglobin).

The most specific laboratory finding for Fanconi anemia is in the metaphase chromosomes of affected individuals. Typical abnormalities include chromatid breaks, gaps, chromosome rearrangements, endoreduplication, or formation of triradials or quadriradials. In an affected patient, the number of abnormalities will dramatically increase after cells have been exposed to the difunctional alkylating agents mitomycin C or diepoxybutane. Because of the low mitotic index often seen in cells from patients with Fanconi anemia, additional methods of diagnosis have been developed using flow cytometry and DNA histograms. After exposure to mitomycin C, Fanconi cells will characteristically accumulate in the $G_2$ phase of the cell cycle.

**Complications:** Recurrent infections, growth hormone deficiency, cryptorchidism, primary testicular failure, hepatomas (may be reversible), peliosis hepatis, unusual sensitivity to chemotherapeutic agents used to prepare for bone marrow transplantation, and severe graft-vs-host disease following bone marrow transplantation.

**Associated Findings:** Acute nonlymphatic leukemia, hepatocellular carcinoma, squamous cell carcinomas. Leukemia is the terminal event in 5–10% of patients with Fanconi anemia. It was formerly thought that Fanconi anemia heterozygotes were at increased risk for developing malignancies. This has now been disproved.

**Etiology:** Autosomal recessive inheritance. Heterogeneity is postulated.

**Pathogenesis:** Fanconi anemia is the most common heritable aplastic anemia. If all cases of childhood aplastic anemia are taken together, approximately one-fifth will be diagnosed as Fanconi anemia. The association between the bone marrow failure and the congenital anomalies is not understood but is presumed to be related to simultaneous developmental events occurring at 25–34 days gestation. Fanconi anemia is possibly a hematopoietic stem cell disorder. Cultures of bone marrow cells from Fanconi patients reveal markedly decreased or absent progenitor cells (CFU-C, CFU-E, BFU-E). The biochemical basis for the enhanced sensitivity to DNA cross-linking agents is unknown, but it is hypothesized to be due to abnormal DNA repair mechanisms. Recent experiments have shown that the subcellular distribution of topoisomerase (a DNA-related enzyme) is different in Fanconi placental cells when compared with normals. In Fanconi patients, the DNA topoisomerase activity is high in the cytoplasm, where it is produced, but low in the nucleus, where it is utilized for DNA repair. Other experiments have shown that mitomycin-C-treated Fanconi cells, when fused with normal fibroblasts, have a decreased number of chromosome abnormalities. This implies production of a clastogenic factor by the Fanconi cells.

**MIM No.:** *22765

**POS No.:** 3234

**Sex Ratio:** M1.9:F1

**Occurrence:** Heterozygote frequency has been estimated at between 1:300 and 1:600. Most of the reported cases have been in whites, although Black, Oriental, Turkish, Arab, and Indian patients have been described. The incidence among white Afrikaans-speaking South Africans is particularly high, with the heterozygote prevalence calculated at about 1:77, and a birth incidence of 1:22,000.

**Risk of Recurrence for Patient's Sib:**
See Part I, *Mendelian Inheritance.*

**Risk of Recurrence for Patient's Child:**
See Part I, *Mendelian Inheritance.* If an affected patient marries a Fanconi heterozygote, half of the offspring will be affected. Risk = 1/300 × 1/2 = 0.16%.

**Age of Detectability:** Rarely present at birth. The onset of pancytopenia is slightly earlier in males than in females. Median age for clinical diagnosis in a male is six years; median age in a female is 7 1/2 years. For males, 90% are diagnosed by age 12 years; in females, 90% are diagnosed by age 14 years. Ultrasound may be helpful in detecting skeletal, renal, or cardiac anomalies.

Diagnosis is available at birth or prenatally. Amniotic fluid cells, fetal blood lymphocytes, and chorionic villus cells, when treated with diepoxybutane, reveal increased chromosome breakage and rearrangements as compared with controls. First trimester prenatal diagnosis based on clastogen-induced chromosomal breakage is now available (Auerbach et al, 1986).

**Gene Mapping and Linkage:** FA (Fanconi anemia) is unassigned.

**Prevention:** None known. Genetic counseling indicated.

**Treatment:** Support with specific transfusions of red cells, white cells, and platelets. Splenectomy is not indicated. Androgen therapy causes definite improvement in blood counts but will have masculinizing side effects. Bone marrow transplantation is a potential form of treatment, although studies have indicated that Fanconi patients are unusually sensitive to chemotherapeutic agents and have a severe problem with graft-vs-host disease.

**Prognosis:** In older studies, an overall 80% mortality by age 12 years. Survival is prolonged with androgen therapy. An association between androgen therapy and the subsequent development of hepatocellular carcinoma has not been proved. Fanconi anemia patients usually die of bleeding, intercurrent infection, or malignancy.

**Detection of Carrier:** In one study, lymphocytes from parents and siblings exhibited a significantly increased diepoxybutane-induced chromosome breakage compared with normal subjects.

**Special Considerations:** This condition should be distinguished from *Thrombocytopenia-multiple malformations-neurologic dysfunction* (Gardner et al, 1983).

**Support Groups:** OR; Eugene; Fanconi Anemia Support Group

**References:**

Fanconi G: Familial constitutional panmyelocytopathy, Fanconi's anemia. I. Clinical aspects. Seminars in Hematology 1967; 4:233–240.

Schroeder TM, et al.: Formal genetics of Fanconi's anemia. Hum Genet 1976; 32:257–288.

Glanz A, Fraser FC: Spectrum of anomalies in Fanconi anemia. J Med Genet 1982; 19:412–416. *

Latts A, et al.: Cytogenetic and flow cytometric studies of cells from patients with Fanconi's anemia. Cytogenet Cell Genet 1982; 33:133–138.

Alter BP, Potter NU: Long-term outcome in Fanconi's anemia: description of 26 cases and review of the literature. In: German J, ed: Chromosome mutation and neoplasia. New York: Alan R. Liss, 1983:43–62. *

Deeg HJ, et al.: Fanconi's anemia treated by allogeneic marrow transplantation. Blood 1983; 61:954–959.

Gardner RJM, et al.: A syndrome of congenital thrombocytopenia with multiple malformations and neurologic dysfunction. J Pediatr 1983; 102:600–603.

Duckworth-Rysiecki G, et al.: Clinical and cytogenetic diversity in Fanconi's anemia. J Med Genet 1984; 21:197–203.

Auerbach AD, et al.: Clastogen-induced chromosomal breakage as a marker for first trimester prenatal diagnosis of Fanconi anemia. Hum Genet 1986; 73:86–88.

Rosendorff J, et al.: Fanconi anemia: another disease of unusually high prevalence in the Afrikaans population of South Africa. Am J Med Genet 1987; 27:793–797.

Schweiger M, et al.: DNA repair in human cells: biochemistry of the hereditary diseases Fanconi's anemia and Cockayne syndrome. Eur J Biochem 1987; 165:235–242.

BI001                                                 **Diana W. Bianchi**

**Panhypopituitarism, X-linked**
  *See DWARFISM, PANHYPOPITUITARY*
**Panic disorder**
  *See MOOD AND THOUGHT DISORDERS*
**Panleukocytic granulation, anomalies**
  *See CHEDIAK-HIGASHI SYNDROME*
**Panner disease (capitellum of humerus)**
  *See JOINTS, OSTEOCHONDRITIS DISSECANS*
**PAPA-Chondroitin sulfate sulfotransferase deficiency**
  *See SPONDYLOEPIPHYSEAL DYSPLASIA, LATE*
**Papillary carcinoma with follicular elements**
  *See CANCER, THYROID, FAMILIAL PAPILLARY CARCINOMA OF*
**Papillary cystadenocarcinoma**
  *See CANCER, THYROID, FAMILIAL PAPILLARY CARCINOMA OF*
**Papilloma of choroid plexus**
  *See CNS NEOPLASMS*
**Papilloma virus infection, congenital susceptibility**
  *See PAPILLOMA VIRUS, CONGENITAL INFECTION*

---

**PAPILLOMA VIRUS, CONGENITAL INFECTION**          **2965**

**Includes:**

> Anogenital warts, congenital
> Condylomata acuminata, congenital
> Fetal effects from papilloma virus
> Laryngeal papillomatosis, juvenile
> Papilloma virus infection, congenital susceptibility
> Recurrent respiratory papillomatosis
> Respiratory papillomatosis, juvenile

**Excludes:**

> Common warts (verruca vulgaris)
> Condylomata lata
> Plane warts (verruca plana)
> Plantar warts (verruca plantaris)

**Major Diagnostic Criteria:** Multiple respiratory papillomas or anogenital condylomata that are either present at birth or detected during infancy or early childhood. Histopathologic examination of excised tissues can confirm the clinical diagnosis. The specific human papillomavirus (HPV) involved can be determined by DNA hybridization studies.

**Clinical Findings:** All areas of the respiratory tract are susceptible to HPV infection. The larynx is the most commonly involved site, but as many as 15% of patients with recurrent respiratory papillomatosis have no apparent laryngeal lesions. Suggestive symptoms may be present from birth, but the diagnosis is not usually made until later. About 15% of patients have onset of their disease during the first year of life, about 30–50% by age five years, but over one third of all patients initially present after age 20 years (adult onset). Presenting symptoms of recurrent respiratory papillomatosis may include hoarseness, abnormal cry, aphonia, stridor or dyspnea. A history of maternal genital warts can be elicited in at least one half of all patients with juvenile-onset disease.

Laryngeal papillomas are usually multiple. They typically regrow after surgical removal, and recurrences may occur within periods as short as 2–3 weeks or as long as several years. DNA hybridization studies have also demonstrated that clinically uninvolved laryngeal sites may harbor a latent HPV infection. Distal extension of papillomas into the trachea has been noted in as many as one third of all patients, but pulmonary involvement is uncommon. Spontaneous remissions of laryngeal papillomas occur in most patients, but their durations are variable.

Laryngeal papillomas can be visualized at endoscopy and the diagnosis confirmed by pathologic examination of excised tissues. Histologically, the lesions are benign squamous papillomas. The presence of koilocytes is indicative of HPV infection. In some patients, HPV particles can be visualized by electron microscopy or detected by immunoperoxidase staining of tissues using antibodies against a genus-specific antigen. DNA hybridization studies are needed to determine the specific HPV type involved.

The moist mucosal surfaces of the anogenital area are also susceptible to HPV infection. The characteristic abnormalities, or condylomata acuminata, are clusters of soft cauliflower-like lesions involving the vulva, perianal area, and, less commonly, the vagina, urethral meatus, or rectum. They may also involve the conjunctiva, mouth, axilla, or umbilicus. A latent HPV infection in clinically and histologically normal sites that are in close proximity to condylomatous lesions may also be present. Condylomata acuminata are uncommon in children and when encountered should arouse the suspicion of sexual abuse. However, several cases with disease onset in the newborn period or early infancy are documented in the literature, suggesting intrauterine or intrapartum transmission. A history of maternal genital warts during pregnancy is commonly elicited. Many condylomata acuminata regress spontaneously.

The diagnosis of condyloma acuminatum is usually based on its typical gross morphology. Cervical lesions are often flat growths and require colposcopy for visualization. The diagnosis is based on characteristic histologic and cytologic features. DNA hybridization is required to establish a specific HPV type as the etiologic agent.

**Complications:** The most feared complication of recurrent respiratory papillomatosis is life-threatening airway obstruction. Malignant transformation of respiratory papillomas is uncommon, but the risk appears higher for patients with prolonged and widespread disease. Although malignant changes are more likely in patients receiving radiation therapy for their disease, this complication also occurs in those not receiving this treatment. Psychosocial complications may include communication difficulties and poor school performance.

Complications of condylomata acuminata may include ulceration, secondary infection, and bleeding. A more serious complication is that of malignant transformation, but the magnitude of this risk is unknown. HPVs have been associated with a variety of genital tract malignancies, including cervical, vulvar, and anorectal carcinomas. Condylomata acuminata may also enlarge during pregnancy to an extent that hampers vaginal delivery. These lesions typically regress after delivery.

**Associated Findings:** None known.

**Etiology:** Both juvenile- and adult-onset respiratory papillomas are associated with infection by HPV types 6 or 11. On the other hand, carcinoma of the larynx may be rarely associated with infection by HPV types 11, 16 or 30.

Condylomata acuminata are most commonly caused by HPV types 6 or 11. HPV types 16, 18, or 31 are found almost exclusively in patients with genital carcinoma.

Recurrent conjunctival papillomatosis has been associated with HPV types 6, 11, and 16.

Associations between chromosome 12 and HPV 18 integration sites have been reported.

**Pathogenesis:** Intrauterine transmission of HPV may occur, since some patients with recurrent respiratory papillomatosis have disease symptoms at birth and at least one newborn with congenital condylomata acuminata has been described in the literature. Viremia is not known to occur with HPV infection, thereby favoring the idea of an ascending route of transmission for these patients. Intrapartum acquisition of HPV appears to be a more significant pathway of infection because over one-half of the patients with juvenile-onset recurrent respiratory papillomatosis have a history of maternal genital warts but only very rarely a history of cesarean delivery. Postnatal transmission of HPV is theoretically possible but unlikely for patients with juvenile-onset respiratory disease. The pathogenesis of adult-onset disease is not understood at the present time. Comparable information for condylomata acuminata presenting in the neonatal period or early infancy is not available.

**MIM No.:** 16796

**Sex Ratio:** Presumably M1:F1, although there appears to be a slight preponderance of males among reported cases.

**Occurrence:** Condylomata acuminata may be found in 0.2% of pregnant women in the United States. However, clinically inapparent cervical HPV infection has been found in as many as 29% of pregnant women in Germany. Foreskins from 70 unselected newborns analyzed by dot blot hybridization revealed that at least 4% contained HPV DNA. About 1,500 new cases of recurrent respiratory papillomatosis are diagnosed each year in the United States.

**Risk of Recurrence for Patient's Sib:** Unknown.

**Risk of Recurrence for Patient's Child:** Unknown.

**Age of Detectability:** Recurrent respiratory papillomatosis may occur at any age, but about one-half of the patients have disease onset by age five years. Condylomata acuminata may be present at birth or first manifest during infancy. Lesions appearing later in childhood or adolescence are due to postnatal acquisition of HPV.

**Gene Mapping and Linkage:** Unknown.

**Prevention:** Delivery by cesarean section for mothers with genital HPV infection would theoretically be helpful, but this has not been studied to date. This method would not prevent cases resulting from intrauterine or postnatal infection by HPV.

**Treatment:** Surgical excision of respiratory papillomas using the carbon dioxide laser. Tracheostomy is sometimes needed to maintain an open airway. Data suggest that the beneficial effect of alpha-interferon in inducing clinical remission is not sustained.

The preferred treatment of condylomata acuminata varies with the age of the patient and extent of the lesions. Carbon dioxide laser therapy, cryosurgery, electrodesiccation and curettage, surgical excision, and podophyllin are commonly used therapeutic modalities. The local injection of interferon alpha-2b or autogenous vaccine has been reported to be beneficial in adults.

**Prognosis:** Respiratory papillomas typically recur after variable periods of time following their removal, thereby necessitating repeated surgical procedures. About one-half of the patients suffer management-related complications such as the development of mucosal webs, hemorrhage, and vocal cord scarring. Extension of disease into the lung parenchyma is rare and carries a poor prognosis, with a mortality rate of about 40%. Spontaneous remissions for variable periods of time are seen in many patients. Malignant transformation is rare but may worsen the prognosis.

The frequency of either spontaneous regression or malignant transformation of anogenital warts is not known.

**Detection of Carrier:** Visual inspection, colposcopy, cytology, and histopathologic examination of biopsy specimens can all be used to detect women with genital HPV infection. DNA hybridization can also detect clinically and histologically inapparent HPV infection in biopsied tissues. Preliminary data indicate that the polymerase chain reaction can be used to increase the frequency of HPV detection in biopsied tissues, swab specimens, and urine from infected individuals.

**Special Considerations:** An accurate estimate of the risk of HPV infection for an infant delivered through an infected birth canal is not available. When one considers the high prevalence of genital HPV infection in pregnant women and the low incidence of clinically apparent recurrent respiratory papillomatosis, the risk appears small. DNA hybridization studies are revolutionizing the understanding of the epidemiology, pathogenesis, and natural history of HPV infection and will undoubtedly resolve many of the currently unanswered questions.

**References:**

Tang C-K, et al.: Congenital condylomata acuminata. Am J Obstet Gynecol 1978; 131:912–913.

De Jong AR, et al.: Condyloma acuminata in children. Am J Dis Child 1982; 136:704–706.

Mounts P, Shah KV: Respiratory papillomatosis: etiological relation to genital tract papillomaviruses. Prog Med Virol 1984; 29:90–114. *

Roman A, Fife K: Human papillomavirus DNA associated with foreskins of normal newborns. J Infect Dis 1986; 153:855–861.

Shah K, et al.: Rarity of cesarean delivery in cases of juvenile-onset respiratory papillomatosis. Obstet Gynecol 1986; 68:795–799.

Byrne JC, et al.: Human papillomavirus-11 DNA in a patient with chronic laryngotracheobronchial papillomatosis and metastatic squamous-cell carcinoma of the lung. New Engl J Med 1987; 317:873–878.

Popescu NC, et al.: Human papillomavirus type 18 DNA is integrated at a single chromosome site in cervical carcinoma cell line SW756. J Virol 1987; 61:1682–1685.

Healy GB, et al.: Treatment of recurrent respiratory papillomatosis with human leukocyte interferon: results of a multicenter randomized clinical trial. New Engl J Med 1988; 319:401–407.

Davis AJ, Emans SJ: Human papilloma virus infection in the pediatric and adolescent patient. J Pediatr 1989; 115:1–9. *

Young LS, et al.: The polymerase chain reaction: a new epidemiological tool for investigating cervical human papillomavirus infection. Br Med J 1989; 298:14–18.

FR039
SE021

**Bishara J. Freij**
**John L. Sever**

**Papillon-Leage syndrome**
*See ORO-FACIO-DIGITAL SYNDROME I*
**Papillon-Lefevre syndrome**
*See HYPERKERATOSIS PALMOPLANTARIS-PERIODONTOCLASIA*
**Parachute mitral valve**
*See VENTRICLE, SINGLE LEFT PAPILLARY MUSCLE*
*also MITRAL VALVE STENOSIS*
**Paradione^, fetal effects of**
*See FETAL TRIMETHADIONE SYNDROME*
**Paraesophageal hernia**
*See HERNIA, HIATAL*
**Paragangliomas of the middle ear and temporal bone**
*See EAR, CHEMODECTOMA OF MIDDLE EAR*
**Paragangliomata**
*See CAROTID BODY TUMOR*
**Parahemophilia**
*See FACTOR V DEFICIENCY*
**Paralysis (cerebral), congenital spastic**
*See CEREBRAL PALSY*
**Paralysis of sixth nerve, congenital**
*See EYE, DUANE RETRACTION SYNDROME*
**Paralysis of vocal cord**
*See VOCAL CORD PARALYSIS*
**Paralysis periodica paramyotonica**
*See PARAMYOTONIA CONGENITA*

## PARALYSIS, HYPERKALEMIC PERIODIC 0794

**Includes:**
Adynamia episodica hereditaria
Hyperkalemic periodic paralysis
Periodic paralysis, II
Periodic paralysis, hyperpotassemic

**Excludes:**
**Paralysis, hypokalemic periodic** (0795)
**Paralysis, normokalemic periodic** (2050)
**Paramyotonia congenita** (0796)

**Major Diagnostic Criteria:** Attacks of paralysis associated with elevated serum potassium. Positive family history.

**Clinical Findings:** The condition is usually first detected by the parents in infancy or in childhood. Affected children have episodes during which they become unusually floppy and move poorly. Onset may be delayed till adulthood, and onset up to 31 years of age has been reported. The frequency of attacks varies between once a week to several mild attacks a day. Most attacks have a short duration, 30–60 minutes. Weakness is usually noticed first in the lower back, thighs, and calves, then spreads to arms and neck. Rarely, there may be difficulty in swallowing and coughing. Clinical myotonia, especially eyelid myotonia, may be a diagnostic clue for the condition. This is characterized by slow opening of the eyelids after forced active closure of the eyes. Myotonic symptoms are not present in all patients.

The paralytic attacks are usually provoked by rest after exercise, but unlike the hypokalemic form, the weakness develops in a shorter period of time (average duration is 30 minutes). One patient became weak when resting after swimming. Sometimes the patients may be able to "walk off" the symptoms early in an attack. This postponement of an attack seems to be only temporary, and the maneuver is sometimes associated with the development of muscle cramps. Factors other than exercise that can precipitate clinical attacks include emotion, cold, hunger, infection, and general anesthesia. This condition may also worsen during pregnancy.

Physical evaluation during the attacks shows variable weakness, usually more prominent in the proximal muscles. Severe flaccid quadriplegia is less frequently seen than in the hypokalemic type. Deep tendon reflexes are diminished or absent in severe attacks.

Physical evaluation between attacks usually shows no abnormality early in life. However, a proximal myopathy with permanent weakness develops later in many patients. The weakness affects pelvic muscles and then spreads to shoulder muscles. Occasionally a wheelchair is needed. Potentially fatal cardiac dysrythmia with sudden death was described in several families with hyperkalemic periodic paralysis.

Laboratory findings include a rise in serum potassium during attacks. Affected persons appear to be hypersensitive to changes in serum potassium concentration, because weakness develops at lower levels than in normal individuals. Between attacks the serum potassium is normal. An abnormally high serum potassium level between attacks suggests secondary rather than primary hyperkalemic periodic paralysis. The electrocardiogram shows an increase in amplitude of precordial T waves during the attacks, consistent with hyperkalemia. Permanent bidirectional ventricular tachydysrythmia was reported in two patients. Electromyography may show myotonic discharges. During an attack, the muscle is inexcitable. The serum creatine kinase may be elevated. Muscle biopsy shows myopathic changes, particularly in advanced cases. Variability in the size of muscle fibers, increased numbers of internal nuclei, vacuoles, and tubular aggregates were described. Decreased potassium levels in the muscle and an increase in the sodium, water, and chloride contents were reported.

Oral administration of potassium chloride (0.10 g per kg body weight) under electrocardiographic monitoring induces a paralytic attack within 90–180 minutes and supports the clinical diagnosis.

**Complications:** Dysphagia with aspiration pneumonitis, and occasionally marked hypoventilation during attacks.

**Associated Findings:** Progressive myopathy with severe weakness may develop late in life.

**Etiology:** Autosomal dominant inheritance with high penetrance in both sexes.

**Pathogenesis:** Undetermined, but may involve an alteration of sodium-potassium ion transport mechanisms across the defective muscle cell membrane. Recent electrophysiologic studies in myotonic and nonmyotonic hyperkalemic periodic paralysis suggest that the failure of propagation of action potentials in the paralytic attacks may be related to the abnormality of the sodium-potassium pump.

**MIM No.:** *17050

**Sex Ratio:** Presumably M1:F1.

**Occurrence:** The hyperkalemic type is the second most frequent of the periodic paralyses. The incidence in Sweden is 0.2:1,000,000. Two Swedish kinships alone accounted for 138 patients in five generations.

**Risk of Recurrence for Patient's Sib:**
See Part I, *Mendelian Inheritance.*

**Risk of Recurrence for Patient's Child:**
See Part I, *Mendelian Inheritance.*

**Age of Detectability:** Usually in infancy or early childhood.

**Gene Mapping and Linkage:** Unknown.

**Prevention:** None known. Genetic counseling indicated.

**Treatment:** The acute attack can be treated with calcium gluconate (0.5–2 g given intravenously), glucose by mouth (2 g per kg of body weight), insulin (15–20 units subcutaneously), or beta-adrenergic agents (1.3 mg metaproterenol inhalation).

Preventive therapy consists of frequent meals of high carbohydrate content; avoidance of fasting, exposure to cold or overexertion, and diuretic agents such as acetazolamide or thiazides. The lowest dose of diuretic required to prevent attack should be used, and the dose should not lower the serum potassium below 3.7 mEq/liter.

**Prognosis:** Generally good for life span, although a very small percentage (less than 1%) of patients may die during a paralytic attack. Myopathic patients with permanent weakness may have a severe motor handicap.

**Detection of Carrier:** By inducing attacks with potassium chloride loading test or by demonstration of myotonia.

**Special Considerations:** Heterogeneity may exist within the clinical entities corresponding to myotonic and nonmyotonic types of hyperkalemic periodic paralysis.

**References:**
Gamstorp I: Adynamia episodica hereditaria. Acta Paediatr Scand 1956; 45(suppl 108):1–126. *
Lehmann-Horn F, et al.: Two cases of adynamia episodica hereditaria: in vitro investigation of muscle cell membrane and contraction parameters. Muscle Nerve 1983; 6:113–120.
Bendheim PE, et al.: Beta-adrenergic treatment of hyperkalemic periodic paralysis. Neurology 1985; 35:746–749.
Gould RJ, et al.: Potentially fatal cardiac dysrythmia and hyperkalemic periodic paralysis. Neurology 1985; 35:1208–1212.
Lehmann-Horn F, et al.: Adynamia episodica hereditaria with myotonia: a non-inactivating sodium current and the effect of extracellular pH. Muscle Nerve 1987; 10:363–374.

I0000                                                   **Victor V. Ionasescu**

## PARALYSIS, HYPOKALEMIC PERIODIC 0795

**Includes:**
    Hypokalemic periodic paralysis
    Periodic paralysis, II
    Periodic paralysis, familial
    Periodic paralysis, hypopotassemic

**Excludes:**
    **Paralysis, hyperkalemic periodic** (0794)
    **Paralysis, normokalemic periodic** (2050)
    **Paramyotonia congenita** (0796)

**Major Diagnostic Criteria:** Attacks of paralysis in conjunction with lowered serum potassium levels. Positive family history.

**Clinical Findings:** This disorder is characterized by attacks of flaccid quadriplegia lasting usually several hours and frequently occurring in the early morning. The muscles of speech, deglutition, and respiration are usually spared. The attacks begin in the second decade of life and are most frequent between the ages of 20 and 35 years, after which they tend to decrease in number and severity, and may completely disappear. The weakness can vary in severity from mild to almost complete paralysis of the neck, trunk, and extremities. Most moderate attacks last 6–24 hours, but severe paralysis may last for 2–3 days or longer. It is characteristic for the lower limbs to be affected first, then the arms, the trunk, and finally the neck. The proximal muscles of the limbs are the first to be affected, while the distal muscles (hands, feet) can move slightly even in severe attacks. The most important predisposing factors are prolonged rest after vigorous exercise and large carbohydrate meals. The plasma potassium falls coincidentally with the development of an attack. Administration of glucose or glucose and insulin leads to hypopotassemia and induces a paralytic attack. Death occurs rarely in an attack.

Examination during an attack shows flaccid paralysis, predominantly in the proximal muscles. The paralyzed muscles fail to respond to direct mechanical or electrical stimulation. The EKG shows bradycardia, prominent U waves, and flattening of the T waves in conjunction with the lowered serum potassium to the level of 2.0 to 2.5 mEq/liter. Muscle biopsy performed during paralytic attack shows multiple vacuoles of the muscle fibers and alterations of the sarcoplasmic reticulum.

Between attacks, patient's strength and serum potassium are within the normal range. Older patients frequently show some degree of proximal limb weakness and atrophy, with nonvacuolar myopathy at biopsy.

**Complications:** During attacks, severe dysphagia with aspiration pneumonitis and respiratory failure from intercostal weakness may occur.

**Associated Findings:** A slowly progressive myopathy with proximal weakness may develop late in life after the paralytic attacks have almost completely disappeared.

**Etiology:** Autosomal dominant inheritance with complete penetrance in males. Cases have been reported in up to six consecutive generations. There is a sex limitation, with frequent failure of manifestation in females in whom the disease, when it occurs, tends to be milder. Less than 10% female patients were reported in several kindreds. For this reason, X-linked recessive inheritance has been discussed in some families in which only male patients were noticed. Hypokalemic periodic paralysis occurs also as a rare, probably genetically determined, complication of thyrotoxicosis.

**Pathogenesis:** A shift of potassium, sodium, chloride and phosphate ions, and water into muscle has been documented during hypopotassemic attacks. Most likely, the fluid and electrolyte movements are caused by a defect in the muscle membrane with increased sodium permeability. Both the surface membrane of muscle and the T tubules, which represent an inward extension of the surface membrane, fail to conduct an action potential during attacks. The abnormal electrolyte shifts and the electrical inexcitability of the muscle fiber may influence the development of the permanent late myopathy.

**MIM No.:** *17040

**Sex Ratio:** M1:F<1

**Occurrence:** The hypokalemic is the most frequent type of periodic paralysis. The incidence in Denmark is 0.8:1,000,000. The association of hypokalemic variant and hyperthyroidism is higher in Japanese and Chinese patients.

**Risk of Recurrence for Patient's Sib:**
    See Part I, *Mendelian Inheritance*. Risk 1:2 to 1:10 for female.

**Risk of Recurrence for Patient's Child:**
    See Part I, *Mendelian Inheritance*. Risk 1:2 to 1:10 for female.

**Age of Detectability:** Usually by the second decade of life.

**Gene Mapping and Linkage:** Unknown.

**Prevention:** None known. Genetic counseling indicated.

**Treatment:** Paralysis is reversible during an attack by oral administration of 10 g potassium chloride for an adult. If the patient shows no signs of recovery after 3 to 4 hours, the dose may be repeated. Preventive therapy consists of a relatively low-sodium (2–3 g per day) and low-carbohydrate (60 to 80 g per day) diet and supplemental oral doses of potassium chloride, 2.5 g per day as 10% aqueous solution. Acetazolamide (up to 1 g per day) is the drug of choice in preventing paralytic attacks. Spironolactone and diazoxide are also used prophylactically.

**Prognosis:** Generally good for life span, but about 2–5% of the patients may die in a severe attack. Permanent late onset myopathy with physical handicap due to weakness and muscle atrophy is relatively common in older patients.

**Detection of Carrier:** Oral administration of glucose (2 g per kg of body weight) combined with 10 to 20 units of crystalline insulin given subcutaneously may precipitate an attack of weakness within 2 to 3 hours in an otherwise asymptomatic carrier.

**References:**
Johnsen T: Familial periodic paralysis with hypokalaemia: experimental and clinical investigations. Dan Med Bull 1981; 28:1–27. *
Rudel R, et al.: Hypokalemic periodic paralysis: in vitro investigation of muscle fiber membrane parameters. Muscle Nerve 1984; 7:110–120.
Buruma OJS, et al.: Familial hypokalemic periodic paralysis: 50 year follow-up of a large family. Arch Neurol 1985; 42:28–31.

I0000
             **Victor V. Ionasescu**

## PARALYSIS, NORMOKALEMIC PERIODIC 2050

**Includes:**
    Normokalemic periodic paralysis
    Periodic paralysis, normopotassemic
    Periodic paralysis, III

**Excludes:**
    **Paralysis, hyperkalemic periodic** (0794)
    **Paralysis, hypokalemic periodic** (0795)
    **Paramyotonia congenita** (0796)

**Major Diagnostic Criteria:** Attacks of paralysis with normal serum potassium levels. Positive family history.

**Clinical Findings:** Twenty-one of 45 members were affected in the kinship originally described. The paralytic attacks began in the first decade and were provoked by rest after exercise, exposure to cold, alcohol in excess and potassium loading. The episodes of weakness occurred at intervals of one to three months lasting from two days to three weeks, often of a severe degree, including quadriplegia and weakness of the muscles of mastication but excluding facial expression, bladder and bowel function, and respiration. Large doses of sodium chloride improved the weakness. The urinary potassium retention, lack of a beneficial effect of glucose, and failure of the serum potassium to increase in attacks distinguished this disease from primary hyperkalemic periodic paralysis.

The diagnosis of normokalemic periodic paralysis was also well documented in another kinship in which a mother and her son were affected. In that family, paralysis was not provoked by lowering the serum potassium to 2 mEq/liter by glucose and insulin or by raising the serum potassium level to 6.6 mEq/liter by oral potassium loading. The resistance to the potassium loading test distinguished this kinship from the previous one.

Physical examination between attacks was normal in all patients. There was no evidence of weakness, myotonia, or changes of reflexes. Weakness during the attacks sometimes involved selective muscles, such as calf muscles and arm extensors. Reflexes were reduced or absent.

Electromyography during a paralytic attack in one patient showed mostly a myopathic pattern (full interference with greatly reduced amplitude). There were several large motor units, which raised the possibility of an associated neurogenic lesion. Motor nerve conduction velocities were normal. Muscle biopsy obtained at the height of an episode of paralysis demonstrated vacuolation of muscle fibers and focal areas of muscle degeneration. Some patients also showed tubular aggregates by electron microscopy, suggesting proliferation of the reticular system of the muscle. Serum creatine kinase was elevated during the paretic attacks in several cases.

There were doubts in the literature about the distinctness of the normokalemic and hyperkalemic types, because some patients with normokalemic periodic paralysis had positive potassium loading test.

**Complications:** Unknown.

**Associated Findings:** None known.

**Etiology:** Autosomal dominant inheritance with complete penetrance.

**Pathogenesis:** A defect in the membrane of the sarcoplasmic reticulum has been postulated.

**MIM No.:** *17060

**Sex Ratio:** Presumably M1:F1.

**Occurrence:** The incidence is 1:100,000 population in the area of Newcastle upon Tyne, England. Undetermined elsewhere, but presumed rare.

**Risk of Recurrence for Patient's Sib:**
See Part I, *Mendelian Inheritance.*

**Risk of Recurrence for Patient's Child:**
See Part I, *Mendelian Inheritance.*

**Age of Detectability:** In the first decade of life.

**Gene Mapping and Linkage:** Unknown.

**Prevention:** None known. Genetic counseling indicated.

**Treatment:** Sodium chloride taken at the onset of an attack will reduce its severity or shorten it. Severe attacks when fully developed may no longer be responsive to this form of therapy. Combination of 9-alpha-fluoro-hydrocortisone and acetazolamide has proved effective in preventing attacks in several cases.

**Prognosis:** Generally good for life span. There were no reports of patients dying during a paralytic attack. The episodic weakness becomes milder and occurs less frequently with age.

**Detection of Carrier:** In families with weakness triggered by potassium chloride, attacks can be induced with the potassium chloride loading test.

**References:**
Poskanzer DC, Kerr DNS: A third type of periodic paralysis with normokalemia and favorable response to sodium chloride. Am J Med 1961; 31:328–342. *
Meyers KR, et al.: Periodic muscle weakness, normokalemia and tubular aggregates. Neurology 1972; 22:269–279. *
Danowski TS, et al.: Clinical and ultrastructural observations in a kindred with normo-hyperkalemic periodic paralysis. J Med Genet 1975; 12:20–28.
Rudel R: The pathophysiologic basis of the myotonias and of the periodic paralyses. In: Engel AG, Banker BQ, eds: Myology. New York: McGraw-Hill, 1986:1297–1319.

I0000                                                      **Victor V. Ionasescu**

**Paralysis, periodica hypokaliemica**
*See PARALYSIS, HYPOKALEMIC PERIODIC*

**Parana hard skin syndrome**
*See SKIN, PARANA HARD SKIN SYNDROME*
**Paramedian lower lip pits-popliteal pterygium**
*See PTERYGIUM SYNDROME, POPLITEAL*
**Paramedian pits of lower lip (isolated trait)**
*See LIP, PITS OR MOUNDS*
**Paramethadione, fetal effects of**
*See FETAL TRIMETHADIONE SYNDROME*
**Paramolar**
*See TEETH, SUPERNUMERARY*

---

## PARAMYOTONIA CONGENITA                                    0796

**Includes:**
Eulenburg disease
Myotonia congenita intermittens
Paralysis periodica paramyotonica
von Eulenburg paramyotonia congenita

**Excludes:**
Myotonia in other syndromes or conditions
**Myotonic dystrophy** (0702)
**Nephrosis, familial type** (0710)
**Paralysis, hyperkalemic periodic** (0794)

**Major Diagnostic Criteria:** Myotonia is induced or aggravated by cold. Positive family history.

**Clinical Findings:** This condition is manifested mainly by myotonia worsened after exposure to cold. There is predilection of the myotonia for facial, lingual, and hand muscles. Myotonia is also aggravated by repeated muscle contraction (paradoxical myotonia). In addition, some of the patients experience attacks of flaccid weakness after exercise or after cold exposure, accompanied by increased serum potassium. The condition is usually evident in infancy, is not progressive, does not affect life expectancy and does not interfere with a reasonably normal social and economic life. Dystrophic features are not present.

Paramyotonia is distinguished from myotonia congenita by the attacks of muscular weakness. The paralytic attacks are quite similar to those that occur in hyperkalemic periodic paralysis. Several authors suggested that the two conditions are identical. However, other authors report cases in which myotonia and weakness were induced in the cold and not accompanied by significant changes in the serum potassium. Therefore, the diagnosis of paramyotonia congenita should be limited only to patients in whom myotonia and paralysis are induced or aggravated by cold with normal serum potassium.

Neurologic evaluation shows myotonic signs and intermittent flaccid weakness with decreased or absent deep tendon reflexes. Patients of three families with paramyotonia congenita had no myotonia in a warm environment.

Electromyography in a cold environment (20°C) showed a significant fall in the amplitude of the compound muscle action potentials (CMAP) obtained from patients with paramyotonia congenita. Cold also induced or worsened a significant decremental response to 2-Hz nerve stimulation and virtually abolished voluntary recruitment of motor unit potentials. None of these changes occurred in patients with myotonia congenita.

**Complications:** Unknown.

**Associated Findings:** Muscle hypertrophy and persistent weakness (myopathy) were reported in older patients.

**Etiology:** Autosomal dominant inheritance with high penetrance in both sexes.

**Pathogenesis:** A muscle membrane defect different from myotonic and nonmyotonic hyperkalemic periodic paralysis has been postulated based on in vitro electrophysiologic studies. In paramyotonia congenita depolarization and paralysis are caused by an abnormal temperature dependence of the Na+ channel kinetics.

**MIM No.:** *16830

**Sex Ratio:** M1:F1

**Occurrence:** Undetermined but presumed rare. Two large families alone account for 17 and 30 affected members across five and six generations respectively.

**Risk of Recurrence for Patient's Sib:**
See Part I, *Mendelian Inheritance.*

**Risk of Recurrence for Patient's Child:**
See Part I, *Mendelian Inheritance.*

**Age of Detectability:** In early childhood, based on clinical and EMG signs of myotonia.

**Gene Mapping and Linkage:** Unknown.

**Prevention:** None known. Genetic counseling indicated.

**Treatment:** Regulation of serum potassium levels by acetazolamide or thiazide diuretics has proved helpful in some families with paramyotonia congenita and hyperkalemia by decreasing the number of paralytic attacks, but it did not change the myotonic findings. Treatment with tocainide (400–1200 mg/day) has been successful in seven patients with paramyotonia congenita.

**Prognosis:** Generally good for life span and function.

**Detection of Carrier:** Demonstration of myotonia, clinically and electromyographically, often at room temperature and always upon exposure to cold.

**Special Considerations:** Heterogeneity of this condition is suggested by the variability of the clinical picture. The molecular genetic basis of the heterogeneity remains unknown.

**References:**

Thrush DC, et al.: Paramyotonia congenita: a clinical, histochemical and pathological study. Brain 1972; 95:537–552. *
Haas A, et al.: Clinical study of paramyotonia congenita with and without myotonia in a warm environment. Muscle Nerve 1981; 4:388–395.
Lehmann-Horn F, et al.: Membrane defects in paramyotonia congenita with and without myotonia in a warm environment. Muscle Nerve 1981; 4:396–406.
Subramony SH, et al.: Distinguishing paramyotonia congenita and myotonia congenita by electromyography. Muscle Nerve 1983; 6:374–379.
Streib EW: Paramyotonia congenita: successful treatment with tocainide: clinical and electrophysiologic findings in seven patients. Muscle Nerve 1987; 10:155–162.

I0000                                    **Victor V. Ionasescu**

**Paranasal sinuses, absent**
*See SINUS, ABSENT PARANASAL*

## PARAPLEGIA, FAMILIAL SPASTIC                    0295

**Includes:**
Spastic paraplegia, hereditary
Spastic paraplegia, pure hereditary
Spastic paraplegia, X-linked, complicated
Strumpell familial spastic paraplegia
Strumpell-Lorrain syndrome

**Excludes:**
Ataxia, Friedreich type (2714)
Ataxia, hereditary
Adrenomyeloneuropathy
Cerebellar ataxia
Cerebral palsy (2931)
Charcot-Marie-Tooth disease
Lison syndrome
Parasagittal intracranial mass
Sjogren syndrome (2101)
Spastic paraplegia, familial, in other syndromes
Spastic paraplegia of perinatal onset
Thoracic spinal cord lesion

**Major Diagnostic Criteria:** Progressive spasticity of the lower extremities with exaggerated deep tendon reflexes and Babinski signs. A positive family history in the autosomal dominant pedigrees is a helpful but not necessary criterion.

**Clinical Findings:** The age of onset is usually in the first decade in the autosomal recessive families. In the autosomal dominant families, there are two groups: type I with age of onset at 13.49 ± 12.25 years and type II with age of onset at 44.9 ± 13.9 years. Intellect is preserved. Dragging of one leg is often the first symptom to be noted. Leg cramps follow, and within 2 to 3 years a scissoring spastic gait emerges. Urinary frequency and urgency occur in 50% of cases. In the older-onset male patients, 60% develop secondary impotence. Their inability to have erections is presumably based on spinal cord pathology, and does not affect biologic reproductive fitness. Increased tone and flexion spasms are frequently reported. Ultimately, one-third of the older patients require wheelchair assistance. Increased deep tendon reflexes and Babinski signs are found in all those affected. Motor weakness occurs late in the illness, and sensory findings are limited to mildly diminished vibratory response below the ankles in 60% of patients. There may be abnormal release of H-reflexes from the small muscle of the foot on tibial nerve stimulation; otherwise, neurophysiologic and X-ray studies are normal. Expressivity of the disease is variable, and mildly affected individuals may be unaware of their problem unless examined by a neurologist. This may be important for counseling issues.

**Complications:** Pes cavus; kyphoscoliosis; hip, knee, and joint contractures, with late-onset entrapment neuropathies.

**Associated Findings:** Late-onset distal wasting of the muscles and urinary tract infections. Patients with the X-linked form frequently have signs of cerebellar dysfunction.

**Etiology:** The majority of reported families show autosomal dominant inheritance. Thirty percent of reported cases are autosomal recessive. Few pedigrees are reported with X-linked inheritance.

**Pathogenesis:** The underlying mechanism is unknown. The predominant neuropathologic lesion is a loss of myelin and axons in the lateral corticospinal tract. The fasciculus gracilis and, to a minor extent, the fasciculus cuneatus are involved at the thoracic and lower cervical levels. Rarely is there involvement of the spinocerebellar and anterior corticospinal tracts.

**MIM No.:** *18260, *27080, *31290

**Sex Ratio:** Probably M1:F1 in non-X-linked cases. M1:F1, M60:F40, and M1:F2 have been reported.

**Occurrence:** Over 200 cases have been reported in the literature.

**Risk of Recurrence for Patient's Sib:**
See Part I, *Mendelian Inheritance.*

**Risk of Recurrence for Patient's Child:**
See Part I, *Mendelian Inheritance.*

**Age of Detectability:** The autosomal recessive form can usually be detected in the first decade. Dominant familial spastic paraplegia is of two forms, one that presents before age 35 years (type I) and one that presents after age 35 years (type II). Spasticity of the lower limbs is more severe in type I families. However, progression is more rapid in the type II families. The few cases described with X-linked recessive inheritance were diagnosed in the first or second decade.

**Gene Mapping and Linkage:** SPG1 (spastic paraplegia, complicated) has been provisionally mapped to Xq27-q28.

**Prevention:** None known. Genetic counseling indicated.

**Treatment:** Dantrolene sodium and baclofen (Lioresal) have been tried with variable success for marked spasticity. Treatment is supportive, with attention to bladder care in those prone to infections.

**Prognosis:** Most patients continue to be gainfully employed and productive in life in spite of their difficulty walking. Life span is not affected.

**Detection of Carrier:** Twenty percent of affected individuals are asymptomatic, but have increased tone and exaggerated reflexes on physical examination. Parents should be examined carefully in all instances.

**Special Considerations:** The variable expressivity of this disease necessitates careful neurologic examination of all family members once a case has been identified. Treatable causes of lower extremity spasticity need to be ruled out, particularly parasagittal masses, thoracic spinal cord tumors, and adrenomyeloneuropathy, which may benefit from dietary therapy.

**References:**
Strümpell A: Über eine bestimmte Form der primaren combinierten Systemerkrankung des Rückenmarks. Arch Psychiatr Nervenkr 1886; 17:217–238.

Behan WMH, Maia M: Strümpell's familial spastic paraplegia: genetics and neuropathology. J Neurol Neurosurg Psychiatry 1974; 37:8–20.

Harding AE: Hereditary "pure" spastic paraplegia: a clinical and genetic study of 22 families. J Neurol Neurosurg Psychiatry 1981; 44:871–888. *

Harding AE: Classification of the hereditary ataxias and paraplegias. Lancet 1983; I:1151–1155.

Kenwrick S, et al.: Linkage analysis of several cloned DNA sequences with the locus of X-linked recessive spastic paraplegia. Am J Hum Genet 1985; 37:A160.

Boustany R-MN, et al.: The autosomal dominant form of "pure" familial spastic paraplegia: clinical findings and linkage analysis of a large pedigree. Neurology 1987; 37(6):910–915. *

B0053                                           **Rose-Mary N. Boustany**

**Parasternal hernia**
  *See DIAPHRAGMATIC HERNIA*
**Parastremmatic dwarfism**
  *See PARASTREMMATIC DYSPLASIA*

---

## PARASTREMMATIC DYSPLASIA                    0798

**Includes:**
  Dwarfism, parastremmatic
  Parastremmatic dwarfism

**Excludes:**
  **Diastrophic dysplasia** (0293)
  **Metatropic dysplasia** (0656)
  **Osteogenesis imperfecta** (0777)

**Major Diagnostic Criteria:** Severe dwarfism with progressive spinal malalignment, short limbs, and rigid joints. On X-ray, the skeleton has a pathognomonic "flocky" appearance due to patchy undermineralization.

**Clinical Findings:** The features are evident at birth, and become progressively more severe. The forehead is high, with brachycephaly and a temporal bulge. The extremities are short, with bilateral genu valgum, bowing of the shins, osseous enlargement of the knees, and contractures of the hip joints. Scoliosis appears in early infancy. Intelligence is normal and there are no visceral ramifications.

On X-ray, the skeleton is grossly undermineralized, coarsely trabeculated, and contains areas of irregular stippling which produces a "flocky" appearance. The vertebral bodies are flattened and irregular, and the pelvic bones are dysplastic. The metaphyses and epiphyses of the tubular bones are severely malformed.

**Complications:** Articular rigidity causes severe handicap, which is accentuated by the effects of spinal cord compression due to progressive spinal malalignment. Cardio-respiratory failure may develop.

**Associated Findings:** None known.

**Etiology:** Presumably autosomal dominant inheritance, with sporadic cases representing new mutations. Neither affected sibs nor parental consanguinity have been recorded. The only report of generation to generation transmission concerns an affected father and daughter. The mother had **Osteogenesis imperfecta**, and the daughter was thought to have inherited both conditions.

**Pathogenesis:** Unknown.

**MIM No.:** 16840

**POS No.:** 3358

**Sex Ratio:** M1:F5 (Observed).

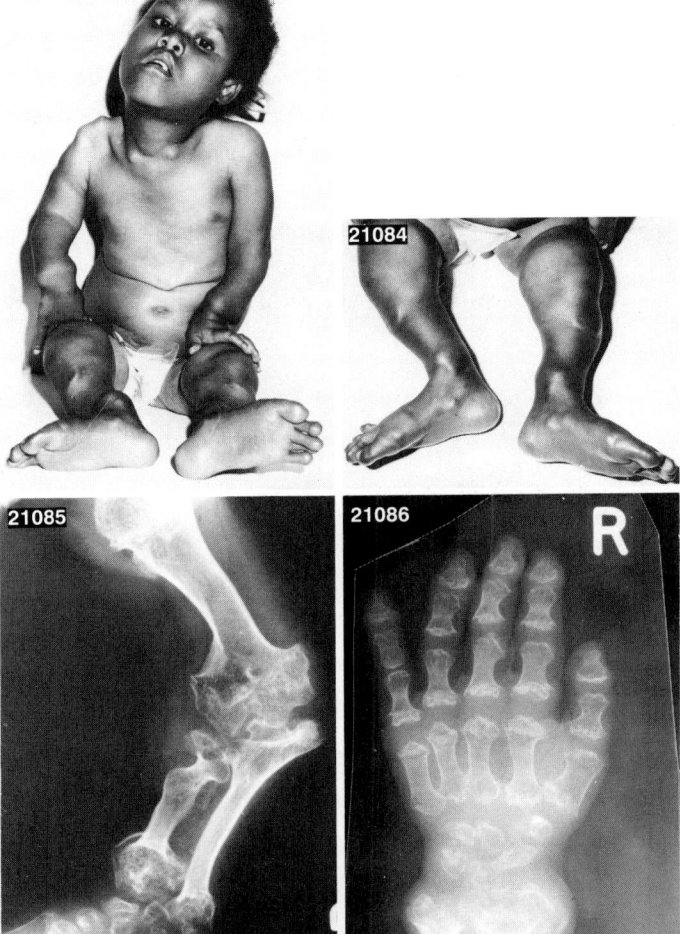

**0798-21083:** An affected girl with dwarfism and malformation of the limbs and trunk. **21084:** The legs of the affected girl show irregular expansion of the shins and ankles. **21085:** X-ray of the arm shows very dysplastic bones with a characteristic "flocky" appearance. **21086:** Hand X-ray shows short tubular bones that are dysplastic with irregular expansion of the metaphyses.

---

**Occurrence:** Six cases have been reported, including four unrelated females, and a father and daughter.

**Risk of Recurrence for Patient's Sib:**
  See Part I, *Mendelian Inheritance.*

**Risk of Recurrence for Patient's Child:**
  See Part I, *Mendelian Inheritance.*

**Age of Detectability:** At birth.

**Gene Mapping and Linkage:** Unknown.

**Prevention:** None known. Genetic counseling indicated.

**Treatment:** Orthopedic correction of limb and spinal malalignment.

**Prognosis:** Progressive physical handicap. Eventual spinal cord compression and cardio-respiratory failure. Intelligence remains unimpaired.

**Detection of Carrier:** Unknown.

**References:**
Rask MR: Morquio-Brailsford osteochondrodystrophy and osteogenesis imperfecta: report of a patient with both conditions. J Bone Joint Surg 1963; 45A:561–570.
Langer LO, et al.: An unusual bone dysplasia: parastremmatic dwarfism. Am J Roentgenol Rad Ther Nuc Med 1970; 110:550–560. *
Horan F, Beighton P: Parastremmatic dwarfism. J Bone Joint Surg 1976; 58B:343–346. * †

BE008                                        Peter Beighton

**Parathormone resistance**
*See PARATHYROID HORMONE RESISTANCE*

---

## PARATHYROID HORMONE RESISTANCE              0830

**Includes:**
>   Albright hereditary osteodystrophy
>   Hypoparathyroidism, resistant (ineffective) hormone
>   Parathormone resistance
>   Pseudohypoparathyroidism, type 1a or 1b (PHP-1a or b)
>   Pseudohypoparathyroidism, type 2 (PHP-2)
>   Pseudo-pseudohypoparathyroidism

**Excludes:**
>   Brachydactyly (0114)
>   Hypoparathyroidism, idiopathic

**Major Diagnostic Criteria:** Either the presence of a characteristic clinical somatotype, referred to as Albright Hereditary Osteodystrophy (AHO), or the demonstration of renal unresponsiveness to parathyroid hormone (PTH) has been considered a sufficient criterion for the diagnosis of pseudohypoparathyroidism (PHP), but the classical description includes both features. At least two biochemical phenotypes (PHP-1 and PHP-2) have been recognized. The major findings are as follows:

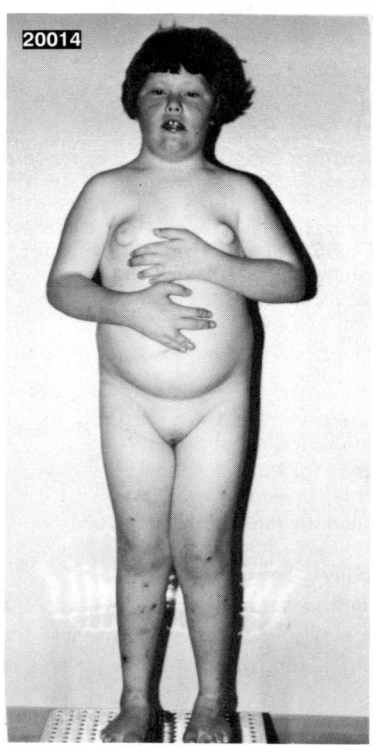

**0830A-20014:** Note characteristic body habitus with truncal obesity, brachydactyly and dysmorphic facies.

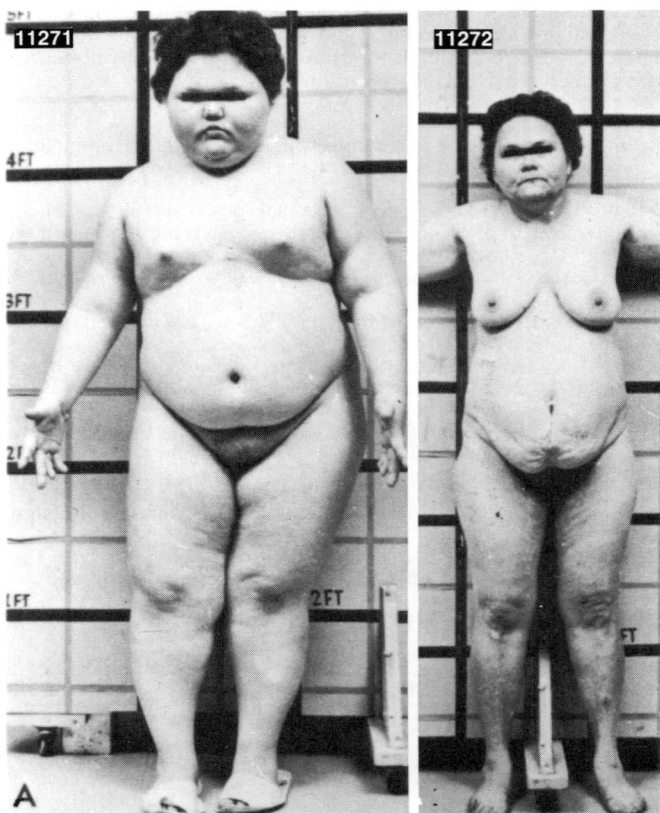

**0830B-11271:** Thirteen-year-old girl with pseudohypoparathyroidism who was the daughter of woman shown in 11272. 11272: Woman with pseudo-pseudohypoparathyroidism.

---

| Feature | PHP-1 | PHP-2 |
|---|---|---|
| Serum | | |
| -calcium | low | low |
| -phosphate | high | normal or high |
| -immunoreactive PTH (iPTH) | high | high |
| Renal response to PTH challenge | | |
| -phosphate excretion | decreased | decreased |
| -3', 5' cyclic AMP (cAMP) excretion | decreased | normal |
| -1,25 $(OH)_2D_3$ synthesis | decreased | ? normal |
| Stimulatory guanine nucleotide nucleotide-binding protein ($G_s$) activity | decreased in some | normal |
| AHO somatotype | present in most | usually absent |

Patients with reduced activity of the $G_s$ (or $N_s$) protein, which is a component of the hormone-sensitive adenylcyclase complex, are subclassified as PHP-1a. Those with normal $G_s$ activity are designated PHP-1b. Normocalcemic individuals with PHP-2 or 2 may be said to have pseudo-pseudohypoparathyroidism (PPHP). They may still show target organ resistance to PTH with or without the $G_s$ protein defect or the AHO somatotype.

**Clinical Findings:** Clinical features of AHO are variable but include short stature, obesity, round face, brachydactyly (particularly the fourth and fifth metacarpals and the distal first phalanx), and mild-to-moderate mental retardation. Other signs of abnormal mineral metabolism include ectopic calcifications in brain (particularly the choroid plexus) and skin, delayed tooth

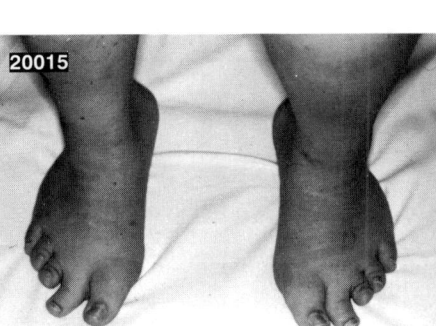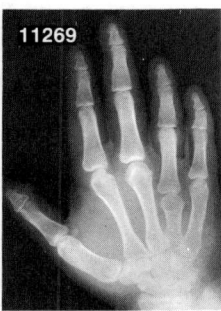

**0830C-20015:** Note brachydactyly; the third, fourth and fifth metatarsals are short. **11269:** Shortened fourth metacarpal.

eruption, enamel hypoplasia, and X-ray features in keeping with hypoparathyroidism. In some patients, isolated skeletal responsiveness to PTH may be inferred from radiographically demonstrable features of hyperparathyroidism (osteitis fibrosa).

**Complications:** Patients may present with hypocalcemic tetany and convulsions. Cataracts and corneal opacities have been described. Moderate to severe hypertension may be found in more than one-half of the adult patients.

**Associated Findings:** In PHP-1a patients, the $G_s$ protein defect is is widespread, and therefore other physiologic functions mediated by the hormone-sensitive adenyl cyclase may also be affected. Thyroid dysfunction may only be evidenced by an exaggerated thyroid-stimulating hormone (TSH) response to thyrotropin-releasing hormone (TRH), but infants with PHP have presented with hypothyroidism. Other hormonal abnormalities include hypergonadotrophic hypogonadism and decreased cAMP responses to glucagon and isoproterenol. Patients with the $G_s$ deficit have anosmia, presumably because a hormone-sensitive adenylcyclase system is required in the transduction of the receptor signal (generated by binding of odiferous molecules) to an electrical impulse in the olfactory neuroepithelial membrane.

**Etiology:** Although considered to be X-linked, many authorities suggest that autosomal dominant inheritance is more compatible with most pedigrees. In PHP-1a, the decrease in Gs activity has been related to an alpha subunit (Gs) deficiency, which is transmitted in an autosomal dominant fashion. In different kindreds, levels of Gs mRNA may be decreased or normal, suggesting further genetic heterogeneity.

**Pathogenesis:** Because there is incomplete concordance between the $G_s$ protein defect and the AHO somatotype or any of the biochemical findings associated with disturbed mineral metabolism, it is suggested that at least one other gene must be involved in the full expression of the PHP phenotype. It has been suggested that the Gs protein defect in the parathyroid gland itself may interfere with synthesis and secretion of PTH, thereby accounting for altered bioactivity of the circulating hormone found in some PHP patients. Multiple forms of the PTH molecule, with agonist or inhibitory activity, may account for some of the temporal and intrafamilial variability that is characteristic of this disorder.

In PHP-1b and PHP-2 individuals, defects in the PTH molecule itself, the PTH receptor, or in the intracellular transduction of the cAMP signal to distal cellular events (e.g. increased 25-hydroxyvitamin D, 1 α hydroxylase activity) have been postulated, but definitive evidence is lacking. The origin of the increased prevalence in females is unknown.

**MIM No.:** *10358, 20333, 30080

**Sex Ratio:** M1:F2.3 (PHP-1 with AHO).

**Occurrence:** Over 50 kindreds documented in the literature.

**Risk of Recurrence for Patient's Sib:**
See Part I, *Mendelian Inheritance.*

**Risk of Recurrence for Patient's Child:**
See Part I, *Mendelian Inheritance.*

**Age of Detectability:** Elevated serum iPTH or decreased RBC $G_s$ activity can be determined shortly after birth. Clinical features (AHO, hypocalcemia, etc.) may not be manifest until later childhood or adulthood.

**Gene Mapping and Linkage:** Unknown.

**Prevention:** None known. Genetic counseling indicated.

**Treatment:** Hypocalcemia associated with decreased circulating 1,25(OH)D levels can be effectively treated with vitamin D or its analogs--dihydrotachysterol, calcitriol [1,25(OH)$_2$D$_3$] or alphacalcidol [1 α (OH)D$_3$]. Adjunctive therapy may include supplemental oral calcium to help normalize serum calcium and thiazides or acetazolamide to reduce calcium excretion. Whether or not very early detection and treatment of associated hypothyroidism will reduce the extent of the mental deficit is not known.

**Prognosis:** Normal life span.

**Detection of Carrier:** Formal testing for $G_s$ activity and delineation of biochemical phenotype may be useful in identifying asymptomatic, clinically normal adults.

**Special Considerations:** Because of the significant clinical, biochemical, and genetic heterogeneity, caution should be exercised in counselling with regard to risks of recurrence or ultimate outcome.

**References:**

Chase LR, et al.: Pseudohypoparathyroidism: defective excretion of 3'–5' CAMP in response to parathyroid hormone. J Clin Invest 1969; 48:1832–1844.

Fitch N: Albright's hereditary osteodystrophy: a review. Am J Med Genet 1982; 11:11–29.

Okano K, et al.: Comparative efficacy of various vitamin D metabolites in the treatment of various types of hypoparathyroidism. J Clin Endocrinol Metab 1982; 55:238–243.

Goltzman DA, et al.: Studies of the multiple molecular forms of bioactive parathyroid hormone and parathyroid hormone-like substances. Recent Prog Horm Res 1986; 42:665–703.

Levine MA, et al.: Activity of the stimulatory guanine nucleotide-binding protein is reduced in erythrocytes from patients with pseudohypoparathyroidism and pseudopseudohypoparathyroidism: biochemical, endocrine, and genetic analysis of Albright's hereditary osteodystrophy in six kindreds. J Clin Endocrinol Metab 1986; 62:497–502.

Radeke HH, et al.: Multiple pre- and postreceptor defects in pseudohypoparathyroidism (a multicenter study with twenty four patients). J Clin Endocrinol Metab 1986; 62:393–402.

Weinstock RS, et al.: Olfactory dysfunction in humans with deficient guamine nucleotide-binding protein. Nature 1986; 322:635–636.

Brickman AS, et al.: Hypertension in pseudohypoparathyroidism type 1. Am J Med 1988; 85:785–792.

Levine MA, et al.: Genetic deficiency of the alpha subunit of the guanine nucleotide-binding protein G(s) as a molecular basis for Albright hereditary osteodystrophy. Proc Nat Acad Sci 1988; 85:617–621.

Spiegel AM: Pseudohypoparathyroidism. In: Scriver CR, et al, eds: The metabolic basis of inherited disease, 6th ed. New York: McGraw-Hill, 1989:2013–2028.

C0016 **David Cole**

**Parathyroid hyperplasia, hereditary**
*See HYPERPARATHYROIDISM, FAMILIAL*
**Parchment right ventricle**
*See VENTRICLE, RIGHT, UHL ANOMALY*

## PARIETAL FORAMINA-CLAVICULAR HYPOPLASIA     2769

**Includes:** Cleidocranial dysplasia-parietal foramina

**Excludes:** **Cleidocranial dysplasia** (0185)

**Major Diagnostic Criteria:** The combination of parietal foramina and clavicular hypoplasia.

**Clinical Findings:** Eckstein and Hoare (1963) described a mother and son with bilateral clavicular hypoplasia and parietal foramina (oval defects in the parietal bone which are covered by skin). Golabi et al (1984) expanded on the phenotype, and described a three generation pedigree with five affected family members. **Megalencephaly** was present in all five. Occipital dermoid with a hair tuft was present in 4/5. Other findings included prominent forehead (2/5), prominent eyes (2/5), midfacial hypoplasia (2/5), short nasal septum (2/5), long philtrum (2/5), thin upper lip (2/5), and small ears or microtia (2/5).

**Complications:** Unknown.

**Associated Findings:** One affected individual also had lacrimal stenosis and epicanthal folds.

**Etiology:** Presumably autosomal dominant inheritance.

**Pathogenesis:** Unknown.

**MIM No.:** 16855

**POS No.:** 3643

**CDC No.:** 755.555

**Sex Ratio:** M1:F1

**Occurrence:** Two families have been reported.

**Risk of Recurrence for Patient's Sib:**
See Part I, *Mendelian Inheritance.*

**Risk of Recurrence for Patient's Child:**
See Part I, *Mendelian Inheritance.*

**Age of Detectability:** At birth, by physical examination.

**Gene Mapping and Linkage:** Unknown.

**Prevention:** None known. Genetic counseling indicated.

**Treatment:** Undetermined, although removal of the hair tuft for cosmetic reasons may be desirable.

**Prognosis:** Excellent. Life span and intellect are not affected.

**Detection of Carrier:** Unknown.

**References:**
Eckstein HB, Hoare RD: Congenital parietal "foramina" associated with faulty ossification of clavicles. Br J Radiol 1963;36:220–221.
Golabi M, et al: Parietal foramina-clavicular hypoplasia. Am J Dis Child 1984; 138:596–599.

T0007                          **Helga V. Toriello**

**Parkes-Weber syndrome**
*See ANGIO-OSTEOHYPERTROPHY SYNDROME*
**Parkinson disease, early onset-mental retardation**
*See X-LINKED MENTAL RETARDATION-BASAL GANGLION DISORDER*
**Parodontopathia acroectodermalis**
*See HYPERKERATOSIS PALMOPLANTARIS-PERIODONTOCLASIA*
**Parotid aplasia or hypoplasia**
*See ALACRIMA-APTYALISM*
**Parotid gland, swelling of**
*See BRANCHIAL CLEFT CYSTS*
**Parotitis associated with Sjogren syndrome**
*See PAROTITIS, PUNCTATE*
**Parotitis of childhood, chronic recurrent**
*See PAROTITIS, PUNCTATE*

## PAROTITIS, PUNCTATE     0799

**Includes:**
Parotitis of childhood, chronic recurrent
Sialangiectasis
Sialectasis
Mikulicz disease
Parotitis associated with Sjogren syndrome

**Excludes:**
Parotid infection, other forms (e.g. viral, sarcoid, bacterial)
**Sjogren syndrome** (2101)

**Major Diagnostic Criteria:** Evidence of punctate sialectasis on sialography. If possible, a tissue examination of the gland should be done to confirm the pathology.

**Clinical Findings:** A unique pathologic process that appears to occur in three different clinical forms:
*Chronic recurrent parotitis of childhood*: Usually misdiagnosed as "recurrent mumps." It is usually not infectious or contagious. Attacks subside about the time of puberty in about 90% of cases.
*Mikulicz disease*: Occurs in adults who have no evidence of systemic disease. In most cases, only the parotid gland is involved. There may be recurrent attacks of parotid swelling or there may be a chronic diffuse enlargement or a discrete mass. Involvement may be unilateral or bilateral.
*Punctate parotitis*: A very frequent, if not a constant, component of **Sjogren syndrome**. The parotitis may be recurrent or may be chronic, diffuse enlargement. Clinically only one gland may be involved, but on X-ray and pathologically, both are affected.
Pathologic and X-ray findings in the parotid gland are similar in all three clinical types. There appear to be three primary histopathologic lesions: hyperplasia of the epithelial and myoepithelial cells of the intralobular ducts, disappearance of acinar structures, and replacement of the glandular parenchyma by a diffuse infiltration of lymphoid cells.
Involvement of larger ducts and gross glandular destruction, with increased fibrosis, is thought to be associated with secondary infection. Occasionally cystic lesions develop from the hyperplastic ducts. In longstanding cases the pathology may undergo involution and fatty replacement.
The classic X-ray findings are demonstrated by sialography in which terminal or punctate sialectasis is seen. Some workers have reported that the lesion then progresses through globular, cavitary, and destructive stages. These may be caused by bacterial infection secondary to reduced salivary flow. Although there is no unanimity of opinion, many feel that the punctate areas are an artifact due to extravasation of contrast material, but nevertheless are a valuable diagnostic sign.

**Complications:** Secondary bacterial infection due to diminution of salivary flow from acinar destruction.

**Associated Findings:** Other manifestations of **Sjogren syndrome**, i.e., xerophthalmia, connective tissue disorders, and lymphoepithelial malignancy.

**Etiology:** This is an inflammatory lesion but not a bacteriologic disease. A chronic viral infection is possible, but this has not been adequately evaluated. Evidence for a genetic etiology in at least some cases is as follows: definite familial incidence, occurrence in very young children, and preliminary studies indicating hereditary factors in **Sjogren syndrome** with which punctate parotitis is usually associated.

**Pathogenesis:** Unknown.

**Sex Ratio:** Varies by clinical type. Chronic recurrent parotitis of childhood, M>1:F1. Mikulicz disease, M1:F>1. See also **Sjogren syndrome**.

**Occurrence:** Undetermined but presumed rare. Seen most frequently during childhood.

**Risk of Recurrence for Patient's Sib:** Unknown.

**Risk of Recurrence for Patient's Child:** Unknown.

**Age of Detectability:** Whenever clinical involvement of the parotid occurs.

**Gene Mapping and Linkage:** Unknown.

**Prevention:** None known. Genetic counseling indicated.

**Treatment:** The type of treatment depends on the gross pathology and severity of clinical symptoms. Mild cases may require only observation and management of secondary infection. Among available treatments are massage of the gland, stimulation of salivary flow by chewing gum or wax, treating infections of the teeth or tonsils, antibiotics for the acute attack, sialography (because the iodides it contains may be beneficial), injection of antibiotics into the duct system, and small doses (800–1,800r) of X-ray therapy, with or without duct ligation. Surgical treatment includes tympanic neurectomy to eliminate the parasympathetic nerve supply to the gland, and either subtotal or total parotidectomy, sparing the facial nerve. The latter treatment is preferred.

**Prognosis:** Chronic recurrent parotitis of childhood subsides around the age of puberty in about 90% of cases. The parotitis of Mikulicz disease and Sjögren syndrome seems to subside spontaneously after a variable length of time.

**Detection of Carrier:** Unknown.

**References:**

Blatt IM. On sialectasis and benign lymphosialadenopathy (the pyogenic parotitis, Goujerot-Sjögren's syndrome, Mikulicz's disease complex), a 10-year study. Laryngoscope 1964; 74:1684–1746.

Bunim JJ. A broader spectrum of Sjögren's syndrome and its pathogenic implications. Ann Rheum Dis 1961; 20:1–10.

Hemenway WG. Chronic punctate parotitis. Laryngoscope 1971; 81:485–509.

Konno A: A study on the pathogenesis of recurrent parotitis in childhood. Ann Otol Rhinol Laryngol 1979; 88(Suppl)63:1–20. *

BE028                                    **LaVonne Bergstrom**

**Paroxysmal polyserositis, familial**
   *See FEVER, FAMILIAL MEDITERRANEAN (FMF)*
**Parry-Romberg syndrome**
   *See HEMIFACIAL ATROPHY, PROGRESSIVE*
**Partial Kearns-Sayre syndrome (PKSS)**
   *See KEARNS-SAYRE DISEASE*
**Partial lipodystrophy-lipoatrophic diabetes-hyperlipidemia**
   *See LIPODYSTROPHY, FAMILIAL LIMB AND TRUNK*
**Partington mental retardation**
   *See X-LINKED MENTAL RETARDATION-DYSTONIC MOVEMENTS OF THE HANDS*
**Parvovirus (B19)-induced fetal aplastic anemia-hydrops fetalis**
   *See FETAL PARVOVIRUS INFECTION*
**Patau syndrome**
   *See CHROMOSOME 13, TRISOMY 13*
**Patent ductus arteriosus**
   *See DUCTUS ARTERIOSUS, PATENT*
**Patent omphalomesenteric duct**
   *See OMPHALOMESENTERIC DUCT ANOMALIES*
**Patent urachus**
   *See URACHAL ANOMALIES*
**Patterson pseudoleprechaunism**
   *See PSEUDOLEPRECHAUNISM, PATTERSON TYPE*
**PBGD deficiency**
   *See PORPHYRIA, ACUTE INTERMITTENT*
**PCB fetopathy**
   *See FETAL EFFECTS OF POLYCHLORINATED BIPHENYL (PCB)*
**PCCA Complementation group**
   *See ACIDEMIA, PROPIONIC*
**PCP, fetal effects**
   *See FETAL EFFECTS FROM ANGEL DUST (PHENCYCLIDINE OR PCP)*
**Pectoralis muscle, absence of**
   *See POLAND SYNDROME*
**Pectum recurvatum**
   *See PECTUS EXCAVATUM*

## PECTUS CARINATUM                                    0801

**Includes:**
   Chicken breast
   Chondrosternal prominence, congenital
   Pigeon breast
   Pyramidal chest
   Sternogladiolar prominence
   Thorax cuneiforme

**Excludes:** Pectus excavatum (0802)

**Major Diagnostic Criteria:** Prominence of sternum with lateral depression of ribs.

**Clinical Findings:** There are three types. *Type I*: "Keel" chest, most common of the three, consists of symmetrical protrusion of the sternum and the costal cartilages. *Type II*: Pouter breast consists of protrusion of the manubrium and the first two sternal cartilages, with depression of the body of the sternum and protrusion of the tip of the xiphoid process. It is the least common of the three. *Type III*: Lateral pectus carinatum consists of asymmetric unilateral protrusion of the anterior chest wall.

The condition is present at birth but may not become obvious until recession of the prominent abdomen in later childhood. There is usually no associated significant limitation of cardiorespiratory function.

**Complications:** Possible psychological effects. Occasionally fatigue, nondescript chest pain, and possibly dyspnea from decreased respiratory excursion of the thorax.

**Associated Findings: Marfan syndrome, Homocystinuria, Mucopolysaccharidosis**, rickets, and various malformation syndromes.

**Etiology:** Unknown.

**Pathogenesis:** Several theories have been proposed. Brodkin believes that the various sternal deformities are the result of failure of the development of muscle in the ventral segment of the diaphragm, and that these portions of the muscle exert a pull on the attached chest wall as a result of the unopposed action of muscles on the other side. Robicsek et al (1979) believe this deformity is due to an overgrowth of the costal cartilages and thus, if the sternum is pushed inward, **Pectus excavatum** results. But, if the sternum is outward, pectus carinatum develops.

**CDC No.:** 754.800

**Sex Ratio:** Presumably M1:F1.

**Occurrence:** Reported as 1:1,660 in the school population of Newark, New Jersey.

**Risk of Recurrence for Patient's Sib:** Unknown.

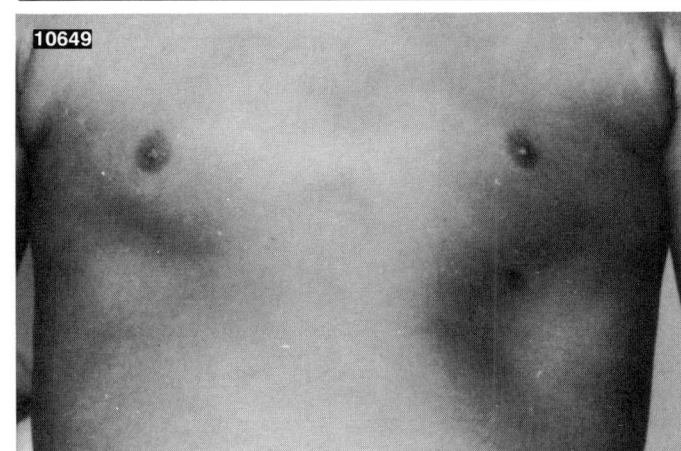

**0801-10649:** Asymmetric pectus carinatum.

**Risk of Recurrence for Patient's Child:** Unknown.

**Age of Detectability:** At birth, by physical examination.

**Gene Mapping and Linkage:** Unknown.

**Prevention:** None known. Genetic counseling indicated.

**Treatment:** Surgery is usually for cosmetic effect and because of the variety of defects, individuality of approach is required. Although it appears that pectus carinatum does not interfere with normal activity, there have been no good reported studies of intrathoracic gas volumes or mechanics of breathing. The deformity is not caused by or related to airway obstruction. It is generally agreed by surgeons that surgical correction should be deferred until the chest wall is stable.

**Prognosis:** Normal for life span and intelligence. Function may depend on severity.

**Detection of Carrier:** Unknown.

**References:**

Ravitch MM: Congenital deformities of the chest wall. In: Benson CD, et al., eds: Pediatric surgery, vol. 1. Chicago: Year Book Medical Publishers, 1962:227.

Pickard LR, et al.: Pectus carinatum: results of surgical therapy. J Ped Surg 1979; 14:228–230.

Robicsek F, et al.: Pectus carinatum. J Thorac Cardiovas Surg 1979; 78:52–61.

Wesselhoeft CW, DeLuca FG: A simplified approach to the repair of pediatric pectus deformities. Ann Thorac Surg 1982; 34:640–646.

J0010                                              **Virginia P. Johnson**

## PECTUS EXCAVATUM             0802

**Includes:**

    Chest, funnel
    Chonechondrosternon
    Funnel chest
    Pectum recurvatum
    Schusterbrust
    Trichterbrust

**Excludes:** Pectus carinatum (0801)

**Major Diagnostic Criteria:** Central depression of the chest at the level of the sternum.

**Clinical Findings:** The anteroposterior diameter of the lower thorax is decreased by the posterior dislocation of the lower sternum, the costal cartilages, and the anterior part of the ribs. The affected portion of the sternum is concavely deformed. The manubrium is generally normal, whereas the xiphoid may extend so far posteriorly as to impinge on the vertebral bodies or the

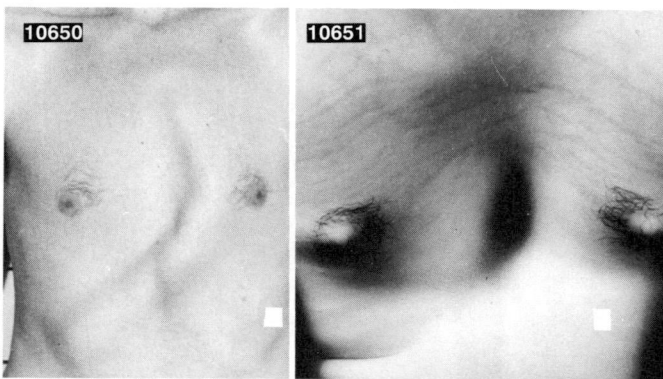

**0802**-10650: Asymmetric pectus excavatum. 10651: Asymmetric pectus excavatum with striae cutis distensae.

paravertebral gutters. The left side of the chest bulges slightly because the heart underlies it very close to the surface.

Children with this anomaly are usually asymptomatic, unless they have primary lung or heart disease. Only occasionally are vague complaints heard about decreased exercise tolerance and chest discomfort. Auscultatory findings may simulate mild pulmonary stenosis and small atrial septal defects. Scalar electrocardiographic and X-ray features may resemble mild right ventricular overload. These are not specific enough to suggest cardiac malformation and are explainable on the basis of heart displacement. Thus cardiac catheterization is often not needed. However, pectus excavatum can reduce the pumping capacity of the heart during upright exercise, and hemodynamic improvement may be achieved with surgery.

**Complications:** Psychologic effects are noted. In the presence of chronic lung disease, congenital or acquired heart conditions, or calcification of cartilages with advanced age, a severe chest deformity can further impair the function of the intrathoracic organs, by dislocation, distortion, compression, or restriction of mobility.

**Associated Findings:** Occurs in association with various syndromes (e.g. **Marfan syndrome**, **Noonan syndrome**), and chronic airway obstruction in infants.

**Etiology:** Possibly autosomal dominant inheritance. There are many sporadic cases.

**Pathogenesis:** Disputed, but the most probable mechanism is an intrinsic failure of osteogenesis. Other theories include a partial weakness of the diaphragm, with the stronger portions causing an asymmetric pull on the chest wall; an abnormally short tendon or fibrous central portion of the diaphragm; and either persistent obstructive respiratory disease causing an increased transpulmonary pressure gradient during respiration, or secondary displacement of the sternum from overgrowth of the costal cartilages, or both.

**MIM No.:** 16930

**CDC No.:** 754.810

**Sex Ratio:** M3:F2 observed.

**Occurrence:** 13–40:10,000.

**Risk of Recurrence for Patient's Sib:**
See Part I, *Mendelian Inheritance.*

**Risk of Recurrence for Patient's Child:**
See Part I, *Mendelian Inheritance.*

**Age of Detectability:** Usually present at birth, often undetected until some months later.

**Gene Mapping and Linkage:** Unknown.

**Prevention:** None known. Genetic counseling indicated.

**Treatment:** Surgical repair of deformity by mobilization and repositioning of the body of the sternum after a subperichondrial resection or morcellation of costal cartilages, or by replacing deformed portions or correcting contours with bone grafts or with prosthetic materials. Temporary internal support with a malleable strut passed transternally is often necessary. The approach to surgical repair depends on individual assessment of the relative significance of physiologic and psychologic indications, and on the balance between operative risks and expectable results. In cases of independent heart or lung diseases, the same factors must be weighed with particular care, and in some cases a more radical approach may be indicated.

**Prognosis:** Probably normal life span. May be progressive or stationary; recurrence after operation not uncommon unless internal strut is used.

**Detection of Carrier:** Unknown.

**References:**

Beiser GD, et al.: Impairment of cardiac function in patients with pectus excavatum with improvement after operative correction. New Engl J Med 1972; 287:267–272.

Haller JA Jr., Turner CS: Diagnosis and operative management of chest wall deformities in children. Surg Clin North Am 1981; 61:1199–1207.

Castile R, et al.: Symptomatic pectus deformities of the chest. Am Rev Respir Dis 1982; 126:564–568.

Wesselhoeft CW, DeLuca FG: A simplified approach to the repair of pediatric pectus deformities. Ann Thorac Surg 1982; 34:640–646.

Cahill JL, et al.: A summary of preoperative and postoperative cardiorespiratory performance in patients undergoing pectus excavatum and carinatum repair. J Ped Surg 1984; 19:430–433.

Leung AKC, Hoo JJ: Familail congenital funnel chest. Am J Med Genet 1987; 26:887–890.

J0010                                                   **Virginia P. Johnson**

**Pedersen hypothesis**
  *See FETAL EFFECTS FROM MATERNAL DIABETES*
**Pee deficiency**
  *See BIOPTERIN SYNTHESIS DEFICIENCY*
**Peg-shaped lateral incisor**
  *See TEETH, ENAMEL HYPOPLASIA*
**Pelizaeus-Merzbacher disease (PMD), connatal type**
  *See PELIZAEUS-MERZBACHER SYNDROME*

---

## PELIZAEUS-MERZBACHER SYNDROME          0803

**Includes:**
  Cerebral sclerosis, diffuse chronic infantile
  Pelizaeus-Merzbacher disease (PMD), connatal type
  Proteolipid protein, myelin
  Leukodystrophy, sudanophilic
  Seitelberg variant, Pelizaeus-Merzbacher syndrome

**Excludes:**
  **Adrenoleukodystrophy, X-linked** (2533)
  **Brain, spongy degeneration** (0115)
  **Cockayne syndrome** (0189)
  **Leukodystrophy, adult onset progressive dominant type** (2975)
  **Leukodystrophy, globoid cell type** (0415)
  Leukodystrophies of nervous system, other
  **Metachromatic leukodystrophies** (0651)
  Nervous system, other degenerative diseases of

**Major Diagnostic Criteria:**  A pattern of involvement of males, with onset around age 4–6 months, and with peculiar pendular nystagmus followed by delay in motor development should strongly suggest the diagnosis. A family history compatible with a pattern of X-linked recessive inheritance is also suggestive.

**Clinical Findings:**  The disease is slowly progressive, with onset usually at 4–6 months of age. The distinctive clinical features are that of a chaotic, pendular nystagmus, often accompanied by shaking movements of the head, combined with hypotonia. Later, choreoathetoid movements develop, and optic atrophy is common. The patients are delayed in early motor milestones and, in the later stage of disease, they often develop contractures and spasticity of the lower limbs. Movements of the arms, particularly fine motor movements, are jerky and clumsy. Speech development may be slightly delayed, but is often within the normal range. Mentation, early in the course of the disease, seems to be relatively normal. Progression is gradual, with increasing involvement of the lower and upper limbs. The nystagmus persists and ataxia becomes a prominent symptom. There is slow progression, and death usually occurs in the third decade.

Renier et al (1981) delineated three variants: the classic type discussed above; a connatal or Seitelberg variant, in which onset is in the neonatal period, the course of the disease is more rapid and severe, and death usually occurs before five years of age; and an intermediate transitional form.

**Complications:**  Progressive neurologic disease. Terminal pneumonia is frequent.

**Associated Findings:**  None known.

**Etiology:**  X-linked recessive inheritance.

**Pathogenesis:**  Probably a defect in the lipophilin constituent of myelin. The pathology is distinctive, with a marked loss of myelin except for relatively well-preserved areas or islands of normal myelin (Tigroid patten). In the severe form (Seitelberg variant), there is more extensive and complete loss of myelin. A similar disorder in the jimpy mouse is due to abnormal synthesis of proteolipid protein associated with an abnormality of the PLP gene resulting in abnormal splicing of the mRNA.

**MIM No.:**  *31208

**Sex Ratio:**  M1:F0

**Occurrence:**  Undetermined but presumed rare. Extensive literature.

**Risk of Recurrence for Patient's Sib:**
  See Part I, *Mendelian Inheritance.*

**Risk of Recurrence for Patient's Child:**
  See Part I, *Mendelian Inheritance.* Affected individuals are not expected to survive to reproduce.

**Age of Detectability:**  Usually by 4–18 months of age. The condition can be diagnosed by magnetic resonance imaging (MRI).

**Gene Mapping and Linkage:**  PLP (proteolipid protein (Pelizaeus-Merzbacher disease)) has been mapped to Xq21.3-q22.

**Prevention:**  None known. Genetic counseling indicated.

**Treatment:**  Unknown.

**Prognosis:**  A slowly progressive leukodystrophy, with few patients surviving the third decade of life.

**Detection of Carrier:**  Unknown.

**Special Considerations:**  This condition was first reported in the German literature prior to the turn of the century.

Closely related processes, with sporadic appearance and without nystagmus as a prominent early sign, but which also have a slowly progressive course compatible with a leukodystrophy, have been observed. Pathologically, these cases do have islands of normal myelin adjacent to areas of marked demyelination.

**References:**
Renier WO, et al.: Connatal Pelizaeus-Merzbacher disease with congenital stridor in two maternal cousins. Acta Neuropath 1981; 54:11–17.
Boulloche J, Aicardi J: Pelizaeus-Merzbacher disease: clinical and nosological study. J Child Neurol 1986; 1:233–239. *
Dautigny A, et al.: The structural gene coding for myelin-associated proteolipid protein is mutated in jimpy mice. Nature 1986; 321:867–869.
Koeppen AH, et al.: Defective biosynthesis of proteolipid protein in Pelizaeus-Merzbacher disease. Ann Neurol 1987; 21:159–170.

GI010                                                   **Herbert Gilmore**

**Pelvofemoral muscular dystrophy**
  *See MUSCULAR DYSTROPHY, LIMB-GIRDLE*
**Pelvospondylitis ossificans**
  *See ANKYLOSING SPONDYLITIS*

---

## PEMPHIGUS, BENIGN FAMILIAL          3255

**Includes:**
  Hailey-Hailey disease
  Skin, pemphigus, benign familial

**Excludes:**
  **Darier disease** (2865)
  Pemphigus vulgaris

**Major Diagnostic Criteria:**  A rash of the intertriginous areas, occurring in early adulthood, and typical histological findings on skin biopsy. These include suprabasal lacunae or fully developed blisters, with acantholysis showing a dilapidated brick wall appearance. Dyskeratotic cells (corps ronds) may be present in the granular layer.

**Clinical Findings:**  A chronic recurrent eruption occurring in the intertriginous areas, especially the axillae and groins. Consists of vesicles on an erythematous base that coalesce to form circinate well defined plaques, sometimes with crusting and exudation. Mucosal lesions appear rarely. Healing occurs spontaneously without scarring. These patients often experience exacerbations during warm weather, associated with sweating and friction. Seventy percent of patients report a positive family history.

**Complications:** Bacterial or candidal contamination are often found. It is felt that these organisms may precipitate exacerbations, although it is possible that they are a secondary phenomenon.

**Associated Findings:** None known.

**Etiology:** Autosomal dominant inheritance.

**Pathogenesis:** The basic defect as seen by electron microscopy is a defect in cellular cohesion. This is thought to arise either due to a defect in the tonofilament-desmosome complex or due to a defect in the synthesis of intercellular substance.

**MIM No.:** *16960

**Sex Ratio:** M1:F1

**Occurrence:** Undetermined but presumed rare.

**Risk of Recurrence for Patient's Sib:**
See Part I, *Mendelian Inheritance.*

**Risk of Recurrence for Patient's Child:**
See Part I, *Mendelian Inheritance.*

**Age of Detectability:** Usually at adolescence or early adulthood.

**Gene Mapping and Linkage:** Unknown.

**Prevention:** None known. Genetic counseling indicated.

**Treatment:** Unknown.

**Prognosis:** Unknown.

**Detection of Carrier:** Unknown.

**References:**
Hailey J, Hailey H: Familial benign chronic pemphigus. Arch Dermatol Syphilol 1939; 39:679–685.
Lever WF: Familial benign pemphigus. In: Dermatology in general medicine. New York: McGraw-Hill, 1987.

GH001                                               **Ruby Ghadially**

**Pena-Shokeir II syndrome**
*See CEREBRO-OCULO-FACIO-SKELETAL SYNDROME*

---

## PENA-SHOKEIR SYNDROME                            2080

**Includes:**
Arthrogryposis multiplex congenita-pulmonary hypoplasia
Fetal akinesia deformation sequence, Pena-Shokeir I phenotype

**Excludes:**
**Cerebro-oculo-facio-skeletal syndrome** (0140)
**Hutterite syndrome, Bowen-Conradi type** (2422)
**Neu-laxova syndrome** (2092)
**Pterygium syndrome, multiple lethal** (2274)

**Major Diagnostic Criteria:** The combination of multiple joint contractures, facial anomalies, and pulmonary hypoplasia. However, these features are really a phenotype that can be produced by decreased fetal movement. The cases which have been reported in the literature represent a heterogeneous group of disorders, on the basis of neuropathic and myopathic evaluations. Nevertheless, as pointed out by Moessing (1983), a typical phenotype is produced with decreased early fetal movement. These same anomalies can be produced by curarizing rats.

**Clinical Findings:** Based on more than 30 cases, the major findings include pulmonary hypoplasia; low-set appearing malformed ears; multiple joint contractures; **Camptodactyly**; clubfeet; **Eye, hypertelorism**; depressed nasal tip; micrognathia; intrauterine growth retardation; and polyhydramnios. Cryptorchidism was seen in all males evaluated. Relatively common features included abnormal placentas, epicanthal folds, highly arched or cleft palate, hypoplastic dermal ridges, webbing across joints, and a short neck.

**Complications:** Most infants have severe respiratory distress at birth because of underdeveloped lungs. Some catch-up growth

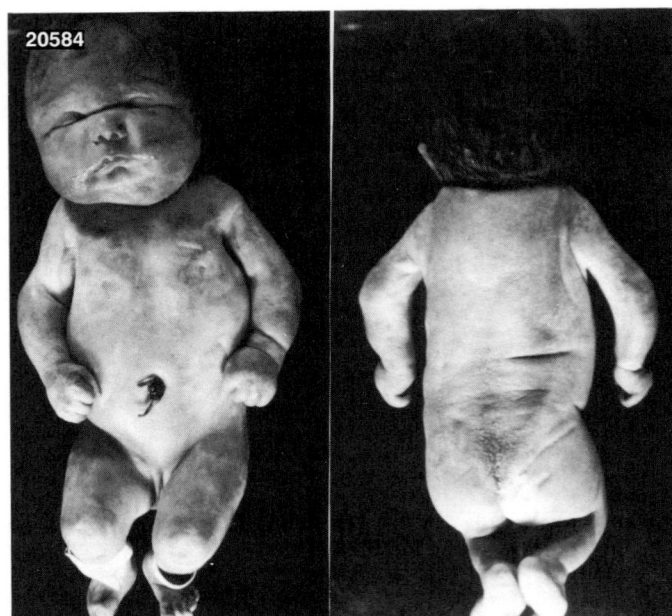

**2080-20584:** Pena-Shokeir syndrome; note multiple joint contractures, and dysmorphic facies. There is also pulmonary hypoplasia.

does appear to be possible. One child survived to 20 months of age.

**Associated Findings:** A few affected infants have had cardiac defects (including hypoplasia, **Aorta, coarctation, Ductus arteriosus, patent**, right ventricular hypertrophy, **Heart, transposition of great vessels**, and cor pulmononale), genitourinary defects (renal microcysts, megaloureter, persistent or cystic urachus, **Hypospadias**, or micropenis), **Cleft palate**, choanal atresia, laryngeal stenosis, microphthalmia, **Optic atrophy, Torticollis**, abnormal lung lobation, pulmonary hemangiomata, thymic hyperplasia, **Adrenal hypoplasia**, islet cell hyperplasia, gastroschisis, intestinal malrotation, **Meckel diverticulum**, anorectal atresia, preaxial **Polydactyly**, absent lower limb, and multiple skin nevi.

**Etiology:** Cases diagnosed as Pena-Shokeir are clearly a heterogeneous group of disorders secondary to several causes, including neurogenic atrophy, anterior horn cell changes, abnormal skeletal musculature, congenital myopathy, and maternal myasthenia gravis. All of these reflect decreased intrauterine movement which produces the common phenotype described in Pena-Shokeir; pulmonary hypoplasia, congenital contractures, depressed nasal tip, micrognathia, and hypertelorism. Many of the specific entities are inherited on an autosomal recessive basis.

**Pathogenesis:** Most, if not all the phenotypic features seen in Pena-Shokeir can be attributed to fetal akinesia or hypokinesia, e.g., lack of in utero movement. Moessinger's (1983) work with rats has shown that the polyhydramnios is associated with decreased or absent swallowing; that the congenital contractures are seen with decreased or absent fetal movement; that the lack of normal fetal respiratory activity is associated with pulmonary hypoplasia; and that the facial anomalies present in these cases are likely to be secondary to decreased facial and jaw movement in utero.

**MIM No.:** *20815

**POS No.:** 3135

**Sex Ratio:** M1:F1

**Occurrence:** Several dozen cases have been reported in the literature.

**Risk of Recurrence for Patient's Sib:**
See Part I, *Mendelian Inheritance.*

**Risk of Recurrence for Patient's Child:**
See Part I, *Mendelian Inheritance.* Affected individuals are not expected to survive to reproduce.

**Age of Detectability:** Prenatal diagnosis with real-time ultrasound is possible, but there may be a risk of missing a case early in the second trimester. Most cases are detected at birth by physical examination.

**Gene Mapping and Linkage:** Unknown.

**Prevention:** None known. Genetic counseling indicated.

**Treatment:** Vigorous physical therapy and pulmonary support during the newborn period give a chance for catch-up growth and survival.

**Prognosis:** Survival depends on the degree of pulmonary hypoplasia. Most affected infants have died soon after birth. Although a few have survived several months, all survivors have had delayed motor development. Mental development has ranged from severly retarded to normal.

**Detection of Carrier:** Unknown.

**Special Considerations:** It bears repeating that Pena-Shokeir is actually a phenotype and represents a heterogeneous group of disorders. Even those cases with decreased numbers of anterior horn cells may be heterogeneous. Within a specific family, however, there is usually a fairly consistent picture, and in all cases there has been decreased intrauterine movement prior to 24 weeks. Herva et al (1985) have reported 16 cases with the Pena-Shokeir phenotype and anterior horn call atrophy, but with severe edema and stillbirth prior to the 35th week of gestation; concluding that this represented a distinct syndrome.

**References:**
Moessinger AC: Fetal akinesia deformation sequence: an animal model. Pediatrics 1983; 72:857–863.
Herva R, et al: A lethal autosomal recessive syndrome of multiple congenital contractures. Am J Med Genet 1985; 20:431–439.
Lindhout D, et al.: The Pena-Shokeir syndrome: report of nine Dutch cases. Am J Med Genet 1985; 21:655–668.
Hall JG: Analysis of the Pena-Shokeir phenotype. Am J Med Genet 1986; 25:99–117. *
Hageman G, et al.: The heterogeneity of the Pena-Shokeir syndrome. Neuropediatrics 1987; 18:45–50.
Davis JE, Kalousek DK: Fetal akinesia deformation sequence in previable fetuses. Am J Med Genet 1988; 29:77–87.
Katzenstein M, Goodman RM: Pre- and postnatal findings in Pena Shokeir I syndrome: case report and a review of the literature. J Craniofac Genet Devel Biol 1988; 8:111–126.
Ohlsson A, et al.: Prenatal sonographic diagnosis of Pena-Shokeir syndrome. Am J Med Genet 1988; 29:59–65.

HA014
T0007

**Judith G. Hall**
**Helga V. Toriello**

**Penchaszadeh-Velasquez-Arwillagi syndrome**
*See NASOPALPEBRAL LIPOMA-COLOBOMA SYNDROME*
**Pendred syndrome**
*See DEAFNESS-GOITER*
**Penicillamine, fetal effects**
*See FETAL D-PENICILLAMINE SYNDROME*
**Penicillamine, fetal effects of**
*See CUTIS LAXA*
**Penis, double (reduplicated)**
*See DIPHALLIA*
**Penis, epispadias**
*See EPISPADIAS*
**Penis, micropenis**
*See ANDROGEN INSENSITIVITY (RESISTANCE), MINIMAL*

## PENTALOGY OF CANTRELL
**3121**

**Includes:**
Cantrell-Haller-Ravitch syndrome
Cantrell pentalogy
Pentalogy syndrome
Peritoneopericardial diaphragmatic hernia
Thoracoabdominal ectopia cordis

**Excludes:**
**Diaphragmatic hernia** (0289)
**Heart, cordis ectopia** (0335)
**Heart, pericardium agenesis** (0805)
**Pectus excavatum** (0802)

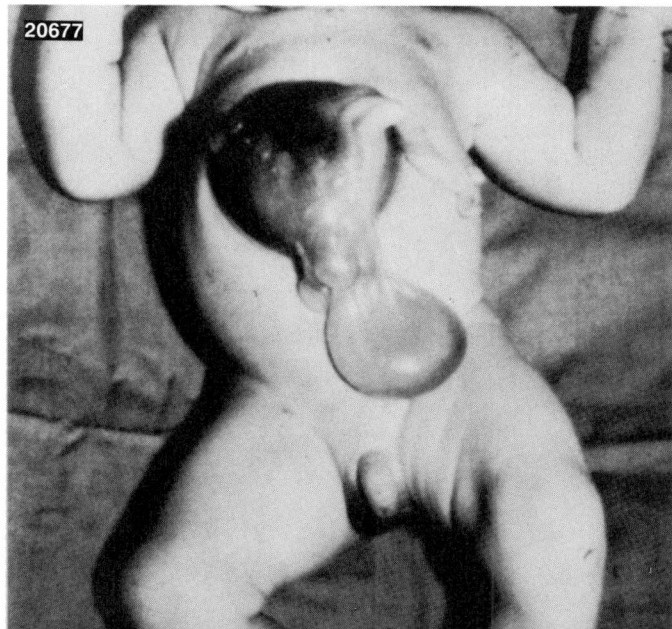

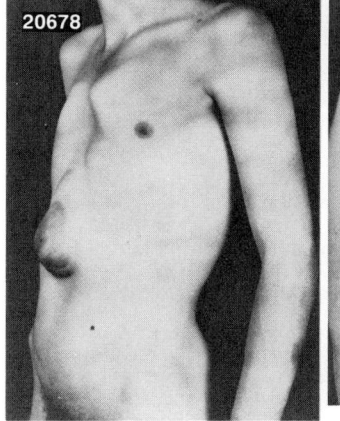 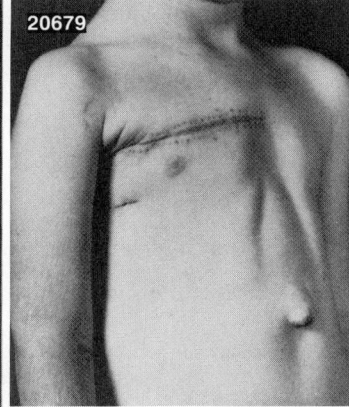

**3121-20677:** Newborn infant with a supraumbilical omphalocele with heart contour visible beneath the skin of the unusually high epigastrium. The child subsequently proved to have tetralogy of Fallot. **20678:** Twenty-year-old male who has tetralogy of Fallot, a broad sternal cleft, diastasis recti, and a supraumbilical hernia covered by thin hyperpigmented skin. **20679:** Two-year-old boy with distal sternal cleft and diastasis recti, shortly after Blalock shunt for tetralogy of Fallot.

**Major Diagnostic Criteria:** Midline, supraumbilical abdominal wall defect; defect of the lower sternum; deficiency of the anterior diaphragm; a defect in the diaphragmatic pericardium; and congenital intracardiac defects. Although a definite diagnosis is made by the presence of all five components, a probable diagnosis is suggested by any four features, and three should prompt consideration of this condition.

**Clinical Findings:** In the full syndrome, there is a distal sternal cleft, an omphalocele-like ventral abdominal defect with diastasis recti, a crescentic midline anterior diaphragmatic defect, a free pericardioperitoneal communication, and an internal cardiac malformation, suggesting a field defect.

The *sternal* defect may range from inconspicuous absence of the xyphoid or shortening to complete clefting or absence. The *abdominal wall* defect may be wide rectus muscle diastasis with the heart often palpable beneath loose hyperpigmented overlying skin. At the other extreme, a huge omphalocele may be present that contains bowel, liver, and the cardiac apex, covered by a translucent membrane. The semilunar *diaphragmatic* defect is unrelated to the more common diaphragmatic defects and is usually relatively small. Occasionally bowel gains entry into the pericardial cavity via the pericardioperitoneal communication. Defects in the *pericardium* typically involve its diaphragmatic aspect. A significant number of patients have a vermiform diverticulum of the left ventricle that may protrude through this communication. Congenital *intracardiac* defects are almost invariably present in the pentalogy and usually include **Atrial septal defects** or **Ventricular septal defect**; tetralogy of Fallot is very common.

Except for some degree of dextrorotation, which is often present, the heart usually lies in normal relationship to the other thoracic viscera. The appearance of ectopia is created by the concomitant defects of the sternum, diaphragm, and abdominal wall, which occasionally leave the heart abnormally exposed. The presence and full extent of the pentalogy may not be readily apparent on initial examination of an infant with a supraumbilical hernia. Several patients have undergone repair of what was assumed to be a simple omphalocele and were only later found to have the pentalogy at the time their cardiac defects were discovered and repaired.

**Complications:** Depend on the severity of the defects and may include rupture of abdominal viscera during delivery, sepsis from peritonitis, cyanosis, congestive heart failure, cardiorespiratory difficulty from visceral herniation into the thorax, and cardiac compression. Most of these complications are currently remediable with surgical therapy. A number of patients have succumbed to respiratory insufficiency secondary to pulmonary hypoplasia. The major morbidity after the newborn period is related to the congenital heart disease. Intelligence is usually normal.

**Associated Findings:** Intestinal malrotation and **Hernia, umbilical** are common. Rarely, severe malformations such as **Exstrophy of cloaca sequence** and neural tube defects may accompany the pentalogy.

**Etiology:** Unknown. Pentalogy of Cantrell is unlikely to be the result of a single gene defect, since, other than one pair of monozygotic twins both with the pentalogy, no cases of affected sibs have been reported. The presence of the pentalogy in only one twin of four reported cases of presumed dizygotic twins suggests that a transmitted maternal infection or toxin is also unlikely.

**Pathogenesis:** A proposed theory postulates that an abnormality must occur prior to or immediately after differentiation of the intraembryonic mesoderm into its splanchnic and somatic layers at about 14–18 days after conception. The diaphragmatic defect results from total or partial failure of the septum transversum to develop from a segment of somatic mesoderm. The pericardium arises from somatic mesoderm immediately adjacent to that from which the septum transversum is derived. The sternum and abdominal wall defects appear to arise from faulty migration of paired mesodermal structures. Since the normal elements of the sternum and abdominal wall are usually present but not fused in affected individuals it is thought that perhaps there is a deficiency

of the ventral paramidline mesoderm into which the migrating premordia of these structures grow.

**POS No.:** 3248

**CDC No.:** 754.820

**Sex Ratio:** M1:F1

**Occurrence:** About 50 cases have been reported in the literature.

**Risk of Recurrence for Patient's Sib:** Unknown. Probably low, since, except for one pair of concordant twins with the pentalogy, no affected sibs have been reported.

**Risk of Recurrence for Patient's Child:** Unknown.

**Age of Detectability:** At birth, or prenatally by ultrasound examination if defects are severe.

**Gene Mapping and Linkage:** Unknown.

**Prevention:** None known. Genetic counseling indicated.

**Treatment:** In most cases in which an **Omphalocele** is present, immediate surgical intervention is mandatory. Repair of sternal, diaphragmatic, and pericardial anomalies are secondary to the problems involved in satisfactory closure of a large omphalocele; however, they are usually most easily corrected at the time of the initial surgery. Recognition and management of the intracardiac lesion is important in infancy. Palliative surgery may be needed early, although a definitive procedure to correct the heart defect is often performed when the child is older.

**Prognosis:** Is primarily determined by the extent of the ventral wall and cardiac defects. May be lethal during the neonatal period. Reports in the literature describe patients with less extensive defects who survived into adulthood without surgical corrective procedures.

**Detection of Carrier:** Unknown.

**Special Considerations:** This specific combination of five anomalies has in the past occasionally been classified as an example of *thoracoabdominal ectopia cordis*. Since the heart defect only appears superficial secondary to the throacoabdominal defects and is not actually ectopic, this association of birth defects should be classified as a separate entity.

Since the pentalogy has been found in two unrelated cases of **Chromosome 18, trisomy 18** and in one case of 45,X/46,XX mosacism, chromosome studies should be considered when evaluating patients with this field defect.

**References:**

Cantrell JR, et al.: A syndrome of congenital defects involving the abdominal wall, sternum, diaphragm, pericardium, and heart. Surg Gynecol Obstet 1958; 107:602–614. * †

Toyama WM: Combined congenital defects of the anterior abdominal wall, sternum, diaphragm, pericardium, and heart: a case report and review of the syndrome. Pediatrics 1972; 50:778–792.

Ravitch MM: Cantrell's pentalogy and notes on diverticulum of the left ventricle. In: Ravitch MM: Congenital deformities of the chest wall and their operative correction. Philadelphia: W.B. Saunders, 1977: 53–77. * †

BR041
BR007

**Christine R. Bryke**
**W. Roy Breg**

**Pentalogy syndrome**
*See PENTALOGY OF CANTRELL*
**Pentazocine induced scleroderma**
*See SCLERODERMA, FAMILIAL PROGRESSIVE*

## PENTOSURIA                                                0804

**Includes:**

L-xylulose reductase deficiency
L-xylulosuria
Xylitol dehydrogenase deficiency

**Excludes:** Alimentary pentosuria

**Major Diagnostic Criteria:** Pentosuric individuals excrete 1–4 gm of L-xylulose per day. Unlike glucose or galactose, xylulose (as well as ketoses such as fructose) reduces Benedict's solution at low temperatures. Consequently, the Lasker and Enklewitz Benedict's test (55° C, 10 minutes) should be used as the first and most convenient diagnostic test. Paper chromatography will provide direct evidence that the urinary sugar is xylulose.

**Clinical Findings:** Pentosuria is not accompanied by any functional disturbances or symptoms other than the daily excretion of gram quantities of the pentose, L-xylulose. The pentose is present in only trace quantities in normal urine. However, presumably as a result of a defect in the liver enzyme system, which acts on this ketopentose, the sugar is poorly metabolized and is largely excreted in the urine. The condition is usually discovered when patients with high levels of urinary sugar are found to be without diabetic symptoms. Analysis of the urine discloses that the reducing sugar is not glucose.

**Complications:** None. Early reports of unusual psychologic manifestations were probably a consequence of the uncertainty of diagnosis and of unnecessary or ineffective attempts at treatment.

**Associated Findings:** **Diabetes mellitus** is occasionally found in pentosuric individuals, but as yet there are no valid data on whether the coincidence of the two conditions is other than rare and random.

**Etiology:** Autosomal recessive inheritance of the enzyme NADP-xylitol (L-xylulose) dehydrogenase. The exception was one study suggesting that in a particular Lebanese family the mechanism of inheritance appeared to be that of a dominant gene with reduced penetrance; subsequent restudy of this family with an improved enzyme assay (Lane and Jenkins, 1985) indicated pseudodominance.

**Pathogenesis:** No specific pathology has been demonstrated. Although it has been stated that the pentosuric condition persists relatively unchanged throughout life, members of one Lebanese family were reported to show pentosuria after earlier urine tests for pentose had been negative. The urinary level of xylulose is not markedly influenced by ordinary variations in diet. A direct test of pentosuric liver has not as yet been possible. Although there is no well-established relationship between pentosuria and diabetes mellitus, there is suggestive evidence that the latter disease may be accompanied by a disturbance in the glucuronate-xylulose pathway. Further work on this possible interrelationship is required. Wang and van Eys (1970) have shown a decrease of NADP-linked xylitol dehydrogenase in red cells of patients with pentosuria.

**MIM No.:** *26080

**Sex Ratio:** M1:F1

**Occurrence:** 1:2,500 births among Ashkenazim. The condition has been encountered almost exclusively in Ashkenazi Jews of Polish-Russian extraction and, occasionally, in individuals of Lebanese descent.

**Risk of Recurrence for Patient's Sib:**
See Part I, *Mendelian Inheritance.*

**Risk of Recurrence for Patient's Child:**
See Part I, *Mendelian Inheritance.*

**Age of Detectability:** In infants, as early as two weeks of age.

**Gene Mapping and Linkage:** Unknown.

**Prevention:** None known. Genetic counseling indicated.

**Treatment:** Unknown.

**Prognosis:** Normal life span.

**Detection of Carrier:** Carriers appear to be capable of handling the normal load of L-xylulose produced in normal metabolism. However, by stressing the glucuronic acid-xylulose metabolic pathway by the administration of a large test dose of D-glucuronolactone, it has been found that the heterozygous carrier of the pentosuric gene is less able than homozygous normal individuals to metabolize the L-xylulose produced from the glucuronolactone.

**Special Considerations:** It is unnecessary to demonstrate that the xylulose is of the L form, since D-xylulosuria has never been reported. However, when desired, the osazone of L-xylulose can be prepared and characterized by its melting point behavior when mixed with D-xylosazone. The derivative mixture melts approximately 40 ° C higher than the separate isomers.

**References:**

Touster O: Pentose metabolism and pentosuria. Am J Med 1959; 26:724–735.
Touster O: Essential pentosuria and the glucuronate-xylulose pathway. Fed Proc 1960; 19:977.
Politzer WM, Fleischmann H: L-xylulosuria in a Lebanese family. Am J Hum Genet 1962; 14:256–260.
Hollmann S, Touster O: Non-glycolytic pathways of metabolism of glucose. New York: Academic Press, 1964:95.
Wang YM, van Eys JO: The enzymatic defect in essential pentosuria. New Engl J Med 1970; 282:892–896.
Lane AB, Jenkins T: Human L-xylulose reductase variation: familial and population studies. Ann Hum Genet 1985; 49:227–235.
Hiatt HH: Pentosuria. In: Scriver CR, et al, eds: The metabolic basis of inherited disease, 6th ed. New York: McGraw-Hill, 1989:481–493.

T0010                                              **Oscar Touster**

**Pepper syndrome**
*See COHEN SYNDROME*

## PEPTIC ULCER DISEASES, NON-SYNDROMIC        2233

**Includes:**

Antral G-cell hyperfunction DU
Combined duodenal and gastric ulcer
Duodenal ulcer (DU)
Gastric ulcer
Hyperpepsinogenemic I duodenal ulcer
Normopepsinogenemic I duodenal ulcer
Rapid gastric emptying duodenal ulcer
Ulcer, duodenal
Ulcer, gastric
Ulcer, peptic

**Excludes:**

**Amyloidoses**
**Endocrine neoplasia, multiple type I** (0350)
Histamine excess (mastocytosis) associated peptic ulcer
**Tremor-duodenal ulcer syndrome** (0963)
**Ulcer-leukonychia-gallstones** (2234)

**Major Diagnostic Criteria:** Endoscopically or X-ray barium study proven ulcer crater, or characteristic scarring of the duodenal bulb.

**Clinical Findings:** The patient usually presents with abdominal pain and is diagnosed by endoscopy or barium X-ray studies, or presents with perforation or upper gastrointestinal bleeding. The pain commonly follows a chronic course with exacerbations and recurrences. There is strong evidence that this disease is a collection of multiple diseases each having distinct underlying mechanisms, but resulting in a similar clinical picture; at least as currently delineated.

**Complications:** Perforation, bleeding, and obstruction.

**Associated Findings:** None known.

**Etiology:** It is clear from family studies demonstrating increased family aggregation, and from twin studies demonstrating increased concordance of disease in monozygotic versus dizygotic twins, that there is a major genetic component or susceptibility to the peptic ulcer diseases.

The etiology appears to be extensively heterogeneous, with dominant inheritance of some specific disorders that predispose to the ulcer diathesis.

Gastric and duodenal ulcers have been found to be distinct disorders by studies that have shown that the increased familial risk for ulcer is site specific. Combined ulcer, i.e., gastric and duodenal, has also been delineated as a distinct entity, through epidemiologic studies showing that the incidence of duodenal and gastric ulcers in the same patient is about twenty times that expected from the relative frequencies of the two disorders in the population.

Heterogeneity of duodenal ulcer disease itself has been shown by family studies. Specific and different pathophysiologic markers that cosegregate with the ulcer disease, some of which have a dominant pattern of inheritance, have been identified.

The most extensive studies have indicated that approximately one-half of the duodenal ulcer population in the Western world have elevated serum pepsinogen I (and total serum pepsinogen as well) and that this hyperpepsinogenemia I is often inherited in a dominant pattern with variable penetrance of the clinical ulcer disease. This physiologically related serum marker appears to identify those who are genetically predisposed to duodenal ulcer disease on the basis of increased pepsin and acid secretion, secondary to an increased mass of chief and parietal cells in the mucosal lining of the body of the stomach.

A subgroup of duodenal ulcer patients with hyperpepsinogenemia I may have it associated with, and possibly due to antral G-cell hyperfunction. These patients have an exaggerated serum gastrin response to feeding and some have an elevated basal acid level.

The remaining one-half of duodenal ulcer patients are normopepsinogenemic I on a familial basis. Rapid gastric emptying has been found to cosegregate with duodenal ulcer in one large family with normopepsinogenemia I duodenal ulcer. This suggests that altered motility leading to an increased acid load to the duodenum is the abnormality resulting in the duodenal ulcer in this family.

Other predisposing familial/inherited factors that have been identified are immunologic associations and gastritis/duodenitis. These suggest autoimmune mechanisms in some subtypes of duodenal ulcer.

Thus duodenal ulcers can have many different predisposing pathophysiological conditions, and the etiology in a given patient can be one or a combination of these abnormalities.

**Pathogenesis:** Multiple distinct factors have been identified. These appear to differ from patient to patient and family to family, and may be multiple in some patients. Excess acid and pepsin secretion, altered gastric motility, and increased gastrin response to a meal are three documented mechanisms. Immunologic derangements and decreased mucosal protection are likely additional mechanisms. Environmental factors include smoking, nonsteroidal inflammatory agents, and possibly the bacterium *campylobacter pyloridis* recently issolated from the stomach and associated with peptic ulcers in some studies.

**MIM No.:** *12685

**Sex Ratio:** M2:F1 in the United States.

**Occurrence:** Estimated at a lifetime prevalence of up to 5% in the United States.

**Risk of Recurrence for Patient's Sib:** Estimated at 10–20%

**Risk of Recurrence for Patient's Child:** Estimated at 10–20%

**Age of Detectability:** Most commonly third to fourth decade of life. Earlier presentations do exist, even in childhood, and may be associated with specific genetic syndromes. Variability of age of onset exists between cultures, suggesting even further heterogeneity.

**Gene Mapping and Linkage:** Unknown.

**Prevention:** None known. Genetic counseling indicated. Recurrence can be prevented by anti-ulcer therapy.

**Treatment:** Treatment is usually symptomatic and empiric but is still very effective. The specific underlying mechanisms for the

peptic ulcer diathesis in a given patient often goes unrecognized. Agents are used that either affect acid secretion or its neutralization: antacids, $H_2$ receptor antagonists; or agents that affect mucosal protection, e.g. sucralfate (a sulfated disaccharide), all have all been shown to be effective in promoting the rate of ulcer healing.

A variety of surgeries (highly selective vagotomy, vagotomy and pyloroplasty, vagotomy and antrectomy) are used for selected patients. We urge that appropriate caution be used before such therapy is performed. It will become increasingly important that attempts are made to identify preoperatively the cause of duodenal ulcer. Specific etiologies might in some cases, e.g. rapid gastric emptying, preclude surgery. Others, such as antral G-cell hyperfunction, might lead to the suggestion of a specific surgery, e.g., antrectomy.

It is likely that identifying the specific components contributing to the ulcer diathesis in a given patient will lead to more specific and efficacious therapy; though at this time this is only true for specific limited subgroups. An example may be prostaglandin agents for non-steroidal anti-inflammatory drug-induced ulcer.

**Prognosis:** Good, especially with recent advances in medical therapy.

**Detection of Carrier:** Hyperpepsinogenemia I can be assayed in serum. This would identify some high-risk individuals in specific families. Antral G-cell hyperfunction can be identified as a predisposing factor in a family member of a patient with this syndrome by demonstrating a markedly enhanced gastric response to a meal. Gastric motility studies can be performed in relatives of those patients found to have rapid gastric emptying. These are markers for specific underlying mechanisms and while they identify individuals at increased risk for disease, these individuals will not necessarily develop the disease, as a wide degree of penetrance exists.

**Special Considerations:** Those families with one clear abnormality, such as hyperplasia of the chief and parietal cells, ascertained by an elevated pepsinogen I or altered gastric motility, allow us to identify the inheritance patterns of peptic ulcer disease susceptibility and are increasing our knowledge regarding specific mechanisms of ulcer development. This will allow us to be more precise in our therapeutic intervention and counseling for prevention. It is clear that the genetic basis is heterogeneous, but this does not preclude the hypothesis of a multifactorial component in expression of some forms of the disease, and the involvement of environmental factors as well.

**References:**

Rotter JI, et al.: Genetic heterogeneity of hyperpepsinogenemic I and normopepsinogenemic I duodenal ulcer disease. Ann Intern Med 1979; 91:372–377. *

Rotter JI: The genetics of peptic ulcer: more than one gene, more than one disease. Progress in Medical Genetics, Vol. IV: Genetics of Gastrointestinal Disease. Philadelphia: W.B. Saunders, 1980:1–58.

Taylor IL, et al.: Family Studies of hypergastrinemic, hyperpepsinogenemic I duodenal ulcer. Ann Intern Med 1981; 95:421–425.

Rotter JI: Peptic Ulcer. In: Emery AE, Rimoin DL: Principles and practice of medical genetics. New York: Churchill Livingstone, 1983:863–878.

Rotter JI, et al.: Pepsinogens and other physiologic markers in genetic studies of peptic ulcer and related disorders. In: Kreuning J, et al, eds: Pepsinogens in man: clinical and genetic advances. New York: Alan R. Liss, 1985:227–244.

Sumii K, et al.: Familial aggregation of duodenal ulcer and an autosomal dominant inheritance of hyperpepsinogenemia I. Hiroshima J Med Sci 1986; 35:171–175.

Andersen LP, et al.: Gastric and duodenal infection caused by C. pyloridis: histopathologic and microbiologic findings. Scand J Gastroenterol 1987; 22:219–224.

Eliakim R, et al.: Duodenal ulcer mucosal injury with nonsteroidal anti-inflammatory drugs. J Clin Gastroenterol 1987; 9:395–399.

ES005

**Theresa J. Escalante**
*Jerome I. Rotter*

**Peptidase D deficiency**
*See PROLIDASE DEFICIENCY*
**Perceptive deafness-corneal dystrophy**
*See CORNEAL DYSTROPHY-SENSORINEURAL DEAFNESS*
**Perceptive hearing loss**
*See DEAFNESS*
**Pericardial constriction-arthritis-camptodactyly**
*See PERICARDITIS-ARTHRITIS-CAMPTODACTYLY*
**Pericardial constriction-growth failure**
*See DWARFISM, MULIBREY TYPE*
**Pericardial defects, congenital**
*See HEART, PERICARDIUM AGENESIS*

---

## PERICARDITIS-ARTHRITIS-CAMPTODACTYLY            2811

**Includes:**
Arthritis-pericarditis-camptodactyly
Camptodactyly-pericarditis-arthritis
Pericardial constriction-arthritis-camptodactyly

**Excludes:**
**Arthritis, rheumatoid** (2517)
**Dwarfism, Mulibrey type** (2081)
**Lupus erythematosus, systemic** (2515)
**Synovitis, familial hypertrophic** (2155)

**Major Diagnostic Criteria:** The combination of constrictive pericarditis, arthritis, and flexion contractures of the fingers.

**Clinical Findings:** In all known cases, **Camptodactyly** affecting thumbs and/or fingers and arthritis with or without synovitis affecting the large joints where present. The arthritis is reportedly not painful. Eight of ten affected children also had restrictive pericarditis. Histologically the pericardium showed fibrosis, which was also noted on synovial biopsy.

In some affected children, elbow, knee, and hip joints had limited movement as well, not always secondary to arthritis or synovitis. Coxa vara was also described in one family.

**Complications:** In some children with restrictive pericarditis, hepatomegaly and jugular vein distension also occurred. These findings disappeared after treatment of the pericarditis.

**Associated Findings:** None known.

**Etiology:** Autosomal recessive inheritance.

**Pathogenesis:** Unknown.

**MIM No.:** *20825

**POS No.:** 4071

**Sex Ratio:** M1:F1

**Occurrence:** One family from Mexico with five affected sibs, one family from Turkey with four affected sibs, and one isolated case from Canada have been reported.

**Risk of Recurrence for Patient's Sib:**
See Part I, *Mendelian Inheritance.*

**Risk of Recurrence for Patient's Child:**
See Part I, *Mendelian Inheritance.*

**Age of Detectability:** In some children, joint limitation was present at birth. In others it occurred in early childhood. Joint enlargement occurred between ages one and eight years; restrictive pericarditis was usually diagnosed within the following two years.

**Gene Mapping and Linkage:** Unknown.

**Prevention:** None known. Genetic counseling indicated.

**Treatment:** Pericardiectomy is indicated. The arthritis was resistant to treatment with corticosteroids or aspirin.

**Prognosis:** Appears to be normal for life span and intelligence.

**Detection of Carrier:** Unknown.

**References:**
Martinez-Lavin M, et al.: A familial syndrome of pericarditis, arthritis, and camptodactyly. New Engl J Med 1983; 309:224–225.
Bulutlar G, et al.: A familial syndrome of pericarditis, arthritis, camptodactyly, and coxa vara. Arthritis Rheum 1986; 29:436–438.
Laxer RM, et al.: The camptodactyly-arthropathy-pericarditis syndrome: case report and literature review. Arthritis Rheum 1986; 29:439–444.

T0007                                              **Helga V. Toriello**

**Pericarditis-arthropathy-camptodactyly (CAP) syndrome**
*See SYNOVITIS, FAMILIAL HYPERTROPHIC*
**Pericardium agenesis**
*See HEART, PERICARDIUM AGENESIS*
**Pericardium, congenital partial or complete absence of**
*See HEART, PERICARDIUM AGENESIS*
**Peridens**
*See TEETH, SUPERNUMERARY*
**Perilymphatic gusher during stapes surgery**
*See DEAFNESS WITH PERILYMPHATIC GUSHER*
**Perinatal conduction system defects**
*See ARRHYTHMIA, CARDIAC CONDUCTION DEFECTS, NEONATAL*
**Perinatal effects of nonsteroidal anti-inflammatory drugs (NSAIDS)**
*See FETAL EFFECTS OF NONSTEROIDAL ANTI-INFLAMMATORY DRUGS (NSAIDS)*
**Perinatal transmission of hepatitis B infection**
*See FETAL EFFECT FROM HEPATITIS B INFECTION*
**Perinatal/neonatal cardiac conduction system defects-arrhythmia**
*See ARRHYTHMIA, CARDIAC CONDUCTION DEFECTS, NEONATAL*
**Perineal anus**
*See ANORECTAL MALFORMATIONS*
**Perinuclear cataract**
*See CATARACT, AUTOSOMAL DOMINANT CONGENITAL*
**Periodic disease**
*See FEVER, FAMILIAL MEDITERRANEAN (FMF)*
**Periodic fever**
*See FEVER, FAMILIAL MEDITERRANEAN (FMF)*
**Periodic neutropenia**
*See NEUTROPENIA, CYCLIC*
**Periodic paralysis, familial**
*See PARALYSIS, HYPOKALEMIC PERIODIC*
**Periodic paralysis, hyperpotassemic**
*See PARALYSIS, HYPERKALEMIC PERIODIC*
**Periodic paralysis, hypopotassemic**
*See PARALYSIS, HYPOKALEMIC PERIODIC*
**Periodic paralysis, II**
*See PARALYSIS, HYPERKALEMIC PERIODIC*
*also PARALYSIS, HYPOKALEMIC PERIODIC*
**Periodic paralysis, III**
*See PARALYSIS, NORMOKALEMIC PERIODIC*
**Periodic paralysis, normopotassemic**
*See PARALYSIS, NORMOKALEMIC PERIODIC*
**Periodic peritonitis**
*See FEVER, FAMILIAL MEDITERRANEAN (FMF)*
**Periodontitis, generalized juvenile**
*See TEETH, PERIODONTITIS, JUVENILE*
**Periodontitis, localized juvenile**
*See TEETH, PERIODONTITIS, JUVENILE*
**Periodontoclasia-hyperkeratosis palmplantaris**
*See HYPERKERATOSIS PALMPLANTARIS-PERIODONTOCLASIA*
**Periodontosis (misnomer)**
*See TEETH, PERIODONTITIS, JUVENILE*
**Periodontosis type Ehlers-Danlos syndrome**
*See EHLERS-DANLOS SYNDROME*
**Periosteal osteosarcoma**
*See OSTEOSARCOMA*
**Peripartum cardiomyopathy (some cases)**
*See CARDIOMYOPATHY, FAMILIAL DILATED*
**Peripheral neuroblastoma**
*See CANCER, EWING SARCOMA*
**Peritoneopericardial diaphragmatic hernia**
*See PENTALOGY OF CANTRELL*
**Perlman syndrome**
*See OVERGROWTH-RENAL HAMARTOMA, PERLMAN TYPE*
**Pernicious anemia, due to defect in intrinsic factor**
*See ANEMIA, PERNICIOUS CONGENITAL*
**Pernicious anemia, juvenile-proteinuria**
*See VITAMIN B(12) MALABSORPTION*
**Peromelia-micrognathia**
*See HYPOGLOSSIA-HYPODACTYLIA*
**Peroneal muscular atrophy, axonal type**
*See NEUROPATHY, HEREDITARY MOTOR AND SENSORY, TYPE I*
**Peroneal muscular atrophy, hypertrophic**
*See NEUROPATHY, HEREDITARY MOTOR AND SENSORY, TYPE I*
**Peroneal muscular atrophy, neuronal**
*See NEUROPATHY, HEREDITARY MOTOR AND SENSORY, TYPE II*

**Peroutka sneeze**
*See ACHOO SYNDROME*
**Peroxisomal biogenesis, disorders of**
*See CEREBRO-HEPATO-RENAL SYNDROME*
**Peroxisomal disorder (one form)**
*See CHONDRODYSPLASIA PUNCTATA, RHIZOMELIC TYPE*
**Peroxisome deficiency**
*See CEREBRO-HEPATO-RENAL SYNDROME*

## PERRAULT SYNDROME 2350

**Includes:**
    Deafness-gonadal dysgenesis
    Gonadal dysgenesis, XX type, with deafness
    Ovarian dysgenesis-sensorineural deafness

**Excludes:**
    **Gonadal dysgenesis, XX type** (0436)
    **Gonadal dysgenesis, XY type** (0437)
    **Turner syndrome** (0977)

**Major Diagnostic Criteria:** 46,XX individuals with infantile female phenotype; streak gonads demonstrated by direct visualization or elevated gonadotropin levels; and sensorineural deafness. Males (46,XY) with normal gonadal function and sensorineural deafness and females (46,XX) with isolated gonadal dysgenesis and normal hearing may be included if they have a positive family history.

**Clinical Findings:** Female individuals with Perrault syndrome have gonadal dysgenesis with an apparently normal (46,XX) chromosomal complement. Both the internal and external genitalia are female, but remain infantile. External genitalia, streak gonads, and endocrine function are indistinguishable from individuals with other types of gonadal dysgenesis, such as 45,X and gonadal dysgenesis, XX type. Hearing loss is usually moderate-to-severe sensorineural deafness and has been documented as early as one year of age. However, one individual had onset of significant hearing loss at age 31 years. Normal hearing has been documented in one female sib who also had gonadal dysgenesis; thus, hearing loss does not appear to be an obligatory manifestation in homozygous females. Male individuals (46,XY) who are sibs of affected females and apparently possess the same genotype have sensorineural hearing loss. However, they appear to have normal gonadal function with normal sexual development. Pallister and Opitz (1979) suggested that the low male-to-female ratio may indicate that hearing loss is not an obligate manifestation in male homozygotes, and thus these individuals have not been detected.

The majority of individuals with Perrault syndrome do not have additional anomalies. However, nine individuals had short stature (height at or below the third centile). Four females had at least one of the following features of **Turner syndrome**: cubitus valgus, congenital lymphedema, short neck, and short fourth and fifth metacarpals. Mental retardation was reported in three affected sibs, one of whom also had a right bundle branch block. Two affected females had lower limb weakness. One of these females was also mentally retarded and had spastic diplegia but also had a history of significant birth trauma. The other individual had ataxia. Both females had limited extraocular eye movements.

Laboratory evaluation of females with Perrault syndrome reveals decreased estrogen levels and increased follicle-stimulating hormone (FSH) and luteinizing hormone (LH) levels. One female also had partial growth hormone deficiency. Streak gonadal biopsy in one patient showed cortical fibrous tissue with absence of primordial follicles. Audiograms in seven patients suggested a pattern of mid-frequency depression and severe loss of high frequencies. Dermatoglyphics were normal in three patients but were mildly abnormal in two patients due to increased ridge count and alteration of main line termination. Bone age was retarded in seven of eight patients studied.

**Complications:** Hypogonadism and infertility in females. Severe speech deficits are common secondary to hearing loss.

**Associated Findings:** Possibly mental retardation, short stature.

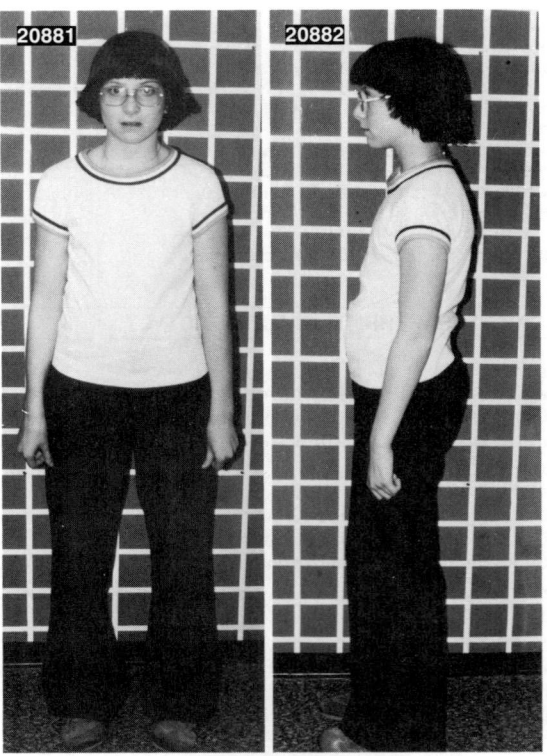

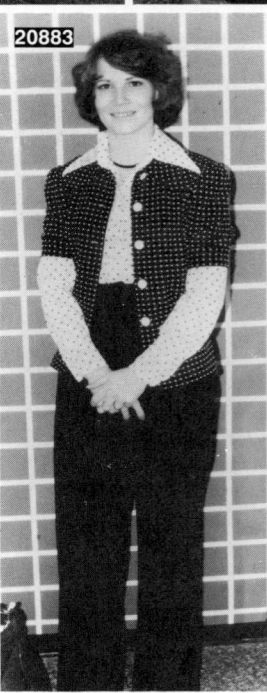

**2350-20881–83:** Perrault syndrome; two sisters who are affected; note the body habitus.

**Etiology:** Autosomal recessive inheritance. Parental consanguinity was reported in two families.

**Pathogenesis:** Gonadal dysgenesis and sensorineural deafness appear to be pleiotropic manifestations of the same gene. It has not been established whether the deafness and the streak gonads are due to a congenital developmental defect or arrest, or to a degenerative process.

**MIM No.:** *23340

**POS No.:** 3764

**Sex Ratio:** Presumably M1:F1; however, in the 21 reported cases the ratio was M1:F6, or M1:F3 if probands are excluded.

**Occurrence:** Nineteen additional individuals in seven families have been reported since Perrault's initial description of two affected sisters in 1951. Two sibships were from western Montana.

**Risk of Recurrence for Patient's Sib:**
See Part I, *Mendelian Inheritance.*

**Risk of Recurrence for Patient's Child:**
See Part I, *Mendelian Inheritance.* 46,XX patients are infertile. 46,XY patients probably have a less than 1% risk in the absence of consanguinity.

**Age of Detectability:** Sensorineural hearing loss can be detected in the first year of life. Diagnosis of Perrault syndrome is usually determined at puberty due to primary amenorrhea and lack of development of secondary sexual characteristics.

**Gene Mapping and Linkage:** Unknown.

**Prevention:** None known. Genetic counseling indicated.

**Treatment:** Estrogen replacement for hypogonadism; specialized educational programs for hearing impairment.

**Prognosis:** Probable normal for life span. Infertility in homozygous females. Varying degrees of hearing and speech deficits. The risk for mental retardation is uncertain.

**Detection of Carrier:** Unknown.

**References:**
Perrault M, et al.: Deux cas de syndrome de Turner avec surdi-multité dans une même fratrie. Bull Mém Soc Méd Hôp Paris 1951; 16:79–84.
Pallister PD, Opitz JM: The Perrault syndrome: autosomal recessive ovarian dysgenesis with facultative, non-sex-limited sensorineural deafness. Am J Med Genet 1979; 4:239–246. *
Bosze P, et al.: Perrault's syndrome in two sisters. Am J Med Genet 1983; 16:237–241.
McCarthy DJ, Opitz JM: Perrault syndrome in sisters. Am J Med Genet 1985; 22:629–631.
Nishi Y, et al.: The Perrault syndrome: clinical report and review. Am J Med Genet 1988; 31:623–629.

M0039
WE005

**Cynthia A. Moore**
**David D. Weaver**

**Persistent ductus arteriosus**
*See DUCTUS ARTERIOSUS, PATENT*
**Persistent frontonasal process**
*See NOSE/NASAL SEPTUM DEFECTS*
**Persistent hypertrophic primary vitreous in OPC dwarfism**
*See DWARFISM, OCULO-PALATO-CEREBRAL TYPE*
**Persistent oviduct syndrome**
*See MULLERIAN DERIVATIVES IN MALES, PERSISTENT*
**Perthes disease**
*See JOINTS, OSTEOCHONDRITIS DISSECANS*
*also HIP, OSTEONECROSIS, CAPITAL FEMORAL EPIPHYSIS*
**Peters anomaly**
*See EYE, ANTERIOR SEGMENT DYSGENESIS*
**Peters anomaly-aortic stenosis-growth and mental retardation**
*See AORTC STENOSIS-CORNEAL CLOUDING-GROWTH AND
    MENTAL RETARDATION*
**Peters anomaly-short limbed dwarfism**
*See DWARFISM (SHORT LIMBED)-PETERS ANOMALY OF THE EYE*
**Peters plus**
*See DWARFISM (SHORT LIMBED)-PETERS ANOMALY OF THE EYE*
*also EYE, ANTERIOR SEGMENT DYSGENESIS*
**Petit mal automatism**
*See SEIZURES, CENTRALOPATHIC*
**Petit mal lapse ("absence")**
*See SEIZURES, CENTRALOPATHIC*
**Petit mal seizures**
*See SEIZURES, CENTRALOPATHIC*
**Petrous pyramid cholesteatoma**
*See EAR, CHOLESTEATOMA OF TEMPORAL BONE*

**Peutz-Jeghers syndrome**
*See INTESTINAL POLYPOSIS, TYPE II*
**Pfeiffer acrocephalopolysyndactyly**
*See ACROCEPHALOPOLYSYNDACTYLY*
**Pfeiffer syndrome**
*See ACROCEPHALOSYNDACTYLY TYPE V*
**PFK, liver type**
*See GLYCOGENOSIS, TYPE VII*
**Phagocytosis, plasma-related defect in**
*See IMMUNODEFICIENCY, PLASMA-ASSOCIATED DEFECT OF
    PHAGOCYTOSIS*
**Phalangeal hypoplasia-gingival fibromatosis**
*See GINGIVAL FIBROMATOSIS-DIGITAL ANOMALIES*
**Pharyngeal cyst or fistula**
*See NECK, BRANCHIAL CLEFT, CYSTS OR SINUSES*
**Pharyngeal muscular dystrophy**
*See MUSCULAR DYSTROPHY, OCULOPHARYNGEAL*
**Pharyngeal pouch syndrome**
*See IMMUNODEFICIENCY, THYMIC AGENESIS*
**Pharyngoesophageal diverticulum**
*See ESOPHAGUS, DIVERTICULUM*
**Pharynx cancer**
*See CANCER, LUNG, FAMILIAL*

## PHARYNX/LARYNX HYPOPLASIA-OMPHALOCELE, SHPRINTZEN-GOLDBERG TYPE                 2774

**Includes:**
Omphalocele-pharynx/larynx hypoplasia, Shprintzen-Goldberg type
Omphalocele with hypoplasia of pharynx and larynx
Shprintzen-Goldberg syndrome

**Excludes:** Beckwith-Wiedemann syndrome (0104)

**Major Diagnostic Criteria:** Omphalocele was found in two of the three cases examined. All known cases have learning disabilities, orbital hypertelorism or telecanthus, downturned oral commisures, hypotonia, scoliosis or kyphosis, reduced pharyngeal circumference, and a hypoplastic larynx.

**Clinical Findings:** Omphalocele and respiratory distress are present at birth. Hypotonia is also present at birth and persists into adult life. The face becomes increasingly dysmorphic with age. Orbital hypertelorism or telecanthus is relatively mild. The lower eye lids are S-shaped. The columella is slightly short, and there is bimaxillary protrusion, giving the nose a broad-based appearance. The oral commisures are downturned. Learning disabilities become apparent at school age. The voice is high pitched, which is secondary to a hypoplastic larynx. The epiglottis is similarly small and immature in configuration. The pharynx is very small, resulting in infantile apnea and frequent respiratory illness. The severity of learning disabilities and neurologic impairment has been variable, but intellectual testing has been within normal limits in all cases.

**Complications:** The constriction of the pharynx and larynx causes severe respiratory distress, especially in the newborn period, often requiring hospitalization and resulting in death in one patient at age four months. Learning disabilities and persistent hypotonia may limit certain activities in school, but cognitive development is not severely impaired. The small larynx causes vocal pitch to be high throughout life. Spinal abnormalities (i.e., scoliosis and lordosis) are probably secondary to hypotonia.

**Associated Findings:** Chronic serious otitis with subsequent mild conductive hearing loss.

**Etiology:** Presumably autosomal dominant inheritance, though there has not been an instance of male-to-male transmission.

**Pathogenesis:** Unknown.

**MIM No.:** 18221

**POS No.:** 4022

**Sex Ratio:** Presumably M1:F1.

**Occurrence:** Reported in a father and three daughters.

**Risk of Recurrence for Patient's Sib:**
See Part I, *Mendelian Inheritance.*

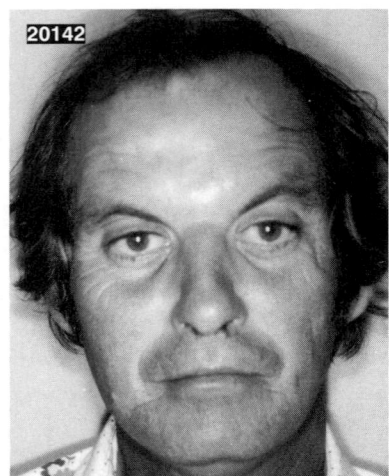

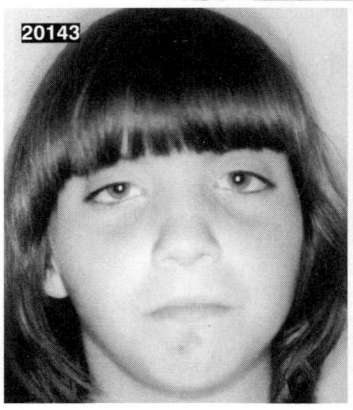
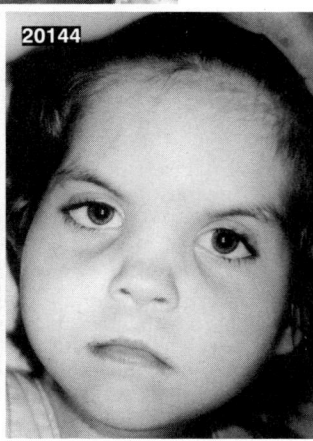

**2774**-20142–44: Subject with his two affected daughters; note epicanthal folds, broad nasal base, short columella, downturned lips and bimaxillary protrusion.

**Risk of Recurrence for Patient's Child:**
See Part I, *Mendelian Inheritance.*

**Age of Detectability:** If **Omphalocele** is present, diagnosis with prenatal ultrasound or fetoscope is possible. If omphalocele is not present, the detection may not occur until laryngeal abnormalities or learning disabilities become apparent during childhood.

**Gene Mapping and Linkage:** Unknown.

**Prevention:** None known. Genetic counseling indicated.

**Treatment:** Surgery for omphalocele as indicated. Laryngeal anomalies do not require intervention. Learning disabilities respond well to educational regimens. Physical therapy for hypotonia is indicated.

**Prognosis:** Normal life span. Hypotonia, high-pitched voice, and appearance are not severe enough to cause major problems, though they may limit certain choices of occupation, as may the learning disabilities.

**Detection of Carrier:** Fiber optic endoscopy of the upper airway is indicated for direct view of pharyngeal dimensions and laryngeal morphology. Testing of peripheral strength and cognitive testing for learning disabilities are possible. Presence of omphalocele should prompt further examination for other features.

**References:**
Shprintzen RJ, Goldberg RB: Dysmorphic facies, omphalocele, laryngeal and pharyngeal hypoplasia, spinal anomalies, and learning

disabilities in a new dominant malformation syndrome. BD:OAS XV(5B). New York: March of Dimes Birth Defects Foundation, 1979:347–353.

SH040
G0008

**Robert J. Shprintzen**
**Rosalie B. Goldberg**

**Phencyclidine, fetal effects**
*See FETAL EFFECTS FROM ANGEL DUST (PHENCYCLIDINE OR PCP)*
**Phenylalanine hydroxylase deficiency**
*See FETAL EFFECTS FROM MATERNAL PKU*
*also PHENYLKETONURIA*
**Phenylketonuria**
*See FETAL EFFECTS FROM MATERNAL PKU*

---

## PHENYLKETONURIA                                    0808

**Includes:**
    Folling disease
    Hyperphenylalaninemia
    Oligophrenia phenylpyruvica
    Phenylalanine hydroxylase deficiency
    PKU1

**Excludes:**
    **Biopterin synthesis deficiency** (2002)
    **Dihydropteridine reductase deficiency** (2001)
    Hyperphenylalanemia, transient

**Major Diagnostic Criteria:** Persistent elevation of blood phenylalanine concentrations above 6 mg/dl with normal or reduced blood tyrosine.

**Clinical Findings:** The major problem in untreated phenylketonuria, and sometimes the only problem, is mental retardation. During the first few weeks of life, there may be severe vomiting and epileptic seizures. Irritability may be seen in infancy. Some children have an eczematoid eruption; others have dry skin. Children may have a "mousy" smell due to phenylacetic acid in the urine and sweat. Although there are exceptions, phenylketonuric individuals tend to have blue eyes, blond hair, and fair skin.

Approximately two-thirds of those with concentrations of phenylalanine in serum above 6 mg/dl will develop moderate-to-severe mental retardation. Neurologic examination in these children may reveal **Microcephaly**, hand posturing with purposeless movements, and increased deep tendon reflexes. Many have abnormal EEG patterns. Some have seizures.

Biochemical characteristics are elevated blood phenylalanine (mean 20 mg/dl with a range of 10–60 mg/dl), urinary excretion of o-hydroxyphenylacetic acid (mean 1.6 μM/g creatinine), and excretion of urinary phenylpyruvic acid, phenyllacticacid and phenylacetylglutamine.

**Complications:** Mental retardation, seizures.

**Associated Findings:** None known.

**Etiology:** Autosomal recessive inheritance.

**Pathogenesis:** Deficiency of liver phenylalanine hydroxylase (PAH) reduces ability to form tyrosine. The accumulation of phenylalanine, phenylpyruvic acid, and other metabolites leads in some way to mental retardation, since prevention of accumulation through dietary restriction of phenylalanine prevents mental retardation.

**MIM No.:** *26160

**POS No.:** 3533

**CDC No.:** 270.100

**Sex Ratio:** M1:F1

**Occurrence:** 1:15,000 live births in the United States. Lower in Blacks and Ashkenazi Jews.

**Risk of Recurrence for Patient's Sib:**
See Part I, *Mendelian Inheritance.*

**Risk of Recurrence for Patient's Child:**
See Part I, *Mendelian Inheritance.* Heterozygous offspring of a

homozygous mother can be mentally retarded (see **Fetal effects from maternal PKU**).

**Age of Detectability:**  At 48 hours, by measurement of blood phenylalanine if protein intake is normal. By the sixth day, the diagnosis should virtually always be clear. The gene for phenylalanine hydroxylase has been cloned, and while the cDNA probe does not recognize the patient with PKU as different from control individuals, there are a number of linked restriction fragment length polymorphisms (RFLPs).

**Gene Mapping and Linkage:**  PAH (phenylalanine hydroxylase) has been mapped to 12q22-q24.2.

**Prevention:**  None known. Genetic counseling indicated.

**Treatment:**  The low-phenylalanine diet is effective in preventing mental retardation. Treatment must be started during the early weeks of life, but this is the logical consequence of the availability of programs of routine neonatal screening in most of the developed countries of the world.

**Prognosis:**  In the untreated patient with mental retardation and seizures, there may be reduced life span. With treatment, the prognosis for life span and intelligence should be excellent.

**Detection of Carrier:**  The cDNA probe and assessment of RFLPs is successful in identifying heterozygotes in an informative family known to be at risk.

**Special Considerations:**  In a collaborative study of newborn screening programs of patients with high concentrations of phenylalanine and normal tyrosine, it was found that about one fourth have had persistent phenylalaninemia between 6 and 19.9 mg/dl, and the remainder have had phenylalaninemia greater than 20 mg/dl. Among untreated patients, normal mental development has been found in almost all of those with phenylalanine concentrations less than 19.9 mg/dl. In treated patients, a diet low in phenylalanine was effective in preventing mental deficiency, particularly if started at less than 30 days of age. A number of terms have been employed in hyperphenylalaninemic patients including phenylketonuria, hyperphenylalanemia, persistent hyperphenylalanemia, phenylalanemia, and atypical phenylketonuria. These patients may represent heterogeneity in the phenylalanine hydroxylase enzyme.

**Support Groups:**
CA; Los Altos; PKU Parents Group
ENGLAND: Kent; Bexley; National Society for Phenylketonuria

**References:**
Lyman FL, ed. Phenylketonuria. Springfield, CC Thomas, 1963.
Berman JL, et al.: Causes for high phenylalanine with normal tyrosine in newborn screening programs. Am J Dis Child 1969; 117:54.
Koch R, et al.: Phenylalaninemia and phenylketonuria. In: Nyhan WL, ed: Heritable disorders of amino acid metabolism. New York: John Wiley & Sons, 1974:109–140.
Shear CS, et al.: Phenylketonuria: experience with diagnosis and management. In: Nyhan WL, ed: Heritable disorders of amino acid metabolism. New York: John Wiley & Sons, 1974:141–159.
Koch R, et al.: Preliminary report on the effects of diet discontinuation in PKU. J Pediatr 1982; 100:870–875.
Güttler F, et al.: Prenatal diagnosis and carrier detection by gene analysis. In: Inherited diseases of amino acid metabolism. Recent progress in the understanding, recognition and management, international symposium in Heidelberg, 1984, Bickel H and Wachtel U, eds., Stuttgart/New York: Georg Thiem Verlag Thieme, 1985:18–36.
Nyhan WL: Diagnostic recognition of genetic disease. Philadelphia, Lea & Febiger, 1987:100–106.

NY000                                      **William L. Nyhan**

**Phenylketonuria II**
*See DIHYDROPTERIDINE REDUCTASE DEFICIENCY*
**Phenylketonuria III**
*See BIOPTERIN SYNTHESIS DEFICIENCY*
**Phenylketonuria VI**
*See BIOPTERIN SYNTHESIS DEFICIENCY*
**Phenylthiocarbamide tasting**
*See TASTING DEFECT, PHENYLTHIOCARBAMIDE*
**Phenylthiourea insensitivity**
*See TASTING DEFECT, PHENYLTHIOCARBAMIDE*

**Phenytoin, fetal effects of**
*See FETAL HYDANTOIN SYNDROME*
*also HOLOPROSENCEPHALY*
**Phenytoin-type embryopathy**
*See FETAL PRIMIDONE EMBRYOPATHY*
**Pheochromocytoma and amyloid-producing medullary thyroid carcinoma**
*See ENDOCRINE NEOPLASIA, MULTIPLE TYPE II*
**Pheochromocytoma-medullary thyroid carcinoma-multiple neuroma**
*See ENDOCRINE NEOPLASIA, MULTIPLE TYPE III*
**Phocomelia**
*See LIMB REDUCTION DEFECTS*
**Phocomelia, deficiency of**
*See HAND, RADIAL CLUB HAND*
**Phocomelia-ectrodactyly-oto-sinus arrhythmia syndrome**
*See LIMB-OTO-CARDIAC SYNDROME*
**Phosphatase, liver alkaline**
*See HYPOPHOSPHATASIA*
**Phosphate-eliminating enzyme, deficiency of**
*See BIOPTERIN SYNTHESIS DEFICIENCY*
**Phosphate-pyrophosphate translocase**
*See GLYCOGENOSIS, TYPE Ic*
**Phosphatidylcholine red cell membrane disorder**
*See ANEMIA, HEMOLYTIC, RED CELL MEMBRANE DEFECTS*
**Phosphoethanolaminuria**
*See HYPOPHOSPHATASIA*
**Phosphofructokinase (PFK) deficiency**
*See GLYCOGENOSIS, TYPE VII*
**Phosphofructokinase, muscle type**
*See GLYCOGENOSIS, TYPE VIII*
**Phosphoglucomutase**
*See GLYCOGENOSES*
**Phosphoglucose isomerase**
*See GLYCOGENOSES*
**Phosphoglucose isomerase inhibitor**
*See GLYCOGENOSIS, TYPE VIII*
**Phosphoglucose isomerase, deficiency of**
*See ANEMIA, GLUCOSE PHOSPHATE ISOMERASE DEFICIENCY*
**Phosphoglucose isomerase, Homberg type**
*See GLYCOGENOSES*
**Phosphoglycerate kinase (PGK) deficiency, erythrocyte**
*See ANEMIA, HEMOLYTIC, ERYTHROCYTE PHOSPHOGLYCERATE KINASE DEFICIENCY*
**Phosphoglycerate kinase, M isozyme**
*See GLYCOGENOSES*
**Phosphoglycerate mutase, M isozyme**
*See GLYCOGENOSES*
**Phosphohexose isomerase, deficiency of**
*See ANEMIA, GLUCOSE PHOSPHATE ISOMERASE DEFICIENCY*

---

**PHOSPHORIBOSYL PYROPHOSPHATE (PRPP) SYNTHETASE ABNORMALITY**                              **0508**

**Includes:**
Ataxia-deafness (sensorineural)-hyperuricemia
Deafness-hyperuricemia-ataxia
Hyperuricemia-deafness (sensorineural)-ataxia
Phosphoribosylpyrophosphate synthetase

**Excludes:**
**Gout** (0441)
**Lesch-Nyhan syndrome** (0588)
Lipodystrophy and neurologic defects

**Major Diagnostic Criteria:**  Progressive spinocerebellar ataxia and sensorineural hearing loss with hyperuricemia. Abnormal hyperactivity of PRPP synthetase.

**Clinical Findings:**  Onset of elevated blood uric acid is in infancy, but may not be recognized until late childhood or at puberty. Similarly, sensorineural hearing loss may be congenital, or it may first be recognized in adolescence or early adult life. Progressive spinocerebellar ataxia, when present, begins later, along with slurred speech. Renal disease and any of the manifestations of **Gout** may occur in the absence of effective treatment. Two adult females with the syndrome have also developed cervicodorsal fat pad ("buffalo hump") without Cushing syndrome and with normal steroid levels. Muscle wasting and weakness are inconstant features. One member of a family studied has developed cardiomyopathy. There is no mental retardation or self-mutilation as in the **Lesch-Nyhan syndrome**.

Audiograms usually show a high-frequency sensorineural loss in the younger affected members, and a sloping sensorineural loss in early adult life. The most severely affected individuals have virtually complete loss of hearing, and this may be congenital. A highly positive SISI (short increment sensitivity index) is found on special testing, indicating cochlear involvement rather than neural or central involvement. Electronystagmography shows changes consistent with a vestibular lesion central to the labyrinth. Petrous pyramid tomography is normal.

Standard renal function tests are normal in the younger affected members. Erythrocyte hypoxanthine-guanine phosphoribosyltransferase levels are normal. Muscle biopsies of affected members with muscle weakness are consistent with a neurogenic myopathy.

**Complications:** Nephrolithiasis, nephropathy, gouty arthritis, tophi.

**Associated Findings:** Congestive heart failure secondary to cardiomyopathy. One patient was reported with limited intelligence and absent lacrimal glands.

**Etiology:** X-linked inheritance.

**Pathogenesis:** Defect of phosphoribosyl pyrophosphate (PRPP) synthetase. This is an unusual defect in that the enzyme is superactive rather than hypoactive. Nevertheless, it may be unstable and short lived. Activities in erythrocytes may accordingly be normal or low. Studies in fibroblasts are usually required. Hyperuricemia results in renal dysfunction and associated symptoms.

**MIM No.:** *31185

**POS No.:** 4266

**Sex Ratio:** M1:F<1

**Occurrence:** Undetermined. Described in a large Mexican-American kindred living in Pueblo, Colorado.

**Risk of Recurrence for Patient's Sib:**
See Part I, *Mendelian Inheritance.*

**Risk of Recurrence for Patient's Child:**
See Part I, *Mendelian Inheritance.*

**Age of Detectability:** Prenatally by enzyme analysis. In infancy by blood uric acid. In childhood by audiometry. Often in adolescence by clinical evaluation.

**Gene Mapping and Linkage:** PRPS1 (phosphoribosyl pyrophosphate synthetase 1) has been mapped to Xq21-q27.

**Prevention:** None known. Genetic counseling indicated.

**Treatment:** Allopurinol will reduce blood uric acid levels and should prevent gout, nephropathy, and nephrolithiasis. However, it has had no retarding or beneficial effects on the deafness, ataxia, muscle weakness, or wasting. Hearing aids and speech training. Treatment for congestive heart failure secondary to cardiomyopathy.

**Prognosis:** Progression of hearing loss, ataxia, and muscle weakness.

**Detection of Carrier:** By PRPP synthetase in cultured fibroblasts.

**References:**
Kelley WN, et al.: A specific enzyme defect in gout assoicated with overproduction of uric acid. Proc Natl Acad Sci USA 1967; 57:1735.
Rosenberg AL, Bartholomew B: Gout and uric acid. Bull Rheum Dis 1969; 19:543.
Rosenberg AL, et al.: Hyperuricemia and neurologic deficits: a family study. New Engl J Med 1970; 282:992–997.
Simmond HA, et al.: An X-linked syndrome characterised by hyperuricaemia, deafness, and neurodevelopmental abnormalities. Lancet 1982; II:68–70.
Becker MA, et al.: Phosphoribosylpyrophosphate synthetase superactivity. Arthritis Rheum 1986; 29:880–888.

BE028
NY000

**LaVonne Bergstrom**
**William L. Nyhan**

**Phosphoribosylpyrophosphate synthetase**
*See PHOSPHORIBOSYL PYROPHOSPHATE (PRPP) SYNTHETASE ABNORMALITY*
**Phosphorylase deficiency glycogen-storage disease of liver**
*See GLYCOGENOSIS, TYPE VI*
**Phosphorylase kinase deficiency of liver**
*See GLYCOGENOSIS, TYPE IXa*
*also GLYCOGEN STORAGE DISEASE, X-LINKED WITH NORMAL HEPATIC ENZYMES*
**Phosphorylase kinase deficiency, generalized**
*See GLYCOGENOSIS, TYPE IXb*
**Photic sneeze reflex**
*See ACHOO SYNDROME*
**Photogenic epilepsy**
*See EPILEPSY, REFLEX*
**Photomyoclonus-deafness-diabetes-nephropathy**
*See DEAFNESS-DIABETES-PHOTOMYOCLONUS-NEPHROPATHY*
**Photosensitivity with defective DNA synthesis**
*See XERODERMA PIGMENTOSUM*
**Photosensitivity, from protoporphyria**
*See PORPHYRIA, PROTOPORPHYRIA*
**Phytanic acid oxidase deficiency**
*See PHYTANIC ACID STORAGE DISEASE*

---

## PHYTANIC ACID OXIDASE DEFICIENCY, INFANTILE TYPE      2278

**Includes:**
    Adrenoleukodystrophy, neonatal (some forms)
    Infantile phytanic acid storage disease
    Pipecolic acidemia (some forms)
    Refsum disease, infantile form

**Excludes:**
    **Adrenoleukodystrophy, X-linked** (2533)
    **Cerebro-hepato-renal syndrome** (0139)
    **Phytanic acid storage disease** (0810)

**Major Diagnostic Criteria:** Retinitis pigmentosa, severe neurosensory deafness, severe developmental delay, peripheral neuropathy, hepatomegaly, facial dysmorphism, simian creases, minor elevation in serum phytanic acid. Serum pipecolic acid and very long chain ($C_{24}$ and $C_{26}$) fatty acids are elevated. Plasmalogen synthesis is impaired. Activities of several enzymes, including phytanic acid oxidase, Acyl-CoA:dihydroxyacetone phosphate acyltransferase and other enzymes now known to be peroxisomal are deficient in several tissues including cultured skin fibroblasts.

**Clinical Findings:** The condition is apparent in infancy, when hepatomegaly (2–5 cm below the costal margin) is noted; several cases have had steatorrhea with a marked bleeding diathesis responsive to Vitamin K. The steatorrhea has resolved spontaneously after some months or years. Most cases have not been

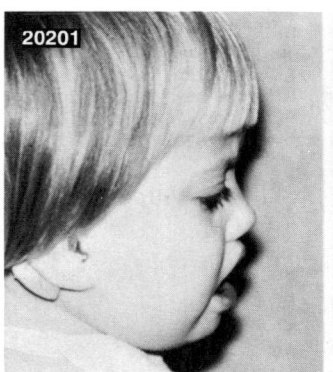
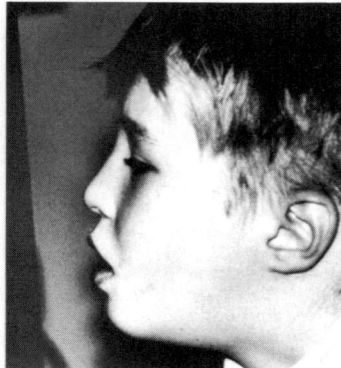

**2278-20201:** Note flattened facies in these two subjects with phytanic oxidase deficiency, infantile type.

investigated in early infancy, so the frequency of the steatorrhea is unclear.

Severe sensorineural hearing loss becomes evident (100%) within the first year, and a severe devlopmental delay is apparent before the first birthday. **Retinitis pigmentosa** has developed within the first two years of life in all cases studied to date. This includes a prominent macular dystrophic component, and is similar to that seen in advanced **Phytanic acid storage disease**. Electroretinography shows severely subnormal rod- and cone-mediated responses. The characteristic facies are considered by some to be reminiscent of **Chromosome 21, trisomy 21**. From the side view, the face is flattened with the nose being rather less prominent than normal. A **Skin crease, single palmer** has been noted in at least five cases. The children are hypotonic, and the tendon reflexes are diminished or absent, consistent with a peripheral neuropathy.

Standard liver function tests are not consistently abnormal, but the liver biopsy is definitely abnormal. On regular microscopy, the architecture of the lobules and hepatocytes is preserved but there is interlobular bridging by bands of fibrous tissue which emanate from the portal triads. On electron microscopy, at least two groups have reported characteristic long, linear, trilaminar membrane bound inclusions within the hepatocytes and probably the Kupffer cells. The composition of these materials is unknown.

*Laboratory Findings*: the level of phytanic acid in the serum is usually elevated (0.5–20mg/dl; normal <0.2 mg/dl) but may occasionally be normal. Pipecolic acid (0.3–3 mg/dl; normal <0.05 mg/dl) has been elevated in all patients in whom it has been measured. The plasma very long chain fatty acids are also elevated, resulting in an increased ratio of hexacosanoate:docosanoate ($C_{26}:C_{22}$) and tetracosanoate:docosanoate ($C_{24}:C_{22}$). Plasmalogen levels are lower than normal; plasma bile acid intermediates may be elevated in some patients.

Multiple enzyme defects are known, including phytanic acid oxidase, dihydroxyacetone phosphate acyltransferase, alkyldihydroxyacetone phosphate synthase, peroxisomal acyl-CoA oxidase, bifunctional protein, and thiolase.

**Complications:** Hemorrhagic episodes, such as cerebral hemorrhage, in the early months due to the bleeding diathesis caused by the malabsorption and steatorrhea. The retinal dystrophy can be severe enough for the patients to be classified as legally blind.

**Associated Findings:** Plasma cholestrol tends to be low, with reduced levels of alpha- and sometimes also beta-lipoproteins in the plasma.

**Etiology:** Presumably autosomal recessive inheritance.

**Pathogenesis:** Early reports emphasized the abnormal levels of phytanic acid in plasma, and it was presumed that the phytanic acid somehow caused the symptoms by a mechanism similar to that in **Phytanic acid storage disease** (Refsum disease). The recent discovery of many other biochemical abnormalities such as elevated pipecolic acid, which is a metabolite of lysine, and the biochemical findings outlined above, all indicate a major defect in peroxisomal function. Not all peroxisomal enzymes are compromised. For example, catalase activity, at least in fibroblasts, is normal, although less than 5% of it is particle bound. There is some debate over whether peroxisomes are absent as in **Cerebro-hepato-renal syndrome** (Zellweger syndrome), or present but diminished in number and metabolic function.

Complementation studies of cell lines from **Cerebro-hepato-renal syndrome**, hyperpipecolicacidemia, and infantile Refsum patients indicate no complementation. Whether this reflects total absence of peroxisomes or allelic mutations is not clear. Conversely, complementation appears to occur with cell fusions of lines from **Cerebro-hepato-renal syndrome** and neonatal adrenoleukodystrophy patients.

The obvious relationship of this disorder to **Cerebro-hepato-renal syndrome** in which serum phytanic acid, pipecolic acid, and very long chain fatty acids are also elevated, and liver peroxisomes are severely deficient, suggests that infantile phytanic acid oxidase deficiency may represent another disorder of peroxisomal function. The cause of the steatorrhea may be from low levels of lipoprotein in the plasma, similar to what is seen in **Abetalipopro-**

teinemia. The facial dysmorphism associated with this syndrome implies that the damage is of prenatal onset.

**Sex Ratio:** Presumably M1:F1.

**Occurrence:** A few dozen cases have been documented.

**Risk of Recurrence for Patient's Sib:**
See Part I, *Mendelian Inheritance.*

**Risk of Recurrence for Patient's Child:**
See Part I, *Mendelian Inheritance.*

**Age of Detectability:** In the neonatal period. Prenatal diagnosis is possible.

**Gene Mapping and Linkage:** Unknown.

**Prevention:** None known. Genetic counseling indicated.

**Treatment:** A phytanic acid restricted diet has been tried in one patient. The diet lowered the phytanic acid level in the plasma and improved the patient's behavior, but did nothing to improve the other symptoms. Therapy for steatorrhea in the early months includes a low lipid diet, probably with medium chain triglycerides and supplements of the fat soluble vitamins. No other specific therapy is currently available.

**Prognosis:** The patients reported to date have all presented similar symptoms in early infancy, and have survived into adolescence with severe and stable developmental delay. It is not known whether there are milder or more severe cases in whom the prognosis may be different.

**Detection of Carrier:** In four obligate heterozygotes, serum phytanic acid was normal, as was the ratio of $C_{26}:C_{22}$ and $C_{24}:C_{22}$ very long chain fatty acids. Thus, carrier detection for infantile phytanic acid oxidase deficiency is not yet possible.

**References:**
Scotto, JM, et al.: Infantile phytanic acid storage disease, a possible variant of Refsum's disease: three cases, including ultrastructural studies of the liver. J Inherit Metab Dis 1982; 5:83–90.
Poulos A, et al.: Infantile Refsum's disease (phytanic acid storage disease): a variant of Zellweger's syndrome? Clin Genet 1984; 26:579–586.
Budden SS, et al.: Dysmorphic syndrome with phytanic acid oxidase deficiency, abnormal very long chain fatty acids, and pipecolic acidemia: studies in four children. J Pediatr 1986; 108:33–39.
Kelley RI, et al.: Neonatal adrenoleukodystrophy: new cases, biochemical studies and differentiation from Zellweger and related peroxisomal polydystrophy syndromes. Am J Med Genet 1986; 23:869–901.
Wanders RJA, et al.: Infantile Refsum disease: deficiency of catalase-containing particles (peroxisomes), alkyldihydroxyacetone phosphate synthase and peroxisomal β-oxidation enzyme proteins. Eur J Pediatr 1986; 145:172–175.
Schutgens RBH, et al.: Peroxisomal disorders: a newly recognized group of genetic diseases. Eur J Pediatr 1986; 144:430–440.
Lazarow PB, Moser HW: Disorders of peroxisome biogenesis. In: Scriver CR, et al, eds: The metabolic basis of inherited disease, 6th ed. New York: McGraw-Hill, 1989:1479–1510.

KE022
BU009

**Nancy G. Kennaway**
**Neil R. M. Buist**

---

**PHYTANIC ACID STORAGE DISEASE**      **0810**

**Includes:**
Heredopathia atactica polyneuritiformis
Phytanic acid oxidase deficiency
Refsum disease

**Excludes:**
**Adrenoleukodystrophy, X-linked** (2533)
**Cerebro-hepato-renal syndrome** (0139)
Elevated pipecolic acid, other syndromes with
**Phytanic acid oxidase deficiency, infantile type** (2278)
Retinal pigmentation without accumulation of phytanic acid
Retinal pigmentation without deficiency in phytanic acid oxidation
Very long chain fatty acids, other syndromes with

**Major Diagnostic Criteria:** Demonstration should be made of abnormal concentrations of phytanic acid in plasma or tissues. The major "clinical triad" consists of retinitis pigmentosa, peripheral neuropathy, and cerebellar ataxia. Cerebrospinal fluid protein level is increased without cells present.

**Clinical Findings:** The clinical features found at the time of reporting are listed here for patients in whom the actual biochemical defect was confirmed. Onset of symptoms is usually before adulthood. Retinal degeneration, with nightblindness, concentric narrowing of visual fields, and an atypical retinal pigmentation are virtually always found. There is peripheral neuropathy in 90% of the patients, with motor weakness, muscular atrophy, loss of deep tendon reflexes, electromyographic evidence of denervation, and loss of superficial sensation to pain, touch, or temperature. Muscle pain, or paresthesias, are infrequent. Other neurologic features include cerebellar signs (75%), nerve deafness (50%), pupillary abnormalities (40%), anosmia (35%), and nystagmus (25%). Cardiac involvement can sometimes be shown, with nonspecific ST-T changes in the precordial EKG or left ventricular enlargement. Cataracts were seen in 40% of the patients, and 60% have some skeletal malformations (shortening of the metatarsals, osteochondritis dissecans, pes cavus, etc). Some patients have ichthyotic skin changes, occasionally florid (trunk, palms, soles). Spinal fluid protein levels are increased in 85% of the patients (55–730 mg/dl; mean: 275), without increased cells present.

**Complications:** Four patients have died suddenly, possibly from cardiac arrhythmias, and two have died with respiratory paralysis. Renal function has been impaired in four patients, and increased urine lipid was noted in one (with severe fatty infiltration of the kidneys).

**Associated Findings:** Aminoaciduria has been reported in two patients, of uncertain relationship to the primary defect.

**Etiology:** Autosomal recessive inheritance, with high consanguinity, and a partial defect in heterozygotes.

**Pathogenesis:** Phytanic acid accumulation has been shown to be secondary to deletion of a phytanic acid oxidizing system, with the specific metabolic block involving the initial α-oxidation. This probably involves specifically an α-hydroxylating system that converts phytanic acid to α-hydroxyphytanic acid.

It is likely that the accumulation of phytanic acid in itself leads to the clinical manifestations of the disease. Animal feeding experiments have been negative, however, and rare instances of moderately elevated plasma phytanic acid levels have been found in parents of patients without clinical signs. It is pertinent that in some patients the course of the illness has been favorably influenced by dietary restriction of phytanic acid.

It is of interest that the nervous system is a natural site of high concentrations of α-hydroxy fatty acids, but skin and nerve tissue from patients analyzed to date have not shown alteration in concentration or composition of these acids.

**MIM No.:** *26650

**POS No.:** 3463

**Sex Ratio:** M1:F1

**Occurrence:** About 100 cases have been documented.

**Risk of Recurrence for Patient's Sib:**
See Part I, *Mendelian Inheritance.*

**Risk of Recurrence for Patient's Child:**
See Part I, *Mendelian Inheritance.*

**Age of Detectability:** The earliest clinical manifestations (e.g. nightblindness) usually occur within the first two decades of life.

**Gene Mapping and Linkage:** Unknown.

**Prevention:** None known. Genetic counseling indicated.

**Treatment:** It is possible to limit the accumulation of phytanic acid and to decrease body stores by a diet from which phytanic acid and its precursors have been removed. Dairy products (butter, milk, cheese) and ruminant fats (beef and sheep) are the major sources, but phytanic acid is widely distributed in foodstuffs, including lipids of marine animals. Phytol in its unesterified form is a precursor for phytanic acid, but when esterified in

the chlorophyll molecule it is apparently minimally absorbed. Plasma phytanate levels have dropped in all patients who have adhered to the special diet, and in none of those adhering has there been a clinical relapse. In four patients follow-up data are now available for up to 10 years; some improvement in symptomatology occurs over the first 6–12 months (excluding cranial nerve manifestations), after which the clinical picture seems to stabilize. Obviously one would anticipate that institution of the diet in childhood would be most advantageous. Repeated plasmapheresis or plasma exchange may also be helpful in depleting body stores of phytanic acid.

Supportive measures for consequences of neuropathy (physiotherapy, orthopedic devices); cataract extraction when indicated.

**Prognosis:** The course of the untreated disease is slowly progressive, with frequent exacerbations and remissions of symptoms (occasionally correlated with intercurrent viral infection). Life expectancy is shortened, but the age at death varies greatly. Expiration in childhood is rare, but death before age 40 years occurred in six of the 33 chemically-established cases. Cardiac and respiratory problems appear to be the major threat to survival.

**Detection of Carrier:** Parents, sibs, and children of known patients are clinically unaffected, and their plasma phytanic acid levels have been normal except in two instances (mothers of patients). Cell cultures from skin biopsies of patients show oxidation of phytanic acid at 1–2% of the normal rate. Cultures from heterozygote individuals have a partial defect, and hence this technique could be used in the detection of heterozygosity.

**References:**
Refsum S: Heredopathia atactica polyneuritiformis; familial syndrome not hitherto described: contribution to clinical study of hereditary diseases of nervous system. Acta Psychiatr Scand 1946; 38 (Suppl.):1.
Steinberg D, et al.: Refsum's disease: a recently characterized lipidosis involving the nervous system. Ann Intern Med 1967; 66:365–395.
Steinberg D, et al.: Refsum's disease: nature of the enzyme defect. Science 1967; 156:1740–1742.
Poulos A, et al.: Patterns of Rufsum's disease: phytanic acid oxidase deficiency. Arch Dis Child 1984; 59:222–229.
Steinberg D: Refsum disease. In: Scriver CR, et al, eds: The metabolic basis of inherited disease, 6th ed. New York: McGraw-Hill, 1989: 1533–1550.

ST012                                      **Daniel Steinberg**
BU009                                      **Neil R. M. Buist**
KE022                                   **Nancy G. Kennaway**

**Pi phenotype ZZ, SZ, Z- and --**
*See ALPHA(1)-ANTITRYPSIN DEFICIENCY*

---

## PICK DISEASE OF THE BRAIN                              3243

**Includes:**
    Brain, lobar atrophy of
    Dementia-lobar atrophy and neuronal cytoplasmic
      inclusions
    Lobar atrophy

**Excludes:**
    **Alzheimer disease**
    **Creutzfeldt-Jakob disease** (3244)
    Multi-infarct dementia
    Subcortical atherosclerotic encephalopathy

**Major Diagnostic Criteria:** A rare degenerative disease of the central nervous system characterized by the insidious onset and slow progression of dementia, frequently with prominent behavioral symptoms and language impairment. It is relentlessly progressive over 2–12 years, leading to death. Brain computerized tomography (CT) or magnetic resonance imaging (MRI) may show characteristic focal or lobar atrophy. There is considerable overlap in clinical symptoms with **Alzheimer disease**, which frequently leads to diagnostic uncertainty. Presumptive clinical diagnosis is confirmed by post-mortem examination of the brain. This demonstrates prominent atrophy in a lobar distribution involving the frontal and/or temporal lobes and distinctive histologic changes of argyrophilic cytoplasmic inclusions (Pick bodies) within neurons and "ballooned" or "inflated" neurons (Pick cells), in the absence of neuritic plaques and neurofibrillary tangles characteristic of Alzheimer disease.

**Clinical Findings:** Symptoms usually begin in the fifth or sixth decade (average age of onset is 54 years), but may occur as early as the third or as late as the ninth decades. The disease is characterized by progressive cognitive deterioration, with specific clinical features reflecting the distribution of the pathologic changes, usually predominantly frontal or temporal lobe involvement. Eighty percent of cases of Pick disease appear to be sporadic while 20% are thought to be familial. There are no consistent differences between the apparently sporadic and familial cases. There is no evidence of differences between maternal and paternal rates of transmission.

The disease can be divided into three stages. The initial stage (usually lasting 1–3 years) is characterized by prominent personality, behavioral, and emotional changes. Judgement is impaired early, insight is lacking and social behavior deteriorates. A wide variety of personality changes can be seen (such as depression, apathy, euphoria and irritability); behavioral changes frequently seen include inappropriate or disinhibited actions, particularly sexual indiscretions. Perhaps the most striking behavioral manifestation is the development of symptoms resembling the Kluver-Bucy syndrome, including emotional blunting, hypersexuality, hyperorality, markedly increased eating, hypermetamorphosis, and visual or auditory agnosia. Language alterations may be noted early but become particularly prominent as the disease progresses.

In the second stage (lasting 3–6 years) cognitive deterioration becomes evident and language disturbance (anomia, verbal stereotypias, impaired comprehension and aphasia) become a dominant feature. It is interesting that memory, calculations, and visuospatial skills remain relatively unimpaired during this phase, which is in contrast to Alzheimer disease where early impairment in these areas is quite characteristic.

In the final stage of Pick disease (lasting 6–12 years), diffuse cognitive deterioration with profound dementia occurs, the person becomes mute or incomprehensible, and a progressive extrapyramidal syndrome usually develops. There is a marked lack of focal motor, sensory or visual signs, such as hemiplegia or visual field deficits. Myoclonus sometimes occurs, but generalized motor seizures are uncommon.

Routine laboratory studies of blood, serum, urine, and cerebrospinal fluid are normal. Vitamin B12 and folate deficiency, neurosyphillis and hypothyroidism should be excluded since they represent potentially treatable causes of dementia. Some investigators have found increased levels of urinary zinc. Neuroimaging studies (brain CT or MRI) may show focal lobar atrophy and provide supportive evidence for the clinical diagnosis as well as serve to exclude other causes of dementia such as multiple infarcts, tumors, and normal pressure **Hydrocephaly**. Positron emission tomography (PET scan) shows hypometabolism of cortical glucose in the anterior frontal and temporal association cortices and is perhaps the best current imaging technique to reliably distinguish Pick disease from Alzheimer disease. The EEG typically remains normal, but may show diffuse, or rarely focal, slowing of the background. Formal neuropsychological evaluation is useful for characterizing the cognitive deficits and quantifying changes as the disease progresses. This may also disclose an anatomical pattern of functional impairment that supports the diagnosis of Pick disease and assists in differentiating it from Alzheimer disease.

**Complications:** Progressive behavioral and cognitive deterioration frequently lead to loss of employment as well as disruption of familial and interpersonal relationships. In the terminal stage of the disease, common complications of the bedridden state such as aspiration pneumonia, urinary tract infections, decubitus ulcers and progressive inanition are seen.

**Associated Findings:** Although it has not been widely investigated, increased urinary excretion of zinc has been found in some patients. An increase in psychiatric symptoms in first degree relatives has been reported.

**Etiology:** Autosomal dominant inheritance with age-dependent penetrance is found in familial cases, which accounts for approximately 20% of the reported cases.

**Pathogenesis:** Unknown. A variety of theories have been proposed, including an axonal disorder with secondary changes in the cell body, a defect in zinc transport by plasma proteins leading to elevated intracortical zinc levels and selective disruption of glutamate function, viral infection, and primary degeneration of the neuronal cell body.

**MIM No.:** 17270

**Sex Ratio:** Probably M1:F1. However, most epidemiologic studies have found a higher overall prevalence and age-specific incidence rates for females (approximately M1:F2).

**Occurrence:** Prevalence is estimated to be less than 1%. The precise incidence and prevalence are unknown since the accurate diagnosis requires pathologic confirmation and the disease is clinically likely to be misdiagnosed as Alzheimer disease.

**Risk of Recurrence for Patient's Sib:**
See Part I, *Mendelian Inheritance*.

**Risk of Recurrence for Patient's Child:**
See Part I, *Mendelian Inheritance*. This risk has not been adequately studied.

**Age of Detectability:** Symptoms may begin as early as the third decade, although the average age of onset is in the fifth or sixth. Pick disease appears to increase in frequency until about age 58; then its frequency decreases until after age 70 its onset becomes rare.

**Gene Mapping and Linkage:** Unknown.

**Prevention:** None known. Genetic counseling indicated.

**Treatment:** There is no effective treatment or cure. Treatment is symptomatic and may include minor and major tranquilizers for control of behavioral symptoms. Supportive medical care, educational and supportive interventions for the family, and symptomatic treatment of complications (e.g. infections, seizures, feeding problems) are provided as indicated. Constantinidis has reported symptomatic improvement in a small number of patients with heavy-metal chelation.

**Prognosis:** The disease progresses over 2–12 years, from the onset of clinical symptoms to the time of death. Decreased life expectancy is observed, with approximately 80% of patients dying within ten years after the onset of the disease.

**Detection of Carrier:** Careful pedigree analysis may allow detection of families and individuals at high risk. There is no laboratory or other test to identify asymptomatic carriers. Groen and Endtz (1982) investigated persons at risk from a large, well-documented family with EEGs and CT scans and found frontal atrophy in four cases out of 12. In one of these cases, clinical signs of Pick disease became manifest a year after the investigation. Formal neuropsychological assessment may detect individuals early in the course of the disease.

**References:**

Malamud N, Waggoner RW: Genealogic and clinicopathologic study of Pick disease. Arch Neurol and Psychiat 1943; 50:288–303.

Sjogren T, et al.: Morbus Alzheimer and morbus Pick: a genetic, clinical, and patho-anatomical study. Acta Psychiat Scand 1952; 82:9–66.

Schenk VWD: Re-examination of a family with Pick's disease. Ann Hum Genet 1959; 23:325–333.

Heston LL: The clinical genetics of Pick's disease. Acta Psychiat Scand 1978; 57:202–206.

Groen JJ, Endtz LJ: Hereditary Pick's disease: second re-examination of a large family and discussion of other hereditary cases, with particular reference to electroencephalography and computerized tomography. Brain 1982; 105:443–459.

Cummings JL, Benson DF: Dementia: a clinical approach. Stoneham, MA: Butterworth Publishing, 1983.

Morris JC, et al.: Hereditary dysphasic dementia and the Pick-Alzheimer spectrum. Ann Neurol 1984; 16:455–466.

Constantinidis J: Heredity and dementia. Gerontol 1986; 32:73–79.
Heston LL, et al.: Pick's disease: clinical genetics and natural history. Arch Gen Psych 1987; 44:409–411.

EA005            **Nancy Lorraine Earl**

**Piebaldism with white forelock**
*See ALBINISM, CUTANEOUS*
**Piebaldness**
*See ALBINISM, CUTANEOUS*
**Piebaldness-deafness**
*See ALBINISM, CUTANEOUS*
**Piebalds**
*See ALBINISM, CUTANEOUS*
**Pierre Robin syndrome**
*See CLEFT PALATE-MICROGNATHIA-GLOSSOPTOSIS*
**Pierre Robin-heart malformation-clubfoot, congenital**
*See CLEFT PALATE-MICROGNATHIA-GLOSSOPTOSIS*
**Pigeon breast**
*See PECTUS CARINATUM*
**Pigment epithelial and choroidal degeneration, dominant central**
*See EYE, MACULAR DYSTROPHY, NORTH CAROLINA TYPE*
**Pigmentary anomaly-colon, aganglionosis**
*See ALBINISM, WAARDENBURG TYPE-HIRSCHSPRUNG AGANGLIONOSIS*
**Pigmentary retinal degeneration**
*See RETINITIS PIGMENTOSA*
**Pigmentary retinitis-congenital amaurosis**
*See RETINA, AMAUROSIS CONGENITA, LEBER TYPE*
**Pigmentation (spotty)-myxomas-endocrine overactivity**
*See NEVI-ATRIAL MYXOMA-MYXOID NEUROFIBROMAS-EPHELIDES*
**Pigmentation-alopecia-polyposis-nail defects**
*See POLYPOSIS-ALOPECIA-PIGMENTATION-NAIL DEFECTS*
**Pigmented adamantinoma**
*See JAW, NEUROECTODERMAL PIGMENTED TUMOR*
**Pigmented ameloblastoma**
*See JAW, NEUROECTODERMAL PIGMENTED TUMOR*
**Pigmented dermatosis, Siemens-Bloch type**
*See INCONTINENTIA PIGMENTI*
**Pigmented epulis, congenital**
*See JAW, NEUROECTODERMAL PIGMENTED TUMOR*
**Pigmented lesions-myxoid neurofibromas-atrial myxoma**
*See NEVI-ATRIAL MYXOMA-MYXOID NEUROFIBROMAS-EPHELIDES*
**Pigmented xerodermoid**
*See XERODERMA PIGMENTOSUM*
**Pigmy, African Baka of central Cameroon**
*See GROWTH DEFICIENCY, AFRICAN PYGMY TYPE*

---

## PILI TORTI-CLEFT LIP/PALATE-SYNDACTYLY     3126

**Includes:**
Cleft lip/palate-syndactyly-pili torti
Syndactyly-cleft lip/palate-pili torti
Zlotogora-Zilberman-Tenenbaum syndrome

**Excludes:**
Cleft lip/palate-ectodermal dysplasia-syndactyly (0179)
Cleft lip/palate-oligodontia-syndactyly-hair defects (2898)
Ectodermal dysplasia, Rapp-Hodgkin type (3056)
Ectrodactyly-ectodermal dysplasia-clefting syndrome (0337)

**Major Diagnostic Criteria:** The combination of pili torti, **Cleft lip** with or without **Cleft palate**, **Syndactyly**, and mental retardation should help to distinguish this syndrome from others.

**Clinical Findings:** Sparse scalp hair, pili torti, downslanting palpebral fissures, malformed protruding ears, cleft lip with or without cleft palate, micrognathia, partial **Syndactyly** of fingers and toes 3–4, single transverse palmar crease (either simian or Sydney line), and severe head lag in infancy. Additional features noted in the older of two reported sib include widely spaced teeth, widely spaced nipples (>97th percentile), and hypoplastic scrotum with cryptorchidism.

This condition has been reported in sibs from one family. A similar condition, **Cleft lip/palate-oligodontia-syndactyly-hair defects**, was also reported in 1987, although the presence of the condition in a mother and daughter, and other clinical differences, suggest that these may be distinct conditions.

**Complications:** Unknown.

**Associated Findings:** None known.

**Etiology:** The presence of this syndrome in sibs of each sex, whose parents are consanguineous, is strongly suggestive of autosomal recessive inheritance.

**Pathogenesis:** Unknown. This condition could be considered an ectodermal dysplasia.

**POS No.:** 4480

**Sex Ratio:** Presumably M1:F1.

**Occurrence:** Two siblings from Israel has been documented.

**Risk of Recurrence for Patient's Sib:**
See Part I, *Mendelian Inheritance.*

**Risk of Recurrence for Patient's Child:**
See Part I, *Mendelian Inheritance.*

**Age of Detectability:** At birth, by physical examination.

**Gene Mapping and Linkage:** Unknown.

**Prevention:** None known. Genetic counseling indicated.

**Treatment:** Supportive, with repair of the cleft lip and palate indicated.

**Prognosis:** Mental retardation is part of the syndrome. Life span is unknown; the younger sib died at age eight months from an illness.

**Detection of Carrier:** Unknown.

**References:**
Zlotogora J, et al.: Cleft lip and palate, pili torti, malformed ears, partial syndactly of fingers and toes, and mental retardation: a new syndrome? J Med Genet 1987; 24:291–293.

T0007            **Helga V. Toriello**

**Pili torti-sensorineural hearing loss**
*See DEAFNESS-PILI TORTI, BJORNSTAD TYPE*
**Pili trianguli et canaliculi**
*See HAIR, UNCOMBABLE-CRYSTALLINE CATARACT*
**Pili trianguli et canaliculi-crystalline cataract**
*See HAIR, UNCOMBABLE-CRYSTALLINE CATARACT*
**Pillay syndrome**
*See DWARFISM (SHORT LIMBED)-PETERS ANOMALY OF THE EYE*
*Also OPHTHALMO-MANDIBULO-MELIC DWARFISM*

---

## PILO-DENTO-UNGULAR DYSPLASIA WITH MICROCEPHALY     2636

**Includes:** Ectodermal dysplasia, pilo-dento-ungular type

**Excludes:**
Ectodermal dysplasia, Christ-Siemens-Touraine type (0333)
Ectodermal dysplasia, Passarge type (3120)
Ectodermal dysplasia, hidrotic (0334)
Tricho-odonto-onychial dysplasia (2889)

**Major Diagnostic Criteria:** Microcephaly, trichodysplasia, onychodysplasia, dental alterations, and gastroesophageal disturbances.

**Clinical Findings:** Thin and sparse scalp hair, synophrys, hypodontia of permanent dentition, dystrophic finger- and toenails, **Microcephaly**, mental retardation, increased deep tendon reflexes, spasticity, scoliosis, advanced bone age, retrognathism, blue sclerae, strabismus, high-arched palate, clinodactyly, dermatoglyphic alterations, nocturnal enuresis, intestinal and respiratory infections, gastroesophageal reflux, esophagus hypotonia, compression of the anterior wall of the upper one-third of the esophagus, and anterior deviation of the trachea.

**Complications:** May gag on solid food and tolerate only liquids.

**Associated Findings:** None known.

**Etiology:** Possibly autosomal recessive inheritance. Parental consanguinity has been reported.

**Pathogenesis:** Unknown.

**POS No.:** 4391

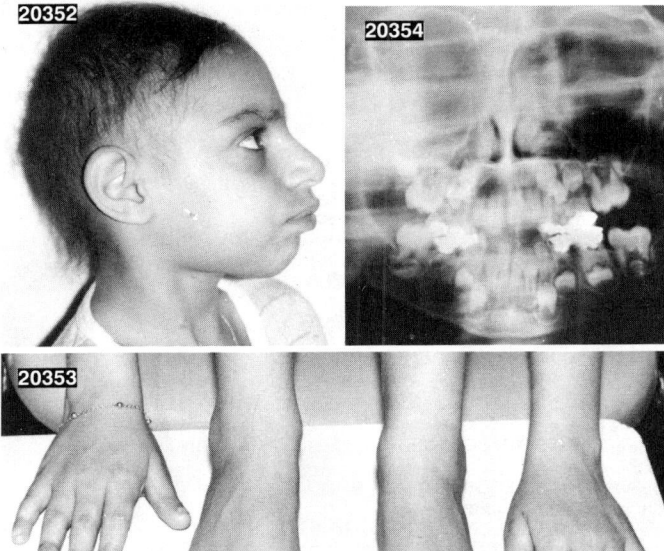

**2636-20352:** Note microcephaly, thin and sparse hair, synophrys, and retrognathism in this affected 6-year-old girl. **20353:** Note dystrophic nails. **20354:** Orthopantomogram at age 6 years; note dental defects.

**Sex Ratio:** Presumably M1:F1.

**Occurrence:** One Brazilian Caucasian girl in a sibship of two, from normal first cousin parents, has been reported.

**Risk of Recurrence for Patient's Sib:**
See Part I, *Mendelian Inheritance*.

**Risk of Recurrence for Patient's Child:**
See Part I, *Mendelian Inheritance*.

**Age of Detectability:** At birth, by physical examination.

**Gene Mapping and Linkage:** Unknown.

**Prevention:** None known. Genetic counseling indicated.

**Treatment:** Use of wigs and dental prosthesis may be cosmetically and psychologically helpful.

**Prognosis:** The only affected person known died at age seven years due to a combination of bone-marrow aplasia (possibly produced by drugs), multiple infections, hemorrhages, and acute anemia.

**Detection of Carrier:** Unknown.

**References:**
Tajara EH, et al.: Displasia pilodentoungular, uma nova sindrome de displasia e malformação. Ciênc Cult (suppl) 1986; 38:894 only.
Tajara EH, et al.: Pilodentoungulardysplasia with microcephaly: a new ectodermal dysplasia/malformation syndrome. Am J Med Genet 1987; 26:153–156.

FR033                                                      **Newton Freire-Maia**

**Pilomatricoma**
*See PILOMATRIXOMA*

---

## PILOMATRIXOMA                                                      2589

**Includes:**
 Calcifying epithelioma of Malherbe
 Cancer, trichomatrical
 Pilomatricoma
 Trichoepithelioma

**Excludes:**
 Calcified hamartomas
 Calcified lymph nodes
 Calcinosis cutis
 Dermoid cysts
 Hemangiomas
 Parotid gland tumors
 Sebaceous adenoma or carcinoma
 Skin and subcutaneous cysts
 Squamous cell carcinomas
 Xanthogranuloma, juvenile

**Major Diagnostic Criteria:** Cytologic evaluation following biopsy, excision, or fine-needle aspiration. Cytologic criteria include 1) presence of cells with large, vesicular nuclei with distinct nucleoli that form clusters or occur singly; and 2) presence of numerous naked nuclei with well-preserved chromatin structure and distinct nucleoli.

**Clinical Findings:** Small, mobile nodules occur in the dermis or subcutaneous tissue, and are usually located in the head and neck. Consistency of the nodules is variable, ranging from cystic, to firm, to stony hard. A reddish-blue mass with areas of yellow-white patches is seen through the overlying layer of skin. Telangiectatic vessels are sometimes present on the overlying skin. Occasionally, overlying skin ruptures, with extrusion of friable granulation or calcified material. Pilomatrixomas are usually well-circumscribed and solitary lesions, but up to 6% are multiple. Average size is 1–3 cm in diameter, but "giant" pilomatrixomas of 15 cm diameter have been reported.

 Pilomatrixomas are often preceded by a history of trauma. Growth is slow and usually asymptomatic. Pain may result from pressure or pinching of the lesion or from secondary infection with bleeding and ulceration. The majority (50–70%) occur in the head and neck region, most frequently on the brow, eyelid, or cheek. No cases have been reported on the palms or soles.

 Modified mammographic techniques have been used to show fine speckled calcification in the lesions. Routine X-ray rarely shows calcifications.

 Histologic appearance is distinctive and allows differentiation from other possible skin lesions. The tumor is made up of irregularly shaped islands of epithelial cells surrounded by a dense fibrous tissue. There are two distinctive cell types: basophilic, and "shadow" or "ghost" cells. The basophilic cells represent immature hair matrix cells and are usually at the periphery. Moving toward the center, there is a transition zone where the cells gradually lose their nuclei. In the center of this area one sees "shadow" or "ghost" cells. These cells have distinct borders but are devoid of their nuclei and display cellular dystrophy and degeneration. The stroma surrounding these cells is made up of granulation tissue with foreign body giant cells. Calcification is present in 75–80% of lesions. Ossification is found in 15–20%. Occasionally, melanin is seen. Aspirates contain only scant cellular granulomatous tissue which is more prevalent on histologic examination. Also, "ghost" or "shadow" cells are more frequently seen singly on cytologic examinations, as opposed to large groups seen on tissue section.

**Complications:** Recurrence is likely if the lesion is not totally excised. There are at least five reported cases of malignant transformation with invasion of local structures.

**Associated Findings:** Multiple pilomatrixomas may be associated with **Intestinal polyposis, type III** and **Myotonic dystrophy.** This association may represent a pleiotropic effect of the myotonic dystrophy gene.

**Etiology:** A benign tumor of hair cell origin.

**Pathogenesis:** First described by Malherbe and Chenantais (1880), who thought the condition originated from sebaceous glands. However, electron microscopy and histochemical studies show that the outer root sheath of the hair follicle is the cell of origin. The calcium deposits that occur in 80% of these lesions are felt to be the result of a dystrophic process. No abnormality in calcium metabolism is present.

**Sex Ratio:** M2:F3

**Occurrence:** The second most common superficial "lump" excised on a child; 1:824 dermatologic pathologic specimens and 1:2,200 surgical pathologic specimens. Most (97%) of the reported cases were Caucasians.

**Risk of Recurrence for Patient's Sib:** Unknown. A familial incidence has been noted in only six cases.

**Risk of Recurrence for Patient's Child:** Unknown.

**Age of Detectability:** While the condition has been identified in neonates, 40% occur in patients less than 10 years of age, and 60% occur in patients less than 20 years of age. The peak incidence is 8–13 years of age.

**Gene Mapping and Linkage:** Unknown.

**Prevention:** None known. Genetic counseling indicated.

**Treatment:** Total excision is needed; and this may need to include overlying skin. Incision and curettage are also advocated.

**Prognosis:** Recurrence is unlikely after adequate surgical excision. Lesions are felt to be benign, but there are reported cases of malignant transformation to a "giant" pilomatrixoma with locally aggressive and invasive behavior. Wide excision is needed in these cases.

**Detection of Carrier:** Unknown.

**Special Considerations:** *Trichoepithelioma* is a tumor similar to the pilomatrixoma. In these tumors, the hair matrix or basophilic cells do not develop into "shadow" cells. Instead, they develop into keratinized areas of "horn cysts." Eosinophils often surround these horn cysts, shown by electron microscope studies to represent immature hair structures. The malignant variant is the *trichomatrical carcinoma*.

**References:**
Malherbe A, Chenantais J: Note sur l'epithelioma calcifie des glands sebaces. Progr Med (Paris) 1880; 8:826–828.
Harper PS: Calcifying epithelioma of Malherbe-Association with myotonic muscular dystrophy. Arch Dermatol 1972; 106:41–44.
Moehlenbeck FW: Pilomatrixoma (calcifying epithelioma). Arch Dermatol 1973; 108:532–534.
Hernandez-Perez E, Cestoni-Parducci RF: Pilomatricoma (calcifying epithelioma): a study of 100 cases in El Salvador. Int J Dermatol 1981; 9:491–494.
Woyke S, et al.: Pilomatrixoma: a pitfall in the aspiration cytology of skin tumors. Acta Cytol 1982; 26:189–194.
Van der Walt JD: Carcinomatous transformation in a pilomatrixoma. Am J Dermatopathol 1984; 6:63–69.
Hawkins DB, Chen WT: Pilomatrixoma of the head and neck in children. Int J Pediatr Otorhinolaryngol 1985; 8:215–223.

MY003
SH050

**Charles M. Myer III**
**Sally Shott**

**Pineal teratomas**
See *TERATOMAS*
**Pinealomas, ectopic**
See *CNS NEOPLASMS*
**Pinna, ectopic placement of pinna**
See *EAR, ECTOPIC PINNA*
**Pinna, hypogenesis of, with associated atresia of external ear**
See *EAR, MICROTIA-ATRESIA*
**Pipecolic acidemia**
See *CEREBRO-HEPATO-RENAL SYNDROME*
**Pipecolic acidemia (some forms)**
See *PHYTANIC ACID OXIDASE DEFICIENCY, INFANTILE TYPE*
**Pits of upper lip**
See *LIP, PITS OR MOUNDS*
**Pitt syndrome**
See *DWARFISM-DYSMORPHIC FACIES-RETARDATION, PITT TYPE*

**Pitt-Rogers-Danks syndrome**
See *DWARFISM-DYSMORPHIC FACIES-RETARDATION, PITT TYPE*
**Pituitary cretinism**
See *THYROTROPIN DEFICIENCY, ISOLATED*
**Pituitary dwarfism II**
See *DWARFISM, LARON*
**Pituitary dwarfism III**
See *DWARFISM, PANHYPOPITUITARY*
**Pituitary dwarfism IV**
See *DWARFISM, PANHYPOPITUITARY*
**Pituitary dwarfism-sella turcica defect**
See *DWARFISM, PITUITARY WITH ABNORMAL SELLA TURCICA*
**Pituitary gland hypoplasia-adrenal hypoplasia, congenital**
See *ADRENAL HYPOPLASIA, CONGENITAL*
**Pityriasis pilaris**
See *SKIN, PITYRIASIS RUBRA PILARIS*
**Pityriasis rubra pilaris**
See *SKIN, PITYRIASIS RUBRA PILARIS*
**PKU**
See *FETAL EFFECTS FROM MATERNAL PKU*
**PKU, atypical**
See *DIHYDROPTERIDINE REDUCTASE DEFICIENCY*
**PKU1**
See *PHENYLKETONURIA*
**Placenta, circumvallate**
See *CIRCUMVALLATE PLACENTA SYNDROME*
**Placental hypoperfusion fetal developmental retardation**
See *FETAL DEVELOPMENTAL RETARDATION WITH MATERNAL HYPERTENSION*
**Placental steroid sulfatase deficiency**
See *ICHTHYOSIS, X-LINKED WITH STEROID SULFATASE DEFICIENCY*
**Plagiocephaly**
See *CRANIOSYNOSTOSIS*

---

**PLAGIOCEPHALY** 2939

**Includes:**
    Head, rhomboid-shaped
    Positional plagiocephaly
    Postural plagiocephaly

**Excludes:**
    **Oculo-auriculo-vertebral anomaly** (0735)
    Craniosynostosis, unilateral coronal
    Craniosynostosis, unilateral lambdoidal

**Major Diagnostic Criteria:** The term *plagiocephaly* is used by some authors to include any asymmetric head shape of any cause. The term is used more specifically here to mean a rhomboid-shaped head with a shift of the cranial base. One side of the face and the contralateral occipital parietal region are flattened, while the opposite sides of the skull seem to bulge. X-rays of the cranial sutures show them to be patent, while CT or MRI scans of the brain demonstrate normal anatomy.

**Clinical Findings:** Generally the infant's head has a normal shape at birth and becomes progressively distorted over the next four months of life as the infant maintains a consistent head posture against his or her mattress and other flat head supports. Then, as the infant develops improved head control, the distortion begins to resolve spontaneously. The head shape usually achieves its maximal resolution by ages 6–8 months. The distinction between positional plagiocephaly from structural facial asymmetry (hemifacial microsomia) may be difficult at times, since the flattened side of the face may be distorted and appear to feature a smaller jaw, abnormal auricle, and decreased unilateral facial movement. The correct diagnosis can be made by noting the overall head shape of plagiocephaly, which is rare in conditions featuring hemifacial microsomia, and then through X-ray assessment of the face.

**Complications:** Plagiocephaly is solely a cosmetic distortion of the skull. The only complication is its failure to resolve spontaneously.

**Associated Findings:** Plagiocephaly is generally associated with congenital muscular torticollis. Presumably the limited neck movement forces the head to remain in limited posture against the mattress. Cervical hemivertebrae or other structural anomalies of

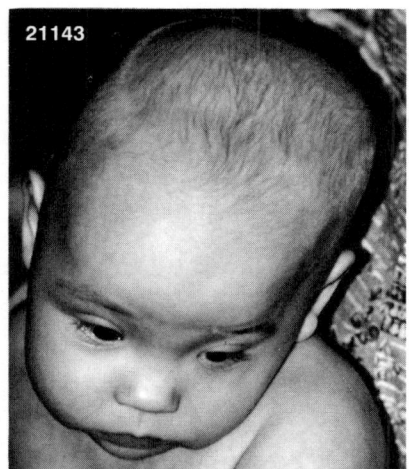

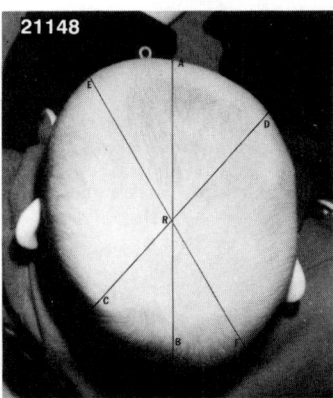
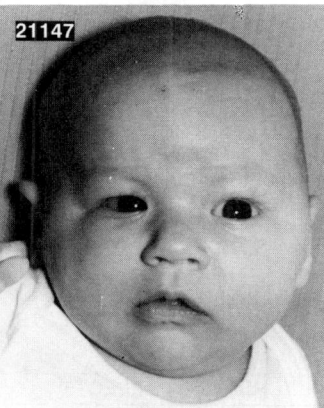

**2939-21143:** An infant with typical positional plagiocephaly. 21148: Positional plagiocephaly is best appreciated from the superior view of the head. The cranium takes on a rhomboid shape with frontal and contralateral occipital flattening (CD) and apparent bulging in the reverse direction (EF). 21147: Characteristic asymmetry of the entire face is seen in full facial view.

neck bones or muscles may also occasionally result in abnormal head shape. Some infants with hypotonia will prefer a single head position and produce a plagiocephalic skull in spite of full passive range in neck movement.

**Etiology:** Postnatal deformation.

**Pathogenesis:** Unknown.

**CDC No.:** 754.050

**Sex Ratio:** M1:F1

**Occurrence:** It is estimated that 8–10:10,000 newborns have some evidence of deformational plagiocephaly.

**Risk of Recurrence for Patient's Sib:** Dependent on the risk of recurrence for the underlying cause of limited head movement.

**Risk of Recurrence for Patient's Child:** Not increased.

**Age of Detectability:** Generally, cosmetically important plagiocephaly is noted by ages 6–8 weeks and progresses to a maximum distortion by age four months.

**Gene Mapping and Linkage:** N/A

**Prevention:** Attempts at increasing neck movement to minimize consistent head positioning is extremely difficult prior to ages 4–6 months. Placing the small infant in a swing, a front- or back-pack, or in other ways maintaining the head in space without any

surface pressure for as many hours a day as is practicable may be a more successful preventive approach.

**Treatment:** The facial asymmetry of deformational plagiocephaly will generally continue to improve for several years and rarely pose a permanent cosmetic problem. The calvarial asymmetry that remains at ages 6–8 months is permanent. If the distortion cannot be easily disguised with hair, corrective treatment can be taken. Lightweight helmets can be fashioned to fit tightly where the head is prominent and allow for brain growth in the areas of normal flattening. Such helmets should be placed between ages 6–8 months to assure that maximum spontaneous recovery occurs while utilizing all remaining brain growth potential to restore head shape. Surgical corrections are possible through calvarectomy, but are rarely needed.

**Prognosis:** Restoration of symmetric head shape can be expected if helmets are employed when spontaneous resolution fails.

**Detection of Carrier:** N/A

**References:**

Dingwall EJ: Artificial cranial deformation. London: John Bale & Sones & Danielsson, 1931.
Clarren SK: Plagiocephaly and torticollis: etiology, natural history, and helmet treatment in 43 patients. J Pediatr 1981; 98:92–95. *
Clarren SK, et al.: Malformations of the cranium. In: Kelley V, ed: Practice of pediatrics. Philadelphia: J.B. Lippincott, 1986. †
Cohen MM, Jr., ed: Craniosynostosis: diagnosis, evaluation and management. New York: Raven, 1986.
Dunne KB, Clarren SK: The origin of prenatal and postnatal deformities. Pediatr Clin North Am 1986; 33:1277–1297.

CL006                        **Sterling K. Clarren**

**Plantar callosities, autosomal dominant painful**
   *See SKIN, PAINFUL PLANTAR CALLOSITIES*
**Plasma cell myeloma**
   *See CANCER, MULTIPLE MYELOMA*
**Plasma cholesteryl ester deficiency, familial**
   *See LECITHIN-CHOLESTEROL ACYL TRANSFERASE DEFICIENCY*
**Plasma cholinesterase, atypical**
   *See CHOLINESTERASE, ATYPICAL*
**Plasma protein S deficiency**
   *See PROTEIN S DEFICIENCY*
**Plasma thromboplastin antecedent (PTA) deficiency**
   *See FACTOR XI DEFICIENCY*
**Plasma thromboplastin component deficiency**
   *See HEMOPHILIA B*
**Plasma transglutaminase**
   *See FACTOR XIII (FIBRIN STABILIZING FACTOR)*

---

**PLASMA, GROUP-SPECIFIC COMPONENT**         **0446**

**Includes:**
    Gc plasma protein component
    Group-specific protein
    Protein Gc
    Vitamin D binding protein (VDBP)

**Excludes:** N/A

**Major Diagnostic Criteria:** The group-specific component is the vitamin D binding protein of human plasma.

**Clinical Findings:** The so-called group-specific component (Gc) is the vitamin D binding protein (VDBP) in the plasma of humans and other mammals. It serves as the transport protein for vitamin $D_3$ and the natural derivatives 25-hydroxy-vitamin D, 1,25-dihydroxy-vitamin D, and 24,25-dihydroxy-vitamin D. It has a single common binding site for these ligands with the greatest affinity for 25-OH-D and $24,25(OH)_2$-D. Thus far, a deficiency of this protein has not been identified. In the various genetic types of vitamin D resistant rickets, as well as in osteogenesis imperfecta, the plasma levels and the vitamin D binding function of this protein are normal. The serum concentration in healthy individuals is approximately 40 mg/dl. There are slight but significant differences in the concentrations among the different genetic Gc types: persons with

Gc 1–1 have on the average higher levels than individuals with Gc 2–1; persons with Gc 2–1 have higher concentrations than individuals with Gc 2–2. Gc is increased in sera of pregnant women. The group-specific component is synthesized in the liver; patients with severe liver diseases tend to have very low Gc serum levels. Gc is also present in cerebrospinal fluid (CSF), ascites fluid, and normal urine.

The vitamin D binding protein Gc is an α(2)-globulin. It has a molecular weight of 50,000 daltons and a sedimentation rate of 4.1 S. It is devoid of lipids. Only the Gc 1 protein has a glycan moiety of 1%. Gc 2 contains no carbohydrate. It consists of a single polypeptide chain. The amino acid sequence and nucleotide sequence of the cDNA has been determined.

Genetic variations were demonstrated first by Hirschfeld in 1959. Three common Gc types were identified by electrophoresis: Gc 1–1, Gc 2–1, and Gc 2–2. They were determined by a pair of autosomal alleles, Gc$^1$ and Gc$^2$. Gc 1–1 has the electrophoertic mobility of a α(2)-globulin; it is electrophoretically heterogeneous and consists of two separable proteins. Gc 2–2 migrates as a slow α(2)-globulin and is homogeneous. Individuals heterozygous for this trait (Gc 2–1) have the products of both alleles in their serum; by electrophoretic procedures three components can be disclosed. For the classification of Gc types, starch-, agarose- and polyacrylamide-gel electrophoresis have also been employed. Recently, isoelectric focusing on polyacrylamide gels followed by immunofixation has been applied for Gc typing. Six common Gc subtypes are designated as 1F-1F, 1F-1S, 1S-1S, 2–1F, 2–1S, and 2–2. They are controlled by three alleles, named Gc$^{1F}$, Gc$^{1S}$, and Gc$^2$.

The practical application of the Gc system is at present restricted to its use as a genetic marker in studies of human populations, in twin studies, and in cases of disputed paternity.

**Complications:**  Unknown.

**Associated Findings:**  None known.

**Etiology:**  Autosomal co-dominant inheritance.

**Pathogenesis:**  Unknown.

**MIM No.:**  *13920

**Sex Ratio:**  M1:F1

**Occurrence:**  Gc$^1$ and Gc$^2$ appear to have a worldwide distribution; both alleles have been disclosed in every population examined. In most populations, Gc$^1$ is more common than Gc$^2$; the frequency of the latter varies from 0.011 in an Australian aborigine tribe from Cundeelee in the Western Desert to 0.385 in a population of Finns from the island of Kokar. In some South American Indian tribes, however, Gc$^2$ is more common than Gc$^1$. Most Caucasian and Asian populations have Gc$^2$ frequencies between 0.20 and 0.30, Black populations have lower Gc$^2$ frequencies between 0.03 and 0.11.

The distribution of the suballeles Gc [1F] and Gc [1S] also shows significant differences between human populations: Europeans tend to have high frequencies for Gc [1S] and low frequencies for Gc [1F], in African populations the opposite is found, whereas Asian populations have similar frequencies for Gc [1F] and Gc [1S]. Useful for anthropological studies is the consideration of the frequencies for Gc [1F] and Gc [2] which permits grouping of populations according to their geographic and/or ethnic origin. The allelic distribution is possibly related to variations in skin pigmentation: small differences in vitamin D-binding have been demonstrated for the different allelic products. It is, therefore, conceivable that differences in the vitamin D transport function of Gc are related to variations in skin pigmentation which in turn are associated with differences in sun shine exposure.

More than 100 genetic variants have, in addition, been identified in the Gc system. These are classified into phenotypes with a double banded and a single banded pattern. The former are mutants of Gc [1], the latter are variants of Gc [2]. Their isoelectric points are either shifted toward the anode or toward the cathode. Some of these variants have been observed only in single families. Others occur in certain populations in appreciable frequencies as, for instance, Gc [1A1] which is found in Australian aborigines and in Melanesians.

**Risk of Recurrence for Patient's Sib:**
See Part I, *Mendelian Inheritance.*

**Risk of Recurrence for Patient's Child:**
See Part I, *Mendelian Inheritance.*

**Age of Detectability:**  In infancy.

**Gene Mapping and Linkage:**  GC (group-specific component (vitamin D binding protein)) has been mapped to 4q12-q13.

**Prevention:**  None known. Genetic counseling indicated.

**Treatment:**  None required.

**Prognosis:**  A recent debate centered on a possible relationship between Gc genotype and genetic susceptibility to acquired immunodeficiency syndrome, concluding that no such association existed (see *New Engl J Med* 1987; 317:630–632).

**Detection of Carrier:**  Unknown.

**References:**

Daiger SP, et al.: Group-specific component (Gc) proteins bind vitamin D and 25-hydroxy-vitamin D. Proc Natl Acad Sci 1975; 72:2076–2080.
Mourant AE, et al.: Sunshine and the geographical distribution of the alleles of the Gc system of plasma proteins. Hum Genet 1976; 33:307–314.
Constans J, et al.: Group-specific component. Report on the First International Workshop. Hum Genet 1979; 48:143–149.
Constans J, et al.: The polymorphism of the vitamin D-binding protein (Gc); isoelectric focusing in 3M urea as additional method for identification of genetic variants. Hum Genet 1983; 65:176–180. *
Yang F, et al.: Human group-specific component (Gc) is a member of the albumin family. Proc Nat Acad Sci 1985; 82:7994–7998. *

CL014                                    **Hartwig Cleve**

**Plasma, plasminogen defects**
*See PLASMINOGEN DEFECTS*

---

## PLASMINOGEN DEFECTS                                    3083

**Includes:**
 Microplasmin
 Plasma, plasminogen defects
 Plasminogen Tochigi

**Excludes:**  N/A

**Major Diagnostic Criteria:**  The plasminogen system is highly polymorphic, with many variant forms having been identified. Variant forms of the proenzyme may be identified by isoelectric focusing, immunoelectrophoresis, and measurements of functional activity in relation to enzyme protein. Most of the known plasminogen variants have no clinical significance; however, several of them have been shown to produce hypercoagulability with thromboembolic complications. Affected individuals in most cases exhibit approximately 50% of normal plasmin activity in their plasma.

**Clinical Findings:**  Reported individuals having the apparently rare variant forms of plasminogen with deficient function have in some cases had severe and recurrent thromboembolic disease. In some families, however, other individuals with the enzyme deficiency have not experienced thrombotic complications, suggesting that other factors may also play a role in the clinical expression of these abnormalities.

**Complications:**  Unknown.

**Associated Findings:**  None known.

**Etiology:**  Autosomal dominant inheritance.

**Pathogenesis:**  Plasminogen is a single-chain protein that circulates in the plasma as an inactive zymogen. Its activation, by cleavage of an Arg-Val bond, converts the molecule to a protease (plasmin) with trypsin-like activity. The principal physiologic role of plasmin is as a fibrinolytic agent. Plasminogen in the blood has been shown to bind to fibrin during its polymerization in the formation of a blood clot. Endothelial cells contain plasminogen activator, which is released in association with thrombus formation. The fibrinolytic action of plasmin is believed to be essential for clot resolution and the re-establishment of the patency of the blood vessels. Diminished plasmin activity resulting from function-deficient mutations presumably interferes with this process and predisposes the affected individuals to thrombotic complications.

**MIM No.:**   *17335

**Sex Ratio:**   M1:F1

**Occurrence:**   All of the function-deficient variants appear to be of rare occurrence.

**Risk of Recurrence for Patient's Sib:**
See Part I, *Mendelian Inheritance.*

**Risk of Recurrence for Patient's Child:**
See Part I, *Mendelian Inheritance.*

**Age of Detectability:**   At birth.

**Gene Mapping and Linkage:**   PLG (plasminogen) has been mapped to 6q26-q27.

**Prevention:**   None known. Genetic counseling indicated.

**Treatment:**   Plasma infusions might be anticipated to replenish deficient plasminogen; however, the efficacy of this form of treatment is as yet unknown. Efforts to manage deficient patients with anticoagulants have in general not been successful.

**Prognosis:**   Most forms are compatible with good health and normal life span. Affected individuals may, however, be at risk for serious thromboembolic complications.

**Detection of Carrier:**   As affected individuals are apparently heterozygous for the abnormality, the disorder is fully expressed in the carrier. Studies of some families, however, have shown the abnormality to be present in some family members who do not exhibit thromboembolic disease.

**References:**

Aoki N, et al.: Abnormal plasminogen: a hereditary molecular abnormality found in a patient with recurrent thrombosis. J Clin Invest 1978; 78:1186–1195.
Wohl RC, et al.: Physiological activation of the human fibrinolytic system. Isolation and characterization of human plasminogen variants Chicago I and Chicago II. J Biol Chem 1979; 254:9063–9069.
Soria J, et al.: Plasminogen Paris I: congenital abnormal plasminogen and its incidence in thrombosis. Thromb Res 1983; 32:229–238.
Miyata T, et al.: Plasminogens Tochigi II and Nagoya: two additional molecular defects with Ala-600→Thr replacement found in plasmin light chain variants. J Biochem 1984; 96:277–287.
Towne JB, et al.: Abnormal plasminogen: a genetically determined cause of hypercoagulability. J Vasc Surg 1984; 1:896–902.
Scharrer IM, et al.: Investigation of a congenital abnormal plasminogen, Frankfurt I, and its relationship to thrombosis. Thromb Haemost 1986; 55:396–401.
Skoda U, et al.: Proposal for the nomenclature of human plasminogen (PLG) polymorphism. Vox Sang 1986; 51:244–248.

H0024                                                      **George R. Honig**

**Plasminogen Tochigi**
See PLASMINOGEN DEFECTS
**Plasmodium vivax malaria**
See MALARIA, VIVAX, SUSCEPTIBILITY TO
**Platelet fibinogen receptor deficiency**
See THROMBASTHENIA, GLANZMANN-NAEGELI TYPE
**Platelet glycoprotein IIb-IIIa deficiency**
See THROMBASTHENIA, GLANZMANN-NAEGELI TYPE
**Platelet, May-Hegglin anomaly**
See LEUKOCYTE, MAY-HEGGLIN ANOMALY
**Platelet/fibronectin abnormality-Ehlers-Danlos syndrome**
See EHLERS-DANLOS SYNDROME
**Platyspondyly-osteosclerosis**
See DYSOSTEOSCLEROSIS
**Pleonosteosis**
See LERI PLEONOSTEOSIS SYNDROME
**Pleura and peritoneum, muscle deficiency between**
See DIAPHRAGM, EVENTRATION

**Plott syndrome**
See VOCAL CORD PARALYSIS
also LARYNGEAL PARALYSIS
also LARYNGEAL ABDUCTOR PARALYSIS-MENTAL RETARDATION
**Poikiloderma atrophicans-cataract**
See ROTHMUND-THOMSON SYNDROME
**Poikiloderma with bullae, Weary type**
See POIKILODERMA, HEREDITARY ACROKERATOTIC, KINDLER-WEARY TYPE

## POIKILODERMA, HEREDITARY ACROKERATOTIC, KINDLER-WEARY TYPE                                                3038

**Includes:**
Acrokeratotic poikiloderma, hereditary
Bullous acrokeratotic poikiloderma of Kindler and Weary
Kindler-Weary syndrome
Poikiloderma with bullae, Weary type

**Excludes:**
**Dyskeratosis congenita** (2024)
**Epidermolysis bullosum, type I** (2560)
Poikiloderma, congenital
**Poikiloderma, sclerosing, hereditary** (3262)
**Rothmund-Thomson syndrome** (2037)
**Urticaria pigmentosa (UP)** (3263)
**Xeroderma pigmentosum** (1005)

**Major Diagnostic Criteria:**   Pigmentary anomaly; vesicopustules in infancy followed by gradually increasing diffuse poikiloderma with striate and reticulate atrophy.

**Clinical Findings:**   The lesions vary with age. During *infancy* vesicopustules or bullae on hands and feet and occasionally the trunk beginning at ages 1–3 months. These lesions resolve in later childhood. From *infancy to five years* transient eczematous eruption in flexural areas with or without pruritus. This lesion resolves by about age five years. *Poikiloderma*: persistent diffuse poikiloderma, especially in the flexural areas and sparing the face, scalp, and ears. This lesions is progressive with striate and reticulate atrophy. Telangiectasia is not a feature. *Acrokeratosis*: keratotic "warty" papules on the hands, feet, knees, and elbows, which persist into adulthood. Families with the putative autosomal accessive type exhibit photosensitivity and intraoral anomalies.

Expression may be incomplete, or more than one gene may be responsible for the complete syndrome: one family in the group reported by Weary et al (1971) had acral blistering and acrokeratoses without eczema and poikiloderma. Photosensitivity and intraoral anomalies exist in the putative autosomal recessive type.

*Histology*: 1) *Vesicles*: in the epidermis, focal spongiosis and microvesicles and areas of hydropic degeneration of the basal cell layer of epidermis and hair follicles; in the dermis, focal lymphohistiocytic inflammatory infiltrates subepidermally, periappendageal, and perivascular and edema. 2) *Poikilodermatous lesions*: epidermal atrophy, pigmentary irregularity, pigmentary incontinence, and mild perivascular infiltration. 3) *Acrokeratotic lesions*: marked localized hyperkeratosis and hypergranulosis; irregular acanthosis; and prominent vessels in upper dermis without inflammatory response.

*Immunology*: elevated IgG levels in affected individuals. Rheumatoid factor was positive in the two oldest patients in the absence of rheumatoid arthritis. Antinuclear factor is of dubious significance.

**Complications:**   Unknown.

**Associated Findings:**   None known.

**Etiology:**   Autosomal dominant inheritance, except in putative type, in which autosomal recessive inheritance in two related Kurdish Jewish sibs has been reported.

**Pathogenesis:**   Unknown.

**MIM No.:**   *17365

**POS No.:**   3382

**Sex Ratio:**   M1:F1

**Occurrence:** About 60 cases have been documented in the literature, including ten persons in one family by Weary et al (1971), 41 persons in six families by Larregue et al (1981), and four cases by Hacham-Zadeh and Garfunkel (1985).

**Risk of Recurrence for Patient's Sib:**
See Part I, *Mendelian Inheritance.*

**Risk of Recurrence for Patient's Child:**
See Part I, *Mendelian Inheritance.*

**Age of Detectability:** During infancy, from ages five weeks to as late as six months.

**Gene Mapping and Linkage:** Unknown.

**Prevention:** None known. Genetic counseling indicated.

**Treatment:** Symptomatic as indicated.

**Prognosis:** Life span does not appear to be reduced; normal intelligence.

**Detection of Carrier:** Unknown.

**Special Considerations:** Genetic heterogeneity may exist, as evidenced by one family within the kindred reported by Weary et al (1971) who had acral blistering and acrokeratosis in the absence of eczema or poikiloderma. Some researchers consider this condition to be a variant of **Epidermolysis bullosum, type I** with mottled pigmentation. Photosensitivity in the putative autosomal recessive disorder may differentiate it as an entity separate from the dominant disorder.

**References:**
Kindler T: Congenital poikiloderma with traumatic bulla formation and progressive cutaneous atrophy. Br J Dermatol 1954; 66:104–111.
Weary PE, et al.: Hereditary acrokeratotic poikiloderma. Arch Dermatol 1971; 103:409–422.
Der Kaloustian VM: Genetic diseases of the skin. Berlin: Springer-Verlag, 1979:122–123.
Larregue M, et al.: Acrokeratose poikilodermique bulleuse et hereditaire de Weary-Kindler. Ann Dermatol Venereol 1981; 103:69–76.
Hacham-Zadeh S, Garfunkel AA: Kindler syndrome in two related Kurdish families. Am J Med Genet 1985; 20:43–48.

WI055                                    **Ingrid M. Winship**

## POIKILODERMA, SCLEROSING, HEREDITARY          3262

**Includes:** Sclerosing poikiloderma, hereditary

**Excludes:**
Poikiloderma, congenital
**Poikiloderma, hereditary acrokeratotic, Kindler-Weary type** (3038)
**Rothmund-Thomson syndrome** (2037)
**Xeroderma pigmentosum** (1005)

**Major Diagnostic Criteria:** *Clinical:* Generalised poikiloderma of the skin, sclerosis of the palms and soles, hyperkeratotic and sclerotic bands in flexures, and clubbing of the fingers.

*Laboratory:* Histology of the skin from antecubital fossae and axillae reveals focal homogenisation of collagen, with a reduction in elastic tissue.

**Clinical Findings:** *Poikiloderma:* A generalised poikiloderma of the skin is accentuated in a flexural distribution, viz. axillae, antecubital and popliteal fossae, as well as the extensor surfaces of the knees, elbows and over the joints of the bands. True poikiloderma, ie hypo-and hyper-pigmentation with telangectasia and atrophy is interspersed with mottled pigmentary change alone.

*Sclerosis:* In addition to poikiloderma, sclerotic changes occur to the skin of the palms and soles; these differ from the changes of scleroderma.

Hyperkeratotic and sclerotic bands in either a reticulate or linear pattern occur in the flexural areas, viz. axillary vault and antecubital and popliteal fossae.

*Clubbing:* Clubbing of the fingers is a consistent feature of this syndrome.

**Complications:** Calcinosis of the tissues in older patients.

**Associated Findings:** Soft systolic murmurs are audible in different areas of the precordium in more than half of affected persons reported.

**Etiology:** Autosomal dominant inheritance.

**Pathogenesis:** A probable heritable disorder of connective tissue.

**MIM No.:** 17370

**Sex Ratio:** M1:F1

**Occurrence:** Rare; Seven affected persons in two unrelated Black families have been reported.

**Risk of Recurrence for Patient's Sib:**
See Part I, *Mendelian Inheritance.*

**Risk of Recurrence for Patient's Child:**
See Part I, *Mendelian Inheritance.*

**Age of Detectability:** Early signs in childhood (±4 years of age).

**Gene Mapping and Linkage:** Unknown.

**Prevention:** None known. Genetic counseling indicated.

**Treatment:** Symptomatic, using keratolytic agents.

**Prognosis:** Life span not affected.

**Detection of Carrier:** Unknown.

**Special Considerations:** This is an extremely rare genodermatosis; however, it would appear that it is indeed an autonomous syndrome.

**References:**
Weary PE, et al.: Hereditary sclerosing poikiloderma. Arch Derm 1969; 100:413–422.
Der Kaloustiaan VM, Kurban AK: Genetic diseases of the skin. Berlin: Springer-Verlag, 1979:122.

WI055                                    **Ingrid M. Winship**

**Poland anomaly**
*See POLAND SYNDROME*
**Poland syndactyly**
*See POLAND SYNDROME*

## POLAND SYNDROME                              0813

**Includes:**
Pectoralis muscle, absence of
Poland anomaly
Poland syndactyly
Poland-Moebius syndrome
Subclavian artery supply disruption sequence (SASDS)
Symbrachydactyly-ipsilateral aplasia of head of pectoralis muscle

**Excludes:**
Symbrachydactyly without associated muscle defect
**Syndactyly** (0923)
Syndactyly as a part of the acrocephalosyndactylies

**Major Diagnostic Criteria:** The association of symbrachydactyly with ipsilateral aplasia of the sternal head of the pectoralis major is diagnostic. The muscle defect is observed clinically as absence of the normal well-developed curved anterior axillary fold.

**Clinical Findings:** The two main components of the syndrome are symbrachydactyly and pectoral muscle defect. Symbrachydactyly is a specific hand malformation, always unilateral, characterized by the association of short digits and syndactyly. The phalanges are short or absent. The middle phalanges are affected more frequently, and in severe cases they are absent or fused with the distal phalanges (terminal symphalangism and assimilation hypoplasia). The distal phalanges are minimally affected and are rarely absent. The thumb is usually least affected. Syndactyly is either partial or complete, usually involving the soft tissues, and is not associated with bone synostosis. Syndactyly frequently involves the index and middle fingers.

The associated muscle defect is ipsilateral aplasia of the sternal

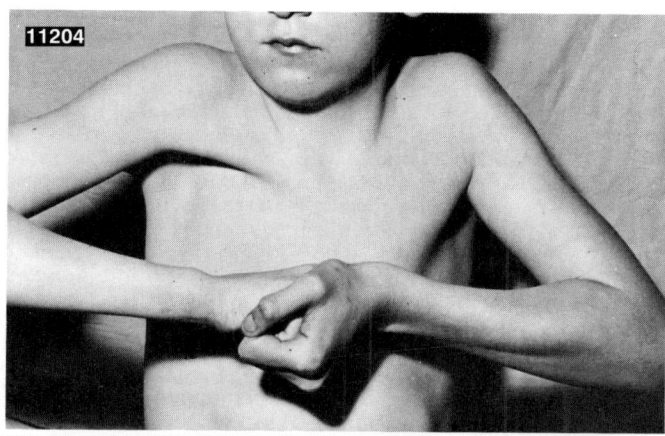

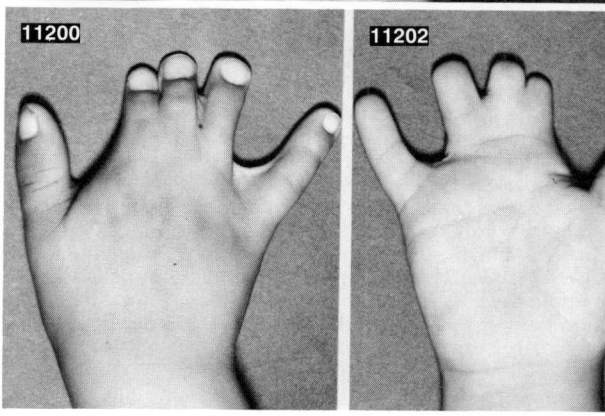

**0813-11204:** Absence of the sternal head of the right pectoral major muscle. **11200-02:** Unilateral digital hypoplasia, brachydactyly and syndactyly.

head of the pectoralis major, while its clavicular head is always present and is sometimes hypertrophied.

Asymmetry of breast development, and ipsilateral absence of the breast and subcutaneous tissue, as well as ipsilateral webbing of the axilla, are sometimes noted.

**Complications:** Defects in pectoralis minor, rectus abdominis, latissimus dorsi, serratus anterior, and intercostal muscles have been reported. Associated bone defects have also been noted; examples are hypoplasia of upper ribs, Sprengel deformity of the scapulae, and shortening of arm and forearm bones.

**Associated Findings:** Ipsilateral hypoplasia of the kidney was noted once. An association with **Diplegia, congenital facial** (Moebius syndrome) has also been suggested.

**Etiology:** Practically all reported cases are sporadic. Some familial patterns have been reported (David and Winter, 1985).

**Pathogenesis:** Bavinck and Winter (1986) have suggested that this and related conditions result from interruption of the early embryonic blood supply in the subclavian arteries, the vertebral arteries and/or their branches. They have suggested the term *subclavian artery supply disruption sequence (SASDS)* for this group of birth defects.

**MIM No.:** 17380, 17375

**POS No.:** 3359

**CDC No.:** 756.800

**Sex Ratio:** M1:F1

**Occurrence:** Among 33 cases with symbrachydactyly, Pol in 1921 found 21 cases with ipsilateral aplasia of the sternal head of the pectoralis major. Among 102 cases with absent sternal head of the pectoralis major, Bing in 1902 found 14 cases with associated symbrachydactyly. Sigiura et al (1962) found one boy with Poland syndactyly among 6,297 Japanese primary school children. In British Columbia, McGillivray and Lowry (1977) found an incidence of 1:32,000 live births. In Brazil, Castilla et al (1980) found 11 cases in 599,109 consecutive newborn infants.

**Risk of Recurrence for Patient's Sib:** Probably not increased.

**Risk of Recurrence for Patient's Child:** Probably not increased.

**Age of Detectability:** At birth, by clinical examination.

**Gene Mapping and Linkage:** Unknown.

**Prevention:** None known. Genetic counseling indicated.

**Treatment:** Surgical correction.

**Prognosis:** Normal life span.

**Detection of Carrier:** Unknown.

**Special Considerations:** At least a dozen instances of the association of the Poland and Moebius syndromes (*Polant-Moebius* syndrome) have been documented (see Stevenson, 1982).

**References:**

Clarkson P: Poland's syndactyly. Guys Hosp Rep 1962; 111:335–346.

McGivillray BC, Lowry RB: Poland syndrome in British Columbia: incidence and reproductive experience of affected persons. Am J Med Genet 1977; 1:65–74.

Temtamy SA, McKusick VA: The genetics of hand malformations. New York: Alan R Liss, for The National Foundation-March of Dimes, 1978.

Castilla EE, et al.: Syndactyly: frequency of specific types. Am J Med Genet 1980; 5:357.

Hegde HR, Shokeir MHK: Posterior shoulder girdle abnormalities with absence of pectoralis major muscle. Am J Med Genet 1982; 13:285–293.

Hester TR, Bostwick J: Poland's syndrome: correction with latissimus muscle transposition. Plast Reconstr Surg 1982; 69:226–233.

Stevenson RE: The Poland-Moebius syndrome. Proc Greenwood Genet Center 1982; 1:26–28.

Suzuki T, et al.: Computed tomography of the pectoralis muscles in Poland's syndrome. Hand 1983; 15:35–41.

David TJ, Winter RM: Familial absence of the pectoralis major, serratus anterior, and latissimus dorsi muscles. J Med Genet 1985; 22:390–392.

Bavinck JNB, Weaver DD: Subclavian artery supply disruption sequence: hypothesis of a vascular etiology for Poland, Klippel-Feil, and Moebius anomalies. Am J Med Genet 1986; 23:903–918.

TE004                                           **Samia A. Temtamy**

**Poland-Moebius syndrome**
 *See POLAND SYNDROME*
**Polar and capsular cataracts**
 *See CATARACT, POLAR AND CAPSULAR*
**Polar cataract**
 *See CATARACT, AUTOSOMAL DOMINANT CONGENITAL*
**Polio, sensitivity to**
 *See POLIO, SUSCEPTIBILITY TO*

---

## POLIO, SUSCEPTIBILITY TO                    3109

**Includes:**

Acute anterior poliomyelitis
Heine-Medin disease
Infantile paralysis
Polio, sensitivity to
Poliomyelitis
Poliovirus receptor
Post-polio syndrome

**Excludes:**

**Amyotrophic lateral sclerosis**
Guillain-Barre syndrome
Infectious meningo-encephalitides
Lyme disease
Motor neuron diseases

**Porphyria**
Sensitivity to other enteroviruses, such as Coxsackie and ECHO
Tick paralysis

**Major Diagnostic Criteria:** *Minor illness*: Polio virus usually causes an asymptomatic infection, but can present as a minor, non-specific systemic illness. Diagnosis at this stage can be made by culturing virus from stool.
*Major illness*: Poliomyelitis begins with upper respiratory and/or GI symptoms, with fever and signs of aseptic meningitis followed by usually asymmetrical paralysis of voluntary muscles. Definitive diagnosis is made by culturing one of the three serotypes of poliovirus from the patient's stool.

**Clinical Findings:** In an epidemic, 90–95% of all poliovirus-infected people are asymptomatic (inapparent). Four to eight percent may suffer a non-specific, abortive illness (minor illness), whereas 1–2% of infections result in neurologic symptoms or signs (major illness).
*Minor illness*: Most patients are asymptomatic, while others have sore throat, abdominal discomfort, vomiting accompanied by minor constitutional symptoms such as low-grade fever, malaise and mild headache. These symptoms last 1–4 days and recede (abortive infection). The incubation period is between 1–5 days.
*Major Illness*: The incubation period for the major illness is usually 4–10 days, rarely 3–35 days. A biphasic course is seen in one-third of 2–10 year-old patients, but is unusual in adults. The symptoms of aseptic meningitis begin with headache, vomiting, irritability and drowsiness. The neck and back may be stiff. The illness may abort at this stage. Paralysis usually develops on the second to fifth day after onset of headache. It may be delayed in children, or conversely, present as one of the initial symptoms. The pre-paralytic phase in adults is more severe than in children. Before onset of paralysis fasiculations may be present and the deep tendon reflexes may be hyperactive.
Spinal poliomyelitis primarily affects muscles of the extremities; the involvement is typically typically asymmetrical and the proximal muscles are more affected than distal. Lower extremities are more frequently involved then upper extremities. Affected muscles are flaccid and the deep tendon reflexes are absent. Atrophy is apparent as early as 5–7 days. When motor neurons of the brainstem are involved (bulbar poliomyelitis), paralysis of pharyngeal and laryngeal muscles is most common; facial muscles may also be involved. Less common is weakness of the muscles of the tongue and of mastication. External oculomotor weakness is rare. Brainstem reticular formation may also be involved, leading to disturbances of breathing, swallowing and cardiovascular control. A few adult patients may develop an encephalitic picture due to extensive involvement of neurons from the hypothalamus to the spinal cord. Such patients often die within 24–72 hours.

**Complications:** Complications of acute paralysis include respiratory failure, decubitus ulcers, and other systemic problems associated with decreased voluntary activity. Chronic complications of paralysis are contractures and weakness of limbs, scoliosis, reduced size or length of a limb, and sometimes persistent respiratory dependence.
A well-documented late complication of poliomyelitis is the occurrence of progressive motor complaints years or decades after the initial infection (*post-polio syndrome*). In some patients the complaints may be limited to joint pain and increased fatiguability, while in others, progressive weakness, atrophy and fasciculations are noted (*post-polio muscular atrophy PPMA*). Mulder's series (see Price and Plum, 1978) of 34 patients had a preponderance of men (M25:F9). Average age of onset of new symptoms was 34 years after recovery from acute poliomyelitis. Onset and involvement of weakness was not limited to limbs originally affected by poliomyelitis. Babinski signs were noted in some patients. The relationship of post-polio muscular atrophy (PPMA) to **Amyotrophic lateral sclerosis** (ALS) is unclear. Norris et al (see Price and Plum 1978) reported 2–8% of patients of adult motor neuron disease to have suffered from previous paralytic poliomyelitis. Poliomyelitis is 200 to 800-fold more common in the adult motor neuron disease group as compared to the general population.

Inflammatory changes in the muscle of patients with PPMA have been described. No evidence of antipolio antibodies has been noted in the CSF of these individuals, though oligoclonal bands may be seen. There is no evidence of persistence of poliovirus infection in these individuals. The speculated mechanisms of PPMA include: 1) Motor neuron damage induced by anti-idiotype antibodies. 2) Progressive decrease in the number of motor neurons as a result of normal aging or shortened lifespan of motor neurons originally damaged by polio infection. 3) A genetic susceptibility to motor neuron damage by poliovirus infection and aging processes, perhaps residing in the poliovirus receptor.

**Associated Findings:** Genetic polymorphisms of the poliovirus receptor have been postulated but not established. Physical signs and symptoms collectively referred to as the poliomyelitic constitution have been reported but never critically verified. Most patients with poliomyelitis have varying degrees of autonomic and sensory symptoms.

**Etiology:** Poliovirus sensitivity is an autosomal dominant trait. Poliomyelitis is transmittted by the three serotypes of the polio virus. Polio virus is an Enterovirus of the family Picornaviridae. It is transmitted by the oral-fecal route. Rarely it has been transmitted iatrogenically by the parenteral route. Family clusters of poliomyelitis have been described. Whether genetic predisposition plays a part in these clusters is unclear. Past studies have claimed that a hereditary factor or an autosomal recessive gene is responsible for paralytic polio. However, scientific documentation is lacking. An initial study reported an increased frequence of HLA-A3 and HLA-A7 histocompatibility antigens in patients with previous poliomyelitis, but a second study could not confirm an association between paralytic polio and HLA-A type. Pregnancy, trauma, increased age, and increased physical activity predispose to paralytic poliomyelitis.

**Pathogenesis:** Lytic poliovirus infection of neurons and the accompanying inflammatory response are the most likely mechanisms of central nervous system damage. Sensitivity to polio virus infection is mediated by a dominant gene localized to the proximal long arm of chromosome 19. The sensitivity is primarily a cell-surface characteristic which is thought to be receptor mediated. Binding studies have shown that the poliovirus receptor is widely present in the central nervous system, and may lie on axon terminals of motor neurons. The virus reaches neurons by hematogenous as well as axonal spread. The worsened severity of paralysis in exercised limbs may be explained by the postulated availability of poliovirus receptors at the neuromuscular junction, leading to axonal spread. Another explanation may be that exercise results in an increase in the number of poliovirus receptors on the motor neurons innervating the exercised limbs. Differences in susceptibility due to age may also be explained in terms of differences in type or number of receptors. However, no differences in the receptor types between different cells or between adult and children have been described, nor has the receptor been isolated or its gene cloned.
The mechanism for the post-polio syndrome or for PPMA is unclear. Persistent poliovirus infection has not been demonstrated in these individuals. Some investigators favor an "overuse" theory. Inflammatory cells have been noted in muscle of these individuals, and in one case, in the spinal cord. It is possible that the mechanism of this syndrome is through antibody directed against the poliovirus receptor on the motor neuron. If the receptor is bound to the antibody and deprived of its natural ligand, the receptor may no longer be able to fulfill its biological role, thereby resulting in motor neuron dysfunction. This theory can be tested by demonstrating receptor-binding antibodies in the sera or CSF of patients with PPMA.

**MIM No.:** *17385

**Sex Ratio:** M1:F1 for poliomyelitis. For PPMA, it has been reported as M2.7:F1 as well as M1:F1.

**Occurrence:** The incidence of poliomyelitis varies with the immune status of the population. In non-immunized populations, it is estimated to be about 1:10,000. Since the introduction of effective programs of vaccination, paralytic poliomyelitis occurs primarily in non-immunized individuals, children with immune deficiency, and susceptible individuals exposed to the vaccine virus, either directly or after fecal passage. Some data suggest attenuated-live virus can revert to a more virulent form in the GI tracts of immunized children; this process has been documented with Poliovirus III. In 1984 there were eight cases of poliomyelitis in the United States, most vaccine-related. In some underdeveloped countries, poliomyelitis continues to be epidemic, mainly due to inadequate immunization programs. Recurrence with a serotype of poliovirus different from the initial infection has occurred.

**Risk of Recurrence for Patient's Sib:** There is no evidence of increased risk of poliomyelitis in siblings, except in non-immunized or immune deficient populations.

**Risk of Recurrence for Patient's Child:** Little risk except in non-immunized or immune deficient populations. A greater risk is to non-immunized adults who come in contact with a child who has recently received the oral vaccine, since the attenuated virus may mutate into a virulent form after passage through the GI tract. Poliovirus sensitivity is an autosomal dominant trait, it is undetermined if receptors resistant to polio virus exist among the human population.

**Age of Detectability:** Poliomyelitis can occur at any age. The incidence and severity is age dependent. The ratio of inapparent to paralytic disease in children is 1000:1, while in adults it is 75:1. No case of *in-utero* poliomyelitis has been convincingly documented.

**Gene Mapping and Linkage:** PVS (poliovirus sensitivity) has been mapped to 19q12-q13.2.

**Prevention:** Paralytic poliomyelitis is preventable by either inactivated (Salk) or live-attenuated (Sabin) poliovirus vaccines. The use of these vaccines has brought about a dramatic decline in the number of paralytic cases in the United States from an average of 21,000 cases per year to just eight in 1984. Problems associated with inactivated vaccine have been generally overcome. The major complication of live-attenuated polio virus is the development of paralytic polio in vaccine recipients and contacts. This risk is low, but vaccine-related cases outnumber naturally occurring ones in immunized populations like the United States.

**Treatment:** Treatment for poliomyelitis is symptomatic. In an epidemic, during the preparalytic period, the patient should remain quiet and rest. Analgesics and hot packs are applied for comfort. In the paralyzed patient, intensive nursing care and positional measures are used to prevent complications. Respiratory support may be needed in case of respiratory failure. Orthopedic and physical therapy measures are instituted for rehabilitation.

There is no treatment for PPMA, although a trial of plasmapheresis for these patients has been proposed, based on the autoantibody theory.

**Prognosis:** Death in poliomyelitis is usually due to respiratory failure. Mortality varies with epidemics and has been reduced due to advanced treatment of complications. In 1916 the mortality was 26.9% in the United States. Patients who survive usually recover considerable motor function. Sixty percent of the eventual recovery occurs in the first three months, 80% in six months and the rest during the next two years. It is likely that improvement occurs due to recovery of sick neurons and due to collateral sprouting of healthy axons, which then innervate the denervated muscle fibers. Muscle fibers may hypertrophy with physical activity and further improve strength.

PPMA, when compared to **Amyotrophic lateral sclerosis**, is a relatively benign disease. In one series, 34 patients were observed for an average of 8.7 years. In only one did the clinical illness cause death.

**Detection of Carrier:** Poliovirus can be excreted for 4–8 weeks after immunization with live-attenuated virus. Some individuals may excrete virus for a prolonged period of time. The virus can be detected by stool culture.

**Special Considerations:** The genetic susceptibility of paralytic poliomyelitis remains unproven. The cause of PPMA as a remote complication of paralytic poliomyelitis remains enigmatic. Persistence of polio virus has not been demonstrated in PPMA or in other motor neuron diseases. What part, if any, the poliovirus receptor plays in inherited motor neuron diseases such as **Amyotrophic lateral sclerosis** and the spinal muscular atrophies is under investigation. As the genes for the poliovirus (sensitivity) receptor and myotonic dystrophy are linked to the same region of chromosome 19, the gene for the poliovirus receptor can be tested as a candidate gene for myotonic dystrophy once it has been cloned.

**References:**
Kovacs E: The biochemistry of poliomyelitis viruses. New York: Macmillan, 1964.
Price RW, Plum F: Handbook of clinical neurology, vol 34. Amsterdam: North Holland Publishing Co., 1978:93–132.
Dalakas MC, et al: A long term follow-up study of patients with post-poliomyelitis neuromuscular symptoms. New Engl J Med 1986; 313:959–963.
Mendelsohn C, et al: Transformation of a human poliovirus receptor gene into mouse cells. Proc Natl Acad Sci 1986; 83:7845–7849.
Siddique T, et al: The poliovirus sensitivity (PVS) gene is on chromosome 19q12-q13.2. Genomics 1988; 3:156–160.

SI032                **Teepu Siddique**
MC039             **Ross McKinney**

**Poliodystrophica cerebri dystrophica**
    *See ALPERS DISEASE*
**Poliomyelitis**
    *See POLIO, SUSCEPTIBILITY TO*
**Poliovirus receptor**
    *See POLIO, SUSCEPTIBILITY TO*
**Polish hereditary amyloidosis**
    *See AMYLOIDOSIS, ASHKENAZI TYPE*
**Pollex varus**
    *See THUMB, CLASPED*
**Pollitt syndrome**
    *See TRICHOTHIODYSTROPHY*
**Polychlorinated biphenyl (PCB), fetal effects of**
    *See FETAL EFFECTS OF POLYCHLORINATED BIPHENYL (PCB)*
**Polycystic disease of infancy and childhood**
    *See KIDNEY, POLYCYSTIC DISEASE, RECESSIVE*
**Polycystic disease of the newborn**
    *See KIDNEY, POLYCYSTIC DISEASE, RECESSIVE*
**Polycystic kidney disease, medullary type**
    *See KIDNEY, NEPHRONOPHTHISIS-MEDULLARY CYSTIC DESEASE*
**Polycystic lipomembranous osteodysplasia-leukoencephalopathy**
    *See OSTEODYSPLASIA, LIPOMEMBRANOUS POLYCYSTIC-DEMENTIA*
**Polycystic ovary disease due to 17-KSR deficiency**
    *See STEROID 17-KETOSTEROID REDUCTASE DEFICIENCY*
**Polycystic renal disease, adult type (Potter type III)**
    *See KIDNEY, POLYCYSTIC DISEASE, DOMINANT*

---

**POLYDACTYLY**                         **0814**

**Includes:**
    Fromont anomaly
    Index finger polydactyly
    Preaxial polydactyly I, II, and III
    Polydactyly of index finger
    Postaxial polydactyly, types A and B
    Thenar hypoplasia
    Thumb polydactyly
    Triphalangeal thumb, opposable

**Excludes:**
    **Chondroectodermal dysplasia** (0156)
    **Chromosome 13, trisomy 13** (0168)
    **Laurence-Moon syndrome** (0578)
    Polydactyly, pre- or postaxial, in complex malformation syndromes
    **Polysyndactyly** (0817)
    **Syndactyly** (0923)

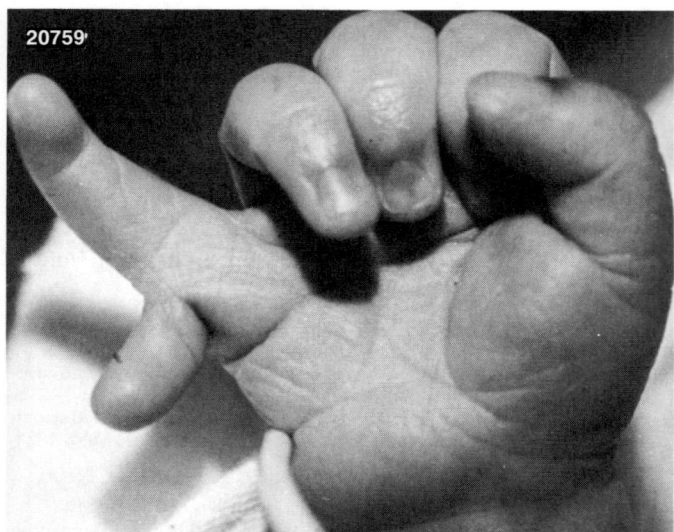

**0814**-20759: Polydactyly, post-axial.

**Major Diagnostic Criteria:** An extra digital triradius is found at the base of the extra digit. When it is a pedunculated postminimus that was surgically removed or fell out spontaneously, the extra triradius in the dermatoglyphics may be the only evidence of postaxial polydactyly.

**Clinical Findings:** In *preaxial polydactyly* the extra digit is on the radial side of the hand. The deformity in polydactyly of the thumb is duplication of all or part of the components of a thumb. In polydactyly of a triphalangeal thumb, the thumb has three phalanges, with duplication of all or part of its components. In polydactyly of the index finger, the thumb is present and the index finger is duplicated. Dermatoglyphic findings in this case are diagnostic, since an extra A triradius and an A line are present, corresponding to the extra index finger. In polysyndactyly, preaxial polydactyly of the toes is associated with variable degrees of syndactyly of the toes and fingers.

In *postaxial polydactyly*, the extra digit is on the ulnar side in the upper limb and the fibular side in the lower limb. Two phenotypic and possibly genetically different varieties exist. In one of them, postaxial polydactyly type A, the extra digit is rather well formed and articulates with the fifty or extra metacarpal. In postaxial polydactyly type B, or pedunculated postminimus, the extra digit is not well formed and is frequently in the form of a skin tag.

**Complications:** Unknown.

**Associated Findings:** None known.

**Etiology:** Usually autosomal dominant inheritance with variable expressivity. Thumb polydactyly is frequently unilateral, and most cases are sporadic with no evidence of inheritance.

**Pathogenesis:** Unknown.

**MIM No.:** *17450, *17460, *17420, 17440

**CDC No.:** 755.0

**Sex Ratio:** M1:F1

**Occurrence:** Postaxial polydactyly is about ten times more frequent in Blacks than in Caucasians. In American whites, incidence figures vary from 1:3,300 to 1:630 live births, and in American Blacks figures vary from 1:300 to 1:100 live births.

**Risk of Recurrence for Patient's Sib:**
See Part I, *Mendelian Inheritance.*

**Risk of Recurrence for Patient's Child:**
See Part I, *Mendelian Inheritance.*

**Age of Detectability:** In utero by fetoscopy (polydactyly), and at birth.

**Gene Mapping and Linkage:** Unknown.

**Prevention:** None known. Genetic counseling indicated.

**Treatment:** Surgical removal of the extra digit.

**Prognosis:** Polydactyly as an isolated malformation does not affect life span.

**Detection of Carrier:** Unknown.

**References:**
Atasu M: Hereditary index finger polysyndactyly: phenotypic, radiological, dermatoglyphic, and genetic findings in a large family. J Med Genet 1976; 13:469–476.

Temtamy SA, McKusick VA: The genetics of hand malformations. New York: Alan R. Liss, for The National Foundation-March of Dimes, 1978.

Ventruto V, et al.: Postaxial polydactyly in two members of the same family. Clin Genet 1980; 18:342–347.

Kucheria K, et al.: An Indian family with postaxial polydactyly in four generations. Clin Genet 1981; 20:36–39.

Graham JM, Jr., et al.: Thumb polydactyly as part of the range of genetic expression for thenar hypoplasia. (Abstract) Am J Hum Genet 1985; 37:A132.

Merlob P, et al.: Familial opposable thriphalangeal thumbs associated with duplication of the big toes. J Med Genet 1985; 22:78–80.

TE004                                                      **Samia A. Temtamy**

**Polydactyly (postaxial)-cortical blindness-growth retardation**
*See BLINDNESS (CORTICAL)-RETARDATION-POSTAXIAL POLYDACTYLY*
**Polydactyly of index finger**
*See POLYDACTYLY*
**Polydactyly of thumbs/hallux-extra phalanges in the thumbs**
*See THUMB, TRIPHALANGEAL-DUPLICATED GREAT TOES*
**Polydactyly, postaxial type A-scalp defects**
*See SCALP DEFECTS-POSTAXIAL POLYDACTYLY*
**Polydactyly, postaxial-median cleft of upper lip**
*See ORO-FACIO-DIGITAL SYNDROME, THURSTON TYPE*
**Polydactyly, preaxial II**
*See THUMB, TRIPHALANGEAL-DUPLICATED GREAT TOES*
**Polydactyly-chondrodystrophy**
*See CHONDROECTODERMAL DYSPLASIA*
**Polydactyly-cleft lip/palate/lingual lump-psychomotor retardation**
*See ORO-PALATAL-DIGITAL SYNDROME, VARADI TYPE*
**Polydactyly-conical teeth-nail dysplasia-short limbs**
*See ACROFACIAL SYNDROME, CURRY-HALL TYPE*

---

## POLYDACTYLY-DISTAL OBSTRUCTIVE UROPATHY          2644

**Includes:**
Postaxial polydactyly-distal obstructive uropathy
Urethral valve, posterior-polydactyly

**Excludes:**
Meckel syndrome (0634)
Postaxial polydactyly as a part of other syndromes

**Major Diagnostic Criteria:** Postaxial polydactyly with or without **Syndactyly** in one or more limbs; posterior urethral valve.

**Clinical Findings:** The association of postaxial polydactyly with distal obstructive uropathy was described in two unrelated stillborn male babies of 36 and 36 1/2 weeks of age respectively. Patient one had Potter sequence involvement (see **Renal agenesis, bilateral** of the face, left postaxial synpolydactyly of the hand, and posterior urethral valve. Patient two had postaxial polydactyly of the left hand and right foot and probable posterior urethral valve.

**Complications:** Patient one had dilation of the proximal portion of the urethra, dilation of the bladder with thickening and a few trabeculations of its wall, bilateral hydroureters, marked bilateral hydronephrosis with renal cystic dysplasia type II-B of Potter, undescended testes, and hypospadias grade I. He also had congestion and complete atelectasis of the lungs. In patient two, catheterization of the urethra was possible for a distance of only 0.5 cm. The bladder was extremely dilated with a smooth wall. Hydroureters were bilateral with no evidence of ureteral stenosis. The kidneys showed marked bilateral hydronephrosis. There was bilateral cryptorchidism. Microscopic examination of the entire penile portion of the urethra failed to show any stenosis. It is likely that the obstruction was caused either by a posterior urethral valve (the abdominal portion of the urethra was not examined) or, less likely, by an anterior urethral stenosis in the region of the glans.

**Associated Findings:** Patient one had patent foramen ovale.

**Etiology:** Unknown.

**Pathogenesis:** Associated anomalies of the genitourinary tract are actually manifestations of the primary defect, namely, posterior urethral valve. Bona fide renal parenchymal malformations with polydactyly suggest the presence of an acrorenal developmental defect (DFD), in and of itself a causally nonspecific malformation. However, since the renal dysplasia in patient one and hydronephrosis in both patients were secondary to distal obstructive uropathy, the association probably does not represent an acrorenal DFD.

**Sex Ratio:** M1:F0. Only males are affected, since a posterior urethral valve is present only in males.

**Occurrence:** Two infants were seen in the months of December 1980 and December 1984 (from a total of approximately 7,502 births).

**Risk of Recurrence for Patient's Sib:** Unknown. Kidney echogram of patient one's brother showed a prominent cystic structure (4.5 ;ts 5 cm) involving the superior aspect of the left kidney. Urologic investigation showed bilateral duplication of the collecting system and ectopic ureterocele with megaureter and hydronephrosis of the left upper pole collecting system. A paternal cousin of the patient had bilateral hydroureters, right more than left.

**Risk of Recurrence for Patient's Child:** Unknown.

**Age of Detectability:** At birth. Prenatal diagnosis is probably possible by routine ultrasonography.

**Gene Mapping and Linkage:** Unknown.

**Prevention:** Prenatal treatment of hydronephrosis may be possible.

**Treatment:** Prenatal treatment of hydronephrosis may be possible.

**Prognosis:** Both known patients were stillborn.

**Detection of Carrier:** Careful clinical and urologic examinations of first degree relatives will help to clarify the spectrum of manifestations.

**Special Considerations:** Because advanced autolysis did not permit good examination of the central nervous system, associated anomalies of the brain could not be definitely excluded.

**References:**
Halal F: Distal obstructive uropathy with polydactyly: a new syndrome? (Letter) Am J Med Genet 1986; 24:753–757.

HA074                                                    **Fahed Halal**

**Polydactyly-ectrodactyly**
  See ECTRODACTYLY-POLYDACTYLY
**Polydactyly-imperforate anus**
  See VATER ASSOCIATION
**Polydactyly-Joubert syndrome**
  See JOUBERT SYNDROME
**Polydactyly-neonatal chondrodystrophy, type I**
  See SHORT RIB-POLYDACTYLY SYNDROME, TYPE I
**Polydactyly-neonatal chondrodystrophy, type II**
  See SHORT RIB-POLYDACTYLY SYNDROME, TYPE II
**Polydactyly-neonatal chondrodystrophy, type III**
  See SHORT RIB-POLYDACTYLY SYNDROME, VERMA-NAUMOFF TYPE
**Polydactyly-obesity-hypogenitalism-iris coloboma**
  See BIEMOND II SYNDROME
**Polydactyly-Robin anomaly-skeletal dysplasia**
  See CLEFT PALATE-DYSMORPHIC FACIES-DIGITAL DEFECTS, MARTSOLF TYPE
**Polydactyly-sex reversal-renal hypoplasia-unilobular lung**
  See SMITH-LEMLI-OPITZ SYNDROME, TYPE II

**Polydactyly-syndactyly-ear lobe syndrome**
  See SYNDACTYLY-POLYDACTYLY-EAR LOBE SYNDROME
**Polydontia**
  See TEETH, SUPERNUMERARY
**Polydysspondyly**
  See SPONDYLOCOSTAL DYSPLASIA
**Polydystrophia oligophrenia**
  See MUCOPOLYSACCHARIDOSIS III

---

## POLYGLANDULAR AUTOIMMUNE SYNDROME     2623

**Includes:**
  Autoimmune polyendocrinopathy-candidiasis-ectodermal dystrophy
  Candidiasis-endocrinopathy syndrome
  Hypoadrenocorticism-hypoparathyroidism-superficial moniliasis
  Moniliasis, familial
  Whitaker syndrome

**Excludes:** Candidiasis, familial chronic mucocutaneous (2117)

**Major Diagnostic Criteria:** Familial occurrence of chronic candidal infection of mucous membranes, skin, and nails. Polyendocrinopathy occurs in roughly one-half of the cases.

**Clinical Findings:** Chronic candidal infection of the oral mucous membranes is almost always evident and usually develops in early childhood, often before age two years. Chronic candidal infection of fingernails and toenails is also frequently present and may result in severe dystrophic changes. Cutaneous disease is somewhat less common and affects primarily the face, hands, and feet. Those severely affected may develop candidal granuloma (thick, hyperkeratotic plaques of the face or nails). Systemic candidiasis is uncommon. In those with endocrinopathy, symptoms and signs of deficient hormone production by the parathyroid, adrenal, and, less commonly, the thyroid, pancreas, stomach, and ovary usually become manifest in the second decade. In rare cases, endocrine abnormalities precede candidiasis by 5–10 years. Endocrinopathy is associated with autoimmunity to the involved gland. Chronic active hepatitis and cirrhosis occur in some patients. Alopecia and tooth hypoplasia are common. Chronic pulmonary disease occasionally develops.

**Complications:** Chronic hoarseness may result from candidal laryngitis. Disfiguring skin lesions may result in psychologic disturbances. Adrenal failure may result in sudden death. Tetany, seizures, cataracts, keratoconjunctivitis, and band keratopathy may occur as a result of hypoparathyroidism. Pancreatic insufficiency can result in steatorrhea and diabetes mellitus. Pernicious anemia and iron deficiency anemia are common.

**Associated Findings:** Thymoma, thymic dysplasia, and splenic agenesis.

**Etiology:** Autosomal recessive inheritance. Multifactorial etiology involving infectious and autoimmune components has also been suggested.

**Pathogenesis:** The frequent occurrence of abnormalities of the cellular immune system, including anergy, hypergammaglobulinemia, selective IgA deficiency, defective *in vitro* nonspecific T suppressor cell activity, impaired *in vitro* production of migration inhibition factor, and autoantibodies to endocrine tissue, have led to the theory that this condition results from an inherited abnormality of the immune system that primarily affects the T lymphocyte, which results in 1) abnormalities of immunoregulation leading to autoimmunity and 2) impaired host resistance to candidal infection.

**MIM No.:** *24030

**Sex Ratio:** M1:F1

**Occurrence:** About 150 cases have been reported, almost one-third from Finland.

**Risk of Recurrence for Patient's Sib:**
  See Part I, *Mendelian Inheritance.*

**Risk of Recurrence for Patient's Child:**
  See Part I, *Mendelian Inheritance.*

**Age of Detectability:** Usually clinically evident in early childhood.

**Gene Mapping and Linkage:** Unknown.

**Prevention:** None known. Genetic counseling indicated.

**Treatment:** Continuous antifungal therapy is usually required. Topical therapy with gentian violet, Mycostatin, and other similar agents is not curative but can prevent progression. Intravenous amphotericin B results in more marked improvement and clearing of lesions, but relapse is invariable. Renal toxicity limits its use. Surgical removal is the only definitive treatment for affected nails. Administration of transfer factor, thymosin, and levamisole have been used with only partial and inconsistent results. Bone marrow transplantation has been used successfully in a single case, but is not recommended because of the risk of graft-versus-host disease. In one study intravenous iron therapy provided a beneficial effect in 8:11 patients. Endocrinopathies must be treated as appropriate to each condition.

**Prognosis:** The outcome depends on the severity of such associated conditions as adrenal insufficiency, hypoparathyroidism, diabetes mellitus, and chronic liver disease. Normal life span is possible.

**Detection of Carrier:** Unknown.

**References:**

Wuepper KD, Fudenberg HH: Moniliasis, "autoimmune" polyendocrinopathy, and immunologic family study. Clin Exp Immunol 1967; 2:71–82.

Blizzard RM, Gibbs JH: Candidiasis: studies pertaining to its association with endocrinopathies and pernicious anemia. Pediatrics 1968; 42:231–237.

Wells RS, et al.: Familial chronic muco-cutaneous candidiasis. J Med Genet 1972; 9:302–310.

Arulanantham K, et al.: Evidence for defective immunoregulation in the syndrome of familial candidiasis endocrinopathy. New Engl J Med 1978; 300:164–168.

Stiehm ER, Fulginiti VA: Immunologic disorders in infants and children, ed 2. Philadelphia: W.B. Saunders, 1980. * †

Ahonen P: Autoimmune polyendocrinopathy-candidiasis-ectodermal dystrophy (APECED): autosomal recessive inheritance. Clin Genet 1985; 27:535–542.

Maclaren NK, Riley WJ: Inherited susceptibility to autoimmune Addison's disease is linked to human leukocyte antigens-DR3 and/or DR4, except when associated with type I autoimmune polyglandular syndrome. J Clin Endocr Metab 1986; 62:455–459.

KA038      **Joseph Kaplan**

**Polyglucosan body disease, adult**
See *SEIZURES, PROGRESSIVE MYOCLONIC, LAFORA TYPE*
**Polykeratosis congenita**
See *NAILS, PACHYONYCHIA CONGENITA*
**Polymastia (polymastie)**
See *BREAST, POLYTHELIA*
**Polymicrogyria**
See *BRAIN, MICROPOLYGYRIA*
**Polymorphous posterior corneal dystrophy**
See *CORNEAL DYSTROPHY, POLYMORPHOUS POSTERIOR*
**Polyneuropathy, familial recurrent**
See *NEUROPATHY, HEREDITARY WITH PRESSURE PALSIES*
**Polyneuropathy-accumulation of neurofilaments**
See *NEUROPATHY, GIANT AXONAL*
**Polyneuropathy-deafness-optic atrophy**
See *DEAFNESS-POLYNEUROPATHY-OPTIC ATROPHY*
**Polyosteochondrite (Turpin and Coste)**
See *EPIPHYSEAL DYSPLASIA, MULTIPLE*
**Polyostotic fibrous dysplasia-skin pigmentation-sexual precocity**
See *FIBROUS DYSPLASIA, POLYOSTOTIC*
**Polyploid phenotype**
See *CHROMOSOME TETRAPLOIDY*
**Polyposis coli, juvenile type**
See *INTESTINAL POLYPOSIS, JUVENILE TYPE*
**Polyposis, familial**
See *INTESTINAL POLYPOSIS, TYPE I*
**Polyposis, Gardner type**
See *INTESTINAL POLYPOSIS, TYPE III*
**Polyposis, intestinal, II**
See *INTESTINAL POLYPOSIS, TYPE II*
**Polyposis, juvenile**
See *INTESTINAL POLYPOSIS, JUVENILE TYPE*

## POLYPOSIS-ALOPECIA-PIGMENTATION-NAIL DEFECTS    3040

**Includes:**

Alopecia-polyposis-pigmentation-nail defects
Cronkhite-Canada syndrome
Gastrointestinal polyposis-ectodermal defects
Pigmentation-alopecia-polyposis-nail defects

**Excludes:**
    **Intestinal polyposis, type II** (2344)
    **Intestinal polyposis, type III** (0536)

**Major Diagnostic Criteria:** Gastrointestinal symptoms (weight loss, vomiting, and diarrhea) associated with hair loss, nail atrophy, and skin hyperpigmentation should suggest the diagnosis.

**Clinical Findings:** Individuals with this condition present with diarrhea, vomiting, anorexia, and sometimes with abdominal pains. Alopecia, nail changes (in the form of loss or dystrophy), and hyperpigmentation of skin or mucosa accompany the gastrointestinal symptoms. X-ray evaluation of the GI tract demonstrates generalized polyposis of the stomach and colon, with occasional involvement of duodenum, rectum, and esophagus. Death usually occurs after a duration of 6–18 months. Onset is at 30–80 years of age. Early descriptions of the polyps have classified them as adenomas, histologically; more recently thay have been characterized as hamartomatous polyps of the juvenile type.

**Complications:** Weight loss, muscle weakness, anemia, and edema all occurred as complications.

**Associated Findings:** Six patients had numbness and tingling, four developed cataracts, two had seizures, and one each had syncope and transient ischemia.

**Etiology:** The cause of this condition is obscure, although it is not thought to be genetic. All reported cases have been sporadic occurrences in otherwise normal families.

**Pathogenesis:** It has been suggested that the ectodermal changes are secondary to an as yet unidentified nutritional deficiency caused by the diffuse polyposis. However, in one patient, the nail changes occurred years before onset of gastrointestinal symptoms, so the ectodermal changes may be concomitant, rather than secondary, findings.

**MIM No.:** 17550

**POS No.:** 3844

**Sex Ratio:** M1:F1

**Occurrence:** More than 50 cases, from all parts of the world, have been reported.

**Risk of Recurrence for Patient's Sib:** Probably not increased.

**Risk of Recurrence for Patient's Child:** Probably not increased.

**Age of Detectability:** Onset of the disorder has been between the ages of 40 and 70 years.

**Gene Mapping and Linkage:** Unknown.

**Prevention:** None known. Genetic counseling indicated.

**Treatment:** Aggressive supportive therapy is recommended over surgical intervention. However, hemicolectomy in one case and partial gastrectomy in another led to apparent recovery.

**Prognosis:** Death usually occurs 6–18 months from the onset of symptoms; however, some patients have survived for 15 years. Death usually occurs in severely symptomatic patients who fail to respond to therapeutic measurers.

**Detection of Carrier:** Unknown.

**Special Considerations:** This condition must be distinguished from the genetic polyposes so that accurate genetic counseling can be provided to relatives.

**References:**

Cronkhite LW, Jr., Canada WJ: Generalized gastrointestinal polyposis: an unusual syndrome of polyposis, pigmentation, alopecia and onychotrophia. New Engl J Med 1955; 252:1011–1015.

Jarnum S, Jensen H: Diffuse gastrointestinal polyposis with ectodermal changes: a case with severe malabsorption and enteric loss of plasma proteins and electrolytes. Gastroenterology 1966; 50:107–118.

Dacruz GMG: Generalized gastrointestinal polyposis: an unusual syndrome of adenomatous polyposis, alopecia, onychorotrophia. Am J Gastroenterol 1967; 47:504–510.

Daniel ES, et al.: The Cronkhite-Canada syndrome: an analysis of clinical and pathologic features and therapy in 55 patients. Medicine 1982; 61:293–309. *

T0007        **Helga V. Toriello**

**Polysaccharide storage cardioskeletal myopathy**
*See MYOPATHY-METABOLIC, GLYCOPROTEIN-GLYCOSAMINOGLYCANS STORAGE TYPE*
**Polyserositis, benign paroxysmal**
*See FEVER, FAMILIAL MEDITERRANEAN (FMF)*
**Polyserositis, recurrent**
*See FEVER, FAMILIAL MEDITERRANEAN (FMF)*
**Polysplenia syndrome**
*See ASPLENIA SYNDROME*

## POLYSYNDACTYLY      0817

**Includes:**
Preaxial polydactyly IV
Preaxial polydactyly of toes associated with syndactyly

**Excludes:**
**Acrocephalosyndactyly**
**Polysyndactyly-dysmorphic craniofacies, Greig type** (2925)
**Syndactyly** (0923)

**Major Diagnostic Criteria:** An extra or duplicated digit occurs with syndactyly (webbing between digits).

**Clinical Findings:** In the feet, preaxial polydactyly or duplication of the first or second toes is associated with syndactyly of various degrees. In the hands, the most common malformation is syndactyly of the third and fourth fingers; the terminal phalanx of the thumb is usually malformed, broad and short, or bifid, and sometimes radially deviated. Pedunculated postminimi is a feature in some families. While the hand malformation is mild and variable, malformation of the feet is constant and nearly uniform.

**Complications:** Unknown.

**Associated Findings:** None known.

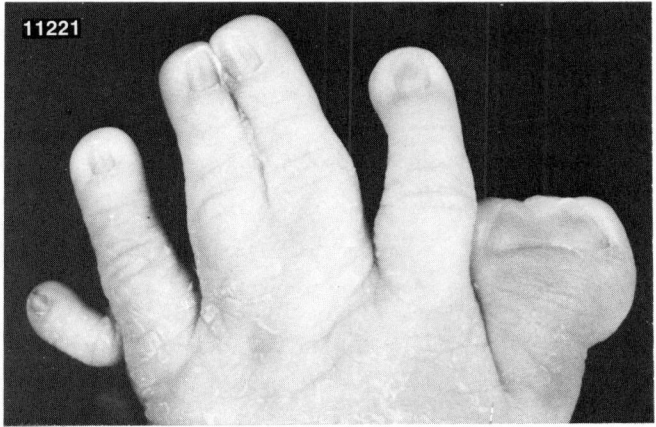

**0817-11221:** Combined pre- and post-axial polysyndactyly.

**Etiology:** Autosomal dominant inheritance with variable expression and complete penetrance.

**Pathogenesis:** Unknown.

**MIM No.:** *17470

**Sex Ratio:** M1:F1

**Occurrence:** Undetermined. Several large kindreds have been reported.

**Risk of Recurrence for Patient's Sib:**
See Part I, *Mendelian Inheritance.*

**Risk of Recurrence for Patient's Child:**
See Part I, *Mendelian Inheritance.*

**Age of Detectability:** At birth.

**Gene Mapping and Linkage:** Unknown.

**Prevention:** None known. Genetic counseling indicated.

**Treatment:** Surgical correction of malformation.

**Prognosis:** Normal life span.

**Detection of Carrier:** Unknown.

**Special Considerations:** Recent research (Baraitser et al, 1983) has pointed out a similarity between polysyndactyly and **Polysyndactyly-dysmorphic craniofacies, Greig type.** The delineation of polysyndactyly as a distinct entity (Temtamy and McKusick, 1978) is, therefore, no longer certain.

**References:**

Goodman RM: A family with polysyndactyly and other anomalies. J Hered 1965; 56:37–38.

Temtamy SA, Loutfy AH: Polysyndactyly in an Egyptian family. BD:OAS X(5). New York: March of Dimes Birth Defects Foundation, 1974:207.

Temtamy SA, McKusick VA: The genetics of hand malformations. New York: Alan R. Liss, 1978.

Baraitser M, et al.: Greig cephalopolysyndactyly: report of 13 affected individuals in three families. Clin Genet 1983; 24:257–265.

Reynolds JF, et al.: Preaxial polydactyly type 4: variability in a large kindred. Clin Genet 1984; 25:267–272.

TE004        **Samia A. Temtamy**

**Polysyndactyly, postaxial-frontonasal dysostosis-cleft lip/palate**
*See ACRO-FRONTO-FACIO-NASAL DYSOSTOSIS*

## POLYSYNDACTYLY-CARDIAC MALFORMATIONS      2815

**Includes:** Heart defects-polysyndactyly

**Excludes:**
**Chondroectodermal dysplasia** (0156)
**Oro-facio-digital syndrome, Mohr type** (0771)
**Polysyndactyly-dysmorphic craniofacies, Greig type** (2925)

**Major Diagnostic Criteria:** The combination of mild facial anomalies, **Syndactyly** of the fingers, duplicated great toes, and cardiac malformations.

**Clinical Findings:** The gestations of all affected individuals were complicated by polyhydramnios; two of the children were stillborn. Facial anomalies in the surviving child included **Eye, hypertelorism** with epicanthal folds, short nose with anteverted nares, long and poorly defined philtrum, micrognathia, posteriorly rotated ears, and creased earlobes. Hirsutism was present on the face and upper trunk. Limb defects were present in all three, and consisted of duplicated great toes (3/3) and **Syndactyly** of fingers 2–5 (2/3). The liveborn child had **Atrial septal defects** and **Ventricular septal defect**; the stillborn children had a single ventricle with a common atrioventricular valve.

**Complications:** Unknown.

**Associated Findings:** A **Urofacial syndrome** was present in one child but may have been a coincidental finding.

**Etiology:** Possibly autosomal recessive inheritance.

**Pathogenesis:** Unknown.

**MIM No.:** 26363

**POS No.:** 3814

**Sex Ratio:** Presumably M1:F1.

**Occurrence:** One sibship of three affected individuals has been reported from France.

**Risk of Recurrence for Patient's Sib:**
See Part I, *Mendelian Inheritance.*

**Risk of Recurrence for Patient's Child:**
See Part I, *Mendelian Inheritance.*

**Age of Detectability:** At birth, although prenatal diagnosis by ultrasound may be possible.

**Gene Mapping and Linkage:** Unknown.

**Prevention:** None known. Genetic counseling indicated.

**Treatment:** Supportive; surgical correction of the cardiac defect may be indicated.

**Prognosis:** Of three reported cases, two were stillborn, and the third died at age 5 1/2 months. Intellectual development is undetermined.

**Detection of Carrier:** Unknown.

**References:**
Bonneau JC, et al.: Polysyndactylie avec cardiopathie complexe a propos de trois cas dans une meme fratrie. J Genet Hum 1983; 31:93–105.

T0007        Helga V. Toriello

---

## POLYSYNDACTYLY-DYSMORPHIC CRANIOFACIES, GREIG TYPE      2925

**Includes:**
Cephalopolysyndactyly syndrome, Greig type
Craniofacial anomalies-polysyndactyly
Frontodigital syndrome
Greig cephalopolysyndactyly syndrome
Skull, peculiar shape-polysyndactyly

**Excludes:**
**Acrocallosal syndrome, Schinzel type** (2263)
Cephalopolysyndactyly syndromes, other
**Eye, hypertelorism** (0504)

**Major Diagnostic Criteria:** Pronounced cutaneous **Syndactyly** of toes and fingers, postaxial **Polydactyly** of toes and fingers, complete or partial duplication of the halluces, and scaphocephaly.

**Clinical Findings:** Craniofacial features include **Megalencephaly**, scaphocephaly, prominent forehead (frontal bossing), and **Eye, hypertelorism** but no overt craniostenosis. Plagiocephaly may occasionally be seen. The most common features of the hands are syndactyly and pedunculated postminimi polydactyly. The syndactyly varies from mild cutaneous webbing to bony fusion. Occasionally, the thumbs may be duplicated or have broad tips. In

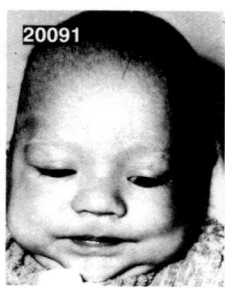 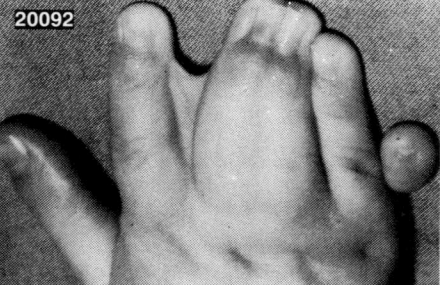

**2925-20091:** Typical craniofacies with high, broad forehead, hypertelorism and broad nasal base. **20092:** Polysyndactyly of the hand.

the feet, the syndactyly is variable and the polydactyly is commonly preaxial, although postaxial polydactyly may be seen. Intelligence is normal in affected individuals, and CT scans show only mild-to-moderate enlargement of the lateral ventricles, basal cisterns, and sylvian fissures.

**Complications:** Palsy of fifth cranial nerve, divergent strabismus, and **Camptodactyly**.

**Associated Findings: Hernia, inguinal.** While mental development is usually normal, mental retardation and absence of corpus callosum has been documented in a small number of patients. Other rare occasional findings include growth retardation and genital hypoplasia. It is undetermined if **Acrocallosal syndrome, Schinzel type** is a distinct entity or a variable expression of the same condition.

**Etiology:** Autosomal dominant inheritance with wide variation in expression. Various chromosomal anomalies have also been suggested.

**Pathogenesis:** The skull congfiguration has led to the suggestion that the cranial features result from basal hypoplasia with compensatory calvarial expansion and retention of an infantile forehead.

**MIM No.:** *17570

**POS No.:** 3489

**Sex Ratio:** M1:F1

**Occurrence:** Unknown. A few dozen cases have been reported, but the features may be so mild that many affected individuals escape notice.

**Risk of Recurrence for Patient's Sib:**
See Part I, *Mendelian Inheritance.*

**Risk of Recurrence for Patient's Child:**
See Part I, *Mendelian Inheritance.*

**Age of Detectability:** Prenatal, by ultrasound observation of polydactyly and macrocephaly.

**Gene Mapping and Linkage:** GCPS (Greig cephalopolysyndactyly syndrome) has been mapped to 7p13.

**Prevention:** None known. Genetic counseling indicated.

**Treatment:** Surgical release of syndactyly and removal of supernumerary digits.

**Prognosis:** Good for life span and general health in the absence of major internal malformations.

**Detection of Carrier:** Unknown.

**References:**
Greig DM: Oxycephaly. Edinb Med J 1928; 33:189–218.
Marshall RE, Smith DW: Frontodigital syndrome: a dominantly inherited disorder with normal intelligence. J Pediatr 1970; 77:129–133. *
Hootnick D, Holmes LB: Familial polysyndactyly and craniofacial anomalies. Clin Genet 1972; 3:128–134. * †
Baraitser M, et al.: Greig cephalopolysyndactyly: report of 13 affected individuals in three families. Clin Genet 1983; 24:257–265. †
Fryns JP, et al.: The Greig polysyndactyly-craniofacial dysmorphism syndrome. Eur J Pediatr 1977; 126:283–287. †
Gallop TR, Fontes LR: The Greig cephalopolysyndactyly syndrome: report of a family and review of the literature. Am J Med Genet 1985; 22:59–68. †
Kruger G, et al.: Greig syndrome in a large kindred due to reciprocal chromosome translocation t(6;7)(q27;p13). Am J Med Genet 1989; 32:411–416.

J0027        Ronald J. Jorgenson
FR030        Jean-Pierre Fryns

**Pompe disease**
*See GLYCOGENOSIS, TYPE IIa*
**Ponstel^, fetal effects**
*See FETAL EFFECTS OF NONSTEROIDAL ANTI-INFLAMMATORY DRUGS (NSAIDS)*
**Popliteal pterygium syndrome**
*See PTERYGIUM SYNDROME, POPLITEAL*
**Popliteal pterygium syndrome, lethal type**
*See PTERYGIUM SYNDROME, POPLITEAL, LETHAL*

**Porcupine man**
  *See NEVUS, EPIDERMAL NEVUS SYNDROME*
**Porencephaly, prenatal**
  *See BRAIN, PORENCEPHALY*
**Porokeratosis of Mibelli**
  *See SKIN, POROKERATOSIS*
**Porokeratosis, linear**
  *See SKIN, POROKERATOSIS*
**Porokeratosis, plantaris**
  *See SKIN, POROKERATOSIS*
**Porphobilinogen deaminase deficiency**
  *See PORPHYRIA, ACUTE INTERMITTENT*
**Porphobilinogen synthase partial deficiency**
  *See DELTA-AMINOLEVULINIC ACID DEHYDRASE DEFICIENCY*

---

## PORPHYRIA CUTANEA TARDA       3064

**Includes:**
  Cutaneous porphyria
  Hepatoerythropoietic porphyria
  Porphyria, hepatocutaneous type
  Porphyria, hepatoerythropoietic
  Uroporphyrinogen decarboxylase deficiency

**Excludes:**
  Porphyria cutanea tarda, sporadic
  **Porphyria** (other)

**Major Diagnostic Criteria:** Characteristic bullous lesions on sun-exposed skin. Laboratory diagnosis requires measurement of porphyrins in both urine and stool. Traditional solvent partition methods demonstrate that uroporphyrin exceeds coproporphyrin in the urine, and coproporphyrin exceeds protoporphyrin in the stool. Chromatographic methods show mainly 8- and 7-carboxylate porphyrins in the urine and an increase of isocoproporphyrin in the stool.

**Clinical Findings:** Blisters form on the sun-exposed areas of the skin, particularly the dorsum of the hands and face. The involved skin is mechanically fragile. Subsequent ulceration and scarring may lead to a scleroderma-like thickening of the skin. Hyperpigmentation and hypertrichosis may also occur. Most patients have evidence of liver disease, with biopsy materials revealing hemosiderosis and lobular inflammatory cellular aggregates. Patients do not have acute photosensitivity and do not have acute porphyric attacks with neurovisceral symptoms.

**Complications:** Increased incidence of hepatocellular carcinoma.

**Associated Findings:** **Lupus erythematosus, systemic** and other autoimmune diseases.

**Etiology:** Autosomal dominant inheritance with variability in expression (the more common sporadic type appears to be the result of environmental injury without any evidence of a genetic component). *Hepatoerythropoietic porphyria* (Toback et al, 1987) is an autosomal recessive disease with less than 10% of normal activity of uroporphyriogen decarboxylase and might represent the homozygous form.

**Pathogenesis:** Fifty percent of normal activity of uroporphyrinogen decarboxylase (E.C. 4.1.1.37) in erythrocytes, liver, and other tissues. Additional agents, especially ethanol or estrogens, are required for overproduction of hepatic porphyrins. Hepatic iron plays a synergistic role in this toxic process by an unknown mechanism. The increased blood porphyrins cause the cutaneous manifestations, perhaps by activating the complement system.

**MIM No.:** *17610

**Sex Ratio:** M1:F1

**Occurrence:** Unknown. The most common porphyria. However, the vast majority of cases are believed to be sporadic, and only a small minority are familial.

**Risk of Recurrence for Patient's Sib:**
  See Part I, *Mendelian Inheritance.*

**Risk of Recurrence for Patient's Child:**
  See Part I, *Mendelian Inheritance.*

**Age of Detectability:** Rarely clinically evident before age 20 years and usually evident after age 40 years. The deficiency in the activity of uroporphyrinogen decarboxylase is detectable throughout life.

**Gene Mapping and Linkage:** UROD (uroporphyrinogen decarboxylase) has been mapped to 1p34.

**Prevention:** None known. Genetic counseling indicated.

**Treatment:** Elimination of potentially precipitating agents, including ethanol, oral iron supplements, oral estrogens, and halogenated aromatic hydrocarbons. Reduction of iron stores by phlebotomy or by subcutaneous desferoxamine infusion. Low-dose chloroquine or hydroxychloroquine is a secondary therapy.

**Prognosis:** Complete remission of symptoms occurs in the majority of patients with therapy. Compatible with a normal life span.

**Detection of Carrier:** Carriers have a 50% deficiency in the activity of uroporphyrinogen decarboxylase in the erythrocytes and liver.

**References:**
Lefkowitch JH, Grossman ME: Hepatic pathology in porphyria cutanea tarda. Liver 1983; 3:19–29.
de Verneuil H, et al.: Enzymatic and immunological studies of uroporphyrinogen decarboxylase in familial porphyria cutanea tarda and hepatoerythropoietic porphyria. Am J Hum Genet 1984; 36:613–622.
Dubart A, et al.: Assignment of human uroporphyrinogen decarboxylase (URO-D) to the p34 band of chromosome 1. Hum Genet 1986; 73(3):277–279.
Rocchi E, et al.: Serum ferritin in the assessment of liver iron overload and iron removal therapy in porphyria cutanea tarda. J Lab Clin Med 1986; 107:36–42.
Sweeney GD: Porphyria cutanea tarda, or the uroporphyrinogen decarboxylase deficiency diseases. Clin Biochem 1986; 19:3–15.
Toback AC, et al.: Hepatoerythropoietic porphyria: clinical, biochemical, and enzymatic studies in a three-generation family lineage. New Engl J Med 1987; 316:645–650.

BR038       **David A. Brenner**

**Porphyria, acute hepatic**
  *See DELTA-AMINOLEVULINIC ACID DEHYDRASE DEFICIENCY*

---

## PORPHYRIA, ACUTE INTERMITTENT       0820

**Includes:**
  PBGD deficiency
  Porphobilinogen deaminase deficiency
  Pyrroloporphyria
  Swedish genetic porphyria
  UPS deficiency

**Excludes:**
  **Delta-aminolevulinic acid dehydrase deficiency** (3091)
  **Porphyria, coproporphyria** (0203)
  **Porphyria, variegate** (0822)

**Major Diagnostic Criteria:** Demonstration of significantly increased porphobilinogen excretion (Watson-Schwartz test), tachycardia, and abdominal pain.

**Clinical Findings:** This condition may exist in a latent form for a lifetime or may be manifest by attacks of neurologic dysfunction. Four known groups of precipitating causes are drugs (barbiturates, sulfonamides, griseofulvin, diphenylhydantoin, and so forth); estrogen and possibly progesterone, oral contraceptives in certain cases; infections; and starvation. Some attacks occur without obvious precipitating factors. In about 10–20% of women with this disease attacks occur in a cyclic pattern, usually beginning about 3 days before menstrual periods.

  The acute attack results from damage in any portion of the nervous system. Signs and symptoms of the acute attack, which are all attributable to autonomic neuropathy, include abdominal pain, constipation (occasionally diarrhea), tachycardia, sweating, labile hypertension, postural hypotension, retinal artery spasm, and vascular spasm in the skin of the limbs. Peripheral neuropathy may be sensory or motor. There may be pain in the back or limbs (more commonly in the legs), which may persist for long periods without motor involvement or may precede motor paralysis. There may be paresthesias, but objective sensory findings are usually absent unless the sensory neuropathy is of long duration. Motor involvement is variable in terms of symmetry, severity, and rate of progress of the process. All peripheral nerves, including cranial, are subject to the neuropathy. CNS manifestations include bulbar paralysis, cerebellar and basal ganglion manifestations, hypothalamic dysfunction, seizures, acute and chronic psychoses, hallucinations, and coma.

Medullary and phrenic nerve involvement may cause respiratory paralysis, which is the most common cause of death. Hyponatremia, sometimes of severe degree, may result from excessive sodium loss from the GI tract or may be associated with the classic findings of the syndrome of inappropriate release of antidiuretic hormone (SIADH). Hypomagnesemia, occasionally sufficient to produce tetany, may accompany the hyponatremia.

The two most significant psychiatric syndromes associated with this disease are organic brain syndrome (irritability, restlessness, confusion, disorientation, hallucinations) and depression. BSP excretion may be normal or decreased during asymptomatic periods, but it is usually impaired during activity of the disease. Other frequent laboratory findings include hypercholesterolemia (40–50% of patients), increased serum PBI and thyroxin-binding globulin (TBG), and hyper-β-lipoproteinemia. During acute attacks, a diabetic glucose tolerance test is often demonstrable.

**Complications:** Chronic pain syndrome (peripheral or abdominal), motor paralysis (including respiratory paralysis), seizures, organic brain syndrome, depression.

**Associated Findings:** None known.

**Etiology:** Autosomal dominant inheritance.

**Pathogenesis:** An increase of delta-aminolevulinic acid synthase and rate-controlling enzyme of the heme biosynthetic pathway has been demonstrated in the livers of patients with this disease. The inherited defect is a decreased level of porphobilinogen deaminase (uroporphyrinogen I synthase). However, it is not clear how these findings relate to the acute attacks of neurologic dysfunction.

**MIM No.:** *17600

**Sex Ratio:** M1:F1.5

**Occurrence:** About 1:66,000 in the British Isles, but in certain areas such as Lapland it is much higher. Probably exceeds 1:66,000 worldwide.

**Risk of Recurrence for Patient's Sib:**
See Part I, *Mendelian Inheritance.*

**Risk of Recurrence for Patient's Child:**
See Part I, *Mendelian Inheritance.*

**Age of Detectability:** The disease is usually not manifest clinically, and is sometimes not evident biochemically before puberty.

**Gene Mapping and Linkage:** PBGD (porphobilinogen deaminase) has been mapped to 11q23.2-qter.

**Prevention:** None known. Genetic counseling indicated.

**Treatment:** Abdominal pain may be relieved by chlorpromazine. Demerol may be useful if chlorpromazine does not completely alleviate pain. The cause of hyponatremia must be determined before it is treated. If caused by primary salt loss from the GI tract, salt replacement is essential. If associated with the findings of the syndrome of inappropriate release of ADH, water restriction has been successful in raising serum sodium levels. The problem has been complicated by the frequent finding of hypovolemia, which, if sufficiently pronounced in the presence of hyponatremia, is an indication for hypertonic saline adminstration. Some patients have responded well to a high-carbohydrate intake-as high as possible (up to 400 g/day or more). Since the response is not uniform or predictable, a high-carbohydrate intake should be attempted in all patients experiencing an attack of an inducible porphyria.

Hematin infusions have been repeatedly shown to curtail an acute attack and have improved the prognosis for all "inducible" porphyrias. It is given at a dose of 2–4 mg/kg for three days (Pierach, 1982).

Supportive care during acute attacks is of great importance. When there is peripheral neuropathy, respiratory paralysis, dysphagia, or coma, careful attention to nursing care, avoidance of aspiration, assisted respiration, early recognition of pneumonia, and physiotherapy are of great importance. Splints and sandbags should be used for wrist- and footdrop.

In those women who experience regularly recurrent attacks in relation to menstrual cycles, administration of oral contraceptive preparations have been useful in preventing attacks. The schedule used is similar to that used for contraception, but the dosage required may or may not be higher. This approach should be used with caution, since experience with it in this type of patient is limited and oral contraceptives sometimes precipitate attacks in women who do not experience the regularly recurring cyclic attacks. A luteinizing hormone-releasing hormone analogue has been shown experimentally to suppress these premenstrual attacks (Anderson et al., 1984).

Prophylaxis is of great importance and involves warning patients and members of their families about avoiding the known precipitating factors.

**Prognosis:** A mortality rate of 24% over a five-year observation period has been reported. In the patient with known disease who has been warned about the precipitating factors, the prognosis is now much improved.

**Detection of Carrier:** In approximately 90% of patients with acute intermittent porphyria, porphobilinogen deaminase (the deficient enzyme) can be found to be decreased in their erythrocytes, thus lending itself very well to carrier detection (Pierach et al., 1987).

*The author wishes to thank Donald P. Tschudy for his contribution to an earlier version of this article.*

**References:**
Wetterberg L: A neuropsychiatric and genetical investigation of acute intermittent porphyria. Stockholm: Bokforlaget, 1968.
Tschudy DP, Lamon JL: Porphyrin metabolism and the porphyrias. In: Bondy PK, Rosenberg LE, ed: Metabolic control and disease. Philadelphia: W.B. Saunders, 1980:939–1008.
Pierach CA: Hematin therapy for the porphyric attack. Semin Liver Disease 1982; 2:125–131.
Anderson KE, et al.: Prevention of cyclical attacks of acute intermittent porphyria with a long-acting agonist of luteinizing hormone-releasing hormone. New Engl J Med 1984; 311:643–645.
Pierach CA, et al.: Red cell porphobilinogen deaminase in the evaluation of acute intermittent porphyria. JAMA 1987; 257:60–61.

PI009                                                      **Claus A. Pierach**

---

**PORPHYRIA, COPROPORPHYRIA**                              **0203**

**Includes:**
Coproporphyrinogen oxidase deficiency
Harderoporphyria

**Excludes:** Hepatic porphyria (other forms)

**Major Diagnostic Criteria:** Increased fecal and urine coproporphyrin with little increase of fecal protoporphyrin. Urinary delta-aminolevulinic acid and porphobilinogen are increased during acute attacks of neurovisceral symptoms.

**Clinical Findings:** Patients present with acute attacks of neurovisceral symptoms similar to those in acute intermittent porphyria. The manifestations of an acute attack may include abdominal pain, neurologic deficits, psychiatric symptoms (hallucinations, depression), and constipation. A minority of patients have photosensitivity, consisting of blistering of the sun-exposed skin. The majority of patients with the inherited defect and biochemical abnormalities are clinically asymptomatic.

**Complications:** Paralysis (rarely progressing to respiratory muscle paralysis), seizures, depression, psychosis, photosensitivity, hypertension.

**Associated Findings:** None known.

**Etiology:** Autosomal dominant inheritance of enzymatic defect. Homozygous cases with more severe clinical manifestations have been reported.

**Pathogenesis:** Enzymatic defect in coproporphyrinogen oxidase (E.C.1.3.3.3). Heterozygotic patients have 50% of the enzymatic activity of controls.

**MIM No.:** *12130

**Sex Ratio:** All patients, M1:F1; symptomatic, M1:F2.5

**Occurrence:** Rarest of the three types of acute hepatic porphyrias. No ethnic predisposition.

**Risk of Recurrence for Patient's Sib:**
See Part I, *Mendelian Inheritance.*

**Risk of Recurrence for Patient's Child:**
See Part I, *Mendelian Inheritance.*

**Age of Detectability:** Decreased activity of coproporphyrinogen oxidase is present at birth; biochemical abnormalities appear postpubescent.

**Gene Mapping and Linkage:** CPO (coproporphyrinogen oxidase) has been mapped to 9.

**Prevention:** Avoidance of precipitating drugs (most commonly phenobarbital, ethanol). Fasting should be avoided. Genetic counseling is indicated.

**Treatment:** Specific treatment of acute attacks includes high-carbohydrate diet and intravenous hematin. Most acute attacks resolve after discontinuing the precipitating drug(s). Specific therapy is the same for all acute hepatic porphyrias and consists of high carbohydrate diet and intravenous hematin.

**Prognosis:** Acute attacks are generally less severe than in acute intermittent porphyria. By avoiding precipitating agents, the disease is compatible with longevity.

**Detection of Carrier:** Decreased activity of coproporphyrinogen oxidase is detectable in cultured fibroblasts, peripheral lymphocytes, and buffy coat preparations. The enzyme activity assay is not widely available. Fecal coproporphyrin levels are elevated in nearly all carriers of the mutant gene.

**References:**
Elder GH, et al.: The primary enzyme defect in hereditary coproporphyria. Lancet 1976; II:1217–1219.
Brodie MJ, et al.: Hereditary coproporphyria: demonstration of the abnormalities in haem biosynthesis in peripheral blood. Q J Med 1977; 46:229–241.
Grandchamp B, et al.: Homozygous case of hereditary coproporphyria. Lancet 1977; II: 1348–1349.
Grandchamp B, et al.: Assignment of the human coproporphyrinogen oxidase to chromosome 9. Hum Genet 1983; 64:180–183.
Nordmann Y, et al.: Harderoporphyria: a variant hereditary coproporphyria. J Clin Invest 1983; 72:1139–1149.
Andrews J, et al.: Hereditary coproporphyria: incidence in a large English family. J Med Genet 1984; 21:341–349.

BR038                                    **David A. Brenner**

## PORPHYRIA, ERYTHROPOIETIC                     **0821**

**Includes:**
Enamel and dentin staining from erythropoietic porphyria
Erythrodontia
Erythropoietic porphyria, congenital
Gunther disease
Hematoporphyria congenita
Uroporphyrinogen III cosynthase deficiency
UROS deficiency

**Excludes:**
Nonporphyric photodermatoses such as xeroderma pigmentosum
Photosensitizing porphyrias

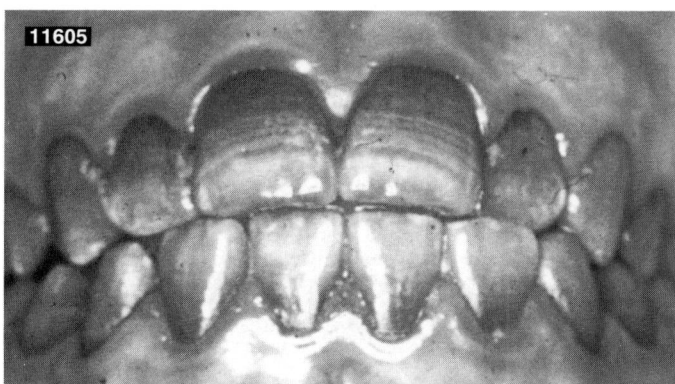

**0821-11605:** Red staining of the teeth.

**Porphyria** (others)
**Teeth, enamel and dentin defects from erythroblastosis fetalis** (0340)

**Major Diagnostic Criteria:** Pink urine, photosensitivity, and hemolysis are the major findings. Demonstration by quantitative methods of greatly increased uroporphyrin I in the urine and fluorescence of red cells and marrow normoblasts. In addition, it is desirable to demonstrate increased erythrocyte uroporphyrin levels by direct analysis. Fluorescence of the teeth should be sought when erythrodontia is not obvious. Clinical pigmentation of teeth may be minimal in some cases, but an extract of ground tooth structure with 0.5 N HCl will normally exhibit brilliant red fluorescence.

**Clinical Findings:** The two organ systems mainly affected are the skin and bone marrow. The onset of symptoms is usually between birth and age 5 years. Pink or red urine may be the first obvious sign. Photosensitivity may manifest in infancy and may cause the child to cry when exposed to sunlight. The vesicles or bullae that appear on the exposed portions of the body often ulcerate and heal, with scarring. Secondary infections in the skin lesions and repeated episodes of ulceration and scarring lead to severe deformities of the nose, ears, eyes, and fingers. Conjunctivitis, keratitis, ectropion, and loss of fingernails and phalanges may occur. Hypertrichosis is often seen on the face and limbs, but areas of alopecia may occur on the scalp. Areas of pigmentation and depigmentation develop in exposed areas.

Hemolysis occurs in the majority of patients with this disease, some of whom can increase red cell production sufficiently to prevent the normochromic anemia seen in others. The more active periods of hemolysis are accompanied by increased fecal urobilinogen, normoblastic hyperplasia of the marrow, and circulating normoblasts. Splenomegaly is present in about 75% of the patients with this disease. Thrombocytopenia, presumably secondary to hypersplenism, and clinically evident jaundice occur rarely.

Bones are red-brown in color and fluoresce red in UV light.

Teeth vary in color from yellow-brown to red-brown to violet. Teeth fluoresce distinctly red in Wood's (UV) light. Both enamel and dentin contain porphyrins. However, higher concentrations are found in dentin.

**Complications:** Varying degrees of deformity of nose, ears, eyes, and fingers. Areas of pigmentation and depigmentation occur on exposed areas. Ectropion, and the loss of nails and terminal phalanges may occur. Areas of alopecia in the scalp and hypertrichosis of the face and limbs. Hemolytic anemia and occasionally hypersplenism.

**Associated Findings:** None known.

**Etiology:** Autosomal recessive inheritance.

**Pathogenesis:** Deficiency of uroporphyrinogen III cosynthetase, which ranges from one-tenth to one-third of normal levels of activity.

Insufficient production or utilization of uroporphyrinogen isomerase resulting in the production of the unusable isomer uroporphyrinogen I. This isomer and its oxidized or decarboxylated products (uroporphyrin I, coproporphyrin I) have a high degree of physical affinity for calcium phosphate and are, therefore, incorporated into the bones and teeth during osteogenesis and odontogenesis. The pigmentation of the teeth is thus dependent primarily upon the level of circulating abnormal porphyrins at the time of initial calcification. In one reported case, a female with proven erythropoietic porphyria gave birth to a basically unaffected infant whose primary teeth, which formed and calcified in utero, were pigmented reddish-brown.

**MIM No.:** *26370

**Sex Ratio:** M1:F1

**Occurrence:** Over 100 cases reported in the literature.

**Risk of Recurrence for Patient's Sib:**
See Part I, *Mendelian Inheritance*.

**Risk of Recurrence for Patient's Child:**
See Part I, *Mendelian Inheritance*.

**Age of Detectability:** Uroporphyrinogen III cosynthetase is expressed in cultured amniotic cells, so prenatal diagnosis is possible. Clinical signs are evident from as early as birth up to age five years at the latest. Probably urinary porphyrin analysis will detect the disease within the first year of life in most cases.

**Gene Mapping and Linkage:** Unknown.

**Prevention:** None known. Genetic counseling indicated.

**Treatment:** Avoidance of light with a wavelength around 4,000 A as much as possible. Use of protective clothing and other protective measures. A sunscreen filter chemically induced in the skin may be useful (see Fusaro et al, 1966 for details). Splenectomy for severe hemolytic anemia has sometimes been useful. Porcelain or acrylic crowns may be useful. Transfusion to suppress erythropoiesis has been reported to be effective.

**Prognosis:** Death usually occurs before middle age.

**Detection of Carrier:** The level of uroporphyrinogen III cosynthetase of carriers is intermediate between normal and homozygotic levels.

*The authors wish to thank Donald P. Tschudy for his contributions to a previous version of this article.*

**References:**
Townes PL: Transplacentally acquired erythrodontia. J Pediatr 1965; 67:600–602.
Fusaro RM, et al.: Sunlight protection in normal skin. Arch Dermatol 1966; 93:106–111.
Deybach JC, et al.: Prenatal exclusion of congenital erythropoietic porphyria (Gunther's disease) in a fetus at risk. Hum Genet 1980; 53:217–221.
Piomelli S, et al.: Complete suppression of the symptoms of congenital erythropoietic porphyria by long-term treatment with high-level transfusions. New Engl J Med 1986; 314:1029–1031.
Pimstone NR, et al.; Therapeutic efficacy of oral charcoal in congenital erythropoietic porphyria. New Engl J Med 1987; 316:390–393.
Tsai SF, et al.: Coupled-enzyme and direct assays for uroporphrinogen III synthase activity in human erythrocytes and cultured lymphoblasts. Anal Biochem 1987; 166:120–133.
Kappas A, et al.: The porphyrias. In: Scriver CR, et al, eds: The metabolic basis of inherited disease, 6th ed. New York: McGraw-Hill, 1989:1305–1366.

BR038
TR003

**David A. Brenner**
**John N. Trodahl**

**Porphyria, hepatocutaneous type**
*See PORPHYRIA CUTANEA TARDA*
**Porphyria, hepatoerythropoietic**
*See PORPHYRIA CUTANEA TARDA*

## PORPHYRIA, PROTOPORPHYRIA 0362

**Includes:**
Erythrohepatic protoporphyria
Erythropoietic protoporphyria (EPP)
Ferrochelatase deficiency
Heme synthase deficiency
Light, sensitivity to
Liver disease-erythrohepatic protoporphyria
Photosensitivity, from protoporphyria
Protoporphyria, erythropoietic
Protoporphyria, porphyria

**Excludes:**
Porphyria cutanea tarda (3064)
Porphyria (others)

**Major Diagnostic Criteria:** The diagnosis of protoporphyria is made by demonstrating an increased level of protoporphyrin in erythrocytes, plasma, and stool. In contrast to lead poisoning and iron deficiency anemia, the increased protoporphyrin in erythrocytes occurs as free protoporphyrin and not the zinc chelate.

**Clinical Findings:** The major clinical manifestation of protoporphyria is photosensitivity. This is usually present from infancy, although patients occasionally have not had symptoms until adolescence or adulthood. They complain of burning, itching, or pain of the skin on exposure to sunlight, sometimes within a few minutes. This is followed by erythema and edema. Vesicles seldom develop unless sun exposure is prolonged. Small, shallow, pitted scars are characteristic. These occur mainly over the nose, cheeks, and backs of the hands. There is also thickening and lichenification of the skin in these areas.

The degree of photosensitivity is variable among patients, even among those in the same family. There is poor correlation between the severity of photosensitivity and the erythrocyte protoporphyrin level.

The other major clinical manifestation of protoporphyria is liver disease. Although the incidence is uncertain, it probably occurs in less than 10% of patients. Jaundice has frequently been the first manifestation of liver disease. This has been followed by a progressive downhill course, leading to death during hepatic failure. Only an occasional patient has recovered after the onset of jaundice. The livers of patients who have died during hepatic failure have been nodular due to cirrhosis and black due to massive deposits of protoporphyrin pigment in hepatobiliary structures. When liver biopsy specimens are examined by polarization microscopy the pigment deposits are birefringent, and by electron microscopy they are seen to contain crystals.

**Complications:** Unknown.

**Associated Findings:** Approximately 20–30% of patients have mild anemia, with hypochromic microcytic indices. There is an increased frequency of cholelithiasis, and some patients require cholecystectomy. Chemical analysis of gallstones has demonstrated the presence of protoporphyrin.

**Etiology:** Autosomal dominant inheritance with variable expression. Some individuals have no clinical manifestations of protoporphyria, but have increased levels of erythrocyte protoporphyrin. They are considered to be clinically unaffected carriers of the gene defect. However, more complex mechanisms of inheritance, in particular a three-allele system, have been postulated on the basis of multiple family studies.

**Pathogenesis:** A reduction in activity of ferrochelatase (also termed *heme synthase* or *protoheme ferrolyase*), which catalyzes the insertion of iron into protoporphyrin to form heme. The enzyme defect is present in all heme-forming tissues. The nature of the abnormality in ferrochelatase has not yet been determined.

As a result of the deficient ferrochelatase activity, protoporphyrin accumulates in excessive amounts. The bone marrow is the major source of the excess protoporphyrin, with a variable contribution from the liver and perhaps other heme-forming tissues.

**MIM No.:** *17700

**Sex Ratio:** M1:F1

**Occurrence:** Protoporphyria occurs in all ethnic groups. The incidence and prevalence have not been precisely determined for any group. It appears to be a relatively common type of porphyria, perhaps second only to porphyria cutanea tarda in frequency. Thus, a reasonable estimate of its prevalence is 1:5,000–10,000 individuals.

**Risk of Recurrence for Patient's Sib:**
See Part I, *Mendelian Inheritance.*

**Risk of Recurrence for Patient's Child:**
See Part I, *Mendelian Inheritance.*

**Age of Detectability:** Usually during infancy due to the photosensitivity, with the average age being approximately 4 years. Occasionally symptoms have not occurred until adolescence or adulthood.

**Gene Mapping and Linkage:** Unknown.

**Prevention:** None known. Genetic counseling indicated.

**Treatment:** Topical sunscreens are ineffective as protective agents against photosensitivity in patients with protoporphyria. However, oral administration of beta-carotene (Solatene) in a dose of 60–180 mg/day reduces photosensitivity in over 80% of patients.

Various therapeutic modalities have been proposed for treatment of hepatobiliary disease in protoporphyria. These include red cell transfusions or the intravenous administration of hematin to suppress erythropoiesis, oral iron therapy (particularly when there is iron deficiency), oral administration of chenodeoxycholic acid to enhance hepatic disposal of protoporphyrin, and oral administration of cholestyramine or activated charcoal to interrupt the enterohepatic circulation of protoporphyrin. None of these therapeutic modalities has been shown in a large group of patients to be the optimal form of therapy. Liver transplantation should be considered for patients with advanced liver disease.

**Prognosis:** Most patients with protoporphyria are expected to have normal life spans. However, patients with progressive liver damage have a poor prognosis.

**Detection of Carrier:** The asymptomatic carrier of the gene defect may be detected by demonstrating an increased level of erythrocyte protoporphyrin. Asymptomatic carriers may also be shown to have diminished ferrochelatase activity in cultured skin fibroblasts and lymphocytes isolated from the blood.

**Special Considerations:** Although serious liver disease appears to occur in less than 10% of patients with protoporphyria, the clinician must be vigilant in observing patients for this complication because of the ominous prognosis. Unfortunately, there is no precise means by which to identify patients who are at risk for this complication. Routine tests of liver function do not provide much information regarding the degree of liver damage since livers can remain mildly abnormal until hepatic decompensation occurs. Any patient with an unexplained abnormality should therefore be observed closely. Patients with high erythrocyte (greater than 1,500 $\mu$g/dl) and plasma (greater than 50 $\mu$g/dl) protoporphyrin levels must also be observed closely. Liver biopsy should be done to assess histology in such patients. Those with hepatocellular necrosis and fibrosis, even if mild, should be considered for therapeutic options outlined above.

An animal model of protoporphyria has been found in cattle. The disease differs from that in humans in that there is a homozygous deficiency of ferrochelatase activity. Cattle manifest photosensitivity but do not develop hepatobiliary disease, limiting their usefulness in studying the pathogenesis and treatment of clinical manifestations of protoporphyria.

**References:**

Magnus IA, et al.: Erythropoietic protoporphyria. A new porphyria syndrome with solar urticaria due to protoporphyrinemia. Lancet 1961; II:448–451.
Bonkowsky HL, et al.: Heme synthetase deficiency in human protoporphyria. Demonstration of the defect in liver and cultured skin fibroblasts. J Clin Invest 1975; 56:1139–1148.
DeLeo VA, et al.: Erythropoietic protoporphyria: 10 years experience. Am J Med 1976; 60:8–22. * †

Bloomer JR: Pathogenesis and therapy of liver disease in protoporphyria. Yale J Biol Med 1979; 52:39–48. †
Went LN, Klasen EC: Genetic aspects of erythropoietic protoporphyria. Ann Hum Genet 1984; 48:105–117.
Bloomer JR, Straka JG: Porphyrin metabolism. In: Arias IM, et al., eds: The liver: biology and pathobiology. New York: Raven, 1988. *

BL023                                                            **Joseph R. Bloomer**

## PORPHYRIA, VARIEGATE                                           0822

**Includes:**
> Mixed porphyria
> Protocoproporphyria
> Protoporphyrinogen oxidase deficiency
> South African porphyria

**Excludes:**
> **Porphyria, acute intermittent** (0820)
> **Porphyria, coproporphyria** (0203)

**Major Diagnostic Criteria:** Increased urinary excretion of porphobilinogen during an acute attack. Increased fecal coproporphyrin and protoporphyrin with normal red cell protoporphyrin.

**Clinical Findings:** This disease may present either cutaneous manifestations of photosensitivity or neurologic aspects identical to those described for acute intermittent porphyria or both.

The skin lesions may be vesicles, bullae, or erosion, with variable degrees of scarring and pigmentation of the skin exposed to sunlight. There may be increased skin fragility. Hypertrichosis on the face or chronic thickening of skin may occur with diffuse yellowish papules. Azotemia and electrolyte abnormalities are frequent and often result from the GI manifestations of the acute attack.

**Complications:** Chronic skin lesions, chronic pain syndrome (peripheral or abdominal), motor paralysis (including respiratory paralysis), seizures, organic brain syndrome, depression.

**Associated Findings:** None known.

**Etiology:** Autosomal dominant inheritance.

**Pathogenesis:** Increased levels of hepatic δ-aminolevulinic acid synthase have been demonstrated, but the relationship of this finding to the attacks of neurologic dysfunction is unknown. The basic genetic defect is probably a protoporphyrinogen oxidase deficiency (Brenner and Bloomer, 1980).

**MIM No.:** *17620

**Sex Ratio:** M1:F1.3 in one series of 66 cases.

**Occurrence:** In the total white population of South Africa it has been estimated as 1:330. Its incidence is probably somewhat less than 1:66,000 in most parts of the world.

**Risk of Recurrence for Patient's Sib:**
See Part I, *Mendelian Inheritance.*

**Risk of Recurrence for Patient's Child:**
See Part I, *Mendelian Inheritance.*

**Age of Detectability:** Usually after puberty.

**Gene Mapping and Linkage:** VP (variegate porphyria (protoporphyrinogen oxidase)) has been provisionally mapped to 14q.

**Prevention:** None known. Genetic counseling indicated.

**Treatment:** Avoidance of sunlight.

Hematin infusions have been repeatedly shown to curtail an acute attack and have improved the prognosis for all "inducible" porphyrias. It is given at a dose of 2–4 mg/kg for three days (Pierach, 1982).

Supportive care during acute attacks is of great importance. When there is peripheral neuropathy, respiratory paralysis, dysphagia, or coma, careful attention to nursing care, avoidance of aspiration, assisted respiration, early recognition of pneumonia, and physiotherapy are of great importance. Splints and sandbags should be used for wrist- and footdrop.

In those women who experience regularly recurrent attacks in relation to menstrual cycles, administration of oral contraceptive preparations have been useful in preventing attacks. The schedule used is similar to that used for contraception, but the dosage required may or may not be higher. This approach should be used with caution, since experience with it in this type of patient is limited and oral contraceptives sometimes precipitate attacks in women who do not experience the regularly recurring cyclic attacks. A luteinizing hormone-releasing hormone analogue has been shown experimentally to suppress these premenstrual attacks (Anderson et al., 1984).

Prophylaxis is of great importance and involves warning patients and members of their families about avoiding the known precipitating factors.

**Prognosis:** Unknown.

**Detection of Carrier:** Increased fecal protoporphyrin was demonstrated in members of one family with the disease (Fromke et al., 1978).

*The author wishes to thank Donald P. Tschudy for his contribution to earlier versions of this article.*

**References:**

Eales L: Porphyria as seen in Cape Town: a survey of 250 patients and some recent studies. S Afr J Lab Clin Med 1963; 9:151–162.

Waldenstrom J, Haeger-Aronsen B: The porphyrias: a genetic problem. Prog Med Genet 1967; 5:58–101.

Fromke VL, et al.: Porphyria variegata: study of a large kindred in the United States. Am J Med 1978; 65:80–88.

Brenner DA, Bloomer JR: The enzymatic defect in variegate porphyria: studies with human cultured skin fibroblasts. New Engl J Med 1980; 302:765–769.

Kushner JP, et al.: Congenital erythropoietic porphyria, diminished activity of uroporphyrinogen decarboxylase and dyserythropoiesis. Blood 1982; 59:725–737.

Mustajoki P, et al.: Homozygous variegate porphyria: a severe skin disease of infancy. Clin Genet 1987; 32:300–305.

PI009                                    **Claus A. Pierach**

**Port-wine stain**
*See NEVUS FLAMMEUS*
**Portal vein atresia**
*See LIVER, VENOUS ANOMALIES*
**Portuguese (Andrade)-type hereditary amyloidosis**
*See AMYLOIDOSIS, TRANSTHYRETIN METHIONINE-30 TYPE*
**Positional plagiocephaly**
*See PLAGIOCEPHALY*
**Post-anesthesia apnea**
*See CHOLINESTERASE, ATYPICAL*
**Post-polio syndrome**
*See POLIO, SUSCEPTIBILITY TO*
**Postaxial acrofacial dysostosis syndrome (POADS)**
*See ACROFACIAL DYSOSTOSIS, POSTAXIAL TYPE*
**Postaxial polydactyly, types A and B**
*See POLYDACTYLY*
**Postaxial polydactyly-dental-vertebral syndrome**
*See HEART-HAND SYNDROME IV*
**Postaxial polydactyly-distal obstructive uropathy**
*See POLYDACTYLY-DISTAL OBSTRUCTIVE UROPATHY*
**Posterior embryotoxon**
*See EYE, ANTERIOR SEGMENT DYSGENESIS*
**Posterior marginal dysplasia of cornea**
*See EYE, ANTERIOR SEGMENT DYSGENESIS*
**Posterior nasal atresia**
*See NOSE, POSTERIOR ATRESIA*
**Posterior polar**
*See CATARACT, AUTOSOMAL DOMINANT CONGENITAL*
**Posterolateral diaphragmatic hernia**
*See DIAPHRAGMATIC HERNIA*
**Postmortem dermatolysis, multiple cysts**
*See FETAL MULTIPLE CYSTS ANOMALY*
**Postural plagiocephaly**
*See PLAGIOCEPHALY*
**Postural torticollis**
*See TORTICOLLIS*
**Potassium-losing nephropathy with low aldosterone**
*See LIDDLE SYNDROME*
**Potassium-sodium disorder of erythrocyte**
*See ANEMIA, HEMOLYTIC, RED CELL MEMBRANE DEFECTS*

**'Potato' nose**
*See NOSE/NASAL SEPTUM DEFECTS*
**Potter syndrome**
*See RENAL AGENESIS, BILATERAL*
**Potter type I infantile polycystic kidney disease**
*See KIDNEY, POLYCYSTIC DISEASE, RECESSIVE*
**Potter type II renal dysplasia**
*See KIDNEY, RENAL DYSPLASIA, POTTER TYPE II*
**Potter type III polycystic kidney disease**
*See KIDNEY, POLYCYSTIC DISEASE, DOMINANT*
**Prader-Labhart-Willi syndrome**
*See PRADER-WILLI SYNDROME*

---

## PRADER-WILLI SYNDROME              0823

**Includes:**
   Hypogenital dystrophy with diabetic tendency
   Hypotonia-hypomentia-hypogonadism-obesity (HHHO)
   Prader-Labhart-Willi syndrome

**Excludes:**
   Adiposogenital dystrophy
   **Alstrom syndrome** (0041)
   **Angelman syndrome** (2086)
   Atonic diplegia and other severe supranuclear hypotonias
   **Cohen syndrome** (2023)
   Hypotonia, other forms of infantile
   **Laurence-Moon syndrome** (0578)
   **Myopathy** (see others)

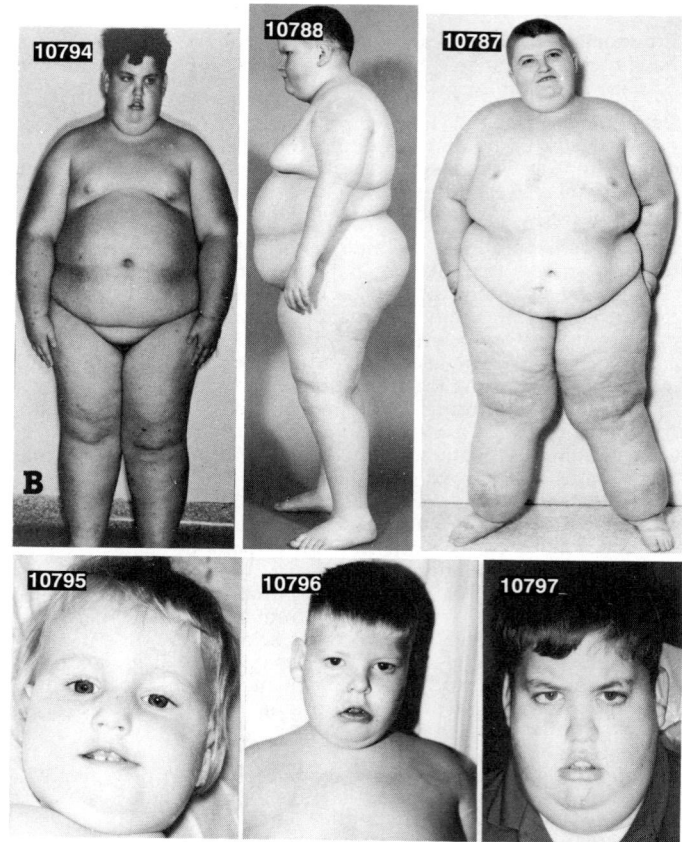

**0823A**-10794, 10788, 10787: Moderate to severe obesity particularly in the trunkal region. 10795–97: Characteristic facies include upslanted palpebral fissures, almond-shaped eyes and full cheeks.

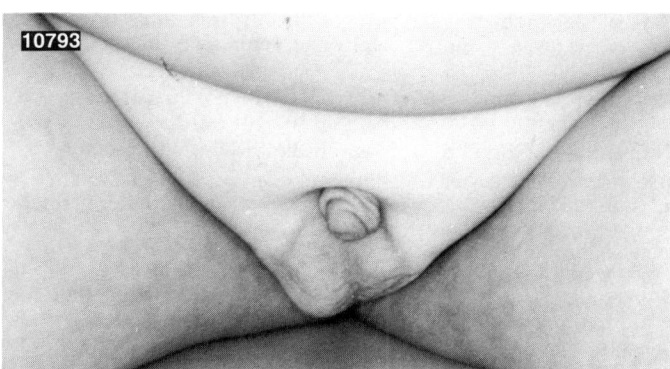

**0823B-10793:** Genital hypoplasia in male with Prader-Willi.

Myotonic dystrophy (0702)
Spinal muscular atrophy (0895)
Williams syndrome (0999)
X-linked mental retardation, Fragile X syndrome (2073)
X-linked mental retardation-short stature-obesity-hypogonadism (3147)

**Major Diagnostic Criteria:** Severe muscular hypo- or atonia, are-flexia, feeding difficulties, and hypothermia characterize the first phase. Micropenis, hypoplastic scrotum, and cryptorchidism are present. Diagnosis of first phase is more difficult for Prader-Willi syndrome (PW) girls, though small or hypoplastic labia minora and clitoris may suggest PW if associated with the above criteria. The second phase is characterized by polyphagia or decreased perception of satiety, delayed psychomotor development, mental subnormality (90% of cases), obesity, short stature, hypogonadism, and behavioral peculiarities.

**Clinical Findings:** A decrease of fetal movements in the last months of pregnancy is sometimes noticed. Breech deliveries occur in 10–40% of the cases. The mean birthweight is several hundred grams less than the average birthweight of term babies. Mean duration of gestation is within the normal range. Some PW

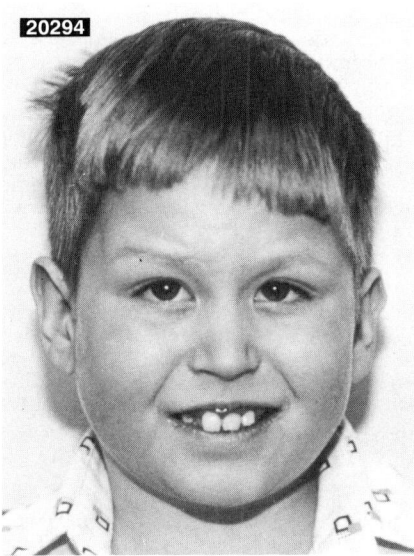

**0823C-20294:** Prader-Willi syndrome; note almond-shaped eyes and full cheeks.

babies are born with dislocated hips and/or talipes valgoplanus. There may also be acromicria (small hands and feet).

The clinical course can be divided into two phases. The first phase is characterized by severe hypotonia or even atonia. There is evidence of facial diplegia with a flat face, a triangular mouth (tented upper lip), and narrow bifrontal diameter. Young infants with PW are almost motionless; Moro response, withdrawal reflex, and tendon reflexes are decreased or absent. Sucking and swallowing reflexes are very poorly developed and usually necessitate feeding by gavage, dropper, spoon, or premature nipple for weeks or even months. There is a tendency to hypothermia in early infancy. Penis and scrotum are hypoplastic; the latter often consists of not more than an area of corrugated skin in the anterior perineum. Testes may be cryptorchid or very small. Female external genitalia may show small or hypoplastic labia minora and clitoris.

Usually after a few months, the PW infants enter the second phase. They become more lively and responsive, and feeding difficulties subside; they become hungry and cry for food. Some PW children have a constant hunger, starting at age 1–6 years (usually age two) forcing them to incessantly seek food. Other PW patients may not seek food, but are unable to recognize satiety and eat as long as food is in sight. As a result, PW children become extremely obese, particularly in the trunk and proximal limbs. In some children forearms and lower legs become obese as well, but hands and feet remain disproportionately small. Longitudinal growth is impaired. Height is almost always below the 50th percentile. The prepubertal growth spurt does not occur, thus growth retardation becomes even more conspicuous at that age.

Psychomotor development is delayed, particularly with motor dependent skills; e.g. sitting and walking. Psychometric tests yield IQs between 20 and 90. A normal IQ is found in 10% of the cases. Some PW adults are able to function at a trainable level, but impaired speech clarity and emotional lability are common problems. PW children show times of exuberant joy, yet they also have excessive outbursts of anger, and temper tantrums that become more severe in the second decade of life to the point where they become unbearable for other family members. Affected children may have mannerisms such as trichotillomania and constant plucking on sores, insect bites, and the like. The muscular hypotonia tends to improve with age. Episodes of incoercible sleep are sometimes observed and may be precipitated by small doses of anorexic drugs such as dexedrine sulfate. Periods of constitutional hyperthermia lasting for days and even weeks are noticed.

Other manifestations are microdontia, dental caries, enamel defects (notably in the first dentition), abnormal saliva (bubbly, viscous, decreased in volume), strabismus, high-arched palate, dry oral mucosa, mesobrachyphalangy, and simian creases. Poorly modeled ears and narrow external ear canals are occasionally encountered. Scoliosis is frequent. Hypopigmentation (fair coloring for their family) occurs in one-half of affected individuals. Osteoporosis, evidenced by radial bone mineral measurement, appears to be a fairly consistent finding. Most PW patients show hypogonadotropic hypogonadism, although hypergonadotropic hypogonadism has been observed. Male PW patients are infertile; the testes are extremely small and show immature and partially hyalinized seminiferous tubules, with decreased or absent spermatogenesis. However, restoration of normal spermatogenesis was noted in at least one patient after he was treated for several months with clomiphene citrate. Leydig cells are present in normal or subnormal number; their maturation is at times inadequate. Plasma testosterone levels are below normal and remain subnormal after clomiphene treatment. Anorchia is found in some cases. The development of secondary sex characteristics in PW males is delayed and incomplete; the voice remains high-pitched.

Female PW patients show either primary or secondary amenorrhea, but are infertile. Menarche, if it occurs, is delayed, though precocious pubarche has been reported. Some females have anovulatory cycles. Estrogenization of the vaginal mucosa varies between moderately decreased and normal. Some cases of hypogonadotropic hypogonadism show normal or more often subnormal responses to clomiphene and luteinizing hormone-releasing hormone. The clomiphene-induced maturation effect may subside after medication is stopped. Secondary sex characteristics of female PW patients vary between incomplete and normal.

Endocrine studies of the pituitary-adrenal and the pituitary-thyroid axes are normal, although mild and inconsistent abnormalities have been reported by some observers. A low somatomedin-C level, and linear growth rate, which respond to growth hormone treatment has been reported. Glucose metabolism disturbance is often found. Normal glucose tolerance is found in young PW patients, while glucose intolerance and insulin hypersensitivity often develop in obese patients. Normal laboratory findings include serum electrolytes, urinalysis, and blood morphology. EEGs are sometimes normal, but nonspecific abnormalities and even paroxysmal discharges such as spike-waves are reported. Muscles show signs of disuse atrophy in some cases.

Recent studies revealed anomalies of chromosome 15 in more than one-half of PW patients. *De novo* deletions of proximal parts of the long arm (del 15q11-q13) are most frequent, at times due to an unbalanced translocation in that region. Less frequently, a 15;15 translocation or an isodicentric chromosome 15 is found. Some of the later may be tetrasomic for 15pter-q11. Thus most chromosomally abnormal PW cases have a common deletion of the "critical" 15q11-q13 region, which may be due to unstable DNA sequences in that region. While there are no clinical differences between PW patients with and without chromosomal anomalies, molecular-genetic studies have isolated more than 10 DNA markers in this same region, including those associated with other variants of mental retardation such as **Angelman syndrome** which also show chromosomal abnormalities, although they may differ with respect to parental origin. A Prader-Willi-like phenotype has also been described in some instances of **X-linked mental retardation, Fragile X syndrome** (Fryns et al, 1988).

The chromosomal deletion has been shown to be paternally derived in almost every case. When the same or similar deletion is in the maternally derived chromosome it has been associated with the **Angelman syndrome** phenotype. Among those patients with Prader-Willi syndrome who do not have a cytogenetically detectable deletion, some have submicroscopic deletions (molecular deletions), others have no detectable paternal contribution and both maternal contributions in the 15q11-q13 region (maternal heterodisomy). These unique findings suggest that genes arising from different sex parents are modified differently prior to conception, and are expressed differently in their offspring (genetic imprinting).

**Complications:** Development of a Pickwickian, or obesity-hypoventilation syndrome, treatable with progesterone. Diabetes mellitus, adult type without tendency to ketosis, appears during second decade or later. Early development of atherosclerosis and glomerulosclerosis occurs. Gastric perforation may occur as a consequence of overeating.

**Associated Findings:** Rumination occurs in 10% to 17% of cases. Seizures (rarely).

**Etiology:** Heterogeneity of PW has been established. Sporadic cases with normal chromosomes may represent apparent autosomal dominant mutations. Recently, a few families with autosomal recessive inheritance have been reported.

**Pathogenesis:** A disturbance within the hypothalamic-pituitary pathway is debated. The few postmortem studies available show no evidence of a microscopic lesion in this area. However, destruction of the ventromedial hypothalamus produces a PW-like picture, with polyphagia and obesity in experimental animals.

**MIM No.:** *17627

**POS No.:** 3361

**CDC No.:** 759.870

**Sex Ratio:** M1:F1

**Occurrence:** About 1:15,000.

**Risk of Recurrence for Patient's Sib:** Estimated at 1:1,000, since most cases are sporadic.

**Risk of Recurrence for Patient's Child:** No PW patient is known to have reproduced.

**Age of Detectability:** At birth or shortly thereafter in male infants. Accurate diagnosis of PW in females is possible in the second phase only.

**Gene Mapping and Linkage:** PWCR (Prader-Willi syndrome chromosome region) has been mapped to 15q11-q12.

**Prevention:** None known. Genetic counseling indicated.

**Treatment:** 1. Passive physiotherapy can prevent disuse atrophy of muscle during the first phase. Active physiotherapy can be initiated as soon as the child reaches the second phase and before activity-limiting obesity develops.

2. Appetite depressants may be tried during the second phase. PW children are hypersensitive to dexedrine sulfate; therefore drug treatment should begin with very small doses. The growth-limiting effect of these drugs only occurs if the dose is higher than 30 mg/day.

3. Gastroplasty has proven to be successful in some cases when other attempts to regulate food intake fail.

4. Patients whose food intake cannot be controlled in the realm of the family, and patients who display severe and disruptive behavioral disorders, may benefit from institutionalization in group homes specializing in PW treatment.

5. To be effective, nutritional behavior modification must begin during the first phase when the child is on a normal caloric intake. The outcome, however, is still uncertain. Support of the family during periods of feeding difficulties and careful communication to them of the expected course of these difficulties should help early acceptance of behavior modification. A low-calorie formula, enough to guarantee adequate but not excessive weight increase, must be designed. Regular feeding hours and habits, such as feeding in the same location and with the same table mat and bib, and an acoustic signal indicating the time of feeding, may allow the regulating of feeding habits and possibly prevent overeating. Early nutritional behavior modification is still experimental, though it appears to be promising.

6. Jaw wiring is not recommended because of possible complications such as aspiration.

7. The greatest problem besides obesity are severe behavior disorders. Residential facilities with specific PW regimens have shown success in dealing with this problem.

8. Depo-Testosterone has been used to treat the microphallus of small boys (25mg IM every three weeks for a total of five injections). Cryptorchidism may respond to hormone therapy, specifically HCG, and should be corrected when the patient is 2–5 years of age, but it is not always possible to bring the testes to the scrotum.

9. Depo-Testosterone given to male adolescents and adults does not remedy the infertility, but may have a beneficial effect on behavior and in the development of secondary sex characteristic.

10. Growth hormone can be used to increase height in some individuals who have documented stimulated or neurosecretory growth hormone secretion.

**Prognosis:** Life expectancy is shortened. Sudden death may occur during the intercurrent infections due to the complicating obesity-hypoventilation syndrome. Early development of diabetic glomerulosclerosis has also been reported. However, some PW patients may reach 50 years of age or more, provided their obesity can be controlled.

**Detection of Carrier:** Unknown.

**Special Considerations:** This condition was first described in 1887 by Langdon-Down, the person who also described Down syndrome, who termed PW "polysarcia". The Prader-Willi Syndrome Association maintains a registry of United States and Canadian patients which currently contains about 1,600 entries.

**Support Groups:** MN; St. Louis Park (6490 Excelsior Blvd., E-102, 55426); Prader-Willi Syndrome Association (PWSA)

**References:**
Niikawa N, Ishikiriyama S: Clinical and cytogenetic studies of the Prader-Willi syndrome: evidence of phenotype-karyotype correlation. Hum Genet 1985; 69:22–27.
Butler M, et al.: Clinical and cytogenetic survey of 39 individuals with Prader-Labhart-Willi syndrome. Am J Med Genet 1986; 23:793–809.

Greenswag LR: Adults with Prader-Willi syndrome. Devel Med Child Neurol 1987; 29:145–152.

Lubinsky M, et al.: Familial Prader-Willi syndrome with normal chromosomes. Am J Med Genet 1987; 28:37–43.

Wiesner GL, et al.: Hypopigmentation in the Prader-Willi syndrome. Am J Hum Genet 1987; 40:431–442.

Fryns JP, et al.: A peculiar subphenotype in the fra(X) syndrome: extreme obesity - short stature - stubby hands and feet - diffuse hyperpigmentation. Clin Genet 1988; 32:388–392.

Greenswag LR, Alexander RC: Management of Prader-Willi syndrome. New York: Springer-Verlag, 1988.

Ledbetter DH, Cassidy SB: The etiology of Prader-Willi syndrome: clinical implications of the chromosome 15 abnormalities. In: Caldwell ML, Taylor RL, eds: Prader-Willi syndrome. New York: Springer-Verlag, 1988.

Knoll JHM, et al.: Angelman and Prader-Willi syndromes share a common chromosome 15 deletion but differ in parental origin of the deletion. Am J Med Genet 1989; 32:285–290.

Nicholls RD, et al.: Restriction fragment length polymorphisms within proximal 15q and their use in molecular cytogenetics and the Prader-Willi syndrome. Am J Med Genet 1989; 33:66–77.

Tantravahi U, et al.: Quantitative calibration and use of DNA probes for investigating chromosome abnormalities in the Prader-Willi syndrome. Am J Med Genet 1989; 33:78–87.

ZE001                                              **Hans Zellweger**

**Prealbumin (TTR) Ala-60 amyloidosis**
  *See AMYLOIDOSIS, APPALACHIAN TYPE*
**Prealbumin (TTR) Ile-33 and/or Gly-49**
  *See AMYLOIDOSIS, ASHKENAZI TYPE*
**Prealbumin defect**
  *See AMYLOIDOSIS, TRANSTHYRETIN METHIONINE-30 TYPE*
**Prealbumin met-111 amyloidosis**
  *See AMYLOIDOSIS, DANISH CARDIAC TYPE*
**Prealbumin Tyr-77 amyloidosis**
  *See AMYLOIDOSIS, ILLINOIS TYPE*
**Prealbumin-84 isoleucine-to-serine**
  *See AMYLOIDOSIS, INDIANA TYPE*
**Preauricular appendages and deafness**
  *See DEAFNESS-EAR PITS*
**Preauricular fistulae**
  *See EAR, PITS*
**Preauricular pit-cervical fistula-hearing loss syndrome**
  *See BRANCHIO-OTO-RENAL DYSPLASIA*
**Preaxial polydactyly I, II, and III**
  *See POLYDACTYLY*
**Preaxial polydactyly IV**
  *See POLYSYNDACTYLY*
**Preaxial polydactyly of toes associated with syndactyly**
  *See POLYSYNDACTYLY*
**Preaxial upper limb deficiency**
  *See HAND, RADIAL CLUB HAND*
**Precalyceal canalicular ectasia**
  *See KIDNEY, MEDULLARY SPONGE KIDNEY*
**Precocious dentition**
  *See TEETH, NATAL OR NEONATAL*
**Precocious periodontitis**
  *See TEETH, PERIODONTITIS, JUVENILE*
**Preductal aortic coarctation**
  *See AORTA, COARCTATION, INFANTILE TYPE*
**Preduodenal portal vein**
  *See LIVER, VENOUS ANOMALIES*
**Preeclampsia, and fetal developmental retardation**
  *See FETAL DEVELOPMENTAL RETARDATION WITH MATERNAL HYPERTENSION*
**Pre-excitation syndromes**
  *See ARRHYTHMIA, WOLFF-PARKINSON-WHITE TYPE*
**Pregnancy-related cholestasis**
  *See INTRAHEPATIC CHOLESTASIS OF PREGNANCY (ICP)*
**Premature alopecia**
  *See HAIR, BALDNESS, COMMON*
**Premaxillary agenesis**
  *See HOLOPROSENCEPHALY*
**Premolar aplasia-hyperhidrosis-canities**
  *See HYPERHIDROSIS-PREMATURE GREYING-PREMOLAR APLASIA*
**Prepyloric membrane**
  *See STOMACH, PYLORIC ATRESIA*
**Presenile dementia, familial**
  *See ALZHEIMER DISEASE, FAMILIAL*

**'Pressure marks' (obsolete)**
  *See NEVUS FLAMMEUS*
**Pressure palsies (hereditary) and neuropathy**
  *See NEUROPATHY, HEREDITARY WITH PRESSURE PALSIES*
**Prieto mental retardation**
  *See X-LINKED MENTAL RETARDATION-SUBCORTICAL ATROPHY-PATELLAR LUXATION*
**Primaquine sensitive anemia**
  *See GLUCOSE-6-PHOSPHATE DEHYDROGENASE DEFICIENCY*
**Primary basilar impression**
  *See BASILAR IMPRESSION, PRIMARY*
**Primary diphallia**
  *See DIPHALLIA*
**Primary hypobetalipoproteinemia**
  *See HYPOBETALIPOPROTEINEMIA*
**Primary hypogonadism**
  *See KLINEFELTER SYNDROME*
**Primary Raynaud phenomenon**
  *See RAYNAUD DISEASE*
**Primary retinal telangiectasia**
  *See RETINA, COATS DISEASE*
**Primidone, fetal effects of**
  *See FETAL PRIMIDONE EMBRYOPATHY*
**Primitive renal tubule syndrome**
  *See RENAL TUBULAR DYSGENESIS*
**Primordial dwarfism**
  *See GROWTH HORMONE DEFICIENCY, ISOLATED*
**Pringle disease**
  *See TUBEROUS SCLEROSIS*
**Prinivil^, possible fetal effects**
  *See FETAL ANGIOTENSIN CONVERTING ENZYME (ACE) INHIBITION RENAL FAILURE*
**Proaccelerin deficiency**
  *See FACTOR V DEFICIENCY*
**Proalbumin Christchurch**
  *See ANALBUMINEMIA*
**Proboscis lateral**
  *See NOSE, PROBOSCIS LATERALIS*
**ProC deficiency**
  *See PROTEIN C DEFICIENCY*
**Procollagen peptidase deficiency**
  *See EHLERS-DANLOS SYNDROME*
**Procollagen protease deficiency**
  *See EHLERS-DANLOS SYNDROME*
**Progenie**
  *See MANDIBULAR PROGNATHISM*

---

## PROGERIA                                        0825

**Includes:**
> Acrogeria
> Aging, accelerated
> Hutchinson-Gilford progeria syndrome
> Progeronanism
> Senile nanism

**Excludes:**
> **Cleidocranial dysplasia** (0185)
> **Cockayne syndrome** (0189)
> **Cutis laxa** (0233)
> "Gerodermata" (various)
> **Leprechaunism** (0587)
> **Mandibuloacral dysplasia** (2082)
> **Oculo-mandibulo-facial syndrome** (0738)
> **Pyknodysostosis** (0846)
> **Seckel syndrome** (0881)
> **Werner syndrome** (0998)

**Major Diagnostic Criteria:** Appearance of accelerated aging, onset of growth failure in the first year of life, weight decreased for height, alopecia, loss of peripheral subcutaneous fat, prominent scalp veins, delayed and abnormal dentition, craniofacial disproportion with small face, micrognathia, prominent eyes, midfacial cyanosis, coxa valga, and normal intelligence.

**Clinical Findings:** The development of an extremely aged appearance is the most striking feature of the syndrome. At birth affected infants may already have suspicious findings ("sclerodermatous skin," midfacial cyanosis, sculptured nose) but are usually

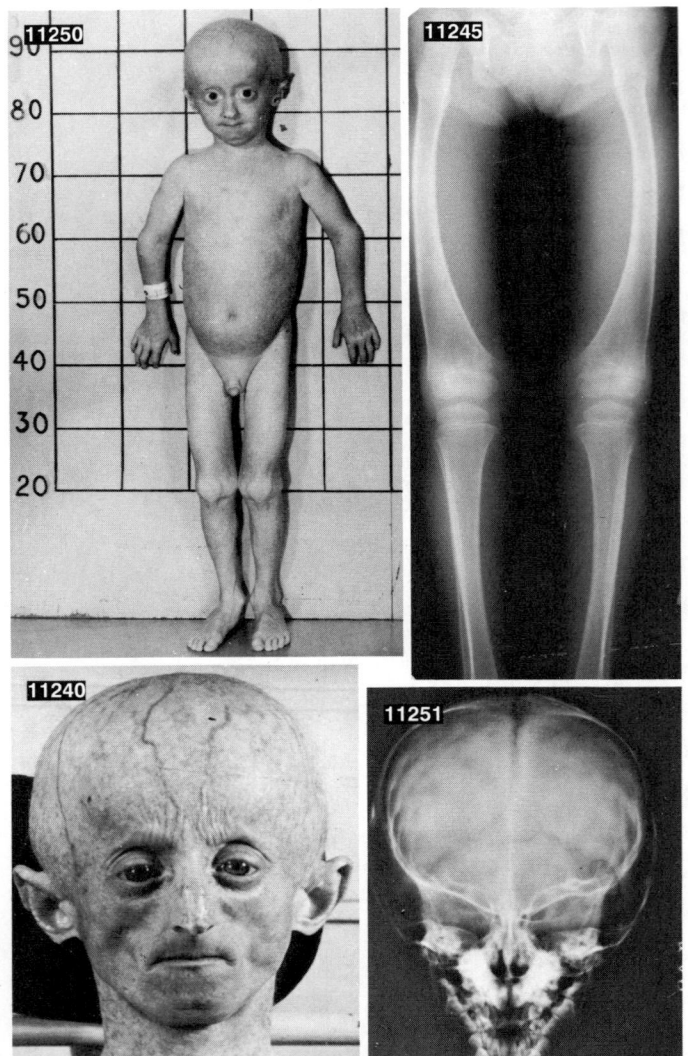

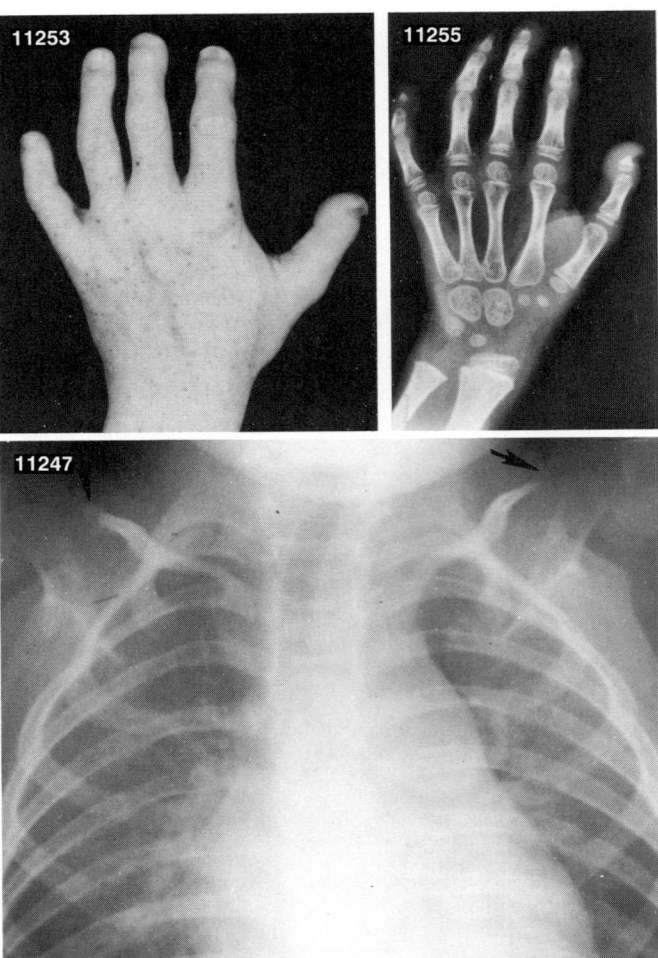

**0825B**-11253: Inability to extend fingers fully, knobby interphalangeal joints, and stubby terminal phalanges of several digits. 11255: Retarded bone age and hypoplastic terminal phalanges. 11247: X-ray of the chest shows osteolysis of the distal clavicles.

**0825A**-11250: Short stature, hairlessness and prominent scalp veins. 11245: Delicate long bones and coxa valga. 11240: Increased prominence of scalp veins and aged appearance in this affected 14-year-old. 11251: X-ray of skull shows open fontanels and small facial bones relative to the calvarium.

considered to be normal appearing infants. During the second six months of life a profound and progressive retardation in weight gain and growth becomes apparent. Growth of the facial bones and mandible also fail, but the cranium remains relatively large. The eyes become prominent. The nose stays small, perhaps beaked, with nasal cartilage contours visible under the thin skin. The mandible continues to grow slowly, resulting in true micrognathia. At about the same time the scalp hair becomes sparse, and the scalp veins become prominent. Eyebrows and eyelashes may disappear during the first and second years of life. The result is total alopecia from the early years on, apart from a few downy, small, white or blond hairs, which may persist throughout life. The effect is to produce what has been called a "plucked-bird appearance."

Concurrent with the failure to gain weight and grow is the gradual disappearance of almost all subcutaneous fat. This absence of subcutaneous fat, along with failure of long bones to grow in girth and in length, results in spindly limbs. The joints, especially the knees, become prominent. Stiffness of joints and limitation of motion develop. This and the invariable coxa valga are the basis for the wide-based "horse-riding stance," usually evident by age two or three years, which adds to the striking appearance. The voice is thin and high-pitched. The clavicles are usually short and thin; the distal one-third frequently becomes radiolucent. The anterior fontanelle remains patent, and there are occasional Wormian bones. The short clavicles are associated with narrow shoulders and pyriform thorax. Abnormalities of nails may become apparent by age two or three years. Nails may be dystrophic, small, and short. The terminal phalanges frequently develop acro-osteolysis and may become radiolucent. The skin develops an aged appearance, being thin, shiny, taut, and dry in some areas and dry, dull, and wrinkled in others. Small, blotchy, brownish pigmentations tend to develop with increasing age. There is a marked delay in dentition, with crowded maloccluded teeth that may be rotated, displaced, or overlapping. There are no ocular abnormalities as in oculomandibulofacial syndrome. Widespread atherosclerosis usually develops. Early death by myocardial infarction or cerebral vascular accident is common. Intelligence is normal or above average.

Excess urinary excretion of hyaluronic acid has been noted. No endocrine or metabolic abnormality has been documented other than an increase in metabolic rate without hyperthyroidism. Growth hormone responses are normal, but insulin tolerance may be increased. Collagen fiber bundles may be disorganized, thickened, and "hyalinized." Extracted collagen has been reported to show decreased solubility and abnormal thermal shrinkage. Chromosomal studies have been normal. There are no consistent abnormalities of serum lipids. Decreased growth capacity of fibroblasts has been variably noted. Abnormalities of DNA repair, HLA antigen expression, and thermolability of enzymes have not been consistently demonstrated.

The condition should be distinguished from *Acrogeria*, a rare condition in which the skin of the hands and feet show signs of premature aging, but there is no alopecia or atherosclerosis (De Groot et al, 1980).

**Complications:** Myocardial infarcts, congestive heart failure, limitation of motion of large and small joints.

**Associated Findings:** Cerebrovascular occlusions secondary to atherosclerosis; hip dislocations; asceptic femoral head necrosis; cephalohematomas; headaches; parathesias.

**Etiology:** In most instances, a sporadic autosomal dominant mutation. In support of this conclusion, there is a significant increase in the average paternal age. Maciel (1988), however, has made a case for autosomal recessive inheritance. A lack of affected sibs is the general rule. Occasional sibships may suggest somatic mosaicism, or stem cell mutation of ovary or testes. Several sets of identical twins have been noted.

**Pathogenesis:** An abnormality of glycosaminoglycan metabolism is suggested by elevated hyaluronic acid excretion. Such an abnormality could alter normal development.

**MIM No.:** 17667, 20120

**POS No.:** 3362

**Sex Ratio:** M1:F1

**Occurrence:** Since it was first described in 1886, approximately 100 cases of progeria have been reported. In the United States, the reported incidence over the past 60 years is about 1:8,000,000, although, since about one-half of cases go unreported, the true incidence may reach 1:4,000,000. In the United States, about 10–15 patients are living at any one time. Cases have been reported from all continents. Several cases have been reported in Black and Oriental populations.

**Risk of Recurrence for Patient's Sib:**
See Part I, *Mendelian Inheritance*. Probably around 1:500 because of the possible somatic mosaicism.

**Risk of Recurrence for Patient's Child:**
See Part I, *Mendelian Inheritance*. No affected individuals are known to have reproduced.

**Age of Detectability:** Generally first to second year of life, but possibly at birth if sclerodermatous skin, glyphic nose, and midfacial cyanosis are present.

**Gene Mapping and Linkage:** Unknown.

**Prevention:** None known. Genetic counseling indicated.

**Treatment:** No specific therapy; small dose aspirin is suggested.

**Prognosis:** General health usually good, with few infections. Physical handicaps due to size are usual. Joint problems are common with increasing age. Psychologic problems related to appearance and self-image are common. The age of nontraumatic death was reported for 18 cases to range from 7 to 27 years, with a median age of 12 years and a mean of 13.4 years. Death was usually due to heart failure.

**Detection of Carrier:** Unknown.

**Special Considerations:** Progeria has been considered a model of apparent accelerated aging, although dementia, cataracts, and tumors, which may be associated with normal aging, are not usually seen. Hyaluronic acid elevation in urine, also seen in **Werner syndrome**, may reflect a basic defect in metabolism.

**Support Groups:** NY; Manhasset (Tel. 516–562–4612); Progeria International Registry

**References:**
DeBusk FL: The Hutchinson-Gilford progeria syndrome. J Pediatr 1972; 80:697–724.
DeGroot WP, et al.: Familial acrogeria (Gottron). Btit J Derm 1980; 103:213–223.
Brown WT, et al.: Progeria, a model disease for the study of accelerated aging In: Woodhead AD, et al., eds: Molecular Biology of Aging. New York: Plenum, 1986:375–396.
Zebrower M, et al.: Urinary hyaluronic acid elevation in Hutchinson-Gilford progeria syndrome. Mech Ageing Dev 1986; 35:39–46.
Dyck JD, et al.: Management of coronary artery disease in Hutchinson-Gilford syndrome. J Pediat 1987; 111:407–410.

BR024
**W. Ted Brown**

**Progeria adultorum**
*See WERNER SYNDROME*

---

## PROGERIA, NEONATAL RAUTENSTRAUCH-WIEDEMANN TYPE      2593

**Includes:**
Progeroid syndrome, neonatal
Rautenstrauch-Wiedemann syndrome
Wiedemann-Rautenstrauch syndrome

**Excludes:**
**Cockayne syndrome** (0189)
**Cutis laxa-growth defect, De Barsy type** (2138)
**Lipodystrophy syndrome, Berardinelli type** (2038)
**Oculo-mandibulo-facial syndrome** (0738)
**Progeria** (0825)

**Major Diagnostic Criteria:** Neonatal progeroid appearance, lipoatrophy, and slow growth.

**Clinical Findings:** Affected children are all small for gestational age and subsequently grow at a slower than average rate. A progeroid appearance is present at birth and consists of macrocephalic appearance, entropion, malar hypoplasia, sparse hair, prominent veins, widened anterior fontanelle, and absence of subcutaneous fat. In all cases, 2–4 incisors were present at birth. These teeth were eventually lost, and subsequent dentition was

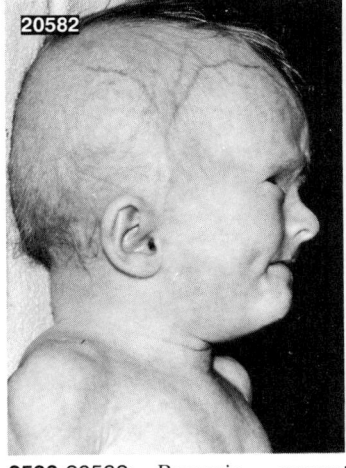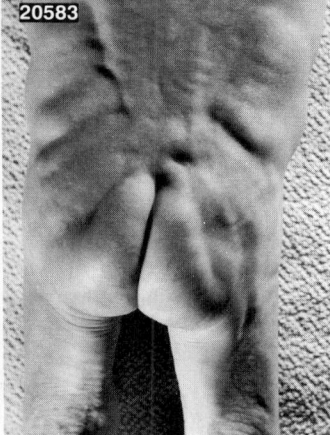

**2593-20582:** Progeria, neonatal Rautenstrauch-Wiedemann type; note hydrocephaloid cranium, prominent venous markings, sparse hair, prominent nose and low-set ears. **20583:** Paradoxical fat accumulation at the buttocks.

delayed. As the children aged, the nose appeared beak-shaped, and paradoxical caudal fat accumulation occurred. Mental retardation is mild to severe. Eyes and digits are normal, although the digits appear long.

**Complications:** May be more prone to feeding difficulties and recurrent respiratory infections.

**Associated Findings:** None known.

**Etiology:** Autosomal recessive inheritance.

**Pathogenesis:** A congenital hypotrophy of subcutaneous fat and mesenchymal tissues. Neuropathologic findings are those of pure sudanophilic leukodystrophy (Martin et al, 1984).

**MIM No.:** *26409

**POS No.:** 3721

**Sex Ratio:** M1:F1

**Occurrence:** Undetermined but presumed rare. All five reported cases have been from Europe.

**Risk of Recurrence for Patient's Sib:**
See Part I, *Mendelian Inheritance.*

**Risk of Recurrence for Patient's Child:**
See Part I, *Mendelian Inheritance.*

**Age of Detectability:** At birth by physical examination.

**Gene Mapping and Linkage:** Unknown.

**Prevention:** None known. Genetic counseling indicated.

**Treatment:** Unknown.

**Prognosis:** Mental retardation is usually present, and ranges from mild to severe. Longevity is unknown; the oldest patient was four years at the time of the last report.

**Detection of Carrier:** Unknown.

**Special Considerations:** One of the patients studied by Rautenstrauch (1977) showed decreased proliferative capacity of the fibroblasts, whereas this was not found in one of Wiedemann's patients (1979). This may indicate that heterogeneity exists, or that decreased proliferation is an inconstant finding, and therefore not of diagnostic value.

**Support Groups:** NY; Staten Island; Progeria International Registry

**References:**
Rautenstrauch T, Snigula F: Progeria: a cell culture study and clinical report of familial incidence. Eur J Pediatr 1977; 124:101–111.
Wiedemann HR: An unidentified neonatal progeroid syndrome: follow-up report. Eur J Pediatr 1979; 130:65–70.
Devos EA, et al.: The Wiedemann-Rautenstrauch or neonatal progeroid syndrome. Eur J Pediatr 1981; 136:245–248. * †
Martin JJ, et al.: The Wiedemann-Rautenstrauch or neonatal progeroid syndrome: neuropathological study of a case. Neuropediatrics 1984; 15:43–48.

T0007                       **Helga V. Toriello**

**Progeroid syndrome of De Barsy**
*See CUTIS LAXA-GROWTH DEFECT, DE BARSY TYPE*

---

## PROGEROID SYNDROME WITH EHLERS-DANLOS FEATURES        3012

**Includes:** Ehlers-Danlos features with progeroid facies

**Excludes:**
**Ehlers-Danlos syndrome** (0338)
**Noonan syndrome** (0720)

**Major Diagnostic Criteria:** Progeroid facies; curly hair; scanty eyebrows and eyelashes; multiple nevi, skin hyperextensibility, bruisability, and fragility; joint hypermobility in digits.

**Clinical Findings:** Mild mental retardation (mean IQ, 60), wrinkled facies, curly and fine hair, scanty eyebrows and eyelashes, telecanthus, periodontitis and multiple caries, low-set and prominent ears, **Pectus excavatum**, winged scapulae, pes planus, skin hyperextensibility and fragility, bruisability, dermatorrhesis, papiraceous scars, multiple nevi, joint hypermobility in digits,

varicose veins, **Hernia, inguinal**, bilateral cryptorchidism. Electron microscopy detects no abnormalities of the skin with exception of a slight distention of intracellular spaces; in the spinous layer the epidermal cells and the collagen bundles are normal.

**Complications:** Unknown.

**Associated Findings:** Mild aortic or pulmonary stenosis, **Brachydactyly** type E, variable stature, hypospadias.

**Etiology:** A *de novo* autosomal dominant mutation has been postulated since all patients were sporadic cases and the paternal age was increased.

This is a distinct nosologic entity that shows variable expression, principally in stature and psychomotor development. In one affected young boy no major handicap was noticed. However, he received psychiatric treatment because of abnormal behavior.

**Pathogenesis:** Probably a primary defect in the synthesis or structure of one of the components of the connective tissue. In one case only half of the amount of a mature proteoglycan was synthesized, and that glycosaminoglycan-free core protein was secreted in fibroblasts (Kreese et al, 1987).

**MIM No.:** 13007

**Sex Ratio:** Presumably M1:F1.

**Occurrence:** About a half-dozen cases have been reported in the literature.

**Risk of Recurrence for Patient's Sib:**
See Part I, *Mendelian Inheritance.*

**Risk of Recurrence for Patient's Child:**
See Part I, *Mendelian Inheritance.*

**Age of Detectability:** During early infancy.

**Gene Mapping and Linkage:** Unknown.

**Prevention:** None known. Genetic counseling indicated.

**Treatment:** Early stimulation; special education.

**Prognosis:** Good for life span; poor for intellectual development.

**Detection of Carrier:** Unknown.

**References:**
Hernández A, et al.: A distinct variant of the Ehlers-Danlos syndrome. Clin Genet 1979; 16:335–339.
Hernández A, et al.: Third case of a distinct variant of the Ehlers-Danlos syndrome. Clin Genet 1981; 20:222–224.
Hernández A, et al.: Ehlers-Danlos features with progeroid facies and mild mental retardation: further delineation of the syndrome. Clin Genet 1986; 30:456–461.
Krusius T, Ruoslahti E: Primary structure of an extracellular matrix proteoglycan core protein deduced from cloned cDNA. Proc Nat Acad Sci 1986; 83:7683–7687.
Kresse H, et al.: Glycosaminoglycan-free small proteoglycan core protein is secreted by fibroblasts from a patient with a syndrome resembling progeroid. Am J Hum Genet 1987; 41:436–453.

HE039                   **Alejandro Hernández**
CA011                   **José María Cantú**

**Progeroid syndrome, neonatal**
*See PROGERIA, NEONATAL RAUTENSTRAUCH-WIEDEMANN TYPE*
**Progeronanism**
*See PROGERIA*
**Progestins, maternal exposure and fetal virilization**
*See FETAL EFFECTS FROM MATERNAL EXTRINSIC ANDROGENS*
**Proglycem^, fetal effects**
*See FETAL EFFECTS FROM MATERNAL VASODILATOR*
**Prognathism, mandibular**
*See MANDIBULAR PROGNATHISM*
**Progonoma**
*See JAW, NEUROECTODERMAL PIGMENTED TUMOR*
**Progressive arthro-ophthalmopathy**
*See ARTHRO-OPHTHALMOPATHY, HEREDITARY, PROGRESSIVE, STICKLER TYPE*
**Progressive bulbar palsy associated with neural deafness (PBPND)**
*See PALSY, PROGRESSIVE BULBAR OF CHILDHOOD*
**Progressive bulbar palsy of childhood (PBPC)**
*See PALSY, PROGRESSIVE BULBAR OF CHILDHOOD*
**Progressive cardiomyopathic lentiginosis**
*See LENTIGINES SYNDROME, MULTIPLE*

Progressive chorea
  See HUNTINGTON DISEASE
Progressive diaphyseal dysplasia
  See DIAPHYSEAL DYSPLASIA
Progressive familial cholestasis
  See JAUNDICE, INTRAHEPATIC CHOLESTATIC, BYLER TYPE
Progressive hypertrophic interstitial neuritis of childhood
  See DEJERINE-SOTTAS DISEASE
Progressive lenticular degeneration
  See HEPATOLENTICULAR DEGENERATION
Progressive muscular dystrophy of childhood
  See MUSCULAR DYSTROPHY, CHILDHOOD
    PSEUDOHYPERTROPHIC
Progressive myoclonus epilepsy without Lafora bodies
  See SEIZURES, PROGRESSIVE MYOCLONIC, UNVERRICHT-
    LUNDBORG TYPE
Progressive systemic sclerosis (PSS)
  See SCLERODERMA, FAMILIAL PROGRESSIVE
Prolapse of laryngeal ventricle
  See LARYNX, VENTRICLE PROLAPSE

---

## PROLIDASE DEFICIENCY                                2616

**Includes:**
  Hyperimidodipeptiduria
  Imidodipeptidase deficiency
  Peptidase D deficiency

**Excludes:** Hyperamidodipeptiduria

**Major Diagnostic Criteria:** Cutaneous ulcers involving the extremities, mostly the legs and feet. Mental retardation is found in a significant percentage of patients. Large quantities of imidodipeptides are excreted in the urine, especially glycylproline. Prolidase activity in erythrocytes, leukocytes, or skin fibroblasts is absent or markedly diminished.

**Clinical Findings:** Skin pathology has been described in about 90% of reported patients, the most prominent lesions being multiple, recurrent ulcers of the lower extremities. Ulcers initially develop in childhood or adolescence and have been reported to appear as early as age 19 months. These scars may be atrophic or sclerotic and can be pigmented or depigmented. Ulcers have been described in two-thirds of reported cases, but their true frequency is probably lower since the diagnosis of prolidase deficiency may not be considered in the absence of these lesions.

Prolidase-deficient individuals may have a variety of other dermatologic lesions, including telangiectasias of the face, shoulders, and hands (40%); scaly erythematous maculopapular lesions (25%); and premature graying of the hair (25%). Few patients had photosensitivity, dry skin, hyperkeratosis of elbows and knees, purpura without underlying hematologic abnormalities, and lymphedema.

Involvement of other organ systems is common. Mild mental retardation is present in more than one-half of the patients. Dysmorphic features, though common, have no specific pattern. Eye examination may disclose hypertelorism, mild ptosis, optic atrophy, or keratitis. A history of recurrent infections such as otitis media or sinusitis has been noted in about 50% of the cases.

Urinary excretion of significant quantities of imidodipeptides, especially glycylproline, is characteristic of this condition. Absence of hyperimidodipeptiduria is strong evidence against the diagnosis of prolidase deficiency. Prolidase activity in erythrocytes, leukocytes, or skin fibroblasts is absent or less than 5% of that of normal controls.

**Complications:** Secondary bacterial infection of ulcerated skin areas.

**Associated Findings:** Obesity, a protuberant abdomen, splenomegaly, joint laxity, deafness, and short stature are present in some patients.

**Etiology:** Autosomal recessive inheritance.

**Pathogenesis:** Prolidase deficiency is the underlying biochemical defect. Prolidase (imidodipeptidase, - EC 3.4.13.9) is an enzyme that splits dipeptides with proline or hydroxyproline at the carboxyl terminal (e.g., glycylproline). Prolidase activity has been

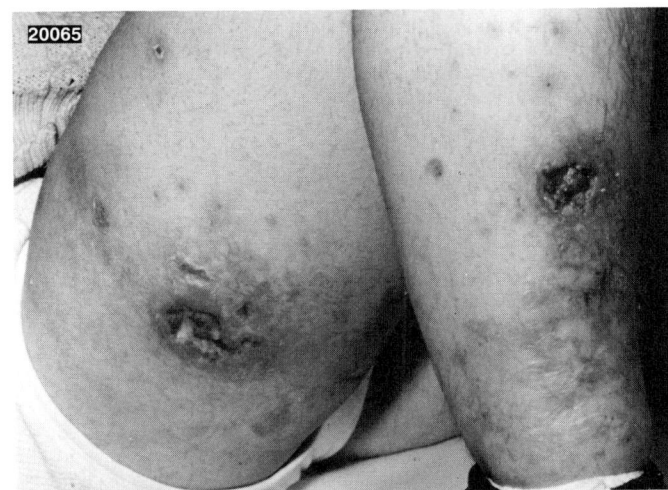

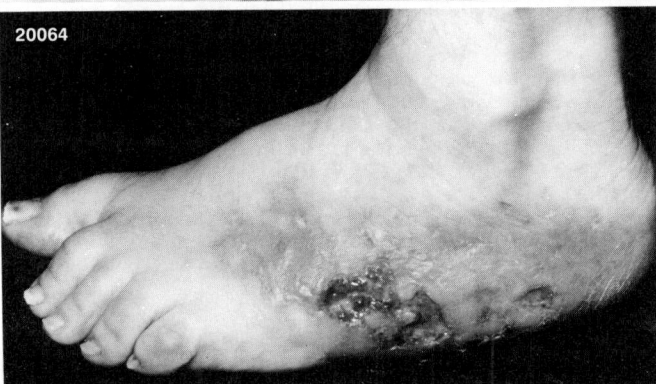

**2616-20064–65:** Note recurrent ulcerations of the leg and foot from prolidase deficiency.

---

detected in all tissues tested in normal individuals. The pathophysiology of the biochemical and clinical abnormalities in prolidase deficiency has not been delineated to date.

**MIM No.:** 26413

**POS No.:** 3767

**Sex Ratio:** M1:F1

**Occurrence:** More than 20 individuals with this condition have been described in the world literature. The patients are from ten different countries: Australia, Belgium, Canada, Denmark, France, Germany, Japan, Lebanon, the United Kingdom, and the United States. One thousand dried blood specimens from Japanese neonates assayed for prolidase activity revealed that about 2% of the samples had intermediate activity consistent with a heterozygote state.

**Risk of Recurrence for Patient's Sib:**
  See Part I, *Mendelian Inheritance.*

**Risk of Recurrence for Patient's Child:**
  See Part I, *Mendelian Inheritance.*

**Age of Detectability:** Prolidase deficiency can be detected in the newborn period by urine screening for imidodipeptide excretion followed by a confirmatory enzyme assay, long before signs or symptoms appear. Ulcers may develop during childhood or adolescence and have been reported to manifest as early as age 19 months. Prenatal diagnosis by amniocentesis or chorionic villus sampling is theoretically possible.

**Gene Mapping and Linkage:** PEPD (peptidase D) has been mapped to 19q12-q13.2.

PEPD has also been mapped to 19p13.2 by in situ hybridization. The gene has been cloned and sequenced. There is a close linkage between PEPD and apolipoprotein C 2 (apo-C2). The condition is linked to **Myotonic dystrophy** and probably linked to the C3-Le-DM-Se-Lu linkage group.

**Prevention:** None known. Genetic counseling indicated.

**Treatment:** Symptomatic treatment of the ulcers. An excellent response to the application of a 5% glycine-5% proline ointment on leg ulcers has been noted in the one patient treated with this modality.

**Prognosis:** Variable. Some patients become bedridden during the second decade of their life because of the severely disabling leg ulcers.

**Detection of Carrier:** Heterozygotes are asymptomatic, do not have imidodipeptiduria, but have reduced erythrocyte prolidase activity compared with normal controls.

**Special Considerations:** There are two main hypotheses for the pathogenesis of the leg ulcers and other manifestations in this condition. One of these attributes the clinical findings to the toxic effects of the imidodipeptides that are not broken down into individual amino acids. The other considers that the skin lesions may be due, to a great extent, to the losses of amino acids in the urine in the form of dipeptides. However, to date both hypotheses lack dependable supportive evidence.

The occurrence of prolidase-like activity about 5% of normal in amount but with a preference for substrate different from normal, in cells homozygous (or compound) for CRM-negative mutations, identified an alternative cleavage activity not encoded at the prolidase locus. Allelic heterogeneity at the major locus, and the amount of alternative peptidase activity encoded elsewhere, appear to be determinants of the associated and heterogeneous clinical phenotype.

**References:**

Der Kaloustian VM, et al.: Prolidase deficiency: an inborn error of metabolism with major dermatological manifestations. Dermatologica 1982; 164:293–304. * †

Freij BJ, et al.: Clinical and biochemical characteristics of prolidase deficiency in siblings. Am J Med Genet 1984; 19:561–571. * †

Arata J, et al.: Effect of topical application of glycine and proline on recalcitrant leg ulcers of prolidase deficiency. Arch Dermatol 1986; 122:626–627.

Freij BJ, Der Kaloustian VM: Prolidase deficiency: a metabolic disorder presenting with dermatologic signs. Int J Dermatol 1986; 25:431–433.

Boright AP, et al.: Prolidase deficiency: biochemical classification of alleles. Am J Med Genet 1989; 44:731–740.

Endo F, et al.: Primary structure and gene localization of human prolidase. J Biol Chem 1989; 264:4476–4481.

Phang JM, Scriver CR: Disorders of proline and hydroxyproline metabolism. In: Scriver CR, et al, eds: The metabolic basis of inherited disease, 6th ed. New York: McGraw-Hill, 1989:577–598.

DE030
FR039

**Vazken M. Der Kaloustian**
**Bishara J. Freij**

**Proline oxidase deficiency**
*See HYPERPROLINEMIA*
**Prominent umbilicus**
*See HERNIA, UMBILICAL*
**Pronation, congenital**
*See RADIAL-ULNAR SYNOSTOSIS*
**Propionic acidemia**
*See ACIDEMIA, PROPIONIC*
**Propionicacidemia I**
*See ACIDEMIA, PROPIONIC*
**Propionyl-CoA-carboxylase deficiency, type I**
*See ACIDEMIA, PROPIONIC*
**Propylthiouracil (PTU) goiter**
*See GOITER, GOITROGEN INDUCED*
**Prostaglandin synthesis inhibition, fetal effects**
*See FETAL EFFECTS OF NONSTEROIDAL ANTI-INFLAMMATORY DRUGS (NSAIDS)*
**Prostatic male urethra, obstruction**
*See URETHRAL VALVES, POSTERIOR*
**Protanopia**
*See COLOR BLINDNESS, RED-GREEN PROTAN SERIES*

**Protean gigantism, Bannayan type**
*See OVERGROWTH, BANNAYAN TYPE*
**Protean gigantism, encephalo-cranio-cutaneous lipomatosis type**
*See PROTEUS SYNDROME*
**Protease inhibitor**
*See ALPHA(1)-ANTITRYPSIN DEFICIENCY*

---

**PROTEIN C DEFICIENCY**      **2918**

**Includes:**

> Heterozygous protein C deficiency
> Homozygous protein C deficiency
> Plasma protein C deficiency
> ProC deficiency
> Purpura fulminans, neonatal
> Thrombophilia, inherited
> Thromboses, and Protein C deficiency
> Thrombotic disease, congenital

**Excludes:**

> **Antithrombin III deficiency** (3066)
> **Fibrinogens, abnormal congenital** (0004)
> **Plasminogen defects** (3083)
> **Protein S deficiency** (2950)
> Vascular plasminogen activator deficiency

**Major Diagnostic Criteria:** Heterozygous protein C deficiency is a familial disorder in which there is an increased risk of thrombosis associated with isolated deficiency of protein C, with levels approximately 50% of normal. Other causes of acquired protein C deficiency, such as vitamin K deficiency, liver disease, or consumptive coagulopathy, must be excluded. Homozygous protein C deficiency is a severe disorder occurring in newborns in whom very low levels (1% of normal or less) of protein C are associated with a purpura fulminans-like syndrome or massive venous thrombosis.

**Clinical Findings:** In families with heterozygous protein C deficiency, levels of approximately 50% of normal protein C may lead to an increased risk of thromboembolic complications. Symptoms usually appear during adolescence or in the young adult and include recurrent thrombophlebitis or pulmonary emboli. In family studies, approximately 75% of protein C-deficient individuals experienced at least one thromboembolic episode. The most frequent site of thrombosis was the deep veins of the lower extremities, occurring in 75% of symptomatic persons. In 40% pulmonary embolism also occurred. Superficial thrombophlebitis was observed in 50%. Mesenteric and cerebral vein thromboses have also been reported. The mean age at which thrombotic events began was 29 years, ranging from 14 to 82 years. Pregnancy, surgery, trauma, parenteral injections, and contraceptive hormones were coexisting risk factors.

Complete (homozygous) deficiency of protein C is associated with purpura fulminans or massive venous thrombosis during the neonatal period. Thus far, there have been a dozen confirmed cases. Usually infants were born to asymptomatic, heterozygous, protein C-deficient parents. Pregnancies were full-term and uncomplicated. The major clinical symptoms included widely distributed purpuric lesions progressing to skin necrosis with bullae formation. Skin biopsy of the hemorrhagic lesions revealed microthrombi and fibrin deposition in capillaries and small vessels. A consumptive coagulopathy was associated with mucosal bleeding, intestinal hemorrhage, hematuria, and intracerebral hemorrhage. Widespread thrombosis included bilateral renal vein, hepatic venous, and inferior vena cava thromboses. Pulmonary emboli and hemorrhagic infarction of the lungs were common findings on autopsy. Cerebral thrombosis and hemorrhage lead to cortical necrosis, hydrocephalus, and seizures. Vitreous hemorrhage leading to cataracts and blindness was seen. The age of onset of lesions varied from 1 to 2 hours to 5 days after birth. Laboratory results were consistent with disseminated intravascular coagulation, including microangiopathic hemolysis, thrombocytopenia, hypofibrinogenemia, increased fibrin split products, and prolonged prothrombin and partial thromboplastin clotting times. Protein C antigen was undetectable or less than one percent in all but three patients. These three infants were reported to have 16–23% antigen, but undetectable protein C activity.

Protein C levels can be measured by assays for antigen or functional activity. Antigen assays include Laurell immunoelectrophoresis, enzyme-linked immunosorbent assay, or radioimmunoassay using either polyclonal rabbit or goat antibodies or monoclonal antibodies. Protein C function can be measured by a variety of methods, depending on its ability to act as an anticoagulant or to act upon a chromogenic substrate. For functional measurement, protein C must first be activated by thrombin (with or without the addition of thrombomodulin) or by a snake venom. Functional assays for protein C are technically more difficult to perform and are not as readily available as the antigenic assay. Normal adult levels of protein C antigen are approximately 65–165% of normal pooled plasma. In normal term infants, protein C antigen, like the other vitamin K proteins, may be reduced to 30% of normal. Protein C may also be secondarily reduced in the postoperative state and in massively obese individuals. Protein C may be elevated during pregnancy. To diagnose hereditary protein C deficiency, liver disease and a vitamin K deficiency must be ruled out. Normal levels of the vitamin K-dependent coagulation factors (Factors VII, IX, and X and prothrombin) should be present.

Plasma levels of protein C may be moderately decreased, secondarily, in persons with consumptive coagulopathy. This diagnosis should be excluded by the presence of normal levels of fibrinogen and platelets with normal fibrin split products in persons with suspected heterozygous protein C deficiency. Although disseminated intravascular coagulation is a feature of the severe homozygous form of protein C deficiency, the marked depression of the protein C level (less than two percent of normal) in association with appropriate family studies will confirm the diagnosis of primary, rather than secondary, protein C deficiency. Other causes of familial thrombosis should be excluded, including abnormalities of fibrinogen or deficiencies of antithrombin III, protein S, plasminogen, or vascular plasminogen activator. The definitive diagnosis of hereditary heterozygous protein C deficiency can only be made with certainty if at least one additional family member is affected. In homozygous protein C deficiency both parents should have reduced levels of protein C antigen or function.

**Complications:** Primarily the sequelae of venous thrombosis. Chronic venous insufficiency may result. Coumarin-induced skin necrosis has also been reported to develop in patients with protein C deficiency within a few days of initiating oral anticoagulant therapy. The lesions usually occur on the lower extremity, the abdominal wall, the breast, or the penis. Lesions progress rapidly to formation of hemorrhagic bullae and full-thickness skin infarction. The cause of coumarin necrosis is explained as resulting from a severe hypercoagulable state following initiation of coumarin therapy due to a rapid fall in protein C levels compared with the clotting factors II, IX, and X because of their different biologic half-lives. Coumarin necrosis may not be avoidable by simultaneous heparin therapy. Complications of homozygous protein C deficiency include sequelae of multiple organ infarct. Renal vein thrombosis has been associated with hypertension and uremia. Cerebral thrombosis or hemorrhage has resulted in developmental retardation, deafness, blindness, and death.

**Associated Findings:** None known.

**Etiology:** Heterozygous protein C deficiency by autosomal dominant inheritance with incomplete penetrance at the clinical level. In most families, the deficient family members show a severe thrombotic tendency in adult life. In homozygous protein C deficiency, both parents would be expected to have a deficiency of protein C. The thrombotic tendency of heterozygotes found by family studies of homozygous newborns is far less severe than in families with heterozygous protein C deficiency. Only six percent have been reported to have experienced venous thrombosis. It has been proposed that, on the basis of clinical manifestations, hereditary protein C deficiency may be divided into two distinct phenotypes: autosomal recessive and autosomal dominant. In the autosomal dominant phenotype, the heterozygotes have recurrent thrombosis during adult life. In the recessive phenotype, heterozygotes have no symptoms and the homozygotes are severely affected with purpura fulminans or massive thrombosis during the neonatal period. There is no clear explanation for the difference between these two apparent phenotypes.

**Pathogenesis:** Protein C is a vitamin K-dependent serine protease zymogen produced in the liver. Upon activation by thrombin, protein C exhibits anticoagulant activity by way of its ability to inactivate clotting factors Va and VIIIa in the presence of protein S, another vitamin K-dependent protein. In addition to this anticoagulant action, activated protein C promotes fibrinolysis probably by inhibiting the inactivator of plasminogen activator. The activation of protein C by thrombin is greatly accelerated if thrombin is first complexed with the endothelial-bound cofactor thrombomodulin. At present two types of protein C deficiency have been described. Type I, in which protein C activity and antigen are equally reduced, probably reflects decreased synthesis of protein C. Type II, in which the biologic activities of protein C are reduced whereas the antigen level is within the normal range, probably reflects production of a dysfunctional protein. Subtypes of type II deficiency may be defined according to the results of a chromogenic functional assay versus the anticoagulant assay. From a clinical standpoint, there appears to be no difference in the two types. In some cases of type II protein C deficiency, an abnormal electrophoretic migration of protein C has been demonstrated.

**MIM No.:** *17686

**Sex Ratio:** M1:F1

**Occurrence:** Prevalence of the autosomal dominant form has been estimated at 1:16,000. Prevalence of the autosomal recessive form in which heterozygotes have no symptoms has been estimated at 1:200–300.

**Risk of Recurrence for Patient's Sib:**
See Part I, *Mendelian Inheritance.*

**Risk of Recurrence for Patient's Child:**
See Part I, *Mendelian Inheritance.*

**Age of Detectability:** Homozygous protein C deficiency can be detected at birth. The diagnosis of heterozygous protein C deficiency should be made cautiously in the young child because of normal low levels of protein C under age six months. Prenatal diagnosis has not been reported.

**Gene Mapping and Linkage:** PROC (protein C (inactivator of coagulation factors Va and VIIIa)) has been mapped to 2q13-q21.

Isolation and characterization of the cDNA coding for human protein C has demonstrated the gene to span 11 kilobases of DNA. The coding and 3' noncoding portion of the gene consists of eight exons and seven introns. There is considerable similarity between the locations of the introns in the genes for protein C and Factor IX. Genotype studies in 14 families with hereditary protein C deficiency revealed a complete deletion of the protein C gene in three families. In two families, changes in Southern blot analysis were produced by either a deletion or insertion of new sequences. Nine families showed no detectable abnormality of the gene. It is likely that most families with protein C deficiency result from a point mutation in the protein C gene. Closely linked Pvu restriction enzyme polymorphism has been demonstrated in two related patients with type I protein C deficiency.

**Prevention:** None known. Genetic counseling indicated.

**Treatment:** In heterozygotes, heparin is effective for treatment of thrombosis. Coumarin therapy is effective in the long-term prevention of venous thromboembolism. Initiation of coumarin therapy has to be monitored carefully because of the risk of coumarin necrosis. Low initial loading doses are recommended to prevent marked and rapid decrease of protein C. Replacement of protein C with fresh-frozen plasma during life-threatening thromboembolism or coumarin necrosis has been reported. Anabolic steroids have been shown to raise protein C levels in heterozygous deficiency. Clinical usefulness of these agents would be expected in type I protein C deficiency only. In the purpura fulminans-like syndrome in homozygous protein C deficiency, infusions of fresh-frozen plasma and prothrombin complex concentrates have been life-saving. Protein C survival in the plasma of these infants has been biphasic, with a first-phase half-life of six hours and a second phase of 10–11 hours. Oral anticoagulant therapy has also been used with success.

**Prognosis:** Heterozygous protein C deficiency is compatible with a long life. Due to the risk of spontaneous recurrence of thrombosis after oral anticoagulation therapy is discontinued, prolonged therapy (possibly for life) is indicated. The ultimate prognosis of homozygous protein C deficiency is extremely guarded. Reported infants who have been maintained on protein C replacement therapy or oral anticoagulant therapy to prevent the catastrophic symptoms of homozygous protein C deficiency. The long-term effects of vitamin K antagonists in children on growth and development are undetermined.

**Detection of Carrier:** In type I heterozygous protein C deficiency, protein C antigen and function would be moderately and proportionately reduced to approximately 50% of normal. In type II protein C heterozygous deficiency, protein C function is reduced to approximately 50% of normal and is associated with normal protein C antigen. In patients on oral anticoagulant therapy, the diagnosis of protein C deficiency may be difficult. Simultaneous measurement of protein C and coagulation factors II and X have been used. If both the ratios of protein C: factor II antigen and protein C: factor X antigen are below 0.5, protein C deficiency may be presumed. This diagnostic determination should be made only after equilibrium of all clotting factors has been reached on oral anticoagulant therapy.

**References:**
Griffin JH, et al.: Deficiency of protein C in congenital thrombotic disease. J Clin Invest 1981; 68:1370–1373.
Crabtree GR, et al.: The range of genotypes underlying human protein C deficiency. Thromb Haemost 1985; 54:56.
Foster DC, et al.: The nucleotide sequence of the gene for human protein C. Proc Natl Acad Sci USA 1985; 82:4673–4677.
Marlar RA: Protein C in thromboembolic disease. Semin Thromb Hemostas 1985; 11:387–393.
Rocchi M, et al.: Mapping of coagulation factors protein C and factor X on chromosome 2 and 13 respectively. Cytogenet Cell Genet 1985; 40:734.
Clouse LH, Comp PC: The regulation of hemostasis: the protein C system. New Engl J Med 1986; 314:1298–1304.
Long GL: Structure and evaluation of the human genes encoding protein C and coagulation factors VII, IX and X. Cold Spring Harbor Symp Quant Biol 1986; 51:525–529.
Pabinger I: Clinical relevance of protein C. Blut 1986; 53:63–75.
Miletich J, et al.: Absence of thrombosis in subjects with heterozygous protein deficiency. New Engl J Med 1987; 317:991–996.
Marlar RA, et al.: Diagnosis and treatment of homozygous protein C deficiency. J Pediatr 1989; 114:528–534.

GR036                                        **Ralph A. Gruppo**

**Protein C inhibitor deficiency**
  See COAGULATION DEFECT, FAMILIAL MULTIPLE FACTORS
**Protein Gc**
  See PLASMA, GROUP-SPECIFIC COMPONENT

## PROTEIN S DEFICIENCY                                   2950

**Includes:**
  Plasma protein S deficiency
  Thromboses, and protein S deficiency

**Excludes:**
  **Antithrombin III deficiency** (3066)
  **Protein C deficiency** (2918)
  Protein S deficiency, acquired

**Major Diagnostic Criteria:** Deep venous thrombosis, which can be recurrent; reduced plasma level of functional protein S.

**Clinical Findings:** Congenital deficiency of functional protein S with associated venous thrombosis. Pulmonary embolism occurs in over half of all patients, and are recurrent in 77% of these. There is no apparent relationship between the level of protein S and the frequency of thrombosis. Patients have been reported who have had severe deficiency of protein S and no history of thrombosis, and there are patients with moderate deficiency who have had recurrent thromboses.

**Complications:** Pulmonary embolism; death from thromboembolic disease.

**Associated Findings:** None known.

**Etiology:** Autosomal dominant inheritance.

**Pathogenesis:** Protein S exists in two forms, as free protein S and as a complex with C4b binding protein (a complement inhibitor protein). The free protein S is the functional protein. This protein S serves as a cofactor for activated protein C. Activated protein C functions as an inhibitor to activated Factors VIII and V.

**MIM No.:** *17688

**Sex Ratio:** M1.6:F1 (estimated).

**Occurrence:** Over a hundred cases have been documented in the literature. Occurrence is estimated to be higher than the number of reported cases would suggest.

**Risk of Recurrence for Patient's Sib:**
  See Part I, *Mendelian Inheritance*.

**Risk of Recurrence for Patient's Child:**
  See Part I, *Mendelian Inheritance*.

**Age of Detectability:** During adolescence.

**Gene Mapping and Linkage:** PROS1 (protein S, alpha) has been mapped to 3p11-q11.2.

**Prevention:** None known. Genetic counseling indicated.

**Treatment:** Coumarin anticoagulants (such as warfarin).

**Prognosis:** Unknown.

**Detection of Carrier:** By protein S levels of about 50% of normal.

**References:**
Comp PC, Esmon CT: Familial protein S deficiency is associated with recurrent thrombosis. J Clin Invest 1984; 74:2082–2088.
Comp PC, Esmon CT: Recurrent venous thromboembolism in patients with a partial deficiency of protein S. New Engl J Med 1984; 311:1525–1528.
Kamiya T, et al.: Inherited deficiency of protein S in a Japanese family with recurrent venous thrombosis: a study of three generations. Blood 1986; 67:406–410.
Engesser L, et al.: Hereditary protein S deficiency: clinical manifestations. Ann Intern Med 1987; 106:677–682.

C0068                                        **James J. Corrigan**

**Protein-losing enteropathy with dilated intestinal lymphatics**
  See INTESTINAL LYMPHANGIECTASIA
**Proteinuria-ocular and facial anomalies-deafness**
  See FACIO-OCULO-ACOUSTIC-RENAL SYNDROME (FOAR SYNDROME)
**Proteinuria-osteolysis**
  See OSTEOLYSIS, CARPAL-TARSAL AND CHRONIC PROGRESSIVE GLOMERULOPATHY
**Proteodermatan sulfate, defective biosynthesis of**
  See EHLERS-DANLOS SYNDROME
**Proteolipid protein, myelin**
  See PELIZAEUS-MERZBACHER SYNDROME

## PROTEUS SYNDROME                                      2382

**Includes:**
  "Elephant man" (possible diagnosis)
  Encephalo-cranio-cutaneous lipomatosis
  Gigantism, hands and feet-nevi-hemihypertrophy-megalencephaly
  Linear sebaceous nevus-mental retardation-seizures
  Organoid nevus syndrome
  Overgrowth, encephalo-cranio-cutaneous lipomatosis type
  Overgrowth, Proteus type
  Protean gigantism, encephalo-cranio-cutaneous lipomatosis type

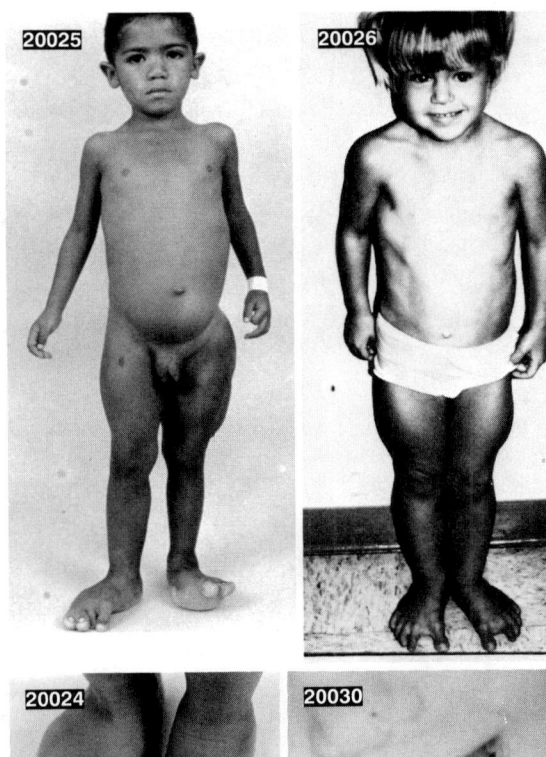

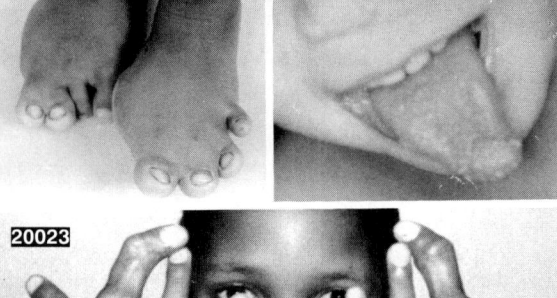

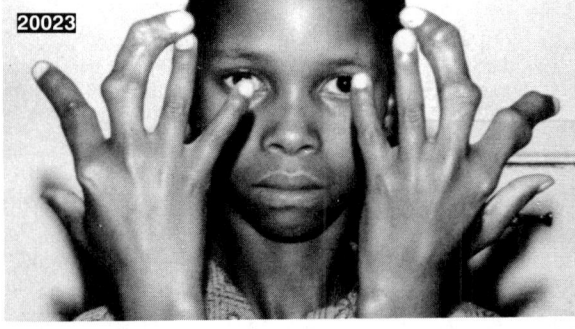

**2382-20025:** Six-year-old boy with asymmetric overgrowth, hypertrophy and syndactyly of the feet, right-sided hypertrophy, lymphangioma of the left thigh, and a right inguinal hernia. **20026:** Five-year-old girl with hemihypertrophy and partial gigantism of the feet. **20024:** Asymmetric hypertrophy of feet with syndactyly; both halluces were surgically removed to improve ambulation. **20030:** Hypertrophy of the tip of the tongue. **20023:** Digital hypertrophy and bizarre angulation.

Schimmelpenning-Feuerstein-Mims syndrome

**Excludes:**
Angiomatosis, cutaneomedullar
Angiomatosis, retinomesencephalic
**Angio-osteohypertrophy syndrome** (0055)
**Enchondromatosis and hemangiomas** (0346)
**Fibrous dysplasia, polyostotic** (0391)

Gingival multiple hamartoma syndrome (0412)
Lipomatosis, diffuse
**Neurofibromatosis** (0712)
**Nevus, blue rubber bleb nevus syndrome** (0113)
**Nevus of Ota** (0716)
**Overgrowth, Bannayan type** (2381)
**Overgrowth, macrocephaly-hemangioma, Riley-Smith type** (2192)
**Sturge-Weber syndrome** (0915)
**Telangiectasia, Osler hemorrhagic** (2021)
**Tuberous sclerosis** (0975)
**Von Hippel-Lindau syndrome** (0995)

**Major Diagnostic Criteria:** Congenital lipomas, occasionally with elements of lymphangioma and/or hemangioma, predominantly subcutaneous, on the cranium and/or intracranially, are essential for the diagnosis. Central nervous system (ectodermal) structural malformations represent a spectrum with frequent eye involvement. **Megalencephaly**, mental retardation, seizures, choristomas, and a variety of other hamartomas further delineate the phenotype, and confirm the diagnosis.

**Clinical Findings:** When present, the **Megalencephaly** is congenital; the head circumference is usually around 2 SD above the mean. Congenital cutaneous hamartomas frequently lead to asymmetry. Partial gigantism secondary to hypertrophy of soft and osseous tissues of the anterior feet and hands in several patients led to the emergence of the Proteus syndrome. Large hamartomas of the soles, predominately lipomatous, were another differentiating sign between Proteus syndrome and the encephalocraniocutaneous lipomatosis.

Until recently, seizures and mental retardation were considered characteristic of encephalocraniocutaneous lipomatosis and not of Proteus syndrome. Additional reported patients, however, seem to bridge the gap between those syndromes. Pigmented intradermal nevi, hyper- and hypopigmented cutaneous streaks, linear verrucose epidermoid nevi, as well as occasional linear subaceous nevi, further delineate the combined phenotype.

On the other hand, the latter clinical features raise the question of whether or not some patients described years ago represent separate entities. The clinical variability of encephalocraniocutaneous lipomatosis appears to be extraordinary, and challenges the current classification of phakomatoses. The symmetric or asymmetric hypertrophy of Proteus syndrome also does not appear to be an unique; i.e., diagnostic clinical feature of the condition.

Ophthalmologic features occasionally noted in patients are anisocoria, heterochromia irides, unilateral microphthalmos, scleral tumor, severe myopia, retinal detachment, cataract, strabismus, and chorioretinitis. Cyst-like alterations of the lungs were observed in two patients. Intelligence is usually normal.

X-ray features include osseous protruberances of the skull, hyperostoses in the external auditory canals and alveolar ridges, irregularly shaped vertebrae, dystrophic intervertebral disks, elongated cervical spine, and kyphoscoliosis.

**Complications:** Excessive localized growth may require surgery to improve function and appearance. The central nervous system malformations frequently lead to the inability to maintain an independent life style. Blindness can complicate the ophthalmologic findings.

**Associated Findings:** Macroorchidism, penile hypertrophy, goiter, early breast development, and congenital dislocation of the hip have been reported in single individuals.

**Etiology:** Unknown. Usually sporadic.

**Pathogenesis:** Possibly faulty embryonic differentiation in the induction, cell migration, and interaction of the cells of the ecto-, meso-, and entoderm. Paracrine growth factors dysregulation appears to play a role in pathogenesis. A somatic cell genetic disorder has also been suggested.

**MIM No.:** 17692

**POS No.:** 3515, 3655

**Sex Ratio:** M1:F1

**Occurrence:** Undetermined. Several dozen cases have been evaluated as possibly having this condition. There appears to be no ethnic predilection.

**Risk of Recurrence for Patient's Sib:** Unknown.

**Risk of Recurrence for Patient's Child:** Unknown.

**Age of Detectability:** At birth for the hamartomas. Several years may be necessary for the emergence of the complete phenotype. Prenatal diagnosis by ultrasound may be possible on the basis of asymmetric hypertrophy of limbs.

**Gene Mapping and Linkage:** Unknown.

**Prevention:** None known. Genetic counseling indicated.

**Treatment:** Orthopedic management of kyphoscoliosis and surgical excision of hamartomas may be performed when clinically indicated.

**Prognosis:** Unknown. A possible malignant potential exists as with other hamartomas.

**Detection of Carrier:** Unknown. First degree relatives should be examined for hamartomas and **Neurofibromatosis**.

**References:**

Gorlin RJ: Proteus syndrome. J Clin Dysmorphol 1984; 2:8–9.

Kousseff BG: Proteus syndrome or another hamartosis. J Clin Dysmorph 1984; 2:23–26.

Lezama DB, Buyse ML: The Proteus syndrome: the emergence of an entity. J Clin Dysmorphol 1984; 2:10–13.

Kousseff BG: Pleiotropy vs heterogeneity in Proteus syndrome. Pediatrics 1986; 78:544–546.

Wiedemann H-R, Burgio GR: Encephalocraniocutaneous lipomatosis and Proteus syndrome. Am J Med Genet 1986; 25:403–404.

Clark RD, et al.: Proteus syndrome: an expanded phenotype. Am J Med Genet 1987; 27:99–117.

Malamitsi-Puchner A, et al.: Severe Proteus syndrome in an 18-month-old boy. Am J Med Genet 1987; 27:119–125.

Viljoen DL, et al.: Proteus syndrome in Southern Africa: natural history and clinical manifestations in six individuals. Am J Med Genet 1987; 27:87–98. †

Cohen MM, Jr: Further diagnostic thoughts about the Elephant Man. Am J Med Genet 1988; 29:777–782.

Kousseff BG, Madan S: The phakomatoses - an hypothesis: paracrine growth regulation disorders? Dysmorph Clin Genet 1988; 2:76–90 †

K0018
VI005

**Boris G. Kousseff**
**Denis L. Viljöen**

**Prothrombin**
*See HYPOPROTHROMBINEMIA*
**Proto-collagen lysyl hydroxylase deficiency**
*See EHLERS-DANLOS SYNDROME*
**Protocoproporphyria**
*See PORPHYRIA, VARIEGATE*
**Proto-oncogene homologous to myelocytomatosis virus**
*See LYMPHOMA, BURKITT TYPE*
**Protoporphyria, erythropoietic**
*See PORPHYRIA, PROTOPORPHYRIA*
**Protoporphyria, porphyria**
*See PORPHYRIA, PROTOPORPHYRIA*
**Protoporphyrinogen oxidase deficiency**
*See PORPHYRIA, VARIEGATE*
**Proximal femoral focal deficiency**
*See FIBULA, CONGENITAL ABSENCE OF*

---

**PRUNE-BELLY SYNDROME**         **2007**

**Includes:**
Abdominal muscles, absence-urinary tract anomaly-cryptorchidism
Abdominal musculature, agenesis, congenital
Eagle-Barrett syndrome

**Excludes:**
**Bladder exstrophy** (3015)
Ventral hernia

**Major Diagnostic Criteria:** Partial or complete absence of abdominal musculature, urinary tract malformations, and bilateral cryp-

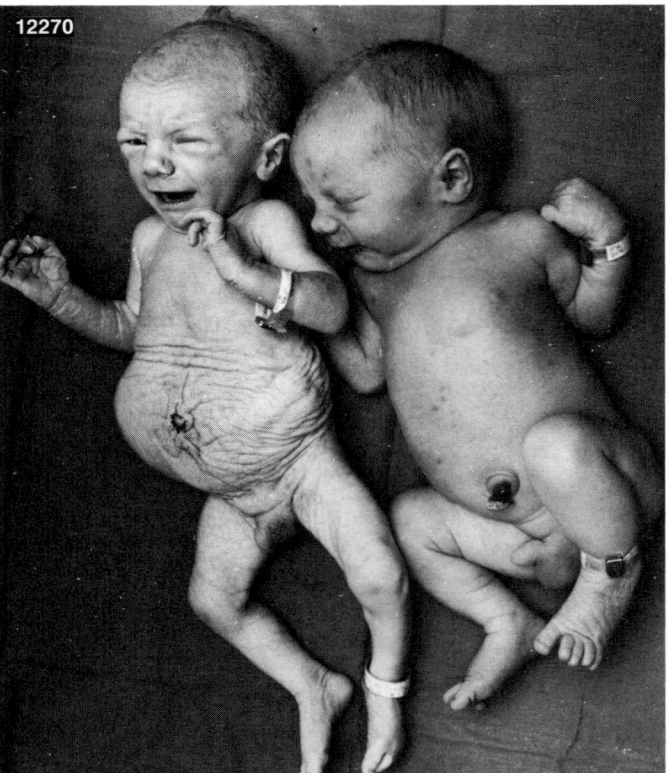

**2007**-12270: Three-day-old monozygotic twins discordant for the abdominal muscle triad. Note the wrinkled and distended abdomen of the affected twin on the left.

torchidism. Confirmation depends on intravenous pyelography (IVP), renal scan and voiding cystourethrogram. Retrograde studies may be necessary in some cases. Urine cultures, renal function tests and biochemical profiles play an important part in the diagnosis and management of the patient.

**Clinical Findings:** This syndrome is recognized at birth, since deficiency of lower and medial parts of the abdominal musculature give the skin the wrinkled appearance of a prune. The fully developed syndrome occurs almost exclusively in males. The defect is quite variable and often asymmetrical, ranging from hypoplasia to complete absence of the abdominal muscles. The lower rectus and oblique muscles are usually intact, pulling the umbilicus cephalad. Ribs are usually flared; Harrison's groove is present.

In the fully developed syndrome the entire genitourinary tract is affected. The kidneys may be dysplastic, cystic, hypoplastic or grossly hydronephrotic. These findings are frequently asymmetric in distribution and kidney function is usually good and does not deteriorate rapidly. Progressive renal failure is the result of chronic urinary tract infection and obstruction uropathy. The dilated and elongated ureters are quite striking on X-ray.

Hydro-ureter or megalo-ureter with poor contractility power are observed by cineradiography. In some cases the ureters are atretic: vesico-urethral reflux is present in most.

The bladder has an enlarged capacity and is trabeculated or megacystic. The apex is attached to the umbilicus; at times the urachus is patent. Although bladder neck obstruction or atresia is rarely reported, this is not a usual finding.

When posterior urethral valves are present, the penile urethra balloons out, often with distention of the prostatic utricle and thickening of the bladder neck. Urachus may be patent allowing leakage of urine through the umbilicus in infants surviving to term. Twenty percent of infants are stillborn; these manifest Potter facies (see **Kidney, polycystic disease, recessive**) and anuria due to renal agenesis. If oliguria is present in the newborn, the survival is poor. Most infants with prune belly syndrome can void normally at birth, but urinary tract infections, and impending chronic renal failure makes early intervention appropriate.

There are milder cases with good renal function in whom surgery can be delayed.

**Complications:** With passage of time the wrinkles flatten out, and the lower abdominal wall bulges in a "pot belly" appearance; this makes it difficult for the child to rise from the supine position. Chronic urinary tract infections eventually lead to uremia.

The time of end stage renal failure depends on the extent of malformations and infection.

When the urinary tract anomaly is severe, such as with complete atresia of the urethra or bilateral renal agenesis oligohydramnios occurs, resulting in multiple compression deformities of the limbs.

Talipes equinovarus and bilateral dislocated hips are the two most common physical abnormalities. Similarly, the hypoplasia of the lungs due to the embarrassment of intrauterine respiratory movements may cause respiratory distress soon after birth. Older children have a tendency to increased respiratory infections.

**Associated Findings:** *Musculoskeletal malformations*: (20–50% of cases): club foot is common. Congenital hip dislocation, skin dimples of elbows, knees, scoliosis, arthrogryposis, **Pectus excavatum** or **Pectus carinatum** hemimelia, myelomeningocele, **Polydactyly**, **Torticollis**, flaired iliac wings, and diastasis of pubis have all been reported.

*Intestinal tract*: imperforate anus is common in the severely affected neonate. Universal mesentery with unattached cecum may cause malrotation of intestines in later life.

*Respiratory tract*: pulmonary hypoplasia with association of oligohydramnios, spontaneous pneumothorax in neonatal period.

*Cardiovascular system*: congenital heart disease is reported in some cases, including **Ductus arteriosus, patent** and septal defects.

*CNS*: craniostenosis and **Microcephaly** have been reported rarely. This may be related to oligohydramnios.

**Etiology:** Undetermined. Discordance was reported seven times, concordance once, in monozygotic twins. One patient was reported to be one of a set of homozygous triplets. The condition has been reported in association with diverse chromosomal anomalies, but most patients have had normal karyotypes.

**Pathogenesis:** The most commonly affected abdominal muscles are the derivatives of the first lumbar myotome, which differentiates between the sixth and tenth week of gestation. Microscopic studies of the muscles show profound alteration, degeneration, and fibrosis.

Two major hypotheses in the pathogenesis of prune belly syndrome exist: one suggests primary distal obstruction in the urinary tract leading to bladder distention and lower abdominal muscular atrophy by duct pressure in early fetal life. The second hypothesis suggests a primary somatic defect in the abdominal musculature. Recent evidence implies that the primary pathogenetic event in the observed pattern of anomalies is overdistension of the fetal abdomen. In some instances, in males particularly, this early distension is associated with urethral obstruction and bladder distension. In the majority of cases, anatomic obstructive lesions could not be identified. In some cases, prune belly results from fetal ascites secondary to various causes.

**MIM No.:** 10010

**POS No.:** 3003

**CDC No.:** 756.720

**Sex Ratio:** M20:F1. Only males have the fully developed syndrome.

**Occurrence:** Over 300 cases have been reported in the English literature.

**Risk of Recurrence for Patient's Sib:** Unknown.

**Risk of Recurrence for Patient's Child:** Unknown. There is no reported case of a prune belly syndrome patient fathering a child.

**Age of Detectability:** At birth. Prenatal diagnosis may be accomplished by ultrasonography after the 20th week of gestation.

**Gene Mapping and Linkage:** Unknown.

**Prevention:** None known. Genetic counseling indicated.

**Treatment:** The primary goal of treatment is the preservation of renal function. This should be directed towards the control of infection and relief of obstruction when present. Surgical management consists of high tubeless urinary diversion, usually pyelostomy, with total reconstruction at the later stage when feasible.

One stage surgery consists of shortening, tapering and reimplantation of ureters, reduction cytoplasty, orchiopexy and plication of abdominal wall. Complete reconstruction of the drainage system and abdominal wall leads to a better prognosis.

**Prognosis:** Survival is related to the level of kidney function. In severe bilateral renal dysplasia, the prognosis is guarded.

Excellent results in children with good renal function and early surgical intervention have been reported.

**Detection of Carrier:** Unknown.

**Special Considerations:** There are only ten reported cases of prune belly syndrome in females. The characteristic urinary tract anomalies are usually missing. Whether these cases represent true prune belly syndrome or are lateral ventral hernias is still debatable.

**References:**

Moine IW, Moine BJ: Prune belly syndrome and fetal ascites. Teratology 1979; 19:111–118.

Pagon RA, et al.: Urethral obstruction malformation complex: a cause of abdominal muscle deficiency and the "prune belly". J Pediatr 1979; 94:900–906.

Woodhouse CRJ, et al.: Prune belly syndrome: report of 47 cases. Arch Dis Child 1982; 57:856–859.

Frydman M, et al.: Chromosome abnormalities in infants with prune belly anomaly. Am J Med Genet 1983; 15:127–135.

Burton BK, Dillard RG: Prune belly syndrome: observations supporting the hypothesis of abdominal overdistension. Am J Med Genet 1984; 17:669–475.

Moerman P, et al.: Pathogenesis of the prune belly syndrome: a functional urethral obstruction caused by prostatic hypoplasia. Pediatrics 1984; 73:470–475.

BI012                                 **Nesrin Bingol**

SA008                                  **Inge Sagel**

**Prurigo Besnier**
*See SKIN, ATOPY, FAMILIAL*

**Pruritus gravidarum**
*See INTRAHEPATIC CHOLESTASIS OF PREGNANCY (ICP)*

---

| **PRURITUS, HEREDITARY LOCALIZED** | **0827** |
|---|---|

**Includes:** Itching, hereditary localized

**Excludes:** Pruritus, non-hereditary

**Major Diagnostic Criteria:** A localized, familial pruritus unassociated with other causes and without significant skin changes.

**Clinical Findings:** Hereditary localized area of pruritus unassociated with any significant skin changes. In the two families reported to date, it occurred on the back. The age of onset is usually in the third decade, but ranges from age four to 41 years.

**Complications:** Unknown.

**Associated Findings:** None known.

**Etiology:** Possibly autosomal dominant or X-linked dominant inheritance.

**Pathogenesis:** Unknown.

**MIM No.:** 17710

**Sex Ratio:** M1:F7 in the reported family. This family also had one male carrier without symptoms who had five affected daughters and two unaffected sons.

**Occurrence:** One kinship reported.

**Risk of Recurrence for Patient's Sib:**
See Part I, *Mendelian Inheritance.*

**Risk of Recurrence for Patient's Child:**
See Part I, *Mendelian Inheritance.*

**Age of Detectability:** Generally in the second to third decade of life.

**Gene Mapping and Linkage:** Unknown.

**Prevention:** None known. Genetic counseling indicated.

**Treatment:** Symptomatic.

**Prognosis:** Normal life span.

**Detection of Carrier:** Unknown.

**References:**
Comings DE, Comings SN: Hereditary localized pruritus. Arch Dermatol 1965; 92:236–237.

C0030

**David E. Comings**

**Psaume syndrome**
*See ORO-FACIO-DIGITAL SYNDROME I*
**Pseudo (platelet-type) von Willebrand disease**
*See VON WILLEBRAND DISEASE*
**Pseudo-arylsulfatase A deficiency**
*See METACHROMATIC LEUKODYSTROPHIES*
**Pseudo-Crouzon disease**
*See CRANIOFACIAL DYSOSTOSIS*
**Pseudo-Hurler disease**
*See G(M1)-GANGLIOSIDOSIS, TYPE 1*
**Pseudo-Hurler polydystrophia**
*See MUCOLIPIDOSIS III*
**Pseudo-pseudohypoparathyroidism**
*See PARATHYROID HORMONE RESISTANCE*

## PSEUDOACHONDROPLASTIC DYSPLASIA          0828

**Includes:**
Gonadal mosaicism in pseudoachondroplasia
Pseudoachondroplastic spondyloepiphyseal dysplasia
Spondyloepiphyseal dysplasia, pseudoachondroplastic type

**Excludes:**
**Achondroplasia** (0010)
**Epiphyseal dysplasia, multiple** (0358)
**Hypochondroplasia** (0510)
**Spondyloepiphyseal dysplasia congenita** (0897)
**Spondyloepiphyseal dysplasia, late** (0898)

**Major Diagnostic Criteria:** Normal at birth. Normal skull, disproportionate short stature, with long trunk and short limbs, and typical vertebral and epiphyseal dysplasia during growth.

**Clinical Findings:** Disproportionate dwarfism with relatively long trunk, short arms and legs, and normal skull and facies; normal-appearing at birth (X-rays taken at birth have been normal); growth retardation and disproportion usually present by two years of age. Growth curve falls off during childhood. Limbs generally shortened; particularly hands and feet. Joint laxity except at elbows. The patient may be knock-kneed or have bowed knees. Trunk relatively long; may be absolutely normal or mildly shortened, with marked lumbar lordosis and mild-to-moderate scoliosis in some individuals. Moderate-to-severe short stature (91.5–137.2 cm adult height). Growth falls off during late childhood and adolescence. X-rays in childhood show oval shape, then moderate flattening of the vertebral bodies, irregularity, and tongue-like projections of central portion of vertebral body; during adolescence, markedly irregular calcification of vertebrae occurs, with partial restoration of normal vertebral form by adulthood. Generalized epiphyseal dysplasia and delay in ossification, particularly in weight bearing joints; capital femoral epiphyses, knees, wrists, and short tubular bones with small, irregular, flat epiphyses, as well as mildly irregular metaphyses during childhood leading to flattening and irregularity of the joint when epiphyses fuse. Faces of affected individuals are similar.

There are no clear differences between the postulated sub-types (I,II,III and IV), although they do differ in apparent inheritance

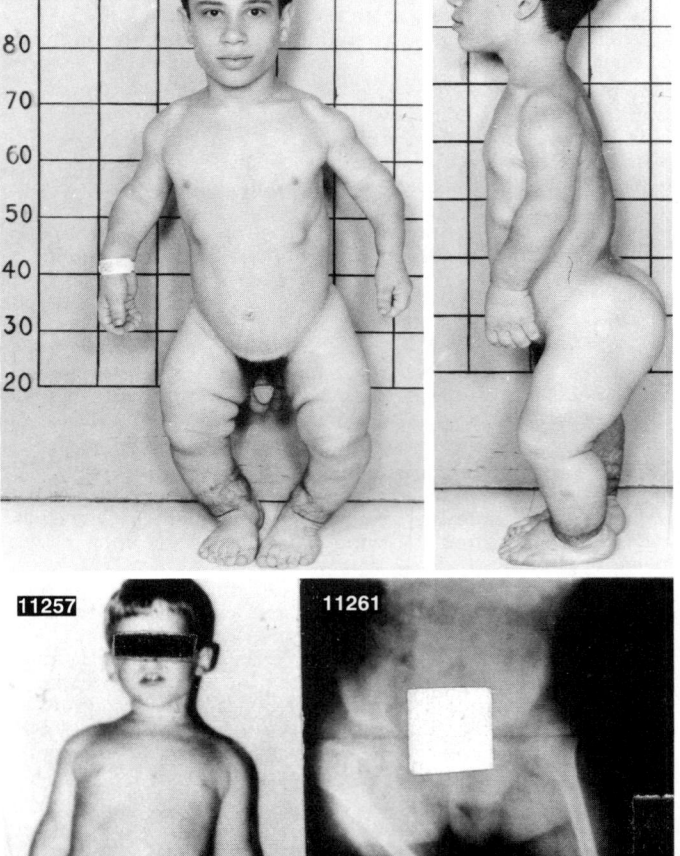

**0828A-11267:** Short stature with short limbs, relatively long trunk and normal skull.   **11268:** Lateral view shows short limbs and exaggerated lumbar lordosis.   **11257–61:** Windswept appearance with knock-knees on right and bow-leg on the left.

patterns and severity. Skeletal, X-ray, and pathologic changes of each sub-type show similar patterns.

**Complications:** Arthritis, particularly hip and knee; scoliosis; ulnar deviation of hand, and joint laxity making functional fixa-

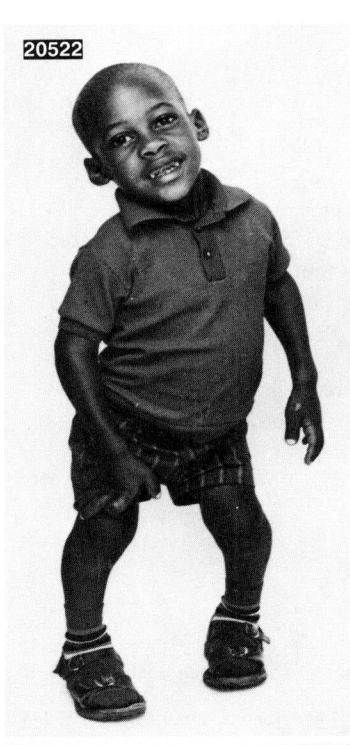

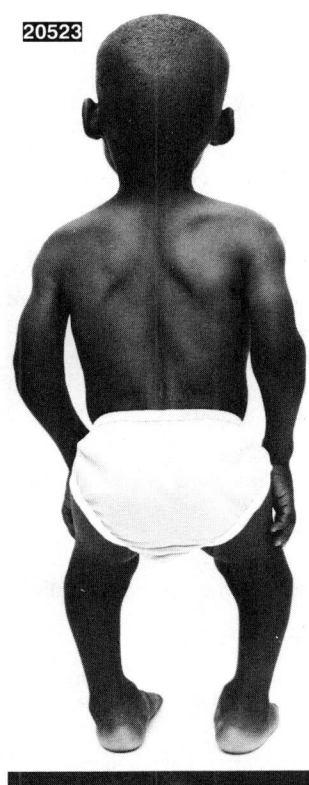

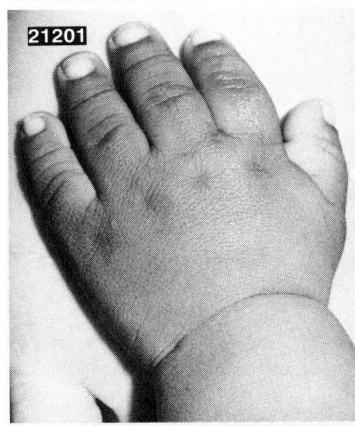

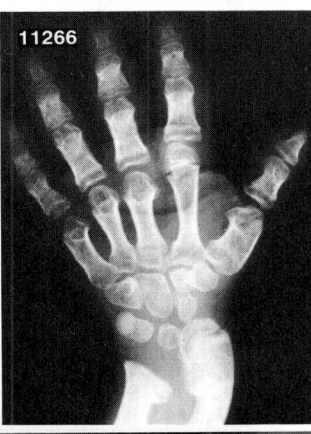

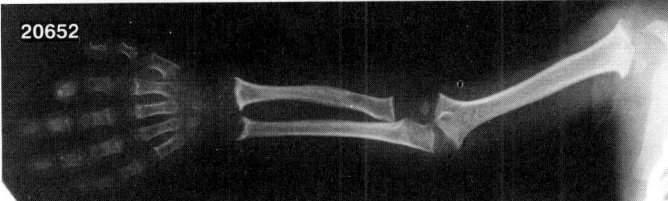

**0828B-20522–23:** Disproportionate short stature with bowed legs and limb deformities. **21201:** Short hand with short digits. **11266:** X-ray of the hand shows abnormality in epiphyseal formation of the distal ulna resulting in relative overgrowth of the radius and ulnar deviation of the hand. The metacarpals and phalanges are all short and stubby. **20652:** X-ray of an affected 4-year-old shows short tubular bones and irregular mushroomed epiphyses.

tion of joints difficult; slow developmental landmarks or waddling gait; social and psychologic adjustments to short stature.

**Associated Findings:** Cord compression has been described.

**Etiology:** Almost all cases have autosomal dominant inheritance or represent new dominant mutations. While penetrance is 100%, fairly marked intrafamilial variability does occur. Some cases previously reported as autosomal recessive inheritance represented parental gonadal mosaicism. A rare condition with autosomal recessive inheritance may, however, exist.

**Pathogenesis:** Accumulation of non-collagenous protein material in the rough endoplasmic reticulum of chondrocytes, and the absence of a specific proteoglycan in cartilage (i.e. not transferred to the Golgi system), appears to be the basic defect.

**MIM No.:** *17715, *17717, *26415, 26416

**POS No.:** 3363

**Sex Ratio:** M1:F1

**Occurrence:** Undetermined, but presumably one-quarter to one-fiftieth as common as **Achondroplasia**.

**Risk of Recurrence for Patient's Sib:**
See Part I, *Mendelian Inheritance.*

**Risk of Recurrence for Patient's Child:**
See Part I, *Mendelian Inheritance.*

**Age of Detectability:** Usually 2–4 years of age. If the parents have a previously affected child, they may suspect the diagnosis at about one year because of short fingers, short arms, or inability to straighten elbow completely.

**Gene Mapping and Linkage:** Unknown.

**Prevention:** None known. Genetic counseling indicated.

**Treatment:** Avoid vigorous athletics, since trauma to joints seems to hasten arthritis. Symptomatic orthopedics for arthritis and bowing. Splinting of wrists and ankles for loose jointedness.

**Prognosis:** Normal for life span and intelligence; fairly severe degenerative arthritis; social, emotional, and vocational problems.

**Detection of Carrier:** Unknown.

**References:**
Maroteaux P, Lamy M: Les formes pseudo-achondroplastiques des dysplasias spondylo-epiphysaires. Presse Med 1959; 67:383–386.
Hall JG: Pseudoachondroplasia. BD:OAS XI(6). Miami: Symposia specialists for The National Foundation-March of Dimes, 1975:187–202. *
Horton WA, et al.: Growth curves for height for diastrophic dysplasia, spondyloepiphyseal dysplasia congenita, and pseudoachondroplasia. Am J Dis Child 1982; 136:316–319.
Stanescu V, et al.: The pathogenetic mechanism in osteochondroplasias. J Bone Joint Surg 1984; 66A:817–836.
Young ID, Moore JR: Severe pseudoachondroplasia with parental consanguinity. J Med Genet 1985; 22:150–153.
Wynne-Davies R, et al.: Pseudoachondroplasia: clinical diagnosis at different ages and comparison of autosomal dominant and recessive types: a review of 32 patients (26 kindreds). J Med Genet 1986; 23:425–434.
Hall JG, et al.: Gonadal mosaicism in pseudoachondroplasia. Am J Med Genet 1987; 28:143–151.

HA014 **Judith G. Hall**

**Pseudoachondroplastic spondyloepiphyseal dysplasia**
*See PSEUDOACHONDROPLASTIC DYSPLASIA*
**Pseudoaldosteronism**
*See LIDDLE SYNDROME*

## PSEUDOAMINOPTERIN SYNDROME 2628

**Includes:** Aminopterin syndrome without aminopterin (ASSA)

**Excludes:** Fetal aminopterin syndrome (0380)

**Major Diagnostic Criteria:** Ocular hypertelorism, ossification defects of cranium, upswept frontal hair pattern, flared eyebrows, and short stature.

**Clinical Findings:** Dysmorphic signs strongly resembling those described in children who were exposed to aminopterin or to methotrexate in early pregnancy (see **Fetal aminopterin syndrome**). Signs include ocular hypertelorism (4/4); bitemporal flattening (3/4); widow's peak with temporal hairline recession and upswept pattern (4/4); arched eyebrows with medial flaring, thinning, and perhaps hypopigmentation laterally (4/4); hypoplastic supraorbital ridges (4/4) with prominent eyeballs (3/4); small palpebral fissures (3/4); prominent nose root (4/4); highly arched or cleft palate (4/4); micrognathia (3/4); and low-set, posteriorly rotated ears (4/4).

The skull is brachycephalic, with incomplete ossification of cranial bones (4/4), delayed fontanelle closure, and synostosis of lambdoid or coronal sutures. Skeletal findings include short stature (4/4), limitation of elbow movement (3/4) with subluxation of radial heads, stenosis of tubular bones, and digital anomalies (3/4). There is mild-to-moderate mental retardation (3/4) and cryptorchidism (3/3).

**Complications:** Unknown.

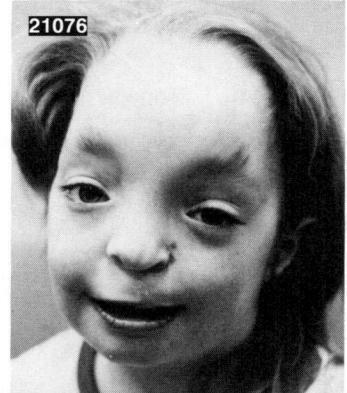

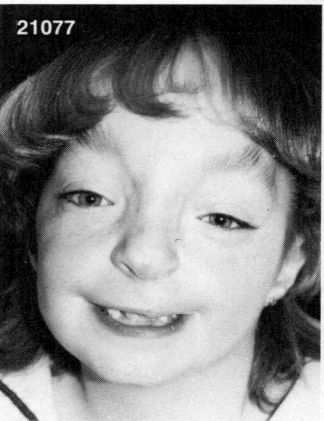 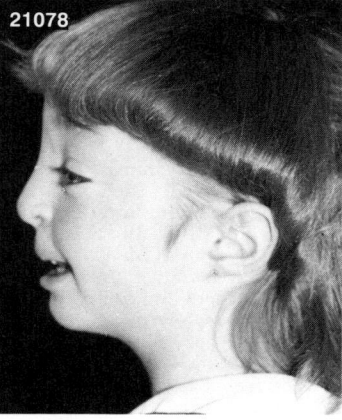

**2628-21076–77:** Note similarity of facial features to those of fetal aminopterin syndrome including ocular hypertelorism, widow's peak, temporal hair recession and upswept pattern, arched eyebrows with medial flaring. **21078:** Lateral view demonstrates the prominent nasal root, micrognathia and low-set ear.

**Associated Findings:** Findings in only one of four patients include **Cleft lip**, **Hydrocephaly**, distal shortening of limbs, and thin long bones with constricted narrow cavities (as in the aminopterin syndrome).

**Etiology:** Possibly autosomal recessive inheritance, if sibs reported by Crane and Heise (1981) represent this condition. One case was found to be mosaic for an apparently symmetrical translocation involving 5q35 and 10q22.

**Pathogenesis:** Unknown.

**Sex Ratio:** Undetermined but presumably M1:F1.

**Occurrence:** Four cases have been reported in the literature.

**Risk of Recurrence for Patient's Sib:** Unknown.

**Risk of Recurrence for Patient's Child:** Unknown.

**Age of Detectability:** At birth. Prenatal detection of some signs may be possible by ultrasound.

**Gene Mapping and Linkage:** Unknown.

**Prevention:** None known. Genetic counseling indicated.

**Treatment:** Surgical management of craniosynostosis, hydrocephalus, possibly hypertelorism, and digital anomalies when indicated.

**Prognosis:** Unknown.

**Detection of Carrier:** Unknown.

**References:**
Shaw EB, Rees EL: Fetal damage due to aminopterin ingestion: follow-up at 17 1/2 years of age. Am J Dis Child 1980; 134:1172–1173.
Crane JP, Heise RL: New syndrome in three affected siblings. Pediatrics 1981; 68:235–237.
Fraser FC, et al.: An aminopterin-like syndrome without aminopterin (ASSAS). Clin Genet 1987; 32:28–34. * †

FR009                                    **F. Clarke Fraser**

**Pseudoaortic stenosis**
*See HEART, SUBAORTIC STENOSIS, MUSCULAR*
**Pseudocholinesterase deficiency**
*See CHOLINESTERASE, ATYPICAL*
**Pseudocholinesterase types E variants**
*See CHOLINESTERASE, ATYPICAL*
**Pseudocholinesterase, E**
*See CHOLINESTERASE, ATYPICAL*
**Pseudocoxalgia**
*See HIP, OSTEONECROSIS, CAPITAL FEMORAL EPIPHYSIS*
**Pseudoglioma of the retina, congenital, bilateral, X-linked**
*See NORRIE DISEASE*
**Pseudohemophilia**
*See VON WILLEBRAND DISEASE*
**Pseudohermaphroditism, familial incomplete male, type 2**
*See STEROID 5 ALPHA-REDUCTASE DEFICIENCY*
**Pseudohermaphroditism, incomplete male, type I**
*See ANDROGEN INSENSITIVITY SYNDROME, INCOMPLETE*
**Pseudohermaphroditism, male internal**
*See MULLERIAN DERIVATIVES IN MALES, PERSISTENT*
**Pseudohermaphroditism, male, steroid 17,20-desmolase deficiency**
*See STEROID 17,20-DESMOLASE DEFICIENCY*
**Pseudohermaphroditism, male gynecomastia**
*See STEROID 17-KETOSTEROID REDUCTASE DEFICIENCY*
**Pseudohermaphroditism-nephron disorder-Wilms tumor**
*See WILMS TUMOR-PSEUDOHERMAPHRODITISM-GLOMERULOPATHY, DENYS-DRASH TYPE*
**Pseudohypertrophic muscular dystrophy**
*See MUSCULAR DYSTROPHY, AUTOSOMAL RECESSIVE PSEUDOHYPERTROPHIC*
**Pseudohypoadrenocorticism**
*See BARTTER SYNDROME*
**Pseudohypoaldosteronism**
*See ALDOSTERONE RESISTANCE*
**Pseudohypoaldosteronism, Persian-Jewish type**
*See ALDOSTERONE RESISTANCE*
**Pseudohypoparathyroidism, type 1a or 1b (PHP-1a or b)**
*See PARATHYROID HORMONE RESISTANCE*
**Pseudohypoparathyroidism, type 2 (PHP-2)**
*See PARATHYROID HORMONE RESISTANCE*
**Pseudohypophosphatasia**
*See HYPOPHOSPHATASIA*

**Pseudoleprechaunism**
*See PSEUDOLEPRECHAUNISM, PATTERSON TYPE*

## PSEUDOLEPRECHAUNISM, PATTERSON TYPE     2626

**Includes:**
    Patterson pseudoleprechaunism
    Pseudoleprechaunism

**Excludes:** Leprechaunism

**Major Diagnostic Criteria:** The combination of normal birth weight, bronzed hyperpigmentation, cutis laxa of large hands and feet, hirsutism, and skeletal dysplasia.

**Clinical Findings:** Findings reported in two affected individuals include normal birth weight (2/2), congenital redundant skin folds (2/2), bronze hyperpigmentation (2/2), hirsutism (2/2), large and beaked nose (2/2), large ears (2/2), large hands and feet with cutis gyrata (2/2), endocrine anomaly (premature adrenarche in one, hyperadrenocorticism in one), severe mental retardation (2/2), seizures (1/2), and skeletal anomalies that include severely delayed bone age (1/2), kyphoscoliosis (1/2), swelling of distal ends of long bones (1/2), genu valgum (1/2), and thickened cranial vault and abnormal metaphyses and diaphyses of the long bones on X-ray (1/2). Abnormal urinary glycosaminoglycan excretion was noted in one patient.

**Complications:** Unknown.

**Associated Findings:** None known.

**Etiology:** Possibly autosomal dominant inheritance.

**Pathogenesis:** Unknown.

**MIM No.:** 16917

**POS No.:** 3494

**Sex Ratio:** M1:F1

**Occurrence:** Two unrelated cases have been reported in the literature.

**Risk of Recurrence for Patient's Sib:**
See Part I, *Mendelian Inheritance.*

**Risk of Recurrence for Patient's Child:**
See Part I, *Mendelian Inheritance.*

**Age of Detectability:** At birth by physical examination.

**Gene Mapping and Linkage:** Unknown.

**Prevention:** None known. Genetic counseling indicated.

**Treatment:** Unknown.

**Prognosis:** One patient died at age seven years. The other patient was age 12 years at the time of the report. Both were severely mentally retarded.

**Detection of Carrier:** Unknown.

**References:**
Patterson JH: Presentation of a patient with leprechaunism. BD:OAS V(4). New York: March of Dimes Birth Defects Foundation, 1969: 117–121.
David TJ, et al.: The Patterson syndrome, leprechaunism, and pseudoleprechaunism. J Med Genet 1981; 18:294–298.

T0007     **Helga V. Toriello**

**Pseudometatropic dwarfism**
*See KNIEST DYSPLASIA*
**Pseudoobstruction, chronic idiopathic intestinal, neuronal type**
*See INTESTINAL PSEUDO-OBSTRUCTION SYNDROMES*
**Pseudopapilledema-macrocephaly-multiple hemangiomata**
*See OVERGROWTH, MACROCEPHALY-HEMANGIOMA, RILEY-SMITH TYPE*
**Pseudopolysystrophy**
*See MUCOLIPIDOSIS III*
**Pseudothalidomide syndrome**
*See ROBERTS SYNDROME*
**Pseudothalidomide-SC syndrome**
*See ROBERTS SYNDROME*
**Pseudotoxoplasmosis syndrome**
*See MICROCEPHALY WITH CHORIORETINOPATHY*

**Pseudovaginal perineoscrotal hypospadias**
*See STEROID 5 ALPHA-REDUCTASE DEFICIENCY*
**Pseudovitamin D-deficiency rickets (PDR)**
*See RESISTANCE TO 1,25 DIHYDROXY VITAMIN D*
**Pseudovitamin D-deficiency rickets (PDR), hereditary**
*See RICKETS, VITAMIN D-DEPENDENT, TYPE I*

## PSEUDOXANTHOMA ELASTICUM     0832

**Includes:**
    Angioid streaks with skin changes
    Elastosis dystrophica
    Groenblad-Strandberg syndrome
    PXE
    Systemic elastorrhexis

**Excludes:** Senile elastosis

**Major Diagnostic Criteria:** Angioid streaks and typical pseudoxanthoma elasticum (PXE) skin changes in the absence of **Bone, Paget disease**. Angioid streaks also occur with Paget disease of bone and with **Anemia, sickle cell**. Encrustation of a normal Bruch membrane by calcium and iron, respectively, may be responsible.

**Clinical Findings:** Changes occur in the skin, eyes, and arteries. The name used for this condition refers to the skin changes which superficially resemble xanthoma and histologically show degeneration of elastic fibers. The skin lesions are usually discernible by the second decade at the latest and are most striking around the neck and in the axilla. The skin of the antecubital area, groin, penis, and periumbilical area may be affected also. The changes consist of yellowish nodular or reticular thickening. The skin about the mouth and chin and in the areas of the nasolabial folds is loose and thickened. The mucosa on the inside of the lower lip may be thickened and yellow, with a superficial vascular network. Not all patients show the chracteristic skin lesions, and scar biopsy may be helpful in establishing the diagnosis in such cases.

In the eyes, the hallmark is angioid streaks: irregular streaking radiating from the disk and lying behind the retinal vessels; so called because of their superficial resemblance to vessels. They are likely to disappear when pressure is applied to the globe. Histologically they can be shown to result from breaks in the Bruch membrane. Hemorrhages also occur in the fundus and threaten vision, especially when they are located in the region of the macula.

Degeneration in the elastic fibers of arteries is accompanied by rupture (especially in the submucosa of the alimentary tract, so that GI bleeding is a major complication in terms of frequency and clinical significance) or occlusion (e.g. in coronary arteries, cerebral arteries, or arteries of limbs).

**Complications:** Blindness, rarely complete. Occlusion of cerebral, coronary, or peripheral arteries with expected clinical results. In pregnant women; deceleration of fetal growth.

**Associated Findings:** None known.

**Etiology:** Autosomal recessive or autosomal dominant inheritance. The autosomal recessive form may be less prone to vascular complications than the autosomal dominant form. Indeed, two distinct autosomal dominant forms may exist. One has severe vascular and ocular changes. The second is accompanied by mild ocular changes, blue sclerae, high palate, and loose jointedness.

**Pathogenesis:** Earliest discernible change in elastic fibers of corium is accretion of calcium salts. Since the fibers, as well as the Bruch membrane, seem to become brittle and fracture, this is presumably a primary disorder of elastic tissue. An inborn error of metabolism with secondary damage to the connective tissue elements (as in **Alkaptonuria** and **Homocystinuria**) is theoretically plausible, but none has been demonstrated.

**MIM No.:** *17785, *26480

**POS No.:** 3346

**Sex Ratio:** Presumably M1:F1 (More females come to medical attention).

**Occurrence:** Several hundred cases have been documented in the literature.

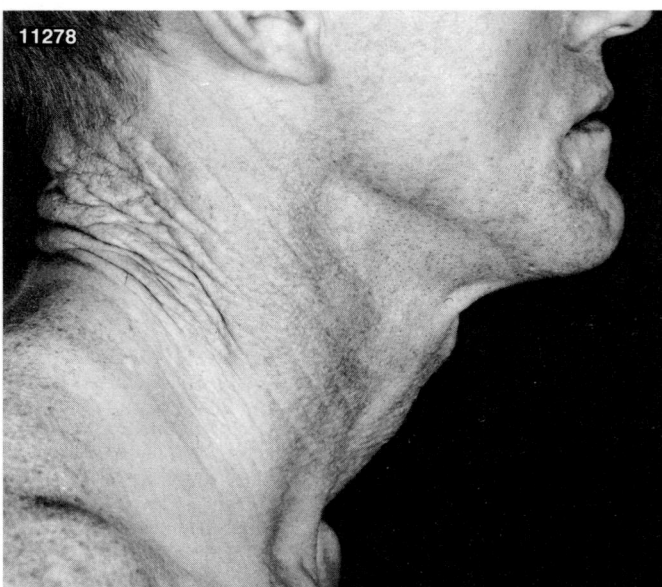

0832A-11278: Note excess and moderately loose skin of neck.

**Risk of Recurrence for Patient's Sib:**
See Part I, *Mendelian Inheritance.*

**Risk of Recurrence for Patient's Child:**
See Part I, *Mendelian Inheritance.*

**Age of Detectability:** Varies; from birth to third or fourth decade.

**Gene Mapping and Linkage:** Unknown.

**Prevention:** None known. Genetic counseling indicated.

**Treatment:** Both vitamin E and vitamin C have been recommended, but there is no evidence of benefit and little rationale for their use. Restriction of calcium intake may be advisable.

**Prognosis:** Normal for intelligence and early function, but life span is significantly reduced by GI bleeding and arterial occlusion.

**Detection of Carrier:** Unknown.

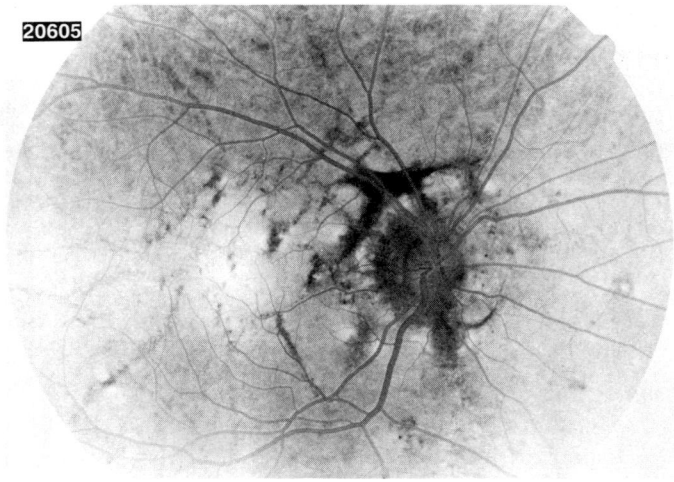

0832B-20605: Pseudoxanthoma elasticum; note angioid streaks in the fundus.

**References:**
McKusick VA: Heritable disorders of connective tissue, 4th ed. St. Louis: C.V. Mosby, 1972.
Pope FM: Autosomal dominant pseudoxanthoma elasticum. J Med Genet 1974; 11:152–157.
Elejalde BR, et al.: Manifestations of pseudoxanthoma elasticum during pregnancy: a case report and review of the literature. Am J Med Genet 1984; 18:755–762.
Remie WA, et al.: Pseudoxanthoma elasticum: high calcium intake in early life correlates with severity. Am J Med Genet 1984; 19:235–244.
Lebwohl M, et al.: Diagnosis of pseudoxanthoma elasticum by scar biopsy in patients without chracteristic skin lesions. New Engl J Med 1987; 317:347–350.
Beighton P, et al.: International nosology of heritable disorders of connective, Berlin, 1986. Am J Med Genet 1988; 29:581–594.

MC023                                    **Victor A. McKusick**

**Psoriasis**
*See SKIN, PSORIASIS VULGARIS*
**Psoriasis-mental retardation, X-linked**
*See X-LINKED MENTAL RETARDATION-PSORIASIS*
**Psoriatic arthritis**
*See ANKYLOSING SPONDYLITIS*
**Psychosine lipidosis**
*See LEUKODYSTROPHY, GLOBOID CELL TYPE*
**PTA deficiency**
*See FACTOR XI DEFICIENCY*
**PTC syndrome**
*See ENDOCRINE NEOPLASIA, MULTIPLE TYPE II*
**PTC taster defect**
*See TASTING DEFECT, PHENYLTHIOCARBAMIDE*

## PTERYGIA-DYSMORPHIC FACIES-SHORT STATURE-MENTAL RETARDATION                           2770

**Includes:**
Face, dysmorphic-pterygia-short stature-mental retardation
Pterygia-mental retardation-distinctive craniofacial features
Short stature-pterygia-dysmophic facies-mental retardation

**Excludes:**
**Arthrogryposes** (0088)
**Arthrogryposis, distal types** (2280)
**Pterygium syndrome**

**Major Diagnostic Criteria:** Shortness, unusual combination of craniofacial anomalies (trigonocephaly; bulging forehead; flat face; posteriorly angulated, low-set ears; and microretrognathia), genital hypoplasia, and multiple pterygia.

**Clinical Findings:** The three known patients presented with severe mental retardation and multiple congenital anomalies. The full clinical expression was present in one female: multiple pterygia (see **Pterygium syndrome, multiple**), **Cleft palate**, and genital hypoplasia. The absence of evident pterygia in the other two known patients precludes classification of this condition as a separate **Pterygium syndrome**.

**Complications:** Unknown.

**Associated Findings:** Hypothyroidism was documented in two of the three patients.

**Etiology:** Possibly autosomal dominant inheritance. The presence of similar facial findings in two grandmothers suggests variable expression and penetrance.

**Pathogenesis:** Unknown.

**MIM No.:** 17798

**POS No.:** 3843

**Sex Ratio:** Three females have been reported.

**Occurrence:** Reported cases consist of three related females who were detected in a survey of 2,000 institutionalized moderately and severely mentally retarded persons.

**Risk of Recurrence for Patient's Sib:**
See Part I, *Mendelian Inheritance.*

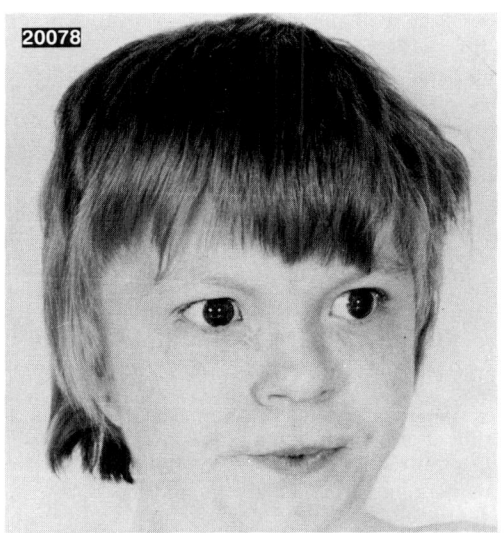

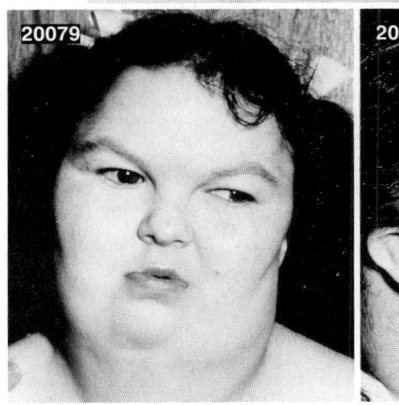
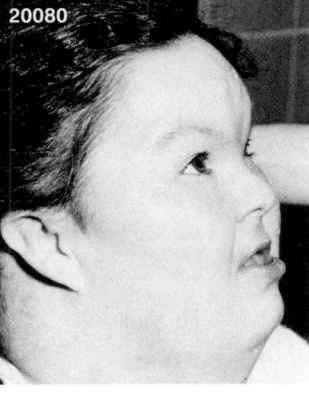

**2770-20078:** Note facies with prominent forehead and flat facies. **20079:** Note prominent forehead and micrognathia. **20080:** Lateral view of face shows prominent forehead, low-set posteriorly rotated ears and microretrognathia.

Pterygium colli
*See NECK, CYSTIC HYGROMA, FETAL TYPE*
Pterygium colli syndrome
*See PTERYGIUM SYNDROME, MULTIPLE*
*also NOONAN SYNDROME*

---

### PTERYGIUM SYNDROME, MULTIPLE　　　2186

**Includes:**
Escobar syndrome
Pterygium colli syndrome
**Excludes:**
**Arthrogryposes** (0088)
**Pterygium syndrome, multiple lethal** (2274)
**Pterygium syndrome, popliteal** (0818)
**Pterygium syndrome, popliteal, lethal** (3233)

**Major Diagnostic Criteria:** Pterygia of the neck, axillae, antecubital fossae, popliteal fossae, intercrural areas, and fingers in combination with multiple joint flexion contractures and crouched stance.

**Clinical Findings:** The most consistent malformations present in the multiple pterygium syndrome include growth retardation (100%), webbing of the neck (100%), antecubital fossae (90%), popliteal fossae (90%), and intercrural area (63%) all of which prevent full extension of arms and legs. Syndactyly (74%) and camptodactyly (84%) of the fingers as well as foot deformities (74%) are common findings. Multiple joint flexion contractures are common (74%) as are epicanthal folds (68%), which give the impression of hypertelorism.

Other findings reported in over 40% of the patients include long philtrum, antimongoloid slanting of the palpebral fissures, low-set ears, micrognathia, eyelid ptosis, cleft palate, down-turned corners of the mouth, rib and vertebral anomalies, scoliosis with or without lordosis, talipes equinovarus and rocker-bottomed feet. Genital anomalies in the male consist of small penis and cryptorchidism, and in the female one may see hypoplastic or absent labia majora.

Malformations less often reported are **Hernia, umbilical** (26%), **Hernia, inguinal** (26%), congenital hip dislocation (21%), and hypoplastic nipples (11%). Rare abnormalities reported in isolated cases include spina bifida occulta, **Cutis laxa**, **Hydrocephaly**, platy-

---

**Risk of Recurrence for Patient's Child:**
See Part I, *Mendelian Inheritance.* No affected individuals are known to have reproduced.

**Age of Detectability:** At birth.

**Gene Mapping and Linkage:** Unknown.

**Prevention:** None known. Genetic counseling indicated.

**Treatment:** Thyroid substitution in patients with associated hypothyroidism. Severe mental retardation and poor motoric prognosis make institutionalization of most patients necessary.

**Prognosis:** Life span does not appear to be affected.

**Detection of Carrier:** Unknown.

**References:**
Hall JG, et al.: The distal arthrogryposes: delineation of new entities - review and nosologic discussion. Am J Med Genet 1982; 11:185–239.
Haspeslagh M, et al.: Mental retardation with pterygia, shortness and distinct facial appearance: a new MCA/MR syndrome. Clin Genet 1985; 28:550–555.

FR030　　　　　　　　　　　　　　　　**Jean-Pierre Fryns**

**Pterygia-mental retardation-distinctive craniofacial features**
*See PTERYGIA-DYSMORPHIC FACIES-SHORT STATURE-MENTAL RETARDATION*

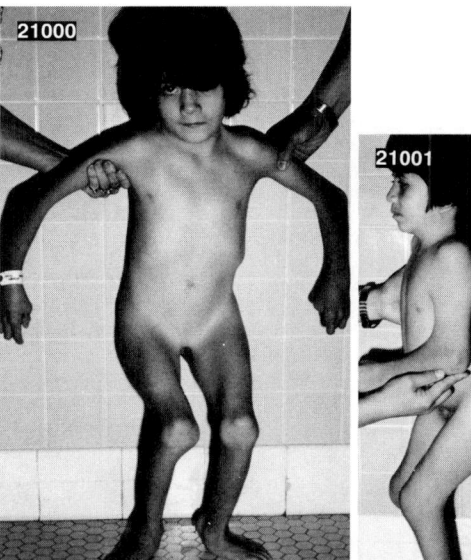
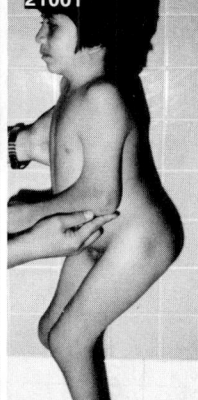

**2186A-21000–01:** Pterygium syndrome, multiple; note restricting pterygia and rocker-bottom feet.

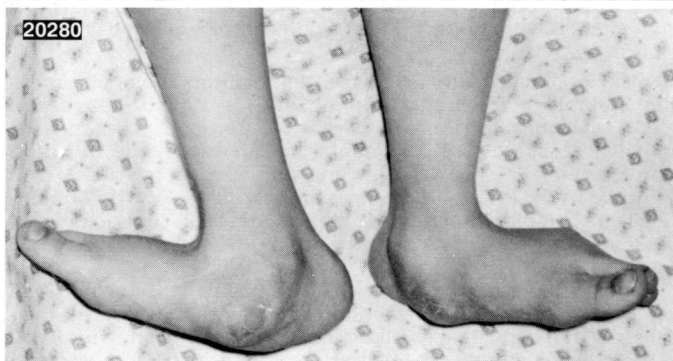

2186B-20279: Digital camptodactyly. 20280: Rocker-bottom feet.

spondyly, clitoromegaly, **Ventricular septal defect**, **Pectus excavatum**, bilateral pulmonary hypoplasia, small heart, absent appendix, and attenuated ascending and transverse colon.

**Complications:** Inability to ambulate independently because of limited extension of the legs. Lack of neck movement due to cervical vertebral fusion.

**Associated Findings:** Progressive joint contractures with fixation and fusion due to lack of movement. Speech difficulties. Psychologic abnormalities may develop due to crippling by the disease in the presence of an otherwise normal IQ.

**Etiology:** Although most cases have been sporadic, occurrences of affected sibs have been reported, lending support to an autosomal recessive pattern of inheritance.

The question of genetic heterogeneity has been raised by reports of a lethal form of multiple pterygium syndrome (see **Pterygium syndrome, multiple lethal**). Gillin and Pryse-Davies (1976) and by Hall (1984) have suggested that two other forms of the syndrome may occur: one with spinal fusion and one with congenital bone fusions.

With the exception of the patient reported by Pashayan et al. (1973) who had 47,XXY/48,XXXY mosaicism, no other chromosomal abnormalities have been reported.

**Pathogenesis:** The origins of the various pterygia are unknown, but biopsy specimens show the presence of muscle degeneration and disorganization of the myofibrils, a finding compatible with muscles not in use.

**MIM No.:** *26500

**POS No.:** 3472

**Sex Ratio:** M1:F1

**Occurrence:** About 50 cases reported in the French, German, and English literature.

**Risk of Recurrence for Patient's Sib:**
See Part I, *Mendelian Inheritance*.

**Risk of Recurrence for Patient's Child:**
See Part I, *Mendelian Inheritance*.

**Age of Detectability:** At birth, with affected individuals showing multiple pterygia and joint flexion contractures. Prenatal diagnosis by ultrasound may be possible.

**Gene Mapping and Linkage:** Unknown.

**Prevention:** None known. Genetic counseling indicated.

**Treatment:** Plastic reconstructive surgery for the cleft palate, popliteal and antecubital fossae pterygia, and the syndactyly. Physical therapy helps to prevent joint fixation.

**Prognosis:** After surgery and with the help of physical therapy, walking and body movements will improve. Life span appears to be normal.

**Detection of Carrier:** Because of phenotypic variation, a careful clinical examination and history of all relatives of an affected patient will help to identify those who are minimally affected.

**Special Considerations:** Major nerves and blood vessels lie free within the pterygia and may be too short for full extension of the extremity. Also, if plastic surgery of the pterygium is attempted and these facts are unrecognized, sectioning of major motor nerves may occur.

**References:**
Pashayan H, et al.: Bilateral aniridia, multiple webs and severe mental retardation in a 47 XXY/48 XXXY mosaic. Clin Genet 1973; 4:126–129.
Gillin ME, Pryse-Davies J: Pterygium syndrome. J Med Genet 1976; 13:249–251.
Escobar V, et al.: Multiple pterygium syndrome. Am J Dis Child 1978; 132:609–611.
Chen H, et al.: Multiple pterygium syndrome. Am J Med Genet 1980; 7:91–102.
Stoll C, et al.: Familial pterygium syndrome. Clin Genet 1980; 18:317–320.
Hall JG, et al.: Limb pterygium syndromes: a review and report of eleven patients. Am J Med Genet 1982; 12:377–409.
Hall JG: The lethal multiple pterygium syndromes.(Editorial) Am J Med Genet 1984; 17:803–807.
Thompson EM, et al.: Multiple pterygium syndrome: evolution of the phenotype. J Med Genet 1987; 24:733–749. *

ES000                                          **Victor Escobar**

---

**PTERYGIUM SYNDROME, MULTIPLE LETHAL          2274**

**Includes:** Lethal multiple pterygium syndrome

**Excludes:**
  **Pena-Shokeir syndrome** (2080)
  **Pterygium syndrome, multiple** (2186)
  **Pterygium syndrome, popliteal, lethal** (3233)

**Major Diagnostic Criteria:** Multiple pterygia with flexion contractures, intrauterine growth retardation, cystic hygroma and/or fetal hydrops, and uniform lethality (12 cases: mean gestational age, 29 menstrual weeks).

**Clinical Findings:** Early in the second trimester some fetuses have appeared normal but subcutaneous edema and cystic hygroma of the neck have been seen, and the ultrasonic measurements have frequently suggested intrauterine growth retardation. Later in gestation, nuchal cystic hygroma and/or fetal hydrops, absent limb movements in the fetus, or polyhydramnios in the mother may be visualized by ultrasound.

Clinically, the multiple pterygia are seen in the chin-to-sternum, cervical, axillary, antecubital, crural, and popliteal regions in association with prominent flexion contractures of the limbs. Nuchal cystic hygroma, generalized fetal hydrops, and loose edematous skin are also observed. Facial dysmorphology has included epicanthal folds, flattened nose, apparently low-set ears, hypertelorism, micrognathia and, occasionally, cleft lip and/or palate.

X-ray studies have revealed microbrachydactyly, a flattened

mandibular angle, absence of the normal cervicothoracic curvature, thiness of the ribs and other bones (some associated with fractures and dislocations), and fusions of the posterior vertebral spinous processes and elbows in the older fetuses.

At autopsy, hypoplastic lungs and heart, and atrophic musculature have been consistently present, and in the fetuses studied, degeneration and paucity of anterior horn motor neurons were observed. One of 46,XY monozygotic twins had female genitalia similar to the sex reversal seen in **Smith-Lemli-Opitz syndrome, type II**.

**Complications:** Malignant hyperthermia was reported in one case (Robinson et al, 1987).

**Associated Findings:** There appear to be several subtypes which are consistent within a family but quite variable between families. One subtype is associated with spinal fusion (Chen et al, 1984), and another with bone fusions (Chen et al, 1984; Van Regemorter, 1984).

**Etiology:** Usually autosomal recessive inheritance, although a few families have shown apparent X-linked inheritance. Sporadic cases have been reported.

**Pathogenesis:** Unknown.

**MIM No.:** 25329, 31215

**POS No.:** 4255

**Sex Ratio:** M1:F1

**Occurrence:** About 200 cases have been observed.

**Risk of Recurrence for Patient's Sib:**
See Part I, *Mendelian Inheritance.*

**Risk of Recurrence for Patient's Child:**
See Part I, *Mendelian Inheritance.* Affected individuals are not expected to survive to reproduce.

**Age of Detectability:** Ultrasound examination has detected affected sibs in families at risk on the basis of **Hydrops fetalis, non-immune,** cystic hygroma on the back of the head and neck, diminished fetal activity, short or fixed limbs, intrauterine growth retardation, and/or by maternal polyhydramnios. Real-time ultrasound will probably detect decreased fetal movement by 10–12 weeks; however, in one of the first families reported, a normal ultrasound examination at 22 menstrual weeks failed to detect an affected fetus.

**Gene Mapping and Linkage:** Unknown.

**Prevention:** None known. Genetic counseling indicated.

**Treatment:** Unknown.

**Prognosis:** Uniformly lethal.

**Detection of Carrier:** Unknown.

**References:**
Hall JG, et al.: Limb pterygium syndromes: a review and report of eleven patients. Am J Med Genet 1982; 12:377–409.
Hall JG: The lethal multiple pterygium syndromes. Am J Med Genet 1984; 17:803–807.
Chen H, et al.: Syndrome of multiple pterygia, camptodactyly, facial anomalies, hypoplastic lungs and heart, cystic hygroma, and skeletal anomalies; delineation of a new entity and review of lethal forms of multiple pterygium syndrome. Am J Med Genet 1984; 17:809–826.
Van Regemorter N, et al.: Lethal multiple pterygium syndrome. Am J Med Genet 1984; 17:827–834.
Herva R, et al.: A lethal autosomal recessive syndrome of multiple congenital contractures. Am J Med Genet 1985; 20:431–439.
Hogge WA, et al.: The lethal multiple pterygium syndromes: is prenatal detection possible? (Letter) Am J Med Genet 1985; 20:441–442.
Martin NJ, et al.: Lethal multiple pterygium syndrome: three consecutive cases in one family. Am J Med Genet 1986; 24:295–304.
Robinson LK, et al.: Lethal multiple pterygium syndrome. Clin Genet 1987; 32:5–9.

DU003         **Peter A. Duncan**
SH009        **Lawrence R. Shapiro**

**2274-20585:** Pterygium syndrome, multiple lethal; note skin webbing at the neck, axillae, antecubital, crural and popliteal areas along with marked edema of the skin and maceration. The nasal bridge was flattened with hypoplastic nasal alae; the ears were low-set and the mouth small.

## PTERYGIUM SYNDROME, POPLITEAL      0818

**Includes:**
> Cleft lip/palate-popliteal pterygium-digital and genital anomalies
> Facio-genito-popliteal syndrome
> Paramedian lower lip pits-popliteal pterygium
> Popliteal pterygium syndrome
> Webbing, popliteal

**Excludes:**
> **Arthrogryposes** (0088)
> **Cleft lip/palate-lip pits or mounds** (0177)
> **Noonan syndrome** (0720)
> **Pterygium syndrome, multiple** (2186)
> **Pterygium syndrome, popliteal, lethal** (3233)
> **Sirenomelia sequence** (3191)

**Major Diagnostic Criteria:** Popliteal webbing (pterygium); pits of lower lip; cleft lip-palate or cleft palate; and genital anomalies.

**Clinical Findings:** Bilateral, rarely unilateral, popliteal pterygium extending from the heel to the ischial tuberosity; intercrural pterygia; cleft lip-palate; and pits or fistulas of the lower lip. Genital anomalies in the male include cryptorchidism and absent or cleft scrotum, and in the female include absence of labia majora and enlarged clitoris. **Syndactyly** of hands or feet, filiform adhesions between the upper and lower lids, and hypoplasia or agenesis of digits may also be present.

**Complications:** Walking difficulties due to limited extension, rotation and abduction of the legs; speech impairment, hearing impairment, and frequent otitis media with conductive hearing loss in patients with cleft palate.

**Associated Findings:** None known.

**Etiology:** Autosomal dominant inheritance with variable expressivity.

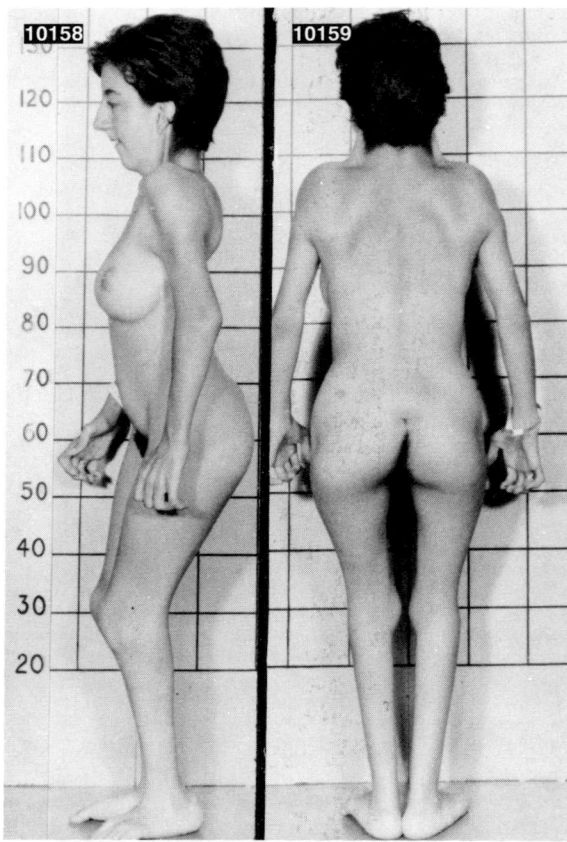

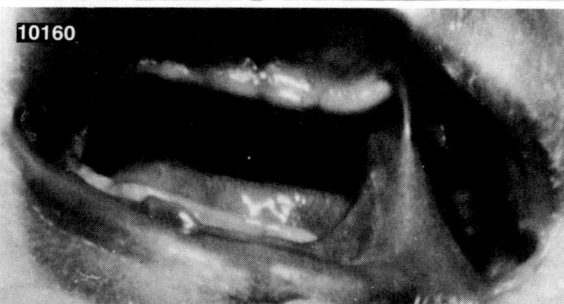

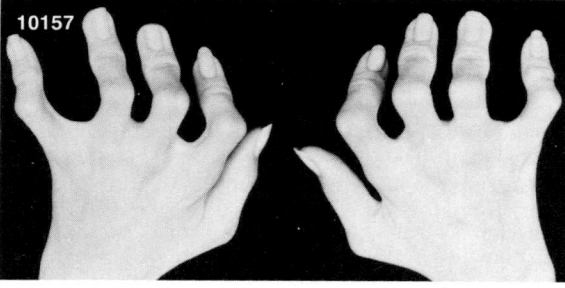

**0818A-10158–59:** Short stature, marked webbed neck, low posterior hairline, flexion contractures of the fingers and knees and foot deformities. **10160:** Soft tissue bands extending from the lower lip to maxillary alveolus at site of incomplete cleft palate. **10157:** Maximal extension of fingers with flexion contractures.

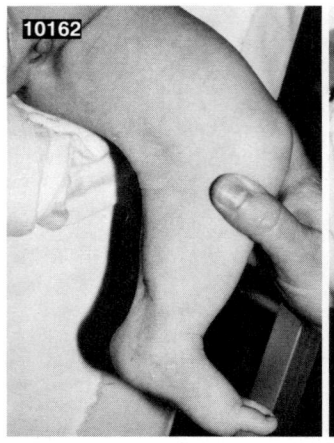

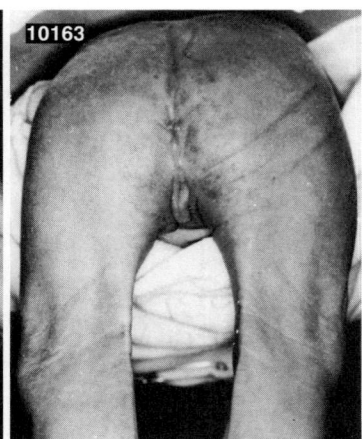

**0818B-10162:** Popliteal ptyergium extending over the popliteal space to the intercrural area with hypoplasia of the labia minora. **10163:** Posterior view of popliteal ptyergium and hypoplasia of the labia minora.

**Pathogenesis:** Unknown.

**MIM No.:** *11950

**POS No.:** 3360

**Sex Ratio:** M1:F1

**Occurrence:** Undetermined. Some 60 cases reported in the literature.

**Risk of Recurrence for Patient's Sib:**
See Part I, *Mendelian Inheritance.*

**Risk of Recurrence for Patient's Child:**
See Part I, *Mendelian Inheritance.*

**Age of Detectability:** At birth.

**Gene Mapping and Linkage:** Unknown.

**Prevention:** None known. Genetic counseling indicated.

**Treatment:** Plastic reparative surgery for cleft lip-palate, lip pits, popliteal pterygium (the sciatic nerve lies free within the pterygium; if plastic surgery of the webbing is attempted and this is not recognized, sectioning of the nerve may occur), ankyloblepharon, and syndactyly; speech therapy. Myringotomy and placement of ventilation tubes if middle ear fluid persists.

**Prognosis:** After surgery, walking will improve as well as speech. General health is not impaired, but disability may be extensive.

**Detection of Carrier:** Unknown.

**References:**
Gorlin RJ, et al.: Popliteal pterygium syndrome: syndrome comprising cleft lip-palate, popliteal and intercrural pterygia, digital and genital anomalies. Pediatrics 1968; 41:503–509.
Bixler D, et al.: Phenotypic variation in the popliteal pterygium syndrome. Clin Genet 1973; 4:220–228.
Escobar V, Weaver, DD: The facio-genito-popliteal syndrome. BD: OAS XIV(6B). New York: March of Dimes Birth Defects Foundation, 1978:185–192.
Pashayan HM, Lewis MB: A family with the popliteal pterygium syndrome. Cleft Palate J 1980; 17:48–51.
Hall J, et al.: Limb pterygium syndromes: a review and report of eleven patients. Am J Med Genet 1982; 12:377–409.
Audino G, et al.: Popliteal pterygium syndrome present with orofacial abnormalities. J Maxellofac Surg 1984; 12:174–177.
Steinberg B, Saunders V: Popliteal pterygium syndrome. Oral Surg 1987; 63:17–20.

**Heddie O. Sedano**

## PTERYGIUM SYNDROME, POPLITEAL, LETHAL     3233

**Includes:**
Bartsocas-Papas syndrome
Popliteal pterygium syndrome, lethal type

**Excludes:**
Pena-Shokeir syndrome (2080)
Pterygium syndrome, multiple (2186)
Pterygium syndrome, multiple lethal (2274)
Pterygium syndrome, popliteal (0818)

**Major Diagnostic Criteria:** Marked popliteal pterygium with cord containing nerve and vessels, synostosis of hand and foot bones, digital hypoplasia, and **Syndactyly.**

**Clinical Findings:** Marked popliteal pterygium with cord containing nerve and vessels, synostosis of hand and foot bones, digital hypoplasia, and **Syndactyly** of the hands and feet. Facial clefts, ectropion, **Eyelid, ankyloblepharon,** hypoplastic nasal tip, filiform bands between the jaws, and corneal anomalies have also been reported.

**Complications:** Unknown.

**Associated Findings:** Supernumerary nipples, hypoplastic external genitalia, and lanugo hair.

**Etiology:** Autosomal recessive inheritance.

**Pathogenesis:** Unknown.

**MIM No.:** *26365

**Sex Ratio:** M1:F1

**Occurrence:** About a half-dozen cases have been reported.

**Risk of Recurrence for Patient's Sib:**
See Part I, *Mendelian Inheritance.*

**Risk of Recurrence for Patient's Child:**
See Part I, *Mendelian Inheritance.*

**Age of Detectability:** At birth. Prenatal diagnosis may be possible by ultrasound.

**Gene Mapping and Linkage:** Unknown.

**Prevention:** None known. Genetic counseling indicated.

**Treatment:** Unknown.

**Prognosis:** Lethal.

**Detection of Carrier:** Unknown.

**References:**
Bartsocas CS, Papas CV: Popliteal pterygium syndrome: evidence for a severe autosomal recessive form. J Med Genet 1972; 9:222–226.
DiStefano G, Romeo MG: La sindrome dello pterigio popliteo. Riv Ped Sic 1974; 29:54–75.
Hall JG, et al.: Limb pterygium syndromes: a review and report of eleven patients. Am J Med Genet 1982; 12:377–409.
Hall JG: The lethal multiple pterygium syndromes. Am J Med Genet 1984; 17:803–807.
Papadia F, et al.: The Bartsocas-Papas syndrome: autosomal recessive form of popliteal pterygium syndrome in a male infant. Am J Med Genet 1984; 17:841–847. * †

DU003
SH009

       **Peter A. Duncan**
      **Lawrence R. Shapiro**

**Pterygoid-levator synkinesis**
*See JAW-WINKING SYNDROME*
**Ptosis and miosis with ophthalmoplegia totalis**
*See OPHTHALMOPLEGIA, TOTAL WITH PTOSIS AND MIOSIS*
**Ptosis, congenital**
*See EYELID, PTOSIS, CONGENITAL*
**Ptosis-epicanthus**
*See EYELID, PTOSIS, CONGENITAL*
**Ptosis-inferior rectus fibrosis, congenital hereditary**
*See EYE, FIBROSIS OF THE EXTRAOCULAR MUSCLES, GENERALIZED*
**Ptosis-superior rectus weakness**
*See EYELID, PTOSIS, CONGENITAL*
**Puberty, incoordinate pattern of in adult male**
*See ANDROGEN INSENSITIVITY (RESISTANCE), MINIMAL*

**Pulmonary arterial stenosis-neonatal liver disease**
*See ARTERIO-HEPATIC DYSPLASIA*
**Pulmonary artery absent, blood supplied by ductus arteriosus**
*See PULMONARY ARTERY, ORIGIN FROM DUCTUS ARTERIOSUS*
**Pulmonary artery origin from contralateral ductus arteriosus**
*See PULMONARY ARTERY, ORIGIN FROM DUCTUS ARTERIOSUS*
**Pulmonary artery origin from ipsilateral ductus arteriosus**
*See PULMONARY ARTERY, ORIGIN FROM DUCTUS ARTERIOSUS*
**Pulmonary artery ring**
*See PULMONARY ARTERY, ORIGIN OF THE LEFT FROM RIGHT PULMONARY ARTERY*
**Pulmonary artery stenosis**
*See PULMONARY ARTERY, COARCTATION*
**Pulmonary artery subclavian steal**
*See AORTA, ISOLATION OF SUBCLAVIAN ARTERY FROM AORTA*
**Pulmonary artery, aberrant left**
*See PULMONARY ARTERY, ORIGIN OF THE LEFT FROM RIGHT PULMONARY ARTERY*

## PULMONARY ARTERY, COARCTATION     0835

**Includes:**
Pulmonary artery stenosis
Pulmonary branch stenosis
Supravalvular pulmonary stenosis

**Excludes:**
Pulmonary artery atresia
Pulmonary hypertension, primary or secondary
Pulmonary stenosis, infundibular
**Pulmonary valve, stenosis** (0839)
Pulmonary vascular disease, occlusive

**Major Diagnostic Criteria:** The characteristic systolic murmurs, heard equally well in both axillae and back as over the base, should suggest the diagnosis, particularly when the patient has **Fetal rubella syndrome, Williams syndrome, Noonan syndrome,** or biliary dysgenesis. Pulmonary artery angiocardiography demonstrates the anatomic constrictions. Differentiation between transient, anatomic, hemodynamic, and syndrome categories is advisable.

**Clinical Findings:** The murmurs of pulmonary artery coarctations are the most common murmurs encountered in the newborn nursery (5% of newborns in one series). In the great majority of cases, these murmurs represent a transient benign condition which disappears with the normal growth and maturation of the pulmonary vascular bed. In a small percentage of cases, the murmurs are produced by the high pulmonary flow of a left-to-right shunt or true anatomic constriction of the pulmonary arteries. In the case of true coarctation the pathologic anatomy varies from a discrete, abrupt narrowing (often at a bifurcation) to a diffuse elongation. Generalized hypoplasia is rarely present in 1 or both main branches. Stenoses often are multiple, but in most cases are only mildly obstructive. Histologically there is intimal thickening and fibrosis with fragmentation of the internal elastic laminae at the site of the obstruction with vein-like dilatation of the distal artery. There may be calcification of the intima in later stages. Four anatomic groups have been described: Type I: in which the stenosis is in the main pulmonary trunk or near its point of bifurcation into the main pulmonary arteries; Type II: stenosis at the bifurcation extending into the left or right branch, or both; Type III: multiple peripheral stenoses; and Type IV: stenosis of the main pulmonary trunk plus peripheral stenoses. Associated cardiac anomalies are common, particularly **Pulmonary valve, stenosis, Ductus arteriosus, patent, Ventricular septal defect, Atrial septal defects,** and **Heart, tetralogy of Fallot.** The likelihood that the coarctations are anatomically significant is greatly increased if the patient has any one of the following syndromes: **Fetal rubella syndrome, Williams syndrome,** or **Noonan syndrome.** In fact, most patients who have severe pulmonary artery coarctations have one of these three syndromes.

The hemodynamic alterations, and consequently the clinical picture, will vary with the degree of obstruction of the pulmonary artery coarctation(s). The presence of an associated lesion will influence the clinical picture. The presence of branch stenosis may be masked by pulmonary valvar or infundibular stenosis, or accentuated by increased pulmonary flow.

The pathophysiology resembles that of pulmonary valve stenosis. With increasing degrees of obstruction there is increased right ventricular hypertension and, consequently, hypertrophy. Certain cases may be progressive and eventually lead to severe and extensive stenosis. Cardiac failure may then occur, resulting in cardiomegaly and right atrial hypertension. A right-to-left shunt across a patent foramen ovale then causes cyanosis.

Continuous murmurs are rarely heard. The usual murmur in pulmonary artery coarctation consists of high-pitched ejection murmur(s) heard in the right axilla, left axilla and back, as well as over the base. There is usually no ejection click and the second heart sound is normal in most cases. The murmurs resemble the peripheral lung murmurs caused by very large atrial level left-to-right shunts. It should be emphasized that, although the great majority of newborns who have murmurs of peripheral pulmonary artery coarctation have a benign, transient condition, these newborns should be followed through sequential visits until the murmurs disappear. If the murmurs are present for more than 3 months, anatomic coarctation or increased pulmonary flow from a shunt should be suspected. Atrial septal defect is not infrequently misdiagnosed as benign pulmonary artery coarctation (until congestive heart failure becomes manifest).

The EKG may be normal in the presence of very mild obstruction. Usually right ventricular hypertrophy of the pressure overload type is present (the degree depending on the severity of the obstruction).

The X-ray findings in isolated pulmonary artery stenosis are not characteristic. With severe bilateral stenosis, the pulmonary arterial vascular workings are diminished. The cardiac silhouette may assume a right ventricular contour, but the pulmonary artery segment is not enlarged.

At cardiac catheterization, a consistent peak systolic pressure gradient within the pulmonary arterial bed of 10mm Hg is consistent with anatomic pulmonary artery coarctation (but may also be found in high pulmonary flow from left-to-right shunts). With severe bilateral stenoses, the morphology of the proximal main pulmonary artery pressure pulse often exhibits a wide pulse pressure characterized by a fast upstroke, a depressed dicrotic notch and a slow diastolic runoff. Indeed, it may show "ventricularization," ie resemble the right ventricular pressure tracing, very similar to that of massive pulmonic valve regurgitation. The degree of right ventricular and right atrial hypertension depends on the severity of the obstruction. In the presence of an associated lesion, the above findings will be changed. For example, an increase in the pressure difference across the coarctation is seen with a large left-to-right shunt.

**Complications:** Right heart failure, right-to-left shunt at atrial level with desaturation and elevated hematocrit, progressive stenosis of coarctations with increasing right ventricular hypertension, pulmonary artery thrombosis, rupture of distal dilated arteries with hemoptysis, and persistent right ventricular hypertension after total correction of the associated cardiac defect (such as tetralogy of Fallot).

**Associated Findings:** Pulmonary artery coarctations are particularly common in certain syndromes. These include **Fetal rubella syndrome, Williams syndrome, Noonan syndrome** and biliary dysgenesis (with or without peculiar facies).

**Etiology:** Multifactorial inheritance is postulated in **Williams syndrome** and in sporadic cases. The condition is found in the autosomal dominant **Noonan syndrome**, following profound teratogenic maternal exposure to rubella virus. and in the biliary dysgenesis syndrome, which may have a teratogenic basis.

**Pathogenesis:** A teratogenic insult (e.g. rubella) may cause a defect in the internal elastic laminae of the artery, producing a localized weakness in the wall in response to pulsatile pressure at systemic levels in utero. Resultant medial damage will then cause intimal hyperplasia and fibrosis.

Other theories include: an inflammatory lesion in an area of turbulent flow (arterial branch) may cause intimal fibrosis, or a

teratogenic insult may cause slowing of the maturation and development of certain segments of the pulmonary vascular bed.

**MIM No.:** *18550

**CDC No.:** 747.380

**Sex Ratio:** M1:F1

**Occurrence:** The occurrence of hemodynamically significant branch stenosis is small: of the order of 1:20,000. The frequency of transient benign disease in the newborn is about 5%. Prevalence varies from higher rates during the rubella pandemic of 1964–65, to lower rates at present.

**Risk of Recurrence for Patient's Sib:**
See Part I, *Mendelian Inheritance*. Varies depending on etiology.

**Risk of Recurrence for Patient's Child:**
See Part I, *Mendelian Inheritance*. Varies depending on etiology.

**Age of Detectability:** In infancy.

**Gene Mapping and Linkage:** Unknown.

**Prevention:** Rubella vaccination for non-pregnant females. Genetic counseling is indicated.

**Treatment:** Arterial reconstruction if stenosis is severe enough and repair is anatomically feasible; lobectomy if multiple peripheral stenoses are localized to one area of the lung. Symptomatic therapy for relief of congestive heart failure.

**Prognosis:** The severity, location, and extent of the stenoses, and the presence or absence of associated syndromes and cardiac defects, determine the prognosis.

**Detection of Carrier:** Varies depending upon etiology.

**References:**
Dunkle LM, Rowe RD: Transient murmur simulating pulmonary artery stenosis in premature infants. Am J Dis Child 1972; 124:666.
Nora JJ, et al.: The Ullrich-Noonan syndrome (Turner phenotype). Am J Dis Child 1974; 127:48. *
Toews WH, et al.: Presentation of atrial septal defect in infancy. JAMA 1975; 234:1250.
Nora JJ, Nora AH. Genetics and counseling in cardiovascular diseases. Springfield: Charles C. Thomas, 1978:105–108.
O'Connor WN, et al.: Supravalvular aortic stenosis: clinical and pathologic observations in six patients. Arch Path Lab Med 1985; 109:179–185.

N0003                                                    **James J. Nora**
N0004                                                    **Audrey H. Nora**

---

## PULMONARY ARTERY, ORIGIN FROM ASCENDING AORTA                                                    0767

**Includes:** Ascending aorta, origin of pulmonary artery

**Excludes:** Pulmonary artery, origin from ductus arteriosus (0768)

**Major Diagnostic Criteria:** Cases of congenital origin of either the right or left pulmonary artery in which the affected lung in actual fact is supplied by a vessel arising from the ascending aorta proximal to the take-off of the first (brachio) cephalic vessel, with or without other cardiac defects.

Diagnosis must be established by cardiac catheterization with angiography in the aortic root, showing a pulmonary artery arising from the ascending aorta.

**Clinical Findings:** Origin of a pulmonary artery from the ascending aorta may occur either on the right or left side. Those on the right tend to be posterior in origin and those on the left anterior. Abnormal origin of one of the pulmonary arteries is usually, not always, contralateral to the aortic arch. The branching pattern of the other aortic arch vessels is usually normal for the situs of the arch. Most commonly the right pulmonary artery is anomalous. With **Heart, tetralogy of Fallot**, the left pulmonary artery is more commonly anomalous, regardless of the sites of the aortic arch.

Symptoms are similar to those of a large left-to-right shunt, and occur in early infancy. Heart failure is common while pulmonary resistances allow a large flow. Elevated pressures in both pulmonary arteries are generally found. If pulmonary resistances increase, as is usual in untreated cases, pulmonary flow will decrease, and eventually cyanosis and hemoptysis will occur, with pulmonary vascular obstructive disease.

The EKG will usually reveal biventricular hypertrophy in early cases, evolving to right ventricular hypertrophy if pulmonary vascular obstructive disease develops. X-ray of the chest may show increased vascularity and cardiomegaly in cases with large left-to-right shunts. Progressive pulmonary vascular obstruction results in decreased heart size and vascularity. Pulmonary function studies may show that the involved lung contributes very little, if any, to gas exchange, although ventilation is normal.

Radioactive isotopes injected intravenously will result in no uptake in the affected side.

**Complications:** Congestive heart failure occurs with large pulmonary blood flow. Hypoxia and hemoptysis result from pulmonary vascular obstructive disease.

**Associated Findings:** If the defect is associated with **Heart, tetralogy of Fallot, Ventricular septal defect,** or **Ductus arteriosus, patent,** complications of those defects may be present.

**Etiology:** Unknown.

**Pathogenesis:** *Anterior type*: In these cases the anomalous pulmonary artery is made up of the left 4th arch (in cases with a right aortic arch), a segment of the dorsal aorta, the distal portion of the left 6th arch, and the left embryonic pulmonary artery. Presumably, in such cases, the segment of the left dorsal aorta between the 6th arch and the 7th intersegmental artery is interrupted, resulting in a left subclavian artery arising anomalously from the descending aorta.

*Posterior type*: The artery is made up of the proximal portion of the 6th arch and the embryonic pulmonary artery. Apparently, at the time of partitioning of the truncus and truncoaortic sac, it was left "stranded." It may therefore be expected to be located always on the right side in situs solitus individuals with either a right or left aortic arch.

**MIM No.:** 12100

**CDC No.:** 747.380

**Sex Ratio:** M1:F1

**Occurrence:** Undetermined but presumed rare.

**Risk of Recurrence for Patient's Sib:** Predicted risk < 1:100. Empiric risk undetermined.

**Risk of Recurrence for Patient's Child:** Predicted risk < 1:100. Empiric risk undetermined.

**Age of Detectability:** In infancy.

**Gene Mapping and Linkage:** Unknown.

**Prevention:** None known. Genetic counseling indicated.

**Treatment:** Surgical anastomosis of the anomalous artery to the main pulmonary trunk, either primarily or with a prosthetic graft, has been successful, and must be undertaken early to avoid pulmonary vascular obstructive disease. Ligation and division of an associated patent ductus arteriosus on the unaffected side is recommended. If associated with tetralogy of Fallot, repair of this defect must also be undertaken.

**Prognosis:** If diagnosis and surgical correction are undertaken early, prognosis is good.

**Detection of Carrier:** Unknown.

**References:**
Netter FH: The Ciba collection of medical illustrations, vol. 5. The heart. New Jersey: Ciba Publications Dept, 1969:162 only.
Cissman NJ: Anomalies of the aortic arch complex. In: Adams FH, Emmanoulides GC, eds: Heart disease in infants, children and adolescents, 3rd ed. Baltimore: Williams & Wilkins, 1983:199–215.

**James J. Nora**

## PULMONARY ARTERY, ORIGIN FROM DUCTUS ARTERIOSUS                  0768

**Includes:**
> Pulmonary artery absent, blood supplied by ductus arteriosus
> Pulmonary artery origin from contralateral ductus arteriosus
> Pulmonary artery origin from ipsilateral ductus arteriosus

**Excludes:**
> Pulmonary artery, absence of, blood not via ductus arteriosus
> **Pulmonary artery, origin from ascending aorta (0767)**

**Major Diagnostic Criteria:** Discrepancy in the vascular pattern between the two lungs may suggest the diagnosis, particularly in patients in whom the symptoms and signs suggest presence of **Heart, tetralogy of Fallot.** Aortic angiography is the procedure of choice in establishing the diagnosis.

**Clinical Findings:** The distal pulmonary artery receives its blood supply not from the pulmonary trunk, but from a ductus arteriosus. Such a ductus arteriosus originates from the aortic arch, if the arch is on the same side, or from the innominate artery if the aortic arch is on the opposite side. There is a tendency for the ductus arteriosus to close at least partially, and thus, as a rule, a large left-to-right shunt is not present. The anomaly is uncommon as an isolated lesion. The clinical findings are largely determined by other cardiovascular anomalies, usually some form of tetralogy of Fallot. Although it most commonly occurs on the left, there have been cases reported on the right side. Recently a case was reported of both pulmonary arteries arising from a normally septated truncus, the right originating from the aorta and the left pulmonary artery from a ductus arteriosus.

If no associated lesions are present, symptoms and signs depend on the magnitude of the left-to-right shunt. If the shunt is small, or if the blood supply to the affected lung is actually decreased, patients are asymptomatic. X-rays of the chest may show discrepancy in the vascularity of the lung fields. If so, the affected lung generally shows a reduced vascular pattern. The unaffected side may show hypervascularity if no significant intracardiac right-to-left shunt is present, such as is seen in cases associated with various forms of tetralogy of Fallot. The lung on the affected side may be smaller than normal. EKG findings are usually determined by associated cardiovascular defects, and may be normal if the anomaly occurs as an isolated lesion.

Pulmonary function tests may show that the involved lung participates very little, if any, in oxygen exchange, although ventilation is normal.

**Complications:** In the unusual case where the lesion is isolated and the ductus arteriosus remains widely patent causing a large left-to-right shunt, congestive heart failure and respiratory infections may occur.

**Associated Findings:** Signs and symptoms of additional lesions such as tetralogy of Fallot may be present.

**Etiology:** Presumably multifactorial inheritance.

**Pathogenesis:** In both forms, the anomaly appears to be due to early obliteration and disappearance of the proximal portion of one or the other sixth arch. The corresponding embryonic pulmonary artery, therefore, will be supplied instead by the distal sixth arch segment, i.e. the ductus arteriosus. In some cases it may be difficult to distinguish the precise origin of the anomalous vessel, i.e. cases of origin of the pulmonary artery from the ascending aorta may occur so close to the innominate artery that a ductal origin is implicated, especially if the origin of the vessel has a narrow caliber.

**MIM No.:** 12100

**CDC No.:** 747.380

**Sex Ratio:** M1:F1

**Occurrence:** Undetermined but presumed rare.

**Risk of Recurrence for Patient's Sib:** Unknown.

**Risk of Recurrence for Patient's Child:** Unknown.

**Age of Detectability:** Depends largely on associated lesions. Can be detected at birth.

**Gene Mapping and Linkage:** Unknown.

**Prevention:** None known. Genetic counseling indicated.

**Treatment:** Surgery might be considered in those cases where the lesion is isolated, and a large left-to-right shunt is present. Anastomosis of the anomalous vessel to the pulmonary trunk may be attempted. In patients who in addition, however, have tetralogy of Fallot, the anomalous vessel may represent the main pulmonary blood supply. Then no such surgical procedure is indicated until complete correction of the tetralogy is accomplished.

**Prognosis:** Depends largely on associated cardiovascular anomalies. If the anomaly is the sole cardiovascular defect, prognosis depends on the magnitude of any left-to-right shunt, and on the pulmonary arteriolar resistance in the affected lung.

**Detection of Carrier:** Unknown.

**References:**
Netter FH: The Ciba collection of medical illustrations, vol. 5. The heart. New Jersey: Ciba Publications Dept, 1969:162 only.
Cissman NJ: Anomalies of the aortic arch complex. In: Adams FH, Emmanoulides GC, eds: Heart disease in infants, children and adolescents, 3rd ed. Baltimore: Williams & Wilkins, 1983:199–215.

N0003                                         **James J. Nora**

## PULMONARY ARTERY, ORIGIN OF THE LEFT FROM RIGHT PULMONARY ARTERY       0766

**Includes:**
Pulmonary artery, aberrant left
Pulmonary artery ring
Pulmonary vascular ring
Vascular ring from aberrant left pulmonary artery

**Excludes:** Vascular rings, other

**Major Diagnostic Criteria:** This anomaly is characterized by the presence of a normal main pulmonary artery which courses undivided toward the right lung. The left pulmonary artery arises from the right pulmonary artery at a point just anterior and to the right of the carina of the trachea. The left pulmonary artery passes toward the left lung, posterior to the right mainstem bronchus, then posteriorly to the trachea and anteriorly to the esophagus. This is the only vascular anomaly which results in a major vessel coming between the trachea and esophagus.

**Clinical Findings:** Respiratory symptoms, which are usually severe, develop in early infancy. Stridor, wheezing, cyanosis, dyspnea, and recurrent respiratory infections may be present. Inspiratory stridor and chest retraction with inspiration are more prominent in this anomaly than in other types of vascular rings with expiratory stridor. Rarely, onset of respiratory symptoms have presented after the second year of life. A few children and adults with this defect have also been reported without respiratory symptoms. Clinical features are due to associated intracardiac defects or associated noncardiac congenital defects.

Chest X-ray may show hyperinflation, atelectasis, or segmental atelectasis of either lung, although the right lung is more often affected. The trachial air column above the carina may appear narrow. Tracheal indentation, anterior bowing of the right mainstem bronchus, and a downward displacement of the carina may be noticed. An anterior and leftward indentation of the barium-filled esophagus near the level of the carina is diagnostic. This finding requires lateral views. Bronchoscopy, although not diagnostic, may reveal extrinsic compression. 2-dimensional echocardiography from the suprasternal notch, computerized axial tomography, and digitally enhanced angiography may aid in the diagnosis. Pulmonary artery angiography is confirmatory. Cardiac catheterization may be required in the evaluation of associated intracardiac defects.

**Complications:** Pulmonary complications are characteristic because a portion of the lung is supplied by a compressed bronchus. Neurologic abnormalities or death may occur as a sequela of hypoxia. Esophageal complications do not occur in this anomaly because the esophagus is not compressed by a ring.

**Associated Findings:** Intracardiac defects are found in about half of the cases. Patent ductus arteriosus (25%), persistent left superior vena cava (20%), **Atrial septal defects** (20%), **Ventricular septal defect** (10%), **aortic valve stenosis, Heart, tetralogy of Fallot, Aorta, coarctation** and aberrant right subclavian artery, persistent atrioventricular canal, single ventricle, and isolation of the left subclavian artery are among the associated defects.

Associated tracheobronchial abnormalities are also found in approximately half of the cases. Complete tracheal rings ("napkin ring cartilage") occur in about 10% of cases. Direct attachment of the right upper lobe bronchus to the trachea (bronchus suus), left epiarterial bronchus, unilateral single-lobed lung, tracheomalacia, and hypoplasia of the distal trachea or bronchus may occur.

Other reported association findings are imperforate anus, **Diaphragmatic hernia**, absent gallbladder, **Biliary atresia**, partial intestinal malrotation, asplenia, **Colon, aganglionosis**, cleft lip and palate, absent left lobe of the thyroid, thymic rests, hemivertebrae, **Aorta, isolation of subclavian artery from aorta**, forearm anomalies, and **Chromosome 21, trisomy 21**.

**Etiology:** Unknown.

**Pathogenesis:** An artery from the pulmonary plexus of the embryonic lung bud normally joins a projection from the ventral part of the aortic sac to form the left pulmonary artery. These vessels and the ventral portion of the left 6th aortic arch eventually form the left pulmonary artery. The dorsal left 6th arch persists as the patent ductus arteriosus. If connection of the pulmonary plexus with the right 6th arch caudal to the lung bud across the midline occurs, the developing left pulmonary artery courses behind the developing tracheobronchial tree.

**MIM No.:** 12100

**CDC No.:** 747.380

**Sex Ratio:** M1:Fl

**Occurrence:** More than 75 cases have been reported. This defect was found in approximately 1.6% of vascular rings in one large series.

**Risk of Recurrence for Patient's Sib:** Unknown. No affected siblings reported.

**Risk of Recurrence for Patient's Child:** Unknown. No affected offspring reported.

**Age of Detectability:** From birth. Death from airway obstruction has occurred as early as the second day of life.

**Gene Mapping and Linkage:** Unknown.

**Prevention:** None known. Genetic counseling indicated.

**Treatment:** Selected cases with mild symptoms may not require surgical intervention. In severe cases, surgical treatment may be effective, although the operative mortality is quite high. Division of the aberrant vessel and reanastomosis to the main pulmonary artery is required in these cases. Aggressive nonoperative management of the patient's pulmonary status is required in the mildly symptomatic patient, as well as in the preoperative stabilization of the severely symptomatic individual.

**Prognosis:** Severely symptomatic individuals have over 90% mortality without operative intervention. Mortality with surgical intervention is also high (38%). Persistent airway symptoms and lack of patency of the repaired left pulmonary artery are commonly found in patients surviving operation.

**Detection of Carrier:** Unknown.

**References:**
Clarkson PM, et al.: Aberrant left pulmonary artery. Am J Dis Child 1967; 113:373–377.
Nora JJ, McNamara DG: Vascular rings and related anomalies. In: Watson H, ed: Pediatric cardiology. St. Louis: C.V. Mosby, 1968: 233–241.

Tan PM, et al.: Aberrant left pulmonary artery. Br Heart J 1968; 30:110–114.
Gumbiner CH, et al.: Pulmonary artery sling. Am J Cardiol 1980; 45:311–315. * †

BR014　　　　　　　　　　　　　　　　　**J. Timothy Bricker**
MC028　　　　　　　　　　　　　　　　　**Dan G. McNamara**

**Pulmonary atresia with hypoplastic right ventricle**
　　*See PULMONARY VALVE, ATRESIA*
**Pulmonary atresia with normal aortic root**
　　*See PULMONARY VALVE, ATRESIA*
**Pulmonary branch stenosis**
　　*See PULMONARY ARTERY, COARCTATION*
**Pulmonary hypertension, familial**
　　*See PULMONARY HYPERTENSION, PRIMARY*

## PULMONARY HYPERTENSION, PRIMARY　　　　2116

**Includes:**
　　Aminorex, effects of
　　Pulmonary hypertension, familial

**Excludes:** Pulmonary hypertension, secondary

**Major Diagnostic Criteria:** Characteristic clinical findings without evidence of underlying amomalies that produce secondary pulmonary hypertension.

**Clinical Findings:** Accentuated pulmonary closure sound with split S2. No significant murmurs or non-specific murmurs. Severe RVH on electrocardiogram, cardiomegaly in advanced cases and increased hilar markings on chest films. Cyanosis in advanced cases. At heart catheterization the pulmonary artery and right ventricular pressures are elevated, often to systemic level, with no evidence of gradients and no findings of structural anomalies of the heart or great vessels.

**Complications:** Congestive heart failure, cyanosis, sudden death.

**Associated Findings:** Has occasionally been found associated with **Raynaud disease**.

**Etiology:** Some families show autosomal dominant inheritance. Certain environmental agents have been implicated, such as in the epidemic of pulmonary hypertension associated with aminorex.

**Pathogenesis:** Progressive occlusive changes with intimal proliferation and medial hypertrophy culminating in the characteristic plexiform lesion of the pulmonary arteries.

**MIM No.:** *17860

**CDC No.:** 747.680

**Sex Ratio:** M1:F1 in childhood. Females predominate among adults.

**Occurrence:** More than 1,000 cases have been reported. This entity represented 1–2% of adults coming to cardiac catheterization at one laboratory.

**Risk of Recurrence for Patient's Sib:**
　　See Part I, *Mendelian Inheritance.*

**Risk of Recurrence for Patient's Child:**
　　See Part I, *Mendelian Inheritance.* Some familial cases occur among sibs without an affected parent.

**Age of Detectability:** Childhood or early adult age.

**Gene Mapping and Linkage:** Unknown.

**Prevention:** Genetic counseling. Removal of environmental hazards such as animorex.

**Treatment:** No consistently effective program is yet available. Oxygen and vasodilators may be used in some selected cases and situations.

**Prognosis:** Guarded to grave.

**Detection of Carrier:** Unknown.

**Support Groups:** Dallas; American Heart Association

**References:**
Kingdon HS, et al.: Familial occurrence of primary pulmonary hypertension. Ann Intern Med 1966; 118:422–426.
Rogge JD, et al.: The familial occurrence of primary pulmonary hypertension. Ann Intern Med 1966; 65:672–684.
Thompson P, McRae C: Familial pulmonary hypertension: evidence of autosomal dominant inheritance. Br Heart J 1970; 32:758–760.
Lloyd JE, et al.: Familial primary pulmonary hypertension: clinical patterns. Am Rev Respir Dis 1984; 129:194–197. *

N0003　　　　　　　　　　　　　　　　　**James J. Nora**
N0004　　　　　　　　　　　　　　　　　**Audrey H. Nora**

**Pulmonary regurgitation due to abnormality of pulmonary valve**
　　*See PULMONARY VALVE, INCOMPETENCE*
**Pulmonary sequestration, extralobar**
　　*See LUNG, LOBE SEQUESTRATION*
**Pulmonary sequestration, intralobar**
　　*See LUNG, LOBE SEQUESTRATION*
**Pulmonary stenoses (peripheral)-brachytelephalangy-deafness**
　　*See KEUTEL SYNDROME*
**Pulmonary stenosis, isolated infundibular**
　　*See VENTRICLE, OBSTRUCTION WITHIN RIGHT VENTRICLE OR ITS OUTFLOW TRACT*
**Pulmonary stenosis-cafe-au-lait spots-mental retardation**
　　*See PULMONIC STENOSIS-CAFE-AU-LAIT SPOTS, WATSON TYPE*
**Pulmonary valve atresia with intact ventricular septum**
　　*See PULMONARY VALVE, ATRESIA*
**Pulmonary valve dysplasia**
　　*See PULMONARY VALVE, STENOSIS*
**Pulmonary valve stenosis with intact ventricular septum**
　　*See PULMONARY VALVE, STENOSIS*
**Pulmonary valve stenosis with normal aortic root**
　　*See PULMONARY VALVE, STENOSIS*

## PULMONARY VALVE, ABSENT　　　　0836

**Includes:**
　　Tetralogy of Fallot with absent pulmonary valve
　　Ventricular septal defect with absent pulmonary valve

**Excludes:** Pulmonary valve, atresia (0837)

**Major Diagnostic Criteria:** A diastolic murmur in the second and third left intercostal space at the sternal border, with enlarged pulmonary artery on X-ray and normal pulmonary vascularity, and a normal EKG, or one showing right ventricular hypertrophy, suggests the diagnosis.
　　Selective pulmonary artery angiocardiography is confirmatory as it will show absence of pulmonary valve tissue or a thickened ridge of tissue with massive reflux of contrast media from the large pulmonary artery into the right ventricle.

**Clinical Findings:** At the site of the pulmonary valve, a ring of nodular tissue is present which has no structural characteristics of a pulmonary valve. Histologically, this tissue is composed of large pale-staining, myxomatous appearing cells. The pulmonary valvar annulus is frequently hypoplastic and therefore stenotic. Because of the pulmonic regurgitation, the right ventricle is enlarged. In addition, the pulmonary trunk and major pulmonary arterial branches are dilated, often appearing aneurysmal. The pulmonary trunk has been studied histologically and found in some cases to present a mosaic of fibers, rather than normal lamellar configuration. In the majority of patients with absent pulmonary valve a **Ventricular septal defect** coexists, usually as part of a **Heart, tetralogy of Fallot** malformation.
　　The clinical findings vary depending upon the type of associated cardiac malformation. In patients with absent pulmonary valve coexisting with ventricular septal defect, the signs and symptoms of congestive cardiac failure occur in infancy. The predominant shunt in infancy is left to right with minimal cyanosis. Pulmonary insufficiency due to isolated absent pulmonary valve usually results in severe congestive heart failure early in infancy or even in utero. Patients with isolated absence of the pulmonary valve are generally asymptomatic until adulthood. The major bronchi may be partially compressed by the aneurysmally

dilated pulmonary arteries which may lead to obstructive emphysema.

Cardiac findings are those of pulmonary stenosis and pulmonary insufficiency. A to-and-fro murmur is present along the left upper sternal border. The systolic portion of the murmur is of the ejection type and may be harsh and loud, especially in those with coexistent cardiac anomalies, whereas it is softer in patients with the isolated anomaly. A diastolic murmur of pulmonary insufficiency is present and its intensity is related to the degree of reflux. The second heart sound is single. A pulmonic systolic ejection click may be present. EKG may be normal if pressures are normal, regurgitation is not gross, and there are no complicating conditions. The EKG of infants with isolated symptomatic absence of the pulmonary valve reveals right ventricular hypertrophy. Among those with coexistent ventricular septal defect, biventricular hypertrophy is observed; and in those with tetralogy of Fallot, right ventricular hypertrophy of pressure overload type. In patients with ventricular septal defect and absent pulmonary valve, generalized cardiomegaly is present on the roentgenogram. The pulmonary trunk and pulmonary vessels, especially the right pulmonary artery, are greatly enlarged and may be misinterpreted as a tumor mass. Tetralogy of Fallot with absent pulmonary valve reveals enlarged pulmonary trunk, but near normal sized cardiac silhouette. With minimal or moderate isolated pulmonary valve anomaly the cardiac size is usually normal, but in symptomatic neonates it is greatly enlarged. The pulmonary trunk is dilated.

A major echocardiographic finding is the inability to image the pulmonary valve. However, a failure to find this structure is relatively weak evidence for diagnosis. Additionally, the right pulmonary artery and right ventricle are usually dilated. Paradoxical septal motion may be present. The tricuspid valve may flutter. The remainder of the echocardiographic examination is normal. Doppler interrogation of the right vantricular outflow area shows the regurgitant flow and the data used to estimate the level of pulmonary artery pressure.

For patients with a ventricular septal defect, additional findings specific for that condition may be present. See **Ventricular septal defect**.

In patients with absent pulmonary valve associated with tetralogy of Fallot, the catheterization data are similar to those of patients with tetralogy of Fallot. Whether the shunt is right to left or left to right depends entirely upon the degree of right ventricular obstruction. In isolated absent pulmonary valve, the right ventricular systolic pressure may be normal or slightly elevated with a small systolic pressure difference across the valve related to increased pulmonary flow. In all cases, the pulmonary arterial pulse pressure contour is characteristic, showing a wide pulse pressure, low diastolic pressure (similar to the right ventricular end diastolic pressure) and a low dicrotic notch. Angiography assists in identifying the presence of associated cardiac malformations. The pulmonary trunk and major pulmonary vessels are greatly dilated and pulsatile. The right ventricular chamber is enlarged and may remain opacified for a prolonged period. The pulmonary valve is not distinct and the pulmonary annulus is narrowed. Pulmonary arteriography reveals reflux of opaque material into the right ventricle.

**Complications:** Congestive cardiac failure, obstructive emphysema.

**Associated Findings:** None known.

**Etiology:** Unknown.

**Pathogenesis:** Unknown.

**Sex Ratio:** M1:F1

**Occurrence:** 2:1,000 in one large series of operated or catherized patients.

**Risk of Recurrence for Patient's Sib:** Unknown.

**Risk of Recurrence for Patient's Child:** Unknown.

**Age of Detectability:** At birth.

**Gene Mapping and Linkage:** Unknown.

**Prevention:** None known. Genetic counseling indicated.

**Treatment:** Congestive cardiac failure and the pulmonary complications must be vigorously treated. Patients with isolated absence of pulmonary valve or with coexistent malformations who are asymptomatic do not require operation. In patients with coexistent congenital cardiac anomalies, particularly ventricular septal defect, management is more difficult and controversial. Several options have been used. Pulmonary arterial banding is a palliative procedure used in some infants with cardiac failure to reduce the left to right shunt, while others would have the ventricular septal defect closed. It may be necessary to simultaneously perform pulmonary angioplasties to reduce the size of the enlarged central pulmonary arteries. Occasionally, the pulmonary valve is replaced.

**Prognosis:** Poor in patients with coexistent defects, with many dying in infancy from congestive cardiac failure complicated by pulmonary disorders. Patients with tetralogy of Fallot may survive relatively symptom free into teens and 20s. Patients with isolated absent pulmonary valve survive until their 70s, although there is increasing evidence that this is not always as benign a condition as once believed. Particularly, in adults who develop unrelated pulmonary diseases resulting in pulmonary hypertension, symptoms may develop because of the increased right ventricular pressure and volume work.

**Detection of Carrier:** Unknown.

**References:**

Miller RA, et al.: Congenital absence of the pulmonary valve: the clinical syndrome of tetralogy of fallot with pulmonary regurgitation. Circulation 1962; 26:266–278.
Venables AW: Absence of the pulmonary valve with ventricular septal defect. Br Heart J 1962; 24:293–296.
Goldberg SJ, et al.: Pediatric and adolescent echocardiography: a handbook. Chicago: Year Book Medical Publishers, 1975.

M0005                                                    **James H. Moller**

---

## PULMONARY VALVE, ATRESIA                              0837

**Includes:**

Atresia of pulmonary valve
Pulmonary atresia with hypoplastic right ventricle
Pulmonary atresia with normal aortic root
Pulmonary valve atresia with intact ventricular septum

**Excludes:**

**Pulmonary valve, stenosis** (0839)
Tetralogy of Fallot with pulmonary valve atresia

**Major Diagnostic Criteria:** Selective right ventricular angiocardiography is needed to establish the pathologic anatomy of pulmonary atresia.

**Clinical Findings:** The pulmonary valve is an imperforate membrane, with two or three small raphae. Right ventricular size in pulmonary atresia with intact ventricular septum is variable, the size corresponding with the size of the tricuspid valve. Small and stenotic tricuspid valves are associated with hypoplastic right ventricle while marked tricuspid insufficiency or Ebstein anomaly of the tricuspid valve occurs with an enlarged right ventricle.

Although the right ventricular infundibulum may be patent to the level of the atretic pulmonary valve, the infundibulum is markedly hypoplastic and may be separated from the atretic pulmonary valve by muscular tissue.

The right ventricle is hypertrophied and endocardial fibroelastosis may coexist. Enlarged myocardial sinusoids may connect to the coronary arterial branches. During systole blood leaves the right ventricle through the sinusoids and flows into the coronary arterial system. An atrial communication is present, usually a patent foramen ovale, or less frequently, an ostium secundum atrial septal defect.

In neonates the patent ductus arteriosus provides the sole source of pulmonary blood flow but it usually closes in the neonatal period. The diameter of the pulmonary trunk varies from normal to hypoplastic and the size does not correlate with the size of the underlying right ventricle. The pulmonary trunk is usually patent to the level of the atretic pulmonary valve and is usually hypoplastic.

Ventricular size has been broadly classified as either hypoplastic or normal. Regardless of the size of the right ventricular cavity, the clinical manifestations are similar. Cyanosis is present at birth or shortly thereafter. If the ductus remains patent, however, only mild cyanosis is present. Cyanosis increases quickly as the ductus closes. The other prominent finding is dyspnea. The signs of cardiac failure are prominent only in patients with tricuspid regurgitation. Physical examination reveals a cyanotic, dyspneic infant with cardiomegaly. The second heart sound is single. In more than half the patients, there is a systolic murmur which is usually soft, and may be related to either the ductus arteriosus or tricuspid regurgitation. The pulmonary vascularity is decreased with markedly ischemic lung fields. There is a tendency for the cardiac silhouette to be larger in patients with an enlarged right ventricle, especially in those with tricuspid insufficiency. The pulmonary arterial segment is concave and the right atrium is greatly enlarged. The upper mediastinum often is narrow and the aortic knob inapparent.

The EKG reveals normal or right axis deviation. This serves to distinguish this condition from tricuspid atresia in which left axis deviation is the rule. Furthermore, a qR pattern in lead aVF suggests pulmonary atresia, whereas such a qR pattern is seen in lead AVL in tricuspid atresia. Right atrial enlargement is present although not always in the first week of life. A few older cases show left atrial enlargement. The precordial leads are useful in distinguishing the 2 types of pulmonary valvar atresia. With a hypoplastic right ventricle, a pattern of "absence of right ventricular forces" is present with an rS in lead V1 and an R in V6. Normal or enlarged right ventricles are associated with classic patterns of right ventricular hypertrophy.

The pulmonary valve can be imaged on echocardiography, but absence of Doppler detected pulmonary flow is inconclusive since the same may exist in cases of pulmonary hypertension in the presence of a patent pulmonary valve. The right ventricular outflow tract usually appears narrowed. In most instances, the aorta will be larger than normal. Right ventricular cavity size depends upon the exact anatomy of a particular patient. Right ventricular hypertrophy almost always is present. If pulmonary blood flow is low, left atrial size is small. If the right pulmonary artery is present, it can be imaged and measured via the suprasternal notch approach.

Cardiac catheterization is useful in establishing the diagnosis. It is not always possible to advance the catheter tip into a hypoplastic right ventricle. The right ventricular pressure is elevated with the peak systolic pressure exceeding the systemic arterial pressure, unless there is marked tricuspid insufficiency, when the right ventricular systolic pressure may be as low as 40 mmHg. Right atrial pressure is elevated and shows large "a" waves. Oxygen saturations on the right side of the heart are low and blood from the left atrium is desaturated. Indicator dilution curves performed from either atrium are practically identical, showing a common pathway of circulation.

Angiocardiography confirms the diagnosis and yields information regarding right ventricular size. The angiocardiogram reveals no passage of contrast material from the right ventricle into the pulmonary artery. Contrast may be seen escaping from the right ventricle either through an insufficient tricuspid valve or through myocardial sinusoids with retrograde filling of coronary arteries. In some cases, opacification of the aortic root occurs as well. Right atrial injections show contrast material flowing from right-to-left atrium, but frequently fail to distinguish this condition from **Tricuspid valve, atresia**. The pulmonary arteries fill by way of a patent ductus arteriosus or enlarged bronchial arteries.

**Complications:** Acidosis secondary to hypoxia, cardiac failure.

**Associated Findings:** None known.

**Etiology:** Undetermined but presumably multifactorial inheritance.

**Pathogenesis:** Probably due to early fusion of the pulmonary valvar primordia.

**CDC No.:** 746.000

**Sex Ratio:** M1:F1

**Occurrence:** Approximately 1:10,000 live births. Prevalence diminishes to only the rare survivors of palliative surgery.

**Risk of Recurrence for Patient's Sib:** Predicted risk: 1:100; Empiric risk: undetermined.

**Risk of Recurrence for Patient's Child:** Affected individuals are not expected to survive to reproduce.

**Age of Detectability:** At birth.

**Gene Mapping and Linkage:** Unknown.

**Prevention:** None known. Genetic counseling indicated.

**Treatment:** Following cardiac catheterization, operation is mandatory. If the right ventricle is of normal size and the infundibulum patent to the level of the pulmonary valve, pulmonary valvotomy can be performed. This may be combined with placement of an outflow tract patch across the pulmonary annulus. When the right ventricle is either hypoplastic and associated with a very stenotic infundibulum or greatly enlarged and associated with massive tricuspid insufficiency, an aortopulmonary shunt should be created and an atrial septostomy performed. Subsequently, in patients with a hypoplastic right ventricle a pulmonary valvotomy should be performed at an early age to reduce the elevated right ventricular systolic pressure.

**Prognosis:** Perioperative use of prostaglandin E1 has dramatically improved the surgical outcome for neonates with pulmonary atresia and intact ventricular septum. The long-term prognosis of these operative survivors has not been determined.

**Detection of Carrier:** Unknown.

**References:**
Zuberbuhler JR, et al.: Morphological variations in pulmonary atresia with intact ventricular septum. Br Heart J 1979; 41:281–288.
Patel RG, et al.: Right ventricular volume determinations in 18 patients with pulmonary atresia and intact ventricular septum. Analysis of factors influencing right ventricular growth. Circulation 1980; 61: 428–440.
Brunlin EA, et al.: Angio-pathological appearances of pulmonary valve in pulmonary atresia with intact ventricular septum. Br Heart J 1982; 47:281–289.
Freedom RM: The morphologic variations of pulmonary atresia with intact ventricular septum: guidelines for surgical intervention. Pediatr Cardiol 1983; 4:183–188.
Freedom RM, et al.: Pulmonary atresia and intact ventricular septum. Scand J Thorac Cardiovasc Surg 1983; 17:1–28.
Smallhorn JF, et al.: Noninvasive recognition of functional pulmonary atresia by echocardiography. Am J Cardiol 1984; 54:925–926.

M0005
BR040

**James H. Moller**
**Elizabeth A. Braunlin**

## PULMONARY VALVE, BICUSPID                              0109

**Includes:** Bicuspid pulmonary valve with or without a raphe

**Excludes:**
    **Pulmonary valve, atresia (0837)**
    **Pulmonary valve, atresia (0837)**

**Major Diagnostic Criteria:** Soft or moderately loud systolic pulmonic ejection murmur unassociated with electrocardiographic or vectorcardiographic abnormalities of any kind may suggest a pulmonary valve lesion.

**Clinical Findings:** Two functional pulmonary valve cusps are present rather than 3. The 2 cusps may be approximately equal in size in which case there usually is no raphe in either sinus of Valsalva. Both sinuses of Valsalva, while larger than normal, are well-formed. More commonly, however, one of the cusps is somewhat larger than the other and contains a raphe which partially divides the sinus of Valsalva into more or less equal sized shallow components. Since by definition neither stenosis nor incompetence is present, the lesion is asymptomatic. Even in nonstenotic bicuspid valves, however, turbulence is usually produced which is responsible for the soft or moderately loud systolic ejection type murmur usually present in these patients. A suprasternal systolic thrill may be present.

The EKG and vectorcardiogram are normal in uncomplicated simple bicuspid pulmonary valve. X-rays of the chest may show minimal "poststenotic" dilatation of the pulmonary trunk. Cross-sectional echocardiography in some instances can show the bicuspid nature of the valve. At cardiac catheterization, no pressure difference is found across the valve and the physiologic findings are normal. A pulmonary arterial angiogram or right ventriculogram may demonstrate the true nature of the anomaly.

**Complications:** Calcification of the bicuspid pulmonary valve is unusual, as is bacterial endocarditis.

**Associated Findings:** A bicuspid pulmonary valve is commonly associated with **Heart, tetralogy of Fallot**, in which case it does not have to be stenotic but may be hypoplastic. Other cardiovascular lesions may be present. Also commonly associated with **Chromosome 18, trisomy 18**.

**Etiology:** Presumably multifactorial inheritance.

**Pathogenesis:** True bicuspid pulmonary valve without a raphe is probably due to absence of one of the pulmonary valve cusp anlagen. This may be the intercalated valve swelling of either of the anlagen derived from the truncus septum. In a bicuspid pulmonary valve with a raphe, all 3 anlagen are present, 2 of these have fused to form a functionally single cusp with 2 poorly developed sinuses of Valsalva separated by a raphe.

**CDC No.:** 746.080

**Sex Ratio:** M1:F1

**Occurrence:** Unknown.

**Risk of Recurrence for Patient's Sib:** Unknown.

**Risk of Recurrence for Patient's Child:** Unknown.

**Age of Detectability:** Probably in early childhood, if all soft pulmonic murmurs are investigated.

**Gene Mapping and Linkage:** Unknown.

**Prevention:** None known. Genetic counseling indicated.

**Treatment:** None if lesion is an isolated one.

**Prognosis:** The prognosis of bicuspid pulmonary valve is excellent, if it occurs as an isolated lesion. If other congenital cardiac defects are present, the prognosis is determined by the associated lesion.

**Detection of Carrier:** Unknown.

**References:**
Koletsky S: Congenital bicuspid pulmonary valve. Arch Pathol 1941; 31:338–353. *
Ford AB, et al.: Isolated congenital bicuspid pulmonary valve: clinical and pathologic study. Am J Med 1956; 20:474–486.
Pierpont MEM, et al.: Chromosomal anomalies. In Pierpont MEM, Moller, JH eds: Genetics of cardiovascular disease. Boston: Martinus Nijhoff, 1987:83–84.

M0005

**James H. Moller**

## PULMONARY VALVE, INCOMPETENCE 0838

**Includes:** Pulmonary regurgitation due to abnormality of pulmonary valve

**Excludes:**
 **Pulmonary valve, absent** (0836)
 Pulmonary valve, secondary incompetence

**Major Diagnostic Criteria:** An early diastolic murmur along the left sternal border with EKG evidence of right ventricular hypertrophy suggests the diagnosis. Pulmonary artery angiocardiography confirms the diagnosis.

**Clinical Findings:** Incompetence of the pulmonary valve results from a structural abnormality of the valve which may be bicuspid, tricuspid or quadricuspid. Functional pulmonary incompetence may also be present in patients with idiopathic dilatation of the pulmonary artery or other lesions which cause dilatation of the pulmonary artery.

Because of incompetence of the pulmonary valve, the right ventricular stroke volume is increased. As a result, the main pulmonary artery, its major branches and the right ventricular chamber are dilated. The degree of dilatation of the right side of the heart is dependent not only upon the degree of pulmonary incompetence but also on the level of pulmonary arterial pressure. If sufficient regurgitation occurs and marked right ventricular dilatation develops, congestive cardiac failure may occur.

The clinical findings are related primarily to the degree of incompetence and the level of pulmonary arterial pressure. Patients with minor degrees of incompetence are asymptomatic. The elevated pulmonary vascular resistance that is normally present in the neonatal period, or that may develop secondarily later in life, tends to augment the degree of regurgitation, thereby imposing an excessive pressure load upon the right ventricle and leading to congestive cardiac failure. Newborn infants with pulmonary insufficiency can thus present with signs of severe cardiac failure. A systolic ejection type murmur is present, which is related to increased right ventricular stroke volume. This murmur is followed by a medium to low-pitched diastolic regurgitant murmur along the left sternal border. The pulmonary component of the second heart sound may be absent if the valve is rudimentary. If both components of the second sound are present, the degree of splitting may be increased because of the increased right ventricular stroke volume. When pulmonary arterial hypertension is present, the pulmonic component is accentuated. A pulmonary ejection click may be present.

Thoracic X-rays in most children show a normal-sized cardiac silhouette with prominent pulmonary trunk and major arterial branches. With severe incompetence or pulmonary hypertension, the right-sided cardiac chambers are enlarged. Cardiac fluoroscopy shows increased pulsations of the pulmonary trunk and main arteries.

The EKG findings may reflect the volume overload on the right ventricle. It may either be normal or reveal mild right ventricular hypertrophy. The latter is manifested as an rSR' pattern in lead $V_1$, a larger than normal S wave in lead $V_6$, and terminal slowing of the QRS electrical forces.

The pulmonary valvular abnormality cannot be visualized by echocardiography. If the insufficiency is of moderate or greater degree, the right ventricular cavity is dilated. In more advanced instances, paradoxical septal motion may be present. Tricuspid flutter has been reported but it is relatively rare. Thickness of the right ventricular wall depends on the level of right ventricular systolic pressure. The right pulmonary artery is usually dilated.

In the presence of significant pulmonary valve incompetence, cardiac catheterization characteristically reveals a wide pulmonary arterial pulse pressure with the diastolic pressure similar to that of right ventricular end diastolic pressure. The dicrotic notch is low. Small systolic pressure gradients may be present between the right ventricle and the pulmonary artery secondary to the increased forward flow.

Angiocardiography shows an enlarged right ventricle especially the infundibulum. The pulmonary trunk is dilated. In severe cases, the main pulmonary arteries may show considerable dilatation as well. Pulmonary arteriography shows retrograde opacification of the right ventricle.

**Complications:** Congestive cardiac failure.

**Associated Findings:** None known.

**Etiology:** Unknown.

**Pathogenesis:** Unknown.

**CDC No.:** 746.020

**Sex Ratio:** M1:F1

**Occurrence:** Less than 1% of all cases of congenital heart defects.

**Risk of Recurrence for Patient's Sib:** Unknown.

**Risk of Recurrence for Patient's Child:** Unknown.

**Age of Detectability:** At birth.

**Gene Mapping and Linkage:** Unknown.

**Prevention:** None known. Genetic counseling indicated.

**Treatment:** If cardiac failure occurs, medical treatment is possible. Surgical therapy is rarely indicated. It could, however, be accomplished by homograft replacement of the pulmonary valve, or other type of valvar prosthesis.

**Prognosis:** Pulmonary valve incompetence has been generally considered a benign condition, but reports of death in the neonatal period and in later life have been reported. Short-term animal studies of surgically induced insufficiency have indicated its benign nature. Longer periods of observation are needed to determine the future course of the child or younger adult with symptom-free isolated pulmonary valvar incompetence.

**Detection of Carrier:** Unknown.

**References:**

Collins NP, et al.: Isolated congenital pulmonic valvular regurgitation; diagnosis by cardiac catheterization and angiocardiography. Am J Med 1960; 28:159–164.

Vlad P, et al.: Congenital pulmonary regurgitation: a report of six autopsied cases. Am J Dis Child 1960; 100:640–641.

Gasul BM, et al.: Congenital isolated pulmonary valvular insufficiency. In: Heart disease in children: diagnosis and treatment. Philadelphia: J.B. Lippincott, 1966:807.

Goldberg SJ, et al.: Pediatric and adolescent echocardiography: a handbook. Chicago: Year Book Medical Publishers, 1975.

Buendia A, et al.: Congenital absence of pulmonary valve leaflets. Br Heart J 1983; 50:31–41. *

Hiraishi S, et al.: Ventricular and pulmonary artery volumes in patients with absent pulmonary valve: factors affecting the natural course. Circulation 1983; 67:183–190.

M0005         **James H. Moller**

**Pulmonary valve, quadricuspid**
*See PULMONARY VALVE, TETRACUSPID*

---

## PULMONARY VALVE, STENOSIS      0839

**Includes:**

> Pulmonary valve dysplasia
> Pulmonary valve stenosis with intact ventricular septum
> Pulmonary valve stenosis with normal aortic root
> Pulmonic stenosis

**Excludes:**

> **Heart, tetralogy of Fallot** (0938)
> Infundibular pulmonic stenosis
> **Pulmonary artery, coarctation** (0835)

**Major Diagnostic Criteria:** A harsh systolic murmur, maximal in the second left intercostal space, with an enlarged main pulmonary artery on X-ray with normal pulmonary vascularity, plus right ventricular hypertrophy on the EKG, indicate the diagnosis. Echocardiography is confirmatory.

**Clinical Findings:** In the majority of patients with pulmonary valvar stenosis, the pulmonary valve is dome-shaped, with partial commissural fusion, resulting in a central circular orifice of variable size. Less frequently, the valve shows no commissural fusion. In the latter form, called pulmonary valvar dysplasia, three distinct cusps and commissures are present, the valvar tissue being greatly thickened and redundant. The sinuses of Valsalva are partly obliterated by tissue composed of large, pale-staining myxomatous-like cells. In this form, pulmonary stenosis results from the mass of valvar tissue encroaching on the pulmonary orifice. Secondary anatomic features of pulmonary valve stenosis include poststenotic dilatation of both the pulmonary trunk and usually also the left pulmonary artery. The right ventricle is hypertrophied in proportion to the severity of the stenosis. With time, two alterations occur in the right ventricle which significantly alter right ventricular function. One of these is the development of myocardial fibrosis and the other is the development of infundibular stenosis. Right atrial enlargement and hypertrophy are present in the more severe cases, and this may be of sufficient degree to open a previously competent patent foramen ovale.

The clinical and laboratory findings are dependent in part upon the severity of the stenosis. The majority of patients with pulmonary valve stenosis are asymptomatic and show normal growth and development. With moderate stenosis, easy fatigability may be present. Congestive cardiac failure and cyanosis (related to a right-to-left atrial shunt) may develop but usually only in patients with severe pulmonary valvar stenosis. These findings may be present in the infant with severe stenosis or may develop gradually in the adult with significant pulmonary valve stenosis. The prominent physical finding is a loud pulmonary systolic ejection murmur, which is usually associated with a thrill along the upper left sternal border and in the suprasternal notch. The murmur is usually introduced by a pulmonic systolic ejection click, but this may be absent in severe cases. Other auscultatory features may be indicative of the severity of the stenosis. With significant pulmonary stenosis, the murmur becomes longer and the peak intensity of the murmur is delayed further into systole. The development or presence of a murmur of tricuspid insufficiency is indicative of severe pulmonary stenosis. The components of the second heart sound are normal in mild stenosis, but with increasing degrees of severity, the pulmonic component becomes delayed and softer, or even inaudible.

Attention must be directed to the general appearance and physical characteristics of the child. They may indicate the etiology of the pulmonary valve stenosis, as in post-rubella syndrome. Children with a dysplastic pulmonary valve are generally small in stature, retarded in sexual development, and have a rather typical triangular shaped face with ptosis, hypertelorism and low-set ears. Pulmonic systolic ejection clicks are rarely heard among these patients. Usually the heart size is normal as is the pulmonary vasculature. There is prominence of the pulmonary trunk and left pulmonary artery. In patients with severe stenosis, the pulmonary artery segment is usually inapparent. With severe or long-standing moderate pulmonary stenosis, the overall cardiac size may be slightly enlarged, representing primarily right ventricular and right atrial enlargement. In patients with cyanosis related to right-to-left atrial shunt, the pulmonary vasculature is diminished, but left atrial enlargement is then present. Combination of decreased pulmonary vascularity and left atrial enlargement should suggest a large right-to-left shunt at atrial level.

In mild pulmonary valvar stenosis, the EKG is normal, or shows only minimal evidence of right ventricular hypertrophy (T wave positive in $V_1$). With more severe stenosis, there is progressively more right axis deviation and right ventricular hypertrophy. Right atrial enlargement may be observed. There is a rough correlation between the height of the R wave in right precordial leads and the severity of the stenosis. In children with dysplastic pulmonary valves, Noonan syndrome with pulmonary stenosis, and rubella patients with stenotic pulmonary valves, the EKG findings of severe right axis deviation (more than +210°) and rS deflections in all precordial leads suggest a degree of right ventricular hypertrophy which is not actually present.

In most instances, the echocardiographic "a" wave amplitude of the pulmonary valve is excessive in some beats; in other beats, the "a" wave appears normal. In some children with pulmonary valvular stenosis, the "a" wave appears normal. Right ventricular anterior wall thickness is related to the severity of the disease. Right ventricular cavity size may vary from small to dilated. If the right ventricular cavity is dilated, paradoxical septal motion may be present even in the absence of a right ventricular volume overload. The right pulmonary artery is usually dilated. Doppler interrogation of the transvacuar jet allows estimation of the gradient.

Cardiac catheterization reveals a systolic pressure difference across the pulmonary valve and there may be a right-to-left shunt at the atrial level. Simultaneous measurement of the cardiac output and the gradient across the pulmonary valve permit calculation of the size of the stenotic pulmonary valvar orifice. Measurement of hemodynamic parameters during exercise permits assessment of right ventricular function. Right ventricular angiography demonstrates a dome-shaped pulmonary valve with a jet of contrast passing through the small central orifice. The angiocardiogram reveals hypertrophy of the right ventricle, especially the crista supraventricularis, which forms the posterior wall of the right ventricular infundibulum. Generally, the infundibulum narrows during systole, but widens significantly during diastole. In patients with a dysplastic pulmonary valve, the valve cusps do not dome and there is no jet. The thickened cusps maintain a fixed position in both diastole and systole; the sinuses of Valsalva are nearly occluded.

**Complications:** Congestive cardiac failure, **Tricuspid valve, insufficiency**, development of myocardial fibrosis, increased hematocrit.

**Associated Findings:** May be seen as part of the **Fetal rubella syndrome**, **Noonan syndrome**, and **Lentigines syndrome, multiple**.

**Etiology:** Multifactorial inheritance in the majority of cases. May be seen as part of the **Fetal rubella syndrome** and the **Lentigines syndrome, multiple**. Variable expressivity is seen in autosomal dominant **Noonan syndrome**.

**Pathogenesis:** Dome-shaped pulmonary valve probably results from fusion of the embryonic valvar cusps. Dysplastic pulmonary valve probably results from failure of reabsorption of the embryonic cusp tissue that normally occurs in the formation of the sinuses of Valsalva.

**MIM No.:** 26550

**CDC No.:** 746.010

**Sex Ratio:** M1:F1

**Occurrence:** Prevalence is approximately 1:1,250 of the general population. About 10% of congenital heart disease.

**Risk of Recurrence for Patient's Sib:** About 2%.

**Risk of Recurrence for Patient's Child:** If mother is affected, empiric risk is about 6.5%. If father is affected, empiric risk is about 1.8%.

**Age of Detectability:** From birth, by clinical examination and cardiac catheterization.

**Gene Mapping and Linkage:** Unknown.

**Prevention:** Genetic counseling is indicated as is rubella vaccination. Special attention must be paid to a possible association with **Noonan syndrome**.

**Treatment:** Medical, symptomatic treatment of congestive cardiac failure, when this is present. The valvar obstruction should be relieved when the calculated pulmonary valve area is less than 0.5 cm²/meter² of body surface area. With a normal cardiac output, this valve area is usually associated with a right ventricular systolic pressure in the range of 75 mm Hg. The traditional approach of operative pulmonary valvotomy has been replaced by an interventional catheter technic -- balloon valve dilatation. This procedure is extremely safe, and leads to excellent relief of the valvar stenosis, except in individuals with a dysplastic pulmonary valve. In patients with significant infundibular stenosis, it may be necessary to resect a portion of the obstructing muscle as well as open the pulmonary valve. In patients with a dysplastic pulmonary valve, the operation involves excision of the valvar tissue or the placement of an outflow patch across the pulmonary annulus.

Infants with severe pulmonary stenosis and cardiomegaly represent surgical emergencies. Prompt performance of diagnostic procedures and pulmonary valvotomy may be lifesaving.

**Prognosis:** Serial cardiac catheterization studies have indicated that beyond infancy patients with mild-to-moderate pulmonary valvar stenosis show no increase in the level of right ventricular pressure. There are suggestions, however, that the incidence of coexistent infundibular pulmonary stenosis increases in each decade of life. As a result, the infundibular stenosis may result in increased levels of right ventricular systolic pressure and complicate operation. With time, right ventricular myocardial fibrosis develops which may significantly alter the compliance and function of the right ventricle. The results of operation in children are excellent and pulmonary valvotomy can be performed successfully at low risk. In adults, particularly those with poor right ventricular function, the operative risk is higher, and the postoperative catheterization data frequently reveal continued poor right ventricular myocardial performance.

**Detection of Carrier:** Unknown.

**References:**
Klinge T, Laursen HB: Familial pulmonary stenosis with underdeveloped or normal right ventricle. Br Heart J 1975; 37:60–64.
Kan JS, et al.: Percutaneous balloon valvuloplasty: a new method for treating congenital pulmonary valve stenosis. New Engl J Med 1982; 307:540–542.
Johnson GL, et al.; Accuracy of combined two-dimensional echocardiography and continuous wave Doppler recordings in the estimation of pressure gradient in right ventricular obstruction. J Am Coll Cardiol 1984; 3:1013–1018.
Trowitzsch E, et al.: Two-dimensional echocardiographic evaluation of right ventricular size function in newborns with severe right ventricular outflow tract obstruction. J Am Coll Cardiol 1985; 6:388–393.
Radtke W: Percutaneous balloon valvotomy of congenital pulmonary stenosis using oversized balloons. J Am Coll Cardiol 1986; 8:909–915.
Nora JJ, Nora AH: Maternal transmission of congenital heart disease. Am J Cardiol 1987; 59:459–463. *
Emmanouilides GC, Baylen BG: Obstructive lesions of the right ventricle and pulmonary arterial tree. In: Adams FH, Emmanouilides GC, eds: Heart disease in infants, children, and adolescents. Baltimore: Williams & Wilkins, 1989.

M0005                                                         **James H. Moller**

## PULMONARY VALVE, TETRACUSPID                                    0840

**Includes:** Pulmonary valve, quadricuspid

**Excludes:** **Pulmonary valve** (other defects)

**Major Diagnostic Criteria:** Selective pulmonary artery angiocardiography is necessary to establish the diagnosis. Even then, exact delineation of a tetracuspid pulmonary valve is difficult. Thus, necropsy is required to definitively document the diagnosis.

**Clinical Findings:** The pulmonary valve has four valve cusps. The cusps may each be of equal size, or one may be smaller. Often it is the supernumerary cusp that is deformed, imperfect or smaller. When present as an isolated anomaly, the right-sided cardiac chambers are normal. If the valve is insufficient, the pulmonary artery and right ventricle may be dilated. Symptoms and signs are only present if the pulmonary valve is incompetent or stenotic.

**Complications:** Pulmonary valve insufficiency, bacterial endocarditis.

**Associated Findings:** None known.

**Etiology:** Unknown.

**Pathogenesis:** Probably results from the formation of an additional intercalated pulmonary valve swelling.

**CDC No.:** 746.080

**Sex Ratio:** M1:F1

**Occurrence:** About 50 autopsy cases reported.

**Risk of Recurrence for Patient's Sib:** Unknown.

**Risk of Recurrence for Patient's Child:** Unknown.

**Age of Detectability:** At birth.

**Gene Mapping and Linkage:** Unknown.

**Prevention:** None known.

**Treatment:** Unknown.

**Prognosis:** Good; the anomaly usually being an incidental finding at necropsy.

**Detection of Carrier:** Unknown.

**References:**
Kissin M: Pulmonary insufficiency with a supernumerary cusp in the pulmonary valve: report of a case with review of the literature. Am Heart J 1936; 12:206–227.
Hurwitz LE, Roberts WC: Quadricuspid semilunar valve. Am J Cardiol 1973; 31:623–626.

Davia JE, et al.: Quardicuspid semilunar valves. Chest 1977; 72:186–189.

M0005                                          **James H. Moller**

**Pulmonary vascular ring**
  See PULMONARY ARTERY, ORIGIN OF THE LEFT FROM RIGHT
    PULMONARY ARTERY
**Pulmonary vein, stenosis of the common**
  See HEART, COR TRIATRIATUM
**Pulmonary venous connection, anomalous (partial)**
  See PULMONARY VENOUS CONNECTION, PARTIAL ANOMALOUS

## PULMONARY VENOUS CONNECTION, PARTIAL ANOMALOUS                                  0841

**Includes:**
  Great veins, transposition of (partial)
  Pulmonary venous connection, anomalous (partial)
  Venous return, anomalous (partial)

**Excludes:** Pulmonary venous connection, total anomalous (0842)

**Major Diagnostic Criteria:** Typical physical examination, electrocardiographic features, and X-ray features of **Atrial septal defects**. Although cardiac catheterization, including selective pulmonary arteriogram, confirms the diagnosis, two-dimensional echocardiography with imaging of pulmonary veins can be diagnostic as well. Computerized tomography also may provide positive identification of partial anomalous pulmonary venous connection (PAPVC).

**Clinical Findings:** *Anatomy:* Partial anomalous pulmonary venous connection occurs when one or more, but not all, of the pulmonary veins connect to the systemic venous circulation instead of the left atrium. Almost every conceivable connection between the pulmonary veins and the proximal systemic veins has been reported. The abnormally draining veins may be either from

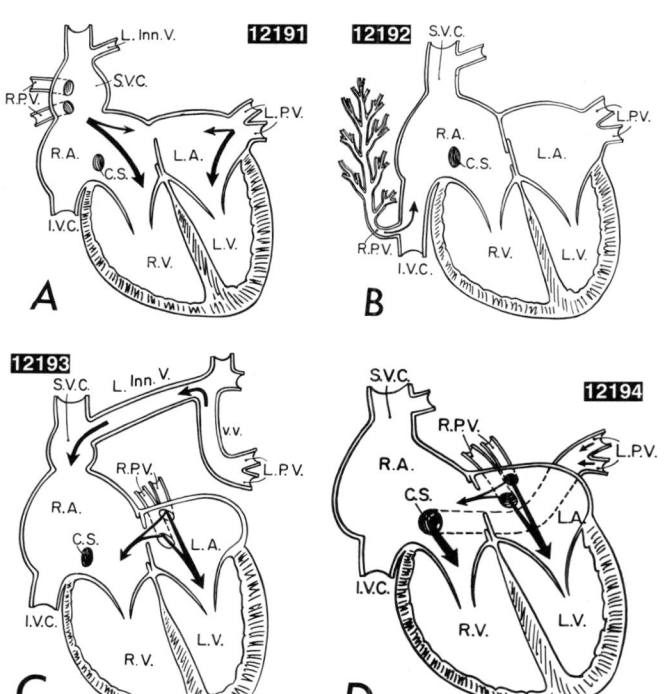

**0841**-12191–94: Common forms of partial anomalous pulmonary venous connection.

the entire right or left lung or from only several segments. Right-sided anomalous pulmonary veins usually empty into the superior vena cava, right atrium, or occasionally into the inferior vena cava and other sites. Anomalous left pulmonary veins usually drain into a left superior vena cava, and occasionally left innominate vein, left subclavian veins, or coronary sinus.

Partial anomalous pulmonary venous connection (PAPVC) is usually associated with an atrial septal defect of the sinus venosus type. Occasionally PAPVC is seen with **Mitral valve stenosis**. Other major associated cardiac anomalies are present in approximately 20% of the cases.

*Physiology:* The fundamental hemodynamic alteration is similar to an atrial septal defect. Increased pulmonary blood flow occurs as a consequence of recirculation through the lungs. The magnitude of the recirculation is determined by: 1) the number of anomalous pulmonary veins, 2) the presence and the size of the atrial septal defect, 3) the pulmonary vascular resistance, and (4) ssociated anomalies. When the atrial septum is intact, the number of anomalously connected veins and the state of the parenchyma determine the amount of blood which drains anomalously. When a single pulmonary vein is anomalously connected, the anomalously draining blood approximates 20% of total pulmonary blood flow. This amount is clinically inapparent. With anomalous drainage of several lobes of the lungs or when PAPVC and atrial septal defect coexist, the hemodynamic picture is similar to that of an uncomplicated atrial septal defect. The left-to-right shunt is usually large.

*Clinical features:* The anomalous connection of one pulmonary vein is inapparent clinically. If all but one of the veins connect anomalously, the clinical features mimic those of total anomalous pulmonary venous connection. Children with PAPVC are usually asymptomatic but may have dyspnea on exertion. Patients presenting with cyanosis in their third and fourth decades occur due to elevated pulmonary vascular resistance.

*Physical findings* are similar to those of **Atrial septal defects**. These include 1) right ventricular lift, 2) when associated with ASD, the $S_2$ is split widely and fixed. When the atrial septum is intact, the $S_2$ is normal, 3) a grade II-III/VI systolic ejection murmur at the upper left sternal border, and 4) a mid-diastolic rumble, due to increased flow across the tricuspid valve. Electrocardiographic findings are similar to those seen in uncomplicated atrial septal defects.

*The chest X-ray* reflects the increased pulmonary blood flow and right ventricular dilatation. Occasionally, a dilated superior vena cava, a crescent-shaped vertical shadow in the right lower lung, or a distended vertical vein may suggest the site of anomalous drainage.

**Complications:** As a consequence of increased pulmonary blood flow, pulmonary vascular hypertension rarely occurs in the third and fourth decade. Pulmonary infections are common in patients with anomalous drainage of the right pulmonary veins to the inferior vena cava associated with pulmonary sequestration (see **Scimitar syndrome**).

**Associated Findings:** Partial anomalous pulmonary venous connection of the right lung is typically a connection of one or more veins from the upper and middle lobes to the superior vena cava and the right atrium near the cavo-atrial junction, usually in association with a sinus venosus type of atrial septal defect. Atrial defects of the fossa ovalis type may also be seen with PAPVC. Partial anomalous pulmonary venous connection occurs in approximately 15% - 25 of cases of cor triatriatum.

Other associated findings include **Mitral valve stenosis**, polysplenia, and **Asplenia syndrome**. Major additional cardiac anomalies are present in approximately 20% of cases of PAPVC. **Turner syndrome** has been reported in association with PAPVC.

**Etiology:** Presumably multifactorial inheritance.

**Pathogenesis:** The lungs arise from a portion of the foregut. Initially pulmonary veins draining the splanchnic plexus and empty into the systemic venous system. If one or more of these pulmonary veins fail to connect with the left atrium, the original drainage into the systemic venous system will persist.

**MIM No.:** 12100

**Sex Ratio:** M1:F1

**Occurrence:** 7:1,000 in the general population; authorities have quoted figures from 6–600:100,000 in the general population. The higher prevalence figure is not compatible with general clinical experience.

**Risk of Recurrence for Patient's Sib:** Unknown.

**Risk of Recurrence for Patient's Child:** Unknown.

**Age of Detectability:** At birth, by echocardiogram or angiography.

**Gene Mapping and Linkage:** Unknown.

**Prevention:** None known. Genetic counseling indicated.

**Treatment:** Exercise restriction is generally not required. Bacterial endocarditis prophylaxis is probably not indicated. Medical therapy may be required. Surgical correction is carried out under cardiopulmonary bypass. The specific procedure to be performed depends on the site of anomalous drainage. An isolated single lobe anomaly is not ordinarily corrected surgically. Timing of surgery is usually at 4–5 years of age, if clinically indicated. Mortality for surgical repair is less than 1%. Most common complications of surgery are superior vena caval obstruction, supraventricular arrhythmias and symptomatic sinus node dysfunction ("sick sinus syndrome").

**Prognosis:** Pathologic studies indicate that patients with one pulmonary vein connected anomalously and with an intact septum have an excelent prognosis with normal life expectancy. The natural history in symptomatic patients seems comparable to those with uncomplicated atrial septal defects. The prognosis is determined by severity of associated anomalies in patients with complicated anatomy.

**Detection of Carrier:** Unknown.

**References:**

Alpert JS, et al.: Anomalous pulmonary venous return with intact atrial septum: diagnosis and pathophysiology. Circulation 1977; 56:870–875.

Price WH, Willey RF: Partial anomalous pulmonary venous drainage in two patients with Turner's syndrome. J Med Genet 1980; 17:133–134.

Whittemore R, et al.: Pregnancy and its outcome in women with and without surgical treatment of congenital heart disease. Am J Cardiol 1982; 50:641–651.

Lucas RV Jr: Anomalous venous connections, pulmonary and systemic. In: Adams FM, Emmanoulides GC, eds: Moss's heart disease in infants, children and adolescents. 3rd ed. Baltimore: Williams & Wilkins, 1983:458–491. *

Rose V, et al.: A possible increase in the incidence of congenital heart defects among the offspring of affected parents. J Am Coll Cardiol 1985; 6:376–382.

Wolf WJ: Diagnostic features and pitfalls in the two-dimensional echocardiographic evaluation of a child with cor triatriatum. Pediatr Cardiol 1986; 6:211–213.

PE019
BR014

**Angel Perez**
**J. Timothy Bricker**

## PULMONARY VENOUS CONNECTION, TOTAL ANOMALOUS · 0842

**Includes:**
Great veins, transposition of (complete)
Pulmonary venous, anomalous return (total)

**Excludes:**
**Pulmonary valve, atresia** (0837)
**Pulmonary valve, stenosis** (0839)
**Pulmonary venous connection, partial anomalous** (0841)
Pulmonary venous connection, subtotal
**Scimitar syndrome** (0879)

**Major Diagnostic Criteria:** Total anomalous pulmonary venous connection (TAPVC) with obstruction: Neonate with intense cyanosis and respiratory distress, X-ray signs of pulmonary venous congestion, and a normal heart size.

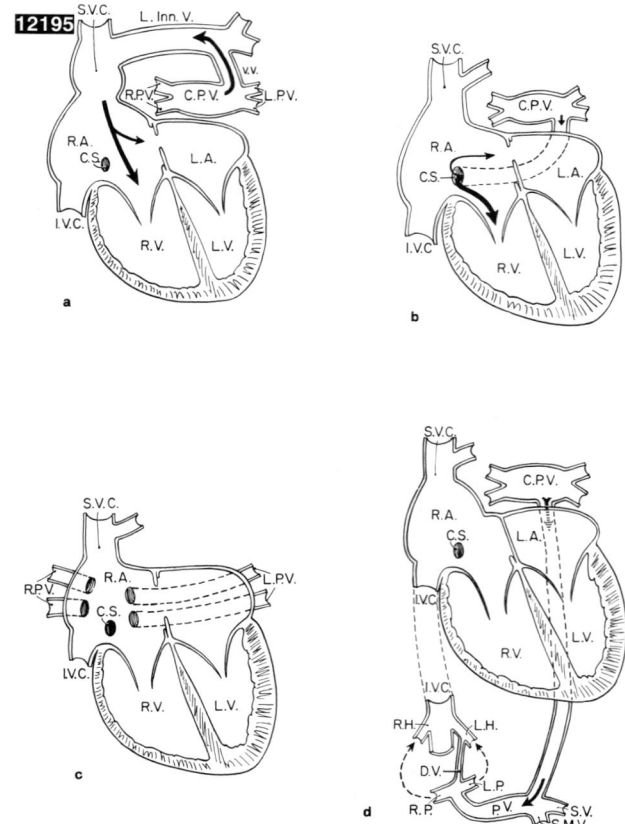

**0842-12195:** Common forms of total anomalous pulmonary venous connection.

TAPVC without obstruction: Infant with cyanosis and signs of congestive heart failure, EKG evidence of right atrial enlargement and right ventricular hypertrophy, and X-ray signs of increased pulmonary blood flow and enlarged right heart structures.

In both forms of TAPVC, selective pulmonary angiography will demonstrate the route of anomalous connection, but in TAPVC with obstruction, pulmonary blood flow may be slowed, and the sites of connection and obstruction not seen until late in levophase. Echocardiography may be diagnostic and angiography is not always required.

**Clinical Findings:** All pulmonary veins drain by abnormal routes directly or indirectly to the right atrium. Interatrial communication, either by atrial septal defect or patent foramen ovale, is therefore an essential component of TAPVC. Approximately 40% of patients with TAPVC have other associated cardiac anomalies. The site of anomalous connection may be classified as (I) supracardiac: to a left vertical vein, left superior vena cava, right superior vena cava or azygous vein, (II) intracardiac: to the coronary sinus or right atrium, (III) infracardiac: to the portal vein, ductus venosus, inferior vena cava or hepatic veins, (IV) mixed: one or more of the above.

The presence or absence of obstruction to pulmonary venous drainage dictates the hemodynamic consequences and therefore the clinical features of TAPVC. Obstruction can occur secondary to a narrow anomalous channel, extrinsic compression of an anomalous channel, interposition of the hepatic sinusoids in infracardiac TAPVC, or a restrictive interatrial communication.

TAPVC with obstruction to pulmonary venous drainage: Pulmonary venous obstruction occurs most often with infracardiac connections but may be secondary to other etiologies as above.

Prenatal changes consisting of increased pulmonary vein and capillary wall thickness may contribute to both pre- and postoperative pulmonary hypertension. Elevated pulmonary resistance and a thickened, non-compliant right ventricle lead to diminished pulmonary blood flow and increased right-to-left atrial shunting. Physical exam therefore reveals cyanosis and respiratory distress at or soon after birth. There are generally no murmurs heard, the pulmonary closure sound is accentuated and the heart is not enlarged. There are rales secondary to pulmonary edema and the liver is enlarged.

X-ray findings are those of pulmonary venous obstruction and pulmonary edema without cardiomegaly. The diffuse reticular pattern of pulmonary vascular markings may resemble those of hyaline membrane disease, but differ in that air bronchograms are absent. Kerley B lines may be seen.

The electrocardiogram usually shows right ventricular hypertrophy, but the QRS axis, atrial and ventricular forces may also be within normal limits for age.

Echocardiograms: two-dimensional echocardiography is a reliable means of diagnosing both the presence and routes of abnormal pulmonary venous connection. In the presence of pulmonary venous obstruction, however, pulmonary blood flow is diminished and the site of connection is more difficult to visualize. Two-dimensional directed Doppler echocardiograms, and more recently, color Doppler flow studies, help identify patterns of blood flow and sites of obstruction. An echo-free space posterior to the left atrium (common pulmonary vein) is a characteristic finding in TAPVC, but may be lacking in some patients with right atrial or mixed connections.

Cardiac catheterization: systemic saturations may be very low secondary to diminished pulmonary blood flow. Streaming of highly saturated renal vein blood can cause confusion in interpretation of inferior vena caval oxygen saturations. Right ventricular pressure is systemic or greater. Right atrial pressure is higher and systemic saturations lower in patients with a restrictive interatrial communication and these patients benefit from balloon atrial septostomy. Pulmonary arteriograms generally require longer film duration (10–15 sec) to allow opacification of pulmonary venous return because of low pulmonary blood flow.

*TAPVC without obstruction to pulmonary venous drainage*: Age of presentation can vary considerably. With postnatal decrease in pulmonary vascular resistance, pulmonary blood flow increases to exceed systemic flow. Patients therefore may be asymptomatic at birth, then develop congestive heart failure, grow poorly and have frequent respiratory infections. Physical exam reveals a variable degree of cyanosis with cardiovascular findings resembling atrial septal defect. An infant may be irritable and poorly nourished. Tachypnea and tachycardia are found as well as a right ventricular heave. The second heart sound is well split with little or no change with respiration and the pulmonary closure sound is accentuated, reflecting pulmonary hypertension. Gallop rhythms are frequent. A grade II-III/VI blowing systolic murmur is audible at the mid-to-upper left sternal border and a diastolic murmur secondary to increased blood flow across the tricuspid valve is present at the lower left sternal border. With anomalous venous connection to the left innominate vein, a venous hum may be present at either upper sternal border. Hepatomegaly is present.

X-ray findings all show increased pulmonary arterial markings and cardiomegaly secondary to right atrial and right ventricular enlargement. The left atrium handles a normal volume of blood and is not enlarged. Occasionally, the chest radiograph allows definition of the route of anomalous drainage. In connection to a left superior vena cava, the "snowman" or "figure of eight" silhouette may be seen, the lower portion formed by the heart and the upper portion formed by the enlarged left SVC-innominate vein - right SVC system. This appearance may be obscured by or confused with a neonatal thymic shadow. Connection to the right SVC may cause dilatation and blurring of the SVC-right atrial junction and connection to the coronary sinus may cause an indentation anteriorly on barium-swallow just below the left atrial shadow.

The EKG invariably shows right atrial enlargement and right ventricular hypertrophy. Approximately half show a qR pattern in the right precordial leads, while the other half show an rR' or rsR'. These findings occur independent of the degree of pulmonary flow or pulmonary arterial pressure.

Echocardiograms: as mentioned previously, two-dimensional Doppler echocardiography is a reliable means of diagnosing TAPVC. Difficulties arise in patients with right atrial isomerism, mixed-type TAPVC and complex cardiac anatomy. The finding of a dilated coronary sinus should lead to searches for anomalous drainage through that structure.

Cardiac catheterization: high oxygen saturations in a systemic vein may allow identification of the site of anomalous connections. Saturations are generally the same in right atrium, right ventricle, pulmonary artery and aorta. Due to the degree of pulmonary to systemic shunting, systemic saturations may be near normal. There may be mild to moderate elevations of both right ventricular and pulmonary artery pressures. Pulmonary arteriograms require large volumes of contrast injected rapidly because of high pulmonary flow. Pulmonary venous opacification is thereby adequate, allowing visualization of the site of connection.

**Complications:** With obstruction, death usually occurs from the first day to the second month. Without obstruction, symptoms of congestive heart failure may begin in infancy. The minority surviving the first year of life generally do not have pulmonary hypertension but are at risk for developing pulmonary vascular disease. Unoperated, overall mortality for TAPVC is 80% in the first year of life.

**Associated Findings:** Other major cardiac defects (excluding interatrial communications) are seen in 5–40%; including transposition of the great arteries, **Ventricular septal defect**, mitral atresia-hypoplastic left heart syndrome, **Tricuspid valve, atresia, Heart, tetralogy of Fallot**, truncus arteriosus, the association of right atrial isomerism with dextrocardia, common AV valve, single ventricle and pulmonary stenosis/atresia.

A low frequency of occurrence of TAPVC has been reported in association with **Heart-hand syndrome, Noonan syndrome, Klippel-Feil anomaly, Cat eye syndrome**, conjoined twins, and agenesis of the right lung and phocomelia. A higher incidence is seen in **Asplenia syndrome**.

**Etiology:** Presumably multifactorial inheritance, although both sporadic geographic clusters in non-related patients and familial recurrences have been reported.

**Pathogenesis:** Embryologically, the inital route of pulmonary venous drainage is through the cardinal veins and the umbilico-vitelline system. Normally, these channels involute after successful anastomosis of pulmonary veins to an outpouching of the sinoatrial portion of the heart. Failure of development of this communication between the common pulmonary vein and left atrium results in TAPVC with persistence of either the cardinal or umbilicovitelline system or both.

**MIM No.:** 10670

**CDC No.:** 747.420

**Sex Ratio:** Reported M3.6:F1 for TAPVC to portal vein. Other sites of connection felt to be M1:F1, but reports show slight male predominance.

**Occurrence:** 1:5,000 live births. 25:1,000 of infants under one year old referred to New England Regional Infant Cardiac Program (NERICP).

**Risk of Recurrence for Patient's Sib:** Unknown.

**Risk of Recurrence for Patient's Child:** Unknown.

**Age of Detectability:** At birth. Fetal echocardiography probably difficult secondary to low pulmonary blood flow in utero.

**Gene Mapping and Linkage:** Unknown.

**Prevention:** None known. Genetic counseling indicated.

**Treatment:** Balloon and blade atrial septostomy improves atrial shunting in TAPVC without obstruction and those with TAPVC and obstruction secondary to a restrictive interatrial communication. This may improve hemodynamics and systemic saturation prior to surgery. Use of prostaglandin E1 is not helpful and in patients with low blood flow secondary to pulmonary venous obstruction could worsen pulmonary edema and exacerbate systemic desaturation.

Some patients without obstruction present later in infancy or childhood and can be managed medically to allow later surgical intervention. Most patients require early surgical correction using hypothermic circulatory arrest.

**Prognosis:** Eighty percent of all unoperated children with TAPVC are dead within the first year of life. Nearly half die in the first three months of life. In TAPVC with obstruction and/or restrictive interatrial communication, death usually occurs in the first weeks of life. In the presence of a large ASD and unobstructed TAPVC, some patients may not present until late childhood or early adulthood. Surgical mortality for the child under one year of age approximates 25–30%, with a mortality closer to 50% for those under one month of age. This is, in part, due to extremely ill neonates with obstruction who present with acidosis and shock. Overall, surgical mortality in the patient over one year of age is less than 5%.

**Detection of Carrier:** Unknown.

**References:**
Nora JJ, Nora AH: Genetics and counseling in cardiovascular diseases. Springfield, IL: Thomas Books, 1978.
Norwood WI, et al.: Total anomalous pulmonary venous connection: surgical considerations. In: Engle ME, ed: Pediatric cardiovascular disease, cardiovascular clinics, 1980:353–364.
Whittemore R, et al.: Pregnancy and its outcome in women with and without surgical treatment of congenital heart disease. Am J Cardiol 1982; 50:641–651.
Lucas RV Jr: Anomalous venous connections, pulmonary and systemic. In: Adams FH, Emmanouilides GS, eds: Heart disease in infants, children and adolescents, 3rd ed. Baltimore: Williams & Wilkins, 1983:458–491. *
Huhta JC, et al.: Cross-sectional echocardiographic diagnosis of total anomalous pulmonary venous connection. Brit Heart J 1985; 53:525–534.
Rose V, et al.: A possible increase in the incidence of congenital heart defects among the offspring of affected parents. J Am Coll Cardiol 1985; 6:376–382.
Solymar L, et al.: Total anomalous pulmonary venous connection in siblings. Acta Paediat Scand 1987; 76:124–127.

PE020
BR014

**James C. Perry**
**J. Timothy Bricker**

**Pulmonary venous return, partial anomalous**
*See SCIMITAR SYNDROME*
**Pulmonary venous, anomalous return (total)**
*See PULMONARY VENOUS CONNECTION, TOTAL ANOMALOUS*
**Pulmonic stenosis**
*See PULMONARY VALVE, STENOSIS*

---

## PULMONIC STENOSIS-CAFE-AU-LAIT SPOTS, WATSON TYPE                                    2776

**Includes:**
Cafe-au-lait spots-pulmonary stenosis
Pulmonary stenosis-café-au-lait spots-mental retardation
Watson syndrome

**Excludes:**
Lentigines syndrome, multiple (0586)
Neurofibromatosis (0712)
Noonan syndrome (0720)

**Major Diagnostic Criteria:** Pulmonic stenosis, cafe-au-lait spots, and limited intelligence inherited in an autosomal dominant fashion.

**Clinical Findings:** Based on 18 patients in four families, pulmonic stenosis occurs in 60%; it may present with exertional dyspnea in childhood or may be a symptomless, incidental finding. Cafe-au-lait spots are found in 100%, but may vary from a few large (more than 5 cm in diameter) spots to about 100 smaller spots. Freckles are common, and axillary freckling occurs. Intelligence has usually

been described as low normal or dull (11/18), but three boys have mild and one girl severe mental retardation. All affected members (3/3) of one family had short adult stature.

**Complications:** Pulmonic stenosis may cause significant exertional dyspnea and cyanosis with right-to-left shunting at the atrial level. One 57-year-old man with pulmonic stenosis and coronary ectasia presented with angina when exerting effort.

**Associated Findings:** One girl has severe soft tissue limitation of movement of her ankles and knees.

**Etiology:** Autosomal dominant inheritance.

**Pathogenesis:** Unknown. The only vascular lesion found clinically, at operation or at autopsy, has been valvular pulmonic stenosis except for the one adult with associated coronary ectasia.

**MIM No.:** *19352

**Sex Ratio:** M1:F1

**Occurrence:** Three families have been described from England, one probable family from France, and one from Canada.

**Risk of Recurrence for Patient's Sib:**
See Part I, *Mendelian Inheritance.*

**Risk of Recurrence for Patient's Child:**
See Part I, *Mendelian Inheritance.*

**Age of Detectability:** At birth, if there are other affected members of the family. Otherwise diagnosis has usually been in mid-childhood.

**Gene Mapping and Linkage:** NF1 (neurofibromatosis 1 (von Recklinghausen disease, Watson disease)) has been mapped to 17q11.2.

**Prevention:** None known. Genetic counseling indicated.

**Treatment:** Pulmonic stenosis is treatable surgically. However, most patients do well without surgical treatment, and two out of three patients have died postoperatively following valvotomy.

**Prognosis:** Unknown. At least two males, one with and one without pulmonic stenosis, have lived into the sixth decade.

**Detection of Carrier:** Clinical examination and cardiac investigation.

**Special Considerations:** Until recently, Watson syndrome has been confused with **Lentigines syndrome, multiple** on the one hand and **Neurofibromatosis** on the other. However, the clinical picture seems sufficiently consistent and different from these two conditions to warrant consideration as a separate disorder.

**References:**
Watson GH: Pulmonary stenosis, cafe-au-lait spots and dull intelligence. Arch of Dis in Child 1967; 42:303–307. * †
Partington MW, et al.: Pulmonary stenosis, cafe au lait spots and dull intelligence: the Watson syndrome revisted. Proc Greenwood Genet Center 1985; 4:105 only.
Allanson JE, Watson GH: Watson syndrome: nineteen years on. Proc Greenwood Genet Center 1987; 6:173 only.

PA026

**M.W. Partington**

**Pulmonic stenosis-congenital nephrosis**
*See NEPHROSIS, CONGENITAL*
**Pulp stones**
*See TEETH, DENTIN DYSPLASIA, CORONAL*
**Pulverulent nuclear cataract**
*See CATARACT, COPPOCK*
**Pulverulent zonular cataract**
*See CATARACT, COPPOCK*
*also CATARACT, AUTOSOMAL DOMINANT CONGENITAL*
**Pupil and lens, ectopic**
*See LENS AND PUPIL, ECTOPIC*
**Pupil shape abnormalities**
*See PUPIL, DYSCORIA*
**Pupil size unequal**
*See PUPIL, ANISOCORIA*

## PUPIL, ANISOCORIA 0058

**Includes:**
Anisocoria
Eye, anisocoria
Pupil size unequal

**Excludes:**
Acquired anisocoria
**Horner syndrome** (0475)
**Rieger syndrome** (2139)

**Major Diagnostic Criteria:** Unequal pupil size greater than 20%.

**Clinical Findings:** Defining the upper limit of normal pupillary inequality at 20%, then 2% of the population have anisocoria ranging from 0.5 to 2.0 mm.

**Complications:** Unknown.

**Associated Findings:** None known.

**Etiology:** Possibly autosomal dominant inheritance. Heterogeneity exists. Other disorders such as iris atrophy and stromal hypoplasia must be excluded as causes.

**Pathogenesis:** Unknown.

**MIM No.:** 10624

**Sex Ratio:** M1:Fl

**Occurrence:** 1:50 live births.

**Risk of Recurrence for Patient's Sib:**
See Part I, *Mendelian Inheritance.*

**Risk of Recurrence for Patient's Child:**
See Part I, *Mendelian Inheritance.*

**Age of Detectability:** In childhood.

**Gene Mapping and Linkage:** Unknown.

**Prevention:** None known. Genetic counseling indicated.

**Treatment:** Unknown.

**Prognosis:** Normal for life span and intelligence. Visual prognosis good.

**Detection of Carrier:** Unknown.

**References:**
Duke-Elder S: System of ophthalmology, vol. 3, part 2. congenital deformities. London: Henry Kimpton, 1964: 592.
Lam BL, et al.: The prevalence of simple anisocoria. Am J Ophthal 1987; 104:69–73.

CR012                                               **Harold E. Cross**

## PUPIL, DYSCORIA 0309

**Includes:**
Dyscoria
Pupil shape abnormalities

**Excludes:**
Corectopia
**Eye, anterior segment dysgenesis** (0439)
**Eye, microphthalmia/coloboma** (0661)
**Eye, pupillary membrane persistence** (0845)
Polycoria
**Pupil, anisocoria** (0058)

**Major Diagnostic Criteria:** Abnormality in the shape of the pupil, in the absence of neoplasia or inflammatory processes with synechiae.

**Clinical Findings:** Abnormally shaped pupils may take the form of a slit (most commonly), hourglass, rectangle or pear. White and Fulton (1937) reported a woman of Russian-Jewish extraction and her daughters with "egg-shaped" pupils. In the absence of malformations of the globe, vision is usually good.

**Complications:** Unknown.

**Associated Findings:** Anterior chamber cleavage syndromes.

**Etiology:** Usually autosomal dominant inheritance. May also occur sporadically.

**Pathogenesis:** Probably related to abnormal "cleavage" of the anterior chamber during embryonic life.

**MIM No.:** 17880

**Sex Ratio:** M1:F1

**Occurrence:** Unknown.

**Risk of Recurrence for Patient's Sib:**
See Part I, *Mendelian Inheritance.*

**Risk of Recurrence for Patient's Child:**
See Part I, *Mendelian Inheritance.*

**Age of Detectability:** At birth.

**Gene Mapping and Linkage:** Unknown.

**Prevention:** None known. Genetic counseling indicated.

**Treatment:** None indicated in the absence of associated ocular malformations.

**Prognosis:** Normal for life and intelligence. Good for vision, if independent of associated ocular malformations.

**Detection of Carrier:** Unknown.

**References:**
White BV Jr., Fulton MN: A rare pupillary defect inherited by identical twins. J Hered 1937; 28:177–179.
Duke-Elder S: System of ophthalmology. vol. 3, part 2. Congenital deformities. London: Henry Kimpton, 1964.
Henkind P, et al.: Mesodermal dysgenesis of the anterior segment: Rieger's anomaly. Arch Ophthalmol 1965; 73:810–817.
Reese AB, Ellsworth RM: The anterior chamber cleavage syndrome. Arch Ophthalmol 1966; 75:307–318.

SU001                                                **Joel Sugar**
G0006                                          **Morton F. Goldberg**

**Pupillary membrane persistence**
*See EYE, PUPILLARY MEMBRANE PERSISTENCE*
**Pupils, fixed, dilated**
*See EYE, IRIDOPLEGIA, FAMILIAL*
**Pure testicular dysgenesis**
*See GONADAL DYSGENESIS, XY TYPE*
**Puretic syndrome**
*See FIBROMATOSIS, JUVENILE HYALINE*
**Purine autism**
*See ADENYLOSUCCINATE MONOPHOSPHATE LYASE DEFICIENCY*
**Purine-nucleoside: orthophosphate ribosyltransferase**
*See IMMUNODEFICIENCY, NUCLEOSIDE-PHOSPHORYLASE DEFICIENCY*
**Purpura fulminans, neonatal**
*See PROTEIN C DEFICIENCY*
**Purtilo syndrome**
*See IMMUNODEFICIENCY, X-LINKED LYMPHOPROLIFERATIVE DISEASE*
**Pustular psoriasis**
*See SKIN, PSORIASIS VULGARIS*
**PXE**
*See PSEUDOXANTHOMA ELASTICUM*
**Pycnodysostosis**
*See PYKNODYSOSTOSIS*
**Pygopagus**
*See TWINS, CONJOINED*

## PYKNODYSOSTOSIS 0846

**Includes:**
Pycnodysostosis
Toulouse-Lautrec (possible diagnosis)

**Excludes:**
**Cleidocranial dysplasia** (0185)
**Osteopetrosis** (see all)

**Major Diagnostic Criteria:** Short stature with craniofacial dysmorphism and pathologic fractures. On X-rays, generalized increased density of the skeleton, delayed closure of the cranial sutures, mandibular hypoplasia, narrowness, partial amputation, or osteolysis of the distal phalanges.

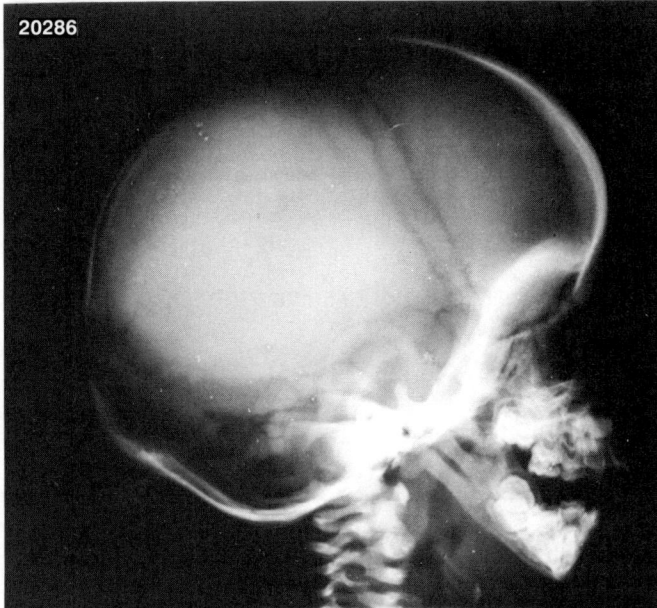

**Clinical Findings:** Patients are of short stature, with a final height of 1.35 to 1.50 m. The head is large with protrusion of the frontal bone; the anterior fontanelle remains largely open, and the chin is small and receding. Usually the sclerae have a bluish color, and dental anomalies with malplacements are frequent. The extremities are short, with a square aspect of the distal phalanges. Abnormal but moderate fragility of bones is usually present.

X-rays show the generally increased density of the skeleton without defective metaphyseal modeling of the long bones. On the hands, the terminal phalanges are narrow, and their distal portion disappears or is replaced by irregular bony fragments (an aspect comparable to that of a local osteolysis). The lack of closure of the anterior fontanelle, marked enlargement of the lambdoid suture, and mandibular hypoplasia are the most striking features. The angle of the mandible is wide so that the entire bone appears to be almost rectilinear. Teeth are irregularly aligned and in the adult total edentia is possible.

**Complications:** The risk of fracture is increased, but the complications of osteopetrosis (nervous compression, anemia) are absent.

**Associated Findings:** In one patient, dyspneic spells occurred as a consequence of mandibular hypoplasia. Spondylolisthesis is also possible.

**Etiology:** Autosomal recessive inheritance.

**Pathogenesis:** Ultrastructural study of growth cartilage reveals the presence of abnormal inclusions in the chondrocytes. These inclusions contain granular material and irregularly interwoven lamellar structure and can be excreted in the cell lacunae. The histochemical characteristics (coloration with Nile blue), and the ultrastructure probably indicate the phospholipid content of the vacuoles (Stanescu et al., 1984).

**MIM No.:** *26580

**POS No.:** 3365

**Sex Ratio:** M1:F1

**Occurrence:** About 30 cases have been documented.

**Risk of Recurrence for Patient's Sib:**
See Part I, *Mendelian Inheritance.*

**Risk of Recurrence for Patient's Child:**
See Part I, *Mendelian Inheritance.*

**Age of Detectability:** Usually during the first five years of life, on the basis of short stature, delayed closure of the anterior fontanelle, or fracture.

**Gene Mapping and Linkage:** Unknown.

**Prevention:** None known. Genetic counseling indicated.

**Treatment:** Orthopedic management of fracture; fixation with expanding intramedullary rods if repetition of tibial fractures.

**Prognosis:** Normal life span. The dwarfism is moderate.

**Detection of Carrier:** Unknown.

**Special Considerations:** There are good reasons to believe that the painter Henri de Toulouse Lautrec suffered from pyknodysostosis.

**References:**
Maroteaux P, Lamy M: La pycnodysostose. Presse Med 1962; 70:999–1002.
Maroteaux P, Lamy M: The malady of Toulouse-Lautrec. J Am Med Assoc 1965; 191:715–717.
Elmore SM, et al.: Pycnodysostosis, with a familial chromosome anomaly. Am J Med 1966; 40:273–282.
Maroteaux P, Fauré C: Pycnodysostosis. Prog Pediatr Radiol 1973; 4:403–413. *
Meredith SC, et al.: Pycnodysostosis: a clinical, pathological and ultramicroscopic study of a case. J Bone Joint Surg 1978; 60A:1122–1128.
Stanescu V, et al.: Pathogenic mechanisms in osteochondrodysplasias. J Bone Joint Surg 1984; 66A:817–836.

**0846-11281:** Pyknodysostosis in cousins; note short stature and craniofacial disproportion. **20286:** Skull X-ray of a 30-month-old male; note lack of closure of the anterior fontanel, marked enlargement of the lamboid suture, and hypoplasia of the mandible, which is almost rectilinear.

**Pierre Maroteaux**

## PYLE DISEASE                                    0847

**Includes:** Metaphyseal dysplasia

**Excludes:** **Craniometaphyseal dysplasia** (0228)

**Major Diagnostic Criteria:** Gross metaphyseal expansion associated with few, if any, clinical manifestations.

**Clinical Findings:** Valgus deformity of the knees may be the only obvious abnormality, but muscular weakness, scoliosis, and bone fragility are sometimes present. In contrast to the mild clinical signs, the X-ray changes are striking. The tubular bones of the legs show gross "Erlenmeyer flask" flaring, particularly in the distal portions of the femora. The long bones of the arms are also undermodeled, and the cortices are generally thin. The skull is virtually normal, apart from a supraorbital prominence. The bones of the pelvis and thoracic cage are expanded.

**Complications:** There may be a mild tendency to fracturing.

**Associated Findings:** None known.

**Etiology:** Autosomal recessive inheritance.

**Pathogenesis:** Unknown.

**MIM No.:** *26590

**POS No.:** 3367

**Sex Ratio:** M1:F1

**Occurrence:** About 20 cases have been documented. The wide geographic distribution includes the United States, Germany, France, South Africa, India, and Saudi Arabia.

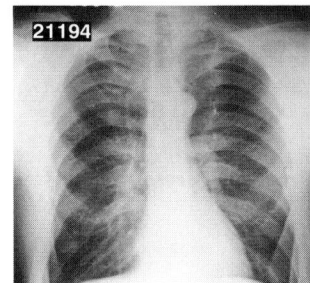
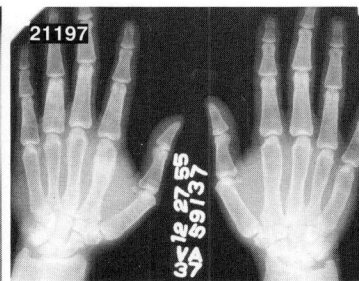
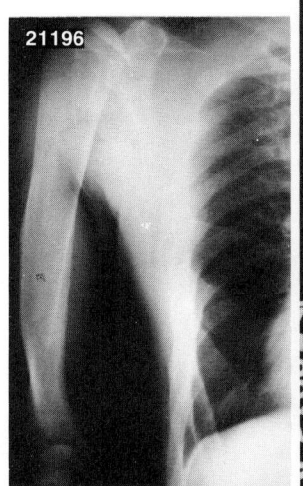
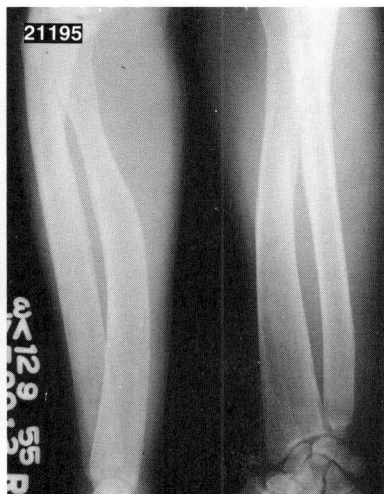
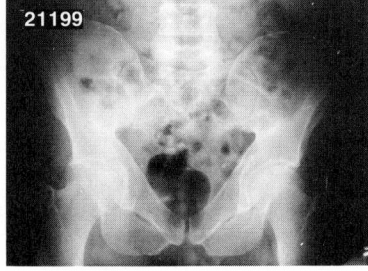
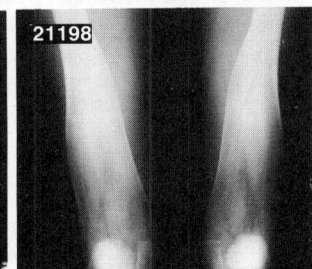

**0847B**-21194: Ribs and clavicles are markedly thickened. 21197: Tubular bones of the hands show marked distal flaring of the metacarpals and proximal flaring of the phalanges. 21196: Humerus is undermodeled in the proximal two-thirds. 21195: Radius and ulna are undermodeled in the distal two-thirds. 21199: Pelvis and ischial bones are thickened. 21198: Femora exhibit most marked "Erlenmeyer flask"-like flare which extends far up the diaphysis.

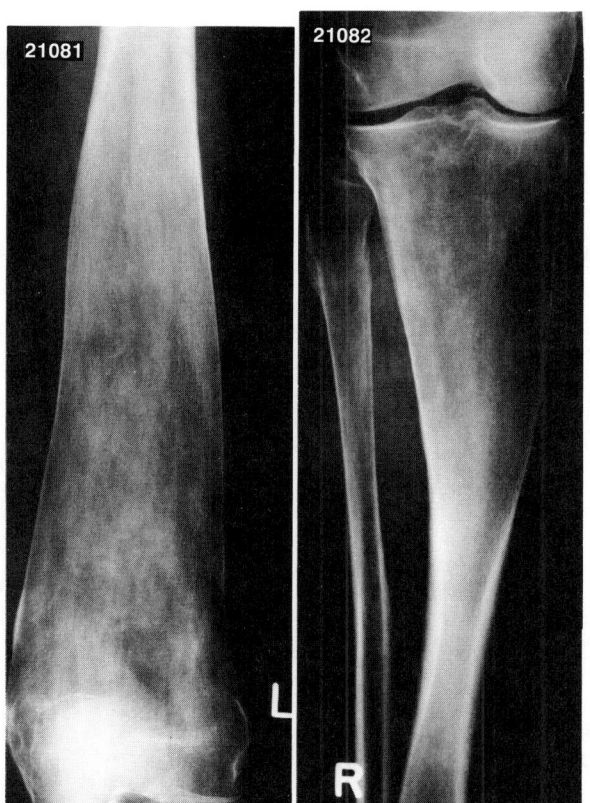

**0847A**-21081: X-ray of the femur of an affected male showing gross Erlenmeyer flask appearance and marked cortical thinning. 21082: The proximal regions of the tibia and fibia are flared and the cortices are thin.

**Risk of Recurrence for Patient's Sib:**
See Part I, *Mendelian Inheritance.*

**Risk of Recurrence for Patient's Child:**
See Part I, *Mendelian Inheritance.*

**Age of Detectability:** In early childhood, by X-ray.

**Gene Mapping and Linkage:** Unknown.

**Prevention:** None known. Genetic counseling indicated.

**Treatment:** Unknown.

**Prognosis:** Intelligence and lifespan are normal. General health is good.

**Detection of Carrier:** Heterozygotes have minor disturbances of modelling in the metaphyses of the tubular bones, especially the distal femora.

**Special Considerations:** This condition is named after Edwin Pyle (1891–1961), an orthopedic surgeon from Waterbury, Connecticut, who published the first case in 1931.

There has been nosologic confusion between Pyle disease and the autosomal recessive form of **Craniometaphyseal dysplasia**. It must be emphasized that these conditions are distinct and separate entities.

**References:**

Pyle E: Case of unusual bone development. J Bone Joint Surg 1931; 13:874–876.

Gorlin RJ, et al.: Pyle's disease (familial metaphyseal dysplasia). J Bone Joint Surg 1970; 52A:345–354.

Raad MS, Beighton P: Autosomal recessive inheritance of metaphyseal dysplasia (Pyle's disease). Clin Genet 1978; 14:251–256. * †

Heselson NG, et al.: The radiological manifestations of metaphyseal dysplasia (Pyle's disease). Brit J Radiol 1979; 52/618:431–440. * †

Beighton P: Pyle disease (metaphyseal dysplasia). J Med Genet 1987; 24:321–324.

BE008                                                      **Peter Beighton**

**Pyloric atresia**
*See STOMACH, PYLORIC ATRESIA*
**Pyloric atresia, hereditary**
*See PYLORODUODENAL ATRESIA, HEREDITARY*
**Pyloric diaphragm, incomplete**
*See STOMACH, PYLORIC ATRESIA*

## PYLORIC STENOSIS                                    0848

**Includes:** Hypertrophic pyloric stenosis, congenital

**Excludes:** Pylorospasm

**Major Diagnostic Criteria:** Nonbilious vomiting and pyloric hypertrophy identified by palpation of a pyloric "tumor." Sonography or upper GI series may be diagnostic when "tumor" cannot be palpated.

**Clinical Findings:** Nonbilious projectile vomiting, characteristically beginning at 2–3 weeks of age, which progresses to almost complete gastric outlet obstruction associated with constipation, weight loss, dehydration, and electrolyte imbalance (hypokalemic alkalosis). Eagerness to nurse after vomiting is common. Visible gastric peristaltic waves proceed from left to right after feeding. The thickened, hypertrophied, muscular pylorus can be palpated in the epigastrium as an olive-sized and olive-shaped movable mass or "tumor." Contrast X-ray studies (using a barium-water mixture) identify an elongated, curved, pyloric channel, with proximal and distal protrusion of the hypertrophied pyloric musculature into the duodenal and gastric lumen to cause the so-called "shoulder" sign. Delayed gastric emptying is not a valid specific diagnostic sign.

**Complications:** Starvation, dehydration, and severe electrolyte imbalance. Jaundice (unusual, less than 3%), with predominance of indirect bilirubin. Hematemesis.

**Associated Findings:** Jaundice (< 3%), gastric ulcer.

**Etiology:** Probably polygenic and sex modified. It is improbable that just one gene makes a major contribution to its genetic liability.

**Pathogenesis:** The hypertrophy of the circular (and some longitudinal) musculature of the pylorus is progressive, to some extent. Variations in mucosal edema account for changes in the degree of obstruction.

**MIM No.:** 17901

**CDC No.:** 750.510

**Sex Ratio:** M4:F1

**Occurrence:** 1:250 births (1:200 males; 1:1,000 females). Most frequent in Caucasians; uncommon in non-Caucasians, rare in Asiatics (especially Chinese). The most common problem requiring abdominal surgery in infancy.

**Risk of Recurrence for Patient's Sib:** If mother was affected, 1:5 (20%) for brothers, and 1:14 (7%) for sisters. If father was affected, 1:20 (5%) for brothers, and 1:40 (21/2 %) for sisters.

**Risk of Recurrence for Patient's Child:** If patient is female, 1:5 (20%) for sons, and 1:14 (7%) for daughters. If patient is male, 1:20 (5%) for sons, and 1:40 (21/2 %) for daughters.

**Age of Detectability:** Usually at 2–4 weeks of age.

**Gene Mapping and Linkage:** Unknown.

**Prevention:** None known. Genetic counseling indicated.

**Treatment:** Laparotomy and Ramstedt pyloromyotomy are curative. Nonsurgical treatment with antispasmodics is generally unsatisfactory.

**Prognosis:** Excellent. Following pyloromyotomy symptoms vanish, and the pyloric hypertrophy disappears. Some evidence suggests a higher incidence of peptic ulcer in later life.

**Detection of Carrier:** Unknown.

**References:**

Carter CO, Evans KA: Inheritance of congenital pyloric stenosis. J Med Genet 1969; 6:233.

Rickham PP, et al., eds: Congenital hypertrophic pyloric stenosis. In: Rickham PP, et al., eds: Neonatal surgery. New York: Appleton-Century-Crofts, 1969:271.

Fried K, et al.: Probable autosomal dominant infantile pyloric stenosis in a large kindred. Clin Genet 1981; 20:328–330.

Spicer RD: Infantile hypertrophic pyloric stenosis: a review. Br J Surg 1982; 69:128–135. *

Tunell WP, Wilson DA: Diagnosis by real time sonograph. J Pediatr Surg 1984; 19:795–199. *

SI004                                               **William K. Sieber**

## PYLORODUODENAL ATRESIA, HEREDITARY          2617

**Includes:**
Duodenal atresia of the first segment, hereditary
Pyloric atresia, hereditary

**Excludes:**
**Intestinal atresia, multiple** (2933)
**Jejunal atresia** (2934)

**Major Diagnostic Criteria:** The pylorus and the first part of the duodenum are reduced to a fibrous band or are obstructed by a diaphragm.

**Clinical Findings:** The pregnancy is complicated by polyhydramnios in about 90% of the cases. The newborn presents with low birth weight in 60% of the cases, and continuous projectile, nonbileous vomiting in 95% of patients. On physical examination, the epigastric region may be distended (in 85%). X-ray studies reveal complete obstruction of the pylorus.

At exploratory laparotomy, there is complete diaphragmatic obstruction (in the majority) or a fibrous band blocking the lumen of the pylorus and the first portion of the duodenum.

**Complications:** If untreated, the patient may die of starvation or perforation of the stomach.

**Associated Findings:** Epidermolysis bullosum associated with complete pyloric atresia was reported in four cases.

**Etiology:** Autosomal recessive inheritance.

**Pathogenesis:** Possibly derangement in the vacuolization of the "solid" stage of the embryonic pylorus.

**MIM No.:** 22340, *26595

**CDC No.:** 751.100

**Sex Ratio:** M1:F1

**Occurrence:** Fewer than 50 patients with the hereditary type have been reported.

**Risk of Recurrence for Patient's Sib:**
See Part I, *Mendelian Inheritance.*

**Risk of Recurrence for Patient's Child:**
See Part I, *Mendelian Inheritance*. The gene frequency of this disorder is very low.

**Age of Detectability:** During the neonatal period.

**Gene Mapping and Linkage:** Unknown.

**Prevention:** None known. Genetic counseling indicated.

**Treatment:** Preferably gastroduodenostomy. Gastrojejunostomy only if gastroduodenostomy is not possible.

**Prognosis:** Excellent with proper surgical intervention.

**Detection of Carrier:** Unknown.

**Special Considerations:** In all cases of pyloroduodenal atresia, it is very important to keep the possibility of the hereditary type in mind for proper counseling of the family. Thus, fetal sonography or postdelivery investigations can be done on time for early surgical intervention, if necessary. This may be life-saving.

**References:**
Mishalany HG, et al.: Familial congenital duodenal atresia. Pediatrics 1970; 46:629–632. *
Bronsther B, et al.: Congenital pyloric atresia: a report of three cases and review of the literature. Surgery 1971; 69:130–136.
Mishalany HG, et al.: Familial congenital duodenal atresia. (Letter) Pediatrics 1971; 47:633–634.
Bar-Maor JA, et al.: Pyloric atresia: a hereditary congenital anomaly with autosomal recessive transmission. J Med Genet 1972; 9:70–72.
Tan KL, Murugasu JJ: Congenital pyloric atresia in siblings. Arch Surg 1973; 106:100–102.
Der Kaloustian VM, et al.: Familial congenital duodenal atresia (cont.). (Letter) Pediatrics 1974; 54:118 only.
Rosenbloom MS, Ratner M: Congenital pyloric atresia and epidermolysis bullosa letalis in premature siblings. J Pediat Surg 1987; 22:374–375.

DE030  
MI039  

**Vazken M. Der Kaloustian**  
**Henry G. Mishalany**

**Pyorrhea-epilepsy-alopecia-mental retardation**
*See ALOPECIA-SEIZURES-MENTAL RETARDATION, SHOKEIR TYPE*
**Pyramidal chest**
*See PECTUS CARINATUM*
**Pyridoxine deficiency induced by isoniazid therapy**
*See NEUROPATHY, HERITABLE ISONIAZIDE TYPE (INH)*
**Pyridoxine dependency**
*See SEIZURES, VITAMIN B(6) DEPENDENCY*
**Pyridoxine-responsive homocystinuria**
*See HOMOCYSTINURIA*
**Pyroglutamic acidemia**
*See ACIDEMIA, PYROGLUTAMIC*
**Pyroglutamic aciduria**
*See ANEMIA, HEMOLYTIC, GLUTATHIONE SYNTHETASE DEFICIENCY*
**Pyropoikilocytosis**
*See ELLIPTOCYTOSIS*
**Pyropoikilocytosis, hereditary**
*See ANEMIA, HEMOLYTIC, RED CELL MEMBRANE DEFECTS*
**Pyrroloporphyria**
*See PORPHYRIA, ACUTE INTERMITTENT*

## PYRUVATE CARBOXYLASE DEFICIENCY WITH LACTIC ACIDEMIA 0850

**Includes:**
Ataxia with lactic acidosis II
Lactic acidemia without hypoxemia
Leigh necrotizing encephalopathy (some cases)

**Excludes:**
Carboxylase deficiency, multiple
**Fructose-1-phosphate aldolase deficiency** (0395)
**Fructose-1,6-diphosphatase deficiency** (0396)
Lactate elevation secondary to other causes
Myopathy, mitochondrial
**Pyruvate dehydrogenase deficiency** (0851)

**Major Diagnostic Criteria:** Neurologic deterioration with lactic and pyruvic acidemia. Demonstration of decreased pyruvate carboxylase activity in cultured skin fibroblasts, leukocytes, or liver confirms the diagnosis.

**Clinical Findings:** Pyruvate carboxylase deficiency has been found in patients who develop severe neonatal lactic acidosis, and those whose clinical disease has a later onset. In the later case, the patient may appear normal at birth and during infancy, but whose development tends to be slow. More serious difficulties become apparent by one year of age. Abnormalities have included "failure to thrive", vomiting, irritability, apathy, inactivity, hypotonia, areflexia, spasticity, cerebellar ataxia, abnormal eye movements, and seizures. The course is usually progressive, with neurologic and intellectual deterioration, and death has occurred within several years. Some children have been diagnosed as having **Encephalopathy, necrotizing** (subacute).

Lactate, pyruvate, and alanine are elevated on most occasions, and the lactate-to-pyruvate ratio is usually in the normal range. In the acute form, the lactate levels may be catastrophically high, and in some instances ammonia, citrulline, proline, and lysine have been described as elevated. Those patients with later onset of obvious symptoms may have lactate levels in the range of 20–40 mg/dl (2–4 mMol/L); levels which do not obviously distort the acid base balance. EEG abnormalities have occurred in some patients. Pyruvate carboxylase activity has been decreased or absent in liver biopsy specimens.

**Complications:** Neurologic and intellectual deterioration. Death, in most instances.

**Associated Findings:** None known.

**Etiology:** Autosomal recessive inheritance.

**Pathogenesis:** Pyruvate carboxylase is important both in gluconeogenesis and in maintaining adequate levels of oxaloacetate to support full activity of the tricarboxylic acid cycle. Hypoglycemia has not been a prominent part of the clinical picture in most patients.

**MIM No.:** *26615

**Sex Ratio:** M1:F1

**Occurrence:** Undetermined but presumed rare. Established literature.

**Risk of Recurrence for Patient's Sib:**
See Part I, *Mendelian Inheritance*.

**Risk of Recurrence for Patient's Child:**
See Part I, *Mendelian Inheritance*. Affected individuals are not expected to survive to reproduce.

**Age of Detectability:** Earliest diagnoses were made within the first several days for the neonatal form, and the first several months for less severely affected patients. Lactate and pyruvate theoretically should be elevated within the first week of life in all patients. Diagnosis is confirmed by liver biopsy or study of cultured skin fibroblasts, and should be positive at birth.

**Gene Mapping and Linkage:** PC (pyruvate carboxylase) has been provisionally mapped to 11q.

**Prevention:** None known. Genetic counseling indicated.

**Treatment:** Thiamine, lipoic acid, glutamine, and aspartic acid in pharmacologic doses have all been reported to be helpful in reducing lactate and pyruvate levels, and in mitigating the symptoms and their rate of progression.

**Prognosis:** Poor. Death usually occurs within several years.

**Detection of Carrier:** Unknown.

**Special Considerations:** The signs and symptoms of this disorder are nonspecific and inconsistent. Primary suspicion is caused by elevated lactate, pyruvate, or alanine, and the diagnosis must be confirmed by liver biopsy. It cannot be readily distinguished from **Pyruvate dehydrogenase deficiency** on clinical or biochemical grounds alone. The assay for pyruvate carboxylase is reported to be difficult and is best performed in a laboratory with experience in the methodology.

Biotin-responsive multiple carboxylase deficiency may present as lactic acidemia due to a predominant deficiency of pyruvate carboxylase. Diagnosis can be confirmed by urinary organic acid analysis.

Lactic acidemia is defined by the presence of a blood lactate in excess of 15 mg/dl and becomes lactic acidosis when compensatory mechanisms are no longer able to maintain the arterial pH in the normal range. Lactate exists in equilibrium with pyruvate and with alanine. The NADH/NAD ratio reflects the ratio of lactate (L) to pyruvate (P). In some instances, the L/P ratio provides a clue to the nature of the primary metabolic error.

Elevation of blood lactate is a laboratory abnormality that may be due to a variety of inherited and acquired conditions. Within each entity, the severity may vary with the nature and degree of the enzyme deficiency. Seizure activity may raise blood and cerebrospinal fluid lactate levels. It is prudent to wait 12–24 hours after the control of electrical seizure activity before assessing lactate and pyruvate.

Because lactate and pyruvate are readily measured in most clinical laboratories, elevations in these compounds may be detected in cases of acidosis, even though the primary cause of the acidosis may be an entirely different disorder. Conversely, significant elevations in both lactate and pyruvate may cause no obvious alteration in plasma bicarbonate and thus be overlooked entirely.

The assessment of patients with elevations of lactate must include measurement of the lactate/pyruvate ratio, urinary lactate excretion, association between lactate and pyruvate levels and meals, plasma and urinary ketone body levels, blood sugar measurement in the fasting and post-prandial state, plasma amino acids, urinary amino and organic acids, and a history for sensitivity to dietary factors or other minor environmental stress. High levels of pyruvate may cause an apparent false-positive test for ketones when using a commercial nitroprusside reagent (Acetest, Ames).

In a decreasing but still significant number of patients with an apparently primary elevation of lactate and pyruvate, no definite enzymatic diagnosis is made. In these instances, some people use empiric dietary therapy or pharmacologic doses of thiamine, biotin, or lipoic acid. False-positive and nonspecific chemical responses to thiamine have been reported.

In most cases in which no enzymatic diagnosis is made, it is most prudent to assume that the inheritance is autosomal recessive. Exceptions include those instances of a similar disease in a parent or those cases of primary myopathy in which autosomal dominant or other inheritance mechanisms may be operating.

### References:

Saudubray JM, et al.: Neonatal congenital lactic acidosis with pyruvate carboxylase deficiency in two siblings. Acta Pediatr Scand 1976; 65:717–724.

Robinson BH, et al.: The genetic heterogeneity of lactic acidosis: occurrence of recognizable inborn errors of metabolism in a pediatric population with lactic acidosis. Pediatr Res 1980; 14:956–962.

Freytag SO, Collier KJ: Molecular cloning of a cDNA for human pyruvate carboxylase. J Biol Chem 1984; 259:12831–12837.

Robinson BH, et al.: The French and North American phenotypes of pyruvate carboxylase deficiency. Am J Hum Genet 1987; 40:50–59.

Robinson BH: Lactic acidemia. In: Scriver CR, et al, eds: The metabolic basis of inherited disease, 6th ed. New York: McGraw-Hill, 1989: 869–888. *

CE001

**Stephen D. Cederbaum**
*John P. Blass*

## PYRUVATE DEHYDROGENASE DEFICIENCY          0851

### Includes:

Alaninuria
Ataxia, intermittent-pyruvate dehydrogenase deficiency
Ataxia, intermittent-pyruvate decarboxylase deficiency
Ataxia with lactic acidosis I
Lactic and pyruvic acidemia with carbohydrate sensitivity
Lactic and pyruvic acidemia with episodic ataxia and
    weakness

### Excludes:

**Fructose-1,6-diphosphatase deficiency** (0396)
Lactic acidosis-persistently increased lactate: pyruvate ratio
Lactic and pyruvic acidemia due to other causes

**Major Diagnostic Criteria:**   Persistent or recurrent pyruvic and usually lactic acidemia. Enzyme deficiency must be confirmed using skin fibroblasts or other tissue.

**Clinical Findings:**   Findings may vary from severe acidosis appearing in the first few days of life to recurrent episodes of ataxia and weakness following upper respiratory infection or other minor stress. Growth retardation has been frequent. Varying permanent neurologic deficits and mental retardation have been seen in most patients. Near-normal resting levels of lactate and pyruvate have been associated with severe neurologic damage in several patients.

Biochemical findings vary from severe lactic acidosis appearing shortly after birth to minimal pyruvic acidemia (1.5–1.8 mg/dl; normally <1.2) 2 hours following a meal high in carbohydrates. In some instances elevation of blood pyruvate levels is seen only during the acute episodes of ataxia and weakness. The blood lactate:pyruvate ratio has almost always been normal (< 20). Alanine excretion of greater than 100 mg/g creatinine is a variable finding and often is present only during acute episodes. Blood alanine has been elevated above 6 mg/dl only with pyruvate values persistently greater than 2.0 mg/dl. Cerebrospinal fluid pyruvate and lactate also have been elevated. Increased lactate in the urine (> 0.7 mg/mg creatine) is seen when blood lactate is 2–4 times normal or more.

**Complications:**   Mental retardation and neurologic damage; in some instances, early death from lactic acidosis.

**Associated Findings:**   None known.

**Etiology:**   Autosomal recessive inheritance.

**Pathogenesis:**   Defective oxidation of pyruvate and deficiency of pyruvate dehydrogenase have been demonstrated in cultured skin fibroblasts, peripheral lymphocytes, muscle, and other visceral tissues. Increased dietary carbohydrates typically precipitate lactic acidosis in the more severely affected patients.

**MIM No.:**   *20880

**Sex Ratio:**   Presumably M1:F1, but males predominate in reported cases.

**Occurrence:**   Over 100 cases have been documented.

**Risk of Recurrence for Patient's Sib:**
    See Part I, *Mendelian Inheritance.*

**Risk of Recurrence for Patient's Child:**
    See Part I, *Mendelian Inheritance.*

**Age of Detectability:**   Shortly after birth, by skin fibroblast assay or other tissue assay. Age at which pyruvate and lactate elevation is detected will probably depend on the nature and severity of the biochemical defect.

**Gene Mapping and Linkage:**   One subunit of the complex has been mapped to the X chromosome; the others are autosomal.

**Prevention:**   None known. Genetic counseling indicated.

**Treatment:**   The disorder is exacerbated by increased carbohydrate intake and improved by increased dietary fat. Avoidance of infection and undue stress is desirable. High doses of thiamine have not yet proven beneficial. Corticosteroid therapy has been reported to abort the acute episodes of ataxia and weakness in several instances.

**Prognosis:**   In most instances irreversible neurologic damage and mental retardation have occurred by the time of diagnosis. The impact of a high-fat diet instituted at an early age has not been assessed. The ultimate risk of permanent neurologic handicap to those patients with only episodic symptoms is unknown.

**Detection of Carrier:**   By analysis of skin fibroblasts. Discrimination incomplete.

**Special Considerations:**   Blood pyruvate levels have always been abnormal following a meal high in carbohydrate. The long-term impact of a high-fat diet has not been determined. Dietary trial for pyruvic and lactic acidemia should be undertaken with care, since other causes of pyruvic acidemia may lead to carbohydrate dependence.

Pyruvate dehydrogenase is a complex of three catalytic and two regulatory enzymes. Deficiency of all three catalytic enzymes, and of the activating enzyme, have been reported. Ultimately, the disorders caused by each defect may be distinguishable clinically and prognostically.

**References:**
Falk RE, et al.: Ketogenic diet in the treatment of pyruvate dehydrogenase deficiency. Pediatrics 1976; 58:713–721.
Robinson BH, et al.: The genetic heterogeneity of lactic acidosis: occurrence of recognizable inborn errors of metabolism in a pediatric population with lactic acidosis. Pediat Res 1980; 14:956–962. *
Prick M, et al.: Pyruvate dehydrogenase deficiency restricted to brain. Neurology 1981; 31:398–404.
McKay N, et al.: Lacticacidemia due to pyruvate dehydrogenase deficiency, with evidence of protein polymorphism in the α-subunit of the enzyme. Eur J Pediat 1986; 144:445–450.
Patel M, Roche T, eds: Alpha ketoacid dehydrogenase complexes: organization, regulation and biochemical aspects. New York: New York Academy of Sciences, 1989.
Robinson BH: Lactic acidemia. In: Scriver CR, et al, eds: The metabolic basis of inherited disease, 6th ed. New York: McGraw-Hill, 1989: 869–888. *

CE001                                    **Stephen D. Cederbaum**
                                              *John P. Blass*

---

## PYRUVATE KINASE DEFICIENCY                           0852

**Includes:**
>     Anemia, hemolytic pyruvate kinase type
>     Pyruvate kinase deficiency of erythrocyte

**Excludes:**
>     Nonspherocytic hemolytic anemias from other enzyme
>         deficiencies
>     Nonspherocytic hemolytic anemias from unstable
>         hemoglobin

**Major Diagnostic Criteria:** Pallor due to hemolytic anemia with reticulocytosis. There is no specific abnormality of erythrocyte morphology. Increased autohemolysis of affected erythrocytes in vitro is usually demonstrable, usually uncorrected by glucose but corrected by adenosine triphosphate (ATP). Erythrocyte 2, 3DPG levels are unusually high, in severely anemic patients reaching levels greater than 3 times normal. Erythrocyte pyruvate kinase activity is reduced, usually to 5–20% of normal. Occasionally, maximal pyruvate kinase activity is normal but the enzyme exhibits unfavorable kinetic properties at low substrate (phosphoenol-pyruvate) concentrations. International standards for biochemical characterization of pyruvate kinase mutants have been developed.

**Clinical Findings:** Signs of excessive hemolysis of varying grades of severity and changing from time to time; chronic hemolytic anemia, hyperbilirubinemia, splenomegaly, reticulocytosis.

**Complications:** Gallstones are secondary to chronic hyperbilirubinemia. Exacerbations of anemia, resulting from transient marrow erythroid hypoplasia, are usually associated with infections. Leg ulcers rarely occur.

**Associated Findings:** Leukocyte pyruvate kinase is normal, but liver pyruvate kinase activity may be reduced.

**Etiology:** Autosomal recessive inheritance.

**Pathogenesis:** The sequence of events preceding hemolysis of pyruvate kinase deficient erythrocytes is poorly understood. Deficient erythrocytes usually have low glycolytic rates in vitro (particularly when compared to control erythrocytes of similar age) and are unable to maintain intracellular ATP levels. However, in vivo erythrocyte ATP levels may be normal. Nevertheless, ATP depletion as a result of inadequate glycolysis is thought to be the central event resulting in premature hemolysis. The almost immediate destruction of a portion of newly formed reticulocytes

in the spleen or elsewhere in the reticuloendothelial system contributes importantly to the observed hemolysis. Molecular variants of erythrocyte pyruvate kinase have been characterized by their abnormal substrate kinetics, but no detailed studies of molecular structure are as yet available.

**MIM No.:**  *26620

**Sex Ratio:**  M1:F1

**Occurrence:** Undetermined but presumed rare. Most affected individuals thus far described have been of European or Amish origin. Extensive literature. An estimated 2.4:1,000 heterozygotes for enzyme deficiency variants.

**Risk of Recurrence for Patient's Sib:**
See Part I, *Mendelian Inheritance.*

**Risk of Recurrence for Patient's Child:**
See Part I, *Mendelian Inheritance.*

**Age of Detectability:** At birth, by assay of erythrocyte pyruvate kinase.

**Gene Mapping and Linkage:** PKLR (pyruvate kinase, liver and RBC) has been provisionally mapped to 1q21.

**Prevention:** None known. Genetic counseling indicated.

**Treatment:** Splenectomy reduces or eliminates the need for blood transfusions in severely anemic patients but is not curative. Anemia persists, but usually a higher hemoglobin level can be maintained. Postsplenectomy reticulocyte counts usually rise rather than fall and may occasionally exceed 90%. Supportive blood transfusions should be given when indicated. Cholecystectomy is indicated if gallstones form.

**Prognosis:** Varies with severity of anemia (e.g. high mortality in early childhood described in unsplenectomized Amish kindred). Most patients survive to adulthood, and mildly anemic patients may expect to have a near-normal life span unless complications (e.g. gallstones) supervene.

**Detection of Carrier:** Carriers are clinically and hematologically normal, but their erythrocyte pyruvate kinase activity is usually one-half the normal level. Alternatively, carriers may have normal enzyme activity, but abnormal substrate kinetics (altered Km of PEP).

**Special Considerations:** Pyruvate kinase deficient reticulocytes are protected from the consequences of their glycolytic defect by the availability of alternate metabolic pathways (oxidative phosphorylation).

Oxidative phosphorylation in such reticulocytes may be inhibited during sequestration in hypoxic, acidic regions of the spleen whereupon glycolysis alone is inadequate to support their increased ATP requirements. The result is ATP depletion which induces a membrane lesion characterized by massive prelytic loss of intracellular potassium and water, cell shrinkage, and increased cell rigidity. The shrunken rigid cell produced is presumed to be susceptible to further sequestration because of difficulty in traversing the 3 micron pores separating splenic cords from sinuses. Eventually, cell lysis occurs. Splenectomy, by removal of a stagnant, hypoxic trap, allows reticulocytes to survive, and partially alleviates the anemia.

**References:**
Keitt AS, Bennett DC: Pyruvate kinase deficiency and related disorders of red cell glycolysis. Am J Med 1966; 41:762–785.
Miwa S: Recommended methods for the characterization of red cell pyruvate kinase variants. Br J Haematol 1979; 43:275–286.
Mentzer WC Jr.: Pyruvate kinase deficiency and disorders of glycolysis. In: Nathan DG, Oski FA, eds: Hematology of infancy and childhood, 3rd ed. Philadelphia: W.B. Saunders, 1987:545–582.
Valentine WN, et al.: Pyruvate kinase and other enzyme deficiency disorders of the erythrocyte. In: Scriver CR, et al, eds: The metabolic basis of inherited disease, 6th ed. New York: McGraw-Hill, 1989: 2341–2366.

ME019                                    **William C. Mentzer, Jr.**

**Pyruvate kinase deficiency of erythrocyte**
*See PYRUVATE KINASE DEFICIENCY*

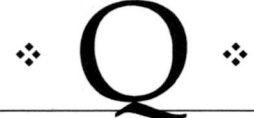

**Quinine, fetal effects of**
   *See OPTIC NERVE HYPOPLASIA*
**Quinoform induced subacute myelo-optico neuropathy (SMON)**
   *See NEUROPATHY, MYELO-OPTICO, SUBACUTE TYPE*
**Quinoid dihydropteridine reductase deficiency**
   *See DIHYDROPTERIDINE REDUCTASE DEFICIENCY*
**Quivering of chin, hereditary**
   *See CHIN, TREMBLING*

# ❖ R ❖

**Rabenhorst syndrome**
  *See VENTRICULAR SEPTAL DEFECT*
**Rabson-Mendenhall syndrome**
  *See LIPODYSTROPHY-COARSE FACIES-ACANTHOSIS NIGRICANS,
    MIESCHER TYPE*
**Rachipagus**
  *See TWINS, CONJOINED*
**Racial lactase deficiency**
  *See LACTASE DEFICIENCY, PRIMARY*
**Radial aplasia-cleft lip/palate**
  *See RADIAL DEFECTS*
**Radial aplasia-craniosynostosis**
  *See CRANIOSYNOSTOSIS-RADIAL APLASIA SYNDROME*

---

## RADIAL DEFECTS                                    0853

**Includes:**
  Deficiency of radial rays and radius and phocomelia
  Phocomelia and radial ray defects
  Radial aplasia-cleft lip/palate
  Radial dysplasia
  Thumb defects

**Excludes:**
  **Craniosynostosis** (0230)
  **Fetal thalidomide syndrome** (0386)
  **Heart-hand syndrome** (0455)
  **Pancytopenia syndrome, Fanconi type** (2029)
  **Thrombocytopenia-absent radius** (0941)
  **Vater association** (0987)
  Ventriculoradial dysplasia

**Major Diagnostic Criteria:** Hypoplasia of the thumb or first metacarpal in the absence of other malformations.

**Clinical Findings:** Several degrees of severity occur. In the mildest form, there is hypoplasia of the first metacarpal often combined with hypoplasia of the thumb. With increasing severity, there is complete loss of the first metacarpal producing a small flail thumb attached to the index finger by soft tissue. The next level of severity is characterized by hypoplasia or aplasia of the radius associated with varying degrees of thumb and first metacarpal hypoplasia (see **Hand, radial club hand**). Both the radius and ulna are absent in the most severe form which is associated with variable radial ray abnormalities and often hypoplasia of the humerus. Approximately 20% of all affected individuals have radial defects alone, of which about two-thirds are unilateral.

A possible variant, *radial aplasia-cleft lip/palate*, has been reported in at least 18 cases (Immeyer, 1967).

**Complications:** Dysfunction of upper limbs related to severity of malformation.

**Associated Findings:** Possibly cleft lip/palate, or this association may constitute a distinct condition.

**Etiology:** If all cases of radial defects with associated anomalies are excluded, most cases are sporadic.

**Pathogenesis:** Suppression of developing limb structures.

**MIM No.:** 17910, 17940

**CDC No.:** 755.280

**Sex Ratio:** M1:F1

**Occurrence:** Undetermined but presumed rare.

**Risk of Recurrence for Patient's Sib:** Undetermined, but probably low.

**Risk of Recurrence for Patient's Child:** Undetermined, but probably low.

**Age of Detectability:** At birth.

**Gene Mapping and Linkage:** Unknown.

**Prevention:** None known. Genetic counseling indicated.

**Treatment:** Surgery may improve function in certain cases.

**Prognosis:** Normal intelligence and life span. Dysfunction is related to severity of deformity.

**Detection of Carrier:** Unknown.

**Special Considerations:** For accurate genetic counseling, as well as proper treatment, it is important to exclude the many complex syndromes in which radial defects occur. In particular, the cardiovascular, GU, and hematologic systems should be carefully examined. Although families have been reported showing autosomal dominant inheritance of isolated radial defects, it is very difficult to completely rule out the more complex syndromes; e.g. **Heart-hand syndrome** with no or only minor heart manifestations.

**References:**
Immeyer F: Lippen-Kiefer-Gaumenspalten bei thalidomidgeschaedigten Kindern. Acta Genet Med Gemellol 1967; 16:244–274.
Carroll RE, Louis DS: Anomalies associated with radial dysplasia. J Pediatr 1974; 84:409–411.
Temtamy SA: On anomalies associated with radial dysplasia. J Pediatr 1974; 85:585 only.

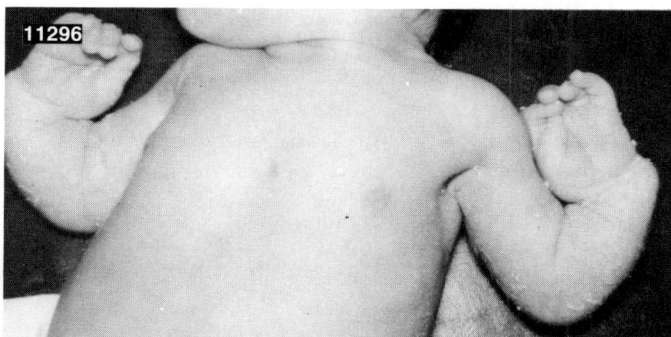

**0853**-11296:   Radial aplasia.

Temtamy SA, McKusick VA: The genetics of hand malformation. New York: Alan R. Liss, 1978.

H0033
H0025

**William A. Horton**
**O.J. Hood**

**Radial deficiency or defect**
*See HAND, RADIAL CLUB HAND*
**Radial dysplasia**
*See HAND, RADIAL CLUB HAND*
*also RADIAL DEFECTS*
**Radial hemimelia**
*See HAND, RADIAL CLUB HAND*
**Radial hypoplasia-deafness-ophthalmoplegia-thrombocytopenia**
*See IVIC SYNDROME*

---

## RADIAL HYPOPLASIA-TRIPHALANGEAL THUMBS-HYPOSPADIAS-DIASTEMA 2772

**Includes:**
    Diastema-radial hypoplasia-triphalangeal thumbs-hypospadias
    Hypospadias-radial hypoplasia-triphalangeal thumbs-diastema
    Schmitt syndrome
    Thumbs, triphalangeal-radial hypoplasia-diastema-hypospadias

**Excludes:**
    **Heart-hand syndrome** (0455)
    **Pancytopenia syndrome, Fanconi type** (2029)
    **Roberts syndrome** (0875)
    **Thrombocytopenia-absent radius** (0941)

**Major Diagnostic Criteria:** In the single described family, all indicated features were present (except hypospadias in the females). The diagnosis should not be entertained in a family unless all the features are present in at least one member or collectively in several family members.

**Clinical Findings:** The hands demonstrate triphalangeal, nonopposable thumbs without flexion creases. Flexion creases are hypoplastic on the second digits. The hands are radially deviated and the forearms are markedly shortened, with limitation in pronation, supination, and extension. Despite the deformities, adults have good manual dexterity and hand-writing skills. In males, the hypospadias consists of a pinpoint meatus on the distal ventral shaft of the penis. A 1–2-mm gap between the upper central incisors (maxillary diastema) is present in all affected individuals; no other dental anomalies were noted.

**Complications:** As with any case of hypospadias, other urinary tract anomalies or obstruction should be investigated, but no urinary complications were noted in the family studied.

**Associated Findings:** None known.

**Etiology:** Autosomal dominant inheritance with complete penetrance and little variability.

**Pathogenesis:** Unknown.

**MIM No.:** 17925

**POS No.:** 3551

**Sex Ratio:** M1:F1

**Occurrence:** One kinship has been reported.

**Risk of Recurrence for Patient's Sib:**
    See Part I, *Mendelian Inheritance.*

**Risk of Recurrence for Patient's Child:**
    See Part I, *Mendelian Inheritance.*

**Age of Detectability:** During the newborn period.

**Gene Mapping and Linkage:** Unknown.

**Prevention:** None known. Genetic counseling indicated.

**Treatment:** Surgical repair of hypospadias. The triphalangeal thumb can be rendered opposable and the radially deviated hand supported by a brace if functionally indicated.

**Prognosis:** Normal life span. Minimal associated disability.

**Detection of Carrier:** By clinical examination.

**References:**
Schmitt E, et al.: An autosomal dominant syndrome of radial hypoplasia, triphalangeal thumbs, hypospadias and maxillary diastema. J Med Genet 1982; 13:63–69.

KE012

**Thaddeus E. Kelly**

**Radial ray hypoplasia syndrome**
*See RADIAL-RENAL-OCULAR SYNDROME*
**Radial rays, deficiency of**
*See HAND, RADIAL CLUB HAND*

---

## RADIAL-RENAL SYNDROME 2771

**Includes:**
    Acro-renal syndrome, Sofer type
    Renal-radial syndrome
    Siegler syndrome
    Sofer syndrome

**Excludes:**
    **Lacrimo-auriculo-dento-digital syndrome** (2180)
    **Pancytopenia syndrome, Fanconi type** (2029)
    **Thrombocytopenia-absent radius** (0941)
    **Vater association** (0987)

**Major Diagnostic Criteria:** Radial aplasia, renal anomalies, and short stature.

**Clinical Findings:** All affected individuals have had bilateral absence or hypoplasia of the radius and absence of the thumbs. In one case the humerus was hypoplastic and the index fingers were absent. Renal anomalies were consistent and included crossed-fused ectopia and unilateral renal agenesis. Vesicoureteral reflux occurred in two cases. The ear was described as malformed in two cases. All affected individuals were below the third percentile for stature. Intellectual development was normal.

**Complications:** Renal failure secondary to reflux nephropathy.

**Associated Findings:** One affected individual has a **Tracheoesophageal fistula** and **Ventricular septal defect**.

**Etiology:** One report was of an affected father and son; the other was of sibs. Therefore, this condition could be heterogeneous and exist in both recessive and dominant forms. Conversely, reduced penetrance or germinal mosaicism could also be the case in one of the parents of the affected sibs.

**Pathogenesis:** Unknown.

**MIM No.:** 17928

**POS No.:** 3633

**Sex Ratio:** M4:F0 (observed).

**Occurrence:** Two families have been reported in the literature. A father and son were reported in Israel, brothers in Utah.

**Risk of Recurrence for Patient's Sib:**
    See Part I, *Mendelian Inheritance.*

**Risk of Recurrence for Patient's Child:**
    See Part I, *Mendelian Inheritance.*

**Age of Detectability:** At birth, although it is likely that prenatal diagnosis by ultrasound is possible.

**Gene Mapping and Linkage:** Unknown.

**Prevention:** None known. Genetic counseling indicated.

**Treatment:** Supportive. Ureteral reimplantation may be indicated.

**Prognosis:** Life span may be affected by the renal anomaly; intellectual development is normal.

**Detection of Carrier:** Unknown.

**References:**
Siegler RL, et al.: Upper limb anomalies and renal disease. Clin Genet 1980; 17:117–119. †

Sofer S, et al.: Radial ray aplasia and renal anomalies in father and son: a new syndrome. Am J Med Genet 1983; 14:151–157. †

T0007                                                           **Helga V. Toriello**

## RADIAL-RENAL-OCULAR SYNDROME                    2643

**Includes:**
>   Acro-renal-ocular syndrome
>   DR syndrome
>   Duane syndrome-radial defects
>   Ferrell-Okihiro-Halal syndrome
>   Okihiro syndrome
>   Radial ray hypoplasia syndrome
>   Thumb-renal-ocular syndrome

**Excludes:**
>   **Acro-renal-mandibular syndrome** (2778)
>   **Anus-hand-ear syndrome** (0072)
>   **Cervico-oculo-acoustic syndrome** (0142)
>   **Eye, Duane retraction syndrome** (3180)
>   **Heart-hand syndrome** (0455)
>   **IVIC syndrome** (3043)
>   **Macular coloboma-brachydactyly** (0621)

**Major Diagnostic Criteria:**   Thumb anomalies include mild (limited motion at the IP joint) to severe hypoplasia or absent thumb and first metacarpal, with **Syndactyly** between digits I-II, or preaxial **Polydactyly**. Renal anomalies include ectopia, fusion, vesicoureteral reflux, bladder diverticulum, recurrent urinary tract infections, hypertension, and mild malrotation. Ocular features consist of **Eye, Duane retraction syndrome**, lid ptosis, uveal coloboma, microcornea, optic nerve coloboma, or choroid atrophy.

**Clinical Findings:**   Seven individuals from three generations of a French-Canadian family had various combinations of acral, renal, and ocular defects (Halal et al, 1984). Three of the seven affected individuals had the complete triad. An eye defect was absent in four individuals. When present, it consisted of bilateral **Eye, Duane retraction syndrome** with unilateral palpebral ptosis (1/7), or bilateral uveal coloboma with unilateral microcornea (1/7), or unilateral coloboma of optic nerve (1/7). Acral anomalies were present in all affected individuals, varying from mild hypoplasia of the tip of the thumbs (but on X-ray, normal distal phalanx) with limited active motion of IP joints (4/7) to moderately severe bilateral hypoplasia of the thumb (1/7), unilateral severe hypoplasia (nonfunctional) of the thumb with hypoplastic first metacarpal (1/7), and preaxial **Polydactyly** type 1 (1/7). Urinary tract anomaly was present in all affected individuals; varying from mild vesicoureteral reflux (1/7) to bladder diverticulum (1/7), renal ectopia (crossed without fusion, 2/7; sacral, 1/7), and mild malrotation (2/7).

   In addition, the family history of an additional adopted boy with the condition indicates no other affected family members; however, the parents were first cousins. The boy had hypoplastic thumbs, **Eye, Duane retraction syndrome** (Duane anomaly), ureteral reflux with posterior urethral valves, hypospadias, membranous imperforate anus, bilateral choanal atresia, small larynx, vocal cord fibrosis, cholesteatoma, a jugular bulb which prolapsed into the middle ear cavity, congenital ossicular chain abnormality, slightly malformed auricles, severe low frequency hearing loss, and moderate hearing loss for the higher frequencies. Average non-verbal intelligence was noted. His WISC-R verbal score showed a pattern consistent with his hearing impairment.

**Complications:**   Functional vision impairment and hearing loss, recurrent urinary tract infections, hypertension, impaired fine motor abilities, and school performance problems.

**Associated Findings:**   Onychodystrophy of toenails (4/7), gastroduodenal ulcer, **Hernia, hiatal**, **Cancer, colorectal**, spina bifida occulta, pulmonic stenosis, preauricular tag, choanal atresia, hearing loss, hypospadias, small larynx, vocal cord fibrosis, jugular bulb prolapse into the middle ear cavity, malformed auricles, cholesteatoma, membranous imperforate anus, and conjunctival dermolipoma.

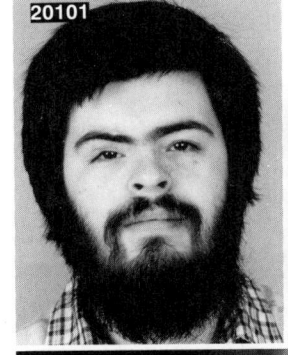
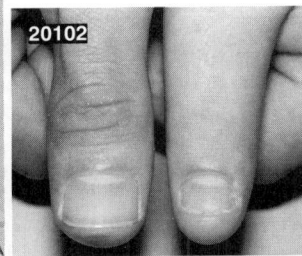
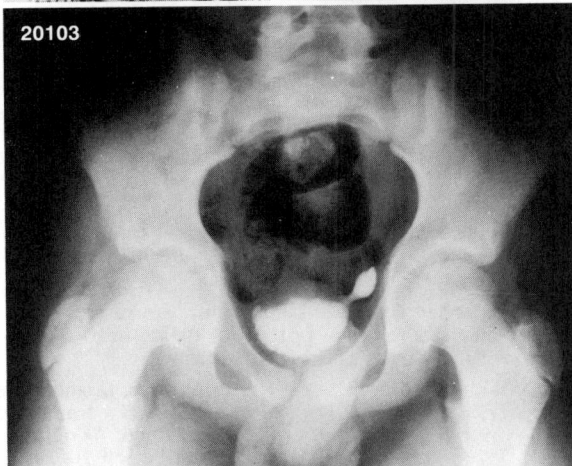
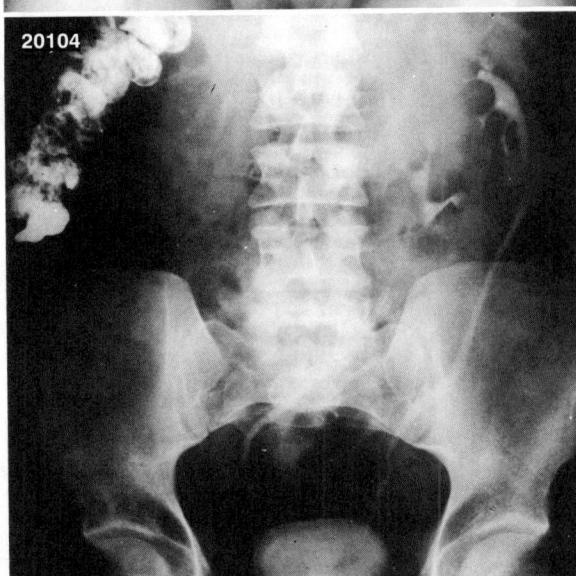

**2643**-20101: Note right palpebral ptosis. 20102: Left, hypoplastic distal portion of the thumb with absent flexion creases; right, normal thumb. 20103: Cystogram showing left paraureteral bladder. 20104: IVP showing crossed renal ectopia without fusion; right, absent kidney.

**Etiology:** Possibly autosomal dominant inheritance with variable expressivity.

**Pathogenesis:** Possibly an incompletely delineated heritable developmental field defect.

**MIM No.:** 10249

**Sex Ratio:** M1:F1

**Occurrence:** Undetermined but presumed rare.

**Risk of Recurrence for Patient's Sib:**
See Part I, *Mendelian Inheritance*.

**Risk of Recurrence for Patient's Child:**
See Part I, *Mendelian Inheritance*.

**Age of Detectability:** Clinically evident at birth. Prenatal diagnosis by ultrasonography appears to be possible.

**Gene Mapping and Linkage:** Unknown.

**Prevention:** None known. Genetic counseling indicated.

**Treatment:** Hand surgery to improve function; early recognition of vision and hearing problems with use of appropriate aids; monitoring for urinary tract infections; surgical management of urinary tract anomalies when appropriate; regular monitoring of blood pressure; and appropriate special education services when needed.

**Prognosis:** Life span appears to be normal. Intelligence is normal; special education may be needed if functional vision or hearing problems are present.

**Detection of Carrier:** Careful clinical thumb examination, since mild hypoplasia of the distal portion of the thumb could be the only apparent manifestation of the syndrome.

**Special Considerations:** The association of **Eye, Duane retraction syndrome** (Duane anomaly) with radial defects was reported previously in two families (Ferrell et al, 1966; Temtamy and McKusick, 1978). In the family reported by Ferrell et al (1966), a father and three of his five children had radial defects that varied in expression from mild hypoplasia of the thenar muscles to absence of the thumb and first metacarpal. The father had radial defects and the Duane anomaly, and the proposita had radial defects and **Atrial septal defects** but did not have the Duane anomaly. A paternal aunt had radial defects and the Duane anomaly, and a paternal uncle had radial malformations only. There was no mention of intravenous pyelogram studies on affected members of the family.

In the family (father and son) reported by Temtamy and McKusick (1978), the father had Duane anomaly with radial defects (bilateral thenar and thumb hypoplasia, with syndactyly of the index finger and unilateral clubhand deformity) and malrotation of both kidneys with partial horseshoe anomaly; his son had apparently normal eyes, bilateral clubhand with absent thumbs, and renal anomalies (absent right kidney, malrotation of left kidney). Associated anomalies were malformed pinnas, pectoral and upper limb hypoplasia, and congenital deafness and facial nerve weakness. Dermatoglyphics in the father showed abnormal flexion creases, absent axial triradius on the left, and distal axial triradius on the right. Temtamy and McKusick (1978) proposed the acronym *DR syndrome* (Duane/radial dysplasia).

More recently, Hayes et al (1985) reported on a child with Duane anomaly, deafness, cervical spine, and radial ray abnormalities. A sister of the proposita had **Oculo-auriculo-vertebral anomaly**, cervical abnormalities, and hypoplasia of the thenar eminence. Four relatives had hypoplasia of the thenar eminence. A fifth had preaxial polydactyly. Duane anomaly was present in two sixth-degree relatives. There was no mention of renal anomaly in any of the affected members. The authors suggested that the disorder be designated the *Okihiro syndrome*, since Okihiro et al (1977) were the first to recognize the constellation of non-ocular abnormalities in a single pedigree.

McDermot and Winter (1987) have also reported a family in which radial defects and Duane anomaly occurred in an autosomal dominant pattern. Anal stenosis was present in one affected individual but no urogenital anomalies were found. Goldblatt and Viljoen (1987) described a father and two daughters with radial ray

hypoplasia, esotropia, and choanal atresia with normal hematologic and renal studies.

Although the constellation of radial, renal and ocular anomalies probably represents a distinct autosomal dominant trait of variable expressivity, the possibility that it may also comprise part of the spectrum of the previously reported syndrome of Duane anomaly with radial defects cannot be excluded.

**References:**
Ferrell RL, et al.: Simultaneous occurrence of the Holt-Oram and the Duane syndrome. J Pediatr 1966; 69:630–634.
Okihiro MM, et al.: Duane syndrome and congenital upper-limb anomalies. Arch Neurol 1977; 34:174–179.
Temtamy S, McKusick VA: The genetics of hand malformations. New York: Alan R. Liss, 1978.
Halal F, et al.: Acro-renal-ocular syndrome: autosomal dominant thumb hypoplasia, renal ectopia, and eye defect. Am J Med Genet 1984; 17:753–762. * †
Hayes A, et al.: The Okihiro syndrome of Duane anomaly, radial ray abnormalities, and deafness. Am J Med Genet 1985; 22:273–280.
Temtamy SA: The DR syndrome or the Okihiro syndrome? (Letter) Am J Med Genet 1986; 25:173–174.
MacDermot K, Winter RM: Radial ray defect and Duane anomaly: report of a family with autosomal dominant trasmission. Am J Med Genet 1987; 27:313–319.
Goldblatt J, Viljoen D: New autosomal dominant radial ray hypoplasia syndrome. Am J Med Genet 1987; 28:647–654.

HA074
M0000
GR000

**Fahed Halal**
**John B. Moeschler**
**John M. Graham, Jr.**

---

## RADIAL-ULNAR SYNOSTOSIS     0854

**Includes:**
Pronation, congenital
Synostosis, radial cubital

**Excludes:**
**Acrocephalosyndactyly type V** (2284)
**Fetal thalidomide syndrome** (0386)
**Humero-radial synostosis** (0477)
**Mandibulofacial dysostosis** (0627)
**Mesomelic dysplasia, Nievergelt type** (0647)
**Poland syndrome** (0813)
Radio-ulnar synostosis as a component of a syndrome
Radio-ulnar synostosis secondary to trauma
**Roberts syndrome** (0875)
**Synostosis, multiple synostosis syndrome** (2312)

**Major Diagnostic Criteria:** Restriction of pronation-supination at the elbow with X-ray evidence of fusion of the proximal radius and ulna.

**Clinical Findings:** Pronation-supination is restricted or absent, and the elbow is often fixed in pronation. Some patients show mild limitation of extension and flexion at the elbow. Sporadic cases may be unilateral or bilateral, whereas familial cases are usually bilateral.

**Complications:** Restriction of pronation-supination.

**Associated Findings:** Other skeletal malformations, including **Craniosynostosis** and congenital hyperthyroidism.

**Etiology:** Most cases are sporadic; about 10% autosomal dominant inheritance (variable expressivity and may occasionally be nonpenetrant, especially in females); occasionally secondary to sex chromosome aneuploidy, notably 48,XXXY and 49,XXXXY.

**Pathogenesis:** Unknown.

**MIM No.:** *17930

**CDC No.:** 755.536

**Sex Ratio:** M2:F1

**Occurrence:** Undetermined. Davenport et al (1924) documented an extensive kindred, and Hansen and Andersen (1970) reported 37 cases.

**Risk of Recurrence for Patient's Sib:**
See Part I, *Mendelian Inheritance.*

**Risk of Recurrence for Patient's Child:**
See Part I, *Mendelian Inheritance.*

**Age of Detectability:** At birth, by clinical examination, and by X-ray when the intervening cartilage has ossified.

**Gene Mapping and Linkage:** Unknown.

**Prevention:** None known. Genetic counseling indicated.

**Treatment:** Rarely surgery may be required to improve the functional position of the forearm.

**Prognosis:** Normal life span.

**Detection of Carrier:** Unknown.

**References:**
Abbott FC: Hereditary congenital dislocations of the radius. Trans Pathol Soc (Lond) 1892; 43:129–139.
Davenport CB, et al.: Radio-ulnar synostosis. Arch Surg 1924; 8:705–762.
Hansen OH, Andersen NO: Congenital radio-ulnar synostosis: report of 37 cases. Acta Orthop Scand 1970; 41:225–230.
Jancu J: Radioulnar synostosis. a common occurrence in sex chromosomal abnormalities. Am J Dis Child 1971; 122:10–11.
Spritz RA: Familial radioulnar synostosis. J Med Genet 1978; 15:160–162.
Cleary JE, Omer GE: Congenital proximal radio-ulnar synostosis: natural history and functional assessment. J Bone Joint Surg 1985; 67A:539–545.

C0066 **J. Michael Connor**

**Radiation embryopathy**
*See FETAL RADIATION SYNDROME*
**Radiation teratogenesis**
*See FETAL RADIATION SYNDROME*
**Radiation, fetal effects of**
*See FETAL RADIATION SYNDROME*
**Radicular dentin dysplasia**
*See TEETH, DENTIN DYSPLASIA, RADICULAR*
**Radius absent-thrombocytopenia**
*See THROMBOCYTOPENIA-ABSENT RADIUS*
**Radius, congenital absence of the**
*See HAND, RADIAL CLUB HAND*
**Radius, deficiency of**
*See HAND, RADIAL CLUB HAND*
**Radix in radice**
*See TEETH, DENS INVAGINATUS*
**Radon gas, fetal effects of**
*See FETAL RADIATION SYNDROME*

---

**RAG SYNDROME** 2578

**Includes:**
Aniridia-Robin sequence-growth delay
Robin sequence-aniridia-growth delay (RAG)

**Excludes:**
**Chromosome 11, partial monosomy 11p** (2245)
**Chromosome 13, monosomy 13q** (0167)
**Progeria** (0825)

**Major Diagnostic Criteria:** Robin sequence with micrognathia and U-shaped cleft palate, absence of the iris bilaterally, and severe growth retardation. Characteristic elfin-like features. The hands are small, with long, pointed fingers and abnormal palmar creases.

**Clinical Findings:** Severe prenatal developmental and growth delay, with reduced amniotic fluid volume and no obvious prenatal fetal movements. The infant has a birth weight of below 1,000 g, but is otherwise strong and healthy. Clinically, characteristic elfin-like facies with aniridia and the Robin anomaly with cleft palate are evident at birth. Weight gain is very slow (less than eight pounds at age two years), and length is short; both parameters being well below the normal percentiles. Chromosomes have been normal. Endocrine findings are normal with normal growth hormone levels.

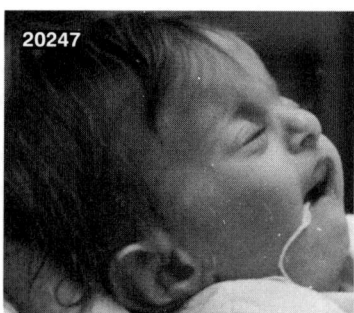
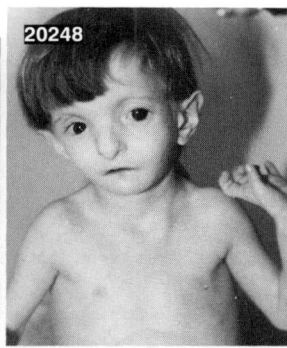
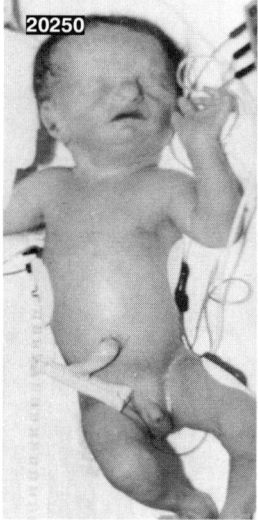
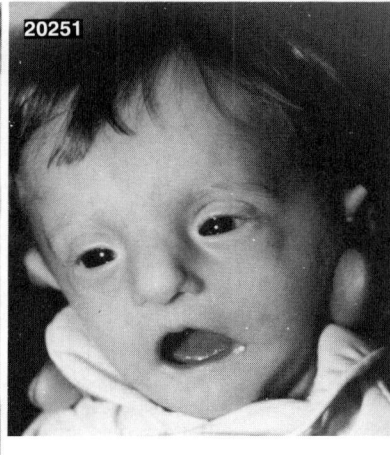

**2578-20247:** Lateral view of proposita with RAG syndrome at age 2 months; note micrognathia. **20248:** Proposita at age 3 years; note unusual triangular facies. **20250:** Younger brother of the proposita at birth. **20251:** Proposita's brother at age 1 year; note the facies are similar to his sister's.

---

Development is very delayed. By age four years, there is no speech; motor skills included standing with support. Only two teeth had erupted in the reported case, although all the dentition appeared to be present. The head circumference was well below normal. Cranial bones were infantile with domes in the center and open sutures. The child was reportedly irritable.

**Complications:** Unknown.

**Associated Findings:** None known.

**Etiology:** Possibly autosomal recessive inheritance.

**Pathogenesis:** Unknown.

**Sex Ratio:** M1:F1

**Occurrence:** One family with two sibs has been described.

**Risk of Recurrence for Patient's Sib:**
See Part I, *Mendelian Inheritance.*

**Risk of Recurrence for Patient's Child:**
See Part I, *Mendelian Inheritance.*

**Age of Detectability:** At birth, or prenatally by ultrasound detection of severe intrauterine growth retardation early in the second trimester.

**Gene Mapping and Linkage:** Unknown.

**Prevention:** None known. Genetic counseling indicated.

**Treatment:** Unknown.

**Prognosis:** Unknown.

**Detection of Carrier:** Unknown.

**References:**

Saal HM, et al.: The RAG syndrome: a new autosomal recessive syndrome with the Robin sequence, aniridia and profound growth retardation and developmental delays. Am J Hum Genet (suppl) 1986; 39:78A.

P0007                                          **Andrew E. Poole**
SA001                                          **Howard M. Saal**

**Ragged red fibers-myoclonic epilepsy**
*See MYOCLONIC EPILEPSY-RAGGED RED FIBERS*
**Ragin' Cajun**
*See JUMPING FRENCHMAN OF MAINE*

---

## RAGWEED POLLEN SENSITIVITY                    3082

**Includes:**

Asthma, ragweed pollen-induced
Hayfever
HLA-A histocompatibility type
Ragweed sensitivity, asymptomatic
Rhinitis, ragweed pollen-induced

**Excludes:**

**Skin, atopy, familial** (3150)
Ragweed oleoresin contact dermatitis

**Major Diagnostic Criteria:** Demonstrable presence of IgE antibody to ragweed pollen components, based on environmental exposure, constitutes ragweed pollen sensitivity. This condition may remain asymptomatic despite annual dispersion of the sensitizer(s) or may manifest as allergic rhinitis or reactive airways disease. Wheal and flare reactions in skin, peaking 15 minutes after intradermal testing with ragweed pollen extracts, indicate allergen-specific, tissue-fixed IgE. Additional, *in vitro* studies, (viz., RAST, ELISA, and other solid-phase immunosorbent tests, as well as leukocyte histamine release) allow assay of specific IgE in serum and tissue fluids. Aerosol challenge, with pollen extracts, of the upper and lower airways can confirm the potential for specific reactivity using patency or secretion-based response parameters. However, a certain clinical diagnosis rests on confirmation of characteristic respiratory symptoms during natural exposure periods.

**Clinical Findings:** Like other atopic individuals (i.e., those prone to synthesize significant IgE following mucosal allergen contact), ragweed-sensitive persons commonly display multiple IgE-based sensitivities, and at least 50% have at least one atopic first-degree relative. Histories of childhood atopic dermatitis with or without gastrointestinal allergy are abnormally frequent. Allergic rhinitis presents as variable nasal obstruction; repetitive sneezing; thin, copious rhinorrhea; and pruritus of eyes, nose, and pharynx. Lacrimation, periorbital swelling, and conjunctival injection often coexist. Symptoms tend to peak shortly after arising, but persist diurnally, often disturbing sleep and contributing to a more or less prominent lassitude. The nasal mucosa commonly reflects prominent edema and venostasis, appearing pale and bluish-gray, and stained mucus often reveals numerous eosinophils. Heightened nasal reactivity is characteristically evident, obstruction and other symptoms readily following chilling, recumbency, and exposure to volatile and particulate irritants. A minority of sensitive persons manifest asthma (bouts of potentially reversible bronchial obstruction and general airway lability) in response to ragweed allergens. In most, sensitivity to additional factors with or without resulting factors, with or without resulting respiratory allergy, is demonstrable. Where ragweed pollen is annually prevalent, symptoms most commonly appear after three to five seasons of exposure. As a result, an onset of pollinosis in childhood is frequent. Spontaneous attenuation of symptoms may occur with advancing age in endemic areas or may continue lifelong.

**Complications:** Because isolated ragweed pollinois lasts, at most, 2–3 months annually, infectious and structural complications are less than in those with perennial symptoms due to diverse sensitivities. However, purulent rhinitis, bronchitis, and sinusitis often complicate pollinosis. In children especially, purulent otitis media or, less commonly, serous otitis reflect accompanying eustachian tube dysfunction. Bouts of intractable, irresistible, repetitive sneezing can pose hazards for operation of vehicles and other machinery requiring constant hand-eye coordination. As in responses to other allergens, ragweed pollinosis confers upper and lower airway hyperreactivity to additional allergens and irritant factors.

**Associated Findings:** A significant minority of ragweed-sensitive persons have experienced skin or gastrointestinal allergy. Most have additional sensitivities with or without resulting respiratory conditions.

**Etiology:** Possibly autosomal dominant inheritance of differential sensitivity. A series of smaller proteins and polypeptides are the sensitizing agents. Of these, antigens E (MW ca. 38,700) constitute 6% of the pollen protein of short (dwarf) ragweed and appears to be its single most important allergen. IgE-reactive materials are eluted at mucous surfaces from intact grains. Additional small micronic and submicronic aerosols carrying pollen allergens occur in nature and may augment exposure.

Genetic associations of several immune response determinants of ragweed pollinosis have been examined. Associations between HLA haplotypes and IgE-mediated skin reactivity to Amb a I (antigen E) of short ragweed in multiple generations of selected kindreds have been reported (Blumenthal and Amos, 1987). However, others (Bias & Marsh, 1975, Marsh et al, 1987) have questioned these conclusions which center on a relatively complex (M.W. 37,800) protein antigen having multiple epitopes. Polygenic factors, or failure of certain family members to express reactivity when studied, has been postulated. More recently, responses to a smaller ragweed pollen component, Amb a V (antigen Ra5); a single chain polypeptide with M.W. *ca* 5,000; have been found strongly associated with Dw 2 and DR2 typing by Marsh et al (1987). Both IgE and IgG reactivity have showed this correlation. Similarly, in persons responding with IgE and IgG to Amb t V of giant ragweed pollen, associations with Dw2 have been described. Most recently Marsh et al (1987) have shown a concordance of response of Amb a VI, (an 11,500 dalton ragweed pollen allergen) and HLA-DR5+ status.

Total IgE level, while not regarded as HLA-assocaited, is a trait for which genetic control is strongly suggested, and high responders appear more prone to pollinosis. The heritability of high and low IgE status has been well supported by twin studies (especially in childhood) by Bazaral et al (1974). In addition, families studied by Gerrard et al (1978) have confirmed the genetic control of IgE, suggesting that high response acts as a recessive trait, although polygenic control seems to be exerted.

**Pathogenesis:** Pollenosis essentially reflects tissue effects of mast cell and basophil secretion following bridging, by allergen, of specific IgE molecules on cell surface receptors. Laboratory-based allergen challenges have confirmed the appearance of proinflammatory mediators, including histamine, prostaglandin $D_2$, sulfidopeptide leukotrienes, and various esterases in nasal washings. Similar events appear to follow bronchial provocation with allergen. Heightened vascular permeability results with tissue edema and hypersecretion by organized glands and goblet cells. In subglottic airways, an intense spasm of mural smooth muscle is associated. Both permeability factors and agents chemotactic for eosinophils and neutrophils follow allergen challenge with immediate (0–90-minute) and late (3–6-hour) appearance peaks. In lower airways, late reactions with neutrophil influx appear to foster bronchial hyperresponsiveness. Nasal hyperreactivity may reflect demonstrated factors including increased mucosal permeability, influxes of mast cells and basophils, and changes in the density of receptors for autonomic neurotransmitters. Additional determinants of symptom severity, including circadian, reflex, and endocrine influences, are suspected.

**MIM No.:** *14280, 17945

**Sex Ratio:** Presumably M1:F1, although an earlier childhood onset in males has been suggested.

**Occurrence:** Rates of sensitization approach or exceed 25% in endemic areas. Symptomatic pollenosis affecting up to 25% of exposed young adults has been observed. Familial clustering of respiratory allergy (including ragweed pollinosis) is prominent, at least 50% of affected persons having one or more first degree relatives with IgE-mediated conditions. However, no simple pattern of inheritance is discernible. Family studies have suggested genetic control(s) of high (vs. normally low) total serum IgE levels. Reported linkage disequilibrium between IgE responsiveness to specific ragweed pollen allergens (E, Ra3, Ra5) and one or more HLA haplotypes also implies a role for immune response genes. In addition, independent transmission of bronchial hyperresponsiveness, a trait promoting asthma, is strongly suggested.

**Risk of Recurrence for Patient's Sib:**
See Part I, *Mendelian Inheritance.*

**Risk of Recurrence for Patient's Child:**
See Part I, *Mendelian Inheritance.*

**Age of Detectability:** Usually during pre-school years in suitably exposed individuals, but may appear later.

**Gene Mapping and Linkage:** HLA-A (major histocompatibility complex, class I) has been mapped to 6p21.3.

**Prevention:** None known. Genetic counseling indicated. While seldom feasible, (geographic) removal of patients from seasonal exposure effectively terminates clinical pollinosis, although asymptomatic sensitivity remains. Patients with severe ragweed-induced rhinitis may have their risk of subsequent asthma diminished by specific (injection) immunotherapy.

**Treatment:** Symptom amelioration by agents that block the release and tissue effects of mast cell-derived mediators has been increasingly successful. H1 antihistamines and topical cromolyn sodium or corticosteroids are mainstays for relief of rhinitis. Asthma often is benefitted by inhaled cromolyn and corticosteroids, as well as by aerosolized and oral bronchodilators; systemic steroids may be required. Immunotherapy with ragweed pollen extracts has proven valuable in hayfever and remains to be critically evaluated in asthma.

**Prognosis:** The proportion of ragweed pollen-sensitive persons who will develop specific symptoms is undefined, but appears large. Determinants of the clinical illness in this risk group remain controversial. However, once pollinosis is established, it tends to recur annually with seasonal exposure. Rhinitis severity seems to augment the small increased risk of de novo asthma in those (initially) with ragweed hayfever alone. A fraction of sensitive persons manifest only asthma over extended periods in response to ragweed pollen.

**Detection of Carrier:** Unknown.

**Special Considerations:** Patients with pollen sensitivity have little, if any, increased risk of adverse reactivity to drugs, radiocontrast media, and hymenoptera (insect) stings when compared with comparable exposed, nonsensitive subjects.

**References:**

Bazaral M, et al.: Genetics of IgE and allergy: serum IgE levels in twins. J Allergy Clin Immunol 1974; 54:288–304.

Blumenthal MN, et al.: Genetic mapping of Ir locus in man: linkage to second locus of HL-A. Science 1974; 184:1301–1303.

Bias WB, Marsh DG: HLA linked antigen E immune response genes: an unproved hypothesis. Science 1975; 188:375–377.

Gerrard JW, et al.: A genetic study of immunoglobulin E. Am J Hum Genet 1978; 30:46–58.

Marsh DG, et al.: HLA-Dw2: a genetic marker for human immune response to short ragweed pollen allergen Ra5. I. Response resulting primarily from natural antigenic exposure. J Exper Med 1982; 155:1439–1451.

Mygind N, Weeke B: Allergic and non-allergic rhinitis. In: Middleton E Jr., et al., eds: Allergy: principles and practice, ed 2. St. Louis: C.V. Mosby, 1983:1101–1117.

Roebber M, et al.: Immunochemical and genetic studies of Amb .t. v (Ra5G), an Ra5G homologue from giant ragweed pollen. J Immunol 1985; 134:3062–3069.

Blumenthal MN, Amos DB: Genetic and immunologic basis of atopic responses. Chest 1987; 91S:176S.

Marsh DG, et al.: Immune responsiveness to Ambrosia artemisiifolia (short ragweed) pollen allergen Amb a VI (Ra6) is associated with HLA-DR5 in allergic humans. Immunogenetics 1987; 26:230–236.

Meyers DA, et al.: Inheritance of total serum IgE (basal levels) in man. Am J Hum Genet 1987; 41:51–62.

S0015                                                   **William R. Solomon**

**Ragweed sensitivity, asymptomatic**
  *See RAGWEED POLLEN SENSITIVITY*
**Ramon syndrome**
  *See GINGIVAL FIBROMATOSIS-CHERUBISM-SEIZURES, RAMON TYPE*
**Ramon syndrome-juvenile rheumatoid arthritis**
  *See GINGIVAL FIBROMATOSIS-CHERUBISM-SEIZURES, RAMON TYPE*
**Ramsay-Hunt syndrome (some cases)**
  *See SEIZURES, PROGRESSIVE MYOCLONIC, UNVERRICHT-LUNDBORG TYPE*
**Ranula congenita**
  *See CYSTIC HYGROMA*
**Raphe, supraumbilical midline-cavernous facial hemangiomas**
  *See HEMANGIOMAS OF THE HEAD AND NECK*
**Rapid gastric emptying-duodenal ulcer**
  *See PEPTIC ULCER DISEASES, NON-SYNDROMIC*
**Rapid isoniazid (INH) inactivation**
  *See ACETYLATOR POLYMORPHISM*
**Rapp-Hodgkin ectodermal dysplasia**
  *See ECTODERMAL DYSPLASIA, RAPP-HODGKIN TYPE*
**Rautenstrauch-Wiedemann syndrome**
  *See PROGERIA, NEONATAL RAUTENSTRAUCH-WIEDEMANN TYPE*

---

## RAYNAUD DISEASE                                        2115

**Includes:**
  Fingers, cold, hereditary
  Primary Raynaud phenomenon
  Raynaud phenomenon

**Excludes:**
  Raynaud phenomenon, secondary
  **Scleroderma, familial progressive** (2154)

**Major Diagnostic Criteria:** Bilateral clinical findings in absence of demonstrable cause of secondary Raynaud phenomenon; duration of symptoms for at least two years.

**Clinical Findings:** Changes in skin color (pallor) and temperature (coolness) mainly involving the hands and feet; excited by cold temperatures and emotional stress.

**Complications:** Raynaud disease, unlike secondary Raynaud phenomenon, is not accompanied by extensive gangrene. Major amputations are never necessary.

**Associated Findings:** Numbness, livido reticulares; rarely, acrocyanosis

**Etiology:** Autosomal dominant and multifactorial inheritance.

**Pathogenesis:** Arteriospasm of unkown cause. Affected individuals have decreased capillary blood flow as compared to unaffected persons.

**MIM No.:** *17960

**Sex Ratio:** M1:F1 in the autosomal dominant form. M1:F>1 in the idiopathic, presumably multifactoria1 form.

**Occurrence:** Undetermined. Lewis and Pickering (1933) reported 23 cases in two working-class British families.

**Risk of Recurrence for Patient's Sib:**
See Part I, *Mendelian Inheritance.*

**Risk of Recurrence for Patient's Child:**
See Part I, *Mendelian Inheritance.*

**Age of Detectability:** Late childhood or early adulthood.

**Gene Mapping and Linkage:** Unknown.

**Prevention:** None known. Genetic counseling indicated.

**Treatment:** Avoidance of cold temperatures and emotional stress. Nifedipine and ketanserin have been used with success.

**Prognosis:** Good.

**Detection of Carrier:** Unknown.

**Special Considerations:** As the nature of this condition has become clearer, there is an emerging consensus that the name should be changed to *Raynaud phenomenon*.

**Support Groups:** Dallas; American Heart Association

**References:**

Allen EV, Brown GE: Raynaud's disease a critical review of minimal requisites for diagnosis. Am J Med Sci 1932; 183:187–200. *

Lewis T, Pickering GW: Observations upon maladies in which the blood supply to digits ceases intermittently or permanently, and upon bilateral gangrene of digits, observations relevant to so-called "Raynauds disease". Clin Sci 1933; 1:327–366. *

Gifford RW Jr, Hines EA Jr: Raynaud's disease among women and girls. Circulation 1957; 16:1012.

White CJ, et al.: Objective benefit of nifedipine in the treatment of Raynauds phenomenon. Am J Med 1986; 80:623–625.

Coffman JD, et al.: International study of ketanserin in Raynaud's phenomenon. Am J Med 1989; 87:264–268.

N0004
N0003

**Audery H. Nora**
**James J. Nora**

**Raynaud phenomenon**
*See RAYNAUD DISEASE*
**Reactive arthritis**
*See ANKYLOSING SPONDYLITIS*
**Reading disorder, developmental**
*See DYSLEXIA*
**Reading disorder, specific**
*See DYSLEXIA*
**Reading epilepsy**
*See EPILEPSY, REFLEX*
**REAR syndrome**
*See ANUS-HAND-EAR SYNDROME*
**Recessive dystrophic epidermolysis bullosa (RDEB)**
*See EPIDERMOLYSIS BULLOSUM, TYPE III*
**Recessive optic atrophy-hearing loss-juvenile diabetes**
*See DIABETES (INSIPIDUS/MELLITUS)-OPTIC ATROPHY-DEAFNESS*
**Rectal aganglionosis**
*See COLON, AGANGLIONOSIS*
**Rectal atresia or stenosis**
*See COLON, ATRESIA OR STENOSIS*
**Rectal duplication**
*See COLON, DUPLICATION*
**Rectoperineal fistula**
*See ANORECTAL MALFORMATIONS*
**Rectus muscle, congenital fibrosis of the inferior**
*See EYE, FIBROSIS OF THE EXTRAOCULAR MUSCLES, GENERALIZED*
**Recurrent erosive corneal dystrophy**
*See CORNEAL DYSTROPHY, RECURRENT EROSIVE*
**Recurrent intrahepatic cholestasis of pregnancy (RICP)**
*See INTRAHEPATIC CHOLESTASIS OF PREGNANCY (ICP)*
**Recurrent respiratory papillomatosis**
*See PAPILLOMA VIRUS, CONGENITAL INFECTION*
**Red cell aregenerative anemia, congenital**
*See ANEMIA, HYPOPLASTIC CONGENITAL*
**Red cell membrane defects**
*See ANEMIA, HEMOLYTIC, RED CELL MEMBRANE DEFECTS*
**Red cell membrane phosphatidylcholine hemolytic anemia**
*See ANEMIA, HEMOLYTIC, ERYTHROCYTE PHOSPHOLIPID DEFECT*
**Red cell permeability defect**
*See ANEMIA, HEMOLYTIC, RED CELL MEMBRANE DEFECTS*
**Red cell phospholipid defect-hemolysis**
*See ANEMIA, HEMOLYTIC, RED CELL MEMBRANE DEFECTS*
**Red palms**
*See SKIN, PALMO-PLANTAR ERYTHEMA*
**Red-fleck retina**
*See RETINA, FLECKED KANDORI TYPE*
**Red-green deutan series color blindness**
*See COLOR BLINDNESS, RED-GREEN DEUTAN SERIES*
**Red-green protan series color blindness**
*See COLOR BLINDNESS, RED-GREEN PROTAN SERIES*
**Reducing body myopathy**
*See MYOPATHY, REDUCING BODY*
**Reduction defects of limb**
*See LIMB REDUCTION DEFECTS*

**Refetoff syndrome**
*See THYROID, HORMONE RESISTANCE*
**Reflux, esophageal**
*See ESOPHAGUS, CHALASIA*
**Refsum disease**
*See PHYTANIC ACID STORAGE DISEASE*
**Refsum disease (some neonatal or infantile forms)**
*See CEREBRO-HEPATO-RENAL SYNDROME*
**Refsum disease, infantile form**
*See PHYTANIC ACID OXIDASE DEFICIENCY, INFANTILE TYPE*
**Regional enteritis/ileitis**
*See INFLAMMATORY BOWEL DISEASE*
**Regional odontodysplasia**
*See TEETH, ODONTODYSPLASIA*
**Reifenstein syndrome**
*See ANDROGEN INSENSITIVITY SYNDROME, INCOMPLETE*
**Reiger anomaly-growth retardation**
*See SHORT SYNDROME*
**Reinclusion of permanent molars, familial**
*See TEETH, MOLAR REINCLUSION*
**Reinhardt-Pfeiffer mesomelic dysostosis**
*See MESOMELIC DYSPLASIA, REINHARDT-PFEIFFER TYPE*
**Reis-Bucklers corneal dystrophy**
*See CORNEAL DYSTROPHY, REIS-BUCKLERS TYPE*
**Reiter syndrome**
*See ANKYLOSING SPONDYLITIS*
**Renal (hyper)uricosuria, isolated**
*See RENAL HYPOURICEMIA*
**Renal 25-hydroxyvitamin D1-hydroxylase deficiency**
*See RICKETS, VITAMIN D-DEPENDENT, TYPE I*
**Renal adysplasia**
*See RENAL AGENESIS, BILATERAL*

---

**RENAL AGENESIS, BILATERAL**                    **0856**

**Includes:**
   Kidneys, absence of
   Kidneys, congenital bilateral absence of
   Potter syndrome
   Renal adysplasia
   Urogenital adysplasia

**Excludes:**
   Potter syndrome associated with infantile polycystic kidney
   Potter syndrome associated with renal dysplasia

**Major Diagnostic Criteria:** Lack of kidneys.

**Clinical Findings:** At birth, infants may show the following features: Potter facies (an appearance of redundant and dehydrated skin, wide-set eyes, prominent fold arising at inner canthus of each eye, "parrot-beak" nose, receding chin, facial expression of an older infant); large, low-set ears with deficient auricular cartilages; no urine output; no kidneys palpable. About 40% of these infants are stillborn, and the majority of those born alive die within four hours. Rarely an infant may survive more than two days, since the condition is incompatible with life.

**Complications:** Death shortly after birth is attributed to asphyxia secondary to pulmonary hypoplasia due to compression of chest from lack of amniotic fluid. Renal failure is usually the other cause of death.

**Associated Findings:** History of oligohydramnios or total absence of amniotic fluid or amnion nodosum. Often premature onset of labor, breech delivery, and birth weight disproportionately low. The patient may have multiple malformations including bilateral pulmonary hypoplasia; genital organ abnormalities such as absence of vas deferens and seminal vesicles or absence of uterus and upper vagina; GI malformations such as anal atresia, absent sigmoid and rectum, and esophageal and duodenal atresia; single umbilical artery; major deformities of lower part of body (sirenomelia) or lower limbs such as clubfoot.

**Etiology:** Bilateral renal agenesis may represent the severe expression of autosomal dominant inheritance of a gene that in its milder expression causes unilateral renal agenesis, double ureter, renal cyst, or hydronephrosis (Roodhooft et al, 1984).

**Pathogenesis:** Unknown.

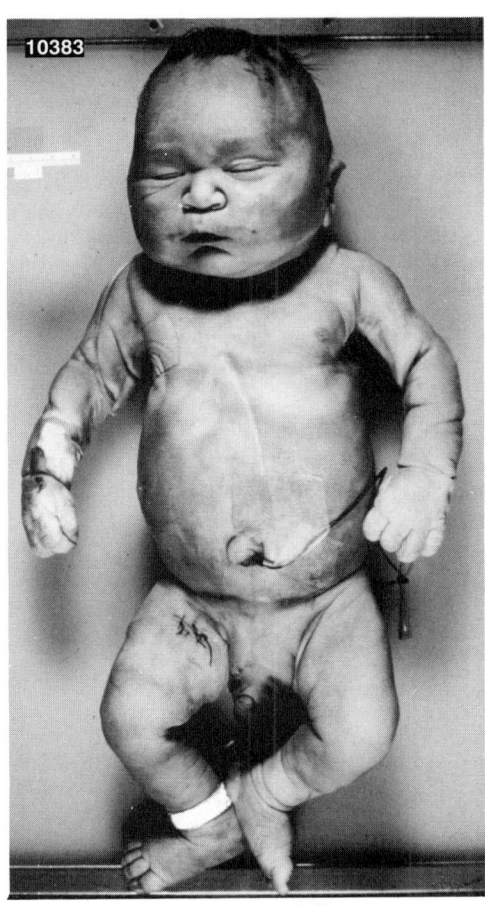

**0856**-10383:   Potter facies, redundant skin and pulmonary hypoplasia secondary to oligohydramnios from bilateral renal agenesis.

**MIM No.:**   *19183
**POS No.:**   3368
**CDC No.:**   753.000
**Sex Ratio:**   M2.5:F1

**Occurrence:**   Estimated at 12:100,000 total births (Carter et al, 1979).

**Risk of Recurrence for Patient's Sib:**
See Part I, *Mendelian Inheritance*. The proportion of sibs affected with bilateral renal agenesis was 6:199 (3.0%) in one study in England (Carter et al, 1979).

**Risk of Recurrence for Patient's Child:**
See Part I, *Mendelian Inheritance*. Affected individuals are not expected to survive to reproduce.

**Age of Detectability:**   Prenatal exam by ultrasound can detect some cases; all others are evident in the neonate.

**Gene Mapping and Linkage:**   Unknown.

**Prevention:**   None known. Genetic counseling indicated.

**Treatment:**   Unknown. Dialysis/renal transplantation is usually not considered because of the pulmonary hypoplasia.

**Prognosis:**   Inevitably fatal.

**Detection of Carrier:**   Unknown.

**Special Considerations:**   Parents and unaffected children have increased risk of having silent genitourinary malformations; especially unilateral renal agenesis (Roodhooft et al, 1984). Parents and

sibs should be screened by ultrasound for asymptomatic malformations.

**Support Groups:**   New York; National Kidney Foundation

**References:**
Potter EL: Bilateral absence of ureters and kidneys: a report of 50 cases. Obstet Gynecol 1965; 25:3–12.
Cain DR, et al.: Familial renal agenesis and total dysplasia. Am J Dis Child 1974; 128:377–380.
Carter CO, et al.: A family study of renal agenesis. J Med Genetics 1979; 16:176–188.
Roodhooft AM, et al.: Familial nature of congenital absence and severe dysgenesis of both kidneys. New Engl J Med 1984; 310:1341–1345. *
Bankier A, et al.: A pedigree study of perinatal lethal renal disease. J Med Genet 1985; 22:104–111.
McPherson E, et al.: Dominantly inherited renal adysplasia. Am J Med Genet 1987; 26:863–872.
Morse RP et al.: Bilateral renal agenesis in three consecutive siblings. Prenatal Diag 1987; 7:573–579.

M0035                                                    **Donald I. Moel**

---

## RENAL AGENESIS, UNILATERAL                               **0857**

**Includes:**
Kidney, congenital solitary
Renal aplasia, unilateral

**Excludes:**
**Renal agenesis, bilateral** (0856)
Renal atrophy, unilateral
Renal dysgenesis, unilateral
Renal hypoplasia, unilateral

**Major Diagnostic Criteria:**   Unilateral renal agenesis is discovered incidentally on X-ray or other examination.

**Clinical Findings:**   The affected infant usually appears normal at birth. Most frequently clinical recognition of unilateral renal agenesis results from an incidental examination during an illness.

Absence of one renal outline, most commonly on the left side; enlarged renal shadow on the opposite side; asymmetry of the outlines of the psoas muscles; renal pelvis of moderate size that does not parallel the degree of parenchymal hypertrophy; ectopy or malrotation of the single kidney in 5–10% of cases. Cystoscopy reveals absence of a ureteral orifice on one side and often absence or deformity of the corresponding half of the interureteral ridge of the trigone. Ultrasonography shows the presence of only one kidney.

**Complications:**   Unless the solitary kidney becomes infected, obstructed, or exposed to toxins, the condition is not clinically significant. Sterility has been noted.

**Associated Findings:**   Usually the ipsilateral ureter is absent or poorly developed; the adrenal gland on the side of anomaly may be absent. Absence or agenesis of the vagina (Mayer-Rokitansky syndrome) is associated with a high rate of urologic abnormalities including renal agenesis, ectopia, fusion anomalies, horseshoe kidneys, duplication anomalies, and ureteroceles. In the male, there may be ipsilateral absence of the testis, vas deferens and/or the seminal vesicles.

A defect in mesodermal development at the primitive streak level is called by the acronym VATER (see **VATER association**). Renal anomalies are also observed in 50% of patients and include renal agenesis, dysplasia or hypoplasia).

**Etiology:**   Possibly autosomal dominant inheritance with variable expressivity and penetrance. In some families, unilateral renal agenesis may be considered a mild expression of a more severe abnormality (i.e. bilateral renal agenesis or dysgenesis).

**Pathogenesis:**   Unknown.

**MIM No.:**   *19183

**CDC No.:**   753.010

**Sex Ratio:**   Presumably M1:F1. Autopsy studies indicate solitary kidney to be more common among males; however, clinical studies indicate it to be more common among females. This apparent difference in sex incidence is attributable to fact that associated complications and other anomalies are more frequently recognized in females.

**Occurrence:** About 1:1,000 infants.

**Risk of Recurrence for Patient's Sib:**
See Part I, *Mendelian Inheritance.*

**Risk of Recurrence for Patient's Child:**
See Part I, *Mendelian Inheritance.*

**Age of Detectability:** During investigation of kidney disease, or as a chance finding.

**Gene Mapping and Linkage:** Unknown.

**Prevention:** None known. Genetic counseling indicated.

**Treatment:** Treatment of infection and/or obstruction in the remaining kidney to preserve renal function. If severely diseased, renal transplantation.

**Prognosis:** Generally good, but depends on remaining kidney function and other associated anomalies.

**Detection of Carrier:** Unknown.

**Support Groups:** New York; National Kidney Foundation

**References:**
Thompson DP, Lynn HB: Genital anomalies associated with solitary kidney. Mayo Clin Proc 1966; 41:538–548.
Emanuel B, et al.: Congenital solitary kidney: a review of 74 cases. Am J Dis Child 1974; 127:17–19.
Carter CO, et al.: A family study of renal agenesis. J Med Genet 1979; 16:176–188.
Uehling DT, et al.: Urologic implications of the VATER association. J Urol 1983; 129:352–354.
Roodhooft AM, et al.: Familial nature of congenital absence and severe dysgenesis of both kidneys. New Engl J Med 1984; 310:1341–1345. *

M0035                                                    **Donald I Moel**

**Renal and X-ray anomalies-midface retraction-hypertrichosis**
*See SCHINZEL-GIEDION SYNDROME*
**Renal aplasia, unilateral**
*See RENAL AGENESIS, UNILATERAL*
**Renal artery stenosis, congenital**
*See ARTERY, RENAL FIBROMUSCULAR DYSPLASIA*

---

## RENAL BICARBONATE REABSORPTIVE DEFECT          0858

**Includes:**
    Bicarbonate-wasting renal tubular acidosis
    Renal tubular acidosis, proximal
    Renal tubular acidosis, rate type
    Renal tubular acidosis, type II
**Excludes:**
    **Renal tubular acidosis** (0862)
    Renal tubular acidosis, type IV
    **Renal tubular syndrome, Fanconi type** (0864)

**Major Diagnostic Criteria:** Hyperchloremic acidosis with reduced renal threshold for bicarbonate-producing bicarbonaturia in the range of 15–25% of the filtered load. Before acidosis is treated, urine pH is less than 6.0. Evidence of a more generalized dysfunction of the proximal tubule (renal Fanconi syndrome) such as amino aciduria, glucosuria, and phosphaturia are absent.

**Clinical Findings:** A small number of children have been reported who exhibit an isolated defect in proximal tubular bicarbonate reabsorption in infancy associated with hyperchloremic metabolic acidosis and failure to thrive. Most cases have been males without a family history of the problem. It is notable that nephrocalcinosis, hypokalemia, hypocitraturia, and metabolic bone disease are absent. These patients have done well on high-dose bicarbonate therapy (15–25 mEq/kg/day), with resolution of acidosis and growth failure.

**Complications:** Failure to thrive, episodes of fever and dehydration.

**Associated Findings:** None reported except in one Norwegian family in which mental retardation, developmental delay, corneal opacities, glaucoma, and hypothyroidism were found in two brothers with pure proximal renal tubular acidosis. It is likely that this family represents a form of the disease different from the sporadic cases.

**Etiology:** Possibly X-linked inheritance. Many cases are sporadic.

**Pathogenesis:** Defective reabsorption of bicarbonate in the proximal tubule leads to bicarbonate loss, sodium wasting, volume contraction, and acidosis.
    There is controversy as to whether proximal tubular carbonic anhydrase activity is normal. Some have speculated that a defect in proximal hydrogen ion secretion or pyruvate carboxylase activity might produce the syndrome. More than one type is likely.

**MIM No.:** 31240

**Sex Ratio:** M1:F0. Nearly all cases have been males.

**Occurrence:** Undetermined but presumed rare.

**Risk of Recurrence for Patient's Sib:**
See Part I, *Mendelian Inheritance.*

**Risk of Recurrence for Patient's Child:**
See Part I, *Mendelian Inheritance.*

**Age of Detectability:** In infancy.

**Gene Mapping and Linkage:** Unknown.

**Prevention:** None known. Genetic counseling indicated.

**Treatment:** Administration of large amounts of sodium bicarbonate (15–25 mEq/kg/day) in divided doses is required to correct acidosis. Polyuria persists.

**Prognosis:** Good with treatment. In most of the sporadic cases, the requirement for bicarbonate therapy has slowly resolved.

**Detection of Carrier:** Unknown.

**Support Groups:** New York; National Kidney Foundation

**References:**
Soriano JR, et al.: Proximal renal tubular acidosis: a defect in bicarbonate reabsorption with normal urinary acidification. Pediatr Res 1967; 1:81–98.
Donckerwolcke RA, et al.: A case of bicarbonate-losing renal tubular acidosis and defective carbonic anhydrase activity. Arch Dis Child 1970; 45:769–773.
Brenes LG, et al.: Familial proximal renal tubular acidosis: a distinct clinical entity. Am J Med 1977; 63:244–252.
Winsnes A, et al.: Congenital, persistent proximal type renal tubular acidosis in two brothers. Acta Paediatr Scand 1979; 68:861–868.
DuBose TD, Jr., Alpern RF: Renal tubular acidosis. In: Scriver CR, et al, eds: The metabolic basis of inherited disease, 6th ed. New York: McGraw-Hill, 1989:2539–2568.

G0052                                                    **Paul Goodyer**

**Renal blastema, nodular or persistent**
*See CANCER, WILMS TUMOR*
**Renal calculi-ulcer-leukonychia**
*See ULCER-LEUKONYCHIA-GALLSTONES*
**Renal cell carcinoma**
*See CANCER, RENAL CELL CARCINOMA*
**Renal disease, polycystic adult type**
*See KIDNEY, POLYCYSTIC DISEASE, DOMINANT*
**Renal disease-deafness-ichthyosis**
*See DEAFNESS-HYPERPROLINURIA-ICHTHYOSIS*
**Renal duplication-hearing loss-external ear anomalies**
*See BRANCHIO-OTO-URETERAL SYNDROME*
**Renal dysplasia, Elejalde type**
*See ACROCEPHALOPOLYDACTYLOUS DYSPLASIA*
**Renal dysplasia-blindness, hereditary**
*See RENAL DYSPLASIA-RETINAL APLASIA, LOKEN-SENIOR TYPE*
**Renal dysplasia-primitive renal tubules**
*See RENAL TUBULAR DYSGENESIS*

## RENAL DYSPLASIA-RETINAL APLASIA, LOKEN-SENIOR TYPE     2687

**Includes:**
> Loken-Senior syndrome
> Nephronophtisis-associated ocular anomalies, familial juvenile
> Renal-retinal dystrophy, familial
> Renal-retinal syndrome
> Renal dysplasia-blindness, hereditary
> Senior-Loken syndrome

**Excludes:**
> **Kidney, nephronophthisis-medullary cystic desease** (3018)
> **Kidney, polycystic disease-cataract-blindness** (3288)
> **Retina, amaurosis congenita, Leber type** (0043)
> **Retinitis pigmentosa** (0869)
> Saldino-Mainzer syndrome

**Major Diagnostic Criteria:** Nephronophthisis (with or without medullary cystic renal disease) and a progressive pigmentary retinal dystrophy, with onset typically in the first year of life.

**Clinical Findings:** In some cases, the progressive pigmentary retinal dystrophy is like those of **Retina, amaurosis congenita, Leber type** and children present with visual impairment in the first year of life. In other cases, the tapetoretinal dystrophy resembles **Retinitis pigmentosa** and develops later. Renal involvement is always insidious in onset. There is a progressive renal insufficiency secondary to abiotrophy of the distal part of the renal tubules, which results in a chronic interstitial nephritis and uremia.

**Complications:** Severely impaired visual acuity secondary to retinal dystrophy and renal failure.

**Associated Findings:** None known.

**Etiology:** Autosomal recessive inheritance. Concordance is observed in monozygotic twins. Consanguinity of the parents is frequent. It has been reported that, in one affected sibship, one child may show only the tapetoretinal dystrophy and another only the nephronophthisis; thus the disease is either due to a gene with pleiotrophic effects and variable expressivity or two closely linked genes, one acting on the renal tubule and the other on the retina.

**Pathogenesis:** May be due to a genetic enzymatic disorder which involves vitamin A metabolism in the retina and changes the metabolism of the retinal tubules. There has been one report of an associated lipidosis.

**MIM No.:** *26690

**POS No.:** 3455

**Sex Ratio:** M1:F1

**Occurrence:** About 150 cases have been documented in the literature.

**Risk of Recurrence for Patient's Sib:**
> See Part I, *Mendelian Inheritance.*

**Risk of Recurrence for Patient's Child:**
> See Part I, *Mendelian Inheritance.*

**Age of Detectability:** If the tapetoretinal dystrophy resembles **Retina, amaurosis congenita, Leber type** with nystagmus, it is detected early in infancy and the electroretinogram is abnormal. Renal function should be followed sequentially to note the abnormality that may not present until later on in the first decade of life.

**Gene Mapping and Linkage:** Unknown.

**Prevention:** None known. Genetic counseling indicated.

**Treatment:** None for the eye; appropriate management of renal failure and its complications. Renal transplant has been performed.

**Prognosis:** The ocular prognosis is poor. Prognosis for renal function is also poor.

**Detection of Carrier:** Scotopic impairment of the ERG in healthy heterozygoes parents has been reported.

**References:**
Senior B: Familial renal-retinal dystrophy. Am J Dis Child 1973;125: 442–447.
François J, et al: Familial juvenile nephronophthisis and associated ocular anomalies (Senior's syndrome): a study of three families. Ophthalmic Paed Genet 1982; 1:97–105.

ME032        **Marilyn B. Mets**

**Renal glucosuria-hyperglycinuria**
*See GLUCOGLYCINURIA*

## RENAL GLYCOSURIA     0861

**Includes:**
> Benign mellituria
> Glucosuria
> Glycosuria, renal
> Renal glycosuria, A and B types
> Renal glycosuria, 0 type

**Excludes:**
> **Diabetes mellitus** (see all)
> **Glucose-galactose malabsorption** (0419)
> **Renal tubular syndrome, Fanconi type** (0864)

**Major Diagnostic Criteria:** The reducing substance in urine is glucose; glycosuria during an otherwise normal oral glucose tolerance test; excretion of > 300 mg glucose per 24 hours on standard carbohydrate diet; and demonstration of reduced renal threshold for glucose by renal titration techniques. Type A renal glycosuria is characterized by reduced threshold and reduced tubular maximum for glucose reabsorption ($T_mG$). Type B renal glycosuria demonstrates reduced threshold, exaggerated "splay", and normal $T_mG$. Type 0 has no threshold or $T_mG$ (tubular glucose reabsorption is completely absent). All three forms have no other proximal or distal tubular abnormalities.

**Clinical Findings:** Asymptomatic glucosuria is not associated with any presenting complaints other than rare episodes of hypoglycemia reported during pregnancy. The condition is usually detected on routine urinalysis.

**Complications:** Iatrogenically induced hypoglycemia in patients misdiagnosed as diabetics and treated with insulin.

**Associated Findings:** None known.

**Etiology:** Autosomal recessive inheritance. Several distinct autosomal mutations are likely.

**Pathogenesis:** Transport defect leads to reduced threshold or reduced $T_m$ for glucose.

**MIM No.:** *23310

**Sex Ratio:** M1:F1

**Occurrence:** Undetermined. Established literature.

**Risk of Recurrence for Patient's Sib:**
> See Part I, *Mendelian Inheritance.*

**Risk of Recurrence for Patient's Child:**
> See Part I, *Mendelian Inheritance.*

**Age of Detectability:** During neonatal period.

**Gene Mapping and Linkage:** Unknown.

**Prevention:** None known. Genetic counseling indicated.

**Treatment:** Unknown.

**Prognosis:** No apparent effect on longevity or health.

**Detection of Carrier:** No reliable means; some carriers do demonstrate mild renal glycosuria.

**Special Considerations:** Early studies using glucose tolerance tests suggested that renal glycosuria is inherited as a dominant trait; recent pedigree analyses using glucose titration techniques indicate that the disorder is inherited in an autosomal recessive fashion and that types A and B renal glycosuria may be found in a single sibship; thus several different mutations affecting one or more glucose transport systems in the kidney may be responsible.

Gut transport system for glucose is not affected in pedigrees studied so far.

**Support Groups:** New York; National Kidney Foundation

**References:**

Elsas LJ, Rosenberg LE: Familial renal glycosuria: a genetic reappraisal of hexose transport by kidney and intestine. J Clin Invest 1969; 48:1845–1854.

Elsas LJ, et al.: Autosomal recessive inheritance of renal glycosuria. Metabolism 1971; 20:968–975.

Oemar BS, et al.: Complete absence of tubular glucose reabsorption: a new type of renal glucosuria (type 0). Clin Nephrol 1987; 27:156–160.

Desjeux, J-F: Congenital selective Na+, D-glucose cotransport defects leading to renal glycosuria and congenital selective intestinal malabsorption of glucose and galactose. In: Scriver CR, et al, eds: The metabolic basis of inherited disease, 6th ed. New York: McGraw-Hill, 1989:2463–2478.

SC050                                                    **Charles R. Scriver**

**Renal glycosuria, 0 type**
  *See RENAL GLYCOSURIA*
**Renal glycosuria, A and B types**
  *See RENAL GLYCOSURIA*
**Renal hamartoma syndrome**
  *See OVERGROWTH-RENAL HAMARTOMA, PERLMAN TYPE*
**Renal hamartomas-nephroblastomatosis-fetal gigantism**
  *See OVERGROWTH-RENAL HAMARTOMA, PERLMAN TYPE*
**Renal histidinura**
  *See HISTIDINURIA*
**Renal hypoplasia-unilobular lung-polydactyly-sex reversal**
  *See SMITH-LEMLI-OPITZ SYNDROME, TYPE II*

---

## RENAL HYPOURICEMIA                                    2005

**Includes:**
  Dalmatian hypouricemia
  Hypouricemia-hypercalciuria-decreased bone density
  Renal (hyper)uricosuria, isolated
  Uric acid urolithiasis

**Excludes:**
  Hypouricemia secondary to antidiuretic hormone, drugs or neoplasm
  **Renal tubular syndrome, Fanconi type** (0864)
  **Transport, renal, defects of** (1501)
  **Xanthine oxidase deficiency** (2411)

**Major Diagnostic Criteria:** 1) serum urate <2 mg/dl (<120 μmol/liter); 2) normal renal excretion of xanthine and absence of other renal tubular abnormalities; 3) increased renal clearance of uric acid (urate/creatinine clearance ratio >0.2).

**Clinical Findings:** There are no characteristic somatic features associated with this condition.

**Complications:** Urolithiasis (calcium urate stones).

**Associated Findings:** Hypercalciuria is not uncommon and may be causally related to increased urate excretion. Other associated conditions include osteoporosis, **Osteopetrosis** (without renal tubular acidosis (RTA)), and infections.

The combination of *hypouricemia, hypercalciuria, and decreased bone density* has been reported in a kindred by Sperling et al (1974).

**Etiology:** Autosomal recessive inheritance. Genetic heterogeneity appears likely, since several different transport defects have been identified.

**Pathogenesis:** Renal handling of urate involves filtration, presecretory reabsorption, secretion, and postsecretory reabsorption. Tests with specific inhibitors of urate secretion (pyrazinamide) and postsecretory reabsorption (probenecid) have been used to show isolated defects in each of these transport pathways. In some cases, a combined defect appears likely.

**MIM No.:** *22015, 24205

**Sex Ratio:** M1:F1

**Occurrence:** Hypouricemia is seen in less than 1% of the population. Two-thirds of these cases are secondary hypouricemia; of the remainder, some may be due to xanthuria or decreased urate synthesis. Published reports suggest an increased frequency in non-Ashkenazi Jewish populations.

**Risk of Recurrence for Patient's Sib:**
  See Part I, *Mendelian Inheritance.*

**Risk of Recurrence for Patient's Child:**
  See Part I, *Mendelian Inheritance.*

**Age of Detectability:** Infants of two to four years of age have been described.

**Gene Mapping and Linkage:** Unknown.

**Prevention:** None known. Genetic counseling indicated.

**Treatment:** Urolithiasis can be avoided with standard regimens, including hydration and alkalinization to increase volume and pH of the urine, and with use of xanthine oxidase inhibitors (allopurinol).

**Prognosis:** A benign disorder, apart from the increased risk of urolithiasis.

**Detection of Carrier:** Urate clearances measured in some obligate heterozygotes are elevated and appear to be intermediate between normals and affected individuals.

**Special Considerations:** The human phenotype is analogous to the well-described autosomal recessive renal hyperuricosuria found in the Dalmatian coachhound. Studies in the latter indicate that transport is also abnormal in erythrocytes.

**Support Groups:** New York; National Kidney Foundation

**References:**

Greene ML, et al.: Hypouricemia due to isolated renal tubular defect: dalmatian dog mutation in man. Am J Med 1972; 53:361–367.

Sperling O, et al.: Hypouricemia, hypercalcinuria, and decreased bone density: a hereditary syndrome. Ann Intern Med 1974; 80:482–487.

Fujiwara Y, et al.: Hypouricemia due to an isolated defect in renal tubular urate reabsorption. Clin Nephrol 1980; 13:44–48.

Takeda E, et al.: Hereditary hypouricemia in children. J Pediatr 1985; 107:71–74.

Sperling O: Hereditary renal hypouricemia. In: Scriver CR, et al, eds: The metabolic basis of inherited disease, 6th ed. New York: McGraw-Hill, 1989:2605–2618.

C0016                                                        **David Cole**

**Renal iminoglycinuria**
  *See IMINOGLYCINURIA*
**Renal medulla, familial disease**
  *See KIDNEY, NEPHRONOPHTHISIS-MEDULLARY CYSTIC DESEASE*

---

## RENAL MESANGIAL SCLEROSIS-EYE DEFECTS          2805

**Includes:**
  Eye defects-diffuse renal mesangial sclerosis
  Mesangial sclerosis, diffuse renal-ocular abnormalities

**Excludes:**
  **Cataract-renal tubular necrosis-encephalopathy, Crome type** (2162)
  **Oculo-cerebro-renal syndrome** (0736)
  **Oculo-reno-cerebellar syndrome** (3050)
  **Renal dysplasia-retinal aplasia, Loken-Senior type** (2687)
  **Wilms tumor-pseudohermaphroditism-glomerulopathy, Denys-Drash type** (3139)

**Major Diagnostic Criteria:** Nephrotic syndrome secondary to diffuse mesangial sclerosis, eye abnormalities, chronic renal failure, and death in early childhood.

**Clinical Findings:** The condition presents in the first year of life with nephrotic syndrome secondary to diffuse mesangial sclerosis and eye abnormalities consisting of nystagmus, optic atrophy, narrowing of retinal arterioles, and abnormal macular areas. Renal failure occurs in early childhood.

**Complications:** Chronic renal failure.

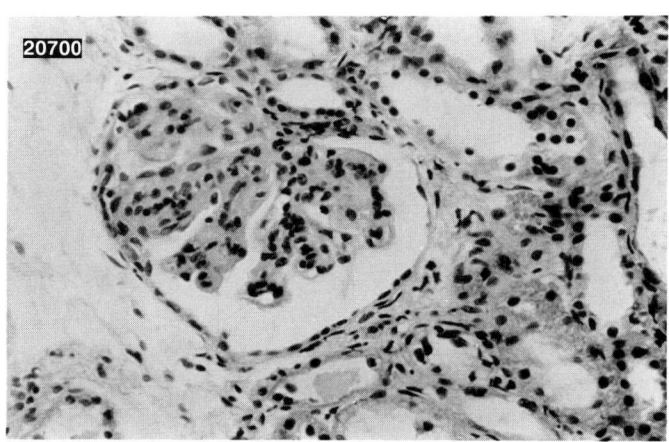

**2805-20700:** Renal mesangial sclerosis-eye defects; renal histology of glomeruli showing diffuse mesangial sclerosis.

**Associated Findings:** Diffuse mesangial sclerosis may be associated with male pseudohermaphroditism, **Cancer, Wilms tumor,** hypertension, and psychomotor retardation. May also be seen in **Wilms tumor-pseudohermaphroditism-glomerulopathy, Denys-Drash type.**

**Etiology:** Possibly autosomal recessive inheritance.

**Pathogenesis:** Possibly an antenatal dysgenetic process.

**MIM No.:** 24966

**Sex Ratio:** Presumably M1:F1

**Occurrence:** This association has been observed in two siblings.

**Risk of Recurrence for Patient's Sib:**
See Part I, *Mendelian Inheritance.*

**Risk of Recurrence for Patient's Child:**
See Part I, *Mendelian Inheritance.*

**Age of Detectability:** Early in the first year of life.

**Gene Mapping and Linkage:** Unknown.

**Prevention:** None known. Genetic counseling indicated.

**Treatment:** Renal transplantation has been performed successfully in patients with diffuse mesangial sclerosis.

**Prognosis:** Chronic renal failure occurs in early childhood.

**Detection of Carrier:** Unknown.

**Support Groups:** New York; National Kidney Foundation

**References:**
Barakat AY, et al.: Diffuse mesangial sclerosis and ocular abnormalities in two siblings. Int J Pediatr Nephrol 1982; 3:33–35. †

BA065
NA009

**Amin Y. Barakat
Samir S. Najjar**

**Renal reabsorption of carnitine, defect in**
*See MYOPATHY-METABOLIC, CARNITINE DEFICIENCY, PRIMARY AND SECONDARY*
**Renal transport defects**
*See TRANSPORT, RENAL, DEFECTS OF*

## RENAL TUBULAR ACIDOSIS 0862

**Includes:**
Deafness (sensorineural)-renal tubular acidosis
Distal renal tubular acidosis
Gradient type renal tubular acidosis
Renal tubular acidosis, classic type
Renal tubular acidosis, type I

**Excludes:**
**Renal bicarbonate reabsorptive defect** (0858)
**Renal tubular acidosis** (0862)
Renal tubular acidosis (incomplete distal), type IV
**Renal tubular acidosis-osteopetrosis syndrome** (3086)
**Renal tubular acidosis-sensorineural deafness** (0863)

**Major Diagnostic Criteria:** Persistent elevation of urinary pH (usually > 6.0) despite acidosis; abnormal distal hydrogen ion secretory capacity reflected by abnormally low urine-to-blood $CO_2$ gradient ($pCO_2 < 35$ mm Hg) despite bicarbonate, sulfate, or phosphate loading or furosemide administration.

**Clinical Findings:** Usually presents in infancy as failure to thrive, hyperchloremic acidosis, hypokalemia, and episodes of vomiting and dehydration. Twenty-five percent may develop a metabolic emergency. In infants, bicarbonaturia may be profound and is the major determinant of the therapeutic sodium bicarbonate requirement; this aspect gradually improves so that, in adults, acidosis is limited to the magnitude of endogenous acid production.

**Complications:** Untreated or partially treated acidosis leads to growth failure, hypercalciuria, hypocitraturia, and nephrocalcinosis by 2–4 years. Hypokalemia and acidosis produce a proximal myopathy and listlessness. Moderate nephrocalcinosis causes interstitial nephritis and sterile pyuria; advanced nephrocalcinosis predisposes to urinary tract infection and occasionally to chronic renal failure.

**Associated Findings:** **Ehlers-Danlos syndrome, Elliptocytosis.** A recessive form associated with progressive nerve deafness has also been identified.

**Etiology:** Autosomal dominant inheritance.

**Pathogenesis:** The distal hydrogen ion secretory defect is independent of transepithelial voltage and availability of urinary buffers. There is some controversy as to whether hypercalciuria is secondary to acidosis or is a direct consequence of the mutation.

**MIM No.:** *17980

**Sex Ratio:** M1:F1

**Occurrence:** Undetermined. Established literature.

**Risk of Recurrence for Patient's Sib:**
See Part I, *Mendelian Inheritance.*

**Risk of Recurrence for Patient's Child:**
See Part I, *Mendelian Inheritance.*

**Age of Detectability:** Usually during the neonatal period; becomes clinically overt by two years of age.

**Gene Mapping and Linkage:** Unknown.

**Prevention:** None known. Genetic counseling indicated.

**Treatment:** Oral sodium bicarbonate 5–15 mEq/kg/day in divided doses is believed to normalize growth, repair hyperkalemia and myopathy, and prevent nephrocalcinosis. Potassium supplementation may be required to avoid hypokalemia and episodes of muscle weakness.

**Prognosis:** Apparently good if compliant with high-dose sodium bicarbonate therapy.

**Detection of Carrier:** Unknown.

**Support Groups:** New York; National Kidney Foundation

**References:**
Rodriquez-Soriano J: The renal regulation of acid-base balance and the disturbances noted in renal tubular acidosis. Pediatr Clin North Am 1971; 18:529–545.
McSherry E, Morris RC, Jr.: Attainment and maintenance of normal

stature with alkali therapy in infants and children with classical renal tubular acidosis. J Clin Invest 1978; 61:509–527.

McSherry E: Renal tubular acidosis in childhood. Kidney Int 1981; 20:799–809.

DuBose TD, Jr., Alpern RF: Renal tubular acidosis. In: Scriver CR, et al, eds: The metabolic basis of inherited disease, 6th ed. New York: McGraw-Hill, 1989:2539–2568.

G0052                                                                    Paul Goodyer

**Renal tubular acidosis, classic type**
   *See RENAL TUBULAR ACIDOSIS*
**Renal tubular acidosis, proximal**
   *See RENAL BICARBONATE REABSORPTIVE DEFECT*
**Renal tubular acidosis, rate type**
   *See RENAL BICARBONATE REABSORPTIVE DEFECT*
**Renal tubular acidosis, type I**
   *See RENAL TUBULAR ACIDOSIS*
**Renal tubular acidosis, type II**
   *See RENAL BICARBONATE REABSORPTIVE DEFECT*

## RENAL TUBULAR ACIDOSIS-OSTEOPETROSIS SYNDROME                                      3086

**Includes:**
   Carbonic anhydrase B
   Carbonic anhydrase II deficiency
   Carbonic anhydrase II, erythrocyte, electrophoretic variant
   Guibaud-Vainsel syndrome
   Marble brain disease
   Osteopetrosis-renal tubular acidosis-cerebral calcification

**Excludes:**
   **Osteopetrosis, benign dominant** (0779)
   **Osteopetrosis, malignant recessive** (0780)
   **Renal bicarbonate reabsorptive defect** (0858)
   **Renal tubular acidosis** (0862)

**Major Diagnostic Criteria:** Metabolic acidosis of varying severity secondary to impaired urinary acidification is present from birth. Osteopetrosis, evident on X-rays, develops by one year of age. Cerebral calcification, most evident on CT scan, appears during the first decade. Additional features are mental retardation, growth failure, abnormal dentition, and bone fractures. Anemia, if present, is usually mild. Diagnosis is established by demonstration of absence of carbonic anhydrase II in erythrocyte lysates. This enzyme deficiency has been demonstrated in every known patient with **Osteopetrosis** and **Renal tubular acidosis**.

**Clinical Findings:** Skeletal X-ray findings include increased bone density, abnormal modeling, transverse banding of metaphyses, fractures, and "bone in bone" appearance. Distal renal tubular acidosis is suggested by metabolic acidosis with hyperchloremia, normal anion gap, and inappropriately alkaline urine pH (over 6.0) without reduction in glomerular filtration rate or elevated urea nitrogen. Bicarbonaturia when plasma $HCO_3-$ is raised to normal levels indicates the presence of a proximal tubular component also. Growth retardation begins after birth, and improves with treatment of the acidosis. Mental retardation is common, and may be severe. Intercranial calcifications are detected by 18 months by CT scan, and later by X-ray. Nephrocalcinosis is absent.

**Complications:** Multiple bone fractures in the first two decades. Episodes of severe hypokalemia may occur. Optic nerve atrophy and other cranial nerve compressions occur.

**Associated Findings:** Restrictive lung disease has been reported.

**Etiology:** Autosomal recessive inheritance.

**Pathogenesis:** Carbonic anhydrase II isozyme (CA II) is absent in erythrocytes. Although not demonstrated in humans, the absence of CAII in renal parenchyma, osteoclasts, and oligodendrial cells is inferred, and presumed to be the basis for the mixed (proximal and distal) renal tubular acidosis, the defect in bone resorption leading to osteopetrosis, and the cerebral calcification.

**MIM No.:** *25973, 11481

**POS No.:** 4170

**Sex Ratio:** M1:F1

**Occurrence:** About 15 kindreds are known, nearly half of which are from Saudi Arabia, Kuwait, and North Africa.

**Risk of Recurrence for Patient's Sib:**
   See Part I, *Mendelian Inheritance*.

**Risk of Recurrence for Patient's Child:**
   See Part I, *Mendelian Inheritance*.

**Age of Detectability:** At birth.

**Gene Mapping and Linkage:** CA2 (carbonic anhydrase II) has been mapped to 8q22.

**Prevention:** None known. Genetic counseling indicated.

**Treatment:** Treatment of renal tubular acidosis with alkali and symptomatic treatment of bone fractures and skeletal deformities.

**Prognosis:** Multiple fractures in childhood, but X-rays and clinical course improve in adolescents. Learning disabilities are usually substantial. Treatment of acidosis improves growth.

**Detection of Carrier:** Possible by demonstrating one-half normal CA II level with normal CA I level in erythrocyte lysate.

**Special Considerations:** Since this disorder may present in infancy, it can be confused with **Osteopetrosis, malignant recessive**. Diagnosis is important because of the much better prognosis in CA II deficiency.

**Support Groups:** New York; National Kidney Foundation

**References:**
Sly WS, et al: Carbonic anhydrase II deficiency identified as the primary defect in the autosomal recessive syndrome of osteopetrosis with renal tubular acidosis and cerebral calcification. Proc Natl Acad Sci USA 1983; 80:2752–2756.

Sly WS, et al: Carbonic anhydrase II deficiency in 12 families with the autosomal recessive syndrome of osteopetrosis with renal tubular acidosis and cerebral calcification. New Engl J Med 1985; 313:139–145.

Ohlsson A, et al: Carbonic anhydrase II deficiency syndrome: recessive osteopetrosis with renal tubular acidosis and cerebral calcification. Pediatrics 1986; 77:371–381.

Sundaram V, et al: Carbonic anhydrase II deficiency: diagnosis and carrier detection using differential enzyme inhibition and inactivation. Am J Hum Genet 1986; 38:125–136.

SL001                                                              William S. Sly

## RENAL TUBULAR ACIDOSIS-SENSORINEURAL DEAFNESS                                         0863

**Includes:**
   Carbonic anhydrase B deficiency
   Deafness, sensorineural-renal tubular acidosis

**Excludes:**
   **Oculo-cerebro-renal syndrome** (0736)
   **Renal tubular acidosis** (0862)
   Renal tubular acidosis with other associated defects

**Major Diagnostic Criteria:** Renal tubular acidosis with a defect in tubular $HCO_3$-resorption and sensorineural hearing loss or deafness.

**Clinical Findings:** At birth or soon thereafter, vomiting, dehydration, polydipsia, polyuria, hyposthenuria, and failure to thrive. Nephrocalcinosis was observed in some cases.

Renal tubular acidosis is a clinical syndrome of disordered renal acidification which is out of proportion to the impairment of glomerular filtration and in which metabolic acidosis results from abnormalities of renal tubular function. This type of renal tubular acidosis is associated with a defect in tubular $HCO_3$-resorption. Deficient carbonic anhydrase B (CA-B) activity in the affected individuals of one family has been suggested; however, repeat evaluations of one of these patients showed normal red cell carbonic anhydrase.

Deafness is variable. In most cases, a sensorineural deafness is present in early childhood. In two sibs the onset of hearing loss was during late childhood, and in two other sibs there was a striking difference in the degree of hearing loss.

**Complications:** Nephrocalcinosis.

**Associated Findings:** Mild mental retardation.

**Etiology:** Autosomal recessive inheritance.

**Pathogenesis:** Unknown.

**MIM No.:** *26730

**POS No.:** 4463

**Sex Ratio:** M5:F4

**Occurrence:** More than 20 cases have been documented in the literature.

**Risk of Recurrence for Patient's Sib:**
See Part I, *Mendelian Inheritance.*

**Risk of Recurrence for Patient's Child:**
See Part I, *Mendelian Inheritance.*

**Age of Detectability:** Early childhood.

**Gene Mapping and Linkage:** CA2 (carbonic anhydrase II) has been mapped to 8q22.

**Prevention:** None known. Genetic counseling indicated.

**Treatment:** Treatment with alkalinizing solutions and high fluid intake. Hearing aid; special training if the hearing loss is severe.

**Prognosis:** Probably normal life span, assuming good medical care.

**Detection of Carrier:** Unknown.

**Support Groups:** New York; National Kidney Foundation

**References:**
Simon H, et al.: The acidification defect in the syndrome of renal tubular acidosis with nerve deafness. Acta Pediatr Scand 1979; 68:291–295.
Cremers CWRJ, et al.: Renal tubular acidosis and sensorineural deafness: an autosomal recessive syndrome. Arch Otolaryngol 1980; 106:287–289.
Dunger DB, et al.: Renal tubular acidosis and nerve deafness. Arch Dis Child 1980; 55:221–225.
Tashian RE, et al.: Inherited variants of human red cell carbonic anhydrase. Hemoglobin 1980; 4:635–651.
Anai T, et al.: Siblings with renal tubular acidosis and nerve deafness: the first family in Japan. Hum Genet 1984; 66:282–285. *

BA033
**James A. Bartley**
*Cor W.R.J. Cremers*

---

## RENAL TUBULAR DYSGENESIS      2608

**Includes:**
    Primitive renal tubule syndrome
    Renal dysplasia-primitive renal tubules
    Renal tubular immaturity
    Renotubular dysgenesis

**Excludes:**
    **Kidney, polycystic disease, recessive** (2003)
    **Kidney, renal dysplasia, Potter type II** (3028)
    **Renal agenesis, unilateral** (0857)

**Major Diagnostic Criteria:** Diagnosis is made by histological findings only. The proximal convoluted tubules are lined with poorly differentiated, crowded cuboidal and columnar epithelial cells which appear abnormally primitive. Normal proximal tubule brush borders are not demonstrated by periodic acid-Schiff stain or by peroxidase-labeled winged pea (Tetragonolobus lotus) lectin, which is a selective marker for proximal tubules. Electron microscopy demonstrates only rare rudimentary brush borders. Glomeruli are normal in appearance, but appear crowded due to a reduced number of tubular cross-sections. The corticomedullary margin is well demarcated, however, the medullary rays are poorly delineated. Renal size may be normal or enlarged.

**Clinical Findings:** Anuria in the neonatal period or prenatal diagnosis of oligohydramnios and inability to demonstrate fetal bladder are often the presenting clinical signs. All published cases have been preterm deliveries.

**Complications:** The neonatal course is complicated by pulmonary hypoplasia. Clinical findings may include Potter facies (see **Renal agenesis, bilateral**), compression deformity of the cranium, and joint contractures.

**Associated Findings:** **Eye, hypertelorism** (one case), **Heart, tetralogy of Fallot** (one case), **Microcephaly** (two cases), and open cranial sutures (three cases), rocker-bottom feet (two cases) and abnormal body proportions (one case).

**Etiology:** Autosomal recessive inheritance.

**Pathogenesis:** The cause of oligohydramnios in these patients is unclear, but the presence of short and undifferentiated tubules might be expected to result in decreased fluid resorption and increased fluid output. Therefore, it seems likely that abnormal glomerular filtration plays a role. No anatomic basis for decreased filtration has been identified, as the glomeruli appear to be histologically normal and well vascularized.

**MIM No.:** *26743

**Sex Ratio:** M8:F4 (observed).

**Occurrence:** Five families have been identified as follows: 1) a nonconsanguineous Chinese mating; 2) first cousin once-removed Sicilian mating; 3) first cousin Egyptian mating; 4) nonconsanguineous American mating of parents of Northern European background; and 5) nonconsanguineous American mating, ethnicity unspecified.

**Risk of Recurrence for Patient's Sib:**
See Part I, *Mendelian Inheritance.*

**Risk of Recurrence for Patient's Child:**
See Part I, *Mendelian Inheritance.* Affected individuals are not expected to survive to reproduce.

**Age of Detectability:** Due to the late onset of oligohydramnios, reliable prenatal diagnosis may not be possible. There have been two cases with amniotic fluid volume at the lower limit of normal at 22 weeks gestation, which progressed to oligohydramnios at 32 weeks gestation. One case presented with oligohydramnios at 26 weeks gestation.

**Gene Mapping and Linkage:** Unknown.

**Prevention:** None known. Genetic counseling indicated.

**Treatment:** Unknown.

**Prognosis:** Lethal.

**Detection of Carrier:** Unknown.

**Support Groups:** New York; National Kidney Foundation

**References:**
Allanson JE, et al.: Possible new autosomal recessive syndrome with unusual renal histopathological changes. Am J Med Genet 1983; 16:57–60.
Voland JR, et al.: Congenital hypernephrotic nephromegaly with tubular dysgenesis: a distinctive inherited renal anomaly. Pediatr Pathol 1985; 4:231–245.
Schwartz BR, et al.: Isolated congenital renal tubular immaturity in siblings. Hum Pathol 1986; 17:1259–1263.
Bernstein J: Congenital malformations of the kidney. In Tisher CC and Brenner BM, (eds): Renal Pathology, vol 2. Philadelphia: J.B. Lipincott, 1989:1278–1304.
Swinford AE, et al.: Renal tubular dysgenesis: delayed onset of oligohydramnios. Am J Med Genet 1989; 32:127–132.

SW007
HI004
**Ann E. Swinford**
**James V. Higgins**

**Renal tubular immaturity**
    *See* RENAL TUBULAR DYSGENESIS
**Renal tubular insufficiency-biliary malformation**
    *See* BILIARY ATRESIA
**Renal tubular necrosis-cataract-encephalopathy**
    *See* CATARACT-RENAL TUBULAR NECROSIS-ENCEPHALOPATHY, CROME TYPE

## RENAL TUBULAR SYNDROME, FANCONI TYPE　　0864

**Includes:**
　Adult Fanconi syndrome
　Fanconi-like syndrome
　Fanconi renotubular syndrome I, childhood and infantile
　　forms
　Fanconi renotubular syndrome II, adult form
　Fanconi syndrome-intestinal malabsorption-galactose
　　intolerance
　Luder-Sheldon syndrome

**Excludes:** Pancytopenia syndrome, Fanconi type (2029)

**Major Diagnostic Criteria:** All aspects of this syndrome reflect impaired renal tubular transport. These include generalized hyperaminoaciduria resembling plasma ultrafiltrate, hypophosphatemia and hyperphosphaturia, low tubular maximum ($T_m$) glucosuria, type II (proximal) renal tubular acidosis with bicarbonate loss, high free water clearance, and high renal clearance of other filtered solutes (e.g., uric acid, potassium). An analogous impairment of intestinal transport may also exist.

The morphologic lesion that affects the proximal tubule, often called a "swan neck lesion," is probably secondary to the functional deficit; it represents atrophy of epithelial cells and loss of volume of proximal tubular mass.

Progressive nephron failure and decreased glomerular filtration can abate phenotypic expression of the Fanconi syndrome in its later stages in some traits (e.g., **Cystinosis**).

**Clinical Findings:** This is a syndrome of many causes, some of which are inherited, yet often unidentified. The clinical manifestations are, in essence, peripheral, being dependent either on the condition causing the syndrome, or on the sequelae of the syndrome itself. The fully expressed syndrome comprises a generalized disturbance of proximal renal tubular transport. The most frequent clinical consequences include hypophosphatemic rickets (phosphate loss), acidosis (bicarbonate loss), weakness (potassium loss), and dehydration (water loss). Growth failure or weight loss may also occur in the uncompensated syndrome.

Time of onset of the trait depends on its cause. Exposure to toxic agents directly precedes most acquired causes, which must be

eliminated before attributing the syndrome to an inherited cause. Inherited traits may produce the Fanconi syndrome either early or late in life; galactosemia and fructosemia produce the syndrome rapidly after the metabolite accumulates in the blood, while prolonged copper accumulation is required in **Hepatolenticular degeneration** before the syndrome is noticed. The recessively inherited Fanconi syndrome associated with **Cystinosis** appears in the first six months of life. The noncystinotic adult idiopathic syndrome may not appear until the fourth decade.

A possible variant, *Luder-Sheldon syndrome* (autosomal dominant), has also been described (Sheldon et al, 1961). A *Fanconi-like* syndrome (Abels and Reed, 1973) also has similarities to yet differences from the recognized Fanconi variants, including multiple cutaneous malignancies.

**Complications:** All clinical manifestions (e.g., rickets or osteomalacia, renal tubular acidosis and dehydration) can be considered as "complications" of the transport defect. Death secondary to uncorrected hypokalemia or dehydration can occur in infants.

**Associated Findings:** Those of the primary trait (e.g., **Cystinosis**, "tyrosinosis," **Hepatolenticular degeneration**) should be considered in their own terms. Death may be the end stage of a number of the primary traits associated with the syndrome.

*Fanconi syndrome-intestinal malabsorption-galactose intolerance* has been reported in a brother and sister of Turkish-Assyrian extraction (Aperia et al, 1981).

**Etiology:** This condition may be acquired or inherited. While autosomal dominant inheritance has been reported, autosomal recessive inheritance of many mutant alleles at numerous autosomal loci determine most of the various forms of the syndrome. Some mutant alleles are easily recognized as primary traits, such as hereditary tyrosinemia, infantile nephropathic cystinosis, galactosemia, fructosemia, and **Hepatolenticular degeneration**. In these, the syndrome is clearly secondary to the expression of the primary trait. Other mutant genes are identifiable only through the presence of the Fanconi syndrome itself, as in the adult idiopathic Fanconi syndrome.

**Pathogenesis:** Impaired *net reabsorption* ability for solute and water across the tubular cell seems to be the fundamental lesion of the syndrome; *affinity* of the solutes for their binding site is apparently not altered. The inhibition of membrane transport is probably linked to specific forms of impaired availability or transduction of metabolic energy for transport.

**MIM No.:** *13460, 22770, 22780, 22781, 22785

**Sex Ratio:** M1:F1

**Occurrence:** Varies with primary cause.

**Risk of Recurrence for Patient's Sib:**
　See Part I, *Mendelian Inheritance.*

**Risk of Recurrence for Patient's Child:**
　See Part I, *Mendelian Inheritance.*

**Age of Detectability:** Varies with primary cause. Prenatal diagnosis is feasible in certain forms (causes), e.g., in cystinosis, hereditary tyrosinemia, and galactosemia.

**Gene Mapping and Linkage:** Unknown.

**Prevention:** Elimination of etiologic factor in acquired forms. Genetic counseling is indicated.

**Treatment:** Offset phenotypic effects of trait; e.g., phosphate supplementation of diet to prevent hypophosphatemia; potassium and bicarbonate replacement to prevent hypokalemia and renal tubular acidosis; high fluid intake to prevent dehydration.

**Prognosis:** Depends upon the cause. Some forms respond better to treatment than do others.

**Detection of Carrier:** This depends on the cause. The syndrome is usually never expressed in carriers, except in unusual pedigrees, such as that described by Ben-Ishay et al. (1961), or by Sheldon et al (1961) where a dominantly inherited trait was identified. Carrier detection is feasible in cases of **Cystinosis** by measurement of cellular lysosomal cystine content, but each cause of Fanconi syndrome must be considered on its own terms (e.g.,

**0864-10480:** Skeletal changes of hypophosphatemia; note grossly deformed chest, foreshortened limbs, limb and joint defects. **10481:** X-ray shows hypophosphatemic rickets with severe nonmineralization with "looser zones" of healing fractures in proximal tibia and fibula.

possible galactosemia; not possible yet, in hereditary tyrosinemia or idiopathic forms).

**Support Groups:** New York; National Kidney Foundation

**References:**
Ben-Ishay D, et al.: Fanconi syndrome with hypouricemia in an adult: family study. Am J Med 1961; 31:793–800.
Sheldon W, et al.: A familial tubular absorption defect of glucose and amino acids. Arch Dis Child 1961; 36:90–95.
Abeles D, Reed WB: Fanconi-like syndrome: immunologic deficiency, pancytopenia, and cutaneous malignancies. Arch Derm 1973; 107:419–423.
Friedman AL, et al.: Autosomal dominant Fanconi syndrome with early renal failure. Am J Med Genet 1978; 2:225–232.
Aperia A, et al.: Familial Fanconi syndrome with malabsorption and galactose intolerance, normal kinase and transferase activity. Acta Paediat Scand 1981; 70:527–533.
Brenton DP, et al.: The adult presenting idiopathic Fanconi syndrome. J Inherit Metab Dis 1981; 4:211–215.
Patrick A, et al.: A family with a dominant form of idiopathic Fanconi syndrome leading to renal failure in adult life. Clin Nephrol 1981; 16:289–292.
Bergeron M, Gougoux A: The renal Fanconi syndrome. In: Scriver CR, et al, eds: The metabolic basis of inherited disease, 6th ed. New York: McGraw-Hill, 1989:2569–2580.

SC050                                              **Charles R. Scriver**

**Renal type amyloidosis**
    *See AMYLOIDOSIS, FAMILIAL VISCERAL*
**Renal-acro-mandibular syndrome**
    *See ACRO-RENAL-MANDIBULAR SYNDROME*
**Renal-branchio-oto dysplasia**
    *See BRANCHIO-OTO-RENAL DYSPLASIA*
**Renal-facio-oculo-acoustic syndrome**
    *See FACIO-OCULO-ACOUSTIC-RENAL SYNDROME (FOAR SYNDROME)*

---

## RENAL-GENITAL-MIDDLE EAR ANOMALIES  0860

**Includes:**
    Genital-renal-middle ear anomalies
    Ear, middle-genitourinary anomalies
    Winter syndrome

**Excludes:**
    Deafness-renal-digital anomalies
    **Nephritis-deafness (sensorineural), hereditary type** (0708)
    **Renal agenesis, bilateral** (0856)
    **Renal agenesis, unilateral** (0857)

**Major Diagnostic Criteria:** Conductive hearing loss, variable renal anomalies, and vaginal atresia.

**Clinical Findings:** Renal abnormalities vary from unilateral hypoplasia to unilateral or bilateral renal agenesis. Vaginal atresia may be associated with normal external genitalia, uterus, fallopian tubes, and ovaries or with extensive internal genital anomalies. Hearing loss is conductive and associated with stenotic external auditory canals. Audiogram shows a conductive loss with a normal bone line. An absent or malformed incus has been described in two patients who had middle ear explorations. Variable features include a beaked nose, micrognathia, low-set small ears, clinodactyly, and mild mental retardation. One sib 47XX +c is presumed **Chromosome X, triplo-X.**

**Complications:** Delayed development of language secondary to the hearing loss. If renal anomalies are extensive enough, they may be incompatible with life. Undiagnosed vaginal atresia can lead to hydrometrocolpos at menarche.

**Associated Findings:** Mild mental retardation, beaked nose, micrognathia, low-set small ears, congenital heart disease, pulmonary hypoplasia.

**Etiology:** Possibly autosomal recessive inheritance with variable expressivity, and possibly sex-influenced. It is not known if there is a form of this syndrome in males.

**Pathogenesis:** Unknown.

**MIM No.:** 26740

**POS No.:** 3376

**Sex Ratio:** M0:F1 (observed).

**Occurrence:** Four, possibly five cases reported, all female.

**Risk of Recurrence for Patient's Sib:**
    See Part I, *Mendelian Inheritance.* Expression of this defect in males is undetermined.

**Risk of Recurrence for Patient's Child:**
    See Part I, *Mendelian Inheritance.* Reproductive fitness undetermined, although those with more severe abnormalities are probably infertile.

**Age of Detectability:** At birth, by clinical examination, although the vaginal atresia and conductive hearing loss may be difficult to detect until later.

**Gene Mapping and Linkage:** Unknown.

**Prevention:** None known. Genetic counseling indicated.

**Treatment:** Middle ear surgery may improve the hearing, although amplification and special training may be necessary prior to middle ear surgery. A vagina may be created by plastic surgery. Other therapy may be required for secondary renal complications.

**Prognosis:** Death may occur in infancy if renal abnormalities are severe, or if associated abnormalities are present. Milder forms are probably compatible with a normal life span.

**Detection of Carrier:** Unknown.

**Special Considerations:** Turner (1970) reported a patient with a narrow external auditory meatus with mild deafness, vaginal atresia, and an absent left kidney. In addition, this patient had crowded dentition, lacrimal duct stenosis, and an anteriorly placed rectum with mild rectal stenosis. This patient may represent an additional example of this syndrome. One affected female is reported to have 47XX+c karyotype that may represent a third X chromosome.

**Support Groups:** New York; National Kidney Foundation

**References:**
Winter JS, et al.: A familial syndrome of renal, genital and middle ear anomalies. J Pediatr 1968; 72:88–93.
Turner G: A second family with renal, vaginal and middle ear anomalies. J Pediatr 1970; 76:641 only.
Franek A: Ein oto-uro-genitales Syndrom Mit Mindervuchs. Monatsschr Kinderheizkd 1982; 130:730–731.
King LA, et al.: Syndrome of genital, renal and middle ear anomalies: a third family and report of a pregnancy. Obstet Gynec 1987; 69:491–493.

*Janet M. Stewart*

**Renal-hepatic-pancreatic dysplasia (one form)**
    *See KIDNEY, POLYCYSTIC DISEASE, RECESSIVE*
**Renal-oculo-cerebellar syndrome**
    *See OCULO-RENO-CEREBELLAR SYNDROME*
**Renal-oculo-cerebro syndrome**
    *See OCULO-CEREBRO-RENAL SYNDROME*
**Renal-radial syndrome**
    *See RADIAL-RENAL SYNDROME*
**Renal-retinal dystrophy, familial**
    *See RENAL DYSPLASIA-RETINAL APLASIA, LOKEN-SENIOR TYPE*
**Renal-retinal syndrome**
    *See RENAL DYSPLASIA-RETINAL APLASIA, LOKEN-SENIOR TYPE*
**Rendu-Osler disease**
    *See TELANGIECTASIA, OSLER HEMORRHAGIC*
**Rendu-Osler-Weber disease**
    *See TELANGIECTASIA, OSLER HEMORRHAGIC*
**Reno-digito-cerebral syndrome**
    *See DIGITO-RENO-CEREBRAL SYNDROME*
**Renotubular dysgenesis**
    *See RENAL TUBULAR DYSGENESIS*
**Renpenning syndrome**
    *See X-LINKED MENTAL RETARDATION, RENPENNING TYPE*
**Reproductive tract injuries in DES daughters**
    *See FETAL DIETHYLSTILBESTROL (DES) EFFECTS*

## RESISTANCE TO 1,25 DIHYDROXY VITAMIN D      2953

**Includes:**
Alopecia-rickets syndrome
Autosomal recessive vitamin D dependency (ARVD)
End-organ unresponsiveness to 1,25 dihydroxycholecalciferol
End-organ unresponsiveness to vitamin D
Hair, development in utero
Hypocalcemic, hypophosphatemic rickets with aminoaciduria
Hypocalcemic rickets, type IIa
Pseudovitamin D-deficiency rickets (PDR)
Rickets-alopecia syndrome
Rickets, hereditary hypocalcemic type IIa
Rickets, vitamin D-dependent, type II
Vitamin D dependency IIa
Vitamin D-dependent rickets, type IIa
Vitamin D-dependent rickets, type IIb

**Excludes:**
**Hypophosphatasia** (0516)
**Hypophosphatemia, non X-linked** (2040)
**Hypophosphatemia, X-linked** (0517)
Pseudohypoparathyroidism
**Rickets, vitamin D-dependent, type I** (0873)

**Major Diagnostic Criteria:** The general features of patients with this defect are rickets or osteomalacia, alopecia, hypocalcemia, secondary hyperparathyroidism, and high serum concentrations of 1,25-dihydroxyvitamin D (1,25[OH]$_2$D), the biologically active form of vitamin D, before or during treatment with calciferols.

**Clinical Findings:** *Resistance to 1,25(OH)$_2$D* is a term applied to a hereditary (and sometimes sporadic) form of hypocalcemic rickets in which there is diminished or absent target tissue responsiveness to the actions of the active form of vitamin D, 1,25(OH)$_2$D. Affected infants appear normal at birth, since fetal mineral homeostasis is determined primarily by maternal calcium and phosphate concentrations. However, serum 1,25(OH)$_2$D levels are probably abnormally high early in life (within the first few weeks). Rickets usually presents prior to age three years; however, some patients presented with osteomalacia as late as age 45 years. All cases with late onset have been eucalcemic. Approximately one-half of the reported cases have total alopecia or sparse hair. Although sometimes present at birth, alopecia is not usually obvious until ages 3–6 months. Alopecia correlates well with the severity of the resistance to 1,25(OH)$_2$D. It is always associated with early age of presentation and is always present in those patients who cannot become normocalcemic with high doses of exogenous calciferols.

Although some patients with alopecia have become normocalcemic with calciferol therapy, none have shown improvement in hair growth. Parental consanguinity has been noted in many of the reported cases, especially those with alopecia. For unknown reasons, there is a striking clustering of cases close to the Mediterranean, even though different cellular defects have been implicated in these cases. Except for patients with alopecia, rickets is the usual presenting complaint.

Clinical manifestations are similar to those of vitamin D-deficiency rickets. Symptoms usually appear before age one year and may occur as early as the first months of life. These include hypotonia, weakness, and growth failure. Motor retardation may be apparent or real. Enamel defects are seen in teeth that calcify postnatally. Pathologic fractures may occur. Later, bony deformities develop. Convulsions or tetany may be the presenting clinical feature. Rickets with a reliable history of adequate intake of vitamin D may be a clue to the diagnosis.

Prominent physical findings are shortness of stature, hypotonia, and the characteristic features of rickets, including thickening of the wrists and ankles, frontal bowing of lower limbs, and positive Trousseau and Chvostek signs.

The X-ray findings are not distinguishable from those associated with other forms of rickets. The diagnosis is documented in the laboratory with hypocalcemia, hypophosphatemia, elevated urinary cyclic AMP, and elevated serum levels of parathyroid hormone, alkaline phosphatase, and 1,25(OH)$_2$D. Serum levels of 25-(OH)D are normal. Pretreatment concentrations of 1,25(OH)$_2$D have ranged from 54 to 966 pg/ml, and from 189 to 4,800 pg/ml during calciferol therapy. Confirmation of the diagnosis requires failure to respond to an adequate trial of supplemental calcium and normal replacement doses of calciferols for three months. Although recent studies have shown an important role for 1,25(OH)$_2$D in regulating immune function, it is not known if resistance to 1,25(OH)$_2$D *per se* in these subjects leads to increased morbidity or mortality from infectious diseases or immune abnormalities. Finally, endocrine studies in several affected patients have indicated that secretion of insulin, TSH, prolactin, growth hormone, and testosterone were either normal or correctable by restoration of eucalcemia with calcium infusions. One affected woman, who was successfully treated with high doses of 1,25(OH)$_2$D, has been reported to become pregnant and bear a normal child.

**Complications:** Bony deformities related to severity of unresponsiveness to calciferol therapy and delay in making diagnosis and initiating treatment.

**Associated Findings:** Alopecia, aminoaciduria, hypotonia, tetany, enamel hypoplasia of teeth that form post-natally.

**Etiology:** Although about one-half of the cases have been sporadic, several kindreds with parental consanguinity and multiple affected children suggests autosomal recessive inheritance.

**Pathogenesis:** This syndrome can be explained on the basis of end-organ resistance to the actions of 1,25(OH)$_2$D. The resistance is due to an abnormality in the receptor for 1,25(OH)$_2$D, or in a post-receptor process. All tissues appear to be affected, although the classic vitamin D target tissues (intestine, bone, and kidney) seem to be the ones primarily responsible for the clinical manifestations of rickets, hypocalcemia, and secondary hyperparathyroidism.

Based on studies in skin fibroblasts cultured from many of the reported kindreds, the lack of tissue responsiveness results from a heterogeneity of at least five defects: 1) Hormone-binding negative. Radioligand binding studies *in vitro* document total lack of functional receptor in about one-half of all the cases, although immunochemical assays demonstrate that a receptor polypeptide is synthesized. 2) Diminished quantity of receptor. Only 10% normal binding capacity with normal receptor affinity has been documented in two kindreds. 3) Reduced affinity of receptor for 1,25(OH)$_2$D. Two kindreds have shown a 20- to 30-fold reduction in the affinity constant for the hormone, but normal receptor binding capacity. 4) Failure of nuclear localization. Cells from two kindreds contained an apparently normal 1,25(OH)$_2$D receptor in soluble extracts, but studies with radioligand in intact cells show no detectable hormone localization to the nucleus as occurs with normal cells. 5) Nuclear uptake-positive resistance.

In three of the four kindreds with the pattern five, receptor elution from DNA-cellulose *in vitro* was abnormal, suggesting that the mutation involved the DNA binding domain of the receptor. Following successful cloning of the vitamin D receptor gene, two kindreds with this pattern have been found to have point mutations in the "zinc finger" loops in the DNA binding region of the receptor gene. Bioassay of fibroblasts from affected patients using induction of an enzyme, 25 hydroxy D-24-hydroxylase or inhibition of cell proliferation by 1,25(OH)$_2$D, has generally correlated well with clinical responsiveness to large doses of calciferols. In the one kindred where osteoblast-like cells were cultured from bone at the time of a surgical procedure, an identical cellular defect was found in the bone cells as was found with fibroblasts, confirming the validity of the fibroblast model system. Finally, lymphocytes, obtained by phlebotomy and activated in culture have also been found to be useful for 1,25(OH)$_2$D receptor and responsiveness studies, recapitulating observations made earlier with fibroblasts.

The frequency of alopecia in the more severely resistant patients suggests a key role for 1,25(OH)$_2$D and its receptor in hair follicle development and/or metabolism *in utero*.

**MIM No.:** 27742, *27744

**Sex Ratio:** Presumably M1:F1.

**Occurrence:** Several kindreds have been reported.

**Risk of Recurrence for Patient's Sib:**
See Part I, *Mendelian Inheritance.*

**Risk of Recurrence for Patient's Child:**
See Part I, *Mendelian Inheritance.*

**Age of Detectability:** Usually the condition is detected in the first 2–3 years of life. Amniotic fluid cells have receptors and a bioresponse to 1,25(OH)$_2$D, thus allowing for the possibility of prenatal diagnosis.

**Gene Mapping and Linkage:** VDR (vitamin D receptor) has been tentatively mapped to 12.

**Prevention:** None known. Genetic counseling indicated.

**Treatment:** In many cases, supplemental 1,25(OH)$_2$D, up to 20 μg daily, along with calcium replacement corrects the hypocalcemia, secondary hyperparathyroidism, and rickets. However, some patients are completely refractory to all forms of calciferol therapy. One unusual patient responded permanently to a short course of treatment with 24,25(OH)$_2$D. One totally resistant patient was treated successfully with prolonged intravenous calcium infusion over several months in the hospital; another was treated with long-term nocturnal calcium infusions.

**Prognosis:** With correction of rickets and hypocalcemia in patients who respond to therapy, the prognosis appears to be good for growth, development, and reproduction. However, the prognosis for totally resistant patients is uncertain.

**Detection of Carrier:** Unknown. Screening of sibs' or parents' fibroblasts *in vitro* has thus far failed to distinguish heterozygotes from normal persons.

**References:**
Marx SJ, et al.: A familial syndrome of decrease in sensitivity to 1,25-dihydroxyvitamin D. J Clin Endocrinol Metab 1978; 47:1303–1310.
Rosen JF, et al.: Rickets with alopecia: an inborn error of vitamin D metabolism. J Pediatrics 1979; 94:729–735. †
Eil C, et al.: A cellular defect in hereditary vitamin-D-dependent rickets type II: defective nuclear uptake of 1,25-dihydroxyvitamin D in cultured skin fibroblasts. New Engl J Med 1981; 304:1588–1591.
Marx SJ, et al.: Hereditary resistance to 1,25-dihydroxyvitamin D. Rec Prog Horm Res 1984; 40:589–615.
Gamblin GT, et al.: Vitamin D-dependent rickets type II: defective induction of 25-hydroxyvitamin D(3)-24-hydroxylase by 1,25-dihydroxyvitamin D$_3$ in cultured skin fibroblasts. J Clin Invest 1985; 75:954–960.
Hirst M, et al.: Vitamin D resistance and alopecia: a kindred with normal 1,25-dihydroxyvitamin D binding, but decreased receptor affinity for deoxyribonucleic acid. J Clin Endocrinol Metab 1985; 60:490–495.
Hochberg L, et al.: Does 1,25-dihydroxyvitamin D participate in the regulation of hormone release from endocrine glands. J Clin Endocrinol Metab 1985; 60:57–61.
Koren R, et al.: Defective binding and function of 1,25-dihydroxyvitamin D3 receptors in peripheral mononuclear cells of patients with end-organ resistance to 1,25-dihydroxyvitamin D. J Clin Invest 1985; 76:2012–2015.
Balsan S, et al.: Long-term nocturnal calcium infusions can cure rickets and promote normal mineralization in hereditary resistance to 1,25-dihydroxyvitamin D. J Clin Invest 1986; 77:1661–1667.
Delvin EE, et al.: Specific 1,25-hydroxycholecalciferol receptors and stimulation of 25-hydroxycholecalciferol-24R hydroxylase in human amniotic cells. Pediatr Res 1987; 21:432–435.
Hughes MR, et al.: Point mutation in the human vitamin D receptor gene associated with hypocalcemic rickets. Science 1988; 242:1702–1705.

EI002           **Charles Eil**

**Respiratory papillomatosis, juvenile**
*See PAPILLOMA VIRUS, CONGENITAL INFECTION*
**Restoril△, fetal effects**
*See FETAL BENZODIAZEPINE EFFECTS*

---

## RESTRICTIVE DERMATOPATHY      2757

**Includes:**
    Contractures-hyperkeratosis
    Hyperkeratosis-contracture syndrome
    Late fetal epidermal dysplasia, type II
    Skin, tight
    Tight skin contracture syndrome

**Excludes:**
    **Ichthyosis**
    **Skin, localized absence of** (0608)

**Major Diagnostic Criteria:** The combination of congenital contractures, hyperkeratosis, and characteristic facial appearance distinguishes this condition from other lethal skin defects.

**Clinical Findings:** All affected infants were born prematurely (31–33 weeks), with the majority of pregnancies complicated by polyhydramnios. Umbilical cords are often short. At birth, all skin had an abnormal appearance, ranging from a hard, shell-like structure, to a translucent, thin skin with prominent vasculature and diffuse erythema. Joint contractures were present in all cases, with knees, elbows, wrists, and ankles generally held in flexion. Fontanelles were wide in almost all cases. Facial anomalies consistently present included apparent hypertelorism; small nose; small, open mouth; micrognathia; and low-set, anomalous ears.

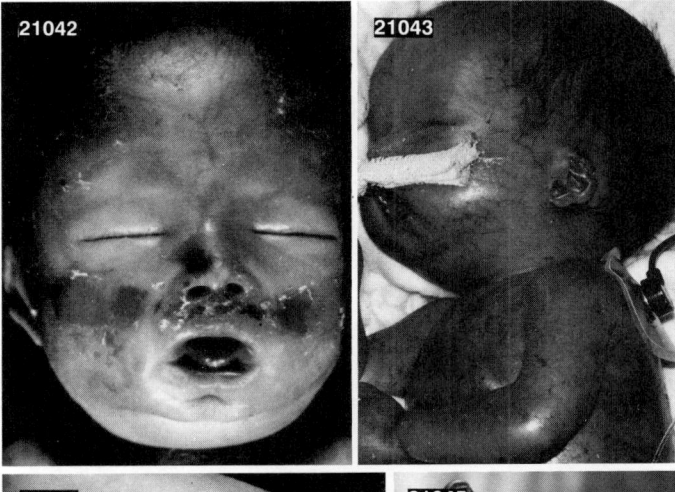
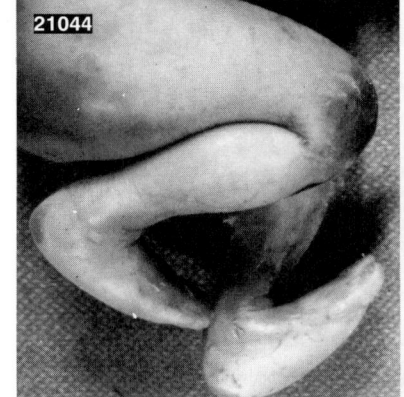
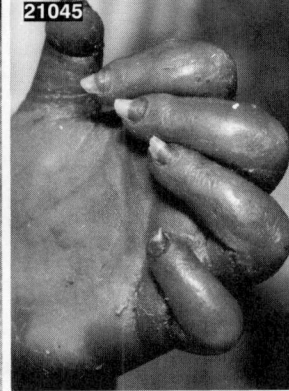

**2757-21042–44:** Restrictive dermatopathy: note small jaw and mouth; pinched, narrow nose; thick, dysplastic ears; relatively large head. All major joints are in a fixed, flexed position with tense, stiff skin which is sloughing in places. **21045:** Camptodactyly of fingers with long, thickened nails.

Occasional anomalies included ectropion and skeletal anomalies, including hypoplastic clavicles, scapulae, and/or long bones.

Histologically, the epidermis is thickened, with hyperkeratosis of the stratum corneum. The pilosebaceous structures and eccrine sweat glands were hypoplastic. The dermis was thinner than normal, with abnormal connective tissue. In cases of Hutterite ethnic origin, muscle immaturity was also noted.

**Complications:** Sepsis was frequently noted. Most of the facial features and contractures are thought to be secondary to fetal hypokinesia, which in turn may be caused by the tight skin.

**Associated Findings:** Present in only one case each were gyral immaturity, choanal atresia, submucous cleft palate, **Ductus arteriosus, patent** with patent foramen ovale, absent adrenal cortex, left ureter duplication, and **Hypospadias**.

**Etiology:** Autosomal recessive inheritance is suggested by the presence of the condition in sibs of both sexes.

**Pathogenesis:** Thought to be a biochemical defect leading to abnormal keratin formation and failure of differentiation.

**MIM No.:** 27521

**POS No.:** 3799

**Sex Ratio:** M1:F1

**Occurrence:** Several sibships have been reported, including two from a Mennonite kindred.

**Risk of Recurrence for Patient's Sib:**
See Part I, *Mendelian Inheritance.*

**Risk of Recurrence for Patient's Child:**
See Part I, *Mendelian Inheritance.*

**Age of Detectability:** At birth, although prenatal diagnosis by amniocentesis or fetoscopy with skin biopsy may be possible.

**Gene Mapping and Linkage:** Unknown.

**Prevention:** None known. Genetic counseling indicated.

**Treatment:** Unknown.

**Prognosis:** All affected infants died soon after birth.

**Detection of Carrier:** Unknown.

**Special Considerations:** There are slight differences in cases of Hutterite origin, e.g., intrauterine growth retardation in Hutterite cases, which may indicate heterogeneity. Furthermore, Stevenson et al (1987) reported a case with virtually identical histologic skin abnormalities, yet a phenotype that was quite different; in their case, the skin seemed to form a cocoon around the fetus, and the facial appearance was different. It is unknown whether this case represents a phenotypic continuum of the same defect, or a distinct condition with similar histology, but different biochemistry.

**References:**
Lowry RB, et al.: Congenital contractures, edema, hyperkeratosis, and intrauterine growth retardation. Am J Med Genet 1985; 22:531–543.
Schuur RE, et al.: A lethal ichthyosis variant with arthrogryposis. Am J Hum Genet 1985; A76.
Toriello HV: Restrictive dermopathy and report of another case. Am J Med Genet 1986; 24:625–629.
Witt DR, et al.: Restrictive dermopathy: a newly recognized autosomal recessive skin dysplasia. Am J Med Genet 1986; 24:631–648.
Stevenson RE, et al.: Cocoon fetus-fetal encasement secondary to ectodermal dysplasia. Proc Greenwood Genet Center 1987; 6:10–15.

T0007                                                    **Helga V. Toriello**

**Rethore syndrome**
  *See CHROMOSOME 9, TRISOMY 9p*
**Reticular dysgenesis**
  *See IMMUNODEFICIENCY, SEVERE COMBINED*
**Reticular pigmented anomaly of flexures**
  *See SKIN CREASES, RETICULATE PIGMENTED FLEXURES, DOWLING-DEGOS TYPE*
**Reticular pigmented dermatosis**
  *See ECTODERMAL DYSPLASIA, NAEGELI TYPE*
**Reticuloendotheliosis, nonlipoid**
  *See LETTERER-SIWE DISEASE*

**Reticulosis, familial histiocytic**
  *See LETTERER-SIWE DISEASE*
  *also IMMUNODEFICIENCY, RETICULOENDOTHELIOSIS WITH EOSINOPHILIA*
**Reticulosis, familial histocytic**
  *See LYMPHOHISTIOCYTOSIS, FAMILIAL ERYTHROPHAGOCYTIC*

---

## RETINA, AMAUROSIS CONGENITA, LEBER TYPE          0043

**Includes:**
   Amaurosis congenita of Leber, types I and II
   Amaurosis of retinal origin, congenital
   Dysgenesis neuroepithelialis retinae
   Pigmentary retinitis-congenital amaurosis
   Retinal aplasia, hereditary
   Retinal blindness, congenital
   Retinal degeneration, congenital
   Retinitis pigmentosa, congenital

**Excludes:**
   **Albinism, ocular** (0032)
   **Color blindness, total** (0198)
   **Nightblindness, congenital stationary, autosomal dominant** (3205)
   **Nightblindness, congenital stationary, autosomal recessive** (3204)
   **Nightblindness, congenital stationary, X-linked recessive** (0718)
   **Renal dysplasia-retinal aplasia, Loken-Senior type** (2687)
   **Retinitis pigmentosa** (0869)

**Major Diagnostic Criteria:** Congenital nystagmus and severely impaired visual function are detected in infancy. The ocular fundi are normal or show optic atrophy with pigmentary disturbances. The photopic and scotopic electroretinograms (ERGs) are severely decreased or extinguished.

**Clinical Findings:** Amaurosis congenita of Leber is a devastating visual disorder of infants first suspected on the basis of severely impaired visual function and congenital nystagmus. Visual acuity usually ranges from "counting fingers" at a few feet to "no light perception" with severe constriction of the visual field. A few patients show 20/100 vision or better and preserved visual fields. At birth, the fundi could appear normal or show optic atrophy, retinal vascular attenuation and pigmentary disturbances. With advancing age, some fundi remain normal while others show progressive changes with "bone spicule" formation, similar to that noted in retinitis pigmentosa. On ERG the photopic and scotopic responses are severely decreased or extinguished. High hyperopia has been suggested as a diagnostic criteria. A small percentage of patients develop cataracts and keratoconus in the second decade. The pleiotropy of the ocular manifestations suggests heterogeneity for isolated amaurosis congenita.

Amaurosis congenita is sometimes a part of a systemic disease associated with a variety of neurological, renal or skeletal abnormalities. The frequency of the association with neurological disorders is controversial. Alstrom found no neurological involvement in 175 patients. In a recent series, Nickel and Hoyt, found one of 31 with psychomotor retardation and 3 with cerebellar hypoplasia. On the other hand, Schappert-Kimmijser et al found 25% of 227 patients and Vaizey found 52% of 21 with significant psychomotor retardation and muscular hypotonia. In a recent series of 43 cases, 10 had mental retardation and other associated systemic findings were noted. Moore and Taylor (1984) have described 3 boys, including 2 brothers, with palsy of saccadic eye movements, suggestive of oculomotor apraxia.

**Complications:** Psychomotor retardation and muscular hypotonia are complications of visual deprivation during childhood development.

**Associated Findings:** *Ocular:* Enophthalmos is frequently present due to repetitive self digital stimulation of the globe causing atrophy of orbital fat. Documentation of decreased total axial length of the globe in a few cases and high hyperopia as a frequent finding suggest that microphthalmia is common. On occasion, macular colobomas and optic disc edema are found.

*Neurologic:* Psychomotor retardation, muscular hypotonia, enlargement of ventricles and cisterns, with widening of cerebral sulci. Cigarette paper scars and increased hyperextensability of skin suggestive of **Ehlers-Danlos syndrome** has been described in one pedigree.

**Etiology:** Autosomal recessive inheritance in some cases, but most are sporadic.

**Pathogenesis:** Undetermined. Some histopathological studies have shown a marked decrease or absence of rod and cone photoreceptors in the retina. Others show immature development or degeneration of photoreceptors.

**MIM No.:** *20400, *20410

**Sex Ratio:** M1:F1

**Occurrence:** Amaurosis congenita of Leber is the diagnosis in 10 to 18% of children in some institutions for the blind in the Netherlands.

**Risk of Recurrence for Patient's Sib:**
See Part I, *Mendelian Inheritance.*

**Risk of Recurrence for Patient's Child:**
See Part I, *Mendelian Inheritance.*

**Age of Detectability:** In infancy.

**Gene Mapping and Linkage:** Unknown.

**Prevention:** None known. Genetic counseling indicated.

**Treatment:** Referral to services for visually impaired to learn non-visual means of communication, and to maximize educational, vocational and social skills.

**Prognosis:** Normal life expectancy. Intelligence is usually normal. Visual handicap leads to a major change in lifestyle.

**Detection of Carrier:** Examination of relatives for evidence of the trait.

**Special Considerations:** Amaurosis congenita has been reported with various congenital renal abnormalities. The ophthalmological manifestations vary: some have congenital blindness with fundus findings consistent with amaurosis congenita while others have acquired visual disturbances with findings more consistent with retinitis pigmentosa. Some authors consider amaurosis congenita associated with renal disease as a separate condition (See **Renal dysplasia-retinal aplasia, Loken-Senior type**).

**References:**
Schappert-Kimmijser J, et al.: Amaurosis congenita (Leber). Arch Ophthalmol 1959; 61:211–218.
Vaizey MJ, et al.: Neurological abnormalities in congenital amaurosis of Leber. Arch Dis Child 1977; 52:399–402.
Nickel B, Hoyt CS: Leber's congenital amaurosis: is mental retardation a frequent associated defect. Arch Ophthalmol 1982; 100:1089–1092.
Foxman SG, et al.: Leber's congenital amaurosis and high hyperopia: a discrete entity. In: Henkind P, ed: Acta 25th International Congress of Ophthalmology. Philadelphia: Lippincott, 1983:85–88.
Moore AT, Taylor SI: A syndrome of congenital retinal dystrophy and saccade palsy - a subset of Leber's amaurosis. Br J Ophthalmol 1984; 68:421–431.
Carr RC, Heckenlively JR: Hereditary pigmentary degenerations of the retina. In: Duane TD, ed: Clinical ophthalmology. vol. 3. Philadelphia: Harper and Row, 1986:9–11.
Schroeder R, et al.: Leber's congenital amaurosis: retrospective review of 43 cases and a new fundus finding in two cases. Arch Ophthal 1987; 105:356–359.

WE035

**Avery H. Weiss**

## RETINA, CAVERNOUS HEMANGIOMA　3176

**Includes:**
　　Angiomas (cavernous) of CNS and retina
　　Cavernoma multiplex
　　Familial cavernous malformations of the CNS and retina
　　　(FCMCR)
　　Gass syndrome
　　Vascular formations, familial

**Excludes:**
　　Retinal capillary hemangioma
　　**Retina, Coats disease** (3135)
　　**Retinal telangiectasia-hypogammaglobulinemia** (0868)
　　**Sturge-Weber syndrome** (0915)
　　**Von Hippel-Lindau syndrome** (0995)

**Major Diagnostic Criteria:** Cavernous hemangiomas of the retina and/or central nervous system. The retinal lesions are best detected by indirect ophthalmoscopy and their diagnosis confirmed by retinal fluorescein angiography. The central nervous system lesions are seen on magnetic resonnance imaging (MRI) and computed tomographic (CT) scanning. These findings may be accompanied by cutaneous angiomas as well as by a family history of other affected individuals.

**Clinical Findings:** In 1940, Weskamp and Cotlier described a neuro-oculo-cutaneous syndrome that consists of cavernous angioma of the central nervous system, cavernous hemangioma of the retina or optic nerve head, and cutaneous angiomas. An affected individual may have either the intracranial or retinal hemangioma, or both. Cutaneous angiomas are a less consistent finding.

Cavernous hemangiomas of the retina rarely cause a decrease in vision and therefore are most often discovered on routine ophthalmoscopic exam. The lesion is usually unilateral and best detected with indirect ophthalmoscopy of the retinal periphery. It has the appearance of a sessile tumor composed of saccular aneurysms filled with dark venous blood looking like a group of grapes projecting from the inner retinal surface. These aneurysms rarely leak and therefore there is no surrounding exudate. Occasionally a lesion will be covered by a gray-white substance suggestive of fibrous tissue or an epiretinal membrane. Spontaneous vitreous hemorrhage can occur particularly from larger lesions. Fluorescein angiography typically shows delayed and incomplete filling of the lesion. Fluorescein caps are highly characteristic and result from sedimentation of the erythrocytes in the dependent portion of the aneurysms. Filling of the angioma is incomplete as a result of thrombosis of some of the aneurysms. The surrounding retinal vasculature appears normal.

The long-term course is believed to be nonprogressive, although some of these lesions clinically appear to have an increase in the size of their associated fibrovascular or epiretinal membranes. The visual acuity is usually unaffected; however, there is a visual field defect corresponding to the location of the retinal lesion.

Cavernous malformations of the central nervous system may be associated with headaches, seizures, or intracranial hemorrhage. There is a high risk of symptomatic disease. One study reporting on 54 patients with FCMCR found that 24 patients (44%) had seizures, while 26 patients (48%) had recognized intracranial hemorrhages of which nine died. These lesions are demonstratable on CT scanning, and may show calcification.

Cutaneous vascular anomalies have been described in association with this syndrome, although it is an inconsistent finding and may be absent in certain pedigrees. Cutaneous hemangiomas are the most typical lesion but a variety of vascular anomalies have been seen in patients with FCMCR.

**Complications:** Headaches, seizures, and strokes are seen in association with the intracranial hemangioma. The retinal lesion does not usually affect vision.

**Associated Findings:** Congenital malformation of the heart and great vessels, and **Nevus, blue rubber bleb nevus syndrome**.

**Etiology:** Autosomal dominant inheritance with high penetrance and variable expressivity.

**Pathogenesis:** This syndrome is considered by some to be a phakomatoses or hamartosis affecting the retina, central nervous system, and skin.

**MIM No.:** *14080

**Sex Ratio:** M1:F1

**Occurrence:** At least 54 patients have been reported from 17 families.

**Risk of Recurrence for Patient's Sib:**
See Part I, *Mendelian Inheritance.*

**Risk of Recurrence for Patient's Child:**
See Part I, *Mendelian Inheritance.*

**Age of Detectability:** These vascular tumors are felt to be congenital and therefore should be present at birth. A retinal cavernous hemangioma was discovered on ophthalmoscopic exam of a full-term baby who had subconjunctival hemorrhages after a prolonged delivery.

**Gene Mapping and Linkage:** Unknown.

**Prevention:** None known. Genetic counseling indicated.

**Treatment:** No treatment required for the retinal lesion.

**Prognosis:** Risk of intracranial hemorrhage or seizures; otherwise life span and lifestyle is unaffected.

**Detection of Carrier:** By fundus and dermatologic exam, as well as neuro-radiologic evaluation.

**Special Considerations:** All first degree relatives of the affected individual are at risk for harboring an intracranial cavernous malformation and should be evaluated. Presymptomatic diagnosis in affected relatives would allow genetic counseling and close monitoring so that prompt treatment can be instituted if symptoms occur.

**References:**

Weskamp C, Cotlier E: Angioma del cerebro y de la retina con malformaciones capilares de la piel. Arch Oftal Buenos Aires, 1940; 15:1–10.

Gass JD: Cavernous Hemangioma of the Retina. Am J Ophthalmol 1971; 71:779–814.

Lewis RA, et al: Cavernous haemangioma of the retina and optic disc: a report of three cases and a review of the literature. Br J Ophthalmol 1975; 59:422–434.

Goldberg RE, et al: Cavernous hemangioma of the retina. Arch Ophthalmology 1979; 97:2321–2324. †

Messmer E, et al: Cavernous hemangioma of the retina: immunohistochemical and ultrastructura observations. Arch Ophthalmol 1984; 102:413–418.

Schwartz AC, et al: Cavernous hemangioma of the retina, cutaneous angiomas, and intracranial vascular lesion by computed tomography and nuclear magnetic resonance imaging. Am J Ophthalmol 1984; 98:483–487.

Dobyns WB, et al: Familial cavernous malformations of the central nervous system and retina. Ann Neurol 1987; 21:578–583. *

SC067
JA016

**Bruce M. Schnall**
**Mohammad S. Jaafar**

---

## RETINA, COATS DISEASE       3135

**Includes:**
Coats disease
Leber miliary aneurysms
Primary retinal telangiectasia
Telangiectasia, congenital retinal

**Excludes:**
Neovascularization, diseases associated with peripheral
**Telangiectasia, Osler hemorrhagic** (2021)
White pupillary reflex (leukocoria), all causes

**Major Diagnostic Criteria:** A predominantly unilateral exudative retinopathy caused by a developmental anomaly (telangiectasia) of retinal vessels. Involved vessels show anomalous capillary branching and connections, capillary enlargement, wider than normal perivascular capillary-free zone, small caliber arterio-

venous shunts, and balloon-shaped structures resembling macroaneurysms on arterioles and even venules, typically in a nonanatomic field of the retina. In the early stages of the disease, the telangiectatic vessels may be invisible on ophthalmoscopy; in later stages, and after intraretinal edema and exudation, the telangiectatic vessels may be visible only using flurescein angiography.

**Clinical Findings:** Coats disease presents in a bimodal age distribution depending on the extent, severity, and size of blood vessels involved. About two-thirds of patients are diagnosed between 18 months and 18 years of age. Up to one-third of patients are 30 years or older before the disease is discovered. Some patients present in the first two years of life, and the disease tends to be more severe in patients younger than four years of age at diagnosis. The peak presentation of diagnosis occurs towards the end of the first decade of life. About three-quarters of patients are males. Approximately one-fourth of cases are discovered on routine ophthalmoscopic examination. Leukocoria (white pupil) is the presenting sign in about one-third of patients, especially infants, and strabismus in about one-sixth of patients.

Disease progression, with subretinal exudation and secondary retinal detachment, correlates with the size of the vessels in the involved vascular bed and the number of retinal quadrants involved. In two-thirds of patients the telangiectasias involve only one quadrant, and in the other third they involve two quadrants; three and four quadrant involvement is rare and associated with poor visual prognosis. The temporal retina is affected preferentially. Subretinal exudation from peripheral lesions tends to pool into the macular area as an elevated mound of yellow material and has been confused with a choroidal tumor or infection or with retinoblastoma. Accurate diagnosis requires thought to the source of the exudation and indirect ophthalmoscopy with 360 degree scleral depression. Cystoid macular edema may develop in patients with either posterior or peripheral telangiectasia and cause decreased visual acuity. Spontaneous regression of the telangiectasia is rare except in advanced stages of the disease.

**Complications:** Serous and exudative retinal detachment; periretinal fibroproliferation; neovascular glaucoma (with total retinal detachment) and cataracts in long-standing disease.

**Associated Findings:** Isolated cases have been reported with a variety of non-specific and inconsistent findings including facial angioma, progressive facial hemiatrophy, **Nephritis-deafness (sensorineural), hereditary type** and **Nevus, epidermal nevus syndrome.** Peripheral retinal vasculopathy similar to Coats disease has been reported in association with **Retinitis pigmentosa** and in a single patient with **De Lange syndrome.** Bilateral Coats-like reaction has been reported in multiple members of a family with muscular dystrophy, deafness, and mental retardation (Small, 1968). Adults with Coats disease have been reported to have elevated serum cholesterol levels.

**Etiology:** An isolated embryologic malformation.

**Pathogenesis:** Unknown. The formation of incompetent and leaky retinal telangiectatic vessels causes the clinical manifestations of the disease.

**MIM No.:** 21635

**Sex Ratio:** In children probably M9:F1; in older patients close to M3:F1.

**Occurrence:** Probably less than 1:5,000.

**Risk of Recurrence for Patient's Sib:** Usually not increased.

**Risk of Recurrence for Patient's Child:** Usually not increased.

**Age of Detectability:** The majority of patients are seen in the first two decades of life, but the disease may be seen at birth or as late as the seventh decade of life.

**Gene Mapping and Linkage:** Unknown.

**Prevention:** None known. Genetic counseling indicated.

**Treatment:** Early treatment of the abnormal vessels by cryotherapy or photocoagulation (argon laser or xenon arc) as soon as the diagnosis is made, in order to prevent the inexorable development of subretinal exudation, macular edema, and exudative retinal detachment. Retinal reattachment surgery is indicated in cases with total exudative retinal detachment. In cases with vitreoretinal traction, vitrectomy, including retinotomy and drainage of subretinal fluid, may be indicated.

**Prognosis:** Good in cases with limited involvement and early treatment, as long as the foveal vasculature is not involved.

**Detection of Carrier:** Affected individuals are detected by indirect ophthalmoscopy and/or fluorescein angiography.

**References:**

Small RG: Coats' disease and muscular dystrophy. Trans Am Acad Ophthalmol Otolaryngol 1968; 72:225–231.

Folk JC, et al: Coats' disease in a patient with Cornelia de Lange syndrome. Am J Ophthalmol 1981; 91:607.

Ridley ME, et al: Coats' disease: evaluation of management. Ophthalmology 1982; 89:1381–1387.

Siegelman S: Coats' disease. In: Retinal diseases: pathogenesis, laser therapy and surgery. Boston: Little Brown, 1984:332–349. *

Gass RDM: Primary or congenital retinal telangiectasis (Leber's miliary aneurysm, Coats' syndrome). In: Stereoscopic Atlas of Macular Diseases. St. Louis: C. V. Mosby, 1987:384–389. *

KA045
TR009

Hassan M. Kattan
Elias I. Traboulsi

**Retina, coloboma**
*See EYE, MICROPHTHALMIA/COLOBOMA*

## RETINA, COMBINED CONE-ROD DEGENERATION 0201

**Includes:**

Cone-rod degeneration, progressive
Cone-rod dystrophy (degeneration)
Retinitis pigmentosa, atypical (some forms)

**Excludes:**

**Choroideremia** (0925)
**Color blindness, blue monocone-monochromatic** (0195)
**Color blindness, total** (0198)
Cone dystrophies (pure)
Drug-induced retinopathies (e.g., thioridazine, chloroquine)
Hyperornithinemia-gyrate atrophy
**Nightblindness, congenital stationary**
**Retina, fundus albipunctatus** (0399)
**Retina, fundus flavimaculatus** (0400)
**Retinitis pigmentosa** (0869)
Retinitis punctata albescens

**Major Diagnostic Criteria:** A heterogeneous group of genetic retinal disorders characterized by a history of progressive loss of the psychophysiologic functions associated with cones to an earlier or more severe degree than rods. Thus, losses of central visual acuity, of color vision, and of tolerance to bright daylight (evidenced as photodysphoria or hemeralopia) are proportionately more obvious than difficulty with night (dim-light) or peripheral vision. Color vision under standard illumination, central and peripheral perimetry, dark adaptometry, and electroretinogram (ERG) may be needed if anamnesis is equivocal. Pigmentary changes in the ocular fundus are not mandatory, for or exclusive of, the diagnosis.

**Clinical Findings:** The term *cone-rod dystrophy* may be confusing, because currently there is no standard nomenclature for genetic disorders of the retina. One usage of the linear order of these attributive nouns emphasizes the clinician's history that the patient loses central or color vision earlier than night or peripheral vision; the other derives from responses to electroretinography. The cone system is tested by light-adapting the retina so that rods are light-saturated and thus will not respond to the flash stimulus, resulting in a characteristic waveform. After the retina has been dark adapted for at least 25 minutes, a dim (blue or white) flash below the cone threshold elicits rod-mediated function. When both the cone and the rod components of these elicited waves are abnormal, the more severely affected is listed first: combined cone-rod dystrophy.

Diminished central vision is usually associated with retinal pigment epithelial alterations within the central 30 degrees of the ocular fundi. Evidence of diffuse cone involvement includes sensitivity/discomfort in daylight (photodysphoria), altered color vision, abnormal contrast sensitivity and central visual field sensitivity, elevated thresholds or altered regeneration times on cone dark adaptation, and reduced amplitudes and prolonged implicit times on ERG. Evidence of diffuse rod involvement is often more subtle and includes peripheral visual losses, abnormally elevated rod thresholds on dark adaptation, and reduced amplitudes and altered implicit times on the rod phases of the ERG.

Combined cone-rod dystrophies must be differentiated from congenital and historically stationary disorders affecting either the cone systems alone (e.g., the cone monochromacies and rod monochromacy) or apparently both the photoreceptors and the neuroepithelial integration (e.g., the congenital stationary night blindnesses and fundus albipunctatus), since both groups may also appear to alter acuity, color, and night visual functions. In addition, they must be distinguished from progressive degenerations of both photoreceptor systems in which the rods are more severely afflicted (rod-cone dystrophies), one subset of which has characteristic ophthalmoscopic retinal changes (the **Retinitis pigmentosa**).

The onset may appear from childhood to late adulthood, with reasonable symmetry of the age of onset among affected members of the same family, especially in recessive variants. The rate of progression and the ultimate severity, as monitored by threshold visual fields or by ERG, are more variable among families with autosomal dominant transmission.

Individuals with autosomal recessive cone-rod dystrophy usually have a decrease in visual acuity during the first two decades of life and may have characteristic "bull's-eye" foveal lesions, which should be differentiated from drug toxicities (e.g., chloroquine), other lipofuscin-storage disorders, or late-onset neuronal ceroid lipofuscinoses.

**Complications:** Unknown.

**Associated Findings:** *Ocular*: posterior cortical cataracts among older individuals; rarely, vitreous syneresis and cells.

*Extraocular*: may occur as part of **Bardet-Biedl syndrome**.

**Etiology:** Autosomal dominant or autosomal recessive inheritance. Numerous sporadic cases have been reported.

**Pathogenesis:** Unknown.

**MIM No.:** *12097

**Sex Ratio:** M1:F1

**Occurrence:** Undetermined. Probably less than one-tenth as common as **Retinitis pigmentosa**.

**Risk of Recurrence for Patient's Sib:**
See Part I, *Mendelian Inheritance*.

**Risk of Recurrence for Patient's Child:**
See Part I, *Mendelian Inheritance*.

**Age of Detectability:** Usually during the second or third decades; later onset does occur.

**Gene Mapping and Linkage:** CORD (cone rod dystrophy (autosomal dominant)) is unassigned.

**Prevention:** None known. Genetic counseling indicated.

**Treatment:** Primary intervention is unavailable. Low-vision aids and visual rehabilitation are appropriate.

**Prognosis:** Visual impairment varies from moderate to considerably less than legal blindness. Most affected individuals cannot maintain a driver's license and do require magnification for reading.

**Detection of Carrier:** At-risk relatives may be examined for minor manifestations or early onset of disease.

**References:**

Krill AE, et al.: The cone degenerations. Doc Ophthalmol 1973; 35:1–80.

Francois J, et al.: Progressive cone dystrophies. Ophthalmologica 1976; 173:81–101.

Grey RHB, et al.: Bull's eye maculopathy with early cone degeneration. Br J Ophthalmol 1977; 61:702–718.

Ferrell RE, et al.: Autosomal dominant cone-rod dystrophy: a linkage study with 17 biochemical and serological markers. Am J Med Genet 1981; 8:363–369.

Marmor MF, et al.: Retinitis pigmentosa: a symposium on terminology and methods of examination. Ophthalmology 1983; 80:126–131.

Rabb MF, et al.: Cone-rod dystrophy: a clinical and histopathologic report. Ophthalmology 1986; 93:1443–1451.

Ripps H, et al.: Progressive cone dystrophy. Ophthalmology 1987; 94:1401–1409.

LE039                                          **Richard Alan Lewis**

## RETINA, CONE DYSTROPHY, X-LINKED                3228

**Includes:** Cone dystrophy, X-linked with tapetal-like sheen

**Excludes:**
   **Color blindness, blue monocone-monochromatic** (0195)
   **Nightblindness, Oguchi type** (0740)

**Major Diagnostic Criteria:** Evidence of major cone dysfunction on electroretinogram (ERG) with normal or only mildly subnormal rod mediated responses.

**Clinical Findings:** Young patients may not be symptomatic. Patients usually present within the first to third decades of life with decreased visual acuity, defective color vision, and myopia. Vision loss may begin in childhood but is not congenital as is the case in **Color blindness, blue monocone-monochromatic**. The visual acuity may be initially as good as 20/25, but in later years may drop to counting fingers or hand motion as macular changes occur. Patients may complain of photophobia or glare sensitivity and may say their vision is best at twilight. Color vision may show either red-green or blue-yellow defects and eventually scotopization on anomaloscope testing similar to that seen in achromatopsia. Nystagmus is not a reported feature.

In all cases the ERG at the earliest age tested has shown generalized loss of cone mediated responses with normal or mildly subnormal rod responses. The EOG light-to-dark ratio may be supernormal early in the disorder but becomes subnormal later in life. Dark adaptometry demonstrates elevation of the cone portion of the curve. Pinckers (1987) believes that the disorder begins as a peripheral cone disorder (abnormal cone ERG with relative preservation of central cone function, including visual acuity) that progresses to a diffuse cone disease (including loss of central cone function). As disease progresses the macular regions develop atrophy of the pigment epithelium and choriocapillaris. At least one form demonstrates a golden-yellow tapetal-like sheen throughout the retina. This sheen appeared to fade somewhat after dark adaptation (the Mizuo-Nakamura phenomenon).

**Complications:** Central or pericentral scotomas develop and enlarge with passing decades. Eventually patients become legally blind, usually from loss of central visual acuity to 20/200 or worse in the better seeing eye. Rod ERG function may be normal or subnormal. It is likely that rod function loss is progressive.

**Associated Findings:** None known.

**Etiology:** X-linked recessive inheritance.

**Pathogenesis:** Unknown.

**MIM No.:** 30402, 30403

**Sex Ratio:** Theoretically M1:F0. Because of carrier manifestations, some women have had significant but usually mild features of the disorder.

**Occurrence:** One of the rarest forms of cone dystrophy, although Pinckers (1987) believes that, because of lack of recognition, X-linked cone dystrophy may be more common than previously realized.

**Risk of Recurrence for Patient's Sib:**
   See Part I, *Mendelian Inheritance.*

**Risk of Recurrence for Patient's Child:**
   See Part I, *Mendelian Inheritance.*

**Age of Detectability:** The electroretinogram has been shown to be abnormal by the end of the first decade of life. The ERG may show abnormality earlier.

**Gene Mapping and Linkage:** COD1 (cone dystrophy 1 (X-linked)) has been provisionally mapped to Xp21.1-p11.3.

**Prevention:** None known. Genetic counseling indicated.

**Treatment:** Routine ophthalmological care, with consideration of low vision aids to regain ability to read as visual acuity decreases. Consider special glasses, such as Corning 550 CPF, which protect rods from excessive light adaptation, and for many patients provide comfort. However, such glasses have not been shown to alter course of the disease.

**Prognosis:** Legal blindness by mid-life. Intelligence, life span, and health are otherwise normal.

**Detection of Carrier:** Carriers usually have normal visual acuity (20/30 or better) but may have subnormal cone ERG responses and abnormal color vision.

**Special Considerations:** Heterogeneity probably exists for X-linked cone dystrophy. It is uncertain whether the disorder described by Heckenlively and Weleber (1986) is the same as that described by Pinckers et al (1981). Heckenlively and Weleber's patients demonstrated a striking tapetal-like sheen. Jacobson et al (1989) reported nine affected males, three of whom showed a bronze-green tapetal-like sheen, and six female carriers from a large four generation family with X-linked cone dystrophy. Fleischman and O'Donnell (1981), described a black kindred with what they call X-linked incomplete achromatopsia. Pinckers believes that Fleischman and O'Donnell's family instead probably represents X-linked cone dystrophy, but that family had gross pathology of the macula not present in Heckenlively's family.

**References:**
Fleischman JA, O'Donnell FE: Congenital X-linked incomplete achromatopsia: evidence for slow progression, carrier fundus findings, and possible genetic linkage with glucose-6-phosphate dehydrogenase locus. Arch Ophthalmol 1981; 99:468–472.

Pinckers A, Timmerman GJMEN: Sex-difference in progressive cone dystrophy I. Ophthalmic Paediatr Genet 1981; 1:17–24.

Pinckers A, et al.: Sex-difference in progressive cone dystrophy II. Ophthalmic Paediatr Genet 1981; 1:25–36. * †

Heckenlively JR, Weleber RG: X-linked recessive cone dystrophy with tapetal-like sheen. Arch Ophthalmol 1986; 104:1322–1328. * †

Pinckers A, Deutman AF: X-linked cone dystrophy: an overlooked diagnosis? Internat Ophthalmol 1987; 10:241–243.

Weleber RG, Eisner A: Cone degeneration ("bull's-eye dystrophies") and color vision defects. In: Newsome DA, ed: Retinal dystrophies and degenerations. New York: Raven Press, 1988:233–256.

Jacobson DM, et al.: X-linked progressive cone dystrophy: clinical characteristics of affected male and female carriers. Ophthalmol 1989; 96:885–895.

WE042                                          **Richard G. Weleber**

**Retina, congenital detachment of**
*See RETINA DYSPLASIA*

## RETINA, CONGENITAL HYPERTROPHY OF RETINAL
## PIGMENT EPITHELIUM                              3134

**Includes:**
   CHRPE, isolated
   CHRPE in adenomatous polyposis (Intestinal polyposis, type III)
   Congenital hypertrophy of the retinal pigment epithelium (CHRPE)
   Retina, pigmentation of, congenital grouped

**Excludes:**
   Adenoma of the retinal pigment epithelium
   Choroidal nevus
   **Intestinal polyposis, type III** (0536)
   Melanocytoma of choroid

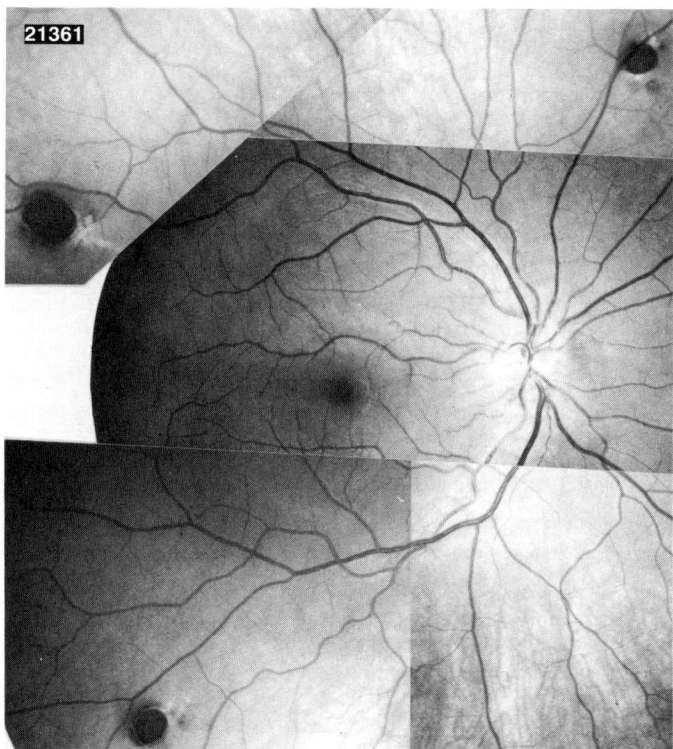

3134-21361: Retina, congenital hypertrophy of the retinal pigment epithelium.

### Retina, grouped hypertrophy of retinal pigment epithelium (3203)

**Major Diagnostic Criteria:** Brown to black, flat, usually solitary, round to oval, sharply demarcated lesions of the ocular fundus at the level of the retinal pigment epithelium.

**Clinical Findings:** Isolated patches of congenital hypertrophy of retinal pigment epithelium (CHRPE) range from isolated dots less than 100 microns up to several disc diameters in size and are densely hyperpigmented (brown to black); they have smooth, sharp margins, and are usually surrounded by a subtle, but sharply defined depigmented halo. These are typically located in the peripheral fundus. With age, small and/or multiple lacunae may develop within the pigmented portion and may enlarge to become confluent and leave a sharp scleral patch in older adults. The frequency of a solitary lesion of any size in one eye in the general population is probably between 1:10 and 1:5. Congenital grouped pigmentation of the retina or "beartracks" (because they resemble animal tracks) are usually unilateral, typically sectoral, pigmented oval patches of CHRPE occurring as clumps of three or four, larger lesions occurring more peripheral to smaller clusters.

The histopathology of both isolated CHRPE and of congenital grouped pigmentation of the retina consists of hypertrophic retinal pigment epithelial cells with agenesis or atrophy of the overlying outer retina.

**Complications:** CHRPE does not affect vision unless it involves the fovea.

**Associated Findings:** Bilateral multiple but isolated and unclustered patches of CHRPE of various sizes and configurations have been found recently to be specific and sensitive markers of adenomatous polyposis in families with familial adenomatous polyposis (see **Intestinal polyposis, type III**). A total of more than three lesions in one or both eyes of an individual at risk indicates probable inheritance of the disease. The pigmented lesions have been observed as early as three months of age (presumably present at birth) and are due apparently to the pleiotropic effects of one gene responsible for familial adenomatous polyposis. These retinal pigment epithelial lesions have not been observed in hereditary colon cancer.

**Etiology:** Undetermined in isolated CHRPE and in congenital grouped pigmentation of the retina.

**Pathogenesis:** Unknown.

**MIM No.:** *17530

**Sex Ratio:** M1:F1

**Occurrence:** Small, solitary, and isolated patches of CHRPE are estimated to occur in 1:10 to 1:5 normal individuals.

**Risk of Recurrence for Patient's Sib:** Unknown.

**Risk of Recurrence for Patient's Child:** Unknown.

**Age of Detectability:** At birth.

**Gene Mapping and Linkage:** Unknown.

**Prevention:** None known. Genetic counseling indicated.

**Treatment:** None necessary.

**Prognosis:** Excellent for vision.

**Detection of Carrier:** Retinal examination with indirect ophthalmoscope.

**Special Considerations:** Because multiple patches of CHRPE are an excellent clinical marker in families with familial adenomatous polyposis, ocular examination with dilated indirect ophthalmoscopy is indicated in families of patients with adenomatous polyposis. If the lesions are present, close monitoring for the development of intestinal polyps and later colon cancer is imperative.

**References:**
Kurz GH, Zimmerman LE: Vagaries of the retinal pigment epithelium. Int Ophthalmol Clin 1962; 2:441–464.
Buettner H: Congenital hypertrophy of the retinal pigment epithelium. Am J Ophthalmol 1975; 79:177–189.
Shields JA, Tso MOM: Congenital grouped pigmentation of the retina: a histopathologic description and report of a case. Arch Ophthalmol 1975; 93:1153–1155.
Blair NP, Trempe CL: Hypertrophy of the retinal pigment epithelium associated with Gardner's syndrome. Am J Ophthalmol 1980; 90:661–667.
Lewis RA, et al.: The Gardner syndrome: significance of ocular features. Ophthalmology 1984; 91:916–925.
Traboulsi EI, Krush AJ, Gardner EJ, et al.: Prevalence and importance of pigmented ocular fundus lesions in Gardner's syndrome. New Engl J Med 1987; 316:661–667.
Baker RH, et al.: Hyperpigmented lesions of the retinal pigment epithelium in familial adenomatous polyposis. Am J Med Genet 1988; 31:427–435.
Lyons LA, et al.: A genetic study of Gardner syndrome and congenital hypertrophy of the retinal pigment epithelium. Am J Hum Genet 1988; 42:290–296.

TR009                                                      **Elias I. Traboulsi**

## RETINA, FLECKED KANDORI TYPE                            2110

**Includes:**
> Fleck retina of Kandori
> Kandori fleck retina
> Red-fleck retina

**Excludes:**
> **Ocular drusen** (0734)
> **Retina, fundus albipunctatus** (0399)
> **Retina, fundus flavimaculatus** (0400)

**Major Diagnostic Criteria:** Typical fundus changes, mild delays in reaching normal dark adaptation final threshold, and normal electrophysiologic testing.

**Clinical Findings:** Characteristic lesions are noted in the equatorial regions of the fundus. These are sharply defined flecks of varying size and shape ranging from the diameter of a retinal vessel to 1.5 times the size of the optic disc. The color has been described by Kandori as "dirty yellow". There are none of the dark pigment spicules seen in primary retinal pigmentary diseases. The disc, macula, vessels and posterior are normal. Fluorescein angiography has shown the flecks to act like pigment epithelial defects, with fluorescence appearing early in the arterial phase, remaining constant in size without leakage into the surrounding retina. Patients followed since 1958 have had no changes in their lesions. This differs from **Retina, fundus flavimaculatus** in which lesions change with time, originally blocking fluorescein and later with destruction of pigment epithelium transmitting fluorescein.

**Complications:** Unknown.

**Associated Findings:** None known.

**Etiology:** One patient was the product of a consanguinous marriage, but the total number of patients is too small to be certain if this is an autosomal recessive disorder.

**Pathogenesis:** No pathologic specimens have been studied but this appears to be a disorder of the retinal pigment epithelium.

**MIM No.:** 22899

**Sex Ratio:** M1:F1

**Occurrence:** Undetermined but presumably rare.

**Risk of Recurrence for Patient's Sib:**
See Part I, *Mendelian Inheritance.*

**Risk of Recurrence for Patient's Child:**
See Part I, *Mendelian Inheritance.*

**Age of Detectability:** In the second decade of life.

**Gene Mapping and Linkage:** Unknown.

**Prevention:** None known. Genetic counseling indicated.

**Treatment:** Night vision aids.

**Prognosis:** Non-progressive or minimally progressive.

**Detection of Carrier:** Unknown.

**References:**
Kandori F: Very rare cases of congenital non-progressive night blindness with fleck retina. Jpn J Ophthalmol 1959; 13:384–386.
Krill AE, Klien BA: Flecked retina syndrome. Arch Ophthalmol 1965; 74:496–508.
Duke-Elder S: System of ophthalmology, vol. 10. St. Louis: C.V. Mosby, 1967:629 only.
Kandori F, et al.: Fleck retina. Am J Ophthalmol 1972; 73:673–685.

W0003                                    **Mitchel L. Wolf**

---

## RETINA, FUNDUS ALBIPUNCTATUS                 0399

**Includes:**
  Fleck retina disease (one form)
  Fundus albipunctatus

**Excludes:**
  Basal laminar drusen
  Canthaxanthine retinopathy
  Cystimers
  Oxalate retinopathy
  Progressive albipunctate dystrophy
  **Retina, flecked Kandori type** (2110)
  Retinitis punctata albescens
  Uyemura syndrome
  Vitamin A deficiency

**Major Diagnostic Criteria:** Typical fundus findings with nightblindness that becomes normal with time and a normal ERG after appropriate adaptation.

**Clinical Findings:** Multiple yellow-white dots, sparing the macula, are seen deep in the retina and are associated with congenital stationary nightblindness. The dots are most dense in the posterior pole and are more scattered towards the periphery. The size of the spots has been described as that of a second order arteriole,

and they are fairly uniform. The retinal vessels and the optic disk remain normal. The dots may fade as the patient advances in age.

Visual functions are well preserved; acuity is normal, color vision is normal and visual fields are full.

Dark adaptometry shows a marked delay in both cone and rod function so that the normal cone threshold, usually achieved at 10 minutes after a standard bleach, is delayed for up to 1 hour and the final rod threshold may not be achieved for 3 hours with a normal of 30 minutes. Electroretinography parallels the course of adaptation so that a normal ERG is recordable after appropriate adaptation but only a cone-dominated ERG is seen if done in a routine fashion. The EOG has a reduced light rise but this, too, becomes normal after prolonged dark adaptation. Kinetic studies of pigment regeneration show marked delays in both rods and cones.

A variant form with faster, but delayed, regeneration has also been reported.

**Complications:** Unknown.

**Associated Findings:** None known.

**Etiology:** While most fleck retina disease is autosomal recessive, this specific form may follow a pattern of autosomal dominant inheritance (Krill, 1977).

**Pathogenesis:** All evidence points to a defect in rate of pigment regeneration with a disturbance in the receptor outer segment-pigment epithelial complex. No histologic examinations have yet been reported.

**MIM No.:** 13688

**Sex Ratio:** M1:F1

**Occurrence:** Undetermined but presumed rare.

**Risk of Recurrence for Patient's Sib:**
See Part I, *Mendelian Inheritance.*

**Risk of Recurrence for Patient's Child:**
See Part I, *Mendelian Inheritance.*

**Age of Detectability:** First decade of life.

**Gene Mapping and Linkage:** Unknown.

**Prevention:** None known. Genetic counseling indicated.

**Treatment:** Night vision pocketscope.

**Prognosis:** Normal life span.

**Detection of Carrier:** Unknown.

**Special Considerations:** The appearance of white dots in the fundus has been reported in vitamin A deficiency and generalized oxalosis. However, these abnormalities have not been seen in fundus albipunctatus patients.

**References:**
Carr RE, et al.: Visual pigment kinetics and adaptation in fundus albipunctatus. Doc Ophthol Proc Ser 1974; 4:193–204.
Franceschetti A, et al.: Chorioretinal heredodegenerations. Springfield: Charles C Thomas, 1974.
Carr RE, et al.: Fluorescein angiography and vitamin A and oxalate levels in fundus albipunctatus. Am J Ophthalmol 1976; 82:549–558.
Krill AE: Hereditary retinal and choroidal diseases: flecked retina diseases, vol 2. Hagerstown, MD: Harper & Row, 1977:739–819.
Marmor MF: Fundus albipunctatus: a clinical study of the fundus lesions, the physiologic defect and the vitamin A metabolism. Doc Ophthal 1977; 43:277–302.
Margolis S, et al.: Variable expressivity in fundus albipunctatus. Ophthalmol 1987; 94:1416–1422.

W0003                                    **Mitchel L. Wolf**

## RETINA, FUNDUS FLAVIMACULATUS  0400

**Includes:**
>  Fundus flavimaculatus with macular degeneration
>  Juvenile macular degeneration, hereditary
>  Macular degeneration and fundus flavimaculatus
>  Stargardt disease

**Excludes:**
>  **Ocular drusen** (0734)
>  **Retina, flecked Kandori type** (2110)
>  **Retina, fundus albipunctatus** (0399)

**Major Diagnostic Criteria:**  Characteristic ophthalmoscopic appearance. Fluorescein angiographic finding may be helpful in diagnosis.

**Clinical Findings:**  This is a group of retinal diseases that include yellow flecks at the level of the pigmented epithelium. Stargardt originally described patients with macular disease in 1909. Even though he included both patients with extensive retinal involvement and patients with little involvement outside the macula, the term "Stargardt disease" is generally used for the more limited macular disease. Franceschetti, in describing his fundus flavimaculatus patients, included another subgroup that had only widespread flecks and no macular involvement; thus, visual acuity was good. His patients with macular involvement and widespread flecks appears to be identical to those described by Stargardt.

Patients are subdivided according to age of onset, retinal involvement and electro-physiological findings:

*Group I is the pure form* of fundus flavimaculatus. It is found in adults, often on routine examination. Despite widespread flecks, these patients initially have good visual acuity and color vision, and normal electro-physiological findings. some patients later develop macular involvement and poor vision.

*Group IIa patients have a childhood onset* of the disease, which remains limited to within the retinal arcades. The ERG and EOG remain normal.

*Group IIb patients also have an early onset of disease, but have widely scattered flecks.* There is early depression of the EOG and photopic ERG. Extensive progressive chorioretinal atrophy involving the macula causes these patients to be more disabled than Group IIa patients.

There have been two families in which Group I disease occurred in the first generation, and severe Group IIb disease occurred in the second generation. This suggests that the Group I disease is the heterozygous form of a subgroup of Group IIb disease.

**Complications:**  Macular degeneration; severe progressive visual loss in some cases.

**Associated Findings:**  None known.

**Etiology:**  Autosomal recessive inheritance is most common for Groups IIa and IIb. Several dominant pedigrees have been reported for Groups I and IIb. Segregation of severe and mild forms of the disease by generation suggests that Group I may be a

heterozygous form of a subgroup of Group IIb. Many Group IIb patients have children and parents with normal retinas. In one series 10/27 cases were classified as familial, so sporadic occurrences likely account for the majority of cases.

**Pathogenesis:**  Histologic studies of eyes from three Group IIb patients have shown accumulation of a lipofuscin-like substance in the pigmented epithelial cells. One Group I patient has shown enlarged RPE cells, but no lipofuscin.

**MIM No.:**  23010

**Sex Ratio:**  M1:F1

**Occurrence:**  At least 50 cases have been documented.

**Risk of Recurrence for Patient's Sib:**
>  See Part I, *Mendelian Inheritance.*

**Risk of Recurrence for Patient's Child:**
>  See Part I, *Mendelian Inheritance.* Autosomal dominant pedigrees have been quite rare.

**Age of Detectability:**  Group I: Uncertain, since usually found on routine exams; visual loss can occur as late as age 65.
  Groups IIa and IIb: Visual loss usually occurs between 8 and 30 years of age.

**Gene Mapping and Linkage:**  Unknown.

**Prevention:**  None known. Genetic counseling indicated.

**Treatment:**  Unknown.

**Prognosis:**  Normal life span; variable vision loss according to subgroup.

**Detection of Carrier:**  By fundus exam.

**References:**

Klein BA, Krill AE: Fundus flavimaculatus, clinical, functional and histopathologic observations. Am J Ophthalmol 1967; 64:3–23.

Merin S, Landau J: Abnormal findings in relatives of patients with juvenile hereditary macular degeneration (Stargardt's disease). Ophthalmologica 1970; 161:1–10.

Krill AE: Krill's hereditary retinal and choroidal diseases. Clinical characteristics. vol. 2. Hagerstown: Harper & Row, 1972. †

Cibis GW, et al.: Dominantly inherited macular dystrophy with flecks (Stargardt). Arch Ophthalmol 1980; 98:1785–1789.

Moloney JBM, et al.: Retinal function in Stargardt's disease and fundus flavimaculatus. Am J Ophthalmol 1983; 96:57–65. *

McDonnel PJ, et al.: Fundus flavimaculatus without maculopathy: a clinicopathologic study. Ophthalmology 1986; 93:116–119.

KI021                                                             **Jane D. Kivlin**

**Retina, giant cyst of**
  *See RETINOSCHISIS*

---

## RETINA, GROUPED HYPERTROPHY OF RETINAL PIGMENT EPITHELIUM  3203

**Includes:**
>  Bear tracks
>  Melanosis retinae
>  Melanosis retinae, congenital grouped
>  Nevoid pigmentation of the retina

**Excludes:**
>  Choroidal nevus
>  **Fetal rubella syndrome** (0384)
>  Malignant melanoma
>  Pigment proliferation secondary to trauma or hemorrhage
>  **Retina, congenital hypertrophy of retinal pigment epithelium** (3134)
>  Sector retinitis pigmentosa

**Major Diagnostic Criteria:**  An asymptomatic congenital disorder occurring most frequently unilaterally. Diagnosis of the condition is usually made during a routine ophthalmoscopic exam.

  Characteristically, the lesion consists of several well defined flat, gray to black colored areas, more often confined to one sector of the fundus. Each pigmented lesion may range in size from 0.1 to 3.0 mm in diameter occurring in groups of 3 to 30 foci. The

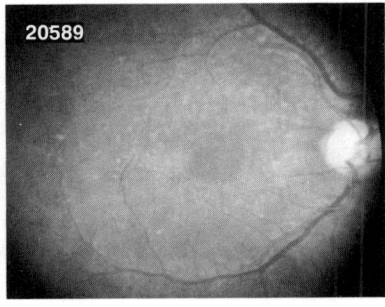
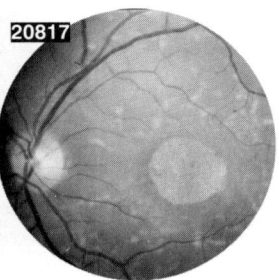

**0400-20589:** Multiple hypopigmented areas of varying shape; visual acuity is 20/100. **20817:** Fundus flavimaculatus with macular degeneration (Stargardt disease).

lesion is commonly larger in the retinal periphery with the surrounding retina being normal. The similarity of grouped hypertrophy of the retinal pigment epithelium to animal footprings has caused them to be termed "bear tracks."

**Clinical Findings:** Grouped hypertrophy of the retinal pigment epithelium should not be confused with **Retina, congenital hypertrophy of retinal pigment epithelium**. In the latter condition, a singular lesion, often surrounded by a thin hypopigmented ring, occurs frequently with depigmented lacunae within the pigmented lesion. The histologic appearance of the two conditions is similar; one being multifocal and the other unifocal.

It is important to note that grouped hypertrophy of the retinal pigment epithelium is a benign lesion. The lesions are nonprogressive and not associated with decrease in vision, visual field defects or electroretinogram change. In addition, no definite associated systemic conditions have been reported.

**Complications:** Unknown.

**Associated Findings:** None known.

**Etiology:** Unknown.

**Pathogenesis:** Unknown.

**Sex Ratio:** M1:F1

**Occurrence:** Undetermined but presumably very uncommon.

**Risk of Recurrence for Patient's Sib:** Presumably low.

**Risk of Recurrence for Patient's Child:** Presumably low.

**Age of Detectability:** At birth.

**Gene Mapping and Linkage:** Unknown.

**Prevention:** None known. Genetic counseling indicated.

**Treatment:** None needed.

**Prognosis:** No association with visual loss. Lesions are nonprogressive.

**Detection of Carrier:** Unknown.

**References:**
Tower P: Congenital grouped pigmentation of the retina. Arch Ophthalmol 1948; 39:536.
Purcell JJ, Shields JA: Hypertrophy with hyperpigmentation of the retinal pigment epithelium. Arch Ophthalmol 1975; 93:1122.
Shields JA, Tso MO: Congenital grouped pigmentation of the retina. Arch Ophthalmol 1975; 93:1153.
Deutman AF: Focal retinal pigment epithelial dystrophies. In: Krill AE, Archer DB, eds.: Krill's hereditary retinal and choroidal diseases, vol 2. Hagerstown: Harper and Row, 1977.
Newsome DA: Pigment epithelial dystrophies. In: Newsome DA, ed.: Retinal dystrophies and degenerations. New York: Raven Press, 1988.

P0025
BE026

**Scott L. Portnoy**
**Donald R. Bergsma**

**Retina, gyrate atrophy**
*See GYRATE ATROPHY OF THE CHOROID AND RETINA*

---

## RETINA, HYALOIDEORETINAL DEGENERATION OF WAGNER 0479

**Includes:**
>Hyaloideoretinal degeneration of Wagner
>Wagner syndrome

**Excludes:**
>Arthro-ophthalmopathy, hereditary, progressive, Stickler type (0090)
>Arthro-ophthalmopathy, Weissenbacher-Zweymuller variant (2424)
>Clefting syndromes
>Retina, vitreoretinopathy, familial exudative (3133)
>Retinal detachments, familial
>Vitreoretinopathy, familial exudative

**Major Diagnostic Criteria:** Mild to moderate myopia, retinal dystrophy, presenile cataracts, vitreous veils, in the absence of retinal detachments.

**Clinical Findings:** Mild nightblindness has its onset in early childhood and is slowly progressive. A mild myopic prescription may be required during early school years, but the visual status will remain stable until the age of 30 to 40 years, when posterior cortical and subcapsular cataracts develop, which in recent years have been successfully removed in the presence of fluid vitreous, vitreous strands and peripheral circumferential vitreous bands. Complications in previous generations included vitreous loss, postoperative hypotony and glaucoma, but not retinal detachments. Only recently has the focus shifted to the progressive retinal dystrophic changes seen in these patients with the development of ring scotomata and night blindness and ultimate blindness in their sixties. On slit lamp examination there is obvious vitreous liquefaction in early life. On fundus examination one observes an at times contiguous, at others interrupted circumferential vitreous band and, emanating from this ring are avascular strands floating freely in the vitreous cavaty. Large areas of chorioretinal dystrophy originating from the disc in a helicoidal pattern are obvious in the older patient.

**Complications:** Large angle kappa with temporal dragging of the macula in some patients, presenile cataracts, glaucoma, retinal dystrophy.

**Associated Findings:** None known.

**Etiology:** Autosomal dominant inheritance.

**Pathogenesis:** The absence of normal vitreous structures suggests an abnormality of type IV collagen. These are, however, not pathognomonic for the condition.

**MIM No.:** *14320

**Sex Ratio:** M1:F1

**Occurrence:** Unknown.

**Risk of Recurrence for Patient's Sib:**
See Part I, *Mendelian Inheritance.*

**Risk of Recurrence for Patient's Child:**
See Part I, *Mendelian Inheritance.*

**Age of Detectability:** Usually not clinically evident until nightblindness is noted in childhood. Mild myopia becomes evident during the early school years, vitreous changes are present during those early years, but not diagnosed unless searched for.

**Gene Mapping and Linkage:** Unknown.

**Prevention:** None known. Genetic counseling indicated.

**Treatment:** Cataract extraction and glaucoma management as indicated. While results have been good, the ultimate vision loss from retinal dystrophic changes cannot be prevented.

**Prognosis:** Life expectancy is normal and there are no extraocular complications. The visual prognosis is guarded.

**Detection of Carrier:** The diagnosis is obvious in all affected if slit lamp and fundus examinations are performed. There have been no skipped generations.

**Special Considerations:** This disease should not be confused with **Arthro-ophthalmopathy, hereditary, progressive, Stickler type**. The patients in Wagner's original family do not have extraocular features and retinal detachments have not occured in any of the affected members. X-ray examinations for epiphyseal changes were normal in five personally examined members, who also had no systemic findings of clefting of the hard or soft palate, nor deafness or subjective joint disease.

This condition has generated an extensive literature and considerable debate, and there is, in fact, no concensus that true Wagner syndrome has ever existed beyond the members of Wagner's original family. A good overview of the debate appears in McKusick's *Mendelian inheritance in Man.*

**References:**
Wagner H: Ein bisher unbekanntes Erbleiden des Auges (Degeneratio hyaloideo-retinalis hereditaria), beobachtet im Kanton Zurich. Klin Monatsbl Augenheilkd 1938; 100:840–857.

Maumenee IH, et al: The Wagner syndrome versus hereditary arthroophthalmopathy. Tr Am Ophth Soc 1982; 80:349–365.

MA054                                                    **Irene H. Maumenee**

## RETINA, MACULAR DEGENERATION, VITELLIRUPTIVE 0622

**Includes:**
    Best disease
    Central cystoid dystrophy
    Exudative detachment of retina, central
    Macular degeneration, polymorphic vitelliruptive
    Macular dystrophy, atypical vitelliform
    Macular pseudocysts
    Vitelliform cysts of macula, congenital
    Vitelliform macular dystrophy
    Vitelliruptive macular degeneration, hereditary

**Excludes:**
    Central serous retinopathy
    Foveomacular vitelliruptive dystrophy, adult type (GASS)
    Progressive foveal dystrophy
    Pseudovitelliform macular degeneration

**Major Diagnostic Criteria:** Typical appearing lesion in younger members of a family with macular degeneration of autosomal dominant inheritance. Abnormal electrooculogram with normal electroretinogram.

**Clinical Findings:** The age of onset of the macular lesion is usually between 5–15 years, but it has been seen as early as one week of age. The typical features of the lesion are seen in early cases. It has been described as looking like "an egg with sunny-side up," at a somewhat later stage like a "scrambled egg," or like a "cystic lesion filled with exudates and precipitates, sometimes with a definite level, resembling a hypopyon." The early lesion is usually yellow or orange in color, elevated, has sharp borders and is frequently almost circular in outline. However, it eventually loses its cystic appearance and the exudate-like material disappears. Rarely, there may be multiple vitelliform lesions in the posterior pole areas. A macular degeneration may then follow which is indistinguishable from other types of macular degenerations. Visual acuity, particularly in the early stages of the disease, is usually better than anticipated from the appearance of the macula. However, deep retinal hemorrhage may occur, probably from the choriocapillaris, with eventual hypertrophic scar formation so that vision can be reduced early in life.

Visual acuity typically remains good until the 4th decade when a secondary macular degeneration frequently occurs. On the other hand, secondary intraretinal macular changes may be minimal and fairly good visual acuity may be maintained throughout life. Visual fields are normal except for central scotoma when acuity is abnormal. Dark adaptation and ERG are usually normal but minimal abnormality has been noted. The electrooculogram is always abnormal.

**Complications:** Intraretinal macular degeneration, macular hemorrhage.

**Associated Findings:** Hyperopia, esotropia, amblyopia (strabismus). Best disease has co-existed with so-called pattern dystrophies of the retinal epithelium in the same families

**Etiology:** Autosomal dominant inheritance with many examples of reduced penetrance and expressivity.

**Pathogenesis:** Three early pathologic reports were from patients who were elderly with extensive choroidal and retinal changes. A recent report from a 29-year-old in the scrambled egg stage showed generalized retinal pigment epithelial (RPE) abnormalities with accumulation of lipofuscin not only in the RPE but also in subretinal macrophages and free in the choroid. Frangieh et al (1982) described the histopathology of the eyes of an 80-year-old lady and postulated that the disease starts in the neurosensory retina, and that the RPE changes are secondary. The electrooculogram is markedly abnormal in all cases tested, even in younger members with early stages of the disease. This finding suggests that a diffuse abnormality of the pigment epithelium exists in this disease even though only the macular area shows ophthalmoscopic changes. With red light, which penetrates the retinal pigment epithelium, the typical lesion of younger subjects is observed. On the other hand, blue light, which does not penetrate beyond the retinal receptors, does not show the typical lesion. Therefore early lesions are probably external to the pigment epithelium. Blue light shows the typical features of the secondary macular degeneration in older subjects indicating its intraretinal location. Fluorescence is not observed with very early lesions; however, after an uncertain period of time, fluorescence characteristic of defective pigment epithelium is seen in the macula and is dependent on the size and position of the original lesion.

**MIM No.:** *15370, *15384

**Sex Ratio:** M1:F1

**Occurrence:** Several large kindreds have been reported, and one study in Sweden traced 250 cases to a single 17th Century source.

**Risk of Recurrence for Patient's Sib:**
    See Part I, *Mendelian Inheritance.*

**Risk of Recurrence for Patient's Child:**
    See Part I, *Mendelian Inheritance.*

**Age of Detectability:** Usually detected between 5–15 years of age, but occasionally may not be noted until the third or even beginning of the fourth decade of life.

**Gene Mapping and Linkage:** Best disease itself has not been mapped, although 6q25 has been suggested as the possible locus (Rivas et al, 1986).

VMD1 (vitelliform macular dystrophy, atypicall) has been provisionally mapped to 8q.

**Prevention:** None known. Genetic counseling indicated.

**Treatment:** Unknown.

**Prognosis:** Life span normal, guarded for vision.

**Detection of Carrier:** A carrier with no macular abnormality can be identified by an abnormal EOG.

**Special Considerations:** Patients with typical vitelliform fusions have been recently reported who have normal EOGs. These patients are not part of a familial disease, have visual loss associated with the lesions, and represent a different entity which has been called "pseudovitelliform degeneration." A late onset dominant disease with small lesions and a mildly abnormal EOG has also been described.

*Macular dystrophy, atypical vitelliform* (Ferrell et al, 1983) has a similar phenotype, and may be simply an allelic mutation.

**References:**
Braley AE, Spivey BE: Hereditary vitelline macular degeneration: a clinical and functional evaluation of a new pedigree with variable expressivity and dominant inheritance. Arch Ophthalmol 1964; 72:743–762.
Krill AE, et al.: Hereditary vitelliruptive macular degeneration. Am J Ophthalmol 1966; 61:1405–1415.
Deutman AF: Electro-oculography in families with vitelliform dystrophy of the fovea: detection of the carrier state. Arch Ophthalmol 1969; 81:305–316.
Frangieh GT, et al.: A histopathologic study of Best's macular dystrophy. Arch Ophthalmol 1982; 100:1115–1121.
Weingeist TA, et al.: Hystopathology of Best's macular dystrophy. Arch Ophthalmol 1982; 100:1108–1114.
Ferrell RE, et al.: Linkage of atypical vitelliform macular dystrophy (VMD-1) to the soluble glutamate pyruvate transaminase (GPT1) locus. Am J Hum Genet 1983; 35:78–84.
Godel V, et al.: Best's vitelliform macular dystrophy. Acta Ophthalmolgica 1986; 175(suppl):1–31. *
Grieffre G, Lodato G: Vitelline dystrophy and pattern dystrophy of the retinal pigment epithelium: concomitant presence in a family. Br J Ophthalmol 1986; 70:526–532.
Rivas FE, et al.: De novo del(6)(q25) associated with macular degeneration. Ann Genet 1986; 29:42–44.
Yoder FE, et al.: Linkage studies of Best's macular dystrophy. Clin Genet 1988; 34:26–30.

W0003                                                    **Mitchel L. Wolf**

**Retina, pigmentation of, congenital grouped**
See *RETINA, CONGENITAL HYPERTROPHY OF RETINAL PIGMENT EPITHELIUM*
**Retina, tapetochoroidal dystrophy**
See *CHOROIDEREMIA*

## RETINA, VITREORETINOPATHY, FAMILIAL EXUDATIVE 3133

**Includes:**

Criswick-Schepens syndrome
Exudative vitreoretinopathy

**Excludes:**

**Arthro-ophthalmopathy, hereditary, progressive, Stickler type** (0090)
Eales disease
**Retina, Coats disease** (3135)
**Retina, hyaloideoretinal degeneration of Wagner** (0479)
**Retinopathy of prematurity** (0872)
**Retinoschisis** (0871)

**Major Diagnostic Criteria:** In the later stages of this ocular disease: organized vitreous membranes and prominent vitreoretinal adhesions, temporal dragging and heterotopia of the macula, peripheral subretinal and intraretinal exudates, and localized retinal detachment. Fluorescein angiography shows disorganization of the architecture and abrupt cessation of the retinal capillary network in the temporal periphery. Fluorescein angiography is essential in establishing the diagnosis of mild cases and asymptomatic family members.

**Clinical Findings:** The fundus changes in advanced familial exudative vitreoretinopathy (FEVR) are most similar to those of **Retinopathy of prematurity** (ROP), with vitreoretinal adhesions, abnormalities of the retinal vasculature, and temporal dragging of the macula. The differentiating features include normal birth weight, absence of a history of prematurity and oxygen administration in FEVR, and the familial (dominant) occurrence of FEVR. Myopia is present in 80% of patients with ROP but is infrequent in FEVR. The severity of the vitreoretinal changes is extremely variable in FEVR and a majority of patients may have normal visual acuity and ocular examination and may only be detected by abnormalities of the peripheral retinal vasculature on wide-field (60–90 degrees) fluorescein angiography; other patients, sometimes in the same family, will have severe bilateral disease with retinal detachment, macular dragging, and poor vision. Both eyes are affected, sometimes with marked asymmetry of the retinal pathology. The disease is generally stable or slowly progressive and may manifest as early as three months of age or be diagnosed as late as 57 years. The severity of the disease does not correlate with advancing patient age. Subretinal exudates are seen in about 15–20% of patients.

**Complications:** Late complications include rubeosis irides, secondary glaucoma, secondary cataract, and band keratopathy. A peripheral "mass-like" appearance has sometimes led to unnecessary enucleation in the mistake diagnosis of **Retinoblastoma.**

**Associated Findings:** Platelet aggregation defects have been detected in all affected members of two families reported by Chaudhuri et al (1983).

**Etiology:** Autosomal dominant inheritance with variability in expression. X-linked inheritance postulated (though unlikely) to be possible in the original report by Criswick and Schepens (1969).

**Pathogenesis:** A defect in peripheral maturation of retinal capillaries has been postulated.

**MIM No.:** *13378, 22723.

**Sex Ratio:** M1:F1

**Occurrence:** About 140 cases have been reported in the world literature; from the United States, Japan, South America, Europe, and (unpublished reports) from the Middle East.

**Risk of Recurrence for Patient's Sib:**
See Part I, *Mendelian Inheritance.*

**Risk of Recurrence for Patient's Child:**
See Part I, *Mendelian Inheritance.*

**Age of Detectability:** Depends on severity of retinal changes. May be as early as three months or as late as the fifth decade. Mean age at diagnosis in one series was ten years.

**Gene Mapping and Linkage:** Unknown.

**Prevention:** None known. Genetic counseling indicated.

**Treatment:** Value of prophylactic cryotherapy is questionable. Vitrectomy and peeling of epiretinal membranes may be performed in very selected cases.

**Prognosis:** Generally good if retinal involvement is mild at initial diagnosis, because of the slowly progressive nature of the disease process.

**Detection of Carrier:** Fluorescein angiography of peripheral fundus should be performed in parents and sibs of affected individuals, and detects silent carriers of the disease.

**References:**
Criswick VG, Schepens CL: Familial exudative vitreoretinopathy. Am J Ophthalmol 1969; 68:578–594.
Gow CLB, Oliver GL: Familial exudative vitreoretinopathy: an expanded view. Arch Ophthalmol 1971; 86:150–155.
Laqua H: Familial exudative vitreoretinopathy. Graefe's Arch Clin Exp Ophthalmol 1980; 213:121–133.
Ober RR, et al.: Autosomal dominant exudative vitreoretinopathy. Br J Ophthalmol 1980; 64:112–120.
Tasman W, et al.: Familial exudative vitreoretinopathy. Trans Am Ophthalmol Soc 1981; 79:211–226. *
Miyakubo H, et al.: Retinal involvement in familial exudative vitreoretinopathy. Ophthalmologica 1982; 185:125–135.
Van Nauhuys CE: Dominant exudative vitreoretinopathy and other vascular developmental disorders of the peripheral retina. The Hague: W Junk Publishers, 1982.
Chaudhuri PR, et al.: Familial exudative vitreoretinopathy associated with familial thrombocytopathy. Br J Ophthalmol 1983; 67:755–758.

TR009                                   **Elias I. Traboulsi**

**Retinal anlage tumor**
See *JAW, NEUROECTODERMAL PIGMENTED TUMOR*
**Retinal anomalies-corneal hypesthesia-deafness-unusual facies**
See *CORNEAL ANESTHESIA-RETINAL DEFECTS-UNUSUAL FACIES-HEART DEFECT*
**Retinal aplasia, hereditary**
See *RETINA, AMAUROSIS CONGENITA, LEBER TYPE*
**Retinal aplasia-cystic kidneys-Joubert syndrome**
See *JOUBERT SYNDROME*
**Retinal blindness, congenital**
See *RETINA, AMAUROSIS CONGENITA, LEBER TYPE*
**Retinal choristoma**
See *JAW, NEUROECTODERMAL PIGMENTED TUMOR*
**Retinal cyst, congenital**
See *RETINOSCHISIS*
**Retinal degeneration, congenital**
See *RETINA, AMAUROSIS CONGENITA, LEBER TYPE*

## RETINAL DYSPLASIA 0866

**Includes:**

Falciform retinal fold
Retina, congenital detachment of
Retinal dysplasia, Reese type
Retinal nonattachment and falciform detachment

**Excludes:**

**Eye, vitreous, persistent hyperplastic primary** (0994)
**Retina, Coats disease** (3135)
**Retina, vitreoretinopathy, familial exudative** (3133)
**Retinoblastoma** (0870)
**Retinopathy of prematurity** (0872)

**Major Diagnostic Criteria:** Retinal dysplasia is a pathologic term referring to the abnormal differentiation of retinal elements, as a result of either genetic or environmental factors. The major histopathologic feature of this disorder is the formation of rosettes by the immature photoreceptor segments. Neural cells forming the rosettes are variably differentiated and are arranged in palisading or radiating formations about a central lumen or space. The retina may appear ophthalmoscopically normal, or may show a variety of topographic abnormalities. The electroretinogram is abnormal and parallels the severity of retinal involvement.

**Clinical Findings:** Retinal dysplasia may be unilateral or bilateral and may appear as an isolated finding or in association with other ocular or systemic abnormalities. The clinical findings are determined primarily by the extent of retinal involvement and usually become evident by early childhood. There is a manifest disturbance of visual function in one or both eyes; nystagmus, strabismus, and abnormal head postures may develop. The retinal findings vary from an isolated fold to total disruption of the retinal structures. The folds generally extend from the optic nerve temporally to the retinal periphery, thus usually involving the macula, and resulting in loss of central vision. In more severe cases, there is marked retinal disruption and cicatrization, with a white mass protruding into the vitreous cavity. Such instances must be differentiated from other conditions causing a white retinal mass.

Visual loss is usually marked but nonprogressive, since retinal damage occur *in utero* and appears not to progress after birth. Visual function and prognosis may, however, be affected by associated ocular abnormalities (*vide infra*).

In genetically determined cases, there may be a positive family history of early visual loss.

**Complications:** The most common complication is visual loss or blindness. Nystagmus and strabismus may occur as a result of visual impairment and macular heterotopia.

**Associated Findings:** Associated ocular abnormalities may include microphthalmos, megalocornea, **Eye, anterior segment dysgenesis**, anterior chamber angle abnormalities with secondary glaucoma, cataract, colobomas of the optic disc or choroid, and optic nerve hypoplasia.

Retinal dysplasia may also occur in association with multiple systemic abnormalities as **Chromosome 13, trisomy 13, Chromosome 18, trisomy 18, Walker-Warburg syndrome**, and **Norrie disease**. There is no correlation between the severity of systemic abnormalities and the extent of retinal dysplasia.

**Etiology:** Retinal dysplasia may occur as an isolated defect, or as a part of many malformation syndromes or chromosomal associated diseases. Autosomal dominant, autosomal recessive, and X-linked recessive inheritance has been reported. Retinal dysplasia has been reported with maternal use of LSD, and has been induced experimentally *in utero* in animal models by radiation, viral infection, and vitamin A deficiency.

**Pathogenesis:** Retinal dysplasia is felt to be a non-specific response of the retina to a variety of noxious influences during various, perhaps critical, periods of its development. Since the retinal pigment epithelium (RPE) is a major organizing factor in the development of normal retinal architecture, any detachment of the sensory retina from the underlying RPE during development results in its disorganization and in dysplasia. Such dysplastic changes do not occur with disruption of the normal sensory retina-pigment epithelium interface after maturation is complete.

**MIM No.:** 18007, *22190, 26640, 31255

**Sex Ratio:** Presumably M1:F1, except in cases of X-linked inheritance.

**Occurrence:** Undetermined.

**Risk of Recurrence for Patient's Sib:**
See Part I, *Mendelian Inheritance.*

**Risk of Recurrence for Patient's Child:**
See Part I, *Mendelian Inheritance.*

**Age of Detectability:** Usually present at birth, but often not clinically evident until several months or years later.

**Gene Mapping and Linkage:** Unknown.

**Prevention:** Avoidance of fetal exposure to LSD, irradiation, and other teratogens. Genetic counseling is indicated.

**Treatment:** Unknown.

**Prognosis:** Poor for vision. Life expectancy and general development depends on associated systemic findings.

**Detection of Carrier:** Visually insignificant mild retinal fold changes have been observed in female carriers of the X-linked recessive form. Iris stromal changes (decreased pigmentation and lack of normal surface markings) were also reported in female carriers, but the significance of these anterior segment changes is unclear as they have not been observed in affected males.

**Special Considerations:** The term retinal dysplasia was once used to designate a specific syndrome of multiple congenital anomalies involving the brain, heart, limbs, mouth and eye, in which the dysplastic retina was one of the most consistent findings. It has since become evident that most of the affected children, including those reported by Reese and diagnosed as having "Reese retinal dysplasia", probably had **Chromosome 13, trisomy 13** or **Walker-Warburg syndrome**. Retinal dysplasia is a pathologic term which is now generally used to refer to the retinal lesion rather than to a specific syndrome, except when inherited as an isolated condition.

*The authors wish to thank Lorenz E. Zimmerman for his suggestions in the preparation of this article.*

**References:**

Reese AB, Straatsma BR: Retinal dysplasia. Am J Ophthalmol 1958; 45:199–211.

Silverstein AM, et al.: The pathogenesis of retinal dysplasia. Am J Ophthalmol 1971; 72:13–21. * †

Lahav M, Albert DM: Clinical and histopathologic classification of retinal dysplasia. Am J Ophthalmol 1973; 75:648–667. * †

Fulton AB, et al.: Human retinal dysplasia. Am J Ophthalmol 1978; 85:690–698. †

Godel V, Goodman RM: X-linked recessive primary retinal dysplasia: clinical findings in affected males and carrier females. Clin Genet 1981; 20:260–266.

Pagon RA, et al.: Autosomal recessive eye and brain anomalies: Warburg syndrome. J Pediatr 1983; 102:542–546.

F0013                                          **David J. Forster**
TR009                                          **Elias I. Traboulsi**
P0024                                          **Robert C. Polomeno**

**Retinal dysplasia, Reese type**
*See RETINAL DYSPLASIA*
**Retinal dystrophy associated with spinocerebellar ataxia**
*See OLIVOPONTOCEREBELLAR ATROPHY, DOMINANT WITH RETINAL DEGENERATION*
**Retinal dystrophy, posterior pole-congenital total hypotrichosis**
*See RETINOPATHY-HYPOTRICHOSIS SYNDROME*

---

**RETINAL FOLD**          **0867**

**Includes:**
Falciform detachment, congenital
Hydrocephaly-retinal nonattachment-falciform fold
Microcephaly-microphthalmia-falciform retinal folds
Retinal septum, congenital

**Excludes:**
Acquired retinal folds secondary to iatrogenic etiologies
Acquired retinal folds secondary to inflammatory disease
Acquired retinal folds secondary to intraocular foreign bodies
**Chromosome 13, trisomy 13** (0168)
**Retina, vitreoretinopathy, familial exudative** (3133)
**Retinopathy of prematurity** (0872)
Rhegmatogenous retinal detachments
**Walker-Warburg syndrome** (2869)

**Major Diagnostic Criteria:** Tractional retinal fold running from the disk to the periphery.

**Clinical Findings:** The folds occur in otherwise normal eyes and are occasionally bilateral. Ophthalmoscopically, they are seen as elevated gray folds or ridges, running from the optic nervehead

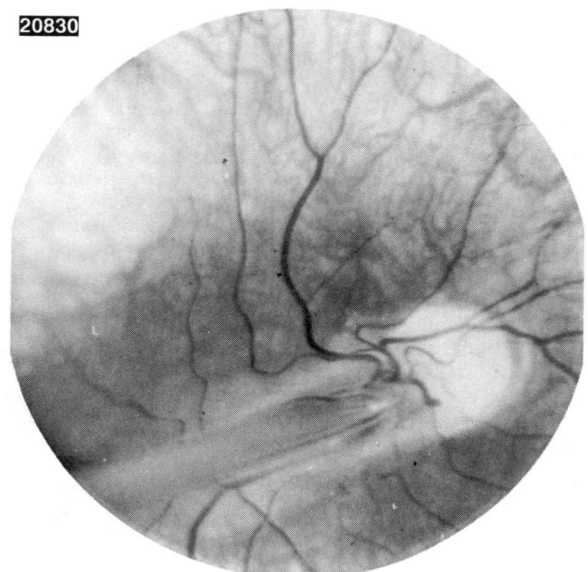

**0867-20830:** Retinal fold.

into the retinal periphery where they commonly expand in a gray fan over the peripheral retina and the pars plana. These folds occur most commonly in the lower temporal quadrant of the retina and, occasionally, send strands forward to the posterior capsule of the lens. Often, there is considerable disturbance in the retinal pigment epithelium along the borders of the fold, and there may be traction or detachment at various places along its course. Remnants of the hyaloid arterial system may be adherent to the surface of the fold. The normal retinal blood vessels appear to be pulled up into this fold, and vessels may be absent from other areas of the retina. Visual acuity is minimal from birth, and the first signs of the condition are strabismus, nystagmus, or, if the folds are bilateral, poor vision.

**Complications:** Cataract formation, traction retinal detachments, and phthisis bulbi have been reported to occur rarely.

**Associated Findings:** **Hydrocephaly**, microphthalmia, congenital dislocation of the hip, mental retardation, **Microcephaly**, hypogenitalism, cryptorchidism.

**Etiology:** May represent a persistence of the posterior primary vitreous, and although this condition may be associated with persistence of the anterior hyperplastic vitreous, it is distinctly different. Pseudogliomas, congenital retinal nonattachment, and retinal dysplasia, have been reported in the second eye of some patients.

In complex syndromes with congenital falciform folds, there are many associated congenital defects in addition to the retinal fold. **Retina, Coats disease** is characterized by retinal telangiectasia and more widespread retinal detachment without a discrete isolated fold. Any inflammatory disease, especially toxoplasmosis and toxocariasis, can cause a retinal fold. In this case, however, the folds run from the area of the granuloma to the retinal periphery and usually do not insert at the disk unless the granuloma is in the peripapillary region.

Retinal falciform folds are characteristic of grade III **Retinopathy of prematurity** (retrolental fibroplasia). Although controversial, some investigators believe that falciform folds may occasionally represent a form of retinopathy of prematurity that occurs without a history of oxygen exposure, prematurity, or low birth weight.

Retinal folds may be the result of retinal detachment surgery secondary to scleral buckling or intraocular gas. Falciform retinal folds may also be a sign of **Retina, vitreoretinopathy, familial exudative**.

Many cases are sporadic, but autosomal dominant, autosomal recessive, and X-linked recessive inheritance has been reported. A syndrome consisting of congenital hydrocephalus, microophthalmia, retinal detachment, or retinal falciform fold, which may or may not be distinct from **Walker-Warburg syndrome**, appears to exist and to be transmitted as an autosomal recessive trait (Warburg, 1978).

**Pathogenesis:** The folds may be caused by a localized persistence of the primary vitreous with adherence of the retina. Other possibilities include an overgrowth of a localized area of the retina, or a difference in the growth rate of the two layers of the optic cup.

**MIM No.:** 18006

**Sex Ratio:** M1:F1

**Occurrence:** Undetermined.

**Risk of Recurrence for Patient's Sib:** Unknown.

**Risk of Recurrence for Patient's Child:** Unknown.

**Age of Detectability:** At birth.

**Gene Mapping and Linkage:** Unknown.

**Prevention:** None known. Genetic counseling indicated.

**Treatment:** Unknown.

**Prognosis:** The condition is static and generally shows no progression. Vision in the involved eye remains static unless the rare complications of detachment or phthisis bulbi occur.

**Detection of Carrier:** Unknown.

**References:**

Mann I: Developmental abnormalities of the eye. Philadelphia: J.B. Lippincott, 1957:200.
Godel V, et al.: Primary retinal dysplasia transmitted as a chromosome-linked recessive disorder. Am J Ophthalmol 1978; 86:221–227.
Warburg M: Hydrocephaly, congenital retinal nonattachment, and congenital falciform fold. Am J Ophthalmol 1978; 85:88–94.
Godel V, et al.: Falciform form of the retina. Can J Ophthalmol 1979; 14:192–194.
Jarmas AL, et al.: Microcephaly, microphthalmia, falciform retinal folds and blindness. Am J Dis Child 1981; 135:930–933.
Young ID, et al.: Microcephaly, microphthalmos, and retinal folds: report of a family. J Med Genet 1987; 24:172–184.

EL007
HA068
WE038

**Robert M. Ellsworth**
**Barrett G. Haik**
**Robert A. Weiss**

**Retinal nonattachment and falciform detachment**
*See RETINAL DYSPLASIA*
**Retinal pigmentary degeneration-microcephaly-mental retardation**
*See RETINOPATHY-MICROCEPHALY-MENTAL RETARDATION*
**Retinal septum, congenital**
*See RETINAL FOLD*

---

## RETINAL TELANGIECTASIA-HYPOGAMMAGLOBULINEMIA
**0868**

**Includes:** Hypogammaglobulinemia-retinal telangiectasia

**Excludes:**
    **Ataxia-telangiectasia** (0094)
    **Retina, Coats disease** (3135)
    Waldenstrom macroglobulinemia

**Major Diagnostic Criteria:** Retinal telangiectasia plus hypogammaglobulinemia.

**Clinical Findings:** Frenkel and Russe (1967) reported two sibs with retinal telangiectasia. The male had absence of IgA and IgM immunoglobulins, and reduction of IgG immunoglobulin. The female had normal immunoglobulin levels but had a deficiency in delayed hypersensitivity. Both individuals had normal karyotypes. Six other unrelated individuals with hypogammaglobulinemia were found to have normal retinal vasculature.

**Complications:** Recurrent infections.

**Associated Findings:** None known.

**Etiology:** Possibly a variant anomaly in segmentation of retinal capillaries.

**Pathogenesis:** Unknown.

**POS No.:** 3913

**Sex Ratio:** Presumably M1:F1.

**Occurrence:** Two siblings reported.

**Risk of Recurrence for Patient's Sib:** Unknown.

**Risk of Recurrence for Patient's Child:** Unknown.

**Age of Detectability:** In infancy.

**Gene Mapping and Linkage:** Unknown.

**Prevention:** None known. Genetic counseling indicated.

**Treatment:** Avoidance of pathogens, treatment of infections as indicated.

**Prognosis:** Unknown.

**Detection of Carrier:** Unknown.

**References:**

Frenkel N, Russe HP: Retinal telangiectasia associated with hypogammaglobulinemia. Am J Ophthalmol 1967; 63:215–220.

G0006　　　　　　　　　　　　　　　　**Morton F. Goldberg**
SU001　　　　　　　　　　　　　　　　　　　　**Joel Sugar**

---

## RETINITIS PIGMENTOSA　　　　　　　　　0869

**Includes:**
　　Pigmentary retinal degeneration
　　Rod-cone dystrophy

**Excludes:**
　　**Choroideremia** (0925)
　　Cone-rod degeneration
　　**Gyrate atrophy of the choroid and retina** (0449)
　　Myopia, malignant
　　**Nightblindness, congenital stationary** (see all)
　　**Retina, fundus albipunctatus** (0399)
　　Retinitis punctata albescens
　　**Usher syndrome** (0983)

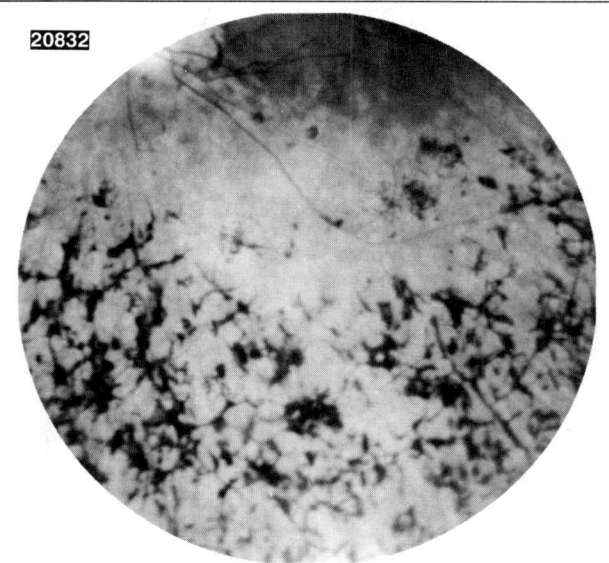

**0869**-20832: Retinitis pigmentosa.

**Major Diagnostic Criteria:** Characteristic impaired rod and cone (photoreceptor) function, and evidence of retinal and pigment epithelial disease by ERG, in the presence or absence of morphologic retinal changes.

**Clinical Findings:** Decreased dim light vision and constricted visual fields are the earliest signs of retinitis pigmentosa (RP), and these may occur prior to the onset of morphologic retinal changes. The common ocular complications which add to the severity of the disease are posterior cortical cataracts and macular involvement, often with cystoid macular edema.

Retinitis pigmentosa may be inherited as a dominant, recessive, or X-linked trait, but 40–50% of affected individuals are isolated cases within their families. *Autosomal recessive* is the most common form, comprising 30–40% of all cases. There is no proof that isolated and recessive forms are the same. Onset is during the first two decades of life, and usually progresses to severe visual loss by the fifth decade.

A slowly progressive adult onset form has been noted with a recordable ERG. This type, although uncommon, is compatible with good visual function. In the more usual cases, the ERG has typically been reported as unrecordable. With the use of a computer-averaged ERG, signals of less than $10\mu$ can be measured easily, and the truly unrecordable ERG is rare.

Some *autosomal dominant* forms also have an onset in the first or second decade, but some may not begin until the fourth or fifth decade. The initial findings are mild, progression is slow, and although night vision and peripheral vision end up severely affected, central vision may be maintained into the sixth or seventh decade. Although complete penetrance is common, some families with variable penetrance have been described, with characteristic changes in the temporal aspects of the ERG. A sectoral form of RP has been documented in some dominant pedigrees, progresses slowly, and is compatible with good function in the normal patches of retina. The sectoral form can masquerade as a nerve fiber bundle defect, or other neurologic visual field deficit, if corresponding pigmentary changes are not noted in the fundus. Dominant cases have been subdivided by their ERG characteristics and these are highly predictive of visual outcome.

The *X-linked* forms are the least common type of RP (8–10%) but tend to be the most severe, with profound visual loss by the fourth decade. The female carriers will often show signs of retinal involvement and may even be symptomatic. Two carrier states are recognized, each unique to a given family, which suggest that there are at least two, not necessarily allelic, genotypes for X-linked RP. Some female carriers show a congenital golden-metallic sheen, which may progress to pigmentary changes in mid-life. In other families, the carriers have normal fundi but develop islands or sectors of pigmentary RP-like degeneration in their mid-30s and 40s.

The typical retinal changes are clumps of pigment resembling bone spicules in the equatorial region, attenuated arterioles, and a waxy somewhat pale disk. The pigment epithelium often develops white dots or diffuse depigmentation easily seen on fluorescein angiography. The pigment dispersion in the retina may take the form of round clumps and, rarely, no pigment clumping is seen. The initial changes are often fine pigment granularity with accumulations over the retinal vessels. Fine salt-and-pepper changes characterized by tiny pigment clumps surrounded by rings of depigmentation help to distinguish the pathologic fundus of early RP from normal blond fundi.

Dark adaptometry invariably shows elevated thresholds in areas of abnormal retina. However, mild and atypical cases may possibly demonstrate normal dark adaptation in some areas of the retina with elevated thresholds elsewhere. The visual field is often first affected in the equatorial region producing an encircling ring-type scotoma which widens toward the periphery and the center with resulting tubular vision. Arcuate or sector defects are also possible. Color vision may be affected. The early changes are tritanopic, and all color perception may be lost in advanced disease. Electrophysiologic studies are abnormal early in the course of the disease. A reduced ERG is the rule, and the early receptor potential (ERP) is also abnormal. Although the rate of progression varies greatly, recent research has carefully examined the natural history in a quantitative fashion. Psychophysical studies comparing rod and cone function across the retina have allowed further subclassification.

**Complications:** Unknown.

**Associated Findings:** *Ocular*: Myopia, macular involvement, cataracts, drusen of the optic nerve, achromatopsia, ophthalmoplegia.

*Extraocular*: The combination of RP and congenital hearing loss is known as **Usher syndrome.** There are a host of genetic disorders with associated RP including **Abetalipoproteinemia, Phytanic acid storage disease, Neuronal ceroid-lipofuscinoses (NCL), Mucopolysaccharidosis** types I-H, I-S, II and III, **Bardet-Biedl syndrome, Olivopontocerebellar atrophy, dominant with retinal degeneration, Renal dysplasia-retinal aplasia, Loken-Senior type,** and **Asphyxiating thoracic dysplasia.**

**Etiology:** Autosomal recessive, autosomal dominant, and X-linked recessive inheritance. The mothers of all males presenting with apparently isolated disease should be examined for X-linked carrier states.

**Pathogenesis:** There is a progressive degeneration of the receptors with associated neuroepithelial atrophy, and glial overgrowth, and an eventual narrowing of the retinal vessels. Depigmentation of the retinal epithelium, with a migration of its pigment into the retina, is characteristic.

The initial site of tissue abnormality is unknown. Both the neuroepithelium, with progressive loss of rods and cones, and the pigment epithelium are abnormal. Degenerated receptors may become partly replaced by neuroglia. The ganglion cells and the nerve fiber layer remain relatively unchanged. The retinal vessels, arterioles, and veins alike, always show marked changes, generally atrophic.

Electron microscopic studies in RP emphasize the relationship between the pigment epithelium and the neural retina. Specimens have been obtained in increasing numbers, and careful studies have been performed on eyes of all genetic subtypes. The question of whether the disease is primary to the receptors or the pigment epithelium has not been conclusively answered.

**MIM No.:** *18010, *26800, 26801, 26802, 26803, *31260, 30320, *31261

**CDC No.:** 362.700

**Sex Ratio:** M1:F1 for all but X-linked forms.

**Occurrence:** Prevalence varies from 1:2,000 to 1:7,000, with an estimated carrier rate of 1:80 to 1:100. An unique form may exist among the Navajo (Heckenlively et al, 1981).

**Risk of Recurrence for Patient's Sib:**
See Part I, *Mendelian Inheritance.*

**Risk of Recurrence for Patient's Child:**
See Part I, *Mendelian Inheritance.*

**Age of Detectability:** Depends on the mode of transmission, with the most frequent onset at the end of the first decade or the beginning of second decade of life.

**Gene Mapping and Linkage:** RP1 (retinitis pigmentosa 1) has been tentatively mapped to 1.
RP2 (retinitis pigmentosa 2) has been mapped to Xp11.4-p11.2.
RP3 (retinitis pigmentosa 3) has been mapped to Xp21.1-p11.4.
CRD (choroidoretinal degeneration) has been mapped to X.

**Prevention:** None known. Genetic counseling indicated.

**Treatment:** Night vision aids and optical field wideners may help some symptoms. Protecting the retina from bright light by sunglasses or occlusion has been advocated, but remains with no substantive proof of benefit. Appropriate therapy for hearing loss may be needed. Vitamin therapy has been associated with slower progression than normal, and treatment trials are being actively investigated.

**Prognosis:** Normal life span unless influenced by an associated systemic problem. There is always impairment of visual fields and night vision, but acuity may be normal.

**Detection of Carrier:** In the X-linked form, the carrier may show a golden glistening "spotty" or "streaky" reflex in the post-equatonal retina area or throughout most of the eyegrounds. This change has been called a "tapetal" reflex. A few carriers will show some of the changes seen in males, but usually, in general, only minimal functional disturbances are noted. Occasionally a mild abnormality, particularly of dark adaptation, is found. Rarely the female carrier will show marked symptoms. The full field ERG and vitreous fluorophotometry have been able to detect a high percentage of carriers. The ERP has also been used to identify carriers. Carriers generally cannot be detected in the autosomal recessive form. Pedigree analysis may reveal obligate carriers.

**Support Groups:**
MD; Baltimore; RP Foundation Fighting Blindness
CANADA: Ontario; Toronto; National Retinitis Pigmentosa Foundation of Canada

**References:**
Merin S, Auerbach E: Retinitis pigmentosa. Surv Ophthalmol 1976; 20:303–346.
Heckenlively J, et al.: Retinitis pigmentosa in the Navajo. Metab Pediat Ophthal 1981; 5:201–206.
Hu D-N: Genetic aspects of retinitis pigmentosa in China. Am J Med Genet 1982; 12:51–56.
Marmor MF, et al.: Retinitis pigmentosa: a symposium on terminology and methods of examination. Ophthalmology 1983; 90:126–131.
Bhattacharya SS, et al.: Close genetic linkage between X-linked RP and a restriction fragment length polymorphism identified by recombinant DNA probe LI.28. Nature 1984; 309:253–255.
Bunker CH, et al.: Prevalence of retinitis pigmentosa in Maine. Am J Ophthalmol 1984; 97:357–365.
Berson EL, et al.: Natural course of RP over a three year interval. Am J Ophthal 1985; 99:240–251.
Fishman GA, et al.: Autosomal dominant retinitus pigmentosa: a method of classification. Arch Ophthal 1985; 103:366–374.
Grohdahl J: Estimation of prognosis and prevalence of retinitus pigmentosa and Usher syndrome in Norway. Clin Genet 1987; 31:255–264.
Heckenlively JR, et al.: Clinical findings and common symptoms in retinitis pigmentosa. Am J Ophthalmol 1988; 105:504–511.
Heckenlively JR: Retinitis pigmentosa. Philadelphia: J.B. Lippincott, 1988.
Pagon RA: Retinitis pigmentosa. Survey of Ophthalmology 1988; 33:137–177.

W0003                                                                    **Mitchel L. Wolf**

**Retinitis pigmentosa, atypical (some forms)**
*See RETINA, COMBINED CONE-ROD DEGENERATION*
**Retinitis pigmentosa, congenital**
*See RETINA, AMAUROSIS CONGENITA, LEBER TYPE*
**Retinitis pigmentosa-hearing loss (sensorineural)**
*See USHER SYNDROME*

## RETINOBLASTOMA                                                          0870

**Includes:**
Cancer, retinoblastoma
Endophytum type retinoblastoma
Exophytum type retinoblastoma
Osteosarcoma, retinoblastoma-related
Trilateral retinoblastoma

**Excludes:**
**CNS neoplasms** (0188)
Diktyoma
Pupil, other causes of white (leukocoria)

**Major Diagnostic Criteria:** Characteristic ophthalmoscopic appearance of a tumor arising in the retina of one or both eyes, usually occurring in an infant less than three years of age. When the tumor is obscured by overlying detachment or inflammatory reaction in the vitreous, neuro-imaging and ultrasonography are useful.

P-32 uptake studies may be useful in special situations, although the injection of P-32 into infants must be regarded with

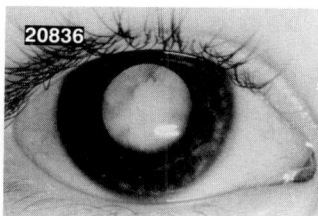

**0870-20834–36:** Typical white "cat's eye" reflex in the affected eye.

great circumspection. Computed axial tomography has been of great value, both in detecting a mass lesion within the eye, and appreciating calcific densities that cannot be demonstrated by other techniques. CT scanning may be useful in detecting extension of tumor into the optic nerve, into the orbit, and into the middle cranial fossa.

Increased levels of lactic acid dehydrogenase have been found in almost all patients with retinoblastoma. The absolute level of this enzyme is increased in the aqueous humor. The aqueous: serum LDH ratio is always greater than one, and there is a fairly characteristic isoenzyme pattern. Aqueous gamma enolase levels may prove to be a more specific marker for cells of neural crest origin.

**Clinical Findings:** The average age at the time of tumor diagnosis is 12 months. The most common presenting sign is a white "cat's eye reflex" in the pupil, and the second most common sign is strabismus. Occasionally, spontaneous necrosis in the tumor will lead to a red, painful eye, with or without secondary glaucoma. In older children, poor vision or vitreous floaters are rarely presenting complaints. Because of a family history, younger sibs should be examined early in life. Consequently about 3% of tumors are identified on routine examination.

In hereditary cases, the tumor arises multifocally in the retina, and at least one-half of all cases have more than one tumor in an involved eye. The tumor arises bilaterally in one-third of all cases. Retinoblastoma occurs in eyes of normal size, and cataract is never seen except as a rare, late complication. The tumor may grow from the retina forward into the vitreous space, the endophytum type, when it can be clearly seen with an ophthalmoscope during the early stages. These tumors usually have a very characteristic creamy-pink color with numerous blood vessels on the surface. The exophytum type, however, grows beneath the retina, in the subretinal potential space. This lesion may be obscured by an overlying detachment, and the borders and surface characteristics cannot be clearly seen.

Two clinical findings are more or less pathognomonic of retinoblastoma. The first is calcification within the tumor which may be seen either with the ophthalmoscope or by X-ray. Approximately 75% of retinoblastomas will show intraocular calcification if the X-rays or CT are properly exposed. When the tumor has achieved a relatively large size, the stroma breaks down and portions of the tumor seeds into the vitreous and may go to the anterior chamber where they may implant on the iris or present as a hypopyon.

**Complications:** *Ocular:* Retinal detachment. Inflammatory reaction due to spontaneous necrosis. Rubeosis iridis. Secondary glaucoma. Phthisis bulbi.

*Systemic complications:* This tumor may spread directly by the optic nerve into the subarachnoid space, and the base of the brain may be seeded with tumor which then produces central nervous system (CNS) symptoms and death. It may also metastasize hematogenously following extension into the choroid. The bone marrow is probably the tissue first invaded, but multiple viscera may be involved later. It is curious that lung parenchyma is rarely involved. If the tumor extends out of the eye into the orbit, it may then spread lympatically to the regional nodes.

**Associated Findings:** The clinical phenotype is usually limited to the retinal tumors, but infants with a detectable defect in the long arm of chromosome 13 have psychomotor retardation and a variety of skeletal defects. About 5% of patients with retinoblastoma have mental retardation, but the vast majority of patients have normal intellectual development.

Patients with the germinal mutation for retinoblastoma seem to have both increased susceptibility to radiation-induced tumors at relatively low dosage levels, and a high incidence (>50%) of second primary neoplasms later in life unrelated to retinoblastoma or the treatment thereof. Osteogenic sarcoma is the most common second tumor, although a variety of other neoplasms have been reported, such as soft tissue sarcomas, and cutaneous malignant melanomas.

Some patients with retinoblastoma have associated ectopic retinoblastoma in the pineal gland or in the parasellar location and are said to have *trilateral retinoblastoma*. When such tumors are considered, a computed tomogram of the head is obtained for a patient with retinoblastoma.

**Etiology:** Autosomal dominant inheritance in 8–10% of cases. About 5–7% of patients demonstrate deletion of the q14 band on the long arm of chromosome 13 in fresh tumor preparations. These may be unilateral or bilateral cases. Only 8% of patients present with a family history at time of diagnosis.

All patients with a family history, all patients with bilateral disease, and all patients with multicentric tumor (even if unilateral) are assumed to have germinal mutations. Approximately 15% of unilateral isolated cases are found to have germinal mutations, but the remainder are not transmitted as would be expected of an autosomal dominant disease. These latter may represent somatic mutations and have one tumor in one eye. Recent information suggests, however, that the molecular defect requires simultaneous alterations at each chromosome 13 locus, this behaving as a "recessive" molecular disease.

**Pathogenesis:** Tumors arise in one or both eyes, probably as photoreceptor precursor cells, and then grow at variable rates, until the globe is entirely filled with tumor. Loss of or mutation of both alleles of the normally present retinoblastoma suppressor oncogene on the long arm of chromosome 13 are needed for a tumor to develop.

**MIM No.:** *18020

**CDC No.:** 190.500

**Sex Ratio:** M1:Fl

**Occurrence:** The tumor now appears to arise in 1:20,000 births. Approximately 200 new cases are seen in the United States each year. Some populations (e.g. Saudi Arabia) appear to have higher prevalence. As more patients with germinal mutations live to reproductive age, an increase in incidence may be expected.

**Risk of Recurrence for Patient's Sib:** With no family history: 1%. With a positive family history: 40%.

**Risk of Recurrence for Patient's Child:** 8–25% if parent had unilateral involvement; almost 40% if parent had bilateral or multicentric retinoblastoma.

**Age of Detectability:** The vast majority of patients are detected before the age of two years. It is extremely unlikely to see the appearance of a new tumor beyond the age of three years. At least two cases with metastatic retinoblastoma at birth are known, and an occasional patient with spontaneous regression has been identified up to the age of 62 years.

**Gene Mapping and Linkage:** RB1 (retinoblastoma 1 (including osteosarcoma)) has been mapped to 13q14.2.

**Prevention:** None known. Genetic counseling indicated.

**Treatment:** Even in isolated cases, *both* parents must have complete medical eye examinations to identify possible spontaneous regression of tumor, which would indicate that the case is "genetic" rather than isolated.

In families with a positive history, all possible effort must be made to examine all children within one week of birth. Supervoltage radiation is the most effective form of treatment, as this tumor is radiocurable. The average tumor dose is 3500–4000r delivered over 3–4 weeks. Radioactive cobalt applicators, light coagulation, diathermy, and cryotherapy are valuable adjunctive measures. Eyes with large tumors, filling more than one-half of the globe, are usually enucleated.

The tumor is sensitive to various chemotherapeutic agents including nitrogen mustard, TEM, thio-TEPA, methotrexate, Cytoxan, actinomycin-D, and vincristine. These agents are not curative, however, and should be used only in conjunction with radiation or in the treatment of as-yet incurable metastatic disease.

**Prognosis:** Overall mortality in the United States is 20%; much higher in less-developed countries. The stage of the disease at the time that diagnosis is made is the most significant factor in the eventual outcome.

For practical purposes, all fatal cases have one or both eyes in group 5 of the Reese-Ellsworth classification. If cases are detected at any earlier stage, and adequate treatment is undertaken, there is virtually no mortality from the primary tumor.

Prognosis appears to be correlate better with size and extent of tumor than with cytologic differentiation.

Several articles have claimed that mortality is greater in Blacks than in Caucasians, but on careful analysis it appears that this is due to the stage of the disease at the time treatment is undertaken.

**Detection of Carrier:** In some families with multiple generations affected, quantitive esterase D levels may be informative. A DNA probe discovered in 1987 will be useful in detecting carriers by demonstrating deletion of 13q14. In all isolated cases, both parents must undergo dilated ophthalmoscopy with a binocular indirect ophthalmoscope and 360 degree scleral depression in a search for spontaneously involuted tumors.

**Special Considerations:** This is a highly malignant hereditary tumor, for which early diagnosis is vital. Leukokoria in infancy must be regarded as the most dangerous sign in all ophthalmology and should lead to thorough investigation for retinoblastoma. Once the tumor has extended outside the eye into the orbit, the chances of cure are slight, and few patients with metastatic retinoblastoma have survived. The differential diagnosis can be quite complex, and the most commonly confused conditions are larval granulomatosis (ocular toxocariasis), **Retina, Coats disease**, angiomatosis retinae, and granulomatous uveitis. Persistent hyperplastic vitreous, retrolental fibroplasia, congenital retinal folds, medullated nerve fibers, and colobomas can usually be identified readily when the children are examined under anesthesia.

The second most common presenting sign is strabismus and all children with this condition should have careful indirect ophthalmoscopic examination of the retina.

**Support Groups:** Atlanta; American Cancer Society

**References:**
Ellsworth RM: The practical management of retino-blastoma. Trans Am Ophthalmol Soc 1969; 67:462.
Reese AB: Tumors of the Eye, 3rd Ed. New York: Harper and Row, 1976.
Zimmerman LE: Retinoblastoma and retinocytoma. In: Spencer WH, ed.: Ophthalmic pathology: an atlas and textbook. Philadelphia: W.B. Saunders. 1985:1292–1351. * †
Cavenee WK, et al.: Prediction of familial predisposition to retinoblastoma. New Engl J Med 1986; 314:1201–1207.
Draper GY, et al.: Second primary neoplasms in patients with retinoblastoma. Br J Cancer 1986; 53:661–671. *
Friend SH, et al.: A human DNA segment with properties of the gene that predispose to retinoblastoma and osteosarcoma. Nature 1986; 323:643–646. *
Fung Y-KT, et al.: Structural evidence for the authenticity of the human retinoblastoma gene. Science 1987; 236:1657–1661.
Wiggs J, et al.: Prediction of the risk of hereditary retinoblastoma, using DNA polymorphisms within the retinoblastoma gene. New Engl J Med 1988; 318:151–157.
Yandell DW, et al.: Oncogenic point mutations in the human retinoblastoma gene: their application to genetic counseling. New Engl J Med 1989; 321:1689–1695.

**Robert M. Ellsworth**

Retinoic acid syndrome
See FETAL RETINOID SYNDROME
Retinoic fetal effects, experimental in animals
See FETAL RETINOID SYNDROME

## RETINOPATHY OF PREMATURITY                    0872

**Includes:**
Fibroplasia retrolental
Retrolental fibroplasia (RLF)

**Excludes:** Retrolental membranes, other causes of

**Major Diagnostic Criteria:** Bilateral retinal pathology that occurs in premature, low-birth-weight children who have usually received supplemental oxygen therapy immediately after birth. Typically, the earliest stages of the disease appear within the first month of life.

*Standard classification for retinopathy of prematurity*
Active stages:
*Stage 1:* Dilatation and tortuosity of retinal vessels.
*Stage 2:* Stage 1 plus neovascularization and some peripheral retinal clouding.
*Stage 3:* Stage 2 plus retinal detachment in the periphery of the fundus. Frequently, a retinal fold develops, extending from the disk to the retinal periphery. Of these folds, approximately 90% occur on the temporal side of the globe. Vitreous hemorrhage often occurs during this stage.
*Stage 4:* Hemispheric or circumferential detachment of the retina.
*Stage 5:* Complete retinal detachment with contracture and organization into a retrolental membrane. Massive vitreous hemorrhage may occur during retinal organization.

Late cicatricial grades:
*Grade I:* A small mass of opaque, gray tissue is present in the retinal periphery with an accompanying localized retinal detachment. In addition, there may be floating gray vitreous opacities with or without a pigment disturbance in the peripheral retina. Myopia is common, but vision may be normal or near normal.
*Grade II:* A mass of opaque, gray tissue, larger than in grade I cicatricial disease, is present in the retinal periphery with an accompanying localized retinal detachment. The disk may show

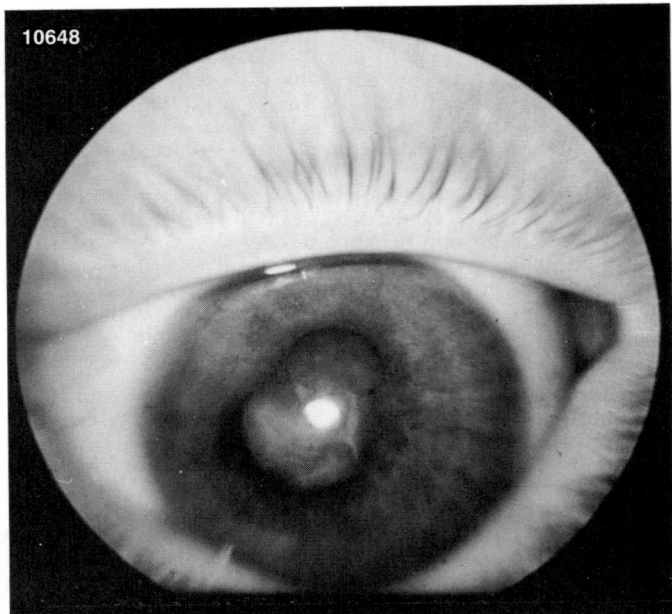

0872-10648:    Retrolental fibroplasia.

moderate distortion, with "dragging" of the major retinal vessels toward the periphery such that they become straighter than usual; this almost always occurs in the temporal direction. In addition, the macula may be displaced with obvious heterotopia. In these cases, the visual acuity ranges from 20/40 to 20/200.

*Grade III*: A large mass of opaque, gray tissue is present in the retina with a fold extending from this mass to the nervehead. When a retinal fold is present, the visual acuity is usually in the 20/200 to hand motion range. As the fold forms, there is often some hemorrhage along its edges; this hemorrhage is associated with a proliferation of the retinal pigment epithelium.

*Grade IV*: Extensive circumferential retinal pathology with a retrolental membrane occupying a portion of the retrolental space. The vision in these eyes is usually limited to hand motion or light perception.

*Grade V*: A total retrolental membrane covering the entire posterior surface of the lens. The entire retina is incorporated into the membrane. These patients have no light perception. Recently, a new, international classification system for retinopathy of prematurity has been proposed by a group of 23 ophthalmologists from 11 countries. This system defines retinopathy of prematurity according to three parameters: location, extent, and stage of the disease.

*A. Location* is defined by specific zones of retinal involvement, using the optic disk as the reference point for the center of each zone:

*Zone 1*: Posterior pole or inner zone. The limits of zone I are defined as two times the distance from the optic nervehead to the center of the macula in all directions (an arc of 60 degrees).

*Zone II*: This zone extends from the edge of zone I peripherally to a point tangential to the nasal ora serrata, extending in a circle to an area near the temporal equator.

*Zone III*: This zone includes the residual retinal crescent anterior to zone II.

*B. Extent* is defined as the specific clock hour position of retinal involvement.

*C. Staging* of the disease reflects the degree of associated vascular abnormalities:

*Stage I*, demarcation line: A relatively flat, white demarcation line separates avascular anterior retina from normal posterior retina. Abnormal branching vessels lead up to the edge of the demarcation line.

*Stage II*, ridge: The demarcation line extends up, as a ridge, out of the plane of the retina; it has height, width, and volume. The ridge may appear to be pink, with vascular tufts apparent posteriorly on the adjacent retina. In addition, vessels from the posterior retina may enter the ridge.

*Stage III*, ridge with extraretinal fibrovascular proliferation: Extraretinal fibrovascular proliferation tissue is present in addition to all of the stage II findings. This extraretinal tissue may be present continuous with, or adjacent to, the posterior aspect of the ridge, or it may develop in the vitreous, perpendicular to the plane of the retina.

*Stage IV*, retinal detachment: Stage III with accompanying secondary exudative with or without traction detachment of the retina.

*Plus disease* is a special subset of the four stages and is used in conjunction when progressive vascular incompetence is present, as evidenced by increasing dilation and tortuosity of the peripheral retinal vessels, engorgement of the iris vasculature, pupillary rigidity, and vitreous haze. When the posterior retinal veins enlarge and the arterioles become tortuous, a "+" is added to the appropriate stage (e.g., stage II+).

**Clinical Findings:** ROP occurs in premature, but generally otherwise normal, infants. These infants are usually born between 26 and 31 weeks gestation, with birth weights ranging from 800 to 1500g. In addition, most of them have received supplemental oxygen. The disease rarely occurs in full-term children of normal birth weight who have not received oxygen therapy. With some exceptions, the disease is bilateral and usually symmetric. There is an active phase early in life, which becomes clinically evident at 3–5 weeks after birth. The earliest sign is constriction of the retinal arterioles, which is followed by venous dilation, increased tortu-

osity, and neovascularization. Subsequently, retinal and vitreous hemorrhages may occur. These hemorrhages typically develop peripherally, particularly in the temporal half of the retina. An exudative phase can occur in which white patches of edema may develop followed by detachment of the peripheral retina. The process may end spontaneously at any stage.

Useful vision may be retained in those patients in whom pathologic changes are limited to peripheral cicatrization. In about 25% of the patients, a progressive cicatricial phase develops from the second to the fifth month of life and is characterized by organization and contracture of the entire retina. The end result is formation of retinal folds or the formation of a dense, gray-white membrane lying behind the lens completely obscuring all view of the fundus. As the retina undergoes progressive contraction, the ciliary processes are drawn into the mass and may be visible around the circumference of the lens without indentation of the globe. Since the retrolental membrane is frequently vascularized, it is possible that progressive traction on this membrane accounts for the hemorrhage that occasionally occurs. The iris is also involved in the process of neovascularization; large radial iris vessels and posterior synechiae are common. Eyes with advanced disease may develop glaucoma transiently; however, the contracture ultimately results in phthisis bulbi. After age six years, the condition of the eyes is usually stationary, although retinal detachments can occur until about age 10 years in patients who have grade III or IV cicatricial retinopathy of prematurity.

**Complications:** Secondary glaucoma may develop during the phase of vasoproliferation or intraocular hemorrhage. Heterochromia may occur as the result of anterior segment hemorrhage. Eccentric fixation may develop as a result of macular ectopia.

**Associated Findings:** High myopia, mental retardation (estimated to be present to some degree in as many as 40% of all cases).

**Etiology:** In premature infants, the retinal vasculature is not fully developed at birth and is abnormally sensitive to the vasoconstrictive effect of ambient oxygen.

**Pathogenesis:** Peripheral retinal hypoxia results from constriction of retinal arterioles. Abnormal surface retinal vessels develop as secondary vasoproliferation occurs in response to this hypoxia. These vessels tend to hemorrhage into the retina and vitreous. When the hemorrhage organizes, secondary traction, detachment of the retina, and ultimate contracture leading to phthisis bulbi can occur. In addition to vasoproliferation, the hypoxia may produce areas of complete vaso-obliteration with considerable capillary endothelial damage.

**Sex Ratio:** M1:F1

**Occurrence:** Undetermined but presumed rare.

**Risk of Recurrence for Patient's Sib:** Presumably not increased.

**Risk of Recurrence for Patient's Child:** Presumably not increased.

**Age of Detectability:** Birth to six weeks of age.

**Gene Mapping and Linkage:** Unknown.

**Prevention:** The ambient oxygen level in the incubator should be kept as low as possible concomitant with the well-being of the infant; in general, at a level of 40% or below. Catheterization of the umbilical artery is useful to monitor the blood $pO_2$ levels. Indirect ophthalmoscopy is not an effective way to monitor oxygen levels, because persistent vitreous haze in premature infants may make visualization difficult and there is very poor correlation between the arterial caliber as viewed with the ophthalmoscope and arterial oxygen tension values. Fluorescein angiography may detect early pathologic changes, but it is not practical in the monitoring of premature infants. Radiation and steroid therapies have been used but without definite effect.

**Treatment:** Light coagulation employed early in the active stages may arrest progression. Cryotherapy may also be useful in obliterating peripheral neovascular tufts in eyes that are technically difficult to treat by photocoagulation. The National Institutes of Health has sponsored an on-going multicenter trial of cryotherapy for retinopathy of prematurity; preliminary results have not been reported to date. Retinal detachment treated by scleral buckling has met with some limited success; however, follow-up has not been long or extensive. Vitamin E supplementation has not been shown to affect the incidence of ROP, but may decrease its severity.

**Prognosis:** Normal for life span. In stages 1 and 2, the active phase may regress spontaneously without serious retinal pathology. The healed grades I and II eyes may have normal maculae and essentially normal vision. In grades III and IV eyes, variable progressive loss of vision may occur as a result of retinal detachments in children aged five to 10 years. In grade V eyes, total loss of vision is typical.

**Detection of Carrier:** Unknown.

**Special Considerations:** In premature infants with an essentially normal cardiovascular system, there is fairly good data indicating that retinal changes will not occur if the ambient oxygen concentration is maintained at a level of 40% or less. The incidence of retinopathy of prematurity is definitely related to prematurity and birth weight.

Retinopathy of prematurity is more frequent and more severe in smaller infants. The rate at which a newborn is weaned from supplemental oxygen therapy does not seem to be related to the occurrence of retinopathy of prematurity. The development of the retina's vascular supply is unique. At the fourth month of gestation, vessels from the embryonic hyaloid system supply the retina. The normal retina does not fully vascularize until shortly after birth in the full-term, normal-birth-weight infant. Perhaps 1% of all cases of retinopathy of prematurity have occurred in infants receiving no significant oxygen therapy. This appears to be related to immaturity of the retinal vessels and peripheral anoxia in the absence of the vasoconstrictive effect of supplemental oxygen. In utero, the arterial oxygen saturation is only 50% or so. It has been suggested that the relative increase in oxygen saturation following birth may stimulate the sensitive premature retinal vessels to cause vasoproliferation and all of the pathologic changes associated with retinopathy of prematurity. Theoretically, a number of factors that can alter oxygen availability to the retina may also contribute to the development of ROP. Some of these factors include packed red blood cell transfusions, sepsis (increased oxygen release by macrophages), low pH, and very low temperatures. Current interest in retinopathy of prematurity centers around infants with the respiratory distress syndrome in whom there is pulmonary pathology and frequently right-to-left shunts. In these infants, the level of ambient oxygen does not reflect arterial oxygen concentration and it is only by monitoring arterial $pO_2$ that we may appreciate the oxygen levels in the retina. Safe limits of oxygen therapy have not been defined but, at the moment, it would seem that retinal $pO_2$ should be maintained at 100 mm Hg or less to avoid retinal pathology.

There is clinical evidence to show that systemic vitamin E therapy may be helpful in preventing the formation of neovascularization extending into the vitreous (stage 2 of active disease). It is thought that vitamin E may prevent free-radical damage to spindle cells (the cells that ultimately align, canalize, and differentiate to form nascent retinal blood vessels). The initiation of vitamin E therapy does not eliminate the occurrence of mild-to-moderate grades of ROP, but it may reduce its severity. However, vitamin E allegedly has multiple potential toxic effects, possibly due to its alteration of normal enzymatic levels.

**References:**
National Society for the Prevention of Blindness (Subcommittee, AB Reese, Chairman): Classification of retrolental fibroplasia. Am J Ophthalmol 1953; 36:1333.
Ashton N, et al.: Effect of oxygen on developing retinal vessels with particular reference to problem of retrolental fibroplasia. Br J Ophthalmol 1964; 38:387.
Patz A: New role of the ophthalmologist in prevention of retrolental fibroplasia. Arch Ophthalmol 1967; 78:565.
Brockhurst RJ, Chishti ML: Cicatrical retrolental fibroplasia: its occurrence without oxygen administration and in full term infants. Albrecht Von Graefes Arch Klin Ophthalmol 1975; 195:113.
Kalina RE, et al.: Retrolental fibroplasia: experience over two decades in one institution. Ophthalmologica 1982; 89:91.
Hittner HM, et al.: Suppression of severe retinopathy of prematurity with vitamin E supplementation. Ophthalmologica 1984; 91:1512–1523.
The Committee for the Classification of Retinopathy of Prematurity: An international classification of retinopathy of prematurity. Arch Ophthalmol 1984; 102:1130–1134.
Topilow HW, et al.: The treatment of advanced retinopathy of prematurity by cryotherapy and scleral buckling surgery. Ophthalmologica 1985; 92:379–387.
Bremer DL, et al.: The efficacy of vitamin E in retinopathy of prematurity. J Pediatr Ophthalmol Strab 1986; 23:132–136.

EL007                        **Robert M. Ellsworth**
WE038                      **Robert A. Weiss**
WU002                          **Gloria Wu**

## RETINOPATHY-HYPOTRICHOSIS SYNDROME    2627

**Includes:**

> Hypotrichosis-retinopathy
> Retinal dystrophy, posterior pole-congenital total hypotrichosis
> Tapetoretinal degeneration-alopecia

**Excludes:** Ectodermal dysplasia-ectrodactyly-macular dystrophy (2793)

**Major Diagnostic Criteria:** Presence of retinal degeneration and hypotrichosis in the absence of ectrodactyly or syndactyly.

**Clinical Findings:** The hypotrichosis is noted during infancy in most cases and may be progressive. In two patients, hypotrichosis appeared in childhood. During childhood or early adolescence, patients manifest progressive decreased vision. The typical retinal changes are atrophy of the retinal epithelium in the posterior pole with pigment deposition in the peripapillar area and macular involvement. There may exist diffuse rarefaction of the retina and increased pigment mobilization in the periphery. Visual field examination may reveal large scotomas. The ERG shows photopic

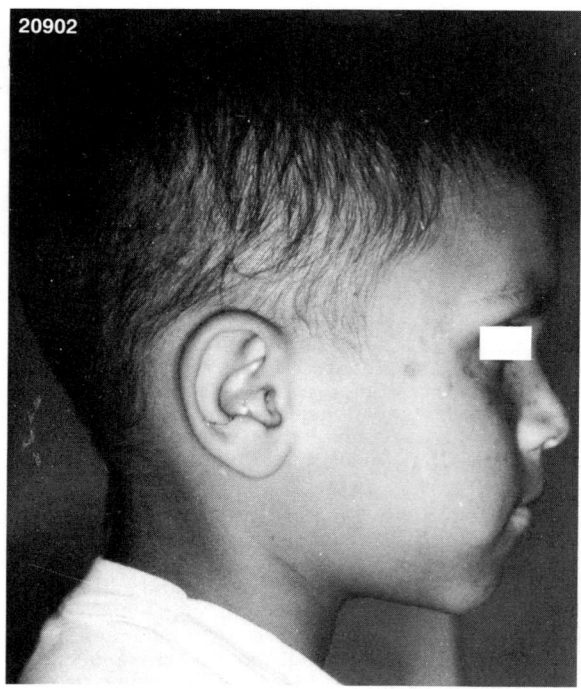

**2627-20902:** Note the pattern and degree of hypotrichosis in this 6-year-old girl with retinopathy-hypotrichosis (RH) syndrome.

involvement; generally preserved for white and orange stimuli but extinct for red and blue stimuli. On testing for color vision, patients will generally show dyschromatopsia.

**Complications:** The retinal dystrophy is progressive and may lead to blindness.

**Associated Findings:** In one Brazilian family with six affected individuals, there was associated acrocyanosis in all cases.

**Etiology:** Presumably autosomal recessive inheritance.

**Pathogenesis:** Unknown.

**POS No.:** 3442, 4428

**Sex Ratio:** Presumably M1:F1. However, 15 of the 20 patients reported have been female.

**Occurrence:** Twenty patients, from eight families, have been observed. Four families (13 patients) are from Brazil, two from Germany, one from Hungary, and one from Sweden.

**Risk of Recurrence for Patient's Sib:**
See Part I, *Mendelian Inheritance.*

**Risk of Recurrence for Patient's Child:**
See Part I, *Mendelian Inheritance.*

**Age of Detectability:** During childhood.

**Gene Mapping and Linkage:** Unknown.

**Prevention:** None known. Genetic counseling indicated.

**Treatment:** Low-vision aids, cosmetic treatment (wig) for hypotrichosis.

**Prognosis:** Normal life span.

**Detection of Carrier:** Unknown.

**References:**

Wagner H: Makulaaffection vergesellchaftet mit Haarabnormität von Lanugotypus, beide vielleicht angeboren bei zwei Geschwistern. Graefes Arch Clin Exp Ophthalmol 1935; 134:71.

Björk A, Jahnberg P: Retinal dystrophy combined with alopecia. Acta Ophthalmol 1975; 53:781.

Kroll P: Beidseitige kongenitale Pigmentblattdystrophie des hinteren Augenpols bei gleichzeitiger Hypotrichosis congenita totalis. Klin Mbl Augenheilkd 1981; 178:118.

Mais FAQ, et al.: Distrofia do epitélio pigmentar retiniano do polo posterior associada com hipotricose congênita difusa. Arq Bras Oftalmol 1984; 47:137.

Pena SDJ, Ribeiro-Goncalves E: Sindrome autossomica recessiva de retinopatia e hipotricose. Ciencia e Cult 1987; 39:741.

PE017                                              **Sergio D.J. Pena**

**Retinopathy-mental retardation**
*See RETINOPATHY-MICROCEPHALY-MENTAL RETARDATION*

## RETINOPATHY-MICROCEPHALY-MENTAL RETARDATION     **2846**

**Includes:**
Mental retardation-retinopathy-microcephaly
Microcephaly-mental retardation-retinopathy
Mirhosseini-Holmes-Walton syndrome
Retinal pigmentary degeneration-microcephaly-mental retardation
Retinopathy-mental retardation

**Excludes:**
**Bardet-Biedl syndrome** (2363)
**Cockayne syndrome** (0189)
**Cohen syndrome** (2023)
**Laurence-Moon syndrome** (0578)
Pigmentary retinopathy in other conditions
**Usher syndrome** (0983)

**Major Diagnostic Criteria:** Severe mental retardation, **Microcephaly**, and retinal pigmentary degeneration.

**Clinical Findings:** Neonatal hypotonia, failure to thrive during infancy, and slow psychomotor development are evident. Impairment of normal growth is probably part of the syndrome.

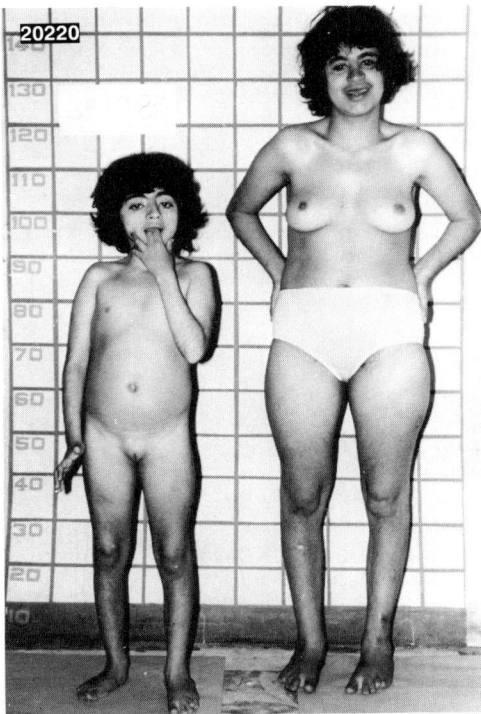

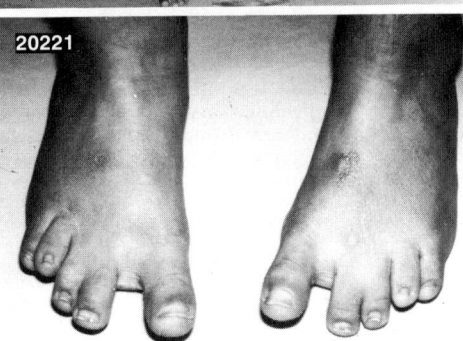

**2846-20220:** Facies with prominent supraorbital ridges, ptosis, short upper lip and short midface as well as the body habitus, short stature and microcephaly. **20221:** Syndactyly of the second and third toes, overlapping fourth toe, and wide gap between the hallux and the second toe.

The physical signs include dolichomicrocephalic skull, small forehead with prominence of the supraorbital ridges, short midface with some mandibular prognathism, bilateral ptosis, highly arched palate, hypoplastic philtrum, malformed teeth (hypoplastic or fused incisors, incisive-like canines), long and slender hands and feet, and scoliosis.

In one sibship, two sisters present bilateral cubitus valgus, genua recurvata, pes valgus, dorsipositioning of the 4th toe, wide gap between the hallux and the 2nd toe, while in the other sibship two brothers had cataracts. One male patient was found to have hypogonadism, probably due to testicular disfunction.

The ophthalmologic evaluation shows normal corneas, atrophy of the optic disc with peripheral pigmentary alteration of the fundi and severe myopic astigmatism. One male patient had both lenses totally cataractous while in the other the lenses had anterior and posterior axial irregular white subcapsular opacities.

The neurologic examination shows muscular strength diminished, muscular tone normal, hyperextensibility of the finger joints, deep tendon reflexes hyperactive, Babinsky sign positive, ataxic-paretic walk, severe retardation of speech and severe mental retardation in the two female patients. The male patients do not have hypertonia or hyperreflexia.

Glucose tolerance test is normal and cytogenetic study shows normal chromosomes (G-banding) in all patients.

**Complications:** Unknown.

**Associated Findings:** None known.

**Etiology:** Probably autosomal recessive inheritance, with possible variable expressivity. It has been suggested this and **Cohen syndrome** may be the same condition.

**Pathogenesis:** Unknown.

**MIM No.:** 26805

**POS No.:** 3540

**Sex Ratio:** M2:F2 (observed).

**Occurrence:** Two brothers in one family and two sisters in another family have been documented. The families were from Brazil and the United States.

**Risk of Recurrence for Patient's Sib:**
See Part I, *Mendelian Inheritance.*

**Risk of Recurrence for Patient's Child:**
See Part I, *Mendelian Inheritance.*

**Age of Detectability:** During childhood.

**Gene Mapping and Linkage:** Unknown.

**Prevention:** None known. Genetic counseling indicated.

**Treatment:** Unknown.

**Prognosis:** Life span is probably not affected.

**Detection of Carrier:** Unknown.

**References:**
Mirhosseini SA, et al.: Syndrome of pigmentary retinal degeneration, cataract, microcephaly, and severe mental retardation. J Med Genet 1972; 9:193–196.
Mendez HMM, et al.: The syndrome of retinal pigmentary degeneration, microcephaly, and severe mental retardation (Mirhosseini-Holmes-Walton syndrome): report of two patients. Am J Med Genet 1985; 22:223–228.

ME039                                    **Heirie Mendez**

---

## RETINOSCHISIS                                    0871

**Includes:**
Juvenile retinoschisis, X-linked
Retinal cyst, congenital
Retina, giant cyst of
Retinoschisis of fovea
Senile retinoschisis, autosomal recessive
Typical retinoschisis, autosomal dominant
Vitreoretinal dystrophy
Vitreous, congenital vascular veils in

**Excludes:** Retinal detachment

**Major Diagnostic Criteria:** Typical retinal findings which fit one of three patterns and are usually easily seen.

**Clinical Findings:** The clinical signs and symptoms usually fit into one of three common pictures:
*Typical retinoschisis* commonly occurs in hyperopic young males; it is frequently bilateral and is often strikingly symmetric. The lesion begins most commonly in the inferior temporal quadrant or, somewhat less commonly, in the superior temporal quadrant, and it appears ophthalmoscopically as a thin, translucent, veil-like membrane extending up as a dome into the vitreous. The translucent membrane contains the retinal vessels and often has small, white dots, which represent glial strands extending across the cystic area. The vitreous is usually fluid, and posterior vitreous detachment is common. The process is often static for many years, although it may be slowly progressive.
*Senile retinoschisis* is related to typical retinoschisis. Senile reti-

noschisis is commonly noted in older patients on routine examination, and it is rarely symptomatic. It is bilateral in approximately 90% of cases, and may develop as a coalescence of peripheral cysts of Blessig. In the early stage, the cystic space is spanned by thin, gray fibers that gradually break, allowing the inner and outer leaves to separate and forming an elevated cyst. In senile retinoschisis, the split retina may extend 360 degrees around the retinal periphery, but it does not commonly progress posteriorly and may remain static for many years.

*Juvenile retinoschisis,* the third clinical variant of retinoschisis, frequently causes serious problems. The area involved by the schisis is very extensive, often including the macula. In some cases the entire retina becomes involved, with subsequent total detachment, preretinal organization, and a poor surgical prognosis. In earlier stages, the areas of schisis often exhibit large holes in the anterior leaf between vessels, and, if breaks develop in both the anterior and posterior leaves of the schisis, a true retinal detachment may occur. These eyes, with a combination of retinoschisis and retinal detachment, are particularly difficult to manage surgically. Patients with juvenile retinoschisis all have foveal retinoschisis, which adds to the visual defect and makes a surgical prognosis for useful vision more questionable. Both macular degeneration and splitting of the retina through the macula may contribute to the visual defect in these patients. The visual field shows a complete scotoma, with a sharp edge in the area of the schisis. On electrophysiologic testing, the electroretinogram (ERG) b wave is markedly depressed, but the a wave is characteristically normal except in severe cases.

**Complications:** Retinal detachment may complicate retinoschisis if holes are present in both the anterior and posterior leaf. Hemorrhage into the vitreous may occur as a result of traction on the retinal vessels, but may be mild and self-limited.

**Associated Findings:** Cystic macular degeneration, hyperopia, astigmatism, strabismus, nystagmus, optic atrophy, posterior cortical cataract, slight posterior capsular opacification, and liquification of the vitreous; rubeosis iridis and neovascular glaucoma have been reported in a case of X-linked juvenile retinoschisis as a complication of retinal detachment.

**Etiology:** Typical retinoschisis, usually by autosomal dominant inheritance. Senile retinoschisis, usually by autosomal recessive inheritance. Juvenile retinoschisis by X-linked recessive inheritance in almost all cases, although autosomal recessive, sporadic, and suspected autosomal dominant pedigrees have been reported.

**Pathogenesis:** Hereditary lamellar splitting in the layers of the retina usually occurs in the plane of the outer plexiform layer in typical and senile retinoschisis and in the nerve fiber layer in juvenile retinoschisis. The juvenile form of the disease may be related to congenital vascular veils in the vitreous, and may be due to a condensation of the vitreous, which was in contact with the inner layers of the optic cup. In addition, it is possible that there is some persistence of the secondary branches of the vasa propria hyaloidae.

In typical retinoschisis, *giant retinal cysts* are evident clinically. These cysts are probably caused by the secretion of hyaluronic acid-sensitive mucopolysaccharides by some of the cells in the inner portion of the retinal cyst. Once retinoschisis has begun because of this secretory mechanism, it may easily spread to peripheral areas of cystoid degeneration and progress posteriorly through normal retina.

Senile retinoschisis, especially the very mild, nonprogressive type, may simply represent a coalescence of peripheral microcysts without the secretory mechanism that appears to cause progression.

**MIM No.:** 18027, *26808, *31270

**Sex Ratio:** M1:F1 in both common and senile types. M1:F>0 for juvenile retinoschisis (female cases, although exceedingly rare, have been reported).

**Occurrence:** Incidence and prevalence of juvenile and typical retinoschisis is undetermined. While incidence of senile retinoschisis is undetermined, its prevalence is 7,000:100,000 (7%) of the population older than age 40 years.

**Risk of Recurrence for Patient's Sib:** See Part I, *Mendelian Inheritance.*

**Risk of Recurrence for Patient's Child:** See Part I, *Mendelian Inheritance.*

**Age of Detectability:** Juvenile retinoschisis may be detected at birth. The more common type of retinal cyst is usually seen in young men. Senile retinoschisis is seen in the fifth, sixth, and seventh decades of life.

**Gene Mapping and Linkage:** RS (retinoschisis) has been mapped to Xp22.2-p22.1.

**Prevention:** None known. Genetic counseling indicated.

**Treatment:** Light coagulation, cryotherapy (with possible drainage of subretinal fluid), vitrectomy for vitreous hemorrhage, and traction are indicated in some cases of juvenile retinoschisis and other selected cases. Since the fluid in the areas of schisis is extremely viscous, it is very difficult to drain by conventional detachment and drainage procedures. In many instances, especially in older adults, there is no or limited progression of the disease and treatment is rarely necessary. While approximately 8.9% of patients with senile retinoschisis develop localized, asymptomatic schisis detachments, the expected incidence of symptomatic progressive retinal detachment in the entire population with senile retinoschisis is only 0.05% (1:2,000). In general, there are three indications for treatment, as follows: 1) Most children with retinoschisis will require treatment; this form of the disease invariably progresses and possibly can be arrested, in some cases, before the macula is threatened. 2) Any patient who has demonstrable holes in both the inner and outer leaves of the schisis needs treatment; it is in these patients that complicated detachments can occur. 3) Patients who have retinal detachment in the fellow eye need treatment.

Two treatment modalities are effective. Light coagulation has been shown to cause collapse of these cysts. There are two rational approaches using light coagulation. The area of the "giant cyst" can be delimited with coagulations, which may function as a barrier to prevent peripheral and posterior spread; however, this barrier cannot be relied on to contain the schisis permanently. If, in addition to a delimiting row of coagulations, the entire area of the schisis is treated, the fluid will often resorb over a period of weeks or months. Apparently the heat has an effect that causes the schisis cavity fluid to resorb. The second approach is cryotherapy; again, the entire area of schisis is treated. At the present state of knowledge, it would seem that either light coagulation or cryotherapy is equally effective.

**Prognosis:** Normal for life span; guarded for vision in the X-linked form.

**Detection of Carrier:** Possibly by RFLP linkage.

**References:**
Mann I, MacRae A: Congenital vascular veils in the vitreous. Br J Ophthalmol 1938; 22:1–10.
Geiser EP, Falls HF: Hereditary retinoschisis. Am J Ophthalmol 1961; 51:1193.
Cibis PA: Retinoschisis: retinal cysts. Trans Am Ophthalmol Soc 1965; 63:417.
Yanoff M, et al.: Histopathology of juvenile retinoschisis. Arch Ophthalmol 1968; 79:49.
Conway BP, Welch RB: X-chromosome linked juvenile retinoschisis with hemorrhagic retinal cyst. Am J Ophthalmol 1977; 83:853.
Hung JY, Hilton GF: Neovascular glaucoma in a patient with X-linked juvenile retinoschisis. Ann Ophthalmol 1980; 12:1054–1055.
Yassur Y, et al.: Autosomal dominant inheritance of retinoschisis. Am J Ophthalmol 1982; 94:338.
Schulman J, et al.: Indications for vitrectomy in congenital retinoschisis. Br J Ophthalmol 1985; 69:482–486.
Byer NE: Long-term natural history study of senile retinoschisis with implications for management. Ophthalmologica 1986; 93:1127–1137.
Dahl N, et al.: DNA linkage analysis of X chromosome linked retinoschisis. (Abstract) Cytogenet Cell Genet 1987; HGM9.

EL007
WE038
WU002

**Robert M. Ellsworth**
**Robert A. Weiss**
**Gloria Wu**

**Retinoschisis of fovea**
    See *RETINOSCHISIS*
**Retinoschisis-early hemeralopia**
    See *EYE, GOLDMANN-FAVRE DISEASE*
**Retraction syndrome**
    See *EYE, DUANE RETRACTION SYNDROME*
**Retrocochlear hearing loss.**
    See *DEAFNESS*
**Retrolental fibroplasia (RLF)**
    See *RETINOPATHY OF PREMATURITY*
**Retromolar**
    See *TEETH, SUPERNUMERARY*
**Retrosternal diaphragmatic hernia**
    See *DIAPHRAGMATIC HERNIA*

## RETT SYNDROME                                         2226

**Includes:**
    Ataxia-dementia-autism
    Autism-dementia-ataxia-loss of purposeful hand use

**Excludes:**
    **Autism, infantile** (2128)
    Cerebellar ataxia
    **Cerebral palsy** (2931)

**Major Diagnostic Criteria:** 1) Normal prenatal, neonatal and early childhood (6–18 months) development and behavior; 2) after initial normal period, deceleration of psychomotor development and then, over a period of up to 18 months, deterioration of mental capacity (dementia with autistic features) and motor abilities, especially purposeful hand use; 3) acquisition of uncoordinated movement (ataxia) of the trunk and limbs, usually with some degree of spasticity and pyramidal tract signs; 4) development of major motor and minor motor seizures, usually associated with characteristic, though not specific EEG abnormalities; 5) subsequent period of more or less stable mental status, but slow and variable progression of the spasticity and seizures; 6) acquired microcephaly; and 7) to date only females have been described with this disorder.

**Clinical Findings:** 1) Normal birth weight, length and head circumference; 2) normal neonatal and early childhood development (6–18 months); 3) the subsequent progressive development of dementia with autistic elements, loss of purposeful hand movements, microcephaly, and later, seizures, generalized spasticity, ataxia, and episodic tachypnea and hyperventilation; 4) the loss of purposeful hand use is accompanied by stereotyped hand movements, usually characterized by flapping and wringing "hand-washing" motions; 5) the episodic hyperventilation, likewise, is highly stereotyped, with tachypnea, expiratory grunting and orofacial grimacing; 6) after the initial decline, a more or less static impoverishment of mental abilities (dementia); 7) more obvious and slow, but highly variable progression of the spasticity, ataxia and seizures; 8) EEG patterns are usually abnormal beyond three years of age. The waking background activity is slow, monotonous and without spatial differentiation, progressing at later ages to decreased voltage and general flattening with occasional bursts of high-amplitude slow waves, focal spikes or bilateral spike-wave complexes. The sleep pattern, on the other hand, shows frequent paroxysmal generalized slow spike-wave complexes; 9) cerebral CT scans may be normal or show nonspecific cortical atrophy; 10) although several of the original cases showed mild to modest hyperammonemia, this has not been a consistent finding.

In general, laboratory data, including karotypes, serum and urine amino acid and organic acid levels, serum and urine levels of copper and ceruloplasmin and other indicators of various types of inborn errors of metabolism, white blood cell and skin fibroblast lysozomal enzyme activities and ultrastructural appearances, have been normal or infrequently and nonspecifically abnormal; CSF catecholamine metabolite (i.e., homovanillic acid, 5-hydroxyindole acetic acid and 3-methoxy-4-hydroxyphenylethylene glycol) levels have been shown to be depressed (Zoghbi et al 1985).

**Complications:** Usually slow, variable progression of the neurological deficits, especially those related to the ataxia, corticospinal tract dysfunction and seizures; at times leading to severe quadriparesis and being wheelchair bound.

**Associated Findings:** None known.

**Etiology:** Uncertain, but limitation of known cases to females, including one pair of half-sisters (related through their mother), raises the possibility of an X-linked mutation (that is lethal in hemizygous males) or an abnormality related to X-chromosome inactivation (vis-a-vis the Lyon Principle). Identical twins are concordant, non-identical twins are discordant.

**Pathogenesis:** Undetermined, with no apparent clues except for the apparent preferential involvement of cerebral gray matter and the diminished levels of CSF catecholamines.

**MIM No.:** 31275

**POS No.:** 3796

**Sex Ratio:** M0:F1

**Occurrence:** Several hundred cases have been reported. Estimated at 1:15,000 in Sweden. Many cases have also been reported from France and Portugal.

**Risk of Recurrence for Patient's Sib:**
See Part I, *Mendelian Inheritance.*

**Risk of Recurrence for Patient's Child:**
See Part I, *Mendelian Inheritance.*

**Age of Detectability:** At six to 48 months of age.

**Gene Mapping and Linkage:** Unknown.

**Prevention:** None known. Genetic counseling indicated.

**Treatment:** Nonspecific supportive and nursing care, physical therapy, and anticonvulsants.

**Prognosis:** The prognosis is poor in terms of neurologic and mental function. Longevity is surely compromised, but accurate estimates are unavailable.

**Detection of Carrier:** Unknown.

**Support Groups:** MD; Fort Washington; International Rett Syndrome Association (IRSA)

**References:**

Rett A: Ueber ein eigenartiges hirnatrophisches Syndrom bei Hyperammoniamie in Kindersalter. Wien Med Wochenschr 1966; 116:723–738.

Hagberg B, et al.: A progressive syndrome of autism, dementia, ataxia and loss of purposeful hand use in girls: Rett's syndrome: report of 35 cases. Am Neurol 1983; 14:471–479.

Kerr A, Stephenson JBP: Rett's syndrome in the west of Scotland. Brit Med Journal 1985; 291:579–582.

Zoghbi HY, et al.: Reduction of biogenic amine levels in the Rett syndrome. N Engl J Med 1985; 313:921–924.

Opitz JM, et al.: The Rett syndrome. Am J Med Genet 1986; 24(suppl 1):1–404.

Tariverdian G, et al.: A monozygotic twin pair with Rett syndrome. Hum Genet 1987; 75:88–90.

Journel H, et al.: Rett phenotype with X/autosome translocation: possible mapping to the short arm of chromosome X. Am J Med Genet 1990; 35:142–147.

Zoghbi HY, et al.: A de novo X;3 translocation in Rett syndrome. Am J Med Genet 1990; 35:148–151.

RI000                                          **Vincent M. Riccardi**

**'Reye syndrome-like' manifestations**
  *See VISCERA, FATTY METAMORPHOSIS*
**Reye-like syndrome, recurrent, due to MCAD**
  *See ACYL-CoA DEHYDROGENASE DEFICIENCY, MEDIUM CHAIN TYPE*

**Rh hump**
  *See TEETH, ENAMEL AND DENTIN DEFECTS FROM ERYTHROBLASTOSIS FETALIS*
**Rh incompatibility**
  *See ERYTHROBLASTOSIS FETALIS*
**Rh null syndrome**
  *See ANEMIA, HEMOLYTIC, RED CELL MEMBRANE DEFECTS*
**Rhabdomyosarcoma**
  *See CANCER, SOFT TISSUE SARCOMA*
**Rheumatoid agglutinators (Raggs)**
  *See ANTIBODIES TO HUMAN ALLOTYPES*
**Rheumatoid arthritis**
  *See ARTHRITIS, RHEUMATOID*
**Rhinitis, ragweed pollen-induced**
  *See RAGWEED POLLEN SENSITIVITY*
**Rhinolalia**
  *See PALATOPHARYNGEAL INCOMPETENCE*
**Rhizomelic chondrodysplasia punctata**
  *See CHONDRODYSPLASIA PUNCTATA, RHIZOMELIC TYPE*
**Rhizomelic dysplasia, familial**
  *See OMODYSPLASIA*

---

## RHIZOMELIC SYNDROME, URBACH TYPE                    2816

**Includes:**
  Skeletal dysplasia, Urbach rhizomelia of humeri
  Urbach skeletal dysplasia with rhizomelia of humeri

**Excludes:**
  **Achondroplasia** (0010)
  **Brachydactyly** (0114)
  **Chondrodysplasia punctata, rhizomelic type** (0154)
  **Epiphyseal dysplasia, multiple** (0358)
  **Omodysplasia** (3280)

**Major Diagnostic Criteria:** Rhizomelia of humeri, **Microcephaly**, saddle nose and congenital heart disease.

**Clinical Findings:** *Craniofacial:* **Microcephaly**; large anterior fontanelle; fine, sparse scalp hair; macroglossia; saddle nose; high-arched palate; micrognathia; short neck.

*Skeletal:* Short stature plus flat, thoracic vertebrae and abnormally shaped epiphyses of long bones; rhizomelia of humeri plus flared epiphyses; kyphosis; dislocated hips plus flat acetabulae; flexion contracture; digitalization of thumb plus bifid distal phalanx; clinodactyly plus hypoplasia of terminal phalanges of hands

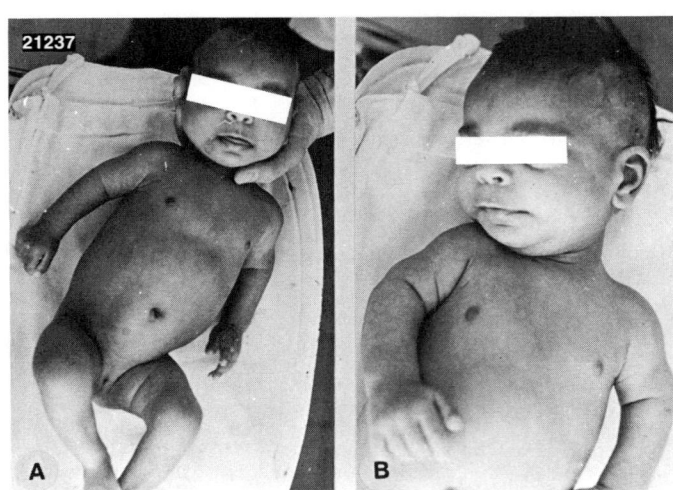

**2816A-21237:** Proband at four months shows microcephaly, macroglossia, short proximal upper extremities, flexion contracture of the knees, micrognathia, saddle nose and digitalization of the right thumb with a broad nail.

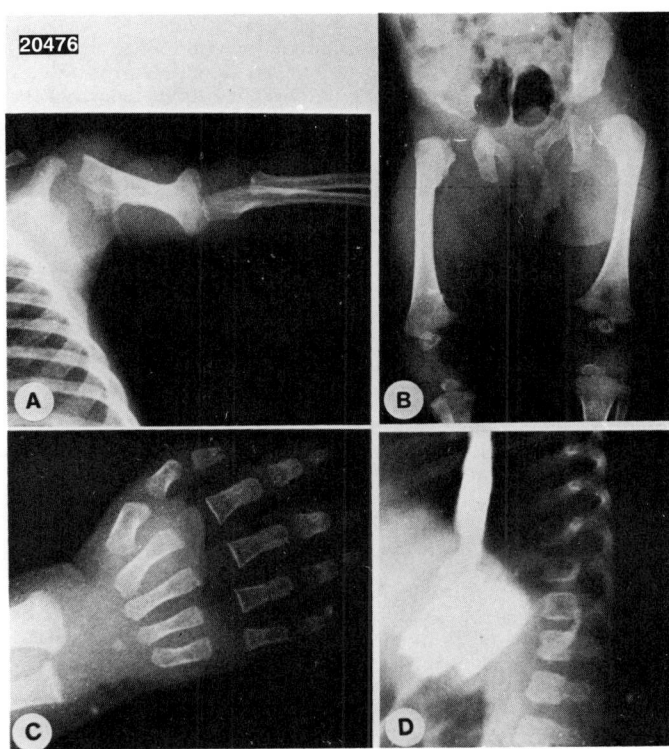

**2816B-20476:** Rhizomelic syndrome: A. Rhizomelia of humerus with flared epiphysis. B. Dislocated hips with flat acetabulae. C. Digitalization of the thumb with bifid distal phalanx. D. Flat thoracic vertebrae.

and feet; prominent calcaneous; additional irregular centers of epiphyses about the knees.

*Other:* Pulmonic stenosis, seborrheic dermatitis, and mental retardation.

**Complications:** Unknown.

**Associated Findings:** Short stature, mental retardation, and congenital heart disease.

**Etiology:** Possibly autosomal recessive inheritance. The parents of the first reported cases were consanguineous, but the precise relationship is not known.

**Pathogenesis:** Unknown.

**MIM No.:** 26825

**POS No.:** 3064

**Sex Ratio:** Presumably M1:F1.

**Occurrence:** Three siblings from one Arab family have been documented.

**Risk of Recurrence for Patient's Sib:**
See Part I, *Mendelian Inheritance.*

**Risk of Recurrence for Patient's Child:**
See Part I, *Mendelian Inheritance.*

**Age of Detectability:** *In utero* by ultrasound at five months gestation.

**Gene Mapping and Linkage:** Unknown.

**Prevention:** None known. Genetic counseling indicated.

**Treatment:** Symptomatic.

**Prognosis:** Unknown.

**Detection of Carrier:** Unknown.

**Special Considerations:** P. Maroteaux has proposed the term **Omodysplasia** based upon the Greek term for humerus, as a name for a disorder of variable expressivity in which hypoplasia of the distal humerus and subluxation of the radial head are major features. Omodysplasia is phenotypically distinct from the syndrome described above.

**References:**
Urbach D, et al.: A new skeletal dysplasia syndrome with rhizomelia of the humeri and other malformations. Clin Genet 1986; 29:83–87.

G0026        **Richard M. Goodman**

**RHS syndrome**
*See SMITH-LEMLI-OPITZ SYNDROME*
**Rib gap defects-micrognathia**
*See CEREBRO-COSTO-MANDIBULAR SYNDROME*
**Ribbing disease**
*See DIAPHYSEAL DYSPLASIA*
**Rice ear wax**
*See EAR, CERUMEN VARIATIONS*
**Richner-Hanhart Syndrome**
*See TYROSINEMIA II, OREGON TYPE*
**Rickets, familial vitamin D-resistant**
*See HYPOPHOSPHATEMIA, X-LINKED*
**Rickets, hereditary hypocalcemic type IIa**
*See RESISTANCE TO 1,25 DIHYDROXY VITAMIN D*

---

**RICKETS, HEREDITARY HYPOPHOSPHATEMIC WITH HYPERCALCIURIA (HHRH)**      **3020**

**Includes:**
HHRH
Hypercalciuria, idiopathic (some forms)
Hypercalciuric rickets
Hypophosphatemic rickets with hypercalciuria

**Excludes:**
**Hypercalciuria, familial idiopathic** (2302)
**Hypophosphatemia, non X-linked** (2040)
**Hypophosphatemia, X-linked** (0517)
Oncogenic hypophosphatemic osteomalacia

**Major Diagnostic Criteria:** Rickets/osteomalacia and elevated serum alkaline phosphatase; low serum phosphorus for age, elevated urine excretion and renal clearance of phosphate, and low TmP/GFR; elevated urine calcium excretion (0.30 g/g creatinine) and intestinal absorption of calcium; elevated plasma 1,25-$(OH)_2D$ for season and age; serum iPTH normal to low normal.

**Clinical Findings:** Onset of the disease is during early childhood in the homozygous phenotype. Signs and symptoms of rickets (in growing persons) and osteomalacia. Hypercalciuria, urinary tract calculi, and nephrolithiasis ("idiopathic hypercalciuria") can be the principal disease in heterozygotes.

**Complications:** Those of rickets/osteomalacia (pseudofractures, deformities, short stature, muscle weakness) and chronic hypercalciuria (urinary calculi and nephrolithiasis).

**Associated Findings:** None known.

**Etiology:** "Incomplete" autosomal recessive inheritance for bone disease. Autosomal dominant inheritance for hypercalciuria.

**Pathogenesis:** All manifestations can be explained by a selective impairment of phosphate reabsorption in the proximal nephron (convoluted segment) causing low serum phosphorus, elevated phosphate clearance, and low TmP/GFR. An adaptive response with increased renal synthesis of 1,25-$(OH)_2D$ causes the high serum hormone value. Increased hormone causes enhanced calcium absorption (intestine) and excretion (kidney), without hyperparathyroidism. Phosphorous deficiency causes defective bone mineralization and growth.

**MIM No.:** *24153

**Sex Ratio:** Presumably M1:F1; M2:F1 observed.

**Occurrence:** Nine members of one Bedouin pedigree have been documented. Other cases have been described in France, Japan, and a Bedouin tribe.

**Risk of Recurrence for Patient's Sib:**
See Part I, *Mendelian Inheritance.*

**Risk of Recurrence for Patient's Child:**
See Part I, *Mendelian Inheritance.*

**Age of Detectability:** Reported cases detected in early childhood. Could be detected as early as infancy.

**Gene Mapping and Linkage:** Unknown.

**Prevention:** None known. Genetic counseling indicated.

**Treatment:** Phosphate supplement in diet (1–2.5 g/day, in childhood, as neutral phosphate salts in four to five divided doses).

**Prognosis:** Excellent for normal mineralization of hard tissues and growth (with early therapy and good compliance). Life long treatment (age-adjusted dosage) is indicated.

**Detection of Carrier:** Carriers (presumed heterozygotes) have elevated urine calcium excretion (the "idiopathic hypercalciuria" phenotype), slightly depressed fasting serum phosphorus, slightly elevated plasma 1,25-$(OH)_2D$ levels (>95 pg/ml), and low normal TmP/GFR (>1.15 SD units below normal mean).

**Special Considerations:** This condition has importance beyond its frequency. The homozygous phenotype has been observed in only nine members of one Bedouin tribe containing 21 presumed (or obligate) heterozygotes (Tieder et al., 1985, 1987) and perhaps also in one Japanese person (Nishiyama et al., 1986) and European cases (Tieder & Stark, 1979; Chen et al, 1989). The phenotype is important because 1) it demonstrates the predicted adaptive response to phosphate depletion (increased renal synthesis of 1,25-$(OH)_2D$); and 2) it identifies a gene product, probably at another cellular location in the proximal nephron different from those controlled by X-linked loci and another autosomal locus which also determine phosphate homeostasis (see **Hypophosphatemia, X-linked** and **Hypercalciuria, familial idiopathic**).

**References:**

Tieder M, Stark H: Forme familiale d'hypercalciurie idiopathique avec nanism, atteinte osseuse et renale chez l'enfant. Helv Paediat Acta 1979; 34:359–367.

Tieder M, et al.: Hereditary hypophosphatemic rickets with hypercalciuria. New Engl J Med 1985; 312:611–617.

Nishiyama S, et al.: A single case of hypophosphatemic rickets with hypercalciuria. J Pediatr Gastroenterol Nutr 1986; 5:826–829.

Tieder M, et al.: "Idiopathic" hypercalciuria and hereditary hypophosphatemic rickets. New Engl J Med 1987; 316:611–617.

Chen C, et al.: Hypercalciuric hypophosphatemic rickets, mineral balance, bone histomorphology, and therapeutic implications of hypercalciuria. Pediatrics 1989; 84:276–280.

SC050                                                  **Charles R. Scriver**

**Rickets, hereditary hypophosphatemic with hypercalciuria (some)**
*See HYPERCALCIURIA, FAMILIAL IDIOPATHIC*

## RICKETS, VITAMIN D-DEPENDENT, TYPE I                    0873

**Includes:**
Autosomal recessive vitamin D-dependency (ARVDD)
Hypocalcemic, hypophosphatemic rickets with aminoaciduria
Pseudovitamin D-deficiency rickets (PDR), hereditary
Renal 25-hydroxyvitamin D1-hydroxylase deficiency
Vitamin D-dependent rickets, hereditary
Vitamin D-dependent rickets, type I
Vitamin D-dependent rickets, type III, aminoaciduria

**Excludes:**
**Cystinosis** (0238)
**Hypophosphatemia, X-linked** (0517)
Hypophosphatemic rickets associated with glucosuria
Hypophosphatemic rickets associated with renal tubular acidosis
**Rickets, hereditary hypophosphatemic with hypercalciuria (HHRH)** (3020)
Rickets, vitamin D-deficient

**Major Diagnostic Criteria:** Radiologic rickets with hypocalcemia, aminoaciduria, and elevated alkaline phosphatase. The vitamin D requirement is usually 20,000 to 100,000 IU daily, considerably greater than that needed to prevent vitamin D-deficiency rickets. Exclusion of other disorders, including intestinal malabsorption, renal insufficiency, and renal tubular abnormalities. Concentrations in blood of 25-hydroxyvitamin D (25-[OH]D) are normal or elevated, and concentrations of 1,25-dihydroxyvitamin D (1,25-[OH]D) are low.

**Clinical Findings:** Clinical manifestations are similar to those of vitamin D-deficiency rickets. Symptoms usually appear before age one year and may occur as early as the first months of life. They include hypotonia, weakness, and growth failure. Motor retardation may be apparent or real. Enamel defects are seen in teeth that calcify postnatally. Pathologic fractures may occur. Later, bony deformities develop. Convulsions or tetany may be the presenting clinical feature. Rickets with a reliable history of adequate intake of vitamin D may be a clue to the diagnosis.

Prominent physical findings are shortness of stature, hypotonia, and the characteristic features of rickets, including thickening of the wrists and ankles, frontal bowing of lower limbs and positive Trousseau and Chvostek signs. X-ray findings are those of classic rickets. They may vary in severity, and they are indistinguishable from those of vitamin D-deficiency rickets.

The serum concentration of calcium is low, and serum phosphate level is low or normal. The levels of alkaline phosphatase and parathyroid hormone are elevated. Generalized aminoaciduria is characteristic.

Urinary cyclic AMP is elevated. GI absorption of calcium is depressed. Antirachitic activity as measured by bioassay is normal. Serum concentrations of 1,25-dihydroxyvitamin $D_3$ are low, while those of 25-(OH)D are normal or elevated.

**Complications:** Rachitic deformities, growth failure.

**Associated Findings:** Hypotonia, muscle weakness, tetany, convulsions. Enamel hypoplasia of teeth that form postnatally.

**Etiology:** Autosomal recessive inheritance.

**Pathogenesis:** A genetic defect in renal 25-hydroxycholecalciferol 1-hydroxylase, the enzyme responsible for the conversion of 25-hydroxyvitamin D to 1,25-dihydroxyvitamin D. This results in an attenuated response to normal amounts of vitamin D and the development of classic rickets and hypocalcemia.

**MIM No.:** *26470

**POS No.:** 3263

**Sex Ratio:** M1:F1

**Occurrence:** Over a half-dozen kindreds reported.

**Risk of Recurrence for Patient's Sib:**
See Part I, *Mendelian Inheritance.*

**Risk of Recurrence for Patient's Child:**
See Part I, *Mendelian Inheritance.*

**Age of Detectability:** Usually before age two years, and as early as the third or fourth month of life.

**Gene Mapping and Linkage:** VDD1 (vitamin D dependency 1) has been provisionally mapped to 12q14.

**Prevention:** None known. Genetic counseling indicated.

**Treatment:** Pharmacologic doses of vitamin D are required, and small physiologic quantities of 1,25-(OH)D or calcitriol are effective. Doses are 0.25 to 2.0 $\mu$g/day. Calcium therapy for hypocalcemic tetany or convulsions. Orthopedic correction of deformities.

**Prognosis:** Treatment results in complete healing of rickets, with normalization of plasma calcium and phosphate concentrations, remission of muscle hypotonia and weakness, and normalization of growth. Continuous treatment is required throughout childhood and probably for life.

**Detection of Carrier:** Unknown.

**References:**

Fraser D, Salter RB: The diagnosis and management of the various types of rickets. Pediatr Clin North Am 1958; 5:417–441.

Prader A, et al.: Eine besondere Form der primaeren Vitamin-D-

resistenten Rachitis mit Hypocalcaemie und autosomal-domi-
nantem Erbgang: die Hereditaere Pseudo-mangelrachitis. Helv Paediatr Acta 1961; 16:452–468.

Fraser D, et al.: Pathogenesis of hereditary vitamin-D-dependent
rickets: an inborn error of vitamin D metabolism involving defective
conversion of 25-hydroxyvitamin D to 1-alpha, 25-dihydroxyvitamin
D. New Engl J Med 1973; 289:817–822.

Balsan S, et al.: 1,25-Dihydroxyvitamin D, and 1,$\alpha$-hydroxyvitamin $D_3$
in children: biologic and therapeutic effects in nutritional rickets and
different types of vitamin D resistance. Pediatr Res 1975; 9:586–593.

Delvin EE, et al.: Vitamin D dependency: replacement therapy with
calcitriol. J Pediatr 1981; 99:26–34.

Liberman UA, et al.: Resistance to 1,25-dihydroxyvitamin D: association with heterogeneous defects in cultured skin fibroblasts. J Clin
Invest 1983; 71:192–200.

Nyhan WL: Diagnostic recognition of genetic disease. Philadelphia:
Lea & Febiger, 1987:253–271. *

NY000　　　　　　　　　　　　　　　　　　　**William L. Nyhan**

**Rickets, vitamin D-dependent, type II**
　*See RESISTANCE TO 1,25 DIHYDROXY VITAMIN D*
**Rickets-alopecia syndrome**
　*See RESISTANCE TO 1,25 DIHYDROXY VITAMIN D*
**Rieger anomaly-lipodystrophy-short stature-diabetes**
　*See LIPODYSTROPHY-RIEGER ANOMALY-SHORT STATURE-
　DIABETES*

---

## RIEGER SYNDROME　　　　　　　　　　　　2139

**Includes:**
　Goniodysgenesis-hypodontia
　Hypodontia-mesoectodermal dysgenesis of iris and cornea
　Iridogoniodysgenesis with somatic anomalies

**Excludes:**
　Axenfeld syndrome
　**Eye, anterior segment dysgenesis** (0439)

**Major Diagnostic Criteria:** Goniodysgenesis and hypodontia.

**Clinical Findings:** Affected individuals have mesodermal dysgenesis of the iris and cornea, congenital absence of the incisors
and occasionally the premolars, and maxillary hypoplasia which is
manifest as a flat midface.

**Complications:** Glaucoma, ectopic pupils.

**Associated Findings:** Failure of involution of the periumbilical
skin.

**Etiology:** Autosomal dominant inheritance.

**Pathogenesis:** Undetermined, although a primary defect in the
mesoderm could explain all features.

**MIM No.:** *18050

**POS No.:** 3380

**Sex Ratio:** M1:F1

**Occurrence:** Undetermined; extensive literature.

**Risk of Recurrence for Patient's Sib:**
　See Part I, *Mendelian Inheritance.*

**Risk of Recurrence for Patient's Child:**
　See Part I, *Mendelian Inheritance.*

**Age of Detectability:** Neonatal period if structural eye defects are
visible, otherwise in early childhood because of visual difficulties
or dental defects.

**Gene Mapping and Linkage:** Unknown.

**Prevention:** None known. Genetic counseling indicated.

**Treatment:** Early diagnosis offers the possibility to ameliorate the
effects of glaucoma. Prostheses for incomplete dentition.

**Prognosis:** Good for life span and intelligence, but deteriorating
vision may lead to total blindness.

**Detection of Carrier:** Unknown.

**Special Considerations:** Since many syndromes have been reported under the heading of Rieger syndrome, there is some
confusion over the physical stigmata that are associated with it. In

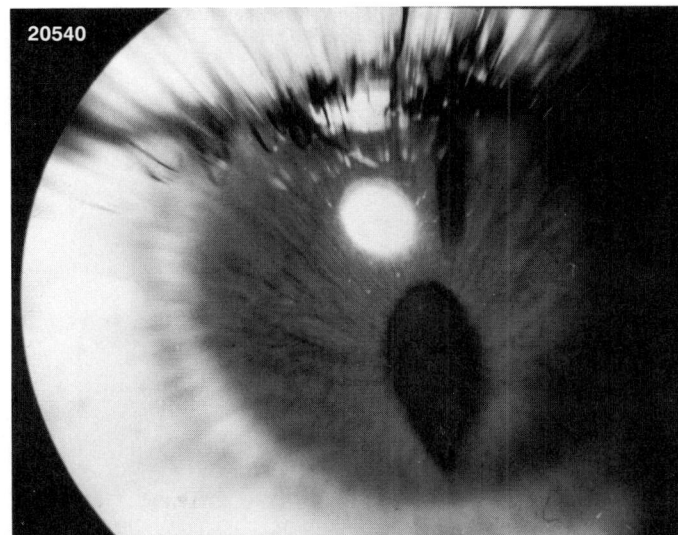

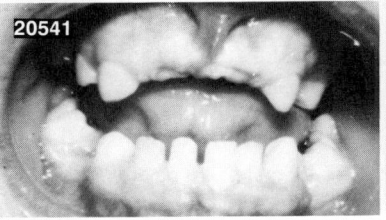 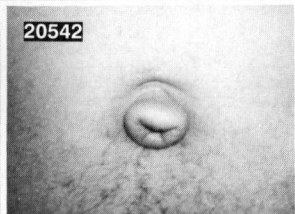

**2139-20540:** Rieger syndrome; note goniodysgenesis with irregular pupil. **20541:** Hypodontia with absence of the incisors.
**20542:** Note failure of involution of the periumbilical skin.

---

one series, for example, a number of patients with failure of
involution of the periumbilical skin were thought to have herniae
and were subjected to surgery unnecessarily.

**References:**

Rieger H: Beiträge zur Kenntniss seltener Mosbildungen der Iris.
Graefe Arch Ophthalmol 1935; 133:602–635.

Alkemade PPH: Dysgenesis mesodermalis of the iris and cornea.
Assen (Netherlands): Van Gorcum, 1969.

Fitch N, Kaback M: The Axenfeld syndrome and the Rieger syndrome.
J Med Genet 1978; 15:30–34.

Jorgenson RJ, et al.: The Rieger syndrome. Am J Med Genet 1978;
2:307–318. * †

Chisholm IA, Chudley AE: Autosomal dominant iridogoniodysgenesis with associated somatic anomalies: four generation family with
Rieger's syndrome. Br J Ophthal 1983; 67:529–534. †

J0027　　　　　　　　　　　　　　　　　　**Ronald J. Jorgenson**

**Right aortic arch types I, II and III**
　*See AORTIC ARCH, RIGHT*
**Right aortic arch-retroesophageal anomalous subclavian artery**
　*See AORTIC ARCH, RIGHT*
**Right atrial myxoma**
　*See MYXOMA, INTRACARDIAC*
**Right coronary artery, anomalous origin from pulmonary artery**
　*See ARTERY, CORONARY, ANOMALOUS ORIGIN FROM
　PULMONARY ARTERY*
**Right ventricular anomalous muscle bundle**
　*See VENTRICLE, DOUBLE CHAMBERED RIGHT*
**Right ventricular hypertrophy-endocardial fibroelastosis**
　*See VENTRICLE, ENDOCARDIAL FIBROELASTOSIS OF RIGHT
　VENTRICLE*
**Right ventricular myxoma**
　*See MYXOMA, INTRACARDIAC*

Right ventricular obstruction by aberrant muscular bands
  *See VENTRICLE, DOUBLE CHAMBERED RIGHT*
Right ventricular subinfundibular obstruction
  *See VENTRICLE, DOUBLE CHAMBERED RIGHT*
Rigid spine syndrome
  *See HAUPTMANN-THANHAUSER SYNDROME*
Riley-Day syndrome
  *See DYSAUTONOMIA I, RILEY-DAY TYPE*
Riley-Smith syndrome
  *See OVERGROWTH, MACROCEPHALY-HEMANGIOMA, RILEY-SMITH TYPE*
Ring 6
  *See CHROMOSOME 6, RING 6*
Ring 9
  *See CHROMOSOME 9, RING 9*
Ring 14
  *See CHROMOSOME 14, RING 14*
Ring 15
  *See CHROMOSOME 15, RING 15*
Ring 18
  *See CHROMOSOME 18, RING 18*
Ring 21
  *See CHROMOSOME 21, RING 21*
Ring 22
  *See CHROMOSOME 22, RING 22*
Ring-like corneal dystrophy
  *See CORNEAL DYSTROPHY, REIS-BUCKLERS TYPE*

---

## ROBERTS SYNDROME          0875

**Includes:**
> Appelt-Gerken-Lenz syndrome
> Bone, absence deformities of long-cleft lip/palate
> Centromere abnormalities-chromatid apposition-Roberts spectrum
> Centromere spreading
> Centromere separation, premature
> Chromosome, abnormal centromere and chromatid apposition
> Limbs, deformities of long bones-cleft lip/palate
> Pseudothalidomide-SC syndrome
> Pseudothalidomide syndrome
> Roberts syndrome spectrum
> SC phocomelia syndrome
> Tetraphocomelia-ocular defects-cleft lip/palate-penile anomalies

**Excludes:**
> **Caudal regression syndrome** (3211)
> **Femoral hypoplasia-unusual facies syndrome** (2027)
> **Fetal thalidomide syndrome** (0386)
> **Heart-hand syndrome** (0455)

**Major Diagnostic Criteria:** Cytogenetic evidence of abnormal centromere and chromatid apposition (ACCA) or "puffing apart" in heterochromatic and centromeric regions of multiple chromosomes, usually most evident in acrocentric chromosomes and the long arms of chromosome Y. Interface nuclear morphology in fibroblasts is often disturbed and shows abnormal nuclear contours (blebbing) and micronuclei. The clinical signs of patients with ACCA are variable. Historically, the term, Roberts syndrome, is applied to patients with severe mid-facial clefting, hypoplastic nasal alae, facial hemangioma, ocular defects (mainly vascularization of the cornea) and absence/shortness-type limb malformations. A more severe spectrum of congenital malformations is found among stillborns, while in milder cases, facial clefts and limb defects are absent. Growth failure is severe in prenatal and postnatal life.

**Clinical Findings:** Among affected stillborns, abnormal brain segmentation, interocular encephaloceles, severe ocular malformations, maxillary agenesis, agenesis of nostrils, severe renal dysplasia, polycystic kidneys, and spina bifida have been found. Severely affected neonates characteristically have hypoplastic alae nasi, severe mid-facial clefts, and severe tetraphocomelia constituting the *Roberts syndrome* phenotype. In children who survive infancy, facial hemangioma, vascularized cornea, or microph-

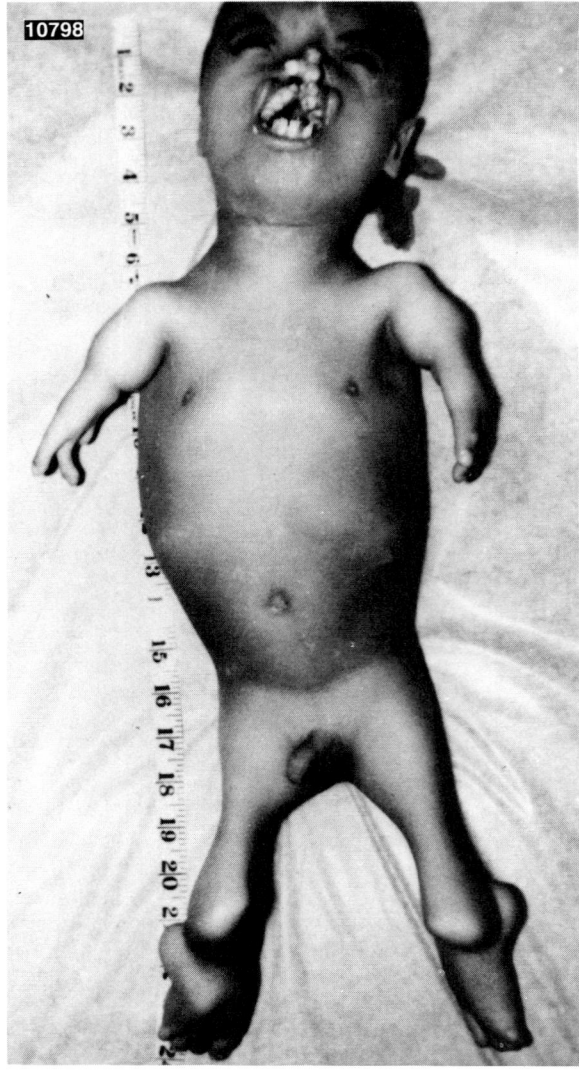

**0875**-10798: Note cleft lip and palate with protrusion of premaxilla and limb defects with shortened and deformed limbs.

---

thalmia, hypoplastic nasal alae (facial clefts are uncommon), micrognathia, mild mental retardation, severe failure to thrive, and milder degrees of tetraphocomelia were described as the *SC Phocomelia* or *Pseudothalidomide syndrome* or phenotype. The mildest clinical spectrum consists of stigmatic facies, vascularized cornea (Peters anomaly; see **Eye, anterior segment dysgenesis**), and mild mental retardation. Growth failure, mental retardation, ocular defects, and prominent penile or clitoral shaft are seen in severely and mildly affected patients.

Birth weight and length can be strikingly subnormal, and subsequent growth drastically lagging. Recorded birth weights of near term infants are illustrative (0.9, 1.04, 1.3, 1.4, 1.6 and 1.8 kg), as are small weights of survivors (at ages seven and 16 years the weight was 7.6 and 5.8 kg, respectively). The limb reduction defects invariably involve all four extremities, tend to be symmetric, and more severe in the upper limbs. The number of fingers is often reduced, radial aplasia or dysplasia is common, and lack of the first metacarpal, thumb, or first phalanx is frequent.

Frontal and interocular encephaloceles, maxillary agenesis, Peters anomaly, severe facial mid-line clefts, agenesis or hypoplastic nostrils, and hypoplastic alae nasi probably reflect the same pathogenesis. One mentally retarded patient with ACCA had no signs of Peters anomaly.

Among survivors, one female had her menarche at 11 years, later married and became pregnant but miscarried in the first trimester. Another female (IQ 70) experienced a full-term pregnancy at the age of 24, delivered a healthy girl, and later developed a malignant melanoma at the age of 32. She was also noted to have hypoplastic iris and scleralization of the peripheral cornea, dysmorphic facies, hypoplasia of the nasal tip, and nasal alae, no facial clefts, and multiple skeletal malformations affecting all limbs; her similarly affected sister died at 43, following a massive stroke.

**Complications:** Prenatal or perinatal death; respiratory and feeding difficulties related to cleft lip and palate; physical limitations due to limb defects; visual difficulties due to ocular malformations resulting from abnormal cleavage of the anterior chamber (Peter Anomaly); mental subnormality.

**Associated Findings:** High mortality among severely affected; mental retardation; failure-to-thrive; and decreased vision. One 23-month-old developed sarcoma botryoides, and a 32-year-old developed malignant melanoma.

**Etiology:** Autosomal recessive inheritance. Clinical heterogeneity is significant.

**Pathogenesis:** Unknown.

**MIM No.:** *26830

**POS No.:** 3378

**Sex Ratio:** M1:F1

**Occurrence:** At least 28 patients from 16 sibships demonstrating ACCA have been reported. Noted in many ethnic groups.

**Risk of Recurrence for Patient's Sib:**
See Part I, *Mendelian Inheritance.*

**Risk of Recurrence for Patient's Child:**
See Part I, *Mendelian Inheritance.*

**Age of Detectability:** Usually at birth, but possible prenatally by elevated maternal serum alpha-fetoprotein or by ultrasound confirming severe fetal failure to thrive, facial clefting, **Microcephaly**, and/or shortened extremeties. Incidental detection of ACCA in amniocytes has also led to the detection of a patient with mild manifestations.

**Gene Mapping and Linkage:** Unknown.

**Prevention:** None known. Genetic counseling indicated.

**Treatment:** Surgical repair of facial and limb defects and corneal grafts; special education.

**Prognosis:** Increased perinatal mortality among those severely affected. Those with milder congenital malformations may not be at risk for a shortened life span.

**Detection of Carrier:** Unknown.

**Special Considerations:** The frequency of ACCA is highest in the heterochromatic procentric region of chromosomes 16, 13–15, 21–22, and long arm of the Y and is strikingly rare in chromosome 11. Such a consistent pattern suggests a constitutive defect common to various chromosomal regions. Utilization of CREST antikinetochore antibodies demonstrated normal antigenicity but unusually large stained kinetochore regions. This suggests the presence of a decondensed or structurally altered kinetochore; a feature noticeable in metaphase but also in interphase cells. Cocultivation of patient and normal fibroblasts did not correct ACCA. Fusion hybrids (patient fibroblasts with Chinese hamster cell lines) apparently supplied the missing gene product needed to correct ACCA.

**References:**
Freeman MVR, et al.: The Roberts syndrome. Clin Genet 1974; 5:1–16.
Hermann J, Opitz JM: The SC phocomelia and the Roberts syndrome, vol. V: nosologic aspects. Eur J Pediatr 1977; 125:117–134.
Wertelecki W, et al.: Abnormal centromere-chromatid aposition (ACCA) and Peters anomaly. Ophthal Pediatr Genet 1985; 6:247–255. †
Krassikoff NE, et al.: Chromatid repulsion associated with Roberts/SC

phocomelia syndrome is reduced in malignant cells and not expressed in interspecies somatic-cell hybrids. Am J Hum Genet 1986; 39:618–630.
Parry DM, et al.: SC phocomelia syndrome, premature centramere separation and congenital cranial nerve paralysis in two sisters, one with malignant melanoma. Am J Med Genet 1986; 24:653–672.
Fryns JP, et al.: The Robert tetraphocomelia syndrome: identical limb defects in two siblings. Ann Genet 1987; 30:243–245.
Romke C, et al.: Roberts syndrome and SC phocamelia: a single genetic entity. Clin Genet 1987; 31:170–177. †
Jabs EW, et al.: Centromere separation and aneuploidy in human mitotic mutants: Roberts syndrome. In: Resnick M, Vig B, eds: Mechanisms of chromosome distribution and aneuploidy. New York: Alan R. Liss, 1989;111–118.
Robins DB, et al.: Prenatal detection of Roberts-SC phocomelia syndrome. Am J Med Genet 1989; 32:390–394.

WE029                                                        **W. Wertelecki**

**Roberts syndrome spectrum**
*See ROBERTS SYNDROME*
**Robertsonian translocation**
*See CHROMOSOME 13, TRISOMY 13*
**Robin anomaly (some)**
*See ARTHRO-OPHTHALMOPATHY, HEREDITARY, PROGRESSIVE, STICKLER TYPE*
**Robin anomaly, isolated**
*See CLEFT PALATE-MICROGNATHIA-GLOSSOPTOSIS*
**Robin sequence**
*See CLEFT PALATE-MICROGNATHIA-GLOSSOPTOSIS*
**Robin sequence with hyperphalangy**
*See DIGITO-PALATAL SYNDROME, STEVENSON TYPE*
**Robin sequence-aniridia-growth delay (RAG)**
*See RAG SYNDROME*

---

**ROBINOW SYNDROME**                                           **0876**

**Includes:**
> Acral dysostosis-facial and genital abnormalities
> Costovertebral segmentation defect-mesomelia
> COVESDEM syndrome
> Dwarfism, mesomelic Robinow type
> Fetal face syndrome
> Mesomelic dysplasia, type Robinow
> Robinow-Silverman-Smith syndrome

**Excludes:**
> **Aarskog syndrome** (0001)
> Mesomelic skeletal dysplasias (other)
> Micropenis, in other conditions

**Major Diagnostic Criteria:** Most patients show at least three of the following four anomalies: the "fetal face," genital hypoplasia, forearm brachymelia, and moderate dwarfing.

**Clinical Findings:** *Fetal face:* So termed because it resembles the face of the fetus at eight weeks. The neurocranium is disproportionately large, while the viscerocranium is hypoplastic. Characteristic features are a bulging forehead; moderate hypertelorism; wide palpebral fissures; a short, upturned nose; and a broad, inverted V-shaped mouth. The facial characteristics become less striking at puberty.

*Genital hypoplasia:* In the male, the penis is often invisible in infancy and childhood unless the surrounding skin is retracted. Testicles are usually of normal size, although frequently undescended. During puberty the glans penis attains normal size, but the shaft remains unduly short. Nevertheless, sexual functioning is possible and procreation has been repeatedly documented. Androgen receptors and 5-α reductase of genital skin fibroblasts have been normal.

In the female, the clitoris and labia minora are hypoplastic. Sexual maturation and reproduction are normal. The pelvis is large enough to permit spontaneous vaginal delivery.

*Forearm brachymelia:* Usually obvious, sometimes demonstrable only by measurement, rarely absent. Mesomelic shortness of the lower extremities is less marked or absent.

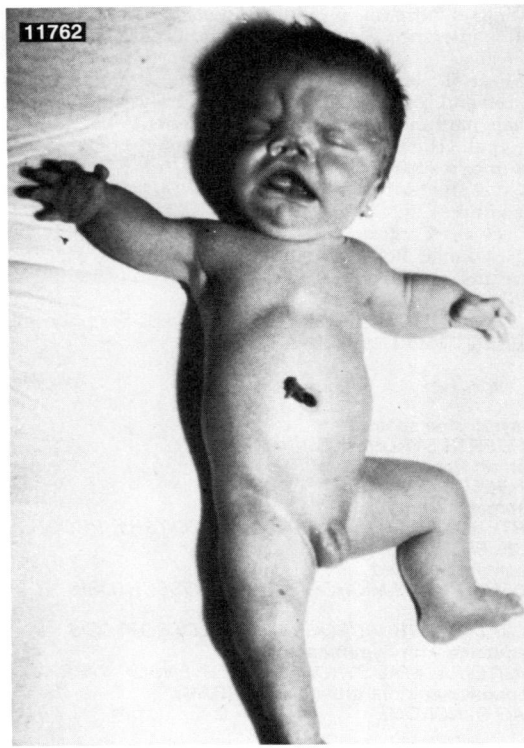

**0876A-11762:** Infant with characteristic triangular facies with broad forehead and forearm brachmelia.

*Moderate dwarfing:* Stature past infancy has ranged from the mean to -8 SD, and has averaged -3.1 SD.

*Intelligence:* Normal in most cases, mildly reduced in some, and severely impaired in a few.

*Common but less frequent findings:* Inguinal hernias, vertebral

**0876B-10801:** Prominent forehead, ocular hypertelorism, short upturned nose, triangular mouth and brachymelia. **10803:** Affected infant shows similar facial features, very short forearms, severe penile hypoplasia.

segmentation defects, radial head dislocation, acromelic brachymelia (short metacarpals and phalanges), bifid or duplicated thumbs or big toes, ankyloglossia, crowding and malalignment of the anterior teeth, gingival hyperplasia, and delayed eruption of permanent teeth.

**Complications:** Scoliosis secondary to vertebral anomalies.

**Associated Findings:** Congenital heart disease (10% or less), cleft lip and palate, dislocated hips, hepatosplenomegaly, hyperostosis.

**Etiology:** Autosomal dominant or recessive inheritance. The two forms are usually distinct clinically and on X-ray. Most sporadic cases can be assigned to one of the two forms, although additional heterogeneity cannot be ruled out.

Patients with the recessive form (once called *Costovertebral segmentation defect with mesomellia,* or *COVESDEM*) tend to be more severely dwarfed, have more extensive vertebral anomalies, and more severe brachymelia. The recessive form is often associated with radio-ulnar dislocation and severe hypoplasia of the proximal radius and distal ulna.

**Pathogenesis:** The association of anomalies suggests a disturbance of embryogenesis around the 8th week.

**MIM No.:** *18070

**POS No.:** 3379

**Sex Ratio:** Probably M1:F1, although males are more likely to be recognized and reported because of the striking penile hypoplasia.

**Occurrence:** About 1:500,000, i.e., about six new cases per year in the United States. Prevalence slightly lower, since 5–10% of patients have died in infancy or early childhood. Some 41 published and 35 unpublished cases have been reviewed.

**Risk of Recurrence for Patient's Sib:**
See Part I, *Mendelian Inheritance.*

**Risk of Recurrence for Patient's Child:**
See Part I, *Mendelian Inheritance.*

**Age of Detectability:** At birth.

**Gene Mapping and Linkage:** Unknown.

**Prevention:** None known. Genetic counseling indicated.

**Treatment:** Orthopedic care for vertebral anomalies. Surgery for undescended testicles and inguinal hernias, orthodontia for dental malalignment, facial reconstruction in selected cases, psychologic support. Testosterone therapy for micropenis has not proven helpful.

**Prognosis:** Facial dysmorphism becomes less striking with age. Sexual functioning and reproduction appear good for both sexes, although male reproduction in the recessive form has not yet been documented.

**Detection of Carrier:** Unknown.

**References:**
Robinow M, et al.: A newly recognized dwarfing syndrome. Am J Dis Child 1969; 117:645–651.
Wadlington WB, et al.: Mesomelic dwarfism with hemivertebrae and small genitalia (the Robinow syndrome). Am J Dis Child 1973; 126:202–205.
Giedion A, et al.: The radiologic diagnosis of the fetal face (Robinow) syndrome (mesomelic dwarfism and small genitalia): report of 3 cases. Helv Paediatr Acta 1975; 30:409–423.
Lee PA, et al.: Robinow's syndrome: partial primary hypogonadism in pubertal boys, with persistence of micropenis. Am J Dis Child 1982; 136:327–330.
Shprintzen RJ, et al.: Male-to-male transmission of Robinow's syndrome: its occurrence in association with cleft lip and cleft palate. Am J Dis Child 1982; 136:594–597.
Bain MD, et al.: Robinow syndrome without mesomelic "brachymelia": report of 5 cases. J Med Genet 1986; 23:350–354.
Robinow M, Markert RJ: The fetal face (Robinow) syndrome: delineation of the dominant and recessive phenotypes. Proc Greenwood Genet Ctr 1988; 7:144 only.

R0004

**Meinhard Robinow**

**Robinow-Silverman-Smith syndrome**
  *See ROBINOW SYNDROME*
**Robinow-Sorauf syndrome**
  *See CRANIOSYNOSTOSIS-FOOT DEFECTS, JACKSON-WEISS TYPE*
**Robinson ectodermal dysplasia-deafness**
  *See ONYCHODYSTROPHY-CONIFORM TEETH-SENSORINEURAL HEARING LOSS*
**Rod body myopathy**
  *See MYOPATHY, NEMALINE*
**Rod monochromatism**
  *See COLOR BLINDNESS, TOTAL*
**Rod-cone dystrophy**
  *See RETINITIS PIGMENTOSA*
**Rogers syndrome**
  *See HEART-HAND SYNDROME IV*
**Rokitansky sequence**
  *See MULLERIAN APLASIA*
**Rokitansky-Kuster-Hauser syndrome**
  *See MULLERIAN APLASIA*
**Rolandic epilepsy**
  *See EPILEPSY, BENIGN CHILDHOOD WITH CENTROTEMPORAL EEG FOCUS (BEC)*
**Rolland-Desbuquois syndrome**
  *See DWARFISM, DYSSEGMENTAL, ROLLAND-DESBUQUOIS TYPE*
**Romano-Ward syndrome**
  *See ARRHYTHMIA, WITH LONG QT INTERVAL WITHOUT DEAFNESS*
**Romberg syndrome**
  *See HEMIFACIAL ATROPHY, PROGRESSIVE*
**Rootless teeth**
  *See TEETH, DENTIN DYSPLASIA, RADICULAR*
**Roots, acquired concrescence of**
  *See TEETH, ROOT CONCRESCENCE*
**Rosenberg-Chutorian syndrome**
  *See DEAFNESS-POLYNEUROPATHY-OPTIC ATROPHY*
**Rosenfeld-Kloepfer syndrome**
  *See PACHYDERMOPERIOSTOSIS*
**Rosewater syndrome**
  *See ANDROGEN INSENSITIVITY SYNDROME, INCOMPLETE*
**Rosselli-Gulienetti syndrome**
  *See CLEFT LIP/PALATE-ECTODERMAL DYSPLASIA-SYNDACTYLY*

---

## ROTHMUND-THOMSON SYNDROME       2037

**Includes:**
> Cataract-poikiloderma atrophicans
> Poikiloderma atrophicans-cataract
> Telangiectasia-pigmentation-cataract syndrome
> Telangiectatic erythema, congenital

**Excludes:**
> **Bloom syndrome** (0112)
> **Cockayne syndrome** (0189)
> **Dermal hypoplasia, focal** (0281)
> **Osteodysplastica gerodermia, Bamatter type** (2099)
> **Werner syndrome** (0998)

**Major Diagnostic Criteria:** Skin atrophy, pigmentation, and telangiectasia appearing from third to sixth month of life; bilateral cataracts appearing from the fourth to the seventh year; hypogonadism with short stature and bony defects.

**Clinical Findings:** Bilateral cataracts developing at about age 4–7 years. The skin is normal at birth but develops cutis telangiectasia and atrophy about the third to sixth month of life, especially in the extensor surfaces of the hands, forearms, legs, thighs, and buttocks, with exposed surfaces being more severely affected. Once the initial inflammatory stage disappears, the affected areas present a combination of pigmentation, depigmentation, atrophy, and telangiectasia. Alopecia has been reported in 35% of the patients. Warty dyskeratosis with malignant transformation has been reported, and 25% of the patients have hypogonadism and nail dystrophy. Over 50% have short stature. A few patients do not have abnormal thumbs. Oral manifestations include microdontia, tooth crown and root malformations, and delayed and ectopic eruption.

**Complications:** Severe vision loss or blindness occurs within a few weeks as a result of the bilateral complete and semisolid eye cataracts. The small tooth roots cause the teeth to exfoliate

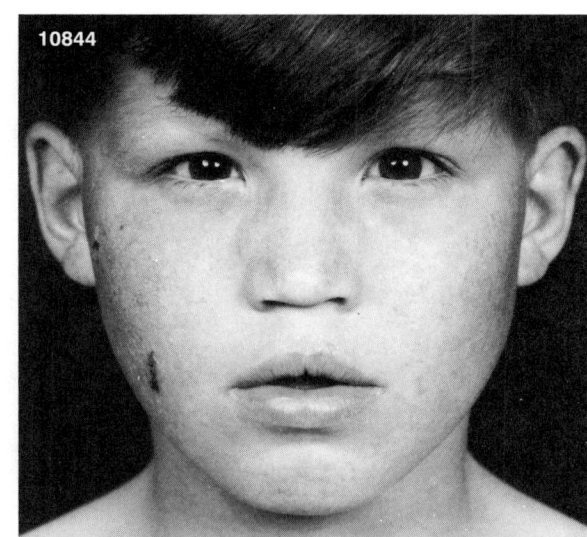

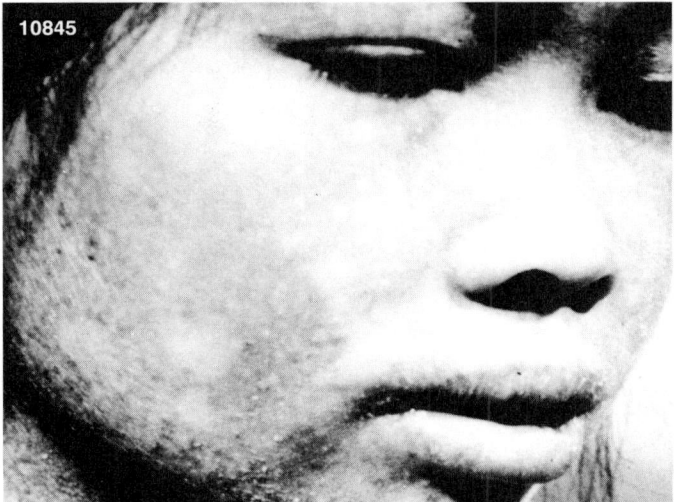

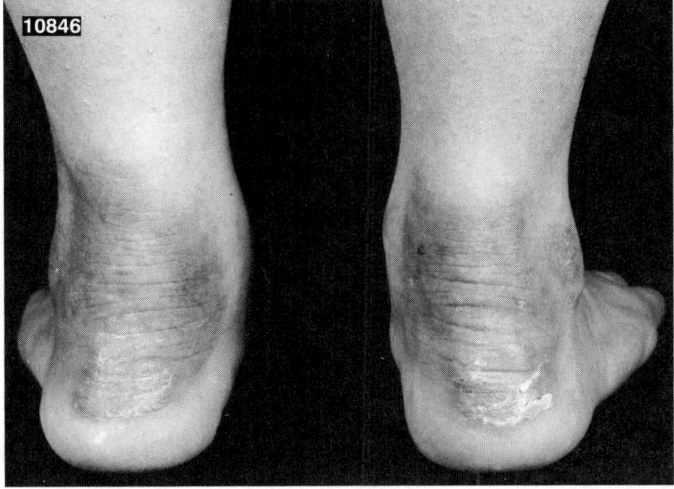

**2037A**-10844–46: Skin atrophy and hyperpigmentation.

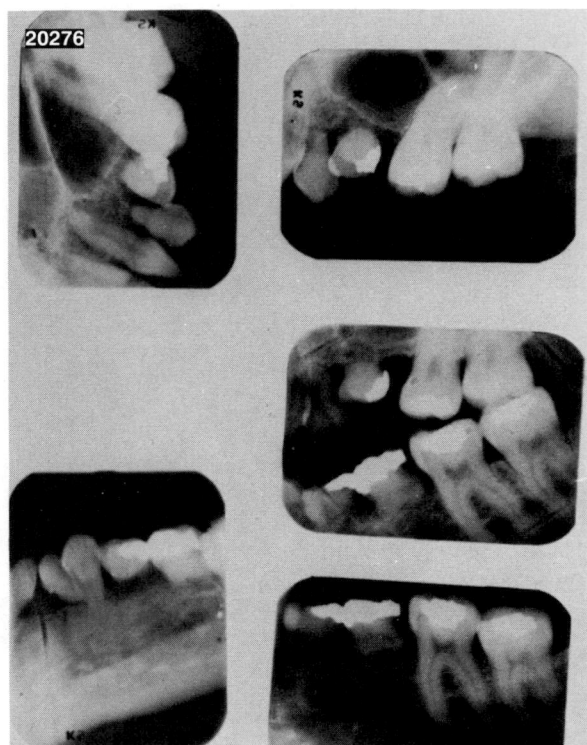

**2037B-20276:** Note short roots and bone loss.

**References:**
Thomson MS: Poikiloderma congenitale. Br J Dermatol 1936; 48:221–234.
Bottomley WK, Box JM: Dental anomalies in the Rothmund-Thomson syndrome. Oral Surg 1976; 41:321–326.
Hall C, et al.: Rothmund-Thomson syndrome with severe dwarfism. Am J Dis Child 1980; 134:165–169. *
Dechenne C, et al.: A Rothmund-Thomson case with hypertension. Clin Genet 1983; 24:266–272.
Starr DG, et al.: Non-dermatological complications and genetic aspects of the Rothmund-Thomson syndrome. Clin Genet 1985; 27:102–104.

ES000 **Victor Escobar**

**Rotor type hyperbilirubinemia**
  *See HYPERBILIRUBINEMIA, CONJUGATED, ROTOR TYPE*
**Roussy-Levy syndrome**
  *See NEUROPATHY, HEREDITARY MOTOR AND SENSORY, TYPE I*
**Rozycki syndrome**
  *See DEAFNESS-VITILIGO-MUSCLE WASTING*
**Rubella malformation syndrome**
  *See FETAL RUBELLA SYNDROME*
**Rubinstein syndrome**
  *See RUBINSTEIN-TAYBI BROAD THUMB-HALLUX SYNDROME*

## RUBINSTEIN-TAYBI BROAD THUMB-HALLUX SYNDROME 0119

**Includes:**
  Brachydactyly-peculiar facies-mental retardation syndrome
  Broad thumb hallux syndrome
  Digitofacial-mental retardation syndrome
  Hallux-broad thumb syndrome
  Michail-Matsoukas-Theodorou-Rubinstein-Taybi syndrome
  Rubinstein syndrome
  Rubinstein-Taylor syndrome

**Excludes:**
  **Acrocephalosyndactyly type I** (0014)
  **Brachydactyly** (0114)

**Major Diagnostic Criteria:** No pathognomonic criterion has been found; however, the finding of broad terminal phalanges of the thumbs and halluces, with or without angulation deformity; characteristic facial appearance with beaked or straight nose, broad nasal bridge, downward slant of palpebral fissures, peculiar "grimacing" smile and mild retrognathia; stature, head circumference, and bone age below the 50th percentile; mental, motor, language, and social retardation and incomplete or delayed descent of testes constitute the clinical syndrome.

**Clinical Findings:** *Developmental Defects*: Mental, motor, social and language retardation (100%); moderate to severe mental retardation (80%); growth defects: stature below 50th percentile (94%); stature at or below 3rd percentile (77%); bone age below 50th percentile (76%); head circumference below 50th percentile (93%); head circumference at or below 10th percentile (85%).
*Cranio-Facial Defects*: Highly arched palate (93%); Downward slanting of palpebral fissures (93%); beaked or straight nose (90%); apparent hypertelorism (85%); mild retrognathia (76%); abnormalities of external ear (74%); peculiar "grimacing" smile (72%); nasal septum extending below alae (72%); broad nasal bridge (71%); large anterior fontanel or delayed closure (64%); thick or highly arched eyebrows (56%); epicanthal folds (54%); prominent forehead (51%); parietal foramina (38%).
*Digital Defects*: Broad terminal phalanges of thumbs and/or halluces (100%); broad terminal phalanges of other fingers (71%); abnormal thumb angulation with proximal (38%); phalanx anomalies; abnormal hallux angulation with anomalies of (20%); proximal phalanx or first metatarsal; duplicated distal phalanx of hallux (14%); duplicated proximal phalanx of hallux (10%).
*Other Skeletal Defects*: Stiff, awkward, unsteady gait (76%); pelvic vertebral anomalies (67%); large foramen magnum (65%); sternal or rib anomalies (56%); overlapping toes (54%); clinodactyly of 5th finger (54%).
*Other Defects*: Incomplete or delayed descent of testes (79%);

prematurely. Blistered skin is frequently associated with sensitivity to sunlight.

**Associated Findings:** None known.

**Etiology:** Autosomal recessive inheritance, although over 70% of the patients have been female. The report of a mother and son with similar findings, however, raises the question of genetic heterogeneity.

**Pathogenesis:** Unknown.

**MIM No.:** *26840

**POS No.:** 3383

**Sex Ratio:** M3:F7

**Occurrence:** At least 65 patients have been documented, all Caucasians.

**Risk of Recurrence for Patient's Sib:**
  See Part I, *Mendelian Inheritance.*

**Risk of Recurrence for Patient's Child:**
  See Part I, *Mendelian Inheritance.*

**Age of Detectability:** Skin lesions develop by the third to sixth month of life, with confirmation as the child develops; eye problems by age 4–7 years.

**Gene Mapping and Linkage:** Unknown.

**Prevention:** None known. Genetic counseling indicated.

**Treatment:** Eye surgery, dental treatment.

**Prognosis:** Life span is within normal limits, unless squamous cell carcinoma is not identified. Reproduction seems to be impaired because of the scanty menstrual cycle in most affected females and juvenile genital organs in males. Nutrition may become important if these patients become edentulous. Early blindness should be anticipated.

**Detection of Carrier:** Unknown.

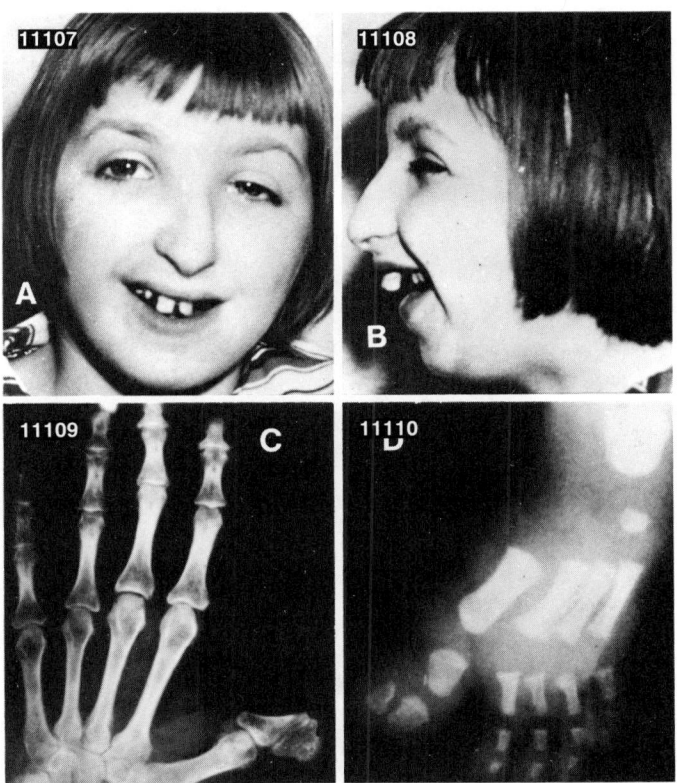

**0119**-11107:   Facies at age 14 years shows downward slanting palpebral fissures, arched eyebrows, ptosis and prominent nose. 11108:  Lateral view of face shows beaked nose with nasal septum extending below alae and micrognathia.   11109:  Triangular and spatulate deformities of proximal and terminal phalanges.   11110:  Broad great toe with duplication of terminal phalanx.

strabismus (72%); EEG abnormalities (67%); hirsutism (64%); refractive error (63%); azygous or other abnormal lung lobation (53%); deep plantar crease in 1st interdigital area (53%); urinary tract disease and/or anomalies (50%); nevus flammeus of forehead, nape of neck or back (46%); simian crease (44%); long eyelashes (44%); congenital heart disease (36%); nasolacrimal duct obstruction (36%); heart murmur (33%); corpus callosum hypoplasia (28%) ptosis (18%); supernumerary nipples (13%).

**Complications:**  Neonatal distress and/or recurrent respiratory tract infections (78%), feeding and swallowing difficulties in infancy (73%), gastroesophageal reflux, weak unusual cry in infancy; urinary tract infections, nephrolithiasis, hydronephrosis/ hydroureter with or without reflux; stiff, awkward, unsteady gait; brisk tendon reflexes in lower limbs; inability to oppose thumb; EEG abnormalities, seizures, meningitis; relative obesity for height particularly involving the lower trunk; irregular crowded teeth, malocclusion; recurrent paronychiae; leukemia, brain tumor (ectopic pinealoma), and intraspinal neurilemoma. Stirt (1982) reported a risk of cardiac arrhythmia with the use of succinylcholine.

**Associated Findings:**  Umbilical hernia, inguinal hernia; eczema, keloids; diabetes or abnormal glucose tolerance test; mild webbing of fingers and/or toes; contracture or dislocation of elbow; short metacarpal, sixth toe on fibular side of foot, hallux valgus, absence or subluxation of patella, coxa valga, genu valgum, valgus foot, pes planus, clubfoot; first degree hypospadias, angulated penis; wide-spaced nipples; short neck; subcortical atrophy, hydrocephalus, cavum septum pellucidum, myelomeningocele; premature

fusion of sternum; coloboma of iris, lens, and/or retina; exophthalmos or enophthalmos, cataract, congenital glaucoma, megalocornea; deviated nasal septum; macroglossia, forked or bifid tongue, bifid uvula, thin upper lip, long philtrum, lack of maxillary prominence with relative prognathism, enamel hypoplasia, talon cusps; stridor, low pitched-husky voice; persistent metopic suture, metopic synostosis, Luckenschädel, hyperostosis frontalis interna, flat occiput, brachycephaly. This list is not intended to be all-inclusive and the significance of many of the findings listed is uncertain.

Dermatoglyphic findings have included increased frequency of arches and decreased frequency of ulnar loops on fingertips, radial loops shifted to fingers other than second, additional triradius on apex of thumb or hallux, rare double pattern on thumbs, somewhat reduced total finger ridge count, large complex pattern in thenar/first interdigital area, hypothenar ulnar loops, distal axial triradius, increased atd angle pattern in second and/or third interdigital area of palm, missing c triradius, distorted and unusually long distal loop or a double loop in hallucal area with laterally displaced f triradius with or without e' triradius.

**Etiology:**  Undetermined. The condition has been reported in several sets of twins, and some familial patterns have been noted. Although multifactorial inheritance has been proposed, Victor McKusick has found this "difficult to accept".

**Pathogenesis:**  Unknown.

**MIM No.:**  26860

**POS No.:**  3384

**CDC No.:**  759.840

**Sex Ratio:**  M1:F1

**Occurrence:**  Simpson and Brissender (1973) estimated the population risk of 3:100,000 in the province of Ontario, Canada. Has been reported in 1:300–500 institutionalized persons with mental retardation over the age of five.

Reported among Caucasians, Orientals (Japanese) and Blacks. 250 cases from 22 countries have been documented.

**Risk of Recurrence for Patient's Sib:**  Undetermined. A 1% risk figure has been suggested by Simpson (1973).

**Risk of Recurrence for Patient's Child:**  Undetermined. No affected individual is know to have reproduced.

**Age of Detectability:**  The syndrome can be detected in the newborn period by characteristic thumb, hallux and facial abnormalities, confirmed by X-ray findings of hands and feet.

**Gene Mapping and Linkage:**  Unknown.

**Prevention:**  None known. Genetic counseling indicated.

**Treatment:**  Interdisciplinary evaluation and management should be considered to deal with the medical, social, psychological, and educational problems. Early management of respiratory and feeding problems. Appropriate medical and surgical care of associated defects, particularly those that require remediation. Antibiotics for infections and anticonvulsants for seizures. Individualized educational plan. Speech and language therapy. Surgery on hallux, particularly with duplication and/or angulation of phalanx may be required to get shoes that will fit properly. Functional results of surgery on angulated thumb deformity have not been published. Avoid obesity in late childhood and adolescence. Management of progressive malocclusion or other dental problems.

**Prognosis:**  Of the 224 cases studied, age range was from one day to 62 years and 21 patients are known to have died. The causes of death and age at the time of death included respiratory distress syndrome (2 days, 8 days), cardiac failure (26 days, 4 months, 5–1/2 months, 2–1/2 years), respiratory infections (14 days, 42 days, 5 months, 18 months, 22 months, 26 months), meningitis (2 weeks), enteritis (2–1/2 years, 6 years), trauma and respiratory infection (9 years), brain tumor (ectopic pinealoma, 14 years), leukemia (25 months, 17 years), aspiration with seizures (33 years), respiratory distress after ventriculo-peritoneal (V-P) shunt (4 months).

**Detection of Carrier:**  Unknown.

**Support Groups:** KA; Smith Center; Rubinstein-Taybi Parent Contact Group

*The Center for Birth Defects Information Services wishes to thank Jack H. Rubinstein for his contributions to a previous version of this article.*

**References:**

Rubinstein JH, Taybi H: Broad thumbs and toes and facial abnormalities: a possible mental retardation syndrome. Am J Dis Child 1963; 105:588–608.

Rubinstein J: The broad thumbs syndrome: progress report 1968. In: Bergsma D, ed: Proceedings conference on the clinical delineation of birth defects, Part II. Malformation syndromes. BD:OAS V(2), 1969:25–41.

Rubinstein JH: Broad thumb-hallux syndrome. In: Swoboda W, Stur O, eds: Proceedings of the international congress of pediatrics, Vienna, Austria, August 29– Sept. 4, 1971, Vienna, Verlag der Wiener Medizinischen Akademie, 1971:471–476.

Simpson NE, Brissender JE: The Rubinstein-Taybi syndrome: familial and dermatoglyphic data. Am J Hum Genet 1973; 25:225–229.

Kajii T, et al.: Monozygotic twins discordant for Rubinstein-Taybi syndrome. J Med Genet 1981; 18:312–314.

Stirt JA: Succinylcholine in Rubinstein-Taybi syndrome (Letter). Anesthesiology 1982; 57:429 (only).

Baraitser M, Preece MA: The Rubinstein-Taybi syndrome: Occurrence in two sets of identical twins. Clin Genet 1983; 23:318–320.

Berry AC: Rubinstein-Taybi syndrome. J Med Genet 1987; 24:562–566.

GR011 **Frank Greenberg**

**Rubinstein-Taylor syndrome**
*See RUBINSTEIN-TAYBI BROAD THUMB-HALLUX SYNDROME*
**Rud syndrome**
*See SEIZURES-ICHTHYOSIS-MENTAL RETARDATION*
**Rudiger syndrome**
*See ECTRODACTYLY-ECTODERMAL DYSPLASIA-CLEFTING SYNDROME*
**Rudimentary uterine horn**
*See MULLERIAN FUSION, INCOMPLETE*
**Rufous albinism**
*See ALBINISM, OCULOCUTANEOUS, RUFOUS TYPE*
**Ruiter-Pompen-Wyers syndrome**
*See FABRY DISEASE*
**Rukavina type hereditary amyloidosis**
*See AMYLOIDOSIS, INDIANA TYPE*
**Russell-Silver syndrome**
*See SILVER SYNDROME*
**Russell-Silver syndrome, X-linked**
*See SILVER SYNDROME, X-LINKED*
**Rutherfurd syndrome**
*See GINGIVAL FIBROMATOSIS-CORNEAL DYSTROPHY*
**Rutledge lethal multiple congenital anomaly syndrome**
*See SMITH-LEMLI-OPITZ SYNDROME, TYPE II*
**Ruvalcaba syndrome**
*See OSTEODYSTROPHY-MENTAL RETARDATION, RUVALCABA TYPE*
**Ruvalcaba-Myhre-Smith syndrome**
*See OVERGROWTH, RUVALCABA-MYHRE-SMITH TYPE*

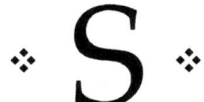

Sabinas brittle hair syndrome
  *See TRICHOTHIODYSTROPHY*
Saccharopine dehydrogenase deficiency
  *See HYPERLYSINEMIA*
Saccharopinuria
  *See HYPERLYSINEMIA*
Sack type Ehlers-Danlos syndrome
  *See EHLERS-DANLOS SYNDROME*
Sacral agenesis
  *See SACROCOCCYGEAL DYSGENESIS SYNDROME*
Sacral agenesis, congenital
  *See CAUDAL REGRESSION SYNDROME*
Sacral defects, anterior
  *See TERATOMA, PRESACRAL-SACRAL DYSGENESIS*
Sacral dysgenesis-presacral teratoma
  *See TERATOMA, PRESACRAL-SACRAL DYSGENESIS*
Sacral meningocele-conotruncal heart defects-head/neck anomalies
  *See MENINGOCELE-CONOTRUNCAL HEART DEFECT, KOUSSEFF TYPE*
Sacral regression
  *See CAUDAL REGRESSION SYNDROME*

## SACROCOCCYGEAL DYSGENESIS SYNDROME                 2380

**Includes:** Sacral agenesis

**Excludes:**
  **Caudal regression syndrome** (3211)
  **Meningomyelocele** (0693)
  **Sirenomelia sequence** (3191)
  **Situs inversus viscerum** (0888)
  **Teratoma, presacral-sacral dysgenesis** (2370)
  **Vater association** (0987)

**Major Diagnostic Criteria:** Sacrococcygeal dysgenesis (agenesis/dysplasia) associated with malformations of the lumbosacral vertebrae, ribs, and terminal spinal cord.

**Clinical Findings:** Most patients with the sacrococcygeal dysgenesis syndrome (SDS) are recognized at birth by the marked tapering of the lower trunk, particularly in the pelvic region, in association with severe hypoplastic lower limb defects. Sacrococcygeal dysgenesis (agenesis and/or dysplasia) is found on X-ray. While 12% of patients have dysmorphic cervicothoracic vertebrae, 51% have their most rostral abnormality in the lumbar spine, with a high ratio (10.5:1) of vertebral agenesis. SDS patients also have high incidences of CNS anomalies and of CNS-related complications such as urinary and anal incontinence (47%) and lower limb paraplegia (20%) which contrast sharply with the complete absence of anatomic malformations in these organ systems. The total associated anomalies in SDS are relatively low (3.3 per patient), as compared to **Sirenomelia sequence** (9.3 per patient), and **Vater association** (6.2 per patient).

Identification of SDS is further aided by concomitant demographic features: maternal diabetes reported in 26% of the patients; situs inversus in 4.6%; and patient survival in 97%. Twinning has a normal incidence of 1.3% in SDS patients.

**Complications:** Neurogenic bladder and sequelae; scoliosis.

**Associated Findings:** None known.

**Etiology:** Unknown. Autosomal dominant inheritance has been suggested in some cases.

**Pathogenesis:** Unknown.

**MIM No.:** 18294

**CDC No.:** 756.170

**Sex Ratio:** M1:F1

**Occurrence:** SDS occurred in 34% of 445 patients identified as having sacrococcygeal dysgenesis.

**Risk of Recurrence for Patient's Sib:** Unknown. Presumed low.

**Risk of Recurrence for Patient's Child:** Unknown. Two families with autosomal dominant transmission have been reported.

**Age of Detectability:** The severe lumbosacrococcygeal and complete sacrococcygeal forms are usually evident at birth, whereas patients with lesions below S3 are frequently not identified until later in life.

**Gene Mapping and Linkage:** Unknown.

**Prevention:** None known. Genetic counseling indicated.

**Treatment:** As indicated by defects, including orthopedic management of spine, pelvis, and lower limb defects, and surveillance for urinary tract complications.

**Prognosis:** Prognosis for life and intellect is dependent on the severity of the associated CNS anomalies. Urinary tract complications are usually either preventable or manageable if diagnosed and treated early in life.

**Detection of Carrier:** Unknown.

**Special Considerations:** In the past, sacrococcygeal dysgenesis syndrome (SDS) has been reported as *sacral agenesis*; however, the term SDS is preferable because not all patients have an absent sacrum, and because of the multi-system involvement.

**References:**
Duhamel B: From the mermaid to anal imperformation: the syndrome of caudal regression. Arch Dis Child 1961; 36:152–155.
Passarge E, Lenz W: Syndrome of caudal regression in infants of diabetic mothers: observations of further cases. Pediatrics 1966; 37:672–675.
Smith DW, et al.: Monozygotic twinning and the Duhamel anomalad (imperforate anus to sirenomelia): a nonrandom association between two aberrations in morphogenesis. BD:OAS XII(5). New York: March of Dimes Birth Defects Foundation, 1976:53–63.
Schinzel AAGL, et al.: Monozygotic twinning and structural defects. J Pediatr 1979; 95:921–930.
Duncan PA, et al.: Distinct caudal regression syndrome identified by associated malformation pattern and demographic features. (Abstract) Proc Greenwood Genet Center 1986; 5:142–143.

DU003                                    **Peter A. Duncan**
SH009                                  **Lawrence R. Shapiro**

**Sacrococcygeal teratoma (benign or malignant)**
  *See TERATOMA, SACROCOCCYGEAL TERATOMA*

**Saddle nose-deafness-myopia-cataract**
*See DEAFNESS-MYOPIA-CATARACT-SADDLE NOSE, MARSHALL TYPE*
**Saethre-Chotzen syndrome**
*See ACROCEPHALOSYNDACTYLY TYPE III*
**Sakati syndrome**
*See ACROCEPHALOPOLYSYNDACTYLY*
**Sakati-Nyhan syndrome**
*See ACROCEPHALOPOLYSYNDACTYLY*
**Saldino-Noonan short rib-polydactyly**
*See SHORT RIB-POLYDACTYLY SYNDROME, TYPE I*

## SALIVARY GLAND LYMPHANGIOMA 2721

**Includes:** Lymphangioma of salivary gland

**Excludes:** Salivary gland, hemangioma (2726)

**Major Diagnostic Criteria:** Based on histologic appearance: lymphangioma simplex has capillary-sized channels; cavernous lymphangioma has dilated lymphatic channels; and cystic hygroma has channels of various sizes.

**Clinical Findings:** Asymptomatic, fluctuant mass located in any of the salivary glands.

**Complications:** May cause upper aerodigestive tract obstruction requiring a tracheotomy. Infection may occur. May result in severe cosmetic deformity.

**Associated Findings:** It is speculated that local infection may precipitate rapid growth.

**Etiology:** Unknown.

**Pathogenesis:** Glandular parenchyma is not replaced but rather it co-exists as islands of normal tissue surrounded by enlarged lymphatic spaces. Occasionally, there is spontaneous regression.

**Sex Ratio:** M1:F>1.

**Occurrence:** Undetermined but presumed rare.

**Risk of Recurrence for Patient's Sib:** Unknown.

**Risk of Recurrence for Patient's Child:** Unknown.

**Age of Detectability:** Commonly seen shortly after birth. More than one-half are present by age one year; 80–90% are present by age two years.

**Gene Mapping and Linkage:** Unknown.

**Prevention:** None known. Genetic counseling indicated.

**Treatment:** Since spontaneous regression is unlikely, surgical excision is the only acceptable mode. Prompt removal is necessary when the potential for airway compromise exists. May require tracheotomy.

**Prognosis:** Good for life span and intelligence. Function is dependent on the presence or absence of complications. Recurrence is uncommon when completely removed.

**Detection of Carrier:** Unknown.

**References:**
Batsakis JG, Regezi JA: Selected controversial lesions of salivary tissues. Otolaryngol Clin North Am 1977; 10:309–328.
Work WP: Cysts and congenital lesions of the parotid glands. Otolaryngol Clin North Am 1977; 10:339–344.
Work WP: Non-neoplastic disorders of the parotid gland. J Otolaryngol 1981; 10:35–40.
Sucupira MS, et al.: Salivary gland imaging and radionuclide dacryocystography in agenesis of salivary glands. Arch Otolaryngol 1983; 109:197–198.

MY003                                                **Charles M. Myer III**
OR005                                                       **Peter Orobello**

**Salivary gland virus infection**
*See FETAL CYTOMEGALOVIRUS SYNDROME*

## SALIVARY GLAND, AGENESIS 2722

**Includes:**
Agenesis of the salivary gland
Mouth, dryness from salivary gland dysfunction
Xerostomia

**Excludes:** Salivary gland, acquired disorders of

**Major Diagnostic Criteria:** Xerostomia (dryness of the mouth) of unknown origin in a child.

**Clinical Findings:** Xerostomia. The diagnosis is confirmed by sodium pertechnetate imaging.

**Complications:** If undetected, sequelae resulting from xerostomia (i.e., poor oral hygiene, dental caries, dysphagia).

**Associated Findings:** The condition is seen in **Sjogren syndrome**.

**Etiology:** Unknown.

**Pathogenesis:** Unknown.

**CDC No.:** 750.230

**Sex Ratio:** Undetermined but presumably M1:F1.

**Occurrence:** Undetermined but presumably rare.

**Risk of Recurrence for Patient's Sib:** Unknown.

**Risk of Recurrence for Patient's Child:** Unknown.

**Age of Detectability:** During childhood.

**Gene Mapping and Linkage:** Unknown.

**Prevention:** None known.

**Treatment:** Early proper oral hygiene; artificial saliva, nutritional supplements, rigorous dental care and frequent dental examinations, and ophthalmologic screening.

**Prognosis:** Good for life span, intelligence and function.

**Detection of Carrier:** Unknown.

**References:**
Batsakis JG, Regezi JA: Selected controversial lesions of salivary tissues. Otolaryngol Clin North Am 1977; 10:309–328.
Work WP: Cysts and congenital lesions of the parotid glands. Otolaryngol Clin North Am 1977; 10:339–344.
Work WP: Non-neoplastic disorders of the parotid gland. J Otolaryngol 1981; 10:35–40.
Sucupira MS, et al.: Salivary gland imaging and radionuclide dacryocystography in agenesis of salivary glands. Arch Otolaryngol 1983; 109:197–198.

MY003                                                **Charles M. Myer III**
OR005                                                       **Peter Orobello**
JA013                                                      **R. Kirk Jackson**

**Salivary gland, branchial cleft cysts**
*See BRANCHIAL CLEFT CYSTS*

## SALIVARY GLAND, DERMOID CYST 2724

**Includes:** Dermoid cyst of the salivary gland

**Excludes:**
**Branchial cleft cysts** (2723)
Dermoid cyst, other
Immunologic diseases
Inflammatory disease, acute and chronic
Neoplastic diseases
Salivary gland, congenital cysts
**Salivary gland, ductal cyst** (2725)
**Salivary gland, hemangioma** (2726)
**Salivary gland lymphangioma** (2721)
Salivary gland, vascular tumors
Traumatic lesions

**Major Diagnostic Criteria:** An isolated mass deep within or near the surface of the parotid gland.

**Clinical Findings:** Isolated mass within the parotid gland which may cause mild ductal compression and secondary parotitis.

**Complications:** Infection, mass effect.

**Associated Findings:** None known.

**Etiology:** Anomalous development resulting in inclusion of all three germinal layers (ectoderm, mesoderm, and endoderm) in a cystic structure.

**Pathogenesis:** Keratinization of squamous epithelium, with associated skin appendages.

**Sex Ratio:** Undetermined but presumably M1:F1.

**Occurrence:** Undetermined but presumably rare.

**Risk of Recurrence for Patient's Sib:** Unknown.

**Risk of Recurrence for Patient's Child:** Unknown.

**Age of Detectability:** Usually during infancy.

**Gene Mapping and Linkage:** Unknown.

**Prevention:** None known. Genetic counseling indicated.

**Treatment:** Subtotal parotidectomy with facial nerve preservation.

**Prognosis:** Good for life span, intelligence, and function. Recurrence is likely unless entirely removed surgically.

**Detection of Carrier:** Unknown.

**References:**
Batsakis JG, Regezi JA: Selected controversial lesions of salivary tissues. Otolaryngol Clin North Am 1977; 10:309–328.
Schuller DE, McCabe BF: Salivary gland neoplasms in children. Otolaryngol Clin North Am 1977; 10:399–412.
Work WP: Cysts and congenital lesions of the parotid glands. Otolaryngol Clin North Am 1977; 10:339–344.
Work WP: Non-neoplastic disorders of the parotid gland. J Otolaryngol 1981; 10:35–40.

MY003
OR005

**Charles M. Myer III**
**Peter Orobello**

### SALIVARY GLAND, DUCTAL CYST                 2725

**Includes:** Ductal cyst of the salivary gland

**Excludes:** Salivary gland, others cysts of the

**Major Diagnostic Criteria:** Unilateral enlargement of the parotid gland during infancy.

**Clinical Findings:** Unilateral parotid enlargement. Sialography may be helpful in identifying the true nature of these lesions.

**Complications:** Repeated infections.

**Associated Findings:** None known.

**Etiology:** Unknown.

**Pathogenesis:** Most likely the result of a congenital retention cyst.

**Sex Ratio:** Undetermined but presumably M1:F1.

**Occurrence:** Undetermined but presumably rare.

**Risk of Recurrence for Patient's Sib:** Unknown.

**Risk of Recurrence for Patient's Child:** Unknown.

**Age of Detectability:** During infancy.

**Gene Mapping and Linkage:** Unknown.

**Prevention:** None known. Genetic counseling indicated.

**Treatment:** None necessary unless there are recurrent infections. Parotidectomy with preservation of the facial nerve is curative and should be performed only if necessary.

**Prognosis:** Good for life span, intelligence, and function. Risk of recurrence is low with complete surgical excision (parotidectomy).

**Detection of Carrier:** Unknown.

**References:**
Batsakis JG, Regezi JA: Selected controversial lesions of salivary tissues. Otolaryngol Clin North Am 1977; 10:309–328.
Work WP: Cysts and congenital lesions of the parotid glands. Otolaryngol Clin North Am 1977; 10:339–344.

Work WP: Non-neoplastic disorders of the parotid gland. J Otolaryngol 1981; 10:35–40.

MY003
OR005

**Charles M. Myer III**
**Peter Orobello**

### SALIVARY GLAND, HEMANGIOMA                 2726

**Includes:** Hemangioma, salivary gland

**Excludes:** Salivary gland lymphangioma (2721)

**Major Diagnostic Criteria:** Asymptomatic tumor of a salivary gland, gradually increasing in size.

**Clinical Findings:** Asymptomatic tumor of a salivary gland, gradually increasing in size, fluctuant to palpation and resulting in facial asymmetry. The tumor is usually confined to the intracapsular portion of the gland, with overlying skin only rarely involved. Enlarges with dependent positioning.

**Complications:** Excessivly rapid growth may result in functional impairment, infection, hemorrhage and/or ulceration.

**Associated Findings:** Other cutaneous hemangiomas may be present.

**Etiology:** Unknown.

**Pathogenesis:** Histologically, a continuum of maturation from capillary or cavernous forms to mixed and hypertrophic forms. The lobular architecture is maintained, but the parenchyma is replaced by endothelial proliferation with vascular differentiation. Acini and ductal structures are unaffected.

**Sex Ratio:** Seen predominantly in females.

**Occurrence:** Found in about 25% of a series of pediatric salivary gland tumors reviewed by Schuller and McCabe (1977).

**Risk of Recurrence for Patient's Sib:** Unknown.

**Risk of Recurrence for Patient's Child:** Unknown.

**Age of Detectability:** Usually discovered shortly after birth.

**Gene Mapping and Linkage:** Unknown.

**Prevention:** None known. Genetic counseling indicated.

**Treatment:** Controversial. Most surgeons prefer not to excise these lesions, since the majority will undergo spontaneous resolution. Excision is indicated with excessively rapid growth or presence of complications.

When appropriate, therapy involves subtotal parotidectomy with facial nerve preservation or total submandibular gland excision. Other methods of therapy include systemic steroids, pressure, and low-dose radiotherapy (not recommended due to possible malignant transformation).

**Prognosis:** Unknown.

**Detection of Carrier:** Unknown.

**References:**
Batsakis JG, Regezi JA: Selected controversial lesions of salivary tissues.
Schuller DE, McCabe BF: Salivary gland neoplasms in children. Otolaryngol Clin North Am 1977; 10:399–412.
Work WP: Cysts and congenital lesions of the parotid glands. Otolaryngol Clin North Am 1977; 10:339–344.
Work WP: Non-neoplastic disorders of the parotid gland. J Otolaryngol 1981; 10:35–40.

MY003
OR003

**Charles M. Myer III**
**Peter Orobello**

## SALIVARY GLAND, MIXED TUMOR      0878

**Includes:**
> Adenoma, hereditary pleomorphic salivary
> Tumor, mixed, of salivary gland

**Excludes:**
> Branchogenic cyst
> Salivary gland tumors (other)

**Major Diagnostic Criteria:** Presence of mixed tumor of salivary gland in more than one member of a family.

**Clinical Findings:** A firm, well-circumscribed mass in the parotid gland without facial nerve involvement is found in the patient in the third decade of life. Excisional biopsy (minimal procedure is submandibular gland excision or lateral parotid lobectomy) reveals pathologic findings of a typical mixed benign tumor. In a series of 401 mixed tumors, Cameron (1959) found three families with tumors affecting more than one member. In one family, brother, sister and father were affected; in another, mother and daughter; and in the third, father and son. In this last family, the diagnosis of the father's tumor was made on clinical grounds, as he refused biopsy or excision. All the offspring were between 21 and 25 years of age.

**Complications:** Tumors rarely show malignant degeneration and rarely metastasize. Involvement of facial nerve with resultant paralysis is rare.

**Associated Findings:** None known.

**Etiology:** Undetermined. Possibly autosomal dominant inheritance.

**Pathogenesis:** Unknown.

**Sex Ratio:** Presumably M1:F1.

**Occurrence:** Undetermined but presumed rare.

**Risk of Recurrence for Patient's Sib:**
> See Part I, *Mendelian Inheritance.*

**Risk of Recurrence for Patient's Child:**
> See Part I, *Mendelian Inheritance.*

**Age of Detectability:** All patients were over 20 years of age at diagnosis.

**Gene Mapping and Linkage:** Unknown.

**Prevention:** None known. Genetic counseling indicated.

**Treatment:** Surgical excision by lateral lobe parotidectomy, total parotidectomy, or submandibular gland excision.

**Prognosis:** Generally good for normal life span, intelligence, and function if proper surgical treatment is employed. Metastases are rare, and untreated mixed tumors usually enlarge slowly.

**Detection of Carrier:** Unknown.

**References:**
Cameron JM: Familial incidence of 'mixed salivary tumors.' Scott Med J 1959; 4:455.

AU005                               **Thomas Aufdemorte**

**Salivary glands and lacrimal puncta, absence of**
*See ALACRIMA-APTYALISM*

## SALLA DISEASE      2041

**Includes:**
> N-acetylneuraminic acid storage disease, infantile (one form)
> Sialic acid storage disease, infantile (one form)
> Sialuria, Finnish type

**Excludes:**
> **Mucolipidosis I** (0671)
> **Sialic acid storage disease, infantile type** (2222)

**Major Diagnostic Criteria:** Both the adult and infantile forms of Salla disease are characterized by alterations in the amount of free (unbound) sialic acid in various tissues and body fluids. Specifically, the urinary concentration of free sialic acid exceeds normal concentrations by 10 to 20 times. Excretion of sialic acid in heterozygotes is normal. Total sialic acid excretion is in the upper range of normal or slightly elevated. Urinary glycosaminoglycan excretion is normal. Cultured skin fibroblasts from affected patients are also characterized by increased levels of free sialic acid. Morphologic evidence of abnormal lysosomal storage occurs in several cell types, including skin biopsy specimens and cultured fibroblasts from patients with the infantile form of the disorder. Activities of the enzymes deficient in other types of lysosomal storage diseases, including sialidase, are normal.

**Clinical Findings:** There appears to be at least two distinct forms of this disease. In the milder form, the so-called Salla disease, affected individuals, born after an uncomplicated pregnancy, appear healthy for the first 6–18 months of life. Signs of progressive CNS deterioration usually appear during the first year. Motor and speech development are delayed; words are often dysarthric, and sentences, if any, are limited to a few words. The stage of moderate-to-severe mental retardation is reached between the ages of five and 10 years, with further deterioration occurring during the second decade. Most individuals have slightly coarse facies. Movements are clumsy, because most patients have ataxia and some muscular hypotonia. The liver and spleen, in general, are not enlarged; the eyes are normal. X-ray findings are limited to a thickened calvarium, while the long bones and vertebrae have a normal structure. The EEG is diffusely abnormal.

In contrast, infantile free sialic acid storage disease is characterized by a more rapid onset of clinical features. Patients with this form of the disease present at or soon after birth with coarse facies, hepatosplenomegaly, clear corneas, hypopigmentation, and diarrhea. The clinical course is one of rapid deterioration, with death in early childhood.

In both forms of the disease vacuolated lymphocytes are seen in the peripheral blood, vacuoles in dermal fibroblasts and histiocytes, as well as in epithelial cells of the blood capillaries, Schwann cells, and the secretory and myoepithelial cells of the sweat glands. Cultured fibroblasts from the infantile form also contain abnormal lysosomes. The activities of several lysosomal enzymes in cultured fibroblasts and in plasma are within normal limites. Urinary excretion of free sialic acid is significantly increased, whereas the total urinary sialic acid excretion is normal.

**Complications:** Unknown.

**Associated Findings:** None known.

**Etiology:** Autosomal recessive inheritance.

**Pathogenesis:** The enlarged storage lysosomes of different cell types (found in skin biopsy material) and the progressive course of the disease clearly indicate that Salla disease should be considered a lysosomal storage disease. Recent evidence strongly suggests that the defect in both Salla and infantile free sialic acid storage disease patients is due to an impairment of normal transport of free sialic acid out of cellular lysosomes as a result of an abnormality of the lysosomal membrane. Moreover, the demonstration of defective sialic acid egress indicates that this disease can be included in a small group of disorders characterized by the defective transport of small molecules across lysosomal membranes. The mechanism responsible for the increased excretion of free sialic acid in these patients remains unclear.

Activities of all lysosomal enzymes studied to date are normal in cultured fibroblasts of the Salla patients.

**MIM No.:** *26874

**Sex Ratio:** M1:F1

**Occurrence:** The milder form of Salla disease has been found almost exclusively in Finland, where close to 40 cases have been reported. In contrast, patients with the infantile form do not appear to have predilection for any particular ethnic group. Evidence to date, however, does suggest that the milder adult form is more common than the infantile form.

**Risk of Recurrence for Patient's Sib:**
> See Part I, *Mendelian Inheritance.*

## Risk of Recurrence for Patient's Child:
See Part I, *Mendelian Inheritance.*

**Age of Detectability:** The age of usual clinical diagnosis is dependent, in large part, on the clinical form of the disorder. In the milder form of Salla disease, delayed development is usually suspected after 6–18 months of age. In contrast, the clinical manifestations of the infantile form are apparent at or very soon after birth. The biochemical abnormalities in all forms of the disease appear to be present throughout life. Prenatal diagnosis has been reported for both forms of the disorder.

**Gene Mapping and Linkage:** Unknown.

**Prevention:** None known. Genetic counseling indicated.

**Treatment:** Supportive.

**Prognosis:** Severe mental retardation before age 10 years seems to be the rule for the milder form of the disease. Additionally, the life span for the mild form of this disorder is probably close to normal, since the oldest living patient is now age 70 years. In contrast, the infantile form of the disorder is characterized by severe mental retardation and death at an early age.

**Detection of Carrier:** Unknown.

**References:**

Aula P, et al.: "Salla disease": a new lysosomal storage disorder. Arch Neurol 1979; 36:88–94.

Renlund M, et al.: Increased urinary excretion of free N-acetyl-neuraminic acid in thirteen patients with Salla disease. Eur J Biochem 1979; 101:245–250.

Hildreth J IV, et al.: N-acetylneuraminic acid accumulation in a buoyant lysosomal fraction of cultured fibroblasts from patients with infantile generalized N-acetylneuraminic acid storage disease. Biochem Biophys Res Commun 1986; 139:838–844.

Jonas AJ: Studies of lysosomal sialic acid metabolism. retention of sialic acid by Salla diseases lysosomes. Biochem Biophys Res Commun 1986; 137:175–181.

Mancini GMS, et al.: Free N-acetylneuraminic acid (NANA) storage disorders: evidence for defective NANA transport across the lysosomal membrane. Hum Genet 1986; 73:214–217.

Paschke E, et al.: Infantile sialic acid storage disease: the fate of biosynthetically labeled N-acetyl-($^3$H)-neuraminic acid in cultured human fibroblasts. Pediatr Res 1986; 20:773–777.

Renlund M, et al.: Defective sialic acid egress from isolated fibroblast lysosomes of patients with Salla disease. Science 1986; 232:59–762.

Renlund M, Aula P: Prenatal detection of Salla disease based upon increased free sialic acid in amniocytes. Am J Med Genet 1987; 28:377–384.

TH021
RE016

George H. Thomas
Martin Renlund

**Salmon patch**
*See NEVUS FLAMMEUS*
**Salonen-Herva-Norio syndrome**
*See HYDROLETHALUS SYNDROME*
**Sandhoff disease**
*See G(M2)-GANGLIOSIDOSIS WITH HEXOSAMINIDASE A AND B DEFICIENCY*
**Sandifer syndrome**
*See TORTICOLLIS*
**Sanfilippo syndrome**
*See MUCOPOLYSACCHARIDOSIS III*
**Santos syndrome**
*See HIRSCHSPRUNG DISEASE-POLYDACTYLY-DEAFNESS*

## SARCOIDOSIS                                                 2966

**Includes:**
> Besnier-Boek-Schaumann disease
> Bilateral hilar involvement
> EN-arthropathy-BHL syndrome
> Mannen-Balcom syndrome

**Excludes:**
> **Cancer, Hodgkin disease, familial** (2352)
> **Lupus erythematosus, systemic** (2515)
> Tuberculous lymphadenitis

**Major Diagnostic Criteria:** Bilateral hilar lymphadenopathy and pulmonary infiltration demonstrated in chest X-ray, elevated serum angiotensin converting enzyme, positive Kveim test, and noncaseating granulomas on biopsy.

**Clinical Findings:** Sarcoidosis is a systemic disease characterized by granulomatous inflammation of almost any organ or tissue, but with a marked predilection for lungs. The onset of the disease is usually between the second and third decades of life. Patients may present with malaise, fever, and dyspnea of insidious onset. In 10–15% of the patients, the onset is acute with erythema nodosum or acute polyarthritis developing in days or weeks, or sudden onset of an infiltrating granulomatous skin rash. Acute-onset sarcoidosis is usually a benign syndrome with a high incidence of spontaneous resolution. Subacute sarcoidosis is often asymptomatic and is initially recognized through health screening or routine chest X-rays. Patients generally have few extrathoracic lesions, and these recover spontaneously. Patients with chronic sarcoidosis patients have both intrathroracic and extrathoracic involvement.

*Extrathoracic sarcoidosis*: may present with symptoms referable to the skin, eyes, peripheral nerves, muscle, liver, or heart. The findings may include skin rash (erythema nodosum and plaque-like), peripheral neuropathy, myopathy, parotid gland enlargement, hepatosplenomegaly, lymphadenopathy, chronic arthritis, and lytic lesions of the bone.

*Laboratory abnormalities*: leukopenia, eosinophilia, and elevated sedimentation rate, hypergammaglobulinemia, hypercalcemia or hypercalciuria, elevated angiotensin-converting enzyme, and positive Kveim test (skin test). Biopsy material shows noncaseating granulomatous inflammation of tissues. Cutaneous changes may be seen in about 40%. Other studies to demonstrate pulmonary involvement include transbronchial lung biopsy and radioactive gallium scan.

*X-ray findings*: bilateral hilar adenopathy, paratracheal adenopathy, and parenchymal reticulonodular infiltrates.

**Complications:** Pulmonary fibrosis, chorioretinitis, congestive heart failure, pericardial effusion, cranial nerve palsies, and nephrolithiasis.

**Associated Findings:** Uveitis, iridocyclitis, peripheral neuropathies, liver and spleen enlargement, myocarditis, myopathies.

**Etiology:** Probably a combination of genetic and environmental factors. It is unclear whether one or several infectious agents are responsible or whether inhalation, ingestion, or dermal contact is the route of exposure. Agents that have been considered are viruses, typical and atypical mycobacteria, fungi, and fine pollen.

**Pathogenesis:** Sarcoidosis is a disorder of widespread, noncaseating granulomas that form in response to an unidentified stimulus. Pulmonary involvement is seen in 90% of the patients. The granulomas are composed of mostly epithelioid cells, but also of giant cells. Activated T lymphocytes and macrophages contribute to granuloma formation. These granulomas are rich in angiotensin-converting enzyme.

**MIM No.:** 18100

**Sex Ratio:** M1:F1.1

**Occurrence:** Sarcoidosis occurs worldwide and affects all ethnic groups. The incidence of sarcoidosis is 11:100,000 in United States, 3–4.5:100,000 in the United Kingdom, and 7:100,000 in Denmark. In the United States, the prevalence of sarcoidosis is much higher in Blacks than in whites.

**Risk of Recurrence for Patient's Sib:** Probably not increased.

**Risk of Recurrence for Patient's Child:** Probably not increased.

**Age of Detectability:** Generally between the second and third decades of life.

**Gene Mapping and Linkage:** Unknown.

**Prevention:** None known. Genetic counseling indicated.

**Treatment:** The preferred therapy for sarcoidosis is corticosteroids. The usual practice is to give 40 mg of prednisone daily for a 2-week period, then gradually tapering to 15 mg for a minimum of 6–8 months. Steroids are indicated in most extrathoracic sarcoidosis. Stage 0 and 1 intrathoracic sarcoidoses do not need treatment.

**Prognosis:** Corticosteroids produce a dramatic therapeutic effect in sarcoidosis. Lifetime, low-dose maintenance therapy may be required in some patients. Persistent prolonged untreated disease is less likely to be reversible.

**Detection of Carrier:** Unknown.

**Special Considerations:** Few familial aggregates have been found. However, no pattern of inheritance has been confirmed. HLA-DR-5 is highly associated with sarcoidosis.

**References:**
Sharma OP, et al.: Familial sarcoidosis: a possible genetic influence. Ann NY Acad Sci 1976; 278:386–400.
Bascom R, Johns CJ: The natural history and management of sarcoidosis. Adv Intern Med 1986; 31:213–241.
James DG: Sarcoidosis: past, present, and future concepts. Clin Dermatol 1986; 4:1–9.
Staton GW Jr., et al.: Comparison of clinical parameters, bronchoalveolar lavage, gallium-67 lung uptake, and serum angiotensin converting enzyme in assessing the activity of sarcoidosis. Sarcoidosis (Italy) 1986; 3:8–10.
Luke RA, et al.: Neurosarcoidosis: the long term clinical course. Neurology 1987; 37:461–463.
Nowack D, Goebel KM: Genetic aspects of sarcoidosis. Arch Intern Med 1987; 147:481–483.

KI016                                        **Smita Kittar**

**Sarcoma family syndrome of Li and Fraumeni (some cases)**
*See CANCER, BREAST, FAMILIAL*
**Sarcosine dehydrogenase complex, deficiency of**
*See SARCOSINEMIA*

---

## SARCOSINEMIA                                        0503

**Includes:**
    Hypersarcosinemia
    Sarcosine dehydrogenase complex, deficiency of
**Excludes:**
    **Acidemia, ethylmalonic-adipic** (2377)
    **Acidemia, glutaric acidemia II, neonatal onset** (2289)

**Major Diagnostic Criteria:** Increased concentration of sarcosine in blood and urine without elevated concentrations of organic acids. Sarcosine levels in patient plasma range from 0.5 to 6.8 mg/dl; sarcosine excretion ranges from 0.13 to 0.84 mg/mg creatinine. Sarcosine is not usually detectable in the body fluids of normal individuals.

**Clinical Findings:** No consistent clinical syndrome has been associated with sarcosinemia. Most patients were initially investigated because of failure to thrive, poor feeding, delayed development, or mental retardation. This has led to a biased increase in patients with these conditions among reported sarcosinemia patients. When an unbiased method, neonatal urine screening, was used, Levy et al. (1984) found four unrelated patients; all had IQs in the normal range. However, one was emotionally disturbed, and one was dyslexic. No dysmorphic or other clinical abnormalities were found. A total of 19 patients from 16 different families have been reported. Of these, eight had normal intelligence, but three of these eight had significant psychiatric problems.

**Complications:** Unknown.

**Associated Findings:** None known.

**Etiology:** Probably autosomal recessive inheritance of an enzyme defect. There is evidence of genetic heterogeneity.

**Pathogenesis:** Sarcosine is not oxidized to glycine. Gerritsen (1972) found a deficiency of the enzyme sarcosine dehydrogenase in the liver of one patient. However, Scott (1974) found a value equal to that of controls in a liver biopsy from his patient. Sarcosine oxidation occurs primarily in the liver and kidney. The dehydrogenase is not present in either fibroblasts or circulating leukocytes.

**MIM No.:** *26890

**Sex Ratio:** Presumably M1:F1.

**Occurrence:** An incidence of 1:350,000 live births was calculated from Massachusetts data.

**Risk of Recurrence for Patient's Sib:**
See Part I, *Mendelian Inheritance.*

**Risk of Recurrence for Patient's Child:**
See Part I, *Mendelian Inheritance.*

**Age of Detectability:** Before age three months by urinalysis.

**Gene Mapping and Linkage:** Unknown.

**Prevention:** None known. Genetic counseling indicated.

**Treatment:** Supportive. Short-term therapy with folic acid was not effective in one patient of Glorieux et al. (1971); however, in the patient of Blom and Fernandes (1979), a decrease in urinary sarcosine excretion was seen after 8 weeks of treatment with high doses of folic acid. Sarcosinemia has been reported to occur in a patient with dietary folic acid deficiency.

**Prognosis:** Normal life span.

**Detection of Carrier:** Not always possible. Oral tolerance tests with sarcosine and dimethylglycine have been done. In some families the excretion of sarcosine from some probable carriers was increased after a sarcosine load. A difference in the ratio of urinary sarcosine to glycine after a sarcosine load has been suggested as another distinguishing criterion.

**Special Considerations:** Sarcosinemia is distinct from **Acidemia, glutaric acidemia II, neonatal onset** in which the activity of a large number of acyl-CoA dehydrogenases are deficient because of the defective activity of the associated electron transporting flavoprotein or its dehydrogenase. In this latter disease, sarcosine and a variety of other organic acids are elevated. In sarcosinemia there is normal excretion of organic acids.

**References:**
Gerritsen T, Waisman HA: Hypersarcosinemia: an inborn error of metabolism. New Engl J Med 1966; 275:66–69. *
Glorieux FH, et al.: Transport and metabolism of sarcosine in hypersarcosinemia and normal phenotypes. J Clin Invest 1971; 50:2313. *
Gerritsen T: Sarcosine dehydrogenase deficiency, the enzyme defect in hypersarcosinemia. Helv Paediatr Acta 1972; 27:33.
Scott CR: Sarcosinemia. In Nyhan WL, ed: Heritable disorders of amino acid metabolism. New York: John Wiley & Sons, 1974:324.
Blom W, Fernandes J: Folic acid dependent hypersarcosinemia. Clin Chem Acta 1979; 91:117.
Levy HL, et al.: Massachusetts metabolic disorders screening program: III. Sarcosinemia. Pediatrics 1984; 74:509. *
Sewell AC, et al.: Sarcosinaemia in a retarded amaurotic child. Europ J Pediat 1986; 144:508–510.

SM020                                        **Margaret L. Smith**

**Sarcotubular myopathy**
*See MYOPATHY, SARCOTUBULAR*
**Sauk syndrome**
*See TAURODONTISM-SHORT ROOTED TEETH-MICROCEPHALIC DWARFISM*
**Say-Barber-Miller syndrome**
*See MICROCEPHALY-RETARDATION-SKELETAL AND IMMUNE DEFECTS*

## SAY-MEYER SYNDROME          3267

**Includes:**
> Trigonocephaly-short stature
> Trigonocephaly-short stature-developmental delay

**Excludes:**
> **C syndrome** (0121)
> **Acrocephalosyndactyly type III** (0229)

**Major Diagnostic Criteria:** The combination of trigonocephaly and growth failure and lack of limb defects should suggest the diagnosis.

**Clinical Findings:** All three affected boys in the one reported family had trigonocephaly, with a prominent vertical ridge on the forehead; **Microcephaly**, short stature; and developmental delay. Additional features include low birthweight (2), prominent eyes (1), hypotelorism (2), epicanthal folds (1), wide nasal bridge (1), beaked nose (1), highly arched palate (1), low-set ears (1), clinodactyly (1), **Hernia, inguinal** (1), and seizures (1). In one child, skull X-rays demonstrated craniosynostosis involving the sagittal, metopic, and left lambdoid sutures; in another the lambdoid and metopic were involved.

**Complications:** Unknown.

**Associated Findings:** None known.

**Etiology:** X-linked recessive inheritance is most likely.

**Pathogenesis:** Unknown.

**MIM No.:** 31432

**Sex Ratio:** M3:F0 (observed).

**Occurrence:** One family from Oklahoma has been documented.

**Risk of Recurrence for Patient's Sib:**
> See Part I, *Mendelian Inheritance.*

**Risk of Recurrence for Patient's Child:**
> See Part I, *Mendelian Inheritance.*

**Age of Detectability:** At birth by the presence of trigonocephaly.

**Gene Mapping and Linkage:** Unknown.

**Prevention:** None known. Genetic counseling indicated.

**Treatment:** Unknown.

**Prognosis:** All three boys had some degree of developmental delay, with the oldest (a 30-year-old) reported as being moderately mentally retarded. His height was 162 cm.

**Detection of Carrier:** Unknown.

**References:**
Say B, Meyer J: Familial syndrome of trigonocephaly associated with short stature and developmental delay. Am J Dis Child 1981; 135:711–712.

T0007            **Helga V. Toriello**

**SBLA syndrome (some cases)**
  *See CANCER, BREAST, FAMILIAL*
**SC phocomelia syndrome**
  *See ROBERTS SYNDROME*
**Scalp cylindroma, types I and II**
  *See SCALP, CYLINDROMAS*
**Scalp defect-ectrodactyly**
  *See LIMB AND SCALP DEFECTS, ADAMS-OLIVER TYPE*
**Scalp defects from fetal exposure**
  *See FETAL EFFECTS FROM METHIMAZOLE AND CARBIMAZOLE*

## SCALP DEFECTS-POSTAXIAL POLYDACTYLY     2922

**Includes:** Polydactyly, postaxial type A-scalp defects

**Excludes:**
> **Chromosome 13, trisomy 13** (0168)
> **Limb and scalp defects, Adams-Oliver type** (0459)
> **Skin, localized absence of** (0608)

**Major Diagnostic Criteria:** Postaxial polydactyly type A combined with a midline skin defect, localized on the vertex or the occipital region, frequently associated with defects of the calvarium or even the meninges. The size of the scalp defect may vary from a 2–3-mm diameter skin defect to a very extensive defect of the whole calvarium.

**Clinical Findings:** A midline scalp defect may occur as an isolated anomaly (see **Skin, localized absence of**) or may be associated with acral reduction anomalies of the limbs (see **Limb and scalp defects, Adams-Oliver type**). At least two reports have dealt with the association of congenital scalp defects and postaxial polydactyly type A.

**Complications:** Unknown.

**Associated Findings:** Scalp defects can be associated with various malformations of the central nervous system. These have been especially well documented after the advent of axial computed tomography, i.e., asymmetric ventricular enlargement and porencephalic cysts localized under the vertex defect.

**Etiology:** Presumably autosomal dominant inheritance with considerable variability in expression and penetrance.

**Pathogenesis:** Unknown.

**MIM No.:** 18125

**POS No.:** 4018

**Sex Ratio:** M1:F1

**Occurrence:** One kindred and one sporadic case have been reported in the literature.

**Risk of Recurrence for Patient's Sib:**
> See Part I, *Mendelian Inheritance.*

**Risk of Recurrence for Patient's Child:**
> See Part I, *Mendelian Inheritance.*

**Age of Detectability:** At birth.

**Gene Mapping and Linkage:** Unknown.

**Prevention:** None known. Genetic counseling indicated.

**Treatment:** Symptomatic.

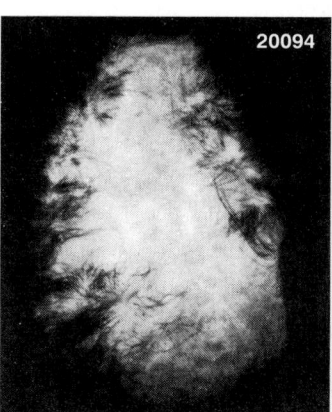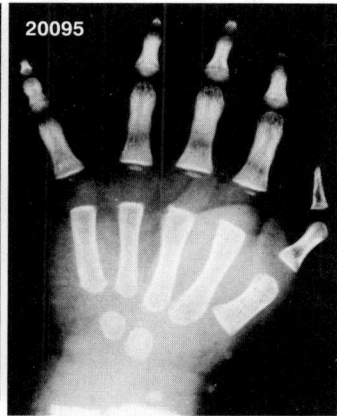

**2922-20094:** Large scalp defect covered by thin atrophic skin.
**20095:** Typical acral reduction defects of the hands.

**Prognosis:** In the first years of life, spontaneous bleeding and granulation of the skin defect occur, and, after the first years of life, the defect is covered by thin, atrophic skin. Calcification and mineralization of the bone defect progressively occur, and after some years the size of the bone defect may become relatively smaller than at birth.

**Detection of Carrier:** Unknown.

**References:**

Fryns JP, Van den Berghe H: Congenital scalp defects associated with postaxial polydactyly. Hum Genet 1979; 49:217–219.

Buttiens M, et al.: Scalp defect associated with postaxial polydactyly: confirmation of a distinct entity with autosomal dominant inheritance. Hum Genet 1985; 71:86–88.

FR030                                               **Jean-Pierre Fryns**

## SCALP, CYLINDROMAS             0235

**Includes:**

Basal cell epithelioma, multiple benign nodular intraepidermal
Cylindromas of the scalp
Cylindromatosis
Endothelioma capitis of Kaposi
Hydradenoma
Hydradenoma, nonpapillary hyalinizing
Neuroepithelioma adenoids
Scalp cylindroma, types I and II
Spiegler-Brooke tumors
Syphonoma
Tomato tumor
Turban tumors of scalp

**Excludes:**

**Epitheliomas, hereditary multiple cystic** (2392)
**Fibromatosis, juvenile hyaline** (0411)

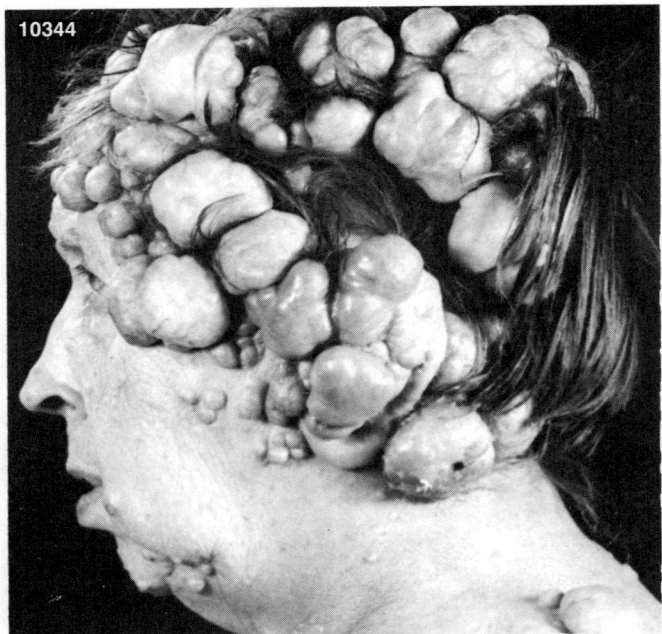

**0235-10344:** Cylindromatosis.

**Major Diagnostic Criteria:** A cylindroma is an epidermal appendage tumor in which differentiation toward apocrine or eccrine structure occurs. It occurs in two forms:

*Type 1:* Multiple sessile or pedunculated dome-shaped, smooth nodules on the scalp with occasional extension to the face, neck, and trunk. These lesions appear in early adulthood and increase in size and number. The size of these dominantly inherited tumors ranges from a few millimeters to several centimeters. They may become extensive on the scalp and give rise to the epithet "turban tumor."

*Type 2:* A solitary tumor of the scalp either sessile or pedunculated. Solitary cylindromas are not inherited.

Histologically, cylindromas, regardless of type, are composed of irregularly shaped islands of epithelial cells separated by a hyaline sheath or cylinder, hence the name, and a narrow band of collagen. These islands are composed of two types of cells, peripheral cells with small dark nuclei, representing undifferentiated cells, and central cells with large, pale nuclei, representing differentiation toward ductal cells.

**Clinical Findings:** These solitary or multiple smooth firm globular tumors of variable size are distinctive in appearance.

**Complications:** Bleeding and infection secondary to trauma can occur with both types of cylindromas. Malignant degeneration with metastatic spread to lymph nodes, viscera, and local extention have been noted with both types. It is to avoid these sequelae, as well as for esthetic consideration, that surgical excision is recommended.

**Associated Findings:** Type 1 cylindromas are commonly associated with multiple trichoepitheliomas.

**Etiology:** *Type 1:* Multiple cylindromas follow a pattern of autosomal dominant inheritance, but the possibility of X-linkage in a small number of families is not completely excluded.

*Type 2:* Solitary cylindromas have no hereditary pattern.

**Pathogenesis:** While histochemical and enzyme histochemical studies have not been convincing, electron microscopy studies and the association with trichoepitheliomas favor an apocrine, rather than an eccrine, differentiation.

**MIM No.:** 12385, 31310

**Sex Ratio:** Type 1, M<1:F1; type 2, M1:F1

**Occurrence:** More than 200 reported cases.

**Risk of Recurrence for Patient's Sib:**
See Part I, *Mendelian Inheritance.*

**Risk of Recurrence for Patient's Child:**
See Part I, *Mendelian Inheritance.*

**Age of Detectability:** Second or third decade of life.

**Gene Mapping and Linkage:** Unknown.

**Prevention:** None known. Genetic counseling indicated.

**Treatment:** Excision.

**Prognosis:** Prognosis is good for both type 1 and type 2 cylindromas, although case reports of malignant degeneration with subsequent metastatic spread argue for careful serial histologic examination of excised tumors. Regular follow-up is desirable.

**Detection of Carrier:** Unknown.

**References:**

Lever WF: Pathogenesis of benign skin tumors of cutaneous appendages and of basal cell epitheliomas. Arch Dermatol Syph 1948; 57:679–724.

Crain RC, et al.: Dermal eccrine cylindroma. Am J Clin Pathol 1961; 35:504–515.

Lyon JB, et al.: Malignant degeneration of turban tumor of the scalp. Trans St. John's Hosp Dermatol 1961; 46:74–77.

Hashimoto K, et al.: Histogenesis of skin appendage tumors. Arch Dermatol 1969; 100:356–369.

Harper PS: Turban tumor (cylindromatosis). BD:OAS; VII(8):338–341. White Plains: March of Dimes-Birth Defects Foundation, 1971. †

C0070                                         **Brian Cook**

Scalp, skull, and limbs; absence defect of Adams-Oliver
*See LIMB AND SCALP DEFECTS, ADAMS-OLIVER TYPE*
Scaphocephaly
*See CRANIOSYNOSTOSIS*
Scapula elevata
*See SPRENGEL DEFORMITY*
Scapuloilioperoneal atrophy-cardiopathy
*See HAUPTMANN-THANHAUSER SYNDROME*
Scarring epidermolysis bullosa
*See EPIDERMOLYSIS BULLOSUM, TYPE III*
Scheibe cochleosaccular degeneration of inner ear
*See EAR, INNER DYSPLASIAS*
Scheie syndrome
*See MUCOPOLYSACCHARIDOSIS I-S*
Scheuermann disease (vertebrae)
*See JOINTS, OSTEOCHONDRITIS DISSECANS*
Schimke X-linked mental retardation syndrome
*See X-LINKED MENTAL RETARDATION-CHOREOATHETOSIS*
Schimmelpenning-Feuerstein-Mims syndrome
*See PROTEUS SYNDROME*
Schindler disease
*See ALPHA-N-ACETYLGALACTOSAMINIDASE DEFICIENCY*
Schinzel syndrome
*See ULNAR-MAMMARY SYNDROME*
Schinzel type acrocallosal syndrome
*See ACROCALLOSAL SYNDROME, SCHINZEL TYPE*

## SCHINZEL-GIEDION SYNDROME 2123

**Includes:**
Face, midface retraction-X-ray and renal anomalies-hypertrichosis
Hypertrichosis-midface retraction-X-ray and renal anomalies
Midface retraction-X-ray and renal anomalies-hypertrichosis
Renal and X-ray anomalies-midface retraction-hypertrichosis

**Excludes:**
**Johanson-Blizzard syndrome** (2026)
**Mucopolysaccharidosis**
**Urofacial syndrome** (2527)

**Major Diagnostic Criteria:** Midface retraction, hypertrichosis, skeletal anomalies, hydronephrosis, and failure to thrive.

**Clinical Findings:** In four reported cases, three involved post-term pregnancy, and polyhydramnios complicated one pregnancy. All affected children have had generalized hypertrichosis; widely patent cranial sutures and fontanelles; hypertelorism; midface retraction; low-set ears; short, broad neck with abundant skin; short forearms and legs; and in examined individuals, skeletal defects on X-ray, including steep short base of the skull, wide occipital synchondrosis, multiple wormian bones, hypoplastic first, and broad other ribs, hypoplastic distal phalanges, and hypoplastic/aplastic pubic bones. Additional features reported in affected individuals include facial hemangioma; high, prominent forehead; choanal stenosis; macroglossia; **Atrial septal defects**; hypoplastic nipples; post-axial polydactyly; narrow, hyperconvex nails; hypoplastic dermal ridges; talipes; and delayed tooth eruption. Genital anomalies are also common, and include short penis with cryptorchidism in males and deep interlabial sulcus in females.

One child died at one day of age; all the surviving children had growth retardation, seizures, and/or abnormal EEG, severe mental retardation, and recurrent apneic spells.

**Complications:** Unknown.

**Associated Findings:** None known.

**Etiology:** Autosomal recessive inheritance.

**Pathogenesis:** Unknown.

**MIM No.:** *26915

**POS No.:** 3025

**Sex Ratio:** Presumably M1:F1

**Occurrence:** About a dozen cases have been observed.

**Risk of Recurrence for Patient's Sib:**
See Part I, *Mendelian Inheritance.*

**Risk of Recurrence for Patient's Child:**
See Part I, *Mendelian Inheritance.*

**Age of Detectability:** At birth, by physical exam.

**Gene Mapping and Linkage:** Unknown.

**Prevention:** None known. Genetic counseling indicated.

**Treatment:** Supportive.

**Prognosis:** Affected individuals are severely retarded; death occurred at age one day, 16.5 months, and 19 months of age in three of four cases reported in the literature. The fourth case was permanently hospitalized at age 10 months.

**Detection of Carrier:** Unknown.

**References:**

Schinzel A, Giedion A: A syndrome of severe midface retraction, multiple skull anomalies, clubfeet, and cardiac and renal malformations in sibs. Am J Med Genet 1978; 1:361–375. * †
Donnai D, Harris R: A further case of a new syndrome including midface retraction, hypertrichosis, and skeletal anomalies. J Med Genet 1979; 16:483–486.
Kelley RI, et al.: Congenital hydronephrosis, skeletal dysplasia, and severe developmental retardation: the Schinzel-Giedion syndrome. J Pediatr 1982; 100:943–946.
Schinzel A: A syndrome of midface retraction, multiple radiological anomalies, renal malformations and hypertrichosis. (Letter) Hum Genet 1982; 62:382 only.

T0007                                                    **Helga V. Toriello**

## SCHISIS ASSOCIATION 2249

**Includes:**
Midline defects
Neural tube defects (some)

**Excludes:**
**Amniotic bands syndrome** (0874)
Chromosomal syndromes with similar phenotypes
**Meningocele** (0642)

**Major Diagnostic Criteria:** A combination of two or more schisis-type defects, i.e., neural tube defects including **Anencephaly**, **Encephalocele**, and spina bifida aperta-cystica (see **Meningomyelocele**); oral clefts including **Cleft lip** with or without **Cleft palate** and posterior cleft palate; **Omphalocele**, exomphalos, gastroschisis, or diaghragmatic defects without other major primary defects.

**Clinical Findings:** Birth weight is low, about 2,000 gm, and mean gestational age is short; about 36 weeks. The distribution of component schisis-type defects is: neural tube defects 42%, oral cleft 27%, omphalocele 19%, and diaphragmatic defects 12%.

**Complications:** About 40% of cases were found in stillborns. Component schisis-type defects provoke a number of secondary consequences and cause an extreme high mortality.

**Associated Findings:** Nearly all component defects have associated anomalies.

**Etiology:** Unknown. Specific polygenic systems may create a liability for different schisis-type defects, and some genes of these systems may participate in governing the closure speed of different developing tissues in general.

**Pathogenesis:** Schisis-type defects are so called *midline defects*, and this developmental field may have poorly buffered morphogenetic properties.

**POS No.:** 4137

**Sex Ratio:** M1:F3; varies with component defects.

**Occurrence:** 10:100,000 total births in Hungary. Owing to high perinatal mortality, prevalences are extremely low following the neonatal period.

**Risk of Recurrence for Patient's Sib:** 3.7%, however, there is a higher fetal death rate in sibs.

**Risk of Recurrence for Patient's Child:** No report exists of a patient having reproduced.

**Age of Detectability:** At birth, prenatal diagnosis including ultrasound examination and amniotic AFP and acetylcholinesterase determination is possible for some components.

**Gene Mapping and Linkage:** Unknown.

**Prevention:** None known. Genetic counseling indicated. Periconceptional multivitamin supplementation may have some benefit.

**Treatment:** No effective measure known in cases involving anencephaly. Surgical intervention in appropriate cases.

**Prognosis:** Usually lethal within the first days of life.

**Detection of Carrier:** Unknown.

**Special Considerations:** Breech presentation and caesarean section in the delivery of index patients are more common. Fetal deaths, miscarriages, and stillbirths have a higher rate in the previous and subsequent pregnancies of index patient's mothers.

**References:**
Czeizel A: Schisis-association. Am J Med Genet 1981; 10:25–34.
Opitz JM: The developmental field concept in clinical genetics. J Pediatr 1982; 101:805–809.

CZ001                                                    **Andrew Czeizel**

**Schizencephaly with head enlargement**
   See *HYDRANENCEPHALY*
**Schizophrenic disorders**
   See *MOOD AND THOUGHT DISORDERS*
**Schlichting syndrome**
   See *CORNEAL DYSTROPHY, POLYMORPHOUS POSTERIOR*
**Schmid metaphyseal dysostosis**
   See *METAPHYSEAL CHONDRODYSPLASIA, TYPE SCHMID*
**Schmid-Fraccaro syndrome**
   See *CAT EYE SYNDROME*
**Schmitt syndrome**
   See *RADIAL HYPOPLASIA-TRIPHALANGEAL THUMBS-HYPOSPADIAS-DIASTEMA*
**Schneckenbecken dysplasia**
   See *SKELETAL DYSPLASIA, SCHNECKENBECKEN TYPE*
**Schnyder crystalline corneal dystrophy**
   See *CORNEAL DYSTROPHY, SCHNYDER CRYSTALLINE*
**Schusterbrust**
   See *PECTUS EXCAVATUM*
**Schwartz-Jampel syndrome**
   See *CHONDRODYSTROPHIC MYOTONIA, SCHWARTZ-JAMPEL TYPE*
**Schwartz-Lelek syndrome (one form)**
   See *CRANIOMETAPHYSEAL DYSPLASIA*
   also *DIAPHYSEAL DYSPLASIA*

---

**SCIMITAR SYNDROME**                                  **0879**

**Includes:**
   Lung, hypoplastic-systemic arterial supply-venous drainage
   Pulmonary venous return, partial anomalous

**Excludes: Pulmonary venous connection, total anomalous** (0842)

**Major Diagnostic Criteria:** A scimitar shadow on chest X-ray in the right hemithorax. Cardiac catheterization must demonstrate the anomalous right pulmonary vein draining caudally into the inferior vena cava. The right lower lobe, in some cases, has received its arterial supply from an anomalous vessel arising from the aorta below the diaphragm.

**Clinical Findings:** Various malformations of the pulmonary venous system have been reported. In the pediatric age group, the scimitar syndrome has been diagnosed most frequently in children being evaluated for recurrent respiratory infections or the presence of the heart in the right chest. In its most complete form, this syndrome consists of: anomalous pulmonary venous connection and drainage of part or the entire lung into the inferior vena cava, hypoplasia of the right lung, hypoplasia of the right pulmonary artery, dextrorotation or dextroposition of the heart; and anomalous subdiaphragmatic systemic arterial supply to the lower

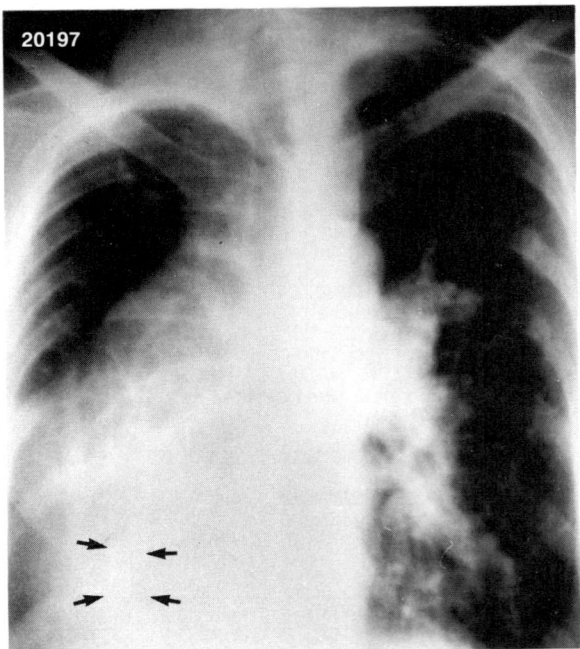

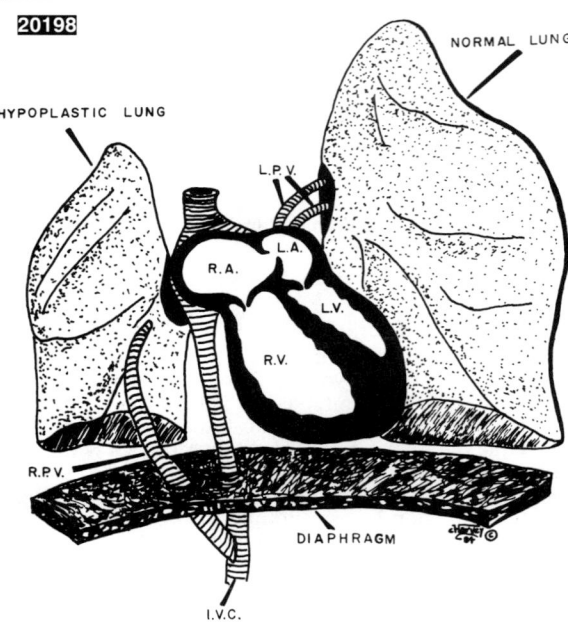

**0879-20197:** Chest X-ray shows cardiac shadow in the right chest (dextro-position) as well as a paracardiac shadow which is "scimitar-shaped" and widens as it approaches the right cardiophrenic angle. **20198:** Diagram shows the constellation of anomalies which produce the scimitar syndrome; note that the right hypoplastic lung and pulmonary vein drain into the inferior vena cava.

---

lobe of the right lung from the aorta or its main branches. The symptoms of this syndrome are related to the degree of hypoplasia of the right lung or associated cardiac anomalies. The presence of the anomalous pulmonary vein of the right lung draining into the inferior vena cava by itself does not usually give rise to symptoms. The diagnosis can be made on plain frontal chest X-ray: in the right hemithorax, a paracardiac shadow which is vertical, gently curved, and increased in width as it approaches the right cardiophrenic angle is seen. The shape of this shadow is similar to the shape of a scimitar. Also, the heart is usually in a dextroposition, and hypoplasia of the right lung in varying degrees may be seen. Bronchogram will demonstrate a variety of anomalies.

**Complications:** Recurrent pneumonia.

**Associated Findings:** Cardiac malformations are common. **Ventricular septal defect, Ductus arteriosus, patent, Heart, tetralogy of Fallot, Aorta, coarctation,** and absent right pulmonary artery have all been reported.

**Etiology:** Presumably multifactorial inheritance.

**Pathogenesis:** Unlike other pulmonary vein anomalies, the scimitar syndrome is accompanied by abnormalities of the right lung of varying degrees of severity. It should probably be considered an abnormal development of the right lung bud, representing a more primitive type of malformation than the usual anomalies of the pulmonary venous system.

**MIM No.:** 10670

**Sex Ratio:** M1:F1 in adults, preponderance of females in pediatric age group.

**Occurrence:** Over 100 cases have been documented.

**Risk of Recurrence for Patient's Sib:** Unknown.

**Risk of Recurrence for Patient's Child:** Unknown.

**Age of Detectability:** In infancy, by X-ray.

**Gene Mapping and Linkage:** Unknown.

**Prevention:** None known. Genetic counseling indicated.

**Treatment:** Antibiotics for recurrent pneumonia. Surgical resection of involved tissue or correction of cardiac anomalies.

**Prognosis:** Dependent on associated cardiac anomalies.

**Detection of Carrier:** Unknown.

**Special Considerations:** The scimitar syndrome is only one of a variety of pulmonary vein anomalies that are diverse in nature and frequently associated with other cardiac malformations. The clinical manifestations are varied but are frequently due to pulmonary venous and arterial hypertension. These anomalies have been classified on an anatomic basis into groups: stenotic lesions, accessory veins, and anomalous connection, either partial or total, in a variety of combinations.

**References:**

Neill CA, et al.: The familial occurrence of hypoplastic right lung with systemic arterial blood supply and venous draining: "Scimitar" syndrome. Bull Johns Hopkins Hosp 1960; 107:1–20.

Jue KL, et al.: Anomalies of great vessels associated with lung hypoplasia: the scimitar syndrome. Am J Dis Child 1966; 111:35–44.

Kiely B, et al.: Syndrome of anomalous venous drainage of the right lung into the inferiorvena cava: a review of 67 reported cases and three new cases in children. Am J Cardiol 1967; 20:102–116.

Nakib A, et al.: Anomalies of the pulmonary veins. Am J Cardiol 1967; 20:77–90.

Oakley D, et al.: Scimitar vein syndrome: report of nine new cases. Am Heart J 1984; 107:596–598.

K0018                                                    **Boris G. Kousseff**

**Sclera (blue)-hydrocephalus-nephrosis-thin skin-growth defect**
  *See NEPHROSIS-HYDROCEPHALUS-THIN SKIN-BLUE SCLERA-GROWTH DEFECT*
**Scleroatrophic and keratotic dermatosis of limbs**
  *See SCLEROTYLOSIS*
**Sclerocornea**
  *See CORNEA PLANA*

## SCLERODERMA, FAMILIAL PROGRESSIVE                    2154

**Includes:**
  Bleomycin induced scleroderma
  CREST syndrome
  L-5-hydroxytryptophan induced scleroderma
  Pentazocine induced scleroderma
  Progressive systemic sclerosis (PSS)
  Sclerosis, familial progressive systemic
  Trichloroethylene induced scleroderma
  Vinyl chloride induced scleroderma

**Excludes:**
  Graft vs host disease
  PSS following cosmetic surgery
  Scleroderma, non-familial
  Shulman syndrome

**Major Diagnostic Criteria:** The American Rheumatism Association (ARA) Scleroderma Criteria Cooperative Study Group suggested the following criteria: 1) proximal scleroderma is the single major criterion (91% sensitivity, 99% specificity); 2) sclerodactyly, pitting scars of fingertips or loss of substance of the finger pad, and bibasilar pulmonary fibrosis contribute as minor criteria; and 3) one major, or two or more minor criteria should be present to diagnose scleroderma.

Skin biopsy is essential to confirm the diagnosis. The characteristic microscopic features of scleroderma are: thickening or atrophy of dermis, thickening of cutis due to accumulation of layers of collagen in the dermis, obliteration of sweat glands and hair follicles, lymphocytic infiltration around sweat glands and roots of hair, hyalinization of walls of subcutaneous arterioles and perivascular infiltration by lymphocytes.

Recent studies on generalized scleroderma suggest the presence of two subsets:

1.) A diffuse cutaneous variety in which there is trunkal and acral skin involvement and early and significant interstital pulmonary fibrosis, renal failure, and diffuse involvement of the GI tract and of the myocardium. The presence of Anti-scl 70 antibody correlates highly with this clinical picture.

2.) A limited cutaneous variety charcterized by severe **Raynaud disease,** acral or no skin involvement, calcinosis, and telangiectasia. This subset is highly correlated with the presence of anti-centromere antibody.

**Clinical Findings:** Hardening of the skin of the hands, palms and chest; leathery feeling of the skin; generalized stiffness; inability to open mouth; polyarthralgia or polyarthritis, or both; blueness of hands and feet (see **Raynaud disease**); difficulty in swallowing; retrosternal chest pain and heartburn; constipation; crampy, abdominal pain.

Laboratory abnormalities that have been described include: elevated sedimentaion rate (ESR), anemia, hypergammaglobulinemia and the presence of antinuclear antibody (ANA) and rheumatoid factor (RF) in the serum.

Capillary nailfold microscopy is a simple procedure which shows characteristic abnormalities in the nailbed capillaries. These include enlargement of capillary loops, loss of capillaries (drop out), disruption of the orderly appearance of the normal capillary bed, and distortion and budding of the capillaries.

Pulmonary function studies show reduced vital capacity and defective diffusion (by carbon monoxide testing). Esophageal manometry shows decreased motility of the lower esophagus and defective functioning of lower esophageal sphincter.

Chest X-ray may show interstitial reticular pattern with prominence of pulmonary arterial segment and dilated heart. Gastrointestinal (GI) series with barium may show distended loops of bowel with air-fluid levels and dilated atonic colon. X-rays of the hands may show thinning of the pulp of the distal phalanges and partial absorption of bony tufts of the terminal phalanges and subcutaneous calcification.

**Complications:** **Raynaud disease,** with loss of fingertips and vasculitic ulcers of the tips of fingers; nodules over extensor aspects of elbows and knees which ulcerate; flexion deformity of fingers; respiratory failure with interstitial lung disease; right heart failure;

pulmonary hypertension; renal hypertension; renal failure; gastrointestinal obstruction.

**Associated Findings:**  None known.

**Etiology:**  Among the various chemicals that are known to induce a clinical picture of scleroderma are vinyl chloride, pentazocine, bleomycin, trichloroethylene and L-5-hydroxytryptophan. Occupational association with mining has been described. Also, recently, a scleroderma-like syndrome has been described from Spain following ingestion of adulterated cooking (rapeseed) oil. Some authors have also cited cases which suggest a genetic susceptibility to this condition.

Clinical, serological and pathological features of progressive systemic sclerosis (PSS) and **Lupus erythematosis, systemic** (SLE) have been described in different members of the same families. A mother with scleroderma, whose daughter had SLE, and a mother with SLE -- whose daughter had scleroderma, have both been described. There has also been a description of identical twins; one with PSS, and one with probable SLE. In another study of eight families containing one member with PSS and another with SLE, concordance for serological features was noted in familial pairs. Seven of the eight pairs in this study did not live in the same household at the onset of their diseases.

**Pathogenesis:**  The etiology of scleroderma remains unknown. Abnormalities of collagen synthesis, collagen metabolism, humoral and cellular immune system, and vasoregulations have all been implicated. Clearly, the fibrosis of the skin and internal organs is due to the overproduction of collagen. There seems to be alterations in the metabolism and turn-over of collagen, and also probably synthesis of abnormal glycoproteins. Increase in quantitative immunoglobulins in the serum, the presence of rheumatoid factor and ANA, peripheral lymphopenia affecting T-cells, presence of T-cells in the tissue infiltrates, and the presence of sensitized lymphocytes in the circulation of patients with progressive systemic sclerosis suggest an immune basis for the pathogenesis of this disease. Also, a serum component capable of producing endothelial injury has been demonstrated in patients with progressive systemic sclerosis.

**MIM No.:**  18175

**Sex Ratio:**  F3:M1

**Occurrence:**  5:10,000,000 per year

**Risk of Recurrence for Patient's Sib:**  Unknown.

**Risk of Recurrence for Patient's Child:**  Unknown.

**Age of Detectability:**  Unknown.

**Gene Mapping and Linkage:**  Unknown. Because the disease is more common in females, some authors have felt that this may be due to a mutant gene or genes on the X chromosome. However, in one report on familial scleroderma, all affected individuals were males, suggesting other inheritance factors.

Older studies have suggested a significant increase in frequency of HLA-A1, B-8, DR3, and DR5. However, more recent studies on large numbers of patients with progressive systemic sclerosis have failed to confirm these associations.

Scleroderma-like illness associated with vinyl chloride exposure is more common in individuals with HLA-DR5 (relative risk 3.5). The risk of progressive systemic sclerosis-like disease for males with DR5 antigen exposed to vinyl chloride is >90%.

**Prevention:**  None known. Genetic counseling indicated.

**Treatment:**  Nearly all patients need supportive therapy to control their **Raynaud disease**, arthritis, espophageal reflux and contractures. Right heart failure and renal disease may require intensive management. Renal failure may require aggressive antihypertensive treatment and renal dialysis. Specific therapy for progressive systemic sclerosis at present is d-Penicillamine.

**Prognosis:**  The natural course is variable. Severe flexion contractures, particularly of the fingers, may be a major problem. Severe **Raynaud disease** may also lead to loss of fingertips or entire fingers and toes. Those with renal disease have the worst prognosis. Patients without visceral involvement may live a reasonably normal life. Prognosis is worse for those with involvement of lungs, kidney or heart at the time of diagnosis.

**Detection of Carrier:**  Unknown.

**Special Considerations:**  An inherited disease of Leghorn chicken, called, 'The University of California at Davis Line 200', has been described. The disease develops early in life with swelling and necrosis of the combs, digits, and the skin of these birds. Later on they develop fibrosis of the esophagus, heart, lungs and the small intestines -- just as in the human disease. These birds also develop antinuclear antibodies, rheumatoid factor, and antibodies to Type II collagen. Under the microscope, the skin shows intense mononuclear cell infiltration, dense deposition of collagen and obliteration of small arteries.

Increased frequency of chromosome breaks has been recognized in many rheumatic diseases. This has been particularly prominent in scleroderma. Chromosome abnormalities have been noted at rates of three times the control values in normals, and also in 95% of the patients examined. Cell cultures of both blood and skin have been shown to demonstrate these abnormalities. In a study of 21 relatives of patients with scleroderma, who also had Raynaud's phenomenon, all showed increased chromosome breaks. Subsequently, six of them developed scleroderma. Sister chromatid exchanges have also been described in scleroderma.

Chromosomal instability has been observed to be significantly increased in such occupations as goldminers with progressive systemic sclerosis. There is also increased chromosomal instability and breakage in patients with progressive systemic sclerosis with no known occupational exposure and in children of patients with progressive systemic sclerosis. These findings, together with the observation that certain chemicals can induce scleroderma-like syndrome, lend support to the concept of predisposition to progressive systemic sclerosis in the presence of certain environmental stimuli. Alternatively, certain chemicals can induce chromosome breaks which may or may not be related to the evolution of clinical disease.

Another interesting feature of this disease is the presence of anticentromere antibody (ACA) which has been noted in one variant of scleroderma called *CREST syndrome*. By special techniques, this antibody has been shown to be directed against the kinetochore discs of the chromosomes. It is occasionally seen in progressive systemic sclerosis also. In one study of 28 patients with scleroderma, fourteen had anticentromere antibody and fourteen did not have this antibody. Major chromosomal anomalies were noted in those with ACA more commonly that in those without ACA.

**Support Groups:**  CA; Watsonville; United Scleroderma Foundation (USF)

**References:**
Greger RE: Familial progressive systemic scleroderma. Arch Dermatol 1975; 111:81–85.
Maricq HR: Widefield capillary microscopy: technique and rating scale for abnormalities seen in scleroderma and related disorders. Arthritis Rheum 1981; 24:1159–1165.
Sheldon WB, et al.: Three siblings with scleroderma (systemic sclerosis) and two with Raynaud's phenomenon from a single kindred. Arthritis Rheum 1981; 24:668–676.
LeRoy E, et al.: Scleroderm (systemic sclerosis): classification, subsets and pathogenisis. (Editorial) J Rheumatol 1988; 15:202–205.
McGregor AR: Familial clustering of scleroderma spectrum disease. Am J Med 1988; 84:1023–1032.
Steen VD, et al.: Clinical correlations and prognosis based on serum autoantibodies in patients with systemic sclerosis. Arthritis Rheum 1988; 31:196–203.

AT002
VA005

**Balu H. Athreya**
**Don C. Van Dyke**

**Sclerosing poikiloderma, hereditary**
*See POIKILODERMA, SCLEROSING, HEREDITARY*
**Sclerosing poliodystrophy, progressive**
*See ALPERS DISEASE*
**Sclerosis, familial progressive systemic**
*See SCLERODERMA, FAMILIAL PROGRESSIVE*
**Sclerosteosis**
*See ENDOSTEAL HYPEROSTOSIS*

## SCLEROSTEOSIS                                           0880

**Includes:**
    Cortical hyperostosis-syndactyly
    Sklerosteose
**Excludes:**
    **Osteopetrosis, benign dominant** (0779)
    **Osteopetrosis, malignant recessive** (0780)
    **Endosteal hyperostosis** (0497)

**Major Diagnostic Criteria:** Gigantism, syndactyly, and X-ray demonstration of sclerosis and hyperostosis of the skull and axial skeleton.

**Clinical Findings:** Mandibular prognathism and frontal prominence become evident by the age of five years. These deformities progress, and in adulthood the face is severely distorted, with dental malocclusion, proptosis, and relative mid-facial hypoplasia. Affected children are tall for their age, and adults with the condition may have gigantism. The majority have partial or total

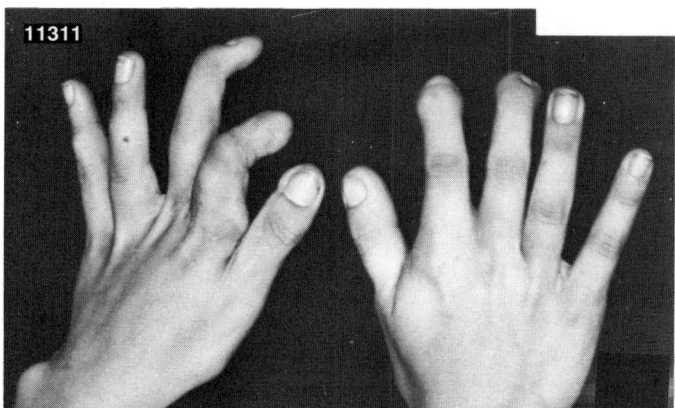

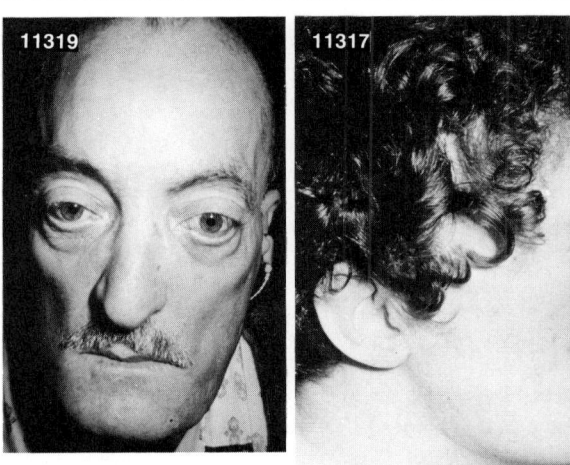

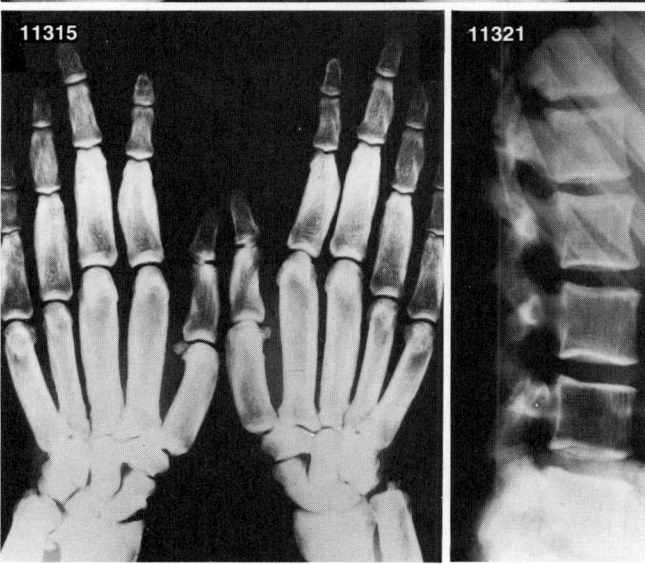

**0880B-**11311:    Syndactyly and radial deviation of 2nd and 3rd fingers and dysplastic nails.    11315:    Sclerosis and lack of diaphyseal constriction.    11321:    Spinal sclerosis and straightening.

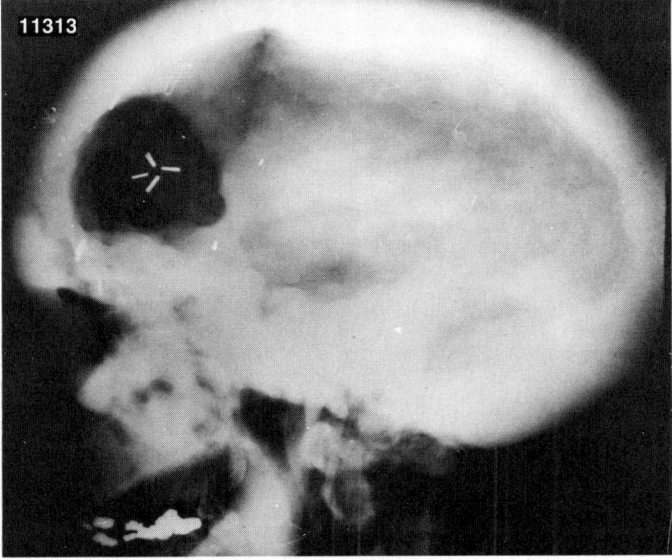

**0880A-**11319:    Asymmetric enlargement of the mandible, facial palsy, proptosis and deafness.    11317:    Profile of face shows broad mandible.    11313:    Massive cranial hyperostosis and thickening of calvaria and skull base. Surgical clips are from a craniotomy.

syndactyly, usually of the second and third fingers, with deviation of the terminal phalanges and hypoplasia of the nails on the corresponding digits. The bones are resistant to trauma and fractures are infrequent. On X-ray, the calvaria is widened and uniformly sclerotic. The base becomes very dense, and the cranial nerve foramina may be obliterated. The sinuses remain patent, and the sella turcica may be expanded. The mandible is dense and massive, with asymmetrical distortion and dental malocclusion. The vertebral end plates and pedicles are sclerotic, but the outlines of the bodies are not disturbed. The clavicles and ribs are widened and dense; the scapulae and pelvis are sclerotic but not expanded. The tubular bones are massive, with cortical hyperostosis and moderate alteration of their external contours.

**Complications:** Transient palsy of the seventh nerve occurs during infancy, and bilateral facial paralysis is usually permanent by adulthood. Progressive bony encroachment upon the middle ear cavities and auditory nerve canals often causes deafness in mid-childhood. Compression of the optic nerves is a late complication. Overgrowth of the calvarium leads to progressive diminution of the capacity of the cranial cavity, with elevation of intracranial pressure. Severe headache due to this mechanism often develops in early adulthood, and several patients have died suddenly from impaction of the medulla oblongata in the foramen magnum.

**Associated Findings:** None known.

**Etiology:** Autosomal recessive inheritance.

**Pathogenesis:** Unknown.

**MIM No.:** *26950

**POS No.:** 3386

**Sex Ratio:** M1:F1

**Occurrence:** About 60 cases have been documented, the majority in the Afrikaner population of South Africa. Sporadic cases, or siblings, have been recorded in the United States (including those from an inbred triracial group from southern Maryland known as the "We-Sorts"), Switzerland, Japan, and Brazil.

**Risk of Recurrence for Patient's Sib:**
See Part I, *Mendelian Inheritance.*

**Risk of Recurrence for Patient's Child:**
See Part I, *Mendelian Inheritance.*

**Age of Detectability:** At birth. Syndactyly or facial palsy in an "at risk" newborn are important diagnostic indicators. X-ray changes are evident by the age of five years.

**Gene Mapping and Linkage:** Unknown.

**Prevention:** None known. Genetic counseling indicated.

**Treatment:** Prophylactic craniectomy in early adulthood is necessary in most affected persons. Decompression of 7th and 8th cranial nerves gives inconsistent results. An external hearing aid may be beneficial. Syndactyly requires cosmetic repair. Orthodontic measures are indicated for dental malalignment.

**Prognosis:** Intelligence and general health are unimpaired. The majority of affected persons develop unilateral or bilateral facial palsy and deafness. Intracranial pressure rises in adulthood, and sudden death from impaction of the medulla oblongata in the foramen magnum is frequent unless circumvented by craniectomy.

**Detection of Carrier:** Heterozygotes have calvarial widening, with loss of distinction between the tables of the skull. The changes are variable in degree and not definitive.

**Special Considerations:** In a mildly affected person with sclerosteosis, the phenotype is very similar to that of severely affected individuals with van Buchem disease (see **Endosteal hyperostosis**). As the Afrikaners are derived from Dutch stock, it is possible that there is some fundamental genetic relationship between these two autosomal recessive disorders.

**References:**
Truswell AS: Osteopetrosis with syndactyly: a morphological variant of Albers-Schonberg's disease. J Bone Joint Surg 1958; 40B:208–218.
Beighton P, The radiology of sclerosteosis. Br J Radiol 1976; 49:934–939. †
Beighton P, et al.: The clinical features of sclerosteosis: a review of the manifestations in twenty-five affected individuals. Ann Intern Med 1976; 84:393–397. †
Beighton P, et al.: Sclerosteosis: an autosomal recessive disorder. Clin Genet 1977; 11:1–7.
Beighton P, Hamersma H: Sclerosteosis in South Africa. S Afr Med J 1979; 55:783–788. * †
Epstein S, et al.: Endocrine function in sclerosteosis. S Afr Med J 1979; 55:1105–1110.
Beighton P, et al.: The syndromic status of sclerosteosis and van Buchem's disease. Clin Genet 1984; 25:175–181. * †

BE008                                    **Peter Beighton**

**Includes:**
Scleroatrophic and keratotic dermatosis of limbs
TYS

**Excludes:** Keratosis palmaris et plantaris of Unna-Thost (3264)

**Major Diagnostic Criteria:** Atrophic fibrosis of the skin of the limbs, nail abnormalities, and keratodermia of the palms and soles in a symmetric distribution.

**Clinical Findings:** The hands are small, erythematous, and covered by thin cracked skin, giving a scleroatrophic appearance. Flattening of the thenar and hypothenar eminences with hyperkeratosis of the palms is present. The fingers are usually streamlined and in a slight flexural position, limiting extension. The nail changes are of the hypoplastic type, presenting with fissures and partial hippocratism. Hypohidrosis may be present. The same changes are exhibited on the feet, occurring symmetrically: acromicria, and keratodermia of the soles, particularly in the pressure points; diffuse erythrodermia; hypohidrosis; and nail abnormalities. The patients are in good health otherwise.

**Complications:** Development of a squamous cell carcinoma within a lesion has been reported by most investigators.

**Associated Findings:** None known.

**Etiology:** Autosomal dominant inheritance.

**Pathogenesis:** Unknown.

**MIM No.:** *18160

**Sex Ratio:** Presumably M1:F1.

**Occurrence:** Several kindreds have been reported (Huriez et al, 1969; Lambert et al, 1978; and Fischer, 1978) with over 50 affected individuals.

**Risk of Recurrence for Patient's Sib:**
See Part I, *Mendelian Inheritance.*

**Risk of Recurrence for Patient's Child:**
See Part I, *Mendelian Inheritance.*

**Age of Detectability:** Usually at birth.

**Gene Mapping and Linkage:** TYS (sclerotylosis) has been provisionally mapped to 4q.

**Prevention:** None known. Genetic counseling indicated.

**Treatment:** Emollient creams can be used to reduce the excessive dryness of the skin.

**Prognosis:** Guarded because of the degeneration of the skin lesions into squamous cell carcinoma usually observed after age 40 years.

**Detection of Carrier:** Unknown.

**References:**
Huriez CL, et al.: Genodermatose sclero-atrophiante et keratodermique des extremites. Ann Dermatol Syphilig 1969; 96:135–146.
Lambert D, et al.: La genodermatose sclero-atrophiante et keratodermique des extremites. Ann dermatol Venereol. 1977; 104:654–657.
Fischer S: La genodermatose scleroatrophiante et keratodermique des extremites (au sujet de trois nouveaux cas familiaux). Ann Dermatol Venereol 1978; 105:1079–1082.
Lambert D, et al.: Genodermatose sclero-atrophiante et Keratodermique des extremites. J Genet Hum 1978; 26:25–31.

MI038                                    **Giuseppe Micali**

**Scoliosis, genetic**
*See SPINE, SCOLIOSIS, IDIOPATHIC*
**Scoto-epilepsy**
*See EPILEPSY, BENIGN OCCIPITAL*
**Scott craniodigital syndrome-mental retardation**
*See CRANIO-DIGITAL SYNDROME-MENTAL RETARDATION, SCOTT TYPE*
**Scrotal tongue**
*See TONGUE, PLICATED*
**Sea-blue histiocyte disease**
*See NIEMANN-PICK DISEASE*

**Sebaceous nevus syndrome**
*See NEVUS, EPIDERMAL NEVUS SYNDROME*
**Seborrheic alopecia**
*See HAIR, BALDNESS, COMMON*

## SECKEL SYNDROME                          0881

**Includes:**
Bird-headed dwarf (obsolete/pejorative)
Bird-headed dwarf, Montreal type
Bird-headed dwarfism, Virchow type
Dwarfism, Seckel type
Microcephalic primordial dwarfism
Nanocephalic dwarf

**Excludes:**
Alopecia-skeletal anomalies-short stature-mental retardation (2782)
Dwarfism, osteodysplastic primordial, Majewski-Ranke type (2582)
Dwarfism, osteodysplastic primordial, Majewski-Winter type (2581)
Microcephaly (0659)

**Major Diagnostic Criteria:** The diagnosis depends upon characteristic craniofacies: small head, large eyes, mental retardation, low birth weight, dwarfism, beaked nose, and other malformations.

**Clinical Findings:** Low birth weight for length of gestation, severe microcephaly, mental retardation, marked postnatal growth retardation, delayed bone age, large eyes, large beaklike nose, narrow face, dysplastic ears, and receding lower jaw. The brain shows a much simplified gross cerebral structure (pongidoid microcephaly), with relatively intact cerebellum.

**Complications:** Premature closure of cranial sutures.

**Associated Findings:** Hypoplastic thumb, dislocation of femoral heads or radial heads, clubfoot, scoliosis, strabismus, and gastrointestinal malformations. Chromosome breakage has been demonstrated in two patients, one of whom had pancytopenia.

**Etiology:** Autosomal recessive inheritance.

**Pathogenesis:** Some patients have had mitomycin C-produced chromosome breakage (Butler et al, 1987), and may account for a subgroup of Seckel cases.

**MIM No.:** *21060, 21070

**POS No.:** 3387

**CDC No.:** 759.820

**Sex Ratio:** M1:F1

**Occurrence:** Estimated at no more than 1:10,000 live births.

**Risk of Recurrence for Patient's Sib:**
See Part I, *Mendelian Inheritance.*

**Risk of Recurrence for Patient's Child:**
See Part I, *Mendelian Inheritance.*

**Age of Detectability:** At birth, or prenatally by serial ultrasound.

**Gene Mapping and Linkage:** Unknown.

**Prevention:** None known. Genetic counseling indicated.

**Treatment:** Unknown.

**Prognosis:** For life: good. For intelligence: mental retardation is a prominent feature of the syndrome. For function: function may be impaired by various anomalies such as dislocated femoral heads, clubfoot, and scoliosis.

**Detection of Carrier:** Unknown.

**Special Considerations:** Fitch et al (1970) described a similar but separate condition with normal birth weight and signs of premature senility which has been designated *bird-headed dwarfism, Montreal type.* Virchow (1896) also described a form of bird-headed dwarfism with low birthweight, but without mental retardation and associated malformations.

**References:**
Virchow R: Vostelling der birmesischen zwerge mit einem Salzburger Riesen. Z Ethnologie 1896 28:524–528.
McKusick VA, et al.: Seckel's bird-headed dwarfism. New Engl J Med 1967; 277:279–286.
Fitch N, et al.: A form of bird-headed dwarfism with features of premature senility. Am J Dis Child 1970; 120:260–264.
Fenolio KR, et al.: Prenatal diagnosis of Seckel syndrome. Am J Hum Genet 1982; 34:88A.
Majewski F, Goecke T: Studies of microcephalic primordial dwarfism: approaches to a delineation of Seckel syndrome. Am J Med Genet 1982; 12:7–21. *
Thompson E, Pembrey M: Seckel syndrome: an overdiagnosed syndrome. J Med Genet 1985; 22:192–201.
Butler MG, et al.: Do some patients with Seckel syndrome have hematological problems and/or chromosome breakage? Am J Med Genet 1987; 27:645–649.
Majoor-Krakauer DF, et al.: Microcephaly, micrognathia, bird-headed dwarfism: prenatal diagnosis of a Seckel-like syndrome. Am J Med Genet 1987; 27:183–188.

GR011

**Frank Greenberg**
*Victor A. McKusick*

**Secondary diphallia**
*See DIPHALLIA*
**Seemanova syndrome**
*See CHROMOSOME INSTABILITY, NIJMEGEN TYPE*
**Segmental tracheal agenesis**
*See TRACHEA, AGENESIS*
**Seip syndrome**
*See LIPODYSTROPHY SYNDROME, BERARDINELLI TYPE*
**Seitelberg variant, Pelizaeus-Merzbacher syndrome**
*See PELIZAEUS-MERZBACHER SYNDROME*
**Seitelberger disease**
*See NEUROAXONAL DYSTROPHY, INFANTILE*
**Seizues, impulsive petit mal**
*See SEIZURES, MYOCLONIC, JUVENILE JANZ TYPE*
**Seizures, benign familial neonatal-infantile**
*See CONVULSIONS, BENIGN FAMILIAL NEONATAL*

## SEIZURES, CENTRALOPATHIC              0135

**Includes:**
Absence seizures
Centralopathic epilepsy
Epilepsy, centralopathic
Epilepsy, centrencephalic
Petit mal seizures
Petit mal automatism
Petit mal lapse ("absence")

**Excludes:**
Akinetic or atonic "drop" seizures
Automatisms and psychopathic behavior
Epilepsy due to focal cortical lesion
Grand mal epilepsy
Myoclonic petit mal
Petit mal grand mal epilepsy
Seizures (other)
Spastic ataxia, Charlevoix-Saguenay type (2566)

**Major Diagnostic Criteria:** The typical, bilaterally synchronous EEG, showing a three per-second spike-and-wave abnormality, is used to identify petit mal epilepsy in the context of concomitant alteration of consciousness.

**Clinical Findings:** There is considerable controversy as to the use of the term "centralopathic epilepsy," particularly since the introduction of the International Classification of the Epilepsies. Petit mal (absence) epilepsy is defined as a seizure disorder characterized by brief lapses in consciousness associated with a typical EEG and the absence of neurologic signs.

The seizure may be so mild that it escapes notice; the child may be observed as inattentive or as daydreaming excessively. Seizures are usually abrupt in onset and may occur frequently for short periods of time. Recurrent seizures can cause loss of concentration and thus deterioration in school performance. The seizures typically begin between the ages of 5 and 10 years and are more common in females. There may be a slight pause, blinking of the eyes, a brief stare, and then resumption of activity. More severe seizures may cause lapses of speech and fluttering of the eyelids. Loss of sphincter control, change in color, and gross motor movements do not occur. At the conclusion of the attack, the patient continues the activity that immediately preceded the seizure. An aura does not occur. The diagnosis is made by the history and the typical EEG finding. Hyperventilation for a period of 3 or 4 minutes is often successful in eliciting a clinical seizure and producing typical EEG changes.

**Complications:** Grand mal seizures are relatively common in patients with petit mal epilepsy. Prolonged grand mal seizures may be associated with airway obstruction and anoxia.

**Associated Findings:** Frequent petit mal seizures can cause deterioration in memory and thus a decline in school performance. Rarely, patients with petit mal epilepsy develop status epilepticus and muteness, which may be misinterpreted as hysteria.

**Etiology:** Autosomal dominant inheritance in some families, although some investigators suggest the interaction of several genetic factors rather than a specific autosomal dominant mode of inheritance.

**Pathogenesis:** Until recently, it was generally accepted that petit mal epilepsy resulted from an abnormality in the subcortical structures, because electrical stimulation of midline areas in the experimental animal and man would often produce the typical EEG abnormality and clinical seizure. More recent studies suggest that petit mal epilepsy results from a cortical disturbance or abnormality, which produces bilateral foci, particularly from the frontal lobes. The delayed age of onset of the seizures may be related to maturation of the brain, including myelination of the corpus callosum and related structures, and the interaction of various neurotransmitters, all of which may be under genetic control.

**MIM No.:** *11710

**Sex Ratio:** M1:F1

**Occurrence:** 1:200.

**Risk of Recurrence for Patient's Sib:**
See Part I, *Mendelian Inheritance*. According to Metrakos and Metrakos (1961, 1966), there is a 50% chance that a patient's sib or offspring will inherit the gene for the spike and wave EEG trait and a 35% chance that the EEG will show a typical three per-second finding sometime during his or her lifetime. There is a 12% chance that the sib or offspring will have a convulsion at some time during his or her lifetime but only an 8% chance that a sib or child of a patient will actually develop petit mal epilepsy.

**Risk of Recurrence for Patient's Child:**
See Part I, *Mendelian Inheritance*. Petit mal epilepsy is probably the result of an autosomal dominant gene, which has low penetrance at birth but gains almost complete penetrance between ages 4 and 16 years and then rather rapidly declines. Twin studies have shown that when one monozygotic twin develops seizures, the chance of the other twin being affected is 80–90%. Dizygotic twins show only a 10% concordance.

**Age of Detectability:** Most readily detected between 4 and 16 years.

**Gene Mapping and Linkage:** Unknown.

**Prevention:** None known. Genetic counseling indicated.

**Treatment:** The use of specific drugs such as ethosuximide, clonazepam, or sodium valproate controls most seizures.
Special education may be necessary for the child with frequent and recurrent seizures that are not responsive to medication.

**Prognosis:** Most patients are seizure-free by age 15 to 20 years and may not require lifelong anticonvulsants.

**Detection of Carrier:** By EEG. Between ages 5 and 15 years approximately 40% of sibs have an abnormal EEG, but they may remain seizure-free clinically. The EEG finding is unusual beyond age 40 years.

**Support Groups:**
MD; Landover; Epilepsy Foundation of America

**References:**
Lennox WG: Heredity of epilepsy as told by relatives and twins. JAMA 1951; 146:529.
Penfield W, Jasper H: Epilepsy and the functional anatomy of the human brain. Boston: Little, Brown, 1954.
Metrakos K, Metrakos JD: Genetics of convulsive disorders: II. Genetic and electroencephalographic studies in centrencephalic epilepsy. Neurology 1961; 11:474–483.
Metrakos JD, Metrakos K: Childhood epilepsy of subcortical ("centrencephalic") origin. Clin Pediatr 1966; 5:536.
Gastaut H: Clinical and electroencephalographical classification of epileptic seizures. Epilepsia 1970; 11:102.
Doose H, et al.: Genetic factors in spike-wave absences. Epilepsia 1973; 14:57.
Newmark ME, Penry JK: Genetics of epilepsy: a review. New York: Raven, 1980.
Commission on Classification and Terminology of the International League Against Epilepsy. Proposal for classification of epilepsies and epileptic syndromes. Epilepsia 1981; 22:489–501.

HA053                                          **Robert H.A. Haslam**

**Seizures, dominant benign neonatal**
*See CONVULSIONS, BENIGN FAMILIAL NEONATAL*

## SEIZURES, FEBRILE                                         2568

**Includes:** Febrile convulsions, simple and complex (complicated)

**Excludes:**
Convulsions, benign familial neonatal (3216)
Convulsions induced by gross abnormality of the brain
Convulsions induced by infections of the central nervous system

**Major Diagnostic Criteria:** Convulsions occurring in the presence of rectal temperature of over 38°C.

**Clinical Findings:** Simple febrile seizures are characterized by generalized and tonic-clonic seizures, usually of brief duration, (1–5 minutes in length). Less frequently, children have focal seizures or postictal Todds paralysis. In 2–3% of cases, the duration of the febrile seizure may last up to 30 minutes, which may indicate preexisting brain pathology. Occurrence of multiple febrile seizures is possible.

**Complications:** No children have died as a direct consequence of febrile seizures per se or their long term neurologic sequelae. However, individuals with febrile seizures of longer duration may be at increased risk to developing status epilepticus. The risk for development of future epilepsy is increased with repeated febrile seizures.

**Associated Findings:** Since infections of the respiratory tract and otitis media, accompanied by high fever, are common in young children (age 5 years or less), over 50% of febrile seizure patients are often seen with these conditions. Associated conditions include roseola, other infectious diseases, and in a small percentage (usually less than 5%) with intracranial infections. Approximately one-third of patients 3–6 years of age demonstrate three-per-second spike-and-wave-paroxysms, although this may not be evident at the time of the convulsion. These paroxysms occur more often in patients with a family history of convulsions.

**Etiology:** Family studies suggest that febrile seizures are a hereditary trait, with the mode of inheritance consistent with multifactorial transmission. However, recent evidence has indicated that transmission in families in which the proband has three or more febrile seizures is consistent with autosomal dominant inheritance. Transmission in families in which the proband has one or two febrile seizures is consistent with a multifactorial model, with a heritability liability of about 70%.

**Pathogenesis:** Unknown. Febrile-like seizures may be produced in laboratory animals by means of high temperature (hyperthermic seizures); however, the temperature increases in the animal models may be inordinately high with respect to those seen in the human patients. In addition, there have been reports of alterations in endorphin metabolism.

**MIM No.:** 12121, 21720

**Sex Ratio:** Presumably M1:F1. However, observed figures are M1.2:F1 for the United States and M1.6:F1 for Japan.

**Occurrence:** Convulsions associated with febrile illness are one of the most common acute neurologic disturbances seen in childhood. The population rate varies with the ethnic group and geographic location. There are high population rates in Japan (6.7%) and uniformly lower rates in Denmark (2.1%) and the United States (2.3%).

**Risk of Recurrence for Patient's Sib:** Overall, 8.0% of sibs will have convulsions with fever. The risk of febrile seizures for sibs is not significantly influenced by the sex of the proband. The greater the number of febrile convulsions in probands, the greater the risk for febrile convulsions in sibs. Complex features (focal seizures, Todds paralysis) in the proband are associated with increased risk for febrile seizures in sibs.

**Risk of Recurrence for Patient's Child:** Nearly 8.4% of children of probands are expected to have a febrile convulsion. Children of female probands, especially sons, have a higher risk than children of male probands. The greater the number of febrile convulsions in probands, the greater the risk for febrile convulsions in the children.

**Age of Detectability:** Usually clinically evident between birth and five years of age.

**Gene Mapping and Linkage:** Unknown.

**Prevention:** Patients with recurrent febrile seizures may be given long-term prophylactic anticonvulsants for one year from the last seizure, two years from the first seizure, or until five years of age.

**Treatment:** There is considerable debate in the literature concerning the utility of treatment for febrile seizures. The use of a loading dose of phenobarbital, at the time of prolonged febrile seizure, has been recommended for control of further febrile seizures, accompanied by clinical evaluation for the presence of structural brain abnormalities. Long-term treatment with phenobarbital does not appear to prevent epilepsy effectively following a febrile seizure. With the complication rate associated with drug usage as great as (or greater than) the risk of epilepsy, the cost/benefit of drug usage needs careful evaluation.

**Prognosis:** Good. However, nearly one-third of all patients with a first febrile seizure will have repeated febrile convulsions.

**Detection of Carrier:** Clinical evaluation and a careful family history.

**Special Considerations:** Patients with febrile seizures have a three-to-six fold increase in risk of epilepsy as compared with the general population. However, the majority of children with febrile seizures do not develop epilepsy. While twin studies of febrile seizures are inconclusive, there appears to be an increase in concordance of febrile seizures in monozygotic twins (31%) versus dizygotic twins (14%), consistent with a genetic as well as an environmental pathogenic mechanism.

**Support Groups:** MD; Landover; Epilepsy Foundation of America

**References:**
Schiottz-Christensen E: Genetic factors in febrile convulsions. Acta Neurol Scandinav 1972; 48:538–546.
van den Berg B: Studies on convulsive disorders in young children: incidence of convulsions among siblings. Develop Med Child Neurol 1974; 16:457–464.
Annegers JF, et al: The risk of epilepsy following febrile convulsions. Neurology 1979; 29:297–303. *
Hauser WA: The risk of seizure disorders among relatives of children with febrile convulsions. Neurology 1985; 35:1268–1273. *
Annegers JF, et al: Prognostic factors for unprovoked seizures after febrile seizures. New Engl J Med 1987; 316:493–498.

Rich SS, et al: Complex segregation analysis of febrile convulsions. Am J Hum Genet 1987; 41:249–257.

RI016
HA073

**Stephen S. Rich**
**W. Allen Hauser**

## SEIZURES, IN FEMALES, JUBERG-HELLMAN TYPE 2479

**Includes:** Juberg-Hellman syndrome

**Excludes:**
**Aicardi syndrome** (2320)
Convulsive disorder-mental retardation, benign familial neonatal
Convulsive disorder with prenatal or early onset, familial
Mental retardation-epilepsy-endocrine disorders

**Major Diagnostic Criteria:** 1) Convulsive disorder with age of onset from six to 18 months; 2) tonic-clonic seizures; 3) mental retardation ranging from profound to mild; and 4) electroencephalograms showing focal, diffuse, or paroxysmal abnormalities, or some combination thereof without unique or consistent patterns.

**Clinical Findings:** Female sex. Convulsive disorder without apparent mental retardation (12/29); convulsive disorder with mental retardation (8/29); asymmetry of the anterior horns (1/29); dilation of lateral ventricles (1/29); **Microcephaly** (1/29); focal electroencephalographic (EEG) abnormality (1/17); diffuse EEG abnormalities (2/17); focal and diffuse EEG abnormalities (2/17); focal and paroxysmal EEG abnormalities (3/17); diffuse and paroxysmal EEG abnormalities (2/17); and focal, diffuse, and paroxysmal EEG abnormalities (2/17).

**Complications:** Postictal paresis, facial asymmetry, and disturbance of gait.

**Associated Findings:** Strabismus, malformation of the hand with **Syndactyly** and digital deficiency.

**Etiology:** Possibly X-linked dominant inheritance with sex-limited expression.

**Pathogenesis:** Unknown.

**MIM No.:** 12125

**Sex Ratio:** M0:F1

**Occurrence:** One kinship originating with 15 affected sisters has been reported.

**Risk of Recurrence for Patient's Sib:**
See Part I, *Mendelian Inheritance.*

**Risk of Recurrence for Patient's Child:**
See Part I, *Mendelian Inheritance.*

**Age of Detectability:** Probably not before six months of age.

**Gene Mapping and Linkage:** Unknown.

**Prevention:** None known. Genetic counseling indicated.

**Treatment:** Anticonvulsant medications such as phenobarbital, diphenylhydantoin sodium, mephobarbital, and primidone. Early childhood educational intervention and special education.

**Prognosis:** Convulsive-free periods may last for years. Mental retardation will vary from mild to profound. Probably normal life span.

**Detection of Carrier:** Unknown.

**Special Considerations:** In the fourth generation, there is an unusually high proportion of affected females (15/18) among the offspring of transmitting males. In addition, 6/7 males with daughters past infancy transmitted the gene. An X-linked dominant gene with limitation of clinical manifestations to females is more likely than autosomal dominant inheritance in this family. The odds ratio is 562:1 favoring X-linked dominant inheritance over autosomal dominant, assuming high but not complete penetrance of either gene.

*The author would like to express his appreciation to Herbert A. Lubs for his help in the follow-up of the family affected with this condition.*

**References:**
Juberg RC, Hellman CD: A new familial form of convulsive disorder and mental retardation limited to females. J Pediatr 1971; 79:726–732. *

JU000                                                    **Richard C. Juberg**

---

## SEIZURES, MYOCLONIC, JUVENILE JANZ TYPE                    2567

**Includes:**

> Epilepsy, juvenile myoclonic, Janz type
> Janz syndrome
> Juvenile myoclonic epilepsy (JME), Janz type
> Myoclonic epilepsy, benign
> Seizues, impulsive petit mal

**Excludes: Seizures** (other)

**Major Diagnostic Criteria:** Isolated bilateral, myoclonic jerks without loss of consciousness, most often of the upper extremities, sometimes also involving lower extremities, that occur usually in the mornings shortly after awakening or after sleep deprivation. Major seizures, generally tonic-clonic, are usually the initial complaint. About 30% of cases also show absence seizures.

**Clinical Findings:** Age of onset is seldom before 10 years. The most common pattern is for myoclonic jerks to start around age 14–15 years. However, patients usually do not recognize jerking as abnormal. Most often, the first tonic-clonic seizure will cause the patient to seek medical help. Patients may comment that they are "clumsy" or "spastic." Often only when asked if they "drop things" in the morning or suddenly "throw things across the room" will the fact that the patient has been having myoclonic jerks emerge. Myoclonic jerks will often start before the first tonic-clonic seizure, but the first occurrences of the two types of seizures may be close together in time. Absence, when it occurs, is almost always of the adolescent type, with a few absence attacks per day.

In almost all cases, the interictal EEG shows bursts of a 4–6-Hz multispike-and-wave pattern, sometimes lasting several seconds. On closed circuit television monitoring, these multispike-and-wave bursts can sometimes be seen to coincide with jerking.

Family history is sometimes positive for generalized epilepsy, either tonic-clonic seizures or absence, and occasionally for juvenile myoclonic epilepsy (JME) itself, but the family history is often negative. Research shows that a high percentage of family members have positive findings on EEG testing. Often, these findings show the same 4–6-Hz multispike-and-wave pattern seen interictally in patients, although jerking is not seen in the clinically unaffected family members. Other EEG abnormalities seen in family members are paroxysmal bursts of 3–5-Hz high-amplitude slowing. Perhaps 17% of sibs over age 20 years show EEG abnormalities, while only 1–5% of the general public show such abnormalities.

JME should be distinguished from the degenerative myoclonic epilepsies, which have a higher recurrence risk and poorer prognosis.

**Complications:** Usual complications of epilepsy. Uncontrolled seizures can be life-threatening and lead to accidents. Jerking can lead to accidents and falls. Complications that result from medications are frequent.

**Associated Findings:** None known.

**Etiology:** Possibly autosomal recessive inheritance with 60% penetrance. A two locus model of inheritance has also been suggested.

**Pathogenesis:** Unknown.

**MIM No.:** 25477

**Sex Ratio:** Presumably M1:F1.

**Occurrence:** Juvenile myoclonic epilepsy is thought to comprise 5–10% of all epilepsies, or a population prevalence of 5–10:10,000. This is probably an underestimate, since people manifesting the myoclonic jerks with no other seizures will seldom seek medical help. The condition affects all ethnic groups.

**Risk of Recurrence for Patient's Sib:** Empiric risk for any form of epilepsy in a sib is about 5–7%. If the sib has an EEG abnormality and is older than age 20 years, risk is apparently not increased. The risk for sibs younger than age 20 years with an EEG abnormality is unknown.

**Risk of Recurrence for Patient's Child:** Unknown.

**Age of Detectability:** Clinical signs start at 10–20 years of age, most frequently around ages 13–15 years. Age when EEG abnormalities start is unknown.

**Gene Mapping and Linkage:** EJM (epilepsy, juvenile myoclonic) has been tentatively mapped to 6p.

**Prevention:** None known. Genetic counseling indicated.

**Treatment:** Valproic acid appears to be 95% effective in controlling both tonic-clonic and myoclonic seizures. Frequently, the EEG signs also disappear with valproic acid treatment. Adverse reactions to valproic acid monotherapy often dictate use of other drugs such as primidone or carbamazepine, but seizures with these medications will sometimes occur.

**Prognosis:** The condition is not progressive, though apparently life-long.

**Detection of Carrier:** Unknown.

**Special Considerations:** Heterogeneity may exist. Reports conflict about the proportions of patients with photosensitivity. Also, some patients have absence seizures while some do not. However, family members with epilepsy (but not JME) have been found to have tonic-clonic seizures without absence in some families, while in other families absence seizures occur without motor involvement. This may point to a similar underlying cause for both types of seizures in families with JME.

JME is frequently misdiagnosed, resulting in the prescription of inappropriate medication. As a result, while medications other than valproic acid will reduce the frequency of seizures, patients often achieve only fair or poor seizure control. In an effort to control seizures, levels of antiepileptic drugs may be increased to the point at which the patient feels constantly drowsy and, since onset is in the teenage years, the patient's education and social adjustment may suffer.

**Support Groups:**

> New York; National Myoclonus Foundation
> MD; Landover; Epilepsy Foundation of America

**References:**
Janz D: Inpulsiv-Petit mal. Dtsch Nervenheilkd 1957; 176:346–86.
Tsuboi T, Christian W: On the genetics of the primary generalized epilepsy with sporadic myoclonias of impulsive petit mal type: a clinical and electroencephalographic study of 399 probands. Humangenetik 1973; 19:155–182.
Delgado-Escueta A, Enrile-Bascal F: Juvenile myoclonic epilepsy of Janz. Neurology 1984; 34:285–294. *
Durner M, et al.: HLA and epilepsie mit impulsive petit mal. In: Speckman EJ, ed: Epilepsie 1987. Rheinbeck: Einhorn Presse, 1988.
Greenberg DA, et al.: Segregation analysis of juvenile myoclonic epilepsy. Genetic Epidemiology 1988; 5:81–94.
Greenberg DA, et al.: Juvenile myoclonic epilepsy (JME) may be linked to the BF and HLA loci on human chromosome 6. Am J Med Genet 1988; 31:185–192. *

GR012                                                    **David A. Greenberg**

---

## SEIZURES, PROGRESSIVE MYOCLONIC, LAFORA TYPE                    2601

**Includes:**

> Epilepsy, myoclonus, Lafora type
> Lafora body disease
> Lafora disease
> Polyglucosan body disease, adult
> Myoclonus epilepsy with Lafora bodies progressive

**Excludes:**

> Action myoclonus-renal failure syndrome
> **Dentatorubropallidoluysian degeneration, hereditary** (3283)
> Dyssynergia cerebellaris myoclonica
> **Gaucher disease** (0406)

Kearns-Sayre disease (2070)
Mucolipidosis I (0671)
Neuronal ceroid-lipofuscinoses (NCL) (0713)
Seizures, myoclonic, juvenile Janz type (2567)
Seizures, progressive myoclonic, Unverricht-Lundborg type
    (2602)

**Major Diagnostic Criteria:** Progressive tonic-clonic seizures starting early in the second decade; myoclonus of variable severity; focal seizures, especially occipital attacks; and relentless cognitive decline. The diagnosis is confirmed by the finding of characteristic Lafora bodies, which may be found in eccrine sweat gland duct cells obtained by skin biopsy and stained for polysaccharides. The storage material is largely composed of complex carbohydrates, which are seen histologically as the typical inclusion bodies.

**Clinical Findings:** The children are initially normal. The first symptoms develop between 11–18 years of age, with a mean age of onset at 14 years. Myoclonic seizures may be virtually continuous or not very striking. Focal occipital seizures occur in about one-half the cases. There is a fairly rapid progressive cognitive decline in all patients. In rare cases, behavioural changes or school failure may be the first symptom, and seizures may be relatively infrequent.

Dysarthria and cerebellar signs appear as the disease progresses. Increased deep tendon reflexes may be found. Both hypotonia and rigidity of the limbs have been described, but spasticity is not seen. Fundoscopic examination is normal.

Death occurs 2–10 years after onset (mean six years), and the mean age at death is twenty years. Four patients are known in whom symptoms began in early adult life with a milder protracted course. These exceptional cases may represent a genetic type separate from the classical form.

The diagnosis may be suspected from the clinical picture. The electroencephalogram shows generalized spike and wave discharges activated by photic stimulation, and progressive slowing of background rhythms. Focal and multifocal posterior epileptiform discharges may also be seen. A modest amount of cerebral atrophy may be shown by neuroradiological studies.

Definitive diagnosis depends on the detection of the characteristic periodic acid Schiff-positive inclusion bodies which are present in various tissues including brain, liver, skeletal and cardiac muscle, and skin. Skin biopsy is the simplest and least invasive diagnostic procedure. Inclusion bodies are reliably found in eccrine sweat gland duct cells. The inclusion bodies consist largely of glucose polymers or polyglucosans with a small variable component of phophate and sulphate groups, and a minor amount of associated protein.

**Complications:** Fairly rapidly progressive pseudodementia, more striking as compared with the other progressive myoclonus epilepsies, is characteristic. The effect of antiepileptic drug toxicity in patients with **Seizures, myoclonic, juvenile Janz type** should be considered in the differential diagnosis.

**Associated Findings:** None known.

**Etiology:** Autosomal recessive inheritance. This has been confirmed by multiple cases in sibships, increased parental consanguinity, and absence of affected relatives in the direct line.

**Pathogenesis:** Unknown.

**MIM No.:** *25478

**Sex Ratio:** M1:F1

**Occurrence:** One of the more common forms of progressive myoclonus epilepsy; over 100 cases have been reported in the world literature. Most common in population groups where there is a high rate of consanguinity, such as in the Island of Réunion, North Africa and Québec, but it is also found in almost every population.

**Risk of Recurrence for Patient's Sib:**
    See Part I, *Mendelian Inheritance.*

**Risk of Recurrence for Patient's Child:**
    See Part I, *Mendelian Inheritance.* Affected individuals are not expected to survive to reproduce.

**Age of Detectability:** Preclinical dianosis can be carried out by skin biopsy in siblings of affected patients. Attempts at isolating a specific oligosaccharide in the urine of patients have failed.

**Gene Mapping and Linkage:** Unknown.

**Prevention:** None known. Genetic counseling indicated.

**Treatment:** Symptomatic treatment of seizures with emphasis on antimyoclonic drugs such as valproic acid and clonazepam, as well as general supportive care.

**Prognosis:** The disease progresses rapidly to severe dementia, quadriplegia, cachexia, and a vegetative state with death at a mean age of 20 years. Survival beyond the age of 25 years is extremely rare.

**Detection of Carrier:** Unknown.

**Special Considerations:** Storage of similar microscopic bodies restricted to processes of neurons and astrocytes has been found in some middle-aged patients with progressive lower and upper motor neuron deficits, marked sensory loss in the legs, neurogenic bladder, and dementia. The stored material may or may not be identical to that seen in Lafora body disease. This disorder is referred to as *adult polyglucosan body disease.*

**Support Groups:**
    New York; National Myoclonus Foundation
    MD; Landover; Epilepsy Foundation of America

**References:**
Lafora GR, Glueck B: Beitrag zur Histopathologie der myoklonischen Epilepsie. Z Gesamte Neurol Psychiatr 1911; 6:1–14.
Carpenter S, et al: Lafora's disease: peroxisomal storage in skeletal muscle. Neurology 1974; 24:531–538. †
Van Heycop ten Ham MW: Lafora disease: a form of progressive myoclonus epilepsy. In: Vinken PJ, Bruyn GW, eds: Handbook of Clinical Neurology, vol 15. Amsterdam: North Holland Publishing, 1974:382–422. *
Robitaille Y, et al: A distinct form of adult polyglucosan body disease with massive involvement of central and peripheral neuronal processes and astrocytes: a report of four cases and a review of the occurrence of polyglucosan bodies in other conditions such as Lafora's disease and normal ageing. Brain 1980; 103:315–336.
Carpenter S, Karpati G: Sweat gland duct cells in Lafora disease: diagnosis by skin biopsy. Neurology 1981; 31:1564–1568. * †
Roger J, et al: Le diagnostic Précoce de la maladie de Lafora: importance des manifestations paroxystiques visuelles et intérêt de la biopsie cutanée. Rev Neurol (Paris) 1983; 139:115–124.
Berkovic SF, Andermann F: The progressive myoclonus epilepsies. In: Pedley TA, Meldrum BS, eds: Recent Advances in Epilepsy. Edinburgh: Churchill Livingstone 1986:157–187. *
Berkovic SF, et al: Progressive myoclonus epilepsies: specific causes and diagnosis. New Eng J Med 1986; 315:296–305. *
Busard HLSM, et al.: Axilla skin biopsy: a reliable test for the diagnosis of Lafora's disease. Ann Neurol 1987; 21:599–601.

AN016                                                          **Eva Andermann**
AN018                                                  **Frederick Andermann**

---

**SEIZURES, PROGRESSIVE MYOCLONIC, UNVERRICHT-LUNDBORG TYPE**                                    **2602**

**Includes:**
    Baltic myoclonus epilepsy
    Dyssynergia cerebellaris myoclonica (some cases)
    Myoclonus epilepsy, Unverricht-Lundborg type
    Progressive myoclonus epilepsy without Lafora bodies
    Ramsay-Hunt syndrome (some cases)
    Unverricht-Lundborg disease

**Excludes:**
    Action myoclonus-renal failure syndrome
    **Dentatorubropallidoluysian degeneration, hereditary** (3283)
    Ekbom syndrome
    **Gaucher disease** (0406)
    **Kearns-Sayre disease** (2070)
    May-White syndrome
    **Mucolipidosis I** (0671)

**Neuronal ceroid-lipofuscinoses (NCL)** (0713)
**Seizures, myoclonic, juvenile Janz type** (2567)
**Seizures, progressive myoclonic, Lafora type** (2601)

**Major Diagnostic Criteria:** Onset between 6–15 years of age; abundant, at times continuous, action and stimulus-sensitive myoclonus; generalized seizures; progressive ataxia with only mild dementia.

**Clinical Findings:** The disorder usually begins at about age 10 years, following a normal infancy and early childhood. The first symptoms are myoclonic jerks or generalized clonic-tonic-clonic seizures, with one following the other within several months or years. Absences and drop attacks occur infrequently. The myoclonic jerks are activated by movement (action myoclonus), and are also sensitive to stimuli such as light, noise and touch. The myoclonus becomes progressively severe, to the point where it interferes with the patients' ability to walk or feed themselves. Major seizures are clonic-tonic-clonic, often occur in the morning, and are not frequent.

Clinical features suggesting occipital onset of the seizures may occasionally be present. Unlike the myoclonus, the generalized seizures are relatively easily controlled by antiepileptic medication.

Dementia develops slowly, with the rate of the decline estimated at approximately one I.Q. point a year. A fixed neurological deficit develops gradually. This includes dysarthria, ataxia, and intention tremor, and is eventually seen in all cases. The disease progresses at a variable rate. In the past, death occurred at a mean age of 24 years; this was probably due to complications of epileptic seizures, unrecognized anticonvulsant toxicity, or respiratory infections due to recumbency and aspiration. Survival to adulthood is usual, some patients reaching the sixth decade. The longer survival is attributed to improved antiepileptic and antimyoclonic symptomatic treatment, in particular the replacement of phenytoin by valproate and clonazepam.

EEG investigations have shown generalized background disturbance and generalized epileptic activity with irregular photosensitive spike and wave or polyspike and wave patterns, and at times occipital focal epileptic discharges. Cortical somatosensory evoked potentials have shown slowing in short-latency median nerve components, suggesting mild involvement of the peripheral and spinal sensory connections, and more severe involvement of the thalamocortical pathways. The slowing increases with progression of the disease. Visual evoked potential latencies are also significantly delayed, but amplitudes are normal. Brainstem auditory evoked potentials show slight but significant prolongation in central conduction time. These findings suggest a multimodel disturbance in sensory projections to cortical areas; however, this may in part be attributed to the effect of anticonvulsant medication. Some cerebellar atrophy is demonstrated by CT scanning of the brain.

The diagnosis is clinical, with key features being the onset, the severity and continous nature of the myoclonus, and the absence of severe or early dementia. No definite biochemical abnormality has been demonstrated, although increased excretion of indican and decreased concentration of plasma tryptophan has been reported. Pathological studies reveal degenerative changes in the brain involving the Purkinje cells, mesial thalamic structures, and inferior olives. There are a few autopsy studies, and the characteristic anatomic picture is still debated.

Singe the diagnosis is clinical, and there is no definite biochemical or pathological marker for this disease, distinction from other types of progressive myoclonus epilepsy may be difficult. In particular, the patients may be diagnosed to suffer from Ramsey Hunt syndrome (dyssynergia cerebellaris myoclonica), in view of the combination of progressive myoclonus epilepsy and spinocerebellar symptoms. However, the Ramsay Hunt syndrome is no longer a useful diagnostic category, since it lacks etiologic specificity.

**Complications:** Related to antiepileptic medication, limitation imposed by the myoclonus, and complications of generalized seizures.

**Associated Findings:** Increased arterial blood pressure has been reported in 14% of patients in Finland.

**Etiology:** Autosomal recessive inheritance. In a series of 93 Finnish patients, Koskiniemi et al (1986) found three affected siblings in three families, two in twenty, and one in forty-four. No parents, offspring, half-siblings, or other family members in the direct line were affected. The parents were consanguineous in 15/68 families, or 22%. Many of the parents of different sibships were related to one another or originated from the same small communities, suggesting a possible founder effect.

**Pathogenesis:** Unknown.

**MIM No.:** *25480

**Sex Ratio:** M1:F1

**Occurrence:** The condition is common in Scandinavia, particularly in Finland, where the incidence has been estimated to exceed 1:20,000. Early cases were reported from Estonia and Sweden. The Finnish patients originate from small rural communities predominantly in the southeast part of Finland and in the adjacent province of East Karelia, which was annexed to Russia following the Second World War.

Eldridge et al (1983) have recently studied 27 patients in 15 families of various ethnic origins in the United States, only two of which had Scandinavian ancestors. There were two Black American families in Eldridge's study. Patients from other countries, including southern Europe, have also been reported.

**Risk of Recurrence for Patient's Sib:**
See Part I, *Mendelian Inheritance*. In the Finnish Study, the proportion of affected siblings over age 15 was calculated to be 0.260 by the *a priori* method, assuming complete truncate ascertainment.

**Risk of Recurrence for Patient's Child:**
See Part I, *Mendelian Inheritance*. Patients only exceptionally have children. Of 15 children of affected parents reported by Lundborg (1912) and by the Finnish group, three died in infancy, and one was mildly retarded. The remainder were healthy. Unfavourable outcomes do not appear to be related to degree of parental illness.

**Age of Detectability:** Children are normal at birth, and their early development is also normal.

**Gene Mapping and Linkage:** Unknown.

**Prevention:** None known. Genetic counseling indicated.

**Treatment:** A poor response to some antiepileptic drugs, mainly phenytoin, has been stressed by Eldridge et al (1983). Optimal treatment at the moment is valproic acid, alone or with clonazepam. Other specific antimyoclonic drugs such as piracetam and 5-hydroxytryptophan have been tried.

**Prognosis:** Average age at death has been 24 years. With improved antiepileptic and supportive treatment, the survival is now much longer, sometimes into the sixth decade.

**Detection of Carrier:** Unknown. In Finland, the heterozygote frequency is estimated as 1:70.

**Special Considerations:** Unverricht-Lundborg disease (Baltic myoclonus), first described by Unverricht in 1891, was the first type of progressive myoclonus epilepsy to be reported. Lundborg recognized the autosomal recessive nature of the disease, and it was the first human disease to be subjected to formal genetic analysis by Weinberg in 1912. However, its existence as a specific entity has only recently been re-confirmed. Reports of the last 90 years contain conflicting and confusing descriptions of clinical and pathological findings in cases regarded as similar to those initially described by Unverricht and Lundborg. Recent studies of patients from the Finnish aggregate by Koskiniemi and coworkers have clarified the features of the disease, and have distinguished it from other causes of progressive myoclonus epilepsy, mainly **Seizures, progressive myoclonic, Lafora type**.

**Support Groups:**
New York; National Myoclonus Foundation
MD; Landover; Epilepsy Foundation of America

**References:**

Unverricht H: Die myoclonie. Leipzig: Franz Deuticke, 1891:1–128.

Lundborg H: Der Erbgang der progressiven Myoklonus-Epilepsie. Z fr die Ges Neur und Psychatrie 1912; 7:353–358.

Koskiniemi M, et al: Progressive myoclonus epilepsy: a clinical and histopathological study. Acta Neurol Scandinav 1974; 50:307–332. *

Norio R, Koskiniemi M: Progressive myoclonus epilepsy: genetic and nosological aspects with special reference to 107 Finnish patients. Clin Genet 1979; 15:382–398. *

Eldridge R, et al: Baltic myoclonus epilepsy: hereditary disorder of childhood made worse by phenytoin. Lancet 1983; 11:838–842. †

Berkovic SF, Andermann F: The progressive myoclonus epilepsies. In: Pedley TA, Meldrum BS, eds: Recent advances in epilepsy, vol 3. Edinbourgh: Churchill Livingstone, 1986:157–187. *

Berkovic SF, et al: Progressive myoclonus epilepsies: specific causes and diagnosis. New Eng J Med 1986; 315:296–305. *

Koskiniemi ML: Baltic myoclonus. In: Fahn S, et al, eds: Myoclonus: advances in neurology, vol 43. New York: Raven Press, 1986:57–64. *

AN016
AN018

**Eva Andermann**
**Frederick Andermann**

---

## SEIZURES, VITAMIN B(6) DEPENDENCY      0991

**Includes:**

Pyridoxine dependency
Vitamin B(6) dependency with convulsions

**Excludes:** Vitamin B(6) deficiency states

**Major Diagnostic Criteria:** There is no specific biochemical or enzymatic phenotype to characterize this convulsive trait. Diagnosis must rest on control of seizures with 10–50 mg pyridoxine HCl intramuscularly, intravenously, or by mouth; positive family history; and no objective evidence for vitamin $B_6$ deficiency.

**Clinical Findings:** This familial convulsive disorder, also called "pyridoxine dependency," is known in at least 14 pedigrees. Symptoms appear in the perinatal period. Although convulsions in utero may occur, most patients develop grand mal seizures during the first week of life; occasionally onset is delayed for several weeks after birth. Hyperirritability, hyperacusis, and feeding difficulties accompany the seizures. The usual anticonvulsant drugs are ineffective. Pyridoxine (or other forms of vitamin $B_6$), given by any route, is the only agent that will control seizures. Electroencephalography can be used to monitor the effect of pyridoxine therapy; the response appears within minutes after administration of the vitamin. The majority of known patients are now severely retarded or have died for want of proper treatment; early treatment with pyridoxine is compatible with normal growth and development. The most important negative features of the syndrome are the absence of any cause or evidence for vitamin $B_6$ deficiency, or other causes for a convulsive disorder.

**Complications:** Retarded development or death.

**Associated Findings:** None known.

**Etiology:** Autosomal recessive inheritance of a mutation putatively affecting the enzymatic synthesis of a neuroregulatory (inhibitor) compound.

**Pathogenesis:** Endogenous metabolism of vitamin $B_6$ and synthesis of the coenzymatically active form, pyridoxal-5-phosphate, from dietary precursors (e.g., pyridoxine) are normal. The immediate clinical response to $B_6$ administration indicates adequate cellular uptake of the vitamin, as well as an intact $B_6$-dependent function awaiting activation. The exaggerated nutritional requirement for the vitamin to sustain normal activity of a particular cellular protein enzyme constitutes the pharmacologic dependency for vitamin $B_6$. It is hypothesized that the mutation may alter the normal relation of glutamic acid decarboxylase (the apoenzyme) with pyridoxal-5-phosphate (the coenzyme); the product of this enzyme's activity is gamma-aminobutyric acid, a presynaptic neuroinhibitor.

**MIM No.:** *26610

**Sex Ratio:** M1:F1

**Occurrence:** Undetermined, but probably more frequent than the limited number of cases in the literature would suggest.

**Risk of Recurrence for Patient's Sib:**
See Part I, *Mendelian Inheritance.*

**Risk of Recurrence for Patient's Child:**
See Part I, *Mendelian Inheritance.*

**Age of Detectability:** In the perinatal period.

**Gene Mapping and Linkage:** GAD (glutamate decarboxylase) has been provisionally mapped to 2.

There are different forms of the enzyme (multiple loci). Deficient brain GAD activity in vitamin B(6) dependency has not been proven.

**Prevention:** None known. Genetic counseling indicated.

**Treatment:** Coenzyme supplementation: vitamin $B_6$ as pyridoxine HCl, pharmacologic dosage (2–50 mg/day); dose must be titrated for individual patient. Dependency is permanent. Febrile conditions and infections may temporarily increase vitamin $B_6$ requirement.

**Prognosis:** Probably good, if treated early. This may require treating the mother with pyridoxine during pregnancy to prevent manifestation of the trait *in utero* in recurrent affected sibs. Late diagnosis and treatment has an 80% risk of retarded development or death.

**Detection of Carrier:** Unknown.

**Special Considerations:** The hereditary nutritional state, broadly termed "vitamin $B_6$ dependency," is a heterogeneous trait involving several distinctive and inherited abnormalities of different apoenzymes. In each case, it is possible that the normal relationship of the apoenzyme with its coenzyme is altered. Precedence for this concept is found in the mutations that affect the pyridoxal-5-phosphate binding site on the $B_6$-requiring enzyme, tryptophan synthetase, in *Neurospora crassa*. Since the original proposal by Scriver that "vitamin $B_6$ dependency with convulsions" is a phenotype reflecting the effect of mutation on a single enzyme (perhaps glutamate decarboxylase), rather than a primary abnormality of vitamin $B_6$ metabolism affecting many apoenzymes, other traits have been proposed as additional forms of "vitamin $B_6$ dependency." Thus, hereditary cystathioninuria, xanthurenicaciduria, and some forms of familial pyridoxine-responsive anemia can each be interpreted as inherited abnormalities of a specific enzyme. Discovery of many other forms of vitamin $B_6$ dependency can be anticipated in view of the many $B_6$-requiring enzyme reactions in amino acid, carbohydrate, and fatty acid metabolism; hyper-β-alaninemia, and some forms of homocystinuria may be further examples. The basis for pyridoxine responsiveness in each trait requires investigation. The glutamic acid decarboxylase in mammalian kidney (it was previously thought to be in brain only) has properties different from the brain enzyme.

**References:**

Bejsovec M, et al.: Familial intrauterine convulsions in pyridoxine dependency. Arch Dis Child 1967; 42:201–207.

Scriver CR, Whelan DT: Glutamic acid decarboxylase (GAD) in mammalian tissue outside the central nervous system, and its possible relevance to hereditary vitamin $B_6$ dependency with seizures. Ann NY Acad Sci 1969; 166:83–96.

Mudd SH: Pyridoxine-responsive genetic disease. Fed Proc 1971; 30:970–976.

Yoshida T, et al.: Vitamin B6 dependency of glutamic acid decarboxylase in the kidney from a patient with vitamin B6 dependent convulsion. Tohoku J Exp Med 1971; 104:195–198.

Bankier A, et al.: Pyridoxine-dependent seizures: a wider clinical spectrum. Arch Dis Child 1983; 58:415–418.

Goutieres F, Aircardi J: Atypical presentations of pyridoxine-dependent seizures: a treatable cause of intractable epilepsy in infants. Ann Neurol 1985; 17:117–120.

SC050

**Charles R. Scriver**

---

**Seizures-adenoma sebaceum-mental retardation**
*See TUBEROUS SCLEROSIS*

**Seizures-hypotonic cerebral palsy-megalocornea-mental retardation**
*See MEGALOCORNEA-MENTAL RETARDATION SYNDROME*

## SEIZURES-ICHTHYOSIS-MENTAL RETARDATION    0741

**Includes:**

Ichthyosis-epilepsy-oligophrenia
Ichthyosis-neurologic disorder-hypogonadism
Oligophrenia-epilepsy-ichthyosis syndrome
Rud syndrome

**Excludes:**

**Sjogren-Larsson syndrome** (2030)
**Xeroderma-mental retardation** (1004)

**Major Diagnostic Criteria:** Seizures, ichthyosis, and mental retardation; the presence of all three apparently being essential. However, the syndrome may be suspected when there is onset of ichthyosis (usually within the first months of life) coupled with somatic and mental retardation. The onset of epilepsy may be delayed beyond the first 10 years of life, but in some instances, it has appeared as early as the first year of life.

**Clinical Findings:** There may be no observable findings at birth. Ichthyosis usually appears during the first two years of life. Ultimate IQ ranges from 30 to 80. Height is variable, with increased frequencies of either short or tall stature.

**Complications:** Severe cases of ichthyosis may show heat prostration in hot weather due to reduced sweating. The only other complications are those secondary to epilepsy and mental retardation.

**Associated Findings:** Retarded somatic development and hypogonadism (probably in most cases); sexual infantilism (about one-half of reported cases). The following conditions have each been reported once: macrocytic anemia, polyneuritis, partial gigantism of long bones, arachnodactyly, retinitis pigmentosa, hyperglycemia, hypothyroidism, macular atrophy, and alopecia totalis. Talipes equinovarus has been reported in some affected individuals.

**Etiology:** Possibly X-linked recessive inheritance.

**Pathogenesis:** The only gross structural defect is the ichthyotic skin. The only reported case that came to autopsy showed CNS changes of a nonspecific nature, typical of those associated with profound mental defect. Functional disorders are mental retardation and epilepsy (or EEG evidence of an epileptic diathesis in most cases in which EEGs were made).

**MIM No.:** 31277

**POS No.:** 3850

**Sex Ratio:** M2:F1

**Occurrence:** About 30 cases reported in the literature.

**Risk of Recurrence for Patient's Sib:**

See Part I, *Mendelian Inheritance.*

**Risk of Recurrence for Patient's Child:**

See Part I, *Mendelian Inheritance.*

**Age of Detectability:** Usually in childhood when all three clinical features are present.

**Gene Mapping and Linkage:** Unknown.

**Prevention:** None known. Genetic counseling indicated.

**Treatment:** Infrequent bathing and cleansing. Use of ointments for the ichthyosis; general treatment measures for epilepsy and mental retardation.

**Prognosis:** Life expectancy is probably shortened. No progressive mental impairment has been noted, but mental retardation appears to vary from severe to mild.

**Detection of Carrier:** Unknown.

**Special Considerations:** The concept of the Rud syndrome involves the perpetuation of what probably began as a translator's error. All complications over the misconceptions about Rud's original case descriptions can be resolved if we call the present syndrome the *Oligophrenia, epilepsy and ichthyosis syndrome,* and do not claim that it is necessarily the same as that described by Rud. See Maldonaldo et al (1975) for a discussion of this neuroichthyoses.

**Support Groups:** MD; Landover; Epilepsy Foundation of America

**References:**
Butterworth T, Strean LP: The ichthyosiform genodermatoses. Postgrad Med. 1965; 37:175–184.
Wells RS, Kerr CB: Genetic classification of ichthyosis. Arch Dermatol 1965; 92:1–6.
Nissley PS, Thomas GH: The Rud syndrome. BD:OAS VII(8). Baltimore: Williams & Wilkins Co. for The National Foundation-March of Dimes, 1971:246–248.
Maldonaldo RR, et al.: Neuroichthyosis with hypogonadism (Rud's syndrome). Int J Dermatol 1975; 14:347–349.
Munke M, et al.: Genetic heterogeneity of the ichthyosis, hypogonadism, mental retardation, and epilepsy syndrome: clinical and biochemical investigations on two patients with Rud syndrome and review of the literature. Eur J Pediat 1983; 141:8–13.
Wisniewski K, et al.: X-linked inheritance of the Rud syndrome. (Abstract) Am J Hum Genet 1985; 37:A83.

MY001    **Terry L Myers**

**Seizures-mental retardation-alopecia**
*See ALOPECIA-SEIZURES-MENTAL RETARDATION, SHOKEIR TYPE*
**Seizures-skin lesions-mental retardation**
*See HYPOMELANOSIS OF ITO*
**Self-healing squamous cell epithelioma, multiple familial**
*See EPITHELIOMA, MULTIPLE SELF-HEALING SQUAMOUS*
**Sella turcica defect-pituitary dwarfism**
*See DWARFISM, PITUITARY WITH ABNORMAL SELLA TURCICA*
**SEMDJL**
*See SPONDYLOEPIMETAPHYSEAL DYSPLASIA-JOINT LAXITY*
**Seminiferous tubule dysgenesis**
*See KLINEFELTER SYNDROME*
**Seminoma**
*See TERATOMAS*
**Senile dementia of the Alzheimer type**
*See ALZHEIMER DISEASE, FAMILIAL*
**Senile dementia, familial**
*See ALZHEIMER DISEASE, FAMILIAL*
**Senile nanism**
*See PROGERIA*
**Senile retinoschisis, autosomal recessive**
*See RETINOSCHISIS*
**Senior-Loken syndrome**
*See RENAL DYSPLASIA-RETINAL APLASIA, LOKEN-SENIOR TYPE*
**Sensenbrenner-Dorst-Owens syndrome**
*See CRANIO-ECTODERMAL DYSPLASIA*
**Sensorimotor neuronopathy-agenesis of the corpus callosum**
*See CORPUS CALLOSUM AGENESIS-SENSORIMOTOR NEUROPATHY, FAMILIAL*
**Sensorineural deafness-chondrodystrophy**
*See CHONDRODYSTROPHY-SENSORINEURAL DEAFNESS, NANCE-INSLEY TYPE*
**Sensorineural hearing loss**
*See DEAFNESS*
**Senter syndrome**
*See ICHTHYOSIFORM ERYTHROKERATODERMA, ATYPICAL WITH DEAFNESS*
**Septal hypertrophy with obstruction, asymmetric**
*See HEART, SUBAORTIC STENOSIS, MUSCULAR*

## SEPTO-OPTIC DYSPLASIA    2018

**Includes:**

De Morsier syndrome
Optic-septo dysplasia

**Excludes:**

**Optic nerve hypoplasia** (0758)
**Thyrotropin deficiency, isolated** (0949)

**Major Diagnostic Criteria:** Two of the three characteristic features of absent septum pellucidum, optic nerve hypoplasia, or hypothalamic hypopituitarism.

**Clinical Findings:** The most common initial symptom is visual impairment with nystagmus as a neonate. The optic disk hypoplasia, bilateral or unilateral, may be difficult to define in infants due to variation in apparent optic disk size. Typically the optic disk is one-third to one-half the normal size, with a cuff-like or double-rim appearance; an outer margin shown by choroidal pigment, an inner hypoplastic margin with relatively large retinal vessels, and pale nerve tissue (Brook et al, 1972). Although blindness is common, visual loss may be mild. Bitemporal hemianopia, if present, is an important clue to defective fibers crossing the optic chiasm. Other findings include coloboma, strabismus, and microphthalmia. Diagnostic studies show normal electroretinogram (ERG) and abnormal visually evoked cortical responses (VER).

Endocrine abnormalities usually become apparent in early childhood, with a drop in growth rate and short stature; however an underlying endocrine deficiency may be responsible for the hypoglycemia with or without seizures, unexplained prolonged hyperbilirubinemia or failure to thrive common in the neonatal period. There is great variability in the multiplicity and severity of endocrine abnormalities. The most common is growth hormone deficiency (93%), followed by ACTH deficiency (57%), hypothyroidism (53%), and diabetes insipidus (Izenberg et al, 1984). Gonadotropin deficiency and sexual precocity have also been described. These hormonal problems are based on hypothalamic dysfunction.

The septum pellucidum is absent in roughly one-half of patients with optic nerve hypoplasia and hypopituitarism (Izenberg et al, 1984). Other CNS abnormalities noted on CT scan or air studies include atrophy of the optic nerve, dilation of the suprasellar and chiasmatic cisterns, enlargement of the pituitary stalk, empty sella, various grades of cortical atrophy, and absent or deficient corpus callosum.

The level of psychomotor development varies greatly from severe mental retardation, to learning disability, to normal mentation.

There is no characteristic craniofacies; however, a few patients had minor malformations; hypertelorism, flat nasal bridge, high-arched palate, and microphthalmus. Septo-optic dysplasia has been described in association with median cleft face syndrome, craniotelencephalic dysplasia, and digital anomalies.

**Complications:** Hypoglycemic seizures due to ACTH or growth hormone deficiency may lead to or aggravate mental retardation.

**Associated Findings:** None known.

**Etiology:** Usually sporadic. Most commonly the firstborn of young mothers.

**Pathogenesis:** Appears to be a developmental field defect affecting midline structures, mainly the optic nerves and chasma, posterior pituitary, anterior hypothalamus, and septum pellucidum. Insult occurs probably at 6 weeks gestation when differentiation of ganglion cells of the eye take place. Septo-optic dysplasia has been assumed to represent the mild end of the spectrum of holoprosencephaly.

**MIM No.:** 18223

**POS No.:** 3398

**Sex Ratio:** M1:F1

**Occurrence:** Undetermined but presumed rare.

**Risk of Recurrence for Patient's Sib:** Unknown. Probably not increased.

**Risk of Recurrence for Patient's Child:** Unknown.

**Age of Detectability:** As early as infancy and as late as the teen years.

**Gene Mapping and Linkage:** Unknown.

**Prevention:** None known. Genetic counseling indicated.

**Treatment:** All cases with optic nerve hypoplasia need follow-up for pituitary endocrine deficiency. There is a lag period of around 3.5 years from the diagnosis of Septo-optic dysplasia to the diagnosis of hypopituitarism. Prevention of recurrent hypoglycemic episodes or seizures should improve overall prognosis. Hormonal replacement therapy may prove beneficial.

**Prognosis:** Depends on other associated CNS pathology, and on the severity and multiplicity of the endocrine deficiency.

**Detection of Carrier:** Unknown.

**References:**

Brook CGD, et al.: Septo-optic dysplasia. Brit Med J 1972; 3:811–813.
Patel H, et al.: Optic nerve hypoplasia with hypopituitarism: septo-optic dysplasia with hypopituitarism. Am J Dis Child 1975; 129:175–180.
Arslanian SA, et al.: Hormonal, metabolic and neuroradiologic abnormalities associated with septo-optic dysplasia. Acta Endocrinol 1984; 107:282–288.
Izenberg I, et al.: The endocrine spectrum of septo-optic dysplasia. Clin Pediatr 1984; 23:632–636.
Blethen SL, Weldon VV: Hypopituitarism and septo-optic "dysplasia" in first cousins. Am J Med Genet 1985; 21:123–129.

J0010                                                    **Virginia P. Johnson**

**Sequeiros-Sack syndrome**
  *See ALOPECIA-SKIN ATROPHY-ANONYCHIA-TONGUE DEFECT*
**Serax^, fetal effects**
  *See FETAL BENZODIAZEPINE EFFECTS*
**Serine 84 amyloidosis**
  *See AMYLOIDOSIS, INDIANA TYPE*
**Sertoli-cell-only syndrome**
  *See GERM CELL APLASIA*

## SERUM ALLOTYPES, HUMAN                                  0476

**Includes:**
  A2m antigens
  Gamma globulin (Gm) antigens
  IgA constant heavy chain locus
  IgG heavy chain loci
  Immunoglobulin Am2
  Immunoglobulin Gm-1
  Immunoglobulin Gm-2
  Immunoglobulin Gm-3
  Immunoglobulin InV (Km)
  Inv (Km) antigens
  Kappa light chain of immunoglobulin

**Excludes:**
  **Immunodeficiency, common variable type (0521)**
  **Immunodeficiency, IgG subclass deficiencies (2947)**

**Major Diagnostic Criteria:** No clinical findings are associated with the presence of these antigens.

**Clinical Findings:** No clinical symptoms are attributable to the presence or absence of Gm or Inv allotypes, but the Am allotypes may be associated with transfusion reactions.

The Gm antigens are found on the heavy chains of IgG and the A2m antigens are found on the heavy chains of IgA2. The Inv(Km) antigens are found on the kappa light chains of the immunoglobulin molecules. Because IgG readily crosses the placenta, an individual's Gm and Inv types cannot ordinarily be determined before 6 months of age. IgA on the other hand does not cross the placenta, hence typing may be done in infants.

**Complications:** Unknown.

**Associated Findings:** None known.

**Etiology:** Normal antigen inheritance as autosomal codominant alleles. The antigens are inherited in different complexes (haplotypes) in each of the several races of man. Accordingly, they are extensively used for human population studies. They may also, in the hands of experts and with caution, be used for paternity testing and for identification of individuals.

**Pathogenesis:** Anti-IgA antibodies may occur as the result of transfusion or of the injection of Ig; possibly also as the result of immunization across the placenta, through a placental rupture.

**MIM No.:** *24050, 14683, *14690, *14691, *14700, *14701, *14702, *14707, *14710, *14711, *14712, *14713, *14716, *14717, *14718, *14720

**Sex Ratio:** M1:F1

**Occurrence:** These normal antigens are present in all races but with different frequencies. Worldwide distribution.

**Risk of Recurrence for Patient's Sib:** As for codominant alleles.

**Risk of Recurrence for Patient's Child:** As for codominant alleles.

**Age of Detectability:** After six months of age.

**Gene Mapping and Linkage:** IGHA1 (immunoglobulin alpha 1) has been mapped to 14q32.33.

IGHA2 (immunoglobulin alpha 2 (A2M marker)) has been mapped to 14q32.33.

IGHJ (immunoglobulin heavy polypeptide, joining region) has been mapped to 14q32.3.

IGHM (immunoglobulin mu) has been mapped to 14q32.33.

IGHV (immunoglobulin heavy polypeptide, variable region (many genes)) has been mapped to 14q32.33.

IGHG1 (immunoglobulin gamma 1 (Gm marker)) has been mapped to 14q32.33.

IGHG2 (immunoglobulin gamma 2 (Gm marker)) has been mapped to 14q32.33.

IGHG3 (immunoglobulin gamma 3 (Gm marker)) has been mapped to 14q32.33.

IGHG4 (immunoglobulin gamma 4 (Gm marker)) has been mapped to 14q32.33.

IGHEP1 (immunoglobulin epsilon pseudogene 1) has been mapped to 14q32.33.

IGHD (immunoglobulin delta) has been mapped to 14q32.33.

IGHE (immunoglobulin epsilon) has been mapped to 14q32.33.

IGKC (immunoglobulin kappa constant region) has been mapped to 2p12.

**Prevention:** Not necessary.

**Treatment:** Not necessary.

**Prognosis:** Normal life span.

**Detection of Carrier:** By means of an agglutination inhibition test.

**References:**

Giblett ER: Genetic markers in the human blood. Oxford: Blackwell Scientific Pub Ltd, 1969.

Steinberg AG: Globulin polymorphisms in man. Annu Rev Genet 1969; 3:25–52.

Grubb R: The genetic markers of human immunoglobulins. New York: Springer-Verlag, 1970.

Steinberg AG, Cook CE: The distribution of human immunoglobin allotypes. Oxford Univ Press, 1981. *

Steinberg AG: Immunoglobulin allotypes. In Atassi MZ, et al, eds: Molecular immunology. New York: Marcel Dekker, 1984:231–253. *

ST013                                    **Arthur G. Steinberg**

**Serum carnosinase deficiency, disorders of**
    *See CARNOSINEMIA*
**Serum ceruloplasmin, low**
    *See HYPOCERULOPLASMINEMIA*
**Serum normal agglutinants (SNaggs)**
    *See ANTIBODIES TO HUMAN ALLOTYPES*
**Serum prothrombin conversion accelerator deficiency**
    *See FACTOR VII DEFICIENCY*
**Setleis syndrome**
    *See ECTODERMAL DYSPLASIA, CONGENITAL FACIAL, SETLEIS TYPE*
**Seventeen-beta-hydroxysteroid dehydrogenase deficiency**
    *See STEROID 17-KETOSTEROID REDUCTASE DEFICIENCY*
**Sever disease (os calcis)**
    *See JOINTS, OSTEOCHONDRITIS DISSECANS*
**Severe combined immunodeficiency (SCID) with leukopenia**
    *See IMMUNODEFICIENCY, SEVERE COMBINED*
**Severe combined immunodeficiency with ADA**
    *See IMMUNODEFICIENCY, ADENOSINE DEAMINASE DEFICIENCY*
**Severe combined immunodeficiency, Nezelof type**
    *See IMMUNODEFICIENCY, NEZELOF TYPE*
**Severe combined immunodeficiency, variant type**
    *See IMMUNODEFICIENCY, NEZELOF TYPE*
**Severe combined immunodeficiency, X-linked (SCIDX)**
    *See IMMUNODEFICIENCY, X-LINKED SEVERE COMBINED*
**Severe combined immunodeficiency-lack of HLA on lymphocytes**
    *See IMMUNODEFICIENCY, SEVERE COMBINED*
**Sex reversal-polydactyly-renal hypoplasia-unilobular lung**
    *See SMITH-LEMLI-OPITZ SYNDROME, TYPE II*
**Sex-linked neurodegenerative disease associated with monilethrix**
    *See MENKES SYNDROME*

**Sexual ateleotic dwarfism**
    *See GROWTH HORMONE DEFICIENCY, ISOLATED*
**Sexual development variations-asymmetry-short stature**
    *See SILVER SYNDROME*
**Sexual headache, benign**
    *See MIGRAINE*
**Sexual maturity (delayed)-short stature-mental retardation**
    *See SHORT STATURE-MENTAL RETARDATION-DELAYED SEXUAL MATURITY*
**Sezary syndrome**
    *See LEUKEMIA/LYMPHOMA, T-CELL*
**Shah-Waardenburg syndrome**
    *See ALBINISM, WAARDENBURG TYPE-HIRSCHSPRUNG AGANGLIONOSIS*
**Shawl scrotum**
    *See AARSKOG SYNDROME*
**Shell teeth**
    *See TEETH, DENTINOGENESIS IMPERFECTA*
**Shokeir syndrome**
    *See ALOPECIA-SEIZURES-MENTAL RETARDATION, SHOKEIR TYPE*
**Short chain acyl-CoA dehydrogenase deficiency (SCAD)**
    *See ACYL-CoA DEHYDROGENASE DEFICIENCY, SHORT CHAIN TYPE*
**Short cord**
    *See UMBILICAL CORD, SHORT*
**Short esophagus, most instances**
    *See HERNIA, HIATAL*
**Short rib-polydactyly syndrome, Majewski type**
    *See SHORT RIB-POLYDACTYLY SYNDROME, TYPE II*
**Short rib-polydactyly syndrome, Naumoff type**
    *See SHORT RIB-POLYDACTYLY SYNDROME, VERMA-NAUMOFF TYPE*
**Short rib-polydactyly syndrome, Saldino-Noonan type**
    *See SHORT RIB-POLYDACTYLY SYNDROME, TYPE I*

---

## SHORT RIB-POLYDACTYLY SYNDROME, TYPE I         0884

**Includes:**

Polydactyly-neonatal chondrodystrophy, type I
Saldino-Noonan short rib-polydactyly
Short rib-polydactyly syndrome, Saldino-Noonan type

**Excludes:**

**Asphyxiating thoracic dysplasia** (0091)
**Chondroectodermal dysplasia** (0156)
Osteochondrodysplasias, other lethal perinatal
**Short rib-polydactyly syndrome, type II** (0883)
**Short rib-polydactyly syndrome, Verma-Naumoff type** (2270)

**Major Diagnostic Criteria:** Lethal congenital dwarfism with marked limb reduction, narrow constricted thorax, short horizontal ribs, post-axial polysyndactyly, multiple systemic abnormalities, hydrops, and characteristic X-ray findings.

**Clinical Findings:** Severe hydrops at birth; marked limb reduction; narrow constricted thorax; pulmonary hypoplasia; protuberant abdomen; postaxial polysyndactyly with short "flipper"-like limbs; nail dysplasia; flat face and occiput resembling "Potter" facies (see **Renal agenesis, bilateral**) associated with oligohydramnios; low-set, flattened, deformed ears; severe cardiovascular abnormalities; gastrointestinal anomalies; gallbladder and cystic duct agenesis; pancreatic cysts and fibrosis; renal agenesis or cystic dysplasia; cloacal atresia (anal, urethral and vaginal); sexual ambiguity (complete suppression of secondary sexual differentiation may result in preponderance of phenotypic females).

X-ray abnormalities include short horizontal ribs; severely shortened tubular bones; marked metaphyseal dysplasia; ragged, pointed ends of tubular bones; longitudinal periosteal spurs projecting from the lateral aspects of the metaphyseal margins; ill-defined corticomedullary differentiation (a distinguishing feature from **Short rib-polydactyly syndrome** types II and III); small, rounded scapulae, small iliac bones with flattened acetabular roofs; vertebral abnormalities; incomplete and irregular ossification of the metacarpal and metatarsal bones and phalanges. Scapular, vertebral and pelvic abnormalities distinguish this condition from **Short rib-polydactyly syndrome** types II and III. Chondro-osseous changes include markedly irregular primary trabeculae. Histopathology is similar to that seen in **Short rib-polydactyly syndrome, Verma-Naumoff type**.

**Complications:** Respiratory insufficiency due to small thoracic cage and decreased pulmonary volume.

**Associated Findings:** None known.

**Etiology:** Autosomal recessive inheritance. Variable, heterogeneous expression and overlapping features with those of **Short rib-polydactyly syndrome** types II and III. Possible explanations for variability and overlapping features include point mutation at different loci, differing allelic mutations at the same locus, or variable expressivity of the same gene mutation.

**Pathogenesis:** Unknown.

**MIM No.:** *26353

**POS No.:** 3390

**Sex Ratio:** An excess of phenotypic females has been observed. Some males have had ambiguous genitalia.

**Occurrence:** About 40 cases have been documented.

**Risk of Recurrence for Patient's Sib:**
See Part I, *Mendelian Inheritance.*

**Risk of Recurrence for Patient's Child:**
See Part I, *Mendelian Inheritance.* Affected individuals are not expected to survive to reproduce.

**Age of Detectability:** At birth, by clinical examination. Prenatal diagnosis is possible by serial ultrasound during second trimester.

**Gene Mapping and Linkage:** Unknown.

**Prevention:** None known. Genetic counseling indicated.

**Treatment:** Unknown.

**Prognosis:** Patients are stillborn or die within hours after birth from respiratory insufficiency and other multiple abnormalities.

**Detection of Carrier:** Unknown.

**References:**
Saldino RM, Noonan CD: Severe thoracic dystrophy with striking micromelia, abnormal osseous development, including the spine and multiple visceral anomalies. Am J Roentgenol 1972; 114:257–263.
Spranger J, et al.: Short rib-polydactyly (SRP) syndromes, types Majewski and Saldino-Noonan. Z Kinderheilk 1974; 116:73–94.
Cherstvoy ED, et al.: Difficulties in classification of the short rib-polydactyly syndrome. Eur J Pediatr 1980; 133:57–61.
Sillence DO: Non-Majewski short rib-polydactyly syndrome. Am J Med Genet 1980; 7:223–229. *
International nomenclature of constitutional diseases of bone, Revision - May 1983. Ann Radiol 1984; 27:275–280.
Bernstein R, et al.: Short rib-polydactyly syndrome: a single or heterogeneous entity? a re-evaluation prompted by four new cases. J Med Genet 1985; 22:46–53.
Yang SS, et al.: Three conditions in neonatal asphyxiating thoracic dysplasia (Jeune) and the short rib-polydactyly syndrome spectrum: a clinicopathologic study. Am J Med Genet 1987; Suppl 3:191–207.
Frzen M, et al.: Comparative histopathology of the growth cartilage in short-rib polydactyly syndromes type I and type II and in chondroectodermal dysplasia. Ann Genet 1988; 31:144–150.

BE043                                    **Renée Bernstein**

---

### SHORT RIB-POLYDACTYLY SYNDROME, TYPE II          0883

**Includes:**
Majewski short rib-polydactyly syndrome
Mohr-Majewski syndrome
Polydactyly-neonatal chondrodystrophy, type II
Short rib-polydactyly syndrome, Majewski type
Skeletal dysplasia, short rib-polydactyly syndrome type II

**Excludes:**
**Asphyxiating thoracic dysplasia** (0091)
**Chondroectodermal dysplasia** (0156)
**Meckel syndrome** (0634)
**Oro-facio-digital syndrome, Mohr type** (0771)

Osteochondrodysplasias, other lethal perinatal
**Short rib-polydactyly syndrome, type I** (0884)
**Short rib-polydactyly syndrome, Verma-Naumoff type** (2270)
**Smith-Lemli-Opitz syndrome, type II** (2635)

**Major Diagnostic Criteria:** Lethal congenital dwarfism with marked limb reduction, narrow constricted thorax, short horizontal ribs, preaxial and postaxial polysyndactyly, systemic abnormalities, hydrops, and characteristic X-ray findings.

**Clinical Findings:** Hydrops at birth; marked limb reduction; narrow constricted thorax; pulmonary hypoplasia; protuberant abdomen; polysyndactyly, preaxial and postaxial; nail dysplasia; craniofacial abnormalities with cleft upper lip or palate; short flat nose; low-set, deformed ears; rudimentary epiglottis; cardiovascular defects; renal dysplasia, polycystic kidneys; gastrointestinal tract anomalies; sexual ambiguity.

X-ray abnormalities include short horizontal ribs; severely shortened tubular bones with disproportionately short ovoid tibiae (the latter distinguishing this condition from **Short rib-polydactyly syndrome** types I and III); moderate metaphyseal dysplasia; clearly demarcated corticomedullary differentiation (distinguishing this condition from **Short rib-polydactyly syndrome, type I**); minimal spurs, normal vertebrae and pelvic bones (also distinguishing this condition from **Short rib-polydactyly syndrome** types I and III). Chondro-osseous changes in proliferative columns and irregularity in columnization is less severe than in types I and II.

**Complications:** Respiratory insufficiency due to small thoracic cage and decreased pulmonary volume.

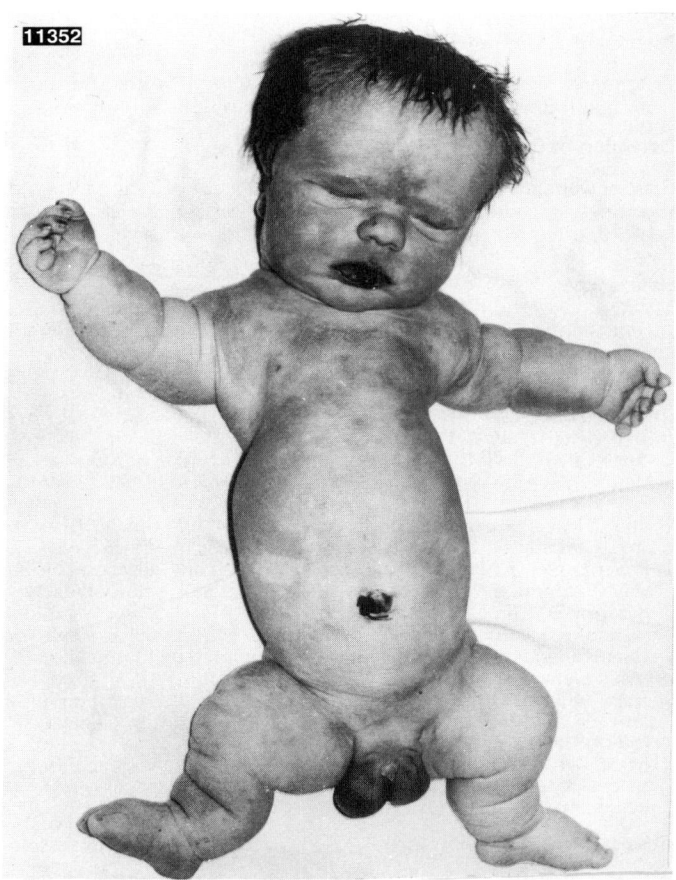

**0883A**-11352: Note shortened limbs, postaxial polydactyly, large head, narrow thorax and hypoplastic penis.

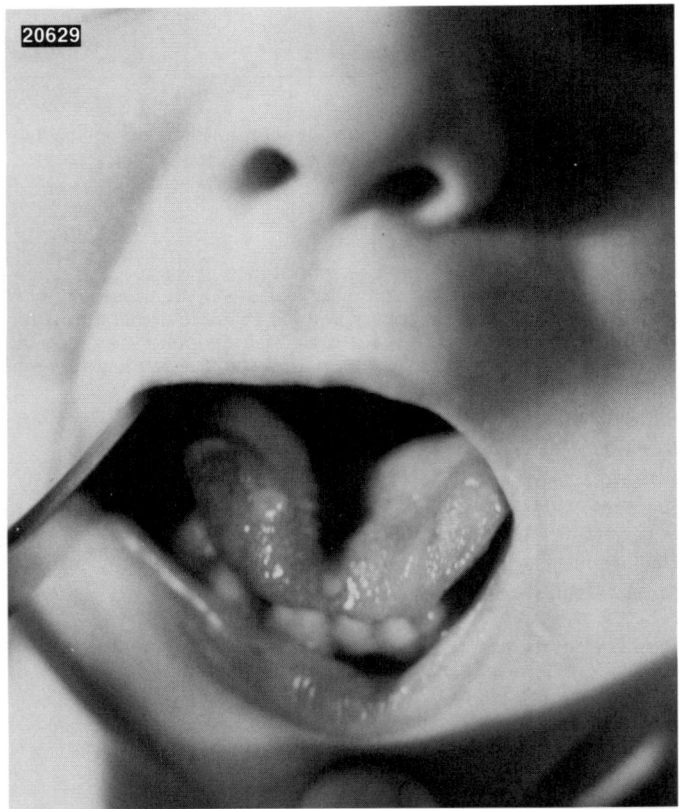

**Associated Findings:** None known.

**Etiology:** Autosomal recessive inheritance. Variable, heterogeneous expression and overlapping features with those of **Short rib-polydactyly syndrome** types I and III. The possible explanations for variability and overlapping features include point mutation at different loci, differing allelic mutations at the same locus, or variable expressivity of the same gene mutation. Silengo et al (1987) has suggested that this condition could be a severe expression of **Oro-facio-digital syndrome, Mohr type**.

**Pathogenesis:** Unknown.

**MIM No.:** *26352

**POS No.:** 3389

**Sex Ratio:** Presumably M1:F1. Some affected males have had ambiguous genitalia.

**Occurrence:** More than 40 cases have been documented in the literature.

**Risk of Recurrence for Patient's Sib:**
See Part I, *Mendelian Inheritance*.

**Risk of Recurrence for Patient's Child:**
See Part I, *Mendelian Inheritance*. Affected individuals are not expected to survive to reproduce.

**Age of Detectability:** At birth, by clinical examination. Prenatal diagnosis is possible by serial ultrasound during second trimester.

**Gene Mapping and Linkage:** Unknown.

**Prevention:** None known. Genetic counseling indicated.

**Treatment:** Unknown.

**Prognosis:** Patients are stillborn or die within hours after birth from respiratory insufficiency and other multiple abnormalities.

**Detection of Carrier:** Unknown.

**Special Considerations:** A transition type between the Mohr and the Majewski syndromes, called *Mohr Majewski syndrome*, has also been reported (Silengo et al, 1987).

**References:**
Majewski F, et al.: Polysyndaktylie, verkürzte gliedmassen und genitalfehlbildungen: kennzeichen cines sellstaendigen syndrome? Z Kinderheilk 1971; 111:118–138.
Spranger J, et al.: Short rib-polysyndactyly (SRP) syndromes, types Majewski and Saldino-Noonan. Z Kinderheilk 1974; 116:73–94.
Chen H, et al.: Short rib-polydactyly syndrome, Majewski type. Am J Med Genet 1980; 7:215–222.
Cooper CP, Hall CM: Lethal short rib-polydactyly syndrome of the Majewski type: a report of three cases. Pediatr Radiol 1982; 144:513–517. *
Walley VM, et al.: Brief clinical report: short rib-polydactyly syndrome, Majewski type. Am J Med Genet 1983; 14:445–452.
Toftager-Larsen K, Benzie RJ: Fetoscopy in prenatal diagnosis of the Majewski and the Saldino-Noonan types of short rib-polydactyly syndromes. Clin Genet 1984; 26:56–60.
Bernstein R, et al.: Short rib-polydactyly syndrome: a single or heterogeneous entity? A re-evaluation prompted by four new cases. J Med Genet 1985; 22:46–53.
Silengo MC, et al.: Oro-facial-digital syndrome II: transition type between the Mohr and the Majewski syndromes. Clin Genet 1987; 31:331–336.
Yang SS, et al.: Three conditions in neonatal asphyxiating thoracic dysplasia (Jeune) and the short rib-polydactyly syndrome spectrum: a clinicopathologic study. Am J Med Genet 1987; Suppl 3:191–207.

BE043                                          **Renée Bernstein**

**Short rib-polydactyly syndrome, type III**
*See SHORT RIB-POLYDACTYLY SYNDROME, VERMA-NAUMOFF TYPE*

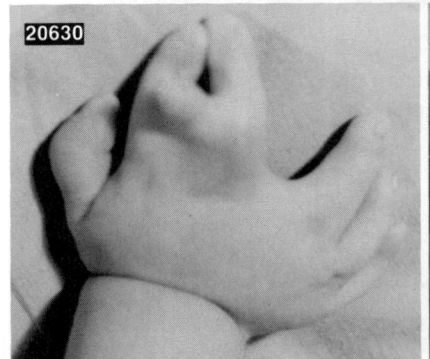
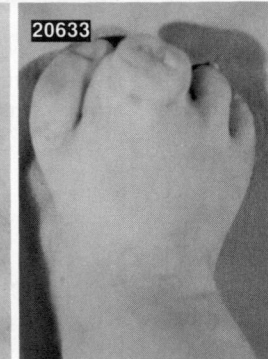
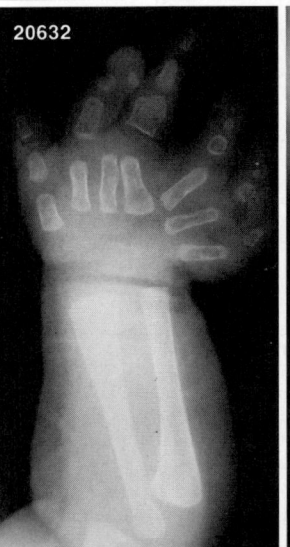
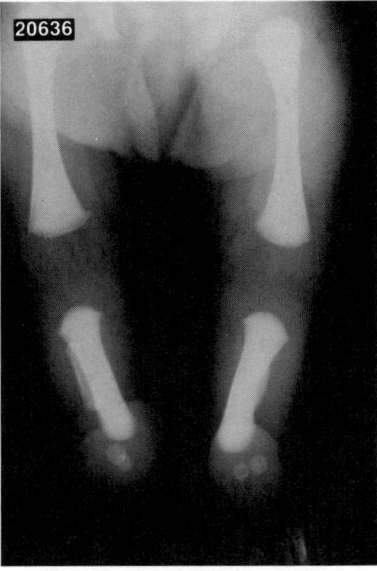

**0883B-20629:** Mohr-Majewski syndrome; note lobate tongue and teeth abnormalities. **20630:** Hand shows pre- and postaxial polydactyly. **20633:** Polysyndactyly of the foot. **20632:** X-ray of the right hand and forearm shows short and stubby radius and ulna, pre- and post-axial polydactyly, alterations in the number and shape of the phalanges, and retarded skeletal age. **20636:** Short and stubby tibia and fibula.

## SHORT RIB-POLYDACTYLY SYNDROME, VERMA-NAUMOFF TYPE
**2270**

**Includes:**
> Naumoff type short-rib polydactyly syndrome
> Polydactyly-neonatal chondrodystrophy, type III
> Short rib-polydactyly syndrome, Naumoff type
> Short rib-polydactyly syndrome, type III
> Skeletal dysplasia-short rib-polydactyly, type III
> Verma-Naumoff short rib-polydactyly

**Excludes:**
> **Asphyxiating thoracic dysplasia** (0091)
> **Chondroectodermal dysplasia** (0156)
> Osteochondrodysplasias, other lethal perinatal

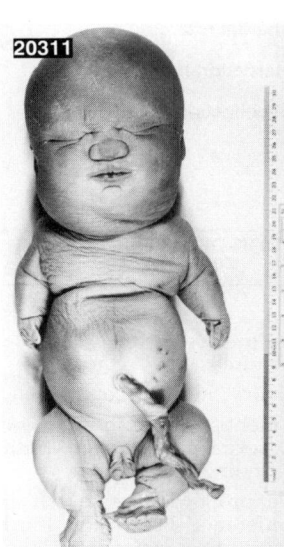
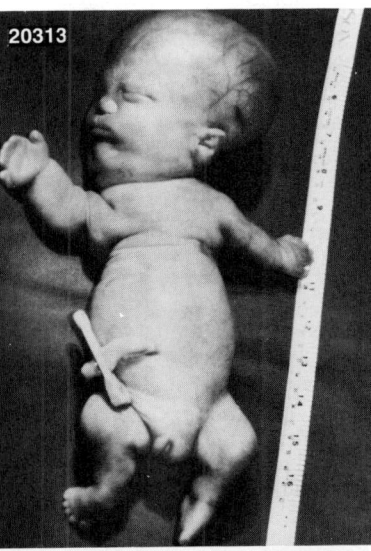

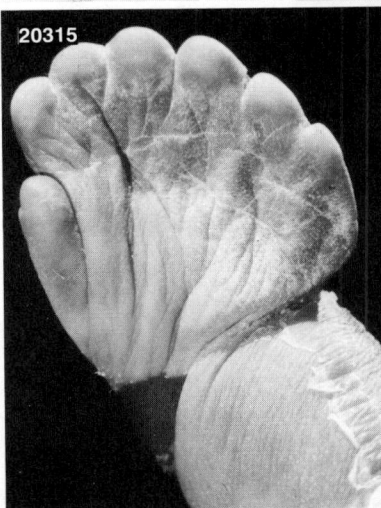
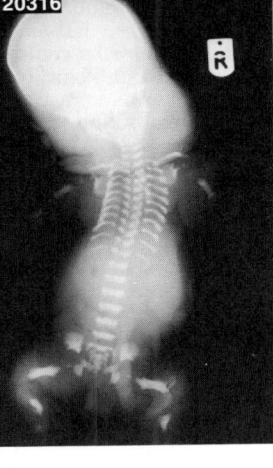

**2270-20311:** Stillborn infant with short-rib polydactyly syndrome type III; note short limbs, narrow thorax, hydropic and flattened facies with frontal bossing and depressed nasal bridge. **20313:** Appearance of a 28-week fetus who is the sib of the infant shown in 20311. **20315:** Pre- and postaxial polydactyly. **20316:** Short horizontal ribs, short tubular bones, widened metaphyses, longitudinal metaphyseal spurs, flat acetabulae and vertebral defects.

**Short rib-polydactyly syndrome, type I** (0884)
**Short rib-polydactyly syndrome, type II** (0883)

**Major Diagnostic Criteria:** Lethal dwarfism with marked limb reduction, narrow constricted thorax, short horizontal ribs, postaxial polysyndactyly, visceral abnormalities (particularly urogenital), hydrops, and characteristic X-ray findings.

**Clinical Findings:** Hydrops at birth; marked limb reduction; narrow constricted thorax; pulmonary hypoplasia; protuberant abdomen; **Polysyndactyly**, usually postaxial; mild nail dysplasia; flat occiput; frontal bossing; depressed nasal bridge ("saddle" nose); "Potter"-like facies, if there is associated oligohydramnios; low-set, flattened, deformed ears; occasional natal teeth and pseudoclefts of gums and lips; variable cardiovascular abnormalities; pancreatic fibrosis; renal dysplasia more common than renal agenesis; cloacal atresia (anal, urethral, and vaginal); and sexual ambiguity. The complete suppression of secondary sexual differentiation may result in preponderance of phenotypic females.

X-ray abnormalities include short, horizontal ribs; severely shortened, tubular bones; metaphyseal dysplasia; widened metaphases; longitudinal metaphyseal spurs; clearly demarcated corticomedullary differentiation (distinguishing feature from **Short rib-polydactyly syndrome, type I**); horizontal, trident lower iliac margins; flat acetabulae; vertebral abnormalities (pelvic and vertebral abnormalities differentiate **Short rib-polydactyly syndrome** (SRPS) types I and III from type II); shortened cranial base (unique to type III). Chondro-osseous changes include shortened or absent zone of proliferative chondrocytes with loss of columnization, and disorganized trabecular formation.

**Complications:** Respiratory insufficiency due to small thoracic cage and decreased pulmonary volume.

**Associated Findings:** None known.

**Etiology:** Autosomal recessive inheritance. Variable, heterogeneous expression and overlapping features with those of **Short rib-polydactyly syndrome** type I and type II. The possible explanations for variability and overlapping features include point mutations at different loci, differing allelic mutations at the same locus, or variable expressivity of the same gene mutation.

**Pathogenesis:** The generalized abnormalities of all organ systems suggest a defect in the regulation of cellular differentiation during early embryogenesis. Cytoplasmic periodic acid-Schiff (PAS) positive, diastase-resistant, inclusion bodies were observed in the chondrocytes of one patient with SRPS type III. These may represent products of abnormal synthesis or impaired secretion into the cartilagenous matrix. Other patients have not shown inclusion bodies.

**MIM No.:** 26351

**POS No.:** 3201

**Sex Ratio:** Based on phenotypic sex: M15:F9 (five males had ambiguous genitalia, and two phenotypic females are known to have a 46,XY karyotype and testes).

**Occurrence:** Over 60 cases have been documented.

**Risk of Recurrence for Patient's Sib:**
See Part I, *Mendelian Inheritance.*

**Risk of Recurrence for Patient's Child:**
See Part I, *Mendelian Inheritance.*

**Age of Detectability:** At birth. Prenatal diagnosis is possible by serial ultrasound during the second trimester.

**Gene Mapping and Linkage:** Unknown.

**Prevention:** None known. Genetic counseling indicated.

**Treatment:** Unknown.

**Prognosis:** Patients are stillborn or die within hours after birth from respiratory insufficiency and other multiple abnormalities.

**Detection of Carrier:** Unknown.

**Special Considerations:** The marked variability in the pattern of anomalies and, to a lesser extent, in X-ray findings, and the considerable overlap of supposedly characteristic features distinguishing the types of **Short rib-polydactyly syndrome** suggests that SRPS is a single syndrome, the different types representing a spectrum of the same pathogenetic mechanisms, which are most severely expressed in SRPS, type I, intermediate in type III, and least severe in type II.

References:
Verma IC, et al.: An autosomal recessive form of lethal chondrodystrophy with severe thoracic narrowing, rhizo-acromelic type of micromelia, polydactyly and genital anomalies. BD:OAS II(6). New York: March of Dimes Birth Defects Foundation, 1975:167–174.
Naumoff P, et al.: Short rib-polydactyly syndrome type 3. Radiology 1977; 122:443–447.
Sillence DO: Non-Majewski short rib-polydactyly syndrome. Am J Med Genet 1980; 7:2223–2229. *
Belloni C, Beluffi G: Short rib-polydactyly syndrome, type Verma-Naumoff. Fortschr Röntgenstr 1981; 134:431–435.
Bernstein R, et al.: Short rib-polydactyly syndrome: a single or heterogeneous entity? A re-evaluation prompted by four new cases. J Med Genet 1985; 22:46–53. †
Sillence D, et al.: Perinatally lethal short rib-polydactyly syndromes: variability in known syndromes. Pediatr Radiol 1987; 17:474–480. *
Yang SS, et al.: Three conditions in neonatal asphyxiating thoracic dysplasia (Jeune) and the short rib-polydactyly syndrome spectrum: a clinicopathologic study. Am J Med Genet 1987; Suppl 3:191–207.
Frzen M, et al.: Comparative histopathology of the growth cartilage in short-rib polydactyly syndromes type I and III and in chondroectodermal dysplasia. Ann Genet 1988; 31:144–150.

BE043 **Renée Bernstein**

**Short stature in the African pygmy**
*See GROWTH DEFICIENCY, AFRICAN PYGMY TYPE*
**Short stature, X-linked, with skin pigmentation**
*See SILVER SYNDROME, X-LINKED*
**Short stature-alopecia-skeletal anomalies-mental retardation**
*See ALOPECIA-SKELETAL ANOMALIES-SHORT STATURE-MENTAL RETARDATION*

## SHORT STATURE-CEREBRAL ATROPHY-KERATOSIS FOLLICULARIS, X-LINKED 2340

**Includes:**
Cerebral atrophy-keratosis follicularis-short stature, X-linked
Keratosis follicularis-dwarfism-cerebral atrophy

**Excludes:**
**Darier disease** (2865)
**Dyskeratosis congenita** (2024)
**Skin, keratosis follicularis spinulosa decalvans** (2867)

**Major Diagnostic Criteria:** Congenital, proportionate, and progressive dwarfism; cerebral atrophy with **Microcephaly**, psychomotor retardation, and convulsions; and keratosis follicularis with alopecia.

**Clinical Findings:** Characteristic features are low birth weight (approximate average 2,415 g), early fetal-like face at birth, delayed somatic and psychomotor development, microcephaly, seizures, delayed dentition, micrognathia, generalized keratosis follicularis with alopecia. X-rays show osteoporosis and delayed bone age; EEG and pneumoencephalogram (PEG) are abnormal.

**Complications:** Microcephaly, psychomotor retardation, and convulsions are probably secondary to cerebral atrophy, whereas alopecia results from the keratosis follicularis.

**Associated Findings:** None known.

**Etiology:** Presumably X-linked recessive inheritance.

**Pathogenesis:** Unknown.

**MIM No.:** 30883

**POS No.:** 3934

**Sex Ratio:** M1:F0

**Occurrence:** Six members of one family have been documented.

**Risk of Recurrence for Patient's Sib:**
See Part I, *Mendelian Inheritance.*

**Risk of Recurrence for Patient's Child:**
See Part I, *Mendelian Inheritance.*

**Age of Detectability:** At birth.

**Gene Mapping and Linkage:** Unknown.

**Prevention:** None known. Genetic counseling indicated.

**Treatment:** Supportive and symptomatic, including anticonvulsant medication and special education.

**Prognosis:** Life expectancy is unknown but probably decreased. Of six reported patients, four were less than six years of age, and two died before two years of age from infections.

**Detection of Carrier:** Unknown.

**References:**
Cantú JM, et al.: A new X-linked recessive disorder with dwarfism, cerebral atrophy, and generalized keratosis follicularis. J Pediatr 1974; 84:564–567. * †

RI015 **Fernando Rivas**
CA011 **José María Cantú**

**Short stature-ear abnormalities-elbow/hip dislocation**
*See AURICULO-OSTEODYSPLASIA*
**Short stature-facial and skeletal defects-mental retardation**
*See KABUKI MAKE-UP SYNDROME*
**Short stature-facial/skeletal anomalies-retardation-macrodontia**
*See KBG SYNDROME*
**Short stature-head/face anomalies-kyphoscoliosis-retardation**
*See COFFIN-LOWRY SYNDROME*
**Short stature-hypolipidemia-leukonychia**
*See HOOFT DISEASE*

## SHORT STATURE-MENTAL RETARDATION-DELAYED SEXUAL MATURITY 2338

**Includes:**
Mental retardation-sexual maturity (delayed)-short stature
Sexual maturity (delayed)-short stature-mental retardation

**Excludes:** Short stature-mental deficiency (in other conditions)

**Major Diagnostic Criteria:** Severe mental retardation, slow growth and maturation, and delayed sexual development with normal laboratory and endocrinologic findings.

**Clinical Findings:** The patients have proportionate dwarfism (height, weight, and cephalic circumference below the third percentile), infantile external genitalia, and severe mental deficiency (IQ: 11–21) with a calm behavior, permanent smile, and inability to communicate by any other means. Since the bone age is also severely delayed (about 5–6 years), the osseous development is somewhat compatible with the somatometric parameters.

The endocrinologic evaluation is normal, including response to specific stimulation. Chromosomal studies demonstrate that this mental retardation syndrome is not associated with **X-linked mental retardation, Fragile X syndrome.**

**Complications:** Unknown.

**Associated Findings:** None known.

**Etiology:** Recessive inheritance, either autosomal or X-linked.

**Pathogenesis:** Unknown.

**Sex Ratio:** M2:F0 (observed).

**Occurrence:** Two cases have been described in the literature.

**Risk of Recurrence for Patient's Sib:**
See Part I, *Mendelian Inheritance.*

**Risk of Recurrence for Patient's Child:**
See Part I, *Mendelian Inheritance.*

**Age of Detectability:** Since the delayed sexual maturation is a major finding, the patients must be older than 15 years of age.

**Gene Mapping and Linkage:** Unknown.

**Prevention:** None known. Genetic counseling indicated.

**Treatment:** Unknown.

**Prognosis:** Poor for independence because of the mental retardation.

**Detection of Carrier:** Unknown.

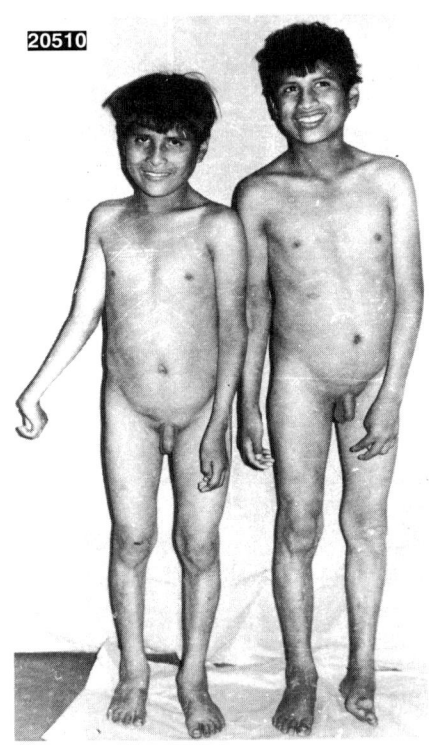

20510

**2338**-20510: Note proportionate short stature in both brothers and the infantile external genitalia.

**References:**
Cantú JM, et al.: Severe mental deficiency, proportionate dwarfism, and delayed sexual maturation: a distinct inherited syndrome. Hum Genet 1980; 56:231–234. *

C0064
CA011

José Sánchez-Corona
José María Cantú

**Short stature-mental retardation-obesity-hypogonadism**
*See X-LINKED MENTAL RETARDATION-SHORT STATURE-OBESITY-HYPOGONADISM*
**Short stature-pterygia-dysmophic facies-mental retardation**
*See PTERYGIA-DYSMORPHIC FACIES-SHORT STATURE-MENTAL RETARDATION*
**Short stature-Rieger anomaly-lipodystrophy-diabetes**
*See LIPODYSTROPHY-RIEGER ANOMALY-SHORT STATURE-DIABETES*
**Short stature-sexual infantilism**
*See TURNER SYNDROME*

## SHORT STATURE-WORMIAN BONES-JOINT DISLOCATIONS 3014

**Includes:**
    Campomelia-wormian bones-blue sclerae-mandibular hypoplasia
    Grant syndrome
    Joint dislocations-wormian bones-short stature
    Osteogenesis imperfecta, possible variant
    Wormian bones-blue sclerae-mandibular hypoplasia-campomelia

**Excludes:** Osteogenesis imperfecta (0777)

**Major Diagnostic Criteria:** The combination of persistent wormian bones, blue sclerae, mandibular hypoplasia, and campomelia should suggest the diagnosis.

**Clinical Findings:** Features common to all three members of the reported family include delayed closure of large anterior fontanelle, blue sclerae, prominent forehead, mandibular hypoplasia, joint hypermobility, and short stature. X-rays demonstrated persistent wormian bones, narrow thorax with or without oddly shaped ribs, shallow glenoid fossae, and upward-bowing clavicles. The proposita also had femoral and tibial bowing in infancy, which improved with age; hypotonia; and multiple joint dislocations. The father had a congenital left clubfoot. Dentition in all was normal; fractures did not occur with increased frequency.

**Complications:** Unknown.

**Associated Findings:** None known.

**Etiology:** Presumably autosomal dominant inheritance.

**Pathogenesis:** A dermal fibroblast culture showed slightly less type I collagen, but not significantly so. Therefore, a connective tissue defect is suggested, but not demonstrated.

**MIM No.:** 13893

**POS No.:** 3854

**Sex Ratio:** M2:F1 (observed).

**Occurrence:** One family with three affected individuals has been reported.

**Risk of Recurrence for Patient's Sib:**
    See Part I, *Mendelian Inheritance.*

**Risk of Recurrence for Patient's Child:**
    See Part I, *Mendelian Inheritance.*

**Age of Detectability:** At birth by physical examination.

**Gene Mapping and Linkage:** Unknown.

**Prevention:** None known. Genetic counseling indicated.

**Treatment:** Supportive.

**Prognosis:** Intelligence, reproductive capability, and life span are normal.

**Detection of Carrier:** Unknown.

**Special Considerations:** Beighton (1981) reported a similar condition with blue sclerae, multiple wormian bones, and lack of fractures; however, the presence of dentinogenesis imperfecta and deafness and the lack of joint hypermobility help to distinguish the two conditions.

**References:**
Beighton P: Familial dentinogenesis imperfecta, blue sclera, and wormian bones without fractures: another type of osteogenesis imperfecta? J Med Genet 1981; 18:124–128.
MacLean JR, et al.: The Grant syndrome: persistent wormian bones, blue sclerae, mandibular hypoplasia, shallow glenoid fossae and campomelia - an autosomal dominant trait. Clin Genet 1986; 29:523–529.

T0007

Helga V. Toriello

## SHORT SYNDROME 2098

**Includes:**
    Growth retardation-Rieger anomaly
    Reiger anomaly-growth retardation

**Excludes:**
    **Eye, anterior segment dysgenesis** (0439)
    **Lipodystrophy-Rieger anomaly-short stature-diabetes** (2834)
    Lipodystrophy, sporadic
    **Silver syndrome** (0887)

**Major Diagnostic Criteria:** Most or all of the following findings are needed to make or suspect the diagnosis: low birth weight with subsequent short stature, liopatrophy of the face and upper limbs, delayed dental eruption, Rieger anomaly, and delayed speech development.
    SHORT syndrome is a mnemonic for S = short stature, H = hyperextensibility or hernia (inguinal), O = ocular depression, R = Rieger anomaly, and T = teething (delayed).

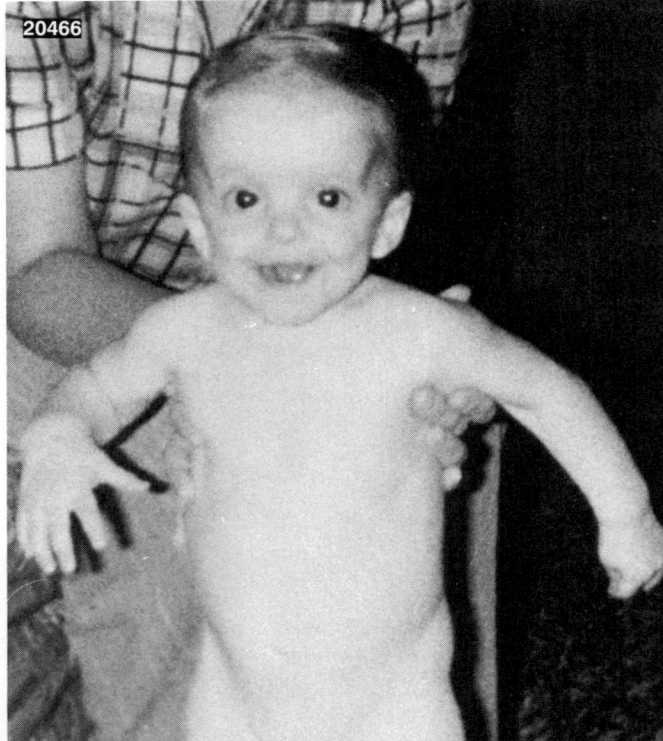

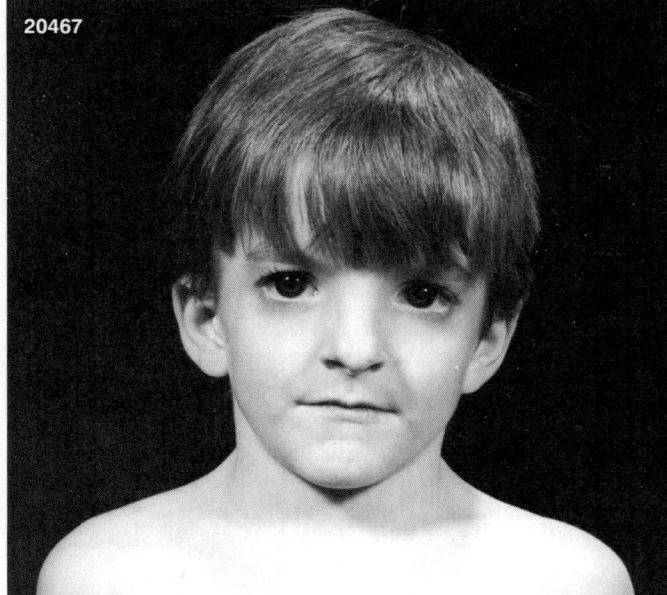

**2098-20466–67:** Reiger anomaly-growth retardation (SHORT syndrome); note triangular facies and hypoplastic nasal alae.

**Clinical Findings:** In the four reported cases, intrauterine growth retardation (3); slow weight gain (3); "triangular" face (4); telecanthus (2); deep-set eyes (4); Rieger anomaly (3); wide nasal bridge (4); hypoplastic alar cartilages (4); micrognathia (4); protuberant pinnae (4); clinodactyly (3); delayed dental eruption (4); lipoatrophy (4); joint hyperextensibility (4); short stature (4); functional cardiac murmur (2); inguinal hernia (2); delayed speech development (4); normal IQ (3); and delayed bone age on X-ray (4).

**Complications:** Frequent infections during infancy have been common.

**Associated Findings:** Sensorineural deafness was present in one patient.

**Etiology:** Probably autosomal recessive inheritance.

**Pathogenesis:** Unknown. Metabolic studies, growth hormone, somatomedin-C, thyroid studies, and banded chromosome studies have all been normal.

**MIM No.:** 26988

**POS No.:** 3496

**Sex Ratio:** M3:F1 (observed)

**Occurrence:** Four cases have been reported.

**Risk of Recurrence for Patient's Sib:**
See Part I, *Mendelian Inheritance.*

**Risk of Recurrence for Patient's Child:**
See Part I, *Mendelian Inheritance.*

**Age of Detectability:** At birth, by physical examination.

**Gene Mapping and Linkage:** Unknown.

**Prevention:** None known. Genetic counseling indicated.

**Treatment:** Screening for hearing ability, treatment of infections, and ocular examination are all indicated.

**Prognosis:** Mentation is normal, life span is unlikely to be impaired.

**Detection of Carrier:** Unknown.

**References:**

Gorlin RJ: A selected miscellany. BD:OAS XI(2). New York: March of Dimes Birth Defects Foundation, 1975:46–48.

Sensenbrenner JA, et al.: A low birthweight syndrome? Reiger syndrome. BD:OAS XI(2). New York: March of Dimes Birth Defects Foundation, 1975:423–426.

Toriello HV, et al.: Report of a case and further delineation of the SHORT Syndrome. Am J Med Genet 1985; 22:311–314.

T0007                                                    **Helga V. Toriello**

**Short-limbed campomelic syndrome, normocephalic type**
*See KYPHOMELIC DYSPLASIA*
**Short-rib syndrome, Beemer type**
*See DWARFISM, SHORT-RIB, BEEMER TYPE*
**Short-segment coarctation**
*See AORTA, COARCTATION, INFANTILE TYPE*

---

## SHOVAL-SOFFER SYNDROME                                  3258

**Includes:**
Male hypogonadism-mental retardation-skeletal anomalies
Skeletal anomalies-male hypogonadism-mental retardation
Testicular deficiency, familial

**Excludes:**
**Bardet-Biedl syndrome** (2363)
**Crandall syndrome** (3257)
**Deafness-pili torti, Bjornstad type** (2015)
**Laurence-Moon syndrome** (0578)

**Major Diagnostic Criteria:** The combination of mental retardation, cervical spine and rib anomalies, and hypogonadism.

**Clinical Findings:** In the two reported affected males, mental retardation and moderate short stature were present. Hypogonadism was present, in that both males had decreased facial and chest hair, breast development, female fat distribution, and small penis and testes. Histologic examination of the testes revealed two types of seminiferous tubules: those affected by true germinal aplasia, and those which were fibrotic. X-ray studies demonstrated rib anomalies, including cervical ribs and/or fusion; and cervical vertebral anomalies, including atlanto-occipital fusion, reversed lordotic curve, and hypertrophic spondylitis.

**Complications:** Unknown.

**Associated Findings:** One patient had a thyroid nodule which was either a cyst or adenoma.

**Etiology:** Possibly X-linked recessive inheritance.

**Pathogenesis:** Unknown.

**MIM No.:** 30750

**Sex Ratio:** M1:F0

**Occurrence:** One family with two affected male sibs has been reported.

**Risk of Recurrence for Patient's Sib:**
See Part I, *Mendelian Inheritance.*

**Risk of Recurrence for Patient's Child:**
See Part I, *Mendelian Inheritance.*

**Age of Detectability:** Unknown. The reported patients were 36 and 47 years at the time of report.

**Gene Mapping and Linkage:** Unknown.

**Prevention:** None known. Genetic counseling indicated.

**Treatment:** Unknown.

**Prognosis:** Prognosis for life span is apparently normal; mental retardation is moderate in severity.

**Detection of Carrier:** Unknown. Some of the female relatives exhibited mild mental retardation.

**References:**
Sohval AR, Soffer LJ: Congenital familial testicular deficiency. Am J Med 1953; 14:328–248.

T0007                                                      **Helga V. Toriello**

**Shprintzen syndrome**
*See VELO-CARDIO-FACIAL SYNDROME*
**Shprintzen-Goldberg syndrome**
*See PHARYNX/LARYNX HYPOPLASIA-OMPHALOCELE,*
*SHPRINTZEN-GOLDBERG TYPE*
*also CRANIOSYNOSTOSIS-ARACHNODACTYLY-HERNIA*
**'Shunt' hyperbilirubinemia**
*See HYPERBILIRUBINEMIA, CONJUGATED*
**Shurtleff syndrome**
*See MARSHALL-SMITH SYNDROME*

## SHWACHMAN SYNDROME                                    0885

**Includes:**
Bone marrow dysfunction-pancreatic insufficiency-short
    stature
Lipomatosis of pancreas, congenital
Metaphyseal dysplasia-pancreatic hypoplasia-marrow
    dysfunction
Pancreatic hypoplasia-marrow dysfunction-metaphyseal
    dysplasia
Shwachman-Bodian syndrome
Shwachman-Diamond-Oski-Khaw syndrome

**Excludes:**
**Cystic fibrosis** (0237)
**Johanson-Blizzard syndrome** (2026)
Pancreatic insufficiency, secondary

**Major Diagnostic Criteria:** Short stature, developmental delay, exocrine pancreatic insufficiency, short ribs with metaphyseal dysplasia, and isolated or combined decreases in red cell, white cell, or platelet counts.

**Clinical Findings:** Patients typically present with either short ribs and bone dysplasia in the newborn period, or developmental delay, short stature, malabsorption, recurrent infections, or hematologic abnormalities in childhood. Pancreatic insufficiency confirmed by quantitative assay of duodenal fluid appears to be the most consistent finding, but is not always accompanied by symptoms. Older patients frequently have normal stool patterns. Short stature, unaffected by nutritional status, is found in most cases, and mild-to-moderate developmental delay is also often evident.

Bone marrow dysfunction is probably always present, but is not always manifested by abnormal peripheral blood counts. Defective granulopoiesis has been demonstrated in vitro in patients who were not neutropenic at the time of the study. Anemia, neutropenia, and thrombocytopenia occur singly or in combination, and can be persistent, cyclic, or intermittent in nature.

Bone dysplasia is common, and may improve with time. The X-ray features are fairly specific, and the lesions found in bone biopsy material appear to differ from other metaphyseal dysplasias.

Saliva production is decreased, but this does not appear to lead to significant clinical symptoms.

**Complications:** Malabsorption of fat and protein, diarrhea, failure to thrive, hypoproteinemia, recurrent bacterial infections, coxa vara deformity, and cirrhosis of the liver. Hearing loss may occur secondary to recurrent otitis media. Leukemia occurs with increased frequency in older patients.

**Associated Findings:** **Colon, aganglionosis,** endocardial fibroelastosis, **Syndactyly,** supernumerary metatarsals, imperforate anus with rectourethral fistula, galactosuria, clitoral hypertrophy, increased circulating fetal hemoglobin, and defective leukocyte mobility.

**Etiology:** Autosomal recessive inheritance. Spontaneous chromosome breakage has been reported in one patient.

**Pathogenesis:** The decreases in bone matrix and pancreatic enzymes, coupled with the presence of inclusions in chondrocytes and pancreatic acinar cells, suggest a defect in polypeptide secretion. This appears to be supported by a decreased production of saliva and salivary amylase, and numerous amorphous particles in the tear layer on slit-lamp examination.

It has been suggested that abnormal polymorphonuclear chemotaxis reflects defective cytoskeletal integrity.

**MIM No.:** *26040

**POS No.:** 3453

**Sex Ratio:** M1:F1

**Occurrence:** The second most common cause of pancreatic insufficiency in childhood. Over 100 cases have been reported.

**Risk of Recurrence for Patient's Sib:**
See Part I, *Mendelian Inheritance.*

**Risk of Recurrence for Patient's Child:**
See Part I, *Mendelian Inheritance.*

**Age of Detectability:** During the newborn or infancy periods.

**Gene Mapping and Linkage:** Unknown.

**Prevention:** None known. Genetic counseling indicated.

**Treatment:** Orally administered pancreatic enzyme replacement improves digestion and absorption of peptides and fats. Early attention to febrile illnesses, including bacterial cultures, is necessary to prevent overwhelming infection. No therapy has been successful in reversing neutropenia, thrombocytopenia, or anemia, but specific replacement of blood components is useful for symptomatic patients. Appropriate orthopedic attention to the metaphyseal dysplasia, especially that involving the hip, may prevent deformity.

**Prognosis:** The long-term prognosis is uncertain. Some patients appear to do very well; others have major difficulties, and death in childhood from overwhelming infection or leukemia is common. The severity of symptoms from the other manifestations of the disorder varies greatly.

**Detection of Carrier:** Unknown.

**References:**
Bodian M, et al.: Congenital hypoplasia of the exocrine pancreas. Acta Paediatr 1964; 53:282–293.
Shwachman H, et al.: The syndrome of pancreatic insufficiency and bone marrow dysfunction. J Pediatr 1964; 65:645–663.
McLennan TW, Steinback HL: Shwachman's syndrome: the broad spectrum of bony abnormalities. Radiology 1974; 112:167–173.
Aggett PJ, et al.: Shwachman's syndrome: a review of 21 cases. Arch Dis Child 1980; 55:331–347. †

Hill RE, et al.: Steatorrhea and pancreatic insufficiency in Shwachman syndrome. Gastroenterology 1982; 83:22–27.

Rothbaum RJ, et al.: Unusual surface distribution of concanavalin A reflects a cytoskeletal defect in neutrophils in Shwachman's syndrome. Lancet 1982; II:800–801.

Tada H, et al.: A case of Shwachman syndrome with increased spontaneous chromosome breakage. Hum Genet 1987; 77:289–291.

DI001            **John H. Di Liberti**
WH007        **Peter F. Whitington**

**Shwachman-Bodian syndrome**
*See SHWACHMAN SYNDROME*
**Shwachman-Diamond-Oski-Khaw syndrome**
*See SHWACHMAN SYNDROME*
**Shy-Magee disease**
*See MYOPATHY, CENTRAL CORE DISEASE TYPE*
**Sialangiectasis**
*See PAROTITIS, PUNCTATE*
**Sialectasis**
*See PAROTITIS, PUNCTATE*
**Sialic acid storage disease, infantile (one form)**
*See SALLA DISEASE*

---

## SIALIC ACID STORAGE DISEASE, INFANTILE TYPE     2222

**Includes:**
  N-acetylneuraminic acid storage disease
  Sialuria, French type
  Sialuria, severe infantile

**Excludes:**
  **Galactosialidosis** (3110)
  **Mucolipidosis I** (0671)
  **Mucolipidosis II** (0672)
  **Mucolipidosis III** (0673)
  **Salla disease** (2041)

**Major Diagnostic Criteria:** Typical clinical findings with early onset accumulation of free sialic acid in tissues, and hypersecretion of free sialic acid in urine.

**Clinical Findings:** Clinical findings are present at birth or soon thereafter and include coarse facies, epicanthus, anteverted nostrils, clear corneas, hypopigmented hair, hepatosplenomegaly, diarrhea, anemia, inactivity, slow growth, and profound developmental impairment.

Abnormalities on X-ray include punctate calcifications of epiphyses and minimal changes of dysostosis multiplex.

Laboratory findings include anemia, clear vacuoles in lymphocytes and other tissues, urinary hypersecretion of free sialic acid, accumulation of free sialic acid in tissues, and nonspecific increase in activities of some lysosomal enzymes.

**Complications:** Unknown.

**Associated Findings:** None known.

**Etiology:** Autosomal recessive inheritance.

**Pathogenesis:** Unknown. Storage of sialic acid in this condition does not appear to be related to a deficiency of a lysosomal hydrolase. A transport defect has been suggested.

**MIM No.:** 26992

**Sex Ratio:** Presumably M1:F1.

**Occurrence:** Less than a dozen cases have been documented.

**Risk of Recurrence for Patient's Sib:**
See Part I, *Mendelian Inheritance*. A family history has been noted in only a few instances; in one the mother of a girl with the syndrome had extreme short stature at birth and extending into adult life, along with precocious sexual development, café-au-lait spots, and mild syndactyly. In another, three affected sibs were reported.

**Risk of Recurrence for Patient's Child:**
See Part I, *Mendelian Inheritance*. No affected individuals have survived to reproduce.

**Age of Detectability:** At birth. Prenatal diagnosis may be possible by quantification of free sialic acid in amniotic fluid and amniocytes.

**Gene Mapping and Linkage:** Unknown.

**Prevention:** None known. Genetic counseling indicated.

**Treatment:** Curative therapy is not available. Supportive therapy has been ineffective. Care for associated symptoms as indicated.

**Prognosis:** Progressive emaciation and loss of environmental contact result in early death.

**Detection of Carrier:** Unknown.

**Special Considerations:** *Sialuria, French type* (Stevenson et al, 1982), observed in a single case, is sialuria of infantile onset and severe manifestations. Free sialic acid is elevated in urine, serum, and cellular cytosol. This condition is distinct from **Sialic acid storage disease, infantile type** and from **Salla disease**.

**References:**

Hancock LW, et al.: Generalized N-acetylneuraminic acid storage disease: quantification and identification of the monosaccharide accumulating in brain and other tissues. Neurochem Res 1982; 38:803–809.

Stevenson RE, et al.: Sialuria: clinical and laboratory features of a severe infantile form. Proc Greenwood Genet Center 1982; 1:73–78.

Tondeur M, et al.: Infantile form of sialic acid storage disorder: clinical, ultrastructural and biochemical studies in two siblings. Eur J Pediatr 1982; 139:142–147.

Stevenson RE, et al.: Sialic acid storage with sialuria: clinical and biochemical features in the severe infantile type. Pediatrics 1983; 72:441–449.

Baumkotter J, et al.: N-acetylneuraminic acid storage disease. Hum Genet 1985; 71:155–159.

Mancini GMS, et al.: Free N-acetylneuraminic acid (NANA) storage disorders. Hum Genet 1986; 73:214–217.

SC053        **Richard J. Schroer**
ST021        **Roger E. Stevenson**

**Sialidase deficiency**
*See MUCOLIPIDOSIS I*
**Sialidosis**
*See MUCOLIPIDOSIS I*
**Sialidosis type II, juvenile-onset form**
*See GALACTOSIALIDOSIS*
**Sialuria, Finnish type**
*See SALLA DISEASE*
**Sialuria, French type**
*See SIALIC ACID STORAGE DISEASE, INFANTILE TYPE*
**Sialuria, severe infantile**
*See SIALIC ACID STORAGE DISEASE, INFANTILE TYPE*
**Siamese twins**
*See TWINS, CONJOINED*
**Sicca syndrome**
*See SJOGREN SYNDROME*
**Sickle cell anemia**
*See ANEMIA, SICKLE CELL*
**Sideroblastic anemia, autosomal recessive**
*See ANEMIA, SIDEROBLASTIC*
**Sideroblastic anemia, congenital hereditary**
*See ANEMIA, CONGENITAL SIDEROBLASTIC, NOT B(6) RESPONSIVE*
**Sideroblastic anemia, hereditary X-linked**
*See ANEMIA, CONGENITAL SIDEROBLASTIC, NOT B(6) RESPONSIVE*
**Sideroblastic anemia, X-linked**
*See ANEMIA, SIDEROBLASTIC*
**Sideroblastic anemia, X-linked-ataxia**
*See ANEMIA, SIDEROBLASTIC*
**Sideroblastic anemia-exocrine pancreatic dysfunction**
*See ANEMIA, SIDEROBLASTIC*
**Sideroblastic anemia-glucose-6-phosphate dehydrogenase deficiency**
*See ANEMIA, SIDEROBLASTIC*
**Sideroblastic anemia-Xg(a) blood group antigen**
*See ANEMIA, SIDEROBLASTIC*
**Sideroblastic hypochromic aplastic anemia, congenital**
*See ANEMIA, CONGENITAL SIDEROBLASTIC, NOT B(6) RESPONSIVE*
**Siderophilin deficiency**
*See ATRANSFERRINEMIA*

**Siemens disease**
    *See MAL DE MELEDA*
**Siemerling-Creutzfeldt disease**
    *See ADRENOLEUKODYSTROPHY, X-LINKED*
**Silent microcephaly**
    *See MICROCEPHALY, ISOLATED AUTOSOMAL DOMINANT TYPE*

## SILVER SYNDROME                                     0887

**Includes:**

Asymmetry, congenital-short stature-sexual development
    variations
Dwarfism, Silver-Russell type
Russell-Silver syndrome
Sexual development variations-asymmetry-short stature
Silver-Russell syndrome

**Excludes:**

Cerebral defects, diffuse static
**Fibrous dysplasia, polyostotic** (0391)
**Hemihypertrophy** (0458)
**Neurofibromatosis** (0712)
**Silver syndrome, X-linked** (2829)
**Turner syndrome** (0977)

**Major Diagnostic Criteria:** Significant skeletal asymmetry, short stature, small size for gestational age, and variations in the clinical and laboratory pattern of sexual development. A combination of three or more of these findings probably should be present for a clinical diagnosis to be made. The presence of several of the minor manifestations (short incurved fifth fingers, triangular facies, turned-down corners of the mouth, café-au-lait spots and syndactyly) tend to make the diagnosis more certain.

**Clinical Findings:** Short stature, significant skeletal asymmetry, variations in the pattern of sexual development, and small size despite being born at term. Other findings include café-au-lait areas of the skin, unusually short and incurved fifth fingers, triangular shape of the face, turned-down corners of the mouth, and syndactyly of the toes. Variable combinations of findings have been reported, and no single finding was noted in all patients.

At birth affected infants are unusually small for gestational age. In those cases in which the pattern of subsequent growth could be evaluated, it usually paralleled the normal growth curve but remained below the third percentile level. The children who were observed into puberty continued to be short. The pattern of puberty and adolescent growth is essentially normal but may occur at a marginally earlier time than normal. Mature height has been described as being comparable to the height reduction at the time the diagnosis was made in earlier childhood. However, some patients have experienced catch-up growth prior to adolescence.

The asymmetry, when present, can be quite variable in extent and degree. In some, one entire side of the body was significantly larger than the other; in others, the extent of the asymmetry was limited and involved only the skull, spine, or all or part of a limb. The asymmetry is probably present at birth, but may not be appreciated for variable periods of time.

Variations in the pattern of sexual development include elevated levels of serum and urinary gonadotropins in prepubertal children of both sexes. Sexual development may be precocious or may occur disproportionately early in relation to other physiologic evidences of maturity. Precocious sexual development is much more likely to occur in affected girls than in boys.

The café-au-lait spots are usually sharply circumscribed, smooth, light brown, and vary in size from less than 1 cm to over 30 cm in diameter. The spots are usually not raised, but in one instance, the entire pigmented area was wrinkled and slightly elevated. The borders of most café-au-lait areas are smooth, but some have jagged edges. Affected children may sweat excessively.

The heads of children with the Silver syndrome may be disproportionately large for the small facial mass ("pseudohydrocephaly"), tapering to a narrow jaw and producing the characteristic triangular-shaped face. The lips are often thin, with the corners of the mouth turned down ("shark mouth"). Delay in the closure of the anterior fontanelle has been noted.

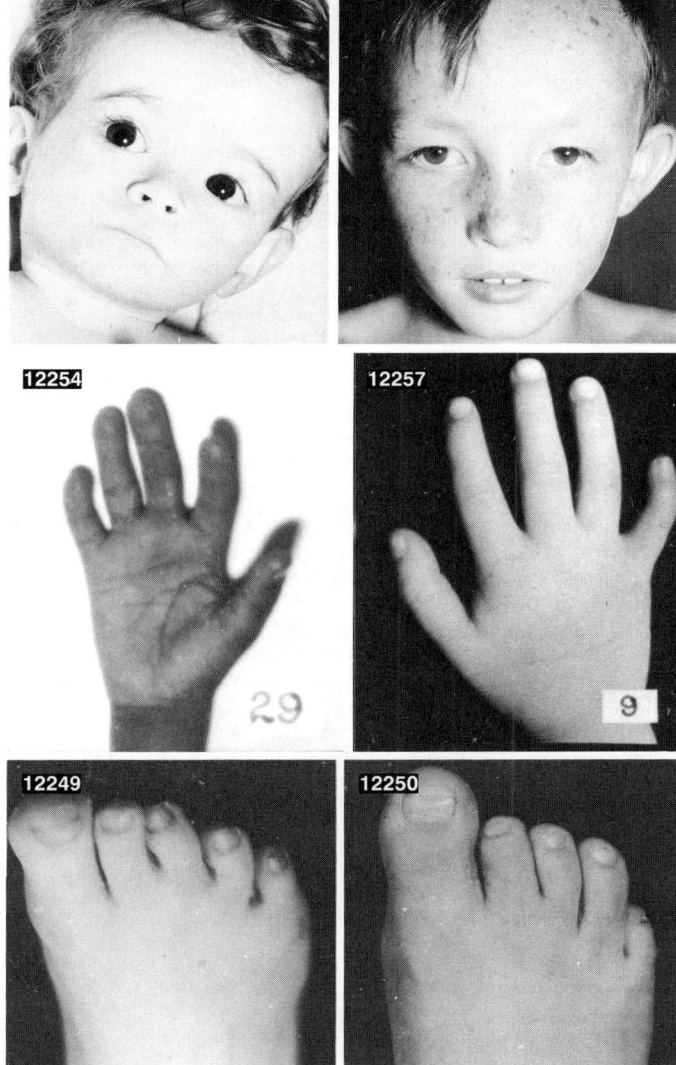

**0887**-12237–36: Typical facies with broad forehead tapering down to a narrow chin with triangular facies. 12254–57: Clinodactyly of the fifth finger. 11249–50: Disproportionate toes and syndactyly of toes 2–3.

Abnormalities of the limbs include incurving of the fifth fingers and variable, usually slight, syndactyly between the second and third toes. Other variations in the size and configuration of the toes are not uncommon. In most cases subcutaneous tissue is sparse. Abnormal genitalia, especially cryptorchidism, are not uncommon. Most affected children have normal intelligence. Bone age is retarded but generally to a lesser degree than height age.

In children who do not exhibit significant skeletal asymmetry or variations in the pattern of sexual development, the combination of small size at birth, shortness of stature, café-au-lait areas of the skin, and unusually short and incurved fifth fingers, is relatively common and may represent a partial form of the syndrome.

Serum gonadotropins and the excretion of urinary gonadotropins may be increased for age. In the first decade, the level of urinary gonadotropins may be increased to that found in normal women during the reproductive period of life. Hypoglycemia has been noted on several occasions. One patient with this syndrome has been described with elevated blood levels of β-hydroxybutyrate and acetoacetate, and massive excretion of these compounds and of $C_6$-$C_{12}$ dicarboxylic acids.

Epiphyseal maturation has been retarded in approximately one-half of the cases. There may be a difference in osseous maturation on the two sides of the body.

In at least two instances, elevated serum levels of growth hormone have been found. In several other cases the serum levels of growth hormone have been decreased, but most children with the syndrome have normal growth hormone values.

Defects of the skeleton, including poorly formed thoracic vertebrae which differed from those seen in the ordinary type of hemivertebra, surface irregularities of the lumbar vertebrae, which resemble those seen in juvenile kyphosis, irregularity and indentation of the metaphyses of the phalanges and hypoplasia, and absence of various phalanges, the sacrum, and the coccyx have all been described.

**Complications:** Although a significant association between **Hemihypertrophy** in children who are not short, and tumors of the kidneys (see **Cancer, Wilms tumor**) and adrenals (see **Cancer, neuroblastoma**) and **adrenal hyperplasia** has been noted, none of the reported cases of the Silver syndrome has been associated with malignancy of the kidneys and adrenals. Asymmetry of the spine and lower limbs may produce disturbances of gait. Precocious puberty may be psychologically disturbing to the child and parents.

**Associated Findings:** Urinary tract abnormalities and cardiac defects have been described in a few cases.

**Etiology:** Possibly autosomal recessive inheritance, or dominant inheritance with incomplete penetrance. An X-linked form has also been reported (see **Silver syndrome, X-linked**).

**Pathogenesis:** The finding of elevated levels of growth hormone in a few cases suggests that the short stature may result in part from a relative unresponsiveness to this hormone. Although growth hormone assays have been normal in most patients studied, several instances of idiopathic growth hormone deficiency, one case of Silver syndrome with growth hormone deficiency in a patient with a craniopharyngioma, and a few cases of elevated levels of growth hormone have been reported. The pathogenesis of both the asymmetry and the other clinical findings is undetermined. Some patients have had diploid-triploid mosaicism during some point in their development.

**MIM No.:** 27005

**POS No.:** 3385

**CDC No.:** 759.820

**Sex Ratio:** M1:F1

**Occurrence:** Close to 200 cases have been documented. All races and ethnic groups appear susceptible.

**Risk of Recurrence for Patient's Sib:**

See Part I, *Mendelian Inheritance*. A family history has been noted in only a few instances; in one the mother of a girl with the syndrome had extreme short stature at birth and extending into adult life, along with precocious sexual development, café-au-lait areas, and mild syndactyly. In another, three affected sibs were reported.

**Risk of Recurrence for Patient's Child:** Unknown.

**Age of Detectability:** Ordinarily at birth, but may not be recognized for several months.

**Gene Mapping and Linkage:** Unknown.

**Prevention:** None known. Genetic counseling indicated.

**Treatment:** Treatment is symptomatic. Corrective shoes, braces, and physical therapy may be necessary, but functional impairment may be minimal despite significant asymmetry. Patients, especially female patients and their parents, should be prepared for the precocious sexual development that may occur. Periodic examination should be carried out to determine the possible presence of a tumor of the kidney or adrenal.

**Prognosis:** Apparently normal for life span. Functional impairment will depend on the degree of asymmetry. In most instances no functional disturbance occurs. Approximately one-third of patients have been reported as showing some degree of mental retardation.

**Detection of Carrier:** Unknown.

**Special Considerations:** Parents of affected individuals and health professionals interested in Silver Syndrome are encouraged to contact the newly-formed ACRSS support Group listed below by writing Lois Vaughan, 5781 Vine Street, Oak Forest, IL, 60452.

**Support Groups:** NJ; Madison (22 Hoyt Street 07940); Association for Children with Russell-Silver Syndrome (ACRSS)

**References:**

Silver HK, et al.: Syndrome of congenital hemihypertrophy, shortness of stature, and elevated urinary gonadotropins. Pediatrics 1953; 368–375. †

Russell A: A syndrome of "intra-uterine dwarfism" recognizable at birth with cranio-facial synostosis, disproportionately short arms, and other anomalies. Proc R Soc Med 1954; 47:1040–1044. †

Silver HK: Asymmetry, short stature, and variations in sexual development: a syndrome of congenital malformations. Am J Dis Child 1964; 107:495–515. *

Tanner JM, et al.: The natural history of the Silver-Russell syndrome: a longitudinal study of thirty-nine cases. Pediatr Res 1975; 9:611–623.

Graham JM Jr., et al.: Diploid-triploid mixoploidy: clinical and cytogenetic aspects. Pediatrics 1981; 68:23–28. †

Gardner L: The lesions of polyploidy: relation to congenital asymmetry and the Russell-Silver syndrome. Am J Dis Child 1982; 136:292–293. †

Nishi Y, et al.: Silver-Russell syndrome and growth hormone deficiency. Acta Pediatr Scand 1982; 71:1035–1036.

Cassidy SB, et al.: Russell-Silver syndrome and hypopituitarism. Am J Dis Child 1986; 140:155–159. †

Davies PSW, et al.: Adolescent growth and pubertal progression in the Silver-Russell syndrome. Arch Dis Child 1988; 63:130–135. †

Willems PJ, et al.: Activation of fatty acid oxidation in the Silver-Russell syndrome and the Brachmann - de Lange syndrome. Am J Med Genet 1988; 30:865–873. †

Duncan PA, et al.: Three-generation dominant transmission of the Silver-Russell syndrome. Am J Med Genet 1990; 35:245–250.

SI012                                                          **Henry K. Silver**

## SILVER SYNDROME, X-LINKED                                            **2829**

**Includes:**

Russell-Silver syndrome, X-linked
Short stature, X-linked, with skin pigmentation
Skin pigmentation-short stature, X-linked

**Excludes:**

**Silver syndrome** (0887)
**Neurofibromatosis** (0712)

**Major Diagnostic Criteria:** Short stature and brown pigmentation of the skin. Males have the clinical appearance of **Silver syndrome**.

**Clinical Findings:** Based on one family with two affected brothers, their mother, and two of her sisters: both males had intrauterine growth retardation, with birth weights of 1,890 and 1,960 g, respectively, at term. The head appeared large and the face triangular. Growth was slow, with both height and weight staying some 2 to 2.5 SD below the mean into middle childhood. One boy had frequent minor infections in infancy and then developed asthma with repeated short admissions to the hospital. Intellectual development was normal.

Abnormal pigmentation of the skin appeared in the second year with a few small spots, some of which were brown and some achromic. Thereafter, over a couple of years, diffuse light-brown pigmentation developed over the lower trunk, arms, and thighs, containing a few achromic and some dark-brown spots. Diffuse depigmentation was seen in the groin. There was no blistering or lichenification, but the achromic areas were easily sunburned.

Nothing abnormal was found in the history of the three affected females, but none achieved an adult height of more than 160 cm whereas their four unaffected sisters were 168 cm tall. All three women had 30 to 50 café-au-lait spots on the trunk and arms with a few achromic spots. All looked similar to each other, with a somewhat large mouth and prominent upper jaw.

**Complications:** Unknown.

**Associated Findings:** The severe asthma seen in one boy may have been coincidental.

**Etiology:** Presumably X-linked inheritance.

**Pathogenesis:** Unknown.

**MIM No.:** 31278

**CDC No.:** 759.820

**Sex Ratio:** M1:F1

**Occurrence:** One family from The Netherlands, living in Canada, has been reported.

**Risk of Recurrence for Patient's Sib:**
See Part I, *Mendelian Inheritance.*

**Risk of Recurrence for Patient's Child:**
See Part I, *Mendelian Inheritance.*

**Age of Detectability:** After the characteristic pigmentation appears in the second year of life.

**Gene Mapping and Linkage:** Unknown.

**Prevention:** None known. Genetic counseling indicated.

**Treatment:** Unknown.

**Prognosis:** Normal life span. Adult height of affected males is likely to be short.

**Detection of Carrier:** Possibly by relatively short stature and café-au-lait spots.

**Special Considerations:** The delineation of this variant of **Silver syndrome** supports the suggestion of others that the syndrome is heterogeneous. Usually the condition is a sporadic event in a family, and many such cases may well not be genetic. Familial cases have been reported and interpreted as indicating autosomal dominant inheritance with incomplete penetrance. Some of these families have shown a pattern of inheritance that is also consistent with X-linked inheritance.

**References:**
Partington MW: X-linked short stature with skin pigmentation: evidence for heterogeneity of the Russell-Silver syndrome. Clin Genet 1986; 29:151–156. * †

PA026                                         **M.W. Partington**

**Silver-Russell syndrome**
*See SILVER SYNDROME*
**Silverman-Handmaker dwarfism**
*See DWARFISM, DYSSEGMENTAL, SILVERMAN-HANDMAKER TYPE*
**Simian crease, incomplete**
*See SKIN CREASE, SINGLE PALMAR*
**Simpson dysmorphia syndrome**
*See SIMPSON-GOLABI-BEHMEL SYNDROME*

---

## SIMPSON-GOLABI-BEHMEL SYNDROME                 2826

**Includes:**
  Bulldog syndrome
  Dysplasia-gigantism syndrome, X-linked
  Golabi-Rosen syndrome
  Overgrowth, Golabi-Rosen type
  Overgrowth-mental retardation syndrome, X-linked
  Simpson dysmorphia syndrome
  X-linked mental retardation-overgrowth syndrome

**Excludes:**
  **Beckwith-Wiedemann syndrome** (0104)
  **Cebebral gigantism** (0137)
  **Marshall-Smith syndrome** (2193)
  **Overgrowth, Ruvalcaba-Myhre-Smith type** (2120)
  **Proteus syndrome** (2382)
  **Weaver syndrome** (2036)

**Major Diagnostic Criteria:** The combination of overgrowth, unusual facial appearance, digital anomalies, and minor skeletal anomalies.

**Clinical Findings:** Six families have been reported. Anomalies present in most affected individuals include pre- and post-natal overgrowth; hypotonia; **Microcephaly; Eye, hypertelorism**; short, broad nose; large mouth with thick lips; submucous cleft or high-arched palate; midline groove or notch of the lower lip, tongue and/or **Hernia, inguinal**; cryptorchidism; broad halluces and thumbs; hypoplastic or absent index fingernails; high palmar pattern intensity; and normal to mildly delayed intellectual and motor development. Occasional abnormalities include hypodontia; pre-auricular dimples or tags; cadiac defects; supernumerary nipples; gastrointestinal abnormalities, including intestinal malrotation or constipation; renal anomalies, including "large", lobulated or cystic kidneys, duplicated renal pelvis, or mild hydronephrosis; postaxial polydactyly; small calf muscles; skin hyperpigmentation; and hyperinsulinemia attributable to an increased number of islets of Langerhans.

A family reported by Opitz et al (1988) included three affected males; the propositus of that family did not have overgrowth and was severely mentally retarded. Behmel et al (1988) suggest that the phenotype in the affected individuals of this family represents the "severe end of the spectrum".

**Complications:** Unknown.

**Associated Findings:** Present in one or two patients each were **Cleft lip, Omphalocele**, ocular coloboma, seizures, and limited extension of elbows and knees.

**Etiology:** Presumably X-linked recessive inheritance.

**Pathogenesis:** Unknown.

**MIM No.:** 30605, 31287

**POS No.:** 3325

**Sex Ratio:** M1:F0

**Occurrence:** Six families and one sporadic case have been described.

**Risk of Recurrence for Patient's Sib:**
See Part I, *Mendelian Inheritance.*

**Risk of Recurrence for Patient's Child:**
See Part I, *Mendelian Inheritance.*

**Age of Detectability:** At birth, by physical exam and presence of overgrowth.

**Gene Mapping and Linkage:** SDYS (Simpson dysmorphia syndrome) has been provisionally mapped to X.

**Prevention:** None known. Genetic counseling indicated.

**Treatment:** Supportive. Surgery may also be indicated.

**Prognosis:** Postnatal mortality is relatively high. In survivors, motor development is essentially normal, although clumsiness is present in childhood. Intellectual development is usually normal or mildly delayed.

**Detection of Carrier:** Carrier females may have some of the pheotypic features, including mild expression of the facial features, **Syndactyly**, hypoplastic index fingernails, and tall stature.

**References:**
Simpson JL, et al.: A previously unrecognized X-linked syndrome of dysmorphia. BD:OAS; XI(2). New York: March of Dimes Birth Defects Foundation, 1973:18–24.
Golabi M, Rosen L: A new X-linked mental retardation overgrowth syndrome. Am J Med Genet 1984; 17:345–358.
Opitz JM: The Golabi-Rosen syndrome. Am J Med Genet 1984; 17:359–366.
Tsukahara M, et al.: A Weaver-like syndrome in a Japanese boy. Clin Genet 1984; 25:73–78.
Behmel A, et al.: A new X-linked dysplasia gigantism syndrome: follow-up in the first family and a second Austrian family. Am J Med Genet 1988; 30:275–285.
Neri G, et al.: Simpson-Golabi-Behmel syndrome: an X-linked encephalo-tropho-schisis syndrome. Am J Med Genet 1988; 30:287–299.

Opitz JM, et al.: Simpson-Golabi-Behmel syndrome: follow-up of the Michigan family. Am J Med Genet 1988; 30:301–308.

T0007

**Helga V. Toriello**

**Sindig-Larsen-Johansson disease (patella)**
See *JOINTS, OSTEOCHONDRITIS DISSECANS*
**Single transverse fold**
See *SKIN CREASE, SINGLE PALMAR*

## SINGLETON-MERTEN SYNDROME 2087

**Includes:**
> Aorta, idiopathic calcification
> Dental and bone defects
> Merten-Singleton syndrome
> Muscle weakness
> Skeletal defects with aortic calcification and muscle weakness

**Excludes:**
> **Ectodermal dysplasia** (see all)
> **Hypophosphatasia** (0516)
> **Mucopolysaccharidosis**
> **Oculo-dento-osseous dysplasia** (0737)
> **Progeria** (0825)
> **Thalassemia** (0939)
> **Xanthomatosis, cerebrotendinous** (2395)

**Major Diagnostic Criteria:** A combination of the following features should be present for a clinical diagnosis of the Singleton-Merten syndrome to be strongly suspected; all were found in the few cases reported: poor physical development, generalized muscular weakness, severe dental dysplasia in deciduous and permanent teeth. X-ray findings showed linear calcification of the proximal aorta and aortic valve; generalized osteoporosis; widened medullary spaces in the metacarpals, metatarsals, and phalanges.

**Clinical Findings:** Pregnancy, delivery, and early postnatal development are normal. The first signs and symptoms appear in infancy (4–24 months). The initial complaint is generalized muscular weakness (100%), which may follow an acute febrile illness (50%). Somatic growth and motor development are delayed (75%), while mental development is normal (100%). Severe dental dysplasia: carious deciduous teeth with premature loss; dysplasia and delayed development of permanent teeth (100%). Generalized osteoporosis is associated with thin cortices, expanded medullary cavities, and poorly defined trabeculae of the short tubular bones of the hands and feet (100%). Progressive calcification of the proximal aorta was apparent on X-ray by 4 to 12 years of age (100%), and calcific aortic valvular stenosis developed in mid to late childhood (100%). Mitral valve calcification was also frequently present (75%). Systolic murmurs were present early in life; however, valvular calcifications were not seen until later. The cardiac abnormalities led to left heart failure, which was the immediate cause of death in all patients.

In addition to the above problems, there may be psoriaform skin eruption in late childhood (50%) and erosion of the terminal phalanges without destructive psoriatic arthritis; soft tissue calcification (50%); calcification of the bursa, proximal radius, and ulna (1/4); and subungual calcification (1/4); hypertension (25%); heart block (25%).

There are no abnormalities in serum calcium, phosphorus, and alkaline phosphatase. Electromyograms are normal. Muscle biopsy shows nonspecific atrophy of the muscle fibers. No metabolic or hematologic disorders have been documented (100%). Death due to left heart failure occurred at 4–18 years of age.

**Complications:** Eye problems (50%): glaucoma and photosensitivity, are presumably related to viral or psoriatic keratitis. Orthopedic deformities (including shallow acetabular fossa, subluxation of femoral head, coxa valga, equinovarus foot deformity) are presumed secondary to generalized muscle weakness. Acro-osteolysis may be a complication of psoriaform eruption.

**Associated Findings:** None known.

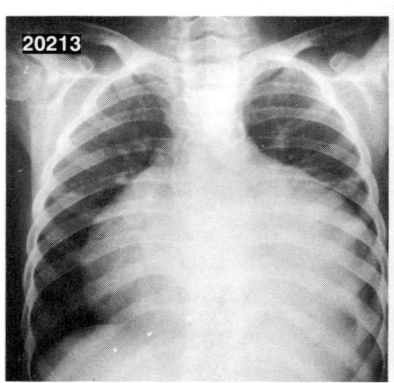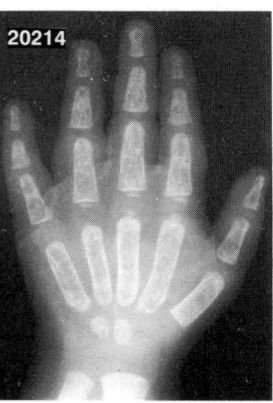

**2087-20213:** The heart is enlarged; there is tubular calcification of the ascending aorta and aortic arch. **20214:** The metacarpals and phalanges are osteoporotic with thinned cortices, accentuated trabeculae, and expansion of the medullary cavities.

**Etiology:** Unknown. Possibly autosomal dominant inheritance.

**Pathogenesis:** The basic pathogenesis of skeletal and cardiovascular changes is unknown. Autopsy findings show extensive calcification of the intima and media of the proximal aorta. There is myocardial degeneration and necrosis without evidence of inflammatory cells.

**MIM No.:** 18225

**POS No.:** 4024

**Sex Ratio:** M1:F3

**Occurrence:** Four cases have been published. Other patients with calcification of the ascending aorta and aortic valve due to idiopathic or infectious aortitis are reported in adults without the skeletal, dental, or muscular stigmata of Singleton-Merten syndrome.

**Risk of Recurrence for Patient's Sib:** All cases have been sporadic.

**Risk of Recurrence for Patient's Child:** No affected individuals have survived to reproduce.

**Age of Detectability:** Usually in infancy (less than age two years) the condition may be suspected clinically by generalized muscle weakness and poor development and abnormal dentition. Systolic murmurs develop early, but cardiovascular calcifications are not seen until four years of age or later. Skeletal changes are present in early infancy.

**Gene Mapping and Linkage:** Unknown.

**Prevention:** None known. Genetic counseling indicated.

**Treatment:** None known; symptomatic treatment of cardiac disease, but there is no experience with valve replacement. Supportive treatment for muscular weakness and complications, including orthopedic deformities.

**Prognosis:** Death from cardiac failure 4–16 years after onset.

**Detection of Carrier:** Unknown.

**References:**
Singleton EB, Merten DF: An unusual syndrome of widened medullary cavities of the metacarpals and phalanges, aortic calcification and abnormal dentition. Pediatr Radiol 1973; 1:2–7. *
McLoughlin MJ, et al.: Idiopathic calcification of the ascending aorta and aortic valve in two young women. Br Heart J 1974; 36:96–100.
Gay B Jr, Kuhn JP: A syndrome of widened medullary cavities of bone, aortic calcification, abnormal dentition, and muscular weakness (the Singleton-Merten syndrome). Radiology 1976; 118:389–395.
Rangaswami N, et al.: Idiopathic linear calcification of the ascending aorta in an adolescent. Am J Dis Child 1979; 133:860–861.

Rosenthal T, et al.: Aortic calcification in young women: a case report. Angiology 1979; 30:53–55.
Theman TE, et al.: Morphological findings in idiopathic calcification of the ascending aorta and aortic valve affecting a young woman. Histopathology 1979; 3:181–190.

ME031                                                          **David F. Merten**

**Sinoatrial block, congenital complete**
*See ARRHYTHMIA, HEART BLOCK, CONGENITAL COMPLETE*

## SINUS, ABSENT PARANASAL                                          0797

**Includes:**

Agenesis of paranasal sinuses, unilateral
Paranasal sinuses, absent
Sinuses, absence of frontal
Sinuses, absence of frontal-microcornea-glaucoma

**Excludes:**  Paranasal sinuses, hypoplastic

**Major Diagnostic Criteria:**  Absence of paranasal sinuses on X-ray, if the patient is past the age at which the sinuses are present on X-rays. (The average age at which the paranasal sinuses become easily identifiable on X-rays is maxillary, one year; frontal, 6–8 years; ethmoid, one year; sphenoid, four years.)

In adults with absence on X-ray of only one sinus, the possibility of neoplastic and inflammatory disease must be eliminated before a diagnosis of agenesis can be assumed. This may necessitate surgical exploration.

**Clinical Findings:**  Transillumination of involved frontal or maxillary sinuses is not possible. However, this is of little help in small children because the sinuses are not large enough normally to transilluminate well. Palpation of the face over the paranasal sinuses will be normal. Examination of the nose may reveal abnormalities of the turbinates on the ipsilateral side of the unilateral agenesis. Waters view, lateral view, Caldwell view, and basal view X-rays will show absence of some or all paranasal sinuses.

**Complications:**  Unknown.

**Associated Findings:**  In one family; microcornea, glaucoma, and absent frontal sinuses.

**Etiology:**  Unknown.

**Pathogenesis:**  Unknown.

**Sex Ratio:**  Presumably M1:F1.

**Occurrence:**  Undetermined but presumed rare.

**Risk of Recurrence for Patient's Sib:**  Unknown.

**Risk of Recurrence for Patient's Child:**  Unknown.

**Age of Detectability:**  At 1–8 years, when paranasal sinuses appear on X-ray.

**Gene Mapping and Linkage:**  Unknown.

**Prevention:**  None known. Genetic counseling indicated.

**Treatment:**  None for absent paranasal sinuses, but in patients with absent frontal sinuses, microcornea, and open-angle glaucoma, insidious blindness may develop unless the glaucoma is treated.

**Prognosis:**  Normal for life span and intelligence.

**Detection of Carrier:**  Unknown.

**Special Considerations:**  There is one reported case of panagenesis of paranasal sinuses and one known case of unilateral absent paranasal sinuses. The case of unilateral agenesis was associated with an ipsilateral hypertrophied middle turbinate resulting in obstruction of the nasal airway on that side. There was also an absence of the inferior turbinate on the same side. A single family presented with *absent frontal sinuses, microcornea, and glaucoma.* In this particular family, no male-to-male transmission was present in the three generations affected; therefore, the type of dominant transmission is unknown.

**References:**
Gob, AS, Acquarelli, MJ: Unilateral absent paranasal sinuses with hypertrophied middle turbinate. West J Med 1966; 7:239–241.
Mocellin, L.: Panagenesis of the paranasal sinuses: report of a case. Arch Otolaryngol 1968; 88:311–314.
Holmes, LB, Walton, DS: Hereditary microcornea, glaucoma and absent frontal sinuses: a family study. J Pediatr 1969; 74:968–972.

GE000                                                        **Robert N. Gebhart**

**Sinuses, absence of frontal**
*See SINUS, ABSENT PARANASAL*
**Sinuses, absence of frontal-microcornea-glaucoma**
*See SINUS, ABSENT PARANASAL*
**Sinusitis-dextrocardia-bronchiectasis syndrome**
*See DEXTROCARDIA-BRONCHIECTASIS-SINUSITIS SYNDROME*
**Sipple syndrome**
*See ENDOCRINE NEOPLASIA, MULTIPLE TYPE II*

## SIRENOMELIA SEQUENCE                                             3191

**Includes:**

Symmelia
Sympodia
Uromelia

**Excludes:**

Caudal regression syndrome (3211)
Vater association (0987)

**Major Diagnostic Criteria:**  Sirenomelia is an anomalous development of the caudal region of the body, with varying degrees of "fusion" of the lower extremities with or without long bones being present.

**Clinical Findings:**  Complete or nearly complete fusion of the lower limbs is the most striking feature of sirenomelia. However, other congenital anomalies usually exist. Hemivertebrae have been observed involving cervical, thoracic and lumbar vertebrae. Spina bifida and meningomyelocele have also been noted. Abnormalities of the pelvis can include fused iliac bones with a poorly formed acetabula. Characteristically a single umbilical artery with hypoplasia of the aorta below the origin of the umbilical artery is present. The external genitalia in males can vary from rudimentary perineal skin tags to almost normal penis and scrotum. Rudimentary ovaries, and anomalous uterus and vagina are occasionally seen in females. Reported urinary tract anomalies include either unilateral or bilateral renal agenesis, renal artery agenesis, renal dysplasia, rudimentary ureters and agenesis of the bladder. Imperforate anus and blind ending rectum are invariably present.

Based on osseous findings, sirenomelia has been classified into seven types: *Type I*, all bones of thigh and lower leg present and unfused; *Type II*, fused fibulae; *Type III*, fibulae absent; *Type IV*, partially fused femora and fused fibulae; *Type V*, partially fused femora; *Type VI*, fused femora and fused tibiae; and *Type VII*, fused femora and absent tibiae. Another classification based on the leg and foot defects include three types: *Symelus* (sympus dipus-two feet), legs almost perfectly united and terminating in a double foot with soles on the anterior surfaces; *Uromelus* (sympus monopus-one foot), incompletely united legs ending in an incomplete single foot with the sole on the anterior surface, and *Sirenomelus* (Sympus apus-no foot), incomplete union of the legs with absence of a distinct foot.

**Complications:**  Unknown.

**Associated Findings:**  Lung hypoplasia is present in a high number of affected cases and is probably due to the associated oligohydramnios. Tracheoesophageal fistula can also be seen. Cardiovascular malformations occur in approximately 25% of the cases and range from **Ventricular septal defect** to acardius amorphus.

**Etiology:**  Unknown. To date all cases have been sporadic. The incidence of the condition in monozygotic twins is increased (100 to 150-fold over that in dizygotic twins or singletons). This suggests that the cause of sirenomelia in twins may be associated with the twinning process itself. The concordance rate in monozygotic twins is low.

**Pathogenesis:** Unknown. Major theories are: *The fusion theory,* the oldest attempt to explain this anomaly, suggests that the lower extremities develop in lateral contact to each other and subsequently become fused. *The classical theory* proposes a deficiency of the caudal axial area in the embryo, allowing the approximation of the side plates from where the limbs develop. The close positioning of the lower limbs permits their fusion with a direct proportional relation between the distance of the lumb buds and the severity of the condition. *The single umbilical artery theory* states that the resulting vascular insufficiency does not allow the normal process of lower limb development. *The vascular steal theory* proposes that sirenomelic malformations result from diversion of the blood flow from caudal structures of the embryo to the placenta. Distal tissues to the steal have demised vascular supply and are arrested or are totally absent at some stage of fetal development. *Extrinsic pressure* is the fifth theory and suggests that any mechanical pressure on the caudal portion of the embryo will impede normal rotation of the limb buds as it has been observed in chick embryos exposed to such influences. Finally, the *neural tube distention theory* has been suggested. Presumably an overdistention of the neural tube in the caudal region expands the roof plate of the tube, displacing and laterally rotating the mesoderm, which allows the fusion of the limb buds.

**POS No.:** 3399

**Sex Ratio:** M2.7:F1

**Occurrence:** From 1.5–4.2:100,000 births. In a series of 331 monozygotic twins, 27 had sirenomelia, with concordance in only two pair.

**Risk of Recurrence for Patient's Sib:** Unknown.

**Risk of Recurrence for Patient's Child:** Affected individuals are not expected to survive to reproduce.

**Age of Detectability:** Second trimester ultrasound findings suggesting this condition include renal agenesis, oligohydramnios, difficulty visualizing the lower extremities or separate legs, and intrauterine growth retardation.

**Gene Mapping and Linkage:** Unknown.

**Prevention:** None known. Genetic counseling indicated.

**Treatment:** Supportive.

**Prognosis:** Poor. The majority of affected individuals are either stillborn or die shortly after birth.

**Detection of Carrier:** Unknown.

**Special Considerations:** A number of investigators have suggested that sirenomelia is a part of the **Caudal regression syndrome**. However, the uniqueness of the clinical findings in sirenomelia justify separation into a separate condition, although there may be a single specific etiological mechanism producing this condition and caudal regression syndrome. At the present time the two most likely mechanisms would be deficiency of caudal mesoderm and vascular disruption. The problem with the vascular etiology theory is that the vascular abnormalities observed in sirenomelia could be secondary to decreased blood flow needs in the caudal region and lower extremities of the embryo, rather than the defects being produced by vascular insufficiency. Aberrant development of the caudal developmental field includes **Vater association, Urorectal septum malformation sequence**, exstrophy of the bladder, exstrophy of the cloaca, **Mullerian aplasia**, sirenomelia, **Caudal regression syndrome**, and cloacal dysgenesis.

**References:**
Stevenson RE, et al.: Vascular steal: the pathogenetic mechanism producing sirenomelia and associated defects of the viscera and soft tissues. Pediatrics 1986; 78:451–457.

Stocker JT, Heifetz SA: Sirenomelia: a morphological study of 33 cases and review of the literature. Perpect Pediatr Pathol 1987; 10:7–50. * †

ES004                                **Luis F. Escobar**
WE005                           **David D. Weaver**
WI063                              **Jeffrey Winn**

**Site-specific colorectal cancer, Lynch syndrome I**
*See CANCER, COLORECTAL*
**Situs inversus intestinalis (complete, partial)**
*See SITUS INVERSUS VISCERUM*

## SITUS INVERSUS VISCERUM           0888

**Includes:** Situs inversus intestinalis (complete, partial)

**Excludes:**
   Dextrocardia
   **Dextrocardia-bronchiectasis-sinusitis syndrome** (0285)

**Major Diagnostic Criteria:** X-ray evaluation of the gastric bubble in the right upper abdomen. Air insufflation of the stomach after passing a nasogastric tube will assist in this diagnostic evaluation. The presence of dextrocardia on the chest X-ray film may be helpful in establishing this diagnosis. In incomplete situs inversus the liver will be palpable in the left upper quadrant of the abdomen on physical examination, whereas in partial situs inversus the liver will be in the normal position. Contrast barium X-ray studies will demonstrate the sigmoid colon to be in the right lower quadrant in cases of complete situs inversus.

**Clinical Findings:** In total situs inversus there is complete transposition of the viscera with the stomach on the left side. Isolated situs inversus of the stomach is extremely rare. Approximately 70% of the patients with situs inversus will have other congenital anomalies of the gastrointestinal tract. Forty percent of affected patients have other major congenital malformations of the heart. Other malformations in this syndrome include clubfeet, choanal atresia, cleft palate, absent humerus, meningomyelocele, and cutaneous hemangioma. Birth weight is only slightly lower than average.

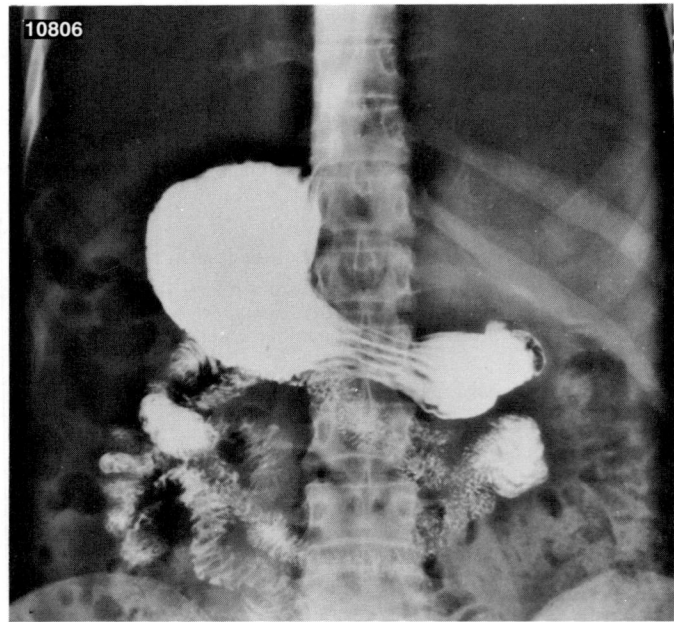

**0888-10806:** Upper GI series showing mirror image positioning of liver, stomach, and intestines in visceral situs inversus.

**Complications:** Complications are determined by the other congenital malformations that accompany situs inversus. Serious complications have resulted from failure to recognize the presence of situs inversus while attempting surgical correction of other visceral malformations.

**Associated Findings:** Congenital heart disease, including **Heart, tetralogy of Fallot**, **Heart, transposition of great vessels**, **Pulmonary valve, stenosis**, septal defects, and others occur twice as frequently when dextrocardia is present. Approximately 50% of the intra-abdominal anomalies require operative correction within the first few months of life. The most common malformations are rotation abnormalities with or without volvulus, **Biliary atresia**, splenic agenesis, duodenal atresia or stenosis, annular pancreas, imperforate anus, anterior portal vein, jejunal atresia and stenosis, gastric duplications, **Colon, aganglionosis**, and left vena cava.

**Etiology:** Possibly autosomal recessive or dominant inheritance. Sporadic cases are frequent.

**Pathogenesis:** Mirror-image transposition of the internal organs may affect thoracic and abdominal viscera together or independently. Because of sequential or dependent organogenesis, a rotational abnormality will affect all subsequent phases of development and associated dependent organs. For example, rotation of the stomach to the right results in transposition of the intestine. The left vitelline and umbilical veins are larger than their mates and have been regarded as determining the early positions of the heart and liver. More recent studies suggest that the rotation of the viscera may depend upon controlling factors in the gut which are operative before the liver bud appears.

**MIM No.:** 27010

**CDC No.:** 759.3

**Sex Ratio:** M6:F4

**Occurrence:** Estimated 1:6,000–8,000 for complete; the partial type is less frequent.

**Risk of Recurrence for Patient's Sib:**
See Part I, *Mendelian Inheritance*. Occurrence has been as high as 50% in some families.

**Risk of Recurrence for Patient's Child:**
See Part I, *Mendelian Inheritance*. Occurrence has been as high as 50% of the offspring.

**Age of Detectability:** Usually within the first few weeks of life, based on the severity of associated malformations.

**Gene Mapping and Linkage:** Unknown.

**Prevention:** None known. Genetic counseling indicated.

**Treatment:** Early recognition and prompt, accurate management of the associated congenital malformations are necessary. The majority of the malformations are very serious, and prompt diagnosis and surgical management are indicated for either intra-abdominal or cardiac lesions. Recognition of situs inversus is imperative for surgical management.

**Prognosis:** Depends on the associated congenital malformations.

**Detection of Carrier:** Unknown.

**References:**

Chib P, et al.: Unusual occurrence of dextrocardia with situs inversus in succeeding generations of a family. J Med Genet 1977; 14:30–32.

Zlotogora J, Elina E: Asplenia and polysplenia syndromes with abnormalities of lateralization in the sibships. J Med Genet 1981; 18:301–302.

Mishalne H, Mahnouski V: Congenital asplenia and anomalies of the gastrointestinal tract. Surgery 1982; January:38–41.

Arnold GL, Bixler D: Probable autosomal recessive inheritance of polysplenia, situs inversus and cardiac defects in an Amish family. Am J Med Genet 1983; 16:35–42.

Niikawa N, et al.: Familial clustering of situs inversus totalis and asplenia and polysplenia syndrome. Am J Med Genet 1983; 16:43–47.

Rott HO: Genetics of Kartagener's syndrome. Eur J Respir Dis 1983; 127:1–4.

Zlotogora J, et al.: Familial situs inversus and congenital heart defects. Am J Med Genet 1987; 26:181–184.

BE049                                                    **Arthur S. Besser**

**Six-pyruvoyl tetrahydropterin synthase deficiency**
*See BIOPTERIN SYNTHESIS DEFICIENCY*

## SJOGREN SYNDROME                                          2101

**Includes:**
> Mikulicz syndrome
> Sicca syndrome

**Excludes:**
> **Parotitis, punctate** (0799)
> **Salivary gland, agenesis** (2722)

**Major Diagnostic Criteria:** Xerostomia and xerophthalmia with (secondary Sjögren syndrome) or without (primary Sjögren syndrome) **Arthritis, rheumatoid** or other autoimmune disease. Also, either unilateral or bilateral salivary gland swelling, usually involving the parotid (80% of primary, 30–40% of secondary). Arthritis is the most frequent initial symptom in secondary Sjögren syndrome. The pathologic hallmark of the disorder is marked lymphocytic infiltration of the salivary glands.

**Clinical Findings:** Primary Sjögren syndrome involves the exocrine glands only, while secondary Sjögren syndrome is associated with a definable autoimmune disease, most commonly **Arthritis, rheumatoid**.

The major clinical manifestations of the disorder affect the eye and the salivary glands. Other systemic findings may also be seen. Ophthalmologic findings are secondary to atrophy of the secretory epithelium of both the major and minor lacrimal glands leading to desiccation of the cornea and conjunctiva (keratoconjunctivitis sicca). The cornea may undergo severe damage. Common symptoms include discomfort and dryness of the eyes, burning, a scratchy or sandy sensation, redness, photophobia, changes in visual acuity, and failure to produce tears.

Salivary gland abnormalities include firm, tender enlargement of one or more parotid or submandibular glands. Salivary glands become atrophic, and saliva becomes deficient in quantity, leading to xerostomia. The lips and oral mucous membranes may also become atrophic. Other common symptoms include difficulty speaking, swallowing, and eating, and loss of taste and smell.

Systemic clinical findings include dry skin, achlorhydria, interstitial pneumonitis, hepatosplenomegaly, **Raynaud disease**, genital dryness, hyposthenuria, myositis, pancreatitis, anemia, lymphadenopathy, dry sparse hair, alopecia, impairment of esophageal motility, and abnormalities of renal tubular function.

Laboratory findings include the presence of polyclonal hypergammaglobulinemia, numerous autoimmune antibodies (both organ-specific and non-organ-specific) and circulating IgG immune complexes, which may include a positive rheumatoid factor (70%) and a positive LE preparation (15–20%). Impaired cell-mediated immunity can be seen. Increased sedimentation rate (67%), anemia (33%), and leukopenia or eosinophilia (25%) can also occur.

Diagnosis of the ophthalmologic components of the disorder is possible by the rose bengal ocular staining technique, which can detect keratoconjunctivitis sicca, and the Schirmer test. The latter test uses filter paper strips placed under the eyelids to measure the quantity of tears secreted, and is the most widely used ocular test for diagnosis.

Sialography or nuclear scanning with technetium 99m can be used to assess salivary gland function.

Confirmation of the diagnosis may be obtained by salivary gland biopsy, which reveals massive lymphoid infiltration, with atrophy of the acinar tissue, and ductal alterations characterized by the formation of epimyoepithelial islands. Labial glands are a convenient source to biopsy. The lymphocytic infiltration is quantifiable and correlates well with the severity of the disease and the clinical manifestations.

**Complications:** Mucosal ulcerations and an increased incidence of dental caries can occur as a result of xerostomia. Xerophthalmia can lead to corneal ulcerations and perforation. An increased incidence of otitis media, bronchitis, pneumonia, pancreatitis, and atrophic gastritis can also be seen. There is also an increased incidence (44 times the expected rate) of lymphoma, usually of the histiocytic or mixed histiocytic-lymphocytic type. Lymphoma is more commonly seen in patients with a history of parotid enlargement, splenomegaly, lymphadenopathy, and/or parotid irradiation.

**Associated Findings:**  Biliary cirrhosis, other liver abnormalities, autoimmune liver disease, laryngeal involvement, membranous glomerulonephritis, nephrocalcinosis, renal insufficiency, uremia, osteomalacia, secondary amyloidosis, and diffuse peripheral neuropathy.

**Etiology:**  Familial occurrence has been infrequently observed. Increased HLA-B8 and HLA-DW3 has been observed in primary Sjögren syndrome.

**Pathogenesis:**  Lymphocyte-mediated destruction of the exocrine glands. Laboratory findings suggest that one of the underlying defects is B-cell hyperreactivity with or without abnormalities of immunoregulation.

**MIM No.:**  27015

**Sex Ratio:**  M1:F9

**Occurrence:**  1:200

**Risk of Recurrence for Patient's Sib:**  Unknown.

**Risk of Recurrence for Patient's Child:**  Unknown.

**Age of Detectability:**  Average age of onset is 50 years, but childhood cases have been reported.

**Gene Mapping and Linkage:**  Unknown.

**Prevention:**  None known. Genetic counseling indicated.

**Treatment:**  Symptomatic. Artificial saliva, artificial tears, antibiotic therapy of infections, good dental hygiene, and analgesics for the pain and tenderness associated with sudden enlargement of the salivary glands.

**Prognosis:**  Varies with severity of the disease and complications.

**Detection of Carrier:**  Unknown.

**References:**
Lichtenfeld JL, et al.: Familial Sjogren's syndrome with associated primary salivary gland lymphoma. Am J Med 1976; 60:286–292.
Shearn MA: Sjogren's syndrome. Med Clin North Am 1977; 61:271–282.
Kassan SS: Increased risk of lymphoma in sicca syndrome. Ann Intern Med 1978; 89:888–892.
Moutsopoulos HM, et al.: Genetic differences between primary and secondary sicca syndrome. New Engl J Med 1979; 301:761–763. *
Moutsopoulos HM, et al.: Sjogren's syndrome (sicca syndrome): current issues. Ann Intern Med 1980; 92:212–226.
Rice DH: Advances in diagnosis and management of salivary gland diseases. West J Med 1984; 140:238–249.
Reveille JD, et al.: Primary Sjogren's syndrome and other autoimmune diseases in families: prevalence and immunogenetic studies in six kindreds. Ann Intern Med 1984; 101:748–756.

IR000                                                    **Mira Irons**

---

## SJOGREN-LARSSON SYNDROME                    2030

**Includes:**
Fatty alcohol:NAD+ oxidoreductase (FAO), deficiency of
Ichthyosis-oligophrenia-spasticity
Oligophrenia-ichthyosis-spasticity
Spasticity-ichthyosis-oligophrenia

**Excludes:**
**Chondrodysplasia punctata**
**Ichthyosis, linearis circumflexa** (2858)
**Phytanic acid storage disease** (0810)
**Seizures-ichthyosis-mental retardation** (0741)

**Major Diagnostic Criteria:**  The triad of congenital ichthyosiform dermatitis, mental deficiency, and spastic paresis of the extremities.

**Clinical Findings:**  In infancy, redness of the skin is first apparent; later, a typical fish-scale appearance (congenital ichthyosiform erythroderma) becomes visible. The areas most affected are the neck, lower abdomen, axillae, and flexures of the elbows.

Almost all patients reported in the literature have been described as retarded, although there are three cases in which the patients have been said to have IQs between 70 and 79 (borderline mental retardation).

Neurologically, the spasticity is usually of the symmetric diplegic type. About 75% of the patients are confined to wheelchairs. Muscle tone is increased in the limbs and in the muscles of the mouth and bulbar region so that speech and feeding may be a problem.

As early as age two years, a degenerative defect in the retinal pigment epithelium can be detected in about 50% of the affected children. These chorioretinal lesions are of varying size in and about the macula.

**Complications:**  Activities of daily living are difficult due to both spasticity and to the limited mental capacities of the patients.

**Associated Findings:**  Seizures, speech disorders, muscular degeneration.

**Etiology:**  Autosomal recessive inheritance.

**Pathogenesis:**  Cultured skin fibroblasts show impaired hexadecanol oxidation due to fatty alcohol:NAD+ oxidoreductase (FAO) deficiency.

**MIM No.:**  *27020

**POS No.:**  3400

**CDC No.:**  757.120

**Sex Ratio:**  M1:F1

**Occurrence:**  Reported from many countries. Sjögren and Larsson (1957) established the syndrome by an exhaustive survey of inhabitants of northern Sweden, which yielded 28 cases in 14 sibships. Incidence in Sweden has been estimated as 6:1,000,000. In Vasterbotten County, Sweden, the prevalence is 8.3:100,000; the gene frequency is 0.01.

**Risk of Recurrence for Patient's Sib:**
See Part I, *Mendelian Inheritance*.

**Risk of Recurrence for Patient's Child:**
See Part I, *Mendelian Inheritance*.

**Age of Detectability:**  The rash can appear in the neonatal period; signs become apparent in the first year of life. Prenatal diagnosis is possible.

**Gene Mapping and Linkage:**  Unknown.

**Prevention:**  None known. Genetic counseling indicated.

**Treatment:**  Symptomatic treatment of skin lesions; infant physical and educational intervention for central nervous system manifestations.

**Prognosis:**  Prognosis depends on the severity of the CNS symptoms. In a wheelchair-bound, severely retarded individual, the prognosis is more guarded than in a less severely affected patient.

**Detection of Carrier:**  By FAO deficiency in skin fibroblasts or leukocytes.

**Special Considerations:**  The dramatic nature of the skin lesions has led to confusion among the many different syndromes presenting with ichthyosis. Sjögren-Larsson is a distinct syndrome, different from the multiple other syndromes with fish-scale appearance of the skin.

**References:**
Sjögren T, Larsson T: Oligophrenia in combination with congenital ichthyosis and spastic disorders: a clinical and genetic study. Acta Psychiatr Neurol Scand (suppl 113) 1957; 32:1–112.
McLennan JE, et al.: Neuropathological correlates in Sjögren-Larsson syndrome. Brain 1974; 97:693.
Jagell S, et al.: Specific changes in the fundus typical for the Sjögren-

Larsson syndrome: an ophthalmological study of 35 patients. Acta Ophthalmol 1980; 58:321–330.

Jagell S, et al.: Sjögren-Larsson syndrome in Sweden: a clinical, genetic and epidemiological study. Clin Genet 1981; 19:233–256.

Jagell S, Linden S: Ichthyosis in the Sjögren-Larsson syndrome. Clin Genet 1982; 21:243–252.

Kousseff BG, et al.: Prenatal diagnosis of Sjogren-Larsson syndrome. J Pediatr 1982; 101:998–1001.

Rizzo WB, et al.: Sjogren-Larsson syndrome: deficient fatty alcohol: NAD+ oxidoreductase (FAO) activity in mixed leukocytes. (Abstract) Am J Hum Genet 1987; 41:A16 only.

C0018            **Mary Coleman**

**Skeletal and facial defects-short stature-mental retardation**
*See KABUKI MAKE-UP SYNDROME*
**Skeletal and laryngeal anomalies-motor and sensory neuropathy**
*See NEUROPATHY, CONGENITAL MOTOR & SENSORY-SKELETAL-LARYNGEAL DEFECTS*
**Skeletal anomalies-joint dislocations-unusual facies**
*See LARSEN SYNDROME*
**Skeletal anomalies-male hypogonadism-mental retardation**
*See SHOVAL-SOFFER SYNDROME*
**Skeletal anomalies-short stature-mental retardation-alopecia**
*See ALOPECIA-SKELETAL ANOMALIES-SHORT STATURE-MENTAL RETARDATION*

## SKELETAL BOWING-CORTICAL THICKENING-BONE FRAGILITY-ICTHYOSIS      2937

**Includes:**
Bone fragility-skeletal bowing-cortical thickening-ichthyosis
Cortical thickening-skeletal bowing-bone fragility-ichthyosis
Ichthyosis-skeletal bowing-cortical thickening-bone fragility
Osteosclerosis-ichthyosis-fractures

**Excludes:**
**Diaphyseal dysplasia** (0290)
**Skeletal dysplasia, Weismann-Netter-Stuhl type** (2542)

**Major Diagnostic Criteria:** Endosteal cortical thickening of the long tubular bones and icthyosis.

**Clinical Findings:** A bone disorder characterized by cortical thickening of the diaphyses of long tubular bones and bowing of the weight-bearing bones. All have had ichthyosis, and three also had an unusual proclivity to fractures. The clinical symptoms were waddling gait, muscle weakness, and leg pains.

**Complications:** Fractures and deformity of long bones.

**Associated Findings:** None known.

**Etiology:** Presumably autosomal dominant inheritance. No male-to-male transmission has been observed, and no affected male has had children; hence, X-linked inheritance cannot be excluded.

**Pathogenesis:** Unknown.

**MIM No.:** 16674

**CDC No.:** 756.480

**Sex Ratio:** M1:F1

**Occurrence:** Six cases in two generations of a family from northern Norway have been documented.

**Risk of Recurrence for Patient's Sib:**
See Part I, *Mendelian Inheritance.*

**Risk of Recurrence for Patient's Child:**
See Part I, *Mendelian Inheritance.*

**Age of Detectability:** During early childhood.

**Gene Mapping and Linkage:** Unknown.

**Prevention:** None known. Genetic counseling indicated.

**Treatment:** Orthopedic correction of deformities.

**Prognosis:** Good, with only moderate handicap.

**Detection of Carrier:** Unknown.

**References:**
Koller M-E, et al.: A familial syndrome of diaphyseal cortical thickening of the long bones, bowed legs, tendency to fracture and ichthyosis. Pediatr Radiol 1979; 8:179–182.

AA002            **Dagfinn Aarskog**

**Skeletal defects with aortic calcification and muscle weakness**
*See SINGLETON-MERTEN SYNDROME*
**Skeletal defects-dysmorphic facies-aural atresia**
*See AURAL ATRESIA-DYSMORPHIC FACIES-SKELETAL DEFECTS*
**Skeletal defects-dysmorphic facies-torsion dystonia**
*See BLEPHARO-NASO-FACIAL SYNDROME*
**Skeletal disorder-deafness**
*See METAPHYSEAL DYSOSTOSIS-DEAFNESS*
**Skeletal dysplasia**
*See DWARFISM*

## SKELETAL DYSPLASIA, 3-M TYPE      2569

**Includes:** Three-M slender-boned nanism

**Excludes:**
**Bloom syndrome** (0112)
**Dwarfism** (other primordial)
**Silver syndrome** (0887)

**Major Diagnostic Criteria:** Low birth weight, short stature, craniofacial dysmorphia, and minor musculoskeletal malformations.

**Clinical Findings:** Low birth weight is a constant feature in postnatal growth deficiency leading to proportionate dwarfism. The head may appear large, but measures at the 50th percentile. The craniofacies is said to be hatchet-shaped with dolichocephaly, triangular face, hypoplastic maxilla, and prominent mouth and chin. The neck is short with prominent trapizii. Sternal abnormalities, winged scapulae, and diastasis recti are common.

On X-ray, the long bones appear slender with diaphyseal constriction and exaggerated modeling. The vertebral bodies may appear long, but reduced in anteroposterior and transverse diameters. The ribs are slender, and the pelvis and iliac wings are small. Bone maturation is delayed.

**Complications:** Unknown.

**Associated Findings:** Spina bifida, short fifth fingers, and hypospadias have been reported.

**Etiology:** Autosomal recessive inheritance.

**Pathogenesis:** Unknown.

**MIM No.:** *27375

**POS No.:** 3613

**CDC No.:** 756.480

**Sex Ratio:** M1:F1

**Occurrence:** Less than two dozen cases have been reported.

**Risk of Recurrence for Patient's Sib:**
See Part I, *Mendelian Inheritance.*

**Risk of Recurrence for Patient's Child:**
See Part I, *Mendelian Inheritance.*

**Age of Detectability:** At birth.

**Gene Mapping and Linkage:** Unknown.

**Prevention:** None known. Genetic counseling indicated.

**Treatment:** Unknown.

**Prognosis:** Good for general health and life span.

**Detection of Carrier:** Subtle facial dysmorphia and slender long bones may be seen in some carriers.

**References:**
Miller JD, et al.: The 3-M syndrome: a heritable low birthweight dwarfism. BD:OAS XI(5). New York: March of Dimes Birth Defects Foundation, 1975:39–47. * †

Cantu JM, et al.: 3-M slender boned nanism. Am J Dis Child 1981; 135:95–98.

Winter RM, et al.: The 3-M syndrome. J Med Genet 1984; 21:124–128. †

Hennekam RCM, et al.: Further delineation of the 3-M syndrome with a review of the literature. Am J Med Genet 1987; 28:195–209.

J0027                                                    **Ronald J. Jorgenson**

**Skeletal dysplasia, acromicric**
*See ACROMICRIC DYSPLASIA*

## SKELETAL DYSPLASIA, BOOMERANG DYSPLASIA          2522

**Includes:**  Boomerang skeletal dysplasia

**Excludes:**  Dwarfism, other lethal neonatal

**Major Diagnostic Criteria:**  Lethal neonatal dwarfism with diagnostic X-ray and characteristic clinical features.

**Clinical Findings:**  This form of neonatal dwarfism is associated with hydramnios, prematurity, and death *in utero* or shortly thereafter. The trunk is shortened with a small chest. All the extremities are shortened and the lower ones are bowed anteriorly. There is equinovarus deformity of the feet. The head is large, with peculiar facial appearances, and a small mandible. The palpebral fissures are horizontal, and there are epicanthal folds. The nose has a broad nasal root, and severe hypoplasia of the septi nasi and lateral cartilages. The nares are small and oval, with a slanted long axis. The philtrum is prominent. X-ray findings include a boomerang-like, triangular, or oval shape of the long bones. The radii and fibulae are missing. Ossification of the cervical and thoracic spine is retarded. In the pelvis, the iliac wings are well developed, but the iliac bodies are hypoplastic and the pubic bones are absent. Moderate to severe hypoplastic/dysplastic changes are present in the feet.

**Complications:**  Intrauterine or neonatal death.

**Associated Findings:**  None known.

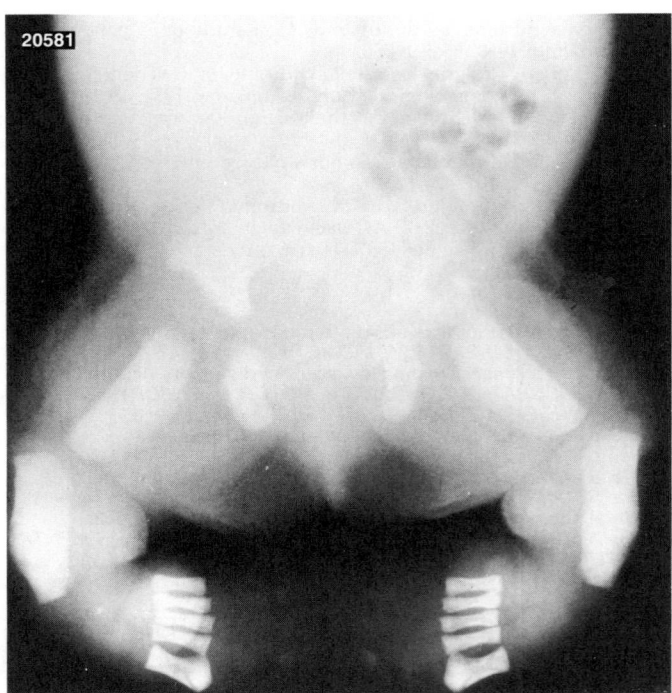

**2522B**-20581:  Boomerang dysplasia; note boomerang-shaped long bones; the pelvis shape is characteristic and one leg bone is missing.

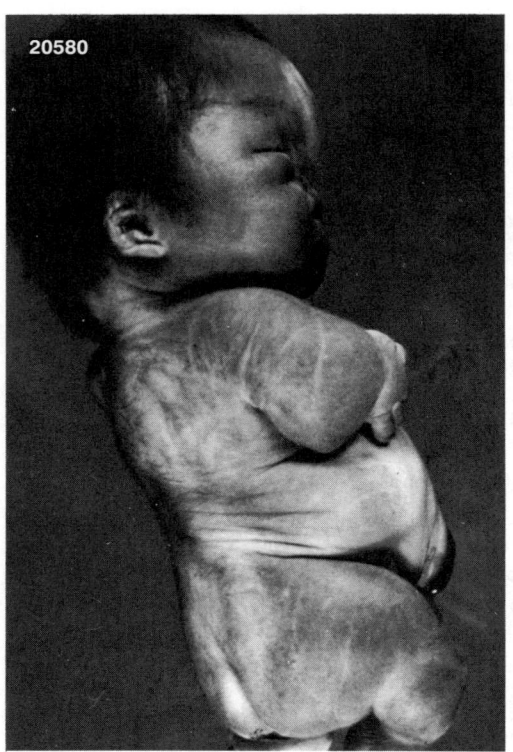

**2522A**-20580:  Boomerang dysplasia; note extreme shortening of the limbs and protrusion of the triangular bones of the extremities.

**Etiology:**  Unknown. Possibly autosomal recessive inheritance.

**Pathogenesis:**  Growth plates are not evenly distributed, and giant cells may be found in the serial sections.

**POS No.:**  3813

**Sex Ratio:**  M3:F0 (observed).

**Occurrence:**  Three cases have been reported in the literature, and at least as many additional cases have been observed.

**Risk of Recurrence for Patient's Sib:**
See Part I, *Mendelian Inheritance.*

**Risk of Recurrence for Patient's Child:**  Affected individuals are not expected to survive to reproduce.

**Age of Detectability:**  At birth. Prenatal diagnosis by ultrasound in the second trimester is possible.

**Gene Mapping and Linkage:**  Unknown.

**Prevention:**  None known. Genetic counseling indicated.

**Treatment:**  Unknown.

**Prognosis:**  Fatal in neonatal period.

**Detection of Carrier:**  Unknown.

**References:**
Kozlowski K, et al.: New forms of neonatal death dwarfism: report of 3 cases. Pediatr Radiol 1981; 10:155–160.
Tenconi R, et al.: Boomerang dysplasia: a new form of neonatal death dwarfism. Fortsch Röntgenstr 1983; 138:378–380.
Kozlowski K, et al.: Boomerang Dysplasia. Brit J Radiol 1985; 58:369–371.

K0021                                                    **K.S. Kozlowski**

## SKELETAL DYSPLASIA, DE LA CHAPELLE TYPE    2631

**Includes:**
de la Chapelle skeletal dysplasia
Neonatal osseous dysplasia I

**Excludes:**
**Achondrogenesis**
**Achondroplasia** (0010)
**Atelosteogenesis** (2521)
**Mesomelic dysplasia, Langer type** (0646)
**Skeletal dysplasia, boomerang dysplasia** (2522)
**Thanatophoric dysplasia** (0940)

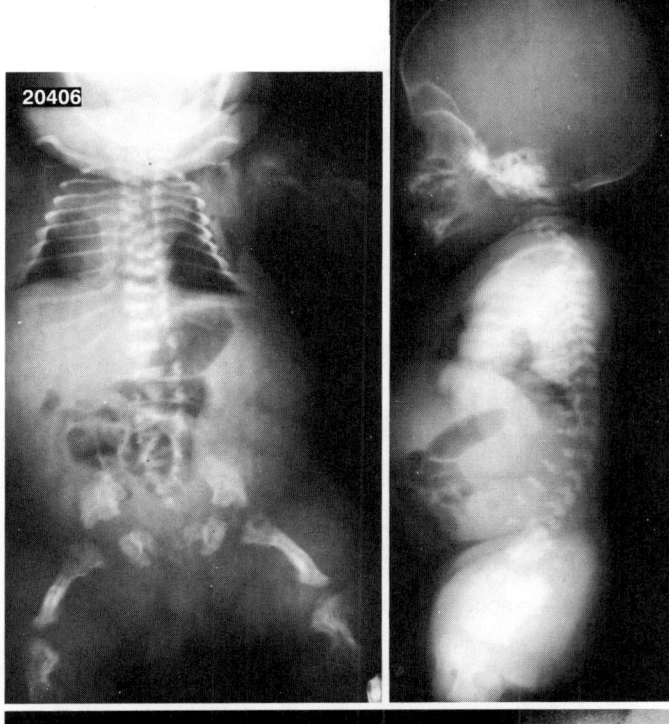

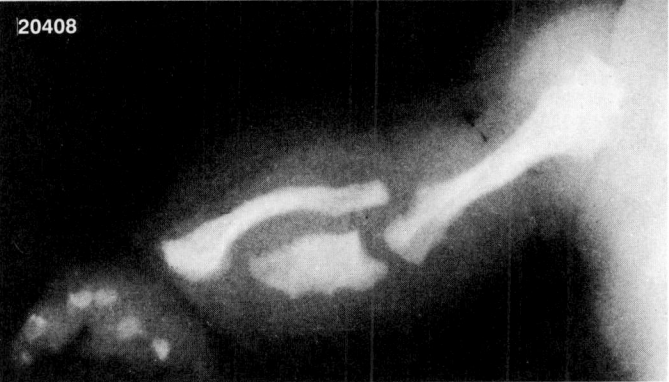

**2631A**-20406:   Note short limbs, platyspondyly, and hypoplastic pelvis.   20407:   Vertebral bodies have small ossification centers with irregular contours and anterior tongue-like projections in the lateral view.   20408:   The ulna is represented by an irregular and almost triangular remnant.

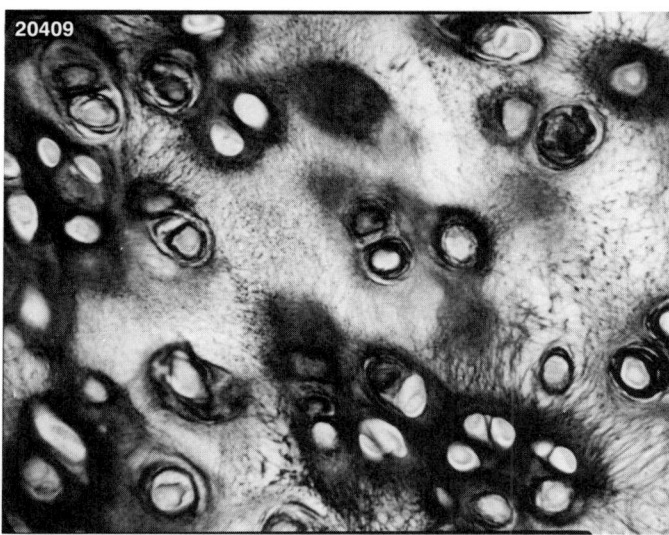

**2631B**-20409:   High-power view of the concentric "lacunar halos" surrounding chondrocytes in the resting zone of skeletal cartilage (methenamine silver nitrate-alcian blue; ×544).

**Major Diagnostic Criteria:**   X-ray features of this lethal neonatal skeletal dysplasia are distinctive and comprise the major diagnostic criteria. The skull, scapulae, and clavicles are not markedly abnormal. However, there is severe spinal deformity with platyspondyly. Vertebral bodies have small ossification centers with irregular contours and anterior tongue-like projections in lateral view. There is a wide cleft between each vertebral body and its respective posterior arch. The acetabulum is flat and horizontal. Bones of the limbs are moderately shortened. Ulnae and fibulae are represented as a very distinctive, almost triangular osseous remnant. The proximal humeral metaphysis is relatively broad. Bones of the hands and digits are small and poorly ossified. "Lacunar halos" have been identified as a distinctive histopathologic feature and have also been seen in some forms of **Achondrogenesis** but not in several other skeletal dysplasias.

**Clinical Findings:**   Affected newborn infants present with immediate apnea. The presence of a dwarfing condition is readily apparent (crown-heel length, 35–40 cm). The head is normocephalic except for **Cleft palate**. The chest is small, and there is moderately severe micromelia with small hands, equinovarus deformity, and widely spaced first and second toes. Scoliosis is sometimes evident from external examination. At autopsy the larynx is seen to be malformed and stenotic, and cartilage from respiratory structures is abnormal. Tracheal and bronchial rings are soft, permitting easy collapse of the major airways. Identification of distinctive "lacunar halos" in skeletal cartilage is aided with methenamine silver nitrate-alcian blue stain.

**Complications:**   Death has occurred at birth in all cases and is attributed to a triad of respiratory tract malformations: laryngeal stenosis, tracheobronchomalacia, and pulmonary hypoplasia.

**Associated Findings:**   Double ossification centers in the phalanges were observed in the original case, but were not present in affected sibs or in an unrelated case. Other abnormalities have been observed, but none of these has been a consistent finding: duplicated renal artery, hydronephrosis, ectopic thymus, multiple endocrine neoplasia, and bifid ureter.

**Etiology:**   Autosomal recessive inheritance.

**Pathogenesis:**   Presumably a defect in the synthesis of a normal component of cartilage, although no biochemical or molecular genetic studies have been reported.

**MIM No.:**   *25605

**POS No.:** 3847

**CDC No.:** 756.480

**Sex Ratio:** M1:F1

**Occurrence:** Four cases from two families have been reported.

**Risk of Recurrence for Patient's Sib:**
See Part I, *Mendelian Inheritance*.

**Risk of Recurrence for Patient's Child:**
See Part I, *Mendelian Inheritance*.

**Age of Detectability:** At birth, or may be detected prenatally by ultrasonography.

**Gene Mapping and Linkage:** Unknown.

**Prevention:** None known. Genetic counseling indicated.

**Treatment:** Attempts at tracheal intubation have failed, apparently due to collapse of floppy tracheal airways, thus obviating attempts at newborn resuscitation.

**Prognosis:** Lethal at birth.

**Detection of Carrier:** Unknown.

**Special Considerations:** There should be no confusion with the term *de la Chapelle syndrome*, which refers to phenotypic males with an apparent 46,XX karyotype resulting from translocation or other mutations of genes determining sex phenotype.

**References:**
de la Chapelle A, et al.: Une rare dysplasia osseuse letale de transmission recessive autosomique. Arch Fr Pediatr 1972; 29:759–770.
Whitley CB, et al.: de la Chapelle dysplasia. Am J Med Genet 1986; 25:29–39.

WH008                                           **Chester B. Whitley**

**Skeletal dysplasia, fibrochondrogenesis**
*See FIBROCHONDROGENESIS*

---

## SKELETAL DYSPLASIA, FUHRMANN TYPE                2696

**Includes:**
    Femoral bowing-fibula aplasia/hypoplasia-poly-, syn-, oligodactyly
    Fibula aplasia/hypoplasia-femoral bowing-poly-, syn-, oligodactyly
    Fuhrmann skeletal dysplasia

**Excludes:**
    Bones, congenital bowing of the long
    **Campomelic dysplasia** (0122)
    **Chondroectodermal dysplasia** (0156)
    **Femoral hypoplasia-unusual facies syndrome** (2027)
    **Fibula, congenital absence of** (2229)
    **Grebe syndrome** (0445)

**Major Diagnostic Criteria:** Aplasia or hypoplasia of the fibulae associated with acromelic duplication or reduction defects and femoral bowing or shortening.

**Clinical Findings:** Fuhrmann et al (1980) described a severe skeletal dysplasia in four full sibs. Variability of expression and asymmetry of the severity of the defects were seen among the affected children. The lower extremities and the pelvis were severely dysplastic, with the upper extremity involvment including postaxial polysyndactyly, cutaneous **Syndactyly, Camptodactyly,** and clinodactyly. The fingernails were variably involved, but the toenails in all the sibs were reduced to scar-like bands of tissue or were absent. The axial skeleton, craniofacies, viscera, and central nervous system were spared. The fourth sib was diagnosed prenatally with ultrasound and aborted at 17–19 weeks gestation. This infant had atypical lobation of the lungs noted at autopsy.

X-ray features included hypoplasia of the pelvic bones, often associated with congenital dislocation of the hips in the more severely affected sibs to slight flaring of the ilia in the mildest case. The femora were bowed or shortened in all cases (asymmetrically in the mildest case). The fibulae were absent during early childhood, but in the one surviving sib rudimentary ossification was

noted at age nine years. The feet demonstrated reduction deformities involving the metatarsals and phalanges and coalescence of the tarsals. The hands demonstrated postaxial hexadactyly, phalangeal hypoplasia, metacarpal coalescence, and interphalangeal ankyloses. The humeri, radii, ulnae, and vertebrae were normal in all sibs.

**Complications:** All sibs had short stature caused by the lower limb deformities. Two of the sibs died of infection in early childhood, but this was thought to be unrelated to their skeletal dysplasia.

**Associated Findings:** None known.

**Etiology:** Presumably autosomal recessive inheritance. The parents were members of a small ethnic minority group from neighboring villages, but consanguinity was not established.

**Pathogenesis:** Chondro-osseous tissue was examined in the abortus. Localized perichondral ossification described as atypical was seen in several sites, but no specific abnormalities of endochondral ossification were found. Reactive ossification with an unusual trabecular pattern was seen at the diaphyseal angulation. Fuhrmann et al (1980) speculated that the pattern of defects was consistent with a developmental field defect.

**MIM No.:** 22893

**POS No.:** 3519

**CDC No.:** 756.480

**Sex Ratio:** M3:F1 (observed).

**Occurrence:** Four sibs of a Turkish-Arabian family working in Germany have been documented.

**Risk of Recurrence for Patient's Sib:**
See Part I, *Mendelian Inheritance*.

**Risk of Recurrence for Patient's Child:**
See Part I, *Mendelian Inheritance*.

**Age of Detectability:** Prenatally.

**Gene Mapping and Linkage:** Unknown.

**Prevention:** None known. Genetic counseling indicated.

**Treatment:** Orthopedic surgery.

**Prognosis:** Unknown.

**Detection of Carrier:** Unknown.

**References:**
Fuhrmann W, et al.: Poly-, syn-, and oligodactyly, aplasia or hypoplasia of fibula, hypoplasia of pelvis and bowing of femora in three sibs-a new autosomal recessive syndrome. Eur J Pediatr 1980; 133:123–129.
Fuhrmann W, et al.: A new autosomal recessive skeletal dysplasia syndrome: prenatal diagnosis and histopathology. In: Papadatos CJ, Bartsocas CS, eds: Skeletal dysplasias. New York: Alan R. Liss, 1982:519–524.

H0025                                              **O.J. Hood**
H0033                                       **William A. Horton**

**Skeletal dysplasia, Grebe type**
*See GREBE SYNDROME*
**Skeletal dysplasia, humerospinal dysostosis**
*See DYSOSTOSIS, HUMEROSPINAL*
**Skeletal dysplasia, Kniest-like**
*See KNIEST-LIKE DYSPLASIA*
**Skeletal dysplasia, kyphomelic dysplasia**
*See KYPHOMELIC DYSPLASIA*
**Skeletal dysplasia, neonatally lethal short-limbed, Glasgow type**
*See THANATOPHORIC DYSPLASIA, GLASGOW TYPE*

## SKELETAL DYSPLASIA, SCHNECKENBECKEN TYPE　　2632

**Includes:**
Chondrodysplasia, lethal neonatal with snail-like pelvis
Schneckenbecken dysplasia
Snail-like pelvis dysplasia

**Excludes:**
**Achondrogenesis, Parenti-Fraccaro type** (0009)
**Achondrogenesis, Houston-Harris type** (2870)
**Achondrogenesis, Langer-Saldino type** (0008)
**Kniest-like dysplasia** (2799)
**Thanatophoric dysplasia** (0940)
**Thanatophoric dysplasia, Glasgow type** (2821)

**Major Diagnostic Criteria:** Lethal neonatal dwarfism with characteristic clinical, X-ray, and histopathologic features.

**Clinical Findings:** This disorder is a form of lethal neonatal dwarfism associated with second trimester polyhydramnios and prematurity. Most published cases were stillborn. On clinical grounds alone, these cases cannot be distinguished from the other known lethal, short-limb dysplasias. The skull is relatively large, with flat face, short trunk, and very short limbs. As shown on X-ray, the skull is normally ossified. The vertebral bodies are hypoplastic and flat. Punctate ossification of a round nature is seen in the lateral projection. There is marked spinal stenosis. The ribs are short and splayed. The iliac wings are "snail-like" (*schneckenbecken* in German) in configuration, with a very unusual medial projection of bone forming the head of the "snail." The ischium is not ossified. The long bones are very short; most had a dumbbell-like appearance without significant metaphyseal abnormalities. There is often ossification of talus and calcaneous.

**Complications:** Intrauterine or neonatal death.

**Associated Findings:** None known.

**2632-20071:** X-ray of an affected fetus showing flattened vertebral bodies, snail-like ilia and dumbbell-shaped long bones. Note the precocious ossification in the ankle.

**Etiology:** Autosomal recessive inheritance.

**Pathogenesis:** Pathologic examination of cartilage has demonstrated resting chondrocytes with round central nucleus and absence of a lacunar space. The matrix often appeared normal. Ultrastructurally, most chondrocytes have their cell membranes immediately adjacent to the interterritorial matrix leaving no lacunar space. The rough endoplasmic reticulum is not dilated.

**MIM No.:** *26925

**POS No.:** 3852

**CDC No.:** 756.480

**Sex Ratio:** M1:F1

**Occurrence:** Nine cases have been documented.

**Risk of Recurrence for Patient's Sib:**
See Part I, *Mendelian Inheritance.*

**Risk of Recurrence for Patient's Child:**
See Part I, *Mendelian Inheritance.*

**Age of Detectability:** At birth, or prenatally by ultrasound.

**Gene Mapping and Linkage:** Unknown.

**Prevention:** None known. Genetic counseling indicated.

**Treatment:** Unknown.

**Prognosis:** Fatal during the neonatal period.

**Detection of Carrier:** Unknown.

**References:**
Rimoin DL: The chondrodystrophies. Adv Hum Genet 1975; 5:1.
Borochowitz Z, et al.: A distinct lethal neonatal chondrodysplasia with snail-like pelvis: Schneckenbecken dysplasia. Am J Med Genet 1986; 25:47–59.
Knowles S, et al.: A new category of lethal short limbed dwarfism. Am J Med Genet 1986; 25:41–46.

B0025　　　　　　　　　　　　　　　**Zvi Borochowitz**

**Skeletal dysplasia, short rib dwarfism, Beemer type**
*See DWARFISM, SHORT-RIB, BEEMER TYPE*
**Skeletal dysplasia, short rib-polydactyly syndrome type II**
*See SHORT RIB-POLYDACTYLY SYNDROME, TYPE II*
**Skeletal dysplasia, Urbach-rhizomelia of humeri**
*See RHIZOMELIC SYNDROME, URBACH TYPE*

## SKELETAL DYSPLASIA, WEISMANN-NETTER-STUHL TYPE　　2542

**Includes:**
Bowing of legs, anterior, with dwarfism
Legs, bowing of anterior-dwarfism
Toxopachyosteose diaphysaire tibio-peroniere
Weismann-Netter-Stuhl syndrome

**Excludes:**
**Campomelic dysplasia** (0122)
**Diaphyseal dysplasia** (0290)
**Femoral hypoplasia-unusual facies syndrome** (2027)
Rickets (all forms)
Syphilitic sabre shins

**Major Diagnostic Criteria:** The diagnosis rests on the X-ray findings: 1) Anterior bowing of tibiae and fibulae, often (35%) associated with lateral bowing of femora, usually bilateral and symmetric, occasionally unilateral. The apex of the tibial curve is at the junction of the middle and lower one-third, and the fibular bowing is slightly lower. The cortex of both bones is thickened throughout, especially on the concave side. The marrow cavity is widened. There is no anterior periosteal overgrowth as in syphilis. There are no signs of present or past rickets. 2) Proportionate short stature (adult stature 120–156 cm). 3) Delayed onset of walking (18 months to five years). 4) Absence of pain, discomfort, or disability. 5) Normal laboratory findings.

**Clinical Findings:** The tibial bowing is readily recognized on inspection and palpation. Most patients state that it has been present as long as they can remember. In a few patients the

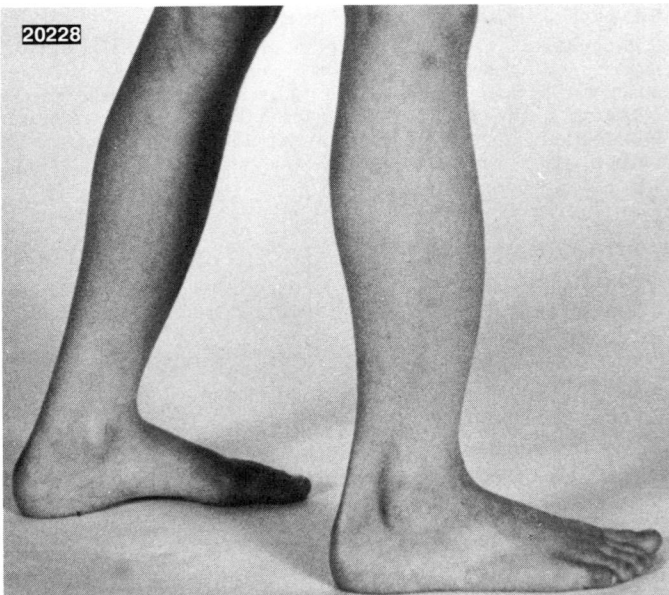

**2542A-20228:** Note the anterior bowing of the tibia.

bowing has been documented at birth, suggesting that onset may be prenatal. No explanation for the delayed onset of walking has been offered. The angulation does not seem to progress with age. Most cases have been discovered incidentally in patients admitted to hospitals for other reasons. Serum calcium, phosphorus, and alkaline phosphatase levels have been normal. Life span is not impaired; the oldest patient was 93 years old at the time of diagnosis. No patient had any discomfort or disability attributable to the bowing. Gait is normal.

Occasional X-ray findings are mild bowing of the radius and sometimes the ulna, square iliac wings, and a horizontal sacrum.

**Complications:** Unknown.

**Associated Findings:** Mental retardation, generally mild, has been reported in 20% of the cases.

**Etiology:** Autosomal or X-linked dominant inheritance. Male-to-male transmission has not been documented. Penetrance is unknown.

**Pathogenesis:** Unknown.

**MIM No.:** 11235

**POS No.:** 3461

**CDC No.:** 756.480

**Sex Ratio:** Presumably M1:F1; observed, M1:F:0.7

**Occurrence:** Forty-one cases have been reported in the literature.

**Risk of Recurrence for Patient's Sib:**
See Part I, *Mendelian Inheritance.*

**Risk of Recurrence for Patient's Child:**
See Part I, *Mendelian Inheritance.*

**Age of Detectability:** Usually at birth.

**Gene Mapping and Linkage:** Unknown.

**Prevention:** None known. Genetic counseling indicated.

**Treatment:** Unknown.

**Prognosis:** Normal life span. No functional impairment except for the delayed onset of walking.

**Detection of Carrier:** Unknown.

**References:**
Weismann-Netter R, Stuhl L: D'une ostéopathie congénitale éventuellement familiale. Presse Med 1954; 62:1618–1621. * †
Keats TE, Alavi SM: Toxopachyostéose diaphysaire tibio-péronière (Weismann-Netter syndrome). Am J Roentgenology 1970; 109:568–574.
Amendola MA, et al.: Weismann-Netter-Stuhl syndrome: toxopachyostéose diaphysaire tibio-péronière. Am J Roentgenology 1980; 135:1211–1215. †

R0004　　　　　　　　　　　　　　　**Meinhard Robinow**

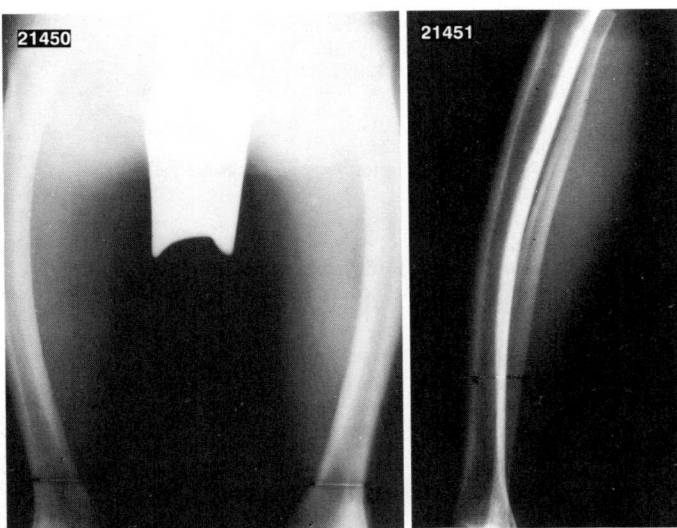

**2542B-21450:** X-ray showing lateral bowing of the femora.
**21451:** X-ray showing anterior bowing of the femora.

**Skeletal dysplasia-Robin anomaly-polydactyly**
　See CLEFT PALATE-DYSMORPHIC FACIES-DIGITAL DEFECTS, MARTSOLF TYPE
**Skeletal dysplasia-short rib-polydactyly, type III**
　See SHORT RIB-POLYDACTYLY SYNDROME, VERMA-NAUMOFF TYPE
**Skeletal dysplasia-sparse hair-dental anomalies**
　See CRANIO-ECTODERMAL DYSPLASIA
**Skeletal malformations-heart disease-conductive hearing loss**
　See MITRAL REGURGITATION-DEAFNESS-SKELETAL DEFECTS
**Skeletal malocclusion, class III**
　See MANDIBULAR PROGNATHISM
**Skeletal maturation (fast)-dysmorphic facies-failure to thrive**
　See MARSHALL-SMITH SYNDROME
**Skeletal-dermo-facio-cardio syndrome**
　See DERMO-FACIO-CARDIO-SKELETAL SYNDROME
**Skeletal-neuro-facio syndrome**
　See FACIO-NEURO-SKELETAL SYNDROME
**Skeleto-branchio-genital syndromes**
　See BRANCHIO-SKELETO-GENITAL SYNDROME
**Skewfoot**
　See FOOT, METATARSUS VARUS
**Skin (thin)-hydrocephalus-nephrosis-blue sclera-growth defect**
　See NEPHROSIS-HYDROCEPHALUS-THIN SKIN-BLUE SCLERA-GROWTH DEFECT
**Skin atrophy, linear**
　See ALOPECIA-SKIN ATROPHY-ANONYCHIA-TONGUE DEFECT
**Skin changes-typical facies-heart defect**
　See CARDIO-FACIAL-CUTANEOUS SYNDROME

## SKIN CREASE, SINGLE PALMAR                   2607

**Includes:**
Crease, single palmar
Four-finger line
Palm, single line
Palmar crease, single transverse
Simian crease, incomplete
Single transverse fold
Sydney line
Transverse crease, single

**Excludes:**
Proximal crease variations
Thenar crease variations

**Major Diagnostic Criteria:**  Fusion of the proximal and distal horizontal creases of the palm.

**Clinical Findings:**  Flexion of the fingers during the second month of gestation normally results in the formation of two horizontal creases, distal and proximal. Fusion of the two lines into a single palmar transverse crease is seen in 2–3% of the adult population. Two lines that approach and are joined by a third line or bridge are called an incomplete single palmar crease. The proximal horizontal palmar crease may traverse the entire palm in a final variant known as a Sydney line. All three findings are related and may be combinatorially found in a single individual.

**Complications:**  Single palmar creases do not affect function of the hand.

**Associated Findings:**  A single palmar crease is commonly associated with **Chromosome 21, trisomy 21** and has been reported to be increased in frequency among premature infants, stillborns, babies dying in the neonatal period, and infants with multiple congenital anomalies, **Fetal rubella syndrome, Chromosome 18, trisomy 18, Smith-Lemli-Opitz syndrome, Rubinstein-Taybi broad thumb-hallux syndrome**, and other conditions.

**Etiology:**  Heterogeneous. A higher frequency is seen in patients with chromosomal anomalies, congenital anomalies, stillbirth, neonatal death and prematurity. Siblings and other first degree relatives have a higher frequency of single palmar creases than expected by chance alone. At least one family has been reported in which the single palmar crease and its variants appears follow autosomal dominant inheritance with decreased penetrance.

**Pathogenesis:**  The single palmar crease is presumed to result from abnormal flexion of the fingers and hand during the first and second months of gestation. Normal infants with single palmar creases have not demonstrated abnormal hand movements or skeletal anomalies.

**Sex Ratio:**  M1:F<1. Among otherwise normal children, there appears to be a higher frequency of the single palmar crease in males. In one pedigree in which the single palmar crease appears to segregate as an autosomal dominant trait, penetrance is 10% in females and 100% in males, suggesting that in this family the single palmar crease is a sex-influenced trait.

**Occurrence:**  The incidence of the single palmar crease in neonates in the American population varies between 3–9%. Only 2–3% of older children and adults are so affected. The decline in prevalence results from the attrition of children with serious congenital abnormalities, and possibly from changes in palmar creases that occur with use of the hand. The prevalence of the single palmar crease varies with ethnic group, ranging as high as 13% in some isolated Chinese subpopulations.

**Risk of Recurrence for Patient's Sib:**  Accurate risks of recurrence in otherwise normal patients are still not determined. Based on a limited number of studies, risk ranges between 14 and 28%, with some variation by sex.

**Risk of Recurrence for Patient's Child:**  14–28% in a normal offspring.

**Age of Detectability:**  Evident by the second month of gestation.

**Gene Mapping and Linkage:**  Unknown.

**Prevention:**  None known. Genetic counseling indicated.

**Treatment:**  Unnecessary, since a single palmar crease will not alone impair the function of the hand of an affected individual.

**Prognosis:**  Because the incidence of the single palmar crease is increased in neonates with complex malformation syndromes, the presence of a single palmar crease should raise the physician's suspicion of abnormality. In the absence of other findings, in the presence of a positive family history of single palmar crease, or when the presence of the single palmar crease is first noted in a normal child of school age, the single palmar crease should be considered to be a normal variant. With the passage of time, the single palmar crease may become an incomplete single palmar crease or separate to form two normal creases.

**Detection of Carrier:**  Clinical examination.

**References:**
Davies PA, Smallpiece V: The single transverse palmar crease in infants and children. Dev Med Child Neurol 1963; 5:491–496.
Johnson CF, Optiz E: The single palmar crease and its clinical significance in a child development clinic: observations and correlations. Clin Pediatr 1971; 10:392–403.
Dar H, et al.: Palmar crease variants and their clinical significance: a study of newborns at risk. Pediatr Res 1977; 11:103–108.

SC058                                        **Harry W. Schroeder, Jr.**

## SKIN CREASES, ABSENT DISTAL INTERPHALANGEAL       2488

**Includes:**  Interphalangeal skin creases, absent distal

**Excludes:**
Interphalangeal crease, single, with deformity of middle phalanx
**Poland syndrome** (0813)
**Symphalangism** (1001)

**Major Diagnostic Criteria:**  Absence of interphalangeal distal creases without any associated malformations.

**Clinical Findings:**  Complete absence of the distal interphalangeal creases of fingers 2, 3, and 4 on the volar and dorsal sides of both hands. There are no nail abnormalities. No bone abnormalities or fusions are found on X-ray examination. Limitation of flexion of the distal interphalangeal joints may be present.

**Complications:**  Difficulties with finger extension have been reported in two cases.

**Associated Findings:**  Mental retardation was present in one case, but may have been fortuitous.

**Etiology:**  Autosomal dominant inheritance with complete penetrance and variable expressivity.

**Pathogenesis:**  One patient presented with absent distal skin creases, **Camptodactyly**, and clinodactyly. This subject was the mother of a child born with preaxial polydactyly type 1 and the **Poland syndrome**. Whether these anomalies represent a mild expression of the Poland syndrome remains to be determined.

**Sex Ratio:**  Presumably M1:F1

**Occurrence:**  Two kindreds have been reported.

**Risk of Recurrence for Patient's Sib:**
See Part I, *Mendelian Inheritance.*

**Risk of Recurrence for Patient's Child:**
See Part I, *Mendelian Inheritance.*

**Age of Detectability:**  Patients have been recognized at ages six and 13 years of age.

**Gene Mapping and Linkage:**  Unknown.

**Prevention:**  None known. Genetic counseling indicated.

**Treatment:**  Unknown.

**Prognosis:**  Good except for two patients in whom decreased flexion of the fingers seemed to be progressive; the patients complained of not being able to play a musical instrument.

**Detection of Carrier:**  Unknown.

**Special Considerations:**  The condition described has some resemblance to a family described with distal symphalangism (Inman et al, 1924; Steinberg and Reynolds, 1948) in which all the patients, except for one (aged three years) presented with bone fusion and absent interphalangeal skin creases.

**References:**
Inman OL et al.: Four generations of symphalangism. J Hered 1924; 15:329–334.
Daniel GH: A case of hereditary anarthrosis of the index finger, with associated abnormalities in the proportion of the fingers. Ann Eugen 1936; 7:281–297.
Steinberg AG, Reynolds EL: Further data on symphalangism. J Hered 1948; 39:23–27.
Fried K, Mundel G: Absence of distal interphalangeal creases of fingers with flexion limitation. J Med Genet 1976; 13:127–130.
Lambert D et al.: Absence of distal interphalangeal fold causing difficulty in extending fingers. J Med Gen 1977; 14:466–467.
Halal F: Minor manifestations in preaxial polydactyly type 1 and Poland complex. Am J Med Genet 1981; 8:221–228.

MJ038                                           **Giuseppe Micali**

**Skin creases, multiple benign circumferential of the limbs**
*See MICHELIN TIRE BABY SYNDROME*

---

**SKIN CREASES, RETICULATE PIGMENTED FLEXURES, DOWLING-DEGOS TYPE**                 **2393**

**Includes:**
Dark dot disease
Dowling-Degos disease (DDD)
Genodermatose en cocarde of Degos
Haber syndrome (some)
Kitamura acropigmentatio reticularis
Reticular pigmented anomaly of flexures

**Excludes:**
Follicular hamartoma, familial multiple
**Skin, acanthosis nigricans** (0005)
**Skin, erythrokeratolysis hiemalis** (2862)

**Major Diagnostic Criteria:** Characteristic, progressive, pigmented maculae in the flexural areas.

**Clinical Findings:** Reticulate pigmented anomaly of the flexures initially affects the axilla and the groin; later in life, other areas, including the intergluteal and inframammary folds, neck, trunk, arms, and wrists, may be involved. The pigmented lesions consist of punctate macules dappled peripherally (2–5 mm); confluence of lesions toward the vault of the axillae and the center of the genitocrural fold is frequent. A shiny and wrinkled appearance of the affected areas sometimes may give an impression of atrophy. Additional signs include the presence of small, pitted, acneform scars around the mouth and scattered dark comedo-like hyperkeratotic follicular lesions on the neck and axillary margins (the so-called *dark dot follicles*). The pigmentation is progressive and asymptomatic; once established, it is thought to be permanent.

**Complications:** In some patients, sun exposure may lead to an exacerbation of the hyperpigmentation. Friction and pressure may also induce pigmentation.

**Associated Findings:** Moderate mental retardation (three cases) and epidermal or trichilemmal cysts (four cases) have been reported. Multiple large seborrheic warts were present in one case.

**Etiology:** Possibly autosomal dominant inheritance with possibly variable penetrance and expressivity.

**Pathogenesis:** Unknown. It is undetermined whether the epidermal proliferation is related to an excess production of melanosomes or a passive retention of melanin.

**MIM No.:** 17985

**Sex Ratio:** M1:F1

**Occurrence:** Undetermined but presumed rare.

**Risk of Recurrence for Patient's Sib:**
See Part I, *Mendelian Inheritance.*

**Risk of Recurrence for Patient's Child:**
See Part I, *Mendelian Inheritance.*

**Age of Detectability:** Possibly during childhood, but the majority of cases are detected during the third to fourth decade of life.

**Gene Mapping and Linkage:** Unknown.

**Prevention:** None known. Genetic counseling indicated.

**Treatment:** Unknown.

**Prognosis:** A benign genodermatosis, but there are cosmetic problems caused by a diffuse hyperpigmentation in some patients.

**Detection of Carrier:** Unknown.

**Special Considerations:** Since it has been noted that Dowling-Degos disease, *Haber syndrome*, and *Kitamura acropigmentatio reticularis* show a very similar histopathologic pattern (epidermal digitate budding, extensive proliferation of the epidermal walls), it has been proposed to include all of these under a spectrum of diseases with different clinical features, but sharing a unique histologic picture.

**References:**
Dowling GB, Freudenthal W: Acanthosis nigricans. Br J Dermatol 1938; 50:467–471.
Degos R, Ossipowski B: Dermatose pigmentaire reticulee des plis. Ann Dermatol Syphilol 1954; 81:147–151.
Howell JB, Freeman RG: Reticular pigmented anomaly of the flexures. Arch Dermatol 1978; 114:400–403.
Jones EW, Grice K: Reticulatd pigmented anomaly of the flexures: Dowling-Degos disease, a new genodermatosis. Arch Dermatol 1978; 114:1150–1157.
Grosshans E, et al.: Ultrastructure of early pigmentary changes in Dowling-Degos disease. J Cutan Pathol 1980; 7:77–87.
Brown WG: Reticulated pigmented anomaly of the flexures: case reports and genetic investigation. Arch Dermatol 1982; 118:490–493.
Kikuchi I, et al.: The broad spectrum of Dowling-Degos disease, including Haber's syndrome: a hereditary abnormal reactivity to stimulation, increasing with age? J Dermatol (Tokyo) 1983; 10:361–375.
Rebora A, Crovato F: The spectrum of Dowling-Degos disease. Br J Dermatol 1984; 110:627–630.
Rebora A, Crovato F: Pigmentatio reticularis faciei et colli. Arch Dermatol 1985; 121:968 only.
Crovato F, Rebora A: Reticulate pigmented anomaly of the flexures associating reticulate acropigmentation. J Am Acad Dermatol 1986; 14:359–361.
Reymond JL, et al.: Dowling-Degos disease (reticulate pigmentation of the flexures) [in French] Ann Dermatol Venereo 1986; 113:249–251

MI038                                           **Giuseppe Micali**

**Skin lesions, papular**
*See SKIN, ELASTOSIS PERFORANS SERPIGINOSA*
**Skin lesions-seizures-mental retardation**
*See HYPOMELANOSIS OF ITO*

---

**SKIN PEELING SYNDROME**                        **2864**

**Includes:**
Deciduous skin, idiopathic
Keratolysis exfoliativa congenita
Skin peeling, familial continual

**Excludes:**
**Ichthyosiform hyperkeratosis, bullous congenital** (2852)
**Ichthyosis, linearis circumflexa** (2858)
Pemphigus foliaceus
**Skin, erythrokeratolysis hiemalis** (2862)
Staphylococcal scalded skin syndrome

**Major Diagnostic Criteria:** Periodic or continuous shedding of whole sheets of stratum corneum. Histopathology demonstrates a split within the lower stratum corneum.

**Clinical Findings:** Ichthyosis is reported in most patients from birth, but the onset may be delayed until late childhood in some cases. All cases exhibit the ability to manually peel large sheets of intact stratum corneum. Palms and soles may be hyperkeratotic but do not peel. Other clinical features, such as the presence or absence of erythroderma, pruritis, easily plucked anagen hairs, or seasonal exacerbation, are variable. Histopathology in patients with erythroderma demonstrates a psoriasiform dermatitis with hyperkeratosis and parakeratosis, while in nonerythrodermic patients the epidermis is unremarkable except for hyperkeratosis. The split occurs within the lower stratum corneum.

**Complications:**  Unknown.

**Associated Findings:**  Short stature. Generalized aminoaciduria with decreased plasma tryptophan levels.

**Etiology:**  Autosomal recessive inheritance is evidenced by reports of consanguinity, more than one affected sib, and absence of vertical transmission. Variability of onset and other clinical features may reflect underlying genetic heterogeneity.

**Pathogenesis:**  Unknown. A generalized aminoaciduria with low plasma tryptophan levels has been reported in some patients. Electron microscopy of the skin in one study demonstrated an intracellular cleavage within the stratum corneum with dense intercellular globular deposits, believed to represent lipid-like material.

**MIM No.:**  *27030

**CDC No.:**  757.900

**Sex Ratio:**  M1:F1

**Occurrence:**  About 20 cases have been reported in the literature, including cases from India, Kuwait, and the United States.

**Risk of Recurrence for Patient's Sib:**
See Part I, *Mendelian Inheritance.*

**Risk of Recurrence for Patient's Child:**
See Part I, *Mendelian Inheritance.*

**Age of Detectability:**  Usually during infancy, but may be delayed until the end of the second decade.

**Gene Mapping and Linkage:**  Unknown.

**Prevention:**  None known. Genetic counseling indicated.

**Treatment:**  Unknown.

**Prognosis:**  Lifelong once established.

**Detection of Carrier:**  Unknown.

**Special Considerations:**  The acquired disorders of pemphigus foliaceus and staphylococcal scalded skin syndrome show cleavage at the stratum granulosum-stratum corneum interface.

**References:**
Kurban AK, Azar HA: Familial continual skin peeling. Br J Dermatol 1969; 81:191–195. * †
Levy SB, Goldsmith LA: The peeling skin syndrome. J Am Acad Dermatol 1982; 7:606–613. * †
Abdel-Hafez K, et al.: Familial continual skin peeling. Dermatologica 1983; 166:22–31.
Silverman AK, et al.: Continual skin peeling syndrome: an electron microscopic study. Arch Dermatol 1986; 122:71–75. †

WI013                                              **Mary L. Williams**

**Skin peeling, familial continual**
*See SKIN PEELING SYNDROME*
**Skin pigmentation-short stature, X-linked**
*See SILVER SYNDROME, X-LINKED*

## SKIN TUMORS, MULTIPLE GLOMUS                             0416

**Includes:**  Glomus tumors, multiple

**Excludes:**
Solitary glomangioma
Solitary glomus tumor

**Major Diagnostic Criteria:**  Positive diagnosis by biopsy. The characteristic histopathologic features are endothelial-lined dilated vascular spaces which are surrounded by one or more layers of the oval glomus tumor (smooth muscle) cells.

**Clinical Findings:**  Multiple flesh-colored to blue nodules in the skin, 0.3 to 3.0 cm in diameter. They may occasionally involve deeper structures such as bone. The lesions are usually regional but may be generalized. The lesions are soft, movable, and sometimes tender. No changes are ordinarily seen in the overlying epidermis.

**Complications:**  Unknown.

**Associated Findings:**  A case has been reported with deformities of the affected limb consisting of hypoplasia with precocious closure of the epiphyses and bradymetacarpia. Another case had some atrophy of the affected limb and (by arteriography) many abnormal ballooning blood vessels at the end of arteries and arteriovenous anastomoses corresponding to tumors.

**Etiology:**  Autosomal dominant inheritance has been seen in several families.

**Pathogenesis:**  Possibly a benign hyperplasia of the normal cutaneous arteriovenous anastomosis.

**MIM No.:**  *13800

**CDC No.:**  757.900

**Sex Ratio:**  M1+:F1

**Occurrence:**  About 50 cases in the medical literature.

**Risk of Recurrence for Patient's Sib:**
See Part I, *Mendelian Inheritance.*

**Risk of Recurrence for Patient's Child:**
See Part I, *Mendelian Inheritance.*

**Age of Detectability:**  The average age of development of the regional type is 29 years and that of the generalized type 40 years. One-third of all cases appear before age 20. Some cases have been apparent at birth.

**Gene Mapping and Linkage:**  Unknown.

**Prevention:**  None known. Genetic counseling indicated.

**Treatment:**  Surgical excision of the lesion.

**Prognosis:**  Normal for life span and intelligence. Functional disability may result from pain or rarely, deformity of the limb. The lesions have no malignant potential.

**Detection of Carrier:**  Unknown.

**References:**
Sluiter JT, Postma C: Multiple glomus tumors of the skin. Acta Dermatol Venereol (Stockh) 1959 39:98.
Gorlin RJ, et al.: Multiple glomus tumor of the pseudocavernous hemangioma type. Arch Derm 1960; 82:776–778.
Gordon B, Hyman AB: Multiple nontender glomus tumors: report of a case with 33 lesions. Arch Dermatol 1961; 83:640.
Goodman TF Jr, Abele DC: Multiple glomus tumors: a clinical and electron microscopic study. Arch Dermatol 1971; 103:11.
Beasley SW, et al.: Hereditary multiple glomus tumours. Arch Dis Child 1986; 61:801–802.

WA046                                              **Silas Wallk**

## SKIN, ACANTHOSIS NIGRICANS                    0005

**Includes:**

    Acanthosis nigricans
    Drug-induced insulin resistance
    Insulin resistance, autosomal dominant type
    Insulin resistance, drug induced type
    Malignant acanthosis nigricans (AN)

**Excludes:**

    Acanthosis nigricans, Hirschowitz type
    Dermatosis papulosa nigra
    Generalized cutaneous papillomatosis
    **Leprechaunism** (0587)

**Major Diagnostic Criteria:** A skin eruption characterized by velvety hyperkeratotic macules, which can be accompanied by various degrees of pigmentation, affecting the entire skin but preferentially the axilla, neck, genitalia, and oral cavity. Acanthosis nigricans (AN) can be accompanied by an internal malignancy, especially an adenocarcinoma of the stomach, or can be associated with insulin resistance, Crouzon Seip, and Beare syndromes; drug

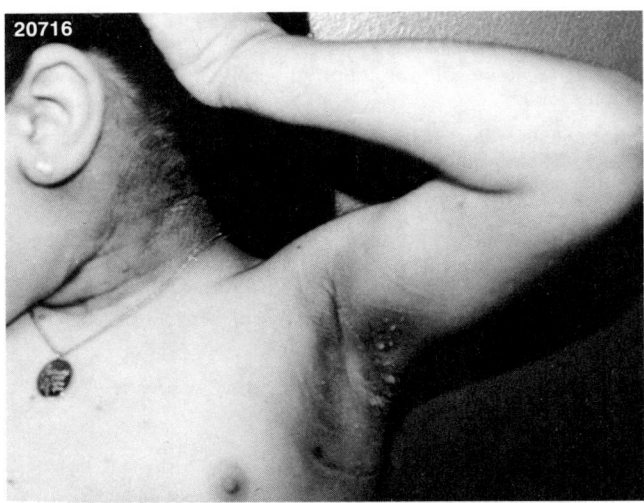

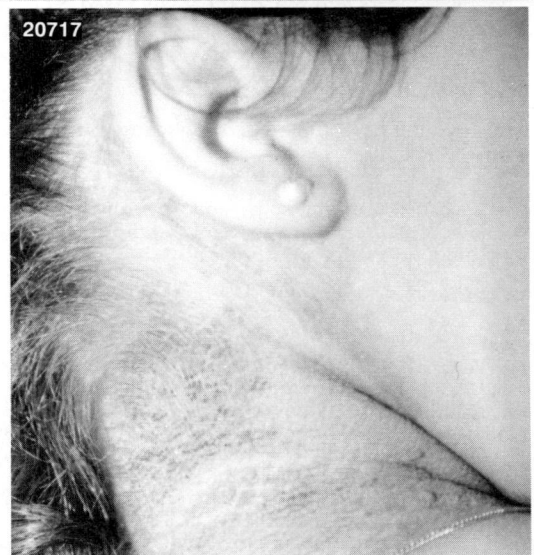

**0005-20716–17:** Acanthosis nigricans; note dark, hyperpigmented, raised lesion in the axilla and the neck.

eruptions and miscellaneous diseases; or it could be inherited as an autosomal dominant.

**Clinical Findings:** The classical presentation consists of dark-brown, velvety, hyperkeratotic macules; there may be slight discoloration or the entire skin may be affected. The body regions affected by AN, in descending order of frequency, are as follows: axillae, neck, genitalia, groin and inner thighs, umbilicus, perianal area, other flexural surfaces, and areolas. Pigmentation of either the axillae or the neck, or both, usually occurs before other areas are involved. Normal skin margins are accentuated.

Multiple, rapidly growing seborrheic keratoses (sign of Leser-Trélat) and florid cutaneous papillomatosis are part of the clinical findings.

About 40% of those cases associated with internal malignancy have oral manifestations, especially of the tongue and lips. The tongue may have hypertrophy and elongation of papillae, deep fissures, and papillomatous growths. Oral lesions are non-pigmented. Lip, buccal mucosa, and palate may be similarly affected. Occasional cases affecting the gingiva may resemble idiopathic fibromatosis. Marked perioral papillomatosis is a frequent finding. Only 15% of cases not associated with internal malignancy have oral manifestations.

In the neoplastic association type, about 75% of the associated tumors are abdominal adenocarcinomas, of which 60% arise in the stomach. Adenocarcinomas of the uterus, pancreas, intestine, and, to a lesser extent, bladder, lung, and breast, can also be associated with AN. These carcinomas have a high degree of malignancy. In about 20% of cases, AN precedes the malignancy by up to 16 years. It parallels the cancer in proportion to the degree of spread; it may regress with radiation therapy or with surgical removal of the tumor, and it may reflourish with recurrence of the adenocarcinoma. Generalized skin hyperpigmentation and pruritus occur in about 40% of cases of the neoplastic association type, and palmar and plantar hyperkeratosis is seen in about 25% of these cases. The vaginal, conjunctival, esophageal, and pharyngeal mucosas can be the site of papillary and verrucous lesions.

The insulin-resistant types have been divided in two groups. Type A (HAIR-AN syndrome) is mostly observed in adolescent or young females, and is characterized by hyperandrogenism, insulin resistance, and AN. Virilization, polycystic ovaries, and accelerated growth are also present. Leprechaunism also falls into this type. Type B is observed in older females with autoimmune disorders. Other endocrinopathies and obesity are also associated with AN, as well as some cases of Bloom, Crouzon, Seip and Beare syndromes. Injection of some drugs, such as nicotinic acid, also may induce AN.

**Complications:** In the neoplastic association type, metastasis and complications due to radiation therapy are expected.

In the insulin-resistant types, complications are derived from the basic defect.

**Associated Findings:** Deep skin margins on the neck can be seen in some patients.

The gingiva, especially the interdental papillae, may become so enlarged as to almost cover the teeth, resembling idiopathic fibromatosis.

**Etiology:** Autosomal dominant or recessive inheritance. It has been suggested that this condition is produced by a peptide or group of peptides. In some patients it is due to genetic defects in insulin receptor pathways.

**Pathogenesis:** It is assumed that the responsible peptides may be produced by the adenocarcinomas and might be present in the endocrinopathies. Growth hormone, adrenocorticotropin and luteinizing hormones have also been thought responsible for the skin changes of AN.

**MIM No.:** *10060, *18730, 20017, *24309, *26970

**CDC No.:** 757.900

**Sex Ratio:** M1:F1 in neoplastic association type; M1:F5 in insulin-resistant types.

**Occurrence:** Some 1,500 cases have been reported to date.

**Risk of Recurrence for Patient's Sib:**
See Part I, *Mendelian Inheritance.*

**Risk of Recurrence for Patient's Child:**
See Part I, *Mendelian Inheritance.*

**Age of Detectability:** More then 80% of affected persons with the neoplastic association type are over 40 years old at the time of onset. Patients with the insulin-resistant types are generally diagnosed during childhood or early adolescence.

**Gene Mapping and Linkage:** Unknown.

**Prevention:** None known. Genetic counseling indicated.

**Treatment:** Neoplastic association type requires oncologic treatment; AN may regress with radiation therapy or with surgical excision of the malignancy involved. Insulin-resistant types will regress with the adequate hormonal treatment.

**Prognosis:** For the neoplastic association type, the mortality rate is 100% and the average survival period after discovery is less than 2 years. For the nonneoplastic association types, the patients have a normal life span.

**Detection of Carrier:** By clinical examination.

**Special Considerations:** Acanthosis nigricans appears not only as a sign of Type A and Type B insulin resistance, but as a sign of the insulin resistance seen in **Leprechaunism.**

**References:**

Rigel DS, Jacobs MI: Malignant acanthosis nigricans: a review. J Dermatol Surg Oncol 1980; 6:923–927.

Andreev VC, et al.: Generalized acanthosis nigricans. Dermatologica 1981; 163:19–24.

Barbieri RL, Ryan KJ: Hyperandrogenism, insulin resistance, and acanthosis nigricans syndrome: a common endocrinopathy with distinct pathophysiologic features. Am J Obstet Gynecol 1983; 147:90–101.

Flier JS: Metabolic importance of acanthosis nigricans. Arch Dermatol 1985; 121:193–194.

Flier JS, et al.: Acanthosis nigricans in obese women with hyperandrogenism: characterization of an insulin-resistant state distinct from the type A and B syndromes. Diabetes 1985; 34:101–107.

SE007 **Heddie O. Sedano**

**Skin, acrokeratosis verruciformis**
*See ACROKERATOSIS VERRUCIFORMIS*

## SKIN, ATOPY, FAMILIAL                                3150

**Includes:**
Allergic diathesis
Allergic rhinitis
Asthma, inherited
Atopic dermatitis
Atopic diathesis with asthma and hayfever
Atopic hypersensitivity
Eczema, atopic
Hayfever, atopic
Prurigo Besnier

**Excludes:**
Croup and Acute epiglotitis
**Cystic fibrosis** (0237)
Hypersensitivity pneumonitis
Infections of the bronchopulmonary system, all
Laryngotracheobronthitis
Lichen simplex chronicus

**Major Diagnostic Criteria:** *Atopic dermatitis:* Usually demonstrates some of the following basic features: pruritis; typical morphology and distribution; flexural lichenification or linearity in adults; facial and extensor involvement in infants and children; chronic or chronically relapsing eczematous dermatitis; personal or family history of atopy (asthma, allergic rhinitis, or atopic dermatitis). Other features include xerosis, immediate skin test reactivity, elevated serum IgE, early age of onset, tendency toward cutaneous infections, tendency towards nonspecific hand or foot derma-

titis, nipple eczema, cheilitis, recurrent conjunctivitis, Dennie-Morgan infraorbital fold, keratoconus, anterior and or posterior subcapsular cataracts, orbital darkening, facial pallor/facial erythema, pityriasis alba, anterior neck folds, itch when sweating, intolerance to wool and lipid solvents, perifollicular accentuation, food intolerance, a course influenced by environmental/emotional factors, and white dermographism.

*Asthma:* 1) presence of significant, obstructive ventilatory abnormality in tests of ventilatory mechanics, 2) presence in some patients of associated cough, chest tightness, wheezing, or dyspnea.

**Clinical Findings:** *Atopic dermatitis:* usually onset is in infancy, occurring frequently at about three months of age. The lesions involve the face at first, but spreading to trunk and extremities does occur. It is always an eczematous inflammation. This may resolve or evolve into the classic pattern of chronic lichenification in antecubital area and popliteal fossa. By the end of the second year of life, many patients have healed, but others continue into the childhood phase, which includes, in addition to face and flexural involvement, involvement of the hands, feet, and sometimes the buttocks and backs of the thighs. The condition is chronic but may alternate between symptom-free intervals and relapses.

*Asthma:* The attacks of infants are generally associated with respiratory infections. Between infections, the infant is generally free of chest symptoms, although some infants may have persistent wheezing.

**Complications:** *Of bronchial asthma:* infections, such as otitis media, sinusitis, bronchitis, pneumonitis, atelectasis, pneumomediastinum and pneumothorax, growth complications, psychologic problems, bronchopulmonary aspergillosis, respiratory failure.

*Of atopic dermatitis:* decreased cell-mediated immunity and malfunctioning chemotaxis are associated with increased occurrence of staphylococcal, viral (including warts, herpes simplex, and molluscum contagiosum), and dermatophytic infections of the skin. Chronically affected areas of the skin may show hyperpigmentation and even depigmentation, related to excessive rubbing and inflammation. Ocular complications include mild conjunctivitis to bilateral cataracts. Cataracts may affect 5–10% of severely affected individuals.

**Associated Findings: Urticaria, dermo-distortive type, Migraine headaches,** drug sensitivity, **Ichthyosis vulgaris,** keratosis pilaris, vitiligo, and **Hair, alopecia areata.**

**Etiology:** Probably autosomal dominant inheritance, with clinical expression dependent on interaction with other factors. Previously, most authors had generally accepted "multifactorial environmental influences on a genetic predisposition". There is also evidence for autosomal recessive inheritance, and for the contribution of several HLA-linked interactive genes.

**Pathogenesis:** For *asthma,* bronchial hyperreactivity. For *atopic eczema,* the role of IgE has been considered in depth, including total serum IgE levels and the propensity to produce IgE in response to common, usually inhaled allergens. Yet patients with agammaglobulinemia do manifest atopic disease. The primary cause of the disease remains unknown. The immunological problems may be secondary to a more pervasive disorder of metabolism.

**MIM No.:** 20920

**Sex Ratio:** *Eczema,* M2:F1 in several studies. Until puberty, *asthma* is approximately twice as common in boys as in girls. The more severe the asthma, the greater preponderance of male over female children. As age increases, there is a reversal of this trend, with female cases predominating in older age groups.

**Occurrence:** *Asthma:* prevalence ranges from a low of 0.06% in Finland, to 1.4% in Sweden, to 8.9% in United States, to 11.4% in Australia.

*Atopic dermatitis:* prevalence is 3.1% among children up to five years of age in England. 19:1,000 among children in United States.

The frequency of eczema in patients with asthma or allergic rhinitis is poorly documented.

The frequency of allergic respiratory symptoms in patients with atopic eczema is approximately 1:3.

**Risk of Recurrence for Patient's Sib:** Multiple factors will determine an individual's risk. One study reported an average risk of 32% if only one other sibling is affected, and the parents are not affected (Kjellman, 1977).

**Risk of Recurrence for Patient's Child:** For atopy, risk figures vary from 15% to 72%, based upon the types of atopy and if one or both parents are affected (Kjellman, 1977).

**Age of Detectability:** *Atopic eczema*: during infancy or early childhood; rarely before six weeks of age.

**Gene Mapping and Linkage:** APY (atopy (allergic asthma and rhinitis)) has been provisionally mapped to 11q12-q13.
There is a possible HLA linkage.

**Prevention:** None known. Genetic counseling indicated.

**Treatment:** *For atopic dermatitis*: topical corticosteroids, tar preparation. Avoidance of extremes in environmental temperature and humidity; avoidance of wool and synthetic fibers on the skin.
*For asthma*: bronchodilators.

**Prognosis:** Although most deaths from *asthma* occur in adults, a significant number do occur in children. Asthma may spontaneously disappear with increasing age after a number of years, and the percentage of patients who continue to have severe disease is relatively low.
*Atopic dermatitis*: figures for persistence of disease vary from 70% in severe cases to 10% overall.
*Allergic rhinitis*: usually persists for many years, and is less likely to remit than asthma.

**Detection of Carrier:** Unknown.

**References:**

Kjellman II: Atopic disease in seven-year-old children: incidence in relation to family history. Acta Paediatr Scand 1977; 66:465–470.
Hanifin JM: Atopic Dermatitis. J Allergy Clin Immunol 1984; 73:211–226.
Saarinen Ulla M: Prophylaxis for atopic disease: role of infant disease. Clin Rev Allergy 1984; 2:151–167.
Borecki IB, et al.: Demonstration of a common major gene with pleiotropic effects on immunoglobulin E levels and allergy. Genet Epidemiol 1985; 2:327–328.
Siegel C: Asthma in infants and children. J Allergy Clin Immunol 1985; 76:1–15.
Rajka G: Natural history and clinical manifestations of atopic dermatitis. Clin Rev Allergy 1986; 4:3–26.
Blumenthal MN, Amos DB: Genetic and Immunologic Basis of atopic responses. Chest 1987; 91:176S–184S.
Cookson WL, Hopkin JM: Dominant and inheritance of atopic immunoglobulin-E responsiveness. Lancet 1988; I:86–88.

FI031 **Cheryl Nagel Fialkoff**

**Skin, atrophy-anonychia-alopecia-tongue defect**
*See ALOPECIA-SKIN ATROPHY-ANONYCHIA-TONGUE DEFECT*

---

## SKIN, CUTANEOUS MELANOSIS, DIFFUSE    2309

**Includes:**
  Cutaneous melanosis (diffuse)
  Hyperpigmentation, familial progressive
  Melanoderma, familial generalized

**Excludes:**
  **Neurocutaneous melanosis** (2014)
  **Skin, hyperpigmentation, familial** (2362)

**Major Diagnostic Criteria:** Diffuse macular pigmentary darkening which intensifies and becomes more widespread over time. Affected individuals are otherwise healthy.

**Clinical Findings:** Children are born with spotted reticulated, striated, and whorled hyperpigmentation including the oral mucosa but sparing palms, soles, conjunctiva (which later become pigmented as the child ages). There is at birth hyperpigmentation of the forehead, lateral face, back, extensor surface of extremities,

and scrotum. Pigmentary darkening and new dark macules develop later (Chernosky et al, 1971). Melanosomes are increased in size and number compared to normal.

**Complications:** Unknown.

**Associated Findings:** None known.

**Etiology:** Possibly X-linked or autosomal dominant inheritance.

**Pathogenesis:** Unknown.

**CDC No.:** 757.900

**Sex Ratio:** Presumably M1:F1

**Occurrence:** Described in at least one kindred.

**Risk of Recurrence for Patient's Sib:**
  See Part I, *Mendelian Inheritance.*

**Risk of Recurrence for Patient's Child:**
  See Part I, *Mendelian Inheritance.*

**Age of Detectability:** As early as childhood.

**Gene Mapping and Linkage:** Unknown.

**Prevention:** None known. Genetic counseling indicated.

**Treatment:** None required.

**Prognosis:** Normal lifespan is expected.

**Detection of Carrier:** Unknown.

**Special Considerations:** A variant is one reported case in a Mexican child born white who then became progressively dark to resemble a black panther with intense Black melanosis of all skin, hair and mucosa (see **Skin, hyperpigmentation, familial**). Melanocyte numbers were normal. Electron microscope showed increased numbers of melanosomes in keratinocytes.

**References:**

Chernosky HE, et al.: Familial Progressive Hyperpigmentation. Arch Derm 1971; 103:581.
Ruiz-Maldonaldo R, et al.: Universal Acquired Melanosis: the Carbon Baby. Arch Derm 1978;114:775.

M0040 **David B. Mosher**

---

## SKIN, CUTANEOUS MELANOSIS: MONGOLIAN SPOT    3206

**Includes:**
  Child spot
  Congenital dermal melanocytosis (CDM)
  Mongolian spot
  Cutaneous melanosis: mongolian spot

**Excludes:**
  **Nevus of Ota** (0716)
  Nevus of Ito

**Major Diagnostic Criteria:** Mongolian spot is a congenital circumscribed melanocytosis which is very common in Orientals and much less so in Caucasians. The sacrum is the classic site of involvement but extra-sacral locations occur.

**Clinical Findings:** There are several types of mongolian spots. The classic or common mongolian spot (MS) occurs over the back and lumbosacral regions; the extra-sacral or aberrant spot which is less frequent occurs elsewhere. There is a well circumscribed variant with sharp discrete margins. A persistent type also occurs ("persistent mongolian spot"). Up to 90% of Asiatics and Amerindians, but less than 10% of Caucasians, are affected. The persistent MS occurs in 3–4%. The classic MS is a blue-green uniformly colored with indistinct, feathered margins and involves the buttock and lumbosacral region bilaterally and not the anus. Lesions may be centimeters in diameter and may cover the entire low back and buttocks. Sharp margins are seen in large lesions. Extra-sacral MS are found on the face or extremities or elsewhere.

A **Cleft lip** - MS type is also described (but not in Caucasians). A special type includes atypical blue nevus type 2, which is an overlap of MS and nevus spots. Overlap with **Nevus flammeus** also occurs.

Studies have shown the dermal melanosis to be present microscopically in the three month fetus and macroscopically at seven months. Pigment density appears greatest at one year and diminishes slowly thereafter; the size of the macule however, reaches maximal dimensions at age two years. Microscopic presence of melanocytes is routine (melanocytes may be DOPA negative). Regression is usually more characteristic of smaller lesions.

**Complications:** Unknown.

**Associated Findings:** None known.

**Etiology:** Unknown.

**Pathogenesis:** Persistence may be related to the presence of a fibrous sheath which is gradually lost and dislodged in a regressing lesion.

**Sex Ratio:** M1:F1

**Occurrence:** Reported in as high as 90% of Asians, but only 10% of Caucasians. Other population groups range between these figures.

**Risk of Recurrence for Patient's Sib:** Presumably not increased.

**Risk of Recurrence for Patient's Child:** Presumably not increased.

**Age of Detectability:** At birth.

**Gene Mapping and Linkage:** Unknown.

**Prevention:** None known. Genetic counseling indicated.

**Treatment:** Cosmetic coverup with Covermark^ (Lydia O'Leary) or Dermablend^ (Flori Roberts). Treatment by laser therapy may be useful in cases of persistent MS.

**Prognosis:** Some 96–97% fade nearly or completely by age ten years.

**Detection of Carrier:** Unknown.

**Special Considerations:** A different type of dermal melanocytosis has been described by Lever in a case of what appeared to be a mongolian spot of the nose at age eight. Extensive dermal melanocytosis was found on biopsy. At age 13, metastatic melanoma was discovered in liver and lymph nodes. Autopsy showed diffuse dermal, visceral and cranial melanosis but only melanophages were present in visceral and cranial tissues.

**References:**
Morooka K: On the Mongolian spot in the Japanese. Acta Anat Jpn 1931; 3:1371.
Hidano A: Persistent Mongolian spot in the adult. Arch Dermatol 1971; 103:680.
Levene A: Disseminated dermal melanocytosis terminating in melanoma: a human condition resembling equine melanotic disease. Br J Derm 1979; 101:197.
Fitzpatrick TB, et al., eds: Dermal melanocytosis (Mongolian spot) in biology and disease of dermal pigmentation. Tokyo: Tokyo Press, 1981:83–94.

M0040 **David B. Mosher**

**Skin, Darier disease**
*See DARIER DISEASE*

---

## SKIN, ELASTOSIS PERFORANS SERPIGINOSA     0339

**Includes:**
Elastoma intrapapillarea perforans verruciforme
Elastosis perforans serpiginosa
Keratosis follicularis serpiginosa
Miescher elastoma
Skin lesions, papular

**Excludes:**
**Skin, Kyrle disease** (0561)
**Skin, porokeratosis** (0819)

**Major Diagnostic Criteria:** Keratotic papules characterized histologically by extrusion of dermal elastic tissue through the epidermis.

**Clinical Findings:** Skin colored, slightly erythematous keratotic papules arranged in arcs, circles, or without particular configuration. These lesions spread peripherally and may become hypopigmented and centrally atrophic. Most frequently observed on the neck and upper extrmities.

**Complications:** Development of keloidal scar following surgical manipulation or electrodesiccation of the skin lesions.

**Associated Findings:** In 26% of the reported cases, elastosis perforans serpiginosa has occurred in association with various heritable disorders such as **Chromosome 21, trisomy 21, Ehlers-Danlos syndrome, Pseudoxanthoma elasticum, Rothmund-Thomson syndrome, Marfan syndrome,** and **Osteogenesis imperfecta.** In several instances, elastosis perforans serpiginosa occurred in patients with **Hepatolenticular degeneration** and **Cystinuria** during treatment with penicillamine.

**Etiology:** Possibly autosomal dominant inheritance.

**Pathogenesis:** Localized increase of dermal elastic fibers with secondary epidermal and follicular epithelial hyperplasia and transepithelial elimination of the elastic fibers through multiple perforating channels.

**MIM No.:** 13010

**CDC No.:** 757.900

**Sex Ratio:** M4:F1

**Occurrence:** Over 120 cases reported.

**Risk of Recurrence for Patient's Sib:**
See Part I, *Mendelian Inheritance.*

**Risk of Recurrence for Patient's Child:**
See Part I, *Mendelian Inheritance.*

**Age of Detectability:** Ninety percent of the patients with elastosis perforans serpiginosa are younger than 30 years of age.

**Gene Mapping and Linkage:** Unknown.

**Prevention:** None known. Genetic counseling indicated.

**Treatment:** Cyrotherapy and tape stripping can be useful therapies. Corticosteroids, local or intralesional, have had little effect. Surgery or electroderscation can result in keloid formation.

**Prognosis:** Normal life expectancy.

**Detection of Carrier:** Unknown.

**References:**
Mehregan AH: Elastosis perforans serpiginosa: a review of the literature and report of 11 cases. Arch Dermatol 1968; 97:381.
Mehregan AH: Perforating dermatoses: a clinicopathologic review. Int J Dermatol 1977; 16:19.
Bardach H, et al.: "Lumpy-bumpy" elastic fibers in the skin and lungs of a patient with a penicillamine-induced elastosis perforans serpiginosa. J Cutan Pathol 1979; 6:243.
Sfar Z, et al.: Deux cas d'elastomes verruciformes apres administration prolongee de D-penicillamine. Ann Dermatol Venereol 1982; 109: 813–814.
Ayala F, Donofrio P: Elastosis perforans serpiginosa: report of a family. Dermatologica 1983; 166:32–37.
Patterson JW: The perforating disorders. J Am Acad Derm 1984; 10:561–581.

S0009 **Lawrence M. Solomon**

---

## SKIN, ERYTHROKERATODERMIA, PROGRESSIVA SYMMETRICA     2863

**Includes:**
Erythematokeratotic phacomatosis
Erythrokeratodermia figurata, congenital familial, in plaques

**Excludes:**
**Giroux-Barbeau syndrome** (2866)
**Skin, erythrokeratodermia, variable** (0361)
**Skin, erythrokeratolysis hiemalis** (2862)
**Skin, pityriasis rubra pilaris** (0811)
**Skin, psoriasis vulgaris** (0833)

**Major Diagnostic Criteria:** Onset in infancy and early childhood of symmetric hyperkeratotic erythematous plaques on head, buttocks, and extremities. **Skin, psoriasis vulgaris** and **Skin, pityriasis rubra pilaris** must be excluded by response to therapy and histopathology.

**Clinical Findings:** Well-demarcated erythematous, hyperkeratotic plaques that are absolutely symmetrically distributed on the head, buttocks, and extremities, but sparing the trunk. The lesions are not present at birth; they begin in infancy, stabilize after 1–2 years, and often partially regress at puberty. The palms and soles may be involved, and the lesions may be pruritic. Histologically, a psoriasiform dermatitis is present, but the disorder differs from psoriasis both in its fixed, absolute symmetry and in its truncal sparing. Moreover, Auspitz sign is absent and Munro microabscesses are not found histologically. Finally, the disorder, unlike psoriasis, is resistant to most topical therapies.

**Complications:** Unknown.

**Associated Findings:** None known.

**Etiology:** Autosomal dominant inheritance with incomplete penetrance and variable expressivity. Several sporadic cases have been reported from consanguineous kindreds, suggesting that a recessive form may also occur.

**Pathogenesis:** Unknown. The epidermis is hyperproliferative. Electron microscopic studies show lipid vacuoles within the stratum corneum and perinuclear swollen mitochondria in stratum granulosum. These findings may not be specific for this disorder, but may reflect the hyperproliferative state.

**CDC No.:** 757.190

**Sex Ratio:** M1:F1

**Occurrence:** Approximately 25 cases have been reported, including ten from Mexico.

**Risk of Recurrence for Patient's Sib:**
See Part I, *Mendelian Inheritance.*

**Risk of Recurrence for Patient's Child:**
See Part I, *Mendelian Inheritance.*

**Age of Detectability:** By early childhood.

**Gene Mapping and Linkage:** Unknown.

**Prevention:** None known. Genetic counseling indicated.

**Treatment:** Responds partially, if at all, to conventional topical therapies. Improvement with oral synthetic retinoids (e.g., etretinate) is reported. However, the risk/benefit ratio of these agents must be carefully considered on an individual basis, particularly their teratogenicity and long-term effects on bones, and treatment should be reserved for disabling cases (see **Fetal retinoid syndrome**).

**Prognosis:** Partial or complete regression may occur at puberty.

**Detection of Carrier:** Careful skin examination coupled with history will help to detect minimally affected family members.

**References:**
Ruiz-Maldonado R, et al.: Erythrokeratodermia progressiva symmetrica: report of 10 cases. Dermatologica 1982; 164:133–141. * †
Nazzaro V, Blanchet-Bardon C: Progressive symmetric erythrokeratoderma: histological and ultrastructural study of patient before and after treatment with etretinate. Arch Dermatol 1986; 122:434–440. †

**Mary L. Williams**

## SKIN, ERYTHROKERATODERMIA, VARIABLE        0361

**Includes:**
  Erythrokeratoderma figurata, congenital familial, in plaques
  Erythrokeratoderma variabilis Mendes da Costa
  Ichthyosis-erythema annulare centrifugum
  Keratosis rubra figurata
  Mendes da Costa syndrome

**Excludes:**
  Erythema, familial annual
  Erythema perstans
  **Ichthyosiform erythrokeratoderma, atypical with deafness** (2861)
  **Skin, erythrokeratodermia, progressiva symmetrica** (2863)

**Major Diagnostic Criteria:** This disorder of cornification is characterized by sharply demarcated, geographic erythemas of shifting configuration and fixed, keratotic plaques bearing no relationship to the variable erythemas in conjunction with characteristic histopathology of laminated hyperkeratosis, acanthosis, and papillomatosis.

**Clinical Findings:** The dermatosis is composed of two parts: first, discrete, irregular configurate patches of erythema that are extremely variable in size, position, duration, and number. These are subject to environmental influences, such as cold, heat, and wind, or to emotional upsets and are relatively transient in nature. Second, there are fixed hyperkeratotic plaques that are sharply demarcated and persistent. These yellow-brown hyperkeratotic plaques have irregular outlines and usually arise on normal skin. In most instances only focal hyperkeratotic plaques are present, but occasionally the hyperkeratosis may be generalized, including the palms and soles. Hair, nails, and mucous membranes are

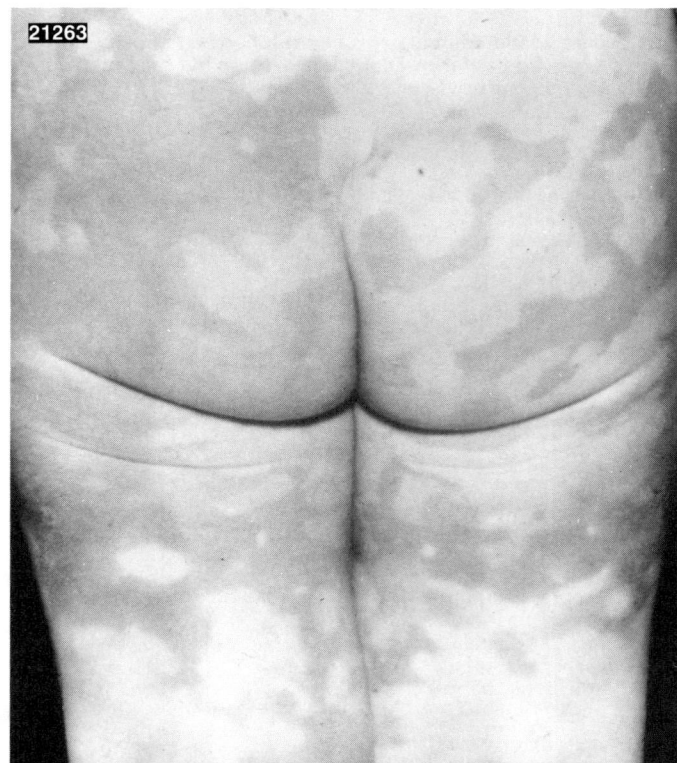

**0361-21263:** Erythrokeratodermia; note the irregular erythematous patches which occur with hyperkeratotic plaques which are not necessarily related to the erythema.

normal. The histopathology of the hyperkeratotic plaques demonstrates marked orthohyperkeratosis and focal parakeratosis with a prominent granular cell layer and severe papillomatosis with suprapapillary thinning. This "church-spire" configuration is characteristic but not diagnostic.

**Complications:** Approximately one-third of the case reports do not mention the presence of erythema. In those cases in which it has been noted, it tends to localize to the face, buttocks, and extensor aspect of the limbs. The hyperkeratotic lesions have a similar distribution, and while they usually develop on normal skin, they may occasionally arise from persistent erythrodermic areas. Their tendency is to persist indefinitely, although rarely they may involve spontaneously. The palms and soles show a variable keratoderma. The Koebner phenomenon (isomorphic response, induction of new lesions at sites of skin trauma) has been elicited in some of these cases. The underlying cause is unknown.

**Associated Findings:** There are isolated reports of perceptive deafness, developmental and growth retardation, and motor dysfunction.

**Etiology:** Usually autosomal dominant inheritance of variable expressivity. The majority of pedigrees are consistent with an autosomal dominant transmission, but other modes of inheritance cannot be excluded in some families. Thorough examination of the parents, sibs, and descendants of an affected individual is important because of the variable expressivity. Some reports describe a generalized hyperkeratosis in conjunction with variable erythrodermas; an autosomal dominant inheritance pattern was documented in one instance.

**Pathogenesis:** Autoradiographic studies reveal a normal epidermal proliferation rate, indicating that this is a "retention type" of hyperkeratosis. Ultrastructural examination reveals decreased numbers of lamellar bodies in the upper stratum spinosum and granular layer and increased numbers of unmyelinated nerves in the papillary dermis. Enzyme histochemical and immunohistochemical investigations have shown a decreased number of epidermal Langerhans cells, a cell of monocyte lineage responsible for antigen recognition and processing.

**MIM No.:** *13320

**CDC No.:** 757.190

**Sex Ratio:** M1:F1

**Occurrence:** Some 150 cases of variable erythrokeratodermia have been reported, the majority being from Europe.

**Risk of Recurrence for Patient's Sib:**
See Part I, *Mendelian Inheritance.*

**Risk of Recurrence for Patient's Child:**
See Part I, *Mendelian Inheritance.*

**Age of Detectability:** At birth in approximately 30% of cases. The majority of the remainder note the onset during the first year of life, but it may be delayed until after the third year of life.

**Gene Mapping and Linkage:** EKV (erythrokeratodermia variabilis) has been provisionally mapped to 1.

**Prevention:** None known. Genetic counseling indicated.

**Treatment:** Topical corticosteroids may be helpful for the erythematous lesions. Palliation of the hyperkeratotic plaques can be achieved with topical retinoic acid, salicylic acid gel, or 5% lactic acid in hydrophilic ointment. Oral synthetic retinoids, particularly etretinate are helpful. Their long-term administration, however, is necessary to control this disorder of cornification, and use of these agents must be carefully considered against their many toxicities.

**Prognosis:** The general tendency is for the process to increase in severity until puberty and then remain stationary or show gradual signs of improvement. The general health remains unaffected.

**Detection of Carrier:** Careful examination of family members.

**References:**
Brown J, Kierland RR: Erythrokeratodermia variabilis: report of 3 cases and review of the literature. Arch Dermatol 1966; 93:194–201. * †

Schellander FG, Fritsch PO: Variable erythrokeratodermia: an unusual case. Arch Dermatol 1969; 100:744–748. †
Cram DL: Erythrokeratoderma variabilis and variable circinate erythrokeratodermis. Arch Dermatol 1970; 101:68–73. * †
Vandersteen PR, Muller SA: Erythrokeratoderma variabilis: an enzyme histochemical and ultrastructural study. Arch Dermatol 1971; 103:362–370.
Gewirtzman GB, et al.: Erythrokeratodermia variabilis. Arch Dermatol 1978; 114:259–261.
Hacham-Zadeh S, Even-Paz Z: Erythrokeratodermia variabilis in a Jewish Kurdish family. Clin Genet 1978; 13:404.
Bond MJ, et al.: Erythrokeratodermia variabilis in a patient followed through the first year of life. Cutis 1982; 30:633. †
Rappaport IP, et al.: Erythrokeratodermia variabilis treated with isotretinoin: a clinical, histological and ultrastructural study. Arch Dermatol 1986; 122:441–445.

WI013                                      **Mary L. Williams**
VA010                                   **Paul R. Vandersteen**

---

## SKIN, ERYTHROKERATOLYSIS HIEMALIS                    2862

**Includes:**
>   Genodermatose en cocarde of Degos
>   Erythrokeratolysis hiemalis
>   Keratolytic winter erythema
>   Oudtshoorn skin

**Excludes:**
>   Erythema, familial annular
>   **Lyme disease** (3212)
>   **Skin creases, reticulate pigmented flexures, Dowling-Degos type** (2393)
>   **Skin, erythrokeratodermia, variable** (0361)
>   **Skin peeling syndrome** (2864)

**Major Diagnostic Criteria:** The combination of cyclic attacks of symmetric erythematous plaques that peel from the center outward in conjunction with characteristic histopathology of spinous cell necrosis.

**Clinical Findings:** This disorder is characterized by cyclic attacks of symmetrically distributed, erythematous plaques that peel full-thickness stratum corneum from the center outward. The onset may begin in infancy or may be delayed until adolescence. The disorder tends to improve by middle age. The disorder is often worse in winter and may be precipitated by fever or surgical operations. Characteristically, the palms and soles are involved, but the disorder of cornification may spill over to dorsal surfaces or occur elsewhere on the body. Histologically, an unusual pattern of necrosis of the spinous cell layers with overlying parakeratosis is present above a zone of basaloid proliferation. As a normal epidermis reforms, the damaged malphigian and corneal layers are lifted outward.

**Complications:** Attacks may be precipitated by fever or surgical operations.

**Associated Findings:** None known.

**Etiology:** Autosomal dominant inheritance with high penetrance.

**Pathogenesis:** Focal necrobiosis of spinous cell layers results in absence of stratum granulosum and parakeratosis. The basal cells underlying these necrobiotic foci proliferate to form six to eight cell layers, and differentiation to spinous cells appears to be blocked.

**CDC No.:** 757.190

**Sex Ratio:** Presumably M1:F1.

**Occurrence:** This disorder has been described primarily in descendants of nineteenth century farmers in the Oudtshoorn district of the Cape of South Africa.

**Risk of Recurrence for Patient's Sib:**
See Part I, *Mendelian Inheritance.*

**Risk of Recurrence for Patient's Child:**
See Part I, *Mendelian Inheritance.*

**Age of Detectability:** Usually clinically evident by adolescence, but may have its onset in infancy.

**Gene Mapping and Linkage:** Unknown.

**Prevention:** None known. Genetic counseling indicated. Avoidance of precipitating factors.

**Treatment:** Unknown.

**Prognosis:** Improves with age. Usually resolved or of trivial severity after middle age.

**Detection of Carrier:** History and clinical examination should allow detection of affected adults.

**References:**
Findlay GH, Morrison JGH: Erythrokeratolysis hiemalis-keratolytic winter erythema or "Oudtshoorn skin": a new epidermal genodermatosis with its histological features. Br J Dermatol 1978; 98:491–495.

WI013                             **Mary L. Williams**

**Skin, generalized folded with an underlying lipomatous nevus**
*See MICHELIN TIRE BABY SYNDROME*

---

## SKIN, HYPERKERATOSIS, FOCAL PALMOPLANTAR AND GINGIVAL        2096

**Includes:**
Gingival hyperkeratosis-hyperkeratosis palmoplantaris
Keratosis, focal palmoplantar and gingival
Palmoplantar hyperkeratosis-gingival hyperkeratosis

**Excludes:**
Hyperkeratosis palmoplantaris-periodontoclasia (0494)
Hyperkeratosis (other)

**Major Diagnostic Criteria:** The combination of hyperkeratosis palmoplantaris and attached gingival hyperkeratosis in a kindred.

**Clinical Findings:** *Skin:* Hyperkeratosis appears around puberty and progresses with age. There is focal-to-widespread hyperkeratosis of the soles of the foot, generally more prominent over the weightbearing areas (the heels, toe pads, and metatarsal heads). These may be painful and can affect ambulation. Hyperkeratosis also occurs on the palms and appears related to trauma. Hyperhidrosis is found in the hyperkeratotic areas. Subungual and circumungual keratin deposits can be found in the toenails at about 4–5 years of age, followed by fingernail changes at ages 8–9 years. Follicular keratoses of the sebaceous areas of the face are common.

*Oral:* Sharply marginated hyperkeratosis involves the labial and lingual attached gingiva. The hard palate, beneath denture-bearing areas, and the lateral bodies or dorsum of the tongue may also be affected. Oral hyperkeratotic areas appear in early childhood and progress in severity with age.

Microscopic examination shows paranuclear bodies in the spinous and granular cell layers of the keratinocytes of the gingival epithelium. Ultrastructure changes show these to be condensed tonofilaments.

**Complications:** Painful hyperkeratosis of the soles may interfere with ambulation.

**Associated Findings:** Many disorders may be associated with hyperkeratosis palmoplantaris. Generalized oral hyperkeratosis, especially of the buccal mucosa, is often reported.

**Etiology:** Autosomal dominant inheritance.

**Pathogenesis:** Unknown.

**MIM No.:** *14873

**CDC No.:** 757.900

**Sex Ratio:** M1:F1

**Occurrence:** Seven kindreds have been documented.

**Risk of Recurrence for Patient's Sib:**
See Part I, *Mendelian Inheritance.*

**Risk of Recurrence for Patient's Child:**
See Part I, *Mendelian Inheritance.*

**Age of Detectability:** During childhood, usually by age five years.

**Gene Mapping and Linkage:** Unknown.

**Prevention:** None known. Genetic counseling indicated.

**Treatment:** Unknown.

**Prognosis:** Good for life span and intelligence; ambulation may be inhibited.

**Detection of Carrier:** By clinical examination.

**References:**
Raphael AL, et al.: Hyperkeratosis of gingival and plantar surfaces. Periodontics 1968; 6:118–120.
Fred HL, et al.: Keratosis palmaris et plantaris. Arch Intern Med 1974; 113:866–871.
Gorlin RJ: Focal palmoplantar and marginal gingival hyperkeratosis in a syndrome. BD:OAS XII(5). New York: March of Dimes Birth Defects Foundation, 1976:239–242.
Roth W, et al.: Hereditary painful callosities. Arch Dermatol 1978; 114:591–592.
Laskaris G, et al.: Focal palmoplantar and oral mucosa hyperkeratosis syndrome: a report concerning five members of a family. Oral Surg 1980; 50:250–253.
Young WG, et al.: Focal palmoplantar and gingival hyperkeratosis syndrome: report of a family, with cytologic, ultrastructural and histochemical findings. Oral Surg 1982; 53:473–482.

G0038                           **Robert J. Gorlin**

**Skin, hyperkeratotic papules or plaques**
*See SKIN, POROKERATOSIS*

---

## SKIN, HYPERPIGMENTATION, FAMILIAL        2362

**Includes:**
"Carbon baby"
Hyperpigmentation, familial progressive
Melanosis, universal
Skin, universal melanosis

**Excludes:**
Acromelanosis progressiva
Dermal melanocytosis
Hyperpigmentation of eyelids
Hyperpigmentation of Fuldauer and Kuijpers
Intestinal polyposis, juvenile type (2259)
Melasma, idiopathic
Neurocutaneous melanosis (2014)
Polyposis-alopecia-pigmentation-nail defects (3040)
Reticulate pigmented anomaly of the flexines
Skin, cutaneous melanosis

**Major Diagnostic Criteria:** *Autosomal dominant:* scattered, hyperpigmented macular spots, streaks, and whorls that gradually enlarge in size and are associated with the development of *de novo* areas of hyperpigmentation. *Autosomal recessive:* normally pigmented skin that develops diffuse hyperpigmentation. Normal vision.

**Clinical Findings:** Two types of familial hyperpigmentation have been described.

*Autosomal dominant:* Multiple macular hyperpigmented spots, streaks, and whorls involving the face, trunk, genitalia, and extensor surfaces of the extremities are present at birth and increase in size with time. New areas of hyperpigmentation develop. The increase in hyperpigmentation is rapid in childhood, but then slows in adolescence and is very slow in adults. The oral-buccal mucosa and conjunctiva are involved, as are the palms and soles, and more than 80% of the body is eventually hyperpigmented, with the remaining skin normally pigmented. Areas of hyperpigmented and normally pigmented skin may give a marbled appearance. The retina is not involved, and vision is normal. No other abnormalities are present. Histologic examination of the skin shows an increase in melanin pigment, particularly in the basal cell layer, by light microscopy and normal melanocytes, with larger, more numerous melanosomes, by electron microscopy.

*Autosomal recessive:* The skin is normally pigmented at birth. A gradual increase in skin pigment starts at ages 4–12 months and progresses to age five years, after which the hyperpigmentation partially recedes. The hyperpigmentation starts with the scalp, the external genitalia and groin, or the abdomen and spreads to involve the face, trunk, and extremities with minimal involvement of the palms and soles. Mucosal pigment is present. The hair is normal or variably pigmented. As the pigment recedes, the child is left with zones of skin, involving large parts of the body, that vary from normal pigmentation to yellow-to-dark pigmentation. Multiple small, white macules develop in the groin and on the trunk, with areas of coalescence. No other abnormalities are present. Histologic examination of the skin shows an increase in number and size of melanocytes in the basal layer and the dermis by light microscopy. The irregularly shaped cells are filled with pigmented melanosomes and can be found in clumps.

**Complications:** Unknown.

**Associated Findings:** None known.

**Etiology:** Autosomal dominant and autosomal recessive inheritance have both been reported.

**Pathogenesis:** Unknown.

**MIM No.:** 14525, *15580

**CDC No.:** 757.900

**Sex Ratio:** Presumably M1:F1.

**Occurrence:** More than a dozen families have been reported.

**Risk of Recurrence for Patient's Sib:**
See Part I, *Mendelian Inheritance.*

**Risk of Recurrence for Patient's Child:**
See Part I, *Mendelian Inheritance.*

**Age of Detectability:** The first year of life.

**Gene Mapping and Linkage:** Unknown.

**Prevention:** None known. Genetic counseling indicated.

**Treatment:** Unknown.

**Prognosis:** Undetermined. Probably normal life span.

**Detection of Carrier:** Unknown.

**Special Considerations:** These two conditions appear to be the result of separate genes affecting melanocyte physiology. A condition called *carbon baby* has been described by Ruiz-Maldonado et al (1978) and may be similar to autosomal recessive familial hyperpigmentation as described above. In the carbon baby, diffuse hyperpigmentation began at age six months and continued until all of the skin and mucous membranes were black, at which time the white undergarments turned gray after being worn. The pigmentation had not receded by age four years. Electron microscopy showed normal melanocyte number with an increase in normal-sized melanosomes. This Mexican boy had two normally pigmented brothers.

**References:**
Wende GW, Bauckus HH: A hitherto undescribed generalized pigmentation of the skin appearing in infancy in brother and sister. J Cutan Genitourinary Dis 1919; 37:685–701.
Carleton A, Biggs R: Diffuse mesodermal pigmentation with congenital cranial abnormality. Br J Derm 1948; 60:10.
Pegum JS: Diffuse pigmentation in brothers. Proc R Soc Med 1955; 48:179–180.
Chernosky ME, et al.: Familial progressive hyperpigmentation. Arch Dermatol 1971; 103:581–591.
Ruiz-Maldonado R, et al.: Universal acquired melanosis. Arch Dermatol 1978; 114:775–778.
Bashito HM, et al.: General dermal melanocytosis. Arch Derm 1981; 117:791.

KI007                    **Richard A. King**

## SKIN, KERATOSIS FOLLICULARIS SPINULOSA DECALVANS                                    2867

**Includes:**
Ichthyosis follicularis
Keratosis follicularis spinulosa decalvans cum ophiasi

**Excludes:**
**Darier disease** (2865)
**Ichthyosiform erythrokeratoderma, atypical with deafness** (2861)

**Major Diagnostic Criteria:** Progressive follicular hyperkeratosis on face and scalp resulting in progressive cicatricial alopecia.

**Clinical Findings:** Noninflammatory follicular hyperkeratosis begins in infancy on the face and progress during childhood to involve the trunk and extremities. In later childhood and adolescence scarring alopecia develops on the eyebrows and scalp. Many patients also develop hyperkeratosis of the palms and soles in adolescence. Photophobia is common and may be due to punctate corneal defects. Atopic diathesis also occurs.

**Complications:** Permanent hair loss due to scarring alopecia develops in most patients.

**Associated Findings:** Photophobia, corneal defects, and atopic diathesis.

**Etiology:** Autosomal dominant inheritance, possibly with more severe manifestations in males. Families with an X-linked pattern of inheritance have also been reported. Sporadic cases have been reported.

**Pathogenesis:** Unknown.

**MIM No.:** *30880

**CDC No.:** 757.900

**Sex Ratio:** M1:F<1. A predominance of males has been reported in the literature.

**Occurrence:** Undetermined. Established literature.

**Risk of Recurrence for Patient's Sib:**
See Part I, *Mendelian Inheritance.*

**Risk of Recurrence for Patient's Child:**
See Part I, *Mendelian Inheritance.*

**Age of Detectability:** In sporadic cases, diagnosis may not be apparent until adolescence when full progression of the disease is evident. In families at risk, facial follicular hyperkeratoses are usually evident in infancy.

**Gene Mapping and Linkage:** Unknown.

**Prevention:** None known. Genetic counseling indicated.

**Treatment:** Topical agents to loosen keratoses (e.g., 5–10% lactic acid) usually are ineffective. Due to their long-term toxicity, use of oral synthetic retinoids should be considered experimental at present.

**Prognosis:** Progressive scarring alopecia; otherwise, normal life span and intelligence.

**Detection of Carrier:** By clinical examination.

**Special Considerations:** In patients with photophobia, **Ichthyosiform erythrokeratoderma, atypical with deafness** should be excluded. An X-linked recessive disorder with more extensive follicular hyperkeratoses, absence of scarring alopecia, absent or atrophic sebaceous glands, and hyperkeratotic plaques of extensor extremities has been delineated by Eramo et al. (1985). Moreover, localized forms of follicular hyperkeratoses with scarring but without photophobia have also been reported.

**References:**
Kuokkanen K: Keratosis follicularis spinulosa decalvans in a family from Northern Finland. Acta Dermatovener (Stockholm) 1941; 51: 156–160.
Rand R, Baden HP: Keratosis follicularis spinulosa decalvans: report of two cases and literature review. Arch Dermatol 1983; 119:22–26.
Eramo LR, et al.: Ichthyosis follicularis with alopecia and photophobia. Arch Dermatol 1985; 121:1167–1174.

WI013                    **Mary L. Williams**

## SKIN, KYRLE DISEASE 0561

**Includes:**
 Hyperkeratosis follicularis et parafollicularis in cutem
  penetrans
 Kyrle disease

**Excludes:**
 Hyperkeratosis lenticularis perstans
 Perforating folliculitis

**Major Diagnostic Criteria:** Follicular and parafollicular hyperkeratotic papules. Kyrle sign; a central keratotic plug which, when removed, leaves a corresponding crater.

**Clinical Findings:** *Distribution:* Widespread, symmetrical, especially arms and legs. Sparing of palms, soles, and mucous membranes.
 *Morphology:* Papules 1–8 mm diameter, follicular or parafollicular, with central hyperkeratotic plug up to 1.5 cm diameter protruding from a crateriform depression. Lesions may be linear or they coalesce into plaques or verrucous streaks. Verrucous streaks usually occur on flexural surfaces.
 *Natural History:* Lesions occur in crops that last several weeks and heal with with minimal or no scarring. The condition is asymptomatic.
 *Pathology:* Epithelial invagination filled by a plug of hyperkeratosis and parakeratosis and containing basophilic cellular debris. Adjacent to plug, epidermis may be acanthotic or atrophic. Granulomatous dermal reaction with infiltrate of neutrophils and lymphocytes and foreign body giant cells. A mild perivascular infiltrate may be seen.

**Complications:** Unknown.

**Associated Findings:** *Ocular:* Posterior subcapsular cataracts. Yellow-brown anterior corneal opacities.
 *Systemic:* Diabetes mellitus, chronic renal failure, cardiac failure, pachyonychia congenita. These conditions usually occur in association with nongenetic Kyrle disease.

**Etiology:** Possibly autosomal dominant inheritance, but most often nongenetic. (No male-male transmission reported.)

**Pathogenesis:** Unknown.

**MIM No.:** 14950

**CDC No.:** 757.900

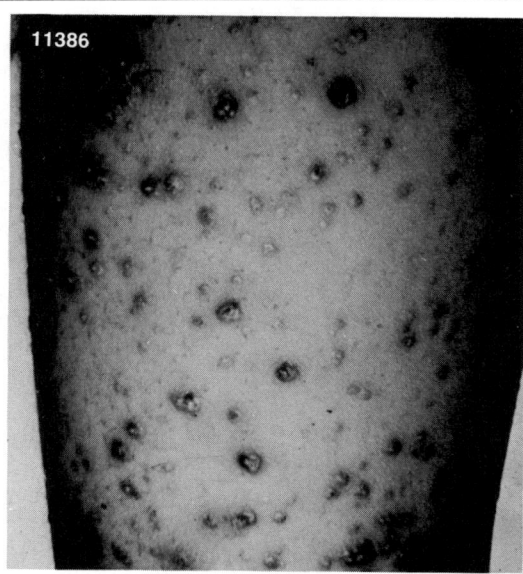

**0561**-11386: Kyrle disease.

**Sex Ratio:** M1:F1

**Occurrence:** Undetermined but presumably rare.

**Risk of Recurrence for Patient's Sib:**
 See Part I, *Mendelian Inheritance.*

**Risk of Recurrence for Patient's Child:**
 See Part I, *Mendelian Inheritance.*

**Age of Detectability:** Onset in third to seventh decade of life.

**Gene Mapping and Linkage:** Unknown.

**Prevention:** None known. Genetic counseling indicated.

**Treatment:** Vitamin A 100,000 units daily; topical keratolytic ointments.

**Prognosis:** Usually good. Associated systemic disease may alter life expectancy.

**Detection of Carrier:** Unknown.

**References:**
Constantine VS, Carter VH: Kyrles disease I. clinical findings in five cases and a review of the literature. Arch Dermatol 1968; 97:624–632.
Constantine VS, Carter VH. Kyrles disease I. histologic findings in five cases and review of the literature. Arch Dermatol 1968; 97:633–639.
Tessler HH, et al.: Ocular findings in a kindred with Kyrle disease. Arch Ophthal 1973; 90:278–280.
Der Kaloustian UM, Kurban AK: Genetic diseases of the skin. Berlin: Springer Verlag, 1979.
Patterson JW: The perforating disorders. J Am Acad Derm 1984; 10:561–581.
Rook A, et al.: Textbook of dermatology, 4th ed. Oxford: Blackwell Scientific Publications, 1986.

WI055                                   **Ingrid M. Winship**

## SKIN, LEIOMYOMAS, MULTIPLE 0890

**Includes:**
 Leiomyomata, hereditary multiple, of skin
 Leiomyomata, multiple cutaneous

**Excludes:** Skin nodules, other

**Major Diagnostic Criteria:** Cutaneous leiomyomata are known to occur as solitary or multifocal skin tumors arising from the pilar arrector muscles of the skin.

**Clinical Findings:** Cutaneous leiomyomata are known to occur as solitary or multifocal skin tumors arising from the pilar arrector muscles of the skin. They are usually less than 15 mm in diameter and appear as a collection of pink to reddish-brown firm intradermal nodules. These benign tumors grow slowly over a period of several years, mostly beginning in late infancy, with new lesions forming as others stabilize. They may occur on any cutaneous surface but most commonly on thighs, lips, and buttocks.

**Complications:** Unknown.

**Associated Findings:** Uterine leiomyomata, occurring before the age of 20 years, were documented in a number of female patients.

**Etiology:** Autosomal dominant inheritance with incomplete penetrance.

**Pathogenesis:** Recently, a severely mentally retarded adult female with chromosome 9p trisomy/18pter monosomy was reported. In addition to a **Chromosome 9, trisomy 9p** phenotype, this patient presented with multiple cutaneous leiomyomata, raising the question whether the occurrence of the chromosomal anomaly and the multiple skin tumors indicates another example of a specific chromosomal deletion (18pter) in a dominantly inherited multiple human tumor.
 Histologic examination identifies the skin lesions as benign tumors of smooth muscle fibers, originating in the pilomotor muscle.

**MIM No.:** *15080

**CDC No.:** 757.900

**Sex Ratio:** M1:F1

**Occurrence:** Undetermined but presumed rare.

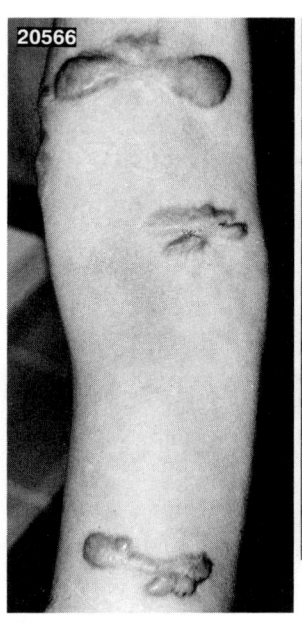
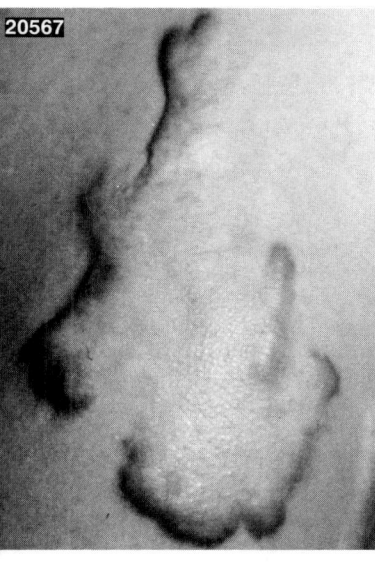

**0890-20566–67:** Note nodular and linear type of multiple cutaneous leiomyomata.

**Risk of Recurrence for Patient's Sib:**
See Part I, *Mendelian Inheritance.*

**Risk of Recurrence for Patient's Child:**
See Part I, *Mendelian Inheritance.*

**Age of Detectability:** About one-half are detectable before 20 years of years.

**Gene Mapping and Linkage:** Unknown.

**Prevention:** None known. Genetic counseling indicated.

**Treatment:** Surgical excision if symptomatic.

**Prognosis:** Normal for life span and health.

**Detection of Carrier:** Unknown.

**References:**
Berendes U, et al.: Segmentary and disseminated lesions in multiple hereditary cutaneous leiomyoma. Hum Genet 1971; 13:81–82.
Engelke H, Christopher E: Leiomyomatosis cutis et uteri. Acta Derm Venereol Stockh 1979; 59(Suppl 85):52–54.
Fryns JP, et al.: 9p Trisomy/18 distal monosomy and multiple cutaneous leiomyomata. Hum Genet 1985; 70:284–286.

FR030                                          **Jean-Pierre Fryns**

## SKIN, LIPOID PROTEINOSIS                                    0599

**Includes:**
Hyalinosis cutis et mucosae
Lipoglycoproteinosis
Lipoproteinosis
Urbach-Wiethe disease

**Excludes: Porphyria, protoporphyria** (0362)

**Major Diagnostic Criteria:** Typical skin and mucosal lesions due to an increased deposition of a hyaline material in the dermis. This deposition may also involve other organs. Hoarseness may be noted early in the course of the condition.

**Clinical Findings:** Skin lesions usually appear during childhood as vesiculopustular lesions on the face and distal extremities. These lesions usually heal with residual depressed acneiform scars. With time, the deposition of hyaline material increases and gradually the susceptible skin and mucosa become irregularly filled with yellowish, pale hyaline deposits in plaques, and papules, nodules on the face and neck. Areas of increased friction (hands, elbows, and knees) are most affected and may be covered with hyperpigmented, hyperkeratotic patches. A characteristic finding is the presence of papules on the eyelid margins, producing "itchy eyes" and a distortion of the eyelashes. However, cutaneous changes may occur on any part of the skin. Patchy alopecia of the scalp or beard is a relatively common finding. The mucous membranes that are most involved include the mouth, larynx, and pharynx. The soft palate may appear thickened and the tongue is often firm and difficult to protrude. Laryngeal examination usually shows a thickened epiglottis, swollen arytenoids, and aryepiglottic folds. Increased stiffness of the vocal cords resulting in hoarseness is a pathognomic sign, often being the first clinical manifestation. Narrowing of the pharynx may occur. An obstruction of the Stensen duct by the infiltrate may cause recurrent parotitis and faulty dentition. Lesions can also be found in the gastrointestinal tract but are usually asymptomatic. Wart-like lesions of unknown origin may be present in the trachea and main bronchi. The neurologic findings are characterized by hippocampal calcifications on either side of the sella turcica or as bilateral calcifications lateral or just above the dorsum sellae. Intracranial calcifications have been found in 52% of the cases. Epilepsy may occur, but seems to be a less common finding than intracranial calcifications as a neurologic sign. The ocular manifestations include moniliform blepharitis (two-thirds of the cases) and, rarely, corneal opacities, glaucoma, and drusen.

**Complications:** Narrowing of the larynx and pharynx may require tracheostomy to ensure adequate ventilation.

**Associated Findings:** Diabetes mellitus, conductive deafness, mental retardation. Severe loss of memory with intact intellect has been reported without involvement of both hippocampi. Pseudomembranous conjunctivitis was present in one case.

**Etiology:** Autosomal recessive inheritance.

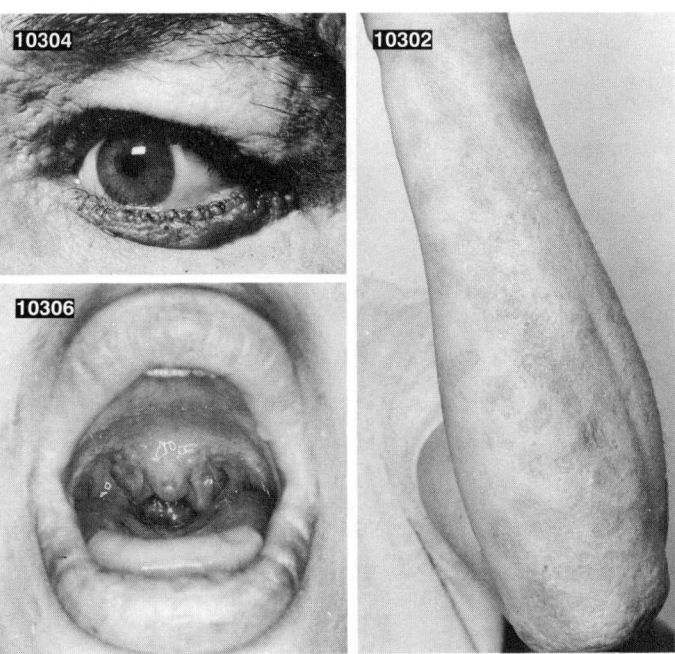

**0599-10304:** Characteristic row of nodules along left lower eyelid. **10306:** Thickening of lip and nodular lesions on pharynx. **10302:** Large atrophic scars on the forearm.

**Pathogenesis:** Biochemical and electron microscopic (EM) studies have shown that the hyaline deposit arises from basal laminae produced by endothelial cells, pericytes, Schwann cells, perineural cells, myofibroblasts, smooth muscle cells, and epithelial cells. The reason for the multilamination of the basal laminae is still obscure. EM studies show that the hyaline substance is composed of a very fine network of procollagen filaments interlinked with amorphous granular material. Recently it was confirmed that the affected dermis contains excessive amounts of matrix glycoproteins and decreased quantities of collagen fibers. Some authors suggest that multilamination may represent either a particular lysosomal storage disease due to single or multiple enzyme defects resulting in defective degradation or a disorder in which cellular activity (fibroblasts and epithelial and endothelial cells) is altered such that fibrous collagens are underproduced and basement membrane collagens overproduced.

**MIM No.:** *24710

**CDC No.:** 757.900

**Sex Ratio:** M1:F1

**Occurrence:** Over 280 cases have been described, and most of the patients appear to be of European descent. Cases have been reported most often in South Africa. It is there that the responsible gene is thought to have been introduced by a German settler and his sister.

**Risk of Recurrence for Patient's Sib:**
See Part I, *Mendelian Inheritance.*

**Risk of Recurrence for Patient's Child:**
See Part I, *Mendelian Inheritance.*

**Age of Detectability:** During the first few years of life. Hoarseness is often present at birth.

**Gene Mapping and Linkage:** Unknown.

**Prevention:** None known. Genetic counseling indicated.

**Treatment:** Carbon dioxide laser treatment of thickened vocal cords has proved to be effective for hoarseness. Anticonvulsants should be prescribed for affected individuals who develop epilepsy. Tracheostomy is necessary in some cases due to laryngeal obstruction.

**Prognosis:** The disease usually runs a chronic and benign course, generally with no shortening of life span.

**Detection of Carrier:** Unknown.

**References:**
Fabrizi G, et al.: Urbach-Wiethe disease: light and electron microscopic study. J Cutan Pathol 1980; 7:8–20.
Bauer EA, et al.: Lipoid proteinosis: in vivo and in vitro evidence for a lysosomal storage disease. J Invest Dermatol 1981; 76:119–125.
Ishibashi A: Hyalinosis cutis et mucosae: defective digestion and storage of basal lamina glycoprotein synthesized by smooth muscle cells. Dermatologica 1982; 165:7–15.
Haneke E, et al.: Hyalinosis cutis et mucosae in siblings. Hum Genet 1984; 68:342–345.
Harper JI, et al.: Lipoid proteinosis: an inherited disorder of collagen metabolism? Br J Dermatol 1985; 113:145–151.
Yakout YM, et al.: Radiological findings in lipoid proteinosis. J Laryngol Otol 1985; 99:259–265.
Barthelemy H, et al.: Lipoid proteinosis with pseudomembranous conjunctivitis. J Am Acad Dermatol 1986; 14:367–371.
Moy LS, et al.: Lipoid proteinosis: ultrastructural and biochemical studies. J Am Acad Dermatol 1987; 16:1193–1201.
Pierard GE, et al.: A clinicopathologic study of six cases of lipoid proteinosis. Am J Dermopathol 1988; 10:300–305.

**Giuseppe Micali**

---

## SKIN, LOCALIZED ABSENCE OF                    0608

**Includes:**
Aplasia cutis congenita (ACC)
Carmi syndrome
Gastrointestinal atresia-aplasia cutis congenital
Localized absence of skin
Skull and scalp, congenital defect

**Excludes:**
Dermal hypoplasia, focal (0281)
Epidermolysis bullosum, type III (2562)
Parietal foramina, symmetric

**Major Diagnostic Criteria:** Localized absence of skin of scalp, trunk and limbs.

**Clinical Findings:** Localized absence of skin at birth. Most commonly seen on scalp, usually at the apex on or near the midline. Presents as ulcer with absence of both skin and hair. Serous membrane may cover subcutaneous tissue. Crusting is followed by healing in a few weeks leaving a fine depressed hairless scar. A similar condition may involve the trunk and limbs, particularly the lower legs.

**Complications:** Underlying skull, meninges and brain may be included in defect.

**Associated Findings:** Unilateral ear anomalies, facial paresis and dermal sinuses may occur. Rarely associated with gastrointestinal atresias or other malformations.

Localized absence of skin occasionally seen in **Chromosome 13, trisomy 13, Chromosome 18, trisomy 18, Chromosome 4, monosomy 4p, Dermal hypoplasia, focal,** recessive dystrophic **Epidermolysis bullosa,** symmetric parietal foramina, **Johanson-Blizzard syndrome** and **Limb and scalp defects, Adams-Oliver type.**

**Etiology:** Autosomal dominant inheritance of a predominantly ''scalp defect''. Autosomal recessive inheritance of some instances of scalp/skull defects, and trunk and limb sites. Most represent isolated cases.

**Pathogenesis:** Localized developmental abnormality of skin. Amniotic adhesions no longer accepted as cause.

**MIM No.:** *10760, 20770, *20773.

**CDC No.:** 757.395

**Sex Ratio:** M1:F1

**Occurrence:** Approximately 250 cases reported.

**Risk of Recurrence for Patient's Sib:**
See Part I, *Mendelian Inheritance.*

**Risk of Recurrence for Patient's Child:**
See Part I, *Mendelian Inheritance.*

**Age of Detectability:** At birth by examination of skin.

**Gene Mapping and Linkage:** Unknown.

**Prevention:** None known. Genetic counseling indicated.

**Treatment:** If defect covers large area, skin grafting may be required.

**Prognosis:** Excellent except in rare patients with associated complications.

**Detection of Carrier:** Unknown.

**References:**
Deekin JH, Caplan RM: Aplasia cutis congenita. Arch Dermatol 1970; 102:386–389.
McMurray BR, et al.: Hereditary aplasia cutis congenita and associated defects: three instances in one family and a survey of reported cases. Clin Pediatr 1977; 16:610–614.
Dubosson J-D, Schneider P: Manifestation familiale d'une aplasie cutanee circonscrite du vertex (ACCV), associele dans un cas a une malformation candiaque. J Genet Hum 1978; 26:351–365.
Anderson CE, et al.: Autosomal dominantly inherited cutis aplasia congenita, ear malformations, right-sided facial paresis, and dermal sinuses. BD:OAS XV(5b) New York: March of Dimes Birth Defects Foundation, 1979:265–270.

Carmi R, et al.: Aplasia cutis congenita in two sibs discordant for pyloric atresia. Am J Med Genet 1982; 11:319–328.

Sybert VP: Aplasia cutis congenita: a report of 12 new families and review of the literature. Pediatr Dermatol 1985; 3:1–14.

Frieden IJ: Aplasia cutis congenita: a clinical review and proposal for classification. J Am Acad Dermat 1986; 14:646–660.

LA007                                                        **Roger L. Ladda**

**Skin, Naegeli syndrome**
*See ECTODERMAL DYSPLASIA, NAEGELI TYPE*

## SKIN, PAINFUL PLANTAR CALLOSITIES                    2895

**Includes:**
>    Brauer keratoderma palmoplantar
>    Buschke-Fischer keratoderma palmoplantar
>    Callosities, painful plantar
>    Plantar callosities, autosomal dominant painful

**Excludes:  Skin** (other defects)

**Major Diagnostic Criteria:**  Noncongenital plantar callosities.

**Clinical Findings:**  Plantar callosities that arise with upright ambulation and persist (these are always present over the pressure points of the soles). Warm and oily feet. Bullae at the edge of the callosities are formed when the patients walk too much, contain a malodorous liquid, and tend to quickly burst. In one large Brazilian kindred (Rachid et al, 1987), no instance of palmar callosities was mentioned even in individuals engaged in heavy manual labor. Osteoarticular X-ray aspects were normal.

**Complications:**  Discomfort and pain during walking.

**Associated Findings:**  None known.

**Etiology:**  Autosomal dominant inheritance.

**Pathogenesis:**  Unknown.

**MIM No.:**  *11414

**CDC No.:**  757.900

**Sex Ratio:**  Presumably M1:F1.

**Occurrence:**  One Caucasian family was verified to have 31 affected persons (13 men and 18 women) in six generations. About 50 cases of possible variants have been reported in the literature.

**Risk of Recurrence for Patient's Sib:**
See Part I, *Mendelian Inheritance.*

**Risk of Recurrence for Patient's Child:**
See Part I, *Mendelian Inheritance.*

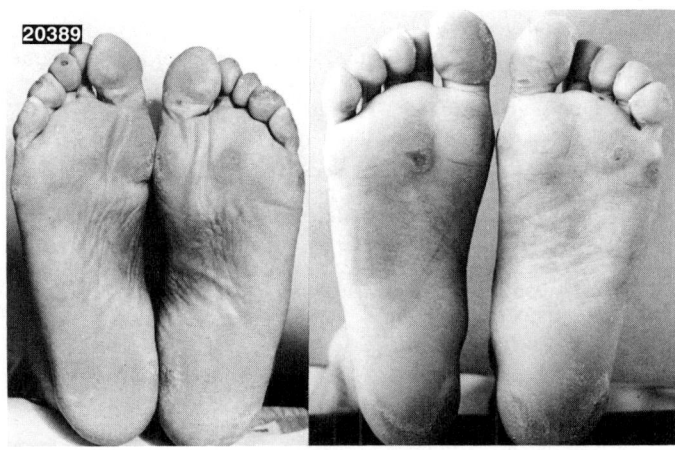

**2895**-20389:  Feet of two patients with plantar callosities.

**Age of Detectability:**  During childhood, after upright ambulation, by physical examination.

**Gene Mapping and Linkage:**  Unknown.

**Prevention:**  None known. Genetic counseling indicated.

**Treatment:**  Hot water and brine alleviate the pain; aromatic tretinoin taken orally may also relieve this genodermatosis.

**Prognosis:**  Normal life span. The callosities and bullae never bleed and tend to regress during winter.

**Detection of Carrier:**  Unknown.

**Special Considerations:**  Some authors consider *Brauer keratoderma palmoplantar, Buschke-Fischer keratoderma palmoplantar,* and other conditions which may or may not involve palmar callosites to be variants of the above described condition. The present author restricts this diagnosis to a condition with *only* plantar callosities.

**References:**
Roth W, et al.: Hereditary painful callosities. Arch Derm 1978; 114: 591–592.

Dupré A, et al.: Treatment of hereditary painful callosities with tretinoin. Arch Dermatol 1979; 115:638–639.

Baden HP, et al.: Hereditary callosities with blisters: report of a family and review. J Am Acad Derm 1984; 11:409–415.

Rachid A, et al.: Autosomal dominant painful plantar callosities. Am J Med Genet 1987; 26:185–187. * †

FR033                                                   **Newton Freire-Maia**

## SKIN, PALMO-PLANTAR ERYTHEMA                         0792

**Includes:**
>    Erythema palmare hereditarium
>    Erythema palmo-plantar
>    Lane disease
>    Palmo-plantar erythema
>    Red palms

**Excludes:**  N/A

**Major Diagnostic Criteria:**  Constant erythema of palmar surfaces of fingers.

**Clinical Findings:**  Constant symmetrical bright mottled erythema over the thenar and hypothenar eminence, palmar surface at the base of the fingers, and the palmar surfaces of the fingers. May involve the soles. Asymptomatic red zone sharply demarcated at wrist crease and side of hands.

**Complications:**  Unknown.

**Associated Findings:**  Keratosis palmaris et plantaris diffusa in certain affected families. May be associated with liver disease, rheumatoid arthritis, chronic immunologic diseases, aging, pregnancy.

**Etiology:**  While McKusick reports observing the trait in successive generations, etiology is still unclear. Possibly of multifactorial etiology.

**Pathogenesis:**  Unknown.

**MIM No.:**  *13300

**CDC No.:**  757.900

**Sex Ratio:**  Presumably M1:F1.

**Occurrence:**  Undetermined but presumed rare.

**Risk of Recurrence for Patient's Sib:**  Unknown.

**Risk of Recurrence for Patient's Child:**  Unknown.

**Age of Detectability:**  Unknown.

**Gene Mapping and Linkage:**  Unknown.

**Prevention:**  None known. Genetic counseling indicated.

**Treatment:**  None required.

**Prognosis:**  Benign asymtomatic condition.

**Detection of Carrier:**  Unknown.

**Special Considerations:** The condition was first described in two patients in 1929. The lesion is indistinguishable from, if not precisely the same phenomenon as, palmar erythema of liver disease, normal pregnancy, rheumatoid arthritis, and perhaps many other diseases. Even such nonspecific states as aging may show red palms. The evidence that it is hereditary is very thin indeed; the heritable etiology of palmar erythema seems to be unfortunately perpetuated from book to book and in published papers since its first casual appearance in 1929.

**References:**
Lane JE: Erytheme palmare hereditarium. Arch Dermatol Syph (Chic) 1929;20:445–448.
Olivier J: Erytheme jpalmo-plantaire hereditarire: maladie de Lane. Arch Belg Derm Syph 1956;12:202–207.
Bland JH, et al.: Palmar erythema and spider angiomata in rheumatoid arthritis. Ann Intern Med 1958;48:1026–1032.

LA007      **Roger L. Ladda**

## SKIN, PARANA HARD SKIN SYNDROME     3051

**Includes:** Parana hard skin syndrome

**Excludes:** Stiff skin syndrome (2629)

**Major Diagnostic Criteria:** Progressive rigidity of skin, commencing in the second to third month of life, with subsequent growth retardation.

**Clinical Findings:** At two to three months of age, the skin and subcutaneous tissue progressively harden, forming an immovable cast. All but the eyelid, neck and ear skin is involved. As the skin hardens, growth decelerates with eventual joint, chest, and abdominal wall immobility. Additional findings include hirsutism, hyperpigmentation of the skin, and enlargement of the parotid glands.

**Complications:** Lichenification of skin in flexure areas and pulmonary insufficiency are the most common complications.

**Associated Findings:** None known.

**Etiology:** The occurrence of this condition in siblings and in an offspring of a consanguineous mating suggests autosomal recessive inheritance.

**Pathogenesis:** Unknown. Histologic studies of the skin have been uninformative.

**MIM No.:** 26053

**POS No.:** 4006

**Sex Ratio:** M1:F1

**Occurrence:** Reported in eight persons from seven families in the Parana region of Brazil.

**Risk of Recurrence for Patient's Sib:**
See Part I, *Mendelian Inheritance.*

**Risk of Recurrence for Patient's Child:**
See Part I, *Mendelian Inheritance.*

**Age of Detectability:** Evident by three months of age.

**Gene Mapping and Linkage:** Unknown.

**Prevention:** None known. Genetic counseling indicated.

**Treatment:** Symptomatic; known treatmens are probably ineffective in preventing the progressive skin hardening.

**Prognosis:** The skin hardening is progressive, death as a result of pulmonary insufficiency appears to be inevitable. Intellect appears unimpaired.

**Detection of Carrier:** Possibly by clinical examination.

**References:**
Cat I, et al: Parana hard-skin syndrome: study of seven families. Lancet 1974; I:215–216.

T0007      **Helga V. Toriello**

**Skin, pemphigus, benign familial**
*See PEMPHIGUS, BENIGN FAMILIAL*

## SKIN, PITYRIASIS RUBRA PILARIS     0811

**Includes:**
    Lichen acuminatus
    Lichen ruber acuminatus
    Pityriasis pilaris
    Pityriasis rubra pilaris

**Excludes:**
    Exfoliative dermatitis-pityriasis rubra pilaris
    **Ichthyosis**
    Keratosis pilaris
    Phrynoderma
    **Skin, erythrokeratodermia, progressiva symmetrica** (2863)
    **Skin, psoriasis vulgaris** (0833)

**Major Diagnostic Criteria:** Pathognomonic black horny follicular plugs on the backs of the fingers; hyperkeratosis of palms and soles. The yellowish or grayish-red to orange or salmon-yellow color of the plaques, with islands of normal skin, and the dry scaliness of the face and scalp, are diagnostic.

**Clinical Findings:** Persistent, dry, horny, acuminate, follicular papules on the dorsal surfaces of the first and second phalanges. These are symmetrically distributed, pinhead in size, brownish-red to rosy-yellow in color, and enclose a dry lusterless atrophic hair in their keratotic centers. The horny central plugs are often capped by a black point. Multiplication and coalescence of papules form plaques, which are symmetrically distributed. The plaques are sharply marginated, with small islands of normal skin within the affected areas. The skin looks like goose flesh and feels like a nutmeg grater.

Nails are dull, rough, brittle, and frequently transversely striated. They are lusterless, and gray or yellow in color. Palms and soles exhibit firm thick reddish-yellow hyperkeratosis, which scales freely, and often become fissured. The face is red, thickened, inelastic, and often there is ectropion of the lower lids.

**Complications:** Unknown.

**Associated Findings:** Liver disease, neuromuscular dysfunction, rheumatism, psoriasis, and hormonal dysfunction.

**Etiology:** Autosomal dominant inheritance with incomplete penetrance. Most cases are sporadic. The herediatry form tends to be less severe and more limited in extent, and does not show lesions at birth.

**Pathogenesis:** Unknown.

**MIM No.:** *17320

**CDC No.:** 757.900

**Sex Ratio:** M1:F1

**Occurrence:** Familial cases reported in a few families.

**Risk of Recurrence for Patient's Sib:**
See Part I, *Mendelian Inheritance.*

**Risk of Recurrence for Patient's Child:**
See Part I, *Mendelian Inheritance.*

**Age of Detectability:** From infancy to 70 years of age, without any significant age predilection.

**Gene Mapping and Linkage:** Unknown.

**Prevention:** None known. Genetic counseling indicated.

**Treatment:** Difficult to evaluate because of natural exacerbations and remissions. Vitamin A by mouth ranging from 50,000 to 200,000 units per day. Metrotrexate has been used. Vitamin A alcohol in Lubriderm^ topically has been used successfully.

**Prognosis:** In 75 patients; 8% resolved completely; 60% improved, 24% remitted and exacerbated, 7% did not change, and 1% became worse.

**Detection of Carrier:** Unknown.

**References:**
Lamar LM, Gaethe G: Pityriasis rubra pilaris. Arch Dermatol 1964; 89:515–522.
Davidson CL Jr., et al.: Pityriasis rubra pilaris: a follow-up study of 57 patients. Arch Dermatol 1969; 100:175–178.

Gross DA, et al.: Pityriasis rubra pilaris: report of a case and analysis of the literature. Arch Dermatol 1969; 99:710–716.

Beamer JE, et al.: Pityriasis rubra pilaris. Cutis 1972; 10:419–421.

MY001                                                          **Terry L. Myers**

## SKIN, POROKERATOSIS                                          0819

**Includes:**

Disseminated superficial actinic porokeratosis (DSAP)
Hyperkeratosis eccentrica
Keratoatrophoderma, chronic progressive
Linear porokeratosis
Porokeratosis, linear
Porokeratosis, plantaris
Porokeratosis of Mibelli
Skin, hyperkeratotic papules or plaques

**Excludes:**

Keratoderma of palms and soles
**Nevus, epidermal nevus syndrome** (0593)

**Major Diagnostic Criteria:** Hyperkeratotic papules or plaques most frequently noted on dorsum of hands and feet. Histologic examination demonstrates cornoid lamella. Biopsy is required to confirm the diagnosis.

**Clinical Findings:** The primary lesion is a small hyperkeratotic papule, which gradually enlarges to form a plaque with a raised wall-like border and a depressed center (crater-like). Some lesions remain small, while others may attain a large size. Any part of the integument, even the mucosa, may be involved. The areas most affected are the hands and feet, especially the dorsal surfaces, and the face and neck.

Since the early classic description of porokeratosis by Mibelli, several clinical variants of the disease have been reported. Most investigators now accept the classification of Chernosky (1967), which includes three subdivisions:

1. *Porokeratosis of Mibelli*, which includes the keratotic verrucous form. These centrifugally spreading patches are surrounded by narrow horny ridges with central atrophy, which produce crater-like lesions.

2. *Disseminated superficial actinic porokeratosis (DSAP)* lesions develop in the third to fourth decade, and occur almost only in the sun-exposed areas of the skin.

3. *Porokeratosis palmaris et plantaris disseminata* occurs first in the second or third decade, on the palmar and plantar surfaces; a rare finding in the other two types of porokeratosis. The lesions spread to other body parts and are not limited to sun-exposed areas. The annular or gyrate plaques have elevated borders.

**Complications:** Malignant degeneration (epidermoid carcinoma) has been reported.

**Associated Findings:** None known.

**Etiology:** Autosomal dominant inheritance, possibly with reduced penetrance in females.

**Pathogenesis:** Undetermined. No relationship to sweat duct, contrary to what is implied by the present name of the disease. Several investigators believe that porokeratosis arises from abnormal clones of keratinocytes, and that the tendency to develop these clones is inherited.

**MIM No.:** *17580, 17585, *17590

**CDC No.:** 757.900

**Sex Ratio:** M2:F1 (observed).

**Occurrence:** Undetermined but presumed rare. Many cases are mild and may escape notice. Wide ethnic distribution.

**Risk of Recurrence for Patient's Sib:**
See Part I, *Mendelian Inheritance.*

**Risk of Recurrence for Patient's Child:**
See Part I, *Mendelian Inheritance.*

**Age of Detectability:** Any age.

**Gene Mapping and Linkage:** Unknown.

**Prevention:** None known. Genetic counseling indicated.

**Treatment:** Excision if feasible. Favorable response to topical 5-fluorouracil has been obtained in some cases of disseminated superficial actinic porokeratosis. Cryosurgery has been found useful for plantar lesions.

**Prognosis:** Normal for life span and intelligence. Involvement of the face may present cosmetic problems. Although characteristically progressive, lesions may spontaneously involute.

**Detection of Carrier:** Unknown.

**Special Considerations:** The name porokeratosis is derived either from the Greek prefix poro (callus) or because Mibelli, the Italian dermatologist who first described the condition, thought that it derived from the sweat glands (pores). A study of cultured fibroblasts from affected areas shows a variety of chromosomal aberrations without any consistent specific abnormality.

**References:**

Chernosky ME, Freeman RG: Disseminated superficial actinic porokeratosis (DSAP). Arch Dermatol 1967; 96:611–624. * †

Mikhail GR, Wertheimer FW: Clinical variants of porokeratosis (Mibelli). Arch Dermatol 1968; 98:124–131. * †

Guss SB, et al.: Porokeratosis plantaris palmaris et disseminata. A third type of porokeratosis. Arch Dermatol 1971; 104:366–373. †

Pirozzi JJ, Rosenthal A: Disseminated superficial actinic porokeratosis: analysis of an affected family. Br J Dermatol 1976; 95:429–432.

Limmer BL: Cryosurgery of porokeratosis plantaris discreta. Arch Dermatol 1979; 115:582–583.

McDonald SG, Peterka ES: Porokeratosis (Mibelli): treatment with topical 5-fluorouracil. J Am Acad Dermatol 1983; 8:107–110.

**0819-10307–08:** Porokeratosis with classic plaque form and dike-like keratotic borders.

MI005                                                        **George R. Mikhail**

## SKIN, PSORIASIS VULGARIS 0833

**Includes:**
> Psoriasis
> Pustular psoriasis

**Excludes:**
> **Ankylosing spondylitis** (2516)
> **Fetal syphilis syndrome** (0385)
> Parapsoriasis
> Pityriasis rosea
> Seborrheic dermatitis
> **Skin, erythrokeratodermia, progressiva symmetrica** (2863)
> **Skin, pityriasis rubra pilaris** (0811)

**Major Diagnostic Criteria:** Lesions of typical morphology and distribution: erythematous scaling plaques, most frequently on elbows, knees, and scalp. When clinical presentation is atypical, histologic confirmation may be necessary.

**Clinical Findings:** *Skin:* erythematous plaques on the skin with silver scale; pinpoint bleeding typically on removal of the scale cases. Distribution is usually generalized with a predisposition for the elbows, knees, scalp, and genitalia. Lesions may be symmetric. Palms and soles may be hyperkeratotic. Koebner phenomenon (isomorphic response) well known. Other morphologies of lesions in psoriasis are erythroderma and pustulosis. Pustular psoriasis may be a medical emergency.

*Nails:* finger- and toenails frequently involved in the form of pitting, dystrophy, and onycholysis.

*Joints:* arthritis, usually asymmetric and more often monoarticular than polyarticular. Five patterns of arthropathy are recognized.

*Onset:* childhood to adulthood.

*Course/Progression:* chronic fluctuating course with remissions and exacerbations.

*Expressivity:* very variable within family members and in each patient in subsequent episodes.

*Histology:* parakeratosis with or without hyperkeratosis; hypogranulosis; uniform elongation of rete ridges or dermal papillae; Munro microabscesses.

**Complications:** Generalized pustular psoriasis may be a medical emergency. This exfoliative erythroderma may be associated with high-output cardiac failure, hypoalbuminemia, and hypothermia.

**Associated Findings:** High uric acid level. β-Hemolytic streptococcus may be associated with guttate psoriasis.

**Etiology:** Multifactorial. Autosomal dominant inheritance with variable penetrance has been reported.

**Pathogenesis:** Lesions are characterized by increased epidermal mitotic rate and decreased cell turnover time, parakeratosis, epidermal hyperplasia, minimal inflammation, and prominent subepidermal capillaries.

Emotional stress plays a large role in the precipitation of psoriasis in susceptible individuals.

Certain drugs are known to aggravate psoriasis, notably indomethacin, β-adrenergic blocking agents, lithium, and antimalarial drugs.

**MIM No.:** *17790

**CDC No.:** 757.900

**Sex Ratio:** M1:F1

**Occurrence:** 3:100 in the United States. Common in Caucasians and infrequent in Blacks.

**Risk of Recurrence for Patient's Sib:** 7.5% if neither parent is affected; 16% if one parent is affected; 50% if both parents are affected.

**Risk of Recurrence for Patient's Child:** 16% if one parent affected; 50% if both parents affected.

**Age of Detectability:** Onset usually in young adulthood, with a range from early childhood to old age.

**Gene Mapping and Linkage:** Certain HLA loci have been linked with psoriasis. HLA-B13, HLA-B17 (worldwide); HLA-BW6, HLA-B37 (restricted to certain population groups); HLA-BW16, HLA-B17, HLA-DW11 (correlate with extensive psoriasis); HLA DW11 (susceptibility to psoriasis is questionable).

**Prevention:** Avoidance of precipitants; e.g., trauma to the skin, emotional stress, and triggering drugs.

**Treatment:** *Topical:* Antimitotic agents include tar derivatives, anthralin derivatives, and corticosteroids. Keratolytic agents include salicylic acid; urea; ultraviolet light A, spectrum 320–400; ultraviolet light B.

*Photochemotherapy:* PUVA-8 methoxypsoralens; 8-MOP + UVA (320–400).

*Systemic:* methotrexate; vitamin A derivatives, retinoids (severe teratogenic effects have been reported with the use of retinoids in early pregnancy. See **Fetal retinoid syndrome**), Corticosteroids probably introduce greater risks than benefits in almost all patients.

**Prognosis:** Life span is normal. IQ not affected. The natural history of psoriasis is one of remissions and exacerbations. With complete clearing of lesions, longstanding remissions may be achieved.

**Detection of Carrier:** Unknown.

**References:**

Abele DC, et al.: Heredity and psoriasis: study of a large family. Arch Derm 1963; 88:38–47.

Watson W, et al.: The genetics of psoriasis. Arch Dermatol 1972; 105:197–207.

Saiag P, et al.: Psoriatic fibroblasts induce hyperproliferation of normal keratinocytes in a skin equivalent model in vitro. Science 1985; 230:669–672.

Dermis DJ: Clinical dermatology, 13th revision. Philadelphia: Harper & Row, 1986.

Rook A, et al.: Textbook of dermatology, ed 4. Oxford: Blackwell, 1986.

WI055                                          **Ingrid M. Winship**

**Skin, stiff skin syndrome**
> *See STIFF SKIN SYNDROME*

**Skin, tight**
> *See RESTRICTIVE DERMATOPATHY*

**Skin, universal melanosis**
> *See SKIN, HYPERPIGMENTATION, FAMILIAL*

## SKIN, VITILIGO 0993

**Includes:**
> Achromia, primary
> Halo nevi
> Leukoderma acquisitum centrifugum of Sutton
> Leukoderma, primary
> Nevus anemicus
> Vitiligo

**Excludes:**
> Achromia secondary to causes of melanocyte destruction
> **Albinism**
> **Deafness-vitiligo-muscle wasting** (0275)
> Depigmentation occurring as a sign of nongenetic disorders
> **Nevus, congenital** (2165)

**Major Diagnostic Criteria:** Progressive, primary melanin depigmentation of skin.

**Clinical Findings:** A small area of normally hyperpigmented skin loses pigmentation. It rapidly enlarges peripherally with sharp margins, reaching a stable size that then may remain static, slowly enlarge and coalesce with other depigmented areas, or repigment.

The condition should be distinguished from *nevus anemicus*, which consists of a patch of pale skin of normal texture, usually on the trunk, described in four generations of a family by Cardose et al (1975).

**Complications:** Sunburn of depigmented skin. Cosmetic defect.

**Associated Findings:** Halo nevus (Chisa, 1965), which may or may not be a part of this condition.

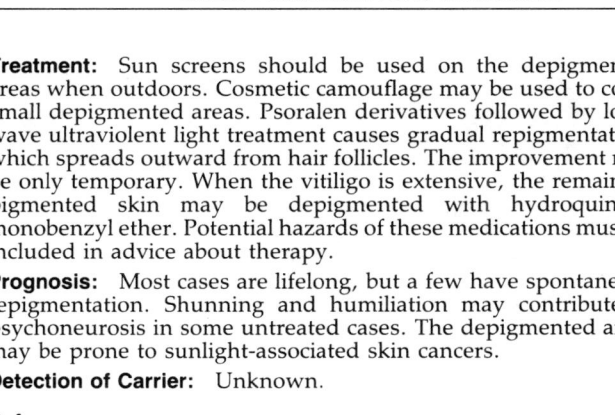

**0993-**11421:  Vitiligo.

**Etiology:**  Presumably polygenic.

**Pathogenesis:**  Melanocytes are absent from the depigmented areas. The mechanism of their loss has not been established.

**MIM No.:**  19320, 23430, 16305

**CDC No.:**  757.900

**Sex Ratio:**  Presumably M1:F1

**Occurrence:**  1:200 has been reported in two studies.

**Risk of Recurrence for Patient's Sib:**  Variable, depending on the number of cases in close relatives and on the amount of inbreeding. Only 2.7% of first degree relatives are found to be affected when all families are considered together. This figure may represent the maximal risk when the patient has no affected relatives. In some reported families, the frequency of affected first degree relatives is nearly 50%. This figure may represent the maximal risk in families with numerous affected relatives and parental consanguinity. The average risk based on polygenic theory should be 6.8%, which may be the approximate risk when the patient has an affected relative or when the patient's parents are consanguineous.

**Risk of Recurrence for Patient's Child:**  Variable, depending on the number of cases in close relatives and on the amount of inbreeding. Only 2.7% of first degree relatives are found to be affected when all families are considered together. This figure may represent the maximal risk when the patient has no affected relatives. In some reported families, the frequency of affected first degree relatives is nearly 50%. This figure may represent the maximal risk in families with numerous affected relatives and parental consanguinity. The average risk based on polygenic theory should be 6.8%, which may be the approximate risk when the patient has an affected relative or when the patient's parents are consanguineous.

**Age of Detectability:**  Any time of life, but about one-half have onset before 20 years of age.

**Gene Mapping and Linkage:**  Unknown.

**Prevention:**  None known. Genetic counseling indicated.

**Treatment:**  Sun screens should be used on the depigmented areas when outdoors. Cosmetic camouflage may be used to cover small depigmented areas. Psoralen derivatives followed by long-wave ultraviolent light treatment causes gradual repigmentation, which spreads outward from hair follicles. The improvement may be only temporary. When the vitiligo is extensive, the remaining pigmented skin may be depigmented with hydroquinone monobenzyl ether. Potential hazards of these medications must be included in advice about therapy.

**Prognosis:**  Most cases are lifelong, but a few have spontaneous repigmentation. Shunning and humiliation may contribute to psychoneurosis in some untreated cases. The depigmented areas may be prone to sunlight-associated skin cancers.

**Detection of Carrier:**  Unknown.

**References:**
Chisa N: Multiple halo nevi in siblings. Arch Derm 1965; 92:404–405.
Cardoso H, et al.: Familial naevus anemicus. (Abstract) Am J Hum Genet 1975; 27:24A only.
Hafez M, et al.: The genetics of vitiligo. Acta Dermatol Venereol (Stockh) 1983; 63:249–251.
Witkop CJ: Abnormalities of pigmentation. In: Emery AEH, Rimoin DL, eds: Principles and practice of medical genetics. New York: Churchill Livingstone, 1983:635 only.
Das SK, et al.: Studies on vitiligo. II. Familial aggregation and genetics. Genet Epidemiol 1985; 2:255–262.

TH017
UR001

**T.F. Thurmon**
**S.A. Ursin**

**Skin, wrinkly skin syndrome**
  *See WRINKLY SKIN SYNDROME*
**Sklerosteose**
  *See SCLEROSTEOSIS*
**Skull and scalp, congenital defect**
  *See SKIN, LOCALIZED ABSENCE OF*
**Skull, peculiar shape-polysyndactyly**
  *See POLYSYNDACTYLY-DYSMORPHIC CRANIOFACIES, GREIG TYPE*
**Sleep disorder**
  *See NARCOLEPSY*
**Sliding hernia**
  *See HERNIA, INGUINAL*
**SLOS (Smith-Lemli-Opitz syndrome)**
  *See SMITH-LEMLI-OPITZ SYNDROME*
**Slow-channel syndrome**
  *See MYASTHENIC SYNDROME, CONGENITAL SLOW CHANNEL TYPE*
**Sly syndrome**
  *See MUCOPOLYSACCHARIDOSIS VII*
**Small cell lymphocytic lymphoma**
  *See LEUKEMIA/LYMPHOMA, B-CELL*
**Small non-cleaved cell lymphoma**
  *See LYMPHOMA, BURKITT TYPE*
**SMED Strudwick**
  *See SPONDYLOEPIMETAPHYSEAL DYSPLASIA, STRUDWICK TYPE*
**Smelling loss, congenital**
  *See ANOSMIA, CONGENITAL*
**Smile, inverted-occult neuropathic bladder**
  *See UROFACIAL SYNDROME*

**SMITH-FINEMAN-MYERS SYNDROME**     **2845**

**Includes:**
  Mental retardation, Smith-Fineman-Myers type
  X-linked mental retardation, Smith-Fineman-Myers type

**Excludes:**  X-linked mental retardation (others)

**Major Diagnostic Criteria:**  Mental retardation with minor physical anomalies; growth and developmental retardation as well as distinctive facial and skeletal signs.

**Clinical Findings:**  The three known male patients were short in stature (less than the 3–10th percentile), severely mentally retarded (a recorded IQ of 21 for a non-familial case), and are lightly

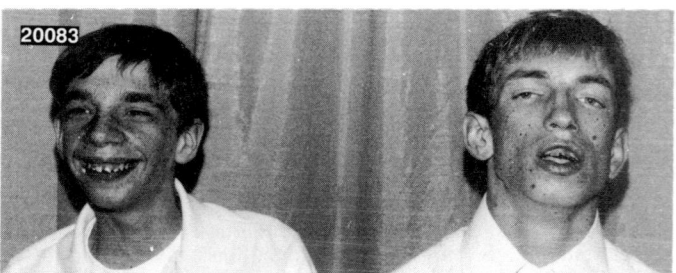

2845-20083: Note the similar facial features in these two unrelated boys.

pigmented with multiple freckles. Facial appearance is most significant for prominence of the maxilla and central incisors with contrasting micrognathia. Other craniofacial findings include dolichocephaly and elongation of the face, upslanting and/or short palpebral fissures, ptosis, strabismus, hyperopia, optic nerve hypoplasia (one case), decreased nasolabial folds, flat philtral pillars, patulous lower lip, and bifid uvula (one case). The facial appearance is reminiscent of patients with **Dubowitz syndrome** or **Marden-Walker syndrome**, but features are more distinctive in these syndromes.

Skeletal features include a thin habitus, minor chest abnormalities such as **Pectus excavatum**, short sternum and rib flaring, bridged palmar creases, femoral anteversion, foot deformities such as hallux valgus, toe **Camptodactyly** and overriding, longitudinal sole creases, metatarsus varus and pes planus, and back changes such as scoliosis and lordosis.

Skeletal X-rays may show delayed bone age, absence of the mastoid process, prominence of the frontal sinuses, overtubulation of the long bones, and scoliosis. Pneumoencephalography of affected brothers showed moderate cortical atrophy but brain biopsies were normal. A brain CAT Scan on an isolated case was essentially normal (thickened calvaria and **Microcephaly**). Metabolic screens and karyotypes were normal.

**Complications:** Psychomotor retardation is severe but non-progressive. There is early delay in attainment of milestones, and later, behavior difficulties and self-stimulation with little capacity for social interaction. Hypotonia and hyperreflexia evolve into hypertonia and spasticity. Mixed seizures developed as early as age 11 months, and were present in all three patients.

**Associated Findings:** Feeding difficulties and infections complicate infancy. The affected brothers were small for gestational age. There was increased fetal and neonatal loss in the family of the isolated case.

**Etiology:** Probably X-linked inheritance (70%) or possibly autosomal recessive inheritance (30%). The family history of an isolated case is suggestive of X-linked inheritance because a sister had a "learning disability" and a maternal aunt had mental retardation attributed to "birth trauma".

**Pathogenesis:** Unknown.

**MIM No.:** 30958

**POS No.:** 3257

**Sex Ratio:** M3:F0 (observed).

**Occurrence:** Three cases have been reported; all male from the United States west, including one pair of affected brothers.

**Risk of Recurrence for Patient's Sib:**
See Part I, *Mendelian Inheritance.*

**Risk of Recurrence for Patient's Child:**
See Part I, *Mendelian Inheritance.*

**Age of Detectability:** The diagnosis in an isolated case would be extremely difficult until clinical features have evolved. When growth and psychomotor retardation with hypotonia have be-

come apparent, recognition of facial and skeletal features, probably by school-age, would allow diagnosis.

**Gene Mapping and Linkage:** Unknown.

**Prevention:** None known. Genetic counseling indicated.

**Treatment:** Anticonvulsants may be required for control of seizures.

**Prognosis:** The three males are institutionalized and are capable of only minimal self-care. Seizures have been controlled with medication. The skeletal features are relatively asymptomatic, although scoliosis is progressive in one patient and may eventually cause pulmonary compromise. Otherwise there is no apparent limitation of life span.

**Detection of Carrier:** Unknown.

**References:**
Smith RD, Fineman RM, Myers GG: Short stature, psychomotor retardation, and unusual facial appearance in two brothers. Am J Med Genet 1980; 7:5–9. * †
Stephenson L, Johnson JP: Smith-Fineman-Myers Syndrome: report of a third case. Am J Med Genet 1985; 22:301–304. * †

J0012                                               **John P. Johnson**

---

## SMITH-LEMLI-OPITZ SYNDROME                                    0891

**Includes:**
RHS syndrome
SLOS (Smith-Lemli-Opitz syndrome)

**Excludes:**
**Meckel syndrome** (0634)
**Smith-Lemli-Opitz syndrome, type II** (2635)

**Major Diagnostic Criteria:** Up to one-half of the infants with Smith-Lemli-Opitz Syndrome (SLOS) manifest prenatal onset of growth retardation (for weight and/or length). Characteristic craniofacial features include microcephaly, narrow high forehead with prominent metopic suture (a high, square "Daniel Webster" forehead), broad nasal bridge, short nose with anteverted nostrils, bilateral epicanthal folds, ptosis, broad maxillary alveolar ridges, cleft of the posterior palate, micrognathia, and abnormally shaped and/or positioned pinnae. Approximately 70% of 46,XY males with SLOS have abnormalities of the external genitalia which include varying degrees of hypospadias, cryptorchidism, and/or frank ambiguous genitalia. Abnormalities of external genitalia in 46,XX females with SLOS have not been reported. The most characteristic limb abnormalities are postaxial polydactyly (seen in 20–30% of cases) and cutaneous syndactyly of toes 2–3 (seen in 75–95% of cases). Relatively nonspecific major malformations occur in a number of other organ systems, including urinary tract defects in approximately 50% (renal hypoplasia, ureteral or urethral constriction, hydronephrosis, cystic kidney disease); congenital heart disease in approximately 20% (endocardial cushion defects, **Heart, tetralogy of Fallot, Ventricular septal defect**); and **Pyloric stenosis** in 15–25% of cases. Detailed neuropathologic information is limited, but characteristic findings include ventriculomegaly plus hypoplasia of the cerebral hemispheres, the cerebellum, and/or the brainstem.

**Clinical Findings:** Postnatal growth retardation and failure to thrive occur in over 90% of individuals with SLOS. Severe feeding problems with regurgitation and poor sucking also occur in over 90% of affected individuals. Hypotonia is frequent in the newborn period, although hypertonia may develop later. Moderate-to-severe mental retardation is to be expected, although one patient with near normal intelligence has been reported. There is currently insufficient information to comment about secondary sexual development or reproductive capacity.

**Complications:** Gastroesophageal reflux and aspiration resulting in bronchopneumonia.

**Associated Findings:** **Colon, aganglionosis** has been reported in several cases.

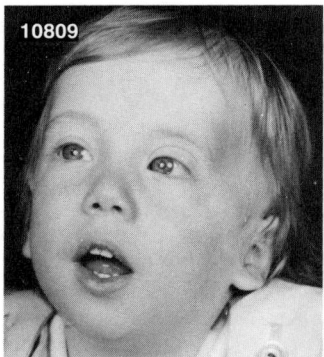
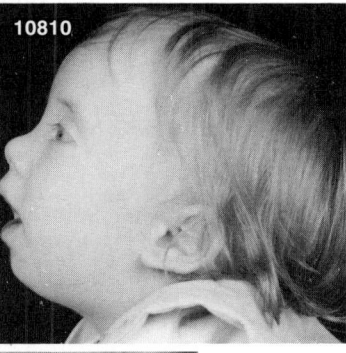

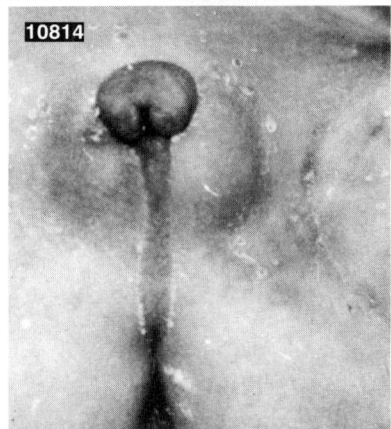

**0891**-10809–10: 18-month-old male with ptosis and small jaw.
10814: Hypospadias and hypoplastic scrotum.

**Etiology:** Autosomal recessive inheritance.

**Pathogenesis:** Unknown.

**MIM No.:** *27040

**POS No.:** 3391

**CDC No.:** 759.820

**Sex Ratio:** Presumably M1:F1. Diagnosed more frequently in males, which probably reflects the greater ease of recognition in the presence of genital abnormalities.

**Occurrence:** Estimated at about 1:40,000.

**Risk of Recurrence for Patient's Sib:**
See Part I, *Mendelian Inheritance.*

**Risk of Recurrence for Patient's Child:**
See Part I, *Mendelian Inheritance.* Most affected individuals do not reproduce.

**Age of Detectability:** In the newborn period. A specific prenatal diagnostic test is not currently available, although ultrasonographic detection of genital anomalies is possible.

**Gene Mapping and Linkage:** Unknown.

**Prevention:** None known. Genetic counseling indicated.

**Treatment:** Unknown.

**Prognosis:** Approximately one-fourth of all affected individuals die within the first two years of life. Most survivors demonstrate moderate to severe mental retardation.

**Detection of Carrier:** Unknown.

**Special Considerations:** The synonym *RSH syndrome* was derived from the surnames of three families originally observed by John Opitz.

**References:**
Smith DW, et al.: A newly recognized syndrome of multiple congenital anomalies. J Pediatr 1964; 64:210–217.
Opitz JM, et al.: The RSH Syndrome. BD:OAS II(2). New York: March of Dimes Birth Defects Foundation, 1969:43–52.
Johnson VP: Smith-Lemli-Opitz syndrome: review and report of two affected siblings. Z Kinderheilk 1975; 119:221–234. *
Lowry RB, Yong SL: Borderline normal intelligence in the Smith-Lemli-Opitz (RSH) syndrome. Am J Med Genet 1980; 5:137–143.
Patterson K, et al.: Hirschsprung disease in a 46,XY phenotypic infant girl with Smith-Lemli-Opitz syndrome. J Pediatr 1983; 103:425–427.
Curry CJR, et al.: Smith-Lemli-Opitz syndrome type II multiple congenital anomalies with male pseudohermaphriditism and frequent early lethality. Am J Med Genet 1987; 26:45–57.
Joseph DB, et al.: Genitourinary abnormalities associated with Smith-Lemli-Opitz syndrome. J Urol 1987; 137:719–721.
Opitz JM, et al.: Smith-Lemli-Opitz (RSH) syndrome bibliography. Am J Med Genet 1987; 28:745–750.

P0021                                        **Barbara Pober**

### SMITH-LEMLI-OPITZ SYNDROME, TYPE II          2635

**Includes:**
  Lung, unilobular-polydactyly-sex reversal-renal hypoplasia
  Polydactyly-sex reversal-renal hypoplasia-unilobular lung
  Renal hypoplasia-unilobular lung-polydactyly-sex reversal
  Rutledge lethal multiple congenital anomaly syndrome
  Sex reversal-polydactyly-renal hypoplasia-unilobular lung

**Excludes:**
  **Aneuploidies** (some)
  **Chondroectodermal dysplasia** (0156)
  **Hydrolethalus syndrome** (2279)
  **Hypothalamic hamartoblastoma syndrome, congenital** (2285)
  **Meckel syndrome** (0634)
  **Oculo-encephalo-hepato-renal syndrome** (3242)
  **Short rib-polydactyly syndrome**
  **Smith-Lemli-Opitz syndrome** (0891)

**Major Diagnostic Criteria:** Three of the following major malformations: **Cleft palate, Polydactyly,** congenital heart disease, cataracts, small tongue, or severe genital ambiguity or pseudohermaphroditism in XY males. A clinical course characterized by frequent early lethality, severe feeding problems, metabolic derangement, and, occasionally, the oligohydramnios sequence. Less frequently seen are **Colon, aganglionosis,** large adrenals, pancreatic islet hypertrophy, unilobated lungs.

**Clinical Findings:** Unlike the **Smith-Lemli-Opitz syndrome** as originally described, Smith-Lemli-Opitz type II is characterized by major structural abnormalities, male pseudohermaphroditism and early death. Pregnancies frequently have been marked by growth retardation and decreased fetal movement, and oligohydramnios has been noted in several instances. Breech presentation occurred in about 50%, and birth asphyxia was extremely common. Three of 43 reported cases died as a consequence of pulmonary hypoplasia secondary to renal agenesis or cystic dysplasia. Congenital heart disease was seen in over 75%, cataracts (50%), postaxial polydactyly (85%), **Cleft palate** (70%), and male pseudohermaphroditism (70%), and genital ambiguity (30%). The incidence of islet cell hyperplasia was approximately 40%, and unilobated lungs were noted in 57% of autopsied cases. Mild **Microcephaly** has been seen in many Smith-Lemli-Opitz type II patients. **Hydrocephaly** and the absence of the corpus callosum have been noted in several patients. Most infants with this presentation have died prior to three months of age. The exact cause of death is frequently not clear, but in those surviving beyond the first few days, poor suck and feeding, projectile vomiting, abdominal distention, profound developmental delay, occasional liver disease, and recurrent respiratory infections are common.

**Complications:** Recurrent respiratory infections, pyloric stenosis, and hepatic dysfunction.

**Associated Findings:** Toe **Syndactyly,** redundant neck skin, short limbs, facial hemangiomata, and joint contractures.

**2635-21508:** Note facial profile with microcephaly and micrognathia. 21509: Polydactyly. 21510: Synda of second and third toes; note also polydactyly.

**Etiology:** Autosomal recessive inheritance.

**Pathogenesis:** The occasional findings of renal cysts, large adrenals and hepatic dysfunction are suggestive of a possible **Peroxisomal** defect. However, initial investigations of long-chain fatty acid levels and plasmalogen synthesis have revealed no abnormalities. The frequency of low estriol levels in late pregnancy, and aberrant sexual differentiation and large adrenals at autopsy, point to a possible defect in fetal adrenal metabolism.

**MIM No.:** *26867

**POS No.:** 3645

**CDC No.:** 759.820

**Sex Ratio:** Presumably M1:F1. The presence of genital ambiguity in affected males has strongly biased the ascertainment of males with this syndrome.

**Occurrence:** Close to 50 that appear to fulfill criteria for the diagnosis have been reported in the literature.

**Risk of Recurrence for Patient's Sib:**
See Part I, *Mendelian Inheritance.*

**Risk of Recurrence for Patient's Child:**
See Part I, *Mendelian Inheritance.* Affected individuals are not expected to survive to reproduce.

**Age of Detectability:** At birth, or prenatally by the 24th week of pregnancy. Ultrasound can be used to assess fetal movement, determine fetal sex, and to assess renal and cardiac function. Amniocentesis for fetal sexing may be appropriate. Measurements of estriols may also be useful but there is no data on these levels in at-risk pregnancies in the second trimester.

**Gene Mapping and Linkage:** Unknown.

**Prevention:** None known. Genetic counseling indicated.

**Treatment:** Surgery for complications such as **Pyloric stenosis** and **Colon, aganglionosis.**

**Prognosis:** Most affected infants have died in the first week of life. The longest survivor died at age 19 months. Severe growth failure and mental retardation have been characteristic in those surviving beyond the first weeks of life.

**Detection of Carrier:** Unknown.

**References:**
Rutledge JC, et al.: A "new" lethal multiple congenital anomaly syndrome. Am J Med Genet 1984; 19:255–264. * †
Donnai D, et al.: The lethal multiple congenital anomaly syndrome of polydactyly, sex reversal, renal hypoplasia, and unilobar lungs. J Med Genet 1986; 23:64–71.
Belmont JW, et al.: Two cases of severe lethal Smith-Lemli-Opitz syndrome. (Letter) Am J Med Genet 1987; 26:65–67.
Curry CJR, et al.: Smith-Lemli-Opitz syndrome-type II: multiple congenital anomalies with male pseudohermaphroditism and frequent early lethality. Am J Med Genet 1987; 26:45–57. *

CU009                                           **Cynthia J.R. Curry**
RU017                                              **Joe C. Rutledge**

**Smith-Magenis syndrome**
*See CHROMOSOME 17, INTERSTITIAL DELETION 17p*
**Smith-McCort dwarfism**
*See DYGGVE-MELCHIOR-CLAUSEN SYNDROME*
**Smith-Strang disease**
*See METHIONINE MALABSORPTION*
**Smoking, cigarette, fetal effects**
*See FETAL EFFECTS OF MATERNAL CIGARETTE SMOKING*
**Snail-like pelvis dysplasia**
*See SKELETAL DYSPLASIA, SCHNECKENBECKEN TYPE*
**Sneezing from light exposure**
*See ACHOO SYNDROME*
**Snow-capped teeth**
*See TEETH, SNOW-CAPPED*
**Solitary polyp syndrome**
*See CANCER, COLORECTAL*
**Somatomedin C deficiency**
*See GROWTH DEFICIENCY, AFRICAN PYGMY TYPE*
**Sorsby syndrome**
*See MACULAR COLOBOMA-BRACHYDACTYLY*
**Sotos syndrome**
*See CEBEBRAL GIGANTISM*
**South African porphyria**
*See PORPHYRIA, VARIEGATE*

**SPASTIC ATAXIA, CHARLEVOIX-SAGUENAY TYPE**     **2566**

**Includes:**
Autosomal recessive spastic ataxia of Charlevoix-Saguenay (ARSACS)
Charlevoix-Saguenay spastic ataxia

**Excludes:**
**Ataxia, Friedreich type** (2714)
**Ataxia-telangiectasia** (0094)
**Ataxia** (others)
**Marinesco-Sjogren syndrome** (2031)
**Optic atrophy, infantile heredofamilial** (0755)
**Paraplegia, familial spastic** (0295)
**Sjogren-Larsson syndrome** (2030)
Troyer syndrome

**Major Diagnostic Criteria:** Onset between 1–2 years of age; spasticity; dysarthria; distal muscle wasting; truncal ataxia; foot deformities; absence of sensory evoked potentials in the lower limbs; nystagmus; retinal striation reminiscent of early **Optic atrophy, Leber type**; and the frequent presence of **Mitral valve prolapse.**

**Clinical Findings:** Although most patients have normal early milestones, none ever walk normally. The parents note unsteadiness and frequent falls when affected children begin to walk. Dysarthria with slurring of speech is always present. Horizontal nystagmus is always present, often with predominance on one side. There is occasionally a more irregular vertical nystagmus. There is also a gross defect of conjugate pursuit ocular movements. These are dysmetric, saccadic, and restricted to the horizontal plane.

Muscle tone is markedly increased in the lower limbs, with polykinetic knee jerks and occasionally clonus at this level. Chaddock and Babinski signs are easily elicited in all cases. Posterior column signs in the lower limbs are found in all patients, with decreased or absent vibration sense in the toes and to a lesser extent at the ankles.

Position sense in the toes is mildly impaired. Cutaneous sensation is normal in all patients. Distal leg atrophy is present in most patients, and this sometimes extends to the anterior compartment of the leg. Pes cavus is frequently seen. Wasting of the small muscles is seen in almost half of the patients. Incontinence of urine or feces is a frequent important feature.

Mean I.Q.'s are in the low normal range, with significant impairment of non-verbal vs. verbal tasks. Visual acuity and fundoscopy are normal, except for striking and markedly increased visibility of the retinal nerve fibers, resembling early stages of **Optic atrophy, Leber type**.

The progression of the disease is relatively slow. The ataxia can be stable for long periods, and then seems to worsen over a period of a few years. Vibration sense gradually diminishes. There are progressive deformities of the feet and hands. The nonverbal performance scales are also negatively correlated with age.

The diagnosis can be suspected from the geographic origin, the early onset of ataxia, the slow progression, and normal or increased deep tendon reflexes in the lower extremities. The main clinical features differentiating these patients from those with classical **Ataxia, Friedreich type** (FA) are constant nystagmus; spasticity with increased deep tendon reflexes; the absence of scoliosis; the presence of retinal striations; incontinence of bladder and/or bowels; absence of hypertrophic cardiomyopathy; and high frequency of **Mitral valve prolapse**.

Motor nerve conduction is slowed in ARSACS, whereas it is normal in FA. Sensory nerve conduction is absent or markedly impaired in both conditions. The EMG shows more signs of denervation in ARSACS, despite the fact that the evolution is slower. The CT scan in ARSACS demonstrates signs of cerebellar atrophy almost limited to the superior parts of the vermis and anterior lobes, whereas in FA, the X-ray signs are variable and less obvious.

Sural nerve biopsy in two patients revealed a severe loss of large myelinated axons contrasting with a normal myelinated fiber density, suggesting a developmental abnormality of peripheral nerve. No diagnostic biochemical abnormalities are known.

**Complications:** Deformities of the feet and hands, including clawing of the toes; pes cavus; equinovarus deformities of the feet, alone or with supination (club feet); marked atrophy of the muscles, leading to claw hands; and internal rotation and scissoring of the lower limbs due to spasticity. Some patients require surgery for Achilles tendon elongation.

**Associated Findings:** None known.

**Etiology:** Autosomal recessive inheritance. This is confirmed by multiple cases in sibships, absence of affected parents or offspring, increased parental consanguinity, and the finding of a common ancestral couple in a number of sibships.

**Pathogenesis:** Unknown.

**MIM No.:** *27055

**Sex Ratio:** M3:F2 (observed, based on 42 patients).

**Occurrence:** Not described outside of the Charlevoix-Saguenay region of Québec, which represents a genetic isolate. The prevalence in this region is unknown. Over 200 cases have been observed.

**Risk of Recurrence for Patient's Sib:**
See Part I, *Mendelian Inheritance*.

**Risk of Recurrence for Patient's Child:**
See Part I, *Mendelian Inheritance*.

**Age of Detectability:** The disease can be suspected soon after the child starts to walk, particularly if there is a positive family history and/or the child originates from the Charlevoix-Saguenay region of Québec.

**Gene Mapping and Linkage:** Unknown.

**Prevention:** None known. Genetic counseling indicated.

**Treatment:** Symptomatic. Lengthening of Achilles tendons and surgical correction of the foot and hand deformities may indicated.

**Prognosis:** The disease is slowly progressive, and survival to the fifth and sixth decade of life is not uncommon. A number of patients have reproduced.

**Detection of Carrier:** Unknown.

**Special Considerations:** It is important to distinguish this very specific and clinically homogeneous form of spastic ataxia from the many similar syndromes that have been previously described, such as Troyer syndrome (Cross and McKusick, 1967).

**Support Groups:**
New York; National Myoclonus Foundation
MD; Landover; Epilepsy Foundation of America

**References:**
Cross HE, McKusick VA: The Troyer syndrome: a recessive form of spastic paraplegia with distal muscle wasting. Arch Neurol 1967; 16:473–485.
Bouchard JP, et al: Autosomal recessive spastic ataxia of Charlevoix-Saguenay. Can J Neuro Sci 1978; 5:61–69. *
Bouchard JP, et al: Electromyography and nerve conduction studies in Friedreich's ataxia and autosomal recessive spastic ataxia of Charlevoix-Saguenay. Can J Neurol Sci 1979; 6:185–189.
Bouchard JP, et al: Electroencephalographic findings in Friedreich's ataxia and autosomal recessive spastic ataxia of Charlevoix-Saguenay (ARSACS). Can J Neurol Sci 1979; 6:191–194.
Dionne J, et al: Oculomotor and vestibular findings in autosomal recessive spastic ataxia of Charlevoix-Saguenay. Can J Neurol Sci 1979; 6:177–184.
Langelier R, et al: Computed tomography of posterior fossa in hereditary ataxias. Can J Neurol Sci 1979; 6:195–198.
Peyronnard JM, et al: The neuropathy of Charlevoix-Saguenay ataxia: an electrophysiological and pathological study. Can J Neurol Sci 1979; 6:199–203.
Barbeau A: A tentative classification of recessively inherited ataxias. Can J Neurol Sci 1982; 9:95–98.

AN016                                                    **Eva Andermann**

---

**Spastic diplegia, from extrinsically caused iodine disorder**
*See CRETINISM, ENDEMIC, AND RELATED DISORDERS*
**Spastic infantile paralysis (cerebral)**
*See CEREBRAL PALSY*
**Spastic paraplegia, hereditary**
*See PARAPLEGIA, FAMILIAL SPASTIC*
**Spastic paraplegia, pure hereditary**
*See PARAPLEGIA, FAMILIAL SPASTIC*
**Spastic paraplegia, X-linked, complicated**
*See PARAPLEGIA, FAMILIAL SPASTIC*
**Spastic paraplegia-palmoplantar hyperkeratosis-retardation**
*See HYPERKERATOSIS PALMOPLANTARIS-SPASTIC PARAPLEGIA-RETARDATION*
**Spastic pseudosclerosis**
*See CREUTZFELDT-JAKOB DISEASE*
**Spasticity-ichthyosis-oligophrenia**
*See SJOGREN-LARSSON SYNDROME*
**Speech fluency disorder**
*See STUTTERING*
**Speech, hypernasal**
*See PALATOPHARYNGEAL INCOMPETENCE*
**Sperocytosis, hereditary**
*See SPHEROCYTOSIS*

---

**SPHEROCYTOSIS**                                                0892

**Includes:**
Anemia, spherocytic, congenital
Minkowski-Chauffard syndrome
Sperocytosis, hereditary

**Excludes:**
**Anemia, hemolytic, red cell membrane defects** (2646)
Anemias, congenital nonspherocytic
**Elliptocytosis** (2665)

**Major Diagnostic Criteria:** Chronic hemolytic anemia of variable severity, with the presence of a variable number of spherocytic and microspherocytic erythrocytes on blood smear. Mean corpuscular hemoglobin concentration (MCHC) often elevated (>34 g/dl). Elevated autohemolysis of erythrocytes upon incubation for 48 hours at 37 degree C, with partial correction in the presence of glucose. Increased sensitivity to lysis of erythrocytes in hypotonic media (osmotic fragility), which is accentuated by incubation for 24 hours at 37 degree C. Absence of erythrocyte autoantibodies.

**Clinical Findings:** The anemia is of variable severity, ranging from normal hemoglobin levels with modestly elevated reticulocytes in some individuals to severe anemia with overt jaundice and markedly elevated reticulocyte counts in others. Severity of anemia is often variable among affected family members. Hemolytic jaundice is common in neonates with hereditary spherocytosis, but the etiology is often not recognized at this age. Anemia is generally more severe in the first year of life, occasionally requiring transfusions, but few patients over age one year require chronic transfusions. Splenomegaly is extremely common (75–100%). A family history of spherocytosis, splenectomies, or cholelithiasis is often elicited. Severely affected individuals may have "hemolytic facies" due to expansion of the medullary spaces in the cranial bones.

**Complications:** The most common potentially life-threatening complications in the individual with an intact spleen are acute exacerbations of anemia. These include aplastic crises characterized by rapidly worsening anemia and reticulocytopenia. The bone marrow shows a marked decrease in erythroid precursors, with a few giant proerythroblasts present. A human parvovirus has been found to cause the majority of aplastic crises and selectively inhibit erythroid cell production in marrow culture. Simultaneous depression of granulocytes and platelets has been reported. Prompt red cell transfusion is generally required. Normal erythrocyte production resumes spontaneously in 7–10 days. Hyperhemolytic crises manifested by worsening anemia, increased jaundice, dark urine, reticulocytosis, and possibly increasing spleen size may be associated with other illnesses such as viral infections. Overt hypersplenism with leukopenia and thrombocytopenia may occur. As many as 50% of patients may develop cholelithiasis or cholecystitis, particularly in the teen and adult years. Other complications of hemolytic anemia such as leg ulcers may occur. Hemochromatosis has been reported, but may represent independent inheritance of an unrelated illness. Following splenectomy, there is an approximately 3% risk for overwhelming postsplenectomy septicemia, which carries a high fatality rate of about 50%. The causative organism is generally pneumococcus. The risk for septicemia exists for an indefinite period following splenectomy.

**Associated Findings:** None known.

**Etiology:** Usually autosomal dominant inheritance, although in about 20% of cases the parents are apparently not affected. In some cases this is due to variable penetrance, since there are some families with hematologically normal parents and more than one affected child. Autosomal recessive inheritance of severe spherocytosis due to partial spectrin deficiency has been reported.

**Pathogenesis:** Hereditary spherocytosis is classified as an inherited erythrocyte membrane protein defect. A variety of biochemical and physiologic abnormalities have been reported in the erythrocytes of these individuals. The most consistent of these is a passive increase in transmembrane sodium leak, which is compensated by increase in ATP-dependent sodium extrusion. Hence, metabolic activity (glucose consumption) is increased, intracellular pH is lower than normal, and 2,3-diphosphoglycerate levels are often depressed. However, the severity of the cation leak does not correlate with the severity of the hemolysis in vivo. The hemolytic process is clearly related to splenic function, since splenectomy usually cures the anemia despite the persistence of the morphologic red cell defect. The spleen is felt to "condition" the red cells so that repetitive passage of a cell through the spleen leads to progressive loss of membrane lipid, with concomitant decrease in surface:volume ratio. The mechanism of this conditioning is unknown. With progressive spherocytic transformation, the cell becomes less deformable, ultimately trapped in the narrow (3 $\mu$m) splenic cords. Increased cell fragmentation under conditions of high shear stress has been seen in some forms of hereditary spherocytosis. Several different membrane protein defects have now been found, consistent with the heterogeneity in clinical severity and inheritance modes. Partial spectrin deficiency with spectrin levels as low as 26–29% of normal has been found in recessively inherited spherocytosis. Interestingly, some degree of spectrin loss may occur in all spherocytosis and correlates with the severity of the hemolysis. Defective binding of spectrin to protein 4.1 in some kindreds with spherocytosis appears to be caused by a defect in the alpha-spectrin V or beta-spectrin IV domain. An abnormal spectrin with increased binding avidity to the cell membrane has also been reported.

**MIM No.:** *18290, *27097

**CDC No.:** 282.000

**Sex Ratio:** M1:F1

**Occurrence:** The most common form of inherited hemolytic anemia in persons of Northern European descent, with a prevalence of 1:5,000. Does occur in other populations.

**Risk of Recurrence for Patient's Sib:**
See Part I, *Mendelian Inheritance.*

**Risk of Recurrence for Patient's Child:**
See Part I, *Mendelian Inheritance.*

**Age of Detectability:** At birth or during early childhood in many cases, although individuals with milder anemia often are discovered as older children or even adults. Prenatal diagnosis has not been reported.

**Gene Mapping and Linkage:** SPH1 (spherocytosis 1 (clinical type II)) has been mapped to 8p21.1-p11.22.
ANK (ankyrin) has been provisionally mapped to 8p21-p11.

**Prevention:** None known. Genetic counseling indicated.

**Treatment:** Splenectomy is definitive treatment. Following splenectomy, red cell survival becomes nearly normal, eliminating the anemia and hemolysis in most individuals. Even severely anemic individuals improve clinically, although the anemia may only be partially relieved. Splenectomy reduces the risks for aplastic and hyperhemolytic crises and gallbladder disease. Because of the risk for postsplenectomy sepsis, careful consideration of splenectomy must be made based on the severity of the anemia. Chronically anemic individuals, particularly those with jaundice, hyperhemolytic events, hypersplenism, poor growth and exercise intolerance, gallbladder disease and so forth, will derive the greatest benefit. Splenectomy is generally deferred until the patient is five years or older due to the unacceptably high incidence of sepsis following splenectomy in infants. Administration of pneumococcal vaccine, preferably prior to splenectomy, as well as prophylactic penicillin administration following splenectomy, may reduce the risk for later sepsis. In the individual with an intact spleen, an aplastic or hyperhemolytic crisis may necessitate red cell transfusion. Folic acid therapy is useful in the recovery phase of aplastic crisis, when transient folate deficiency may occur. Symptomatic gallbladder disease may require cholecystectomy.

**Prognosis:** Following splenectomy, spherocytosis is generally compatible with a normal life-style, although about 2% of these individuals will succumb to overwhelming bacterial infection.

**Detection of Carrier:** In dominantly inherited spherocytosis, most heterozygotes are clinically affected. Occasionally, a parent may have a detectable increase in passive red cell sodium flux without evidence of spherocytes, possibly representing incomplete penetrance. In the recessive form of spherocytosis, reduced red cell spectrin occurs in heterozygotes, but such testing is currently available only on an experimental basis.

**Special Considerations:** The presence of spherocytes on a blood smear indicates a population of cells with reduced surface:volume ratio and may result from a variety of congenital or acquired illnesses. Such cells may exhibit increased osmotic fragility, regardless of their origin. Therefore, until definitive tests for intrinsic red cell membrane abnormalities become clinically available, the diagnosis of hereditary spherocytosis can only be made when due consideration is given to other causes of spherocyte formation. For example, hereditary spherocytosis in the neonate may be difficult to distinguish from erythroblastosis fetalis due to a maternal-fetal ABO incompatibility. A further difficulty in establishing the diagnosis of hereditary spherocytosis in the newborn is that neonatal red cells ordinarily exhibit *decreased* osmotic fragility compared to erythrocytes from older individuals. A diagnosis of spherocytosis in a neonate should always be confirmed by retesting at age six months or older.

**References:**
Wiley JS: Co-ordinated increase of sodium leak and sodium pump in hereditary spherocytosis. Br J Haematol 1972; 22:529–542.
Agre P, et al.: Deficient red cell spectrin in severe, recessively inherited spherocytosis. New Engl J Med 1982; 306:1155–1161.
Goodman SR, et al.: Identification of the molecular defect in the erythrocyte membrane skeleton of some kindreds with hereditary spherocytosis. Blood 1982; 60:772–784.
Burke BE, Shotton DM: Erythrocyte membrane skeleton abnormalities in hereditary spherocytosis. Br J Haematol 1983; 54:173–187.
Agre P, et al.: Partial deficiency of erythrocyte spectrin in hereditary spherocytosis. Nature 1985; 314:380–383.
Becker PS, Lux SE: Hereditary spherocytosis and related disorders. Clin Hematol 1985; 14:15–43.
Chilicote RR, et al.: Association of red cell spherocytosis with deletion of the short arm of chromosome 8. Blood 1987; 69:156–159.

LA041                                   **Richard J. Labotka**

**Spherocytosis, hereditary**
*See ANEMIA, HEMOLYTIC, RED CELL MEMBRANE DEFECTS*

---

## SPHEROPHAKIA-BRACHYMORPHIA SYNDROME          0893

**Includes:**
   Mesodermal dysmorphodystrophy, brachymorphic type, congenital
   Weill-Marchesani syndrome

**Excludes:**  Short stature, constitutional-dislocated lens and pupil

**Major Diagnostic Criteria:**  Congenital spherophakia, with or without dislocated lenses, and short stature.

**Clinical Findings:**  Characterized by microspherophakia and progressive dislocation of the lens in patients of pyknic habitus. The height is usually below the third percentile. The patients show brachycephaly, pug nose, depressed nasal bridge, and short pudgy hands and feet. There may be articular stiffness and limitation of extension. Affected persons have marked myopia.

**Complications:**  Acute pupillary block glaucoma.

**Associated Findings:**  Subvalvular fibromuscular aortic stenosis was reported in one 11-year-old girl.

**Etiology:**  Presumably autosomal recessive inheritance with partial expression in the heterozygote, although dominant inheritance has been suggested in some pedigrees.

**Pathogenesis:**  Undetermined. Acute glaucoma may arise through several mechanisms. The anterior displacement of the lens may block the pupil and hinder the aqueous flow. In this case dilation of the pupil may relieve the symptoms. Glaucoma may also arise as a complication of a dislocated lens through irritation of the ciliary body. Complete luxation into the anterior chamber is occasionally seen, and may lead to corneal decompensation.

**MIM No.:**  *27760

**POS No.:**  3043

**CDC No.:**  743.310

**Sex Ratio:**  M1:F1

**Occurrence:**  1:100,000, with world-wide distribution.

**Risk of Recurrence for Patient's Sib:**
   See Part I, *Mendelian Inheritance.*

**Risk of Recurrence for Patient's Child:**
   See Part I, *Mendelian Inheritance.*

**Age of Detectability:**  At birth, if suspected.

**Gene Mapping and Linkage:**  Unknown.

**Prevention:**  None known. Genetic counseling indicated.

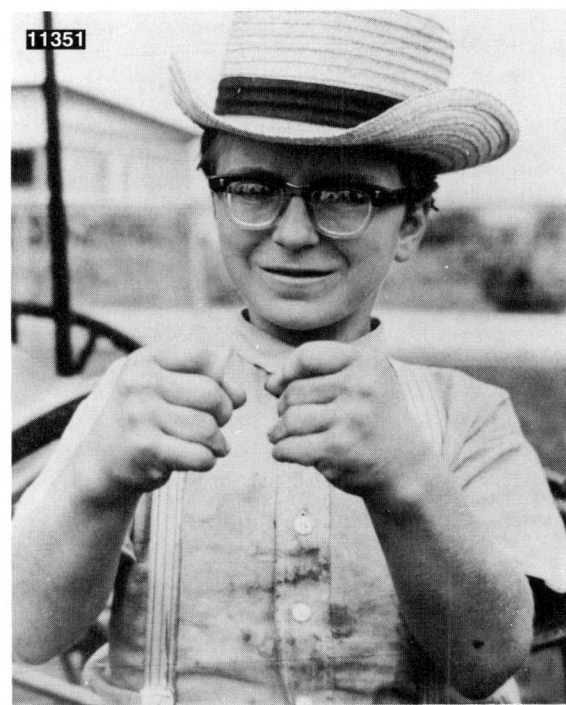

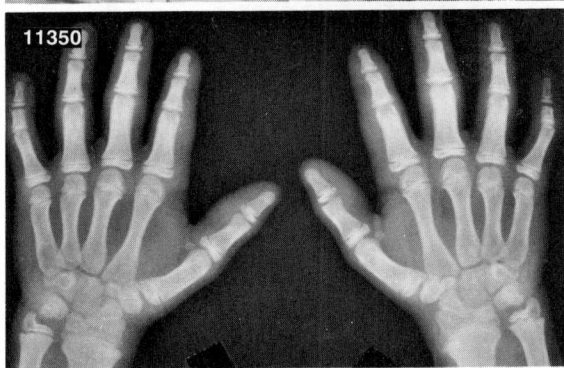

**0893**-11351:   Pug nose, short hands with knobby joints, and restriction in flexion.   11350:   All bones are short, especially middle phalanges of 5th fingers.

**Treatment:**  Control of intraocular pressure; prophylactic iridotomy or lens extraction if glaucoma present.

**Prognosis:**  Good for life span and intelligence, reduced visual function.

**Detection of Carrier:**  By clinical examination, looking for a distinctly short pyknic habitus without the ocular findings in first degree relatives.

**References:**
Kloepfer HW, Rosenthal JW: Possible genetic carriers in the spherophakia - brachymorphia syndrome. Am J Hum Genet 1955; 7:398–425.
Rennert OM: The Marchesani syndrome: a brief review. Am J Dis Child 1969; 117:703–705.
Jensen AD, et al.: Ocular complications in the Weill-Marchesani syndrome. Am J Ophthal 1974; 77:261–269.
Ferrier S, et al.: Le syndrome de Marchesani (spherophakie-brachymorphie). Helv Paediatr Acta 1980; 35:185–198.

Young ID, et al.: Weill-Marchesani syndrome in a mother and son. Clin Genet 1986; 30:475–480.

MA054                                                    Irene H. Maumenee

**Sphingomyelin lipidosis**
*See NIEMANN-PICK DISEASE*
**Sphingomyelinase deficiency**
*See NIEMANN-PICK DISEASE*
**Spiegler-Brooke tumors**
*See EPITHELIOMAS, HEREDITARY MULTIPLE CYSTIC
also SCALP, CYLINDROMAS*
**Spielmeyer-Sjogren disease (juvenile NCL)**
*See NEURONAL CEROID-LIPOFUSCINOSES (NCL)*
**Spielmeyer-Vogt disease (juvenile NCL or JNCL)**
*See NEURONAL CEROID-LIPOFUSCINOSES (NCL)*
**Spina bifida cystica with paralysis**
*See MENINGOMYELOCELE*
**Spina bifida cystica without neurologic deficit**
*See MENINGOCELE*
**Spina bifida-anencephaly**
*See BRAIN, ARNOLD-CHIARI MALFORMATION*
**Spinal achnoid cysts-distichiasis-lymphedeme, hereditary**
*See DISTICHIASIS-LYMPHEDEMA SYNDROME*
**Spinal and bulbar muscular atrophy**
*See SPINAL MUSCULAR ATROPHY*
**Spinal ataxia, heredofamilial**
*See ATAXIA, FRIEDREICH TYPE*
**Spinal cord cavitation**
*See SYRINGOMYELIA*

## SPINAL CORD, NEURENTERIC CYST                        0894

**Includes:**
Cyst of the spinal cord associated with posterior mediastinal cyst
Neurenteric cyst of spinal cord

**Excludes:** Diastematomyelia (0292)

**Major Diagnostic Criteria:** Progressive neurologic deficit consisting of weakness and sensory loss from pressure on the spinal cord of a cyst demonstrated by sonography or myelography.

**Clinical Findings:** Depending upon the level of the persisting embryonic defect, a progressive neurologic loss occurs, as well as a paralysis of the legs, bladder, and bowel. Sensory loss is present in the newborn or during the first few years of life. If there is an associated posterior mediastinal cyst, cardiothoracic symptoms are present. There is generally no skin lesion over the area of the affected spinal cord. Butterfly vertebrae are also seen.

**Complications:** Failure to sweat below the level of the lesion; temperature control is difficult.

**Associated Findings:** Bowel duplications, mediastinal or cervical cysts; diastematomyelia.

**Etiology:** Unknown.

**Pathogenesis:** There is a persistent connection between the alimentary tract and the midline neural structures with this mesodermal defect. One hypothesis is that primitive notocordal plate tissue carries entoderm into the vertebral canal, and enterogenous cysts occur within the spinal canal in the lower cervical or upper thoracic level. The association of enterogenous cysts with vertebral anomalies suggests errors in embryonic development. A midline ectoendodermal adhesion obstructing the axial mesoderm and persisting as a neurenteric connection through the vertebral defect in the second week of life is postulated. During the third week the axial mesoderm would have to either split or detour in order to pass the ectoendodermal adhesion. This might result in defects in the vertebral bodies, with the adhesion remaining as a postnatal cyst and a diastematomyelia or band between the alimentary canal and spinal cord.

**CDC No.:** 742.580

**Sex Ratio:** Presumably M1:F1.

**Occurrence:** Undetermined but presumed rare.

**Risk of Recurrence for Patient's Sib:** Unknown.

**Risk of Recurrence for Patient's Child:** Unknown.

**Age of Detectability:** Unknown.

**Gene Mapping and Linkage:** Unknown.

**Prevention:** None known.

**Treatment:** Surgical excision or drainage of the spinal cyst is possible. If a cyst is present in the mediastinum or neck, it may be removed during a secondary operation. Prevention of kidney disease secondary to bladder paralysis.

**Prognosis:** Depends on the degree of paralysis and the rapidity of onset.

**Detection of Carrier:** Unknown.

**References:**
Bale PM: A congenital intraspinal gastroenterogenous cyst and diastematomyelia. J Neurol Neurosurg Psychiatry 1973; 36:1011.

SH007                                                    Kenneth Shapiro

**Spinal dysraphism syndrome**
*See LIPOMENINGOCELE*

## SPINAL MUSCULAR ATROPHY                              0895

**Includes:**
Bulbospinal muscular atrophy, X-linked
Finkel late-adult spinal muscular atrophy
Kennedy disease
Kugelberg-Welander disease
Muscular atrophy, adult spinal
Muscular atrophy, juvenile spinal
Muscular atrophy, spinal, intermediate type
Spinal and bulbar muscular atrophy
Spinal muscular atrophy, benign-hypertrophy of calves
Spinal muscular atrophy, childhood isolated
Spinal muscular atrophy, distal type
Spinal muscular atrophy, facioscapulohumeral type
Spinal muscular atrophy, infantile acute form
Spinal muscular atrophy, infantile chronic form
Spinal muscular atrophy, proximal, adult type
Spinal muscular atrophy, type I
Spinal muscular atrophy, type II
Spinal muscular atrophy, type III
Spinal muscular atrophy, type IV
Werdnig-Hoffmann disease

**Excludes:**
**Amyotrophic lateral sclerosis** (2067)
**Charcot-Marie-Tooth disease**
**G(M2)-gangliosidosis with hexosaminidase A and B deficiency** (0433)
**G(M2)-gangliosidosis with hexosaminidase A deficiency** (0434)
Guillain-Barre syndrome
Hypotonia, benign congenital
**Muscular atrophy, spinal and bulbar, X-linked Kennedy type** (2493)
**Muscular dystrophy** (see all)

**Major Diagnostic Criteria:** Hypotonia, weakness, and decreased or absent deep tendon reflexes with characteristic electromyogram (EMG) and muscle biopsy findings.

**Clinical Findings:** A number of forms of spinal muscular atrophy (SMA) have been described, with the infantile type I (*Werdnig-Hoffmann*) and juvenile type III (*Kugelberg-Welander*) being perhaps the best recognized.

In the infantile form (*type I*), symptoms may begin in utero with decreased fetal movement, at birth, or in the first months of life. Hypotonia, weakness, decreased spontaneous activity, and decreased or absent deep tendon reflexes are some of the first signs. There is no sensory loss. Intercostal muscles are nearly always involved, while the diaphragm is spared, resulting in "paradoxic" respirations. Common findings include muscle atrophy; fasciculations, particularly of the tongue; and a characteristic "frog" position with abducted hips and flexed knees. There is a failure to attain age-appropriate motor milestones. The course is rapidly progressive, with death occurring within 1 to 2 years of diagnosis, usually due to pulmonary infection or respiratory insufficiency.

In the juvenile form (*type III*), onset is usually after the second year and may occur as late as adolescence or adulthood. The course may be slowly progressive, but is often static, and there may be slight improvement with age. The proximal muscles are affected first, and may initially mimic Duchenne muscular dystrophy. A fine tremor of outstretched arms is often present. Life span may be normal. Intellectual development is normal.

An intermediate form (*chronic childhood spinal muscular atrophy, type II*), probably genetically distinct from the juvenile form, presents in infancy usually between six to 24 months, and has a prolonged course extending over several years.

Both slowly progressive and rapidly progressive adult onset forms have been recognized.

Other, probably distinct, forms known as distal SMAs involve only distal muscles and have a slow clinical progression.

Laboratory findings include normal cerebrospinal-fluid. Muscle enzymes are usually normal but may be mildly elevated in the juvenile form. Electromyogram (EMG) shows a denervation pattern with large amplitude, polyphasic potentials of long duration, reduced interference pattern on voluntary movement, and fibrillation potentials at rest. Nerve conduction times are normal or minimally prolonged. Muscle biopsy shows groups of angular atrophied fibers interspersed with large bundles of exclusively type I (usually) or type II fibers. "Type grouping" can be demonstrated with appropriate histochemical stains. Atrophy of anterior horn cells of the spinal cord and peripheral nerve degeneration are seen.

Electron microscopic findings include disorganized fibrils, filaments, and sarcomeres, as well as mitochondrial changes, nuclear clumping, and areas of regeneration.

In several families, hexosaminidase deficiency (see **G(M2)-gangliosidosis**) has been associated with clinical and laboratory findings of SMA.

**Complications:**  Recurrent lower respiratory infection, scoliosis, osteoporosis, and other orthopedic deformities.

**Associated Findings:**  Urinary incontinence, cardiomyopathy, cardiac arrhythmia, arthrogryposis. One family was reported in which weakness was confined mainly to the face and pectoral girdle musculature (Fenichel et al, 1967). Hausmanowa-Petrusewicz (1984) reported an absence of tonsillar tissue.

**Etiology:**  Autosomal recessive inheritance (most cases of types I, II, and III) is most common, but some cases of types II and III, many cases of adult onset type IV, and some of the distal varieties are by autosomal dominant inheritance. For an X-linked form, see **Muscular atrophy, spinal and bulbar, X-linked Kennedy type**.

**Pathogenesis:**  Degeneration of anterior horn cells of the spinal cord and brain stem, with subsequent distinctive changes in the associated muscles.

**MIM No.:**  15859, *15860, 18296, 18297, *18298, *25330, *25340, *25355, 27112, 27115

**CDC No.:**  335.000

**Sex Ratio:**  Presumably M1:F1. Males are more frequently reported, although males with the juvenile form may be less severely involved. This accounts, in part, for the belief that some cases may be X-linked.

**Occurrence:**  Incidence 4:100,000 live births in northeast England (infantile form). Prevalence 12:1,000,000 in northeast England (juvenile form). The Kugelberg-Welander form has been frequently reported in an inbred Scottish population and on Reunion Island.

**Risk of Recurrence for Patient's Sib:**
See Part I, *Mendelian Inheritance*.

**Risk of Recurrence for Patient's Child:**
See Part I, *Mendelian Inheritance*.

**Age of Detectability:**  Before two years of age in the infantile form; two years to adulthood in the juvenile form. An adult form with onset in the fifth or sixth decade has been reported (Jansen et al, 1986).

**Gene Mapping and Linkage:**  SBMA (spinal and bulbar muscular atrophy (Kennedy disease)) has been mapped to Xq13-q22.

**Prevention:**  None known. Genetic counseling indicated.

**Treatment:**  Physical therapy, respiratory care, scrupulous treatment of respiratory infections, and orthopedic care.

**Prognosis:**  In the infantile and adult forms: death within one to two years of onset. In the juvenile form: prolonged survival and sometimes normal life span.

**Detection of Carrier:**  Unknown.

**Special Considerations:**  The nosology of the spinal muscular atrophies has provoked considerable discussion. Several genetic and clinical entities are readily recognized, but there are several other forms. Pearn (1978) distinguished at least ten separate SMA syndromes and postulates 15 or more mutant genes. Until basic defects are identified, distinctions remain imprecise. Although age of onset, clinical course, pattern of muscle involvement, and mode of inheritance are useful distinguishing characteristics for prognosis and counseling purposes, they must be interpreted carefully, since overlapping may occur among the various forms. Families are known in which different members are affected by clinically distinct forms of SMA. Bouwsma et al (1986), Zerres et al (1987), and others have supported Becker's allelic model as an explanation for some unusual pedigrees.

**Support Groups:**
New York; Muscular Dystrophy Association (MDA)
IL; Highland Park (P.O. Box 1465); Families of Spinal Muscular Atrophy

**References:**
Fenichel GM, et al.: Neurogenic atrophy simulating facioscapulohumeral dystrophy. Arch Neurol 1967; 17:257–260.
Emery AEH: The nosology of the spinal muscular atrophies. J Med Genet 1971; 8:481–494.
Pearn JH: Incidence, prevalence and gene frequency studies of childhood spinal muscular atrophy. J Med Genet 1978; 15:409–433.
Johnson WG: Hexosaminidase deficiency: a cause of recessively inherited motor neuron diseases. Adv Neurol 1982; 36:159–164.
Hausmanowa-Petrusewicz I, et al.: Chronic proximal spinal muscular atrophy of childhood and adolescence: sex influence. J Med Genet 1984; 21:447–450.
Hausmanowa-Petrusewicz I, et al.: Chronic proximal spinal muscular atrophy of childhood and adolescence: problems of classification and genetic counseling. J Med Genet 1985; 22:350–353.
Bouwsma G, et al.: Unusual pedigree pattern in seven families with spinal muscular atrophy. Clin Genet 1986; 30:145–149.
Jansen PHP, et al.: A rapidly progressive autosomal dominant scapulohumeral form of spinal muscular atrophy. Ann Neurol 1986; 20:538–540.
Zerres K, et al.: Becker's allelic model to explain unusual pedigrees with spinal muscular atrophy. (Letter) Clin Genet 1987; 31:276–277.

BA039                                                **Louis E. Bartoshesky**

**Spinal muscular atrophy, benign-hypertrophy of calves**
See SPINAL MUSCULAR ATROPHY
**Spinal muscular atrophy, childhood isolated**
See SPINAL MUSCULAR ATROPHY
**Spinal muscular atrophy, distal type**
See SPINAL MUSCULAR ATROPHY
**Spinal muscular atrophy, facioscapulohumeral type**
See SPINAL MUSCULAR ATROPHY
**Spinal muscular atrophy, infantile acute form**
See SPINAL MUSCULAR ATROPHY
**Spinal muscular atrophy, infantile chronic form**
See SPINAL MUSCULAR ATROPHY
**Spinal muscular atrophy, proximal, adult type**
See SPINAL MUSCULAR ATROPHY
**Spinal muscular atrophy, type I**
See SPINAL MUSCULAR ATROPHY
**Spinal muscular atrophy, type II**
See SPINAL MUSCULAR ATROPHY

**Spinal muscular atrophy, type III**
   See SPINAL MUSCULAR ATROPHY
**Spinal muscular atrophy, type IV**
   See SPINAL MUSCULAR ATROPHY
**Spinal muscular atrophy-hypertrophy of the calves**
   See MUSCULAR ATROPHY, SPINAL AND BULBAR, X-LINKED
      KENNEDY TYPE
**Spine, rigid spine syndrome**
   See HAUPTMANN-THANHAUSER SYNDROME

## SPINE, SCOLIOSIS, IDIOPATHIC                      3003

**Includes:**
   Discogenic scoliosis
   Scoliosis, genetic

**Excludes:**
   Scoliosis, paralytic
   Scoliosis associated with other disorders

**Major Diagnostic Criteria:** Spinal curvature with associated rotation that is *structural*. Curvature may or may not be progressive in both growing and skeletally mature individuals. The abnormality is confirmed by X-ray of the spine taken in the erect position.

**Clinical Findings:** Trunk asymmetry with curvature of the spine in the thoracic, thoracolumbar, or lumbar regions, the right thoracic pattern being the most commmon. The most frequent type of idiopathic scoliosis is classified as *adolescent* with onset at more than two years of age. Two other types of scoliosis are seen; *infantile* is seen from birth to age three years and is typically a left thoracic curve. The curvatures may be resolving or progressive. *Juvenile idiopathic scoliosis* is diagnosed from ages three to ten years.

Typically, in the adolescent idiopathic group, the patients are taller and heavier than their peers without scoliosis. The natural history and risk of progression are intimately involved with skeletal maturity or its lack, and the adolescent growth spurt. It has been shown that increase in the rate of progression of curves does occur during the adolescent growth spurt, although the reasons for this are not clear. Conversely, an adolescent who is at or near skeletal maturity and who has a relatively small curve is at very little risk for progression of the curve.

**Complications:** With some curvatures, significant cosmetic deformity occurs, including trunk shift, waist asymmetry, pelvic obliquity, rib hump, uneven shoulders, and asymmetric neck line. Large curvatures in the thoracic spine are associated with restrictive lung disease. Pain and neurologic deficits can be found in older individuals, particularly with larger curves. Continued progression of curving can occur in skeletally mature individuals with larger curves (i.e., greater than 45 degrees).

**Associated Findings:** Some degree of ligamentous laxity, **Mitral valve prolapse**.

**Etiology:** The cause of idiopathic scoliosis is unclear, but vestibular system dysfunction, posterior spinal cord column malfunction, and abnormalities in vibratory sense can be implicated. Other findings not clearly determined to be causes are abnormal collagen, hormonal abnormalities, and muscle abnormalities.

**Pathogenesis:** Initial curving and deformity occurs through the soft tissues. With further progression, rotation and other secondary deformities (e.g., rib hump) develop. With further increase in size, secondary changes in vertebrae (e.g., wedging) can occur.

**MIM No.:** 18180

**CDC No.:** 754.200

**Sex Ratio:** M1:F4–7. From school screening data, small curves (less than 20 degrees) are seen equally among boys and girls. Larger curves (greater than 20 degrees) occur more frequently in girls.

**Occurrence:** The prevalence of scoliosis has been studied using chest and school screening data. Chest X-rays are accurate for thoracic curves but do not show the lumbar spine and thus underestimate the incidence (1.9% for curves greater than 10 degrees). School screening data reveal an incidence 1.1 to 3.2%.

**Risk of Recurrence for Patient's Sib:** Probably greater than general population. Although there is some controversy about this, a positive family history occurred with twice the frequency in children with progressive curves compared with that in children with stable curves.

**Risk of Recurrence for Patient's Child:** Unknown. Probably greater than that of the general population.

**Age of Detectability:** *Infantile,* birth to three years; *juvenile,* 3–10 years; *adolescent,* greater than ten years.

**Gene Mapping and Linkage:** Unknown.

**Prevention:** None known. Genetic counseling indicated.

**Treatment:** Observation is recommended for small curves (i.e., less than 25 degrees) in growing children. For progressive curves of 25 to 40–45 degrees, nonoperative treatment (e.g., a brace) is advised to prevent curve progression. For curves greater than 45 degrees and for those that progress despite bracing, surgery is recommended to correct the curve and to prevent further progression. Various approaches (e.g., anterior vs. posterior) and types of instrumentation (e.g., Harrington, C-D, Zielke) are available.

**Prognosis:** The importance of detection is to prevent severe curve progression. The predictive factors for progression in growing children are curve size, the Risser sign, and the skeletal age at diagnosis. Other important factors are menstrual history and curve pattern. Curve progression in adults relates primarily with size and pattern of curve.

**Detection of Carrier:** By clinical examination.

**Support Groups:**
   CA; Orange; Scoliosis Research Society
   MA; Belmont; National Scoliosis Foundation
   NY; Manhasset; The Scoliosis Association

**References:**
Bobechko WP, et al.: Electrospinal instrumentation for scoliosis: current status. Orthop Clin North Am 1979; 10:927–941.
Carr WA, et al.: Treatment of idiopathic scoliosis in the Milwaukee brace. J Bone Joint Surg 1980; 62A:599–612.
Weinstein SL, et al.: Idiopathic scoliosis. J Bone Joint Surg 1981; 63A:702–712.
Axelgaard J, et al.: Correction of spinal curvatures by transcutaneous electrical muscle stimulation. Spine 1983; 8:463–481.
Bunnell WP: The natural history of idiopathic scoliosis. 19th Ann Meet SRS, Orlando, FL: 1984.
Lonstein JE, Carlson JM: The prediction of curve progression in untreated idiopathic scoliosis during growth. J Bone Joint Surg 1984; 66A:1061–1071.
Smith MK, et al.: Idiopathic scoliosis and mitral valve prolapse. J Fam Pract 1984; 19:2, 229.
Bradford DS, Hensinger RM: The pediatric spine. New York: Thieme, 1985.
Bradford DS, et al.: Moe's textbook of scoliosis and other spinal deformities, ed 2. Philadelphia: W.B. Saunders, 1987.
Connor JM, et al.: Genetic aspects of early childhood scoliosis. Am J Med Genet 1987; 27:419–424.

LU015                                          **John P. Lubicky**

## SPINE, SPONDYLOLISTHESIS AND SPONDYLOLYSIS    3004

**Includes:**
   Dysplastic spondylolisthesis and spondylolysis
   Isthmic spondylolisthesis and spondylolysis
   Spondylolisthesis, spine
   Spondylolysis, spine

**Excludes:**
   Spondylolisthesis; degenerative, traumatic, and pathologic
   Spondylolysis; degenerative, traumatic, and pathologic

**Major Diagnostic Criteria:** *Spondylolysis* is a defect in the pars interarticularus, resulting in a discontinuity of the body and pedicle with the remainder of the neural arch. This is confirmed by oblique X-rays of the vertebrae, tomography, or computed tomography (CT) with reconstruction. *Spondylolisthesis* is the slipping forward of one vertebrae onto another. This is confirmed by lateral erect X-rays. Isthmic spondylolisthesis is the forward shift of the cranial vertebrae on the inferior one in association with either a lytic defect of the pars or an elongation of an intact pars interarticularus. *Dysplastic spondylolisthesis* is the forward shift of the upper vertebrae on a lower vertebrae in association with a congenital deficiency of the facet articulation that allows the slippage to occur. These conditions are confirmed by plain X-ray and by tomography or CT scans. The degree of spondylolisthesis is graded according to the percentage of slip.

*Grade I* is a slippage of 0–25%, *grade II* is a slippage of 25–50%, *grade III* is a slippage of 50–75%, and *grade IV* is a slippage greater than 75%. Spondyloptosis is the complete displacement of the upper vertebrae anterior to the vertebrae below. The percentage of slip is the ratio of the millimeters of displacement of the olisthetic vertebrae over the width of the C5 vertebrae as measured in the standing lateral X-ray. The slip angle is determined by a line drawn parallel to the inferior end-plate of the olisthetic vertebrae and a line drawn perpendicular to the posterior cortex of the vertebrae below.

**Clinical Findings:** Symptoms are generally uncommon during childhood and adolescence. If present, symptoms fall into two categories. The first is mild low back pain or aching in the low back and buttocks related to activities and is generally decreased with rest. The second form of presentation is low back pain with an associated significant radicular component into the posterior thigh and occasionally into the calves. The second form of presentation is generally not associated with the grade I slips. In the higher grades of slippage, an observable and palpable step-off can be felt at the level of spondylolisthesis. Occasionally in the symptomatic patient pressure over the involved arch may reproduce the patient's symptoms. The patient with a high degree of slip has a more characteristic clinical presentation. The sacrum becomes more vertical secondary to pelvic rotation, creating heart-shaped buttocks on examination. The lumbar spine goes into a secondary hyperlordotic position. The hip joints are forced into hyperextension, and the knees remain flexed. Varying degrees of spasm of the hamstrings are generally present. These deformities are thought to be due to the hyperkyphotic deformity of the olisthetic vertebrae.

Neurologic deficits may be present. These generally involve the L5 root, but may involve all of the sacral roots in severe cases. Scoliosis may be associated with spondylolisthesis. This is not a structural curve in the early stages, but may develop some structural characteristics in time. Spina bifida occulta is seen in over 90% of children with spondylolitic spondylolisthesis and in over 70% of adolescents.

**Complications:** Hyperlordosis of the lumbar spine with associated hamstring tightness can be seen in high-degree slips. The exact cause of hamstring tightness is not known. The abnormal gait pattern associated with these findings is described as stiff leg short-strided. A radiculopathy may be seen, including motor weakness in the rare patient. In the rare dysplastic spondylolisthesis, a low cauda equina syndrome may be seen. This generally is not found in the spondylolitic spondylolistheses.

**Associated Findings:** Generally there are no associated findings other than the X-ray findings of spina bifida occulta and scoliosis.

**Etiology:** Family studies suggest that spondylolitic spondylolisthesis is an inherited trait. The exact mode of transmission has not been defined. Most investigators believe the inheritance pattern to be either autosomal dominant with reduced penetrance, multifactorial, or genetic heterogeneity with multiple Mendelian traits.

**Pathogenesis:** Development of the spondylolitic defect probably takes place in an area of dysplasia in the cartilagenous model of the arch. Assumption of the upright position is probably associated with the development of the actual defect. Spondylolysis has not been identified in the person who does not leave the recumbent position. There is excess stress to the area of the pars, which may be associated with a stress fracture of the pars.

**MIM No.:** 18420

**CDC No.:** 756.130

**Sex Ratio:** M2:F1

**Occurrence:** Six percent of the Caucasian population have X-ray evidence of spondylolysis as an adult: 8% in males and 4% in females. The frequency in various ethnic groups has been reported to be less than 3% in Blacks and greater than 50% in Eskimos. The high frequency in the Eskimo population may be due to the posture assumed while performing many of their tasks.

**Risk of Recurrence for Patient's Sib:**
See Part I, *Mendelian Inheritance.*

**Risk of Recurrence for Patient's Child:**
See Part I, *Mendelian Inheritance.*

**Age of Detectability:** The youngest reported patient was four months old. Most patients are first seen in early childhood at ages 5–6. Many cases are not clinically evident throughout life.

**Gene Mapping and Linkage:** Unknown.

**Prevention:** None known. Genetic counseling indicated.

**Treatment:** Most patients are asymptomatic and require no treatment. Patients with grade I and II slips are allowed full activities. Patients with grade III and IV slips should be followed with serial X-rays, and, if progression of the slip is documented, fusion should be performed. Patients with symptoms are generally treated with rest followed by appropriate stretching and strengthening exercises for the trunk and lower extremities. A brace may be useful at times in controlling symptoms. Patients who present with significant hamstring tightness and pain and who do not respond to the above regimen usually respond to fusion. The question of reduction of severe degrees of slips, i.e., grades III and IV, is controversial. Those patients with a high slip angle should attempt to reduce at least the slip angle by postural means at the time of fusion.

**Prognosis:** Good in most patients. Pain and deformity can usually be helped by surgical intervention, if needed.

**Detection of Carrier:** Unknown.

**References:**

Taillard W: Le spondylolisthesis chez l'enfant et l'adolescent (Etude de 50 cas). Acta Orthop Scand 1954; 24:115–144.

Wiltse LL: The etiology of spondylolisthesis. J Bone Joint Surg 1962; 44A:539–560.

Neugebauer FL: The classic: a new contribution to the history and etiology of spondyl-olisthesis. Clin Orthop 1976; 117:4–22.

Wynn-Davies R, Scott JHS: Inheritance and spondylolisthesis: a radiographic family survey. J Bone Joint Surg 1979; 61B(3):301–305.

Fredrickson D, et al.: The natural history of spondylolysis and spondylolisthesis. J Bone Joint Surg 1984; 66A:669–707.

FR041                               **Bruce E. Fredrickson**
LU015                                **John P. Lubicky**

**Spinocerebella ataxia with dysmorphism**
*See ATAXIA-DYSMORPHIC FACIES-TRICHODYSPLASIA*
**Spinocerebellar ataxia with dementia and amyloid plaques**
*See GERSTMANN-STRAUSSLER SYNDROME*
**Spinocerebellar ataxia-sideroblastic anemia**
*See ANEMIA, SIDEROBLASTIC*

---

## SPINOCEREBELLAR DEGENERATION-CORNEAL DYSTROPHY     2619

**Includes:**
Corneal-cerebellar syndrome
Corneal dystrophy-spinocerebellar degeneration

**Excludes:**
**Amyloidosis, Finnish type (2145)**
**Ataxia, Friedreich type (2714)**
**Corneal dystrophy, endothelial (0208)**
**Fabry disease (0373)**
**Mucopolysaccharidosis**

**Major Diagnostic Criteria:** Moderate mental retardation, bilateral corneal opacification starting in the second year of life and leading to severe visual impairment, and slowly progressive cerebellar abnormalities with variable dorsal column and upper motor neuron involvement.

**Clinical Findings:** Corneal opacification is noted during the second year of life and is slowly progressive. During the third decade, recurrent eye pain may start, along with photophobia, foreign body sensation, and lacrimation. Visual acuity is reduced to counting fingers at one meter and to noticing hand motion.

Neurologically, the following may be present: unsteady tandem gait, head tremor, ataxia on finger-to-nose and heel-to-shin tests, exaggeration of myotatic tendon reflexes in the upper and lower limb, hyperreflexia, slight increase in the muscle tone, with fairly good muscle power. Sensory findings are normal. Eye movements are normal, without nystagmus. Plantar reflexes may be extensor or flexor. IQ is 50–60.

The EEG may reveal localized or diffuse slow waves or prominent, high-voltage waves. Nerve conduction studies may show delayed motor conduction in the peroneal nerve and delayed distal latency. Electromyography and audiometry are normal. There may be a slight increase in alpha-1, alpha-2 serum protein fractions and an increase in IgG, IgA, and IgM.

Histologic examination shows findings of corneal dystrophy, including corneal edema, thickening of Descemet membrane, and degenerative pannus. High-resolution light and electron microscopy of muscle shows variation in muscle fiber size and subsarcolemmal mitochondrial aggregates intermixed with lysosomes and lipid droplets, myelin figures, and increased thickness of the basement membrane of capillaries. A moderate degree of glycogen, giant mitochondria with dense, crystalline, filamentous inclusions may be seen. The sural nerve shows an increase in connective tissue between fibers and reduction in the number of myelinated nerve fibers.

**Complications:** Unknown.

**Associated Findings:** Cervical lordosis, lumbar rotoscoliosis, or severe osteoarthritis of the hip joint may be found.

**Etiology:** Autosomal recessive inheritance. The two sisters reported with this condition had consanguineous parents.

**Pathogenesis:** Unknown.

**MIM No.:** 27131

**POS No.:** 3534

**Sex Ratio:** Presumably M1:F1.

**Occurrence:** Two sisters were reported from Lebanon.

**Risk of Recurrence for Patient's Sib:**
See Part I, *Mendelian Inheritance.*

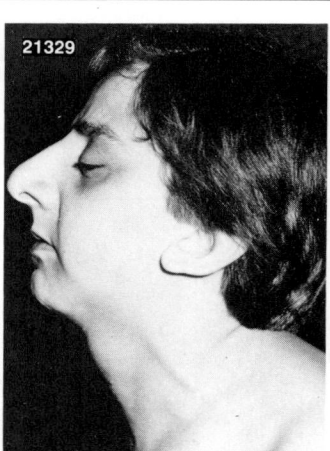 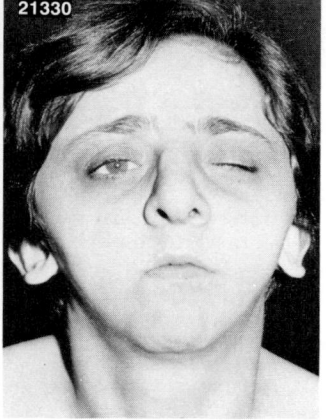

**2619-21329–30:** Facial view shows corneal dystrophy and ptosis.

**Risk of Recurrence for Patient's Child:**
See Part I, *Mendelian Inheritance.*

**Age of Detectability:** The corneal opacities begin during the second year of life, and the neurologic findings appear toward the end of the first decade of life.

**Gene Mapping and Linkage:** Unknown.

**Prevention:** None known. Genetic counseling indicated.

**Treatment:** Corneal grafting can be performed. However, vision cannot be improved more than 20/100 because of amblyopia.

**Prognosis:** Normal life span. However, both the decreased vision and the neurologic problems are disabling and limit the independence of the patient.

**Detection of Carrier:** Unknown.

**References:**
Der Kaloustian VM, et al.: Familial spinocerebellar degeneration with corneal dystrophy. Am J Med Genet 1985; 20:325–339.

DE030                                **Vazken M. Der Kaloustian**

**Spinopontine atrophy**
*See MACHADO-JOSEPH DISEASE*
**Spirochete, fetal effects of maternal Lyme disease**
*See FETAL EFFECTS FROM LYME DISEASE*

---

## SPLEEN, CONGENITAL ISOLATED HYPOSPLENIA          2600

**Includes:**
Hyposplenia, congenital isolated
Splenic agenesis, isolated congenital

**Excludes:** Asplenia syndrome (0092)

**Major Diagnostic Criteria:** The presence of Howell-Jolly bodies in an infant with repeated infections or on routine examination should make the physician suspicious of congenital splenic hypoplasia or agenesis. Other findings in the blood smear are polycythemia, Heinz bodies, siderocytes, target cells, and normablasts. A chest X-ray in an older infant or child may demonstrate an absence of the splenic shadow. Absence or hyposplenia can be confirmed with radioisotope imaging of the spleen.

**Clinical Findings:** With the absence of other congenital anomalies, splenic hypoplasia or agenesis will present with repeated episodes of sepsis, usually of the upper respiratory tract or lungs.

**Complications:** Persistent or recurrent, difficult-to-treat infections may cause death.

**Associated Findings:** **Mucopolysaccharidosis** has been reported in one series of patients with congenital hyposplenia.

**Etiology:** Possibly autosomal recessive inheritance, although autosomal dominant inheritance has also been suggested. Consanguinity was present in the sibship reported by Kevy et al (1968)

**Pathogenesis:** Compression or a stretching force on the developing splenic artery at about the fourth week of gestation may prevent the spleen from developing. At birth the spleen is noted to weigh 1g or less.

**MIM No.:** *27140

**CDC No.:** 759.010

**Sex Ratio:** M1:F1

**Occurrence:** Undetermined but presumed rare. Familial patterns have been reported in one sibship and two generations of another family.

**Risk of Recurrence for Patient's Sib:**
See Part I, *Mendelian Inheritance.*

**Risk of Recurrence for Patient's Child:** Unknown.

**Age of Detectability:** Usually within the first few weeks to the first few months of life.

**Gene Mapping and Linkage:** Unknown.

**Prevention:** None known. Genetic counseling indicated.

**Treatment:** Early recognition and prompt diagnosis and treatment of sepsis will save the patient's life. Prophylactic antibiotics and vaccination for *Pneumococcus* and *Haemophilus* infections after age two years should be implemented.

**Prognosis:** Depends on early recognition and treatment of sepsis. In a series of patients with the asplenic syndrome, there is an improved survival with asplenia or hyposplenia.

**Detection of Carrier:** Unknown.

**References:**

Kevy SV, et al.: Hereditary splenic hypoplasia. Pediatrics 1968; 42:752–758.

Gray SW, Skandalakis JE: Embryology for surgeons. Philadelphia: W.B. Saunders, 1972.

Dehner LP: Pediatric surgical pathology. St. Louis: C.V. Mosby, 1975.

Biggar WD, Remirez RA: Congenital asplenia: immunologic assessment and a clinical review of eight surviving patients. Pediatrics 1981; 67:548–551.

Monie IW: The asplenia syndrome: an explanation for absence of the spleen. Teratology 1982; 25:215–219.

Gates AJ, Black SH: Isolated congenital hyposplenia (ICH) in two generations of a non-consanguineous family. (Abstract) Am J Hum Genet 1986; 39:A61 only.

BE049                                                    **Arthur S. Besser**

---

## SPLEEN, CYSTS                                                    0240

**Includes:**
>    Cysts, true, benign
>    Epidermoid cysts
>    Epithelial cysts
>    Mesothelial cysts-squamous metaplasia

**Excludes:**
>    Cystic lymphangioma
>    Degenerative (post-traumatic) cysts
>    Dermoid tumor with cystic degeneration
>    Parasitic cyst
>    Polycystic hemangioma
>    Serous cyst
>    Splenic capsular fusion with pancreatic pseudocyst

**Major Diagnostic Criteria:** Cyst (usually unilocular) of spleen with lining consisting of a single cell layer of flattened cells, most likely mesothelium.

**Clinical Findings:** Cysts are minimal or absent in early life despite the assumption that splenic cysts have congenital origin. Splenic cysts have not been identified in series of autopsies of stillbirths, infants and children. They produce symptoms only when they cause splenic enlargement as a result of fluid accumulation within the cyst lumen. The most common presenting symptom is dull left upper quadrant pain. Next most common is a mass in the left upper quadrant. Other presentations include rupture (up to 25% in some series), dyspnea and early satiety due to gastric compression. Overt abdominal protuberance has been described.

The X-ray triad of a normal intraveneous pyelogram, inferior displacement of the splenic flexure of the colon and medial displacement of the left gastric border is diagnostic of splenic enlargement. Imaging techniques reveal the cystic nature of the lesion. Ultrasound, computerized tomography and radionucleide liver-spleen scan ($^{99m}$Tc-sulfocolloid or $^{198}$Au) are each capable of determining the nature and size of splenic cysts. The histologic type is confirmed at surgical splenectomy.

The cyst is often large - ranging from 6 to more than 30 cm in diameter. It has a thin squamous epithelial-like lining and contains sero-sanguious to toothpaste-like fluid ranging in color from light yellow to dark brown. The wall is occasionally calcified. Cysts most often involve the upper pole of the spleen.

**Complications:** Rupture of the cyst with intraperitonal hemorrhage is the most common and life-threatening complication. Splenic cyst rarely has been associated with hypersplenism.

**Associated Findings:** None known.

**Etiology:** Unknown.

**Pathogenesis:** The most likely mechanism is inclusion of primative coelomic mesothelium into the splenic primordium during early organogenesis. Against this hypothesis is the fact that the splenic primordium arises as a specialized condensation of mesenchyme within the leaves of the dorsal mesogastrium and therefore is not open to inclusions from a mesothelial surface. An alternative hypothesis is invagination of capsular surface mesothelium during later development. Against this, it is interesting to note that cysts have not been reported in accessory spleens despite their incidence of up to 35% in adult autopsies. In either case, the mesothelial remnant undergoes squamous metaplasia to form the characteristic epithelial lining. The lining secretes fluid into the cystic lumen producing the expanded cyst which is clinically evident.

**CDC No.:** 759.080

**Sex Ratio:** M1:F1.5–10

**Occurrence:** Fewer than 200 splenic cysts reported.

**Risk of Recurrence for Patient's Sib:** Not increased.

**Risk of Recurrence for Patient's Child:** Not increased.

**Age of Detectability:** Six months to seventy years (usually in second to fourth decade) by clinical examination.

**Gene Mapping and Linkage:** Unknown.

**Prevention:** None known. Genetic counseling indicated.

**Treatment:** Surgical cystectomy is needed. Because of the risk of hemorrhage from the spleen, total splenectomy has been successfully performed for treatment of cysts. Subtotal splenectomy is recommended because of the risk of post-splenectomy sepsis or reduced immune competence.

**Prognosis:** Excellent unless rupture and hemorrhage occur or surgical therapy is complicated by hemorrhage.

**Detection of Carrier:** Unknown.

**References:**

Bostick WL, Lucia SP: Nonparasitic, noncancerous cystic tumors of the spleen. AMA Arch Pathol 1949; 47:215–222.

Fowler RH: Collective review: non-parasitic cystic tumors of the spleen. Int Abstr Surg (Surg Gynec Obstet) 1953; 96:209–227.

Browne MK: Epidermoid cysts of the spleen. Brit J Surg 1963; 50:838–841.

Hoffman E: Non-parasitic splenic cysts. Am J Surg 1968; 93:765–770.

Blank E, Cambell JR: Epidermoid cysts of the spleen. Pediatrics 1973; 51:75–84.

Ough YD, et al.: Mesothelial cysts of the spleen with squamous metaplasia. Am J Clin Pathol 1981; 75:666–669.

Dachman AH, et al.: Nonparasitic spleen cysts: a report of 52 cases with radiologic-pathologic correlation. Am J Roentgen 1986; 147:537–542.

Khan AH, et al.: Partial splenectomy for benign cystic lesions of the spleen. J Pediatr Surg 1986; 21:749–752.

SH054                                                  **Douglas R. Shanklin**
WH007                                                  **Peter F. Whitington**
                                                        *John R. Esterly*

**Splenic agenesis**
>    *See ASPLENIA SYNDROME*

**Splenic agenesis, isolated congenital**
>    *See SPLEEN, CONGENITAL ISOLATED HYPOSPLENIA*

## SPLENOGONADAL FUSION-LIMB DEFECT 3053

**Includes:**
> Limb deficiency-splenogonadal fusion
> Micrognathia-limb deficiency-splenogonadal fusion
> Splenogonadal fusion, isolated

**Excludes:**
> Hypoglossia-hypodactylia (0451)

**Major Diagnostic Criteria:** The combination of terminal transverse limb defects and splenogonadal fusion.

**Clinical Findings:** Lower limb involvement, ranging from unilateral missing lower leg to total absence of both legs. Upper limbs were also involved (13/17), with severity ranging from missing fingers on one hand to total lack of both arms. Orofacial anomalies also occur, with micrognathia (7/17) the most common finding. Anal atresia or stenosis occurred in three cases.

**Complications:** Bowel obstruction, **Hernia, inguinal**, and cryptorchidism.

**Associated Findings:** Reported in one affected individual each were plagiocephaly, misshapen and posteriorly rotated ears, anodontia, V-shaped palate, congenital heart defect, unilateral diaphragmatic agenesis, **Diaphragmatic hernia**, polymicrogyria, and bifid vertebrae C6-T3.

**Etiology:** Unknown. No familial cases have been reported; no affected individuals have reproduced. Autosomal dominant inheritance has therefore not been ruled out.

**Pathogenesis:** Unknown. Several theories have been proposed to explain the co-occurrence of splenogonadal fusion and limb defects; none entirely satisfactory.

**MIM No.:** 18330

**POS No.:** 4025

**Sex Ratio:** M15:F2 observed.

**Occurrence:** Seventeen cases have been reported in the literature.

**Risk of Recurrence for Patient's Sib:**
> See Part I, *Mendelian Inheritance.*

**Risk of Recurrence for Patient's Child:**
> See Part I, *Mendelian Inheritance.*

**Age of Detectability:** At birth, although prenatal diagnosis is theoretically possible.

**Gene Mapping and Linkage:** Unknown.

**Prevention:** None known. Genetic counseling indicated.

**Treatment:** Supportive.

**Prognosis:** Although 8/14 individuals died within the first year of life or were stillborn, two other individuals were aged 10 and 15 years at the time of last report. The ten-year-old was mildly mentally retarded; the 15-year-old was of apparently normal intellect.

**Detection of Carrier:** Unknown.

**Special Considerations:** It has been suggested by Pauli and Greenlaw (1982) that splenogonadal fusion-limb defect and **Hypoglossia-hypodactylia** may have a similar, if not identical, pathogenesis and therefore represent different expressions of the same basic defect. It is also suggested that splenogonadal fusion without limb defects is pathogenetically related to splenogonadal fusion with limb defects, and simply represent differences in the timing of the occurrence of the initial insult.

**References:**
Putschar WGJ, Manion WC: Splenic-gonadal fusion. Am J Path 1956; 32:15–35.
Hives JR, Eggum PR: Splenic-gonadal fusion causing bowel obstruction. Arch Surg 1961; 83:887–889.
Pauli RM, Greenlaw A: Limb deficiency and splenogonadal fusion. Am J Med Genet 1982; 13:81–90. †
Gouw ASH, et al.: The spectrum of spleno-gonadal fusion. Eur J Pediatr 1985; 144:316–323.

Helga V. Toriello

T0007

**Splenomegaly-gingival fibromatosis-digital anomalies**
> See *GINGIVAL FIBROMATOSIS-DIGITAL ANOMALIES*
**Split hand and split foot with mandibular hypoplasia**
> See *ACRO-RENAL-MANDIBULAR SYNDROME*
**Split hand deformity-mandibulofacial dysostosis**
> See *ACROFACIAL DYSOSTOSIS, NAGER TYPE*
**Split notocord syndrome**
> See *DIASTEMATOMYELIA*
**Split-hand deformity**
> See *ECTRODACTYLY*
**Spondylitis deformans**
> See *ANKYLOSING SPONDYLITIS*

## SPONDYLOCOSTAL DYSOSTOSIS-VISCERAL DEFECTS-DANDY WALKER CYST 2924

**Includes:**
> Dandy-Walker cyst-spondylocostal dysostosis-visceral defects
> Micromelia (lethal)-spondylocostal dysostosis-skeletal anomalies
> Visceral defects-Dandy-Walker cysts-spondylocostal dysostosis

**Excludes: Achondrogenesis**

**Major Diagnostic Criteria:** Severe micromelia, **Cleft palate**, rockerbottom feet, generalized **Brachydactyly**, **Hydrocephaly** with **Corpus callosum agenesis** and Dandy-Walker cyst, pulmonary hypoplasia, intestinal malrotation, right heart hypoplasia, dysplastic small kidneys, stenosis of the ureterovesicular junction, and uterovaginal duplication.

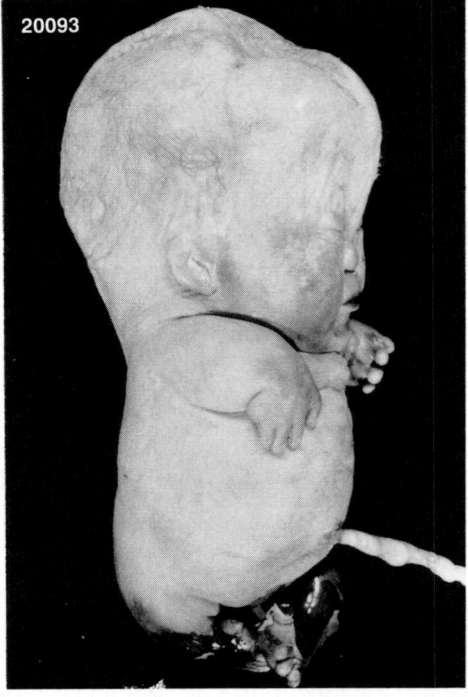

**2924-20093:** Micromelic dwarfism with marked hydrocephaly, short trunk and narrow chest.

**Clinical Findings:** Based on two cases; severe micromelia, **Cleft palate**, rocker-bottom feet, generalized **Brachydactyly**, **Hydrocephaly** with **Corpus callosum agenesis** and Dandy-Walker cyst, pulmonary hypoplasia, intestinal malrotation, right heart hypoplasia, dysplastic small kidneys, stenosis of the ureterovesicalar junction, and uterovaginal duplication.

**Complications:** Unknown.

**Associated Findings:** In addition to the short-limbed dwarfism and the spondylocostal dysostosis, identical external and internal malformations were present in both stillborns. Polyhydramnios was evident in the third trimester of pregnancy.

**Etiology:** Two isolated patients have been reported. As for other types of lethal short-limbed dwarfism, autosomal recessive inheritance is possible.

**Pathogenesis:** Histologic examination of the growth plates revealed that the reserve cartilage was hypercellular, often with clumping of the resting chrondrocytes into lacunae containing three to four cells. The cartilage matrix and the individual chondrocytes appeared normal. The endochondral ossification was disturbed, with markedly narrowed zones of proliferation and hypertrophy.

**POS No.:** 3659

**Sex Ratio:** M1:F1 (based on the two known patients).

**Occurrence:** Undetermined but presumably rare. Two patients have been reported.

**Risk of Recurrence for Patient's Sib:**
See Part I, *Mendelian Inheritance.*

**Risk of Recurrence for Patient's Child:**
See Part I, *Mendelian Inheritance.* Affected individuals are not expected to survive to reproduce.

**Age of Detectability:** Prenatal ultrasound diagnosis is, in principle, feasible in the second trimester of pregnancy by the presence of short-limbed dwarfism, central nervous system malformations, and polyhydramnios.

**Gene Mapping and Linkage:** Unknown.

**Prevention:** None known. Genetic counseling indicated.

**Treatment:** Supportive.

**Prognosis:** Lethal syndrome due to the short-limbed dwarfism, short trunk, narrow chest, and severity of the central nervous system malformations.

**Detection of Carrier:** Unknown.

**References:**
Shih LY, et al.: Dwarfism associated with prenatal ventriculomegaly. Prenatal Diagn 1983; 3:69–73.
Moerman PH, et al.: A new lethal chondrodysplasia with spondylocostal dysostosis, multiple internal anomalies and Dandy-Walker cyst. Clin Genet 1985; 27:160–164.

FR030                                                    **Jean-Pierre Fryns**

**Spondylocostal dysplasia**
*See SPONDYLOTHORACIC DYSPLASIA*

---

## SPONDYLOCOSTAL DYSPLASIA                                    0896

**Includes:**
    Costovertebral segmentation anomalies
    Hemivertebrae, autosomal dominant multiple
    Jarcho-Levin syndrome
    Polydysspondyly

**Excludes:**
    **Facial cleft, lateral** (0374)
    **Incontinentia pigmenti** (0526)
    **Klippel-Feil anomaly** (2032)
    **Larsen syndrome** (0570)
    **Nevoid basal cell carcinoma syndrome** (0101)
    **Oculo-auriculo-vertebral anomaly** (0735)
    **Spondylothoracic dysplasia** (0900)

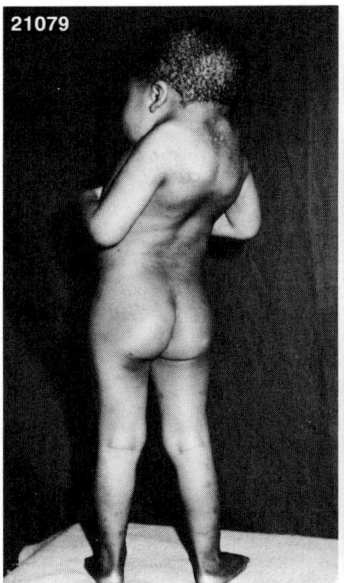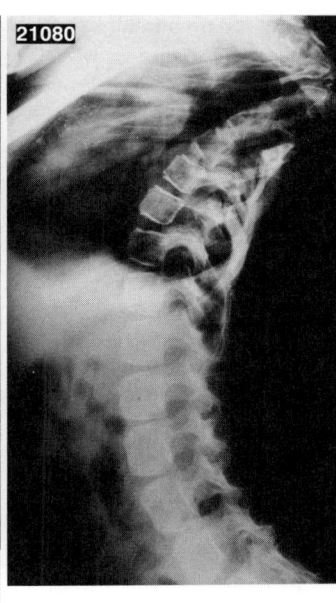

**0896-21079:** An affected girl aged 5 years. Her neck is short and she has a lumbar lordosis and mild dorsal kyphoscoliosis. **21080:** Lateral X-ray of the spine showing unusually tall vertebral bodies in the upper lumbar and lower thoracic regions.

---

**Major Diagnostic Criteria:** A shortened trunk associated with segmentation anomalies of the vertebrae and ribs, with a normal skull and limbs.

**Clinical Findings:** Short-trunked dwarfism associated with multiple anomalies of the vertebrae and ribs. The skull and limbs are normal. The upper/lower segment ratio is decreased for age, and the arm span is greater than the height. The neck is thick and short, and rotary movements are limited. Patients are usually asymptomatic in childhood, but increasing limitation of motion of the spine with back pain can occur in adults. X-rays show gross disorganization of vertebral segmentation, with a reduced number of vertebrae, fused or "block" vertebrae, hemivertebrae and sagitally cleft or "butterfly" vertebrae. The ribs and their vertebral pedicles are reduced in number, and many of those present are hypoplastic or fused. The bones of the skull and limbs are normal.

A relatively mild form of recessively inherited spondylocostal dysplasia has also been reported which is difficult to distinguish clinically from dominant spondylocostal dysplasia.

**Complications:** Increasing limitation of spinal movement, which may be associated with back pain and referred pain secondary to nerve root compression.

**Associated Findings:** None known.

**Etiology:** Usually autosomal dominant inheritance, although a milder recessive form has also been reported. In one report of a similar condition in a mother and daughter, both carried a 14–15 chromosome translocation.

**Pathogenesis:** Unknown.

**MIM No.:** *12260

**POS No.:** 3390, 3410, 3393

**Sex Ratio:** M1:F1

**Occurrence:** About a dozen families have been reported.

**Risk of Recurrence for Patient's Sib:**
See Part I, *Mendelian Inheritance.*

**Risk of Recurrence for Patient's Child:**
See Part I, *Mendelian Inheritance.*

**Age of Detectability:** At birth, by clinical and X-ray examination.

**Gene Mapping and Linkage:** Unknown.

**Prevention:** None known. Genetic counseling indicated.

**Treatment:** The effects of bracing or spinal fusion to prevent scoliosis and nerve root compression have not been systematically evaluated.

**Prognosis:** Normal life span.

**Detection of Carrier:** By clinical examination of first degree relatives.

**References:**

Van de Sar A: Hereditary multiple hemivertebrae. Docum Med Geogr Trop 1952; 4:23–28.

Rimoin DL, et al.: Spondylocostal dysplasia: a dominantly inherited form of short-trunked dwarfism. Am J Med 1968; 45:948–953.*†

Ayme S, Preus M: Spondylocostal/spondylothoracic dysostosis: the clinical basis for prognosticating and genetic counseling. Am J Med Genet 1986; 24:599–606.

Lorenz P, Rupprecht E: Spondylocostal dysostosis: dominant type. Am J Med Genet 1990; 35:219–221.†

B0025

Zvi Borochowitz
*David L. Rimoin*

**Spondylodysplasia with pure brachyolmia**
*See BRACHYOLMIA, HOBAEK TYPE*
**Spondylodysplasia, dominant type**
*See BRACHYOLMELIA, DOMINANT TYPE*
**Spondylodysplasia, Maroteaux type**
*See BRACHYOLMELIA, MAROTEAUX TYPE*
**Spondyloenchondrodysplasia**
*See SPONDYLOMETAPHYSEAL DYSPLASIA WITH ENCHONDROMATOUS CHANGES*

## SPONDYLOEPIMETAPHYSEAL DYSPLASIA          2313

**Includes:**

Spondyloepimetaphyseal dysplasia, Irapa type (SEMDIT)
Spondyloepimetaphyseal dysplasia, Minnesota type
Spondylometepiphyseal dysplasia (SMED)
Spondylometaepiphyseal dysplasia

**Excludes:**

**Metaphyseal chondrodysplasia** (all)
**Spondyloepimetaphyseal dysplasia, Strudwick type** (3059)
**Spondyloepiphyseal dysplasia congenita** (0897)
**Spondyloepimetaphyseal dysplasia-joint laxity** (2244)
**Spondyloepiphyseal dysplasia, late** (0898)

**Major Diagnostic Criteria:** Disproportionate short stature with X-ray changes involving the spine, epiphyses, and metaphyses.

**Clinical Findings:** The term *spondyloepimetaphyseal dysplasia* (SEMD) is used broadly to include any skeletal dysplasia involving the spine, epiphyses, and metaphyses. Several clinical syndromes meeting this criterion have been reported. This article will focus on two specific conditions:

The *Irapa type* of SEMD was first described by Arias et al. in 1976. Three Mexican sibs with the same entity were described by Hernandez et al (1980). Like **Spondyloepimetaphyseal dysplasia, Strudwick type**, these children have severe short-trunk dwarfism with platyspondyly, **Pectus carinatum**, increased lumbar lordosis, genu valga, and pes planus. Features distinguishing Irapa type include short metacarpals and metatarsals with a relatively spared second metatarsal.

SEMD, *Minnesota type*, has been identified in 26 individuals from 19 families. This disorder was not clinically recognized until ages 1–2 years, although X-ray changes were present at birth. The extremities and trunk became noticeably short between ages 1–2 years. The neck is short and the chest is barrel shaped. Hip and knee flexion contractures, genu valga, and pes planus develop in early childhood. Kyphoscoliosis is progressive and requires surgery in the more severe cases. Odontoid hypoplasia to aplasia has been noted in all individuals, and some require cervical spine fusion. Whether life span is altered is not known, but respiratory insufficiency does occur.

X-ray findings of the Minnesota-type SEMD include marked platyspondyly with mild-to-moderate kyphoscoliosis, odontoid hypoplasia to aplasia, wide and short proximal femora, irregular ossification centers at the knee, marked metaphyseal widening and irregularity, and flat epiphyses.

SEMD, Minnesota type, has been previously misclassified as a variant of **Pseudoachondroplastic dysplasia** or, occasionally, as **Mucopolysaccharidosis IV**. Unlike the other SEMDs, clinical recognition usually occurs between ages one and two years, but X-ray changes are present in the newborn.

**Complications:** Severe scoliosis and cord compression are consequences of the vertebral malformations. Myopia was found in one patient, but ophthalmologic evaluations were not done routinely. The vitreoretinal degeneration and retinal detachments of SED congenita do not appear to be a feature of these disorders. Inguinal and umbilical hernias have occurred, and they probably reflect the underlying connective tissue disorder.

**Associated Findings:** Midface hemangioma, bilateral congenital hydronephrosis.

**Etiology:** Families with unaffected parents and multiple affected sibs have been reported with SEMDIT, suggesting autosomal recessive inheritance.

SEMD, Minnesota type, by autosomal dominant inheritance. Four families with parent-to-child transmission have been documented. Sporadic cases have also been reported.

**Pathogenesis:** Biochemical alterations in type II collagen have been reported in three cases of unclassified SEMD.

**MIM No.:** *27165

**Sex Ratio:** M1:F1 (Minnesota type). Arias et al. (1976) observed a predominance of affected males in their Irapa population.

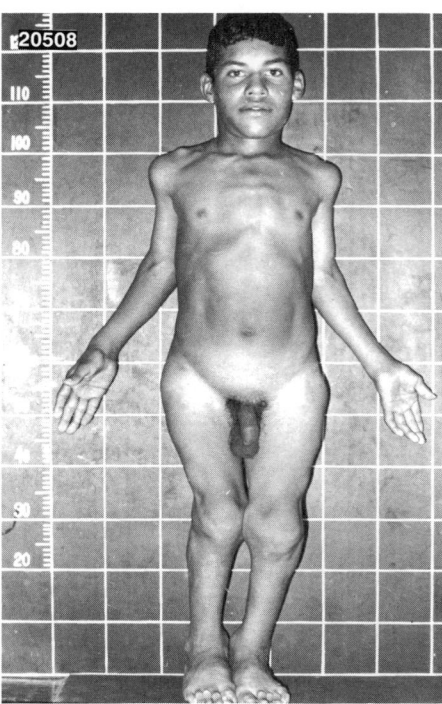

2313-20508: Spondyloepimetaphyseal dysplasia; note disproportionate short stature, rhizomelic shortening of the limbs and a semiflexed posture.

**Occurrence:** At least 19 reported cases of SEMDIT; and 26 cases SEMD, Minnesota type. Unclassified SEMD has also been reported.

**Risk of Recurrence for Patient's Sib:**
See Part I, *Mendelian Inheritance.*

**Risk of Recurrence for Patient's Child:**
See Part I, *Mendelian Inheritance.*

**Age of Detectability:** SEMDIT is clinically detectable at birth; SEMD, Minnesota type, is detectable during the first 1–2 years of life.

**Gene Mapping and Linkage:** Unknown.

**Prevention:** None known. Genetic counseling indicated.

**Treatment:** Symptomatic management of orthopedic complications. Special attention must be paid to the potential of cervical vertebral abnormalities and secondary cord compression.

**Prognosis:** The natural history has not been well delineated. The most serious complications are cord compression and respiratory insufficiency. Only one of the cases of Anderson et al. (1982) was mentally retarded; this was a child with congenital hydronephrosis who underwent multiple surgeries very early in infancy. On the whole, intelligence is normal.

**Detection of Carrier:** Unknown.

**Special Considerations:** Genetic heterogeneity undoubtedly exists in this group of patients. This is evidenced by the existence of not only of clinically distinct types of SEMD, but also of multiple persons with short stature and X-ray changes involving the spine, epiphyses, and metaphyses who do not fit into any currently accepted classification. Families have been observed that conform to both autosomal dominant and autosomal recessive modes of inheritance. Thus, genetic counseling in this condition must cover the possibilities of either dominant or recessive inheritance. In addition, the potential of metaphyseal involvement later in life should be considered in any infant in whom the diagnosis is made.

**References:**

Murdoch JL, Walker BA: A "new" form of spondylometaphyseal dysplasia. BD:OAS V(4). New York: March of Dimes Birth Defects Foundation, 1969:368–370.

Arias S, et al.: Irapa osteochondrodysplastic dwarfism: an ethnic marker gene for a subgroup or polymorphic differentiation in one locus. Exerpta Med Int Congress Ser 1976; 397:173 only.

Hernandez A, et al.: Autosomal recessive spondylo-epi-metaphyseal dysplasia (Irapa type) in a Mexican family: delineation of the syndrome. Am J Med Genet 1980; 5:179–188.

Arias S: Osteochondrodysplasia Irapa type: an ethnic marker gene in two subcontinents. Am J Med Genet 1981; 8:251–253.

Spranger JW, Maroteaux P: Genetic heterogeneity of spondyloepiphyseal dysplasia congenita? Am J Med Genet 1982; 13:241–242.

Murray L, et al.: Abnormal type II collagen in the spondyloepi- and spondyloepimetaphyseal dysplasias. Clin Res 1985; 33:118a.

FR005                                    **Clair A. Francomano**

**Spondyloepimetaphyseal dysplasia, Irapa type (SEMDIT)**
*See SPONDYLOEPIMETAPHYSEAL DYSPLASIA*
**Spondyloepimetaphyseal dysplasia, Minnesota type**
*See SPONDYLOEPIMETAPHYSEAL DYSPLASIA*

---

## SPONDYLOEPIMETAPHYSEAL DYSPLASIA, STRUDWICK TYPE                3059

**Includes:**
> Dappled metaphysis syndrome
> SMED Strudwick
> Spondylometaphyseal dysplasia, Brazilian type
> Spondylometaepiphyseal dysplasia, Strudwick type
> Spondylometaepiphyseal dysplasia congenita
> Strudwick syndrome

**Excludes:**
> **Spondyloepimetaphyseal dysplasia** (2313)
> **Spondyloepimetaphyseal dysplasia-joint laxity** (2244)

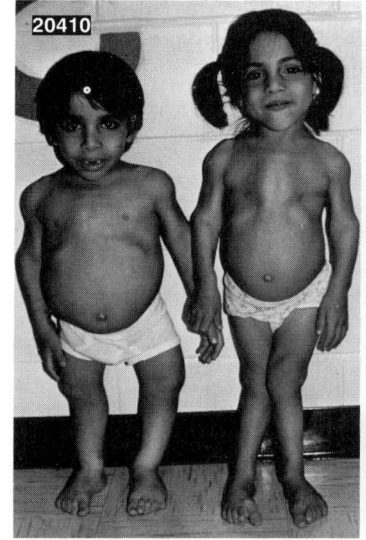
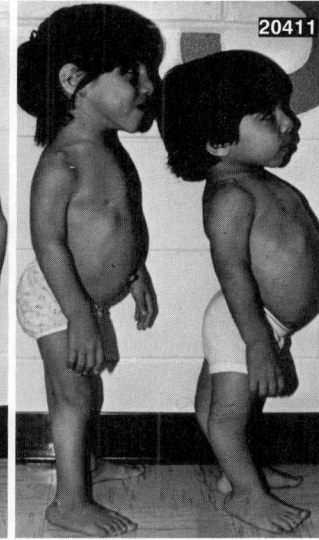
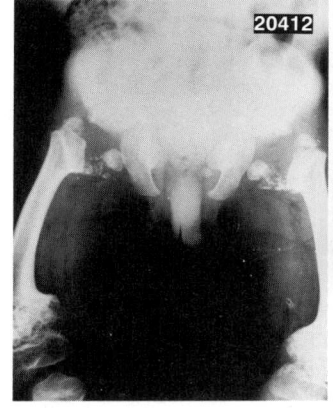
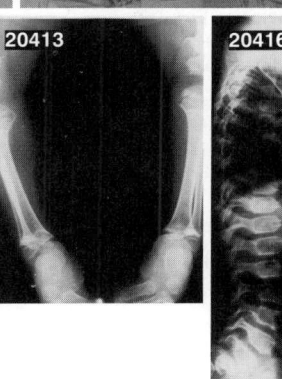
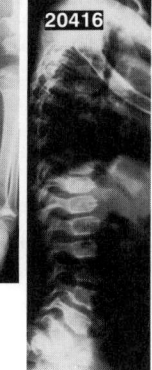

**3059**-20410: Spondylometepiphyseal dysplasia, Strudwick type; note short trunk-short limb type of short stature with normal facies and genua valga. 20411: Lateral view shows lordosis and pectus carinatum. 20412: Hypoplastic pelvis, coxa vara with wide, irregular metaphyses and shortened femurs in the brother. 20413: Tibiae vara, metepiphyseal changes. 20416: Hypoplastic flattened vertebrae with anterior beaking, and accentuated lordosis.

---

**Spondyloepiphyseal dysplasia congenita** (0897)
**Spondylometaphyseal chondrodysplasia, Kozlowski type** (0899)

**Major Diagnostic Criteria:** Short trunk-short limb dwarfism with delayed epiphyseal maturation present at birth. The face appears normal. Exacerbated lordosis, scoliosis, genua valga, **Pectus carinatum**, and pes planus appear later.

**Clinical Findings:** The most common major and characteristic features are the disproportionate short stature at birth and normal-appearing skull and facies. A **Cleft palate** may be present. Clubfeet, hernias, dislocated hips, and hydronephrosis are additional nonspecific anomalies. With age, lordosis, scoliosis, pectus carinatum with rib flaring and Harrison groove, knock knees, and pes planus appear. With exertion, arthralgias are common.

X-ray findings include epiphyseal delay at birth and club-shaped femora; ribs with splayed, bulbous anterior ends; hypoplastic olecranon and odontoid and fragmented appearance of the epiphyses during infancy and early childhood. Metaphyseal "dappling" of alternating osteosclerosis and radiolucencies appears usually after age three years. It starts on the proximal femur and subsequently involves the proximal humeri, distal radii, ulnae, and both ends of tibiae and fibulae. The dappling is greater in the ulna than in the radius and in the fibula compared with the tibia; this is in contrast to other metaphyseal dysplasias. Platyspondyly is almost always present after age one year. Pear-shaped vertebrae are seen as a result of posterior hypoplasia of vertebral bodies. Scoliosis is usually a late sign, after age ten years.

In a few patients with the condition, chondro-osseous studies have shown abnormal iliac crest growth plate. Clustering of chondrocytes in the proliferative and hypertrophic zones with short osseous trabeculae arising at irregular intervals were noted. Inclusion bodies were observed in many chondrocytes. Costochondral junction study in a patient showed hypocellularity of the growth plate with very few hypertrophic or proliferative cells.

Electron microscope studies of cartilage have shown chondrocytes with dilated rough endoplasmic reticulum, filled with granular material. The matrix appeared normal.

**Complications:** Genua valga may be so severe that it limits ambulation and requires surgery. Amortization of the hip is another complication. The hypoplastic odontoid could lead to C1-C2 dislocation and cord compression. The **Cleft palate** leads to recurrent ear infections and possible conductive hearing loss.

**Associated Findings:** Myopia, hydronephrosis, **Mitral valve prolapse**, and hemangioma have been reported on occasion.

**Etiology:** Probably autosomal recessive inheritance.

**Pathogenesis:** The abnormalities of the growth plate with hypocellularity are probably responsible for the stunted growth. The inclusion bodies in the chondrocytes suggest metabolic rearrangement most likely involving the collagen (Murray & Rimoin, 1985), but the exact pathogenetic mechanism remains unknown.

**MIM No.:** 27167

**POS No.:** 3561

**Sex Ratio:** M1:F1

**Occurrence:** Fewer than 30 cases have been reported.

**Risk of Recurrence for Patient's Sib:**
See Part I, *Mendelian Inheritance.*

**Risk of Recurrence for Patient's Child:**
See Part I, *Mendelian Inheritance.*

**Age of Detectability:** At birth or during infancy. Prenatal diagnosis should be possible.

**Gene Mapping and Linkage:** Unknown.

**Prevention:** None known. Genetic counseling indicated.

**Treatment:** Palliative corrective surgery for the orthopedic deformities.

**Prognosis:** As in the other severe skeletal dysplasias, life span may be shortened; accurate data, however, are not available.

**Detection of Carrier:** Unknown.

**Special Considerations:** The eponym Strudwick is derived from the prototype patient seen at Johns Hopkins Hospital.

**References:**
Murdoch JL, Walker BA: A "new" form of spondylometaphyseal dysplasia. BD:OAS V(4). New York: March of Dimes Birth Defects Foundation, 1969:368–370.
Diamond L: Spondylometaphyseal dysplasia (Brazilian type). BD:OAS X(12). New York: March of Dimes Birth Defects Foundation, 1974: 412–415.
Anderson CE, et al.: Spondylometaepiphyseal dysplasia, Strudwick type. Am J Med Genet 1982; 13:243–256.
Spranger JW, Maroteaux P: Genetic heterogeneity of spondyloepiphyseal dysplasia congenita? Am J Med Genet 1982; 13:241–242.
Kousseff BG, Nichols P: Autosomal recessive spondylometepiphyseal dysplasia, type Strudwick. Am J Med Genet 1984; 17:547–550.
Murray LW, Rimoin DL: Type II collagen abnormalities in the spondyloepi- and spondyloepimetaphyseal dysplasias. (Abstract) Am J Hum Genet 1985; 37:A13.

K0018                                    **Boris G. Kousseff**

---

## SPONDYLOEPIMETAPHYSEAL DYSPLASIA-JOINT LAXITY                    2244

**Includes:**
Joint laxity-spondyloepimetaphyseal dysplasia
SEMDJL

**Excludes:**
Skeletal dysplasias and joint laxity syndromes, other
**Spondyloepimetaphyseal dysplasia** (2313)
**Spondyloepimetaphyseal dysplasia, Strudwick type** (3059)

**Major Diagnostic Criteria:** X-ray evidence of generalized spondyloepimetaphyseal dysplasia, hypermobility, and characteristic facies.

**Clinical Findings:** Dwarfism; articular hypermobility; spinal malalignment; thoracic asymmetry; elbow deformity (bilateral dislocation of the radial heads); foot deformity (bilateral talipes equinovarus). *Facies:* oval face, long upper lip, protuberant eyes, variable blue sclera. *Hands:* spatulate terminal phalanges, especially of the thumbs, gross joint laxity permitting abnormal positioning. *Skin:* soft, doughy texture with some hyperelasticity.

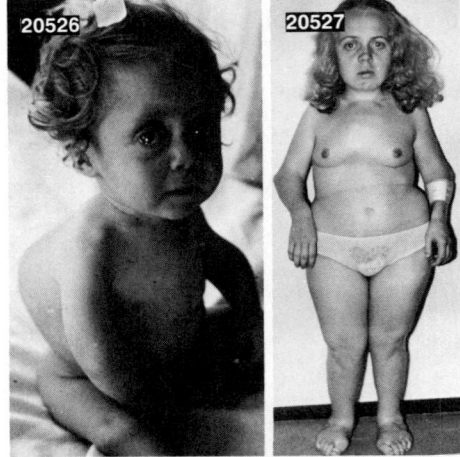

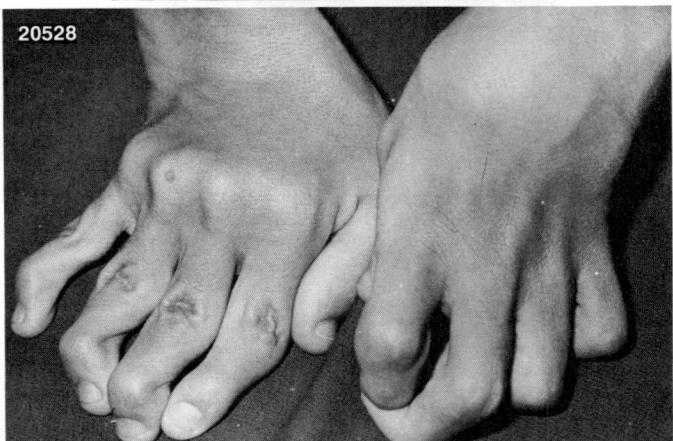

**2244-20526:** Spondyloepimetaphyseal dysplasia-joint laxity; note this 2-year-old girl with characteristic facies, elbow deformity due to dislocation of the radial heads and kyphosis. **20527:** Short stature, dislocation of the radial heads, genu valgum, pes planus and the characteristic facies with prominent eyes and a long upper lip. **20528:** Unusual hand positioning as a result of gross joint laxity. The terminal phalanges are spatulate.

**Complications:** Spinal cord compression, cardio-respiratory failure.

**Associated Findings: Cleft palate;** (31%); high palate (12%); cardiac defect (**Ventricular septal defect, Atrial septal defects,** MI) (28%); genu valgus (weight bearing) (80%); **Hip, congenital dislocated** (27%), **Myopia, congenital.**

**Etiology:** Autosomal recessive inheritance.

**Pathogenesis:** Possibly a structural defect in collagen.

**MIM No.:** *27164

**POS No.:** 4257

**Sex Ratio:** M1:F1

**Occurrence:** Twenty known cases, all in the Afrikaner population of South Africa. 1:40,000 live births. The condition is potentially lethal. Several of the affected families have German antecedents and it is possible that the gene reached the Afrikaner population (Dutch ancestry) from Germanic sources.

**Risk of Recurrence for Patient's Sib:**
See Part I, *Mendelian Inheritance.*

**Risk of Recurrence for Patient's Child:**
See Part I, *Mendelian Inheritance.*

**Age of Detectability:** At birth, or possibly by ultrasound in second trimester.

**Gene Mapping and Linkage:** Unknown.

**Prevention:** None known. Genetic counseling indicated. Antenatal recognition of limb or spine malalignment may be possible in early pregnancy by ultrasonic monitoring.

**Treatment:** Surgical stabilization of progressive spinal malalignment is indicated in the majority of patients. This operation is difficult, and long-term results are indifferent. Orthopedic measures may be required for congenital dislocation of hips, talipes equinovarus and genu valgum following weight bearing.

**Prognosis:** Only two of the 20 known patients have survived to early adulthood. Eight have died during childhood and the 10 survivors all have significant handicap.

**Detection of Carrier:** Unknown.

**References:**
Beighton P, Kozlowski K: Spondylo-epimetaphyseal dysplasia with joint laxity and severe, progressive kyphoscoliosis. Skel Radiol 1980; 5:205–212.
Beighton P, et al.: Spondylo-epimetaphyseal dysplasia with joint laxity and severe, progressive kyphoscoliosis. S Afr Med J 1983; 64:772–775.
Beighton P, et al.: The manifestations and natural history of spondylo-epimetaphyseal dysplasia with joint laxity. Clin Genet 1984; 26:308–317.
Kozlowski K, Beighton P: Radiographic features of spondylo-epimetaphyseal dysplasia with joint laxity and severe, progressive kyphoscoliosis: review of 19 cases. Fortschr Röntgenstr 1984; 141:337–341.
Beighton P, et al.: International nosology of heritable disorders of connective tissue, Berlin, 1986. Am J Med Genet 1988; 29:581–594.

BE008 **Peter Beighton**

---

## SPONDYLOEPIPHYSEAL DYSPLASIA CONGENITA     0897

**Includes:** Dwarfism, short-trunk with retarded ossification

**Excludes:**
   Mucopolysaccharidosis IV (0678)
   Spondyloepiphyseal dysplasia, late (0898)
   Spondyloepiphyseal dysplasia (others)

**Major Diagnostic Criteria:** Short-trunk type of dwarfism; retarded ossification of the vertebral bodies and proximal femur; coxa vara; and normally shaped hand bones.

**Clinical Findings:** Flat face, myopia or retinal detachment (approximately 50% of cases); muscular hypotonia in infancy; occasionally cleft palate or clubfoot; short-trunk type of dwarfism,

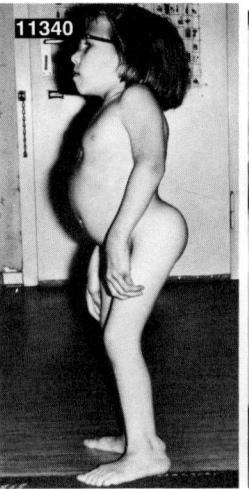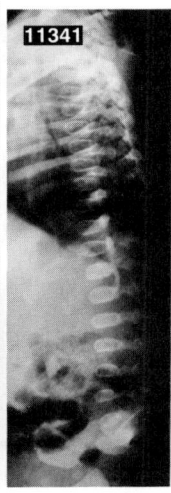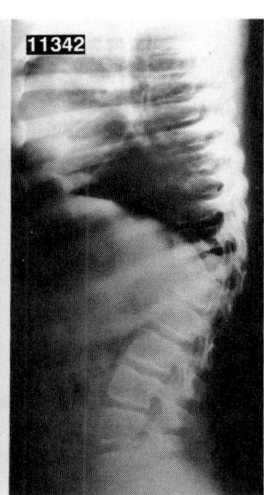

**0897-11340:** Short trunk dwarfism, lumbar lordosis which is accentuated. Facies are flat and glasses are worn to correct myopia. **11341:** At age 2 months: flat vertebral bodies, dorsal wedging of thoracic and upper lumbar bodies. **11342:** At age 13 years: platyspondyly in dorsal spine and kyphosis.

---

barrel-chest, genu valga or vara; waddling gait; and normal-sized hands and feet.

X-rays show retarded ossification of the spine and proximal femora with flattened, anteriorly pointed vertebral bodies; lack of ossification of the pubic and ischial bones in young infants; grossly retarded or absent ossification of the femoral head and neck in older patients; severe varus deformity of the femoral neck; varying degrees of epiphyseal and metaphyseal irregularities of the long tubular bones; and retarded ossification of the hand bones which are normally shaped.

A number of patients with clinical and X-ray features of spondyloepiphyseal dysplasia have been described who died at or shortly after birth. Histologically, these patients seem to differ from those with bona fide spondyloepiphyseal dysplasia congenita, exhibiting features reminiscent of hypochondrogenesis. At least one patient with these histologic features is known to have survived to the age of 12 years and at that age had more severe bone changes than other patients with spondyloepiphyseal dysplasia congenita. In particular, there was considerable involvement of the metaphyses at the knees and wrists, and the hand bones were not entirely normal. The condition is probably heterogenous.

**Complications:** Retinal detachment may lead to blindness. Premature and severe arthritic changes occur in the hips. Hypoplasia of the odontoid process of C2 and lax ligaments predispose to atlantoaxial instability and spinal cord compression. Kyphoscoliosis, hyperextensible finger joints, and joint dislocation.

**Associated Findings:** Recurrent otitis has been observed. Moderate sensorineural hearing loss (30–60 db), especially marked in high tones. Associated ocular findings include myopia, strabismus, cataracts, buphthalmos, and secondary glaucoma.

**Etiology:** Autosomal dominant inheritance with considerable variability in phenotypic expression. Sporadic cases are common.

**Pathogenesis:** Histologic studies show a hypocellular matrix and a lack of column formation, with an irregular array of broad, short spicules of calcified cartilage and bone. Electron microscopic examination of cartilage reveals widely distended cisterns of rough endoplasmic reticulum in the chondrocytes.

Murray and Rimoin (1985) found abnormal mobility of type II collagen cyanogen bromide peptides which may be a consequence of excessive posttranslation modification which in turn results from impediments in the formation of the collagen helix.

Lee et al (1989) identified a structural defect in collagen, type II (COL2A1) among the members of a large family with spondyloepiphyseal dysplasias.

**MIM No.:** *18390

**POS No.:** 3394

**CDC No.:** 756.460

**Sex Ratio:** M1:F1

**Occurrence:** Estimated at about 1:100,000.

**Risk of Recurrence for Patient's Sib:**
See Part I, *Mendelian Inheritance.*

**Risk of Recurrence for Patient's Child:**
See Part I, *Mendelian Inheritance.*

**Age of Detectability:** At birth.

**Gene Mapping and Linkage:** COL2A1 (collagen, type II, alpha 1) has been mapped to 12q14.3.

**Prevention:** None known. Genetic counseling indicated.

**Treatment:** Early correction of clubfoot deformity, closure of cleft palate; prevention of retinal detachment by regular ophthalmologic examinations and coagulation of early retinal tears. Careful neurologic examinations to detect early signs of cervical cord compression. Symptomatic orthopedic care.

**Prognosis:** The patients reach adulthood and may reproduce. The adult height varies between 84 and 128 cm. Mental development is normal. Patients who die at or shortly after birth probably have a different disorder.

**Detection of Carrier:** The phenotype is usually well expressed and easily detectable by clinical and X-ray studies.

**References:**

Macpherson RI: Spondyloepiphyseal dysplasia congenita. Pediatr Radiol 1980; 9:217–224.

Spranger J, Langer LO: Spondyloepiphyseal dysplasia congenita. Radiology 1980; 94:313–322.

Wynne-Davies R, Hall C: Two clinical variants of spondylo-epiphyseal congenita. J Bone Joint Surg 1982; 64B:435–441.

Harrod MJE, et al.: Genetic heterogeneity in spondyloepiphyseal dysplasia congenita. Am J Med Genet 1984; 18:311–320.

Murray TG, et al.: Spondyloepiphyseal dysplasia congenita: light and electron microscope studies of the eye. Arch Ophthal 1985; 103:407–411.

Murray TG, Rimoin DL: Type II collagen abnormalities in the spondyloepi- and spondyloepimetaphyseal dysplasias. (Abstract) Am J Hum Genet 1985; 37:A13.

Lee B, et al.: Identification of the molecular defect in a family with spondyloepiphyseal dysplasia. Science 1989; 244:978–980.

MY001                                    **Terry L. Myers**
SP007                               **Jürgen W. Spranger**

**Spondyloepiphyseal dysplasia tarda, Toledo type**
*See SPONDYLOEPIPHYSEAL DYSPLASIA, LATE*

## SPONDYLOEPIPHYSEAL DYSPLASIA, LATE      0898

**Includes:**
Chondroitin sulfate sulfotransferase deficiency
Chondro-osteodystrophy
Dwarfism, dysplasia spondyloepiphysaria tarda
Dysplasia spondyloepiphysaria tarda
PAPA-Chondroitin sulfate sulfotransferase deficiency
Spondyloepiphyseal dysplasia, X-linked form
Spondyloepiphyseal dysplasia tarda, Toledo type

**Excludes:**
Mucopolysaccharidosis IV (0678)
Spondyloepiphyseal dysplasia congenita (0897)
Spondyloepiphyseal dysplasia-mental retardation (3127)

**Major Diagnostic Criteria:** Short trunk dwarfism, with characteristic spinal and hip involvement, of late childhood or early adolescence onset. Skeletal X-rays confirm the diagnosis.

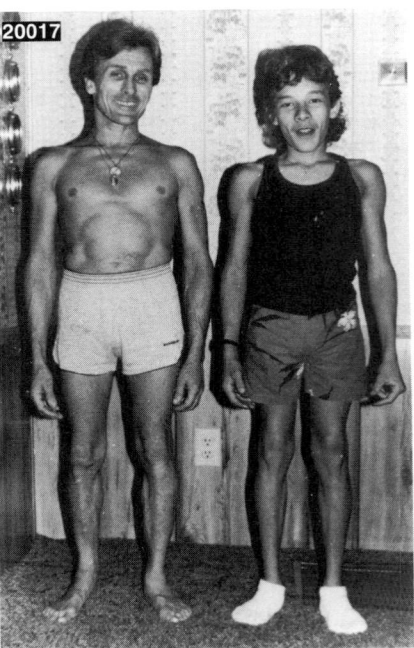

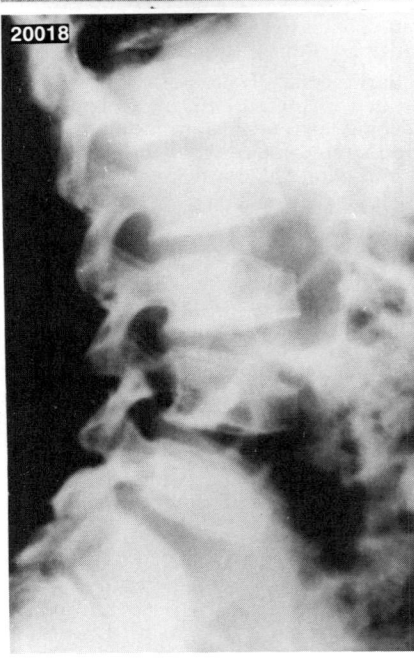

**0898A-20017:** Uncle and nephew with short-spine type of disproportionate short stature; limb lengths are relatively normal. **20018:** Characteristic humped-up platyspondylotic vertebral bodies on this lateral view of the lumbar spine.

**Clinical Findings:** In the typical case, disproportionate short stature secondary to vertebral loss of height. Adult height ranges from 130–155 cm. Premature osteoarthrosis, primarily of the spine and hips, frequently leads to restricted mobility. Less frequently, shoulders, knees and ankles are involved. Laboratory studies are usually normal. Skeletal X-rays rays show flattening of the vertebral bodies with a hump-shaped build-up of ivory-like bone in the central and posterior portions of the superior and inferior plates. There is a complete lack of visible bone in the areas of the ring

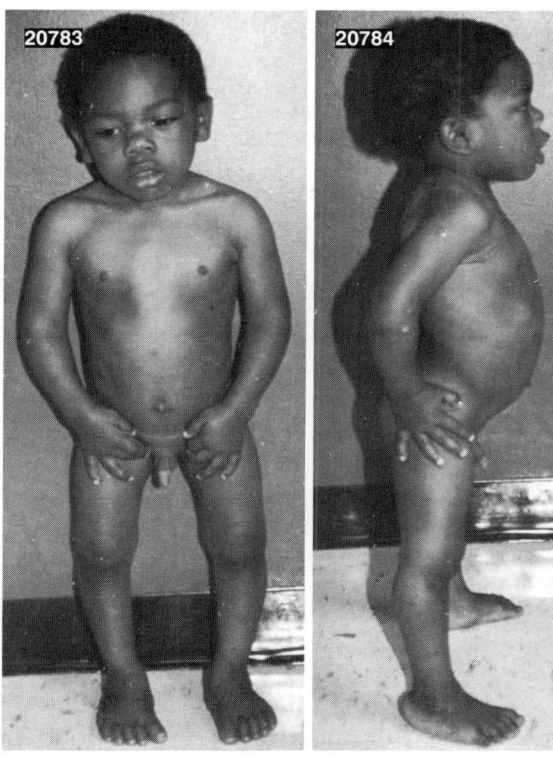

**0898B-20783-84:** Spondyloepiphyseal dysplasia; note short trunk, bowed legs, mild lordosis.

apophyses (projection from vertebrae). The disk spaces appear narrow, and at first glance may appear calcified, but the calcification is actually part of the vertebral body itself. Premature disk generation does occur. The platyspondyly extends throughout the thoracic and cervical spine to the C 2 level with less marked involvement of the end plates. The thoracic cage appears increased in both transverse and anteroposterior diameters. The bony pelvis is small. The acetabuli are deep and the femoral necks short. Mild dysplastic changes are seen in all large joints, especially the hips. Premature osteoarthosis of the hips, with extensive cyst formation, may develop in the third or fourth decade. The bones of the hands appear normal.

In addition to the more common X-linked form of this condition, a few families have been described with an autosomal dominant form. other cases have been reported with an autosomal recessive form which has been termed *chondro-osteodystrophy*. A *Toledo type* variant of the recessive form, with corneal opacity and anomalies of urinary mucopolysaccharides, is sometimes called *(PAPA)-Chondroitin sulfate sulfotransferase deficiency* (Toledo, 1978).

**Complications:** Premature osteoarthrosis of the hips almost always occurs in adulthood, and may lead to disabling pain and restricted mobility. Pain in the back and shoulders is also reported.

**Associated Findings:** One patient has been reported with poikiloderma and lymphoma. Deutan color blindness segregated with this condition in the three affected males of one family. A large kindred with numerous affected individuals included two males with protan color blindness.

**Etiology:** Usually X-linked recessive inheritance with variable expressivity and almost complete penetrance. Autosomal dominant and recessive inheritance has also been reported.

**Pathogenesis:** Unknown.

**MIM No.:** *31340, *27160, *27163, *18410

**POS No.:** 3395

**CDC No.:** 756.460

**Sex Ratio:** M1:F0 in the X-linked form. Presumably M1:F1 in the dominant and recessive forms.

**Occurrence:** Undetermined. Reported in several kindreds and ethnic groups.

**Risk of Recurrence for Patient's Sib:**
See Part I, *Mendelian Inheritance.*

**Risk of Recurrence for Patient's Child:**
See Part I, *Mendelian Inheritance.*

**Age of Detectability:** Late childhood or early adolescence, by short trunk dwarfism and typical skeletal X-rays.

**Gene Mapping and Linkage:** SEDL (spondyloepiphyseal dysplasia, late) has been provisionally mapped to Xp22.

**Prevention:** None known. Genetic counseling indicated.

**Treatment:** Palliative; physical therapy for the joint stiffness and pain. Total hip replacement is considered for severely disabled patients.

**Prognosis:** Normal life span and intelligence. Premature osteoarthrosis may lead to disabling pain and restricted mobility in mid or late adulthood.

**Detection of Carrier:** Clinical examination of first degree relatives.

**References:**
Maroteaux P, et al.: La dysplasie spondylo-epiphysaire tardive. Presse Med 1957; 65:1205–1208.
Langer LO: Spondyloepiphyseal dysplasia tarda. Radiology 1964; 82:833–839.
Bannerman RM, et al.: X-linked spondyloepiphyseal dysplasia tarda: clinical and linkage data. J Med Genet 1971; 8:291–301.
Spranger J, Langer LO: Spondyloepiphyseal dysplasia. BD:OAS X(9). Miami: Symposia Specialists for The National Foundation March of Dimes, 1974:19.
Toledo SPA, et al.: Recessively inherited, late onset, spondylar dysplasia and peripheral corneal opacity with anomalies in urinary mucopolysaccharides. Am J Med Genet 1978; 2:385–395.
Kousseff BG, et al.: Spondyloepiphyseal dysplasia tarda and deutan color blindness in a family. (Abstract) 7th Internat Congress of Hum Genet, Berlin, 1986:258.

K0018        **Boris G. Kousseff**

**Spondyloepiphyseal dysplasia, pseudoachondroplastic type**
*See PSEUDOACHONDROPLASTIC DYSPLASIA*
**Spondyloepiphyseal dysplasia, X-linked form**
*See SPONDYLOEPIPHYSEAL DYSPLASIA, LATE*

## SPONDYLOEPIPHYSEAL DYSPLASIA-MENTAL RETARDATION      3127

**Includes:** Mental retardation-spondyloepiphyseal dysplasia

**Excludes:** Spondyloepiphyseal dysplasia, late (0898)

**Major Diagnostic Criteria:** The combination of **Spondyloepiphyseal dysplasia, late** with mental retardation, particularly in a female, helps to distinguish this condition from others.

**Clinical Findings:** Normal birth weights and lengths with normal or near-normal early development in one patient and delayed milestones in the remaining two known patients. Physical examinations done when these affected females were adults demonstrated short stature (<3rd percentile), joint limitation, and mild-to-moderate mental retardation. X-ray studies revealed absent dens epistrophei (2/3), platyspondyly (3/3), anterior protrusion in the lumbar region (3/3), flared iliac bones with short sacrosciatic notch (3/3), coxa valga (3/3), and abnormal epiphyses of the femur and humerus (3/3).

**Complications:** Degenerative joint changes.

**Associated Findings:** None known.

**Etiology:** Probably autosomal recessive inheritance.

**Pathogenesis:** Unknown.

**MIM No.:** 27162

**POS No.:** 4280

**Sex Ratio:** M0:F3 (observed).

**Occurrence:** Reported in three sisters in an inbred Bedouin family.

**Risk of Recurrence for Patient's Sib:**
See Part I, *Mendelian Inheritance*.

**Risk of Recurrence for Patient's Child:**
See Part I, *Mendelian Inheritance*.

**Age of Detectability:** Probably during late childhood.

**Gene Mapping and Linkage:** Unknown.

**Prevention:** None known. Genetic counseling indicated.

**Treatment:** Orthopedic intervention may be indicated.

**Prognosis:** Mental retardation is present. Life span is unknown, although unlikely to be significantly affected.

**Detection of Carrier:** Unknown.

**References:**
Kohn G, et al.: Spondyloepiphyseal dysplasia tarda: a new autosomal recessive variant with mental retardation. J Med Genet 1987; 24:366–377.

T0007                                                          **Helga V. Toriello**

**Spondyloepiphyseal-spondyloperipheral dysplasia**
*See SPONDYLOPERIPHERAL DYSPLASIA*
**Spondylohumerofemoral hypoplasia, giant cell**
*See ATELOSTEOGENESIS*
**Spondylolisthesis, spine**
*See SPINE, SPONDYLOLISTHESIS AND SPONDYLOLYSIS*
**Spondylolysis, spine**
*See SPINE, SPONDYLOLISTHESIS AND SPONDYLOLYSIS*
**Spondylometaepiphyseal dysplasia**
*See SPONDYLOEPIMETAPHYSEAL DYSPLASIA*
**Spondylometaepiphyseal dysplasia congenita**
*See SPONDYLOEPIMETAPHYSEAL DYSPLASIA, STRUDWICK TYPE*
**Spondylometaepiphyseal dysplasia, Strudwick type**
*See SPONDYLOEPIMETAPHYSEAL DYSPLASIA, STRUDWICK TYPE*

## SPONDYLOMETAPHYSEAL CHONDRODYSPLASIA, KOZLOWSKI TYPE                                   0899

**Includes:**
Chondrodysplasia, spondylometaphseal, Kozlowski type
Dwarfism, Kozlowski type
Kozlowski chondrodysplasia, spondylometaphyseal

**Excludes:**
**Metatropic dysplasia** (0656)
**Mucopolysaccharidosis IV** (0678)
**Spondyloepimetaphyseal dysplasia**
Spondylometaphyseal chondrodysplasias, other types

**Major Diagnostic Criteria:** Short stature and X-ray signs of platyspondyly and metaphyseal osteochondrodysplasia.

**Clinical Findings:** Progressive, moderate short stature with predominant shortening of the trunk, waddling gait, kyphosis, and normal head. Adult height is about 140 cm. X-rays show generalized platyspondyly with unique shape of the vertebral bodies, metaphyseal osteochondrodysplasia, and retarded carpal and tarsal bone age.

**Complications:** Kyphosis; scoliosis; early, severe osteoarthritic changes.

**Associated Findings:** None known.

**Etiology:** Autosomal dominant and autosomal recessive inheritance has been reported.

**Pathogenesis:** Undetermined. Fibrous appearance of cartilage matrix.

**MIM No.:** 18425, *27166

**POS No.:** 3396

**Sex Ratio:** M1:F1

**Occurrence:** Over a dozen possible cases have been reported, but diagnostic classifications are still tentative.

**Risk of Recurrence for Patient's Sib:**
See Part I, *Mendelian Inheritance*.

**Risk of Recurrence for Patient's Child:**
See Part I, *Mendelian Inheritance*.

**Age of Detectability:** Preschool, by X-ray features.

**Gene Mapping and Linkage:** Unknown.

**Prevention:** None known. Genetic counseling indicated.

**Treatment:** Physiotherapy, orthopedic treatment.

**Prognosis:** Normal life span.

**Detection of Carrier:** Unknown.

**Special Considerations:** A number of patients with spine and metaphyseal dysplastic changes have been described who differ from the standard profile of this condition in X-ray appearance and distribution of the lesions. Although an attempt has been made to divide these cases into certain subtypes, their classification is still in question.

**References:**
Kozlowski K, et al.: La dysostose spondylo-metaphysaire. Presse Med 1967; 75:2769–2774.
Kozlowski K: Spondylo-metaphyseal dysplasia. Prog Pediatr Radiol 1973; 4:229–308.
Kozlowski K: Metaphyseal and spondylo-metaphyseal dysplasias. Clin Orthop 1976; 114:83–93.
Kozlowski K, et al.: Spondylo-metaphyseal dysplasias (Report of a case of common type and three pairs of siblings of "new varieties"). Austr Radiol 1976; 20:154–164.
Schorr S, et al.: Spondyloenchondrodysplasia. Radiology 1976; 118: 133–139.
Kozlowski K, et al.: Spondylo-metaphyseal dysplasia (report of a case of common type and three cases of "new varieties"). Röfo 1979; 130:222–230.
Kozlowski K, et al.: Spondylo-metaphyseal dysplasia (Report of 7 cases and essay of classification). In: Papadatos CJ, Bartsocas CS, eds: Skeletal dysplasias. New York: Alan R. Liss, 1982:89–101.
Ouadfel-Meziane A, et al.: Sponndylometaphyseal dysplasia: report of three familial cases. Ann Genet 1987; 30:216–220.

K0021                                                          **K.S. Kozlowski**

## SPONDYLOMETAPHYSEAL DYSPLASIA WITH ENCHONDROMATOUS CHANGES                             2595

**Includes:** Spondyloenchondrodysplasia

**Excludes:**
**Enchondromatosis** (0345)
**Enchondromatosis and hemangiomas** (0346)
Enchondromatosis with irregular vertebral lesions
**Metachondromatosis** (0650)
**Mucopolysaccharidosis IV** (0678)
**Spondyloepimetaphyseal dysplasia, Strudwick type** (3059)
**Spondylometaphyseal chondrodysplasia, Kozlowski type** (0899)
**Spondylometaphyseal dysplasia** (other)

**Major Diagnostic Criteria:** Disproportionate short stature with short trunk and limbs. Typical radiolucencies in the metaphyses, which extend into the shafts of the long bones. Spinal changes mainly confined to the posterior part of the vertebral bodies with severe platyspondyly. With time, irregular end-plates become apparent. Calcification of the basal ganglia, spasticity, and mental retardation may be variably present.

**Clinical Findings:** Birth length may be normal. Low birth weight was observed in the patients reported by Schorr et al (1976). Short stature probably becomes apparent only in the second year, but X-ray changes are already present at age six months. The growth rate is slow, with normal pubertal spurt. Patients may reach 150 cm, but most patients will probably be shorter. Kyphosis with increased lumbar lordosis is frequent and affects final height. The wrists, elbows, and knees appear widened, and joint and limb pains may be present. There may be difficulties in psychosocial adaptation. Mental retardation and spasticity are variably present.

The typical X-ray changes include radiolucent "masses" resembling enchondromas, which extend from the irregular metaphyses into the shafts of the long bones. The distal ulna and proximal fibula seem more severely affected than the corresponding radius and tibia. The elbow is almost spared, and the hips are moderately involved. In the spine similar radiolucencies are confined mainly to the posterior part of the vertebral bodies around the growth plate, as evidenced by computerized tomographic (CT) studies. Severe platyspondyly is present, but the vertebral bodies are not widened and present a cut-off anterior border. The iliac crests and sacrum are also involved. Three out of five patients who had brain CT scans showed calcification of the basal ganglia, not apparent on a plain skull X-ray.

At age six months, rachitic-like metaphyseal changes were already present. At age 31 months, typical radiolucencies were seen, and with time sclerotic streaks tend to appear and extend into the shafts of the long bones.

In the spine, irregularities of the end-plates tend to appear, and in the second decade a typical appearance of "vertebra within a vertebra" may develop.

**Complications:** Kyphosis, increased lumbar lordosis, and genu valgus.

**Associated Findings:** Three patients had mental retardation. Four patients had neurological manifestations ranging from spasticity of the lower limbs to quadriparesis.

**Etiology:** Autosomal recessive inheritance.

**Pathogenesis:** It has been suggested that the changes are cartilagenous in nature, but there is no histopathological evidence to support this view. A needle iliac crest biopsy did not enter a cartilagenous island. By light microscope, the chondrocytes showed non-specific changes only. Electron microscope studies showed inclusions within the rough endoplasmatic reticulum similar to those seen in **Kniest dysplasia.**

**MIM No.:** *27155

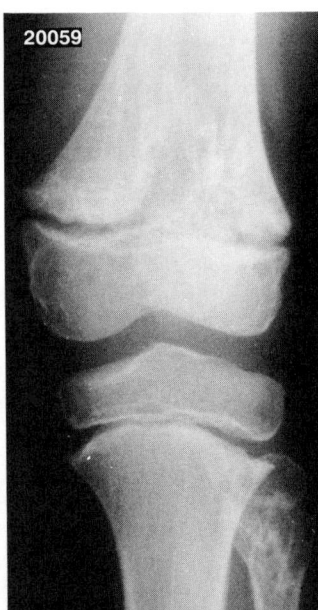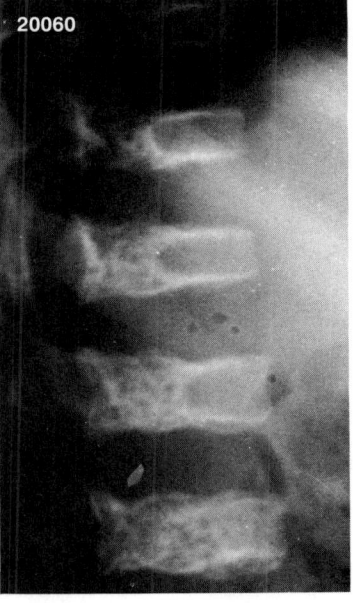

**2595-20059:** Metaphyseal changes are seen in this knee X-ray.
**20060:** Flattened and narrowed vertebral bodies.

**POS No.:** 4026

**Sex Ratio:** Presumably M1:F1.

**Occurrence:** Two sibs were reported by Schorr et al (1976), two patients by Sauvegrain et al (1982). The total number of reported patients is under twenty. Frydman et al studied six patients including two pairs of sibs. Two of the reported families are Iraqi Jews (four patients), and three are Palestinian Arabs (four patients). Menger et al (1989) reported on four patients and reviewed other reports.

**Risk of Recurrence for Patient's Sib:**
See Part I, *Mendelian Inheritance.*

**Risk of Recurrence for Patient's Child:**
See Part I, *Mendelian Inheritance.*

**Age of Detectability:** Clinically evident in the second year of life. X-ray changes were already present at age six months and probably earlier.

**Gene Mapping and Linkage:** Unknown.

**Prevention:** None known. Genetic counseling indicated.

**Treatment:** Physical therapy to prevent spine deformities. Analgesics for joint and limb pains. Psychologic support as indicated. Limb lengthening procedures may be appropriate.

**Prognosis:** Probably normal life span. Physical handicaps are related to the short stature and to the severity of kyphosis. Sauvegrain et al (1982), Menger et al (1989) and Frydman et al each observed one patient with mental retardation. Neurological manifestations ranging from spasticity to quadriparesis were seen in four patients.

**Detection of Carrier:** Unknown.

**Special Considerations:** The mother of two affected sibs and her sister and nephew had a stature below the third percentile without evidence of skeletal involvement (Frydman et al, 1986). This observation may indicate that the abnormal gene may have some effect in the heterozygote.

Other types of spondylometaphyseal dysplasia with enchondromatous-like changes also exist (i.e. see Sauvegrain et al, 1982).

**References:**

Schorr S, et al.: Spondyloenchondrodysplasia. Radiology 1976; 118: 133–139.

Sauvegrain J, et al.: Chondromes multiples avec atteinte rachidienne. Spondylo-enchondroplasie et autres formes. J Radiol 1982; 61:495–501.

Frydman M, et al.: Spondylometaphyseal dysplasia with "enchondromatous-like" changes: a distinctive type. 7th International Congress of Human Genetics, Berlin, September 22–26, 1986:257.

Menger H, et al.: Spondyloenchondrodysplasia. J Med Genet 1989; 26:93–99.

FR034                                            **Moshe Frydman**

**Spondylometaphyseal dysplasia, Brazilian type**
*See SPONDYLOEPIMETAPHYSEAL DYSPLASIA, STRUDWICK TYPE*
**Spondylometepiphyseal dysplasia (SMED)**
*See SPONDYLOEPIMETAPHYSEAL DYSPLASIA*

---

**SPONDYLOPERIPHERAL DYSPLASIA**      **3054**

**Includes:**
Spondyloepiphyseal-spondyloperipheral dysplasia
Spondyloperipheral dysplasia with short ulna

**Excludes:**
**Acromesomelic dysplasia**
**Brachydactyly** (0114)
**Exostoses-anetodermia-brachydactyly type E** (2764)
Pseudohypoparathyroidism
Pseudo-pseudohypoparathyroidism

**Major Diagnostic Criteria:** The combination of brachydactyly E, shortened long bones, and vertebral defects should suggest the diagnosis.

**Clinical Findings:** The hand and foot abnormalities, when present, are consistent with brachydactyly E, with short, broad metacarpals and metatarsals, short distal phalanges, and short fifth finger middle phalanges. Most affected individuals have short stature at or below the 10th percentile, with normal facial features. Spine and long bone anomalies are variable, ranging from no vertebral or long bone involvement to short or absent distal ulnae, humeri, tibiae, and femora. Coxarthrosis and epiphyseal dysplasia of the humerus have also been described. The spine anomalies are described as biconcavity with or without platyspondyly.

**Complications:** Joint and back pain and limitation of supination of various joints are relatively common complications; subchronic synovitis may also occur.

**Associated Findings:** None known.

**Etiology:** Autosomal dominant inheritance seems more likely than autosomal recessive, in that Sybert et al (1979) reported affected individuals in five generations.

**Pathogenesis:** Unknown.

**MIM No.:** 27170

**POS No.:** 4027

**Sex Ratio:** M1:F1

**Occurrence:** Three families have been reported, two in the United States and one in Czechoslovakia. A single case from South Africa has also been reported.

**Risk of Recurrence for Patient's Sib:**
See Part I, *Mendelian Inheritance.*

**Risk of Recurrence for Patient's Child:**
See Part I, *Mendelian Inheritance.*

**Age of Detectability:** During childhood.

**Gene Mapping and Linkage:** Unknown.

**Prevention:** None known. Genetic counseling indicated.

**Treatment:** Supportive, with orthopedic treatment possibly indicated.

**Prognosis:** Life span and intellect are apparently normal.

**Detection of Carrier:** Unknown.

**References:**
Kelly TE, et al.: An unusual familial spondyloepiphyseal dysplasia: "spondyloperipheral dysplasia." I: BD:OAS XIII(3B). New York: March of Dimes Birth Defects Foundation, 1977:149–165.
Sybert VP, et al.: Variable expression in a dominantly inherited skeletal dysplasia with similarities to brachydactyly E and spondyloepiphyseal-spondyloperipheral dysplasia. Clin Genet 1979; 15; 160–166. * †
Vanek J: Spondyloperipheral dysplasia. J Med Genet 1983; 20:117–121. †
Goldblatt J, Behari D: Unique skeletal dysplasia with absence of the distal ulnae. Am J Med Genet 1987; 28:625–630.

T0007                                   **Helga V. Toriello**

**Spondyloperipheral dysplasia with short ulna**
*See SPONDYLOPERIPHERAL DYSPLASIA*

---

## SPONDYLOTHORACIC DYSPLASIA                               0900

**Includes:**
  Costovertebral dysplasia
  Hemivertebrae, autosomal recessive multiple
  Jarcho-Levin syndrome
  Occipito-facial-cervico-thoracic-abdomino-digital dysplasia
  Spondylocostal dysplasia
  Vertebral anomalies
**Excludes:**
  **Robinow syndrome** (0876)
  **Spondylocostal dysplasia** (0896)
**Major Diagnostic Criteria:** Severe vertebral dysplasia and fusion giving markedly short trunk and "crab-like" appearance on X-ray.

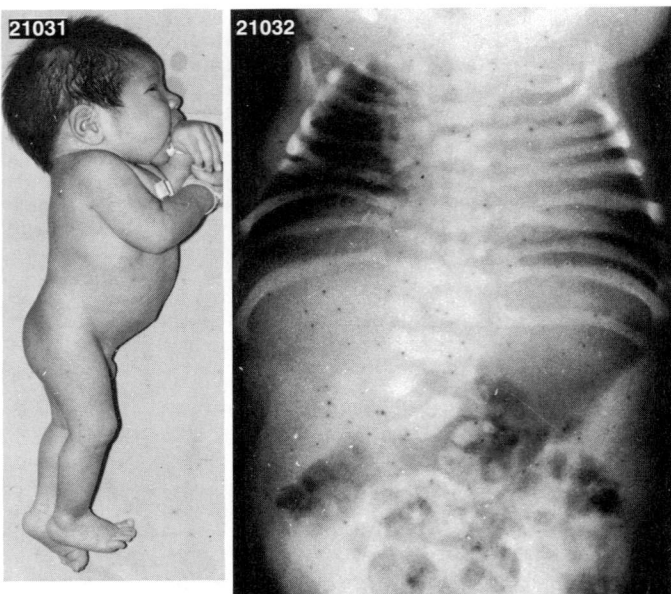

0900-21031: Spondylothoracic dysplasia; note short trunk and protuberant abdomen. 21032: Chest X-ray shows crab-like chest deformity from vertebral and rib anomalies.

---

**Clinical Findings:** Congenital short trunk with protuberant abdomen and relatively long limbs, which may be of normal length. The trunk is short because of anomalous vertebral development (hemivertebrae, partially absent vertebral bodies, fused vertebrae) and incomplete segmentation of the ribs. The thorax has a bizarre "crab-like" appearance on X-ray, with ribs splaying out from fused vertebrae. The neck is short, also because of anomalous vertebrae, with a low posterior hairline and limited movement. The occiput is prominent. The facies are round, somewhat puffy, with the chin resting on the chest. Long fingers and toes, even hammer toes, have been reported. Many patients have hernias. Nonskeletal anomalies reported include bilobed bladder, hydronephrosis, cerebral polygyria, anal atresia, submucous cleft palate, single umbilical artery, bilateral hydroceles, and inguinal hernia.

**Complications:** Affected children often die in infancy as a result of pulmonary insufficiency and pneumonia.

**Associated Findings:** None known.

**Etiology:** Autosomal recessive inheritance. Consanguinity, and affected sibs of both sexes, have been reported.

**Pathogenesis:** These particular spinal and rib anomalies probably have their origin in early embryonic development during vertebral segmentation; about the fourth to six week. Secondary anomalies in trunk and thorax shape occur.

**MIM No.:** *27730

**POS No.:** 3410

**Sex Ratio:** M16:F11 (observed).

**Occurrence:** 27 infants have been reported in 17 families. Most patients have been Puerto Rican.

**Risk of Recurrence for Patient's Sib:**
See Part I, *Mendelian Inheritance.*

**Risk of Recurrence for Patient's Child:**
See Part I, *Mendelian Inheritance.* Affected individuals are not expected to survive to reproduce.

**Age of Detectability:** At birth. Prenatal diagnosis by ultrasound should be possible.

**Gene Mapping and Linkage:**  Unknown.

**Prevention:**  None known. Genetic counseling indicated.

**Treatment:**  Respiratory support.

**Prognosis:**  Most reported cases have died in infancy.

**Detection of Carrier:**  Clinical examination of first degree relatives.

**Special Considerations:**  Less severe vertebral segmentation anomalies have been reported in similar but different conditions with autosomal dominant and recessive inheritance.

**References:**

Perez-Comas A, et al.: Occipito-facial-cervico-thoracic-abdomino-digital dysplasia. Jarcho-Levin syndrome of vertebral anomalies: a report of six cases and a review of the literature. J Pediatr 1974; 85:388–391.

Poor MA, et al.: Nonskeletal malformations in one of three siblings with Jarcho-Levin syndrome of vertebral anomalies. J Pediatr 1983; 103:270–272.

Cassidy SB, et al.: Natural history of Jarcho-Levin syndrome. (Abstract) Proc Greenwood Genet Center 3:92–94.

Young ID, Moore JR: Spondylocostal dysostosis. J Med Genet 1984; 21:68–69.

HA014                                    **Judith G. Hall**

**Sponge kidney**
 *See KIDNEY, MEDULLARY SPONGE KIDNEY*
**Spongioblastoma multiforme**
 *See CANCER, GLIOMA, FAMILIAL*
**Spongy glioneuronal dystrophy**
 *See ALPERS DISEASE*
**Spoon nails**
 *See NAILS, KOILONYCHIA*
**Sporadic Burkitt lymphoma**
 *See LYMPHOMA, BURKITT TYPE*
**'Spotted bones'**
 *See OSTEOPOIKILOSIS*
**Spotted corneal dystrophy**
 *See CORNEAL DYSTROPHY, MACULAR TYPE*
**Sprengel anomaly-hydrocephalus-costovertebral dysplasia**
 *See HYDROCEPHALUS-COSTOVERTEBRAL DYSPLASIA-SPRENGEL ANOMALY*

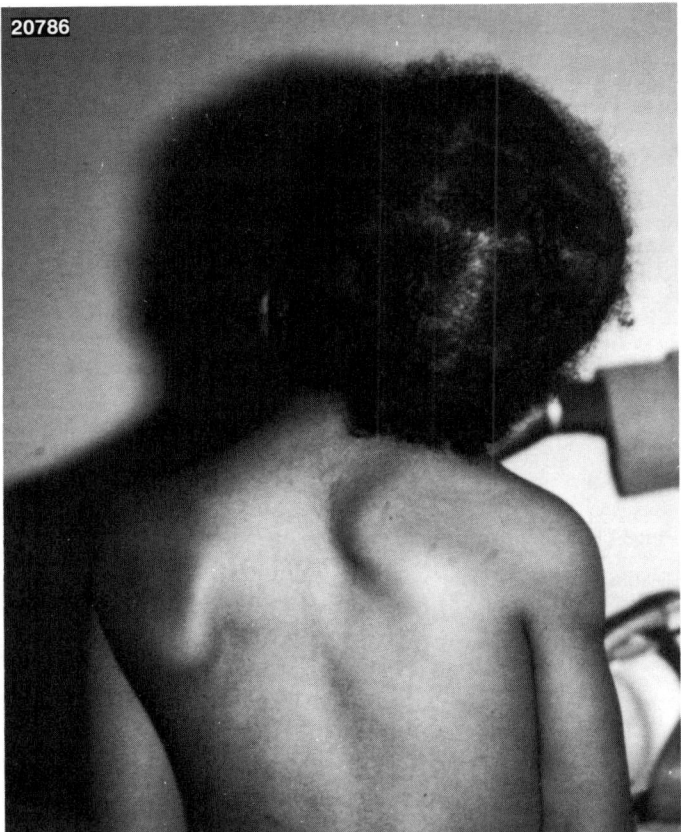

0901-20786:  Sprengel deformity; note high, triangular scapula.

## SPRENGEL DEFORMITY                    0901

**Includes:**
 High scapula
 Scapula elevata

**Excludes:**  Klippel-Feil anomaly (2032)

**Major Diagnostic Criteria:**  Clinical or X-ray evidence of elevated scapula.

**Clinical Findings:**  The scapula is located higher than its usual T2 - T7 position and is usually hypoplastic, having the "fetal shape" of an equilateral triangle. It lies closer to the midline, producing a lump in the web of the neck, and is rotated such that the glenoid fossa faces downward, restricting abduction of the affected arm. Involvement may be bilateral. A communication of bone, cartilage, or fibrous tissue between the scapula and adjacent vertebrae is found in 25–50% of patients. Over one-half the cases (67%) have associated skeletal anomalies or shoulder muscle hypoplasia.

Among those families showing autosomal dominant transmission, some demonstrate the scapula deformity alone in all affected members, while in other families the entire spectrum of associated anomalies may be found, with wide variation among affected members.

**Complications:**  Limitation of motion (elevation) of ipsilateral arm, related to degree of scapular deformity.

**Associated Findings:**  Scoliosis, hemivertebrae, fused vertebrae, spina bifida occulta, cervical ribs, missing ribs, fused ribs, chest deformities, situs inversus, clavicular anomalies, cleft palate, and hypoplasia of the muscles of the shoulder girdle.

**Etiology:**  Most cases occur sporadically, but autosomal dominant inheritance has been reported.

**Pathogenesis:**  The defect presumably results from failure of the mesenchymal anlage of the scapula to descend from its cervical position to the normal thoracic position during the second month of gestation.

**MIM No.:**  *18440

**CDC No.:**  755.556

**Sex Ratio:**  Presumably M1:F1. M1:F2 observed in sporadic cases.

**Occurrence:**  About 20 families have been reported.

**Risk of Recurrence for Patient's Sib:**
 See Part I, *Mendelian Inheritance*. Low risk for sporadic cases.

**Risk of Recurrence for Patient's Child:**
 See Part I, *Mendelian Inheritance*.

**Age of Detectability:**  At birth, or during childhood.

**Gene Mapping and Linkage:**  Unknown.

**Prevention:**  None known. Genetic counseling indicated.

**Treatment:**  Surgery may not be needed in mild cases; however, in those severely affected, both function and cosmetic appearance can be improved by reconstructive surgery. This usually involves removal of the omovertebral communication and excision of the superomedial part of the scapula.

Conservative treatment, including exercise, passive stretching and voluntary elevation of the unaffected scapula, has been used but appears to be of little value.

**Prognosis:** Life span and intelligence are normal. Functional disability is related to degree of scapula deformity and associated anomalies.

**Detection of Carrier:** Unknown.

**References:**

Otter GD: Bilateral Sprengel's syndrome with situs inversus totalis. Acta Orthopaedica Scand 1970; 41:402–410.

Wilson MG, et al.: Dominant inheritance of Sprengel's deformity. J Pediatr 1971; 79:818–821.

Cavendish ME: Congenital elevation of the scapula. J Bone Joint Surg [Br] 1972; 54B:395–408.

Chung SM, Nissenbaum MM: Congenital and developmental defects of the shoulder. Orthop Clin North Am 1975; 6:381–392.

Hodgson SV, Chiu DC: Dominant transmission of Sprengel's shoulder and cleft palate. J Med Genet 1981; 18:263–265.

H0033
H0025

**William A. Horton**
**O.J. Hood**

**Sprue**
  *See GLUTEN-SENSITIVE ENTEROPATHY*
**Spun-glass hair and crystalline cataract**
  *See HAIR, UNCOMBABLE-CRYSTALLINE CATARACT*
**Stable Factor deficiency**
  *See FACTOR VII DEFICIENCY*
**Stale fish syndrome**
  *See TRIMETHYLAMINURIA*
**Stammering**
  *See STUTTERING*
**Stanescu osteosclerosis**
  *See CRANIOFACIAL DYSOSTOSIS-DIAPHYSEAL HYPERPLASIA*
**Stapes ankylosis and perilymphatic gusher-deafness**
  *See DEAFNESS WITH PERILYMPHATIC GUSHER*
**Stapes fixation-deafness**
  *See DEAFNESS WITH PERILYMPHATIC GUSHER*
**Stapes fixation-oligodontia-cleft palate**
  *See CLEFT PALATE-STAPES FIXATION-OLIGODONTIA*
**Stargardt disease**
  *See RETINA, FUNDUS FLAVIMACULATUS*
**Startle disease**
  *See HYPEREKPLEXIA*
**Startle syndromes**
  *See JUMPING FRENCHMAN OF MAINE*
**Stationary nightblindness with high myopia congenital**
  *See NIGHTBLINDNESS, CONGENITAL STATIONARY, X-LINKED RECESSIVE*
**Stationary nightblindness with normal fundus congenital**
  *See NIGHTBLINDNESS, CONGENITAL STATIONARY, AUTOSOMAL RECESSIVE*
**Stature, short**
  *See DWARFISM*
**Status Bonnevie-Ullrich**
  *See NOONAN SYNDROME*
**Steatocystoma-pachyonychia congenita**
  *See PACHYONYCHIA CONGENITA-STEATOCYSTOMA MULTIPLEX*
**Steely hair disease**
  *See MENKES SYNDROME*
**Steinert disease**
  *See MYOTONIC DYSTROPHY*
**Stenosis at the conus elasticus**
  *See LARYNX, ATRESIA*
**Stenosis of anterior nares**
  *See NOSE, ANTERIOR ATRESIA*
**Stenosis of aqueduct of Sylvius**
  *See HYDROCEPHALY*
**Stenosis of ostium infundibulum**
  *See VENTRICLE, OBSTRUCTION WITHIN RIGHT VENTRICLE OR ITS OUTFLOW TRACT*
**Stenosis, combined subglottic**
  *See SUBGLOTTIC STENOSIS*
**Stenosis, hard subglottic**
  *See SUBGLOTTIC STENOSIS*
**Stenosis, soft subglottic**
  *See SUBGLOTTIC STENOSIS*
**Stenosis, subglottic**
  *See SUBGLOTTIC STENOSIS*
**Stephens syndrome (ophthalmoplegia-ataxia-peripheral neuropathy)**
  *See KEARNS-SAYRE DISEASE*

## STERNAL MALFORMATION-VASCULAR DYSPLASIA ASSOCIATION 3055

**Includes:**
  Hemangiomata-cleft sternum
  Leiber sternal clefts and telangiectasia/hemangiomas
  Vascular dysplasia-sternal malformation association

**Excludes:**
  Cleft sternum without associated anomalies
  **Heart, cordis ectopia** (0335)
  **Pentalogy of Cantrell** (3121)

**Major Diagnostic Criteria:** The combination of cleft sternum and hemangiomata.

**Clinical Findings:** The sternal defect ranged in severity from cleft of the upper one-third to cleft of the entire sternum. Hemangiomas usually affect the face, neck, and chin. Most were present at birth, although in one case the hemangioma did not become noticeable until age three months. In most cases, the vascular lesions are limited to the skin; however, one child also had a respiratory tract hemangioma, and a second had an intra-abdominal hemangioma.

**Complications:** Infection is the most common complication. If internal hemangiomas are present, site-dependent complications such as respiratory compromise and gastrointestinal bleeding can also occur.

**Associated Findings:** Micrognathia was present in two individuals; absent pericardium and unilateral **Cleft lip** were found in one individual each.

**Etiology:** Only one pair of affected sibs has been described; all other cases have been sporadic. Multifactorial inheritance or heterogeneity has not been ruled out.

**Pathogenesis:** A midline defect affecting mesodermal structure and proliferation of angioblastic tissue has been postulated. The components of this anomaly are thought to arise between 8–10 weeks of gestation.

**POS No.:** 3504

**Sex Ratio:** Presumably M1:F1.

**Occurrence:** About 15 cases have been reported.

**Risk of Recurrence for Patient's Sib:** Among 15 patients, two were sibs. Risk may therefore be small, but not neglible.

**Risk of Recurrence for Patient's Child:** Unknown.

**Age of Detectability:** At birth.

**Gene Mapping and Linkage:** Unknown.

**Prevention:** None known. Genetic counseling indicated.

**Treatment:** Surgical correction of the sternal defect may be indicated; corticosteroids may stop the progression of the hemangiomas; treatment of complications, such as infection, is also indicated.

**Prognosis:** Barring any complications, prognosis for normal growth, intellectual development, and life span is good.

**Detection of Carrier:** Unknown.

**References:**

Hague KN: Isolated asternia: an independent entity. Clin Genet 1984; 25:362–365.

Hersh JH, et al.: Sternal malformation/vascular dysplasia association. Am J Med Genet 1985; 21:177–186.

Opitz JM: Editorial comment on the papers by Hersh et al. and Kaplan et al. on sternal cleft. Am J Med Genet 1985; 21:201–202.

T0007

**Helga V. Toriello**

**Sternocleidomastoid torticollis**
  *See TORTICOLLIS*
**Sternogladiolar prominence**
  *See PECTUS CARINATUM*
**Sternomastoid torticollis**
  *See TORTICOLLIS*

## STEROID 3 BETA-HYDROXYSTEROID DEHYDROGENASE DEFICIENCY                     0909

**Includes:**   Adrenal hyperplasia II

**Excludes:**   Adrenal steroidogenesis, other enzyme deficiencies in

**Major Diagnostic Criteria:**   Ambiguous genitalia in both males and females, vomiting, dehydration, and low serum sodium and chloride constitute the major manifestations. Elevated 17-ketosteroid (17-KS) excretion, predominately dehydroepiandrosterone (DHEA) or its derivatives, preponderance of δ5 urinary steroid compounds, mild virilization in females or under-masculinization in males, and suppression of abnormal steroids with exogenous glucocorticoids.

**Clinical Findings:**   This is a rare form of congenital adrenal hyperplasia (CAH) in which the enzyme defect occurs early in adrenal steroidogenesis and affects the mineralocorticoid, glucocorticoid, and sex steroid pathways. Thus, in severe enzyme deficiency, salt loss, hyponatremia, hyperkalemia, vomiting, and dehydration are characteristic. In patients with partial defects, mineralocorticoid deficiency may not become apparent without stress, but hyponatremia becomes manifest during salt deprivation, particularly during withdrawal of supplemental glucocorticoids. Gradation in the severity of salt loss occurs even in affected sibs emphasizing the clinical heterogeneity in this syndrome,

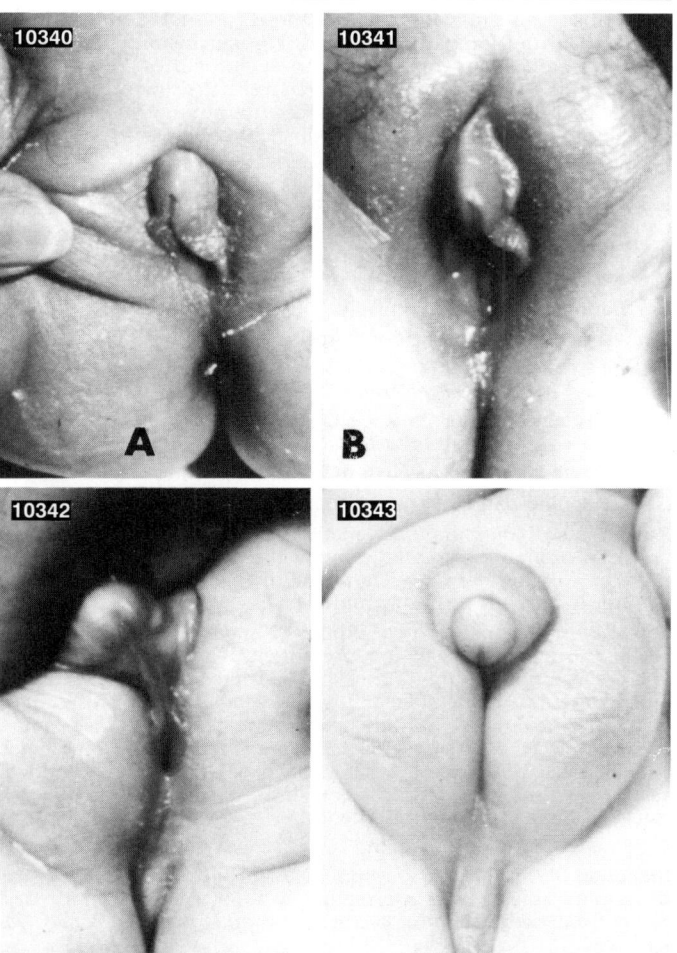

**0909-10340–41:**   Mild clitoral hypertrophy and pubic hair development in a female.   **10342–43:**   Bifid scrotum, severe hypospadias, and small phallus in a male.

which has been diagnosed in a 40-year-old woman. The external genitalia show variable degrees of abnormality in both males and females. Males have hypospadias, often perineal or second degree in type, and a bifid scrotum, with or without cryptorchidism. Females have labial fusion; clitoral hypertrophy, which is often mild; and mild but progressive hirsutism. This inadequate masculinization in males and mild virilization in females results from the accumulation and defective conversion of DHEA, a weak androgen, to androstenedione and, subsequently, to testosterone.

Laboratory tests reveal a high urinary excretion of 17-ketosteroids in which DHEA or its metabolites predominate. 17-hydroxycorticosteroids and aldosterone excretion are typically low but may be normal in patients with partial defects, where plasma cortisol and cortisol production rates have been shown to be within the normal range. Pregnenolone and its derivatives (δ5-pregnenetriol; 16α-hydroxy pregnenolone, 17α hydroxy pregnenolone) rather than pregnanolone derivatives (pregnanetriol), predominate in urine, reflecting the lack of enzyme isomerase activity required to shift the double bond from the C5-C6 position in the B-ring, to the C4-C5 position in the A ring of the steroid nucleus. The enzyme defect also occurs in the fetal testes (and ovary) and persists into later life, so that the response to exogenous (and presumably endogenous) gonadotropin is subnormal. However, in individuals with partial defects, there is evidence for increasing 3β-HSD activity with age, the enzyme activity being extra-adrenal, and probably hepatic in origin. Consequently, with increasing age, a large amount of pregnanetriol may appear in the urine, but this does not represent the coexistence of a double enzyme defect in 3β-HSD and 21-hydroxy activity. It should be noted that in severe enzyme deficiency, six of the seven initially reported patients died despite adequate glucocorticoid and salt replacement. The adrenal glands are hypertrophied, and histologically they appear laden with lipid.

**Complications:**   Salt loss, dehydration, hypoglycemia, and death may occur. Involvement of the gonads may preclude spontaneous puberty or fertility.

**Associated Findings:**   None known.

**Etiology:**   Autosomal recessive inheritance.

**Pathogenesis:**   The enzyme defect appears to affect the adrenals, as well as the gonads. There is a difference in the timing of maximal enzyme activity in the testis and ovary. Thus 3β-HSD activity in the testes is maximal at about the third intrauterine month, whereas in the ovaries and adrenal glands it becomes maximal at about the fourth month. Consequently, the abnormalities in male external genitalia are more severe.

An animal model of 3β-HSD deficiency has been produced in rats by the administration of a C-19 substrate analog to the mother. Partial prevention of hypospadias in affected male rats has been achieved by testosterone administration in utero; the anatomic defect in affected female offspring was prevented by *in utero* administration of corticosterone.

**MIM No.:**   *20181

**CDC No.:**   255.200

**Sex Ratio:**   M1:F1

**Occurrence:**   About a dozen cases have been documented.

**Risk of Recurrence for Patient's Sib:**
See Part I, *Mendelian Inheritance.*

**Risk of Recurrence for Patient's Child:**
See Part I, *Mendelian Inheritance.*

**Age of Detectability:**   May be detected from birth to adult life; most frequently in the first years of life, by virtue of salt loss, with ambiguity of external genitalia. Antenatal diagnosis has not been demonstrated.

**Gene Mapping and Linkage:**   HSDB3 (hydroxy-delta 5-steroid dehydrogenase, 3 beta- and steroid delta-isomerase) has been provisionally mapped to 1p13-p11.

**Prevention:**   None known. Genetic counseling indicated.

**Treatment:**   Treatment with glucocorticoid and mineralocorticoids should be instituted early, particularly in view of the reported high mortality in severely affected patients. Because the defect affects the gonads, replacement with sex steroids at puberty will be required. Surgical correction of hypospadias or clitoromegaly may be required.

**Prognosis:** Normal life span in patients with partial defects; death has been reported in severely affected infants despite adequate replacement therapy. Reproductive function will be impaired.

**Detection of Carrier:** Unknown.

**Special Considerations:** MN; Wrenshall (c/o Diana Johnson, 10 Co Hwy 4); Congenital Adrenal Hyperplasia Group

**References:**

Goldman AS: Experimental congenital adrenocortical hyperplasia: persistent postnatal deficiency in activity of 3β-hydroxysteroid dehydrogenase produced *in utero*. J Clin Endocrinol 1967; 27:1041.

Zachmann M, et al.: Unusual type of congenital adrenal hyperplasia probably due to deficiency of 3β-hydroxysteroid dehydrogenase. case report of a surviving girl with steroid studies. J Clin Endocrinol 1970; 30:719.

Bongiovanni AM, et al.: Urinary excretion of pregnanetriol and δ5-pregnenetriol in two forms of congenital adrenal hyperplasia. J Clin Invest 1971; 50:2751.

Kenny FM, et al.: Partial 3β-hydroxysteroid dehydrogenase (3βHSD) deficiency in a family with congenital adrenal hyperplasia: evidence for increasing 3β-HSD activity with age. Pediatrics 1971; 48:756.

Zachmann M, et al.: 3 β-hydroxysteroid dehydrogenase deficiency: follow-up study in a girl with pubertal bone age. Hormone Res 1979; 11:292–302.

Rosenfeld RL, et al.: Pubertal presentation of congenital δ5–3β-hydroxysteroid dehydrogenase deficiency. J Clin Endocrinol Metab 1980; 51:345.

Miller WL, Levine LS: Molecular and clinical advance in congenital adrenal hyperplasia. J Pediat 1987; 111:1–17.

White PC, et al.: Congenital adrenal hyperplasia. New Engl J Med 1987; 316:1519 (first part) and 1580 (second part).

New MI, et al.: The adrenal hyperplasias. In: Scriver CR, et al, eds: The metabolic basis of inherited disease, 6th ed. New York: Mc-Graw-Hill, 1989:1881–1918.

SP004                                                              **Mark A. Sperling**

---

## STEROID 5 ALPHA-REDUCTASE DEFICIENCY          3062

**Includes:**

Genital ambiguity, pseudovaginal perineoscrotal hypospadias
Male pseudohermaphroditism due to 5 alpha-reductase deficiency
Pseudohermaphroditism, familial incomplete male, type 2
Pseudovaginal perineoscrotal hypospadias

**Excludes:**

Genital ambiguity in XY males, external (other)
Receptor-dependent androgen-responsive defects
Testis differentiation defects
Testosterone production defects

**Major Diagnostic Criteria:** Perineal hypospadias with separate urethral and vaginal openings within a urogenital sinus. The testes are usually cryptorchid. At puberty, there is impressive genital and somatic virilization, without gynecomastia. Plasma testosterone is normal or elevated, but its level in relation to 5α-dihydrotestosterone is high. Plasma luteinizing hormone is high; follicle stimulating hormone may be high. Urinary 5α-reduced metabolites of testosterone and of various other C-19 and C-21 steroids are low. Decreased or defective 5α-reductase activity in fresh tissue slices or cultured genital skin fibroblasts.

**Clinical Findings:** The infant is born with external genitalia that are predominantly feminine in character, but is otherwise well. Plasma testosterone level is normal or elevated basally and augments normally in response to a course of human chorionic gonadotropin. In either case the plasma testosterone: 5α-dihy-

drotestosterone ratio is higher than normal. The epididymes, vasa deferentia, and seminal vesicles (all Wolffian duct derivatives) are present, but the prostate is impalpable or hypoplastic. Müllerian duct derivatives are absent. At puberty, the voice deepens, skeletal muscle development is normal, the phallus grows, the scrotum becomes rugose and pigmented, pubic hair growth is impressive, and the testes often descend. Spermatogenesis may be near normal in testes that have not been cryptorchid. The subjects have erections and ejaculates. They do not have temporal hairline recession, facial and body hair are less than normal, and acne is rare. Despite a female sex-of-rearing, subjects have a remarkable tendency to adopt a male sexual identity and orientation at puberty.

**Complications:** None, except those in the psychosexual sphere, and particularly if inadequate reinforcement of the female sex-of-rearing allows affected subjects to adopt a male identity at puberty.

**Associated Findings:** None known.

**Etiology:** Autosomal recessive inheritance.

**Pathogenesis:** 5α-reductase is the enzyme responsible for converting testosterone to 5α-dihydrotestosterone (DHT). Deficient activity of the enzyme in androgen target tissues yields a phenotype that distinguishes testosterone-dependent from DHT-dependent events in male sexual development. Since Wolffian differentiation is normal, it is testosterone-dependent. Indeed, 5α-reductase enzyme activity does not appear in Wolffian-derived structures until they have passed their critical period in differentiation. Contrarily, masculinization of the neutral external genital primordia and prostate morphogenesis are DHT dependent. Hence their development is blocked. Not surprisingly, 5α-reductase enzyme activity appears in these structures before their critical period of differentiation. The fact that growth and maturation of the external genitalia occur at puberty suggests that these structures acquire a degree of responsiveness to testosterone that they lack in utero. The elevated plasma level of luteinizing hormone suggests that DHT is important for negative feedback of LH release. The absence of clinical features in female homozygotes means that testosterone is sufficient for normal female sexual development.

**MIM No.:** *26460

**Sex Ratio:** M1:F1 biochemically, but M1:F0 clinically.

**Occurrence:** Uncommon, but precise data are unavailable.

**Risk of Recurrence for Patient's Sib:**
See Part I, *Mendelian Inheritance.*

**Risk of Recurrence for Patient's Child:**
See Part I, *Mendelian Inheritance.*

**Age of Detectability:** At birth in XY homozygotes.

**Gene Mapping and Linkage:** Unknown.

**Prevention:** None known. Genetic counseling indicated. In theory, DHT replacement could prevent the dysmorphogenesis, but there is no way, currently, to detect affected male fetuses early enough to use this form of prophylaxis.

**Treatment:** Diagnosis in early infancy and an early decision on sex-of-rearing are basic to good treatment. If a male sex-of-rearing is chosen, topical application of DHT cream to the external genitalia will facilitate staged surgical reconstruction in the male direction. At puberty, intramuscular testosterone in doses sufficient to raise the plasma DHT level into the normal range have been beneficial. An excessively high level of DHT must be avoided as it reduces the plasma testosterone level secondarily and thereby causes loss of libido and impotence.

**Prognosis:** Normal life span.

**Detection of Carrier:** Asymptomatic male and female carriers are often detectable by their intermediately abnormal levels of urinary 5α-reduced metabolites of testosterone and other C-19 or C-21 steroids.

**Special Considerations:** Measurement and characterization of 5α-reductase activity in cultured genital skin fibroblasts may be useful for ruling out the diagnosis. However, the normal level of

5α-reductase activity in these cells is very variable. In some laboratories, the lower level of normal is at the limit of sensitivity of the assay. Hence, in these laboratories such cells cannot be used to rule in the diagnosis. Normal cultured nongenital skin fibroblasts are even more likely to have very low levels of 5α-reductase activity. They should not be used for ruling in the diagnosis.

The remarkable tendency for affected subjects, reared as females, to adopt a male sexual identity at puberty indicates that exposure of the brain to testosterone prenatally, in early postnatal life, and at puberty is sufficient to overcome a female sex-of-rearing, unless the latter is strongly reinforced.

### References:

Peterson RE, et al.: Male pseudohermaphroditism due to steroid 5α-reductase deficiency. Am J Med 1977; 62:170–191.

Pinsky L, et al.: 5α-reductase activity of genital and non-genital skin fibroblasts from patients with 5α-reductase deficiency, androgen insensitivity, or unknown forms of male pseudohermaphroditism. Am J Med Genet 1978; 1:407–416.

Imperato-McGinley J, et al.: Androgens and the evolution of male-gender identity among male pseudohermaphrodites with 5α-reductase deficiency. New Engl J Med 1979; 300:1233–1237.

Imperato-McGinley J, et al.: Steroid 5α-reductase deficiency in a 65 year old male pseudohermaphrodite: the natural history, ultrastructure of the testes and evidence for inherited enzyme heterogeneity. J Clin Endocrinol Metab 1980; 50:15–22.

Price P, et al.: High dose androgen therapy in male pseudohermaphroditism due to 5α-reductase deficiency and disorders of the androgen receptor. J Clin Invest 1984; 74:1496–1508.

Imperato-McGinley J, et al.: Decreased urinary C19 and C21 steroid 5α-metabolites in parents of male pseudohermaphrodites with 5α-reductase deficiency: detection of carriers. J Clin Endocrinol Metab 1985; 60:553–558.

Imperato-McGinley J, et al.: The diagnosis of 5α-reductase deficiency in infancy. J Clin Endocrinol Metab 1986; 63:1313–1318.

PI005      **Leonard Pinsky**

---

### STEROID 11 BETA-HYDROXYLASE DEFICIENCY     0902

**Includes:**
> Adrenal hyperplasia IV
> Adrenogenital syndrome with hypertension
> Hypertensive form of adrenal hyperplasia
> P450C11B1, deficiency of

**Excludes:** Enzyme deficiencies in adrenal steroid biosynthesis, other

**Major Diagnostic Criteria:** Progressive virilization, excessive 17-KS and 17-OHCS excretion, and markedly elevated concentration of compound-S in plasma or urine which is suppressed during glucocorticoid replacement.

**Clinical Findings:** Progressive virilization and all the sequelae of excessive androgen formation, including ambiguity of the external genitalia in genetic and gonadal females, as described for 21-hydroxylase deficiency. However, salt loss, hyponatremia, and hyperkalemia do not occur. Hypertension may occur but is not universally present, suggesting a spectrum in the severity of enzyme deficiency. The enzyme involved catalyzes the conversion of 11-deoxycortisol (compound-S) to cortisol (compound-F) in the glucocorticoid pathway, and deoxycorticosterone (DOC) to corticosterone (compound-B) in the mineralocorticoid pathway. Consequently, the plasma concentrations of compound-S and DOC are elevated, as are the respective urinary excretion products, whereas plasma and urinary cortisol and aldosterone may be diminished. Urinary excretion of 17-ketosteroids is elevated, reflecting excessive adrenal androgen production, which is unaffected by the enzyme block and stimulated by excessive ACTH that results from inadequate cortisol secretion. Urinary 17-hydroxy-corticosteroids (17-OHCS) are also elevated since compound-S and its urinary metabolite, tetrahydro-S, both contain the 17, 21 dihydroxy, 20 keto grouping, which reacts in the standard 17-OHCS measurements. Pregnanetriol excretion in urine may be modestly elevated.

Salt restriction is not associated with a rise in aldosterone, even after suppression of DOC by administered cortisol, suggesting that the same enzyme is involved in both glucocorticoid and mineralocorticoid pathways. Plasma renin levels are low. Mild cases may present in adult life and simulate the Stein-Leventhal syndrome.

**Complications:** Ambiguity of the external genitalia may result in false gender assignment in genetic females; lack of electrolyte disturbances may delay the diagnosis in males. Progressive virilization, premature epiphyseal closure, and final short stature, as well as preclusion of normal puberty and fertility may result from the untreated condition. Hypertension is a direct result of excessive production of DOC, a potent mineralocorticoid.

**Associated Findings:** Gynecomastia has been described in an affected male infant.

**Etiology:** Autosomal recessive inheritance.

**Pathogenesis:** The enzyme block prevents the normal synthesis of cortisol, resulting in excessive ACTH stimulation and adrenal hyperplasia. The androgenic pathway is unaffected by the block; consequently, production of dehydroepiandrosterone, androstenedione, and testosterone is increased, producing virilization, rapid growth, and accelerated bone maturation. DOC also is secreted in large quantities, resulting in salt and water retention, volume expansion, and hypertension, with low renin secretion. Both the enzymatic block and the suppressed renin contribute to low aldosterone secretion.

A block in 11-hydroxylation may occur in some adrenocortical carcinomas, thus totally simulating the clinical features and plasma and urinary steroid patterns observed with the congenital enzyme deficiency. However, under these circumstances glucocorticoid replacement will not suppress the oversecretion of the specific steroids. The possibility of carcinoma must always be considered in "late onset" cases. Metapyrone (SU4885) is a drug that also blocks 11-hydroxylation; use is made of this agent in studying the intactness of the hypothalamic-pituitary-adrenal axis.

**MIM No.:** *20201

**CDC No.:** 255.200

**Sex Ratio:** M1:F1

**Occurrence:** Undetermined but presumed rare. About 40 cases reported in Jews of Moroccan and Iranian extraction.

**Risk of Recurrence for Patient's Sib:**
> See Part I, *Mendelian Inheritance.*

**Risk of Recurrence for Patient's Child:**
> See Part I, *Mendelian Inheritance.*

**Age of Detectability:** From birth to adult life. Intrauterine diagnosis has been demonstrated, based on maternal urine or amniotic fluid hormone measurements.

**Gene Mapping and Linkage:** CYP11B1 (cytochrome P450, subfamily XIB, polypeptide 1 (steroid 11-beta-hydroxylase)) has been mapped to 8q21-q22.

CYP11B2 (cytochrome P450, subfamily XIB, polypeptide 2 (steroid 11-beta-hydroxylase)) has been provisionally mapped to 8q21-q22.

**Prevention:** None known. Genetic counseling indicated.

**Treatment:** Replacement therapy with cortisol arrests virilization and restores blood pressure to normal. Intrauterine diagnosis is theoretically feasible, as is intrauterine therapy with cortisol to minimize virilization. Primary and definitive surgical repair may be required for ambiguous genitalia in genetic females.

**Prognosis:** Normal for life span, reproduction, and intelligence when diagnosed early and appropriate treatment is instituted.

**Detection of Carrier:** Theoretically, via levels of compound-S achieved after ACTH stimulation, but in practice this has not proven useful. Unlike the 21-hydroxylase defect, there is no association with the HLA system that would permit identification of the heterozygote, or antenatal diagnosis or detection of an unrecognized homozygote (see **Steroid 21-hydroxylase deficiency**).

**Special Considerations:** MN; Wrenshall (c/o Diana Johnson, 10 Co Hwy 4); Congenital Adrenal Hyperplasia Group

**References:**
McLaren NK, et al.: Gynecomastia with congenital virilizing adrenal hyperplasia (11-β-hydroxylase deficiency). J Pediat 1975; 86:597.
Cathelineau G, et al.: Adrenocortical 11β-hydroxylation defect in adult women with post menarchial onset of symptoms. J Clin Endocrinol Metab 1980; 51:287.
Pang S, et al.: Hormonal studies in obligate heterozygotes and siblings of patients with 11β-hydroxylase deficiency congenital adrenal hyperplasia. J Clin Endocrinol Metab 1980; 50:586.
Rosler A, et al.: Clinical variability of congenital adrenal hyperplasia due to 11-beta-hydroxylase deficiency. Hormone Res 1982; 16:133–141.
Zachmann M, et al.: Clinical and biochemical variability of congenital adrenal hyperplasia due to 11β-hydroxylase deficiency: a study of 25 patients. J Clin Endocrinol Metab 1983; 56:222.
Hochberg Z, et al.: Growth and pubertal development in patients with congenital adrenal hyperplasia due to 11-beta-hydroxylase deficiency. Am J Dis Child 1985; 139:771–776.
Miller WL, Levine LS: Molecular and clinical advance in congenital adrenal hyperplasia. J Pediat 1987; 111:1–17.
White PC, et al.: Congenital adrenal hyperplasia. New Engl J Med 1987; 316:1519 (first part) and 1580 (second part).
New MI, et al.: The adrenal hyperplasias. In: Scriver CR, et al, eds: The metabolic basis of inherited disease, 6th ed. New York: McGraw-Hill, 1989:1881–1918.

SP004                                           **Mark A. Sperling**

---

## STEROID 17 ALPHA-HYDROXYLASE DEFICIENCY          0903

**Includes:**
Adrenal hyperplasia V
Hypertensive congenital adrenal hyperplasia

**Excludes:**
Adrenal hyperplasia, other forms
**Hyperaldosteronism, familial glucocorticoid suppressible** (0484)

**Major Diagnostic Criteria:** Diminished 17-hydroxylated steroids and sex steroids, hypertension, and lack of secondary sexual characteristics in phenotypic females or males with ambiguous genitalia. Secretion of DOC (deoxycorticosterone) is elevated but can be suppressed with administration of glucocorticoids. The cortisol response to ACTH and the sex steroid hormone responses to chorionic gonadotropin are diminished or absent.

**Clinical Findings:** Hypertension and the absence of secondary sexual characteristics. The enzyme defect prevents the formation of cortisol or any of its 17-hydroxylated precursors, as well as the formation of sex steroids, the latter defect apparently shared by the gonad. Mineralocorticoid formation is not affected.

In females, there is no ambiguity of the external genitalia at birth, but secondary sexual characteristics (breasts, and pubic and axillary hair) fail to develop and primary amenorrhea may be the presenting complaint. Acute abdominal pain secondary to infarction of cystic enlarged ovaries has been reported in sibs. As might be expected from a defect interfering with adrenal and testicular androgen formation and thus male sexual differentiation, genotypic males have congenitally ambiguous genitalia. The penis is small or rudimentary, hypospadias is present, and the labia majora fail to fuse, creating a shallow vagina. Cryptorchidism may be present.

Laboratory tests reveal hypokalemic alkalosis, low cortisol concentrations in plasma or 17-OHCS excretion in urine, and low-to-absent 17-ketosteroids (17-KS), estrogens, and testosterone. Plasma ACTH levels are elevated, and there is no response or a subnormal response in serum cortisol, or urinary 17-OHCS, or 17-KS following administration of ACTH. Similarly there is little or no gonadal response to administration of chorionic gonadotropin. Endogenous serum gonadotropin concentrations are high in older

individuals. In contrast, circulating corticosterone (compound-B) and deoxycorticosterone (DOC) levels are elevated. Plasma renin is low, as is aldosterone, suggesting salt and water retention and volume expansion by DOC, with resultant suppression of the renin/angiotensin/aldosterone pathway. This is confirmed by finding normal renin and aldosterone concentrations after suppressive doses of glucocorticoids. Partial defects with normokalemia have been described, but hypertension, diminished or absent sexual hair, and amenorrhea have been characteristic in all females, who consequently present in the mid-to-late teen years. In genetic males with the complete defect, the external genitalia will be entirely female, and diagnosis can be delayed until puberty, unless hypertension and hypokalemia are recognized. Males with the partial defect will be recognized earlier by virtue of ambiguity of the external genitalia.

A defect in 17-hydroxylation has been found in an infant with a corticosterone-secreting adrenal tumor nonsuppressible by glucocorticoids. Glucocorticoid-responsive hyperaldosteronism should and can be differentiated because 17-hydroxy corticosteroids and 17-ketosteroids are intermittently elevated.

**Complications:** Hypertension and hypokalemia result from excessive DOC secretion. Phenotypically normal female external genitalia in genetic males may result in false gender assignment. Impaired sexual development and fertility occur in both sexes.

**Associated Findings:** None known.

**Etiology:** Autosomal recessive or possibly X-linked recessive inheritance.

**Pathogenesis:** A defect in 17-hydroxylation affecting adrenal and gonadal steroidogenesis.

**MIM No.:** *20211

**CDC No.:** 255.200

**Sex Ratio:** M1:F1

**Occurrence:** At least 40 cases have been reported in the literature.

**Risk of Recurrence for Patient's Sib:**
See Part I, *Mendelian Inheritance.*

**Risk of Recurrence for Patient's Child:**
See Part I, *Mendelian Inheritance.* Fertility impaired.

**Age of Detectability:** From birth to adult life; most frequently in the second decade as a result of lack of pubertal development. Antenatal diagnosis has not yet been demonstrated.

**Gene Mapping and Linkage:** CYP17 (cytochrome P450, subfamily XVII (steroid 17-alpha-hydroxylase)) has been provisionally mapped to 10.

**Prevention:** None known. Genetic counseling indicated.

**Treatment:** Therapy with replacement doses of glucocorticoids returns blood pressure and serum potassium level to normal; it corrects inhibition of the renin/angiotensin/aldosterone pathway. Estrogen therapy in females and testosterone treatment in males brings about normal secondary sexual development. Corrective surgery may be necessary in males with ambiguity of the external genitalia.

**Prognosis:** Normal for life span and intelligence, but fertility may be impaired. Malignant hypertension may develop if the condition is not treated.

**Detection of Carrier:** Hypertension and mild elevation of aldosterone partially suppressible by glucocorticoids were reported in the mother of an affected patient in whom the 17-hydroxylase defect seemed limited to the adrenal.

**References:**
Weinstein RL, et al.: Deficient 17-hydroxylation in a corticosterone producing adrenal tumor from an infant with hemihypertrophy and visceromegaly. J Clin Endocrinol 1970; 30:457.
DeLange WE, et al.: Primary amenorrhea with hypertension due to 17-hydroxylase deficiency. Acta Med Scand 1973; 193:565.
Waldhäusl W, et al.: Combined 17α-and 18-hydroxylase deficiency associated with complete male pseudohermaphroditism and hypoaldosteronism. J Clin Endocrinol Metab 1978; 46:236.

Yazaki K, et al.: Hypokalemic myopathy associated with 17-alpha-hydroxylase deficiency: a case report. Neurology 1982; 32:94–97.

Morimoto I, et al.: An autopsy case of 17α-hydroxylase deficiency with malignant hypertension. J Clin Endocrinol Metab 1983; 56:915.

Miller WL, Levine LS: Molecular and clinical advance in congenital adrenal hyperplasia. J Pediat 1987; 111:1–17.

White PC, et al.: Congenital adrenal hyperplasia. New Engl J Med 1987; 316:1519 (first part) and 1580 (second part).

New MI, et al.: The adrenal hyperplasias. In: Scriver CR, et al, eds: The metabolic basis of inherited disease, 6th ed. New York: McGraw-Hill, 1989:1881–1918.

SP004                                                   **Mark A. Sperling**

## STEROID 17,20-DESMOLASE DEFICIENCY      **0904**

**Includes:** Pseudohermaphroditism, male, steroid 17,20-desmolase deficiency

**Excludes:**
Enzymatic defects in testosterone biosynthesis, other
**Steroid 3 beta-hydroxysteroid dehydrogenase deficiency** (0909)
**Steroid 17 alpha-hydroxylase deficiency** (0903)

**Major Diagnostic Criteria:** The condition is to be considered in an infant with ambiguous genitalia, low to absent 17-ketosteroids and with no response to HCG or ACTH stimulation. Other steroids are normal and adrenals and gonads are present. The karyotype is 46,XY. The testicular tissue is unable to convert precursors at the 17,20-desmolase step.

**Clinical Findings:** The hallmark of this syndrome is ambiguous genitalia in genetic males. Although long suspected, the condition has only recently been described. The propositi were male cousins with ambiguous genitalia and XY karyotype. A maternal uncle had been reared as a female; his karyotype was XY, testicles had been surgically removed, and a rudimentary uterus was present as well as one fallopian tube. Excretion of all androgens, including dehydroepiandrosterone and testosterone, was minimal or undetectable, even after administration of human chorionic gonadotropin (HCG) at a dose of G5,000 U/m² for 5 days. In contrast, secretion of glucocorticoids and mineralocorticoids was essentially normal. In vitro, testicular tissue from an affected patient readily converted 17-ketosteroids to testosterone, excluding 17-ketoreductase deficiency, but testosterone could not be formed from other precursors such as pregnenolone, progesterone, or their 17-hydroxylated equivalents. Thus, the defect appears to be at the 17,20-desmolase step. Infertility is to be expected in these individuals. Affected females have normal internal and external genitalia and failure of pubertal development, with infertility due to inability to form estrogen. With a complete defect, genetic males may have female external genitalia.

**Complications:** Infertility.

**Associated Findings:** None known.

**Etiology:** Autosomal recessive inheritance. Until recently, lack of reports of affected females made it difficult to rule out X-linked inheritance.

**Pathogenesis:** The clinical features are explicable on the basis of 17,20-desmolase deficiency affecting the adrenal and gonad.

**MIM No.:** *30915

**CDC No.:** 255.200

**Sex Ratio:** Presumably M1:F1, although most cases reported to date have been male.

**Occurrence:** Undetermined but presumably rare.

**Risk of Recurrence for Patient's Sib:**
See Part I, *Mendelian Inheritance.*

**Risk of Recurrence for Patient's Child:**
See Part I, *Mendelian Inheritance.* Fertility is severely impaired.

**Age of Detectability:** Birth to adult life. Males are likely to present in the perinatal period because of ambiguous genitalia; females

will present because of failure to develop secondary sexual changes.

**Gene Mapping and Linkage:** TDD (testicular 17,20-desmolase deficiency) has been mapped to X.

Other researchers believe that the same polypeptide subserves this condition and **Steroid 17 alpha-hydroxylase deficiency**, and CYP17 (cytochrome P450, steroid 17-alpha-hydroxylase) has been provisionally mapped to 10.

**Prevention:** None known. Genetic counseling indicated.

**Treatment:** In females, treatment with estrogen should permit sexual development but will not restore fertility. In males with severe ambiguity of genitalia, plastic reconstruction of female external genitalia, removal of testes, and rearing in the female role would seem to be indicated, since construction of adequate male genitalia and repair of hypospadias may be technically impossible. When ambiguity is less severe, plastic repair of external genitalia, and treatment with testosterone to bring about pubertal changes at the appropriate time are indicated.

**Prognosis:** Normal life span, but fertility is severely impaired.

**Detection of Carrier:** Unknown.

**References:**
Zachmann M, et al.: Testicular 17,20-desmolase deficiency causing male pseudohermaphroditism. Acta Endocrinol [Suppl] (Copen) 1971; 155:65–80.

Zachmann M, et al.: Steroid 17,20-desmolase deficiency: a new cause of male pseudohermaphroditism. Clin Endocrinol 1972; 1:369–385.

Goebelsmann U: Male pseudohermaphroditism consistent with 17, 20-desmolase deficiency. Gynecol Invest 1976; 7:138–156.

Zachmann M, et al.: Two types of male pseudohermaphroditism due to 17,20-desmolase deficiency. J Clin Endocrinol Metab 1982; 55:487.

Larrea F, et al.: Hypergonadotrophic hypogonadism in an XX female subject due to 17,20 steriod desmolase deficiency. Acta Endrocrinol 1983; 103:400.

Miller WL, Levine LS: Molecular and clinical advance in congenital adrenal hyperplasia. J Pediat 1987; 111:1–17.

New MI, et al.: The adrenal hyperplasias. In: Scriver CR, et al, eds: The metabolic basis of inherited disease, 6th ed. New York: McGraw-Hill, 1989:1881–1918.

SP004                                                   **Mark A. Sperling**

## STEROID 17-KETOSTEROID REDUCTASE DEFICIENCY      **2299**

**Includes:**
Male pseudohermaphroditism due to 17-KSR deficiency
Neutral 17-beta-hydroxysteroid oxidoreductase deficiency
Polycystic ovary disease due to 17-KSR deficiency
Pseudohermaphroditism, male-gynecomastia
Seventeen-beta-hydroxysteroid dehydrogenase deficiency

**Excludes:**
**Androgen insensitivity syndrome, incomplete** (0050)
Enzymatic defects in testosterone biosynthesis, other
**Gonadal dysgenesis, XY type** (0437)
**Steroid 5 alpha-reductase deficiency** (3062)

**Major Diagnostic Criteria:** Elevated androstenedione (δ⁴)A to testosterone ratio in plasma in a 46,XY male with female or ambiguous external genitalia. Similar laboratory criteria apply to a female with clinical features of polycystic ovary disease (PCOD).

**Clinical Findings:** Affected males usually appear to be phenotypic females at birth, although some degree of ambiguity may be present. Testes may or may not be present in the inguinal canal. At puberty, virilization takes place normally. Although the enzyme deficiency leads to deficient testosterone and hence dihydrotestosterone production, Wolffian structures are present, indicating that less testosterone is necessary for this developmental step than for masculinization of the external genitalia. Testicular biopsy material from adults shows absent or markedly decreased spermatogenesis and marked peritubular sclerosis. Serum gonadotropin levels are high. At puberty, males may develop gynecomastia. The diagnosis is uncommonly made prior to puberty unless a sib is affected. Some women with polycystic ovary disease (PCOD) have been found to have the enzyme deficiency in the ovary. Serum testosterone level in females may be proportionately higher because nongonadal peripheral 17-ketosteroid reductase (KSR) enzymatic activity is intact and by inference is a separate enzyme. The sclerocystic ovaries apparently result from deficient ovarian estradiol production (derived normally from testosterone) with a secondary LH increase and cystic changes. Definite diagnosis in either sex would require demonstration of absent or deficient 17-KSR activity in gonadal tissue.

**Complications:** Psychosocial problems may develop in males because of sexual ambiguity and confusion in gender assignment.

**Associated Findings:** Testicular carcinoma has been reported in a male with persistent cryptorchidism.

**Etiology:** Probably autosomal recessive inheritance, given that some families have been consanguineous. Most reports are of affected males, because of the genital ambiguity. Depending on the severity of the enzyme defect, affected females could go undetected.

**Pathogenesis:** The clinical features in both sexes are explicable on the basis of deficient gonadal ($\delta^4$)A to testosterone conversion.

**MIM No.:** *26430

**CDC No.:** 255.200

**Sex Ratio:** Probably M1:F1, if careful sibship studies are made, although ascertainment through genital ambiguity yields far more affected males.

**Occurrence:** Undetermined but presumably rare. Large kinships were reported in an inbred Arab community in Israel. A Venezuelan sibship and about a dozen other widely distributed cases have been reported.

**Risk of Recurrence for Patient's Sib:**
See Part I, *Mendelian Inheritance.*

**Risk of Recurrence for Patient's Child:**
See Part I, *Mendelian Inheritance.* Males are infertile. Because of the rarity of the condition, the risk to fertile females is negligible.

**Age of Detectability:** From birth to adulthood, with most males being diagnosed at puberty. Many females are likely undiagnosed or otherwise categorized as having PCOD.

**Gene Mapping and Linkage:** Unknown.

**Prevention:** None known. Genetic counseling indicated.

**Treatment:** Males reared as females should have gonadectomy and reconstructive genital surgery is necessary. Estrogen therapy will be required for life. Females may require therapy for PCOD. Some males have switched gender roles at puberty with success, analogous to men with **Steroid 5 alpha-reductase deficiency.**

**Prognosis:** Normal life span with impaired fertility. Cryptorchid testes may become malignant.

**Detection of Carrier:** Unknown.

**References:**

Saez JM, et al.: Familial male pseudohermaphroditism with gynecomastia due to testicular 17-ketosteroid reductase defect. I. Study in vivo. J Clin Endocrinol 1971; 32:604–610.

Lanes R, et al.: Sibship with 17-ketosteroid reductase (17-KSR) deficiency and hypothyroidism: lack of linkage of histocompatibility leucocyte antigen and 17-KSR loci. J Clin Endocrinol Metab 1983; 57:190–196.

Balducci R, et al.: Familial male pseudohermaphroditism with gynecomastia due to 17-beta-hydroxysteroid dehydrogenase deficiency: a report of 3 cases. Clin Endocrinol 1985; 23:439–444.

Pang S, et al.: Hirsuitism, polycystic ovarian disease, and ovarian 17-ketosteroid reductase deficiency. New Engl J Med 1987; 316:1295–1301.

Ecksteria B, et al.: The nature of the defect in familial male pseudohermaphroditism in males of Gaza. J Clin Endocrinol Metab 1989; 68:477–485.

**R. Neil Schimke**

## STEROID 18-HYDROXYLASE DEFICIENCY 0905

**Includes:**
Adrenal 18-hydroxylase deficiency
Aldosterone deficiency I
Corticosterone methyl oxidase type I deficiency

**Excludes:**
**Adrenal hypoaldosteronism of infancy, transient isolated** (0023)
**Adrenal hypoplasia, congenital** (0024)
Angiotensin-unresponsive hypoaldosteronism
**Steroid 18-hydroxysteroid dehydrogenase deficiency** (0906)

**Major Diagnostic Criteria:** Infants with this condition have clinical features of hypoaldosteronism with vomiting, dehydration, hyponatremia, and hyperkalemia. There are no abnormalities in the production of glucocorticoids and sex steroids, but there is overproduction of corticosterone and little or no 18-OH corticosterone.

**Clinical Findings:** These patients characteristically present in infancy with features of mineralocorticoid deficiency: dehydration, vomiting, failure to thrive, hyponatremia, and hyperkalemia. The original report concerned three cousins from an inbred family: two girls and one boy, all with normal external genitalia. There was no abnormal hyperpigmentation. Investigation revealed normal urinary excretion of 17-hydroxycorticosteroids and 17-ketosteroids, with a normal response to stimulation by ACTH. Aldosterone excretion was undetectable, and there was no response to ACTH or salt deprivation. However, urinary excretion of corticosterone and its metabolites was markedly increased, whereas only small amounts of 11-deoxycorticosterone (DOC) were detected, even after ACTH stimulation, and 18-hydroxycorticosterone or its metabolites were absent. The defect therefore involves the 18-hydroxylation step from corticosterone to 18-OH corticosterone; the second to last step in aldosterone biosynthesis. The adrenal gland of one affected patient showed a poorly developed zona glomerulosa and a hypertrophied juxtaglomerular apparatus. Despite the severe reduction in aldosterone synthesis, patients on a normal salt intake can maintain marginal sodium balance with serum sodiums of 120–130 mEq/liter; salt deprivation is poorly tolerated. There is an excellent response to supplementation with salt and a mineralocorticoid. As with other defects involving aldosterone secretion, there is an amelioration of the salt-losing tendency with increasing age, so that electrolyte balance can be maintained by a high salt intake without addition of mineralocorticoid, although the basic biochemical defect persists. Milder forms of this entity also exist, since hypoaldosteronism and increased excretion of corticosterone consistent with an 18-hydroxylase defect has been reported in young adults. The possibility that transient hypoaldosteronism of infancy represents a maturational delay in 18-hydroxylation has been separately discussed (see **Adrenal hypoaldosteronism of infancy, transient isolated.**)

**Complications:** In newborns, death may result from failure to replace fluids, salt, and mineralocorticoid.

**Associated Findings:** None known.

**Etiology:** Autosomal recessively inheritance.

**Pathogenesis:** The final two steps in aldosterone biosynthesis involve the hydroxylation of carbon 18 of corticosterone followed by oxidation (dehydrogenation) of the same carbon to produce aldosterone. Since cortisol and sex steroid synthesis is unaffected, there is no elevation in ACTH or hyperpigmentation, and the external genitalia are normal. Although large quantities of corticosterone and some DOC are produced, they are weak mineralocorticoids relative to aldosterone. Hyponatremia, hyperkalemia, and volume depletion ensue, with an attempt to stimulate aldosterone via the renin-angiotensin system, thus accounting for renal juxtaglomerular hyperplasia. The reduced or absent 18-hydroxycorticosterone, with overproduction of corticosterone, confirms the locus of the defect. More recently, the traditional concepts concerning the final two steps of aldosterone biosynthesis from corticosterone have been revised. Although a two-step, mixed oxidation-reduction reaction is likely, the actual intermediate may not be 18-hydroxycorticosterone itself. Thus, the suggested terminology for the defects in the two biosynthetic steps for aldosterone are corticosterone methyloxidase defects types 1 and 2. When corticosterone only is elevated, (and not suppressible by exogenous glucocorticoid to distinguish it from 17-hydroxylase deficiency) the defect is type 1. When the defect is characterized by overproduction of both corticosterone and 18-hydroxycorticosterone, the defect is type 2.

**MIM No.:** *20340

**CDC No.:** 255.200

**Sex Ratio:** M1:F1

**Occurrence:** At least six cases reported; three from common ancestry.

**Risk of Recurrence for Patient's Sib:**
See Part I, *Mendelian Inheritance.*

**Risk of Recurrence for Patient's Child:**
See Part I, *Mendelian Inheritance.*

**Age of Detectability:** Usually in the newborn period or in the first year of life, but milder defects may be detected at any age.

**Gene Mapping and Linkage:** Unknown.

**Prevention:** None known. Genetic counseling indicated.

**Treatment:** Treatment with salt supplementation and a mineralocorticoid, such as DOC, is necessary in the first few years of life. Later, patients appear able to maintain normal electrolyte balance by adjusting their sodium intake without mineralocorticoid supplements.

**Prognosis:** Excellent for life span, intelligence, and reproduction if electrolyte disturbance is recognized and appropriately treated.

**Detection of Carrier:** Unknown.

**Special Considerations:** Hypoaldosteronism, with apparent selective inhibition of the 18-hydroxylation step has been reported after prolonged administration of heparin. In adults over 40 years of age with hypoaldosteronism and biochemical findings compatible with defective aldosterone synthesis, cardiovascular complications of hypokalemia have been a prominent presenting feature.

**References:**
Rösler A, et al.: The nature of the defect in a salt-wasting disorder in Jews of Iran. J Clin Endocrinol Metab 1977; 44:279.
Veldhuis JD: Inborn error in the terminal step of aldosterone biosynthesis: corticosterone methyl oxidase type II deficiency in a North American pedigree. New Engl J Med 1980; 303:117.
Rosler A: The natural history of salt-wasting disorders of adrenal and renal origin. J Clin Endocrinol Metab 1984; 59:689.
Miller WL, Levine LS: Molecular and clinical advance in congenital adrenal hyperplasia. J Pediat 1987; 111:1–17.
White PC, et al.: Congenital adrenal hyperplasia. New Engl J Med 1987; 316:1519 (first part) and 1580 (second part).
New MI, et al.: The adrenal hyperplasias. In: Scriver CR, et al, eds: The metabolic basis of inherited disease, 6th ed. New York: McGraw-Hill, 1989:1881–1918.

SP004                                   **Mark A. Sperling**

## STEROID 18-HYDROXYSTEROID DEHYDROGENASE DEFICIENCY                               0906

**Includes:**
Adrenal 18-hydroxysteroid dehydrogenase deficiency
Aldosterone deficiency II
Corticosterone methyl oxidase type II deficiency

**Excludes:**
**Adrenal hypoaldosteronism of infancy, transient isolated** (0023)
**Adrenal hypoplasia, congenital** (0024)
Angiotensin-unresponsive hypoaldosteronism
**Steroid 18-hydroxylase deficiency** (0905)

**Major Diagnostic Criteria:** Varying degrees of severity of vomiting and dehydration accompanied by salt loss and hyperkalemia are the early manifestations of this syndrome. The genitalia are normal. The condition is due to hypoaldosteronism, with elevated

production of 18-hydroxycorticosterone and normal cortisol and sex steroid levels.

**Clinical Findings:** This defect is identical in its chemical findings to that caused by **Steroid 18-hydroxylase deficiency**. Growth failure, with hyponatremia and hyperkalemia that ameliorate with increasing age, and hypoaldosteronism, are its hallmarks. The genitalia are normal and the response to salt and mineralocorticoid supplementation is excellent.

**Complications:** The degree of salt loss and hyperkalemia will determine the extent of early complications.

**Associated Findings:** None known.

**Etiology:** Autosomal recessive inheritance.

**Pathogenesis:** Identical to that described for **Steroid 18-hydroxylase deficiency** except that the defect involves the final step in aldosterone biosynthesis. Biochemically, the defect involves the final oxidation (dehydrogenation) of 18-hydroxycorticosterone to aldosterone. Thus, the steroid patterns differ only in that production of 18-hydroxycorticosterone is increased, but that of aldosterone remains low, despite stimuli such as ACTH. As indicated for the 18-hydroxylase deficiency syndrome, the term methyloxidase defect type II has been suggested to describe this condition, which is characterized by overproduction of both corticosterone and 18-hydroxycorticosterone.

**MIM No.:** *20341

**CDC No.:** 255.200

**Sex Ratio:** M1:F1

**Occurrence:** Over 25 cases document. Most frequent in Iranian Jews.

**Risk of Recurrence for Patient's Sib:**
See Part I, *Mendelian Inheritance.*

**Risk of Recurrence for Patient's Child:**
See Part I, *Mendelian Inheritance.*

**Age of Detectability:** Usually in the newborn period or in the first year of life, but milder defects may be detected at any age.

**Gene Mapping and Linkage:** Unknown.

**Prevention:** None known. Genetic counseling indicated.

**Treatment:** Treatment with salt supplementation and a mineralocorticoid, such as DOC, is necessary in the first few years of life. Later, patients appear able to maintain normal electrolyte balance by adjusting their sodium intake without mineralocorticoid supplements.

**Prognosis:** Excellent, if treatment with mineralocorticoid and salt is instituted.

**Detection of Carrier:** Unknown.

**References:**
Rösler A, et al.: The nature of the defect in a salt-wasting disorder in Jews of Iran. J Clin Endocrinol Metab 1977; 44:279–291.
Veldhuis JD, et al.: Inborn error in the terminal step of aldosterone biosynthesis: corticosterone methyloxidase type II deficiency in a North American pedigree. New Engl J Med 1980; 303:117–121.
Rösler A: The natural history of salt-wasting disorders of adrenal and renal origin. J Clin Endocrinol Metab 1984; 59:689.
Miller WL, Levine LS: Molecular and clinical advance in congenital adrenal hyperplasia. J Pediat 1987; 111:1–17.
White PC, et al.: Congenital adrenal hyperplasia. New Engl J Med 1987; 316:1519 (first part) and 1580 (second part).
New MI, et al.: The adrenal hyperplasias. In: Scriver CR, et al, eds: The metabolic basis of inherited disease, 6th ed. New York: McGraw-Hill, 1989:1881–1918.

SP004                                   **Mark A. Sperling**

**Steroid 18-oxidation, delayed biochemical maturation of**
*See ADRENAL HYPOALDOSTERONISM OF INFANCY, TRANSIENT ISOLATED*

## STEROID 20–22 DESMOLASE DEFICIENCY    0907

**Includes:**

    Adrenal hyperplasia I

    Lipoid adrenal hyperplasia with male
        pseudohermaphroditism

    P450 side-chain cleavage enzyme, deficiency of

**Excludes:** Adrenal hyperplasia, other forms

**Major Diagnostic Criteria:** Vomiting, hyperkalemia, dehydration, and shock in a neonate with low serum sodium and chloride are the earliest manifestations. Males may have ambiguous genitalia. There is virtual absence of all steroids in their urine or blood. Definitive diagnosis is not feasible without performing stimulation tests with ACTH and HCG; both should be abnormal, without a rise in pregnenolone. A presumptive diagnosis can be made if the adrenals show the characteristic histology.

**Clinical Findings:** This defect affects the critical initial reaction in the conversion of cholesterol to pregnenolone, a step involving cleavage of the cholesterol side chain from carbon 20 to carbon 22. The entire cleavage process, although termed a desmolase, may represent a series of enzyme reactions shared by the adrenal and gonad and mediated by a P450 enzyme catalyzing side-chain cleavage (P450 SCC). Because of the early site in the assembly of all steroids, salt and water loss, and glucocorticoid insufficiency are universal findings. The external genitalia are normal in females, but males may have ambiguity, supporting the contention that the gonad is affected and thus precludes masculinization during fetal life. Laboratory investigation reveals virtual absence of urinary steroids, including pregnenolone, and low secretion rates of cortisol and aldosterone. Extended survival is possible, but death is frequent, despite seemingly adequate replacement with glucocorticoids, mineralocorticoids, and salt. At necropsy, the adrenals are markedly enlarged, and the cells are distended with cholesterol. Consanguinity has been frequent in the parents of affected individuals.

**Complications:** Death is frequent, even with adequate therapy.

**Associated Findings:** None known.

**Etiology:** Autosomal recessive inheritance.

**Pathogenesis:** The clinical features are explicable from the site and severity of the enzyme block affecting the adrenal and gonad, and the deficiency of glucocorticoids, mineralocorticoids, and sex steroids. The specific process, known as cholesterol side-chain

cleavage, is catalyzed by a specific form of cytochrome P-450; P450 (CSS), which is localized to the inner mitochondrial membrane.

**MIM No.:** *20171

**CDC No.:** 255.200

**Sex Ratio:** M1:F1

**Occurrence:** About 35 cases, with about a dozen surviving, have been documented in the literature.

**Risk of Recurrence for Patient's Sib:**
    See Part I, *Mendelian Inheritance.*

**Risk of Recurrence for Patient's Child:**
    See Part I, *Mendelian Inheritance.* Surviving affected individuals will probably be infertile.

**Age of Detectability:** Usually in the newborn period as a result of salt loss or ambiguous genitalia. Antenatal diagnosis has not been demonstrated.

**Gene Mapping and Linkage:** CYP11A (cytochrome P450, subfamily XIA) has been mapped to 15.

**Prevention:** None known. Genetic counseling indicated.

**Treatment:** Early recognition and replacement therapy with glucocorticoid, mineralocorticoid, and salt are essential for survival. Replacement therapy with estrogen or testosterone will be required to achieve secondary sexual characteristics in those reaching the age of puberty. In genetic males with severe ambiguity of the external genitalia, closely resembling those of a female, plastic reconstruction to achieve male characteristics is, at best, difficult. Consideration should therefore be given to raising the individual as a female with appropriate surgical correction of the external genitalia.

**Prognosis:** Prognosis has been poor in severely affected individuals. Infertility is likely in those surviving to adult life.

**Detection of Carrier:** Unknown.

**Special Considerations:** Aminoglutethimide, a toxic drug used rarely to inhibit steroidogenesis in adrenal carcinoma, acts by inhibiting the desmolase system and experimentally can simulate lipoid adrenal hyperplasia.

**Support Groups:** MN; Wrenshall (c/o Diana Johnson, 10 Co Hwy 4); Congenital Adrenal Hyperplasia Group

**References:**

Camacho AM, et al.: Congenital adrenal hyperplasia due to a deficiency of one of the enzymes involved in biosynthesis of pregnenolone. J Clin Endocrinol 1968; 28:153–161.

Moragas A, Ballabriga A: Congenital lipoid hyperplasia of the fetal adrenal gland. Helv Paediatr Acta 1969; 24:226.

Kirkland RT: Congenital lipoid adrenal hyperplasia in an eight-year-old phenotypic female. J Clin Endocrinol Metab 1973; 36:488–496.

Miller WL, Levine LS: Molecular and clinical advance in congenital adrenal hyperplasia. J Pediat 1987; 111:1–17.

Nebert DW, et al.: The P450 gene superfamily: recommended nomenclature. DNA 1987; 6:1–11.

White PC, et al.: Congenital adrenal hyperplasia. New Engl J Med 1987; 316:1519 (first part) and 1580 (second part).

New MI, et al.: The adrenal hyperplasias. In: Scriver CR, et al, eds: The metabolic basis of inherited disease, 6th ed. New York: McGraw-Hill, 1989:1881–1918.

SP004                                             **Mark A. Sperling**

## STEROID 21-HYDROXYLASE DEFICIENCY    0908

**Includes:**

    Adrenal hyperplasia III

    Adrenal hyperplasia-1, congenital virilizing

    Female pseudohermaphroditism

    Macrogenitosomia praecox

    Male pseudo-precocious puberty

**Excludes:** Adrenal steroidogenesis, other enzyme deficiencies in

**Major Diagnostic Criteria:** Elevated 17-ketosteroids (17-KS) and pregnanetriol excretion or markedly elevated plasma 17α-hydroxyprogesterone (50–450 times normal) and ACTH levels in patients

**0907-21392:** Simplified scheme of steroidogenesis in the adrenal gland.

with progressive virilization from birth. Abnormal steroid secretion must be suppressed following glucocorticoid administration.

Affected female infants show a variable degree of masculinization; males appear normal, but the external genitalia may be hyperpigmented in both sexes. Vomiting and dehydration may occur in the salt-losing variety.

**Clinical Findings:** This is the most common variant of congenital adrenal hyperplasia (CAH) resulting from a defect in the enzyme that catalyzes the conversion of progesterone or 17α-hydroxy progesterone to deoxycorticosterone or 11-deoxycortisol, respectively; a step requiring hydroxylation of the carbon at the 21 position of the steroid nucleus. The androgen pathway is not blocked, so the fetus is exposed to excessive androgens from about the third month of intrauterine life. Consequently, newborn females show variable degrees of masculinization of the external genitalia, ranging from mild clitoral hypertrophy to complete labioscrotal fusion simulating a scrotum, male phallus with urethra opening at its tip, absence of palpable gonads within the "scrotal sac," and presence of a prostate. However, ovaries and a uterus are present and the chromosomal sex is female. Excessive skin pigmentation may be present around the genitalia or nipples, reflecting increased ACTH (MSH). In newborn males no abnormality is apparent, although some may have phallic enlargement. However, progressive virilization occurs in both sexes, resulting in rapid initial growth; accelerated bone age development, with premature fusion of epiphyses and final short stature, progressive clitoral or penile enlargement, early development of pubic and axillary hair, acne, hirsutism, voice changes, male habitus, and male gender identification. Males have been referred to as an infant "Hercules." Untreated females fail to undergo pubertal changes due to suppression of gonadotropins by androgen excess. In males, the same mechanism prevents testicular enlargement, allowing differentiation from true precocious puberty secondary to ectopic or inappropriate pituitary gonadotropin secretion. However, rarely, there may be adrenal rests within the testes, subject to ACTH stimulation, which may result in symmetric or nodular testicular enlargement and suggest precocious puberty or testicular neoplasia. In females with ambiguous genitalia the diagnosis is usually established in infancy or early childhood; occasional cases have been identified in the second decade and as late as the sixth decade of life. Complete external virilization of newborn females may delay diagnosis and lead to false gender assignment with consequent psychologic sequelae.

Patients with partial or mild defects in 21-hydroxylase deficiency have normal serum electrolytes and may have normal levels of cortisol and aldosterone production, the latter rising with a low salt diet. The serum cortisol response to ACTH may be minimal, indicating existing maximal stimulation by endogenous ACTH. Adrenal capacity is limited, however, since many of these patients develop salt loss during stress or during diagnostic sodium restriction, with hyponatremia, hyperkalemia, vomiting, severe dehydration, and vascular collapse.

Complete or severe 21-hydroxylase deficiency manifests itself early in the neonatal period with vomiting, renal salt loss, hyponatremia, hyperkalemia, and dehydration. A misdiagnosis of pyloric stenosis may be made in newborn males; death of an older sib in infancy, particulary during stress, may be recorded.

There is no direct correlation between the degree of virilization or external genital ambiguity and completeness of the 21-hydroxylase defect. However, plasma and urinary cortisol and its metabolites are decreased, as is aldosterone; salt restriction is poorly tolerated and does not produce further increments in aldosterone secretion.

The clinical division of patients into "salt-losers" and "non-salt losers" is relatively arbitrary, and it is highly likely that the mild and severe forms represent a spectrum of a single enzyme deficiency, although debate on this issue continues. All affected subjects display abnormalities in sodium balance, ranging from borderline depletion, detectable by elevated levels of plasma renin activity in the simple virilizers, to overt salt-loss and hypovolemia in the clinical salt-losers. There is a high degree of correlation among the degree of salt-loss, plasma renin activity and ACTH levels, suggesting a relationship between the renin-angiotensin system and the pituitary-adrenal axis. These findings have important clinical implications because they suggest that both salt-losers and simple virilizers would benefit from treatment with mineralocorticoids for optimal hormonal control of the disease, including suppression of excessive androgen production with lower than conventionally recommended doses of glucocorticoids. Independent studies confirm these concepts. It is therefore strongly recommended that all patients with the 21-hydroxylase deficiency receive some mineralocorticoid supplement in addition to glucocorticoid therapy.

Irrespective of clinical type, all affected patients have elevated urinary excretion of 17-ketosteroids and pregnanetriol, the excretory product of 17α-hydroxyprogesterone. Plasma levels of these substances as well as testosterone, derived from peripheral conversion of androgen precursors, are elevated. Urinary 17-hydroxycorticosteroids or plasma cortisol may be low or normal, depending on the severity of the block.

**Complications:** Lack of cortisol and aldosterone may result in hypoglycemia, and severe electrolyte disturbances with dehydration and shock, particularly during stress. Ambiguity of genitalia may result in false gender assignment for genetic females. Progressive virilization, early epiphyseal closure with short stature, preclusion of normal pubertal changes, and infertility are direct sequelae of the untreated condition, or of poor patient compliance. Adenomatous changes within the adrenal or adrenal rest tissue in distant sites, such as testes, may also occur with inadequate treatment.

**Associated Findings:** Renal anomalies have been associated with this syndrome.

**Etiology:** Autosomal recessive inheritance.

**Pathogenesis:** The pathogenesis of all the features is explicable from the site and severity of the enzyme block, deficiency of cortisol or aldosterone, and oversecretion of androgens. In about 95% of cases, 21-hydroxylation is impaired in the zona fasciculata of the adrenal cortex so that 17-hydroxyprogesterone is not converted to 11-deoxycortisol. ACTH levels increase, resulting in excess cortisol precursors which are shunted into excessive production of androgens, resulting in virilization.

**MIM No.:** *20191

**CDC No.:** 255.200

**Sex Ratio:** M1:F1

**Occurrence:** Varies with geographic locale: 1:500 in certain Eskimos, 1:5,000 in Switzerland, 1:15,000 in the United States Caucasians.

**Risk of Recurrence for Patient's Sib:**
See Part I, *Mendelian Inheritance.*

**Risk of Recurrence for Patient's Child:**
See Part I, *Mendelian Inheritance.*

**Age of Detectability:** Molecular probes can now be used to establish the diagnosis in the fetus. Successful antenatal detection and neonatal screening have been reported. Amniotic fluid screening shows elevated 17-alpha-hydroxyprogesterone, delta-4-androstenedione, and pregnanetriol levels; maternal serum screening after 34 weeks shows increased concentration of 17-

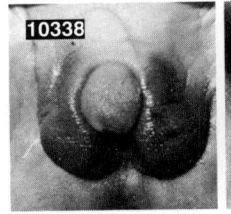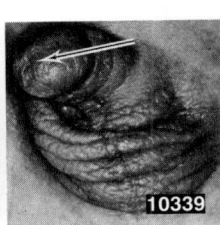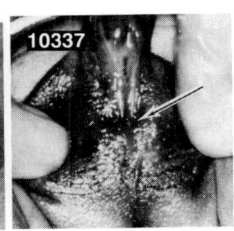

**0908-10337–39:** Complete and incomplete virilization of the external genitalia in genetic females.

alpha-hydroxyprogesterone; a genetic linkage with HLA-B antigens is determined on cultured amniotic fluid cells.

**Gene Mapping and Linkage:** CYP21 (cytochrome P450, subfamily XXI) has been mapped to 6p21.3.

**Prevention:** Diagnosis of an affected female early in gestation by molecular probes or HLA typing permits attempts at preventing virilization by high-dose glucocorticoid therapy to the mother.

**Treatment:** Replacement therapy with cortisol arrests the progressive virilization. A mineralocorticoid (DOC or 9α-fluorohydrocortisone), with additional salt intake, may be necessary in the salt-losing form; a mineralocorticoid should also be provided for non-salt-losers. Supplemental cortisol is necessary during acute stress. Antenatal diagnosis, with cortisol injections into the amniotic fluid or fetus, may minimize virilization.

Initial plastic surgical repair of ambiguous genitalia is achieved between the first to third years of life in order to permit appropriate gender identification and sex rearing. Definitive plastic repair can be achieved after puberty. Psychologic counseling may be required for parents and in late-diagnosed cases with ambiguous genitalia.

It is generally agreed that if diagnosis is missed for the first 3–4 years, a completely virilized female with penile urethra and apparent cryptorchidism should be perpetuated in male rearing and identification.

**Prognosis:** Normal for life span, reproduction, and intelligence, when diagnosed early and appropriately treated.

**Detection of Carrier:** Urinary pregnanetriol excretion after ACTH infusion has been reported to be elevated in the parents of affected children when compared with controls. This test has not been commonly employed. The close linkage between the gene for 21-hydroxylase deficiency and the HLA-B locus provides a method for detection of carriers or for prenatal diagnosis once an index case is established. cDNA probes can be used to detect carriers.

**Support Group:** MN; Wrenshall (c/o Diana Johnson, 10 Co Hwy 4); Congenital Adrenal Hyperplasia Group.

**References:**

Migeon CJ, et al.: The attenuated form of congenital adrenal hyperplasia as an allelic form of 21-hydroxylase deficiency. J Clin Endocrinol Metab 1980; 51:647–649.

Kohn B, et al.: Late-onset steroid-21-hydroxylase deficiency: a variant of classical congenital adrenal hyperplasia. J Clin Endocrinol Metab 1982; 55:817–827.

Hughes IA, et al.: Prenatal diagnosis of congenital adrenal hyperplasia. J Med Genet 1987; 24:344–347.

Miller WL, Levine LS: Molecular and clinical advance in congenital adrenal hyperplasia. J Pediat 1987; 111:1–17.

Mulaikal R, et al.: Fertility rates in female patients with congenital adrenal hyperplasia due to 21-hydroxylase deficiency. New Engl J Med 1987; 316:178–182.

White PC, et al.: Congenital adrenal hyperplasia. New Engl J Med 1987; 316:1519–1524 (first part) and 1580–1586 (second part).

Killeen AA, et al.: Diagnosis of classical steroid 21-hydroxylase deficiency using an HLA-B locus-specific DNA-probe. Am J Med Genet 1988; 29:703–712.

Miller WL: Gene conversions, deletions and polymorphisims in congenital adrenal hyperplasia. Am J Hum Genet 1988; 42:4–7.

New MI, et al.: The adrenal hyperplasias. In: Scriver CR, et al, eds: The metabolic basis of inherited disease, 6th ed. New York: McGraw-Hill, 1989:1881–1918.

Pang S, et al.: Prenatal treatment of congenital adrenal hyperplasia due to 21-hydroxylase deficiency. New Engl J Med 1990; 322:111–115.

SP004                                            **Mark A. Sperling**

**Steroid sulfatase deficiency disease (SSDD)**
*See ICHTHYOSIS, X-LINKED WITH STEROID SULFATASE DEFICIENCY*

## STEROID, BINDING GLOBULIN ABNORMALITIES 0222

**Includes:**
    CBG-transcortin abnormalities
    Corticosteroid-binding globulin abnormalities
    Corticosteroid-binding globulin, decreased
    Corticosteroid-binding globulin, increased
    Transcortin deficiency

**Excludes:**
    Disease-induced changes in CBG
    Drug-induced changes in CBG

**Major Diagnostic Criteria:** No known signs or symptoms accompany this biochemical variant. Low or elevated total plasma cortisol with a normal amount of free cortisol are found in plasma and urine in the absence of disease or drugs affecting CBG. Measurement of free cortisol in urine, or determination of binding capacity of plasma for radioactively labeled cortisol akin to the T3 resin uptake test may be required.

**Clinical Findings:** Congenital abnormalities in cortisol-binding globulin (CBG) do not reflect a disease state and are not associated with any abnormality in adrenal function or symptomatology. They are detected as laboratory findings in individuals who have low or high concentrations of cortisol in plasma, but are otherwise normal. However, the laboratory findings may suggest hyper- or hypofunction of the adrenal and spur unnecessary investigations.

**Complications:** Unknown.

**Associated Findings:** None known.

**Etiology:** CBG deficiency is familial and transmitted by autosomal dominant or X-linked recessive inheritance. CBG excess is also familial but the mode of transmission is uncertain. The most common cause of CBG excess is pregnancy and estrogen-containing medication.

**Pathogenesis:** Cortisol-binding globulin (CBG-transcortin) is a plasma glycoprotein with high affinity for cortisol as well as progesterone, deoxycorticosterone, corticosterone and some synthetic glucocorticoids. About 75% of plasma cortisol is reversibly bound by CBG, 15% is bound to albumin, and about 10% remains free and biologically active, being constantly replenished from CBG. Decreased CBG is associated with a low total cortisol, and increased CBG with a high total cortisol; in both circumstances, free cortisol remains normal, urinary excretion of free cortisol is also normal, and cortisol production and the response to ACTH remain normal. In liver disease and nephrotic syndrome, CBG, and consequently total cortisol, are low; in pregnancy and with estrogen therapy CBG and total cortisol are high.

**MIM No.:** 12250

**Sex Ratio:** M1:F<1 in CBG deficiency; M1:F1 in CBG excess

**Occurrence:** About a dozen familial cases documented; 8 in three generations of one family.

**Risk of Recurrence for Patient's Sib:**
    See Part I, *Mendelian Inheritance*. For CBG excess, undetermined.

**Risk of Recurrence for Patient's Child:**
    See Part I, *Mendelian Inheritance*. For CBG excess, undetermined.

**Age of Detectability:** At birth.

**Gene Mapping and Linkage:** Unknown.

**Prevention:** None known. Genetic counseling indicated.

**Treatment:** Not required.

**Prognosis:** Excellent.

**Detection of Carrier:** Unknown.

**References:**

Doe RP, et al.: Familial decrease in corticosteroid-binding globulin. Metabolism 1965; 14:940.

Lohrenz FN, et al.: Adrenal function and serum protein concentrations in a kindred with decreased corticosteroid-binding globulin (CBG) concentration. J Clin Endocrinol Metab 1967; 27:966.

Lohrenz FN, et al.: Idiopathic or genetic elevation of corticosteroid-binding globulin? J Clin Endocrinol Metab 1968; 28:1073–1075.

Hadjian AJ, et al.: Cortisol binding to proteins in plasma in the human neonate and infant. Pediatr Res 1975; 9:40.

Derncor P, et al.: Unexplained high transcortin levels in patients with various hematological disorders and their relatives: a connection between these high transcortin levels and HLA antigen B 12. J Clin Endocrinol Metab 1980; 50:421.

Dunn JF, et al.: Transport of steroid hormones: binding of 21 endogenous steroids to both testosterone-binding globulin and corticosteroid-binding globulin in human plasma. J Clin Endocrinol Metab 1981; 53:58.

Pugeat MM: Transport of steroid hormones: interaction of 70 drugs with testosterone-binding globulin and corticosteroid-binding globulin in human plasma. J Clin Endocrinol Metab 1981; 53:69.

SP004                                           **Mark A. Sperling**

**Stevenson syndrome**
*See DIGITO-PALATAL SYNDROME, STEVENSON TYPE*
**Stickler syndrome**
*See ARTHRO-OPHTHALMOPATHY, HEREDITARY, PROGRESSIVE, STICKLER TYPE*
**Stiff man syndrome (obsolete; pejorative)**
*See HALLERVORDEN-SPATZ DISEASE*

---

## STIFF SKIN SYNDROME                          2629

**Includes:**
  Fascial dystrophy
  Skin, stiff skin syndrome

**Excludes:**
  **Arthrogryposis**
  **Dwarfism-stiff joints** (2033)
  **Hallervorden-Spatz disease** (2526)
  **Kuskokwin syndrome** (0560)
  Lipomatosis, systemic
  **Neck/face, lipomatosis** (0601)
  Sclerema
  **Scleroderma, familial progressive** (2154)
  **Skin, parana hard skin syndrome** (3051)

**Major Diagnostic Criteria:** Thick, indurated skin over most of the body associated with firm muscles, joint stiffness, and contractures present from birth or early childhood.

**Clinical Findings:** Features are limited to the soft tissues and are usually present from birth. Skin has rock hard consistency without evidence of atrophy or vascular change. Central areas, buttocks, shoulders, and proximal limbs are more severely affected. Underlying muscles appear firm but have normal strength. Joint stiffness and contractures may occur. Viscera are not affected.

**Complications:** Limitation at joints, impaired ventilation secondary to chest wall involvement.

**Associated Findings:** None known.

**Etiology:** Autosomal dominant inheritance.

**Pathogenesis:** Basic metabolic defect. The inital report of increased dermal glycosaminoglycan deposition has not been confirmed. Abnormal production and extracellular organization of collagen in the fascia has been identified in one patient.

**MIM No.:** *18490

**POS No.:** 3469

**Sex Ratio:** M1:F1

**Occurrence:** About a dozen families have been reported.

**Risk of Recurrence for Patient's Sib:**
  See Part I, *Mendelian Inheritance.*

**Risk of Recurrence for Patient's Child:**
  See Part I, *Mendelian Inheritance.*

**Age of Detectability:** At birth or during the early years.

**Gene Mapping and Linkage:** Unknown.

**Prevention:** None known. Genetic counseling indicated.

**Treatment:** Unknown.

**Prognosis:** Undetermined. The degree of incapacitation appears minimal in the reported cases.

**Detection of Carrier:** Unknown.

**References:**
Esterly ND, McKusick VA: Stiff skin syndrome. Pediatrics 1971; 47:360–369.

Singer HS, et al.: The stiff skin syndrome: new genetic and biochemical investigations BD:OAS XIII(3B). New York: March of Dimes Birth Defects Foundation, 1977:254–255.

Jablonska S, et al.: Congenital fascial dystrophy: a noninflammatory disease of fascia: the stiff skin syndrome. Pediatr Derm 1984; 2:87–97.

ST021                                           **Roger E. Stevenson**

**Stiff baby syndrome, hereditary**
*See HYPEREKPLEXIA*
**Stiff man syndrome, congenital**
*See HYPEREKPLEXIA*
**Stilbestrol-R, fetal effects**
*See FETAL DIETHYLSTILBESTROL (DES) EFFECTS*
**Stilling-Turk-Duane syndrome**
*See EYE, DUANE RETRACTION SYNDROME*
**Stimulus-evoked epilepsy**
*See EPILEPSY, REFLEX*
**Stippled epiphyses**
*See CHONDRODYSPLASIA PUNCTATA, X-LINKED DOMINANT TYPE*
**Stomach cancer**
*See CANCER, GASTRIC FAMILIAL*

---

## STOMACH, DIVERTICULUM                         0911

**Includes:** Gastric diverticulum, congenital

**Excludes:**
  Gastric cysts
  **Stomach, duplication** (0912)

**Major Diagnostic Criteria:** There are no consistent symptoms or signs, and diagnosis is made by X-ray findings using contrast material.

**Clinical Findings:** No characteristic clinical findings are present. Usually X-ray diagnosis shows an outpouching from juxtacardiac posterior gastric wall involving all layers of the gastric wall. occurs. This may occur near the pylorus in the presence of a high small bowel obstruction, probably as an acquired lesion.

**Complications:** Severe vomiting. In one instance, intussusception of the diverticulum resulted in gangrenous perforation and peritonitis.

**Associated Findings:** None known.

**Etiology:** Unknown.

**Pathogenesis:** May originate as a duplication, or result from pressure effects of pyloric or duodenal obstruction.

**CDC No.:** 750.740

**Sex Ratio:** Presumably M1:F1.

**Occurrence:** Undetermined. Usually asymptomatic and discovered by chance X-ray, at gastroscopy or operation, or incidentally at necropsy.

**Risk of Recurrence for Patient's Sib:** Unknown.

**Risk of Recurrence for Patient's Child:** Unknown.

**Age of Detectability:** At any age.

**Gene Mapping and Linkage:** Unknown.

**Prevention:** None known.

**Treatment:** Surgical excision rarely indicated.

**Prognosis:** Unknown.

**Detection of Carrier:** Unknown.

**References:**
Ogur GL, Kolarsick AJ: Gastric diverticula in infancy. J Pediatr 1951; 39:723.

Burke MB: Gastric diverticula in childhood: a report of two cases and a review of the literature. J Singapore Paediatr Soc 1965; 7:101–106.

SI004     **William K. Sieber**

## STOMACH, DUPLICATION     0912

**Includes:**
     Cardioduodenal duct
     Gastric enterocystoma
     Stomach, reduplication of

**Excludes:**
     Dorsal enteric remnants
     Ectopic pancreas involving gastric wall
     **Esophagus, duplication** (0368)
     **Meckel diverticulum** (0633)
     Mediastinal gastric cysts
     **Stomach, diverticulum** (0911)

**Major Diagnostic Criteria:** Palpable abdominal mass with X-ray evidence of origin from the gastric wall. Usually gastric origin can be established only at operation. Sonography and technetium scan may identify gastric lining of cystic mass.

**Clinical Findings:** May present as an asymptomatic upper abdominal mass, a mass with vomiting or GI bleeding; may simulate pyloric stenosis (with symptoms beginning at birth and an easily palpable pyloric "tumor"); or may present as diffuse peritonitis due to rupture of the duplication. An abdominal mass is almost always palpable. X-ray studies with contrast material sometimes clarify the diagnosis but usually demonstrate only pressure effects along the greater curvature and obstruction. These findings, with depression of the splenic flexure, are suggestive of gastric duplication.

**Complications:** Pyloric obstruction, rupture of the duplication and resulting generalized peritonitis, sepsis, and autodigestion with erosion into surrounding viscera may cause gastrocolic fistula and other bizarre fistulizations.

**Associated Findings:** Carcinomatous degeneration of the duplication, usually solitary; occasionally there are other duplications of alimentary tract.

**Etiology:** Possibly error of recanalization.

**Pathogenesis:** Embryonic, possible persistence of solid stage, with failure of coalescence of the vacuoles that form lumen.

**CDC No.:** 750.750

**Sex Ratio:** M1:F8 (observed on one series).

**Occurrence:** About 65 cases have been reported in the literature.

**Risk of Recurrence for Patient's Sib:** Unknown.

**Risk of Recurrence for Patient's Child:** Unknown.

**Age of Detectability:** Often during the neonatal period, by physical examination, but small cysts may be detected only if they become symptomatic in later life.

**Gene Mapping and Linkage:** Unknown.

**Prevention:** None known. Genetic counseling indicated.

**Treatment:** Laparotomy and surgical excision of the duplication and the associated site of attachment to the normal gastric wall may require simple excision, or subtotal or even total gastrectomy. Internal drainage by anastomosis of the cyst to the true gastric lumen has relieved symptoms.

**Prognosis:** Excellent when surgically removed. Carcinoma has been reported in long-standing duplications.

**Detection of Carrier:** Unknown.

**References:**
Kremer RM, et al.: Duplication of the stomach. J Pediatr Surg 1970; 5:360–364.
Pruksapang C, et al.: Gastric duplications. J Pediatr Surg 1979; 14:83–85.
Spence RK, et al.: Coexistent gastric duplication and accessory pan-

creas: clinical manifestations, embryogenesis, and treatment. J Pediatr Surg 1986; 21:68–70.

SI004     **William K. Sieber**

## STOMACH, HYPOPLASIA     0913

**Includes:** Microgastria

**Excludes:** Agastrica

**Major Diagnostic Criteria:** Stomach hypoplasia is diagnosed by upper GI examination and is always associated with failure of rotation of the stomach, without differentiation into fundus, body, and pyloric areas. The esophagus is usually dilated and takes over some storage function.

**Clinical Findings:** Vomiting, hematemesis, malnutrition, and secondary anemia are noted at birth, and these intensify.

**Complications:** Malnutrition.

**Associated Findings:** None known.

**Etiology:** Unknown.

**Pathogenesis:** Unknown.

**CDC No.:** 750.780

**Sex Ratio:** Presumably M1:F1.

**Occurrence:** Undetermined but presumed arre.

**Risk of Recurrence for Patient's Sib:** Unknown.

**Risk of Recurrence for Patient's Child:** Unknown.

**Age of Detectability:** Usually in neonatal period, by X-ray exam.

**Gene Mapping and Linkage:** Unknown.

**Prevention:** None known. Genetic counseling indicated.

**Treatment:** Continuous slow feeding. Surgical enlargement of stomach and correction of reflux may be helpful in selected patients.

**Prognosis:** General poor health has been the rule, with early death in most. Two cases followed for long periods slowly developed a functional stomach.

**Detection of Carrier:** Unknown.

**References:**
Blank E, et al.: Congenital microgastria: a case report with a 26 year follow-up. Pediatrics 1973; 51:1037.
Hochberger, et al.: Congenital microgastria: a follow-up observation over six years. Pediatr Radiol 1974; 2:207.
Anderson KD, Guzzetta PC: Treatment of congenital microgastria and dumping syndrome. J Pediatr Surg 1983; 18:747.
Mandell GA, et al.: A case of microgastria in association with splenic-gonadal fusion. Pediatr Radiol 1983; 13:95–98.

SI004     **William K. Sieber**

## STOMACH, PYLORIC ATRESIA     0910

**Includes:**
     Antral atresia
     Antral web
     Aplasia of pylorus, congenital
     Fibromuscular atresia of antrum
     Gastric atresia
     Gastric outlet obstruction, incomplete
     Prepyloric membrane
     Pyloric atresia
     Pyloric diaphragm, incomplete

**Excludes:**
     Duodenal atresia (supraampullary)
     **Duodenum, atresia or stenosis** (0300)
     **Pyloric stenosis** (0848)
     **Pyloroduodenal atresia, hereditary** (2617)

**Major Diagnostic Criteria:** Nonbilious vomiting with X-ray identification of the antrum as the site of obstruction. Often identified only at time of surgery.

**Clinical Findings:** Nonbilious vomiting in a new born infant having a scaphoid lower abdomen and a distended stomach. Maternal hydramnios is common. X-ray examination examination discloses only a large air-filled stomach with no second "bubble." Incomplete diaphragms can be identified only by upper GI series, or by gastroscopy. In such infants partial obstruction produces clinical findings identical with pyloric stenosis, but originating at birth.

**Complications:** Hypokalemic alkalosis, dehydration, starvation.

**Associated Findings:** Two non-inherited cases had **Chromosome 21, trisomy 21. Epidermolysis bullosum** associated with complete pyloric atresia was reported in four cases.

**Etiology:** Partial obstruction, as discussed in this article, is of undetermined etiology. Complete atresia by autosomal recessive inheritance (see **Pyloroduodenal atresia, hereditary**).

**Pathogenesis:** Error of recanalization of the gastric lumen.

**CDC No.:** 750.780

**Sex Ratio:** M11:F15 (observed).

**Occurrence:** 1:1,000,000 births; about 1% of reported gastrointestinal atresias.

**Risk of Recurrence for Patient's Sib:** Unknown.

**Risk of Recurrence for Patient's Child:** Unknown.

**Age of Detectability:** From birth to as late as adulthood.

**Gene Mapping and Linkage:** Unknown.

**Prevention:** None known. Genetic counseling indicated.

**Treatment:** Laparotomy, gastroduodenostomy, gastrojejunostomy, or excision of pyloric membrane have all been successful in relieving the obstruction. When associated with **Epidermolysis bullosum, type II**, no treatment is advised.

**Prognosis:** Good.

**Detection of Carrier:** Unknown.

**References:**
Bronsther B, et al.: Congenital pyloric atresia: a report of three cases and a review of the literature. Surg 1971; 69:130–136.
Woolley MM, et al.: Congenital partial gastric antral obstruction. Ann Surg 1974; 180:265–271.
Weitzel A, et al.: Two cases of pyloric atresia. Z Kinderchir 1984; 39:396–398.
Rosenbloom MS, Ratner M: Congenital pyloric atresia and epidermolysis bullosa letalis in premature siblings. J Pediat Surg 1987; 22:374–376.

SI004                                    **William K. Sieber**

**Stomach, reduplication of**
*See STOMACH, DUPLICATION*

## STOMACH, TERATOMA                           0914

**Includes:**
Dermoid cyst of stomach
Gastric teratoma
Tridermal gastric teratoma
Tridermic teratoma of stomach

**Excludes:** N/A

**Major Diagnostic Criteria:** Large upper abdominal mass with calcification by X-ray suggests the diagnosis. Confirmed only by gross and microscopic pathology.

**Clinical Findings:** Abdominal mass. GI bleeding is sometimes present (3 of 17 cases). X-ray studies characteristically show areas of calcification in large, bulky tumors that may cause gastric obstruction. Respiratory difficulty and intestinal obstruction may be present secondary to pressure from the large abdominal mass.

**Complications:** Gastric bleeding and/or obstruction, respiratory distress due to increased intra-abdominal pressure.

**Associated Findings:** None known.

**Etiology:** Unknown.

**Pathogenesis:** Unknown.

**POS No.:** 3399

**CDC No.:** 750.780

**Sex Ratio:** M1:F>0.

**Occurrence:** About 30 cases have been reported; all but one being male.

**Risk of Recurrence for Patient's Sib:** Undetermined but apparently small.

**Risk of Recurrence for Patient's Child:** Undetermined but apparently small.

**Age of Detectability:** Usually at birth or during infancy.

**Gene Mapping and Linkage:** Unknown.

**Prevention:** None known. Genetic counseling indicated.

**Treatment:** Surgical excision of the tumor by partial or total gastrectomy.

**Prognosis:** Fifteen of 16 patients recovered following surgical resection of the tumor.

**Detection of Carrier:** Unknown.

**References:**
DeAngelis VR: Gastric teratoma in a newborn infant: total gastrectomy with survival. Surgery 1969; 66:794–795.
Ohgami H, et al.: Gastric teratoma in infancy and childhood: report of three cases and review of literature. Jpn J Surg 1973; 3:218–220.
Haley T, et al.: Gastric teratoma with gastrointestinal bleeding. J Pediatr Surg 1976; 21:949–950.
Purvis JM, et al.: Gastric teratoma: first reported case in a female. J Pediatr Surg 1979; 14:86–88.

SI004                                    **William K. Sieber**

**Stomach-duodenum-small intestine-rectum, duplication of**
*See INTESTINAL DUPLICATION*
**Stomatitis areata migrans**
*See TONGUE, GEOGRAPHIC*
**Stomatocytosis, hereditary**
*See ANEMIA, HEMOLYTIC, RED CELL MEMBRANE DEFECTS*

## STORAGE DISEASE, NEUTRAL LIPID TYPE          2859

**Includes:**
Chanarin-Dorfman syndrome
Chanarin syndrome
Cornification, disorder of, neutral lipid storage type (DOC 12)
Ichthyotic neutral lipid storage disease
Ichthyosiform erythroderma with leukocyte vacuolization
Neutral lipid storage disease with ichthyosis
Triglyceride storage disease-impaired fatty acid oxidation

**Excludes:**
**Cholesteryl ester storage disease** (0151)
**Ichthyosis, congenital erythrodermic** (2855)
**Myopathy-metabolic, carnitine deficiency, primary and secondary** (0124)
**Myopathy-metabolic, carnitine palmityl transferase deficiency** (0125)
**Phytanic acid storage disease** (0810)
**Wolman disease** (1003)

**Major Diagnostic Criteria:** Affected patients exhibit a generalized ichthyosiform erythroderma in conjunction with lipid vacuoles in circulating granulocytes and monocytes. Lipid storage is widespread in tissues and can also be demonstrated in skin, muscle, or liver biopsy material or within cultured fibroblasts.

**Clinical Findings:** Generalized ichthyosis, myopathy, and vacuolated leukocytes. Clinically, the disorder of cornification most closely resembles **Ichthyosis, congenital erythrodermic** of mild-to-moderate severity. Some patients have also exhibited atopic-like dermatitis.

Prominent lipid vacuoles are seen in virtually every circulating granulocyte and monocyte, and the diagnosis can be established readily by direct examination of a peripheral blood smear. Lipid vacuoles are also present within numerous cell types, including those of the skin, where vacuoles are found within dermal cells and within the basal and granular cell layers of the epidermis. Lipid vacuoles are also present within cells of the gastrointestinal epithelia, skeletal muscle, and liver. Despite widespread evidence of tissue lipid storage, serum lipid levels are usually normal and systemic manifestations may be subtle. Myopathy may be discovered only upon detailed testing, but serum muscle enzyme levels are elevated. All patients who have undergone liver biopsy have exhibited severe fatty change, but this may not be reflected in liver function studies. Both neurosensory deafness and cataracts are present in some patients. Mild developmental delay and growth retardation may also be features of this syndrome.

**Complications:** Liver dysfunction, weakness, and intolerance to fasting.

**Associated Findings:** Atopic-like dermatitis occurs in some patients.

**Etiology:** Autosomal recessive inheritance.

**Pathogenesis:** Since electron microscopy demonstrates non-membrane-enclosed lipid droplets, the disorder is unlikely to be a lysosomal storage disease. The stored lipid is triglyceride. Studies on cultured cells *in vitro* suggest a novel defect in fatty acid metabolism distinct from other known abnormalities of triglyceride metabolism, including Wolman disease (acid lipase deficiency) and carnitine deficiency. Some investigators have suggested an impairment of long-chain fatty acid oxidation, but this has been disputed by others.

Electron microscopic studies of epidermis have shown a unique abnormality of lamellar body structure in which the normal lamellae are disrupted by electron-lucent, globular inclusions. These distortions may be responsible for the abnormality in cohesion in this disorder.

**MIM No.:** *27563

**POS No.:** 4111

**Sex Ratio:** Presumably M1:F1; observed, M8:F6.

**Occurrence:** Fourteen patients with this syndrome have been reported; the majority of these were of Middle Eastern or Mediterranean descent.

**Risk of Recurrence for Patient's Sib:**
See Part I, *Mendelian Inheritance.*

**Risk of Recurrence for Patient's Child:**
See Part I, *Mendelian Inheritance.*

**Age of Detectability:** Usually evident at birth. Prenatal diagnosis has not been attempted but may be possible if amniocytes also store lipid or by fetal blood sampling if fetal leukocytes store lipid.

**Gene Mapping and Linkage:** Unknown.

**Prevention:** None known. Genetic counseling indicated.

**Treatment:** No specific therapy is recognized.

**Prognosis:** Probably normal for life span. Visual and hearing deficits or myopathy may be disabling. Intelligence may be normal or impaired.

**Detection of Carrier:** Carriers exhibit similar lipid vacuoles within some of their eosinophils.

**Special Considerations:** A peripheral blood smear from all patients with generalized ichthyosis should be examined because systemic symptoms may not be pronouced in these patients.

**References:**

Dorfman ML, et al.: Ichthyosiform dermatosis with system lipidosis. Arch Dermatol 1974; 110:261–266.
Chanarin I, et al.: Neutral lipid storage disease: a new disorder of lipid metabolism. Br Med J 1975; 1:553–555. *
Elias PM, Williams ML: Neutral lipid storage disease with ichthyosis: defective lamellar body contents and intercellular dispersion. Arch Dermatol 1985; 121:1000–1008. †
Williams ML, et al.: Ichthyosis and neutral lipid storage disease. Am J Med Genet 1985; 20:711–726. * †
Williams ML, et al.: Neutral lipid storage disease with ichthyosis: lipid content and metabolism in fibroblasts. J Inherit Metab Dis 1988; 11:131–143.

WI013                                          **Mary L. Williams**

**'Stork bite' mark**
*See NEVUS FLAMMEUS*
**Strabismus, Duane type**
*See EYE, DUANE RETRACTION SYNDROME*
**Straight-chain C6-C10-omega-dicarboxylic aciduria**
*See ACYL-CoA DEHYDROGENASE DEFICIENCY, MEDIUM CHAIN TYPE*
**Strangulated hernia**
*See HERNIA, INGUINAL*
**Straussler disease**
*See GERSTMANN-STRAUSSLER SYNDROME*
**Strawberry nevus**
*See HEMANGIOMAS OF THE HEAD AND NECK*
**Streblodactyly**
*See CAMPTODACTYLY*
**Streblomicrodactyly**
*See CAMPTODACTYLY*
**Streeter bands**
*See AMNIOTIC BANDS SYNDROME*
**Streptomycin, fetal effects**
*See FETAL AMINOGLYCOSIDE OTOTOXICITY*
**Streptomycin-sensitivity deafness**
*See DEAFNESS, STREPTOMYCIN-SENSITIVITY*
**Striatonigral degeneration, autosomal dominant**
*See MACHADO-JOSEPH DISEASE*
**Stridor, congenital**
*See LARYNGOMALACIA*
**Stroke-like episodes**
*See MYOPATHY, MITOCHONDRIAL-ENCEPHALOPATHY-LACTIC ACIDOSIS-STROKE*
**Stromal dystrophy of the cornea, congenital hereditary**
*See CORNEAL DYSTROPHY, STROMAL, CONGENITAL HEREDITARY*
**Strudwick syndrome**
*See SPONDYLOEPIMETAPHYSEAL DYSPLASIA, STRUDWICK TYPE*
**Strumpell familial spastic paraplegia**
*See PARAPLEGIA, FAMILIAL SPASTIC*
**Strumpell-Lorrain syndrome**
*See PARAPLEGIA, FAMILIAL SPASTIC*
**Stuart-Prower Factor deficiency**
*See FACTOR X DEFICIENCY*
**'Stub thumb'**
*See BRACHYDACTYLY*

## STURGE-WEBER SYNDROME                      0915

**Includes:**

Encephalofacial angiomatosis
Encephalotrigeminal angiomatosis
Fourth phacomatosis
Meningeal capillary angiomatosis

**Excludes:**

**Neurofibromatosis** (0712)
**Tuberous sclerosis** (0975)
**Von Hippel-Lindau syndrome** (0995)

**Major Diagnostic Criteria:** Port-wine angioma of the face following the distribution of the trigeminal nerve and accompanied by seizures and intracranial calcifications.

**Clinical Findings:** Capillary angioma over the first or all of the three divisions of the fifth cranial nerve is always present at birth. There may be glaucoma on the side of the angioma due to the outflow occlusion of the angle. Generalized seizures begin at 1–2 years of age. Intracranial calcifications do not appear until after 2 years of age, although CT scans may demonstrate calcification earlier. The skull is smaller on the side of the abnormality; 15% of affected individuals have bilateral angiomas and bilateral neurologic involvement.

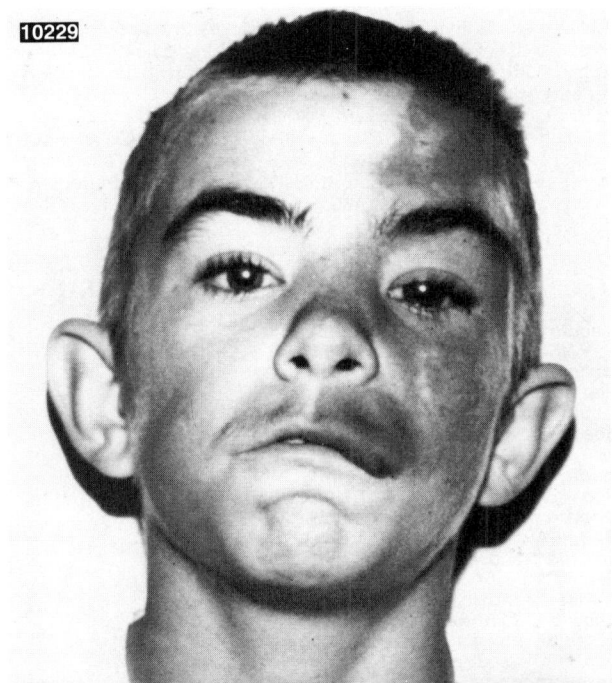

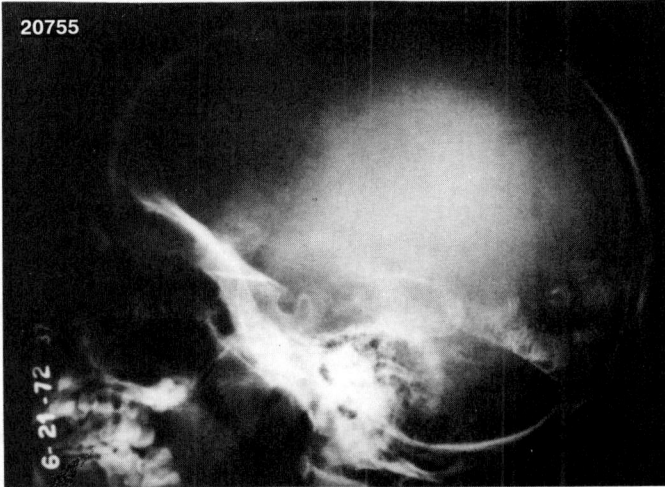

**0915**-10229: Typical unilateral distribution of port wine stain. 20755: Skull X-ray shows double contour or "railroad track" pattern of intercranial calcifications.

**Complications:** Seizures, mental retardation.

**Associated Findings:** Sometimes associated with **Angio-osteohypertrophy syndrome**. **Nevus of Ota** has been reported.

**Etiology:** Unknown.

**Pathogenesis:** The intracranial calcifications are not in blood vessel walls, but in the second and third layers of cortex, presumably due to tissue anoxia. The calcifications consist of characteristic serpiginous double tracks. An alternate explanation for calcification is transudation of protein through abnormal vessels and calcium binding. Degeneration of neurons and gliosis follows. The homolateral eye may be enlarged because of congenital glaucoma (buphthalmos). The iris of such an eye may remain blue, although the normal eye is brown, due to angiomatosis of the choroid. Hemiplegia is present, in many cases opposite the

side of the nevus. Hemianopsia is frequently found in patients who can be tested.

**MIM No.:** 18530

**POS No.:** 3397

**CDC No.:** 759.610

**Sex Ratio:** Presumably M1:F1.

**Occurrence:** Undetermined but presumed rare.

**Risk of Recurrence for Patient's Sib:** Unknown.

**Risk of Recurrence for Patient's Child:** Unknown.

**Age of Detectability:** Facial lesions determine the diagnosis at birth. In patients diagnosed on the basis of seizures, one-half were diagnosed before one year of age.

**Gene Mapping and Linkage:** Unknown.

**Prevention:** None known. Genetic counseling indicated.

**Treatment:** In uncontrolled seizure states, cortical resection or hemispherectomy is indicated. Results of this therapy are reasonably good.

**Prognosis:** Normally progressive. If seizures become frequent, mental retardation occurs. Normal development may occur in slowly progressive patients or in those without major CNS involvement.

**Detection of Carrier:** Unknown.

**References:**

Weber FP: Notes on association of extensive haemangiomatous naevus of skin with cerebral (meningeal) haemangioma, especially cases of facial vascular naevus with contralateral hemiplegia. Proc R Soc Med 1929; 22:25.

Furukawa T, et al.: Sturge-Weber and Klippel-Trenaunay syndrome with nevus of Ota and Ito. Arch Derm 1970; 102:640–645.

Boltshauser E, et al.: Sturge-Weber syndrome with bilateral intracranial calcification. J Neurol Neurosurg Psychiatry 1976; 39:429.

Hoffman HJ, et al.: Hemispherectomy for Sturge-Weber syndrome. Child Brain 1979; 5:223.

SH007                                          **Kenneth Shapiro**

---

**STUTTERING**                                          **3060**

**Includes:**
    Dysfluency
    Speech fluency disorder
    Stammering

**Excludes:** Cluttering

**Major Diagnostic Criteria:** The diagnosis of stuttering is based on a purely behavioral analysis. In fact, the disorder is essentially defined by its symptoms, or, in other words, the symptoms and the disease are synonymous. Stuttering is generally defined as the interruption of the normal flow of speech by repetitions or prolongations of whole words or parts of words or by prolonged silences (or "blocks"), which may be accompanied by a struggle response, ticks, and grimaces.

**Clinical Findings:** Stuttering has been noted to begin most often in early childhood (at ages 4–5 years) and at that point tends to be characterized by easy repetitions of parts of words or whole words. Struggle behavior (visible and audible blockings of speech with accompanying grimacing) and increased severity of stuttering begins to occur later in childhood and continues to worsen through adolescence unless treated successfully. Males are far more likely to stutter than are females, and a strong familial pattern has been reported. To date, no specific structural phenotype has been documented.

   A number of studies have shown physiologic responses associated with stuttering, such as increased anxiety levels and altered EEG patterns (e.g., increased beta wave production versus alpha waves), but many investigators believe that much of the physiologic response is secondary to the altered speech pattern, and the stress it causes the stutterer. To date, no physiologic phenotype has been demonstrated conclusively. Many other structural, physiologic, medical, and behavioral disorders have been hypothesized, but none have been scientifically confirmed.

Stuttering may be inconsistent. For example, many stutterers will be more dysfluent in certain environments or situations. Most stutterers are fluent when singing.

**Complications:** Stutterers may withdraw from situations demanding strong communication skills. They may also develop strong anxiety responses in situations that center around communicative ability, such as telephone conversation, meeting strangers, and other social interactions. Struggle responses appear later in the stutterer and are generally thought to be operantly learned behaviors.

**Associated Findings:** Though dysfluent speech may occur in individuals with a variety of neurogenic disorders such as **Neurofibromatosis**, stuttering generally occurs as an isolated findings in individuals who are reportedly otherwise normal.

**Etiology:** A number of hypotheses have been forwarded regarding the etiology of stuttering, including autosomal dominant inheritance, purely environmental factors, X-linked recessive inheritance, and sex-modified transmission of an autosomal dominant trait. At present, multifactorial inheritance seems to provide the best model for the majority of stutterers, though etiologic heterogeneity cannot be ruled out. In fact, it has not been established that all stuttering is in fact the same disorder, thus raising questions about the validity of considering it a "disease" versus merely a "symptom" of an underlying biologic dysfunction.

**Pathogenesis:** Unknown.

**MIM No.:** 18445

**Sex Ratio:** Reports range from M2:F1 to M10:F1. The most likely figure is approximately M4:F1.

**Occurrence:** Childhood dysfluency has been reported in up to 5% of males and 2% of females, although the incidence of fully expressed stuttering in the general population is undetermined. The condition is relatively common and known to occur in all cultures. An estimated prevalence of 0.7 has been reported. Stuttering is said to be unusually frequent in the Japanese, low in Polynesians, and almost completely absent in American Indians.

**Risk of Recurrence for Patient's Sib:** If neither parent is affected, males, 18%; females, 2%. If father is affected, males, 26%; females, 12%. If mother is affected, males, 33%; females, <1%.

**Risk of Recurrence for Patient's Child:** For males, 22%; females, 9%

**Age of Detectability:** After onset of speech, but not usually until past three years of age.

**Gene Mapping and Linkage:** Unknown.

**Prevention:** None known. Genetic counseling indicated.

**Treatment:** Speech therapy.

**Prognosis:** Life span is normal. Speech therapy is often, though not always, effective.

**Detection of Carrier:** Unknown.

**Special Considerations:** Stuttering may not be a single disorder, but rather a symptom of many possible biologically based problems of speech or voice coordination. However, its organic basis cannot be refuted, and extrinsic or environmental factors may be contributory, but not pathogenetic.

**References:**
Young A: Onset, prevalence, ar.l recovery from stuttering. J Speech Hear Disord 1975; 40:49–58.
Kidd KK: A genetic perspective on stuttering. J Fluence Disord 1977; 2:259–269.
Kidd KK, et al.: Vertical transmission of susceptibility to stuttering with sex-modified expression. Proc Natl Acad Sci USA 1978; 78:606–610.
Kidd KK, et al.: The possible causes of the sex ratio in stuttering and its implications. J Fluency Disord 1978; 3:13–23.
Chakravartti R, et al.: Hereditary factors in stammering. J Genet Hum 1979; 27:319–328.
Kidd KK, et al.: Familial stuttering patterns are not related to one measure of severity. J Speech Hear Res 1980; 23:539–545.
Cox NJ, Kidd KK: Can recovery from stuttering be considered a genetically milder subtype of stuttering? Behav Genet 1983; 13:129–139.
Cox NJ, et al.: Segregation analyses of stuttering. Genet Epidemiol 1984; 1:245–253.
Cox NJ, et al.: Some environmental factors and hypotheses for stuttering in families with several stutterers. J Speech Hear Res 1984; 27:543–548.

SH040
SA045

**Robert J. Shprintzen**
**Vicki L. Sadewitz**

**Subacute myelo-optico neuropathy (SMON)**
See NEUROPATHY, MYELO-OPTICO, SUBACUTE TYPE
**Subacute necrotizing encephalomyelopathy (SNE)**
See ENCEPHALOPATHY, NECROTIZING
**Subacute spongiform encephalopathy**
See CREUTZFELDT-JAKOB DISEASE
also GERSTMANN-STRAUSSLER SYNDROME
**Subaortic stenosis, discrete**
See HEART, SUBAORTIC STENOSIS, FIBROUS
**Subaortic stenosis, fibrous**
See HEART, SUBAORTIC STENOSIS, FIBROUS
**Subaortic stenosis, idiopathic hypertrophic**
See HEART, SUBAORTIC STENOSIS, MUSCULAR
**Subaortic stenosis, muscular**
See HEART, SUBAORTIC STENOSIS, MUSCULAR
**Subclavian artery supply disruption sequence (SASDS)**
See POLAND SYNDROME
**Subclavian artery, anomalous origin of contralateral**
See ARTERY, ANOMALOUS ORIGIN OF CONTRALATERAL SUBCLAVIAN
**Subclavian artery, isolation from aorta**
See AORTA, ISOLATION OF SUBCLAVIAN ARTERY FROM AORTA
**Subcostosternal hernia**
See DIAPHRAGMATIC HERNIA
**Subendocardial fibroelastosis, right ventricular**
See VENTRICLE, ENDOCARDIAL FIBROELASTOSIS OF RIGHT VENTRICLE
**Suberylglycinuria**
See ACYL-CoA DEHYDROGENASE DEFICIENCY, MEDIUM CHAIN TYPE

## SUBGLOTTIC HEMANGIOMA                    0918

**Includes:** Hemangioma, subglottic

**Excludes:**
Respiratory distress from other causes
**Subglottic stenosis** (0919)

**Major Diagnostic Criteria:** The clinical history and typical endoscopic appearance are considered sufficiently diagnostic for therapy, pending biopsy confirmation.

**Clinical Findings:** Because these hemangiomas are located subglottically affected infants typically have a history of dyspnea and inspiratory stridor which may become biphasic, yet the cry and voice remain clear. The fluctuating character of the respiratory distress, varying from day to day or even hour to hour, particularly with crying or exertion, is considered strongly diagnostic. The absence of marked temperature elevation, leukocytosis, and pharyngeal inflammation distinguish this disease from tracheobronchitis. Cutaneous hemangioma, particularly of the head and neck, should prompt immediate suspicion of a similar lesion in the subglottis in any child with respiratory distress; however about one-half of all patients will have no external hemangioma.

Soft tissue X-rays of the neck are generally nonspecific, although larger lesions may be seen on airway films. Typically, there is an asymmetric narrowing in the subglottis. Barium swallow may show posterior displacement of the esophagus from the air column in the subglottic area. Laryngoscopy and bronchoscopy allow visualization of the hemangioma, which usually appears as a sessile mass between the true vocal cord and the lower limit of the cricoid cartilage located in the posterolateral portion of the subglottis. The color varies from pink to blue; depending on the lesion's vascularity and relative depth beneath the mucosa. Such hemangiomas are readily compressible, differentiating them from other tumors of the larynx. Biopsy is generally condemned as dangerous and unnecessary because hemorrhage may be very difficult to control.

**Complications:** Acute respiratory failure or "sudden death" in about one-half of cases.

**Associated Findings:** Failure to gain weight; a characteristic of chronic respiratory obstruction.

**Etiology:** Unknown.

**Pathogenesis:** Usually a cavernous hemangioma with mature endothelium on only one side of the subglottic area, but may circumscribe the entire lumen.

**Sex Ratio:** M1:F2 (observed).

**Occurrence:** Between 1913 and 1986, 356 cases of infantile subglottic hemangioma were reported in the English literature.

The actual incidence has been difficult to establish because autopsy gross examination of infants succumbing to acute respiratory failure from this disease reveals no abnormality of the trachea or larynx. This finding is explained by the submucosal locations of these tumors, and when emptied of blood the lumen contour is restored with normal-appearing mucosa. With the recent increased awareness of this lesion, some centers advocate routine sections of the larynx and trachea in all cases of "sudden death" of unknown etiology in infants.

**Risk of Recurrence for Patient's Sib:** Unknown.

**Risk of Recurrence for Patient's Child:** Unknown.

**Age of Detectability:** Usually asymptomatic at birth. However, over 90% will develop symptoms before age three months.

**Gene Mapping and Linkage:** Unknown.

**Prevention:** None known. Genetic counseling indicated.

**Treatment:** Systemic steroids have produced dramatic regression of tumors in two to four weeks; and recurrence has been controlled by a second course of steroids. Excision of the tumor by laryngofissure is reserved for those tumors requiring tracheostomy that have not regressed after serveral years. Laser excision may be appropriate before attempting an open procedure. Smaller lesions may be treated with the carbon dioxide laser.

Tracheostomy is necessary with moderate-to-severe respiratory distress. Low-dose irradiation or injection of sclerosing agents are probably ineffective and may be dangerous to the developing larynx.

**Prognosis:** The lesions usually cease growth by age nine months, followed by gradual regression. A normal life span is expected if the patient survives infancy.

**Detection of Carrier:** Unknown.

**Special Considerations:** The association with cutaneous hemangioma and hemangioma of other organs is well documented. This includes hemangioma of the parotid gland, mediastinum, abdominal viscera, central nervous system, and retina. With multiple hemangiomas, there may be sufficient shunting of blood from the arterial to the venous system to cause right heart failure. Thrombocytopenia may result from the trapping of platelets within a large hemangioma.

**References:**
Calcaterra VC: An evaluation of the treatment of subglottic hemangioma. Laryngoscope 1968; 78:195.
Cohen SR: Unusual lesions of the larynx, trachea and bronchial tree. Ann Otol Rhinol Laryngol 1969; 78:476.
Cracovaner AJ: Anomalies of the larynx. In: Maloney WH, ed: Otolaryngology. Hagerstown: Harper and Row, 1969:42.
Choa OI, et al.: Subglottic hemangioma in children. J Laryngol Otol 1986; 100:447–454.
Shikhani AH, et al.: Infantile subglottic hemangiomas: an update. Ann Otol Rhinol Laryngol 1986; 95:336–347.

**Thomas Aufdemorte**

## SUBGLOTTIC STENOSIS 0919

**Includes:**
    Stenosis, combined subglottic
    Stenosis, hard subglottic
    Stenosis, soft subglottic
    Stenosis, subglottic

**Excludes:** Acquired subglottic stenosis

**Major Diagnostic Criteria:** Stridor and cyanosis due to a developmental defect of the conus elasticus or the cricoid cartilage, which produces stenosis (when the infant's transverse subglottic diameter is less than 4 mm). The diagnosis is made by endoscopic examination.

**Clinical Findings:** Symptoms are variable according to the degree of stenosis, the presence of other anomalies, and superimposed infection. Symptoms may begin at birth with stridor and cyanosis. Other infants will be asymptomatic until superimposed low-grade infections cause recurrent bouts of respiratory difficulty, commonly misdiagnosed as croup. Lateral X-ray of the neck may show a decrease in anteroposterior (AP) diameter of the subglottic airway. Direct laryngoscopy and bronchoscopy are the most important studies for establishing the diagnosis. In the infant's larynx the subglottic region is cone-shaped and the smallest part of the larynx. The cricoid cartilage is somewhat funnel-shaped, with an AP diameter greater than that of the trachea. Later development produces the ring-shaped cricoid.

*Soft stenosis:* Narrowing of the normally cone-shaped conus elasticus produces a diffuse stenosis. This "hypertrophy" is composed of increased amounts of connective tissue and large dilated mucous glands, with a normal epithelial covering.

*Hard stenosis:* Caused by the cricoid cartilage, the lumen is compressed in inward "overgrowth" of its cartilaginous walls.

*Combined stenosis:* A subglottic stenosis can be caused by both soft (conus elasticus) and hard (cricoid cartilage) components.

**Complications:** Airway obstruction, exercise intolerance.

**Associated Findings:** None known.

**Etiology:** Unknown.

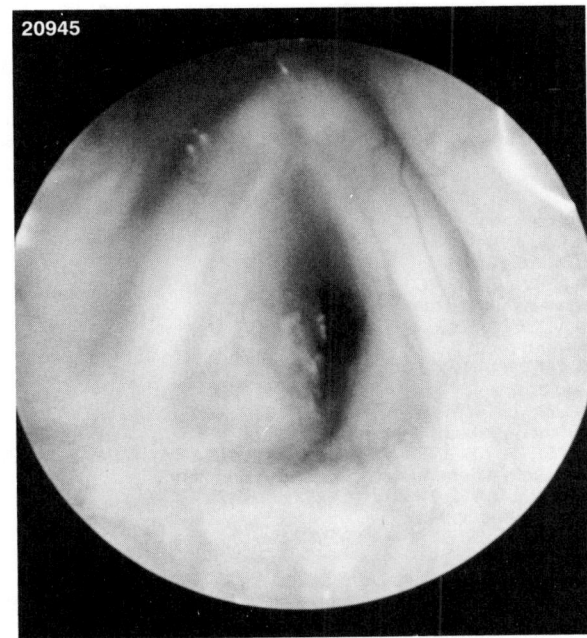

**0919-20945:** Subglottic stenosis.

**Pathogenesis:** Possible hypotheses include failure of the lateral infraglottic branchial fused masses to recanalize (soft stenosis) or recanalization after chondrification centers for the cricoid cartilage appear. An alternate theory suggests developmental arrest and formation of the stenosis from mesodermal elements.

**Sex Ratio:** M1:F1

**Occurrence:** Undetermined but presumed rare.

**Risk of Recurrence for Patient's Sib:** Unknown.

**Risk of Recurrence for Patient's Child:** Unknown.

**Age of Detectability:** Usually at or shortly after birth, but may not be detected until infant develops a respiratory infection or "croup". May become apparent following intubation if the child cannot be extubated or develops an obstruction.

**Gene Mapping and Linkage:** Unknown.

**Prevention:** None known. Genetic counseling indicated.

**Treatment:** In very mild stenosis no treatment is needed, other than aggressive therapy of upper respiratory infections. Functionally significant stenosis will require a tracheotomy until laryngeal growth produces an adequate airway. In Holinger's series of 53 infants with subglottic stenosis (1967), 39 required tracheotomy because of progressive respiratory difficulty.

**Prognosis:** Good if mild or if recognized and promptly treated. It is presently thought that most or all of these stenoses will "cure" themselves with growth. If the condition is severe and untreated, the patient may die of acute upper airway obstruction. A marginal airway may become inadequate during a respiratory infection. If tracheotomy is required, there is significant morbidity and mortality in infants and young children.

**Detection of Carrier:** Unknown.

**References:**

Holinger PH, et al.: Congenital anomalies of the larynx. Ann Otol Rhinol Laryngol 1954; 63:581–606.
Cavanagh F: Congenital laryngeal web. Proc R Soc Med 1965; 58:272–277.
Holinger PH, Brown WT: Congenital webs, cysts, laryngoceles, and other anomalies of the larynx. Ann Otol Rhinol Laryngol 1967; 76:744–752.
Cotton RT, Myer III, CM: Contemporary surgical management of laryngeal stenosis in children. Am J Otolaryngol 1984; 5:360–368.

MY003                                          **Charles M. Myer III**

**Subglottic web**
  See LARYNX, WEB
**Subluxation of lens**
  See LENS, ECTOPIC
**Subluxed nasal septum, congenital**
  See NOSE, DISLOCATED NASAL SEPTUM
**Submerged teeth**
  See TEETH, ANKYLOSED
**SUC syndrome**
  See UMBILICAL CORD, SHORT UMBILICAL CORD SYNDROME
**Succedaneous teeth, agenesis of**
  See TEETH, PEGGED OR ABSENT MAXILLARY LATERAL INCISOR
**Succinic semialdehyde dehydrogenase deficiency**
  See ACIDEMIA, GAMMA-HYDROXYBUTYRIC
**Succinylcholine apnea**
  See CHOLINESTERASE, ATYPICAL
**Sucrase insufficiency**
  See SUCRASE-ISOMALTASE DEFICIENCY
**Sucrase intolerance, congenital**
  See SUCRASE-ISOMALTASE DEFICIENCY
**Sucrase-alpha dextrinase insufficiency**
  See SUCRASE-ISOMALTASE DEFICIENCY

## SUCRASE-ISOMALTASE DEFICIENCY                    0920

**Includes:**
  Anisomaltasia
  Asucrosia
  Disaccharide intolerance I
  Isomaltase insufficiency
  Isomaltase-sucrase deficiency
  Sucrase-alpha dextrinase insufficiency
  Sucrase insufficiency
  Sucrase intolerance, congenital
  Sucrose-isomaltose malabsorption, congenital

**Excludes:**
  **Lactase deficiency, congenital** (0566)
  **Lactase deficiency, primary** (0567)
  Secondary sucrase-isomaltase deficiency

**Major Diagnostic Criteria:** Fermentative diarrhea from the earliest time of sucrose, dextrin, or starch ingestion, which disappears when these foods are eliminated and which does not occur with feedings of monosaccharides or lactose. Deliberate feeding of measured doses of sucrose, isomaltose, or palatinose yields flat serum glucose curve, abdominal discomfort, and explosive stool of pH below 5.0. The disaccharide can usually be identified in blood, urine, and stool after feeding for a tolerance test. If one is certain that the condition is congenital, these criteria may suffice if the patient's condition precludes peroral biopsy. However, demonstration of normal intestinal histology and decreased or absent sucrase and isomaltase activity is essential in most instances.

**Clinical Findings:** Symptoms of fermentative diarrhea and failure to thrive begin with initial ingestion of sucrose or dextrins. This would be virtually at birth in infants on modified milk formulas, or with weaning and introduction of sucrose or fruits containing sucrose. Severity of symptoms varies among individuals, but they are usually more severe in infants and young children. In most patients sucrosuria is present on ingestion of this disaccharide. Symptoms clear as soon as the offending disaccharide is removed from the diet. Patients with intolerance to sucrose are virtually universally described as simultaneously intolerant to isomaltose, the 1–6α-linked diglucose, which is found at the branching points of polysaccharide molecules (dextrins, starches).

The stool is fluid and frothy from contained gas, as it is passed. The pH of fresh stool is always below 5.0 if sucrose or dextrins have been ingested, and it may contain reducing sugars (glucose or fructose). These monosaccharides and sucrose or isomaltose may be identified in the stool by chromatography. Ingestion of a standard dose of sucrose (1.5–2.0 g/kg or 45–60 m/m²) always results in a flat 3-hour "tolerance curve" for serum glucose, or with increased breath hydrogen excretion. The test dose almost universally produces clinical discomfort and explosive diarrhea during the observation period.

The Zurich group initially demonstrated that all patients with sucrose intolerance were also intolerant to isomaltose. It is this defect that causes the inability to tolerate dextrins and starches in young infants. Since adequate supplies of isomaltose are not available to demonstrate the flat absorption curve in routine loading tests, palatinose (1–6α-linked glucose and fructose), a bacterial product, is substituted. This disaccharide is split by the same α-glycosidase as is isomaltose. In addition to sucrosemia and sucrosuria, patients with this deficiency of sucrase-isomaltase demonstrate isomaltose in blood and urine after dextrin and starch feedings, and also palatinose in these fluids after its ingestion for tolerance testing.

The importance of the isomaltase deficiency is variously regarded by different authors. In our own experience, patients must remain on a sucrose-free diet for life to avoid symptoms. However, starches appear to be tolerated in reasonably normal amounts, once patients are beyond the early months of life. This is probably because isomaltose makes up only approximately 10% of the average starch molecule.

Peroral biopsy specimen of the upper small intestinal mucosa is histologically normal, but it contains decreased sucrase and isomaltase activities when these are compared with the activities of maltases 1 and 2 (not maltase 3, 4, and 5) and of lactase, or when assayed in relation to unit weight, or to protein content of the tissue.

**Complications:** Dehydration, electrolyte, and acid-base disturbance in almost all cases. Failure to thrive or death in all cases, if correct diagnosis is not made and treatment is not instituted early enough.

**Associated Findings:** Renal calculi.

**Etiology:** Autosomal recessive inheritance of sucrase and isomaltase deficiency. The combined deficiencies of two enzymes (sucrase-isomaltase) is unusual in genetic defects. It has been suggested that a common regulator gene, or inhibitor, is shared by both enzyme molecules. More probably, they are not separate but represent two activity centers of the same molecule. Gray (1975) suggests that the defect be viewed, for this reason, as sucrase-$\alpha$ dextrinase deficiency, since free isomaltose is not present in the intestinal lumen.

**Pathogenesis:** Ingested sucrose or isomaltose, which results from amylolytic action on polysaccharides, are not hydrolyzed to the component monosaccharides in the upper small intestine, as in normal individuals, and pass undigested to the colon. In this organ these disaccharides are hydrolyzed and fermented. The resultant mixture contains two and three carbon volatile acids, glucose, fructose (if sucrose has been ingested), and often the undigested disaccharide(s). The increase in osmolarity of the colonic contents induces a net flux of water to the lumen. A combination of the irritant effect of the excessive fermentation, increased colonic gas, and distension of the bowel walls by the increase in fluid, results in explosive passage of the loose stool.

**MIM No.:** *22290

**Sex Ratio:** Presumably M1:F1.

**Occurrence:** As high as 1:100 in Greenland Eskimos, and probably increased in Alaskan Eskimos. 2:1,000 in North Americans. Intestinal sucrase deficiency is a cause of diarrhea in adults.

**Risk of Recurrence for Patient's Sib:**
See Part I, *Mendelian Inheritance.*

**Risk of Recurrence for Patient's Child:**
See Part I, *Mendelian Inheritance.*

**Age of Detectability:** In early infancy, by loading with sucrose and isomaltose or palatinose and assay of enzymes in intestinal mucosal biopsy specimen.

**Gene Mapping and Linkage:** SI (sucrase-isomaltase) has been provisionally mapped to 3q25-q26.

**Prevention:** None known. Genetic counseling indicated.

**Treatment:** Avoidance of sucrose in diet. Dextrins and starches should also be avoided in very young infants. Toddlers and older children tolerate these quite well, but sucrose is either never tolerated, or, in some instances, may begin to be taken without concomitant symptoms in the second decade of life.

Fluid and electrolyte support may be necessitated during the diarrheal activity in undiagnosed infants.

**Prognosis:** Normal life span, if patient is diagnosed and treated. In many patients, the symptoms disappear with aging. In a few instances, if not recognized in infancy, patients may die of severe inanition and electrolyte disturbances.

**Detection of Carrier:** Although some parents have been demonstrated to have decreased sucrase-isomaltase activities in peroral biopsy specimens, the tolerance of such individuals for loading with the appropriate disaccharides is usually better than that of children. This confusing finding cannot yet be interpreted to mean either that they represent heterozygote carriers or that they are affected but have undergone the improvement in clinical symptomatology, which is characteristic with growing out of childhood.

**References:**
Prader A, Auricchio S: Defects of intestinal disaccharide absorption. Ann Rev Med 1965; 16:345–385.

Davidson M: Disaccharide intolerance. Pediatr Clin North Am 1967; 14:93–107.
Antonowicz I, et al.: Congenital sucrase-isomaltase deficiency. Pediatrics 1972; 49:847–853.
Gray GM: Carbohydrate digestion and absorption. New Engl J Med 1975; 292:1225–1230.
Gray GM, et al.: Sucrase-isomaltase deficiency. New Engl J Med 1976; 294:750–753.
Harms H-K, et al.: Enzyme-substitution therapy with yeast saccharomyces cerevisiae in congenital sucrase-isomaltase deficiency. New Engl J Med 1987; 316:1306–1309.
Lloyd ML, Olsen WA: A study of the molecular pathology of sucrase-isomaltase deficiency. New Engl J Med 1987; 316:438–442.

DA017                                        **Murray Davidson**

**Sucrose-isomaltose malabsorption, congenital**
*See SUCRASE-ISOMALTASE DEFICIENCY*
**Sudden infant death syndrome (SIDS), one theory of**
*See MYOPATHY, MALIGNANT HYPERTHERMIA*
**Sugarman syndrome**
*See ORO-FACIO-DIGITAL SYNDROME, SUGARMAN TYPE*
**Sugio-Kajii syndrome**
*See TRICHO-RHINO-PHALANGEAL SYNDROME, TYPE III*
**Sulcus mentalis**
*See FACE, CHIN FISSURE*

---

## SULFATASE DEFICIENCY, MULTIPLE                2860

**Includes:**
Mucosulfatidosis
Sulfatidosis, juvenile, Austin type

**Excludes:**
**Metachromatic leukodystrophies** (0651)
**Mucopolysaccharidosis**

**Major Diagnostic Criteria:** Early onset developmental delay; hepatomegaly; ichthyosis developing after 2–3 years of age; dysostosis multiplex; and deficiency of two or more sulfatases demonstrated in biologic fluids and/or cultured skin fibroblasts.

**Clinical Findings:** Most patients come to medical attention during the first two years of life for evaluation of delayed development and/or mild to moderate organomegaly. In a few carefully studied cases, slow development was documented from infancy. Severe acrocyanosis may occur intermittantly. On physical exam there may be mildly coarsened facial features. Mild corneal clouding is sometimes detected by slit lamp exam but is not severe enough to be detected with the hand ophthalmoscope. Some patients have exhibited vertical nystagmus. There is usually moderate hepatomegaly or hepatosplenomegaly, camptodactyly, and limited extension of the elbows and hips. The deep tendon reflexes are absent or reduced. The characteristic ichthyotic skin rash which usually is not present until 2–3 years of life, waxes and wanes and is particularly prominent over the trunk.

The peripheral leukocytes often have abnormal granulation. X-rays reveal dysostosis multiplex. There is mild to moderate mucopolysacchariduria and sulfatiduria. Urinary arylsulfatase A is deficient. Nerve conduction velocities are slow.

**Complications:** Seizures have occurred in several reported cases.

**Associated Findings:** Some patients have had broad thumbs and great toes.

**Etiology:** Autosomal recessive inheritance.

**Pathogenesis:** The primary defect responsible for this deficiency of at least seven sulfatases including six lysosomal and one microsomal enzyme is not known. Complementation studies in somatic cell hybrids indicate that the structural genes for these sulfatases are intact. A defect in a shared regulatory or stabilizing factor or a defect in a common co-factor or post-translational modification could account for the biochemical phenotype of multiple enzymatic deficiencies. The observations that cultured skin fibroblasts from multiple sulfatase deficiency patients express near normal levels of sulfatase activity under certain culture conditions and that several of the sulfatases in these cells have markedly reduced half-lives supports the notion of a defect in a shared stabilizing factor.

The sulfatases which have been shown to be deficient in this disorder and the disease associated with specific deficiency of each are shown below:

| SULFATASE | ASSOCIATED SYNDROME |
|---|---|
| Iduronate sulfatase | *Mucopolysaccharidosis II* |
| Heparan N-sulfatase | *Mucopolysaccharidosis III* (Sanfilippo A) |
| N-acetylglucosamine 6-sulfatase | *Mucopolysaccharidosis III* (Sanfilippo D) |
| Galactose 6-sulfatase | *Mucopolysaccharidosis IV* |
| N-acetylgalactosamine 4-sulfatase (arylsulfatase B) | *Mucopolysaccharidosis VI* |
| Arylsulfatase A | *Metachromatic leukodystrophies* |
| Steroid sulfatase (arylsulfatase C) | *Ichthyosis, X-linked with steroid sulfatase deficiency* |

Certain aspects of the clinical phenotype can be attributed mainly to deficiency of one particular sulfatase by comparison with the phenotypes of the inherited isolated sulfatase deficiencies. For example, the ichthyosis resembles that of isolated steroid sulfatase deficiency, the peripheral nerve involvement resembles that of arylsulfatase A deficiency and the dysostosis multiplex resembles that observed in deficiencies of iduronate sulfatase, heparan N-sulfatase, N-acetylglucosamine 6-sulfatase and N-acetylgalactosamine 4-sulfatase.

**MIM No.:**  *27220

**Sex Ratio:**  M1:F1

**Occurrence:**  Fewer than 25 cases have been reported. Some reports of **Mucopolysaccharidosis II** in females may actually represent this disorder.

**Risk of Recurrence for Patient's Sib:**
See Part I, *Mendelian Inheritance.*

**Risk of Recurrence for Patient's Child:**
See Part I, *Mendelian Inheritance.* No affected individuals are known to have reproduced.

**Age of Detectability:**  Clinically evident within the first few months of life. Biochemical abnormalities are present *in utero.*

**Gene Mapping and Linkage:**  Unknown.

**Prevention:**  None known. Genetic counseling indicated.

**Treatment:**  Unknown.

**Prognosis:**  Life span of reported cases ranged from a few months to 12 years.

**Detection of Carrier:**  Some but not all heterozygotes have had reduced levels of one or more sulfatases, but this is so variable as to be unreliable.

**References:**
Austin JH: Studies of metachromatic leukodystrophy. Arch Neurol 1973; 28:258–264.
Fluharty AL, et al.: Arylsulfatase A modulation with pH in multiple sulfatase deficiency disorder fibroblasts. Am J Hum Genet 1979; 31:574–580.
Burk RD, et al.: Early manifestations of multiple sulfatase deficiency. J Pediatr 1984; 104:574–578.
Fedde K, Horwitz AL: Complementation of multiple sulfatase deficiency in somatic cell hybrids. Am J Hum Genet 1984; 36:623–633.
Steckel F, et al.: Synthesis and stability of arylsulfatase A and B in fibroblasts from multiple sulfatase deficiency. Eur J Biochem 1985; 151:141–145.
Steckel F, et al.: Multiple sulfatase deficiency: degradation of arylsulfatase A and B after endocytosis in fibroblasts. Eur J Biochem 1985; 151:147–152.
Horwitz AL, et al.: Rapid degradation of steroid sulfatase in multiple sulfatase deficiency. Biochem Biophys Res Comm 1986; 135:389–396.

**David Valle**

**Sulfatide lipidosis**
See METACHROMATIC LEUKODYSTROPHIES
**Sulfatidosis, juvenile, Austin type**
See SULFATASE DEFICIENCY, MULTIPLE
**Sulfatidosis, juvenile, Austin type (Some forms)**
See MUCOPOLYSACCHARIDOSIS II
**Sulfatidosis, juvenile, Austin type (some forms)**
See METACHROMATIC LEUKODYSTROPHIES
**Sulfite oxidase/xanthine dehydrogenase/aldehyde oxidase deficiency**
See MOLYBDENUM CO-FACTOR DEFICIENCY
**Sulfo-iduronate sulfatase deficiency**
See MUCOPOLYSACCHARIDOSIS II
**Sulfocysteinuria**
See ACIDURIA, SULFITE OXIDASE DEFICIENCY
**Sulfonamides, fetal effects of**
See OPTIC NERVE HYPOPLASIA
**Summerskill disease**
See CHOLESTASIS, INTRAHEPATIC, RECURRENT BEGIN
**Summerskill-Tygstrup disease**
See CHOLESTASIS, INTRAHEPATIC, RECURRENT BEGIN
**Summitt syndrome**
See ACROCEPHALOPOLYSYNDACTYLY
**Superior vena cava syndrome**
See CANCER, THYMOMA
**Supernumerary puncta and canaliculi**
See EYELID, PUNCTA AND CANALICULI, SUPERNUMERARY
**Supraaortic stenosis**
See AORTIC STENOSIS, SUPRAVALVAR
**Supraglottic web**
See LARYNX, WEB
**Supramitral ring**
See MITRAL VALVE STENOSIS
**Suprapineal recess**
See BRAIN, MIDLINE CAVES
**Supraumbilical (paraumbilical) hernia**
See HERNIA, UMBILICAL
**Supravalvar aortic stenosis**
See WILLIAMS SYNDROME
also AORTIC STENOSIS, SUPRAVALVAR
**Supravalvular pulmonary stenosis**
See PULMONARY ARTERY, COARCTATION
**Supraventricular tachycardia paroxysmal**
See ARRHYTHMIA, SUPRAVENTRICULAR TACHYCARDIAS, CONGENITAL
**Supraventricular tachycardias, congenital**
See ARRHYTHMIA, SUPRAVENTRICULAR TACHYCARDIAS, CONGENITAL
**Surdocardiac syndrome**
See CARDIO-AUDITORY SYNDROME
**Sutural cataract**
See CATARACT, AUTOSOMAL DOMINANT CONGENITAL
**Suxamethonium sensitivity**
See CHOLINESTERASE, ATYPICAL

## SWEATING, GUSTATORY 0448

**Includes:**
    Auriculotemporal syndrome
    Frey syndrome
    Gustatory sweating
    Hyperhidrosis, gustatory

**Excludes:**
    Parotid duct fistula
    Postencephalitic gustatory sweating
    Posttraumatic and postoperative gustatory sweating
    Syringomyelia (0924)

**Major Diagnostic Criteria:**  A lifelong history of facial and neck sweating, with or without flushing, during or after eating, in a person who has no medically or surgically induced neurologic deficits. A strong positive family history is usually present.

**Clinical Findings:**  At the time of or just after eating or drinking, perspiration of the face and neck is noted. The face and neck areas may show associated flushing. No increase of sweating or flushing is noted in other areas of the body. The symptoms appear with any food or beverage, but there are no symptoms or findings to suggest specific food allergy. There is no history of trauma or surgery in the area, nor of encephalitis or neurologic deficits. Generally the symptoms have been lifelong or date from infancy; often a family history can be obtained.

**Complications:** Social embarrassment or in extreme cases withdrawal from social contacts might occur.

**Associated Findings:** None known.

**Etiology:** Probably autosomal dominant inheritance.

**Pathogenesis:** Unknown.

**MIM No.:** 14410

**Sex Ratio:** M>1:F1 (observed).

**Occurrence:** Undetermined. The known cases have been in American Blacks as reported by Mailander (1967); and 3 generations of Zuni Indians with the syndrome have been studied by Jacobs. However, there is no reason to believe that other ethnic groups might not also be affected.

**Risk of Recurrence for Patient's Sib:**
See Part I, *Mendelian Inheritance.*

**Risk of Recurrence for Patient's Child:**
See Part I, *Mendelian Inheritance.*

**Age of Detectability:** In infancy.

**Gene Mapping and Linkage:** Unknown.

**Prevention:** None known. Genetic counseling indicated.

**Treatment:** Intratympanic section of Jacobsen nerve (ninth cranial nerve) might be successful in interrupting the efferent innervation to the parotid gland. This is postulated on the theory that aberrant autonomic innervation occurs. It is thought that the sweat glands and blood vessels of the skin are innervated by parasympathetic rather than sympathetic fibers. A topical preparation, such as 3% scopolamine cream, may be useful in instances where the sweating is not profuse. In mild cases simple assurance to the patient that he does not have a serious or life-threatening disorder may be sufficient. Intracranial section of the 9th cranial nerve is not justified for this benign disease. X-ray therapy of the skin would require near-cancerocidal doses to destroy the sweat glands and also is not indicated. In some instances, elevation of a skin flap overlying the parotid gland is useful.

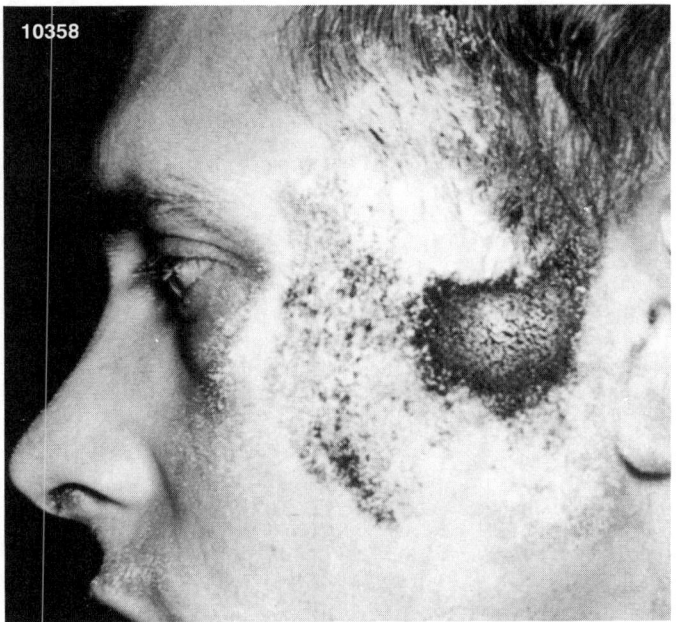

0448-10358: Gustatory sweating.

**Prognosis:** Good for normal life span. Total function of the patient is limited only if he tends to withdraw from society.

**Detection of Carrier:** Unknown.

**Special Considerations:** As pointed out by Mailander, the incidence of this disorder may be higher than reported since affected individuals may tend to deny the symptoms or withdraw from society. Also, in both ethnic groups in which this condition has been described there is a tendency to ignore such physical complaints or at least not to bring them to medical attention. Often this is an incidental finding when the patient is receiving medical care for an unrelated problem. An erroneous diagnosis of parotid fistula or neuropsychiatric disease is often made and proper therapy not instituted.

*The author wishes to thank Kent F. Jacobs for his help in preparing this article.*

**References:**
Mailander JC: Hereditary gustatory sweating. J Am Med Assoc 1967; 201:203–204.

BE028                                                        **LaVonne Bergstrom**

**Sweaty feet syndrome**
   *See ACIDEMIA, ISOVALERIC*
**Swedish genetic porphyria**
   *See PORPHYRIA, ACUTE INTERMITTENT*
**Swedish type distal myopathy**
   *See MUSCULAR DYSTROPHY, DISTAL*
**Swedish-type hereditary amyloidosis**
   *See AMYLOIDOSIS, TRANSTHYRETIN METHIONINE-30 TYPE*
**Swiss type hereditary amyloidosis**
   *See AMYLOIDOSIS, INDIANA TYPE*
**Swiss-cheese cartilage syndrome**
   *See KNIEST DYSPLASIA*
**Swyer syndrome**
   *See GONADAL DYSGENESIS, XY TYPE*
**Sydney line**
   *See SKIN CREASE, SINGLE PALMAR*
**Sylvian seizures**
   *See EPILEPSY, BENIGN CHILDHOOD WITH CENTROTEMPORAL EEG FOCUS (BEC)*
**Symbrachydactyly-ipsilateral aplasia of head of pectoralis muscle**
   *See POLAND SYNDROME*
**Symmelia**
   *See SIRENOMELIA SEQUENCE*
**Symphalangism**
   *See SYNOSTOSIS*

**SYMPHALANGISM**                                                    **1001**

**Includes:**
   Cushing symphalangism
   Deafness (conduction)-multiple synostoses
   Deafness-symphalangism, Herrmann type
   Facio-audio-osymphalangism
   Herrmann symphalangism-brachydactyly syndrome
   Synostoses, multiple-brachydactyly
   Synostoses (multiple)-conduction deafness
   Symphalangism, C.S. Lewis type
   Symphalangism-brachydactyly
   Symphalangism, distal
   Symphalangism, proximal
   Thumbs, stiff
   WL symphalangism-brachydactyly syndrome

**Excludes:**
   **Brachydactyly** (0114)
   **Diastrophic dysplasia** (0293)
   **Poland syndrome** (0813)
   **Skin creases, absent distal interphalangeal** (2488)
   **Synostosis** (1522)

**Major Diagnostic Criteria:** *Symphalangism* refers to general ankylosis of the joints of fingers or toes. Several forms exist, and many of these are or appear to be inherited. In addition, the condition

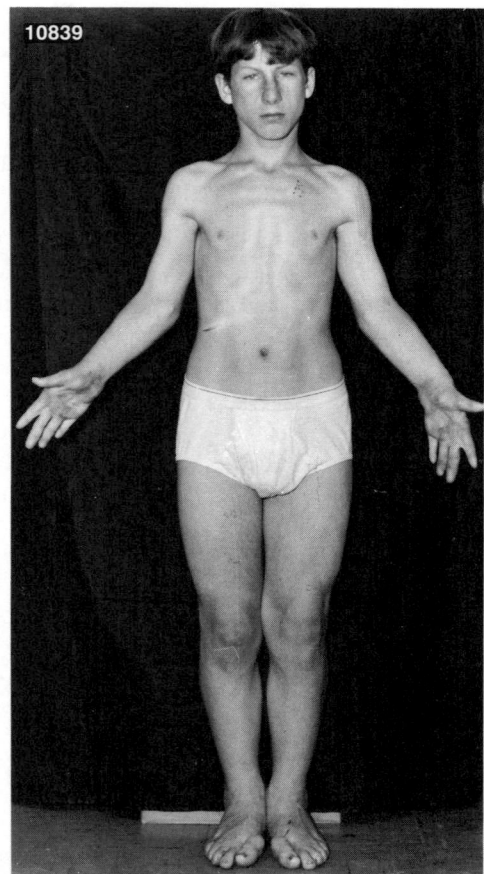

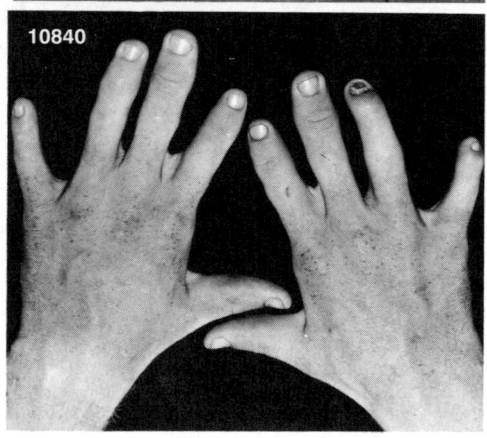

**1001A**-10839: Characteristic facies with long nose and thin upper lip. 10840: Proximal symphalangism and brachydactyly.

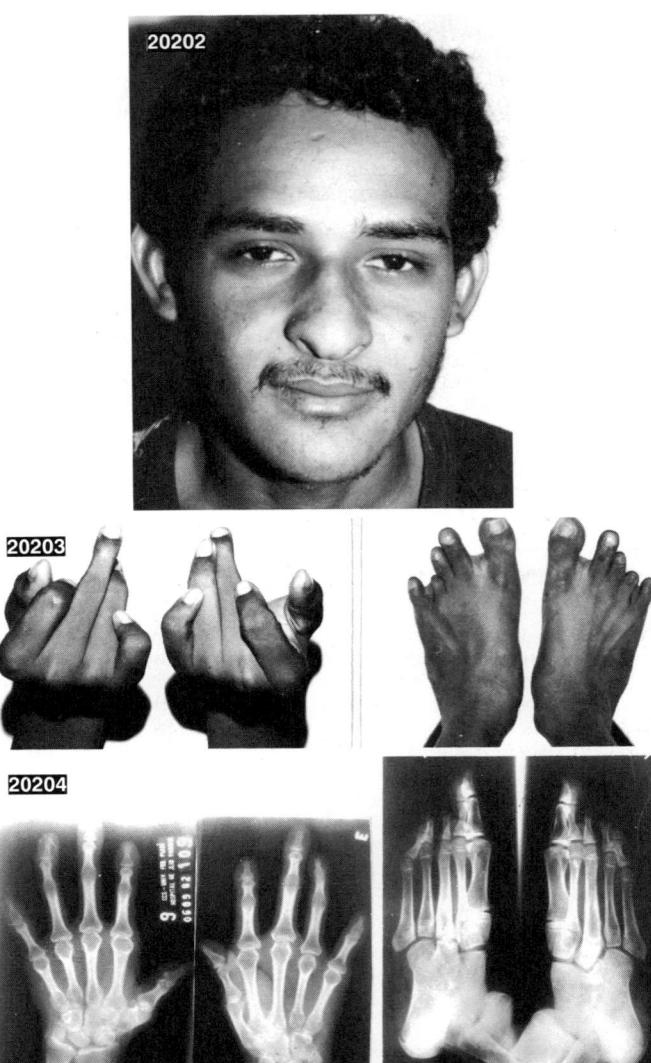

**1001B**-20202: Typical facies with hypoplastic nasal alae and short upper lip. 20203: Note symphalangism, clinodactyly, absence of part of the toes, and a wide gap between the first and second toes. 20204: X-rays of the hands and feet show symphalangism, carpal and tarsal synostosis, partial synostosis of the first and second metacarpals, tarsometatarsal synostosis, and agenesis of the phalanges.

can be observed in combination with other findings including brachydactyly, deafness, and other hand and foot anomalies.

The *Symphalangism-brachydactyly syndrome* (also known as *Deafness-symphalangism, Herrmann type, Synostoses, multiple-brachydactyly*, and the *WL symphalangism-brachydactyly syndrome*, is a specific disorder consisting of 1) Symphalangism, proximal, 100%; 2) Brachydactyly, especially involving the thumb and great toe, 100%; 3) Prominent cylindrical nose with hypoplastic alae nasi, 100%; 4) Carpal and tarsal coalitions, 100%; 5) Hypoplastic/absent

middle phalanges, 100%; 6) Cubitus valgus or limited range of motion at the elbow, 86%; 7) Conductive deafness, 72+%.

**Clinical Findings:** C.S. Lewis suffered from a specific form of symphalangism to which he attributed his decision to became an author (Lewis, 1955, p. 12). This "still thumbs" variant has also been observed in association with brachydactyly and mental retardation.

Both *distal* (Matthews et al, 1987) and *proximal* (Cremers et al, 1985) symphalangism have been described. Learman et al (1981) reported an Arabic kindred with proximal symphalangism and syndactyly, clinodactyly, hypoplasia of the thenar and hypothenar eminences, and unique dermatoglyphics.

*Cushing symphalangism*, which involves absence of the proximal interphalangeal joints, has been traced back, perhaps erroneously, to the Earl of Shrewsbury in the 15th century. Conductive hearing loss has also been reported in this condition (Cremers, et al, 1985).

*Multiple synostoses* is a feature of the *WL symphalangism-brachydactyly syndrome*, so designated by Herrmann (1974) from the names of the two husbands of the mother of the children described in his account. The syndrome itself was first reported by W.G. Fuhrmann in a 1966 issue of *Humangenetik*.

This pleiotropic syndrome is characterized by proximal symphalangism, brachydactyly, absence of distal portions of digits, dermatoglyphic abnormalities, shortness of first metacarpals/metatarsals, synostosis of carpal/tarsal bones, dislocation of the head of the radius, conductive hearing deficit, and a particular facial appearance. The face is long and narrow, with a prominent, long, hemicylindrical nose and a thin upper lip. The hearing deficit is apparently due to ankylosis of the stapes. Patients are of normal height but may have abnormal body proportions due to short arms. The syndrome shows considerable intrafamily variability. In early infancy, symphalangism may be apparent clinically (stiffness, absence of flexion and extension creases at the joint) but not on X-ray.

**Complications:** Limited joint mobility in fingers, wrists, elbows and feet; gait abnormalities.

**Associated Findings:** Strabismus, radial head dislocation, radiohumeral synostosis, and mild cutaneous syndactyly.

**Etiology:** Autosomal dominant inheritance.

**Pathogenesis:** Unknown.

**MIM No.:** 18565, *18570, 18575, *18580, *18640, *18650

**POS No.:** 3402

**Sex Ratio:** M1:F1

**Occurrence:** About 20 cases of WL symphalangism-brachydactyly syndrome have been reported from about six families, including one from Japan. A large Brazilian kindred with 28 cases of WL or a closely related condition was reported by da-Silva et al (1984). There is an extensive literature on other variants of symphalangism, but no consensus on their occurrence.

**Risk of Recurrence for Patient's Sib:**
See Part I, *Mendelian Inheritance.*

**Risk of Recurrence for Patient's Child:**
See Part I, *Mendelian Inheritance.*

**Age of Detectability:** Usually at birth.

**Gene Mapping and Linkage:** Unknown.

**Prevention:** None known. Genetic counseling indicated.

**Treatment:** The abnormalities of the arms, hands, and feet do not usually require surgical procedures. Patients with symphalangism should have a hearing evaluation (which may need to be repeated) to rule out a hearing deficit and a comprehensive skeletal survey to rule out further skeletal abnormalities. Hearing aids, stapedectomy, and insertion of a prosthesis may improve hearing.

**Prognosis:** Symphalangism, carpal synostoses and hearing loss are slowly progressive.

**Detection of Carrier:** Possibly by clinical examination of first degree relatives.

**References:**
Lewis CS: Surprised by joy. New York: Harcourt, Brace and World, 1955.
Maroteaux P, et al.: La maladie des synotoses multiples. Nouv Presse Med 1972; 1:3041–3047.†
Herrmann J: Symphalangism and brachydactyly syndrome: report of the *WL* symphalangism-brachydactyly syndrome: review of literature and classification. BD:OAS X(5). Miami: Symposia Specialists for The National Foundation-March of Dimes, 1974:23–53. †
Learman Y, et al.: Symphalangism with multiple anomalies of the hands and feet. Am J Med Genet 1981; 10:245–255.
Higashi K, Inoue S: Conductive deafness, symphalangism, and facial abnormalities: the WL syndrome in a Japanese family. Am J Med Genet 1983; 16:105–109. †
da-Silva EO, et al.: Multiple synostosis syndrome: study of a large Brazilian kindred. Am J Med Genet 1984; 18:237–247.

Cremers C, et al.: Proximal symphalangia and stapes ankylosis. Arch Otolaryng 1985; 111:765–767.
Hurvitz SA, et al.: The facio-audio-symphalangism syndrome: report of a case and review of the literature. Clin Genet 1985; 28:61–68.
Matthews S, et al.: Distal symphalangism with involvement of the thumbs and great toes. Clin Genet 1987; 32:375–378.

LU001
R0007
HE023
DA025

**Mark Lubinsky**
**Luther K. Robinson**
**Jürgen Herrmann**
**Elias O. da-Silva**

**Symphalangism, C.S. Lewis type**
*See SYMPHALANGISM*
**Symphalangism, distal**
*See SYMPHALANGISM*
**Symphalangism, proximal**
*See SYMPHALANGISM*
**Symphalangism-brachydactyly**
*See SYMPHALANGISM*
**Sympodia**
*See SIRENOMELIA SEQUENCE*
**Syncephalus**
*See TWINS, CONJOINED*
**Syncope and QT prolongation without deafness**
*See ARRHYTHMIA, WITH LONG QT INTERVAL WITHOUT DEAFNESS*

---

# SYNDACTYLY                                              0923

**Includes:**
Metacarpal 4–5 fusion
Syndactyly type I (zygodactyly)
Syndactyly type II (synpolydactyly)
Syndactyly type III (ring and little finger syndactyly)
Syndactyly type IV (Haas type and Cenani-Lenz type)
Syndactyly type V (with metacarpal and metatarsal fusion)

**Excludes:**
**Acrocephalosyndactyly type I** (0014)
**Amniotic bands syndrome** (0874)
**Poland syndrome** (0813)
Syndactyly with multifactorial inheritance

**Major Diagnostic Criteria:** Syndactyly indicates webbing between digits. Genetic types may be identified by determining if the abnormalities fit into a known characteristic patterns, and identifying similarly affected relatives.

**Clinical Findings:** In *syndactyly, type I* (zygodactyly), there is usually webbing between the 3rd and 4th fingers, either complete

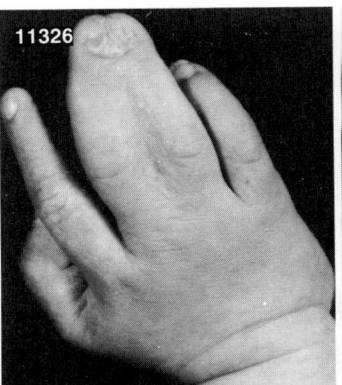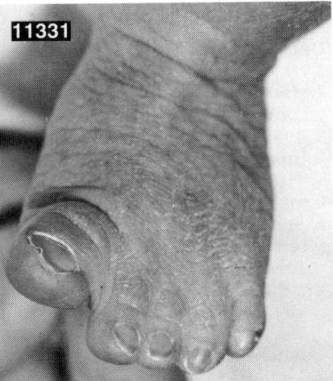

**0923-11326:** Syndactyly with bony fusion between fingers 3 and 4. **11331:** Complete syndactyly between toes 2, 3 and 4, and partial syndactyly between hallux and 2nd toe.

reaching to the nails, or partial, and occasionally associated with fusion of the distal phalanges of these fingers. Other fingers are sometimes also involved, but the 3rd and 4th fingers are the most commonly affected. In the feet, there is usually webbing between the 2nd and 3rd toes, either complete or partial.

In *syndactyly, type II* (synpolydactyly), there is usually syndactyly of the 3rd and 4th fingers associated with polydactyly of all components or of part of the 4th finger in the web. In the feet, there is polydactyly of the 5th toe.

In *syndactyly, type III* (ring and little finger syndactyly), syndactyly between the ring and the little fingers is usually complete and bilateral. The 5th finger is short, with absent or rudimentary middle phalanx. Feet are usually not affected in this type. This type of syndactyly is the hand malformation in oculodentoosseous dysplasia.

In *syndactyly, type IV* (Haas type) there is complete cutaneous fusion of the fingers, giving the hands a cup-like appearance. In Cenani-Lenz type the complete syndactyly is associated with bizarre disorganization of metacarpals and phalanges; the radius and ulna are either fused, short, or rudimentary. Feet are similarly affected.

In *syndactyly, type V*, there is an associated metacarpal and metatarsal fusion. The metacarpals and metatarsals most commonly fused are the 3rd and 4th or the 4th and 5th. Soft tissue syndactyly usually affects the 3rd and 4th fingers and the 2nd and 3rd toes. Syndactyly is usually more extensive and complete.

**Complications:** Unknown.

**Associated Findings:** None known.

**Etiology:** Autosomal dominant inheritance of most types. Fusion of metacarpals 4–5 is inherited as an X-linked recessive trait in some families. Cenani-Lenz syndactyly by autosomal recessive inheritance.

**Pathogenesis:** Unknown.

**MIM No.:** *18590, *18600, *18610, 18620, *18630, *21278, *30963

**CDC No.:** 755.1

**Sex Ratio:** M1:F1

**Occurrence:** Syndactyly type I (zygodactyly) is the most common, with an incidence of 1:3,000 live births in North Americans.

**Risk of Recurrence for Patient's Sib:**
See Part I, *Mendelian Inheritance.*

**Risk of Recurrence for Patient's Child:**
See Part I, *Mendelian Inheritance.*

**Age of Detectability:** At birth.

**Gene Mapping and Linkage:** MF4 (metacarpal 4–5 fusion) has been mapped to X.

**Prevention:** None known. Genetic counseling indicated.

**Treatment:** Surgical intervention.

**Prognosis:** Normal life span.

**Detection of Carrier:** Unknown.

**References:**
Haas SL: Bilateral complete syndactylism of all fingers. Am J Surg 1940; 50:363–366.
Johnston O, Kirby VV: Syndactyly of the ring and little finger. Am J Hum Genet 1955; 7:80–82.
Cross HE, et al.: Type II syndactyly. Am J Hum Genet 1968; 20:368–380.
Holmes LB, et al.: Metacarpal 4–5 fusion with X-linked recessive inheritance. Am J Hum Genet 1972; 24:562–568.
Temtamy SA, McKusick VA: The genetics of hand malformations. BD:OAS IV(3). New York: march of Dimes Birth Defects Foundation, 1978.
Castila EE, et al.: Syndactyly: frequency of specific types. Am J Med Genet 1980; 5:357–364.
Pfeiffer RA, Meisel-Stosiek M: Present nosology of the Cenani-Lenz type of syndactyly. Clin Genet 1982; 21:74–79.
Robinow M, et al.: Syndactyly type V. Am J Med Genet 1982; 11:475–482.
Merlob P, Grunebaum M: Type II syndactyly or synpolydactyly. J Med Genet 1986; 23:237–241.

TE004

**Samia A. Temtamy**

**Syndactyly type I (zygodactyly)**
*See* SYNDACTYLY
**Syndactyly type II (synpolydactyly)**
*See* SYNDACTYLY
**Syndactyly type III (ring and little finger syndactyly)**
*See* SYNDACTYLY
**Syndactyly type IV (Haas type and Cenani-Lenz type)**
*See* SYNDACTYLY
**Syndactyly type V (with metacarpal and metatarsal fusion)**
*See* SYNDACTYLY

## SYNDACTYLY, CENANI TYPE      2976

**Includes:**
Cenani-Lenz syndactyly
Cenani syndactylism

**Excludes:**
**Acrocephalosyndactyly**
**Poland syndrome** (0813)
**Syndactyly** (other)
Syndactyly associated with congenital constriction rings
Syndactyly with multifactorial inheritance

**Major Diagnostic Criteria:** Complete syndactyly of the digits, giving a mitten-like appearance to the hands. Fusion of all the carpal bones and disorganization of the metacarpals and phalanges.

**Clinical Findings:** The fingers are enclosed in the webbing and are deformed. The digits in some appear pea-shaped. Radioulnar synostosis is common, and the radius and ulna may be short or rudimentary. The feet may be similarly affected.

**Complications:** Unknown.

**Associated Findings:** None known.

**Etiology:** Autosomal recessive inheritance.

**Pathogenesis:** Unknown.

**MIM No.:** *21278

**POS No.:** 3887

**Sex Ratio:** M1:F1

**Occurrence:** About a dozen cases have been documented.

**Risk of Recurrence for Patient's Sib:**
See Part I, *Mendelian Inheritance.*

**Risk of Recurrence for Patient's Child:**
See Part I, *Mendelian Inheritance.*

**Age of Detectability:** At birth. Prenatal ultrasonography may detect this condition.

**Gene Mapping and Linkage:** Unknown.

**Prevention:** None known. Genetic counseling indicated.

**Treatment:** Surgical intervention.

**Prognosis:** Normal life span.

**Detection of Carrier:** Unknown.

**References:**
Cenani A, Lenz W: Total Syndaktylie und totale radioulnare Synostose bei zwei Bruedern. Ein Beitrag zur Genetik der Syndaktylien. Z Kinderheilkd 1967; 101:181–190.
Drohm D, et al.: Totale syndaktylie mit mesomeler Armverkerzung, radioulnaeren und metacarpalen Synostosen und Disorganisation der Phalangen ("Cenani-Syndaktylie"). Klin Paediatr 1976; 188:359–365.
Temtamy SA, McKusick VA: The genetics of hand malformations. New York: Alan R. Liss, 1978:320–322.
Dodinval P: Oligodactyly and multiple synostoses of the extremities: two case in sibs. Hum Genet 1979; 48:183–189.

Pfeiffer RA, Meisel-Stosiek M: Present nosology of the Cenani-Lenz type of syndactyly. Clin Genet 1982; 21:74–79.

HE006 **Jacqueline T. Hecht**

**Syndactyly-anophthalmos**
*See ANOPHTHALMIA-LIMB ANOMALIES*
**Syndactyly-cleft lip/palate-ectodermal dysplasia**
*See CLEFT LIP/PALATE-ECTODERMAL DYSPLASIA-SYNDACTYLY*
**Syndactyly-cleft lip/palate-oligodontia-hair defects**
*See CLEFT LIP/PALATE-OLIGODONTIA-SYNDACTYLY-HAIR DEFECTS*
**Syndactyly-cleft lip/palate-pili torti**
*See PILI TORTI-CLEFT LIP/PALATE-SYNDACTYLY*
**Syndactyly-cryptophthalmos**
*See FRASER SYNDROME*

## SYNDACTYLY-MICROCEPHALY-MENTAL RETARDATION, FILIPPI TYPE          2820

**Includes:**
Filippi syndrome
Microcephaly-syndactyly-mental retardation, Filippi type

**Excludes:**
**Aarskog syndrome** (0001)
**Blepharo-naso-facial syndrome** (2088)
**Cranio-digital syndrome-mental retardation, Scott type** (2831)
**KBG syndrome** (0554)
**Syndactyly**, type I (zigodactyly) syndromes, other
**Tricho-rhino-phalangeal syndrome, type II** (0967)
**Waardenburg syndromes** (0997)

**Major Diagnostic Criteria:** Unusual facial appearance, **Microcephaly**, retarded somatic and mental development, inability to speak, and **Syndactyly** type I of fingers and toes.

**Clinical Findings:** Growth retardation and low birth weight. Height, weight, and head size are generally below the third percentile. Broad and prominent nasal root and diminished alar flare give an unusual facial appearance. Striking **Syndactyly** of fingers 3 and 4, clinodactyly of finger 5, and **Syndactyly** of toes 2,3, and 4 are present; however, one girl showed an absence of finger syndactyly and presence of bilateral simian creases.

Mental retardation is severe to mild: with IQ between 30 and 60. Prepubertal genitalia with bilateral cryptorchidism and incomplete descent of testes are present in males. Inarticulate sounds or some utterance of sounds are recorded with no hearing deficit. Skeletal X-rays show moderately retarded bone age (two years below normal) in one male; brachymesophalangy of the fifth fingers; and syndactyly, limited to the soft tissues. Chromosomes have been normal (G and Q bands).

**Complications:** Defective speech and language development.

**Associated Findings:** None known.

**Etiology:** Possibly autosomal recessive inheritance with some variability in expression.

**Pathogenesis:** Unknown.

**MIM No.:** 27244

**POS No.:** 3725

**Sex Ratio:** Presumably M1:F1; M2:F1 observed.

**Occurrence:** Three of eight sibs (two boys and one girl) of healthy, unrelated parents from Italy have been documented.

**Risk of Recurrence for Patient's Sib:**
See Part I, *Mendelian Inheritance.*

**Risk of Recurrence for Patient's Child:**
See Part I, *Mendelian Inheritance.*

**Age of Detectability:** In early infancy.

**Gene Mapping and Linkage:** Unknown.

**Prevention:** None known. Genetic counseling indicated.

**Treatment:** Training in language through auditory or manual learning techniques, and oral speech training.

**Prognosis:** Normal life span. Mental retardation is severe to mild.

**Detection of Carrier:** Unknown.

**References:**
Filippi G: Unusual facial appearance, microcephaly, growth and mental retardation, and syndactyly: a new syndrome? Am J Med Genet 1985; 22:821–824.

FI030 **Giorgio Filippi**

## SYNDACTYLY-POLYDACTYLY-EAR LOBE SYNDROME          3042

**Includes:**
Ear lobe-syndactyly-polydactyly syndrome
Goldberg-Pashayan syndrome
Polydactyly-syndactyly-ear lobe syndrome

**Excludes:**
**Polydactyly** (isolated)
**Polysyndactyly-dysmorphic craniofacies, Greig type** (2925)
Zygodactyly

**Major Diagnostic Criteria:** The combination of **Polydactyly** of hands and sometimes feet, **Syndactyly** of the toes, and minor earlobe anomalies should suggest the diagnosis.

**Clinical Findings:** Ten affected individuals from a single family have been described. Earlobe anomalies consisted of a deep, horizontal groove (7/10) or a nodule (2/10). Five individuals had bilateral postaxial polydactyly of the hands, with the extra digit ranging from a soft tissue nubbin to a well-formed finger. Foot anomalies included hallux syndactyly (6/10), syndactyly of toes 2–3 (5/10), preaxial polydactyly (7/10), MTP delta phalanx (4/10), and accessory metatarsal (4/10), occurring alone or in combination. However, only four individuals had all three anomalies (earlobe, foot, and hand); the other six had only one or two of the above-listed findings.

**Complications:** Unknown.

**Associated Findings:** None known.

**Etiology:** Autosomal dominant inheritance. This condition was originally reported in three generations of one kindred, with male-to-male transmission occurring twice.

**Pathogenesis:** Unknown.

**MIM No.:** *18635

**POS No.:** 3901

**Sex Ratio:** M1:F1

**Occurrence:** One United States family with ten affected members has been reported.

**Risk of Recurrence for Patient's Sib:**
See Part I, *Mendelian Inheritance.*

**Risk of Recurrence for Patient's Child:**
See Part I, *Mendelian Inheritance.*

**Age of Detectability:** At birth by the presence of hand and foot anomalies.

**Gene Mapping and Linkage:** Unknown.

**Prevention:** None known. Genetic counseling indicated.

**Treatment:** Surgical removal of extra digits or release of syndactyly, if indicated.

**Prognosis:** Life span and intellect are not affected.

**Detection of Carrier:** Unknown.

**References:**
Goldberg MJ, Pashayan HM: Hallux syndactyly, ulnar polydactyly, abnormal ear lobes: a new syndrome. BD:OAS XII(5). New York: March of Dimes Birth Defects Foundation, 1976:255–266.

T0007 **Helga V. Toriello**

**Syngnathism, congenital**
  *See CLEFT PALATE-PERSISTENCE OF BUCCOPHARYNGEAL MEMBRANE*
**Synkinetic ptosis**
  *See JAW-WINKING SYNDROME*
**Synopthalmia**
  *See CYCLOPIA*
**Synostoses (multiple)-conduction deafness**
  *See SYMPHALANGISM*
**Synostoses, multiple-brachydactyly**
  *See SYMPHALANGISM*

---

## SYNOSTOSIS                                        1522

**Includes:**  Symphalangism

Synostosis denotes the presence of bony fusions that cause limitation of joint movement, eg. extension, flexion, supination and pronation. The long bones of the upper extremities are most often affected but carpals, tarsals, and phalanges can also be involved. Synostosis specifically denotes either fusion of sutures, as in the calvarium or fusion of two long bones as in **Radial-ulnar synostosis**. *Symphalangism* describes fusion of the phalanges and coalition refers to fusion of the carpal or tarsal bones. Bony fusions may be difficult to detect in the newborn or in early childhood but decreased range of movement and reduction of the joint space on X-ray are suggestive of synostosis.

Bony fusions can occur from trauma or arise secondarily from abnormal bone growth such as that occuring in **Exostoses, multiple cartilaginous**. In this condition, the bony outgrowths can cause bridging and synostosis which leads to bony deformation and decreased range of joint movement. Bony fusions may be isolated abnormalities or part of single gene and chromosomal syndromes. For example, **Radial-ulnar synostosis** is an autosomal dominant condition, but radioulnar synostosis also commonly occurs in the 48,XXXY, 49,XXXXY and **Acrofacial dysostosis, Nager type**. Multiple joints can be involved such as that seen in **Synostosis, multiple synostosis syndrome** where symphalangism, carpal and tarsal coalitions and occasionally radiohumeral synostosis occur. Symphalangism is also present in dwarfing conditions such as **Diastrophic dysplasia** and **Kniest dysplasia**.

The pathogenesis of bony fusions is unknown. Atrophy and fibrosis of the supernator and pronator muscles and thickened interosseous membranes have been found in the radioulnar synostosis suggesting longterm joint immobility. Isolated unilateral synostosis generally is not genetic, but bilateral involvement usually has a genetic etiology. Indeed **Radial-ulnar synostosis** is an autosomal dominant condition; and autosomal recessive and dominant patterns of inheritance have been reported for conditions associated with radiohumeral synostosis. When synostosis occurs as part of a condition, recurrence of the bony abnormality is related to the frequency that it occurs in the condition and the recurrence of the condition.

Treatment of bony fusions is limited. Surgery is generally not recommended except where there is a possibility of obtaining a more functional fixed position of an extremity. Physical therapy early in life is not recommended for dwarfing conditions as it may cause the fusions to worsen.

HE006                                    **Jacqueline T. Hecht**

**Synostosis, humero-radial**
  *See HUMERO-RADIAL SYNOSTOSIS*
**Synostosis, radial cubital**
  *See RADIAL-ULNAR SYNOSTOSIS*
**Synotia-agnathia-microstomia**
  *See AGNATHIA-MICROSTOMIA-SYNOTIA*

## SYNOVITIS, FAMILIAL HYPERTROPHIC                  2155

**Includes:**
  Arthritis, "E" family
  Arthropathy-camptodactyly syndrome
  Camptodactyly-arthropathy syndrome
  Jacobs syndrome
  Pericarditis-arthropathy-camptodactyly (CAP) syndrome

**Excludes:**
  **Arthritis, rheumatoid** (2517)
  Thumbs, trigger

**Major Diagnostic Criteria:**  1) Onset soon after birth of trigger thumbs followed by flexion contractures of other proximal interphalangeal joints; 2) development of painless effusions at large joints (especially knees, wrists and ankles) during early childhood; 3) no fever, rash, iritis, visceromegaly, nodules, leucocytosis, systemic illness; 4) normal growth and development; 5) no radiographic destructive changes; femoral necks unusually broad and with varus deformity (present in three other families; not commented on in other reported cases; 6) distinctive microscopic pathology with large hypertrophic avascular synovial villi with giant cells but no underlying inflammation. Some villi are lined by or replaced by fibrin-like material; 7) similar findings in affected tendon sheaths extend into the underlying tendons causing tight adhesions of tendon sheaths to tendons. These are difficult to lyse. A large amount of fibrous tissue is seen in underlying normal tendons.

**Clinical Findings:**  Trigger thumbs are the first manifestation noted during the first few months of life, followed soon thereafter by flexion contractures in the proximal interphalangeal joints of other fingers. A diagnosis of tenosynovitis is made and tendon sheath releases are often performed. Joint effusions are then noted at the knee and typical pathologic findings have been demonstrated in biopsy material taken from the knee as early as age 20 months. Synovial "pouches" become apparent at the wrists and effusions are apparent in the ankle joints. While the children have no pain at first, during the second decade pain and morning stiffness become more apparent and progressive limitations are noted at the hips with exaggerated lumbar lordosis.

In early childhood the erythrocyte sedimentation rate (ESR) is normal, but in one affected family the ESR was elevated during later childhood. Elevation of the ESR has not been noted in other families.

There is a paucity of X-ray findings in childhood, but in three families there was a striking varus deformity of the femoral necks.

**Complications:**  During the third decade of life one affected individual developed extraordinary chondrocalcinosis with progressively increasing amounts of calcium being demonstrable on X-ray in joint spaces. This patient had increasingly frequent attacks of pseudogout. One of her sibs was said to have a similar problem, although this could not be demonstrated on X-ray.

**Associated Findings:**  Acute pericarditis, and in some cases constrictive pericarditis, has been seen as a feature of this syndrome in three recent reports; one patient had a brief attack of pericarditis thought to be tuberculous.

**Etiology:**  Although the number of affected individuals in each reported family (6/11;3/5;3/3;2/2) suggested autosomal dominant inheritance with absence of the disease in any parent being explained by incomplete penetrance, affected individuals in the oldest family now have seven unaffected children. This observation, plus the absence of disease in the parents, and the fact that at least initially the disease was only recognized when multifamily cases presented, now makes recessive inheritance much more likely. Of the 14 reported cases only three were male, but all families had a predominance of female children.

**Pathogenesis:**  Possibly a chemical defect affecting synovial lining cells. There are no reports of attempts to grow the cells in tissue culture.

**MIM No.:**  *20825

**Sex Ratio:** M1:F5 original reports; M4:F7 patients with pericarditis.

**Occurrence:** About two dozen cases have been reported.

**Risk of Recurrence for Patient's Sib:**
See Part I, *Mendelian Inheritance.*

**Risk of Recurrence for Patient's Child:**
See Part I, *Mendelian Inheritance.*

**Age of Detectability:** May be suspected at two months of age; diagnosis possible in the second year in a first case in a family, but by two months of age in subsequent cases.

**Gene Mapping and Linkage:** Unknown.

**Prevention:** None known. Genetic counseling indicated.

**Treatment:** Diagnosis enables avoidance of hazardous medications prescribed for juvenile rheumatoid arthritis, including corticosteroids which have been administered to many affected children. Appropriate surgery (finger tendon releases) can be performed and inappropriate surgery (open synovial biopsies) can be avoided. In later life if chondrocalcinosis appears with symptoms of pseudogout treatment can be tailored to maneuvers appropriate for crystal arthropathy rather than rheumatoid arthritis, gout or infection.

**Prognosis:** Normal function is the rule throughout childhood but tendon sheath releases are required for satisfactory use and appearance of fingers. More severely affected individuals develop rather severe limitation of motion of the hips which is progressive during the second and third decades and disability may be expected to increase thereafter.

**Detection of Carrier:** The mother of the index family always had an elevated erythrocyte sedimentation rate and developed increasing but undefined arthritic complaints during the fifth decade of life.

**Special Considerations:** It remains to be determined whether this disorder is to be included as one of the forms of familial pyrophosphate arthropathy; however, none of the described forms begin in early childhood or have the markers of the disease observable in all of these children. It is possible that the crystal arthritis seen in the one older individual, and perhaps developing in others, is a non-specific secondary effect of the defect rather than a clue to etiology and pathogenesis of the disorder.

A similar disorder, *Familial arthritis and camptodactyly* (Malleson et al.: Arthritis Rheum 1981; 24:1199–1204) is distinguished by biopsy evidence of inflammation in the synovium, a finding strikingly absent in all reported cases of familial hypertrophic synovitis.

**References:**
Athreya BH, Schumacher HR: Pathologic features of a familial arthropathy associated with congenital flexion contractures of fingers. Arthritis Rheum 1978; 21:429–437.
Malleson P, et al.: Familial arthritis and camptodactyly. Arthritis Rheum 1981; 24:1199–1204.
Jacobs JC: Pediatric rheumatology for the practitioner. New York: Springer-Verlag, 1982:151–154.
Martinez-Lavin M, et al.: A familial syndrome of pericarditis arthritis and camptodactyly. New Engl J Med 1983; 309:224–225.
Ochi T, et al.: The pathology of the involved tendons in patients with familial arthropathy and congenital camptodactyly. Arthritis Rheum 1983; 26:896–900.
Bulutlar G, et al.: A familial syndrome of pericarditis, arthritis, camptodactyly, and coxa vera. Arthritis Rheum 1986; 29:436–438.
Laxer RM, et al.: The camptodactyly-arthropathy-pericarditis syndrome: case report and literature review. Arthritis Rheum 1986; 29:439–444.

JA012                                              **Jerry C. Jacobs**

**Synovitis-granulomatous-uveitis-cranial neoropathies, familial**
*See GRANULOMATOSIS-POLYSYNOVITIS, FAMILIAL SYSTEMIC*
**Syphilis, prenatal**
*See FETAL SYPHILIS SYNDROME*
**Syphonoma**
*See SCALP, CYLINDROMAS*

---

## SYRINGOMYELIA                                    0924

**Includes:**
Gliosis
Spinal cord cavitation
**Excludes:**
Intramedullary spinal cord tumor
**Myopathy**
**Neuropathy**

**Major Diagnostic Criteria:** Progressive muscular atrophy of the upper extremities associated with anesthesia and trophic changes.

**Clinical Findings:** Syringomyelia most commonly involves the cervical enlargement of the spinal cord. The pathologic process of cavitation most frequently originates in the region of the anterior white commissure. The symptoms and signs result from expanding cavitation and subsequent gliosis.

Rapidly progressive scoliosis is relatively common. Atrophy and weakness of the intrinsic hand muscles may be the first finding, but progressive wasting of arm, trunk, and neck musculature follows. The upper limbs are flaccid and areflexic. The corticospinal tracts are often compromised, so that spasticity, weakness, hyperreflexia, and extensor plantar responses are noted in the lower limbs.

Sensory symptoms, particularly loss of pain and temperature sensation, are the result of destruction of the lateral spinothalamic tracts. Analgesia is usually more apparent than tactile anesthesia. Trophic changes include Charcot joints, abnormalities of perspiration, and skin ulceration. The most frequent age of presentation is during the third and fourth decades.

Cervical spine X-rays may show widening of the interpediculate distance, particularly in the sagittal diameter. Bony erosion is rare. The CSF protein may be elevated. Myelography frequently shows an abnormally enlarged spinal cord. CT may demonstrate the lesion, but MRI is the procedure of choice to demonstrate the location and extent of cystic lesion.

**Complications:** Poser (1956) examined 245 cases of syringomyelia and found a 16% incidence of associated intramedullary tumors. Mild trauma to the cord has been reported to cause bleeding within the cavity followed by marked deterioration in function. Syringobulbia may occur due to upward extension of the process from the cervical spinal cord into the medulla producing lower cranial nerve abnormalities and bulbar signs causing aspiration, pneumonia, and death.

**Associated Findings:** Spina bifida, **Klippel-Feil anomaly**, cervical ribs, **Brain, Arnold-Chiari malformation, Hydrocephaly**, webbed fingers, abnormal hair distribution, basilar impression and invagination, and hypospadias.

**Etiology:** Both autosomal dominant and autosomal recessive inheritance have been suggested, with little evidence. Most cases are non-familial.

**Pathogenesis:** Syringomyelia may be the result of an abnormality of embryogenesis. The abnormality may be the result of an arrest in the development of the spinal cord before complete differentiation of gray and white matter occurs. An alternate theory suggests that during development of the cord there is a failure of the normal migration of spongioblasts from the central canal region. These cells later develop the capability of proliferating and causing cavitation. Netsky (1953) suggested that syringomyelia is the result of developmental anomalies of the intramedullary blood supply, which leads to infarction, gliosis, and cavity formation.

**MIM No.:** 18670, 27248

**CDC No.:** 336.000

**Sex Ratio:** M1:F1

**Occurrence:** Hundreds of cases have been reported.

**Risk of Recurrence for Patient's Sib:** Unknown.

**Risk of Recurrence for Patient's Child:** Unknown.

**Age of Detectability:** Usually between the ages of 20 and 40 years, primarily by physical examination, CT, and myelography.

The condition may be detected in infancy, particularly when a spinal MRI is obtained in connection with evaluation for an associated spina bifida, occult dysraphism, and craniovertebral anomalies.

**Gene Mapping and Linkage:** Unknown.

**Prevention:** None known. Genetic counseling indicated.

**Treatment:** Laminectomy and appropriate drainage of the rapidly enlarging cavity is indicated in the presence of progressive neurologic signs. Trophic skin changes require treatment.

**Prognosis:** Slowly progressive. Bulbar paralysis may lead to chronic aspiration and death. Has been fatal in over one-half of all cases.

**Detection of Carrier:** Unknown.

**References:**

Jackson M: Familial lumbosacral syringomyelia and the significance of developmental errors of the spinal cord and column. Med J Aust 1949; 1:433.

Netsky M: Syringomyelia: a clinical pathologic study. Arch Neurol Psychiatry 1953; 70:741.

Poser CM: Relationship between syringomyelia and neoplasm. Springfield: Charles C Thomas, 1956.

Bentley SJ, et al.: Familial syringomyelia. J Neurol Neurosurg 1975; 38:346–349.

Dichiro G, et al.: Computerized axial tomography in syringomyelia. New Engl J Med 1975; 292:13.

Gimenez-Roldan S, et al.: Familial communicating syringomyelia. J Neuro Sci 1978; 36:135–146.

HA053                                    **Robert H.A. Haslam**

**Systemic carnitine deficiency due to MCAD**
  See *ACYL-CoA DEHYDROGENASE DEFICIENCY, MEDIUM CHAIN TYPE*

**Systemic elastorrhexis**
  See *PSEUDOXANTHOMA ELASTICUM*

**Systemic G(M2)-gangliosidosis**
  See *G(M2)-GANGLIOSIDOSIS WITH HEXOSAMINIDASE A AND B DEFICIENCY*

**Systemic lupus erythematosis (SLE)**
  See *LUPUS ERYTHEMATOSUS, SYSTEMIC*

# ❖ T ❖

**T-cell antigen receptor, alpha subunit (TCRA)**
*See LEUKEMIA/LYMPHOMA, T-CELL*
**T-cell chronic lymphocytic leukemia**
*See LEUKEMIA/LYMPHOMA, T-CELL*
**T-cell leukemia/lymphoma, adult**
*See LEUKEMIA/LYMPHOMA, T-CELL*
**T-cell prolymphocytic leukemia**
*See LEUKEMIA/LYMPHOMA, T-CELL*
**T-lymphocyte deficiency**
*See IMMUNODEFICIENCY, NEZELOF TYPE*
**Tabatznik syndrome**
*See HEART-HAND SYNDROME II*
**Tabes of Friedreich**
*See ATAXIA, FRIEDREICH TYPE*
**Tachycardia, junctional**
*See ARRHYTHMIA, SUPRAVENTRICULAR TACHYCARDIAS, CONGENITAL*
**Takahara syndrome**
*See ACATALASEMIA*
**Talipes calcaneovalgus**
*See FOOT, CONGENITAL CLUBFOOT*
**Talipes equinovarus, congenital idiopathic**
*See FOOT, TALIPES EQUINOVARUS (TEV)*
**Tangier disease**
*See ANALPHALIPOPROTEINEMIA*
**Tapazole∧, fetal effects**
*See FETAL EFFECTS FROM METHIMAZOLE AND CARBIMAZOLE*
**Tapetochoroidal dystrophy, progressive**
*See CHOROIDEREMIA*
**Tapetoretinal degeneration-alopecia**
*See RETINOPATHY-HYPOTRICHOSIS SYNDROME*
**TAR syndrome**
*See THROMBOCYTOPENIA-ABSENT RADIUS*
**Tarsomegaly**
*See DYSPLASIA EPIPHYSEALIS HEMIMELICA*
**Tarui disease**
*See GLYCOGENOSIS, TYPE VII*
**Taste blindness**
*See TASTING DEFECT, PHENYLTHIOCARBAMIDE*
**Taste threshold to bitter compounds containing the N-C-S group**
*See TASTING DEFECT, PHENYLTHIOCARBAMIDE*

---

## TASTING DEFECT, PHENYLTHIOCARBAMIDE          0809

**Includes:**
Phenylthiocarbamide tasting
Phenylthiourea insensitivity
PTC taster defect
Taste blindness
Taste threshold to bitter compounds containing the N-C-S group

**Excludes:** Taste threshold to other substances, hereditary differences.

**Major Diagnostic Criteria:** Inability to taste dilute phenylthiocarbamide (PTC). There is a bimodal population curve for detecting increasing concentrations of PTC. Tasters can detect bitterness at 50 parts per million (ppm), whereas nontasters can detect only concentrations of about 400 ppm.

**Clinical Findings:** The threshold for the bitter taste of substances containing the N-C=S group, such as phenylthiocarbamide, propylthiouracil, and naturally occurring goitrogens, such as goitrin, is bimodal in many populations. The only other substance which elicits this bimodal threshold is anetholtrithione.

Goitrin or other thioureas occur in cabbage, kale and rutabaga in quantities too dilute to evoke a bitter taste. When eaten in excess, they may cause goiters by inhibiting both iodide organification and iodotyrosine coupling in thyroglobulin. This is especially true for small animals and human infants fed milk from cows eating large quantities of these or similar foods. The goitrogenic effect is independent of the taster status of the individual.

**Complications:** Unknown.

**Associated Findings:** Tasters having the HLA-B8 antigen have a six-fold greater incidence of Graves' disease, whereas nontasters are more likely to be hypothyroid, with nodular goiter. Most athyrotic cretins are nontasters.

Depression is more common among tasters according to a subjective test of depression severity (Beck's Depression Inventory). There is an increased incidence of nontasters associated with **Diabetes mellitus**.

Congenital cataracts, aphakic retinal detachment, and both convergent and divergent squint are associated with a higher incidence of nontasters. There is also an increased incidence of nontasters in people with primary simple **Glaucoma**, and of tasters in people with closed angle glaucoma; individuals with congenital glaucoma are more likely to be tasters.

Some studies indicate an increased incidence of nontasters among alcoholics, but the effect of alcohol on taste sensitivity in general is unknown.

**Etiology:** Homozygosity of a recessive gene, t. Individuals who are heterozygous (Tt) and homozygous for T are tasters.

**Pathogenesis:** Unknown.

**MIM No.:** *17120

**Sex Ratio:** M1:F1

**Occurrence:** About 30% among individuals of western European descent; lower or almost non-existent in some African, Chinese, American Indian, Brasilian Indian and Eskimo populations. The highest gene frequency of t (0.76) was reported among the Kayastha Indian community, but their smoking and eating habits may predispose them to general taste insensitivity.

**Risk of Recurrence for Patient's Sib:** 25% if neither parent is a nontaster; 50% if one parent is a nontaster; 100% if both parents are nontasters.

**Risk of Recurrence for Patient's Child:** 100% if spouse is a nontaster; 50% if spouse is heterozygous; 0% if spouse is TT.

**Age of Detectability:** In infancy. There is a slight diminution of taste sensitivity with advancing age.

**Gene Mapping and Linkage:** PTC (phenylthiocarbamide tasting) is ULG1.

Linked to Kell with a lod score of 10.78 for a theta = 0.045.

**Prevention:** None known. Genetic counseling indicated.

**Treatment:** Appropriate treatment for associated conditions is required.

**Prognosis:** Excellent.

**Detection of Carrier:** Taster parent or taster child of an affected individual. There is no reliable distinction between TT and Tt individuals, although heterozygotes have somewhat diminished thresholds.

**Special Considerations:** Some associations have been single studies of limited population groups. Although statistical significance has been demonstrated, panethnicity has not. The odor of PTC solutions may contribute to taste perception.

**References:**

Harris H, Kalmus H: The measurement of taste sensitivity to phenylthiourea (PTC). Ann Eugen 1949; 15:24–31.
Conneally PM, et al.: Linkage relations of the loci for Kell and phenylthiocarbamide (PTC) taste sensitivity. Hum Hered 1976; 26:267–271.
Farid NR, et al.: HLA and phenylthiocarbamide (PTC) tasting in autoimmune thyroid disease. Tissue Antigens 1977; 10:414–416.
David R, Jenkins T: Genetic markers in glaucoma. Brit J Ophthalm 1980; 64:227–231.
Padma T, Murty JS: Association of genetic markers with some eye diseases. Acta Anthropogenetica 1983; 7:1–12.
Swinson RP: Genetic markers and alcoholism. Recent developments in Alcoholism 1983; 1:9–24.
Whittemore PB: Phenylthiocarbamide (PTC) tasting and reported depression. J Clin Psychol 1986; 42:260–263.

VI006
KA006

Jaclyn M. Vidgoff
Hans Kalmus

**Taurodontism**
*See TEETH, TAURODONTISM*

---

## TAURODONTISM-SHORT ROOTED TEETH-MICROCEPHALIC DWARFISM 3232

**Includes:**

Dwarfism, microcephalic-taurodontism-short rooted teeth
Sauk syndrome
Teeth, short rooted-taurodontism-microcephalic dwarfism

**Excludes:**

**Angelman syndrome** (2086)
**Beckwith-Wiedemann syndrome** (0104)
**Bloom syndrome** (0112)
**Chromosome XXY, XXYY, and XXXXY syndromes with taurodontism**
**Cockayne syndrome**
**De Lange syndrome** (0242)
**Meckel syndrome** (0634)
**Neu-laxova syndrome** (2092)
**Oculo-cerebro-facial syndrome, Kaufman type** (2179)
**Rubinstein-Taybi broad thumb-hallux syndrome** (0119)
**Seckel syndrome** (0881)
**Teeth, taurodontism** (0926)
**Tricho-dento-osseous syndrome** (0965)
**Tricho-rhino-phalangeal syndrome**

**Major Diagnostic Criteria:** Taurodontism and short rooted teeth in conjunction with microcephalic dwarfism.

**Clinical Findings:** Low-birth-weight (1,040–2,068), small placental, microcephalic dwarfism. The facies are small and delicate. The nose is thin but not prominently beaked. The eyes are proportional in size to the face, and the ear lobes are distinct. The mandible is usually small with a class II occlusion and maxillary overbite, and the chin is not small or retruded. There is no cleft palate.

This syndrome is characterized by the dentition. There is true microdontia. The teeth are small in proportion to the small face. The incisors do not meet at contact points. The enamel is of normal thickness relative to the booth size. The teeth have been reported to be mobile and can shed spontaneously.

On X-ray, the molars are taurodont and may contain pulpal calcifications. The roots of the anterior teeth are short and may be foreshortened by external resorption. Periapical radiolucent areas develop on anterior teeth with apical resorption without a history of trauma.

**Complications:** The most obvious complications are the premature loss of teeth, progressive malposition of teeth, and the development of diastemas between teeth. Affected individuals are retarded but usually shy and passive.

**Associated Findings:** Class II malocclusion and pulpal calcifications.

**Etiology:** Possibly autosomal recessive inheritance. In all instances, parents and parental relatives have been unaffected. Karyotypes have been 46,XY in male patients. G-banded karyotypes, chromosomal breakage, and sister chromatid exchanges have been normal.

**Pathogenesis:** Unknown.

**Sex Ratio:** M3:F1

**Occurrence:** The condition has been documented in four cases; American Caucasians, French-Canadians, and Japanese.

**Risk of Recurrence for Patient's Sib:**
See Part I, *Mendelian Inheritance*. Observed figure is 40%.

**Risk of Recurrence for Patient's Child:** Unknown. Affected individuals have not been known to reproduce.

**Age of Detectability:** After the age of seven for the permanent dentition, by radiographic examination.

**Gene Mapping and Linkage:** Unknown.

**Prevention:** None known. Genetic counseling indicated.

**Treatment:** Routine oral hygiene.

**Prognosis:** Unknown.

**Detection of Carrier:** Unknown.

**References:**

Sauk JJ, et al.: Taurodontism, diminished root formation and microcephalic dwarfism. Oral Surg 1973; 36:231–235.
Gardner DG, Girgis B: Taurodontism, short roots, and external resorption, associated with short stature and a small head. Oral Surg 1977; 44:271–273.
Tsuchiya H, et al.: Analysis of the dentition and orofacial skeleton in Seckel's bird-headed dwarfism. J Max-Fac Surg 1981; 9:170–175.

SA029
WI043

John J. Sauk
Carl J. Witkop, Jr.

**Taussig-Bing syndrome**
*See VENTRICLE, DOUBLE-OUTLET RIGHT WITH ANTERIOR SEPTAL DEFECT*
**Tay syndrome**
*See TRICHOTHIODYSTROPHY*
**Tay-Sachs disease**
*See G(M2)-GANGLIOSIDOSIS WITH HEXOSAMINIDASE A DEFICIENCY*
**Tay-Sachs with visceral involvement**
*See G(M1)-GANGLIOSIDOSIS, TYPE 1*
**TC2 deficiency**
*See TRANSCOBALAMIN II DEFICIENCY*
**Tear duct, blocked**
*See NASOLACRIMAL DUCT OBSTRUCTION*
**Teeth (anomalies)-skeletal dysplasia-sparse hair**
*See CRANIO-ECTODERMAL DYSPLASIA*
**Teeth (conical)-polydactyly-nail dysplasia-short limbs**
*See ACROFACIAL SYNDROME, CURRY-HALL TYPE*
**Teeth (coniform)-onychodystrophy-deafness**
*See ONYCHODYSTROPHY-CONIFORM TEETH-SENSORINEURAL HEARING LOSS*
**Teeth (pseudoanodontia)-growth retardation-alopecia**
*See GROWTH RETARDATION-ALOPECIA-PSEUDOANODONTIA-OPTIC ATROPHY*
**Teeth retention**
*See TEETH, IMPACTED*

## TEETH, AMELOGENESIS IMPERFECTA         0046

**Includes:**

Amelogenesis imperfecta, hypocalcification type
Amelogenesis imperfecta, hypomaturation type
Amelogenesis imperfecta, hypoplastic type
Amelogenesis imperfecta, pigmented hypomaturation type
Enamel hypoplasia, hereditary
Enamel, hypoplastic-hypocalcified with taurodontism
Enamel, hypoplastic-hypomaturation
Enamel, hypoplastic-hypomaturation-taurodontism
Microdontia, generalized

**Excludes:**

Enamel defects associated with extrinsic causes
Enamel defects associated with generalized diseases
Enamel defects associated with syndromes
Isolated taurodontism-trichodentoosseous, isolated
**Teeth, enamel hypoplasia** (0342)
**Teeth, snow-capped** (2136)

**Major Diagnostic Criteria:** All or most teeth have defective enamel and other possible causes have been eliminated.

**Clinical Findings:** Clinical, X-ray and histologic features vary according to type of amelogenesis. Both primary and permanent dentitions are affected unless otherwise noted. Anterior open bite is common in the severe hypoplastic and hypocalcified types. Several types have been deliniated:

*Type I, Hypoplastic* The enamel does not develop to normal thickness. On X-ray, the enamel contrasts normally from dentin.

*Type IA, The hypoplastic, pitted autosomal dominant type* has enamel with random pits from pinpoint to pinhead size, located primarily on labial or buccal surfaces in permanent teeth, often arranged in rows and columns. Some teeth may appear normal in both dentitions.

*Type IB, The hypoplastic, local autosomal dominant type* may affect only primary teeth or teeth in both dentitions. Pits and grooves of hypoplastic enamel occur in a horizontal fashion across the middle third of the tooth. All or only some teeth show this defect. Most frequently affected are the incisors, premolars, or primary molars.

*Type IC, The hypoplastic, local autosomal recessive type* is more severe than the dominant type. Nearly all teeth are affected in both dentitions. Type IC has been described by Chosack et al (1979).

*Type ID, The hypoplastic, smooth autosomal dominant type,* in which the enamel is generally thin so the crowns frequently do not meet at contact points. The enamel is hard, glossy, smooth, and varies from white to yellow-brown in color, except at contact points, where it may be hypocalcified and stained. X-rays show a thin layer of enamel outlining the crown. Unerupted teeth that undergo intraalveolar resorption are frequent. Small calcified bodies

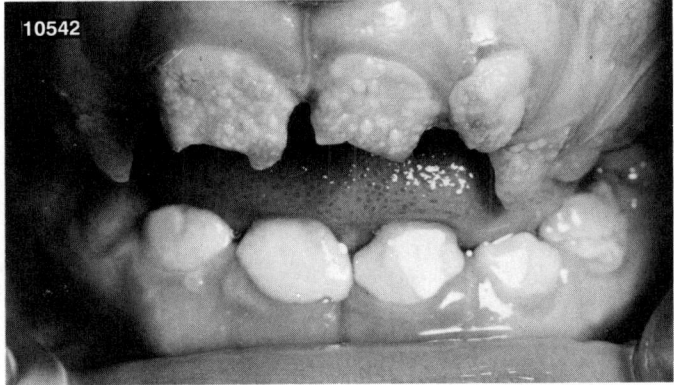

**0046-10542:** Amelogenesis imperfecta, hypocalcified type.

may be seen adjacent to unerupted teeth. Anterior open bite occurs in about 50%.

*Type IE, The hypoplastic, smooth X-linked dominant type* affects males who have enamel that is thin, brown to yellow-brown, smooth, and shiny. Carrier females have alternating vertical bands of normal and abnormal enamel (Lyon effect). X-rays of male teeth show a thin layer of enamel outlining the crowns. Unerupted teeth with resorption of crowns are less frequently seen here than in types ID, IF, IG, and IIA. Anterior open bite occurs in most males and in about one-half of affected females. X-rays of female teeth show vertical banding of the enamel.

*Type IF, The hypoplastic, rough autosomal dominant type* is associated with a thin, brown, very hard enamel, which has a granular vitreous surface. Contact between adjacent teeth is lacking. On X-ray, the teeth are outlined by a thin layer of enamel. There is high contrast between the enamel and dentin. Unerupted teeth with resorption of crowns may occur. Anterior open bite occurs in about 50% of cases.

*Type IG, The enamel agenesis autosomal recessive type* has a rough, granular tooth surface and is light yellow-brown in color. Adjacent teeth lack contact. There is no X-ray evidence of enamel, and many teeth are unerupted and partially resorbed in the alveolus. On microscopic examination the only evidence of enamel is the laminated agate-like vitreous calcification on the dentin surface. Anterior open bite occurs frequently, 9:11. It is not known if this type is different from enamel agenesis and nephrocalcinosis.

*Type II, Hypomaturation* The enamel is of normal thickness but has a mottled appearance, is slightly softer than normal enamel, and chips from the crown. On X-ray, the enamel has approximately the same radiodensity as dentin.

*Type IIA, The hypomaturation, pigmented autosomal recessive type* has enamel that is clear to cloudy, mottled, agar-brown in color, and of normal thickness. The enamel fractures from the dentin and is softer than normal, admitting a probe point under pressure. X-rays show lack of contrast between enamel and dentin. Unerupted teeth with resorption of the crowns are uncommon. Anterior open bite occurs infrequently.

*Type IIB, The hypomaturation, X-linked recessive type.* In affected males, the enamel of the primary teeth is ground glass white, whereas the enamel of the permanent teeth is mottled yellow. The enamel is soft and will admit the point of a probe under pressure. The condition Lyonizes in females, where the primary teeth have random alternating vertical bands of abnormal ground glass white enamel with bands of translucent enamel. The permanent teeth have random alternating vertical bands of either opaque white or opaque yellow enamel with bands of translucent normal enamel. Transillumination aids the diagnosis in females. In males, the X-ray contrast between enamel and dentin is reduced in comparison with normal enamel; in females, no defects are observed.

*Type IIC and IID* See **Teeth, snow-capped.**

*Type III, Hypocalcified* The enamel initially develops normal thickness, is orange-yellow at eruption, and consists of poorly calcified matrix, which is rapidly lost, leaving dentin cores. On X-ray, the enamel is less radiopaque than dentin.

*Type IIIA, The hypocalcified, autosomal dominant type* is characterized by unerupted and newly erupted teeth covered by a light yellow-brown to orange-colored enamel of normal thickness. After eruption, the enamel becomes brown to black from food stains. It is friable, soft, and rapidly lost by attrition. By 10–12 years of age, only dentin cores remain. The cervical enamel may be better calcified. It is associated with anterior open bite frequently (22:26). The teeth are sensitive to temperature changes. On X-ray, the enamel is less radiopaque than the dentin. The crowns have a moth-eaten appearance with a radiodense line of calcified enamel at the cervical edge. Teeth accumulate heavy deposits of calculus.

*Type IV, Hypoplastic-hypocalcified with taurodontism* The enamel is less than normal in thickness and mottled. Molar teeth have a taurodontic shape. On X-ray, the enamel has approximately the same radiodensity as dentin.

*Type IVA, The hypoplastic-hypomaturation type* associated with taurodontic molar teeth is distinct from the **Tricho-dento-osseous**

**syndrome**, lacking the nail, hair, and bone changes of the latter. The enamel is mottled, has a yellow-brown color, and is pitted and thin. Large pulp chambers may occur in single rooted teeth. On X-ray, the enamel is thin and rough and has about the same radiodensity as dentin.

**Complications:** Among 50 patients: psychologic distress may occur or be aggravated by unsightly teeth 40/50; early tooth loss 46/50; prone to periodontal disease 25/50; sensitivity to hot and cold 24/50; pulpal exposure from attrition 8/50.

**Associated Findings:** Anterior open bite was found in 22/26 with the hypocalcified autosomal dominant type; in 22/22 men and in 18/30 women with the hypoplastic, smooth X-linked dominant type; and in 15/29 with the hypoplastic rough autosomal dominant type.

**Etiology:** Inherited as autosomal dominant, autosomal recessive, or X-linked depending upon type. It is not known whether the autosomal traits and the X-linked traits represent genes at different loci or if they represent alleles.

**Pathogenesis:** Structural defects in enamel formation. The primary protein defect is unknown. In the hypoplastic forms there is a failure of ameloblasts to lay down an enamel matrix of full thickness. It is my opinion that in the thin enamel type the defect is primarily in the ameloblast, while in the pitted forms there may be a vascular defect of the enamel organ. In the hypocalcified types full thickness of the enamel matrix is produced but fails to calcify normally. Scanning electron microscopy shows a defect in the so-called enamel sheath in hypomaturation types. Degeneration of the end-stage enamel organ is associated with resorption of unerupted tooth crowns.

**MIM No.:** *10450, *10453, 13090, *20470, *30110, *30120

**Sex Ratio:** Autosomal dominant and recessive types M1:F1; X-linked dominant type M1:F2; X-linked recessive type M1:F0 (if females who have a mild defect detectable by special examination are included, M1:F2).

**Occurrence:** 1:16,000 in North American Caucasians.

**Risk of Recurrence for Patient's Sib:**
See Part I, *Mendelian Inheritance.*

**Risk of Recurrence for Patient's Child:**
See Part I, *Mendelian Inheritance.*

**Age of Detectability:** At the time of eruption of teeth; 1–2 years by visual examination.

**Gene Mapping and Linkage:** AIH2 (amelogenesis imperfecta 2, hypocalcification (autosomal dominant)) has been tentatively mapped to unassigned.
AIH1 (amelogenesis imperfecta 1, hypomaturation or hypoplastic (?=AMG & AMGS)) has been mapped to Xp22.
AMG (amelogenin (?=AMGS & AIH)) has been mapped to Xp22.31-p22.1.
Types IE and IIB are X-chromosomal.

**Prevention:** None known. Genetic counseling indicated.

**Treatment:** Excellent results in all types with full crown restorations and composite resins for less severe types. Orthodontic procedure for open bite. Desensitizing toothpaste may be used.

**Prognosis:** Early loss of teeth by attrition, pulp exposure, and periodontal disease if untreated. With restoration, normal life span of teeth can be maintained.

**Detection of Carrier:** In the recessive type this is not possible. In the X-linked recessive type, alternating vertical stripes of normal translucent enamel and opaque yellow-white abnormal enamel occur, which can best be seen on transillumination.

**Special Considerations:** Dental restoration at an early age is recommended to avoid psychosocial trauma. Nearly all patients (80 of the 100 patients seen to date) have shown marked psychosocial affects from their unsightly teeth. With treatment there has been a marked improvement in their personality and social relations with others; however, a few individuals who had used their defect to elicit attention from family members had negative reactions after restoration.

**References:**
Witkop CJ Jr, Rao SR: Inherited defects in tooth structure. BD:OAS 1971:VII(7):153–184. †
Winter GB, Brook AH: Enamel hypoplasia and anomalies of the enamel. Dent Clin North Am 1975; 19:3–24. †
Witkop CJ Jr, Sauk JJ Jr: Defects of enamel. In: Stewart RE, Prescott GH, eds: Oral facial genetics. St. Louis: CV Mosby Co., 1976:151–226. * †
Chosack A, et al.: Amelogenesis imperfecta among Israeli Jews and the description of a new type of local hypoplastic autosomal recessive amelogenesis imperfecta. Oral Surg 1979; 47:148–156. †
Congleton J, Burkes EJ: Amelogenesis imperfecta with taurodontism. Oral Surg 1979; 48:540–544. †
Escobar VH, et al.: A clinical, genetic, and ultrastructural study of snow-capped teeth: amelogenesis imperfecta, hypomaturation type. Oral Surg 1981; 52:607–614. †

WI043                                    **Carl J. Witkop, Jr.**

---

## TEETH, ANKYLODONTIA, MULTIPLE HERITABLE TYPE     2243

**Includes:**
Ankylodontia, multiple heritable type
Dental eruption, arrested
Eruption failure of the permanent dentition
Hypercementosis

**Excludes:** N/A

**Major Diagnostic Criteria:** Malocclusion characterized by partial eruption of the permanent dentition; percussion dullness of the teeth; X-ray hypercementosis, and absence of periodontal ligament space.

**Clinical Findings:** Malocclusion characterized by partial eruption of the permanent dentition; percussion dullness of the teeth; X-ray hypercementosis, and absence of periodontal ligament space.

**Complications:** Unknown.

**Associated Findings:** None known.

**Etiology:** Autosomal dominant inheritance with high penetrance.

**Pathogenesis:** Unknown.

**Sex Ratio:** M1:F1

**Occurrence:** Six cases from two families have been reported.

**Risk of Recurrence for Patient's Sib:**
See Part I, *Mendelian Inheritance.*

**Risk of Recurrence for Patient's Child:**
See Part I, *Mendelian Inheritance.*

**Age of Detectability:** After six years of age.

**Gene Mapping and Linkage:** Unknown.

**Prevention:** None known. Genetic counseling indicated.

**Treatment:** Unknown. Orthodontic therapy ineffective.

**Prognosis:** Masticatory function compromised; difficult dental extractions.

**Detection of Carrier:** Clinical examination confirmed by X-ray.

**References:**
Humerfelt A, Reitan K: Effects of hypercementosis on the movability of teeth during orthodontic treatment. Angle Orthod 1966; 36:179–189.
Shokeir MHK: Complete failure of eruption of all permanent teeth: an autosomal dominant disorder. Clin Genet 1974; 5:322–326.
Israel H: Early hypercementosis and arrested dental eruption: heritable multiple ankylodontia. J Craniofac Genet Dev Biol 1984; 4:243–246.

IS002                                         **Harry Israel**

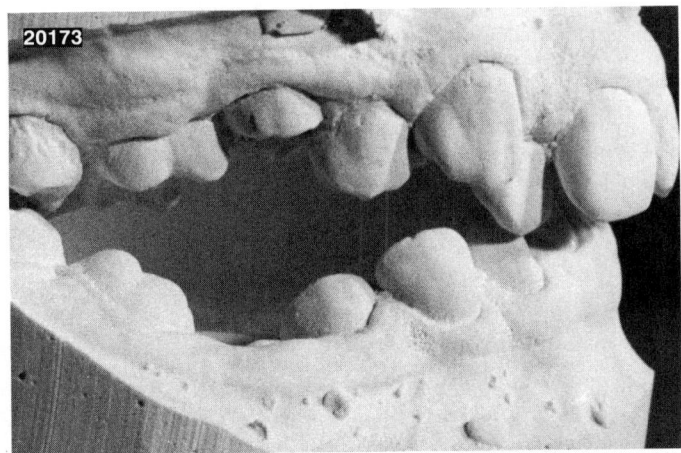

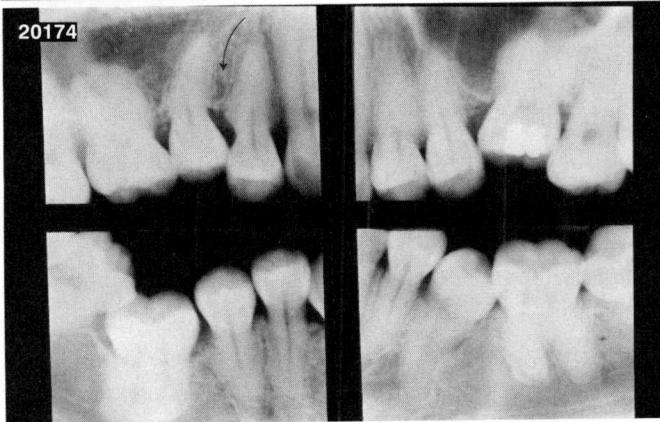

**2243**-20173: The extreme degree of arrested dental development has created severe malocclusion. 20174: Hypercementosis and reduction of the periodontal ligament spaces are evident throughout. The arrow defines an especially obvious site.

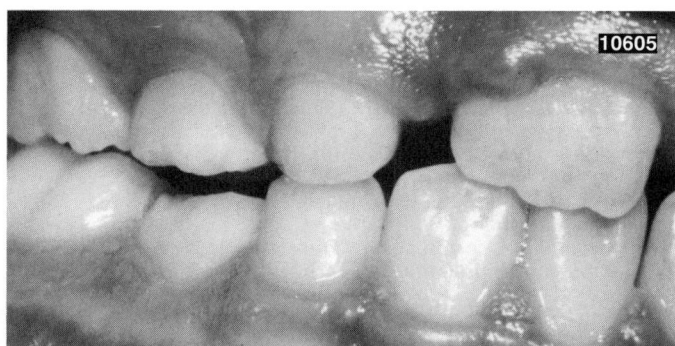

**0927-10605:** Ankylosed mandibular first primary molar.

---

## TEETH, ANKYLOSED                                     0927

**Includes:**
    Ankylosed teeth
    Submerged teeth

**Excludes:**
    Teeth, dens invaginatus (0276)
    Teeth, dilacerated (0929)
    Teeth, fused (0930)
    Teeth, geminated (0931)
    Teeth, impacted (0932)
    Teeth, molar reinclusion (2137)
    Teeth, root concrescence (0928)

**Major Diagnostic Criteria:** The occlusal surface of the affected tooth is situated below the plane of occlusion, and the tooth lacks mobility to manual rocking.

**Clinical Findings:** A fusion of tooth cementum and bone, occurring anywhere along path of eruption, either before or after emergence of tooth into the mouth. The condition may affect any tooth, but the mandibular first primary molar is most frequently involved. Ankylosis becomes clinically apparent by 1) occlusal plane of tooth beneath the plane of occlusion of adjacent teeth, 2) clinical crown height less than that of adjacent teeth, and 3) immobility to manual rocking. A solid sound on percussion and X-ray evidence of partial obliteration of periodontal ligament are nonessential criteria for diagnosis. The interproximal alveolar bone height is below that of adjacent unaffected teeth.

**Complications:** Difficulty extracting the affected tooth, noneruption of succedaneous tooth, supereruption of opposing tooth/teeth, tipping of adjacent teeth, loss of arch length, and possible development of malocclusion or local periodontal pathology.

**Associated Findings:** Subsequent to dental caries, there may be pulpal exposure, periapical infection, granuloma, cyst formation, and loss of teeth, followed by possible drifting and development of malocclusion. On occasion, ankylosis of primary teeth may be associated with congenitally missing succedaneous teeth. Lack of alveolar bone height may predispose to local periodontal pathology. Enamel opacity, hypoplasia, and malformed teeth in association with ankylosed molars have been reported in the permanent dentition.

**Etiology:** Undetermined, but a genetic or congenital gap in periodontal ligament is cited as an intrinsic causative factor. Chemical or thermal irritation, disturbed local metabolism, infection, local mechanical trauma, and reimplantation of evulsed tooth are cited as extrinsic causative factors.

**Pathogenesis:** The affected tooth has an area of cemental root resorption repaired by osteoid-like tissue which is continuous with alveolar bone. Periodontal ligament may become increasingly obliterated in affected area.

**Sex Ratio:** M1:F1

**Occurrence:** Reported in a United States study to affect 6.9% of primary molar teeth; very rare in secondary teeth unless they are traumatized. The prevalence in other world population groups is reported to range from 14.2% to 35.2%.

**Risk of Recurrence for Patient's Sib:** Significantly increased over population incidence.

**Risk of Recurrence for Patient's Child:** Unknown.

**Age of Detectability:** When adjacent teeth have reached occlusal plane, by clinical or X-ray examination.

**Gene Mapping and Linkage:** Unknown.

**Prevention:** Avoidance of extrinsic causative factors.

**Treatment:** Extraction of affected tooth, artificial restoration of proximal and occlusal contacts, or leaving tooth undisturbed. In some instances extraction may be delayed and the tooth utilized as a space maintainer until the succedaneous tooth is ready to erupt. Presence of succedaneous tooth should be established prior to extracting the affected tooth. Extraction of an ankylosed tooth usually requires vertical sectioning of the tooth and surgical removal of each section. Affected mandibular first primary molars are likely to exfoliate normally, and early extraction is not indicated. Affected maxillary and mandibular second primary molars tend to become severely affected, with marked absence of alveolar bone growth, and they do not exfoliate normally. Such teeth should be extracted.

**Prognosis:** *Treated*: Excellent. If there is no succedaneous tooth, a partially restored ankylosed tooth can serve well indefinitely. Periodic replacement of the restoration may be required as changes occur in surrounding alveolar bone. Alveolar bone height will always be lower than that of adjacent unaffected teeth.

*Untreated*: Tooth will not erupt to the plane of occlusion and surrounding alveolar bone height will not develop. Mandibular first primary molars are likely to exfoliate normally. Maxillary and mandibular second primary molars tend to become severely affected and tend not to exfoliate normally. In addition, there may be complications as listed above. The condition does not appear to affect longevity of patient.

**Detection of Carrier:** Unknown.

**References:**

Via WF: Submerged deciduous molars: familial tendencies. J Am Dent Assoc 1964; 69:127–129.

Biederman WB: The problem of the ankylosed tooth. Dent Clin North Am 1968; 24:409–424.

Brearley LJ, McKibben DH Jr: Ankylosis of primary molar teeth. I. Prevalence and characteristics. II: a longitudinal study. J Dent Child 1973; 40:54–63.

Darling AI, Levers BGH: Submerged human deciduous molars and ankylosis. Arch Oral Biol 1973; 18:1021–1040.

Messer LB, Cline JT: Ankylosed primary molars: results and treatment recommendations from an eight-year longitudinal study. Pediatr Dent 1980; 2:37–47.

Koyoumdjisky-Kaye E, Steigman S: Ethnic variability in the prevalence of submerged primary molars. J Dent Res 1982; 61:1401–1404.

MC021

**D. H. McKibben, Jr.**
*Louise Brearley Messer*

---

## TEETH, ANODONTIA, PARTIAL OR COMPLETE     2134

**Includes:**
> Hypodontia
> Oligodontia, isolated
> Teeth, congenitally missing

**Excludes:**
> Anodontia associated with syndromes, diseases, or extrinsic causes
> **Ectodermal dysplasia** (all)
> Hypodontia in/from syndromes, diseases, or extrinsic causes
> Oligodontia, not isolated
> Schizodontism
> **Teeth, ankylosed** (0927)
> **Teeth, impacted** (0932)
> **Teeth, microdontia** (0660)
> **Teeth, pegged or absent maxillary lateral incisor** (0934)
> **Teeth, root concrescence** (0928)

**Major Diagnostic Criteria:** Congenital absence of one or more teeth in the primary or the permanent dentition in the absence of associated systemic malformations.

**Clinical Findings:** Congenital agenesis of one or more teeth may occur in both the deciduous and permanent dentitions, although it appears more often in the permanent teeth. The most commonly affected teeth are the third molars: one, two, or all of them may be absent. The maxillary lateral incisors and second mandibular bicuspids are also frequently missing. The mandibular lateral incisors and first molars are rarely affected.

When deciduous teeth are involved, the succedaneous permanent teeth will usually be missing as well. Various degrees and combinations as to right or left side may occur within individuals and within kindreds. Because of the missing teeth, occlusion is usually defective in these children. An oral soft tissue examination generally shows no abnormalities. X-ray examination must be carried out to confirm the agenesis and a detailed dental history obtained in order to rule out extractions and trauma.

A positive family history for one or more missing teeth in combination with the lack of an environmental insult to explain causation are usual. In many kindreds, congenital absence of teeth and microdontia occur simultaneously either in the same individual, or in different individuals i.e., one person will have microdontia and another has agenesis. This finding suggested that microdontia and hypodontia/anodontia were expressions of the same genetic character and may constitute phenotypic variations of a continuous spectrum of tooth size diminution.

**Complications:** The most obvious complications are malocclusion, drifting of teeth, diastemas between present teeth. In severe cases, the patients are almost edentulous and their facial appearance becomes an important factor. Nutritional deficiencies might occur in these children, since they are unable to chew.

The most commonly mentioned finding in children with severe hypodontia is their psychologic status. The lack of teeth gives them an undesirable facial profile. Several reports show these children to be shy, secluded, and isolated from their peers. Fortunately, the number of severely affected children is low. Most affected individuals only have one or two missing teeth.

**Associated Findings:** Possibly microdontia.

**Etiology:** Family studies suggest that hypodontia/anodontia is a hereditary trait, although the mode of transmission is unclear. Many investigators consider hypodontia to be the result of a single gene, often transmitted as an autosomal dominant with incomplete penetrance and variable expressivity, or as an X-linked dominant phenotype. Others consider it to be a multifactorial trait. The best data suggested that hypodontia was an autosomal dominant phenotype. These data have been reanalyzed twice, using different methods. The autosomal dominant hypothesis was confirmed in one, while in the other, a multifactorial model provided a better fit to the data.

**Pathogenesis:** Absence of tooth development is the major reason hypodontia occurs, but why teeth fail to develop is unclear. However, destruction of the dental lamina, space limitations, and competition for minimum nutritional requirements causing regressions and agenesis, functional abnormalities of the dental epithelium, and failure of induction of the underlying mesenchyme have all been implicated in the production of hypodontia.

**MIM No.:** *10660, *20678, 31350

**Sex Ratio:** Presumably M1:F1. (M1:F1.3 observed).

**Occurrence:** Varies among different populations. The prevalence of hypodontia of the secondary dentition of Caucasians ranged from 2.3 to 9.6%; Hawaiians, 1.7%; American Blacks, 2.0%; Japanese, 1.1%; and Chinese, 0.15%. The frequency of the individual teeth involved also varies: the third molars are the most commonly affected teeth, followed by maxillary lateral incisors, then lower mandibular bicuspids.

The incidence of anodontia is 0.5% of Swedish children. Hypodontia is found in the primary dentition of 5% of Japanese children; and in between 0.1 and 0.7% of Caucasians.

**Risk of Recurrence for Patient's Sib:**
> See Part I, *Mendelian Inheritance*. Empiric risk is 0.82.

**Risk of Recurrence for Patient's Child:**
> See Part I, *Mendelian Inheritance*.

**Age of Detectability:** After eight years of age for the permanent dentition, by X-ray examination.

**Gene Mapping and Linkage:** Unknown.

**Prevention:** None known. Genetic counseling indicated.

**Treatment:** Prosthetic replacement and orthodontic treatment.

**Prognosis:** Normal life span. Patients adapt quite well to the use of prosthetic devices.

**Detection of Carrier:** Examination of relatives for evidence of the trait.

**Special Considerations:** The term, "hypodontia" should be used to describe the absence of one or more teeth. The term "oligodontia" is commonly used in the literature and is intended in many cases to be used interchangeably with hypodontia. However, the term oligodontia should be reserved for those instances when hypodontia is part of a multi-system condition or syndrome. Furthermore, the term oligodontia may be used preferably to describe the absence of numerous teeth (compared with relatively fewer teeth implied by the use of the term hypodontia). Anodontia, the complete absence of teeth, is the most extreme example of oligodontia.

Although hypodontia seems to be a hereditary trait which more likely follows an autosomal dominant inheritance pattern, its phenotypic expression in members of the same family is variable.

The ratios of affected to normal individuals are also variable and suggest that, although this is a genetic trait, environmental effects and gene-gene interaction also play a significant role in its production and expression.

**References:**

Dahlberg AA: Inherited congenital absence of six incisors, deciduous and permanent. J Dent Res 1937; 16:59–62.

Juarez CK, Spence A: The genetics of hypodontia. J Dent Res 1974; 53:781–783.

Graber LW: Congenital absence of teeth: a review with emphasis on inheritance patterns. J Am Dent Assoc 1978; 96:266–275.

Burzynski N, Escobar V: Classification and genetics of numeric anomalies of the dentition. BD:OAS XIX(1). New York: March of Dimes Birth Defects Foundation, 1983:95–106.

Witkop CJ, Jr.: Agenesis of succedaneous teeth: an expression of the homozygous state of the gene for the pegged or missing maxillary lateral incisor trait. Am J Med Genet 1987; 26:431–436.

ES000                                          **Victor Escobar**

**Teeth, anterior permanent, flame-shaped pulp chambers**
   *See TEETH, DENTIN DYSPLASIA, CORONAL*
**Teeth, carnivore-like**
   *See TEETH, LOBODONTIA*
**Teeth, congenital**
   *See TEETH, NATAL OR NEONATAL*
**Teeth, congenitally missing**
   *See TEETH, ANODONTIA, PARTIAL OR COMPLETE*
**Teeth, conical, multiple**
   *See TEETH, LOBODONTIA*
**Teeth, conical-clefting-ectropion**
   *See CLEFTING-ECTROPION-CONICAL TEETH*
**Teeth, connate**
   *See TEETH, FUSED*

## TEETH, DEFECTS FROM TETRACYCLINE                   0341

**Includes:**
   Brown teeth
   Enamel and dentin defects from tetracycline
   Grey teeth
   Tetracycline discoloration of enamel and dentin
   Yellow teeth

**Excludes:**
   **Teeth, amelogenesis imperfecta** (0046)
   **Teeth, dentinogenesis imperfecta** (0279)
   **Teeth, enamel and dentin defects from erythroblastosis fetalis** (0340)

**Major Diagnostic Criteria:** Yellow, brown or grey discoloration of teeth, distributed in horizontal bands and exhibiting yellow fluorescence under ultraviolet light.

**Clinical Findings:** Yellow, brown or grey discoloration of enamel and dentin of teeth. Seen most frequently in primary dentition. In severe cases, some enamel of primary molars and cuspids and secondary incisors and molars may be hypoplastic or missing. Incidence is variable, depending upon use of tetracyclines in community in early years of child's life and length of period of administration. Exposure to sunlight may change yellow color to brownish grey. In ultraviolet light affected areas fluoresce pale to bright yellow, although fluorescence may be lost in teeth whose color has changed to brownish grey.

**Complications:** Attrition of the hypoplastic tooth structure.

**Associated Findings:** Staining of bones.

**Etiology:** Tetracycline administered during the period of tooth calcification. Primary dentition is affected when drug is given

during the last 2 months of intrauterine life to 9 months of age. The anterior teeth of the secondary dentition may be affected if administration occurs between birth and 5 years. The degree of involvement depends on total dose. Where this exceeds 100 mg/kg (30–35 mg/kg/day) in first few months of life, discoloration and hypoplasia of enamel of primary dentition can be expected in 90% or more cases. Where drug is given to premature infants shortly after birth, hypoplasia of enamel is more likely to occur.

Involvement of secondary dentition is less common and unlikely with a normal single course of administration but may affect severely the anterior teeth if drug is given over a period of months during the first 5 years of life.

Tetracycline hydrochloride, demethylchlortetracycline and chlortetracycline produce a yellower discoloration than oxytetracycline which causes a paler creamy color. Incidence with long acting new tetracyclines not known.

**Pathogenesis:** Tetracycline is deposited in developing dentin and enamel.

**Sex Ratio:** M1:F1

**Occurrence:** Variable. Depends upon the use of tetracyclines in the community. Prevalence varies with year and age of children. When last studied in the United States, in children 4–12 years of age, 1:24 (urban) and 1:71 (rural) in 1964 and 1:7 (urban) in 1966. Use of tetracycline in pregnant women has since been discontinued.

When total dose exceeds 100 mg/kg in the first 12 months, discoloration and hypoplasia of primary dentition occurs in at least 90% of cases. Dose required to produce changes in secondary dentition not known.

**Risk of Recurrence for Patient's Sib:** Related directly to tetracycline exposure.

**Risk of Recurrence for Patient's Child:** Related directly to tetracycline exposure.

**Age of Detectability:** After eruption of teeth.

**Gene Mapping and Linkage:** N/A

**Prevention:** Do not give tetracycline in any form during last 2 months of pregnancy or during first 5 years of life.

**Treatment:** In general, no treatment. Esthetic crowns may be considered for older children with severe discoloration or hypoplasia of anterior secondary teeth.

**Prognosis:** No effect on general health. Teeth may change color and become either darker or lighter with exposure to sunlight. Psychosocial problems may develop in person with severely stained and hypoplastic teeth.

**Detection of Carrier:** Unknown.

**References:**

Wallman IS, Hilton HB: Teeth pigmented by tetracycline. Lancet 1962; I:827.

Witkop CJ Jr, Wolf RO: Hypoplasia and intrinsic staining of enamel following tetracycline therapy. JAMA 1963; 185:100.

WA015                                          **I.S. Wallman**

## TEETH, DENS INVAGINATUS                            0276

**Includes:**
   Dens invaginatus
   Dens telescopes
   Dilated composite odontome
   Gestant odontome
   Radix in radice

**Excludes:**
   Dens evaginatus
   **Teeth, lobodontia** (0607)

**Major Diagnostic Criteria:** An anomalous invagination of tooth structure, involving the crown or root, in which the outer surface of enamel or cementum is continuous with the inner layer. Diagnosis confirmed by X-ray.

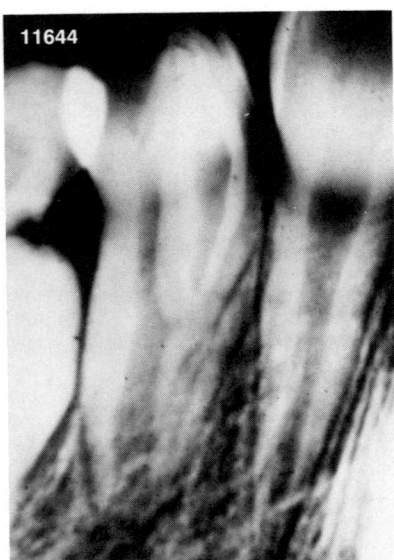

**0276-11644:** X-ray shows "tooth within a tooth" appearance.

**Clinical Findings:** This is a relatively common dental anomaly that is often bilateral. The maxillary permanent dentition is usually affected: most commonly the lateral incisors and less frequently the central incisors, premolars, and molars. It is occasionally found in mandibular permanent teeth, usually premolars. It has been reported in supernumerary teeth and is exceedingly rare in the deciduous dentition. Most cases of dens invaginatus involve the crown. Clinically the crown may be normal or conical, peg-, or barrel-shaped, with a pit or groove on the lingual/occlusal surface. X-ray examination is necessary for accurate diagnosis and management and is especially beneficial prior to tooth eruption.

The invagination may have a direct communication with the pulp chamber or it may have a thin wall of dental hard tissue. This area is susceptible to the accumulation of debris and bacterial invasion with subsequent pulpal necrosis. Pulpal necrosis may occur in the newly erupted tooth.

Classification of dens invaginatus is as follows:

Type 1: confined to tooth crown, an accentuated lingual pit may be considered a minor form.

Type 2: involves crown and root.

Type 3: involves crown and root and has a periapical or periodontal foramen.

On X-ray examination there are small, inverted, pear-shaped areas of enamel within the pulp cavity, which may extend to the apex in the more severe forms. This often suggests the appearance of a tooth within a tooth. The more severe forms are likely to be associated with dilation of the tooth.

**Complications:** Pulpal necrosis may occur before root formation is complete. A periapical abscess, cyst, or granuloma may occur.

**Associated Findings:** Has been reported in association with **Teeth, microdontia** and **Teeth, taurodontism** with **Teeth, dentinogenesis imperfecta**, and with ameloblastoma.

**Etiology:** Possibly autosomal dominant inheritance.

**Pathogenesis:** One or more invaginations of the enamel organ or Hertwig's epithelial root sheath into the dental papilla of the developing tooth. It is theorized that these invaginations may result from focal growth retardation or proliferation or from increased external pressure.

**MIM No.:** 12530

**Sex Ratio:** M1:F1

**Occurrence:** 0.04–10% is reported incidence (3% of 3,000 Swedish children and 1.7% of Saudi Arabians). Prevalence is 0.25–5.2%.

**Risk of Recurrence for Patient's Sib:** See Part I, *Mendelian Inheritance*. Observed frequency, 32%.

**Risk of Recurrence for Patient's Child:** See Part I, *Mendelian Inheritance*. Observed frequency, 43%.

**Age of Detectability:** Prior to eruption by X-ray examination.

**Gene Mapping and Linkage:** Unknown.

**Prevention:** None known. Genetic counseling indicated.

**Treatment:** Eruption of a tooth exhibiting dens invaginatus may be anticipated if detected by X-ray. Upon eruption, or after removal of the soft tissue just prior to eruption, the invagination on the labial/occlusal surface may be prophylactically sealed or a dental restoration placed.

Teeth with pulpal necrosis may require apexification if root formation is incomplete, conventional root canal therapy with or without apicoectomy and retrograde restoration, or, in the extreme case, extraction.

**Prognosis:** Prophylactic dental restoration will prevent pulpal necrosis in most cases. Once pulpal involvement occurs the tooth may be retained in the majority of cases by using a variety of endodontic procedures. In addition to the pulpal considerations, anomalous crown shapes may compromise periodontal health and require restorative procedures. Extraction is necessary in only the rare case today.

**Detection of Carrier:** Unknown.

**References:**

Oehlers FAC: Dens invaginatus (dilated composite odontome). I. variations of the invagination process and associated crown forms. Oral Surg 1957; 10:1204–1218.

Grahnen H: Dens invaginatus I. A clinical, roentgenological and genetic study of permanent upper lateral incisors. Odontol Rev 1959; 10:115–137.

Ferguson FS: Successful apexification technique in an immature tooth with dens in dente. Oral Surg 1980; 49:356–359.

De Smit A, Demaut L: Nonsurgical endodontic treatment of invaginated teeth. J Endodont 1982; 8:506–511.

Ruprecht A, et al.: The incidence of dental invagination. J Pedodont 1986; 10:265–272.

ZU002                                          **Susan L. Zunt**

## TEETH, DENTIN DYSPLASIA, CORONAL          0277

**Includes:**

Coronal dentin dysplasia
Dentin dysplasia, coronal
Dentin dysplasia, type II
Pulp stones
Teeth, anterior permanent, flame-shaped pulp chambers
Teeth, pulpal dysplasia
Teeth, thistle-shaped pulp chambers

**Excludes:**

**Branchio-skeleto-genital syndrome** (0118)
Calcinosis
**Dentino-osseous dysplasia** (0280)
**Ehlers-Danlos syndrome** (0338)
Fibrous dysplasia of dentin
**Osteogenesis imperfecta** (0777)
**Teeth, dentin dysplasia, radicular** (0278)
**Teeth, dentinogenesis imperfecta** (0279)
**Teeth, odontodysplasia** (0739)

**Major Diagnostic Criteria:** Opalescent, brownish-blue primary teeth and normal-appearing permanent teeth. On X-ray, primary teeth have obliterated pulp chambers; anterior permanent teeth have flame- or thistle-shaped pulp chambers; molars have bow-tie-shaped pulp chambers.

Must be differentiated from **Teeth, dentinogenesis imperfecta** in which teeth of both dentitions are opalescent.

**Clinical Findings:** Primary teeth are brownish-blue with a translucent opalescent sheen and are identical in appearance with teeth seen in **Teeth, dentinogenesis imperfecta (0279)**. Permanent teeth are

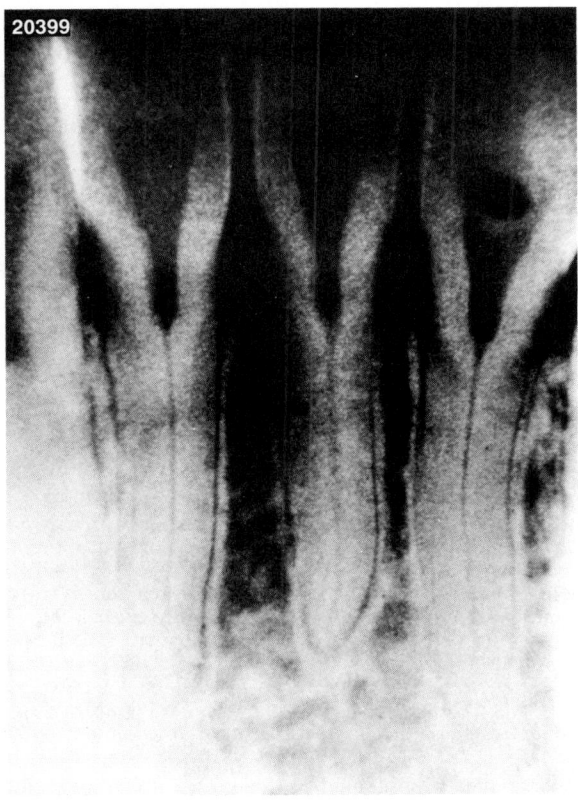

**0277A-20399:** Thistle-tube pulps in dentin dysplasia.

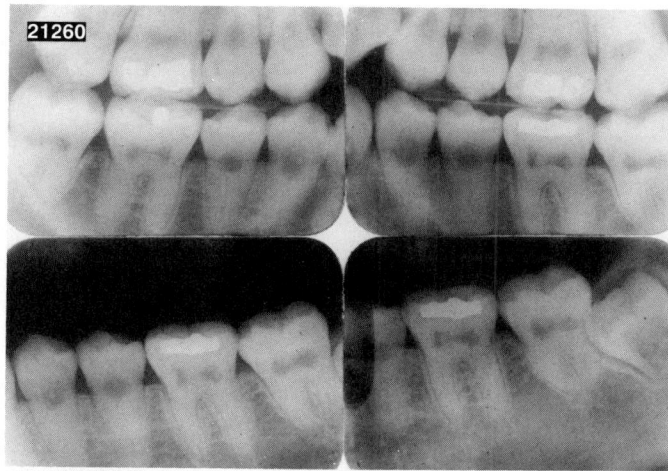

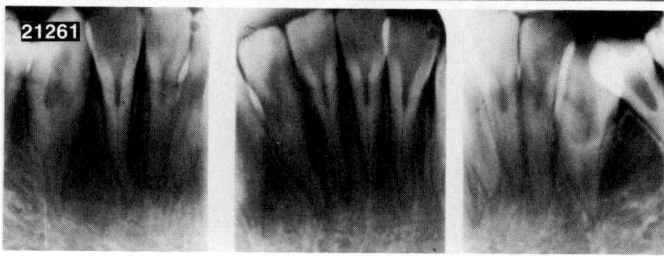

**0277C-21260–61:** Dentin dysplasia, coronal; permanent molars have bow-tie–shaped chambers and premolars and incisors have large flame-shaped chambers with flat apical floors. Teeth are of normal color.

normal in color, size, and shape. By X-ray, the primary teeth have obliterated pulp chambers and reduced root canals. Anterior permanent teeth have flame-shaped pulp chambers, often with a radicular extension with or without pulp stones. Molar teeth have bow-tie-shaped pulp chambers. Root formation in permanent teeth is usually normal. Primary teeth abrade rapidly.

**Complications:** Crowns of primary teeth rapidly lost by attrition.

**Associated Findings:** None known.

**Etiology:** Autosomal dominant inheritance.

**Pathogenesis:** Undetermined. The dentin of primary teeth is amorphous, resembling a gray granular gelatin with vestiges of tubule formation. The permanent teeth coronally have normal tubular dentin. The radicular dentin has a transition zone in which tubular, atubular, and fibrous dentin is admixed. Osteo- and

tubular denticles may occur in the pulp chamber, which is flame-shaped. With age, the pulp chamber becomes partially obliterated in permanent teeth.

**MIM No.:** *12542

**Sex Ratio:** M1:F1

**Occurrence:** Rare. Approximately 80 kindreds have been reported or are known.

**Risk of Recurrence for Patient's Sib:**
See Part I, *Mendelian Inheritance.*

**Risk of Recurrence for Patient's Child:**
See Part I, *Mendelian Inheritance.*

**Age of Detectability:** At age nine to 18 months, upon eruption of primary teeth by visual and X-ray examination.

**Gene Mapping and Linkage:** Unknown.

**Prevention:** None known. Genetic counseling indicated.

**Treatment:** Crowning of primary teeth. Resin bonded restorations.

**Prognosis:** Premature loss of teeth may be slightly increased.

**Detection of Carrier:** Unknown.

**Special Considerations:** Pulpal dysplasia is a different condition. It has been seen in two families, and the individuals who have this condition have an associated growth and developmental retardation which is not associated with **Teeth, dentin dysplasia, coronal.**

**References:**
Shields EP, et al.: A proposed classification for heritable human dentine defects with a description of a new entity. Arch Oral Biol 1973; 18:543–553.
Giansanti JS, Allen JD: Dentin dysplasia, type II, or dentin dysplasia, coronal type. Oral Surg 1974; 38:911–917.

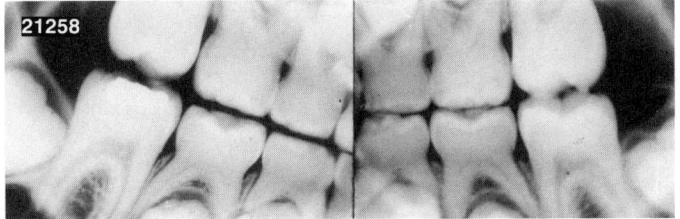

**0277B-21258:** Dentin dysplasia, coronal; primary teeth have obliterated pulp chambers shown in the primary molars. Primary teeth are an opalescent brown color and resemble those seen in dentinogenesis imperfecta both clinically and radiographically.

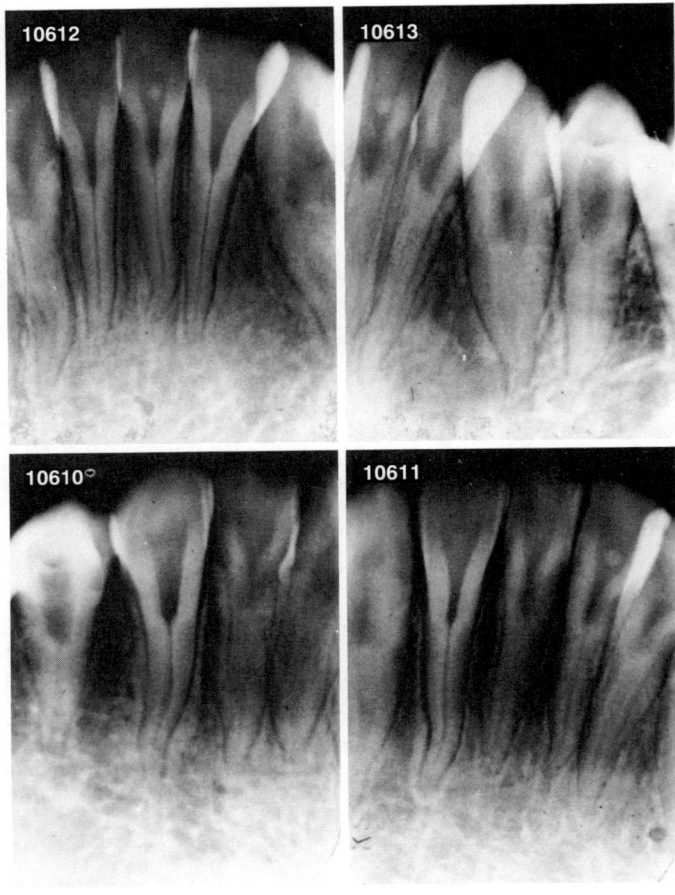

0277D-10610–13:   Thistle-shaped pulp chambers.

Witkop CJ Jr: Hereditary defects of dentin. Dent Clin North Am 1975; 19:25–45.
Melnick M, et al.: Dentin dysplasia, type II: a rare autosomal dominant disorder. Oral Surg 1977; 44:592–599. * †

WI043                                        **Carl J. Witkop, Jr.**

## TEETH, DENTIN DYSPLASIA, RADICULAR          **0278**

**Includes:**
> Dentin dysplasia, radicular
> Dentin dysplasia, type I
> Nonopalescent opalescent dentine
> Radicular dentin dysplasia
> Rootless teeth

**Excludes:**
> **Branchio-skeleto-genital syndrome** (0118)
> Calcinosis
> **Dentino-osseous dysplasia** (0280)
> **Ehlers-Danlos syndrome** (0338)
> Fibrous dysplasia of dentin
> **Osteogenesis imperfecta** (0777)
> **Teeth, dentin dysplasia, coronal** (0277)
> **Teeth, dentinogenesis imperfecta** (0279)
> **Teeth, odontodysplasia** (0739)

**Major Diagnostic Criteria:**   Generally, teeth are normal in color, but on X-ray examinations they lack pulp chambers or have

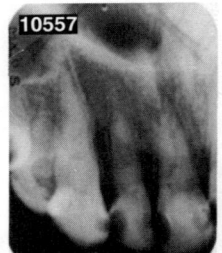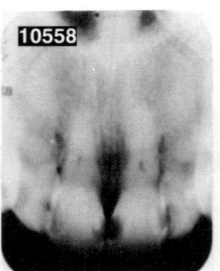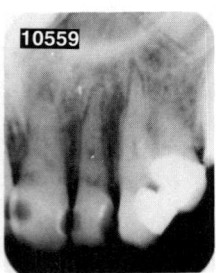

0278A-10557–59:   Radicular dentin dysplasia.

half-moon-shaped pulp chambers and short or abnormally shaped roots.

**Clinical Findings:**   Both dentitions are affected. Teeth are usually normal in color and contour of crowns but may have a bluish-brown hue. Teeth are frequently malaligned in arch with a history of drifting. X-ray changes include absent or half-moon-shaped pulp chambers in 100%, short or abnormally shaped roots in 80%, radiolucent areas around roots in 20%. Coronal dentin and enamel are histologically normal. Radicular and pulp areas filled with foci of dentin formed in the dental papilla surrounded by dentin formed from the normal root development. The histologic picture resembles a stream flowing around boulders. Vascular channels cap the foci of dentin formed in the papilla. Periapical lesions are radicular cysts. Teeth may exfoliate spontaneously or with minor trauma.

**Complications:**   Spontaneous exfoliation of teeth, premature loss of teeth, and destruction of jaws by cyst expansion.

**Associated Findings:**   None known.

**Etiology:**   Autosomal dominant inheritance. Five of 30 propositi have had normal parents, which may indicate either genetic heterogeneity, variable expressivity, or high mutation rate.

**Pathogenesis:**   A defect in the epithelial root sheath, in which epithelial cells invade the dental papilla and induce mesenchymal cells at many foci to undergo transformation to odontoblasts. These odontoblasts lay down multiple areas of dentin, which fuse and become surrounded by a layer of more normal radicular

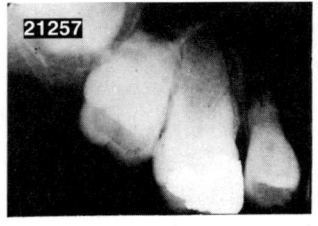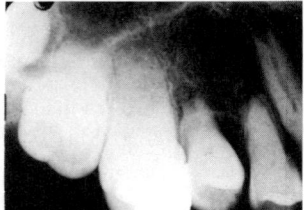
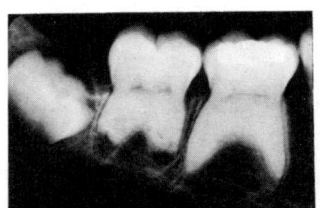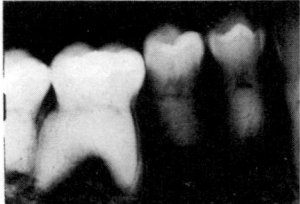

0278B-21257:   Radicular dentin dysplasia; pulp chambers are obliterated except for a crescent-shaped area below the coronal dentin. Roots are short and some are surrounded by a radiolucent area in the bone.

dentin, resulting in complete or nearly complete obliteration of pulp chambers, root canals, and short abnormal roots. Epithelial rests undergo cystic degeneration, forming periapical cysts.

**MIM No.:** *12540

**Sex Ratio:** M1:F1

**Occurrence:** 1:50,000 among North American Caucasians.

**Risk of Recurrence for Patient's Sib:**
See Part I, *Mendelian Inheritance.*

**Risk of Recurrence for Patient's Child:**
See Part I, *Mendelian Inheritance.*

**Age of Detectability:** By X-ray examination at time of eruption of teeth, age 9 to 18 months.

**Gene Mapping and Linkage:** Unknown.

**Prevention:** None known. Genetic counseling indicated.

**Treatment:** Prosthetic replacement of teeth, extraction, and surgical treatment of cysts.

**Prognosis:** No apparent effect on life span. Usually complete loss of teeth by third to fourth decades.

**Detection of Carrier:** Unknown.

**Special Considerations:** Clinically and histologically identical teeth also occur in dentino-osseous dysplasia and in the branchio-skeleto-genital syndrome. This type of dentin dysplasia also occurs in the tricho-onycho-dental syndrome, which has hair, nail, and enamel defects. A similar but less severe dentin defect also occurs in some types of Ehlers-Danlos syndrome, enamel and interradicular dentin dysplasia, tumoral calcinosis with hyperphosphatemia, and in dermatomyositis.

**References:**

Bruszt P: Sur deux cas de dysplasie dentinaire. Bull Group Int Rech Sci Stomatol Odontol 1969; 12:107–119.

Witkop CJ Jr, Rao S: Inherited defects in tooth structure. In BD:OAS; VII(7). Baltimore: William & Wilkins, 1971, 153–184. *

Sauk JJ Jr, et al.: An electron optic analysis and explanation for the etiology of dentinal dysplasia. Oral Surg 1972; 33:763–771. *

Shields ED, et al.: Heritable defects in dentine; description, differentiation and classification. Arch Oral Biol 1973; 18:543–553.

Witkop CJ Jr: Hereditary defects of dentin. Dent Clin North Am 1975; 19:25–45. †

Melnick M, et al.: Dentin dysplasia type I: a scanning electron microscope analysis of the primary dentition. Oral Surg 1980; 50:335–339.

WI043                                 **Carl J. Witkop, Jr.**

## TEETH, DENTINOGENESIS IMPERFECTA      0279

**Includes:**
>   Dentinogenesis imperfecta, Brandywine type
>   Dentinogenesis imperfecta, Mayflower type
>   Dentinogenesis imperfecta, Shields type II, III
>   Opalescent dentin
>   Shell teeth
>   Teeth, hereditary brown

**Excludes:**
>   **Branchio-skeleto-genital syndrome** (0118)
>   Calcinosis
>   **Dentino-osseous dysplasia** (0280)
>   **Ehlers-Danlos syndrome** (0338)
>   Fibrous dysplasia of dentin
>   **Osteogenesis imperfecta** (0777)
>   **Teeth, dentin dysplasia, coronal** (0277)
>   **Teeth, dentin dysplasia, radicular** (0278)
>   **Teeth, odontodysplasia** (0739)

**Major Diagnostic Criteria:** Lack of any pulp chambers on X-ray examination in opalescent teeth of both dentitions.

**Clinical Findings:** Two types of dentinogenesis may exist: a milder form frequently tracing ancestry to descendants of the Mayflower (DI type II) and a more severe form, the Brandywine type (DI, type III). The phenotypes frequently overlap, and DI, type III may only be a stage in development of DI, type II.

All teeth in both dentitions are affected. Teeth are bluish-brown to brown in color with opalescent sheen. Crowns are bulbous-shaped. Enamel hypoplasia occurs in about 20%. The enamel fractures and easily abrades so the teeth wear rapidly, and, in adults, only roots may remain. Lack of history of repeated fractures and absence of other signs of osteogenesis imperfecta.

Pulp chambers and root canals are absent on X-ray examination. A few patients may show normal or large chambers or canals in primary teeth as a variation in expressivity. Short, thin roots.

Histologically, there are scanty, atypical tubules of varying width and length and globular dentin. Lack of scalloping occurs in most cases at the dentinoenamel junction. Cell remnants are embedded in dentin.

**Complications:** There is secondary hypoplasia of the alveolar process, probably from loss of occlusal tooth surface, resulting in large gingivae and alveolar ridges. Premature loss of teeth results from attrition, pulp exposure, and fractures of crown. Occasional periapical cyst formation occurs, but less frequently than that seen in dentin dysplasia.

**Associated Findings:** None known.

**Etiology:** Autosomal dominant inheritance with low mutation rate and with variable expression.

**Pathogenesis:** A defect in odontoblasts, which form a defective periodic acid Schiff (PAS)-positive matrix. Odontoblasts differentiate and lay down 1–2 mm of fairly normal-appearing tubules adjacent to the dentinoenamel junction. This layer of odontoblasts degenerates, and, new layer differentiates from mesenchyme and lays down 1–2 mm of atypical dentin. This process continues until tooth is completely filled. The dentin matrix does not calcify properly, lacking phosphophoryn, a calcium-binding protein. Abnormal peripulpal dentin contains reticulin and type III collagen, normally not present except in the mantle layer.

**MIM No.:** *12549, 12550

**Sex Ratio:** M55:F45. Several large studies of over 600 affected persons and their normal sibs have shown a consistent and statistically significant deviation of the expected 1:1 ratio.

**Occurrence:** Prevalence 1:8,000 in the general North American population. Occurs in isolates in higher prevalence. Highest known, Brandywine isolate of Maryland, 1:15. Reported nearly exclusively in people of Caucasian ancestry, especially tracing ancestry to France. Unreported in pure Black, Asiatic, or Australoid populations.

**Risk of Recurrence for Patient's Sib:**
See Part I, *Mendelian Inheritance.*

**Risk of Recurrence for Patient's Child:**
See Part I, *Mendelian Inheritance.*

**Age of Detectability:** Upon eruption of teeth at age 9–18 months, by visual and X-ray examination.

**Gene Mapping and Linkage:** DGI1 (dentinogenesis imperfecta 1) has been mapped to 4q12-q23.

**Prevention:** None known. Genetic counseling indicated.

**Treatment:** Crowning usually fails unless teeth are well formed. Children aged 4–15 years: Do not extract teeth. Place full denture prosthesis over teeth to maintain alveolar ridge. Adults: Full-mouth extraction and prosthetic replacements. Caution! Teeth are soft and crush under forceps pressure. Extract by elevation. Recommend treatment at early age, as the unsightly teeth affect psychosocial development. Alveolectomy may be needed in older children and adults prior to prosthetic replacement.

**Prognosis:** No effect on life span. Early loss of teeth. Risk of alveolar infection. Untreated cases can be associated with social difficulties.

**Detection of Carrier:** Unknown.

**Special Considerations:** Genetic heterogeneity may exist in this category. Shields et al (1973) feel that the Brandywine triracial isolate type with an occasional child showing large pulp chambers in primary teeth is a different disease than that found in most families. Studies to date have not shown definitive collagen, glycosaminoglycan, or phosphophoryn differences in the Brandywine type and what these authors term dentinogenesis imperfecta, type II (hereditary opalescent dentin), or in a similar tooth defect in **Osteogenesis imperfecta** (DI type I).

An occasional variation in the expressivity of this gene is encountered in kindreds of the classic disease. These variants usually affect primary teeth, which demonstrate normal-sized or very large pulp chambers (*shell teeth*). Sections reveal a reduced or absent layer of odontoblasts on the pulpal surface in these instances. Several reports of isolated cases have designated such cases as a separate entity; however, permanent teeth of relatives usually show the classic disease picture. Must be differentiated from dentin dysplasia, which usually has a remnant of pulp chamber visible on X-ray examination.

Two large studies indicate that there is a significantly increased reproductive fitness of 30–35% of affected individuals over their unaffected sibs and the population from which they were derived. Among a triracial isolate, all of the excess was attributable to excess male reproduction and among North American Caucasians to excess female reproduction, possibly indicating psychosocial factors involved with unsightly teeth.

**References:**

Witkop CJ Jr, et al.: Medical and dental findings in the Brandywine isolate. Ala J Med Sci 1966; 3:382–403.
Witkop CJ Jr: Manifestations of genetic disease in the human pulp. Oral Surg 1971; 32:278–316. * †
Shields ED, et al.: A proposed classification for heritable human dentine defects with a description of a new entity. Arch Oral Biol 1973; 18:543–553.
Sauk JJ, et al.: Immunohistochemical localization of type III collagen in the dentin of patients with osteogenesis imperfecta and hereditary opalescent dentin. J Oral Pathol 1980; 9:210–220.
Takagi Y, Veis A: Matrix protein difference between human normal and dentinogenesis imperfecta dentin. In: Veis A, ed: The chemistry and biology of mineralized connective tissue, vol 22. New York: Elsevier North Holland, 1981:233–243.
Ball SP, et al.: Linkage between dentinogenesis imperfecta and Gc. Ann Hum Genet 1982; 46:35–40.
Levin LS, et al.: Dentinogenesis imperfecta in the Brandywine isolate. Oral Surg Oral Med Oral Path 1983; 56:267–274.

WI043

Carl J. Witkop, Jr.

---

## TEETH, DIASTEMA, MEDIAN INCISAL          0291

**Includes:**
> Diastema, dental medial
> Median incisal diastema
> Midline diastema

**Excludes:** Teeth, microdontia (0660)

**Major Diagnostic Criteria:** A space of 1 mm or greater between normal sized maxillary central incisors. The labial frenum may be observed to extend into the incisive papilla so that tugging on the labial frenum results in blanching of the interdental papilla.

**Clinical Findings:** A true diastema is caused by a persistent tectolabial frenum following the eruption of the permanent teeth. It does not spontaneously recede. True diastema occurs in approximately 10% of individuals without an abnormally positioned labial frenum. Conversely, a marginally situated labial frenum without diastema can be observed. Physiologic spacing of mixed dentition at an early age is not true median diastema. Mandibular central incisors may show diastema too.

**Complications:** Undetermined. Orthodontic closure of the interincisal diastema is not mechanically difficult, but the stability of the closure has been problematic.

**Associated Findings:** Median diastema is a frequent finding in individuals with mental retardation.

**Etiology:** Hereditary factors are suggested; possibly autosomal dominant inheritance. Forty-three percent of all subjects with diastema had similarly affected parents and sibs. Twin studies

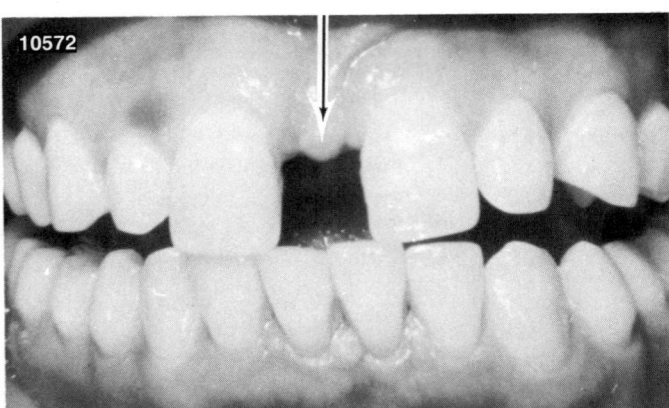

0291-10572: Diastema.

---

show a high concordance rate among monozygotic and a low rate among dizygotic twins. Single gene inheritance is most likely. Anterior teeth spacing or separation may also be caused by a larger arch size, abnormal tongue posture, discrepancy in tooth size, missing lateral incisors, or the presence of supernumeraries.

**Pathogenesis:** The tectolabial frenum consists of two parts: a connective tissue septum in the maxillary suture, which separates the upper dental ridge in median sagittal plane, and the frenular plate, which corresponds to the somewhat later-appearing labial frenum. The deciduous incisor buds are separated during the rise of the septum, which, under normal conditions, regresses or involutes. In most cases, involution of the septum occurs at the same time as resorption of the frenular plate. Any discrepancy in timing will result in a diastema.

**MIM No.:** 12590

**Sex Ratio:** Higher prevalence in females at age 6 years, but the opposite is seen at age 14 years (possibly because girls mature earlier than boys).

**Occurrence:** True diastema occurs in approximately ten percent of individuals without an abnormally positioned labial frenum. Ninety-seven percent of 6-year-old children exhibit a maxillary midline diastema followed by a sharp decrease in occurrence (45% of 9-year-olds, 9% of 16-year-olds) due to eruption of permanent maxillary anterior teeth. Diastemas greater than 0.5 mm were found in 22.33% of the adult subjects (aged 18 to 60 years).

**Risk of Recurrence for Patient's Sib:**
> See Part I, *Mendelian Inheritance*.

**Risk of Recurrence for Patient's Child:**
> See Part I, *Mendelian Inheritance*.

**Age of Detectability:** After the complete eruption of the dentition has occurred (for deciduous teeth, around three years ± 6 months; for permanent teeth, about 21 years ± 6 months, including third molars).

**Gene Mapping and Linkage:** Unknown.

**Prevention:** None known. Genetic counseling indicated.

**Treatment:** As a general rule, if a diastema persists after the maxillary canines erupt, then a frenectomy with or without space closure is considered. It is best to perform a frenectomy after orthodontic space closure since the scar tissue that forms after the surgical procedure is more resilient than the original frenum. If the diastema exceeds 4 to 5 mm prior to canine eruption, the probability is high that bodily tooth movement will be necessary to accomplish closure and root paralleling.

**Prognosis:** Excellent.

**Detection of Carrier:** Unknown.

**References:**
Banker CA, et al.: Alternative methods for the management of persistent maxillary central diastema. Gen Dent 1982; 30:136–139.
Teo CS: Maxillary median diastema: aetiology and incidence. Singapore Dent J 1983; 8:59–63.
McVay TJ, Latta GH, Jr: Incidence of the maxillary midline diastema in adults. J Prosthet Dent 1984; 52:809–811.

PA047                                             **Raj-Rajendra A. Patel**

## TEETH, DILACERATED                          **0929**

**Includes:** Dilacerated teeth

**Excludes:**
    **Teeth, ankylosed** (0927)
    **Teeth, fused** (0930)
    **Teeth, geminated** (0931)
    **Teeth, impacted** (0932)
    **Teeth, root concrescence** (0928)
    **Teeth, supernumerary** (0936)
    Twinning of teeth

**Major Diagnostic Criteria:** Clinical or X-ray evidence of displacement of tooth crown due to abnormal curvature in development.

**Clinical Findings:** Displacement of the tooth crown in relation to root, characterized by clinically obvious malalignment of varying severity. Hard and soft tissues of the crown or root may show defective formation. The crown may show hypoplasia or hypocalcification. Appearance on X-ray depends upon severity of the condition and the spatial relationship of oral tissues, X-ray film, and beam. The most frequently affected teeth in descending order

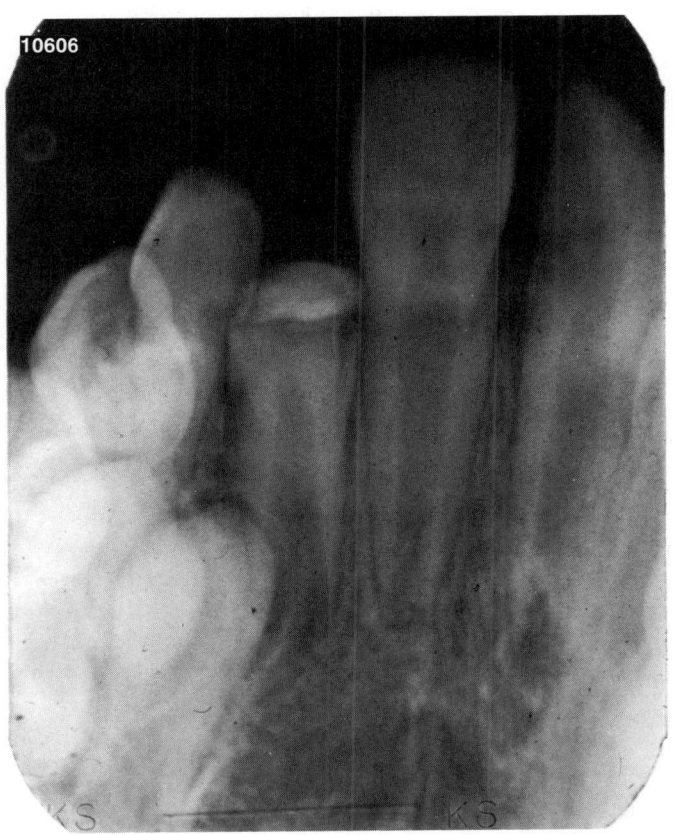

**0929-10606:** Intraoral radiograph of a dilacerated crown of maxillary permanent lateral incisor.

of involvement are: 1) mandibular third molars, 2) maxillary bicuspids, 3) mandibular secondary incisors, and 4) maxillary secondary incisors. Primary teeth are very rarely affected.

**Complications:** Psychosocial problems may arise due to unesthetic anterior affected tooth/teeth; dental caries may occur in hypoplastic defects, if present; continued root formation may be arrested; affected tooth or associated teeth may not erupt; and infection, dentigerous cyst formation, and ameloblastomatous change may develop in relation to an unerupted dilacerated tooth/teeth.

**Associated Findings:** Subsequent to dental caries, there may be pulpal exposure, periapical infection, granuloma, cyst formation, and loss of teeth followed by possible drifting and development of malocclusion.

**Etiology:** Trauma to developing tooth, prior to completion of root formation, results in coronal displacement. Displacement of crown or the developing root(s) may occur 1) during traumatic intrusion or extrusion of primary teeth; 2) during removal of primary teeth; 3) in cases of tooth size-arch size discrepancy resulting in tooth crowding; and 4) subsequent to pressure from adjacent pathologic processes (e.g. cyst).

**Pathogenesis:** At the point of crown-root deflection, enamel or dentin may exhibit abnormal matrix formation or calcification. Crown enamel and dentin may show hypoplasia or hypocalcification. Root apex may exhibit arrested cellular differentiation.

**Sex Ratio:** M1:F1

**Occurrence:** Undetermined but presumed rare.

**Risk of Recurrence for Patient's Sib:** Unknown.

**Risk of Recurrence for Patient's Child:** Unknown.

**Age of Detectability:** Variable, depending upon time of individual tooth formation. Condition is detectable on X-ray during early crown or root formation.

**Gene Mapping and Linkage:** Unknown.

**Prevention:** Avoidance of trauma to unerupted or erupting teeth; careful surgical removal of primary teeth, and early diagnosis and treatment of pathologic processes adjacent to dental structures.

**Treatment:** Orthodontic correction of tooth size-arch size deficiencies to avoid dental crowding. Other therapy may include removal of involved tooth and fabrication of prosthetic replacement, if indicated. Where possible, appropriate restoration of tooth structure to provide function, or, if asymptomatic and acceptable to the patient, leave undisturbed. Endodontic therapy, if indicated, is difficult to perform satisfactorily. Root fracture may occur during extraction of involved tooth.

**Prognosis:** Prognosis of condition depends upon severity of crown-root malalignment, extent of tooth eruption, and condition of clinical crown. With increasing severity of any of these factors, the prognosis of involved tooth worsens. Unless pathology such as infection, dentigerous cyst formation, and ameloblastomatous change develop in relation to an unerupted, dilacerated tooth, the condition does not interfere with longevity.

**Detection of Carrier:** Unknown.

**References:**
Large ND: Anomalies of the teeth and regressive alterations of the teeth. In: Tiecke RW, ed: Oral pathology. 1st ed. New York: McGraw-Hill, 1965:233.
Shafer WG, et al.: A textbook of oral pathology, 3rd ed. Philadelphia: W.B. Saunders, 1974:37.
Stewart RE, et al.: Pediatric dentistry, 1st ed. St. Louis: Mosby, 1982:99–100.

WA011                             **Paul O. Walker**
SC054                             **Mary E. Schwind**

**Teeth, double**
    *See TEETH, FUSED*
**Teeth, double shoveling**
    *See TEETH, INCISORS, SHOVEL-SHAPED*

## TEETH, ENAMEL AND DENTIN DEFECTS FROM ERYTHROBLASTOSIS FETALIS　　0340

**Includes:**
Blueberry muffin rash
Enamel shelf teeth
Erythroblastosis fetalis and staining of enamel and dentin
Hemolytic disease of newborn
Rh hump

**Excludes:**
**Teeth, amelogenesis imperfecta** (0046)
**Teeth, defects from tetracycline** (0341)
**Teeth, odontodysplasia** (0739)

**Major Diagnostic Criteria:** Primary teeth with green, brown, or blue hue and history of parental blood group incompatibilities.

**Clinical Findings:** Intrinsic staining of enamel and dentin of the deciduous teeth occurs with or without enamel hypoplasia. The stain ranges from green, brown, black, or yellow to blue or a mixture of any of these. Orange stain has also been demonstrated. The green stain does not affect the crowns of the deciduous teeth uniformly. The centrals are completely discolored, but the lateral incisors, cuspid, and molars may be only partially stained. Enamel hypoplasia results in defects involving the incisal edges of the anterior teeth and the middle of the crown of the cuspids, where a typical ring-like defect, called *Rh hump*, appears. Icterus gravis, hydrops fetalis, and anemia of the newborn with erythroblastosis represent different grades of clinical severity of the same syndrome of hemolytic anemia affecting the fetus. Chalky enamel surface seen in fluorosis, yellow tetracycline stain observed in permanent teeth, red fluorescence seen in porphyria, and green stain common in other forms of neonatal jaundice must be all considered in the differential diagnosis.

**Complications:** Possible psychosocial complex may arise due to unesthetic appearance of primary teeth. Dental caries may occur in hypoplastic defects, if present.

**Associated Findings:** Dermal erythropoiesis (2 to 8 mm in size, bluish, red, or magenta macules, and infiltrated papules, known as *blueberry muffin rash*). If they begin in early childhood, other hereditary hemolytic diseases such as **Anemia, sickle cell** and **Thalassemia** may result in pigmentation of the permanent teeth.

**Etiology:** Hemolysed erythrocytes liberate hemosiderin pigment, which may become deposited in developing dentin matrices. Ameloblasts apparently are damaged by bilirubin deposited in the dental organ, producing enamel hypoplasia in some cases.

**Pathogenesis:** Hemolytic anemia develops in the infants when an Rh-positive fetus is nurtured in the womb of an Rh-negative mother who has developed anti-Rh antibodies previously. When the antibodies pass the placental membrane and enter the fetal circulation, they agglutinate fetal erythrocytes, bind complement, and cause hemolysis. The same immunologic lesion may evolve as a consequence of ABO isoantigen incompatibility, in which the fetus is A, B, or AB and the mother lacks A or B isoantigens.

**CDC No.:** 282.000

**Sex Ratio:** M1:F1

**Occurrence:** Erythroblastosis fetalis actually occurs in about 10% of pregnancies, but the observed rate is only 0.5%. The low incidence may be explained by the inability of the mother to form antibodies in the presence of an Rh-positive fetus, failure of transplacental transfer of the antigen, or a low level of antibodies in the peripheral blood. Only 22% of patients with ABO incompatibility present enamel hypoplasia. The Rh hump occurs in 1: 2,000 children.

**Risk of Recurrence for Patient's Sib:** If Rh immune globulin is administered to the mother, sensitization is 1% or less; if not administered, risk increases with successive pregnancies.

**Risk of Recurrence for Patient's Child:** Rh incompatibility occurs in 1:200 pregnancies.

**Age of Detectability:** At eruption of primary teeth (First deciduous tooth, central incisor, erupts at around 6 to 7 months).

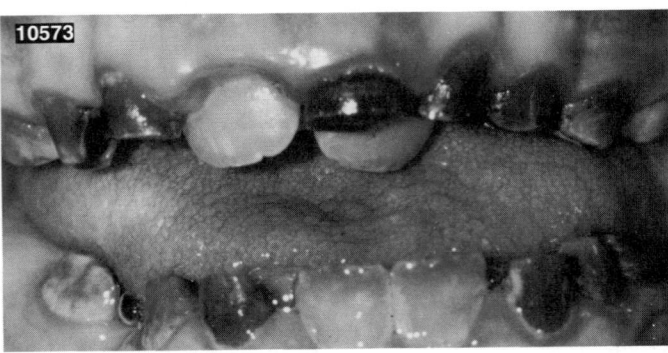

**0340**-10573:　Bilirubin staining of teeth.

**Gene Mapping and Linkage:** Rhesus blood group locus on chromosome 1 (1p32–1pter). ABO blood group locus on chromosome 9 (9pter-9q33).

**Prevention:** Administer Rh immune globulin (RhIG) to unsensitized Rh-negative women after abortion, amniocentesis, ectopic pregnancy, or delivery of an Rh-positive infant.

**Treatment:** Since it affects only the deciduous teeth, the defect presents only a temporary cosmetic problem; esthetics and function may be restored by complete coverage with crowns.

**Prognosis:** Excellent once the oral condition has been treated. Untreated, unesthetic primary teeth may predispose toward childhood psychopathology. Dental caries may occur in hypoplastic defects, if present. Perinatal mortality rate in alloimmunization twin pregnancies is about 9.2%.

**Detection of Carrier:** Parental blood grouping and Rh determination will identify the potential in children to develop this condition.

**References:**
Shafer WG, et al.: A textbook of oral pathology, ed 4. Philadelphia: W.B. Saunders, 1983.
Frigoletto FD, et al.: Ultrasonographic fetal surveillance in the management of the isoimmunized pregnancy. N Engl J Med 1986; 315:430–432.

PA047　　　　　　　　　　　　　　　　**Raj-Rajendra A. Patel**

## TEETH, ENAMEL HYPOPLASIA　　0342

**Includes:**
Enamel aplasia, chronologic
Hutchinson incisors
Intrauterine and neonatal enamel hypoplasia
Mulberry molars
Peg-shaped lateral incisor
Turner tooth

**Excludes:**
Heritable disorders of enamel and dentin
Hypoplastic defects of enamel from exanthematous disease
**Porphyria, erythropoietic** (0821)
**Teeth, amelogenesis imperfecta** (0046)
**Teeth, defects from tetracycline** (0341)
**Teeth, enamel and dentin defects from erythroblastosis fetalis** (0340)

**Major Diagnostic Criteria:** A quantitative defect of enamel visually and morphologically identified as involving the surface of the enamel (an external defect) and associated with a reduced thickness of enamel.

**Clinical Findings:** The defective enamel may occur as (1) shallow or deep pits, or rows of pits arranged horizontally in a linear fashion across the tooth surface or generally distributed over the whole or part of the enamel surface; (2) small or large, wide or narrow grooves; (3) partial or complete absence of enamel over small or considerable areas of dentin.

**Complications:** Dental caries is more likely to occur in hypoplastic enamel.

**Associated Findings:** A qualitative defect of enamel identified visually as an abnormality in the translucency (opacity) of enamel, characterized by a white or discolored (cream, brown, yellow) area, due to hypoplastic enamel.

**Etiology:** Several systemic factors are associated with enamel hypoplasia, as follows:
*Birth trauma:* Breech presentation, multiple pregnancy, caesarian section, prolonged labor.
*Infections; maternal, postnatal:* Syphilis, rubella, measles, chicken pox, scarlet fever, pneumonia, and gastrointestinal infections such as *Salmonella* gastroenteritis.
*Maternal metabolic diseases:* Hypoxia, toxemia of pregnancy, diabetes.
*Perinatal metabolic diseases:* Hyperbilirubinemia, neonatal asphyxia, hypocalcemia, prematurity complications, hypopituitarism.
*Postnatal metabolic diseases:* Hypothyroidism, hypoparathyroidism, congenital cardiac diseases, gastrointestinal malabsorption, nephrotic syndrome, chronic renal failure, biliary atresia.
*Nutritional disorders, maternal, perinatal, and postnatal:* Vitamin D deficiency, celiac disease.
*Chemicals, maternal, perinatal, and postnatal:* Tetracycline, thalidomide, lead intoxication, excessive fluoride.

**Pathogenesis:** Uncertain, but the mechanism appears to involve multifactorial events. Offending agent possibly damages the ameloblasts directly. The lesion appears to be a defect of matrix growth and maturation, probably involving a partial and momentary failure of the operating cycle of an ameloblast. Faulty formation of enamel matrix due to degenerative changes in the ameloblastic layer results in enamel hypoplasia.

**Sex Ratio:** Presumably M1:F1

**Occurrence:** The incidence of at least one tooth with defective enamel in normal children is approximately 63%. However, enamel hypoplasia of primary teeth is found in 21% of children born with low birth weight (<1,500 g). The prevalence of all acquired enamel defects according to Pindborg (1982) is about 14% in primary teeth and between 3% and 15% in permanent teeth.

**Risk of Recurrence for Patient's Sib:** Low, provided no environmental insults are present.

**Risk of Recurrence for Patient's Child:** Low, provided no environmental insults are present.

**Age of Detectability:** Defects can be seen in areas corresponding to both prenatal and postnatal tooth formation. Diagnosis is made by visual, clinical, and X-ray examination for primary teeth at ages 2–5 years, and for permanent teeth at ages 6–7 years.

**Gene Mapping and Linkage:** N/A

**Prevention:** Maintain proper nutritional status during pregnancy; prevent maternal infections, metabolic diseases, toxemia of pregnancy, and febrile childhood diseases.

**Treatment:** Regular topical applications of fluoride on defective enamel increase resistance to dental decay. Shallow pits and grooves can be filled with sealants; deeper defects, with composite restorative material. Full crown coverage is desirable for severe cases.

**Prognosis:** Depends on severity of enamel defect. Some defects weaken the enamel structurally, and others create difficult restorative or cosmetic problems. In the most severe cases teeth are extracted.

**Detection of Carrier:** Unknown.

**Special Considerations:** Chronic fetal distress, as manifested by a significantly subnormal birth weight, is almost always associated with severe damage to the enamel organ. Postnatal enamel is more susceptible to disturbances in mineralization than is prenatal enamel.

**References:**

Ainamo J, Cutress TW: An epidemiological index of developmental defects of dental enamel (DDE Index). Int Dent J 1982; 32:159–167.
Pindborg JJ: Aetiology of developmental enamel defects not related to fluorosis. Int Dent J 1982; 32:123–134. *
Noren JG: Enamel structure in deciduous teeth from low-birth-weight infants. Acta Odontol Scand 1983; 41:355–362.
Daculsi G, et al.: High-resolution study by transmission electron microscopy of a microhypoplasia of the human enamel surface. Arch Oral Biol 1984; 29:210–203.
Sarnat H, Moss SJ: Diagnosis of enamel defects. NY State Dent J. 1985; 51:103–104. *
Seow WK: Oral complications of premature birth. Aust Dent J, 1986; 31:23–29.

PA047 **Raj-Rajendra A. Patel**

**Teeth, enlarged**
*See TEETH, MACRODONTIA*

## TEETH, EPULIS, CONGENITAL      0360

**Includes:**

    Epulis, congenital
    Gingival granular cell tumor, congenital
    Granular cell epulis, congenital
    Granular cell fibroblastoma, congenital
    Granular cell myoblastoma, congenital
    Granular cell tumor (WHO terminology)

**Excludes:**

    Granular cell myoblastoma
    Granular cell neurofibroma

**Major Diagnostic Criteria:** Soft tissue mass of the anterior maxilla or mandible that is present at birth. Ninety percent occur in females. Diagnosis requires histologic confirmation.

**Clinical Findings:** Uncommon, benign soft tissue nodule present in newborns, including the premature infant. Usually a solitary lesion, occasionally multiple (10%). Usually in the incisor or canine region of the maxilla or mandible (ratio: 2 maxilla : 1 mandible). Usually a broad-based soft tissue nodule, but may be pedunculated. Usually covered with intact, normal-appearing mucosa, but may be ulcerated. Size: 1–2 cm diameter average, range 0.3–7.5 cm. Some tumors will regress in size if untreated, but this is not always the case.
*Histology:* Sheets of uniform granular cells with a delicate plexiform capillary network and stromal fibroblasts. Lack of both a prominent neural component and psuedoepitheliomatous hyperplasia of the overlying squamous epithelium differentiates this from granular cell tumors (granular cell myoblastoma). Occasional nests of odontogenic epithelium may be observed. Cytoplasmic PAS-positive, diastase-resistant granules are present. Immunohistochemical studies have been negative for S-100 protein, carcinoembryonic antigen, and estrogen receptors.
*X-ray findings:* Occasional speckled calcifications.

**Complications:** May interfere with nursing and breathing. Rarely affects the developing dentition. Polyhydramnios resulting from obstructed fetal swallowing.

**Associated Findings:** None known.

**Etiology:** Unknown.

**Pathogenesis:** Controversy persists as to whether this lesion is a hamartoma or a neoplasm and as to the histogenesis. Fuhr and Krogh (1972) reviewed the major theories of origin, which included neurogenic, myogenic, fibroblastic, histiocytic, and odontogenic. Several investigators have suggested that the congenital epulis of the newborn represents a degenerative process of mesenchymal tissue that may be hormonally moderated, i.e., by estrogen. Ultrastructural and immunohistochemical studies are suggestive of a mesenchymal origin for this tumor.
The congenital epulis of the newborn is thought by most investigators to be a separate and distinct clinicohistopathologic entity and not a type of granular cell tumor (granular cell myo-

blastoma). Granular cell tumors exhibit strong ultrastructural and immunohistochemical evidence of neurogenic origin.

**Sex Ratio:** M1:F9

**Occurrence:** About 200 cases in the world literature.

**Risk of Recurrence for Patient's Sib:** No familial tendency reported.

**Risk of Recurrence for Patient's Child:** Unknown.

**Age of Detectability:** Present at birth. Has been seen in premature infants, and intrauterine ultrasonographic detection at 35 weeks has been reported.

**Gene Mapping and Linkage:** Unknown.

**Prevention:** None known. Genetic counseling indicated.

**Treatment:** Conservative surgical excision, avoiding the developing dentition, is the treatment of choice. Tumors removed later in the neonatal period have been reported to be smaller, with histologic evidence suggestive of involution. Spontaneous regression and regression of incompletely excised tumors are not uncommon.

**Prognosis:** Excellent for health and life span. Recurrence has not been reported of this benign tumor. Rarely, the developing deciduous dentition may be affected. There are occasional reports of continued difficulty in breathing following surgical excision. There is no evidence of malignant transformation, a malignant counterpart, or metastasis.

**Detection of Carrier:** Unknown.

**References:**

Custer RP, Fust JA: Congenital epulis. Am J Clin Pathol 1952; 22:1044–1053.

Fuhr AH, Krogh PH: Congenital epulis of the newborn. J Oral Surg 1972; 30:30–35.

Lack EE, et al.: Gingival granular cell tumors of the newborn. Am J Surg Pathol 1981; 5:37–46.

Lack EF, et al.: Gingival granular cell tumor of the newborn ("congenital epulis"): ultrastructural observations relating to histogenesis. Hum Pathol 1982; 13:686–689.

Lifshitz MS, et al.: Congenital granular cell epulis. Cancer 1984; 153:1845–1848.

Rainy JB, Smith IJ: Congenital epulis of the newborn. J Pediatr Surg 1984; 19:305–306.

ZU002                                    **Susan L. Zunt**

**Teeth, fetal**
*See TEETH, NATAL OR NEONATAL*

---

**TEETH, FUSED**                                    **0930**

**Includes:**
   Incisor, single upper central
   Maxillary incisor, single central
   Teeth, connate
   Teeth, double

**Excludes:**
   **Teeth, dens invaginatus** (0276)
   **Teeth, ankylosed** (0927)
   **Teeth, root concrescence** (0928)
   **Teeth, geminated** (0931)

**Major Diagnostic Criteria:** A developmental anomaly consisting of the union of two or more normally separate teeth by confluent dentin or, rarely, enamel. X-ray evidence is required to confirm the diagnosis.

**Clinical Findings:** More common in primary than permanent dentition. Usually involves two normally separate teeth, or a tooth plus a supernumerary. The usual primary location is at the anterior mandible, while the location in permanent teeth is usually the anterior maxilla or mandible. May be unilateral or bilateral. Fusion of primary teeth is often followed by hypodontia in the permanent successors. Clinical examination reveals a wide tooth often with a longitudinal groove. X-ray films are necessary

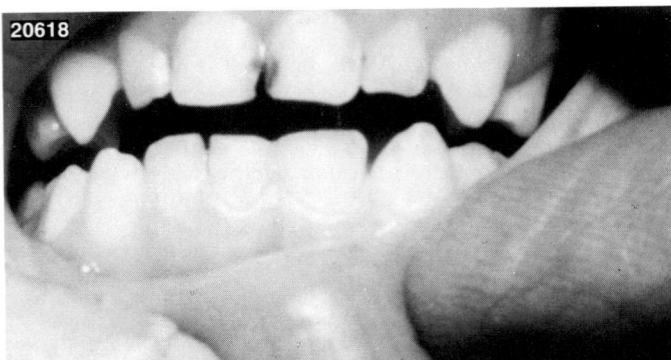

**0930-20618:** Teeth, fused; note fusion of the central and lateral incisors.

---

to establish the diagnosis and dental management. The root canals may be separate or fused.

**Complications:** Esthetics may be compromised when anterior teeth are involved. This may result in psychological problems. Dental caries may develop in the longitudinal groove. Fused primary teeth may influence the permanent dentition by retarding eruption, dental arch space discrepancy and malocclusion. The abnormal shape of fused teeth may predispose to periodontal disease.

**Associated Findings:** Increased incidence in **Fetal thalidomide syndrome**. Winter et al (1988) reported single upper central incisor as a feature of a possible "new" ectodermal dysplasia. Found in humans with abnormal brain development, and the mouse with hypervitaminosis A, trypan blue injection, and riboflavin deficiency.

**Etiology:** Possibly autosomal recessive or autosomal dominant inheritance with incomplete penetrance. May result from external pressure or forces causing contact between developing tooth buds.

**Pathogenesis:** Union of two separate developing tooth buds. The degree of fusion, incomplete to complete, is dependent on the stage at which the contact occurs.

**MIM No.:** 14725, 27300

**Sex Ratio:** M1:F1

**Occurrence:** Approximately 1:100 incidence; prevalence is approximately 0.6% of the Caucasian population; higher in the Japanese (2.5%) and American Indian. Primary dentition: 0.5–2.5%. Permanent dentition: 1%.

**Risk of Recurrence for Patient's Sib:** Unknown. Higher than general population.

**Risk of Recurrence for Patient's Child:** Unknown. Higher than general population.

**Age of Detectability:** Before eruption, by X-ray.

**Gene Mapping and Linkage:** Unknown.

**Prevention:** None known. Genetic counseling indicated.

**Treatment:** Children with fusion of primary teeth require dental evaluation for esthetics, caries prevention and treatment, and dental arch space management. Attempts to maintain the primary fused tooth may be important if the permanent successor is missing. The treatment of fused teeth in the permanent dentition may involve several dental therapeutic modalities, including orthodontics, endodontics, and prosthodontics. Some fused teeth may be separated. In some cases it may be necessary to extract the fused teeth and recommend prosthetic replacement.

**Prognosis:** Depends on the degree of confluence of dentin and pulp, and the morphology and X-ray features.

**Detection of Carrier:** Unknown.

**References:**

Brook AH, Winter GB: Double teeth: a retrospective study of "geminated" and "fused" teeth in children. Br Dent J 1970; 129:123–130.

McKibben DR, Brearley LJ: Radiographic determination of the prevalence of selected dental anomalies of children. J Dent Child 1971; 38:390–398.

Jarvinen S, et al.: Epidemiologic study of joined primary teeth in Finnish children. Community Dent Oral Epidemiol 1980; 8:201–202.

Delany GM, Goldblatt LI: Fused teeth: a multidisciplinary approach to treatment. J Am Dent Assoc 1981; 103:732–734.

Bazan MT: Fusion of maxillary incisors across the midline: clinical report. Pediatr Dent 1983; 5:220–221.

Gregg TA: Surgical division and pulpotomy of a double incisor tooth. Br Dent J 1985; 159:254–256.

Winter RM, et al.: Sparse hair, short stature, hypoplastic thumbs, single upper central incisor and abnormal skin pigmentation: a possible "new" form of ectodermal dysplasia. Am J Med Genet 1988; 29:209–216.

ZU002                                            **Susan L. Zunt**

## TEETH, GEMINATED             0931

**Includes:** Geminated teeth

**Excludes:**
Teeth, ankylosed (0927)
Teeth, dens invaginatus (0276)
Teeth, dilacerated (0929)
Teeth, fused (0930)
Teeth, impacted (0932)
Teeth, root concrescence (0928)

**Major Diagnostic Criteria:** An enlarged bifid or cloven crown on a single root. Number of teeth normally in the arch is neither increased nor decreased.

**Clinical Findings:** Single tooth structure with two completely or incompletely separated crowns that have a single root and a single or partially divided pulp chamber. Clinical crown may exhibit hypoplasia or hypocalcification of enamel or dentin. There is a normal number of teeth in the affected area. The condition is usually limited to mandibular (primary or secondary) incisors.

**Complications:** Delayed eruption of affected or succedaneous tooth. Unesthetic anterior teeth may predispose toward psychopathology. Dental caries may occur in hypoplastic defects, if present. Abnormal coronal morphology may predispose toward malocclusion or periodontal pathology.

**Associated Findings:** Subsequent to dental caries, there may be pulpal exposure, periapical infection, granuloma, cyst formation, and loss of teeth, with possible drifting and resultant malocclusion.

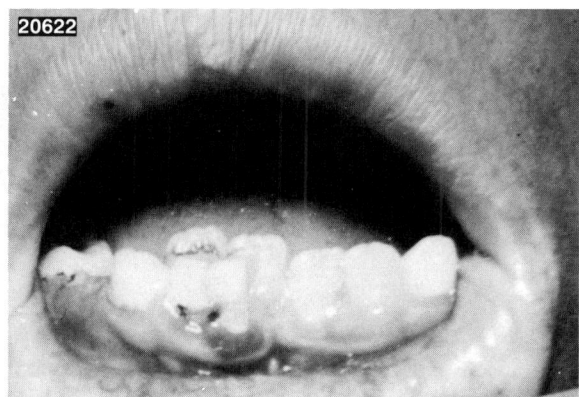

**0931-20622:** Teeth, geminated primary lateral incisors.

**Etiology:** Undetermined. Some cases appear familial.

**Pathogenesis:** Invagination of dental lamina of tooth germ, resulting in double crown, ranging in morphology from an accessory cusp to bifid appearance.

**Sex Ratio:** Presumably M1:F1

**Occurrence:** Undetermined but presumed rare.

**Risk of Recurrence for Patient's Sib:** Unknown.

**Risk of Recurrence for Patient's Child:** Unknown.

**Age of Detectability:** Variable, depending upon age of calcification of the affected tooth. Detected preeruptively on X-ray or posteruptively on clinical examination.

**Gene Mapping and Linkage:** Unknown.

**Prevention:** None known. Genetic counseling indicated.

**Treatment:** Extract affected tooth (presence of succedaneous tooth should be ascertained prior to removing affected primary tooth). Endodontic therapy may be difficult, if root canal is partially divided. It is not always possible to differentiate between gemination and a case in which there has been fusion between a normal tooth and a supernumerary tooth); appropriate restoration of tooth crown, if possible; removal of minimally affected part of crown; or leave tooth undisturbed.

**Prognosis:** Depends on the extent and location of coronal separation, the extent of occlusal disharmony, and the periodontal condition of the affected tooth. A minimally involved tooth with good occlusion and a healthy periodontium has an excellent prognosis. Affected teeth with malocclusion or periodontal pathology have poor prognosis. The condition does not appear to affect life span.

**Detection of Carrier:** Unknown.

**References:**

Large ND: Anomalies of the teeth and regressive alterations of the teeth. In: Tiecke RW, ed: Oral pathology, ed 1. New York: McGraw-Hill, 1965:235 only.

Shafer WG, et al.: A textbook of oral pathology, ed 3. Philadelphia: W.B. Saunders, 1974:35–36.

Stewart RE, et al.: Pediatric dentistry, ed 1. St. Louis: Mosby, 1982:100 only.

WA011                                   **Paul O. Walker**
SC054                                **Mary E. Schwind**

**Teeth, ghost**
*See TEETH, ODONTODYSPLASIA*
**Teeth, hereditary brown**
*See TEETH, DENTINOGENESIS IMPERFECTA*
**Teeth, hypoplastic enamel**
*See AMELO-CEREBRO-HYPOHIDROTIC SYNDROME*
**Teeth, immature**
*See TEETH, NATAL OR NEONATAL*

## TEETH, IMPACTED             0932

**Includes:**
Impacted teeth
Teeth retention
Dentes incluses

**Excludes:**
Teeth, ankylosed (0927)
Teeth, dens invaginatus (0276)
Teeth, dilacerated (0929)
Teeth, fused (0930)
Teeth, geminated (0931)
Teeth, root concrescence (0928)

**Major Diagnostic Criteria:** A tooth that is completely or partially unerupted and is positioned against another tooth, bone, or soft tissue so that its further eruption is unlikely. Unerupted teeth include embedded and impacted teeth, which are not seen clinically but are quite apparent on X-ray.

**Clinical Findings:** Any tooth may become impacted; most commonly involved are the third molars, followed by cuspids. The pericoronal space becomes an ideal trap for bacteria, food residue, and cell debris. The dentist often finds pericoronitis associated with a partially erupted mandibular third molar. In the upper jaw, impacted teeth have been found in the vicinity of the maxillary sinus and, occasionally, in the nose. Lower wisdom teeth may be located in the ascending ramus, at the base of the mandible, in the condylar neck, and in the coronoid process.

**Complications:** An impacted tooth may cause infection, resorption of the adjacent roots, idiopathic pain, trismus, and, due to lack of function in arch, may produce loss of arch length and malocclusion.

**Associated Findings:** Supernumerary teeth occur in 0.3%-3.8% of the population.

**Etiology:** A logical explanation for impacted teeth is the gradual evolutionary reduction in the size of the human mandible and maxilla. The modern diet does not require a decided effort in mastication, and thus growth stimulus of the jaws is lost. Impactions occur because of malpositioning of the tooth bud or obstruction in the path of eruption. Local causative factors include lack of space due to underdeveloped jaws, malocclusion of adjacent teeth, prolonged retention with or without premature loss of primary teeth, and local pathosis such as supernumerary teeth, cysts, and odontogenic tumor. Rare syndromic conditions may also show impactions, such as **Cleidocranial dysplasia, Intestinal polyposis, type III, Craniosynostosis, Progeria, Achondroplasia,** and **Teeth, amelogenesis imperfecta.** The etiology of tooth impaction is related to an arch-length deficiency, except for maxillary cuspid palatal impaction.

**Pathogenesis:** Undetermined. It is possible that malposition of the tooth follicle can lead to the premature exhaustion of the eruptive forces, and to a malposition of the erupted tooth.

**MIM No.:** 30828

**Sex Ratio:** Impacted canines occur more frequently among females than among males (M1:F2.5).

**Occurrence:** Impacted teeth are an increasingly common problem. Andreasen et al. (1986) summarized incidence figures mentioned in various studies: The overall incidence of all impactions reported in 1961 is 16.7%. In a recent study done in 1985, 96.5% of the patients showed X-ray evidence of one or more unerupted or impacted teeth; 98% of these were third molar impactions, 0.9–2% were cuspids, and 0.27% were first premolars. These surveys were performed in the United States.

**Risk of Recurrence for Patient's Sib:** Not increased except in unusual familial cases.

**Risk of Recurrence for Patient's Child:** Not increased except as part of an associated syndrome.

**Age of Detectability:** Following calcification of tooth crown, by X-ray.

**Gene Mapping and Linkage:** Unknown.

**Prevention:** Extraction of supernumerary teeth in the pathway of eruption facilitates spontaneous eruption. Mechanical space maintainers should be used after premature loss of teeth.

**Treatment:** Surgical removal of impacted teeth. More than 55% of extractions are done between the ages of 16 and 25 years, when indicated.

**Prognosis:** There is no association between impacted teeth and systemic disease.

**Detection of Carrier:** Possibly by clinical examination in familial cases.

**References:**
Mercuri LG, O'Neill R: Multiple impaced and supernumerary teeth in sisters. Oral Surg 1980; 50:293 only.
Goldberg MH, et al.: Complications after mandibular third molar surgery: a statistical analysis of 500 consecutive procedures in private practice. J Am Dent Assoc 1985; 111:227–229.
Tetsch P, Wagner W: Operative extraction of wisdom teeth. Littleton, CO: PSG, 1985.

Andreasen JO, et al.: Oral health care: more than caries and periodontal disease. A survey of epidemiological studies on oral disease. Int Dent J 1986; 36:207–214.
Nitzan DW, et al.: The effect of aging on tooth morphology: a study on impacted teeth. Oral Surg 1986; 61:54–60.

PA047                                          **Raj-Rajendra A. Patel**

---

### TEETH, INCISORS, SHOVEL-SHAPED                 2135

**Includes:**
    Incisors, barrel-shape
    Teeth, double shoveling
    Teeth, semi-shovel

**Excludes:**
    Teeth, crown malformations (other)
    **Teeth, pegged or absent maxillary lateral incisor (0934)**

**Major Diagnostic Criteria:** Incisor teeth with prominent elevation or hypertrophy of the marginal ridges, enclosing the lingual fossa.

**Clinical Findings:** Elevation or hypertrophy of the marginal ridges enclosing the lingual fossa is the characteristic feature of shovel-shaped incisors. The enamel is not hypertrophied on the marginal ridges; dentin is also involved in their formation. Bilateral symmetry is usually seen and, when central upper incisors are affected, the lateral incisors are commonly affected. As a result of the high marginal ridges sometimes being extremely elevated, a so-called barrel-shaped incisor can be seen. There is a prominent, common variant called double shovel-shape, in which the labial marginal ridges are also strongly elevated. These teeth tend to look wide and large for the patient's mouth. Sometimes the mandibular incisors and canines can also be affected, but the lingual fossa is never as prominent as it is in the maxillary incisors.

**Complications:** Unknown.

**Associated Findings:** Because of the enlargement of the marginal ridges, the lingual fossa becomes accentuated and a deep pit can be seen there. As a result, caries is a common complication which often is not detected until too late, after pulpal exposure has occurred.

**Etiology:** Undetermined. Several models for explaining genetic control of shoveling have been proposed: 1) Autosomal dominant inheritance with variable expressivity, 2) two autosomal alleles without dominance, and 3) polygenic inheritance.

The extent to which genetic factors determine the degree of shovel shapes has been studied by considering different familial correlations. The parent-offspring correlations, when compared to the full-sib correlation, suggest that there is no dominance deviation in the variation of shoveling. They also suggest that about 68% of the variation seen in shoveling can be explained by the additive effect of genes.

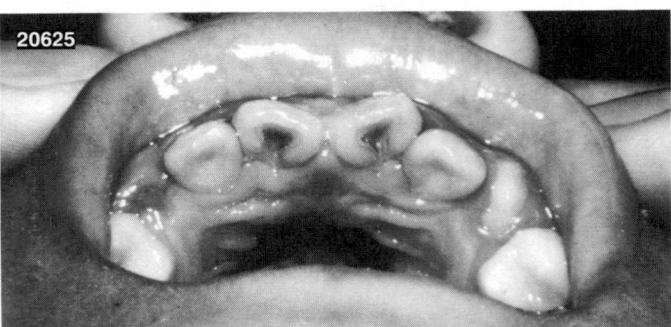

**2135-20625:** Teeth, incisors, shovel-shaped; note also mesiopalatal rotation.

**Pathogenesis:** Primate incisors display a cingulum formed by a mesial, a cervical and a distal marginal tuberculum. In a shovel-shaped tooth, the marginal ridges are well developed and the median ridge is reduced.

**MIM No.:** 14740

**Sex Ratio:** M1:F1

**Occurrence:** Depends on the population being studied. For Caucasians, an average incidence over several populations is 37.9%; for Japanese, 95.5%; and for the American Indian, 99.0%.

**Risk of Recurrence for Patient's Sib:**
See Part I, *Mendelian Inheritance.*

**Risk of Recurrence for Patient's Child:**
See Part I, *Mendelian Inheritance.*

**Age of Detectability:** As soon as the incisors erupt in the mouth; about six to seven years of age.

**Gene Mapping and Linkage:** Unknown.

**Prevention:** None known. Genetic counseling indicated.

**Treatment:** Pulpal complications due to caries should be prevented by doing prophylactic restorations of the lingual fossa when indicated.

**Prognosis:** Normal life span.

**Detection of Carrier:** By oral examination.

**References:**

Lee GTR, Goose DH: The inheritance of dental traits in a Chinese population in the United Kingdom. J Med Genet 1972; 9:336–339.

Kirveskari P: Morphological traits in the permanent dentition of the living skolt lapps. Proceedings of the Finnish Dental Society 1974; (Suppl II)70.

Portin P, Alvesalo L: The inheritance of shovel shape incisors in maxillary incisors. Am J Phys Anthrop 1974; 41:59–62.

Blanco R, Chakraborti R: Genetics of shovel-shaped maxillary central incisors. Am J Phys Anthrop 1976; 44:233–236.

Escobar V, et al.: Genetic structure of the Queckchi Indians. Hum Hered 1979; 29:134–142.

ES000                        **Victor Escobar**

---

## TEETH, LOBODONTIA          0607

**Includes:**
Lobodontia
Teeth, carnivore-like
Teeth, conical, multiple
"Wolf teeth"

**Excludes:**
Hypodontia
**Teeth, dens invaginatus** (0276)
**Teeth, enamel hypoplasia** (0342)
**Teeth, microdontia** (0660)

**Major Diagnostic Criteria:** Multiple dental anomalies of the teeth resulting in a dentition resembling that of a carnivore.

**Clinical Findings:** Multiple anomalies of the teeth resulting in a dentition resembling that of a carnivore. All observed cases have had multitubercular molar crowns, generalized reduction of crown size, accentuation of mesiobuccal cusps of molars and buccal cusps of premolars, accentuation of cingulum of premolars and incisors, suppression in height of other molar and premolar cusps and large diastemata in upper and lower canine regions. Some, but not all cases, have in addition, multiple dens in dente or deep palatal invaginations, single conical molar roots, agenesis of teeth, ectopic eruption of teeth, and shovel-shaped incisors.

**Complications:** Pulpal inflammation, degeneration and periapical involvement in teeth with dens in dente.

**Associated Findings:** None known.

**Etiology:** Autosomal dominant inheritance.

**Pathogenesis:** Undetermined. The morphologic alterations peculiar to this entry are genetically determined, and clinical com-

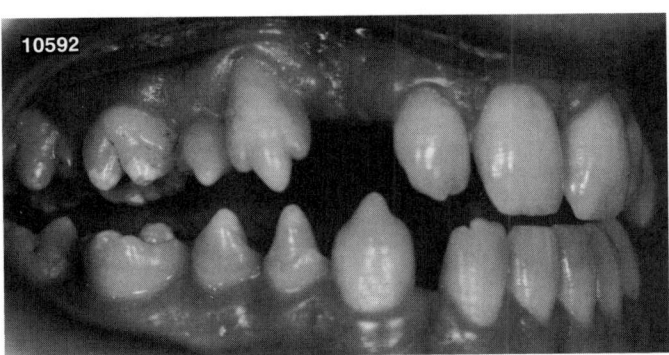

**0607-10592:** Note cone-shaped mandibular premolars and fang-like maxillary canine.

plications such as pulpal degeneration in teeth with dens in dente probably occur after eruption into the oral cavity.

**MIM No.:** *18700

**Sex Ratio:** Presumably M1:F1 (observed M7:F5).

**Occurrence:** Estimated to be less than 1:1,000,000. Three kindreds have been documented.

**Risk of Recurrence for Patient's Sib:**
See Part I, *Mendelian Inheritance.*

**Risk of Recurrence for Patient's Child:**
See Part I, *Mendelian Inheritance.*

**Age of Detectability:** At two years by clinical and X-ray examination of deciduous teeth.

**Gene Mapping and Linkage:** Unknown.

**Prevention:** None known. Genetic counseling indicated.

**Treatment:** Root canal therapy for teeth with dens in dente; use of occlusal sealants following eruption. Occlusal table should be restored, and cusps preserved.

**Prognosis:** Apparently normal life span.

**Detection of Carrier:** Unknown.

**References:**

Robbins IM, Keene HJ: Multiple morphologic dental anomalies: report of a case. Oral Surg 1964; 17:683–690.

Mayhall JT: Analysis of dental form regression syndrome. IADR program and abstract #373, 1967.

Shuff RY: A patient with multiple conical teeth. Dent Practit 1972; 22:414–417.

Brook AN, Winder M: Lobodontia: a rare inherited dental anomaly. Br Dent J 1979; 147:213–215.

Dahlberg AA: Rationale of identification based on biological factors of the dentition. Am J Forensic Med Pathol 1984; 5(4).

DA002             **Albert A. Dahlberg**
KE003                **Harris J. Keene**

**Teeth, localized arrested development**
*See TEETH, ODONTODYSPLASIA*

---

## TEETH, MACRODONTIA          0617

**Includes:**
Megadontia
Teeth, enlarged

**Excludes:**
Conjoined teeth
**Hemihypertrophy** (0458)
**Teeth, fused** (0930)

**Major Diagnostic Criteria:** Teeth are significantly larger than normal. Mesiodistal and buccolingual measurements exceed range of normal variation.

**Clinical Findings:** Teeth that are larger than normal can be classified as follows: (1) True-generalized or generalized proportional macrodontia is a condition in which all teeth are larger than normal. It has been associated with pituitary gigantism and hemihypertrophy. (2) Relative-generalized or generalized disproportional macrodontia is the result of the presence of normal or slightly larger than normal teeth in small jaws. This disparity in size gives the illusion of macrodontia. (3) Localized macrodontia is a condition in which one or a few large teeth exist in relation to an otherwise normal dentition and body size. It usually involves the mandibular third molar. True macrodontia of a single tooth should not be confused with conjoined teeth or fusion of teeth, in which early in odontogenesis, the union of two or more teeth results in a single large tooth. In hemihypertrophy of the face, a variant of this localized macrodontia may occasionally be seen in which the teeth of the involved side are considerably larger than those of the unaffected side.

**Complications:** Crowding and irregular alignment of the dentition (malocclusion) result when relative-generalized macrodontia occurs. Large teeth may get impacted and may later show dentigerous cyst formation.

**Associated Findings:** Macrodontia occurs in syndromes in which there may be numerous other features such as mental retardation, hypogonadism, midface hypoplasia, and limb deformities, among others. For example: **KBG syndrome, Klinefelter syndrome,** and **Sturge-Weber syndrome.**

**Etiology:** The size of teeth is only one variable in a complex system of craniofacial development, the components of which generally show a continuous size variation. Twin studies have established a genetic component in tooth size variability. Family studies have demonstrated consistently that important environmental effects are superimposed upon genetic effects to determine tooth size. From animal experimentation, these environmental influences were shown to be largely maternal, such as cytoplasmic inheritance, prenatal uterine environment (influenced by maternal diet), and postnatal maternal effects. No genetic basis for tooth size asymmetry has been detected, and tooth pairs (e.g., maxillary canines, mandibular first premolars) may be assumed to be under identical genetic control with respect to size. Asymmetry is thus considered to be the result of a phenotypic environmental disturbance during tooth development.

**Pathogenesis:** Secretion of an abnormally high level of growth hormone may result in increased size of all body tissues, including teeth and jaws. This is apparently what happens in true-generalized macrodontia associated with pituitary gigantism.

**Sex Ratio:** M1:F1

**Occurrence:** Undetermined.

**Risk of Recurrence for Patient's Sib:** Probably very low.

**Risk of Recurrence for Patient's Child:** Probably very low.

**Age of Detectability:** At the time of eruption of deciduous and permanent teeth.

**Gene Mapping and Linkage:** Unknown.

**Prevention:** None known. Genetic counseling indicated.

**Treatment:** No treatment is necessary or indicated except in cases where there is malocclusion, or when impacted teeth are present. Then, extraction and orthodontic treatment is recommended.

**Prognosis:** Excellent.

**Detection of Carrier:** Unknown.

**References:**
Harzer W: A hypothetical model of genetic control of tooth-crown growth in man. Arch Oral Biol 1987; 32:159–162.

PA047                                            **Raj-Rajendra A. Patel**

## TEETH, MESIOPALATAL TORSION OF CENTRAL INCISORS                    2133

**Includes:**
>    Counterwing teeth
>    Incisors, mesiopalatal torsion of central
>    Incisors, rotation of upper central
>    Mesiolabial rotation of upper central incisors
>    Mesiopalatal rotation of upper central incisors
>    Wing teeth

**Excludes:**
>    Bite, open
>    **Teeth, supernumerary** (0936)
>    Teeth, crowding

**Major Diagnostic Criteria:** The upper central incisors must be in a correct alignment within the dental arch, with the distal part of the crown rotated labially, bringing the mesial part to a palatal position in the absence of crowding.

**Clinical Findings:** Mesiopalatal rotation of upper central incisors presents as a rotation of the upper central incisors within their bony sockets. The distal part of the crown is rotated labially, bringing the mesial part to a lingual position. The reverse position or mesiolabial rotation also occurs. This latter position gives the impression of a pointed prominence to the upper incisor region. The teeth shapes are normal, and they are correctly positioned in the maxillary dental arch.

**Complications:** Malocclusion.

**Associated Findings:** Although this condition usually occurs as an isolated finding, its presence suggests malocclusion and esthetic disharmony.

**Etiology:** Risk of recurrence figures have been derived from a study of 166 families. A segregation analysis suggests an autosomal dominant trait, with variable expression and a penetrance of 84%.

**Pathogenesis:** Fetal material suggests that the rotation of the incisors as seen clinically in erupted teeth is a continuation of a rotation seen during early embryonic development. One can then hypothesize that the mechanism for rotation of the incisors from the position seen in fetal life to the adult position is defective and does not allow for this movement. Linkage studies have placed this trait in close association with blood group P and chromosome 6. This linkage association lends support to the existence of this trait as a separate genetic entity.

**MIM No.:** 14735

**Sex Ratio:** M1:F1

**Occurrence:** Incidence and prevalence depend on the population studied. In the average American Indian, 23–44%; among

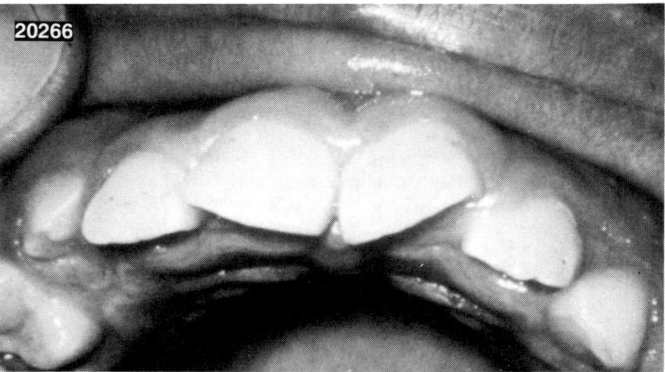

**2133-20266:** Note winged teeth resulting from the mesiopalatal torsion of the central incisors.

Caucasions, 6%; Chinese 5.2%; Japanese, 5.6%, and Hawaiians, 22%.

**Risk of Recurrence for Patient's Sib:** Empiric risk: 58% if one parent is affected; 40% if both parents are normal.

**Risk of Recurrence for Patient's Child:** Empiric risk :40%.

**Age of Detectability:** After the teeth erupt in the mouth.

**Gene Mapping and Linkage:** Linkage studies have placed this trait in close association with blood group P on chromosome 6.

**Prevention:** None known. Genetic counseling indicated.

**Treatment:** Interceptive orthodontics. In older children and adult patients, orthodontic treatment can be performed if the degree of rotation is severe enough to require treatment. However, one should bear in mind that tooth rotations around their axes are one of the most difficult orthodontic problems, since teeth tend to revert to their original position once the orthodontic appliances have been removed.

**Prognosis:** An association with several other traits characteristic of Indian populations has been reported, especially **Teeth, incisors, shovel-shaped**. Because of the deep lingual fossae, these teeth are more susceptible to caries and pulpal involvement. Otherwise, longevity of the tooth is not affected.

**Detection of Carrier:** By oral examination.

**References:**

Escobar V, et al.: The inheritance of bilateral rotation of maxillary central incisors. Am J Phys Anthrop 1976; 45:109–116.

Escobar V: A genetic study of upper central incisor rotation (wing teeth) in the Pima Indians. PhD thesis, Department of Medical Genetics. Indianapolis: Indiana University School of Medicine, 1979.

ES000                                                    **Victor Escobar**

---

## TEETH, MICRODONTIA                                           **0660**

**Includes:**
>    Microdontia
>    Teeth, small

**Excludes:**
>    **Chondroectodermal dysplasia** (0156)
>    **Chromosome 21, trisomy 21** (0171)
>    Ectodermal dysplasia, anhidrotic
>    **Eye, anterior segment dysgenesis** (0439)
>    **Fetal radiation syndrome** (0383)
>    **Incontinentia pigmenti** (0526)
>    **Teeth, amelogenesis imperfecta** (0046)
>    **Teeth, pegged or absent maxillary lateral incisor** (0934)

**Major Diagnostic Criteria:** The involved tooth or teeth must be small enough to be outside the usual limits of variation.

**Clinical Findings:** The involved tooth or teeth are small in size, well beyond usual limits of variation. Microdontia is manifested in 2 forms: true generalized microdontia which is extremely rare, occurring in some cases of pituitary dwarfism and, secondly, microdontia involving a single tooth or groups of teeth. The latter commonly affects the lateral incisors and maxillary molars and, along with the reduction in size, these teeth often exhibit a change in shape.

**Complications:** Cosmetic problem may have psychologic effects.

**Associated Findings:** Microdontia of the whole dentition may occur in syndromes, for example, **Chromosome 21, trisomy 21**, congenital heart disease, and pituitary dwarfism.

Microdontia may occur as a partial manifestation in a number of conditions including: **Cleft lip**, **Turner syndrome**, focal dermal hypoplasia, lipoid proteinosis, some forms of **Mucopolysacchari-dosis**, **Oculo-auriculo-vertebral anomaly**, progeria, **Craniofacial dysostosis**, **Ehlers-Danlos syndrome**, **Sturge-Weber syndrome**, **Teeth, odontodysplasia**, **Osteogenesis imperfecta**, **Teeth, dentinogenesis imperfecta**, oculomandibulodyscephaly, and monilethrix. Small cone-shaped teeth may occur in many syndromes in which teeth are missing, especially those generally classed as **Ectodermal dysplasia**.

The most common form of microdontia (1.2 to 3.2% of general population) are peg maxillary lateral incisors. This is a discrete genetic trait which is manifest as either peg or missing maxillary lateral incisors. This tooth is also found in microform in **Acrocephalopolysyndactyly** (type III). Loss of the central mamelon of developing incisors in patients with congenital syphilis results in small screwdriver-shaped teeth. Absent or small mandibular incisors are nearly a constant feature of the **Hypoglossia-hypodactylia**. Microdontia of a specific tooth, the maxillary second primary molar, occurs in **Williams syndrome**.

**Etiology:** A hypothesis proposed by Harzer (1987) states 1) autosomal and X-linked genes determine the basic structures of tooth germ, whereas additional genes may promote size compensations during early odontogenesis; and 2) the tooth germ and the surrounding bone structures are genetically interdependent with regard to size determination so that there is a growth hierarchy. In one study, an association between hypodontia and microdontia was established. These findings may be explained as a multifactorial model having a continuous scale, related to tooth number and size, with thresholds. Reduced or hypoplastic maxillary laterals are a variable expression of the gene for congenitally missing lateral incisors. The genetic contribution to variation of mesiodistal diameter is greater both for individual teeth and tooth groups than it is to buccolingual diameter. However, there is a general decrease in heritability from anterior to posterior in the upper jaw and no clear trend in the lower jaw.

**Pathogenesis:** Unknown. Some disturbance impending on the full development of the tooth germ or germs involved either by disturbing enamel organ development or secondarily by faulty formation of dentin or enamel.

**Sex Ratio:** M1:F1.6

**Occurrence:** Prevalence of microdontia for males is 1.9%, for females is 3.1%, and for both sexes is 2.5%. True generalized microdontia is rare. Individual microdontia is more common, reaching 4% for third molars.

**Risk of Recurrence for Patient's Sib:** Incidence among first degree relatives of all probands is 29.1%.

**Risk of Recurrence for Patient's Child:** Unknown.

**Age of Detectability:** At eruption of teeth by dental examination.

**Gene Mapping and Linkage:** Unknown.

**Prevention:** None known. Genetic counseling indicated.

**Treatment:** Requires a collective effort in preventive dentistry, restorative dentistry, oral surgery, orthodontics, and prosthodontics.

**Prognosis:** Excellent for isolated microdontia.

**Detection of Carrier:** Unknown.

**References:**

Steinberg AG, et al.: Hereditary generalized microdontia. J Dent Res 1961; 40:58.

Shafer WG, et al.: A textbook of oral pathology, 2nd ed. Philadelphia, W.B. Saunders, Co., 1963:34.

Woof CM: Missing maxillary lateral incisors: a genetic study. Am J Hum Genet 1971; 23:289.

Freire-Maia N, Pinheiro M: Ectodermal dysplasias: a clinical and genetic study. New York: Alan R Liss, 1984.

Harzer W: A hypothetical model of genetic control of tooth-crown growth in man. Arch Oral Biol 1987; 32:159–162.

WI043                                              **Carl J. Witkop, Jr.**
PA047                                              **Raj-Rajendra A. Patel**

## TEETH, MOLAR REINCLUSION        2137

**Includes:**
Ankylosis of teeth
Dental ankylosis
Molars, reincluded
Reinclusion of permanent molars, familial

**Excludes:**
**Teeth, dilacerated** (0929)
**Teeth, impacted** (0932)

**Major Diagnostic Criteria:** Molar teeth which, during or after a period of active eruption, stop their relative occlusal movement and remain below the occlusal plane.

**Clinical Findings:** Teeth are considered to be reincluded if, after a short period of active eruption and occlusal function, they fail to maintain their occlusal position in relation to other teeth. This leads to the false impression that they are depressed (being reincluded) into the jawbone while, in fact, they are remaining stationary while their neighbors continue to move occlusally. The only affected teeth so far appear to be both upper and lower molars, which present clinically as a posterior open bite. Although ankylosis (fusion of cementum to alveolar bone) has been blamed for the occurrence of "submerged teeth," this is not a finding in patients with familial reinclusion of permanent molars. Linkage studies, using blood and serum groups as markers, have provisionally assigned the "molar reinclusion" gene to the same linkage group as the gene locus of blood group P.

**Complications:** Unknown.

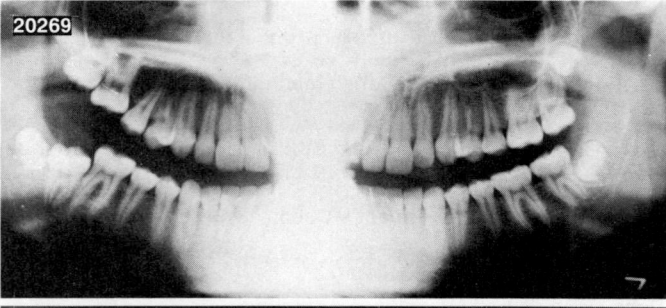

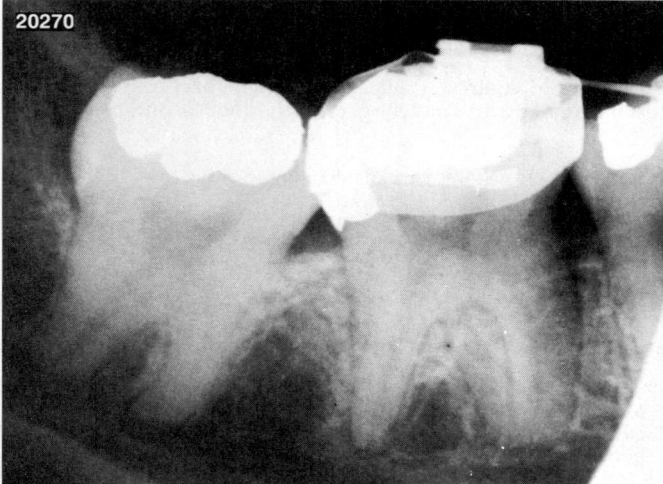

**2137-20269:** Submerged upper and lower molars. 20270: Note the presence of the peridontal ligament in this close-up of the same teeth as shown in 20269.

**Associated Findings:** Supereruption of opposing teeth with tipping of adjacent teeth and development of malocclusion. Reported patients have been identified because of an open posterior bite on the affected site.

When the infraocclusion is severe, soft tissue covers these teeth again. Since they did break through the epithelium initially, an epithelial-lined tract occurs which communicates the tooth with the oral cavity. This raises the possibility of local periodontal pathology.

**Etiology:** Twelve families regarded as examples of a genetic entity different from tooth ankylosis suggest autosomal dominant inheritance.

**Pathogenesis:** The primary biochemical defect which prevents these teeth from reaching their normal position in the dental arch is unknown. However, tooth ankylosis as a result of environmental or congenital injury to the periodontal membrane has been suggested as the etiologic factor. Yet, histologic and scanning electron microscopy studies have failed to reveal any indications of ankylosis. Proffitt and Vig (1981) suggest that a primary defect in the periodontal ligament or its vascular supply may be involved.

**MIM No.:** *15795

**Sex Ratio:** M1:F1

**Occurrence:** Nine families are from the Netherlands, two from the United States, and one from India have been documented. However, scattered in the literature on ankylosed teeth, one can find references of familial cases which may represent this condition.

**Risk of Recurrence for Patient's Sib:**
See Part I, *Mendelian Inheritance.*

**Risk of Recurrence for Patient's Child:**
See Part I, *Mendelian Inheritance.*

**Age of Detectability:** In the late teens, when adjacent teeth have reached their final occlusal plane.

**Gene Mapping and Linkage:** Unknown.

**Prevention:** None known. Genetic counseling indicated.

**Treatment:** Orthodontic treatment may be successful in correcting this condition, since tooth ankylosis is not present. However, Proffitt and Vig (1981) suggest that orthodontic treatment of such teeth can produce ankylosis. Surgical removal of bone and soft tissue covering the teeth have proved successful when inducing eruption of these molars. At least one case is known in which teeth did not erupt in spite of orthodontic treatment, and had to be surgically removed.

**Prognosis:** Treated, the prognosis is good. Orthodontic treatment may bring these teeth into normal occlusion. Once this has happened, surrounding alveolar bone will develop. Since there appear to be no other associated findings, life span is not affected.

**Detection of Carrier:** Unknown.

**Special Considerations:** Orthodontic treatment should always be attempted. If ineffective because of the possibility of undetectable ankylosis, surgical luxation of the tooth might be attempted. This has been suggested to permit resumption of eruption by breaking the bony bridge.

**References:**
Biederman W: Etiology and treatment of tooth ankylosis. Am J Ortho 1962; 48:670–684.
Bosker H, Nijenhuis LW: Possible linkage between a gene causing reinclusion of molar I and blood group P. Cytogenet Cell Genet 1975; 14:255–256.
Bosker H, et al.: Familial reinclusion of permanent molars. Clin Genet 1978; 13:314–320.
Kapoor AK, et al.: Bilateral posterior open bite. Oral Surg 1981; 52:21–22.
Poffitt WR, Vig KL: Primary failure of eruption: a possible cause of posterior open bite. Am J Ortho 1981; 80:173–190.

ES000                 **Victor Escobar**

## TEETH, NATAL OR NEONATAL                                    0933

**Includes:**
  Precocious dentition
  Teeth, congenital
  Teeth, fetal
  Teeth, immature
  Teeth, present at birth

**Excludes:** Inclusion cysts of the oral mucosa in the newborn (3236)

**Major Diagnostic Criteria:** One or two teeth are present at birth or in first month of life.

**Clinical Findings:** Natal teeth are present at birth (75%). Neonatal teeth appear in the first 30 days of life (25%). Usually, one or two natal/neonatal teeth are seen in the anterior mandibular incisor area (85%).

A dental X-ray may be helpful in determining the maturity of the natal/neonatal tooth and whether it represents early eruption of a deciduous (90%) or a supernumerary (10%) tooth. The parent can hold the infant and positioned dental X-ray film during the exposure.

Natal teeth are slightly more common in females than males. The natal tooth's structure may resemble primary teeth, but it is more often a small, chalky white to yellow, conical structure with enamel defects. These teeth are often hypomineralized, cartilaginous in texture, and wear or fracture easily. Most natal/neonatal teeth are in the anterior mandibular incisor area (85%). Seventy percent of natal/neonatal teeth are firm in the alveolus, while 30% are mobile. These mobile teeth may be immature anomalous dental structures with little or no root development that may exfoliate in 10–15 days if untreated. Some of the initially mobile teeth will become firm if left in situ. A localized swelling of the alveolar mucosa is observed overlying neonatal teeth.

Failure of root formation with disruption of Hertwig epithelial root sheath, a large vascular dental pulp, irregular dentin, and cementum hypoplasia or agenesis have also been reported.

**Complications:** With teeth present, these complications include sublingual and/or lingual frenula ulceration resulting in feeding

difficulties and irritability, as well as laceration or irritation of nursing mother's nipples. There is a potential for aspiration or swallowing (the latter has little clinical significance) of mobile natal/neonatal teeth, but neither has been reported.

With extraction, neonatal hypoprothrombinemia or bleeding defects should be excluded. Excessive hemorrhage has been reported following extraction, including one infant who had received vitamin K at birth. Lost space in the dental arch may be significant. Rarely, extraction may damage the underlying developing permanent tooth.

**Associated Findings:** Facial clefts, **Cyclopia, Pachyonychia congenita-steatocystoma multiplex, Oculo-mandibulo-facial syndrome,** and **Chondroectodermal dysplasia.**

A few unique syndromes have been identified with natal teeth as a feature (Harris et al, 1976; McDonald and Reed, 1982).

**Etiology:** Undetermined. Familial tendency identified in 15–24% of reported cases.

**Pathogenesis:** Superficial location of a developing tooth is the most accepted theory.

**MIM No.:** 18705

**CDC No.:** 520.600

**Sex Ratio:** M1:F>1

**Occurrence:** 1:2,000–6,000 live births

**Risk of Recurrence for Patient's Sib:** Overall risk in the absence of established inheritance pattern is 15%.

**Risk of Recurrence for Patient's Child:** Overall risk in the absence of established inheritance pattern is 15%.

**Age of Detectability:** Natal teeth: at birth; neonatal teeth: within 30 days of birth.

**Gene Mapping and Linkage:** Unknown.

**Prevention:** None known. Genetic counseling indicated.

**Treatment:** If the natal/neonatal teeth are causing the infant discomfort, refusal to eat, ulceration or they exhibit incomplete immature development with excessive mobility, extracton can be accomplished with topical or local anesthesia. Supernumerary teeth should be extracted in most cases. Natal/neonatal teeth that are components of the deciduous dentition should be maintained for as long as possible.

Dental evaluation by a pedodontist is strongly recommended.

**Prognosis:** Immature, mobile, supernumerary natal or neonatal teeth often require extraction. If these teeth are part of the normal complement of deciduous teeth, an attempt should be made to maintain them. Often the mobility will decrease as root development proceeds.

The presence of natal/neonatal teeth may herald significant dental arch space management problems. Dental consultation with a pediatric dentist is recommended.

In general, the patient has a good medical prognosis if natal/neonatal teeth are an isolated finding. Modification of the prognosis results with the presence of the less frequently associated conditions.

**Detection of Carrier:** Unknown.

**Special Considerations:** The nursing mother may be at risk for injury, although this may resolve with continued breast feeding, i.e., the child becomes conditioned not to bite.

Among the Chinese, the presence of natal teeth is considered very bad luck and the parents may require reassurance.

King Louis XIV and other significant historical figures were born with teeth (Bodenhoff and Gorlin, 1963).

**References:**
Bodenoff J, Gorlin RJ: Natal and neonatal teeth: folklore and fact. Pediatrics 1963; 32:1087–1098.
Harris DJ, et al.: Natal teeth, patent ductus arteriosus and intestinal pseudo-obstruction: a lethal syndrome in the newborn. Clin Genet 1976; 9:479–482.
Anneroth G, et al.: Clinical, histologic and microradiographic study of natal, neonatal and preerupted teeth. Scand J Dent Res 1978; 86:58–66.

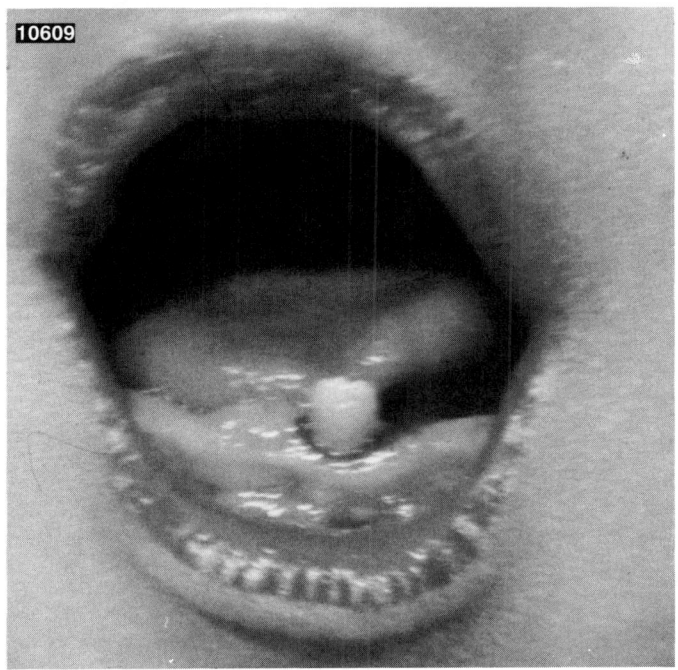

**0933-10609:** Natal tooth.

McDonald RM, Reed WB: Natal teeth and steatocystoma multiplex complicated by hidradenitis suppurative. Arch Dermatol 1982; 112: 1132–1134.

Ronk SL: Multiple immature teeth in a newborn. J Pedod 1982; 6:254–260.

McDonald RE, Avery DR: Dentistry for the child and adolescent, 4th ed. St. Louis: C.V. Mosby, 1983:114–116.

Leung AKC: Natal teeth. Am J Dis Child 1986; 140:249–251.

ZU002                                    **Susan L. Zunt**

## TEETH, ODONTOBLASTIC DYSPLASIA, FOCAL          2109

**Includes:**
> Dentin dysplasia type III
> Odontoblastic dysplasia, focal

**Excludes:**
> **Dentino-osseous dysplasia** (0280)
> **Osteogenesis imperfecta** (0777)
> **Teeth, dentin dysplasia, coronal** (0277)
> **Teeth, dentin dysplasia, radicular** (0278)
> **Teeth, dentinogenesis imperfecta** (0279)
> **Teeth, odontodysplasia** (0739)

**Major Diagnostic Criteria:** Extensive pulp stone formation in all permanent teeth which are otherwise clinically and on X-ray within normal limits.

**Clinical Findings:** Extensive pulp stones are present in the pulp chambers and/or canals of all permanent teeth. The root canals in many anterior teeth are distorted in proximity to these pulpal masses. Pulp stone formation in posterior teeth is so extensive that only a very thin radiolucent line distinguishes the pulpal wall boundaries. All permanent teeth are normal in size, shape, color, enamel hardness, vitality (electrical) and radiographic dentin-enamel contrast. Light and scanning electron microscopy reveal the pulp stones to be true denticles composed of a chaotic array of dysplastic dentinal tubules attached to the floor of the pulp chamber. Similar but separate excrescences of dysplastic dentin are identified on the dentinal walls of the pulp canals. Histologically, the bulk of the enamel, dentin and cementum are within normal limits.

**Complications:** Unknown.

**Associated Findings:** None known.

**Etiology:** Unknown.

**Pathogenesis:** Appears to be a primary dentin defect in which the dysplastic pulpal masses originate from circumscribed groups of odontoblasts at the pulpal wall which produce chaotic dentin.

**Sex Ratio:** Presumably M1:F1.

**Occurrence:** Only one case has been reported.

**Risk of Recurrence for Patient's Sib:** Unknown.

**Risk of Recurrence for Patient's Child:** Unknown.

**Age of Detectability:** In young adulthood.

**Gene Mapping and Linkage:** Unknown.

**Prevention:** None known. Genetic counseling indicated.

**Treatment:** None necessary.

**Prognosis:** Unknown.

**Detection of Carrier:** Unknown.

**Special Considerations:** Focal odontoblastic dysplasia shares with **Teeth, dentin dysplasia, coronal** extensive pulp stone formation in all teeth present. However, differences between the reported cases exist relative to the apparent site of origin of the pulp stones, dentition involved, shape of pulp chamber and crowns, and associated stature and mental defects. It may be that these two conditions will be found to be variations of the same process.

**References:**
Eastman JR, et al.: Focal odontoblastic dysplasia: dentin dysplasia type III? Oral Surg 1977; 44:909–914.

G0009                                **Lawrence I. Goldblatt**

## TEETH, ODONTODYSPLASIA          0739

**Includes:**
> Odontodysplasia
> Odontogenesis imperfecta
> Odontogenic dysplasia
> Regional odontodysplasia
> Teeth, ghost
> Teeth, localized arrested development
> Unilateral dental malformation

**Excludes:**
> **Teeth, amelogenesis imperfecta** (0046)
> **Teeth, dentin dysplasia, coronal** (0277)
> **Teeth, dentin dysplasia, radicular** (0278)
> **Teeth, dentinogenesis imperfecta** (0279)
> Teeth, shell

**Major Diagnostic Criteria:** Segments of primary or permanent dentition exhibit hypoplasia and hypocalcification of enamel and dentin. Affected teeth show reduced radiodensity (described as

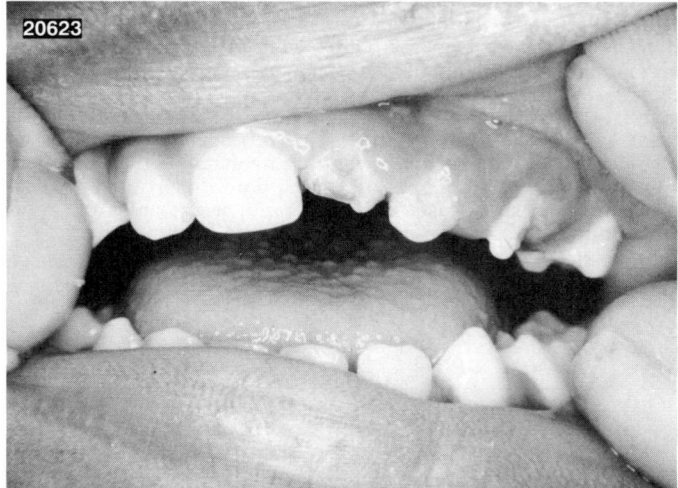

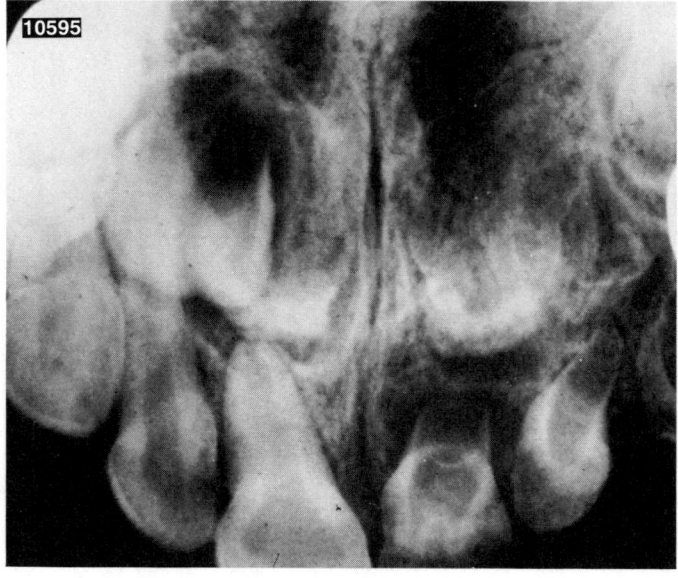

0739-20623–10595:  Teeth, odontodysplasia.

"ghostly") and abnormally large pulp chambers with calcific inclusions.

**Clinical Findings:** Dysgenesis of enamel, dentin, and pulp, with hypoplasia and hypocalcification of enamel and dentin. Primary or secondary teeth may be affected independently, with only a portion of the teeth being involved. It is unlikely that the succedaneous tooth will be formed normally if the primary tooth is involved. Condition appears to occur more frequently in the maxillary arch; it affects the primary teeth equally, but the incisors and cuspids of the permanent teeth are more commonly involved. Affected teeth may remain unerupted, with associated enlarged follicles. Affected teeth are characterized by defective formation of both enamel and dentin, and are 1) smaller than normal, 2) of abnormal morphology, and 3) delayed or partially erupted. Histologically, there may be calcifications within the pulp or follicle. Corpuscular structures comprising concentric layers of collagenous connective tissue may occur in the follicle.

X-rays show reduced radiodensity and abnormally large pulpal chambers with calcific inclusions and short or hypoplastic roots. Root formation may be near-normal or much delayed.

**Complications:** Delayed eruption of primary or secondary teeth. Unesthetic anterior teeth may predispose to psychosocial concerns. Dental caries may occur in hypoplastic defects. Brittleness of teeth may predispose to coronal fractures.

**Associated Findings:** Subsequent to dental caries, there may be pulpal exposure, periapical infection, granuloma, cyst formation, and loss of teeth with possible drifting and resultant malocclusion.

**Etiology:** Undetermined. Both prenatal and early postnatal influences appear to be important. Intrinsic causative factors suggested are localized viral infection, abnormal vascular supply, localized tissue ischemia, and somatic mutation. Trauma or ionizing radiation do not appear to be tenable causes.

**Pathogenesis:** Initial event unknown; affected teeth show thin, hypoplastic, and hypocalcified enamel exhibiting irregular, aprismatic, matrix formation, with embedded cellular debris. Dentin shows tubular irregularity, with amorphous clefts of debris. The pulp may exhibit inflammation and calcific inclusions. The dental follicle may show corpuscular structures comprising concentric layers of collagenous connective tissue and calcifications. There may be delayed root formation, with large pulp chambers and root canals.

**Sex Ratio:** Estimated M1:F2

**Occurrence:** About 65 reported cases.

**Risk of Recurrence for Patient's Sib:** Probably not increased.

**Risk of Recurrence for Patient's Child:** Probably not increased.

**Age of Detectability:** Detected pre-eruptively by X-ray, or post-eruptively by clinical examination.

**Gene Mapping and Linkage:** Unknown.

**Prevention:** None known.

**Treatment:** Removal of affected primary teeth. Removal of affected, pulpally-involved secondary teeth and fabrication of artificial replacements for function and esthetics. An affected secondary tooth bud may be removed, attached to soft tissue of affected primary tooth, during extraction. Teeth may fracture readily. Affected teeth may be associated with a firm, painless, soft tissue swelling of the labial and lingual gingiva.

**Prognosis:** Treated: excellent for primary dentition, but succedaneous teeth may be involved. Untreated: associated complications may occur. Oral condition does not appear to interfere with patient's longevity.

**Detection of Carrier:** Unknown.

**References:**

Lustmann J, et al.: Odontodysplasia report of two cases and review of the literature. Oral Surg 1975; 39:781–793.

Herold RCB, et al.: Abnormal tooth tissue in human odontodysplasia. Oral Surg 1976; 42:357–365.

Bixler D: Heritable disorders affecting dentin. In: Stewart RE, Prescott GH, eds: Oral and facial genetics. St. Louis: C.V. Mosby, 1976:242–244.

Walton L, et al.: Odontodysplasia: report of three cases with vascular nevi overlying the adjacent stem of the face. Oral Surg 1978; 46:676–684.

WA011
SC054

**Paul O. Walker**
**Mary E. Schwind**

## TEETH, PEGGED OR ABSENT MAXILLARY LATERAL INCISOR    0934

**Includes:**

Lateral incisors, absence of
Maxillary lateral incisor, hypodontia of
Maxillary lateral incisor, pegged or missing
Succedaneous teeth, agenesis of

**Excludes:**

**Chromosome 21, trisomy 21** (0171)
Hypodontia-cleft lip
**Teeth, anodontia, partial or complete** (2134)
**Teeth, microdontia** (0660)
Teeth, pegged or absent associated with other syndromes

**Major Diagnostic Criteria:** Small maxillary lateral incisors.

**Clinical Findings:** The maxillary lateral incisor teeth may be small, peg-shaped, or congenitally missing. Various degrees and combinations as to right or left side may occur within individuals and within kindreds. Teeth in both dentitions may be affected, but the secondary teeth are most commonly affected.

**Complications:** Diastema of maxillary central incisors, or diastema between the canines and central incisors. Drifting of teeth.

**Associated Findings:** Congenital absence of premolar teeth (10–20%), and a higher incidence of pegged or congenitally missing third molar.

**Etiology:** Usually autosomal dominant inheritance.

While the trait shows an autosomal dominant inheritance pattern, the expression shows a threshold effect for missing teeth, i.e. below a certain size the pegged tooth gene seems to be expressed as a missing tooth and does not show smaller and smaller pegged teeth. At the other end of the continuum of tooth size, kindred studies show persons with normal-sized lateral incisiors who apparently can pass the gene to offspring. The ratio between pegged and missing teeth varies by population: Swedes 1:1, United States Caucasians 1:1, Orientals 1:0.09. In United States Caucasians, a 2:1 preference for the left side is reported. Several families have been observed in which both parents had pegged permanent maxillary lateral incisors, and the children had severe oligodontia involving primarily agenesis of succedaneous permanent teeth. These kindreds are compatible with the hypothesis of the homozygous expression of the gene.

**Pathogenesis:** Absence or reduction in the size of tooth germ.

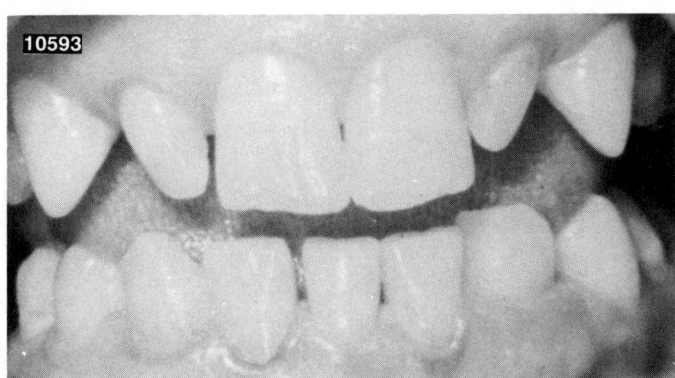

**0934-10593:** Peg-shaped maxillary lateral incisors.

**MIM No.:** *15040

**Sex Ratio:** Presumably M1:F1 (M1:F1.4 observed).

**Occurrence:** 1–3:100 in Caucasions and 6–7:100 in Orientals.

**Risk of Recurrence for Patient's Sib:**
See Part I, *Mendelian Inheritance.*

**Risk of Recurrence for Patient's Child:**
See Part I, *Mendelian Inheritance.*

**Age of Detectability:** Six to eight years of age, for permanent dentition.

**Gene Mapping and Linkage:** Unknown.

**Prevention:** None known. Genetic counseling indicated.

**Treatment:** Prosthetic replacement and orthodontic treatment.

**Prognosis:** Normal life span.

**Detection of Carrier:** Unknown.

**References:**

Witkop CJ Jr.: Studies of intrinsic disease in isolates with observations on penetrance and expressivity of certain anatomical traits. In: Pruzansky S, ed: Congenital anomalies of the face and associated structures. Springfield: Charles C Thomas, 1961:291–368.

Meskin LH, Gorlin RJ: Agenesis and peg-shaped permanent maxillary lateral incisors. J Dent Res 1963; 42:1476–1479.

Grahnen H: Hypodontia in the permanent dentition. Odont Rev 1965; 7(suppl 3):419–421.

Sutter J: L'Atteinte des incisives latérales supérieures. étude d'une mutation à l'échelle démographique. Paris: Presse Univ Fr, 1966.

Woolf CM: Missing maxillary lateral incisors: a genetic study. Am J Hum Genet 1971; 23:289–296.

Witkop CJ Jr: Agenesis of succedaneous teeth: an expression of the homozygous state of the gene for the pegged or missing maxillary lateral incisor trait. Am J Med Genet 1987; 26:431–436. †

WI043                                    **Carl J. Witkop, Jr.**

---

### TEETH, PERIODONTITIS, JUVENILE          0806

**Includes:**
Bone atrophy, diffuse
Cementopathia, deep
Precocious periodontitis
Periodontitis, generalized juvenile
Periodontitis, localized juvenile
Periodontosis (misnomer)

**Excludes:**
Acatalasemia (0006)
Agranulocytosis

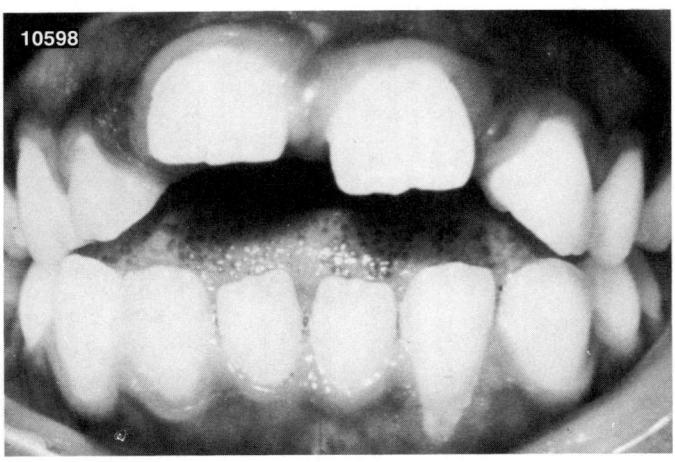

**0806A**-10598:   Malpositioned teeth in periodontosis.

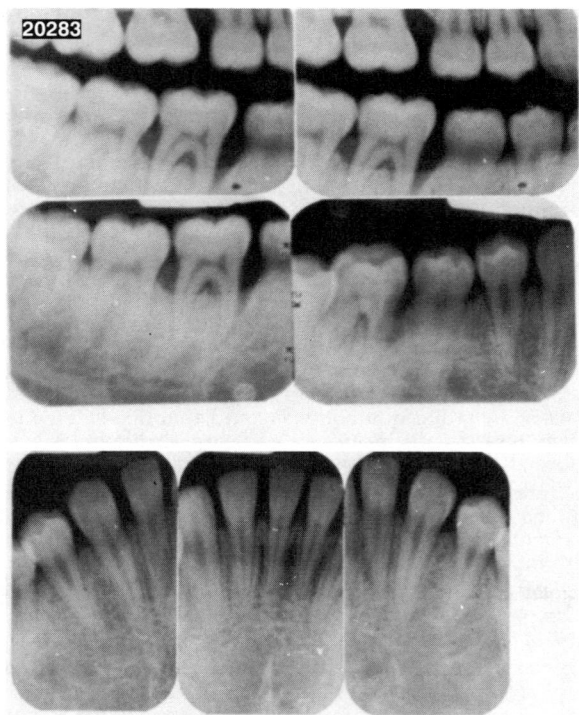

**0806B**-20283:   Note periodontal bone destruction in central incisors and first molars of both arches in a 20-year-old white female.

---

Chediak-Higashi syndrome (0143)
Chromosome 21, trisomy 21 (0171)
Compromised blood supply
Diabetes mellitus, insulin dependent type (0549)
Histiocytosis
Hypergammaglobulinemia IgE
Hyperkeratosis palmoplantaris-periodontoclasia (0494)
Hypophosphatasia (0516)
Hypovitaminosis D
Lazy leukocyte syndrome
Leukemia
Neutropenia, cyclic (0714)

**Major Diagnostic Criteria:** Rapid idiopathic loss of connective tissue attachment and alveolar bone at more than one tooth in the permanent and sometimes the deciduous dentition in children. Destruction of the alveolar bone is initiated in the incisor and first molar areas, but may extend into the adjacent alveolus later in the disease, causing migration and loss of teeth. There are insufficient local irritants in the mouth to account for the degree of alveolar bone destruction, and no other associated anomalies are present.

Conditions that need to be present to confirm the diagnosis of juvenile periodontitis include 1) good general health as determined by a physical examination, including a chest X-ray, CBC and WBC, urinalysis, sedimentation rate, hemoglobin, and hematocrit; 2) bone loss of 2 mm or more around more than one tooth, detectable on X-ray; 3) local irritants absent or not commensurate with amount of bone loss. 4) age of less than 30 years.

**Clinical Findings:** Juvenile periodontitis is a rapidly progressive periodontal disease seen in adolescents who are otherwise in good health. The age of detection is usually around 11–13 years, but it has been shown that the defect is also present in the primary dentition.

In the early stages of the disease, only the first molars and incisors are affected (localized periodontitis), but as the disease progresses the periodontal tissues of other teeth become involved until the whole dentition is affected (generalized or postjuvenile periodontitis). Two types of generalized juvenile periodontitis have been suggested to exist: a chronic disseminated and slowly progressive disease and an acute disseminated and rapidly progressive condition.

In the initial stages, the disease is a painless condition that is followed by tooth migration and mobility in the apparent absence of inflammation. The gingival tissues appear to be normal in size, color, and texture, but upon gentle probing severe loss of attachment and bleeding is evident. Despite the deep periodontal pockets present at one or more proximal surfaces of affected teeth, gingival tissues usually remain positioned nearly normal in relation to the cementoenamel junction. The amount of periodontal destruction observed cannot be accounted for by the minimal amounts of supragingival and subgingival calculus deposits found. Often, a heavy sulcular fluid is present, giving the appearance of an exudate. Caries have been reported to be minimal in these patients. Periapical X-rays show a bilateral pattern of bone loss involving mainly the incisors and first molars. Destruction of the interdental septa is vertical, angular, or arc-like rather than horizontal. On the first molars, alveolar resorption is seen frequently on the mesial aspect of the root.

**Complications:** Rapid progression and premature loss of teeth in a relatively young individual with severe alveolar bone destruction. The incidence of recurrence after treatment is high if a frequent and strict maintenance schedule is not followed.

**Associated Findings:** Alveolar ridge destruction may cause difficulties wearing lower dentures due to poor retention. For treatment to be successful, there is a strong need for optimal oral hygiene by the patient.

**Etiology:** The etiology of juvenile periodontitis is unclear. Bacterial, genetic, and immunologic theories have been proposed to explain this condition.

Using anaerobic culturing techniques, two main bacteria associated with juvenile periodontitis have consistently been identified: 1) *Actinobacillus actinomycetemcomitans (Aa)* and 2) several species of *Capnocytophaga*. *Capnocytophaga* is capable of reducing neutrophil chemotaxis as well as phagocytosis. *Aa* can alter neutrophil phagocytotic function and cell morphology. Most young patients subjected to an infection develop antibodies to associated bacteria, but may demonstrate an arrested localized form of juvenile periodontitis into adulthood. Those who do not develop sufficient antibody levels will progress into the generalized form. Recently, Genco (1986) has shown that in about 70% of patients with localized juvenile periodontitis the polymorphonuclear neutrophil leukocytes (PMNs) have a decreased number of surface receptor sites for circulating antibodies. This defect seems to be familial, effectively reduces chemotaxis, and is often present prior to the onset of periodontitis. The question still remains, nevertheless, as to whether the PMN defect is caused by the bacteria or by a genetic factor that allows the bacteria more easily to infect susceptible individuals. The answer may depend on the fact that after periodontal treatment, the PMN activity of juvenile periodontitis patients returns to normal levels, suggesting the possibility that no genetic predisposition is required to contract the disease.

Evidence to support the heritable nature of juvenile periodontitis relies on the important role that individual patient susceptibility seems to play in the production of the disease, on particular associations of juvenile periodontitis with certain blood groups, on specific human leukocyte antigen (HLA) associations which if present suggest a role for genes at the major histocompatibility locus (MHC), and on the recent provisional assignment to a locus on the long arm of chromosome 4. Both autosomal dominant and autosomal recessive, as well as X-linked dominant, patterns of inheritance have been proposed to explain the transmission of juvenile periodontitis. The consensus, however, is that bacterial cross colonization plays a major role in the familial distribution of juvenile periodontitis, making a genetic pattern (if any) more difficult to identify.

**Pathogenesis:** The histopathologic changes observed have been correlated by different authors with the clinical sequence of events. First, degeneration of the principal fibers of the periodontal membrane occurs. The membrane widens, and bone is resorbed. Capillary proliferation is observed, and loose connective tissue develops. The epithelial attachment does not proliferate, and no inflammatory response is observed. As the disease progresses, proliferation of epithelial attachment and mild cellular infiltrate by plasma cells occur. Finally, the epithelial attachment separates from the roots, and deep pockets develop.

The cementum is thin and may present areas of resorption. The alveolar bone is irregular, and evidence of idiopathic osteoblastic activity and osteoclastic resorption is present. The spongiosa may be replaced by fibrous tissue.

Studies of PMN motility show abnormally low levels of PMN chemotaxis-directed migration. Microbiologic analysis shows predominant populations of *A. actinomycetemcomitans*, *Bacteroides ochraceus*, and gram-positive cocci and rods. The results of serum antibody titers (IgG, IgM, and IgA) in patients with juvenile periodontitis show increased antibody activity (IgG) to *A. actinomycetemcomitans* but low antibody levels to *B. gingivalis*, while the opposite is true for adult-onset periodontitis. Juvenile periodontitis patients also had impaired lymphocyte blastogenic responses to selected gram-negative organisms. They also have neutrophilic granulocytes in the circulating blood, with an impaired capacity to react to chemotactic stimuli. This neutrophil dysfunction may be caused by a cell-associated defect of long duration. These findings, together with available culture data, imply that localized juvenile periodontitis and juvenile periodontitis are microbiologically distinct diseases.

Circulating antibodies to antigens of pathogenic strains of *A. actinomycetemcomitans* have been found in a large percentage of localized juvenile periodontitis patients and in a small percentage of generalized juvenile periodontitis patients. Those patients who develop high levels of antibodies will demonstrate an arrested localized form of juvenile periodontitis into adulthood, whereas those who do not will progress into a more severe generalizd form of the acute disseminated form. This suggests that there may be a genetically controlled host resistance or susceptibility to the disease.

**MIM No.:** *17065, 26095

**Sex Ratio:** Reported to be in the range M1:F1 to M1:F41, but most studies consider that the true ratio is around M1:F3.

**Occurrence:** Varies with geographic areas and with populations, being higher for populations of African and Middle Eastern descent. The relative frequency in the United States is 0.02% for whites, 0.8% for Blacks, and 0.2% for Asians.

**Risk of Recurrence for Patient's Sib:** Empiric risk based on observed ratio is 0.17%.

**Risk of Recurrence for Patient's Child:** Unknown.

**Age of Detectability:** Usually about ages 11–13 years, when severe idiopathic bone loss can be detected in X-rays of incisors and first molars of otherwise healthy children.

**Gene Mapping and Linkage:** JPD (juvenile periodontitis) has been provisionally mapped to 4.

**Prevention:** None known. Genetic counseling indicated.

**Treatment:** About two-thirds of the patients with localized disease respond favorably to conventional periodontal treatment, involving 1) administration of tetracycline 250 mg qid for 2 weeks prior to surgery, 2) excision of the deepened pockets, 3) root curettage with removal of granulation tissue after flap elevation, and 4) plaque control. After surgery, the patients are instructed to rinse with chlorhexidine mouth wash for 2 minutes, twice a day, for the first 2 weeks after surgery. Professional tooth cleaning is carried out by a dental hygienist or dentist once every 3 months.

Treatment of localized juvenile periodontitis results in resolution of gingival inflammation, substantial gain in attachment, and refilling of bone in the angular defects. These patients are prone to recurrence, especially during the first 2 years after treatment. Treatment for the generalized form of juvenile periodontitis is less effective but is recommended, since some arresting of the disease process does occur.

**Prognosis:** The disease usually progresses with early loss of teeth. Treatment is necessary to arrest the disease process.

**Detection of Carrier:** Prior to ages 11–13 years, when the initial signs usually occur, it is not possible to detect individuals at risk for juvenile periodontitis. The discovery that neutrophil chemotaxis deficiency often precedes localized juvenile periodontitis may help to identify those children under age 12 years who are not yet affected.

**Special Considerations:** As the descriptive criteria for juvenile periodontitis have become more specific, diagnostic technology has been developed to confirm the diagnosis with blood studies, immunologic studies, and bacterial analyses. Despite these advances, confusion remains among clinicians on the use of the terms *periodontosis* and *juvenile periodontitis*. The term *periodontosis* was coined in 1942 by Orban and Weinmann to designate a condition seen in young individuals who had very little calculus for the amount of alveolar bone destruction seen and seemed to be essentially noninflammatory. Contemporary observers, however, had difficulty differentiating this type of periodontal disease from other forms in which additional findings were being observed. As a result, in 1963, the term *juvenile periodontitis* was created to identify other forms of periodontal disease in which an environmental component was observed. Despite this separation, much confusion and skepticism about the existence of a disease entity called *periodontosis* remained, and at the 1966 World Workshop in periodontics the American Academy of Periodontology issued the statement that "There is insufficient evidence to identify periodontosis as a specific disease entity. . . ." By consensus, the Academy agreed to place the word *periodontosis* in parentheses after the term juvenile periodontitis. Although every so often the terms are still used interchangeably, the name *juvenile periodontitis* is more accurate than *periodontosis* because current evidence suggests an associated bacterial etiology and because insufficient information exists to show a definitive genetic pattern of inheritance.

**References:**
Fourel J: Periodontosis: a periodontal syndrome. J Periodontol 1972; 43:240–255.
Melnick M, et al.: Periodontosis: a phenotypic and genetic analysis. Oral Surg 1976; 42:32–41.
Cullinan MO, et al.: The distribution of HLA-A and B antigens in patients and their families with periodontosis. J Periodont Res 1980; 15:177–184.
Lindhe J, Slots J: Juvenile periodontitis (periodontosis). In: Lindhe J, ed: Textbook of clinical periodontology. Philadelphia: W.B. Saunders, 1983:188–201.
Saxen L, Nevalinna HR: Autosomal recessive inheritance of juvenile periodontitis: test of a hypothesis. Clin Genet 1984; 25:332–335.
Long JC, et al.: Segregation analysis of early onset periodontitis. Am J Hum Genet 1985; 37:A200.
Page RC, et al.: Clinical and laboratory studies of a family with high prevalence of juvenile periodontitis. J Periodontol 1985; 56:602–610.
Roulton D, et al.: Linkage analysis of dentinogenesis imperfecta and juvenile periodontitis: creating a 5 point map of 4q. Am J Hum Genet 1985; 37:A206.
Genco R: New genetic evidence for juvenile periodontitis. Dentistry Today 1986; 4:1.
Beaty TH, et al.: Genetic analysis of juvenile periodontitis in families ascertained through an affected proband. Am J Hum Genet 1987; 40:443–452.

ES000
M0044

**Victor Escobar**
**Regan L. Moore**

**Teeth, poor eruption-corneal dystrophy-gingival fibromatosis**
*See GINGIVAL FIBROMATOSIS-CORNEAL DYSTROPHY*
**Teeth, present at birth**
*See TEETH, NATAL OR NEONATAL*
**Teeth, pulpal dysplasia**
*See TEETH, DENTIN DYSPLASIA, CORONAL*

## TEETH, ROOT CONCRESCENCE 0928

**Includes:**
Cementum, environmental defects in
Concrescence of roots of teeth
Roots, acquired concrescence of
True concrescence

**Excludes:**
**Teeth, ankylosed** (0927)
**Teeth, dilacerated** (0929)
**Teeth, fused** (0930)
**Teeth, geminated** (0931)
**Teeth, impacted** (0932)

**Major Diagnostic Criteria:** The roots of two or more teeth are united by cementum after the formation of the crowns. Only if this condition has occurred during tooth development is it called *true concrescence*. A union of two teeth by cementum after the completion of root formation is termed *acquired concrescence*. In both cases, there is no interdential combination and the crowns are not affected. Diagnosis can frequently be established by X-ray examination.

**Clinical Findings:** The most common location for true concrescence is between the second and third molars in the maxilla. Concrescence may occur in both impacted and erupted teeth. Concrescence is almost impossible to detect clinically, since the crowns of affected teeth appear clinically normal.

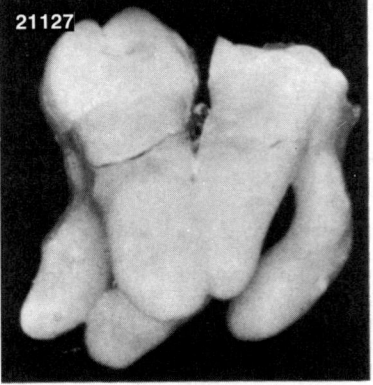

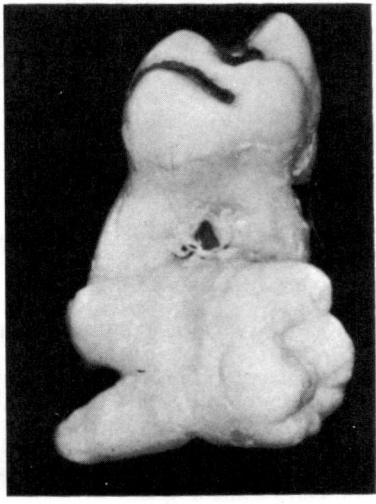

**0928-21127:** Concrescence of the molars.

**Complications:** 1) Delayed eruption of teeth as a consequence of root resorption or ankylosis of the root surface to the underlying bone. 2) Delayed eruption of succedaneous teeth. 3) Involved teeth often have periodontal involvement.

**Associated Findings:** None known.

**Etiology:** Undetermined. One hypothesis poses either a lack of space or dislocation of tooth germs as probable causes. No genetic inheritance has been established. True concrescence between maxillary second and third molars occurs in an arch where lack of space is most common. Etiology of acquired concrescence includes hypercementosis associated with either chronic infections or other systemic diseases such as Paget disease of bone.

**Pathogenesis:** Two elements must be fulfilled. First is the close approximation of the roots of adjacent teeth. This may result from simple crowding or from the constant changing of positions during the eruptive process. Second is the deposition of additional cementum. Union of the cementum of teeth is usually in the apical two-thirds of the root and is of an acellular type. Concrescence may occur before or after teeth have erupted. Microscopically, affected teeth are found to have separate pulp canals and roots.

**Sex Ratio:** M1:F1.

**Occurrence:** Undetermined. The prevalence of supernumerary teeth in Caucasian populations ranges between 0.15 and 1%. Ninety percent or more occur in the maxilla.

**Risk of Recurrence for Patient's Sib:** Unknown.

**Risk of Recurrence for Patient's Child:** Unknown.

**Age of Detectability:** Since crowns are not affected, concrescence of roots is not usually detected clinically. Concrescence may be observed on X-ray when the tooth involved or the region is X-rayed for other diagnostic purposes.

**Gene Mapping and Linkage:** Unknown.

**Prevention:** None known. Genetic counseling indicated.

**Treatment:** Concrescence alone does not require treatment, because the affected teeth are normal except for the union of cemental tissue. If these teeth are either in malocclusion or impacted, extraction is indicated.

**Prognosis:** If the teeth are fully erupted into good occlusion with healthy periodontium, prognosis is excellent. The condition is clinically not significant unless one of the attached teeth is to be extracted.

**Detection of Carrier:** Unknown.

**References:**
Eversole LR: Clinical outline of oral pathology: diagnosis and treatment, ed 2. Philadelphia: Lea & Febiger, 1984. †
Mader CL: Concrescence of teeth: a potential treatment hazard. Gen Dent 1984; 32:52–55.
Braham RL, Morris ME: Textbook of pediatric dentistry, ed 2. Baltimore: Williams & Wilkins, 1985. *

PA047                                                                    Raj-Rajendra A. Patel

**Teeth, semi-shovel**
See TEETH, INCISORS, SHOVEL-SHAPED
**Teeth, short rooted-taurodontism-microcephalic dwarfism**
See TAURODONTISM-SHORT ROOTED TEETH-MICROCEPHALIC DWARFISM
**Teeth, small**
See TEETH, MICRODONTIA

## TEETH, SNOW-CAPPED                                    2136

**Includes:**
Amelogenesis imperfecta, hypomaturation type
Snow-capped teeth

**Excludes:**
**Teeth, amelogenesis imperfecta** (0046)
Fluorosis

**Major Diagnostic Criteria:** Areas of white-opaque enamel on incisal third of all teeth associated with areas of brown pigmentation.

**Clinical Findings:** On clinical examination, affected teeth have a smooth surface, which is hard and resists penetration by a sharp instrument. The enamel appears normal and does not chip away from the dentin. The defect in the enamel seems to be limited to the incisal and occlusal third of the teeth, with areas of defective enamel either opaque white or brownish in color. The pattern of severity varies from individual to individual, but in every affected individual all permanent teeth are clinically affected. The junction between clinically normal and abnormal enamel is well defined. The condition seems to be present at eruption, and both the primary and secondary dentitions are affected. Some patients present with tooth sensitivity to heat, cold, touch, and sweet. No unusual X-rays findings occur.

**Complications:** As in other amelogenesis imperfectas, the unsightly teeth may produce psychological changes in the child's personality.

**Associated Findings:** Difficulties in chewing, since some of the patients have tooth sensitivity to touch and/or sweets.

**Etiology:** X-linked recessive inheritance.

**Pathogenesis:** Low magnification SEM examination shows porosities of variable size distributed randomly over the abnormal enamel surface. Interestingly enough, if the tooth is etched with HCL and the prismless layer of the enamel is removed, the underlying enamel appears to have a normal structure. This confirms previous suggestions that the genetic defect is limited to the prismless layer of the enamel.

**MIM No.:** *30110

**Sex Ratio:** M1:F0. A few females are mildly affected.

**Occurrence:** Prevalence of 1:2,000 for the general population has been suggested without definitive data.

**Risk of Recurrence for Patient's Sib:**
See Part I, *Mendelian Inheritance.*

**Risk of Recurrence for Patient's Child:**
See Part I, *Mendelian Inheritance.*

**Age of Detectability:** Visual examination after eruption of teeth.

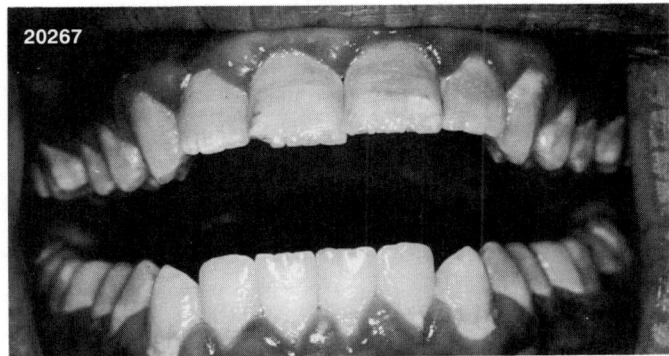

**2136-20267:** Note the "snow-capped" appearance of the teeth on the incisal third of all teeth. This is characteristically seen in amelogenesis imperfecta hypomaturation type III.

**Gene Mapping and Linkage:** AIH1 (amelogenesis imperfecta 1, hypomaturation or hypoplastic (?=AMG & AMGS)) has been mapped to Xp22.

**Prevention:** None known. Genetic counseling indicated.

**Treatment:** Unknown.

**Prognosis:** Excellent. No effect on life span.

**Detection of Carrier:** Unknown.

**Special Considerations:** No data regarding the biochemical defect in snow-capped teeth have been published, nor have sufficient numbers of families been reported to permit complete characterization of gene expression. However, both intra- and interfamilial variation is present in this trait. The differential diagnosis should always include fluorosis. However, while fluorosis is usually bright and shiny, snow-capped teeth enamel is dull and white.

**References:**

Witkop CJ Jr, Sauk JJ Jr: Defects of enamel. In: Stewart RE, Prescott GH, eds: Oral facial genetics. St. Louis: C.V. Mosby, 1976.
Escobar V, et al.: A clinical, genetic, and ultrastructural study of snow-capped teeth: amelogenesis imperfecta, hypomaturation type. Oral Surg 1981; 52:609–614.

ES000                                           **Victor Escobar**

---

## TEETH, SUPERNUMERARY                                    0936

**Includes:**
- Distomolar
- Hyperodontia
- Mesiodens
- Paramolar
- Peridens
- Polydontia
- Retromolar
- Teeth, supplementary

**Excludes:**
- **Cleidocranial dysplasia** (0185)
- **Intestinal polyposis, type III** (0536)
- Odontomas

**Major Diagnostic Criteria:** Teeth in addition to those of the normal series (20 deciduous and 32 permanent teeth). Supernumerary teeth (ST) are usually abnormal in size and shape and may or may not erupt (remain impacted). They usually have no deciduous precursor and no replacing tooth. Morphologic features include diminutive, blunted, conical, and multicusped teeth.

**Clinical Findings:** ST may develop in any tooth-bearing area, but occur most frequently in the anterior and molar regions of the maxilla and the premolar region of the mandible either unilaterally or bilaterally. ST are usually single, but multiple ST have been reported and are unusual in the deciduous dentition. The number of supernumerary primary teeth is underestimated, so it is likely that many teeth exfoliate without being recognized as ST. Most common of all ST is a *mesiodens* between maxillary central incisors. The majority have conical crowns and short roots. A *paramolar* arises alongside the maxillary molars and is usually buccally placed, whereas a *distomolar* (or a *retromolar*) develops distal to a third molar. A *peridens* is one that has erupted outside the dental arches, e.g., into the nose, which termed a *nasal tooth*. Other locations include palate, orbit, coronoid process, and maxillary antrum. The ratio of frequency of all ST in the maxilla versus in the mandible is 8:1, and that of unerupted to erupted is 5:1.

**Complications:** Malocclusion, ectopic or delayed eruption, and impaction and resorption of adjacent teeth due to the presence of ST have been observed. The possibility of ameloblastoma formation in the walls of the follicle exists. It is speculated that cysts such as the median alveolar, median mandibular, lateral periodontal, and even globulomaxillary cysts are variants of a supernumerary primordial cyst.

**Associated Findings:** ST may be associated with facial cleft. They are also seen in syndromes such as **Cleidocranial dysplasia, Oro-facio-digital syndrome, Cherubism, Klippel-Feil anomaly, Cataract-brachydactyly-oto-dental defects, Fabry disease, Chondroectodermal dysplasia, Incontinentia pigmenti,** and **Tricho-rhino-phalangeal syndrome.** The incidence of concurrent hyperodontia and hypodontia ranges from 8–41:10,000.

**Etiology:** It has been suggested that ST develop from a third tooth bud arising from the dental lamina near the permanent tooth bud, or possibly from splitting of the permanent bud itself. This latter view is somewhat unlikely, since the associated permanent teeth are usually normal in all respects. In some cases there appears to be a hereditary tendency for the development of ST. Mesiodens has been reported as transmitted by autosomal dominant inheritance with lack of penetrance. It has been suggested that hyperodontia is controlled by a number of different loci, and a polygenic scheme should be considered.

**Pathogenesis:** It is contended that supernumerary buds originate either from an occasional accessory proliferation of the dental lamina or from whorls of epithelial cells that persist from the breaking up of epithelial cords. These epithelial clusters also have the potential to produce tooth-like tumors (odontomas) and cyst linings, as determined by the stage of differentiation of enamel organ.

**MIM No.:** 18710

**Sex Ratio:** M2:F1. In one pedigree (Finn, 1967) all 14 females were affected while the three males were not.

**Occurrence:** Prevalence of ST among males is 2.4%, among females is 1.7%, and for both sexes is 2.1%. Incidence among first degree relatives of all probands is 19.7%. Overall frequency of ST ranges from 0.3–3.8%. Hyperodontia is seen in approximately 0.5% of children. Occurrence of supernumerary premolars is 1:10,000 individuals. Multiple ST occur in 14% of all cases that have ST.

**Risk of Recurrence for Patient's Sib:**
See Part I, *Mendelian Inheritance*. Probably not increased, except in association with a syndrome, or in the rare familial instance. Careful examination of relatives is indicated.

**Risk of Recurrence for Patient's Child:**
See Part I, *Mendelian Inheritance*. In sporadic, isolated ST, there is no increased risk.

**Age of Detectability:** Often diagnosed for the first time at ages 6–8 years by routine, full-mouth X-rays.

**Gene Mapping and Linkage:** Unknown.

**Prevention:** None known. Genetic counseling indicated.

**Treatment:** Extraction is the recommended course of treatment for ST. However, a success rate of 95% with autologous transplantation of ST has been reported.

**Prognosis:** Excellent. In certain cases there is no immediate indication for surgical removal. However, the patient should receive a regular clinical and X-ray examination.

**Detection of Carrier:** Possibly by clinical examination.

**References:**
Finn SB: Clinical pedodontics. Philadelphia: W.B. Saunders, 1967.
Grover PS, Lorton L: The incidence of supernumerary teeth. Gen Dent 1984; 32:224–227.

PA047                                    **Raj-Rajendra A. Patel**

**Teeth, supplementary**
*See TEETH, SUPERNUMERARY*

## TEETH, TAURODONTISM                                    0926

**Includes:**
"Bull teeth"
Hypertaurodontism
Hypotaurodontism
Mesotaurodontism
Taurodontism

**Excludes:**
Hyperphosphatasia-mental retardation, Mabry type
**Hypophosphatemia, X-linked** (0517)
**Teeth, amelogenesis imperfecta** (0046)
**Teeth, odontodysplasia** (0739)
**Teeth, taurodontism** (0926)
**Tricho-dento-osseous syndrome** (0965)

**Major Diagnostic Criteria:** Multirooted teeth with vertically enlarged pulp chambers and apical displacement of the furcation of the roots.

**Clinical Findings:** The large pulp chambers of taurodontic teeth ("bull teeth") are most striking in the molars. The crowns of teeth appear normal. The condition is detected on X-ray. The furcations of the roots of molar and premolar teeth are displaced apically. The body and root of the teeth have a block rectangular shape. This is a relatively frequent trait particularly among Eskimos, American Indians, Bantus, and extinct hominids (Neanderthal). Classified on extent of the apical displacement of the furcation of roots as hypotaurodontism, mesotaurodontism, and hypertaurodontism.

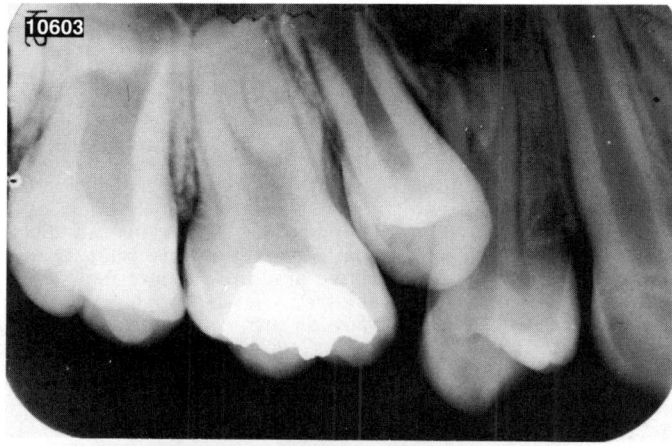

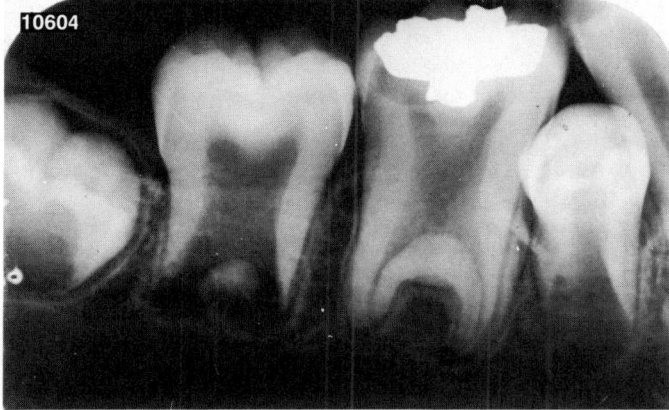

**0926**-10603–04:  Taurodontism.

**Complications:** When occurring with associated syndromes, pulp exposures with abcess formation and tooth loss are frequent.

**Associated Findings:** Taurodont teeth occur in X chromosome aneuploidy (90%); other chromosome abnormalities, e.g. **Chromosome 21, trisomy 21** (55%); other autosomal translocations and trisomy; **Oto-dental dysplasia**; **Tricho-dento-osseous syndrome, Amelo-onycho-hypohidrotic syndrome**, and **Oro-facio-digital syndrome, Mohr type.** Moller et al (see Gorlin et al, 1975) reported taurodontia in combination with absent teeth and sparse hair, as well as other findings often seen in hypohidrotic forms of **Ectodermal dysplasia.**

Teeth with large pulp chambers occur in **Hypophosphatemia, X-linked**, vitamin-D-refractory rickets (including renal types such as **Renal tubular syndrome, Fanconi type**), in the shell teeth variant of **Teeth, dentinogenesis imperfecta**; and in **Teeth, odontodysplasia**, and internal resorption. The anthropologic explanation for the high frequency of this trait in certain populations past and present is that it has a selective value; where teeth are used as tools (skin tanning), the taurodont tooth is less liable to pulp exposure from attrition than the cynodont tooth.

**Etiology:** Probably multifactorial inheritance, if not associated with syndrome of other known inheritance. Of the 22 completely examined kindreds, 19 show no affected parents, and none of the parents are known to be consanguinous. Twelve of the 21 have other affected sibs. Genetic heterogeneity is likely, and evidence for either dominant or recessive transmission is suggested in some kindreds when the condition is a part of an associated syndrome.

**Pathogenesis:** The primary alteration is unknown. The Hertwig epithelial root sheath fails to invaginate at the proper point below the crown to form roots in multirooted teeth, resulting in teeth with large pulp chambers such that the distance from the bifurcation or trifurcation of roots to the cementoenamel junction is greater than the occlusal-cervical distance. When associated with chromosomal anomalies, taurodontism probably reflects a defect in genetic homeostasis due to altered cell division and induction timing.

**MIM No.:**  27270, 27298

**Sex Ratio:**  M1:F1

**Occurrence:**  At least hypotaurodontism occurs in about 2:100 in the Caucasian population of the United States. Occurs in all races. Occurs in higher frequencies among Eskimos (20%) and Aleuts; in African Boskopoid, and Australoid (30%). Frequently noted in fossil hominid remains, particularly Neanderthal (20–60%). Found in 90% of X-chromosomal aneuploid patients, and in 55% of **Chromosome 21, trisomy 21** patients.

**Risk of Recurrence for Patient's Sib:**  Based on 24 North American Caucasian propositi and corrected for ascertainment: 22%.

**Risk of Recurrence for Patient's Child:**  Unknown.

**Age of Detectability:**  From three to 12 years of age, by X-ray examination.

**Gene Mapping and Linkage:**  Unknown.

**Prevention:**  None known. Genetic counseling indicated.

**Treatment:**  Taurodontic teeth frequently have pulp horns approaching the dentino-enamel junction. Pulp may be exposed when abrasion of the enamel exposes pulp horn at the dentin level. Teeth may require onlay capping to prevent pulp exposure, abcess formation, and tooth loss.

**Prognosis:**  Normal life span.

**Detection of Carrier:**  Unknown.

**References:**
Witkop CJ Jr: Manifestations of genetic diseases in the human pulp. Oral Surg 1971; 32:278–316. * †
Gorlin RJ, et al.: A selected miscellany. BD:OAS XI(2). New York: March of Dimes Birth Defects Foundation, 1975:39–50.
Jaspers MT, Witkop CJ Jr: Taurodontism, an isolated trait associated with syndromes and X-chromosomal aneuploidy. Am J Hum Genet 1980; 32:396–413. * †
Jaspers MT: Taurodontism in the Down syndrome. Oral Surg 1981; 51:632–636.

Jorgenson RJ: The conditions manifesting taurodontism. Am J Med Genet 1982; 11:435–442.

Witkop CJ, et al.: Taurodontism: an anomaly of teeth reflecting disruptive developmental homeostasis. Am J Med Genet 1988; 4:85–97.

WI043 **Carl J. Witkop, Jr.**

**Teeth, thistle-shaped pulp chambers**
*See TEETH, DENTIN DYSPLASIA, CORONAL*
**Tegison^, fetal effects of**
*See FETAL RETINOID SYNDROME*
**Tegretal^, fetal exposure**
*See FETAL CARBAMAZEPINE EXPOSURE*
**Tel-Hashomer camptodactyly syndrome**
*See CAMPTODACTYLY SYNDROME, TEL HASHOMER TYPE*
**Telangiectasia macularis eruptiva perstans**
*See URTICARIA PIGMENTOSA (UP)*
**Telangiectasia, congenital retinal**
*See RETINA, COATS DISEASE*

---

## TELANGIECTASIA, OSLER HEMORRHAGIC      2021

**Includes:**

> Hemorrhagic telangiectasia, hereditary
> Osler disease
> Osler-Weber-Rendu disease
> Rendu-Osler disease
> Rendu-Osler-Weber disease

**Excludes:**

> **Ataxia-telangiectasia** (0094)
> Calcinosis-Raynaud-scleroderma-telangiectasia (CRST)
> **Fabry disease** (0373)
> **Nevus, blue rubber bleb nevus syndrome** (0113)
> Telangiectasia, hereditary benign

**Major Diagnostic Criteria:** The classic triad consists of cutaneous or mucosal telangiectasias; recurrent nasal or gastrointestinal hemorrhage with normal coagulation factors; and a positive family history. About 20% of patients have a negative family history.

**Clinical Findings:** The majority of patients have telangiectasias of the skin and mucous membranes. The telangiectasias appear as red to purple 2 mm to 2 cm papules or nodules that blanch with pressure. Additionally, there may be spider-like forms consisting of a central dot with radiating venules. The most common locations for the telangiectasias are the face, oral and nasopharyngeal membranes, tips of the digits, subungual and periungual areas, palms, and soles. The frequency of patients demonstrating telangiectasias increases with age, to 90% by sixty years of age. The most common complaint, however, is epistaxis, which occurs in 78% of affected patients. Roughly one third of this group have had nasal hemorrhage severe enough to require tranfusion. The second most common complaint (44%) is gastrointestinal hemorrhage secondary to intestinal telangiectasias.

The usual onset is in the fifth decade of life, although bleeding has been reported in infancy. Liver abnormalities (30%) have been reported, including hepatic telangiectasias, passive hepatic congestion, arteriovenous fistulas, connective tissue formation with fibrosis, and atypical cirrhosis. Vascular malformations of the brain and spinal cord are relatively common (27%). Presenting symptoms may be headache, recurrent syncope, diplopia, vertigo, visual or auditory disturbances, dysarthria, or paresthesias. Approximately 20% of affected patients have hemoptysis secondary to pulmonary arteriovenous malformations. These may be demonstrable on standard chest X-rays. Vascular malformations of the retina, thyroid, heart, spleen, pancreas, kidneys, prostate, cervix, bladder, urethra, diaphragm, vertebrae, aorta, and other major arteries have been reported.

**Complications:** Anemia requiring tranfusions; high-output cardiac failure secondary to anemia or systemic arteriovenous shunt; cyanosis secondary to large pulmonary arteriovenous malformations; polycythemia; transient ischemic attacks; stroke; seizures; brain abscess (almost all associated with pulmonary arteriovenous malformations); and portal-systemic encephalopathy.

There have been several reports of a lethal homozygous form of this condition in which affected infants rapidly develop generalized telangiectasia and die within the first few months of life.

**Associated Findings:** Duodenal ulcer, **Von Willebrand disease**, cleidocranial dysostosis, and hepatocellular carcinoma.

**Etiology:** Autosomal dominant inheritance.

**Pathogenesis:** Hereditary hemorrhagic telangiectasia is a generalized vascular dysplasia. The telangiectasias are small collections of thin-walled blood vessels without muscular or elastic layers. Because of the lack of supporting connective tissue, these vessels are easily subject to traumatic or spontaneous rupture. On electron microscopy, the affected vessels have been shown to be dilated venules. Erythrocytes extravasate through gaps in the vascular endothelial cell junctions. These gaps are caused by defective overlapping of the endothelial cytoplasmic villi. Microthrombi are present within these gaps and are presumed to be necessary for closure of the endothelial junction. Additional abnormalities have been demonstrated in the perivascular tissues: abnormally large fibrils, increased amounts of amorphous material, and marked edema. It is not known whether the endothelial junction gap is due primarily to an intrinsic abnormality in the endothelial cell or whether it is secondary to defects in the periendothelial support structure.

**MIM No.:** *18730

**POS No.:** 3760

**Sex Ratio:** M1:F1

**Occurrence:** 1-2:100,000. Has been reported in all races, but is most common in Caucasians.

**Risk of Recurrence for Patient's Sib:**
See Part I, *Mendelian Inheritance.*

**Risk of Recurrence for Patient's Child:**
See Part I, *Mendelian Inheritance.*

**Age of Detectability:** The median age at diagnosis is 44 years. Fifty percent of patients develop epistaxis in first decade of life.

**Gene Mapping and Linkage:** Unknown.

**Prevention:** None known. Genetic counseling indicated.

**Treatment:** Mainly supportive and not curative. Trauma to the oral mucosa should be avoided, and a very soft toothbrush should be used. Local treatment in the form of compression, cauterization, vasoconstriction, or lubrication is the most common means of controlling bleeding. Tranfusion and iron supplementation are prescribed for severe hemorrhage. Systemic estrogen has been

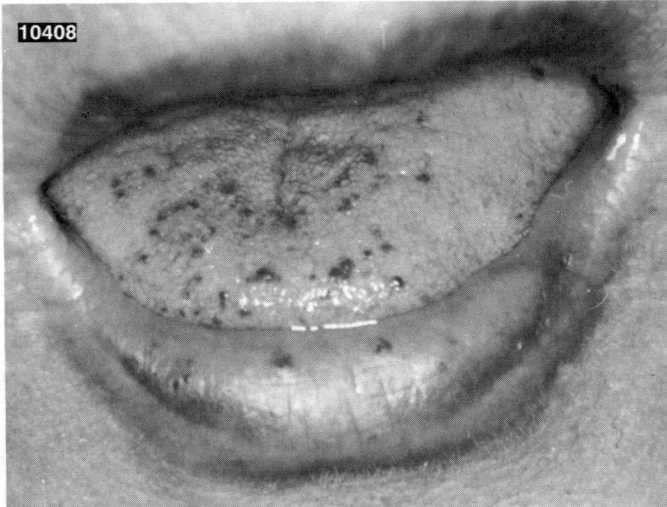

**2021-10408:** Telangiectasia on the tongue.

given with limited success as treatment for recurrent epistaxis. On electron microscopy, estrogen has been shown to re-establish continuity of the endothelium of affected vessels. For severe epistaxis, septal dermoplasty is advocated. This protects vessels from trauma by the application of a split-thickness skin graft over superficial nasal vessels. In symptomatic patients (with cyanosis, polycythemia, brain abscess, hemothorax, or severe hemoptysis), pulmonary arteriovenous fistulas have been treated with surgical excision or balloon embolization. Gastrointestinal hemorrhage rarely responds to electrocautery. Surgical removal of intestinal telangiectatic areas is not recommended, except in cases of life-threatening bleeding. Cerebral arteriovenous malformations have been treated with surgery, embolization, and proton beam irradiation.

**Prognosis:** Except in severe cases, patients with this disorder generally lead normal lives. Rarely, patients may have frequent and severe bleeding episodes.

**Detection of Carrier:** Unknown.

**Special Considerations:** *Calcinosis-Raynaud-scleroderma-telangiectasia (CRST)*, a probable collagen vascular disease, is a phenocopy of this condition, and may also be familial (Frayha et al, 1977).

**Support Groups:**
CA; Palo Alto; Hereditary Hemorrhagic Telangiectasia Foundation (HHTF)
MA; Amherst (c/o Dr. Bruce Jacobson, Biochemistry Dept., Univ. of Mass.); Hereditary Hemorrhagic Telangiectasia Registry

**References:**

Hodgson CH, et al.: Hereditary hemorrhagic telangiectasia and pulmonary arteriovenous fistula. New Engl J Med 1959; 261:625–636.
Hashimoto K, et al.: Hereditary hemorrhagic telangiectasia. An electron microscopy study. Oral Surg 1972; 34:751–762.
Frayha RA, et al.: Familial CRST syndrome with sicca complex. J Rheumatol 1977; 4:53–58.
Martini A: The liver in hereditary hemorrhagic telangiectasia: an inborn error of vascular structure with multiple manisfestations. Gut 1978; 19:531–537.
Roman G, et al.: Neurological manifestations of hereditary hemorrhagic telangiectasia (Rendu-Osler-Weber disease): report of two cases and review of the literature. Ann Neurol 1978; 4:130–144.
Bartolucci EG, et al.: Oral manifestations of hereditary hemorrhagic telangiectasia. J Periodontol 1982; 53:163–167.
Reilly PJ, et al.: Clinical manifestations of hereditary hemorrhagic telangiectasia. Am J Gastroenterol 1984; 79:363–367.
Cooke DAP: Renal arteriovenous malformation demonstrated angiographically in hereditary haemorrhagic telangiectasia (Rendu-Osler-Weber disease). J Roy Soc Med 1986; 79:744–746.
Plauchu H, et al.: Age-related clinical profile of hereditary hemorrhagic telangiectasia in an epidemiologically recruited population. Am J Med Genet 1989; 32:291–297.

BI001                                            **Diana W. Bianchi**

**Telangiectasia-pigmentation-cataract syndrome**
*See ROTHMUND-THOMSON SYNDROME*
**Telangiectatic erythema, congenital**
*See ROTHMUND-THOMSON SYNDROME*
**Telangiectatic osteosarcoma**
*See OSTEOSARCOMA*
**Telecanthus**
*See BLEPHAROPTOSIS-BLEPHAROPHIMOSIS-EPICANTHUS INVERSUS-TELECANTHUS*
**Telecanthus with associated abnormalities**
*See HYPERTELORISM-HYPOSPADIAS SYNDROME*

## TELECANTHUS, HEREDITARY                      2425

**Includes:**
Eyes, interpupillary distance
Face, interpupillary distance
Juberg-Hirsch syndrome

**Excludes:**
**Hypertelorism-hypospadias syndrome** (0505)
**Hypertelorism-microtia-facial cleft-conductive deafness** (0506)

**Major Diagnostic Criteria:** 1) Telecanthus (separation of the medial canthi more than 2 SD from mean for age, sex, and ethnic group); 2) dacryostenosis; 3) dacryagogatresia; 4) cleft lip and palate; 5) occult cleft lip; 6) asymmetric nares, 7) hypodontia.

**Clinical Findings:** Telecanthus (8/9); dacryostenosis or dacryagogatresia (3/9); occult cleft lip (2/9); cleft lip and palate (1/9); epicanthi (2/9); iridic coloboma (1/9); anisocoria (1/9); strabismus (2/9); asymmetric, external nares (4/9); hypoplastic columella nasi (3/9); rectangular uvula (1/9); bifid uvula (1/9); anomalous teeth (2/9); congenital absence of mandibular teeth (2/9); congenital absence of maxillary teeth (3/9). Sphenoidal bone abnormality, such as heaviness or asymmetry, may be seen, as well as the central hiatus of the maxillary and palatal bones seen with the palatal defect.

**Complications:** A speech defect may be associated with palatal deficiency. Severe dental crowding with anterior and posterior crossbite may result from a palatal defect. Malocclusion may accompany congenital absence of teeth.

**Associated Findings:** Penile chordee was present in one male. Clinodactyly of the 3rd, 4th, and 5th digits was present in one male.

**Etiology:** Autosomal dominant inheritance with incomplete penetrance and variable expressivity.

**Pathogenesis:** Unknown.

**MIM No.:** 18735

**Sex Ratio:** M3:F6 (observed in one kindred).

**Occurrence:** One kindred reported.

**Risk of Recurrence for Patient's Sib:**
See Part I, *Mendelian Inheritance.*

**Risk of Recurrence for Patient's Child:**
See Part I, *Mendelian Inheritance.*

**Age of Detectability:** At birth.

**Gene Mapping and Linkage:** Unknown.

**Prevention:** None known. Genetic counseling indicated.

**Treatment:** Plastic and reconstructive surgery, orthodontics, ophthalmologic surgery, speech therapy.

**Prognosis:** Normal life span.

**Detection of Carrier:** By physical examination.

**References:**

Pryor H.B.: Objective measurement of interpupillary distance. Pediatrics 1969; 44:973–977.
Juberg RC, Hirsch R: Expressivity of heritable telecanthus in five generations of a kindred. Am J Hum Genet 1971; 23:547–554. * †
Juberg RC, et al.: Normal values for intercanthal distance of 5 to 11-year-old American blacks. Pediatrics 1975; 55:431–436.

JU000                                            **Richard C. Juberg**

**Telecanthus-hypospadias syndrome**
*See HYPERTELORISM-HYPOSPADIAS SYNDROME*
**Temazepam, fetal effects**
*See FETAL BENZODIAZEPINE EFFECTS*
**Temporal bone cholesteatoma**
*See EAR, CHOLESTEATOMA OF TEMPORAL BONE*
**Temporal "forceps marks" scarring and unusual facies**
*See ECTODERMAL DYSPLASIA, CONGENITAL FACIAL, SETLEIS TYPE*
**Temporal lobe, agenesis**
*See BRAIN, ARACHNOID CYSTS*

**Tenosynovitis, progressive-contractures-systemic involvement**
  *See ARTHRITIS-ARTERITIS SYNDROME*
**Terata Anacatadidymus**
  *See TWINS, CONJOINED*
**Terata Anadidymus**
  *See TWINS, CONJOINED*
**Terata Catadidymus**
  *See TWINS, CONJOINED*
**Teratoid cyst of the orbit, congenital**
  *See EYE, ORBITAL TERATOMA, CONGENITAL*
**Teratoid tumor of head or neck**
  *See NECK/HEAD, DERMOID CYST OR TERATOMA*
**Teratologic syndrome of visceral heterotaxy**
  *See ASPLENIA SYNDROME*
**Teratoma**
  *See ORAL DERMOIDS*

## TERATOMA, PRESACRAL-SACRAL DYSGENESIS    2370

**Includes:**
  Hemisacrum, familial type II
  Meningocele, anterior sacral
  Sacral defects, anterior
  Sacral dysgenesis-presacral teratoma

**Excludes:**
  Sacral defect with anterior sacral meningocele, X-linked
  **Teratoma, sacrococcygeal teratoma** (0877)

**Major Diagnostic Criteria:**  Presacral teratoma plus sacral defect, or a positive family history and a sacral defect.

**Clinical Findings:**  This variable dominant disorder may differ from family to family. Classically, it includes presacral teratoma, sacral dysgenesis, sacral dimple, and anal stenosis as primary anomalies. Anterior meningocele and tethered cord may also be seen in some cases, and teratoma may be absent. Many affected individuals are asymptomatic.

**Complications:**  Constipation, retrorectal abcess, meningitis, and functional urinary tract anomalies ranging from reflux to neurogenic bladder. Malignant degeneration can occur but is relatively infrequent, with a rate estimated at 5%.

**Associated Findings:**  None known.

**Etiology:**  Autosomal dominant inheritance with variable expression.

**Pathogenesis:**  It is tempting to ascribe the clinical findings associated with the teratoma to a physical effect of the mass during development. However, the teratoma is not always present even when these other findings are. For example, one family investigated had two members with teratomas and sacral findings, one with an anterior meningocele, and another with severe anal stenosis and sacral anomaly; the latter two without any evidence of teratoma. This would therefore seem to suggest a dominant variable developmental field defect, probably acting at the stage of determination, rather than morphogenesis.

**MIM No.:**  *17645

**POS No.:**  4155

**Sex Ratio:**  M1:F1

**Occurrence:**  About ten families have been reported.

**Risk of Recurrence for Patient's Sib:**
  See Part I, *Mendelian Inheritance.*

**Risk of Recurrence for Patient's Child:**
  See Part I, *Mendelian Inheritance.*

**Age of Detectability:**  Prenatal detection has been accomplished using ultrasound.

**Gene Mapping and Linkage:**  Unknown.

**Prevention:**  None known. Genetic counseling indicated.

**Treatment:**  Physical anomalies should be treated surgically as needed. Although the teratomas are generally benign, the still present risk for malignancy is enough to warrant their removal. The possibility of a tethered cord, meningitis, or neurological deficits should be cause for rapid intervention, but family members may be reluctant to have surgery for asymptomatic findings. Surgical treatment of urinary tract problems may be necessary. Appropriate chemotherapy and other treatment for malignancy is indicated.

**Prognosis:**  If complications do not arise, prognosis is excellent. Most complications are manageable or avoidable.

**Detection of Carrier:**  X-ray of the sacral area and ultrasound of the pelvis.

**Special Considerations:**  The frequency of teratomas in different families seems to vary. These may very well represent different alleles, and it is possible that the teratoma may not occur at all, or only very rarely, in some kindreds.

**Support Groups:**  Atlanta; American Cancer Society

**References:**
Ashcraft KW, et al.: Familial presacral teratomas. BD:OAS XI(5). New York: March of Dimes Birth Defects Foundation, 1975:143–146.
Bolande RP: Childhood tumors and their relationship to birth defects. In: Mulvihill JJ, et al, ed: Genetics of human cancer. New York: Raven Press, 1977:43–75.
Durkin-Stamm MV, et al.: An unusual dysplasia-malformation-cancer syndrome in two patients. Am J Med Genet 1978; 1:279–289.
Yates VD, et al.: Anterior sacral defects: an autosomal dominantly inherited condition. J Pediatr 1983; 102:239–242.
Welch JP, Aterman K: The syndrome of caudal dysplasia: a review, including etiologic considerations and evidence of heterogeneity. Pediat Pathol 1984; 2:313–327.

LU001                                                **Mark Lubinsky**

## TERATOMA, SACROCOCCYGEAL TERATOMA    0877

**Includes:**
  Currarime triad
  Sacrococcygeal teratoma (benign or malignant)

**Excludes:**
  Sacromeningocele
  **Teratoma, presacral-sacral dysgenesis** (2370)

**Major Diagnostic Criteria:**  Most frequently seen as a tumor projecting at the sacrococcygeal area. Lobulated tumor mass in presacral space. Histopathologic confirmation is required.

All teratomas include cellular elements derived from embryonic ectoderm, endoderm, and mesoderm. The most common tissues observed in the mature (benign) form of teratoma are those of the respiratory, gastro-intestinal, and nervous systems, and are clearly recognizable as to cell type and organ system. Fully developed limbs, segments of normal intestine, and well-formed teeth have been found in benign tumors. The incidence of calcification with benign tumors is 35%. Incomplete maturation of various components is observed in immature teratomas, while neoplastic tissue, usually adenocarcinomas (53%), is identified in patients with malignant teratomas.

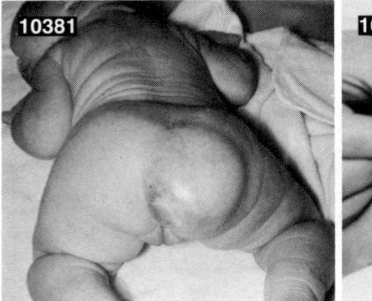 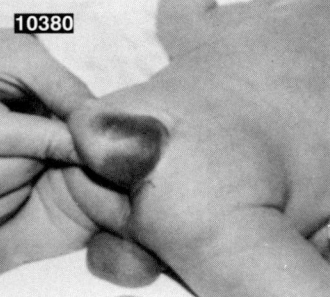

**0877**-10381–80:    Sacrococcygeal teratoma.

**Clinical Findings:** Sacrococcygeal teratomas are classified by their location. The most common type (47%) is predominantly external (sacrococcygeal), with only a minimal presacral component; type 2 (34%) tumors present externally but with a significant intrapelvic extension; type 3 (9%) are apparent externally, but the predominant mass is pelvic and extends into the abdomen; the type 4 (10%) tumor is entirely presacral with no external presentation. The visible tumor presents as a lobulated mass, bulging into the perineum, distorting and displacing the anus and external genitalia to a more anterior position. The tumors are composed of both solid and cystic areas, and are enclosed within a fibrous capsule. The extent of presacral extension can be ascertained by rectal digital examination and plain X-rays demonstrating anterior displacement of the rectal gas column. The majority (76%) of sacrococcygeal teratomas present within the first two months of life, at which time the incidence of pelvic obstructive symptoms, including bowel and bladder dysfunction, is 7%, and the risk of malignancy is 10.1%. Symptoms are present in 80% of infants when the teratoma is discovered after two months of age, and the incidence of malignancy in this group is 91.7%.

**Complications:** Ulceration and infection; ulceration and hemorrhage may occur in association with hemangiomatous component; malignancy (related to age of first detection: newborn and first two months of life 10.1%; after first two months 91.7%).

**Associated Findings:** None known.

**Etiology:** Unknown.

**Pathogenesis:** A sacrococcygeal teratoma begins as a zone of totipotent cells derived from the distal primitive streak and remnants of Hensen node. These undergo disorganized growth in contiguity with the developing coccygeal area.

Benign tumors, while arising from the sacrococcygeal region, have both an intrapelvic and external perineal component. Approximately 6% will grow outward and be pedunculated in appearance. The malignant tumors are primarily intrapelvic in location.

**MIM No.:** *17645

**CDC No.:** 238.040

**Sex Ratio:** M1:F3

**Occurrence:** 1:40,000 live births. One ten-year national study identified 105 cases.

**Risk of Recurrence for Patient's Sib:** Unknown.

**Risk of Recurrence for Patient's Child:** Unknown.

**Age of Detectability:** At birth or under two months of age in 76%; older than two months, 24%. Prenatally, there is increased amniotic fluid alpha-fetoprotein; ultrasound shows soft-tissue mass attached to lower pole of fetus and hydramnios; amniography shows soft-tissue mass with smooth encapsulated outline.

**Gene Mapping and Linkage:** Unknown.

**Prevention:** None known. Genetic counseling indicated.

**Treatment:** Treatment is operative removal of the tumor with reconstruction of the perineal region. Since these tumors are intimately associated with the perichondrium of the coccyx, coccygectomy is mandatory to avoid local recurrence of the tumors. The entire mass can be excised through a perineal incision in most patients; a combined abdominosacral procedure is necessary to remove all the intrapelvic component of large dumbbell-shaped tumors.

Reexcision of recurrent tumors, plus radiotherapy and chemotherapy, if recurrence is malignant.

**Prognosis:** Overall operative mortality is 4%. *Benign teratoma* cure following complete excision of tumor with coccygectomy has been 100%. Recurrence rate without coccygectomy is 31.3%. *Malignant teratoma:* 60% die within 10 months of operation; only 11% survive without apparent residual disease.

**Detection of Carrier:** Unknown.

**Special Considerations:** A syndrome of presacral teratoma with anorectal stenosis and recognizable sacral defect, sometimes called *Currarime triad*, has been described in 17 individuals from six kindreds (Yates et al, 1983).

**Support Groups:** Atlanta; American Cancer Society

**References:**

Donnellan WA, Swenson O: Benign and malignant sacrococcygeal teratomas. Surgery 1968; 64:834–846.
Dillard BM, et al.: Sacrococcygeal teratoma in children. J Pediatr Surg 1970; 5:53–59.
Altman RP, et al.: Sacrococcygeal teratoma: American Academy of Pediatrics surgical section survey for 1973. J Pediatr Surg 1974; 9:389–398.
Noseworthy J, et al.: Sacrococcygeal germ cell tumors in childhood: an updated experience with 118 patients. J Pediatr Surg 1981; 16:358–364.
Yates VD, et al.: Anterior sacral defects: an autosomal dominantly inherited condition. J Pediat 1983; 102:239–242.

T0009                        **Robert J. Touloukian**

## TERATOMAS                              2919

**Includes:**

> Dermoid cyst
> Epignathus
> Pineal teratomas
> Seminoma
> Testical tumors

**Excludes:**

> Fetus in fetu
> Hamartomas
> Mixed tumors

**Major Diagnostic Criteria:** Teratomas are tumors formed from totipotent cells with ectodermal, mesodermal, and endodermal derivatives. The dermoid, or hair-filled cyst, of the ovary is a teratoma variant with well-differentiated skin appendages.

**Clinical Findings:** Derivatives of skin, teeth, respiratory mucosa, alimentary mucosa, various endocrine glands, and the central nervous system are common constituents of teratomas. They differ from hamartomas, which represent proliferation of tissue appropriate to the region of origin, and choristomas with tissue not normally found in the region of origin by virtue of their tissue heterogeneity. Teratomas occur most often in a para-axial, gonadal, or midline location from the brain to sacral area. Based on a survey of 142 cases in infants and children, the primary sites for teratomas included the sacrococcyx (84 cases), ovaries (15), testicles (15), mediastinum (14), retroperitoneum (7), cervix (3), gastrointestinal tract (1), palate (epignathus; 1), vagina (1), and uterine cervix (1). Teratomas are classified histologically as benign (mature adult tissue only), immature (embryonic tissue present but not malignant tissue), and malignant (frankly malignant tissue present in addition to mature or embryonic tissue). By these criteria, malignancy occurred in 40 of the 142 cases cited above (28%) and was highly correlated with elevated serum alpha-fetoprotein. Some authors cite a high incidence of maligant degeneration in benign teratomas as justification for aggressive therapy.

Sacrococcygeal teratomas present most commonly in infancy. About one-half are benign. There is a poor prognosis for malignant tumors, especially in older patients. Ovarian and testicular teratomas are usually detected in the first two years of life. Ovarian teratomas are more likely to be malignant in children, while the reverse is true of testicular teratomas. Most mediastinal teratomas occur in adults, while retroperitoneal teratomas are restricted almost exclusively to early childhood. Gastric, orbital, pulmonary, cardiac, and hepatic teratomas have been reported as rarities.

**Complications:** Nonresectable malignant teratomas are usually fatal despite radiation or chemotherapy. Fetal epignathous tumors may cause polyhydramnios. Ovarian teratomas may present with abdominal pain and vomiting after torsion.

**Associated Findings:** Fetal teratomas may cause or be associated with congenital malformations, such as **Hydrocephaly** with intracranial tumors, urogenital anomalies, or **Meningomyelocele** with sacrococcygeal tumors. In addition to adjacent malformations that might occur secondary to tumor compression, a general increased incidence (nine percent of patients) of noncontiguous congenital malformations has been reported.

**Etiology:** While most teratomas are sporadic, several families with an autosomal dominant predisposition to ovarian dermoid cysts have been reported. These families, plus the existence of mouse mutations that cause a high incidence of either ovarian or testicular teratomas, suggest genetic factors as part of the etiology of teratomas. Hereditary teratomas may be underreported because of their benign phenotype or spontaneous regression.

The bilaterality, early onset, and familial occurrence of ovarian teratomas suggest that chromosome deletions or genetic mutations will eventually be demonstrated for these and other teratomas.

**Pathogenesis:** While the presence of vertebral organization may be used to distinguish the fetus in fetu from teratomas, a relationship of both to twinning has been hypothesized. Ovarian teratomas may be viewed as an example of parthenogenesis through self-fertilization; one report postulates failure of extrusion of the second polar body at meiosis. Consistent chromosomal rearrangements or oncogene mutations have not yet been defined in teratomas.

**MIM No.:** 27312, 27330.

**CDC No.:** 238.000

**Sex Ratio:** M1:F2–3 for sacrococcygeal teratomas; M1:F1 for nongonadal tumors.

**Occurrence:** Teratomas constitute approximately three percent of childhood tumors.

**Risk of Recurrence for Patient's Sib:** Undetermined but presumably rare.

**Risk of Recurrence for Patient's Child:** Undetermined but presumably rare.

**Age of Detectability:** Teratomas are the most common neoplasms in newborns and may be detected prenatally by ultrasonography or maternal serum alpha-fetoprotein measurement.

**Gene Mapping and Linkage:** Unknown.

**Prevention:** None known. Genetic counseling indicated.

**Treatment:** Extirpation of accessible, benign lesions is recommended to prevent malignant degeneration. Malignant lesions are removed surgically followed by radiotherapy with or without regimens of chemotherapy, including vincristine, adriamycin, actinomycin D, cyclophosphamide, and bleomycin.

**Prognosis:** Prognosis ranges from survival averaging sixteen months for malignant sacrococcygeal teratoma, to excellent for benign or contained lesions.

**Detection of Carrier:** Unknown.

**Support Groups:** Atlanta; American Cancer Society

**References:**

Warkany J: Congenital malformations. Chicago: Yearbook Medical, 1971:1239–1246.

Hecht F, et al.: Ovarian teratomas and genetics of germ-cell formation. Lancet 1976; II:1311.

Chervenak FA, et al.: Diagnosis and management of fetal teratomas. Obstet Gynecol 1985; 66:666–671.

Siman A, et al.: Familial occurrence of mature ovarian teratomas. Obstet Gynecol 1985; 66:278–279.

Billmire DF, Grosfeld JL: Teratomas in childhood: analysis of 142 cases. J Pediatr Surg 1986; 21:548–551.

von der Maase H, et al.: Carcinoma in situ of contralateral testis in patients with testicular germ cell cancer: study of 27 cases in 500 patients. Brit Med J 1986; 293:1398–1401.

WI024                                                            **Golder N. Wilson**

**Teratomas of the orbit**
*See NECK/HEAD, DERMOID CYST OR TERATOMA*

**Terminal longitudinal defects**
*See LIMB REDUCTION DEFECTS*
**Terminal transverse defects**
*See LIMB REDUCTION DEFECTS*
**Teschler-Nicola/Killian syndrome**
*See PALLISTER-KILLIAN MOSAIC SYNDROME*
**Testes, congenital absence of**
*See ANORCHIA*
**Testical tumors**
*See TERATOMAS*
**Testicular deficiency, familial**
*See SHOVAL-SOFFER SYNDROME*
**Testicular feminization, complete**
*See ANDROGEN INSENSITIVITY SYNDROME, COMPLETE*
**Testicular feminization, incomplete type**
*See ANDROGEN INSENSITIVITY SYNDROME, INCOMPLETE*
**Testicular regression syndrome**
*See AGONADIA*
*also ANORCHIA*
**Testicular regression, embryonic**
*See ANORCHIA*
*also AGONADIA*
**Testis-determining factor, X-chromosomal**
*See GONADAL DYSGENESIS, XY TYPE*
**Testosterones, maternal exposure and fetal virilization**
*See FETAL EFFECTS FROM MATERNAL EXTRINSIC ANDROGENS*
**Tethered fetus syndrome**
*See UMBILICAL CORD, SHORT UMBILICAL CORD SYNDROME*
**Tetracycline discoloration of enamel and dentin**
*See TEETH, DEFECTS FROM TETRACYCLINE*
**Tetralogy of Fallot**
*See HEART, TETRALOGY OF FALLOT*
**Tetralogy of Fallot with absent pulmonary valve**
*See PULMONARY VALVE, ABSENT*
**Tetramelic deficiencies-ectodermal dysplasia-deformed ears**
*See ODONTO-TRICHOMELIC SYNDROME*
**Tetramelic monodactyly**
*See ECTRODACTYLY*
**Tetraphocomelia-ocular defects-cleft lip/palate-penile anomalies**
*See ROBERTS SYNDROME*
**Tetraphocomelia-thrombocytopenia syndrome**
*See THROMBOCYTOPENIA-ABSENT RADIUS*
**TEV**
*See FOOT, TALIPES EQUINOVARUS (TEV)*

---

## THALASSEMIA                                                    0939

**Includes:**

Cooley anemia
Hemoglobin Lepore syndromes
Mediterranean anemia
Microcythemia

**Excludes:**

**Anemia, congenital sideroblastic, not B(6) responsive** (2659)
**Anemia, sideroblastic** (1518)
Hematologic disease from iron or other nutritional deficiency
**Seizures, vitamin B(6) dependency** (0991)

**Major Diagnostic Criteria:** Pallor, microcytic anemia, and jaundice, which vary with the type of thalassemia. Most clinically significant forms of $\beta$ thalassemia are accompanied by "compensatory" changes, expressed as an increase in the percentage of hemoglobins $A_2$ and/or F. Forms of $\alpha$ thalassemia associated with moderate-to-severe clinical disease often are accompanied by the presence of abnormal hemoglobins composed entirely of non-$\alpha$ chains. These include hemoglobin H ($\beta_4$) and hemoglobin Barts ($\gamma_4$).

**Clinical Findings:** All clinically significant forms of thalassemia are accompanied by anemia and erythrocyte microcytosis. Enlargement of the liver and/or spleen may also be present. Anemia may vary from very mild to a degree of severity sufficient to require periodic transfusions in order to sustain life. Clinical features of major forms of thalassemia by type include:

$\beta$ *Severe* ($\beta^0$) *heterozygous:* Possible splenomegaly and mild icterus.

$\beta$ *Severe* ($\beta^0$) *homozygous:* Pallor, jaundice, bone deformities with

**Table 0939-1**  Clinical and Hematologic Features of the Major Forms of Thalassemia

| Type | Hemoglobin findings | Hematologic changes | Clinical features |
|---|---|---|---|
| **Heterozygous** | | | |
| $\beta$ Severe ($\beta^0$)(high $A_2$) | $A_2$, 3.5%–7.5%<br>F, 1%–6% | Erythrocyte microcytosis and hypochromia, mild-to-moderate anemia | Possible splenomegaly and mild icterus |
| $\beta$ Mild ($\beta^+$)(high $A_2$) | $A_2$, 3.5%–7.5% | Erythrocyte microcytosis and hypochromia, mild or absent anemia | Usually none |
| $\beta$ Silent carrier | $A_2$ and F normal (F-containing cells sometimes detectable by slide elution test) | Hematologically normal | None |
| $\beta\delta$ (high F) | $A_2$, normal or low<br>F, 5%–20% | Erythrocyte microcytosis and hypochromia, mild or absent anemia | Usually none |
| $\gamma\delta\beta$ | Normal | Newborn: microcytosis, hemolytic anemia with normoblastemia<br>Adult: same as heterozygous $\beta^0$ | Newborn: hemolytic disease with splenomegaly<br>Adult: same as heterozygous $\beta^0$ |
| $\alpha$ Severe ($\alpha_1$)(-,-) | Adult: normal<br>Newborn: Barts, 5%–10% | Erythrocyte microcytosis and hypochromia, mild anemia | Usually none |
| $\alpha$ Mild ($\alpha_2$)(-,$\alpha$)<br>($\alpha$ Silent carrier) | Adult: normal<br>Newborn: Barts, 1%–2% | Usually normal | Usually none |
| $\alpha_1/\alpha_2$ compound Heterozygous (Hb H disease)(-,-/-,$\alpha$) | H ($\beta_4$), 5%–25%<br>Barts ($\gamma_4$), 1%–3% | Erythrocyte hypochromia, poikilocytosis, anisocytosis; inclusion bodies demonstrable by supravital staining; moderate anemia | Pallor, jaundice, hepatosplenomegaly |
| **Homozygous** | | | |
| $\beta$ Severe ($\beta^0$) | F, 30%–95% | Markedly abnormal red cell morphology with microcytosis and hypochromia, nucleated red cells, severe anemia | Pallor, jaundice, bone deformities with abnormal facies, hepatosplenomegaly, usually transfusion-dependent |
| $\beta$ Mild ($\beta^+$) | F, 40%–80% | Poikilocytosis, anisocytosis, target cells; moderate anemia | Pallor, hepatosplenomegaly, jaundice; transfusions not usually required |
| $\beta\delta$ (high F) | F, 100% | Poikilocytosis, anisocytosis, hypochromia, microcytosis; mild-to-moderate anemia | Mild jaundice, hepatosplenomegaly usually present |
| $\alpha$ Severe ($\alpha_1$)(-,-/-,-) | Barts, 80%–90%<br>A and F, absent | Red cell hypochromia, anisocytosis, poikilocytosis; severe anemia | Hydrops fetalis with severe edema, hepatosplenomegaly, congestive heart failure; usually still-birth or death within first 24 hr. |
| $\alpha$ Mild ($\alpha_2$)(-,$\alpha$/-,$\alpha$) | (same findings as heterozygous $\alpha_1$)(see above) | | |

abnormal facies, hepatosplenomegaly, usually transfusion-dependent.

*β Mild (β+) homozygous:* Pallor, hepatosplenomegaly, jaundice; transfusions not usually required.

*βδ heterozygous:* Usually clinically normal.

*βδ homozygous:* Pallor, hepatosplenomegaly.

*α0 (-,-) heterozygous:* Usually normal.

*α+ (-,α) heterozygous:* Usually normal.

*Hemoglobin H disease (-,-/-,α):* Pallor, jaundice, hepatosplenomegaly.

*α0 homozygous (-,-/-,-):* Hydrops fetalis with severe edema, hepatosplenomegaly, congestive heart failure, usually stillbirth or death within 24 hours after birth.

Hematologic changes of major forms of thalassemia by type include:

*β Severe (β0) heterozygous:* Erythrocyte microcytosis and hypochromia, mild-to-moderate anemia; increased levels of hemoglobin $A_2$ and hemoglobin F.

*β Severe (β0) homozygous:* Markedly abnormal red cell morphology with marked hypochromia, nucleated red cells, severe anemia; hemoglobin F 80–95%.

*β Mild (β+) homozygous:* Poikilocytosis, anisocytosis, target cells, moderate anemia; hemoglobin F 40–80%.

*βδ heterozygous:* Erythrocyte microcytosis and hypochromia, mild or absent anemia; hemoglobin $A_2$ normal or low with hemoglobin F 5–20%.

*βδ homozygous:* Poikilocytosis, anisocytosis, hypochromia, microcytosis, moderate anemia; hemoglobin F 100%.

*α0 (-,-) heterozygous:* Usually normal.

*α+ (-,α) heterozygous:* Usually normal.

*Hemoglobin H disease (-,-/-,α):* Erythrocyte hypochromia, poikilocytosis, anisocytosis, inclusion bodies demonstrable by supravital staining, moderate anemia; hemoglobin H ($\beta_4$) 5–25%.

*α0 homozygous (-,-/-,-):* Red cell hypochromia, anisocytosis, poikilocytosis, severe anemia; hemoglobin Barts 80–90%.

**Complications:** *Anemia:* "Ineffective erythropoiesis" is characteristic of severe forms of thalassemia. The bone marrow erythroid elements are greatly increased, and utilization of iron and other erythropoietic nutrients is accelerated significantly, but inadequate numbers of mature erythrocytes are released into the peripheral blood. This series of events is thought to result from intramedullary destruction of erythroid precursors. In addition to the disordered erythropoiesis in these conditions, a major hemolytic component is also present, attributed to enhanced reticuloendothelial trapping of erythrocytes as a result of inclusion body formation. The red cell inclusions represent precipitated globin material, resulting from the unbalanced synthesis of complementary ($\alpha$ and non-$\alpha$) globin chains of hemoglobin.

*Enlargement of liver and spleen:* These changes result from several associated features of thalassemia. These include extramedullary hematopoiesis, congestive changes related to anemia and myocardial dysfunction, and proliferation of reticuloendothelial elements due to hemosiderin deposition.

*Cortical thinning of bone with associated fractures and deformities:* These changes appear to be related to the massive expansion of erythroid bone marrow.

*Iron overload:* As a result of chronic anemia, patients with thalassemia absorb considerably increased quantities of iron. For this reason, and particularly because of the large quantities of iron that are derived from blood transfusions, these patients often develop severe complications, including liver dysfunction with cirrhosis; pancreatic iron loading, which in some cases is associated with overt diabetes; and myocardial dysfunction, which, not infrequently, leads to the development of intractable arrhythmias and death.

**Associated Findings:** None known.

**Etiology:** Autosomal recessive inheritance. All of the thalassemia disorders represent biosynthetic defects, which result in a deficiency of synthesis of one or more of the globin chains of hemoglobin. More than 75 distinct molecular abnormalities give rise to thalassemia. These include partial or total deletion of the globin genes; mutations involving the promoter regions of the genes; mutations involving splice junction regions at exon-intron boundaries; mutations causing abnormal splicing of the mRNA precursors; "nonsense" mutations, which cause premature termination of globin chain synthesis; and mutations involving translation initiation and termination codons. A number of structurally abnormal hemoglobins are also expressed with the thalassemia phenotype. These include hemoglobin E, the Lepore hemoglobins, and a group of hyper-unstable variants.

**Pathogenesis:** The genetic abnormalities that underlie these conditions result in a biosynthetic deficiency of the affected globin chain(s), with an accompanying decrease in the concentration of hemoglobin in the erythroid cells due to the globin deficiency. As an additional consequence, a relative excess of the noninvolved globin chain is produced within the hemoglobin-synthesizing cells. Because uncombined globin chains are unstable in solution, this globin material undergoes intracellular precipitation, leading to inclusion body formation. This, in turn, leads to greatly accelerated cellular destruction, with a major hemolytic process that may aggravate the primary degree of anemia.

**MIM No.:** 27350

**Sex Ratio:** M1:F1

**Occurrence:** The thalassemias occur predominantly in tropical and subtropical areas of Europe, Africa, and Asia. In regions of high gene frequency, an occurrence of greater than 1:100 births has been documented. All forms of thalassemias are uncommon in Northern European and in Western Hemispheric native populations. The prevalence is highly variable, depending on the population group.

**Risk of Recurrence for Patient's Sib:**
See Part I, *Mendelian Inheritance.*

**Risk of Recurrence for Patient's Child:**
See Part I, *Mendelian Inheritance.*

**Age of Detectability:** All forms of $\alpha$ thalassemia are fully expressed and detectable at birth. Antenatal detection in the second trimester fetus can be accomplished by fetal blood sampling or by restriction endonuclease mapping studies using fetal cells derived from amniotic fluid. This can be accomplished as early as 8–10 weeks by chorionic villus biopsy.

The $\beta$ thalassemias are normally not clinically expressed until 3–6 months of age. Detection at birth and prenatal detection in the first or second trimester fetus are accomplished by globin synthesis studies, by DNA analysis, or in appropriate families by linkage studies with a DNA polymorphism.

**Gene Mapping and Linkage:** The $\alpha$-globin locus has been mapped to 16p13.3, and the $\beta$-globin locus to 11p15.5. Several mutant hemoglobin $\alpha$-chain genes have been shown to exist in close linkage with $\alpha$-thalassemia gene deletions. These include Hb G Philadelphia (68 Lys), Hb Q (65 His), Hb Hasharon (47 His), Hb Nigeria (81 Cys), Hb J Tongariki (115 Asp), and Hb J Capetown (92 Gln). A $\beta$-chain mutant, Hb Vicksburg (75 deleted), appears to be linked to a $\beta$-thalassemia gene.

**Prevention:** None known. Genetic counseling indicated.

**Treatment:** In patients with severe $\beta$ thalassemia, periodic transfusions may be required to sustain life. Use of transfusions containing "neocytes" or young red blood cells with a longer life span may allow reduction of the numbers of transfusions required. By application of "hypertransfusion" regimens, whereby transfusions are administered to a sufficient degree and at frequent intervals so as to maintain a near-normal hemoglobin concentration in the blood, many of the secondary complications, particularly cardiac dysfunction and skeletal changes can be largely prevented. This form of therapy, however, serves to increase the degree of iron storage. Treatment that minimizes iron storage is becoming important in the treatment of thalassemias requiring transfusions. Desferrioxamine is given by long-term infusion via a mechanical pump. Bone marrow transplantation, when successful, is curative.

**Prognosis:** The application of intensive transfusion therapy in patients with severe $\beta$ thalassemia has greatly improved the quality of life for these patients, but the increased iron burden that this form of therapy produces has come to represent the major cause of death of these patients, as a result of cardiac or hepatic failure. Median survival for the transfusion-dependent thalassemia patient has been approximately 20 years, but the introduction of improved methods of chelation therapy holds promise that increased survival will be achieved.

**Detection of Carrier:** Most forms of heterozygous $\alpha$ and $\beta$ thalassemia are accompanied by microcytosis, mild anemia, and morphologic abnormalities of the erythrocytes. "Silent-carrier" forms of these disorders have also been identified, and these individuals may have no apparent hematologic abnormality. Heterozygous $\beta$ thalassemia can be confirmed by the findings of elevated levels of hemoglobins $A_2$ or F. The heterozygous forms of $\alpha$ thalassemia, on the other hand, typically have no abnormality of hemoglobin composition. These usually require an investigation of family members and studies of globin chain synthesis or restriction endonuclease mapping studies for confirmation of the diagnosis. Some of the forms of hereditary persistence of fetal hemoglobin may be difficult to distinguish from heterozygous $\beta$-thalassemia syndromes.

**Special Considerations:** The hemoglobin Lepore syndromes are caused by hemoglobin types containing abnormal non-$\alpha$ chains that are hybrid molecules which contain parts of the fused $\delta$-globin and $\beta$-globin chains. These mutant hemoglobins produce the clinical and hematologic features of a thalassemia syndrome. When present in combination with a gene for $\beta$ thalassemia, these syndromes may present as severe, transfusion-dependent thalassemia. The Lepore hemoglobins are identified by electrophoresis and exhibit a mobility, at alkaline pH, similar to that of sickle hemoglobin. Hemoglobin Constant Spring, an extended $\alpha$ chain variant, produces the phenotype of $\alpha$ thalassemia, and has been observed in a large percentage of individuals with Hb H disease. Its electrophoretic mobility at alkaline pH is slower than that of Hb $A_2$.

**Support Groups:**
New York; Cooley's Anemia Blood and Research Foundation for Children
New York; Cooley's Anemia Foundation, Inc.
NY; Douglaston; AHEPA Cooley's Anemia Foundation

**References:**

Propper RD, et al.: Continuous subcutaneous administration of desferrioxamine in patients with iron overload. New Engl J Med 1977; 297:418–423.

Propper RD, et al.: New approaches to the transfusion management of thalassemia. Blood 1980; 55:55–60.

Weatherall DJ, Clegg JB: The thalassemia syndromes, 3rd ed. Oxford: Blackwell Scientific Publications, 1981.

Modell B, Berdoukas V: The clinical approach to thalassemia. London: Grune & Stratton, 1984.

Honig GR, Adams JG III: Human hemoglobin genetics. Vienna: Springer-Verlag, 1986.

Lucarelli G, et al.: Marrow transplantation in patients with advanced thalassemia. New Engl J Med 1987; 316:1050–1055.

Weatherall DF, et al.: The hemoglobinopathies. In: Scriver CR, et al, eds: The metabolic basis of inherited disease. New York: McGraw-Hill, 1989:2281–2340.

H0024                                                    **George R. Honig**

**Thalidomide external ear malformation**
*See EAR, MICROTIA-ATRESIA*
**Thalidomide, fetal effects**
*See FETAL THALIDOMIDE SYNDROME*
**Thanatophoric dwarfism**
*See THANATOPHORIC DYSPLASIA*

---

## THANATOPHORIC DYSPLASIA                                0940

**Includes:**

Dwarfism, thanatophoric
Thanatophoric dwarfism

**Excludes:**

**Asphyxiating thoracic dysplasia** (0091)
**Craniosynostosis, Kleeblattschadel type** (0555)
Dwarfism, short-limb, other forms in the newborn
**Skeletal dysplasia, Schneckenbecken type** (2632)
**Thanatophoric dysplasia, Glasgow type** (2821)

**Major Diagnostic Criteria:** Severe neonatal short-limb dwarfism with characteristic X-ray features, including vertebral and pelvic abnormalities, and a narrow thorax with short cupped ribs and irregular metaphyses.

**Clinical Findings:** Birth length ranges from 36 to 46 cm. Limbs are very short and extend away from an essentially normal-sized trunk with thighs abducted and externally rotated. The fingers are very short and conically shaped. The head is relatively large, with a prominent forehead and depressed nasal bridge. The thorax is small, and respiratory distress occurs. Hypotonia and numerous skin folds are present; the primitive reflexes are absent. Death within the first few days is usual, although survival for over six months has been reported.

X-ray findings include vertebral bodies that have a small vertical diameter, with the narrowest area in the middle of the body in both anteroposterior (AP) and lateral projections. The intervertebral spaces are large. The posterior vertebral elements are well ossified. The interpediculate distance is narrowed in the mid or lower lumbar spine. The ilia have a short vertical dimension. The transverse diameter is greater than the vertical. The inferior margin of the ilia is horizontal and the sacrosciatic notches small. The pubic and ischial bones are broad and short. The thorax is narrow in both AP and transverse diameters, with short ribs, the ends of which are cupped. The long bones are very short; relatively broad, and bowed with irregular, spur-like flaring of the metaphyses. Hand and foot bones are very short and broad. There are no abnormal laboratory findings. The presence of a cloverleaf skull probably reflects variability, rather than heterogeneity.

**Complications:** Most reported affected infants die of respiratory complications. On autopsy, some have showed an impression on the spinal cord made by the small foramen magnum.

**Associated Findings:** Hydrocephaly has been reported.

**Etiology:** Probably polygenic inheritance, with a high rate of new dominant mutations. Gross changes of thanatophoric dwarf-

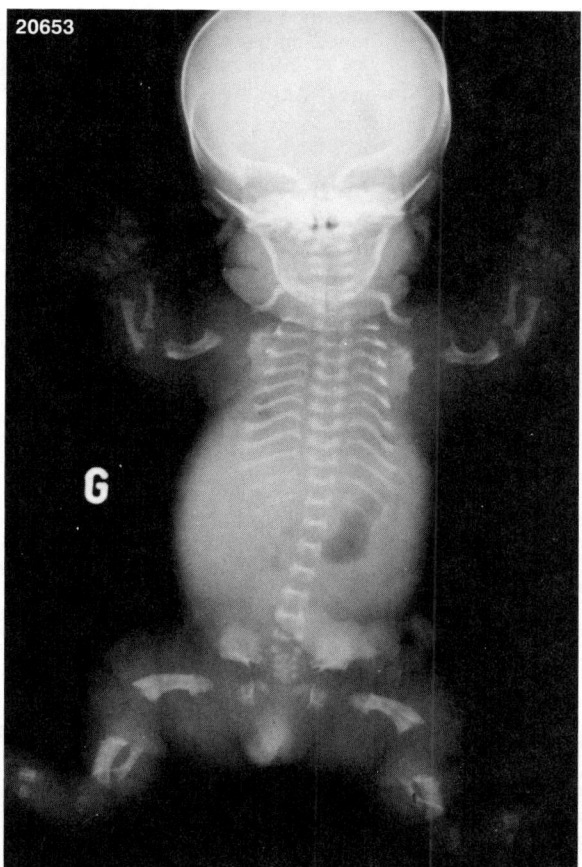

**0940-20653:** Thanatophoric dysplasia in a newborn; note short long bones and ribs, flattening of the vertebral bodies, and horizontal acetabular roofs.

---

ism appear similar but more marked than those of heterozygous achondroplasia. Presumed cases of homozygous achondroplasia have gross deformity intermediate between those of thanatophoric dwarfism and heterozygous achondroplasia. No infant with changes of thanatophoric dwarfism has been born to a couple with one achondroplastic mate. Although several kindreds have been reported where two or more siblings are affected by "thanatophoric dysplasia," analysis of X-rays and chondroosseous histopathology has demonstrated that they do not have this entity, except for two affected sibs with the additional feature of cloverleaf skull. All other documented cases of thanatophoric dysplasia have been sporadic.

**Pathogenesis:** Characteristic generalized disruption of growth plate with persistant mesenchymal-like tissue.

**MIM No.:** *18760

**POS No.:** 3411

**CDC No.:** 756.447

**Sex Ratio:** Presumably M1:F1.

**Occurrence:** 1:42,000. Most affected individuals die in infancy.

**Risk of Recurrence for Patient's Sib:**

See Part I, *Mendelian Inheritance.* The empiric risk has been computed at 2%.

**Risk of Recurrence for Patient's Child:**

See Part I, *Mendelian Inheritance.* Affected individuals are not expected to survive to reproduce.

**Age of Detectability:** At birth, by X-ray. Prenatally, by ultrasonography showing shortened limbs, small chest, relatively large head with thickened scalp, protuberant abdomen, hydramnios.

**Gene Mapping and Linkage:** Unknown.

**Prevention:** None known. Genetic counseling indicated.

**Treatment:** Unknown.

**Prognosis:** Fatal in first year of life, usually in first week.

**Detection of Carrier:** Unknown.

**References:**

Maroteaux P, et al.: Le nanisme thanatophore. Presse Med 1967; 75:2519–2524.
Langer LO Jr, et al.: Thanatophoric dwarfism: a condition confused with achondroplasia in the neonate, with brief comments on achondrogenesis and homozygous achondroplasia. Radiology 1969; 92: 285–294.
Rimoin DL: The chondrodystrophies. Adv Hum Genet 1975; 5:1–118.
Maroteaux P, et al.: The lethal chondrodysplasias. Clin Orthop 1976; 114:31–45.
Nissenbaum M, et al.: Thanatophoric dwarfism: two case reports and survey of the literature. Can Pediatr 1977; 16:690–697.
Elejalde BR, de Elejalde MM: Thanatophoric dysplasia: fetal manifestations and prenatal diagnosis. Am J Med Genet 1985; 22:669–683.
Martinez-Frias ML, et al.: Thanatophoric dysplasia: an autosomal dominant condition. Am J Med Genet 1988; 31:815–820.

B0025
LA016

**Zvi Borochowitz**
**Leonard O. Langer, Jr.**
*David L. Rimoin*

## THANATOPHORIC DYSPLASIA, GLASGOW TYPE     2821

**Includes:** Skeletal dysplasia, neonatally lethal short-limbed, Glasgow type

**Excludes:**
   **Skeletal dysplasia** (other)
   **Thanatophoric dysplasia** (0940)

**Major Diagnostic Criteria:** Severe neonatal short-limb dwarfism with characteristic X-ray features.

**Clinical Findings:** Birth length about 36 cm, with severe micromelia. The head is relatively normal, but facies are flattened. Neonatal death occurs from respiratory insufficiency. Cataracts and unexplained hepatosplenomegaly were present in one child.

   X-ray findings include shortness of all long bones, with curved femora, moderate rib shortness, a short skull base, hypoplastic mandible, hypoplasia of the ilia, pubic, and ischial bones, and mild platyspondyly.

**Complications:** Neonatal death due to respiratory insufficiency.

**Associated Findings:** Polyhydramnios may occur.

**Etiology:** Possibly autosomal recessive inheritance.

**Pathogenesis:** Marked disturbance of enchondral ossification with reduced numbers of proliferating and hypertrophic chondrocytes, irregular thickness and reduction in number of advancing cartilaginous columns in the metaphysis, and a fine zone of mesenchymal tissue blocking off the epiphyseal plate from the marrow cavity.

**MIM No.:** 27368

**Sex Ratio:** Presumably M1:F1.

**Occurrence:** Two females sibs from the West of Scotland have been documented.

**Risk of Recurrence for Patient's Sib:**
   See Part I, *Mendelian Inheritance.*

**Risk of Recurrence for Patient's Child:**
   See Part I, *Mendelian Inheritance.* Affected individuals are not expected to survive to reproduce.

**Age of Detectability:** During the second trimester by ultrasonic measurement of long bone lengths.

**Gene Mapping and Linkage:** Unknown.

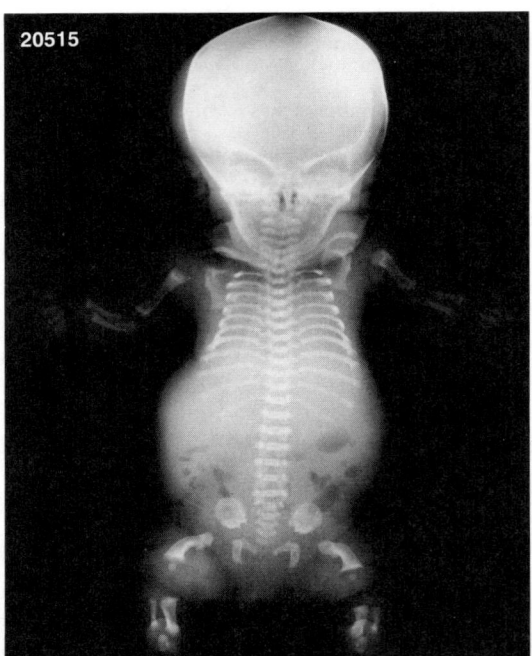

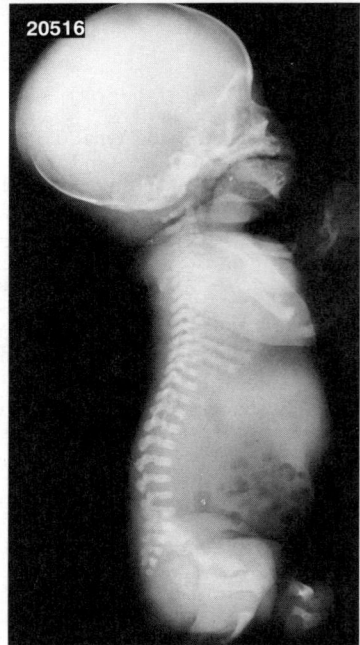

**2821-20515–16:** Thanatophoric dysplasia, Glasgow type: note short limbs with curved femora, and small pelvic bones. Lateral view demonstrates platyspondyly and micrognathia.

**Prevention:** None known. Genetic counseling indicated.

**Treatment:** Unknown.

**Prognosis:** Fatal during the newborn period.

**Detection of Carrier:** Unknown.

**Special Considerations:** Differentiation from **Thanatophoric dysplasia** is vital in view of the high recurrence risk for this condition. Short curved "telephone-receiver" femora are seen in both conditions, but other X-ray features, notably the spinal changes, serve to distinguish between the two conditions.

**References:**
Connor JM, et al.: Lethal neonatal chondrodysplasias in the West of Scotland 1970–1983 with a description of a thanatophoric, dysplasialike, autosomal recessive disorder, Glasgow variant. Am J Med Genet 1985; 22:243–253. * †

C0066

**J. Michael Connor**

**Thenar hypoplasia**
*See POLYDACTYLY*
**Thiamine-responsive MSUD**
*See MAPLE SYRUP URINE DISEASE*
**Thick lips-oral mucosa**
*See ACROMEGALOID FACIAL APPEARANCE SYNDROME*
**Thiemann disease (phalangeal epiphyses)**
*See JOINTS, OSTEOCHONDRITIS DISSECANS*
**Third and fourth pharyngeal pouch syndrome**
*See IMMUNODEFICIENCY, THYMIC AGENESIS*
**Thode mental retardation**
*See X-LINKED MENTAL RETARDATION-Xq DUPLICATION*
**Thompson-Baraitser syndrome**
*See OCULO-ENCEPHALO-HEPATO-RENAL SYNDROME*
**Thomsen congenital myotonia**
*See MYOTONIA CONGENITA*
**Thoracic aorta, coarctation of lower**
*See AORTA, COARCTATION*
**Thoracic dysplasia, asphyxiating**
*See ASPHYXIATING THORACIC DYSPLASIA*

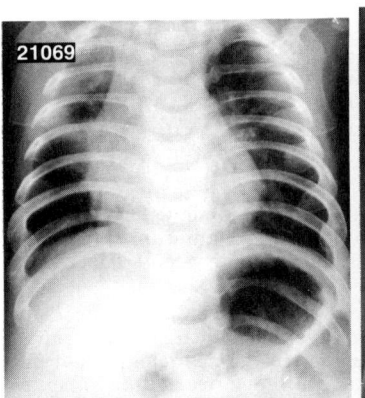
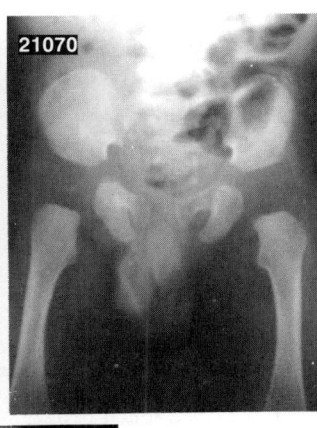

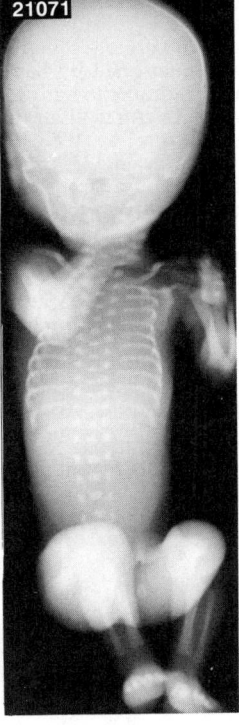

## THORACIC DYSPLASIA-HYDROCEPHALUS          **3129**

**Includes:** Hydrocephaly-thoracic dysplasia

**Excludes:** Asphyxiating thoracic dysplasia (0091)

**Major Diagnostic Criteria:** Hydrocephaly with a narrow thorax and short ribs.

**Clinical Findings:** The condition has been described in two sibs, one liveborn and one diagnosed prenatally. Present in both were **Hydrocephaly**, narrow thorax with short ribs, and short limbs, with the shortness being primarily rhizomelic. Mental retardation was present in the living child, and is also likely a component of this condition.

**Complications:** Death from respiratory insufficiency.

**Associated Findings:** None known.

**Etiology:** Possibly autosomal recessive inheritance.

**Pathogenesis:** Unknown.

**MIM No.:** 27373

**POS No.:** 4191

**Sex Ratio:** Presumably M1:F1.

**Occurrence:** Two sibs from a family of Pakistani ethnic origin has been documented.

**Risk of Recurrence for Patient's Sib:**
See Part I, *Mendelian Inheritance.*

**Risk of Recurrence for Patient's Child:**
See Part I, *Mendelian Inheritance.*

**Age of Detectability:** At birth. Prenatal diagnosis using ultrasound is possible.

**Gene Mapping and Linkage:** Unknown.

**Prevention:** None known. Genetic counseling indicated.

**Treatment:** Shunting of **Hydrocephaly**.

**Prognosis:** Poor. The liveborn child died at age 18 months.

**Detection of Carrier:** Unknown.

**References:**
Winter RM, et al.: A previously undescribed syndrome of thoracic dysplasia and communicating hydrocephalus in two sibs, one diagnosed prenatally by ultrasound. J Med Genet 1987; 24:204–206.

T0007

**Helga V. Toriello**

**3129-21069:** Chest X-ray at 4 months shows short, horizontal ribs and narrow thorax. **21070:** Iliac bones are small and there is mild metaphyseal flaring of the femora. **21071:** Postmortem X-ray of an affected 19-week-old fetus shows short, horizontal, angulated ribs.

**Thoracic tracheoesophageal fistula, congenital isolated H-type**
*See TRACHEOESOPHAGEAL FISTULA*
**Thoracic tracheoesophageal fistula-esophageal atresia**
*See TRACHEOESOPHAGEAL FISTULA*
**Thoracic-pelvic-phalangeal dystrophy**
*See ASPHYXIATING THORACIC DYSPLASIA*
**Thoracoabdominal ectopia cordis**
*See PENTALOGY OF CANTRELL*
**Thoracolaryngopelvic dysplasia**
*See THORACOPELVIC DYSOSTOSIS*
**Thoracopagus**
*See TWINS, CONJOINED*

## THORACOPELVIC DYSOSTOSIS 2775

**Includes:**
    Barnes syndrome
    Thoracolaryngopelvic dysplasia

**Excludes: Asphyxiating thoracic dysplasia** (0091)

**Major Diagnostic Criteria:** Characteristic X-ray features are short ribs; small, round ileum with a small and shallow sciatic notch; and poor development of the acetabulum. Significant respiratory distress in the neonatal period improves with age. A constricted pelvis is noted in adults.

**Clinical Findings:** Infants usually present with a small chest and respiratory distress of variable severity, which is rarely fatal. Respiratory suppport may be needed in the neonatal period, but milder cases improve with age and achieve near-normal respiratory function, a much better outcome than would be anticipated from the neonatal state. The chest remains narrow, and lung volumes may be reduced.

Laryngeal hypoplasia of variable severity is may also be noted. Although this was not mentioned by Bankier and Danks (1983), the small larynx in the child came to light by difficult intubation for an anesthetic at a later date. A small larynx has been a feature in the other reports, and Burn et al (1986) rightly pointed out that this condition may be the same as that of *thoracolaryngopelvic dysplasia*, originally reported by Barnes et al (1969).

The two adult women who were reported had a constricted pelvis, necessitating delivery of infants by cesarean section. Stature has been in the normal range. Other reported skeletal changes include slight difference in lower limb length, high clavicles, narrow thoracic cage, and mild thoracic scoliosis. The facies and other organs appear normal, and intelligence is in the normal range.

**Complications:** Unknown.

**Associated Findings:** None known.

**Etiology:** Possibly autosomal dominant inheritance.

**Pathogenesis:** Unknown.

**MIM No.:** 18777

**POS No.:** 3606

**Sex Ratio:** Presumably M1:F1.

**Occurrence:** Three families have been reported.

**Risk of Recurrence for Patient's Sib:**
See Part I, *Mendelian Inheritance.*

**Risk of Recurrence for Patient's Child:**
See Part I, *Mendelian Inheritance.*

**Age of Detectability:** During the newborn period.

**Gene Mapping and Linkage:** Unknown.

**Prevention:** None known. Genetic counseling indicated.

**Treatment:** Respiratory support, including artificial ventilation, may be necessary during the neonatal period. Mild cases improve and need no further respiratory treatment. Operative intervention has been reported in more severe cases, splitting the sternum and inserting bone grafts. This, together with more lengthy ventilatory support, achieved improvement, but death from respiratory failure and cor pulmonale have occurred in childhood. Tracheostomy has been used for severe laryngeal hypoplasia. Women are advised of the need of delivery by cesarean section because of constricted pelvis.

**Prognosis:** Good for those who survive the respiratory distress during the neonatal period without operative intervention.

**Detection of Carrier:** Clinical and X-ray examination.

**References:**
Barnes ND, et al.: Thoracic dystrophy. Arch Dis Child 1969; 44:11–17.
Bankier A, Danks DM: Thoracic-pelvic dysostosis: a "new" autosomal dominant form. J Med Genet 1983; 20:276–279.
Burn J, et al.: Autosomal dominant thoracolaryngopelvic dysplasia: Barnes syndrome. J Med Genet 1986; 23:345–349.

BA062                **Agnes Bankier**

**Thorax cuneiforme**
   *See PECTUS CARINATUM*
**Thost-Unna disease**
   *See KERATOSIS PALMARIS ET PLANTARIS OF UNNA-THOST*
**Three methylcrotonyl-CoA carboxylase deficiency, isolated**
   *See ACIDURIA, BETA-METHYL-CROTONYL-GLYCINURIA*
**Three-jointed thumb**
   *See THUMB, TRIPHALANGEAL*
**Three-M slender-boned nanism**
   *See SKELETAL DYSPLASIA, 3 M TYPE*
**Three-methylcrotonylglycinuria**
   *See ACIDURIA, BETA-METHYL-CROTONYL-GLYCINURIA*
**Thrombasthenia**
   *See THROMBASTHENIA, GLANZMANN-NAEGELI TYPE*

## THROMBASTHENIA, GLANZMANN-NAEGELI TYPE 2683

**Includes:**
    Diacyclothrombopathia IIb-IIIa
    Glanzmann thrombasthenia
    Glycoprotein complex IIb-IIIa, deficiency of
    Platelet fibinogen receptor deficiency
    Platelet glycoprotein IIb-IIIa deficiency
    Thrombasthenia
    Thrombocytopathic purpura

**Excludes:**
    **Albinism, oculocutaneous, Hermansky-Pudlak type** (0033)
    Bernard-Soulier giant platelet syndrome
    Gray platelet syndrome
    Platelet release abnormality
    **Von Willebrand disease** (0996)

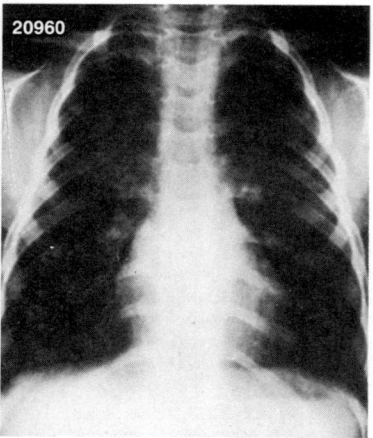
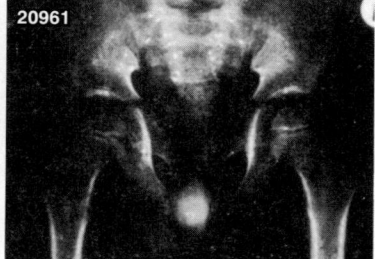

**2775-20959:** Thoracopelvic dysostosis; note short ribs in an affected infant. **20960:** "Bell-shaped" thorax in an older child. **20961:** Narrow pelvic inlet in the adult; note short, round ileum, and shallow sciatic notch.

**Major Diagnostic Criteria:** A hemorrhagic disorder characterized by low or normal platelet number; prolonged bleeding time; abnormal platelet aggregation responses to ADP, epinephrine, and collagen; abnormal clot retraction; and deficient platelet fibrinogen.

**Clinical Findings:** A lifelong bleeding diathesis. The hemorrhagic disorder varies in severity among families from a relatively mild disease manifesting with prolonged bleeding only at surgery or severe injury to a more aggressive hemorrhagic disorder characterized by purpurae and mucosal bleeding not associated with obvious trauma.

**Complications:** Those arising from the hemorrhagic manifestations of the disease. Bleeds can be exsanguinating when affecting an oral, nasal, or gastrointestinal mucosal site. Internal hemorrhages may involve vital structures or musculoskeletal limb structures.

**Associated Findings:** None known.

**Etiology:** Usually autosomal recessive inheritance, with infrequent "dominant pedigrees" possibly reflecting a heterozygous expression.

**Pathogenesis:** A platelet membrane defect identified with this disorder involving the platelet membrane glycoprotein complex IIb/IIIa (GP IIb/IIIa). Two subgroups have been documented. This classification is based on the low levels of GP IIIa with virtual absence of GP IIb and bound fibrinogen in subgroup type I and the reduced levels of GP IIb/IIIa in subgroup II. This subgroup is associated with limited amounts of fibrinogen binding. Variations have also been described on the basis of the extent of fibrinogen bound within the alpha granules.

**MIM No.:** *27380, 18780

**Sex Ratio:** M1:F1

**Occurrence:** The prevalence of this disease is higher in populations in which consanguinity is more likely. Established literature; considered second most frequent bleeding disorder in Jordan.

**Risk of Recurrence for Patient's Sib:**
See Part I, *Mendelian Inheritance.*

**Risk of Recurrence for Patient's Child:**
See Part I, *Mendelian Inheritance.*

**Age of Detectability:** At birth.

**Gene Mapping and Linkage:** GP2B (glycoprotein IIb (IIb/IIIa complex, platelet, CD41B)) has been mapped to 17q21.32.

**Prevention:** None known. Genetic counseling indicated.

**Treatment:** Platelet transfusion.

**Prognosis:** Depends on the severity of the hemorrhagic diathesis. In its severest form, prognosis is guarded.

**Detection of Carrier:** Quantitation of GP IIb/IIIa is not a routinely available procedure, but has the potential to detect the heterozygous state.

**References:**
Stormorken H, et al.: Diagnosis of heterozygotes in Glanzmann's thrombasthenia. Thromb Haemost 1982; 48:217–221.
George JN, et al.: Molecular defects in interactions of platelet with the vessel wall. New Engl J Med 1984; 311:1084–1098.
Giltay JC, et al.: Normal synthesis and expression of endothelial IIb/IIIa in Glanzmann's thrombasthenia. Blood 1987; 69:809–812.
Nurden AT, et al.: A variant of Glanzmann's thrombasthenia with abnormal glycoprotein IIb-IIIa complexes in the platelet membrane. J Clin Invest 1987; 79:962–969.
Nurden AT: Platelet membrane glycoproteins and their clinical aspects. In: Verstraete M, et al., eds: Thrombosis and haemostasis. Leuven: University Press, 1987:93–125.

G0055                          **Edward Gomperts**

**Thrombocytopathic purpura**
*See THROMBASTHENIA, GLANZMANN-NAEGELI TYPE*

---

## THROMBOCYTOPENIA-ABSENT RADIUS     0941

**Includes:**
> Amegakaryocytic thrombocytopenia-bilateral absence of the radii
> Megakaryocytopenia-radius aplasia
> Radius absent-thrombocytopenia
> TAR syndrome
> Tetraphocomelia-thrombocytopenia syndrome
> Thrombocytopenia-bilateral absence of the radii

**Excludes:**
> **Chromosome 18, trisomy 18** (0160)
> **Fetal thalidomide syndrome** (0386)
> **Heart-hand syndrome** (0455)
> **Pancytopenia syndrome, Fanconi type** (2029)

**Major Diagnostic Criteria:** Thrombocytopenia < 100,000 platelets/cubic mm. Bilateral absence of radius.

**Clinical Findings:** *Hematologic:* The affected newborn often has purpura, nosebleeds, bloody stools, and hematemesis. Thrombocytopenia probably 100% at some time. More than 90% have

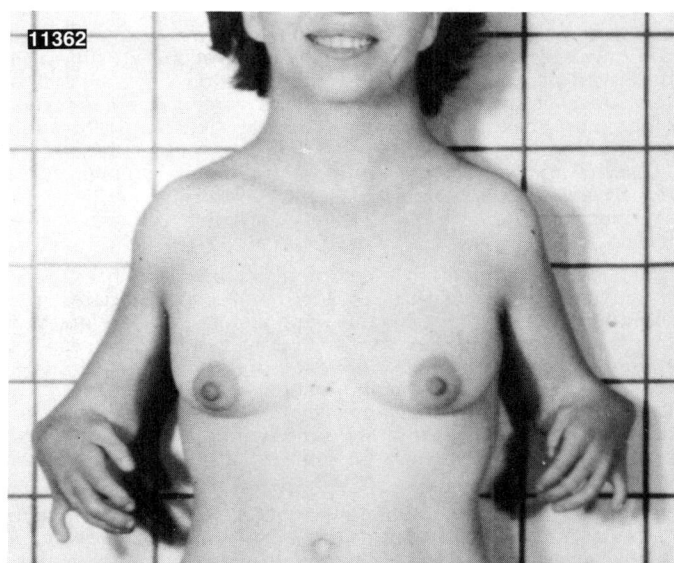

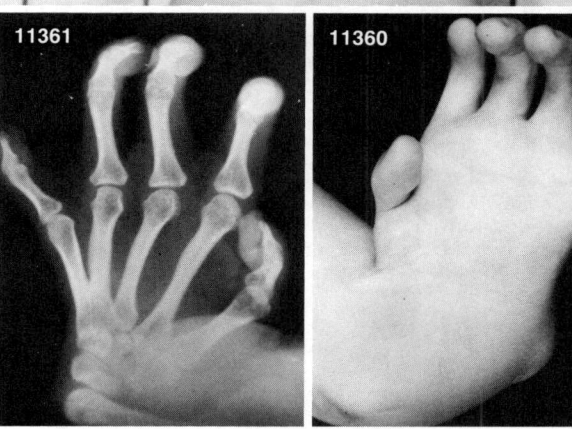

0941-11362: Symmetric, short upper limbs with radial deviation of hands and hypoplastic shoulder girdle. 11361: Absent radius and middle phalanx of 5th finger. 11360: Short forearm, radial deviation of hand, syndactyly, flexion contractures and abduction of 5th finger.

symptoms in the first four months of life. Megakaryocytes are small, basophilic, vacuolated, and nongranulated when thrombocytopenia is present. Thrombocytopenia is episodic, probably sometimes precipitated by stress, infections, and surgery. Platelet counts, often 15,000–30,000 in infancy, improve to almost normal range by adulthood. Platelet aggregation and survival are reduced.

Leukemoid reactions are recorded in 60–70% of patients during the first year of life. White blood counts may exceed 35,000, with a shift to left; and thrombocytopenia is worse during such reactions. The patient often has hepatosplenomegaly during leukemoid reaction.

Eosinophilia is recorded in bone marrow and peripheral smears in more than one-half of the patients.

Anemia, particularly during the first year of life, may have a hemolytic component or be related to blood loss. The frequency of anemia is undetermined.

*Skeletal*: The radius is always absent bilaterally. Hands are probably abnormal in all cases, with limited extension, radial deviation, hypoplastic carpals and phalanges, but thumbs always present. If the thumbs are absent, some other diagnosis must be considered. The muscles that normally attach to the radius attach instead to the wrist and pull it radially, leading to radial subluxation of the wrist. The ulnas are probably somewhat shorter and malformed in all cases; and absent bilaterally in 20%, unilaterally in 8%. The humerus is abnormal in at least one-half of the cases; absent in 5%, resulting in phocomelia. Other anomalies include dislocated hips, tibial torsion, subluxation of knees, stiff knee, dislocated patella, overriding fifth toe, rib and spine anomalies, hypoplasia of mandible and maxilla, and, rarely, severe reduction of leg long bones (giving tetraphocomelia). Short stature for family is frequent.

*Cardiac anomalies* are present in 30%; the most common being **Heart, tetralogy of Fallot** and **Atrial septal defects**.

Other anomalies are rare; mental retardation with intracranial bleeds, and glaucoma.

**Complications:** Significant symptomatic bleeding because of thrombocytopenia; death in 35–40%, almost all associated with bleeding, particularly intracranial, and almost all before one year of age; delayed motor development because of hand deformities, eventually good function, nerve compression, and arthritis at older age because of hand malformation; subluxation of wrist and knees may need splinting. Congestive failure secondary to heart defects and anemia; abnormal dermatoglyphics present in all cases, increased frequency of simian lines, decreased flexion creases.

**Associated Findings:** Mental retardation seen in 7% probably secondary to intracranial bleeding; cow milk allergy may be related and precipitates episodes of thrombocytopenia, eosinophilia, leukemoid reactions, and hemolysis; diarrheal illness common during the first year of life. *Tetraphocomelia*, simulating **Fetal thalidomide syndrome**, was reported in one infant (Anyane-Yeboa et al, 1985).

**Etiology:** Autosomal recessive inheritance. No increased consanguinity has been reported.

**Pathogenesis:** Undetermined. Gene action must occur early in gestation, between fourth and eighth weeks, to affect radial formation, blood-forming elements, and chambers of the heart. The condition may be fatal intrauterinely in some affected male embryos, since the M:F ratio is less than expected.

**MIM No.:** *27400

**POS No.:** 3412

**CDC No.:** 759.840

**Sex Ratio:** M5:F7 observed, possibly due to the condition being fatal intrauterinely in some affected males.

**Occurrence:** Over 100 cases are known, with no specific geographic or ethnic group distribution.

**Risk of Recurrence for Patient's Sib:**
See Part I, *Mendelian Inheritance*. Intra and interfamilial variabil-

ity present with regard to extent of skeletal, hematologic, and cardiac involvement.

**Risk of Recurrence for Patient's Child:**
See Part I, *Mendelian Inheritance*. Patients are fertile and no patient-to-child transmission has yet been observed.

**Age of Detectability:** At birth, or prenatally from the 16 weeks by ultrasound.

**Gene Mapping and Linkage:** Unknown.

**Prevention:** None known. Genetic counseling indicated.

**Treatment:** Avoid infections, stress and surgery during first year, because these may precipitate severe thrombocytopenia. Supportive hematologic; i.e., platelet transfusions from a single donor if possible, whole blood transfusions; corrective orthopedic, braces for forearms early, surgery if indicated; elimination of cow's milk during infancy if indicated; cardiac care as indicated.

**Prognosis:** Appears to be good if the child survives the first year. May need strenuous supportive therapy for thrombocytopenia during the first year. Women have heavy menses. Probably normal life span, if patient survives childhood.

**Detection of Carrier:** Unknown.

**Special Considerations:** The possibility that this condition represents a genetic compound (e.g. one Fanconi anemia gene and one as-yet-undefined gene that could be lethal in homozygous states) would explain the lack of consanguinity in a rare recessive disorder. There is an interesting report from Turkey (Altay et al, 1975) of a possibly affected man fathering a son with classic Fanconi anemia.

**Support Groups:** NJ; Linwood; Thrombocytopenia Absent Radius Syndrome (TARSA)

**References:**
Hall JG, et al.: Thrombocytopenia with absent radius (TAR). Medicine 1969; 48:411–439.
Altay C, et al.: Fanconi's anemia in offspring of patient with congenital radial and carpal hypoplasia. New Engl J Med 1975; 293:151.
Ray R, et al.: Brief clinical report: lower limb anomalies in the thrombocytopenia absent-radius (TAR) syndrome. Am J Med Genet 1980; 7:523–528.
Stephens TD: Muscle abnormalities associated with radial aplasia. Teratology 1983; 27:1–6.
Anyane-Yeboa K, et al.: Tetraphocomelia in the syndrome of thrombocytopenia with absent radii. Am J Med Genet 1985; 20:571–576.
Hall JG: Thrombocytopenia and absent radius (TAR) syndrome. J Med Genet 1987; 24:79–83.

HA014                                                          **Judith G. Hall**

**Thrombocytopenia-bilateral absence of the radii**
See *THROMBOCYTOPENIA-ABSENT RADIUS*
**Thrombocytopenia-Dohle bodies in neutrophils**
See *LEUKOCYTE, MAY-HEGGLIN ANOMALY*
**Thrombocytopenia-hemangioma syndrome**
See *HEMANGIOMA-THROMBOCYTOPENIA SYNDROME*

---

**THROMBOCYTOPENIC PURPURA AND LIPID HISTIOCYTOSIS**                                0942

**Includes:**
    Idiopathic thrombocytopenic purpura
    Lipid histiocytosis of spleen
    Lipidosis-thrombocytopenia-angiomata of the spleen
    Thrombocytopenic purpura, autoimmune

**Excludes:**
    Follicular lipoidosis
    **Gaucher disease** (0406)
    Lipid histiocytosis associated with diabetes
    Lipid histiocytosis associated with hyperlipemic states
    Lipid histiocytosis associated with malignancy
    Lipid histiocytosis associated with thalassemia
    Sea-blue histiocyte syndrome
    Sphingolipidoses other

**Major Diagnostic Criteria:** Thrombocytopenia and histologic demonstration of splenic histiocytosis.

**Clinical Findings:** The general findings are those usual for chronic, so-called *idiopathic thrombocytopenic purpura (ITP)* (Karpatkin 1985); easy bruising, cutaneous petechiae and ecchymoses, epistaxis, and other mucous membrane hemorrhages. The platelet count is low, and antiplatelet antibodies can be demonstrated in the serum of 70% or more of ITP patients. The serum lipids are normal. Bone marrow shows increased megakaryocytes; lipid histiocytes in the marrow are rare. The spleen is usually not enlarged clinically.

The process of lipid histiocytosis occurring in patients with ITP can be recognized only upon examination of the extirpated spleen, rarely on bone marrow examination. In various studies it has been reported to be present in 2–30% of splenectomized cases. Although the incidence of this phenomenon has increased sharply since the introduction of corticosteroid therapy for ITP, the true nature of this relationship is not known. On direct analysis, the splenic lipids are found to be generally increased, perhaps somewhat more prominently in the phospholipid fraction. Increased destruction of formed blood elements is thought to be pertinent, with platelet breakdown the most likely source of the sequestered lipid material.

**Complications:** Hemorrhage.

**Associated Findings:** Postsplenectomy infection.

**Etiology:** Unknown. The possible role of corticosteroids is undetermined.

**Pathogenesis:** Lipid-containing vacuolated histiocytes are found in the splenic pulp. By electron microscopy, these can be seen to contain osmiophilic lamellated inclusions in the cytoplasm.

**MIM No.:** 18803

**Sex Ratio:** M1:F1

**Occurrence:** Undetermined but presumed rare. Observed mainly in Caucasians.

**Risk of Recurrence for Patient's Sib:** Unknown.

**Risk of Recurrence for Patient's Child:** Unknown.

**Age of Detectability:** From three years of age to adulthood, based on experience to date from the examination of splenic specimens.

**Gene Mapping and Linkage:** Unknown.

**Prevention:** None known. Genetic counseling indicated.

**Treatment:** Management of purpura or hemorrhage.

**Prognosis:** Dependent on control of hemorrhage.

**Detection of Carrier:** Unknown.

*The author wishes to thank the late Lottie Strauss for her contributions to an earlier version of this article.*

**References:**
Saltzstein SL: Phospholipid accumulation in histiocytes of splenic pulp associated with thrombocytopenic purpura. Blood 1961; 18:73–88.
Hill JM, et al.: Secondary lipidosis of spleen associated with thrombocytopenia and other blood dyscrasias treated with steroids. Am J Clin Pathol 1963; 39:607–615.
Quinton S, et al.: Histiocytosis of spleen, lymph node, and bone marrow, associated with thrombocytopenia, splenomegaly and splenic angiomata. Am J Clin Pathol 1967; 47:484–489.
Tavassole M, McMillan R: Structure of the spleen in idiopathic thrombocytopenic purpura. Am J Clin Pathology 1975; 64:180–191.
Cohn J, Tygstrup I: Foamy histiocytosis of the spleen in patients with chronic thrombocytopenia. Scand J Hematol 1976; 16:33–37.
Luk SC, et al.: Platelet phagocytosis in the spleen of patients with idiopathic thrombocytopenic purpura (ITP). Histopathology 1980; 4:127–136.
Karpatkin S: Autoimmune thrombocytopenic purpura. Sem Hemat 1985; 22:260–288.
Diebold J, Audoin J: Association of splenoma, peliosis, and lipid histiocytosis in spleen or accessory spleen removed in two patients with chronic idiopathic thrombocytopenic purpura after long term treatment with steroids. Path Res Practice 1988; 183:446–452.

QU007                                          **Stephen J. Qualman**

---

Thrombocytopenic purpura, autoimmune
 *See THROMBOCYTOPENIC PURPURA AND LIPID HISTIOCYTOSIS*
Thrombophilia due to deficiency of AT III, hereditary
 *See ANTITHROMBIN III DEFICIENCY*
Thrombophilia, inherited
 *See PROTEIN C DEFICIENCY*
Thromboses, and protein S deficiency
 *See PROTEIN S DEFICIENCY*
Thrombotic disease, congenital
 *See PROTEIN C DEFICIENCY*
Thrombotic microangiopathy, familial
 *See HEMOLYTIC-UREMIC SYNDROME*
Thrombotic thrombocytopenic purpura, familial
 *See HEMOLYTIC-UREMIC SYNDROME*
Thumb defects
 *See RADIAL DEFECTS*
Thumb extensors, aplastic or hypoplastic
 *See THUMB, CLASPED*
Thumb polydactyly
 *See POLYDACTYLY*

---

## THUMB, ADDUCTED THUMB SYNDROME     2075

**Includes:**
 Adducted thumb syndrome
 Thumbs, congenital clasped

**Excludes:**
 **Arthrogryposis, distal types** (2280)
 **Cranio-carpo-tarsal dysplasia, whistling face type** (0223)
 **Thumb, clasped** (0175)
 **X-linked mental retardation-clasped thumb** (2291)

**Major Diagnostic Criteria:** The combination of craniostenosis, microcephaly, cleft palate, swallowing difficulty, and adducted thumbs should suggest the diagnosis.

**Clinical Findings:** Breech delivery (2/9); feeding difficulties in the neonatal period (9/9); respiratory difficulties in the neonatal period (6/9); hypotonia (4/9); hirsutism (5/9); craniosynostosis or craniostenosis (6/9); microcephaly (8/9); prominent occiput (5/9); ophthalmoplegia (5/9); downslanting palpebral fissures (3/9); cleft soft palate/bifid uvula/high-arched palate (8/95); micrognathia (3/9); low-set, poorly formed ears (8/9); laryngomalacia (2/9); pectus excavatum (3/9); adducted thumbs (9/9); **Foot, talipes equinovarus (TEV)** or calcaneovalgus (8/9); torticollis (2/9); other joint contractures (4/9); radial arch hypothenar pattern (3/9); muscle fibrillations (4/9); seizures (6/9); and mental retardation (5/9).

X-ray findings have included hypoplastic metacarpals and clubbed ribs. Autopsies have revealed dysmyelination of the central nervous system.

**Complications:** Pneumonia was a frequent complication.

**Associated Findings:** Each of the following was present in only one patient: epicanthal folds, distichiasis, entropion, short first metacarpal, **Ventricular septal defect**, and **Hernia, inguinal**.

**Etiology:** Probably autosomal recessive inheritance.

**Pathogenesis:** Most of the findings, including the facial features, are secondary to the CNS defects. Christian et al (1971) suggested that the basic defect could be abnormal lipid synthesis or an abnormal structural protein necessary to myelin synthesis. However, the basic defect is unknown.

**MIM No.:** *20155

**POS No.:** 3591

**CDC No.:** 755.500

**Sex Ratio:** Presumably M1:F1.

**Occurrence:** Nine cases have been reported; three from an Amish kindred.

**Risk of Recurrence for Patient's Sib:**
 See Part I, *Mendelian Inheritance.*

**Risk of Recurrence for Patient's Child:**
 See Part I, *Mendelian Inheritance.*

**Age of Detectability:** At birth by physical examination and lack of thumb extension during Moro reflex.

**Gene Mapping and Linkage:** Unknown.

**Prevention:** None known. Genetic counseling indicated.

**Treatment:** Supportive care.

**Prognosis:** Poor. Six patients died during the first year of life. One living child was two years at the time of the report and had an IQ of 90; a second living child was four years and was severely retarded (not yet able to stand or crawl).

**Detection of Carrier:** Unknown.

**References:**
Christian JC, et al.: The adducted thumbs syndrome. Clin Genet 1971; 2:95–103.
Fitch N, Levy EP: Adducted thumb syndromes. Clin Genet 1975; 8:190–198. *
Majoor-Krakaver O, Weicker H: Das ''adducted-thumb-syndrome'', poster session 17. Tagung der Gesellschaft fur anthropologie und Humangenetik Gottingen 1981; 23:269.
Kunze J, et al.: Adducted thumb syndrome: report of a new case and a diagnostic approach. Eur J Pediatr 1983; 141:122–126. *

T0007                                    **Helga V. Toriello**

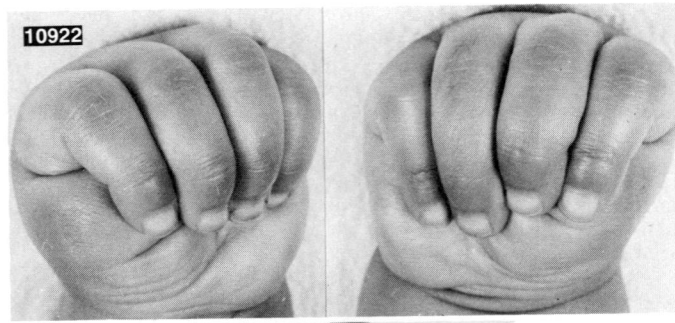

---

## THUMB, CLASPED                                    **0175**

**Includes:**
Adducted thumbs
Extensor pollicis brevis or longus
Extensor pollicis longus, congenital absence of
Pollex varus
Thumb-clutched hand
Thumb extensors, aplastic or hypoplastic
Thumb, flexion adduction deformity of
Ulnar deviation of fingers syndrome

**Excludes:**
**Arthrogryposes** (0088)
''Cortical'' thumbs
**Cranio-carpo-tarsal dysplasia, whistling face type** (0223)
**Radial defects** (0853)
**Thumb, adducted thumb syndrome** (2075)
**X-linked mental retardation-clasped thumb** (2291)

**Major Diagnostic Criteria:** An isolated inability to extend the thumb, secondary to hypoplasia or aplasia of the extensor muscles and tendons.

**Clinical Findings:** An isolated aplasia or hypoplasia, usually bilateral, of the extensor muscles and tendons of the thumb, resulting in persistently flexed or adducted first metacarpals bilaterally; proximal phalanx of the thumb is flexed forward and partially subluxed. Most common defect involves the extensor pollicis brevis, with an accompanying impairment of extension at the metacarpophalangeal joint. Defects of the extensor pollicis longus have also been described.

Since persistent adduction of the thumb may result from any imbalance in extension and flexion forces, due to structural or neurologic defects, it may be observed in conjunction with generalized joint abnormalities or as part of other distinct syndromes.

**Complications:** Without treatment, atrophy of the intrinsic thumb muscles and soft tissue contractures occur, resulting in limited function.

**Associated Findings:** Ulnar deviation or flexion deformities of other fingers, excessively long 4th and 5th digits, congenital dislocation of hip, scoliosis, torticollis, foot deformities.

**Etiology:** Possibly X-linked inheritance.

**Pathogenesis:** Unknown.

**MIM No.:** 31410

**CDC No.:** 755.500

**Sex Ratio:** M27:F15 (observed)

**Occurrence:** At least 42 cases have been reported in the literature.

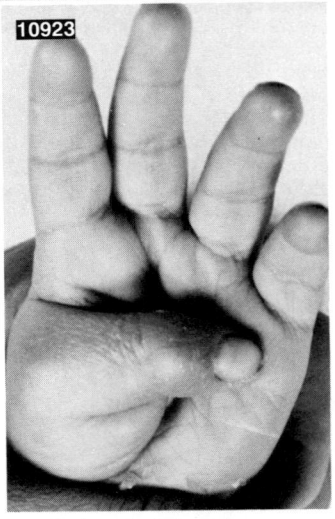

**0175-10922:** Clasped thumb deformity at age 1 year. **10923:** Clasped thumb in an older child.

---

**Risk of Recurrence for Patient's Sib:**
See Part I, *Mendelian Inheritance.*

**Risk of Recurrence for Patient's Child:**
See Part I, *Mendelian Inheritance.*

**Age of Detectability:** At birth or during infancy.

**Gene Mapping and Linkage:** Unknown.

**Prevention:** None known. Genetic counseling indicated.

**Treatment:** Early splinting of the thumb in extension and adduction may give good results. Unresponsive or untreated cases may need surgery for release of soft tissues or tendon transplants or transfers.

**Prognosis:** Mild-to-moderate impairment in function, improved with early treatment.

**Detection of Carrier:** Unknown.

**Special Considerations:** Adducted thumbs may occur with other phalangeal extensor defects and with clubfeet, with an apparent dominant inheritance, or in generalized arthrogryposis. Hypoplasia of the radial ray or neurologic impairment may result in an adducted thumb, as seen in X-linked hydrocephalus. It has also been noted in **Thumb, adducted thumb syndrome** with cleft palate, microencephaly, and dysmyelination; and in **X-linked mental retardation-clasped thumb** with aphasia and shuffling gait; and in **Cranio-carpo-tarsal dysplasia, whistling face type.** In familial trigger thumb, the defect is bilateral and the flexion is at the interphalangeal joint, not at the metacarpophalangeal joint.

**References:**
Weckesser EC, et al.: Congenital clasped thumb (congenital flexion-adduction deformity of the thumb). A syndrome, not a specific entity. J Bone Joint Surg 1968; 50A:1417–1428.
Fitch N, Levy EP. Adducted thumb syndromes. Clin Genet 1975; 8:190–198.
Anderson TE, Breed AL: Congenital clasped thumb and the Moro reflex (letter). J Pediat 1981; 99:664–665.
Wood VE: Congenital thumb deformities. Clin Orthop 1985; 195:7–25.

AT002
VA005

**Balu H. Athreya**
**Don C. Van Dyke**

**Thumb, congenital clasped-mental retardation**
*See X-LINKED MENTAL RETARDATION-CLASPED THUMB*
**Thumb, flexion adduction deformity of**
*See THUMB, CLASPED*
**Thumb, long-brachydactyly syndrome**
*See BRACHYDACTYLY-LONG THUMB SYNDROME*

---

## THUMB, TRIPHALANGEAL                              2276

**Includes:**
Delta phalanx
Hyperphalangeal thumb
Three-jointed thumb
Triphalangeal thumb, nonopposable

**Excludes:**
Phalangeal duplication of the thumb
Pseudotriphalangism

**Major Diagnostic Criteria:** Triphalangeal thumb (TPT) is a type of hyperphalangy in which a middle extra phalanx is interposed between the two normal phalanges of the thumb.

**Clinical Findings:** In general, TPT appears elongated, with three phalanges and an additional interphalangeal joint. Ulnar deviation at the terminal phalanx is common. Typically, an extra set of skin creases overlies the additional interphalangeal joint. A narrow first web space may be detrimental to the functional ability of the thumbs, as they lose dexterity. An enlarged first web space is uncommon. Horizontal patterns of dermal ridges are present in the thenar region. TPT may be unilateral or bilateral (in the majority of cases). In general, unilateral TPT is sporadic and bilateral is familial.

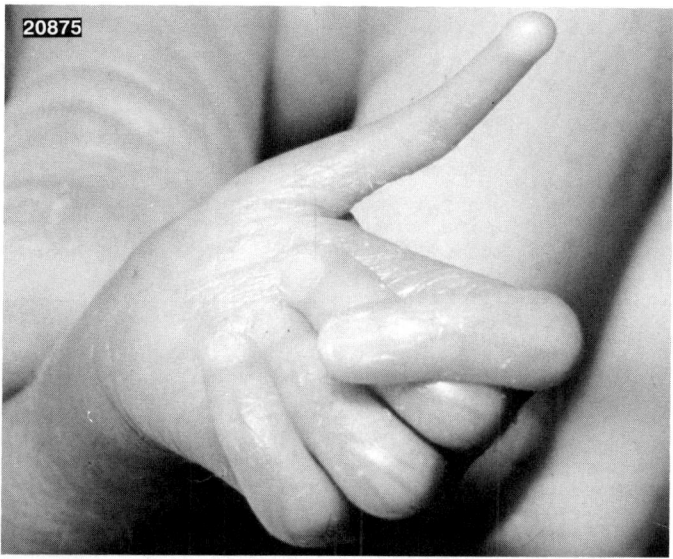

**2276-20875:** Thumb, triphalangeal; note finger-like thumb.

There are two types of TPT. *True TPT*: a four-fingered hand with TPT; and a *Finger-like TPT*: a five-fingered hand. True TPT usually has a normal position, with a normal thenar muscle; it is an opposable thumb having an almost normal rotation. A finger-like TPT lies at the same plane as the other digits, has a hypoplastic or absent thenar muscle, and functionally is a nonopposable thumb, with restriction of movement at the distal interphalangeal joint.

On X-ray, a TPT appears elongated, with an additional middle phalanx and interphalangeal joint. The extra phalanx may have three shapes: a small, triangular phalanx called *delta phalanx*; a rectangular shape; or a normal, regular phalanx. The shape of the abnormal phalanx is a definite factor in the direction of the deviation of the distal phalanx. The "delta phalanx" routinely causes deviation. Usually the distal phalanx has an ulnar deviation. Radial deviation *varus thumb* is very rare.

Patients with a small ossicle (delta phalanx) as a middle phalanx usually have opposable thumbs, but when the middle phalanx is rectangular or regular, opposition is generally very difficult. A true opposable TPT has a first metacarpal slightly shorter than usual, and its epiphyseal plate is at the proximal end, similar to the phalanges (as in the normal thumb). The finger-like nonopposable TPT has a long first metacarpal, and its epiphyseal plate is at the distal end.

**Complications:** Without treatment, the supernumerary component tends to displace the normal components and to increase the deviation of the terminal phalanx, resulting in limited function. The hand becomes less efficient, both in heavy manual work and in more delicate activities.

**Associated Findings:** **Polydactyly** of the thumb or other digits, **Syndactyly**, radial hypoplasia, and split hand. Polydactyly of the big toe or the fifth toe, split foot, dislocation of the patella, and tibial hypoplasia have also been reported. Extraskeletal associated anomalies include congenital heart disease, iris coloboma, hypoplasia of the lacrimal puncta, deafness, cleft lip and/or palate, imperforate anus, anemia, thrombocytopenia, **Hypomelanosis of Ito**, and mental retardation.

**Etiology:** May be sporadic, familial, or part of a complex malformation syndrome. The sporadic occurrence of TPT is relatively uncommon.

The wedge-shaped delta phalanx is more frequently sporadic and also more frequently unilateral. Two-thirds have a positive family history, typically of autosomal dominant inheritance with marked penetrance and variable expressivity. The inheritance of TPT in a syndrome depends on the specific syndrome in which it appears.

**Pathogenesis:** Unknown.

**MIM No.:** 19060

**CDC No.:** 755.500

**Sex Ratio:** M1:F1

**Occurrence:** The general incidence of all types of TPT has been estimated at 1:25,000.

**Risk of Recurrence for Patient's Sib:**
See Part I, *Mendelian Inheritance.*

**Risk of Recurrence for Patient's Child:**
See Part I, *Mendelian Inheritance.*

**Age of Detectability:** At birth.

**Gene Mapping and Linkage:** Unknown.

**Prevention:** None known. Genetic counseling indicated.

**Treatment:** The treatment of a true opposable TPT is mainly connected with the angular deformity. With minimal angulation, minimal or slight impaired function, and without associated anomalies, there is no need for treatment. However, most cases of true TPT require extirpation of the extra phalanx.

The nonopposable, finger-like TPT is a difficult functional problem, which must be corrected by surgery. Pollicization with large dorsal flaps, or metacarpal osteotomy or metacarpal removal, has been performed. TPT associated with other local anomalies (especially polydactyly) is a major surgical problem. The treatment must be early (by the age of two years); frequently a better result is obtained by removing the TPT, even if function appears better than in the biphalangeal thumb.

**Prognosis:** Isolated (nonsyndromatic) true TPT has a good functional prognosis. The nonopposable, finger-like TPT function can be improved by surgery, but functional results are not always satisfactory. Life span is normal in both types.

**Detection of Carrier:** Unknown.

**Special Considerations:** TPT has been described in the literature as part of numerous syndromes, but many of these descriptions are incomplete, and the type of thumb anomaly is not precisely defined. In the reports with a good description, the TPT was of a nonopposable finger-like type and not a true opposable TPT.

**References:**

Swanson AB, Brown KS: Hereditary triphalangeal thumb. J Hered 1962; 53:259–265.

Miura T: Triphalangeal thumb. Plastic Reconstr Surg 1976; 58:587–594. †

Theander G, Carstam N: Triphalangism and pseudotriphalangism of the thumb in children. Acta Radiol 1979; 20:223–232. *

Wood VE: Treatment of the triphalangeal thumb. Clin Orthop Rel Res 1979; 120:188–200. *

Lamb DW, et al.: Five-fingered hand associated with partial or complete tibial absence and pre-axial polydactyly. J Bone Joint Surg 1983; 65B:60–63.

Qazi Q, Kassner EG: Triphalangeal thumb. J Med Genet 1988; 25:505–520.

ME034
RE025

**Paul Merlob**
**Salomon H. Reisner**

**Thumb, triphalangeal-acrofacial dysostosis-cleft lip/palate**
*See ACROFACIAL DYSOSTOSIS-CLEFT LIP/PALATE-
TRIPHALANGEAL THUMB*

---

## THUMB, TRIPHALANGEAL-BRACHYECTRODACTYLY 2884

**Includes:**

Brachyectrodactyly-triphalangeal thumb
Ectrodactyly-brachydactyly-triphalangeal thumb
Triphalangeal thumb-brachyectrodactyly syndrome

**Excludes:**

**Anus-hand-ear syndrome** (0072)
**Deafness-onycho-osteo-dystrophy-retardation-seizures (DOORS)** (0262)
**Ectrodactyly** (0336)
**Fetal thalidomide syndrome** (0386)
**Heart-hand syndrome** (0455)
**Vater association** (0987)

**Major Diagnostic Criteria:** **Thumb, triphalangeal**, with or without **Polydactyly** and index fingernail dysplasia associated with **Ectrodactyly** or **Brachydactyly** and/or **Syndactyly** of the toes.

**Clinical Findings:** The typical hand malformations are triphalangy of the thumbs and index fingernail dysplasia. The foot anomalies range from true split foot to variable hypoplasia of toe 3 with or without syndactyly. A wide variability in clinical expression has been observed in the familial cases. One affected individual had normal hands and minimal brachydactyly of toe 3. The nail dysplasia of the index finger has proved to be the only feature of the syndrome in two affected relatives of a typical patient. Careful examination of all the family members of a given case is therefore essential.

**Complications:** Orthopedic problems may be anticipated in patients with severe foot involvement.

**Associated Findings:** None known.

**Etiology:** Autosomal dominant inheritance with variability of clinical expression. The mutation rate is unknown; two of 23 cases are sporadic and possibly result from a fresh gene mutation.

**Pathogenesis:** The combination of absence deformities, such as ectrodactyly, with duplication anomalies, such as triphalangeal thumb and polydactyly, has been induced in experimental animals by teratogen exposure. In mice, interchangeability between

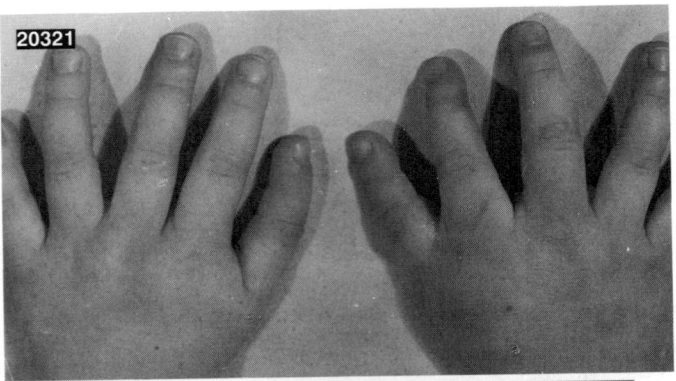

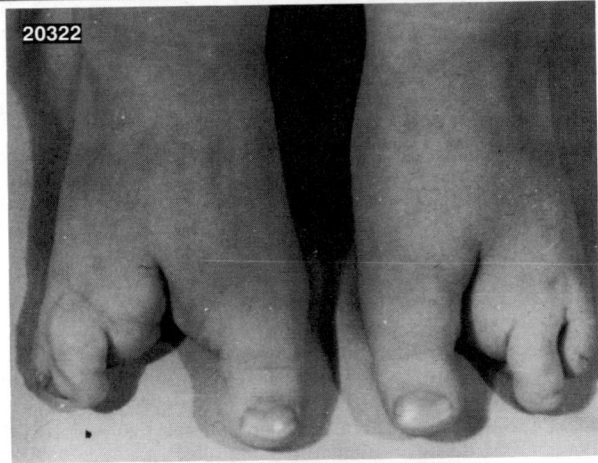

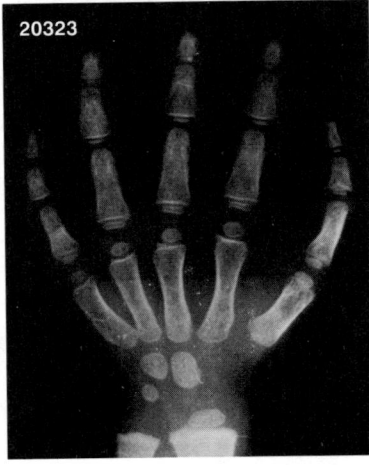

**2884-20321:** Note finger-like thumb; the preaxial polydactyly of the right hand has been surgically corrected. **20322:** Ectrosyndactyly of the feet. **20323:** Hand X-ray shows triphalangeal thumb.

polydactyly and oligodactyly has been observed in genetically induced malformations as well. In humans, **Fetal thalidomide syndrome** represents the best example of limb malformations in which reductional and duplication anomalies occur, depending on the time of exposure to the teratogen.

In this syndrome, the hand malformation is almost always of the duplication type, whereas in the feet only absence anomalies are seen. This suggests that the gene mutation affects the limb development at a definite stage, although the actual mechanism is still unknown.

**MIM No.:** 19068

**POS No.:** 3962

**Sex Ratio:** M8:F15 (observed).

**Occurrence:** Twenty-three cases have been reported in the literature.

**Risk of Recurrence for Patient's Sib:**
See Part I, *Mendelian Inheritance.*

**Risk of Recurrence for Patient's Child:**
See Part I, *Mendelian Inheritance.*

**Age of Detectability:** At birth. Cases with reduced clinical expression may be detected only by familial studies.

**Gene Mapping and Linkage:** Unknown.

**Prevention:** None known. Genetic counseling indicated.

**Treatment:** Orthopedic management of foot deformities; plastic surgery may be indicated.

**Prognosis:** Normal life span.

**Detection of Carrier:** By clinical examination.

**References:**

Carnevale A, et al.: A new syndrome of thriphalangeal thumbs and brachy-ectrodactyly. Clin Genet 1980; 18:244–252. * †
Majewski F, et al.: Triphalangeal thumb ectrodactyly in a sporadic case. Clin Genet 1981; 20:310–314.
Cirillo Silengo M, et al.: Triphalangeal thumb and brachyectrodactyly syndrome: confirmation of autosomal dominant inheritance. Clin Genet 1987; 31:13–18.

SI033
FR040

**Margherita C. Silengo
Piergiorgio Franceschini**

## THUMB, TRIPHALANGEAL-DUPLICATED GREAT TOES     2277

**Includes:**

Hyperphalangism of thumbs-duplication of thumbs and big toes
Polydactyly of thumbs/hallux-extra phalanges in the thumbs
Polydactyly, preaxial II
Triphalangeal thumbs-duplication of great toes
Triphalangeal thumb, opposable

**Excludes:**

**Thumb, triphalangeal** (2276)
**Thumb, triphalangeal-brachyectrodactyly** (2884)
**Tibial hypoplasia/aplasia-ectrodactyly** (2388)

**Major Diagnostic Criteria:** A triphalangeal thumb with duplication of big toes in a familial nonsyndromic association.

**Clinical Findings:** The abnormality appears only in the thumbs and great toes. The thumbs have all the characteristics of a true triphalangeal thumb. They appear long, with three phalanges, an additional interphalangeal joint, and an extra set of skin creases. Ulnar deviation of the terminal phalanx is common. The position of the thumb, the thenar region, and the first webspace are normal. The thumbs are opposable, although there is restriction in movement at the distal interphalangeal joint. The other fingers are normal. The great toes are duplicated, with cutaneous **Syndactyly.** The other four toes are normal.

On X-ray, the thumbs appear elongated, with an additional middle phalanx and interphalangeal joint. The middle extra phalanx of the thumbs at birth may be composed of two small ossification centers. The first metacarpal is shorter than usual, with the epiphyseal plate at its proximal end. Hexadactyly with five metatarsals is noted on X-rays of the feet. The first metatarsal is more distally placed than usual, is very large, and has a broad distal end. The great toes are duplicated and composed of two separate phalangeal bones. Cutaneous syndactyly is visible between the duplicated parts of the great toes. The rest of the skeletal survey shows no abnormalities.

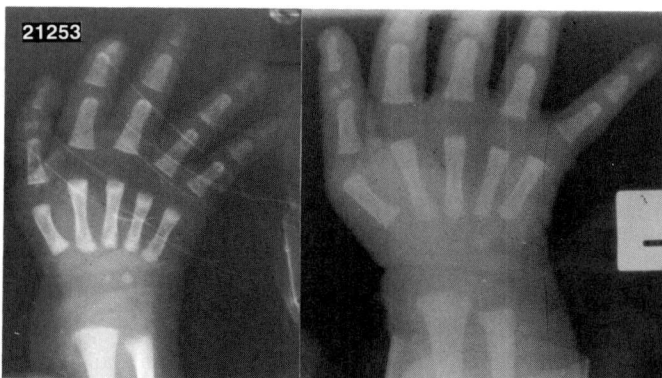

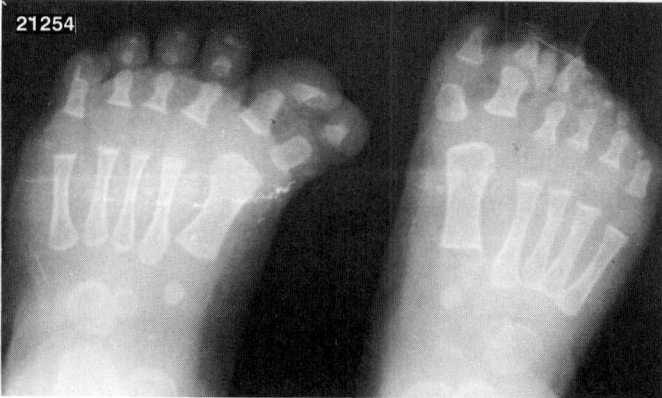

**2277-21253:** Bilateral triphalangeal thumbs. **21254:** Bilateral duplication of the great toes.

This is the typical presentation of this thumb-hallux association. However, there is great variability in expression between the patients and within the same patient. Some patients have a finger-like thumb in place of a true triphalangeal thumb; others have both types, a true triphalangeal thumb on one hand and a finger-like thumb in the other one.

**Complications:** Without treatment, the hand may become less efficient, both in heavy manual work and in more delicate activities.

**Associated Findings:** None known.

**Etiology:** Autosomal dominant inheritance with marked penetrance and great variability in expression.

**Pathogenesis:** Unknown.

**MIM No.:** *17450

**POS No.:** 4201

**CDC No.:** 755.500

**Sex Ratio:** Presumably M1:F1 (M3:F4 observed).

**Occurrence:** About five kinships have been documented.

**Risk of Recurrence for Patient's Sib:**
See Part I, *Mendelian Inheritance.*

**Risk of Recurrence for Patient's Child:**
See Part I, *Mendelian Inheritance.*

**Age of Detectability:** At birth.

**Gene Mapping and Linkage:** Unknown.

**Prevention:** None known. Genetic counseling indicated.

**Treatment:** A true triphalangeal thumb needs extirpation of the extra phalanx, while a finger-like thumb will be corrected by pollicization. Duplication of the great toes should be treated before the child begins walking. Amputation of the most medial toe, together with removal of the wide metatarsal head, is indicated.

**Prognosis:** Normal life span. Without early and adequate treatment, functional impairment with worsening restriction of movement.

**Detection of Carrier:** Unknown.

**References:**
Manoiloff EO: A rare case of hereditary hexadactylism. Am J Phys Anthropol 1931; 15:503–508.
Hefner RA: Hereditary polydactyly associated with extra phalanges in the thumb. J Hered 1940; 31:25–27.
Komai T, et al.: A Japanese kindred of hyperphalangism of thumbs and duplication of thumbs and big toe. Folia Hered Pathol 1953; 2:307–312.
Temtamy S, McKusick VA: The genetics of hand malformations. New York: Alan R. Liss, 1978.
Merlob P, et al.: Familial opposable triphalangeal thumbs associated with duplication of the big toes. J Med Genet 1985; 22:78–80. * †

ME034
GR038
RE025

Paul Merlob
Michael Grunebaum
Salomon H. Reisner

**Thumb-clutched hand**
  See THUMB, CLASPED
**Thumb-renal-ocular syndrome**
  See RADIAL-RENAL-OCULAR SYNDROME
**Thumbs, congenital clasped**
  See THUMB, ADDUCTED THUMB SYNDROME
**Thumbs, stiff**
  See SYMPHALANGISM
**Thumbs, triphalangeal-hypoplastic anemia**
  See ANEMIA, HYPOPLASTIC-TRIPHALANGEAL THUMBS, AASE-SMITH TYPE
**Thumbs-onychodystrophy-distal osteodystrophy-seizure-retardation**
  See DEAFNESS-ONYCHO-OSTEO-DYSTROPHY-RETARDATION-SEIZURES (DOORS)
**Thurston syndrome**
  See ORO-FACIO-DIGITAL SYNDROME, THURSTON TYPE
**Thymic Agenesis**
  See IMMUNODEFICIENCY, THYMIC AGENESIS
**Thymic agenesis from maternal exposure to retinoids**
  See FETAL RETINOID SYNDROME
**Thymic alymphoplasia**
  See IMMUNODEFICIENCY, X-LINKED SEVERE COMBINED
**Thymic aplasia**
  See IMMUNODEFICIENCY, THYMIC AGENESIS
  also IMMUNODEFICIENCY, NEZELOF TYPE
**Thymic dysplasia with normal immunoglobulins**
  See IMMUNODEFICIENCY, NEZELOF TYPE
**Thymic epithelial hypoplasia**
  See IMMUNODEFICIENCY, X-LINKED SEVERE COMBINED
**Thymoma with "acquired" combined immunodeficiency**
  See AGAMMAGLOBULINEMIA-THYMOMA SYNDROME
**Thymoma, familial**
  See CANCER, THYMOMA
**Thymoma-agammaglobulinemia syndrome**
  See AGAMMAGLOBULINEMIA-THYMOMA SYNDROME
**Thymus and parathyroids, congenital absence of the**
  See IMMUNODEFICIENCY, THYMIC AGENESIS
**Thyroglobulin synthesis, defect in**
  See THYROID, THYROGLOBULIN DEFECTS
**Thyroglobulin, absent**
  See THYROID, THYROGLOBULIN DEFECTS

---

**THYROGLOSSAL DUCT REMNANT**                    **0945**

**Includes:**
  Duct, thyroglossal remnant
  Lingual thyroid
  Thyroglossal duct, cyst or sinus
**Excludes:**
  **Branchial cleft cysts** (2723)
  **Nasopharyngeal cysts** (0706)
  **Neck/head, dermoid cyst or teratoma** (0283)
  Lipoma
  Suppurative lesions

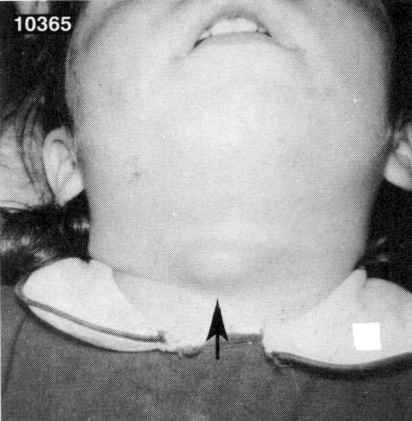

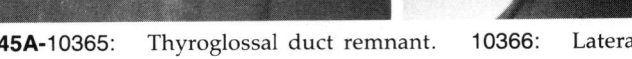

**0945A**-10365:  Thyroglossal duct remnant.  **10366:**  Lateral view.

---

**Major Diagnostic Criteria:** Lingual mass, or midline neck cyst or mass, moving with deglutition or tongue protrusion, with or without associated infection.

**Clinical Findings:** Midline or slightly lateral solid or cystic mass or sinus in the anterior neck, located anywhere from the tongue base to the suprasternal region. A thyroglossal cyst may be present laterally in the neck or into the larynx. A tract from the cyst to the foramen cecum may remain patent, allowing cyst fluid to drain into the mouth. When this occurs the cyst may become smaller. However, in most cases, the duct is closed and persists as a fibrous cord that may be palpated from the neck mass to the center of the hyoid bone. A sinus opening onto the anterior neck may occasionally discharge a few drops of fluid. When the patient swallows or protrudes the tongue, the cyst may appear to move upward in the neck.

The thyroglossal duct, cyst, and tract are remnants of the

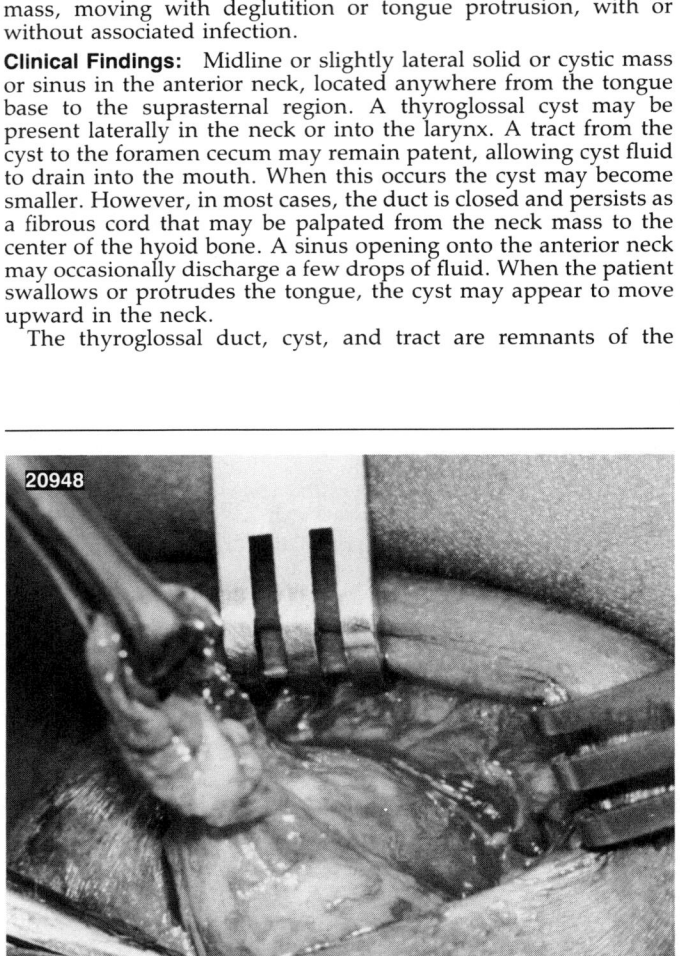

**0945B**-20948:  Thyroglossal duct cyst.

embryologic descent of the developing thyroid gland from the pharynx to the neck. In some instances several tiny ducts may be found. Rarely descent does not occur and a mass at the foramen cecum may not be a thyroglossal duct cyst, but a lingual thyroid.

An $I^{125}$ thyroid scan should be done in the case of lingual mass. If the lingual thyroid is the only thyroid tissue in the body; the radioactive isotope uptake will be in the area of the base of the tongue. Most patients with a lingual thyroid are euthyroid, although in a series of cretins 63.6% had ectopic thyroid. The majority of patients are asymptomatic. 65–70% have no other thyroid tissue. Diagnosis may be made by fine needle aspiration for cytology.

Grossly the lingual thyroid is hemispheric, about 2 cm in diameter, pink, and covered by squamous epithelium through which vascular markings are visible. The most common histology is fetal or microvillar adenomatous pattern, closely followed by normal thyroid microscopic appearance. The thyroglossal cyst and duct may be lined with squamous, ciliated respiratory, pseudo-stratified columnar, columnar, cuboidal, or transitional epithelium. More than one type of epithelium may be present. Subepithelial aggregations of lymphocytes may be seen. The epithelial lining may be replaced by fibrous tissue. Thyroid follicles may be seen in 2–36% of specimens. The contents may be mucoid, grumous, or pasty.

**Complications:** Infection (50%); recurrence (15–20%); osteomyelitis of hyoid bone; airway obstruction.

**Associated Findings:** Papillary adenocarcinoma (less than 100 reported cases).

**Etiology:** Unknown.

**Pathogenesis:** Failure of the thyroglossal anlage to descend to the normal location of the thyroid gland. Persistence of a cystic dilation of embryonic thyroglossal duct.

**CDC No.:** 759.220

**Sex Ratio:** M1:F4–5

**Occurrence:** 31 cases in 86,000 consecutive admissions to Mayo Clinic. In a series of routine autopsies, 10% had ectopic thyroid tissue.

**Risk of Recurrence for Patient's Sib:** Unknown.

**Risk of Recurrence for Patient's Child:** Unknown.

**Age of Detectability:** Usually in early childhood, by physical examination.

**Gene Mapping and Linkage:** Unknown.

**Prevention:** None known. Genetic counseling indicated.

**Treatment:** En bloc surgical excision of cyst and a core of tissue in continuity with the middle one-third of hyoid bone and to the foramen cecum (Sistrunk, 1920). Treatment of infection with antibiotics. Primary excision is recommended rather than incision and drainage. Medical treatment consists of $I^{131}$ ablation of the lingual thyroid followed by hormonal suppression. However, excision of the lingual thyroid and implantation of slices into the sternocleidomastoid muscle has been successful. Surgical treatment may be reserved for cases where hemorrhage, cystic degeneration, suspected malignancy, or failure of medical therapy has occurred.

Endotracheal intubation or tracheotomy may be needed if the airway is obstructed. For carcinoma of the thyroglossal remnant; total thyroidectomy, bilateral neck explorations, followed by $I^{131}$ and hormonal suppression.

**Prognosis:** Good if adequately excised.

**Detection of Carrier:** Unknown.

**References:**
Sistrunk WE: The surgical treatment of cysts of the thyroglossal tract. Ann Surg 1920; 71:121–122. *

Swan H, et al.: Autotransplantation of the lingual thyroid. Arch Surg 1958; 76:458–464.

Sadé J, Rosen G: Thyroglossal cysts and tracts: a histological and histochemical study. Ann Otol Rhinol Laryngol 1968; 77:139–145.

Ward PH, Strahan RW, et al.: The many faces of thyroglossal duct. Trans Am Acad Ophth & Otol 1970; 74:310–318 *.

Weider DJ, Parker W: Lingual thyroid: review, case reports and therapeutic guidelines, Ann Otol Rhinol Laryngol 1977; 86:841–848.

Hawkins DB, et al.: Cysts of the thyroglossal duct. Laryngoscope 1982; 92:1254–1258.

BE028                                           **LaVonne Bergstrom**

**Thyroglossal duct, cyst or sinus**
*See THYROGLOSSAL DUCT REMNANT*
**Thyroid 1, transforming sequence**
*See CANCER, THYROID, FAMILIAL PAPILLARY CARCINOMA OF*
**Thyroid hormone organification defect IIB**
*See DEAFNESS-GOITER*
**Thyroid hormone, familial resistance to**
*See THYROID, HORMONE RESISTANCE*
**Thyroid hormone, generalized tissue resistance to**
*See THYROID, HORMONE RESISTANCE*
**Thyroid hormone, insensitivity to**
*See THYROID, HORMONE RESISTANCE*
**Thyroid hormone, partial resistance to**
*See THYROID, HORMONE RESISTANCE*
**Thyroid hormone, pituitary resistance to**
*See THYROID, HORMONE RESISTANCE*
**Thyroid hormone, refractoriness to**
*See THYROID, HORMONE RESISTANCE*
**Thyroid hormone, target hormone resistance to**
*See THYROID, HORMONE RESISTANCE*
**Thyroid hormonogenesis, genetic defect in**
*See DEAFNESS-GOITER*
**Thyroid hormonogenesis, genetic defect in, I**
*See THYROID, IODIDE TRANSPORT DEFECT*
**Thyroid hormonogenesis, genetic defect in, IIA**
*See THYROID, PEROXIDASE DEFECT*
**Thyroid hormonogenesis, genetic defect in, IV**
*See THYROID, IODOTYROSINE DEIODINASE DEFICIENCY*
**Thyroid hormonogenesis, genetic defect in, V**
*See THYROID, THYROGLOBULIN DEFECTS*
**Thyroid organification defects (some types)**
*See THYROID, PEROXIDASE DEFECT*
**Thyroid peroxidase deficiency**
*See THYROID, PEROXIDASE DEFECT*

---

## THYROID, DYSGENESIS                                           0946

**Includes:**
Agoitrous cretinism
Agoitrous hypothyroidism
Athyreotic hypothyroidism
Athyrosis
Cretinism, agoitrous
Cretinism, athyreotic
Cretinism, sporadic nongoitrous
Cryptothyroidism

**Excludes:**
Cretinism, endemic (3167)
Thyroid dyshormonogenesis, all forms
Thyroid, iodotyrosine deiodinase deficiency (0543)
Thyroid, peroxidase defect (0947)
Thyrotropin deficiency, isolated (0949)
Thyrotropin unresponsiveness (0948)

**Major Diagnostic Criteria:** Cord blood or filter paper spot T4 concentration $< 7$ μg/dl and TSH concentration $> 60$ μU/ml. After one week of age, serum T4 is below the range for age and TSH $> 10$ μU/ml. Serum T3 concentrations are variable. Thyroidal radioiodine uptake and scan may be confirmatory.

**Clinical Findings:** Infants with thyroid dysgenesis may have ectopic or hypoplastic thyroid tissue or total thyroid agenesis. Thus, there is a spectrum of severity of thyroid hormone deficiency. Some thyroid tissue is present in as many as 70–80% of cases. Infants with inadequate thyroid tissue are born with low (hypothyroid) circulating levels of thyroxine (T4) and high TSH concentrations. Significant but low levels of T4 usually are present in infants with residual functioning thyroid tissue, and serum TSH levels are increased. Thyroid scanning techniques are not sensitive enough to detect small volumes of residual tissue in some infants, but significant circulating concentrations of triiodothyronine (T3) during the neonatal period in the face of low serum T4 concentrations suggest the presence of residual functioning thyroid tissue. Significant levels of circulating thyroglobulin also indicate the presence of thyroid tissue.

Although signs and symptoms of hypothyroidism may occur in the newborn period, the clinical diagnosis is difficult and is made early (before 8–12 weeks) in only 30% of affected infants. Suggestive early signs and symptoms include a large posterior fontanel, prolonged "physiologic" hyperbilirubinemia, mild myxedema of the face and neck, respiratory distress in a full-term infant, hypothermia (< 35.5° C rectal), bradycardia (rate < 100), constipation, lethargy, poor feeding, noisy breathing, and persistent nasal stuffiness. The more classic signs and symptoms of macroglossia, abdominal distention, umbilical hernia, hypotonia, dry hair and skin, puffy facies, and hoarse cry appear later in infancy and indicate prolonged hypothyroidism. In children, delayed growth, delayed skeletal maturation, and delayed dental development are the most sensitive indicators of thyroid hormone deficiency. Hypofunction of a variety of organ systems may be detected by careful study but offer only nonspecific, secondary evidence for thyroid hormone deficiency. Congenital hypothyroidism leads to intellectual deficit and clinical brain dysfunction if thyroid replacement therapy is not begun before 45 days of age; 95% of infants begun on treatment before this time develop normal intellect, whereas only 10% or less develop normally if treatment is delayed beyond one year.

**Complications:** Mental retardation, growth retardation, delayed bone and dental maturation.

**Associated Findings:** Nearly all athyreotic cretins are PTC nontasters.

**Etiology:** Usually sporadic. A few familial cases have been described, associated with maternal autoimmune thyroid disease. Also a few cases have occurred after administration of therapeutic doses of radioiodine for treatment of thyrotoxicosis. In these cases, the pregnancy was of 10–20 weeks duration at the time of therapy, and pregnancy was not suspected.

**Pathogenesis:** Failure of normal embryologic development of the thyroid gland primordium. Hypoplasia may be associated with ectopy or residual thyroid gland tissue, which may be located at the base of the tongue, between the base of the tongue and the hyoid bone, or between the hyoid bone and the normal position below the thyroid cartilage. Ectopic location of residual thyroid tissue occurs in 60–80% of cases. Residual tissue is hyperplastic with a high cell/colloid ratio and little visible colloid. The reduced volume of thyroid tissue results in deficiency of T4 secretion and compensatory increase in secretion of TSH from the pituitary gland. T3 secretion may be increased from the intensely stimulated residual tissue, and the normal or near-normal serum T3 levels offer some protection against severe thyroid hormone deficiency.

**MIM No.:** *21870

**POS No.:** 3521

**CDC No.:** 759.210

**Sex Ratio:** M1:F4

**Occurrence:** 1:5,526 in whites; 1:32,377 in blacks.

**Risk of Recurrence for Patient's Sib:** Very small. There is some evidence to suggest that the risk may be increased if the mother has a high titer of antithyroid, and particularly TSH receptor, antibody.

**Risk of Recurrence for Patient's Child:** Very small.

**Age of Detectability:** At birth, by cord blood or filter paper spot screening for T4 and TSH concentrations.

**Gene Mapping and Linkage:** Unknown.

**Prevention:** Avoidance of radioiodine treatment of thyrotoxicosis in pregnancy. Counseling for women with high thyroid antibody titer.

**Treatment:** Treatment with thyroid hormone to prevent complications.

**Prognosis:** Normal life span with early diagnosis and treatment; mental deficiency and growth retardation without therapy. The prognosis for mental development becomes poorer as treatment is delayed.

**Detection of Carrier:** Unknown.

**References:**
Dussault JH, et al.: Thyroid function in neonatal hypothyroidism. J Pediatr 1976; 89:541.
Klein AH, et al.: Neonatal thyroid function in congenital hypothyroidism. J Pediatr 1976; 89:545.
Brown AL, et al.: Racial differences in the incidence of congenital hypothyroidism. J Pediatr 1981; 99:934–936.
New England Congenital Hypothyroidism Collaborative. Neonatal hypothyroid screening: status of patients at 6 years. J Pediatr 1985; 107:915–919.
Rovet J, et al.: Intellectual outcome in children with fetal hypothyroidism. J Pediatr 1987; 110:700–704.
Muir A, et al.: Thyroid scanning, ultrasound and serum thyroglobulin in determining the origin of congenital hypothyroidism. Am J Dis Child 1988; 142:214–216.
New England Congenital Hypothyroidism Collaborative: Elementary school performance of children with congenital hypothyroidism. J Pediatr 1990; 116:27–32.

FI017 **Delbert A. Fisher**

**Thyroid, familial papillary carcinoma**
*See CANCER, THYROID, FAMILIAL PAPILLARY CARCINOMA OF*

## THYROID, HORMONE RESISTANCE                    0257

**Includes:**
   Refetoff syndrome
   Thyroid hormone, familial resistance to
   Thyroid hormone, generalized tissue resistance to
   Thyroid hormone, insensitivity to
   Thyroid hormone, partial resistance to
   Thyroid hormone, pituitary resistance to
   Thyroid hormone, refractoriness to
   Thyroid hormone, target hormone resistance to
   Thyrotropin secretion, inappropriate

**Excludes:**
   **Cretinism, endemic** (3167)
   **Deafness-goiter** (0249)
   **Epiphyseal dysplasia, multiple** (0358)
   Euthyroid hyperthyroxinemia
   Familial dysalbuminemic hyperthyroxinemia (FDH)
   Graves disease, neonatal
   Inborn errors of thyroid hormone synthesis
   Thyrotropin-secreting pituitary adenoma
   **Thyrotropin unresponsiveness** (0948)
   **Thyroxine-binding globulin defects** (0950)

**Major Diagnostic Criteria:** Goiter and thyroid overactivity associated with high levels of free (protein-unbound) circulating thyroid hormone, non-suppressed thyrotropin (thyroid stimulating hormone, TSH), absence of thyrotoxicosis and diminished response to exogenous thyroid hormone.

**Clinical Findings:** The first description of this defect was in three siblings of consanguineous parents, who presented with deaf-mutism, delayed bone maturation, goiter, high levels of protein-bound iodine and the absence of stigmata of thyrotoxicosis. Subsequent case reports have shown a heterogeneity of features in terms of growth, bone maturation, hearing and mental development, as well as in the severity of the defect. Most patients have small goiters but none have ophthalmopathy or dermopathy typical of Graves' disease. The hallmark is elevated levels of circulating thyroid hormone (thyroxine and triiodothyronine), in the presence of eumetabolism, with normal concentration of thyroxine-binding globulin and non-suppressed thyrotropin. Both thyroxine and triiodothyronine are the L-isomers. Free thyroxine in blood is elevated. The 24-hour thyroidal radioiodide uptake is high and is non suppressible with replacement doses of thyroid hormone. The extrathyroidal thyroxine and triiodothyronine pools and their rates of degradation are elevated. Penetration of thyroxine into tissues and its conversion to triiodothyronine are normal. Circulating thyrotropin levels are normal or just above the normal range and increase in response to the administration of thyrotropin-releasing hormone. Thyroid-stimulating immunoglobulins are absent as are thyroglobulin and thyroid microsomal antibodies. Administration of replacement doses of thyroid hormone fail to supress the response of thyrotropin to thyrotropin-releasing hormone. Glucocorticoids and dopaminergic drugs, given in usual doses, produce their suppressive effect on thyrotropin. Some patients have demonstrable abnormalities of their nuclear receptor for thyroid hormone.

**Complications:**  Probably deafness, bony dysgenesis and sequelae of hypothyroidism in patients given treatment aimed to reduce the circulating thyroid hormone level.

**Associated Findings:**  Sensorineural hearing loss has been described in several cases and may be a complication of hypothyroidism during early life. Other abnormalities, probably not related to thyroid hormone activity have been observed less frequently. These are: winged scapulae, vertebral abnormalities, pigeon breat, prurigo Besnier, congenital ichthyosis and bull's eye type macular atrophy.

**Etiology:**  Possibly represents the manifestation of a number of defects beginning at the interaction of thyroid hormone with its receptor and encompassing all subsequent steps leading to the expression of thyroid hormone action. The defect may be familial (30 families) or sporadic (7 cases). Both autosomal recessive and autosomal dominant modes of inheritance have been suggested. Consanguinity is known to have occurred in 4 families. Some cases may represent *de novo* mutations.

**Pathogenesis:**  The condition appears to be a congenital metabolic defect of resistance to the action of thyroid hormone which affects tissues to a variable degree and that has been partially compensated by the production of excess hormone. Since thyroid hormone is probably essential for normal embryonic development and post-natal growth and maturation, complete thyroid hormone unresponsiveness by all tissues would presumably be incompatible with life. In some cases there may be demonstrable abnormalities at the level of the nuclear thyroid hormone receptor. The latter probably represents one of a spectrum of biochemical abnormalities responsible for the observed resistance to the hormone. Bioassys in cultured skin fibroblasts from affected subjects have not been always diagnostic. However, recent work has shown that in fibroblasts from 6 out of 7 patients with resistance to thyroid hormone, triiodothyronine suppressed fibronectin synthesis clearly less than in fibroblasts from normal subjects. The test may prove to be useful in the tissue diagnosis of the defect.

**MIM No.:**  *18857, *27430

**POS No.:**  3910

**Sex Ratio:**  M1:F1

**Occurrence:**  Undetermined; 120 cases have been reported affecting individuals with a wide spectrum of ethnic backgrounds.

**Risk of Recurrence for Patient's Sib:**
See Part I, *Mendelian Inheritance.*

**Risk of Recurrence for Patient's Child:**
See Part I, *Mendelian Inheritance.*

**Age of Detectability:**  Infancy, although often not detected until adulthood. The diagnosis can be made at any age on the basis of a small goiter with elevated serum thyroid hormone levels in the presence of euthyroidism and non-suppressed thyrotropin.

**Gene Mapping and Linkage:**  Unknown.

**Prevention:**  None known. Genetic counseling indicated.

**Treatment:**  Avoid all treatment designed to correct the hyperthyroidism and thus normalize the thyroid hormone levels in serum. Treatment with supraphysiologic doses of thyroid hormone is reserved for patients with hypometabolism and growth retardation and for patients who have received therapy causing irrevers-

ible reduction of the hormonal reserve of the thyroid gland. Special training for deaf-mutism.

**Prognosis:**  Variable but life span is probably normal. Thyroid hormone deprivation during early age may result in diminished mental and physical development.

**Detection of Carrier:**  Unknown.

**Special Considerations:**  The distinguishing features of this syndrome includes thyrotropin-mediated elevation of circulating levels of free thyroid hormone in the presence of clinical euthyroidism. Isolated tissue responses suggestive of hypothyroidism may be present, especially during early life. Administration of replacement doses of thyroid hormone fails to suppress thyrotropin, and supraphysiologic doses fail to induce signs of thyrotoxicity or produce the normal metabolic responses to thyroid hormone excess. Uptake of thyroid hormone and conversion of thyroxine to triiodothyronine are normal. A variant of the syndrome with resistance to thyroid hormone selective to the pituitary gland has been described. In the latter condition, patients have thyrotropin induced thyrotoxicosis with hypermetabolism. A condition with little clinical significance but which can be confused with thyrotoxicosis is familial dysalbuminemic hyperthyroxinemia (FDH). FDH has several subtypes and is frequent in Hispanics of Puerto Rican origin (Ruiz et al, 1982).

**References:**

Refetoff S, et al.: Familial syndrome combining deaf-mutism, stippled epiphyses, goiter and abnormally high PBI: Possible target organ refractoriness to thyroid hormone. J Clin Endocrinol Metab 1967; 27:279–294.

Refetoff S, et al.: Studies of a sibship with apparent hereditary resistance to the intracellular action of thyroid hormone. Metabolism 1972; 21:723–756.

Bernal J, et al.: Abnormalities of triiodothyronine binding to lymphocyte and fibroblast nuclei from patients with peripheral resistance to thyroid hormone action. J Clin Endocrinol Metab 1978; 47:1266–1272.

Brooks MH, et al.: Familial thyroid hormone resistance. Am J Med 1981; 71:414–421.

Weintraub BD, et al.: Inappropirate secretion of thyroid stimulating hormone. Ann Intern Med 1981; 95:339–351.

Refetoff S: Syndromes of thyroid hormone resistance. Am J Physiol 1982; 243:E88–E98.

Eil C, et al.: Nuclear binding of [125]-triiodothyronine in dispersed cultured skin fibroblasts from patients with resistance to thyroid hormone. J Clin Endocrinol Metab 1982; 55:502–510.

Ruiz M, et al.: Familial dysalbuminemic hyperthyroxinemia: a syndrome that can be confused with thyrotoxicosis. New Engl J Med 1982; 306:635–639.

Ceccarelli P, et al.: Resistance to thyroid hormone diagnosed by the reduced response of fibroblasts to the triiodothyronine-induced suppression of fibronectin synthesis. J Clin Endocrinol Metab 1987; 65:242–246.

RE007                                               **Samuel Refetoff**
EI002                                                      **Charles Eil**

---

**THYROID, IODIDE TRANSPORT DEFECT**                          **0542**

**Includes:**
> Goiter, familial (some forms)
> Hypothyroidism, congenital (some forms)
> Iodide accumulation, transport or trapping defect
> Iodide transport defect, partial
> Thyroid hormonogenesis, genetic defect in, I

**Excludes:**
> **Goiter, goitrogen induced** (0435)
> **Thyroid, dysgenesis** (0946)
> **Thyroid, iodotyrosine deiodinase deficiency** (0543)
> **Thyrotropin unresponsiveness** (0948)
> Other types of thyroid dyshormonogenesis

**Major Diagnostic Criteria:**  Congenital hypothyroidism, or compensated hypothyroidism; an absent or very reduced RAI uptake in the presence of normal or increased serum TSH levels, and low salivary to plasma iodide ratio. Known goitrogens must be absent from the diet.

**Clinical Findings:** Patients are generally hypothyroid, usually presenting during infancy with developmental, growth, and skeletal retardation. Other signs of congenital hypothyroidism, such as lethargy, constipation, macroglossia, dry skin, umbilical hernia, and cretinoid facies may be present. Goiter may be evident at birth, but usually appears in early childhood. Laboratory findings include a low T4 with a low radioactive iodine (RAI) uptake with no increase after exogenous TSH administration. The defect may be complete or partial, indicating genetic heterogeneity.

**Complications:** Congenital hypothyroidism, with mental and physical retardation.

**Associated Findings:** Occasionally mechanical airway obstruction secondary to a large goiter.

**Etiology:** Autosomal recessive inheritance. Heterogeneity in the iodide transport defect exists. Three patients with a defect in thyroidal iodide transport but with some residual concentrating ability of their salivary glands and gastric mucosa have been described. Clinically, they are congenitally hypothyroid, and the defect in these cases also appears to be transmitted as an autosomal recessive trait. Whether they represent a different mutation at the same gene locus involved in the complete defect, or a separate basic defect of iodide transport, is unknown.

**Pathogenesis:** The transport defect may be due either to an altered postulated membrane iodide receptor or carrier, or an altered energy supply to this active transport system.

**MIM No.:** *27440

**Sex Ratio:** M1:F1

**Occurrence:** Presumably rare. However, since the defect can be treated with a high iodide intake, it may not be apparent in areas of high dietary iodide intake.

**Risk of Recurrence for Patient's Sib:**
See Part I, *Mendelian Inheritance.*

**Risk of Recurrence for Patient's Child:**
See Part I, *Mendelian Inheritance.*

**Age of Detectability:** Clinical symptoms of congenital hypothyroidism are usually apparent during the first one-half year of life. Occasionally goiter is present at birth. Serum T4 or TSH screening may be diagnostic at birth.

**Gene Mapping and Linkage:** Unknown.

**Prevention:** None known. Genetic counseling indicated.

**Treatment:** Early replacement therapy with thyroxine to prevent hypothyroidism. Iodide therapy also has been successfully utilized. Surgical removal of goiter if airway obstruction is present. Educational programs for the problem of mental retardation.

**Prognosis:** Prevention of mental retardation is dependent on early treatment in infancy.

**Detection of Carrier:** Unknown.

**References:**
Medeivos-Neto, G.A. et al.: Partial defect of iodide trapping mechanism in two siblings with congenital goiter and hypothyroidism. J Clin Endocrinol Metab 1972; 35:370–377.
Stanbury, J.B. and Chapman, E.M.: Congenital hypothyroidism with goiter. Absence of an iodide-concentrating mechanism. Lancet 1960 I:1162–1165.
Stanbury, J.B.: Familial goiter. In: Wyngaarden JB, Fredrickson DS, eds: The metabolic basis of inherited disease, 4th ed. New York: McGraw-Hill, 1978:206–239.
Couch RM, et al.: Congenital hypothyroidism caused by defective iodide transport. J Pediatr 1985; 106:950–953.
Wolff J: Congenital goiter with defective iodide transport. Endocrin Rev 1983; 4:240–254.
Couch RM, et al.: Congenital hypothyroidism caused by defective iodide transport. J Pediatr 1985; 106:950–953.

**R. Neil Schimke**

---

## THYROID, IODOTYROSINE DEIODINASE DEFICIENCY     0543

**Includes:**
Deiodinase deficiency
Goiter, familial (some forms)
Hypothyroidism, congenital (some forms)
Iodotyrosine dehalogenase deficiency
Iodotyrosine deiodinase deficiency, partial
Iodotyrosine deiodinase deficiency, peripheral
Thyroid hormonogenesis, genetic defect in, IV
Thyroidal deiodination deficiency

**Excludes:**
Goiter, goitrogen induced (0435)
Thyroid, dysgenesis (0946)
Thyroid, iodide transport defect (0542)
Other types of thyroid dyshormonogenesis

**Major Diagnostic Criteria:** Congenital hypothyroidsim, or compensated hypothyroidism with a rapid and high thyroid uptake and turnover of RAI; no deiodination of injected, labeled MIT (monoiodotyrosine) or DIT (diiodotyrosine); and probably MIT and DIT and their derivatives in abnormally high concentration in plasma and urine.

**Clinical Findings:** Patients with the complete form of iodotyrosine deiodinase deficiency, presumably homozygous for the trait, have the typical clinical appearance of congenital hypothyroidism. There is a variable age of onset in the development of goiter, that may be present at birth, but usually develops during childhood. Clinical laboratory findings are a low serum T4 with a rapid and high uptake and turnover of radioactive iodine. MIT and DIT and their derivatives are probably present in abnormally high concentrations in the plasma and urine. Exogenous intravenous administration of MIT or DIT results in their excretion unchanged in the urine, indicating deficient peripheral deiodination of these compounds as well.

Some presumedly heterozygous relatives of these patients, especially females, have goiters but are euthyroid. They display a partial impairment in peripheral deiodination when given exogenous DIT intravenously.

**Complications:** Congenital hypothyroidism, with resultant mental and growth retardation.

**Associated Findings:** Occasionally airway obstruction due to an enlarged goiter.

**Etiology:** Autosomal recessive inheritance. Homozygous state manifesting congenital hypothyroidism; heterozygotes, especially females, may manifest euthyroid goiter.

**Pathogenesis:** The iodotyrosine deiodinase enzyme is not involved in the direct synthesis of $T_4$ or $T_3$, but functions as a salvage mechanism for iodide recovery from thyroglobulin-bound MIT and DIT not utilized in synthesis. A defect in this enzyme results in continued loss of iodinated precursors and depletion of available iodine stores, with resultant hypothyroidism. Consistent with this is the observation that replacement therapy with a large excess of iodide can reestablish a euthyroid state.

**MIM No.:** *27480

**Sex Ratio:** M1:F1

**Occurrence:** Undetermined. Since iodide therapy can ameliorate the disorder, it may not be clinically apparent in areas with a high dietary iodide intake.

**Risk of Recurrence for Patient's Sib:**
See Part I, *Mendelian Inheritance.*

**Risk of Recurrence for Patient's Child:**
See Part I, *Mendelian Inheritance.*

**Age of Detectability:** Symptoms of congenital hypothyroidism usually are apparent during the first half-year of life, usually with goiter. Serum T4 screening should detect this at birth.

**Gene Mapping and Linkage:** Unknown.

**Prevention:** None known. Genetic counseling indicated.

**Treatment:** Early replacement therapy with thyroxine to prevent congenital hypothyroidism. Iodide treatment has been successful, although large doses are often necessary. Surgical removal of a goiter may be necessary, due to pressure symptoms. Educational programs for the problem of mental retardation.

**Prognosis:** Good, with early treatment of hypothyroidism. Poor mental development, if treated late.

**Detection of Carrier:** Intravenous radioiodine-labeled diiodotyrosine (DIT) test may distinguish the heterozygous state.

**Special Considerations:** Heterogeneity of iodotyrosine deiodinase defects has become apparent. Patients have been described with a partial deiodination deficiency, a deficient thyroidal deiodination with normal peripheral deiodination, and a peripheral defect with a normal thyroidal iodotyrosine deiodinase activity. Clinically, these patients usually have been euthyroid with goiter. The genetic etiology of each of these types is unclear. They may represent other mutations at the same locus, or at a different locus, perhaps affecting different tissue isoenzymes or enzyme subunits.

**References:**
Stanbury, JB, et al.: Familial goiter and related disorders. In: Stanbury JB, et al. eds: The Metabolic Basis of Inherited Disease, 5th Ed. New York: McGraw-Hill, 1983:231–269.

SC016                                                    **R. Neil Schimke**

---

## THYROID, PEROXIDASE DEFECT                               0947

**Includes:**
  Goiter, familial
  Hypothyroidism, congenital
  Iodide peroxidase deficiency
  Thyroid organification defects (some types)
  Thyroid peroxidase deficiency
  Thyroid hormonogenesis, genetic defect in, IIA

**Excludes:**
  **Deafness-goiter** (0249)
  Hashimoto thyroiditis
  Thyroglobulin synthesis, abnormal
  **Thyroid, dysgenesis** (0946)
  Thyroid dyshormonogenesis, other
  Thyroid nonperoxidase deficient organification defects,
    other

**Major Diagnostic Criteria:** Hypothyroidism or compensated hypothyroidism, with a rapid discharge of radioiodine after administration of thiocyanate or perchlorate. In addition, *in vitro* demonstration of defective peroxidase activity.

**Clinical Findings:** Clinical heterogeneity is apparent in patients with thyroid peroxidase deficiency. One group, congenitally hypothyroid, presents in early infancy or childhood with mental, growth, and skeletal retardation, and a typical cretinoid appearance. The appearance of goiter is variable, but it usually appears during early childhood. Clinical laboratory findings include a low serum thyroxine, and patients demonstrate a rapid discharge of radioactive iodine, of variable amounts, from the thyroid after oral administration of thiocyanate or perchlorate. This indicates an abnormally large pool of inorganic iodide in the thyroid; this iodide is not organically bound to thyroglobulin, whereas in the normal individual virtually no iodide is dischargeable. Other conditions, such as Hashimoto thyroiditis, or a hyperactive thyroid remnant, may result in a partial perchlorate discharge and must be differentiated by other tests.

Another group of patients have presented with goiter but are clinically and chemically euthyroid. They demonstrate a partial radioactive iodine discharge with perchlorate or thiocyanate administration. These patients usually can be distinguished clinically from the **Deafness-goiter** syndrome by the presence of normal hearing.

**Complications:** Mental and physical retardation due to congenital hypothyroidism.

**Associated Findings:** Occasionally, airway obstruction secondary to a large goiter.

**Etiology:** Usually autosomal recessive inheritance. The genetics of a partial defect, with euthyroid goiter, is unclear; though dominant inheritance has been postulated in some families.

**Pathogenesis:** Thyroid peroxidase, in the presence of the necessary substrates, functions to oxidize inorganic iodide and transfer it to organically bound iodine. Several defects in peroxidase enzymatic activity have been defined. In the first, there is a quantitatively decreased activity that cannot be restored by the addition of hematin, the prosthetic group of the enzyme. This defect has been found among the group of patients with congenital hypothyroidism who also demonstrate complete *in vivo* perchlorate discharge.

A second defect is the peroxidase apoenzyme prosthetic group defect. No in vitro peroxidase activity is present; however, upon the addition of hematin, its prosthetic group, enzymatic activity is partially restored. Thus this defect appears to affect the binding site and thereby the affinity of the apoenzyme for its prosthetic group. These patients demonstrate only partial impairment of organification in vivo. These patients have shown a spectrum of severity; some compensated and euthyroid, and some hypothyroid.

Defects in iodide organification may result from a defect in the peroxidase enzyme. In addition, a defective thyroglobulin molecule, a defective hydrogen peroxide generating system, or abnormal cytoarchitecture may also result in impaired organification. Such defects may be responsible for the organification failure in non-peroxidase-deficient conditions, such as **Deafness-goiter**. In addition, many of the original patients described with organification defects may prove to have a peroxidase enzyme defect or a separate organification defect.

The thyroid microsomal antigen involved in autoimmune thyroid disease is, at least in part, thyroid peroxidase (TPO) (Seto et al, 1987).

**MIM No.:** *27450

**Sex Ratio:** M1:F1 in the congenital hypothyroid group. Among those patients with euthyroid goiter, there is a predominance of females.

**Occurrence:** Unknown.

**Risk of Recurrence for Patient's Sib:**
  See Part I, *Mendelian Inheritance.*

**Risk of Recurrence for Patient's Child:**
  See Part I, *Mendelian Inheritance.*

**Age of Detectability:** Clinically, symptoms of hypothryoidism are usually apparent during early infancy. Goiter may be present in infancy, but usually is not apparent until childhood. Serum thyroxine or TSH screening may detect hypothyroidism at birth.

**Gene Mapping and Linkage:** TPO (thyroid peroxidase) has been mapped to 2pter-p12.

**Prevention:** None known. Genetic counseling indicated.

**Treatment:** Early treatment with thyroid replacement if hypothyroid, and to reduce size of the goiter. Educational programs for problems of mental retardation.

**Prognosis:** Good in euthyroid goiter. Poor for mental development in congenital hypothyroidism, unless treated in early infancy.

**Detection of Carrier:** Unknown.

**References:**
Seto P, et al.: Isolation of a complementary DNA clone for thyroid microsomal antigen. J Clin Invest 1987; 80:1205–1208.
Dumont JE, et al.: Thyroid disorders. In: Scriver CR, et al, eds: The metabolic basis of inherited disease, 6th ed. New York: McGraw-Hill, 1989:1843–1880. *
New England Congenital Hypothyroidism Collaborative: Elementary school performance of children with congenital hypothyroidism. J Pediatr 1990; 116:27–32.

SC016                                                    **R. Neil Schimke**

## THYROID, THYROGLOBULIN DEFECTS      3061

**Includes:**

Goiter, congenital
Goitrous hypothyroidism
Hypothyroidism, congenital
Thyroglobulin, absent
Thyroglobulin synthesis, defect in
Thyroid hormonogenesis, genetic defect in, V

**Excludes:**

**Deafness-goiter** (0249)
**Thyroid, dysgenesis** (0946)
Thyroid dyshormonogenesis (other)
Thyroid organification defects

**Major Diagnostic Criteria:** Congenital primary hypothyroidism or compensated primary hypothyroidism with a normal thyroid scan; increased radioiodine uptake; absent or abnormal thyroglobulin by thyroid biopsy.

**Clinical Findings:** Infants are usually detected by thyroid screening with a low-normal or low thyroxine (T4) level and elevated serum TSH. A thyroid scan with [123]I or technetium reveals a normal or enlarged thyroid gland. A serum thyroglobulin measurement by radioimmunoassay may show a low or absent level. A perchlorate discharge test usually will be negative but can be positive in patients with a thyroglobulin defect. Infants are usually treated with T4 until ages 2–3 years or later, when a definitive workup to define the defect can be conducted off T4 replacement with no risk to brain development. If untreated, these infants develop growth retardation, a cretinoid appearance, delayed skeletal growth and maturation, and mental retardation.

Definitive characterization of the defect requires thyroid radioiodine uptake studies to document increased uptake and turnover of radioiodine, testing for labeled monoiodotyrosine (MIT) and diodotyrosine (DIT) in urine to exclude a thyroid iodotyrosine deiodinase defect, a perchlorate discharge test to exclude a peroxidase system defect, and thyroid biopsy. Histologic examination reveals hyperplasia with decreased or absent colloid and decreased or absent thyroglobulin by immunohistochemistry studies. Labeled aminoacid incorporation studies of thyroid tissue *in vitro* show little or no thyroglobulin. Measurements of thyroglobulin mRNA will help to resolve the level of the defect. A labeled cDNA probe can be used to test for the presence of the thyroglobulin gene.

**Complications:** Mental and physical retardation due to congenital hypothyroidism.

**Associated Findings:** If untreated, large goiter.

**Etiology:** Defects associated with both autosomal dominant and autosomal recessive inheritance have been identified.

**Pathogenesis:** The thyroid gland synthesizes thyroglobulin (TG) as substrate for iodothyronine (T4 and T3) biosynthesis. Thyroglobulin, which provides the tyrosyl residues for iodotyrosine synthesis, is an iodinated glycoprotein with a molecular weight approximating 660,000 daltons and a sedimentation coefficient of 19.4 (19S). It is composed of two 12S subunits each of which is comprised of two to four peptide chains. The predominant protein in thyroid colloid is 19S TG, and the thyroid gland normally contains 50–100 mg TG for every 1g of gland. MIT, DIT, T3 and T4 are present within TG as iodoaminoacyl residues that can be cleaved by proteolytic enzymes. The tyrosyl residues, which are the iodine acceptors of TG, comprise about three percent of the weight of the protein, and about two-thirds of these are spatially oriented to be susceptible to iodination. Synthesis of T4 and T3 does not occur in the absence of thyroglobulin synthesis, and, if the thyroglobulin molecule is abnormal in structure, MIT and DIT might not be spatially oriented for coupling.

Thyroglobulin synthesis could be deficient due to a gene deletion, a gene defect leading to defective transcription, a post-transcription translation defect, or production of an abnormal thyroglobulin. Patients have been reported with reduced or absent thyroglobulin, low molecular weight thyroglobulin, a thyroglobulin-like protein that was incompletely glycosylated, a thyro-

globulin that was resistant to iodination, and an abnormal intracellular transport of thyroglobulin into the colloid space. These patients often secrete other iodinated proteins into blood (such as iodoalbumin) and excrete iodinated aminoacids (iodohistidine) in urine.

**MIM No.:** *18845, 27490

**Sex Ratio:** M1:F1

**Occurrence:** Undetermined but presumed rare.

**Risk of Recurrence for Patient's Sib:**
See Part I, *Mendelian Inheritance.*

**Risk of Recurrence for Patient's Child:**
See Part I, *Mendelian Inheritance.*

**Age of Detectability:** At birth, by elevated TSH level.

**Gene Mapping and Linkage:** TG (thyroglobulin) has been mapped to 8q24.

**Prevention:** None known. Genetic counseling indicated.

**Treatment:** Early treatment with thyroid replacement, if hypothyroid, to reduce size of the goiter. Educational programs for problems of mental retardation.

**Prognosis:** Good if treated in early infancy.

**Detection of Carrier:** Unknown.

**References:**

Desai KB, et al.: Familial goiter with absence of thyroglobulin and synthesis of thyroid hormones from thyroidal albumin. J Endocrinol 1974; 60:389–397.
Monaco F, et al.: Isolation and characterization soluble and particulate thyroid iodoproteins in human congenital goiter. Horm Res 1974; 5:141–155.
Lissitzky S, et al.: Defective thyroglobulin export as a cause of congenital goiter. Clin Endocrinol 1975; 4:363–392.
Dinsart C, et al.: Thyroglobulin complimentary DNA as a means to investigate congenital goiters with impaired thyroglobulin synthesis. Ann Endocrinol 1979; 39:133 only.
Silva JE, et al.: Low molecular weight thyroglobulin leading to a goiter in a 12 year old girl. J Clin Endocrinol Metab 1984; 58:526–534.
Dumont JE, et al.: Thyroid disorders. In: Scriver CR, et al, eds: The metabolic basis of inherited disease, 6th ed. New York: McGraw-Hill, 1989:1843–1880. *

FI017                             **Delbert A. Fisher**

**Thyroid-stimulating hormone, resistance to**
*See THYROTROPIN UNRESPONSIVENESS*
**Thyroidal deiodination deficiency**
*See THYROID, IODOTYROSINE DEIODINASE DEFICIENCY*

## THYROTOXICOSIS      3230

**Includes:**

Graves disease
Hyperthyroidism

**Excludes:**

Euthyroid hyperthyroxinemia
HCG-related hyperthyroidism
Hyperthyroidism as part of Hashimoto disease
Iatrogenic hyperthyroidism
Jod-Basedow disease
Pituitary resistance to thyroxine, selective
Toxic adenoma
Toxic multinodular goiter (some)
TSH-producing tumor with hyperthyroidism

**Major Diagnostic Criteria:** Elevated serum levels of T4 and T3, and elevated radioiodine uptake in the thyroid, along with depressed serum TSH level. Thyroid enlargement is generally but not invariably present, particularly in the elderly. Symptoms vary.

**Clinical Findings:** The classic clinical picture consists of hyperactivity, nervousness, and tremor in a patient with a smooth, symmetrically enlarged thyroid gland. The patient is often hyperreflexic, irritable, and has lost weight despite a voracious appetite.

Heat intolerance and increased sweating may be evident as well. Graves ophthalmopathy, onycholysis and pretibial myxedema may be present, or may occur in the absence of clinical thyrotoxicosis. The typical laboratory findings are elevated serum levels of T4 and T3, and elevated radioiodine uptake in the thyroid, along with depressed serum TSH level. Severe, untreated Graves disease may eventuate in thyroid storm with extreme muscle weakness, hyperpyrexia, and cardiovascular collapse. The ophthalmopathy usually accompanies the hyperthyroid state, but there is no correlation regarding relative severity. Moreover, the ocular changes may preceed overt thyrotoxicosis, or even occur many years after the thyroid has been successfully treated.

**Complications:** Untreated disease may result in extreme cachexia secondard to the hypermetabolic state and gastrointestinal hypermotility. High output heart failure may occur. Menstrual irregularities may be present. In young children, growth may be impaired. Enlargement of extraocular muscles, when ophthalmopathy is present, results in restrictive strabismus, and crowding of structures in the orbit may lead to compressive optic neuropathy.

**Associated Findings:** Other autoimmune endocrine diseases may preceed, occur with, or succeed Graves disease, the most common being **Diabetes mellitus** and idiopathic autoimmune Addison disease. Associated conditions also include myasthenia gravis, pernicious anemia and, periodic paralysis (the latter being reported most commonly in Japanese patients).

**Etiology:** Multifactorial inheritance pattern.

**Pathogenesis:** Graves disease is the prototype of an autoimmune disease. The thyrotoxicosis is secondary to circulating thyroid stimulating immunoglobulins (TSI) that arise presumably because of some defect in immune surveillance. There is an association with HLA antigens, particularly B8 and D3 in North America and Europe. In Japan, the association is with B35/D12. As with other autoimmune diseases, the consensus is that multilocus genetic factors interact with some environmental component, probably viral, to produce the disease. Graves disease may be etiologically heterogenous. The ophthalmopathy is likely related to crossreactivity of the TSI with some component of the extra ocular muscles, possibly the acetylcholine receptor.

**MIM No.:** 27500

**Sex Ratio:** M1:F5

**Occurrence:** 30–50:100,000 in females, 6–8:100,000 in males. The lifetime risk is about 5% for females and 1% for males.

**Risk of Recurrence for Patient's Sib:** Average risk about 5%. If a female relative is HLA identical with an affected individual, this risk is probably about 15%. The risk for male sibs is correspondingly lower.

**Risk of Recurrence for Patient's Child:** Unknown. Probably about the same as sibling risk overall, although impressive pedigrees consistent with sex-influenced autosomal dominant patterns have been reported. These may be due to reporting bias in conjunction with a common disease. Neonatal Graves disease is due to transplacental passage of TSI (pseudodominant inheritance).

**Age of Detectability:** At any point over the lifetime.

**Gene Mapping and Linkage:** Unknown.

**Prevention:** None known. Genetic counseling indicated.

**Treatment:** Oral thionamides, radioactive iodine, and thyroidectomy are all appropriate treatment modalities. Steroids may be useful in early ophthalmopathy. Radiation therapy or decompression of the orbit surgically may be necessary if compressive neuropathy occurs.

**Prognosis:** Excellent for thyroid disease. Not predictible insofar as ocular complications are concerned.

**Detection of Carrier:** Unknown.

**References:**
Adams DD, et al.: On the nature of the genes influencing the prevalence of Graves' disease. Life Sci 1983; 31:3–13.
Brennan MD, Gorman C: Thyroid dysfunction and ophthalmopathy.

In: Gorman CA, et al, eds: The eye and orbit in thyroid disease. New York: Raven Press, 1984:49–58.
Solomon DH: Treatment of Graves' hyperthyroidism. In: Ingbar SH, Braverman LE, eds: Wermer's the thyroid, 5th ed. Philadelphia: J.B. Lippencott, 1986:987–1014.
Utiger RD: Treatment of Graves' ophthalmopathy. New Engl J Med 1989; 321:1403–1405.

SC016                                                                    **R. Neil Schimke**

---

## THYROTROPIN DEFICIENCY, ISOLATED                    0949

**Includes:**
> Hypothalamic hypothyroidism
> Isolated TSH deficiency
> Pituitary cretinism
> Thyrotropin, biologically inactive

**Excludes:**
> **Cretinism, endemic** (3167)
> Cretinism, sporadic nonendemic
> **Dwarfism, panhypopituitary** (0303)
> **Immunodeficiency, thymic agenesis** (0943)
> **Parathormone resistance** (0830)
> **Thyroid, dysgenesis** (0946)

**Major Diagnostic Criteria:** Documentation of low circulating thyroid-stimulating hormone (TSH) and thyroxine concentrations. An isolated TSH deficiency is often a component of pseudohypoparathyroidism (see **Parathormone resistance**), and proper genetic counseling requires exclusion of this latter disorder.

**Clinical Findings:** The severity of (TSH) deficiency and secondary hypothyroidism varies; but in most cases the symptoms are mild, and the diagnosis is not made until adulthood. The symptoms are usually vague and not suggestive of thyroid disease, i.e. dizziness, weakness, constipation, angina pectoris, and so on. Severely affected individuals may rarely manifesting mental retardation, hypometabolism, dry puffy skin, husky voice, and delayed dental and skeletal maturation have been described. The diagnosis is established by confirming both low serum TSH and thyroxine levels.

**Complications:** Dependent upon severity of secondary hypothyroidism. Untreated severe disease will lead to profound mental and physical retardation.

**Associated Findings:** None known.

**Etiology:** Almost all cases have been sporadic, but there have been at least two pairs of female sibs reported from a consanguineous mating, which suggests autosomal recessive inheritance.

**Pathogenesis:** Various defects in the hypothalamic-pituitary axis have been postulated, and both hypothalamic and pituitary primary defects probably exist.

**MIM No.:** 27510

**Sex Ratio:** M1:F1

**Occurrence:** More than a dozen cases have been reported; many of them Japanese.

**Risk of Recurrence for Patient's Sib:**
> See Part I, *Mendelian Inheritance.*

**Risk of Recurrence for Patient's Child:**
> See Part I, *Mendelian Inheritance.*

**Age of Detectability:** Although usually not suspected until adulthood, the condition may be diagnosed at birth.

**Gene Mapping and Linkage:** Unknown.

**Prevention:** None known. Genetic counseling indicated.

**Treatment:** Replacement therapy with thyroxine.

**Prognosis:** Depends on severity of secondary hypothyroidism.

**Detection of Carrier:** Unknown.

**References:**
Odell WD: Isolated deficiencies of anterior pituitary hormones, symptoms and diagnosis. J Am Med Assoc 1966; 197:1006–1016.

Miyai D, et al.: Familial isolated thyrotropin deficiency with cretinism. New Engl J Med 1971; 285:1043–1048.

Rimoin DL, Schimke RN: Genetic disorders of the endocrine glands. St. Louis: C.V. Mosby, 1971:11–65.

Kohno H, et al.: Pituitary cretinism in two sisters. Arch Dis Child 1980; 55:725–727.

H0033 **William A. Horton**
H0025 **O.J. Hood**

## Thyrotropin secretion, inappropriate
*See THYROID, HORMONE RESISTANCE*

---

## THYROTROPIN UNRESPONSIVENESS 0948

**Includes:**

Hypothyroidism, congenital
Thyroid-stimulating hormone, resistance to
TSH resistance

**Excludes:**

**Thyroid, dysgenesis** (0946)
Thyroid dyshormonogenesis, other
**Thyrotropin deficiency, isolated** (0949)

**Major Diagnostic Criteria:** Congenital hypothyroidism with an elevated serum thyroid-stimulating hormone (TSH), a normal-sized thyroid, normal radiodine (RAI) uptake, and lack of response to exogenous thyrotropin administration.

**Clinical Findings:** Mental and growth retardation and other typical stigmata of congenital hypothyroidism. The thyroid gland is of normal size. Clinical laboratory findings include low serum thyroxine, markedly elevated serum TSH, and normal baseline RAI uptake. Administration of exogenous TSH does not increase serum thyroxine, RAI uptake, or glandular size. *In vitro* study of thyroid slices reveal no stimulation with the addition of TSH.

**Complications:** Congenital hypothyroidism, with accompanying mental and growth retardation.

**Associated Findings:** None known.

**Etiology:** Possibly autosomal recessive inheritance.

**Pathogenesis:** Thyrotropin has multiple effects on the thyroid, including stimulating cell division and thyroglobulin synthesis. An altered thyrotropin receptor site, or a defect in a subsequent step, such as a second messenger system, may be responsible for this disorder.

**MIM No.:** 27520

**Sex Ratio:** Presumably M1:F1.

**Occurrence:** About a dozen cases have been reported.

**Risk of Recurrence for Patient's Sib:**
See Part I, *Mendelian Inheritance*.

**Risk of Recurrence for Patient's Child:**
See Part I, *Mendelian Inheritance*.

**Age of Detectability:** Clinically, symptoms of congenital hypothyroidism are usually apparent during the first one-half year of life. Newborn serum thyroxine or TSH screening may suggest the disorder at birth. Complete delineation requires *in vitro* study.

**Gene Mapping and Linkage:** TSHR (thyroid stimulating hormone receptor) has been provisionally mapped to 22q11-q13.

**Prevention:** None known. Genetic counseling indicated.

**Treatment:** Early thyroxine replacement. Educational programs for problems of mental retardation.

**Prognosis:** Poor for mental and physical development if not treated early; however, this may be improved with early detection and therapy.

**Detection of Carrier:** Unknown.

**References:**
Dumont JE, et al.: Thyroid disorders. In: Scriver CR, et al, eds: The metabolic basis of inherited disease, 6th ed. New York: McGraw-Hill, 1989:1843–1880.

SC016 **R. Neil Schimke**

## Thyrotropin, biologically inactive
*See THYROTROPIN DEFICIENCY, ISOLATED*
## Thyroxine-binding capacity of serum, increase or decrease
*See THYROXINE-BINDING GLOBULIN DEFECTS*
## Thyroxine-binding globulin (TBG) of serum
*See THYROXINE-BINDING GLOBULIN DEFECTS*

---

## THYROXINE-BINDING GLOBULIN DEFECTS 0950

**Includes:**

Thyroxine-binding capacity of serum, increase or decrease
Thyroxine-binding globulin (TBG) of serum

**Excludes:**

Thyroxine-binding capacity of serum, acquired variation
Thyroxine-binding capacity of serum, chemically indiced variation

**Major Diagnostic Criteria:** Persistent high or low levels of thyroxine-binding globulin (TBG) or serum thyroxine in the absence of drug administration, and demonstration of a familial pattern.

**Clinical Findings:** No clinical disease or associated congenital abnormality has been observed in patients with familial excess or deficiency of TBG. The abnormalities produce either an increase or decrease in serum thyroid hormone concentrations and alter the pool sizes and half-time of disappearance of radioiodine-labeled thyroid hormones in the extrathyroidal pools. The rates of peripheral utilization of thyroid hormones, however, are normal. Normal circulating concentrations of TBG range from about 2–5 mg/dl; values of 2–9 mg/dl are seen in the newborn. Normal serum thyroxine (T4 concentrations range from 4.5 to 12.5 µg/dl; values in the newborn are 7–17 µg/dl. Patients with absent TBG have T4 levels in the hypothyroid range without evidence of hypothyroidism. Patients with low levels of TBG have low or low-normal TBG levels with low or low-normal serum T4 concentrations. TBG levels in adult patients with increased TBG range from 5 to 10 mg/dl, and T4 values from 13 to 25 µg/dl. Serum TSH values are normal.

At least six variants have been described: including TBG-A found in 40% of Australian aborigines; TBG-S found in Blacks, Eskimos, Melanesians, Polynesians, and Indonesians, but not in Caucasians; and the TBG-Gary; TBG-Quebec; TBG-Montreal; and the heat-stable TBG-Chicago (Murata et al, 1986; Takamatsu and Refetoff, 1986).

**Complications:** Unknown.

**Associated Findings:** Retarded mental and motor development has been reported.

**Etiology:** Presumably X-linked dominant or codominant inheritance of a biochemical defect, although autosomal dominant inheritance has been reported. The defect probably represent mutations at a single X-linked locus.

**Pathogenesis:** TBG, like glucose-6-phosphate dehydrogenase (see **Glucose-6-phosphate dehydrogenase deficiency**), is subject to both genetically determined increases and decreases in its concentration. The genetic defect presumably results in abnormal binding of T4 with or without alteration in the rate of hepatic TBG synthesis. Thorson et al (1966) presented evidence for two thyroid-binding globulins, thus creating the potential for heterogeneity in both high and low TBG.

**MIM No.:** *31420, *18860

**Sex Ratio:** While a sex-linked condition, intermediate TBG levels are seen in females.

**Occurrence:** At least 1:5,000 births (1:2,800 males). TBG excess is the rarer condition, with only a dozen or so kinships reported.

**Risk of Recurrence for Patient's Sib:**
See Part I, *Mendelian Inheritance.*

**Risk of Recurrence for Patient's Child:**
See Part I, *Mendelian Inheritance.*

**Age of Detectability:** For absent TBG: at birth by measuring serum thyroxine or TBG-binding capacity. For decreased or increased TBG: at one month by measuring serum thyroxine or TBG-binding capacity.

**Gene Mapping and Linkage:** TBG (thyroxin binding globulin) has been mapped to Xq21-q22.

**Prevention:** None known. Genetic counseling indicated.

**Treatment:** Early recognition is important in order to prevent unnecessary treatment for hypothyroidism.

**Prognosis:** Normal life span.

**Detection of Carrier:** By reduced levels of TBG or serum thyroxine.

**References:**

Thorson SC, et al.: Evidence for the existence of two thyroxine-binding globulin moieties. J Clin Endocr 1966; 26:181–188.

Rivas ML, et al.: Genetic variants of thyroxine-binding globulin (TBG). BD:OAS VII(6). New York: March of Dimes Birth Defects Foundation, 1971:34–41.

Hodgson SF, Wahner HW: Hereditary increased thyroxin binding globulin capacity. Proc Mayo Clinic 1972; 47:720–724.

Refetoff S, et al.: Study of four new kindreds with inherited thyroxine-binding globulin abnormalities. J Clin Invest 1972; 51:848–867.

Bigazzi M, et al.: Inherited X-chromosome linked thyroxin binding gloubin deficiency in a homozygous female. J Endocr Invest 1980; 4:349–352.

Grimald S, et al.: Polymorphism of human thyroxin-binding globulin. J Clin Endocr Metab 1983; 57:1186–1192.

Murata Y, et al.: Inherited abnormality of thyroxin-binding globulin with no demonstrable thyroxin-binding activity and high serum levels of denatured thyroxin-binding globulin. New Engl J Med 1986; 314:694–699.

Takamatsu J, Refetoff S: Inherited heat-stable variant thyroxin-binding globulin (TBG-Chicago). J Clin Endocr Metab 1986; 63:1140–1144.

Jenkins MB, Steffes MW: Congenital thyroxin binding globulin deficiency: incidence and inheritance. Hum Genet 1987; 77:80–84.

FI017                                       **Delbert A. Fisher**

**Tibia, absence of, with polydactyly**
*See MESOMELIC DYSPLASIA, WERNER TYPE*
**Tibia, bilateral aplasia of with polydactyly and absent thumbs**
*See MESOMELIC DYSPLASIA, WERNER TYPE*
**Tibia, hypoplasia of, with polydactyly**
*See MESOMELIC DYSPLASIA, WERNER TYPE*
**Tibial aplasia**
*See TIBIAL APLASIA/HYPOPLASIA*

## TIBIAL APLASIA/HYPOPLASIA         2387

**Includes:**
    Tibial aplasia
    Tibial hemimelia
    Tibial hypoplasia

**Excludes:**
    **Mesomelic dysplasia, Werner type** (0649)
    **Mesomelic dysplasia** (other)
    Tibial hemimelia-fibular and ulnar dimelia
    Tibial hemimelia-fibular dimelia-mirror feet (diplopodia)
    **Tibial hypoplasia/aplasia-ectrodactyly** (2388)

**Major Diagnostic Criteria:** Abnormalities limited to unilateral or bilateral tibial hypoplasia/aplasia with or without hypoplasia/aplasia of preaxial bones of the foot.

**Clinical Findings:** Isolated tibial hemimelia is characterized in X-rays by unilateral or bilateral tibial hypoplasia or aplasia with or without preaxial hypoplasia or aplasia of bones of the feet. Affected individuals do not have other skeletal or nonskeletal

abnormalities. Delayed and difficult ambulation and short stature are the primary clinical problems.

**Complications:** Clubfoot, fibular dislocation, fibular curving, and fibular hypertrophy or hyperplasia.

**Associated Findings:** None known.

**Etiology:** Both autosomal dominant and autosomal recessive inheritance, as well as sporadic cases, have been identified.

**Pathogenesis:** Unknown.

**MIM No.:** 27522

**CDC No.:** 755.365

**Sex Ratio:** M1:F1

**Occurrence:** Undetermined but presumed rare.

**Risk of Recurrence for Patient's Sib:**
See Part I, *Mendelian Inheritance.*

**Risk of Recurrence for Patient's Child:**
See Part I, *Mendelian Inheritance.*

**Age of Detectability:** At birth. Prenatal diagnosis may be possible by ultrasound.

**Gene Mapping and Linkage:** Unknown.

**Prevention:** None known. Genetic counseling indicated.

**Treatment:** Orthopedic devices, surgery, and rehabilitation.

**Prognosis:** Good, with adjustment to physical disability.

**Detection of Carrier:** Unknown.

**Special Considerations:** Tibial hypoplasia and tibial aplasia (agenesis) are separated clinically by X-ray findings, but a radiolucent cartilaginous tibial anlage may later ossify or may be detected at surgery. The presence or absence of any tibia may influence the choice of orthopedic surgery and devices and determine the ultimate form and function of the affected limb.

Tibial hemimelia may be the only manifestation of **Tibial hypoplasia/aplasia-ectrodactyly**, or may represent a separate entity.

Most cases of isolated tibial hemimelia are sporadic, but there are families with both vertical and horizontal transmission. Unaffected parents have had multiple children with isolated tibial hemimelia that has subsequently segregated as an autosomal dominant suggesting germinal mosaicism. There is no method of identifying the isolated case as autosomal dominant, autosomal recessive, or sporadic.

**References:**

Clark MW: Autosomal dominant inheritance of tibial meromelia: report of a kindred. J Bone Joint Surg 1975; 57A:262–264. †

Jones D, et al.: Congenital aplasia and dysplasia of the tibia with intact fibula: classification and management. J Bone Joint Surg 1978; 60B:31–39. †

Schroer RJ, Meyer LC: Autosomal dominant tibial hypoplasia-aplasia. Proc Greenwood Genet Center 1983; 2:27–31. * †

McKay M, et al.: Isolated tibial hemimelia in sibs: an autosomal-recessive disorder? Am J Med Genet 1984; 17:603–607. * †

Richieri-Costa A: Tibial hemimelia-cleft lip/palate in a Brazilian child born to consanguineous parents. Am J Med Genet 1987; 28:325–329. †

SC053                                     **Richard J. Schroer**

**Tibial aplasia/hypoplasia-ectrodactyly**
*See TIBIAL HYPOPLASIA/APLASIA-ECTRODACTYLY*
**Tibial hemimelia**
*See TIBIAL APLASIA/HYPOPLASIA*
**Tibial hemimelia-split hand/split foot**
*See TIBIAL HYPOPLASIA/APLASIA-ECTRODACTYLY*
**Tibial hypoplasia**
*See TIBIAL APLASIA/HYPOPLASIA*

## TIBIAL HYPOPLASIA/APLASIA-ECTRODACTYLY    2388

**Includes:**
    Ectrodactyly-tibial hemimelia
    Gollop-Wolfgang syndrome
    Hypoplasia/aplasia of tibia and/or ulna with split-hand/split
      foot
    Tibial aplasia/hypoplasia-ectrodactyly
    Tibial hemimelia-split hand/split foot

**Excludes:**
    **Ectrodactyly** (0336)
    **Ectrodactyly-ectodermal dysplasia-clefting syndrome** (0337)
    **Limb and scalp defects, Adams-Oliver type** (0459)
    **Tibial aplasia/hypoplasia** (2387)

**Major Diagnostic Criteria:** Split hand/split foot and tibial or ulnar hypoplasia/aplasia.

**Clinical Findings:** Split hand/split foot and long bone hypoplasia/ aplasia are associated in the same individual or members of the same family. The split hand may be severe or isolated 3–4 syndactyly. Tibial and ulnar are the most common long bone deficiencies. The tibial (preaxial) deficiency may be isolated hypoplasia of the hallux. More severe limb deficiencies, peromelia and transverse hemimelia, have been reported.

**Complications:** Dislocations and contractures of knees and elbows; club foot.

**Associated Findings: Polydactyly**, distal hypoplasia, duplication or bifurcation of femur, and hypoplasia of patella.

**Etiology:** Autosomal dominant and autosomal recessive inheritance have been reported.

**Pathogenesis:** Unknown.

**MIM No.:** *18360

**POS No.:** 3974

**CDC No.:** 755.250, 755.365, 755.350

**Sex Ratio:** M1:F1

**Occurrence:** Undetermined but presumed rare.

**Risk of Recurrence for Patient's Sib:**
    See Part I, *Mendelian Inheritance.*

**Risk of Recurrence for Patient's Child:**
    See Part I, *Mendelian Inheritance.*

**Age of Detectability:** At birth.

**Gene Mapping and Linkage:** Unknown.

**Prevention:** None known. Genetic counseling indicated.

**Treatment:** Orthopedic devices, surgery, and rehabilitation.

**Prognosis:** Good, with adjustment to physical disability.

**Detection of Carrier:** Unknown.

**Special Considerations:** The majority of familial cases of split-hand/split-foot and tibial and/or ulnar deficiency are consistent with autosomal dominant inheritance. Nonpenetrance and variable expressivity including isolated syndactyly or isolated hypoplastic great toes have been reported. Tibial deficiency and ulnar deficiencies have been reported both separately and together in different families. Autosomal recessive inheritance, suggested by affected children of normal parents, is questionable because of the marked variability of expression, including nonpenetrance of the autosomal dominant variety. Split-hand/split-foot with long bone aplasia may be a severe manifestation of isolated split-hand/split-foot, or may represent one or more etiologically separate entities.

**References:**
Temtamy S, McKusick V: The genetics of hand malformations. New York: Alan R. Liss Inc, 1978:53–71. †
Bujdoso G, Lenz W: Monodactylous splithand-splitfoot: a malformation occurring in three distinct genetic types. Eur J Pediatr 1980; 133:207–215. †
Majewski F, et al.: Aplasia of tibia with split-hand/split-foot deformity:

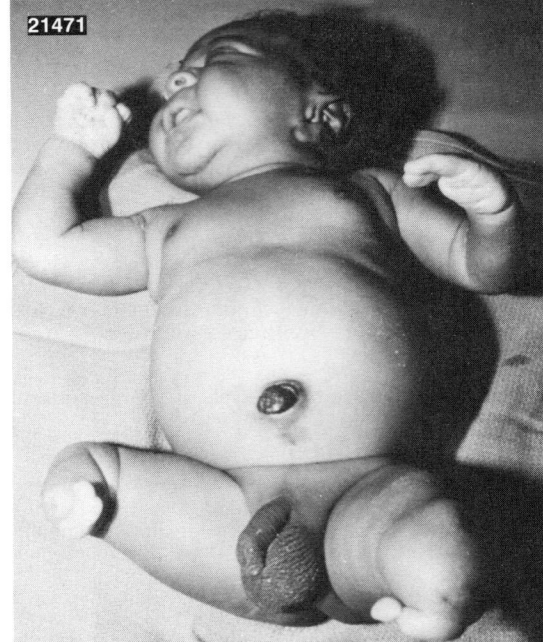

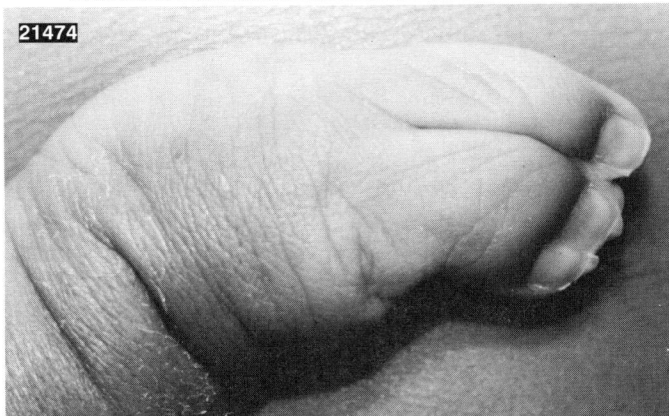

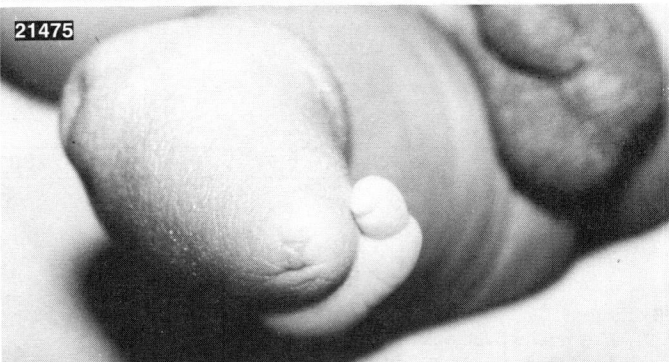

**2388A-21471:** Normal head and trunk measurements with normal external genitalia. There are severe limb reduction defects with a hypoplastic left forearm. **21474:** There are three digits on the left hand with syndactyly. **21475:** Note the skin dimples, malformed digits and hypoplastic distal segment of the right leg.

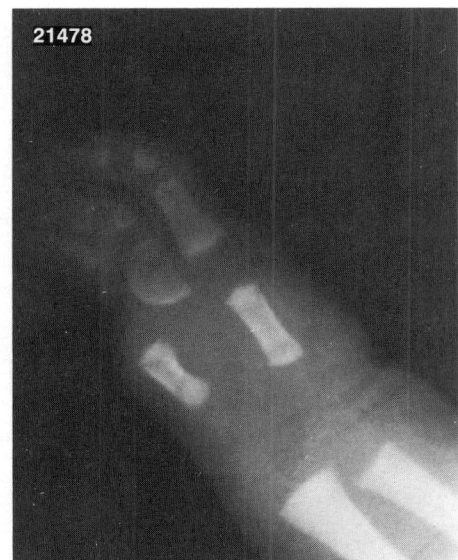

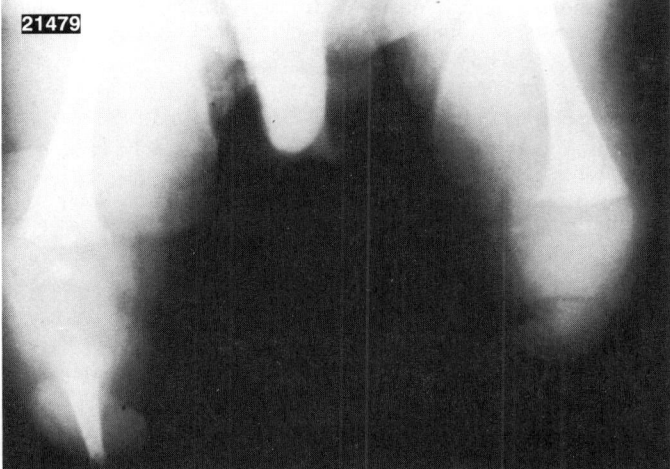

**2388B-21478:** X-ray shows deformity of the left hand with fusion of the proximal phalanges into a block and three digit syndactyly. **21479:** X-ray shows hypoplastic right tibia and aplasia of the left tibia and fibula. The left femoral epiphysis is similarly hypoplastic compared to the right.

report of six families with 35 cases and considerations about variability and penetrance. Hum Genet 1985; 70:136–147. * †

Schroer RJ: Split-hand/split-foot. Proc Greenwood Genet Center 1986; 5:65–75. †

Richieri-Costa A, et al.: Tibial hemimelia: report on 37 new cases, clinical and genetic considerations. Am J Med Genet 1987; 27:867–884. * †

SC053

**Richard J. Schroer**

**Tick-borne meningopolyneuritis.**
See FETAL EFFECTS FROM LYME DISEASE
**Tics, multiple motor and vocal**
See TOURETTE SYNDROME
**Tight skin contracture syndrome**
See RESTRICTIVE DERMATOPATHY
**TKCR syndrome**
See CERVICO-DERMO-GU SYNDROME, GOEMINNE TYPE
**Tobramycin, fetal effects**
See FETAL AMINOGLYCOSIDE OTOTOXICITY

**Tobrex△, fetal effects**
See FETAL AMINOGLYCOSIDE OTOTOXICITY
**Toe, recurring fibroma**
See DIGITAL FIBROMA, RECURRING IN INFANTS & CHILDREN
**Toes, polysyndactyly-Hirschsprung disease-cardiac defect**
See HIRSCHSPRUNG DISEASE-CARDIAC DEFECT
**Tomaculous neuropathy**
See NEUROPATHY, HEREDITARY WITH PRESSURE PALSIES
**Tomato tumor**
See SCALP, CYLINDROMAS
**Tongue curling**
See TONGUE, FOLDING OR ROLLING
**Tongue gigantism**
See MACROGLOSSIA

---

### TONGUE, ANKYLOGLOSSIA 0061

**Includes:**
   Ankyloglossia
   Tongue-tie
   Tongue, pseudocleft

**Excludes:**
   **Hypoglossia-hypodactylia** (0451)
   Palatoglossal adhesion

**Major Diagnostic Criteria:** Tongue movement is restricted so that with the mouth opened to its fullest extent, effort to raise the tongue tip fails to bring it above the level of a line between the commissures of the mouth. Upon forward protrusive effort the tip of the tongue demonstrates a central groove.

**Clinical Findings:** A variation of the lingual frenum resulting in an elevated and short band-like structure adherent at a higher than normal position of attachment on the alveolar ridge behind the central incisors causing a restriction of elevation and protrusion of tongue.

**Complications:** Some varieties may produce spacing of mandibular central incisors, periodontal disease, and some limitations in cleansing excursions of the tongue. There is no interference with infant nursing or later masticatory functions. If any disorder in speech is produced by ankyloglossia, it is extremely minor.

**Associated Findings:** None known.

**Etiology:** Possibly autosomal dominant inheritance.

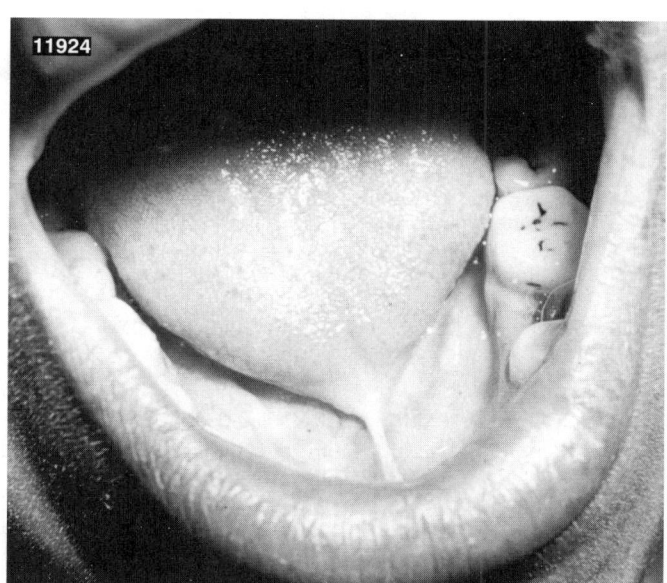

**0061-11924:** Ankyloglossia.

**Pathogenesis:** A developmental variation in the lingual frenum of the tongue such that the fibrous band of the midline raphe of the tongue, which anteriorly forms the lingual frenum, attaches anteriorly to tongue tip and high onto the alveolar process.

**MIM No.:** 10628

**CDC No.:** 750.000

**Sex Ratio:** M1:F1

**Occurrence:** Estimated at 1:330. Familial cases reported in the Dutch and German literature.

**Risk of Recurrence for Patient's Sib:** Unknown.

**Risk of Recurrence for Patient's Child:** Unknown.

**Age of Detectability:** At birth.

**Gene Mapping and Linkage:** Unknown.

**Prevention:** None known. Genetic counseling indicated.

**Treatment:** A decision for surgical release should be based upon associated dental disorders or dental prosthetic needs. The speech benefits of a release procedure should not be overestimated since they are probably insignificant. However, affected musical wind instrument players may benefit from surgical release.

**Prognosis:** Excellent.

**Detection of Carrier:** Unknown.

**References:**

McEnery ET, Gaines FP: Tongue-tie in infants and children. J Pediatr 1941; 18:252.

Stucke K: Zur frage der verkürzung der zungenbänochens. Aertgl Wschr 1946; 1:259.

Keizer D: Dominant erfeljik ankyloglosson. Ned Tijdschr Geneeskd 1952; 96:2203–2205.

Wilson RA, et al.: Ankyloglossia superior: palatoglossal adhesion in the newborn infant. Pediatrics 1963; 31:1051.

Witkop CJ Jr, Barros L: Oral and genetic studies of Chileans, 1960. I. Oral anomalies Am J Phys Anthropol 1963; 21:15.

Block JR: The role of the speech clinician in determining indications for frenulotomy in cases of ankyloglossia. NY State Dent J 1968; 34:479.

Young EC, et al.: Examining for tongue-tie. Clin Pediatr 1979; 18:298.

Nevin NC, et al.: Ankyloglossum superious syndrome. J Oral Surg 1980; 50:254.

HA067            **James R. Hayward**

**Tongue, bifid**
*See TONGUE, CLEFT*

## TONGUE, CLEFT        0952

**Includes:**
Tongue, bifid
Tongue, trifid

**Excludes:**
Hypoglossia-hypodactylia (0451)
Oro-facio-digital syndrome I (0770)
Tongue, ankyloglossia (0061)
Tongue, pseudocleft

**Major Diagnostic Criteria:** Tongue divided into two or more lobes.

**Clinical Findings:** True cleft of the tongue divides the tongue into two or more lobes, in contrast to pseudocleft tongue in which the body appears to be divided into two lobes due to the pull of a short frenum. Cleft tongue may be part of a continuum of cleft mandible. However, both occur as isolated conditions.

**Complications:** The cleft does not usually interfere with speech unless associated with cleft lip and/or palate.

**Associated Findings:** Cleft lip, cleft palate, cleft mandible, heart defects, polydactyly, cryptorchidism, strabismus, absent hyoid, facial asymmetry, polypoid growth attached to tongue apex, and cervical webbing.

**Etiology:** All reported cases appear to have been sporadic.

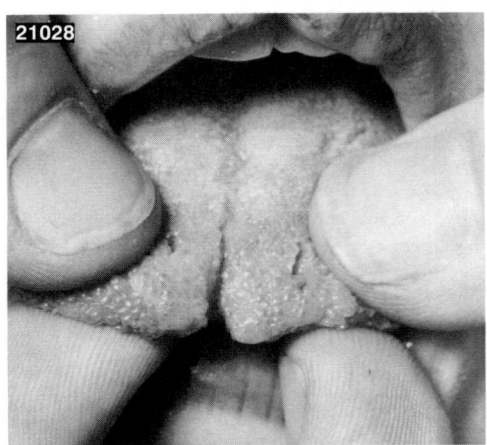

0952-21028: Cleft tongue.

**Pathogenesis:** Failure of fusion during embryogenesis of lateral tongue processes from a defect involving the first branchial arch.

**CDC No.:** 750.140

**Sex Ratio:** M5:F7 (observed).

**Occurrence:** Less than two dozen cases reported.

**Risk of Recurrence for Patient's Sib:** Presumably low, since condition is usually sporadic.

**Risk of Recurrence for Patient's Child:** Presumably low, since condition is usually sporadic.

**Age of Detectability:** At birth.

**Gene Mapping and Linkage:** Unknown.

**Prevention:** None known. Genetic counseling indicated.

**Treatment:** Surgical repair.

**Prognosis:** Isolated cleft tongue does not seem to interfere with longevity. Prognosis appears to be dependent upon associated defects.

**Detection of Carrier:** Unknown.

**References:**

Hubinger HL: Bifid tongue: report of case. J Oral Surg 1952; 10:64–66. †

Gorlin R, et al.: Syndromes of the head and neck, ed 2. New York: McGraw-Hill, 1976:178–179.

WE013          **Bernd Weinberg**

## TONGUE, FISSURED       0953

**Includes:**
Fissured tongue
Lingua fissurata types I, II, and III

**Excludes:**
Tongue, cleft (0952)
Tongue, geographic (0954)
Tongue, plicated (0956)

**Major Diagnostic Criteria:** Multiple fissures on the tongue, other than the normal variation of a single shallow, central fissure at the insertion of the median raphe.

**Clinical Findings:** Many persons have one or two superficial midline fissures which are normal variations of the mucosal insertion of the median raphe of the tongue. Fissured tongue can be of several types arising from a variety of causes:

*Type I*: A deep central furrow, which probably represents a part of a continuum of normal midline raphe on one hand, and cleft tongue at the other.

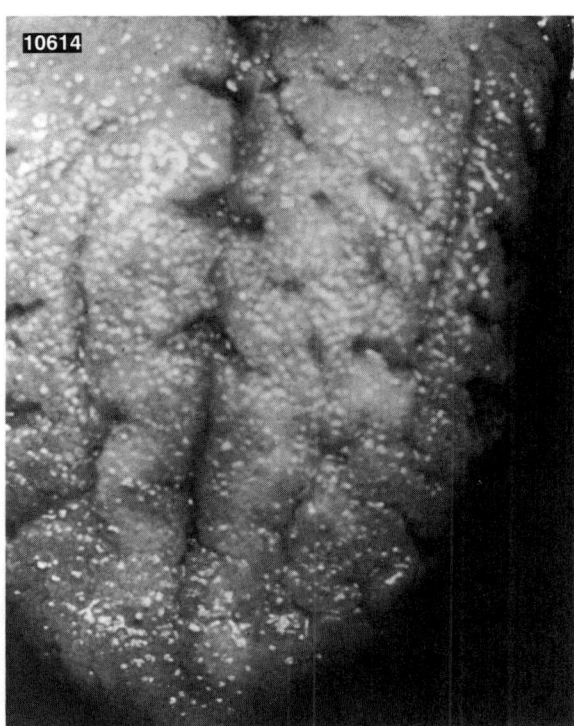

**0953-10614:** Fissured tongue.

*Type II*: Multiple narrow fissures running parallel or obliquely at right angles to the midline raphe.

*Type III*: Deep, broad fissures parallel to the midline raphe in which the lingual papillae are absent and the base has a dense band of connective tissue scar. May be distinguished from **Tongue, plicated** by age and size distribution.

**Complications:** Unknown.

**Associated Findings:** Type III fissures are associated with cleft palate. May be governed by the same gene as **Tongue, geographic** and **Tongue, plicated**.

**Etiology:** Possibly autosomal dominant inheritance. It has been suggested that familial cases may be caused by the same gene responsible for **Tongue, geographic** and **Tongue, plicated**. Some cases may be caused by intrauterine infections.

**Pathogenesis:** *Type I*: Fissures represent incomplete fusion of the lateral halves of the tongue or binding of the mucosa to the central raphe of the tongue.

*Type II*: Unknown, but are probably acquired. When congenital they may be secondary to intrauterine infections, such as syphilis, and when they develop postnatally they are probably associated with a wide variety of infections and malnutrition.

*Type III*: Found in some patients with cleft palate including submucous clefts and is thought to be due to a misplacement of tongue-palatal shelf relationship during palatal development. Normally, initial palatal development takes place such that the palatal shelves grow downward between the lateral borders of the tongue and the cheek, and then snap into a horizontal relationship with each other. These fissures appear to result from the inferior borders (which become the midline margins after snapping into horizontal relationship) of the palatal shelves developing on the surface of the tongue instead of lateral to the tongue borders.

**MIM No.:** 13740

**CDC No.:** 750.180

**Sex Ratio:** M1:F1 in all three types.

**Occurrence:** Prevalence of Types I and II combined is about 1:20 over all age groups. Type III, about 1:10 to 1:8 cases with cleft palate.

**Risk of Recurrence for Patient's Sib:** Unknown.

**Risk of Recurrence for Patient's Child:** Unknown.

**Age of Detectability:** Type III: at birth. Type I and some Type II: from infancy to adulthood, by clinical examination.

**Gene Mapping and Linkage:** Unknown.

**Prevention:** None known. Genetic counseling indicated.

**Treatment:** Unknown.

**Prognosis:** Excellent for life and function.

**Detection of Carrier:** Unknown.

**References:**

Biegert J: Anthropologisch-erbbiologische unterschung der menschlichen zunge. Z Morph Anthrop 1954; 46:371–399. *
Witkop CJ Jr, Barros L: Oral and genetic studies of Chileans, 1960. I. oral anomalies. Am J Phys Anthropol 1963; 21:15–24.
Gorlin RJ: Developmental anomalies of face and oral structures. In: Gorlin RJ, Goldman HM, eds: Thoma's oral pathology, vol. I. 6th ed. St. Louis: C.V. Mosby, 1970:30–95.

WI043                                    **Carl J. Witkop, Jr.**

---

## TONGUE, FOLDING OR ROLLING          0951

**Includes:**
   Cloverleaf tongue
   Tongue curling

**Excludes:  Tongue, ankyloglossia (0061)**

**Major Diagnostic Criteria:** Ability to fold back the tongue or to roll the tongue so as to form a tube.

**Clinical Findings:** Ability to fold the tongue tip back upon itself or to roll or curl the sides of the tongue inward to form a tube. Both movements are performed by the intrinsic muscles of the tongue with no mechanical assistance. The two abilities are independent of each another.

*Cloverleaf tongue*, a possible variant, consists of the ability to fold the tongue in a particular cloverleaf configuration (Whitney, 1950).

**Complications:** Unknown.

**Associated Findings:** None known.

**Etiology:** Undetermined. Some researchers have suggested autosomal dominant inheritance, but other studies have refuted this conclusion.

**Pathogenesis:** Dependent upon genetic characteristics enabling unusual movement of the intrinsic muscles of the tongue.

**MIM No.:** 18930, 12910

**CDC No.:** 750.180

**Sex Ratio:** Presumably M1:F1. The ability to roll the tongue has been found in 63% of males and 66.84% of females. In males, this skill appears to be associated with the ability to move the ears.

**Occurrence:** In a sample of black individuals it was found that 70.79% of males could roll or curl their tongues but not fold it back upon itself, that 2.10% of the males could fold but not roll their tongues, and that 10.27% could both fold and roll their tongues. In the same sample it was found that 65.25% of females could roll but not fold, that 2.44% could fold but not roll, and that 17.26% could both fold and roll their tongues.

In a sample of various groups to determine the ability to roll the tongue, the following percentages were obtained: American whites 65.62, Chinese 62.2, Dutch 65.98, Jewish, 53.33.

**Risk of Recurrence for Patient's Sib:** Unknown.

**Risk of Recurrence for Patient's Child:** Unknown.

**Age of Detectability:** Early childhood.

**Gene Mapping and Linkage:** Unknown.

**Prevention:** N/A

**Treatment:** None required.

**Prognosis:** Normal for life span and intelligence with no known functional disability. No investigations have been made into a possible relationship between this ability and speech function.

**Detection of Carrier:** Unknown.

**References:**

Urbanowski A, Wilson J: Tongue curling. J Hered 1947; 38:365–366.

Hsu TC: Tongue upfolding; a newly reported heritable character in man. J Hered 1948; 39:187–188.

Liu T, Hsu T: Tongue-folding and tongue-rolling in a sample of the Chinese population. J Hered 1949; 40:19–21.

Whitney DD: Clover-leaf tongues. J Hered 1950; 41:176 only.

Lee JW: Tongue-folding and tongue-rolling in an American Negro population sample. J Hered 1955; 46:289–291.

Hernandez M: La movilidad del pabellon auditivo. Trab Anthropol 1980; 18:199–203.

MY003
**Charles M. Myer III**

## TONGUE, GEOGRAPHIC     0954

**Includes:**

> Annulus migrans
> Glossitis, benign migratory
> Lingua plicata
> Stomatitis areata migrans
> Tongue, wandering rash of

**Excludes:**

> **Ankylosing spondylitis** (2516)
> Erythema multiforme
> **Glossitis, median rhomboid** (0417)
> Glossitis, resulting from nutritional deficiencies
> Lichen planus
> Lingual lesions of aphthae
> Pemphigus
> Syphilis
> **Tongue, fissured** (0953)
> **Tongue, plicated** (0956)
> Tuberculosis

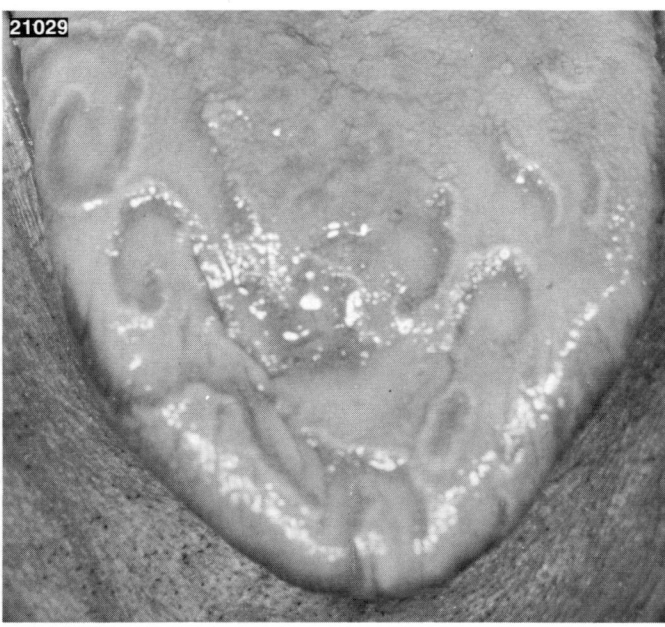

**0954-21029:** Geographic tongue.

**Major Diagnostic Criteria:** The diagnosis is readily made from the striking appearance of discrete, smooth, red patches on the silver-gray, rough, dorsal surface of the tongue. "Migration" or evanescence of the patches over a period of days is diagnostic in otherwise doubtful cases. Rarely, the pattern may seem static for days or weeks, but even here, biopsy is seldom necessary to rule out other lesions.

**Clinical Findings:** Characteristic lesions are discrete, reddened, smooth, irregularly shaped patches on the dorsal and lateral surfaces of the anterior two-thirds of the tongue. The borders are often slightly raised and white or pale yellow in color. The pattern often resembles the configuration of a map; hence, the term "geographic" tongue. The lesions usually "migrate" by healing on one border while advancing on another. They tend to undergo exacerbations and regressions, and may often be completely absent for varying periods of time. About one-fourth of affected persons have tenderness, burning; occasionally, these symptoms are severe.

**Complications:** Unknown.

**Associated Findings:** It has been suggested that this condition may be associated with some of the same genes responsible for **Tongue, fissured** and **Tongue, plicated**. A history of allergy was found in 40% of the cases. A few cases have been reported in which identical lesions have appeared on other areas of the oral mucosa (*stomatitis areata migrans*) and even on the skin (*annulus migrans*).

**Etiology:** Familial occurrence best explained by multifactorial inheritance. Nutritional deficiency and infection are unlikely factors. Emotional stress is a contributing factor. Allergy seems worthy of investigation, as total and allergen-related serum IgE levels are higher in affected individuals.

**Pathogenesis:** Lesions progress through three stages: acute inflammation; chronic inflammation and desquamation; and regeneration and recornification. All three may be present in different areas of a given lesion.

Microscopically, the early lesions or advancing borders of older lesions show acute inflammation of the superficial mucosa, with intercellular edema and neutrophilic infiltration of the epithelium. The central areas are noncornified, with flattened or atrophic papillae, and show chronic inflammation. Many lesions show a striking resemblance to pustular psoriasis. In general, other laboratory tests are of no known diagnostic value.

**MIM No.:** 13740

**CDC No.:** 750.180

**Sex Ratio:** M1:F1

**Occurrence:** The incidence is somewhat higher than the prevalence because lesions are evanescent in many affected individuals. Prevalence is 1:83 among whites and Blacks between five and 70 years of age in surveys of several thousand people, each involving school children or dental patients in the United States. Higher occurrences have been reported in Japan and Israel, but these represent incidence rather than prevalence, and were conducted in wartime when nutritional deficiencies and stress were likely to have caused tongue lesions easily confused with those of geographic tongue.

**Risk of Recurrence for Patient's Sib:** Empirical risk 11%; higher if one or more parents are affected.

**Risk of Recurrence for Patient's Child:** Empirical risk 14%.

**Age of Detectability:** Has been observed in infants.

**Gene Mapping and Linkage:** Unknown.

**Prevention:** None known. Genetic counseling indicated.

**Treatment:** Reassurance. Soothing mouth wash for symptoms.

**Prognosis:** No effect on life span.

**Detection of Carrier:** Unknown.

**References:**

Redman RS, et al.: Psychological component in the etiology of geographic tongue. J Dent Res 1966; 45:1403–1408.

Richardson ER: Incidence of geographic tongue and median rhomboid glossitis in 3,319 Negro college students. Oral Surg 1968; 26:623–625.

Redman RS, et al.: Hereditary component in the etiology of geographic tongue. Am J Hum Genet 1972; 24:124–133.

Hume WJ: Geographic stomatitis: a critical review. J Dent 1975; 3:25–43. *

Eidelman E, et al.: Scrotal tongue and geographic tongue: polygenic and associated traits. Oral Surg 1976; 42:591–596. *

Marks R, Czary D: Geographic tongue: sensitivity to the environment. Oral Surg 1984; 58:156–159.

RE003                                    **Robert S. Redman**

**Tongue, isolated congenital enlarged**
  *See MACROGLOSSIA*
**Tongue, large and protruding**
  *See MACROGLOSSIA*
**Tongue, median cleft**
  *See CLEFTS, LOWER MEDIAN LIP, MANDIBLE AND TONGUE*
**Tongue, pigmented fungiform papillae of**
  *See TONGUE, PIGMENTED PAPILLAE*

## TONGUE, PIGMENTED PAPILLAE          0955

**Includes:**
  Tongue, prominent pigmented papillae of
  Tongue, pigmented fungiform papillae of

**Excludes:**
  **Intestinal polyposis**
  Pigmentation, mucocutaneous
  Pigmentation, physiologic
  Tongue pigmentation

**Major Diagnostic Criteria:** Long-term history of presence of pigmented fungiform papillae of tongue. It is important to differentiate this condition from **Intestinal polyposis, type II.**

**Clinical Findings:** Brown to brownish-red pigmentation localized to tips of fungiform papillae. Lesions located primarily on tip and lateral margins of tongue. Occasionally, brown macules, 1–2 mm in diameter, on soft palate; distribution extending to junction of hard and soft palate. Routine blood and urine laboratory studies, serum electrolytes, and X-ray films of the chest and skull are normal.

**Complications:** Unknown.

**Associated Findings:** None known.

**Etiology:** Autosomal recessive inheritance, with about 89% penetrance in adults.

**Pathogenesis:** Undetermined. The pigmentary defect is present at birth and persists through life. The pigmentation is limited to the fungiform papillae of the tongue, with the occasional exception of pigmented macules of the soft palate. There is no correlation between this condition and the state of nutrition of the mother or the patient.

**MIM No.:** *27525

**CDC No.:** 750.180

**Sex Ratio:** M1:F9 (observed).

**Occurrence:** 1:12 African Blacks; 1:50 African whites. No data is available for other populations.

**Risk of Recurrence for Patient's Sib:**
  See Part I, *Mendelian Inheritance.*

**Risk of Recurrence for Patient's Child:**
  See Part I, *Mendelian Inheritance.*

**Age of Detectability:** Usually within first three months of life, by clinical observation. Rarely seen in the newborn.

**Gene Mapping and Linkage:** Unknown.

**Prevention:** None known. Genetic counseling indicated.

**Treatment:** None required.

**Prognosis:** Normal for life span, intelligence, and function.

**Detection of Carrier:** Unknown.

**References:**
Kaplin EJ, W'srand MB: The clinical tongue. Lancet 1961; I:1094.
Koplon BS, Hurley HJ: Prominent pigmented papillae of the tongue. Arch Dermatol 1967; 95:394.
Rao DC, Lew R: Complex segregation analysis of tongue pigmentation. Hum Hered 1978; 28:317–320.

AU005                                    **Thomas Aufdemorte**

**Tongue, Pleomorphic lipoma**
  *See NECK/FACE, LIPOMATOSIS*

## TONGUE, PLICATED                       0956

**Includes:** Scrotal tongue

**Excludes:**
  **Cheilitis granulomatosa, Melkersson-Rosenthal type** (2083)
  **Chromosome 21, trisomy 21** (0171)

**Major Diagnostic Criteria:** Lingual papillae are divided into multiple groups by definite shallow fissures.

**Clinical Findings:** The tongue has a wrinkled or cerebriform appearance. The papillae of the tongue are divided into multiple groups or islands by definite small shallow fissures, which may not be apparent without folding the tongue so the surface mucosa is stretched. The small fissures involve the dorsal mucosa, including the edges of the tongue. **Tongue, geographic** may be superimposed giving a patchy or map-like appearance, with areas showing relatively short, smooth-appearing mucosa surrounded by longer white papillae at the borders. The two conditions are associated in about 20% of cases. The condition is asymptomatic.

**Complications:** Unknown.

**Associated Findings:** Plicated tongue occurs in **Cheilitis granulomatosa, Melkersson-Rosenthal type,** and in about 30% of patients with **Chromosome 21, trisomy 21.** Hanhart (1934) reported a 47% frequency in psychotic patients. The autosomal dominant form is associated with migraine headaches in some families.

**Etiology:** While many kindreds show autosomal dominant inheritance, it is not known if all cases are inherited. In most

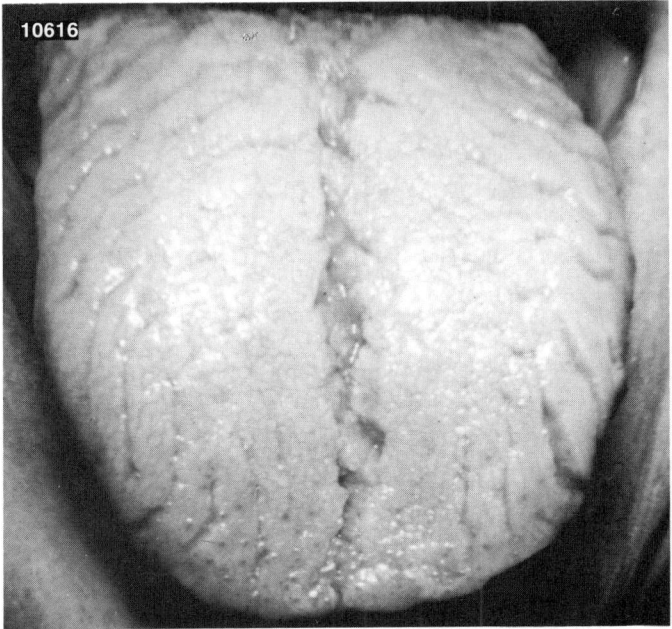

**0956**-10616:   Plicated tongue.

instances, this is probably an age-related developmental polygenic anomaly. Since plicated tongue and **Tongue, Geographic** occur together with high frequency in first degree relatives, the mode of inheritance of each remains unclear and suggests etiologic heterogeneity and/or genes in common to both traits.

**Pathogenesis:** Undetermined. Condition is rare before age four years. Cerebriform pattern becomes more pronounced around puberty. One study showed a inconclusive association with blood group O. An association between plicated tongue and persons with low serum vitamin A levels has not been substantiated in later studies.

**MIM No.:** 13740

**CDC No.:** 750.180

**Sex Ratio:** M2.24:F1.68.

**Occurrence:** Prevalence 1:20 to 1:12 in all age groups combined. Shows increasing frequency with age, from about 1:100 in children to 1:8 in adults over 40. Rare before age four years.

**Risk of Recurrence for Patient's Sib:**
See Part I, *Mendelian Inheritance.*

**Risk of Recurrence for Patient's Child:**
See Part I, *Mendelian Inheritance.*

**Age of Detectability:** Frequency and severity of plicated tongue increases with age. Most cases are detectable by 12 years of age, by clinical examination.

**Gene Mapping and Linkage:** Unknown.

**Prevention:** None known. Genetic counseling indicated.

**Treatment:** None indicated. Vitamin A has been used with questionable success.

**Prognosis:** Excellent. Does not reduce longevity.

**Detection of Carrier:** Unknown.

**References:**
Hanhart E: Die faltenzunge (lingua plicata) als stigma nervöser mind-
    erwertigkeit. Verh Schweiz Naturforsch Ges 1934; 115:432–433.
Witkop CJ Jr, Barros L: Oral and genetic studies of Chileans 1960. I.
    Oral anomalies. Am J Phys Anthropol 1963; 21:15–24.
Gorlin RJ: Developmental anomalies of face and oral structures. In:
    Gorlin RJ, Goldman HM, eds: Thoma's oral pathology, 6th ed. vol.
    1. St. Louis: C.V. Mosby, 1970:30–95. †
Eidelman E, et al.: Scrotal tongue and geographic tongue: polygenic
    and associated traits. Oral Surg 1976; 42:591–596. *

WI043                                         **Carl J. Witkop, Jr.**

**Tongue, prominent pigmented papillae of**
    *See TONGUE, PIGMENTED PAPILLAE*
**Tongue, trifid**
    *See TONGUE, CLEFT*
**Tongue, wandering rash of**
    *See TONGUE, GEOGRAPHIC*
**Tongue-tie**
    *See TONGUE, ANKYLOGLOSSIA*
**Tooth and nail syndrome**
    *See HYPODONTIA-NAIL DYSGENESIS*
**Tooth-hair-bone-nail dysplasia**
    *See TRICHO-DENTO-OSSEOUS SYNDROME*
**Toothless man of Sind**
    *See ECTODERMAL DYSPLASIA, CHRIST-SIEMENS-TOURAINE TYPE*

---

## TORSION DYSTONIA                           0957

**Includes:** Dystonia musculorum deformans

**Excludes:**
    **Cerebral palsy** (2931)
    Dystonia, drug induced
    Dystonic lipidosis
    **Hallervorden-Spatz disease** (2526)
    **Hepatolenticular degeneration** (0469)
    **Huntington disease** (0478)
    Hysteria
    **Niemann-Pick disease** (0717)

Parkinsonism, early onset
    **X-linked mental retardation-basal ganglion disorder** (2841)

**Major Diagnostic Criteria:** The diagnosis is clinical, and is suspected by the appearance of involuntary movement or posturing of one part of the body; often plantar flexion inversion movement of a foot combined with a pattern of progression. Family history may assist the diagnosis.

**Clinical Findings:** The disease has at least two hereditary types: autosomal recessive, and autosomal dominant. The autosomal recessive type has been described in Ashkenazi Jews with an earlier age of onset and a more rapid course. The dystonic posturing of the extremity is at first intermittent but gradually becomes constant. The symptoms spread to other extremities, eventually the neck and the trunk. The affected limbs assume a fixed, continuously maintained, abnormal attitude upon which athetotic fluctuations are superimposed later in the progression of the disease.

Autosomal dominant torsion dystonia has been reported mostly in non-Jewish families, particularly those from Sweden and French Canada. It has a more variable age of onset. It fluctuates in course and has more involvement of the axial musculature. In one-fourth of these patients, torticollis is the initial symptom.

The disease is a progressive movement disorder. Symptoms may be worse under stress. The movements may be triggered by the motion of any other part of the body or ultimately may appear spontaneously. Extrapyramidal movements cease during sleep.

**Complications:** Activities of daily living can be limited due to the involuntary movements and the dystonic posturing of the extremities. Eventually arthritis may develop in the affected limbs.

**Associated Findings:** The vast majority of patients have normal mental intelligence and are fully aware of their condition as they gradually become functionally handicapped in the motor area.

**Etiology:** Autosomal recessive or autosomal dominant inheritance.

**Pathogenesis:** Norepinephrine concentrations are markedly and consistently decreased in the lateral and posterior hypothalamus, mammillary body, subthalamic nucleus, and locus ceruleus. The cause of the neurochemical abnormality is undetermined.

**MIM No.:** *12810, *22450

**Sex Ratio:** M1:F1

**Occurrence:** In the autosomal recessive form, 1:20,000 live births are reported in Ashkenazi Jewish families.

**Risk of Recurrence for Patient's Sib:**
See Part I, *Mendelian Inheritance.*

**Risk of Recurrence for Patient's Child:**
See Part I, *Mendelian Inheritance.*

**Age of Detectability:** In the autosomal recessive type, onset is between four and 16 years of age. In the autosomal dominant type, there is a greater variation in the age of detectability.

**Gene Mapping and Linkage:** DYT1 (dystonia, torsion 1 (autosomal dominant)) has been provisionally mapped to 9q32-q34.
    DYT2 (dystonia, torsion 2 (autosomal recessive)) is unassigned.

**Prevention:** None known. Genetic counseling indicated.

**Treatment:** A number of treatment modalities are available, but there is no consistently successful treatment. The most frequently used modalities include stereotactic surgery, L-dopa, bromocriptine, baclofen, lissuride, and diazepam.

**Prognosis:** Eventually the patients become bedridden and exhausted by constant muscular activity. The usual cause of death is intercurrent infection.

**Detection of Carrier:** Unknown.

**Support Groups:**
    CA; Beverly Hills; Dystonia Medical Research Foundation
    NY; Melville; Dystonia Foundation
    CANADA: BC; Vancouver; Dystonia Medical Research Foundation

**References:**

Eldridge R: The torsion dystonias: literature review and genetic and clinical studies. Neurology 1970; 20:1–78.

Marsden CD, et al.: Natural history of idiopathic torsion dystonia. Adv Neurol 1976; 14:177–187.

Zilber N, et al.: Inheritance of ideopathic torsion dystonia among Jews. J Med Genet 1984; 21:13–20.

Hornykiewicz O, et al.: Brain neurotransmitters in dystonia musculorum deformans. New Engl J Med 1986; 315:347–353.

C0018                                                    **Mary Coleman**

**Torsion dystonia-skeletal and facial defects**
*See BLEPHARO-NASO-FACIAL SYNDROME*

## TORTICOLLIS                                                    2940

**Includes:**

Muscular torticollis
Postural torticollis
Sandifer syndrome
Sternocleidomastoid torticollis
Sternomastoid torticollis
Wryneck

**Excludes:**

Cervical hemivertebrae
**Cervico-dermo-gu syndrome, Goeminne type** (2174)
**Klippel-Feil anomaly** (2032)
**Oculo-auriculo-vertebral anomaly** (0735)

**Major Diagnostic Criteria:** The affected sternocleidomastoid muscle is shortened so that the head is tipped forward and the chin is pointed away from the affected muscle. The muscle may feel hard or woody. A mass may be palpated in the body of the muscle in about 20% of cases.

**Clinical Findings:** Typically, the head is held in a neutral posture at birth, but tips into the wry position over the subsequent days or weeks. The active range of neck motion may vary with muscle shortening and will become intermittently more severe when the child is irritated, fatigued, or ill. Torticollis will generally remain persistent until ages 4–6 months and will then spontaneously, slowly improve. The pathology of the muscle mass discloses fibrous reaction without hemorrhage. The presence or size of the mass has no prognostic significance.

**Complications:** Torticollis often precedes the progressive development of a rhomboidal head shape with flattening of the face ispilateral to the shortened neck muscle and contralateral flattening of the occipitoparietal area (see **Plagiocephaly**).

Although there is some speculation that persistent torticollis affects overall gross motor development, no studies have clearly demonstrated this to be the case.

**Associated Findings:** Torticollis may be associated with other prenatal deformities, including scoliosis, metatarsus adductus, calcaneovalgus, and possibly dislocated hip. Hypotonia and other intrinsic neuromuscular disorders that predispose fetuses to constraint may be found.

**Etiology:** Congenital deformation without genetic predisposition is the usual situation. However, several multigeneration pedigrees have been reported, variably suggesting autosomal dominant, recessive, and polygenic inheritance.

**Pathogenesis:** There is general agreement that congenital torticollis is produced as a prenatal injury to the sternocleidomastoid muscle. The precise mechanism(s) of that injury are undetermined.

**MIM No.:** 18960

**CDC No.:** 756.860

**Sex Ratio:** M1:F1

**Occurrence:** Estimated at 6:10,000 live births, although some authors believe subtle damage to the sternomastoid is found in as many as 200:10,000 infants.

**Risk of Recurrence for Patient's Sib:**
See Part I, *Mendelian Inheritance*. Generally, deformities occur through an interaction of increased fetal size, decreased intrauterine space, and decreased fetal movement. Each pregnancy must be assessed for contributing factors.

**Risk of Recurrence for Patient's Child:**
See Part I, *Mendelian Inheritance*. Undetermined but presumed low unless familial.

**Age of Detectability:** Usually evident within the first 2–4 weeks of life.

**Gene Mapping and Linkage:** Unknown.

**Prevention:** None known. Genetic counseling indicated.

**Treatment:** Generally, torticollis resolves spontaneously by 6–12 months of life. When wryneck is persistent after 9–12 months of life, physical therapy will usually resolve the situation. In rare cases, a surgical release of the muscle after age three years may be necessary.

**Prognosis:** Normal neck movement can generally be expected.

**Detection of Carrier:** Careful clinical evaluation of the maternal pelvis and uterus may detect problems predisposing to constraining the fetus, and family histories may help to identify the rare families with multiply affected members.

**Special Considerations:** *Sandifer syndrome*, first described in 1969, is the rare association of GE reflux-torticollis to the left (Sutcliffe, 1969; Ramenofsky et al, 1978). Its cause is unknown, but since the wry neck resolves with the correction of reflux it is assumed to be neurologic.

**References:**

Sutcliffe J: Torsion spasms and abnormal postures in children with hiatus hernia: Sandifer's syndrome. Prog Pediatr Radiol 1969; 2:190–197.

Dunn PM: Congenital sternomastoid torticollis: an intrauterine postural deformity. Arch Dis Child 1974; 49:824–825.

Clark RN: Diagnosis and management of torticollis. Pediatr Ann 1976; 5:43–60.

Ramenofsky ML, et al.: Gastroesophageal reflux and torticollis. J Bone Joint Surg 1978; 60-A:1140–1141.

Clarren SK: Plagiocephaly and torticollis: etiology, natural history, and helmet treatment in 43 patients. J Pediatr 1981; 98:92–95.

Smith DW: Recognizable patterns of human deformities. Philadelphia: W.B. Saunders, 1981. * †

Dunne KB, Clarren SK: The origin of prenatal and postnatal deformities. Pediatr Clin North Am 1986; 33:1277–1297. †

Thompson F, et al.: Familial congenital muscular torticollis: case report and review of the literature. Clin Orthop Rel Res 1986; 202:193–196.

CL006                                            **Sterling K. Clarren**

**Torticollis-keloids-cryptorchidism-renal dysplasia**
*See CERVICO-DERMO-GU SYNDROME, GOEMINNE TYPE*
**Torus mandibular**
*See MANDIBLE, TORUS MANDIBULARIS*
**Torus palatinus**
*See PALATE, TORUS PALATINUS*
**Total anomalous hepatic venous return**
*See LIVER, VENOUS ANOMALIES*
**Total cataract**
*See CATARACT, AUTOSOMAL DOMINANT CONGENITAL*
**Total lipodystrophy-acromegaloid gigantism**
*See LIPODYSTROPHY SYNDROME, BERARDINELLI TYPE*
**Toulouse-Lautrec (possible diagnosis)**
*See PYKNODYSOSTOSIS*
**Toumaala-Haapanen syndrome**
*See OCULO-OSTEO-CUTANEOUS SYNDROME, TOUMAALA-HAAPANEN TYPE*
**Touraine-Solente-Gole syndrome**
*See PACHYDERMOPERIOSTOSIS*

## TOURETTE SYNDROME                                    2305

**Includes:**
    Gilles de la Tourette syndrome
    Tics, multiple motor and vocal

**Excludes:**
    **Hallervorden-Spatz disease** (2526)
    **Hepatolenticular degeneration** (0469)
    **Huntington disease** (0478)
    Klazomania
    Tardive dyskinesia
    **Torsion dystonia** (0957)

**Major Diagnostic Criteria:** Tourette syndrome (TS) is clinically diagnosed on the basis of the presence of multiple motor tics (e.g., eye blinks, facial grimaces, head jerks, shoulder shrugs, arm movements, trunk movements) and multiple vocal tics (e.g. throat clearing, sniffing, hissing, coughing, sucking, yelping, ejaculation of inappropriate words or phrases including coprolalia). The onset is usually before age 21 years, and the symptoms must persist for at least one year.

**Clinical Findings:** Motor tics typically appear well before vocal tics. The motor tics usually show a rostral-caudal progression, so that tics involving the face and head usually precede those involving the trunk or extremeties. Symptoms vary in their complexity, frequency, and degree of social role dysfunction they produce. In most cases this is a lifelong chronic illness, with symptoms waxing and waning over time.

**Complications:** Coprolalia develops in approximately one-third of the patients. This and other severe symptoms can be socially disabling. Although not life threatening, this illness can markedly limit the individual's choices for a satisfying and productive life.

**Associated Findings:** Over one-half of the patients seen in a clinic will have attention problems that can interfere with school work. In addition, a large percentage (50–75%) will also develop obsessions and compulsions. In fact, in later life the obsessions and compulsions may be the most troublesome features of the illness.

**Etiology:** Autosomal dominant inheritance with incomplete penetrance, although a substantial number of patients (10–35%) do not have a positive family history and appear to be isolated cases.

**Pathogenesis:** Unknown.

**MIM No.:** *13758

**Sex Ratio:** Approximately M3:F1.

**Occurrence:** The incidence has been estimated to be between 1:2,000 and 1:3,000 for males, and between 1:5,000 and 1:10,000 for females, but most investigators believe that this syndrome tends to be underdiagnosed.

**Risk of Recurrence for Patient's Sib:**
    See Part I, *Mendelian Inheritance*. Tourette syndrome, 10%; chronic multiple tics, 20%; obsessive compulsive disorders, 10%.

**Risk of Recurrence for Patient's Child:**
    See Part I, *Mendelian Inheritance*.

**Age of Detectability:** The age of onset can range from two to 21 years, with mean onset at seven years of age.

**Gene Mapping and Linkage:** GTS (Gilles de la Tourette syndrome) is unassigned.

**Prevention:** None known. Genetic counseling indicated.

**Treatment:** Currently haloperidol is frequently used to control symptoms; a number of other medications, including pimozide, piperidine, clonazepam, and clonidine have also been tried with variable results.

**Prognosis:** Chronic lifelong illness in most cases.

**Detection of Carrier:** Unknown.

**Special Considerations:** This syndrome is particularly difficult to diagnose, since a wide variety of symptoms can usher in the syndrome.

**Support Groups:**
    NY; Bayside; Tourette Syndrome Association (TSA)
    AUSTRALIA: Victoria; Elsternick; Tourette Syndrome Association of Australia
    CANADA: Ontario; Willowdale; Tourette Syndrome Foundation of Canada
    DENMARK: Lyngby; Tourette Syndrome Association of Denmark
    ENGLAND: Essex; Ilford; Tourette Syndrome Association of Great Britain
    THE NETHERLANDS: Rhood; Tourette Syndrome Association of The Netherlands

**References:**
Comings DE, Comings BG: Tourette syndrome: clinical and psychological aspects of 250 cases. Am J Hum Genet 1985; 37:435–450.
Pauls DL, Leckman JF: The inheritance of Gilles de la Tourette's syndrome and associated behaviors: evidence for autosomal dominant transmission. New Engl J Med 1986; 315:993–997.
Shapiro AK, et al.: Gilles de la Tourette Syndrome, 2nd ed. New York: Raven Press, 1988.

PA048
C0018
        **David Pauls**
        **Mary Coleman**

**Townes-Brocks syndrome**
    *See ANUS-HAND-EAR SYNDROME*
**Toxopachyosteose diaphysaire tibio-peroniere**
    *See SKELETAL DYSPLASIA, WEISMANN-NETTER-STUHL TYPE*
**Toxoplasmosis, infantile**
    *See FETAL TOXOPLASMOSIS SYNDROME*

## TRACHEA, AGENESIS                                    2848

**Includes:**
    Segmental tracheal agenesis
    Tracheal aplasia
    Tracheal atresia

**Excludes:**
    **Tracheal agenesis-multiple anomaly association** (2849)
    Tracheal stenosis

**Major Diagnostic Criteria:** Congenital absence of all or part of the trachea.

**Clinical Findings:** Tracheal agenesis manifests at birth with severe respiratory distress and difficulty with resuscitation. Many cases are born at or near term after uncomplicated pregnancies. Occasionally polyhydramnios or intrauterine growth retardation may lead to fetal assessment and diagnosis of associated anomalies, though the tracheal agenesis is not usually suspected before birth. There may be complete or, less commonly, partial absence of the trachea. Several classifications of tracheal agenesis subtypes have been described. The classification of Floyd et al (1962) documents three main types: *type I*, in which part of the distal trachea is preserved and communicates with the esophagus; *type II*, in which the main stem bronchi are connected below the normal carina by an interbronchial segment communicating by a fistula to the esophagus; and *type III*, in which the main stem bronchi enter the esophagus separately. Rarer forms include those with complete pulmonary agenesis and segmental defects. Type II is the most common form, seen in approximately 60% of cases.

    In the more than 50 cases of tracheal agenesis reported to date, the defect has usually been fatal within a few hours, though operations aimed at stabilizing the child and providing a permanent airway have been attempted. The longest survival reported is six weeks.

**Complications:** This condition has been uniformly fatal.

**Associated Findings:** Associated anomalies in the respiratory system include **Larynx, atresia** (15%) and **Lung, aberrant lobe** (20%). Over 80% of reported cases have had major anomalies in other systems, especially the cardiovascular (65%), genitourinary (45%), gastrointestinal (30%), and musculoskeletal (30%) systems. Central nervous system and craniofacial anomalies are rarely reported.

**Etiology:** Unknown.

**Pathogenesis:** Presumably involves faulty development of the tracheobronchial tree. The laryngotracheal groove develops as a ventral projection of the floor of the foregut caudal to the pharyngeal pouches. The lung buds develop as this outgrowth extends caudally. Along the lateral margins of the outgrowth, the tracheoesophageal grooves form, grow inward, and join in a caudocephalad direction to produce the tracheoesophageal septum. Failure of the cephalic portion of the laryngotracheal groove to form would result in total or partial absence of the trachea, though the bronchi and lungs would remain. Incomplete fusion of the tracheoesophageal folds would allow abnormal persistence of communication between the trachea or bronchi and the esophagus.

**Sex Ratio:** M1.5:F1 for all reported cases, but M3:F1 for isolated tracheal agenesis.

**Occurrence:** Over 50 cases have been reported in the world literature, and the defect has been seen in all ethnic groups. A population-based survey in Manitoba indicated an incidence of approximately 1:80,000 live births.

**Risk of Recurrence for Patient's Sib:** Presumably low. No recurrences have been documented, although detailed family studies have not been undertaken.

**Risk of Recurrence for Patient's Child:** Defect has been lethal in all cases.

**Age of Detectability:** At or soon after birth. May go unrecognized as tracheal agenesis if postmortem examination is not carried out.

**Gene Mapping and Linkage:** Unknown.

**Prevention:** None known. Genetic counseling indicated.

**Treatment:** Surgical intervention has been attempted in several patients. Initial therapy has involved utilization of the esophagus as a conduit to the bronchi or insertion of an endobronchial tube. Survival has varied from 23 hours to six weeks. Definitive repair will be complicated by lack of suitable homologous or prosthetic tracheal replacements and is unlikely to be successful until a graft is available that can provide suitable ciliated epithelium, withstand normal pressure changes, and allow for normal growth and development. In most cases survival is jeopardized by the presence of other serious birth defects, especially complex congenital heart anomalies.

**Prognosis:** With currently available therapy, this condition is lethal.

**Detection of Carrier:** Unknown.

**References:**
Floyd J, et al.: Agenesis of the trachea. Am Rev Respir Dis 1962; 86:557–560.
Hopkinson JM: Congenital absence of the trachea. J Pathol 1972; 107:63–66. †
Buchino JJ, et al.: Tracheal agenesis: a clinical approach. J Pediatr Surg 1982; 17:132–137.
Evans JA, et al.: Tracheal agenesis and associated malformations: a comparison with tracheoesophageal fistula and the VACTERL association. Am J Med Genet 1985; 21:21–34.*

EV001                                        **Jane A. Evans**

**Tracheal agenesis association**
*See TRACHEAL AGENESIS-MULTIPLE ANOMALY ASSOCIATION*

## TRACHEAL AGENESIS-MULTIPLE ANOMALY ASSOCIATION      2849

**Includes:**
Tracheal agenesis association
Tracheal-renal-alimentary-cardiovascular-limb association

**Excludes:**
**Trachea, agenesis** (2848)
**Vater association** (0987)

**Major Diagnostic Criteria:** Presence of tracheal agenesis should alert the physician to the possibility of associated anomalies, especially in the cardiovascular, genitourinary, gastrointestinal, and musculoskeletal systems. Although not recognized as a specific syndrome, a child with tracheal agenesis and a major anomaly in one or more of these additional systems may be an example of a specific tracheal-renal-alimentary-cardiovascular-limb association.

**Clinical Findings:** Over 80% of reported cases of tracheal agenesis have additional major anomalies. The most common of these are **Lung, aberrant lobe** (26%), imperforate anus (see **Anorectal malformations**) (21%), **Ventricular septal defect** (33%), **Atrial septal defects** (21%), single umbilical artery (29%), and single kidney (21%). **Larynx, atresia,** duodenal atresia (see **Duodenum, atresia or stenosis**), pancreatic anomalies, cystic dysplastic kidney, aberrant internal genitalia, and radial ray defects are also relatively common (10–20%).

This association has obvious similarities to **Vater association**, but differs in the nature and frequency of anomalies. In particular, defects of the axial skeleton and external genital anomalies are relatively rare (<10%) in the tracheal agenesis association, and the heart defects tend to be more complex (e.g., **Heart, truncus arteriosus**, **Heart, transposition of great vessels**, hypoplastic left heart).

Patients with the tracheal-renal-alimentary-cardiovascular-limb association rarely have defects in other systems. However, tracheal agenesis has also been seen in one patient with sirenomelia (see **Sirenomelia sequence**), and infants with total absence of the pulmonary system have had other major anomalies, including neural tube defects, urethral atresia, and hemimelia.

Children with tracheal agenesis and other major anomalies are frequently premature (50% are less than 37 weeks gestation), and approximately 20% show intrauterine growth retardation. Polyhydramnios has been noted in some cases with associated duodenal atresia. In many, however, multiple anomalies are not suspected until birth, when the tracheal agenesis causes severe respiratory distress and difficulty with resuscitation. All cases have been fatal within a few hours or days, although surgical intervention has allowed survival to a maximum of six weeks.

**Complications:** Death at or shortly after birth.

**Associated Findings:** None known.

**Etiology:** Unknown.

**Pathogenesis:** Unknown. Several potential mechanisms could explain the pattern of anomalies observed in some of the patients. For example, some cases with aberrant lung lobation, congenital heart defects and spleen anomalies may represent defects of laterality similar to the asplenia/polysplenia spectrum. Review of patients with bilateral right or left sidedness has shown an increased incidence of defects, such as tracheoesophageal anomalies, gastric hypoplasia, agenesis of the gallbladder, annular pancreas, duodenal stenosis, imperforate anus, **Kidney, horseshoe**, and hydroureter, that are also seen in the tracheal agenesis association.

At least two cases of tracheal agenesis with associated anomalies have been seen in one of monozygous twins; the co-twins were normal. It is possible in these cases that the multiple anomalies have a basis in vascular interchange between twins.

A third mechanism may, as with **Vater association**, involve disorganization and faulty migration of cells from the primitive streak, though this hypothesis is purely speculative at this time. The tracheal agenesis association probably represents a polytopic field defect.

**POS No.:** 3405

**Sex Ratio:** Approximately M1.2:F1.

**Occurrence:** Over 40 cases of tracheal agenesis with other major defects have been reported. About 20 of these involve children with tracheal agenesis and two or more other anomalies seen in the more restricted tracheal-renal-alimentary-cardiovascular-limb association. Incidence is approximately 1:100,000.

**Risk of Recurrence for Patient's Sib:** Probably low, although detailed family studies have not been carried out. The published reports of tracheal agenesis patients document two cases of **Anencephaly** and one of **Ventricular septal defect** among 43 sibs, suggesting a possible susceptibility to midline defects in these families.

**Risk of Recurrence for Patient's Child:** No affected individuals have survived to reproduce.

**Age of Detectability:** At birth, when obvious external anomalies such as radial ray defects and imperforate anus may also be noted. The precise nature of the tracheal anomaly and other internal defects may only become apparent at postmortem examination.

**Gene Mapping and Linkage:** Unknown.

**Prevention:** None known. Genetic counseling indicated.

**Treatment:** Attempts have been made to treat the tracheal agenesis surgically, but survival beyond age six weeks has not been achieved. Long-term survival is unlikely until suitable tracheal replacements are available, and will in many cases be complicated by congenital heart defects and other associated anomalies.

**Prognosis:** All patients have died by age six weeks.

**Detection of Carrier:** Careful histories documenting relatives with other midline defects may help to indicate families at increased risk.

**References:**
Fonkalsrud EW, et al.: Surgical treatment of tracheal agenesis. J Thorac Cardiovasc Surg 1963; 45:520–525.
McNie DJM, Pryse-Davies J: Tracheal agenesis. Arch Dis Child 1970; 45:143–144.
Hopkinson JM: Congenital absence of the trachea. J Pathol 1972; 107:63–66. †
Evans JA, et al.: Tracheal agenesis and associated malformations: a comparison with tracheoesophageal fistula and the VACTERL association. Am J Med Genet 1985; 21:21–34. *

EV001                                            **Jane A. Evans**

**Tracheal aplasia**
 *See TRACHEA, AGENESIS*
**Tracheal atresia**
 *See TRACHEA, AGENESIS*
**Tracheal lobe**
 *See LUNG, ABERRANT LOBE*
**Tracheal-renal-alimentary-cardiovascular-limb association**
 *See TRACHEAL AGENESIS-MULTIPLE ANOMALY ASSOCIATION*
**Tracheo-laryngo-esophageal cleft**
 *See LARYNGO-TRACHEO-ESOPHAGEAL CLEFT*

---

**TRACHEOESOPHAGEAL FISTULA**           **0960**

**Includes:**
 Cervical tracheoesophageal fistula, congenital isolated H-type
 Esophageal atresia-tracheoesophageal fistula
 Thoracic tracheoesophageal fistula, congenital isolated H-type
 Thoracic tracheoesophageal fistula-esophageal atresia

**Excludes:**
 Bronchopulmonary foregut malformations-esophageal communication
 Intralobar sequestration-esophageal communications
 Tracheoesophageal fistula acquired due to caustic ingestion
 Tracheoesophageal fistula acquired due to surgery
 Tracheoesophageal fistula acquired due to trauma

**Major Diagnostic Criteria:** Repeated bouts of pneumonia and gastric dilation suggest a tracheoesophageal fistula. Contrast material swallowed with careful positioning under fluoroscopic control may demonstrate the fistula. Tamponading of the distal esophagus by balloon catheter may force the contrast material (barium or metriziamide) through the fistula. Esophagobronchoscopy with installation of methylene blue into the endotracheal tube under anesthesia is necessary if contrast studies do not demonstrate the fistula.

**Clinical Findings:** Repeated episodes of aspiration syndrome or pneumonia and choking or coughing when feeding are almost always present. Liquids cause greater difficulty than solids. The repeated episodes of bronchopneumonia beginning early in life are diffuse, patch-like infiltrates. Marked abdominal distention occurs following crying and coughing. The distention is due to air escaping through the fistula into the GI tract.

**Complications:** Aspiration and suffocation. Repeated episodes of pneumonitis and sepsis. Failure to thrive. Chronic pulmonary insufficiency and disability.

**Associated Findings:** None known.

**Etiology:** Van Staey et al (1984), after studying 33 pedigrees, concluded that "with the exception of [cases attributable to] chromosomal or of a known monogenic or teratogenic syndrome, the recurrence risk fit into a multifactorial scheme."

**Pathogenesis:** Failure of closure of laryngotracheal groove. Continued passage of saliva or food from the esophagus through the fistula into the bronchus causes chemical pneumonitis with subsequent sepsis, death, or chronic pulmonary insufficiency.

**MIM No.:** 18996

**CDC No.:** 750.3

**Sex Ratio:** M1:F1

**Occurrence:** 1:75,000 to 1:100,000 live births.

**Risk of Recurrence for Patient's Sib:** Unknown.

**Risk of Recurrence for Patient's Child:** Unknown.

**Age of Detectability:** Newborn through early infancy. The diagnosis is usually established by one year of age.

**Gene Mapping and Linkage:** Unknown.

**Prevention:** None known. Genetic counseling indicated.

**Treatment:** In patients with a cervical esophageal fistula, which occurs in about two-thirds of the cases, suture ligation and division of the fistula can be performed in the cervical region through a neck exploration under general anesthesia. A right thoracotomy is performed for thoracic fistulas with suture ligation and division of the fistula.

**Prognosis:** Excellent, if the diagnosis is made before chronic lung disease or disability occurs.

**Detection of Carrier:** Unknown.

**References:**
Ravitch M, et al.: Pediatric surgery, ed 3. Chicago: Yearbook Medical, 1979.
Van Staey M, et al.: Familial congenital esophageal atresia: personal case report and a review of the literature. Hum Genet 1984; 66:260–266.
Welch K, et al.: Pediatric surgery, ed 4. Chicago: Yearbook Medical, 1986.

BE049                                            **Arthur S. Besser**

**Tracheoesophageal fistula with or without esophageal atresia**
 *See ESOPHAGUS, ATRESIA AND TRACHEOESOPHAGEAL FISTULA*

## TRACHEOMALACIA                                    2505

**Includes:**  Tracheomalacia, secondary

**Excludes:**
**Bronchomalacia** (2995)
Chondromalacia, congenital
**Larsen syndrome, lethal type** (2800)
Polychondritis

**Major Diagnostic Criteria:**  Bronchoscopy is essential for definitive diagnosis. Bronchoscopic findings include weak cartilaginous support of the trachea with anterior-posterior expiratory collapse, anterior-posterior inspiratory collapse with exertion, and a widened posterior membranous wall. When it is associated with tracheoesophageal fistula, the tracheal cartilages have an indented half-circle shape, and the posterior membranous wall is widened.

**Clinical Findings:**  Clinical features vary from mild to severe depending on the location, length, and degree of airway collapse. Features include inspiratory and/or expiratory stridor, wheezing, cough (sometimes barking), hyperextension of the neck, recurrent respiratory infections, difficulty clearing endobronchial secretions, sometimes reflex apnea, respiratory distress, croup, and cyanosis.

Patients with tracheoesophageal fistula have a 30% incidence of secondary tracheomalacia. In mild cases, symptoms begin about age 5–6 months. Moderate cases develop during the first 2–6 months. In severe cases, symptoms of stridor at rest, and occasionally cardiac arrest, develop during the first two months of life.

Primary tracheomalacia in premature infants is noted after extubation. In mature, normal infants, severe symptoms may develop in the first few weeks of life.

**Complications:**  Reflex apnea, respiratory arrest, cardiac arrest, and recurrent pneumonia.

**Associated Findings:**  Primary tracheomalacia is seen in premature infants, otherwise normal infants, and in association with **Chondrodysplasia**.

Secondary tracheomalacia is associated with **Tracheoesophageal fistula**, innominate artery "compression", vascular ring, and congenital cyst or tumor.

**Etiology:**  Endoscopic evaluations suggest congenital disease for primary tracheomalacia. The cartilage to muscle ratio of 2:1 is grossly abnormal (the normal ratio is 4.5 to 1). See also **Tracheoesophageal fistula**.

**Pathogenesis:**  Unknown. When associated with innominate artery compression, it is not known if the artery is in an abnormal location producing localized tracheomalacia, or if normally positioned artery compresses a soft trachea.

**CDC No.:**  748.320

**Sex Ratio:**  Undetermined but presumably M1:F1.

**Occurrence:**  Undetermined but presumed rare.

**Risk of Recurrence for Patient's Sib:**  Unknown.

**Risk of Recurrence for Patient's Child:**  Unknown.

**Age of Detectability:**  During the first few weeks or months of life.

**Gene Mapping and Linkage:**  Unknown.

**Prevention:**  None known. Genetic counseling indicated.

**Treatment:**  For severe innominate artery compression, suspension of artery from posterior sternum, or reimplantation.

**Prognosis:**  Excellent for mild to moderate cases. Fair to good for severe cases.

**Detection of Carrier:**  Unknown.

**References:**
Baxter JD, Dunbar JS: Tracheomalacia. Ann Otol Rhinol Laryngol 1963; 72:1013–1023.
Cogbill TH, et al.: Primary tracheomalacia. Ann Thorac Surg 1983; 35:538–541.

Benjamin B: Tracheomalacia in infants and children. Ann Otol Rhinol Laryngol 1984; 93:438–442.

HU015                                              **Richard Hubbell**
MY003                                          **Charles M. Myer III**

**Tracheomalacia, secondary**
*See TRACHEOMALACIA*
**Tragus, of ear, absent**
*See EAR, ABSENT TRAGUS*
**Tranebjaerg mental retardation**
*See X-LINKED MENTAL RETARDATION-PSORIASIS*
**Tranquilizer, fetal effects (some)**
*See FETAL BENZODIAZEPINE EFFECTS*

## TRANSCOBALAMIN II DEFICIENCY                   2624

**Includes:**
Transcobalamin II, hereditary abnormal (TC2)
Vitamin B(12) binding protein defects

**Excludes:**
**Anemia, pernicious congenital** (2656)
**Vitamin B(12) malabsorption** (0992)

**Major Diagnostic Criteria:**  Failure to thrive; irritability; beefy red, smooth tongue; macrocytic anemia; occasionally pancytopenia. Immunologic alteration may predispose to infection. Serum $B_{12}$ levels are typically normal, but have been reported to be low. Diagnosis is established by demonstrating absent transcobalamin II by immunologic means or by demonstrating nonfunctional transcobalamin II (TC II) in binding or delivery assays.

**Clinical Findings:**  Children have presented with clinical signs from several weeks to several months of age. Part of the variability in the age of presentation has resulted from variable use of oral vitamin supplements. Either folate or vitamin $B_{12}$ orally can delay manifestations of the disease.

Children present with symptoms and signs as a result of either anemia or infection. Pallor, weakness, and irritability are common. Diarrhea, pneumonia, and failure to thrive have been reported. Laboratory evaluation reveals megaloblastic anemia: red cells are macrocytic, and neutrophils are hypersegmented. Bone marrow aspiration typically shows severe megaloblastic changes in both the erythroid and myeloid series. Two patients have been reported with erythroid hypoplasia or aplasia. The marrow picture can be confused with leukemia or myelodysplastic syndrome (preleukemia).

**Complications:**  Administration of folate may improve the anemia associated with TC II deficiency, but will exacerbate neurologic impairment. Two patients so treated developed severe neurologic impairment, one with associated mental retardation.

**Associated Findings:**  Immunodeficiency has been reported in two patients. One exhibited agammaglobulinemia and inability to make antibody to specific antigenic challenge. The second presented with *Pneumocystis carinii* pneumonia and exhibited failure to produce antibody to specific antigenic stimuli. In both cases, therapeutic doses of cobalamin led to complete restoration of immune function.

**Etiology:**  Autosomal recessive inheritance. More commonly, children inherit an allele from each parent, which results in production of no immunologically or functionally detectable TC II. One patient inherited one silent allele and one allele that coded for a protein that was immunologically reactive as TC II but that could not function in vitamin $B_{12}$ transport.

**Pathogenesis:**  Lack of functional TC II results in severe impairment in availability of vitamin $B_{12}$ metabolites to cells.

**MIM No.:**  *27535

**Sex Ratio:**  M1:F1 (six girls and four boys have been described).

**Occurrence:**  Ten cases have been documented in the literature.

**Risk of Recurrence for Patient's Sib:**
See Part I, *Mendelian Inheritance.*

**Risk of Recurrence for Patient's Child:**
See Part I, *Mendelian Inheritance.*

**Age of Detectability:** Cord blood can be used to assay for TC II.

**Gene Mapping and Linkage:** TCN2 (transcobalamin II; macrocytic anemia) has been mapped to 22q.

**Prevention:** None known. Genetic counseling indicated.

**Treatment:** Pharmacologic doses of cyanocobalamin or hydroxycobalamin completely correct the defect. Cobalamin circulates in plasma either free or bound to albumin and reaches tissues in adequate levels. Lifetime treatment is required. Most patients have been treated with intramuscular cobalamins. A single patient has been maintained exclusively on oral hydroxycobalamin but there are theoretical concerns about this approach. Treated patients grow and develop normally.

**Prognosis:** With prompt diagnosis and treatment, life span is normal. Delayed diagnosis or inadvertent administration of folate may result in neurologic impairment or mental retardation.

**Detection of Carrier:** Heterozygotes will have 50% of the immunologic or functional TC II detectable in normal individuals.

**References:**
Hakami N, et al.: Neonatal megaloblastic anemia due to inherited transcobalamin II deficiency in two siblings. New Engl J Med 1971; 285:1163–1170. *
Hitzig WH: Hereditary transcobalamin-II deficiency: clinical findings in a new family. J Pediatr 1974; 85:622–628.
Seligman PA, et al.: Studies of a patient with megaloblastic anemia and an abnormal transcobalamin II. New Engl J Med 1980; 303:1209–1212.
Hall CA: Congenital disorders of vitamin B12 transport and their contributions to concepts. Yale J Biol Med 1981; 54:485–495.
Meyers PA, Carmel R: Hereditary transcobalamin II deficiency with subnormal serum cobalamin levels. Pediatrics 1984; 74:866–871.
Rosenblatt DS, et al.: Expression of transcobalamin II by amniocytes. Prenatal Diag 1987; 7:35–39.

ME040                                                          **Paul Meyers**

**Transcobalamin II, hereditary abnormal**
*See TRANSCOBALAMIN II DEFICIENCY*
**Transcortin deficiency**
*See STEROID, BINDING GLOBULIN ABNORMALITIES*
**Transformation gene:ONC:MYC**
*See LYMPHOMA, BURKITT TYPE*
**Transformational migraine**
*See MIGRAINE*
**Transfusion, twin-to-twin**
*See FETAL MONOZYGOUS MULTIPLE PREGNANCY DYSPLACENTATION EFFECTS*
**Transient migraine accompaniments**
*See MIGRAINE*
**Translocase 1 deficiency**
*See GLYCOGENOSIS, TYPE Ib*
**Translocase 2 deficiency**
*See GLYCOGENOSIS, TYPE Ic*
**Transport defect involving folate malabsorption**
*See FOLATE MALABSORPTION*

## TRANSPORT, RENAL, DEFECTS OF                      1501

**Includes:** Renal transport defects

The human body is composed of organs and systems. They, in turn, contain cells that have subcellular compartments. Membranes delineate these different spaces. Chemical composition differs in each membrane-defined compartment. Control of the molecular traffic across membranes is one mechanism by which specific composition of particular compartments is achieved.

Disorders of transfer across plasma membranes are more common, but there are confirmed Mendelian disorders affecting transport across *intra*cellular membranes. **Cystinosis, Salla Disease**, and a form of Vitamin B12-dependent methylmalonic aciduria each have impaired lysosomal efflux; of cystine (the disulfide), sialic acid, and free cobalamin (cblF complementation group) respec-

tively. **Glycogenosis, Type Ib** is a disorder of glucose-6-phosphate transfer across endoplasmic reticulum.

Transmembrane transport of molecules is accomplished by several processes that achieve and maintain the distributions of freely soluble substances on opposite sides of membranes. Diffusion does not do this; gated channels, ion gradient or voltage-coupled carriers, and receptor-mediated endocytotic processes can. The ability of mediated processes to recognize specific ions, substrates, and ligands is a function of their macromolecular component(s). Their specificity is determined by the genes that encode the polypeptide component of the transporter or channel. It follows that mutations at loci coding for structural components of transport systems may modify the associated functions (inborn errors of transport).

As a general principle, mutations affecting brush-border membrane systems are not expressed in parenchymal cells. On the other hand, basolateral membrane transporters in epithelial cells and plasma membrane transporters of parenchymal cells serve homologous functions (fluxes between extracellular and intracellular fluids), and one might expect a mutation affecting a carrier in the basolateral membrane to be expressed also in parenchymal cells (and vice versa). The defect in efflux on the cationic amino acid carrier in lysinuric-protein intolerance is an example: the mutant phenotype is expressed in basolateral membranes of kidney and small intestine and the plasma membrane of skin fibroblasts.

A major stimulus for the recognition of "inborn errors of transport" was awareness first of renal glucosuria and then of various renal hyperaminoacidurias. Many renal transport disorders have counterparts in intestinal absorption. Refinements in the classification of renal transport systems lead to a topologic view of transport systems in the nephron. Systems in brush-border and basolateral membranes have different roles to play and different specificities for substrates. Systems in convoluted and straight segments of proximal nephron are likely to have different properties, even when they transport the same substrate or group of substrates (see Table 1501–1). The relative importance of the transport system in the maintenance of metabolic homeostasis determines the extent of the phenotypic effect of the mutation affecting it.

A partial classification of mendelian disorders of membrane transport is given in Tables 1501–1 and 1501–2. Most of the phenotypes listed are disorders of carriers and channels for low-molecular weight organic substrates and ions.

**References:**
Scriver CR, et al, eds: The metabolic basis of inherited disease, 6th ed. New York: McGraw-Hill, 1989:

SC050                                                    **Charles R. Scriver**

**Transposition of great vessels**
*See HEART, TRANSPOSITION OF GREAT VESSELS*
**Transposition of liver**
*See LIVER, TRANSPOSITION*
**Transsuccinylase (E2) deficiency**
*See ACIDEMIA, 2-OXOGLUTARIC*
**Transthyretin (prealbumin) Ala-60 amyloidosis**
*See AMYLOIDOSIS, APPALACHIAN TYPE*
**Transthyretin (prealbumin) Ile-33 and/or Gly-49**
*See AMYLOIDOSIS, ASHKENAZI TYPE*
**Transthyretin (prealbumin) met-111 amyloidosis**
*See AMYLOIDOSIS, DANISH CARDIAC TYPE*
**Transthyretin (prealbumin) Tyr-77 amyloidosis**
*See AMYLOIDOSIS, ILLINOIS TYPE*
**Transthyretin abnormality**
*See AMYLOIDOSIS, TRANSTHYRETIN METHIONINE-30 TYPE*
**Transthyretin amyloidoses**
*See AMYLOIDOSES*
**Transthyretin-84 isoleucine-to-serine**
*See AMYLOIDOSIS, INDIANA TYPE*
**Transverse crease, single**
*See SKIN CREASE, SINGLE PALMAR*
**Transverse terminal defects of limb**
*See AMNIOTIC BANDS SYNDROME*
**Transverse vaginal septum**
*See VAGINAL SEPTUM, TRANSVERSE*

**Table 1501·1** Mendelian Disorders of Amino Acid Transport

| Name | Amino Acid Affected | Kidney Site (Putative)[a] Segment[b] | Kidney Site (Putative)[a] Membrane[c] | Other organs | Inheritance |
|---|---|---|---|---|---|
| Classical **Cystinuria** | Cystine, Lysine Ornithine, Arginine | PS | BBM | Intestine (some pedigrees) | AR (incompletely recessive for some alleles) |
| Isolated **Cystinuria** | Cyst(e)ine | PC | BBM | | AR |
| **Hyperdibasic aminoaciduria**-1 | Lysine, Ornithine, Arginine | PC | BBM | Intestine | AD |
| **Hyperdibasic aminoaciduria**-2 | Lysine, Ornithine, Arginine | PC/PS | BLM | Fibroblast Intestine Liver(?) | AR |
| **Hyperlysinuria, isolated** | Lysine | PS(?) | BBM(?) | Intestine | AR |
| **Hartnup disorder** | Neutrals (excluding iminoacids & glycine) | PC | BBM | Intestine | AR |
| Familial **Iminoglycinuria** | Proline, Hydroxyproline, Glycine | PC(?) | BBM(?) | Intestine | AR (incompletely recessive for some alleles) |
| Isolated **Histidinuria** | Histidine | PS(?) | BBM(?) | Intestine (some pedigrees) | AR |
| **Aciduria, dicarboxylic aminoaciduria** | Glutamic & aspartic acids | PC | BBM | | AR |
| **Methionine malabsorption** | Methionine | | | Intestine | AR(?) |
| **Tryptophan malabsorption** | Tryptophan | | | Intestine | AR(?) |
| **Cystinosis** | Cystine (disulphide) | | | Lysosome (efflux) | AR |
| Fanconi Syndrome(s) Primary & Secondary forms[d] | Amino acids (all), other organic substrates and electrolytes | PC,PS(?) BBM, BLM? | | | AR (many loci) |

[a]Site refers to proximal nephron segment (convoluted or straight) and membrane (brush-border or basolateral). In no case has there been confirmation by direct measurement of site affected.
[b]PC, proximal convoluted segment; PS, proximal straight segment.
[c]BBM, brush-border membrane; BLM, basolateral membrane.
[d]Fanconi syndromes (secondary Mendelian forms) include **Cystinosis, Fructose-1-phosphate aldolase deficiency, Galactosemia, Tyrosinemia, Hepatolenticular degeneration, Oculo-cerebro-renal syndrome,** and **Rickets, Vitamin D-dependent, type I.**

**Table 1501·2** Other Mendelian Disorders of Membrane Transport

| Name | Substrate Affected | Tissue Affected | Inheritance |
|---|---|---|---|
| Renal **glycosuria** | Glucose | Kidney (PC?[a]) | AR (multiple alleles) |
| **Glucose-galactose malabsorption** | Glucose, galactose | Kidney (PS?) Intestine | AR |
| **Salla disease** | Sialic acid | Lysosome (efflux) | AR |
| **Glycogenosis, Type I** | Glucose-6-P | Endoplasmic reticulum (?) | AR |
| **Renal hypouricemia** | Uric acid | Kidney (Proximal & distal tubule sites) | AR (multiple loci?, alleles) |
| **Hypophosphatemia, X-linked** | Phosphate | i. Kidney, (bone?) ii. Kidney, inner ear, (bone?) | XL Dominant (2 loci)[b] |
| **Hypophosphatemia, non X-linked** | Phosphate | Kidney | AD (and AR) (alleles?) |
| **Bartter Syndrome** | Chloride (primary) Potassium (secondary) | Kidney (Henle loop, thick ascending limb?) | AR |
| **Hypomagnesemia, primary** | Mg$^{2+}$ | Kidney, intestine | AR & XLD forms |
| **Renal tubular acidosis** | H$^+$ | Kidney (distal tubule) | AD |
| **Renal bicarbonate reabsorptive defect** | HCO$_3^-$ | Kidney (Proximal tubule) | XLD AR (forms) (various loci? & alleles?) |
| **Thyroid, iodide transport defect** | I$^-$ | Thyroid, salivary glands | AR |
| **Diarrhea, congenital chloride** | Cl$^-$ | Intestine | AR |
| **Diabetes insipidus, vasopressin resistant** | H$_2$O | Kidney (collecting duct) | XLR |
| **Hypercholesteremia** | LDL-Cholesterol | Parenchymal cells (Plasma membrane receptor) | AD |
| **Vitamin B(12) malabsorption** | Vitamin B$_{12}$ | Intestine | AR |
| **Vitamin B(12) lysosomal transport defect** | Free B$_{12}$ | Lysosome (efflux) | AR |
| **Folate malabsorption** | Folic acid | Intestine, (other tissues?) | AR |
| **Myopathy-metabolic, carnitine deficiency** | Carnitine | Kidney (other tissues?) | AR |

[a]PC, PS: See Table 1501-1
[b]Corresponding loci in mouse are *Hyp* and *Gy*.

**Tranxene**△**, fetal effects**
   *See FETAL BENZODIAZEPINE EFFECTS*
**Trapezoidocephaly-synostosis syndrome**
   *See ANTLEY-BIXLER SYNDROME*
**Treacher Collins syndrome**
   *See MANDIBULOFACIAL DYSOSTOSIS*
**Treacher Collins-Franceschetti syndrome**
   *See MANDIBULOFACIAL DYSOSTOSIS*
**Treacher Collins mandibulofacial dysostosis, recessive type**
   *See MANDIBULOFACIAL DYSOSTOSIS, TREACHER-COLLINS TYPE, RECESSIVE*
**Tremor, benign essential**
   *See TREMOR, HEREDOFAMILIAL*

## TREMOR, HEREDOFAMILIAL       0964

**Includes:**  Tremor, benign essential

**Excludes:**
   **Hepatolenticular degeneration** (0469)
   **Huntington disease** (0478)
   **Multiple sclerosis, familial** (2598)
   Parkinson disease
   **Tremor-duodenal ulcer syndrome** (0963)

**Major Diagnostic Criteria:**  A symmetric familial tremor is present in an otherwise healthy individual in whom medical and neurologic causes of the tremor have been excluded.

**Clinical Findings:**  The tremor is most commonly noted between the ages of 40 and 50 years. Although rarely documented at the age extremes, essential tremor may begin in the neonate and the elderly. The tremor begins in the hands and arms in a symmetric fashion. It then may involve the facial muscles and tongue. When the tremor involves the head and neck, it has been termed "senile" tremor. If severe, dysarthria may result. The trunk and legs are least commonly involved. The tremor is more pronounced during movement and maintenance of postures against gravity, diminishes at rest and disappears during sleep. Fatigue and emotion may enhance the tremor, and alcohol may relieve it. The tremor is of variable amplitude; the frequency is 3–12 per second. The tremor may be progressive or remain unchanged throughout life. Remissions are rare. There are no associated neurologic signs in the majority of patients.

**Complications:**  Approximately 20% eventually develop rigidity of varying degrees.

**Associated Findings:**  None known.

**Etiology:**  Autosomal dominant inheritance with complete penetrance by the age of 70.

**Pathogenesis:**  Many theories have been advanced: 1) autosomal dominant tremor is a monosymptomatic form of Parkinson disease. Larsson and Sjögren's large study (1960) did not support this view; 2) Minor (1936) suggested the tremor was a triad which included fecundity and longevity. 3) More recent experimental studies have suggested an abnormality of monoamines in the rubro-olivo-cerebello-rubral tracts. No consistent neuropathology has been described.

**MIM No.:**  *19030

**Sex Ratio:**  M1:F1

**Occurrence:**  In Sweden, it has been estimated that the gene frequency is 1:10,000. In the parish of Xa-sjö, the gene frequency approaches 1:22.

**Risk of Recurrence for Patient's Sib:**
   See Part I, *Mendelian Inheritance.*

**Risk of Recurrence for Patient's Child:**
   See Part I, *Mendelian Inheritance.*

**Age of Detectability:**  Tremor is usually evident by the fifth decade of life.

**Gene Mapping and Linkage:**  Unknown.

**Prevention:**  None known. Genetic counseling indicated.

**Treatment:**  If tremor is severe, appropriate job placement may be helpful. Most patients with autosomal dominant tremor do not seek medical advice. Many patients report that the tremor is mitigated by ethanol. Propanolol, a β-adrenergic blocking agent, and primidone may be effective. The primidone effect is felt to be from a metabolite, phenylethylmalonamide.

**Prognosis:**  Good for life span. Function affected by degree of tremor and rigidity.

**Detection of Carrier:**  Unknown.

**References:**

Minor L: Heredo-familiare nervenkrankheiten ohne anatomischen befundi: das erbleiche zittern. In: Bumke O, Foerster O, eds: handbuch der neurologie. Berlin: Springer, 1936; 16:974–1005.

Critchley M: Observations on essential heredofamilial tremor. Brain 1949; 72:113–139.

Larsson M, Sjögren H: Essential tremor: a clinical and genetic population study. Acta Psychiatry Scand 1960; 144 (Suppl 36):1–176.

Marshall J: Observations on essential tremor. J Neurol Neurosurg Psychiatry 1962; 25:112–125.

Vanasse M, et al.: Shuddering attacks in children: an early clinical manifestation of essential tremor. Neurology 1976; 26:1027–1030.

O'Brien MD, et al.: Benign familial tremor treated with primidone. Br Med J 1981; 282:178–180.

HA053               **Robert H.A. Haslam**
MC035               **Ross McLeod**

## TREMOR-DUODENAL ULCER SYNDROME    0963

**Includes:**
   Duodenal ulcer-tremor syndrome
   Tremor-nystagmus-duodenal ulcer

**Excludes:**
   **Narcolepsy** (3287)
   Tremor of head-nystagmus
   **Tremor, heredofamilial** (0964)
   Tremor of limbs-nystagmus
   Tremor of other etiology

**Major Diagnostic Criteria:**  Slowly progressive "essential" tremor, "congenital" nystagmus, and duodenal ulceration.

**Clinical Findings:**  Nystagmus is present from birth or is noted in childhood (4–8 years). Rotary nystagmus occurs at rest, intensified by lateral gaze, and accompanied by refractive errors. Slowly progressive tremor starts in childhood, but more often after puberty, involving fingers, hands, shoulders, and head; it is increased with fatigue or emotional upset, but temporarily alleviated by alcohol. Signs of cerebellar dysfunction may be present, i.e., slight ataxia, unsteadiness, incoordination, and clumsiness. Symptoms and signs of duodenal ulceration usually appear later in life but may precede the neurologic syndrome. Unusual need for sleep, with a narcolepsy-like propensity for falling asleep, is noted in some patients.

**Complications:**  Complaints and bleeding from duodenal ulceration. Physical handicap from increasing tremor and from cerebellar dysfunction. Social and mental deterioration because of alcoholism and physical disability have been reported.

**Associated Findings:**  None known.

**Etiology:**  Autosomal dominant inheritance with fairly uniform expressivity. In a few patients, partial manifestations were noted.

**Pathogenesis:**  The presence of cerebellar signs in severely affected persons may point to a possible pathogenetic relationship to the genetic cerebellar atrophies. The combination of neurologic dysfunction, duodenal ulceration, and narcolepsy is explained by some disturbance of the autonomic nervous system.

**MIM No.:**  *19031

**POS No.:**  4166

**Sex Ratio:**  M2:F1 (observed in the family reported)

**Occurrence:**  The syndrome was reported in a family of Swedish-Finnish descent.

**Risk of Recurrence for Patient's Sib:**
   See Part I, *Mendelian Inheritance.*

**Risk of Recurrence for Patient's Child:**
See Part I, *Mendelian Inheritance.*

**Age of Detectability:** In childhood or adolescence.

**Gene Mapping and Linkage:** Unknown.

**Prevention:** None known. Genetic counseling indicated.

**Treatment:** Dietary treatment and surgery for duodenal ulceration; prevention of alcoholism; physiotherapy.

**Prognosis:** Life expectancy usually is normal; the neurologic syndrome is slowly progressive. Some patients are incapacitated early in life by tremor and ataxia.

**Detection of Carrier:** Possibly by clinical examination of first degree relatives.

**References:**
Neuhäuser G, et al.: Essential tremor, nystagmus and duodenal ulceration. a "new" dominantly inherited condition. Clin Genet 1976; 9:81–91.
Rotter JL, Rimoin DL: The genetic syndromology of peptic ulcer. Am J Med Genet 1981; 10:315–321.

NE012                                          **Gerhard Neuhäuser**

**Tremor-nystagmus-duodenal ulcer**
*See TREMOR-DUODENAL ULCER SYNDROME*
**Trevor disease**
*See DYSPLASIA EPIPHYSEALIS HEMIMELICA*
**Triazolam, fetal effects**
*See FETAL BENZODIAZEPINE EFFECTS*
**Trichloroethylene induced scleroderma**
*See SCLERODERMA, FAMILIAL PROGRESSIVE*

---

**TRICHO-DENTO-OSSEOUS SYNDROME**                         **0965**

**Includes:**
    Bone-hair-nail-tooth dysplasia
    Enamel hypoplasia-taurodontism-tight hair-cortical
        sclerosteosis
    Hair-bone-nail-tooth dysplasia
    Nail-hair-bone-tooth dysplasia
    Tooth-hair-bone-nail dysplasia

**Excludes:**
    **Amelo-onycho-hypohidrotic syndrome** (0045)
    **CHANDS** (3039)
    **Tricho-dermodysplasia-dental defects** (2903)
    **Tricho-odonto-onychial dysplasia** (2889)

**Major Diagnostic Criteria:** Enamel dysplasia, taurodontism (see **Teeth, taurodontism**), excessively curly hair in infancy, and excessively radiodense bones.

**Clinical Findings:** The enamel of both primary and secondary teeth is thin, soft, and yellowish brown in color. The molars are taurodont in form. Tooth eruption may be delayed or some teeth may be congenitally missing. The teeth have large pulp chambers and often become abscessed within the first years of life.

The hair in infancy is curly but not woolly, and the lashes and eyebrows are long. In some cases the hair tends to straighten with age. The nails are thin and show splitting of the superficial layers; sometimes only a few toenails show the defect.

Multiple fractures due to sclerosis of cortical bone occurs in about 30% of cases. The base of the skull, mastoids, and zones of provisional calcification in the long bones are the areas most commonly involved.

**Complications:** Attrition of teeth, with exposure of pulps and abscess formation and premature loss of teeth.

**Associated Findings:** Mandibular prognathism and a shallow nasal bridge is found in some families.

**Etiology:** Autosomal dominant inheritance. Three variants have been documented.

**Pathogenesis:** A defect in ectodermal cells involving the morpho-differentiation of tooth, hair, and nail form and structure.

**MIM No.:** *19032

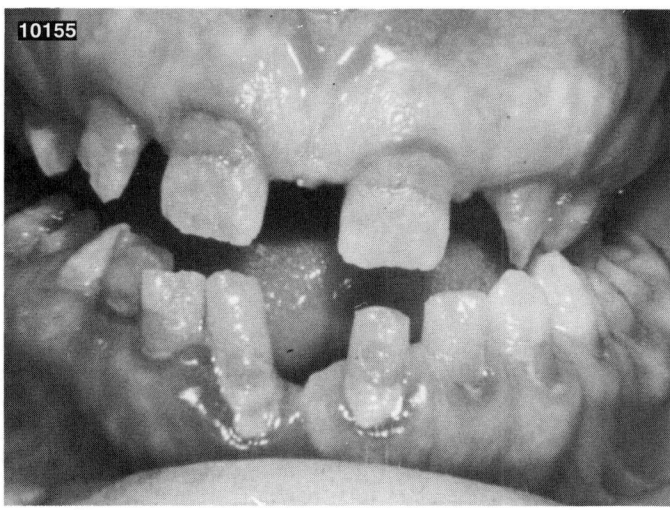

0965-10155:   Enamel dysplasia.

---

**POS No.:**   3414

**Sex Ratio:**   M1:F1

**Occurrence:** About a dozen kindreds reported; some possibly of Irish extraction.

**Risk of Recurrence for Patient's Sib:**
See Part I, *Mendelian Inheritance.*

**Risk of Recurrence for Patient's Child:**
See Part I, *Mendelian Inheritance.*

**Age of Detectability:** At six months to one year of age, at tooth eruption.

**Gene Mapping and Linkage:** Unknown.

**Prevention:** None known. Genetic counseling indicated.

**Treatment:** Early restoration of teeth, and prosthetic replacement of lost or congenitally missing teeth.

**Prognosis:** Does not affect life span. Premature loss of teeth in untreated case.

**Detection of Carrier:** Mildly affected individuals may be found by clinical examination.

**Special Considerations:** The features that differentiate the three types of tricho-dento-osseous (TDO) syndrome are that the long bones are predominantly involved in TDO-I, the cranial bones are predominantly involved in TDO-III, while both are involved in TDO-II. Furthermore, the hair is woolly and easily detachable in TDO-II.

**References:**
Robinson GC, et al.: Hereditary enamel hypoplasia: its association with characteristic hair structure. Pediatrics 1966; 37:498–502.
Lichtenstein J, et al.: The tricho-dento-osseous (TDO) syndrome. Am J Hum Genet 1972; 24:569–582. * †
Jorgenson RJ, Warson RW: Dental anomalies in the trich-dento-osseous syndrome. Oral Surg 1973; 36:693–700. †
Quattromani F, et al.: Clinical heterogeneity in the tricho-dento-osseous syndrome. Hum Genet 1983; 64:116–121.
Shapiro SD, et al.: Tricho-dento-osseous syndrome: heterogeneity or clinical variability. Am J Med Genet 1983; 16:225–236. *

J0027                                      **Ronald J. Jorgenson**
                                           *Hermine M. Pashayan*

## TRICHO-DERMODYSPLASIA-DENTAL DEFECTS          2903

**Includes:**
Dental defects-trichodermodysplasia
Ectodermal dysplasia, tricho-dermodysplasia-dental defects
Trichodermodysplasia-dental alterations

**Excludes:**
**Dermo-odontodysplasia** (2763)
**Ectodermal dysplasia** (anhidrotic types)
**Ectodermal dysplasia, hidrotic** (0334)
**Odonto-onychodermal dysplasia** (2618)

**Major Diagnostic Criteria:** Trichodysplasia, dental anomalies, and skin alterations.

**Clinical Findings:** Fine, dry, slow-growing, brittle, and lusterless hair; generalized hypotrichosis; delayed eruption of deciduous teeth; hypodontia of both dentitions; small and peg-shaped upper central incisors; recurrent epistaxis; palmoplantar keratosis; facial wens; café-au-lait spots on the back; and bilateral inward (tibial) deflection of the fourth toes.

**Complications:** Unknown.

**Associated Findings:** Dystrophic toenails; partial absence of the alveolar wall of the mandible (one patient); and retroverted uterus (one patient).

**Etiology:** Autosomal dominant or possibly X-linked dominant inheritance. A mother and her only two children (one girl and one boy) were described.

**Pathogenesis:** Defective formation of several derivatives of the embryonic ectoderm suggests that this condition must be classified as an ectodermal dysplasia.

**POS No.:** 4226

**Sex Ratio:** Presumably M1:F1; M1:F2 observed.

**Occurrence:** Three members of one Brazilian family have been documented.

**Risk of Recurrence for Patient's Sib:**
See Part I, *Mendelian Inheritance.*

**Risk of Recurrence for Patient's Child:**
See Part I, *Mendelian Inheritance.*

**Age of Detectability:** During childhood, by physical examination.

**Gene Mapping and Linkage:** Unknown.

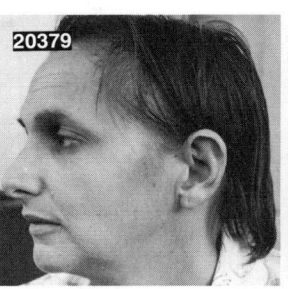
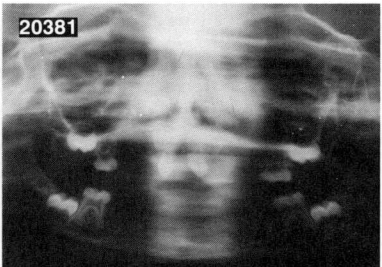
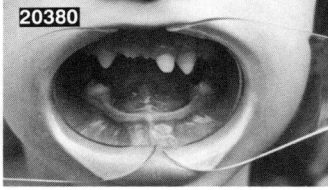
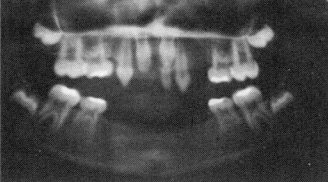

**2903-20379:** Affected woman at 36 years of age; note scalp hypotrichosis, sparse eyebrows (especially the distal 2/3), and facial wens. **20381:** Orthopantomogram of an affected boy at 4 years of age. **20380:** Oral findings in an affected girl at age 7 years.

**Prevention:** None known. Genetic counseling indicated.

**Treatment:** Prosthetic replacement and orthodontic treatment.

**Prognosis:** Life span is not affected.

**Detection of Carrier:** Unknown.

**Special Considerations:** The vertebral problems presented by the mother do not seem to be a part of the condition, since they are also present in her own mother but not in the other members of the kindred.

**References:**
Freire-Maia N: Ectodermal dysplasias. Hum Hered 1971; 21:309–312.
Freire-Maia N: Ectodermal dysplasias revisited. Acta Genet Med Gemellol 1977; 26:121–131.
Freire-Maia DV, et al.: Tricodermodisplasia com alterações dentárias. Ciênc Cult (suppl) 1985; 37:746.
Pinheiro M, et al.: Trichodermodysplasia with dental alterations: an apparently new genetic ectodermal dysplasia of the tricho-odonto-onychial subgroup. Clin Genet 1986; 29:332–336.

PI008                                            **Marta Pinheiro**

## TRICHO-ODONTO-ONYCHIAL DYSPLASIA          2889

**Includes:** Ectodermal dysplasia, tricho-odonto-onychial type

**Excludes:**
**Ectodermal dysplasia, Christ-Siemens-Touraine type** (0333)
**Ectodermal dysplasia, hidrotic** (0334)
**Odonto-onychodysplasia-alopecia** (2890)
**Tricho-dermodysplasia-dental defects** (2903)

**Major Diagnostic Criteria:** Alopecia at the parietal region, generalized hypotrichosis, dental abnormalities, onychodystrophy, and skin alterations.

**Clinical Findings:** Dry, brittle, and sparse scalp hair at the temporal and occipital regions; alopecia at the parietal region; scanty eyebrows, eyelashes, and axillary and pubic hair; enamel hypoplasia leading to secondary anodontia; dystrophic finger- and toenails; yellowish or brownish toenails; extranumerary nipples; dermatoglyphics with palmar and digital ridge dissociation; palmoplantar keratosis; xeroderma on limbs; pigmented nevi; ephelides, actinic keratosis, papules, and crusts on scalp; skull deficiency (6 x 8 cm) in the frontoparietal region of one patient.

**Complications:** Psychologic problems due to partial alopecia; feeding problems due to dental loss.

**Associated Findings:** None known.

**Etiology:** Probably autosomal recessive inheritance.

**Pathogenesis:** Defective formation of several derivatives of the embryonic ectoderm suggests that this condition must be classified as an ectodermal dysplasia.

**MIM No.:** 27545

**POS No.:** 3603

**Sex Ratio:** Presumably M1:F1; M0:F4 observed.

**Occurrence:** Four sisters in one Brazilian sibship of 13 have been documented.

**Risk of Recurrence for Patient's Sib:**
See Part I, *Mendelian Inheritance.*

**Risk of Recurrence for Patient's Child:**
See Part I, *Mendelian Inheritance.*

**Age of Detectability:** At birth, by physical examination.

**Gene Mapping and Linkage:** Unknown.

**Prevention:** None known. Genetic counseling indicated.

**Treatment:** Early aggressive dental care to reduce spread of caries and avoid decay; wigs are cosmetically and psychologically helpful. Skull deficiency in one patient required plastic surgery, skin grafts, and flap rotation of skin.

**Prognosis:** Normal for life span.

**Detection of Carrier:** Unknown.

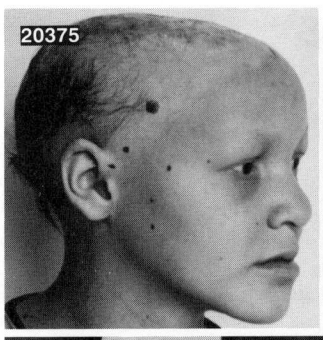
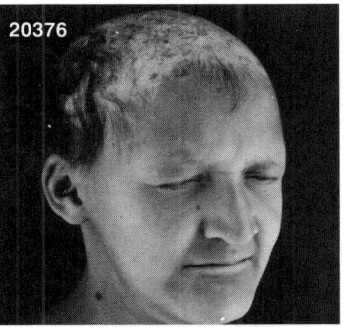
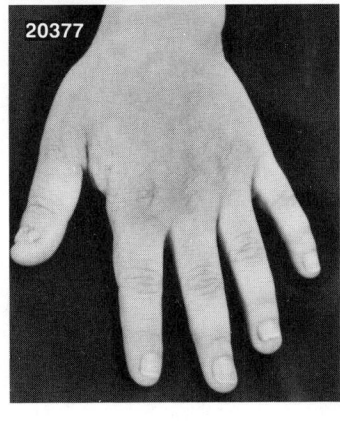
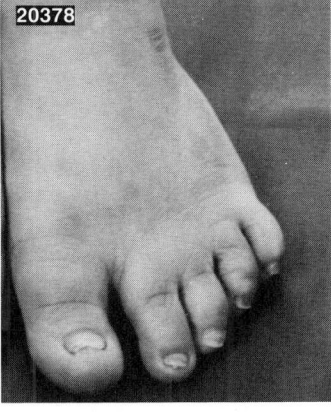

**2889**-20375: Affected 16-year-old female; note the extensive area of alopecia on the top of the head with only a peripheral fringe of hair in the temporal and occipital regions. She had a skull deficiency that measured 6 × 8 cm in the fronto-parietal region which was also traumatically altered. Note also the absence of eyebrows and lashes, mandibular prognathism, and a large number of pigmented nevi. 20376: Affected 22-year-old woman; note central alopecia with hypotrichosis of the peripheral fringe, eyebrows, and lashes as well as ephelides, actinic keratosis, papules and crusts on the scalp. 20377: Dystrophic nails. 20378: Dystrophic toenails.

**References:**
Pinheiro M, et al.: Trichodontoonychial dysplasia: a new meso-ectodermal dysplasia. Am J Med Genet 1983; 15:67–70.

PI008            **Marta Pinheiro**

**Tricho-onycho-dysplasia-neutropenia**
*See ONYCHO-TRICHODYSPLASIA-NEUTROPENIA*

## TRICHO-ONYCHODYSPLASIA-XERODERMA      2892

**Includes:**
Ectodermal dysplasia, tricho-onychodysplasia-xeroderma type
Onycho-trichodysplasia-xeroderma
Xeroderma-tricho-onychodysplasia

**Excludes:**
**Ectodermal dysplasia, hidrotic** (0334)
**Odonto-onychodysplasia-alopecia** (2890)
**Tricho-dermodysplasia-dental defects** (2903)
**Trichodysplasia-xeroderma** (2894)

**Major Diagnostic Criteria:** Hair and nail alterations, and xeroderma.

**Clinical Findings:** Absent hair and nails at birth, but normal hair later; dystrophic fingernails and toenails; mild-to-severe generalized xeroderma with permanent and abundant scaling over the entire body; tendency to fissures in hands and feet.

**Complications:** Psychologic problems due to skin alterations.

**Associated Findings:** None known.

**Etiology:** Probably autosomal recessive inheritance. Parental consanguinity has been noted.

**Pathogenesis:** Defective formation of some derivatives of the embryonic ectoderm and absence of malformations show that this condition is a pure ectodermal dysplasia.

**Sex Ratio:** Presumably M1:F1.

**Occurrence:** One Caucasian Brazilian 23-year-old boy belonging to a sibship of five from nonconsanguineous parents has been reported. One of his sisters, who died at age three months, was reported to have been equally affected. He also has a first and second cousin, the daughter of first cousins, who was reported more severely affected.

**Risk of Recurrence for Patient's Sib:**
See Part I, *Mendelian Inheritance.*

**Risk of Recurrence for Patient's Child:**
See Part I, *Mendelian Inheritance.*

**Age of Detectability:** At birth, by physical examination.

**Gene Mapping and Linkage:** Unknown.

**Prevention:** None known. Genetic counseling indicated.

**Treatment:** Avoidance of exposure to the sun, ordinary xeroderma care.

**Prognosis:** Normal life span.

**Detection of Carrier:** The mother of two affected individuals presented discrete xeroderma.

**References:**
Freire-Maia N, et al.: Trichoonychodysplasia with xeroderma: an apparently hitherto undescribed pure ectodermal dysplasia. Rev Bras Genet 1985; 8:775–778.

PI008            **Marta Pinheiro**

**Tricho-rhino-auriculo-phalangeal multiple exostoses dysplasia**
*See TRICHO-RHINO-PHALANGEAL SYNDROME, TYPE II*
**Tricho-rhino-phalangeal syndrome, dominant type I**
*See TRICHO-RHINO-PHALANGEAL SYNDROME, TYPE I*
**Tricho-rhino-phalangeal syndrome, recessive form**
*See TRICHO-RHINO-PHALANGEAL SYNDROME, TYPE I*

## TRICHO-RHINO-PHALANGEAL SYNDROME, TYPE I      0966

**Includes:**
Tricho-rhino-phalangeal syndrome, dominant type I
Tricho-rhino-phalangeal syndrome, recessive form

**Excludes:**
Dysostosis, other forms of radiographic peripheral
**Tricho-rhino-phalangeal syndrome, type II** (0967)
**Tricho-rhino-phalangeal syndrome, type III** (2847)

**Major Diagnostic Criteria:** Short stature, with deformities of the joints of the fingers and hands, characteristic X-ray changes, sparse scalp hair, pear-shaped nose, and long philtrum.

**Clinical Findings:** Short stature (variable: adult heights have ranged from 99 cm for females to 162 cm for males). Sparse, slowly growing scalp hair; eyebrows heavier medially than laterally; long philtrum; and a pear-shaped nose (of variable severity). There is usually a deformity at the proximal interphalangeal (IP) joints of hands.

*X-ray findings:* Cone-shaped epiphyses of phalanges, with ivory epiphyses (in 75%); premature fusion of involved epiphyses to the shaft. There is a scattered pattern of involvement, with middle phalanges most commonly involved. The metacarpals may be short (frontal projection). No abnormal laboratory findings.

**Complications:** Thin hair, crooked fingers, and misshaped nose may be of cosmetic concern to affected individual, especially females. **Hip, osteonecrosis, capital femoral epiphysis** has been reported and several adults, with compatible residual deformity.

**Associated Findings:** Progressive arthritic changes of the dorsal spine, elbows, and fingers may occur in midlife.

**Etiology:** Usually autosomal dominant inheritance with great variability of expression, but autosomal recessive inheritance has also been reported. Recent reports have documented complex

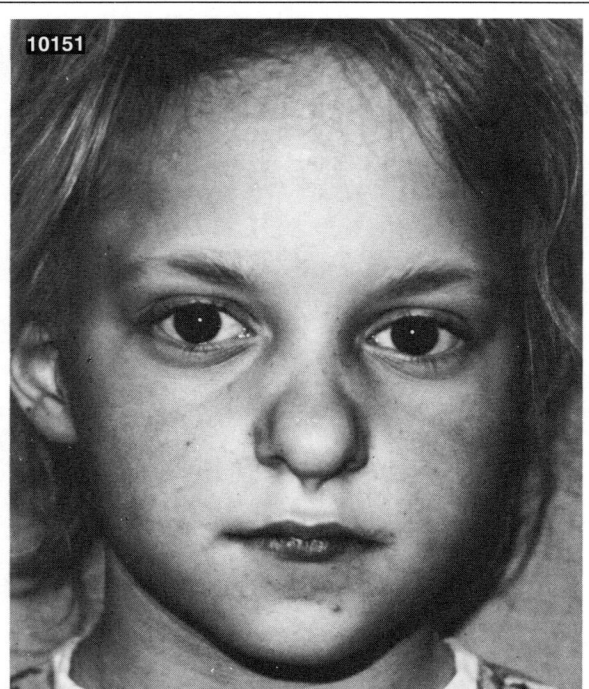

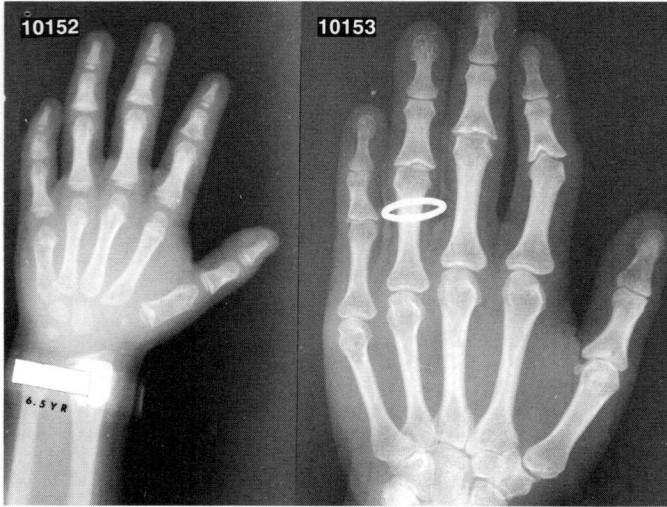

**0966-10151:** Typical facies with bulbous, pear-shaped nose with prominent philtrum. **10152:** Typical cone and ivory epiphyses in child's X-ray. **10153:** In adult, some residual deformity from old cones.

chromosomal rearrangements which have been linked to a deleted segment; 8q24.12 (Buhler et al, 1987).

**Pathogenesis:** Unknown.

**MIM No.:** *19035, 27550

**POS No.:** 3415

**Sex Ratio:** Presumably M1:F1.

**Occurrence:** Over a dozen kindreds have been reported, including several of Japanese extraction.

**Risk of Recurrence for Patient's Sib:**
See Part I, *Mendelian Inheritance.*

**Risk of Recurrence for Patient's Child:**
See Part I, *Mendelian Inheritance.*

**Age of Detectability:** In late childhood, by a combination of X-ray and clinical methods.

**Gene Mapping and Linkage:** A link to 8q24.12 has been suggested (Buhler et al, 1987).

**Prevention:** None known. Genetic counseling indicated.

**Treatment:** A wig, if thin hair is of concern to the affected individual. Treatment for **Hip, osteonecrosis, capital femoral epiphysis** if this occurs.

**Prognosis:** Normal life span.

**Detection of Carrier:** Possibly by clinical examination of first degree relatives.

**References:**

Giedion A: Cone-shaped epiphyses of the hands and their diagnostic value: the tricho-rhino-phalangeal syndrome. Ann Radiol (Paris) 1967; 10:322–329.

Giedion A, et al.: Autosomal dominant transmission of the tricho-rhino-phalangeal syndrome. Helv Paediat Acta 1973; 28:249–259.

Pashayan H, et al.: The tricho-rhino-phalangeal syndrome. Am J Dis Child 1974; 127:257–261.

McCloud DJ, Solomon LM: The tricho-rhino-phalangeal syndrome. Brit J Derm 1977; 96:403–407.

Peltola J, Kuokkanen K: Tricho-rhino-phalangeal syndrome in five succesive generations: report on a family in Finland. Acta Derm Venerol 1978; 58:65–68.

Sugiura Y: Tricho-rhino-phalangeal syndrome associated with Perthes-disease-like bone change and spondylolisthesis. Jpn J Hum Genet 1978; 23:23–30.

Ferrandez A, et al.: The trichorhinophalangeal syndrome: report of 4 familial cases belonging to 4 generations. Helv Paediat Acta 1980; 35:559–567.

Howell CJ, Wynne-Davies R: The tricho-rhino-phalangeal syndrome: a report of 14 cases in 7 kindreds. J Bone Joint Surg 1986; 68B:311–314.

Buhler EM, et al.: A final word on the tricho-rhino-phalangeal syndromes. Clin Genet 1987; 31:273–275.

B0025
LA016

**Zvi Borochowitz**
**Leonard O. Langer, Jr.**
*David L. Rimoin*

---

## TRICHO-RHINO-PHALANGEAL SYNDROME, TYPE II          0967

**Includes:**
>    Acrodysplasia with exostoses
>    Giedion-Langer syndrome
>    Langer-Giedion syndrome
>    Tricho-rhino-auriculo-phalangeal multiple exostoses dysplasia

**Excludes:**
**Exostoses, multiple cartilaginous** (0685)
**Metachondromatosis** (0650)
**Tricho-rhino-phalangeal syndrome, type I** (0966)
**Tricho-rhino-phalangeal syndrome, type III** (2847)

**Major Diagnostic Criteria:** Bulbous nose, cone epiphyses, and multiple exostoses.

**Clinical Findings:** Craniofacial features include a broad nasal bridge; a bulbous, pear-shaped nose with tented, thickened alae;

prominent elongated philtrum; apparent mandibular micrognathia; thin upper lip; and large, laterally protruding ears. Scalp hair is thin, but eyebrows may be normal or even bushy laterally. There is mild microcephaly in 60%, mild-to-severe mental retardation in 70% of affected individuals, with disproportionate speech delay in at least one-half, and multiple cartilaginous exostoses with onset before the fifth year. The exostoses are present in the same distribution as in **Exostoses, multiple cartilaginous**, although some observers consider them to be quite different. They usually increase in number until skeletal maturation, and may lead to asymmetric limb growth. Spinal curvature may be seen. Ribs may be thin. Short stature of postnatal onset, cone-shaped epiphyses of the Giedion type 12 with clinobrachydactyly, and redundant or loose skin, which improves with age, are seen.

Other features seen in some patients include laxity or hypermobility of joints and hypotonia; changes in capital femoral epiphyses (see **Hip, osteonecrosis, capital femoral epiphysis**); exotropia, ptosis, ocular hypertelorism; winged scapulae; fractures; pigmented nevi increasing with age; recurrent respiratory infections; hearing deficit; colobomata of iris; partial syndactyly of 4th and 5th fingers; heart anomalies; and GU anomalies.

**Complications:**  Compression of nerves or vessels, and limitation of movement or asymmetric growth of limbs, may occur secondary to exostoses.

**Associated Findings:**  Respiratory infections and fractures.

**Etiology:**  All cases have been sporadic except one father/daughter pair and one pair of like-sexed twins. No consanguinity or advanced parental age have been observed. Buhler et al (1987) concluded that the condition is due to a chromosomal deletion in the segment 8q24.11 to 8q24.13.

**Pathogenesis:**  Facial and nose shape, epiphyseal changes, and exostoses are probably due to abnormal growth of endochondrial bone; however, a common mechanism to explain the hair abnormalities and mental retardation is undetermined.

**MIM No.:**  15023

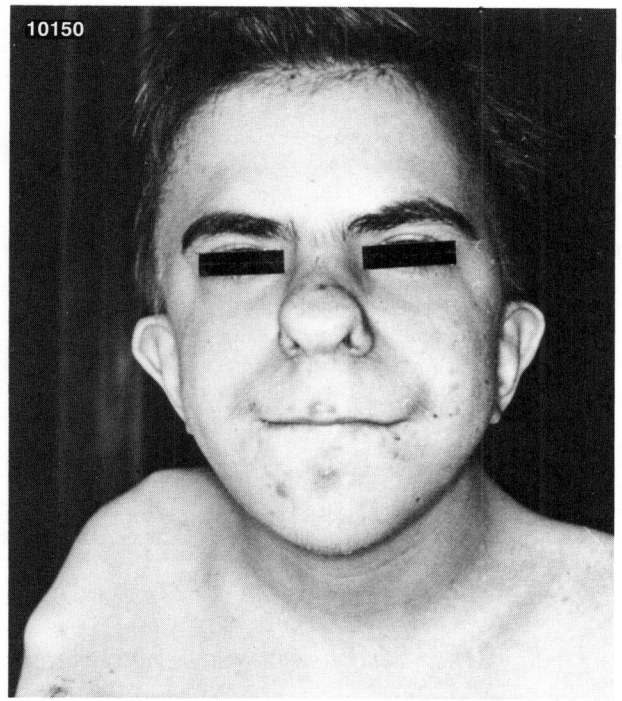

**0967-10150:**  Characteristic nose, bushy eyebrows and long philtrum.

**POS No.:**  3416

**Sex Ratio:**  M3:F1

**Occurrence:**  About 50 cases have been reported in the literature.

**Risk of Recurrence for Patient's Sib:**  Unknown.

**Risk of Recurrence for Patient's Child:**  Apparently low.

**Age of Detectability:**  At birth for facial characteristics; epiphyseal changes by three years of age, exostosis by five years of age.

**Gene Mapping and Linkage:**  LGCR (Langer-Giedion syndrome chromosome region) has been mapped to 8q24.11-q24.13.

**Prevention:**  None known. Genetic counseling indicated.

**Treatment:**  Orthopedic excision of impinging exostoses; special school for developmental delay, with emphasis on speech development.

**Prognosis:**  Depends on degree of mental retardation, if present.

**Detection of Carrier:**  Unknown.

**Special Considerations:**  It is important to distinguish this disorder from **Tricho-rhino-phalangeal syndrome, type I** and **Exostoses, multiple cartilaginous** because of the poorer prognosis, sporadic nature, frequent mental retardation, and other complications seen in this condition, as well as possible translocation carriers in the family if a chromosomal deletion is present.

**References:**
Murachi S, et al.: Familial tricho-rhino-phalangeal syndrome type II. Clin Genet 1981; 19:149–155.
Langer LO Jr, et al.: The tricho-rhino-phalangeal syndrome. Am J Med Genet 1984; 19:81–111.
Buhler EM, et al.: A final word on the tricho-rhino-phalangeal syndromes. Clin Genet 1987; 31:273–275.

HA014                                          **Judith G. Hall**

---

### TRICHO-RHINO-PHALANGEAL SYNDROME, TYPE III          2847

**Includes:**  Sugio-Kajii syndrome

**Excludes:**
    **Acrodysostosis** (0016)
    **Osteodystrophy-mental retardation, Ruvalcaba type** (2076)
    Peripheral dysostosis, other forms of
    **Tricho-rhino-phalangeal syndrome, type I** (0966)
    **Tricho-rhino-phalangeal syndrome, type II** (0967)

**Major Diagnostic Criteria:**  Clinical features of **Tricho-rhino-phalangeal syndrome, type I** plus a severe form of generalized shortness of all phalanges, metacarpals and metatarsals.

**Clinical Findings:**  Craniofacial dysmorphology (6/6) including somewhat light-colored sparse hairs, hypoplastic alae nasi, pear-shaped nose, a long, broad and prominent philtrum, protruding upper lip, malar hypoplasia, prominent maxilla, delayed eruption of teeth, and malocclusion is almost identical to that of **Tricho-rhino-phalangeal syndrome, type I**. Cone-shaped epiphyses of phalanges with premature fusion of the epiphysis and clinodactyly are common (3/4, an infant excluded). Characteristic findings which may differ from **Tricho-rhino-phalangeal syndrome, type I** include severe short stature (4/5), broad hip in post-adolescent female patients (3/3), osteochondritis of the spine (2/3), and severely short and stubby fingers with shortness of all metacarpals, metatarsals and phalanges (5/5), the end of which appears a mushroom shape on X-ray films. There is no mental retardation (6/6).

**Complications:**  Limitation of joint movements, **Pectus carinatum**, and thoracic scoliosis are sometimes seen.

**Associated Findings:**  None known.

**Etiology:**  Autosomal dominant inheritance with variability in expression.

**Pathogenesis:**  Unknown.

**POS No.:**  4413

**Sex Ratio:**  M2:F4 (observed).

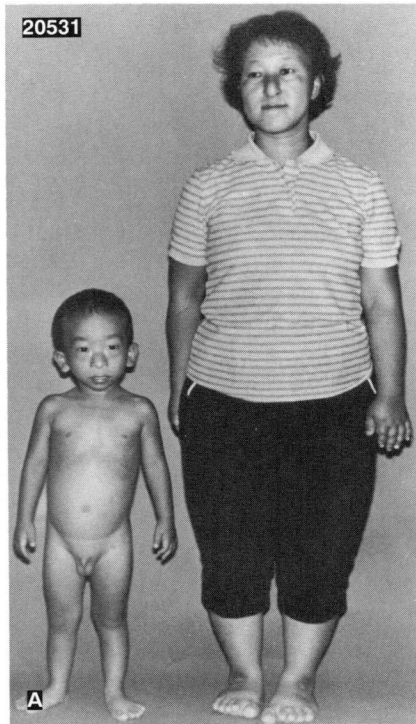

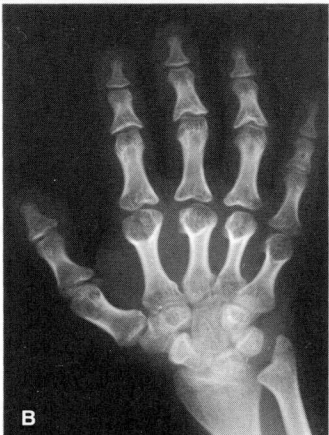

**2847-20531:** Tricho-rhino-phalangeal syndrome, type III; A. Note affected mother and son with characteristic facies, short stature and short stubby fingers. B. X-ray of the hand shows shortened phalanges and metacarpals.

**Occurrence:** Six affected Japanese have been documented; five from a family and one sporadic case.

**Risk of Recurrence for Patient's Sib:**
See Part I, *Mendelian Inheritance.*

**Risk of Recurrence for Patient's Child:**
See Part I, *Mendelian Inheritance.*

**Age of Detectability:** Possibly in early infancy.

**Gene Mapping and Linkage:** Unknown.

**Prevention:** None known. Genetic counseling indicated.

**Treatment:** As with **Tricho-rhino-phalangeal syndrome, type I.**

**Prognosis:** Normal life span.

**Detection of Carrier:** Unknown.

**References:**
Sugio Y, Kajii T: Ruvalcaba syndrome: autosomal dominant inheritance. Am J Med Genet 1984; 19:741–753. †
Niikawa N, Kamei T: The Sugio-Kajii syndrome: proposed tricho-rhino-phalangeal syndrome type III. Am J Med Genet 1986; 24:759–760. * †

NI010                                    **Norio Niikawa**

## TRICHODENTAL DYSPLASIA WITH REFRACTIVE ERRORS                                    2813

**Includes:**
    Ectodermal dysplasia, euhidrotic-refractive errors
    Kopysc syndrome
    Trichodental dysplasia-hyperopia

**Excludes:**
    **Ectodermal dysplasia**
    **Hair, atrichia congenita** (2346)
    **Hair, hypotrichosis** (3151)
    **Tricho-dento-osseous syndrome** (0965)
    **Tricho-dermodysplasia-dental defects** (2903)

**Major Diagnostic Criteria:** The combination of abnormally shaped teeth, hypotrichosis, and hyperopia, with normal nails and sweating.

**Clinical Findings:** Sparse, brittle scalp hair; broad nose; cone-shaped teeth (both deciduous and permanent affected); and skin anomalies consisting of perifollicular papules affecting the trunk and limbs and reticular hyperpigmentation on the neck nape. In each case, hyperopia was diagnosed at age six years. One patient also had astigmatism and amblyopia. Microscopic examination of hair revealed pili annulati (alternating light and dark rings of pigmentation).

**Complications:** Unknown.

**Associated Findings:** None known.

**Etiology:** Probably autosomal recessive inheritance.

**Pathogenesis:** One of the ectodermal dysplasias, although the basic genetic defect is unknown.

**MIM No.:** 26202

**Sex Ratio:** Presumably M1:F1.

**Occurrence:** Reported in a brother and sister in one family from Poland.

**Risk of Recurrence for Patient's Sib:**
See Part I, *Mendelian Inheritance.*

**Risk of Recurrence for Patient's Child:**
See Part I, *Mendelian Inheritance.*

**Age of Detectability:** During the first year of life by the presence of thin scalp hair and cone-shaped teeth.

**Gene Mapping and Linkage:** Unknown.

**Prevention:** None known. Genetic counseling indicated.

**Treatment:** Correction of the ocular defect is indicated. Dental or orthodontic treatment may also be indicated.

**Prognosis:** Life span and intellect are apparently unaffected.

**Detection of Carrier:** Unknown.

**References:**
Kopysc Z, et al.: A new syndrome in the group of euhidrotic ectodermal dysplasia: pilodental dysplasia with refractive errors. Hum Genet 1985; 70:376–378.

T0007                                    **Helga V. Toriello**

**Trichodental dysplasia-hyperopia**
    *See TRICHODENTAL DYSPLASIA WITH REFRACTIVE ERRORS*
**Trichodermodysplasia-dental alterations**
    *See TRICHO-DERMODYSPLASIA-DENTAL DEFECTS*
**Trichodysplasia hereditary**
    *See HAIR, HYPOTRICHOSIS*

**Trichodysplasia-dysmorphic facies-ataxia**
*See ATAXIA-DYSMORPHIC FACIES-TRICHODYSPLASIA*

## TRICHODYSPLASIA-XERODERMA        2894

**Includes:** Xeroderma-trichodysplasia

**Excludes: Hair, hypotrichosis** (3151)

**Major Diagnostic Criteria:** Trichodysplasia with structural changes, and xeroderma.

**Clinical Findings:** Variable degree of scalp hypotrichosis (from almost alopecia to an apparently normal amount of hair with a small alopetic area); coarse, brittle, slow-growing, and excessively dry scalp hair; irregularly sparse eyebrows; short and scanty

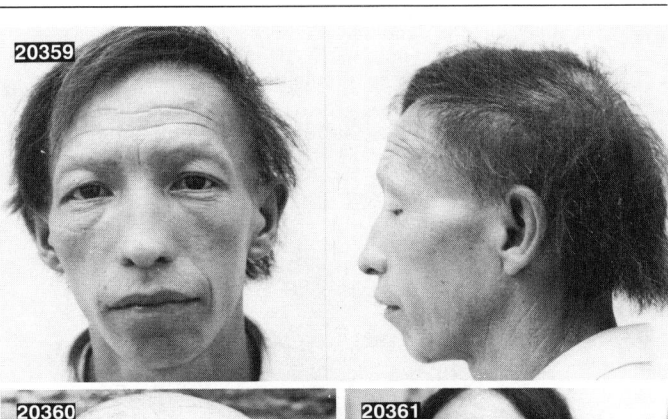
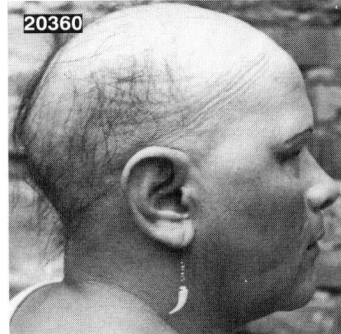
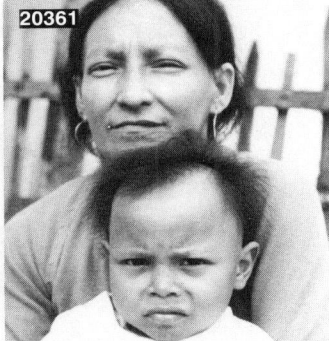
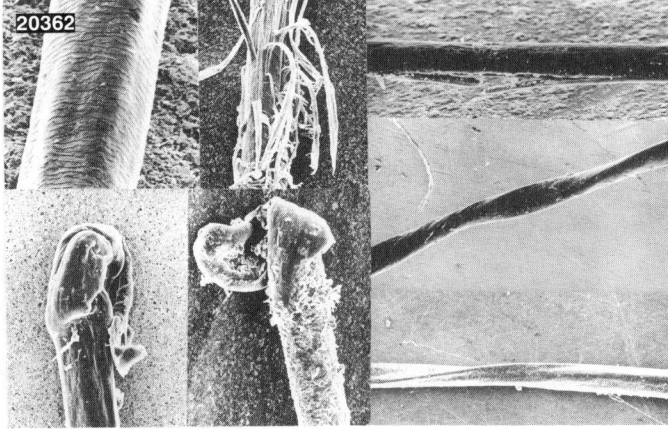

**2894-20359–61:** Note varying degrees of hypotrichosis involving the scalp, eyebrows and lashes. **20362:** Scanning electron micrograph showing defects of the hair shafts: longitudinal grooves, peeling, longitudinal splitting, dystrophic bulb, scaling and pili torti.

eyelashes; absent beard; sparse axillary and pubic hair; scalp hair shafts with pili torti, scaling, longitudinal grooves, longitudinal splitting, and peeling; variable degree of universal xeroderma.

**Complications:** Psychologic problems due to hair alterations.

**Associated Findings:** None known.

**Etiology:** Probably autosomal dominant inheritance with variable expression. The many instances of male-to-male transmission and the presence of normal daughters of affected men rule out X-linked dominant inheritance.

**Pathogenesis:** Probably a defect in ectodermal cells involving the morphodifferentiation of skin and hair structure.

**MIM No.:** 19036

**POS No.:** 4440

**Sex Ratio:** Presumably M1:F1; M36:F29 observed.

**Occurrence:** A Brazilian family of mixed Portuguese, Paraguayan, Bolivian and Amerindian origin was verified to have 65 affected members in five generations.

**Risk of Recurrence for Patient's Sib:**
See Part I, *Mendelian Inheritance.*

**Risk of Recurrence for Patient's Child:**
See Part I, *Mendelian Inheritance.*

**Age of Detectability:** At birth, by physical examination.

**Gene Mapping and Linkage:** Unknown.

**Prevention:** None known. Genetic counseling indicated.

**Treatment:** Use of wigs is cosmetically and psychologically helpful; skin emollients.

**Prognosis:** Normal life span.

**Detection of Carrier:** Unknown.

**References:**
Pinheiro M, Freire-Maia N: Trichodysplasia-xeroderma: an autosomal dominant condition. Clin Genet 1987; 31:62–67.

PI008                  **Marta Pinheiro**

**Trichoepithelioma**
*See PILOMATRIXOMA*
**Trichoepitheliomas, multiple**
*See EPITHELIOMAS, HEREDITARY MULTIPLE CYSTIC*

## TRICHOMEGALY-RETARDATION-DWARFISM-RETINAL PIGMENTARY DEGENERATION        2294

**Includes:**
Eyelashes (long)-mental retardation
Oliver-McFarlane syndrome

**Excludes:**
**Albinism, ocular** (0032)
**Albinism, oculocutaneous**
**Bardet-Biedl syndrome** (2363)
**Ectodermal dysplasia**
Trichomegaly, congenital

**Major Diagnostic Criteria:** Long and sparse eyelash and eyebrow hair, pigmentary degeneration of the retina, growth retardation.

**Clinical Findings:** Intrauterine growth retardation is present, and postnatal growth is slow, with poor weight gain and eventual short stature. Bone maturation is delayed. Frontal and occipital bossing are present. Long eyelash (up to 40 mm) and eyebrow hair is present at birth or within the first year. The eyelashes can be curved and sparse. Diffuse retinal pigmentary degeneration is present by age two years, and visual acuity is reduced to 20/200 or more. Nystagmus may be present. The electroretinogram is absent, and the pigmentary degeneration lacks the characteristic bone corpuscles found in **Retinitis pigmentosa.**

Scalp hair is sparse (i.e., patchy or frontal alopecia) in the first decade of life, and total scalp alopecia has been noted in a 37-year-old patient. A scalp skin biopsy from one patient showed degenerating hair follicles with lymphocytic histiocytic infiltration, typical of alopecia areata. Slow dental eruption was present in one patient, resulting in small, discolored teeth at age 30 months, while dentition was normal in one four-year-old patient. Cryptorchidism and hypogonadism with lack of secondary sexual characteristics has been described in the two reported adult cases. Developmental delay and mental retardation have been present in three of six cases, normal intelligence in one of six, and no developmental information for one of six. Gait ataxia, generalized clumsiness, and titubation of the head, associated with cerebellar atrophy demonstrated by computed tomography of the head, were present in the 37-year-old patient. Neurologic problems other than those involving the visual system were not described in the remaining five reported cases.

Nonbanded chromosome analyses were normal in three cases. An abnormality, possibly representing partial 13q trisomy resulting from a familial translocation was reported in one case in 1972.

**Complications:** Progressive reduction in visual acuity resulting from retinal pigmentary degeneration.

**Associated Findings:** Hypothyroidism (2/6) and growth hormone deficiency (1/6) have been described. The sella was described as "empty" in the 37-year-old male with hypothyroidism and growth hormone deficiency.

**Etiology:** Unknown. The six reported cases have been sporadic with no affected sibs.

**Pathogenesis:** Unknown.

**MIM No.:** 27540

**POS No.:** 3442

**CDC No.:** 270.200

**Sex Ratio:** 5M:1F (observed).

**Occurrence:** A half-dozen cases have been documented.

**Risk of Recurrence for Patient's Sib:** Unknown.

**Risk of Recurrence for Patient's Child:** Unknown. Both reported adults had hypogonadism and absent testes and are presumed to be sterile.

**Age of Detectability:** At birth or within the first year of life.

**Gene Mapping and Linkage:** Unknown.

**Prevention:** None known. Genetic counseling indicated.

**Treatment:** Hormone therapy for endocrine deficiencies.

**Prognosis:** Unknown. Adult cases were reported at ages 19 and 37 years.

**Detection of Carrier:** Unknown.

**References:**
Oliver GL, McFarlane DC: Congenital trichomegaly. Arch Ophthalmol 1965; 74:169–171.
Cant JS: Ectodermal dysplasia. J Pediatr Ophthalmol 1967; 4:13–17.
Corby DG, et al.: Trichomegaly, pigmentary degeneration of the retina, and growth retardation. Am J Dis Child 1971; 121:344–345.
Delleman JW, Van Walbeek K: The syndrome of trichomegaly, tapetoretinal degeneration and growth disturbances. Ophthalmologica 1975; 171:313–315.
Patton MA, et al.: Congenital trichomegaly, pigmentary retinal degeneration, and short stature. Am J Ophthalmol 1986; 101:490–491.
Sampson JR, et al.: Oliver McFarlane syndrome: a 25 year follow-up. Am J Med Genet 1989; 34:199–201. †

KI007                                              **Richard A. King**

**Trichopoliodystrophy**
*See MENKES SYNDROME*
**Trichorrhexis nodosa syndrome**
*See TRICHOTHIODYSTROPHY*

## TRICHOTHIODYSTROPHY                                    2559

**Includes:**
   Amish brittle hair syndrome
   Hair-brain syndrome
   Hair defect-photosensitivity-mental retardation
   Hair, sparse, short, thin and brittle
   Hair, "tiger tail"
   Ichthyosis-trichothiodystrophy
   Pollitt syndrome
   Sabinas brittle hair syndrome
   Tay syndrome
   Trichorrhexis nodosa syndrome
   Trichothiodystrophy-ichthyosis
   Trichothiodystrophy-neuro-cutaneous syndrome

**Excludes:**
   **Cockayne syndrome** (0189)
   **Ichthyosis, linearis circumflexa** (2858)
   **Marinesco-Sjogren syndrome** (2031)
   **Oculo-mandibulo-facial syndrome** (0738)

**Major Diagnostic Criteria:** A group of related conditions involving brittle hair with reduced sulfur content; and other possible

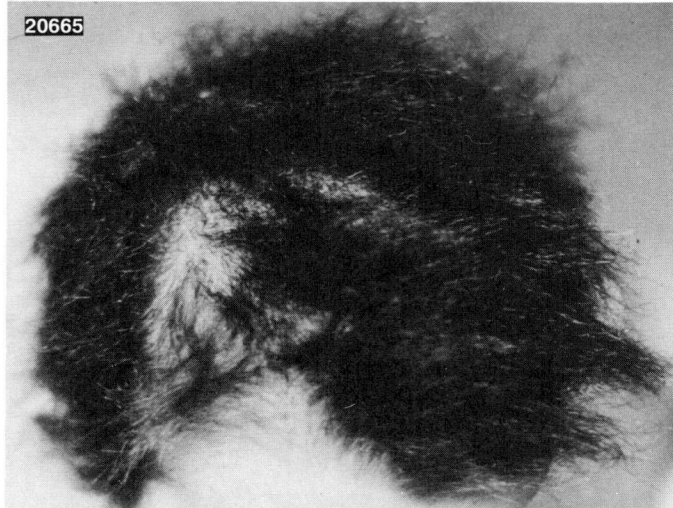

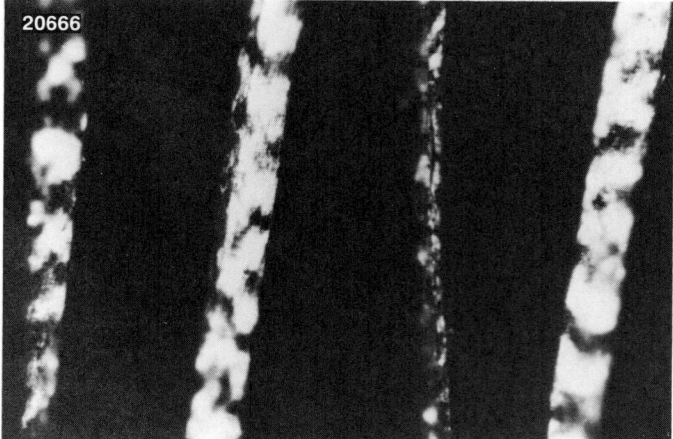

2559-20665: Sparse, stubbly and easily broken scalp hair. 20666: "Zig-zag" pattern of dark and bright zones demonstrated by polarizing microscopy of the hair shaft.

associated features including mental retardation, short stature, decreased fertility, ichthyosis, photosensitivity, and peculiar face.

**Clinical Findings:**  Delivery is frequently preterm. Birth weight is low for pregnancy age. Physical development is definitely slow. Short stature; **Microcephaly**; mild, nonprogressive mental impairment; poor motor coordination, and unsteady gait may be seen. Some patients show signs of neurologic abnormality (ataxia, intention tremor). Neurosensory hearing loss and cataract are rarely reported. Face is peculiar, with receding chin and small nose. Ichthyosis or ichthyosiform erythroderma are common.

The most dramatic and consistent findings are the hair abnormalities. The hair is sparse, short, thin, and brittle. Analysis with light, polarizing, and scanning electron microscopy shows pili torti, trichoschisis, trichorrhexis nodosa, and a peculiar pattern of alternating dark and bright bands, giving a "tiger tail" appearance. Nails are frequently dysplastic. Cystine and cysteic acid of hair and nails content is lower (50%) than normal. Postpubertal patients have delayed and reduced development of secondary sexual characters. Fertility is reduced.

In about one-half of the reported families, the patients present a marked sensitivity to sunlight and photophobia; freckle-like lesions in the sun-exposed areas usually occur. Cultured cells from these patients are hypersensitive to UVC light and are defective in the repair of UV-induced DNA damage. This defect is due to the presence of the same mutation responsible for **Xeroderma pigmentosum**, complementation group D as demonstrated by complementation analysis of UDS in hybrid cells.

**Complications:**  Susceptibility to infections.

**Associated Findings:**  None known.

**Etiology:**  Usually autosomal recessive inheritance.

**Pathogenesis:**  The reduced content of sulfur-rich matrix proteins may account for the hair shaft disruption; however, the pathogenetic mechanisms of this and other symptoms are unknown.

**MIM No.:**  *21139, 23403, *23405, *24217, 27555

**POS No.:**  3456

**Sex Ratio:**  M1:F1

**Occurrence:**  At least sixty-nine patients, belonging to 38 families, have been reported. In ten of these families, the parents of affected individuals are apparently unrelated; consanguinity data are missing on five families. In the remaining 23 families consanguinity has been demonstrated and accounts for the high prevalence of the syndrome in specific regions (northern Indiana, Sabinas, Mexico, and northeastern Italy, where 25, 12, and four patients, respectively, can be traced to common ancestors).

**Risk of Recurrence for Patient's Sib:**
See Part I, *Mendelian Inheritance.*

**Risk of Recurrence for Patient's Child:**
See Part I, *Mendelian Inheritance.*

**Age of Detectability:**  Early infancy; prenatal diagnosis of the DNA repair defect can be performed in pregnancies at-risk for trichothiodystrophy associated with **Xeroderma pigmentosum** D.

**Gene Mapping and Linkage:**  Unknown.

**Prevention:**  None known. Genetic counseling indicated. Prevention of actinic damage by avoiding sunlight in patients with photosensitivity.

**Treatment:**  As indicated for infections or other symptomatic problems. Lubricants for hair. Avoid use of dyes, straighteners, permanents, and hot combs.

**Prognosis:**  Varies with the specific symptoms. Reduced life span, intelligence, and sexual function have been reported.

**Detection of Carrier:**  Unknown.

**Special Considerations:**  The notable finding regarding trichothiodystrophy is the association with **Xeroderma pigmentosum**. Studies of DNA repair performed on patients displaying photosensitivity showed a reduced capacity to repair UV-induced DNA damage caused by XP, complementation group D, mutation. Unexpectedly in trichothiodystrophy patients, precancerous skin lesions and tumors, which characterize the pathology of age-matched xeroderma pigmentosum, complementation group D, patients have never been observed. The association of xeroderma pigmentosum and trichothiodystrophy in more than one patient in a kindred and in different unrelated families could indicate a linkage between the loci involved in the two syndromes.

The various acronyms PIBIDS, IBIDS, and BIDS have been used to designate combinations of photosensitivity, ichthyosis, brittle hair, impaired intelligence, decreased fertility, and short stature.

**References:**
Tay CH: Ichthyosiform erythroderma, hair shaft abnormalities, and mental and growth retardation. Arch Dermatol 1971; 104:4–13.
Jackson CE, et al.: Brittle hair with short stature, intellectual impairment and decreased fertility: an autosomal recessive syndrome in an Amish kindred. Pediatrics 1974; 54:201–207.
Happle R, et al.: The Tay syndrome (congenital ichthyosis with trichothiodystrophy). Eur J Pediatr 1984; 141:149–152.
Price VH, et al.: Trichothiodystrophy: sulfur-deficient brittle hair as a marker for a neuroectodermal symptom complex. Arch Dermatol 1984; 116:1375–1384.
Stefanini M, et al.: Xeroderma pigmentosum (complementation group D mutation) is present in patients affected by trichothiodystrophy with photosensitivity. Hum Genet 1986; 74:107–112.

NU002                                           **Fiorella Nuzzo**
B0051                                           **Carla Borrone**

**Trichothiodystrophy-ichthyosis**
*See TRICHOTHIODYSTROPHY*
**Trichothiodystrophy-neuro-cutaneous syndrome**
*See TRICHOTHIODYSTROPHY*
**Trichothiodystrophy-sun sensitivity**
*See XERODERMA PIGMENTOSUM*
**Trichterbrust**
*See PECTUS EXCAVATUM*
**Tricuspid incompetence**
*See TRICUSPID VALVE, INSUFFICIENCY*
**Tricuspid regurgitation**
*See TRICUSPID VALVE, INSUFFICIENCY*

---

**TRICUSPID VALVE, ATRESIA**                           **0968**

**Includes:**
> Atresia of tricuspid valve
> Atretic atrioventricular (AV) valve of the right atrium
> Heart, tricuspid valve atresia
> Ventricle, hypoplasia of right

**Excludes:**
> **Pulmonary valve, atresia** (0837)
> **Tricuspid valve, stenosis** (0970)
> Ventricular inversion when valve of the left atrium is atretic

**Major Diagnostic Criteria:**  Although tricuspid atresia is a great mimicker of other forms of cyanotic heart disease, the following findings are virtually pathognomonic in a patient who exhibits cyanosis: reversed Q loop in the horizontal plane (deeper Q waves in lead $V_5$ than $V_6$), diminished vascularity by X-ray and left axis deviation and the two aforementioned signs, plus the added X-ray finding of juxtaposition of the atrial appendages.

A selective right atriogram is the procedure of choice to confirm the diagnosis. All cases reveal the typical sequence of opacification: right atrium, left atrium, left ventricle. In cases with normally related great vessels and transposition with noninversion, there is a clear zone, termed "right ventricular window," just below and medial to the lower margin of the right atrium. In patients with inversion, the right ventricular window is absent because the right ventricle is located superiorly and anteriorly. A selective left ventriculogram is recommended for precise location of the origin of the great arteries, the type of obstruction to pulmonary flow if present, the contractile state of the left ventricle, the position of the right ventricle, and the size of **Ventricular septal defect**.

Includes cases with ventricular inversion in which the atretic right atrioventricular (AV) valve is bicuspid or mitral-like and the functioning left AV valve is tricuspid. Thus, the term "tricuspid atresia" is retained for all cases in which the AV valve of the right atrium is atretic, regardless of its anatomy.

**Clinical Findings:** Despite considerable variation in the anatomic and physiologic manifestations from case to case, certain features are common to all: atresia of the AV valve of the right atrium; patent atrial septum; an enlarged mitral orifice; a hypertrophied left ventricle which functions as a single ventricle; and a rudimentary and essentially nonfunctioning right ventricle. Tricuspid atresia is divided into two main categories according to the relationship of the aorta and the pulmonary trunk: those with normally related great vessels and those with transposition of the great vessels. Tricuspid atresia with transposition may be subdivided into two additional categories: those with and without inversion of the ventricles. Regardless from which morphologic ventricle the pulmonary trunk arises, obstruction to pulmonary flow occurs under the following circumstances: atresia of the pulmonary valve with the pulmonary arteries perfused through a patent ductus arteriosus or via bronchial arteries: stenosis of the pulmonary valve; a narrowed subpulmonary tract or a combination of the latter two. Among cases with normally related great vessels, obstruction to pulmonary flow may occur because of a small ventricular septal defect. Lastly, patients with transposition may exhibit the additional abnormality, double outlet right ventricle. The aorta is anterior and arises from a rudimentary right ventricle, while the pulmonary trunk arises partially or entirely from the right ventricle. Regardless, the left AV valve tissue is not in continuity with either semilunar valve. Juxtaposition of the atrial appendages-levoposition of the right atrial appendage occurs in a relatively high percentage of cases with transposition and noninversion. A right aortic arch is present in 7–8% of cases. Dextrocardia or dextroversion, with atria in situs solitus position, also occurs with increased frequency especially where there is shunt vascularity.

The hemodynamic alterations, and consequently the clinical manifestations, will vary according to the magnitude of pulmonary flow, the position of the great vessels and the type of ventricular arrangement, inversion or noninversion. Whatever the anatomic type, in all cases of tricuspid atresia there is a right-to-left shunt at the atrial level. The right atrium becomes enlarged and hypertrophied since it functions as the sole pumping chamber for blood from the venae cavae. It pushes all the systemic venous blood through either the foramen ovale or through an atrial septal defect. The right ventricle is usually so diminutive as to be functionally ineffective. Consequently, the left ventricle becomes the single propelling chamber for delivery of blood into both great arteries. As the left atrium is the common mixing chamber into which all the saturated (pulmonary venous) and desaturated (systemic venous) blood is poured, the peripheral arterial saturation depends on the relative amounts of each. Other factors that diminish peripheral arterial saturation are ventricular failure and obstruction to aortic flow.

The presence of cyanosis, the EKG and the thoracic X-ray are the vital clinical data. The auscultatory findings are of little help. Cyanosis is common to most patients. Those with decreased pulmonary flow may exhibit hypoxic spells as well. In patients with increased pulmonary flow, cyanosis may be clinically absent. Congestive heart failure often occurs during infancy, especially when pulmonary flow is increased. Older children exhibit the usual stigmata of the cyanotic child: clubbing, growth retardation and frequent bouts of bronchitis. EKG evidence of left axis deviation is present in at least 90% of the cases. The exceptions are usually patients with excess pulmonary flow in whom a normal axis may be present. Usual signs are left ventricular hypertrophy and diminished or absent signs of right ventricular activity. Pure right ventricular hypertrophy is never seen. Patients with normally related great vessels show Q waves in the left precordial leads, whereas those with transposition rarely show Q waves in the left precordial leads. The presence of deeper Q waves in the lead $V_5$ than $V_6$ in a cyanotic patient is virtually pathognomonic of tricuspid atresia with normally related great vessels. The thoracic roentgenogram is extremely variable, and may mimic virtually any form of cyanotic heart disease. The pulmonary flow may be excessive (uncommon), normal (rare), or diminished (common).

The classic and most common variety resembles **Heart, tetralogy of Fallot**. There are certain roentgen findings, when occurring in a cyanotic patient, that are suggestive of tricuspid atresia: juxtaposition of the atrial appendages, dextroversion or dextrocardia (in whom the atria are situs solitus), and right aortic arch which occurs in approximately 7–8% of cases.

The echocardiogram shows an absent tricuspid valve (although motion of the right atrial floor can be confused as valve), dilation of the left ventricular cavity, a small right ventricular cavity and a thickened right ventricular anterior wall. Caution must be exercised as this is a diagnosis of exclusion.

Cardiac catheterization will confirm the presence of a right-to-left shunt at the atrial level, degree of peripheral arterial desaturation, and often the presence or absence of obstruction to pulmonary flow, if the catheter is placed within the pulmonary trunk.

**Complications:** Death may occur from congestive heart failure and pneumonia, clubbing, severe hypoxic spells, growth retardation, or frequent bouts of bronchitis.

**Associated Findings:** None known.

**Etiology:** Presumably multifactorial inheritance.

**Pathogenesis:** The formation of the right AV valve probably occurs during the 4th intrauterine week. Although embryogenesis is not fully understood, normal rotation of the ventricular septum probably fails and the right AV orifice is sacrificed, so that the embryologic AV valve results in an enlarged mitral valve at the expense of an atretic tricuspid valve.

**MIM No.:**    27720

**CDC No.:**    746.100

**Sex Ratio:**    Presumably M1:F1

**Occurrence:**    Approximately 1:5,000 live births. Prevalence < 1 in 5,000 in the pediatric population.

**Risk of Recurrence for Patient's Sib:**    Estimated at about 1%.

**Risk of Recurrence for Patient's Child:**    Unknown. Reproductive fitness is greatly diminished.

**Age of Detectability:**    From birth, by selective angiocardiography.

**Gene Mapping and Linkage:**    Unknown.

**Prevention:**    None known. Genetic counseling indicated.

**Treatment:**    In patients with obstruction to pulmonary flow, procedures are aimed at increasing pulmonary blood flow, which can be accomplished by a side-to-side anastomosis of the ascending aorta to the right pulmonary artery (Waterson-Cooley shunt) or by the creation of a subclavian artery-pulmonary artery shunt (Blalock-Taussig operation). In older children, an anastomosis between the superior vena cava and the distal right pulmonary artery (Glenn procedure) is preferred by some. Those patients with excess flow to the pulmonary arteries may require a banding to decrease pulmonary flow and prevent hyperresistant changes occurring in the vasculature. Some of these, plus patients with only a moderate degree of obstruction to pulmonary flow, may be managed medically. A few such patients reach adult age. Symptomatic therapy for congestive heart failure and pneumonia may be necessary.

**Prognosis:**    The prognosis closely depends upon the anatomic type and in particular, the magnitude of pulmonary blood flow. Most individuals, regardless of type, expire during infancy unless palliative surgery is performed. Those with some form of severe pulmonary stenosis expire due to severe hypoxia; those with excess pulmonary flow expire secondary to congestive heart failure, pneumonia, etc. Those individuals who survive infancy without palliation do so because they developed high pulmonary vascular resistance, or there is only a moderate degree of obstruction to pulmonary flow, regardless of origin of the pulmonary trunk.

**Detection of Carrier:**    Unknown.

**References:**
Glenn WW, et al.: Circulatory bypass of the right side of the heart. VI. shunt between superior vena cava and distal right pulmonary

artery: report of clinical application in 38 cases. Circulation 1965; 31:172.

Elliott LP, et al.: The roentgenology of tricuspid atresia. Semin Roentgenol 1968; 3:399.

Meyer RA, Kaplan S: Echocardiography in the diagnosis of hypoplasia of the left or right ventricles in the neonate. Circulation 1972; 46:55.

Rosenthal A, Dick M: Tricuspid atresia. In: Adams FH, Emmanoullides GC, eds: Heart disease in infants, children, and adolescents, 3rd ed. Baltimore: Williams & Wilkins Co., 1983:271–283. *

EL004

**Larry P. Elliott**
*Irwin F. Hawkins, Jr.*

## Tricuspid valve, downward displacement
*See TRICUSPID VALVE, EBSTEIN ANOMALY*

---

## TRICUSPID VALVE, EBSTEIN ANOMALY                    0332

**Includes:**
> Ebstein anomaly of tricuspid valve
> Eskatlith^, fetal effects
> Lithium, fetal effects
> Lithobid^, fetal effects
> Lithone^, fetal effects
> Tricuspid valve, downward displacement

**Excludes:**
> Ebstein anomaly in cases of ventricular inversion
> **Fetal lithium effects** (2732)
> Other forms of congenital tricuspid valve incompetence

**Major Diagnostic Criteria:**  In the acyanotic individual, selective angiocardiography or cardiac catheterization with the intracavitary electrode catheter are necessary to establish a definitive diagnosis. The diagnosis of Ebstein anomaly becomes mandatory in the cyanotic individual who has bouts of tachycardia with decreased pulmonary vascular markings on chest X-rays, an ECG showing either large P waves, a prolonged PR interval and a precordial QRS pattern suggesting RBBB or having no definite criteria for either right or left ventricular hypertrophy, or the type B WPW pattern.

**Clinical Findings:**  The pathology of Ebstein anomaly is extremely variable. The two characteristic features are redundancy of valve tissue and adherence of a variable portion of the septal and posterior cusps to the right ventricular wall. Redundancy involves all cusps, although the anterior cusp is always much less affected. The area of adherence may be small, in which case the true origin of the cusps at the atrioventricular annulus is close to the apparent origin; or it may extend all the way down to the ring formed by the parietal band, crista supraventricularis, septal and moderator bands and anterior papillary muscle. That portion of the ventricle between the annulus and the apparent origin of the valve is said to be "atrialized," as it more or less forms a common chamber with the right atrium. The myocardium of the atrialized portion of the right ventricle may be fairly well developed in mild forms of the anomaly. In severe forms it may be fibrous. Both the pathology and pathophysiology are variable. In rare cases of Ebstein anomaly, the valve mechanism may function almost normally. With increasing severity of the anomaly, there is valvar insufficiency and/or stenosis. In time, right atrial pressure is elevated, the right atrium becomes markedly enlarged and a right-to-left shunt is established through an anatomically patent foramen ovale or, rarely, an atrial septal defect.

The malformation may be so pronounced as to cause intrauterine or neonatal death. Symptoms and signs are commonly present during the first month of life, particularly cyanosis, murmurs, congestive heart failure and bouts of tachycardia. Symptoms in the older child and adult are dyspnea on exertion, profound weakness or fatigue, cyanosis, bouts of tachycardia and in the terminal stages, cardiac failure. Auscultation is variable. Often the widely split components of the first sound are followed by a systolic murmur, two widely split components of the second sound and frequently a prominent third or fourth sound, producing a "triple" or "quadruple" rhythm. A diastolic murmur may surround either S₃ or S₄, or both.

The EKG either shows a right bundle branch block pattern or the Wolff-Parkinson-White (type B) pattern often with right atrial enlargement and a prolonged PR interval. The vectorcardiogram classically shows P loop changes of right atrial enlargement and slowing of the terminal rightward, superior and anterior QRS forces consistent with RBBB. The radiologic features in infancy are variable ranging from slight to massive cardiac enlargement and often resemble severe pulmonic stenosis with an intact ventricular septum and a right-to-left shunt. In patients of all age groups, certain X-ray features are seen: there are varying degrees of right heart enlargement; the pulmonary artery segment is usually inapparent; no left atrial enlargement; the aortic knob is normal or small; pulmonary vascular markings are normal or decreased, and even with chronic congestive heart failure, pleural effusion is not seen.

The M-mode echocardiogram shows dilation of the right ventricular cavity and delayed tricuspid closure with respect to mitral diastolic closure. The tricuspid valve excursion is exaggerated and its echo representation is displaced leftward. Many patients have paradoxic septal motion. The 2-dimensional echocardiogram will demonstrate the "displaced" tricuspid valve.

Cardiac catheterization, to be diagnostic, must demonstrate that a portion of the right ventricle functions as the right atrium. When, with an intracavitary electrode catheter, right ventricular muscle potentials are recorded in the presence of a right atrial pressure, the diagnosis is established. The hemodynamic findings depend on whether there is tricuspid insufficiency, or stenosis, or both. In cyanotic individuals, the right-to-left shunt is localized to the atrial level. Angiocardiography is best performed in the right ventricle. This outlines clearly the enlarged right atrium, the atrialized right ventricle and the functional right ventricle. The true and apparent annulus divide the inferior margin of the cardiac border in the AP view into three distinct compartments.

**Complications:**  Cerebral abscess, thromboembolic phenomena and organ pathology secondary to chronic congestive failure.

**Associated Findings:**  These most commonly are a ventricular septal defect or pulmonary stenosis or atresia. Extracardiac anomalies are rare.

**Etiology:**  Multifactorial inheritance. Lithium has been proposed as a specific environmental trigger (see **Fetal lithium effects**).

**Pathogenesis:**  Ebstein anomaly is probably an abnormality of the process of undermining of the embryonic right ventricular myocardium which normally leads to the formation of the tricuspid valve apparatus. In Ebstein anomaly, it remains incomplete and never reaches the annulus. Thus, the normal development of chordae and papillary muscles does not take place, or remains abortive. The relatively normal development of the anterior cusp is probably related to its very early liberation.

**MIM No.:**  22470

**CDC No.:**  746.200

**Sex Ratio:**  M1:F1

**Occurrence:**  Approximately 1:200 births with congenital heart disease. Risk of congenital heart disease, most often Ebstein anomaly, is 10% for infants of mothers taking lithium in the first weeks of pregnancy. Prevalence 1:50,000 to 1:20,000 in the pediatric population.

**Risk of Recurrence for Patient's Sib:**  Empiric risk 1.0%

**Risk of Recurrence for Patient's Child:**  Unknown.

**Age of Detectability:**  From birth, particularly with selective right ventricular angiocardiography or the intracavitary electrode catheter.

**Gene Mapping and Linkage:**  Unknown.

**Prevention:**  Genetic counseling is indicated. Mothers on lithium should review options with a knowledgeable counselor.

**Treatment:**  Replacement of abnormal tricuspid valve with a prosthesis, appropriate drugs or electrical conversion for bouts of tachycardia. Symptomatic therapy for congestive heart failure. Antibiotic therapy for cerebral abscess.

**Prognosis:** Variable, depending on the degree of pathologic anatomy and resultant distortion of physiology. Ebstein anomaly may cause neonatal death or be compatible with a normal life span.

**Detection of Carrier:** Unknown.

**References:**

Donegan CC Jr, et al.: Familial Ebstein's anomaly of the tricuspid valve. Am Heart J 1968; 75:375–379.

Nora JJ, et al.: Lithium, Ebstein's anomaly, and other congenital heart defects. Lancet 1974; II:594–595. *

Park JM, et al.: Ebstein's anomaly of the tricuspid valve associated with prenatal exposure to lithium carbonate. Am J Dis Child 1980; 134:704–708.

Silverman NH, Snider AR: Two-dimensional echocardiography in congenital heart disease. Connecticut: Appleton-Century-Crofts, 1982.

Van Mierop LHS, et al.: Anomalies of the tricuspid valve resulting in stenosis or incompetence. In: Adams FH, et al., eds: Heart disease in infants, children, and adolescents, ed 3. Baltimore: Williams & Wilkins, 1983. *

Pierard LA, et al.: Persistent atrial standstill in familial Ebstein's anomaly. Brit Heart J 1985; 53:594–597.

N0003            **James J. Nora**

## TRICUSPID VALVE, INSUFFICIENCY      0969

**Includes:**

Heart, tricuspid valve insufficiency
Tricuspid incompetence
Tricuspid regurgitation

**Excludes:**

**Heart, endocardial cushion defects** (0347)
Tricuspid insufficiency secondary to bacterial/fungal endocarditis
Tricuspid insufficiency secondary to Ebstein anomaly
Tricuspid insufficiency secondary to rheumatic heart disease
Tricuspid insufficiency secondary to trauma
Tricuspid valve insufficiency, transient neonatal

**Major Diagnostic Criteria:** Cyanosis, dyspnea, and cardiomegaly are present. Angiocardiography is the procedure of choice with cine- or biplane angiograms from the right ventricle demonstrating reflux into the right atrium. The normally inserted tricuspid valve distinguishes this lesion from **Tricuspid valve, Ebstein anomaly.** Other diagnoses within the differential include **Pulmonary valve, stenosis, Pulmonary valve, atresia** with tricuspid insufficiency with a normally sized right ventricle.

**Clinical Findings:** The pathologic anatomy in congenital tricuspid insufficiency varies. It may be due to a primary malformation (dysplasia) of the valve, shortened chordae tendineae, or defective papillary muscles with fibrosis. In some cases, the septal cusp remains adherent to the ventricular septum.

Isolated congenital tricuspid insufficiency is an extremely rare cardiac lesion. The most common presenting signs and symptoms include dyspnea, cyanosis, cardiomegaly and right-sided congestive heart failure. A pulsatile, enlarged liver and neck vein distention with prominent v waves have been observed.

A loud pansystolic murmur is invariably heard along the lower right or left sternal border with transmission to the back. The increase in intensity on inspiration is of tricuspid origin. An associated mid and late diastolic rumble represents relative tricuspid stenosis.

The X-ray findings are dependent on the severity of the lesion. In the symptomatic patient, the usual findings include massive cardiac enlargement with either normal or diminished vascularity of the lung fields. The right atrium is huge and in postmortem studies is 2–3 times the normal size. The right ventricular cavity is also increased in size.

The EKG commonly shows tall, peaked P waves, particularly in lead II, right axis deviation, and a $q^R$ or $rs^{R'}$ pattern over the right precordium, indicating right atrial enlargement and right ventricular hypertrophy. Also seen in some cases is a right bundle branch block pattern.

The echocardiogram in the Ebstein abnormality is described elsewhere (see **Tricuspid valve, Ebstein anomaly**). In tricuspid insufficiency, it shows a dilated right ventricle, and septal motion may be paradoxic.

Selective right ventricular angiocardiography demonstrates reflux of contrast material into the right atrium during ventricular systole. A right-to-left atrial shunt through a patent foramen ovale is often an associated finding.

The right atrial mean pressure is invariably elevated; and the right atrial pressure pulse has a systolic plateau with a prominent V wave and a rapid y descent. In the symptomatic neonate, right ventricular pressure is often at systemic levels, and is associated with pulmonary hypertension.

**Complications:** Most infants improve with digitalis, diuretics, and oxygen as the pulmonary vascular resistance falls. Follow-up of many of these children has shown relatively normal hemodynamics with mild tricuspid insufficiency.

**Associated Findings:** None known.

**Etiology:** Unknown.

**Pathogenesis:** Undetermined, but probably due to the abnormal or incomplete elaboration of the septal cusp of the tricuspid valve. This may be adherent to the septum, or possess only very short chordae tendineae.

**CDC No.:** 746.105

**Sex Ratio:** Presumably M1:F1

**Occurrence:** About 20 cases reported in the world literature.

**Risk of Recurrence for Patient's Sib:** Unknown.

**Risk of Recurrence for Patient's Child:** Unknown.

**Age of Detectability:** From birth, by selective angiocardiography.

**Gene Mapping and Linkage:** Unknown.

**Prevention:** None known. Genetic counseling indicated.

**Treatment:** Those instances of functional tricuspid insufficiency revert to normal when the underlying abnormality is corrected. Oxygen, which dilates the pulmonary vascular bed and thus results in a lowering of pulmonary vascular resistance, has a role in management. Surgical intervention has rarely been attempted, and usually has a fatal outcome.

Symptomatic therapy may be a treatment for right-sided congestive heart failure including digitalization and diuretics, and oxygen.

**Prognosis:** Unknown.

**Detection of Carrier:** Unknown.

**References:**

Reisman M, et al.: Congenital tricuspid insufficiency: a cause of massive cardiomegaly and heart failure in the neonate. J Pediatrics 1965; 66:869–876.

Ahn AJ, Segal BL: Isolated tricuspid insufficiency: clinical features, diagnosis and management. Prog Cardiovasc Dis 1966; 9:166–193. *

Goldberg SJ, et al.: Pediatric and adolescent echocardiography. Chicago: Year Book Medical Publishers, 1975.

HE014          **William E. Hellenbrand**
BE029          **Michael A. Berman**
TA002          **Norman S. Talner**

## TRICUSPID VALVE, STENOSIS 0970

**Includes:** Heart, narrowing of tricuspid orifice

**Excludes:**
Tricuspid stenosis from large atrial level shunts
Tricuspid stenosis secondary to rheumatic heart disease
Tricuspid stenosis secondary to right atrial myxomas
**Tricuspid valve, atresia** (0968)
**Tricuspid valve, Ebstein anomaly** (0332)

**Major Diagnostic Criteria:** The clinical, X-ray, and electrocardiographic manifestations of tricuspid stenosis with right ventricular hypoplasia are often identical to those of **Tricuspid valve, atresia**. Two dimensional echocardiography with Doppler analysis and/or cardiac catheterization with selective angiocardiography are needed to differentiate these two anomalies.

**Clinical Findings:** Isolated tricuspid stenosis is extremely rare, with few proven cases reported in the literature. With moderate-to-severe tricuspid stenosis, right atrial hypertension occurs, resulting in hypertrophy and dilatation of the chamber. Atrial dilatation promotes continued patency of the foramen ovale which allows for right atrial decompression but results in systemic venous blood gaining access to the systemic arterial circulation. The majority of children with congenital tricuspid stenosis have diminished pulmonary flow and may present in early infancy with cyanosis. Cyanotic spells associated with paroxysmal dyspnea may occur in these patients within the first six months of life. Enough blood may bypass the right ventricle through a large atrial communication such that there is insufficient flow across the tricuspid valve to produce a detectable murmur. When right atrial to right ventricular blood flow is of sufficient magnitude, atrial contraction may be reflected as a presystolic precordial impulse at the left sternal border, a jugular venous ''a'' wave, or a hepatic presystolic pulsation. A short mid-to-late diastolic rumble can only rarely be appreciated. Other murmurs will reflect associated lesions, particularly pulmonary stenosis, ventricular septal defect, or patent ductus arteriosus.

X-rays of the chest reveal decreased pulmonary vascularity and signs of an enlarged right atrium. The plain films cannot be distinguished from the **Heart, tetralogy of Fallot**, **Tricuspid valve, Ebstein anomaly**, and certain forms of **Tricuspid valve, atresia**.

The most constant findings on electrocardiography are peaked ''P'' waves, indicating right atrial enlargement. QRS axis and signs of left ventricular hypertrophy are variable, depending on the degree of right ventricular hypoplasia.

The two-dimensional echocardiogram shows a narrowed tricuspid valve orifice and a small, or even hypoplastic, right ventricular cavity. In severe forms, tricuspid valve motion may be absent and thus be indistinguishable from tricuspid atresia. In such circumstances Doppler analysis may be able to demonstrate flow through the valve, thus excluding tricuspid atresia.

Cardiac catheterization helps to confirm the diagnosis of tricuspid stenosis as well as to further evaluate associated defects. Passage of the catheter from the right atrium to the right ventricle on occasion may be difficult since the preferred pathway is into the left atrium. Simultaneous right atrial and right ventricular tracings should demonstrate a diastolic pressure difference, but such simultaneous records are rarely obtained. Generally, pullback tracings from the right ventricle to the right atrium are used for detection of the pressure difference.

Selective right atrial and right ventricular angiocardiography aid in the demonstration of the abnormality and associated defect(s). Frequently, the right atrial injection will show thickening of the valve and right-to-left atrial shunt.

**Complications:** Cyanosis, secondary to right-to-left shunt via a patent foramen ovale or associated **Atrial septal defects**. Systemic venous congestion manifested by peripheral edema and ascites. Infrequently, a superior vena caval type of syndrome may develop.

**Associated Findings:** None known.

**Etiology:** Unknown.

**Pathogenesis:** Probably due to partial fusion of the tricuspid valve primordia at an early age.

**CDC No.:** 746.100

**Sex Ratio:** Presumably M1:F1.

**Occurrence:** 3:1,000 cases of autopsied congenital heart disease.

**Risk of Recurrence for Patient's Sib:** Unknown. Strong familial tendency reported, but no accurate recurrence risk is known.

**Risk of Recurrence for Patient's Child:** Unknown.

**Age of Detectability:** From birth, with echocardiography and/or selective angiocardiography. Prenatal diagnosis may be possible through the use of fetal echocardiography and Doppler analysis.

**Gene Mapping and Linkage:** Unknown.

**Prevention:** None known. Genetic counseling indicated.

**Treatment:** Valvotomy or prosthetic valve replacement. Associated lesions must be considered individually. Infants with cyanosis and right ventricular hypoplasia or other lesions (e.g. pulmonary artery hypoplasia), which are not amenable to immediate surgical correction, may benefit from a systemic to pulmonary artery anastomosis. The use of an atrial-to-pulmonary artery conduit (Fontan procedure) or right atrial-right ventricular outflow conduit has been suggested for patients surviving infancy who are not candidates for valve reconstruction or replacement.

**Prognosis:** Influenced primarily by the severity of the stenosis, degree of right ventricular hypoplasia, and the nature of associated intracardiac abnormalities.

**Detection of Carrier:** Possibly by echocardiography and Doppler analysis.

**References:**
Calleja HB, et al.: Congenital tricuspid stenosis. Am J Card 1960; 6:821–829.
Medd WE, et al.: Isolated hypoplasia of the right ventricle and tricuspid valve in siblings. Br Heart J 1961; 23:25–30.
Dabachi F, et al.: Hypoplasia of the right ventricle and tricuspid valve in siblings. J Pediatr 1967; 71:869–874.
Dimich I, et al.: Congenital tricuspid stenosis-case treated by heterograft replacement of the tricuspid valve. Am J Cardiol 1973; 31:89–92.
Bharati S, et al.: Anatomic variations in underdeveloped right ventricle related to tricuspid atresia and stenosis. J Thoracic Cardiovasc Surg 1976; 72:383–400.
Van Mierop LHS, et al.: Ebstein's anomaly. In: Moss' heart disease in infants, children and adolescents, 4th ed. Baltimore: William and Wilkins, 1989.

RI012                                      **Richard E. Ringel**
HE014                              **William E. Hellenbrand**
BR039                                        **Joel I. Brenner**
BE029                                   **Michael A. Berman**

**Tridermal gastric teratoma**
*See STOMACH, TERATOMA*
**Tridermic teratoma of stomach**
*See STOMACH, TERATOMA*
**Tridermoma of head or neck**
*See NECK/HEAD, DERMOID CYST OR TERATOMA*
**Tridione△, fetal effects of**
*See FETAL TRIMETHADIONE SYNDROME*
**Triglyceride storage disease-impaired fatty acid oxidation**
*See STORAGE DISEASE, NEUTRAL LIPID TYPE*

## TRIGONENCEPHALY, AUTOSOMAL DOMINANT TYPE    3030

**Includes:**
Craniosynostosis of metopic sutures
Metopic suture synostosis

**Excludes:**
**C syndrome** (0121)
**Say-Meyer syndrome** (3267)

**Major Diagnostic Criteria:** Trigonocephaly with normal mental development and positive family history should suggest the diagnosis.

**Clinical Findings:** In six affected individuals from the same family, trigonocephaly limited to metopic suture involvement was present. In the two examined individuals, an S-curved lower lid (2/2), **Microcephaly** (1/2), short inner canthal distance (1/2), and preauricular skin tag (1/2) were also present. Mental development in all affected individuals was normal.

**Complications:** Unknown.

**Associated Findings:** An omphalocele was present in one affected individual.

**Etiology:** Possibly autosomal dominant inheritance with variable expressivity and possible reduced penetrance.

**Pathogenesis:** Unknown.

**MIM No.:** 19044

**CDC No.:** 754.070

**Sex Ratio:** M5:F1 (observed).

**Occurrence:** One family from Israel has been reported.

**Risk of Recurrence for Patient's Sib:**
See Part I, *Mendelian Inheritance.*

**Risk of Recurrence for Patient's Child:**
See Part I, *Mendelian Inheritance.*

**Age of Detectability:** Possibly at birth or during infancy, by the abnormal skull shape.

**Gene Mapping and Linkage:** Unknown.

**Prevention:** None known. Genetic counseling indicated.

**Treatment:** Unknown.

**Prognosis:** Life span and intellectual development appear to be unimpaired.

**Detection of Carrier:** Unknown.

**References:**
Frydman M, et al.: Trigonocephaly: a new familial syndrome. Am J Med Genet 1984; 18:55–59.

T0007            **Helga V. Toriello**

**Trigonocephaly "C" syndrome**
*See C SYNDROME*
**Trigonocephaly-short stature**
*See SAY-MEYER SYNDROME*
**Trigonocephaly-short stature-developmental delay**
*See SAY-MEYER SYNDROME*
**Trihydroxycoprostanic acidemia**
*See ACIDEMIA, TRIHYDROXYCOPROSTANIC*
**Trimethadione, fetal effects of**
*See FETAL TRIMETHADIONE SYNDROME*

## TRIMETHYLAMINURIA    3241

**Includes:**
Fish odor syndrome
Stale fish syndrome

**Excludes:** N/A

**Major Diagnostic Criteria:** Excretion of trimethylamine in urine.

**Clinical Findings:** A prominent odor of rotting fish, particularly in areas of active sweating, such as the axillae and feet. This may become more severe after puberty. There are no physical manifestations, however severe psychosocial problems have been described, such as aggressive behavior, poor school performance, and depression.

**Complications:** Unknown.

**Associated Findings:** One patient has been described with **Noonan syndrome**, neutropenia, anemia, splenomegaly, and an intermittent fishy odor, and with elevated levels of trimethylamine in the urine.

**Etiology:** Autosomal recessive inheritance.

**Pathogenesis:** Trimethylamine is normally formed in man, in the gut, by the action of bacteria on ingested choline (from eggs, liver, legumes) and trimethylamine-oxide (from some species of salt water fish). It is then transported to the liver and oxidized to form trimethylamine oxide, which is then excreted in the urine. Patients with this disorder have diminished activity of hepatic trimethylamine-n-oxide synthetase, causing accumulation of trimethylamine, which is responsible for the fishy odor.

**MIM No.:** *27570

**Sex Ratio:** M1:F1

**Occurrence:** Eighteen cases have been reported in the literature. A random study of 169 people, however, detected two carriers, suggesting that the condition may be more common than initially thought.

**Risk of Recurrence for Patient's Sib:**
See Part I, *Mendelian Inheritance.*

**Risk of Recurrence for Patient's Child:**
See Part I, *Mendelian Inheritance.*

**Age of Detectability:** Can be variable, depending on ingestion of substrates. Two cases have been reported in which the odor was present from infancy, while the mother was breast feeding and had eaten eggs or fish.

**Gene Mapping and Linkage:** Unknown.

**Prevention:** None known. Genetic counseling indicated.

**Treatment:** Usually dietary restriction of fish and choline containing foods eliminates the odor. However, two patients have also required antibiotics to reduce intestinal bacterial degradation of choline and trimethylamine.

**Prognosis:** Excellent.

**Detection of Carrier:** Oral challenge with 600 mg. of trimethylamine can detect partial impairment of N-oxidation in carriers.

**References:**
Humbert JR, et al.: Trimethylaminuria: the fish-odour syndrome. Lancet 1970; II:770–771.
Higgins T, et al.: Trimethylamine-n-oxide synthesis: a human variant. Biochem Med 1972; 6:392–396.
Calvert GD: Trimethylaminuria and inherited Noonan Syndrome. Lancet 1973; I:320–321.
Lee CWG, et al.: Trimethylaminuria: fishy odors in children. New Eng J Med 1976; 295:937–938.
Danks DM, et al.: Trimethylaminuria: diet does not always control the fishy odor. New Eng J Med 1976; 295:962 only.
Todd WA: Psychosocial problems as the major complication of an adolescent with trimethylaminuria. J Pediatr 1979; 94:936–937.
Nyhan WL: Abnormalities in amino acid metabolism in clinical medicine. Stanford, CT: Appleton-Century-Crofts, 1984:360–362.
Shelley ED, Shelley WB: The fish-odour syndrome: trimethylaminuria. J Am Med Asso 1984; 251:253–255.

Al-Waiz, et al.: Trimethylaminuria (fish-odour syndrome): an inborn error of oxidative metabolism. Lancet 1987; II:634–635.

Al Waiz, et al.: Trimethylaminuria (fish-odour syndrome): a study of an affected family. Clin Sci 1988; 74:231–236.

MA095                                                                    **Deborah L. Marsden**

**Triose phosphate isomerase deficiency**
  See ERYTHROCYTE TRIOSEPHOSPHATE ISOMERASE DEFICIENCY
**Triosephosphate isomerase deficiency**
  See ERYTHROCYTE TRIOSEPHOSPHATE ISOMERASE DEFICIENCY
**Triphalangeal thumb, nonopposable**
  See THUMB, TRIPHALANGEAL
**Triphalangeal thumb, opposable**
  See POLYDACTYLY
**Triphalangeal thumb-brachyectrodactyly syndrome**
  See THUMB, TRIPHALANGEAL-BRACHYECTRODACTYLY
**Triphalangeal thumb, opposable**
  See THUMB, TRIPHALANGEAL-DUPLICATED GREAT TOES
**Triphalangeal thumbs-duplication of great toes**
  See THUMB, TRIPHALANGEAL-DUPLICATED GREAT TOES
**Triphalangeal thumbs-onychodystrophy and digital malformations**
  See DEAFNESS-TRIPHALANGEAL THUMBS-ONYCHODYSTROPHY
**Triphalangeal thumbs-radial hypoplasia-diastema-hypospadias**
  See RADIAL HYPOPLASIA-TRIPHALANGEAL THUMBS-
    HYPOSPADIAS-DIASTEMA
**Triple nares**
  See NOSE/NASAL SEPTUM DEFECTS
**Trismus-pseudocamptodactyly**
  See CAMPTODACTYLY-TRISMUS SYNDROME
**Trisomy 13-15 syndrome**
  See CHROMOSOME 13, TRISOMY 13
**Trisomy D1 syndrome**
  See CHROMOSOME 13, TRISOMY 13
**Trisomy G syndrome**
  See CHROMOSOME 21, TRISOMY 21
**Trisomy, ovulation induction**
  See OVULATION INDUCTION TRISOMY
**Tritan defect, incomplete**
  See COLOR BLINDNESS, YELLOW-BLUE TRITAN
**Tritanomaly**
  See COLOR BLINDNESS, YELLOW-BLUE TRITAN
**Tritanopia**
  See COLOR BLINDNESS, YELLOW-BLUE TRITAN
**Troxidone embryopathy**
  See FETAL TRIMETHADIONE SYNDROME
**True agonadism**
  See AGONADIA
**True concrescence**
  See TEETH, ROOT CONCRESCENCE
**True esophageal diverticulum**
  See ESOPHAGUS, DIVERTICULUM
**True Klinefelter syndrome**
  See KLINEFELTER SYNDROME
**True median cleft**
  See LIP, MEDIAN CLEFT OF UPPER
**True transposition of great vessels**
  See HEART, TRANSPOSITION OF GREAT VESSELS
**Truncus arteriosus (persistent) types I-III**
  See HEART, TRUNCUS ARTERIOSUS
**Trypsin-1**
  See TRYPSINOGEN DEFICIENCY

---

**TRYPSINOGEN DEFICIENCY**                                          **0973**

**Includes:**
  Isolated trypsinogen deficiency
  Trypsin-1

**Excludes:**
  **Cystic fibrosis** (0237)
  **Intestinal enterokinase deficiency** (0533)
  Secondary pancreatic exocrine insufficiency
  **Shwachman syndrome** (0885)

**Major Diagnostic Criteria:** Malabsorption and protein calorie malnutrition cause failure to thrive, edema, and anemia in infancy. Demonstration of trypsinogen deficiency is required. Basal and secretin-stimulated duodenal aspirates contain subnormal activities of peptidases but normal amylase and lipase. After incubation with enterokinase, there is no increase in trypsin activity. After incubation with bovine trypsin, there is normal activity of carboxypeptidase, chymotrypsin, and elastase but no augmentation of tryptic activity. The maneuvers indicate an absence of pancreatic trypsinogen.

**Clinical Findings:** Reported patients presented in infancy with failure to thrive, hypoproteinemia, edema, and anemia, i.e., the pattern of protein-calorie malnutrition. Generalized malabsorption was evident in each. There was no evidence for serum protein loss in urine or stool. Fecal nitrogen and fat excretion were increased. Pancreatic exocrine function was characteristically disturbed.

Confusion may occur in two circumstances: 1) the severely malnourished infant with generalized pancreatic exocrine dysfunction and subnormal activities of all exocrine enzymes; 2) trypsinogen activation may be accomplished by incubation with bovine trypsin (4° C for 16 hours) in some patients. This test is not reliable and should not be used to diagnose absence of trypsinogen. Enterokinase alone should be used in the incubation as a pro-enzyme activator.

**Complications:** Protein malabsorption, hypoproteinemia, edema, secondary pancreatic exocrine dysfunction, generalized malabsorption, failure to grow and gain weight, and anemia.

**Associated Findings:** None known.

**Etiology:** Autosomal recessive inheritance.

**Pathogenesis:** Normal trypsinogen is secreted by the pancreas and is converted within the intestinal lumen to trypsin. Trypsin, in turn, activates other propeptidases to their active enzymatic forms. Deficiency of trypsinogen results in subnormal activities of all peptidases. Lipase and amylase are secreted as active enzymes, and are not deficient in trypsinogen deficiency disease.

**MIM No.:** *27600

**Sex Ratio:** M2:F1

**Occurrence:** About a half-dozen cases have been documented.

**Risk of Recurrence for Patient's Sib:**
  See Part I, *Mendelian Inheritance.*

**Risk of Recurrence for Patient's Child:**
  See Part I, *Mendelian Inheritance.*

**Age of Detectability:** In infancy.

**Gene Mapping and Linkage:** TRY1 (trypsin 1) has been mapped to 7q32-qter.

**Prevention:** None known. Genetic counseling indicated.

**Treatment:** Provision of pancreatic enzymes by oral replacement; elemental diets are useful in providing nutrition in infancy.

**Prognosis:** Excellent.

**Detection of Carrier:** Unknown.

**References:**
Townes PL: Trypsinogen deficiency disease. J Pediatr 1965; 66:275–285.
Morris MD, Fisher DA: Trypsinogen deficiency disease. Am J Dis Child 1967; 114:203–208.
Townes PL, et al.: Further observations on trypsinogen deficiency disease: report of a second case. J Pediatr 1967; 71:220–224.
Emi M, et al.: Cloning, characterization and nucleotide sequences of two cDNAs coding human pancreating trypsinogens. Gene 1986; 41:305–310.

WH007                                                              **Peter F. Whitington**

## TRYPTOPHAN MALABSORPTION 0974

**Includes:**
Blue diaper syndrome
Hypercalcemia, familial with nephrocalcinosis and
indicanuria

**Excludes:**
**Hartnup disorder** (0453)
Intestinal malabsorption syndromes
**Phenylketonuria** (0808)

**Major Diagnostic Criteria:** Severe prolonged hypercalcemia can be provoked by L-tryptophan in affected probands. There is excess tryptophan in the feces of the patient. Tryptophan derivatives increased in the urine (e.g., indoleacetic acid, indolelactic acid, indolylacetyl glutamine, indole acetamide, and indican) are of intestinal origin. These derivatives are secondary to retention of tryptophan in the intestinal lumen.

Blue staining of diapers is caused by indigotin, presumably formed by enzymatic conversion of indolic compounds in urine. The source of the urinary enzyme(s) may be from damaged renal tissue. Fecal *Pseudomonas aeruginosa* contamination of urine on diaper may produce a phenocopy.

Plasma tryptophan concentration is normal; the rise following oral L-tryptophan load (100 mg/kg) is less than normal.

Renal clearance of tryptophan is normal under endogenous conditions.

**Clinical Findings:** Hypercalcemia and nephrocalcinosis are associated with a defect in intestinal absorption of L-tryptophan. Two brothers had a similar clinical course involving failure to thrive, recurrent unexplained fever, infections, irritability, and constipation. Bluish discoloration of the diapers was observed continuously from early infancy. The first-born died after a mastoidectomy; the second was alive at 44 months. The vitamin D intake was 1,400 units daily in both patients (maximum RDA: 400 units), but no clinical signs of the infantile hypercalcemia syndrome were apparent.

**Complications:** Hypercalcemia, producing nephrocalcinosis. The defect in tryptophan absorption is, in some undetermined way, correlated with the occurrence of hypercalcemia.

**Associated Findings:** None known.

**Etiology:** Undetermined, but possibly autosomal recessive or X-linked recessive inheritance of a biochemical defect.

**Pathogenesis:** Proposed deficiency of substrate-specific intestinal membrane transport system for L-tryptophan.

**MIM No.:** 21100

**Sex Ratio:** In the only reported pedigree, there were two affected male siblings, one female sib with no symptoms (but "occasionally blue diapers"), and one normal male sib.

**Occurrence:** One family has been reported.

**Risk of Recurrence for Patient's Sib:**
See Part I, *Mendelian Inheritance.*

**Risk of Recurrence for Patient's Child:**
See Part I, *Mendelian Inheritance.*

**Age of Detectability:** In infancy.

**Gene Mapping and Linkage:** Unknown.

**Prevention:** None known. Genetic counseling indicated.

**Treatment:** Reduced protein intake; advisable to limit vitamin D intake to 400 units/day. Treatment for hypercalcemia; avoidance of dietary alkali and high milk intake is prudent.

**Prognosis:** Limited if hypercalcemia is complicated by nephrocalcinosis.

**Detection of Carrier:** Both parents in the only reported pedigree were free of abnormal biochemical manifestations or clinical symptoms.

**Special Considerations:** The indoluria may resemble that present in **Hartnup disorder**, but a specific hyperaminoaciduria distinguishes the latter trait. Indoluria also occurs in phenylketonuria, apparently because phenylalanine competes with tryptophan for intestinal absorption. In neither primary disease is there hypercalcemia. Tryptophan malabsorption and indoluria accompany many forms of intestinal malabsorption.

**References:**
Drummond KN, et al.: The blue diaper syndrome: familial hypercalcemia with nephrocalcinosis and indicanuria. A new familial disease, with definition of the metabolic abnormality. Am J Med 1964; 37:928–948.
Michael AF, et al.: Tryptophan metabolism in man. J Clin Invest 1964; 43:1730–1746.
Libit SA, et al.: Fecal Pseudomonas aeruginosa as a cause of the blue diaper syndrome. J Pediatr 1972; 81:546–560.

SC050

**Charles R. Scriver**

**TSH resistance**
*See THYROTROPIN UNRESPONSIVENESS*
**Tuberculosis, INH inactivation peripheral neuropathy**
*See NEUROPATHY, HERITABLE ISONIAZIDE TYPE (INH)*
**Tuberose sclerosis**
*See TUBEROUS SCLEROSIS*

## TUBEROUS SCLEROSIS 0975

**Includes:**
Adenoma sebaceum-seizures-mental retardation
Bourneville syndrome
Epiloia
Mental retardation-seizures-adenoma sebaceum
Pringle disease
Seizures-adenoma sebaceum-mental retardation
Tuberose sclerosis

**Excludes:** **Neurofibromatosis** (0712)

**Major Diagnostic Criteria:** Adenoma sebaceum, seizures, and mental retardation constitute the classic symptom complex. There are many variations of the disease, even within the same family.

**Clinical Findings:** Tuberous sclerosis is a multisystem disease classically characterized by the triad of adenoma sebaceum, epilepsy, and mental retardation. Many variations have been documented. The disease may present in infancy with infantile spasms and tufts of white hair or faintly depigmented nevi, which are shaped in the form of an ash leaf and vary in size. These nevi are differentiated from vitiligo by the presence of melanocytes in the lesion, although the number of pigmented melanocytes is lower than in adjacent normomelanotic skin. Depigmented nevi are often difficult to appreciate, but ultraviolet light (a Wood lamp) may be helpful in their identification. In the preschool child the most common symptom is epilepsy. Although the seizures are primarily generalized tonic-clonic, focal motor, complex partial, and petit mal variants have been observed. Mental retardation of a moderate to severe degree occurs in about one-half of the cases.

Skin lesions are present in the majority of cases and include adenoma sebaceum, shagreen plaques, subungual fibromata, depigmented nevi, subcutaneous nodules, and café-au-lait spots in decreasing frequency. In the very young infant only the depigmented nevi or hair patch may be present. Retinal tumors consisting of mulberry lesions and plaques of glia (phakoma) have been noted in as many as 70%. Oral lesions include gingival fibromas and small enamel pits on the teeth, and the iris may have hypopigmented spots. Attention is brought to their disease by the complications of tuberous sclerosis or family members with tuberous sclerosis.

CT scan of the brain shows cerebral calcification, most frequently subependymally in the walls of the third and lateral ventricles, especially in the region of the basal ganglia. Subependymal nodules can be seen on MRI in the majority of patients. Skull X-rays demonstrate intracranial calcification in approximately 50%. The EEG is not characteristic. X-rays of the hands reveal cystic areas of rarefaction, particularly in the phalanges (30–60%). A chest X-ray may rarely demonstrate symmetric coarse markings, which appear as multiple cysts. Occasionally an intravenous pyelogram or abdominal CT will suggest a renal mass

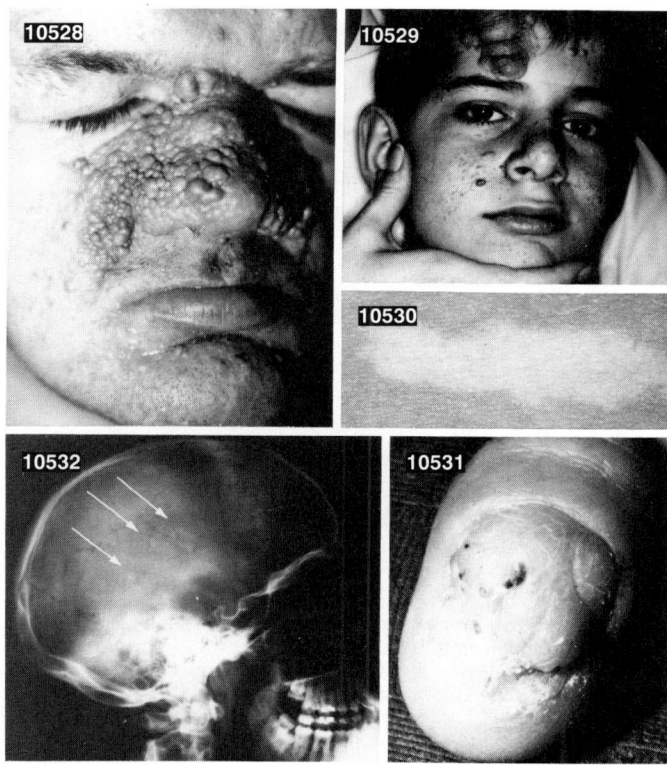

**0975A-10528:** Angiofibromas. **10529:** Polypoid fibrous masses on forehead. **10530:** Patch of vitiligo. **10531:** Subungual fibroma. **10532:** Skull X-ray showing intracranial calcifications.

(angiomyolipoma), or a renal ultrasound will detect polycystic kidneys. Facial adenoma sebaceum are actually angiofibromas, with consistent histologic features and on biopsy show a benign hamartomatous tumor composed of many cellular elements, including sebaceous glands, smooth muscle, blood vessels, and hair follicles.

**Complications:** Infrequently, the cerebral glial nodules undergo malignant transformation to a giant cell astrocytoma. More commonly the nodules may by their position or growth cause obstruction of the CSF pathway and an increase in intracranial pressure secondary to hydrocephalus. Optic atrophy may be the end result. Other eye complications include congenital blindness, cataract, and chorioretinitis. The rupture of a cyst within the lung parenchyma may produce a pneumothorax. More commonly, progressive dyspnea, hemoptysis, and pulmonary hypertension occur if the lung is involved. Tumors located within the kidney can cause obstruction, leading to pyelonephritis and uremia, and true polycystic kidneys can be rarely associated. Up to one-half may have rhabdomyomas of the heart which can be detected in the fetus at risk by echocardiogram.

**Associated Findings:** None known.

**Etiology:** Autosomal dominant inheritance, although it has been estimated that as many as 85% of the cases are the result of new mutations. Paternal age is not increased.

**Pathogenesis:** Unknown.

**MIM No.:** *19110

**POS No.:** 3417

**CDC No.:** 759.500

**Sex Ratio:** M1:F1

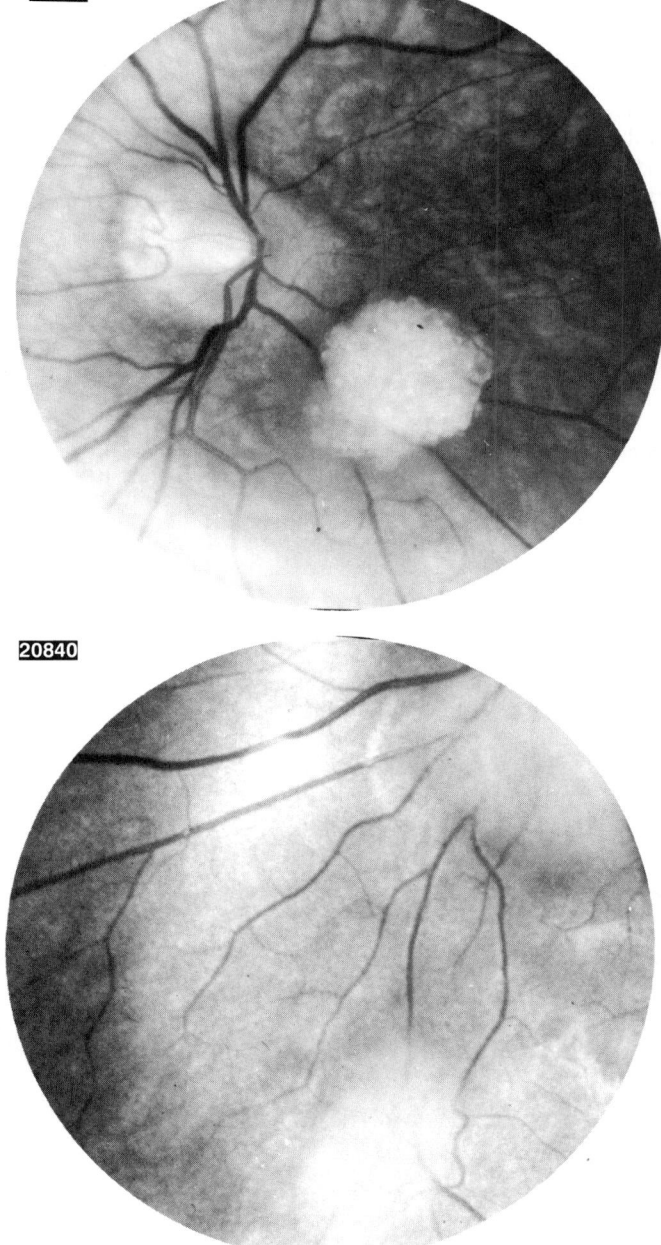

**0975B-20838:** Classical phakoma (mulberry). **20840:** Flat, smooth phakoma.

**Occurrence:** 1:10,000 to 1:50,000 in all populations and ethnic groups studied.

**Risk of Recurrence for Patient's Sib:**
See Part I, *Mendelian Inheritance*.

**Risk of Recurrence for Patient's Child:**
See Part I, *Mendelian Inheritance*. The most severe cases do not reproduce because of death at an early age.

**Age of Detectability:** Shortly after birth, when the combination of infantile spasms and depigmented skin lesions is present. Calcifications and/or subependymal masses seen on CT scan may be confirmatory. At age two to five years, by physical examination and appropriate X-rays. Prenatal diagnosis has been reported (Journel et al, 1986).

**Gene Mapping and Linkage:**  TSC1 (tuberous sclerosis 1) has been provisionally mapped to 9q.

Exclusion of linkage to 9p has been demonstrated for some families (Kandt et al, 1989).

**Prevention:**  None known. Genetic counseling indicated.

**Treatment:**  Anticonvulsants for the treatment of seizures. Dermatologic cosmetic procedures for facial angiofibromas. Occasional surgical removal of a strategically placed glial nodule of the brain. Treatment of the complications.

**Prognosis:**  Asymptomatic patients with skin lesions and normal intelligence probably have a normal life span in the absence of renal failure or brain tumors. This is in contrast to severely retarded children with infantile spasms who probably have a progressive course with early death.

**Detection of Carrier:**  Unknown.

**Special Considerations:**  Careful investigation of first degree relatives of those affected should be undertaken prior to genetic counseling. This should include examination for pitted enamel hypoplasia (Lygidakis and Lindenbaum, 1987), of skin for cutaneous lesions, examination by an ophthalmologist for retinal phakomata, and CT scan of cranium and possibly kidneys. If these investigations are negative, the recurrence risk is low for subsequent sibs, in keeping with a new mutation. Two rare cases of affected sibs with unaffected parents have been reported.

**Support Groups:**
MA; Rockland; American Tuberous Sclerosis Association
IL; Winfield; National Tuberous Sclerosis Association
AUSTRALIA: NSW; Bulli; The Australian Tuberous Sclerosis Society
THE NETHERLANDS: Duiven; Stichting Tubereuze Sclerosis Nederland
SCOTLAND: Glasgow; Tuberous Sclerosis Association of Great Britain

**References:**
Monaghan HP, et al.: Tuberous sclerosis complex in children. Am J Dis Child 1981 135:912–917.
Baraitser M: The genetics of neurological disorders. New York: Oxford University Press, 1982.
Gutman I, et al.: Hypopigmented iris spot: an early sign of tuberous sclerosis. Am Acad Ophthalmol 1982; 89:1155–1159.
Cassidy SB, et al.: Family studies in tuberous sclerosis. J Am Med Assoc 1983; 249:1302–1304.
Sugita K, et al.: Tuberous sclerosis: report of two cases studied by computerized cranial tomography within one week after birth. Brain Dev 1985; 7:438–443.
Journel H, et al.: Prenatal diagnosis of familial tuberous sclerosis following detection of cardiac rhabdomyoma by ultrasound. Prenatal Diagnosis 1986; 6:283–289.
Fryer AE, et al.: Forehead plaque: a presenting skin sign in tuberous sclerosis. Arch Dis Child 1987; 62:292–304.
Grether P, et al.: Wilms' tumor in an infant with tuberous sclerosis. Ann Genet 1987; 30:183–185.
Hall JG, Byers PH: Genetics of tuberous sclerosis. (Letter) Lancet 1987; 28:751 only.
Lygidakis NA, Lindenbaum RH: Pitted enamel hypoplasia in tuberous sclerosis patients and first degree relatives. Clin Genet 1987; 32:216–221.
Roach ES, et al.: Magnetic resonance imaging in tuberous sclerosis. 1987; 44:301–303.
Gomez MR, ed: Tuberous sclerosis, 2nd ed. New York: Raven Press, 1988.
Kandt RS, et al.: Absence of linkage of tuberous sclerosis to the ABO blood group locus. Exp. Neurol 1989; 104:223–228.

HA053                                              **Robert H.A. Haslam**

**Tubular ectasia**
*See KIDNEY, MEDULLARY SPONGE KIDNEY*
**Tubular male pseudohermaphroditism**
*See MULLERIAN DERIVATIVES IN MALES, PERSISTENT*

**Tubular nostril congenital**
*See NOSE, PROBOSCIS LATERALIS*

## TUBULAR STENOSIS                                0976

**Includes:**
Dwarfism-congenital medullary stenosis
Dwarfism-cortical thickening of tubular bones
Hypocalcemia-dwarfism-cortical thickening of tubular bones
Kenny-Caffey syndrome
Kenny disease
Medullary stenosis, congenital
Tubular stenosis, Kenny type

**Excludes:**
Cleidocranial dysplasia (0185)
Osteopetrosis, benign dominant (0779)
Osteopetrosis, malignant recessive (0780)
Parathormone resistance (0830)
Pyknodysostosis (0846)
Silver syndrome (0887)

**Major Diagnostic Criteria:**  Proportionate dwarfism; ophthalmologic abnormalities; epidsodic hypocalcemia; and characteristic X-ray findings, including cortical thickening and medullary stenosis of the long bones.

**Clinical Findings:**  Small stature is often of prenatal origin. The anterior fontanel is usually quite large in early childhood, very late in closing, and associated with a widely split metopic suture. The forehead is prominent and appears especially so because the eyes are usually small. Hyperopia is characteristically present, and strabismus or pseudopapilledema may occur. Intelligence is usually normal.

Episodes of hypocalcemia and hyperphosphatemia often are present in infancy but may occur at any age. Such episodes may be precipitated by illness or surgery, and may cause tetany or seizures.

X-ray features are distinctive: narrow long bone diaphyses, with narrowing of the marrow cavities and thickening of the cortex. The metaphyses are overfunnelized, and there is absence of the diploic space in the skull. Skeletal maturation during childhood is delayed. Vertebrae, round bones, and facial bones are normal.

**Complications:**  Episodes of hypocalcemic tetany or seizures may occur, especially in infancy or during periods of stress.

**Associated Findings:**  Idiopathic hypoparathyroidism and other parathyroid anomalies. Abnormal hearing and dental anomalies have been reported.

**Etiology:**  Autosomal dominant inheritance with variable expressivity.

**Pathogenesis:**  Unknown.

**MIM No.:**  *12700

**POS No.:**  3086

**Sex Ratio:**  M1:F1

**Occurrence:**  About 20 cases have been reported, all Caucasian.

**Risk of Recurrence for Patient's Sib:**
See Part I, *Mendelian Inheritance.*

**Risk of Recurrence for Patient's Child:**
See Part I, *Mendelian Inheritance.*

**Age of Detectability:**  In infancy.

**Gene Mapping and Linkage:**  Unknown.

**Prevention:**  None known. Genetic counseling indicated.

**Treatment:**  Vitamin D and calcium have been used succesfully to treat symptomatic hypocalcemia.

**Prognosis:**  Apparently good for normal life span and intelligence, although one patient died unexpectantly at 19 years of age. Adult height has been 121–155 cm in affected females.

**Detection of Carrier:**  Unknown.

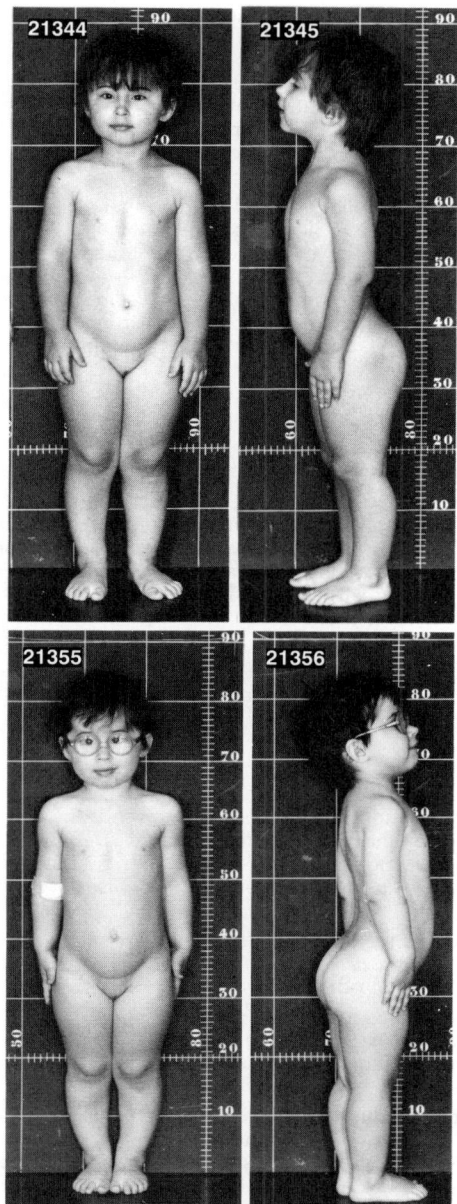

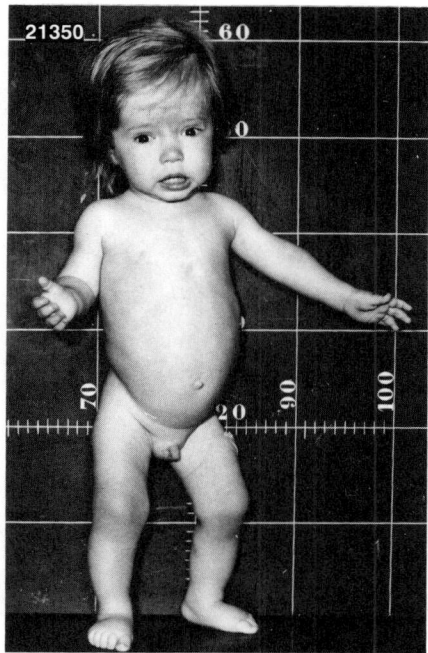

**0976B-**21350: Affected 1½-year-old male; note marked short stature, macrocephaly, and prominent forehead.

**0976A-**21344–56: Affected girls at 6½ (upper) and 6 years (lower) of age; note marked short stature, macrocephaly, mildly dysmorphic facies and microphthalmos.

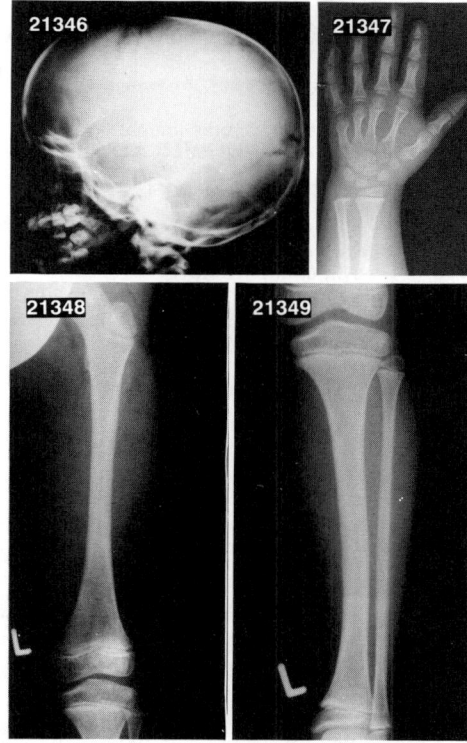

**0976C-**21346–49: X-ray findings show large skull with open anterior fontanel, absent diploic space and prominent forehead, medullary stenosis, mild brachymetacarpism, and cortical thickening of tubular bones.

**References:**
Kenny FM, Linarelli L: Dwarfism and cortical thickening of tubular bones. Am J Dis Child 1966; 111:201–207.
Caffey J: Congenital stenosis of medullary spaces in tubular bones and calvaria in two proportionate dwarfs - mother and son; coupled with transitory hypocalcemic tetany. Am J Roentgenol 1967; 100:1–11.
Boynton JR, et al.: Ocular findings in Kenny's syndrome. Arch Ophthalmol 1979; 97:896–900.
Lee WK, et al.: The Kenny-Caffey syndrome: growth retardation and hypocalcemia in a young boy. Am J Med Genet 1983; 14:773–782.
Larsen JL, et al.: Unusual cause of short stature. Am J Med 1985; 78:1025–1032.
Fanconi S, et al.: Kenny syndrome: evidence for idiopathic hypopara-

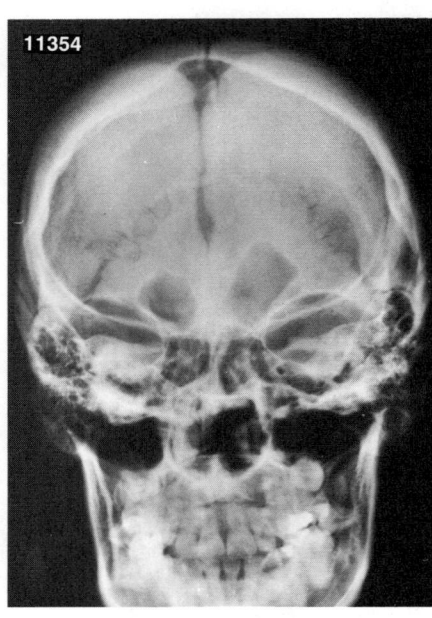
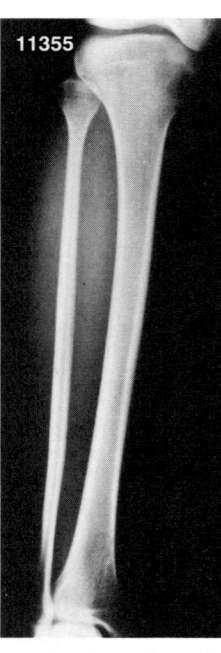

**0976D-11354:** Markedly thickened bony calvaria with wide open anterior fontanel and unfused metopic suture. **11355:** Stenosis of the diaphyseal portion of long bones, medullary canals severely constricted; in the fibula, almost obliterated.

thyroidism in two patients and for abnormal parathyroid hormone in one. J Pediatr 1986; 109:469–475.

FR017                                                    **J.M. Friedman**

**Tubular stenosis, Kenny type**
*See TUBULAR STENOSIS*
**Tubulointerstitial nephropathy, chronic idiopathic**
*See KIDNEY, NEPHRONOPHTHISIS-MEDULLARY CYSTIC DESEASE*
**Tuftsin deficiency**
*See IMMUNODEFICIENCY, TUFTSIN DEFICIENCY TYPE*
**Tumor, juxtavagal**
*See CAROTID BODY TUMOR*
**Tumor, mixed, of salivary gland**
*See SALIVARY GLAND, MIXED TUMOR*
**Tumors of the central nervous system, site-specific aggregation**
*See CANCER, NEUROEPITHELIAL AND MENINGEAL*
**Tune deafness**
*See DEAFNESS, TUNE*
**Turban tumors**
*See EPITHELIOMAS, HEREDITARY MULTIPLE CYSTIC*
**Turban tumors of scalp**
*See SCALP, CYLINDROMAS*
**Turbinate deformity**
*See NOSE, TURBINATE DEFORMITY*

---

**TURCOT SYNDROME**                                              **2739**

**Includes:**
 Brain tumor-adenomatous polyposis syndrome
 Central nervous system tumors-polyposis of colon
 Colon (familial polyposis)-CNS tumors
 Glioma-polyposis

**Excludes:**
 Brain tumors-small numbers of colorectal adenomas in the
  young
 **Cancer, glioma, familial** (2839)
 **Intestinal polyposis, type I** (0535)
 **Intestinal polyposis, type III** (0536)

**Major Diagnostic Criteria:** Central nervous system tumor (medulloblastoma, glial cell tumor, or pituitary adenoma) in a patient affected with or at risk for adenomatous polyposis syndrome. These histopathologic types of brain tumors appear to be one of the several extraintestinal manifestations of **Intestinal polyposis, type I** which is characterized >100 colorectal adenomas, autosomal dominant inheritance, and a chromosomal marker on 5q21-q22.

**Clinical Findings:** The clinical findings are those of a brain tumor, with the neurologic manifestations dependent on the anatomic site. Clinical evidence of the brain tumor can either precede or follow onset of manifestations of adenomatous polyposis syndrome. Examination of parents, sibs, and offspring for evidence of adenomatous polyposis syndrome, including its extracolonic manifestations, may confirm the familial nature of the illness. However, affected members of the same family may demonstrate different patterns of extracolonic disease.

**Complications:** The clinical picture is usually dominated by the manifestations of the brain tumor. Colorectal carcinoma can result from polyposis if a preventive colectomy is not performed.

**Associated Findings:** Other extracolonic manifestations of adenomatous polyposis syndrome may be present, including epidermal inclusion cysts, **Retina, congenital hypertrophy of retinal pigment epithelium**, occult radio-opaque jaw lesions, and carcinomas of the thyroid and other extracolonic sites. Café-au-lait spots have been reported in several patients.

**Etiology:** **Intestinal polyposis, type I** is an autosomal dominantly inherited condition. Extracolonic manifestations, including brain tumors, are variable components of undetermined etiology.

**Pathogenesis:** Unknown.

**MIM No.:** *27630

**Sex Ratio:** M1:F1

**Occurrence:** Adenomatous polyposis syndrome (see **Intestinal polyposis, type I**) has an incidence of about 1:7,500 to 1:22,000 live births. Turcot syndrome occurs in less than 5% of pedigrees with adenomatous polyposis. Fewer than 100 cases have been documented.

**Risk of Recurrence for Patient's Sib:**
 See Part I, *Mendelian Inheritance*. For brain tumor, uncertain; rare sibs with Turcot syndrome have been reported.

**Risk of Recurrence for Patient's Child:**
 See Part I, *Mendelian Inheritance*. No cases of brain tumor in offspring of a patient with Turcot syndrome have been reported in the literature.

**Age of Detectability:** Adenomatous polyposis syndrome may be detectable *in utero* by use of the recently described chromosomal markers. Some clinical markers are apparent in childhood (elevated colonic mucosal ornithine decarboxylase activity, **Retina, congenital hypertrophy of retinal pigment epithelium**, presence of occult radio-opaque jaw lesions). The brain tumor may present clinically before or after the manifestations of adenomatous polyposis syndrome.

**Gene Mapping and Linkage:** APC (adenomatosis polyposis coli) has been mapped to 5q21-q22.

**Prevention:** None known. Genetic counseling indicated.

**Treatment:** Appropriate therapy for **Intestinal polyposis, type I** and brain tumor.

**Prognosis:** Outcome usually depends on results of the therapy of the brain tumor.

**Detection of Carrier:** N/A

**Special Considerations:** The literature contains reports of sibs with brain tumors and small numbers of colorectal adenomas occurring at a young age (Baughman syndrome). The relationship of this syndrome to Turcot syndrome must await the results of DNA studies.
 Although the eponym *Turcot syndrome* is used after the 1959 publication of J. Turcot et al., the first patient with this syndrome was reported in the literature in 1949 by H.W. Crail.

**Support Groups:** Atlanta; American Cancer Society

**References:**
Crail HW: Multiple primary malignancies arising in the rectum, brain, and thyroid. Naval Medical Bulletin 1949; 49:123–128.
Turcot J, et al.: Malignant tumors of the central nervous system associated with familial polyposis of the colon: report of two cases. Dis Colon Rectum 1959; 2:465–468.
Baughman FA Jr., et al.: The glioma-polyposis syndrome. New Engl J Med 1969; 281:1345–1346.
Bodmer WF, et al.: Localization of the gene for familial polyposis on chromosome 5. Nature 1987; 328:614–616.
Costa OL, et al.: Turcot syndrome: autosomal dominant or recessive transmission? Dis Colon Rectum 1987; 30:391–394.
Jarvis L, et al.: Turcot's syndrome: a review. Dis Colon Rectum 1988; 31:907–914.

HA078          **Stanley R. Hamilton**

**Turner phenotype with normal karyotype**
*See NOONAN SYNDROME*

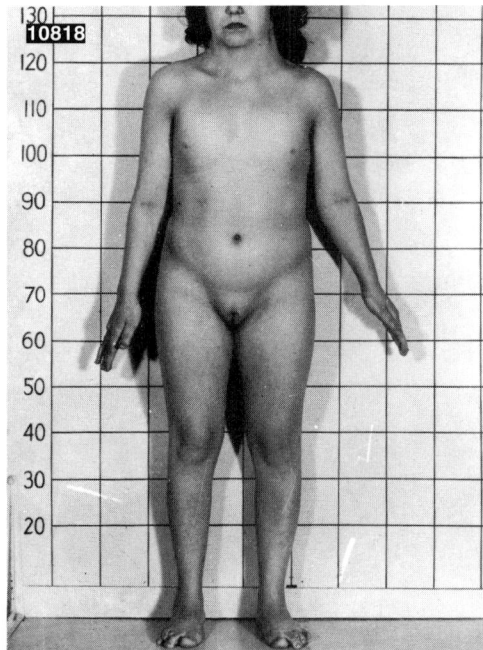

## TURNER SYNDROME      0977

**Includes:**
> Chromosome X, monosomy X
> Chromosome 45,X syndrome
> Mosaic Turner syndrome
> Short stature-sexual infantilism
> Ullirch-Turner syndrome

**Excludes:**
> **Chromosome 22, trisomy mosaicism** (2478)
> **Gonadal dysgenesis, XX type** (0436)
> **Gonadal dysgenesis, XY type** (0437)
> **Noonan syndrome** (0720)

**Major Diagnostic Criteria:** A female should be tested for the diagnosis of Turner syndrome if during the newborn period she has edema of the hands and feet and excessive skin of the neck or if during childhood she has short stature, left-sided cardiac or aortic problems, particularly coarctation or dilation of the aorta. During the teenage period, the diagnosis should be suspected if there is delayed adolescence and primary amenorrhea, particularly if associated with short stature. In each of these situations, a karyotype should be obtained to establish or exclude Turner syndrome.

Since features found in the Turner syndrome are also seen in other conditions, a chromosomal analysis demonstrating partial or complete monosomy X or monosomy X mosaicism is mandatory to make the diagnosis. Cytogenetic analyses from several tissue sources may be necessary to detect a mosaic form of Turner syndrome. A buccal smear is not an adequate laboratory test to diagnose Turner syndrome and should never be used.

**Clinical Findings:** The frequency of the cardinal clinical features of Turner syndrome are small stature, often evident at birth (100%); ovarian dysgenesis with concomitant amenorrhea and sterility (>90%); lymphedema, with puffiness of the dorsum of the hands and feet, often noted at birth (40%); broad chest, sometimes with pectus excavatum, with widely spaced and often hypoplastic or inverted nipples (>80%); anomalous ears, most often prominent (80%); low posterior hairline with short-appearing neck (80%); narrow maxilla (palate) (80%); micrognathia (>70%); cubitus valgus (70%); narrow, hyperconvex, and deeply set nails (70%); renal anomalies (the most common being horseshoe kidney and double or cleft renal pelvis) (60%); redundant skin of the neck or webbed neck (50%); short metacarpals and metatarsals of the fourth digits (50%); pigmented nevi (50%); hearing impairment (50%); cardiac and aortic defects, including bicuspid aortic valves and coarctation, dilation, and rupture of the aorta (20–40%); and unexplained hypertension (27%).

Less common features of Turner syndrome include ptosis of the eyelids, hypertelorism, and vertebral and other skeletal anomalies. Dermatoglyphic features include an increase in hypothenar patterns, a distally placed palmar axial triradius, and large fin-

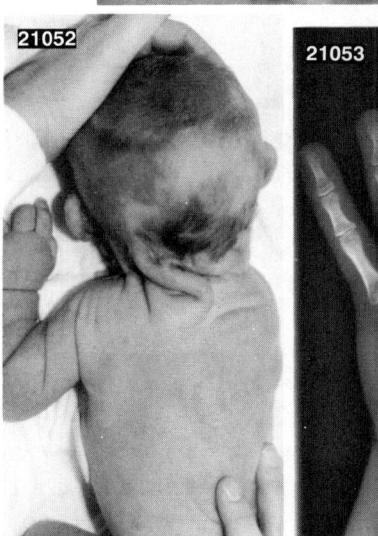
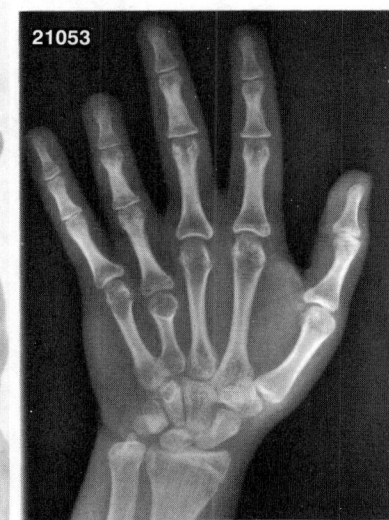

**0977A-10818:** Female with 45,X karyotype and webbed neck, shield-like chest, cubitus valgus and sexual infantilism. **21052:** Newborn infant with 45,X karyotype and cystic hygroma. **21053:** Hand X-ray of an adult with short 4th metacarpal and a resulting short 4th finger.

gertip patterns, most commonly whorls, with an increase in total ridge count. A transverse palmar crease (simian crease) is seen more often than in the general population. Secondary amenorrhea occurs infrequently and generally early.

Hypoplastic left heart syndrome occurs more frequently in Turner syndrome and may represent the extreme of the left-sided heart lesions seen in these patients. In addition, the incidence of congenital heart disease in Turner syndrome patients with webbing of the neck appears to be increased. For instance, Clark (1984) found that 30% of 106 patients with neck webbing had congenital heart disease, while only 9% of 87 patients without the webbing had a significant heart defect. One explanation for this is that

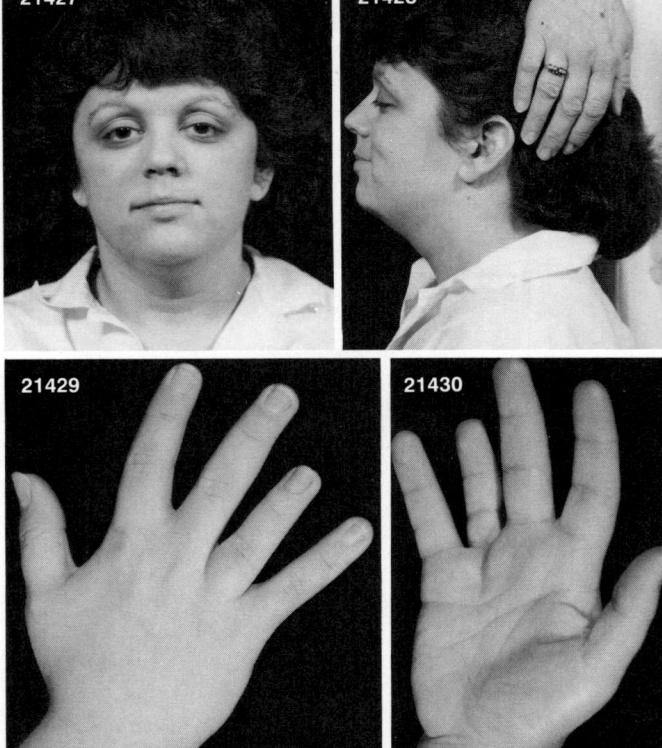

**0977B-21427–28:** AP and lateral views of a 24-year-old woman with 45,X/46,Xr(X)/46, X,i(Xq). This patient has a high arched palate, but does not have neck webbing. **21429:** Right hand shows short 4th finger due to a short 4th metacarpal. **21430:** Palm of the right hand shows a rearrangement of the creases of the base of the 4th finger.

45,X/46,XX, in which case the effects of the monosomic cell line may be mitigated by the normal cell line. In addition, structural abnormalities of the X chromosome may produce partial monosomy of either the p or q arms or both. When one of the short arms is deleted, the Turner phenotype is invariably present, while normal gonadal development and function is generally preserved. However, this function is lost if the deletion extends to the proximal region of Xp11. Monosomy for Xq produces gonadal dysgenesis when the breakpoint is at or proximal to Xq21, with about one-half of the patients showing signs of Turner syndrome. Pure gonadal dysgenesis has been observed when the breakpoint is at or distal to Xq22 (Passarge and Schmidt, 1983).

### Karyotypes found in patients with Turner syndrome

| Karyotype | Description | Percent of cases |
|---|---|---|
| 45,X | Complete monosomy X | 57 % |
| 46,X,i(Xq) and mosaics with i(xq) | Isochromosome of the long arm of the X chromosome (monosomy Xp) | 17 % |
| Mosaics 45,X/46XX; 45,X/47,XXX; etc | Mosaic monosomy | 12 % |
| 45,X/46XY | Mosaic monosomy X with Y-bearing cell line | 4 % |
| Other (del(Xp), r(X), mosaics) | Xp monosomy, ring X | 10 % |

**Pathogenesis:** Monosomy X may occur as a result of nondisjunction during gametogenesis in either the mother or the father, or it may be the result of errors in mitosis after fertilization. An increased incidence of Turner syndrome births among older mothers has not been demonstrated. In fact, in testable cases, the paternal-derived sex chromosome is more often missing than the maternal X chromosome. This would suggest that a meiotic error in spermatogenesis or a loss of the paternal X or Y chromosome through mitotic error is the more usual cause.

It is unclear why either deletions of the short arm of an X chromosome or a missing X chromosome produces the Turner phenotype. It is clear that monosomy X is highly lethal prenatally, since cytogenetic investigations of spontaneous abortions indicate that more than 95% of Turner conceptuses do not reach term.

With regard to oogenesis and development of ovaries in Turner syndrome, evaluation of 45,X embryos and fetuses has shown that ovarian development is normal. Subsequently, the rate of degeneration of the primary oocytes appears to be increased over that in 46,XX females. Consequently, by puberty there are few, if any, oocytes remaining in the ovaries of Turner individuals. However, there is the occasional Turner female who develops secondary sexual characteristics and menses and may be fertile. In these women, the germ cell attrition rate is most likely less, and oocytes are present at puberty and beyond. These cases may represent the extreme end of the spectrum of germ cell degeneration, or they may be cases of Turner mosaicism. Turner mosaics frequently have normal puberty, are often fertile, but have earlier onset of menopause.

Patients with 45,X/46,XY mosaicism may have clitoral enlargement at birth and virilize to an extent at puberty. The pathogenesis of gonadal tumors in these individuals is not understood.

The lymphedema seen in Turner syndrome results from atresia, hypoplasia, and delayed development of the lymphatic system. The edema seen in fetuses is frequently profound and may be detected prenatally by ultrasound as hydrops fetalis or cystic hygroma.

**POS No.:** 3104

**CDC No.:** 758.610, 758.600

**Sex Ratio:** M0:F1

**Occurrence:** A minimum estimate of 1:5,000 live births.

**Risk of Recurrence for Patient's Sib:** Very low unless an identical twin.

lymphedema compresses the ascending aorta, altering the intracardiac blood flow.

Earlier studies suggested an increased incidence in mental retardation among females with Turner syndrome. It is now recognized that this is not the case, but affected individuals may have a deficiency in spatial ability that will affect their performance on standard IQ tests. Verbal skills are reportedly normal.

In general, no single one of the above clinical findings is found in every patient, and, likewise, no one patient exhibits every clinical feature listed.

**Complications:** Coarctation, hypertension, and aortic dilation may require treatment. Aortic dissection may develop as a result of the aortic dilation and may be lethal if not treated promptly. Females with 45,X or 45,X/46,XX karyotypes are generally not considered at increased risk for gonadal neoplasias. However, with 45,X/46,XY mosaicism, the Y-bearing cell line does predispose these patients to these neoplasias. Thus, any Turner syndrome patient with a Y chromosome cell line must have her gonads surgically removed.

Psychologic problems may result from sexual infantilism, short stature, primary amenorrhea, and sterility.

**Associated Findings:** Turner females may have an increase incidence of thyroiditis, diabetes mellitus, and collagen-vascular disease.

**Etiology:** The most frequent karyotype in Turner syndrome is 45,X, i.e. complete monosomy X. Mosaic individuals may be

**Risk of Recurrence for Patient's Child:** More than 99% of Turner syndrome patients are sterile. A study of pregnancies among women with 45,X and various mosaic karyotypes identified 54 pregnancies that resulted in 16 miscarriages, one termination, 12 abnormal children, three stillborns, and 22 normal live-born. The abnormalities included neural tube defects, **Chromosome 21, trisomy 21**, and Turner syndrome mosaicism. These observations may represent biases in ascertainment in that most of these children were first identified at birth as having congential or chromosomal abnormalities that resulted in the chromosomal analysis of their mothers. As might be expected, the reproductive record of Turner women who were identified first is better than those recognized retrospectively.

**Age of Detectability:** Prenatally through adulthood.

**Gene Mapping and Linkage:** See *Gene Map*.

**Prevention:** None known. Genetic counseling indicated.

**Treatment:** Cyclic estrogen replacement therapy is usually begun in the second decade of life in patients lacking sexual development. The therapy should be delayed for as long as possible to allow for maxium growth in height. However, much delay may not be possible for psychologic reasons if the girl is disturbed because she is not maturing at the same rate as her peers. Some authorities recommend the use of anabolic steroids for several years prior to the onset of estrogen therapy in an effort to increase the growth rate. More recent studies report the use of synthetic human growth hormone with encouraging preliminary results. In one study, administering human growth hormone in conjunction with anabolic steroids produced the greatest growth response.

Surgical intervention may be necessary for cardiovascular and renal anomalies, ptosis of the eyelids, and webbing of the neck. Surgical removal of any remaining gonadal tissue is indicated if a Y-bearing cell line is present. Vision and hearing defects may need to be corrected, and orthondontic treatment for dental malocclusion may be necessary. Supportive counseling or psychotherapy may be necessary because of short stature, lack of sexual development, and sterility. If learning disabilities occur, special education may be required.

Although the vast majority of women with Turner syndrome have been incapable of reproduction, they usually have normal uteruses. There are now cases reported in which embryos were transplanted in the uteruses of the Turner individuals who then carried the resulting pregnancies to term. Appropriate prepregnancy and intrapregnancy hormonal support was needed in each case.

**Prognosis:** Life span is presumably normal if there are no cardiovascular and renal anomalies, hypertension, and gonadal tumors, or if these conditions are treated.

**Detection of Carrier:** Unknown.

**Special Considerations:** The clinical features listed are based on cases with 45,X karyotypes. If a 46,XX cell line exists, these features may mitigate the effects of the monosomy X cell line. Thus, the frequency of sexual development, menses, and fertility is greater in the mosaic female, and other physical problems may be absent or less severe. Additionally, the mean ultimate height of mosaic patients is greater than that of nonmosaic Turner syndrome patients.

In nonmosaic patients with 46, X,i(Xq) karyotype, the phenotype is not significantly different from that seen in nonmosaic monosomy X. The severity of the phenotypic alterations in 46,X,r(X) and 46,X,del(Xp) patients may roughly correlate with the extent of deletion of the short arm of X. A deletion of the long arm of the X chromosome does produce gonadal dysgenesis, with resulting sexual infantilism, amenorrhea, and sterility. While the majority of patients with Xq deletions do not exhibit the typical phenotypic features of Turner syndrome, there are reported patients with short stature and the somatic features of Turner syndrome who have Xq deletions. Phenotypic variation appears to correlate with the break point on the long arm.

**Support Groups:**
CA; Sacramento; Turner's Syndrome Society of Sacramento
MD; Baltimore; Human Growth Foundation
NJ; Somerset; Turner's Syndrome Support Group
CANADA: Ontario; Downsview; Turner's Syndrome Society

**References:**
Turner HH: A syndrome of infantilism, congenital webbed neck, and cubitus valgus. Endocrinology 1938; 23:566. *
Palmer CG, Reichmann A: Chromosomal and clinical findings in 100 females with Turner syndrome. Hum Genet 1976; 35:35–49.
Simpson JL: Disorders of sexual differentiation. Chicago: Year Book Medical Publishers, 1977:259–302. *
Dewhurst J: Fertility in 47,XXX and 45,X patients. J Med Genet 1978; 15:132–135.
Passarge P, Schmidt A: Functional consequences of X-chromosome loss in the human female. In: Sandberg A, ed: Cytogenetics of the mammalian X chromosome, Part B: X chromosome anomalies and their clinical manifestations. New York: Alan R. Liss, 1983:301–320.
Bender B, et al.: Cognitive development of unselected girls with complete and partial X monosomy. Pediatrics 1984; 73:175–182.
Clark EB: Neck web and congenital heart defects: a pathogenic association in 45 X-O turner syndrome? Teratology 1984, 29:355–361.
Hassold T, et al.: Determination of the parental origin of sex-chromosome monosomy using restriction fragment length polymorphisms. Am J Hum Genet 1985; 37:965–972.
Lin AE, et al.: Aortic dilation, dissection, and rupture in patients with Turner syndrome. J Pediatr 1986; 109:820–826.
Rosenfeld RG, et al.: Methionyl human growth hormone and oxandrolone in Turner syndrome: preliminary results of a prospective randomized trial. J Pediatr 1986; 109:936–943. *
Knudtzon J, Aarskog D: 45,X/46,XY mosaicism: a clinical review and report of ten cases. Eur J Pediatr 1987; 146:266–271.
Massarano AA, et al.: Ovarian ultrasound appearances in Turner syndrome. J Pediatr 1989; 114:568–573.

DA029
WE005

**Margaret A. Davee**
**David D. Weaver**

**Turner syndrome phenotype**
*See NECK, CYSTIC HYGROMA, FETAL TYPE*
**Turner syndrome, familial**
*See NOONAN SYNDROME*
**Turner tooth**
*See TEETH, ENAMEL HYPOPLASIA*
**Turner-Kieser syndrome**
*See NAIL-PATELLA SYNDROME*
**Turricephaly**
*See CRANIOSYNOSTOSIS*
**Twin-to-twin transfusion**
*See FETAL MONOZYGOUS MULTIPLE PREGNANCY DYSPLACENTATION EFFECTS*

---

**TWINS, CONJOINED**                                                    **0202**

**Includes:**
Conjoined twins
Craniopagus
Dicephalus
Diprosopus
Dipygus
Ischiopagus
Monozygotic twins, conjoined
Omphalopagus
Pygopagus
Rachipagus
Siamese twins
Syncephalus
Terata anacatadidymus
Terata anadidymus
Terata catadidymus
Thoracopagus

**Excludes:** Parasitic twinning

**Major Diagnostic Criteria:** Fusion of some portion of monovular or monozygotic twins.

**Clinical Findings:** Diagnosis evident by physical examination. The visceral conjunction between the co-twins requires X-ray,

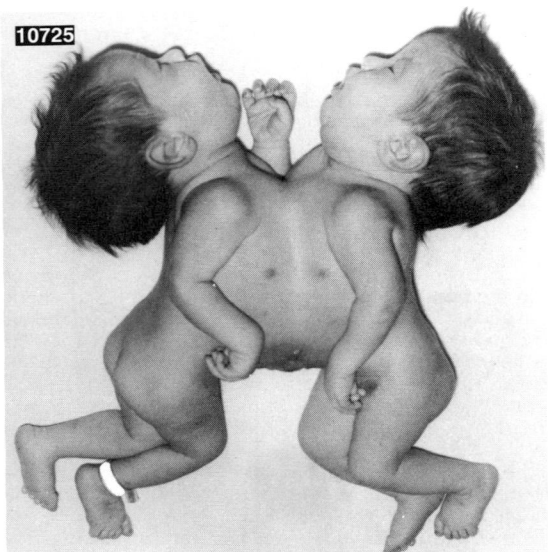

0202A-10725: Lateral view of thoracopagus twins.

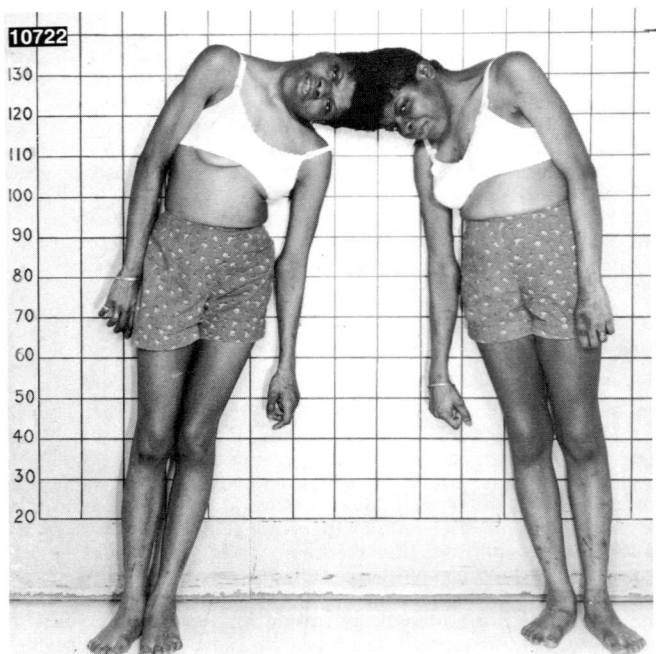

isotope and ultrasound techniques to outline anatomic and functional interdependence. Diagnosis can be made in utero by the use of X-ray or ultrasound techniques. Common types of fusion include:

Terata catadidymus - fusion caudally
Diprosopus - single trunk and limbs, varying duplication of face and head
Dicephalus - single trunk and limbs, duplication of head
Ischiopagus - Fusion at ischia, the axis of the 2 bodies being at 180° - 6% +
Pygopagus - fusion in sacral region - 19% +
Terata anadidymus - fusion in cephalic region
Dipygus - fusion limited to region proximal to pelvis
Syncephalus - Single head, separation below head
Craniopagus - fusion at the head - 2% +
Terata anacatadidymus - fusion in midportion of body
Thoracopagus - fusion in sternal region - 74% +
Omphalopagus - fusion in abdominal region
Rachipagus - fusion back to back in sagittal plane, fusion limited to upper trunk and cervical region
Rudolph et al (1967) reviewed 117 cases; the basic problem in thoracopagus is whether separate hearts allow surgery. In ischiopagus, pygopagus and craniopagus decisions need to be made concerning which twin will benefit from single shared organs.

**Complications:** All cases with conjoined hearts have died with or without the aid of surgery. Unexplained postoperative deaths have occurred, therefore, careful postoperative monitoring is required.

**Associated Findings:** Nearly all cases of dicephalus and diprosopus have associated neural tube defects.

**Etiology:** Conjoined twins are the product of a single ovum. They are monovular or monozygotic twins. Teratogenesis occurs by incomplete fission during the process of twinning. While monozygotic twinning is considered uninfluenced by genetic factors, Harvey et al (1977) has reported on ten families with multiple pairs of monozygotic twins. Derom et al (1987) has reported a significant increase in the frequency of zygotic splitting producing monozygotic twins and triplets after artificial induction of ovulation.

**Pathogenesis:** According to Zimmermann (1967), the morula becomes a blastocyst on day 6 of ovulation age. Within this vesicle, 0.2–0.3 mm in length, the inner cell mass develops at one

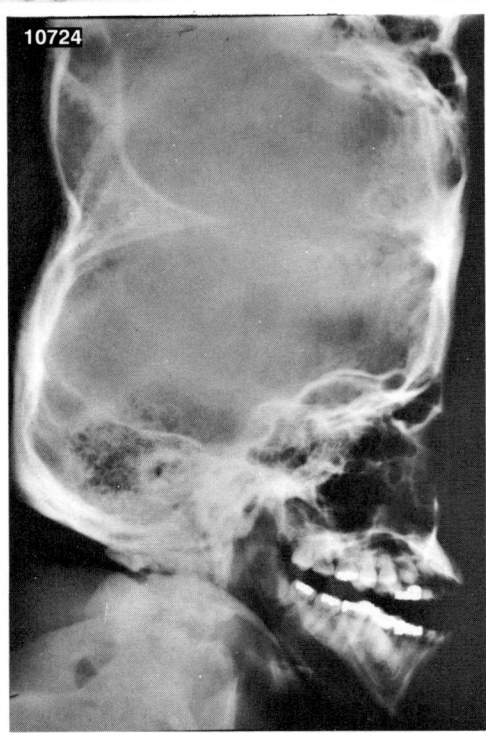

0202B-10722: Conjoined craniophagus twins at 23 years of age.
10724: Lateral view of skulls showing bony fusion and projecting bony shelf.

pole. The inner cell mass is totipotent for morphogenesis and organogenesis. For a short time, this cell mass has the potentialities of forming a single or dual embryologic primordium or germinal disk. The caudal end, appearing between 15 and 18 days of embryonic age, represents the primitive streak which is the primordium of all intraembryogenic mesoderm. Terata are the result either of disordered morphogenesis or organogenesis. By day 20 the process of either normal twinning or conjoined twinning will be initiated. The end of the 3rd week of development age marks the end of the period of incomplete fission. The anomalous twinning can occur at any point of incomplete division of the inner cell mass accounting for the variations in types of conjoined twins.

**MIM No.:**  27641

**CDC No.:**  759.4

**Sex Ratio:**  M3:F7

**Occurrence:**  0.06:1000 live births in India and Africa; 0.004:1000 live births in Europe and the Americas. Prevalence rare.

**Risk of Recurrence for Patient's Sib:**  Undetermined but presumably rare.

**Risk of Recurrence for Patient's Child:**  Undetermined but presumably rare.

**Age of Detectability:**  At birth or prenatally.

**Gene Mapping and Linkage:**  Unknown.

**Prevention:**  None known. Genetic counseling indicated.

**Treatment:**  Extent of cardiac anomalies not detectable before 8 weeks of fetal development. The presence of twins with a single fetal EKG is the most serious condition.

Surgical separations have been successfully performed on all conjoined twins with exception of those thoracopagus with conjoined hearts. Although experience is scanty, it is probable that other anomalies of fission can be managed by existing rehabilitation procedures.

**Prognosis:**  Although conjoined twins have lived as long as 63 years without separation, surgical separation is the management of choice. Psychologic studies of unoperated twins reveal serious limitations to the quality of life. The rehabilitation of any postoperative defects due to incomplete fission of shared organs and tissues is vital to the success of the surgical approach. The general experience has been that optimal surgical management requires a well-rehearsed surgical and pediatric team. In the absence of a single heart, the procedure should not be carried out under emergency conditions. At present, there are no survivors following division of a single heart, however, it is expected that this will become possible with continuing advances in cardiovascular surgery.

**Detection of Carrier:**  Unknown.

**Special Considerations:**  Steps in evaluation of operability: 1) Physical examination to differentiate thoracopagus and omphalopagus twins; operative separation of omphalopagus twins. 2) EKG with standard leads to determine ventricular independence; operative separation of those with separate QRS complexes (25%). 3) Angiography with physiologic study to determine great vessel and atrial communication; operative separation of conjoined atrium (10%) and 4) Ethical considerations; e.g. whether only one twin can survive with existing shared ventricular structure (68%).

**Support Groups:**
  RI; Providence; The Twins Foundation
  MD; Rockville; National Organization of Mothers of Twin Clubs

**References:**
Nichols BL, et al.: General clinical management of thoracopagus twins. In: Bergsma D, ed: Conjoined twins. BD:OAS 1967; III(1):28. White Plains: The National Foundation-March of Dimes.

Rudolph AJ, et al.: Obstetric management of conjoined twins. In Bergsma D, ed: Conjoined twins. BD:OAS 1967; III(1):38. White Plains: The National Foundation-March of Dimes.

Zimmermann AA: Embryologic and anatomic considerations of conjoined twins. In Bergsma D, ed: Conjoined twins. BD:OAS 1967; III(1):18. White Plains: The National Foundation-March of Dimes.

Harvey MAS, et al.: Familial monozygotic twinning. J Pediat 1977; 90:246–248.

Benirscke K, et al.: Conjoined twins: nosology and congenital malformations. BD:OAS 1978; XIV(6A):179. White Plains: The National Foundation-March of Dimes.

Edmonds LD, Layde PM: Conjoined twins in the United States, 1970–1977. Teratology 1982; 25:301.

Derom C, et al.: Increased monozygotic twinning rate after ovulation induction. Lancet 1987; I:1236–1238.

Cunniff C, et al.: Laterality defects in conjoined twins. Am J Med Genet 1988; 31:669–677.

NI003                                        **Buford L. Nichols**

---

**TWINS, CONJOINED, TERATOGENICITY          2928**

**Includes:**
  Clomaphene ovulation induction and conjoined twins
  Griseofulvin exposure and conjoined twins
  Valproic acid and conjoined twins

**Excludes:**  Fetal effects (other)

**Major Diagnostic Criteria:**  Possible teratogenic exposure causing conjoined twinning.

**Clinical Findings:**  Several suspicious periconceptional drug exposures have been reported with conjoined twinning. Two cases of conjoined twins with periconceptional maternal griseofulvin exposure have been separately reported to the Food and Drug Administration. Griseofulvin is an orally administered agent for fungus infections, usually epidermal. Because of the rarity of conjoined twins (about 1:20,000 pregnancies), and the infrequency of maternal first trimester griseofulvin exposure (about 1:2,000), this coincidence is unlikely to have occurred by chance. Both of the outcomes with griseofulvin exposure were thoracopagus, which consitute about 18% of conjoined twins. Record studies of 86 other cases of conjoined twins did not find a griseofulvin exposure, but this is inadequate to rule out an association, because of the rarity of griseofulvin exposure.

Seven cases of conjoined twinning have been reported with clomaphene ovulation induction (two published). Only one set occurred in cohort studies totalling 5,519 clomaphene inductions. This indicates this is a rare occurrence with clomaphene induction. Clomaphene is a much more frequent pregnancy exposure than griseofulvin. Two of the clomaphene exposed cases were detected among 61 conjoined twins in two birth defect registries. Case control study of conjoined twins is necessary to determine if clomaphene exposure is more frequent than expected.

One set of conjoined twins with associated spina bifida has been reported to FDA with maternal exposure to an antiepileptic combination including valproic acid. Valproic acid is known to be associated with spina bifida, and spina bifida is known to be associated with conjoined twinning.

**Complications:**  Unknown.

**Associated Findings:**  None known.

**Etiology:**  Where a drug teratogen is associated with conjoined twinning, the etiology could be either the agent or the indication for which the agent is given. Subfertility for which clomaphene is given could be the actual true association. In this case, an association may be found with subfertility management other than clomaphene. Epilepsy for which valproic acid is given, or fungus infections for which griseofulvin is given, have less causal plausibility.

**Pathogenesis:**  Interference with completion of twinning fission of blastula from 15–20 days following ovulation. Griseofulvin is known to be an animal teratogen. It affects microtubules, which have a role in spindle formation. Other agents having such an effect include vincristine, podophyllotoxin, and colchicine.

**Sex Ratio:**  Presumably M1:F1.

**Occurrence:**  For these suspicious exposures, data is inadequate to establish that conjoined twinning is a result of exposure, but adequate to show that association is infrequent.

**Risk of Recurrence for Patient's Sib:**  Unknown.

**Risk of Recurrence for Patient's Child:**  Unknown.

**Age of Detectability:**  Prenatal detection by ultrasound is possible.

**Gene Mapping and Linkage:** Unknown.

**Prevention:** Because griseofulvin treatment is seldom urgent, use should be avoided in early pregnancy. With accidental exposure, most outcomes are likely to be normal.

**Treatment:** Unknown.

**Prognosis:** Unknown.

**Detection of Carrier:** N/A

**Special Considerations:** The FDA Division of Drug Experience urges exposure inquiries and reports on any conjoined twins.

*This article expresses the views of the author and is not an official statement of the Food and Drug Administration.*

**References:**

Carlson DH, et al.: Cephalothoracopagus syncephalus: prenatal roentgenographic diagnosis. Pediat Radiol 1975; 3:50–52.

Edmunds LD, Layde PM: Conjoined twins in the U.S., 1970–1977. Teratology 1982; 25:301–308.

Brenbridge AN, Teja K: Sonographic findings in the prenatal diagnosis of cephalothoracopagus syncephalus. J Reprod Med 1987; 32:59–62.

Knudsen LB: No association between griseofulvin and conjoined twinning. Lancet 1987; II:1097.

Rosa FW, et al.: Griseofulvin teratology including two thoracopagus conjoined twins. Lancet 1987; I:171. *

R0018                                               **Franz W. Rosa**

**Twins, parasitic conjoined without spinal columns**
  *See LIMBS, SUPERNUMERARY*
**Two-Chambered right ventricle**
  *See VENTRICLE, DOUBLE CHAMBERED RIGHT*
**Two-oxoglutaric aciduria**
  *See ACIDEMIA, 2-OXOGLUTARIC*
**Tylosis**
  *See KERATOSIS PALMARIS ET PLANTARIS OF UNNA-THOST*
**Tylosis with malignancy**
  *See HOWEL EVANS SYNDROME*
**Typical retinoschisis, autosomal dominant**
  *See RETINOSCHISIS*
**Typus degenerativus Amstelodamensis**
  *See DE LANGE SYNDROME*
**Typus Edinburgensis**
  *See EDINBURGH MALFORMATION SYNDROME*
**Tyrosinase negative oculocutaneous albinism**
  *See ALBINISM, OCULOCUTANEOUS, TYROSINASE NEGATIVE*
**Tyrosinase positive oculocutaneous albinism**
  *See ALBINISM, OCULOCUTANEOUS, TYROSINASE POSITIVE*
**Tyrosine 77 amyloidosos**
  *See AMYLOIDOSIS, ILLINOIS TYPE*
**Tyrosine aminotransferase deficiency**
  *See TYROSINEMIA II, OREGON TYPE*
**Tyrosine transaminase deficiency**
  *See TYROSINEMIA II, OREGON TYPE*
**Tyrosinemia and tyrosyluria, hereditary**
  *See TYROSINEMIA I*

## TYROSINEMIA I                                    0978

**Includes:**
  Four-hydroxyphenylpyruvic acid oxidase deficiency
  Fumarylacetoacetase deficiency
  Hepatorenal tyrosinemia
  Tyrosinemia and tyrosyluria, hereditary
  Tyrosinemia III
  Tyrosinosis, acute and chronic

**Excludes:**
  Tyrosinemia and tyrosyluria associated with disease states
  Tyrosinemia and tyrosyluria, transient of newborn
  **Tyrosinemia II, Oregon type** (2009)

**Major Diagnostic Criteria:** Clinical evidence of hepatic cellular damage and renal tubular defect, in association with hypertyrosinemia and a distinctive aminoaciduria. There is persistent elevation of the concentration of tyrosine in plasma above 3 mg/dl with normal or slightly elevated levels of plasma phenylalanine,

(phenylalanine/tyrosine ratio less than 1.0) and urinary hyperexcretion of tyrosyl compounds (p-hydroxyphenyllactic, p-hydroxyphenylpyruvic, and p-hydroxyphenylacetic acids) in the fasting state. Concentrations of alpha-fetoprotein in the blood are elevated. The currently accepted diagnostic feature is the excretion of large amounts of succinylacetone in the urine.

Differential diagnosis should include hereditary fructose intolerance, galactosemia, neonatal hepatitis, and congenital CMV infection.

Transient tyrosinemia of the newborn also presents with elevated concentrations of tyrosine in plasma, along with normal or slightly elevated phenylalanine and tyrosyluria. This condition appears to have no significant clinical sequelae. The elevation of tyrosine and tyrosyluria in this condition occur within the first 2 weeks of life and usually persists for one to two months, but it may persist for longer periods. The alteration of tyrosine metabolism seen in this condition is indicative of delayed maturation of liver enzyme systems and not a true inborn error of metabolism. It is more apt to occur in immature infants who ingest high-protein formula without vitamin C. Administration of high doses of vitamin C results in rapid return to normal of elevated plasma tyrosine levels. See **Tyrosinemia II, Oregon type**.

**Clinical Findings:** There are two variant patterns: acute and chronic.

The *acute form* is represented by most of the reported patients. Onset of symptoms occurs under one year of age. The presenting symptoms frequently are general manifestations such as temperature elevation, lethargy, and irritability; failure to thrive, however, has been the presenting complaint in nearly all cases. Hepatomegaly with or without abdominal distention, jaundice, or hepatic cirrhosis, has been found in more than 80% of patients. Vomiting, edema, ascites, and peculiar odor occur in at least one-half of the cases. Progressive hepatic failure may result in jaundice, anemia, ecchymosis, hemorrhage, melena, hematuria hypoproteinemia, diarrhea and, as noted in nearly one-third of patients, often in the terminal stage, demise is rapid.

The *chronic form* of hereditary tyrosinemia has been reported in a relatively small number of patients. Symptoms develop secondary to renal tubular dysfunction, and patients present with rickets and a less severe degree of hepatic cirrhosis. Most of these patients died under ten years of age; exceptions include a few recently reported patients between the ages of 12 and 20 years, several of whom have benefited from dietary treatment and hepatic transplantation.

Mental retardation and neurologic abnormalities are not constant findings.

Biochemical determinations in affected persons with acute or chronic hereditary tyrosinemia show elevated plasma levels of tyrosine above 3 mg/dl, with range of 3–12 mg/dl, (normal: < 1 mg/dl) and constant hyperexcretion of tyrosyl compounds (p-hydroxyphenyllactic acid, p-hydroxyphenylpyruvic acid, and p-hydroxyphenylacetic acid) in the fasting state. Increased levels of succinylacetone and succinylacetic acid in serum and urine, and increased urinary excretion of δ-aminolevulinic acid have been reported in the majority of recent cases.

Plasma levels of phenylalanine are usually not elevated.

Other significant urinary findings are a generalized aminoaciduria; hyperphosphaturia; proteinuria; and the presence of reducing substances, usually glucose.

Hypophosphatemia; reduced prothrombin-proconvertin index; hypoglycemia; elevated concentrations of alpha-fetoprotein; and elevated methionine in serum are frequent laboratory findings, particularly in terminal stages of hepatic failure.

X-rays demonstrate the characteristic bony changes of rickets.

**Complications:** Hepatic cirrhosis, resulting in hepatic failure and death in over 80% of cases; a complex renal tubular defect, producing a generalized aminoaciduria; hypophosphatemic rickets, more common in chronic form of hereditary tyrosinemia; and a coagulation defect, evidenced by ecchymosis, melena, hematuria, and prothrombin abnormality in about one-third of the cases.

**Associated Findings:**  Hepatoma (hepatocarcinoma) has been reported in over 30% of patients with tyrosinemia I who survive beyond two years of age; evidence suggests this is due to factors other than cirrhosis. The median age of death is reported to be five years, with a range from four to 25 years.

A few individuals have been reported with intermittent attacks of severe pain in the abdomen and legs, hypertensive crisis, and increased urinary excretion of δ-aminolevulinic acid.

A single case of diabetes mellitus has been reported. There is theoretical speculation that hyperkalemia, hypophosphatemia, and hypermethioninemia may contribute to pancreatic dysfunction; pancreatic islet cell hyperplasia and hypoglycemia have been observed. Tyrosinemia I has been reported in a child with partial monosomy 4p-.

**Etiology:**  Autosomal recessive inheritance. Specific data are not available to answer whether or not the observed impairment of enzyme activity of p-hydroxyphenylpyruvic acid oxidase, or of fumarylacetoacetase, represents the primary expression of the abnormal gene. Finding acute and chronic cases in a single family strengthens the hypothesis that there is one disease process, which has variable clinical manifestations.

The one individual with "tyrosinosis" reported by Medes appears to represent a different inborn error of metabolism, with the enzymatic block resulting in hyperexcretion of p-hydroxyphenylpyruvic acid, which is greater than the excretion of other tyrosyl compounds. This strongly suggests that the site of the block was in p-hydroxyphenylpyruvic acid oxidase, but the disorder is clearly different from that found in patients with "hereditary tyrosinemia." Medes' patient had myasthenia gravis but was essentially unaffected by the biochemical abnormality (tyrosinosis). A patient with mild retardation, seizures, abnormal EEG, and CT scan associated with defective activity of p-hydroxyphenylpyruvic acid oxidase and normal tyrosine aminotransferase and fumarylacetoacetase activities has been reported. This patient may represent the same disorder described by Medes, although the case has been cataloged as a new varient of hypertyrosinemia; *Tyrosinemia III* or *Four-hydroxyphenylpyruvic acid oxidase deficiency*.

**Pathogenesis:**  Several enzyme defects have been established in hepatic, renal and other organ tissues in affected patients. A marked deficiency of the enzyme p-hydroxyphenylpyruvic acid oxidase in hepatic and renal tissues has been reported whenever enzyme assays have been determined. This enzyme defect results in tyrosinemia and tyrosyluria. Data suggest that the decreased enzyme activity of p-HPPA oxidase found in this disorder may be secondary to liver disease, rather than causitive.

A deficiency of the enzyme fumarylacetoacetic acid hydrolase (fumarylacetoacetase), catalyzing the last step in the degradation of tyrosine, has been documented. This enzyme activity is markedly deficient in hepatic and renal tissue of affected patients, as well as in lymphocytes, skin fibroblasts, and cultured amniotic fluid cells. The resultant accumulation of its metabolites, succinylacetoacetate, succinylacetone, and furmarylacetone, partially explain multiple other enzyme deficiencies observed in this disease. These data have led to the suggestion that fumarylacetoacetase deficiency may be the primary enzyme defect in the pathogenesis of this disorder.

Methionine adenosyltransferase, cystathionine synthase, and tyosine aminotransferase (TAT) are reportedly decreased in the liver of patients with this condition.

The molecular defect of this disorder remains unclear. Clinical and biochemical variability observed in these patients point to the possibility that it may be due to a defect in a regulatory gene common for p-hydroxyphenylpyruvic acid oxidase and fumarylacetoacetase.

**MIM No.:**  *27670, *27671

**Sex Ratio:**  M1:F1

**Occurrence:**  Varies among different populations. An estimated 146:100,000 live births, and an estimated 1 carrier for every 14 persons has been determined in an isolated French Canadian population, as compared to an overall incidence of 8:100,000 in the French Canadian population of Quebec. Newborn screening in Norway and Sweden established a prevalence of 1:120,000 and 1:100,000 respectively. Approximately 100 cases, acute and chronic form, have been reported in the literature; most during the past 25 years.

**Risk of Recurrence for Patient's Sib:**
See Part I, *Mendelian Inheritance.*

**Risk of Recurrence for Patient's Child:**
See Part I, *Mendelian Inheritance.* Affected individuals are not expected to survive to reproduce.

**Age of Detectability:**  *Acute form*: hyperexcretion of tyrosyl compounds in urine and elevated plasma tyrosine has been reported as early as 2–3 weeks of age in one patient with a known affected sib.

*Chronic form*: onset of symptoms reported as early as six months of age, but most cases detected between one and three years of age.

Recent studies demonstrate increased succinylacetone in urine and serum at birth, and prenatally in amniotic fluid; activity of fumarylacetoacetase measured in cultured amniotic fibroblast cells is decreased (<5% of controls) in affected fetuses, thus allowing prenatal diagnosis. The feasibilty of enzymatic diagnosis in chorionic villus has been suggested. The δ-aminolevulinate dehydratase-inhibition test, an indirect measure of succinylacetone, provides another method for prenatal diagnosis in at-risk families.

**Gene Mapping and Linkage:**  FAH (fumarylacetoacetate) has been provisionally mapped to 15q23-q25.

**Prevention:**  None known. Genetic counseling indicated.

**Treatment:**  Low phenylalanine - low tyrosine diets have been tried, and some improvement in biochemical and clinical aspects of the disorder have been reported. Dietary treatment should begin early in life, and careful monitoring of plasma tyrosine, phenylalanine, and methionine is advised, with use of currently recommended formula, because of the high methionine concentrations. Cholestasis was reported in one patient, possibly associated with hypermethioninemia, suggesting the need to monitor serum bile acids as well.

Hepatic transplant, reported in several patients, offers the best opportunity for survival. Replacement of the liver corrects the hepatic enzyme deficiency, but kidney and other tissues remain potentially affected. Renal tubular dysfunction has reportedly continued after otherwise successful liver transplantation.

Supportive and symptomatic treatment for GI disturbances, electrolyte imbalance, hypoglycemia, anemia, bleeding, and rickets.

**Prognosis:**  *Untreated acute form*: Most patients die before one year of age, and frequently within one month after the onset of symptoms.

*Untreated chronic form*: Few patients are reported to have survived beyond ten years of age.

*Treated patients* on restricted phenylalanine-tyrosine diets may have an increased life expectancy, but data on long-term follow-up are inadequate. There is improvement of general symptoms, including disappearance of acidosis and ascites. The renal tubular lesion and rickets improve, and a growth spurt may occur. Significant improvement of liver disease has been recorded, but results are highly variable and possibly depend on the extent of prior irreversible hepatic damage, acute vs. chronic form, or on yet undetermined pathologic factors. Even when restrictive diets are started early in life, outcomes suggest that diet alone is not effective in preventing serious and fatal progression of liver and renal disease.

Hepatic transplantation appears to correct the enzyme defect, but renal and other tissue deficiencies persist in renal lesions of variable severity.

**Detection of Carrier:**  Levels of fumarylacetoacetase in red blood cells, lymphocytes, and fibroblasts of parents yield intermediate enzyme values, consistent with heterozygosity.

**Special Considerations:**  Tyrosinemia, tyrosinosis, and tyrosyluria have been interchangeably used in the literature to describe conditions with increased tyrosine in blood and urine, but it has become increasingly clear that a number of different conditions are described under these names. Some are probably true inborn errors of metabolism, and some represent maturational delay.

Several variant forms of hereditary hypertyrosinemia have been reported; patients demonstrating tyrosinemia, tyrosyluria, reduced p-hydroxyphenylpyruvic acid oxidase, and normal fumarylacetoacetase activity without hepatorenal dysfunction, or oculodermal lesions but with varied neurological symptoms, and normal FAH enzyme levels. One patient has been reported to have intermittent CNS symptoms associated with deficient activity of hepatic four-hydroxyphenylpyruvate dioxygenase; and two children with severe metabolic acidosis excreted unique tyrosine metabolites, hawkinsin, and four-hydroxycyclo-hexylacetic acid in urine (see **Hawkinsinuria**).

**References:**

Halvorsen S, et al.: Tyrosinosis: a study of 6 cases. Arch Dis Child 1966; 41:238–249. †

Shear CS, et al.: Tyrosinosis and tyrosinemia. In: Nyhan WL, ed: Amino acid metabolism and genetic variation. New York: McGraw-Hill, 1967:97–114. †

Gartner JC, et al.: Orthotopic liver transplantation in children: two-year experience with 47 patients. Pediatrics 1984; 74:140–145.

Nyhan WL: The tyrosinemias. In: Nyhan WL, ed: Abnormalities in amino acid metabolism in clinical medicine. Norwalk, CT: Appleton-Century-Crofts, 1984:149–169. *

Berger R: Biochemical aspects of type I hereditary tyrosinemia. In Bickel H, Wachtel U, eds: Inherited diseases of amino acid metabolism: recent progress in the understanding, recognition and management. New York: Thieme, 1985:191–202.

Kvittingen EA, et al.: Prenatal diagnosis of hereditary tyrosinemia by determination of fumarylacetoacetase in cultured amniotic fluid cells. Pediatr Res 1985; 19:334–337.

Starzl TE, et al.: Changing concepts: liver replacement for hereditary tyrosinemia and hepatoma. J Pediatr 1985; 106:604–606.

Tuchman M, et al.: Contribution of extrahepatic tissues to biochemical abnormalities in hereditary tyrosinemia type I. J Pediatr 1987; 110:399–403.

Goldsmith LA, Laberge C: Tyrosinemia and related disorders. In: Scriver CR, et al, eds: The metabolic basis of inherited disease, 6th ed. New York: McGraw-Hill, 1989:547–562. *

SH017
NY000

**Carol S. Shear**
**William L. Nyhan**

---

# TYROSINEMIA II, OREGON TYPE            2009

**Includes:**
Cytosolic tyrosine transaminase deficiency
Keratosis palmoplantaris-corneal dystrophy
Oculocutaneous tyrosinemia or tyrosinosis
"Oregon type" tyrosinosis
Richner-Hanhart Syndrome
Tyrosine aminotransferase deficiency
Tyrosine transaminase deficiency
Tyrosinemia with eye and skin lesions, familial
Tyrosinemia-plantar and palmar keratosis-ocular keratitis

**Excludes:**
**Tyrosinemia I** (0978)
Tyrosinemia and tyrosyluria, transient of the newborn
Tyrosinemia and tyrosyluria associated with disease states

**Major Diagnostic Criteria:** The diagnosis should be considered in patients with persistent elevation of the concentration of tyrosine in plasma (.1-.6mg/100dl) hyperexcretion of tyrosine, and tyrosyluria. The additional presence of the characteristic oculocutaneous lesions is diagnostic. Hepatic and renal functions are normal.

**Clinical Findings:** The predominant clinical features of the disease are ocular keratitis, hyperkeratosis and erosions of palms, soles, fingertips and toes. Mental retardation is commonly seen. The association of these clinical abnormalities with tyrosinemia, tyrosinuria, and tyrosyluria comprise this disorder. There is variable expressivity among patients described which suggests genetic heterogeneity.

Ocular symptoms such as photophobia, hyperlacrimation, redness and pain are present as early as two weeks of age. Most affected patients develop keratitis early in the first year of life, although onset is variable. A few patients have not manifested symptoms until eight or nine years of age, and others have not had any evidence of eye disease. The ocular lesions are mostly limited to the corneal epithelium and have been described as dendritic keratitis. Nonspecific inflammatory changes of the cornea and conjunctiva have been described, as well as corneal nebulae, and superficial or deep corneal ulcers. Patients have been misdiagnosed as having herpes-simplex keratitis. Fluorescein staining is absent or minimal. Cultures have been negative for herpes-simplex virus, bacteria and fungi. Treatment with topical antibiotics, corticosteroids or lubricants has been ineffective. Chronic eye disease in the untreated patient may result in cataracts, corneal scarring and opacification, nystagmus, exotropia, and visual impairment.

Skin lesions usually appear weeks or months after the onset of eye symptoms and may be painful. Initially, pinpoint papular lesions appear on fingers, toes, palms and soles; later they increase in size (5–10mm) and become hyperkeratotic. Some lesions are punctate erosions which may become crusted, hyperkeratotic, erythematous or pustular. Most often, the lesions are found on the distal phalanges or thenar and hypothenar eminences. The distribution may be linear. The skin lesions may clear spontaneously or worsen independent of topical or systemic therapies or other environmental factors. Many reported patients have been described as moderately to severely retarded. Others have demonstrated educational delay and behavioral abnormalities, presumably secondary to visual impairment. Microcephaly has been noted in at least four patients. Two patients displayed growth retardation and seizures; one patient reported had multiple congenital anomalies.

In affected patients the elevated concentrations of tyrosine in plasma range from 16–62mg/dl. Increased urinary excretion of tyrosine exceeds 2.5mg/mg creatine and has been reported as high as 3.2mg. p-tyramine, n-acetyltyrosine, p-hydroxyphenyllactic acid, p-hydroxyphenylacetic acid, and p-hydroxyphenylpyruvic acid may be found in the urine.

**Complications:** The chronic, inflammatory ocular lesions may result in corneal clouding, cataracts or glaucoma, and may lead to visual impairment or blindness. Subungual hyperkeratosis can produce separation of the nails and painful plantar lesions may limit or interfere with walking. **Microcephaly**, growth retardation, hyperactivity, aberrant behavior, and self-mutilation also have been reported.

**Associated Findings:** None known.

**Etiology:** Autosomal recessive inheritance.

**Pathogenesis:** Deficiency of cytoplasmic hepatic tyrosine aminotransferase (L-tyrosine-2-oxyglutarate aminotransferase) has been reported. This enzyme catalyzes the conversion of tyrosine to p-hydroxyphenylpyruvic acid (p-HPPA). Hepatic tyrosine aminotransferase is found in the mitochondria and in the cytoplasm; only the cytoplasmic enzyme is deficient. Patients with tyrosinemia II generally have higher concentrations of tyrosine in plasma than do patients with **Tyrosinemia I**.

A causal relationship has been demonstrated between the hypertyrosinemia of the eye and skin in that a low tyrosine-low phenylalanine diet which lowers the level of tyrosine in plasma results in healing lesions. Conversely, an increase in blood tyrosine is followed by recurrence of the lesions. Experiments with an animal model have demonstrated parallel findings of epithelial corneal and dermal lesions. Rats fed excessive diets of tyrosine developed focal corneal lesions in which the presence of bifringent needle-shaped crystals, resembling tyrosine crystals, were demonstrated (electron and polarizing microscopy). The crystals may be responsible for cell disruption, and the release of lysosomal enzymes causing the acute inflammatory response seen in the corneal epithelium. Similar histologic changes have been observed in dermal lesions. Tyrosine crystals placed in the skin or peritoneal cavity do not produce an inflammatory response. However, it has been postulated that when tyrosine crystallizes within the cells, an inflammatory response is initiated. Increased synthesis of tonofibrils and keratohyalin, and large numbers of micro-tubules, have been observed. The reason for the predilection of lesions for ocular and volar epithelium in humans with tyrosinemia II and in rats with experimental tyrosinemia is unknown.

**MIM No.:** *27660

**Sex Ratio:** M1:F1

**Occurrence:** About 50 patients have been reported since this syndrome recognized in the early 1960s. Affected patients have been of Italian, Norwegian, Anglo-Saxon and American Black ethnic origin.

**Risk of Recurrence for Patient's Sib:**
See Part I, *Mendelian Inheritance*.

**Risk of Recurrence for Patient's Child:**
See Part I, *Mendelian Inheritance*.

**Age of Detectability:** Hypertyrosinemia may be present in the first few weeks of life. Onset of clinical symptoms is highly variable. Ocular lesions may occur as early as two weeks, often within 3–6 months or later, followed by skin lesions.

**Gene Mapping and Linkage:** TAT (tyrosine aminotransferase) has been mapped to 16q22.1.

**Prevention:** None known. Genetic counseling indicated.

**Treatment:** Dietary restriction: low phenylalanine - low tyrosine diet appears uniformly successful. Blood levels of tyrosine in treated patients are preferably maintained below 10mg/dl. If the diet is stopped, symptoms recur.

**Prognosis:** The oculocutaneous lesions respond readily to the dietary restrictions of tyrosine and phenylalanine.

Two young children, less than three years of age at the time of the report, born to an untreated woman with oculocutaneous tyrosinemia, have had normal physical and psychomotor development.

**Detection of Carrier:** Unknown. Oral tyrosine load tests have not succeeded in differentiating carriers from control.

**Special Considerations:** An oculocutaneous disorder described by Richner and Hanhart in 1938 appears to be identical to this disorder. Some of the earlier reported patients with *Richner-Hanhart Syndrome* have been studied and the presence of an abnormality in tyrosine metabolism has been confirmed (Balato et al, 1986).

**References:**
Richner H: Hornhautaffektion bei keratoma palmare et plantare hereditarium. Klin Monatsbl Augenheilkd 1938; 100:580–588.
Bardelli MM, et al.: Familial tyrosinemia with eye and skin lesions. presentation of two cases. Ophthalmologica (Basel) 1977; 175:5–9.
Faull KF, et al.: Metabolic studies on two patients with nonhepatic tyrosinemia using deurated tyrosine loads. Pediatr Res 1977; 11:631–637.
Goldsmith LA, et al.: Hepatic enzymes of tyrosine metabolism in tyrosinemia II. J Invest Dermatol 1979; 73:500–522.
Ney D, et al.: Dietary management of oculocutaneous tyrosinemia in an 11-year-old child. Am J Dis Child 1983; 137:995–1000.
Balato N, et al.: Tyrosinemia type II in two cases previously reported as Richner-Hanhart syndrome. Dermatoloaica 1986; 173:66–74.
Nyhan WL, Sakati NA: Oculocutaneous tyrosinemia. In: Nyhan WL, ed: Diagnostic recognition of genetic disease. Philadelphia: Lea & Febiger, 1987:112–119. *

SH017
NY000

**Carol S. Shear**
**William L. Nyhan**

**Tyrosinemia III**
*See TYROSINEMIA I*
**Tyrosinemia with eye and skin lesions, familial**
*See TYROSINEMIA II, OREGON TYPE*
**Tyrosinemia-plantar and palmar keratosis-ocular keratitis**
*See TYROSINEMIA II, OREGON TYPE*
**Tyrosinosis, acute and chronic**
*See TYROSINEMIA I*
**TYS**
*See SCLEROTYLOSIS*

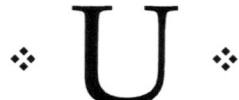

‖ **'U'-shaped hearing loss**
*See DEAFNESS (SENSORINEURAL), MIDFREQUENCY*
**UDP-galactose-epimerase deficiency**
*See GALACTOSE EPIMERASE DEFICIENCY*
**UDP-glucuronosyltransferase deficiency, type I**
*See UDP-GLUCURONOSYLTRANSFERASE, SEVERE DEFICIENCY TYPE I*

---

## UDP-GLUCURONOSYLTRANSFERASE, SEVERE DEFICIENCY TYPE I                      0961

**Includes:**
Crigler-Najjar syndrome, type I
Hyperbilirubinemia, Crigler-Najjar type
Jaundice without bilirubin glucuronide in bile
UDP-glucuronosyltransferase deficiency, type I

**Excludes:**
Hyperbilirubinemia, conjugated (3009)
Hyperbilirubinemia, conjugated, Rotor type (3237)
Hyperbilirubinemia, transient familial neonatal (3238)
Hyperbilirubinemia, unconjugated (0487)

**Major Diagnostic Criteria:** Persistent physiologic jaundice of newborn in the absence of hemolysis, serum unconjugated bilirubin concentration in excess of 20 mg/dl, and virtual absence of bilirubin glucuronides in bile.

**Clinical Findings:** Lifelong nonhemolytic unconjugated hyperbilirubinemia with serum bilirubin concentrations of approximately 15–40 mg/dl (mean, approximately 24 mg/dl). Approximately 75% of affected individuals develop kernicterus during the neonatal period and die in infancy. Survivors may show varied clinical signs of bilirubin encephalopathy. Rarely, signs of kernicterus develop for the first time at or after puberty, usually in association with infection.

Hepatic UDP-glucuronosyltransferase activity with bilirubin as a substrate is undetectable. Activity toward some other substrates, including 4-methylumbelliferone and o-aminophenol, is markedly decreased. Urinary excretion of glucuronides after ingestion of menthol, salicylamide, and n-acetyl-p-aminophenol is decreased to 25% of normal. Fecal urobilinogen excretion is 40–50% of normal.

Serum transaminase, alkaline phosphatase, albumin, and bile salt levels are normal. Gallbladder is normally visualized by oral cholecystography. Morphologic examination of the liver reveals no abnormality except occasional canalicular "bile plugs." Bile contains variable amounts of unconjugated bilirubin. Excretion of unconjugated bilirubin is increased during phototherapy.

**Complications:** Kernicterus occurs in the vast majority of cases and has a variety of neurologic sequelae.

**Associated Findings:** None known.

**Etiology:** Autosomal recessive inheritance of an enzyme defect.

**Pathogenesis:** Severe inherited deficiency of UDP-glucuronosyltransferase activity toward bilirubin. The clinical disorder results from the toxic effect of unconjugated bilirubin, particularly on the central nervous system.

**MIM No.:** *21880

**CDC No.:** 277.400

**Sex Ratio:** M1:F1

**Occurrence:** About 70 cases have been reported in the literature.

**Risk of Recurrence for Patient's Sib:**
See Part I, *Mendelian Inheritance.*

**Risk of Recurrence for Patient's Child:**
See Part I, *Mendelian Inheritance.* Patients often do not live to child-bearing age.

**Age of Detectability:** Second to third week of life.

**Gene Mapping and Linkage:** Unknown.

**Prevention:** None known. Genetic counseling indicated.

**Treatment:** Exchange transfusion or plasmapheresis during the neonatal period may prevent kernicterus. Maintenance therapy includes phototherapy. Exposure to visible light results in geometric or structural isomerization of bilirubin, which permits its biliary excretion without conjugation.

Recently, liver transplantation has been performed in a few patients. This results in a rapid decrease in serum bilirubin levels.

Patients should not receive drugs, such as sulfonamides or warfarin, that compete with bilirubin for binding sites on albumin, thereby possibly precipitating kernicterus. Phenobarbital administration has no long-lasting effect on serum bilirubin levels in this condition.

**Prognosis:** Approximately 75% of affected individuals die during the first five years of life from kernicterus or infection. Survival during the neonatal period is improving by the efficient use of plasmapheresis and phototherapy. Liver transplantation may markedly improve the prognosis in older children.

**Detection of Carrier:** Oral menthol tolerance test (1–2 g for young adults) is useful in distinguishing carriers from normal controls. Urinary menthol glucuronide excretion is quantitated in urine collected for 5 hours after menthol ingestion. Control subjects excrete 39 ± 7.2% of ingested menthol as urinary menthol glucuronide during this period. Heterozygous carriers excrete only about 18% of the given dose during the test period.

**Special Considerations:** Kernicterus is precipitated by coexisting conditions such as hypoxia, acidosis, sepsis, and prematurity, and is therefore not an obligatory or specific manifestation of this disorder. Because of therapeutic implications, UDP-glucuronosyltransferase deficiency type I must be differentiated from **Hyperbilirubinemia, unconjugated.**

The Gunn strain of mutant Wistar rat has the type I defect.

**References:**
Crigler JF Jr., Najjar VA: Congenital familial nonhemolytic jaundice with kernicterus. Pediatrics 1952; 10:169–179.
Childs B, et al.: Glucuronic acid conjugation by patients with familial nonhemolytic jaundice and their relatives. Pediatrics 1959; 23:903–913.

Arias IM: Chronic unconjugated hyperbilirubinemia without overt signs of hemolysis in adolescents and adults. J Clin Invest 1962; 41:2233–2245.

Wolkoff AW, et al.: Crigler-Najjar syndrome (type I) in an adult male. Gastroenterology 1979; 76:840–848.

Shevell MI, et al.: Crigler-Najjar syndrome I: treatment by home phototherapy followed by orthotopic hepatic transplantation. J Pediatr 1987; 110:429–431.

CH036 **Jayanta Roy Chowdhury**

## UDP-glucuronosyltransferase, severe deficiency type II
*See HYPERBILIRUBINEMIA, UNCONJUGATED*
## UDPG-glycogen transferase
*See GLYCOGEN SYNTHETASE DEFICIENCY*
## Uhl anomaly
*See VENTRICLE, RIGHT, UHL ANOMALY*
## Ulcer, duodenal
*See PEPTIC ULCER DISEASES, NON-SYNDROMIC*
## Ulcer, gastric
*See PEPTIC ULCER DISEASES, NON-SYNDROMIC*
## Ulcer, peptic
*See PEPTIC ULCER DISEASES, NON-SYNDROMIC*
## Ulcer, peptic/hiatal hernia-cafe-au-lait-hypertelorism-myopia
*See GASTROCUTANEOUS SYNDROME*

## ULCER-LEUKONYCHIA-GALLSTONES                2234

**Includes:**
> Duodenal ulcer-leukonychia-gallstones
> Leukonychia totalis
> Leukonychia-ulcer-gallstones
> Renal calculi-ulcer-leukonychia

**Excludes:**
> **Amyloidoses** (1502)
> Histamine excess syndrome (mastocytosis associated)
> **Knuckle pads-leukonychia-deafness** (0558)
> **Endocrine neoplasia, multiple type I** (0350)
> **Nails, leukonychia** (0589)
> **Tremor-duodenal ulcer syndrome** (0963)

**Major Diagnostic Criteria:** White nails, duodenal ulcer, and/or cholelithiasis.

**Clinical Findings:** The clinical picture is recognized when the patient has the combination of leukonychia totalis (white nails), and duodenal ulcer or gallstones. One patient might not have all characteristics present, but is considered likely to be affected if he has one of the characteristics and is a first degree relative to a patient with the complete syndrome. The leukonychia is reportedly present from birth and affects all nails in those patients with the abnormality. Leukonychia has often been considered an incidental finding, but has been noted to be familial.

Limited clinical experience, and limited number of cases makes it difficult to describe a distinct clinical course. The cases reported do not appear to be distinct in their presentation from other patients with gallstones and peptic ulcer, in terms of age of onset or complications.

**Complications:** Gastric cancer has been reported in one relative, occurring after gastrectomy for an ulcer. Since gastric cancer is generally increased secondary to the peptic ulcer surgery, it is unknown at this time if there is a specific increased evidence of gastric cancer in this syndrome. At this time it would be prudent to suggest close follow up in those patients who have undergone gastrectomy for treatment of their duodenal ulcer.

As regards to other complications, perforation has been reported in one case. Pancreatitis has also been reported in two patients in the literature. The complete history is not available and it is not known if this was a complication of cholelithiasis.

**Associated Findings:** Renal calculi and sebaceous cyst in association with leukonychia have been reported by Bushkell and Gorlin in a father and son with leukonychia, cysts, and renal calculi. In their review of inherited leukonychia they found one family with 16/19 family members (including the proband) with multiple sebaceous cysts as the only additional feature. One other case was

reported to have peptic ulcer disease and leukonychia, but no sebaceous cysts, or renal calculi. In the three cases with leukonychia and renal calculi and sebaceous cysts, one (age 50) had pancreatitis, one (age 58) had gallbladder disease, and the third was 27 years old, and had not manifested peptic ulcer or gallbladder disease. It is entirely possible that all these features, leukonychia, gallstones, peptic ulcer disease, sebaceous cysts, and renal calculi are all related, and are really one syndrome. This is supported by the tentative evidence that suggests a relationship between renal calculi and duodenal ulcer in specific families.

**Etiology:** Autosomal dominant inheritance with variable penetrance.

**Pathogenesis:** Unknown.

**MIM No.:** *15160

**Sex Ratio:** M1:F1

**Occurrence:** Undetermined but presumed rare. Several kindreds have been documented.

**Risk of Recurrence for Patient's Sib:**
> See Part I, *Mendelian Inheritance.*

**Risk of Recurrence for Patient's Child:**
> See Part I, *Mendelian Inheritance.*

**Age of Detectability:** Usually in the third or fourth decade when ulcer or cholelithiasis symptoms present. Leukonychia has been reportedly present from birth.

**Gene Mapping and Linkage:** Unknown.

**Prevention:** None known. Genetic counseling indicated.

**Treatment:** Increased surveillance in the offspring with leukonychia for symptoms of peptic ulcer disease and cholelithiasis, and standard medical symptomatic therapy. Post-gastrectomy patients will need appropriate follow up.

**Prognosis:** There is no evidence that the prognosis differs markedly from the patients with non-syndromic peptic ulcer disease or cholelithiasis.

**Detection of Carrier:** Possibly by leukonychia (white nails) in first degree relatives.

**References:**
Albright SD, Wheeler CE: Leukonychia. Arch Dermatol 1964; 90:392–399.

Bushkell LL, Gorlin RJ: Leukonychia totalis, multiple sebaceous cysts, and renal calculi. Arch Dermatol 1975; 111:899–901.

Rotter JI: The genetics of peptic ulcer: more than one gene, genetics of gastrointestinal disease. Philadelphia: W.B. Saunders, 1980:1–58.

Ingegno AP, Yatto RP: Hereditary white nails (leukonychia totalis) duodenal ulcer and gallstones. NY State J of Med 1982; 82:1797–1800.

Rotter JI: Peptic ulcer. In: Emery AE, Rimoin DL, eds: Principles and practice of medical genetics. New York: Churchill Livingstone, 1983:863–878.

ES005 **Theresa J. Escalante**
*Jerome I. Rotter*

## Ulcerative colitis
*See INFLAMMATORY BOWEL DISEASE*
## Ulcerative proctitis
*See INFLAMMATORY BOWEL DISEASE*
## Ullirch-Turner syndrome
*See TURNER SYNDROME*
## Ullrich syndrome
*See NOONAN SYNDROME*
## Ullrich-Noonan syndrome
*See NOONAN SYNDROME*
## Ulna and fibula, hypoplasia of
*See MESOMELIC DYSPLASIA, REINHARDT-PFEIFFER TYPE*
## Ulnar and fibular absence with severe limb deficiency
*See LIMB DEFECT WITH ABSENT ULNA/FIBULA*
## Ulnar deviation of fingers syndrome
*See THUMB, CLASPED*
## Ulnar drift, congenital
*See HAND, ULNAR DRIFT*
## Ulnar polydactyly-Hirschsprung disease
*See HIRSCHSPRUNG DISEASE-CARDIAC DEFECT*

## ULNAR-MAMMARY SYNDROME 0981

**Includes:**
Mammary-ulnar syndrome
Pallister syndrome
Schinzel syndrome

**Excludes:**
**Mesomelic dysplasia, Nievergelt type** (0647)
**Mesomelic dysplasia, Reinhardt-Pfeiffer type** (0648)

**Major Diagnostic Criteria:** Combination of absent, hypoplastic, or duplicated ulnar ray structures, with hypoplastic and nonfunctional apocrine and mammary glands, and growth and pubertal delay.

**Clinical Findings:** This is a complex malformation syndrome with variable expression, characteristically involving a combination of upper limb and mammary gland defects. The abnormalities of the upper limbs may be quite asymmetric. They include clinodactyly; camptodactyly; hexadactyly; and shortness/absence of phalanges/metacarpals of the ulnar digits, of carpal bones, and of the ulna. The thumb, radius, humerus and shoulder girdle may also be involved. The apocrine-mammary defects include absence of body odor and axillary sweating, and developmental functional failure of mammary glands and nipples.

**Complications:** Physical limitations due to upper limb defects, inability to nurse, and delayed adolescence.

**Associated Findings:** Scoliosis, absence of teeth, bifid uvula, imperforate hymen, bicornate uterus, cryptorchidism, anal stenosis/atresia, and growth retardation (with late catch-up of growth) and pubertal delay.

**Etiology:** Autosomal dominant inheritance with variability of expression.

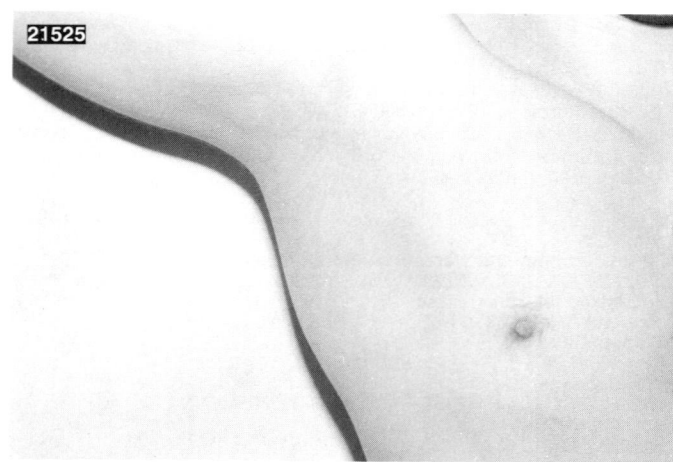

**0981B-21525:** Total absence of axillary hair, and small nipples.

**Pathogenesis:** Unknown.

**MIM No.:** *18145

**POS No.:** 3420

**Sex Ratio:** M1:F1

**Occurrence:** Some 16 cases in four families have been documented.

**Risk of Recurrence for Patient's Sib:**
See Part I, *Mendelian Inheritance.*

**Risk of Recurrence for Patient's Child:**
See Part I, *Mendelian Inheritance.*

**Age of Detectability:** At birth.

**Gene Mapping and Linkage:** Unknown.

**Prevention:** None known. Genetic counseling indicated.

**Treatment:** Orthopedic surgery for upper limb malformations; plastic surgery for breast and nipple hypoplasia; hymenotomy; orchiopexy.

**Prognosis:** Good.

**Detection of Carrier:** Variability of gene expression may be such that very minimally affected persons may have severely affected offspring. The hand malformation may be totally absent.

**References:**
Gonzalez CH, et al.: Studies of malformation syndromes of man 42B: mother and son affected with the ulnar-mammary syndrome type Pallister. Eur J Pediatr 1976; 123:225–235.
Pallister PD, et al.: Studies of malformation syndromes in man 42: a pleiotropic dominant mutation affecting skeletal, sexual and apocrine-mammary development. BD:OAS XII(5). New York: Alan R. Liss, for The National Foundation-March of Dimes, 1976:247–254.
Hecht JT, Scott CI, Jr.: The Schinzel syndrome in a mother and daughted. Clin Genet 1984; 25:63–67.
Schinzel A: Ulnar-mammary syndrome. J Med Genet 1987; 24:778–781.
Schinzel A, et al.: The ulnar-mammary syndrome: an autosomal dominant pleiotropic gene. Clin Genet 1987; 32:160–168. (Erratum: Clin Genet 1987; 32:425 only).

HE023
PA010

**Jürgen Herrmann**
**Philip D. Pallister**

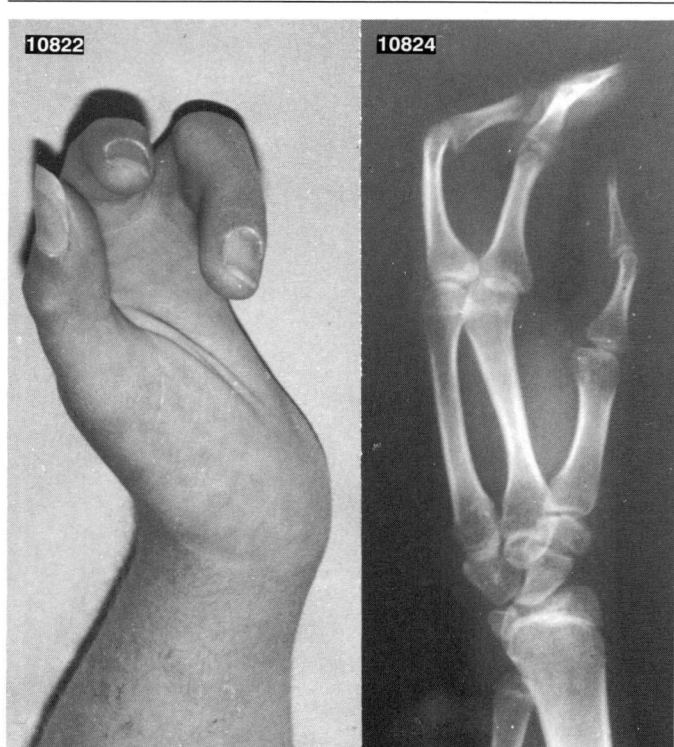

**0981A-10822–24:** Hypoplasia of distal ulna and absence of ulnar ray derivatives including lateral carpals, 4th and 5th metacarpals, and phalanges.

**Umbilical arteries, multiple**
*See UMBILICAL CORD, MULTIPLE VESSELS*
**Umbilical cord (giant), associated with patent urachus**
*See URACHAL ANOMALIES*
**Umbilical cord agenesis**
*See UMBILICAL CORD, SHORT UMBILICAL CORD SYNDROME*
**Umbilical cord aplasia**
*See UMBILICAL CORD, SHORT UMBILICAL CORD SYNDROME*

**Umbilical cord deformation sequence**
*See UMBILICAL CORD, LONG*
**Umbilical cord hernia**
*See OMPHALOCELE*
**Umbilical cord looping**
*See UMBILICAL CORD, LONG*
**Umbilical cord torsion (coarctation)**
*See UMBILICAL CORD, LONG*
**Umbilical cord true knot**
*See UMBILICAL CORD, LONG*

---

## UMBILICAL CORD, LONG                    2956

**Includes:**
    Umbilical cord deformation sequence
    Umbilical cord looping
    Umbilical cord torsion (coarctation)
    Umbilical cord true knot

**Excludes:**
    **Neu-Laxova syndrome** (2092)
    **Umbilical cord, short** (2955)
    **Umbilical cord, short umbilical cord syndrome** (2957)

**Major Diagnostic Criteria:** In abortuses, a long cord measures in excess of 2.5 times the crown-rump length. In preterm infants, the umbilical cord measures 2 SD or more above the mean length as corrected for sex. At term gestation, the cord length exceeds 80 cm; cords measuring more than 300 cm have been detected.

**Clinical Findings:** During the prenatal period, polyhydramnios is usually, but not always, present. Ultrasonographic visualization is possible (but is usually unreliable) after the first trimester. During parturition, cord prolapse, along with mechanical compression (compromise) of the fetal circulation may occur. The latter condition results in changes in fetal heart rate and ultimately leads to fetal distress (hypoxia). Umbilical vein thromboses and cord entanglements (body loops, knots) are much more common in long cords. True knots are common in long cords and increase the blood pressure required to maintain normal fetal perfusion. Constrictive loops around a fetal part (neck, arm, shoulder, trunk) rarely may impart deep grooves in the underlying fetal tissues and may lead to significant structural deformation.

**Complications:** Long cords are significantly (p <0.001) prone to accidents (loops, knots, prolapse). The long cord accident rate is 60%. The incidence of anomalies (velamentous insertion, hematoma, vein thrombosis, single umbilical artery, and torsion) is also increased in the fetus with a long cord (19%) compared with normal (14%) and short (17%) cords. Long cords are prone to coiling (looping), true knot formation (0.4–0.5% of deliveries), and cord prolapse at delivery. Following large volume amniocentesis, long cords are at greater risk for knot and loop formations. In each of these conditions, the fetal vascular supply may be compromised. The incidence of frequent variable decelerations of the baseline fetal heart rate is significantly increased in fetuses with long cords (p <0.05) as are FHR patterns, suggesting fetal distress (p <0.05).

**Associated Findings:** Twinning, polyhydramnios, abdominal pregnancy, fetal hyperkinesia, fetal hypertension (e.g., maternal drugs: amphetamines, cocaine, xanthines), and fetal growth retardation.

**Etiology:** Undetermined but presumably nongenetic.

**Pathogenesis:** Current theories include excessive fetal movement (hyperkinesia), excessive stretch during development (e.g., polyhydramnios, abdominal pregnancy), and fetal hypertension.

**Sex Ratio:** M1:F1

**Occurrence:** Long cords are seen in 11% of abortus specimens. Long cords occur in 7% of all deliveries. In pregnancies complicated by polyhydramnios, as many as 12% of cords may be classified as long.

**Risk of Recurrence for Patient's Sib:** Presumably low.

**Risk of Recurrence for Patient's Child:** Unknown.

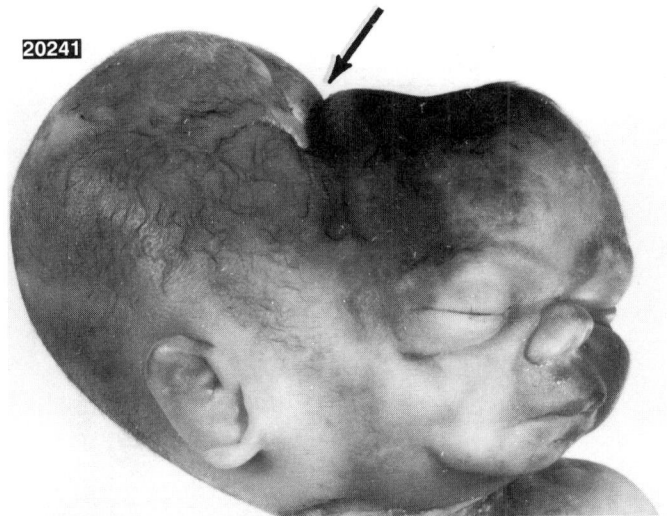

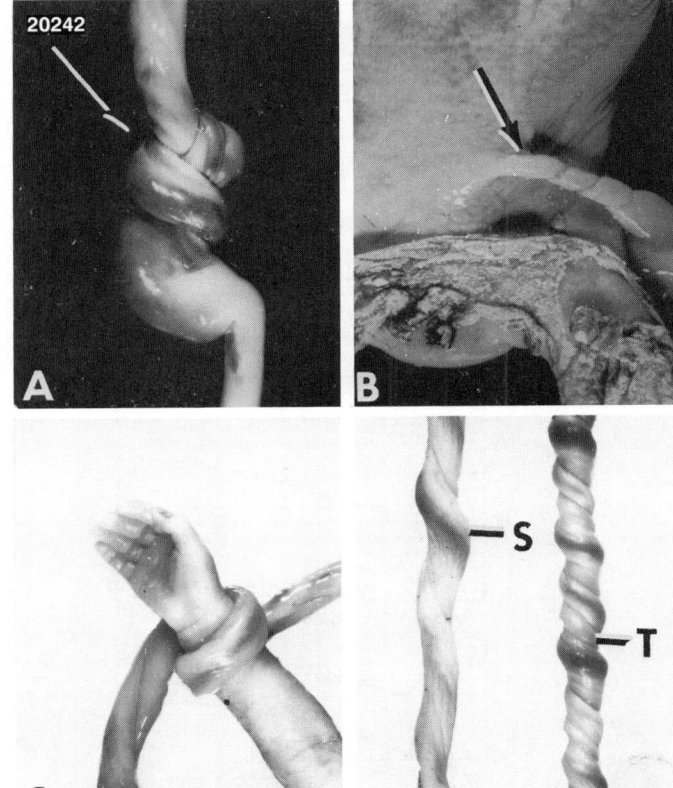

**2956A-20241:** Newborn with an 80 cm long umbilical cord showing significant deformation of the skull due to an umbilical cord loop (arrow). **20242:** Abnormalities associated with "long umbilical cord": A. True knot with vascular compression; B. Torsion of cord near fetal abdomen (arrow); C. Cord loop around fetal arm; D. Long cords showing normal (left hand) vascular spiral (S) as opposed to cord twists (T).

---

**Age of Detectability:** Possibly evident on fetal ultrasound after 12 weeks gestation or shortly thereafter. Most are not detected until delivery.

**Gene Mapping and Linkage:** Unknown.

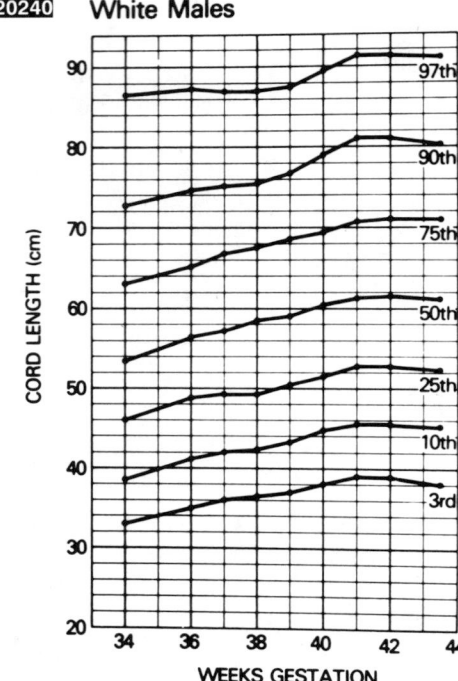

**20240** White Males

CORD LENGTH (cm) / WEEKS GESTATION

97th
90th
75th
50th
25th
10th
3rd

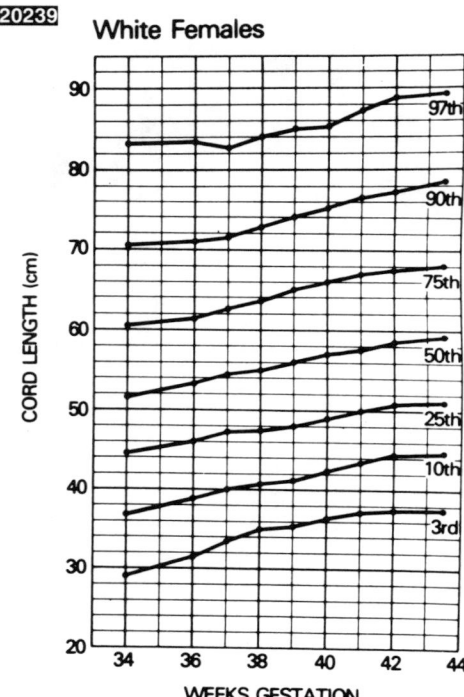

**20239** White Females

CORD LENGTH (cm) / WEEKS GESTATION

97th
90th
75th
50th
25th
10th
3rd

**2956B-20240:** Umbilical cord length by gestational age in US white males (Mills et al). **20239:** Umbilical cord length by gestational age in US white females (Mills et al).

**Prevention:** No known methods currently available except when maternal drugs induce fetal hypertension (e.g., amphetamines, cocaine, xanthines). In the latter cases, drugs should be discontinued.

**Treatment:** None necessary except that during delivery efforts should be directed toward preventing compromise of the fetal vascular supply; fetal monitoring is indicated.

**Prognosis:** Excellent if complications of hypoxia are avoided during intrauterine development at delivery.

**Detection of Carrier:** Unknown.

**References:**

Javert CT, Barton B: Congenital and acquired lesions of the umbilical cord and spontaneous abortion. Am J Obstet Gynecol 1952; 63:1065–1077.

Rayburn WF, et al.: Umbilical cord length and intrapartum complications. Obstet Gynecol 1981; 57:450–452.

Mossenger AC, et al.: Umbilical cord length as an index of fetal activity: experimental study and clinical implications. Pediatr Res 1982; 16:109–112.

Mills JL, et al.: Standards for measuring umbilical cord length. Placenta 1983; 4:423–426.

BL002 **Will Blackburn**

---

**UMBILICAL CORD, MULTIPLE VESSELS** **2576**

**Includes:**
Umbilical arteries, multiple
Umbilical veins, multiple

**Excludes:** Umbilical vein, persistent right

**Major Diagnostic Criteria:** Multiple umbilical arteries and veins.

**Clinical Findings:** Duplicated umbilical vessels have been reported in both normal infants and infants with major or multiple congenital anomalies.

**Complications:** None directly from the duplicated vessels, but as in babies with single umbilical artery, the extent of the complications in infants with multiple umbilical cord vessels depends on the severity of the associated congenital malformations.

**Associated Findings:** None known.

**Etiology:** Unknown.

**Pathogenesis:** Abnormal division of the umbilical vessels within the Wharton's jelly portion of the cord at 3–5 weeks gestation.

**Sex Ratio:** M1:F1

**Occurrence:** Karchmer et al (1966) examined the umbilical cords of 40 malformed infants. From this population, two were identified with cords containing three umbilical arteries.

**Risk of Recurrence for Patient's Sib:** Unknown.

**Risk of Recurrence for Patient's Child:** Unknown.

**Age of Detectability:** At birth.

**Gene Mapping and Linkage:** Unknown.

**Prevention:** None known. Genetic counseling indicated.

**Treatment:** Unknown.

**Prognosis:** Unknown.

**Detection of Carrier:** Unknown.

**References:**

Karchmer S, et al.: Anomalies del cordon umbilical y coexistencia de malformaciones congenitas. Ginecologia y Obstetricia de Mexico 1966; 21:831–837.

Painter D, Russell P: Four-vessel umbilical cord associated with multiple congenital anomalies. Obstet Gynecol 1977; 50:505–507.

Beck R, Naulty CM: A human umbilical cord with four arteries. Clin Pediatr 1985; 24:118–119.

EL013 **Sami B. Elhassani**

## UMBILICAL CORD, SHORT                                                       2955

**Includes:**
    Fetal constraint
    Short cord

**Excludes:**
    Cerebroarthrodigital syndrome
    **Umbilical cord, long** (2956)
    **Umbilical cord, short umbilical cord syndrome** (2957)

**Major Diagnostic Criteria:**  Short umbilical cords measure more than 10 cm but less than 35.5 cm at term delivery.

**Clinical Findings:**  The umbilical cord attains most of its growth during the first and second trimesters; a slow rate of growth is attained during the third trimester and postterm periods. Short umbilical cords measure more than 10 cm but less than 35.5 cm at term delivery. Short cords during the fetal period are those with lengths in the lower 6th percentile corrected for sex and gestational age. The cord, although short, is usually structurally normal. The surface amnion may show signs of amnion nodosum and other structural abnormalities. A slight reduction of cord length has been associated with **Chromosome 21, trisomy 21** and infants born to mothers with hypertension. Unfortunately, intrauterine diagnosis is difficult.

**Complications:**  A cord length of 35.5 cm is thought to be necessary for the normal progression of a vaginal delivery. Short cords are susceptible to traumatic traction or avulsion and fetal exsanguination during vaginal delivery. Short cords are at increased risk for failure of fetal descent, uterine inversion, placental abruption, abnormal fetal heart rate (63%), and cord anomalies (17%).

**Associated Findings:**  Short cords are most often associated with conditions that produce intrauterine constraint (e.g., oligohydramnios, uterine anomalies, or deformations), fetal constraint (e.g., amniotic bands-adhesions, skin disease), fetal limb anomalies (e.g., amelia, **Sirenomelia sequence**, arthrogryposis), and fetal hypokinesia (e.g., CNS and neuromuscular diseases). Body wall defects are common (cyllosomus, pleurosomus, omphalocele) as are signs of fetal compression (Potter facies, thoracic and lung hypoplasia, abnormal limb position, and limb deformations). Fetal renal disease (e.g., renal agenesis, dysplasia, or cystic disease) is common. Both genetic and nongenetic syndromes are also encountered.

### Table 1   Factors Associated with Short Umbilical Cord

Intrauterine Environmental Constraint
    Oligohydramnios
        Fetal Oliguria-Anuria
        Amnionic Fluid Leakage
    **Amniotic bands syndrome**
    Uterine Malformations-Deformations
    Multiple Pregnancy
Fetal Cutaneous Constraint
    Restrictive Dermopathy
    **Skin, localized absence of**
    Congenital **Contractures**
    **Epidermolysis bullosum**
    **Stomach, pyloric atresia**
Fetal Cutaneous Constraint + Hypokinesia
    "Cocoon" Fetus
    **Neu-Laxova syndrome**
    **Ectrodactyly**
    **Pterygium syndrome**
Fetal Hypokinesia
    Chromosome Abnormalities
        **Chromosome 21, trisomy 21**
            (mild degrees of cord shortening)
        **Chromosome triploidy**
        **Prader-Willi syndrome** (possibly)
    Lissencephaly-Associated Syndromes
        **Neu-Laxova syndrome**

**Pena-Shokeir syndrome**
**Cerebro-oculo-facio-skeletal syndrome**
**Cerebro-hepato-renal syndrome**
**Lissencephaly syndrome**
**Muscular dystrophy, congenital with mental retardation**
Neuromuscular
    **Spinal muscular atrophy** (prenatal)
    **Muscular dystrophy, congenital with mental retardation**
Limb Anomalies
    Amelia
    **Arthrogryposes**
    **Cranio-carpo-tarsal dysplasia, whistling face type**
    Acardiac Fetus
Maternal Hypertension
    (mild degrees of cord shortening)
Fetal Hypotension
Maternal Drugs
Acardiac Fetus

**Etiology:**  Both genetic and nongenetic associations have been reported.

**Pathogenesis:**  A variety of conditions are known to promote umbilical cord growth (fetal blood pressure, fetal movement, and cord stretch or increased tension); hence, most theories embrace the concept that short cords are due to situations leading to reduced stretch (e.g., constraint syndromes), reduced fetal movement, or reduced fetal blood pressure.

**Sex Ratio:**  Variable due to diverse associations.

**Occurrence:**  About 0.8 to 1.2% of all umbilical cords are short.

**Risk of Recurrence for Patient's Sib:**  Variable depending on nature of etiology and pathogenesis.

**Risk of Recurrence for Patient's Child:**  Unknown.

**Age of Detectability:**  Usually evident by the end of the second trimester and by ultrasonography during the third trimester. Most commonly noted in association with reduced fundal height (e.g., oligohydramnios).

**Gene Mapping and Linkage:**  Unknown.

**Prevention:**  In conditions in which oligohydramnios is due to obstruction of the lower urinary tract (posterior urethral bands, urethral stenosis, or agenesis), the placement of an intrauterine catheter to drain urine continuously into the amniotic cavity prevents progressive renal degeneration and enhances lung growth by expanding the amniotic fluid volume.

**Treatment:**  Cesarean section delivery may be indicated because of risk for umbilical cord laceration or avulsion during vaginal delivery.

**Prognosis:**  Variable depending on provoking condition. Short umbilical cord is associated with decreased Apgar scores, the need for resuscitation at delivery, hypotonia, jittery-tremorous newborns, and subsequent psychomotor abnormalities.

**Detection of Carrier:**  Only possible when associated with known genetic conditions.

**References:**
Purola E: The length and insertion of the umbilical cord. Ann Chir Gynaecol Fenn 1968; 57:621–622.
Punnett HH, et al.: Syndrome of ankylosis, facial anomalies and pulmonary hypoplasia. J Pediatr 1974; 85:375–377.
Miller ME, et al.: Short umbilical cord: its origin and relevance. Pediatrics 1981; 67:618–621.
Moessinger AC, et al.: Umbilical cord length as an index of fetal activity: experimental study and clinical implications. Pediatr Res 1982; 16:109–112.
Mills JL, et al.: Standards for measuring umbilical cord length. Placenta 1983; 4:423–426.
Naeye RL: Umbilical cord length: clinical significance. J Pediatr 1985; 107:278–281.

BL002                                                                 **Will Blackburn**

## UMBILICAL CORD, SHORT UMBILICAL CORD SYNDROME                           2957

**Includes:**
  Acordia
  Flying fetus syndrome
  SUC syndrome
  Tethered fetus syndrome
  Umbilical cord agenesis
  Umbilical cord aplasia

**Excludes:**
  Acardiac twin
  Amniotic adhesions
  **Amniotic bands syndrome** (0874)
  Amniotic rupture sequence
  Single umbilical artery
  **Umbilical cord, long** (2956)
  **Umbilical cord, short** (2955)

**Major Diagnostic Criteria:** The amniotic sac is intact, and amniotic bands (adhesions) are absent; the fetus is almost directly apposed or tethered to the placenta. The umbilical cord and sometimes its structures are extremely short, measuring 10 cm or less at term gestation. A single umbilical artery is usually present. An abdominal wall defect (omphalocele) is present and may lie in direct contact with the amniotic surface of the placental plate. The fetal trunk (spine) is sharply bent in the direction of umbilical cord tethering, which results in pleurosomus- or cyllosoma-like deformations.

Deformations of the extremities are present (e.g., clubfoot, abnormal rotation, or asymmetry). Internal anomalies are always present (e.g., diaphragmatic hernia, gastrointestinal, or genitourinary). SUC syndrome infants look alike; infants with amniotic rupture sequence also have very short umbilical cords but do not look alike.

**Clinical Findings:** Clinical signs appear by the end of the first trimester and include decreased fundal height, decreased fetal growth, and reduced amniotic fluid volume. Ultrasonography reveals close approximation of fetus and placenta and usually no visible umbilical cord. The fetus is progressively bent (pleurosomus; "flying fetus") in the direction of tethering, and body orientation (position) does not change as pregnancy proceeds. Reduced fetal movement (hypokinesia) is present. Sirenoid malformations have been reported in a few cases.

At birth, the placenta and fetus are delivered together, but occasionally the placenta may be avulsed from the fetus. Inspection reveals undeveloped body stalk elements (short, "naked" umbilical vessels surrounded by little or no Wharton jelly) and close approximation of placenta, fetal membranes, and fetal body wall elements (e.g., omphalocele membrane). X-ray studies reveal skeletal abnormalities (kyphoscoliosis, pleurosomus, pelvic hypoplasia, fused or abnormal ribs), signs of diaphragmatic hernia (persistent pleuroperitoneal canal), and severe, asymmetric, thoracic hypoplasia.

**Complications:** Due to fetal tethering, fetal descent during parturition does not occur; abnormal fetal presentation is the rule. Abruptio placenta and inversion of the uterus may occur. During vaginal delivery, avulsion of the placenta and funicular hemorrhage are common. Affected infants usually survive to term and are remarkably well developed; respiratory distress due to pulmonary hypoplasia is noted immediately after birth and is a common cause of death.

**Associated Findings:** Necropsy studies reveal internal anomalies involving the skeletal, gastrointestinal, and genitourinary systems.

**Etiology:** Unknown. Genetic mechanisms have not been described.

**Pathogenesis:** Current theories include a generalized failure in body stalk growth with subsequent failure of umbilical artery growth. When sirenoid malformations are present a "vascular steal" mechanism has been considered.

**Sex Ratio:** M1:F1

**Occurrence:** Unknown. Necropsy studies reveal an incidence of 1:600 necropsies.

**Risk of Recurrence for Patient's Sib:** Presumably low.

**Risk of Recurrence for Patient's Child:** Affected individuals do not survive to reproduce.

**Age of Detectability:** Usually at 12–14 weeks gestation.

**Gene Mapping and Linkage:** Unknown.

**Prevention:** None known. Genetic counseling indicated.

**Treatment:** Delivery by cesarean section is recommended due to high risk for placental vessel avulsion, fetal exsanguination, and abnormal fetal presentation. No treatment is currently available.

**Prognosis:** All patients have died shortly after birth due to respiratory insufficiency. A few have died *in utero*.

**Detection of Carrier:** Unknown.

**References:**
Gruenwald P, Mayberger HW: Differences in abnormal development of monozygotic twins. Arch Pathol 1960; 70:685–695.
Miller ME, et al.: Short umbilical cord: its origin and relevance. Pediatrics 1981; 67:618–621.
Barr M, Heidelberger KP: Short umbilical cord: cause or effect of fetal anomalies? Proc Greenwood Genet Center 1983; 2:100–101.
Blackburn WR, Cooley NR, Jr.: Short umbilical cord syndrome: an anomaly complex recognizable during the prenatal period. Clin Res 1984; 32:884A.

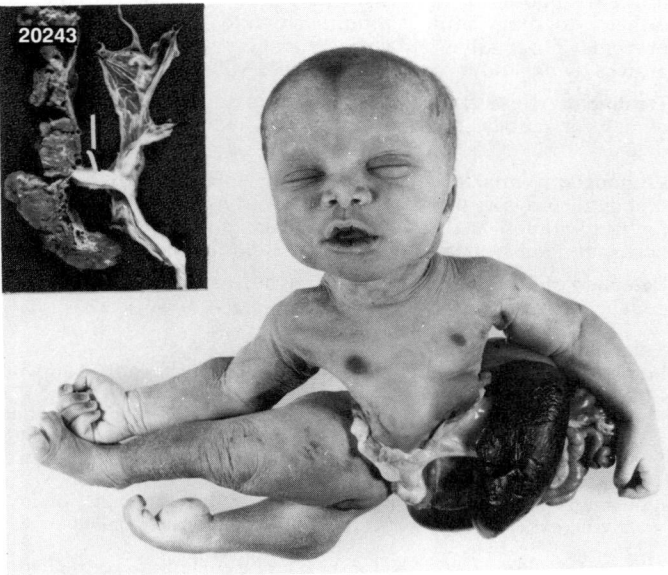

**2957-20243:** Newborn with short umbilical cord syndrome. Note the short cord (inset, arrow) and the infant's pleurosomus deformation. The omphalocele membrane is in close approximation to the fetal surface of the placenta (inset).

BL002                                                                       **Will Blackburn**

## UMBILICAL CORD, SINGLE ARTERY    2500

**Includes:**  Artery, umbilical cord, single

**Excludes:**  Umbilical vessel defects, other

**Major Diagnostic Criteria:**  Absence of one of the two umbilical arteries during routine newborn physical examination. Because 14% of infants with single umbilical artery die perinatally, and the incidence of major anomalies in those who die is 53%, a thorough physical as well as an earlier and a closer than usual follow-up examination should be performed.

**Clinical Findings:**  While the occurrence of single umbilical artery by itself is a benign condition, the pathologic clinical signs are related to associated malformations. Such malformations include those of skeletal, gastrointestinal, cardiovascular and nervous systems. The condition is also frequently found in babies with **Chromosome 13, trisomy 13** and **Chromosome 18, trisomy 18**.

**Complications:**  The extent of the complications is dependent on the severity of the congenital anomalies associated with single umbilical artery.

**Associated Findings:**  None known.

**Etiology:**  Single umbilical artery has been said to be associated with a variety of high-risk pregnancies such as advanced maternal age, high parity, multiple gestation, diabetes, intrauterine growth retardation, and reduced placental weight.

**Pathogenesis:**  It is not known whether absence of the second umbilical artery is due to primary aplasia or atrophy. Monie (1970) reported the presence of single umbilical artery in normal human embryos 3–4 mm in length; therefore, the finding of the condition at birth may be due to the persistence of the normally transient single umbilical artery.

**CDC No.:**  747.500

**Sex Ratio:**  M1:F1

**Occurrence:**  Single umbilical artery is one of the most common congenital malformations, occurring in about 1% of neonates. Microscopic examination of the umbilical cord of 48 affected infants showed no significant differences in congenital anomalies or neonatal mortality between infants with agenesis of one of their arteries and infants with arterial obliteration.

**Risk of Recurrence for Patient's Sib:**  Unknown.

**Risk of Recurrence for Patient's Child:**  Unknown.

**Age of Detectability:**  At birth, or prenatally by ultrasound imaging.

**Gene Mapping and Linkage:**  Unknown.

**Prevention:**  None known. Genetic counseling indicated.

**Treatment:**  Unknown.

**Prognosis:**  Unknown.

**Detection of Carrier:**  Unknown.

**Special Considerations:**  Because 10.3% of malformed fetuses and 17.1% of chromosomally abnormal fetuses have single umbilical artery, karyotyping of malformed newborns with single umbilical artery is advisable. The following are recommended for babies with single umbilical artery: 1) thorough physical examination, with special attention to intra-abdominal masses, dysmorphic features of the face, and anomalies of the hands and feet. 2) prenatal counseling, emphasizing the expected normal development of the majority of infants with single umbilical artery. 3) earlier and closer than usual follow-up examination, again with special attention to the abdomen, face, hands, and feet. 4) special procedures (invasive or noninvasive) not indicated at the time of the diagnosis should be reserved for the detection of additional anomalies, particularly a suspected intra-abdominal mass.

**References:**

Monie IW: Genesis of single umbilical artery. Am J Obstet Gynecol 1970; 108:400–405.
Collaborative Perinatal Study of the National Institute of Neurologic Diseases and Stroke: Women and their Pregnancies. DHEW publication No. (NIH) 73–379. Washington, D.C.: U.S. Department of Health, Education, and Welfare, 1972.
Altshuler G, et al.: Single umbilical artery: correlation of clinical status and umbilical cord histology. Am J Dis Child 1975; 129:697 only.
Bjoro K, Jr: Vascular anomalies of the umbilical cord: obstetric implications. Early Human Development 1983; 8:118–127.
Heifetz SA: Single umbilical artery: a statistical analysis of 237 autopsy cases and review of the literature. Perspect Pediatr Pathol 1984; 8:345–377.
Byrne J, Blanc WA: Malformations and chromosome anomalies in spontaneously aborted fetuses with single umbilical artery. Am J Obstet Gynecol 1985; 151:340–342.

EL013                                                      **Sami B. Elhassani**

**Umbilical hernia**
   See HERNIA, UMBILICAL
**Umbilical polyp**
   See OMPHALOMESENTERIC DUCT ANOMALIES
**Umbilical veins, multiple**
   See UMBILICAL CORD, MULTIPLE VESSELS
**Ump synthase deficiency**
   See ACIDEMIA, OROTIC
**Uncombable hair and crystalline cataract**
   See HAIR, UNCOMBABLE-CRYSTALLINE CATARACT
**Ungual ectodermal dysplasia**
   See ECTODERMAL DYSPLASIA, HIDROTIC
**Unilateral dental malformation**
   See TEETH, ODONTODYSPLASIA
**Univentricular heart of the left ventricular type**
   See VENTRICLE, SEPTUM DEXTROPOSITION AND DOUBLE INLET LEFT VENTRICLE
**Unna nevus**
   See NEVUS FLAMMEUS
**Unusual facies-growth/mental retardation-microcephaly-cleft palate**
   See WEAVER-WILLIAMS SYNDROME
**Unverricht-Lundborg disease**
   See SEIZURES, PROGRESSIVE MYOCLONIC, UNVERRICHT-LUNDBORG TYPE
**Upper limb cardiovascular syndrome**
   See HEART-HAND SYNDROME
**UPS deficiency**
   See PORPHYRIA, ACUTE INTERMITTENT

## URACHAL ANOMALIES    2573

**Includes:**
   Bladder diverticulum, superior
   Patent urachus
   Umbilical cord (giant), associated with patent urachus
   Urachal cyst or sinus

**Excludes:**
   **Omphalomesenteric duct anomalies** (2574)
   **Umbilical cord, long** (2956)
   Umbilical cord tumors

**Major Diagnostic Criteria:**  Urine discharges from the umbilicus. The diagnosis may be confirmed by injecting a radiopaque material into the umbilical orifice, thus outlining the patency of the urachal lumen or by introducing a colored dye into the bladder through a urethral catheter.

**Clinical Findings:**  *Completely patent urachus:* a small or giant umbilical bud which discharges urine. Radiopaque material injected into the umbilical orifice demonstrates the patent urachal tract. Bladder outlet obstruction may be an associated anomaly; a voiding cystourethrogram is advisable.
*Urachal cyst:* a superficial infraumbilical midline mass with a high susceptibility to infection. The diagnosis is frequently made by physical examination. In addition, a cystogram should be obtained to determine if there is any communication with the bladder.
*Urachal sinus:* urine discharges from the umbilical stump. Sometimes the urachal sinus can be felt as a thick cord beneath the skin coursing toward the bladder. Contrast studies should be obtained to outline the sinus tract.

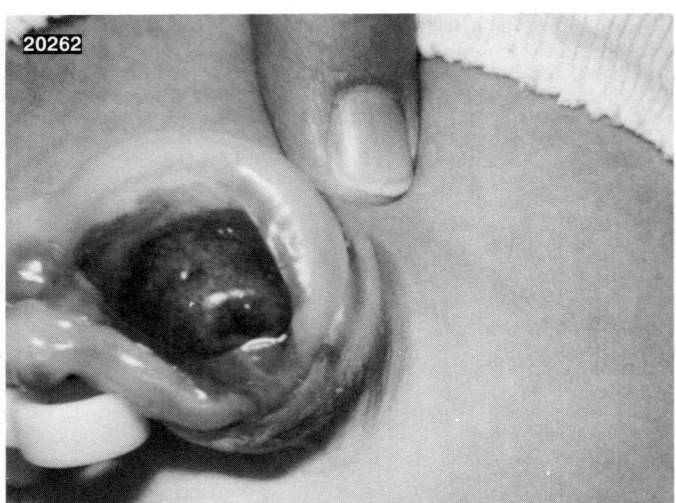

**2573-20262:** Patent urachus; note the orifice in the umbilical stump.

*Urachal diverticulum*: usually asymptomatic; it can be demonstrated only by cystogram.

**Complications:** Recurrent infections are likely in all untreated urachal malformations.

**Associated Findings:** None known.

**Etiology:** Persistence of the embryonic luminal communication between the bladder and the umbilicus.

**Pathogenesis:** Failure of the normal obliteration of the distal allantois may result in any of the four types of urachal anomalies.

**Sex Ratio:** M2:F1

**Occurrence:** 1:629 births.

**Risk of Recurrence for Patient's Sib:** Unknown.

**Risk of Recurrence for Patient's Child:** Unknown.

**Age of Detectability:** The majority of urachal anomalies are detected at birth. Occasionally, a patent urachus is not recognized until after the cord has fallen off and urine escapes from the umbilicus. This rare clinical manifestation is usually associated with a giant umbilical cord.

**Gene Mapping and Linkage:** Unknown.

**Prevention:** None known. Genetic counseling indicated.

**Treatment:** Excision of the urachal tract is the treatment of choice to avoid recurrent urinary tract infections.

**Prognosis:** Unknown.

**Detection of Carrier:** Unknown.

**References:**
Ente G, Penzer PH: Giant umbilical cord associated with patent urachus. Am J Dis Child 1970; 120:82–83.

EL013                                    **Sami B. Elhassani**

**Urachal cyst or sinus**
  *See URACHAL ANOMALIES*
**Urachal defects from fetal exposure**
  *See FETAL EFFECTS FROM METHIMAZOLE AND CARBIMAZOLE*
**Urbach skeletal dysplasia with rhizomelia of humeri**
  *See RHIZOMELIC SYNDROME, URBACH TYPE*
**Urbach-Wiethe disease**
  *See SKIN, LIPOID PROTEINOSIS*
**Urea cycle disorders**
  *See HYPERAMMONEMIA*
**Ureteral-vesical reflux**
  *See VESICO-URETERAL REFLUX*

**Ureterovesical stenosis**
  *See EPIDERMOLYSIS BULLOSUM, TYPE II*
**Urethral valve, posterior-polydactyly**
  *See POLYDACTYLY-DISTAL OBSTRUCTIVE UROPATHY*

## URETHRAL VALVES, POSTERIOR                    2407

**Includes:** Prostatic male urethra, obstruction

**Excludes:**
  Urethral diverticula
  Urethral polyps
  Urethral strictures

**Major Diagnostic Criteria:** Visualization of posterior valves by voiding cystourethrogram.

**Clinical Findings:** Congenital obstruction of the prostatic urethra. Presenting findings include decreased urinary stream (25%), distended bladder (67%), urinary infection (50%), abdominal distention (30%), renal failure (33%), papable kidneys (50%), hematuria (10%), failure to thrive (50%), fever of unknown origin (25%), vomiting and diarrhea (33%), and hypertension (5%).

Symptoms may manifest in early infancy, but may go undetected until later in infancy or childhood.

**Complications:** Urinary infections, hydronephrosis, bladder neck hypertrophy, vesicoureteral reflux, renal failure, hypertension.

**Associated Findings:** Obstruction of the ureteropelvic or ureterovesicular junction, rectal prolapse, renal dysplasia, renal agenesis, and pulmonary hypoplasia.

**Etiology:** Unknown.

**Pathogenesis:** Posterior valves may arise from 1) an embryonic remnant of the urogenital membrane, 2) an anomalous junction of the Wollfian duct and the prostatic utricle, 3) persistence of the Wollfian ducts, or 4) fusion of the epithelial colliculus with the roof of the posterior urethra.

**CDC No.:** 753.600

**Sex Ratio:** M1:F0

**Occurrence:** Undetermined but presumed rare.

**Risk of Recurrence for Patient's Sib:** Presumably low.

**Risk of Recurrence for Patient's Child:** Unknown.

**Age of Detectability:** The majority of patients present during the first year of life, with one-third given medical assistance within the first three months. However, posterior valves may go undetected until later in childhood or even in adulthood. Prenatal ultrasonography may expedite early detection and treatment.

**Gene Mapping and Linkage:** Unknown.

**Prevention:** None known. Genetic counseling indicated.

**Treatment:** The objectives of management include establishing adequate drainage of the urinary tract and removal of the lesion. Surgical strategies vary depending on the severity of the obstruction or the age of the patient. Adequate urinary drainage may be accomplished by inserting an indwelling bladder catheter or may require a suprapubic or upper urinary tract diversion. Removal of valves is usually performed by transurethral endoscopic fuguration.

**Prognosis:** Unknown.

**Detection of Carrier:** Unknown.

**Special Considerations:** Early detection and surgical intervention can greatly improve the prognosis by reducing the morbidity and mortality associated with urinary infections and acute renal failure. Additionally, early intervention can reduce the incidence of chronic renal failure and end-stage kidney disease caused by posterior valves. In recent years, in utero detection of hydronephrosis by prenatal ultrasound may lead to early diagnosis and management in the immediate post natal period. Fetal surgery has been recently attempted, but this procedure still remains experimental.

**References:**
Mayor G, et al.: Renal function in obstructive uropathy: long-term effect of reconstructive surgery. Pediatrics 1975; 56:740–747.
Harrison MR, et al.: Fetal surgery for congenital hydronephrosis. New Engl J Med 1982; 306:591–593.
Warshaw BL, et al.: Prognostic features in infants with obstructive uropathy due to posterior urethral valves. J Urol 1985; 133:240–242.
Hulbert WC, et al.: Current views on posterior urethral valves. Ped Annal 1988; 17:31–36.

HY001                                     **Leonard C. Hymes**

**Uric acid metabolism-central nervous system disorder**
See LESCH-NYHAN SYNDROME
**Uric acid urolithiasis**
See RENAL HYPOURICEMIA
**Uridine diphosphate galactose 4'-epimerase deficiency**
See GALACTOSE EPIMERASE DEFICIENCY
**Urinary reflux, primary, congenital, or idiopathic**
See VESICO-URETERAL REFLUX
**Urinary tract and digital defects-nephrosis-deafness**
See NEPHROSIS-DEAFNESS-URINARY TRACT AND DIGITAL DEFECTS

---

## UROFACIAL SYNDROME                          2527

**Includes:**
Bladder (dysplastic)-hydronephrosis-hydroureter-grimacing facies
Facial palsy, partial-urinary abnormalities*
Hydronephrosis-dysmorphic facies, Ochoa type
Hydronephrosis-hydroureter-dysplastic bladder-grimacing facies
Ochoa syndrome
Smile, inverted-occult neuropathic bladder

**Excludes:**
Hydronephrosis due to posterior urethral valves
Hydronephrosis due to ureteral stenosis
Hydronephrosis without facial abnormalities
**Kidney, polycystic disease, dominant** (0859)
**Kidney, polycystic disease, recessive** (2003)
**Renal agenesis, bilateral** (0856)

**Major Diagnostic Criteria:** The condition should be considered in all newborns and children who present with hydronephrosis and pyelonephritis, usually bilateral. There are two characteristics that differentiate this condition from other types of pyelonephritis and hydronephrosis: the peculiar appearance of the face and occult neuropathic bladder, with retention and severe bladder changes in the absence of neurologic or obstructive problems. At first it is difficult to recognize the characteristic facies, but, once known, it becomes diagnostic; and children with it should undergo a complete evaluation of the urinary tract. Most children show hydronephrosis and hydroureter, which vary from mild to severe including trabeculation, diverticula, vesicoureteral reflux, urinary tract infections, and spastic posterior urethra.

Some patient have impaired growth, but others have normal growth and psychomotor development. About 60% have constipation.

**Clinical Findings:** Appearance of the face is usually diagnostic. Noticeable at birth, it can be easily recognized through life. It is most noticeable when the patient smiles or laughs.

Early signs of the condition are diurnal and nocturnal enuresis (20% have both). Urinary tract infections were found in all patients. Hypertension developed in 13.8% of the patients reported by Ochoa and Gorlin (1987). Six (14%) had severe renal failure with uremia. Urodynamic evaluation of the bladder showed a hypertonic, hyperreflexic bladder, with uninhibited contractions of the detrusor. The bladder is macroscopically abnormal, with diverticulae and trabeculation; some are even congenital. It is suspected that there is a histologic abnormality producing the noted defects and also the hypertrophic neck of the bladder. It is likely that these changes induce ureteral reflux and

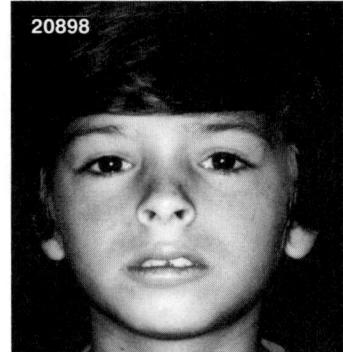
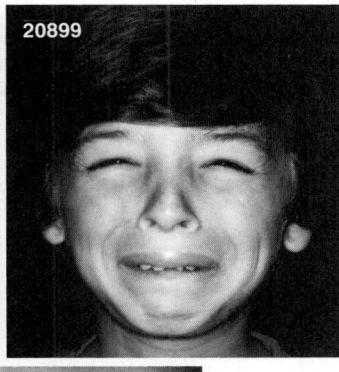
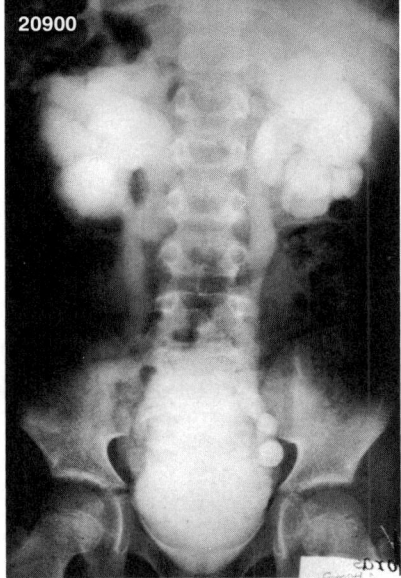

**2527-20898:** Note normal facial expression. **20899:** Grimace or inverted facial expression when laughing. **20900:** IVP shows bilateral hydronephrosis and a trabeculated bladder.

---

retention of urine, with the consequent infections, hydronephrosis, and hydroureter.

**Complications:** Urinary tract abnormalities, constipation, infections, hydronephrosis, renal failure, enuresis, retention of urine. Renal failure is probably the most concerning of the complications and could be prevented by early diagnosis and surgical treatment of the urinary tract obstruction.

**Associated Findings:** Neural tube defects, spina bifida occulta, **Meningocele**. Cryptorchidism was found in all affected males and may be causally related to the syndrome. One patient had psychomotor developmental delay, which does not appear to be a major constituent of the condition since all others have normal intellectual performance.

**Etiology:** Autosomal recessive inheritance, although some researchers believe that dominant inheritance cannot be fully ruled out. The extent of consanguinity is a topic of debate.

**Pathogenesis:** It is likely that there is a generalized abnormality of the neural tissue of the bladder and perhaps of the ureters and urethra that induces urine retention, ureteral reflux, dilation infection, dilated ureters, hydronephrosis, and pyelonephritis with renal failure. The earliest manifestations that we have seen are in newborns or children, but given the severity of the lesions seen in newborns, it is possible that the condition affects the fetus and produces severe damage to the urinary tract with the consequent oligohydramnios and pulmonary hypoplasia, although there have been no reports of an affected fetus.

About two-thirds of the patients have constipation, which may be a manifestation of the abnormality of the neural tissue of the abdominal viscera.

**MIM No.:** *23673

**POS No.:** 4264

**Sex Ratio:** M1.25:F1

**Occurrence:** Twenty-three families with 36 affected children (reported by Ochoa and Gorlin, 1987) and 19 probable cases recognized by case histories are known to be affected in Colombia. Reports exist of at least three other families, two in the United States and one in England.

**Risk of Recurrence for Patient's Sib:**
See Part I, *Mendelian Inheritance.*

**Risk of Recurrence for Patient's Child:**
See Part I, *Mendelian Inheritance.*

**Age of Detectability:** At birth, or possibly the condition can be detected in utero by sonography of the GU tract.

**Gene Mapping and Linkage:** Unknown.

**Prevention:** None known. Genetic counseling indicated.

**Treatment:** There is no specific treatment for the tissue and neural defect of this condition. Treatment is geared to correct the urinary tract obstruction and to cure the infection to prevent chronic renal failure. In some cases reconstructive surgery of the ureters and the ureterovesicular junction, ureterostomies, and ileal derivations are necessary depending on the severity of the compromise of the bladder. If severe renal damage has occurred, peritoneal dialysis, hemodialysis, and even kidney transplant are permanent therapeutic approaches, but the limitations imposed by the abnormal bladder need to be kept in mind when planning for these types of procedures.

**Prognosis:** The prognosis depends greatly on 1) the severity of the lesions at the time of diagnosis, 2) the degree of impairment of the renal function, 3) the success of the surgical correction of the anatomic defects, and 4) the presence of other malformations, such as meningocele, which could make the complications more severe and more difficult to treat. The rate of death in childhood or in the early teen years appears to be high in the severe cases, but long survival of the mild ones is a distinct possibility.

**Detection of Carrier:** Unknown.

**Special Considerations:** It is likely that this is a common syndrome, affecting many of those children who have hydronephrosis and hydroureter with an abnormal bladder, but that it is not accurately diagnosed because most physicians dealing with these malformations of the urinary tract are not aware of the association of such malformations with the peculiar facies.

**References:**
Elajalde BR: Genetic and diagnostic considerations in three families with abnormalities of facial expression and congenital urinary obstruction: "the Ochoa syndrome." Am J Med Genet 1979; 3:97–108.
Ochoa B, Gorlin RJ: Urofacial (Ochoa) syndrome. Am J Med Genet 1987; 27:661–667.

EL002                                                    **B. Rafael Elejalde**
EL014                                  **Maria Mercedes de Elejalde**

**Urogenital adysplasia**
    *See RENAL AGENESIS, BILATERAL*
**Urolithiasis, 2,8-dihydroxyadenine (DHA)**
    *See ADENINE PHOSPHO-RIBOSYL-TRANSFERASE (APRT)*
    *DEFICIENCY*
**Uromelia**
    *See SIRENOMELIA SEQUENCE*
**Uroporphyrinogen decarboxylase deficiency**
    *See PORPHYRIA CUTANEA TARDA*
**Uroporphyrinogen III cosynthase deficiency**
    *See PORPHYRIA, ERYTHROPOIETIC*

## URORECTAL SEPTUM MALFORMATION SEQUENCE    3161

**Includes:**
    Cloacal dysgenesis with female virilization
    Cloacal membrane, persistence of

**Excludes:**
    **Androgen insensitivity syndrome, incomplete** (0050)
    Androgen steroidogenesis, disorders of
    **Prune-belly syndrome** (2007)
    Sex chromosome abnormalities
    **Steroid 21-hydroxylase deficiency** (0908)
    **Vater association** (0987)

**Major Diagnostic Criteria:** Presence of a phallus-like structure (1.5 to 2 cm long), absent labia, no perineal openings (no anus, urethra, or introitus), vesicovaginorectal fistula, oligohydramnios, normal chromosomes, and normal adrenal gland function.

**Clinical Findings:** All of the reported cases had normal female karyotype (46,XX) in association with ambiguous genitalia. The abnormalities of the genitalia consisted of a phallus-like perineal structure, no urethral or vaginal openings, imperforate anus, vesicovaginorectal communication, and Mullerian duct defects. Urinary abnormalities, including renal agenesis or dysplasia, hydronephrosis, severe bladder dilation, or absence of the urethra were present in about 70% of the cases. Even with urethral agenesis, abdominal distention was seen in only 29% of the cases; its absence probably owes to absorption of fetal urine in the colon after passage through the vesicovaginorectal fistula. Ninety-four percent of the patients had abnormalities of the uterus and vagina. The ovaries were grossly and histologically normal. A history of oligohydramnios was usually present.

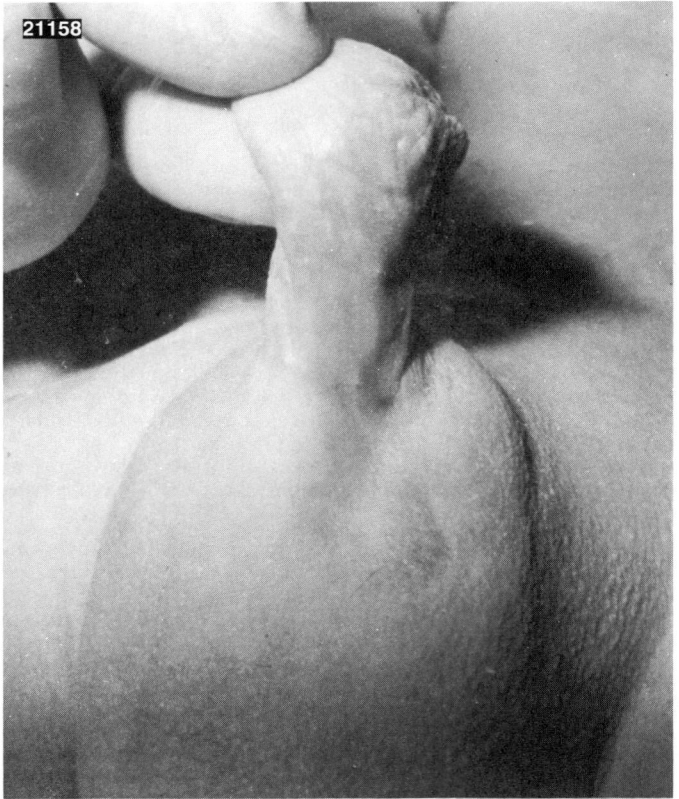

3161-21158: Note the phallus-like structure and a perineum without urethral or vaginal opening.

**Complications:** Most newborns die within the first 48 hours of life from severe respiratory distress secondary to lung hypoplasia or, rarely, pulmonary edema. The lung hypoplasia probably results from the oligohydramnios. Acute renal failure may be present in those cases in which renal abnormalities have severely compromised kidney function. Chronic renal failure has developed as late as age three years. Abdominal distension also may be caused by GI tract obstruction and may require surgical intervention.

**Associated Findings:** Persistent urachus, sacral agenesis, clinodactyly of the fifth finger, tracheoesophageal fistula, malrotation of the gut, and absent left radius and sometimes the thumb have been reported.

**Etiology:** All reported cases have been sporadic.

**Pathogenesis:** The cloaca is the most distal portion of the embryonic hindgut. By the sixth week of the development of a coronal sheet of mesenchyme, the urorectal septum, proliferates caudally and makes contact with the cloacal membrane, thus dividing the cloaca into an anterior cavity, the urogenital sinus, and a posterior one, the rectum and upper anal canal. The cloacal membrane, as a result of its fusion with the urorectal septum, is divided into the urogenital diaphragm ventrally and the anal membrane dorsally. These two membranes normally break down, leaving the urogenital sinus and anal canal connected to the outside (amniotic cavity). Recently, Escobar et al (1987) hypothesized that this condition is the result of failure of the urorectal septum to divide the cloacal cavity properly or to fuse with the cloacal membrane. These deficiencies lead to persistence of the cloacal cavity and membrane, with abnormal differentiation of both the internal and external genitalia and anal ampulla. The cause of phallic growth is undetermined.

**Sex Ratio:** M0:F1. This condition has only been recognized in females. In males, persistence of the cloaca may not be recognized, because it is diagnosed either as **Vater association** or urethral obstruction sequence with imperforate anus.

**Occurrence:** Between 1959 and 1987, nineteen cases were reported in the literature.

**Risk of Recurrence for Patient's Sib:** Presumably less than one percent.

**Risk of Recurrence for Patient's Child:** There are no reports of a pregnancy in an affected individual.

**Age of Detectability:** Prenatal diagnosis has been accomplished by ultrasound detection of a septated cystic structure in the fetal pelvis, no detectable bladder, fetal hydronephrosis, and oligohydramnios. The condition may be detected clinically at, or shortly after birth.

**Gene Mapping and Linkage:** Unknown.

**Prevention:** None known. Genetic counseling indicated.

**Treatment:** Surgery is usually required to alleviate the imperforate anus and urethral obstruction. Later, in surviving children, reconstructive surgery of the genitourinary system is needed. Respiratory distress, if present, may require intensive respiratory support.

**Prognosis:** Stillborn cases have been reported. Long-term survival of affected individuals is unusual. Seventy-six percent die of respiratory complications or renal failure during the first month of life. Chronic renal failure may lead to premature death in those who survive infancy.

**Detection of Carrier:** Unknown.

**Special Considerations:** Although this phenotype is distinctive, chromosomal analysis in the neonatal period should be done to distinguish this condition from males with ambiguous genitalia and from chromosomal aberrations.

**References:**

Lubinsky M: Female pseudohermaphroditism and associated anomalies. Am J Med Genet 1980; 6:123–136.

Wenstrup R, Pagon R: Female pseudohermaphroditism with anorectal, mullerian duct, and urinary tract malformations: report of four cases. J Pediatr 1985; 107:771–775.

Escobar LF, et al.: Urorectal septum malformation sequence: report of six cases and embryological analysis. Am J Dis Child 1987; 141:1021–1024. *

ES004
WE005
BI017

**Luis F. Escobar**
**David D. Weaver**
**David Bixler**

**UROS deficiency**
*See PORPHYRIA, ERYTHROPOIETIC*

---

**URTICARIA PIGMENTOSA (UP)**      **3263**

**Includes:**

Mast cell disease
Mastocytosis
Telangiectasia macularis eruptiva perstans

**Excludes:**

**Urticaria**
**Xeroderma pigmentosum** (1005)

**Major Diagnostic Criteria:** Hyperpigmented macules or papules on the skin. Dariers sign: erythema and edema of skin lesions in response to trauma. Histology of the skin: mast cell infiltrate in the upper third of the dermis; occasionally nodular aggregates of mast cells extend into the subcutaneous fat and eosinophils are scattered within the infiltration.

**Clinical Findings:** Four clinical forms of urticaria pigmentosa exist: (1) Localized; mastocytoma. (2) Generalized: (a) maculopapular; (b) telangiectasia macularis eruptiva perstans; (c) erythrodermic, diffuse.

In addition, systemic mastocytosis may occur; organs involved include bone, gastrointestinal tract, lymphatic systems, spleen and liver.

The skin lesions present as multiple red-brown macules and papules distributed on the trunk and occasionally the limbs. Multiple nodular, lichenoid and plaquelike lesions may be seen, and a rare bullous variety exists.

Ten percent of cases are solitary; a mastocytoma is a red-brown, pink or yellow nodule.

*Telangiectasia macularis eruptiva perstans*, a confluent pattern of telangiectatic and hyperpigmented macules, is a rare variant.

Symptoms of UP are a wheal and flare response to skin trauma, pruritis and flushing. Most patients are asymptomatic. Flushing is precipitated by exercise, hot baths, stress, cold exposure and drugs (especially aspirin and codeine).

**Complications:** Unknown.

**Associated Findings:** None known.

**Etiology:** Autosomal dominant inheritance, possibly with reduced expressivity.

**Pathogenesis:** The accumulation of mast cells in various organs of the body is the hallmark of mastocytosis. Degranulation of mast cells leads to release of chemical mediators into the skin and other tissues, which results in increased vascular permeability and smooth muscle constriction, and affects leucocyte migration and platelet ulceration.

**MIM No.:** 15480

**Sex Ratio:** M1:F1

**Occurrence:** Some 150 cases were seen at the Mayo clinic between 1917 and 1952 (Klaus, 1962). Most affected persons are Caucasians. Familial cases are rare; approximately 50 cases reported in world literature.

**Risk of Recurrence for Patient's Sib:**

See Part I, *Mendelian Inheritance*. Reduced expressivity is possible.

**Risk of Recurrence for Patient's Child:**

See Part I, *Mendelian Inheritance*. Reduced expressivity is possible.

**Age of Detectability:** Urticaria pigmentosa usually presents in childhood.

**Gene Mapping and Linkage:** Unknown.

**Prevention:** None known. Genetic counseling indicated.

**Treatment:** Symptomatic treatment with antihistamines is recomended. Ketotifen may be of use as a mast cell stabiliser.

**Prognosis:** In the absence of systemic involvement, life span is normal.

**Detection of Carrier:** Unknown.

**Special Considerations:** As many as 50 familial cases of urticaria pigmentosa have been recorded. Uniovular twins have been concordant for UP in all but two reported families (Selamonowitz et al, 1970). The inheritance in these families has been autosomal dominant. However, it is important to note that the majority of urticaria pigmentosa or mastocytosis of any type is not familial.

**References:**

Klaus SN, Winkelmann RK: Course of urticaria pigmentosa in children. Arch Derm 1962; 86:68–71.

Shaw JM: Genetic aspects of urticaria pigmentosa. Arch Derm 1968; 97:137–138.

Selamonowitz VJ, et al.: Uniovular twins discordant for cutaneous mastocytosis. Arch Derm 1970; 102:34–41.

Di Bacco RS, De Leo VA: Mastocytosis and the mast cell. J Am Acad Derm 1982; 7:709–722.

Fowler JF, et al.: Familial urticaria pigmentosa. Arch Derm 1986; 122:80–81.

WI055      **Ingrid M. Winship**

**Urticaria syndromes, acquired**
*See COLD HYPERSENSITIVITY*

## URTICARIA, DERMO-DISTORTIVE TYPE     3124

**Includes:**

Dermodistortive urticaria
Vibratory angioedema

**Excludes:**

**Angioedema, hereditary** (0054)
Dermographia
Pressure urticaria

**Major Diagnostic Criteria:** The presence of physical urticaria secondary to stretching or vibration of the skin is sufficient to suggest the diagnosis.

**Clinical Findings:** The rather sudden (i.e., within a few minutes) appearance of transient, pruritic, erythematous wheals in areas of skin exposed to repetitive vibratory or stretching stimulation characterizes the disorder. These wheals usually disappear within one hour. If extensive stimulation is present, systemic manifestations such as faintness, facial flushing, and headache appear.

**Complications:** Unknown.

**Associated Findings:** None known.

**Etiology:** Probably autosomal dominant inheritance with a high degree of penetrance.

**Pathogenesis:** Unknown. Histamine may be the mediator of the responses.

**MIM No.:** 12563

**Sex Ratio:** Presumably M1:F1.

**Occurrence:** One family of Christian Lebanese ethnic origin has been reported.

**Risk of Recurrence for Patient's Sib:**
See Part I, *Mendelian Inheritance.*

**Risk of Recurrence for Patient's Child:**
See Part I, *Mendelian Inheritance.*

**Age of Detectability:** Symptoms can occur soon after birth.

**Gene Mapping and Linkage:** Unknown.

**Prevention:** None known. Genetic counseling indicated.

**Treatment:** Unknown. Avoidance of precipitating stimuli is beneficial.

**Prognosis:** Good. Although annoying, this condition does not affect life span or intelligence.

**Detection of Carrier:** Unknown.

**Special Considerations:** Dermodistortive urticaria and vibratory angioedema could be the same condition.

**References:**

Epstein PA, Kidd KK: Dermo-distortive urticaria: an autosomal dominant dermatologic disorder. Am J Med Genet 1981; 9:307–315.

Epstein PA, et al.: Genetic linkage analysis of dermo-distortive urticaria. Am J Med Genet 1981; 9:317–321.

T0007      **Helga V. Toriello**

## URTICARIA-DEAFNESS-AMYLOIDOSIS     0982

**Includes:**

Amyloidosis-deafness-urticaria
Deafness-urticaria-amyloidosis
Muckle-Wells syndrome

**Excludes:**

**Amyloidoses** (other)
**Fever, familial mediterranean (FMF)** (2161)

**Major Diagnostic Criteria:** Include "aguey bouts" with characteristic skin rash, progressive perceptive deafness, nephropathy, and typical perireticulin amyloidosis.

**Clinical Findings:** During adolescence "aguey bouts" (chills, fever, malaise) make their appearance and recur continually thereafter. Over the next two to four decades perceptive deafness appears and progresses; finally nephropathy appears and leads to death. The "aguey bouts" recur every three weeks or so, lasting 24 to 48 hours. They are accompanied by malaise, a geographic urticarial rash, no particular alteration of leukocytes, but with hyperglobulinemia and raised sedimentation rate. Pes cavus, short metacarpals, short stature, and some skin thickening are usually present. Nephropathy is of the sclerotic amyloid variety, combining predominantly azotemic manifestations with substantial proteinuria. Permanganate-sensitive amyloid deposition is also present in other parts of the body in the pattern characteristic of typical (i.e., perireticulin) amyloidosis plus pulmonary parenchymal involvement. Antigenically, the deposits consist of AA protein alone. The changes in the ear include degeneration of the organ of Corti and vestibular sensory epithelium, atrophy of the cochlear nerve, and ossification of the basilar membrane.

Deafness always develops, and the condition is transmitted as an autosomal dominant. It thus differs from **Fever, familial mediterranean (FMF)**, which does not include deafness and is autosomal recessive. It also differs from the deafness in other forms of hereditary but dominantly nephropathic amyloidosis, and all of the other types of hereditary **Amyloidosis**.

**Complications:** Loss of libido and eventually uremic renal failure (seen in all but one case).

**Associated Findings:** Glaucoma was reported in two patients.

**Etiology:** Autosomal dominant inheritance with incomplete penetrance.

**Pathogenesis:** Unknown.

**MIM No.:** *19190

**POS No.:** 3130

**Sex Ratio:** Presumably M1:F1 (M1.3:F1 observed).

**Occurrence:** Eight families with this condition have been described, the most recent in 1988 (Messier), as well as six sporadic cases. In addition, three families have been described with what appears to be an incomplete variant, comprising all the features of the clinical syndrome but lacking amyloidosis. Finally, a family with *dominantly* inherited **Fever, familial mediterranean (FMF)**, which included neither deafness nor urticaria, was reported by Bergman and Warmenius (1968).

**Risk of Recurrence for Patient's Sib:**
See Part I, *Mendelian Inheritance.*

**Risk of Recurrence for Patient's Child:**
See Part I, *Mendelian Inheritance.*

**Age of Detectability:** In early adolescence, at clinical appraisal of "aguey bouts" which are an initial manifestations. The full syndrome not established before the third decade of life.

**Gene Mapping and Linkage:** Unknown.

**Prevention:** None known. Genetic counseling indicated.

**Treatment:** From an early age, hearing aids, auditory and speech training, and lip-reading instruction may be helpful. Eventually, the usual supportive therapy or more radical treatment for renal failure will be required.

**Prognosis:** Usually death from uremia during the fifth or sixth decade.

**Detection of Carrier:** Possibly by clinical examination of first degree relatives.

**References:**
Muckle TJ, Wells MV: Urticaria, deafness and amyloidosis: a new heredo-familial syndrome. Q J Med 1962; 31:235–248.

Bergman F, Warmenius S: Familial perireticular amyloidosis in a Swedish family. Am J Med 1968; 45:601–606.

Alexander F, Atkins EL: Familial renal amyloidosis: case reports, literature review and classification. Am J Med 1975; 59:121–128.

Letosa RM, et al.: Sindrome de Muckle-Wells: estudio de una familia. Rev Clin Española 1978; 149:93–96.

Muckle TJ: The Muckle-Wells syndrome: a review. Br J Dermatol 1979; 100:87–92. *

Sweeney PJ, et al.: Muckle-Wells syndrome: first Irish case. J Irish Coll Phys Surg 1979; 9:68 only.

Messier G, et al.: Overt or occult renal amyloidosis in the Muckle-Wells syndrome. Siciety de Nephrologie des Paris, 1988.

MU002                                    **Thomas J. Muckle**

---

## USHER SYNDROME                                    0983

**Includes:**
Deafness (sensorineural)-retinitis pigmentosa
Hallgren syndrome
Retinitis pigmentosa-hearing loss (sensorineural)

**Excludes:**
**Alstrom syndrome** (0041)
**Cockayne syndrome** (0189)
**Cockayne syndrome, type II** (2787)
Enzyme deficiencies, disorders with multiple peroxisomal
**Fetal rubella syndrome** (0384)
**Nephritis-deafness (sensorineural), hereditary type** (0708)
**Phytanic acid oxidase deficiency, infantile type** (2278)
**Phytanic acid storage disease** (0810)

**Major Diagnostic Criteria:** Sensorineural hearing loss and **Retinitis pigmentosa.** May be documented by electrophysiologic methods.

**Clinical Findings:** The cardinal manifestations of sensorineural hearing loss and retinitis pigmentosa are variable in time of onset and severity, leading most observers to comment on heterogeneity in Usher syndrome. While two separate classification schemes have been devised to group families according to severity (Merin et al., 1974; Gorlin et al., 1979), other studies have found considerable intrafamilial variability for both otic and optic manifestations (Bateman et al., 1980). Over 90% of patients have profound congenital deafness, with onset of retinitis pigmentosa by age 10 years. The minority will have either severe congenital deafness with retinitis manifested in the second decade or progressive hearing loss with retinitis appearing around puberty. The ophthalmologic findings may be characteristic with pallor of the optic nerve, arteriolar narrowing, and "bone spicule" concretions of pigment. Recently, the possibility of biochemical diagnosis has been raised by finding a decreased content of polyunsaturated fatty acids in plasma phospholids from patients with Usher syndrome.

**Complications:** Several investigators comment on a typical psychosis in Usher syndrome patients; when mental deficiency and psychosis are present, the disorder is termed *Hallgren syndrome.* Labyrinthine ataxia is relatively frequent and necessitates discrimination from Refsum disease (see **Phytanic acid storage disease**) by phytanic acid measurement. Posterior sublenticular cataracts are a later complication. Since Usher syndrome accounts for 6–10% of the congenitally deaf population, all hearing-impaired individuals under age 25 years should be screened for decreasing dark adaptation or peripheral vision. Early recognition of such individuals allows social and vocational preparation for life as a deaf and blind adult.

**Associated Findings:** Abnormalities of nasal cilia and sperm axonemes have been described.

**Etiology:** Unsually autosomal recessive inheritance; a rare X-linked form was suggested by two pairs of affected brothers whose mothers were sisters.

**Pathogenesis:** The abnormalities in nasal cilia, sperm, and photoreceptor axonemes provides one potential route for gene expression; serum fatty acid abnormalities in Usher syndrome, and various peroxisomal disorders having retinitis with deafness, provides another.

**MIM No.:** *27690, 31265

**POS No.:** 3421

**Sex Ratio:** M1:F1

**Occurrence:** Prevalence has been estimated at 3.6–5:100,000 (Grondahl, 1987). A prevalence of 3:1,000 normal individuals was estimated in Denmark. Clusters of patients have been reported in Berlin (Mainly Jews), Finland, Norway (particularly among Lapps), and Louisiana (French Cajuns).

**Risk of Recurrence for Patient's Sib:**
See Part I, *Mendelian Inheritance.*

**Risk of Recurrence for Patient's Child:**
See Part I, *Mendelian Inheritance.*

**Age of Detectability:** In most patients, profound sensorineural hearing loss is recognized at birth or during infancy. Less than 10% will have progressive hearing loss recognized in the first decade. Retinitis pigmentosa may not be diagnosed until after puberty.

**Gene Mapping and Linkage:** GC (group-specific component (vitamin D binding protein)) has been mapped to 4q12-q13.

**Prevention:** None known. Genetic counseling indicated.

**Treatment:** Special education, cataract removal.

**Prognosis:** Life span is normal, but severe deafness and blindness are anticipated in most patients. The sensorineural hearing loss is described as stable by most observers, but some reports describe deterioration with age.

**Detection of Carrier:** One report cites the presence of gyrate atrophy in heterozygotes.

**Special Considerations:** Usher syndrome is undoubtedly a heterogenous group of autosomal recessive disorders, to be further delineated by clinical, metabolic, and DNA marker studies.

**References:**
Usher CH: Bowman's lecture: on a few hereditary eye affections. Trans Ophthalmol Soc UK 1935; 55:164–245.

Merin S, et al.: Usher's and Hallgren's syndromes. Acta Genet Med Gemellol 1974; 23:45–55.

Gorlin RJ, et al.: Usher's syndrome type III. Arch Otolaryngol 1979; 105:353–354.

Bateman JB, et al.: Heterogeneity of retinal degeneration and hearing impairment syndromes. Am J Ophthalmol 1980; 90:755–767. †

Boughman JA, et al.: Usher syndrome: definition and estimate of prevalence from two high-risk populations. J Chronic Dis 1983; 36:595–603.

Bazan NG, et al.: Decreased content of docosahexanoate and arachidonate in plasma phospholipids in Usher's syndrome. Biochem Biophys Res Commun 1986; 141:600–604.

Hunter DG, et al.: Abnormal sperm and photoreceptor axonemes in Usher's syndrome. Arch Ophthalmol 1986; 104:385–389.

Shinkawa H, Nadol JB, Jr.: Histopathology of the inner ear in Usher's syndrome as observed by light and electron microscopy. Ann Otol Rhinol Laryng 1986; 95:313–318.

Grondahl J: Estimation of prognosis and prevalence of retinitis pigmentosa and Usher syndrome in Norway. Clin Genet 1987; 31:225–264.

WI024                                            **Golder N. Wilson**

**Uterine hernia syndrome**
*See MULLERIAN DERIVATIVES IN MALES, PERSISTENT*
**Uterine inguinal hernia syndrome**
*See MULLERIAN DERIVATIVES IN MALES, PERSISTENT*
**Uterus arcuatus**
*See MULLERIAN FUSION, INCOMPLETE*
**Uterus bicornus**
*See MULLERIAN FUSION, INCOMPLETE*
**Uterus bicornus unicollis**
*See MULLERIAN FUSION, INCOMPLETE*
**Uterus bilocularis**
*See MULLERIAN FUSION, INCOMPLETE*
**Uterus bipartitus**
*See MULLERIAN FUSION, INCOMPLETE*
**Uterus didelphys**
*See MULLERIAN FUSION, INCOMPLETE*
**Uterus pseudodidelphys**
*See MULLERIAN FUSION, INCOMPLETE*
**Uterus subseptus**
*See MULLERIAN FUSION, INCOMPLETE*
**Uterus unicornus**
*See MULLERIAN FUSION, INCOMPLETE*
**Uterus, congenital absence of**
*See MULLERIAN APLASIA*
**Uterus-limb syndrome**
*See LIMB, UPPER HYPOPLASIA-MULLERIAN DUCT DEFECTS*
**Uveal coloboma**
*See EYE, MICROPHTHALMIA/COLOBOMA*

## UVULA, CLEFT                            0184

**Includes:**
    Bifid uvula
    Uvula, split

**Excludes:**
    **Cleft lip** (0178)
    **Cleft palate** (0180)

**Major Diagnostic Criteria:** Mid-line separation of uvula.

**Clinical Findings:** Cleft uvula varies from a notching of uvula to complete cleft of uvula extending to the posterior border of the soft palate.

**Complications:** Hypernasality.

**Associated Findings:** Submucous cleft palate.

**Etiology:** Multifactorial inheritance, although an autosomal dominant form may exist.

**Pathogenesis:** Failure of complete fusion of the uvular portion of the medial halves of the soft palate during embryogenesis.

**MIM No.:** 19210

**CDC No.:** 749.080

**Sex Ratio:** M1.2:F1

**Occurrence:** One percent among Caucasians, 10% among Mongolians including American Indians.

**Risk of Recurrence for Patient's Sib:** About ten percent without an affected parent, 30% with an affected parent.

**Risk of Recurrence for Patient's Child:** About ten percent.

**Age of Detectability:** At birth.

**Gene Mapping and Linkage:** Unknown.

**Prevention:** None known. Genetic counseling indicated.

**Treatment:** Surgical correction is seldom needed, but available.

**Prognosis:** Normal life expectancy.

**Detection of Carrier:** Unknown.

**Special Considerations:** Some cases of cleft uvula may be microforms of cleft palate. In persons with cleft uvula the complete removal of the adenoid pad during tonsillectomy and adenoidectomy may produce hypernasal speech.

**References:**

Meskin LH, et al.: Abnormal morphology of the soft palate. I. the prevalence of cleft uvula. Cleft Palate J 1964; 1:342–346. *

Meskin LH, et al.: Abnormal morphology of the soft palate. II. the genetics of cleft uvula. Cleft Palate J 1965; 2:40–45. *

Richardson ER: Cleft uvula: incidence in negroes. Cleft Palate J 1970; 7:669–672.

Chosack A, Eidelman E: Cleft uvula: prevalence and genetics. Cleft Palate J 1987; 5:63–67.

J0027                                 **Ronald J. Jorgenson**

**Uvula, split**
*See UVULA, CLEFT*

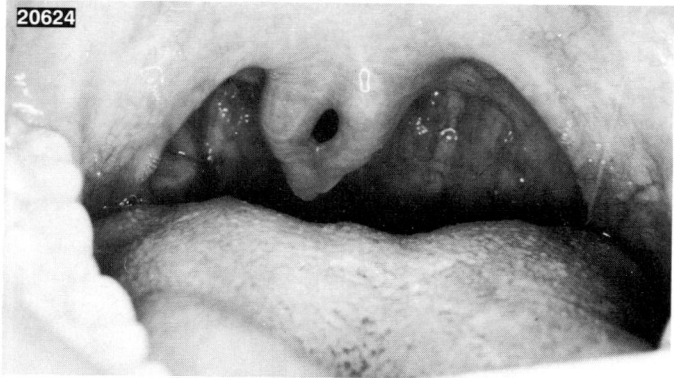

**0184-20624:** Cleft uvula.

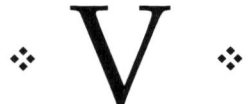

**VACTEL association**
*See VATER ASSOCIATION*
**VACTERL association**
*See VATER ASSOCIATION*
**Vagina, absence, congenital (one form)**
*See VAGINAL ATRESIA*
**Vagina, congenital absence of**
*See MULLERIAN APLASIA*
**Vaginal atresia**
*See MULLERIAN APLASIA*

## VAGINAL ATRESIA                                      0984

**Includes:**  Vagina, absence, congenital (one form)

**Excludes:**
    **Hymen, imperforate** (0483)
    **Mullerian aplasia** (0682)
    Pseudohermaphroditism, all forms of male and female
    **Renal-genital-middle ear anomalies** (0860)
    **Vaginal septum, transverse** (0985)

**Major Diagnostic Criteria:**  Atresia of the lower vagina in a female (46,XX) with a normal upper vagina, uterus, external genitalia, and ovaries.

**Clinical Findings:**  The lower one-fifth to one-third of the vagina is replaced by 2–3 cm of fibrous tissue. The remaining (superior) portion of the vagina is well differentiated. External genitalia are normal for females. The uterine cervix and corpus, fallopian tubes, and ovaries are likewise normal. Usually somatic anomalies are not present, although renal anomalies have been reported. At puberty female secondary sexual development is normal, except for absence of menses.

    Vaginal atresia should be differentiated from **Mullerian aplasia**, a condition in which the cephalad portion of the vagina and the uterus are absent. Some authors group both these conditions under "congenital absence of vagina." In addition, an autosomal recessive trait characterized by vaginal atresia, renal hypoplasia or agenesis, and middle ear anomalies (see **Renal-genital-middle ear anomalies**) has been described.

**Complications:**  Menstrual products cannot pass because of the atretic lower vagina. Hydrometrocolpos may lead to amenorrhea, as well as abdominal pain or palpable masses as the result of accumulation of fluid.

**Associated Findings:**  Renal anomalies have been reported.

**Etiology:**  Undetermined. Familial aggregates are very rare. Limitation of the defect to a single organ system is compatible with polygenic/multifactorial inheritance.

**Pathogenesis:**  The caudal portion of the vagina is formed from invagination of the urogenital sinus, whereas the cephalad portion is of müllerian origin. In vaginal atresia the urogenital sinus presumably fails to contribute the caudal portion of the vagina.

**CDC No.:**  752.410

**Sex Ratio:**  M0:F1

**Occurrence:**  Occurs in perhaps 5–10% of females said to have "absence of the vagina", as opposed to **Mullerian aplasia** which is more common.

**Risk of Recurrence for Patient's Sib:**  Probably not greater than 1–5% for female sib to be affected, assuming multifactorial etiology.

**Risk of Recurrence for Patient's Child:**  No more than 1–5% for a female child to be affected, assuming multifactorial etiology.

**Age of Detectability:**  Usually at puberty, when hydrometrocolpos causes primary amenorrhea. Occasionally mucocolpos occurs in neonates.

**Gene Mapping and Linkage:**  Unknown.

**Prevention:**  None known. Genetic counseling indicated.

**Treatment:**  Surgical extirpation of the fibrous tissue. The thickness of atretic portion precludes simple incisional drainage.

**Prognosis:**  Normal life span; normal fertility.

**Detection of Carrier:**  Unknown.

**References:**
Dennison WM, Bacsich P: Imperforate vagina in the newborn: neonatal hydrocolpos. Arch Dis Child 1961; 36:156–160.
Simpson JL: Disorders of sexual differentiation: etiology and clinical delineation. New York: Academic Press, 1976:345–346.
Jones HW Jr, Rock JA: Reparative and constructive surgery of the female generative tract. Baltimore: Williams & Wilkins, 1983:161–164.

SI018                               **Joe Leigh Simpson**

## VAGINAL SEPTUM, TRANSVERSE                         0985

**Includes:**
    Hydrometrocolpos-postaxial polydactyly-congential heart anomalies
    Kaufman-McKusick syndrome
    McKusick-Kaufman syndrome
    Transverse vaginal septum

**Excludes:**
    **Chondroectodermal dysplasia** (0156)
    **Hymen, imperforate** (0483)
    **Mullerian aplasia** (0682)
    **Mullerian fusion, incomplete** (0684)
    **Vaginal atresia** (0984)
    Vaginal septum, longitudinal

**Major Diagnostic Criteria:**  Transverse vaginal septum, with or without a perforation, in a 46,XX individual with normal ovaries, normal external genitalia, and otherwise normal müllerian derivatives.

**Clinical Findings:**  Transverse septa are usually located near the junction of the upper one-third and lower two-thirds of the vagina; however, septa may be present in the middle or lower one-third. These septa are about 1 cm thick and may or may not have a perforation. A perforation, if present, is usually central in location; however, it may occasionally be eccentric. The external genitalia, uterine cervix, uterine corpus, fallopian tubes, and ovaries are normal. The most frequent presenting symptom is primary amenorrhea. Hydrometrocolpos or hematometrocolpos may be noted on pelvic examination. No somatic abnormalities are present. At puberty normal secondary sexual development occurs.

Longitudinal vaginal septa, sagittal or coronal, have been reported, but these septa represent an entity different from transverse vaginal septa. Longitudinal septa rarely produce clinical problems.

**Complications:** If no perforation is present, mucus and menstrual fluid cannot be expelled and, hence, hydrometrocolpos may develop. Coital difficulties or abnormalities of the second stage of labor have been reported.

**Associated Findings:** Polydactyly and cardiac anomalies have been associated with transverse vaginal septum, but usually no associated anomalies are present.

**Etiology:** Although autosomal recessive inheritance appears to be responsible for transverse vaginal septa in the Amish, heritable tendencies have not been verified in other ethnic groups. Whether the presence of polydactyly and/or heart anomalies indicates a separate condition (*Kaufman-McKusick syndrome*) has not been determined.

**Pathogenesis:** Vaginal septa probably result from failure of the urogenital sinus derivatives and the müllerian duct derivatives to fuse or canalize properly in order to form a normal vagina. Although this explanation is accepted by most investigators, the situation may be more complex. Some data suggest that abnormal mesodermal proliferation may occur.

**MIM No.:** *23670

**CDC No.:** 752.380

**Sex Ratio:** M0:F1

**Occurrence:** At least six families, and many individual cases (some associated with consanguinity), have been documented.

**Risk of Recurrence for Patient's Sib:**
See Part I, *Mendelian Inheritance*. In the Amish 1:4 for 46,XX sibs; 1:8 for all sibs. In other ethnic groups, similar risk figures may or may not be appropriate.

**Risk of Recurrence for Patient's Child:**
See Part I, *Mendelian Inheritance*. Some forms could be inherited in polygenic/multifactorial fashion, in which case the risk is estimated at less than 5%.

**Age of Detectability:** Usually at puberty, because of primary amenorrhea with or without hydrometrocolpos, or hematometrocolpos. Occasionally mucocolpos is noted at birth, and Farrell et al (1986) described prenatal diagnosis. Some affected patients have been detected because of coital difficulties or abnormalities during labor.

**Gene Mapping and Linkage:** Unknown.

**Prevention:** None known. Genetic counseling indicated.

**Treatment:** Surgical extirpation or creation of an opening in the septum if no perforation is present; enlargement of the perforation may be necessary if the opening is very small.

**Prognosis:** Normal life span.

**Detection of Carrier:** Glandular hypospadias and prominent scrotal raphe are claimed by some to be manifestations in the male.

**References:**
McKusick VA, et al.: Recessive inheritance of a congenital malformation syndrome. J Am Med Asso 1968; 204:113–116.
Simpson JL: Disorders of sexual differentiation: etiology and clinical delineation. New York: Academic Press, 1976:348–351.
Sarto GE, Simpson JL: Abnormalities of the Müllerian and Wolffian duct systems. BD:OAS XIV(6c). New York: Alan R. Liss, for The National Foundation-March of Dimes, 1978:37–55.
Robinow M, Shaw A: The McKusick/Kaufman syndrome: recessively inherited vaginal atresia, hydrometrocolpos, uterovaginal duplications, anorectal anomalies, postaxial polydactyly, and congenital heart disease. J Pediatr 1979; 94:776–778.
Suidan FG, Azoury RS: The transverse vaginal septum: a clinicopathologic evaluation. Obstet Gynecol 1979; 54:278–283.
Goecke T, et al.: Hydrometrocolpos, postaxial polydactyly, congenital heart disease, and anomalies of the gastrointestinal and genitourinary tracts. Eur J Pediatr 1981; 136:297–305.
Jones HW Jr, Rock JA: Reparative and constructive surgery of the female generative tract. Baltimore: Williams & Wilkins, 1983:158–164.
Pinsky L: Origin of the "associated" anomalies in Kaufman-McKusick syndrome. (Letter) Am J Med Genet 1983; 14:791–792.
Farrell SA, et al.: Abdominal distension in Kaufman-McKusick syndrome. Am J Med Genet 1986; 25:205–210.

SI018                                              **Joe Leigh Simpson**

**Valine transaminase deficiency**
*See HYPERVALINEMIA*
**Valinemia**
*See HYPERVALINEMIA*
**Valium^, fetal effects**
*See FETAL BENZODIAZEPINE EFFECTS*
**Vallecular cyst**
*See EPIGLOTTIS, VALLECULAR CYST*
**Valproate sensitivity**
*See ORNITHINE TRANSCARBAMYLASE DEFICIENCY*
**Valproic acid and conjoined twins**
*See TWINS, CONJOINED, TERATOGENICITY*
**Valproic acid, fetal damage from**
*See FETAL VALPROATE SYNDROME*
**Valproic acid, fetal effects**
*See MENINGOMYELOCELE*
**Valvar aortic stenosis**
*See AORTIC VALVE STENOSIS*
**Van Allen type amyloidosis**
*See AMYLOIDOSIS, IOWA TYPE*
**Van Bogaert spongy degeneration of the CNS**
*See BRAIN, SPONGY DEGENERATION*
**Van Buchem disease**
*See ENDOSTEAL HYPEROSTOSIS*

---

## VAN DEN BOSCH SYNDROME                        0986

**Includes:** Anhidrosis-mental retardation-eye and skeletal defects

**Excludes:**
   Choroideremia (0925)
   Ectodermal dysplasia, Christ-Siemens-Touraine type (0333)
   X-linked mental retardation (1509)

**Major Diagnostic Criteria:** Anhidrosis, mental retardation, choroideremia, acrokeratosis verruciformis, and winged scapulae.

**Clinical Findings:** Anhidrosis associated with mental deficiency; delayed somatic growth; ophthalmologic abnormalities (horizontal nystagmus, myopia, choroideremia, abnormal retinogram); winged scapulae; acrokeratosis verruciformis; and bronchial and skin infections.

**Complications:** Hyperthermia, intolerance to heat, and bronchial and skin infections.

**Associated Findings:** None known.

**Etiology:** X-linked recessive inheritance.

**Pathogenesis:** Unknown.

**MIM No.:** *31450

**POS No.:** 3424

**Sex Ratio:** M1:F0

**Occurrence:** Described in a single Dutch kindred.

**Risk of Recurrence for Patient's Sib:**
See Part I, *Mendelian Inheritance*.

**Risk of Recurrence for Patient's Child:**
See Part I, *Mendelian Inheritance*.

**Age of Detectability:** In neonatal period.

**Gene Mapping and Linkage:** A small deletion on the long arm of the X-chromosome could explain the concurrence of the different components of this syndrome, which have been described as isolated X-linked traits.

**Prevention:** None known. Genetic counseling indicated.

**Treatment:** Avoid high environmental temperature, encourage hydration; special education as needed.

**Prognosis:** Unknown.

**Detection of Carrier:** Possibly altered sweat pores in carrier.

**References:**
Van Den Bosch, J: A new syndrome in three generations of a Dutch family. Ophthalmologica 1959; 137:422–423.

WI021                                    **R.S. Wilroy, Jr.**

**van der Woude syndrome**
   See *CLEFT LIP/PALATE-LIP PITS OR MOUNDS*
**Van Gelderen syndrome**
   See *ALOPECIA-SKELETAL ANOMALIES-SHORT STATURE-MENTAL RETARDATION*
**Van Lohuizen syndrome**
   See *CUTIS MARMORATA*
**Varadi-Papp syndrome**
   See *ORO-PALATAL-DIGITAL SYNDROME, VARADI TYPE*
**Varicella embryopathy**
   See *FETAL EFFECTS FROM VARICELLA-ZOSTER*
**Varicella-zoster, fetal effects**
   See *FETAL EFFECTS FROM VARICELLA-ZOSTER*
**Vascular anomalies-congenital heart defects-distichiasis**
   See *DISTICHIASIS-HEART DEFECT-PERIPHERAL VASCULAR DISEASE/ANOMALIES*
**Vascular dysplasia-sternal malformation association**
   See *STERNAL MALFORMATION-VASCULAR DYSPLASIA ASSOCIATION*
**Vascular formations, familial**
   See *RETINA, CAVERNOUS HEMANGIOMA*
**Vascular malformations of middle ear**
   See *EAR, OSSICLE AND MIDDLE EAR MALFORMATIONS*
**Vascular malformations, familial**
   See *HEMANGIOMAS OF THE HEAD AND NECK*
**Vascular tumors hemangioid cell derivation-spontaneous hemorrhage**
   See *HEMANGIOMA-THROMBOCYTOPENIA SYNDROME*
**Vasolidator, fetal effects**
   See *FETAL EFFECTS FROM MATERNAL VASODILATOR*
**Vasopressin-resistant**
   See *DIABETES INSIPIDUS, VASOPRESSIN RESISTANT TYPES I AND II*
**Vasotec^, fetal effects**
   See *FETAL ANGIOTENSIN CONVERTING ENZYME (ACE) INHIBITION RENAL FAILURE*
**Vasquez syndrome**
   See *X-LINKED MENTAL RETARDATION-GROWTH-HEARING AND GENITAL DEFECTS*

---

## VATER ASSOCIATION                                    0987

**Includes:**
   Imperforate anus-polydactyly syndrome
   Polydactyly-imperforate anus
   VACTEL association
   VACTERL association

**Excludes:**
   **Anus-hand-ear syndrome** (0072)
   **Charge association** (2124)
   **Heart-hand syndrome** (0455)
   **MURCS association** (2406)
   **Renal agenesis, unilateral** (0857)
   **Tracheal agenesis-multiple anomaly association** (2849)

**Major Diagnostic Criteria:** The VATER association is diagnosed, according to the criteria of Quan and Smith (1973), on the basis of the presence of three of five designated VATER ascertainment abnormalities: *V*ertebral dysgenesis, *A*nal atresia, *T*racheoesophageal fistula with *E*sophageal atresia, and *R*enal and *R*adial limb dysgenesis in the absence of a chromosome aberration.

**Clinical Findings:** While many additional malformations are observed in VATER patients, and result in a high average number of anomalies (seven to eight) per patient, central system abnormalities are minimally increased and mental retardation is only an occasional problem. The malformations are widely distributed throughout the body, with approximately two-thirds located in the lower body segment, notably those of the distal intestinal and genitourinary tracts, lumbosacrococcygeal vertebrae, pelvis, and lower limbs. Anomalies observed in the upper body segment include esophageal atresia with or without tracheoesophageal fistula, radial limb dysgenesis, heart, proximal intestinal tract, rib, and respiratory tract abnormalities. Hypersegmentation (13–14 ribs and/or thoracic vertebrae; 6–7 lumbar vertebrae) occurs in approximately 10% of VATER patients.

**Complications:** Respiratory, cardiac, and renal failure can be severe in VATER patients neonatally.

**Associated Findings:** Monozygotic twinning is increased (6%), while maternal diabetes and situs inversus have low incidences when compared with those of patients with the **Sacrococcygeal dysgenesis syndrome**.

**Etiology:** Nearly all cases have been sporadic, although a few familial cases have been reported (Auchterlonie and White, 1982).

**Pathogenesis:** Unknown.

**MIM No.:** 19235

**POS No.:** 3425

**Sex Ratio:** M1:F1

**Occurrence:** About 250 cases have been documented. Probably underreported, since patients previously identified to have only multiple anomalies can now be diagnosed as having the VATER association.

**Risk of Recurrence for Patient's Sib:** Minimal, except in familial cases.

**Risk of Recurrence for Patient's Child:** Unknown.

**Age of Detectability:** At birth or shortly thereafter.

**Gene Mapping and Linkage:** Unknown.

**Prevention:** None known. Genetic counseling indicated.

**Treatment:** Surgical correction or medical management of spine, limb, cardiovascular, urinary, intestinal, and other malformations as indicated.

**Prognosis:** The overall survival of 46 VATER patients was 72% (Weaver et al., 1986) but the series did not include fetal deaths or stillbirths. The prognosis of each VATER patient will depend on the particular combination and severity of abnormalities present, and on the availability of surgical and medical correction.

**Detection of Carrier:** Unknown.

**Special Considerations:** VATER is an acronym used to identify a sporadic, nonrandom association of specified abnormalities. It is probably best to confine the designation of VATER association to patients who rigidly meet the original criteria of Quan and Smith (1973).

**References:**
Quan L, Smith DW: The VATER association, vertebral defects, anal atresia, T-E fistula with esophageal atresia, radial and renal dysplasia: a spectrum of associated defects. J Pediatr 1973; 82:104–107.
Smith DW, et al.: Monozygotic twinning and the Duhamel anomalad (imperforate anus to sirenomelia); a non-random association between two aberrations in morphogenesis. BD:OAS XII(5). New York: March of Dimes Birth Defects Foundation, 1976:53–63.
Auchterlonie IA, White MP: Recurrence of the VATER association within a sibship. Clin Genet 1982; 21:122–124.
Khoury MJ, et al.: A population study of the VACTERL association: evidence for its etiologic heterogeneity. Pediatrics 1983; 71:815–820.
Duncan PA, et al.: Distinct caudal regression syndrome identified by associated malformation pattern and demographic features. (Abstract) Proc Greenwood Genet Center 1986; 5:142 only.
Weaver DD, et al.: The VATER association: analysis of 46 patients. Am J Dis Child 1986; 140:225–229.
Duncan PA, Shapiro LR: Seronomelia and VATER association: possi-

ble interrelated disorders with common embryologic pathogenesis. Dysmorphol Clin Genet 1988; 2:96–103.

DU003
SH009

Peter A. Duncan
Lawrence R. Shapiro

**Vein of Galen aneurysm**
*See CNS ARTERIOVENOUS MALFORMATION*

## VELO-CARDIO-FACIAL SYNDROME                    2129

**Includes:** Shprintzen syndrome
**Excludes:**

Arthro-ophthalmopathy, hereditary, progressive, Stickler type (0090)
Cardio-auditory syndrome (0123)
Cleft palate-micrognathia-glossoptosis (0182)
Fetal alcohol syndrome (0379)
G syndrome (0401)
Hypertelorism-hypospadias syndrome (0505)
Immunodeficiency, thymic agenesis (0943)
Myotonic dystrophy (0702)
Tricho-rhino-phalangeal syndrome
Vena cava, persistent left superior joined to coronary sinus (0807)

**Major Diagnostic Criteria:** Numerous physical, psychological, and behavioral findings have been documented in this common syndrome of clefting. However, with the exception of some of the

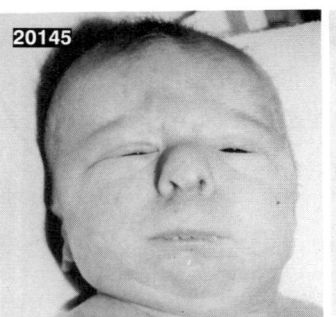

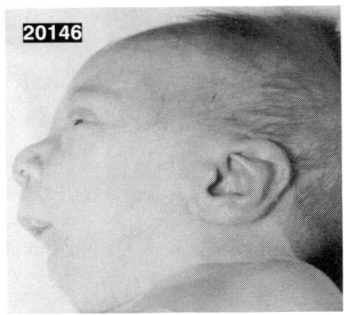

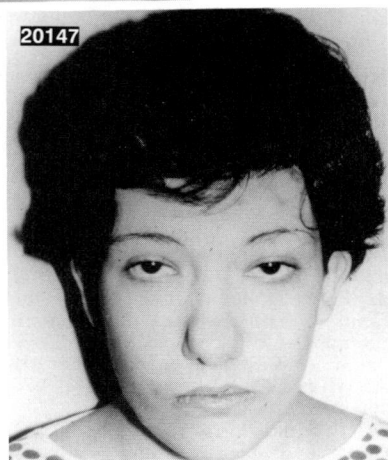

**2129-20145:** Note prominent nose with squared nasal root, long philtrum and mild facial asymmetry. **20146:** Lateral view of the face; the micrognathia is not characteristic and is an associated finding in this infant. **20147:** Adult subject; note prominent nose with squared root and narrow alar base.

cardiac anomalies and **Cleft palate**, the majority of anomalies associated with this syndrome are minor and occur with frequency in the general population. However, the following combination of anomalies should lead to a strong suspicion of this syndrome:

1) cleft, submucous cleft, or occult submucous cleft of the secondary palate, or hypernasal speech, 2) **Ventricular septal defect** (VSD) alone or in combination with other cardiac anomalies, including **Aortic arch, right** and **Heart, tetralogy of Fallot**, 3) learning disabilities or mental retardation, hypotonia, and mildly delayed developmental milestones, 4) relatively small stature, 5) relatively small head circumference, often **Microcephaly**, 6) slender, tapered hands and digits, often hyperextensible, 7) retrognathia, 8) characteristic facies, including a prominent nose with a large, squared nasal root and narrow alar base, malar flatness, vertical maxillary excess, long philtrum, and open-mouth posture, bluish suborbital venous congestion (often referred to as "allergic shiners"), occasional mild facial asymmetry, 9) small auricles, often with thickened helical rims, occasionally asymmetrical with one slightly larger than the other, 10) cephalometric X-rays show platybasia (obtuse angulation of the cranial base) with relatively normal mandibular morphology, 11) frequent upper respiratory illness with apparent immunologic deficiency, 12) tortuous retinal vessels and occasionally other eye anomalies, including microphthalmia and ocular coloboma, 13) medial displacement of the internal carotid arteries in the posterior pharyngeal wall, 14) absent or small thymus, tonsils or adenoids, and 15) hypocalcemia and hypotonia in infancy.

**Clinical Findings:** Birth weight is usually normal. Growth often proceeds normally during infancy and young childhood, though "failure to thrive" has been reported in approximately 25% of affected neonates. This has been associated with obstructive apnea in a number of neonates. Obstructive apnea has been seen in affected neonates and is precipitated by both retrognathia and pharyngeal hypotonia. Hypocalcemia has been reported in approximately 10% of known cases. In several of these cases, hypocalcemia has occurred in association with absent thymus and right sided aortic arch, thus leading to the diagnosis of **Immunodeficiency, thymic agenesis** occurring in association with velo-cardio-facial syndrome. As the children get older, growth is constant though they tend to remain relatively small, usually falling between the second and twenty-fifth percentile.

Developmental milestones are usually mildly delayed, though they may be barely within normal limits. Nearly all of the reported cases have been "floppy babies" remaining relatively hypotonic throughout childhood. However, intellectual impairment is generally not evident in preschool years. Language development is often mildly delayed and speech is almost always characterized by hypernasality, with or without overt clefting of the palate. With advancing age, especially after entering school where more abstract reasoning becomes necessary, learning disabilities and perhaps even mild intellectual impairment become apparent. The majority of the children require some type of special class placement or supplementary educational services, especially in earlier school years, but are eventually "mainstreamed" and graduate from high school. Several affected individuals have also completed college. However, the range of IQ scores in secondary school age children with this syndrome is reported at 69–87 on a performance scale (with mean scores of 79 and 70 respectively).

Hypernasal speech has been observed in nearly all documented cases to date, whether obtained from cleft palate centers or cardiac clinics. Hypernasality has been related to both the frequent occurrence of **Cleft palate** (including submucous and occult submucous cleft palate) and to hypotonia of the pharynx. It is of interest to note that obstructive sleep apnea has been reported following pharyngeal flap surgery, including one reported case of sudden death one month postoperatively. Surgical risk is also increased by the observation of medial displacement of the internal carotid arteries in approximately 25% of cases examined nasopharyngoscopically.

Patients have displayed a very characteristic personality. They have a bland affect, are disinhibited, impulsive, and very affectionate.

Based upon approximately 150 cases clinical findings can be summarized as learning disabilities (100%); **Cleft palate** including submucous and occult submucous cleft palate (98%); hypernasal speech and high pitched voice (98%); pharyngeal hypotonia (90%); retrognathia (87%); cardiac anomalies (80%), including **Ventricular septal defect** (65%), **Aortic arch, right** (35%), **Heart, tetralogy of Fallot** (21%), aberrant left subclavian artery (20%), and a variety of associated cardiac anomalies which occurred in less than 10% of reported cases.

Characteristic facies, including in any combination: "long face" with vertical maxillary excess (85%), prominent nose with squared nasal root and narrow alar base and resultant compromise of the nasal airway (75%), long philtrum and upper lip (70%), malar flatness (70%), narrow palpebral fissures (65%), blue suborbital venous congestion, or "allergic shiners" (50%), and abundant scalp hair (50%); obtuse angulation of the cranial base, or platybasia (75%); intermittent conductive hearing loss secondary to frequent serous otitis media and cleft palate (75%); small auricles and minor auricular anomalies, including thickened helical folds (60%); slender hands and tapered digits, generally small by measurement (60%); tortuous retinal vessels (50%); small or absent tonsils and adenoids (50%); mental retardation (40%); **Microcephaly** (40%); small stature (30%); medial displacement of the internal carotid arteries (25%); **Hernia, inguinal** (25%); **Hernia, umbilical** (20%); scoliosis (15%); **Cleft palate-micrognathia-glossoptosis** (15%); hypospadias (10% of affected males); absent thymus (approximately 10%); hypocalcemia (approximately 10%);

With the exception of cardiac X-rays (chest films, cardiac catheterizations, echocardiograms, etc.), X-ray findings to date have been limited to cephalometry which has shown anomalies of the basicranium (platybasia) and videofluoroscopic phonation studies of the pharynx which has shown hypotonia of the pharyngeal walls in approximately 80% of the cases examined.

**Complications:** Obstructive sleep apnea has been frequently observed in nearly half of the cases who were seen as neonates for the first time. There were several factors contributing to this upper airway compromise, including retrognathia, pharyngeal (and generalized) hypotonia, and severe constriction of the nose. Several patients have developed obstructive sleep apnea following pharyngeal flap surgery to relieve hypernasal speech. Palatal and other surgery may be complicated by cardiac anomalies. Medial displacement of the internal carotid arteries may also lead to bleeding complications during pharyngeal surgery. A small number of infants have died because of the severity of their cardiac anomalies.

**Associated Findings:** **Holoprosencephaly**, diastasis recti, synophrys, sensori-neural hearing loss, and cryptorchidism.

**Etiology:** Autosomal dominant inheritance.

**Pathogenesis:** The numerous vascular anomalies may point towards a major effect on the circulatory system. Numerous patients have had karyotypes and no chromosome anomalies have been found. Similarly, numerous biochemical tests have been performed because of early failure to thrive, but no metabolic or immunologic factors have been found with the exception of absent thymic hormone in patients with absent thymus. Cleft palate is clearly a primary feature of the syndrome and is not secondary to retrognathism. Retrognathia is caused by posterior displacement of the temporomandibular joint which is related to the flattening of the cranial base (platybasia). The mandible is morphologically normal. Similarly, the prominence of the nasal root and the malar deficiency which result in the characteristic facies are caused by the abnormal flexion of the cranial base and the abnormal arrangement and orientation of the facial bones.

Neurologic investigations have failed to show any identifiable abnormalities within the brain to account for hypotonia, learning disabilities, or mental retardation. However, it should be noted that nearly all patients have relatively small head circumferences with approximately 40% of the patients being microcephalic. Small stature is a primary feature of the syndrome and is not secondary to cardiac anomalies.

**MIM No.:** *19243

**POS No.:** 3132

**Sex Ratio:** M1:F1

**Occurrence:** Common syndrome of clefting, comprising as much as 5% of the population of individuals with cleft palate without cleft lip. At least 150 cases have been observed.

**Risk of Recurrence for Patient's Sib:**
See Part I, *Mendelian Inheritance.*

**Risk of Recurrence for Patient's Child:**
See Part I, *Mendelian Inheritance.*

**Age of Detectability:** Can be detected at birth if the association of cleft palate and cardiac anomalies is present, or if **Cleft palate-micrognathia-glossoptosis** or **Immunodeficiency, thymic agenesis** is present. Characteristic facies may not be apparent until later in childhood. Speech disorders, language impairment, and learning disabilities are valuable aids in the diagnosis of this syndrome, but are also not evident until at least 2–3 years of age.

**Gene Mapping and Linkage:** Unknown.

**Prevention:** None known. Genetic counseling indicated.

**Treatment:** Symptomatic treatment for cardiac, palatal, speech, hearing, and learning problems can be very effective. If patient feels it is necessary, aesthetic surgery (rhinoplasty, maxillary and mandibular osteotomies) can remove facial stigmata. Early failure to thrive is most often related to obstructive apnea and is best temporarily relieved by placement of a nasopharyngeal tube. Several patients have required glossopexy which was usually divided by six months of age.

**Prognosis:** Life span is normal. All documented cases to date have had learning disabilities, especially in the areas of mathematics and reading comprehension. Forty percent of documented cases have been mildly mentally retarded. However, the prognosis for normal social functioning is good.

**Detection of Carrier:** Unknown.

**Special Considerations:** This syndrome is one of the most common syndromes of clefting, but because affected children are not severely dysmorphic, diagnosis may be difficult. However, identification is important because of special treatment considerations for speech, language, and learning deficits. Early identification can lead to the interception of anticipated learning disabilities and more effective educational management.

**References:**
Strong WB: Familial syndrome of right-sided aortic arch, mental deficiency, and facial dysmorphism. J Pediatr 1968; 73:882–888.
Shprintzen RJ, et al.: A new syndrome involving cleft palate, cardiac anomalies, typical facies, and learning disabilities: velo-cardio-facial syndrome. Cleft Palate J 1978; 15:56–62.
Young D, et al.: Cardiac malformations in the velocardiofacial syndrome. Am J Cardiol, 1980; 46:643–648.
Shprintzen RJ, et al.: The velo-cardio-facial syndrome: a clinical and genetic analysis. Pediatrics 1981; 67:167–172.
Aruystas M, Shprintzen RJ: Craniofacial morphology in the velo-cardio-facial syndrome. J Craniofac Genet Dev Biol 1984; 4:39–45.
Golding-Kishner K, Weller G: Velo-cardio-facial syndrome: language and psychological profiles. J Craniofacial Genet Devel Biol 1985; 5:259–266.
Williams MA, et al.: Male-to-male transmission of the velo-cardio-facial syndrome: a case report and review of 60 cases. J Craniofacial Genet Devel Biol, 1985; 5:175–180.
Wraith JE, et al.: Velo-cardio-facial syndrome presenting as holoprosencephaly. Clin Genet 1985; 27:408–410.
Beemer FA, et al.: Additional eye findings in a girl with velo-cardio-facial syndrome. Am J Med Genet 1986; 24:541–542.
Williams MA, et al.: Adenoid hypoplasia in the velo-cardio-facial syndrome. J Craniofac Genet Devel Biol 1987; 7:23–26.

SH040                                        **Robert J. Shprintzen**

**Velopharyngeal incompetence**
*See PALATOPHARYNGEAL INCOMPETENCE*
**Velopharyngeal insufficiency**
*See PALATOPHARYNGEAL INCOMPETENCE*
**Vena cava connecting to right atrium via coronary sinus**
*See VENA CAVA, PERSISTENT LEFT SUPERIOR JOINED TO CORONARY SINUS*

## VENA CAVA, ABSENT HEPATIC SEGMENT 0528

**Includes:**
> Azygos continuation of inferior vena cava
> Inferior vena cava, absent
> Inferior vena cava, absent hepatic segment
> Infrahepatic interruption of inferior vena cava

**Excludes:** N/A

**Major Diagnostic Criteria:** As an isolated defect, absence of the hepatic segment of the inferior vena cava (IVC) gives rise to no symptoms. Associated cardiac defects are frequently present and signs and symptoms are dependent on the specific abnormalities. The condition is frequently present in the polysplenia syndrome.

**Clinical Findings:** In this condition the IVC is absent between the renal veins and the hepatic veins. The systemic venous drainage from below the interruption is via an enlarged azygos vein to the superior vena cava. Less often, the hemiazygos vein is the alternative venous pathway and empties into a persistent left superior vena cava.

The anomaly by itself does not alter hemodynamics and is not responsible for symptomatology. It may be identified on X-ray by absence of the IVC density at the cardiophrenic angle in the lateral view. The collateral route of flow to the right SVC by the azygos vein creates a large rounded density seen in the right lung field just above the SVC-RA junction. This anomaly is almost invariably present when the radiograph shows the stomach in a malposed position. In other words, if the thoracic contents are in their usual position (situs solitus) and the stomach is right-sided, or if the thoracic contents indicate situs inversus and the stomach is left-sided, absent hepatic segment of the IVC is present until proven otherwise.

This may occur as an isolated anomaly, but usually there are associated cardiovascular defects. It is particularly common as part of the polysplenia syndrome.

**Complications:** Inadvertent ligation of the azygos vein may lead to death. During cardiopulmonary bypass, the surgeon must recognize and deal with the altered systemic venous drainage.

**Associated Findings:** Multiple spleens, abnormal cardiac situs, isolated abdominal situs inversus.

**Etiology:** Unknown.

**Pathogenesis:** Hypoplasia or aplasia of the anastomosis that normally develops between right subcardinal and proximal vitelline venous systems (renal and posthepatic segments of the IVC).

**CDC No.:** 747.480

**Sex Ratio:** Presumably M1:F1

**Occurrence:** About 1:100 patients with congenital heart disease. Rare in the absence of congenital cardiac disease.

**Risk of Recurrence for Patient's Sib:** Unknown.

**Risk of Recurrence for Patient's Child:** Unknown.

**Age of Detectability:** From birth by selective angiography.

**Gene Mapping and Linkage:** Unknown.

**Prevention:** None known. Genetic counseling indicated.

**Treatment:** Unknown.

**Prognosis:** In the rare situation where there are no associated cardiac anomalies, longevity is normal. Interruption of the IVC with azygos continuation does not influence the prognosis of other conditions.

**Detection of Carrier:** Unknown.

**References:**
Anderson RC, et al.: Anomalous inferior vena cava with azygos continuation (infrahepatic interruption of the inferior vena cava): report of 15 new cases. J Pediatr 1961; 59:370.
Lucas RV Jr.: Anomalous venous connection, pulmonary and systemic. In: Adams FH, Emmanouilides GC, eds: Heart disease in infants, children, and adolescents. Baltimore: Williams & Wilkins, 1983:486–488.

LU003 **Russell V. Lucas, Jr.**

## VENA CAVA, PERSISTENT LEFT SUPERIOR JOINED TO CORONARY SINUS 0807

**Includes:** Vena cava connecting to right atrium via coronary sinus

**Excludes:**
> Vena cava, persistent left superior connecting to left atrium
> **Pulmonary venous connection, total anomalous** (0842)

**Major Diagnostic Criteria:** A persistent left superior vena cava (LSVC) is virtually always an incidental finding. Angiography or catheter passage confirms the diagnosis.

**Clinical Findings:** In this anomaly, a persistent LSVC connects to the coronary sinus. The physiology is normal. Its importance lies in the frequent coexistence of other congenital cardiac defects and in the technical complications it may engender during cardiac catheterization or cardiac surgery. From the junction of the left subclavian and left internal jugular veins the LSVC descends vertically in front of the aortic arch. A short distance from its origin, it receives the superior left intercostal vein, then passes in front of the left pulmonary hilum. It receives the hemiazygos vein, penetrates the pericardium and crosses the posterior wall of the left atrium obliquely, receives the greater cardiac vein and enters the coronary sinus.

The coronary sinus and its right atrial ostium are larger than normal. As a rule, the persistent LSVC is part of a bilateral superior caval system. Rarely the RSVC may be absent.

X-ray features: The shadow of the LSVC may be seen along the left upper border of the mediastinum. Diagnosis may be confirmed by passage of a cardiac catheter into the LSVC via the left subclavian vein or by way of the coronary sinus from the heart.

**0528-12167:** Absent hepatic segment of inferior vena cava. Two views.

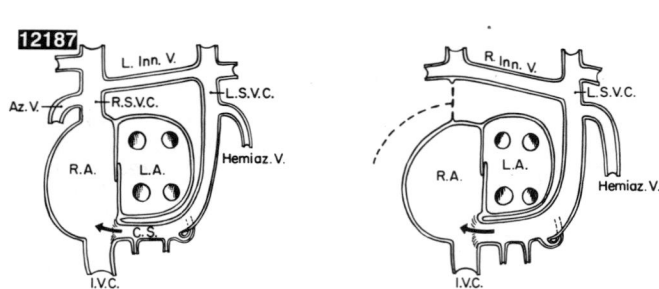

**0807-12187:** Diagrams illustrating persistent left superior vena cava connected to coronary sinus.

Echocardiographic features: The enlarged coronary sinus may produce an abnormal echo in the left atrium. This echo is similar to the left atrial echoes produced by TAPVC to coronary sinus and cor triatriatum.

**Complications:** Utilization of the LSVC for catheter passage in a right heart study may interfere with the satisfactory completion of the procedure. At operation, ligation of the LSVC may be fatal when the RSVC is absent. Cannulation of the LSVC via the coronary sinus is necessary during cardiopulmonary bypass.

**Associated Findings:** Heart, **tetralogy of Fallot, Ventricular septal defect,** sinus venosus atrial septal defect, cyanotic congenital cardiac defects, particularly those with malposition of the heart or abdominal viscera. A high incidence of leftward P axis is found in patients with persistent LSVC.

**Etiology:** Unknown.

**Pathogenesis:** Embryologically, persistence of the LSVC is a consequence of simple failure of obliteration of the left common cardinal vein.

**CDC No.:** 747.410

**Sex Ratio:** Presumably M1:F1.

**Occurrence:** Prevalence 1:330 in the general population. 1:30 in patients with congenital heart disease.

**Risk of Recurrence for Patient's Sib:** Unknown.

**Risk of Recurrence for Patient's Child:** Unknown.

**Age of Detectability:** From birth, by catheterization or angiography.

**Gene Mapping and Linkage:** Unknown.

**Prevention:** None known. Genetic counseling indicated.

**Treatment:** Unknown.

**Prognosis:** Excellent when occurring as an isolated anomaly.

**Detection of Carrier:** Unknown.

**References:**
Winter FS: Persistent left superior cava: survey of the world literature and report of 30 additional cases. Angiology 1954; 5:90. *
Lucas RV Jr., Schmidt R: Anomalous venous connection, pulmonary and systemic. In: Adams FH, Emmanouilides GC, eds: Heart disease in infants, children, and adolescents, 3rd ed. Baltimore: Williams & Wilkins, 1983:482–484. *

LU003                                        **Russell V. Lucas, Jr.**

**Venezuelan equine encephalitis (VEE)**
*See FETAL VENEZUELAN EQUINE ENCEPHALITIS INFECTION*
**Venous aneurysm of external ear, pulsating**
*See EAR, ARTERIOVENOUS FISTULA*
**Venous return, anomalous (partial)**
*See PULMONARY VENOUS CONNECTION, PARTIAL ANOMALOUS*
**Ventricle, anomalous muscle bundle of right**
*See VENTRICLE, OBSTRUCTION WITHIN RIGHT VENTRICLE OR ITS OUTFLOW TRACT*

## VENTRICLE, DIVERTICULUM                          0988

**Includes:**
Aneurysm, congenital left ventricular
Diverticular aneurysm of the left ventricle
Diverticulosis of the left ventricle
Diverticulum of left ventricle
Diverticulum of right ventricle

**Excludes:**
Arrhythmogenic right ventricular dysplasia
Ventricular aneurysm due to Chagas' disease
Ventricular aneurysm due to ischemic cardiac disease
Ventricular aneurysm due to open heart surgical procedures

**Major Diagnostic Criteria:** Although acceptable resolution for diagnosis could be expected with two-dimensional echocardiography, digital subtraction X-ray with peripheral intravenous injec-

tion, or with nuclear magnetic resonance imaging, the current standard for diagnosis is contrast ventriculography. Angled angiographic views may be required, depending upon the size and location of the diverticulum. Criteria for diagnosis with noninvasive imaging may be established as greater experience with these rare defects is accumulated.

**Clinical Findings:** Clinical manifestations are related to the size of the diverticulum and to its anatomic location. A subxiphoid, palpable pulsating mass in the epigastrium may be due to an apical left ventricular diverticulum with associated midline defects of the diaphragm or anterior abdominal wall. Usually, however, there are not physical findings specifically suggesting the presence of a ventricular diverticulum and murmurs are uncommon. Congestive cardiac failure, peripheral emboli, ventricular arrhythmias including ventricular tachycardia and ventricular fibrillation, and sudden death due to arrhythmia or aneurysm rupture are among the other presentations of a ventricular diverticulum. A congenital left ventricular diverticular aneurysm may also present as an asymptomatic abnormality on routine chest X-ray or electrocardiography in a healthy, asymptomatic adult. Atypical chest pain syndromes and endocarditis have been attributed to LV diverticulae.

Electrocardiographic findings are frequent but not diagnostic. Left ventricular hypertrophy, left ventricular strain, T wave abnormalities, ST segment elevation, and "pseudoinfarction" patterns have been described.

Symptoms and findings may be present due to associated cardiovascular anomalies.

**Complications:** Rupture of ventricular diverticulum; arrhythmias, including ventricular tachycardia or ventricular fibrillation; sudden death from rupture or arrhythmias; infective endocarditis; and peripheral embolic and congestive cardiac failure are among the possible complications.

**Associated Findings:** Congenital coronary anomalies, pericardial defects, midline defects of the diaphragm or anterior abdominal wall, and omphalocele have been reported. Associated congenital cardiac anomalies can include single ventricle, **Atrial septal defects, Ventricular septal defect, Aorta, coarctation, Ductus arteriosus, patent.**

**Etiology:** Unknown.

**Pathogenesis:** Possibilities include focal myocarditis occurring during intrauterine development, or a focal ischemic myocardial event occurring during fetal development.

**Sex Ratio:** Presumably M1:F1.

**Occurrence:** Less than 1:200,000 births (less than 0.05% of congenital heart disease). The incidence of mild and unrecognized cases, however, is obviously unknown.

**Risk of Recurrence for Patient's Sib:** Unknown.

**Risk of Recurrence for Patient's Child:** Unknown.

**Age of Detectability:** From birth, by ventriculography

**Gene Mapping and Linkage:** Unknown.

**Prevention:** None known. Genetic counseling indicated.

**Treatment:** Resection of a large diverticulum is likely to be required. Surgical repair of associated midline or intracardiac congenital defects may be required. Medical or surgical treatment of a patient with arrhythmias due to a diverticulum may be required.

**Prognosis:** Without treatment, the presence of a large diverticulum is associated with death in infancy in the majority of cases. The prognosis may be limited by the type of associated anomalies in those cases with other congenital cardiovascular defects in addition to ventricular diverticulum.

**Detection of Carrier:** Unknown.

**References:**
Powell SJ: Diverticulum of the left ventricle: case report with special reference to electrocardiographic findings. Am Heart J 1958; 55:518–522.
Edget JW, et al.: Diverticulum of the heart: part of the syndrome of

congenital cardiac and midline thoracic and abdominal defects. Am J Cardiol 1969; 24:580–583.

Norton JB, et al.: Congenital diverticulum of the left ventricle. Am J Dis Child 1973; 126:702–704.

Treistman B, et al.: Diverticular aneurysm of left ventricle. Am J Cardiol 1973; 32:119–123. *

Baltaxe HA, et al.: Diverticulosis of the left ventricle. AJR 1979; 133:257–261. *

Fellows CL, et al.: Ventricular dysrhythmias associated with congenital left ventricular aneurysms. Am J Cardiol 1986; 57:997–999.

JE006                                      **Larry S. Jefferson**
BR014                                   **J. Timothy Bricker**

## VENTRICLE, DOUBLE CHAMBERED RIGHT       2414

**Includes:**

    Anomalous muscle bundle of the right ventricle
    Anomalous right ventricular muscles
    Double chambered right ventricle
    Obstructing muscular bands of the right ventricle
    Obstruction within the right ventricular body
    Right ventricular anomalous muscle bundle
    Right ventricular obstruction by aberrant muscular bands
    Right ventricular subinfundibular obstruction
    Two-chambered right ventricle

**Excludes:**

    Combined valvular and infundibular stenosis
    **Heart, tetralogy of Fallot** (0938)
    Infundibular stenosis, primary
    **Pulmonary valve, stenosis** (0839)
    Subvalvular pulmonary stenosis

**Major Diagnostic Criteria:** A holosystolic ejection-type murmur usually best localized to the mid-precordial region coupled with the electrocardiographic finding of right ventricular hypertrophy usually isolated to the far right ($V_4R$–$V_3R$) precordial leads are indicative of the diagnosis. The vectorcardiogram further supports the electrocardiographic features and the phonocardiogram allows positive identification of the appearance of the murmur. Echocardiographic and Doppler studies allow noninvasive positioning of the obstruction and gradient determination. Cardiac catheterization and angiocardiography confirm the diagnosis invasively but are not positively necessary.

**Clinical Findings:** The anatomical configuration is generally considered to be of two types. In both the right ventricle is divided by muscular elements into a high pressure inflow and low pressure outflow chamber. A low type of obstruction is produced when the muscular structure arises at or near the apical region of the right ventricle and courses obliquely to approximate a point superior to the tricuspid valve annulus. In the high type the obstruction encircles the right ventricle in a more circumferential fashion just superior to the tricuspid annulus and below the usual position of the supraventricular crest.

The nature of these structures has been debated with earlier reports considering the low type of obstruction to be secondary to hypertrophy of the moderator band. However, electro-physiologic studies following surgical resection of this structure have failed to confirm specific alterations in the right ventricular excitation sequence casting doubt upon this consideration. Nonetheless the appearance with detailed angiographic study as well as at the time of surgery is that of muscular structures at least approximating the expected positions of both the moderator band and the septomarginal band in the respective types, involving hypertrophy of each component to greater or lesser degree to cause the varying appearances.

The age at presentation is highly variable due both to a wide spectrum of severity of obstruction and to the natural history of a tendency for the obstruction to be progressive with time. It has rarely been diagnosed in infancy but with improved non-invasive diagnostic techniques this may change. Additionally, the condition is frequently associated with other cardiac abnormalities which not infrequently are discovered before the obvious signs of double chambered right ventricle are identified.

Symptoms and clinical findings are dependent upon both the severity of obstruction and associated defects. The patients are usually acyanotic, but extreme obstruction combined with an appropriately positioned large ventricular septal defect may cause sufficient right to left shunt to result in cyanosis. The presence of a systolic murmur with characteristic phonocardiographic appearance and a highly specific electro-vectorcardiographic pattern usually allow inclusion of the diagnosis on clinical grounds. The murmur is of holosystolic duration with ejection appearance. It is therefore unusual for the more common forms of right ventricular outlet obstruction; similarly it is unlike the murmur generated by ventricular septal defect to which it is similar in duration.

The position of the murmur, which is best localized to the midprecordial area, is also unlike that of these more common congenital cardiac malformations. The principal electrocardiographic feature is a displacement of the right ventricular hypertrophy pattern further rightward so that it is usually only seen in the right chest leads $V_3R$-$V_4R$; also frequently seen is failure to find evidence for right ventricular hypertrophy both in lead aVR and the left precordial leads. The vectorcardiogram confirms this unusual appearance which has been shown to likely be due to displacement of a segment of hypertrophied myocardium localized to the superomedial aspect of the right ventricle. Of note is the fact that associated abnormalities have not been shown to alter either the auscultatory-phonocardiographic findings or the electro-vectorcardiographic appearance.

The two-dimensional echocardiogram is usually indicative of hypertrophy of the obstructing muscular structures but by itself does not positively diagnose the abnormality. Combining the two-dimensional echocardiogram with Doppler flow mapping will usually allow both positioning of the level of obstruction and calculation of its degree.

Invasive study can be largely eliminated by appropriately combining the non-invasive evaluations but still may be necessary for the delineation of the presence and severity of associated malformations.

Once the anatomy is clearly defined, surgical relief is quite straightforward and is indicated when the lesion is hemodynamically significant.

**Complications:** The usual problems resulting from congenital cardiac lesions must be considered. Foremost amongst these is endocarditis. Others include progression to higher grades of obstruction with occasional production of cyanosis, brain abscess, and rarely right ventricular failure. Surgical complications include difficulty with tricuspid valvular chordal attachments when the obstructive elements are resected.

**Associated Findings:** Other forms of congenital cardiac malformations are frequent, occurring in at least 75% of reported cases. The principal association is with **Ventricular septal defect**. **Chromosome 21, trisomy 21** has also been described.

**Etiology:** Presumably multifactorial inheritance.

**Pathogenesis:** Only the trabecular component of the right ventricle is involved with uniform sparing of the outlet zone. There thus appears to be a primary defect in the formation of trabecular components of the right ventricle and may represent malformation of normally occurring structures.

**Sex Ratio:** M1:F1

**Occurrence:** Less than 0.5% of all congenital cardiac abnormalities.

**Risk of Recurrence for Patient's Sib:** Unknown.

**Risk of Recurrence for Patient's Child:** Unknown.

**Age of Detectability:** At birth.

**Gene Mapping and Linkage:** Unknown.

**Prevention:** None known. Genetic counseling indicated.

**Treatment:** Primary surgical resection of the obstructing elements, and repair of associated defects. Use of non-invasive methodology should allow earlier detection and enhance management. Echo-Doppler investigation for gradient determination would be expected to reduce need for cardiac catheterization in most instances.

**Prognosis:** Depends on the severity of obstruction and its progression. Patients with low grade obstruction may not require surgery at any time, but will require non-invasive follow-up to determine progression. Corrective surgery for those hemodynamically significant should result in normal life span.

**Detection of Carrier:** Unknown.

**References:**

Fellows KE, et al.: Angiography of obstructing muscular bands of the right ventricle. Am J Roentgenol 1972; 128:249–256.

Byrum CJ, et al.: Excitation of the double chamber right ventricle: electrophysiologic and anatomic correlation. Am J Cardiol 1982; 49:1254–1258.

Folger GM Jr: Electro-vectorcardiographic features of double-chambered right ventricle. Eur Heart J 1984; 5:1043–1053.

Folger GM Jr: Right ventricular outflow pouch associated with double-chambered right ventricle. Am Heart J 1985; 109:1044–1049.

Folger GM Jr: The right ventricular pouch: a proposed explanation for the electro-vectorcardiographic pattern of double chambered right ventricle. Angiology 1986; 37:483–486.

El Tohami ETA, et al.: The murmur of double-chambered right ventricle: phonocardiographic evaluation. Clin Cardiol 1987; 10:309–315.

F0002                                                    **Gordon M. Folger, Jr.**

## VENTRICLE, DOUBLE OUTLET LEFT                          0581

**Includes:**

> Double outlet l. ventricle-atresia of r. ventricular infundibulum
> Double outlet left ventricle-pulmonary stenosis
> Double outlet left ventricle-ventricular septal defect
> Left ventricle, double outlet

**Excludes:**

> Great vessels arising from a common left or primitive ventricle
> Ventricle, double outlet right, with ventricular inversion.

**Major Diagnostic Criteria:** The origin of both the pulmonary artery and aorta are entirely or predominantly above the left ventricle.

**Clinical Findings:** This rare anomaly occurs when both the pulmonary artery and the aorta arise entirely or predominantly above the morphological left ventricle. Both semilunar valves may have fibrous continuity with the mitral valve. The right ventricle may be normally formed, but may be hypoplastic with infundibular atresia. The atria and viscera are usually in solitus arrangement, with concordant relation of the atria and ventricles. The semilunar valves may be in the same coronal plane, or the aortic valve level may be anterior or posterior to the pulmonary valve level. The aorta is usually to the right of the pulmonary trunk. The ventricular septal defect (VSD) may be subaortic or subpulmonic in location or confluent with both great vessels.

The presence or absence of pulmonary stenosis largely determines the clinical course. Cyanosis is prominent with significant pulmonary stenosis and VSD, and the clinical picture may be indistinguishable from that of tetralogy of Fallot. Clinical signs in this group include a prominent ejection systolic murmur due to pulmonary stenosis, and an accentuated single second heart sound at the base. EKGs show right axis deviation and right ventricular hypertrophy. Chest X-ray shows slight cardiac enlargement and decreased pulmonary vascular markings.

In contrast, patients with VSD but without pulmonary stenosis are relatively acyanotic initially and present with congestive cardiac failure. Pulmonary artery hypertension with increased pulmonary blood flow is clinically evident. The precordium is hyperactive, and the second heart sound is split with pulmonary closure accentuation. A pansystolic murmur is present at the lower left sternal border, sometimes with a prominent mid-diastolic flow murmur. EKG shows combined ventricular hyper-

trophy. The chest X-ray shows a large heart with increased pulmonary vascularity. These findings may suggest the diagnosis of transposition of the great arteries with VSD.

Hemodynamic data from the published cases showed a systolic pressure gradient at the pulmonary or subpulmonary valve level in 4 cases; right ventricular infundibular atresia was present in 1 patient, and no obstruction was present in the remaining 2. Right ventricular hypertension was present in all patients. In the infant with an intact ventricular septum, the right ventricular peak systolic pressure was greater than the systemic level. The observation of almost identical oxygen saturations in the aorta, pulmonary artery and left ventricle in a cyanotic patient suspected clinically as having tetralogy of Fallot, seems to be an important clue to the diagnosis of double outlet left ventricle with pulmonary stenosis.

Selective biplanar angiography with injections into both the right and left ventricle establishes the diagnosis by demonstrating both vessels arising predominantly to the left of the septum above the morphological left ventricle, and establishes the presence or absence of pulmonary or subpulmonary stenosis, the presence or absence of a VSD, and the status of the atrio-ventricular valves.

At surgery, external inspection of the position of the great arteries has not been helpful in suggesting the diagnosis of double outlet left ventricle, since the great arteries may be similar in appearance to that seen in patients with tetralogy of Fallot, or they may be malposed in a manner similar to that noted in complete transposition of the great arteries or double outlet right ventricle. However, careful analysis of arterioventricular connections during cardiopulmonary bypass can establish the diagnosis.

**Complications:** Congestive heart failure, pulmonary hypertension, cyanosis.

**Associated Findings:** VSD, pulmonary stenosis, right ventricular infundibular atresia, tricuspid valve stenosis, atresia or straddling.

**Etiology:** Unknown.

**Pathogenesis:** Van Praagh postulated abnormal conal growth resulting in essentially no conal tissue beneath both the great vessels, which leaves them in a side-by-side position above the left ventricle with both semilunar valves in fibrous continuity with the mitral valve. Anderson emphasized rather an absorptive process involving both the right and left ventricular conus.

**Sex Ratio:** M1.5:F1, based on 111 cases.

**Occurrence:** Van Praagh and Weinberg (1983) reviewed 111 well-documented cases based upon personal examinations and the literature.

**Risk of Recurrence for Patient's Sib:** Unknown. Predictably low risk because of the rarity of the lesion.

**Risk of Recurrence for Patient's Child:** Unknown.

**Age of Detectability:** From birth.

**Gene Mapping and Linkage:** Unknown.

**Prevention:** None known. Genetic counseling indicated.

**Treatment:** *Palliative surgery:* systemic-pulmonary artery shunt for cyanotic infants with diminished pulmonary blood flow; pulmonary artery banding for acyanotic infants with markedly increased pulmonary blood flow.

*Corrective surgery* for both groups: intraventricular diversion of blood from right ventricle to pulmonary artery with patch repair of VSD; radical reconstruction with pericardial tunnel or extracardiac valve-bearing conduit from right ventricle to pulmonary artery and patch closure of VSD; Fontan-type procedure when coexistent tricuspid atresia.

**Prognosis:** Following intracardiac repair, patients reported alive and improved.

**Detection of Carrier:** Unknown.

**References:**

Pacifico AD, et al.: Surgical treatment of double-outlet left ventricle. Circulation 1973; III-19, 23, 47–48.

Bharati S, et al.: Morphologic spectrum of double outlet left ventricle and its surgical significance. Circulation 1977; 56:43.

Van Praagh R, Weinberg PM: Double outlet left ventricle. In: Moss AJ, et al., eds: Heart disease in infants, children, and adolescents. 3rd ed. Baltimore: Williams & Wilkins, 1983:370–385. *

N0003

**James J. Nora**

## VENTRICLE, DOUBLE-OUTLET RIGHT WITH ANTERIOR SEPTAL DEFECT                                                      0297

**Includes:**

Taussig-Bing syndrome
Ventricular septal defect-double outlet right ventricle

**Excludes:**

**Heart, transposition of great vessels** (0962)
**Ventricle, double-outlet right with posterior septal defect** (0298)

**Major Diagnostic Criteria:**  Clinical evidence of cyanosis, cardiomegaly, heart failure, increased pulmonary arterial vascularity and biventricular hypertrophy in an infant who also demonstrates, on plain chest roentgenogram, gross enlargement of the relatively normally situated main pulmonary artery is suggestive of DORV with anterior VSD. The exact anatomic diagnosis depends upon 2-D echocardiography and selective angiocardiography.

**Clinical Findings:**  Double outlet right ventricle (DORV) with anterior ventricular septal defect (VSD) is that cardiac malformation in which both the aorta and pulmonary artery arise entirely from the right ventricle. The only outlet from the left ventricle is via a large VSD anterior to or above the crista supraventricularis. This position of the VSD is just inferior to the pulmonary artery. Thus, the pulmonary artery overrides the defect to a varying extent, but arises in otherwise normal fashion from the right ventricular infundibulum. The pulmonary trunk and aorta are normally interrelated externally. However, the aortic valve is displaced to the right and lies higher than normal at about the same level as the pulmonic valve in both the cross-sectional and coronal body planes. Thus, the aortic valve cannot be in continuity with the anterior leaflet of the mitral valve. Right ventricular infundibular obstruction is not seen, but pulmonic valvar stenosis occurs rarely.

Clinical features mimic complete transposition of the great arteries with a VSD. The position of the VSD beneath the pulmonic valve results in selective streaming of left ventricular (oxygenated) blood into the pulmonary artery. The aorta receives primarily right ventricular (desaturated) blood. Thus, the patient is cyanotic from birth, although this may be mild in early infancy. Heart failure, chronic respiratory infections and growth retardation are usually present. A harsh systolic murmur is present at the upper left sternal border but is usually not accompanied by a thrill. The second sound is narrowly split or single and the pulmonic component is accentuated. A diastolic murmur of pulmonic insufficiency is occasionally heard. The EKG shows right axis deviation, right atrial enlargement and biventricular hypertrophy. Plain chest roentgenograms demonstrate markedly increased pulmonary vascularity of a shunt type, a prominent pulmonary artery segment, cardiomegaly involving both ventricles and left atrial enlargement. This is one of the few admixture lesions that is overtly cyanotic with a normally positioned pulmonary artery segment.

Since a great anatomic spectrum exists in this lesion, the echocardiographic differential diagnosis for DORV includes abnormalities in the tetralogy/truncus group as well as those in the transposition group. Identification of septal-aortic override or septal-pulmonic override with mitral semilunar discontinuity is essential for making this diagnosis. It was initially reported that an anterior displacement of the posterior great vessel from the mitral valve was diagnostic of this disorder. However, it has recently been pointed out that great difficulties arise in demonstrating this anterior-posterior displacement. Further, the presence of a subaortic or subpulmonic conus separating this posterior great vessel semilunar valve from the mitral valve is at least as important in delineating these malformations as is the anterior-posterior displacement. Secondary characteristics involving abnormal great

vessel orientation may be of use in defining this group. See also **Heart, tetralogy of Fallot.**

Cardiac catheterization and angiocardiography are necessary to establish the precise anatomy. Significant systemic arterial desaturation is present, and pulmonary artery oxygen saturation exceeds systemic artery saturation. This is in contrast to DORV with a posterior VSD. Catheter position may suggest the abnormal location of the aortic valve. Selective right ventricular angiography will demonstrate denser opacification of the aorta than of the pulmonary artery, while selective left ventricular angiography will demonstrate the VSD and denser opacification of the pulmonary artery than of the aorta. Angiocardiography also demonstrates the abnormal position of the aortic valve and its lack of relation to anterior leaflet of the mitral valve.

**Complications:**  Chronic heart failure, frequent respiratory infection, growth failure, and cyanosis may cause early death. With increasing age, pulmonary vascular disease will occur.

**Associated Findings:**  None known.

**Etiology:**  Presumably multifactorial inheritance.

**Pathogenesis:**  Failure of transfer of the posterior great artery (aorta) to the left ventricle results in DORV. The pathogenesis of the VSD is variable, but apparently is due to faulty development in both the conus septum and the muscular ventricular septum. Recently it has been appreciated that neural crest cells contribute importantly to cardiac morphogenesis. In fact, experimental removal of certain regions of the cranial neural crests causes double outlet right ventricle.

**MIM No.:**  12100, 14050

**Sex Ratio:**  M1:F1

**Occurrence:**  Less than 1:100 cases of congenital heart disease.

**Risk of Recurrence for Patient's Sib:**  Unknown.

**Risk of Recurrence for Patient's Child:**  Unknown.

**Age of Detectability:**  From birth.

**Gene Mapping and Linkage:**  Unknown.

**Prevention:**  None known. Genetic counseling indicated.

**Treatment:**  In infancy, palliative surgery may be necessary. Creation of an atrial septal defect and pulmonary artery banding will increase the amount of intracardiac mixing and thus increase the supply of oxygenated blood to the aorta. The total complex is now amenable to surgical correction by use of either senning procedure, or the Mustard procedure, originally designed for complete transposition of the great arteries. The atrial portion of the operation is performed as usual. The VSD is closed by a patch in such a way as to transfer the pulmonary artery to the left ventricle. Anatomic correction by use of the vatene procedure can also be considered.

Other therapy as necessary for congestive heart failure and pulmonary infection.

**Prognosis:**  Overall prognosis is poor with pulmonary arteriolar vascular disease being a common early complication. Survival beyond childhood without surgery is unlikely. With successful corrective surgery, prognosis is favorable.

**Detection of Carrier:**  Unknown.

**References:**

Van Praagh R: What is the Taussig-Bing malformation? Circulation 1968; 38:445–449.

Sridaromont S, et al.: Double-outlet right ventricle: anatomic and angiographic correlations. Mayo Clinic Proceedings 1978; 53:555–577.

Hagler DJ, et al.: Double-outlet right ventricle: wide-angle two-dimensional echocardiograph observations. Circulation 1981; 63:419–428. †

Wilcox BR, et al.: Surgical anatomy of double-outlet right ventricle with situs solitus and atrioventricular concordance. J Thorac Cardiovasc Surg 1981; 82:405–417.

Hagler DJ, et al.: Double-outlet right ventricle. In: Adams FH, Emmanouiledes GC, eds: Moss' heart disease in infants, children and adolescents, 3rd ed. Baltimore: Williiams & Wilkins, 1983:351–369. * †

Pacifico AD, et al.: Intra-ventricular tunnel repair for Taussig-Bing heart and related cardiac anomalies. Circulation 1986; 74:53–66. * †
Kirby ML: Cardiac morphogenesis: recent research advances. Pediatr Res 1987; 21:219–224.

GE013                                                         **Ira H. Gessner**

## VENTRICLE, DOUBLE-OUTLET RIGHT WITH POSTERIOR SEPTAL DEFECT                    0298

**Includes:**  Great vessels from right ventricle-posterior septal defect

**Excludes:**
>   **Heart, tetralogy of Fallot** (0938)
>   **Heart, transposition of great vessels** (0962)
>   **Ventricle, double-outlet right with anterior septal defect** (0297)
>   **Ventricular septal defect** (0989)

**Major Diagnostic Criteria:**  Clinical evidence of a large left-to-right ventricular level shunt with pulmonary hypertension and a superiorly oriented, counterclockwise frontal plane (QRS) loop should arouse suspicion of double outlet right ventricle (DORV) with posterior ventricular septal defect (VSD) and no pulmonic stenosis. Selective angiography and/or comprehensive 2-D echocardiograph can establish a correct diagnosis. DORV with posterior VSD and pulmonic stenosis simulates tetralogy of Fallot almost exactly. The presence of marked right atrial enlargement and of atrioventricular conduction delay would suggest DORV with pulmonic stenosis, but selective angiocardiography and/or 2-D echocardiograph can establish the exact anatomy.

**Clinical Findings:**  DORV with posterior VSD is that cardiac malformation in which both the aorta and pulmonary artery arise entirely from the right ventricle. The only outlet from the left ventricle is via a large VSD which is posteriorly located, i.e. below the crista supraventricularis. The pulmonary trunk and aorta are normally interrelated externally. However, the aortic valve is displaced to the right and lies higher than normal at about the same level as the pulmonic valve in both the cross-sectional and coronal body planes. The displaced aortic valve causes lack of continuity between the anterior leaflet of the mitral valve and the aortic valve. Obstruction to flow into the pulmonary artery is common due to right ventricular infundibular hypertrophy. Subaortic obstruction is rarely seen.

Clinical features are determined by the degree of pulmonic obstruction. Without pulmonic obstruction, the clinical features closely resemble a large VSD with right ventricular hypertension. Poor growth, frequent respiratory infection and heart failure are present in infancy. A precordial systolic thrill and a grade IV/VI harsh systolic murmur along the lower left sternal border, a narrowly split and accentuated second sound, and an apical diastolic murmur of increased mitral valve flow indicate the presence of a large VSD with elevated right ventricular pressure. Cyanosis is usually minimal or absent because the posterior location of the VSD allows left ventricular output to be directed through the VSD towards the aortic valve; thus significant mixing in the right ventricle may not occur. With time, pulmonary arteriolar disease may develop resulting in increased pulmonary vascular resistance. Cyanosis will then become a prominent feature. The EKG demonstrates left atrial enlargement and biventricular hypertrophy. A distinctive EKG feature commonly seen is marked left axis deviation and superior counterclockwise frontal plane QRS forces, similar to that seen in an endocardial cushion defect. Plain chest X-rays demonstrate a large pulmonary artery segment, increased pulmonary vascularity of the shunt type, left atrial enlargement and cardiomegaly, findings which are not specific for this malformation. In the presence of significant pulmonic obstruction, the clinical features mimic those of tetralogy of Fallot and indeed may be indistinguishable. Cyanosis is present from early infancy. A left lower parasternal systolic thrill and murmur and a single second sound are found. There is no mitral flow murmur.

The EKG frequently demonstrates right atrial enlargement and always shows right ventricular hypertrophy of the type commonly seen in tetralogy of Fallot. In DORV with pulmonary stenosis, right axis deviation is seen and the QRS forces are directed inferiorly. Delayed atrioventricular conduction time and intraventricular conduction delay are commonly seen. Right atrial enlargement and delayed atrioventricular conduction are unusual in tetralogy of Fallot, providing one of the few distinguishing clinical features between these two malformations. Plain chest X-rays demonstrate decreased pulmonary arterial vascularity, a prominent aorta, mild cardiomegaly involving the right heart, a small right ventricular outflow tract with absence of a pulmonary artery segment, and no left atrial enlargement; these features are commonly seen in tetralogy of Fallot as well.

Since a great anatomic spectrum exists in this lesion, the echocardiographic differential diagnosis for DORV includes abnormalities in the tetralogy/truncus group as well as those in the transposition group. Identification of septal-aortic override or septal-pulmonic override with mitral semilunar discontinuity is essential for making this diagnosis. It was initially reported that an anterior displacement of the posterior great vessel from the mitral valve was diagnostic of this disorder. However, it has recently been pointed out that great difficulties arise in demonstrating this anterior-posterior displacement. Further, the presence of a subaortic or subpulmonic conus separating this posterior great vessel semilunar valve from the mitral valve is at least as important in delineating these malformations as is the anterior-posterior displacement. Doppler echocardiograph can be used to quantitate pulmonic stenosis, if present. Secondary characteristics involving abnormal great vessel orientation may be of use in defining this group. See also **Heart, tetralogy of Fallot**.

Cardiac catheterization and selective angiocardiography are necessary to establish the precise anatomic and hemodynamic diagnosis. Without pulmonic obstruction, the catheterization findings are those of a large VSD with equal pressures in the left and right ventricles. Mild systemic arterial desaturation is usually seen, although, as mentioned above, streaming of left ventricular blood into the aorta may be so precise that little systemic arterial desaturation is found. Systemic arterial oxygen saturation is significantly greater than pulmonary oxygen saturation. Position of the catheter in the great vessels may suggest the abnormal location of the aortic valve. Selective right and left ventricular angiography will demonstrate the exact anatomic situation; a lack of continuity of the mitral valve with a semilunar valve, a large posterior VSD and the abnormal location of the aortic valve. In the presence of pulmonic obstruction, the catheterization findings are similar to tetralogy of Fallot. Again, catheter localization of the aortic valve may suggest its abnormal position. However, selective right ventricular angiography is necessary to differentiate between these 2 malformations.

**Complications:**  Without pulmonic stenosis, chronic heart failure, frequent respiratory infections and poor growth occur. Eventual development of pulmonary vascular disease is common. With pulmonic stenosis, hypoxic spells may occur.

**Associated Findings:**  None known.

**Etiology:**  Presumably multifactorial inheritance.

**Pathogenesis:**  Failure of transfer of the posterior great artery (aorta) to the left ventricle results in DORV. The conus septum fails to develop properly and a large VSD results. If the conus septum is displaced anteriorly and becomes hypertrophied, infundibular (pulmonic) obstruction results. Recently, it has been appreciated that neural crest cells contribute importantly to cardiac morphogenesis. Indeed, experimental removal of certain regions of the cranial neural crest causes double outlet right ventricle.

**MIM No.:**  12100, 14050

**Sex Ratio:**  M1:F1

**Occurrence:**  Less than 1:100 cases of congenital heart defects.

**Risk of Recurrence for Patient's Sib:**  Unknown.

**Risk of Recurrence for Patient's Child:**  Unknown.

**Age of Detectability:**  From birth.

**Gene Mapping and Linkage:**  Unknown.

**Prevention:** None known. Genetic counseling indicated.

**Treatment:** Corrective surgery may be accomplished by construction of a tunnel from the VSD to the root of the aorta. If present, infundibular hypertrophy can be resected. When the aorta is too far removed from the VSD for correction, pulmonary artery banding may be performed as a palliative procedure in the absence of infundibular obstruction. Symptomatic therapy for congestive heart failure and pneumonia may be indicated.

**Prognosis:** Poor; survival is enhanced by a moderate degree of pulmonic obstruction.

**Detection of Carrier:** Unknown.

**Special Considerations:** DORV may occur in association with the fundamental ventricular abnormality: ventricular inversion. In that instance, since the anatomic right ventricle is located on the left, both great arteries arise from the left-sided right ventricle.

Complete transposition of the great vessels may occur together with DORV. In that situation, the aorta is located to the left and slightly anteriorly arising from the right ventricular infundibulum. The pulmonary artery arises to the right and posterior of the aorta with lack of continuity between the mitral valve and the pulmonic valve. The physiology is similar to the ordinary case of complete transposition of the great vessels with a VSD.

**References:**

Sridaromont S, et al.: Double-outlet right ventricle: anatomic and angiographic correlations. Mayo Clinic Proceedings 1978; 53:555–577. * †

Hagler DJ, et al.: Double-outlet right ventricle: wide-angle two-dimensional echocardiograph observations. Circulation 1981; 63: 419–428. †

Wilcox BR, et al.: Surgical anatomy of double-outlet right ventricle with situs solitus and atrioventricular concordance. J Thorac Cardiovasc Surg 1981; 82:405–417.

Hagler DJ, et al.: Double-outlet right ventricle. In: Adams FH, Emmanouiledes GC, eds: Moss' heart disease in infants, children and adolescents, 3rd ed. Baltimore: Williiams & Wilkins, 1983:351–369. * †

Kirby ML: Cardiac morphogenesis: recent research advances. Pediatr Res 1987; 21:219–224.

GE013

**Ira H. Gessner**

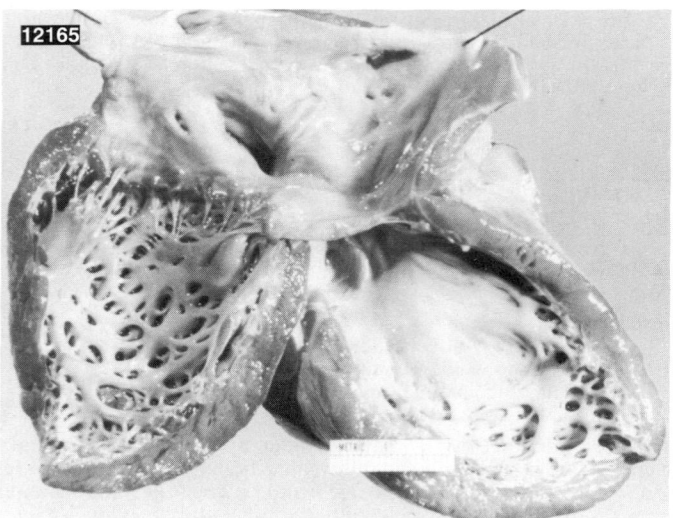

---

## VENTRICLE, ENDOCARDIAL FIBROELASTOSIS OF LEFT VENTRICLE

**0348**

**Includes:**

> Endocardial fibroelastosis (EFE) of left ventricle
> Myocardial hypertrophy-endocardial fibroelastosis
> Ventricular, left, endocardial fibrosis fibroelastosis
> Ventricular, left, endocardial sclerosis
> Ventricular, left, subendocardial fibroelastosis

**Excludes:**

> Cardiomyopathy, nonobstructive
> **Carnitine deficiency, systemic** (2121)
> Myocarditis
> **Ventricle, endocardial fibroelastosis of right ventricle** (0349)
> **Ventricle, endomyocardial fibrosis of left** (0353)

**Major Diagnostic Criteria:** EKG evidence of extreme left ventricular hypertrophy and T-wave changes, radiographic findings of cardiomegaly with enlargement of the left ventricle and left atrium and hemodynamic and angiographic evidence of altered left ventricular performance with mitral insufficiency. When the above findings occur in a young infant, this diagnosis must be considered.

**Clinical Findings:** This is a condition in which the endocardium of the left ventricle is thickened and noncompliant. Symptoms usually occur in the first 12 months of life, infrequently after 1 year of age or before the first month. Evidence of cardiac decompensation with rapid onset in a previously healthy infant is the characteristic finding in all clinically recognized cases. With progression, if untreated, the terminal state is peripheral collapse accompanied by greyish cyanosis and feeble pulses. Auscultation

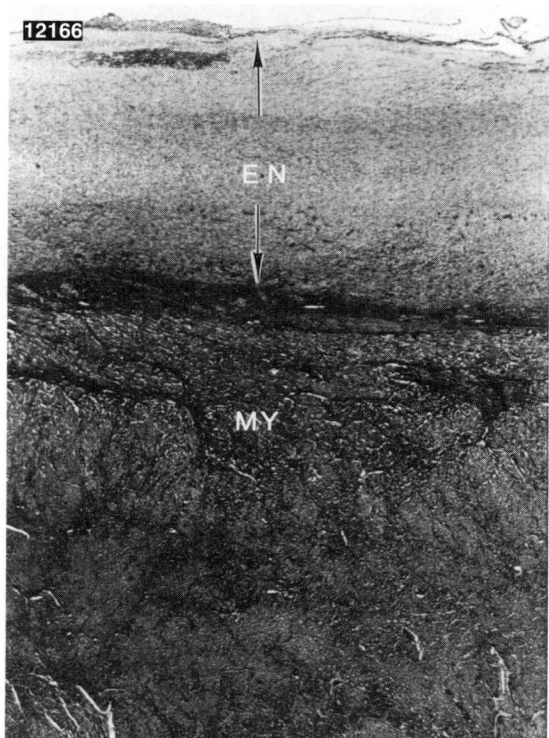

**0348-12165:** Gross anatomy of endocardial fibroelastosis of the left ventricle. **12166:** Photomicrograph of section of the left ventricle illustrating endocardial fibroelastosis. The endocardium is greatly thickened (between arrows EN) and is comprised principally of fibrous-appearing tissue. The myocardium (MY) is also hypertrophied.

---

of the heart while decompensation is present may reveal only tachycardia and a gallop rhythm. Gross cardiac enlargement is uniformly present. With compensation, a murmur of mitral insufficiency is not uncommonly present and may be clinically obvious in 30–50% of the patients. Most affected infants have accentuated 3rd and 4th heart sounds. The 1st and 2nd sounds may be normal.

Laboratory Findings: The EKG is considered typical and usually forms the basis of the clinical diagnosis. The principal findings are extreme left ventricular hypertrophy with flattening or inversion of the left precordial T waves. These findings occur in 80–90% of patients. X-rays uniformly reveal the heart to be enlarged, particularly the left atrium and ventricle. Evidence of pulmonary venous hypertension or obstruction is invariably present. The functional disorder apparent at cardiac catheterization and angiography is progressive failure of the left ventricle to maintain an adequate contractile state. There is a decrease in left heart output and an increase in left ventricular end systolic, as well as in end diastolic volumes. The result is extreme left ventricular dilatation and failure, although a small number of cases, probably less than 10%, may reveal a nondilated left ventricle. This functional disturbance may be due to the altered endocardium which limits contractility or alters metabolism of the myocardium by reducing the oxygen supply to the subendocardial layer. Valvar regurgitation, principally mitral, due to primary involvement, as well as left ventricular dilatation, demonstrable with left ventricular angiography, further adds to the left ventricular work load. Physiologically, left ventricular end diastolic pressure rises and peak dp/dt falls as myocardial contractility is further embarrassed. Myocardial failure ensues. Left atrial pressure rises as does pulmonary venous pressure.

Echocardiography, at present, cannot routinely differentiate this disease from other forms of congestive cardiomyopathy. The left ventricular and septal walls may be abnormally thickened but the endocardial surface may appear normal. However, it has been demonstrated that dense echoes from thickened endocardium may be identified in certain cases. The wall motion is poor and the left ventricular cavity is usually dilated. The mitral valve motion is attenuated, and the anterior posterior leaflets are seen together. The anterior leaflet is seemingly displaced posteriorly and does not reach the septum in diastole. The left atrium is dilated to a greater or lesser extent, depending upon the degree of left heart failure or mitral insufficiency. Of perhaps greater importance is the ability of the echocardiogram to exclude other abnormalities with similar presentation which may be more amenable to definitive therapy, such as **Artery, coronary, anomalous origin from pulmonary artery**.

Pathologic Anatomy: Grossly, the left ventricle is dilated and thickened. The chordae tendineae of the mitral valve are shortened. The endocardium of the left ventricle and, occasionally, of the left atrium, is thickened and presents as a glistening, pearly-white lining of the chamber. The mitral valve usually presents a similar appearance. The aortic valve may also be involved. Microscopically, the fundamental pathologic change is the thickened endocardium composed principally of elastic tissue but with an increased amount of collagenous tissue. However, wide variation in the amounts of these elements has been noted to occur. The condition may thus be less specific and more heterogeneous than previously supposed. Myocardial alterations have also been reported with a decrease in the ratio of capillary to myocardial fiber volume. Electron microscopic studies have indicated the composition of the thickened endocardium to be principally fibrin, but this information lacks confirmation by other investigators.

**Complications:** Congestive heart failure with coincident failure to thrive and difficult feeding are the principal complications. The decompensation, often amenable initially to therapy with digitalis preparations, frequently becomes intractable with death occurring in 75% by the end of the first year of life. Systemic thromboembolic phenomena represent a serious but little emphasized complication. Emboli from the left ventricle have been reported within all major systemic arterial systems and pulmonary emboli have been reported originating from the right ventricle.

**Associated Findings:** Associated cardiovascular defects, principally those causing overload of the left ventricle are recognized. Thus, coarctation of the aorta, aortic stenosis and mitral insufficiency are the leading associated abnormalities seen.

**Etiology:** No specific etiologic agent is known to cause the condition, although a number of agents have been implicated. Originally, the abnormality was thought to be the result of intrauterine infection and was considered a fetal endocarditis. More recently, a number of investigators have reported serologic

and cultural evidence for extrauterine or intrauterine infection with Coxsackie as well as other enteroviruses. A relationship to mumps virus has been suggested because of a reportedly high incidence of positive skin tests to mumps antigen in individuals with endocardial fibroelastosis. However, the initial observation of this relationship has not been confirmed by other investigators.

Evidence of obstruction to the cardiac lymphatics has also been reported, further suggesting an inflammatory etiology. A familial incidence is recognized suggesting a hereditary cause. Secondary EFE, occurring with aortic atresia, mitral valvar disease, usually regurgitation, aortic stenosis and aortic coarctation all suggest overload of the left ventricle as a contributing factor. It is not known, however, whether the EFE in these circumstances is identical to that seen with the isolated lesion.

**Pathogenesis:** The mode of origin and development of this entity is not known. Whether it develops as a response to one of a number of possible agents over a period of time, or is a basic congenital abnormality of the endocardial surface of the heart, has not been determined. Furthermore, it has not been ascertained whether the lesion is a static one, present as an inherent endocardial defect throughout most of intrauterine and early extrauterine life, or whether if it becomes progressively more severe until it causes left ventricular failure and often death. Thus, if the defect is not progressive, or if progression should be halted, "mild" or subclinical cases might occur. The result would be that the abnormality would be of such a low-grade severity that symptoms might not be produced. Because the lesion is rarely, if ever, accurately diagnosed in an asymptomatic state, and even if entertained in such a state, cannot be definitely proven, the occurrence of sequential structural changes remains conjectural.

**MIM No.:** *30530, 22600

**CDC No.:** 425.300

**Sex Ratio:** M0.6:Fl

**Occurrence:** Approximately 1:6000 live births. Appears to have a higher incidence in colder climates and is less commonly encountered in the tropics. Apparently the incidence has decreased in the past decade in North America.

**Risk of Recurrence for Patient's Sib:** Empirical risk 3.8%.

**Risk of Recurrence for Patient's Child:** Unknown.

**Age of Detectability:** Most commonly within the 1st year of life, infrequent before the 1st month and after the 2nd year. Ventricular enlargement may be detected on ultrasound in the 3rd trimester.

**Gene Mapping and Linkage:** EFE2 (endocardial fibroelastosis 2) has been provisionally mapped to X.

**Prevention:** None known. Genetic counseling indicated.

**Treatment:** Treatment is strictly supportive with efforts to control congestive heart failure. General experience shows that the infant so treated has greater longevity and may survive this disease.

**Prognosis:** An estimated 50% or greater of diagnosed and treated patients will survive an indefinite period of time. As soon as the disease produces congestive heart failure, the prognosis without treatment is poor and the infant cannot be expected to survive.

**Detection of Carrier:** Unknown.

**References:**

Sellers FJ, et al.: The diagnosis of primary endocardial fibroelastosis. Circulation 1964; 29:49–59.

Mitchell SC, et al.: An epidemiologic assessment of primary endocardial fibroelastosis. Am J Cardiol 1966; 18:859–866.

Chen S, et al.: Endocardial fibroelastosis: family studies with special reference to counseling. J Pediatr 1971; 79:385–392–392. *

Westwood M, et al.: Heredity in primary endocardial fibroelastosis. Br Heart J 1975; 37:1077–1084. *

Factor SM: Endocardial fibroelastosis: myocardial and vascular alterations associated with viral-like nuclear particles. Am Heart J 1978; 96:791–801.

Van Der Hauwaert LG, et al.: Long-term echocardiographic assessment of dilated cardiomyopathy in children. Am J Cardiol 1983; 52:1066–1071.

Hodgson S, et al.: Endocardial fibroelastosis: possible X-linked inheritance. J Med Genet 1987; 24:210–214.

F0002                                                                   **Gordon M. Folger, Jr.**

---

## VENTRICLE, ENDOCARDIAL FIBROELASTOSIS OF RIGHT VENTRICLE                                                  0349

**Includes:**

Endocardial fibroelastosis (EFE) of right ventricle
Right ventricular hypertrophy-endocardial fibroelastosis
Subendocardial fibroelastosis, right ventricular
Ventricular, right, endocardial fibroelastosis

**Excludes:**

Cardiomyopathy, nonobstructive
Cardiomyopathy, obstructive of right ventricle
Endomyocardial sclerosis
Myocarditis
**Ventricle, endocardial fibroelastosis of left ventricle** (0348)
**Ventricle, endomyocardial fibrosis of right** (0354)

**Major Diagnostic Criteria:** Angiocardiography of the right ventricle demonstrates the small contracted right ventricle. Two-dimensional echocardiograph should suggest the possibility.

**Clinical Findings:** A rare condition of the right ventricle in which the endocardium is thickened and noncompliant. Although dilation has been observed, the right ventricle is usually contracted and constricted. Most cases have been described as occurring with other right heart malformations, with no more than ten cases of the primary type reported. When EFE of the right ventricle occurs as a primary lesion, it may present findings similar to hypoplasia of the right ventricle with cyanosis, evidence of systemic venous engorgement and reduced pulmonary blood flow.

Laboratory Findings: The EKG pattern is similar to that seen with hypoplasia of the right ventricle in other causes. Radiographically the heart is enlarged, the apex tilted up and the pulmonary conus segment is absent. The pulmonary vasculature is reduced. The findings at cardiac catheterization, as with the other laboratory findings, are similar to those seen in pulmonary atresia or extreme stenosis. The right ventricle is diminutive and there is a massive right-to-left shunt at the atrial level.

Pathology: Isolated primary EFE of the right ventricle such as is seen in the left ventricular form is extremely unusual. In this condition, no obstruction to the otherwise normal right ventricle occurs. The gross appearance, however, is identical to the condition as it occurs as a primary lesion of the left ventricle revealing an opaque white endocardium which is thickened on cut section as well as tough and fibrous. The right ventricle, however, is contracted rather than dilated.

Microscopic: The endocardial layer is increased many times its normal thickness with abundance of elastic fibers and an increase in collagenous tissue. The subendocardial-myocardial junction usually shows a few degenerative muscle fibers.

**Complications:** Congestive heart failure, right-to-left atrial shunt, hypoxemia and acidosis.

**Associated Findings:** The condition is nearly always associated with other intracardiac anomalies, principally pulmonary atresia or extreme stenosis with intact ventricular septum.

**Etiology:** Undetermined. Familial occurrence in 3 generations has been described.

**Pathogenesis:** Unknown.

**MIM No.:** *30560, 22600

**CDC No.:** 425.300

**Sex Ratio:** Presumably M1:F1

**Occurrence:** Less than ten cases of the primary type have been substantiated.

**Risk of Recurrence for Patient's Sib:** Unknown.

**Risk of Recurrence for Patient's Child:** Unknown.

**Age of Detectability:** Generally during early infancy, rarely after 2–3 months.

**Gene Mapping and Linkage:** Unknown.

**Prevention:** None known. Genetic counseling indicated.

**Treatment:** Palliative systemic venous to right pulmonary artery anastomosis to improve pulmonary blood flow and reduce right heart work load. Symptomatic therapy for congestive heart failure.

**Prognosis:** Death in early infancy is nearly inevitable with survival seldom more than a few months unless a palliative procedure is carried out.

**Detection of Carrier:** Unknown.

**References:**

Andersen DN, Kelly J: Endocardial fibroelastosis; endocardial fibroelastosis associated with congenital malformations of the heart. Pediatrics 1956; 18:513–521.
Morgan AD, et al.: Endocardial fibroelastosis of the right ventricle in the newborn: presenting the clinical picture of the hypoplastic right heart syndrome. Am J Cardiol 1966; 18:933–937. *
Larson JE, et al.: Isolated endocardial fibroelastosis of the right ventricle associated with pulmonary hypertension. Am Heart J 1984; 107:1286–1290.

F0002                                                                   **Gordon M. Folger, Jr.**

---

## VENTRICLE, ENDOMYOCARDIAL FIBROSIS OF LEFT                                        0353

**Includes:**

African cardiopathy
Cardiopathy, constrictive
Davies disease
Endomyocardial fibrosis (EMF) of left ventricle

**Excludes:**

Endocardial fibroelastosis-primary myocardial hypertrophy
**Ventricle, endocardial fibroelastosis of left ventricle** (0348)
**Ventricle, endomyocardial fibrosis of right** (0354)

**Major Diagnostic Criteria:** Hemodynamic data showing malfunction of the left ventricle and angiocardiography demonstrating reduction of myocardial contractility are the principal features. Angiographic demonstration of apical filling defects in the left ventricle, as well as mitral regurgitation, are usually present. Two-dimensional echocardiograph identifies the findings of left ventricular restrictive disease.

**Clinical Findings:** Similar to those of endomyocardial fibrosis of the right ventricle. Cardiomegaly is uncommon as this is a restrictive heart disease. Likewise, displacement of the apical impulse is unusual, and it is rarely prominent or heaving. With pulmonary hypertension secondary to mitral regurgitation and advanced left ventricular disease, an accentuated pulmonary component of the second heart sound may be present. A prominent third heart sound is a constant finding and an opening snap may be detected in 1/3 to 1/2 of the cases. A characteristic apical systolic murmur occupying early systole has been reported due to early phase mitral insufficiency with mitral competency occurring in late systole.

Laboratory Findings: Eosinophilia may occur but may be secondary to parasitic infestation. Gamma globulin levels are often elevated. The EKG tracing may be normal and is reportedly rarely helpful. With advanced disease hypertrophy of the left atrium may be seen, and with the development of significant pulmonary hypertension, right atrial hypertrophy and right ventricular hypertrophy develop. Enlargement of the heart is usually present. With pulmonary hypertension, right atrial and ventricular enlargement are usually detectable and left atrial enlargement may be apparent. Pulmonary venous congestion is a frequent finding. Elevation of the left atrial pressure and the left ventricular end diastolic pressure are the usual findings. Pulmonary hypertension is found in nearly 50% of the patients studied but this varies with the degree of left ventricular disease. The left ventricular chamber is frequently small with constant apical filling defects. Contractility is greatly reduced. The left atrium is enlarged and mitral regurgitation is usually present. The echocardiographic findings of small left ventricle and left atrial dilatation indicate the restrictive nature of the abnormality. Apical obliteration of the ventricle by thickened endocardium may be diagnostic of the condition.

Pathologic Anatomy: Grossly, there is a recurring pattern of fibrotic endocardial lesions occurring in two areas - one on the posterior wall of the left ventricle involving the endocardium in the area behind the posterior leaflet of the mitral valve, the chordae of the posterior mitral leaflet and a portion of the endocardium of the outflow tract; and 1 located at the apex of the ventricle tapering toward the endocardium of the septum to terminate at the bases of the posterior papillary muscles. Microscopic findings are the same as endomyocardial fibrosis of right ventricle.

**Complications:**  The development of severe pulmonic hypertension secondary to reduced left ventricular compliance and mitral regurgitation is the principal complication. With pulmonary hypertension, right atrial and ventricular dilatation may occur with the possibility of pulmonary embolic phenomena. Congestive heart failure is a frequent finding and the common cause of death.

**Associated Findings:**  None known.

**Etiology:**  Unknown.

**Pathogenesis:**  Unknown.

**Sex Ratio:**  M1:F1

**Occurrence:**  Unknown.

**Risk of Recurrence for Patient's Sib:**  Unknown.

**Risk of Recurrence for Patient's Child:**  Unknown.

**Age of Detectability:**  Generally early adult life to middle age, rarely in childhood.

**Gene Mapping and Linkage:**  Unknown.

**Prevention:**  None known. Genetic counseling indicated.

**Treatment:**  Anticongestive measures restore compensation for varying periods of time, but the outcome is uniformly fatal, usually in early middle age.

A growing number of cases surgically treated employing endomyocardectomy and replacement of both atrioventricular valves with very satisfactory results has given rise to optimism in the care of some of these patients.

**Prognosis:**  Poor, with death from the condition occurring uniformly.

**Detection of Carrier:**  Unknown.

**Special Considerations:**  For related details, see also **Ventricle, endomyocardial fibrosis of right**.

**References:**
Cockshott WP: Angiocardiography of endomyocardial fibrosis. Br J Radiol 1965; 38:192–200.
Connor DH, et al.: Endomyocardial fibrosis in Uganda (Davies' disease). I. An epidemiologic, clinical and pathologic study. Am Heart J 1967; 74:687–709.
Connor DH, et al.: Endomyocardial fibrosis in Uganda (Davies' disease). II. An epidemiologic, clinical and pathologic study. Am Heart J 1968; 75:107–124.
Gonzales-Lavin L, et al.: Endomyocardial fibrosis: diagnosis and treatment. Am Heart J 1983; 105:699–705.
Fawzy ME, et al.: Endomyocardial fibrosis: report of eight cases. J Am Coll Cardiol 1985; 5:983–988. *

**Gordon M. Folger, Jr.**

## VENTRICLE, ENDOMYOCARDIAL FIBROSIS OF RIGHT    0354

**Includes:**
African cardiopathy
Cardiopathy, constrictive
Davies disease
Endomyocardial fibrosis (EMF) of right ventricle

**Excludes:**
Endocardial fibroelastosis-primary myocardial hypertrophy
**Ventricle, endocardial fibroelastosis of right ventricle** (0349)
**Ventricle, endomyocardial fibrosis of left** (0353)

**Major Diagnostic Criteria:**  Hemodynamic changes consist principally of evidence for right ventricular dysfunction with elevation of right atrial pressure and right ventricular end diastolic pressures. Cardiac angiography reveals reduction in right ventricular contractility. Echocardiography reveals the findings of restrictive cardiomyopathy of any cause.

**Clinical Findings:**  A disorder of the cardiac connective tissues characteristically occurring among native of equatorial Africa in which the ventricular endocardium and subendocardial layers, as well as the supportive tissue of the ventricular wall, are thickened and rendered noncompliant. Increased numbers of Caucasians and non-African Blacks are being recognized with the condition around the world.

Characteristically, evidence of right heart failure occurs insidiously. The involved individual is almost invariably a Negro in the early adult years, although children as young as 2 years have been reported to have the condition. Ascites is the most striking feature. Peripheral edema may be present but much less prominent. Hepatosplenomegaly is common with a pulsatile liver frequently present. The cardiac findings consist of enlargement of the heart detectable in 50–60% of patients; a right ventricular lift occurs in approximately half of the patients; an accentuated third heart sound is found in nearly all patients; and the murmur of tricuspid insufficiency is found in 15–25% of cases. Pericardial effusion is common, occurring in nearly 50% of reported cases.

Laboratory Findings: Eosinophilia of significance occurs in some individuals but may be secondary to coexisting parasitic infestation. Elevated gamma globulin levels are commonly encountered. The QRS axis is usually normal. QRS voltages are generally normal or decreased with hypertrophy patterns uncommon. Atrial hypertrophy occurs in approximately 50% of individuals and is more often a P mitral configuration or a pattern suggesting hypertrophy of both atria. Less commonly, right atrial enlargement alone is noted. Characteristic or diagnostic EKG patterns have not been reported. Atrial fibrillation occurs at some time in approximately one-third of cases. Endomyocardial fibrosis is a restrictive heart disease; therefore, gross cardiomegaly is usually due either to enlargement of the right atrium or to the coexistence of a pericardial effusion. Dilatation of the right ventricular infundibular area is, however, a frequent radiographic as well as angiographic finding. Intracardiac calcification may be visualized. Elevation of the right ventricular end diastolic pressure is a constant finding. The right ventricular pressure curve closely resembles that of constrictive pericarditis even though that condition does not coexist. The cardiac output may be normal or reduced. By cardiac angiography, reduced contractility of the right ventricle and a degree of tricuspid insufficiency are common findings. The right ventricular body may appear nearly obliterated with only the dilated infundibular area remaining cavitary. Similarly, the 2-dimensional echocardiograph appearance of apical obliteration of the ventricle by thickened endocardium may be diagnostic.

Pathologic Anatomy: The gross appearance of the heart is that of extreme enlargement of the right atrium, a contracted right ventricle, particularly the apical area with dilatation of the right ventricular outflow area. Significant right ventricular hypertrophy is uncommon. Endocardial fibrosis characteristically is more severe at the apical portion of the right ventricle, usually extending to encase the papillary muscles but sparing the chordae tendineae and the tricuspid valve leaflets. Mural thrombi are often present in the right atrium and may occur in the right ventricle. Calcification in the fibrotic areas occurs occasionally. The microscopic findings are a swollen appearance of the connective tissues of the endocardium and underlying myocardial interstices. The earlier finding that these tissues contain elevated amounts of acid mucopolysaccharide has not been found to be specific for endomyocardial fibrosis. Distinct increase in cardiac muscle fiber size is recognized. Inflammatory changes are not observed.

**Complications:** Congestive heart failure is a uniform finding and the principal cause of death. Pulmonary emboli secondary to thrombi in the right atrium and ventricle are a major complication.

**Associated Findings:** None known.

**Etiology:** No definite etiologic agent has been identified. A number of agents, however, capable of instituting an autoimmune reaction have been considered. Included in these have been infectious agents, toxins and dietary idiosyncracy; none of which have been positively implicated. However, the distribution of the lesion to very specific areas within the heart, and in no other place, and the inability to find immunologically competent cells in areas undergoing change have cast some doubt upon an immunologic origin. Malnutrition has been considered but appears unlikely. Some similarities to rheumatic fever have caused consideration of this disease as the cause of the changes seen but this, too, is unproven.

**Pathogenesis:** Undetermined, but currently thought to be secondary to an autoimmune mechanism.

**Sex Ratio:** M1:F1

**Occurrence:** Undetermined. Found in native African Blacks, much less frequently in Blacks from other world areas. Rare in non-Black populations.

**Risk of Recurrence for Patient's Sib:** Unknown.

**Risk of Recurrence for Patient's Child:** Unknown.

**Age of Detectability:** The disease is seen occasionally in children as young as 2 years, but its clinical onset is more commonly in a young adult.

**Gene Mapping and Linkage:** Unknown.

**Prevention:** None known. Genetic counseling indicated.

**Treatment:** Anticongestive measures restore compensation for varying periods of time, but it appears that the outcome is uniformly fatal. A growing number of cases surgically treated employing endomyocardectomy and replacement of both atrioventricular valves with very satisfactory results has given rise to optimism in the care of some of these patients.

**Prognosis:** Poor, with death from the condition occurring uniformly, usually in the age range from early adulthood to early middle age.

**Detection of Carrier:** Unknown.

**References:**
Cockshott WP: Angiocardiography of endomyocardial fibrosis. Br J Radiol 1965; 38:192–200.
Connor DH, et al.: Endomyocardial fibrosis in Uganda (Davies' disease). I. An epidemiologic, clinical and pathologic study. Am Heart J 1967; 74:687–709.
Connor DH, et al.: Endomyocardial fibrosis in Uganda (Davies' disease). II. An epidemiologic, clinical and pathologic study. Am Heart J 1968; 75:107–124.
Somers K, et al.: Clinical features of endomyocardial fibrosis in the right ventricle. Br Heart J 1968; 30:322–331.
Gonzalez-Lavin L, et al.: Endomyocardial fibrosis: diagnosis and treatment. Am Heart J 1983; 105:699–705. *
Fawzy ME, et al.: Endomyocardial fibrosis: report of eight cases. J Am Coll Cardiol 1985; 5:983–988.

F0002                                          **Gordon M. Folger, Jr.**

**Ventricle, functional obstruction of left**
*See HEART, SUBAORTIC STENOSIS, MUSCULAR*
**Ventricle, hypoplasia of right**
*See TRICUSPID VALVE, ATRESIA*

## VENTRICLE, OBSTRUCTION WITHIN RIGHT VENTRICLE OR ITS OUTFLOW TRACT                                    0731

**Includes:**
 Pulmonary stenosis, isolated infundibular
 Stenosis of ostium infundibulum
 Ventricle, anomalous muscle bundle of right
 Ventricle, two-chambered right
 Ventricular muscle bands, aberrant right

**Excludes:**
 Heart, tetralogy of Fallot (0938)
 Pulmonary valve, stenosis (0839)

**Major Diagnostic Criteria:** A pulmonary ejection murmur with EKG evidence of right ventricular hypertrophy should suggest the diagnosis. Angiocardiography confirms the diagnosis.

**Clinical Findings:** Four anatomic types of infundibular pulmonary stenosis have been identified: 1) a fibrous band at the site of the juncture of the infundibulum and right ventricle (stenosis of os infundibulum); 2) diffuse narrowing of the infundibulum by thickened myocardium; 3) anomalous muscle bundles which are proximal to the infundibulum. These bundles are hyperplastic muscle bands passing from the area near the septal leaflet of the tricuspid valve to the anterior ventricular wall. Also, the moderator band may be hyperplastic; and 4) as part of a diffuse idiopathic myocardial hypertrophy in which the hypertrophied ventricular septum obstructs the lumen of the right ventricular outflow tract. Since the location of the right ventricular outflow obstruction varies, differences in the size of the distal or infundibular chamber and the proximal right ventricular cavity result. The right ventricle proximal to the obstruction is hypertrophied, as is the right atrium. Unlike cases with stenosis of pulmonary valve, the pulmonary artery is not dilated.

Infundibular stenosis may also occur secondary to severe stenosis of the pulmonary valve. Here, also, the clinical features vary with the degree of right ventricular outflow obstruction. With mild stenosis, the patients are asymptomatic; in those with severe stenosis, easy fatigability and at times right-sided congestive cardiac failure occur. Cyanosis may be present in the latter group, if a right-to-left shunt occurs through an anatomically patent foramen ovale. A pulmonic systolic ejection murmur is present. It may be located lower along the left sternal border than in valvar stenosis, particularly when the obstruction is located low in the right ventricle. The murmur is longer, and the peak intensity later in severe stenosis. Likewise, the degree of splitting of the second heart sound increases with increasing severity, and the intensity of the pulmonary component is diminished. In contrast to valvar pulmonic stenosis, an ejection click is uncommon.

X-rays of infundibular stenosis are similar to those of valvar pulmonary stenosis, except that poststenotic dilatation of the pulmonary trunk or left pulmonary artery is not usually present.

The EKG demonstrates right ventricular hypertrophy, the severity of which is directly related to the degree of stenosis. Progression of EKG evidence of right ventricular hypertrophy is more frequently observed in this condition than in stenosis of the pulmonary valve.

The outflow tract of the right ventricle is seen by echocardiography, but its precise character is difficult to assess. In this condition, right ventricular and septal hypertrophy occur. In some instances, an abnormal muscle band may be visualized. The pulmonary valve frequently has an early but incomplete closure followed by reopening.

Cardiac catheterization typically reveals a systolic pressure gradient within the right ventricle, although this may be missed if the obstruction is located close to the pulmonary valve. In patients with anomalous muscle bundle, the pressure gradient may be found close to the tricuspid valve. Since the obstruction is generally caused by myocardial tissue, it is dynamic in nature. With exercise or isoproterenol infusion, the degree of obstruction may increase, thereby reducing the effective right ventricular outflow area. The right ventricular end diastolic and right atrial pressures may be elevated, and in severe cases, a right-to-left shunt exists at the atrial level.

Biplane right ventriculography confirms the diagnosis. This demonstrates the muscular narrowing in the infundibular area. Although the obstruction is visualized throughout the cardiac cycle, it is more marked during systole than diastole, again indicating its dynamic nature. Whereas most pulmonary outflow obstructions are best visualized in the lateral projection, an anomalous muscle bundle is best seen in the anteroposterior projection. Since the muscle bundles' course is primarily in an anteroposterior direction, they are seen end on as circular nonopacified areas low in the right ventricle. The pulmonary valve is normal and poststenotic dilatation of the pulmonary artery is usually not present.

**Complications:** Right-sided cardiac failure, myocardial fibrosis, bacterial endocarditis, **Tricuspid valve, insufficiency**.

**Associated Findings:** None known.

**Etiology:** Unknown.

**Pathogenesis:** Anomalous or hyperplastic muscle bundles may be due to incomplete involution of the embryonic right ventricular trabeculae.

**Sex Ratio:** M1:F1

**Occurrence:** Undetermined. Less than 1% of congenital cardiac defects.

**Risk of Recurrence for Patient's Sib:** Unknown.

**Risk of Recurrence for Patient's Child:** Unknown.

**Age of Detectability:** From birth.

**Gene Mapping and Linkage:** Unknown.

**Prevention:** None known.

**Treatment:** If stenosis is severe, surgical excision may be necessary.

**Prognosis:** Data regarding the natural history of these conditions are scanty. There is, however, one report describing serial cardiac catheterizations. It shows that anomalous muscle bundles become more obstructive with time. The other forms are also believed to be progressive, but there is little evidence to support this.

**Detection of Carrier:** Unknown.

**References:**

Lucas RV Jr, et al.: Anomalous muscle bundle of the right ventricle: hemodynamic consequences and surgical considerations. Circulation 1962; 25:443–455.

Hartmann AF Jr, et al.: Development of right ventricular obstruction by aberrant muscular bands. Circulation 1964; 30:679–685.

Rowland TW, et al.: Double-chamber right ventricle: experience with 17 cases. Am Heart J 1975; 89:455–462.

Baumstark A, et al.: Combined double chambered right ventricle and discrete subaortic stenosis. Circulation 1978; 57:299–302.

Emmanouilides GC, Baylen BG: Primary infundibular stenosis. In: Emmanouilides GC, ed: Heart disease in infants, children, and adolescents. Baltimore: Williams & Wilkins, 1983.

M0005                                                    **James H. Moller**

---

**VENTRICLE, RIGHT, UHL ANOMALY**                        **0979**

**Includes:**
    Parchment right ventricle
    Uhl anomaly
    Ventricular myocardium, aplasia of right

**Excludes:**
    **Tricuspid valve, Ebstein anomaly** (0332)
    **Ventricle, endomyocardial fibrosis of right** (0354)
    Ventricle, hypoplastic right

**Major Diagnostic Criteria:** The diagnosis may be suspected clinically from the marked cardiomegaly, reduced pulmonary vascular markings, feeble heart tones without significant murmurs and the EKG findings described below. It is established by echocardiography or angiocardiography which demonstrates the enormous but thin-walled and poorly contracting right ventricle devoid of trabeculae, and the normal location of the tricuspid orifice.

**Clinical Findings:** The pathologic anatomy is characterized by enormous dilatation of the heart, chiefly of the right atrium and right ventricle, and virtual absence of muscle fibers in the wall of the right ventricle. The right atrium is dilated and thick-walled due to hypertrophy and endocardial fibroelastosis. The foramen ovale is often patent; the tricuspid valve is normal. The wall of the grossly dilated right ventricle is thin, translucent and parchment-like, ranging in thickness from 1–2 mm. Its endocardial surface is opaque white due to fibroelastosis. The trabeculae are deficient and flat, the papillary muscles and chordae tendineae are thin and delicate. The crista supraventricularis is likewise flat and hypoplastic. On microscopic examination, the right ventricular wall consists solely of a thickened endocardial layer, showing fibroelastosis, and a subjacent epicardial layer with increased fatty and connective tissue. No intervening muscle fibers are observed between these two layers except, occasionally, a few islands of myocardial cells in areas adjoining the pulmonary ring, tricuspid annulus or diaphragmatic surface. The pulmonary valve is normal but the pulmonary trunk and main branches appear hypoplastic. The left atrium and left ventricle are normal or may reveal hypertrophy with fibroelastosis. The coronary vessels appear normal, as do the systemic and pulmonary veins. The positional relationship of the pulmonary trunk and aorta is normal. The basic physiologic abnormality consists of failure of the right ventricle to function as a pump for the pulmonary circulation. It behaves as a passive reservoir for blood coming from the right atrium, and as such, is a constantly overloaded chamber, which accounts for its enormously dilated state. Pumping is accomplished by right atrial contraction, and cardiac output is accordingly low.

The clinical picture is characterized by heart failure in infancy or early childhood, marked cardiomegaly, feeble heart tones with gallop rhythm and the absence of murmurs. The increased cardiac dullness is unaccompanied by any significant precordial heave or apical impulse. Heart failure is chiefly right-sided, manifested by hepatomegaly, peripheral edema and normal lung findings.

The chest X-rays reveal an enormous cardiac shadow with reduced pulmonary vascular markings. In the frontal projection, there is increased convexity of the right heart border due to right atrial enlargement, and extension of the left heart border to the lateral chest wall caused by the pronounced dilatation of the right ventricle. The pulmonary artery segment is inconspicuous. In the lateral as well as in the right and left anterior oblique projections, there is marked extension of the cardiac borders anteriorly and posteriorly, giving an impression of combined ventricular enlargement. The prominent posterior heart border is, however, mainly due to the posterior displacement of the heart from the right heart dilatation.

The EKG commonly shows broad, peaked and tall P waves due to right atrial enlargement, and small amplitude QRS complexes in the chest lead tracings without a definite ventricular hypertrophy pattern. In addition, the vectorcardiogram reveals counterclockwise posteriorly oriented horizontal QRS loop with the initial forces directed leftwards and anteriorly.

The two-dimensional echocardiogram shows gross enlargement of the right atrium, normal position of the tricuspid valve, and marked dilatation of the right ventricle, with minimum or absent contractions. Doppler flow analysis may reveal normal findings across the tricuspid valve, but normal flow pattern across the pulmonary valve. Unlike **Tricuspid valve, Ebstein anomaly**, an atrial systole-coincident diastolic opening of the pulmonary valve is observed. In Ebstein disease, the septal motion may be paradoxic, whereas in the Uhl anomaly it has been reported to be normal.

At cardiac catheterization, the right atrial presystolic "a" wave is high and of approximately the same magnitude as the right ventricular and pulmonary arterial systolic pressures. Slight systemic arterial oxygen unsaturation may be observed if right-to-left shunting across a patent foramen ovale is present. Angiocardiography is diagnostic. It characteristically reveals gross enlargement of the right ventricle with generalized thinness of its wall, absence of trabeculae, normal location of the tricuspid orifice and prolonged emptying time. Small shunting across a patent foramen ovale may or may not be demonstrated following opacification of the right atrium. The pulmonary trunk and main branches appear hypoplastic.

**Complications:** Congestive heart failure and death occur in infancy or early childhood.

**Associated Findings:** An additional abnormality of the left ventricle such as endocardial fibroelastosis or myofibrosis, may be present, and this promotes earlier onset of the intractable heart failure.

**Etiology:** Unknown.

**Pathogenesis:** Possibly a congenital defect of the primordium of the right ventricular myocardium.

**Sex Ratio:** Presumably M1:F1.

**Occurrence:** Less than 1:100,000 births; under 0.1% of congenital heart disease.

**Risk of Recurrence for Patient's Sib:** Unknown.

**Risk of Recurrence for Patient's Child:** Unknown.

**Age of Detectability:** From birth, by echocardiograph or by cardiac catheterization and angiocardiography.

**Gene Mapping and Linkage:** Unknown.

**Prevention:** None known. Genetic counseling indicated.

**Treatment:** Superior vena cava - right pulmonary artery anastomosis or some other type of right heart bypass surgery, in those with heart failure but without associated left ventricular myocardial disease, to decompress the right heart and improve the pulmonary circulation. Other measures include symptomatic therapy for congestive heart failure.

**Prognosis:** Poor. In the usual cases where there is almost total absence of the right ventricular myocardium, death from heart failure occurs during infancy. Survival for several years is possible when the myocardial defect is not extensive.

**Detection of Carrier:** Unknown.

**References:**

Arcilla RA, Gasul BM: Congenital aplasia or marked hypoplasia of the myocardium of the right ventricle (Uhl's anomaly): clinical angiocardiographic and hemodynamic findings. J Pediatr 1961; 58:381–388. *

Cumming GR, et al.: Congenital aplasia of the myocardium of the right ventricle (Uhl's anomaly). Am Heart J 1965; 70:671–676.

French JW, et al.: Echocardiographic findings in Uhl's anomaly: demonstration of diastolic pulmonary valve opening. Am J Cardiol 1975; 36:349–353.

AR001                        **René A. Arcilla**

## VENTRICLE, SEPTUM DEXTROPOSITION AND DOUBLE INLET LEFT VENTRICLE      0286

**Includes:**

  Cor triloculare biatriatum

  Dextroposition of ventricular septum-double inlet left ventricle

  Double inlet left ventricle with ventricular inversion

  Double inlet left ventricle without ventricular inversion

  Holmes heart

  Univentricular heart of the left ventricular type

  Ventricle, single with rudimentary outflow chamber

**Excludes:**

  **Mitral valve atresia** (0665)

  **Tricuspid valve, atresia** (0968)

  Other forms of functional single ventricle

**Major Diagnostic Criteria:** Clinical evidence of a large left-to-right shunt in a mildly cyanotic infant with electrovectorcardiographic evidence of severe left ventricular hypertrophy should suggest the possibility of double inlet left ventricle with noninversion of the ventricles. Similar clinical findings in the presence of electrovectorcardiographic evidence of right ventricular hypertrophy as evidenced by significant Q waves in lead $V_1$, plus similar deep Q waves in standard lead III and lead aVF, should suggest the possibility of double inlet left ventricle with inversion of the ventricles. Cardiac catheterization and selective angiocardiography will confirm the exact anatomic situation.

**Clinical Findings:** Double inlet left ventricle is that cardiac malformation in which both atrioventricular valves open into a large ventricular chamber which morphologically resembles a left ventricle. The left A-V valve communicates exclusively with this large left ventricle. The right A-V valve may also communicate exclusively with the large left ventricle but may override a hypoplastic ventricular septum and open partially into a more or less rudimentary right ventricle. Double inlet left ventricle is usually, but not necessarily, associated with transposition of the great arteries in which case the aorta arises from the rudimentary right ventricle which consists only of a rightward and anteriorly placed infundibular chamber. In the rare instance when the great arteries are normally related (and the ventricles are not inverted), the complex is known as the Holmes heart. The atrial septum is usually intact, although small atrial septal defects may occur. A ventricular septal defect is always present as the route of communication from the large single ventricle to the rudimentary right ventricular infundibular chamber. If the ventricular septal defect is small, there may be functional obstruction to the aorta. Pulmonic or subpulmonic obstruction may also be present, ranging from mild stenosis to complete atresia.

The anatomic complex double inlet left ventricle may also occur in the presence of ventricular inversion. In that condition the large ventricular chamber, which has the internal morphology of a left ventricle and which receives both A-V valves, is located on the right side. The apex of the heart (in situs solitus) usually points to the left, but dextroversion may be present. The pulmonary trunk almost always arises from the main chamber. The left A-V valve may override the ventricular septum in some cases. The hypoplastic right ventricular infundibular chamber is placed leftward, superiorly and anteriorly and gives origin to the aorta. The ventricular septum lies in the sagittal plane. As with noninversion, pulmonic or subpulmonic obstruction may be present.

Clinical features are usually those of a large left-to-right shunt with bidirectional intracardiac mixing and are similar for both inversion and noninversion of the ventricles. In the absence of pulmonary stenosis, cyanosis is initially mild. With increased pulmonary vascular resistance, cyanosis will increase. A harsh systolic murmur and systolic thrill are present along the left sternal border and the second sound is single or narrowly split with accentuation of the pulmonic component. A mitral diastolic flow murmur is common and congestive heart failure is frequently present. When pulmonic or subpulmonic obstruction is present, the clinical findings depend upon the degree of obstruction. When mild, the findings may be unchanged. When severe, cyanosis is prominent, the murmurs may be insignificant, and the second sound is single. When obstruction to aortic outflow is present, the clinical picture frequently mimics aortic atresia or severe coarctation of the aorta and survival beyond a few months of life is unlikely.

The electrovectorcardiographic features depend upon whether inversion or noninversion of the ventricles is present. Regardless of the type of single ventricle, there is almost invariably an alteration of the initial cardiac vectors from the anticipated normal. Additional features suggest noninversion from inversion. With noninversion, the EKG and the vectorcardiogram demonstrate marked left ventricular hypertrophy. The mean frontal QRS axis ranges from +25° to +75° and the initial QRS forces are directed leftward and anteriorly, recording little or no Q wave in any of the usual chest leads ($V_3R$ to $V_7$). The major QRS forces are shifted leftward and posteriorly resulting in rS complexes in lead $V_1$ and Rs complexes in lead $V_6$. Left and right atrial enlargement are frequently present. When pulmonic obstruction is present, the EKG is relatively unchanged except that right atrial enlargement is more marked. In the presence of ventricular inversion, the EKG and vectorcardiogram are quite different. As in ventricular inversion with two ventricles, the initial QRS forces are directed leftward, superiorly and usually posteriorly, resulting in Q waves in standard lead III, lead aVF and lead $V_1$. However, the major portion of the QRS forces is directed rightward and anteriorly, indicating anterior chamber hypertrophy, and resulting in qRs complexes in lead $V_1$ and RS complexes in $V_6$. The QRS axis in the frontal plane is directed somewhat to the right between 100° and 135°. Cardiac arrhythmias, especially varying degrees of atrioventricular block, are more common in the presence of ventricular inversion. As is the case with noninversion, atrial hypertrophy may be present and when pulmonic obstruction is significant, right atrial enlargement is more marked.

The echocardiographic diagnosis of this disorder requires demonstration that two separate atrioventricular valves exist without an intervening ventricular septum. Differential diagnosis of the various forms of single ventricle, as well as some forms of complete atrioventricular canal, is extremely difficult echocardiographically. Nevertheless, the demonstration of the transposed great vessel relationship in the presence of two atrioventricular valves and the absence of an intervening ventricular septal echo may suggest a diagnosis of single ventricle. An additional important feature is the identification of a small outflow tract anteriorly located but unrelated to an atrioventricular valve. It has been reported by some authors that double-inlet left ventricle can be demonstrated reliably with the 2-dimensional echocardiogram, and that this assists in the identification of the type of major ventricular chamber, whether left, right, or undifferentiated.

Chest X-ray findings depend upon the degree of pulmonic obstruction and the position of the right ventricular infundibulum. In the usual case without pulmonic obstruction, there is prominent shunt type vascularity, generalized cardiomegaly, biatrial enlargement and mediastinal findings suggestive of transposition of the great arteries. When pulmonic obstruction is significant, pulmonary arterial vascularity appears normal or decreased, and heart size is normal or slightly enlarged. Chest X-rays may suggest the presence of ventricular inversion by the position of the great arteries and the bulge of the infundibular chamber on the left upper border of the cardiac shadow.

Cardiac catheterization demonstrates a lack of significant shunting at the atrial level, based on fully saturated left atrial blood and no significant oxygen increase in the right atrium. Ventricular and peripheral arterial oxygen values show mild desaturation and are about equal. Selective angiocardiography is necessary to demonstrate the precise anatomy. The presence of ventricular inversion is apparent by the position of the infundibular chamber and the orientation of the ventricular septum. The interrelationship of the great arteries is of little value in distinguishing inversion from noninversion. Angiocardiography will demonstrate the presence of two independent atrioventricular valves entering a large single ventricle, which communicates with a rudimentary right ventricular infundibular chamber.

**Complications:**  Persistent cardiac failure and repeated pulmonary infections frequently prove fatal. When pulmonic obstruction is significant, hypoxic complications may occur. Aortic obstruction may result in low cardiac output, poor systemic perfusion, and death within the first few months of life.

**Associated Findings:**  None known.

**Etiology:**  Probably multifactorial inheritance.

**Pathogenesis:**  Probably due to a failure of alignment of the right portion of the atrioventricular canal with the primitive right ventricle. Thus, the right ventricle does not develop and functions only as an outlet chamber. The reason for the high degree of association of double inlet left ventricle with transposition of the great arteries is unknown.

**Sex Ratio:**  M2:F1

**Occurrence:**  Less than 1:100 cases of congenital heart defects.

**Risk of Recurrence for Patient's Sib:**  Unknown.

**Risk of Recurrence for Patient's Child:**  Unknown.

**Age of Detectability:**  From birth.

**Gene Mapping and Linkage:**  Unknown.

**Prevention:**  None known. Genetic counseling indicated.

**Treatment:**  Palliative procedures such as pulmonary artery banding, or systemic-pulmonary artery shunt in the presence of severe pulmonic stenosis, may prolong life. Other therapy as necessary for congestive heart failure and pneumonia.

**Prognosis:**  Poor; survival into adulthood possible with moderate pulmonic obstruction. Most cases die early in life.

**Detection of Carrier:**  Unknown.

**References:**
Van Praagh R, et al.: Diagnosis of the anatomic types of single or common ventricle (Review). Am J Cardiol 1965; 15:345.
De la Cruz MV, Miller BL: Double-inlet left ventricle: two pathological specimens with comments on the embryology and on its relation to single ventricle. Circulation 1968; 37:249.
Goldberg SJ, et al.: Pediatric and adolescent echocardiography. Chicago: Year Book Medical Publishers, 1975.
Seward J, et al.: Preoperative and postoperative echocardiographic observations in common ventricle. Circulation 1975; 52 (Suppl II):46.
Gessner IH, et al.: The vectorcardiogram in double inlet left ventricle, with and without ventricular inversion. In: Hoffman I, ed: Vectorcardiography. Amsterdam: North Holland Publishing Co, 1976.
Foale R, et al.: Double-inlet ventricle. Two dimensional echocardiographic findings (abstr). Circulation 1980; 62:III-332.

GE013                                    Ira H. Gessner
EL004                                    Larry P. Elliott
MI020                                    B. Lynn Miller

## VENTRICLE, SINGLE LEFT PAPILLARY MUSCLE    0582

**Includes:**
   Left ventricle, single papillary muscle
   Parachute mitral valve

**Excludes:**  Mitral stenosis, other anatomic forms of congenital

**Major Diagnostic Criteria:**  Short of direct visualization, this parachute deformity is best demonstrated by two-dimensional echocardiograph. Its hemodynamic significance is best assessed by cardiac catheterization.

**Clinical Findings:**  In its pure form, this entity consists of a mitral valve with normal leaflets and commissures. The chordae tendineae, however, are thickened, shortened and converge into a single or nearly single papillary muscle, much as the shrouds of a parachute, hence the descriptive name. While the leaflets and commissures are normal, the short, thickened chordae tendineae with their single point of insertion may severely compromise the effective mitral valve orifice as blood must flow through the interchordal spaces. In addition, the normal mobility of the leaflets is lacking because of the thickened chordae. The clinical manifestations, then, are those of mitral stenosis.

The symptomatology is quite variable and dependent on the presence, or absence, of associated lesions. In general, however, symptoms lead to a diagnosis of congenital heart disease early in life. Dyspnea, congestive heart failure and pulmonary infections are common presenting complaints. Right ventricular hypertrophy can usually be detected during physical examination. A systolic murmur at the apex and accentuated first and second sounds are frequent auscultatory findings. The classic diastolic murmur of mitral stenosis is variable. If a diastolic murmur is present, it may be secondary to increased flow from an associated left-to-right shunt lesion. However, if the murmur has a presystolic accentuation, anatomic mitral valve obstruction should be suspected. Unlike acquired mitral stenosis, the opening snap is an infrequent finding. Either an associated obstructive lesion or congestive heart failure may mask the characteristic murmur.

The chest film may show pulmonary venous obstruction and an enlarged heart with discrete left atrial enlargement. The cardiogram will reflect right-sided enlargement and left atrial enlargement. It cannot be overemphasized, however, that the characteristic physical and laboratory findings may be masked by coexisting lesions.

Coexisting left heart lesions have been stressed in most case reports. These include supravalvar stenosing ring of the mitral valve, aortic stenosis, subaortic stenosis and coarctation of the aorta. Additionally, fibroelastotic changes in the left heart are not uncommon. In at least three cases, however, right ventricular outflow tract obstruction, either at the pulmonic valve or below, has been reported.

Two-dimensional echocardiograph generally delineates the architecture of the mitral valve quite well. Additionally, Doppler interrogation of the transmitral flow will indicate whether there is hemodynamic obstruction.

Cardiac catheterization data usually will show elevated pulmonary artery and pulmonary arterial wedge pressures secondary to obstruction; however, a simultaneous comparison of left atrial pressure with left ventricular diastolic pressure is mandatory to confirm a pressure difference across the valve. As with the clinical findings, catheterization data may be misleading because of associated defects.

**Complications:** Frequent pulmonary infections, growth failure and death from congestive heart failure.

**Associated Findings:** None known.

**Etiology:** Unknown.

**Pathogenesis:** Unknown.

**Sex Ratio:** Presumably M1:F1

**Occurrence:** Undetermined. About eight percent of congenital mitral stenosis is accompanied by this parachute deformity.

**Risk of Recurrence for Patient's Sib:** Unknown.

**Risk of Recurrence for Patient's Child:** Unknown.

**Age of Detectability:** In the neonatal period by clinical evaluations, echocardiography and cardiac catheterizations.

**Gene Mapping and Linkage:** Unknown.

**Prevention:** None known. Genetic counseling indicated.

**Treatment:** Symptomatic therapy for congestive heart failure and respiratory infections, with operative intervention for the severe forms.

**Prognosis:** Depends on the associated lesions. Most patients are severely symptomatic and die in early childhood. Recently, several successful valve replacements have been reported in children in whom the associated cardiac lesions were not severe. The long-term prognosis for the operative children is not known.

**Detection of Carrier:** Unknown.

**Special Considerations:** Congenital mitral stenosis is a very rare lesion. The parachute deformity of the mitral valve is only one form. Undoubtedly there are reported cases of congenital mitral stenosis which include this deformity. Its frequency as a cause of hemodynamic abnormality is not now known. Its significance is related to the inability to correct this lesion with conservative valvotomy. Thus, a decision for the necessity of surgical intervention must include the probability of mitral valve replacement.

**References:**
Shone JD, et al.: The developmental complex of "parachute mitral valve," supravalvular ring of left atrium, subaortic stenosis and coarctation of aorta. Am J Cardiol 1963; 11:714–725. * †
Terzaki AK, et al.: Successful surgical treatment for "parachute mitral valve" complex: report of 2 cases. J Thorac Cardiovasc Surg 1968; 56:1–10.
Simon AL, et al.: The angiographic features of a case of parachute mitral valve. Am Heart J 1969; 77:809–813.
Glancy DL, et al.: Parachute mitral valve: further observations and associated lesions. Am J Cardiol 1971; 27:309–313.
Ruckman NR, et al.: Anatomic types of congenital mitral stenosis: report of 49 autopsy cases with consideration of diagnosis and surgical implications. Am J Cardiol 1978; 42:592–601. * †
Grenadier E, et al.: Two-dimensional echo Doppler study of congenital disorder of the mitral valve. Am Heart J 1984; 107:319–325.

MI019                                          **Robert H. Miller**

**Ventricle, single with rudimentary outflow chamber**
*See VENTRICLE, SEPTUM DEXTROPOSITION AND DOUBLE INLET LEFT VENTRICLE*
**Ventricle, two-chambered right**
*See VENTRICLE, OBSTRUCTION WITHIN RIGHT VENTRICLE OR ITS OUTFLOW TRACT*

## VENTRICLES, INVERTED WITH TRANSPOSITION OF GREAT ARTERIES                    0540

**Includes:**
> Atrioventricular discordance with ventriculoarterial discordance
> Corrected transposition of great vessels/arteries
> Inverted transposition of great arteries
> L-transposition with situs solitus
> Ventricular inversion with L-transposition (L-TGV)

**Excludes:**
> Common ventricle with inversion of infundibular chamber
> Double inlet left ventricle
> D-transposition
> **Heart, transposition of great vessels** (0962)
> L-transposition with rudimentary ventricle
> Single ventricle with L-transposition
> **Ventricles, inverted without transposition of great arteries** (0541)

**Major Diagnostic Criteria:** Ventricular inversion with L-transposition confirmed by two-dimensional echocardiography or by contrast ventriculography.

**Clinical Findings:** The hemodynamic findings in ventricular inversion with L-TGV define this malformation. The systemic venous blood enters a normally placed right atrium and then passes to the smooth-walled left ventricle through a bicuspid atrioventricular valve which has fibrous continuity with the pulmonary valve. Blood is ejected into a posterior, medial, and rightward pulmonary trunk before passing into the lungs. The pulmonary venous return empties into a normal left atrium before passage across a tricuspid atrioventricular valve (which is commonly abnormal) to the coarsely trabeculated right ventricle. Finally blood is ejected into the anterior and leftward aorta. The tricuspid atrioventricular valve and aortic valve are separated by the crista supraventricularis and the aortic valve is in a superior position when compared with the pulmonic valve, a reversal of the usual positions. Thus, in this malformation there is atrioventricular discordance and ventriculoarterial discordance. The coronary artery distribution is also abnormal with the right coronary artery arising above the right aortic sinus and giving origin of the anterior descending branch. The left coronary artery arises above the left sinus and traverses posteriorly giving rise to the conal branch and posterior descending artery. Also notable is the malposition of the ventricular conduction system with the AV node, His bundle and bundle branches mirror image in distribution. As a result these patients may have varying degrees of atrioventricular block. Disturbances in conduction/rhythm occur in approximately 60% of patients. Complete heart block occurs in 20–55% of patients while first degree atrioventricular block is seen in 60% of cases. Supraventricular tachycardia, atrial fibrillation, and Wolff-Parkinson-White syndrome may also occur.

The symptoms and physical findings in these patients are generally related to their associated lesions. When no associated malformations are found, these patients may live normal lives with essentially normal life expectancy. In those patients with associated lesions, 75 percent have symptoms in the first month of life. The associated lesions are generally large ventricular septal defects, with or without pulmonary artery obstruction, and the presenting symptoms include those of heart failure with large left-to-right shunts or cyanosis and apnea with pulmonary artery obstruction and right-to-left shunts. Physical examination commonly demonstrates a loud second sound which is frequently palpable at the midleft sternal border and is due to the anatomic position of the semilunar valves. The loudness of this sound is thus due to the proximity of the anterior aortic valve to the chest wall and occurs with aortic valve closure. The pulmonic component is not heard. A soft systolic ejection murmur at the mid-left sternal border from turbulence with ejection into the pulmonary artery is heard in patients without associated defects. Left AV valve (tricuspid) lesions are frequent and generally cause insufficiency, heard as a holosystolic murmur at the lower left sternal border. When pulmonic stenosis is present, a harsh systolic ejection murmur may be auscultated at the mid or lower left sternal border. A ventricular septal defect may cause a harsh murmur at the lower left sternal border.

Commonly associated malformations in this anomaly include: 1) ventricular septal defects in up to 80% of cases. These are generally large, perimembranous defects. Other types of VSDs such as supracristal, muscular, or "swiss-cheese" defects may be seen less commonly; 2) pulmonic stenosis in approximately 70% of patients. The area of stenosis can be either valvar or subvalvar; 3) systemic atrioventricular valve insufficiency in approximately 30% of patients, most of which have Ebstein-like malformation that can also obstruct the right ventricular outflow; 4) rhythm disturbances. Much less commonly associated malformations include: 5) atrial septal defect, 6) patent ductus arteriosus, 7) malpositions of cardiac apex, such as dextroversion, mirror-image dextrocardia, or levoversion; 8) coarctation of the aorta; 9) mitral or tricuspid atresia; 10) situs inversus viscera. Anomalies of pulmonary and systemic venous return are rarely associated.

The chest radiograph of patients with ventricular inversion, L-transposition, and no associated defects may be normal. However, non-diagnostic findings may be noted. A narrow mediastinum with a "straight left heart border" can occur with absence of the pulmonary artery knob or bump, due to the anterior position of the aorta. Occasionally there is hilar prominence of a right pulmonary artery segment which appears elevated with respect to the left. This is the so-called "waterfall" appearance of the right hilus. Cardiomegaly, increased pulmonary vascular markings, and left atrial enlargement may be present. These may be secondary to left-to-right shunt or left AV valve insufficiency. When predominant right-to-left shunting occurs, a prominent left upper heart border bulge may occur due to ascending aorta dilation. If situs solitus and dextroversion are present, the diagnosis of ventricular inversion and L-transposition is correct in approximately 80%.

Electrocardiographic findings include abnormal reversal of the precordial Q wave pattern and clockwise rotation of the frontal plane QRS loops. Left axis deviation is common and both ventricular and atrial enlargement may occur. Rhythm disturbances include first degree AV block, complete AV block, atrial fibrillation, and Wolff-Parkinson-White syndrome.

Echocardiography may be diagnostic with two-dimensional and Doppler examination. The parasternal short axis view can demonstrate the rightward, posterior and medial pulmonary artery and leftward and anterior aorta, as well as right-sided mitral valve. The apical or subxiphoid four-chamber view may show ventricular septal and atrial septal anatomy, respectively, as well as the AV valve anatomy. A trabeculated left-sided ventricle with an infundibular chamber leftward and anteriorly may be demonstrated. Flow patterns of AV valve insufficiency and direction of shunts may be shown by Doppler.

Cardiac catheterization and angiography will show the catheter course from venous ventricle to the posterior, medial pulmonary artery and from systemic ventricle to the anterior aorta. Ventriculography demonstrate the side-by-side position of the ventricles and ventricular septal orientation. The venous ventricle is generally triangular in shape. The systemic trabeculated ventricle is rounded and leftward with an infundibular chamber which is bordered superiorly by the crista supraventricularis. The pulmonary trunk is midline while the aorta is superior and leftward. The shunts and valvar insufficiency may also be ascertained at catheterization. Coronary artery pattern can be outlined by selective aortography.

**Complications:** Most commonly includes conduction defects, left AV valve insufficiency, and congestive heart failure. Other complications include bacterial endocarditis and recurrent pneumonia.

**Associated Findings:** Associated cardiovascular anomalies are common. These include: 1) ventricular septal defects; 2) pulmonary stenosis; 3) left atrioventricular valve insufficiency with Ebstenoid malformation; 4) malposition of the cardiac apex; 5) rhythm disturbances; 6) atrial septal defects; 7) patent ductus arteriosus; 8) coarctation of aorta; 9) mitral atresia; 10) tricuspid

atresia and situs inversus of the viscera. Anomalies of systemic or pulmonary venous return may be encountered rarely.

**Etiology:** Multifactorial inheritance.

**Pathogenesis:** Abnormal rotation of the bulboventricular loop during the third to fourth week of gestation. De la Cruz et al. proposed bulboventricular loop twisting leftward instead of rightward with lack of spiral rotation of the conotruncal septum as the major abnormality. Grant proposed this defect to be a disturbance of "polarity" of conotruncal development with the primary defect being the formation of L-loop in situs solitus and D-loop in situs inversus, with secondary loss of truncal septum coiling.

**MIM No.:** 12100

**Sex Ratio:** M1.6:F1

**Occurrence:** About 1:22,000 live births.

**Risk of Recurrence for Patient's Sib:** Estimated at 1.5%.

**Risk of Recurrence for Patient's Child:** Unknown.

**Age of Detectability:** From birth by echocardiography and angiography. Fetal echocardiography is becoming able to diagnose anatomy and rhythm disturbance.

**Gene Mapping and Linkage:** Unknown.

**Prevention:** None known. Genetic counseling indicated.

**Treatment:** Treatment of fetal complete AV block is presently being studied and pacemaker placement shortly after birth is technically feasible if required. Repair of the ventricular septal defect, pulmonic stenosis, and AV valve insufficiency (repair or prosthesis) may be necessary in some cases. Permanent pacemaker implantation may also be required.

**Prognosis:** This is dependent on associated malformations. Those patients with no associated defects potentially have normal life expectancy. Sudden death due to dysrhythmias may occur. Approximately 60% of patients with associated cardiac anomalies die in the first year of life or in late adolescence due to chronic cardiac failure. Surgical therapy is more difficult technically with the right coronary artery course across the pulmonary outflow tract.

**Detection of Carrier:** Unknown.

**References:**
Van Praagh R, Van Praagh S: Isolated ventricular inversion. a consideration of the morphogenesis, definition, and diagnosis of nontransposed and transposed great arteries. Am J Cardiol 1966; 17:395–406.
Allwork SP, et al.: Congenitally corrected transposition of the great arteries. morphologic study of 32 cases. Am J Cardiol 1976; 38:910–923. *
Van Praagh R, et al.: Anatomically corrected malposition of the great arteries (S.D.L.). Circulation 1975; 51:20–31.
Westerman GR, et al.: Corrected transposition and repair of associated intracardiac defects. Circulation 1982; 66(Suppl I):1–197.

BR014
T0014

**J. Timothy Bricker**
**Jeffrey A. Towbin**

---

## VENTRICLES, INVERTED WITHOUT TRANSPOSITION OF GREAT ARTERIES     0541

**Includes:**
   Inversion of ventricles without reversal of arterial trunks
   Ventricular inversion, isolated

**Excludes:** Ventricles, inverted with transposition of great arteries (0540)

**Major Diagnostic Criteria:** Ventricles inverted without transposition of great arteries. Selective arterial and venous ventriculography are essential to the anatomic confirmation of this entity.

**Clinical Findings:** The atria, ventricles and their atrioventricular valves are identical to those described for inversion of the ventricles with transposition of the great vessels. Systemic venous blood enters a normally located right atrium and passes through a morphologic mitral valve into a morphologic left ventricle. The aorta, however, arises posteriorly and to the right of the pulmonary artery from the right-sided morphologic left ventricle. The pulmonary veins empty into a normally located left atrium. Blood passes through a morphologic tricuspid valve into a morphologic right ventricle from which the pulmonary trunk arises anteriorly and to the left of the aorta. The right coronary artery arises above the right lateral aortic valve sinus and gives rise to the anterior descending coronary artery. The left coronary artery arises above the left aortic valve sinus and gives rise to the left marginal artery and distal circumflex coronary artery. As in essentially all forms of inversion with 2 ventricles, the coronary artery pattern is inverted. From the side, the great vessels do not appear transposed because the aorta is posterior to the pulmonary trunk. In the frontal view, the aorta lies to the left of the pulmonary trunk, and its ascending portion may be convex to the left. Thus, anatomically, the great vessels are not considered transposed because the anterior leaflet of the mitral valve is in continuity with aortic valve tissue.

As the hemodynamics are the same as in complete transposition of the great arteries, patients having this entity have similar signs and symptoms. In other words, the aorta arises from the venous ventricle and the pulmonary trunk arises from the arterial ventricle. Maintenance of life depends primarily on the associated defects. With only a patent foramen ovale or small atrial septal defect, cyanosis is apparent at birth, and congestive heart failure and poor weight gain occur early in life. A soft systolic murmur, grade 2/6 or less, is heard and the second heart sound is single. If a large ventricular septal defect (VSD) is also present, allowing good mixing of the arterial and venous streams and also an increased pulmonary blood flow, cyanosis is minimal; but congestive heart failure, repeated respiratory infections and poor weight gain are commonly seen. Such patients have a loud systolic murmur and thrill along the lower left sternal border and a diastolic flow murmur over the midprecordium and apex.

The ideal set of associated anomalies is a large VSD and an appropriate degree of pulmonary stenosis. The VSD allows excellent mixing at the ventricular level, and the pulmonary stenosis prevents volume overload of the heart and congestive heart failure. Such patients have a normal sized heart, a single component of S₂ and a harsh systolic murmur along the left sternal border. These patients have mild-to-moderate cyanosis at rest, increasing with activity. With age, cyanosis gradually increases, exercise tolerance decreases and clubbing develops. Besides VSD and various types of right ventricular outflow tract obstruction, patent ductus arteriosus and right aortic arch have been observed.

Analysis of the electrovectorcardiogram shows that the initial QRS forces are directed abnormally to the left and slightly anteriorly. The QRS loop shows slowing of ventricular depolarization, but the pattern of the intraventricular block is not classic right or left heart block. This QRS loop is so inscribed as to record either a QR or R complex in the right precordial leads. This QR pattern, in itself, always suggests inversion of the ventricles. The axis varies from mild right axis deviation to mild left axis deviation.

The echocardiographic demonstration of a right-sided mitral valve and a left-sided tricuspid valve in the presence of ventricular inversion is extremely difficult. Single-crystal findings have appeared unreliable although it has been reported that tricuspid valves can be identified by their lack of semilunar continuity and mitral valves by the presence of semilunar continuity. This is an extremely difficult differential to achieve. High resolution real-time cross-sectional echocardiographic systems can differentiate the morphology of tricuspid and mitral valves as well as their relationship to the atrioventricular septum for the determination of the ventricular situs. The abnormal orientation of ventricles as well as the ventricular septum in this disorder sometimes makes the M-mode differential diagnosis between these disorders and forms of single ventricle extremely difficult.

Chest X-rays are identical to cases with inversion of the ventricles with transposition. With large communications between the 2 circulations, the pulmonary vascularity is prominent and of the shunt type. In the presence of a severe degree of obstruction to pulmonary blood flow, pulmonary vascularity is diminished. There is a relatively higher incidence of right aortic arch.

Cardiac catheterization provides data similar to that obtained in cases of complete transposition of the great arteries. Ventricular angiocardiography is identical to that described for inversion of the ventricles. The diagnosis is based upon the site of origin of the great vessels and the relationship of the right AV valve with aortic valvar tissue. In the AP view, the aorta appears transposed in that it arises to the left of the pulmonary trunk. In the lateral view, however, the great vessels appear normally related. The aorta arises posterior to the pulmonary trunk and there is a fibrous continuity between the anterior leaflet of the right-sided bicuspid AV valve and the aortic valve. The pulmonary trunk arises from the right ventricular infundibulum. The pulmonary valve is superior and anterior to the aortic valve. Associated intracardiac or extracardiac anomalies will be defined in the conventional manner. Another important angiocardiographic finding is the anterior descending coronary artery arising from the right coronary artery as is typical in all cases with the basic ventricular arrangement of inversion of the ventricles with or without transposition of the great arteries.

**Complications:** Congestive heart failure, recurrent respiratory infections, growth failure are the common complications in infancy. In older individuals, polycythemia and its sequelae are the rule.

**Associated Findings:** None known.

**Etiology:** Unknown.

**Pathogenesis:** Inversion of the ventricles without transposition of the great arteries is due to two embryologic errors: inversion of the bulboventricular loop and that pathologic abnormality which, occurring with a normally developing loop, will result in transposition of the great arteries.

**MIM No.:** 12100

**Sex Ratio:** Presumably M1:F1

**Occurrence:** Undetermined. Less than a dozen cases reported.

**Risk of Recurrence for Patient's Sib:** Unknown.

**Risk of Recurrence for Patient's Child:** Unknown.

**Age of Detectability:** From birth, by selective ventriculography.

**Gene Mapping and Linkage:** Unknown.

**Prevention:** None known. Genetic counseling indicated.

**Treatment:** Palliative surgery in infancy varies with the hemodynamic state. With marked increased pulmonary blood flow, pulmonary artery banding and creation of an atrial septal defect are advised. In those patients with inadequate mixing, a balloon catheter atrial septostomy or Blalock-Hanlon procedure is advisable. With severe right ventricular outflow tract obstruction, a shunt procedure may be indicated. Corrective surgery using the Mustard procedure and correcting the associated defects is feasible.

Therapy for congestive heart failure and upper respiratory infections.

**Prognosis:** Depends on the associated defects. Best prognosis is when a large VSD and moderate pulmonic stenosis are present. Because of the paucity of cases reported or recognized, no further statements can be made in regard to morbidity, mortality or life expectancy.

**Detection of Carrier:** Unknown.

**References:**

Van Praagh R, Van Praagh S: Isolated ventricular inversion: a consideration of the morphogenesis, definition and diagnosis of nontransposed and transposed great arteries. Am J Cardiol 1966; 17:395.

Van Mierop LHS: The heart. In: Netter FH, ed: Ciba collection of medical illustrations. vol. 5. Summit, N.J.: Ciba Publishing, 1969: 118.

Solinger R, et al.: Deductive echocardiographic analysis in infants with congenital heart disease. Circulation 1974; 50:1072.

Henry WL, et al.: Evaluation of atrial ventricular valve morphology in congenital heart disease by real-time cross-sectional echocardiography. Circulation 1975; 50(suppl II):120.

Silverman NH, Snider AR: Two-dimensional echocardiography in congenital heart disease. Connecticut: Appleton-Century-Crofts, 1982.

EL004
SC013

**Larry P. Elliott**
**Gerold L. Schiebler**
*L.H.S. Van Mierop*

**Ventricular cyst of larynx**
See *LARYNGOCELE*
**Ventricular fibrillation with prolonged Q-T interval**
See *ARRHYTHMIA, WITH LONG QT INTERVAL WITHOUT DEAFNESS*
**Ventricular hypertrophy, hereditary**
See *HEART, SUBAORTIC STENOSIS, MUSCULAR*
**Ventricular inversion with L-transposition**
See *VENTRICLES, INVERTED WITH TRANSPOSITION OF GREAT ARTERIES*
**Ventricular inversion, isolated**
See *VENTRICLES, INVERTED WITHOUT TRANSPOSITION OF GREAT ARTERIES*
**Ventricular muscle bands, aberrant right**
See *VENTRICLE, OBSTRUCTION WITHIN RIGHT VENTRICLE OR ITS OUTFLOW TRACT*
**Ventricular myocardium, aplasia of right**
See *VENTRICLE, RIGHT, UHL ANOMALY*
**Ventricular preexcitation**
See *ARRHYTHMIA, WOLFF-PARKINSON-WHITE TYPE*

## VENTRICULAR SEPTAL DEFECT                    0989

**Includes:**
Aneurysm of membranous septum with one or more perforations
Cranioacrofacial syndrome
Eisenmenger complex
Membranous septal defect
Muscular septum, defects in various portions of
Rabenhorst syndrome
Ventricular septal defect, supracristal

**Excludes:**
**Heart, endocardial cushion defects** (0347)
**Heart, tetralogy of Fallot** (0938)

**Major Diagnostic Criteria:** For patients with small defects who are asymptomatic and have normal X-ray and EKG, the hallmark of diagnosis is the characteristic VSD murmur. For symptomatic patients and those who have evidence of abnormal hemodynamic overloads, cardiac catheterization can confirm the diagnosis and establish the hemodynamic state. Most defects 3 mm in diameter can be diagnosed with cross section echocardiography.

**Clinical Findings:** The position of single or multiple defects of the ventricular septum is variable; however, the associated hemodynamic changes are due primarily to the size of the defect. Clinical assessment should be made on the basis of size of the defect, the magnitude of the left-to-right shunt, and the resistance to blood flow through the lungs. The spectrum of clinical findings can be divided into 3 categories: small ventricular septal defects, moderate-to-large defects with large pulmonary blood flow and mild-to-moderate elevation of pulmonary vascular resistance, and large ventricular septal defects with marked elevation of pulmonary vascular resistance and normal-to-diminished pulmonary blood flow.

*Small Ventricular Defects* have minimal hemodynamic changes and clinical manifestations are inapparent. A harsh systolic murmur along the lower left sternal border is the characteristic finding. Components of the second sound are usually normal. The X-ray findings demonstrate a normal sized heart with normal pulmonary vascularity. The EKG usually is normal or has early biventricular hypertrophy pattern. Some patients, however, demonstrate left axis deviation which possibly is due to an associated anomaly of the left ventricular conduction system. An aneurysm of the membranous septum causes no symptoms unless large enough to obstruct right ventricular outflow.

*Moderate-to-Large Ventricular Defect* with increased pulmonary blood flow and mild-to-moderate elevation of pulmonary vascular resistance: the clinical manifestations are primarily determined by the magnitude of pulmonary blood flow. Congestive heart failure occurs in approximately one-third of these patients between 1–3 months of age. After 12–16 months of age, large left-to-right shunts are usually tolerated without severe heart failure. The usual systolic murmur is located along the left sternal border and is usually decrescendo in nature. An early faint diastolic blow in the pulmonic area is rarely present as a result of pulmonary insufficiency. There is an apical diastolic murmur of increased mitral flow across the mitral valve. The second sound is loud and usually closely split in those patients with high pulmonary artery pressure. The X-ray demonstrates cardiomegaly and increased pulmonary vascularity commensurate with the magnitude of the left-to-right shunt. In infants, associated pulmonary venous congestion may be evident. Left atrial enlargement usually is present. The EKG demonstrates combined ventricular hypertrophy and left atrial enlargement as a rule.

*Large Ventricular Septal Defect* with high pulmonary vascular resistance and approximately normal pulmonary blood flow: the major hemodynamic overload is right ventricular hypertension, which is tolerated well throughout early childhood. There are no symptoms throughout infancy and cyanosis is rare until later childhood. Growth proceeds normally. There is no VSD murmur; however, there is frequently a pulmonic ejection murmur in the second left interspace which may be associated with an early diastolic blow of pulmonary insufficiency. The second sound is loud and single. Apical diastolic murmurs are absent. The roentgenographic findings demonstrate a normal to minimally enlarged heart, right ventricular hypertrophy, prominent main pulmonary artery segment and increased hilar markings. There is pronounced contrast between the prominent central pulmonary arterial vessels and the diminished markings in the outer third of the lung field in some cases. The EKG demonstrates right ventricular hypertrophy and right axis deviation. Left atrial and left ventricular hypertrophy are absent. Cardiac catheterization will confirm the presence of a defect, the magnitude of shunting present, the pulmonary vascular resistance and the work load on the left ventricle. Oxygen saturation data and indicator dilution curves are important in assessing systemic and pulmonary blood flow, detection of the site of shunt and evaluating bidirectional shunts.

Echocardiograph is useful to estimate the size of the defect, the degree of left atrial and ventricular enlargement, and to identify any associated defects.

**Complications:** Death from congestive heart failure and pneumonia; especially in infancy. Bacterial endocarditis. Development of high pulmonary vascular resistance. Aortic insufficiency occasionally occurs.

**Associated Findings:** An increasingly wide range of associated findings are being reported, including complex syndromes and chromosomal anomalies.

**Etiology:** Presumably multifactorial inheritance. A high prevalence has been noted in association with chromosomal trisomies.

**Pathogenesis:** Failure of closure of the subaortic portion of ventricular septum, with anomalous development of any one or several components, i.e. embryonic muscular septum, the endocardial cushions, and conal swellings. Muscular defects may be due to failure of increasing muscle mass to obliterate intratrabecular spaces.

**MIM No.:** 12285

**CDC No.:** 745.4

**Sex Ratio:** M1:F1

**Occurrence:** Incidence 1:400 full-term live births; slightly higher in prematures.

**Risk of Recurrence for Patient's Sib:** About 3%.

**Risk of Recurrence for Patient's Child:** If mother is affected, the empiric risk is about 9.5%. If the father is affected, the empiric risk is about 2%.

**Age of Detectability:** From birth, by cardiac catheterization or echocardiography. Murmur usually detectable by three weeks of age.

**Gene Mapping and Linkage:** Unknown.

**Prevention:** None known. Genetic counseling indicated.

**Treatment:** Definitive surgery recommended for moderate and large defects with increased pulmonary blood flow. Medical therapy for congestive heart failure and pneumonia prior to surgery.

**Prognosis:** Patients with small defects have excellent prognosis. Without proper medical or surgical therapy, infants with heart failure have poor prognosis. Those who survive infancy with large defects and high pulmonary pressure have good prognosis during childhood. However, some with high pulmonary artery pressure develop further increases in pulmonary vascular resistance and the Eisenmenge syndrome with increased age.

**Detection of Carrier:** Unknown.

**Special Considerations:** The natural history of ventricular defects may involve dynamic changes in the physiologic state of the patient with time. This is also the most common congenital heart defect. Small defects present little physiologic overload, and these patients do well. Also, up to 80% of small ventricular defects may spontaneously close during infancy. Infants with large defects and marked increase in pulmonary blood flow may follow one of several courses between the age of six months to four years: the defect may become smaller and thereby diminish the left-to-right shunt; the size of the defect may remain constant with little change in pulmonary vascular resistance, and thereby the patient may maintain marked increased pulmonary blood flow with associated overload on the left ventricle.

After 12–18 months of age, congestive heart failure may spontaneously improve in the face of an unchanging pulmonary blood flow; in patients with large defects and marked pulmonary blood flow, hypertrophy of the infundibulum may occur with development of pulmonary stenosis; large defects may not change in size and pulmonary vascular resistance may gradually increase with ultimate reduction in pulmonary blood flow. It is this latter group which may progress from the infant picture of large pulmonary blood flow and heart failure, to the childhood state of markedly elevated pulmonary resistance (*Eisenmenger* syndrome). Note: Eisenmenger *syndrome* clinically refers to a physiologic state in which the pulmonary vascular resistance is equal to or exceeds that of the systemic vascular resistance. Eisenmenger *complex* refers specifically to a particular type of large ventricular septal defect; infracristal ventricular septal defect with overriding aorta without infundibular stenosis, which embryologically results from a hypoplasia of the conus septum.

**References:**
Hoffman JI, Rudolph AM: The natural history of ventricular septal defects in infancy. Am J Cardiol 1965; 16:634–653.
Rudolph AM: The effects of postnatal circulatory adjustments in congenital heart disease. Pediatrics 1965; 36:763–772.
Grosse FR: The Rabenhorst-syndrome: a cardio-acral-facial syndrome. Z Kinderheilk 1974; 117:109–114.
Goldberg SJ, et al.: Pediatric and adolescent echocardiography, 2nd ed. Chicago: Year Book Medical Publishers, 1980:307–328.
Nora JJ, Nora AH: Maternal transmission of congenital heart disease. Am J Cardiol 1987; 59:459–463. *
Graham TP, et al.: Defects of the ventricular septum. In: Adams FH, et al., eds: Heart disease in infants, children, and adolescents, 4th ed. Baltimore: Williams & Wilkins, 1989:189–209. *

GR002                                                    **Thomas P. Graham**

**Ventricular septal defect with absent pulmonary valve**
    *See PULMONARY VALVE, ABSENT*
**Ventricular septal defect, endocardial cushion defect type**
    *See HEART, ENDOCARDIAL CUSHION DEFECTS*
**Ventricular septal defect, supracristal**
    *See VENTRICULAR SEPTAL DEFECT*
**Ventricular septal defect-double outlet right ventricle**
    *See VENTRICLE, DOUBLE-OUTLET RIGHT WITH ANTERIOR SEPTAL DEFECT*
**Ventricular septal defect-Hirschsprung disease**
    *See HIRSCHSPRUNG DISEASE-CARDIAC DEFECT*

**Ventricular, left, endocardial fibrosis fibroelastosis**
    *See VENTRICLE, ENDOCARDIAL FIBROELASTOSIS OF LEFT VENTRICLE*
**Ventricular, left, endocardial sclerosis**
    *See VENTRICLE, ENDOCARDIAL FIBROELASTOSIS OF LEFT VENTRICLE*
**Ventricular, left, subendocardial fibroelastosis**
    *See VENTRICLE, ENDOCARDIAL FIBROELASTOSIS OF LEFT VENTRICLE*
**Ventricular, right, endocardial fibroelastosis**
    *See VENTRICLE, ENDOCARDIAL FIBROELASTOSIS OF RIGHT VENTRICLE*
**Ventriculomegaly**
    *See HYDROCEPHALY*
**Verma-Naumoff short rib-polydactyly**
    *See SHORT RIB-POLYDACTYLY SYNDROME, VERMA-NAUMOFF TYPE*

---

## VERMIS AGENESIS                                              2106

**Includes:**
    Cerebellar vermis agenesis
    Cerebello-parenchymal disorder IV

**Excludes:**
    **Cerebellar agenesis** (2011)
    **Hydrocephaly** (0481)
    **Joubert syndrome** (2908)

**Major Diagnostic Criteria:** Patients with agenesis of the vermis may be asymptomatic or show hypotonia, ataxia and incoordination. Pneumoencephalogram or CT scan show an enlarged IV ventricle.

**Clinical Findings:** Hypotonia, nystagmus, tremor, and ataxia are present.

**Complications:** Unknown.

**Associated Findings: Meningocele, Encephalocele,** agenesis of corpus callosum, cranioschisis, and heterotopias may be present.

**Etiology:** Unknown.

**Pathogenesis:** Failure of fusion of the cerebellar crest is thought to result in agenesis of the vermis. This fusion begins rostrally and the anterior part of the vermis is formed before the posterior portion. Thus, partial agenesis of the anterior vermis does not occur. The insult leading to complete agenesis occurs earlier during development than that resulting in agenesis of the posterior vermis.

**MIM No.:** *21330

**CDC No.:** 742.230

**Sex Ratio:** Unknown.

**Occurrence:** Unknown.

**Risk of Recurrence for Patient's Sib:** Unknown.

**Risk of Recurrence for Patient's Child:** Unknown.

**Age of Detectability:** In infancy, if symptomatic.

**Gene Mapping and Linkage:** Unknown.

**Prevention:** None known. Genetic counseling indicated.

**Treatment:** Undetermined.

**Prognosis:** Variable.

**Detection of Carrier:** Unknown.

**References:**
Rubinstein HS, Freeman W: Cerebellar agenesis. J Nerv Ment Dis 1940; 92:489–502.
Andermann E, et al.: Three familial midline malformation syndromes of the central nervous system: "agenesis of the corpus callosum and anterior horn cell disease; agenesis of the cerebellar vermis; and atrophy of the cerebellar vermis." BD:OAS XI(2). New York: March of Dimes Birth Defects Foundation, 1975:269.
Macchi G, Bentivoglio M: Agenesis of hypoplasia of cerebellar structures. In: Vinken PJ, Bruyn GW, eds: Congenital malformations of

the brain and skull, part 1: Handbook of clinical neurology. Amsterdam: North Holland, 1977:367–393.

GA018                                      **Bhuwan P. Garg**

**Vertebral anomalies**
*See SPONDYLOTHORACIC DYSPLASIA*
**Vertebral body hypoplasia-lethal short-limbed dwarfism**
*See DWARFISM, LETHAL, SHORT-LIMBED PLATYSPONDYLIC TYPE*
**Vesical exstrophy**
*See BLADDER EXSTROPHY*
**Vesical-ureteral reflux (VUR)**
*See VESICO-URETERAL REFLUX*

## VESICO-URETERAL REFLUX                     2408

**Includes:**
Ureteral-vesical reflux
Urinary reflux, primary, congenital, or idiopathic
Vesical-ureteral reflux (VUR)

**Excludes:**  Reflux secondary to obstructive uropathy

**Major Diagnostic Criteria:**  The presence of vesicoureteral reflux is an objective X-ray sign diagnosed by voiding cystogram, i.e., the retrograde flow of urine into the ureter(s) during micturition. Additional studies may include urine cultures, serum electrolytes, intravenous pyelography, renal sonography, radionuclide techniques, and cystoscopy.

**Clinical Findings:**  Reflux predisposes to infections of the urinary tract. Severe cases may develop pyelonephritis, hydronephrosis, and scarring of renal parenchyma, which may lead to hypertension and sometimes renal failure. The severity of reflux is graded by voiding cystogram and is based on the level of retrograde urine flow within the upper urinary tract, the presence of hydronephrosis, and the degree of ureteral distension and tortuosity.

**Complications:**  Cystitis, pyelonephritis, hydronephrosis, renal scarring, hypertension, and renal failure.

**Associated Findings:**  Reflux may be secondary to obstructive uropathy (**Urethral valves, posterior**, ureteral duplications) or neurogenic bladder, but these entities are excluded from the present discussion of primary vesicoureteral reflux.

**Etiology:**  Reflux may be familial but without a consistent pattern of inheritance.

On the basis of a family in which three brothers and their maternal grandmother were affected, Middleton et al (1975) concluded that an X-linked form may exist. None of three sisters were affected. Van den Abbeele et al (1987) reported reflux in 27 of 60 (45%) asymptomatic siblings of patients with known reflux.

Chapman et al (1985) applied complex segregation analysis to data from 88 families with at least one person with this condition. They concluded that a single major locus is the most important causal factor. The mutant allele was estimated to be dominant, with a frequency of about 0.1%. As adults, about 45% of persons with the gene would have vesico-ureteral reflux and/or reflux nephropathy, and 15% develop renal failure, compared to 0.05% and 0.001% respectively, for persons without the gene.

**Pathogenesis:**  Congenital or idiopathic reflux may be a heterogenous entity arising from a shortened intravesicular ureter or, an abnormally positioned ureteral orifice.

**MIM No.:**  19300, 31455

**CDC No.:**  753.880

**Sex Ratio:**  M1:F8

**Occurrence:**  Reported in 20–30% of school-aged females with infections of the urinary tract. This disorder is rare in Blacks.

**Risk of Recurrence for Patient's Sib:**
See Part I, *Mendelian Inheritance.*

**Risk of Recurrence for Patient's Child:**
See Part I, *Mendelian Inheritance.*

**Age of Detectability:**  During infancy or in preschool and school-aged children.

**Gene Mapping and Linkage:**  Unknown.

**Prevention:**  None known. Genetic counseling indicated.

**Treatment:**  Early detection and management is mandatory if recurrent infections and renal injury are to be prevented. Mild reflux is usually managed with prophylactic antibiotics and may resolve later in childhood or adolescence. Surgical reimplantation of the refluxing ureter(s) is recommended for moderate-to-severe degrees of reflux. Surgery may also be required in mildly affected patients who continue to have urinary tract infections despite the use of prophylactic antibiotics.

**Prognosis:**  The prevention of pyelonephritis and scarring of renal parenchyma are the prime objectives of management. Mild cases, with either no or minimal degrees of hydronephrosis, may resolve spontaneously in later childhood. Treatment is directed at preventing infection with prophylactic antibiotics until reflux resolves. In more severe cases, with moderate-to-severe hydronephrosis and tortuous distended ureters, antireflux surgery is usually advocated.

**Detection of Carrier:**  Unknown.

**References:**
Winberg J, et al.: Epidemiology of symptomatic urinary tract infections in childhood. Acta Paediatr Scand 1974; 252:S1–20. *
Middleton GW, et al.: Sex-linked familial reflux. J Urol 1975; 114:36–39.
Ransley PG, et al.: Vesicoureteral reflux: continuing surgical dilemma. Urology 1978; 12:246–255. *
Lyon RP, et al.: Treatment of vescoureteral reflux. Urology 1980; 16:38–46.
Smellie JM, et al.: Children with urinary tract infection: a comparison of those with and those without vesicoureteral reflux. Kidney Int 1981; 20:717–722. *
Woodard JR: Vesicoureteral reflux: a surgical perspective. Am J Kidney Dis 1983; 3:136–138.
Chapman CJ, et al.: Vesicoureteral reflux: segregation analysis. Am J Med Genet 1985; 20:577–584.
Van den Abbeele AD, et al.: Vesicoureteral reflux in asymptomatic siblings of patients with known reflux: radionuclide cystography. Pediatrics 1987; 79:147–153.

HY001                                      **Leonard C. Hymes**

**Vesiculocephaly**
*See COLPOCEPHALY*
**Viljoen rhizomelic dysplasia**
*See OMODYSPLASIA*
**Vinyl chloride induced scleroderma**
*See SCLERODERMA, FAMILIAL PROGRESSIVE*
**Virilization of the female from maternal extrinsic androgens**
*See FETAL EFFECTS FROM MATERNAL EXTRINSIC ANDROGENS*

## VISCERA, FATTY METAMORPHOSIS            0990

**Includes:**
Acyl-CoA dehydrogenase deficiency (some)
Carnitine deficiency, primary systemic (some)
Fatty acid oxidation disorders
Hepatic carnitine palmitoyl transferase deficiency (some)
Hypoglycemic nonketotic dicarboxylic aciduria (some)
Liver, steatosis of
"Reye syndrome-like" manifestations
Viscera, steatosis of, familial
White liver disease

**Excludes:**
**Alpha(1)-antitrypsin deficiency** (0039)
**Carnitine deficiency, systemic** (2121)
**Cerebro-hepato-renal syndrome** (0139)
Collagen storage disease
**Cystic fibrosis** (0237)
**Diabetes mellitus**
**Fructose-1-phosphate aldolase deficiency** (0395)
**Galactosemia** (0403)
**Hepatolenticular degeneration** (0469)
Histiocytosis

**Hyperlipoproteinemia, combined** (0496)
Jamaican vomiting sickness (hypoglycin A intoxication)
Lipidosis
**Phytanic acid oxidase deficiency, infantile type** (2278)
**Phytanic acid storage disease** (0810)
Reye syndrome
**Tyrosinemia**
Viscera, toxic, nutritional, and inflammatory steatosis of
**Wolman disease** (1003)

**Major Diagnostic Criteria:** A group of inborn errors of mitochondrial beta oxidation of fatty acids, most often characterized by acute attacks of vomiting, hypoketotic hypoglycemia, and acidosis, with a variable age of onset and variable degrees of hepatic, CNS, cardiac, and skeletal muscle manifestations. Pathologic findings include various degrees of fatty infiltration of liver parenchymal cells, renal tubular epithelium, myocardium, and skeletal muscle. Gas chromatography mass spectrometry (GCMS) analysis of serum and urine shows excessive accumulation and excretion of secondary metabolites of saturated fatty acids. The diagnosis is confirmed by the demonstration of decreased ability of cultured fibroblasts, mononuclear leukocytes, or liver cells and their mitochondria to oxidize radiolabeled fatty acids or, in the case **Acidemia, glutaric acidemia II, neonatal onset**, by the detection of deficiency of electron transfer flavoprotein (ETF) or electron transfer flavoprotein: ubiquinone oxidoreductase (ETF:QO) in fibroblasts, using the techniques of enzymatic assay or immunoblotting. In the case **Carnitine deficiency, systemic**, the finding of primary low serum and tissue carnitine levels is diagnostic.

**Clinical Findings:** A considerable variation exists in the clinical presentation and biochemical picture according to the type and severity of the enzyme defect. The most severe acute cases present in the neonatal period or during infancy with poor feeding, vomiting, "sweaty feet" odor (in **Acidemia, glutaric acidemia II, neonatal onset**), hepatomegaly, hyperbilirubinemia, cardiac arrhythmias, apnea, hypotonia, seizures, and lethargy progressing to coma and death. Less severe cases usually present at a later age with intermittent "Reye syndrome-like" attacks that are provoked by fasting stress and include vomiting, hepatomegaly, elevated liver enzymes, hyperammonemia, and encephalopathy. The episodes usually respond favorably to appropriate treatment, and only negligible symptoms are observed between attacks. The mildest cases are characterized by a chronic course with cardiomyopathy and/or skeletal muscle weakness. Although not the rule, most acute catastrophic cases are caused by **Acyl-CoA dehydrogenase deficiency, long chain type, Acyl-CoA dehydrogenase deficiency, medium chain type, Acidemia, glutaric acidemia II, neonatal onset**, or by **Carnitine deficiency, systemic**. The acute fatal cases are usually characterized by multisystemic fatty infiltration, whereas in milder cases only the liver, myocardium, or skeletal muscle are affected. The fatty changes in liver cells are usually of a macrovesicular type.

Biochemical features that are common to all these disorders during acute attacks include abnormal liver function tests, nonketotic hypoglycemia, metabolic acidosis, carnitine deficiency (primary or secondary), and the overproduction of omega (dicarboxylic acids) and omega-1 oxidation products of fatty acids identified by GCMS analysis of serum and urine. The latter compounds include adipic, suberic, and sebacic acids ($C_6$-$C_{10}$-dicarboxylic acids), 5(OH)hexanoic acid, 7(OH)octanoic acid, 9(OH)decanoic acid, hexanoylglycine, and suberylglycine in medium- and long-chain **Acyl-CoA dehydrogenase deficiency** and in **Carnitine deficiency, systemic**; all the above along with ethylmalonic acid, isobutyric acid, 2 methylbutyric acid, isovaleric and glutaric acids and their glycine conjugates, and sometimes sarcosine, are found in **Acidemia, glutaric acidemia II, neonatal onset**. No abnormal organic aciduria has been reported in hepatic carnitine palmitoyl tranferase deficiency.

A family history of death of sibs or clinical episodes suggestive of defective fatty acid oxidation usually exists. The clinical expression and the severity of the specific enzyme defect within a family are consistent, which suggests a complete penetrance.

**Complications:** Survivors of the acute episodes may develop permanent brain damage, severe hypotonia, and abnormal psychomotor development. The milder cases exhibit cardiomegaly, myopathy, or are free of symptoms.

**Associated Findings:** Acidemia, glutaric acidemia II, neonatal onset with deficient ETF:QO has been associated with congenital anomalies, including polycystic kidneys, renal dysgenesis, **Kidney, polycystic disease infantile potter type I**, anomalies of the abdominal wall and external genitalia, and cerebral malformations.

**Etiology:** Autosomal recessive inheritance. Only one family exhibiting an X-linked recessive mode of inheritance has been reported.

**Pathogenesis:** A defective transport of long-chain fatty acids into the mitochondria is responsible for the derangement in fatty acid oxidation in **Carnitine deficiency, systemic** and hepatic carnitine palmitoyl transferase deficiency. It is not clear whether the primary abnormality in the former is reduced carnitine biosynthesis, abnormal gastrointestinal absorption, a renal tubular defect with loss of carnitine in the urine, or abnormal carnitine transport into tissues.

Seven mitochondrial flavin adenine dinucleotide (FAD) requiring acyl-dehydrogenases, i.e., those specific for dimethylglycine, glutaryl-CoA, isovaleryl-CoA, isobutyryl CoA and 2-methylbutyryl CoA, short-chain acyl-CoA, medium-chain acyl-CoA, and long-chain acyl-CoA, appear to be defective in multiple acyl-CoA dehydrogenase deficiency. The primary biochemical abnormality is a deficiency of either ETF or ETF:QO, which are responsible for the transfer of electrons from the flavoprotein acyl-CoA dehydrogenases to the mitochondrial respiratory chain. In some patients the dehydrogenase specific for sarcosine is also involved.

In the isolated medium-chain or long-chain **Acyl-CoA dehydrogenase deficiency**, the defect is at the level of $C_6$-$C_{12}$ or $C_{12}$-$C_{18}$ chain mitochondrial beta oxidation, respectively.

**MIM No.:** *22810

**Sex Ratio:** M1:F1

**Occurrence:** Thus far, about 20 kinships have been documented.

**Risk of Recurrence for Patient's Sib:**
See Part I, *Mendelian Inheritance.*

**Risk of Recurrence for Patient's Child:**
See Part I, *Mendelian Inheritance.*

**Age of Detectability:** In neonatal period for severe cases; milder cases can be diagnosed at any age.

**Gene Mapping and Linkage:** Unknown.

**Prevention:** None known. Genetic counseling indicated.

**Treatment:** During acute attacks, intravenous glucose and mannitol, mechanical ventilation, muscle relaxants, and intracranial pressure monitoring. Riboflavin or carnitine administration during acute episodes have only been successful in a few cases. Medical and supportive therapy for chronic cardiomyopathy and skeletal myopathy. Chronic carnitine treatment for **Carnitine deficiency, systemic**.

**Prognosis:** The acute catastrophic cases, especially those associated with **Acyl-CoA dehydrogenase deficiency, long chain type, Acyl-CoA dehydrogenase deficiency, medium chain type, and Acidemia, glutaric acidemia II, neonatal onset**, usually result in rapid deterioration and death, despite aggressive treatment. Survivors may develop permanent brain damage. Milder cases may have acute episodes during fasting, or may suffer from cardiac or skeletal muscle abnormalities, but usually have normal life span and normal intelligence.

**Detection of Carrier:** Intermediate levels of acyl-CoA dehydrogenase activity or, in the case of **Acidemia, glutaric acidemia II, neonatal onset**, intermediate ETF/ETF:QO activity in cultured fibroblasts or mononuclear leukocytes. No conclusions on the detection of carriers in **Carnitine deficiency, systemic** or hepatic carnitine palmitoyl transferase deficiency have been formulated.

**Special Considerations:** The fasting-induced nonketotic hypoglycemia observed in this group of disorders is a result of the defective oxidation of fatty acids, which normally produces ketone bodies during fasting and increases gluconeogenesis flux by providing the acetyl-CoA and the reducing equivalents (NADH) necessary for gluconeogenesis. The carnitine deficiency found in all acyl-CoA dehydrogenase deficiency disorders is due to the sequestration of carnitine as acyl-carnitine. The origin of the excessive accumulation of fatty acid metabolites in the beta oxidation disorders is the alternative omega and omega-1 oxidation of fatty acids to dicarboxylic acids and omega-1 hydroxy-monocarboxylic acids, respectively, in the microsomes (cytochrome P-450 system), further beta oxidation of these compounds in the peroxisomes, and alternative glycine conjugation. The accumulated fatty acid metabolites are toxic and probably contribute directly to the hepatocerebral toxicity by uncoupling oxidative phosphorylation and by interfering with neuronal membrane function.

In *Mendelian Inheritance in Man* (McKusick, 1988), a heterogenous group of case reports, published in the medical literature between 1964 and 1984, is summarized under the histologic, descriptive heading "Fatty Metamorphosis of Viscera." No detailed biochemical studies, specifically GCMS analysis and enzymatic studies, were performed in any, but one, of those cases. Based on analysis of the cases and the knowledge gathered over the last decade concerning the biochemical lesions and abnormal metabolic blocks in fatty acid degradation, it seems reasonable to conclude that most, if not all, of these case reports belong to the group of inherited inborn errors of mitochondrial fatty acid oxidation described here. Increased awareness of these inherited conditions, especially in patients presenting with "Reye syndrome-like" manifestations, and performance of detailed metabolic investigations will probably result in the detection of many other cases.

**References:**

Gregersen N, et al.: Suberylglycine excretion in the urine from a patient with dicarboxylic aciduria. Clin Chim Acta 1976; 70:417–425.
Chesney RW, et al.: A three-month-old infant with seizures, hypoglycemia, and apnea. Am J Med Genet 1983; 16:373–388.
Goodman SI, Frerman FE: Glutaric acidaemia type II (multiple acyl-CoA dehydrogenation deficiency). J Inherit Metab Dis 1984; 7:33–37.
Coates PM, et al.: Genetic deficiency of medium-chain acyl coenzyme A dehydrogenase: studies in cultured skin fibroblasts and peripheral mononuclear leukocytes. Pediatr Res 1985; 19:671–676.
Gregersen N: The acyl-CoA dehydrogenation deficiencies. Scand J Clin Lab Invest 1985; (suppl 174):45:1–60.
Rebouche CJ, Paulson DJ: Carnitine metabolism and function in humans. Ann Rev Nutr 1986; 6:41–66.
Moon A, Rhead WJ: Complementation analysis of fatty acid oxidation disorders. J Clin Invest 1987; 79:59–64.
Roe CR, Coates PM: Acyl-CoA dehydrogenase deficiencies. In: Scriver CR, et al, eds: The metabolic basis of inherited disease, 6th ed. New York: McGraw-Hill, 1989:889–914.

ZE004
CH038
**Israel Zelikovic**
**Russell W. Chesney**

**Viscera, steatosis of, familial**
*See VISCERA, FATTY METAMORPHOSIS*
**Visceral defects-Dandy-Walker cysts-spondylocostal dysostosis**
*See SPONDYLOCOSTAL DYSOSTOSIS-VISCERAL DEFECTS-
DANDY WALKER CYST*
**Visceral myopathy, familial**
*See MEGACYSTIS-MEGADUODENUM SYNDROME*
**Visceral myopathy, hereditary hollow**
*See MEGACYSTIS-MEGADUODENUM SYNDROME*
**Visceral myopathy-external ophthalmoplegia**
*See MUSCULAR DYSTROPHY, OCULO-GASTROINTESTINAL*
**Visceral neuropathy**
*See INTESTINAL PSEUDO-OBSTRUCTION SYNDROMES*
**Visceromegaly-umbilical hernia-macroglossia**
*See BECKWITH-WIEDEMANN SYNDROME*
**Vitamin A megadose, retinol or retinaldehyde fetal effects of**
*See FETAL RETINOID SYNDROME*
**Vitamin B binding protein**
*See TRANSCOBALAMIN II DEFICIENCY*
**Vitamin B dependency with convulsions**
*See SEIZURES, VITAMIN B(6) DEPENDENCY*

**Vitamin B lysosomal release defect**
*See VITAMIN B(12) LYSOSOMAL TRANSPORT DEFECT*
**Vitamin B storage disease**
*See VITAMIN B(12) LYSOSOMAL TRANSPORT DEFECT*

## VITAMIN B(12) LYSOSOMAL TRANSPORT DEFECT      2994

**Includes:**

Cobalamin, defect in lysosomal release of
Cobalamin F disease
Methylmalonicaciduria due to B(12) release defect
Vitamin B(12) lysosomal release defect
Vitamin B(12) storage disease

**Excludes:**

Acidemia, methylmalonic (0658)
Combined methylmalonic aciduria-homocystinuria diseases
Methylcobalamin deficiency (2605)
Transcobalamin II deficiency (2624)

**Major Diagnostic Criteria:** Methylmalonic aciduria responsive to therapy with vitamin $B_{12}$; decreased whole cell synthesis of adenosyl-$B_{12}$ and methyl-$B_{12}$ in the presence of elevated unmetabolized vitamin $B_{12}$ in lysosomes. Complementation with cbl C and cbl D fibroblast lines.

**Clinical Findings:** Stomatitis, glossitis, multifocal seizures, hypotonia, developmental delay, feeding difficulties.

**Complications:** Unknown.

**Associated Findings:** In one unpublished case, sudden infant death.

**Etiology:** Presumably autosomal recessive inheritance.

**Pathogenesis:** Defect in transfer of free vitamin $B_{12}$ from lysosomes to cytoplasm.

**MIM No.:** 27738

**Sex Ratio:** Presumably M1:F1 (M0:F2 observed).

**Occurrence:** The index case and one additional unrelated patient have been documented since the condition was discovered in 1985.

**Risk of Recurrence for Patient's Sib:**
See Part I, *Mendelian Inheritance.*

**Risk of Recurrence for Patient's Child:**
See Part I, *Mendelian Inheritance.*

**Age of Detectability:** During the neonatal period. One unaffected sib of the proband was diagnosed prenatally.

**Gene Mapping and Linkage:** Unknown.

**Prevention:** None known. Genetic counseling indicated.

**Treatment:** The proband was treated with oral and intramuscular vitamin $B_{12}$.

**Prognosis:** Unknown.

**Detection of Carrier:** Unknown.

**Special Considerations:** Although homocystinuria and megaloblastic anemia was not detected in the original proband, the second patient did have both, as would be expected based on the combined deficiency in methyl-$B_{12}$ and adenosyl-$B_{12}$.

**References:**

Rosenblatt DS, et al.: Defect in vitamin B-12 release from lysosomes: newly described inborn error of vitamin B-12 metabolism. Science 1985; 228:1319–1321.
Rosenblatt DS, et al.: New disorder of vitamin $B_{12}$ metabolism (cobalamin F) presenting as methylmalonic aciduria. Pediatrics 1986; 78:51–54.
Watkins D, Rosenblatt DS: Failure of lysosomal release of vitamin $B_{12}$: a new complementation group causing methylmalonic aciduria (cbl F). Am J Hum Genet 1986; 39:404–408.
Shih VE, et al.: Defective lysosomal release of vitamin B12: hereditary cobalamin metabolic disorder associated with sudden death. Am J Med Genet 1989; 33:555–563.

WA053
R0052
**David Watkins**
**David S. Rosenblatt**

## VITAMIN B(12) MALABSORPTION  0992

### Includes:
Anemia, pernicous, juvenile
Cobalamin malabsorption
Ileal B(12) transport deficiency
Imerslund-Grasbeck syndrome
Malabsorption of vitamin B(12) (two types)
Pernicious anemia, juvenile-proteinuria

### Excludes:
**Anemia, pernicious congenital** (2656)
Anemia, pernicious, due to deficiency of extrinsic factor
Blind loop syndrome
Diphyllobothrium latum infestation
**Folate malabsorption** (2166)
**Transcobalamin II deficiency** (2624)

**Major Diagnostic Criteria:** Demonstration of vitamin $B_{12}$ deficiency by abnormal Schilling test, reduced serum vitamin $B_{12}$ concentration, and increased excretion of methylmalonic acid and/or homocystine in the urine. Absence of serum antibodies to intrinsic factor and gastric parietal cells. Normal gastric mucosa.

Gastric juice analysis and response to ingested intrinsic factor distinguish three forms of congenital $B_{12}$ malabsorption. Patients with deficiency of intrinsic factor (see **Anemia, pernicious congenital**) will respond clinically and chemically to ingestion of normal gastric juice or to administered intrinsic factor and $B_{12}$. Patients with functionally impaired intrinsic factor and those with ileal transport defect will have immunologically detectable intrinsic factor in gastric aspirate. Patients with functionally abnormal intrinsic factor will respond to exogenous normal intrinsic factor, while those with the transport defect will not. Patients with $B_{12}$ malabsorption due to specific ilial "receptor site" defect (*Imerslund-Grasbeck syndrome*) will respond only to parenteral administration of physiologic amounts (1 $\mu$g/day) of vitamin $B_{12}$.

**Clinical Findings:** Megaloblastic anemia noted during the first 1–3 years of life (100%): one group of children lacks gastric intrinsic factor; a second group has an immunologically identifiable, functionally defective intrinsic factor; a third group lacks the ileal transport mechanism for vitamin $B_{12}$.

**Complications:** Combined system disease of the central nervous system (CNS).

**Associated Findings:** Permanent proteinuria is noted in nearly one-half of patients with ileal transport defect. This form of the disorder is also called the *Imerslund-Gräsbeck* syndrome.

**Etiology:** Autosomal recessive inheritance of a defect affecting either the synthesis of gastric intrinsic factor or the specific vitamin $B_{12}$ transport system in the terminal ileum.

**Pathogenesis:** Deficiency of vitamin $B_{12}$ leads to megaloblastic anemia, methylmalonic aciduria, and CNS disease.

**MIM No.:** *26110

**Sex Ratio:** M1:F1

**Occurrence:** Over 50 cases have been documented; half in Finland.

**Risk of Recurrence for Patient's Sib:**
See Part I, *Mendelian Inheritance.*

**Risk of Recurrence for Patient's Child:**
See Part I, *Mendelian Inheritance.*

**Age of Detectability:** At one to two years of age.

**Gene Mapping and Linkage:** Unknown.

**Prevention:** None known. Genetic counseling indicated.

**Treatment:** Parenteral administration of vitamin $B_{12}$ (1 $\mu$g/day); blood transfusions may be required initially.

**Prognosis:** Good, if treatment initiated before permanent CNS damage ensues.

**Detection of Carrier:** Not well defined; both parents of a single patient with ileal transport defect were reported to have moderate impairment of vitamin $B_{12}$ absorption, without anemia.

**Special Considerations:** The existence of this condition provides strong evidence for single gene control of synthesis of gastric intrinsic factor, and for an ileal "receptor" in the vitamin $B_{12}$ transport process.

### References:
McIntyre OR, et al.: Pernicious anemia in childhood. New Engl J Med 1965; 272:981–986.
Mohamed SD, et al.: Juvenile familial megaloblastic anaemia due to selective malabsorption of vitamin $B_{12}$: a family study and a review of the literature. Q J Med 1966; 35:433–453.
Donaldson RH: Mechanisms of malabsorption of cobalamin. In: Babior BM, ed.: Cobalamin biochemistry and pathophysiology. New York: John Wiley & Sons, 1975:335.
Sennett C, et al.: Transmembrane transport of cobalamin in prokaryotic and eukaryotic cells. Ann Rev Biochem 1981; 50:1053–1086.
Broch H, et al.: Imerslund-Grasbeck anemia: a long-term follow-up study. Acta Paediat Scand 1984; 73:248–253.
Heisel, MA et al.: Congenital pernicious anemia: report of seven patients with studies of the extended family. J Pediatr 1984; 105:564–568.

FL001

**David B. Flannery**
*Leon E. Rosenberg*

**Vitamin D binding protein (VDBP)**
*See PLASMA, GROUP-SPECIFIC COMPONENT*
**Vitamin D dependency IIa**
*See RESISTANCE TO 1,25 DIHYDROXY VITAMIN D*
**Vitamin D-dependent rickets, hereditary**
*See RICKETS, VITAMIN D-DEPENDENT, TYPE I*
**Vitamin D-dependent rickets, type I**
*See RICKETS, VITAMIN D-DEPENDENT, TYPE I*
**Vitamin D-dependent rickets, type IIa**
*See RESISTANCE TO 1,25 DIHYDROXY VITAMIN D*
**Vitamin D-dependent rickets, type IIb**
*See RESISTANCE TO 1,25 DIHYDROXY VITAMIN D*
**Vitamin D-dependent rickets, type III, Aii-aminoaciduria**
*See RICKETS, VITAMIN D-DEPENDENT, TYPE I*
**Vitamin K-antagonist embryopathy**
*See FETAL WARFARIN SYNDROME*
**Vitelliform cysts of macula, congenital**
*See RETINA, MACULAR DEGENERATION, VITELLIRUPTIVE*
**Vitelliform macular dystrophy**
*See RETINA, MACULAR DEGENERATION, VITELLIRUPTIVE*
**Vitelline cyst**
*See OMPHALOMESENTERIC DUCT ANOMALIES*
**Vitelline duct anomalies**
*See OMPHALOMESENTERIC DUCT ANOMALIES*
**Vitelline duct, remnant**
*See MECKEL DIVERTICULUM*
**Vitelliruptive macular degeneration, hereditary**
*See RETINA, MACULAR DEGENERATION, VITELLIRUPTIVE*
**Vitiligo**
*See SKIN, VITILIGO*
**Vitiligo-deafness-muscle wasting**
*See DEAFNESS-VITILIGO-MUSCLE WASTING*
**Vitreoretinal dysplasia, X-linked**
*See NORRIE DISEASE*
**Vitreoretinal dystrophy**
*See RETINOSCHISIS*
**Vitreous, congenital vascular veils in**
*See RETINOSCHISIS*
**Vitreous, persistent hyperplastic primary (PHPV)**
*See EYE, VITREOUS, PERSISTENT HYPERPLASTIC PRIMARY*
**Vocal cord dysfunction**
*See LARYNGEAL PARALYSIS*
**Vocal cord dysfunction, adductor type**
*See VOCAL CORD PARALYSIS*
**Vocal cord dysfunction, familial**
*See LARYNGEAL ABDUCTOR PARALYSIS-MENTAL RETARDATION*
**Vocal cord paralysis**
*See LARYNGEAL PARALYSIS*

## VOCAL CORD PARALYSIS                                    2506

**Includes:**
Gerhardt syndrome
Laryngeal abductor paralysis
Paralysis of vocal cord
Plott syndrome
Vocal cord dysfunction, adductor type

**Excludes:**
Arytenoid fixation
Glottic scarring, posterior
**Laryngeal paralysis** (3080)
Vocal cord paralysis, acquired
Vocal cord web

**Major Diagnostic Criteria:** Flexible laryngoscopy demonstrates abductor paralysis of the vocal cords with paramedian positioning. May be unilateral or bilateral.

**Clinical Findings:** Symptoms of upper airway obstruction with stridor, abnormal voice or cry, a tendency for aspiration, and recurrent chest infections. Unilateral vocal cord paralysis is often undetected because of the relative paucity of symptoms.

**Complications:** Airway obstruction may be life threatening with bilateral vocal cord paralysis. Aspiration and recurrent chest infections with unilateral obstruction may also precipitate chronic problems.

**Associated Findings:** When vocal cord paralysis results from central pathology, such as Arnold-Chiari malformation (see **Anencephaly**), **Hydranencephaly** is a common occurrence. Brainstem abnormalities are also seen frequently.

May be seen with central neurologic defects which commonly affect both vocal cords, including **Meningomyelocele**, anterior horn cell degeneration, or cerebral degeneration or concussion.

**Etiology:** Congenital forms are associated with birth trauma; forceps delivery or prolonged second stage labor (80% are unilateral, with the left side involved more commonly than the right). Birth anoxia; often with resultant brainstem damage( most commonly bilateral). Idiopathic; involving an equal number of bilateral and unilateral cases. Autosomal dominant and X-linked inheritance have been reported. Holinger et al (1976) reported that paralyses are 55% congenital, 40% acquired, and 5% idiopathic.

**Pathogenesis:** Central neurologic pathology affects the vagal nuclei contained within the nucleus ambiguus, and results most frequently in bilateral paralysis. Peripheral neurologic trauma most frequently results in unilateral vocal cord paralysis secondary to recurrent laryngeal nerve damage.

**Sex Ratio:** M1:F:<1 (slight male preponderance).

**Occurrence:** The third most common congenital laryngeal anomaly, following **Laryngomalacia** and **Subglottic stenosis**.

**Risk of Recurrence for Patient's Sib:** Varies with etiology.

**Risk of Recurrence for Patient's Child:** Varies with etiology.

**Age of Detectability:** Often at birth, but may not be apparent for several weeks or months depending on onset of symptoms.

**Gene Mapping and Linkage:** Unknown.

**Prevention:** In cases of surgical trauma, careful dissection with identification of recurrent and superior laryngeal nerves will avoid the problem. Minimizing birth trauma will also decrease the frequency of such lesions.

**Treatment:** Maintain the airway and treat the precipitating pathology. Careful evaluation of the likelihood of spontaneous recovery should be made.

Unilateral vocal cord paralysis rarely causes major respiratory symptoms. Intermittent stridor, weak cry, and a tendency to chest infections may be seen. Underlying pathology should be treated and paralysis managed expectantly. Vocal cord injection to medialize the cord may be appropriate.

Bilateral vocal cord paralysis nearly always requires a tracheotomy for relief of obstruction. Further management should be based on likelihood of recovery. Many methods of vocal cord lateralization have been described as methods for improving the airway.

**Prognosis:** Outlook for spontaneous recovery depends on the etiology. Emery and Fearon (1984) report 100% recovery from birth trauma and acquired idiopathic causes; 60% recovery from peripheral trauma and central neurologic pathology; 20% recovery from congenital idiopathic causes; and 0% from birth anoxia.

**Detection of Carrier:** Unknown.

**References:**
Plott D: Congenital laryngeal-abductor paralysis due to nucleus ambiguus dysgenesis in three brothers. New Engl J Med 1964; 271:593–597.
Holinger LD, et al.: Etiology of bilateral abductor vocal cord paralysis. Ann Otol Rhinol Laryngol 1976; 85:428–436.
Cohen SR, et al.: Laryngeal paralysis in children: a long term retrospective study. Ann Otol Rhinol Laryngol 1982; 91:417–424.
Gundfast KM, Milmoe G: Congenital hereditary bilateral abductor vocal cord paralysis. Ann Otol Rhinol Laryngol 1982; 91:564–566.
Emery P, Fearon B: Vocal cord palsy in pediatric practice: a review of 71 cases. Int J Pediatr Otorhinolaryng 1984; 8:147–154.
Cunningham MJ, et al.: Familial vocal cord dysfunction. Pediatrics 1985; 76:750–753.

MY003
OR005

**Charles M. Myer III**
**Peter Orobello**

**Vogt cephalosyndactyly**
*See ACROCEPHALOSYNDACTYLY TYPE I*
**Vohwinkel syndrome**
*See DEAFNESS-KERATOPACHYDERMIA-DIGITAL CONSTRICTIONS*
**Volvulus of midgut**
*See INTESTINAL ROTATION, INCOMPLETE*
**von Bechterew disease**
*See ANKYLOSING SPONDYLITIS*
**von Eulenburg paramyotonia congenita**
*See PARAMYOTONIA CONGENITA*
**von Gierke disease**
*See GLYCOGENOSIS, TYPE Ia*

## VON HIPPEL-LINDAU SYNDROME                              0995

**Includes:**
Hemangiomatosis, multiple
Lindau disease

**Excludes:** Cerebellar tumor

**Major Diagnostic Criteria:** A retinal or cerebellar hemangioblastoma in a patient with a positive family history is indicative of the condition, or the presence of a retinal and central nervous system (CNS) hemangioblastoma in the same patient, is diagnostic.

**Clinical Findings:** The age of onset varies, but is most common in the fourth decade. There is no age at which individuals at risk can be assumed to be unaffected. The lesions are most frequent in the peripheral retina but may be seen at the disk border or macula, producing complaints of visual disturbance, particularly blurred vision. The lesion is raised, red, and globular. It is fed by a dilated arteriole and drained by a tortuous vein. The retinal lesions are multiple in about one-third of the patients. They may undergo calcification and ossification.

Hemangioblastomas involving the CNS are most common in the posterior fossa. They may be situated in the cerebellar hemispheres, vermis, or the medulla. They may be multiple; most are cystic. An intermittent occipital headache is a frequent early symptom. Vomiting, vertigo, ataxia, nystagmus, dysarthria, and dysmetria are common findings. Mental changes may accompany an increase in intracranial pressure.

The spinal cord is frequently involved, primarily in the cervical and thoracic segments. The hemangioblastoma is usually intramedullary and posterior, producing loss of sensation and proprioception. A spastic paraparesis develops with progressive cord compression.

Approximately 15% of cerebellar hemangioblastomas are associated with polycythemia. A skull X-ray may show signs of

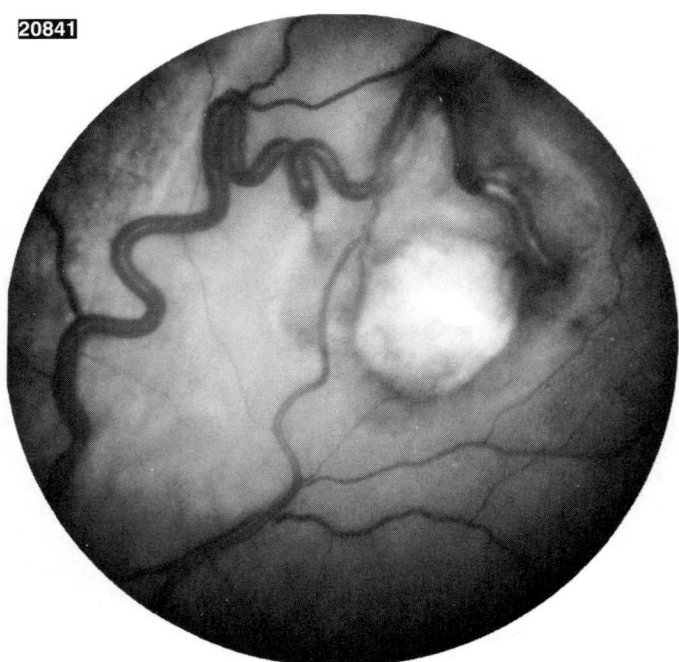

**0995-20841:** Von Hippel-Lindau syndrome; retina.

---

increased intracranial pressure. Computed axial tomography (CT) with contrast enhancement is extremely useful in the localization of the tumor. Vertebral angiography is the study of choice to define clearly the extent and vascular supply of a posterior fossa hemangioblastoma. A myelogram and selective segmental angiogram of the spinal cord will identify a spinal cord tumor. Intravenous pyelogram, renal angiography, and CT scan are used to demonstrate renal or adrenal lesions. The CT scan may also show pancreatic lesions.

**Complications:** The retinal lesions are usually progressive. Exudation occurs at the site of the tumor, causing retinal detachment and eventual blindness. Cataracts and glaucoma may occur as well. The posterior fossa hemangioblastomas produce hydrocephalus by distortion of the aqueduct of Sylvius. Herniation of the cerebellar tonsils can result. Syringomyelia has occasionally been noted in association with a spinal cord hemangioblastoma. Hypertensive crises may complicate an associated pheochromocytoma; renal carcinomas may metastasize. Diabetes mellitus can result from pancreatic involvement.

**Associated Findings:** Renal, pancreatic, hepatic, and epididymal cysts; renal carcinoma; pheochromocytoma; angiomatosis of liver, ovary, and skin; tumors of epididymis.

**Etiology:** Autosomal dominant inheritance. Most cases (80–93%) are sporadic.

**Pathogenesis:** Nervous tissue is secondarily damaged by expanding vascular hamartomatous tumors. One suggestion is that the retinal tumors result from malformation of the mesenchyma in the third month of fetal life, when the retina is vascularized and a mesenchymal plate is formed in the roof of the fourth ventricle.

**MIM No.:** *19330

**POS No.:** 3676

**CDC No.:** 759.620

**Sex Ratio:** M1:F1

**Occurrence:** 1:50,000 to 1:60,000

**Risk of Recurrence for Patient's Sib:**
See Part I, *Mendelian Inheritance.*

**Risk of Recurrence for Patient's Child:**
See Part I, *Mendelian Inheritance.*

**Age of Detectability:** Usually by the fourth decade of life, by the presence of retinal and CNS hemangioblastomas.

**Gene Mapping and Linkage:** VHL (von-Hippel Lindau syndrome) has been mapped to 3p.

**Prevention:** None known. Genetic counseling indicated.

**Treatment:** If a retinal tumor is found, photocoagulation or cryocoagulation is the treatment of choice. Diathermy or cryocoagulation may be effective if the lesion is extensive. Follow-up fundus examinations are necessary, as new or recurrent retinal angiomas may occur. Enucleation may be necessary. Treatment of the CNS lesions is surgical, and consideration should be given to surgical removal of a tumor before irreversible CNS damage has occurred.

Once a diagnosis has been made, the patient's entire family should be carefully studied, including annual examination of the retina by indirect ophthalmoscopy from the age of six years, and thorough neurologic examination. Blindness may be prevented if retinal tumors are detected and treated early. CT scanning of the abdomen is the most sensitive screen for renal cysts and carcinoma and pancreatic tumors and cysts, and should occur biennially beginning at 20 years of age. Elevated urinary vanillylmandelic acid (VMA) and serum catecholamine levels suggest a pheochromocytoma. Screening should start at ten years of age. Finally, biennial cranial CT of at risk relatives should begin at 15 years of age.

**Prognosis:** Usually slowly progressive. Patients tend to die of increased intracranial pressure secondary to the CNS hemangioblastomas.

**Detection of Carrier:** Unknown.

**Special Considerations:** The finding of polycythemia in some patients with von Hippel-Lindau disease is of considerable interest. It has been shown that the cyst fluid from some cerebellar hemangioblastomas has a definite erythropoietic stimulator effect, measured by the red cell incorporation of $^{59}Fe$ in these patients.

The kidney is known to be the principal site of erythropoietin production. Some cystic renal carcinomas produce erythropoietin. Histologically cerebellar hemangioblastomas and renal carcinomas have many similarities. The reappearance of polycythemia following successful removal of a CNS hemangioblastoma might, therefore, suggest a recurrence of the CNS tumor or the development of a renal cell carcinoma.

**References:**

Melmon KL, Rosen SW: Lindau's disease: a review of the literature and study of a large kindred. Am J Med 1964; 36:595–617.

Horton WA, et al.: Von Hippel-Lindau disease: clinical and pathological manifestations in nine families with 50 affected members. Arch Intern Med 1976; 136:769–777.

Levine E, et al.: CT screening of the abdomen in von Hippel-Lindau disease. Am J Roentgenology (Baltmore) 1982; 139:505–510.

Ionasescu V, Zellweger H: Genetics in neurology. New Yoek: Raven Press, 1983.

Go RCP, et al.: Segregation and linkage analyses of von Hippel-Lindau disease among 220 descendants from one kindred. Am J Hum Genet 1984; 36:131–142.

Huson SM, et al.: Cerebellar haemangioblastoma and von Hippel-Lindau disease. Brain 1986; 109:1297–1310.

HA053                                                              **Robert H.A. Haslam**

---

**Von Mayer-Rokitansky-Kuster anomaly**
*See MULLERIAN APLASIA*
**von Recklinghausen disease**
*See NEUROFIBROMATOSIS*

## VON WILLEBRAND DISEASE                                          0996

**Includes:**

Pseudohemophilia
Pseudo (platelet-type) von Willebrand disease
von Willebrand-like disorders

**Excludes:** Hemophilia A (0461)

**Major Diagnostic Criteria:** Prolonged bleeding time (template method) and decreased Factor VIII activity are the most commonly accepted criteria. Ristocetin cofactor activity and von Willebrand protein are often abnormally low. The results of all of these studies may vary in a single individual and among affected members of a family. Particularly in the more common type I and type II von Willebrand disease, the bleeding time may sporadically become normal in a patient who usually has a prolonged bleeding time. Depressed baseline Factor VIII coagulant activity may be elevated into the normal range by stress or pregnancy. The von Willebrand protein normally occurs in multimeric form, and analysis of the protein multamers by SDS-agarose gel electrophoresis or by crossed immunoelectrophoresis is often required to distinguish among the various types and subtypes of von Willebrand disease.

**Clinical Findings:** Menorrhagia, epistaxis, and excessive bleeding after minor mouth injuries, lacerations, and loss of deciduous teeth, as well as bruising after mild trauma. Patients with the lowest activities of Factor VIII, particularly those with type III von Willebrand disease, have the greatest tendency to easy bruising, periarticular hemorrhages, and other manifestations characteristic of classic hemophilia (see **Hemophilia A**).

A number of distinct types of von Willebrand disease have been characterized. Zimmerman and Ruggeri (1987) list seven: types I, IIA, IIB, IIC, IID, IIE, and III. A large variety of subtypes have also been described (Ruggeri and Zimmerman, 1987).

**Complications:** Increased risk of bleeding following surgery, dental procedures, and acute trauma. Severe cases may develop permanent joint changes similar to those seen in **Hemophilia A**.

**Associated Findings:** None known.

**Etiology:** Autosomal dominant (types I, IIA, IIB, IID, and IIE) and autosomal recessive (types IIC and III) inheritance.

**Pathogenesis:** *Type I*: This is the most frequent form of von Willebrand disease. A characteristic finding is a proportional decrease in factor VIII coagulant activity (VIII-C) and von Willebrand factor. The multimeric composition of von Willebrand factor, as determined by electrophoresis in agarose gel, is characteristically normal.

*Type IIA*: As with all of the Type II variants, Type IIA is characterized by an absence of the large von Willebrand factor multimers. Ristocetin cofactor activity is markedly reduced, although the von Willebrand factor protein level may be normal. Factor VIII-C activity is often disproportionately higher than the von Willebrand factor protein level. The bleeding time of affected individuals is consistently prolonged.

*Type IIB*: The most characteristic finding is an increase over normal of ristocetin-induced platelet aggregation in platelet-rich plasma. Both von Willebrand factor and factor VIII-C levels are decreased or may be normal.

*Type IIC*: Distinctive findings, demonstrable by agarose gel electrophoresis of plasma, include a marked increase in the smallest multimer component as well as a repeating doublet pattern. The levels of factor VIII-C and von Willebrand factor protein are characteristically normal.

*Types IID and IIE*: Autosomal dominant forms that differ from types IIA and IIB by the presence of unique structural abnormalities of individual multimers demonstrable by SDS-agar electrophoresis.

*Type III*: The von Willebrand factor in this rare recessive form is markedly decreased or absent, and affected individuals exhibit severe bleeding manifestations. Factor VIII-C, although also greatly decreased, nevertheless has at least some measurable activity.

**MIM No.:** *19340, 27748

**CDC No.:** 286.400

**Sex Ratio:** M1:F1

**Occurrence:** Discovered by E.A. von Willebrand on the Aland Islands between Sweden and Finland in 1931, the current incidence is estimated at 30–50:1,000,000.

**Risk of Recurrence for Patient's Sib:**
See Part I, *Mendelian Inheritance*. Manifestations within a single family can vary markedly.

**Risk of Recurrence for Patient's Child:**
See Part I, *Mendelian Inheritance*. Manifestations within a single family can vary markedly.

**Age of Detectability:** Probably at birth, though more often only when accidental injury precipitates bleeding episodes, as in early childhood.

**Gene Mapping and Linkage:** F8VWF (coagulation factor VIII VWF (von Willebrand factor)) has been mapped to 12pter-p12.

**Prevention:** None known. Genetic counseling indicated.

**Treatment:** Cryoprecipitated Factor VIII, fresh plasma, and fresh frozen plasma all will elevate circulating Factor VIII levels (usually more than can be accounted for by the activity of the amount of Factor VIII administered) and reduce the risk of bleeding following surgical and dental procedures. Factor VIII concentrate raises the level of Factor VIII but does not correct the bleeding time because it does not contain von Willebrand factor.

Treatment with any of the agents above may be required to stop persistent bleeding, most frequently epistaxis. If one dose does not suffice, treatment intervals of 24 hours can be employed since severity of bleeding is generally correlated with Factor VIII activity, and the response of the Factor VIII level to therapy is frequently more prolonged than the average T 1/2 of 12 hours observed in classic hemophilia. The correction in bleeding time and platelet function is shorter, with a T 1/2 closer to 6–12 hours. Aspirin should be avoided because it prolongs the bleeding time in these patients.

1-deamino-8-d-arginine vasopressin (desmopressin, DDAVP), a vasopressin analog, may raise the factor VIII and ristocetin cofactor levels, correct the bleeding time, and prevent or treat clinical bleeding in patients with most forms of type I and type IIA von Willebrand disease. Desmopressin is usually not effective in type II or III von Willebrand disease, and is contraindicated in patients with types IIB or platelet-related disease, in whom this treatment may produce thrombocytopenia.

**Prognosis:** Few patients are substantially handicapped by the defect. However, patients with severe disease may have significant episodes of bleeding throughout their life, and excessive bleeding in female patients is likely with childbirth.

**Detection of Carrier:** Screening procedures include template bleeding time, level of Factor VIII procoagulant activity, Factor VIII related antigen, and von Willebrand factor, not all of which are consistently abnormal in all patients.

**Special Considerations:** Because of the risk of transfusion-induced hepatitis B, administration of hepatitis B vaccine is recommended as soon as diagnosis of von Willebrand disease is made.

Acquired forms of von Willebrand-like disorders have also been described in association with **Lupus erythematosis, systemic**; malignancies; and lymphoproliferative disorders. Immunoglobulin inhibitors directed against the factor VIII complex appear to mediate these disorders.

Weiss et al (1982) described a platelet-related form of pseudo-von Willebrand disease in four members, from four generations, of a family whose platelets underwent aggregation by human FVIII/VWF in the absence of ristocetin.

**References:**

Ruggeri ZM, et al.: Heightened interaction between platelets and factor VIII von Willebrand factor in a new subtype of von Willebrand disease. New Engl J Med 1980; 302:1047–1051.

Weiss HJ, et al.: Pseudo-von Willebrand's disease. New Engl J Med 1982; 306:326–333.

Zimmerman TS, et al.: Factor VIII/von Willebrand factor. Progr in Hemat 1983; 13:279–309.

Ruggeri ZM, Zimmerman TS: Von Willebrand factor and von Willebrand disease. Blood 1987; 70:895–904.

Zimmerman TS, Ruggeri ZM: Von Willebrand disease. Hum Path 1987; 18:140–152.

H0024                                                **George R. Honig**

**von Willebrand-like disorders**
  *See VON WILLEBRAND DISEASE*
**Voorhoeve disease**
  *See OSTEOPATHIA STRIATA*
**Vrolik disease**
  *See OSTEOGENESIS IMPERFECTA*
**VSR syndrome**
  *See CONTRACTURES, HERRMANN-OPITZ ARTHROGRYPOSIS
  TYPE*

# ❖ W ❖

**W Syndrome**
 *See PALLISTER-W SYNDROME*
**Waardenburg syndrome variant**
 *See ALBINISM, WAARDENBURG TYPE-HIRSCHSPRUNG*
  *AGANGLIONOSIS*
**Waardenburg syndrome, type I (dystopia canthorum present)**
 *See WAARDENBURG SYNDROMES*
**Waardenburg syndrome, type II (dystopia canthorum not present)**
 *See WAARDENBURG SYNDROMES*
**Waardenburg syndrome, type III (Klein-Waardenburg limb anomalies)**
 *See WAARDENBURG SYNDROMES*

## WAARDENBURG SYNDROMES　　　　　　　0997

**Includes:**
 Hirschsprung disease-pigmentary anomaly
 Klein-Waardenburg syndrome
 Limb anomalies (upper)-Waardenburg syndrome
 Waardenburg-ocular albinism
 Waardenburg syndrome, type I (dystopia canthorum
  present)
 Waardenburg syndrome, type II (dystopia canthorum not
  present)
 Waardenburg syndrome, type III (Klein-Waardenburg limb
  anomalies)

**Excludes:**
 **Acrocephalosyndactyly type I** (0014)
 **Albinism, cutaneous** (0031)
 **Albinism, cutaneous-deafness** (0030)
 **Albinism, Waardenburg type-hirschsprung aganglionosis** (2823)
 **Anophthalmia-limb anomalies** (3172)
 **Eye, hypertelorism** (0504)
 Heterochromia irides, acquired
 **Oro-facio-digital syndrome**

**Major Diagnostic Criteria:** 1) Dystopia canthorum (lateral displacement of medial canthi, including inferior lacrimal puncta, with normal interpupillary distance), 80–99%; 2) broad nasal bridge usually with lack of frontonasal angle and bulbous nose with hypoplastic alae nasi, 80%; 3) synophrys (confluent eyebrows), 50%; 4) heterochromia irides, 25%; 5) poliosis (white forelock), 20–40%; 6) congenital deafness, 20%.

**Clinical Findings:** Dystopia canthorum (present in type I, absent in type II); synophrys; heterochromia irides (sometimes restricted to single segment of one eye; if heterochromia is absent, irides are often bright blue in color), may include albinotic fundi, normal-to-subnormal electroretinogram. Deafness may be unilateral or bilateral, sensorineural type, and vestibular function may be impaired; type II has a higher frequency of deafness than type I, and those showing deafness are more likely to demonstrate other stigmata of the syndrome. Poliosis, may be present at birth, then disappear and reappear later; often premature graying of hair, eyelashes, and eyebrows as early as age seven years. Vitiligo in 15% of cases, usually found on arms and face. In type III, there are

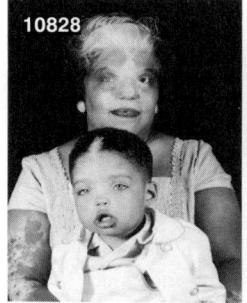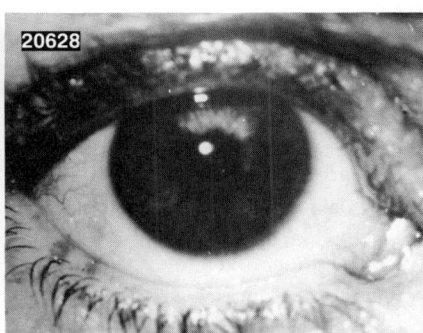
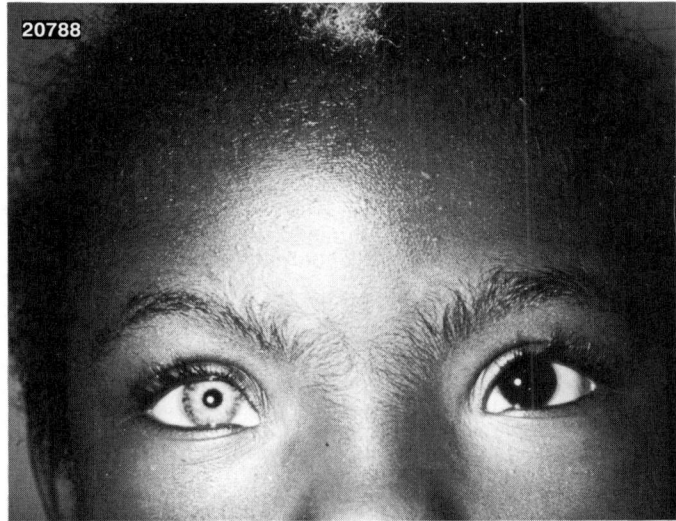

**0997-10828:** Son has blue irides; mother's right eye is blue; both have dystopia canthorum and patchy depigmentation of skin and limbs. **20628:** Close-up of heterochromia of the iris. **20788:** White forelock, heterochromia of the iris, and lateral displacement of the puncta.

bilateral defects of the upper limbs, including hypoplasia, contractures, carpal fusion, and syndactyly.

**Complications:** Primarily related to deafness, undiagnosed deafness sometimes leading to pseudomental retardation; poor lacrimal conduction; occasional glaucoma.

**Associated Findings:** Craniosynostosis, high-arched or cleft palate, blepharophimosis (type III), glaucoma, hydrophthalmos, true esotropia (20% of cases), anophthalmia with limb malformations, upper limb-pectoral girdle arthromyodysplasia (type III), Sprengel deformity (winged scapula), Hirschsprung megacolon or atretic disorders of the GI tract (type I and II), unilateral ptosis and the Marcus Gunn phenomenon (type II), congenital heart disease, **Ventricular septal defect, Meningocele,** spina bifida.

**Etiology:** Autosomal dominant inheritance with variable expression; type I penetrance, 85%; heterogeneity proposed by Hageman and Delleman (1977). A possible recessive variant has been documented in five families (see **Albinism, Waardenburg type-Hirschsprung aganglionosis.**

**Pathogenesis:** Defect of migration of neural crest cells has been hypothesized.

**MIM No.:** 14882, *19350, 19351, 27758

**POS No.:** 3426

**CDC No.:** 759.800

**Sex Ratio:** M1:F1

**Occurrence:** 1:20,000 to 1:40,000; 3% of congenitally deaf children have this syndrome.

**Risk of Recurrence for Patient's Sib:**
See Part I, *Mendelian Inheritance.*

**Risk of Recurrence for Patient's Child:**
See Part I, *Mendelian Inheritance.*

**Age of Detectability:** Unknown.

**Gene Mapping and Linkage:** WS1 (Waardenburg syndrome, type 1) has been tentatively mapped to 9q34.

**Prevention:** None known. Genetic counseling indicated.

**Treatment:** Early recognition and treatment of deafness or ocular complications.

**Prognosis:** Compatible with normal life span; mental retardation is not a characteristic.

**Detection of Carrier:** Affected persons often have only subtle signs, and are recognized in retrospect after a more severely affected relative is investigated.

**References:**
Waardenburg, PJ: A new syndrome combining developmental anomalies of the eyelids, eyebrows, and nose root, with pigmentary defects of the iris and head hair and with congenital deafness. Am J Hum Genet 1951; 3:195–253.
Arias S: Genetic heterogeneity in the Waardenburg syndrome. BD: OAS VII(4). New York: March of Dimes Birth Defects Foundation, 1971:87–101.
Hageman MJ, Delleman JW: Heterogeneity in Waardenburg syndrome. Am J Hum Genet 1977; 29:468–485.
Francois J: Waardenburg's memorial lecture: Waardenburg's syndrome. Int Ophthalmol 1982; 5:3–13.
Goodman RM, et al.: Upper limb involvement in the Klein Waardenburg syndrome. Am J Med Genet 1982; 11:425–433.
Klein D: Historical background and evidence for dominant inheritance of the Klein-Waardenburg syndrome (type III). Am J Med Genet 1983; 14:231–239.
Preus M, et al.: Waardenburg syndrome: penetrance of major signs. Am J Med Genet 1983; 15:383–388.

GA025                                              **Arthur R. Garrett**

**Waardenburg-ocular albinism**
  *See* WAARDENBURG SYNDROMES
**Waardenburg-Shah syndrome**
  *See* ALBINISM, WAARDENBURG TYPE-HIRSCHSPRUNG
     AGANGLIONOSIS
**Waardengurg anophthalmia syndrome**
  *See* ANOPHTHALMIA-LIMB ANOMALIES
**Wackenheim syndrome**
  *See* DYSOSTOSIS, CHEIROLUMBAR
**Wagner syndrome**
  *See* RETINA, HYALOIDEORETINAL DEGENERATION OF WAGNER
**Waisman syndrome**
  *See* X-LINKED MENTAL RETARDATION-BASAL GANGLION
     DISORDER

**Includes:**
  Cerebroocular dysgenesis
  Cerebroocular dysplasia-muscular dystrophy
  Cerebro-oculo-muscular syndrome
  Chemke syndrome
  HARD syndrome
  HARD +/-E syndrome
  Hydrocephalus-agyria-retinal dysplasia
  Lissencephaly syndrome II
  Muscular dystrophy-cerebrooculocal dysplasia
  Pagon syndrome
  Warburg syndrome

**Excludes:**
  **Craniotelencephalic dysplasia** (2791)
  **Lissencephaly syndrome** (0603)
  **Muscular dystrophy, congenital with mental retardation** (2705)
  **Retinal fold** (0867)

**Major Diagnostic Criteria:** Agyria (or polymicrogyria) with pebbled surface, absent cortical layers, striking glial and vascular proliferation, and white matter edema. Other features include retinal and cerebellar malformations and congenital muscular dystrophy.

**Clinical Findings:** Among 63 documented patients: type II lissencephaly (61/61); cerebellar malformations (58/58); retinal abnormalities (49/49); congenital muscular dystrophy (25/25); **Hydrocephaly** (60/62); anterior chamber dysgenesis (53/58); vermis hypoplasia (40/40); Dandy-Walker malformation (16/49); posterior encephalocele (19/63); cleft lip/palate (9/63); **Microcephaly** (8/51); and microphthalmia (28/53).

**Complications:** Seizures.

**Associated Findings:** Hypoplasia of corpus callosum and/or septum pellucidum. Coloboma (8/36). Elevated serum creatine kinase levels. Congenital contractures.

**Etiology:** Autosomal recessive inheritance.

**Pathogenesis:** Unknown.

**MIM No.:** *23667

**POS No.:** 3656

**CDC No.:** 742.240

**Sex Ratio:** M25:F34 (observed).

**Occurrence:** About sixty cases have been reported in the literature.

**Risk of Recurrence for Patient's Sib:**
See Part I, *Mendelian Inheritance.*

**Risk of Recurrence for Patient's Child:**
See Part I, *Mendelian Inheritance.* Affected individuals are not expected to survive to reproduce.

**Age of Detectability:** At birth. Has been successfully detected prenatally by high resolution ultrasound based on the presence of fetal hydrocephaly in pregnancies at risk.

**Gene Mapping and Linkage:** Unknown.

**Prevention:** None known. Genetic counseling indicated.

**Treatment:** Supportive.

**Prognosis:** Most affected infants have decreased life span (median survival nine months), although some patients have been known to survive for several years. Median survival was between 4–9 months. Usually associated with significant mental impairment.

**Detection of Carrier:** Unknown.

**Special Considerations:** Walker-Warburg syndrome has also been designated as the HARD -/+E syndrome (Hydrocephaly, Agyria, Retinal Dysplasia, with or without Encephalocele).

**References:**
Pagon R, et al.: Hydrocephalus, agyria, retinal dysplasia, encephalocele (HARD+/-E) syndrome: an autosomal recessive condition.

BD:OAS XIV(6B). New York: March of Dimes Birth Defects Foundation, 1978:233–241.

Pagon R, et al.: Autosomal recessive eye and brain abnormalities: Warburg syndrome. J Pediatr 1983; 102:542–546. *

Dobyns WB, et al.: Syndromes with lissencephaly II: Walker-Warburg and cerebro-oculo-muscular syndromes and a new syndrome with type II lissencephaly. Am J Med Genet 1985; 22:157–195. * †

Crowe C, et al.: The prenatal diagnosis of the Walker-Warburg Syndrome. Prenat Diagn 1986; 6:177–185.

Dobyns WB, et al.: Diagnostic criteria for Walker-Warburg syndrome. Am J Med Genet 1989; 32:195–210. * †

GR011                                                    **Frank Greenberg**

**Walt Disney dwarfism**
 *See OSTEODYSPLASTICA GERODERMIA, BAMATTER TYPE*
**Warburg syndrome**
 *See WALKER-WARBURG SYNDROME*
**Ward-Romano syndrome**
 *See ARRHYTHMIA, WITH LONG QT INTERVAL WITHOUT DEAFNESS*
**Warfarin, fetal effects of**
 *See FETAL WARFARIN SYNDROME*
**Warkany Syndrome**
 *See CHROMOSOME 8, TRISOMY 8*
**Watson syndrome**
 *See PULMONIC STENOSIS-CAFE-AU-LAIT SPOTS, WATSON TYPE*

---

## WEAVER SYNDROME                                          2036

**Includes:** Weaver-Smith syndrome

**Excludes:**
 **Beckwith-Wiedemann syndrome** (0104)
 **Cebebral gigantism** (0137)
 **Marshall-Smith syndrome** (2193)
 **Simpson-Golabi-Behmel syndrome** (2826)

**Major Diagnostic Criteria:** Excessive growth of pre- or postnatal onset, characteristic facial features and advanced osseous maturation. The carpal bone development is frequently more advanced than the general skeleton.

**Clinical Findings:** Based on 27 cases, the pertinent features of this syndrome include:

### Major Features of Weaver Syndrome Patients

|  | Number/Total | Percentage |
|---|---|---|
| *Excessive Growth* | | |
| Postnatally | 25/25 | 100 |
| Prenatally | 18/25 | 72 |
| *Performance* | | |
| Motor delay | 11/11 | 100 |
| Hoarse and/or low-pitched cry | 17/19 | 90 |
| Developmental delay or mental retardation | 20/25 | 80 |
| Excessive appetite | 5/7 | 71 |
| Hypertonia | 15/22 | 68 |
| Spasticity | 4/11 | 36 |
| Hypotonia | 4/22 | 18 |
| Seizures | 3/20 | 15 |
| *Craniofacial* | | |
| Micrognathia | 21/21 | 100 |
| Ocular hypertelorism | 22/23 | 96 |
| Large ears | 22/23 | 96 |
| Increased bifrontral diameter | 19/20 | 95 |
| Telecanthus | 18/19 | 95 |
| Long and accentuated philtrum | 18/23 | 78 |
| Macrocephaly | 17/22 | 77 |
| Dysplastic ears | 8/15 | 53 |
| Strabismus | 3/6 | 50 |
| Depressed nasal bridge | 9/21 | 43 |
| Down-slanting palpebral fissures | 7/19 | 37 |
| Flat occiput | 5/13 | 38 |

|  | Number/Total | Percentage |
|---|---|---|
| Epicanthal folds | 2/15 | 13 |
| *Extremities* | | |
| Prominent finger pads | 11/12 | 92 |
| Deeply set, narrow or hyperconvexed nails | 11/13 | 85 |
| Limited extension of ankles, wrists, elbows, hips, or knees | 10/12 | 83 |
| Broad thumbs | 7/10 | 70 |
| Hyperextensibility of fingers | 4/5 | 80 |
| Camptodactyly | 13/18 | 72 |
| Talipes equinovarus | 6/10 | 60 |
| *Skeleton* | | |
| Carpal bone age increased | 16/17 | 94 |
| Flared metaphyses, especially the distal femora and ulnae | 18/21 | 86 |
| Advanced general osseous maturation | 16/20 | 80 |
| Mottled or irregular epiphyses | 4/9 | 44 |
| Scoliosis or kyphosis | 4/9 | 44 |
| Short ribs | 2/6 | 33 |
| *Others* | | |
| Umbilical hernia | 15/15 | 100 |
| Inguinal hernia | 8/8 | 100 |
| Excessive and loose skin of the neck or extremities | 13/14 | 93 |
| Cryptorchidism | 6/10 | 60 |
| Excessive or prolonged hyper-bilirubinemia | 2/4 | 50 |
| Thin and/or fine scalp hair | 2/3 | 67 |

The excessive growth is present either at birth or has its onset during infancy. Mental deficiency, when present, is usually mild but ranges from mild to profound. Five individuals are reported to have had normal intellectual function. Most characteristics show considerable variation in the degree of expression. Speech difficulty, particularly dysphasia, may be common. The mean birth lengths for 14 term males and seven term females were 4.94 kg and 3.87 kg, respectively; mean birth lengths for eight term males and five term females were 56.4 cm and 54 cm, respectively, and the mean occipitofrontal circumferences (OFC) of six term males and four term females were 38.7 cm and 35.3 cm, respectively. All values for males are at or above the 97th percentile while length and weight for females is at the 90th percentile and the OFC is at about the 85th percentile.

**Complications:** Dystocia may occur because of the macrocephaly and/or macrosomia. The megalocephaly is associated with ventriculomegaly which may lead to the impression of hydrocephalus and unnecessary ventricular shunting.

**Associated Findings:** Features present in two or more of 27 patients with this condition and which are not listed above include spasticity, speech difficulty or no speech, **Eyelid, ptosis, congenital**, prominent lips, maxillary hypoplasia, short neck, inverted nipples, hyperextensibility of fingers, hemangioma, hirsutism, platyspondyly, and anterior wedging of vertebrae. Those found in only one individual are hyperactivity, delayed menarche, amenorrhea, **Myopia, congenital**, **Ear, auditory canal atresia**, widely spaced and irregularly aligned teeth, delayed eruption of permanent teeth, **Ductus arteriosus, patent**, **Ventricular septal defect**, **Hypospadias**, **Pectus excavatum**, hexadactyly, short fourth metatarsals, tapered fingers, large hands and feet, dislocated hips, simian crease, multiple dermal nevi, cervical spinal stenosis, Wormian bones, increased bone density, and hypothyroidism.

**Etiology:** Unknown.

**Pathogenesis:** Many features of this syndrome result from excessive growth. The cause of the overgrowth is unknown; no consistent endocrinological disturbance has been found. A pregnancy-related growth factor is unlikely since several infants have

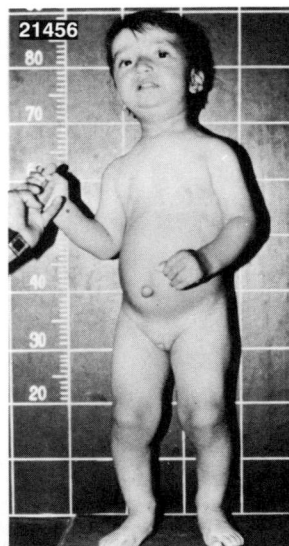

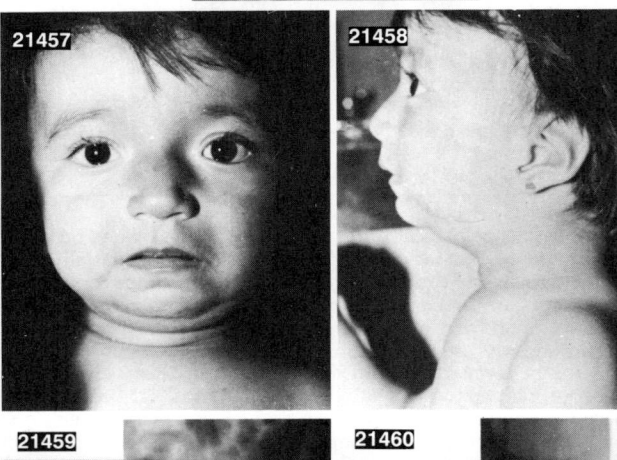

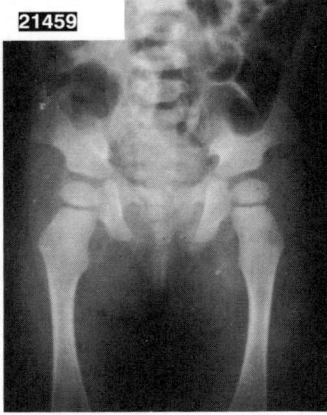

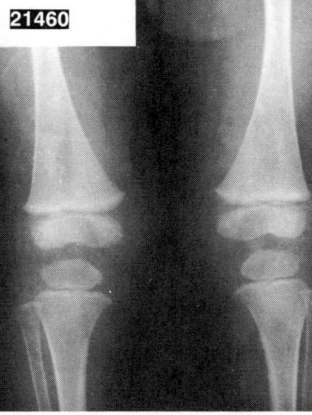

**2036**-21456: General view shows tall stature. 21457: Close-up shows increased bifrontal diameter, ocular hypertelorism. 21458: Lateral view of the face shows prominent occiput, enlarged ears and micrognathia. 21459–60: X-rays show accelerated maturation and widened femora.

not shown the accelerated growth until after birth and in most the excessive growth rate has continued for years.

**POS No.:** 3429
**Sex Ratio:** M17:F7

**Occurrence:** Twenty-seven cases have been documented in the literature.

**Risk of Recurrence for Patient's Sib:** All cases have been sporadic.

**Risk of Recurrence for Patient's Child:** Unknown.

**Age of Detectability:** At birth.

**Gene Mapping and Linkage:** Unknown.

**Prevention:** None known. Genetic counseling indicated.

**Treatment:** Cesarean section for significant dystocia, appropriate orthopedics.

**Prognosis:** Functional impairment will depend on degree of mental dysfunction and severity of orthopedic problems. Life span is not known to be altered.

**Detection of Carrier:** Unknown.

**Special Considerations:** This condition most likely is separate from the **Marshall-Smith syndrome** that also has accelerated osseous maturation, increased linear growth, and developmental delay. Patients with the latter condition lack the characteristic facial features of Weaver syndrome, usually have a poor weight gain, possess broad middle phalanges of the 3–5 fingers, and often die during infancy.

Roussounis and Crawford (1983) reported siblings whom they believed had Weaver syndrome. However, not enough data are presented to justify this conclusion. A patient reported by Tsukahara et al. is now thought to have **Simpson-Golabi-Behmel syndrome** (Kajii and Tsukahara, 1984).

**References:**
Weaver DD, et al.: A new overgrowth syndrome with accelerated skeletal maturation, unusual facies, and camptodactyly. J Pediatr 1974; 84:547–552. * †
Fitch N: The syndromes of Marshall and Weaver. J Med Genet 1980; 17:174–178
Majewski F, et al.: The Weaver syndrome: a rare type of primordial overgrowth. Eur J Pediatr 1981; 137:277–282.
Weisswichert PH, et al.: Accelerated bone maturation syndrome of the Weaver type. Eur J Paediatr 1981; 137:329–333.
Roussounis SH, Crawford MJ: Siblings with Weaver syndrome. J Pediatr 1983; 102:595–597
Kajii T, Tsukahara M: The Golabi-Rosen syndrome. Am J Med Genet 1984; 19:819 only.
Ardinger HH, et al.: Further delineation of the Weaver syndrome. J Pediatr 1986; 108:228–235. * †
Greenberg F, et al.: Weaver syndrome: the changing phenotype in an adult. Am J Med Genet 1989; 33:127–129.

WE005
RA023

**David D. Weaver**
**Maria A. Ramos-Arroyo**

**Weaver-Smith syndrome**
*See WEAVER SYNDROME*

---

**WEAVER-WILLIAMS SYNDROME**                    **2195**

**Includes:**
  Cleft palate-growth/mental retardation-microcephaly-unusual facies
  Growth/mental retardation-microcephaly-unusual facies-cleft palate
  Microcephaly-growth/mental retardation-unusual facies-cleft palate
  Unusual facies-growth/mental retardation-microcephaly-cleft palate

**Excludes:**
  **Cockayne syndrome** (0189)
  **Marden-Walker syndrome** (0629)
  **Oro-cranio-digital syndrome** (0769)
  **Seckel syndrome** (0881)

**Major Diagnostic Criteria:** Based on only two cases, criteria include severe **Microcephaly**, growth and mental retardation, unusual facies, **Cleft palate** and delayed skeletal maturation.

**Clinical Findings:** The physical characteristics shared by a brother and sister from a nonconsanguineous marriage included severe to profound mental retardation, severe microcephaly (occipitofrontal circumferences were 5 to 6 SDs below the mean), weight deficiency associated with little subcutaneous fat, diminished muscle mass, cupped and hypoplastic ears, orbital hypertelorism, midfacial hypoplasia, malformed and small teeth, cleft palate, down-turned and small mouth, clinodactyly of fingers, generalized hypoplasia of bone and delayed skeletal maturation. Neither had comprehensible speech. Features present only in the brother were moderate hearing deficit, preauricular pit, micrognathia and a long skinny neck. The sister had strabismus, prognathism, a short neck, seizures, spasticity and hemiparesis, findings which were not present in the brother. The adult height of the brother (161 cm) was just below the third percentile. Birth length and weight in both were normal.

**Complications:** Unknown.

**Associated Findings:** None known.

**Etiology:** Possibly autosomal recessive inheritance.

**Pathogenesis:** Unknown.

**POS No.:** 4046

**Sex Ratio:** M1:F1 (observed).

**Occurrence:** A brother and sister have been reported.

**Risk of Recurrence for Patient's Sib:**
See Part I, *Mendelian Inheritance.*

**Risk of Recurrence for Patient's Child:**
See Part I, *Mendelian Inheritance.*

**Age of Detectability:** At birth.

**Gene Mapping and Linkage:** Unknown.

**Prevention:** None known. Genetic counseling indicated.

**Treatment:** Unknown.

**Prognosis:** Affected individuals will probably have mental retardation. This condition may be compatible with a normal life span.

**Detection of Carrier:** Unknown.

**References:**
Weaver DD, Williams CPS: A syndrome of microcephaly, mental retardation, unusual facies, cleft palate and weight deficiency. BD:OAS XIII(3B). New York: March of Dimes Birth Defects Foundation, 1977:69–84.

WE005                                          **David D. Weaver**

**Webbing, popliteal**
*See PTERYGIUM SYNDROME, POPLITEAL*
**Weemaes chromosome breakage syndrome**
*See CHROMOSOME INSTABILITY, NIJMEGEN TYPE*
**Weill-Marchesani syndrome**
*See SPHEROPHAKIA-BRACHYMORPHIA SYNDROME*
**Weismann-Netter-Stuhl syndrome**
*See SKELETAL DYSPLASIA, WEISMANN-NETTER-STUHL TYPE*
**Weissenbacher-Zweymuller variant of arthro-ophthalmopathy**
*See ARTHRO-OPHTHALMOPATHY, WEISSENBACHER-
    ZWEYMULLER VARIANT*
**Welander type of muscular dystrophy**
*See MUSCULAR DYSTROPHY, DISTAL*
**Werdnig-Hoffmann disease**
*See SPINAL MUSCULAR ATROPHY*
**Wermer syndrome**
*See ENDOCRINE NEOPLASIA, MULTIPLE TYPE I*

## WERNER SYNDROME                                      0998

**Includes:**
Aging, premature (one form)
Progeria adultorum

**Excludes:**
**Mandibuloacral dysplasia** (2082)
**Progeria** (0825)
**Rothmund-Thomson syndrome** (2037)
**Scleroderma, familial progressive** (2154)

**Major Diagnostic Criteria:** Growth arrests at puberty, and cataracts develop in the second or third decade. Premature graying and balding; scleroderma-like involvement of limbs; marked diminution of muscle mass and subcutaneous tissue of limbs; chronic, slowly healing ulcerations over pressure points of feet and ankles; beak-shaped nose; premature development of arteriosclerosis, diabetes mellitus, hypogonadism, and localized soft tissue calcifications.

**Clinical Findings:** Features first become apparent between ages 15 and 30 years, with habitus of premature aging, shortness of stature, beaked nose, premature graying of hair with alopecia, diabetes mellitus, and cataract formation. There is atrophy with loss of subcutaneous tissue and tightness of the limbs. Circumscribed keratosis and ulcers develop on the skin, persisting over pressure points on the limbs. Poor muscular development and localized soft tissue calcifications are noted in the limbs. Ocular findings, usually noted in the second or third decade, include bilateral juvenile cataracts, macular degeneration, retinitis pigmentosa, and chorioretinitis. Diabetes mellitus and hypogonadism are the two most frequent endocrine abnormalities. Endocrine studies have failed to establish other deficiencies. Sterility, impotence, irregular or absent menses, loss of libido, high-pitched voice, mild gynecomastia, and scant, if any, pubic, axillary, and trunk hair are present. Intelligence was described in 22 cases: Ten of these were noted to be retarded. X-rays reveal osteoporosis, osteomyelitis-type lesions, neurotrophic bone changes in the feet, flat feet and gross foot deformities, osteoarthritis of peripheral

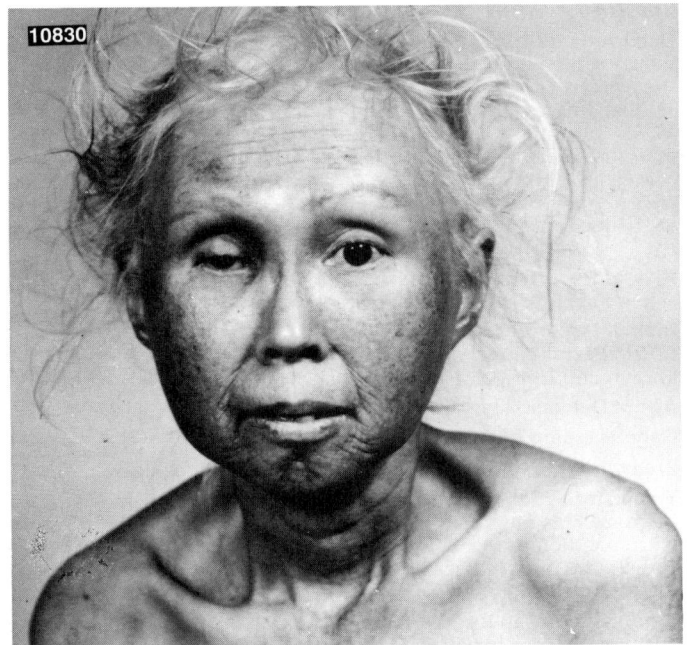

**0998-10830:** 48-year-old female with prematurely aged appearance.

joints, and spondylotic deformities of the spine. Signs of generalized arteriosclerosis are prominent, with diminished or absent peripheral pulses in the lower limbs, and angina with myocardial infarction is seen. Many cases may go undiagnosed.

**Complications:** Myocardial infarction, congestive heart failure, ulcerations of limbs, blindness secondary to cataracts; 10% develop neoplasms with a high frequency of sarcomas.

**Associated Findings:** None known.

**Etiology:** Autosomal recessive inheritance.

**Pathogenesis:** Pathologically, patients have shown generalized arteriosclerosis and coronary artery disease. Cardiac findings include calcification of coronary arteries and valves and either typical myocardial infarction or multifocal myocardial fibrosis. Endocrine organs have shown no specific histologic changes except testicular atrophy. Microscopic changes in the skin have included atrophy of the epidermis, thickening of the corium with fibrous tissue, and atrophy or rete pegs. A striking increase in the incidence of neoplasia has been noted and includes melanotic sarcoma, sarcoma of the uterus, fibroliposarcoma, hepatoma, carcinoma of the female breast, and osteogenic sarcoma. Resemblances to progeria in children suggest that the Werner syndrome may represent a later expression of progeria. The scleroderma-type skin lesions, the sclerotic lesions in other organs, and the high incidence of mesenchymal tumors suggest an aberration in connective tissue metabolism. Elevated levels of hyaluronic acid excretion in urine has been reported in many cases from Japan. This suggests that an abnormality in glycosaminoglycan metabolism, a connective tissue component, may be related to the pathogenesis of the disease. Tissue culture studies indicate a striking diminution of the growth potential of fibroblasts in vitro, suggesting that this is a manifestation of senescence at the cellular level. Although there are many resemblances of Werner syndrome to the aging process, important differences exist. In Werner syndrome, there is usually no clinical or pathologic resemblance to senile dementia or to the brain changes noted with aging. Also, while neoplasms are common in old age, the types seen in Werner syndrome (sarcomas, other connective tissue neoplasm, and other unusual tumors) are different from those frequently encountered with advancing age.

**MIM No.:** *27770

**POS No.:** 3765

**Sex Ratio:** M1:F1

**Occurrence:** Estimated to be 1:50,000 to 1:1,000,000. Many cases may be undiagnosed. Only five to ten living patients are known in the United States.

Over 150 cases have been reported in the world literature since 1904. The condition has been observed in Caucasians, Orientals, and Blacks; it has been reported in North and South America, the Middle East, and Japan, particularly in Caucasians of Jewish ancestry and in Sardinia. As many as 100 cases have been reported in the Japanese literature, probably related to higher consanguinity.

**Risk of Recurrence for Patient's Sib:**
See Part I, *Mendelian Inheritance.*

**Risk of Recurrence for Patient's Child:**
See Part I, *Mendelian Inheritance.* Fertility is diminished; 0.4 known children per patient on the average.

**Age of Detectability:** Detectable clinically by 15 to 30 years of age.

**Gene Mapping and Linkage:** Unknown.

**Prevention:** None known. Genetic counseling indicated.

**Treatment:** Cataracts are surgically resected when mature. **Diabetes mellitus** is usually mild and responds to diet or oral hypoglycemic therapy. Conventional treatments are indicated for arteriosclerotic heart disease, congestive heart failure, cutaneous ulcers, and malignancy.

**Prognosis:** Many patients survive to the fourth and fifth decades, and a few survive to the sixth and seventh decades. Death is usually caused by malignancy or arteriosclerotic heart disease. Functional impairment from medical complications generally occurs 15–20 years after the onset. Generalized arteriosclerosis and scleroderma-type skin changes are progressive and irreversible.

**Detection of Carrier:** Increased frequency of premature graying in relatives suggests that heterozygotes may have partial expression.

**Special Considerations:** There is a striking decrease in the growth potential of fibroblasts in Werner syndrome. Thus, the patient's fibroblasts behave *in vitro* as do those of aged individuals. Cultured skin fibroblasts have a remarkably reduced life span, and there is a slow rate of DNA elongation.

A high frequency of clonally derived chromosomal aberrations termed *verigated translocation mosaicism*, has been seen in cultured fibroblasts. This suggests that Werner syndrome may be considered to be one of several chromosome breakage syndromes, including **Bloom syndrome, Ataxia telangiectasia,** and **Pancytopenia syndrome, Fanconi type.** The elevated excretion of hyaluronic acid could be due to a defect in glycosaminoglycan metabolism, which might explain many of the apparent abnormalities of connective tissue seen in Werner syndrome.

**References:**

Epstein CJ, et al.: Werner's syndrome: a review of its symptomatology, natural history, pathologic features, genetics and relationship to the natural aging process. Medicine 1966; 45:177–222.

Salk D: Werner's syndrome: a review of recent research with an analysis of connective tissue metabolism, growth control of cultured cells, and chromosomal aberrations. Hum Genet 1982; 62:1–15.

Brown WT: Werner's syndrome. In: German J, ed: Chromosome mutation and neoplasia. New York: Alan R. Liss, 1983:85–93.

Salk D, et al.: Werner's syndrome and human aging. advances in experimental medicine and biology, vol 190. New York: Plenum, 1985.

Bauer EA, et al.: Diminished response of Werner's syndrome fibroblasts to growth factors PDGF and FGF. Science 1986; 234:1240–1243.

BR024                                                          **W. Ted Brown**

**Weyers acrofacial dysostosis**
*See ACROFACIAL DYSOSTOSIS*
*also ACROFACIAL SYNDROME, CURRY-HALL TYPE*

**Weyers oligodactyly**
*See HAND, ULNAR AND FIBULAR RAY DEFICIENCY, WEYERS TYPE*

**Whelan syndrome**
*See ORO-FACIO-DIGITAL SYNDROME, WHELAN TYPE*

**Whistling face syndrome**
*See CRANIO-CARPO-TARSAL DYSPLASIA, WHISTLING FACE TYPE*

**Whitaker Negroes**
*See ECTODERMAL DYSPLASIA, CHRIST-SIEMENS-TOURAINE TYPE*

**Whitaker syndrome**
*See POLYGLANDULAR AUTOIMMUNE SYNDROME*

**White folded dysplasia of mucosa**
*See MUCOSA, WHITE FOLDED DYSPLASIA*

**White liver disease**
*See VISCERA, FATTY METAMORPHOSIS*

**White sponge nevus of Cannon**
*See MUCOSA, WHITE FOLDED DYSPLASIA*

**Wieacker syndrome**
*See CONTRACTURES-MUSCLE ATROPHY-OCULOMOTOR APRAXIA*

**Wieacker-Wolff syndrome**
*See CONTRACTURES-MUSCLE ATROPHY-OCULOMOTOR APRAXIA*

**Wiedemann-Rautenstrauch syndrome**
*See PROGERIA, NEONATAL RAUTENSTRAUCH-WIEDEMANN TYPE*

**Wiedmann-Beckwith syndrome**
*See BECKWITH-WIEDEMANN SYNDROME*

**Wildermuth ear**
*See EAR, PROMINENT ANTHELIX*

**Wildervack syndrome**
*See EYE, DUANE RETRACTION SYNDROME*

**Wildervanck syndrome**
*See CERVICO-OCULO-ACOUSTIC SYNDROME*

# WILLIAMS SYNDROME                                    0999

**Includes:**

Elfin faces-hypercalcemia
Hypercalcemia-peculiar facies-supravalvular aortic stenosis
Supravalvar aortic stenosis
Williams-Beuren syndrome

**Excludes:**

**Aortic stenosis, supravalvar** (0078)
Hypercalcemia without facial or cardiac anomalies

**Major Diagnostic Criteria:** Typical facies with full lips, broad nasal bridge, broad nasal tip and anteverted nares; with or without growth and mental deficiency; and supravalvular aortic or pulmonary arterial stenosis. Infantile hypercalcemia may be present.

**Clinical Findings:** More frequent features include mild short stature, sometimes low birth weight (median of 2.7 kg with range of 1.5–4.0 kg); mild to moderate mental retardation, short attention span with distractibility, hyperverbal speech, loquacious behavior during childhood, with severe behavior problems in one-sixth of patients, IQ most commonly 40–70 (average IQ=56); broad maxilla and mouth with full prominent "cupid's bow" upper lip, anteverted nares with full nasal tip, full pouting cheeks and open mouth with tendency toward inner epicanthic folds, small mandible, prominent ears, and unusual stellate patterning in the iris; and supravalvular aortic stenosis or hypoplasia, peripheral pulmonary artery stenosis, or septal defect in about 75% the patients. There may also be renal artery stenosis with hypertension, hypoplasia of the aorta, and other arterial anomalies. Rarely, may present in infancy with coarse facial features, hepatosplenomegaly, and hernias suggestive of a lysosomal storage disease which resolves with age.

**Complications:** Renal disease and calcinosis secondary to hypercalcemia. Sudden death has been reported in a few cases.

**Associated Findings:** Hoarse voice, hyperacusis, strabismus, craniosynostosis, hypodontia, inguinal hernia, kyphosis, kyphoscoliosis, joint contractures and joint limitation, radioulnar synostosis, mitral insufficiency, elevated serum cholesterol and hypercalcemia during infancy (8–18 months), with symptoms and signs such as hypotonia, constipation, anorexia, vomiting, polyuria, polydipsia, renal insufficiency, vicarious calcification, and transient facial palsy. Bladder diverticulae are usually only evident by means of excretory urography. Diverticulitis of the bowel has been

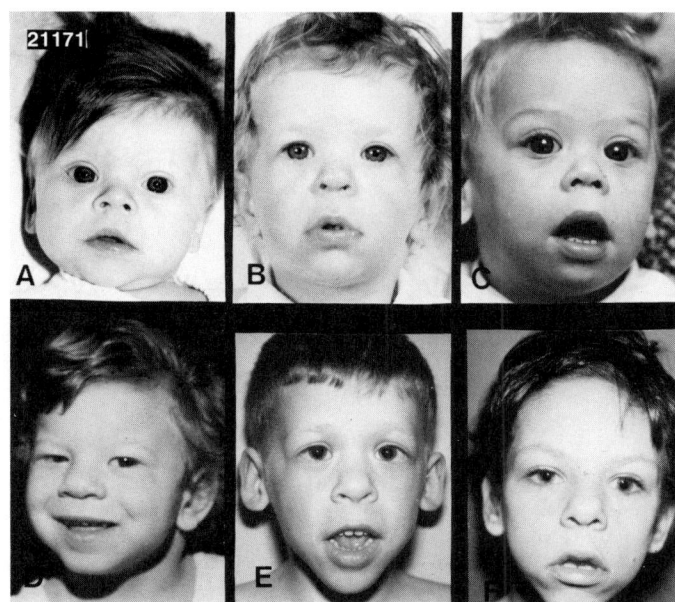

**0999B-**21171:  Note the characteristic facies in these unrelated children.

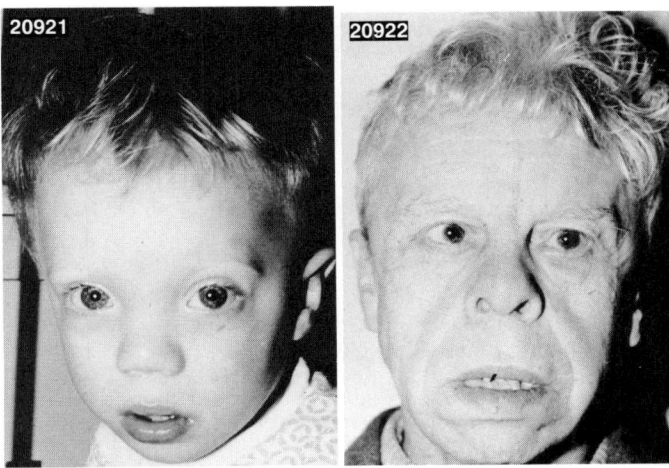

**0999A-**20921:  Williams syndrome in a 2-year-old boy with typical facies; speckled iris, prominent, wide-set eyes, full cheeks, and prominent open mouth.   **20922:**  The typical facies are still evident in this 65-year-old male with Williams syndrome.

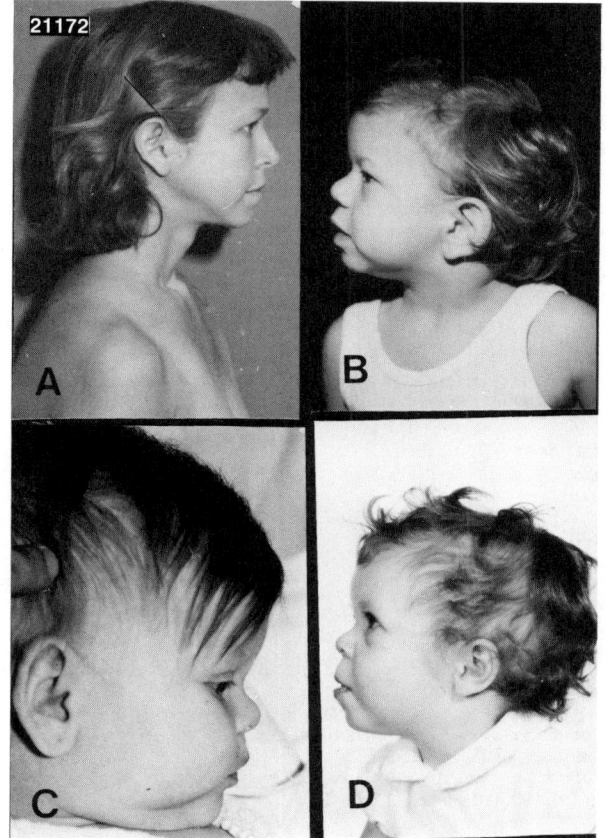

**0999C-**21172:  Lateral view of facies shows full cheeks.

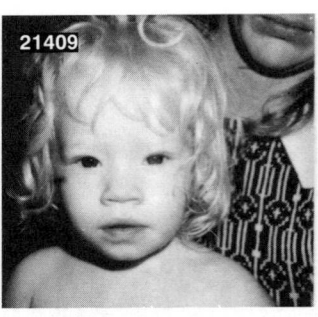 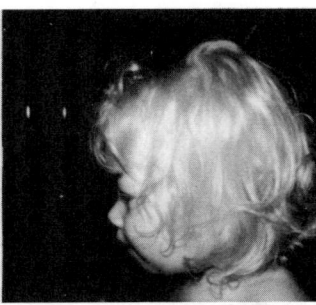

**0999D-21409:** Note broad forehead, flat nasal bridge and full cheeks.

described in adults. Recurrence of hypercalcemia has been reported in adults. Autism has been reported.

**Etiology:** Usually a sporadic occurrence, although autosomal dominant inheritance has been suggested, with most cases representing new mutations.

**Pathogenesis:** Possibly a defect in calcitonin production, release or activity (Culler, 1985). An abnormal synthesis or degradation of 1,25-(OH)2D has been suggested (Burn, 1986).

**MIM No.:** *19405

**POS No.:** 3427

**Sex Ratio:** Presumably M1:F1.

**Occurrence:** The incidence has been estimated as 1:10,000 (Grimm and Wesselhoeft, 1980).

**Risk of Recurrence for Patient's Sib:**
See Part I, *Mendelian Inheritance.* Usually sporadic.

**Risk of Recurrence for Patient's Child:**
See Part I, *Mendelian Inheritance.*

**Age of Detectability:** From birth to early childhood.

**Gene Mapping and Linkage:** WMS (William syndrome) has been tentatively mapped to 4q33-qter.

**Prevention:** None known. Genetic counseling indicated.

**Treatment:** When hypercalcemia still exists, elimination of vitamin D from the diet and limitation of calcium intake should be considered. Cardiac surgery may be indicated for severe cardiac defects. Individualized educational programs; physical, occupational, and speech therapy may be indicated.

**Prognosis:** Variable. No average life span can be inferred from existing data.

**Detection of Carrier:** Unknown.

**Support Groups:** TX; Klein; Williams Syndrome Association

**References:**
Williams JCP, et al.: Supravalvular aortic stenosis. Circulation 1961; 24:1311–1318.
Bennett FC, et al.: The Williams elfin facies syndrome. Pediatrics 1978; 61:303–306.
Grimm T, Wesselhoeft H: The genetic aspects of Williams-Beuren syndrome and the isolated form of the supravalvular aortic stenosis; investigation of 128 families. Z Kardiol 1980; 69:168–172.
Preus M: The Williams syndrome: objective definition and diagnosis. Clin Genet 1984; 25:422–428.
Culler FL, et al.: Impaired calcitonin secretion in patients with Williams syndrome. J Pediatr 1985; 107:720–723.
Burn J: Williams syndrome. J Med Genet 1986; 23:389–395.
Biesecker LG, et al.: Renal insufficiency in Williams syndrome. Am J Med Genet 1987; 28:131–135.
Maisuls H, et al.: Cardiovascular finding in the Williams-Beuren syndrome. Am Heart J 1987; 114:897–899.

BU040
GR011

**Merlin G. Butler**
**Frank Greenberg**

---

**Williams-Beuren syndrome**
See *WILLIAMS SYNDROME*
**Williams-Campbell syndrome**
See *BRONCHOMALACIA*
**Wilms tumor**
See *CANCER, WILMS TUMOR*
**Wilms tumor-aniridia**
See *CHROMOSOME 11, PARTIAL MONOSOMY 11p*
**Wilms tumor-aniridia syndrome**
See *ANIRIDIA*
**Wilms tumor-aniridia-gonadoblastoma-mental retardation (WAGR)**
See *CHROMOSOME 11, PARTIAL MONOSOMY 11p*

## WILMS TUMOR-PSEUDOHERMAPHRODITISM-GLOMERULOPATHY, DENYS-DRASH TYPE 3139

**Includes:**
Denys-Drash syndrome
Drash syndrome
Gonadal differentiation (abnormal)-nephropathy-Wilms tumor
Nephropathy-pseudohermaphroditism-Wilms tumor
Pseudohermaphroditism-nephron disorder-Wilms tumor
Wilms tumor-pseudohermaphroditism-nephropathy

**Excludes:** Colon, atresia or stenosis (0193)

**Major Diagnostic Criteria:** Gonadal dysfunction usually consisting of male pseudohermaphroditism, glomerulopathy, and **Cancer, Wilms tumor.** According to Habib et al (1985) the syndrome includes patients with either male pseudohermaphroditism or Wilms tumor when associated with the renal histologic lesion of diffuse mesangial sclerosis.

**Clinical Findings:** The renal disease presents with proteinuria with or without nephrotic syndrome, hypertension, hematuria, and progressive renal insufficiency leading to end-stage renal disease in infancy. The external genitalia are frequently ambiguous, most patients being male pseudohermaphrodites. Wilms tumor occurs in about 55% of cases and may be diagnosed years after the appearance of kidney disease.

**Complications:** Chronic renal failure. Dysgenetic gonads carry 20–30% risk of malignancy.

**Associated Findings:** Hydronephrosis, vesicoureteral reflux, urogenital abnormalities.

**Etiology:** Usually sporadic.

**Pathogenesis:** May be due to defective embryogenesis of the urogenital ridge.

**MIM No.:** 19408

**POS No.:** 4227

**Sex Ratio:** M1:F>0. The majority of reported patients are male pseudohermaphrodites; however, the syndrome has been also described in females.

**Occurrence:** About 30 cases have been documented in the literature.

**Risk of Recurrence for Patient's Sib:** Undetermined, but probably small.

**Risk of Recurrence for Patient's Child:** Undetermined, but probably small.

**Age of Detectability:** Usually during early infancy.

**Gene Mapping and Linkage:** Unknown.

**Prevention:** None known. Genetic counseling indicated.

**Treatment:** Since Wilms tumor develops in 55% of patients, bilateral nephrectomy is advised once end-stage renal disease sets in. Removal of gonadal tissue is also advised during the same procedure to avoid malignant transformation. Renal transplantation has been performed successfully.

**Prognosis:** Untreated patients usually die in infancy.

**Detection of Carrier:** Unknown.

**Special Considerations:** This syndrome should be considered in any infant with ambiguous genitalia. Diffuse mesangial sclerosis is the usual histologic lesion in this syndrome, but it may also be a form of infantile nephrotic syndrome, sometimes associated with eye abnormalities (see **Renal mesangial sclerosis-eye defects**).

**Support Groups:** New York; National Kidney Foundation

**References:**

Denys P, et al.: Association d'un syndrome anotomopatholgique de psuedohermaphroditisme masculin, d'une tumeur de Wilms, d'une nephropathie parenchymateuse et d'une mosaicisme XX/XY. Arch Fr Pediatr 1967; 24:729–739.

Drash A, et al.: A syndrome of pseudohermaphroditism, Wilms' tumor, hypertension, and degenerative renal disease. J Pediatr 1970; 76:585–593.

Barakat AY, et al.: Pseudohermaphroditism, nephron disorder and Wilms' tumor: a unifying concept. Pediatrics 1974; 54:366–369.

Habib R, et al.: The nephropathy associated with male pseudohermaphroditism and Wilms' tumor (Drash syndrome): a distinctive glomerular lesion-report of 10 cases. Clin Nephrol 1985; 24:269–278.

Barakat AY: Nomenclature of Drash syndrome. (Letter) Clin Nephrol 1988; 29:107 only.

BA065                                           **Amin Y. Barakat**

**Wilms tumor-pseudohermaphroditism-nephropathy**
*See WILMS TUMOR-PSEUDOHERMAPHRODITISM-GLOMERULOPATHY, DENYS-DRASH TYPE*
**Wilson disease**
*See HEPATOLENTICULAR DEGENERATION*

---

## WINCHESTER SYNDROME                          1000

**Includes:**
"Arthritis-like" condition-short stature
Connective tissue disorder-joint stiffening-short stature
Winchester-Grossman syndrome

**Excludes:**
Arthritis mutilans
**Arthritis, rheumatoid** (2517)
Asymbolia
**Charcot-Marie-Tooth disease**
Gorham disease
**Mucolipidosis**
**Mucopolysaccharidosis**
**Osteolysis** (1521)
Reticulohistiocytosis, multicentric

**Major Diagnostic Criteria:** Short stature, joint stiffening with severe flexion contractures, peripheral corneal opacities, skin thickening, X-ray features of progressive carpotarsal osteolysis, and progressive destruction of small joints. Light and electron microscopic evaluation of thickened skin confirms the diagnosis.

**Clinical Findings:** Winchester syndrome begins before age two years, heralded by symmetric polyarthralgias of large and small joints. Swelling and pain with limitation of motion develop within the first two years of life without associated localized erythema, warmth, or other constitutional symptoms. Intermittent polyarthralgias continue throughout childhood and lead to flexion contractures of the fingers, elbows, hips, knees and ankles. Areas of skin become thickened and leathery, and gradually develop hyperpigmentation and a hypertrophic appearance. Five of seven patients have had coarsened facial features. Peripheral corneal opacities are noted by mid-childhood. Linear growth is retarded from early, childhood leading to dwarfism. Although motor development is retarded, intelligence is normal.

X-rays reveal generalized osteoporosis and progressive osteolysis of carpal and tarsal bones, sometimes with complete resorption by the second decade. Progressive intra- and periarticular erosions of small joints may simulate severe juvenile rheumatoid arthritis; bony anklyosis may develop.

Skin biopsies of affected areas have revealed fibroblastic hyperplasia and, at a later age, abnormal collagen bundle architecture in the deep dermis. Characteristic ultrastructural dilation of mitochondria is observed in fibroblasts. The carpal bones appear to be replaced by dense fibrous tissue, and sections of bone disclose a paucity of trabeculae; growth plates appear normal.

**Complications:** Severe progressive flexion contractures of major and minor joints lead to immobile "claw hands", and nonambulation that may lead to almost complete disability. Fractures are more common as a result of osteoporosis.

**Associated Findings:** The lips and gingiva may appear hypertrophic.

**Etiology:** Autosomal recessive inheritance.

**Pathogenesis:** Joint contractures, skin thickening, abnormal dermal collagen, and corneal opacities may be due to abnormal fibroblast function. Dwarfism, osteolysis, and osteoporosis appear to be secondary to excessive bone resorption.

**MIM No.:** *27795

**POS No.:** 3428

**Sex Ratio:** Presumably M1:F1 (M3:F4 observed in seven cases).

**Occurrence:** Undetermined. Recorded cases have occurred in Puerto Rican, Mexican, Indian, and Iranian families.

**Risk of Recurrence for Patient's Sib:**
See Part I, *Mendelian Inheritance.*

**Risk of Recurrence for Patient's Child:**
See Part I, *Mendelian Inheritance.*

**Age of Detectability:** Usually by one year of age; before two years of age.

**Gene Mapping and Linkage:** Unknown.

**Prevention:** None known. Genetic counseling indicated.

**Treatment:** Serial casting, continuous passive range of motion machines, or other orthopedic procedures to decrease flexion contractures may be of some benefit.

**Prognosis:** Normal intelligence, but with significant functional disability.

**Detection of Carrier:** Possibly by clinical examination of first degree relatives.

**Special Considerations:** The coarsened facies, thickened skin, corneal clouding, dwarfism, and joint contractures suggest a mucopolysaccharoid storage disease or mucolipidosis. However, the absence of mucopolysacchariduria and presence of rheumatoid-like small joint destruction and carpotarsal osteolysis distinguishe the Winchester syndrome from these latter conditions, as does the absence of lysosomal vacuolization in fibroblasts and chondrocytes. The Winchester syndrome may be differentiated from juvenile **Arthritis, rheumatoid** by the lack of prominent constitutional symptoms, normal erythrocyte sedimentation rate, negative antinuclear antibody and rheumatoid factor, and by extra-skeletal manifestations, particularly the skin changes.

**References:**

Winchester P, et al.: A new acid mucopolysaccharidosis with skeletal deformities simulating rheumatoid arthritis. Am J Roentgenol Radium Ther Nucl Med 1969; 106:121–128.

Brown SI, Kuwabara T: Peripheral corneal opacification and skeletal deformities: a newly recognized acid mucopolysaccharidosis simulating rheumatoid arthritis. Arch Ophthal 1970; 83:667–677.

Hollister DW, et al.: The Winchester syndrome: a nonlysosomal connective tissue disease. J Pediatr 1974; 84:701–709. *

Cohen AH, et al.: The skin in Winchester syndrome. Arch Dermatol 1975; 111:230–236.

Nabai H, et al.: Winchester syndrome: report of a case from Iran. J Cutan Pathol 1977; 4:281–285.

Irani A, et al.: The Winchester syndrome: a case report. Indian Pediatr 1978; 15:861–863.

G0043                                           **Donald P. Goldsmith**

**Winchester-Grossman syndrome**
*See WINCHESTER SYNDROME*
**Wind blown hand**
*See HAND, ULNAR DRIFT*
**Wind-mill vain hand**
*See HAND, ULNAR DRIFT*

**Windmill vane hand syndrome**
  See *CRANIO-CARPO-TARSAL DYSPLASIA, WHISTLING FACE TYPE*
**Wing teeth**
  See *TEETH, MESIOPALATAL TORSION OF CENTRAL INCISORS*
**Winter syndrome**
  See *RENAL-GENITAL-MIDDLE EAR ANOMALIES*
**Wiskott-Aldrich syndrome**
  See *IMMUNODEFICIENCY, WISKOTT-ALDRICH TYPE*
**WL symphalangism-brachydactyly syndrome**
  See *SYMPHALANGISM*
**Wolcott-Rallison syndrome**
  See *EPIPHYSEAL DYSPLASIA, MULTIPLE-DIABETES MELLITUS*
**Wolf syndrome**
  See *CHROMOSOME 4, MONOSOMY 4p*
**Wolf teeth**
  See *TEETH, LOBODONTIA*
**Wolf-Hirschhorn syndrome**
  See *CHROMOSOME 4, MONOSOMY 4p*
**Wolff syndrome**
  See *ALBINISM, CUTANEOUS*
**Wolff-Parkinson-White syndrome**
  See *ARRHYTHMIA, WOLFF-PARKINSON-WHITE TYPE*
**Wolfram syndrome**
  See *DIABETES (INSIPIDUS/MELLITUS)-OPTIC ATROPHY-DEAFNESS*

---

## WOLMAN DISEASE                                    1003

**Includes:**
  LIPA deficiency
  Lysosomal acid lipase deficiency
  Wolman disease-hypolipoproteinemia-acanthocytosis
  Xanthomatosis, familial-involvement and calcification of
    adrenals

**Excludes:**
  **Analphalipoproteinemia** (0048)
  **Biliary atresia** (0110)
  **Cholesteryl ester storage disease** (0151)
  **Lipogranulomatosis** (0598)
  **Niemann-Pick disease** (0717)

**Major Diagnostic Criteria:** The diagnosis can be considered certain in a young infant with hepatosplenomegaly, steatorrhea, enlarged and calcified adrenals, foam cells in the marrow, and vacuolization of lymphocytes. Death usually occurs in infancy. Substantiation of the diagnosis depends on demonstration of deficient acid lipase activity in leukocytes and cultured skin fibroblasts.

**Clinical Findings:** Characteristically, infants present with poor weight gain, vomiting, and loose, frequent stools in the early weeks of life. Symmetrically enlarged, calcified adrenals are seen to have a diffuse punctate pattern of calcification on X-ray examination of the abdomen. Anemia occurs in early infancy. Chronic nutritional failure becomes increasingly severe in spite of all special management efforts (handicapped by foam cell infiltration in the intestinal villi), and the patients die by ages 2–9 months with wasting and infection. Neuromuscular development is retarded, but mostly in a secondary fashion, with neuronal changes of limited distribution when present at all (retina, sympathetic ganglia, myenteric plexus). There is moderate enlargement of the liver and spleen, organs in which the fundamental lipid-laden foam cell diathesis is well visualized: Neutral fat accumulation and cholesterol (80–90% esterified) is marked. Liver cholesterol levels have varied from 3 to 9% of the net weight and spleen; phospholipid levels are normal. Foam cells are found in the bone marrow, and there is prominent vacuolization of the circulating agranulocytes. The possibility has now been raised that some children with this basic syndrome may have a considerably later expression of the GI symptoms, longer survival, and less evident calcification of the adrenals.

**Complications:** Chronic nutritional failure, and possibly some degree of adrenocortical insufficiency. A positive balance for nutrients and electrolytes, with a margin for support of general development, is extremely difficult to achieve.

**Associated Findings:** On several occasions, serum alphalipoprotein levels have been found to be very low, although not comparable to those in **Analphalipoproteinemia**.

  *Wolman disease-hypolipoproteinemia-acanthocytosis*, described by Eto and Kitagawa (1970), is a possible variant unique in its hypolipoproteinemia and acanthocytosis.

**Etiology:** Autosomal recessive inheritance. There is deficient activity of lysosomal acid lipase in cultured fibroblasts, leukocytes, amniocytes, liver, spleen, lymph node, and aortic tissue. With natural substrates the enzyme activity is less than 10% of control. Electrophoresis separates acid lipase into three bands. In Wolman disease there is absence of the least anodal (A) band. This isoenzyme appears to function both as a cholesterol ester hydrolase and triacylglycerol hydrolase, and its deficient activity in Wolman disease leads to lysosomal accumulation of cholesteryl esters and to a lesser extent of triglycerides.

**Pathogenesis:** The enlargement of liver, spleen, adrenal, and lymph nodes is a consequence of cholesteryl ester and triglyceride accumulation. The adrenal calcification may be a consequence of necrosis and cell infiltrates demonstrated in the fetal adrenal gland of a closely related condition: cholesterol ester storage disease. The degree of cholesteryl ester storage probably is sufficient to lead to cellular malfunction. The lysosomal cholesteryl esterase normally hydrolyzes the cholesteryl esters, which enter the cell via the "Brown and Goldstein" LDL pathway, and the deficient activity of this enzyme in Wolman disease compromises the critical control mechanisms associated with this pathway. These effects probably account for the plasma lipoprotein abnormalities and premature atherosclerosis associated with cholesteryl ester storage disease, in which there is deficiency of the same enzyme. These changes may not be observed in Wolman disease, probably due to their short life span.

**MIM No.:** *27800, 27810

**Sex Ratio:** M1:F1

**Occurrence:** Forty-two cases reported to date. No predilection in any particular group.

**Risk of Recurrence for Patient's Sib:**
  See Part I, *Mendelian Inheritance*.

**Risk of Recurrence for Patient's Child:**
  See Part I, *Mendelian Inheritance*. No affected individuals are known to have reproduced.

**Age of Detectability:** In infancy, clinically. Calcification of the adrenals has been detected within the first few days of life on several occasions, and it should be visible on abdominal X-rays of the mother in later pregnancy. Prenatal diagnosis (lipase studies on cultured fetal cells) has been done.

**Gene Mapping and Linkage:** LIPA (lipase A, lysosomal acid (Wolman disease)) has been mapped to 10.

**Prevention:** None known. Genetic counseling indicated.

**Treatment:** Very unsatisfactory to date. Simplified, high-calorie, high-protein feedings, or low-residue feedings, have not been adequate to allow reasonable weight gain and have been limited by the diarrhea and vomiting. Adrenal corticosteroid supplements have been regularly used. No useful effects have been identified from cholestyramine, d-thyroxine, clofibrate, or medium-chain triglyceride treatments. In the future, enzyme replacement therapy or gene therapy may become feasible. Such approaches are made more hopeful by the absence of significant central nervous system involvement in Wolman disease and by the fact that the acid lipase has been purified and does carry the mannose-6-phosphate ligand, which allows for receptor-mediated targeting to the lysosome.

**Prognosis:** The usual (infant) patients have expired, in spite of all therapeutic efforts, at ages 1.5 to 9 months, rarely a few months longer. Reports now exist of children with milder symptoms and of later onset who are surviving into middle or late childhood.

**Detection of Carrier:** Leukocytes or cultured skin fibroblasts of carriers have approximately one-half of the normal activity of acid lipase. This detection is facilitated by a recently developed fluorometric assay.

**Special Considerations:** **Cholesteryl ester storage disease** is allelic with Wolman disease. Patients with cholesterol ester storage disease are mildly disabled and may live to midadulthood or longer. They have liver disease and premature arteriosclerosis. The relationship between Wolman disease and cholesterol ester storage disease is not clear. Patients with intermediate degrees of severity have been reported. One patient with cholesteryl ester storage disease has shown adrenal calcification, while a patient with Wolman disease lacked it.

**References:**
Crocker AC, et al.: Wolman's disease: three new patients with a recently described lipidosis. Pediatrics 1965; 35:627–640.
Eto Y, Kitagawa T: Wolman disease with hypolipoproteinemia and acanthocytosis: clinical and biochemical observations. J Pediatr 1970; 77:862–867.
Coates PM, et al.: Prenatal diagnosis of Wolman disease. Am J Med Genet 1978; 2:397–407.
Koch G, et al.: Assignment of LIPA, associated with human lipase deficiency to human chromosome 10 and comparative assignment to mouse chromosome 19. Somatic Cell Genet 1981; 7:345–358.
Nigre A, et al.: New spectrophotometric assays of acid lipase and their use in the diagnosis of Wolman and cholesteryl ester storage disease. Anal Biochem 1985; 145:398–405.
Cagle PT, et al.: Clinicopathological conference: pulmonary hypertension in an 18-year-old girl with cholesteryl ester storage disease (CESD). Am J Med Genet 1986; 24:711–722.
Schmitz G, Assmann G: Acid lipase deficiency: Wolman disease and cholesteryl ester storage disease. In: Scriver CR, et al, eds: The metabolic basis of inherited disease, 6th ed. New York: McGraw-Hill, 1989:1623–1644. *

M0038                                      **Hugo Moser**

**Wolman disease-hypolipoproteinemia-acanthocytosis**
   *See WOLMAN DISEASE*
**Word blindness, congenital**
   *See DYSLEXIA*
**Wormian bones-blue sclerae-mandibular hypoplasia-campomelia**
   *See SHORT STATURE-WORMIAN BONES-JOINT DISLOCATIONS*

---

**WRINKLY SKIN SYNDROME**                     **2907**

**Includes:** Skin, wrinkly skin syndrome

**Excludes:**
   **Cutis laxa** (0233)
   **Cutis laxa-growth defect, De Barsy type** (2138)
   **Ehlers-Danlos syndrome** (0338)
   **Osteodysplastica gerodermia, Bamatter type** (2099)

**Major Diagnostic Criteria:** Universal features are wrinkly skin of the dorsum of the hands and feet, wrinkly skin of the abdomen, an increased number of palmar and plantar creases, a prominent venous pattern of the skin, and hypoelasticity of the wrinkly skin.

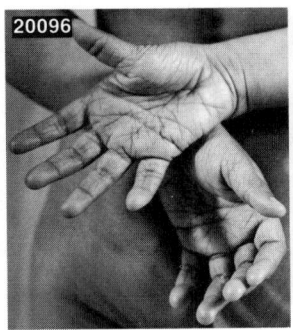 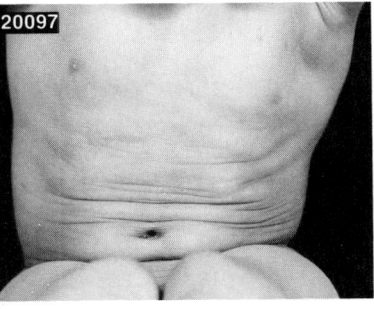

**2907-20096:** Increased palmar creases and aged appearance of the skin in this 5-year-old. **20097:** Transverse wrinkling of the abdomen in a 5-year-old.

**Clinical Findings:** The skin findings are present at birth. Progression of the skin findings is unknown; however, described cases do not display the generalized hypoelasticity of **Cutis laxa** or the generalized wrinkling of the skin and aged facial appearance of **Osteodysplastica gerodermia, Bamatter type.** Congenital hip dysplasia (7/7) joint hyperextensibility (5/6), and spinal deformity (6/7) are frequent features. Hypotonia (5/5), **Microcephaly** (4/5), and psychomotor retardation (4/6) occur with sufficient frequency to indicate that this syndrome has significant extracutaneous manifestations. Skin biopsy specimens have been normal in two patients, but one patient showed a decreased number and length of elastic fibers in the wrinkled as opposed to nonwrinkled skin.

**Complications:** Altered gait due to hip dysplasia and spinal deformities.

**Associated Findings:** Failure to thrive, short stature, myopia, chorioretinitis, congenital heart disease.

**Etiology:** Autosomal recessive inheritance, with consanguinity noted in all cases.

**Pathogenesis:** Some aspects may be due to disordered elastic metabolism.

**MIM No.:** *27825

**POS No.:** 3978

**Sex Ratio:** Presumably M1:F1. M2:F7 observed.

**Occurrence:** About a dozen cases have been documented in the literature.

**Risk of Recurrence for Patient's Sib:**
   See Part I, *Mendelian Inheritance.*

**Risk of Recurrence for Patient's Child:**
   See Part I, *Mendelian Inheritance.*

**Age of Detectability:** At birth.

**Gene Mapping and Linkage:** Unknown.

**Prevention:** None known. Genetic counseling indicated.

**Treatment:** Orthopedic management of hip dysplasia and spinal deformities.

**Prognosis:** Life span undetermined. The degree of mental retardation is also undetermined.

**Detection of Carrier:** Unknown. Carriers are not known to have any clinical manifestations.

**References:**
Gazit E, et al.: The wrinkly skin syndrome: a new heritable disorder of connective tissue. Clin Genet 1973; 4:186–192. * †
Goodman RM, et al.: The wrinkly skin syndrome and cartilage-hair hypoplasia (a new variant ?) in sibs of the same family. In: Papadatos CJ, Bartsocas CS, eds: Skeletal dysplasias. New York: Alan R. Liss, 1982:205–214.
Karrar ZA, et al.: Cutis laxa, intrauterine growth retardation, and bilateral dislocation of the hips: a report of five cases. In: Papadatos CJ, Bartsocas CS, eds: Skeletal dysplasia. New York: Alan R. Liss, 1982:215–221.
Karrar ZA, et al.: The wrinkly skin syndrome: a report of two siblings from Saudi Arabia. Clin Genet 1983; 23:308–310.
Casamassima AC, et al.: The wrinkly skin syndrome: phenotype and additional manifestations. Am J Med Genet 1987; 27:885–893. * †

CA035                           **Anthony C. Casamassima**

**Wryneck**
   *See TORTICOLLIS*
**WT limb-blood syndrome**
   *See WT SYNDROME*

## WT SYNDROME 3145

**Includes:**

Blood-limb syndrome
Fanconi-like radioulnar hypoplasia-hypoplastic anemia
Limb-blood syndrome
WT limb-blood syndrome

**Excludes:** Pancytopenia syndrome, Fanconi type (2029)

**Major Diagnostic Criteria:** Upper limb malformations, especially radial ray defects, in conjunction with hypoplastic anemia, with variable age of onset.

**Clinical Findings:** Abnormalities of upper extremities, including radioulnar synostosis; digitalized hypoplastic, or absent thumbs; and clinodactyly with or without **Camptodactyly** (usually of the fifth fingers). The anemia is usually chronic megaloblastic anemia with variable intensity and course. Increased mean corpuscular volume (MCV) can precede anemia by years. Bone marrow is usually hypoplastic, with megaloblastic changes in red cell precursors. In some families, pancytopenia is seen. Individuals presenting with severe hypoplastic anemia have decreased life span, often dying within six months to four years of onset of symptoms. Increased chromosome breakage has not been reported.

**Complications:** Transfusion-dependent treatment for chronic anemia may lead to iron overload, causing organ dysfunction such as congestive heart failure or cirrhosis of the liver. Congestive heart failure is often responsible for death. Affected individuals with pancytopenia may have bleeding and an increased incidence of infection secondary to neutropenia.

**Associated Findings:** History of easy bruising may precede development of severe hematologic symptoms. In one family reported with WT syndrome, short stature, sensorineural deafness, a characteristic facial appearance (high forehead, midface hypoplasia, upturned nose, and prominant ears) and hyperpigmentation were observed.

**Etiology:** Autosomal dominant inheritance with variable expression and virtually complete penetrance.

**Pathogenesis:** Unknown.

**MIM No.:** 19435

**POS No.:** 4053

**Sex Ratio:** Presumably M1:F1; M1.14:F1 (observed).

**Occurrence:** Three United States families have been documented; two in the Midwest, one in the Rocky Mountains.

**Risk of Recurrence for Patient's Sib:**
See Part I, *Mendelian Inheritance.*

**Risk of Recurrence for Patient's Child:**
See Part I, *Mendelian Inheritance.*

**Age of Detectability:** Limb anomalies are apparent at birth. Hematologic problems are variable in age of onset.

**Gene Mapping and Linkage:** Unknown.

**Prevention:** None known. Genetic counseling indicated.

**Treatment:** Symptomatic treatment of anemia.

**Prognosis:** Variable, depending on the severity of hematologic symptoms. For severe hypoplastic anemia, death often occurs within six months to 3–4 years of symptom onset.

**Detection of Carrier:** By physical examination and CBC and red blood cell MCV.

**Special Considerations:** The condition derives its name from the first two families described; the W. and the T. families. This condition should be distinguished from **Pancytopenia syndrome, Fanconi type** (Fanconi anemia), which is also associated with refractory anemia and radial ray defects. Families reported to have Fanconi anemia and an increased incidence of leukemia and congenital anomalies in nonanemic (or non-Fanconi syndrome) relatives may actually represent the WT syndrome.

**References:**

Gonzalez CH, et al.: The WT syndrome-a "new" autosomal dominant pleiotropic trait of radial/ulnar hypoplasia with high risk of bone marrow failure and/or leukemia. BD:OAS XIII(3B). New York: March of Dimes Birth Defects Foundation, 1977:31–38.

Smith ACM, et al.: WT syndrome: a third family. Am J Hum Genet 1987; 41:A84.

SM016 **Ann C.M. Smith**

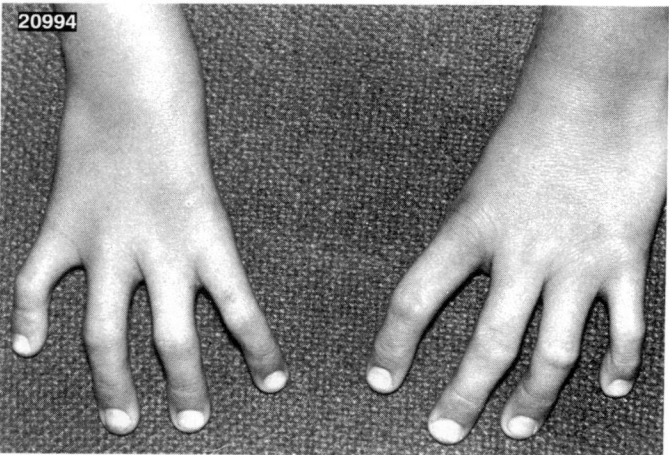

**3145**-20992: WT syndrome; note high forehead, upturned nose and prominent ears. This 13-year-old male has sensorineural deafness. 20993: Lateral view of the face shows midface hypoplasia. 20994: Bilateral absence of the thumbs.

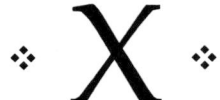

**X-linked adult onset spinobulbar muscular atrophy**
*See MUSCULAR ATROPHY, SPINAL AND BULBAR, X-LINKED KENNEDY TYPE*
**X-linked adult spinal muscular atrophy**
*See MUSCULAR ATROPHY, SPINAL AND BULBAR, X-LINKED KENNEDY TYPE*
**X-linked copper malabsorption**
*See MENKES SYNDROME*
**X-linked fragile site**
*See X-LINKED MENTAL RETARDATION, FRAGILE X SYNDROME*

## X-LINKED MENTAL RETARDATION                    1509

The concept of X-linked mental retardation has evolved continuously over the last 50 years. (Penrose, 1938) first suggested that the more frequent occurence of mental retardation in males, compared to females, was not due to a number of X-linked genes but to social factors. It now appears that about a third of mental retardation in males may be explainable on the basis of X-linked genes. This concept was later reviewed and confirmed by Morton, et al (1977) and Herbst (1980), and others who suggested that a total of seven to nineteen specific disorders accounted for this sex difference. In the 1960's, Lehrke (1974) also promulgated the idea of the significance of X-linked genes in mental retardation. Progress in understanding X-linked mental retardation was delayed not only by the absence of laboratory diagnosis for these entities, but, at least in retrospect, by the frequent occurence of mildly affected females in many families which obscured the expected pedigree pattern of pure X-linked recessive inheritance. The few publications in this area were generally referenced under the term "non-specific X-linked mental retardation". These included the reports by Martin and Bell (1943) and Renpenning et al (1962). No specific clinical findings within these families were reported in either paper.

In 1969, Lubs reported the marker X, now known as the fragile X, in a family with mental retardation in four males. Giraud et al (1976) and Harvey et al (1977) reported additional cases. At the same time Sutherland (1977) demonstrated the requirements for low folate and low thymidine in culture media for consistent detection of the fragile X. This opened the door to repeatable and planned studies of X-linked mental retardation. The family originally reported by Martin and Bell (1943) was restudied by Richards et al (1981) and proved to have the fragile X. Although *Martin-Bell syndrome* has often been used to describe the fragile X syndrome, it is a confusing reference since neither the clinical features nor the fragile X were observed in the original report and the more descriptive term "fragile X" is preferred.

Most studies have shown that only 30–40% of unselected families with X-linked mental retardation have the fragile X. Nine members of the family reported by Renpenning et al (1962) were restudied by Fox et al (1980). This family proved not to have the fragile X chromosome but did show a moderately consistent pattern of findings, including low mean measurements for height, weight, head circumference and testicular volume, and probably

represents a distinct syndrome. No laboratory tests yet exist for the remaining entities. Very likely, certain of the apparently similar disorders described below will be delineated as clinical entities by linkage and localization studies and others will prove to be overlapping descriptions of a syndrome described under several names by different authors. Only in twelve of the syndromes reported to date have two or more families been reported. The syndromes described by Atkins et al (1985) and by Clark et al (1987), for example, are listed as separate entities although their facial features are quite similar. The "distinguishing features" of hypertelorism and short stature in the Atkins family (compared to hypotelorism and normal stature in the Clark-Baraitser family) may have been familial since other family members had similar findings.

Table 1509–1 presents a working summary of disorders that have been included in the category of non-specific X-linked mental retardation but now have emerging, more specific, features. It does not include all possible entities. X-linked disorders with mental retardation and obvious clinical manifestations, such as hydrocephaly or blindness, are not generally included in this classification. About 80 X-linked disorders may include mental retardation as one manifestation.

**References:**
Penrose LS: A clinical and genetic study of 1,280 cases of mental defect. Special Rep Ser No. 229, London, Med Res Council, 1938.
Martin JP, Bell J: A pedigree of mental defect showing sex-linkage. J Neurol Psychiatr 1943; 6:154–157.
Renpenning H, et al.: Familial sex-linked mental retardation. Can Med Assoc J 1962; 87:954–956.
Giraud F, et al.: Constitutional chromosomal breakage. Hum Genet 1969; 34:125–136.
Lubs HA: A marker-X chromosome. Am J Hum Genet 1969; 21:231–244.
Lehrke RG: X-linked mental retardation and verbal disability. New York, Intercontinental Medical Book Corporation, 1974. BDOAS X:1–100 (Publication of PhD thesis of the same title, University of Wisconsin, 1968).
Harvey J, et al.: Familial X-linked mental retardation with an X chromosome abnormality. J Med Genet 1977; 14:46–50.
Morton N, et al.: Colchester revisited: a genetic study of mental defect. J Med Genet 1977; 14:1–9.
Sutherland GR: Fragile sites on human chromosomes: demonstration of their dependence on the type of tissue culture medium. Science 1977; 197:265–266.
Fox P, et al.: X-linked mental retardation: Renpenning revisited. Am J Med Genet 1980; 7:491–495.
Herbst DS, Miller JR: Non-specific X-linked mental retardation. II. The frequency in British Columbia. Am J Med Genet 1980; 7:461–469.
Richards BW, et al.: Fragile X-linked mental retardation: the Martin-Bell syndrome. J Ment Defic Res 1981; 25:253–256.
Atkin JF, et al.: A new X-linked mental retardation syndrome. Am J Med Genet 1985; 21:697–705.

**Table 1509-1   Selected X-linked Mental Retardation Syndromes**

| Condition | Distinctive Features | Other Features |
|---|---|---|
| **TWO OR MORE FAMILIES REPORTED** | | |
| X-linked mental retardation, Fragile X syndrome | Fragile X diagnostic<br>Large testes<br>Connective tissue abnormalities with hyperextension, pectus & floppy mitral valve | May have narrow faces, with hypoplastic midface late in childhood with prominent ears. Approximately 1/3 females retarded or dull |
| X-linked mental retardation, Renpenning type | Small head, short stature<br>Small testes (each 2–25 %ile) | All features are highly variable & may fall in normal range in some family members |
| X-linked mental retardation, Marfanoid habitus type | Tall (>90 %ile), thin<br>Connective tissue abnormalities with pectus & long, thin hands. Long, narrow face with thin, high nasal bridge, small chin.<br>Large testes (≥90 %ile) | Agenesis corpus callosum in some |
| Simpson-Golabi-Behmel syndrome | Striking coarse facies<br>Macrostomia<br>Pre + postnatal overgrowth<br>Coccygeal skin tags<br>Midline notching lower lip | Submucous cleft<br>Bone anomalies<br>Cystic kidney<br>Hepatosplenomegaly<br>Early death in some |
| X-linked mental retardation-growth-hearing and genital defects | Small stature & delayed bone age. Mild-severe deafness. Small scrotum & penis. Cryptorchidism | Severe mental retardation<br>Small palpebral fissures<br>Flat nasal bridge<br>Poor survival |
| X-linked mental retardation-clasped thumb | Bilateral absence of extensor pollicis brevis tendons with thumb flexion deformity | Usually normal appearance<br>May have growth retardation, lordosis & microcephaly |
| X-linked mental retardation-Xq duplication | Growth deficiency<br>Short stature (below 3rd %ile)<br>Somatomedin C deficiency<br>Delayed bone age<br>Peculiar face | Small palpebral fissure<br>Bilateral ptosis<br>Tented upper lip<br>Full lower lip<br>Down turned corners of mouth |
| FG syndrome, Opitz-Kaveggia type | Hypotonia<br>Slow motor development<br>Short stature<br>Abnormal skull/relative macrocephaly<br>High, prominent forehead<br>Frontal cowlick<br>Micrognathia<br>Muscle weakness | Hypertelorism/telecanthus<br>Abnormal (mostly anti-mongoloid) palpebral slant<br>Long philtrum<br>High, arched palate<br>Abnormal dermatoglyphics<br>Striking personality |
| Coffin-Lowry syndrome | Downslanting palpebral fissures<br>Mild hypertelorism<br>Prominent brow<br>Broad nose<br>Microcephaly<br>Short stature<br>Unusual facial appearance | Thick, soft skin<br>Large hands with tapering fingers |
| Smith-Fineman-Myers syndrome | Micrognathia<br>Narrow face<br>Patulous lower lip | Minor foot deformities<br>Hyperreflexia<br>Seizures |
| X-linked mental retardation-choreoathetosis | Choreoathetosis in first year; often constant. Later spasticity, ophthalmoplegia & deafness. Postnatal growth retardation & microcephaly. | Appears normal at birth<br>Later sunken eyes & pinched lower nose |
| Borjeson-Forssman-Lehmann syndrome | Short stature (<3 %ile)<br>Narrow palpebral fissures<br>Large ears, hypogonadism<br>Seizures | Obesity and swelling of subcutaneous face, hypometabolism, short upturned nose |
| **SINGLE FAMILY REPORTED** | | |
| X-linked mental retardation, Atkin type | Short stature<br>Hypertelorism<br>Broad nose and coarse facies<br>Large testes (? familial) | Large, square forehead<br>May have large head & ears. (? familial) |

**Table 1509-1 (continued)** Selected X-linked Mental Retardation Syndromes

| Condition | Distinctive Features | Other Features |
| --- | --- | --- |
| X-linked mental retardation, Clark-Baraitser type | Normal stature<br>Hypotelorism<br>Broad nose & coarse facies<br>Large testes | Large head (males) & square forehead |
| X-linked mental retardation, Golabi-Ito-Hall type | Postnatal growth deficiency and micro-cephaly<br>Narrow, triangular face<br>Anteverted ears<br>Upslanted palpebral fissures<br>Laterally displaced inner canthi | Epicanthal folds<br>ASD<br>Brittle, dry hair |
| X-linked mental retardation-craniofacial abnormalities-club foot | Peculiar facies (coarse)<br>Microcephaly<br>Large anterior fontanel<br>Club foot deformity<br>Early death | Epicanthic folds<br>Flat nasal bridge<br>Anteverted nostrils<br>Abnormal teeth<br>Hypotonia |
| Seizures, in females, Juberg-Hellman type | Probably X-linked dominant inheritance. Expression limited to females. Seizures with onset 6–18 months. Half also re-tarded. | |
| X-linked mental retardation-basal ganglion disorder | Persistent frontal lobe reflexes, cogwheel rigidity, abnormal gait & Parkinsonian tremor. Frontal bossing & large head. | Strabismus<br>Seizures |
| X-linked mental retardation-skeletal dysplasia | Ridging of metopic suture<br>Fused & hemi-vertebrae<br>Scoliosis & sacral hypoplasia<br>Short mid-phalanges<br>Abducens palsy | Antimongoloid slant & epicanthic folds<br>Broad nasal bridge |
| Contractures-muscle atrophy-oculo-motor apraxia | Weakness of upper and lower limbs<br>Distal muscle atrophy<br>Dyspraxia of the eye, face and tongue muscles<br>Swallowing difficulties | Overlap of toes<br>Manifestations apparently more restricted to ner-vous system |
| X-linked mental retardation-psoriasis | Delayed psychomotor development<br>Normal growth<br>Ataxic gait<br>Seizures | Apparent hypertelorism<br>Large ears, macrostomia<br>Long philtrum |
| X-linked mental retardation-dystonic movements of hands | Normal growth<br>Dysarthria | No special facial features |
| X-linked mental retardation-subcorti-cal atrophy-patellar luxation | Facial dysmorphia<br>Clinodactily<br>Ear malformations<br>High nasal bridge<br>Patella luxation<br>Febrile convulsion<br>Abnormalities of fundus of eye | Abnormal teeth<br>Skin dimple of lower back<br>Limb malformation |
| Hyperkeratosis palmoplantaris-spas-tic paraplegia-retardation | Pes cavus deformity<br>Abnormal gait | Peculiar face (may be familial) |
| X-linked mental retardation-muscular weakness-awkward gait | Severe MR<br>Hypotonia<br>Joint contractures<br>Delayed, clumsy walking<br>Awkward, wide-base gait | Hyporeflexia<br>Marked speech defect<br>No special facial features described |
| Short stature-cerebral atrophy-kera-tosis follicularis, X-linked | Delayed somatic growth<br>Microcephaly<br>Seizures | Absence of hair and eyelashes<br>Micrognathia<br>Delayed dentition |
| X-linked mental retardation-short stature-obesity-hypogonadism | Moderate to Severe MR<br>Mild obesity—infancy onset<br>Distinct facial features<br>Short neck | Bitemporal narrowing<br>Almond-shaped palpebral fissures<br>Flat nasal bridge<br>Inverted V-shaped upper lip<br>Short upper lip |

Clark RD, Baraitser M: A new X-linked mental retardation syndrome. (Letter) Am J Med Genet 1987; 26:13–15.

LU002
AR011

**Herbert A. Lubs**
**J. Fernando Arena**

**X-linked mental retardation with fragile X**
*See X-LINKED MENTAL RETARDATION, FRAGILE X SYNDROME*

---

## X-LINKED MENTAL RETARDATION, ATKIN TYPE    2840

**Includes:** Atkin-Flaitz X-linked mental retardation
**Excludes:**
  **X-linked mental retardation, Clark-Baraitser type** (2640)
  **X-linked mental retardation** (other)

**Major Diagnostic Criteria:** Expected findings include moderate-to-severe mental retardation in males and normal intelligence or mild mental retardation in females, short stature, **Megalencephaly**, and coarse facial features.

**Clinical Findings:** Affected individuals have a facial appearance similar to that found in **Coffin-Lowry syndrome**, including large, square forehead; prominent supraorbital ridges; **Eye, hypertelorism**; downslanting palpebral fissure; and broad nasal tip with anteverted nostrils. Other features include **Megalencephaly**, micrognathia, and large ears.

All affected males have moderate-to-severe mental retardation, with developmental delays being noted within the first year of life. Females show mild mental retardation. Twenty-seven percent (3/11) have seizures. Most have a congenial personality, though aggressive behavior has also been exhibited.

Orodental findings include microdontic maxillary lateral inci-

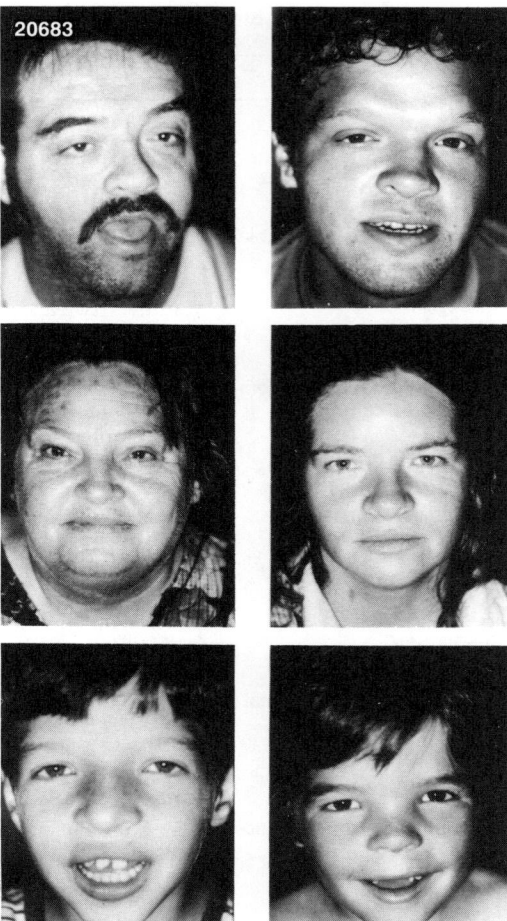

**2840B-20683:** Faces of representative affected relatives; note Coffin-Lowry-like facies.

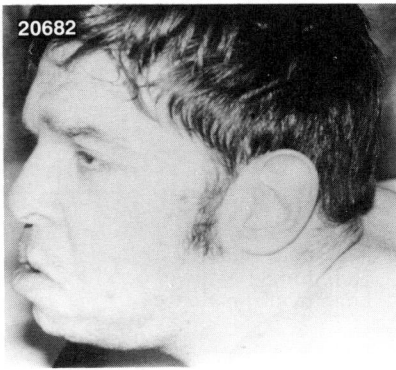

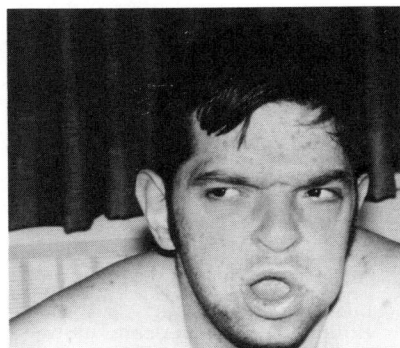

**2840A-20682:** X-linked mental retardation, Atkin type; note coarse facial features similar to that found in the Coffin-Lowry syndrome with prominent supraorbital ridge, broad nasal tip with anteverted nares and thick lower lip.

sors, diastema between maxillary central incisors, palatal torus, and exaggerated median furrow of the tongue.

Other findings include short stature, obesity, and macroorchidism.

**Complications:** Unknown.

**Associated Findings:** None known.

**Etiology:** X-linked inheritance. There is no male-to-male transmission; however, none of the known affected males have reproduced. Women are mildly affected or unaffected.

**Pathogenesis:** Unknown.

**MIM No.:** *30953

**Sex Ratio:** M11:F3 (observed). Limited data suggest that if this is an X-linked condition, females may be affected more often than expected due to lyonization.

**Occurrence:** One kinship with 14 affected members has been documented.

**Risk of Recurrence for Patient's Sib:**
  See Part I, *Mendelian Inheritance*.

**Risk of Recurrence for Patient's Child:**
  See Part I, *Mendelian Inheritance*.

**Age of Detectability:** Within the first year of life, if family history is positive.

**Gene Mapping and Linkage:**  MRX1 (mental retardation, X-linked 1 (non-dysmorphic)) has been mapped to Xp11-q13.

**Prevention:**  None known. Genetic counseling indicated.

**Treatment:**  Treatment of seizures if present, or behavior therapy if needed.

**Prognosis:**  Normal life span.

**Detection of Carrier:**  Unknown.

**Special Considerations:**  Some described features may be familial. The macrocephaly may still be a component of the syndrome as, relatively, the heads are larger than unaffected relatives'. The macroorchidism is likely to be a component of the syndrome, as the average testicular volume in affected individuals is greater than that of unaffected individuals in the same family.

**References:**
Atkin JF, et al.: A new X-linked mental retardation syndrome. Am J Med Genet 1985; 21:697–705.

AT004                                    **Joan F. Atkin**

**X-linked mental retardation, Chudley-Lowry-Hoar type**
*See X-LINKED MENTAL RETARDATION-SHORT STATURE-OBESITY-HYPOGONADISM*

## X-LINKED MENTAL RETARDATION, CLARK-BARAITSER TYPE       2640

**Includes:**  Clark-Baraitser X-linked mental retardation

**Excludes:**
    **Borjeson-Forssman-Lehmann syndrome** (2272)
    **Coffin-Lowry syndrome** (0190)
    **X-linked mental retardation** (other)

**Major Diagnostic Criteria:**  **Megalencephaly**, mental retardation of a mild-to-moderate degree, and obesity are present. Affected males have macroorchidism.

**Clinical Findings:**  Affected males are more severely retarded than females; however, both share the facial features of hypotelorism, prominent supraorbital ridges, broad nasal base, thick lower lip, and large ears. Diastema of upper central incisors and small upper lateral incisors are seen. Obesity is moderate, and stature is normal. **Megalencephaly** is present only in males.

**Complications:**  Unknown.

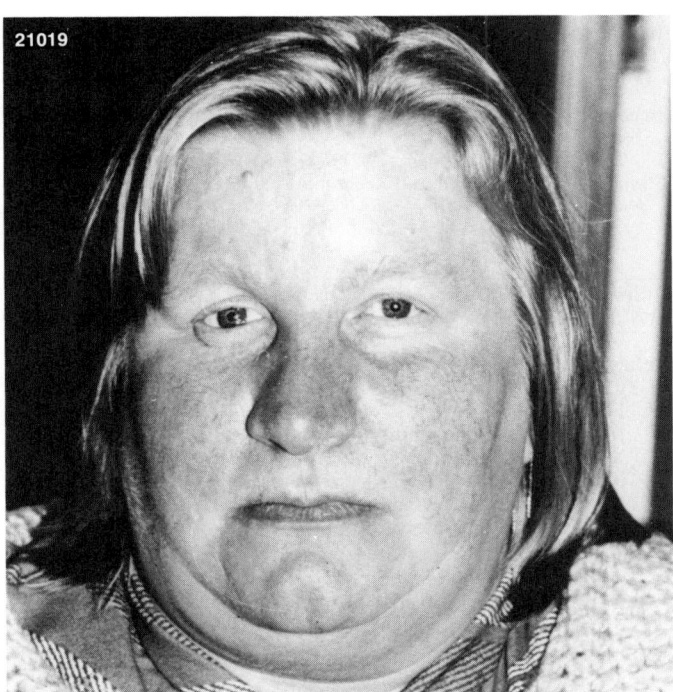

**2640B**-21019:  Mildly retarded and obese mother of sons shown in 21020 & 21021.

**Associated Findings:**  None known.

**Etiology:**  In one family, a mildly affected woman bore two moderately retarded sons and three normal children, including one daughter. This is compatible with X-linked inheritance with decreased expression in the female; however, autosomal dominant inheritance cannot be ruled out.

**Pathogenesis:**  Unknown.

**MIM No.:**  *30953

**Sex Ratio:**  M2:F1 (observed).

**Occurrence:**  One family has been reported in the literature.

**Risk of Recurrence for Patient's Sib:**
    See Part I, *Mendelian Inheritance.*

**Risk of Recurrence for Patient's Child:**
    See Part I, *Mendelian Inheritance.*

**Age of Detectability:**  Evident during early childhood by mental retardation and recognizable facies.

**Gene Mapping and Linkage:**  MRX1 (mental retardation, X-linked 1 (non-dysmorphic)) has been mapped to Xp11-q13.

**Prevention:**  None known. Genetic counseling indicated.

**Treatment:**  Unknown.

**Prognosis:**  Apparently normal life span, mild-to-moderate mental retardation.

**Detection of Carrier:**  Clinical examination of females for evidence of the trait is indicated.

**Special Considerations:**  Many similarities exist between this condition and **X-linked mental retardation, Atkin type**. The differences, that those affected who were reported by Atkin were shorter and had **Eye, hypertelorism**, were considered significant by some but not all observers.

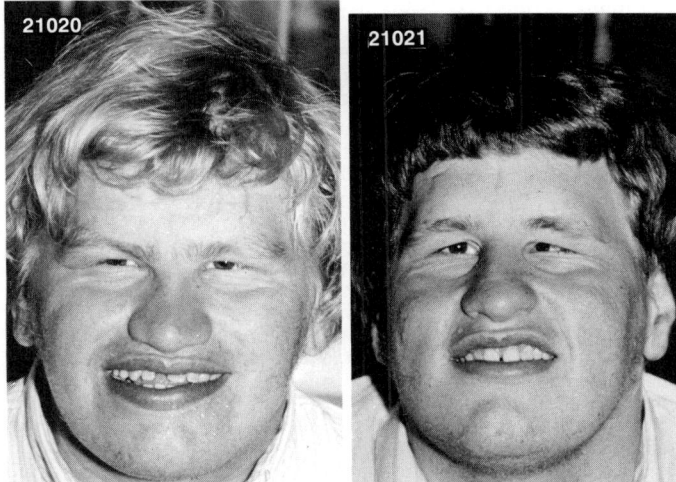

**2640A**-21020–21:  X-linked mental retardation, Clark-Baraitser type; two moderately retarded affected brothers.

**References:**
Clark RD, Baraitser M: A new X-linked mental retardation syndrome. (Letter) Am J Med Genet 1987; 26:13–15.

CL004
BA058

**Robin Dawn Clark**
**Michael Baraitser**

**X-linked mental retardation, Fitzsimmons type**
*See HYPERKERATOSIS PALMOPLANTARIS-SPASTIC PARAPLEGIA-RETARDATION*

---

## X-LINKED MENTAL RETARDATION, FRAGILE X SYNDROME
**2073**

**Includes:**
Chromosome, Marker X
Fragile X chromosome
Martin-Bell X-linked mental retardation
Mental retardation, X-linked-marXq28
X-linked fragile site
X-linked mental retardation-macroorchidism
X-linked mental retardation with fragile X

**Excludes:**
**X-linked mental retardation, Renpenning type** (2920)
X-linked mental retardation without the fragile X chromosome

**Major Diagnostic Criteria:** The definitive diagnosis depends upon finding the fragile X chromosome. Males with the fragile X

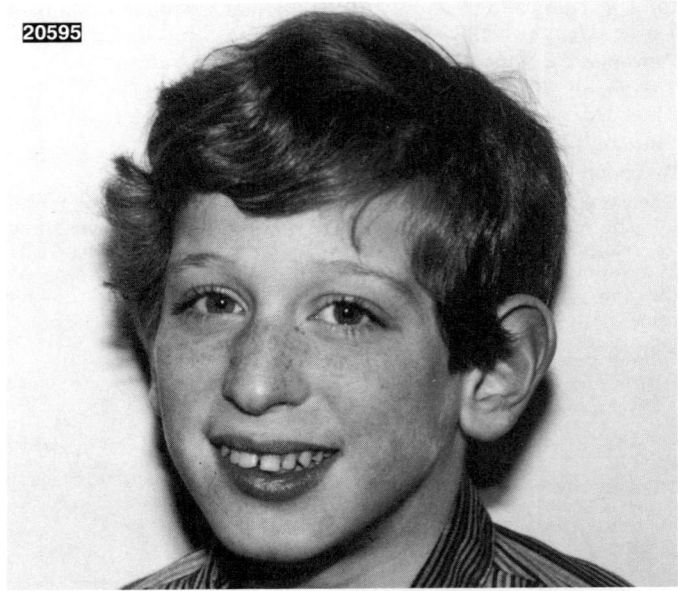

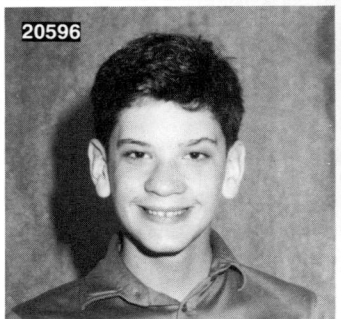
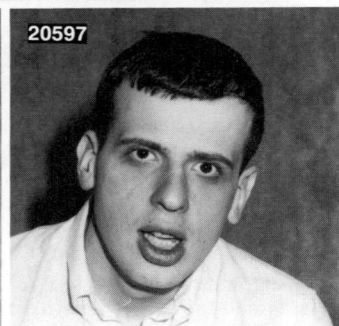

**2073B**-20595–97: Chromosome X, Fragile X syndrome; note long face with prominent ears and nose, large mouth and thick lips.

---

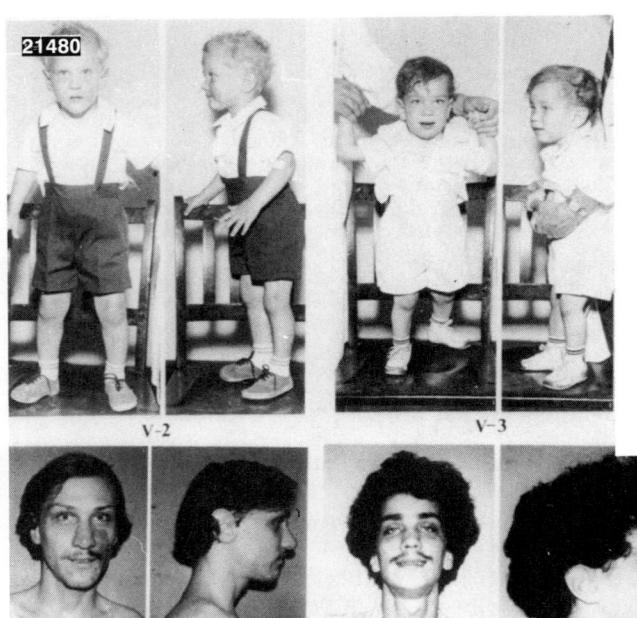

**2073A**-21480: Original siblings with fragile X described by Lubs (1969). Sib 1 on left at age 3 and 18. Sib 2 at right at 18 mo. and age 17. Both had low set, posteriorly angulated and slightly large ears and broadly based stance. Heads in both at age 17 and 18 are narrower than their normal brother's and father's (not shown). Ears and jaws have changed little in 15 years, although face is longer and more narrow in Sib 2. There is slight pectus and similar size nevus in Sib 1, age 3 and 18.

(abbreviated fra(X)) tend to have mental retardation, large testes and minor connective tissue manifestations. Females are usually of normal intelligence but may be mildly retarded with minor abnormalities. There is often a family history of mental retardation which follows an X-linked pattern of inheritance, but an increasingly large proportion of sporadic cases are now being recognized.

**Clinical Findings:** The degree of mental retardation in affected males varies from borderline normal to severe.

Unusually large testes (megalotestes or macroorchidism) are found in 80–90% of affected males after puberty. Testicular function is normal. Affected males may have one or both testes of normal size and there is some overlap with normal male testicular size. Prior to puberty, large testes are usually not present but have been described. Large testes (≥30 ml) are sometimes found in retarded males without the fragile X.

Craniofacial features which may be found in affected males are large head, prominent forehead, large ears, and a facies which becomes increasingly long and thin with age. The appearance of a long face is due to a shortening of the interzygomatic distance by about 1 cm. The mandible also becomes particularly prominent in some males after age 20.

Possible connective tissue manifestions include hyperextension of fingers in the majority of children, mild-to-severe pectus excavatum and floppy mitral valve in 80% over age 18 (ordinarily without complications). Occasionally long fingers and hand abnormalities are present. Fine skin and a high-arched palate also have been described.

Behavior is variable. Many are hyperactive, particularly during clinic visits and during the younger years. Management is usually possible at home.

Diagnosis of the fragile X in newborns and young infants on purely clinical criterial is currently difficult. Large, posteriorly rotated ears with minimal folding may be the only physical sign.

Clinical findings in female carriers: Appearance and intelligence are usually normal. A third of carriers have mild mental retardation. A long face has been described in affected carriers and connective tissue manifestations may occur. Increased twinning and fertility have been reported.

**Complications:**  Autistic-like behavior occurs in 5–10% of males. Seizures may occur.

**Associated Findings:**  None known.

**Etiology:**  X-linked inheritance. In affected males, the X chromosome shows a lightstaining gap or fragile site at Xq27.3 in 4–60% cells. The distal portion of Xq may appear bisatellated. A gene at or very closely linked to this fragile site is responsible for the abnormalities in this syndrome. The gene behaves neither as a pure X-linked recessive or dominant gene and may be best described as semi-dominant with decreased penetrance in males.

The fragility of the X, which has not been demonstrated *in vivo*, is probably unrelated to these abnormalities and serves primarily as a marker for the responsible gene. In interspecies somatic cell hybrids, however, crossing-over occurs at the fragile cell hybrids, and may play a role in the pathogenosis of the abnormalities in man.

Males who express neither the clinical nor the cytogenetic manifestations occur and transmit the gene. This may occur in as many as 20% of males with this gene. Nearly all male and female siblings of such transmitting males are normal, as are their obligate carrier daughters. Several mechanisms, including inactivation of the locus during meiosis in certain females, and a stepwise premutation and mutation due to unequal crossing over have been postulated to explain these males. All mothers of sporadic cases are not, as once thought, carriers. Increasingly frequent diagnosis of sporadic cases on clinical grounds will require a new analysis of these data in the future. Isolation of the gene itself will ultimately permit resolution of these uncertainties and an explanation of the unusual genetic mechanisms.

**Pathogenesis:**  Unknown.

**MIM No.:**  *30955

**POS No.:**  3324

**Sex Ratio:**  M1.0:F0.7

**Occurrence:**  It is estimated that mental retardation due to the fra(X) occurs in at least 1:2,000 male births and is only slightly less frequent in females. The incidence is sufficient to class the fragile X as the most common inherited cause of mental retardation in males.

**Risk of Recurrence for Patient's Sib:**  If mother is a carrier and has a normal intelligence at least 40% and probably 50% of male sibs are affected. One-half of daughters receive the chromosome, and 30–40% will be retarded, for a net risk of 15–20%. The risk of having a retarded female offspring may be higher for retarded heterozygotes.

If fra(X) studies fail to demonstrate any female carriers in the family, current data indicate that a quarter of male siblings and 7–8% of male cousins are affected. It should not be assumed that all mothers of affected, sporadic males are carriers.

**Risk of Recurrence for Patient's Child:**  Few affected males have reproduced. Unaffected carrier males have no risk of affected sons. All daughters are obligate carriers but the risk of retardation is very low. The risks described above for obligate female carriers also hold for their daughters' offspring.

**Age of Detectability:**  An affected male has not yet been diagnosed at birth on clinical grounds alone. During infancy and early childhood, developmental delay and large ears may permit the diagnosis to be suspected. The fragile X chromosome itself in males can be detected cytogenetically at anytime from lymphocytes. Many reports of the prenatal diagnosis of the fragile X in males have been published.

**Gene Mapping and Linkage:**  FRAXA (fragile site, folic acid type, rare, fra(X)(q27.3)) has been mapped to Xq27.3.

**Prevention:**  None known. Genetic counseling indicated.

**Treatment:**  Speech therapy as well as early infant stimulation may be indicated. Psychological consultation in managing hyperactivity and autistic behavior may be helpful. Blind trials with folic acid or folate derivatives have not demonstrated significant improvement in either intelligence or behavior.

**Prognosis:**  Mental retardation is reported in all fragile X expressing males, and in about 30–40% of carrier females.

**Detection of Carrier:**  Blood (lymphocytes) must be cultured in a low-folate and low-thymidine medium such as medium 199 to demonstrate the fragile X. Alternatively, a folate antagonist such as methotrexate or FUdr which blocks thymidylate synthetase can be used. Many obligate carriers show no or a very low, frequency of fragile X positive cells. The demonstration of the fragile X in skin fibroblasts is sometimes difficult. In intelligent female carriers, the fragile X may be hard to detect because the frequency of the fragile X is usually low.

**Special Considerations:**  Chromosome studies to detect the fragile X must be done under special culture medium conditions as described above. Ordinary culture conditions with complete medium obscure the expression of the fragile X. Therefore, if a male is suspected of having the fragile X and has not had special cytogenetic studies designed to screen for the fragile X, chromosome studies must be repeated under correct conditions. These conditions include medium 199 or the addtion of FUdr or methotrexate. The proportion of cells expressing the fragile X varies and 50–100 should be examined. Care should be taken to distinguish the Xq27.3 fragile site from the similar but non-risk bearing fragile site at Xq27.2.

The fragile X can occur in normal males who can transmit it, but not show it cytogenetically. Prenatal diagnosis is still difficult and should only be undertaken in laboratories with significant experience in the detection of the fragile X. Detection of the fragile X from fetal blood from periumbilical blood may be the prenatal diagnostic procedure of choice.

Linkage studies of the fragile X site with DNA markers are available and of use in carrier testing and genetic counseling, but several problems currently limit their usefulness for prenatal diagnosis. The gene order from proximal to distal is DXS51 (a DNA marker), F9 (factor IX), fragile X DXS52 (a DNA marker) and DX515 (still another DNA marker). The recombinational distances currently average about 7% from DXS51 to F9, 22% from F9 to fra(X), 13% from fra(X) to DXS52 and 2% from DXS52 to DXS15. There appears to be genetic heterogeneity with tight linkage (about 18%) between F9 and fra(X) in some families and loose linkage (about 35%) in others. Because of these relatively large recombination distances, the final decision regarding of the fragile X is still best made by its cytogenetic demonstration.

*The authors wish to thank Thomas W. Glover and Grant R. Sutherland for their contributions to an earlier version of this article.*

**Support Groups:**
  NJ; Bridgeton; National Fragile X Support Group
  CO; Denver; The Fragile X Foundation

**References:**
Lubs HA: A marker X chromosome. Am J Hum Genet 1969; 21:231–244.
Sutherland GR: Heritable fragile sites on human chromosomes. I. Factors affecting expression in lymphocyte culture. Am J Hum Genet 1979; 31:125–135.
Jacobs PA, et al: X-linked mental retardations: a study of 7 families. Am J Med Genet 1980; 7:471–489.
Turner G, et al: Heterozygous expression of X-linked mental retardation and X-chromosome marker fra (X)(q27). New Engl J Med 1980; 303:662–664.
Turner G, et al: X-linked mental retardation, macro-orchidism, and the Xq27 fragile site. J Pediatr 1980; 96:837–841.

Sutherland GR: The fragile X chromosome. Int Rev Cytol 1983; 81:107–141.

Sutherland GR, Hecht F: Fragile sites on human chromosomes. New York: Oxford University Press, 1985.

Brown WT, et al.: Multilocus analysis of the fragile X syndrome. Hum Genet 1988; 78:201–205.

Fryns JP, et al.: A peculiar subphenotype in the fra (X) syndrome: extreme obesity - short stature - stubby hands and feet - diffuse hyperpigmentation. Clin Genet 1988; 32:388–392.

Schwartz CE, et al.: Fragile X monograph. Proc Greenwood Genet Ctr 1988; 7:76–117.

Spano LM, Opitz JM: Bibliography on X-linked mental retardation, the fragile X and related subjects. Am J Med Genet 1988; 30:31–60.

Bridge PJ, Lillicrap DP: Molecular diagnosis of the fragile X [Fra (X)] syndrome: calculation of risks based on flanking DNA markers in small phase-unknown families. Am J Med Genet 1989; 33:92–99.

LU002                                                          Herbert A. Lubs
HE007                                                          Frederick Hecht

## X-LINKED MENTAL RETARDATION, GOLABI-ITO-HALL TYPE                                                    3199

**Includes:** Golabi-Ito-Hall syndrome

**Excludes:** X-linked mental retardation (other)

**Major Diagnostic Criteria:** Mental retardation, postnatal growth deficiency, postnatal **Microcephaly**, narrow triangular face, anteverted ears, upslanted palpebral fissures, epicanthal folds.

**Clinical Findings:** Mental retardation (one with IQ estimated at 23); postnatal growth deficiency (3/3) noted during the first year of life; postnatal **Microcephaly** (3/3); narrow triangular face (2/3); anteverted ears (3/3); mild hearing loss (1/3); up-slanted palpebral fissures with epicanthal folds (3/3) and laterally displaced inner canthi (2/3). Thin upper lip appeared to be present in (3/3) photographs. Congenital heart defect (**Atrial septal defects** in one case, questionable in the second). Brittle, dry hair (2/3); asymmetric chest (1/3), and chest malformation (1/3). Hypospadias (1/3).

Pertinent normal features include normal testicular size (two prepubertal, one postpubertal), normal results of urine amino acid analysis (two cases reported), and normal chromosomes (one case reported).

**Complications:** One case developed petit mal seizures.

**Associated Findings:** Possible congenital heart defect.

**Etiology:** X-linked recessive inheritance.

**Pathogenesis:** Unknown.

**MIM No.:** *30953

**POS No.:** 3590

**Sex Ratio:** M3:F0 (observed).

**Occurrence:** Three individuals in one Caucasian family (two boys, sons of sisters, and their mother's brother) have been clinically evaluated or had their hospital records reviewed.

**Risk of Recurrence for Patient's Sib:**
See Part I, *Mendelian Inheritance.*

**Risk of Recurrence for Patient's Child:**
See Part I, *Mendelian Inheritance.*

**Age of Detectability:** During the first year of life.

**Gene Mapping and Linkage:** MRX1 (mental retardation, X-linked 1 (non dysmorphic)) has been mapped to Xp11-q13.

**Prevention:** None known. Genetic counseling indicated.

**Treatment:** Unknown.

**Prognosis:** Normal life span is presumed; however, three suspected cases reported in the same family died before ten years of age.

**Detection of Carrier:** Unknown.

**References:**
Golabi M, et al: A new X-linked multiple congenital anomalies/mental retardation syndrome. Am J Med Genet 1984; 17:367–374.

AR011                                                          J. Fernando Arena
LU002                                                          Herbert A. Lubs

### X-linked mental retardation, Holmes-Gang type
*See X-LINKED MENTAL RETARDATION-CRANIOFACIAL ABNORMALITIES-CLUB FOOT*

## X-LINKED MENTAL RETARDATION, MARFANOID HABITUS TYPE                                                2921

**Includes:** Marfanoid habitus and X-linked mental retardation

**Excludes:**
**Aicardi syndrome** (2320)
**Corpus callosum agenesis** (0220)
**Facio-neuro-skeletal syndrome** (2339)
**FG syndrome**
**X-linked mental retardation** (other)

**Major Diagnostic Criteria:** The combination of psychomotor retardation (usually moderate) with a relatively tall, thin (Marfanoid) habitus; a long, thin face; a high-arched palate; and joint hyperextensibility in one or more persons consistent with X-linked inheritance.

**Clinical Findings:** The first four males described were from one kindred. All were retarded (IQ range, 40–60) with tall stature (>75th percentile), a large head (>90th percentile), a high-arched palate, small mandible, and hypernasal speech. Three are asthenic (height ≤50th percentile) with long narrow faces and joint hyperextensibility. Despite long fingers, none showed true arachnodactyly or an increased arm span. Other features included **Pectus excavatum** (noted in two) and **Atrial septal defects** (in one case), and large testes (≥ 90th percentile in three).

All test negative for **X-linked mental retardation, Fragile X syndrome**. Complete **Corpus callosum agenesis** was seen in one patient, with partial absence in his brother. One had seizures. Three were poorly coordinated, and all four had attention deficits. Behavior was otherwise variable, showing jocularity, aggressiveness, dependency, and autistic-like mannerisms.

Two further pairs of retarded male siblings (IQ: 56–70), who share similar craniofacial features and the slender, Marfanoid habitus have been reported (Fryns & Buttiens, 1987). These individuals differ, however, in that only one measures below the 75th percentile in height, three show a HC ≤ 50th percentile, and two have short palates with hypernasality. Arm spans exceed height and halluces are short in all, while two have kyphosis and one has kyphoscoliosis. X-rays show an occasional shortening of some metacarpals, metatarsals, and/or proximal phalanges. Testes are normal in two and small in two, with elevated follicle-stimulating hormone levels in one of these. Behavior varies from normal to shy or hyperactive.

All four mothers are of normal intelligence; one has an increased arm span. A female sib from the original kindred had a low-average IQ and was tall and thin with a high-arched palate, retro-micrognathia, and a high-pitched, hypernasal voice. She has had a son who is reported to be "slow," but has not been evaluated.

**Complications:** Seizures; dental malocclusion and hypernasal speech secondary to craniofacial disproportion and possible velopharyngeal insufficiency; and aggressive or autistic-like behavior.

**Associated Findings:** It is unclear whether the agenesis of the corpus callosum and the septal defect are an intrinsic part of the syndrome or are associated findings.

**Etiology:** X-linked recessive inheritance, but one presumed carrier female has mild morphologic changes as well as lower than expected intellectual function.

**Pathogenesis:** The abnormal gene presumably has a deleterious effect on brain and connective tissue development.

**MIM No.:** 30952

**POS No.:** 3705

**Sex Ratio:** For significant retardation, the ratio is probably M1: F0, but mild manifestations may be seen in an unknown, but probably small, number of female carriers.

**Occurrence:** Eight males from three kindreds have been documented.

**Risk of Recurrence for Patient's Sib:**
See Part I, *Mendelian Inheritance.*

**Risk of Recurrence for Patient's Child:**
See Part I, *Mendelian Inheritance.*

**Age of Detectability:** Hypotonia and hyperextensibility may be noticeable at birth, especially in a family at risk. Abnormalities of the corpus callosum should likewise be detectable. However, this family was not identified until psychomotor retardation had persisted for several years.

**Gene Mapping and Linkage:** Unknown.

**Prevention:** None known. Genetic counseling indicated.

**Treatment:** Usual intervention for secondary complications, e.g., anticonvulsants, orthodontics, as well as exceptional student education and various therapy modalities as indicated.

**Prognosis:** Normal life span is presumed. Vocational training has permitted two affected males to be employed under supervision. No progressive cardiovascular symptoms secondary to the apparent connective tissue involvement, except for a questionable prolapsed mitral valve, have been detected.

**Detection of Carrier:** Female first degree relatives of affected males, who have a Marfanoid habitus, lower than anticipated intelligence, with or without evidence of alterations in the corpus callosum, are probably carriers.

**References:**
Lujan JE, et al.: A form of X-linked mental retardation with marfanoid habitus. Am J Med Genet 1984; 17:311–322. †
Fryns JP, Buttiens M: X-linked mental retardation with marfanoid habitus. Am J Med Genet 1987; 28:267–274. †

CA016

**Mary Esther Carlin**

## X-LINKED MENTAL RETARDATION, RENPENNING TYPE 2920

**Includes:** Renpenning syndrome

**Excludes:** X-linked mental retardation (other)

**Major Diagnostic Criteria:** Small head, small testes, and short stature in a pedigree with X-linked mental retardation.

**Clinical Findings:** All manifestations are variable. Most individuals have severe mental retardation (IQ less than 45 or unmeasurable), a head circumference ranging from the second to the 20th percentile, height less than the 20th percentile, and small testes (usually less than the 25th percentile). One individual with a small head, small testes, and short stature had an IQ of 87. Striking changes occur with age. A relatively normal appearance may be replaced by a marked angulation of the face, loss of facial fat, and development of a somewhat triangular facial appearance. In one kindred, two of four affected individuals showed hyperextensibility of fingers without pectus or other connective tissue signs. Aggressive behavior and repetitive speech are frequently described. The majority have been institutionalized. Laboratory tests for **X-linked mental retardation, Fragile X syndrome** are negative.

**Complications:** Unknown.

**Associated Findings:** None known.

**Etiology:** X-linked recessive inheritance.

**Pathogenesis:** Unknown.

**MIM No.:** *30950, 30954

**Sex Ratio:** M1:F0

**Occurrence:** At least three kindreds have been reported, including a Dutch Mennonite pedigree from Alberta and Saskatchewan.

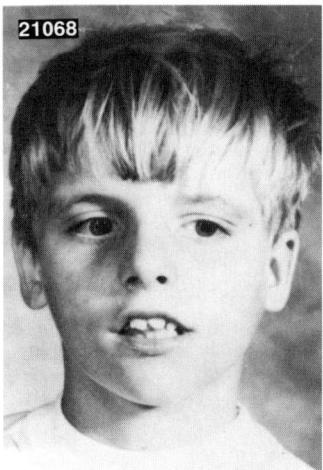
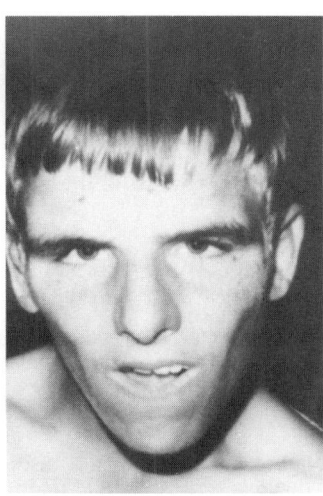
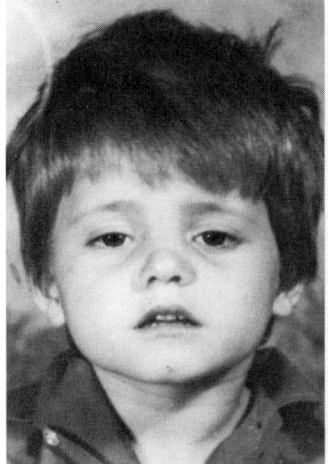
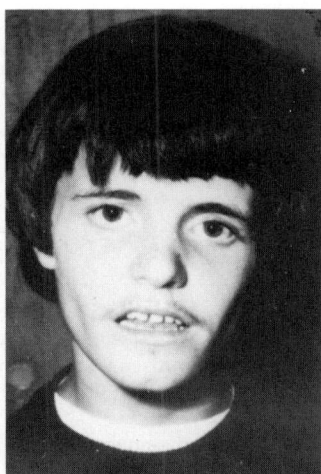

**2920**-21068: Siblings showing changes in facial appearance with increasing angulation and loss of facial fat with age (sibling 1, aged 12 and 25, upper row, and sibling 2, aged 5 and 20 years, lower row).

**Risk of Recurrence for Patient's Sib:**
See Part I, *Mendelian Inheritance.*

**Risk of Recurrence for Patient's Child:**
See Part I, *Mendelian Inheritance.*

**Age of Detectability:** No data are available for head or testicular size at birth. Since appearance may not become obviously abnormal until the late teens, early diagnosis will probably be difficult unless small head and body size or delayed development are observed in a member of a family with X-linked mental retardation.

**Gene Mapping and Linkage:** MRX2 (mental retardation, X-linked 2) has been provisionally mapped to Xp22.3-p22.2.

**Prevention:** None known. Genetic counseling indicated.

**Treatment:** Unknown.

**Prognosis:** Normal life span is presumed, with severe retardation most frequent. One individual with a low-normal IQ is known. No major organ complications have been reported.

**Detection of Carrier:** Only for obligate carriers known from pedigree.

**Special Considerations:** The original family report by Renpenning et al (1962) demonstrated only nonspecific mental retardation. A restudy by Fox et al in 1980 delineated the major diagnostic criteria and demonstrated the absence of the fragile X. In the interim, the term *Renpenning syndrome* came to be used synonymously with *nonspecific mental retardation*. This practice should be discontinued, and the term *Renpenning syndrome* should be confined to the context of this specific condition.

**References:**

Renpenning HJ, et al.: Familial sex-linked mental retardation. Can Med Assoc J 1962; 87:954–956.
Fox P, et al.: X-linked mental retardation: Renpenning revisited. Am J Med Genet 1980; 7:491–495.
Sutherland GR, et al.: Linkage studies with the gene for an X-linked syndrome of mental retardation, microcephaly and spastic diplegia (MRX2). Am J Med Genet 1988; 30:493–508.

LU002                                                                 **Herbert A. Lubs**

**X-linked mental retardation, Schimke type**
*See X-LINKED MENTAL RETARDATION-CHOREOATHETOSIS*
**X-linked mental retardation, Scott type**
*See CRANIO-DIGITAL SYNDROME-MENTAL RETARDATION, SCOTT TYPE*
**X-linked mental retardation, Smith-Fineman-Myers type**
*See SMITH-FINEMAN-MYERS SYNDROME*
**X-linked mental retardation, Urban type (possibly)**
*See X-LINKED MENTAL RETARDATION-SHORT STATURE-OBESITY-HYPOGONADISM*
**X-linked mental retardation, Vasquez type (possibly)**
*See X-LINKED MENTAL RETARDATION-SHORT STATURE-OBESITY-HYPOGONADISM*

## X-LINKED MENTAL RETARDATION-BASAL GANGLION DISORDER                                           2841

**Includes:**
Basal ganglion disorder-mental retardation
Parkinson disease, early onset-mental retardation
Waisman syndrome

**Excludes:**
**Contractures-muscle atrophy-oculomotor apraxia** (2832)
**Microcephaly** (0659)
**X-linked mental retardation, Atkin type** (2840)
**X-linked mental retardation, Fragile X syndrome** (2073)
**X-linked mental retardation, Renpenning type** (2920)
**X-linked mental retardation** (other)

**Major Diagnostic Criteria:** **Megalencephaly** with increased, nonprogressive, fronto-occipital circumference and frontal bossing; average stature; no macroorchidism. Neurologic symptomatology includes cogwheel rigidity, postural changes, parkinsonian tremors, and shuffling gait. Seizures may be present.

**Clinical Findings:** Clinical signs manifest in early childhood in the form of psychomotor delays, particularly in areas of speech and language; **Megalencephaly** (on X-ray the calvaria was larger than the facial bones); hyperactivity and seizures in some of the affected boys. There were no signs of dysmorphism, testicular size was normal, and physical appearance resembled that of unaffected family members.

The onset of neurologic symptomatology varied from age two years to later in childhood; all affected males gradually developed tremors, mild choreoathetoid movements, upper and lower limb rigidity of the cogwheel type, and shuffling gait.

In adulthood, persistent frontal lobe reflexes were present, with resting appendicular axial tremors at 3–6 cycles per second. There was paucity of movement, and gait was slow and stooped with poor recovery of balance. Speech was characterized by hypokinetic dysarthria. Affect was appropriate. IQ ranged from 30 to 70 in affected family members.

It is unclear whether the disorder is very slowly progressive or whether differences occurring with age are attributable to neurologic change rather than time progression. The oldest affected male in the family is currently in his late 50s and is not thought to be deteriorating.

Cytogenetic evaluation has been normal in all affected individuals.

**Complications:** Seizures ranging from grand mal to EEG abnormalities. Affected individuals have difficulty living independently but are able to function with a moderate degree of supervision.

**Associated Findings:** Two of the affected males had eye abnormalities, consisting of a partial iris coloboma in one and of thinning of the right cornea with a tear in the Descemet membrane in the other.

**Etiology:** Presumably X-linked recessive inheritance.

**Pathogenesis:** The neurologic signs are indicative of basal ganglia impairment. No pathologic evaluation has been done on any affected individual.

**MIM No.:** 31151

**Sex Ratio:** M13:F:1 (observed). There was one minimally affected female in the described family.

**Occurrence:** One kindred has been documented in the literature.

**Risk of Recurrence for Patient's Sib:**
See Part I, *Mendelian Inheritance*.

**Risk of Recurrence for Patient's Child:**
See Part I, *Mendelian Inheritance*. No affected males are known to have reproduced.

**Age of Detectability:** During early infancy, by developmental delays and macrocephaly.

**Gene Mapping and Linkage:** The gene has been linked (lod score >5.0) to Xq27-qter markers, DXS52, DXS15, F8, DXS134

**Prevention:** None known. Genetic counseling indicated.

**Treatment:** Early childhood special education. L-dopa has been tried experimentally and did not result in measurable improvement.

**Prognosis:** Life span appears to unaffected, and progression, if present, is extremely slow. The oldest living affected individual is in his 50s.

**Detection of Carrier:** Unknown.

**Support Groups:**
New York; American Parkinson Disease Association
New York; Parkinson's Disease Foundation
Chicago; United Parkinson Foundation (UPF)
CA; Newport Beach; Parkinson's Educational Program (PEP USA)
FL; Miami; National Parkinson Foundation

**References:**

Laxova R, et al.: An X-linked recessive basal ganglia disorder with mental retardation. Am J Med Genet 1985; 21:681–689.

LA033                                                                 **Renata Laxova**

## X-LINKED MENTAL RETARDATION-CHOREOATHETOSIS                                            2830

**Includes:**
Choreoathetosis-mental retardation, X-linked
Schimke X-linked mental retardation syndrome
X-linked mental retardation, Schimke type

**Excludes:**
**Borjeson-Forssman-Lehmann syndrome** (2272)
**Lesch-Nyhan syndrome** (0588)
**Paraplegia, familial spastic** (0295)
**X-linked mental retardation, Fragile X syndrome** (2073)
**X-linked mental retardation, Renpenning type** (2920)
**X-linked mental retardation-growth-hearing and genital defects** (2480)
**X-linked mental retardation** (other)

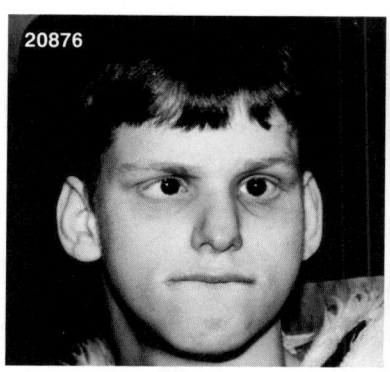 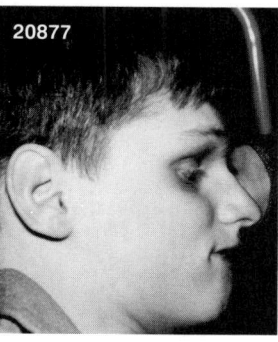

**2830-20876–77:** X-linked mental retardation-choreoathetosis.

**Major Diagnostic Criteria:** Childhood onset of choreoathetosis, mental and growth retardation, and postnatal **Microcephaly.**

**Clinical Findings:** Hypotonia is evident at birth. Choreoathetosis begins in the first year of life; followed later by progressive spasticity. Head circumference is normal at birth, but postnatal **Microcephaly** develops in the first few months. Growth velocity likewise decelerates early. Strabismus is common, and the eyes are sunken. Nerve deafness is present. Feeding difficulties have been noted. Mental retardation is profound.

**Complications:** Progressive inanition, bronchopneumonia, and contractures.

**Associated Findings:** None known.

**Etiology:** Presumably X-linked recessive inheritance.

**Pathogenesis:** Unknown. One autopsied case showed cystic changes in basal ganglia, spongy degeneration, calcification and gliosis in the thalamus and globus pallidus, and a marked loss of Purkinje cells in the cerebellum.

**MIM No.:** 31284

**Sex Ratio:** M1:F0

**Occurrence:** Four cases from two kinships have been reported in the literature.

**Risk of Recurrence for Patient's Sib:**
See Part I, *Mendelian Inheritance.*

**Risk of Recurrence for Patient's Child:**
See Part I, *Mendelian Inheritance.*

**Age of Detectability:** During the first few months of life.

**Gene Mapping and Linkage:** Unknown.

**Prevention:** None known. Genetic counseling indicated.

**Treatment:** Supportive.

**Prognosis:** Survival dependent on intensity of supportive care. The oldest male died in his 20s.

**Detection of Carrier:** Unknown.

**References:**
Schimke RN, et al.: A new X-linked syndrome comprising progressive basal ganglion dysfunction, mental and growth retardation, external ophthalmoplegia, postnatal microcephaly, and deafness. Am J Med Genet 1984; 17:323–332.

SC016 **R. Neil Schimke**

## X-LINKED MENTAL RETARDATION-CLASPED THUMB 2291

**Includes:**
Adducted thumb-mental retardation
Bianchine-Lewis syndrome
Gareis-Mason syndrome
Mental retardation-aplasia-shuffling gait-adducted thumbs (MASA)
Thumb, congenital clasped-mental retardation
X-linked mental retardation-clasped-thumb syndrome

**Excludes:**
Thumb, adducted thumb syndrome (2075)
Thumb, clasped (0175)
X-linked mental retardation, Fragile X syndrome (2073)
X-linked mental retardation, Renpenning type (2920)
X-linked mental retardation (other)

**Major Diagnostic Criteria:** Congenital flexion-adduction contractures of the thumbs with hypoplastic thenar musculature, and mental retardation.

**Clinical Findings:** *Musculoskeletal abnormalities:* Thumb contractures (13/13) which are variable in severity, and most often symmetric, with hypoplastic thenar eminence. Mild short stature (8/13); lordosis and/or kyphosis (8/13); pes planus (3/13); pes cavus

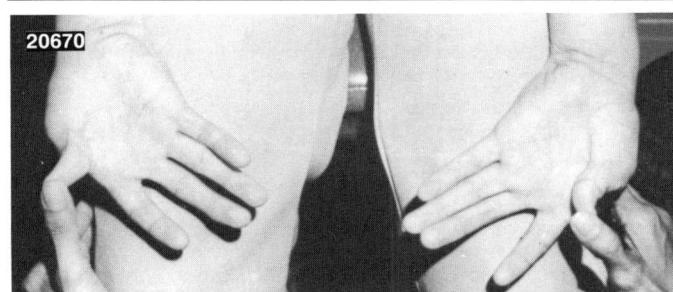

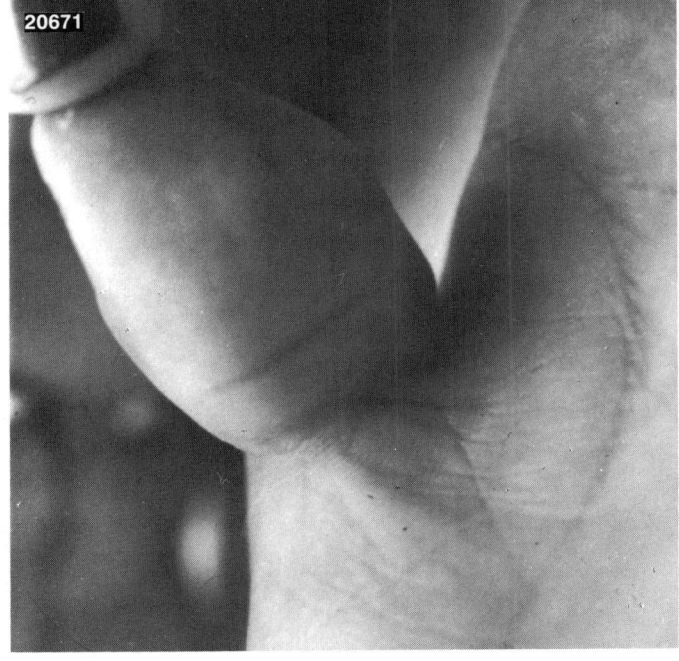

**2291-20670–71:** Mental retardation-clasped thumb syndrome, Mason-Gareis type; note adducted thumbs with hypoplastic thenar musculature in full view and close up.

(1/13); calcaneovalgus deformity (1/13); and flexion contracture of the second finger (1/13).

*CNS abnormalities*: Mental retardation (13/13); Lower extremity spasticity (5/13) (an additional two had shuffling gait and hyperactive lower extremity deep tendon reflexes); **Microcephaly** (4/13). Speech abnormalities are variable: All kindreds have individuals with speech abnormalities; the most severely affected was apparently aphasic when examined at eight years of age. Developmental milestones range from severely delayed to normal for the first three years. Developmental history and intelligence of obligate carrier females have not been examined.

*Pertinent normal features*: Testicular size is normal in postpubertal males. Facial features are normal with no malar or maxillary hypoplasia, enlarged ears, or prominent chin. Chromosomes are normal in all kindreds; one kindred has been evaluated at the sub-band level (maximally "stretched"), and three kindreds tested negative for the presence of **X-linked mental retardation, Fragile X syndrome**.

Unlike the cortical thumbing seen in children with **Cerebral palsy**, and the prenatal contractures seen in the varying **Arthrogryposis**, the contractures associated with this condition are present at birth and are anatomically abnormal, with complete extension impossible.

**Complications:** Pincer grasp may be compromised.

**Associated Findings:** **Heart, tetralogy of Fallot** with a double aortic arch, and a peripheral pulmonic stenosis; hairy nevus.

**Etiology:** X-linked recessive inheritance, with carrier female at risk, presumably from Lyonization. In the four kindreds described, there have been no instances of male-to-male inheritance (in at least three generations), and in three families, four obligate carrier females had affected children with two spouses.

**Pathogenesis:** Unknown.

**MIM No.:** 30335, 30925

**POS No.:** 3432

**Sex Ratio:** M41:F2 (observed).

**Occurrence:** Four kindreds have been reported; two Mexican-American, and two Anglo-American. Forty-one affected males and two affected females have been documented, with 20 obligate carriers and 35 females at 50% risk of carrier status.

**Risk of Recurrence for Patient's Sib:**
See Part I, *Mendelian Inheritance*.

**Risk of Recurrence for Patient's Child:**
See Part I, *Mendelian Inheritance*.

**Age of Detectability:** Abduction and extension of the thumb may be seen in the fetus prior to 16 weeks gestation with diagnostic ultrasound. The diagnosis should be approached with great caution, since normal fetuses hold their fingers flexed and thumb flexed and adducted for prolonged periods of time. Mildly affected fetuses with little limitation of extension will not be detectable. The thenar muscle dysplasia is presumed to occur during organogenesis, although this presumption is not proven, and in fact may occur later in pregnancy.

**Gene Mapping and Linkage:** Unknown.

**Prevention:** None known. Genetic counseling indicated.

**Treatment:** Individuals in two families have shown hypoplastic or absent extensor pollicis brevis and longus tendons. Physical therapy alone has not helped mobility and function of affected thumbs. The thumb anomaly may be treatable with orthopedic surgery in some cases.

**Prognosis:** Normal life span is presumed, with a range of developmental delay from none to severe; mental retardation varies from mild to profound, and some individuals appear to be in the dull normal range. Kyphosis, scoliosis, and lumbar lordosis may develop, as well as spastic lower extremities.

**Detection of Carrier:** Unknown.

**Special Considerations:** Clasped thumbs from congenitally hypoplastic extensor muscles have been described as an isolated anomaly, and also as associated with X-linked recessive hydro-

cephalus from aqueductal stenosis (see **Hydrocephaly**). These conditions must be differentiated by appropriate diagnostic tests.

**References:**
Bianchine JW, Lewis RC: The MASA syndrome: a new heritable mental retardation syndrome. Clin Genet 1974; 5:298–306. *
Gareis FJ, Mason JD: X-linked mental retardation associated with bilateral clasp thumb anomaly. Am J Med Genet 1984; 17:333–338.
Yeatman GW: Mental retardation-clasped thumb syndrome. Am J Med Genet 1984; 17:339–344.
Roberts RM, Lewandowski RC: X-linked mental retardation-clasped thumb syndrome (Gareis-Mason syndrome): further delineation of the phenotype. (Abstract) Dysmorphol Clin Genet 1987; 1:75 only.

R0003                                **Richard M. Roberts**

**X-linked mental retardation-clasped-thumb syndrome**
*See X-LINKED MENTAL RETARDATION-CLASPED THUMB*

## X-LINKED MENTAL RETARDATION-CRANIOFACIAL ABNORMALITIES-CLUB FOOT     3200

**Includes:**
    Holmes-Gang syndrome
    X-linked mental retardation, Holmes-Gang type

**Excludes:**
    **FG syndrome**
    **X-linked mental retardation** (other)

**Major Diagnostic Criteria:** Retarded psychomotor development. Peculiar facies with epicanthic folds; flat nasal bridge and anteverted nostrils; low-set ears; and thin upper lip. Club foot deformity and early death.

**Clinical Findings:** Retarded psychomotor development (3/3); **Microcephaly** (1/3); narrow skull (1/3); large anterior fontanel (3/3); low-set ears (3/3); epicanthal folds (3/3); flat nasal bridge (3/3); short nose with anteverted nostrils (2/3); club foot deformity (3/3); and early death before the second year of life (two at six months; one at 16 months). Autopsy findings in two cases revealed small brain (2/2), kidney hypoplasia and dysplasia (1/2), and hyperplasia and immaturity of pancreatic islet (1/2). The severity of the mental retardation in this disorder is underscored by the fact that none of the three males had any meaningful response to his environment.

**Complications:** Three cases died before the second year of life from infection.

**Associated Findings:** Oligohydramnios, abnormal teeth, hypotonia and a harsh, grating cry were present in one patient.

**Etiology:** Presumably X-linked recessive inheritance.

**Pathogenesis:** Unknown.

**MIM No.:** *30953

**POS No.:** 4082

**Sex Ratio:** M1:F0

**Occurrence:** Three individuals in one Caucasian family (one boy and two of his mother's brothers) have been clinically evaluated or had their hospital records reviewed.

**Risk of Recurrence for Patient's Sib:**
See Part I, *Mendelian Inheritance*.

**Risk of Recurrence for Patient's Child:**
See Part I, *Mendelian Inheritance*.

**Age of Detectability:** During the first year of life.

**Gene Mapping and Linkage:** MRX1 (mental retardation, X-linked 1 (non-dysmorphic)) has been mapped to Xp11-q13.

**Prevention:** None known. Genetic counseling indicated.

**Treatment:** Unknown.

**Prognosis:** The three reported cases died during the first 16 months of life.

**Detection of Carrier:** The two reported obligate carriers had normal intelligence and appearance.

**References:**

Holmes LB, Gang DL: An X-linked mental retardation syndrome with craniofacial abnormalities, microcephaly and club foot. Am J Med Genet 1984; 17:375–382.

AR011                              **J. Fernando Arena**
LU002                              **Herbert A. Lubs**

## X-LINKED MENTAL RETARDATION-DYSTONIC MOVEMENTS OF THE HANDS                              3251

**Includes:**

Hands, dystonic movements-mental retardation, X-linked
Partington mental retardation

**Excludes:   X-linked mental retardation** (other)

**Major Diagnostic Criteria:**   Mild-to-moderate mental retardation; episodic dystonic movements of the hands; dysarthria; normal height; normal head circumference and facial features.

**Clinical Findings:**   Mild to moderate mental retardation (10/10); dystonic spasms of hands (9/9); dysarthria (7/8); normal height (6/6); normal head circumference (5/6); normal facial features (6/6); postural flexion and abnormal gait (4/6); seizures (2/6); strabismus (1/1); spastic quadriplegia (1/1); death during infancy (2/10).

**Complications:**   Unknown.

**Associated Findings:**   None known.

**Etiology:**   Presumably X-linked recessive inheritance.

**Pathogenesis:**   Unknown.

**Sex Ratio:**   M10:F0 observed.

**Occurrence:**   One family with ten affected males has been reported.

**Risk of Recurrence for Patient's Sib:**

See Part I, *Mendelian Inheritance*.

**Risk of Recurrence for Patient's Child:**

See Part I, *Mendelian Inheritance*.

**Age of Detectability:**   During childhood.

**Gene Mapping and Linkage:**   DNA markers DXS41 (p99.6), DXS206 (SJ2.3), DXS84 (p754 and p754–11), DXS (p58.1), DXYS1 (pDP34) and DXS52 (St14) were highly informative. The maximum lod score was 2.11 at O of 0.00 for DXS41. This represents odds in favor of linkage of more than 100:1. These markers are spread between Xp21 and Xcen. The regional localization for the gene for this type of XLMR is likely therefore to be Xpter→Xp21.

**Prevention:**   None known. Genetic counseling indicated.

**Treatment:**   Unknown.

**Prognosis:**   Unknown.

**Detection of Carrier:**   Unknown.

**References:**

Partington M W, et al.: X-linked mental retardation with dystonic movements of the hands. Am J Med Genet 1988; 30:251–262.

AR011                              **J. Fernando Arena**
LU002                              **Herbert A. Lubs**

## X-LINKED MENTAL RETARDATION-GROWTH-HEARING AND GENITAL DEFECTS                              2480

**Includes:**

Juberg-Marsidi mental retardation
Mental retardation-growth/hearing/genital defects, X-linked
Microcephaly, X-linked
Vasquez syndrome

**Excludes:**

**Paraplegia, familial spastic** (0295)
**X-linked mental retardation, Fragile X syndrome** (2073)
**X-linked mental retardation** (other)

**Major Diagnostic Criteria:**   1) Mental retardation, severe; 2) growth retardation; 3) delayed bone age; 4) deafness; 5) ocular

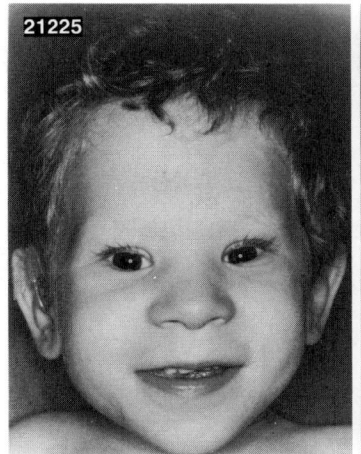
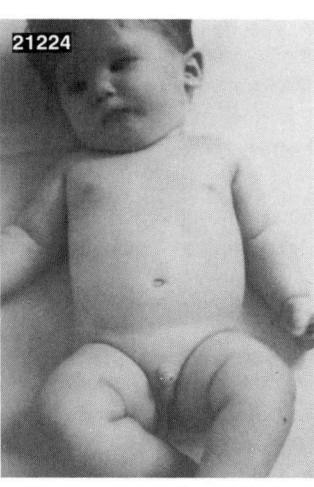

**2480A-21225:**   The proband at 2 8/12 years; note the high forehead, small palpebral fissures, and flat nasal bridge.   **21224:** The proband's younger uncle at age 10 months; note the esotropia and microgenitalism.

abnormalities; 6) flat nasal bridge; 7) microgenitalism, small scrotum with cryptorchidism, and small penis; 8) onychodystrophy of fingers and toes.

**Clinical Findings:**   Birth weight <2,500 g (3/3); birth length <50 cm (3/3); growth <3rd percentile (3/3); bone age retarded (3/3); hearing impairment, mild to severe (3/3); narrow palpebral fissures (2/3); strabismus (2/3); epicanthi (1/3); light retinal pigmentation (2/3); flat nasal bridge (3/3); cryptorchidism (3/3); rudimentary scrotum (3/3); small penis (3/3); and severe mental retardation (3/3).

The *Vasquez syndrome* (Vasquez et al, 1979) has additional features of obesity and gynecomastia.

**Complications:**   Those commonly associated with severe mental retardation.

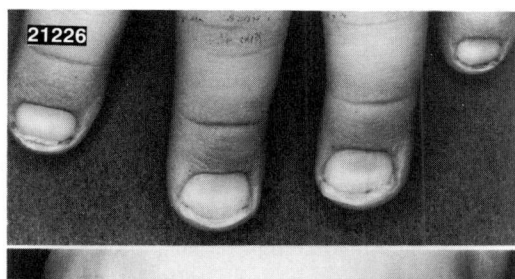
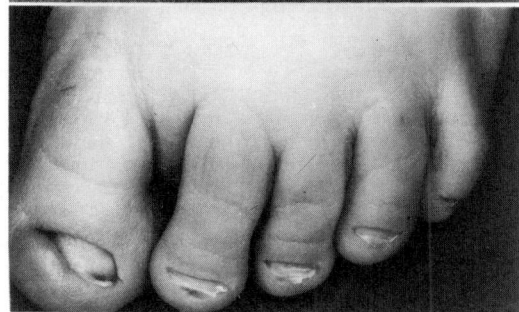

**2480B-21226:**   Note the flat, broad concave fingernails and dysplastic, ingrown toenails.

**Associated Findings:** High forehead, hemicerebral atrophy, dysplastic ears, highly arched palate.

**Etiology:** X-linked recessive inheritance.

**Pathogenesis:** Unknown.

**MIM No.:** *30959

**POS No.:** 3584

**Sex Ratio:** M3:F0 (observed from one kindred).

**Occurrence:** One kindred each has been reported from Ohio and France.

**Risk of Recurrence for Patient's Sib:**
See Part I, *Mendelian Inheritance.*

**Risk of Recurrence for Patient's Child:**
See Part I, *Mendelian Inheritance.*

**Age of Detectability:** In the neonatal period, by clinical findings.

**Gene Mapping and Linkage:** Unknown.

**Prevention:** None known. Genetic counseling indicated.

**Treatment:** Early childhood educational intervention and special education.

**Prognosis:** Less than normal life span, perhaps less than 10 years.

**Detection of Carrier:** Unknown.

**References:**
Vasquez SB, et al.: X-linked hypogonadism, gynecomastia, mental retardation, short stature, and obesity: a new syndrome. J Pediatr 1979; 94:56–60.
Juberg RC, Marsidi I: A new form of X-linked mental retardation with growth retardation, deafness, and microgenitalism. Am J Hum Genet 1980; 32:714–722. * †
Mattei JF, et al.: X-linked mental retardation, growth retardation, deafness and microgenitalism: a second familial report. Clin Genet 1983; 23:70–74.

JU000  **Richard C. Juberg**

**X-linked mental retardation-hypotonia**
*See X-LINKED MENTAL RETARDATION-MUSCULAR WEAKNESS-AWKWARD GAIT*
**X-linked mental retardation-macroorchidism**
*See X-LINKED MENTAL RETARDATION, FRAGILE X SYNDROME*
**X-linked mental retardation-muscular atrophy**
*See X-LINKED MENTAL RETARDATION-MUSCULAR WEAKNESS-AWKWARD GAIT*

---

## X-LINKED MENTAL RETARDATION-MUSCULAR WEAKNESS-AWKWARD GAIT     3249

**Includes:**
Allan-Herndon-Dudley (limber neck) mental retardation
Muscular atrophy-mental retardation, X-linked
Neck, limber-mental retardation
X-linked mental retardation-hypotonia
X-linked mental retardation-muscular atrophy

**Excludes:** X-linked mental retardation (other)

**Major Diagnostic Criteria:** Severe mental retardation; muscular weakness with moderate atrophy; delayed walking (clumsy attempts at walking between the ages of 3–4 years). Awkward, wide-based, incoordinate gait; marked speech deficit (unintelligible mumbling or gibberish); delayed and poor control of bowel and bladder functions. No evidence of sexual potency. No special facial features described.

**Clinical Findings:** Based on 24 affected males in the only pedigree described (22 with some clinical information and eight examined in detail): severe mental retardation (21/22); unable to walk or walking with great difficulty (15/22); unable to talk or talked poorly (13/22). Speech ability was not mentioned in nine cases. Muscle atrophy (4/22).

**Complications:** Moderate contractures of hamstring tendons are frequent, and more severe contractures are present in those patients who do little or no walking.

**Associated Findings:** None known.

**Etiology:** Presumably X-linked recessive inheritance.

**Pathogenesis:** Unknown.

**MIM No.:** 30960

**Sex Ratio:** M24:F0

**Occurrence:** One family with 24 affected males has been reported.

**Risk of Recurrence for Patient's Sib:**
See Part I, *Mendelian Inheritance.*

**Risk of Recurrence for Patient's Child:**
See Part I, *Mendelian Inheritance.*

**Age of Detectability:** After six months of age. At that time, it is noticed that the patients seem weak and are unable to hold up their heads. "Limber neck" is the term used by the affected family to describe the condition at this age.

**Gene Mapping and Linkage:** Unknown.

**Prevention:** None known. Genetic counseling indicated.

**Treatment:** Unknown.

**Prognosis:** The disease is not progressive. The physical condition of the patients remains the same over a period of years. Affected individuals usually die of intercurrent infections. Age of death in seven cases: one during the first decade; three during the second decade; one during the third decade; and one during the fifth decade.

**Detection of Carrier:** Unknown.

**References:**
Allan W, et al.: Some examples of the inheritance of mental deficiency: apparently sex-linked idiocy and microcephaly. Am J Ment Defic 1944; 48:325–334.

AR011
LU002  **J. Fernando Arena**
**Herbert A. Lubs**

**X-linked mental retardation-overgrowth syndrome**
*See SIMPSON-GOLABI-BEHMEL SYNDROME*

---

## X-LINKED MENTAL RETARDATION-PSORIASIS     3252

**Includes:**
Psoriasis-mental retardation, X-linked
Tranebjaerg mental retardation

**Excludes:** X-linked mental retardation (other)

**Major Diagnostic Criteria:** Mental retardation; seizures (onset during first five years of life); psoriasis (onset from neonatal period to 11 years of age).

**Clinical Findings:** Delayed psycomotor development with severe mental retardation (4/4); seizures (4/4); psoriasis (4/4); hypotonia (4/4); long face (4/4); high forehead (4/4); **Eye, hypertelorism** (4/4); broad nasal bridge (4/4); long philtrum (4/4); mouth-breathing facial changes and macrostomia (4/4); prominent lower lips (4/4); mild prognathism (4/4); large, anteverted ears (4/4); ataxic gait (2/4); strabismus (2/4); normal prometaphase chromosomes analysis without fragile X (3/3).

**Complications:** Unknown.

**Associated Findings:** Scoliosis (1/4); retarded bone age (1/4).

**Etiology:** Presumably X-linked recessive inheritance.

**Pathogenesis:** Unknown.

**Sex Ratio:** M4:F0 observed.

**Occurrence:** One family with four affected males has been reported.

**Risk of Recurrence for Patient's Sib:**
See Part I, *Mendelian Inheritance.*

**Risk of Recurrence for Patient's Child:**
 See Part I, *Mendelian Inheritance.*
**Age of Detectability:** During infancy.
**Gene Mapping and Linkage:** Unknown.
**Prevention:** None known. Genetic counseling indicated.
**Treatment:** Unknown.
**Prognosis:** Unknown.
**Detection of Carrier:** Unknown.

**References:**
Tranebjaerg, et al.: X-linked mental retardation associated with psoriasis: a new syndrome? Am J Med Genet 1988; 30:263–273.

AR011
LU002

J. Fernando Arena
Herbert A. Lubs

## X-LINKED MENTAL RETARDATION-SHORT STATURE-OBESITY-HYPOGONADISM      3147

**Includes:**
 Short stature-mental retardation-obesity-hypogonadism
 X-linked mental retardation, Chudley-Lowry-Hoar type
 X-linked mental retardation, Urban type (possibly)
 X-linked mental retardation, Vasquez type (possibly)
 Young-Hughes syndrome
**Excludes:**
 **Bardet-Biedl syndrome** (2363)
 **Borjeson-Forssman-Lehmann syndrome** (2272)
 **Dwarfism-dysmorphic facies-retardation, Pitt type** (2814)
 **Prader-Willi syndrome** (0823)
 **X-linked mental retardation** (other)

**Major Diagnostic Criteria:** Mental retardation in a male with moderate short stature, obesity, and hypogonadism.

**Clinical Findings:** Developmental delay and hypotonia is noted early, usually by 6–9 months of age. Growth parameters show moderate short stature, mild to moderate obesity and hypogonadism beyond puberty. The phallus is normal sized with evidence of small testes. Cryptorchidism has been noted in some affected individuals. The families described by Young & Hughes (1982) and Chudley et al (1988) had hypergonadotropic hypogonadism. The upper extremities may appear shortened distally. **Camptodactyly** was present in some boys, but this is not a consistent feature. Dermatoglyphic analysis in the family reported by Chudley et al (1988) showed a low total finger ridge count with normal palmar creases.

The facial features in affected males were distinct in the cases reported by Chudley et al (1988); consisting of almond-shaped eyes, bitemporal narrowing of the forehead, flat nasal bridge, and a short philtrum with elevated upper lip in the shape of an inverted V. The mouth was large with a high arched palate. The neck was short. The report by Young & Hughes (1982) described a multigeneration family of affected males with a distinctive face with macrostomia, and a thin upper lip and ocular squints; different from the facies in the family reported by Chudley et al (1988). Affected males in the Young & Hughes family had unusual skin diseases, with ichthyosis in one and chronic, atopic and sun-sensitive skin afflictions in the three others.

The diagnosis of **Prader-Willi syndrome** was considered and excluded in all of the affected individuals.

**Complications:** Unknown.

**Associated Findings:** Genu valgum and pes planus were seen in the older boys. One boy was born with bilateral dislocated hips. In males who were possibly affected, one died of possible congenital heart disease in infancy and the other died of complications of a seizure disorder. Chronic skin disease in some males.

**Etiology:** X-linked recessive inheritance.

**Pathogenesis:** Unknown.

**POS No.:** 3585

**Sex Ratio:** M1:F0

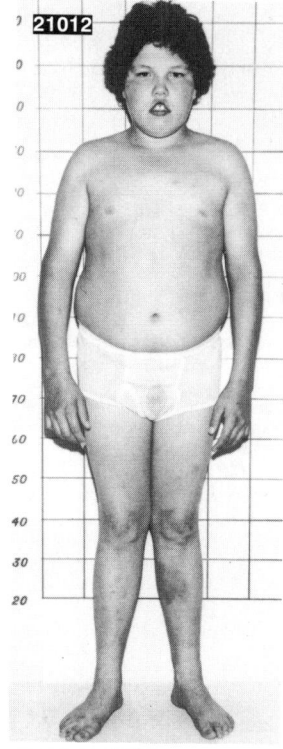

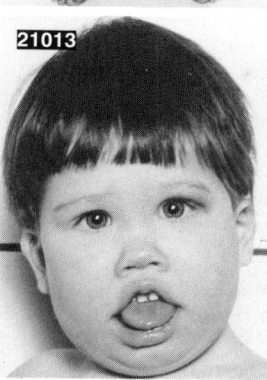

**3147-21012:** Note relative short stature, obesity, typical facial features, genu valgum and flat feet. **21013:** Affected young male; note inverted "V"-shaped upper lip and flat nasal bridge.

**Occurrence:** Three members of two Canadian families have been reported, and other families with similar conditions have also been documented.

**Risk of Recurrence for Patient's Sib:**
 See Part I, *Mendelian Inheritance.*

**Risk of Recurrence for Patient's Child:**
 See Part I, *Mendelian Inheritance.*

**Age of Detectability:** Can be suspected in early infancy.

**Gene Mapping and Linkage:** Based on the family reported by Chudley et al (1988), the gene is possibly located in proximal Xp or Xq region since linkage excluded in distal regions of Xp and Xq. RFLP studies support X chromosome transmission. Since the clinical features in the reported families are not identical, there may be genetic heterogeneity for this disorder with more than one loci on the X chromosome.

**Prevention:** None known. Genetic counseling indicated.

**Treatment:** Correction of limb deformities and ocular squints as required. Cryptorchidism by hormonal or surgical intervention.

**Prognosis:** Unknown. Several of the affected males appear healthy. The oldest described was in his mid-40's. Mental retardation is significant.

**Detection of Carrier:** Unknown.

**References:**

Borjeson M, et al.: An X-linked recessively inherited syndrome characterized by grave mental deficiency, epilepsy and endocrine disorder. Acta Med Scand 1962; 171:12–21. †

Urban MD, et al.: Familial syndrome of mental retardation, short stature, contractures of the hands and genital anomalies. J Pediatr 1979; 94:52–55. †

Vasquez SB, et al.: X-linked hypogonadism, gynecomastia, mental retardation, short stature and obesity: a new syndrome. J Pediatr 1979; 94:56–60. †

Young ID, Hughes HE: Sex-linked mental retardation, short stature, obesity and hypogonadism: report of a family. J Ment Defic Res 1982; 26:153–162. * †

Opitz JM, Sutherland GR: Conference report: International Workshop on the Fragile X and X-Linked Mental Retardation. Am J Med Genet 1984; 17:5–94.

Chudley AE, et al.: Mental retardation, distinct facial changes, short stature, obesity and hypogonadism: a new X-linked mental retardation syndrome. Am J Med Genet 1988; 31:741–751. * †

CH030
L0010

**Albert E. Chudley**
**R. Brian Lowry**

---

## X-LINKED MENTAL RETARDATION-SKELETAL DYSPLASIA 2904

**Includes:**
Abducens palsy-skeletal dysplasia-mental retardation
Christian syndrome
Joint defects with X-linked mental retardation

**Excludes:**
**Aarskog syndrome** (0001)
**Coffin-Lowry syndrome** (0190)
**FG syndrome, Opitz-Kaveggia type** (0754)
**G syndrome** (0401)
**Hypertelorism-hypospadias syndrome** (0505)
**X-linked mental retardation, Fragile X syndrome** (2073)
**X-linked mental retardation, Renpenning type** (2920)
**X-linked mental retardation** (other)

**Major Diagnostic Criteria:** Moderate mental retardation in males with short stature and skeletal anomalies.

**Clinical Findings:** Among the skeletal findings are ridging of metopic suture, fusion of cervical vertebrae, thoracic hemivertebrae, scoliosis, sacral hypoplasia, and short middle phalanges. Abducens palsy occurred in 4/4. Carrier females are mentally normal but may (3/5) show fusion of cervical vertebrae, shortened middle phalanges (3/5), or glucose intolerance (3/5).

**Complications:** Unknown.

**Associated Findings:** Glucose intolerance (3/4) and imperforate anus (1/4) have been found.

**Etiology:** X-linked recessive inheritance.

**Pathogenesis:** Unknown.

**MIM No.:** 30962

**POS No.:** 4222

**Sex Ratio:** M1:F0 (the full syndrome is seen only in males).

**Occurrence:** Reported in four male first cousins in three sibships connected through females.

**Risk of Recurrence for Patient's Sib:**
See Part I, *Mendelian Inheritance*.

**Risk of Recurrence for Patient's Child:**
See Part I, *Mendelian Inheritance*.

**Age of Detectability:** At birth, or prenatally by linked restriction fragment length polymorphisms.

**Gene Mapping and Linkage:** MRSD (mental retardation-skeletal dysplasia) has been provisionally mapped to Xq27-q28.

**Prevention:** None known. Genetic counseling indicated.

**Treatment:** Special education.

**Prognosis:** Apparently consistent with a normal life span.

**Detection of Carrier:** RFLP linkage. Examination of female relatives for skeletal abnormalities.

**References:**

Christian JC, et al.: X-linked skeletal dysplasia with mental retardation. Clin Genet 1977; 11:128–136.

Dlouhy SR, et al.: Localization of the gene for a syndrome of X-linked skeletal dysplasia and mental retardation to Xq27-qter. Hum Genet 1987; 75:136–139.

H0003
CH029
DL000

**M.E. Hodes**
**Joe C. Christian**
**S.R. Dlouhy**

---

## X-LINKED MENTAL RETARDATION-SUBCORTICAL ATROPHY-PATELLAR LUXATION 3248

**Includes:** Prieto mental retardation

**Excludes:** **X-linked mental retardation** (other)

**Major Diagnostic Criteria:** Mental retardation; facial dysmorphia (low-set malformed ears, prominent nose with high nasal bridge, retrognathia); abnormal growth of teeth (double row of lower incisors in two cases); skin dimple at the lower back; clinodactyly; patella luxation; malformation of lower limbs; abnormal fundus of the eye (partial papillar atrophy); and subcortical atrophy.

**Clinical Findings:** Based on eight males of the same family: mental retardation (8/8) with subcortical atrophy (6/6); facial dysmorphia (8/8) with prominent nose (5/8), which may have been familial, and retrognathia (4/8); clinodactyly (8/8); ear malformation (7/8); subcortical atrophy (6/8); febrile convulsion (6/8); abnormalities of fundus of eye (5/8); skin dimple at lower back (5/8); patellar luxation (5/8); limb malformation (5/8); abnormal teeth (4/8); bilateral coxa valga (3/8); cranial asymmetry (2/3); and **Eye, hypertelorism** (1/8).

**Complications:** Unknown.

**Associated Findings:** None known.

**Etiology:** Presumably X-linked recessive inheritance.

**Pathogenesis:** Unknown.

**MIM No.:** 30961

**Sex Ratio:** M8:F0

**Occurrence:** One family with eight affected males has been reported in the literature.

**Risk of Recurrence for Patient's Sib:**
See Part I, *Mendelian Inheritance*.

**Risk of Recurrence for Patient's Child:**
See Part I, *Mendelian Inheritance*.

**Age of Detectability:** During the first year of life.

**Gene Mapping and Linkage:** Unknown.

**Prevention:** None known. Genetic counseling indicated.

**Treatment:** Unknown.

**Prognosis:** Unknown.

**Detection of Carrier:** Unknown.

**References:**

Prieto F, et al.: X-linked dysmorphia syndrome with mental retardation. Clin Genet 1987; 32:326–334.

AR011
LU002

**J. Fernardo Arena**
**Herbert A. Lubs**

## X-LINKED MENTAL RETARDATION-XQ DUPLICATION 3250

**Includes:**
Chromosome Xq duplication-mental retardation, X-linked
Thode mental retardation

**Excludes:** X-linked mental retardation (other)

**Major Diagnostic Criteria:** Severe intellectual handicap; marked short stature; unusual facial appearance characterized by epicanthic folds, ptosis, small palpebral fissures, tented upper lip, and downturned corners of the mouth. Partial duplication of long arm of X (q13.1-q21.1) must be demonstrated.

**Clinical Findings:** In the report by Thode et al (1988) all three affected males had a characteristic and very similar facial appearance, including small palpebral fissures, bilateral epicanthic folds, ptosis, tented upper lip, and down-turned corners of the mouth. Mid-line depression of the chin was present (2/3), as were bilateral **Hernia, inguinal** (2/3). All had high or impalpable testes, and a 15 degree bent knee posture. Short stature and delayed bone age was present in each. The clinical findings were similar in an earlier report by Vejerslev et al (1985), and in an unpublished report by Leonard.

**Complications:** Unknown.

**Associated Findings:** All had low somatomedin C levels. In two, there was a normal growth hormone level, but an elevated growth hormone level was present in the third. The relationship of this duplication and somatomedin C (which has been mapped to chromosome 11p15) is unclear. Gene dosage effect was shown functionally in one affected and two carriers using PKG determinations and a c-DNA probe for this region. In carrier females, the abnormal X was late replicating and their phenotype was normal.

**Etiology:** Duplication of X (q13.1-q21.1).

**Pathogenesis:** Unknown.

**Sex Ratio:** M3:F0 observed.

**Occurrence:** Three affected families have been reported.

**Risk of Recurrence for Patient's Sib:**
See Part I, *Mendelian Inheritance*.

**Risk of Recurrence for Patient's Child:**
See Part I, *Mendelian Inheritance*.

**Age of Detectability:** Prenatally or at birth.

**Gene Mapping and Linkage:** Duplication of X (q13.1-q21.1).

**Prevention:** None known. Genetic counseling indicated.

**Treatment:** Unknown.

**Prognosis:** Limited, with severe mental retardation.

**Detection of Carrier:** By chromosome studies.

**References:**
Steinbach P, et al.: Tandem duplication dup (dx) (q13q22) in a male proband inherited from the mother showing mosaicism of X-inactivation. Hum Genet 1980; 54:309–313.
Vejerslev LO, et al.: Inherited tandem duplication dup (X) (q131-q212) in a male proband. Clin Genet 1985; 27:276–281.
Thode A, et al.: A new syndrome with mental retardation, short stature and an Xq duplication. Am J Med Genet 1988; 30:239–250.

LU002                             **Herbert A. Lubs**
AR011                         **J. Fernando Arena**

**X-linked mixed deafness syndrome**
*See DEAFNESS WITH PERILYMPHATIC GUSHER*
**Xanax^, fetal effects**
*See FETAL BENZODIAZEPINE EFFECTS*
**Xanthine dehydrogenase/sulfite oxidase/aldehyde oxidase deficiency**
*See MOLYBDENUM CO-FACTOR DEFICIENCY*

## XANTHINE OXIDASE DEFICIENCY 2411

**Includes:** Xanthinuria

**Excludes:** **Molybdenum co-factor deficiency** (2412)

**Major Diagnostic Criteria:** Low serum uric acid (generally < 1 mg/dl, 0.06 mmol/L), low urinary uric acid (generally <50 mg/24 hr, 3 mmol/24 hr) with increased urinary excretion of xanthine and hypoxanthine (oxypurines > 200 mg/24 hr, 12 mmol/24 hr). Some patients develop xanthine stones in the renal tract (40%).

**Clinical Findings:** No specific clinical findings other than the formation of urinary tract stones in some patients. Low serum uric acid (generally < 1 mg/dl, 0.06 mmol/L), low urinary uric acid (generally <50 mg/24 hr, 3 mmol/24 hr) with increased urinary excretion of xanthine and hypoxanthine (oxypurines > 200 mg/24 hr, 1.2 mmol/24 hr).

**Complications:** Unknown.

**Associated Findings:** Pheochromocytoma, hemochromatosis. Xanthinuria has been associated with sulfite oxidase deficiency but this is a different defect associated with **Molybdenum co-factor deficiency**. A myopathy and recurrent polyarthritis has been observed in 6% of cases.

**Etiology:** Autosomal recessive inheritance.

**Pathogenesis:** Deficiency of the enzyme xanthine oxidase E.C.1.2.3.2.

**MIM No.:** *27830

**Sex Ratio:** M1:F1

**Occurrence:** At least 58 cases have been documented in the literature, including a Black male.

**Risk of Recurrence for Patient's Sib:**
See Part I, *Mendelian Inheritance*.

**Risk of Recurrence for Patient's Child:**
See Part I, *Mendelian Inheritance*.

**Age of Detectability:** Generally not until adult life.

**Gene Mapping and Linkage:** Unknown.

**Prevention:** None known. Genetic counseling indicated.

**Treatment:** Increased fluid intake to lead to dilution of urine would help in those patients who form renal calculi. Otherwise, none is required.

**Prognosis:** Normal life span. A few patients may be affected by renal stones.

**Detection of Carrier:** Unknown.

**References:**
Dent CE, Philpot GR: Xanthinuria: an inborn error (or deviation) of metabolism. Lancet 1954; I:182–185.
Avazian JH: Xanthinuria and hemochromatosis. New Engl J Med 1964; 270:18–22.
Engelman K, et al.: Clinical, physiological and biochemical studies of a patient with xanthinuria and pheochromocytoma. Am J Med 1964; 37:839–861.
Crawhall JC, et al.: Separation and quantitation of oxypurines by isocratic high pressure liquid chromatography: application to xanthinuria and the Lesch-Nyhan syndrome. Biochem Med 1983; 30:261–270.
Carpenter TO, et al.: Hereditary xanthinuria presenting in infancy with nephrolithiasis. J Pediatr 1986; 109:307–309.
Mateos FA, et al.: Hereditary xanthinuria: evidence for enhanced hypoxanthine salvage. J Clin Invest 1987; 79:847–852.
Holmes EW, Wyngaarden JB: Hereditary xanthinuria. In: Scriver CR, et al, eds: The metabolic basis of inherited disease, 6th ed. New York: McGraw-Hill, 1989:1085–1094.

CR006                           **John C. Crawhall**

**Xanthinuria**
*See XANTHINE OXIDASE DEFICIENCY*
**Xanthism**
*See ALBINISM, OCULOCUTANEOUS, RUFOUS TYPE*
**Xanthoma tuberosum multiplex**
*See HYPERCHOLESTEREMIA*

## XANTHOMATOSIS, CEREBROTENDINOUS            2395

**Includes:**
> Cerebral cholesterinosis
> Cerebrotendinous xanthomatosis
> Cholestanalosis

**Excludes:** N/A

**Major Diagnostic Criteria:** Achilles tendon xanthomatosis, progressive neurologic disease (mental retardation, dementia, spinal cord paresis, cerebellar ataxia, and peripheral neuropathy), and cataracts appear most frequently. The diagnosis is confirmed chemically by finding an elevated plasma cholestanol level (>1 mg/dl) in combination with a low or normal plasma cholesterol concentration (<220 mg/dl); increased quantities of C-27 bile alcohol glucuronides are excreted in bile and urine and circulate in plasma.

**Clinical Findings:** Achilles tendon xanthomas (95%) develop during the second decade. Cataracts (80%) are often present at this time. Neurologic impairment: dementia (90%), spinal cord paresis (95%), and cerebellar ataxia (90%) begin in the second or third decades. Mental retardation (50%) as evidenced by poor school performance is present in one-half of the patients and appears when the affected child enters school. The neurologic diseases progress without remission so that by the fifth decade vital brain functions controlling speech and swallowing become impaired. Because of associated coronary atherosclerosis, fatal myocardial infarctions (10%) have developed. Since the clinical presentation varies among affected family members, it is essential to look for the biochemical abnormalities (plasma cholestanol and plasma, bile, and urine bile alcohol glucuronides) in all sibs. Pulmonary insufficiency (5%) and endocrine hypofunction (3%) have also been noted. Chemically, elevated plasma cholestanol levels in combination with low or normal plasma cholesterol concentrations are diagnostic for cerebrotendinous xanthomatosis (CTX). Increased cholestanol is also present in xanthomas, nerve tissue (brain and peripheral nerve), and bile. Defective hepatic bile acid synthesis is manifested by reduced biliary chenodeoxycholic acid and by the excretion of C-27 bile alcohol glucuronides (bile acid precursors) in bile and urine.

Most subjects with CTX show neurologic dysfunction with dementia, weakness, loss of coordination, and spasticity. As the disease evolves, the neurologic complications worsen. Cataracts affect vision, coronary atherosclerosis leads to angina pectoris and myocardial infarction, pulmonary nodules, shortness of breath, and dyspnea may develop.

**Complications:** Unknown.

**Associated Findings:** Hypothyroidism and hypoadrenalism have been detected infrequently. Severe osteoporosis and an increased number of bone fractures have been noted, and urinary calculi appear more frequently.

**Etiology:** Autosomal recessive inheritance. The basic defect involves incomplete oxidation of the side chain in the conversion of cholesterol to bile acids. The precise enzymatic defect in bile acid synthesis remains controversial, because the mechanism of side chain cleavage in bile acid synthesis has not been defined quantitatively.

**Pathogenesis:** Reduced synthesis of the two primary bile acids cholic acid and chenodeoxycholic acid leads to deficient enterohepatic bile acid pools. As a result, hepatic cholesterol synthesis is increased. Cholestanol, the 5α-dihydro derivative of cholesterol, is overproduced and is derived from cholesterol directly via the diversion of the bile acid precursor 7α-hydroxycholesterol. Both cholesterol and cholestanol are incorporated into plasma lipoproteins and transported in plasma to various tissues. Because of bile acid synthesis defects, the bile alcohols with 27 carbons and the hydroxyl groups at C-3, C-7, and C-12 resemble cholic acid but contain incompletely oxidized side chains. In addition, hydroxy groups at C-25 accumulate as glucuronides, and these bile alcohol glucuronides are excreted in bile and urine and thus circulate in plasma. It has been hypothesized that the deposition of cholesterol and cholestanol in the central nervous system results from

damage to the blood-brain barrier caused by plasma bile alcohol glucuronides.

Although defective side chain oxidation in cholic acid synthesis exists and large quantities of bile alcohol glucuronides are found, the exact enzymatic defect cannot be defined until the quantitative mechanism of the side chain oxidation in cholic acid synthesis is determined. Two pathways are known (microsomal 25-hydroxylation and mitochondrial 26-hydroxylation), and both may actually produce cholic acid in humans.

**MIM No.:** *21370

**POS No.:** 4379

**Sex Ratio:** Presumably M1:F1, although females have been reported more frequently.

**Occurrence:** Undetermined, although all populations, including Caucasians, Blacks, and Orientals, have been affected. There is a particularly high occurrence in Sephardic Jews in Israel.

**Risk of Recurrence for Patient's Sib:**
See Part I, *Mendelian Inheritance*. Although 1:4 is expected, family studies suggest a greater number of affected sibs.

**Risk of Recurrence for Patient's Child:**
See Part I, *Mendelian Inheritance*.

**Age of Detectability:** Usually clinically evident by ages 20–30 years, when tendon xanthomas, cataracts, and neurologic disease present.

**Gene Mapping and Linkage:** Unknown.

**Prevention:** None known. Genetic counseling indicated.

**Treatment:** Replacing chenodeoxycholic acid in the enterohepatic circulation of affected persons will inhibit abnormal bile acid synthesis. To date, in 14 of 17 persons treated with chenodeoxycholic acid (750 mg/day), improved neurologic function and lower plasma and cerebrospinal fluid cholestanol levels occurred. However, it is important to emphasize that the earlier the treatment is started (the younger the patient treated), the better the effect. For example, an older patient (aged 74 years) with long-standing neurologic disease is not likely to improve. In contrast, the recognition of the diagnosis before neurologic damage and the institution of treatment will likely prevent the onset of the disease.

**Prognosis:** In patients with mild neurologic disease, treatment with chenodeoxycholic acid (750 mg/day) has prevented further progression of the disease, and in some cases has reversed it.

**Detection of Carrier:** Unknown.

**References:**
Salen G: Cholestanol deposition in cerebrotendinous xanthomatosis: a possible mechanism. Ann Intern Med 1971; 75:843–851.
Berginer VM, et al.: Long-term treatment of cerebrotendinous xanthomatosis with chenodeoxycholic acid. New Engl J Med 1984; 311: 1649–1652.
Berginer VM, et al.: Pregnancy in women with cerebrotendinous xanthomatosis. Am J Med Genet 1988; 31:11–16.
Bjorkhem I, Skrede S: Familial diseases with storage of sterols other than cholesterol: cerebrotendinous xanthomatosis and phytosterolemia. In: Scriver CR, et al, eds: The metabolic basis of inherited disease, 6th ed. New York: McGraw-Hill, 1989:1283–1303.

SA041                                                    **Gerald Salen**

**Xanthomatosis, familial-involvement and calcification of adrenals**
*See WOLMAN DISEASE*
**Xanthous negros**
*See ALBINISM, OCULOCUTANEOUS, RUFOUS TYPE*
**Xerocytosis, hereditary**
*See ANEMIA, HEMOLYTIC, RED CELL MEMBRANE DEFECTS*

## XERODERMA PIGMENTOSUM                                    1005

**Includes:**

Angioma pigmentosum et atrophicum
Kaposi dermatosis
Photosensitivity with defective DNA synthesis
Pigmented xerodermoid
Trichothiodystrophy-sun sensitivity
Xeroderma pigmentosum with normal DNA repair rates

**Excludes:**

**Cockayne syndrome** (0189)
Genodermatoses with defective DNA repair, other
Genodermatoses with malignancy, other
Genodermatoses with ultraviolet hypersensitivity, other
**Nevoid basal cell carcinoma syndrome** (0101)
**Trichothiodystrophy** (2559)
**Xeroderma pigmentosum-mental retardation** (1004)

**Major Diagnostic Criteria:**  Infantile onset of photosensitivity, and/or freckling, and photophobia. Early development of skin and eye cancers. Cellular hypersensitivity to killing by ultraviolet radiation, accompanied by defective DNA repair.

**Clinical Findings:**  *Skin:* Changes are seen almost exclusively on sun exposed skin. Early acute photosensitivity with blistering on minimal sun exposure (seen in about one-half of patients) and/or freckling in response to ultraviolet light (50% by age 18 months); subsequent poikiloderma (increased pigment, decreased pigment, atrophy, and telangiectasia); development of premalignant and benign skin tumors (actinic keratoses, angiomas, and keratoacanthomas); development of malignant skin tumors (2,000-fold in-

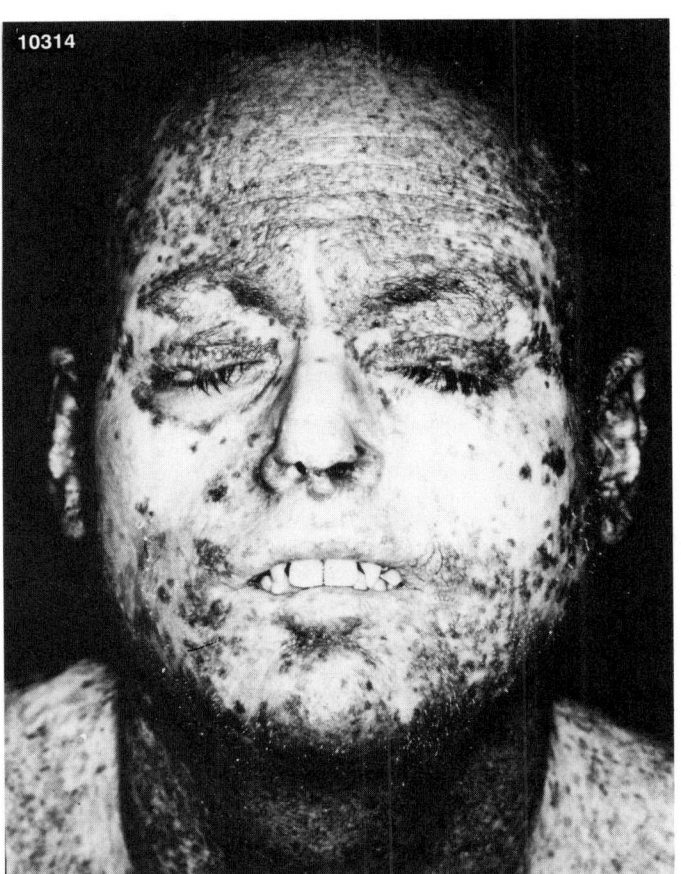

**1005-10314:**   Marked skin changes of xeroderma pigmentosum.

creased frequency by age 20 years). Basal cell and squamous cell carcinomas (50% of tumor patients by age eight years), multiple tumors are common, with >90% on face, head, or neck; malignant melanoma (3–50% of different series); rarely, sarcomas.

*Eyes:* Symptoms limited to ultraviolet-exposed (anterior) portion of the eye include photophobia (reported for 21% of patients, median age two years); conjunctivitis; keratitis; ectropion, entropion of lids; benign tumors (conjunctival inflammatory masses, papillomas); and malignant neoplasms (2,000-fold increased frequency by age 20 years). Symptoms associated with the anterior eye and lids include epitheliomas, basal cell carcinomas, and melanomas.

*Oral:* Rarely, squamous cell carcinoma of tip of tongue.

*Laboratory findings:* Cellular hypersensitivity to killing, and hypermutability to ultraviolet radiation and certain chemical carcinogens such as benzo-a-pyrene (found in cigarette smoke). Defective DNA repair, with a range of residual repair levels observed among patients extending from undetectable to normal. These defects can be demonstrated in cultured fibroblasts, lymphocytes, amniotic fluid cells, and *in vivo* epidermis. Nine excision repair complementation groups have been identified, plus a "variant" form with defective post-replication repair.

**Complications:**  Metastasis of melanoma, squamous cell carcinoma; loss of eyelid; corneal opacification.

**Associated Findings:**  Rarely, internal neoplasms (including four cases of primary brain tumors) have been reported. Two patients have been reported with clinical findings and laboratory tests characteristic of both XP and **Cockayne syndrome**.

**Etiology:**  Autosomal recessive inheritance. Consanguinity reported in 30% of cases. Multiple laboratory forms have been identified, probably with different defects in DNA repair.

**Pathogenesis:**  Failure to repair DNA damage after ultraviolet exposure. Probably defective ultraviolet repair endonuclease(s). Ultraviolet-induced somatic mutations are believed to result in the neoplasms. Eight sub-types have been identified, termed complementation groups A through I.

**MIM No.:**  *27870, *27871, *27872, *27873, *27874, 27875, *27876, *27878, *27879, 27881

**CDC No.:**  757.360

**Sex Ratio:**  M1:F1

**Occurrence:**  Estimated to be 1:250,000 in the United States, 1:40,000 in Japan, and relatively high in Egypt, Tunisia, and wherever consanguinity is high. Approximately 1,000 English language cases have been reported.

**Risk of Recurrence for Patient's Sib:**
See Part I, *Mendelian Inheritance.*

**Risk of Recurrence for Patient's Child:**
See Part I, *Mendelian Inheritance.* Patients have been reported with clinically normal children.

**Age of Detectability:**  *Skin sun sensitivity or freckling:* One-half by 18 months of age, 75% by four years of age, and 95% by 15 years of age. Photophobia can be seen in the neonate. Pigmented xerodermoid with "variant" type repair defects has adult onset of symptoms following extensive sun exposure. All cell types tested, including fetal cells, have a DNA repair defect (excision repair or post-replication repair). Prenatal diagnosis has been reported based on DNA repair studies of cultured amniotic fluid cells.

**Gene Mapping and Linkage:**  XPAC (fast kinetic complementation DNA repair in xeroderma pigmentosum, group A) has been provisionally mapped to 1q.

XPF (xeroderma pigmentosum, complementation group F) has been provisionally mapped to 15.

**Prevention:**  None known. Genetic counseling indicated.

**Treatment:**  Early diagnosis, rigorous protection from ultraviolet radiation and chemical carcinogens such as those present in cigarette smoke, use of physical sunscreens (glasses, long hair, double layers of clothing); use of topical sunscreens (with at least Sun Protection Factor [SPF] 15), baseline photography of skin; regular examination of skin and eyes by parent and physician;

early excision of tumors. For extensive skin disease, prophylactic dermatome shaving, dermabrasion, or excision and grafting of the entire face has been reported. Corneal transplantation may be indicated. Experimental studies with oral retinoids have been demonstrated to prevent new neoplasms, but the dosage required has been toxic.

**Prognosis:** Survival is generally reduced due to neoplasms, but depends on the form of the disorder and extent of ultraviolet exposure. Five percent of 830 cases reported in the literature were more than 45 years of age, and seven were over 64 years of age. A 70% probability of survival was attained at age 40 years; a 28 year reduction in comparison with the United States general population. However, the few patients who have been diagnosed early in life and rigorously protected from ultraviolet exposure did not develop the severe cutaneous abnormalities.

**Detection of Carrier:** Most carriers are clinically normal, although there is a suggested increase in skin cancer risk. A few carriers have been reported with abnormal polyADP ribose metabolism, plasminogen activator levels, or increased chromosome breakage following X-ray *in vitro*. At present, there is no laboratory test that will consistently detect XP carriers.

**Special Considerations:** The Xeroderma Pigmentosum Registry (c/o Dept of Pathology, Room C520, Medical Science Building, CMDNJ-New Jersey Medical School, 100 Bergen St, Newark, NJ 07103) collects information on xeroderma pigmentosum patients and provides educational material to physicians.

**Support Groups:** NJ; Newark; Xeroderma Pigmentosum Registry

**References:**

Robbins JH, et al.: Xeroderma pigmentosum: an inherited disease with sun sensitivity, multiple cutaneous neoplasms, and abnormal DNA repair. Ann Intern Med 1974; 80:221–248. †

Kraemer KH, et al.: DNA repair protects against cutaneous and internal neoplasia: evidence from studies of xeroderma pigmentosum. Carcinogenesis 1984; 5:511–514.

Kraemer KH, Slor H: Xeroderma pigmentosum. Clin Dermatol 1985; 3:33–69. †

Kraemer KH: Heritable diseases with increased sensitivity to cellular injury. In: Fitzpatrick TB, et al., eds: Dermatology in general medicine. New York: McGraw Hill, 1987:1791–1796. †

Kraemer KH, et al.: Xeroderma pigmentosum: cutaneous, ocular and neurologic abnormalities in 830 published cases. Arch Dermatol 1987; 123:241–250. *

Kraemer KH, et al.: Prevention of skin cancer in xeroderma pigmentosum with the use of oral isotretinoin. New Engl J Med 1988; 318:1633–1637.

Cleaver J, Kraemer KH: Xeroderma pigmentosum. In: Scriver CR, et al, eds: The metabolic basis of inherited disease, 6th ed. New York: McGraw-Hill, 1989:2949–2973.

KR019                                    **Kenneth H. Kraemer**

**Xeroderma pigmentosum with normal DNA repair rates**
*See XERODERMA PIGMENTOSUM*

---

## XERODERMA PIGMENTOSUM-MENTAL RETARDATION    1004

**Includes:**
DeSanctis-Cacchione syndrome
Mental retardation-xeroderma pigmentosum
Xeroderma pigmentosum-neurologic abnormalities

**Excludes:**
**Cockayne syndrome** (0189)
Photodermatoses with neurologic disease, other
**Trichothiodystrophy** (2559)
**Xeroderma pigmentosum** (1005)

**Major Diagnostic Criteria:** Cutaneous and ocular abnormalities of **Xeroderma pigmentosum** (XP), plus one or more neurologic abnormalities. Cellular hypersensitivity to killing by ultraviolet radiation accompanied by defective DNA repair.

**Clinical Findings:** Skin and eye abnormalities of **Xeroderma pigmentosum**: photosensitivity, freckling, and photophobia with sub-

sequent neoplasia. Onset may be earlier and more severe than is observed in **Xeroderma pigmentosum** patients without neurologic abnormalities.

In addition, one or more of the following neurologic abnormalities (minimal percentages based on case reports of 154 patients with xeroderma pigmentosum and neurologic abnormalities): progressive mental deterioration, low intelligence (80%); microcephaly (25%); progressive sensorineural deafness (20%); hyporeflexia or areflexia (20%); spasticity, late onset of ataxia and choreoathetoid movements, abnormal electroencephalogram (11%); and neuropathic electromyogram, loss of neurons in cerebral cortex, and demyelination of dorsal columns. Most patients have only a few neurologic abnormalities, such as hyporeflexia and progressive hearing loss. Onset of neurologic symptoms may be in early infancy, or (in 5% or more) delayed until after five to ten years of age.

Some patients may have dwarfism (15%), retarded bone age, and/or immature sexual development (12%).

**Complications:** Skin and eyes: as in **Xeroderma pigmentosum**. Neurological: in severe cases, loss of ability to walk and talk.

**Associated Findings:** Rarely, internal neoplasms.

The rare *DeSanctis-Cacchione syndrome* consists of xeroderma pigmentosum and most of the neurologic abnormalities listed above, with the addition of dwarfism and immature sexual development.

**Etiology:** Probably autosomal recessive inheritance. Consanguinity has been reported in 30%. Multiple molecular forms are likely, probably with different defects in DNA repair.

**Pathogenesis:** Failure to repair DNA damage after ultraviolet light exposure. The defect is demonstrated in cultured fibroblasts, lymphocytes, and *in vivo* epidermis.

Probably defective ultraviolet repair endonuclease(s). Of nine excision repair complementation groups, five have patients with neurologic abnormalities. Patients in group A may have severe neurologic involvement, or only minimal involvement. Patients in group D generally have later onset of neurologic degeneration, if at all. Two patients have xeroderma pigmentosum plus **Cockayne syndrome** (one in group B and the other in group H). Residual repair rates range from undetectable to 50% of normal in patients with neurologic abnormalities.

**MIM No.:** 27880

**POS No.:** 3431

**CDC No.:** 757.360

**Sex Ratio:** M1:F1

**Occurrence:** Prevalence of **Xeroderma pigmentosum** is estimated at 1:250,000 in the United States; 1:40,000 in Japan. Approximately 200 English language cases have been reported with neurological abnormalities, representing about 20% of the total **Xeroderma pigmentosum** cases reported (the proportion is higher in Japan).

**Risk of Recurrence for Patient's Sib:**
See Part I, *Mendelian Inheritance*. Generally, multiple affected sibs have similar manifestations, however, one kindred was reported with two children with XP, but only the older with neurologic abnormalities.

**Risk of Recurrence for Patient's Child:**
See Part I, *Mendelian Inheritance*. Of 152 patients reported in a literature survey, none had children.

**Age of Detectability:** Prenatal diagnosis of xeroderma pigmentosum has been reported based on DNA repair studies of cultured amniotic fluid cells. Skin sun sensitivity or freckling is seen in one-half by six months of age, in 75% by 18 months of age, and in 95% by five years of age. Photophobia is seen in the neonate. Neurological abnormalities usually appear in early childhood, but may have their onset in the second decade of life.

**Gene Mapping and Linkage:** Unknown.

**Prevention:** None known. Genetic counseling indicated.

**Treatment:** *Skin and eyes*: early diagnosis, rigorous protection from ultraviolet radiation and chemical carcinogens such as those present in cigarette smoke, use of physical sunscreens (glasses, long hair, double layers of clothing), use of topical sunscreens (with Sun Protection Factor 15+), baseline photography of skin; regular examination of skin and eyes by parent and physician, and early excision of tumors. For extensive skin disease, prophylactic dermatome shaving, dermabrasion, or excision and grafting of the entire face has been reported. Corneal transplantation may be indicated. Experimental studies with oral retinoids have been shown to prevent new neoplasms, but the doses used have been toxic. *Neurological*: hearing aids may be beneficial.

**Prognosis:** Survival of patients with xeroderma pigmentosum is generally reduced. Prognosis depends on the form of the disorder and the extent of ultraviolet exposure. Ten percent of 152 cases were less than 30 years old. The survival probability is not significantly different from that of patients with **Xeroderma pigmentosum** without neurological abnormalities.

**Detection of Carrier:** Carriers of xeroderma pigmentosum are generally clinically normal. There is a possibility of increased skin cancer risk. A few carriers have been reported with abnormal polyADP ribose metabolism, plasminogen activator levels, or *in vitro* hypersensitivity to X-ray-induced chromosome breakage.

**Special Considerations:** The Xeroderma Pigmentosum Registry (c/o Dept of Pathology, Room C520, Medical Science Building, CMDNJ-New Jersey Medical School, 100 Bergen St, Newark, NJ 07103) is collecting information on xeroderma pigmentosum patients, and provides educational material to physicians.

**Support Groups:** NJ; Newark; Xeroderma Pigmentosum Registry

**References:**

Robbins JH, et al.: Xeroderma pigmentosum: an inherited disease with sun sensitivity, multiple cutaneous neoplasms, and abnormal DNA repair. Ann Intern Med 1974; 80:221–248. †

Kraemer KH, Slor H: Xeroderma pigmentosum. Clin Dermatol 1985; 3:33–69. †

Kraemer KH: Heritable diseases with increased sensitivity to cellular injury. In: Fitzpatrick TB, et al., eds: Dermatology in general medicine. New York: McGraw Hill, 1987:1791–1796. †

Kraemer KH, et al.: Xeroderma pigmentosum: cutaneous, ocular and neurologic abnormalities in 830 published cases. Arch Dermatol 1987; 123:241–250. *

Kraemer KH, et al.: Prevention of skin cancer in xeroderma pigmentosum with the use of oral isotretinoin. New Engl J Med 1988; 318:1633–1637.

Cleaver JE, Kraemer KH: Xeroderma pigmentosum. In: Scriver CR, et al, eds: The metabolic basis of inherited disease, 6th ed. New York: McGraw-Hill, 1989:2949–2973.

KR019                                    **Kenneth H. Kraemer**

**Xeroderma pigmentosum-neurologic abnormalities**
*See XERODERMA PIGMENTOSUM-MENTAL RETARDATION*
**Xeroderma-tricho-onychodysplasia**
*See TRICHO-ONYCHODYSPLASIA-XERODERMA*
**Xeroderma-trichodysplasia**
*See TRICHODYSPLASIA-XERODERMA*
**Xerostomia**
*See SALIVARY GLAND, AGENESIS*
**Xk-related chronic granulomatous disease**
*See GRANULOMATOUS DISEASE, CHRONIC X-LINKED*
**XX form of pure gonadal dysgenesis**
*See GONADAL DYSGENESIS, XX TYPE*
**XX Gonadal dysgenesis**
*See GONADAL DYSGENESIS, XX TYPE*
**XX-XY Turner phenotype**
*See NOONAN SYNDROME*
**XY form of pure gonadal dysgenesis**
*See GONADAL DYSGENESIS, XY TYPE*
**XY gonadal agenesis syndrome**
*See ANORCHIA*
*also AGONADIA*
**XY gonadal dysgenesis**
*See GONADAL DYSGENESIS, XY TYPE*
**Xylitol dehydrogenase deficiency**
*See PENTOSURIA*

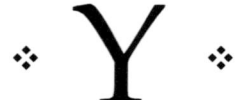

Yellow mutant oculocutaneous albinism
*See ALBINISM, OCULOCUTANEOUS, YELLOW MUTANT*
Yellow nail syndrome with familial late-onset lymphedema
*See LYMPHEDEMA II*
Yellow teeth
*See TEETH, DEFECTS FROM TETRACYCLINE*
Yellow-blue color defect
*See COLOR BLINDNESS, YELLOW-BLUE TRITAN*
Young-Hughes syndrome
*See X-LINKED MENTAL RETARDATION-SHORT STATURE-OBESITY-HYPOGONADISM*
Yucheng, congenital
*See FETAL EFFECTS OF POLYCHLORINATED BIPHENYL (PCB)*

## YUNIS-VARON SYNDROME                               2405

**Includes:**
Cleidocranial dysplasia-micrognathia-no thumb-distal aphalangia
Cleidocranial dysplasia-micrognathia, Yunis-Varon type
Micrognathia-cleidocranial dysplasia

**Excludes:  Cleidocranial dysplasia** (0185)

**Major Diagnostic Criteria:** 1) Craniofacial disproportion; 2) micrognathia; 3) absent or hypoplastic clavicles, thumbs and great toes; 4) aphalangia of fingers or toes with short or absent metacarpals and metatarsal bones; 5) sparse hair; and 6) postnatal short stature.

**Clinical Findings:** The mean birth weight (2.3 kg) is below average, but body length and head circumference are within normal limits. There is craniofacial disproportion, with marked micrognathia leading to feeding difficulties and failure to thrive. In the one child surviving infancy, growth retardation was progressive and extreme, with relative **Microcephaly**, developmental delay, and moderate mental retardation. The anterior fontanelle is widely open. Hair is sparse, with thin or absent eyebrows and eyelashes. The ears protrude and have a simple pattern. The lips are thin. The clavicles, thumbs, and first toes may be absent or hypoplastic. Fingers and toes may show **Syndactyly** and absent phalanges, and the metacarpals and metatarsals may be short or absent.

The pattern of X-ray findings is distinctive. Cardiac arrhythmia and cardiac enlargement may occur. Routine biochemical tests and chromosomal karyotypes have been normal.

**Complications:** Death in infancy, presumably from feeding and respiratory difficulties or unrecognized cardiomyopathy.

**Associated Findings:** None known.

**Etiology:** Autosomal recessive inheritance.

**Pathogenesis:** Unknown.

**MIM No.:** *21634

**POS No.:** 3485

**CDC No.:** 755.555

**Sex Ratio:** M3:F4

**Occurrence:** Seven patients from five families; one Canadian, one Australian, and three 3 Columbian, have been documented.

**Risk of Recurrence for Patient's Sib:**
See Part I, *Mendelian Inheritance.*

**Risk of Recurrence for Patient's Child:**
See Part I, *Mendelian Inheritance.*

**Age of Detectability:** At birth. In theory this condition should be detectable *in utero.*

**Gene Mapping and Linkage:** Unknown.

**Prevention:** None known. Genetic counseling indicated.

**Treatment:** Scrupulous attention to feeding in early infancy; comparable to that in the Pierre Robin sequence. Cardiac arrythmia was controlled by phenytoin in one patient.

**Prognosis:** Deaths occurred on the first day of life and on days 22, 35, 50, and 65. One survivor spent the first 10 weeks of his life in hospital, but thereafter fed well. He showed progressive growth failure, with a height at 4 1/4 years of age of 84 cm; 19 cm or over four standard deviations below the mean for his age. His head circumference (42 cm) was some six standard deviations below average. Development was slow with a developmental quotient of about 40.

Another survivor has normal intelligence, with growth on the third centile. Cardiomegaly has persisted to age three years.

**Detection of Carrier:** Unknown.

**References:**
Yunis E, Varon H: Cleidocranial dysostosis, severe micrognathism, bilateral absence of thumbs and first metatarsal bone and distal aphalangia: a new genetic syndrome. Am J Dis Child 1980; 134:649–653. * †
Hughes HE, Partington MW: The syndrome of Yunis and Varon: report of a further case. Am J Med Genet 1983; 14:539–544. †
Partington MW: Cardiomyopathy added to the Yunis-Varon syndrome. Proc Greenwood Genet Ctr 1988; 7:224–225.

PA026                                           **M.W. Partington**

Yusho, congenital
*See FETAL EFFECTS OF POLYCHLORINATED BIPHENYL (PCB)*

# ❖ Z ❖

**Zayid-Farraj syndrome**
*See DERMATOARTHRITIS, FAMILIAL HISTIOCYTIC*
**Zellweger syndrome**
*See CEREBRO-HEPATO-RENAL SYNDROME*
**Zestril^, possible fetal effects**
*See FETAL ANGIOTENSIN CONVERTING ENZYME (ACE)
INHIBITION RENAL FAILURE*
**Zimmermann-Laband syndrome**
*See GINGIVAL FIBROMATOSIS-DIGITAL ANOMALIES*
**Zinsser-Cole-Engman syndrome**
*See DYSKERATOSIS CONGENITA*
**Zlotogora-Zilberman-Tenenbaum syndrome**
*See PILI TORTI-CLEFT LIP/PALATE-SYNDACTYLY*
**Zollinger-Ellison syndrome (some cases)**
*See ENDOCRINE NEOPLASIA, MULTIPLE TYPE I*
**Zonana syndrome**
*See OVERGROWTH, BANNAYAN TYPE*
**Zonular cataract**
*See CATARACT, AUTOSOMAL DOMINANT CONGENITAL*
**Zwerchfell eventration**
*See DIAPHRAGM, EVENTRATION*
**Zypokowski-Margolis syndrome**
*See ALBINISM, CUTANEOUS*

# GENE MAP TABLE BY SYMBOL NAME

| SYMBOL | MARKER NAME | MAP LOCATION | NO | ARTICLE TITLE |
|---|---|---|---|---|
| AACT | alpha-1-antichymotrypsin | 14q32.1 | 3279 | ALPHA-1-ANTICHYMOTRYPSIN DEFICIENCY |
| ABO | ABO blood group | 9q34.1-q34.2 | 0340 | TEETH, ENAMEL AND DENTIN DEFECTS FROM ERYTHROBLASTOSIS FETALIS |
| ACAD | acyl-Coenzyme A dehydrogenase, multiple | X | 2289 | ACIDEMIA, GLUTARIC ACIDEMIA II |
| ACADL | acyl-Coenzyme A dehydrogenase, long chain | unassigned | 2228 | ACYL-CoA DEHYDROGENASE DEFICIENCY, LONG CHAIN TYPE |
| ACADM | acyl-Coenzyme A dehydrogenase, C-4 to C-12 straight-chain | 1p31 | 2324 | ACYL-CoA DEHYDROGENASE DEFICIENCY, MEDIUM CHAIN TYPE |
| ACADS | acyl-Coenzyme A dehydrogenase, C-2 to C-3 short chain | 12q22-qter | 2323 | ACYL-CoA DEHYDROGENASE DEFICIENCY, SHORT CHAIN TYPE |
| AD1 | Alzheimer disease 1 | 21pter-q21 | 2354 | ALZHEIMER DISEASE, FAMILIAL |
| ADA | adenosine deaminase | 20q13.11 or 20q13.2-qter | 2196 | IMMUNODEFICIENCY, ADENOSINE DEAMINASE DEFICIENCY |
| ADFN | albinism-deafness syndrome | Xq25-q27 | 0030 | ALBINISM, CUTANEOUS-DEAFNESS |
| ADH1 | alcohol dehydrogenase (class I), alpha polypeptide | 4q21-q23 | 3074 | ALCOHOL INTOLERANCE |
| ADH2 | alcohol dehydrogenase (class I), beta polypeptide | 4q21-q23 | 3074 | ALCOHOL INTOLERANCE |
| ADH3 | alcohol dehydrogenase (class I), gamma polypeptide | 4q21-q23 | 3074 | ALCOHOL INTOLERANCE |
| ADSL | adenylosuccinate lyase | 22 | 3113 | ADENYLOSUCCINATE MONOPHOSPHATE LYASE DEFICIENCY |
| AGA | aspartylglucosaminidase | 4q21-qter | 2042 | ASPARTYLGLUCOSAMINURIA |
| AGMX1 | agammaglobulinemia, X-linked 1 (Bruton) | Xq21.33-q22 | 0027 | IMMUNODEFICIENCY, AGAMMAGLOBULINEMIA, X-LINKED, INFANTILE |
| AGS | Alagille syndrome | 20p12-p11 | 2084 | ARTERIO-HEPATIC DYSPLASIA |
| AHC | adrenal hypoplasia, congenital | Xp21.3-p21.2 | 0024 | ADRENAL HYPOPLASIA, CONGENITAL |
| AHH | aryl hydrocarbon hydroxylase | 2pter-q31 | 2747 | CANCER, LUNG, FAMILIAL |
| AIC | Aicardi syndrome | Xp22 | 2320 | AICARDI SYNDROME |
| AIED | Aland island eye disease (Forsius-Eriksson ocular albinism | Xp21.3-p21.2 | 3183 | FORSIUS-ERIKSSON SYNDROME |
| AIH1 | amelogenesis imperfecta 1, hypomaturation or hypoplastic (?=AMG & AMGS) | Xp22 | 0046 | TEETH, AMELOGENESIS IMPERFECTA |
| AIH1 | amelogenesis imperfecta 1, hypomaturation or hypoplastic (?=AMG & AMGS) | Xp22 | 2136 | TEETH, SNOW-CAPPED |
| AIH2 | amelogenesis imperfecta 2, hypocalcification (autosomal dominant) | unassigned | 0046 | TEETH, AMELOGENESIS IMPERFECTA |
| AK1 | adenylate kinase 1 | 9q34.1-q34.2 | 2660 | ANEMIA, ADENYLATE KINASE DEFICIENCY |
| AK2 | adenylate kinase 2 | 1p34 | 2660 | ANEMIA, ADENYLATE KINASE DEFICIENCY |
| AK3 | adenylate kinase 3 | 9p24-p13 | 2660 | ANEMIA, ADENYLATE KINASE DEFICIENCY |
| ALAD | aminolevulinate, delta-, dehydratase | 9q34 | 3091 | DELTA-AMINOLEVULINIC ACID DEHYDRASE DEFICIENCY |
| ALB | albumin | 4q11-q13 | 0047 | ANALBUMINEMIA |
| ALD | adrenoleukodystrophy | Xq28 | 2533 | ADRENOLEUKODYSTROPHY, X-LINKED |
| ALDH2 | aldehyde dehydrogenase 2, mitochondrial | 12q24.2 | 3074 | ALCOHOL INTOLERANCE |
| ALDOA | aldolase A, fructose-bisphosphate | 16q22-q24 | 2662 | ERYTHROCYTE ALDOLASE-A DEFICIENCY |
| ALDOB | aldolase B, fructose bisphosphate | 9q21.3-q22.2 | 0395 | FRUCTOSE-1-PHOSPHATE ALDOLASE DEFICIENCY |
| ALPL | alkaline phosphatase, liver/bone/kidney | 1p36.1-p34 | 0516 | HYPOPHOSPHATASIA |
| ALS | amyotrophic lateral sclerosis | unassigned | 2069 | AMYOTROPHIC LATERAL SCLEROSIS, FAMILIAL ADULT AND JUVENILE TYPES |
| ALS | amyotrophic lateral sclerosis | unassigned | 2067 | AMYOTROPHIC LATERAL SCLEROSIS |
| AMG | amelogenin (?=AMGS & AIH) | Xp22.31-p22.1 | 0046 | TEETH, AMELOGENESIS IMPERFECTA |
| AMH | anti-Mullerian hormone | 19p13.3 | 0683 | MULLERIAN DERIVATIVES IN MALES, PERSISTENT |
| AN1 | aniridia 1 | 2p | 0057 | ANIRIDIA |
| AN2 | aniridia 2 without Wilms' tumor, GU abnormalities, and M.R. | 11p13 | 0057 | ANIRIDIA |
| AN2 | aniridia 2 without Wilms' tumor, GU abnormalities, and M.R. | 11p13 | 2245 | CHROMOSOME 11, PARTIAL MONOSOMY 11p |
| ANCR | Angelman syndrome chromosome region | 15q11-q12 | 2086 | ANGELMAN SYNDROME |

| SYMBOL | MARKER NAME | MAP LOCATION | NO | ARTICLE TITLE |
|---|---|---|---|---|
| ANK | ankyrin | 8p21-p11 | 0892 | SPHEROCYTOSIS |
| ANK | ankyrin | 8p21-p11 | 2646 | ANEMIA, HEMOLYTIC, RED CELL MEMBRANE DEFECTS |
| AOM | arthroophthalmopathy, progressive (Stickler syndrome) | 12q14 | 2424 | ARTHRO-OPHTHALMOPATHY, WEISSENBACHER-ZWEYMULLER VARIANT |
| AOM | arthroophthalmopathy, progressive (Stickler syndrome) | 12q14 | 0090 | ARTHRO-OPHTHALMOPATHY, HEREDITARY, PROGRESSIVE, STICKLER TYPE |
| APC | adenomatosis polyposis coli | 5q21-q22 | 0536 | INTESTINAL POLYPOSIS, TYPE III |
| APC | adenomatosis polyposis coli | 5q21-q22 | 0535 | INTESTINAL POLYPOSIS, TYPE I |
| APC | adenomatosis polyposis coli | 5q21-q22 | 2739 | TURCOT SYNDROME |
| APOA1 | apolipoprotein A-I | 11q23-q24 | 3165 | APOLIPOPROTEIN A-I AND C-III DEFICIENCY STATES |
| APOA1 | apolipoprotein A-I | 11q23-q24 | 3096 | HYPOALPHALIPOPROTEINEMIA |
| APOA4 | apolipoprotein A-IV | 11q23-qter | 3096 | HYPOALPHALIPOPROTEINEMIA |
| APOB | apolipoprotein B (including Ag(x) antigen) | 2p24-p23 | 3227 | APO B-100, DEFECTIVE, FAMILIAL |
| APOB | apolipoprotein B (including Ag(x) antigen) | 2p24-p23 | 0002 | ABETALIPOPROTEINEMIA |
| APOB | apolipoprotein B (including Ag(x) antigen) | 2p24-p23 | 2646 | ANEMIA, HEMOLYTIC, RED CELL MEMBRANE DEFECTS |
| APOC1 | apolipoprotein C-I | 19q13.2 | 3096 | HYPOALPHALIPOPROTEINEMIA |
| APP | amyloid beta (A4) precursor protein | 21qq21.2 | 2354 | ALZHEIMER DISEASE, FAMILIAL |
| APR | apolipoprotein receptor | 12q13-q14 | 3165 | APOLIPOPROTEIN A-I AND C-III DEFICIENCY STATES |
| APR | apolipoprotein receptor | 12q13-q14 | 0048 | ANALPHALIPOPROTEINEMIA |
| APRT | adenine phosphoribosyltransferase | 16q24 | 3104 | ADENINE PHOSPHO-RIBOSYL-TRANSFERASE (APRT) DEFICIENCY |
| APY | atopy (allergic asthma and rhinitis) | 11q12-q13 | 3150 | SKIN, ATOPY, FAMILIAL |
| AR | androgen receptor (dihydrotestosterone receptor; testicular feminization) | Xq12 | 2954 | ANDROGEN INSENSITIVITY (RESISTANCE), MINIMAL |
| AR | androgen receptor (dihydrotestosterone receptor; testicular feminization) | Xq12 | 0049 | ANDROGEN INSENSITIVITY SYNDROME, COMPLETE |
| AR | androgen receptor (dihydrotestosterone receptor; testicular feminization) | Xq12 | 0050 | ANDROGEN INSENSITIVITY SYNDROME, INCOMPLETE |
| ARG1 | arginase, liver | 6q23 | 0086 | ARGININEMIA |
| ARSA | arylsulfatase A | 22q13.31-qter | 0651 | METACHROMATIC LEUKODYSTROPHIES |
| ARSB | arylsulfatase B | 5p11-q13 | 0679 | MUCOPOLYSACCHARIDOSIS VI |
| ARVP | arginine vasopressin (neurophysin II) | 20 | 2611 | DIABETES INSIPIDIS, NEUROHYPOPHYSEAL TYPE |
| ASB | anemia, sideroblastic/hypochromic | X | 1518 | ANEMIA, SIDEROBLASTIC |
| ASL | argininosuccinate lyase | 7pter-q22 | 0087 | ACIDURIA, ARGININOSUCCINIC |
| ASMD | anterior segment mesenchymal dysgenesis | 4q | 0439 | EYE, ANTERIOR SEGMENT DYSGENESIS |
| ASS | argininosuccinate synthetase | 9q34-qter | 0174 | CITRULLINEMIA |
| AT3 | antithrombin III | 1q23-q25.1 | 3066 | ANTITHROMBIN III DEFICIENCY |
| ATA | ataxia telangiectasia (complementation group A) | 11q22-q23 | 0094 | ATAXIA-TELANGIECTASIA |
| ATN | albinism, tyrosinase-negative (?=TYR) | ULG5 | 0034 | ALBINISM, OCULOCUTANEOUS, TYROSINASE NEGATIVE |
| ATS | Alport syndrome | Xq21.3-q24 | 0708 | NEPHRITIS-DEAFNESS (SENSORINEURAL), HEREDITARY TYPE |
| B2M | beta-2-microglobulin | 15q21-q22.2 | 3106 | AMYLOIDOSIS, HEMODIALYSIS-RELATED |
| BCEI | breast cancer, estrogen-inducible sequence expressed in | 21q22.3 | 2351 | CANCER, BREAST, FAMILIAL |
| BCH | benign chorea | unassigned | 2306 | CHOREA, BENIGN FAMILIAL |
| BCL1 | B cell CLL/lymphoma 1 | 11q13.3 | 3097 | LEUKEMIA/LYMPHOMA, B CELL |
| BCL2 | B cell CLL/lymphoma 2 | 18q21.3 | 3097 | LEUKEMIA/LYMPHOMA, B CELL |
| BCL2 | B cell CLL/lymphoma 2 | 18q21.3 | 3107 | LYMPHOMA, NON-HODGKIN |
| BCP | blue cone pigment | 7q22-qter | 0199 | COLOR BLINDNESS, YELLOW-BLUE TRITAN |

| SYMBOL | MARKER NAME | MAP LOCATION | NO | ARTICLE TITLE |
|---|---|---|---|---|
| BCR | breakpoint cluster region | 22q11 | 3092 | LEUKEMIA, CHRONIC MYELOID (CML) |
| BDM | behavior disorder modifier | X | 1532 | MOOD AND THOUGHT DISORDERS |
| BFLS | Borjeson-Forssman-Lehmann syndrome | Xq26-q27 | 2272 | BORJESON-FORSSMAN-LEHMANN SYNDROME |
| BPGM | 2,3-bisphosphoglycerate mutase | 7q31-q34 | 2664 | ERYTHROCYTE, DIPHOSPHOGLYCERATE MUTASE (2,3) DEFICIENCY |
| BTS | Batten disease | 16 | 0713 | NEURONAL CEROID-LIPOFUSCINOSES (NCL) |
| BWS | Beckwith-Wiedemann syndrome | 11pter-p15.4 | 0104 | BECKWITH-WIEDEMANN SYNDROME |
| C1NH | complement component 1 inhibitor (angioedema, hereditary) | 11q12-q13.1 | 0054 | ANGIOEDEMA, HEREDITARY |
| C1QA | complement component 1, q subcomponent, alpha polypeptide | 1p | 3210 | COMPLEMENT COMPONENT 1, DEFICIENCY OF |
| C1QB | complement component 1, q subcomponent, beta polypeptide | 1p | 3210 | COMPLEMENT COMPONENT 1, DEFICIENCY OF |
| C1R | complement component 1, r subcomponent | 12p13 | 3210 | COMPLEMENT COMPONENT 1, DEFICIENCY OF |
| C1S | complement component 1, s subcomponent | 12p13 | 3210 | COMPLEMENT COMPONENT 1, DEFICIENCY OF |
| C2 | complement component 2 | 6p21.3 | 2201 | COMPLEMENT COMPONENT 2, DEFICIENCY OF |
| C3 | complement component 3 | 19p13.3-p13.2 | 2219 | COMPLEMENT COMPONENT 3, DEFICIENCY OF |
| C4A | complement component 4A | 6p21.3 | 2220 | COMPLEMENT COMPONENT 4, DEFICIENCY OF |
| C4B | complement component 4B | 6p21.3 | 2220 | COMPLEMENT COMPONENT 4, DEFICIENCY OF |
| C4BP | complement component 4 binding protein | 1q32 | 2220 | COMPLEMENT COMPONENT 4, DEFICIENCY OF |
| CA2 | carbonic anhydrase II | 8q22 | 0863 | RENAL TUBULAR ACIDOSIS-SENSORINEURAL DEAFNESS |
| CA2 | carbonic anhydrase II | 8q22 | 3086 | RENAL TUBULAR ACIDOSIS-OSTEOPETROSIS SYNDROME |
| CAE | cataract, zonular pulverulent (FY-linked) | 1q21-q25 | 2342 | CATARACT, AUTOSOMAL DOMINANT CONGENITAL |
| CAE | cataract, zonular pulverulent (FY-linked) | 1q21-q25 | 3174 | CATARACT, COPPOCK |
| CAT | catalase | 11p13 | 0006 | ACATALASEMIA |
| CBBM | color blindness, blue monochromatic | Xq28 | 0195 | COLOR BLINDNESS, BLUE MONOCONE-MONOCHROMATIC |
| CBS | cystathionine-beta-synthase | 21q22.3 | 0474 | HOMOCYSTINURIA |
| CCA | congenital contractual arachnodactyly | unassigned | 0085 | ARACHNODACTYLY, CONTRACTURAL BEALS TYPE |
| CCAT | cataract, congenital | ULG3 | 3173 | CATARACT, HUTTERITE |
| CCT | cataract, congenital, total | X | 0132 | CATARACT, CORTICAL AND NUCLEAR |
| CD11A | antigen CD11A (p180), lymphocyte function-associated antigen 1 | 16p13.1-p11 | 2970 | GRANULOCYTE GLYCOPROTEIN CD11/CD18 DEFICIENCY |
| CD13 | antigen CD13 (p150) | 15q25-qter | 2970 | GRANULOCYTE GLYCOPROTEIN CD11/CD18 DEFICIENCY |
| CD18 | lymphocyte function-associated antigen 1; macrophage antigen | 21q22.3 | 2970 | GRANULOCYTE GLYCOPROTEIN CD11/CD18 DEFICIENCY |
| CDPX | chondrodysplasia punctata | Xp22.32 | 2730 | CHONDRODYSPLASIA PUNCTATA, X-LINKED DOMINANT TYPE |
| CECR | cat eye syndrome chromosome region | 22pter-q11 | 0544 | CAT EYE SYNDROME |
| CF | cystic fibrosis | 7q31-q32 | 0237 | CYSTIC FIBROSIS |
| CHE1 | cholinesterase (serum) 1 | 3q26-qter | 0152 | CHOLINESTERASE, ATYPICAL |
| CHE2 | cholinesterase (serum) 2 | 2q | 0152 | CHOLINESTERASE, ATYPICAL |
| CLG | collagenase, epidermolysis bullosa, dystrophic, (autosomal recessive) | 11q21-q22 | 2562 | EPIDERMOLYSIS BULLOSUM, TYPE III |
| CLS | Coffin-Lowry syndrome | Xp22.2-p22.1 | 0190 | COFFIN-LOWRY SYNDROME |
| CMM | cutaneous malignant melanoma/dysplastic nevus | 1p36 | 2318 | CANCER, MALIGNANT MELANOMA, FAMILIAL |
| CMM | cutaneous malignant melanoma/dysplastic nevus | 1p36 | 2165 | NEVUS, CONGENITAL NEVOMELANOCYTIC |
| CMT1 | Charcot-Marie-Tooth neuropathy 1 | 1q | 2104 | NEUROPATHY, HEREDITARY MOTOR AND SENSORY, TYPE I |

| SYMBOL | MARKER NAME | MAP LOCATION | NO | ARTICLE TITLE |
|---|---|---|---|---|
| CMT2 | Charcot-Marie-Tooth neuropathy 2 | 17p13.1-q12 | 2104 | NEUROPATHY, HEREDITARY MOTOR AND SENSORY, TYPE I |
| CMTX | Charcot-Marie-Tooth neuropathy, X-linked | Xq11-q13 | 2104 | NEUROPATHY, HEREDITARY MOTOR AND SENSORY, TYPE I |
| COD1 | cone dystrophy 1 (X-linked) | Xp21.1-p11.3 | 3228 | RETINA, CONE DYSTROPHY, X-LINKED |
| COL1A1 | collagen, type I, alpha 1 | 17q21.3-q22 | 0777 | OSTEOGENESIS IMPERFECTA |
| COL1A2 | collagen, type I, alpha 2 | 7q21.3-q22.1 | 0777 | OSTEOGENESIS IMPERFECTA |
| COL2A1 | collagen, type II, alpha 1 | 12q14.3 | 0897 | SPONDYLOEPIPHYSEAL DYSPLASIA CONGENITA |
| CORD | cone rod dystrophy (autosomal dominant) | unassigned | 0201 | RETINA, COMBINED CONE-ROD DEGENERATION |
| CP | ceruloplasmin | 3q23-q25 | 3077 | HYPOCERULOPLASMINEMIA |
| CPO | coproporphyrinogen oxidase | 9 | 0203 | PORPHYRIA, COPROPORPHYRIA |
| CPP | ceruloplasmin pseudogene | 8q21.13-q23.1 | 3077 | HYPOCERULOPLASMINEMIA |
| CPS1 | carbamoyl phosphate synthetase 1, mitochondrial | 2p | 3022 | CARBAMOYL PHOSPHATE SYNTHETASE DEFICIENCY |
| CRD | choroidoretinal degeneration | X | 0869 | RETINITIS PIGMENTOSA |
| CRD | choroidoretinal degeneration | X | 0925 | CHOROIDEREMIA |
| CRS | craniosynostosis | 7p21 | 0230 | CRANIOSYNOSTOSIS |
| CSNB1 | congenital stationary night blindness 1 | Xp21.1-p11.23 | 0718 | NIGHTBLINDNESS, CONGENITAL STATIONARY, X-LINKED RECESSIVE |
| CTH | cystathionase | 16 | 0236 | CYSTATHIONINURIA |
| CTM | cataract, Marner | 16 | 2342 | CATARACT, AUTOSOMAL DOMINANT CONGENITAL |
| CTM | cataract, Marner | 16 | 0132 | CATARACT, CORTICAL AND NUCLEAR |
| CYBB | cytochrome b-245, beta polypeptide (chronic granulomatous disease) | Xp21.1 | 0443 | GRANULOMATOUS DISEASE, CHRONIC X-LINKED |
| CYP1 | cytochrome P450, subfamily I (aromatic compound-inducible) | 15q22-q24 | 2747 | CANCER, LUNG, FAMILIAL |
| CYP11A | cytochrome P450, subfamily XIA | 15 | 0907 | STEROID 20-22 DESMOLASE DEFICIENCY |
| CYP11B1 | cytochrome P450, subfamily XIB, polypeptide 1 (steroid 11-beta-hydroxylase) | 8q21-q22 | 0902 | STEROID 11 BETA-HYDROXYLASE DEFICIENCY |
| CYP11B2 | cytochrome P450, subfamily XIB, polypeptide 2 (steroid 11-beta-hydroxylase) | 8q21-q22 | 0902 | STEROID 11 BETA-HYDROXYLASE DEFICIENCY |
| CYP17 | cytochrome P450, subfamily XVII (steroid 17-alpha-hydroxylase) | 10 | 0903 | STEROID 17 ALPHA-HYDROXYLASE DEFICIENCY |
| CYP19 | cytochrome P450, subfamily XIX (aromatization of androgens) | 15q21 | 2308 | GYNECOMASTIA DUE TO INCREASED AROMATASE ACTIVITY, FAMILIAL |
| CYP21 | cytochrome P450, subfamily XXI | 6p21.3 | 0908 | STEROID 21-HYDROXYLASE DEFICIENCY |
| DBH | dopamine beta-hydroxylase (dopamine beta-monooxygenase) | 9q34 | 2883 | DOPAMINE BETA-HYDROXYLASE DEFICIENCY, CONGENITAL |
| DES | desmin | 2 | 3072 | MYOPATHY OR CARDIOMYOPATHY DUE TO DESMIN DEFECT |
| DFN3 | deafness, conductive, with fixed stapes | Xq13-q21.2 | 3116 | DEAFNESS WITH PERILYMPHATIC GUSHER |
| DGCR | DiGeorge syndrome chromosome region | 22q11.21-q11.23 | 0943 | IMMUNODEFICIENCY, THYMIC AGENESIS |
| DGI1 | dentinogenesis imperfecta 1 | 4q12-q23 | 0279 | TEETH, DENTINOGENESIS IMPERFECTA |
| DHOF | dermal hypoplasia, focal | X | 0281 | DERMAL HYPOPLASIA, FOCAL |
| DIA1 | diaphorase (NADH) (cytochrome b-5 reductase) | 22q13.31-qter | 2682 | METHEMOGLOBINEMIA, NADH-DEPENDENT DIAPHORASE DEFICIENCY |
| DIR | diabetes insipidus, renal | Xq28 | 0287 | DIABETES INSIPIDUS, VASOPRESSIN RESISTANT TYPES I AND II |
| DKC | dyskeratosis congenita | Xq27-q28 | 2024 | DYSKERATOSIS CONGENITA |
| DM | dystrophia myotonia | 19q13.2-q13.3 | 0702 | MYOTONIC DYSTROPHY |
| DMD | muscular dystrophy, Duchenne and Becker types | Xp21.3-p21.1 | 0689 | MUSCULAR DYSTROPHY, CHILDHOOD PSEUDOHYPERTROPHIC |

| SYMBOL | MARKER NAME | MAP LOCATION | NO | ARTICLE TITLE |
|---|---|---|---|---|
| DMD | muscular dystrophy, Duchenne and Becker types | Xp21.3-p21.1 | 0687 | MUSCULAR DYSTROPHY, ADULT PSEUDOHYPERTROPHIC |
| DTS | diphtheria toxin sensitivity | 5q23 | 3079 | DIPHTHERIA, SUSCEPTIBILITY TO |
| DYT1 | dystonia, torsion 1 (autosomal dominant) | 9q32-q34 | 0957 | TORSION DYSTONIA |
| DYT2 | dystonia, torsion 2 (autosomal recessive) | unassigned | 0957 | TORSION DYSTONIA |
| EBDCT | epidermolysis bullosa dystrophica (Cockayne-Touraine) | unassigned | 2560 | EPIDERMOLYSIS BULLOSUM, TYPE I |
| EBN | epilepsy, benign neonatal | 20q | 3216 | CONVULSIONS, BENIGN FAMILIAL NEONATAL |
| EBR3 | epidermolysis bullosa progressiva | ULG4 | 2562 | EPIDERMOLYSIS BULLOSUM, TYPE III |
| EBS1 | epidermolysis bullosa simplex (Ogna) | 8 | 2560 | EPIDERMOLYSIS BULLOSUM, TYPE I |
| EDA | ectodermal dysplasia, anhidrotic (hypohydrotic) | Xq12-q13.1 | 0333 | ECTODERMAL DYSPLASIA, CHRIST-SIEMENS-TOURAINE TYPE |
| EFE2 | endocardial fibroelastosis 2 | X | 0348 | VENTRICLE, ENDOCARDIAL FIBROELASTOSIS OF LEFT VENTRICLE |
| EJM | epilepsy, juvenile myoclonic | 6p | 2567 | SEIZURES, MYOCLONIC, JUVENILE JANZ TYPE |
| EKV | erythrokeratodermia variabilis | 1 | 0361 | SKIN, ERYTHROKERATODERMIA, VARIABLE |
| EL1 | elliptocytosis 1 (Rh-linked); band 4.1 protein | 1pter-p34 | 2646 | ANEMIA, HEMOLYTIC, RED CELL MEMBRANE DEFECTS |
| EL1 | elliptocytosis 1 (Rh-linked); band 4.1 protein | 1pter-p34 | 2665 | ELLIPTOCYTOSIS |
| EMD | Emery-Dreifuss muscular dystrophy | Xq27.3-q28 | 2491 | EMERY-DREIFUSS SYNDROME |
| EPB3 | erythrocyte surface protein band 3 | 17q21-qter | 2646 | ANEMIA, HEMOLYTIC, RED CELL MEMBRANE DEFECTS |
| ETFA | electron transfer flavoprotein, alpha polypeptide (glutaric aciduria II) | 15q23-q25 | 2377 | ACIDEMIA, ETHYLMALONIC-ADIPIC |
| F10 | coagulation factor X | 13q34 | 2670 | FACTOR X DEFICIENCY |
| F11 | coagulation factor XI | 4q35 | 2671 | FACTOR XI DEFICIENCY |
| F12 | coagulation factor XII (Hageman) | 5q33-qter | 2672 | FACTOR XII DEFICIENCY |
| F13A1 | coagulation factor XIII, A1 polypeptide | 6p25-p24 | 2673 | FACTOR XIII (FIBRIN STABILIZING FACTOR) |
| F2 | coagulation factor II (prothrombin) | 11p11-q12 | 2679 | HYPOPROTHROMBINEMIA |
| F2L | coagulation factor II (prothrombin)-like | Xpter-q25 | 2679 | HYPOPROTHROMBINEMIA |
| F2L | coagulation factor II (prothrombin)-like | Xpter-q25 | 2674 | COAGULATION DEFECT, FAMILIAL MULTIPLE FACTORS |
| F5 | coagulation factor V | 1q21-q25 | 2668 | FACTOR V DEFICIENCY |
| F7 | coagulation factor VII | 13q34 | 2669 | FACTOR VII DEFICIENCY |
| F8C | coagulation factor VIIIc, procoagulant component (hemophilia A) | Xq28 | 0461 | HEMOPHILIA A |
| F8VWF | coagulation factor VIII VWF (von Willebrand factor) | 12pter-p12 | 0996 | VON WILLEBRAND DISEASE |
| F9 | coagulation factor IX (Christmas disease) | Xq26.3-q27.1 | 0462 | HEMOPHILIA B |
| FA | Fanconi anemia | unassigned | 2029 | PANCYTOPENIA SYNDROME, FANCONI TYPE |
| FAH | fumarylacetoacetate | 15q23-q25 | 0978 | TYROSINEMIA I |
| FGA | fibrinogen, A alpha polypeptide | 4q28 | 2661 | AFIBROGINEMIA, CONGENITAL |
| FGA | fibrinogen, A alpha polypeptide | 4q28 | 0004 | FIBRINOGENS, ABNORMAL CONGENITAL |
| FGB | fibrinogen, B beta polypeptide | 4q28 | 2661 | AFIBROGINEMIA, CONGENITAL |
| FGB | fibrinogen, B beta polypeptide | 4q28 | 0004 | FIBRINOGENS, ABNORMAL CONGENITAL |
| FGDY | faciogenital dysplasia (Aarskog syndrome) | Xq13 | 0001 | AARSKOG SYNDROME |
| FGG | fibrinogen, gamma polypeptide | 4q28 | 2661 | AFIBROGINEMIA, CONGENITAL |
| FGG | fibrinogen, gamma polypeptide | 4q28 | 0004 | FIBRINOGENS, ABNORMAL CONGENITAL |
| FH | fumarate hydratase | 1q42.1 | 2599 | ACIDURIA, FUMARIC |
| FMD | facioscapulohumeral muscular dystrophy | unassigned | 2049 | MUSCULAR DYSTROPHY, FACIO-SCAPULO-HUMERAL |
| FRAXA | fragile site, folic acid type, rare, fra(X)(q27.3) | Xq27.3 | 2073 | X-LINKED MENTAL RETARDATION, FRAGILE X SYNDROME |
| FRDA | Friedreich ataxia | 9q13-q21.1 | 2714 | ATAXIA, FRIEDREICH TYPE |
| FUCA1 | fucosidase, alpha-L- 1, tissue | 1p35-p34 | 0398 | FUCOSIDOSIS |

| SYMBOL | MARKER NAME | MAP LOCATION | NO | ARTICLE TITLE |
|---|---|---|---|---|
| FY | Duffy blood group | 1q21-q25 | 3065 | MALARIA, VIVAX, SUSCEPTIBILITY TO |
| G6PD | glucose-6-phosphate dehydrogenase | Xq28 | 0420 | GLUCOSE-6-PHOSPHATE DEHYDROGENASE DEFICIENCY |
| GAA | glucosidase, alpha; acid | 17q23 | 0011 | GLYCOGENOSIS, TYPE IIa |
| GAA | glucosidase, alpha; acid | 17q23 | 2873 | GLYCOGENOSIS, TYPE IIb |
| GAD | glutamate decarboxylase | 2 | 0991 | SEIZURES, VITAMIN B(6) DEPENDENCY |
| GALC | galactosylceramidase | 17 | 0415 | LEUKODYSTROPHY, GLOBOID CELL TYPE |
| GALE | UDP-galactose-4-epimerase | 1p36-p35 | 0357 | GALACTOSE EPIMERASE DEFICIENCY |
| GALK | galactokinase | 17q23-q25 | 0402 | GALACTOKINASE DEFICIENCY |
| GALT | galactose-1-phosphate uridyltransferase | 9p13 | 0403 | GALACTOSEMIA |
| GBA | glucosidase, beta; acid | 1q21 | 0406 | GAUCHER DISEASE |
| GC | group-specific component (vitamin D binding protein) | 4q12-q13 | 0983 | USHER SYNDROME |
| GC | group-specific component (vitamin D binding protein) | 4q12-q13 | 0446 | PLASMA, GROUP-SPECIFIC COMPONENT |
| GCP | green cone pigment (color blindness, deutan) | Xq28 | 0196 | COLOR BLINDNESS, RED-GREEN DEUTAN SERIES |
| GCPS | Greig cephalopolysyndactyly syndrome | 7p13 | 2925 | POLYSYNDACTYLY-DYSMORPHIC CRANIOFACIES, GREIG TYPE |
| GGT1 | gamma-glutamyltransferase 1 | 22q11.1-q11.2 | 0422 | GLUTATHIONURIA |
| GH1 | growth hormone 1 | 17q22-q24 | 0447 | GROWTH HORMONE DEFICIENCY, ISOLATED |
| GK | glycerol kinase deficiency | Xp21.3-p21.2 | 2310 | GLYCEROL KINASE DEFICIENCY |
| GLA | galactosidase, alpha | Xq21.3-q22 | 0373 | FABRY DISEASE |
| GLB1 | galactosidase, beta 1 | 3pter-p21 | 3215 | G(M1)-GANGLIOSIDOSIS, TYPE 3 |
| GLB1 | galactosidase, beta 1 | 3pter-p21 | 0431 | G(M1)-GANGLIOSIDOSIS, TYPE 1 |
| GLI | glioma-associated oncogene homolog (zinc finger protein) | 12q13 | 2839 | CANCER, GLIOMA, FAMILIAL |
| GM2A | GM2 ganglioside activator protein | 5 | 0434 | G(M2)-GANGLIOSIDOSIS WITH HEXOSAMINIDASE A DEFICIENCY |
| GNPTA | UDP-N-acetylgluco.-lysosomal-enzyme N-acetylglucosaminephosphotrans. | 4q21-q23 | 0673 | MUCOLIPIDOSIS III |
| GNPTA | UDP-N-acetylgluco.-lysosomal-enzyme N-acetylglucosaminephosphotrans. | 4q21-q23 | 0672 | MUCOLIPIDOSIS II |
| GNS | N-acetylglucosamine-6-sulfatase (Sanfilippo disease IIID) | 12q14 | 0677 | MUCOPOLYSACCHARIDOSIS III |
| GP2B | glycoprotein IIb (IIb/IIIa complex, platelet, CD41B) | 17q21.32 | 2683 | THROMBASTHENIA, GLANZMANN-NAEGELI TYPE |
| GPI | glucose phosphate isomerase | 19q13.1 | 2750 | ANEMIA, GLUCOSE PHOSPHATE ISOMERASE DEFICIENCY |
| GPX1 | glutathione peroxidase 1 | 3q11-q12 | 2675 | ANEMIA, HEMOLYTIC, GLUTATHIONINE PEROXIDASE DEFICIENCY |
| GRL | glucocorticoid receptor | 5q31-q32 | 2952 | GLUCOCORTICOID RESISTANCE |
| GSL | galactosialidosis | 20 | 3110 | GALACTOSIALIDOSIS |
| GSR | glutathione reductase | 8p21.1 | 2676 | ANEMIA, HEMOLYTIC, GLUTATHIONE REDUCTASE DEFICIENCY |
| GTS | Gilles de la Tourette syndrome | unassigned | 2305 | TOURETTE SYNDROME |
| GUD | genitourinary dysplasia component of WAGR | 11p13 | 2742 | CANCER, WILMS TUMOR |
| GUD | genitourinary dysplasia component of WAGR | 11p13 | 2245 | CHROMOSOME 11, PARTIAL MONOSOMY 11p |
| GUSB | glucuronidase, beta | 7q21.2-q22 | 0680 | MUCOPOLYSACCHARIDOSIS VII |
| HBB | hemoglobin, beta | 11p15.5 | 0886 | ANEMIA, SICKLE CELL |
| HD | Huntington disease | 4pter-p16.3 | 0478 | HUNTINGTON DISEASE |
| HEXA | hexosaminidase A (alpha polypeptide) | 15q23-q24 | 0434 | G(M2)-GANGLIOSIDOSIS WITH HEXOSAMINIDASE A DEFICIENCY |
| HEXB | hexosaminidase B (beta polypeptide) | 5q13 | 0433 | G(M2)-GANGLIOSIDOSIS WITH HEXOSAMINIDASE A AND B DEFICIENCY |
| HFE | hemochromatosis | 6p21.3 | 0460 | HEMOCHROMATOSIS, IDIOPATHIC |
| HHG | hypergonadotropic hypogonadism | ULG5 | 0556 | KLINEFELTER SYNDROME |
| HHH | hyperornithinemia-hyperammonemia-homocitrullinuria | 13q34 | 3169 | HYPERORNITHINEMIA-HYPERAMMONEMIA-HOMOCITRULLINURIA |

| SYMBOL | MARKER NAME | MAP LOCATION | NO | ARTICLE TITLE |
|---|---|---|---|---|
| HIGM1 | hyper IgM syndrome | Xq24-q27 | 2524 | IMMUNODEFICIENCY, X-LINKED WITH HYPER IgM |
| HIS | histidase | 12 | 0472 | HISTIDINEMIA |
| HK1 | hexokinase 1 | 10q22 | 2678 | ANEMIA, HEMOLYTIC, ERYTHROCYTE HEXOKINASE DEFICIENCY |
| HLA-A | major histocompatibility complex, class I | 6p21.3 | 3082 | RAGWEED POLLEN SENSITIVITY |
| HOAC | hypoacusis 2 (autosomal recessive) | UlG4 | 0271 | DEAFNESS (SENSORINEURAL), RECESSIVE PROFOUND |
| HOMG | hypomagnesemia, secondary hypocalcemia | X | 0514 | HYPOMAGNESEMIA, PRIMARY |
| HP | haptoglobin | 16q22.1 | 0452 | HAPTOGLOBIN |
| HPRT | hypoxanthine phosphoribosyltransferase | Xq26 | 0588 | LESCH-NYHAN SYNDROME |
| HPRT | hypoxanthine phosphoribosyltransferase | Xq26 | 0441 | GOUT |
| HPT | hypoparathyroidism | Xq26-q27 | 0515 | HYPOPARATHYROIDISM, FAMILIAL |
| HSAS | hydrocephalus, stenosis of the aqueduct of Sylvius | X | 0481 | HYDROCEPHALY |
| HSDB3 | hydroxy-delta 5-steroid dehydrogenase, 3 beta- and steroid delta-i somerase | 1p13-p11 | 0909 | STEROID 3 BETA-HYDROXYSTEROID DEHYDROGENASE DEFICIENCY |
| HV1S | herpes simplex virus type 1 sensitivity | 3 or 11p11-qter | 2988 | FETAL HERPES SIMPLEX VIRUS INFECTION |
| HVBS4 | hepatitis B virus integration site 4 | 2 | 3008 | FETAL EFFECT FROM HEPATITIS B INFECTION |
| HVBS8 | hepatitis B virus integration site 8 | 17p12-p11.2 | 3008 | FETAL EFFECT FROM HEPATITIS B INFECTION |
| HYP | hypophosphatemia, vitamin D resistant rickets | Xp22.2-p22.1 | 0517 | HYPOPHOSPHATEMIA, X-LINKED |
| IC1 | ichthyosis 1, (autosomal recessive); congenital ichthyosiform erythroderma | unassigned | 2853 | ICHTHYOSIS, LAMELLAR RECESSIVE |
| IC1 | ichthyosis 1, (autosomal recessive); congenital ichthyosiform erythroderma | unassigned | 2855 | ICHTHYOSIS, CONGENITAL ERYTHRODERMIC |
| IDS | iduronate 2-sulfatase (Hunter syndrome) | Xq27.3-q28 | 0676 | MUCOPOLYSACCHARIDOSIS II |
| IDUA | iduronidase, alpha-L- | 22pter-q11 | 0675 | MUCOPOLYSACCHARIDOSIS I-S |
| IDUA | iduronidase, alpha-L- | 22pter-q11 | 0674 | MUCOPOLYSACCHARIDOSIS I-H |
| IF | complement component I | 4q24-q25 | 2219 | COMPLEMENT COMPONENT 3, DEFICIENCY OF |
| IFNA | interferon, alpha (leukocyte) | 9p22-p13 | 3090 | INTERFERON DEFICIENCY |
| IFNB1 | interferon, beta 1, fibroblast | 9p22 | 3090 | INTERFERON DEFICIENCY |
| IFNB3 | interferon, beta 3, fibroblast | 2p23-qter | 3090 | INTERFERON DEFICIENCY |
| IFNG | interferon, gamma | 12q24.1 | 3090 | INTERFERON DEFICIENCY |
| IFNR | interferon production regulator | 16 | 3090 | INTERFERON DEFICIENCY |
| IGF1 | insulin-like growth factor 1 | 12q23 | 3100 | GROWTH DEFICIENCY, AFRICAN PYGMY TYPE |
| IGHA1 | immunoglobulin alpha 1 | 14q32.33 | 0476 | SERUM ALLOTYPES, HUMAN |
| IGHA1 | immunoglobulin alpha 1 | 14q32.33 | 0521 | IMMUNODEFICIENCY, COMMON VARIABLE TYPE |
| IGHA2 | immunoglobulin alpha 2 (A2M marker) | 14q32.33 | 0476 | SERUM ALLOTYPES, HUMAN |
| IGHA2 | immunoglobulin alpha 2 (A2M marker) | 14q32.33 | 0521 | IMMUNODEFICIENCY, COMMON VARIABLE TYPE |
| IGHD | immunoglobulin delta | 14q32.33 | 0521 | IMMUNODEFICIENCY, COMMON VARIABLE TYPE |
| IGHD | immunoglobulin delta | 14q32.33 | 0476 | SERUM ALLOTYPES, HUMAN |
| IGHE | immunoglobulin epsilon | 14q32.33 | 0521 | IMMUNODEFICIENCY, COMMON VARIABLE TYPE |
| IGHE | immunoglobulin epsilon | 14q32.33 | 0476 | SERUM ALLOTYPES, HUMAN |
| IGHEP1 | immunoglobulin epsilon pseudogene 1 | 14q32.33 | 0521 | IMMUNODEFICIENCY, COMMON VARIABLE TYPE |
| IGHEP1 | immunoglobulin epsilon pseudogene 1 | 14q32.33 | 0476 | SERUM ALLOTYPES, HUMAN |
| IGHG1 | immunoglobulin gamma 1 (Gm marker) | 14q32.33 | 0476 | SERUM ALLOTYPES, HUMAN |
| IGHG1 | immunoglobulin gamma 1 (Gm marker) | 14q32.33 | 2947 | IMMUNODEFICIENCY, IgG SUBCLASS DEFICIENCIES |
| IGHG1 | immunoglobulin gamma 1 (Gm marker) | 14q32.33 | 0521 | IMMUNODEFICIENCY, COMMON VARIABLE TYPE |
| IGHG2 | immunoglobulin gamma 2 (Gm marker) | 14q32.33 | 0476 | SERUM ALLOTYPES, HUMAN |
| IGHG2 | immunoglobulin gamma 2 (Gm marker) | 14q32.33 | 0521 | IMMUNODEFICIENCY, COMMON VARIABLE TYPE |
| IGHG2 | immunoglobulin gamma 2 (Gm marker) | 14q32.33 | 2947 | IMMUNODEFICIENCY, IgG SUBCLASS DEFICIENCIES |

| SYMBOL | MARKER NAME | MAP LOCATION | NO | ARTICLE TITLE |
|---|---|---|---|---|
| IGHG3 | immunoglobulin gamma 3 (Gm marker) | 14q32.33 | 2947 | IMMUNODEFICIENCY, IgG SUBCLASS DEFICIENCIES |
| IGHG3 | immunoglobulin gamma 3 (Gm marker) | 14q32.33 | 0476 | SERUM ALLOTYPES, HUMAN |
| IGHG3 | immunoglobulin gamma 3 (Gm marker) | 14q32.33 | 0521 | IMMUNODEFICIENCY, COMMON VARIABLE TYPE |
| IGHG4 | immunoglobulin gamma 4 (Gm marker) | 14q32.33 | 0476 | SERUM ALLOTYPES, HUMAN |
| IGHG4 | immunoglobulin gamma 4 (Gm marker) | 14q32.33 | 2947 | IMMUNODEFICIENCY, IgG SUBCLASS DEFICIENCIES |
| IGHG4 | immunoglobulin gamma 4 (Gm marker) | 14q32.33 | 0521 | IMMUNODEFICIENCY, COMMON VARIABLE TYPE |
| IGHJ | immunoglobulin heavy polypeptide, joining region | 14q32.3 | 0476 | SERUM ALLOTYPES, HUMAN |
| IGHJ | immunoglobulin heavy polypeptide, joining region | 14q32.3 | 0521 | IMMUNODEFICIENCY, COMMON VARIABLE TYPE |
| IGHM | immunoglobulin mu | 14q32.33 | 0476 | SERUM ALLOTYPES, HUMAN |
| IGHM | immunoglobulin mu | 14q32.33 | 0521 | IMMUNODEFICIENCY, COMMON VARIABLE TYPE |
| IGHV | immunoglobulin heavy polypeptide, variable region (many genes) | 14q32.33 | 0476 | SERUM ALLOTYPES, HUMAN |
| IGJ | immunoglobulin J polypeptide | 4q21 | 3073 | LEUKEMIA, ACUTE LYMPHOCYTIC, FAMILIAL |
| IGKC | immunoglobulin kappa constant region | 2p12 | 0476 | SERUM ALLOTYPES, HUMAN |
| IGKC | immunoglobulin kappa constant region | 2p12 | 0521 | IMMUNODEFICIENCY, COMMON VARIABLE TYPE |
| IL6 | interleukin 6 | 7p21-p14 | 3090 | INTERFERON DEFICIENCY |
| IP1 | incontinentia pigmenti 1 | Xp11.21-cen | 0526 | INCONTINENTIA PIGMENTI |
| IVD | isovaleryl Coenzyme A dehydrogenase | 15q14-q15 | 0547 | ACIDEMIA, ISOVALERIC |
| JPD | juvenile periodontitis | 4 | 0806 | TEETH, PERIODONTITIS, JUVENILE |
| KAL | Kallmann syndrome | Xp22.32 | 2301 | KALLMANN SYNDROME |
| KMS | Kabuki make-up syndrome | unassigned | 2355 | KABUKI MAKE-UP SYNDROME |
| KRT19 | keratin 19 | 17q21-q23 | 2675 | ANEMIA, HEMOLYTIC, GLUTATHIONINE PEROXIDASE DEFICIENCY |
| LCAT | lecithin-cholesterol acyltransferase | 16q22.1 | 2646 | ANEMIA, HEMOLYTIC, RED CELL MEMBRANE DEFECTS |
| LCAT | lecithin-cholesterol acyltransferase | 16q22.1 | 0580 | LECITHIN-CHOLESTEROL ACYL TRANSFERASE DEFICIENCY |
| LCO | liver cancer oncogene | 2q14-q21 | 1505 | CANCER, FAMILIAL |
| LCT | lactase | 2 | 0566 | LACTASE DEFICIENCY, CONGENITAL |
| LDHA | lactate dehydrogenase A | 11p15.1-p14 | 0568 | LACTATE DEHYDROGENASE ISOZYMES |
| LDHB | lactate dehydrogenase B | 12p12.2-p12.1 | 0568 | LACTATE DEHYDROGENASE ISOZYMES |
| LDHC | lactate dehydrogenase C | 11 | 0568 | LACTATE DEHYDROGENASE ISOZYMES |
| LDLR | low density lipoprotein receptor (familial hypercholesterolemia) | 19p13.2-p13.1 | 0488 | HYPERCHOLESTEREMIA |
| LGCR | Langer-Giedion syndrome chromosome region | 8q24.11-q24.13 | 0967 | TRICHO-RHINO-PHALANGEAL SYNDROME, TYPE II |
| LGMD2 | limb girdle muscular dystrophy 2 (autosomal recessive) | unassigned | 0691 | MUSCULAR DYSTROPHY, LIMB-GIRDLE |
| LIPA | lipase A, lysosomal acid (Wolman disease) | 10 | 0151 | CHOLESTERYL ESTER STORAGE DISEASE |
| LIPA | lipase A, lysosomal acid (Wolman disease) | 10 | 1003 | WOLMAN DISEASE |
| LOX | lysyl oxidase; ?cutis laxa-X; ?Ehlers-Danlos V | X | 0338 | EHLERS-DANLOS SYNDROME |
| LOX | lysyl oxidase; ?cutis laxa-X; ?Ehlers-Danlos V | X | 3219 | OCCIPITAL HORN SYNDROME |
| LPL | lipoprotein lipase | 8p22 | 0489 | HYPERCHYLOMICRONEMIA |
| LYP | lymphoproliferative syndrome | Xq25-q26 | 2210 | IMMUNODEFICIENCY, X-LINKED LYMPHOPROLIFERATIVE DISEASE |
| MAA | microphthalmia or anophthalmia and associated anomalies | X | 3171 | LENZ MICROPHTHALMIA SYNDROME |
| MAFD1 | major affective disorder 1 | 11p15.5 | 1532 | MOOD AND THOUGHT DISORDERS |
| MAFD2 | major affective disorder 2 | Xq27-q28 | 1532 | MOOD AND THOUGHT DISORDERS |
| MANB | mannosidase, alpha B, lysosomal | 19cen-q13.1 | 2079 | MANNOSIDOSIS |
| MDCR | Miller-Dieker syndrome chromosome region | 17p13.3 | 0603 | LISSENCEPHALY SYNDROME |

| SYMBOL | MARKER NAME | MAP LOCATION | NO | ARTICLE TITLE |
|---|---|---|---|---|
| MEN1 | multiple endocrine neoplasia 1 | 11q12-q13 | 0350 | ENDOCRINE NEOPLASIA, MULTIPLE TYPE I |
| MEN2A | multiple endocrine neoplasia IIA | 10p11.2-q11.2 | 0351 | ENDOCRINE NEOPLASIA, MULTIPLE TYPE II |
| MEN2B | multiple endocrine neoplasia IIB | 10pter-q11.2 | 0352 | ENDOCRINE NEOPLASIA, MULTIPLE TYPE III |
| MF4 | metacarpal 4-5 fusion | X | 0923 | SYNDACTYLY |
| MFS | Marfan syndrome | unassigned | 0630 | MARFAN SYNDROME |
| MGC1 | megalocornea 1 (X-linked) | Xq12-q26 | 0637 | CORNEA, MEGALOCORNEA |
| MHAM | multiple hamartoma (Cowden syndrome) | unassigned | 0412 | GINGIVAL MULTIPLE HAMARTOMA SYNDROME |
| MJD | Machado-Joseph disease | unassigned | 2996 | MACHADO-JOSEPH DISEASE |
| MLR | mineralocorticoid receptor (aldosterone receptor) | 4q31 | 0829 | ALDOSTERONE RESISTANCE |
| MNK | Menkes syndrome | Xcen-q13 | 0643 | MENKES SYNDROME |
| MPO | myeloperoxidase | 17q21.3-q23 | 2214 | IMMUNODEFICIENCY, MYELOPEROXIDASE DEFICIENCY TYPE |
| MRSD | mental retardation-skeletal dysplasia | Xq27-q28 | 2904 | X-LINKED MENTAL RETARDATION-SKELETAL DYSPLASIA |
| MRX1 | mental retardation, X-linked 1 (non dysmorphic) | Xp11-q13 | 2640 | X-LINKED MENTAL RETARDATION, CLARK-BARAITSER TYPE |
| MRX1 | mental retardation, X-linked 1 (non dysmorphic) | Xp11-q13 | 3199 | X-LINKED MENTAL RETARDATION, GOLABI-ITO-HALL TYPE |
| MRX1 | mental retardation, X-linked 1 (non dysmorphic) | Xp11-q13 | 2840 | X-LINKED MENTAL RETARDATION, ATKIN TYPE |
| MRX1 | mental retardation, X-linked 1 (non dysmorphic) | Xp11-q13 | 3200 | X-LINKED MENTAL RETARDATION-CRANIOFACIAL ABNORMALITIES-CLUB FOOT |
| MRX2 | mental retardation, X-linked 2 | Xp22.3-p22.2 | 2920 | X-LINKED MENTAL RETARDATION, RENPENNING TYPE |
| MSS | Marinesco-Sjogren syndrome | ULG5 | 2031 | MARINESCO-SJOGREN SYNDROME |
| MTM1 | myotubular myopathy 1 | Xq27-q28 | 0695 | MYOPATHY, MYOTUBULAR |
| MUT | methylmalonyl Coenzyme A mutase | 6p21 | 0658 | ACIDEMIA, METHYLMALONIC |
| MYC | avian myelocytomatosis viral (v-myc) oncogene homolog | 8q24 | 3089 | LYMPHOMA, BURKITT TYPE |
| NAGA | acetylgalactosaminidase, alpha-N- | 22q13-qter | 3254 | ALPHA-N-ACETYLGALACTOSAMINIDASE DEFICIENCY |
| NBCCS | nevoid basal cell carcinoma syndrome | 1p | 0101 | NEVOID BASAL CELL CARCINOMA SYNDROME |
| NCF1 | neutrophil cytosolic factor 1 | 10 | 0443 | GRANULOMATOUS DISEASE, CHRONIC X-LINKED |
| NDP | Norrie disease (pseudoglioma) | Xp11.4-p11.3 | 0721 | NORRIE DISEASE |
| NEU | neuraminidase | 10pter-q23 or 6 | 0671 | MUCOLIPIDOSIS I |
| NF1 | neurofibromatosis 1 (von Recklinghausen disease, Watson disease) | 17q11.2 | 2776 | PULMONIC STENOSIS-CAFE-AU-LAIT SPOTS, WATSON TYPE |
| NF1 | neurofibromatosis 1 (von Recklinghausen disease, Watson disease) | 17q11.2 | 0712 | NEUROFIBROMATOSIS |
| NF2 | neurofibromatosis 2 (bilateral acoustic neuroma) | 22q11-q13.1 | 0012 | ACOUSTIC NEUROMATA |
| NHS | Nance-Horan syndrome (congenital cataracts and dental anomalies) | Xp22.3-p21.1 | 2119 | CATARACTS-OTO-DENTAL DEFECTS |
| NM | neutrophil migration | 7q22-qter | 2970 | GRANULOCYTE GLYCOPROTEIN CD11/CD18 DEFICIENCY |
| NP | nucleoside phosphorylase | 14q11.2 | 0729 | IMMUNODEFICIENCY, NUCLEOSIDE-PHOSPHORYLASE DEFICIENCY |
| NPS1 | nail patella syndrome 1 | 9q34 | 0704 | NAIL-PATELLA SYNDROME |
| OA1 | ocular albinism 1 (Nettleship-Falls) | Xp22.3 | 0032 | ALBINISM, OCULAR |
| OAT | ornithine aminotransferase | 10q26 | 0449 | GYRATE ATROPHY OF THE CHOROID AND RETINA |
| OCRL | oculocerebrorenal syndrome of Lowe | Xq25-q26.1 | 0736 | OCULO-CEREBRO-RENAL SYNDROME |
| OFD1 | oral-facial-digital syndrome I | X | 0770 | ORO-FACIO-DIGITAL SYNDROME I |
| OI4 | osteogenesis imperfecta type IV | 7q21.3-q22.1 | 0777 | OSTEOGENESIS IMPERFECTA |
| OPA1 | optic atrophy (autosomal dominant) | unassigned | 3069 | OPTIC ATROPHY, KJER TYPE |

| SYMBOL | MARKER NAME | MAP LOCATION | NO | ARTICLE TITLE |
|---|---|---|---|---|
| OPD | otopalatodigital syndrome | X | 2258 | OTO-PALATO-DIGITAL SYNDROME, II |
| OPD | otopalatodigital syndrome | X | 0786 | OTO-PALATO-DIGITAL SYNDROME, I |
| OPEM | ophthalmoplegia, external, with myopia | X | 0750 | OPHTHALMOPLEGIA EXTERNA-MYOPIA |
| OT | prepro-oxytocin (neurophysin I) | 20 | 2611 | DIABETES INSIPIDIS, NEUROHYPOPHYSEAL TYPE |
| OTC | ornithine carbamoyltransferase | Xp21.1 | 3023 | ORNITHINE TRANSCARBAMYLASE DEFICIENCY |
| PAH | phenylalanine hydroxylase | 12q22-q24.2 | 0808 | PHENYLKETONURIA |
| PAH | phenylalanine hydroxylase | 12q22-q24.2 | 2236 | FETAL EFFECTS FROM MATERNAL PKU |
| PALB | prealbumin | 18q11.2-q12.1 | 2881 | AMYLOIDOSIS, APPALACHIAN TYPE |
| PALB | prealbumin | 18q11.2-q12.1 | 2141 | AMYLOIDOSIS, TRANSTHYRETIN METHIONINE-30 TYPE |
| PALB | prealbumin | 18q11.2-q12.1 | 2880 | AMYLOIDOSIS, ASHKENAZI TYPE |
| PALB | prealbumin | 18q11.2-q12.1 | 2143 | AMYLOIDOSIS, DANISH CARDIAC TYPE |
| PALB | prealbumin | 18q11.2-q12.1 | 2882 | AMYLOIDOSIS, ILLINOIS TYPE |
| PALB | prealbumin | 18q11.2-q12.1 | 2142 | AMYLOIDOSIS, INDIANA TYPE |
| PBGD | porphobilinogen deaminase | 11q23.2-qter | 0820 | PORPHYRIA, ACUTE INTERMITTENT |
| PBT | piebald trait | 4q12-q21 | 0031 | ALBINISM, CUTANEOUS |
| PC | pyruvate carboxylase | 11q | 0850 | PYRUVATE CARBOXYLASE DEFICIENCY WITH LACTIC ACIDEMIA |
| PCCA | propionyl Coenzyme A carboxylase, alpha polypeptide | 13q22-q34 | 0826 | ACIDEMIA, PROPIONIC |
| PEPD | peptidase D | 19q12-q13.2 | 2616 | PROLIDASE DEFICIENCY |
| PFKL | phosphofructokinase, liver type | 21q22.3 | 0428 | GLYCOGENOSIS, TYPE VII |
| PFKM | phosphofructokinase, muscle type | 1cen-q32 | 0428 | GLYCOGENOSIS, TYPE VII |
| PFKM | phosphofructokinase, muscle type | 1cen-q32 | 0429 | GLYCOGENOSIS, TYPE VIII |
| PGK1 | phosphoglycerate kinase 1 | Xq13 | 2657 | ANEMIA, HEMOLYTIC, ERYTHROCYTE PHOSPHOGLYCERATE KINASE DEFICIENCY |
| PHK | phosphorylase kinase deficiency, liver (glycogen storage disease type VIII) | X | 0430 | GLYCOGENOSIS, TYPE IXa |
| PHK | phosphorylase kinase deficiency, liver (glycogen storage disease type VIII) | X | 2303 | GLYCOGEN STORAGE DISEASE, X-LINKED WITH NORMAL HEPATIC ENZYMES |
| PHKA | phosphorylase kinase, alpha | Xq12-q13 | 0430 | GLYCOGENOSIS, TYPE IXa |
| PHKA | phosphorylase kinase, alpha | Xq12-q13 | 2303 | GLYCOGEN STORAGE DISEASE, X-LINKED WITH NORMAL HEPATIC ENZYMES |
| PHP | panhypopituitarism | X | 0303 | DWARFISM, PANHYPOPITUITARY |
| PI | alpha-1-antitrypsin (protease inhibitor) | 14q32.1 | 0039 | ALPHA(1)-ANTITRYPSIN DEFICIENCY |
| PKD1 | polycystic kidney disease 1 (autosomal dominant) | 16p13 | 0859 | KIDNEY, POLYCYSTIC DISEASE, DOMINANT |
| PKLR | pyruvate kinase, liver and RBC | 1q21 | 0852 | PYRUVATE KINASE DEFICIENCY |
| PLG | plasminogen | 6q26-q27 | 3083 | PLASMINOGEN DEFECTS |
| PLP | proteolipid protein (Pelizaeus-Merzbacher disease) | Xq21.3-q22 | 0803 | PELIZAEUS-MERZBACHER SYNDROME |
| PROC | protein C (inactivator of coagulation factors Va and VIIIa) | 2q13-q21 | 2918 | PROTEIN C DEFICIENCY |
| PROS1 | protein S, alpha | 3p11-q11.2 | 2950 | PROTEIN S DEFICIENCY |
| PRPS1 | phosphoribosyl pyrophosphate synthetase 1 | Xq21-q27 | 0508 | PHOSPHORIBOSYL PYROPHOSPHATE (PRPP) SYNTHETASE ABNORMALITY |
| PRPS1 | phosphoribosyl pyrophosphate synthetase 1 | Xq21-q27 | 0441 | GOUT |
| PTC | phenylthiocarbamide tasting | ULG1 | 0809 | TASTING DEFECT, PHENYLTHIOCARBAMIDE |
| PTS | 6-pyruvyltetrahydropterin synthase | unassigned | 2002 | BIOPTERIN SYNTHESIS DEFICIENCY |
| PVS | poliovirus sensitivity | 19q12-q13.2 | 3109 | POLIO, SUSCEPTIBILITY TO |
| PWCR | Prader-Willi syndrome chromosome region | 15q11-q12 | 0823 | PRADER-WILLI SYNDROME |
| PYGL | phosphorylase, glycogen; liver (Hers disease, glycogen storage disease type VI) 14q11.2-q24.3 | | 0427 | GLYCOGENOSIS, TYPE VI |
| PYGM | phosphorylase, glycogen (McArdle syndrome) | 11q12-q13.2 | 2877 | GLYCOGENOSIS, TYPE V |
| QDPR | quinoid dihydropteridine reductase | 4p15.3 | 2001 | DIHYDROPTERIDINE REDUCTASE DEFICIENCY |
| RB1 | retinoblastoma 1 (including osteosarcoma) | 13q14.2 | 0870 | RETINOBLASTOMA |

| SYMBOL | MARKER NAME | MAP LOCATION | NO | ARTICLE TITLE |
|---|---|---|---|---|
| RCP | red cone pigment (color blindness, protan) | Xq28 | 0197 | COLOR BLINDNESS, RED-GREEN PROTAN SERIES |
| RH | Rhesus blood group | 1p36.2-p34 | 3063 | ERYTHROBLASTOSIS FETALIS |
| RP1 | retinitis pigmentosa 1 | 1 | 0869 | RETINITIS PIGMENTOSA |
| RP2 | retinitis pigmentosa 2 | Xp11.4-p11.2 | 0869 | RETINITIS PIGMENTOSA |
| RP3 | retinitis pigmentosa 3 | Xp21.1-p11.4 | 0869 | RETINITIS PIGMENTOSA |
| RS | retinoschisis | Xp22.2-p22.1 | 0871 | RETINOSCHISIS |
| SBMA | spinal and bulbar muscular atrophy (Kennedy disease) | Xq13-q22 | 0895 | SPINAL MUSCULAR ATROPHY |
| SBMA | spinal and bulbar muscular atrophy (Kennedy disease) | Xq13-q22 | 2493 | MUSCULAR ATROPHY, SPINAL AND BULBAR, X-LINKED KENNEDY TYPE |
| SCA1 | spinal cerebellar ataxia (olivopontocerebellar ataxia) | 6p24-p21.3 | 0742 | OLIVOPONTOCEREBELLAR ATROPHY, DOMINANT MENZEL TYPE |
| SCIDX1 | severe combined immunodeficiency, X-linked 1 | Xq13-q21.1 | 0524 | IMMUNODEFICIENCY, X-LINKED SEVERE COMBINED |
| SCZD2 | schizophrenia disorder 2 | unassigned | 1532 | MOOD AND THOUGHT DISORDERS |
| SDYS | Simpson dysmorphia syndrome | X | 2826 | SIMPSON-GOLABI-BEHMEL SYNDROME |
| SEDL | spondyloepiphyseal dysplasia, late | Xp22 | 0898 | SPONDYLOEPIPHYSEAL DYSPLASIA, LATE |
| SI | sucrase-isomaltase | 3q25-q26 | 0920 | SUCRASE-ISOMALTASE DEFICIENCY |
| SMPD1 | sphingomyelin phosphodiesterase 1, acid lysosomal | 17 | 0717 | NIEMANN-PICK DISEASE |
| SPG1 | spastic paraplegia, complicated | Xq27-q28 | 0295 | PARAPLEGIA, FAMILIAL SPASTIC |
| SPH1 | spherocytosis 1 (clinical type II) | 8p21.1-p11.22 | 0892 | SPHEROCYTOSIS |
| SPH1 | spherocytosis 1 (clinical type II) | 8p21.1-p11.22 | 2646 | ANEMIA, HEMOLYTIC, RED CELL MEMBRANE DEFECTS |
| STS | steroid sulfatase (microsomal) | Xp22.32 | 2532 | ICHTHYOSIS, X-LINKED WITH STEROID SULFATASE DEFICIENCY |
| TAL1 | T cell acute lymphoblastic leukemia 1 | 11p15 | 3095 | LEUKEMIA/LYMPHOMA, T-CELL |
| TAT | tyrosine aminotransferase | 16q22.1 | 2009 | TYROSINEMIA II, OREGON TYPE |
| TBG | thyroxin binding globulin | Xq21-q22 | 0950 | THYROXINE-BINDING GLOBULIN DEFECTS |
| TCD | tapeto-choroidal dystrophy, progressive choroidemia | Xq21.1-q21.2 | 0925 | CHOROIDEREMIA |
| TCN2 | transcobalamin II; macrocytic anemia | 22q | 2624 | TRANSCOBALAMIN II DEFICIENCY |
| TCRA | T cell receptor, alpha (V,D,J,C) | 14q11.2 | 3095 | LEUKEMIA/LYMPHOMA, T-CELL |
| TDD | testicular 17,20-desmolase deficiency | X | 0904 | STEROID 17,20-DESMOLASE DEFICIENCY |
| TDF | testis determining factor | Yp11.3 | 0437 | GONADAL DYSGENESIS, XY TYPE |
| TG | thyroglobulin | 8q24 | 3061 | THYROID, THYROGLOBULIN DEFECTS |
| TKC | torticollis, keloids, cryptorchidism and renal dysplasia | Xq28-qter | 2174 | CERVICO-DERMO-GU SYNDROME, GOEMINNE TYPE |
| TPI1 | triosephosphate isomerase 1 | 12p13 | 2686 | ERYTHROCYTE TRIOSEPHOSPHATE ISOMERASE DEFICIENCY |
| TPO | thyroid peroxidase | 2pter-p12 | 0947 | THYROID, PEROXIDASE DEFECT |
| TRY1 | trypsin 1 | 7q32-qter | 0973 | TRYPSINOGEN DEFICIENCY |
| TSC1 | tuberous sclerosis 1 | 9q | 0975 | TUBEROUS SCLEROSIS |
| TSHR | thyroid stimulating hormone receptor | 22q11-q13 | 0948 | THYROTROPIN UNRESPONSIVENESS |
| TST1 | transforming sequence, thyroid 1 | 10q11.2 | 2641 | CANCER, THYROID, FAMILIAL PAPILLARY CARCINOMA OF |
| TYR | tyrosinase | 11q14-q21 | 0034 | ALBINISM, OCULOCUTANEOUS, TYROSINASE NEGATIVE |
| TYS | sclerotylosis | 4q | 3076 | SCLEROTYLOSIS |
| UMPS | uridine monophosphate synthetase | 3cen-q21 | 0772 | ACIDEMIA, OROTIC |
| UROD | uroporphyrinogen decarboxylase | 1p34 | 3064 | PORPHYRIA CUTANEA TARDA |
| VDD1 | vitamin D dependency 1 | 12q14 | 0873 | RICKETS, VITAMIN D-DEPENDENT, TYPE I |
| VDR | vitamin D receptor | 12 | 2953 | RESISTANCE TO 1,25 DIHYDROXY VITAMIN D |
| VHL | von-Hippel Lindau syndrome | 3p | 0995 | VON HIPPEL-LINDAU SYNDROME |
| VMD1 | vitelliform macular dystrophy, atypical | 8q | 0622 | RETINA, MACULAR DEGENERATION, VITELLIRUPTIVE |

| SYMBOL | MARKER NAME | MAP LOCATION | NO | ARTICLE TITLE |
|---|---|---|---|---|
| VP | variegate porphyria (protoporphyrinogen oxidase) | 14q | 0822 | PORPHYRIA, VARIEGATE |
| VWS | Van der Woude syndrome | 1q32-q41 | 0177 | CLEFT LIP/PALATE-LIP PITS OR MOUNDS |
| WAGR | Wilms tumor, aniridia, genitourinary abnormalities, and MR | 11p13 | 0057 | ANIRIDIA |
| WAGR | Wilms tumor, aniridia, genitourinary abnormalities, and MR | 11p13 | 2742 | CANCER, WILMS TUMOR |
| WAS | Wiskott-Aldrich syndrome | Xp11.4-p11.21 | 0523 | IMMUNODEFICIENCY, WISKOTT-ALDRICH TYPE |
| WMS | William syndrome | 4q33-qter | 0999 | WILLIAMS SYNDROME |
| WND | Wilson disease | 13q14.2-q21 | 0469 | HEPATOLENTICULAR DEGENERATION |
| WS1 | Waardenburg syndrome, type 1 | 9q34 | 0997 | WAARDENBURG SYNDROMES |
| WT1 | Wilms tumor 1 | 11p13 | 2742 | CANCER, WILMS TUMOR |
| WT2 | Wilms tumor 2 | unassigned | 2742 | CANCER, WILMS TUMOR |
| XK | Kell blood group precursor (McLeod phenotype) | Xp21.1 | 2646 | ANEMIA, HEMOLYTIC, RED CELL MEMBRANE DEFECTS |
| XPAC | fast kinetic complementation DNA repair in xeroderma pigmentosum, group A | 1q | 1005 | XERODERMA PIGMENTOSUM |
| XPF | xeroderma pigmentosum, complementation group F | 15 | 1005 | XERODERMA PIGMENTOSUM |
| ZWS | Zellweger syndrome | 7q11 | 0139 | CEREBRO-HEPATO-RENAL SYNDROME |

# GENE MAP PICTORIALS BY CHROMOSOME

| SYMBOL | MARKER NAME | CHROMOSOME | MAP LOCATION | NO | ARTICLE TITLE |
|---|---|---|---|---|---|
| EKV | erythrokeratodermia variabilis | | 1 | 0361 | SKIN, ERYTHROKERATODERMIA, VARIABLE |
| RP1 | retinitis pigmentosa 1 | | 1 | 0869 | RETINITIS PIGMENTOSA |
| PFKM | phosphofructokinase, muscle type | | 1cen-q32 | 0428 | GLYCOGENOSIS, TYPE VII |
| PFKM | phosphofructokinase, muscle type | | 1cen-q32 | 0429 | GLYCOGENOSIS, TYPE VIII |
| NBCCS | nevoid basal cell carcinoma syndrome | | 1p | 0101 | NEVOID BASAL CELL CARCINOMA SYNDROME |
| C1QA | complement component 1, q subcomponent, alpha polypeptide | | 1p | 3210 | COMPLEMENT COMPONENT 1, DEFICIENCY OF |
| C1QB | complement component 1, q subcomponent, beta polypeptide | | 1p | 3210 | COMPLEMENT COMPONENT 1, DEFICIENCY OF |
| HSDB3 | hydroxy-delta 5-steroid dehydrogenase, 3 beta- and steroid delta-i somerase | | 1p13-p11 | 0909 | STEROID 3 BETA-HYDROXYSTEROID DEHYDROGENASE DEFICIENCY |
| ACADM | acyl-Coenzyme A dehydrogenase, C-4 to C-12 straight-chain | | 1p31 | 2324 | ACYL-CoA DEHYDROGENASE DEFICIENCY, MEDIUM CHAIN TYPE |
| AK2 | adenylate kinase 2 | | 1p34 | 2660 | ANEMIA, ADENYLATE KINASE DEFICIENCY |
| UROD | uroporphyrinogen decarboxylase | | 1p34 | 3064 | PORPHYRIA CUTANEA TARDA |
| FUCA1 | fucosidase, alpha-L-1, tissue | | 1p35-p34 | 0398 | FUCOSIDOSIS |
| CMM | cutaneous malignant melanoma/dysplastic nevus | | 1p36 | 2165 | NEVUS, CONGENITAL NEVOMELANOCYTIC |
| CMM | cutaneous malignant melanoma/dysplastic nevus | | 1p36 | 2318 | CANCER, MALIGNANT MELANOMA, FAMILIAL |
| GALE | UDP-galactose-4-epimerase | | 1p36-p35 | 0357 | GALACTOSE EPIMERASE DEFICIENCY |
| ALPL | alkaline phosphatase, liver/bone/kidney | | 1p36.1-p34 | 0516 | HYPOPHOSPHATASIA |
| RH | Rhesus blood group | | 1p36.2-p34 | 3063 | ERYTHROBLASTOSIS FETALIS |
| EL1 | elliptocytosis 1 (Rh-linked); band 4.1 protein | | 1pter-p34 | 2646 | ANEMIA, HEMOLYTIC, RED CELL MEMBRANE DEFECTS |
| EL1 | elliptocytosis 1 (Rh-linked); band 4.1 protein | | 1pter-p34 | 2665 | ELLIPTOCYTOSIS |
| XPAC | fast kinetic complementation DNA repair in xeroderma pigmentosum, group A | | 1q | 1005 | XERODERMA PIGMENTOSUM |
| CMT1 | Charcot-Marie-Tooth neuropathy 1 | | 1q | 2104 | NEUROPATHY, HEREDITARY MOTOR AND SENSORY, TYPE I |
| GBA | glucosidase, beta; acid | | 1q21 | 0406 | GAUCHER DISEASE |
| PKLR | pyruvate kinase, liver and RBC | | 1q21 | 0852 | PYRUVATE KINASE DEFICIENCY |
| CAE | cataract, zonular pulverulent (FY-linked) | | 1q21-q25 | 2342 | CATARACT, AUTOSOMAL DOMINANT CONGENITAL |
| F5 | coagulation factor V | | 1q21-q25 | 2668 | FACTOR V DEFICIENCY |
| FY | Duffy blood group | | 1q21-q25 | 3065 | MALARIA, VIVAX, SUSCEPTIBILITY TO |
| CAE | cataract, zonular pulverulent (FY-linked) | | 1q21-q25 | 3174 | CATARACT, COPPOCK |
| AT3 | antithrombin III | | 1q23-q25.1 | 3066 | ANTITHROMBIN III DEFICIENCY |
| C4BP | complement component 4 binding protein | | 1q32 | 2220 | COMPLEMENT COMPONENT 4, DEFICIENCY OF |
| VWS | Van der Woude syndrome | | 1q32-q41 | 0177 | CLEFT LIP/PALATE-LIP PITS OR MOUNDS |
| FH | fumarate hydratase | | 1q42.1 | 2599 | ACIDURIA, FUMARIC |
| LCT | lactase | | 2 | 0566 | LACTASE DEFICIENCY, CONGENITAL |
| GAD | glutamate decarboxylase | | 2 | 0991 | SEIZURES, VITAMIN B(6) DEPENDENCY |
| HVBS4 | hepatitis B virus integration site 4 | | 2 | 3008 | FETAL EFFECT FROM HEPATITIS B INFECTION |
| DES | desmin | | 2 | 3072 | MYOPATHY OR CARDIOMYOPATHY DUE TO DESMIN DEFECT |
| AN1 | aniridia 1 | | 2p | 0057 | ANIRIDIA |
| CPS1 | carbamoyl phosphate synthetase 1, mitochondrial | | 2p | 3022 | CARBAMOYL PHOSPHATE SYNTHETASE DEFICIENCY |
| IGKC | immunoglobulin kappa constant region | | 2p12 | 0476 | SERUM ALLOTYPES, HUMAN |
| IGKC | immunoglobulin kappa constant region | | 2p12 | 0521 | IMMUNODEFICIENCY, COMMON VARIABLE TYPE |
| IFNB3 | interferon, beta 3, fibroblast | | 2p23-qter | 3090 | INTERFERON DEFICIENCY |
| APOB | apolipoprotein B (including Ag(x) antigen) | | 2p24-p23 | 0002 | ABETALIPOPROTEINEMIA |
| APOB | apolipoprotein B (including Ag(x) antigen) | | 2p24-p23 | 2646 | ANEMIA, HEMOLYTIC, RED CELL MEMBRANE DEFECTS |

1

2

| SYMBOL | MARKER NAME | CHROMOSOME | MAP LOCATION | NO | ARTICLE TITLE |
|---|---|---|---|---|---|
| APOB | apolipoprotein B (including Ag(x) antigen) | | 2p24-p23 | 3227 | APO B-100, DEFECTIVE, FAMILIAL |
| TPO | thyroid peroxidase | | 2pter-p12 | 0947 | THYROID, PEROXIDASE DEFECT |
| AHH | aryl hydrocarbon hydroxylase | | 2pter-q31 | 2747 | CANCER, LUNG, FAMILIAL |
| CHE2 | cholinesterase (serum) 2 | | 2q | 0152 | CHOLINESTERASE, ATYPICAL |
| PROC | protein C (inactivator of coagulation factors Va and VIIIa) | | 2q13-q21 | 2918 | PROTEIN C DEFICIENCY |
| LCO | liver cancer oncogene | | 2q14-q21 | 1505 | CANCER, FAMILIAL |
| HV1S | herpes simplex virus type 1 sensitivity | **3** | 3 or 11p11-qter | 2988 | FETAL HERPES SIMPLEX VIRUS INFECTION |
| UMPS | uridine monophosphate synthetase | | 3cen-q21 | 0772 | ACIDEMIA, OROTIC |
| VHL | von-Hippel Lindau syndrome | | 3p | 0995 | VON HIPPEL-LINDAU SYNDROME |
| PROS1 | protein S, alpha | | 3p11-q11.2 | 2950 | PROTEIN S DEFICIENCY |
| GLB1 | galactosidase, beta 1 | | 3pter-p21 | 0431 | G(M1)-GANGLIOSIDOSIS, TYPE 1 |
| GLB1 | galactosidase, beta 1 | | 3pter-p21 | 3215 | G(M1)-GANCLIOSIDOSIS, TYPE 3 |
| GPX1 | glutathione peroxidase 1 | | 3q11-q12 | 2675 | ANEMIA, HEMOLYTIC, GLUTATIONINE PEROXIDASE DEFICIENCY |
| CP | ceruloplasmin | | 3q23-q25 | 3077 | HYPOCERULOPLASMINEMIA |
| SI | sucrase-isomaltase | | 3q25-q26 | 0920 | SUCRASE-ISOMALTASE DEFICIENCY |
| CHE1 | cholinesterase (serum) 1 | | 3q26-qter | 0152 | CHOLINESTERASE, ATYPICAL |
| JPD | juvenile periodontitis | **4** | 4 | 0806 | TEETH, PERIODONTITIS, JUVENILE |
| QDPR | quinoid dihydropteridine reductase | | 4p15.3 | 2001 | DIHYDROPTERIDINE REDUCTASE DEFICIENCY |
| HD | Huntington disease | | 4pter-p16.3 | 0478 | HUNTINGTON DISEASE |
| ASMD | anterior segment mesenchymal dysgenesis | | 4q | 0439 | EYE, ANTERIOR SEGMENT DYSGENESIS |
| TYS | sclerotylosis | | 4q | 3076 | SCLEROTYLOSIS |
| ALB | albumin | | 4q11-q13 | 0047 | ANALBUMINEMIA |
| GC | group-specific component (vitamin D binding protein) | | 4q12-q13 | 0446 | PLASMA, GROUP-SPECIFIC COMPONENT |
| GC | group-specific component (vitamin D binding protein) | | 4q12-q13 | 0983 | USHER SYNDROME |
| PBT | piebald trait | | 4q12-q21 | 0031 | ALBINISM, CUTANEOUS |
| DGI1 | dentinogenesis imperfecta 1 | | 4q12-q23 | 0279 | TEETH, DENTINOGENESIS IMPERFECTA |
| IGJ | immunoglobulin J polypeptide | | 4q21 | 3073 | LEUKEMIA, ACUTE LYMPHOCYTIC, FAMILIAL |
| GNPTA | UDP-N-acetylglucoso.-lysosomal-enzyme N-acetylglucosaminephosphotrans. | | 4q21-q23 | 0672 | MUCOLIPIDOSIS II |
| GNPTA | UDP-N-acetylglucoso.-lysosomal-enzyme N-acetylglucosaminephosphotrans. | | 4q21-qter | 0673 | MUCOLIPIDOSIS III |
| ADH1 | alcohol dehydrogenase (class I), alpha polypeptide | | 4q21-q23 | 3074 | ALCOHOL INTOLERANCE |
| ADH2 | alcohol dehydrogenase (class I), beta polypeptide | | 4q21-q23 | 3074 | ALCOHOL INTOLERANCE |
| ADH3 | alcohol dehydrogenase (class I), gamma polypeptide | | 4q21-q23 | 3074 | ALCOHOL INTOLERANCE |
| AGA | aspartylglucosaminidase | | 4q21-qter | 2042 | ASPARTYLGLUCOSAMINURIA |
| IF | complement component I | | 4q24-q25 | 2219 | COMPLEMENT COMPONENT 3, DEFICIENCY OF |
| FGA | fibrinogen, A alpha polypeptide | | 4q28 | 0004 | FIBRINOGENS, ABNORMAL CONGENITAL |
| FGB | fibrinogen, B beta polypeptide | | 4q28 | 0004 | FIBRINOGENS, ABNORMAL CONGENITAL |
| FGG | fibrinogen, gamma polypeptide | | 4q28 | 0004 | FIBRINOGENS, ABNORMAL CONGENITAL |
| FGA | fibrinogen, A alpha polypeptide | | 4q28 | 2661 | AFIBROGINEMIA, CONGENITAL |
| FGB | fibrinogen, B beta polypeptide | | 4q28 | 2661 | AFIBROGINEMIA, CONGENITAL |
| FGG | fibrinogen, gamma polypeptide | | 4q28 | 2661 | AFIBROGINEMIA, CONGENITAL |
| MLR | mineralocorticoid receptor (aldosterone receptor) | | 4q31 | 0829 | ALDOSTERONE RESISTANCE |
| WMS | William syndrome | | 4q33-qter | 0999 | WILLIAMS SYNDROME |

| SYMBOL | MARKER NAME | CHROMOSOME | MAP LOCATION | NO | ARTICLE TITLE |
|---|---|---|---|---|---|
| F11 | coagulation factor XI | | 4q35 | 2671 | FACTOR XI DEFICIENCY |
| GM2A | GM2 ganglioside activator protein | | 5 | 0434 | G(M2)-GANGLIOSIDOSIS WITH HEXOSAMINIDASE A DEFICIENCY |
| ARSB | arylsulfatase B | | 5p11-q13 | 0679 | MUCOPOLYSACCHARIDOSIS VI |
| HEXB | hexosaminidase B (beta polypeptide) | | 5q13 | 0433 | G(M2)-GANGLIOSIDOSIS WITH HEXOSAMINIDASE A AND B DEFICIENCY |
| APC | adenomatosis polyposis coli | | 5q21-q22 | 0535 | INTESTINAL POLYPOSIS, TYPE I |
| APC | adenomatosis polyposis coli | | 5q21-q22 | 0536 | INTESTINAL POLYPOSIS, TYPE III |
| APC | adenomatosis polyposis coli | | 5q21-q22 | 2739 | TURCOT SYNDROME |
| DTS | diphtheria toxin sensitivity | | 5q23 | 3079 | DIPHTHERIA, SUSCEPTIBILITY TO |
| GRL | glucocorticoid receptor | | 5q31-q32 | 2952 | GLUCOCORTICOID RESISTANCE |
| F12 | coagulation factor XII (Hageman) | | 5q33-qter | 2672 | FACTOR XII DEFICIENCY |
| EJM | epilepsy, juvenile myoclonic | | 6p | 2567 | SEIZURES, MYOCLONIC, JUVENILE JANZ TYPE |
| MUT | methylmalonyl Coenzyme A mutase | | 6p21 | 0658 | ACIDEMIA, METHYLMALONIC |
| HFE | hemochromatosis | | 6p21.3 | 0460 | HEMOCHROMATOSIS, IDIOPATHIC |
| CYP21 | cytochrome P450, subfamily XXI | | 6p21.3 | 0908 | STEROID 21-HYDROXYLASE DEFICIENCY |
| C2 | complement component 2 | | 6p21.3 | 2201 | COMPLEMENT COMPONENT 2, DEFICIENCY OF |
| C4A | complement component 4A | | 6p21.3 | 2220 | COMPLEMENT COMPONENT 4, DEFICIENCY OF |
| C4B | complement component 4B | | 6p21.3 | 2220 | COMPLEMENT COMPONENT 4, DEFICIENCY OF |
| HLA-A | major histocompatibility complex, class I | | 6p21.3 | 3082 | RAGWEED POLLEN SENSITIVITY |
| SCA1 | spinal cerebellar ataxia (olivopontocerebellar ataxia) | | 6p24-p21.3 | 0742 | OLIVOPONTOCEREBELLAR ATROPHY, DOMINANT MENZEL TYPE |
| F13A1 | coagulation factor XIII, A1 polypeptide | | 6p25-p24 | 2673 | FACTOR XIII (FIBRIN STABILIZING FACTOR) |
| ARG1 | arginase, liver | | 6q23 | 0086 | ARGININEMIA |
| PLG | plasminogen | | 6q26-q27 | 3083 | PLASMINOGEN DEFECTS |
| GCPS | Greig cephalopolysyndactyly syndrome | | 7p13 | 2925 | POLYSYNDACTYLY-DYSMORPHIC CRANIOFACIES, GREIG TYPE |
| CRS | craniosynostosis | | 7p21 | 0230 | CRANIOSYNOSTOSIS |
| IL6 | interleukin 6 | | 7p21-p14 | 3090 | INTERFERON DEFICIENCY |
| ASL | argininosuccinate lyase | | 7pter-q22 | 0087 | ACIDURIA, ARGININOSUCCINIC |
| ZWS | Zellweger syndrome | | 7q11 | 0139 | CEREBRO-HEPATO-RENAL SYNDROME |
| GUSB | glucuronidase, beta | | 7q21.2-q22 | 0680 | MUCOPOLYSACCHARIDOSIS VII |
| COL1A2 | collagen, type I, alpha 2 | | 7q21.3-q22.1 | 0777 | OSTEOGENESIS IMPERFECTA |
| OI4 | osteogenesis imperfecta type IV | | 7q21.3-q22.1 | 0777 | OSTEOGENESIS IMPERFECTA |
| BCP | blue cone pigment | | 7q22-qter | 0199 | COLOR BLINDNESS, YELLOW-BLUE TRITAN |
| NM | neutrophil migration | | 7q22-qter | 2970 | GRANULOCYTE GLYCOPROTEIN CD11/CD18 DEFICIENCY |
| CF | cystic fibrosis | | 7q31-q32 | 0237 | CYSTIC FIBROSIS |
| BPGM | 2,3-bisphosphoglycerate mutase | | 7q31-q34 | 2664 | ERYTHROCYTE, DIPHOSPHOGLYCERATE MUTASE (2,3) DEFICIENCY |
| TRY1 | trypsin 1 | | 7q32-qter | 0973 | TRYPSINOGEN DEFICIENCY |
| EBS1 | epidermolysis bullosa simplex (Ogna) | | 8 | 2560 | EPIDERMOLYSIS BULLOSUM, TYPE I |
| ANK | ankyrin | | 8p21-p11 | 0892 | SPHEROCYTOSIS |
| ANK | ankyrin | | 8p21-p11 | 2646 | ANEMIA, HEMOLYTIC, RED CELL MEMBRANE DEFECTS |
| GSR | glutathione reductase | | 8p21.1 | 2676 | ANEMIA, HEMOLYTIC, GLUTATHIONE REDUCTASE DEFICIENCY |

| SYMBOL | MARKER NAME | CHROMOSOME | MAP LOCATION | NO | ARTICLE TITLE |
|---|---|---|---|---|---|
| SPH1 | spherocytosis 1 (clinical type II) | | 8p21.1-p11.22 | 0892 | SPHEROCYTOSIS |
| SPH1 | spherocytosis 1 (clinical type II) | | 8p21.1-p11.22 | 2646 | ANEMIA, HEMOLYTIC, RED CELL MEMBRANE DEFECTS |
| LPL | lipoprotein lipase | | 8p22 | 0489 | HYPERCHYLOMICRONEMIA |
| VMD1 | vitelliform macular dystrophy, atypicall | | 8q | 0622 | RETINA, MACULAR DEGENERATION, VITELLIRUPTIVE |
| CYP11B1 | cytochrome P450, subfamily XIB, polypeptide 1 (steroid 11-beta-hydroxylase) | | 8q21-q22 | 0902 | STEROID 11 BETA-HYDROXYLASE DEFICIENCY |
| CYP11B2 | cytochrome P450, subfamily XIB, polypeptide 2 (steroid 11-beta-hydroxylase) | | 8q21-q22 | 0902 | STEROID 11 BETA-HYDROXYLASE DEFICIENCY |
| CPP | ceruloplasmin pseudogene | | 8q21.13-q23.1 | 3077 | HYPOCERULOPLASMINEMIA |
| CA2 | carbonic anhydrase II | | 8q22 | 0863 | RENAL TUBULAR ACIDOSIS-SENSORINEURAL DEAFNESS |
| CA2 | carbonic anhydrase II | 8 | 8q22 | 3086 | RENAL TUBULAR ACIDOSIS-OSTEOPETROSIS SYNDROME |
| TG | thyroglobulin | | 8q24 | 3061 | THYROID, THYROGLOBULIN DEFECTS |
| MYC | avian myelocytomatosis viral (v-myc) oncogene homolog | | 8q24 | 3089 | LYMPHOMA, BURKITT TYPE |
| LGCR | Langer-Giedion syndrome chromosome region | | 8q24.11-q24.13 | 0967 | TRICHO-RHINO-PHALANGEAL SYNDROME, TYPE II |
| CPO | coproporphyrinogen oxidase | | 9 | 0203 | PORPHYRIA, COPROPORPHYRIA |
| GALT | galactose-1-phosphate uridylyltransferase | | 9p13 | 0403 | GALACTOSEMIA |
| IFNB1 | interferon, beta 1, fibroblast | | 9p22 | 3090 | INTERFERON DEFICIENCY |
| IFNA | interferon, alpha (leukocyte) | | 9p22-p13 | 3090 | INTERFERON DEFICIENCY |
| AK3 | adenylate kinase 3 | | 9p24-p13 | 2660 | ANEMIA, ADENYLATE KINASE DEFICIENCY |
| TSC1 | tuberous sclerosis 1 | | 9q | 0975 | TUBEROUS SCLEROSIS |
| FRDA | Friedreich ataxia | | 9q13-q21.1 | 2714 | ATAXIA, FRIEDREICH TYPE |
| ALDOB | aldolase B, fructose bisphosphate | | 9q21.3-q22.2 | 0395 | FRUCTOSE-1-PHOSPHATE ALDOLASE DEFICIENCY |
| DYT1 | dystonia, torsion 1 (autosomal dominant) | | 9q32-q34 | 0957 | TORSION DYSTONIA |
| NPS1 | nail patella syndrome 1 | | 9q34 | 0704 | NAIL-PATELLA SYNDROME |
| WS1 | Waardenburg syndrome, type 1 | | 9q34 | 0997 | WAARDENBURG SYNDROMES |
| DBH | dopamine beta-hydroxylase (dopamine beta-monooxygenase) | | 9q34 | 2883 | DOPAMINE BETA-HYDROXYLASE DEFICIENCY, CONGENITAL |
| ALAD | aminolevulinate, delta-, dehydratase | 9 | 9q34 | 3091 | DELTA-AMINOLEVULINIC ACID DEHYDRASE DEFICIENCY |
| ASS | argininosuccinate synthetase | | 9q34-qter | 0174 | CITRULLINEMIA |
| ABO | ABO blood group | | 9q34.1-q34.2 | 0340 | TEETH, ENAMEL AND DENTIN DEFECTS FROM ERYTHROBLASTOSIS FETALIS |
| AK1 | adenylate kinase 1 | | 9q34.1-q34.2 | 2660 | ANEMIA, ADENYLATE KINASE DEFICIENCY |
| LIPA | lipase A, lysosomal acid (Wolman disease) | | 10 | 0151 | CHOLESTERYL ESTER STORAGE DISEASE |
| NCF1 | neutrophil cytosolic factor 1 | | 10 | 0443 | GRANULOMATOUS DISEASE, CHRONIC X-LINKED |
| CYP17 | cytochrome P450, subfamily XVII (steroid 17-alpha-hydroxylase) | | 10 | 0903 | STEROID 17 ALPHA-HYDROXYLASE DEFICIENCY |
| LIPA | lipase A, lysosomal acid (Wolman disease) | | 10 | 1003 | WOLMAN DISEASE |
| MEN2A | multiple endocrine neoplasia IIA | | 10p11.2-q11.2 | 0351 | ENDOCRINE NEOPLASIA, MULTIPLE TYPE II |
| MEN2B | multiple endocrine neoplasia IIB | | 10pter-q11.2 | 0352 | ENDOCRINE NEOPLASIA, MULTIPLE TYPE III |
| NEU | neuraminidase | 10 | 10pter-q23 or 6 | 0671 | MUCOLIPIDOSIS I |

| SYMBOL | MARKER NAME | CHROMOSOME | MAP LOCATION | NO | ARTICLE TITLE |
|---|---|---|---|---|---|
| TST1 | transforming sequence, thyroid 1 | | 10q11.2 | 2641 | CANCER, THYROID, FAMILIAL PAPILLARY CARCINOMA OF |
| HK1 | hexokinase 1 | | 10q22 | 2678 | ANEMIA, HEMOLYTIC, ERYTHROCYTE HEXOKINASE DEFICIENCY |
| OAT | ornithine aminotransferase | | 10q26 | 0449 | GYRATE ATROPHY OF THE CHOROID AND RETINA |
| LDHC | lactate dehydrogenase C | | 11 | 0568 | LACTATE DEHYDROGENASE ISOZYMES |
| F2 | coagulation factor II (prothrombin) | | 11p11-q12 | 2679 | HYPOPROTHROMBINEMIA |
| CAT | catalase | | 11p13 | 0006 | ACATALASEMIA |
| AN2 | aniridia 2 without Wilms' tumor, GU abnormalities, and M.R. | | 11p13 | 0057 | ANIRIDIA |
| WAGR | Wilms tumor, aniridia, genitourinary abnormalities, and MR | | 11p13 | 0057 | ANIRIDIA |
| AN2 | aniridia 2 without Wilms' tumor, GU abnormalities, and M.R. | | 11p13 | 2245 | CHROMOSOME 11, PARTIAL MONOSOMY 11p |
| GUD | genitourinary dysplasia component of WAGR | | 11p13 | 2245 | CHROMOSOME 11, PARTIAL MONOSOMY 11p |
| GUD | genitourinary dysplasia component of WAGR | | 11p13 | 2742 | CANCER, WILMS TUMOR |
| WAGR | Wilms tumor, aniridia, genitourinary abnormalities, and MR | | 11p13 | 2742 | CANCER, WILMS TUMOR |
| WT1 | Wilms tumor 1 | | 11p13 | 2742 | CANCER, WILMS TUMOR |
| TAL1 | T cell acute lymphoblastic leukemia 1 | | 11p15 | 3095 | LEUKEMIA/LYMPHOMA, T-CELL |
| LDHA | lactate dehydrogenase A | | 11p15.1-p14 | 0568 | LACTATE DEHYDROGENASE ISOZYMES |
| HBB | hemoglobin, beta | | 11p15.5 | 0886 | ANEMIA, SICKLE CELL |
| MAFD1 | major affective disorder 1 | | 11p15.5 | 1532 | MOOD AND THOUGHT DISORDERS |
| BWS | Beckwith-Wiedemann syndrome | | 11pter-p15.4 | 0104 | BECKWITH-WIEDEMANN SYNDROME |
| PC | pyruvate carboxylase | | 11q | 0850 | PYRUVATE CARBOXYLASE DEFICIENCY WITH LACTIC ACIDEMIA |
| MEN1 | multiple endocrine neoplasia I | | 11q12-q13 | 0350 | ENDOCRINE NEOPLASIA, MULTIPLE TYPE I |
| APY | atopy (allergic asthma and rhinitis) | | 11q12-q13 | 3150 | SKIN, ATOPY, FAMILIAL |
| C1NH | complement component 1 inhibitor (angioedema, hereditary) | | 11q12-q13.1 | 0054 | ANGIOEDEMA, HEREDITARY |
| PYGM | phosphorylase, glycogen (McArdle syndrome) | | 11q12-q13.2 | 2877 | GLYCOGENOSIS, TYPE V |
| BCL1 | B cell CLL/lymphoma 1 | | 11q13.3 | 3097 | LEUKEMIA/LYMPHOMA, B CELL |
| TYR | tyrosinase | | 11q14-q21 | 0034 | ALBINISM, OCULOCUTANEOUS, TYROSINASE NEGATIVE |
| CLG | collagenase, epidermolysis bullosa, dystrophic, (autosomal recessive) | | 11q21-q22 | 2562 | EPIDERMOLYSIS BULLOSUM, TYPE III |
| ATA | ataxia telangiectasia (complementation group A) | | 11q22-q23 | 0094 | ATAXIA-TELANGIECTASIA |
| APOA1 | apolipoprotein A-I | | 11q23-q24 | 3096 | HYPOALPHALIPOPROTEINEMIA |
| APOA1 | apolipoprotein A-I | | 11q23-q24 | 3165 | APOLIPOPROTEIN A-I AND C-III DEFICIENCY STATES |
| APOA4 | apolipoprotein A-IV | | 11q23-qter | 3096 | HYPOALPHALIPOPROTEINEMIA |
| PBGD | porphobilinogen deaminase | | 11q23.2-qter | 0820 | PORPHYRIA, ACUTE INTERMITTENT |
| HIS | histidase | | 12 | 0472 | HISTIDINEMIA |
| VDR | vitamin D receptor | | 12 | 2953 | RESISTANCE TO 1,25 DIHYDROXY VITAMIN D |
| LDHB | lactate dehydrogenase B | | 12p12.2-p12.1 | 0568 | LACTATE DEHYDROGENASE ISOZYMES |
| TPI1 | triosephosphate isomerase 1 | | 12p13 | 2686 | ERYTHROCYTE TRIOSEPHOSPHATE ISOMERASE DEFICIENCY |
| C1R | complement component 1, r subcomponent | | 12p13 | 3210 | COMPLEMENT COMPONENT 1, DEFICIENCY OF |
| C1S | complement component 1, s subcomponent | | 12p13 | 3210 | COMPLEMENT COMPONENT 1, DEFICIENCY OF |

**11**

| SYMBOL | MARKER NAME | CHROMOSOME | MAP LOCATION | NO | ARTICLE TITLE |
|---|---|---|---|---|---|
| F8VWF | coagulation factor VIII VWF (von Willebrand factor) | | 12pter-p12 | 0996 | VON WILLEBRAND DISEASE |
| GLI | glioma-associated oncogene homolog (zinc finger protein) | | 12q13 | 2839 | CANCER, GLIOMA, FAMILIAL |
| APR | apolipoprotein receptor | | 12q13-q14 | 0048 | ANALPHALIPOPROTEINEMIA |
| APR | apolipoprotein receptor | | 12q13-q14 | 3165 | APOLIPOPROTEIN A-I AND C-III DEFICIENCY STATES |
| AOM | arthroophthalmopathy, progressive (Stickler syndrome) | 12 | 12q14 | 0090 | ARTHRO-OPHTHALMOPATHY, HEREDITARY, PROGRESSIVE, STICKLER TYPE |
| GNS | N-acetylglucosamine-6-sulfatase (Sanfilippo disease IIID) | | 12q14 | 0677 | MUCOPOLYSACCHARIDOSIS IIID |
| VDD1 | vitamin D dependency 1 | | 12q14 | 0873 | RICKETS, VITAMIN D-DEPENDENT, TYPE I |
| AOM | arthroophthalmopathy, progressive (Stickler syndrome) | | 12q14 | 2424 | ARTHRO-OPHTHALMOPATHY, WEISSENBACHER-ZWEYMULLER VARIANT |
| COL2A1 | collagen, type II, alpha 1 | | 12q14.3 | 0897 | SPONDYLOEPIPHYSEAL DYSPLASIA CONGENITA |
| PAH | phenylalanine hydroxylase | | 12q22-q24.2 | 0808 | PHENYLKETONURIA |
| PAH | phenylalanine hydroxylase | | 12q22-q24.2 | 2236 | FETAL EFFECTS FROM MATERNAL PKU |
| ACADS | acyl-Coenzyme A dehydrogenase, C-2 to C-3 short chain | | 12q22-qter | 2323 | ACYL-CoA DEHYDROGENASE DEFICIENCY, SHORT CHAIN TYPE |
| IGF1 | insulin-like growth factor 1 | | 12q23 | 3100 | GROWTH DEFICIENCY, AFRICAN PYGMY TYPE |
| IFNG | interferon, gamma | | 12q24.1 | 3090 | INTERFERON DEFICIENCY |
| ALDH2 | aldehyde dehydrogenase 2, mitochondrial | | 12q24.2 | 3074 | ALCOHOL INTOLERANCE |
| RB1 | retinoblastoma 1 (including osteosarcoma) | | 13q14.2 | 0870 | RETINOBLASTOMA |
| WND | Wilson disease | 13 | 13q14.2-q21 | 0469 | HEPATOLENTICULAR DEGENERATION |
| PCCA | propionyl Coenzyme A carboxylase, alpha polypeptide | | 13q22-q34 | 0826 | ACIDEMIA, PROPIONIC |
| F7 | coagulation factor VII | | 13q34 | 2669 | FACTOR VII DEFICIENCY |
| F10 | coagulation factor X | | 13q34 | 2670 | FACTOR X DEFICIENCY |
| HHH | hyperornithinemia-hyperammonemia-homocitrullinuria | | 13q34 | 3169 | HYPERORNITHINEMIA-HYPERAMMONEMIA-HOMOCITRULLINURIA |
| VP | variegate porphyria (protoporphyrinogen oxidase) | | 14q | 0822 | PORPHYRIA, VARIEGATE |
| NP | nucleoside phosphorylase | | 14q11.2 | 0729 | IMMUNODEFICIENCY, NUCLEOSIDE-PHOSPHORYLASE DEFICIENCY |
| TCRA | T cell receptor, alpha (V,D,J,C) | | 14q11.2 | 3095 | LEUKEMIA/LYMPHOMA, T-CELL |
| PYGL | phosphorylase, glycogen; liver (Hers disease, glycogen storage disease type VI) | | 14q11.2-q24.3 | 0427 | GLYCOGENOSIS, TYPE VI |
| PI | alpha-1-antitrypsin (protease inhibitor) | 14 | 14q32.1 | 0039 | ALPHA(1)-ANTITRYPSIN DEFICIENCY |
| AACT | alpha-1-antichymotrypsin | | 14q32.1 | 3279 | ALPHA-1-ANTICHYMOTRYPSIN DEFICIENCY |
| IGHJ | immunoglobulin heavy polypeptide, joining region | | 14q32.3 | 0476 | SERUM ALLOTYPES, HUMAN |
| IGHJ | immunoglobulin heavy polypeptide, joining region | | 14q32.3 | 0521 | IMMUNODEFICIENCY, COMMON VARIABLE TYPE |
| IGHA1 | immunoglobulin alpha 1 | | 14q32.33 | 0476 | SERUM ALLOTYPES, HUMAN |
| IGHA2 | immunoglobulin alpha 2 (A2M marker) | | 14q32.33 | 0476 | SERUM ALLOTYPES, HUMAN |
| IGHD | immunoglobulin delta | | 14q32.33 | 0476 | SERUM ALLOTYPES, HUMAN |
| IGHE | immunoglobulin epsilon | | 14q32.33 | 0476 | SERUM ALLOTYPES, HUMAN |
| IGHEP1 | immunoglobulin epsilon pseudogene 1 | | 14q32.33 | 0476 | SERUM ALLOTYPES, HUMAN |
| IGHG1 | immunoglobulin gamma 1 (Gm marker) | | 14q32.33 | 0476 | SERUM ALLOTYPES, HUMAN |
| IGHG2 | immunoglobulin gamma 2 (Gm marker) | | 14q32.33 | 0476 | SERUM ALLOTYPES, HUMAN |
| IGHG3 | immunoglobulin gamma 3 (Gm marker) | | 14q32.33 | 0476 | SERUM ALLOTYPES, HUMAN |
| IGHG4 | immunoglobulin gamma 4 (Gm marker) | | 14q32.33 | 0476 | SERUM ALLOTYPES, HUMAN |
| IGHM | immunoglobulin mu | | 14q32.33 | 0476 | SERUM ALLOTYPES, HUMAN |

| SYMBOL | MARKER NAME | CHROMOSOME | MAP LOCATION | NO | ARTICLE TITLE |
|---|---|---|---|---|---|
| IGHV | immunoglobulin heavy polypeptide, variable region (many genes) | | 14q32.33 | 0476 | SERUM ALLOTYPES, HUMAN |
| IGHA1 | immunoglobulin alpha 1 | | 14q32.33 | 0521 | IMMUNODEFICIENCY, COMMON VARIABLE TYPE |
| IGHD | immunoglobulin delta | | 14q32.33 | 0521 | IMMUNODEFICIENCY, COMMON VARIABLE TYPE |
| IGHA2 | immunoglobulin alpha 2 (A2M marker) | | 14q32.33 | 0521 | IMMUNODEFICIENCY, COMMON VARIABLE TYPE |
| IGHE | immunoglobulin epsilon | | 14q32.33 | 0521 | IMMUNODEFICIENCY, COMMON VARIABLE TYPE |
| IGHEP1 | immunoglobulin epsilon pseudogene 1 | | 14q32.33 | 0521 | IMMUNODEFICIENCY, COMMON VARIABLE TYPE |
| IGHG1 | immunoglobulin gamma 1 (Gm marker) | | 14q32.33 | 0521 | IMMUNODEFICIENCY, COMMON VARIABLE TYPE |
| IGHG2 | immunoglobulin gamma 2 (Gm marker) | | 14q32.33 | 0521 | IMMUNODEFICIENCY, COMMON VARIABLE TYPE |
| IGHG3 | immunoglobulin gamma 3 (Gm marker) | | 14q32.33 | 0521 | IMMUNODEFICIENCY, COMMON VARIABLE TYPE |
| IGHG4 | immunoglobulin gamma 4 (Gm marker) | | 14q32.33 | 0521 | IMMUNODEFICIENCY, COMMON VARIABLE TYPE |
| IGHM | immunoglobulin mu | | 14q32.33 | 0521 | IMMUNODEFICIENCY, COMMON VARIABLE TYPE |
| IGHV | immunoglobulin heavy polypeptide, variable region (many genes) | | 14q32.33 | 0521 | IMMUNODEFICIENCY, COMMON VARIABLE TYPE |
| IGHG1 | immunoglobulin gamma 1 (Gm marker) | | 14q32.33 | 2947 | IMMUNODEFICIENCY, IgG SUBCLASS DEFICIENCIES |
| IGHG2 | immunoglobulin gamma 2 (Gm marker) | | 14q32.33 | 2947 | IMMUNODEFICIENCY, IgG SUBCLASS DEFICIENCIES |
| IGHG3 | immunoglobulin gamma 3 (Gm marker) | | 14q32.33 | 2947 | IMMUNODEFICIENCY, IgG SUBCLASS DEFICIENCIES |
| IGHG4 | immunoglobulin gamma 4 (Gm marker) | | 14q32.33 | 2947 | IMMUNODEFICIENCY, IgG SUBCLASS DEFICIENCIES |
| CYP11A | cytochrome P450, subfamily XIA | | 15 | 0907 | STEROID 20-22 DESMOLASE DEFICIENCY |
| XPF | xeroderma pigmentosum, complementation group F | | 15 | 1005 | XERODERMA PIGMENTOSUM |
| PWCR | Prader-Willi syndrome chromosome region | | 15q11-q12 | 0823 | PRADER-WILLI SYNDROME |
| ANCR | Angelman syndrome chromosome region | | 15q11-q12 | 2086 | ANGELMAN SYNDROME |
| IVD | isovaleryl Coenzyme A dehydrogenase | | 15q14-q15 | 0547 | ACIDEMIA, ISOVALERIC |
| CYP19 | cytochrome P450, subfamily XIX (aromatization of androgens) | | 15q21 | 2308 | GYNECOMASTIA DUE TO INCREASED AROMATASE ACTIVITY, FAMILIAL |
| B2M | beta-2-microglobulin | | 15q21-q22.2 | 3106 | AMYLOIDOSIS, HEMODIALYSIS-RELATED |
| CYP1 | cytochrome P450, subfamily I (aromatic compound-inducible) | | 15q22-q24 | 2747 | CANCER, LUNG, FAMILIAL |
| HEXA | hexosaminidase A (alpha polypeptide) | **15** | 15q23-q24 | 0434 | G(M2)-GANGLIOSIDOSIS WITH HEXOSAMINIDASE A DEFICIENCY |
| FAH | fumarylacetoacetate | | 15q23-q25 | 0978 | TYROSINEMIA I |
| ETFA | electron transfer flavoprotein, alpha polypeptide (glutaric aciduria II) | | 15q23-q25 | 2377 | ACIDEMIA, ETHYLMALONIC-ADIPIC |
| CD13 | antigen CD13 (p150) | | 15q25-qter | 2970 | GRANULOCYTE GLYCOPROTEIN CD11/CD18 DEFICIENCY |
| CTM | cataract, Marner | | 16 | 0132 | CATARACT, CORTICAL AND NUCLEAR |
| CTH | cystathionase | | 16 | 0236 | CYSTATHIONINURIA |
| BTS | Batten disease | | 16 | 0713 | NEURONAL CEROID-LIPOFUSCINOSES (NCL) |
| CTM | cataract, Marner | | 16 | 2342 | CATARACT, AUTOSOMAL DOMINANT CONGENITAL |
| IFNR | interferon production regulator | | 16 | 3090 | INTERFERON DEFICIENCY |
| PKD1 | polycystic kidney disease 1 (autosomal dominant) | | 16p13 | 0859 | KIDNEY, POLYCYSTIC DISEASE, DOMINANT |
| CD11A | antigen CD11A (p180), lymphocyte function-associated antigen 1 | | 16p13.1-p11 | 2970 | GRANULOCYTE GLYCOPROTEIN CD11/CD18 DEFICIENCY |
| ALDOA | aldolase A, fructose-bisphosphate | | 16q22-q24 | 2662 | ERYTHROCYTE ALDOLASE-A DEFICIENCY |
| HP | haptoglobin | | 16q22.1 | 0452 | HAPTOGLOBIN |
| LCAT | lecithin-cholesterol acyltransferase | **16** | 16q22.1 | 0580 | LECITHIN-CHOLESTEROL ACYL TRANSFERASE DEFICIENCY |
| TAT | tyrosine aminotransferase | | 16q22.1 | 2009 | TYROSINEMIA II, OREGON TYPE |

| SYMBOL | MARKER NAME | CHROMOSOME | MAP LOCATION | NO | ARTICLE TITLE |
|---|---|---|---|---|---|
| LCAT | lecithin-cholesterol acyltransferase | | 16q22.1 | 2646 | ANEMIA, HEMOLYTIC, RED CELL MEMBRANE DEFECTS |
| APRT | adenine phosphoribosyltransferase | | 16q24 | 3104 | ADENINE PHOSPHO-RIBOSYL-TRANSFERASE (APRT) DEFICIENCY |
| GALC | galactosylceramidase | | 17 | 0415 | LEUKODYSTROPHY, GLOBOID CELL TYPE |
| SMPD1 | sphingomyelin phosphodiesterase 1, acid lysosomal | | 17 | 0717 | NIEMANN-PICK DISEASE |
| HVBS8 | hepatitis B virus integration site 8 | | 17p12-p11.2 | 3008 | FETAL EFFECT FROM HEPATITIS B INFECTION |
| CMT2 | Charcot-Marie-Tooth neuropathy 2 | | 17p13.1-q12 | 2104 | NEUROPATHY, HEREDITARY MOTOR AND SENSORY, TYPE I |
| MDCR | Miller-Dieker syndrome chromosome region | | 17p13.3 | 0603 | LISSENCEPHALY SYNDROME |
| NF1 | neurofibromatosis 1 (von Recklinghausen disease, Watson disease) | | 17q11.2 | 0712 | NEUROFIBROMATOSIS |
| NF1 | neurofibromatosis 1 (von Recklinghausen disease, Watson disease) | **17** | 17q11.2 | 2776 | PULMONIC STENOSIS-CAFE-AU-LAIT SPOTS, WATSON TYPE |
| KRT19 | keratin 19 | | 17q21-q23 | 2675 | ANEMIA, HEMOLYTIC, GLUTATIONINE PEROXIDASE DEFICIENCY |
| EPB3 | erythrocyte surface protein band 3 | | 17q21-qter | 2646 | ANEMIA, HEMOLYTIC, RED CELL MEMBRANE DEFECTS |
| COL1A1 | collagen, type I, alpha 1 | | 17q21.3-q22 | 0777 | OSTEOGENESIS IMPERFECTA |
| MPO | myeloperoxidase | | 17q21.3-q23 | 2214 | IMMUNODEFICIENCY, MYELOPEROXIDASE DEFICIENCY TYPE |
| GP2B | glycoprotein IIb (IIb/IIIa complex, platelet, CD41B) | | 17q21.32 | 2683 | THROMBASTHENIA, GLANZMANN-NAEGELI TYPE |
| GH1 | growth hormone 1 | | 17q22-q24 | 0447 | GROWTH HORMONE DEFICIENCY, ISOLATED |
| GAA | glucosidase, alpha; acid | | 17q23 | 0011 | GLYCOGENOSIS, TYPE IIa |
| GAA | glucosidase, alpha; acid | | 17q23 | 2873 | GLYCOGENOSIS, TYPE IIb |
| GALK | galactokinase | | 17q23-q25 | 0402 | GALACTOKINASE DEFICIENCY |
| PALB | prealbumin | | 18q11.2-q12.1 | 2141 | AMYLOIDOSIS, TRANSTHYRETIN METHIONINE-30 TYPE |
| PALB | prealbumin | | 18q11.2-q12.1 | 2142 | AMYLOIDOSIS, INDIANA TYPE |
| PALB | prealbumin | | 18q11.2-q12.1 | 2143 | AMYLOIDOSIS, DANISH CARDIAC TYPE |
| PALB | prealbumin | **18** | 18q11.2-q12.1 | 2880 | AMYLOIDOSIS, ASHKENAZI TYPE |
| PALB | prealbumin | | 18q11.2-q12.1 | 2881 | AMYLOIDOSIS, APPALACHIAN TYPE |
| PALB | prealbumin | | 18q11.2-q12.1 | 2882 | AMYLOIDOSIS, ILLINOIS TYPE |
| BCL2 | B cell CLL/lymphoma 2 | | 18q21.3 | 3097 | LEUKEMIA/LYMPHOMA, B CELL |
| BCL2 | B cell CLL/lymphoma 2 | | 18q21.3 | 3107 | LYMPHOMA, NON-HODGKIN |
| MANB | mannosidase, alpha B, lysosomal | | 19cen-q13.1 | 2079 | MANNOSIDOSIS |
| LDLR | low density lipoprotein receptor (familial hypercholesterolemia) | | 19p13.2-p13.1 | 0488 | HYPERCHOLESTEREMIA |
| AMH | anti-Mullerian hormone | **19** | 19p13.3 | 0683 | MULLERIAN DERIVATIVES IN MALES, PERSISTENT |
| C3 | complement component 3 | | 19p13.3-p13.2 | 2219 | COMPLEMENT COMPONENT 3, DEFICIENCY OF |
| PEPD | peptidase D | | 19q12-q13.2 | 2616 | PROLIDASE DEFICIENCY |
| PVS | poliovirus sensitivity | | 19q12-q13.2 | 3109 | POLIO, SUSCEPTIBILITY TO |

| SYMBOL | MARKER NAME | CHROMOSOME | MAP LOCATION | NO | ARTICLE TITLE |
|---|---|---|---|---|---|
| GPI | glucose phosphate isomerase | | 19q13.1 | 2750 | ANEMIA, GLUCOSE PHOSPHATE ISOMERASE DEFICIENCY |
| APOC1 | apolipoprotein C-I | | 19q13.2 | 3096 | HYPOALPHALIPOPROTEINEMIA |
| DM | dystrophia myotonia | | 19q13.2-q13.3 | 0702 | MYOTONIC DYSTROPHY |
| ARVP | arginine vasopressin (neurophysin II) | 20 | 20 | 2611 | DIABETES INSIPIDIS, NEUROHYPOPHYSEAL TYPE |
| OT | prepro-oxytocin (neurophysin I) | | 20 | 2611 | DIABETES INSIPIDIS, NEUROHYPOPHYSEAL TYPE |
| GSL | galactosialidosis | | 20 | 3110 | GALACTOSIALIDOSIS |
| AGS | Alagille syndrome | | 20p12-p11 | 2084 | ARTERIO-HEPATIC DYSPLASIA |
| EBN | epilepsy, benign neonatal | | 20q | 3216 | CONVULSIONS, BENIGN FAMILIAL NEONATAL |
| ADA | adenosine deaminase | | 20q13.11 or 20q13.2-qter | 2196 | IMMUNODEFICIENCY, ADENOSINE DEAMINASE DEFICIENCY |
| AD1 | Alzheimer disease 1 | 21 | 21pter-q21 | 2354 | ALZHEIMER DISEASE, FAMILIAL |
| APP | amyloid beta (A4) precursor protein | | 21q21.2 | 2354 | ALZHEIMER DISEASE, FAMILIAL |
| PFKL | phosphofructokinase, liver type | | 21q22.3 | 0428 | GLYCOGENOSIS, TYPE VII |
| CBS | cystathionine-beta-synthase | | 21q22.3 | 0474 | HOMOCYSTINURIA |
| BCEI | breast cancer, estrogen-inducible sequence expressed in | | 21q22.3 | 2351 | CANCER, BREAST, FAMILIAL |
| CD18 | lymphocyte function-associated antigen 1; macrophage antigen | | 21q22.3 | 2970 | GRANULOCYTE GLYCOPROTEIN CD11/CD18 DEFICIENCY |
| ADSL | adenylosuccinate lyase | 22 | 22 | 3113 | ADENYLOSUCCINATE MONOPHOSPHATE LYASE DEFICIENCY |
| CECR | cat eye syndrome chromosome region | | 22pter-q11 | 0544 | CAT EYE SYNDROME |
| IDUA | iduronidase, alpha-L- | | 22pter-q11 | 0674 | MUCOPOLYSACCHARIDOSIS 1-H |
| IDUA | iduronidase, alpha-L- | | 22pter-q11 | 0675 | MUCOPOLYSACCHARIDOSIS 1-S |
| TCN2 | transcobalamin II; macrocytic anemia | | 22q | 2624 | TRANSCOBALAMIN II DEFICIENCY |
| BCR | breakpoint cluster region | | 22q11 | 3092 | LEUKEMIA, CHRONIC MYELOID (CML) |
| TSHR | thyroid stimulating hormone receptor | | 22q11-q13 | 0948 | THYROTROPIN UNRESPONSIVENESS |
| NF2 | neurofibromatosis 2 (bilateral acoustic neuroma) | | 22q11-q13.1 | 0012 | ACOUSTIC NEUROMA |
| GGT1 | gamma-glutamyltransferase 1 | | 22q11.1-q11.2 | 0422 | GLUTATHIONURIA |
| DGCR | DiGeorge syndrome chromosome region | | 22q11.21-q11.23 | 0943 | IMMUNODEFICIENCY, THYMIC AGENESIS |
| NAGA | acetylgalactosaminidase, alpha-N- | | 22q13-qter | 3254 | ALPHA-N-ACETYLGALACTOSAMINIDASE DEFICIENCY |
| ARSA | arylsulfatase A | | 22q13.31-qter | 0651 | METACHROMATIC LEUKODYSTROPHIES |
| DIA1 | diaphorase (NADH) (cytochrome b-5 reductase) | | 22q13.31-qter | 2682 | METHEMOGLOBINEMIA, NADH-DEPENDENT DIAPHORASE DEFICIENCY |
| CCT | cataract, congenital, total | | X | 0132 | CATARACT, CORTICAL AND NUCLEAR |
| DHOF | dermal hypoplasia, focal | | X | 0281 | DERMAL HYPOPLASIA, FOCAL |
| PHP | panhypopituitarism | | X | 0303 | DWARFISM, PANHYPOPITUITARY |
| LOX | lysyl oxidase; ?cutis laxa-X; ?Ehlers-Danlos V | | X | 0338 | EHLERS-DANLOS SYNDROME |
| EFE2 | endocardial fibroelastosis 2 | | X | 0348 | VENTRICLE, ENDOCARDIAL FIBROELASTOSIS OF LEFT VENTRICLE |

| SYMBOL | MARKER NAME | CHROMOSOME | MAP LOCATION | NO | ARTICLE TITLE |
|---|---|---|---|---|---|
| PHK | phosphorylase kinase deficiency, liver (glycogen storage disease type VIII) | | X | 0430 | GLYCOGENOSIS, TYPE IXa |
| HSAS | hydrocephalus, stenosis of the aqueduct of Sylvius | | X | 0481 | HYDROCEPHALY |
| HOMG | hypomagnesemia, secondary hypocalcemia | | X | 0514 | HYPOMAGNESEMIA, PRIMARY |
| OPEM | ophthalmoplegia, external, with myopia | | X | 0750 | OPHTHALMOPLEGIA EXTERNA-MYOPIA |
| OFD1 | oral-facial-digital syndrome I | | X | 0770 | ORO-FACIO-DIGITAL SYNDROME I |
| OPD | otopalatodigital syndrome | | X | 0786 | OTO-PALATO-DIGITAL SYNDROME, I |
| CRD | choroidoretinal degeneration | | X | 0869 | RETINITIS PIGMENTOSA |
| TDD | testicular 17,20-desmolase deficiency | | X | 0904 | STEROID 17,20-DESMOLASE DEFICIENCY |
| MF4 | metacarpal 4-5 fusion | | X | 0923 | SYNDACTYLY |
| CRD | choroidoretinal degeneration | | X | 0925 | CHOROIDEREMIA |
| ASB | anemia, sideroblastic/hypochromic | | X | 1518 | ANEMIA, SIDEROBLASTIC |
| BDM | behavior disorder modifier | | X | 1532 | MOOD AND THOUGHT DISORDERS |
| OPD | otopalatodigital syndrome | | X | 2258 | OTO-PALATO-DIGITAL SYNDROME, II |
| ACAD | acyl-Coenzyme A dehydrogenase, multiple | | X | 2289 | ACIDEMIA, GLUTARIC ACIDEMIA II |
| PHK | phosphorylase kinase deficiency, liver (glycogen storage disease type VIII) | | X | 2303 | GLYCOGEN STORAGE DISEASE, X-LINKED WITH NORMAL HEPATIC ENZYMES |
| SDYS | Simpson dysmorphia syndrome | | X | 2826 | SIMPSON-GOLABI-BEHMEL SYNDROME |
| MAA | microphthalmia or anophthalmia and associated anomalies | | X | 3171 | LENZ MICROPHTHALMIA SYNDROME |
| LOX | lysyl oxidase; ?cutis laxa-X; ?Ehlers-Danlos V | | X | 3219 | OCCIPITAL HORN SYNDROME |
| MNK | Menkes syndrome | | Xcen-q13 | 0643 | MENKES SYNDROME |
| MRX1 | mental retardation, X-linked 1 (non dysmorphic) | | Xp11-q13 | 2640 | X-LINKED MENTAL RETARDATION, CLARK-BARAITSER TYPE |
| MRX1 | mental retardation, X-linked 1 (non dysmorphic) | | Xp11-q13 | 2840 | X-LINKED MENTAL RETARDATION, ATKIN TYPE |
| MRX1 | mental retardation, X-linked 1 (non dysmorphic) | | Xp11-q13 | 3199 | X-LINKED MENTAL RETARDATION, GOLABI-ITO-HALL TYPE |
| MRX1 | mental retardation, X-linked 1 (non dysmorphic) | | Xp11-q13 | 3200 | X-LINKED MENTAL RETARDATION-CRANIOFACIAL ABNORMALITIES-CLUB FOOT |
| IP1 | incontinentia pigmenti 1 | | Xp11.21-cen | 0526 | INCONTINENTIA PIGMENTI |
| RP2 | retinitis pigmentosa 2 | | Xp11.4-p11.2 | 0869 | RETINITIS PIGMENTOSA |
| WAS | Wiskott-Aldrich syndrome | | Xp11.4-p11.21 | 0523 | IMMUNODEFICIENCY, WISKOTT-ALDRICH TYPE |
| NDP | Norrie disease (pseudoglioma) | | Xp11.4-p11.3 | 0721 | NORRIE DISEASE |
| CYBB | cytochrome b-245, beta polypeptide (chronic granulomatous disease) | | Xp21.1 | 0443 | GRANULOMATOUS DISEASE, CHRONIC X-LINKED |
| XK | Kell blood group precursor (McLeod phenotype) | | Xp21.1 | 2646 | ANEMIA, HEMOLYTIC, RED CELL MEMBRANE DEFECTS |
| OTC | ornithine carbamoyltransferase | | Xp21.1 | 3023 | ORNITHINE TRANSCARBAMYLASE DEFICIENCY |
| CSNB1 | congenital stationary night blindness 1 | | Xp21.1-p11.23 | 0718 | NIGHTBLINDNESS, CONGENITAL STATIONARY, X-LINKED RECESSIVE |
| COD1 | cone dystrophy 1 (X-linked) | | Xp21.1-p11.3 | 3228 | RETINA, CONE DYSTROPHY, X-LINKED |
| RP3 | retinitis pigmentosa 3 | | Xp21.1-p11.4 | 0869 | RETINITIS PIGMENTOSA |
| DMD | muscular dystrophy, Duchenne and Becker types | | Xp21.3-p21.1 | 0687 | MUSCULAR DYSTROPHY, ADULT PSEUDOHYPERTROPHIC |
| DMD | muscular dystrophy, Duchenne and Becker types | | Xp21.3-p21.1 | 0689 | MUSCULAR DYSTROPHY, CHILDHOOD PSEUDOHYPERTROPHIC |
| AHC | adrenal hypoplasia, congenital | | Xp21.3-p21.2 | 0024 | ADRENAL HYPOPLASIA, CONGENITAL |
| GK | glycerol kinase deficiency | | Xp21.3-p21.2 | 2310 | GLYCEROL KINASE DEFICIENCY |
| AIED | Aland island eye disease (Forsius-Eriksson ocular albinism) | | Xp21.3-p21.2 | 3183 | FORSIUS-ERIKSSON SYNDROME |
| AIH1 | amelogenesis imperfecta 1, hypomaturation or hypoplastic (?=AMG & AMGS) | | Xp22 | 0046 | TEETH, AMELOGENESIS IMPERFECTA |

X

| SYMBOL | MARKER NAME | CHROMOSOME | MAP LOCATION | NO | ARTICLE TITLE |
|---|---|---|---|---|---|
| SEDL | spondyloepiphyseal dysplasia, late | | Xp22 | 0898 | SPONDYLOEPIPHYSEAL DYSPLASIA, LATE |
| AIH1 | amelogenesis imperfecta 1, hypomaturation or hypoplastic (?=AMG & AMGS) | | Xp22 | 2136 | TEETH, SNOW-CAPPED |
| AIC | Aicardi syndrome | | Xp22 | 2320 | AICARDI SYNDROME |
| CLS | Coffin-Lowry syndrome | | Xp22.2-p22.1 | 0190 | COFFIN-LOWRY SYNDROME |
| HYP | hypophosphatemia, vitamin D resistant rickets | | Xp22.2-p22.1 | 0517 | HYPOPHOSPHATEMIA, X-LINKED |
| RS | retinoschisis | | Xp22.2-p22.1 | 0871 | RETINOSCHISIS |
| OA1 | ocular albinism 1 (Nettleship-Falls) | | Xp22.3 | 0032 | ALBINISM, OCULAR |
| NHS | Nance-Horan syndrome (congenital cataracts and dental anomalies) | | Xp22.3-p21.1 | 2119 | CATARACTS-OTO-DENTAL DEFECTS |
| MRX2 | mental retardation, X-linked 2 | | Xp22.3-p22.2 | 2920 | X-LINKED MENTAL RETARDATION, RENPENNING TYPE |
| AMG | amelogenin (?=AMGS & AIH) | | Xp22.31-p22.1 | 0046 | TEETH, AMELOGENESIS IMPERFECTA |
| KAL | Kallmann syndrome | | Xp22.32 | 2301 | KALLMANN SYNDROME |
| STS | steroid sulfatase (microsomal) | | Xp22.32 | 2532 | ICHTHYOSIS, X-LINKED WITH STEROID SULFATASE DEFICIENCY |
| CDPX | chondrodysplasia punctata | | Xp22.32 | 2730 | CHONDRODYSPLASIA PUNCTATA, X-LINKED DOMINANT TYPE |
| F2L | coagulation factor II (prothrombin)-like | | Xpter-q25 | 2674 | COAGULATION DEFECT, FAMILIAL MULTIPLE FACTORS |
| F2L | coagulation factor II (prothrombin)-like | | Xpter-q25 | 2679 | HYPOPROTHROMBINEMIA |
| CMTX | Charcot-Marie-Tooth neuropathy, X-linked | | Xq11-q13 | 2104 | NEUROPATHY, HEREDITARY MOTOR AND SENSORY, TYPE I |
| AR | androgen receptor (dihydrotestosterone receptor; testicular feminization) | | Xq12 | 0049 | ANDROGEN INSENSITIVITY SYNDROME, COMPLETE |
| AR | androgen receptor (dihydrotestosterone receptor; testicular feminization) | | Xq12 | 0050 | ANDROGEN INSENSITIVITY SYNDROME, INCOMPLETE |
| AR | androgen receptor (dihydrotestosterone receptor; testicular feminization) | | Xq12 | 2954 | ANDROGEN INSENSITIVITY (RESISTANCE), MINIMAL |
| PHKA | phosphorylase kinase, alpha | | Xq12-q13 | 0430 | GLYCOGENOSIS, TYPE IXa |
| PHKA | phosphorylase kinase, alpha | | Xq12-q13 | 2303 | GLYCOGEN STORAGE DISEASE, X-LINKED WITH NORMAL HEPATIC ENZYMES |
| EDA | ectodermal dysplasia, anhidrotic (hypohydrotic) | | Xq12-q13.1 | 0333 | ECTODERMAL DYSPLASIA, CHRIST-SIEMENS-TOURAINE TYPE |
| MGC1 | megalocornea 1 (X-linked) | | Xq12-q26 | 0637 | CORNEA, MEGALOCORNEA |
| FGDY | faciogenital dysplasia (Aarskog syndrome) | | Xq13 | 0001 | AARSKOG SYNDROME |
| PGK1 | phosphoglycerate kinase 1 | | Xq13 | 2657 | ANEMIA, HEMOLYTIC, ERYTHROCYTE PHOSPHOGLYCERATE KINASE DEFICIENCY |
| SCIDX1 | severe combined immunodeficiency, X-linked 1 | | Xq13-q21.1 | 0524 | IMMUNODEFICIENCY, X-LINKED SEVERE COMBINED |
| DFN3 | deafness, conductive, with fixed stapes | | Xq13-q21.2 | 3116 | DEAFNESS WITH PERILYMPHATIC GUSHER |
| SBMA | spinal and bulbar muscular atrophy (Kennedy disease) | | Xq13-q22 | 0895 | SPINAL MUSCULAR ATROPHY |
| SBMA | spinal and bulbar muscular atrophy (Kennedy disease) | | Xq13-q22 | 2493 | SPINAL MUSCULAR ATROPHY, SPINAL AND BULBAR, X-LINKED KENNEDY TYPE |
| TBG | thyroxin binding globulin | | Xq21-q22 | 0950 | THYROXINE-BINDING GLOBULIN DEFECTS |
| PRPS1 | phosphoribosyl pyrophosphate synthetase 1 | | Xq21-q27 | 0441 | GOUT |
| PRPS1 | phosphoribosyl pyrophosphate synthetase 1 | | Xq21-q27 | 0508 | PHOSPHORIBOSYL PYROPHOSPHATE (PRPP) SYNTHETASE ABNORMALITY |
| TCD | tapeto-choroidal dystrophy, progressive choroidemia | | Xq21.1-q21.2 | 0925 | CHOROIDEREMIA |
| GLA | galactosidase, alpha | | Xq21.3-q22 | 0373 | FABRY DISEASE |
| PLP | proteolipid protein (Pelizaeus-Merzbacher disease) | | Xq21.3-q22 | 0803 | PELIZAEUS-MERZBACHER SYNDROME |

| SYMBOL | MARKER NAME | CHROMOSOME | MAP LOCATION | NO | ARTICLE TITLE |
|---|---|---|---|---|---|
| ATS | Alport syndrome | | Xq21.3-q24 | 0708 | NEPHRITIS-DEAFNESS (SENSORINEURAL), HEREDITARY TYPE |
| AGMX1 | agammaglobulinemia, X-linked 1 (Bruton) | | Xq21.33-q22 | 0027 | IMMUNODEFICIENCY, AGAMMAGLOBULINEMIA, X-LINKED, INFANTILE |
| HIGM1 | hyper IgM syndrome | | Xq24-q27 | 2524 | IMMUNODEFICIENCY, X-LINKED WITH HYPER IgM |
| LYP | lymphoproliferative syndrome | | Xq25-q26 | 2210 | IMMUNODEFICIENCY, X-LINKED LYMPHOPROLIFERA-TIVE DISEASE |
| OCRL | oculocerebrorenal syndrome of Lowe | | Xq25-q26.1 | 0736 | OCULO-CEREBRO-RENAL SYNDROME |
| ADFN | albinism-deafness syndrome | | Xq25-q27 | 0030 | ALBINISM, CUTANEOUS-DEAFNESS |
| HPRT | hypoxanthine phosphoribosyltransferase | | Xq26 | 0441 | GOUT |
| HPRT | hypoxanthine phosphoribosyltransferase | | Xq26 | 0588 | LESCH-NYHAN SYNDROME |
| HPT | hypoparathyroidism | | Xq26-q27 | 0515 | HYPOPARATHYROIDISM, FAMILIAL |
| BFLS | Borjeson-Forssman-Lehmann syndrome | | Xq26-q27 | 2272 | BORJESON-FORSSMAN-LEHMANN SYNDROME |
| F9 | coagulation factor IX (Christmas disease) | | Xq26.3-q27.1 | 0462 | HEMOPHILIA B |
| SPG1 | spastic paraplegia, complicated | | Xq27-q28 | 0295 | PARAPLEGIA, FAMILIAL SPASTIC |
| MTM1 | myotubular myopathy 1 | | Xq27-q28 | 0695 | MYOPATHY, MYOTUBULAR |
| MAFD2 | major affective disorder 2 | | Xq27-q28 | 1532 | MOOD AND THOUGHT DISORDERS |
| DKC | dyskeratosis congenita | | Xq27-q28 | 2024 | DYSKERATOSIS CONGENITA |
| MRSD | mental retardation-skeletal dysplasia | | Xq27-q28 | 2904 | X-LINKED MENTAL RETARDATION-SKELETAL DYSPLASIA |
| FRAXA | fragile site, folic acid type, rare, fra(X)(q27.3) | | Xq27.3 | 2073 | X-LINKED MENTAL RETARDATION, FRAGILE X SYNDROME |
| IDS | iduronate 2-sulfatase (Hunter syndrome) | | Xq27.3-q28 | 0676 | MUCOPOLYSACCHARIDOSIS II |
| EMD | Emery-Dreifuss muscular dystrophy | | Xq27.3-q28 | 2491 | EMERY-DREIFUSS SYNDROME |
| CBBM | color blindness, blue monochromatic | | Xq28 | 0195 | COLOR BLINDNESS, BLUE MONOCONE-MONOCHROMATIC |
| GCP | green cone pigment (color blindness, deutan) | | Xq28 | 0196 | COLOR BLINDNESS, RED-GREEN DEUTAN SERIES |
| RCP | red cone pigment (color blindness, protan) | | Xq28 | 0197 | COLOR BLINDNESS, RED-GREEN PROTAN SERIES |
| DIR | diabetes insipidus, renal | | Xq28 | 0287 | DIABETES INSIPIDUS, VASOPRESSIN RESISTANT TYPES I AND II |
| G6PD | glucose-6-phosphate dehydrogenase | | Xq28 | 0420 | GLUCOSE-6-PHOSPHATE DEHYDROGENASE DEFICIENCY |
| F8C | coagulation factor VIIIc, procoagulant component (hemophilia A) | | Xq28 | 0461 | HEMOPHILIA A |
| ALD | adrenoleukodystrophy | | Xq28 | 2533 | ADRENOLEUKODYSTROPHY, X-LINKED |
| TKC | torticollis, keloids, cryptorchidism and renal dysplasia | | Xq28-qter | 2174 | CERVICO-DERMO-GU SYNDROME, GOEMINNE TYPE |
| TDF | testis determining factor | | Yp11.3 | 0437 | GONADAL DYSGENESIS, XY TYPE |

# BIRTH DEFECT-NUMBER-TO-PRIME NAME INDEX

0001 AARSKOG SYNDROME
0002 ABETALIPOPROTEINEMIA
0003 EYE, CRYPTOPHTHALMOS WITH OTHER
      MALFORMATIONS
0004 FIBRINOGENS, ABNORMAL CONGENITAL
0005 SKIN, ACANTHOSIS NIGRICANS
0006 ACATALASEMIA
0007 ACETYLATOR POLYMORPHISM
0008 ACHONDROGENESIS, LANGER-SALDINO TYPE
0009 ACHONDROGENESIS, PARENTI-FRACCARO TYPE
0010 ACHONDROPLASIA
0011 GLYCOGENOSIS, TYPE IIa
0012 ACOUSTIC NEUROMATA
0013 ACROCEPHALOPOLYSYNDACTYLY
0014 ACROCEPHALOSYNDACTYLY TYPE I
0015 ACRODERMATITIS ENTEROPATHICA
0016 ACRODYSOSTOSIS
0017 ACROFACIAL DYSOSTOSIS
0018 ACROMEGALOID PHENOTYPE-CUTIS VERTICIS
      GYRATA-CORNEAL LEUKOMA
0019 ACROMESOMELIC DYSPLASIA, CAMPAILLA-
      MARTINELLI TYPE
0020 ACROMESOMELIC DYSPLASIA, MAROTEAUX-
      MARTINELLI-CAMPAILLA TYPE
0021 ACRO-OSTEOLYSIS, DOMINANT TYPE
0022 ACROPECTOROVERTEBRAL DYSPLASIA
0023 ADRENAL HYPOALDOSTERONISM OF INFANCY,
      TRANSIENT ISOLATED
0024 ADRENAL HYPOPLASIA, CONGENITAL
0025 ADRENOCORTICAL UNRESPONSIVENESS TO ACTH,
      HEREDITARY
0026 ADRENOCORTICOTROPIC HORMONE DEFICIENCY,
      ISOLATED
0027 IMMUNODEFICIENCY, AGAMMAGLOBULINEMIA,
      X-LINKED, INFANTILE
0028 AGNATHIA-MICROSTOMIA-SYNOTIA
0029 AGONADIA
0030 ALBINISM, CUTANEOUS-DEAFNESS
0031 ALBINISM, CUTANEOUS
0032 ALBINISM, OCULAR
0033 ALBINISM, OCULOCUTANEOUS, HERMANSKY-
      PUDLAK TYPE
0034 ALBINISM, OCULOCUTANEOUS, TYROSINASE
      NEGATIVE
0035 ALBINISM, OCULOCUTANEOUS, TYROSINASE
      POSITIVE
0036 ALBINISM, OCULOCUTANEOUS, YELLOW MUTANT
0037 ALKAPTONURIA
0038 HAIR, ALOPECIA AREATA
0039 ALPHA(1)-ANTITRYPSIN DEFICIENCY
0040 ACIDEMIA, 3-KETOTHIOLASE DEFICIENCY
0041 ALSTROM SYNDROME
0042 BREAST, AMASTIA
0043 RETINA, AMAUROSIS CONGENITA, LEBER TYPE
0044 AMELO-CEREBRO-HYPOHIDROTIC SYNDROME
0045 AMELO-ONYCHO-HYPOHIDROTIC SYNDROME
0046 TEETH, AMELOGENESIS IMPERFECTA
0047 ANALBUMINEMIA
0048 ANALPHALIPOPROTEINEMIA
0049 ANDROGEN INSENSITIVITY SYNDROME, COMPLETE
0050 ANDROGEN INSENSITIVITY SYNDROME,
      INCOMPLETE
0051 ANEMIA, HYPOPLASTIC CONGENITAL
0052 ANENCEPHALY
0053 AORTIC SINUS OF VALSALVA, ANEURYSM
0054 ANGIOEDEMA, HEREDITARY
0055 ANGIO-OSTEOHYPERTROPHY SYNDROME
0057 ANIRIDIA

0058 PUPIL, ANISOCORIA
0059 EYE, ANISOMETROPIA
0060 EYELID, ANKYLOBLEPHARON
0061 TONGUE, ANKYLOGLOSSIA
0062 PANCREAS, ANNULAR
0063 ARTERY, ANOMALOUS ORIGIN OF
      CONTRALATERAL SUBCLAVIAN
0064 ARTERY, CORONARY, ANOMALOUS ORIGIN FROM
      PULMONARY ARTERY
0065 ECTRODACTYLY-ANONYCHIA
0066 NAILS, ANONYCHIA, HEREDITARY
0067 EYE, ANOPHTHALMIA
0068 ANORCHIA
0069 ANORECTAL MALFORMATIONS
0070 ANOSMIA, CONGENITAL
0071 ANTIBODIES TO HUMAN ALLOTYPES
0072 ANUS-HAND-EAR SYNDROME
0073 AORTA, COARCTATION
0074 AORTIC ARCH, CERVICAL
0075 AORTIC ARCH, DOUBLE
0076 AORTIC ARCH INTERRUPTION
0077 AORTIC ARCH, RIGHT
0078 AORTIC STENOSIS, SUPRAVALVAR
0079 AORTIC VALVE ATRESIA
0080 AORTIC VALVE STENOSIS
0081 AORTIC VALVE, TETRACUSPID
0082 AORTICO-LEFT VENTRICULAR TUNNEL
0083 AORTICO-PULMONARY SEPTAL DEFECT
0084 LENS, APHAKIA
0085 ARACHNODACTYLY, CONTRACTURAL BEALS TYPE
0086 ARGININEMIA
0087 ACIDURIA, ARGININOSUCCINIC
0088 ARTHROGRYPOSES
0090 ARTHRO-OPHTHALMOPATHY, HEREDITARY,
      PROGRESSIVE, STICKLER TYPE
0091 ASPHYXIATING THORACIC DYSPLASIA
0092 ASPLENIA SYNDROME
0093 ATAXIA-HYPOGONADISM SYNDROME
0094 ATAXIA-TELANGIECTASIA
0095 ATRANSFERRINEMIA
0096 ATRIAL SEPTAL DEFECTS
0097 EAR, AUDITORY CANAL ATRESIA
0098 AURICULO-OSTEODYSPLASIA
0099 HAIR, BALDNESS, COMMON
0100 BARTTER SYNDROME
0101 NEVOID BASAL CELL CARCINOMA SYNDROME
0102 ECTODERMAL DYSPLASIA, BASAN TYPE
0103 BASILAR IMPRESSION, PRIMARY
0104 BECKWITH-WIEDEMANN SYNDROME
0105 BERLIN SYNDROME
0106 ACIDURIA, BETA-MERCAPTOLACTATE-CYSTEINE
      DISULFIDURIA
0107 ACIDURIA, BETA-METHYL-CROTONYL-GLYCINURIA
0108 AORTIC VALVE, BICUSPID
0109 PULMONARY VALVE, BICUSPID
0110 BILIARY ATRESIA
0111 BLEPHAROCHALASIS-DOUBLE LIP-NONTOXIC
      GOITER
0112 BLOOM SYNDROME
0113 NEVUS, BLUE RUBBER BLEB NEVUS SYNDROME
0114 BRACHYDACTYLY
0115 BRAIN, SPONGY DEGENERATION
0116 GLYCOGENOSIS, TYPE IV
0117 NECK, BRANCHIAL CLEFT, CYSTS OR SINUSES
0118 BRANCHIO-SKELETO-GENITAL SYNDROME
0119 RUBINSTEIN-TAYBI BROAD THUMB-HALLUX
      SYNDROME
0120 BRONCHIAL ATRESIA

0121 C SYNDROME
0122 CAMPOMELIC DYSPLASIA
0123 CARDIO-AUDITORY SYNDROME
0124 MYOPATHY-METABOLIC, CARNITINE DEFICIENCY, PRIMARY AND SECONDARY
0125 MYOPATHY-METABOLIC, CARNITINE PALMITYL TRANSFERASE DEFICIENCY
0126 CARNOSINEMIA
0127 CAROTID BODY TUMOR
0128 OSTEOLYSIS, CARPAL-TARSAL AND CHRONIC PROGRESSIVE GLOMERULOPATHY
0129 OSTEOLYSIS, RECESSIVE CARPAL-TARSAL
0130 EYE, CARUNCLE ABERRATIONS
0131 CATARACT-ICHTHYOSIS
0132 CATARACT, CORTICAL AND NUCLEAR
0133 CATARACT, POLAR AND CAPSULAR
0134 MYOPATHY, CENTRAL CORE DISEASE TYPE
0135 SEIZURES, CENTRALOPATHIC
0137 CEREBRAL GIGANTISM
0138 CEREBRO-COSTO-MANDIBULAR SYNDROME
0139 CEREBRO-HEPATO-RENAL SYNDROME
0140 CEREBRO-OCULO-FACIO-SKELETAL SYNDROME
0141 EAR, CERUMEN VARIATIONS
0142 CERVICO-OCULO-ACOUSTIC SYNDROME
0143 CHEDIAK-HIGASHI SYNDROME
0144 LIP, CHEILITIS GLANDULARIS
0145 EAR, CHEMODECTOMA OF MIDDLE EAR
0146 FACE, CHIN FISSURE
0147 CHIN, TREMBLING
0148 DIARRHEA, CONGENITAL CHLORIDE
0149 BILE DUCT CHOLEDOCHAL CYST
0150 EAR, CHOLESTEATOMA OF TEMPORAL BONE
0151 CHOLESTERYL ESTER STORAGE DISEASE
0152 CHOLINESTERASE, ATYPICAL
0153 CHONDRODYSPLASIA PUNCTATA, MILD SYMMETRIC TYPE
0154 CHONDRODYSPLASIA PUNCTATA, RHIZOMELIC TYPE
0155 CHONDRODYSTROPHIC MYOTONIA, SCHWARTZ-JAMPEL TYPE
0156 CHONDROECTODERMAL DYSPLASIA
0157 CHROMOSOME 8, TRISOMY 8
0158 CHROMOSOME 18, MONOSOMY 18p
0159 CHROMOSOME 18, MONOSOMY 18q
0160 CHROMOSOME 18, TRISOMY 18
0161 CHROMOSOME 11, PARTIAL TRISOMY 11q
0162 CHROMOSOME 11, MONOSOMY 11q
0163 CHROMOSOME 5, MONOSOMY 5p
0164 CHROMOSOME 4, MONOSOMY 4p
0165 CHROMOSOME 14, PARTIAL TRISOMY 14q
0167 CHROMOSOME 13, MONOSOMY 13q
0168 CHROMOSOME 13, TRISOMY 13
0169 CHROMOSOME TRIPLOIDY
0170 CHROMOSOME 21, MONOSOMY 21
0171 CHROMOSOME 21, TRISOMY 21
0172 CHROMOSOME 22, MONOSOMY 22
0173 CHROMOSOME MOSAICISM, 45,X/46,XY TYPE
0174 CITRULLINEMIA
0175 THUMB, CLASPED
0176 CLEFT LIP/PALATE-FILIFORM FUSION OF EYELIDS
0177 CLEFT LIP/PALATE-LIP PITS OR MOUNDS
0178 CLEFT LIP
0179 CLEFT LIP/PALATE-ECTODERMAL DYSPLASIA-SYNDACTYLY
0180 CLEFT PALATE
0181 CLEFT PALATE-PERSISTENCE OF BUCCOPHARYN-GEAL MEMBRANE
0182 CLEFT PALATE-MICROGNATHIA-GLOSSOPTOSIS
0183 CLEFT PALATE-STAPES FIXATION-OLIGODONTIA
0184 UVULA, CLEFT
0185 CLEIDOCRANIAL DYSPLASIA
0186 CNS ARTERIOVENOUS MALFORMATION
0187 CIRCUMVALLATE PLACENTA SYNDROME

0188 CNS NEOPLASMS
0189 COCKAYNE SYNDROME
0190 COFFIN-LOWRY SYNDROME
0191 OCULAR MOTOR APRAXIA, COGAN CONGENITAL TYPE
0192 COLON, AGANGLIONOSIS
0193 COLON, ATRESIA OR STENOSIS
0194 COLON, DUPLICATION
0195 COLOR BLINDNESS, BLUE MONOCONE-MONOCHROMATIC
0196 COLOR BLINDNESS, RED-GREEN DEUTAN SERIES
0197 COLOR BLINDNESS, RED-GREEN PROTAN SERIES
0198 COLOR BLINDNESS, TOTAL
0199 COLOR BLINDNESS, YELLOW-BLUE TRITAN
0200 ARTERY, BRACHIOCEPHALIC AND CONTRALATERAL CAROTID, COMMON ORIGIN
0201 RETINA, COMBINED CONE-ROD DEGENERATION
0202 TWINS, CONJOINED
0203 PORPHYRIA, COPROPORPHYRIA
0204 HEART, COR TRIATRIATUM
0205 CORNEA PLANA
0206 CORNEAL DYSTROPHY-SENSORINEURAL DEAFNESS
0207 CORNEAL DYSTROPHY, ENDOTHELIAL, CONGENITAL HEREDITARY
0208 CORNEAL DYSTROPHY, ENDOTHELIAL
0209 CORNEAL DYSTROPHY, GRANULAR
0210 CORNEAL DYSTROPHY, JUVENILE EPITHELIAL MEESMANN TYPE
0211 CORNEAL DYSTROPHY, LATTICE TYPE
0212 CORNEAL DYSTROPHY, MACULAR TYPE
0213 CORNEAL DYSTROPHY, POLYMORPHOUS POSTERIOR
0214 CORNEAL DYSTROPHY, RECURRENT EROSIVE
0215 CORNEAL DYSTROPHY, REIS-BUCKLERS TYPE
0216 CORNEAL DYSTROPHY, SCHNYDER CRYSTALLINE
0217 ARTERY, CORONARY CALCINOSIS
0218 ARTERY, CORONARY, ARTERIOVENOUS FISTULA
0219 ARTERY, SINGLE CORONARY
0220 CORPUS CALLOSUM AGENESIS
0221 CORTICAL HYPEROSTOSIS, INFANTILE
0222 STEROID, BINDING GLOBULIN ABNORMALITIES
0223 CRANIO-CARPO-TARSAL DYSPLASIA, WHISTLING FACE TYPE
0224 CRANIO-DIAPHYSEAL DYSPLASIA
0225 CRANIOFACIAL DYSOSTOSIS
0226 CRANIOFACIAL DYSOSTOSIS-DIAPHYSEAL HYPERPLASIA
0227 CRANIOFACIAL DYSSYNOSTOSIS
0228 CRANIOMETAPHYSEAL DYSPLASIA
0229 ACROCEPHALOSYNDACTYLY TYPE III
0230 CRANIOSYNOSTOSIS
0231 CRANIOSYNOSTOSIS-RADIAL APLASIA SYNDROME
0232 EAR, CRYPTOTIA
0233 CUTIS LAXA
0234 CYCLOPIA
0235 SCALP, CYLINDROMAS
0236 CYSTATHIONINURIA
0237 CYSTIC FIBROSIS
0238 CYSTINOSIS
0239 CYSTINURIA
0240 SPLEEN, CYSTS
0241 EAR, DARWIN TUBERCLE
0242 DE LANGE SYNDROME
0243 DEAFNESS, PFAENDLER TYPE
0245 DEAFNESS-ATOPIC DERMATITIS
0246 DEAFNESS-DIABETES
0247 DEAFNESS-EAR PITS
0249 DEAFNESS-GOITER
0250 METAPHYSEAL DYSOSTOSIS-DEAFNESS
0251 DEAFNESS-MYOPIA
0252 DEAFNESS-ONYCHODYSTROPHY
0253 DEAFNESS-OPTIC NERVE ATROPHY, PROGRESSIVE
0254 DEAFNESS-MALFORMED, LOW-SET EARS

0255 DEAFNESS-DIABETES-PHOTOMYOCLONUS-NEPHROPATHY
0256 DEAFNESS, DOMINANT LOW-FREQUENCY
0257 THYROID, HORMONE RESISTANCE
0258 DEAFNESS-HYPERPROLINURIA-ICHTHYOSIS
0259 DEAFNESS-KERATOPACHYDERMIA-DIGITAL CONSTRICTIONS
0261 DEAFNESS-MYOPIA-CATARACT-SADDLE NOSE, MARSHALL TYPE
0262 DEAFNESS-ONYCHO-OSTEO-DYSTROPHY-RETARDATION-SEIZURES (DOORS)
0263 KEUTEL SYNDROME
0265 DEAFNESS-DIVERTICULITIS-NEUROPATHY
0266 DEAFNESS (SENSORINEURAL)-DYSTONIA
0267 DEAFNESS (SENSORINEURAL), MIDFREQUENCY
0268 DEAFNESS-POLYNEUROPATHY-OPTIC ATROPHY
0269 DEAFNESS (SENSORINEURAL), PROGRESSIVE HIGH-TONE
0270 DEAFNESS (SENSORINEURAL), RECESSIVE EARLY-ONSET
0271 DEAFNESS (SENSORINEURAL), RECESSIVE PROFOUND
0272 DEAFNESS, STREPTOMYCIN-SENSITIVITY
0273 DEAFNESS, TUNE
0274 DEAFNESS, UNILATERAL INNER EAR
0275 DEAFNESS-VITILIGO-MUSCLE WASTING
0276 TEETH, DENS INVAGINATUS
0277 TEETH, DENTIN DYSPLASIA, CORONAL
0278 TEETH, DENTIN DYSPLASIA, RADICULAR
0279 TEETH, DENTINOGENESIS IMPERFECTA
0280 DENTINO-OSSEOUS DYSPLASIA
0281 DERMAL HYPOPLASIA, FOCAL
0282 DERMO-CHONDRO-CORNEAL DYSTROPHY, FRANCOIS TYPE
0283 NECK/HEAD, DERMOID CYST OR TERATOMA
0284 EYE, DERMOLIPOMA
0285 DEXTROCARDIA-BRONCHIECTASIS-SINUSITIS SYNDROME
0286 VENTRICLE, SEPTUM DEXTROPOSITION AND DOUBLE INLET LEFT VENTRICLE
0287 DIABETES INSIPIDUS, VASOPRESSIN RESISTANT TYPES I AND II
0288 DIAPHRAGM, EVENTRATION
0289 DIAPHRAGMATIC HERNIA
0290 DIAPHYSEAL DYSPLASIA
0291 TEETH, DIASTEMA, MEDIAN INCISAL
0292 DIASTEMATOMYELIA
0293 DIASTROPHIC DYSPLASIA
0294 ACIDURIA, DICARBOXYLIC AMINOACIDURIA
0295 PARAPLEGIA, FAMILIAL SPASTIC
0296 DISTICHIASIS
0297 VENTRICLE, DOUBLE-OUTLET RIGHT WITH ANTERIOR SEPTAL DEFECT
0298 VENTRICLE, DOUBLE-OUTLET RIGHT WITH POSTERIOR SEPTAL DEFECT
0299 DUBOWITZ SYNDROME
0300 DUODENUM, ATRESIA OR STENOSIS
0301 CONTRACTURE, DUPUYTREN
0302 DWARFISM, LARON
0303 DWARFISM, PANHYPOPITUITARY
0304 DWARFISM, PITUITARY WITH ABNORMAL SELLA TURCICA
0306 DYGGVE-MELCHIOR-CLAUSEN SYNDROME
0307 DYSAUTONOMIA I, RILEY-DAY TYPE
0308 DYSCHONDROSTEOSIS
0309 PUPIL, DYSCORIA
0310 DYSOSTEOSCLEROSIS
0311 DYSPLASIA EPIPHYSEALIS HEMIMELICA
0312 EAR, ABSENT TRAGUS
0313 EAR, ARTERIOVENOUS FISTULA
0314 EAR, CUPPED
0315 EAR, INNER DYSPLASIAS
0316 EAR, ECTOPIC PINNA

0317 EAR, EXCHONDROSIS
0318 EAR, EXOSTOSES
0319 EAR, HAIRY
0320 EAR, LOBE, ABSENT
0321 EAR LOBE, CLEFT
0322 EAR LOBE, PIT
0323 EAR LOBE, ATTACHED
0324 EAR LOBE, HYPERTROPHIC THICKENED
0325 EAR, LONG, NARROW, POSTERIORLY ROTATED
0326 EAR, LOP
0327 EAR, LOW-SET
0328 EAR, MOZART TYPE
0329 EAR, PITS
0330 EAR, PROMINENT ANTHELIX
0331 EAR, SMALL WITH FOLDED-DOWN HELIX
0332 TRICUSPID VALVE, EBSTEIN ANOMALY
0333 ECTODERMAL DYSPLASIA, CHRIST-SIEMENS-TOURAINE TYPE
0334 ECTODERMAL DYSPLASIA, HIDROTIC
0335 HEART, CORDIS ECTOPIA
0336 ECTRODACTYLY
0337 ECTRODACTYLY-ECTODERMAL DYSPLASIA-CLEFTING SYNDROME
0338 EHLERS-DANLOS SYNDROME
0339 SKIN, ELASTOSIS PERFORANS SERPIGINOSA
0340 TEETH, ENAMEL AND DENTIN DEFECTS FROM ERYTHROBLASTOSIS FETALIS
0341 TEETH, DEFECTS FROM TETRACYCLINE
0342 TEETH, ENAMEL HYPOPLASIA
0343 ENCEPHALOCELE
0344 ENCEPHALOPATHY, NECROTIZING
0345 ENCHONDROMATOSIS
0346 ENCHONDROMATOSIS AND HEMANGIOMAS
0347 HEART, ENDOCARDIAL CUSHION DEFECTS
0348 VENTRICLE, ENDOCARDIAL FIBROELASTOSIS OF LEFT VENTRICLE
0349 VENTRICLE, ENDOCARDIAL FIBROELASTOSIS OF RIGHT VENTRICLE
0350 ENDOCRINE NEOPLASIA, MULTIPLE TYPE I
0351 ENDOCRINE NEOPLASIA, MULTIPLE TYPE II
0352 ENDOCRINE NEOPLASIA, MULTIPLE TYPE III
0353 VENTRICLE, ENDOMYOCARDIAL FIBROSIS OF LEFT
0354 VENTRICLE, ENDOMYOCARDIAL FIBROSIS OF RIGHT
0355 EYELID, EPIBLEPHARON
0357 GALACTOSE EPIMERASE DEFICIENCY
0358 EPIPHYSEAL DYSPLASIA, MULTIPLE
0359 EPITHELIOMA, MULTIPLE SELF-HEALING SQUAMOUS
0360 TEETH, EPULIS, CONGENITAL
0361 SKIN, ERYTHROKERATODERMIA, VARIABLE
0362 PORPHYRIA, PROTOPORPHYRIA
0363 ESOPHAGUS, ACHALASIA
0364 ESOPHAGUS, ATRESIA
0365 ESOPHAGUS, ATRESIA AND TRACHEOESOPHAGEAL FISTULA
0366 ESOPHAGUS, CHALASIA
0367 ESOPHAGUS, DIVERTICULUM
0368 ESOPHAGUS, DUPLICATION
0369 ESOPHAGUS, STENOSIS
0370 EAR, EUSTACHIAN TUBE DEFECTS
0371 EYELID, ECTROPION, CONGENITAL
0372 EYELID, ENTROPION
0373 FABRY DISEASE
0374 FACIAL CLEFT, LATERAL
0375 FACIAL CLEFT, OBLIQUE
0376 DIPLEGIA, CONGENITAL FACIAL
0377 PALSY, CONGENITAL FACIAL
0378 PALSY, LATE-ONSET FACIAL, FAMILIAL
0379 FETAL ALCOHOL SYNDROME
0380 FETAL AMINOPTERIN SYNDROME
0381 FETAL CYTOMEGALOVIRUS SYNDROME
0382 FETAL HYDANTOIN SYNDROME
0383 FETAL RADIATION SYNDROME

0384 FETAL RUBELLA SYNDROME
0385 FETAL SYPHILIS SYNDROME
0386 FETAL THALIDOMIDE SYNDROME
0387 FETAL TOXOPLASMOSIS SYNDROME
0388 FETAL TRIMETHADIONE SYNDROME
0389 FETAL WARFARIN SYNDROME
0390 FIBROUS DYSPLASIA, MONOSTOTIC
0391 FIBROUS DYSPLASIA, POLYOSTOTIC
0393 FINGERPRINTS, ABSENT
0394 FRONTOMETAPHYSEAL DYSPLASIA
0395 FRUCTOSE-1-PHOSPHATE ALDOLASE DEFICIENCY
0396 FRUCTOSE-1,6-DIPHOSPHATASE DEFICIENCY
0397 FRUCTOSURIA
0398 FUCOSIDOSIS
0399 RETINA, FUNDUS ALBIPUNCTATUS
0400 RETINA, FUNDUS FLAVIMACULATUS
0401 G SYNDROME
0402 GALACTOKINASE DEFICIENCY
0403 GALACTOSEMIA
0404 GALLBLADDER, ANOMALIES
0405 GASTROSCHISIS
0406 GAUCHER DISEASE
0407 GINGIVAL FIBROMATOSIS
0408 GINGIVAL FIBROMATOSIS-CORNEAL DYSTROPHY
0409 GINGIVAL FIBROMATOSIS-DIGITAL ANOMALIES
0410 GINGIVAL FIBROMATOSIS-HYPERTRICHOSIS
0411 FIBROMATOSIS, JUVENILE HYALINE
0412 GINGIVAL MULTIPLE HAMARTOMA SYNDROME
0413 GINGIVAL FIBROMATOSIS-DEPIGMENTATION-
     MICROPHTHALMIA
0414 GLAUCOMA, CONGENITAL
0415 LEUKODYSTROPHY, GLOBOID CELL TYPE
0416 SKIN TUMORS, MULTIPLE GLOMUS
0417 GLOSSITIS, MEDIAN RHOMBOID
0418 GLUCOGLYCINURIA
0419 GLUCOSE-GALACTOSE MALABSORPTION
0420 GLUCOSE-6-PHOSPHATE DEHYDROGENASE
     DEFICIENCY
0421 ACIDEMIA, GLUTARIC ACIDEMIA I
0422 GLUTATHIONURIA
0423 GLUTEN-SENSITIVE ENTEROPATHY
0424 GLYCOGEN SYNTHETASE DEFICIENCY
0425 GLYCOGENOSIS, TYPE Ia
0426 GLYCOGENOSIS, TYPE III
0427 GLYCOGENOSIS, TYPE VI
0428 GLYCOGENOSIS, TYPE VII
0429 GLYCOGENOSIS, TYPE VIII
0430 GLYCOGENOSIS, TYPE IXa
0431 G(M1)-GANGLIOSIDOSIS, TYPE 1
0432 G(M1)-GANGLIOSIDOSIS, TYPE 2
0433 G(M2)-GANGLIOSIDOSIS WITH HEXOSAMINIDASE A
     AND B DEFICIENCY
0434 G(M2)-GANGLIOSIDOSIS WITH HEXOSAMINIDASE A
     DEFICIENCY
0435 GOITER, GOITROGEN INDUCED
0436 GONADAL DYSGENESIS, XX TYPE
0437 GONADAL DYSGENESIS, XY TYPE
0438 GONADOTROPIN DEFICIENCIES
0439 EYE, ANTERIOR SEGMENT DYSGENESIS
0440 GORLIN-CHAUDHRY-MOSS SYNDROME
0441 GOUT
0443 GRANULOMATOUS DISEASE, CHRONIC X-LINKED
0444 NOSE, GRANULOSIS RUBRA NASI
0445 GREBE SYNDROME
0446 PLASMA, GROUP-SPECIFIC COMPONENT
0447 GROWTH HORMONE DEFICIENCY, ISOLATED
0448 SWEATING, GUSTATORY
0449 GYRATE ATROPHY OF THE CHOROID AND RETINA
0450 MUSCLE WASTING OF HANDS-SENSORINEURAL
     DEAFNESS
0451 HYPOGLOSSIA-HYPODACTYLIA
0452 HAPTOGLOBIN
0453 HARTNUP DISORDER

0454 ARRHYTHMIA, HEART BLOCK, CONGENITAL
     COMPLETE
0455 HEART-HAND SYNDROME
0456 HEMANGIOMA-THROMBOCYTOPENIA SYNDROME
0458 HEMIHYPERTROPHY
0459 LIMB AND SCALP DEFECTS, ADAMS-OLIVER TYPE
0460 HEMOCHROMATOSIS, IDIOPATHIC
0461 HEMOPHILIA A
0462 HEMOPHILIA B
0463 LIVER, AGENESIS
0464 LIVER, ARTERIAL ANOMALIES
0465 LIVER, CYST, SOLITARY
0466 LIVER, HEMANGIOMATOSIS
0467 LIVER, ACCESSORY LOBE
0468 LIVER, VENOUS ANOMALIES
0469 HEPATOLENTICULAR DEGENERATION
0470 CONTRACTURES, HERRMANN-OPITZ
     ARTHROGRYPOSIS TYPE
0471 HERNIA, HIATAL
0472 HISTIDINEMIA
0473 HOLOPROSENCEPHALY
0474 HOMOCYSTINURIA
0475 HORNER SYNDROME
0476 SERUM ALLOTYPES, HUMAN
0477 HUMERO-RADIAL SYNOSTOSIS
0478 HUNTINGTON DISEASE
0479 RETINA, HYALOIDEORETINAL DEGENERATION OF
     WAGNER
0480 HYDRANENCEPHALY
0481 HYDROCEPHALY
0482 HYDROXYPROLINEMIA
0483 HYMEN, IMPERFORATE
0484 HYPERALDOSTERONISM, FAMILIAL
     GLUCOCORTICOID SUPPRESSIBLE
0486 HYPERBETA-ALANINEMIA
0487 HYPERBILIRUBINEMIA, UNCONJUGATED
0488 HYPERCHOLESTEROLEMIA
0489 HYPERCHYLOMICRONEMIA
0490 HYPERCYSTINURIA
0491 HYPERDIBASIC AMINOACIDURIA
0492 HYPERGLYCINEMIA, NON-KETOTIC
0493 HYPERHIDROSIS-PREMATURE GREYING-PREMOLAR
     APLASIA
0494 HYPERKERATOSIS PALMOPLANTARIS-
     PERIODONTOCLASIA
0495 HYPERLIPOPROTEINEMIA, BROAD BETA TYPE
0496 HYPERLIPOPROTEINEMIA, COMBINED
0497 ENDOSTEAL HYPEROSTOSIS
0498 HYPEROSTOSIS FRONTALIS INTERNA
0499 HYPERPARATHYROIDISM, FAMILIAL
0500 HYPERTRIGLYCERIDEMIA
0501 HYPERLIPOPROTEINEMIA V
0502 HYPERPROLINEMIA
0503 SARCOSINEMIA
0504 EYE, HYPERTELORISM
0505 HYPERTELORISM-HYPOSPADIAS SYNDROME
0506 HYPERTELORISM-MICROTIA-FACIAL
     CLEFT-CONDUCTIVE DEAFNESS
0507 HAIR, HYPERTRICHOSIS, LANUGINOSA
0508 PHOSPHORIBOSYL PYROPHOSPHATE (PRPP)
     SYNTHETASE ABNORMALITY
0509 HYPERVALINEMIA
0510 HYPOCHONDROPLASIA
0511 HYPODONTIA-NAIL DYSGENESIS
0512 HYPOGLYCEMIA, FAMILIAL NEONATAL
0514 HYPOMAGNESEMIA, PRIMARY
0515 HYPOPARATHYROIDISM, FAMILIAL
0516 HYPOPHOSPHATASIA
0517 HYPOPHOSPHATEMIA, X-LINKED
0518 HYPOSPADIAS
0520 IMINOGLYCINURIA
0521 IMMUNODEFICIENCY, COMMON VARIABLE TYPE
0522 IMMUNODEFICIENCY, SEVERE COMBINED

0523 IMMUNODEFICIENCY, WISKOTT-ALDRICH TYPE
0524 IMMUNODEFICIENCY, X-LINKED SEVERE COMBINED
0525 IMMUNOGLOBULIN A DEFICIENCY
0526 INCONTINENTIA PIGMENTI
0527 ARTERY, INDEPENDENT ORIGIN OF IPSILATERAL VERTEBRAL
0528 VENA CAVA, ABSENT HEPATIC SEGMENT
0529 HERNIA, INGUINAL
0530 EAR, ANEURYSM OF INTERNAL CAROTID ARTERY
0531 INTESTINAL ATRESIA OR STENOSIS
0532 INTESTINAL DUPLICATION
0533 INTESTINAL ENTEROKINASE DEFICIENCY
0534 INTESTINAL LYMPHANGIECTASIA
0535 INTESTINAL POLYPOSIS, TYPE I
0536 INTESTINAL POLYPOSIS, TYPE III
0537 INTESTINAL ROTATION, INCOMPLETE
0538 MUCOSA (ORAL/EYE), INTRAEPITHELIAL DYSKERATOSIS, BENIGN
0539 CHERUBISM
0540 VENTRICLES, INVERTED WITH TRANSPOSITION OF GREAT ARTERIES
0541 VENTRICLES, INVERTED WITHOUT TRANSPOSITION OF GREAT ARTERIES
0542 THYROID, IODIDE TRANSPORT DEFECT
0543 THYROID, IODOTYROSINE DEIODINASE DEFICIENCY
0544 CAT EYE SYNDROME
0545 INTESTINAL ILEUS, ISOLATED MECONIUM ILEUS
0546 AORTA, ISOLATION OF SUBCLAVIAN ARTERY FROM AORTA
0547 ACIDEMIA, ISOVALERIC
0548 JAW-WINKING SYNDROME
0549 DIABETES MELLITUS, INSULIN DEPENDENT TYPE
0550 DIABETES (INSIPIDUS/MELLITUS)-OPTIC ATROPHY-DEAFNESS
0552 EYE, KERATOCONUS
0553 EYE, KERATOPATHY, BAND-SHAPED
0554 KBG SYNDROME
0555 CRANIOSYNOSTOSIS, KLEEBLATTSCHADEL TYPE
0556 KLINEFELTER SYNDROME
0557 KNIEST DYSPLASIA
0558 KNUCKLE PADS-LEUKONYCHIA-DEAFNESS
0559 NAILS, KOILONYCHIA
0560 KUSKOKWIN SYNDROME
0561 SKIN, KYRLE DISEASE
0562 EAR, LABYRINTH APLASIA
0563 LACRIMAL CANALICULUS ATRESIA
0564 LACRIMAL GLAND, ECTOPIC
0565 LACRIMAL SAC FISTULA
0566 LACTASE DEFICIENCY, CONGENITAL
0567 LACTASE DEFICIENCY, PRIMARY
0568 LACTATE DEHYDROGENASE ISOZYMES
0569 LACTOSE INTOLERANCE
0570 LARSEN SYNDROME
0571 LARYNX, ATRESIA
0572 LARYNX, CYSTS
0573 LARYNX, VENTRICLE PROLAPSE
0574 LARYNX, WEB
0575 LARYNGOCELE
0576 LARYNGOMALACIA
0577 LARYNGO-TRACHEO-ESOPHAGEAL CLEFT
0578 LAURENCE-MOON SYNDROME
0579 OPTIC ATROPHY, LEBER TYPE
0580 LECITHIN-CHOLESTEROL ACYL TRANSFERASE DEFICIENCY
0581 VENTRICLE, DOUBLE OUTLET LEFT
0582 VENTRICLE, SINGLE LEFT PAPILLARY MUSCLE
0583 LENS AND PUPIL, ECTOPIC
0584 LENS, ECTOPIC
0585 LENTICONUS
0586 LENTIGINES SYNDROME, MULTIPLE
0587 LEPRECHAUNISM
0588 LESCH-NYHAN SYNDROME
0589 NAILS, LEUKONYCHIA

0590 LIDDLE SYNDROME
0591 OCULAR DERMOIDS
0592 LIMB-OTO-CARDIAC SYNDROME
0593 NEVUS, EPIDERMAL NEVUS SYNDROME
0594 LIP, DOUBLE
0595 LIP, MEDIAN CLEFT OF UPPER
0596 LIP, PITS OR MOUNDS
0597 LIPASE, CONGENITAL ABSENCE OF PANCREATIC
0598 LIPOGRANULOMATOSIS
0599 SKIN, LIPOID PROTEINOSIS
0600 LIPOMAS, FAMILIAL SYMMETRIC
0601 NECK/FACE, LIPOMATOSIS
0602 LIPOMENINGOCELE
0603 LISSENCEPHALY SYNDROME
0604 LIVER, HAMARTOMA
0605 HEPATIC FIBROSIS, CONGENITAL
0606 LIVER, TRANSPOSITION
0607 TEETH, LOBODONTIA
0608 SKIN, LOCALIZED ABSENCE OF
0610 ARRHYTHMIA, WITH LONG QT INTERVAL WITHOUT DEAFNESS
0611 LUNG, ABERRANT LOBE
0612 LUNG, LOBE SEQUESTRATION
0613 ALVEOLAR RIDGES, LYMPHANGIOMA
0614 LYMPHEDEMA I
0615 LYMPHEDEMA II
0616 HYPERLYSINEMIA
0617 TEETH, MACRODONTIA
0618 MACROGLOSSIA
0619 EAR, MACROTIA
0621 MACULAR COLOBOMA-BRACHYDACTYLY
0622 RETINA, MACULAR DEGENERATION, VITELLIRUPTIVE
0623 EYELID, MADAROSIS
0626 MANDIBULAR PROGNATHISM
0627 MANDIBULOFACIAL DYSOSTOSIS
0628 MAPLE SYRUP URINE DISEASE
0629 MARDEN-WALKER SYNDROME
0630 MARFAN SYNDROME
0631 MAXILLA, MEDIAN ALVEOLAR CLEFT
0632 McDONOUGH SYNDROME
0633 MECKEL DIVERTICULUM
0634 MECKEL SYNDROME
0635 FACE, MEDIAN CLEFT FACE SYNDROME
0636 CLEFTS, LOWER MEDIAN LIP, MANDIBLE AND TONGUE
0637 CORNEA, MEGALOCORNEA
0638 MEGALOCORNEA-MENTAL RETARDATION SYNDROME
0639 OPTIC DISK, MELANOCYTOMA
0640 EYE, MELANOSIS OCULI, CONGENITAL
0641 MELORHEOSTOSIS
0642 MENINGOCELE
0643 MENKES SYNDROME
0645 MESENTERIC CYSTS
0646 MESOMELIC DYSPLASIA, LANGER TYPE
0647 MESOMELIC DYSPLASIA, NIEVERGELT TYPE
0648 MESOMELIC DYSPLASIA, REINHARDT-PFEIFFER TYPE
0649 MESOMELIC DYSPLASIA, WERNER TYPE
0650 METACHONDROMATOSIS
0651 METACHROMATIC LEUKODYSTROPHIES
0652 METAPHYSEAL CHONDRODYSPLASIA, TYPE JANSEN
0653 METAPHYSEAL CHONDRODYSPLASIA, TYPE McKUSICK
0654 METAPHYSEAL CHONDRODYSPLASIA, TYPE SCHMID
0655 METAPHYSEAL CHONDRODYSPLASIA WITH THYMOLYMPHOPENIA
0656 METATROPIC DYSPLASIA
0657 METHIONINE MALABSORPTION
0658 ACIDEMIA, METHYLMALONIC
0659 MICROCEPHALY
0660 TEETH, MICRODONTIA
0661 EYE, MICROPHTHALMIA/COLOBOMA

0663 LENS, MICROSPHEROPHAKIA
0664 EAR, MICROTIA-ATRESIA
0665 MITRAL VALVE ATRESIA
0666 MITRAL VALVE INSUFFICIENCY
0667 MITRAL REGURGITATION-DEAFNESS-SKELETAL DEFECTS
0668 MITRAL VALVE PROLAPSE
0669 MITRAL VALVE STENOSIS
0670 ALOPECIA-EPILEPSY-OLIGOPHRENIA, MOYNAHAN TYPE
0671 MUCOLIPIDOSIS I
0672 MUCOLIPIDOSIS II
0673 MUCOLIPIDOSIS III
0674 MUCOPOLYSACCHARIDOSIS I-H
0675 MUCOPOLYSACCHARIDOSIS I-S
0676 MUCOPOLYSACCHARIDOSIS II
0677 MUCOPOLYSACCHARIDOSIS III
0678 MUCOPOLYSACCHARIDOSIS IV
0679 MUCOPOLYSACCHARIDOSIS VI
0680 MUCOPOLYSACCHARIDOSIS VII
0681 MUCOSA, WHITE FOLDED DYSPLASIA
0682 MULLERIAN APLASIA
0683 MULLERIAN DERIVATIVES IN MALES, PERSISTENT
0684 MULLERIAN FUSION, INCOMPLETE
0685 EXOSTOSES, MULTIPLE CARTILAGINOUS
0687 MUSCULAR DYSTROPHY, ADULT PSEUDOHYPER-TROPHIC
0688 MUSCULAR DYSTROPHY, AUTOSOMAL RECESSIVE PSEUDOHYPERTROPHIC
0689 MUSCULAR DYSTROPHY, CHILDHOOD PSEUDOHYPERTROPHIC
0690 MUSCULAR DYSTROPHY, DISTAL
0691 MUSCULAR DYSTROPHY, LIMB-GIRDLE
0692 MUSCULAR DYSTROPHY, OCULOPHARYNGEAL
0693 MENINGOMYELOCELE
0695 MYOPATHY, MYOTUBULAR
0696 MYOPATHY, NEMALINE
0699 MYOPIA, CONGENITAL
0700 MYOSITIS OSSIFICANS PROGRESSIVA
0701 MYOTONIA CONGENITA
0702 MYOTONIC DYSTROPHY
0703 ECTODERMAL DYSPLASIA, NAEGELI TYPE
0704 NAIL-PATELLA SYNDROME
0705 NASOLACRIMAL DUCT OBSTRUCTION
0706 NASOPHARYNGEAL CYSTS
0707 NOSE, NASOPHARYNGEAL STENOSIS
0708 NEPHRITIS-DEAFNESS (SENSORINEURAL), HEREDITARY TYPE
0709 NEPHROSIS, CONGENITAL
0710 NEPHROSIS, FAMILIAL TYPE
0711 JAW, NEUROECTODERMAL PIGMENTED TUMOR
0712 NEUROFIBROMATOSIS
0713 NEURONAL CEROID-LIPOFUSCINOSES (NCL)
0714 NEUTROPENIA, CYCLIC
0715 NEVUS FLAMMEUS
0716 NEVUS OF OTA
0717 NIEMANN-PICK DISEASE
0718 NIGHTBLINDNESS, CONGENITAL STATIONARY, X-LINKED RECESSIVE
0720 NOONAN SYNDROME
0721 NORRIE DISEASE
0722 NOSE/NASAL SEPTUM DEFECTS
0723 NOSE, ANTERIOR ATRESIA
0724 NOSE, BIFID
0725 NOSE, DUPLICATION
0726 NOSE, GLIOMA
0727 NOSE, POSTERIOR ATRESIA
0728 NOSE, TRANSVERSE GROOVE
0729 IMMUNODEFICIENCY, NUCLEOSIDE-PHOSPHORYLASE DEFICIENCY
0731 VENTRICLE, OBSTRUCTION WITHIN RIGHT VENTRICLE OR ITS OUTFLOW TRACT

0732 FACIO-OCULO-ACOUSTIC-RENAL SYNDROME (FOAR SYNDROME)
0734 OCULAR DRUSEN
0735 OCULO-AURICULO-VERTEBRAL ANOMALY
0736 OCULO-CEREBRO-RENAL SYNDROME
0737 OCULO-DENTO-OSSEOUS DYSPLASIA
0738 OCULO-MANDIBULO-FACIAL SYNDROME
0739 TEETH, ODONTODYSPLASIA
0740 NIGHTBLINDNESS, OGUCHI TYPE
0741 SEIZURES-ICHTHYOSIS-MENTAL RETARDATION
0742 OLIVOPONTOCEREBELLAR ATROPHY, DOMINANT MENZEL TYPE
0743 OLIVOPONTOCEREBELLAR ATROPHY, DOMINANT SCHUT-HAYMAKER TYPE
0744 OLIVOPONTOCEREBELLAR ATROPHY, DOMINANT WITH OPHTHALMOPLEGIA
0745 OLIVOPONTOCEREBELLAR ATROPHY, DOMINANT WITH RETINAL DEGENERATION
0746 OLIVOPONTOCEREBELLAR ATROPHY, LATE-ONSET
0747 OLIVOPONTOCEREBELLAR ATROPHY, RECESSIVE FICKLER-WINKLER TYPE
0748 OMPHALOCELE
0750 OPHTHALMOPLEGIA EXTERNA-MYOPIA
0751 OPHTHALMOPLEGIA, FAMILIAL STATIC
0752 OPHTHALMOPLEGIA, PROGRESSIVE EXTERNAL
0753 OPHTHALMOPLEGIA, TOTAL WITH PTOSIS AND MIOSIS
0754 FG SYNDROME, OPITZ-KAVEGGIA TYPE
0755 OPTIC ATROPHY, INFANTILE HEREDOFAMILIAL
0756 OPTIC DISK PITS
0757 OPTIC DISK, TILTED
0758 OPTIC NERVE HYPOPLASIA
0759 OPTICO-COCHLEO-DENTATE DEGENERATION
0760 ORAL DERMOIDS
0761 ORBITAL AND PERIORBITAL DERMOID CYSTS
0762 ORBITAL CEPHALOCELES
0763 ORBITAL NERVE GLIOMA
0764 ORBITAL HEMANGIOMA
0765 ORBITAL AND PERIORBITAL LYMPHANGIOMA
0766 PULMONARY ARTERY, ORIGIN OF THE LEFT FROM RIGHT PULMONARY ARTERY
0767 PULMONARY ARTERY, ORIGIN FROM ASCENDING AORTA
0768 PULMONARY ARTERY, ORIGIN FROM DUCTUS ARTERIOSUS
0769 ORO-CRANIO-DIGITAL SYNDROME
0770 ORO-FACIO-DIGITAL SYNDROME I
0771 ORO-FACIO-DIGITAL SYNDROME, MOHR TYPE
0772 ACIDEMIA, OROTIC
0773 EAR, OSSICLE AND MIDDLE EAR MALFORMATIONS
0774 JOINTS, OSTEOCHONDRITIS DISSECANS
0775 OSTEODYSPLASTY
0776 OSTEOECTASIA
0777 OSTEOGENESIS IMPERFECTA
0778 OSTEOPATHIA STRIATA
0779 OSTEOPETROSIS, BENIGN DOMINANT
0780 OSTEOPETROSIS, MALIGNANT RECESSIVE
0781 OSTEOPOIKILOSIS
0782 OSTEOPOROSIS, JUVENILE IDIOPATHIC
0783 OSTEOPOROSIS-PSEUDOGLIOMA SYNDROME
0784 OTO-DENTAL DYSPLASIA
0785 OTO-OCULO-MUSCULO-SKELETAL SYNDROME
0786 OTO-PALATO-DIGITAL SYNDROME, I
0787 OTOSCLEROSIS
0788 PACHYDERMOPERIOSTOSIS
0789 NAILS, PACHYONYCHIA CONGENITA
0790 PALATE, FISTULA
0791 PALLISTER-W SYNDROME
0792 SKIN, PALMO-PLANTAR ERYTHEMA
0793 PANCREATITIS, HEREDITARY
0794 PARALYSIS, HYPERKALEMIC PERIODIC
0795 PARALYSIS, HYPOKALEMIC PERIODIC
0796 PARAMYOTONIA CONGENITA

0797 SINUS, ABSENT PARANASAL
0798 PARASTREMMATIC DYSPLASIA
0799 PAROTITIS, PUNCTATE
0800 DUCTUS ARTERIOSUS, PATENT
0801 PECTUS CARINATUM
0802 PECTUS EXCAVATUM
0803 PELIZAEUS-MERZBACHER SYNDROME
0804 PENTOSURIA
0805 HEART, PERICARDIUM AGENESIS
0806 TEETH, PERIODONTITIS, JUVENILE
0807 VENA CAVA, PERSISTENT LEFT SUPERIOR JOINED
     TO CORONARY SINUS
0808 PHENYLKETONURIA
0809 TASTING DEFECT, PHENYLTHIOCARBAMIDE
0810 PHYTANIC ACID STORAGE DISEASE
0811 SKIN, PITYRIASIS RUBRA PILARIS
0812 IMMUNODEFICIENCY, PLASMA-ASSOCIATED
     DEFECT OF PHAGOCYTOSIS
0813 POLAND SYNDROME
0814 POLYDACTYLY
0815 BREAST, POLYTHELIA
0817 POLYSYNDACTYLY
0818 PTERYGIUM SYNDROME, POPLITEAL
0819 SKIN, POROKERATOSIS
0820 PORPHYRIA, ACUTE INTERMITTENT
0821 PORPHYRIA, ERYTHROPOIETIC
0822 PORPHYRIA, VARIEGATE
0823 PRADER-WILLI SYNDROME
0824 NOSE, PROBOSCIS LATERALIS
0825 PROGERIA
0826 ACIDEMIA, PROPIONIC
0827 PRURITUS, HEREDITARY LOCALIZED
0828 PSEUDOACHONDROPLASTIC DYSPLASIA
0829 ALDOSTERONE RESISTANCE
0830 PARATHYROID HORMONE RESISTANCE
0832 PSEUDOXANTHOMA ELASTICUM
0833 SKIN, PSORIASIS VULGARIS
0834 EYELID, PTOSIS, CONGENITAL
0835 PULMONARY ARTERY, COARCTATION
0836 PULMONARY VALVE, ABSENT
0837 PULMONARY VALVE, ATRESIA
0838 PULMONARY VALVE, INCOMPETENCE
0839 PULMONARY VALVE, STENOSIS
0840 PULMONARY VALVE, TETRACUSPID
0841 PULMONARY VENOUS CONNECTION, PARTIAL
     ANOMALOUS
0842 PULMONARY VENOUS CONNECTION, TOTAL
     ANOMALOUS
0844 EYELID, PUNCTA AND CANALICULI,
     SUPERNUMERARY
0845 EYE, PUPILLARY MEMBRANE PERSISTENCE
0846 PYKNODYSOSTOSIS
0847 PYLE DISEASE
0848 PYLORIC STENOSIS
0849 ACIDEMIA, PYROGLUTAMIC
0850 PYRUVATE CARBOXYLASE DEFICIENCY WITH
     LACTIC ACIDEMIA
0851 PYRUVATE DEHYDROGENASE DEFICIENCY
0852 PYRUVATE KINASE DEFICIENCY
0853 RADIAL DEFECTS
0854 RADIAL-ULNAR SYNOSTOSIS
0856 RENAL AGENESIS, BILATERAL
0857 RENAL AGENESIS, UNILATERAL
0858 RENAL BICARBONATE REABSORPTIVE DEFECT
0859 KIDNEY, POLYCYSTIC DISEASE, DOMINANT
0860 RENAL-GENITAL-MIDDLE EAR ANOMALIES
0861 RENAL GLYCOSURIA
0862 RENAL TUBULAR ACIDOSIS
0863 RENAL TUBULAR ACIDOSIS-SENSORINEURAL
     DEAFNESS
0864 RENAL TUBULAR SYNDROME, FANCONI TYPE
0866 RETINAL DYSPLASIA
0867 RETINAL FOLD

0868 RETINAL TELANGIECTASIA-HYPOGAMMAGLOBU-
     LINEMIA
0869 RETINITIS PIGMENTOSA
0870 RETINOBLASTOMA
0871 RETINOSCHISIS
0872 RETINOPATHY OF PREMATURITY
0873 RICKETS, VITAMIN D-DEPENDENT, TYPE I
0874 AMNIOTIC BANDS SYNDROME
0875 ROBERTS SYNDROME
0876 ROBINOW SYNDROME
0877 TERATOMA, SACROCOCCYGEAL TERATOMA
0878 SALIVARY GLAND, MIXED TUMOR
0879 SCIMITAR SYNDROME
0880 SCLEROSTEOSIS
0881 SECKEL SYNDROME
0882 CAMPTODACTYLY-TRISMUS SYNDROME
0883 SHORT RIB-POLYDACTYLY SYNDROME, TYPE II
0884 SHORT RIB-POLYDACTYLY SYNDROME, TYPE I
0885 SHWACHMAN SYNDROME
0886 ANEMIA, SICKLE CELL
0887 SILVER SYNDROME
0888 SITUS INVERSUS VISCERUM
0890 SKIN, LEIOMYOMAS, MULTIPLE
0891 SMITH-LEMLI-OPITZ SYNDROME
0892 SPHEROCYTOSIS
0893 SPHEROPHAKIA-BRACHYMORPHIA SYNDROME
0894 SPINAL CORD, NEURENTERIC CYST
0895 SPINAL MUSCULAR ATROPHY
0896 SPONDYLOCOSTAL DYSPLASIA
0897 SPONDYLOEPIPHYSEAL DYSPLASIA CONGENITA
0898 SPONDYLOEPIPHYSEAL DYSPLASIA, LATE
0899 SPONDYLOMETAPHYSEAL CHONDRODYSPLASIA,
     KOZLOWSKI TYPE
0900 SPONDYLOTHORACIC DYSPLASIA
0901 SPRENGEL DEFORMITY
0902 STEROID 11 BETA-HYDROXYLASE DEFICIENCY
0903 STEROID 17 ALPHA-HYDROXYLASE DEFICIENCY
0904 STEROID 17,20-DESMOLASE DEFICIENCY
0905 STEROID 18-HYDROXYLASE DEFICIENCY
0906 STEROID 18-HYDROXYSTEROID DEHYDROGENASE
     DEFICIENCY
0907 STEROID 20-22 DESMOLASE DEFICIENCY
0908 STEROID 21-HYDROXYLASE DEFICIENCY
0909 STEROID 3 BETA-HYDROXYSTEROID
     DEHYDROGENASE DEFICIENCY
0910 STOMACH, PYLORIC ATRESIA
0911 STOMACH, DIVERTICULUM
0912 STOMACH, DUPLICATION
0913 STOMACH, HYPOPLASIA
0914 STOMACH, TERATOMA
0915 STURGE-WEBER SYNDROME
0916 HEART, SUBAORTIC STENOSIS, FIBROUS
0917 HEART, SUBAORTIC STENOSIS, MUSCULAR
0918 SUBGLOTTIC HEMANGIOMA
0919 SUBGLOTTIC STENOSIS
0920 SUCRASE-ISOMALTASE DEFICIENCY
0921 ACIDURIA, SULFITE OXIDASE DEFICIENCY
0922 ARRHYTHMIA, SUPRAVENTRICULAR
     TACHYCARDIAS, CONGENITAL
0923 SYNDACTYLY
0924 SYRINGOMYELIA
0925 CHOROIDEREMIA
0926 TEETH, TAURODONTISM
0927 TEETH, ANKYLOSED
0928 TEETH, ROOT CONCRESCENCE
0929 TEETH, DILACERATED
0930 TEETH, FUSED
0931 TEETH, GEMINATED
0932 TEETH, IMPACTED
0933 TEETH, NATAL OR NEONATAL
0934 TEETH, PEGGED OR ABSENT MAXILLARY LATERAL
     INCISOR
0936 TEETH, SUPERNUMERARY

0938 HEART, TETRALOGY OF FALLOT
0939 THALASSEMIA
0940 THANATOPHORIC DYSPLASIA
0941 THROMBOCYTOPENIA-ABSENT RADIUS
0942 THROMBOCYTOPENIC PURPURA AND LIPID
    HISTIOCYTOSIS
0943 IMMUNODEFICIENCY, THYMIC AGENESIS
0944 AGAMMAGLOBULINEMIA-THYMOMA SYNDROME
0945 THYROGLOSSAL DUCT REMNANT
0946 THYROID, DYSGENESIS
0947 THYROID, PEROXIDASE DEFECT
0948 THYROTROPIN UNRESPONSIVENESS
0949 THYROTROPIN DEFICIENCY, ISOLATED
0950 THYROXINE-BINDING GLOBULIN DEFECTS
0951 TONGUE, FOLDING OR ROLLING
0952 TONGUE, CLEFT
0953 TONGUE, FISSURED
0954 TONGUE, GEOGRAPHIC
0955 TONGUE, PIGMENTED PAPILLAE
0956 TONGUE, PLICATED
0957 TORSION DYSTONIA
0958 MANDIBLE, TORUS MANDIBULARIS
0959 PALATE, TORUS PALATINUS
0960 TRACHEOESOPHAGEAL FISTULA
0961 UDP-GLUCURONOSYLTRANSFERASE, SEVERE
    DEFICIENCY TYPE I
0962 HEART, TRANSPOSITION OF GREAT VESSELS
0963 TREMOR-DUODENAL ULCER SYNDROME
0964 TREMOR, HEREDOFAMILIAL
0965 TRICHO-DENTO-OSSEOUS SYNDROME
0966 TRICHO-RHINO-PHALANGEAL SYNDROME, TYPE I
0967 TRICHO-RHINO-PHALANGEAL SYNDROME, TYPE II
0968 TRICUSPID VALVE, ATRESIA
0969 TRICUSPID VALVE, INSUFFICIENCY
0970 TRICUSPID VALVE, STENOSIS
0971 HERMAPHRODITISM, TRUE
0972 HEART, TRUNCUS ARTERIOSUS
0973 TRYPSINOGEN DEFICIENCY
0974 TRYPTOPHAN MALABSORPTION
0975 TUBEROUS SCLEROSIS
0976 TUBULAR STENOSIS
0977 TURNER SYNDROME
0978 TYROSINEMIA I
0979 VENTRICLE, RIGHT, UHL ANOMALY
0981 ULNAR-MAMMARY SYNDROME
0982 URTICARIA-DEAFNESS-AMYLOIDOSIS
0983 USHER SYNDROME
0984 VAGINAL ATRESIA
0985 VAGINAL SEPTUM, TRANSVERSE
0986 VAN DEN BOSCH SYNDROME
0987 VATER ASSOCIATION
0988 VENTRICLE, DIVERTICULUM
0989 VENTRICULAR SEPTAL DEFECT
0990 VISCERA, FATTY METAMORPHOSIS
0991 SEIZURES, VITAMIN B(6) DEPENDENCY
0992 VITAMIN B(12) MALABSORPTION
0993 SKIN, VITILIGO
0994 EYE, VITREOUS, PERSISTENT HYPERPLASTIC
    PRIMARY
0995 VON HIPPEL-LINDAU SYNDROME
0996 VON WILLEBRAND DISEASE
0997 WAARDENBURG SYNDROMES
0998 WERNER SYNDROME
0999 WILLIAMS SYNDROME
1000 WINCHESTER SYNDROME
1001 SYMPHALANGISM
1002 ARRHYTHMIA, WOLFF-PARKINSON-WHITE TYPE
1003 WOLMAN DISEASE
1004 XERODERMA PIGMENTOSUM-MENTAL
    RETARDATION
1005 XERODERMA PIGMENTOSUM
1500 MYOPATHIES
1501 TRANSPORT, RENAL, DEFECTS OF

1502 AMYLOIDOSES
1503 ECTODERMAL DYSPLASIAS
1504 EPILEPSY, FAMILIAL
1505 CANCER, FAMILIAL
1506 DWARFISM
1507 GLYCOGENOSES
1508 IMMUNODEFICIENCIES
1509 X-LINKED MENTAL RETARDATION
1511 ICHTHYOSIS
1512 DEAFNESS
1514 CATARACTS
1516 ALBINISM
1517 FOOT, CONGENITAL CLUBFOOT
1518 ANEMIA, SIDEROBLASTIC
1519 HYPERAMMONEMIA
1521 OSTEOLYSIS
1522 SYNOSTOSIS
1525 COMPLEMENT COMPONENT, ALTERNATIVE
    PATHWAYS, DEFICIENCIES OF
1532 MOOD AND THOUGHT DISORDERS
2001 DIHYDROPTERIDINE REDUCTASE DEFICIENCY
2002 BIOPTERIN SYNTHESIS DEFICIENCY
2003 KIDNEY, POLYCYSTIC DISEASE, RECESSIVE
2004 KIDNEY, HORSESHOE
2005 RENAL HYPOURICEMIA
2006 CARBOXYLASE DEFICIENCY, HOLOCARBOXYLASE
    DEFICIENCY TYPE
2007 PRUNE-BELLY SYNDROME
2008 EPISPADIAS
2009 TYROSINEMIA II, OREGON TYPE
2010 ALBINISM, OCULAR, AUTOSOMAL RECESSIVE TYPE
2011 CEREBELLAR AGENESIS
2012 COLPOCEPHALY
2013 MIETENS-WEBER SYNDROME
2014 NEUROCUTANEOUS MELANOSIS
2015 DEAFNESS-PILI TORTI, BJORNSTAD TYPE
2016 MUSCULAR DYSTROPHY, OCULO-
    GASTROINTESTINAL
2017 EPIPHYSEAL DYSPLASIA, MULTIPLE, RECESSIVE
    TARDA TYPE
2018 SEPTO-OPTIC DYSPLASIA
2019 LIMB REDUCTION-ICHTHYOSIS
2020 GELEOPHYSIC DWARFISM
2021 TELANGIECTASIA, OSLER HEMORRHAGIC
2022 HAJDU-CHENEY SYNDROME
2023 COHEN SYNDROME
2024 DYSKERATOSIS CONGENITA
2025 COFFIN-SIRIS SYNDROME
2026 JOHANSON-BLIZZARD SYNDROME
2027 FEMORAL HYPOPLASIA-UNUSUAL FACIES
    SYNDROME
2028 ANEMIA, HYPOPLASTIC-TRIPHALANGEAL THUMBS,
    AASE-SMITH TYPE
2029 PANCYTOPENIA SYNDROME, FANCONI TYPE
2030 SJOGREN-LARSSON SYNDROME
2031 MARINESCO-SJOGREN SYNDROME
2032 KLIPPEL-FEIL ANOMALY
2033 DWARFISM-STIFF JOINTS
2034 ONYCHODYSTROPHY-CONIFORM TEETH-
    SENSORINEURAL HEARING LOSS
2035 CARDIOFACIAL SYNDROME-ASYMMETRIC FACIES
2036 WEAVER SYNDROME
2037 ROTHMUND-THOMSON SYNDROME
2038 LIPODYSTROPHY SYNDROME, BERARDINELLI TYPE
2039 DISTICHIASIS-LYMPHEDEMA SYNDROME
2040 HYPOPHOSPHATEMIA, NON X-LINKED
2041 SALLA DISEASE
2042 ASPARTYLGLUCOSAMINURIA
2043 CHROMOSOME 22, SUPERNUMERARY DER 22,
    T(11:22)
2044 NEUROPATHY, HERITABLE ISONIAZIDE TYPE (INH)
2045 PALSY, PROGRESSIVE BULBAR OF CHILDHOOD
2047 NEUROPATHY, MYELO-OPTICO, SUBACUTE TYPE

2049 MUSCULAR DYSTROPHY, FACIO-SCAPULO-HUMERAL
2050 PARALYSIS, NORMOKALEMIC PERIODIC
2052 MYOPATHY-CATARACT-GONADAL DYSGENESIS
2054 DEJERINE-SOTTAS DISEASE
2056 MYOPATHY, DISPROPORTIONATE FIBER TYPE I
2058 MYOPATHY, MYOGLOBINURIA-ABNORMAL GLYCOLOSIS, HEREDITARY TYPE
2059 MYOPATHY, FAMILIAL LYSIS OF TYPE I FIBERS
2062 MYOPATHY, REDUCING BODY
2063 MYOPATHY, SARCOTUBULAR
2067 AMYOTROPHIC LATERAL SCLEROSIS
2068 AMYOTROPHIC LATERAL SCLEROSIS, GUAM TYPE
2069 AMYOTROPHIC LATERAL SCLEROSIS, FAMILIAL ADULT AND JUVENILE TYPES
2070 KEARNS-SAYRE DISEASE
2071 NEUROPATHY, HEREDITARY RECURRENT BRACHIAL
2073 X-LINKED MENTAL RETARDATION, FRAGILE X SYNDROME
2075 THUMB, ADDUCTED THUMB SYNDROME
2076 OSTEODYSTROPHY-MENTAL RETARDATION, RUVALCABA TYPE
2078 OCULO-OSTEO-CUTANEOUS SYNDROME, TOUMAALA-HAAPANEN TYPE
2079 MANNOSIDOSIS
2080 PENA-SHOKEIR SYNDROME
2081 DWARFISM, MULIBREY TYPE
2082 MANDIBULOACRAL DYSPLASIA
2083 CHEILITIS GRANULOMATOSA, MELKERSSON-ROSENTHAL TYPE
2084 ARTERIO-HEPATIC DYSPLASIA
2085 NASO-DIGITO-ACOUSTIC SYNDROME, KEIPERT TYPE
2086 ANGELMAN SYNDROME
2087 SINGLETON-MERTEN SYNDROME
2088 BLEPHARO-NASO-FACIAL SYNDROME
2092 NEU-LAXOVA SYNDROME
2093 DENTO-FACIO-SKELETAL DEFECTS, ACKERMAN TYPE
2095 ECTODERMAL DYSPLASIA, CONGENITAL FACIAL, SETLEIS TYPE
2096 SKIN, HYPERKERATOSIS, FOCAL PALMOPLANTAR AND GINGIVAL
2098 SHORT SYNDROME
2099 OSTEODYSPLASTICA GERODERMIA, BAMATTER TYPE
2100 ACROFACIAL DEFECTS, EMERY-NELSON TYPE
2101 SJOGREN SYNDROME
2102 LERI PLEONOSTEOSIS SYNDROME
2103 BLEPHAROPTOSIS-BLEPHAROPHIMOSIS-EPICANTHUS INVERSUS-TELECANTHUS
2104 NEUROPATHY, HEREDITARY MOTOR AND SENSORY, TYPE I
2105 NEUROPATHY, HEREDITARY MOTOR AND SENSORY, TYPE II
2106 VERMIS AGENESIS
2107 HISTIDINURIA
2108 NEUROPATHY, HEREDITARY WITH PRESSURE PALSIES
2109 TEETH, ODONTOBLASTIC DYSPLASIA, FOCAL
2110 RETINA, FLECKED KANDORI TYPE
2112 ARRHYTHMIA, FROM MATERNAL AUTOIMMUNE DISEASE, CONGENITAL
2113 ACIDEMIA, GAMMA-HYDROXYBUTYRIC
2114 ACIDEMIA, 3-HYDROXY-3-METHYLGLUTARIC
2115 RAYNAUD DISEASE
2116 PULMONARY HYPERTENSION, PRIMARY
2117 CANDIDIASIS, FAMILIAL CHRONIC MUCOCUTANEOUS
2118 PALATOPHARYNGEAL INCOMPETENCE
2119 CATARACTS-OTO-DENTAL DEFECTS
2120 OVERGROWTH, RUVALCABA-MYHRE-SMITH TYPE
2122 ARTHRITIS-ARTERITIS SYNDROME
2123 SCHINZEL-GIEDION SYNDROME

2124 CHARGE ASSOCIATION
2125 ANTLEY-BIXLER SYNDROME
2126 ACROFACIAL DYSOSTOSIS, POSTAXIAL TYPE
2127 CRANIO-ECTODERMAL DYSPLASIA
2128 AUTISM, INFANTILE
2129 VELO-CARDIO-FACIAL SYNDROME
2130 CHROMOSOME 12, PARTIAL TRISOMY 12p
2131 CHROMOSOME 15, PARTIAL TRISOMY DISTAL 15q
2132 CHROMOSOME 2, PARTIAL TRISOMY 2p
2133 TEETH, MESIOPALATAL TORSION OF CENTRAL INCISORS
2134 TEETH, ANODONTIA, PARTIAL OR COMPLETE
2135 TEETH, INCISORS, SHOVEL-SHAPED
2136 TEETH, SNOW-CAPPED
2137 TEETH, MOLAR REINCLUSION
2138 CUTIS LAXA-GROWTH DEFECT, DE BARSY TYPE
2139 RIEGER SYNDROME
2140 COLD HYPERSENSITIVITY
2141 AMYLOIDOSIS, TRANSTHYRETIN METHIONINE-30 TYPE
2142 AMYLOIDOSIS, INDIANA TYPE
2143 AMYLOIDOSIS, DANISH CARDIAC TYPE
2144 AMYLOIDOSIS, IOWA TYPE
2145 AMYLOIDOSIS, FINNISH TYPE
2146 AMYLOIDOSIS, ICELANDIC TYPE
2147 AMYLOIDOSIS, CORNEAL
2149 AMYLOIDOSIS, OHIO TYPE
2150 AMYLOIDOSIS, FAMILIAL VISCERAL
2151 DEAFNESS-TRIPHALANGEAL THUMBS-ONYCHODYSTROPHY
2154 SCLERODERMA, FAMILIAL PROGRESSIVE
2155 SYNOVITIS, FAMILIAL HYPERTROPHIC
2157 INFLAMMATORY DISEASE, NEONATAL BATES-LORBER TYPE
2158 DERMATOARTHRITIS, FAMILIAL HISTIOCYTIC
2160 MYXOMA, INTRACARDIAC
2161 FEVER, FAMILIAL MEDITERRANEAN (FMF)
2162 CATARACT-RENAL TUBULAR NECROSIS-ENCEPHALOPATHY, CROME TYPE
2163 HIP, CONGENITAL DISLOCATED
2164 FOOT, TALIPES EQUINOVARUS (TEV)
2165 NEVUS, CONGENITAL NEVOMELANOCYTIC
2166 FOLATE MALABSORPTION
2167 ACROFACIAL DYSOSTOSIS, NAGER TYPE
2168 GLYCOGENOSIS, TYPE Ib
2169 BIEMOND II SYNDROME
2170 CHARLIE M SYNDROME
2172 FACIAL DYSMORPHIA-JOINT HYPEREXTENSIBILITY SYNDROME
2173 NEUROECTODERMAL SYNDROME, FLYNN-AIRD TYPE
2174 CERVICO-DERMO-GU SYNDROME, GOEMINNE TYPE
2175 GROWTH DEFICIENCY-FACIAL DEFECTS-BRACHYDACTYLY
2176 GROWTH-MENTAL DEFICIENCY, MYHRE TYPE
2177 HERRMANN-PALLISTER-OPITZ SYNDROME
2178 HOOFT DISEASE
2179 OCULO-CEREBRO-FACIAL SYNDROME, KAUFMAN TYPE
2180 LACRIMO-AURICULO-DENTO-DIGITAL SYNDROME
2181 LETTERER-SIWE DISEASE
2184 CRANIOSYNOSTOSIS-FIBULAR APLASIA, LOWRY TYPE
2185 CRANIO-FRONTO-NASAL DYSPLASIA
2186 PTERYGIUM SYNDROME, MULTIPLE
2187 NEPHROSIS-HYDROCEPHALUS-THIN SKIN-BLUE SCLERA-GROWTH DEFECT
2188 OCULO-OTO-NASAL MALFORMATIONS WITH OSTEO-ONYCHO DYSPLASIA
2189 PALLISTER-KILLIAN MOSAIC SYNDROME
2191 CAMPTODACTYLY SYNDROME, GUADALAJARA TYPE II

2192 OVERGROWTH, MACROCEPHALY-HEMANGIOMA, RILEY-SMITH TYPE
2193 MARSHALL-SMITH SYNDROME
2194 DIGITO-PALATAL SYNDROME, STEVENSON TYPE
2195 WEAVER-WILLIAMS SYNDROME
2196 IMMUNODEFICIENCY, ADENOSINE DEAMINASE DEFICIENCY
2197 IMMUNODEFICIENCY, AGRANULOCYTOSIS, INFANTILE KOSTMANN TYPE
2198 HYDROPS FETALIS, NON-IMMUNE
2201 COMPLEMENT COMPONENT 2, DEFICIENCY OF
2210 IMMUNODEFICIENCY, X-LINKED LYMPHOPROLIFER-ATIVE DISEASE
2211 IMMUNODEFICIENCY, HYPER IgE TYPE
2214 IMMUNODEFICIENCY, MYELOPEROXIDASE DEFICIENCY TYPE
2215 NEUTROPENIA, BENIGN FAMILIAL
2216 IMMUNODEFICIENCY, NEZELOF TYPE
2217 IMMUNODEFICIENCY, TUFTSIN DEFICIENCY TYPE
2219 COMPLEMENT COMPONENT 3, DEFICIENCY OF
2220 COMPLEMENT COMPONENT 4, DEFICIENCY OF
2222 SIALIC ACID STORAGE DISEASE, INFANTILE TYPE
2224 BRANCHIO-OTO-RENAL DYSPLASIA
2226 RETT SYNDROME
2227 OSTEODYSPLASIA, LIPOMEMBRANOUS POLYCYSTIC-DEMENTIA
2228 ACYL-CoA DEHYDROGENASE DEFICIENCY, LONG CHAIN TYPE
2229 FIBULA, CONGENITAL ABSENCE OF
2230 HAWKINSINURIA
2231 CHROMOSOME 9, PARTIAL MONOSOMY 9p
2232 INFLAMMATORY BOWEL DISEASE
2233 PEPTIC ULCER DISEASES, NON-SYNDROMIC
2234 ULCER-LEUKONYCHIA-GALLSTONES
2235 MAXILLONASAL DYSPLASIA, BINDER TYPE
2236 FETAL EFFECTS FROM MATERNAL PKU
2237 OSTEOPATHIA STRIATA-CRANIAL SCLEROSIS-MEGALENCEPHALY
2238 CHROMOSOME TETRAPLOIDY
2239 HIP, DYSPLASIA, NAMAQUALAND TYPE
2240 OPSISMODYSPLASIA
2241 OVERGROWTH-RENAL HAMARTOMA, PERLMAN TYPE
2242 FACES SYNDROME
2243 TEETH, ANKYLODONTIA, MULTIPLE HERITABLE TYPE
2244 SPONDYLOEPIMETAPHYSEAL DYSPLASIA-JOINT LAXITY
2245 CHROMOSOME 11, PARTIAL MONOSOMY 11p
2246 CARDIOMYOPATHY-GENITAL DEFECTS
2249 SCHISIS ASSOCIATION
2250 AMYLOIDOSIS, FAMILIAL CUTANEOUS
2251 MUCOLIPIDOSIS IV
2252 NECK, CYSTIC HYGROMA, FETAL TYPE
2253 OSTEOPETROSIS, MILD RECESSIVE
2254 FETAL BRAIN DISRUPTION SEQUENCE
2255 CAMPTODACTYLY
2256 CAMPTODACTYLY SYNDROME, TEL HASHOMER TYPE
2257 CAMPTODACTYLY SYNDROME, GUADALAJARA TYPE I
2258 OTO-PALATO-DIGITAL SYNDROME, II
2259 INTESTINAL POLYPOSIS, JUVENILE TYPE
2260 FETAL D-PENICILLAMINE SYNDROME
2261 FETAL RETINOID SYNDROME
2263 ACROCALLOSAL SYNDROME, SCHINZEL TYPE
2264 HYPOMELANOSIS OF ITO
2265 FRYNS SYNDROME
2266 MENINGOCELE-CONOTRUNCAL HEART DEFECT, KOUSSEFF TYPE
2267 DIGITO-TALAR DYSMORPHISM
2270 SHORT RIB-POLYDACTYLY SYNDROME, VERMA-NAUMOFF TYPE

2271 FRASER SYNDROME
2272 BORJESON-FORSSMAN-LEHMANN SYNDROME
2273 ACROFACIAL SYNDROME, CURRY-HALL TYPE
2274 PTERYGIUM SYNDROME, MULTIPLE LETHAL
2275 CONTRACTURES, CONGENITAL LETHAL FINNISH TYPE
2276 THUMB, TRIPHALANGEAL
2277 THUMB, TRIPHALANGEAL-DUPLICATED GREAT TOES
2278 PHYTANIC ACID OXIDASE DEFICIENCY, INFANTILE TYPE
2279 HYDROLETHALUS SYNDROME
2280 ARTHROGRYPOSIS, DISTAL TYPES
2281 ARTHROGRYPOSIS, AMYOPLASIA TYPE
2284 ACROCEPHALOSYNDACTYLY TYPE V
2285 HYPOTHALAMIC HAMARTOBLASTOMA SYNDROME, CONGENITAL
2286 GLYCEROL INTOLERANCE SYNDROME
2287 EYE, IRIDOPLEGIA, FAMILIAL
2288 HIP, OSTEONECROSIS, CAPITAL FEMORAL EPIPHYSIS
2289 ACIDEMIA, GLUTARIC ACIDEMIA II
2291 X-LINKED MENTAL RETARDATION-CLASPED THUMB
2292 HAND, ULNAR AND FIBULAR RAY DEFICIENCY, WEYERS TYPE
2293 GROWTH RETARDATION-ALOPECIA-PSEUDOANODONTIA-OPTIC ATROPHY
2294 TRICHOMEGALY-RETARDATION-DWARFISM-RETINAL PIGMENTARY DEGENERATION
2295 CUTIS VERTICUS GYRATA
2296 CUTIS MARMORATA
2297 FETAL DIETHYLSTILBESTROL (DES) EFFECTS
2298 LEYDIG CELL HYPOPLASIA
2299 STEROID 17-KETOSTEROID REDUCTASE DEFICIENCY
2300 HYPOGONADOTROPIC HYPOGONADISM
2301 KALLMANN SYNDROME
2302 HYPERCALCIURIA, FAMILIAL IDIOPATHIC
2303 GLYCOGEN STORAGE DISEASE, X-LINKED WITH NORMAL HEPATIC ENZYMES
2304 OTO-SPONDYLO-MEGAEPIPHYSEAL DYSPLASIA
2305 TOURETTE SYNDROME
2306 CHOREA, BENIGN FAMILIAL
2307 ARTERY, RENAL FIBROMUSCULAR DYSPLASIA
2308 GYNECOMASTIA DUE TO INCREASED AROMATASE ACTIVITY, FAMILIAL
2309 SKIN, CUTANEOUS MELANOSIS, DIFFUSE
2310 GLYCEROL KINASE DEFICIENCY
2311 DISTICHIASIS-HEART DEFECT-PERIPHERAL VASCULAR DISEASE/ANOMALIES
2313 SPONDYLOEPIMETAPHYSEAL DYSPLASIA
2314 HAIR, HYPERTRICHOSIS, X-LINKED
2315 GINGIVAL FIBROMATOSIS-DEAFNESS, JONES TYPES
2316 MEGACYSTIS-MEGADUODENUM SYNDROME
2317 INTESTINAL HYPOPERISTALSIS, MEGACYSTIS-MICROCOLON TYPE
2318 CANCER, MALIGNANT MELANOMA, FAMILIAL
2319 MEGALENCEPHALY
2320 AICARDI SYNDROME
2322 DEAFNESS-HYPOGONADISM
2323 ACYL-CoA DEHYDROGENASE DEFICIENCY, SHORT CHAIN TYPE
2324 ACYL-CoA DEHYDROGENASE DEFICIENCY, MEDIUM CHAIN TYPE
2325 CHROMOSOME 1, MONOSOMY 1q
2326 DIABETES MELLITUS, MATURITY ONSET OF THE YOUNG (MODY)
2327 DIABETES MELLITUS, NON-INSULIN DEPENDENT TYPE
2328 DIABETES MELLITUS, MUTANT INSULIN TYPES
2330 INTESTINAL PSEUDO-OBSTRUCTION SYNDROMES
2331 ONYCHO-TRICHODYSPLASIA-NEUTROPENIA
2332 OSTEOCHONDRODYSPLASIA WITH HYPERTRICHOSIS

2333 MICROCEPHALY WITH CHORIORETINOPATHY
2334 MICROCEPHALY, ISOLATED AUTOSOMAL DOMINANT TYPE
2335 CHROMOSOME 9, TETRASOMY 9p
2336 CHROMOSOME 18, TETRASOMY 18p
2337 DERMO-FACIO-CARDIO-SKELETAL SYNDROME
2338 SHORT STATURE-MENTAL RETARDATION-DELAYED SEXUAL MATURITY
2339 FACIO-NEURO-SKELETAL SYNDROME
2340 SHORT STATURE-CEREBRAL ATROPHY-KERATOSIS FOLLICULARIS, X-LINKED
2341 ATAXIA-DYSMORPHIC FACIES-TRICHODYSPLASIA
2342 CATARACT, AUTOSOMAL DOMINANT CONGENITAL
2343 CANCER, COLORECTAL
2344 INTESTINAL POLYPOSIS, TYPE II
2345 DEAFNESS-MALFORMED EARS-MENTAL RETARDATION
2346 HAIR, ATRICHIA CONGENITA
2348 CHROMOSOME 2, TRISOMY DISTAL 2q
2349 CHROMOSOME 2, MONOSOMY OF MEDIAL 2q
2350 PERRAULT SYNDROME
2351 CANCER, BREAST, FAMILIAL
2352 CANCER, HODGKIN DISEASE, FAMILIAL
2354 ALZHEIMER DISEASE, FAMILIAL
2355 KABUKI MAKE-UP SYNDROME
2356 ALBINISM-BLACK LOCKS-DEAFNESS
2357 ALBINISM, OCULOCUTANEOUS, BROWN TYPE
2358 ALBINISM, OCULOCUTANEOUS, RUFOUS TYPE
2359 ALBINOIDISM
2360 HYPOPIGMENTATION-IMMUNE DEFECT, GRISCELLI TYPE
2361 NEUROECTODERMAL MELANOLYSOSOMAL SYNDROME
2362 SKIN, HYPERPIGMENTATION, FAMILIAL
2363 BARDET-BIEDL SYNDROME
2364 OCULO-FACIAL SYNDROME, BENCZE TYPE
2365 ABRUZZO-ERICKSON SYNDROME
2366 CHONDRODYSTROPHY-SENSORINEURAL DEAFNESS, NANCE-INSLEY TYPE
2368 ORO-PALATAL-DIGITAL SYNDROME, VARADI TYPE
2369 DONLAN SYNDROME
2370 TERATOMA, PRESACRAL-SACRAL DYSGENESIS
2371 JAUNDICE, INTRAHEPATIC CHOLESTATIC, BYLER TYPE
2374 CANCER, PANCREAS, FAMILIAL ADENOCARCINOMA OF
2377 ACIDEMIA, ETHYLMALONIC-ADIPIC
2380 SACROCOCCYGEAL DYSGENESIS SYNDROME
2381 OVERGROWTH, BANNAYAN TYPE
2382 PROTEUS SYNDROME
2385 FETAL EFFECTS FROM MATERNAL HYPERTHERMIA
2386 HYPOBETALIPOPROTEINEMIA
2387 TIBIAL APLASIA/HYPOPLASIA
2388 TIBIAL HYPOPLASIA/APLASIA-ECTRODACTYLY
2390 NEUROPATHY, CONGENITAL SENSORY WITH ANHIDROSIS
2392 EPITHELIOMAS, HEREDITARY MULTIPLE CYSTIC
2393 SKIN CREASES, RETICULATE PIGMENTED FLEXURES, DOWLING-DEGOS TYPE
2394 HYPERAPOBETALIPOPROTEINEMIA
2395 XANTHOMATOSIS, CEREBROTENDINOUS
2396 CAMPTODACTYLY-CLEFT PALATE-CLUB FOOT, GORDON TYPE
2397 HIP, CONGENITAL COXA VARA
2398 ACANTHOCYTOSIS-NEUROLOGIC DEFECTS
2400 HYDATIDIFORM MOLE
2401 ARRHYTHMIA, CARDIAC CONDUCTION DEFECTS, NEONATAL
2402 DIGITAL FIBROMA, RECURRING IN INFANTS & CHILDREN
2403 APLASIA CUTIS CONGENITA-GASTROINTESTINAL ATRESIA

2404 HOMOCYSTINURIA, N(5,10) METHYLENE TETRAHYDROFOLATE DEFICIENCY TYPE
2405 YUNIS-VARON SYNDROME
2406 MURCS ASSOCIATION
2407 URETHRAL VALVES, POSTERIOR
2408 VESICO-URETERAL REFLUX
2409 HAND, RADIAL CLUB HAND
2410 HAND, ULNAR DRIFT
2411 XANTHINE OXIDASE DEFICIENCY
2412 MOLYBDENUM CO-FACTOR DEFICIENCY
2414 VENTRICLE, DOUBLE CHAMBERED RIGHT
2415 GALLBLADDER, AGENESIS
2419 CHARCOT MARIE TOOTH DISEASE-DEAFNESS
2421 DYSEQUILIBRIUM SYNDROME
2422 HUTTERITE SYNDROME, BOWEN-CONRADI TYPE
2423 LIPODYSTROPHY-COARSE FACIES-ACANTHOSIS NIGRICANS, MIESCHER TYPE
2424 ARTHRO-OPHTHALMOPATHY, WEISSENBACHER-ZWEYMULLER VARIANT
2425 TELECANTHUS, HEREDITARY
2426 CHROMOSOME 1, TRISOMY 1q32-qter
2428 CHROMOSOME 1, TRISOMY 1q25-1q32
2429 CHROMOSOME 1, MONOSOMY 1q4
2430 CHROMOSOME 3, TRISOMY 3q2
2431 CHROMOSOME 3, MONOSOMY 3p2
2432 CHROMOSOME 3, TRISOMY 3p2
2433 CHROMOSOME 4, TRISOMY 4p
2434 CHROMOSOME 4, TRISOMY DISTAL 4q
2435 CHROMOSOME 4, MONOSOMY DISTAL 4q
2436 CHROMOSOME 5, TRISOMY 5p
2437 CHROMOSOME 5, TRISOMY 5q3
2438 CHROMOSOME 6, TRISOMY 6p2
2439 CHROMOSOME 6, TRISOMY 6q2
2440 CHROMOSOME 6, RING 6
2442 CHROMOSOME 7, TRISOMY 7q2-3
2443 CHROMOSOME 7, MONOSOMY 7q3
2444 CHROMOSOME 7, MONOSOMY 7q2
2445 CHROMOSOME 7, MONOSOMY 7q1
2446 CHROMOSOME 7, TRISOMY 7p2
2447 CHROMOSOME 7, MONOSOMY 7p2
2449 CHROMOSOME 8, TRISOMY 8p
2450 CHROMOSOME 8, MONOSOMY 8p2
2451 CHROMOSOME 9, TRISOMY 9p
2452 CHROMOSOME 9, TRISOMY 9
2453 CHROMOSOME 9, TRISOMY 9q3
2454 CHROMOSOME 9, RING 9
2455 CHROMOSOME 10, TRISOMY 10q2
2456 CHROMOSOME 10, TRISOMY 10p
2457 CHROMOSOME 10, MONOSOMY 10p
2458 CHROMOSOME 10, MONOSOMY 10q2
2459 CHROMOSOME 11, TRISOMY 11p
2461 CHROMOSOME 12, MONOSOMY 12p
2462 CHROMOSOME 12, TRISOMY 12q2
2463 CHROMOSOME 13, TRISOMY DISTAL 13q
2464 CHROMOSOME 13, TRISOMY 13q1
2465 CHROMOSOME 13, MONOSOMY 13q3
2466 CHROMOSOME 14, TRISOMY 14q
2467 CHROMOSOME 14, RING 14
2468 CHROMOSOME 15, RING 15
2469 CHROMOSOME 16, TRISOMY 16p
2470 CHROMOSOME 16, TRISOMY 16q
2471 CHROMOSOME 17, TRISOMY 17q2
2472 CHROMOSOME 18, TRISOMY 18q2
2473 CHROMOSOME 18, RING 18
2474 CHROMOSOME 19, TRISOMY 19q
2475 CHROMOSOME 20, TRISOMY 20p
2476 CHROMOSOME 21, RING 21
2477 CHROMOSOME 22, RING 22
2478 CHROMOSOME 22, TRISOMY MOSAICISM
2479 SEIZURES, IN FEMALES, JUBERG-HELLMAN TYPE
2480 X-LINKED MENTAL RETARDATION-GROWTH-HEARING AND GENITAL DEFECTS
2486 ACHEIROPODY

2487 APROSOPIA
2488 SKIN CREASES, ABSENT DISTAL INTERPHALANGEAL
2491 EMERY-DREIFUSS SYNDROME
2492 KING SYNDROME
2493 MUSCULAR ATROPHY, SPINAL AND BULBAR,
    X-LINKED KENNEDY TYPE
2494 LIMBS, SUPERNUMERARY
2495 FETAL METHYLMERCURY EFFECTS
2496 FETAL VALPROATE SYNDROME
2497 FETAL ACQUIRED IMMUNE DEFICIENCY SYNDROME
    (AIDS) INFECTION
2498 FETAL EFFECTS FROM MATERNAL DIABETES
2499 FETAL EFFECTS FROM VARICELLA-ZOSTER
2500 UMBILICAL CORD, SINGLE ARTERY
2501 LUNG, CONGENITAL LOBAR ADENOMATOSIS
2502 OSTEOFIBROUS DYSPLASIA OF TIBIA AND FIBULA
2505 TRACHEOMALACIA
2506 VOCAL CORD PARALYSIS
2508 CRANIODIAPHYSEAL DYSPLASIA, LENZ-MAJEWSKI
    TYPE
2509 FETAL MULTIPLE CYSTS ANOMALY
2510 FETAL EFFECTS FROM MATERNAL CARBON
    MONOXIDE EXPOSURE
2511 CRANIOSYNOSTOSIS-FOOT DEFECTS,
    JACKSON-WEISS TYPE
2512 MAXILLOFACIAL DYSOSTOSIS
2513 CHROMOSOME 17, INTERSTITIAL DELETION 17p
2514 HEMANGIOMAS OF THE HEAD AND NECK
2515 LUPUS ERYTHEMATOSUS, SYSTEMIC
2516 ANKYLOSING SPONDYLITIS
2517 ARTHRITIS, RHEUMATOID
2518 CHROMOSOME 6, MONOSOMY DISTAL 6q
2519 CHROMOSOME 16, MONOSOMY 16q
2520 IMMUNODEFICIENCY WITH CENTROMERIC
    INSTABILITY
2521 ATELOSTEOGENESIS
2522 SKELETAL DYSPLASIA, BOOMERANG DYSPLASIA
2523 FOOT, METATARSUS VARUS
2524 IMMUNODEFICIENCY, X-LINKED WITH HYPER IgM
2526 HALLERVORDEN-SPATZ DISEASE
2527 UROFACIAL SYNDROME
2528 ACROCEPHALOPOLYDACTYLOUS DYSPLASIA
2532 ICHTHYOSIS, X-LINKED WITH STEROID SULFATASE
    DEFICIENCY
2533 ADRENOLEUKODYSTROPHY, X-LINKED
2534 ICHTHYOSIS VULGARIS
2535 CHROMOSOMES, COMPLEX REARRANGEMENTS
2536 CHROMOSOME 1, TRISOMY-MONOSOMY 1 MOSAIC
2537 CHROMOSOME 22, MONOSOMY 22q
2538 CHROMOSOME, NUCLEOLAR ORGANIZER REGION,
    TRANSLOCATION
2539 CHROMOSOME 14, MONOSOMY 14q (q24.3-q32.1)
2540 CHROMOSOME 20, PERICENTRIC INVERSION
2542 SKELETAL DYSPLASIA, WEISMANN-NETTER-STUHL
    TYPE
2543 CHROMOSOME 6, MONOSOMY PROXIMAL 6q
2544 CHROMOSOME 5, MONOSOMY 5q INTERSTITIAL
2547 CHROMOSOME 14, TRISOMY 14 MOSAIC
2548 CHROMOSOME 15, TRISOMY 15q1
2550 CHROMOSOME 18, TRISOMY 18p AND q11
2551 CHROMOSOME INSTABILITY, NIJMEGEN TYPE
2552 CHROMOSOME XYY
2553 CHROMOSOME 7, MOSAIC TRISOMY 7
2554 CHROMOSOME 4, RING 4
2556 MARTSOLF SYNDROME
2558 HAIR, UNCOMBABLE-CRYSTALLINE CATARACT
2559 TRICHOTHIODYSTROPHY
2560 EPIDERMOLYSIS BULLOSUM, TYPE I
2561 EPIDERMOLYSIS BULLOSUM, TYPE II
2562 EPIDERMOLYSIS BULLOSUM, TYPE III
2563 BRANCHIO-OCULO-FACIAL SYNDROME
2564 ACIDEMIA, MEVALONIC
2565 ACIDEMIA, 2-OXOGLUTARIC

2566 SPASTIC ATAXIA, CHARLEVOIX-SAGUENAY TYPE
2567 SEIZURES, MYOCLONIC, JUVENILE JANZ TYPE
2568 SEIZURES, FEBRILE
2569 SKELETAL DYSPLASIA, 3-M TYPE
2570 HAND-FOOT-GENITAL SYNDROME
2571 OSTEOGLOPHONIC DYSPLASIA
2572 NEVI-ATRIAL MYXOMA-MYXOID NEUROFIBROMAS-
    EPHELIDES
2573 URACHAL ANOMALIES
2574 OMPHALOMESENTERIC DUCT ANOMALIES
2575 HERNIA, UMBILICAL
2576 UMBILICAL CORD, MULTIPLE VESSELS
2578 RAG SYNDROME
2579 CLEFT PALATE-DYSMORPHIC FACIES-DIGITAL
    DEFECTS, MARTSOLF TYPE
2580 FOUNTAIN SYNDROME
2581 DWARFISM, OSTEODYSPLASTIC PRIMORDIAL,
    MAJEWSKI-WINTER TYPE
2582 DWARFISM, OSTEODYSPLASTIC PRIMORDIAL,
    MAJEWSKI-RANKE TYPE
2584 DWARFISM, MICROCEPHALIC PRIMORDIAL WITH
    CATARACTS
2585 ORO-FACIO-DIGITAL SYNDROME, BARAITSER-BURN
    TYPE
2586 ORO-FACIO-DIGITAL SYNDROME, WHELAN TYPE
2587 CARDIO-FACIAL-CUTANEOUS SYNDROME
2588 EPIGLOTTIS, VALLECULAR CYST
2589 PILOMATRIXOMA
2590 ECTODERMAL DYSPLASIA, HAY-WELLS TYPE
2591 BIOTINIDASE DEFICIENCY
2592 ORO-FACIO-DIGITAL SYNDROME, THURSTON TYPE
2593 PROGERIA, NEONATAL RAUTENSTRAUCH-
    WIEDEMANN TYPE
2595 SPONDYLOMETAPHYSEAL DYSPLASIA WITH
    ENCHONDROMATOUS CHANGES
2596 OSTEOLYSIS, ESSENTIAL
2597 NOSE, CHOANAL ATRESIA-LYMPHEDEMA
2598 MULTIPLE SCLEROSIS, FAMILIAL
2599 ACIDURIA, FUMARIC
2600 SPLEEN, CONGENITAL ISOLATED HYPOSPLENIA
2601 SEIZURES, PROGRESSIVE MYOCLONIC, LAFORA
    TYPE
2602 SEIZURES, PROGRESSIVE MYOCLONIC,
    UNVERRICHT-LUNDBORG TYPE
2603 FETAL EFFECTS FROM MATERNAL COCAINE ABUSE
2604 ALACRIMA-APTYALISM
2605 METHYLCOBALAMIN DEFICIENCY
2606 HYPOVENTILATION, CONGENITAL CENTRAL
    ALVEOLAR TYPE
2607 SKIN CREASE, SINGLE PALMAR
2608 RENAL TUBULAR DYSGENESIS
2610 GINGIVAL FIBROMATOSIS-CHERUBISM-SEIZURES,
    RAMON TYPE
2611 DIABETES INSIPIDIS, NEUROHYPOPHYSEAL TYPE
2614 LIPODYSTROPHY, FAMILIAL LIMB AND TRUNK
2615 HEMIFACIAL ATROPHY, PROGRESSIVE
2616 PROLIDASE DEFICIENCY
2617 PYLORODUODENAL ATRESIA, HEREDITARY
2618 ODONTO-ONYCHODERMAL DYSPLASIA
2619 SPINOCEREBELLAR DEGENERATION-CORNEAL
    DYSTROPHY
2623 POLYGLANDULAR AUTOIMMUNE SYNDROME
2624 TRANSCOBALAMIN II DEFICIENCY
2626 PSEUDOLEPRECHAUNISM, PATTERSON TYPE
2627 RETINOPATHY-HYPOTRICHOSIS SYNDROME
2628 PSEUDOAMINOPTERIN SYNDROME
2629 STIFF SKIN SYNDROME
2631 SKELETAL DYSPLASIA, DE LA CHAPELLE TYPE
2632 SKELETAL DYSPLASIA, SCHNECKENBECKEN TYPE
2634 GENITO-PALATO-CARDIAC SYNDROME
2635 SMITH-LEMLI-OPITZ SYNDROME, TYPE II
2636 PILO-DENTO-UNGULAR DYSPLASIA WITH
    MICROCEPHALY

2638 HAND, LOCKING DIGITS-GROWTH DEFECT
2639 MICROCEPHALY-LYMPHEDEMA
2640 X-LINKED MENTAL RETARDATION, CLARK-BARAITSER TYPE
2641 CANCER, THYROID, FAMILIAL PAPILLARY CARCINOMA OF
2642 MICHELIN TIRE BABY SYNDROME
2643 RADIAL-RENAL-OCULAR SYNDROME
2644 POLYDACTYLY-DISTAL OBSTRUCTIVE UROPATHY
2646 ANEMIA, HEMOLYTIC, RED CELL MEMBRANE DEFECTS
2647 ANEMIA, HEINZ BODY
2650 ANEMIA, DYSERYTHROPOIETIC, TYPE III
2651 ANEMIA, DYSERYTHROPOIETIC, TYPE I
2652 ANEMIA, DYSERYTHROPOIETIC, TYPE II
2656 ANEMIA, PERNICIOUS CONGENITAL
2657 ANEMIA, HEMOLYTIC, ERYTHROCYTE PHOSPHOGLYCERATE KINASE DEFICIENCY
2659 ANEMIA, CONGENITAL SIDEROBLASTIC, NOT B(6) RESPONSIVE
2660 ANEMIA, ADENYLATE KINASE DEFICIENCY
2661 AFIBROGINEMIA, CONGENITAL
2662 ERYTHROCYTE ALDOLASE-A DEFICIENCY
2664 ERYTHROCYTE, DIPHOSPHOGLYCERATE MUTASE (2,3) DEFICIENCY
2665 ELLIPTOCYTOSIS
2666 EOSINOPHILIA, FAMILIAL
2667 ANEMIA, HEMOLYTIC, ERYTHROCYTE PHOSPHOLIPID DEFECT
2668 FACTOR V DEFICIENCY
2669 FACTOR VII DEFICIENCY
2670 FACTOR X DEFICIENCY
2671 FACTOR XI DEFICIENCY
2672 FACTOR XII DEFICIENCY
2673 FACTOR XIII (FIBRIN STABILIZING FACTOR)
2674 COAGULATION DEFECT, FAMILIAL MULTIPLE FACTORS
2675 ANEMIA, HEMOLYTIC, GLUTATIONINE PEROXIDASE DEFICIENCY
2676 ANEMIA, HEMOLYTIC, GLUTATHIONE REDUCTASE DEFICIENCY
2677 ANEMIA, HEMOLYTIC, GLUTATHIONE SYNTHETASE DEFICIENCY
2678 ANEMIA, HEMOLYTIC, ERYTHROCYTE HEXOKINASE DEFICIENCY
2679 HYPOPROTHROMBINEMIA
2681 LEUKOCYTE, MAY-HEGGLIN ANOMALY
2682 METHEMOGLOBINEMIA, NADH-DEPENDENT DIAPHORASE DEFICIENCY
2683 THROMBASTHENIA, GLANZMANN-NAEGELI TYPE
2686 ERYTHROCYTE TRIOSEPHOSPHATE ISOMERASE DEFICIENCY
2687 RENAL DYSPLASIA-RETINAL APLASIA, LOKEN-SENIOR TYPE
2688 IMMUNODEFICIENCY, RETICULOENDOTHELIOSIS WITH EOSINOPHILIA
2689 CANCER, RENAL CELL CARCINOMA
2690 DWARFISM, DYSSEGMENTAL, ROLLAND-DESBUQUOIS TYPE
2691 HYPEROSTOSIS, WORTH TYPE
2692 DYSOSTOSIS, CHEIROLUMBAR
2694 FIBROCHONDROGENESIS
2695 OSTEOMESOPYKNOSIS
2696 SKELETAL DYSPLASIA, FUHRMANN TYPE
2698 DYSOSTOSIS, HUMEROSPINAL
2699 EPIPHYSEAL DYSPLASIA, MULTIPLE RIBBING TYPE
2701 NEUROAXONAL DYSTROPHY, INFANTILE
2702 LUNG, BRONCHOGENIC CYST
2703 LUNG, EMPHYSEMA CONGENITAL LOBAR
2705 MUSCULAR DYSTROPHY, CONGENITAL WITH MENTAL RETARDATION
2706 MUSCULAR DYSTROPHY, CONGENITAL WITH ARTHROGRYPOSIS

2707 MYOPATHY-METABOLIC, MITOCHONDRIAL CYTOCHROME C OXIDASE DEFICIENCY
2709 MYOPATHY-METABOLIC, MYOADENYLATE DEAMINASE DEFICIENCY
2710 MYOPATHY, MALIGNANT HYPERTHERMIA
2711 ALBINISM, OCULOCUTANEOUS, MINIMAL PIGMENT TYPE
2712 ALEXANDER DISEASE
2714 ATAXIA, FRIEDREICH TYPE
2716 ACROMICRIC DYSPLASIA
2718 NOSE, ANTERIOR STENOSIS
2719 NOSE, DISLOCATED NASAL SEPTUM
2720 NOSE, TURBINATE DEFORMITY
2721 SALIVARY GLAND LYMPHANGIOMA
2722 SALIVARY GLAND, AGENESIS
2723 BRANCHIAL CLEFT CYSTS
2724 SALIVARY GLAND, DERMOID CYST
2725 SALIVARY GLAND, DUCTAL CYST
2726 SALIVARY GLAND, HEMANGIOMA
2730 CHONDRODYSPLASIA PUNCTATA, X-LINKED DOMINANT TYPE
2731 FETAL VENEZUELAN EQUINE ENCEPHALITIS INFECTION
2732 FETAL LITHIUM EFFECTS
2733 FETAL EFFECTS OF POLYCHLORINATED BIPHENYL (PCB)
2734 FETAL EFFECTS FROM MATERNAL EXTRINSIC ANDROGENS
2736 CANCER, NEUROBLASTOMA
2739 TURCOT SYNDROME
2742 CANCER, WILMS TUMOR
2743 CANCER, SEBACEOUS GLAND TUMOR-MULTIPLE VISCERAL CARCINOMA
2744 CANCER, MULTIPLE MYELOMA
2745 CANCER, THYMOMA
2746 CANCER, GASTRIC FAMILIAL
2747 CANCER, LUNG, FAMILIAL
2748 CANCER, NEUROEPITHELIAL AND MENINGEAL
2749 CANCER, SOFT TISSUE SARCOMA
2750 ANEMIA, GLUCOSE PHOSPHATE ISOMERASE DEFICIENCY
2752 OCULO-CEREBRO-CUTANEOUS SYNDROME
2754 KYPHOMELIC DYSPLASIA
2755 MICROCEPHALY-HIATUS HERNIA-NEPHROSIS, GALLOWAY TYPE
2756 ACROMEGALOID FACIAL APPEARANCE SYNDROME
2757 RESTRICTIVE DERMATOPATHY
2758 CATARACT-MICROCORNEA SYNDROME
2759 CLEFTING-ECTROPION-CONICAL TEETH
2760 CORNEO-DERMATO-OSSEOUS SYNDROME
2761 CRANIOFACIAL-DEAFNESS-HAND SYNDROME
2762 DEAFNESS-EAR DEFECTS-FACIAL PALSY
2763 DERMO-ODONTODYSPLASIA
2764 EXOSTOSES-ANETODERMIA-BRACHYDACTYLY TYPE E
2765 ALOPECIA-ANOSMIA-DEAFNESS-HYPOGONADISM, JOHNSON TYPE
2766 DWARFISM, LETHAL, SHORT-LIMBED PLATYSPONDYLIC TYPE
2767 FACIAL CLEFTING SYNDROME, GYPSY TYPE
2768 METAPHYSEAL DYSPLASIA-MAXILLARY HYPOPLASIA-BRACHYDACTYLY
2769 PARIETAL FORAMINA-CLAVICULAR HYPOPLASIA
2770 PTERYGIA-DYSMORPHIC FACIES-SHORT STATURE-MENTAL RETARDATION
2771 RADIAL-RENAL SYNDROME
2772 RADIAL HYPOPLASIA-TRIPHALANGEAL THUMBS-HYPOSPADIAS-DIASTEMA
2774 PHARYNX/LARYNX HYPOPLASIA-OMPHALOCELE, SHPRINTZEN-GOLDBERG TYPE
2775 THORACOPELVIC DYSOSTOSIS
2776 PULMONIC STENOSIS-CAFE-AU-LAIT SPOTS, WATSON TYPE

2777 ABLEPHARON-MACROSTOMIA
2778 ACRO-RENAL-MANDIBULAR SYNDROME
2779 ACRO-FRONTO-FACIO-NASAL DYSOSTOSIS
2780 AGNATHIA-HOLOPROSENCEPHALY
2781 ALBINISM-MICROCEPHALY-DIGITAL DEFECTS
2782 ALOPECIA-SKELETAL ANOMALIES-SHORT
     STATURE-MENTAL RETARDATION
2783 ALOPECIA-MENTAL RETARDATION
2784 ANOPHTHALMIA-LIMB ANOMALIES
2785 AREDYLD SYNDROME
2786 HYDROCEPHALUS-HEART DEFECT-DENSE BONES,
     BEEMER TYPE
2787 COCKAYNE SYNDROME, TYPE II
2789 BLINDNESS (CORTICAL)-RETARDATION-POSTAXIAL
     POLYDACTYLY
2790 CRANIOSYNOSTOSIS-MENTAL RETARDATION-
     CLEFTING SYNDROME
2791 CRANIOTELENCEPHALIC DYSPLASIA
2792 DIGITO-RENO-CEREBRAL SYNDROME
2793 ECTODERMAL DYSPLASIA-ECTRODACTYLY-
     MACULAR DYSTROPHY
2794 ECTRODACTYLY-POLYDACTYLY
2795 CEREBRO-NEPHRO-OSTEODYSPLASIA, HUTTERITE
     TYPE
2796 HYPOGONADISM-DIABETES-ALOPECIA-DEAFNESS-
     RETARDATION-EKG ANOMALIES
2797 HYPOGONADISM-PARTIAL ALOPECIA
2799 KNIEST-LIKE DYSPLASIA
2800 LARSEN SYNDROME, LETHAL TYPE
2801 LYMPHEDEMA-HYPOPARATHYROIDISM
2802 MANDIBULOFACIAL DYSOSTOSIS, TREACHER
     COLLINS TYPE, RECESSIVE
2805 RENAL MESANGIAL SCLEROSIS-EYE DEFECTS
2807 DIGITAL DEFECTS-NODULAR ERYTHEMA-
     EMACIATION, NAKAJO TYPE
2808 DWARFISM, OCULO-PALATO-CEREBRAL TYPE
2809 CLEFT PALATE-OMPHALOCELE
2810 OTO-ONYCHO-PERONEAL SYNDROME
2811 PERICARDITIS-ARTHRITIS-CAMPTODACTYLY
2812 DWARFISM (SHORT LIMBED)-PETERS ANOMALY OF
     THE EYE
2813 TRICHODENTAL DYSPLASIA WITH REFRACTIVE
     ERRORS
2814 DWARFISM-DYSMORPHIC FACIES-RETARDATION,
     PITT TYPE
2815 POLYSYNDACTYLY-CARDIAC MALFORMATIONS
2816 RHIZOMELIC SYNDROME, URBACH TYPE
2818 DWARFISM, SHORT-RIB, BEEMER TYPE
2819 AORTIC STENOSIS-CORNEAL CLOUDING-GROWTH
     AND MENTAL RETARDATION
2820 SYNDACTYLY-MICROCEPHALY-MENTAL
     RETARDATION, FILIPPI TYPE
2821 THANATOPHORIC DYSPLASIA, GLASGOW TYPE
2822 LIMB DEFECT WITH ABSENT ULNA/FIBULA
2823 ALBINISM, WAARDENBURG TYPE-HIRSCHSPRUNG
     AGANGLIONOSIS
2824 ALBINISM, OCULAR-LATE-ONSET-SENSORINEURAL
     DEAFNESS, X-LINKED
2825 BRANCHIAL ARCH SYNDROME, X-LINKED
2826 SIMPSON-GOLABI-BEHMEL SYNDROME
2828 HYPERKERATOSIS PALMOPLANTARIS-SPASTIC
     PARAPLEGIA-RETARDATION
2829 SILVER SYNDROME, X-LINKED
2830 X-LINKED MENTAL RETARDATION-
     CHOREOATHETOSIS
2831 CRANIO-DIGITAL SYNDROME-MENTAL
     RETARDATION, SCOTT TYPE
2832 CONTRACTURES-MUSCLE ATROPHY-OCULOMOTOR
     APRAXIA
2833 ECTODERMAL DYSPLASIA-ADRENAL CYST
2834 LIPODYSTROPHY-RIEGER ANOMALY-SHORT
     STATURE-DIABETES

2836 CORNEAL ANESTHESIA-RETINAL DEFECTS-
     UNUSUAL FACIES-HEART DEFECT
2838 MICROCEPHALY, AUTOSOMAL RECESSIVE WITH
     NORMAL INTELLIGENCE
2839 CANCER, GLIOMA, FAMILIAL
2840 X-LINKED MENTAL RETARDATION, ATKIN TYPE
2841 X-LINKED MENTAL RETARDATION-BASAL
     GANGLION DISORDER
2842 ALOPECIA-SKIN ATROPHY-ANONYCHIA-TONGUE
     DEFECT
2845 SMITH-FINEMAN-MYERS SYNDROME
2846 RETINOPATHY-MICROCEPHALY-MENTAL
     RETARDATION
2847 TRICHO-RHINO-PHALANGEAL SYNDROME, TYPE III
2848 TRACHEA, AGENESIS
2849 TRACHEAL AGENESIS-MULTIPLE ANOMALY
     ASSOCIATION
2851 AMYLOIDOSIS, FAMILIAL LICHEN
2852 ICHTHYOSIFORM HYPERKERATOSIS, BULLOUS
     CONGENITAL
2853 ICHTHYOSIS, LAMELLAR RECESSIVE
2854 ICHTHYOSIS, LAMELLAR DOMINANT
2855 ICHTHYOSIS, CONGENITAL ERYTHRODERMIC
2856 ICHTHYOSIS, HARLEQUIN FETUS
2857 ICHTHYOSIS HYSTRIX, CURTH-MACKLIN TYPE
2858 ICHTHYOSIS, LINEARIS CIRCUMFLEXA
2859 STORAGE DISEASE, NEUTRAL LIPID TYPE
2860 SULFATASE DEFICIENCY, MULTIPLE
2861 ICHTHYOSIFORM ERYTHROKERATODERMA,
     ATYPICAL WITH DEAFNESS
2862 SKIN, ERYTHROKERATOLYSIS HIEMALIS
2863 SKIN, ERYTHROKERATODERMIA, PROGRESSIVA
     SYMMETRICA
2864 SKIN PEELING SYNDROME
2865 DARIER DISEASE
2866 GIROUX-BARBEAU SYNDROME
2867 SKIN, KERATOSIS FOLLICULARIS SPINULOSA
     DECALVANS
2868 MYOPATHY-METABOLIC, GLYCOPROTEIN-
     GLYCOSAMINOGLYCANS STORAGE TYPE
2869 WALKER-WARBURG SYNDROME
2870 ACHONDROGENESIS, HOUSTON-HARRIS TYPE
2871 GLYCOGENOSIS, TYPE Ic
2873 GLYCOGENOSIS, TYPE IIb
2874 GLYCOGENOSIS, TYPE IIc
2875 GLYCOGENOSIS, TYPE IId
2877 GLYCOGENOSIS, TYPE V
2878 GLYCOGENOSIS, TYPE IXb
2879 GLYCOGENOSIS, TYPE IXc
2880 AMYLOIDOSIS, ASHKENAZI TYPE
2881 AMYLOIDOSIS, APPALACHIAN TYPE
2882 AMYLOIDOSIS, ILLINOIS TYPE
2883 DOPAMINE BETA-HYDROXYLASE DEFICIENCY,
     CONGENITAL
2884 THUMB, TRIPHALANGEAL-BRACHYECTRODACTYLY
2885 LIMB, REDUCTION DEFORMITIES OF UPPER LIMBS
2887 ODONTO-TRICHOMELIC SYNDROME
2889 TRICHO-ODONTO-ONYCHIAL DYSPLASIA
2890 ODONTO-ONYCHODYSPLASIA-ALOPECIA
2892 TRICHO-ONYCHODYSPLASIA-XERODERMA
2894 TRICHODYSPLASIA-XERODERMA
2895 SKIN, PAINFUL PLANTAR CALLOSITIES
2897 NEURO-FACIO-DIGITO-RENAL SYNDROME
2898 CLEFT LIP/PALATE-OLIGODONTIA-SYNDACTYLY-
     HAIR DEFECTS
2903 TRICHO-DERMODYSPLASIA-DENTAL DEFECTS
2904 X-LINKED MENTAL RETARDATION-SKELETAL
     DYSPLASIA
2905 PACHYONYCHIA CONGENITA-STEATOCYSTOMA
     MULTIPLEX
2906 HAIR, MONILETHRIX
2907 WRINKLY SKIN SYNDROME
2908 JOUBERT SYNDROME

2909 AORTA, COARCTATION, INFANTILE TYPE
2910 DIPHALLIA
2912 MYASTHENIC SYNDROME, CONGENITAL SLOW CHANNEL TYPE
2913 MYASTHENIC SYNDROME, FAMILIAL INFANTILE TYPE
2915 CRANIOSYNOSTOSIS-ARACHNODACTYLY-HERNIA
2918 PROTEIN C DEFICIENCY
2919 TERATOMAS
2920 X-LINKED MENTAL RETARDATION, RENPENNING TYPE
2921 X-LINKED MENTAL RETARDATION, MARFANOID HABITUS TYPE
2922 SCALP DEFECTS-POSTAXIAL POLYDACTYLY
2924 SPONDYLOCOSTAL DYSOSTOSIS-VISCERAL DEFECTS-DANDY WALKER CYST
2925 POLYSYNDACTYLY-DYSMORPHIC CRANIOFACIES, GREIG TYPE
2926 FETAL EFFECTS FROM METHIMAZOLE AND CARBIMAZOLE
2927 FETAL EFFECTS FROM MATERNAL VASODILATOR
2928 TWINS, CONJOINED, TERATOGENICITY
2929 FETAL BENZODIAZEPINE EFFECTS
2930 FETAL BARBITURATE EFFECTS
2931 CEREBRAL PALSY
2932 LIMB, UPPER HYPOPLASIA-MULLERIAN DUCT DEFECTS
2933 INTESTINAL ATRESIAS, MULTIPLE
2934 JEJUNAL ATRESIA
2935 DWARFISM, DYSSEGMENTAL, SILVERMAN-HANDMAKER TYPE
2936 HYDROCEPHALUS-COSTOVERTEBRAL DYSPLASIA-SPRENGEL ANOMALY
2937 SKELETAL BOWING-CORTICAL THICKENING-BONE FRAGILITY-ICTHYOSIS
2938 KNEE, GENU RECURVATUM
2939 PLAGIOCEPHALY
2940 TORTICOLLIS
2941 EYELID, COLOBOMA
2944 BRAIN, ARNOLD-CHIARI MALFORMATION
2945 ERYTHROCYTE, LACTATE TRANSPORTER DEFECT
2946 LYMPHOHISTIOCYTOSIS, FAMILIAL ERYTHROPHAGOCYTIC
2947 IMMUNODEFICIENCY, IgG SUBCLASS DEFICIENCIES
2950 PROTEIN S DEFICIENCY
2952 GLUCOCORTICOID RESISTANCE
2953 RESISTANCE TO 1,25 DIHYDROXY VITAMIN D
2954 ANDROGEN INSENSITIVITY (RESISTANCE), MINIMAL
2955 UMBILICAL CORD, SHORT
2956 UMBILICAL CORD, LONG
2957 UMBILICAL CORD, SHORT UMBILICAL CORD SYNDROME
2958 FETAL MONOZYGOUS MULTIPLE PREGNANCY DYSPLACENTATION EFFECTS
2960 FETAL EFFECTS OF MATERNAL CIGARETTE SMOKING
2961 FETAL DEVELOPMENTAL RETARDATION WITH MATERNAL HYPERTENSION
2962 FETAL ANGIOTENSIN CONVERTING ENZYME (ACE) INHIBITION RENAL FAILURE
2965 PAPILLOMA VIRUS, CONGENITAL INFECTION
2966 SARCOIDOSIS
2967 ACIDURIA, 3-METHYLGLUTACONIC TYPE I
2968 ACIDURIA, 3-METHYLGLUTACONIC TYPE II
2970 GRANULOCYTE GLYCOPROTEIN CD11/CD18 DEFICIENCY
2975 LEUKODYSTROPHY, ADULT-ONSET PROGRESSIVE DOMINANT TYPE
2976 SYNDACTYLY, CENANI TYPE
2977 CUTIS LAXA-DELAYED DEVELOPMENT-LIGAMENTOUS LAXITY
2979 FRONTO-FACIO-NASAL DYSPLASIA
2980 FETAL PARVOVIRUS INFECTION

2981 GASTROCUTANEOUS SYNDROME
2982 FETAL PRIMIDONE EMBRYOPATHY
2984 GAMMA-AMINOBUTYRIC ACID (GABA) TRANSAMINASE DEFICIENCY
2986 FETAL EFFECTS FROM ANGEL DUST (PHENCYCLIDINE OR PCP)
2988 FETAL HERPES SIMPLEX VIRUS INFECTION
2990 HYPERLYSINURIA, ISOLATED
2991 FETAL CARBAMAZEPINE EXPOSURE
2992 FETAL AMINOGLYCOSIDE OTOTOXICITY
2993 OVULATION INDUCTION TRISOMY
2994 VITAMIN B(12) LYSOSOMAL TRANSPORT DEFECT
2995 BRONCHOMALACIA
2996 MACHADO-JOSEPH DISEASE
2998 BRAIN, PORENCEPHALY
2999 BRAIN, MICROPOLYGYRIA
3000 BRAIN, MIDLINE CAVES
3001 BRAIN, SCHIZENCEPHALY
3002 BRAIN, ARACHNOID CYSTS
3003 SPINE, SCOLIOSIS, IDIOPATHIC
3004 SPINE, SPONDYLOLISTHESIS AND SPONDYLOLYSIS
3005 DYSLEXIA
3006 CHROMOSOME X, TRIPLO-X
3007 CHROMOSOME X, POLY-X
3008 FETAL EFFECTS FROM HEPATITIS B INFECTION
3009 HYPERBILIRUBINEMIA, CONJUGATED
3010 ICHTHYOSIS-CHEEK-EYEBROW SYNDROME
3012 PROGEROID SYNDROME WITH EHLERS-DANLOS FEATURES
3013 NEUROPATHY, CONGENITAL MOTOR & SENSORY-SKELETAL-LARYNGEAL DEFECTS
3014 SHORT STATURE-WORMIAN BONES-JOINT DISLOCATIONS
3015 BLADDER EXSTROPHY
3018 KIDNEY, NEPHRONOPHTHISIS-MEDULLARY CYSTIC DISEASE
3019 KIDNEY, MEDULLARY SPONGE KIDNEY
3020 RICKETS, HEREDITARY HYPOPHOSPHATEMIC WITH HYPERCALCIURIA (HHRH)
3022 CARBAMOYL PHOSPHATE SYNTHETASE DEFICIENCY
3023 ORNITHINE TRANSCARBAMYLASE DEFICIENCY
3026 NEPHROSIS-NERVE DEAFNESS-HYPOPARATHY-ROIDISM, BARAKAT TYPE
3028 KIDNEY, RENAL DYSPLASIA, POTTER TYPE II
3029 AASE-SMITH SYNDROME
3030 TRIGONENCEPHALY, AUTOSOMAL DOMINANT TYPE
3031 ALOPECIA-SEIZURES-MENTAL RETARDATION, SHOKEIR TYPE
3032 CORPUS CALLOSUM AGENESIS-SENSORIMOTOR NEUROPATHY, FAMILIAL
3033 ANGIOLIPOMATOSIS
3034 BIEMOND I SYNDROME
3035 BRACHYDACTYLY-LONG THUMB SYNDROME
3036 BRACHYOLMELIA, HOBAEK TYPE
3037 BRANCHIO-OTO-URETERAL SYNDROME
3038 POIKILODERMA, HEREDITARY ACROKERATOTIC, KINDLER-WEARY TYPE
3039 CHANDS
3040 POLYPOSIS-ALOPECIA-PIGMENTATION-NAIL DEFECTS
3041 EDINBURGH MALFORMATION SYNDROME
3042 SYNDACTYLY-POLYDACTYLY-EAR LOBE SYNDROME
3043 IVIC SYNDROME
3044 DERMATO-OSTEOLYSIS, KIRGHIZIAN TYPE
3045 LARYNGEAL ABDUCTOR PARALYSIS-MENTAL RETARDATION
3046 DEAFNESS-NEPHRITIS-MACROTHROMBOPATHIA
3047 MUSCLE-EYE-BRAIN SYNDROME
3048 EPIPHYSEAL DYSPLASIA, MULTIPLE-DIABETES MELLITUS
3049 NASOPALPEBRAL LIPOMA-COLOBOMA SYNDROME
3050 OCULO-RENO-CEREBELLAR SYNDROME

3051 SKIN, PARANA HARD SKIN SYNDROME
3052 ACRO-OSTEOLYSIS, NEUROGENIC
3053 SPLENOGONADAL FUSION-LIMB DEFECT
3054 SPONDYLOPERIPHERAL DYSPLASIA
3055 STERNAL MALFORMATION-VASCULAR DYSPLASIA ASSOCIATION
3056 ECTODERMAL DYSPLASIA, RAPP-HODGKIN TYPE
3058 ORO-FACIO-DIGITAL SYNDROME, SUGARMAN TYPE
3059 SPONDYLOEPIMETAPHYSEAL DYSPLASIA, STRUDWICK TYPE
3060 STUTTERING
3061 THYROID, THYROGLOBULIN DEFECTS
3062 STEROID 5 ALPHA-REDUCTASE DEFICIENCY
3063 ERYTHROBLASTOSIS FETALIS
3064 PORPHYRIA CUTANEA TARDA
3065 MALARIA, VIVAX, SUSCEPTIBILITY TO
3066 ANTITHROMBIN III DEFICIENCY
3068 ACROKERATOELASTOIDOSIS
3069 OPTIC ATROPHY, KJER TYPE
3072 MYOPATHY OR CARDIOMYOPATHY DUE TO DESMIN DEFECT
3073 LEUKEMIA, ACUTE LYMPHOCYTIC, FAMILIAL
3074 ALCOHOL INTOLERANCE
3076 SCLEROTYLOSIS
3077 HYPOCERULOPLASMINEMIA
3079 DIPHTHERIA, SUSCEPTIBILITY TO
3080 LARYNGEAL PARALYSIS
3081 BONE, PAGET DISEASE
3082 RAGWEED POLLEN SENSITIVITY
3083 PLASMINOGEN DEFECTS
3086 RENAL TUBULAR ACIDOSIS-OSTEOPETROSIS SYNDROME
3089 LYMPHOMA, BURKITT TYPE
3090 INTERFERON DEFICIENCY
3091 DELTA-AMINOLEVULINIC ACID DEHYDRASE DEFICIENCY
3092 LEUKEMIA, CHRONIC MYELOID (CML)
3095 LEUKEMIA/LYMPHOMA, T-CELL
3096 HYPOALPHALIPOPROTEINEMIA
3097 LEUKEMIA/LYMPHOMA, B-CELL
3100 GROWTH DEFICIENCY, AFRICAN PYGMY TYPE
3101 OSTEOSARCOMA
3103 MENTAL RETARDATION, HEMOGLOBIN H RELATED
3104 ADENINE PHOSPHO-RIBOSYL-TRANSFERASE (APRT) DEFICIENCY
3106 AMYLOIDOSIS, HEMODIALYSIS-RELATED
3107 LYMPHOMA, NON-HODGKIN
3109 POLIO, SUSCEPTIBILITY TO
3110 GALACTOSIALIDOSIS
3112 CANCER, EWING SARCOMA
3113 ADENYLOSUCCINATE MONOPHOSPHATE LYASE DEFICIENCY
3116 DEAFNESS WITH PERILYMPHATIC GUSHER
3118 CHOLESTASIS-LYMPHEDEMA, AAGENAES TYPE
3120 ECTODERMAL DYSPLASIA, PASSARGE TYPE
3121 PENTALOGY OF CANTRELL
3122 NEPHROSIS-DEAFNESS-URINARY TRACT AND DIGITAL DEFECTS
3124 URTICARIA, DERMO-DISTORTIVE TYPE
3126 PILI TORTI-CLEFT LIP/PALATE-SYNDACTYLY
3127 SPONDYLOEPIPHYSEAL DYSPLASIA-MENTAL RETARDATION
3128 LIMB REDUCTION-MENTAL RETARDATION
3129 THORACIC DYSPLASIA-HYDROCEPHALUS
3130 AURAL ATRESIA-DYSMORPHIC FACIES-SKELETAL DEFECTS
3131 MICROCEPHALY-RETARDATION-SKELETAL AND IMMUNE DEFECTS
3132 MENTAL RETARDATION-HEART DEFECTS-BLEPHAROPHIMOSIS
3133 RETINA, VITREORETINOPATHY, FAMILIAL EXUDATIVE

3134 RETINA, CONGENITAL HYPERTROPHY OF RETINAL PIGMENT EPITHELIUM
3135 RETINA, COATS DISEASE
3137 EYE, GOLDMANN-FAVRE DISEASE
3138 CRYOGLOBULINEMIA
3139 WILMS TUMOR-PSEUDOHERMAPHRODITISM-GLOMERULOPATHY,DENYS-DRASH TYPE
3140 NEUROPATHY, GIANT AXONAL
3141 GRANULOMATOSIS-POLYSYNOVITIS, FAMILIAL SYSTEMIC
3142 FOOT, VERTICAL TALUS
3143 BRACHYOLMELIA, MAROTEAUX TYPE
3144 BRACHYOLMELIA, DOMINANT TYPE
3145 WT SYNDROME
3146 KIDNEY, GLOMERULOCYSTIC
3147 X-LINKED MENTAL RETARDATION-SHORT STATURE-OBESITY-HYPOGONADISM
3148 HEMOLYTIC-UREMIC SYNDROME
3150 SKIN, ATOPY, FAMILIAL
3151 HAIR, HYPOTRICHOSIS
3155 LIVER, CONGENITAL CYSTIC DILATATION OF INTRAHEPATIC DUCTS
3158 OPTIC DISK, MORNING GLORY ANOMALY
3159 EYE, ORBITAL TERATOMA, CONGENITAL
3161 URORECTAL SEPTUM MALFORMATION SEQUENCE
3163 GERM CELL APLASIA
3165 APOLIPOPROTEIN A-I AND C-III DEFICIENCY STATES
3166 COLLAGENOMA, MULTIPLE CUTANEOUS, FAMILIAL
3167 CRETINISM, ENDEMIC, AND RELATED DISORDERS
3169 HYPERORNITHINEMIA-HYPERAMMONEMIA-HOMOCITRULLINURIA
3170 N-ACETYLGLUTAMATE SYNTHETASE DEFICIENCY
3171 LENZ MICROPHTHALMIA SYNDROME
3173 CATARACT, HUTTERITE
3174 CATARACT, COPPOCK
3176 RETINA, CAVERNOUS HEMANGIOMA
3179 BROWN SYNDROME
3180 EYE, DUANE RETRACTION SYNDROME
3183 FORSIUS-ERIKSSON SYNDROME
3184 CORNEA, CENTRAL CLOUDY DYSTROPHY OF FRANCOIS
3185 EYE, FIBROSIS OF THE EXTRAOCULAR MUSCLES, GENERALIZED
3186 EYE, LIGNEOUS CONJUNCTIVITIS
3190 FACIO-CARDIOMELIC DYSPLASIA, LETHAL
3191 SIRENOMELIA SEQUENCE
3193 EXSTROPHY OF CLOACA SEQUENCE
3194 FETAL EFFECTS FROM MATERNAL LEAD EXPOSURE
3195 HYPERGONADOTROPIC HYPOGONADISM WITH CARDIOMYOPATHY
3197 ACROFACIAL DYSOSTOSIS-CLEFT LIP/PALATE-TRIPHALANGEAL THUMB
3198 CORNEAL DYSTROPHY, STROMAL, CONGENITAL HEREDITARY
3199 X-LINKED MENTAL RETARDATION, GOLABI-ITO-HALL TYPE
3200 X-LINKED MENTAL RETARDATION-CRANIOFACIAL ABNORMALITIES-CLUB FOOT
3201 LIVER, POLYCYSTIC AND MULTICYSTIC DISEASE, ADULT TYPE
3203 RETINA, GROUPED HYPERTROPHY OF RETINAL PIGMENT EPITHELIUM
3204 NIGHTBLINDNESS, CONGENITAL STATIONARY, AUTOSOMAL RECESSIVE
3205 NIGHTBLINDNESS, CONGENITAL STATIONARY, AUTOSOMAL DOMINANT
3206 SKIN, CUTANEOUS MELANOSIS: MONGOLIAN SPOT
3210 COMPLEMENT COMPONENT 1, DEFICIENCY OF
3211 CAUDAL REGRESSION SYNDROME
3212 FETAL EFFECTS FROM LYME DISEASE
3214 ICHTHYOSIS-COLOBOMA-HEART DEFECT-DEAFNESS-MENTAL RETARDATION
3215 G(M1)-GANGLIOSIDOSIS, TYPE 3

3216 CONVULSIONS, BENIGN FAMILIAL NEONATAL
3217 EPILEPSY, BENIGN CHILDHOOD WITH
　　　CENTROTEMPORAL EEG FOCUS (BEC)
3218 EPILEPSY, BENIGN OCCIPITAL
3219 OCCIPITAL HORN SYNDROME
3220 ARTICULAR HYPERMOBILITY, FAMILIAL
3221 ANEMIA, HEMOLYTIC, GAMMA-GLUTAMYL/
　　　CYSTEINE SYNTHETASE DEFICIENCY
3222 MICROVILLUS INCLUSION DISEASE
3223 MIGRAINE
3224 MYOPATHY, MITOCHONDRIAL-ENCEPHALOPATHY-
　　　LACTIC ACIDOSIS-STROKE
3225 MYOCLONIC EPILEPSY-RAGGED RED FIBERS
3226 LIPID TRANSPORT DEFECT OF INTESTINE
3227 APO B-100, DEFECTIVE, FAMILIAL
3228 RETINA, CONE DYSTROPHY, X-LINKED
3229 ACHOO SYNDROME
3230 THYROTOXICOSIS
3232 TAURODONTISM-SHORT ROOTED TEETH-
　　　MICROCEPHALIC DWARFISM
3233 PTERYGIUM SYNDROME, POPLITEAL, LETHAL
3234 CARDIOMYOPATHY, FAMILIAL DILATED
3235 ANIRIDIA-CEREBELLAR ATAXIA-MENTAL
　　　DEFICIENCY
3236 MUCOSA, ORAL INCLUSION CYSTS OF THE
　　　NEWBORN
3237 HYPERBILIRUBINEMIA, CONJUGATED, ROTOR TYPE
3238 HYPERBILIRUBINEMIA, TRANSIENT FAMILIAL
　　　NEONATAL
3239 EPILEPSY, REFLEX
3240 ATTENTION-DEFICIT HYPERACTIVITY DISORDER
　　　(ADHD)
3241 TRIMETHYLAMINURIA
3242 OCULO-ENCEPHALO-HEPATO-RENAL SYNDROME
3243 PICK DISEASE OF THE BRAIN
3244 CREUTZFELDT-JAKOB DISEASE
3245 GERSTMANN-STRAUSSLER SYNDROME
3246 HAUPTMANN-THANHAUSER SYNDROME
3248 X-LINKED MENTAL RETARDATION-SUBCORTICAL
　　　ATROPHY-PATELLAR LUXATION
3249 X-LINKED MENTAL RETARDATION-MUSCULAR
　　　WEAKNESS-AWKWARD GAIT
3250 X-LINKED MENTAL RETARDATION-Xq DUPLICATION
3251 X-LINKED MENTAL RETARDATION-DYSTONIC
　　　MOVEMENTS OF THE HANDS
3252 X-LINKED MENTAL RETARDATION-PSORIASIS

3254 ALPHA-N-ACETYLGALACTOSAMINIDASE
　　　DEFICIENCY
3255 PEMPHIGUS, BENIGN FAMILIAL
3256 ACROKERATOSIS VERRUCIFORMIS
3257 CRANDALL SYNDROME
3258 SHOVAL-SOFFER SYNDROME
3259 OPHTHALMO-MANDIBULO-MELIC DWARFISM
3260 HYPEREKPLEXIA
3261 ALPERS DISEASE
3262 POIKILODERMA, SCLEROSING, HEREDITARY
3263 URTICARIA PIGMENTOSA (UP)
3264 KERATOSIS PALMARIS ET PLANTARIS OF
　　　UNNA-THOST
3265 HEART-HAND SYNDROME II
3266 HEART-HAND SYNDROME III
3267 SAY-MEYER SYNDROME
3268 HIRSCHPRUNG DISEASE-MICROCEPHALY-
　　　COLOBOMA
3269 HIRSCHSPRUNG DISEASE-POLYDACTYLY-DEAFNESS
3270 JUMPING FRENCHMAN OF MAINE
3271 ISAACS-MERTENS SYNDROME
3272 HEART-HAND SYNDROME IV
3273 NEVO SYNDROME
3274 MUTCHINICK SYNDROME
3275 ACIDEMIA, TRIHYDROXYCOPROSTANIC
3276 CHOLESTASIS, INTRAHEPATIC, RECURRENT BENIGN
3277 BILE DUCTS, INTERLOBULAR, NONSYNDROMIC
　　　PAUCITY
3278 INTRAHEPATIC CHOLESTASIS OF PREGNANCY (ICP)
3279 ALPHA-1-ANTICHYMOTRYPSIN DEFICIENCY
3280 OMODYSPLASIA
3281 FETAL EFFECTS OF NONSTEROIDAL
　　　ANTI-INFLAMMATORY DRUGS (NSAIDS)
3282 EYE, MACULAR DYSTROPHY, NORTH CAROLINA
　　　TYPE
3283 DENTATORUBROPALLIDOLUYSIAN DEGENERATION,
　　　HEREDITARY
3284 CYSTIC HYGROMA
3285 LIMB REDUCTION DEFECTS
3286 HIRSCHSPRUNG DISEASE-CARDIAC DEFECT
3287 NARCOLEPSY
3288 KIDNEY, POLYCYSTIC DISEASE-CATARACT-
　　　BLINDNESS
3289 MAL DE MELEDA
3290 HOWEL-EVANS SYNDROME

# MIM-NUMBER-TO-PRIME-NAME INDEX

|  | 10005 | AARSKOG SYNDROME |
|  | 10010 | PRUNE-BELLY SYNDROME |
| * | 10030 | LIMB AND SCALP DEFECTS, ADAMS-OLIVER TYPE |
| * | 10050 | ACANTHOCYTOSIS-NEUROLOGIC DEFECTS |
| * | 10060 | SKIN, ACANTHOSIS NIGRICANS |
| * | 10065 | ALCOHOL INTOLERANCE |
| * | 10080 | ACHONDROPLASIA |
| * | 10100 | ACOUSTIC NEUROMATA |
|  | 10112 | ACROCEPHALOPOLYSYNDACTYLY |
| * | 10120 | ACROCEPHALOSYNDACTYLY TYPE I |
| * | 10140 | ACROCEPHALOSYNDACTYLY TYPE III |
| * | 10160 | ACROCEPHALOPOLYSYNDACTYLY |
| * | 10160 | ACROCEPHALOSYNDACTYLY TYPE V |
|  | 10180 | ACRODYSOSTOSIS |
| * | 10185 | ACROKERATOELASTOIDOSIS |
| * | 10190 | ACROKERATOSIS VERRUCIFORMIS |
| * | 10210 | ACROMEGALOID PHENOTYPE-CUTIS VERTICIS GYRATA-CORNEAL LEUKOMA |
| * | 10215 | ACROMEGALOID FACIAL APPEARANCE SYNDROME |
|  | 10237 | ACROMICRIC DYSPLASIA |
|  | 10240 | ACRO-OSTEOLYSIS, DOMINANT TYPE |
|  | 10249 | RADIAL-RENAL-OCULAR SYNDROME |
| * | 10250 | HAJDU-CHENEY SYNDROME |
| * | 10250 | OSTEOLYSIS, ESSENTIAL |
| * | 10251 | ACROPECTOROVERTEBRAL DYSPLASIA |
| * | 10260 | ADENINE PHOSPHO-RIBOSYL-TRANSFERASE (APRT) DEFICIENCY |
| * | 10270 | IMMUNODEFICIENCY, ADENOSINE DEAMINASE DEFICIENCY |
| * | 10300 | ANEMIA, ADENYLATE KINASE DEFICIENCY |
| * | 10302 | ANEMIA, ADENYLATE KINASE DEFICIENCY |
| * | 10303 | ANEMIA, ADENYLATE KINASE DEFICIENCY |
| * | 10305 | ADENYLOSUCCINATE MONOPHOSPHATE LYASE DEFICIENCY |
|  | 10330 | HYPOGLOSSIA-HYPODACTYLIA |
| * | 10358 | PARATHYROID HORMONE RESISTANCE |
| * | 10360 | ANALBUMINEMIA |
|  | 10370 | ALCOHOL INTOLERANCE |
|  | 10372 | ALCOHOL INTOLERANCE |
|  | 10373 | ALCOHOL INTOLERANCE |
|  | 10375 | ALCOHOL INTOLERANCE |
| * | 10385 | ERYTHROCYTE ALDOLASE-A DEFICIENCY |
| * | 10390 | HYPERALDOSTERONISM, FAMILIAL GLUCOCORTICOID SUPPRESSIBLE |
|  | 10400 | HAIR, ALOPECIA AREATA |
| * | 10413 | ALOPECIA-SEIZURES-MENTAL RETARDATION, SHOKEIR TYPE |
| * | 10417 | ALPHA-N-ACETYLGALACTOSAMINIDASE DEFICIENCY |
| * | 10420 | NEPHRITIS-DEAFNESS (SENSORINEURAL), HEREDITARY TYPE |
| * | 10430 | ALZHEIMER DISEASE, FAMILIAL |
| * | 10450 | TEETH, AMELOGENESIS IMPERFECTA |
| * | 10453 | TEETH, AMELOGENESIS IMPERFECTA |
| * | 10457 | AMELO-ONYCHO-HYPOHIDROTIC SYNDROME |
| * | 10476 | ALZHEIMER DISEASE, FAMILIAL |
| * | 10480 | AMYLOIDOSIS, TRANSTHYRETIN METHIONINE-30 TYPE |
|  | 10490 | AMYLOIDOSIS, APPALACHIAN TYPE |
|  | 10490 | AMYLOIDOSIS, INDIANA TYPE |
|  | 10500 | AMYLOIDOSIS, DANISH CARDIAC TYPE |
| * | 10510 | AMYLOIDOSIS, IOWA TYPE |
| * | 10512 | AMYLOIDOSIS, FINNISH TYPE |
| * | 10515 | AMYLOIDOSIS, ICELANDIC TYPE |
| * | 10520 | AMYLOIDOSIS, FAMILIAL VISCERAL |
| * | 10521 | AMYLOIDOSIS, OHIO TYPE |
| * | 10525 | AMYLOIDOSIS, FAMILIAL LICHEN |
|  | 10527 | AMYLOIDOSIS, TRANSTHYRETIN METHIONINE-30 TYPE |
| * | 10540 | AMYOTROPHIC LATERAL SCLEROSIS |
| * | 10540 | AMYOTROPHIC LATERAL SCLEROSIS, FAMILIAL ADULT AND JUVENILE TYPES |
| * | 10540 | AMYOTROPHIC LATERAL SCLEROSIS, GUAM TYPE |
|  | 10555 | AMYOTROPHIC LATERAL SCLEROSIS |
|  | 10555 | AMYOTROPHIC LATERAL SCLEROSIS, FAMILIAL ADULT AND JUVENILE TYPES |
|  | 10558 | CANCER, COLORECTAL |
| * | 10560 | ANEMIA, DYSERYTHROPOIETIC, TYPE III |
|  | 10565 | ANEMIA, HYPOPLASTIC CONGENITAL |
| * | 10610 | ANGIOEDEMA, HEREDITARY |
| * | 10620 | ANIRIDIA |
| * | 10621 | ANIRIDIA |
| * | 10621 | CHROMOSOME 11, PARTIAL MONOSOMY 11p |
|  | 10622 | ANIRIDIA |
|  | 10624 | PUPIL, ANISOCORIA |
|  | 10625 | CLEFT LIP/PALATE-FILIFORM FUSION OF EYELIDS |
|  | 10626 | ECTODERMAL DYSPLASIA, HAY-WELLS TYPE |
|  | 10628 | TONGUE, ANKYLOGLOSSIA |
| * | 10630 | ANKYLOSING SPONDYLITIS |
| * | 10660 | TEETH, ANODONTIA, PARTIAL OR COMPLETE |
|  | 10670 | PULMONARY VENOUS CONNECTION, TOTAL ANOMALOUS |
|  | 10670 | SCIMITAR SYNDROME |
|  | 10690 | ECTRODACTYLY-ANONYCHIA |
|  | 10700 | NAIL-PATELLA SYNDROME |
|  | 10720 | ANOSMIA, CONGENITAL |
| * | 10725 | EYE, ANTERIOR SEGMENT DYSGENESIS |
| * | 10728 | ALPHA-1-ANTICHYMOTRYPSIN DEFICIENCY |
| * | 10730 | ANTITHROMBIN III DEFICIENCY |
| * | 10740 | ALPHA(1)-ANTITRYPSIN DEFICIENCY |
| * | 10748 | ANUS-HAND-EAR SYNDROME |
| * | 10755 | AORTIC ARCH INTERRUPTION |
| * | 10760 | SKIN, LOCALIZED ABSENCE OF |
|  | 10766 | HYPOALPHALIPOPROTEINEMIA |
| * | 10768 | APOLIPOPROTEIN A-I AND C-III DEFICIENCY STATES |
| * | 10768 | HYPOALPHALIPOPROTEINEMIA |
| * | 10769 | HYPOALPHALIPOPROTEINEMIA |
| * | 10771 | HYPOALPHALIPOPROTEINEMIA |
| * | 10773 | APO B-100, DEFECTIVE, FAMILIAL |
| * | 10791 | GYNECOMASTIA DUE TO INCREASED AROMATASE ACTIVITY, FAMILIAL |
|  | 10805 | ARTHRITIS-ARTERITIS SYNDROME |
|  | 10811 | ARTHROGRYPOSES |
|  | 10811 | ARTHROGRYPOSIS, AMYOPLASIA TYPE |
|  | 10812 | ARTHROGRYPOSIS, DISTAL TYPES |
|  | 10813 | ARTHROGRYPOSIS, DISTAL TYPES |
|  | 10820 | MUSCLE WASTING OF HANDS-SENSORINEURAL DEAFNESS |
| * | 10830 | ARTHRO-OPHTHALMOPATHY, HEREDITARY, PROGRESSIVE, STICKLER TYPE |
| * | 10830 | ARTHRO-OPHTHALMOPATHY, WEISSENBACHER-ZWEYMULLER VARIANT |
| * | 10833 | CANCER, LUNG, FAMILIAL |
|  | 10872 | ATELOSTEOGENESIS |
| * | 10876 | EAR, AUDITORY CANAL ATRESIA |
| * | 10880 | ATRIAL SEPTAL DEFECTS |
| * | 10900 | AURICULO-OSTEODYSPLASIA |
| * | 10915 | MACHADO-JOSEPH DISEASE |
| * | 10920 | HAIR, BALDNESS, COMMON |
| * | 10927 | ANEMIA, HEMOLYTIC, RED CELL MEMBRANE DEFECTS |

* 10940 NEVOID BASAL CELL CARCINOMA SYNDROME
  10950 BASILAR IMPRESSION, PRIMARY
* 10970 AMYLOIDOSIS, HEMODIALYSIS-RELATED
  10973 AORTIC VALVE, BICUSPID
  10974 NOSE, BIFID
  10990 BLEPHAROCHALASIS-DOUBLE LIP-NONTOXIC
        GOITER
  11005 BLEPHARO-NASO-FACIAL SYNDROME
* 11010 BLEPHAROPTOSIS-BLEPHAROPHIMOSIS-
        EPICANTHUS INVERSUS-TELECANTHUS
* 11070 MALARIA, VIVAX, SUSCEPTIBILITY TO
* 11170 ERYTHROBLASTOSIS FETALIS
* 11220 NEVUS, BLUE RUBBER BLEB NEVUS SYNDROME
* 11230 HYPERHIDROSIS-PREMATURE
        GREYING-PREMOLAR APLASIA
  11235 SKELETAL DYSPLASIA, WEISMANN-NETTER-
        STUHL TYPE
  11243 BRACHYDACTYLY-LONG THUMB SYNDROME
* 11250 BRACHYDACTYLY
* 11260 BRACHYDACTYLY
* 11270 BRACHYDACTYLY
* 11300 BRACHYDACTYLY
* 11310 BRACHYDACTYLY
* 11320 BRACHYDACTYLY
* 11330 BRACHYDACTYLY
  11340 BIEMOND I SYNDROME
  11350 BRACHYOLMELIA, DOMINANT TYPE
* 11360 NECK, BRANCHIAL CLEFT, CYSTS OR SINUSES
  11362 BRANCHIO-OCULO-FACIAL SYNDROME
* 11365 BRANCHIO-OTO-RENAL DYSPLASIA
  11370 BREAST, AMASTIA
* 11371 CANCER, BREAST, FAMILIAL
* 11380 ICHTHYOSIFORM HYPERKERATOSIS, BULLOUS
        CONGENITAL
* 11400 CORTICAL HYPEROSTOSIS, INFANTILE
* 11414 SKIN, PAINFUL PLANTAR CALLOSITIES
* 11420 CAMPTODACTYLY
* 11430 CAMPTODACTYLY-CLEFT PALATE-CLUB FOOT,
        GORDON TYPE
* 11440 CANCER, BREAST, FAMILIAL
* 11440 CANCER, FAMILIAL
* 11440 CANCER, GASTRIC FAMILIAL
* 11440 CANCER, SEBACEOUS GLAND
        TUMOR-MULTIPLE VISCERAL CARCINOMA
* 11440 CANCER, SOFT TISSUE SARCOMA
  11448 CANCER, BREAST, FAMILIAL
  11450 CANCER, COLORECTAL
  11462 DERMO-FACIO-CARDIO-SKELETAL SYNDROME
  11481 RENAL TUBULAR ACIDOSIS-OSTEOPETROSIS
        SYNDROME
  11515 CARDIO-FACIAL-CUTANEOUS SYNDROME
* 11520 CARDIOMYOPATHY, FAMILIAL DILATED
  11525 COLLAGENOMA, MULTIPLE CUTANEOUS,
        FAMILIAL
  11547 CAT EYE SYNDROME
* 11550 ACATALASEMIA
* 11565 CATARACT, POLAR AND CAPSULAR
* 11570 CATARACT, AUTOSOMAL DOMINANT
        CONGENITAL
* 11570 CATARACT, CORTICAL AND NUCLEAR
* 11580 CATARACT, AUTOSOMAL DOMINANT
        CONGENITAL
* 11580 CATARACT, CORTICAL AND NUCLEAR
* 11590 CATARACT, AUTOSOMAL DOMINANT
        CONGENITAL
* 11590 CATARACT, CORTICAL AND NUCLEAR
  11610 CATARACT, AUTOSOMAL DOMINANT
        CONGENITAL
  11610 CATARACT, CORTICAL AND NUCLEAR
* 11615 CATARACT-MICROCORNEA SYNDROME
* 11620 CATARACT, AUTOSOMAL DOMINANT
        CONGENITAL
* 11620 CATARACT, COPPOCK

* 11630 CATARACT, AUTOSOMAL DOMINANT
        CONGENITAL
* 11630 CATARACT, CORTICAL AND NUCLEAR
* 11640 CATARACT, AUTOSOMAL DOMINANT
        CONGENITAL
* 11640 CATARACT, CORTICAL AND NUCLEAR
* 11660 CATARACT, AUTOSOMAL DOMINANT
        CONGENITAL
* 11660 CATARACT, POLAR AND CAPSULAR
  11670 CATARACT, AUTOSOMAL DOMINANT
        CONGENITAL
  11670 CATARACT, CORTICAL AND NUCLEAR
* 11680 CATARACT, AUTOSOMAL DOMINANT
        CONGENITAL
* 11680 CATARACT, CORTICAL AND NUCLEAR
* 11692 GRANULOCYTE GLYCOPROTEIN CD11/CD18
        DEFICIENCY
* 11700 MYOPATHY, CENTRAL CORE DISEASE TYPE
* 11710 SEIZURES, CENTRALOPATHIC
* 11755 CEREBRAL GIGANTISM
* 11755 NEVO SYNDROME
  11765 CEREBRO-COSTO-MANDIBULAR SYNDROME
* 11770 HYPOCERULOPLASMINEMIA
* 11780 EAR, CERUMEN VARIATIONS
* 11810 KLIPPEL-FEIL ANOMALY
* 11820 NEUROPATHY, HEREDITARY MOTOR AND
        SENSORY, TYPE I
* 11821 NEUROPATHY, HEREDITARY MOTOR AND
        SENSORY, TYPE II
* 11822 NEUROPATHY, HEREDITARY MOTOR AND
        SENSORY, TYPE I
* 11830 CHARCOT MARIE TOOTH DISEASE-DEAFNESS
  11833 LIP, CHEILITIS GLANDULARIS
* 11840 CHERUBISM
* 11845 ARTERIO-HEPATIC DYSPLASIA
* 11865 CHONDRODYSPLASIA PUNCTATA, MILD
        SYMMETRIC TYPE
* 11870 CHOREA, BENIGN FAMILIAL
* 11900 FACE, CHIN FISSURE
* 11930 CLEFT LIP/PALATE-LIP PITS OR MOUNDS
* 11950 PTERYGIUM SYNDROME, POPLITEAL
  11954 CLEFT PALATE
  11957 CLEFT PALATE
  11958 CLEFTING-ECTROPION-CONICAL TEETH
* 11960 CLEIDOCRANIAL DYSPLASIA
  11980 FOOT, TALIPES EQUINOVARUS (TEV)
* 11990 FOOT, CONGENITAL CLUBFOOT
  12000 AORTA, COARCTATION
  12000 AORTA, COARCTATION, INFANTILE TYPE
* 12010 COLD HYPERSENSITIVITY
* 12015 OSTEOGENESIS IMPERFECTA
* 12016 OSTEOGENESIS IMPERFECTA
* 12020 EYE, MICROPHTHALMIA/COLOBOMA
  12040 MACULAR COLOBOMA-BRACHYDACTYLY
  12050 LIP, PITS OR MOUNDS
* 12055 COMPLEMENT COMPONENT 1, DEFICIENCY OF
* 12057 COMPLEMENT COMPONENT 1, DEFICIENCY OF
* 12058 COMPLEMENT COMPONENT 1, DEFICIENCY OF
* 12070 COMPLEMENT COMPONENT 3, DEFICIENCY OF
* 12079 COMPLEMENT COMPONENT 4, DEFICIENCY OF
* 12081 COMPLEMENT COMPONENT 4, DEFICIENCY OF
* 12082 COMPLEMENT COMPONENT 4, DEFICIENCY OF
* 12083 COMPLEMENT COMPONENT 4, DEFICIENCY OF
* 12097 RETINA, COMBINED CONE-ROD
        DEGENERATION
* 12098 GRANULOCYTE GLYCOPROTEIN CD11/CD18
        DEFICIENCY
  12100 MITRAL VALVE INSUFFICIENCY
  12100 MITRAL VALVE STENOSIS
  12100 PULMONARY ARTERY, ORIGIN FROM
        ASCENDING AORTA
  12100 PULMONARY ARTERY, ORIGIN FROM DUCTUS
        ARTERIOSUS

12100 PULMONARY ARTERY, ORIGIN OF THE LEFT FROM RIGHT PULMONARY ARTERY
12100 PULMONARY VENOUS CONNECTION, PARTIAL ANOMALOUS
12100 VENTRICLE, DOUBLE-OUTLET RIGHT WITH ANTERIOR SEPTAL DEFECT
12100 VENTRICLE, DOUBLE-OUTLET RIGHT WITH POSTERIOR SEPTAL DEFECT
12100 VENTRICLES, INVERTED WITH TRANSPOSITION OF GREAT ARTERIES
12100 VENTRICLES, INVERTED WITHOUT TRANSPOSITION OF GREAT ARTERIES
12102 ISAACS-MERTENS SYNDROME
* 12105 ARACHNODACTYLY, CONTRACTURAL BEALS TYPE
* 12120 CONVULSIONS, BENIGN FAMILIAL NEONATAL
12121 SEIZURES, FEBRILE
* 12125 SEIZURES, IN FEMALES, JUBERG-HELLMAN TYPE
* 12130 PORPHYRIA, COPROPORPHYRIA
* 12140 CORNEA PLANA
* 12150 CORNEAL DYSTROPHY, REIS-BUCKLERS TYPE
* 12170 CORNEAL DYSTROPHY, ENDOTHELIAL, CONGENITAL HEREDITARY
* 12180 CORNEAL DYSTROPHY, SCHNYDER CRYSTALLINE
* 12182 CORNEAL DYSTROPHY, RECURRENT EROSIVE
* 12190 CORNEAL DYSTROPHY, GRANULAR
* 12200 CORNEAL DYSTROPHY, POLYMORPHOUS POSTERIOR
* 12210 CORNEAL DYSTROPHY, JUVENILE EPITHELIAL, MEESMANN TYPE
* 12220 CORNEAL DYSTROPHY, LATTICE TYPE
* 12240 CORNEAL DYSTROPHY, RECURRENT EROSIVE
12243 CORNEAL ANESTHESIA-RETINAL DEFECTS-UNUSUAL FACIES-HEART DEFECT
12244 CORNEO-DERMATO-OSSEOUS SYNDROME
12247 DE LANGE SYNDROME
12250 STEROID, BINDING GLOBULIN ABNORMALITIES
* 12260 SPONDYLOCOSTAL DYSPLASIA
* 12275 HIP, CONGENITAL COXA VARA
12285 VENTRICULAR SEPTAL DEFECT
12288 CRANIOFACIAL-DEAFNESS-HAND SYNDROME
12290 CRANIOFACIAL DYSOSTOSIS-DIAPHYSEAL HYPERPLASIA
12292 CRANIO-FRONTO-NASAL DYSPLASIA
* 12300 CRANIOMETAPHYSEAL DYSPLASIA
* 12310 CRANIOSYNOSTOSIS
12315 CRANIOSYNOSTOSIS-FOOT DEFECTS, JACKSON-WEISS TYPE
* 12340 CREUTZFELDT-JAKOB DISEASE
* 12350 CRANIOFACIAL DYSOSTOSIS
* 12355 CRYOGLOBULINEMIA
12357 EYELID, ANKYLOBLEPHARON
* 12370 CUTIS LAXA
12385 SCALP, CYLINDROMAS
* 12420 DARIER DISEASE
12440 EAR, DARWIN TUBERCLE
* 12448 ONYCHODYSTROPHY-CONIFORM TEETH-SENSORINEURAL HEARING LOSS
* 12450 DEAFNESS-KERATOPACHYDERMIA-DIGITAL CONSTRICTIONS
* 12470 DEAFNESS (SENSORINEURAL), MIDFREQUENCY
* 12480 DEAFNESS (SENSORINEURAL), PROGRESSIVE HIGH-TONE
* 12490 DEAFNESS, DOMINANT LOW-FREQUENCY
12500 DEAFNESS, UNILATERAL INNER EAR
* 12510 DEAFNESS-EAR PITS
12525 DEAFNESS-OPTIC NERVE ATROPHY, PROGRESSIVE
* 12527 DELTA-AMINOLEVULINIC ACID DEHYDRASE DEFICIENCY
12530 TEETH, DENS INVAGINATUS

* 12537 DENTATORUBROPALLIDOLUYSIAN DEGENERATION, HEREDITARY
* 12540 TEETH, DENTIN DYSPLASIA, RADICULAR
* 12542 TEETH, DENTIN DYSPLASIA, CORONAL
* 12544 DENTINO-OSSEOUS DYSPLASIA
* 12548 MOOD AND THOUGHT DISORDERS
* 12549 TEETH, DENTINOGENESIS IMPERFECTA
12550 TEETH, DENTINOGENESIS IMPERFECTA
* 12552 CARDIOFACIAL SYNDROME-ASYMMETRIC FACIES
* 12554 FINGERPRINTS, ABSENT
* 12563 URTICARIA, DERMO-DISTORTIVE TYPE
12564 DERMO-ODONTODYSPLASIA
* 12566 MYOPATHY OR CARDIOMYOPATHY DUE TO DESMIN DEFECT
* 12570 DIABETES INSIPIDIS, NEUROHYPOPHYSEAL TYPE
* 12580 DIABETES INSIPIDUS, VASOPRESSIN RESISTANT TYPES I AND II
* 12585 DIABETES MELLITUS, MATURITY ONSET OF THE YOUNG (MODY)
12590 TEETH, DIASTEMA, MEDIAN INCISAL
* 12605 DIGITO-TALAR DYSMORPHISM
* 12605 HAND, ULNAR DRIFT
12607 ALBINOIDISM
* 12615 DIPHTHERIA, SUSCEPTIBILITY TO
12620 MULTIPLE SCLEROSIS, FAMILIAL
* 12630 DISTICHIASIS
12632 DISTICHIASIS-HEART DEFECT-PERIPHERAL VASCULAR DISEASE/ANOMALIES
* 12660 OCULAR DRUSEN
12670 OCULAR DRUSEN
* 12680 EYE, DUANE RETRACTION SYNDROME
* 12685 PEPTIC ULCER DISEASES, NON-SYNDROMIC
* 12690 CONTRACTURE, DUPUYTREN
* 12700 TUBULAR STENOSIS
* 12720 DWARFISM-STIFF JOINTS
* 12730 DYSCHONDROSTEOSIS
* 12755 DYSKERATOSIS CONGENITA
* 12760 MUCOSA (ORAL/EYE), INTRAEPITHELIAL DYSKERATOSIS, BENIGN
* 12770 DYSLEXIA
12780 DYSPLASIA EPIPHYSEALIS HEMIMELICA
* 12810 TORSION DYSTONIA
12830 EAR, EXOSTOSES
12840 EAR, MOZART TYPE
12850 EAR, MOZART TYPE
12850 EAR, SMALL WITH FOLDED-DOWN HELIX
* 12860 EAR, CUPPED
* 12860 EAR, MACROTIA
* 12870 EAR, PITS
12880 EAR, LOP
12890 EAR LOBE, ATTACHED
* 12898 EAR LOBE, HYPERTROPHIC THICKENED
12900 EAR LOBE, PIT
12910 TONGUE, FOLDING OR ROLLING
* 12920 ECTODERMAL DYSPLASIA, BASAN TYPE
* 12940 ECTODERMAL DYSPLASIA, RAPP-HODGKIN TYPE
* 12950 ECTODERMAL DYSPLASIA, HIDROTIC
12955 ECTODERMAL DYSPLASIA-ADRENAL CYST
* 12960 LENS, ECTOPIC
12983 ECTRODACTYLY-ECTODERMAL DYSPLASIA-CLEFTING SYNDROME
12985 EDINBURGH MALFORMATION SYNDROME
* 12990 ECTRODACTYLY-ECTODERMAL DYSPLASIA-CLEFTING SYNDROME
* 13000 EHLERS-DANLOS SYNDROME
13001 EHLERS-DANLOS SYNDROME
13002 EHLERS-DANLOS SYNDROME
* 13005 EHLERS-DANLOS SYNDROME
13006 EHLERS-DANLOS SYNDROME

13007 PROGEROID SYNDROME WITH EHLERS-DANLOS FEATURES
* 13008 EHLERS-DANLOS SYNDROME
13009 EHLERS-DANLOS SYNDROME
13010 SKIN, ELASTOSIS PERFORANS SERPIGINOSA
* 13045 ANEMIA, HEMOLYTIC, RED CELL MEMBRANE DEFECTS
13045 ELLIPTOCYTOSIS
* 13050 ANEMIA, HEMOLYTIC, RED CELL MEMBRANE DEFECTS
* 13050 ELLIPTOCYTOSIS
* 13060 ANEMIA, HEMOLYTIC, RED CELL MEMBRANE DEFECTS
* 13060 ELLIPTOCYTOSIS
* 13065 BECKWITH-WIEDEMANN SYNDROME
13071 LUNG, EMPHYSEMA CONGENITAL LOBAR
13090 TEETH, AMELOGENESIS IMPERFECTA
* 13110 ENDOCRINE NEOPLASIA, MULTIPLE TYPE I
13130 DIAPHYSEAL DYSPLASIA
* 13140 EOSINOPHILIA, FAMILIAL
13145 EYELID, EPIBLEPHARON
13146 EYELID, EPIBLEPHARON
* 13170 EPIDERMOLYSIS BULLOSUM, TYPE III
* 13175 EPIDERMOLYSIS BULLOSUM, TYPE III
* 13180 EPIDERMOLYSIS BULLOSUM, TYPE I
13185 EPIDERMOLYSIS BULLOSUM, TYPE III
13188 EPIDERMOLYSIS BULLOSUM, TYPE I
* 13190 EPIDERMOLYSIS BULLOSUM, TYPE I
* 13195 EPIDERMOLYSIS BULLOSUM, TYPE I
13196 EPIDERMOLYSIS BULLOSUM, TYPE I
* 13200 EPIDERMOLYSIS BULLOSUM, TYPE III
13209 EPILEPSY, BENIGN OCCIPITAL
13210 EPILEPSY, REFLEX
13230 EPILEPSY, REFLEX
* 13240 EPIPHYSEAL DYSPLASIA, MULTIPLE
* 13240 EPIPHYSEAL DYSPLASIA, MULTIPLE RIBBING TYPE
* 13270 EPITHELIOMAS, HEREDITARY MULTIPLE CYSTIC
* 13280 EPITHELIOMA, MULTIPLE SELF-HEALING SQUAMOUS
* 13300 SKIN, PALMO-PLANTAR ERYTHEMA
* 13319 GIROUX-BARBEAU SYNDROME
* 13320 SKIN, ERYTHROKERATODERMIA, VARIABLE
13345 CANCER, EWING SARCOMA
13345 CANCER, NEUROEPITHELIAL AND MENINGEAL
* 13350 EAR, EXCHONDROSIS
13369 EXOSTOSES-ANETODERMIA-BRACHYDACTYLY TYPE E
* 13370 EXOSTOSES, MULTIPLE CARTILAGINOUS
* 13378 RETINA, VITREORETINOPATHY, FAMILIAL EXUDATIVE
13410 PALSY, CONGENITAL FACIAL
* 13420 PALSY, LATE-ONSET FACIAL, FAMILIAL
13443 COAGULATION DEFECT, FAMILIAL MULTIPLE FACTORS
13451 COAGULATION DEFECT, FAMILIAL MULTIPLE FACTORS
13452 COAGULATION DEFECT, FAMILIAL MULTIPLE FACTORS
13454 COAGULATION DEFECT, FAMILIAL MULTIPLE FACTORS
* 13457 FACTOR XIII (FIBRIN STABILIZING FACTOR)
* 13460 RENAL TUBULAR SYNDROME, FANCONI TYPE
13478 FEMORAL HYPOPLASIA-UNUSUAL FACIES SYNDROME
* 13482 AFIBROGINEMIA, CONGENITAL
* 13482 FIBRINOGENS, ABNORMAL CONGENITAL
* 13483 AFIBROGINEMIA, CONGENITAL
* 13483 FIBRINOGENS, ABNORMAL CONGENITAL
* 13485 AFIBROGINEMIA, CONGENITAL
* 13485 FIBRINOGENS, ABNORMAL CONGENITAL
* 13510 MYOSITIS OSSIFICANS PROGRESSIVA
13530 GINGIVAL FIBROMATOSIS

13540 GINGIVAL FIBROMATOSIS-HYPERTRICHOSIS
* 13550 GINGIVAL FIBROMATOSIS-DIGITAL ANOMALIES
* 13555 GINGIVAL FIBROMATOSIS-DEAFNESS, JONES TYPES
13558 ARTERY, RENAL FIBROMUSCULAR DYSPLASIA
* 13570 EYE, FIBROSIS OF THE EXTRAOCULAR MUSCLES, GENERALIZED
13590 COFFIN-SIRIS SYNDROME
* 13600 FINGERPRINTS, ABSENT
* 13630 NEUROECTODERMAL SYNDROME, FLYNN-AIRD TYPE
* 13655 EYE, MACULAR DYSTROPHY, NORTH CAROLINA TYPE
* 13680 CORNEAL DYSTROPHY, ENDOTHELIAL
* 13685 ACIDURIA, FUMARIC
13686 ACIDURIA, FUMARIC
13688 RETINA, FUNDUS ALBIPUNCTATUS
13704 GALLBLADDER, AGENESIS
13710 IMMUNOGLOBULIN A DEFICIENCY
* 13715 GAMMA-AMINOBUTYRIC ACID (GABA) TRANSAMINASE DEFICIENCY
13727 GASTROCUTANEOUS SYNDROME
13740 TONGUE, FISSURED
13740 TONGUE, GEOGRAPHIC
13740 TONGUE, PLICATED
13744 GERSTMANN-STRAUSSLER SYNDROME
13755 NEVUS, CONGENITAL NEVOMELANOCYTIC
* 13758 TOURETTE SYNDROME
* 13780 CANCER, GLIOMA, FAMILIAL
13792 KIDNEY, GLOMERULOCYSTIC
* 13800 SKIN TUMORS, MULTIPLE GLOMUS
* 13804 GLUCOCORTICOID RESISTANCE
13807 GLUCOGLYCINURIA
* 13830 ANEMIA, HEMOLYTIC, GLUTATHIONE REDUCTASE DEFICIENCY
13850 IMINOGLYCINURIA
13890 GOUT
13893 SHORT STATURE-WORMIAN BONES-JOINT DISLOCATIONS
13900 NOSE, GRANULOSIS RUBRA NASI
* 13920 PLASMA, GROUP-SPECIFIC COMPONENT
13921 GROWTH-MENTAL DEFICIENCY, MYHRE TYPE
* 13925 GROWTH HORMONE DEFICIENCY, ISOLATED
13950 EAR, HAIRY
13975 ACROFACIAL DEFECTS, EMERY-NELSON TYPE
* 14000 HAND-FOOT-GENITAL SYNDROME
* 14010 HAPTOGLOBIN
14020 HAPTOGLOBIN
* 14035 HAWKINSINURIA
* 14040 ARRHYTHMIA, HEART BLOCK, CONGENITAL COMPLETE
* 14045 HEART-HAND SYNDROME III
14050 VENTRICLE, DOUBLE-OUTLET RIGHT WITH ANTERIOR SEPTAL DEFECT
14050 VENTRICLE, DOUBLE-OUTLET RIGHT WITH POSTERIOR SEPTAL DEFECT
14070 ANEMIA, HEINZ BODY
* 14080 HEMANGIOMAS OF THE HEAD AND NECK
* 14080 RETINA, CAVERNOUS HEMANGIOMA
14085 HEMANGIOMAS OF THE HEAD AND NECK
14100 HEMANGIOMA-THROMBOCYTOPENIA SYNDROME
14130 HEMIFACIAL ATROPHY, PROGRESSIVE
* 14135 OCULO-FACIAL SYNDROME, BENCZE TYPE
14140 OCULO-AURICULO-VERTEBRAL ANOMALY
14175 MENTAL RETARDATION, HEMOGLOBIN H RELATED
* 14190 ANEMIA, SICKLE CELL
14234 DIAPHRAGMATIC HERNIA
14240 HERNIA, HIATAL
14242 FETAL HERPES SIMPLEX VIRUS INFECTION
* 14245 FETAL HERPES SIMPLEX VIRUS INFECTION

| | | |
|---|---|---|
| * | 14260 | ANEMIA, HEMOLYTIC, ERYTHROCYTE HEXOKINASE DEFICIENCY |
| | 14267 | HIP, DYSPLASIA, NAMAQUALAND TYPE |
| | 14270 | HIP, CONGENITAL DISLOCATED |
| * | 14273 | DERMATOARTHRITIS, FAMILIAL HISTIOCYTIC |
| * | 14280 | RAGWEED POLLEN SENSITIVITY |
| * | 14290 | HEART-HAND SYNDROME |
| * | 14300 | HORNER SYNDROME |
| | 14305 | HUMERO-RADIAL SYNOSTOSIS |
| * | 14310 | HUNTINGTON DISEASE |
| * | 14320 | RETINA, HYALOIDEORETINAL DEGENERATION OF WAGNER |
| | 14325 | HYDROCEPHALUS-COSTOVERTEBRAL DYSPLASIA-SPRENGEL ANOMALY |
| * | 14350 | HYPERBILIRUBINEMIA, UNCONJUGATED |
| * | 14387 | HYPERCALCIURIA, FAMILIAL IDIOPATHIC |
| | 14389 | HYPERCHOLESTEROLEMIA |
| | 14410 | SWEATING, GUSTATORY |
| * | 14425 | HYPERLIPOPROTEINEMIA, COMBINED |
| | 14440 | HYPERCHOLESTEROLEMIA |
| | 14450 | HYPERLIPOPROTEINEMIA, BROAD BETA TYPE |
| | 14460 | HYPERTRIGLYCERIDEMIA |
| | 14465 | HYPERLIPOPROTEINEMIA V |
| | 14470 | CANCER, RENAL CELL CARCINOMA |
| * | 14475 | HYPEROSTOSIS, WORTH TYPE |
| | 14480 | HYPEROSTOSIS FRONTALIS INTERNA |
| | 14525 | SKIN, HYPERPIGMENTATION, FAMILIAL |
| * | 14540 | EYE, HYPERTELORISM |
| * | 14541 | G SYNDROME |
| * | 14560 | KING SYNDROME |
| * | 14560 | MYOPATHY, MALIGNANT HYPERTHERMIA |
| * | 14570 | HAIR, HYPERTRICHOSIS, LANUGINOSA |
| * | 14575 | HYPERTRIGLYCERIDEMIA |
| * | 14590 | DEJERINE-SOTTAS DISEASE |
| | 14595 | HYPOBETALIPOPROTEINEMIA |
| | 14600 | HYPOCHONDROPLASIA |
| | 14615 | HYPOMELANOSIS OF ITO |
| | 14616 | LIMB, UPPER HYPOPLASIA-MULLERIAN DUCT DEFECTS |
| * | 14630 | HYPOPHOSPHATASIA |
| | 14635 | HYPOPHOSPHATEMIA, NON X-LINKED |
| | 14645 | HYPOSPADIAS |
| | 14650 | DOPAMINE BETA-HYDROXYLASE DEFICIENCY, CONGENITAL |
| | 14651 | HYPOTHALAMIC HAMARTOBLASTOMA SYNDROME, CONGENITAL |
| * | 14655 | HAIR, HYPOTRICHOSIS |
| * | 14659 | ICHTHYOSIS HYSTRIX, CURTH-MACKLIN TYPE |
| * | 14660 | NEVUS, EPIDERMAL NEVUS SYNDROME |
| * | 14670 | ICHTHYOSIS VULGARIS |
| * | 14672 | ICHTHYOSIS-CHEEK-EYEBROW SYNDROME |
| | 14675 | ICHTHYOSIS, LAMELLAR DOMINANT |
| | 14680 | ICHTHYOSIFORM HYPERKERATOSIS, BULLOUS CONGENITAL |
| | 14683 | IMMUNODEFICIENCY, COMMON VARIABLE TYPE |
| | 14683 | SERUM ALLOTYPES, HUMAN |
| * | 14690 | IMMUNODEFICIENCY, COMMON VARIABLE TYPE |
| * | 14690 | SERUM ALLOTYPES, HUMAN |
| * | 14691 | IMMUNODEFICIENCY, COMMON VARIABLE TYPE |
| * | 14691 | SERUM ALLOTYPES, HUMAN |
| * | 14700 | IMMUNODEFICIENCY, COMMON VARIABLE TYPE |
| * | 14700 | SERUM ALLOTYPES, HUMAN |
| * | 14701 | IMMUNODEFICIENCY, COMMON VARIABLE TYPE |
| * | 14701 | SERUM ALLOTYPES, HUMAN |
| * | 14702 | IMMUNODEFICIENCY, COMMON VARIABLE TYPE |
| * | 14702 | SERUM ALLOTYPES, HUMAN |
| | 14706 | IMMUNODEFICIENCY, HYPER IgE TYPE |

| | | |
|---|---|---|
| * | 14707 | IMMUNODEFICIENCY, COMMON VARIABLE TYPE |
| * | 14707 | SERUM ALLOTYPES, HUMAN |
| * | 14710 | IMMUNODEFICIENCY, COMMON VARIABLE TYPE |
| * | 14710 | IMMUNODEFICIENCY, IgG SUBCLASS DEFICIENCIES |
| * | 14710 | SERUM ALLOTYPES, HUMAN |
| * | 14711 | IMMUNODEFICIENCY, COMMON VARIABLE TYPE |
| * | 14711 | IMMUNODEFICIENCY, IgG SUBCLASS DEFICIENCIES |
| * | 14711 | SERUM ALLOTYPES, HUMAN |
| * | 14712 | IMMUNODEFICIENCY, COMMON VARIABLE TYPE |
| * | 14712 | IMMUNODEFICIENCY, IgG SUBCLASS DEFICIENCIES |
| * | 14712 | SERUM ALLOTYPES, HUMAN |
| * | 14713 | IMMUNODEFICIENCY, COMMON VARIABLE TYPE |
| * | 14713 | IMMUNODEFICIENCY, IgG SUBCLASS DEFICIENCIES |
| * | 14713 | SERUM ALLOTYPES, HUMAN |
| * | 14716 | IMMUNODEFICIENCY, COMMON VARIABLE TYPE |
| * | 14716 | SERUM ALLOTYPES, HUMAN |
| * | 14717 | IMMUNODEFICIENCY, COMMON VARIABLE TYPE |
| * | 14717 | SERUM ALLOTYPES, HUMAN |
| * | 14718 | IMMUNODEFICIENCY, COMMON VARIABLE TYPE |
| * | 14718 | SERUM ALLOTYPES, HUMAN |
| | 14720 | IMMUNODEFICIENCY, COMMON VARIABLE TYPE |
| * | 14720 | SERUM ALLOTYPES, HUMAN |
| | 14725 | TEETH, FUSED |
| | 14735 | TEETH, MESIOPALATAL TORSION OF CENTRAL INCISORS |
| | 14740 | TEETH, INCISORS, SHOVEL-SHAPED |
| * | 14744 | GROWTH DEFICIENCY, AFRICAN PYGMY TYPE |
| | 14748 | INTRAHEPATIC CHOLESTASIS OF PREGNANCY (ICP) |
| * | 14757 | INTERFERON DEFICIENCY |
| * | 14762 | INTERFERON DEFICIENCY |
| * | 14764 | INTERFERON DEFICIENCY |
| * | 14766 | INTERFERON DEFICIENCY |
| * | 14775 | IVIC SYNDROME |
| | 14777 | ALOPECIA-ANOSMIA-DEAFNESS-HYPOGONADISM, JOHNSON TYPE |
| * | 14779 | LEUKEMIA, ACUTE LYMPHOCYTIC, FAMILIAL |
| * | 14780 | AASE-SMITH SYNDROME |
| * | 14790 | ARTICULAR HYPERMOBILITY, FAMILIAL |
| * | 14790 | EHLERS-DANLOS SYNDROME |
| | 14792 | KABUKI MAKE-UP SYNDROME |
| * | 14795 | KALLMANN SYNDROME |
| * | 14805 | KBG SYNDROME |
| * | 14840 | KERATOSIS PALMARIS ET PLANTARIS OF UNNA-THOST |
| * | 14873 | SKIN, HYPERKERATOSIS, FOCAL PALMOPLANTAR AND GINGIVAL |
| | 14880 | CRANIOSYNOSTOSIS, KLEEBLATTSCHADEL TYPE |
| | 14882 | WAARDENBURG SYNDROMES |
| | 14886 | KLIPPEL-FEIL ANOMALY |
| | 14887 | KLIPPEL-FEIL ANOMALY |
| * | 14890 | KLIPPEL-FEIL ANOMALY |
| | 14900 | ANGIO-OSTEOHYPERTROPHY SYNDROME |
| * | 14920 | KNUCKLE PADS-LEUKONYCHIA-DEAFNESS |
| * | 14930 | NAILS, KOILONYCHIA |
| * | 14940 | HYPEREKPLEXIA |
| | 14950 | SKIN, KYRLE DISEASE |
| * | 14970 | LACRIMAL CANALICULUS ATRESIA |
| * | 14970 | NASOLACRIMAL DUCT OBSTRUCTION |

* 14973 LACRIMO-AURICULO-DENTO-DIGITAL
         SYNDROME
* 15000 LACTATE DEHYDROGENASE ISOZYMES
* 15010 LACTATE DEHYDROGENASE ISOZYMES
* 15015 LACTATE DEHYDROGENASE ISOZYMES
  15016 LACTATE DEHYDROGENASE ISOZYMES
  15022 LACTOSE INTOLERANCE
  15023 TRICHO-RHINO-PHALANGEAL SYNDROME,
         TYPE II
* 15025 LARSEN SYNDROME
* 15026 LARYNGEAL PARALYSIS
* 15027 LARYNGEAL PARALYSIS
  15028 LARYNGOMALACIA
  15030 LARYNX, ATRESIA
* 15040 TEETH, PEGGED OR ABSENT MAXILLARY
         LATERAL INCISOR
  15060 HIP, OSTEONECROSIS, CAPITAL FEMORAL
         EPIPHYSIS
  15060 JOINTS, OSTEOCHONDRITIS DISSECANS
* 15080 SKIN, LEIOMYOMAS, MULTIPLE
  15105 CRANIODIAPHYSEAL DYSPLASIA,
         LENZ-MAJEWSKI TYPE
* 15110 LENTIGINES SYNDROME, MULTIPLE
* 15120 LERI PLEONOSTEOSIS SYNDROME
* 15140 LEUKEMIA/LYMPHOMA, B-CELL
* 15141 LEUKEMIA, CHRONIC MYELOID (CML)
* 15143 LEUKEMIA/LYMPHOMA, B-CELL
* 15143 LYMPHOMA, NON-HODGKIN
* 15151 GRANULOCYTE GLYCOPROTEIN CD11/CD18
         DEFICIENCY
* 15160 NAILS, LEUKONYCHIA
* 15160 ULCER-LEUKONYCHIA-GALLSTONES
  15163 LIP, PITS OR MOUNDS
* 15166 LIPODYSTROPHY, FAMILIAL LIMB AND TRUNK
  15168 LIPODYSTROPHY-RIEGER ANOMALY-SHORT
         STATURE-DIABETES
  15180 NECK/FACE, LIPOMATOSIS
* 15190 LIPOMAS, FAMILIAL SYMMETRIC
  15270 ARRHYTHMIA, FROM MATERNAL
         AUTOIMMUNE DISEASE, CONGENITAL
  15270 LUPUS ERYTHEMATOSUS, SYSTEMIC
* 15280 INTESTINAL LYMPHANGIECTASIA
* 15295 MICROCEPHALY-LYMPHEDEMA
* 15310 LYMPHEDEMA I
* 15320 LYMPHEDEMA II
  15330 LYMPHEDEMA II
* 15337 GRANULOCYTE GLYCOPROTEIN CD11/CD18
         DEFICIENCY
* 15340 DISTICHIASIS-LYMPHEDEMA SYNDROME
* 15348 OVERGROWTH, BANNAYAN TYPE
  15350 OVERGROWTH, MACROCEPHALY-
         HEMANGIOMA, RILEY-SMITH TYPE
* 15363 MACROGLOSSIA
* 15365 DEAFNESS-NEPHRITIS-MACROTHROMBOPATHIA
* 15370 RETINA, MACULAR DEGENERATION,
         VITELLIRUPTIVE
* 15384 RETINA, MACULAR DEGENERATION,
         VITELLIRUPTIVE
  15435 FACIAL CLEFTING SYNDROME, GYPSY TYPE
  15440 ACROFACIAL DYSOSTOSIS, NAGER TYPE
* 15450 MANDIBULOFACIAL DYSOSTOSIS
  15460 JAW-WINKING SYNDROME
* 15470 MARFAN SYNDROME
  15474 MARFAN SYNDROME
  15475 MARFAN SYNDROME
* 15478 DEAFNESS-MYOPIA-CATARACT-SADDLE NOSE,
         MARSHALL TYPE
  15480 URTICARIA PIGMENTOSA (UP)
* 15500 MAXILLOFACIAL DYSOSTOSIS
  15505 MAXILLONASAL DYSPLASIA, BINDER TYPE
* 15510 LEUKOCYTE, MAY-HEGGLIN ANOMALY
* 15531 INTESTINAL PSEUDO-OBSTRUCTION
         SYNDROMES

* 15531 MEGACYSTIS-MEGADUODENUM SYNDROME
* 15560 CANCER, MALIGNANT MELANOMA, FAMILIAL
* 15560 NEVUS, CONGENITAL NEVOMELANOCYTIC
* 15580 SKIN, HYPERPIGMENTATION, FAMILIAL
* 15590 CHEILITIS GRANULOMATOSA,
         MELKERSSON-ROSENTHAL TYPE
  15595 MELORHEOSTOSIS
* 15623 MESOMELIC DYSPLASIA, WERNER TYPE
  15625 METACHONDROMATOSIS
* 15640 METAPHYSEAL CHONDRODYSPLASIA, TYPE
         JANSEN
* 15650 METAPHYSEAL CHONDRODYSPLASIA, TYPE
         SCHMID
  15651 METAPHYSEAL DYSPLASIA-MAXILLARY
         HYPOPLASIA-BRACHYDACTYLY
* 15652 FOOT, METATARSUS VARUS
* 15655 KNIEST DYSPLASIA
* 15658 MICROCEPHALY, ISOLATED AUTOSOMAL
         DOMINANT TYPE
  15659 MICROCEPHALY WITH CHORIORETINOPATHY
* 15661 MICHELIN TIRE BABY SYNDROME
* 15685 CATARACT, AUTOSOMAL DOMINANT
         CONGENITAL
* 15685 CATARACT, POLAR AND CAPSULAR
  15730 MIGRAINE
* 15770 MITRAL VALVE PROLAPSE
  15780 MITRAL REGURGITATION-DEAFNESS-SKELETAL
         DEFECTS
  15790 DIPLEGIA, CONGENITAL FACIAL
* 15795 TEETH, MOLAR REINCLUSION
* 15800 HAIR, MONILETHRIX
  15825 CHROMOSOME MOSAICISM, 45,X/46,XY TYPE
* 15830 CAMPTODACTYLY-TRISMUS SYNDROME
  15832 CANCER, SEBACEOUS GLAND
         TUMOR-MULTIPLE VISCERAL CARCINOMA
  15833 MULLERIAN APLASIA
* 15835 GINGIVAL MULTIPLE HAMARTOMA SYNDROME
  15859 SPINAL MUSCULAR ATROPHY
* 15860 SPINAL MUSCULAR ATROPHY
* 15890 MUSCULAR DYSTROPHY, FACIO-SCAPULO-
         HUMERAL
  15920 HAUPTMANN-THANHAUSER SYNDROME
  15942 EYE, IRIDOPLEGIA, FAMILIAL
* 16015 MYOPATHY, MYOTUBULAR
* 16050 MUSCULAR DYSTROPHY, DISTAL
  16055 MYOPATHY-CATARACT-GONADAL DYSGENESIS
  16057 MYOPATHY-METABOLIC, GLYCOPROTEIN-
         GLYCOSAMINOGLYCANS STORAGE TYPE
* 16070 MYOPIA, CONGENITAL
* 16080 MYOTONIA CONGENITA
* 16090 MYOTONIC DYSTROPHY
* 16098 NEVI-ATRIAL MYXOMA-MYXOID
         NEUROFIBROMAS-EPHELIDES
* 16100 ECTODERMAL DYSPLASIA, NAEGELI TYPE
* 16120 NAIL-PATELLA SYNDROME
* 16140 NARCOLEPSY
* 16150 NOSE, TRANSVERSE GROOVE
* 16180 MYOPATHY, NEMALINE
* 16210 NEUROPATHY, HEREDITARY RECURRENT
         BRACHIAL
* 16220 NEUROFIBROMATOSIS
* 16222 NEUROFIBROMATOSIS
  16224 NEUROFIBROMATOSIS
  16226 NEUROFIBROMATOSIS
  16227. NEUROFIBROMATOSIS
  16229 NOONAN SYNDROME
* 16230 ENDOCRINE NEOPLASIA, MULTIPLE TYPE III
* 16235 NEURONAL CEROID-LIPOFUSCINOSES (NCL)
* 16250 NEUROPATHY, HEREDITARY WITH PRESSURE
         PALSIES
* 16270 NEUTROPENIA, BENIGN FAMILIAL
  16280 NEUTROPENIA, CYCLIC

| | | |
|---|---|---|
| | 16282 | GRANULOCYTE GLYCOPROTEIN CD11/CD18 DEFICIENCY |
| | 16305 | SKIN, VITILIGO |
| * | 16310 | NEVUS FLAMMEUS |
| | 16320 | NEVUS, EPIDERMAL NEVUS SYNDROME |
| * | 16340 | MESOMELIC DYSPLASIA, NIEVERGELT TYPE |
| * | 16350 | NIGHTBLINDNESS, CONGENITAL STATIONARY, AUTOSOMAL DOMINANT |
| * | 16370 | BREAST, POLYTHELIA |
| * | 16395 | NOONAN SYNDROME |
| | 16400 | NOSE/NASAL SEPTUM DEFECTS |
| * | 16405 | IMMUNODEFICIENCY, NUCLEOSIDE-PHOSPHORYLASE DEFICIENCY |
| | 16418 | OCULO-CEREBRO-CUTANEOUS SYNDROME |
| * | 16420 | OCULO-DENTO-OSSEOUS DYSPLASIA |
| | 16421 | OCULO-AURICULO-VERTEBRAL ANOMALY |
| * | 16430 | MUSCULAR DYSTROPHY, OCULOPHARYNGEAL |
| * | 16440 | OLIVOPONTOCEREBELLAR ATROPHY, DOMINANT MENZEL TYPE |
| * | 16450 | OLIVOPONTOCEREBELLAR ATROPHY, DOMINANT WITH RETINAL DEGENERATION |
| * | 16460 | OLIVOPONTOCEREBELLAR ATROPHY, DOMINANT SCHUT-HAYMAKER TYPE |
| * | 16470 | OLIVOPONTOCEREBELLAR ATROPHY, DOMINANT WITH OPHTHALMOPLEGIA |
| | 16475 | OMPHALOCELE |
| * | 16490 | DWARFISM (SHORT LIMBED)-PETERS ANOMALY OF THE EYE |
| * | 16490 | OPHTHALMO-MANDIBULO-MELIC DWARFISM |
| * | 16500 | OPHTHALMOPLEGIA, FAMILIAL STATIC |
| | 16510 | KEARNS-SAYRE DISEASE |
| | 16510 | OPHTHALMOPLEGIA, PROGRESSIVE EXTERNAL |
| | 16513 | OPHTHALMOPLEGIA, PROGRESSIVE EXTERNAL |
| * | 16550 | OPTIC ATROPHY, KJER TYPE |
| | 16555 | OPTIC NERVE HYPOPLASIA |
| * | 16580 | JOINTS, OSTEOCHONDRITIS DISSECANS |
| | 16600 | ENCHONDROMATOSIS |
| | 16600 | ENCHONDROMATOSIS AND HEMANGIOMAS |
| * | 16620 | OSTEOGENESIS IMPERFECTA |
| * | 16621 | OSTEOGENESIS IMPERFECTA |
| * | 16622 | OSTEOGENESIS IMPERFECTA |
| | 16623 | OSTEOGENESIS IMPERFECTA |
| | 16624 | OSTEOGENESIS IMPERFECTA |
| | 16625 | OSTEOGLOPHONIC DYSPLASIA |
| * | 16630 | OSTEOLYSIS, CARPAL-TARSAL AND CHRONIC PROGRESSIVE GLOMERULOPATHY |
| | 16645 | OSTEOMESOPYKNOSIS |
| * | 16650 | OSTEOPATHIA STRIATA-CRANIAL SCLEROSIS-MEGALENCEPHALY |
| * | 16660 | OSTEOPETROSIS, BENIGN DOMINANT |
| * | 16670 | OSTEOPOIKILOSIS |
| | 16674 | SKELETAL BOWING-CORTICAL THICKENING-BONE FRAGILITY-ICTHYOSIS |
| * | 16675 | OTO-DENTAL DYSPLASIA |
| * | 16680 | OTOSCLEROSIS |
| * | 16690 | ELLIPTOCYTOSIS |
| | 16710 | PACHYDERMOPERIOSTOSIS |
| * | 16720 | NAILS, PACHYONYCHIA CONGENITA |
| | 16721 | PACHYONYCHIA CONGENITA-STEATOCYSTOMA MULTIPLEX |
| | 16725 | BONE, PAGET DISEASE |
| | 16750 | PALATOPHARYNGEAL INCOMPETENCE |
| * | 16773 | NASOPALPEBRAL LIPOMA-COLOBOMA SYNDROME |
| | 16775 | PANCREAS, ANNULAR |
| * | 16780 | PANCREATITIS, HEREDITARY |
| | 16787 | MOOD AND THOUGHT DISORDERS |
| | 16796 | PAPILLOMA VIRUS, CONGENITAL INFECTION |
| * | 16800 | CAROTID BODY TUMOR |
| * | 16800 | EAR, CHEMODECTOMA OF MIDDLE EAR |
| * | 16830 | PARAMYOTONIA CONGENITA |
| | 16840 | PARASTREMMATIC DYSPLASIA |
| | 16855 | PARIETAL FORAMINA-CLAVICULAR HYPOPLASIA |
| | 16910 | DUCTUS ARTERIOSUS, PATENT |
| | 16917 | PSEUDOLEPRECHAUNISM, PATTERSON TYPE |
| | 16930 | PECTUS EXCAVATUM |
| * | 16950 | LEUKODYSTROPHY, ADULT-ONSET PROGRESSIVE DOMINANT TYPE |
| * | 16950 | MULTIPLE SCLEROSIS, FAMILIAL |
| * | 16960 | PEMPHIGUS, BENIGN FAMILIAL |
| * | 17040 | PARALYSIS, HYPOKALEMIC PERIODIC |
| * | 17050 | PARALYSIS, HYPERKALEMIC PERIODIC |
| * | 17060 | PARALYSIS, NORMOKALEMIC PERIODIC |
| * | 17065 | TEETH, PERIODONTITIS, JUVENILE |
| | 17110 | IMMUNODEFICIENCY, PLASMA-ASSOCIATED DEFECT OF PHAGOCYTOSIS |
| * | 17120 | TASTING DEFECT, PHENYLTHIOCARBAMIDE |
| * | 17140 | ENDOCRINE NEOPLASIA, MULTIPLE TYPE II |
| | 17148 | LIMB-OTO-CARDIAC SYNDROME |
| * | 17176 | HYPOPHOSPHATASIA |
| * | 17186 | GLYCOGENOSIS, TYPE VII |
| * | 17240 | ANEMIA, GLUCOSE PHOSPHATE ISOMERASE DEFICIENCY |
| | 17250 | DEAFNESS-DIABETES-PHOTOMYOCLONUS-NEPHROPATHY |
| | 17270 | PICK DISEASE OF THE BRAIN |
| * | 17280 | ALBINISM, CUTANEOUS |
| * | 17310 | GROWTH HORMONE DEFICIENCY, ISOLATED |
| * | 17320 | SKIN, PITYRIASIS RUBRA PILARIS |
| * | 17335 | PLASMINOGEN DEFECTS |
| * | 17365 | POIKILODERMA, HEREDITARY ACROKERATOTIC, KINDLER-WEARY TYPE |
| | 17370 | POIKILODERMA, SCLEROSING, HEREDITARY |
| | 17375 | POLAND SYNDROME |
| | 17380 | POLAND SYNDROME |
| * | 17385 | POLIO, SUSCEPTIBILITY TO |
| * | 17390 | KIDNEY, POLYCYSTIC DISEASE, DOMINANT |
| * | 17400 | KIDNEY, NEPHRONOPHTHISIS-MEDULLARY CYSTIC DISEASE |
| | 17405 | LIVER, POLYCYSTIC AND MULTICYSTIC DISEASE, ADULT TYPE |
| * | 17420 | POLYDACTYLY |
| | 17430 | ORO-FACIO-DIGITAL SYNDROME, THURSTON TYPE |
| | 17440 | POLYDACTYLY |
| * | 17450 | POLYDACTYLY |
| * | 17450 | THUMB, TRIPHALANGEAL-DUPLICATED GREAT TOES |
| * | 17460 | POLYDACTYLY |
| * | 17470 | POLYSYNDACTYLY |
| | 17480 | FIBROUS DYSPLASIA, POLYOSTOTIC |
| * | 17490 | INTESTINAL POLYPOSIS, JUVENILE TYPE |
| * | 17510 | INTESTINAL POLYPOSIS, TYPE I |
| * | 17520 | INTESTINAL POLYPOSIS, TYPE II |
| * | 17530 | INTESTINAL POLYPOSIS, TYPE III |
| * | 17530 | RETINA, CONGENITAL HYPERTROPHY OF RETINAL PIGMENT EPITHELIUM |
| | 17550 | POLYPOSIS-ALOPECIA-PIGMENTATION-NAIL DEFECTS |
| * | 17570 | POLYSYNDACTYLY-DYSMORPHIC CRANIOFACIES, GREIG TYPE |
| | 17578 | BRAIN, PORENCEPHALY |
| * | 17580 | SKIN, POROKERATOSIS |
| | 17585 | SKIN, POROKERATOSIS |
| * | 17590 | SKIN, POROKERATOSIS |
| * | 17600 | PORPHYRIA, ACUTE INTERMITTENT |
| * | 17610 | PORPHYRIA CUTANEA TARDA |
| * | 17620 | PORPHYRIA, VARIEGATE |
| * | 17627 | PRADER-WILLI SYNDROME |
| | 17630 | AMYLOIDOSIS, APPALACHIAN TYPE |
| | 17630 | AMYLOIDOSIS, ASHKENAZI TYPE |
| | 17630 | AMYLOIDOSIS, DANISH CARDIAC TYPE |
| | 17630 | AMYLOIDOSIS, ILLINOIS TYPE |
| | 17630 | AMYLOIDOSIS, INDIANA TYPE |

17630 AMYLOIDOSIS, TRANSTHYRETIN METHIONINE-30 TYPE
* 17645 TERATOMA, PRESACRAL-SACRAL DYSGENESIS
* 17645 TERATOMA, SACROCOCCYGEAL TERATOMA
17667 PROGERIA
* 17670 MANDIBULAR PROGNATHISM
* 17686 PROTEIN C DEFICIENCY
* 17688 PROTEIN S DEFICIENCY
17692 PROTEUS SYNDROME
* 17693 HYPOPROTHROMBINEMIA
* 17700 PORPHYRIA, PROTOPORPHYRIA
17710 PRURITUS, HEREDITARY LOCALIZED
* 17715 PSEUDOACHONDROPLASTIC DYSPLASIA
* 17717 PSEUDOACHONDROPLASTIC DYSPLASIA
17720 LIDDLE SYNDROME
* 17740 CHOLINESTERASE, ATYPICAL
* 17750 CHOLINESTERASE, ATYPICAL
17773 ALDOSTERONE RESISTANCE
* 17785 PSEUDOXANTHOMA ELASTICUM
* 17790 SKIN, PSORIASIS VULGARIS
17798 PTERYGIA-DYSMORPHIC FACIES-SHORT STATURE-MENTAL RETARDATION
* 17830 EYELID, PTOSIS, CONGENITAL
* 17860 PULMONARY HYPERTENSION, PRIMARY
17880 PUPIL, DYSCORIA
17890 EYE, PUPILLARY MEMBRANE PERSISTENCE
17901 PYLORIC STENOSIS
17910 HAND, RADIAL CLUB HAND
17910 RADIAL DEFECTS
17925 RADIAL HYPOPLASIA-TRIPHALANGEAL THUMBS-HYPOSPADIAS-DIASTEMA
17928 RADIAL-RENAL SYNDROME
* 17930 RADIAL-ULNAR SYNOSTOSIS
17940 RADIAL DEFECTS
17945 RAGWEED POLLEN SENSITIVITY
* 17960 RAYNAUD DISEASE
* 17965 ANEMIA, HEMOLYTIC, RED CELL MEMBRANE DEFECTS
* 17970 ANEMIA, HEMOLYTIC, ERYTHROCYTE PHOSPHOLIPID DEFECT
* 17970 ANEMIA, HEMOLYTIC, RED CELL MEMBRANE DEFECTS
* 17980 RENAL TUBULAR ACIDOSIS
17985 SKIN CREASES, RETICULATE PIGMENTED FLEXURES, DOWLING-DEGOS TYPE
18006 RETINAL FOLD
18007 RETINAL DYSPLASIA
* 18010 RETINITIS PIGMENTOSA
* 18020 RETINOBLASTOMA
18027 RETINOSCHISIS
18030 ARTHRITIS, RHEUMATOID
* 18050 RIEGER SYNDROME
* 18070 ROBINOW SYNDROME
18075 CRANIOSYNOSTOSIS-FOOT DEFECTS, JACKSON-WEISS TYPE
* 18080 NEUROPATHY, HEREDITARY MOTOR AND SENSORY, TYPE I
18087 OSTEODYSTROPHY-MENTAL RETARDATION, RUVALCABA TYPE
18089 OVERGROWTH, RUVALCABA-MYHRE-SMITH TYPE
* 18090 GINGIVAL FIBROMATOSIS-CORNEAL DYSTROPHY
* 18092 ALACRIMA-APTYALISM
18100 SARCOIDOSIS
18125 SCALP DEFECTS-POSTAXIAL POLYDACTYLY
* 18135 HAUPTMANN-THANHAUSER SYNDROME
18144 JOINTS, OSTEOCHONDRITIS DISSECANS
* 18145 ULNAR-MAMMARY SYNDROME
18150 MOOD AND THOUGHT DISORDERS
* 18160 SCLEROTYLOSIS
18175 SCLERODERMA, FAMILIAL PROGRESSIVE
18180 SPINE, SCOLIOSIS, IDIOPATHIC

18221 PHARYNX/LARYNX HYPOPLASIA-OMPHALOCELE, SHPRINTZEN-GOLDBERG TYPE
18223 SEPTO-OPTIC DYSPLASIA
18225 SINGLETON-MERTEN SYNDROME
* 18260 PARAPLEGIA, FAMILIAL SPASTIC
* 18290 ANEMIA, HEMOLYTIC, RED CELL MEMBRANE DEFECTS
* 18290 SPHEROCYTOSIS
18294 CAUDAL REGRESSION SYNDROME
18294 SACROCOCCYGEAL DYSGENESIS SYNDROME
18296 SPINAL MUSCULAR ATROPHY
18297 SPINAL MUSCULAR ATROPHY
* 18298 SPINAL MUSCULAR ATROPHY
18330 SPLENOGONADAL FUSION-LIMB DEFECT
* 18360 ECTRODACTYLY
* 18360 TIBIAL HYPOPLASIA/APLASIA-ECTRODACTYLY
18370 ACROFACIAL DYSOSTOSIS, NAGER TYPE
* 18390 SPONDYLOEPIPHYSEAL DYSPLASIA CONGENITA
* 18410 SPONDYLOEPIPHYSEAL DYSPLASIA, LATE
18420 SPINE, SPONDYLOLISTHESIS AND SPONDYLOLYSIS
18425 SPONDYLOMETAPHYSEAL CHONDRODYSPLA-SIA, KOZLOWSKI TYPE
* 18440 SPRENGEL DEFORMITY
18445 STUTTERING
18485 HYPEREKPLEXIA
* 18490 STIFF SKIN SYNDROME
* 18500 ANEMIA, HEMOLYTIC, RED CELL MEMBRANE DEFECTS
* 18501 ANEMIA, HEMOLYTIC, RED CELL MEMBRANE DEFECTS
18515 DEAFNESS, STREPTOMYCIN-SENSITIVITY
18530 STURGE-WEBER SYNDROME
* 18550 AORTIC STENOSIS, SUPRAVALVAR
* 18550 PULMONARY ARTERY, COARCTATION
18565 SYMPHALANGISM
* 18570 SYMPHALANGISM
18575 SYMPHALANGISM
* 18580 SYMPHALANGISM
* 18590 SYNDACTYLY
* 18600 SYNDACTYLY
* 18610 SYNDACTYLY
18620 SYNDACTYLY
* 18630 SYNDACTYLY
* 18635 SYNDACTYLY-POLYDACTYLY-EAR LOBE SYNDROME
* 18640 SYMPHALANGISM
* 18650 SYMPHALANGISM
* 18658 GRANULOMATOSIS-POLYSYNOVITIS, FAMILIAL SYSTEMIC
18670 SYRINGOMYELIA
* 18688 LEUKEMIA/LYMPHOMA, T-CELL
* 18700 TEETH, LOBODONTIA
18705 TEETH, NATAL OR NEONATAL
18710 TEETH, SUPERNUMERARY
* 18730 SKIN, ACANTHOSIS NIGRICANS
* 18730 TELANGIECTASIA, OSLER HEMORRHAGIC
18735 TELECANTHUS, HEREDITARY
18750 HEART, TETRALOGY OF FALLOT
* 18760 THANATOPHORIC DYSPLASIA
18777 THORACOPELVIC DYSOSTOSIS
18780 THROMBASTHENIA, GLANZMANN-NAEGELI TYPE
18803 THROMBOCYTOPENIC PURPURA AND LIPID HISTIOCYTOSIS
18840 IMMUNODEFICIENCY, THYMIC AGENESIS
* 18845 THYROID, THYROGLOBULIN DEFECTS
18855 CANCER, THYROID, FAMILIAL PAPILLARY CARCINOMA OF
* 18857 THYROID, HORMONE RESISTANCE
* 18860 THYROXINE-BINDING GLOBULIN DEFECTS

18874 MESOMELIC DYSPLASIA, WERNER TYPE
* 18877 MESOMELIC DYSPLASIA, WERNER TYPE
18930 TONGUE, FOLDING OR ROLLING
* 18950 HYPODONTIA-NAIL DYSGENESIS
18960 TORTICOLLIS
* 18970 MANDIBLE, TORUS MANDIBULARIS
* 18970 PALATE, TORUS PALATINUS
18996 ESOPHAGUS, ATRESIA AND TRACHEOESOPH-
AGEAL FISTULA
18996 TRACHEOESOPHAGEAL FISTULA
* 19008 LYMPHOMA, BURKITT TYPE
* 19010 CHIN, TREMBLING
* 19030 TREMOR, HEREDOFAMILIAL
* 19031 TREMOR-DUODENAL ULCER SYNDROME
* 19032 TRICHO-DENTO-OSSEOUS SYNDROME
* 19035 TRICHO-RHINO-PHALANGEAL SYNDROME,
TYPE I
19036 TRICHODYSPLASIA-XERODERMA
19044 TRIGONENCEPHALY, AUTOSOMAL DOMINANT
TYPE
* 19045 ERYTHROCYTE TRIOSEPHOSPHATE ISOMERASE
DEFICIENCY
19060 THUMB, TRIPHALANGEAL
19068 THUMB, TRIPHALANGEAL-BRACHYECTRODAC-
TYLY
* 19090 COLOR BLINDNESS, YELLOW-BLUE TRITAN
* 19110 TUBEROUS SCLEROSIS
19115 IMMUNODEFICIENCY, TUFTSIN DEFICIENCY
TYPE
* 19120 DEAFNESS, TUNE
19140 MESOMELIC DYSPLASIA, REINHARDT-PFEIFFER
TYPE
* 19148 HAIR, UNCOMBABLE-CRYSTALLINE CATARACT
* 19183 RENAL AGENESIS, BILATERAL
* 19183 RENAL AGENESIS, UNILATERAL
19190 URTICARIA-DEAFNESS-AMYLOIDOSIS
19200 MULLERIAN FUSION, INCOMPLETE
19205 MULLERIAN FUSION, INCOMPLETE
19210 UVULA, CLEFT
19235 VATER ASSOCIATION
19243 VELO-CARDIO-FACIAL SYNDROME
* 19250 ARRHYTHMIA, WITH LONG QT INTERVAL
WITHOUT DEAFNESS
* 19260 HEART, SUBAORTIC STENOSIS, MUSCULAR
19300 VESICO-URETERAL REFLUX
19320 SKIN, VITILIGO
* 19325 INTESTINAL ROTATION, INCOMPLETE
* 19330 VON HIPPEL-LINDAU SYNDROME
* 19340 VON WILLEBRAND DISEASE
* 19350 WAARDENBURG SYNDROMES
19351 WAARDENBURG SYNDROMES
* 19352 PULMONIC STENOSIS-CAFE-AU-LAIT SPOTS,
WATSON TYPE
* 19353 ACROFACIAL DYSOSTOSIS
* 19353 ACROFACIAL SYNDROME, CURRY-HALL TYPE
* 19370 CRANIO-CARPO-TARSAL DYSPLASIA,
WHISTLING FACE TYPE
* 19390 MUCOSA, WHITE FOLDED DYSPLASIA
* 19405 WILLIAMS SYNDROME
19407 ANIRIDIA
* 19407 CANCER, WILMS TUMOR
19408 WILMS TUMOR-PSEUDOHERMAPHRODITISM-
GLOMERULOPATHY,DENYS-DRASH TYPE
19420 ARRHYTHMIA, WOLFF-PARKINSON-WHITE TYPE
19435 WT SYNDROME
* 19438 ANEMIA, HEMOLYTIC, RED CELL MEMBRANE
DEFECTS
* 20010 ABETALIPOPROTEINEMIA
* 20010 ANEMIA, HEMOLYTIC, RED CELL MEMBRANE
DEFECTS
20011 ABLEPHARON-MACROSTOMIA
* 20015 ACANTHOCYTOSIS-NEUROLOGIC DEFECTS
20017 SKIN, ACANTHOSIS NIGRICANS

* 20040 ESOPHAGUS, ACHALASIA
* 20050 ACHEIROPODY
* 20060 ACHONDROGENESIS, HOUSTON-HARRIS TYPE
* 20060 ACHONDROGENESIS, PARENTI-FRACCARO TYPE
* 20061 ACHONDROGENESIS, HOUSTON-HARRIS TYPE
* 20061 ACHONDROGENESIS, LANGER-SALDINO TYPE
* 20070 GREBE SYNDROME
20090 METAPHYSEAL CHONDRODYSPLASIA WITH
THYMOLYMPHOPENIA
20097 DENTO-FACIO-SKELETAL DEFECTS, ACKERMAN
TYPE
20098 ACRO-RENAL-MANDIBULAR SYNDROME
20099 ACROCALLOSAL SYNDROME, SCHINZEL TYPE
* 20100 ACROCEPHALOPOLYSYNDACTYLY
20102 ACROCEPHALOPOLYSYNDACTYLY
* 20110 ACRODERMATITIS ENTEROPATHICA
* 20110 NEUROPATHY, MYELO-OPTICO, SUBACUTE
TYPE
20118 ACRO-FRONTO-FACIO-NASAL DYSOSTOSIS
20120 PROGERIA
* 20125 ACROMESOMELIC DYSPLASIA,
CAMPAILLA-MARTINELLI TYPE
* 20125 ACROMESOMELIC DYSPLASIA,
MAROTEAUX-MARTINELLI-CAMPAILLA TYPE
* 20130 ACRO-OSTEOLYSIS, NEUROGENIC
20140 ADRENOCORTICOTROPIC HORMONE
DEFICIENCY, ISOLATED
* 20145 ACYL-CoA DEHYDROGENASE DEFICIENCY,
MEDIUM CHAIN TYPE
* 20146 ACYL-CoA DEHYDROGENASE DEFICIENCY,
LONG CHAIN TYPE
* 20147 ACYL-CoA DEHYDROGENASE DEFICIENCY,
SHORT CHAIN TYPE
* 20155 THUMB, ADDUCTED THUMB SYNDROME
* 20171 STEROID 20-22 DESMOLASE DEFICIENCY
* 20181 STEROID 3 BETA-HYDROXYSTEROID
DEHYDROGENASE DEFICIENCY
* 20191 STEROID 21-HYDROXYLASE DEFICIENCY
* 20201 STEROID 11 BETA-HYDROXYLASE DEFICIENCY
* 20211 STEROID 17 ALPHA-HYDROXYLASE DEFICIENCY
* 20220 ADRENOCORTICAL UNRESPONSIVENESS TO
ACTH, HEREDITARY
20240 AFIBROGINEMIA, CONGENITAL
* 20250 IMMUNODEFICIENCY, SEVERE COMBINED
20265 AGNATHIA-HOLOPROSENCEPHALY
* 20270 IMMUNODEFICIENCY, AGRANULOCYTOSIS,
INFANTILE KOSTMANN TYPE
* 20292 IMMUNODEFICIENCY, SEVERE COMBINED
* 20310 ALBINISM, OCULOCUTANEOUS, TYROSINASE
NEGATIVE
* 20320 ALBINISM, OCULOCUTANEOUS, TYROSINASE
POSITIVE
20328 ALBINISM, OCULOCUTANEOUS, MINIMAL
PIGMENT TYPE
* 20329 ALBINISM, OCULOCUTANEOUS, BROWN TYPE
* 20330 ALBINISM, OCULOCUTANEOUS,
HERMANSKY-PUDLAK TYPE
* 20331 ALBINISM, OCULAR, AUTOSOMAL RECESSIVE
TYPE
20332 ALBINISM, OCULOCUTANEOUS, YELLOW
MUTANT
20333 PARATHYROID HORMONE RESISTANCE
20334 ALBINISM-MICROCEPHALY-DIGITAL DEFECTS
* 20340 STEROID 18-HYDROXYLASE DEFICIENCY
* 20341 STEROID 18-HYDROXYSTEROID
DEHYDROGENASE DEFICIENCY
20345 ALEXANDER DISEASE
* 20350 ALKAPTONURIA
20355 ALOPECIA-SKELETAL ANOMALIES-SHORT
STATURE-MENTAL RETARDATION
20360 ALOPECIA-EPILEPSY-OLIGOPHRENIA,
MOYNAHAN TYPE
* 20365 ALOPECIA-MENTAL RETARDATION

*  20370  ALPERS DISEASE
*  20375  ACIDEMIA, 3-KETOTHIOLASE DEFICIENCY
   20378  NEPHRITIS-DEAFNESS (SENSORINEURAL),
          HEREDITARY TYPE
*  20380  ALSTROM SYNDROME
*  20400  RETINA, AMAUROSIS CONGENITA, LEBER TYPE
*  20410  RETINA, AMAUROSIS CONGENITA, LEBER TYPE
*  20420  NEURONAL CEROID-LIPOFUSCINOSES (NCL)
*  20430  NEURONAL CEROID-LIPOFUSCINOSES (NCL)
   20450  NEURONAL CEROID-LIPOFUSCINOSES (NCL)
*  20470  TEETH, AMELOGENESIS IMPERFECTA
*  20487  AMYLOIDOSIS, CORNEAL
*  20510  AMYOTROPHIC LATERAL SCLEROSIS
*  20510  AMYOTROPHIC LATERAL SCLEROSIS, FAMILIAL
          ADULT AND JUVENILE TYPES
*  20520  AMYOTROPHIC LATERAL SCLEROSIS
*  20520  AMYOTROPHIC LATERAL SCLEROSIS, FAMILIAL
          ADULT AND JUVENILE TYPES
   20525  AMYOTROPHIC LATERAL SCLEROSIS
   20525  AMYOTROPHIC LATERAL SCLEROSIS, FAMILIAL
          ADULT AND JUVENILE TYPES
*  20530  ANALBUMINEMIA
*  20540  ANALPHALIPOPROTEINEMIA
   20560  ANEMIA, HYPOPLASTIC-TRIPHALANGEAL
          THUMBS, AASE-SMITH TYPE
   20590  ANEMIA, HYPOPLASTIC CONGENITAL
   20595  ANEMIA, CONGENITAL SIDEROBLASTIC, NOT
          B(6) RESPONSIVE
   20650  ANENCEPHALY
   20655  ANGIOLIPOMATOSIS
   20670  ANIRIDIA-CEREBELLAR ATAXIA-MENTAL
          DEFICIENCY
   20675  ANIRIDIA-CEREBELLAR ATAXIA-MENTAL
          DEFICIENCY
*  20678  TEETH, ANODONTIA, PARTIAL OR COMPLETE
*  20680  NAILS, ANONYCHIA, HEREDITARY
*  20690  EYE, ANOPHTHALMIA
   20692  ANOPHTHALMIA-LIMB ANOMALIES
   20700  ANOSMIA, CONGENITAL
   20741  ANTLEY-BIXLER SYNDROME
   20750  ANORECTAL MALFORMATIONS
   20770  SKIN, LOCALIZED ABSENCE OF
*  20773  APLASIA CUTIS CONGENITA-GASTROINTESTI-
          NAL ATRESIA
*  20773. SKIN, LOCALIZED ABSENCE OF
   20778  AREDYLD SYNDROME
*  20780  ARGININEMIA
*  20790  ACIDURIA, ARGININOSUCCINIC
   20795  ANENCEPHALY
   20795  BRAIN, ARNOLD-CHIARI MALFORMATION
*  20800  ARTERY, CORONARY CALCINOSIS
*  20815  PENA-SHOKEIR SYNDROME
*  20820  KUSKOKWIN SYNDROME
*  20825  PERICARDITIS-ARTHRITIS-CAMPTODACTYLY
*  20825  SYNOVITIS, FAMILIAL HYPERTROPHIC
*  20840  ASPARTYLGLUCOSAMINURIA
*  20850  ASPHYXIATING THORACIC DYSPLASIA
   20853  ASPLENIA SYNDROME
*  20880  PYRUVATE DEHYDROGENASE DEFICIENCY
*  20890  ATAXIA-TELANGIECTASIA
   20891  ATAXIA-TELANGIECTASIA
   20920  SKIN, ATOPY, FAMILIAL
   20930  ATRANSFERRINEMIA
   20977  AURAL ATRESIA-DYSMORPHIC
          FACIES-SKELETAL DEFECTS
   20985  AUTISM, INFANTILE
*  20988  HYPOVENTILATION, CONGENITAL CENTRAL
          ALVEOLAR TYPE
*  20990  BARDET-BIEDL SYNDROME
   20997  HYDROCEPHALUS-HEART DEFECT-DENSE
          BONES, BEEMER TYPE
   21000  OPTIC ATROPHY, INFANTILE HEREDOFAMILIAL

*  21020  ACIDURIA, BETA-METHYL-CROTONYL-
          GLYCINURIA
   21021  ACIDURIA, BETA-METHYL-CROTONYL-
          GLYCINURIA
*  21025  HYPERAPOBETALIPOPROTEINEMIA
   21030  NEUROPATHY, CONGENITAL SENSORY WITH
          ANHIDROSIS
   21035  BIEMOND II SYNDROME
   21040  NOSE, BIFID
   21050  BILIARY ATRESIA
   21055  BILIARY ATRESIA
*  21060  SECKEL SYNDROME
   21070  SECKEL SYNDROME
   21072  DWARFISM, OSTEODYSPLASTIC PRIMORDIAL,
          MAJEWSKI-RANKE TYPE
   21073  DWARFISM, OSTEODYSPLASTIC PRIMORDIAL,
          MAJEWSKI-WINTER TYPE
*  21090  BLOOM SYNDROME
   21100  TRYPTOPHAN MALABSORPTION
*  21118  HUTTERITE SYNDROME, BOWEN-CONRADI TYPE
   21120  FRASER SYNDROME
   21135  KYPHOMELIC DYSPLASIA
   21137  OCULO-OSTEO-CUTANEOUS SYNDROME,
          TOUMAALA-HAAPANEN TYPE
   21138  BRANCHIO-SKELETO-GENITAL SYNDROME
*  21139  TRICHOTHIODYSTROPHY
   21145  BRONCHOMALACIA
*  21150  PALSY, PROGRESSIVE BULBAR OF CHILDHOOD
*  21160  JAUNDICE, INTRAHEPATIC CHOLESTATIC,
          BYLER TYPE
*  21175  C SYNDROME
   21191  CAMPTODACTYLY SYNDROME, GUADALAJARA
          TYPE I
   21192  CAMPTODACTYLY SYNDROME, GUADALAJARA
          TYPE II
*  21196  CAMPTODACTYLY SYNDROME, TEL HASHOMER
          TYPE
*  21197  CAMPOMELIC DYSPLASIA
   21198  CANCER, LUNG, FAMILIAL
*  21205  CANDIDIASIS, FAMILIAL CHRONIC
          MUCOCUTANEOUS
   21211  CARDIOMYOPATHY, FAMILIAL DILATED
   21212  CARDIOMYOPATHY-GENITAL DEFECTS
*  21214  MYOPATHY-METABOLIC, CARNITINE
          DEFICIENCY, PRIMARY AND SECONDARY
*  21216  MYOPATHY-METABOLIC, CARNITINE
          DEFICIENCY, PRIMARY AND SECONDARY
*  21220  CARNOSINEMIA
*  21240  CATARACT-ICHTHYOSIS
*  21250  CATARACT, HUTTERITE
   21260  CATARACT, CORTICAL AND NUCLEAR
   21270  CATARACT, CORTICAL AND NUCLEAR
   21272  MARTSOLF SYNDROME
   21275  GLUTEN-SENSITIVE ENTEROPATHY
*  21278  SYNDACTYLY
*  21278  SYNDACTYLY, CENANI TYPE
*  21284  ATAXIA-HYPOGONADISM SYNDROME
*  21300  CEREBELLAR AGENESIS
*  21330  JOUBERT SYNDROME
*  21330  VERMIS AGENESIS
*  21370  XANTHOMATOSIS, CEREBROTENDINOUS
*  21410  CEREBRO-HEPATO-RENAL SYNDROME
   21415  CEREBRO-OCULO-FACIO-SKELETAL SYNDROME
   21430  KLIPPEL-FEIL ANOMALY
   21435  CHANDS
*  21440  NEUROPATHY, HEREDITARY MOTOR AND
          SENSORY, TYPE I
*  21445  HYPOPIGMENTATION-IMMUNE DEFECT,
          GRISCELLI TYPE
*  21450  CHEDIAK-HIGASHI SYNDROME
*  21470  DIARRHEA, CONGENITAL CHLORIDE
   21480  CHARGE ASSOCIATION
   21480  NOSE, POSTERIOR ATRESIA

* 21490 CHOLESTASIS-LYMPHEDEMA, AAGENAES TYPE
* 21495 ACIDEMIA, TRIHYDROXYCOPROSTANIC
  21500 CHOLESTERYL ESTER STORAGE DISEASE
* 21510 CHONDRODYSPLASIA PUNCTATA, RHIZOMELIC TYPE
* 21515 CHONDRODYSTROPHY-SENSORINEURAL DEAFNESS, NANCE-INSLEY TYPE
* 21515 OTO-SPONDYLO-MEGAEPIPHYSEAL DYSPLASIA
  21555 CIRCUMVALLATE PLACENTA SYNDROME
* 21570 CITRULLINEMIA
  21590 CLEFT LIP
  21610 ORO-CRANIO-DIGITAL SYNDROME
  21630 CLEFT PALATE-STAPES FIXATION-OLIGODONTIA
* 21634 YUNIS-VARON SYNDROME
  21635 RETINA, COATS DISEASE
* 21640 COCKAYNE SYNDROME
  21641 COCKAYNE SYNDROME, TYPE II
* 21650 OCULAR MOTOR APRAXIA, COGAN CONGENITAL TYPE
* 21655 COHEN SYNDROME
  21682 EYE, MICROPHTHALMIA/COLOBOMA
* 21690 COLOR BLINDNESS, TOTAL
* 21695 COMPLEMENT COMPONENT 1, DEFICIENCY OF
* 21700 COMPLEMENT COMPONENT 2, DEFICIENCY OF
* 21703 COMPLEMENT COMPONENT 3, DEFICIENCY OF
  21709 EYE, LIGNEOUS CONJUNCTIVITIS
  21710 AMNIOTIC BANDS SYNDROME
  21710 LIMB AND SCALP DEFECTS, ADAMS-OLIVER TYPE
  21720 EPILEPSY, FAMILIAL
  21720 SEIZURES, FEBRILE
* 21730 CORNEA PLANA
  21740 CORNEAL DYSTROPHY-SENSORINEURAL DEAFNESS
* 21750 EYE, KERATOPATHY, BAND-SHAPED
* 21770 CORNEAL DYSTROPHY, ENDOTHELIAL, CONGENITAL HEREDITARY
* 21780 CORNEAL DYSTROPHY, MACULAR TYPE
* 21800 CORPUS CALLOSUM AGENESIS-SENSORIMOTOR NEUROPATHY, FAMILIAL
  21801 BLINDNESS (CORTICAL)-RETARDATION-POSTAXIAL POLYDACTYLY
* 21830 CRANIO-DIAPHYSEAL DYSPLASIA
* 21833 CRANIO-ECTODERMAL DYSPLASIA
  21835 CRANIOFACIAL DYSSYNOSTOSIS
* 21840 CRANIOMETAPHYSEAL DYSPLASIA
* 21850 CRANIOSYNOSTOSIS
* 21850 CRANIOSYNOSTOSIS-FOOT DEFECTS, JACKSON-WEISS TYPE
  21855 CRANIOSYNOSTOSIS-FIBULAR APLASIA, LOWRY TYPE
* 21860 CRANIOSYNOSTOSIS-RADIAL APLASIA SYNDROME
  21865 CRANIOSYNOSTOSIS-MENTAL RETARDATION-CLEFTING SYNDROME
  21867 CRANIOTELENCEPHALIC DYSPLASIA
* 21870 THYROID, DYSGENESIS
* 21880 UDP-GLUCURONOSYLTRANSFERASE, SEVERE DEFICIENCY TYPE I
* 21890 CATARACT-RENAL TUBULAR NECROSIS-ENCEPHALOPATHY, CROME TYPE
* 21900 EYE, CRYPTOPHTHALMOS WITH OTHER MALFORMATIONS
* 21900 FRASER SYNDROME
* 21910 CUTIS LAXA
* 21915 CUTIS LAXA-GROWTH DEFECT, DE BARSY TYPE
* 21920 CUTIS LAXA-DELAYED DEVELOPMENT-LIGAMENTOUS LAXITY
  21925 CUTIS MARMORATA
  21930 CUTIS VERTICUS GYRATA
* 21950 CYSTATHIONINURIA
* 21970 CYSTIC FIBROSIS

* 21975 CYSTINOSIS
* 21980 CYSTINOSIS
* 21990 CYSTINOSIS
* 22010 CYSTINURIA
* 22011 MYOPATHY-METABOLIC, MITOCHONDRIAL CYTOCHROME C OXIDASE DEFICIENCY
* 22015 RENAL HYPOURICEMIA
  22020 HYDROCEPHALY
* 22040 CARDIO-AUDITORY SYNDROME
* 22050 DEAFNESS-ONYCHO-OSTEO-DYSTROPHY-RETARDATION-SEIZURES (DOORS)
* 22050 DEAFNESS-ONYCHODYSTROPHY
* 22050 DEAFNESS-TRIPHALANGEAL THUMBS-ONYCHODYSTROPHY
* 22070 DEAFNESS (SENSORINEURAL), RECESSIVE PROFOUND
* 22080 DEAFNESS (SENSORINEURAL), RECESSIVE PROFOUND
  22100 DEAFNESS, PFAENDLER TYPE
  22120 DEAFNESS-MYOPIA
* 22130 DEAFNESS-MALFORMED EARS-MENTAL RETARDATION
* 22130 DEAFNESS-MALFORMED, LOW-SET EARS
* 22130 EAR, LOW-SET
* 22135 DEAFNESS-VITILIGO-MUSCLE WASTING
  22140 DEAFNESS-DIVERTICULITIS-NEUROPATHY
  22160 DEAFNESS (SENSORINEURAL), RECESSIVE EARLY-ONSET
  22170 DEAFNESS-ATOPIC DERMATITIS
* 22177 OSTEODYSPLASIA, LIPOMEMBRANOUS POLYCYSTIC-DEMENTIA
* 22180 DERMO-CHONDRO-CORNEAL DYSTROPHY, FRANCOIS TYPE
  22181 DERMATO-OSTEOLYSIS, KIRGHIZIAN TYPE
  22188 LARSEN SYNDROME
* 22190 RETINAL DYSPLASIA
  22210 DIABETES MELLITUS, INSULIN DEPENDENT TYPE
* 22230 DIABETES (INSIPIDUS/MELLITUS)-OPTIC ATROPHY-DEAFNESS
  22250 DIASTEMATOMYELIA
* 22260 DIASTROPHIC DYSPLASIA
* 22269 HYPERDIBASIC AMINOACIDURIA
* 22270 HYPERDIBASIC AMINOACIDURIA
  22273 ACIDURIA, DICARBOXYLIC AMINOACIDURIA
  22276 DIGITO-RENO-CEREBRAL SYNDROME
* 22280 ERYTHROCYTE, DIPHOSPHOGLYCERATE MUTASE (2,3) DEFICIENCY
* 22290 SUCRASE-ISOMALTASE DEFICIENCY
* 22300 LACTASE DEFICIENCY, CONGENITAL
* 22310 LACTASE DEFICIENCY, PRIMARY
* 22336 DOPAMINE BETA-HYDROXYLASE DEFICIENCY, CONGENITAL
* 22337 DUBOWITZ SYNDROME
  22340 DUODENUM, ATRESIA OR STENOSIS
  22340 PYLORODUODENAL ATRESIA, HEREDITARY
* 22380 DYGGVE-MELCHIOR-CLAUSEN SYNDROME
* 22390 DYSAUTONOMIA I, RILEY-DAY TYPE
* 22405 DYSEQUILIBRIUM SYNDROME
* 22410 ANEMIA, DYSERYTHROPOIETIC, TYPE II
* 22412 ANEMIA, DYSERYTHROPOIETIC, TYPE I
  22423. DYSKERATOSIS CONGENITA
* 22430 DYSOSTEOSCLEROSIS
  22440 DWARFISM, DYSSEGMENTAL, ROLLAND-DESBUQUOIS TYPE
  22441 DWARFISM, DYSSEGMENTAL, SILVERMAN-HANDMAKER TYPE
* 22450 TORSION DYSTONIA
  22470 TRICUSPID VALVE, EBSTEIN ANOMALY
* 22490 ECTODERMAL DYSPLASIA, CHRIST-SIEMENS-TOURAINE TYPE
* 22490 ECTODERMAL DYSPLASIA, PASSARGE TYPE

22500    CLEFT LIP/PALATE-ECTODERMAL DYSPLASIA-SYNDACTYLY
* 22520    LENS AND PUPIL, ECTOPIC
* 22528    ECTODERMAL DYSPLASIA-ECTRODACTYLY-MACULAR DYSTROPHY
22529    ECTRODACTYLY-POLYDACTYLY
22530    ECTRODACTYLY
22531    EHLERS-DANLOS SYNDROME
22532    EHLERS-DANLOS SYNDROME
* 22535    EHLERS-DANLOS SYNDROME
22536    EHLERS-DANLOS SYNDROME
* 22540    EHLERS-DANLOS SYNDROME
22541    EHLERS-DANLOS SYNDROME
22545    ANEMIA, HEMOLYTIC, RED CELL MEMBRANE DEFECTS
* 22550    CHONDROECTODERMAL DYSPLASIA
22600    VENTRICLE, ENDOCARDIAL FIBROELASTOSIS OF LEFT VENTRICLE
22600    VENTRICLE, ENDOCARDIAL FIBROELASTOSIS OF RIGHT VENTRICLE
* 22620    INTESTINAL ENTEROKINASE DEFICIENCY
* 22645    EPIDERMOLYSIS BULLOSUM, TYPE III
* 22650    EPIDERMOLYSIS BULLOSUM, TYPE III
* 22660    EPIDERMOLYSIS BULLOSUM, TYPE III
22665    EPIDERMOLYSIS BULLOSUM, TYPE II
* 22670    EPIDERMOLYSIS BULLOSUM, TYPE II
22673    EPIDERMOLYSIS BULLOSUM, TYPE II
22675    AMELO-CEREBRO-HYPOHIDROTIC SYNDROME
22675    EPILEPSY, FAMILIAL
22680    EPILEPSY, FAMILIAL
22685    EPILEPSY, FAMILIAL
* 22690    EPIPHYSEAL DYSPLASIA, MULTIPLE, RECESSIVE TARDA TYPE
22695    EPIPHYSEAL DYSPLASIA, MULTIPLE, RECESSIVE TARDA TYPE
* 22698    EPIPHYSEAL DYSPLASIA, MULTIPLE-DIABETES MELLITUS
22720    HYPOGONADOTROPIC HYPOGONADISM
22723.    RETINA, VITREORETINOPATHY, FAMILIAL EXUDATIVE
* 22726    ECTODERMAL DYSPLASIA, CONGENITAL FACIAL, SETLEIS TYPE
22727    FACIO-CARDIOMELIC DYSPLASIA, LETHAL
22729    FACIO-OCULO-ACOUSTIC-RENAL SYNDROME (FOAR SYNDROME)
* 22730    COAGULATION DEFECT, FAMILIAL MULTIPLE FACTORS
22731    COAGULATION DEFECT, FAMILIAL MULTIPLE FACTORS
* 22740    FACTOR V DEFICIENCY
* 22750    FACTOR VII DEFICIENCY
* 22760    FACTOR X DEFICIENCY
* 22765    PANCYTOPENIA SYNDROME, FANCONI TYPE
22770    RENAL TUBULAR SYNDROME, FANCONI TYPE
22780    RENAL TUBULAR SYNDROME, FANCONI TYPE
22781    RENAL TUBULAR SYNDROME, FANCONI TYPE
22785    RENAL TUBULAR SYNDROME, FANCONI TYPE
* 22800    LIPOGRANULOMATOSIS
* 22810    VISCERA, FATTY METAMORPHOSIS
22820    FIBULA, CONGENITAL ABSENCE OF
22830    GONADOTROPIN DEFICIENCIES
22830    HYPOGONADOTROPIC HYPOGONADISM
* 22852    FIBROCHONDROGENESIS
* 22860    FIBROMATOSIS, JUVENILE HYALINE
22893    SKELETAL DYSPLASIA, FUHRMANN TYPE
22899    RETINA, FLECKED KANDORI TYPE
* 22905    FOLATE MALABSORPTION
22907    GONADOTROPIN DEFICIENCIES
* 22930    ATAXIA, FRIEDREICH TYPE
22931    ATAXIA, FRIEDREICH TYPE
* 22940    FRONTO-FACIO-NASAL DYSPLASIA
* 22960    FRUCTOSE-1-PHOSPHATE ALDOLASE DEFICIENCY

* 22970    FRUCTOSE-1,6-DIPHOSPHATASE DEFICIENCY
* 22980    FRUCTOSURIA
* 22985    FRYNS SYNDROME
* 23000    FUCOSIDOSIS
23010    RETINA, FUNDUS FLAVIMACULATUS
* 23020    GALACTOKINASE DEFICIENCY
* 23035    GALACTOSE EPIMERASE DEFICIENCY
* 23040    GALACTOSEMIA
* 23045    ANEMIA, HEMOLYTIC, GAMMA-GLUTAMYL/CYSTEINE SYNTHETASE DEFICIENCY
* 23050    G(M1)-GANGLIOSIDOSIS, TYPE 1
23060    G(M1)-GANGLIOSIDOSIS, TYPE 2
23065    G(M1)-GANGLIOSIDOSIS, TYPE 3
* 23074    GROWTH RETARDATION-ALOPECIA-PSEUDOANODONTIA-OPTIC ATROPHY
* 23080    GAUCHER DISEASE
23090    GAUCHER DISEASE
23100    GAUCHER DISEASE
* 23105    GELEOPHYSIC DWARFISM
* 23107    OSTEODYSPLASTICA GERODERMIA, BAMATTER TYPE
23109    HYDATIDIFORM MOLE
* 23130    GLAUCOMA, CONGENITAL
* 23160    GLUCOSE-GALACTOSE MALABSORPTION
* 23167    ACIDEMIA, GLUTARIC ACIDEMIA I
* 23168    ACIDEMIA, ETHYLMALONIC-ADIPIC
* 23170    ANEMIA, HEMOLYTIC, GLUTATIONINE PEROXIDASE DEFICIENCY
23180    ANEMIA, HEMOLYTIC, GLUTATHIONE REDUCTASE DEFICIENCY
* 23190    ANEMIA, HEMOLYTIC, GLUTATHIONE SYNTHETASE DEFICIENCY
* 23195    GLUTATHIONURIA
* 23200    ACIDEMIA, PROPIONIC
23210    GLYCOGENOSIS, TYPE IId
* 23220    GLYCOGENOSIS, TYPE Ia
23222    GLYCOGENOSIS, TYPE Ib
23224    GLYCOGENOSIS, TYPE Ic
* 23230    GLYCOGENOSIS, TYPE IIa
* 23230    GLYCOGENOSIS, TYPE IIb
23233    GLYCOGENOSIS, TYPE IIc
* 23240    GLYCOGENOSIS, TYPE III
* 23250    GLYCOGENOSIS, TYPE IV
* 23260    GLYCOGENOSIS, TYPE V
* 23270    GLYCOGENOSIS, TYPE VI
* 23280    GLYCOGENOSIS, TYPE VII
* 23280    GLYCOGENOSIS, TYPE VIII
* 23310    RENAL GLYCOSURIA
* 23330    GONADAL DYSGENESIS, XX TYPE
* 23340    PERRAULT SYNDROME
23342    GONADAL DYSGENESIS, XY TYPE
23344    LEYDIG CELL HYPOPLASIA
23350    GORLIN-CHAUDHRY-MOSS SYNDROME
* 23370    GRANULOMATOUS DISEASE, CHRONIC X-LINKED
* 23400    FACTOR XII DEFICIENCY
23403    TRICHOTHIODYSTROPHY
* 23405    TRICHOTHIODYSTROPHY
23410    OCULO-MANDIBULO-FACIAL SYNDROME
23420    HALLERVORDEN-SPATZ DISEASE
23430    SKIN, VITILIGO
23440    ANGELMAN SYNDROME
* 23450    HARTNUP DISORDER
23470    ARRHYTHMIA, CARDIAC CONDUCTION DEFECTS, NEONATAL
23470    ARRHYTHMIA, HEART BLOCK, CONGENITAL COMPLETE
23500    HEMIHYPERTROPHY
* 23520    HEMOCHROMATOSIS, IDIOPATHIC
23540    HEMOLYTIC-UREMIC SYNDROME
23560    HERMAPHRODITISM, TRUE
23570    ANEMIA, HEMOLYTIC, ERYTHROCYTE HEXOKINASE DEFICIENCY

|   |   |   |
|---|---|---|
|   | 23575 | HIRSCHSPRUNG DISEASE-CARDIAC DEFECT |
| * | 23580 | HISTIDINEMIA |
| * | 23583 | HISTIDINURIA |
|   | 23600 | CANCER, HODGKIN DISEASE, FAMILIAL |
| * | 23610 | CYCLOPIA |
| * | 23610 | HOLOPROSENCEPHALY |
| * | 23620 | HOMOCYSTINURIA |
| * | 23625 | HOMOCYSTINURIA, N(5,10) METHYLENE TETRAHYDROFOLATE DEFICIENCY TYPE |
| * | 23627 | METHYLCOBALAMIN DEFICIENCY |
|   | 23630 | HOOFT DISEASE |
| * | 23640 | HUMERO-RADIAL SYNOSTOSIS |
|   | 23645 | CEREBRO-NEPHRO-OSTEODYSPLASIA, HUTTERITE TYPE |
|   | 23660 | HYDROCEPHALY |
| * | 23667 | WALKER-WARBURG SYNDROME |
| * | 23668 | HYDROLETHALUS SYNDROME |
| * | 23670 | VAGINAL SEPTUM, TRANSVERSE |
| * | 23673 | UROFACIAL SYNDROME |
|   | 23675 | HYDROPS FETALIS, NON-IMMUNE |
| * | 23700 | HYDROXYPROLINEMIA |
|   | 23710 | HYMEN, IMPERFORATE |
| * | 23730 | CARBAMOYL PHOSPHATE SYNTHETASE DEFICIENCY |
|   | 23731 | N-ACETYLGLUTAMATE SYNTHETASE DEFICIENCY |
|   | 23740 | HYPERBETA-ALANINEMIA |
| * | 23745 | HYPERBILIRUBINEMIA, CONJUGATED, ROTOR TYPE |
| * | 23750 | HYPERBILIRUBINEMIA, CONJUGATED |
|   | 23755 | HYPERBILIRUBINEMIA, CONJUGATED |
| * | 23780 | HYPERBILIRUBINEMIA, CONJUGATED |
| * | 23790 | HYPERBILIRUBINEMIA, TRANSIENT FAMILIAL NEONATAL |
|   | 23820 | HYPERCYSTINURIA |
| * | 23830 | HYPERGLYCINEMIA, NON-KETOTIC |
|   | 23832 | KLINEFELTER SYNDROME |
| * | 23860 | HYPERCHYLOMICRONEMIA |
| * | 23870 | HYPERLYSINEMIA |
| * | 23897 | HYPERORNITHINEMIA-HYPERAMMONEMIA-HOMOCITRULLINURIA |
| * | 23900 | OSTEOECTASIA |
| * | 23910 | ENDOSTEAL HYPEROSTOSIS |
|   | 23920 | HYPERPARATHYROIDISM, FAMILIAL |
| * | 23950 | HYPERPROLINEMIA |
| * | 23951 | HYPERPROLINEMIA |
| * | 23980 | HYPERTELORISM-MICROTIA-FACIAL CLEFT-CONDUCTIVE DEAFNESS |
|   | 23985 | OSTEOCHONDRODYSPLASIA WITH HYPERTRICHOSIS |
| * | 24020 | ADRENAL HYPOPLASIA, CONGENITAL |
| * | 24030 | POLYGLANDULAR AUTOIMMUNE SYNDROME |
| * | 24050 | IMMUNODEFICIENCY, COMMON VARIABLE TYPE |
| * | 24050 | SERUM ALLOTYPES, HUMAN |
| * | 24060 | GLYCOGEN SYNTHETASE DEFICIENCY |
| * | 24080 | HYPOGLYCEMIA, FAMILIAL NEONATAL |
| * | 24108 | HYPOGONADISM-DIABETES-ALOPECIA-DEAFNESS-RETARDATION-EKG ANOMALIES |
|   | 24109 | HYPOGONADISM-PARTIAL ALOPECIA |
| * | 24120 | BARTTER SYNDROME |
| * | 24150 | HYPOPHOSPHATASIA |
| * | 24151 | HYPOPHOSPHATASIA |
| * | 24153 | RICKETS, HEREDITARY HYPOPHOSPHATEMIC WITH HYPERCALCIURIA (HHRH) |
|   | 24175 | HYPOSPADIAS |
| * | 24190 | HAIR, ATRICHIA CONGENITA |
|   | 24205 | RENAL HYPOURICEMIA |
| * | 24210 | ICHTHYOSIS, CONGENITAL ERYTHRODERMIC |
| * | 24210 | ICHTHYOSIS, LAMELLAR RECESSIVE |
|   | 24215 | ICHTHYOSIFORM ERYTHROKERATODERMA, ATYPICAL WITH DEAFNESS |
| * | 24217 | TRICHOTHIODYSTROPHY |
| * | 24230 | ICHTHYOSIS, CONGENITAL ERYTHRODERMIC |
| * | 24230 | ICHTHYOSIS, LAMELLAR RECESSIVE |
| * | 24250 | ICHTHYOSIS, HARLEQUIN FETUS |
| * | 24260 | IMINOGLYCINURIA |
| * | 24270 | IMMUNODEFICIENCY, NEZELOF TYPE |
|   | 24286 | IMMUNODEFICIENCY WITH CENTROMERIC INSTABILITY |
| * | 24309 | LIPODYSTROPHY-COARSE FACIES-ACANTHOSIS NIGRICANS, MIESCHER TYPE |
| * | 24309 | SKIN, ACANTHOSIS NIGRICANS |
| * | 24315 | INTESTINAL ATRESIA OR STENOSIS |
| * | 24315 | INTESTINAL ATRESIAS, MULTIPLE |
| * | 24318 | INTESTINAL PSEUDO-OBSTRUCTION SYNDROMES |
|   | 24330 | CHOLESTASIS, INTRAHEPATIC, RECURRENT BENIGN |
| * | 24340 | ACETYLATOR POLYMORPHISM |
| * | 24340 | NEUROPATHY, HERITABLE ISONIAZIDE TYPE (INH) |
|   | 24345 | ANOSMIA, CONGENITAL |
| * | 24350 | ACIDEMIA, ISOVALERIC |
| * | 24360 | JEJUNAL ATRESIA |
| * | 24370 | IMMUNODEFICIENCY, HYPER IgE TYPE |
| * | 24380 | JOHANSON-BLIZZARD SYNDROME |
|   | 24410 | JUMPING FRENCHMAN OF MAINE |
| * | 24420 | KALLMANN SYNDROME |
| * | 24440 | DEXTROCARDIA-BRONCHIECTASIS-SINUSITIS SYNDROME |
| * | 24445 | OCULO-CEREBRO-FACIAL SYNDROME, KAUFMAN TYPE |
|   | 24450 | EYE, KERATOCONUS |
|   | 24485 | KERATOSIS PALMARIS ET PLANTARIS OF UNNA-THOST |
| * | 24500 | HYPERKERATOSIS PALMOPLANTARIS-PERIODONTOCLASIA |
| * | 24515 | KEUTEL SYNDROME |
| * | 24519 | KNIEST-LIKE DYSPLASIA |
| * | 24520 | LEUKODYSTROPHY, GLOBOID CELL TYPE |
|   | 24521 | MENINGOCELE-CONOTRUNCAL HEART DEFECT, KOUSSEFF TYPE |
|   | 24534 | ERYTHROCYTE, LACTATE TRANSPORTER DEFECT |
| * | 24560 | LARSEN SYNDROME |
|   | 24565 | LARSEN SYNDROME, LETHAL TYPE |
|   | 24580 | LAURENCE-MOON SYNDROME |
|   | 24590 | ANEMIA, HEMOLYTIC, RED CELL MEMBRANE DEFECTS |
| * | 24590 | LECITHIN-CHOLESTEROL ACYL TRANSFERASE DEFICIENCY |
| * | 24620 | LEPRECHAUNISM |
| * | 24640 | LETTERER-SIWE DISEASE |
| * | 24645 | ACIDEMIA, 3-HYDROXY-3-METHYLGLUTARIC |
|   | 24650 | BERLIN SYNDROME |
| * | 24660 | LIPASE, CONGENITAL ABSENCE OF PANCREATIC |
|   | 24670 | LIPID TRANSPORT DEFECT OF INTESTINE |
| * | 24710 | SKIN, LIPOID PROTEINOSIS |
| * | 24720 | LISSENCEPHALY SYNDROME |
|   | 24741 | LYMPHEDEMA-HYPOPARATHYROIDISM |
| * | 24795 | HYPERLYSINURIA, ISOLATED |
|   | 24800 | MEGALENCEPHALY |
| * | 24825 | HYPOMAGNESEMIA, PRIMARY |
| * | 24830 | MAL DE MELEDA |
| * | 24837 | MANDIBULOACRAL DYSPLASIA |
|   | 24839 | MANDIBULOFACIAL DYSOSTOSIS, TREACHER COLLINS TYPE, RECESSIVE |
| * | 24850 | MANNOSIDOSIS |
| * | 24860 | MAPLE SYRUP URINE DISEASE |
| * | 24870 | MARDEN-WALKER SYNDROME |
|   | 24877 | FACIO-NEURO-SKELETAL SYNDROME |
| * | 24880 | MARINESCO-SJOGREN SYNDROME |
|   | 24895 | McDONOUGH SYNDROME |
| * | 24900 | MECKEL SYNDROME |

* 24910 FEVER, FAMILIAL MEDITERRANEAN (FMF)
  24920 COLON, AGANGLIONOSIS
* 24921 INTESTINAL HYPOPERISTALSIS, MEGACYSTIS-MICROCOLON TYPE
* 24931 MEGALOCORNEA-MENTAL RETARDATION SYNDROME
  24940 NEUROCUTANEOUS MELANOSIS
  24942 OSTEODYSPLASTY
  24960 MIETENS-WEBER SYNDROME
  24962 MENTAL RETARDATION-HEART DEFECTS-BLEPHAROPHIMOSIS
  24963 MUTCHINICK SYNDROME
* 24965 ACIDURIA, BETA-MERCAPTOLACTATE-CYSTEINE DISULFIDURIA
  24966 RENAL MESANGIAL SCLEROSIS-EYE DEFECTS
  24967 HEART-HAND SYNDROME IV
  24970 MESOMELIC DYSPLASIA, LANGER TYPE
  25000 METACHROMATIC LEUKODYSTROPHIES
* 25010 METACHROMATIC LEUKODYSTROPHIES
  25020 METACHROMATIC LEUKODYSTROPHIES
* 25025 METAPHYSEAL CHONDRODYSPLASIA, TYPE McKUSICK
  25042 METAPHYSEAL DYSOSTOSIS-DEAFNESS
  25045 EXOSTOSES-ANETODERMIA-BRACHYDACTYLY TYPE E
* 25060 METATROPIC DYSPLASIA
* 25080 METHEMOGLOBINEMIA, NADH-DEPENDENT DIAPHORASE DEFICIENCY
* 25090 METHIONINE MALABSORPTION
* 25095 ACIDURIA, 3-METHYLGLUTACONIC TYPE I
* 25095 ACIDURIA, 3-METHYLGLUTACONIC TYPE II
* 25100 ACIDEMIA, METHYLMALONIC
* 25117 ACIDEMIA, MEVALONIC
* 25120 MICROCEPHALY
  25124 MICROCEPHALY-RETARDATION-SKELETAL AND IMMUNE DEFECTS
* 25126 CHROMOSOME INSTABILITY, NIJMEGEN TYPE
* 25126 MICROCEPHALY, AUTOSOMAL RECESSIVE WITH NORMAL INTELLIGENCE
* 25127 MICROCEPHALY WITH CHORIORETINOPATHY
* 25130 MICROCEPHALY-HIATUS HERNIA-NEPHROSIS, GALLOWAY TYPE
  25175 LENS, MICROSPHEROPHAKIA
* 25180 EAR, MICROTIA-ATRESIA
* 25210 ORO-FACIO-DIGITAL SYNDROME, MOHR TYPE
* 25215 MOLYBDENUM CO-FACTOR DEFICIENCY
  25220 HAIR, MONILETHRIX
* 25240 MUCOLIPIDOSIS I
* 25250 MUCOLIPIDOSIS II
* 25260 MUCOLIPIDOSIS III
* 25265 MUCOLIPIDOSIS IV
* 25280 MUCOPOLYSACCHARIDOSIS I-H
* 25280 MUCOPOLYSACCHARIDOSIS I-S
* 25290 MUCOPOLYSACCHARIDOSIS III
* 25292 MUCOPOLYSACCHARIDOSIS III
* 25293 MUCOPOLYSACCHARIDOSIS III
* 25294 MUCOPOLYSACCHARIDOSIS III
* 25300 MUCOPOLYSACCHARIDOSIS IV
  25301 MUCOPOLYSACCHARIDOSIS IV
* 25320 MUCOPOLYSACCHARIDOSIS VI
* 25322 MUCOPOLYSACCHARIDOSIS VII
* 25325 DWARFISM, MULIBREY TYPE
* 25326 BIOTINIDASE DEFICIENCY
* 25327 CARBOXYLASE DEFICIENCY, HOLOCARBOXY-LASE DEFICIENCY TYPE
* 25328 MUSCLE-EYE-BRAIN SYNDROME
  25329 PTERYGIUM SYNDROME, MULTIPLE LETHAL
* 25330 SPINAL MUSCULAR ATROPHY
  25331 CONTRACTURES, CONGENITAL LETHAL FINNISH TYPE
* 25340 SPINAL MUSCULAR ATROPHY
* 25355 SPINAL MUSCULAR ATROPHY
* 25360 MUSCULAR DYSTROPHY, LIMB-GIRDLE

* 25370 MUSCULAR DYSTROPHY, AUTOSOMAL RECESSIVE PSEUDOHYPERTROPHIC
* 25380 MUSCULAR DYSTROPHY, CONGENITAL WITH MENTAL RETARDATION
* 25390 MUSCULAR DYSTROPHY, CONGENITAL WITH ARTHROGRYPOSIS
  25400 MYOPATHY-CATARACT-GONADAL DYSGENESIS
* 25415 ANOSMIA, CONGENITAL
  25420 MYASTHENIC SYNDROME, CONGENITAL SLOW CHANNEL TYPE
* 25421 MYASTHENIC SYNDROME, FAMILIAL INFANTILE TYPE
  25450 CANCER, MULTIPLE MYELOMA
* 25460 IMMUNODEFICIENCY, MYELOPEROXIDASE DEFICIENCY TYPE
* 25475 MYOPATHY-METABOLIC, MYOADENYLATE DEAMINASE DEFICIENCY
  25477 SEIZURES, MYOCLONIC, JUVENILE JANZ TYPE
* 25478 SEIZURES, PROGRESSIVE MYOCLONIC, LAFORA TYPE
* 25480 SEIZURES, PROGRESSIVE MYOCLONIC, UNVERRICHT-LUNDBORG TYPE
* 25511 MYOPATHY-METABOLIC, CARNITINE PALMITYL TRANSFERASE DEFICIENCY
* 25512 MYOPATHY-METABOLIC, CARNITINE PALMITYL TRANSFERASE DEFICIENCY
* 25515 MYOPATHY, MYOGLOBINURIA-ABNORMAL GLYCOLOSIS, HEREDITARY TYPE
  25516 MYOPATHY, FAMILIAL LYSIS OF TYPE I FIBERS
  25517 MYOPATHY-CATARACT-GONADAL DYSGENESIS
  25520 MYOPATHY, MYOTUBULAR
* 25531 MYOPATHY, DISPROPORTIONATE FIBER TYPE I
  25550 MYOPIA, CONGENITAL
  25560 MUSCULAR DYSTROPHY, CONGENITAL WITH ARTHROGRYPOSIS
* 25570 MYOTONIA CONGENITA
* 25580 CHONDRODYSTROPHIC MYOTONIA, SCHWARTZ-JAMPEL TYPE
* 25596 MYXOMA, INTRACARDIAC
  25598 NASO-DIGITO-ACOUSTIC SYNDROME, KEIPERT TYPE
  25599 OTO-OCULO-MUSCULO-SKELETAL SYNDROME
* 25600 ENCEPHALOPATHY, NECROTIZING
* 25603 MYOPATHY, NEMALINE
  25604 DIGITAL DEFECTS-NODULAR ERYTHEMA-EMACIATION, NAKAJO TYPE
* 25605 SKELETAL DYSPLASIA, DE LA CHAPELLE TYPE
* 25610 KIDNEY, NEPHRONOPHTHISIS-MEDULLARY CYSTIC DISEASE
  25620 NEPHROSIS-DEAFNESS-URINARY TRACT AND DIGITAL DEFECTS
* 25630 NEPHROSIS, CONGENITAL
  25634 NEPHROSIS-NERVE DEAFNESS-HYPOPARATHYROIDISM, BARAKAT TYPE
  25635 NEPHROSIS, FAMILIAL TYPE
* 25650 ICHTHYOSIS, LINEARIS CIRCUMFLEXA
* 25652 NEU-LAXOVA SYNDROME
* 25654 GALACTOSIALIDOSIS
* 25655 MUCOLIPIDOSIS I
* 25660 NEUROAXONAL DYSTROPHY, INFANTILE
  25669 NEURO-FACIO-DIGITO-RENAL SYNDROME
  25670 CANCER, NEUROBLASTOMA
* 25671 NEUROECTODERMAL MELANOLYSOSOMAL SYNDROME
* 25673 NEURONAL CEROID-LIPOFUSCINOSES (NCL)
* 25680 NEUROPATHY, CONGENITAL SENSORY WITH ANHIDROSIS
* 25685 NEUROPATHY, GIANT AXONAL
* 25720 NIEMANN-PICK DISEASE
* 25722 NIEMANN-PICK DISEASE
* 25725 NIEMANN-PICK DISEASE
* 25727 NIGHTBLINDNESS, CONGENITAL STATIONARY, AUTOSOMAL RECESSIVE

25730 CHROMOSOME 13, TRISOMY 13
25730 CHROMOSOME 18, TRISOMY 18
25730 KLINEFELTER SYNDROME
25735 NECK, CYSTIC HYGROMA, FETAL TYPE
25770 OCULO-AURICULO-VERTEBRAL ANOMALY
* 25780 GINGIVAL FIBROMATOSIS-DEPIGMENTATION-MICROPHTHALMIA
25791 DWARFISM, OCULO-PALATO-CEREBRAL TYPE
* 25797 OCULO-RENO-CEREBELLAR SYNDROME
25798 ODONTO-ONYCHODERMAL DYSPLASIA
* 25810 NIGHTBLINDNESS, OGUCHI TYPE
* 25830 OLIVOPONTOCEREBELLAR ATROPHY, RECESSIVE FICKLER-WINKLER TYPE
25832 CLEFT PALATE-OMPHALOCELE
* 25836 ONYCHO-TRICHODYSPLASIA-NEUTROPENIA
* 25840 OPHTHALMOPLEGIA, TOTAL WITH PTOSIS AND MIOSIS
25845 OPHTHALMOPLEGIA, PROGRESSIVE EXTERNAL
25848 OPSISMODYSPLASIA
25865 DEAFNESS-POLYNEUROPATHY-OPTIC ATROPHY
* 25870 OPTICO-COCHLEO-DENTATE DEGENERATION
* 25885 ORO-FACIO-DIGITAL SYNDROME, SUGARMAN TYPE
25886 ORO-FACIO-DIGITAL SYNDROME, BARAITSER-BURN TYPE
* 25887 GYRATE ATROPHY OF THE CHOROID AND RETINA
* 25890 ACIDEMIA, OROTIC
25892 ACIDEMIA, OROTIC
25927 OSTEODYSPLASTY
* 25940 OSTEOGENESIS IMPERFECTA
25941 OSTEOGENESIS IMPERFECTA
* 25942 OSTEOGENESIS IMPERFECTA
25950 OSTEOSARCOMA
25960 OSTEOLYSIS, RECESSIVE CARPAL-TARSAL
25961 OSTEOLYSIS, ESSENTIAL
* 25970 OSTEOPETROSIS, MALIGNANT RECESSIVE
25971 OSTEOPETROSIS, MILD RECESSIVE
25972 OSTEOPETROSIS, MALIGNANT RECESSIVE
* 25973 OSTEOPETROSIS, MALIGNANT RECESSIVE
* 25973 RENAL TUBULAR ACIDOSIS-OSTEOPETROSIS SYNDROME
25975 OSTEOPOROSIS, JUVENILE IDIOPATHIC
* 25977 OSTEOPOROSIS-PSEUDOGLIOMA SYNDROME
25978 OTO-ONYCHO-PERONEAL SYNDROME
26013 NAILS, PACHYONYCHIA CONGENITA
26035 CANCER, PANCREAS, FAMILIAL ADENOCARCINOMA OF
* 26040 SHWACHMAN SYNDROME
26050 CNS NEOPLASMS
26053 SKIN, PARANA HARD SKIN SYNDROME
* 26080 PENTOSURIA
26095 TEETH, PERIODONTITIS, JUVENILE
* 26100 ANEMIA, PERNICIOUS CONGENITAL
* 26110 VITAMIN B(12) MALABSORPTION
26154 DWARFISM (SHORT LIMBED)-PETERS ANOMALY OF THE EYE
* 26155 MULLERIAN DERIVATIVES IN MALES, PERSISTENT
* 26160 FETAL EFFECTS FROM MATERNAL PKU
* 26160 PHENYLKETONURIA
* 26163 DIHYDROPTERIDINE REDUCTASE DEFICIENCY
* 26164 BIOPTERIN SYNTHESIS DEFICIENCY
26170 ANEMIA, HEMOLYTIC, ERYTHROCYTE PHOSPHOGLYCERATE KINASE DEFICIENCY
* 26175 GLYCOGENOSIS, TYPE IXb
26180 CLEFT PALATE-MICROGNATHIA-GLOSSOPTOSIS
26200 CRANDALL SYNDROME
26200 DEAFNESS-PILI TORTI, BJORNSTAD TYPE
26202 TRICHODENTAL DYSPLASIA WITH REFRACTIVE ERRORS
* 26219 LIPODYSTROPHY-COARSE FACIES-ACANTHOSIS NIGRICANS, MIESCHER TYPE

26235 DWARFISM-DYSMORPHIC FACIES-RETARDATION, PITT TYPE
* 26240 GROWTH HORMONE DEFICIENCY, ISOLATED
* 26250 DWARFISM, LARON
* 26260 DWARFISM, PANHYPOPITUITARY
* 26270 DWARFISM, PITUITARY WITH ABNORMAL SELLA TURCICA
26310 KIDNEY, POLYCYSTIC DISEASE-CATARACT-BLINDNESS
* 26320 HEPATIC FIBROSIS, CONGENITAL
* 26320 KIDNEY, POLYCYSTIC DISEASE, RECESSIVE
* 26320 LIVER, CONGENITAL CYSTIC DILATATION OF INTRAHEPATIC DUCTS
26351 SHORT RIB-POLYDACTYLY SYNDROME, VERMA-NAUMOFF TYPE
* 26352 SHORT RIB-POLYDACTYLY SYNDROME, TYPE II
* 26353 SHORT RIB-POLYDACTYLY SYNDROME, TYPE I
26354 HEART-HAND SYNDROME IV
26363 POLYSYNDACTYLY-CARDIAC MALFORMATIONS
26365 PTERYGIUM SYNDROME, POPLITEAL, LETHAL
26370 PORPHYRIA, ERYTHROPOIETIC
26375 ACROFACIAL DYSOSTOSIS, POSTAXIAL TYPE
* 26409 PROGERIA, NEONATAL RAUTENSTRAUCH-WIEDEMANN TYPE
26413 PROLIDASE DEFICIENCY
* 26415 PSEUDOACHONDROPLASTIC DYSPLASIA
26416 PSEUDOACHONDROPLASTIC DYSPLASIA
* 26430 STEROID 17-KETOSTEROID REDUCTASE DEFICIENCY
* 26435 ALDOSTERONE RESISTANCE
* 26460 STEROID 5 ALPHA-REDUCTASE DEFICIENCY
* 26470 RICKETS, VITAMIN D-DEPENDENT, TYPE I
* 26480 PSEUDOXANTHOMA ELASTICUM
* 26490 FACTOR XI DEFICIENCY
* 26500 PTERYGIUM SYNDROME, MULTIPLE
26550 PULMONARY VALVE, STENOSIS
26560 NEPHROSIS, CONGENITAL
* 26570 FIBROMATOSIS, JUVENILE HYALINE
* 26580 PYKNODYSOSTOSIS
26585 GROWTH DEFICIENCY, AFRICAN PYGMY TYPE
* 26590 PYLE DISEASE
* 26595 PYLORODUODENAL ATRESIA, HEREDITARY
* 26610 SEIZURES, VITAMIN B(6) DEPENDENCY
* 26613 ACIDEMIA, PYROGLUTAMIC
26614 ANEMIA, HEMOLYTIC, RED CELL MEMBRANE DEFECTS
26614 ELLIPTOCYTOSIS
* 26615 PYRUVATE CARBOXYLASE DEFICIENCY WITH LACTIC ACIDEMIA
* 26620 PYRUVATE KINASE DEFICIENCY
26627 GINGIVAL FIBROMATOSIS-CHERUBISM-SEIZURES, RAMON TYPE
26640 RETINAL DYSPLASIA
* 26650 PHYTANIC ACID STORAGE DISEASE
* 26690 RENAL DYSPLASIA-RETINAL APLASIA, LOKEN-SENIOR TYPE
* 26700 OVERGROWTH-RENAL HAMARTOMA, PERLMAN TYPE
* 26730 RENAL TUBULAR ACIDOSIS-SENSORINEURAL DEAFNESS
26740 RENAL-GENITAL-MIDDLE EAR ANOMALIES
* 26743 RENAL TUBULAR DYSGENESIS
* 26750 IMMUNODEFICIENCY, SEVERE COMBINED
* 26770 IMMUNODEFICIENCY, RETICULOENDOTHELIO-SIS WITH EOSINOPHILIA
* 26770 LYMPHOHISTIOCYTOSIS, FAMILIAL ERYTHROPHAGOCYTIC
* 26800 RETINITIS PIGMENTOSA
26801 RETINITIS PIGMENTOSA
26802 RETINITIS PIGMENTOSA
26803 RETINITIS PIGMENTOSA
26805 RETINOPATHY-MICROCEPHALY-MENTAL RETARDATION

*  26808  RETINOSCHISIS
*  26810  EYE, GOLDMANN-FAVRE DISEASE
   26825  RHIZOMELIC SYNDROME, URBACH TYPE
*  26830  ROBERTS SYNDROME
*  26840  ROTHMUND-THOMSON SYNDROME
   26860  RUBINSTEIN-TAYBI BROAD THUMB-HALLUX
           SYNDROME
*  26867  SMITH-LEMLI-OPITZ SYNDROME, TYPE II
   26870  HYPERLYSINEMIA
*  26874  SALLA DISEASE
*  26880  G(M2)-GANGLIOSIDOSIS WITH
           HEXOSAMINIDASE A AND B DEFICIENCY
*  26890  SARCOSINEMIA
   26895  MYOPATHY, SARCOTUBULAR
*  26915  SCHINZEL-GIEDION SYNDROME
*  26925  SKELETAL DYSPLASIA, SCHNECKENBECKEN
           TYPE
*  26950  SCLEROSTEOSIS
   26960  NIEMANN-PICK DISEASE
*  26970  LIPODYSTROPHY SYNDROME, BERARDINELLI
           TYPE
*  26970  SKIN, ACANTHOSIS NIGRICANS
   26986  DWARFISM, SHORT-RIB, BEEMER TYPE
   26988  SHORT SYNDROME
   26992  SIALIC ACID STORAGE DISEASE, INFANTILE
           TYPE
   27005  SILVER SYNDROME
   27010  SITUS INVERSUS VISCERUM
   27015  SJOGREN SYNDROME
*  27020  SJOGREN-LARSSON SYNDROME
*  27030  SKIN PEELING SYNDROME
*  27040  SMITH-LEMLI-OPITZ SYNDROME
*  27055  SPASTIC ATAXIA, CHARLEVOIX-SAGUENAY
           TYPE
*  27080  PARAPLEGIA, FAMILIAL SPASTIC
*  27097  ANEMIA, HEMOLYTIC, RED CELL MEMBRANE
           DEFECTS
*  27097  SPHEROCYTOSIS
   27112  SPINAL MUSCULAR ATROPHY
   27115  SPINAL MUSCULAR ATROPHY
   27127  ATAXIA-DYSMORPHIC FACIES-
           TRICHODYSPLASIA
   27131  SPINOCEREBELLAR DEGENERATION-CORNEAL
           DYSTROPHY
*  27140  SPLEEN, CONGENITAL ISOLATED HYPOSPLENIA
   27153  BRACHYOLMELIA, HOBAEK TYPE
*  27155  SPONDYLOMETAPHYSEAL DYSPLASIA WITH
           ENCHONDROMATOUS CHANGES
*  27160  SPONDYLOEPIPHYSEAL DYSPLASIA, LATE
   27162  SPONDYLOEPIPHYSEAL DYSPLASIA-MENTAL
           RETARDATION
*  27163  SPONDYLOEPIPHYSEAL DYSPLASIA, LATE
*  27164  SPONDYLOEPIMETAPHYSEAL DYSPLASIA-JOINT
           LAXITY
*  27165  SPONDYLOEPIMETAPHYSEAL DYSPLASIA
*  27166  SPONDYLOMETAPHYSEAL CHONDRODYSPLA-
           SIA, KOZLOWSKI TYPE
   27167  SPONDYLOEPIMETAPHYSEAL DYSPLASIA,
           STRUDWICK TYPE
   27170  SPONDYLOPERIPHERAL DYSPLASIA
*  27190  BRAIN, SPONGY DEGENERATION
   27195  HEART, SUBAORTIC STENOSIS, FIBROUS
*  27198  ACIDEMIA, GAMMA-HYDROXYBUTYRIC
*  27220  METACHROMATIC LEUKODYSTROPHIES
*  27220  MUCOPOLYSACCHARIDOSIS II
*  27220  SULFATASE DEFICIENCY, MULTIPLE
*  27230  ACIDURIA, SULFITE OXIDASE DEFICIENCY
   27235  ACROCEPHALOPOLYSYNDACTYLY
   27244  SYNDACTYLY-MICROCEPHALY-MENTAL
           RETARDATION, FILIPPI TYPE
   27248  SYRINGOMYELIA
   27270  TEETH, TAURODONTISM

*  27275  G(M2)-GANGLIOSIDOSIS WITH
           HEXOSAMINIDASE A DEFICIENCY
*  27280  G(M2)-GANGLIOSIDOSIS WITH
           HEXOSAMINIDASE A DEFICIENCY
   27298  TEETH, TAURODONTISM
   27300  TEETH, FUSED
   27312  TERATOMAS
   27325  AGONADIA
   27325  ANORCHIA
   27330.  TERATOMAS
   27340  ODONTO-TRICHOMELIC SYNDROME
   27341  ECTRODACTYLY
   27350  THALASSEMIA
   27367  CRANIOSYNOSTOSIS, KLEEBLATTSCHADEL
           TYPE
   27368  THANATOPHORIC DYSPLASIA, GLASGOW TYPE
   27373  THORACIC DYSPLASIA-HYDROCEPHALUS
*  27375  SKELETAL DYSPLASIA, 3-M TYPE
*  27380  THROMBASTHENIA, GLANZMANN-NAEGELI
           TYPE
*  27400  THROMBOCYTOPENIA-ABSENT RADIUS
   27415  HEMOLYTIC-UREMIC SYNDROME
   27423  AGAMMAGLOBULINEMIA-THYMOMA
           SYNDROME
   27423  CANCER, THYMOMA
*  27430  THYROID, HORMONE RESISTANCE
*  27440  THYROID, IODIDE TRANSPORT DEFECT
*  27450  THYROID, PEROXIDASE DEFECT
*  27460  DEAFNESS-GOITER
*  27480  THYROID, IODOTYROSINE DEIODINASE
           DEFICIENCY
   27490  THYROID, THYROGLOBULIN DEFECTS
   27500  THYROTOXICOSIS
   27510  THYROTROPIN DEFICIENCY, ISOLATED
   27520  THYROTROPIN UNRESPONSIVENESS
   27521  RESTRICTIVE DERMATOPATHY
   27522  TIBIAL APLASIA/HYPOPLASIA
*  27525  TONGUE, PIGMENTED PAPILLAE
*  27535  TRANSCOBALAMIN II DEFICIENCY
   27540  TRICHOMEGALY-RETARDATION-DWARFISM-
           RETINAL PIGMENTARY DEGENERATION
   27545  TRICHO-ODONTO-ONYCHIAL DYSPLASIA
   27550  TRICHO-RHINO-PHALANGEAL SYNDROME,
           TYPE I
   27555  TRICHOTHIODYSTROPHY
*  27563  STORAGE DISEASE, NEUTRAL LIPID TYPE
   27565  ACIDEMIA, TRIHYDROXYCOPROSTANIC
*  27570  TRIMETHYLAMINURIA
*  27600  TRYPSINOGEN DEFICIENCY
*  27630  TURCOT SYNDROME
   27641  FETAL MONOZYGOUS MULTIPLE PREGNANCY
           DYSPLACENTATION EFFECTS
   27641  TWINS, CONJOINED
*  27660  TYROSINEMIA II, OREGON TYPE
*  27670  TYROSINEMIA I
*  27671  TYROSINEMIA I
   27682  LIMB DEFECT WITH ABSENT ULNA/FIBULA
*  27690  USHER SYNDROME
   27700  MULLERIAN APLASIA
*  27710  HYPERVALINEMIA
   27717  ORO-PALATAL-DIGITAL SYNDROME, VARADI
           TYPE
   27720  TRICUSPID VALVE, ATRESIA
*  27730  SPONDYLOTHORACIC DYSPLASIA
   27732  MUSCULAR DYSTROPHY, OCULO-
           GASTROINTESTINAL
   27738  VITAMIN B(12) LYSOSOMAL TRANSPORT
           DEFECT
   27742  RESISTANCE TO 1,25 DIHYDROXY VITAMIN D
*  27744  RESISTANCE TO 1,25 DIHYDROXY VITAMIN D
   27748  VON WILLEBRAND DISEASE
   27758  ALBINISM, WAARDENBURG TYPE-
           HIRSCHSPRUNG AGANGLIONOSIS

27758 WAARDENBURG SYNDROMES
* 27760 SPHEROPHAKIA-BRACHYMORPHIA SYNDROME
* 27770 WERNER SYNDROME
27772 CRANIO-CARPO-TARSAL DYSPLASIA, WHISTLING FACE TYPE
* 27790 HEPATOLENTICULAR DEGENERATION
* 27795 WINCHESTER SYNDROME
* 27800 WOLMAN DISEASE
27810 WOLMAN DISEASE
* 27825 WRINKLY SKIN SYNDROME
* 27830 XANTHINE OXIDASE DEFICIENCY
* 27840 ALBINISM, OCULOCUTANEOUS, RUFOUS TYPE
* 27870 XERODERMA PIGMENTOSUM
* 27871 XERODERMA PIGMENTOSUM
* 27872 XERODERMA PIGMENTOSUM
* 27873 XERODERMA PIGMENTOSUM
* 27874 XERODERMA PIGMENTOSUM
* 27875 XERODERMA PIGMENTOSUM
* 27876 XERODERMA PIGMENTOSUM
* 27878 XERODERMA PIGMENTOSUM
* 27879 XERODERMA PIGMENTOSUM
27880 XERODERMA PIGMENTOSUM-MENTAL RETARDATION
27881 XERODERMA PIGMENTOSUM
* 30010 ADRENOLEUKODYSTROPHY, X-LINKED
* 30020 ADRENAL HYPOPLASIA, CONGENITAL
* 30025 ADRENOCORTICAL UNRESPONSIVENESS TO ACTH, HEREDITARY
* 30030 IMMUNODEFICIENCY, AGAMMAGLOBULINE-MIA, X-LINKED, INFANTILE
* 30040 IMMUNODEFICIENCY, X-LINKED SEVERE COMBINED
* 30050 ALBINISM, OCULAR
* 30060 FORSIUS-ERIKSSON SYNDROME
30065 ALBINISM, OCULAR-LATE-ONSET-SENSORINEURAL DEAFNESS, X-LINKED
* 30070 ALBINISM, CUTANEOUS-DEAFNESS
30080 PARATHYROID HORMONE RESISTANCE
* 30100 IMMUNODEFICIENCY, WISKOTT-ALDRICH TYPE
* 30105 NEPHRITIS-DEAFNESS (SENSORINEURAL), HEREDITARY
* 30110 TEETH, AMELOGENESIS IMPERFECTA
* 30110 TEETH, SNOW-CAPPED
* 30120 TEETH, AMELOGENESIS IMPERFECTA
* 30122 AMYLOIDOSIS, FAMILIAL CUTANEOUS
* 30130 ANEMIA, SIDEROBLASTIC
30131 ANEMIA, SIDEROBLASTIC
30141 ANENCEPHALY
* 30150 FABRY DISEASE
30170 ANOSMIA, CONGENITAL
30180 ANORECTAL MALFORMATIONS
30190 BORJESON-FORSSMAN-LEHMANN SYNDROME
30195 BRANCHIAL ARCH SYNDROME, X-LINKED
* 30220 CATARACT, CORTICAL AND NUCLEAR
30230 CATARACT, CORTICAL AND NUCLEAR
* 30235 CATARACTS-OTO-DENTAL DEFECTS
30238 DIGITO-PALATAL SYNDROME, STEVENSON TYPE
30270 METACHROMATIC LEUKODYSTROPHIES
* 30280 NEUROPATHY, HEREDITARY MOTOR AND SENSORY, TYPE I
30290 CHARCOT MARIE TOOTH DISEASE-DEAFNESS
* 30295 CHONDRODYSPLASIA PUNCTATA, X-LINKED DOMINANT TYPE
30296 CHONDRODYSPLASIA PUNCTATA, X-LINKED DOMINANT TYPE
* 30310 CHOROIDEREMIA
30311 CHOROIDEREMIA
30320 CHOROIDEREMIA
30320 RETINITIS PIGMENTOSA
30335 X-LINKED MENTAL RETARDATION-CLASPED THUMB
* 30360 COFFIN-LOWRY SYNDROME

30365 COLON, ATRESIA OR STENOSIS
30370 COLOR BLINDNESS, BLUE MONOCONE-MONOCHROMATIC
* 30380 COLOR BLINDNESS, RED-GREEN DEUTAN SERIES
* 30390 COLOR BLINDNESS, RED-GREEN PROTAN SERIES
30400 COLOR BLINDNESS, YELLOW-BLUE TRITAN
30402 RETINA, CONE DYSTROPHY, X-LINKED
30403 RETINA, CONE DYSTROPHY, X-LINKED
30405 AICARDI SYNDROME
* 30410 CORPUS CALLOSUM AGENESIS
30411 CRANIO-FRONTO-NASAL DYSPLASIA
30412 OTO-PALATO-DIGITAL SYNDROME, II
* 30415 EHLERS-DANLOS SYNDROME
* 30415 OCCIPITAL HORN SYNDROME
30420 CUTIS VERTICUS GYRATA
30430 ANOSMIA, CONGENITAL
30435 DEAFNESS-HYPOGONADISM
* 30440 DEAFNESS WITH PERILYMPHATIC GUSHER
* 30480 DIABETES INSIPIDUS, VASOPRESSIN RESISTANT TYPES I AND II
* 30490 DIABETES INSIPIDIS, NEUROHYPOPHYSEAL TYPE
* 30500 DYSKERATOSIS CONGENITA
30505 DEAFNESS (SENSORINEURAL)-DYSTONIA
* 30510 ECTODERMAL DYSPLASIA, CHRIST-SIEMENS-TOURAINE TYPE
* 30520 EHLERS-DANLOS SYNDROME
* 30530 VENTRICLE, ENDOCARDIAL FIBROELASTOSIS OF LEFT VENTRICLE
* 30540 AARSKOG SYNDROME
* 30545 FG SYNDROME, OPITZ-KAVEGGIA TYPE
* 30560 DERMAL HYPOPLASIA, FOCAL
* 30560 VENTRICLE, ENDOCARDIAL FIBROELASTOSIS OF RIGHT VENTRICLE
* 30562 FRONTOMETAPHYSEAL DYSPLASIA
* 30570 GERM CELL APLASIA
* 30590 GLUCOSE-6-PHOSPHATE DEHYDROGENASE DEFICIENCY
* 30595 ACIDEMIA, GLUTARIC ACIDEMIA II
* 30600 GLYCOGEN STORAGE DISEASE, X-LINKED WITH NORMAL HEPATIC ENZYMES
* 30600 GLYCOGENOSIS, TYPE IXa
30605 SIMPSON-GOLABI-BEHMEL SYNDROME
* 30610 GONADAL DYSGENESIS, XY TYPE
* 30640 GRANULOMATOUS DISEASE, CHRONIC X-LINKED
* 30670 HEMOPHILIA A
30680 HEMOPHILIA A
* 30690 HEMOPHILIA B
* 30700 HYDROCEPHALY
* 30703 GLYCEROL KINASE DEFICIENCY
30715 HAIR, HYPERTRICHOSIS, X-LINKED
30740 ATAXIA-HYPOGONADISM SYNDROME
30750 SHOVAL-SOFFER SYNDROME
* 30760 HYPOMAGNESEMIA, PRIMARY
* 30770 HYPOPARATHYROIDISM, FAMILIAL
* 30780 HYPOPHOSPHATEMIA, X-LINKED
30781 HYPOPHOSPHATEMIA, X-LINKED
* 30800 GOUT
* 30800 LESCH-NYHAN SYNDROME
30805 LIMB REDUCTION-ICHTHYOSIS
* 30810 ICHTHYOSIS, X-LINKED WITH STEROID SULFATASE DEFICIENCY
* 30823 IMMUNODEFICIENCY, X-LINKED WITH HYPER IgM
* 30824 IMMUNODEFICIENCY, X-LINKED LYMPHOPROLIFERATIVE DISEASE
30828 TEETH, IMPACTED
* 30830 INCONTINENTIA PIGMENTI
* 30870 KALLMANN SYNDROME

* 30880 SKIN, KERATOSIS FOLLICULARIS SPINULOSA DECALVANS
30883 SHORT STATURE-CEREBRAL ATROPHY-KERATOSIS FOLLICULARIS, X-LINKED
30885 LARYNGEAL ABDUCTOR PARALYSIS-MENTAL RETARDATION
30885 LARYNGEAL PARALYSIS
30890 OPTIC ATROPHY, LEBER TYPE
* 30900 OCULO-CEREBRO-RENAL SYNDROME
* 30915 STEROID 17,20-DESMOLASE DEFICIENCY
* 30920 MOOD AND THOUGHT DISORDERS
30925 X-LINKED MENTAL RETARDATION-CLASPED THUMB
* 30930 CORNEA, MEGALOCORNEA
* 30935 OSTEODYSPLASTY
* 30940 MENKES SYNDROME
* 30950 X-LINKED MENTAL RETARDATION, RENPENNING TYPE
30952 X-LINKED MENTAL RETARDATION, MARFANOID HABITUS TYPE
* 30953 X-LINKED MENTAL RETARDATION, ATKIN TYPE
* 30953 X-LINKED MENTAL RETARDATION, CLARK-BARAITSER TYPE
* 30953 X-LINKED MENTAL RETARDATION, GOLABI-ITO-HALL TYPE
* 30953 X-LINKED MENTAL RETARDATION-CRANIOFACIAL ABNORMALITIES-CLUB FOOT
30954 X-LINKED MENTAL RETARDATION, RENPENNING TYPE
* 30955 X-LINKED MENTAL RETARDATION, FRAGILE X SYNDROME
30956 HYPERKERATOSIS PALMOPLANTARIS-SPASTIC PARAPLEGIA-RETARDATION
30958 SMITH-FINEMAN-MYERS SYNDROME
* 30959 X-LINKED MENTAL RETARDATION-GROWTH-HEARING AND GENITAL DEFECTS
30960 X-LINKED MENTAL RETARDATION-MUSCULAR WEAKNESS-AWKWARD GAIT
30961 X-LINKED MENTAL RETARDATION-SUBCORTICAL ATROPHY-PATELLAR LUXATION
30962 X-LINKED MENTAL RETARDATION-SKELETAL DYSPLASIA
* 30963 SYNDACTYLY
30970 EYE, MICROPHTHALMIA/COLOBOMA
* 30980 LENZ MICROPHTHALMIA SYNDROME
* 30990 MUCOPOLYSACCHARIDOSIS II
* 31020 MUSCULAR DYSTROPHY, ADULT PSEUDOHYPERTROPHIC
* 31020 MUSCULAR DYSTROPHY, CHILDHOOD PSEUDOHYPERTROPHIC
* 31030 EMERY-DREIFUSS SYNDROME
* 31040 MYOPATHY, MYOTUBULAR
31046 MYOPIA, CONGENITAL
* 31050 NIGHTBLINDNESS, CONGENITAL STATIONARY, X-LINKED RECESSIVE
* 31060 NORRIE DISEASE
31098 OMPHALOCELE
* 31100 OPHTHALMOPLEGIA EXTERNA-MYOPIA
31107 DEAFNESS-POLYNEUROPATHY-OPTIC ATROPHY
* 31120 ORO-FACIO-DIGITAL SYNDROME I
* 31125 ORNITHINE TRANSCARBAMYLASE DEFICIENCY

31128 OSTEOPATHIA STRIATA
* 31130 OTO-PALATO-DIGITAL SYNDROME, I
31145 PALLISTER-W SYNDROME
31151 X-LINKED MENTAL RETARDATION-BASAL GANGLION DISORDER
* 31180 ANEMIA, HEMOLYTIC, ERYTHROCYTE PHOSPHOGLYCERATE KINASE DEFICIENCY
31185 GOUT
* 31185 PHOSPHORIBOSYL PYROPHOSPHATE (PRPP) SYNTHETASE ABNORMALITY
31190 CLEFT PALATE-MICROGNATHIA-GLOSSOPTOSIS
* 31200 DWARFISM, PANHYPOPITUITARY
* 31208 PELIZAEUS-MERZBACHER SYNDROME
31210 ANDROGEN INSENSITIVITY SYNDROME, INCOMPLETE
31215 PTERYGIUM SYNDROME, MULTIPLE LETHAL
31230 ANDROGEN INSENSITIVITY (RESISTANCE), MINIMAL
31230 ANDROGEN INSENSITIVITY SYNDROME, INCOMPLETE
31240 RENAL BICARBONATE REABSORPTIVE DEFECT
31255 RETINAL DYSPLASIA
* 31260 RETINITIS PIGMENTOSA
* 31261 RETINITIS PIGMENTOSA
31265 USHER SYNDROME
* 31270 RETINOSCHISIS
31275 RETT SYNDROME
31277 SEIZURES-ICHTHYOSIS-MENTAL RETARDATION
31278 SILVER SYNDROME, X-LINKED
31284 X-LINKED MENTAL RETARDATION-CHOREOATHETOSIS
31285 EMERY-DREIFUSS SYNDROME
31286 CRANIO-DIGITAL SYNDROME-MENTAL RETARDATION, SCOTT TYPE
31287 SIMPSON-GOLABI-BEHMEL SYNDROME
* 31290 PARAPLEGIA, FAMILIAL SPASTIC
31310 EPITHELIOMAS, HEREDITARY MULTIPLE CYSTIC
31310 SCALP, CYLINDROMAS
* 31320 MUSCULAR ATROPHY, SPINAL AND BULBAR, X-LINKED KENNEDY TYPE
* 31340 SPONDYLOEPIPHYSEAL DYSPLASIA, LATE
31350 TEETH, ANODONTIA, PARTIAL OR COMPLETE
31360 HYPERTELORISM-HYPOSPADIAS SYNDROME
* 31370 ANDROGEN INSENSITIVITY (RESISTANCE), MINIMAL
* 31370 ANDROGEN INSENSITIVITY SYNDROME, COMPLETE
* 31370 ANDROGEN INSENSITIVITY SYNDROME, INCOMPLETE
31410 THUMB, CLASPED
* 31420 THYROXINE-BINDING GLOBULIN DEFECTS
* 31430 CERVICO-DERMO-GU SYNDROME, GOEMINNE TYPE
31432 SAY-MEYER SYNDROME
* 31450 VAN DEN BOSCH SYNDROME
* 31455 VESICO-URETERAL REFLUX
* 31458 CONTRACTURES-MUSCLE ATROPHY-OCULOMOTOR APRAXIA
31460 CERVICO-OCULO-ACOUSTIC SYNDROME
* 31485 ANEMIA, HEMOLYTIC, RED CELL MEMBRANE DEFECTS

# POSSUM-NUMBER-TO-PRIME-NAME INDEX

3001 AARSKOG SYNDROME
3003 PRUNE-BELLY SYNDROME
3004 ACHONDROGENESIS, LANGER-SALDINO TYPE
3004 ACHONDROGENESIS, PARENTI-FRACCARO TYPE
3006 ACHONDROPLASIA
3007 ACROCEPHALOSYNDACTYLY TYPE I
3008 ACROCEPHALOPOLYSYNDACTYLY
3008 ACROCEPHALOSYNDACTYLY TYPE V
3010 ACROCEPHALOPOLYSYNDACTYLY
3010 ACROCEPHALOSYNDACTYLY TYPE III
3011 ACRODYSOSTOSIS
3012 ACROFACIAL DYSOSTOSIS
3013 ACRO-OSTEOLYSIS, DOMINANT TYPE
3013 HAJDU-CHENEY SYNDROME
3014 ACROMESOMELIC DYSPLASIA, CAMPAILLA-
     MARTINELLI TYPE
3015 ACROMESOMELIC DYSPLASIA, MAROTEAUX-
     MARTINELLI-CAMPAILLA TYPE
3016 ACROPECTOROVERTEBRAL DYSPLASIA
3017 CAMPTODACTYLY-TRISMUS SYNDROME
3018 AICARDI SYNDROME
3019 ARTERIO-HEPATIC DYSPLASIA
3020 ALSTROM SYNDROME
3021 AMELO-CEREBRO-HYPOHIDROTIC SYNDROME
3022 AMELO-ONYCHO-HYPOHIDROTIC SYNDROME
3023 FABRY DISEASE
3025 SCHINZEL-GIEDION SYNDROME
3026 ANUS-HAND-EAR SYNDROME
3027 ARACHNODACTYLY, CONTRACTURAL BEALS TYPE
3028 ACIDURIA, ARGININOSUCCINIC
3029 OCULO-CEREBRO-FACIAL SYNDROME, KAUFMAN
     TYPE
3030 ARTHRO-OPHTHALMOPATHY, HEREDITARY,
     PROGRESSIVE, STICKLER TYPE
3030 ARTHRO-OPHTHALMOPATHY, WEISSENBACHER-
     ZWEYMULLER VARIANT
3031 BLEPHAROCHALASIS-DOUBLE LIP-NONTOXIC
     GOITER
3032 ASPHYXIATING THORACIC DYSPLASIA
3033 ATAXIA-TELANGIECTASIA
3035 AURICULO-OSTEODYSPLASIA
3036 BECKWITH-WIEDEMANN SYNDROME
3038 DEAFNESS-PILI TORTI, BJORNSTAD TYPE
3039 BLEPHARO-NASO-FACIAL SYNDROME
3040 BLOOM SYNDROME
3041 HYPERHIDROSIS-PREMATURE GREYING-PREMOLAR
     APLASIA
3042 BRACHYDACTYLY
3043 SPHEROPHAKIA-BRACHYMORPHIA SYNDROME
3044 OCULO-OSTEO-CUTANEOUS SYNDROME,
     TOUMAALA-HAAPANEN TYPE
3045 CRANIODIAPHYSEAL DYSPLASIA, LENZ-MAJEWSKI
     TYPE
3046 BRANCHIO-SKELETO-GENITAL SYNDROME
3047 NASO-DIGITO-ACOUSTIC SYNDROME, KEIPERT TYPE
3048 C SYNDROME
3049 CAMPOMELIC DYSPLASIA
3051 CAMPTODACTYLY SYNDROME, TEL HASHOMER
     TYPE
3053 OSTEOLYSIS, CARPAL-TARSAL AND CHRONIC
     PROGRESSIVE GLOMERULOPATHY
3054 ACROCEPHALOPOLYSYNDACTYLY
3055 CEBEBRAL GIGANTISM
3056 CEREBRO-COSTO-MANDIBULAR SYNDROME
3057 CEREBRO-HEPATO-RENAL SYNDROME
3059 CERVICO-OCULO-ACOUSTIC SYNDROME
3060 CHEDIAK-HIGASHI SYNDROME

3061 METAPHYSEAL CHONDRODYSPLASIA, TYPE
     McKUSICK
3062 CHONDRODYSTROPHY-SENSORINEURAL DEAFNESS,
     NANCE-INSLEY TYPE
3064 CHONDRODYSPLASIA PUNCTATA, RHIZOMELIC
     TYPE
3064 RHIZOMELIC SYNDROME, URBACH TYPE
3065 CHONDRODYSPLASIA PUNCTATA, MILD
     SYMMETRIC TYPE
3066 CHONDROECTODERMAL DYSPLASIA
3067 CHROMOSOME 3, TRISOMY 3p2
3069 CHROMOSOME 4, MONOSOMY 4p
3070 CHROMOSOME 4, TRISOMY 4p
3071 CHROMOSOME 4, TRISOMY DISTAL 4q
3072 CHROMOSOME 4, MONOSOMY DISTAL 4q
3073 CHROMOSOME 5, MONOSOMY 5p
3075 CHROMOSOME 6, TRISOMY 6p2
3077 CHROMOSOME 8, TRISOMY 8
3078 CHROMOSOME 8, TRISOMY 8p
3079 CHROMOSOME 9, TRISOMY 9p
3080 CHROMOSOME 9, TRISOMY 9
3081 CHROMOSOME 9, PARTIAL MONOSOMY 9p
3083 CHROMOSOME 10, TRISOMY 10q2
3084 CHROMOSOME 10, TRISOMY 10p
3085 CHROMOSOME 10, MONOSOMY 10p
3086 TUBULAR STENOSIS
3087 CHROMOSOME 11, MONOSOMY 11q
3088 CHROMOSOME 12, PARTIAL TRISOMY 12p
3090 CHROMOSOME 13, TRISOMY 13
3091 CHROMOSOME 13, MONOSOMY 13q3
3094 CHROMOSOME 18, TRISOMY 18
3095 CHROMOSOME 18, MONOSOMY 18p
3096 CHROMOSOME 18, MONOSOMY 18q
3098 ORO-FACIO-DIGITAL SYNDROME, SUGARMAN TYPE
3099 CHROMOSOME 20, TRISOMY 20p
3100 CHROMOSOME 21, TRISOMY 21
3101 DWARFISM, PANHYPOPITUITARY
3104 TURNER SYNDROME
3105 CHROMOSOME X, POLY-X
3106 CHROMOSOME X, POLY-X
3107 KLINEFELTER SYNDROME
3112 CHROMOSOME 1, MONOSOMY 1q
3113 LAURENCE-MOON SYNDROME
3114 CHROMOSOME TRIPLOIDY
3115 CHROMOSOME TETRAPLOIDY
3118 CHROMOSOME 1, MONOSOMY 1q4
3121 ENCHONDROMATOSIS
3122 CHROMOSOME 7, MONOSOMY 7q1
3124 CHROMOSOME 12, TRISOMY 12q2
3125 CHROMOSOME 13, MONOSOMY 13q
3126 CHROMOSOME 1, TRISOMY 1q32-qter
3130 URTICARIA-DEAFNESS-AMYLOIDOSIS
3131 OSTEODYSTROPHY-MENTAL RETARDATION,
     RUVALCABA TYPE
3132 VELO-CARDIO-FACIAL SYNDROME
3133 BRANCHIO-OTO-RENAL DYSPLASIA
3134 LISSENCEPHALY SYNDROME
3135 PENA-SHOKEIR SYNDROME
3136 CEREBRO-OCULO-FACIO-SKELETAL SYNDROME
3137 ECTODERMAL DYSPLASIA, RAPP-HODGKIN TYPE
3138 ORO-CRANIO-DIGITAL SYNDROME
3139 CLEFT LIP/PALATE-FILIFORM FUSION OF EYELIDS
3140 CLEFT LIP/PALATE-LIP PITS OR MOUNDS
3141 CLEFT LIP/PALATE-ECTODERMAL DYSPLASIA-
     SYNDACTYLY
3143 ACROFACIAL DYSOSTOSIS
3143 ACROFACIAL DYSOSTOSIS, NAGER TYPE
3145 CLEFT PALATE-STAPES FIXATION-OLIGODONTIA

3146 CLEIDOCRANIAL DYSPLASIA
3147 ORO-FACIO-DIGITAL SYNDROME, BARAITSER-BURN TYPE
3149 COCKAYNE SYNDROME
3149 COCKAYNE SYNDROME, TYPE II
3150 COFFIN-LOWRY SYNDROME
3151 COFFIN-SIRIS SYNDROME
3152 COHEN SYNDROME
3153 CORNEAL DYSTROPHY-SENSORINEURAL DEAFNESS
3154 CORPUS CALLOSUM AGENESIS
3155 GINGIVAL MULTIPLE HAMARTOMA SYNDROME
3156 CRANIO-CARPO-TARSAL DYSPLASIA, WHISTLING FACE TYPE
3157 CRANIO-DIAPHYSEAL DYSPLASIA
3159 CRANIOFACIAL DYSOSTOSIS-DIAPHYSEAL HYPERPLASIA
3160 CRANIOFACIAL DYSSYNOSTOSIS
3161 MANDIBULOACRAL DYSPLASIA
3162 CRANIOMETAPHYSEAL DYSPLASIA
3165 CRANIOSYNOSTOSIS-RADIAL APLASIA SYNDROME
3166 ARTHROGRYPOSIS, DISTAL TYPES
3166 CAMPTODACTYLY-CLEFT PALATE-CLUB FOOT, GORDON TYPE
3170 CRANIO-ECTODERMAL DYSPLASIA
3171 CRANIOSYNOSTOSIS-FIBULAR APLASIA, LOWRY TYPE
3172 MENINGOCELE-CONOTRUNCAL HEART DEFECT, KOUSSEFF TYPE
3173 GORLIN-CHAUDHRY-MOSS SYNDROME
3175 HERRMANN-PALLISTER-OPITZ SYNDROME
3178 GINGIVAL FIBROMATOSIS-DEPIGMENTATION-MICROPHTHALMIA
3179 EYE, CRYPTOPHTHALMOS WITH OTHER MALFORMATIONS
3179 FRASER SYNDROME
3180 CUTIS LAXA
3181 CUTIS LAXA-DELAYED DEVELOPMENT-LIGAMENTOUS LAXITY
3181 CUTIS LAXA-GROWTH DEFECT, DE BARSY TYPE
3182 CHARLIE M SYNDROME
3183 DE LANGE SYNDROME
3184 EXOSTOSES, MULTIPLE CARTILAGINOUS
3185 DIASTROPHIC DYSPLASIA
3187 DUBOWITZ SYNDROME
3188 DYGGVE-MELCHIOR-CLAUSEN SYNDROME
3189 DYSAUTONOMIA I, RILEY-DAY TYPE
3190 DYSCHONDROSTEOSIS
3191 DYSKERATOSIS CONGENITA
3193 MYOTONIC DYSTROPHY
3194 METAPHYSEAL DYSOSTOSIS-DEAFNESS
3196 DEAFNESS-OPTIC NERVE ATROPHY, PROGRESSIVE
3196 DEAFNESS-POLYNEUROPATHY-OPTIC ATROPHY
3198 DEAFNESS-HYPERPROLINURIA-ICHTHYOSIS
3199 DEAFNESS-KERATOPACHYDERMIA-DIGITAL CONSTRICTIONS
3200 DEAFNESS-MYOPIA-CATARACT-SADDLE NOSE, MARSHALL TYPE
3201 SHORT RIB-POLYDACTYLY SYNDROME, VERMA-NAUMOFF TYPE
3202 EXOSTOSES-ANETODERMIA-BRACHYDACTYLY TYPE E
3204 DERMAL HYPOPLASIA, FOCAL
3205 DERMO-CHONDRO-CORNEAL DYSTROPHY, FRANCOIS TYPE
3206 DIAPHYSEAL DYSPLASIA
3207 DWARFISM, LARON
3208 ECTODERMAL DYSPLASIA, CHRIST-SIEMENS-TOURAINE TYPE
3209 ECTODERMAL DYSPLASIA, HIDROTIC
3210 ECTRODACTYLY
3211 ECTRODACTYLY-ECTODERMAL DYSPLASIA-CLEFTING SYNDROME
3212 EHLERS-DANLOS SYNDROME

3213 ACROFACIAL DEFECTS, EMERY-NELSON TYPE
3214 EPIPHYSEAL DYSPLASIA, MULTIPLE
3215 NEVUS, EPIDERMAL NEVUS SYNDROME
3218 FETAL ALCOHOL SYNDROME
3219 FETAL AMINOPTERIN SYNDROME
3220 FETAL CYTOMEGALOVIRUS SYNDROME
3221 FETAL HYDANTOIN SYNDROME
3222 FETAL RUBELLA SYNDROME
3223 FETAL SYPHILIS SYNDROME
3224 FETAL THALIDOMIDE SYNDROME
3225 FETAL TOXOPLASMOSIS SYNDROME
3227 FETAL WARFARIN SYNDROME
3228 FACIO-CARDIOMELIC DYSPLASIA, LETHAL
3229 MUSCULAR DYSTROPHY, FACIO-SCAPULO-HUMERAL
3230 BLEPHAROPTOSIS-BLEPHAROPHIMOSIS-EPICANTHUS INVERSUS-TELECANTHUS
3232 FEMORAL HYPOPLASIA-UNUSUAL FACIES SYNDROME
3233 MYOSITIS OSSIFICANS PROGRESSIVA
3234 PANCYTOPENIA SYNDROME, FANCONI TYPE
3236 FRONTOMETAPHYSEAL DYSPLASIA
3237 HAND-FOOT-GENITAL SYNDROME
3238 FUCOSIDOSIS
3239 G SYNDROME
3240 MICROCEPHALY WITH CHORIORETINOPATHY
3241 GLYCOGEN STORAGE DISEASE, X-LINKED WITH NORMAL HEPATIC ENZYMES
3241 GLYCOGENOSIS, TYPE III
3241 GLYCOGENOSIS, TYPE IXa
3241 GLYCOGENOSIS, TYPE IXb
3241 GLYCOGENOSIS, TYPE IXc
3241 GLYCOGENOSIS, TYPE Ia
3241 GLYCOGENOSIS, TYPE Ib
3241 GLYCOGENOSIS, TYPE Ic
3241 GLYCOGENOSIS, TYPE V
3241 GLYCOGENOSIS, TYPE VI
3241 GLYCOGENOSIS, TYPE VII
3241 GLYCOGENOSIS, TYPE VIII
3242 G(M1)-GANGLIOSIDOSIS, TYPE 1
3242 G(M1)-GANGLIOSIDOSIS, TYPE 2
3243 OSTEODYSPLASTICA GERODERMIA, BAMATTER TYPE
3244 G(M2)-GANGLIOSIDOSIS WITH HEXOSAMINIDASE A AND B DEFICIENCY
3244 G(M2)-GANGLIOSIDOSIS WITH HEXOSAMINIDASE A DEFICIENCY
3245 ALBINISM, OCULOCUTANEOUS, HERMANSKY-PUDLAK TYPE
3247 HEART-HAND SYNDROME
3248 HEART, CORDIS ECTOPIA
3248 PENTALOGY OF CANTRELL
3250 LIMB AND SCALP DEFECTS, ADAMS-OLIVER TYPE
3251 HEPATOLENTICULAR DEGENERATION
3252 CONTRACTURES, HERRMANN-OPITZ ARTHROGRYPOSIS TYPE
3253 HOMOCYSTINURIA
3253 HOMOCYSTINURIA, N(5,10) METHYLENE TETRAHYDROFOLATE DEFICIENCY TYPE
3254 HUMERO-RADIAL SYNOSTOSIS
3256 ENDOSTEAL HYPEROSTOSIS
3257 SMITH-FINEMAN-MYERS SYNDROME
3258 HYPERTELORISM-HYPOSPADIAS SYNDROME
3259 HYPERTELORISM-MICROTIA-FACIAL CLEFT-CONDUCTIVE DEAFNESS
3260 HYPOCHONDROPLASIA
3261 HYPODONTIA-NAIL DYSGENESIS
3262 HYPOPHOSPHATASIA
3263 HYPOPHOSPHATEMIA, X-LINKED
3263 RICKETS, VITAMIN D-DEPENDENT, TYPE I
3265 INCONTINENTIA PIGMENTI
3266 CHERUBISM
3267 CAT EYE SYNDROME

3269 JOHANSON-BLIZZARD SYNDROME
3270 KBG SYNDROME
3271 CRANIOSYNOSTOSIS, KLEEBLATTSCHADEL TYPE
3272 KNIEST DYSPLASIA
3273 ANGIO-OSTEOHYPERTROPHY SYNDROME
3274 KLIPPEL-FEIL ANOMALY
3275 LARSEN SYNDROME
3276 BARDET-BIEDL SYNDROME
3277 LENTIGINES SYNDROME, MULTIPLE
3277 LENZ MICROPHTHALMIA SYNDROME
3278 LEPRECHAUNISM
3279 LESCH-NYHAN SYNDROME
3280 LIMB-OTO-CARDIAC SYNDROME
3283 ACROFACIAL DYSOSTOSIS
3283 MANDIBULOFACIAL DYSOSTOSIS
3283 MANDIBULOFACIAL DYSOSTOSIS,
     TREACHER-COLLINS TYPE, RECESSIVE
3284 MARDEN-WALKER SYNDROME
3285 MARFAN SYNDROME
3286 McDONOUGH SYNDROME
3287 MECKEL SYNDROME
3288 FACE, MEDIAN CLEFT FACE SYNDROME
3290 MENKES SYNDROME
3292 MESOMELIC DYSPLASIA, LANGER TYPE
3293 MESOMELIC DYSPLASIA, NIEVERGELT TYPE
3294 LIMB DEFECT WITH ABSENT ULNA/FIBULA
3294 MESOMELIC DYSPLASIA, REINHARDT-PFEIFFER TYPE
3295 MESOMELIC DYSPLASIA, WERNER TYPE
3296 METAPHYSEAL CHONDRODYSPLASIA, TYPE JANSEN
3298 METAPHYSEAL CHONDRODYSPLASIA, TYPE SCHMID
3299 METAPHYSEAL CHONDRODYSPLASIA WITH
     THYMOLYMPHOPENIA
3300 METATROPIC DYSPLASIA
3301 MICROCEPHALY
3303 MITRAL REGURGITATION-DEAFNESS-SKELETAL
     DEFECTS
3304 ALOPECIA-EPILEPSY-OLIGOPHRENIA, MOYNAHAN
     TYPE
3305 MUCOLIPIDOSIS I
3306 MUCOLIPIDOSIS II
3307 MUCOLIPIDOSIS III
3308 MUCOPOLYSACCHARIDOSIS I-H
3309 MUCOPOLYSACCHARIDOSIS II
3310 MUCOPOLYSACCHARIDOSIS III
3311 MUCOPOLYSACCHARIDOSIS IV
3312 MUCOPOLYSACCHARIDOSIS I-S
3313 MUCOPOLYSACCHARIDOSIS VI
3314 MUCOPOLYSACCHARIDOSIS VII
3316 MARSHALL-SMITH SYNDROME
3317 MIETENS-WEBER SYNDROME
3318 DWARFISM-STIFF JOINTS
3319 ENDOCRINE NEOPLASIA, MULTIPLE TYPE III
3323 GINGIVAL FIBROMATOSIS-HYPERTRICHOSIS
3324 X-LINKED MENTAL RETARDATION, FRAGILE X
     SYNDROME
3325 SIMPSON-GOLABI-BEHMEL SYNDROME
3326 NEU-LAXOVA SYNDROME
3328 DWARFISM, MULIBREY TYPE
3330 MAXILLONASAL DYSPLASIA, BINDER TYPE
3331 NAIL-PATELLA SYNDROME
3332 NEUROFIBROMATOSIS
3333 NEURONAL CEROID-LIPOFUSCINOSES (NCL)
3334 NIEMANN-PICK DISEASE
3335 NOONAN SYNDROME
3336 NORRIE DISEASE
3338 FACIO-OCULO-ACOUSTIC-RENAL SYNDROME (FOAR
     SYNDROME)
3339 OCULO-AURICULO-VERTEBRAL ANOMALY
3340 OCULO-CEREBRO-RENAL SYNDROME
3341 OCULO-DENTO-OSSEOUS DYSPLASIA
3342 OCULO-MANDIBULO-FACIAL SYNDROME
3345 DWARFISM, OSTEODYSPLASTIC PRIMORDIAL,
     MAJEWSKI-RANKE TYPE

3346 PSEUDOXANTHOMA ELASTICUM
3347 ORO-FACIO-DIGITAL SYNDROME I
3348 ORO-FACIO-DIGITAL SYNDROME, MOHR TYPE
3349 OSTEOGENESIS IMPERFECTA
3351 OTO-OCULO-MUSCULO-SKELETAL SYNDROME
3352 OTO-PALATO-DIGITAL SYNDROME, I
3354 OSTEODYSPLASTY
3355 ODONTO-TRICHOMELIC SYNDROME
3357 PALLISTER-W SYNDROME
3358 PARASTREMMATIC DYSPLASIA
3359 POLAND SYNDROME
3360 PTERYGIUM SYNDROME, POPLITEAL
3361 PRADER-WILLI SYNDROME
3362 PROGERIA
3363 PSEUDOACHONDROPLASTIC DYSPLASIA
3365 PYKNODYSOSTOSIS
3367 PYLE DISEASE
3368 KIDNEY, POLYCYSTIC DISEASE, RECESSIVE
3368 KIDNEY, RENAL DYSPLASIA, POTTER TYPE II
3368 RENAL AGENESIS, BILATERAL
3369 PACHYDERMOPERIOSTOSIS
3370 HEMIFACIAL ATROPHY, PROGRESSIVE
3371 CLEFT PALATE-MICROGNATHIA-GLOSSOPTOSIS
3372 LARSEN SYNDROME, LETHAL TYPE
3373 FIBROUS DYSPLASIA, POLYOSTOTIC
3374 OSTEOPETROSIS, MALIGNANT RECESSIVE
3376 RENAL-GENITAL-MIDDLE EAR ANOMALIES
3378 ROBERTS SYNDROME
3379 ROBINOW SYNDROME
3380 RIEGER SYNDROME
3382 POIKILODERMA, HEREDITARY ACROKERATOTIC,
     KINDLER-WEARY TYPE
3383 ROTHMUND-THOMSON SYNDROME
3384 RUBINSTEIN-TAYBI BROAD THUMB-HALLUX
     SYNDROME
3385 SILVER SYNDROME
3386 SCLEROSTEOSIS
3387 DWARFISM, OSTEODYSPLASTIC PRIMORDIAL,
     MAJEWSKI-WINTER TYPE
3387 SECKEL SYNDROME
3388 ARTHROGRYPOSIS, DISTAL TYPES
3389 SHORT RIB-POLYDACTYLY SYNDROME, TYPE II
3390 SHORT RIB-POLYDACTYLY SYNDROME, TYPE I
3390 SPONDYLOCOSTAL DYSPLASIA
3391 SMITH-LEMLI-OPITZ SYNDROME
3393 SPONDYLOCOSTAL DYSPLASIA
3394 SPONDYLOEPIPHYSEAL DYSPLASIA CONGENITA
3395 SPONDYLOEPIPHYSEAL DYSPLASIA, LATE
3396 SPONDYLOMETAPHYSEAL CHONDRODYSPLASIA,
     KOZLOWSKI TYPE
3397 STURGE-WEBER SYNDROME
3398 SEPTO-OPTIC DYSPLASIA
3399 CAUDAL REGRESSION SYNDROME
3399 SIRENOMELIA SEQUENCE
3399 STOMACH, TERATOMA
3400 SJOGREN-LARSSON SYNDROME
3402 SYMPHALANGISM
3403 CHONDRODYSTROPHIC MYOTONIA,
     SCHWARTZ-JAMPEL TYPE
3405 TRACHEAL AGENESIS-MULTIPLE ANOMALY
     ASSOCIATION
3407 ECTODERMAL DYSPLASIA, CONGENITAL FACIAL,
     SETLEIS TYPE
3410 SPONDYLOCOSTAL DYSPLASIA
3410 SPONDYLOTHORACIC DYSPLASIA
3411 THANATOPHORIC DYSPLASIA
3412 THROMBOCYTOPENIA-ABSENT RADIUS
3414 TRICHO-DENTO-OSSEOUS SYNDROME
3415 TRICHO-RHINO-PHALANGEAL SYNDROME, TYPE I
3416 TRICHO-RHINO-PHALANGEAL SYNDROME, TYPE II
3417 TUBEROUS SCLEROSIS
3419 DIGITO-TALAR DYSMORPHISM
3420 ULNAR-MAMMARY SYNDROME

3421 USHER SYNDROME
3424 VAN DEN BOSCH SYNDROME
3425 VATER ASSOCIATION
3426 WAARDENBURG SYNDROMES
3427 WILLIAMS SYNDROME
3428 WINCHESTER SYNDROME
3429 WEAVER SYNDROME
3430 CORTICAL HYPEROSTOSIS, INFANTILE
3431 XERODERMA PIGMENTOSUM-MENTAL
     RETARDATION
3432 X-LINKED MENTAL RETARDATION-CLASPED THUMB
3436 LIPOGRANULOMATOSIS
3437 NEUROECTODERMAL SYNDROME, FLYNN-AIRD
     TYPE
3438 MARINESCO-SJOGREN SYNDROME
3439 LIPODYSTROPHY SYNDROME, BERARDINELLI TYPE
3439 LIPODYSTROPHY, FAMILIAL LIMB AND TRUNK
3442 RETINOPATHY-HYPOTRICHOSIS SYNDROME
3442 TRICHOMEGALY-RETARDATION-DWARFISM-
     RETINAL PIGMENTARY DEGENERATION
3446 DIGITO-RENO-CEREBRAL SYNDROME
3449 DEAFNESS-MALFORMED, LOW-SET EARS
3453 SHWACHMAN SYNDROME
3455 RENAL DYSPLASIA-RETINAL APLASIA,
     LOKEN-SENIOR TYPE
3456 TRICHOTHIODYSTROPHY
3457 LIMB REDUCTION-ICHTHYOSIS
3459 GELEOPHYSIC DWARFISM
3460 HOLOPROSENCEPHALY
3461 SKELETAL DYSPLASIA, WEISMANN-NETTER-STUHL
     TYPE
3462 ANGELMAN SYNDROME
3463 PHYTANIC ACID STORAGE DISEASE
3464 CATARACTS-OTO-DENTAL DEFECTS
3469 STIFF SKIN SYNDROME
3471 HYPOTHALAMIC HAMARTOBLASTOMA SYNDROME,
     CONGENITAL
3472 PTERYGIUM SYNDROME, MULTIPLE
3478 AGNATHIA-HOLOPROSENCEPHALY
3478 AGNATHIA-MICROSTOMIA-SYNOTIA
3480 CHARGE ASSOCIATION
3485 YUNIS-VARON SYNDROME
3486 MUSCLE WASTING OF HANDS-SENSORINEURAL
     DEAFNESS
3487 ACROFACIAL DYSOSTOSIS
3487 ACROFACIAL DYSOSTOSIS, POSTAXIAL TYPE
3489 POLYSYNDACTYLY-DYSMORPHIC CRANIOFACIES,
     GREIG TYPE
3490 ONYCHO-TRICHODYSPLASIA-NEUTROPENIA
3491 CHEILITIS GRANULOMATOSA, MELKERSSON-
     ROSENTHAL TYPE
3492 OCULO-FACIAL SYNDROME, BENCZE TYPE
3494 PSEUDOLEPRECHAUNISM, PATTERSON TYPE
3496 LIPODYSTROPHY-RIEGER ANOMALY-SHORT
     STATURE-DIABETES
3496 SHORT SYNDROME
3497 MARTSOLF SYNDROME
3502 BORJESON-FORSSMAN-LEHMANN SYNDROME
3504 STERNAL MALFORMATION-VASCULAR DYSPLASIA
     ASSOCIATION
3506 OCULO-CEREBRO-CUTANEOUS SYNDROME
3508 BRACHYDACTYLY-LONG THUMB SYNDROME
3509 FETAL EFFECTS FROM ANGEL DUST
     (PHENCYCLIDINE OR PCP)
3511 FRONTO-FACIO-NASAL DYSPLASIA
3512 CRANIOSYNOSTOSIS-FOOT DEFECTS,
     JACKSON-WEISS TYPE
3515 PROTEUS SYNDROME
3516 DIABETES (INSIPIDUS/MELLITUS)-OPTIC
     ATROPHY-DEAFNESS
3519 SKELETAL DYSPLASIA, FUHRMANN TYPE
3521 THYROID, DYSGENESIS
3524 ECTODERMAL DYSPLASIA, HAY-WELLS TYPE

3525 HYPOMELANOSIS OF ITO
3526 OVERGROWTH, RUVALCABA-MYHRE-SMITH TYPE
3527 NEVOID BASAL CELL CARCINOMA SYNDROME
3528 ICHTHYOSIFORM ERYTHROKERATODERMA,
     ATYPICAL WITH DEAFNESS
3529 AREDYLD SYNDROME
3530 FETAL EFFECTS FROM VARICELLA-ZOSTER
3532 FETAL EFFECTS FROM MATERNAL HYPERTHERMIA
3533 FETAL EFFECTS FROM MATERNAL PKU
3533 PHENYLKETONURIA
3534 SPINOCEREBELLAR DEGENERATION-CORNEAL
     DYSTROPHY
3535 MURCS ASSOCIATION
3536 ALBINISM, OCULOCUTANEOUS, BROWN TYPE
3536 ALBINISM, OCULOCUTANEOUS, RUFOUS TYPE
3536 ALBINISM, OCULOCUTANEOUS, TYROSINASE
     NEGATIVE
3536 ALBINISM, OCULOCUTANEOUS, TYROSINASE
     POSITIVE
3536 ALBINISM, OCULOCUTANEOUS, YELLOW MUTANT
3537 HYPOGLOSSIA-HYPODACTYLIA
3540 RETINOPATHY-MICROCEPHALY-MENTAL
     RETARDATION
3541 KABUKI MAKE-UP SYNDROME
3542 NASOPALPEBRAL LIPOMA-COLOBOMA SYNDROME
3546 LACRIMO-AURICULO-DENTO-DIGITAL SYNDROME
3548 MUCOLIPIDOSIS IV
3549 ALOPECIA-MENTAL RETARDATION
3551 RADIAL HYPOPLASIA-TRIPHALANGEAL
     THUMBS-HYPOSPADIAS-DIASTEMA
3552 ATELOSTEOGENESIS
3555 ACROCALLOSAL SYNDROME, SCHINZEL TYPE
3556 OVERGROWTH, BANNAYAN TYPE
3561 SPONDYLOEPIMETAPHYSEAL DYSPLASIA,
     STRUDWICK TYPE
3562 ALOPECIA-SKELETAL ANOMALIES-SHORT
     STATURE-MENTAL RETARDATION
3565 ELEJALDE SYNDROME
3566 FG SYNDROME, OPITZ-KAVEGGIA TYPE
3567 HYDROLETHALUS SYNDROME
3570 ANTLEY-BIXLER SYNDROME
3578 GINGIVAL FIBROMATOSIS-DEAFNESS, JONES TYPES
3580 ECTODERMAL DYSPLASIA-ECTRODACTYLY-
     MACULAR DYSTROPHY
3581 DEAFNESS-ONYCHODYSTROPHY
3582 OTO-ONYCHO-PERONEAL SYNDROME
3584 X-LINKED MENTAL RETARDATION-GROWTH-
     HEARING AND GENITAL DEFECTS
3585 X-LINKED MENTAL RETARDATION-SHORT
     STATURE-OBESITY-HYPOGONADISM
3586 DWARFISM, SHORT-RIB, BEEMER TYPE
3588 BRANCHIO-OTO-URETERAL SYNDROME
3589 MUSCLE-EYE-BRAIN SYNDROME
3590 X-LINKED MENTAL RETARDATION,
     GOLABI-ITO-HALL TYPE
3591 THUMB, ADDUCTED THUMB SYNDROME
3593 JOUBERT SYNDROME
3595 ALOPECIA-ANOSMIA-DEAFNESS-HYPOGONADISM,
     JOHNSON TYPE
3596 HYPERKERATOSIS PALMOPLANTARIS-SPASTIC
     PARAPLEGIA-RETARDATION
3598 CHROMOSOME 21, MONOSOMY 21
3599 LYMPHEDEMA-HYPOPARATHYROIDISM
3600 MICROCEPHALY, ISOLATED AUTOSOMAL
     DOMINANT TYPE
3601 CRANIOFACIAL-DEAFNESS-HAND SYNDROME
3603 TRICHO-ODONTO-ONYCHIAL DYSPLASIA
3604 DERMATO-OSTEOLYSIS, KIRGHIZIAN TYPE
3606 THORACOPELVIC DYSOSTOSIS
3608 FRYNS SYNDROME
3609 ODONTO-ONYCHODERMAL DYSPLASIA
3610 ACROFACIAL DYSOSTOSIS

3612 HYPOGONADISM-DIABETES-ALOPECIA-DEAFNESS-RETARDATION-EKG ANOMALIES
3613 SKELETAL DYSPLASIA, 3 M TYPE
3614 CARDIOFACIAL SYNDROME-ASSYMETRIC FACIES
3615 LERI PLEONOSTEOSIS SYNDROME
3618 BRANCHIO-OCULO-FACIAL SYNDROME
3621 AMNIOTIC BANDS SYNDROME
3622 FACES SYNDROME
3623 BRANCHIAL ARCH SYNDROME, X-LINKED
3624 FETAL RETINOID SYNDROME
3627 CARDIO-FACIAL-CUTANEOUS SYNDROME
3628 CHROMOSOME 22, SUPERNUMERARY DER 22, T(11:22)
3630 OTO-SPONDYLO-MEGAEPIPHYSEAL DYSPLASIA
3631 GROWTH-MENTAL DEFICIENCY, MYHRE TYPE
3632 ACROFACIAL SYNDROME, CURRY-HALL TYPE
3633 RADIAL-RENAL SYNDROME
3638 INTESTINAL POLYPOSIS, TYPE II
3639 CRANIOTELENCEPHALIC DYSPLASIA
3640 GROWTH RETARDATION-ALOPECIA-PSEUDOANODONTIA-OPTIC ATROPHY
3642 FIBROCHONDROGENESIS
3643 PARIETAL FORAMINA-CLAVICULAR HYPOPLASIA
3644 HYDROCEPHALUS-HEART DEFECT-DENSE BONES, BEEMER TYPE
3645 SMITH-LEMLI-OPITZ SYNDROME, TYPE II
3646 DWARFISM-DYSMORPHIC FACIES-RETARDATION, PITT TYPE
3647 HYPERKERATOSIS PALMOPLANTARIS-PERIODONTOCLASIA
3648 OVERGROWTH-RENAL HAMARTOMA, PERLMAN TYPE
3649 OPSISMODYSPLASIA
3650 FETAL VALPROATE SYNDROME
3652 DISTICHIASIS-HEART DEFECT-PERIPHERAL VASCULAR DISEASE/ANOMALIES
3655 PROTEUS SYNDROME
3656 WALKER-WARBURG SYNDROME
3658 CONTRACTURES, CONGENITAL LETHAL FINNISH TYPE
3659 SPONDYLOCOSTAL DYSOSTOSIS-VISCERAL DEFECTS-DANDY WALKER CYST
3660 CARDIO-AUDITORY SYNDROME
3661 ACROMEGALOID FACIAL APPEARANCE SYNDROME
3662 CUTIS VERTICUS GYRATA
3664 ARTHROGRYPOSIS, AMYOPLASIA TYPE
3667 CLEFTING-ECTROPION-CONICAL TEETH
3669 CRANIOSYNOSTOSIS-ARACHNODACTYLY-HERNIA
3673 ANGIOLIPOMATOSIS
3675 KEUTEL SYNDROME
3676 VON HIPPEL-LINDAU SYNDROME
3678 CHROMOSOME 6, MONOSOMY PROXIMAL 6q
3679 BRACHYOLMELIA, DOMINANT TYPE
3679 BRACHYOLMELIA, MAROTEAUX TYPE
3679 BRACHYOLMIA, HOBAEK TYPE
3682 FACIAL CLEFTING SYNDROME, GYPSY TYPE
3683 CHROMOSOME 1, TRISOMY 1q25-1q32
3684 CHROMOSOME 1, MONOSOMY 1q
3685 CHROMOSOME 2, MONOSOMY OF MEDIAL 2q
3686 CHROMOSOME 2, TRISOMY DISTAL 2q
3687 CHROMOSOME 3, MONOSOMY 3p2
3688 CHROMOSOME 3, TRISOMY 3q2
3689 CHROMOSOME 6, TRISOMY 6q2
3690 CHROMOSOME 13, TRISOMY 13q1
3690 CHROMOSOME 13, TRISOMY DISTAL 13q
3691 CHROMOSOME 8, MONOSOMY 8p2
3693 CHROMOSOME 2, PARTIAL TRISOMY 2p
3695 ACRO-FRONTO-FACIO-NASAL DYSOSTOSIS
3696 CHROMOSOME 16, TRISOMY 16p
3697 CHROMOSOME 11, PARTIAL MONOSOMY 11p
3698 FACIO-NEURO-SKELETAL SYNDROME
3701 BIEMOND II SYNDROME
3702 CHROMOSOME 18, TETRASOMY 18p

3703 CHROMOSOME 22, TRISOMY MOSAICISM
3705 X-LINKED MENTAL RETARDATION, MARFANOID HABITUS TYPE
3710 OTO-PALATO-DIGITAL SYNDROME, II
3711 OSTEOPOROSIS-PSEUDOGLIOMA SYNDROME
3712 CHROMOSOME 16, TRISOMY 16q
3714 DYSEQUILIBRIUM SYNDROME
3717 CEREBRO-NEPHRO-OSTEODYSPLASIA, HUTTERITE TYPE
3720 ANENCEPHALY
3720 ENCEPHALOCELE
3720 MENINGOCELE
3720 MENINGOMYELOCELE
3721 PROGERIA, NEONATAL RAUTENSTRAUCH-WIEDEMANN TYPE
3723 CATARACT-MICROCORNEA SYNDROME
3725 SYNDACTYLY-MICROCEPHALY-MENTAL RETARDATION, FILIPPI TYPE
3728 DYSOSTEOSCLEROSIS
3732 CARDIOMYOPATHY-GENITAL DEFECTS
3733 DEAFNESS-ONYCHO-OSTEO-DYSTROPHY-RETARDATION-SEIZURES (DOORS)
3734 MEGALOCORNEA-MENTAL RETARDATION SYNDROME
3741 LIPODYSTROPHY-COARSE FACIES-ACANTHOSIS NIGRICANS, MIESCHER TYPE
3742 DYSPLASIA EPIPHYSEALIS HEMIMELICA
3744 DISTICHIASIS-LYMPHEDEMA SYNDROME
3747 KEARNS-SAYRE DISEASE
3754 MICROCEPHALY-LYMPHEDEMA
3755 GREBE SYNDROME
3757 NEUROCUTANEOUS MELANOSIS
3759 ENCHONDROMATOSIS AND HEMANGIOMAS
3760 TELANGIECTASIA, OSLER HEMORRHAGIC
3763 DEXTROCARDIA-BRONCHIECTASIS-SINUSITIS SYNDROME
3764 PERRAULT SYNDROME
3765 WERNER SYNDROME
3766 INTESTINAL POLYPOSIS, TYPE III
3767 PROLIDASE DEFICIENCY
3768 CHOLESTASIS-LYMPHEDEMA, AAGENAES TYPE
3771 GROWTH HORMONE DEFICIENCY, ISOLATED
3775 METACHROMATIC LEUKODYSTROPHIES
3780 CYSTINOSIS
3781 ACIDEMIA, METHYLMALONIC
3784 MAPLE SYRUP URINE DISEASE
3787 GLYCOGENOSIS, TYPE IIb
3787 GLYCOGENOSIS, TYPE IIc
3787 GLYCOGENOSIS, TYPE IId
3789 GALACTOSEMIA
3792 CYSTIC FIBROSIS
3795 OSTEOPATHIA STRIATA
3796 RETT SYNDROME
3797 ATAXIA, FRIEDREICH TYPE
3799 RESTRICTIVE DERMATOPATHY
3800 PALLISTER-KILLIAN MOSAIC SYNDROME
3805 ALBINISM-MICROCEPHALY-DIGITAL DEFECTS
3809 GONADAL DYSGENESIS, XX TYPE
3809 GONADAL DYSGENESIS, XY TYPE
3812 HUTTERITE SYNDROME, BOWEN-CONRADI TYPE
3813 SKELETAL DYSPLASIA, BOOMERANG DYSPLASIA
3814 POLYSYNDACTYLY-CARDIAC MALFORMATIONS
3816 BIEMOND I SYNDROME
3818 ACROCEPHALOPOLYSYNDACTYLY
3819 ACRO-RENAL-MANDIBULAR SYNDROME
3821 NEPHROSIS-NERVE DEAFNESS-HYPOPARATHY-ROIDISM, BARAKAT TYPE
3822 ECTODERMAL DYSPLASIA, BASAN TYPE
3827 BERLIN SYNDROME
3829 AASE-SMITH SYNDROME
3829 ANEMIA, HYPOPLASTIC-TRIPHALANGEAL THUMBS, AASE-SMITH TYPE

3830 INTESTINAL HYPOPERISTALSIS, MEGACYSTIS-MICROCOLON TYPE
3832 CUTIS MARMORATA
3835 CLEFT PALATE-OMPHALOCELE
3839 ACROMEGALOID PHENOTYPE-CUTIS VERTICIS GYRATA-CORNEAL LEUKOMA
3843 PTERYGIA-DYSMORPHIC FACIES-SHORT STATURE-MENTAL RETARDATION
3844 POLYPOSIS-ALOPECIA-PIGMENTATION-NAIL DEFECTS
3845 CHANDS
3846 NEPHROSIS-HYDROCEPHALUS-THIN SKIN-BLUE SCLERA-GROWTH DEFECT
3847 SKELETAL DYSPLASIA, DE LA CHAPELLE TYPE
3849 IVIC SYNDROME
3850 SEIZURES-ICHTHYOSIS-MENTAL RETARDATION
3852 SKELETAL DYSPLASIA, SCHNECKENBECKEN TYPE
3854 SHORT STATURE-WORMIAN BONES-JOINT DISLOCATIONS
3855 DEAFNESS-VITILIGO-MUSCLE WASTING
3864 DEAFNESS-NEPHRITIS-MACROTHROMBOPATHIA
3870 ORO-FACIO-DIGITAL SYNDROME, THURSTON TYPE
3872 ACROMICRIC DYSPLASIA
3875 MENTAL RETARDATION-HEART DEFECTS-BLEPHAROPHIMOSIS
3887 SYNDACTYLY, CENANI TYPE
3890 CERVICO-DERMO-GU SYNDROME, GOEMINNE TYPE
3896 LIMB, UPPER HYPOPLASIA-MULLERIAN DUCT DEFECTS
3897 APLASIA CUTIS CONGENITA-GASTROINTESTINAL ATRESIA
3899 MICROCEPHALY-RETARDATION-SKELETAL AND IMMUNE DEFECTS
3901 SYNDACTYLY-POLYDACTYLY-EAR LOBE SYNDROME
3905 GASTROCUTANEOUS SYNDROME
3910 THYROID, HORMONE RESISTANCE
3911 CORPUS CALLOSUM AGENESIS-SENSORIMOTOR NEUROPATHY, FAMILIAL
3913 RETINAL TELANGIECTASIA-HYPOGAMMAGLOBU-LINEMIA
3917 EPIPHYSEAL DYSPLASIA, MULTIPLE-DIABETES MELLITUS
3919 ABLEPHARON-MACROSTOMIA
3921 MAXILLOFACIAL DYSOSTOSIS
3923 CLEFT PALATE-DYSMORPHIC FACIES-DIGITAL DEFECTS, MARTSOLF TYPE
3926 MYOPATHY-CATARACT-GONADAL DYSGENESIS
3930 KYPHOMELIC DYSPLASIA
3934 SHORT STATURE-CEREBRAL ATROPHY-KERATOSIS FOLLICULARIS, X-LINKED
3941 OSTEOCHONDRODYSPLASIA WITH HYPERTRICHOSIS
3947 METAPHYSEAL DYSPLASIA-MAXILLARY HYPOPLASIA-BRACHYDACTYLY
3948 EDINBURGH MALFORMATION SYNDROME
3956 CATARACT-RENAL TUBULAR NECROSIS-ENCEPHALOPATHY, CROME TYPE
3959 AMYLOIDOSIS, CORNEAL
3959 AMYLOIDOSIS, FINNISH TYPE
3962 THUMB, TRIPHALANGEAL-BRACHYECTRODACTYLY
3966 CHROMOSOME 18, TRISOMY 18q2
3974 TIBIAL HYPOPLASIA/APLASIA-ECTRODACTYLY
3978 WRINKLY SKIN SYNDROME
3980 FETAL TRIMETHADIONE SYNDROME
3985 MICROCEPHALY-HIATUS HERNIA-NEPHROSIS, GALLOWAY TYPE
3989 DENTINO-OSSEOUS DYSPLASIA
3990 HEART-HAND SYNDROME
3993 DWARFISM, OCULO-PALATO-CEREBRAL TYPE
3995 OCULO-RENO-CEREBELLAR SYNDROME
3996 MUSCULAR DYSTROPHY, OCULO-GASTROINTESTINAL
3999 ATAXIA-HYPOGONADISM SYNDROME

4004 OSTEOGLOPHONIC DYSPLASIA
4006 SKIN, PARANA HARD SKIN SYNDROME
4008 LARYNGEAL ABDUCTOR PARALYSIS-MENTAL RETARDATION
4015 METACHONDROMATOSIS
4018 SCALP DEFECTS-POSTAXIAL POLYDACTYLY
4022 PHARYNX/LARYNX HYPOPLASIA-OMPHALOCELE, SHPRINTZEN-GOLDBERG TYPE
4024 SINGLETON-MERTEN SYNDROME
4025 SPLENOGONADAL FUSION-LIMB DEFECT
4026 SPONDYLOMETAPHYSEAL DYSPLASIA WITH ENCHONDROMATOUS CHANGES
4027 SPONDYLOPERIPHERAL DYSPLASIA
4046 WEAVER-WILLIAMS SYNDROME
4053 WT SYNDROME
4057 ABRUZZO-ERICKSON SYNDROME
4061 CATARACT-ICHTHYOSIS
4071 PERICARDITIS-ARTHRITIS-CAMPTODACTYLY
4077 DYSOSTOSIS, HUMEROSPINAL
4082 X-LINKED MENTAL RETARDATION-CRANIOFACIAL ABNORMALITIES-CLUB FOOT
4093 DEAFNESS-GOITER
4100 ALBINISM, WAARDENBURG TYPE-HIRSCHSPRUNG AGANGLIONOSIS
4111 STORAGE DISEASE, NEUTRAL LIPID TYPE
4114 CORNEO-DERMATO-OSSEOUS SYNDROME
4115 DEAFNESS-HYPOGONADISM
4118 ECTODERMAL DYSPLASIA, NAEGELI TYPE
4120 ALBINISM, CUTANEOUS-DEAFNESS
4120 ALBINISM, OCULAR-LATE-ONSET-SENSORINEURAL DEAFNESS, X-LINKED
4132 ACROCEPHALOPOLYSYNDACTYLY
4137 SCHISIS ASSOCIATION
4153 ECTRODACTYLY-POLYDACTYLY
4155 TERATOMA, PRESACRAL-SACRAL DYSGENESIS
4162 FOUNTAIN SYNDROME
4166 TREMOR-DUODENAL ULCER SYNDROME
4170 RENAL TUBULAR ACIDOSIS-OSTEOPETROSIS SYNDROME
4181 NAILS, PACHYONYCHIA CONGENITA
4183 KING SYNDROME
4183 MYOPATHY, MALIGNANT HYPERTHERMIA
4187 DWARFISM, MICROCEPHALIC PRIMORDIAL WITH CATARACTS
4191 THORACIC DYSPLASIA-HYDROCEPHALUS
4201 THUMB, TRIPHALANGEAL-DUPLICATED GREAT TOES
4209 GENITO-PALAT0-CARDIAC SYNDROME
4211 GINGIVAL FIBROMATOSIS-CHERUBISM-SEIZURES, RAMON TYPE
4216 KALLMANN SYNDROME
4218 HYDROCEPHALUS-COSTOVERTEBRAL DYSPLASIA-SPRENGEL ANOMALY
4222 X-LINKED MENTAL RETARDATION-SKELETAL DYSPLASIA
4226 TRICHO-DERMODYSPLASIA-DENTAL DEFECTS
4227 WILMS TUMOR-PSEUDOHERMAPHRODITISM-GLOMERULOPATHY, DENYS-DRASH TYPE
4229 NEVUS, BLUE RUBBER BLEB NEVUS SYNDROME
4239 FACIAL DYSMORPHIA-JOINT HYPEREXTENSIBILITY SYNDROME
4249 OSTEOPATHIA STRIATA-CRANIAL SCLEROSIS-MEGALENCEPHALY
4255 PTERYGIUM SYNDROME, MULTIPLE LETHAL
4257 SPONDYLOEPIMETAPHYSEAL DYSPLASIA-JOINT LAXITY
4259 MEGACYSTIS-MEGADUODENUM SYNDROME
4260 GINGIVAL FIBROMATOSIS-CORNEAL DYSTROPHY
4262 OSTEODYSPLASIA, LIPOMEMBRANOUS POLYCYSTIC-DEMENTIA
4264 UROFACIAL SYNDROME
4265 NOSE, CHOANAL ATRESIA-LYMPHEDEMA

4266 PHOSPHORIBOSYL PYROPHOSPHATE (PRPP) SYNTHETASE ABNORMALITY
4267 KNUCKLE PADS-LEUKONYCHIA-DEAFNESS
4277 ICHTHYOSIS-CHEEK-EYEBROW SYNDROME
4280 SPONDYLOEPIPHYSEAL DYSPLASIA-MENTAL RETARDATION
4281 DWARFISM, DYSSEGMENTAL, SILVERMAN-HANDMAKER TYPE
4282 DWARFISM, DYSSEGMENTAL, ROLLAND-DESBUQUOIS TYPE
4283 KUSKOKWIN SYNDROME
4299 CHONDRODYSPLASIA PUNCTATA, X-LINKED DOMINANT TYPE
4313 CAMPTODACTYLY SYNDROME, GUADALAJARA TYPE I
4315 FETAL METHYLMERCURY EFFECTS
4318 ABETALIPOPROTEINEMIA
4325 HYPOGONADISM-PARTIAL ALOPECIA
4328 MUSCULAR DYSTROPHY, OCULOPHARYNGEAL
4335 NEVI-ATRIAL MYXOMA-MYXOID NEUROFIBROMAS-EPHELIDES
4336 NEURO-FACIO-DIGITO-RENAL SYNDROME
4340 NEPHROSIS-DEAFNESS-URINARY TRACT AND DIGITAL DEFECTS
4341 LARYNGO-TRACHEO-ESOPHAGEAL CLEFT
4357 ECTRODACTYLY-ANONYCHIA
4364 ACANTHOCYTOSIS-NEUROLOGIC DEFECTS
4366 ACIDEMIA, MEVALONIC

4369 CHROMOSOME 7, MONOSOMY 7p2
4374 CHROMOSOME INSTABILITY, NIJMEGEN TYPE
4375 IMMUNODEFICIENCY WITH CENTROMERIC INSTABILITY
4379 XANTHOMATOSIS, CEREBROTENDINOUS
4384 CHARCOT MARIE TOOTH DISEASE-DEAFNESS
4385 EMERY-DREIFUSS SYNDROME
4389 CHROMOSOME 14, TRISOMY 14 MOSAIC
4391 PILO-DENTO-UNGULAR DYSPLASIA WITH MICROCEPHALY
4404 MICHELIN TIRE BABY SYNDROME
4412 CAMPTODACTYLY SYNDROME, GUADALAJARA TYPE II
4413 TRICHO-RHINO-PHALANGEAL SYNDROME, TYPE III
4418 HAIR, UNCOMBABLE-CRYSTALLINE CATARACT
4428 RETINOPATHY-HYPOTRICHOSIS SYNDROME
4430 DEAFNESS-EAR DEFECTS-FACIAL PALSY
4440 TRICHODYSPLASIA-XERODERMA
4456 GRANULOMATOSIS-POLYSYNOVITIS, FAMILIAL SYSTEMIC
4457 OSTEOMESOPYKNOSIS
4463 RENAL TUBULAR ACIDOSIS-SENSORINEURAL DEAFNESS
4480 PILI TORTI-CLEFT LIP/PALATE-SYNDACTYLY
4483 DWARFISM (SHORT LIMBED)-PETERS ANOMALY OF THE EYE
4499 FETAL EFFECTS FROM MATERNAL DIABETES
4510 KNIEST-LIKE DYSPLASIA

## CDC-NUMBER-TO-PRIME-NAME INDEX

090.000 FETAL SYPHILIS SYNDROME
171.800 CANCER, EWING SARCOMA
189.000 CANCER, WILMS TUMOR
190.500 RETINOBLASTOMA
191.000 CANCER, GLIOMA, FAMILIAL
191.000 CNS NEOPLASMS
194.000 CANCER, NEUROBLASTOMA
214.800 LIPOMAS, FAMILIAL SYMMETRIC
237.700 NEUROFIBROMATOSIS
238.000 TERATOMAS
238.040 TERATOMA, SACROCOCCYGEAL TERATOMA
239.200 CYSTIC HYGROMA
239.200 NECK, BRANCHIAL CLEFT, CYSTS OR SINUSES
239.200 NECK, CYSTIC HYGROMA, FETAL TYPE
239.200 NECK/HEAD, DERMOID CYST OR TERATOMA
251.200 HYPOGLYCEMIA, FAMILIAL NEONATAL
255.200 STEROID 3 BETA-HYDROXYSTEROID
        DEHYDROGENASE DEFICIENCY
255.200 STEROID 11 BETA-HYDROXYLASE DEFICIENCY
255.200 STEROID 17 ALPHA-HYDROXYLASE DEFICIENCY
255.200 STEROID 17,20-DESMOLASE DEFICIENCY
255.200 STEROID 17-KETOSTEROID REDUCTASE
        DEFICIENCY
255.200 STEROID 18-HYDROXYLASE DEFICIENCY
255.200 STEROID 18-HYDROXYSTEROID DEHYDROGENASE
        DEFICIENCY
255.200 STEROID 20-22 DESMOLASE DEFICIENCY
255.200 STEROID 21-HYDROXYLASE DEFICIENCY
257.800 ANDROGEN INSENSITIVITY SYNDROME,
        COMPLETE
270.100 PHENYLKETONURIA
270.200 ALBINISM, CUTANEOUS
270.200 ALBINISM, OCULAR
270.200 ALBINISM, OCULAR, AUTOSOMAL RECESSIVE
        TYPE
270.200 ALBINISM, OCULOCUTANEOUS, BROWN TYPE
270.200 ALBINISM, OCULOCUTANEOUS,
        HERMANSKY-PUDLAK TYPE
270.200 ALBINISM, OCULOCUTANEOUS, MINIMAL
        PIGMENT TYPE
270.200 ALBINISM, OCULOCUTANEOUS, RUFOUS TYPE
270.200 ALBINISM, OCULOCUTANEOUS, TYROSINASE
        NEGATIVE
270.200 ALBINISM, OCULOCUTANEOUS, TYROSINASE
        POSITIVE
270.200 ALBINISM, OCULOCUTANEOUS, YELLOW
        MUTANT
270.200 ALBINISM-BLACK LOCKS-DEAFNESS
270.200 TRICHOMEGALY-RETARDATION-DWARFISM-
        RETINAL PIGMENTARY DEGENERATION
270.300 MAPLE SYRUP URINE DISEASE
270.600 ACIDURIA, ARGININOSUCCINIC
270.700 HYPERGLYCINEMIA, NON-KETOTIC
271.000 GLYCOGEN STORAGE DISEASE, X-LINKED WITH
        NORMAL HEPATIC ENZYMES
271.000 GLYCOGEN SYNTHETASE DEFICIENCY
271.000 GLYCOGENOSIS, TYPE Ia
271.000 GLYCOGENOSIS, TYPE Ib
271.000 GLYCOGENOSIS, TYPE Ic
271.000 GLYCOGENOSIS, TYPE IIa
271.000 GLYCOGENOSIS, TYPE IIb
271.000 GLYCOGENOSIS, TYPE IId
271.000 GLYCOGENOSIS, TYPE III
271.000 GLYCOGENOSIS, TYPE IV
271.000 GLYCOGENOSIS, TYPE V
271.000 GLYCOGENOSIS, TYPE VI
271.000 GLYCOGENOSIS, TYPE VII
271.000 GLYCOGENOSIS, TYPE VIII

271.000 GLYCOGENOSIS, TYPE IXa
271.000 GLYCOGENOSIS, TYPE IXb
271.000 GLYCOGENOSIS, TYPE IXc
277.000 CYSTIC FIBROSIS
277.010 CYSTIC FIBROSIS
277.400 HYPERBILIRUBINEMIA, CONJUGATED
277.400 HYPERBILIRUBINEMIA, CONJUGATED, ROTOR
        TYPE
277.400 HYPERBILIRUBINEMIA, TRANSIENT FAMILIAL
        NEONATAL
277.400 HYPERBILIRUBINEMIA, UNCONJUGATED
277.400 UDP-GLUCURONOSYLTRANSFERASE, SEVERE
        DEFICIENCY TYPE I
277.510 MUCOPOLYSACCHARIDOSIS I-H
277.620 ALPHA(1)-ANTITRYPSIN DEFICIENCY
277.630 CHOLINESTERASE, ATYPICAL
279.200 IMMUNODEFICIENCY, SEVERE COMBINED
279.200 IMMUNODEFICIENCY, X-LINKED SEVERE
        COMBINED
282.000 SPHEROCYTOSIS
282.000 TEETH, ENAMEL AND DENTIN DEFECTS FROM
        ERYTHROBLASTOSIS FETALIS
282.100 ELLIPTOCYTOSIS
282.200 GLUCOSE-6-PHOSPHATE DEHYDROGENASE
        DEFICIENCY
282.600 ANEMIA, SICKLE CELL
286.000 HEMOPHILIA A
286.000 HEMOPHILIA B
286.400 VON WILLEBRAND DISEASE
330.100 G(M1)-GANGLIOSIDOSIS, TYPE 1
330.100 G(M1)-GANGLIOSIDOSIS, TYPE 2
330.100 G(M2)-GANGLIOSIDOSIS WITH HEXOSAMINIDASE
        A AND B DEFICIENCY
330.100 G(M2)-GANGLIOSIDOSIS WITH HEXOSAMINIDASE
        A DEFICIENCY
335.000 SPINAL MUSCULAR ATROPHY
336.000 SYRINGOMYELIA
352.600 DIPLEGIA, CONGENITAL FACIAL
362.700 RETINITIS PIGMENTOSA
425.300 VENTRICLE, ENDOCARDIAL FIBROELASTOSIS OF
        LEFT VENTRICLE
425.300 VENTRICLE, ENDOCARDIAL FIBROELASTOSIS OF
        RIGHT VENTRICLE
426.705 ARRHYTHMIA, WOLFF-PARKINSON-WHITE TYPE
427.900 ARRHYTHMIA, SUPRAVENTRICULAR
        TACHYCARDIAS, CONGENITAL
427.900 ARRHYTHMIA, WITH LONG QT INTERVAL
        WITHOUT DEAFNESS
520.600 TEETH, NATAL OR NEONATAL
524.080 CLEFT PALATE-MICROGNATHIA-GLOSSOPTOSIS
550.000 HERNIA, INGUINAL
550.100 HERNIA, INGUINAL
550.900 HERNIA, INGUINAL
553.100 HERNIA, UMBILICAL
658.800 AMNIOTIC BANDS SYNDROME
740.0   ANENCEPHALY
741     MENINGOMYELOCELE
742.0   ENCEPHALOCELE
742.100 MICROCEPHALY
742.230 VERMIS AGENESIS
742.240 LISSENCEPHALY SYNDROME
742.240 WALKER-WARBURG SYNDROME
742.260 HOLOPROSENCEPHALY
742.280 BRAIN, MICROPOLYGYRIA
742.280 BRAIN, MIDLINE CAVES
742.280 BRAIN, SCHIZENCEPHALY
742.3   HYDROCEPHALY
742.320 HYDRANENCEPHALY

| | |
|---|---|
| 742.400 | MEGALENCEPHALY |
| 742.410 | BRAIN, PORENCEPHALY |
| 742.420 | BRAIN, ARACHNOID CYSTS |
| 742.480 | BRAIN, ARNOLD-CHIARI MALFORMATION |
| 742.520 | DIASTEMATOMYELIA |
| 742.580 | SPINAL CORD, NEURENTERIC CYST |
| 742.800 | JAW-WINKING SYNDROME |
| 742.810 | DYSAUTONOMIA I, RILEY-DAY TYPE |
| 743.000 | EYE, ANOPHTHALMIA |
| 743.100 | EYE, MICROPHTHALMIA/COLOBOMA |
| 743.200 | GLAUCOMA, CONGENITAL |
| 743.220 | CORNEA, MEGALOCORNEA |
| 743.300 | LENS, APHAKIA |
| 743.310 | LENS, MICROSPHEROPHAKIA |
| 743.310 | SPHEROPHAKIA-BRACHYMORPHIA SYNDROME |
| 743.325 | CATARACT, POLAR AND CAPSULAR |
| 743.326 | CATARACT, AUTOSOMAL DOMINANT CONGENITAL |
| 743.326 | CATARACT, CORTICAL AND NUCLEAR |
| 743.330 | LENS, ECTOPIC |
| 743.380 | LENTICONUS |
| 743.420 | ANIRIDIA |
| 743.430 | EYE, MICROPHTHALMIA/COLOBOMA |
| 743.440 | LENS AND PUPIL, ECTOPIC |
| 743.480 | EYE, ANTERIOR SEGMENT DYSGENESIS |
| 743.520 | OPTIC DISK PITS |
| 743.520 | OPTIC DISK, MELANOCYTOMA |
| 743.520 | OPTIC DISK, MORNING GLORY ANOMALY |
| 743.520 | OPTIC DISK, TILTED |
| 743.520 | OPTIC NERVE HYPOPLASIA |
| 743.580 | EYE, VITREOUS, PERSISTENT HYPERPLASTIC PRIMARY |
| 743.600 | BLEPHAROPTOSIS-BLEPHAROPHIMOSIS-EPICANTHUS INVERSUS-TELECANTHUS |
| 743.600 | EYELID, PTOSIS, CONGENITAL |
| 743.610 | EYELID, ECTROPION, CONGENITAL |
| 743.620 | EYELID, ENTROPION |
| 743.630 | DISTICHIASIS |
| 743.630 | EYE, CRYPTOPHTHALMOS WITH OTHER MALFORMATIONS |
| 743.630 | EYELID, EPIBLEPHARON |
| 743.635 | BLEPHAROPTOSIS-BLEPHAROPHIMOSIS-EPICANTHUS INVERSUS-TELECANTHUS |
| 743.635 | EYELID, ANKYLOBLEPHARON |
| 743.636 | EYELID, COLOBOMA |
| 743.640 | LACRIMAL CANALICULUS ATRESIA |
| 743.660 | LACRIMAL GLAND, ECTOPIC |
| 743.660 | LACRIMAL SAC FISTULA |
| 744.010 | EAR, MICROTIA-ATRESIA |
| 744.020 | EAR, OSSICLE AND MIDDLE EAR MALFORMATIONS |
| 744.030 | EAR, INNER DYSPLASIAS |
| 744.030 | EAR, LABYRINTH APLASIA |
| 744.090 | DEAFNESS-EAR PITS |
| 744.200 | EAR, MACROTIA |
| 744.230 | EAR, ECTOPIC PINNA |
| 744.230 | EAR, EXCHONDROSIS |
| 744.230 | EAR, EXOSTOSES |
| 744.230 | EAR, LOBE, ABSENT |
| 744.230 | EAR, LOP |
| 744.230 | EAR, MOZART TYPE |
| 744.230 | EAR, PROMINENT ANTHELIX |
| 744.245 | EAR, LOW-SET |
| 744.246 | EAR, LONG, NARROW, POSTERIORLY ROTATED |
| 744.250 | EAR, EUSTACHIAN TUBE DEFECTS |
| 744.280 | EAR, CRYPTOTIA |
| 744.280 | EAR, DARWIN TUBERCLE |
| 744.280 | EAR, SMALL WITH FOLDED-DOWN HELIX |
| 744.400 | BRANCHIAL CLEFT CYSTS |
| 744.900 | CYSTIC HYGROMA |
| 744.900 | NECK, CYSTIC HYGROMA, FETAL TYPE |
| 745.000 | HEART, TRUNCUS ARTERIOSUS |
| 745.010 | AORTICO-PULMONARY SEPTAL DEFECT |

| | |
|---|---|
| 745.1 | HEART, TRANSPOSITION OF GREAT VESSELS |
| 745.2 | HEART, TETRALOGY OF FALLOT |
| 745.4 | VENTRICULAR SEPTAL DEFECT |
| 745.5 | ATRIAL SEPTAL DEFECTS |
| 745.6 | HEART, ENDOCARDIAL CUSHION DEFECTS |
| 746.000 | PULMONARY VALVE, ATRESIA |
| 746.010 | PULMONARY VALVE, STENOSIS |
| 746.020 | PULMONARY VALVE, INCOMPETENCE |
| 746.080 | PULMONARY VALVE, BICUSPID |
| 746.080 | PULMONARY VALVE, TETRACUSPID |
| 746.100 | TRICUSPID VALVE, ATRESIA |
| 746.100 | TRICUSPID VALVE, STENOSIS |
| 746.105 | TRICUSPID VALVE, INSUFFICIENCY |
| 746.200 | TRICUSPID VALVE, EBSTEIN ANOMALY |
| 746.300 | AORTIC VALVE STENOSIS |
| 746.400 | AORTIC VALVE, BICUSPID |
| 746.480 | AORTIC VALVE ATRESIA |
| 746.500 | MITRAL VALVE STENOSIS |
| 746.505 | MITRAL VALVE ATRESIA |
| 746.600 | MITRAL VALVE INSUFFICIENCY |
| 746.800 | DEXTROCARDIA-BRONCHIECTASIS-SINUSITIS SYNDROME |
| 746.820 | HEART, COR TRIATRIATUM |
| 746.850 | HEART, PERICARDIUM AGENESIS |
| 746.870 | ARRHYTHMIA, HEART BLOCK, CONGENITAL COMPLETE |
| 746.880 | ARRHYTHMIA, CARDIAC CONDUCTION DEFECTS, NEONATAL |
| 746.880 | ARRHYTHMIA, FROM MATERNAL AUTOIMMUNE DISEASE, CONGENITAL |
| 746.880 | HEART, CORDIS ECTOPIA |
| 746.885 | ARTERY, CORONARY, ARTERIOVENOUS FISTULA |
| 747.000 | DUCTUS ARTERIOSUS, PATENT |
| 747.1 | AORTA, COARCTATION |
| 747.1 | AORTA, COARCTATION, INFANTILE TYPE |
| 747.215 | AORTIC ARCH INTERRUPTION |
| 747.220 | AORTIC STENOSIS, SUPRAVALVAR |
| 747.230 | AORTIC ARCH, RIGHT |
| 747.240 | AORTIC SINUS OF VALSALVA, ANEURYSM |
| 747.250 | AORTIC ARCH, DOUBLE |
| 747.290 | AORTICO-LEFT VENTRICULAR TUNNEL |
| 747.380 | PULMONARY ARTERY, COARCTATION |
| 747.380 | PULMONARY ARTERY, ORIGIN FROM ASCENDING AORTA |
| 747.380 | PULMONARY ARTERY, ORIGIN FROM DUCTUS ARTERIOSUS |
| 747.380 | PULMONARY ARTERY, ORIGIN OF THE LEFT FROM RIGHT PULMONARY ARTERY |
| 747.410 | VENA CAVA, PERSISTENT LEFT SUPERIOR JOINED TO CORONARY SINUS |
| 747.420 | PULMONARY VENOUS CONNECTION, TOTAL ANOMALOUS |
| 747.480 | LIVER, VENOUS ANOMALIES |
| 747.480 | VENA CAVA, ABSENT HEPATIC SEGMENT |
| 747.500 | UMBILICAL CORD, SINGLE ARTERY |
| 747.610 | ARTERY, RENAL FIBROMUSCULAR DYSPLASIA |
| 747.680 | PULMONARY HYPERTENSION, PRIMARY |
| 747.800 | CNS ARTERIOVENOUS MALFORMATION |
| 748.000 | NOSE, ANTERIOR ATRESIA |
| 748.000 | NOSE, ANTERIOR STENOSIS |
| 748.000 | NOSE, POSTERIOR ATRESIA |
| 748.110 | NOSE, DUPLICATION |
| 748.120 | NOSE, BIFID |
| 748.180 | NOSE, GLIOMA |
| 748.180 | NOSE, GRANULOSIS RUBRA NASI |
| 748.180 | NOSE, NASOPHARYNGEAL STENOSIS |
| 748.180 | NOSE, TRANSVERSE GROOVE |
| 748.180 | NOSE, TURBINATE DEFORMITY |
| 748.185 | NOSE, PROBOSCIS LATERALIS |
| 748.2 | LARYNX, WEB |
| 748.300 | LARYNGOCELE |
| 748.300 | LARYNGOMALACIA |
| 748.300 | LARYNX, ATRESIA |

748.300 LARYNX, VENTRICLE PROLAPSE
748.320 TRACHEOMALACIA
748.350 BRONCHIAL ATRESIA
748.380 LARYNX, CYSTS
748.385 LARYNGO-TRACHEO-ESOPHAGEAL CLEFT
748.390 LARYNGO-TRACHEO-ESOPHAGEAL CLEFT
748.480 LUNG, BRONCHOGENIC CYST
748.520 LUNG, LOBE SEQUESTRATION
748.580 LUNG, CONGENITAL LOBAR ADENOMATOSIS
748.580 LUNG, EMPHYSEMA CONGENITAL LOBAR
748.690 LUNG, ABERRANT LOBE
749.0 CLEFT PALATE
749.080 UVULA, CLEFT
749.1 CLEFT LIP
749.190 CLEFTS, LOWER MEDIAN LIP, MANDIBLE AND
         TONGUE
749.2 CLEFT LIP
750.000 TONGUE, ANKYLOGLOSSIA
750.110 HYPOGLOSSIA-HYPODACTYLIA
750.120 MACROGLOSSIA
750.140 CLEFTS, LOWER MEDIAN LIP, MANDIBLE AND
         TONGUE
750.140 TONGUE, CLEFT
750.180 TONGUE, FISSURED
750.180 TONGUE, FOLDING OR ROLLING
750.180 TONGUE, GEOGRAPHIC
750.180 TONGUE, PIGMENTED PAPILLAE
750.180 TONGUE, PLICATED
750.210 PALATOPHARYNGEAL INCOMPETENCE
750.230 SALIVARY GLAND, AGENESIS
750.260 LIP, PITS OR MOUNDS
750.270 LIP, CHEILITIS GLANDULARIS
750.270 LIP, DOUBLE
750.280 MANDIBLE, TORUS MANDIBULARIS
750.3 TRACHEOESOPHAGEAL FISTULA
750.300 ESOPHAGUS, ATRESIA
750.310 ESOPHAGUS, ATRESIA AND TRACHEOESOPH-
         AGEAL FISTULA
750.340 ESOPHAGUS, STENOSIS
750.420 ESOPHAGUS, DIVERTICULUM
750.430 ESOPHAGUS, DUPLICATION
750.480 ESOPHAGUS, ACHALASIA
750.480 ESOPHAGUS, CHALASIA
750.510 PYLORIC STENOSIS
750.600 HERNIA, HIATAL
750.740 STOMACH, DIVERTICULUM
750.750 STOMACH, DUPLICATION
750.780 STOMACH, HYPOPLASIA
750.780 STOMACH, PYLORIC ATRESIA
750.780 STOMACH, TERATOMA
751.000 OMPHALOMESENTERIC DUCT ANOMALIES
751.010 MECKEL DIVERTICULUM
751.1 INTESTINAL ATRESIA OR STENOSIS
751.100 INTESTINAL ATRESIAS, MULTIPLE
751.100 PYLORODUODENAL ATRESIA, HEREDITARY
751.190 JEJUNAL ATRESIA
751.230 ANORECTAL MALFORMATIONS
751.240 ANORECTAL MALFORMATIONS
751.3 COLON, AGANGLIONOSIS
751.490 INTESTINAL ROTATION, INCOMPLETE
751.600 LIVER, AGENESIS
751.610 HEPATIC FIBROSIS, CONGENITAL
751.610 LIVER, CYST, SOLITARY
751.610 LIVER, POLYCYSTIC AND MULTICYSTIC DISEASE,
         ADULT TYPE
751.620 LIVER, ACCESSORY LOBE
751.620 LIVER, ARTERIAL ANOMALIES
751.620 LIVER, HAMARTOMA
751.620 LIVER, HEMANGIOMATOSIS
751.620 LIVER, TRANSPOSITION
751.630 GALLBLADDER, AGENESIS
751.640 GALLBLADDER, ANOMALIES
751.650 BILIARY ATRESIA

751.660 BILE DUCT CHOLEDOCHAL CYST
751.720 PANCREAS, ANNULAR
751.780 PANCREATITIS, HEREDITARY
751.810 INTESTINAL DUPLICATION
751.880 INFLAMMATORY BOWEL DISEASE
751.880 INTESTINAL ENTEROKINASE DEFICIENCY
751.880 INTESTINAL HYPOPERISTALSIS,
         MEGACYSTIS-MICROCOLON TYPE
751.880 INTESTINAL LYMPHANGIECTASIA
751.880 INTESTINAL POLYPOSIS, JUVENILE TYPE
751.880 INTESTINAL PSEUDO-OBSTRUCTION SYNDROMES
751.880 JAUNDICE, INTRAHEPATIC CHOLESTATIC, BYLER
         TYPE
752.380 VAGINAL SEPTUM, TRANSVERSE
752.410 VAGINAL ATRESIA
752.430 HYMEN, IMPERFORATE
752.600 HYPERTELORISM-HYPOSPADIAS SYNDROME
752.600 HYPOSPADIAS
752.610 EPISPADIAS
752.700 HERMAPHRODITISM, TRUE
752.710 GONADAL DYSGENESIS, XY TYPE
752.720 GONADAL DYSGENESIS, XX TYPE
752.800 ANORCHIA
752.860 DIPHALLIA
753.000 RENAL AGENESIS, BILATERAL
753.010 RENAL AGENESIS, UNILATERAL
753.110 KIDNEY, POLYCYSTIC DISEASE, RECESSIVE
753.120 KIDNEY, POLYCYSTIC DISEASE, DOMINANT
753.140 KIDNEY, NEPHRONOPHTHISIS-MEDULLARY
         CYSTIC DISEASE
753.150 KIDNEY, MEDULLARY SPONGE KIDNEY
753.150 KIDNEY, NEPHRONOPHTHISIS-MEDULLARY
         CYSTIC DISEASE
753.320 KIDNEY, HORSESHOE
753.500 BLADDER EXSTROPHY
753.600 URETHRAL VALVES, POSTERIOR
753.880 VESICO-URETERAL REFLUX
754.020 NOSE, DISLOCATED NASAL SEPTUM
754.050 PLAGIOCEPHALY
754.070 TRIGONENCEPHALY, AUTOSOMAL DOMINANT
         TYPE
754.200 SPINE, SCOLIOSIS, IDIOPATHIC
754.300 HIP, CONGENITAL DISLOCATED
754.430 KNEE, GENU RECURVATUM
754.500 FOOT, TALIPES EQUINOVARUS (TEV)
754.520 FOOT, METATARSUS VARUS
754.735 FOOT, VERTICAL TALUS
754.800 PECTUS CARINATUM
754.810 PECTUS EXCAVATUM
754.820 PENTALOGY OF CANTRELL
754.840 HAND, RADIAL CLUB HAND
754.880 HAND, LOCKING DIGITS-GROWTH DEFECT
754.880 HAND, ULNAR DRIFT
755.0 ECTRODACTYLY-POLYDACTYLY
755.0 POLYDACTYLY
755.1 SYNDACTYLY
755.2 LIMB REDUCTION-ICHTHYOSIS
755.2 LIMB, UPPER HYPOPLASIA-MULLERIAN DUCT
         DEFECTS
755.250 ECTRODACTYLY
755.250 ECTRODACTYLY-POLYDACTYLY
755.250 TIBIAL HYPOPLASIA/APLASIA-ECTRODACTYLY
755.280 RADIAL DEFECTS
755.350 ECTRODACTYLY
755.350 TIBIAL HYPOPLASIA/APLASIA-ECTRODACTYLY
755.365 TIBIAL APLASIA/HYPOPLASIA
755.365 TIBIAL HYPOPLASIA/APLASIA-ECTRODACTYLY
755.380 FEMORAL HYPOPLASIA-UNUSUAL FACIES
         SYNDROME
755.440 HAND, ULNAR AND FIBULAR RAY DEFICIENCY,
         WEYERS TYPE
755.500 CAMPTODACTYLY
755.500 THUMB, ADDUCTED THUMB SYNDROME

755.500 THUMB, CLASPED
755.500 THUMB, TRIPHALANGEAL
755.500 THUMB, TRIPHALANGEAL-DUPLICATED GREAT
TOES
755.510 DIGITO-TALAR DYSMORPHISM
755.510 HAND, ULNAR AND FIBULAR RAY DEFICIENCY,
WEYERS TYPE
755.536 RADIAL-ULNAR SYNOSTOSIS
755.555 CLEIDOCRANIAL DYSPLASIA
755.555 PARIETAL FORAMINA-CLAVICULAR HYPOPLASIA
755.555 YUNIS-VARON SYNDROME
755.556 SPRENGEL DEFORMITY
755.616 FOOT, VERTICAL TALUS
755.660 HIP, CONGENITAL COXA VARA
755.660 HIP, DYSPLASIA, NAMAQUALAND TYPE
755.800 ARTHROGRYPOSES
755.800 ARTHROGRYPOSIS, AMYOPLASIA TYPE
755.800 ARTHROGRYPOSIS, DISTAL TYPES
755.810 LARSEN SYNDROME
755.810 LARSEN SYNDROME, LETHAL TYPE
756.000 CRANIOSYNOSTOSIS
756.030 CRANIOSYNOSTOSIS, KLEEBLATTSCHADEL TYPE
756.040 CRANIOFACIAL DYSOSTOSIS
756.040 CRANIOFACIAL DYSOSTOSIS-DIAPHYSEAL
HYPERPLASIA
756.045 MANDIBULOFACIAL DYSOSTOSIS
756.045 MANDIBULOFACIAL DYSOSTOSIS, TREACHER
COLLINS TYPE, RECESSIVE
756.046 OCULO-MANDIBULO-FACIAL SYNDROME
756.055 ACROCEPHALOSYNDACTYLY TYPE I
756.056 ACROCEPHALOSYNDACTYLY TYPE III
756.057 ACROCEPHALOSYNDACTYLY TYPE V
756.057 CRANIOSYNOSTOSIS-FOOT DEFECTS,
JACKSON-WEISS TYPE
756.060 OCULO-AURICULO-VERTEBRAL ANOMALY
756.080 LIMB AND SCALP DEFECTS, ADAMS-OLIVER TYPE
756.085 EYE, HYPERTELORISM
756.085 HYPERTELORISM-HYPOSPADIAS SYNDROME
756.110 KLIPPEL-FEIL ANOMALY
756.130 SPINE, SPONDYLOLISTHESIS AND
SPONDYLOLYSIS
756.170 SACROCOCCYGEAL DYSGENESIS SYNDROME
756.400 ASPHYXIATING THORACIC DYSPLASIA
756.410 ENCHONDROMATOSIS
756.420 ENCHONDROMATOSIS AND HEMANGIOMAS
756.430 ACHONDROPLASIA
756.445 DIASTROPHIC DYSPLASIA
756.446 METATROPIC DYSPLASIA
756.447 THANATOPHORIC DYSPLASIA
756.450 METAPHYSEAL CHONDRODYSPLASIA WITH
THYMOLYMPHOPENIA
756.450 METAPHYSEAL CHONDRODYSPLASIA, TYPE
JANSEN
756.450 METAPHYSEAL CHONDRODYSPLASIA, TYPE
McKUSICK
756.450 METAPHYSEAL CHONDRODYSPLASIA, TYPE
SCHMID
756.450 METAPHYSEAL DYSPLASIA-MAXILLARY
HYPOPLASIA-BRACHYDACTYLY
756.460 SPONDYLOEPIPHYSEAL DYSPLASIA CONGENITA
756.460 SPONDYLOEPIPHYSEAL DYSPLASIA, LATE
756.470 EXOSTOSES, MULTIPLE CARTILAGINOUS
756.470 EXOSTOSES-ANETODERMIA-BRACHYDACTYLY
TYPE E
756.480 CRANIODIAPHYSEAL DYSPLASIA,
LENZ-MAJEWSKI TYPE
756.480 SKELETAL BOWING-CORTICAL THICKENING-
BONE FRAGILITY-ICTHYOSIS
756.480 SKELETAL DYSPLASIA, 3-M TYPE
756.480 SKELETAL DYSPLASIA, DE LA CHAPELLE TYPE
756.480 SKELETAL DYSPLASIA, FUHRMANN TYPE
756.480 SKELETAL DYSPLASIA, SCHNECKENBECKEN TYPE

756.480 SKELETAL DYSPLASIA, WEISMANN-NETTER-
STUHL TYPE
756.500 OSTEOGENESIS IMPERFECTA
756.510 FIBROUS DYSPLASIA, POLYOSTOTIC
756.520 CHONDROECTODERMAL DYSPLASIA
756.525 CHONDROECTODERMAL DYSPLASIA
756.530 CORTICAL HYPEROSTOSIS, INFANTILE
756.540 OSTEOPETROSIS, BENIGN DOMINANT
756.540 OSTEOPETROSIS, MALIGNANT RECESSIVE
756.540 OSTEOPETROSIS, MILD RECESSIVE
756.550 DIAPHYSEAL DYSPLASIA
756.560 OSTEOPOIKILOSIS
756.570 EPIPHYSEAL DYSPLASIA, MULTIPLE
756.570 EPIPHYSEAL DYSPLASIA, MULTIPLE RIBBING TYPE
756.570 EPIPHYSEAL DYSPLASIA, MULTIPLE, RECESSIVE
TARDA TYPE
756.575 CHONDRODYSPLASIA PUNCTATA, MILD
SYMMETRIC TYPE
756.575 CHONDRODYSPLASIA PUNCTATA, RHIZOMELIC
TYPE
756.580 OSTEOCHONDRODYSPLASIA WITH
HYPERTRICHOSIS
756.580 OSTEODYSPLASTY
756.580 OSTEOECTASIA
756.580 OSTEOFIBROUS DYSPLASIA OF TIBIA AND FIBULA
756.580 OSTEOGLOPHONIC DYSPLASIA
756.580 OSTEOLYSIS, CARPAL-TARSAL AND CHRONIC
PROGRESSIVE GLOMERULOPATHY
756.580 OSTEOLYSIS, ESSENTIAL
756.580 OSTEOLYSIS, RECESSIVE CARPAL-TARSAL
756.580 OSTEOMESOPYKNOSIS
756.580 OSTEOPATHIA STRIATA
756.580 OSTEOPATHIA STRIATA-CRANIAL
SCLEROSIS-MEGALENCEPHALY
756.580 OSTEOPOROSIS, JUVENILE IDIOPATHIC
756.580 OSTEOPOROSIS-PSEUDOGLIOMA SYNDROME
756.610 DIAPHRAGMATIC HERNIA
756.620 DIAPHRAGM, EVENTRATION
756.700 OMPHALOCELE
756.710 GASTROSCHISIS
756.720 PRUNE-BELLY SYNDROME
756.800 POLAND SYNDROME
756.830 NAIL-PATELLA SYNDROME
756.850 EHLERS-DANLOS SYNDROME
756.860 TORTICOLLIS
756.880 MYOPATHY OR CARDIOMYOPATHY DUE TO
DESMIN DEFECT
756.880 MYOPATHY, CENTRAL CORE DISEASE TYPE
756.880 MYOPATHY, DISPROPORTIONATE FIBER TYPE I
756.880 MYOPATHY, FAMILIAL LYSIS OF TYPE I FIBERS
756.880 MYOPATHY, MALIGNANT HYPERTHERMIA
756.880 MYOPATHY, MITOCHONDRIAL-
ENCEPHALOPATHY-LACTIC ACIDOSIS-STROKE
756.880 MYOPATHY, MYOGLOBINURIA-ABNORMAL
GLYCOLOSIS, HEREDITARY TYPE
756.880 MYOPATHY, MYOTUBULAR
756.880 MYOPATHY, NEMALINE
756.880 MYOPATHY, SARCOTUBULAR
756.880 MYOPATHY-CATARACT-GONADAL DYSGENESIS
756.880 MYOPATHY-METABOLIC, CARNITINE
DEFICIENCY, PRIMARY AND SECONDARY
756.880 MYOPATHY-METABOLIC, CARNITINE PALMITYL
TRANSFERASE DEFICIENCY
756.880 MYOPATHY-METABOLIC, GLYCOPROTEIN-
GLYCOSAMINOGLYCANS STORAGE TYPE
756.880 MYOPATHY-METABOLIC, MITOCHONDRIAL
CYTOCHROME C OXIDASE DEFICIENCY
756.880 MYOPATHY-METABOLIC, MYOADENYLATE
DEAMINASE DEFICIENCY
757.000 LYMPHEDEMA I
757.000 LYMPHEDEMA II
757.100 ICHTHYOSIS, HARLEQUIN FETUS
757.120 SJOGREN-LARSSON SYNDROME

| | |
|---|---|
| 757.190 | GIROUX-BARBEAU SYNDROME |
| 757.190 | ICHTHYOSIFORM HYPERKERATOSIS, BULLOUS CONGENITAL |
| 757.190 | ICHTHYOSIS HYSTRIX, CURTH-MACKLIN TYPE |
| 757.190 | ICHTHYOSIS, CONGENITAL ERYTHRODERMIC |
| 757.190 | ICHTHYOSIS, LAMELLAR DOMINANT |
| 757.190 | ICHTHYOSIS, LAMELLAR RECESSIVE |
| 757.190 | ICHTHYOSIS, LINEARIS CIRCUMFLEXA |
| 757.190 | SKIN, ERYTHROKERATODERMIA, PROGRESSIVA SYMMETRICA |
| 757.190 | SKIN, ERYTHROKERATODERMIA, VARIABLE |
| 757.190 | SKIN, ERYTHROKERATOLYSIS HIEMALIS |
| 757.195 | ICHTHYOSIS VULGARIS |
| 757.197 | ICHTHYOSIFORM ERYTHROKERATODERMA, ATYPICAL WITH DEAFNESS |
| 757.330 | EPIDERMOLYSIS BULLOSUM, TYPE I |
| 757.330 | EPIDERMOLYSIS BULLOSUM, TYPE II |
| 757.330 | EPIDERMOLYSIS BULLOSUM, TYPE III |
| 757.340 | BERLIN SYNDROME |
| 757.340 | ECTODERMAL DYSPLASIA, BASAN TYPE |
| 757.340 | ECTODERMAL DYSPLASIA, CHRIST-SIEMENS-TOURAINE TYPE |
| 757.340 | ECTODERMAL DYSPLASIA, HIDROTIC |
| 757.346 | ECTODERMAL DYSPLASIA, CONGENITAL FACIAL, SETLEIS TYPE |
| 757.346 | ECTODERMAL DYSPLASIA, HAY-WELLS TYPE |
| 757.346 | ECTODERMAL DYSPLASIA-ADRENAL CYST |
| 757.350 | INCONTINENTIA PIGMENTI |
| 757.360 | XERODERMA PIGMENTOSUM |
| 757.360 | XERODERMA PIGMENTOSUM-MENTAL RETARDATION |
| 757.370 | CUTIS LAXA |
| 757.380 | NEVUS FLAMMEUS |
| 757.380 | NEVUS OF OTA |
| 757.380 | NEVUS, BLUE RUBBER BLEB NEVUS SYNDROME |
| 757.380 | NEVUS, CONGENITAL NEVOMELANOCYTIC |
| 757.380 | NEVUS, EPIDERMAL NEVUS SYNDROME |
| 757.390 | CUTIS MARMORATA |
| 757.395 | SKIN, LOCALIZED ABSENCE OF |
| 757.400 | HAIR, ALOPECIA AREATA |
| 757.400 | HAIR, ATRICHIA CONGENITA |
| 757.410 | HAIR, MONILETHRIX |
| 757.450 | HAIR, HYPERTRICHOSIS, LANUGINOSA |
| 757.450 | HAIR, HYPERTRICHOSIS, X-LINKED |
| 757.480 | HAIR, BALDNESS, COMMON |
| 757.500 | NAILS, ANONYCHIA, HEREDITARY |
| 757.516 | NAILS, PACHYONYCHIA CONGENITA |
| 757.520 | NAILS, KOILONYCHIA |
| 757.530 | NAILS, LEUKONYCHIA |
| 757.600 | BREAST, AMASTIA |
| 757.650 | BREAST, POLYTHELIA |
| 757.680 | GYNECOMASTIA DUE TO INCREASED AROMATASE ACTIVITY, FAMILIAL |
| 757.900 | DARIER DISEASE |
| 757.900 | ECTODERMAL DYSPLASIA, NAEGELI TYPE |
| 757.900 | SKIN PEELING SYNDROME |
| 757.900 | SKIN TUMORS, MULTIPLE GLOMUS |
| 757.900 | SKIN, ACANTHOSIS NIGRICANS |
| 757.900 | SKIN, CUTANEOUS MELANOSIS, DIFFUSE |
| 757.900 | SKIN, ELASTOSIS PERFORANS SERPIGINOSA |
| 757.900 | SKIN, HYPERKERATOSIS, FOCAL PALMOPLANTAR AND GINGIVAL |
| 757.900 | SKIN, HYPERPIGMENTATION, FAMILIAL |
| 757.900 | SKIN, KERATOSIS FOLLICULARIS SPINULOSA DECALVANS |
| 757.900 | SKIN, KYRLE DISEASE |
| 757.900 | SKIN, LEIOMYOMAS, MULTIPLE |
| 757.900 | SKIN, LIPOID PROTEINOSIS |
| 757.900 | SKIN, PAINFUL PLANTAR CALLOSITIES |
| 757.900 | SKIN, PALMO-PLANTAR ERYTHEMA |
| 757.900 | SKIN, PITYRIASIS RUBRA PILARIS |
| 757.900 | SKIN, POROKERATOSIS |
| 757.900 | SKIN, PSORIASIS VULGARIS |

| | |
|---|---|
| 757.900 | SKIN, VITILIGO |
| 758.0 | CHROMOSOME 21, TRISOMY 21 |
| 758.1 | CHROMOSOME 13, TRISOMY 13 |
| 758.2 | CHROMOSOME 18, TRISOMY 18 |
| 758.300 | CHROMOSOME 21, MONOSOMY 21 |
| 758.310 | CHROMOSOME 5, MONOSOMY 5p |
| 758.320 | CHROMOSOME 4, MONOSOMY 4p |
| 758.330 | CHROMOSOME 13, MONOSOMY 13q |
| 758.340 | CHROMOSOME 18, MONOSOMY 18q |
| 758.350 | CHROMOSOME 18, MONOSOMY 18p |
| 758.500 | CHROMOSOME 8, TRISOMY 8 |
| 758.520 | CHROMOSOME 22, TRISOMY MOSAICISM |
| 758.585 | CHROMOSOME TETRAPLOIDY |
| 758.586 | CHROMOSOME TRIPLOIDY |
| 758.600 | TURNER SYNDROME |
| 758.610 | TURNER SYNDROME |
| 758.7 | KLINEFELTER SYNDROME |
| 758.800 | CHROMOSOME MOSAICISM, 45,X/46,XY TYPE |
| 758.990 | BRANCHIO-OCULO-FACIAL SYNDROME |
| 758.990 | CHROMOSOME 1, MONOSOMY 1q |
| 758.990 | CHROMOSOME 1, MONOSOMY 1q4 |
| 758.990 | CHROMOSOME 1, TRISOMY 1q25-1q32 |
| 758.990 | CHROMOSOME 1, TRISOMY 1q32-qter |
| 758.990 | CHROMOSOME 2, MONOSOMY OF MEDIAL 2q |
| 758.990 | CHROMOSOME 2, PARTIAL TRISOMY 2p |
| 758.990 | CHROMOSOME 2, TRISOMY DISTAL 2q |
| 758.990 | CHROMOSOME 3, MONOSOMY 3p2 |
| 758.990 | CHROMOSOME 3, TRISOMY 3p2 |
| 758.990 | CHROMOSOME 3, TRISOMY 3q2 |
| 758.990 | CHROMOSOME 4, MONOSOMY DISTAL 4q |
| 758.990 | CHROMOSOME 4, RING 4 |
| 758.990 | CHROMOSOME 4, TRISOMY 4p |
| 758.990 | CHROMOSOME 4, TRISOMY DISTAL 4q |
| 758.990 | CHROMOSOME 5, MONOSOMY 5q INTERSTITIAL |
| 758.990 | CHROMOSOME 5, TRISOMY 5p |
| 758.990 | CHROMOSOME 5, TRISOMY 5q3 |
| 758.990 | CHROMOSOME 6, MONOSOMY DISTAL 6q |
| 758.990 | CHROMOSOME 6, MONOSOMY PROXIMAL 6q |
| 758.990 | CHROMOSOME 6, RING 6 |
| 758.990 | CHROMOSOME 6, TRISOMY 6p2 |
| 758.990 | CHROMOSOME 6, TRISOMY 6q2 |
| 758.990 | CHROMOSOME 7, MONOSOMY 7p2 |
| 758.990 | CHROMOSOME 7, MONOSOMY 7q1 |
| 758.990 | CHROMOSOME 7, MONOSOMY 7q2 |
| 758.990 | CHROMOSOME 7, MONOSOMY 7q3 |
| 758.990 | CHROMOSOME 7, MOSAIC TRISOMY 7 |
| 758.990 | CHROMOSOME 7, TRISOMY 7p2 |
| 758.990 | CHROMOSOME 7, TRISOMY 7q2-3 |
| 758.990 | CHROMOSOME 8, MONOSOMY 8p2 |
| 758.990 | CHROMOSOME 8, TRISOMY 8p |
| 758.990 | CHROMOSOME 9, PARTIAL MONOSOMY 9p |
| 758.990 | CHROMOSOME 9, RING 9 |
| 758.990 | CHROMOSOME 9, TETRASOMY 9p |
| 758.990 | CHROMOSOME 9, TRISOMY 9 |
| 758.990 | CHROMOSOME 9, TRISOMY 9p |
| 758.990 | CHROMOSOME 9, TRISOMY 9q3 |
| 758.990 | CHROMOSOME 10, MONOSOMY 10p |
| 758.990 | CHROMOSOME 10, MONOSOMY 10q2 |
| 758.990 | CHROMOSOME 10, TRISOMY 10p |
| 758.990 | CHROMOSOME 10, TRISOMY 10q2 |
| 758.990 | CHROMOSOME 11, MONOSOMY 11q |
| 758.990 | CHROMOSOME 11, PARTIAL MONOSOMY 11p |
| 758.990 | CHROMOSOME 11, PARTIAL TRISOMY 11q |
| 758.990 | CHROMOSOME 11, TRISOMY 11p |
| 758.990 | CHROMOSOME 12, MONOSOMY 12p |
| 758.990 | CHROMOSOME 12, PARTIAL TRISOMY 12p |
| 758.990 | CHROMOSOME 12, TRISOMY 12q2 |
| 758.990 | CHROMOSOME 13, MONOSOMY 13q3 |
| 758.990 | CHROMOSOME 13, TRISOMY 13q1 |
| 758.990 | CHROMOSOME 13, TRISOMY DISTAL 13q |
| 758.990 | CHROMOSOME 14, MONOSOMY 14q (q24.3-q32.1) |
| 758.990 | CHROMOSOME 14, PARTIAL TRISOMY 14q |
| 758.990 | CHROMOSOME 14, RING 14 |

| | |
|---|---|
| 758.990 | CHROMOSOME 14, TRISOMY 14 MOSAIC |
| 758.990 | CHROMOSOME 14, TRISOMY 14q |
| 758.990 | CHROMOSOME 15, PARTIAL TRISOMY DISTAL 15q |
| 758.990 | CHROMOSOME 15, RING 15 |
| 758.990 | CHROMOSOME 15, TRISOMY 15q1 |
| 758.990 | CHROMOSOME 16, MONOSOMY 16q |
| 758.990 | CHROMOSOME 16, TRISOMY 16p |
| 758.990 | CHROMOSOME 16, TRISOMY 16q |
| 758.990 | CHROMOSOME 17, INTERSTITIAL DELETION 17p |
| 758.990 | CHROMOSOME 17, TRISOMY 17q2 |
| 758.990 | CHROMOSOME 18, RING 18 |
| 758.990 | CHROMOSOME 18, TETRASOMY 18p |
| 758.990 | CHROMOSOME 18, TRISOMY 18p AND q11 |
| 758.990 | CHROMOSOME 18, TRISOMY 18q2 |
| 758.990 | CHROMOSOME 19, TRISOMY 19q |
| 758.990 | CHROMOSOME 20, PERICENTRIC INVERSION |
| 758.990 | CHROMOSOME 20, TRISOMY 20p |
| 758.990 | CHROMOSOME 21, RING 21 |
| 758.990 | CHROMOSOME 22, MONOSOMY 22 |
| 758.990 | CHROMOSOME 22, MONOSOMY 22q |
| 758.990 | CHROMOSOME 22, RING 22 |
| 758.990 | CHROMOSOME 22, SUPERNUMERARY DER 22, T(11:22) |
| 758.990 | CHROMOSOME INSTABILITY, NIJMEGEN TYPE |
| 758.990 | CHROMOSOME X, POLY-X |
| 758.990 | CHROMOSOME X, TRIPLO-X |
| 758.990 | CHROMOSOME XYY |
| 758.990 | CHROMOSOME, NUCLEOLAR ORGANIZER REGION, TRANSLOCATION |
| 758.990 | CHROMOSOMES, COMPLEX REARRANGEMENTS |
| 759.000 | ASPLENIA SYNDROME |
| 759.010 | SPLEEN, CONGENITAL ISOLATED HYPOSPLENIA |
| 759.080 | SPLEEN, CYSTS |
| 759.110 | ADRENAL HYPOPLASIA, CONGENITAL |
| 759.210 | THYROID, DYSGENESIS |
| 759.220 | THYROGLOSSAL DUCT REMNANT |
| 759.3 | SITUS INVERSUS VISCERUM |
| 759.4 | TWINS, CONJOINED |
| 759.500 | TUBEROUS SCLEROSIS |
| 759.600 | INTESTINAL POLYPOSIS, TYPE II |
| 759.610 | STURGE-WEBER SYNDROME |
| 759.620 | VON HIPPEL-LINDAU SYNDROME |
| 759.630 | INTESTINAL POLYPOSIS, TYPE III |
| 759.800 | CRANIO-CARPO-TARSAL DYSPLASIA, WHISTLING FACE TYPE |
| 759.800 | NOONAN SYNDROME |
| 759.800 | ORO-FACIO-DIGITAL SYNDROME I |
| 759.800 | ORO-FACIO-DIGITAL SYNDROME, BARAITSER-BURN TYPE |
| 759.800 | ORO-FACIO-DIGITAL SYNDROME, MOHR TYPE |
| 759.800 | ORO-FACIO-DIGITAL SYNDROME, THURSTON TYPE |
| 759.800 | ORO-FACIO-DIGITAL SYNDROME, WHELAN TYPE |
| 759.800 | WAARDENBURG SYNDROMES |
| 759.820 | BARDET-BIEDL SYNDROME |
| 759.820 | COCKAYNE SYNDROME |
| 759.820 | COCKAYNE SYNDROME, TYPE II |
| 759.820 | DE LANGE SYNDROME |
| 759.820 | LAURENCE-MOON SYNDROME |
| 759.820 | SECKEL SYNDROME |
| 759.820 | SILVER SYNDROME |
| 759.820 | SILVER SYNDROME, X-LINKED |
| 759.820 | SMITH-LEMLI-OPITZ SYNDROME |
| 759.820 | SMITH-LEMLI-OPITZ SYNDROME, TYPE II |
| 759.840 | ANGIO-OSTEOHYPERTROPHY SYNDROME |
| 759.840 | HEART-HAND SYNDROME |
| 759.840 | RUBINSTEIN-TAYBI BROAD THUMB-HALLUX SYNDROME |
| 759.840 | THROMBOCYTOPENIA-ABSENT RADIUS |
| 759.860 | ARTHRO-OPHTHALMOPATHY, HEREDITARY, PROGRESSIVE, STICKLER TYPE |
| 759.860 | MARFAN SYNDROME |
| 759.870 | BECKWITH-WIEDEMANN SYNDROME |
| 759.870 | CEREBRO-COSTO-MANDIBULAR SYNDROME |
| 759.870 | CEREBRO-HEPATO-RENAL SYNDROME |
| 759.870 | INTESTINAL ILEUS, ISOLATED MECONIUM ILEUS |
| 759.870 | LEPRECHAUNISM |
| 759.870 | MENKES SYNDROME |
| 759.870 | NEPHRITIS-DEAFNESS (SENSORINEURAL), HEREDITARY TYPE |
| 759.870 | PRADER-WILLI SYNDROME |
| 759.890 | HEMIHYPERTROPHY |
| 759.890 | MECKEL SYNDROME |
| 760.710 | FETAL ALCOHOL SYNDROME |
| 760.750 | FETAL HYDANTOIN SYNDROME |
| 771.090 | FETAL RUBELLA SYNDROME |
| 771.210 | FETAL CYTOMEGALOVIRUS SYNDROME |
| 771.210 | FETAL TOXOPLASMOSIS SYNDROME |

# ILLUSTRATION CREDITS BY PUBLISHER[1]

**Academic Press**
New chromosome syndromes, 1977:245-272, 21498

**Acta Geneticae Medical et Gemellologiae**
1970:19:421-424, 20475

**American Journal of Diseases of Children**
1976, 10715
1966:112:79-81, 10758
1972:123:254-258, 11008
1972:123:254-258, 11009
1964:107:49, 12236
1964:107:49, 12237
1964:107:49, 12249
1964:107:49, 12250
1964:107:49, 12254
1964:107:49, 12257
1984:138:821, 20175
1984:138:821, 20176
1984:138:821, 20177
1984:138:821, 20178
1984:138:821, 20179
1984:138:821, 20180
1974:127:408-409, 20577
1974:127:408-409, 20578
1976:130:1244, 21499
1974:127:408-409, 20579
1975:129:360-362, 21123
1987:141:1021-1024, 21158
1981:135:729-731, 21161
1970:120:255-257, 21165
1970:120:255-257, 21166
1970:120:255-257, 21167
1980:134:285-289, 21174
1971:122:443, 21328

**American Journal of Human Genetics**
1972:24:189-213, 21507
1975:27:521-527, 20419
1980:32:714-722, 21224
1980:32:714-722, 21225
1981:33:455, 21416
1981:33:455, 21417
1981:33:455, 21418
1972:24:189-213, 21497
1972:24:189-213, 21501
1972:24:189-213, 21502
1972:24:189-213, 21506

**American Journal of Medical Genetics**
1987:27:943-952, 20050
1987:27:943-952, 20051
1983:14:335-346, 20066
1983:14:335-346, 20067
1983:14:335-346, 20068
1983:14:335-346, 20069
1983:14:335-346, 20070
1987:26:207-215, 20298
1987:26:207-215, 20299
1987:26:207-215, 20300
1987:26:207-215, 20301
1984:18:781-788, 20305
1984:18:781-788, 20306
1982:11:329-336, 20363
1982:11:329-336, 20364
1978:1:291-299, 20391
1978:1:291-299, 20392
1978:1:291-299, 20393
1978:1:291-299, 20394
1978:1:291-299, 20395
1986:25:29-39, 20406
1986:25:29-39, 20407
1986:25:29-39, 20408
1986:25:29-39, 20409
1983:15:29-38, 20418
1984:18:671, 20458

1984:18:671, 20459
1984:18:671, 20460
1984:18:671, 20461
1985:21:137-142, 20462
1985:21:137-142, 20463
1986:25:1-8, 20464
1986:25:1-8, 20465
1985:22:311-314, 20466
1985:22:311-314, 20467
1985:431-439, 20477
1985:431-439, 20478
1985:431-439, 20479
1980:5:179-188, 20508
1985:22:243-253, 20515
1985:22:243-253, 20516
1984:19:653-664, 20519
1984:19:653-664, 20520
1985:20:597-606, 20539
1984:19:487-499, 20554
1984:19:487-499, 20555
1987:26:217-220, 20559
1986:25:537-541, 20562
1986:25:537-541, 20563
1983:16:213-224, 20584
1984:17:809-826, 20585
1980:7:75-83, 20588
1985:22:685, 20593
1985:22:685, 20594
1982:12:327-331, 20626
1986:25:467-471, 20680
1986:25:467-471, 20681
1985:21:697-705, 20682
1985:21:697-705, 20683
1983:14:225-229, 20685
1983:14:225-229, 20686
1983:14:225-229, 20688
1983:14:225-229, 20689
1985:20:283-294, 20866
1985:20:283-294, 20867
1985:20:283-294, 20870
1985:20:283-294, 20872
1987:27:661-667, 20898
1987:27:661-667, 20899
1987:27:661-667, 20900
1985:21:669-680, 20938
1985:21:669-680, 20939
1985:21:669-680, 20940
1985:21:669-680, 20941
1985:21:669-680, 20942
1984:19:307, 20970
1984:19:307, 20971
1987:28:297-302, 20990
1982:11:185-239, 22125
1987:28:297-302, 20991
1980:7:91-102, 21000
1980:7:91-102, 21001
1987:26:13-15, 21019
1987:26:13-15, 21020
1987:26:13-15, 21021
1985:22:501-512, 21040
1985:22:531-543, 21042
1985:22:531-543, 21043
1985:22:531-543, 21044
1985:22:531-543, 21045
1986:SUP2:53-63, 21050
1986:SUP2:53-63, 21051
1985:21:569-574, 21066
1984:19:161-169, 21073
1982:11:185-239, 21124
1982:11:383-395, 21280
1982:11:383-395, 21281
1982:11:383-395, 21282
1982:11:383-395, 21283
1983:14:335-346, 21314
1983:14:335-346, 21316

1. The illustration number, in numeric order, as it appears in the text, follows the Publisher citation.

1983:14:335-346, 21317
1983:14:335-346, 21318
1983:14:335-346, 21323
1985:20:325-339, 21329
1985:20:325-339, 21330
1986:2:53-63, 21369
1986:2:53-63, 21370
1987:28:303-309, 21373
1987:28:303-309, 21374
1979:3:269-279, 21375
1979:3:65-80, 21386
1979:3:65-80, 21387
1979:3:65-80, 21388
1979:3:65-80, 21389
1979:3:65-80, 21390
1979:3:65-80, 21391
1985:21:417-432, 21393
1985:21:417-432, 21394
1985:21:417-432, 21396
1985:21:417-432, 21397
1983:14:501-511, 21411
1983:14:501-511, 21412
1983:14:501-511, 21413
1983:14:501-511, 21414
1987:26:207-215, 21421
1987:26:207-215, 21422
1985:20:159-163, 21423
1985:20:159-163, 21424
1985:20:159-163, 21425
1984:19:487, 21426
1984:19:369-377, 21431
1984:19:369-377, 21432
1981:9:139-146, 21445
1981:9:139-146, 21446
1981:9:139-146, 21447
1981:9:139-146, 21448
1988:29:573-579, 21450
1988:29:573-579, 21451
1984:17:133-144, 21480
1989:32:461-467, 21481
1989:32:461-467, 21482
1989:32:461-467, 21483

## American Journal of Medicine
1973:54:793-800, 21234
1973:54:793-800, 21235
1973:54:793-800, 21236

## American Journal of Ophthalmology
1988:105:40-45, 21272

## American Journal of Physical Anthropology
1976:45:109-116, 20266

## Annales de Genetique
1978:21:247-251, 21340
1979:22:165-167, 20514

## Annals of Internal Medicine
1987:106:538-545, 20405
1976:84:393-397, 11311
1976:84:393-397, 11313
1976:84:393-397, 11315
1976:84:393, 11317
1976:84:393, 11319
1976:84:393, 11321
1987:106:538-545, 20404

## Annals of Otology, Rhinology & Laryngology
1979:88:100-104, 21067

## Applied Neurophysiology
1963:23:1, 10218

## Archives of Dermatology
1966:93:194-201, 21263
1970:101:699, 10295

## Archives of Ophthalmology
1986:104:61-64, 21159
1986:104:61-64, 21160

## Archives of Otolaryngology
1973:98:124-128, 21011

## Birth Defects Original Article Series
1974:10:41-50, 10675
1974:10:41-50, 10676
1974:10:41-50, 10677
1974:10:167-170, 10709
1974:10:22, 10902
1974:10:22, 10903
1974:10:22, 10904
1974:10:23, 10905
1974:10:23, 10906
1974:10:23, 10907
1976:12:309, 10908
1974:10:337, 10910
1974:10:25, 10911
1974:10:25, 10912
1974:10:25, 10913
1974:10:337, 10914
1974:10:337, 10915
1974:10:216, 10922
1974:10:216, 10923
1977:13:53-67, 20547
1977:13:53-67, 20548
1977:13:53-67, 20549
1977:13:53-67, 20552
1977:13:53-67, 20553
1976:12:275-278, 20571
1977:13:167, 21454
1976:12:275-278, 20572
1978:14:287-78, 21187
1978:14:287-78, 21188
1978:14:287-78, 21189
1969:5:79-95, 21194
1969:5:79-95, 21195
1969:5:79-95, 21196
1969:5:79-95, 21197
1969:5:79-95, 21198
1969:5:79-95, 21199
1975:11:30-33, 21294
1975:11:30-33, 21295
1975:11:30-33, 21296
1975:11:30-33, 21297
1975:11:30-33, 21298
1975:11:30-33, 21299
1977:13:167, 21452
1977:13:167, 21453

## Bulletin of the Johns Hopkins Hospital
1964:114:402-411, 10711

## Charles C. Thomas
10108

## Clinical Genetics
1974:5:294, 10714
1976:16:1-18, 21368
1974:5:1, 10798
1984:25:68-72, 20154
1983:24:140-146, 20272
1983:24:140-146, 20273
1983:24:140-146, 20274
1985:27:414, 20346
1985:27:414, 20347
1981:19:321-330, 20480
1981:19:321-330, 20481
1981:19:321-330, 20482
1981:19:321-330, 20483
1981:19:321-330, 20484
1980:17:209-212, 20509
1985:28:251-254, 20513
1984:26:308-317, 20526
1984:26:308-317, 20527
1984:26:308-317, 20528
1987:32:28-34, 21076
1987:32:28-34, 21077
1987:32:28-34, 21078
1981:19:23-25, 21079
1981:19:23-25, 21080
1978:14:251-256, 21081
1978:14:251-256, 21082
1974:5:363-367, 21089
1974:5:363-367, 21090
1980:18:413-416, 21149
1980:18:413-416, 21150

1981:20:1-5, 21153
1981:20:1-5, 21154
1974:5:127-132, 21155
1974:5:127-132, 21156
1976:10:319-324, 21164
1976:10:319-324, 21168
1976:10:319-324, 21169
1976:10:319-324, 21170
1984:25:422-448, 21171
1984:25:422-448, 21172
1983:23:376-379, 21218
1986:29:83-87, 21237
1981:19:202-206, 21334
1981:19:202-206, 21335
1976:16:1-18, 21362
1976:16:1-18, 21363
1976:16:1-18, 21364
1976:16:1-18, 21365
1976:16:1-18, 21366
1976:16:1-18, 21367

**Dental Clinics of North America**
1975:19:1-27, 10613
1975:19:1-27, 10610
1975:19:1-27, 10611
1975:19:1-27, 10612

**Dermatologica**
1982:164:293-304, 20064
1982:164:293-304, 20065

**Dysmorphology and Clinical Genetics**
1987:1:17-20, 20188
1987:1:17-20, 20189
1987:1:17-20, 20190
1987:1:142-144, 20586
1987:1:142-144, 20587
1988:2:104-108, 20601
1988:2:104-108, 20602
1988:2:104-108, 20603
1984:2(4):29-30, 20794
1984:2(4):29-30, 20795
1989:3, 21456
1989:3, 21457
21458
21459
21460
1989:3:103-107, 21461
1989:3:103-107, 21462
1989:3:103-107, 21463
1989:3:103-107, 21464
1989:3:103-107, 21465
1989:3:103-107, 21466
1989:3:28-32, 21471
1989:3:28-32, 21474
1989:3:28-32, 21475
1989:3:28-32, 21478
1989:3:28-32, 21479
1989:4:97-102, 21515
1989:4:97-102, 21516
1989:4:97-102, 21517
1990:4, 21518
1990:4, 21519
1989:3:61-64, 21525

**Editions Medecine et Hygiene**
1969:17:45-52, 21064
1969:17:45-52, 21063

**European Journal of Pediatrics**
1982:138:301-303, 20072
1979:130:65, 20582
1979:130:65, 20583

**Helvetica Paediatrica Acta**
1980:35:243-251, 21293
1980:35:243-251, 21289
1980:35:243-251, 21290
1980:35:243-251, 21291
1980:35:243-251, 21292

**Human Genetics**
1985:69:243-245, 20161
1985:69:243-245, 20162
1976:31:219-225, 20403

1980:56:231-234, 20510
1978:40:231-234, 20511
1977:36:243-247, 20512
1981:57:210-213, 21157
1978:40:311-324, 21240
1978:40:311-324, 21241
1978:40:311-324, 21243
1978:40:311-324, 21244
1978:40:311-324, 21247
1979:50:241-246, 21249
1979:47:233-237, 21338
1979:47:233-237, 21339
1979:48:151-156, 21384
1979:48:151-156, 21385

**Humangenetik**
1975:29:233-241, 21343
1973:19:341-343, 21173
1975:29:233-241, 21341
1975:29:233-241, 21342

**Internationale Stiftung Mozarteum**
21442

**Journal of Bone and Joint Surgery**
1975:57:542, 10716
1972:54:509, 21217
1975:57:542, 10717
1976:58B:343-346, 21083
1976:58B:343-346, 21084
1976:58B:343-346, 21085
1976:58B:343-346, 21086

**Journal of Clinical Dysmorphology**
1985:3:2-9, 20252

**Journal of Medical Genetics**
1970:7:11-19, 10345
1985:22:46-53, 20311
1985:22:46-53, 20313
1985:22:46-53, 20315
1985:22:46-53, 20316
1986:32:355-359, 20675
1986:32:355-359, 20676
1974:11:287-291, 20873
1974:11:287-291, 20874
1983:20:277, 20959
1983:20:277, 20960
1973:42:428-434, 21288
1983:20:277, 20961
1985:22:36-38, 21054
1987:24:204-206, 21069
1987:24:204-206, 21070
1987:24:204-206, 21071
1987:24:9-13, 21091
1987:24:9-13, 21092
1987:24:9-13, 21093
1988:25:157-163, 21175
1988:25:157-163, 21176
1981:18:129-133, 21250
1981:18:129-133, 21251
1981:18:129-133, 21252
1985:22:78-80, 21253
1985:22:78-80, 21254
1977:14:144-147, 21255
1977:14:144-147, 21256

**Journal of Neurosurgical Sciences**
1983:59:215-228, 20308
1983:59:215-228, 20309
1983:58:89-102, 21126
1983:59:215-228, 20310

**Journal of Pediatric Ophthalmology and Strabismus**
1988:25:93-98, 20591

**Journal of Pediatrics**
1960:56:778, 10737
1960:56:778, 10738
1960:56:778, 10739
1960:56:778, 10740
1960:56:778, 10741
1975:86:388, 21470
1960:56:778, 10742
1970:77:856, 20977

1975:87:280-284, 20999
1987:110:747-750, 21145
1987:110:747-750, 21146
1981:98:92-95, 21148
1971:79:450-455, 21151
1971:79:450-455, 21152
1969:74:755-762, 21158
1969:74:755-762, 21159
1969:74:755-762, 21160
1969:74:755-762, 21164
1986:109:469-475, 21344
1986:109:469-475, 21345
1986:109:469-475, 21346
1986:109:469-475, 21347
1986:109:469-475, 21348
1986:109:469-475, 21349
1986:109:469-475, 21350
1986:109:469-475, 21355
1986:109:469-475, 21356

**Klinische Paediatrie**
1973:185:181-186, 21062
1973:185:181-186, 21061

**Lea & Febiger**
Nyhan, WL: Diagnostic recognition, 1987:126, 20183
Nyhan, WL: Diagnostic recognition, 1987:142, 20184
Diagnosis and treatment 2nd ed., 1984, 21127

**Minerva Pediatrica**
1967:19:2187, 10444

**Neurology**
1967:17:961, 12228
1967:17:961, 12229
1967:17:961, 12230
1967:17:961, 12231
1967:17:961, 12232
1967:17:961, 12233

**Neuropediatrics**
1980:11:291-297, 20350

**New England Journal of Medicine**
1986:314:1542-1546, 21131
1986:314:1542-1546, 21130

**Oral Surgery**
1964:17:683-690, 10592
1964:18:409-418, 10603
1964:18:409-418, 10604

**Pediatric Clinics of North America**
1986:33:1277-1297, 21143
1986:33:1277-1297, 21144

**Pediatric Dentistry**
1985:7:326-328, 20281
1985:7:326-328, 20282

**Pediatric Radiology**
1981:10:155-160, 20580
1981:10:155-160, 20581
1980:10:46-50, 21219
1980:10:46-50, 21220
1980:10:46-50, 21221

**Pediatrics**
1971:48:756-765, 10340
1971:48:756-765, 10341
1971:48:756-765, 10342
1971:47:610-612, 21142
1971:48:756-765, 10343
1978:61:12-15, 21136
1978:61:12-15, 21139
1978:61:12-15, 21140

**Pergamon Press**
1961, 10123

**Plastic and Reconstructive Surgery**
1971:48:542-500, 10543
1971:48:542-500, 10544
1971:48:542-500, 10545

**Postgraduate Medical Journal**
1977:53:507-515, 21222

**Radiology**
1970:95:129-134, 20862
1970:95:129-134, 20863
1970:95:129-134, 20864
1970:95:129-134, 20865

**South African Medical Journal**
1979:21:659-665, 21087
1979:21:659-665, 21088
1979:21:659-665, 21223

**Springer-Verlag**
Wackenheim, A: Cheirolumbar dysostosis, 1980, 20331
Wackenheim, A: Cheirolumbar dysostosis, 1980, 20332
Wackenheim, A: Cheirolumbar dysostosis, 1980, 20333
Wackenheim, A: Cheirolumbar dysostosis, 1980, 20334
Wackenheim, A: Cheirolumbar dysostosis, 1980, 20335
Wackenheim, A: Cheirolumbar dysostosis, 1980, 20336
Wackenheim, A: Cheirolumbar dysostosis, 1980, 20337
Wackenheim, A: Cheirolumbar dysostosis, 1980, 20338
Wackenheim, A: Cheirolumbar dysostosis, 1980, 20339
Wackenheim, A: Cheirolumbar dysostosis, 1980, 20340
Wackenheim, A: Cheirolumbar dysostosis, 1980, 20341
Wackenheim, A: Cheirolumbar dysostosis, 1980, 20342
Wackenheim, A: Cheirolumbar dysostosis, 1980, 20343

**St. Justine Clinic of Medical Genetics**
10374

**Surgery in Gynecology and Obstetrics**
1958:107:602-614, 20677
1958:107:602-614, 20678
1958:107:602-614, 20679

**Syndrome Identification**
1977:5:14-18, 20052
1977:5:14-18, 20053
1977:5:14-18, 20054
1977:5:14-18, 20055
1977:5:14-18, 20056
1987:26:551-556, 20564
1987:26:551-556, 20565

**University of Minnesota Dermatology**
10307

**W.B. Saunders**
Smith, DW: Recognizable patterns of human malformation, 1982:228., 20279
Smith, DW: Recognizable patterns of human malformation, 1982:228, 20280
Smith, DW: Recognizable patterns of human malformation, 3rd Ed., 1982:439, 20518
Smith, DW: Recognizable patterns of human malformation, 3rd ed., 1982:439, 20521
Smith, DW: Recognizable patterns of human malformation, 4th ed., 1988:605, 20573
Smith, DW: Recognizable patterns of human malformation, 4th ed., 1988:605, 20574

**Year Book Medical Publishers**
Current Problems in Surgery, 1966, 10370
Current Problems in Surgery, 1966, 10371

**Z Kinderheilkd**
1975:120:1, 20558
1968:102:1-4, 20448
1968:102:1-4, 20449
1968:102:1-4, 20450
1968:102:1-4, 20451
1968:102:1-4, 20452
1968:102:1-4, 20453
1975:120:231, 20556

# ILLUSTRATION CREDITS BY CONTRIBUTOR

**Dagfinn Aarskog**
20350, 20418, 20977, 20978, 20979

**Louise C. Abbott**
10613

**Albert M. Abrams**
10610, 10611, 10612

**Kirk Aleck**
20445, 20447

**Judith Allanson**
21091, 21092, 21093

**Rudolph Angermuller**
21442

**Holly Hutchison Ardinger**
20518, 20519, 20520, 20521

**Joan F. Atkin**
20682, 20683

**Gerald D. Aurbach**
11269, 11271, 11272

**Biagio Azzarelli**
20929

**Michael Baraitser**
21002, 21003, 21006, 21007, 21009, 21010

**Amin Y. Barakat**
20700

**Bruce J. Bart**
10239, 10240, 10314, 11386, 11421

**Christos S. Bartsocas**
10479

**Harold N. Bass**
21398, 21400, 21401

**J. Bronwyn Bateman**
20016, 20842, 21273, 21274, 21275, 21276, 21277

**Arthur L. Beaudet**
10718, 10719, 21470

**Frits A. Beemer**
20344, 20345

**Peter Beighton**
10716, 10717, 11311, 11313, 11315, 11317, 11319, 11321, 11640, 11646, 20522, 20523, 20526, 20527, 20528, 21073, 21079, 21080, 21081, 21082, 21083, 21084, 21085, 21086, 21087, 21088, 21089, 21090, 21201, 21207, 21210, 21211, 21214, 21215, 21217, 21218, 21219, 21220, 21221, 21222, 21223

**Renee Bernstein**
20311, 20313, 20315, 20316

**Diana W. Bianchi**
20222, 21313

**Josette W. Bianchine**
10649, 10995

**David Bixler**
10160, 10162, 10163, 10636, 21014

**F. Owen Black**
21011

**Will Blackburn**
20235, 20236, 20237, 20238, 20239, 20240, 20241, 20242, 20243

**E.M. Bleeker-Wagemakers**
20156, 20157, 20158, 20159

**Zvi Borochowitz**
20001, 20002, 20003, 20071, 20082, 20468, 20604, 21402, 21403, 21443

**Sylvia S. Bottomley**
20614, 20615, 20616

**Jack Brown**
21263

**Kenneth S. Brown**
20628

**W. Ted Brown**
20595, 20596, 20597

**Merlin G. Butler**
20601, 20602, 20603

**Mary Louise Buyse**
10383, 10573

**Jose-Maria Cantu**
20161, 20162, 20163, 20508, 20510, 20513, 20514, 21031, 21032, 21033

**J. Aidan Carney**
20225

**Nancy J. Carpenter**
20215, 20216

**Anthony C. Casamassima**
20096, 20097

**Florence Char**
20701, 20702, 20704, 20705, 20706, 20707, 20710, 20711, 20712, 20713, 20715, 20716, 20717, 20719, 20720, 20721, 20722, 20723, 20724, 20725, 20726, 20729, 20730, 20731, 20734, 20735, 20737, 20738, 20739, 20740, 20741, 20742, 20744, 20745, 20746, 20747, 20748, 20749, 20750, 20752, 20755, 20756, 20757, 20759, 20763, 20764, 20765, 20766, 20768, 20769, 20770, 20771, 20772, 20773, 20774, 20775, 20776, 20779, 20780, 20783, 20784, 20786, 20788, 20790, 20791, 20792, 20793, 20794, 20795

**Harold Chen**
20195, 20196, 20584, 20585, 21000, 21001, 21038, 21039, 21405, 21406, 21407, 21408, 21409, 21410, 21411, 21412, 21413, 21414

**Albert E. Chudley**
21013

**Robin Dawn Clark**
21019, 21020, 21021

**Sterling K. Clarren**
20588, 21143, 21144, 21147, 21148

**David Cogan**
10220

**M. Michael Cohen**
10008, 10032, 10044, 10045, 10046, 10047, 10048, 10093, 10094, 10095, 10096, 10097, 10098, 10143, 10144, 10145, 10216, 10229, 10242, 10243, 10251, 10253, 10254, 10435, 10436, 10437, 10438, 10439, 10440, 10441, 10528, 10529, 10530, 10531, 10532, 10582, 10583, 10614, 10673, 10674, 10793, 10794, 10795, 10796, 10797, 10916, 10917, 10928, 10930, 10931, 10932, 10949, 10951, 11131, 11132, 11149, 11150, 11151, 11307, 11309, 12204, 12205

**David E.C. Cole**
20014, 20015

**J. Michael Connor**
20515, 20516

**Linda F. Cooper**
21145, 21146

**Maria P. de A. Coutinho**
20878, 20878, 20879, 20879, 20880, 20880

**F. Susan Cowchock**
20626

**Cor W.R.J. Cremers**
21067, 21184

**Harold E. Cross**
12168, 21036, 21037

**Cynthia J. Curry**
21508, 21509, 21510

**Bernard D'Souza**
20903, 20904, 20905, 20906, 20933, 20934, 20935, 20936

**Elias O. da-Silva**
20202, 20203, 20204, 20560, 20561

**David M. Danks**
11008, 11009, 20655, 20656, 20657, 20658, 20659, 20660, 20959, 20960, 20961, 20962, 20963, 20964, 20965, 20967, 20968, 20970, 20971, 20974

**Margaret Davee**
21053, 21427, 21428, 21429, 21430

**F.L. DeBusk**
11240, 11245, 11247

**William DeMyer**
10218, 12228, 12229, 12230, 12231, 12232, 12233

**Joao Monteiro de Pina-Neto**
20062, 20063

**J.W. Delleman**
20797, 20798, 20803, 20805, 20806, 20807, 20808, 20809, 20810, 20811, 20812, 20816, 20817, 20818, 20819, 20820, 20827, 20828, 20830, 20832, 20834, 20836, 20838, 20840, 20841

**Vazken M. Der Kaloustian**
20064, 20065, 20066, 20067, 20068, 20069, 20070, 21314, 21316, 21317, 21318, 21323, 21328, 21329, 21330

**Peter J. Dignan**
21384, 21385

**Alan E. Donnenfeld**
20136, 20137, 20138, 21481, 21482, 21483

**John P. Dorst**
11017

**Peter A. Duncan**
20571, 20572, 20573, 20574

**Paolo Durand**
10444

**Jesse E. Edwards**
12150

**B. Rafael Elejalde**
20547, 20548, 20549, 20552, 20553, 20554, 20555, 21362, 21363, 21364, 21365, 21366, 21367, 21368, 21386, 21387, 21388, 21389, 21390, 21391, 21393, 21394, 21396, 21397

**Sami B. Elhassani**
20257, 20258, 20259, 20261, 20262, 20263, 20264, 20265

**Nabil I. Elsahy**
10543, 10544, 10545

**Gerald M. English**
10362

**Charles J. Epstein**
10830

**Marianne P. Eronen**
20288, 20289, 20290, 20291, 20292

**Luis F. Escobar**
21158

**Victor Escobar**
20266, 20267, 20269, 20270, 20272, 20273, 20274, 20276, 20279, 20280, 20281, 20282, 20283

**Carla Evans**
20844, 20845, 20846, 20847, 20848, 20849

**L.R. Eversole**
21127

**Sergio Fanconi**
21344, 21345, 21346, 21347, 21348, 21349, 21350, 21355, 21356

**Malcolm A. Ferguson-Smith**
10818

**G. Filippi**
11145

**Wayne H. Finley**
21161

**Naomi Fitch**
20606, 20988, 20989

**J.S. Fitzsimmons**
20575, 20576

**David B. Flannery**
20517, 20570

**Gordon M. Folger**
12165, 12166

**Piergiorgio Franceschini**
20629, 20630, 20632, 20633, 20636

**Uta Francke**
21452, 21453, 21454, 21497, 21498, 21499, 21501, 21502, 21506, 21507

**F. Clarke Fraser**
21076, 21077, 21078

**Joseph F. Fraumeni**
10743

**Ademar Freire-Maia**
20419

**Newton Freire-Maia**
20352, 20353, 20354, 20355, 20363, 20364, 20365, 20366, 20370, 20372, 20373, 20374, 20389, 20420, 20421, 20425, 20426, 20427, 20428, 20429, 20430, 20475

**Jaime L. Frias**
20496, 20497, 20498, 20499, 20500, 20501, 20502, 20503, 20504, 20505, 21294, 21295, 21296, 21297, 21298, 21299, 21515, 21516, 21517

**Moshe Frydman**
20059, 20060, 20346, 20347, 20348, 20349

**Jean-Pierre Fryns**
20019, 20021, 20022, 20031, 20032, 20033, 20038, 20039, 20040, 20041, 20078, 20079, 20080, 20081, 20088, 20089, 20090, 20091, 20092, 20093, 20094, 20095, 20131, 20470, 20471, 20472, 20473, 20562, 20563, 20564, 20565, 20566, 20567, 20850, 20851, 20852, 20853, 20854, 20855, 20907, 20908, 20909, 20910, 20911, 20912, 20913, 20914, 20915, 20917, 20918, 20919, 20920, 20921, 20922, 20923, 20924, 20925, 20926, 20928, 21046, 21047, 21048, 21049, 21404

**Atsuko Fujimoto**
20050, 20051, 20193, 20194, 20873, 20874

**Lawrence Gans**
21237

**Diana Garcia-Cruz**
20185, 20511, 20512, 21456, 21457, 21458, 21459, 21460

**Bhuwan P. Garg**
12200, 12201

**Kenneth L. Garver**
21162, 21163, 21164, 21168, 21169, 21170

**Mark C. Gebhardt**
20569

**Ekkart Genee**
21063, 21064

**James German**
21116

**Ronald E. Gier**
10120, 10121, 10122

**Enid F. Gilbert-Barness**
20485, 20486, 20487

**Mitchell S. Golbus**
21288

**Morton F. Goldberg**
10402, 10403, 10627, 10640, 10646

**Donald Goldsmith**
20488, 20489

**Stanley Goldstein**
20866, 20867, 20870, 20872

**Thomaz Rafael Gollop**
20685, 20686, 20688, 20689, 20692, 20693, 20694, 20695

**Richard M. Goodman**
10868, 10869, 10873, 10874, 20328, 20329, 20476

**Hymie Gordon**
10302, 10304, 10306

**Robert J. Gorlin**
10119, 10133, 10135, 10136, 10148, 10149, 10321, 10322, 10323, 10324, 10325, 10326, 10358, 10427, 10430, 10737, 10738, 10739, 10740, 10741, 10742, 12271, 20898, 20899, 20900, 20975, 20976, 21194, 21195, 21196, 21197, 21198, 21199

**John M. Graham**
21050, 21051, 21369, 21370

**Frank Greenberg**
20293, 20294, 20295, 20296, 20297

**Fahed Halal**
20100, 20101, 20102, 20103, 20104, 20106, 20107, 20108, 20109, 20122, 20123, 20124, 20128

**Bryan D. Hall**
10099, 10101, 10102, 10150, 10659, 21174, 21187, 21188, 21189

**Judith G. Hall**
11360, 11361, 11362, 21123, 21124, 21126, 22125

**Carol Haynes**
20517

**Jurgen Herrmann**
10009, 10675, 10676, 10677, 10709, 10744, 10746, 10747, 10748, 10749, 10822, 10824, 10839, 10840

**Riitta Herva**
20477, 20478, 20479, 20480, 20481, 20482, 20483, 20484

**Reba Michels Hill**
20599, 20600

**Richard Hoefnagel**
10408, 10620, 10787, 11200, 11202, 11204

**Georg Hoffmann**
20181, 20182

**Thomas M. Holder**
10370, 10371

**Lewis B. Holmes**
10726

**George R. Honig**
20164

**H. Eugene Hoyme**
20980, 20981, 20982

**Alasdair G.W. Hunter**
21240, 21241, 21243, 21244, 21247, 21278, 21279, 21280, 21281, 21282, 21283, 21375

**Victor Ionasescu**
20013, 20305, 20306, 20308, 20309, 20310

**Harry Israel**
20173, 20174

**Elizabeth J. Ives**
12270

**Ian Jeffries**
20875

**Jan E. Jirasek**
10382

**John P. Johnson**
20083, 20613

**Virginia P. Johnson**
20593, 20594, 20607, 20608, 20609, 20610, 20611, 20612

**Ronald J. Jorgenson**
10030, 10155, 10245, 10247, 10274, 10276, 10514, 10572, 10593, 10597, 10598, 10609, 10617, 10920, 10967, 11057, 11089, 11103, 11104

**Ronald J. Jorgenson**
20396, 20397, 20399, 20401, 20402

**Ronald J. Jorgenson**
20540, 20541, 20542

**Richard C. Juberg**
10130, 21155, 21156, 21157, 21158, 21159, 21160, 21164, 21224, 21225, 21226, 21416, 21417, 21418

**Stephen G. Kahler**
20667, 20668, 20669

**Stephen G. Kaler**
20244, 20245, 20246, 21518, 21519

**Raymond S. Kandt**
20351

**James R. Kasser**
20884, 20885, 20886

**Donald Kaufman**
21097

**Robert L. Kaufman**
10257, 10259, 10260, 10979, 10980, 10982

**Harris J. Keene**
10592

**Thaddeus E. Kelly**
10922, 10923

**Nancy G. Kennaway**
20201

**Kenneth R. Kenyon**
11073

**Yukio Kitano**
20698, 20699

**Jane Kivlin**
20589, 21159, 21160

**Steven E. Kopits**
11257, 11261

**Boris G. Kousseff**
20017, 20018, 20026, 20030, 20042, 20043, 20044, 20045, 20046, 20047, 20048, 20049, 20197, 20198, 20199, 20200, 20410, 20411, 20412, 20413, 20416, 21255, 21256, 21303, 21304, 21305, 21306, 21307, 21308, 21309

**K.S. Kozlowski**
20577, 20578, 20579, 20580, 20581

**Celeste M. Krauss**
20210, 20211, 20212, 21423, 21424, 21425

**Dhavendra Kumar**
20154

**Jurgen Kunze**
20072, 20996, 20997, 20998

**A. Kurtz**
20627

**Michael Edison Labhard**
20169, 20170, 20171, 20172

**Roger L. Ladda**
21132, 21133, 21134, 21136, 21139, 21140, 21185, 21186

**Charlotte Z. Lafer**
20490, 20491, 20492

**Leonard O. Langer**
21113, 21114, 21115

**Lawrence G. Leichtman**
20188, 20189, 20190

**Richard Alan Lewis**
20637, 20638, 20639, 20640, 20896

**Raymond M. Lewkonia**
21072

**Richard Lindenberg**
20930, 20931, 20932

**R.B. Lowry**
11026, 11027, 21012, 21040, 21042, 21043, 21044, 21045

**Herbert A. Lubs**
21068, 21480

**Russell V. Lucas**
12156, 12167, 12187, 12191, 12192, 12193, 12194, 12195

**Philip M. Marden**
10758

**Pierre Maroteaux**
20284, 20285, 20286, 20287, 20647, 20648, 20649, 20650, 20651, 20652, 20653, 20654, 21022, 21023, 21024, 21025, 21026, 21027

**John T. Martsolf**
20052, 20053, 20054, 20055, 20056, 20391, 20392, 20393, 20394, 20395

**Victor A. McKusick**
10123, 10207, 10238, 10261, 10262, 10292, 10296, 10297, 10298, 10308, 10320, 10344, 10359, 10389, 10390, 10411, 10452, 10480, 10481, 10489, 10490, 10492, 10493, 10498, 10505, 10506, 10507, 10508, 10509, 10515, 10650, 10651, 10656, 10657, 10722, 10724, 10752, 10806, 10809, 10810, 10828, 10844, 10845, 10846, 10851, 10852, 10864, 10865, 10881, 10886, 10887, 10888, 10889, 10890, 10891, 10892, 10893, 10894, 10895, 10897, 10908, 10918, 10936, 10953, 10954, 10955, 10956, 10957, 10978, 11003, 11013, 11028, 11029, 11031, 11032, 11038, 11040, 11041, 11044, 11045, 11046, 11047, 11049, 11052, 11053, 11054, 11070, 11071, 11085, 11086, 11087, 11088, 11090, 11153, 11154, 11155, 11181, 11250, 11251, 11253, 11255, 11267, 11268, 11278, 11281, 11326, 21270

**Peter Meinecke**
21065, 21300, 21301, 21302, 21433, 21434, 21435, 21461, 21462, 21463, 21464, 21465, 21466, 21525

**Heirie M.M. Mendez**
20220, 20221

**Paul Merlob**
21253, 21254

**David F. Merten**
20213, 20214

**Lawrence H. Meskin**
10546

**Louise Brearley Messer**
10605, 10606

**Virginia V. Michels**
20110, 20252

**Joyce A. Mitchell**
21268

**Cynthia A. Moore**
21035

**Merle E. Morris**
12158, 12159

**Gabriel Mortimer**
20493, 20494

**John E. Murphy**
20403

**Charles M. Myer**
20943, 20945, 20948, 20949, 20950, 20951, 20953, 20954, 20955, 20956, 20958

**George Nager**
10131, 10132

**Samir S. Najjar**
20207

**Giovanni Neri**
20057, 20058, 20529, 20530, 21373, 21374

**Richard Neu**
21142

**Gerhard Neuhauser**
20556, 20558

**Buford L. Nichols**
10725, 11082

**Pat Nichols**
20111, 20112, 20117, 20119

**Norio Niikawa**
20217, 20531

**Sirkka-Liisa Noponen**
20477, 20478, 20479, 20480, 20481, 20482, 20483, 20484

**James J. Nora**
12139

**Fiorella Nuzzo**
20665, 20666

**William L. Nyhan**
12169, 20183, 20184

**John M. Opitz**
10763, 10764, 10765, 10814, 11331, 12211, 12224, 12225, 21431, 21432

**B.A. Paes**
21471, 21474, 21475, 21478, 21479

**Philip D. Pallister**
10782, 10783, 10784, 20881, 20882, 20883

**Michael W. Partington**
20454

**Sharon G. Paryani**
21130, 21131

**Eberhard Passarge**
10626, 11352

**Michael A. Patton**
20298, 20299, 20300, 20301, 21421, 21422

**Sergio D.J. Pena**
20902

**Rudolf A. Pfeiffer**
21177, 21178, 21182

**Marta Pinheiro**
20359, 20360, 20361, 20362, 20367, 20368, 20369, 20375, 20376, 20377, 20378, 20379, 20380, 20381, 20386, 20387, 20388

**Leonard Pinsky**
21098, 21099, 21100

**Andrew E. Poole**
20247, 20248, 20250, 20251

**Andrew K. Poznanski**
10151, 10152, 10153, 20862, 20863, 20864, 20865

**Marilyn Preus**
10705, 10706, 10714, 10715, 21171, 21172

**Zvonimir Puretic**
20008, 20009, 20010

**David T. Purtilo**
20404, 20405

**Qutub H. Qazi**
20061, 21165, 21166, 21167

**Mark M. Ravitch**
20677, 20678, 20679

**Salomon H. Reisner**
10134

**J. Marc Rhoads**
21484

**Arthur R. Rhodes**
20205, 20206

**David L. Rimoin**
10316, 10319, 10332, 10333, 10334, 10348, 10350, 10351, 10472, 10473, 10474, 10939, 10940, 10941, 10942, 10988, 10989, 10990, 10991, 10992, 10993, 11266

**Richard M. Roberts**
20670, 20671, 20672, 20673, 20674

**Meinhard Robinow**
10467, 10477, 10478, 10801, 10803, 11058, 11060, 11762, 20175, 20176, 20177, 20178, 20179, 20180, 20228, 20590, 21104, 21105, 21106, 21266, 21267, 21445, 21446, 21447, 21448, 21450, 21451

**Luther K. Robinson**
20455, 20456

**Karol Rondou**
20031, 20032, 20033, 20038, 20039, 20040, 20041, 20078, 20079, 20080, 20081, 20091, 20092, 20093, 20094, 20095, 20470, 20471, 20472, 20473, 20562, 20563, 20564, 20565, 20566, 20567, 20850, 20851, 20852, 20853, 20854, 20855, 20907, 20908, 20909, 20910, 20911, 20912, 20913, 20914, 20915, 20917, 20918, 20919, 20920, 20921, 20922, 20923, 20924, 20925, 20926, 20928, 21046, 21047, 21048, 21049

**Allen Root**
20253, 20254, 20255, 20256

**Jack H. Rubinstein**
11107, 11108, 11109, 11110

**Carlos Ruiz**
20330

**R.H.A. Ruvalcaba**
21149, 21150, 21151, 21152, 21153, 21154

**George H. Sack**
20938, 20939, 20940, 20941, 20942

**Carlos F. Salinas**
21521, 21522, 21523, 21524

**Riitta Salonen**
20458, 20459, 20460, 20461

**Jose Sanchez-Corona**
20509

**Burhan Say**
20675, 20676, 21173

**R. Neil Schimke**
10625, 10750, 10757, 11221, 20876, 20877

**Albert A.G.L. Schinzel**
20132, 20133, 20134, 20135, 21286, 21287, 21289, 21290, 21291, 21292, 21293

**Jerry A. Schneider**
20532

**C. Ronald Scott**
21018

**Charles I. Scott**
10157, 10158, 10159, 11010, 11012, 11093, 11094, 11098, 11350, 11351

**John H. Seashore**
21527

**Robert E. Sharkey**
10118, 10365, 10366, 10381, 11296, 12311

**L.J. Sheffield**
20168

**Robert J. Shprintzen**
20139, 20140, 20141, 20142, 20143, 20144, 20145, 20146, 20147, 20148, 20149, 20150, 20151, 20152, 20153

**M. Cirillo Silengo**
20321, 20322, 20323

**Henry K. Silver**
12236, 12237, 12249, 12250, 12254, 12257

**Dharmdeo N. Singh**
20664

**William S. Sly**
11099, 11100

**Ann C.M. Smith**
20992, 20993, 20994

**Morton E. Smith**
20887, 20888

**John Stuart Soeldner**
21249

**Lawrence Solomon**
20223, 20224

**Annemarie Sommer**
21075

**Mark A. Sperling**
10337, 10338, 10339, 10340, 10341, 10342, 10343, 21392

**Jurgen W. Spranger**
10455, 10457, 10458, 10459, 10902, 10903, 10904, 10905, 10906, 10907, 10911, 10912, 10913, 11023, 11024, 11025, 11340, 11341, 11342, 21426

**Roger E. Stevenson**
20191, 20192, 20985, 20986, 20987, 21102, 21103, 21109, 21110, 21111, 21262

**Hartmut Stoess**
20661, 20662, 20663

**Claude Stoll**
20165, 20166, 20167, 20431, 20433, 20434, 20435, 20438, 20439, 20440, 20598

**Charles Strom**
20559

**Gerald I. Sugarman**
10910, 10914, 10915

**Robert Suskind**
10295

**Kutay Taysi**
20086, 20087

**A.S. Teebi**
21054, 21056, 21057, 21058, 21059

**Helga Toriello**
20462, 20463, 20464, 20465, 20466, 20467

**Robert J. Touloukian**
10367, 10368, 10369, 10377, 10380

**Philip L. Townes**
10963

**Elias Traboulsi**
20533, 20591, 20592, 21272, 21361

**Catherine Turleau**
20901, 21334, 21335, 21336, 21337, 21338, 21339, 21340, 21341, 21342, 21343

**L. H. S. Van Mierop**
10235, 10236

**Denis Viljoen**
20004, 20005, 20006, 20007, 20011, 20023, 20024, 20025, 20074, 20075, 20076, 20077, 20605

**Auguste Wackenheim**
20331, 20332, 20333, 20334, 20335, 20336, 20337, 20338, 20339, 20340, 20341, 20342, 20343

**Thomas A. Waldmann**
10745

**Colin E. Wallis**
20586, 20587

**Mette Warburg**
10644, 10648

**John Waterson**
20535, 20536

**David D. Weaver**
20226, 20227, 21035, 21052

**Avery Weiss**
21118, 21119, 21120, 21121, 21122

**Chester B. Whitley**
20406, 20407, 20408, 20409

**Peter Wieacker**
20539

**Hans-Rudolph Wiedemann**
20448, 20449, 20450, 20451, 20452, 20453, 20582, 20583, 21061, 21062

**Charles A. Williams**
20495, 20990, 20991

**R.S. Wilroy**
12163, 12164, 21420

**Golder N. Wilson**
21175, 21176

**Miriam G. Wilson**
11354, 11355

**A.M. Winchester**
10345, 10355

**Ingrid Winship**
20641, 20642, 20643, 20644, 20645, 20646

**Robin M. Winter**
21066, 21069, 21070, 21071, 21250, 21251, 21252

**Carl J. Witkop**
10128, 10542, 10557, 10558, 10559, 10590, 10594, 10595, 10596, 10603, 10604, 10616, 10618, 11605, 11620, 11644, 11924, 20617, 20618, 20620, 20622, 20623, 20624, 20625, 21028, 21029, 21030, 21257, 21258, 21259, 21260, 21261

**Beverly Phyllis Wood**
11034, 11036, 11037

**Yoshifumi Yamamoto**
20680, 20681

**Elaine H. Zackai**
20999

**Ismail Zayid**
21234, 21235, 21236

**Hans Zellweger**
10788

**Janice Zunich**
21419